EXPERT

2018

ICD-10-CM Expert for Hospitals

The complete official code set

Codes valid October 1, 2017 through September 30, 2018

POWER UP YOUR CODING with Optum360, your trusted coding partner for 32 years. **Visit optum360coding.com.**

Publisher's Notice

The *ICD-10-CM Expert for Hospitals: The Complete Official Code Set* is designed to be an accurate and authoritative source regarding coding and every reasonable effort has been made to ensure accuracy and completeness of the content. However, Optum360 makes no guarantee, warranty, or representation that this publication is accurate, complete or without errors. It is understood that Optum360 is not rendering any legal or other professional services or advice in this publication and that Optum360 bears no liability for any results or consequences that may arise from the use of this book.

Acknowledgments

Lauri Gray, RHIT, CPC, AHIMA-approved ICD-10-CM/PCS Trainer, *Product Manager*

Karen Schmidt, BSN, *Technical Director*

Anita Schmidt, BS, RHIT, AHIMA-approved ICD-10-CM/PCS Trainer, *Clinical Technical Editor*

Anne Kenney, BA, MBA, CCA, CCS, *Clinical Technical Editor*

Karen Krawzik, RHIT, CCS, AHIMA-approved ICD-10-CM/PCS Trainer, *Clinical Technical Editor*

Peggy Willard, CCS, AHIMA-approved ICD-10-CM/PCS Trainer, *Clinical Technical Editor*

Leanne Patterson, CPC, *Clinical Technical Editor*

Stacy Perry, *Manager, Desktop Publishing*

Lisa Singley, *Project Manager*

Tracy Betzler, *Senior Desktop Publishing Specialist*

Hope M. Dunn, *Senior Desktop Publishing Specialist*

Katie Russell, *Desktop Publishing Specialist*

Kate Holden, *Editor*

Our Commitment to Accuracy

Optum360 is committed to producing accurate and reliable materials.

To report corrections, please visit www.optum360coding.com/accuracy or email accuracy@optum.com. You can also reach customer service by calling 1.800.464.3649, option 1.

Copyright

Property of Optum360, LLC. Optum360 and the Optum360 logo are trademarks of Optum360, LLC. All other brand or product names are trademarks or registered trademarks of their respective owner.

© 2017 Optum360, LLC. All rights reserved.

Made in the USA
ISBN 978-1-62254-398-4

Anita Schmidt, BS, RHIT, AHIMA-approved ICD-10-CM/PCS Trainer

Ms. Schmidt has expertise in Level I Adult and Pediatric Trauma hospital coding, specializing in ICD-9-CM, ICD-10-CM/PCS, DRG, and CPT coding. Her experience includes analysis of medical record documentation, assignment of ICD-10-CM and PCS codes, DRG validation, as well as CPT code assignments for same-day surgery cases. She has conducted coding training and auditing, including DRG validation, conducted electronic health record training, and worked with clinical documentation specialists to identify documentation needs and potential areas for physician education. Most recently she has been developing content for resource and educational products related to ICD-10-CM and ICD-10-PCS. Ms. Schmidt is an AHIMA-approved ICD-10-CM/PCS trainer, and is an active member of the American Health Information Management Association (AHIMA) and the Minnesota Health Information Management Association (MHIMA).

Anne Kenney, BA, MBA, CCA, CCS

Ms. Kenney has expertise in ICD-10-CM/PCS, ICD-9-CM, DRG, and CPT coding. Most recently she has been developing content for ICD-10-CM and ICD-10-PCS applications. Her prior experience in a major teaching hospital includes assignment of ICD-9-CM codes and DRGs, CPT code assignments, and determining physician evaluation and management levels for inpatient, emergency department, and observation cases. Ms. Kenney is an active member of the American Health Information Management Association (AHIMA) and the Minnesota Health Information Management Association (MHIMA).

Peggy Willard, CCS, AHIMA-approved ICD-10-CM/PCS Trainer

Ms. Willard's expertise is ICD-10-CM and PCS including in-depth analysis of medical record documentation, ICD-10-CM/PCS code and DRG assignment. In recent years she has been responsible for the creation and development of several print products and e-books designed to assist with appropriate application of ICD-10-CM and PCS coding system. Ms. Willard has several years of prior experience in Level I Adult and Pediatric Trauma hospital coding, specializing in ICD-9-CM, DRG, and CPT coding with emphasis in conducting coding audits, and conducting coding training for coding staff and clinical documentation specialists. Ms. Willard is an active member of the American Health Information Management Association (AHIMA) and the Minnesota Health Information Management Association (MHIMA).

OPTUM 360°®

CODING TOOLS THIS
EFFICIEN
ARE BUILT FOR **CODING PROFESSIONALS**

MedicalReferenceEngine.com is the precision coding solution for **searching regulatory content.**

POWERFUL

Robust Medicare content. Search this essential repository of up-to-date national and local regulations and policy from CMS. Also included are dozens of Optum360® reference books.

Powerful lookup tools. CodeLogic™ search engine technology allows you to search across all three code sets simultaneously. View LCD/NCD, lay descriptions, illustrations and Internet Only Manual references for each code.

EFFICIENT

Flexible customization options. Set bookmarks to easily locate previously viewed documents. Save frequently performed searches. Create multiple search preferences to easily toggle between criteria when working on numerous projects.

Access forms and fee schedules. Easily find Medicare fee schedules and frequently used forms.

ACCURATE

Continuously adding pertinent content. Search with confidence for the most up-to-date regulatory information needed to achieve compliance.

Customized email alerts. Maintain compliance with alerts to newly updated rules and regulations.

Includes
20+
essential Optum360 references, plus regulatory content.

SCHEDULE A DEMO TODAY

 CLICK
optum360coding.com/mre

 CALL
1-800-464-3649, option 1

© 2017 Optum360, LLC. All rights reserved. WF342211 4/17

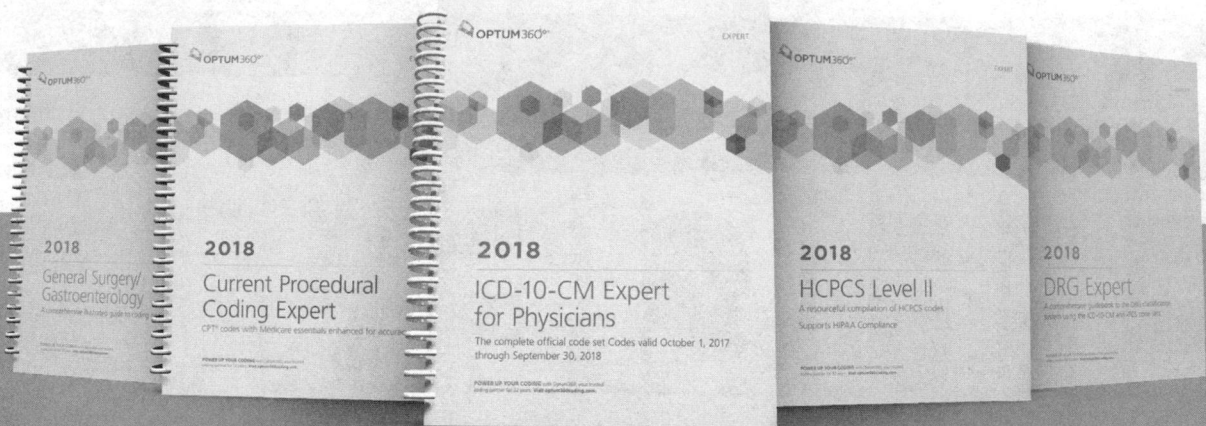

Keep your go-to coding resources up to date.

Stay current and compliant with our 2018 edition code books.
With more than 30 years in the coding industry, Optum360® is proud to
be your trusted resource for coding, billing and reimbursement resources.
Our 2018 editions include tools for ICD-10-CM/PCS, CPT®, HCPCS, DRG,
specialty-specific coding and much more.

SAVE UP TO 25% ON ADDITIONAL CODING RESOURCES

Visit us at optum360coding.com
and enter promo code **FOBA18ED**
to save 25%.

Call 1-800-464-3649, option 1,
and be sure to mention promo
code **FOBA18ED** to save 20%.

CPT is a registered trademark of the American Medical Association.

Excludes custom fee and bookstore items, data files, online coding tools and educational courses. Cannot be combined with any other offer. Offer not valid for
Partner or Medallion accounts. © 2017 Optum360, LLC. All rights reserved. WF345835 SPRJ3632

A modern approach to CDI matches the pace of change in health care.

The move to value-based care increases the need for accuracy in clinical documentation—across every patient and payer.

A modern CDI approach makes the work of CDI specialists more efficient by automatically reviewing every patient record and prioritizing those that require intervention.

Using case-finding logic and state-of-the-art natural language processing, Optum CDI 3D connects clinical indicators to identify records with gaps or deficiencies and enables timely documentation improvement, cleaner claims, faster reimbursement and accurate reporting.

Optum CDI 3D, together with Optum's market-leading Enterprise CAC, provides unmatched capabilities in a single, fully integrated CDI and coding solution.

Modernizing your CDI program starts here.
Visit optum360.com/CDI3D to learn more.

OPTUM CDI 3D

- Automates 100-percent record review and identifies clinical documentation improvement opportunities

- Identifies co-morbidities, HACs and patient safety indicators

- Streamlines the query loop between CDIS and physicians

- Enhances code assignment efficiency, compliance and quality reporting

Visit: optum360.com/CDI3D
Email: optum360@optum.com

© 2017 Optum360, LLC. All rights reserved. 2/17
U.S. Patent Nos. 6,915,254; 7,908,552; 8,682,823; 8,731,954; and other patents pending

Let Optum360 help you find the best product for your needs.

Together with you, Optum360® can help drive financial results across your organization with industry-leading resources that cut through the complexity of medical coding challenges.

Let us help you find the best coding solution, at the best price.

Contact your Medallion representative directly or call Customer Service at 1-800-464-3649, option 1.

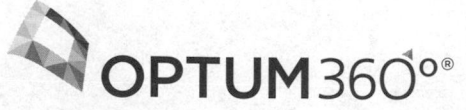

© 2017 Optum360, LLC. All rights reserved. WF351448 SPRJ3539 4/17

OPTUM 360°®

Optum360 **Learning**

Earn your CEUs with US

You've worked hard for your coding credentials, and now you need an easy way to maintain your certification.

Optum360® offers the most complete training in the marketplace, designed to address exactly what you and your organization need. We offer eLearning courses you can take online at your desk; you can invite a specialist to your office for on-the-job preparation; or ask our consulting professionals to create a tailor-made program specific for your organization.

Our strategy is simple — education must be concise, relevant and accurate. Choose the delivery method that works best for you:

- **eLearning:** Web-based courses offered at the most convenient times for your learners. eLearning courses are interactive, task-focused and developed around practical scenarios. These self-paced courses include "try-it" functionality, knowledge checks and downloadable resources.

- **Instructor-led training (ILT):** On-site or remote courses, built specifically for your organization.

- **Webinars:** Online courses, geared toward a broad market of learners, delivered in a live or recorded setting.

- **Podcasts and videos:** Physician-focused online courses available when and where convenient.

NO MATTER HOW YOU CHOOSE TO EARN YOUR CEUs, OPTUM360 IS HERE TO HELP YOU.

VISIT
optum360coding.com/learning

CALL
1-800-464-3649, option 1

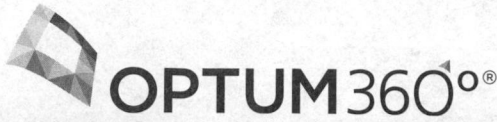

RE NEW

It's time to renew your Optum360 coding tools.

2018 ICD-10-CM Expert for Physicians

2018 Current Procedural Coding Expert

2018 HCPCS Level II

SAVE UP TO 25%*

when you renew your 2018 coding essentials.

ITEM #	TITLE INDICATE THE ITEMS YOU WISH TO PURCHASE	QUANTITY	PRICE PER PRODUCT	TOTAL
			Subtotal	
	(AK, DE, HI, MT, NH & OR are exempt)		Sales Tax	
	1 item $10.95 • 2–4 items $12.95 • 5+ CALL		Shipping & Handling	
			TOTAL AMOUNT ENCLOSED	

Save up to 25% when you renew.

PROMO CODE: RENEW18B

Visit **optum360coding.com** and enter the promo code above.

Call **1-800-464-3649, option 1,** and mention the promo code above.

Fax this order form with purchase order to **1-801-982-4033.** *Optum360 no longer accepts credit cards by fax.*

Mail this order form with payment and/or purchase order to: **Optum360, PO Box 88050, Chicago, IL 60680-9920.** *Optum360 no longer accepts credit cards by mail.*

Name _____

Address _____
_____

Customer Number _____ Contact Number _____

○ CHECK ENCLOSED (PAYABLE TO OPTUM360)

○ BILL ME   ○ P.O.# _____

( ) _____
Telephone
( ) _____
Fax
_____ @ _____
E-mail

Optum360 respects your right to privacy. We will not sell or rent your email address or fax number to anyone outside Optum360 and its business partners. If you would like to remove your name from Optum360 promotions, please call 1-800-464-3649, option 1.

*Save 20% when you order by phone, fax or mail; save 25% when you order online. Save 15% on AMA and custom fee products. Offer excludes digital coding tools, workers' comp and bookstore products.

© 2017 Optum360, LLC. All rights reserved. WF337935 SPRJ3517

Contents

© 2017 Optum360, LLC

Preface

ICD-10-CM Official Preface

This FY 2018 update of the International Statistical Classification of Diseases and Related Health Problems, 10th revision, Clinical Modification (ICD-10-CM) is being published by the United States government in recognition of its responsibility to promulgate this classification throughout the United States for morbidity coding. The International Statistical Classification of Diseases and Related Health Problems, 10th Revision (ICD-10), published by the World Health Organization (WHO), is the foundation of ICD-10-CM. ICD-10 continues to be the classification used in cause-of-death coding in the United States. The ICD-10-CM is comparable with the ICD-10. The WHO Collaborating Center for the Family of International Classifications in North America, housed at the Centers of Disease Control and Prevention's National Center for Health Statistics (NCHS), has responsibility for the implementation of ICD and other WHO-FIC classifications and serves as a liaison with the WHO, fulfilling international obligations for comparable classifications and the national health data needs of the United States. The historical background of ICD and ICD-10 can be found in the Introduction to the International Classification of Diseases and Related Health Problems (ICD-10), 2010, World Health Organization, Geneva, Switzerland.

ICD-10-CM is the United States' clinical modification of the World Health Organization's ICD-10. The term "clinical" is used to emphasize the modification's intent: to serve as a useful tool in the area of classification of morbidity data for indexing of health records, medical care review, and ambulatory and other health care programs, as well as for basic health statistics. To describe the clinical picture of the patient the codes must be more precise than those needed only for statistical groupings and trend analysis.

Characteristics of ICD-10-CM

ICD-10-CM far exceeds its predecessors in the number of concepts and codes provided. The disease classification has been expanded to include health-related conditions and to provide greater specificity at the 6th and 7th character level. The 6th and 7th characters are not optional and are intended for use in recording the information documented in the clinical record.

ICD-10-CM extensions, interpretations, modifications, addenda, or errata other than those approved by the Centers for Disease Control and Prevention are not to be considered official and should not be utilized. Continuous maintenance of the ICD-10- CM is the responsibility of the aforementioned agencies. However, because the ICD-10-CM represents the best in contemporary thinking of clinicians, nosologists, epidemiologists, and statisticians from both public and private sectors, when future modifications are considered, advice will be sought from all stakeholders.

All official authorized addenda since the last complete update (October 1, 2017) have been included in this revision. For more detailed information please see the complete official authorized addenda to ICD-10-CM, including the "ICD-10-CM Official Guidelines for Coding and Reporting," and a description of the ICD-10-CM updating and maintenance process.

What's New for 2018

Official Updates

The National Center for Health Statistics (NCHS), a section of the Centers for Disease Control and Prevention (CDC), is the agency charged with maintaining and updating ICD-10-CM. The 2018 official addendum was posted to the Centers for Medicare and Medicaid Services (CMS) website on June 13, 2017, identifying the changes to the ICD-10-CM code set for fiscal 2018. A summary of changes is provided below:

- 360 new codes added

- 226 code descriptions revised

- 34 codes changed from valid to invalid

Note: Validity changes are the result of new codes being added to the classification, changing a previously valid code to an invalid code, creating a new subcategory

A04.7	Enterocolitis due to Clostridium difficile
C96.2	Malignant mast cell tumor
D47.Ø	Histiocytic and mast cell tumors of uncertain behavior
E85.8	Other amyloidosis
H54.Ø	Blindness, both eyes
H54.11	Blindness, right eye, low vision left eye
H54.12	Blindness, left eye, low vision right eye
H54.2	Low vision, both eyes
H54.41	Blindness, right eye, normal vision left eye
H54.42	Blindness, left eye, normal vision right eye
H54.51	Low vision, right eye, normal vision left eye
H54.52	Low vision, left eye, normal vision right eye
I27.2	Other secondary pulmonary hypertension
KØ6.Ø	Gingival recession
K56.5	Intestinal adhesions [bands] with obstruction (postprocedural) (postinfection)
K56.6Ø	Unspecified intestinal obstruction
K56.69	Other intestinal obstruction
K91.3	Postprocedural intestinal obstruction
M48.Ø6	Spinal stenosis, lumbar region
N63	Unspecified lump in breast
OØØ.1Ø	Tubal pregnancy without intrauterine pregnancy
OØØ.11	Tubal pregnancy with intrauterine pregnancy
OØØ.2Ø	Ovarian pregnancy without intrauterine pregnancy
OØØ.21	Ovarian pregnancy with intrauterine pregnancy
P29.3	Persistent fetal circulation
P83.8	Other specified conditions of integument specific to newborn
P91.8	Other specified disturbances of cerebral status of newborn
Q53.11	Abdominal testis, unilateral
Q53.21	Abdominal testis, bilateral
TØ7	Unspecified multiple injuries
T14.8	Other injury of unspecified body region
T14.9Ø	Injury, unspecified
T14.91	Suicide attempt
Z36	Encounter for antenatal screening of mother

- 122 codes deleted from the classification

SØ6.1X7D	Traumatic cerebral edema with loss of consciousness of any duration with death due to brain injury prior to regaining consciousness, subsequent encounter
SØ6.1X7S	Traumatic cerebral edema with loss of consciousness of any duration with death due to brain injury prior to regaining consciousness, sequela
SØ6.1X8D	Traumatic cerebral edema with loss of consciousness of any duration with death due to other cause prior to regaining consciousness, subsequent encounter
SØ6.1X8S	Traumatic cerebral edema with loss of consciousness of any duration with death due to other cause prior to regaining consciousness, sequela
SØ6.2X7D	Diffuse traumatic brain injury with loss of consciousness of any duration with death due to brain injury prior to regaining consciousness, subsequent encounter
SØ6.2X7S	Diffuse traumatic brain injury with loss of consciousness of any duration with death due to brain injury prior to regaining consciousness, sequela
SØ6.2X8D	Diffuse traumatic brain injury with loss of consciousness of any duration with death due to other cause prior to regaining consciousness, subsequent encounter
SØ6.2X8S	Diffuse traumatic brain injury with loss of consciousness of any duration with death due to other cause prior to regaining consciousness, sequela
SØ6.3Ø7D	Unspecified focal traumatic brain injury with loss of consciousness of any duration with death due to brain injury prior to regaining consciousness, subsequent encounter
SØ6.3Ø7S	Unspecified focal traumatic brain injury with loss of consciousness of any duration with death due to brain injury prior to regaining consciousness, sequela
SØ6.3Ø8D	Unspecified focal traumatic brain injury with loss of consciousness of any duration with death due to other cause prior to regaining consciousness, subsequent encounter
SØ6.3Ø8S	Unspecified focal traumatic brain injury with loss of consciousness of any duration with death due to other cause prior to regaining consciousness, sequela
SØ6.317D	Contusion and laceration of right cerebrum with loss of consciousness of any duration with death due to brain injury prior to regaining consciousness, subsequent encounter
SØ6.317S	Contusion and laceration of right cerebrum with loss of consciousness of any duration with death due to brain injury prior to regaining consciousness, sequela
SØ6.318D	Contusion and laceration of right cerebrum with loss of consciousness of any duration with death due to other cause prior to regaining consciousness, subsequent encounter
SØ6.318S	Contusion and laceration of right cerebrum with loss of consciousness of any duration with death due to other cause prior to regaining consciousness, sequela
SØ6.327D	Contusion and laceration of left cerebrum with loss of consciousness of any duration with death due to brain injury prior to regaining consciousness, subsequent encounter

S06.327S   Contusion and laceration of left cerebrum with loss of consciousness of any duration with death due to brain injury prior to regaining consciousness, sequela

S06.328D   Contusion and laceration of left cerebrum with loss of consciousness of any duration with death due to other cause prior to regaining consciousness, subsequent encounter

S06.328S   Contusion and laceration of left cerebrum with loss of consciousness of any duration with death due to other cause prior to regaining consciousness, sequela

S06.337D   Contusion and laceration of cerebrum, unspecified, with loss of consciousness of any duration with death due to brain injury prior to regaining consciousness, subsequent encounter

S06.337S   Contusion and laceration of cerebrum, unspecified, with loss of consciousness of any duration with death due to brain injury prior to regaining consciousness, sequela

S06.338D   Contusion and laceration of cerebrum, unspecified, with loss of consciousness of any duration with death due to other cause prior to regaining consciousness, subsequent encounter

S06.338S   Contusion and laceration of cerebrum, unspecified, with loss of consciousness of any duration with death due to other cause prior to regaining consciousness, sequela

S06.347D   Traumatic hemorrhage of right cerebrum with loss of consciousness of any duration with death due to brain injury prior to regaining consciousness, subsequent encounter

S06.347S   Traumatic hemorrhage of right cerebrum with loss of consciousness of any duration with death due to brain injury prior to regaining consciousness, sequela

S06.348D   Traumatic hemorrhage of right cerebrum with loss of consciousness of any duration with death due to other cause prior to regaining consciousness, subsequent encounter

S06.348S   Traumatic hemorrhage of right cerebrum with loss of consciousness of any duration with death due to other cause prior to regaining consciousness, sequela

S06.357D   Traumatic hemorrhage of left cerebrum with loss of consciousness of any duration with death due to brain injury prior to regaining consciousness, subsequent encounter

S06.357S   Traumatic hemorrhage of left cerebrum with loss of consciousness of any duration with death due to brain injury prior to regaining consciousness, sequela

S06.358D   Traumatic hemorrhage of left cerebrum with loss of consciousness of any duration with death due to other cause prior to regaining consciousness, subsequent encounter

S06.358S   Traumatic hemorrhage of left cerebrum with loss of consciousness of any duration with death due to other cause prior to regaining consciousness, sequela

S06.367D   Traumatic hemorrhage of cerebrum, unspecified, with loss of consciousness of any duration with death due to brain injury prior to regaining consciousness, subsequent encounter

S06.367S   Traumatic hemorrhage of cerebrum, unspecified, with loss of consciousness of any duration with death due to brain injury prior to regaining consciousness, sequela

S06.368D   Traumatic hemorrhage of cerebrum, unspecified, with loss of consciousness of any duration with death due to

other cause prior to regaining consciousness, subsequent encounter

S06.368S   Traumatic hemorrhage of cerebrum, unspecified, with loss of consciousness of any duration with death due to other cause prior to regaining consciousness, sequela

S06.377D   Contusion, laceration, and hemorrhage of cerebellum with loss of consciousness of any duration with death due to brain injury prior to regaining consciousness, subsequent encounter

S06.377S   Contusion, laceration, and hemorrhage of cerebellum with loss of consciousness of any duration with death due to brain injury prior to regaining consciousness, sequela

S06.378D   Contusion, laceration, and hemorrhage of cerebellum with loss of consciousness of any duration with death due to other cause prior to regaining consciousness, subsequent encounter

S06.378S   Contusion, laceration, and hemorrhage of cerebellum with loss of consciousness of any duration with death due to other cause prior to regaining consciousness, sequela

S06.387D   Contusion, laceration, and hemorrhage of brainstem with loss of consciousness of any duration with death due to brain injury prior to regaining consciousness, subsequent encounter

S06.387S   Contusion, laceration, and hemorrhage of brainstem with loss of consciousness of any duration with death due to brain injury prior to regaining consciousness, sequela

S06.388D   Contusion, laceration, and hemorrhage of brainstem with loss of consciousness of any duration with death due to other cause prior to regaining consciousness, subsequent encounter

S06.388S   Contusion, laceration, and hemorrhage of brainstem with loss of consciousness of any duration with death due to other cause prior to regaining consciousness, sequela

S06.4X7D   Epidural hemorrhage with loss of consciousness of any duration with death due to brain injury prior to regaining consciousness, subsequent encounter

S06.4X7S   Epidural hemorrhage with loss of consciousness of any duration with death due to brain injury prior to regaining consciousness, sequela

S06.4X8D   Epidural hemorrhage with loss of consciousness of any duration with death due to other causes prior to regaining consciousness, subsequent encounter

S06.4X8S   Epidural hemorrhage with loss of consciousness of any duration with death due to other causes prior to regaining consciousness, sequela

S06.5X7D   Traumatic subdural hemorrhage with loss of consciousness of any duration with death due to brain injury before regaining consciousness, subsequent encounter

S06.5X7S   Traumatic subdural hemorrhage with loss of consciousness of any duration with death due to brain injury before regaining consciousness, sequela

S06.5X8D   Traumatic subdural hemorrhage with loss of consciousness of any duration with death due to other cause before regaining consciousness, subsequent encounter

S06.5X8S Traumatic subdural hemorrhage with loss of consciousness of any duration with death due to other cause before regaining consciousness, sequela

S06.6X7D Traumatic subarachnoid hemorrhage with loss of consciousness of any duration with death due to brain injury prior to regaining consciousness, subsequent encounter

S06.6X7S Traumatic subarachnoid hemorrhage with loss of consciousness of any duration with death due to brain injury prior to regaining consciousness, sequela

S06.6X8D Traumatic subarachnoid hemorrhage with loss of consciousness of any duration with death due to other cause prior to regaining consciousness, subsequent encounter

S06.6X8S Traumatic subarachnoid hemorrhage with loss of consciousness of any duration with death due to other cause prior to regaining consciousness, sequela

S06.817D Injury of right internal carotid artery, intracranial portion, not elsewhere classified with loss of consciousness of any duration with death due to brain injury prior to regaining consciousness, subsequent encounter

S06.817S Injury of right internal carotid artery, intracranial portion, not elsewhere classified with loss of consciousness of any duration with death due to brain injury prior to regaining consciousness, sequela

S06.818D Injury of right internal carotid artery, intracranial portion, not elsewhere classified with loss of consciousness of any duration with death due to other cause prior to regaining consciousness, subsequent encounter

S06.818S Injury of right internal carotid artery, intracranial portion, not elsewhere classified with loss of consciousness of any duration with death due to other cause prior to regaining consciousness, sequela

S06.827D Injury of left internal carotid artery, intracranial portion, not elsewhere classified with loss of consciousness of any duration with death due to brain injury prior to regaining consciousness, subsequent encounter

S06.827S Injury of left internal carotid artery, intracranial portion, not elsewhere classified with loss of consciousness of any duration with death due to brain injury prior to regaining consciousness, sequela

S06.828D Injury of left internal carotid artery, intracranial portion, not elsewhere classified with loss of consciousness of any duration with death due to other cause prior to regaining consciousness, subsequent encounter

S06.828S Injury of left internal carotid artery, intracranial portion, not elsewhere classified with loss of consciousness of any duration with death due to other cause prior to regaining consciousness, sequela

S06.897D Other specified intracranial injury with loss of consciousness of any duration with death due to brain injury prior to regaining consciousness, subsequent encounter

S06.897S Other specified intracranial injury with loss of consciousness of any duration with death due to brain injury prior to regaining consciousness, sequela

S06.898D Other specified intracranial injury with loss of consciousness of any duration with death due to other cause prior to regaining consciousness, subsequent encounter

S06.898S Other specified intracranial injury with loss of consciousness of any duration with death due to other cause prior to regaining consciousness, sequela

S06.9X7D Unspecified intracranial injury with loss of consciousness of any duration with death due to brain injury prior to regaining consciousness, subsequent encounter

S06.9X7S Unspecified intracranial injury with loss of consciousness of any duration with death due to brain injury prior to regaining consciousness, sequela

S06.9X8D Unspecified intracranial injury with loss of consciousness of any duration with death due to other cause prior to regaining consciousness, subsequent encounter

S06.9X8S Unspecified intracranial injury with loss of consciousness of any duration with death due to other cause prior to regaining consciousness, sequela

S63.13 Subluxation and dislocation of proximal interphalangeal joint of thumb

S63.131 Subluxation of proximal interphalangeal joint of right thumb

S63.131A Subluxation of proximal interphalangeal joint of right thumb, initial encounter

S63.131D Subluxation of proximal interphalangeal joint of right thumb, subsequent encounter

S63.131S Subluxation of proximal interphalangeal joint of right thumb, sequela

S63.132 Subluxation of proximal interphalangeal joint of left thumb

S63.132A Subluxation of proximal interphalangeal joint of left thumb, initial encounter

S63.132D Subluxation of proximal interphalangeal joint of left thumb, subsequent encounter

S63.132S Subluxation of proximal interphalangeal joint of left thumb, sequela

S63.133 Subluxation of proximal interphalangeal joint of unspecified thumb

S63.133A Subluxation of proximal interphalangeal joint of unspecified thumb, initial encounter

S63.133D Subluxation of proximal interphalangeal joint of unspecified thumb, subsequent encounter

S63.133S Subluxation of proximal interphalangeal joint of unspecified thumb, sequela

S63.134 Dislocation of proximal interphalangeal joint of right thumb

S63.134A Dislocation of proximal interphalangeal joint of right thumb, initial encounter

S63.134D Dislocation of proximal interphalangeal joint of right thumb, subsequent encounter

S63.134S Dislocation of proximal interphalangeal joint of right thumb, sequela

S63.135 Dislocation of proximal interphalangeal joint of left thumb

S63.135A Dislocation of proximal interphalangeal joint of left thumb, initial encounter

S63.135D Dislocation of proximal interphalangeal joint of left thumb, subsequent encounter

S63.135S Dislocation of proximal interphalangeal joint of left thumb, sequela

S63.136 Dislocation of proximal interphalangeal joint of unspecified thumb

S63.136A	Dislocation of proximal interphalangeal joint of unspecified thumb, initial encounter
S63.136D	Dislocation of proximal interphalangeal joint of unspecified thumb, subsequent encounter
S63.136S	Dislocation of proximal interphalangeal joint of unspecified thumb, sequela
S63.14	Subluxation and dislocation of distal interphalangeal joint of thumb
S63.141	Subluxation of distal interphalangeal joint of right thumb
S63.141A	Subluxation of distal interphalangeal joint of right thumb, initial encounter
S63.141D	Subluxation of distal interphalangeal joint of right thumb, subsequent encounter
S63.141S	Subluxation of distal interphalangeal joint of right thumb, sequela
S63.142	Subluxation of distal interphalangeal joint of left thumb
S63.142A	Subluxation of distal interphalangeal joint of left thumb, initial encounter
S63.142D	Subluxation of distal interphalangeal joint of left thumb, subsequent encounter
S63.142S	Subluxation of distal interphalangeal joint of left thumb, sequela
S63.143	Subluxation of distal interphalangeal joint of unspecified thumb
S63.143A	Subluxation of distal interphalangeal joint of unspecified thumb, initial encounter
S63.143D	Subluxation of distal interphalangeal joint of unspecified thumb, subsequent encounter
S63.143S	Subluxation of distal interphalangeal joint of unspecified thumb, sequela
S63.144	Dislocation of distal interphalangeal joint of right thumb
S63.144A	Dislocation of distal interphalangeal joint of right thumb, initial encounter
S63.144D	Dislocation of distal interphalangeal joint of right thumb, subsequent encounter
S63.144S	Dislocation of distal interphalangeal joint of right thumb, sequela
S63.145	Dislocation of distal interphalangeal joint of left thumb
S63.145A	Dislocation of distal interphalangeal joint of left thumb, initial encounter
S63.145D	Dislocation of distal interphalangeal joint of left thumb, subsequent encounter
S63.145S	Dislocation of distal interphalangeal joint of left thumb, sequela
S63.146	Dislocation of distal interphalangeal joint of unspecified thumb
S63.146A	Dislocation of distal interphalangeal joint of unspecified thumb, initial encounter
S63.146D	Dislocation of distal interphalangeal joint of unspecified thumb, subsequent encounter
S63.146S	Dislocation of distal interphalangeal joint of unspecified thumb, sequela

Proprietary Updates

The following proprietary features have also been added:

- 150+ new definitions that describe, in lay terms, a specific condition or disease process

- 50+ new illustrations

- Updated *AHA Coding Clinic* references through second quarter 2017

- Updated pharmacology list

- New HCC icon identifying CMS hierarchical condition category (CMS-HCC) codes

- New appendix outlining the Medicare Advantage risk-adjustment model

- Updated coding examples in the chapter-specific guideline sections, specific to the inpatient setting

- New POA Exempt list, provided as a searchable data file, available at Optum360coding.com

Introduction

History of ICD-10-CM

The ICD-10-CM classification system was developed by the National Center for Health Statistics (NCHS) as a clinical modification to the ICD-10 system developed by the World Health Organization (WHO), primarily as a unique system for use in the United States for morbidity and mortality reporting. Although ICD-10 replaced ICD-9 for use in coding and classifying of mortality data from death certificates beginning January 1, 1999, ICD-10-CM implementation was postponed many years until legislation to replace ICD-9-CM, volumes 1 and 2, with ICD-10-CM was approved.

ICD-10 is the copyrighted product of the World Health Organization (WHO), which has authorized the development of a clinical modification (CM) of ICD-10 for use in the United States. However, all modifications to the ICD-10 must conform to WHO conventions for ICD. The development of ICD-10-CM included comprehensive evaluation by a Technical Advisory Panel and extensive consultation with physician groups, clinical coders, and other industry experts.

The ICD-10-CM draft and crosswalk between ICD-9-CM and ICD-10-CM were made available on the Centers for Medicare and Medicaid Services (CMS) website for public comment. The initial public comment period extended from December 1997 through February 1998. A field test for ICD-10-CM was conducted in the summer of 2003 jointly by the American Hospital Association (AMA) and the American Health Information Management Association (AHIMA). Public comments and suggestions were reviewed and additional modifications to ICD-10-CM were made. Revisions were made to ICD-10-CM based on the established update process for ICD-10-CM (the ICD-10-CM Coordination and Maintenance Committee) and the World Health Organization's ICD-10 (the Update and Revision Committee).

These revisions to ICD-10-CM have included:

- Information relevant to ambulatory and managed care encounters
- Expanded injury codes
- Creation of combination diagnosis/symptom codes to reduce the number of codes needed to fully describe a condition
- The addition of 6th and 7th character classifications
- Incorporation of common 4th and 5th character classifications
- Classifications specific to laterality
- Classification refinement for increased data granularity

This new structure allows for further expansion than was possible with the ICD-9-CM classification system.

The Department of Health and Human Services (HHS) published the final rule regarding the adoption of both ICD-10-CM and ICD-10-PCS in the January 16, 2009, *Federal Register* (45 CFR part 162 [CMS—0013—F]). The initial compliance date for implementation of ICD-10-CM and ICD-10-PCS as a replacement for ICD-9-CM was set at October 1, 2013. On April 17, 2012, the Department of Health and Human Services (HHS) released a notice to postpone the date by which certain health care entities have to comply with International Classification of Diseases, 10th Revision diagnosis and procedure codes (ICD-10). The compliance date for implementation of ICD-10-CM and ICD-10-PCS as a replacement for ICD-9-CM was changed to October 1, 2014. On April 1, 2014, Congress enacted the Protecting Access to Medicare Act of 2014, which contained a provision to delay the implementation of ICD-10-CM/PCS by at least one year, prohibiting the Department of Health and Human Services (HHS) from adopting the ICD-10-CM/PCS code sets as the mandatory standard until October 1, 2015. Eventually, the ICD-10-CM/PCS code sets were implemented in their entirety on October 1, 2015, and ICD-9-CM, volumes 1 and 2, were retired.

ICD-10-CM for Hospitals: The Complete Official Code Set

ICD-10-CM for Hospitals: The Complete Official Code Set 2018 includes many of the enhancements described below in direct response to requests from our subscribers.

As you review the content, you will find the following:

- Optum360 Exclusive feature — Check Placeholder Alert symbol, indicating the need for one or more "filler" X character assignments in the 5th and/or 6th character position to appropriately assign a required character in the 7th character position

- Optum360 Exclusive feature — Key word differentiation by the use of a green font that highlights the differentiating terms in similar code descriptions in a given category

- Optum360 Exclusive feature — Exclusive *following* references and Check Additional Character symbol in the indexes. The *following* references (designed and used exclusively by Optum360) help coders locate those alphanumeric codes that are out of sequence in the tabular section.

- Optum360 Exclusive feature — Exclusive shaded guides in the index that help users easily follow the indent levels for the subterms under a main term

- Illustrations throughout the tabular list and at the back of the book that feature anatomy and terminology included in the ICD-10-CM classification system

- Optum360 Exclusive feature — Detailed muscle/tendon tables that correspond with codes in chapters 13 and 19

- The complete ICD-10-CM Official Guidelines for Coding and Reporting, published by the U.S. Department of Health and Human Services and approved by the cooperating parties (American Health Information Management Association, National Center for Health Statistics, Centers for Medicare and Medicaid Services, American Hospital Association)

- Optum360 Exclusive feature — Official chapter-specific guidelines with coding examples specific to the hospital setting at the beginning of each chapter

- Exclusive color coding, symbols, and footnotes that alert coders to coding and reimbursement issues, including the majority of the Medicare code edits and identification of conditions that significantly affect DRG assignment

- A searchable data file for complication and comorbidity (CC) exclusions with a reference beneath applicable codes to make it easier to determine complications and comorbidities excluded from a particular principal diagnosis

- All official ICD-10-CM codes, indexes, notes, footnotes, and symbols

- Icons and definitions to differentiate between the two types of Excludes notes

- Check 4th, 5th, 6th, and 7th character symbols that identify codes that require the addition of a 4th, 5th, 6th, or 7th character for code specificity and validity

- Color coding and symbol legend at the bottom of each page

Please review "How to Use *ICD-10-CM Expert for Hospitals*" in this manual to learn about the features that will help you assign and report correct codes, ensuring appropriate reimbursement.

How to Use ICD-10-CM Expert for Hospitals 2018

This International Classification of Diseases, 10th Revision, Clinical Modification (ICD-10-CM) is being published by the United States Government in recognition of its responsibility to promulgate this classification throughout the United States for morbidity coding. This code book represents an adaptation of ICD-10 that was created specifically for use in the United States. Revisions to ICD-10-CM will be made based on the established update process for ICD-10-CM (the ICD-10-CM Coordination and Maintenance Committee) and the World Health Organization's ICD-10 (the Update and Revision Committee).

Use of Official Sources

The *ICD-10-CM Expert for Hospitals* contains the official U.S. Department of Health and Human Services, Tenth Revision, Clinical Modification (ICD-10-CM) codes, effective for the current year.

Much of the color coding and many of the symbols and footnotes that identify coding and reimbursement issues are derived from official federal government sources, including Medicare Code Editor (MCE), version 34, ICD-10 MS-DRG Definitions Manual Files, version 34, and the *Federal Register,* volume 82, number 81, April 28, 2017 ("Hospital Inpatient Prospective Payment Systems for Acute Care Hospitals and the Long-Term Care Hospital Prospective Payment System and Proposed Policy Changes and Fiscal Year 2018 Rates; Proposed Rule").

For the most current files related to IPPS please refer to the following:

https://www.cms.gov/Medicare/Medicare-Fee-for-Service-Payment/AcuteInpatientPPS/IPPS-Regulations-and-Notices.html.

Steps to Correct Coding

1. Before beginning to use this code book, review section I.A., "Conventions for the ICD-10-CM," and section I.B., "General Coding Guidelines," of the ICD-10-CM Official Guidelines for Coding and Reporting.

2. Look up the main term in the alphabetic index and scan the subterm entries as appropriate. Review continued lines and additional subterms that may appear in the next column or on the next page.

3. Note all parenthetical terms (nonessential modifiers) that help in code selection but do not affect code assignment. Shaded vertical guidelines in the index are provided to help determine the indentation level for each subterm in relation to the main terms.

4. Pay close attention to the following instructions in the index:

    – "See," "see also," and "see category" cross-references

    – "With"/"without" notes

    – "Omit code" notes

    – "Due to" subterms

    – Other instructions found in note boxes, such as "code by site"

    – *Following* references and Check Additional Character symbol in the indexes. The *following* references (designed and used exclusively by Optum360) help coders locate those alphanumeric codes that are out of sequence in the tabular section.

5. Do not code from the alphabetic index without verifying the accuracy of the code in the Tabular List. Locate the code in the alphanumerically arranged Tabular List.

6. To determine the appropriateness of the code selection and proper coding, read all instructional material:

    – "Includes" and both types of "Excludes" notes

    – "Use additional code" and "code first underlying disease" instructions

    – "Code also"

    – 4th, 5th, and 6th character requirements and 7th character extension requirements

    – CC Exclusions

    – Age and sex symbols

7. Consult the official ICD-10-CM guidelines, which govern the use of specific codes. These guidelines provide both general and chapter-specific coding guidance.

8. Confirm and assign the correct code.

Organization

This book is organized in the following manner:

Introduction

The introductory material in this book includes the ICD-10-CM Official Preface, the history of ICD-10-CM as well as an overview of the classification system.

Official ICD-10-CM Conventions and Guidelines

This section provides an explanation of the conventions and guidelines regulating the appropriate assignment and reporting of ICD-10-CM codes. This coding guidance is presented by the National Center for Health Statistics (NCHS), a governmental agency of the Centers for Disease Control and Prevention (CDC), within the United States Department of Health and Human Services (DHHS).

Alphabetic Index to Diseases

The Alphabetic Index to Diseases is arranged in alphabetic order by disease — by specific illness, injury, eponym, abbreviation, or other descriptive diagnostic term. The index also lists diagnostic terms for other reasons for encounters with health care professionals.

Neoplasm Table

The Neoplasm Table provides the proper code based upon histology of the neoplasm and site.

Table of Drugs and Chemicals

The Table of Drugs and Chemicals lists the drug and the specific codes that identify the drug and the intent. No additional external cause of injury and poisoning code is assigned in ICD-10-CM.

Index to External Causes

The Alphabetic Index to External Causes of injuries is arranged in alphabetic order by main term indicating the event.

Tabular List of Diseases

ICD-10-CM codes and descriptors are arranged numerically within the Tabular List of diseases within 21 separate chapters according to body system or nature of injury and disease. Classifications which were previously considered supplemental to ICD-9-CM (e.g., V codes and E codes) are incorporated into the Tabular Listing of ICD-10-CM as individual chapters. Chapters 20, "External Causes of Morbidity," and 21, "Factors Influencing Health Status and Contact with Health Services," include chapter-specific guidelines.

Appendixes

The resources described below have been included as appendixes for the *ICD-10-CM Expert for Hospitals: The Complete Official Code Set.* These resources further instruct the inpatient coder on the appropriate application of the ICD-10-CM code set.

Appendix A: 10 Steps to Correct Coding

This step-by-step tutorial walks the coder through the process of locating the correct code in the alphabetic index and verifying it in the tabular section while following applicable conventions and guidelines. Detailed examples are provided and explained along with advice for proper sequencing.

Appendix B: Valid 3-character ICD-10-CM Codes

The user may consult this table to confirm that no further specificity, such as the use of 4th, 5th, 6th, or 7th characters or placeholders (X), is necessary. All ICD-10-CM codes that are valid at the three-character level are listed.

Appendix C: Pharmacology List 2018

This reference is a comprehensive but not all-inclusive list of pharmacological agents used to treat acute and/or chronic conditions. Drugs are listed in alphabetical order by their brand and/or generic names along with their drug action and indications for which they may commonly be prescribed. Some drugs have also been mapped to their appropriate long-term drug use Z code.

Appendix D: Z Codes for Long-Term Drug Use with Associated Drugs

This resource correlates Z codes that are used to identify current long-term drug use with a list of drugs that are typically categorized to that class of drug.

Note: These tables are not all-inclusive but list some of the more commonly used drugs.

Appendix E: Major Complication and Comorbidity (MCC) Code List

This is a full listing of conditions considered to be major complications and/or comorbidities that when present as a secondary diagnosis may affect DRG assignment under the Medicare Severity DRG (MS-DRG) system.

Appendix F: Complication and Comorbidity (CC) Code List

This is a full listing of conditions considered to be complications and/or comorbidities that when present as a secondary diagnosis may affect DRG assignment under the MS-DRG system.

Appendix G: Lists of Principal Diagnoses That Are Their Own CC and Their Own MCC

This listing displays those ICD-10-CM combination codes that may function as their own CC or MCC when sequenced as a principal diagnosis based on the MS-DRG system.

Appendix H: Present on Admission (POA) Tutorial

This tutorial walks the coder through the process of assigning the appropriate present-on-admission (POA) indicator for inpatient codes based on the POA reporting guidelines. Detailed scenarios for a variety of situations are provided and discussed.

Appendix I: Hospital Acquired Conditions

This comprehensive table displays codes that identify conditions that are considered reasonably preventable when occurring during the hospital admission and may prevent the case from grouping to a higher-paying MS-DRG. Many of these HACs are conditional and are based on reporting the specific diagnosis code(s) in combination with certain procedure codes, which are also noted in this table.

Appendix J: Centers for Medicare & Medicaid Services (CMS) Hierarchical Condition Categories (HCC) (CMS-HCC)

This resource provides the framework behind CMS's Medicare Advantage (MA) program, a risk-adjustment model developed as a means of compensating health care plans with large numbers of Medicare Part C beneficiaries. It includes a brief synopsis of the evolution of the program from its inception; insight into the various elements needed to predict risk, including the principles used to develop the hierarchical condition categories (HCCs), one of the fundamental components of the risk adjustment model; and a description of the audit process used to ensure the accuracy of payments made to MA plans.

Illustrations

This section includes illustrations of normal anatomy with ICD-10-CM specific terminology.

ICD-10-CM Hospital Data Files

To save space in this coding manual and provide more comprehensive references for the user, Optum360 has provided searchable data files for certain features in this manual. These data files can be accessed at the following:

http://www.optum360coding.com/ProdcutUpdates/

Two data files are available for FY 2018; the titles and passwords to each of these are provided below:

- CC Exclusions Data File

  Title: "2018 ICD-10-CM for Hospitals CC Excludes Data File"

  Password: OptumCCExcl18

- POA Exempt Data File

  Title: "2018 ICD-10-CM for Hospitals POA Exemption Data File"

  Password: OptumPOAExempt18

Overview of ICD-10-CM Official Conventions

This is an overview of the ICD-10-CM official conventions, which are general rules for the use of the classification system, independent of the guidelines. The official conventions and instructions of the classification, which take precedence over the guidelines, are incorporated within the alphabetic index and tabular list as instructional notes and are applicable regardless of the health care setting. For the full version of the official conventions, see the ICD-10-CM Official Guidelines for Coding and Reporting, section I.A., which is included in this book.

Format

ICD-10-CM is divided into two main parts: the index, an alphabetical list of terms and their corresponding code, and the Tabular List, a sequential, alphanumeric list of codes divided into chapters based on body system or condition. The index contains the Index to Diseases and Injuries (main index) and the Index to External Causes of Injury. Also included in the main Index is the Neoplasm Table and a Table of Drugs and Chemicals.

The Tabular List contains categories, subcategories, and valid codes. ICD-10-CM is an alphanumeric classification system. The 1st character of a three-character category is a letter. The 2nd and 3rd characters may be numbers or alpha characters. A three-character category without further subclassification is equivalent to a valid three-character code. Subcategories are either four or five characters. Subcategory characters include either letters or numbers. Codes may be three, four, five, six, or seven characters in length, in which each level of subdivision after a category is a subcategory. The final level of subdivision is a valid code. The final character in a code may be either a letter or a number.

The ICD-10-CM uses the letter "X" as a placeholder. A placeholder "X" is used as a 5th character placeholder at certain six character codes to allow for future expansion, without disturbing the 6th character structure. For instance, an initial encounter for accidental poisoning by penicillin is coded to T36.ØX1A. The "X" in the 5th character position is a placeholder, or filler character.

Similarly, certain categories have applicable 7th character extensions. In these cases, the 7th character extension is required for all codes within the category, or as otherwise instructed in the tabular list notations. 7th character extensions must always be the last character in the data field. If a code is not a full six characters in length, a dummy placeholder "X" must be used to fill in the empty characters when a 7th character extension is required.

Punctuation

[ ]   In the Tabular List, brackets are used to enclose synonyms, alternative wording, or explanatory phrases. In the index, brackets are used to identify manifestation codes.

( )   Parentheses are used in both the index and tabular list to enclose nonessential modifiers; supplementary words that may be present or absent in the statement of a disease or procedure without affecting the code number to which it is assigned.

:   Colons are used in the tabular list after an incomplete term that needs one or more of the modifiers following the colon to make it assignable to a given category.

Abbreviations

NEC

The abbreviation NEC, "Not elsewhere classifiable" represents "other specified" in the ICD-10-CM. An Index entry that states NEC directs the coder to an "other specified" code in the Tabular List. Codes titled "Other" or "Other specified" in the Tabular List (usually a code with a 4th or 6th character 8 and 5th character 9) are for use when the information in the medical record provides detail for which a specific code does not exist.

NOS

The abbreviation NOS, "Not otherwise specified," in the Tabular List may be interpreted as "unspecified." Codes in the Tabular List with "Unspecified" in the title (usually a code with a 4th or 6th character 9 and 5th character Ø) are for use when the information in the medical record is insufficient to assign a more specific code.

Typeface

Boldface

Boldface type is used for main term entries in the alphabetic index, and all codes and descriptions in the Tabular List.

General Notes

The following conventions and notes appear only in the Tabular List of Diseases:

Includes Notes

The word INCLUDES appears immediately under certain categories to further define, clarify, or give examples of the content of a code category.

Inclusion Terms

Lists of inclusion terms are included under certain codes. These terms indicate some of the conditions for which that code number may be used. Inclusion terms may be synonyms with the code title, or, in the case of "other specified" codes, the terms may also provide a list of various conditions included within a classification code. The inclusion terms are not exhaustive. The index may provide additional terms that may also be assigned to a given code.

Excludes Notes

ICD-10-CM has two types of excludes notes. Each note has a different definition for use. However, they are similar in that they both indicate that codes excluded from each other are independent of each other.

Excludes 1

An EXCLUDES1 note is a "pure" excludes. It means "NOT CODED HERE!" An Excludes 1 note indicates mutually exclusive codes: two conditions that cannot be reported together. For example, a congenital form of a disease may not be reported with the acquired form of the same condition. The code excluded should never be reported with the applicable codes listed above the excludes notation.

An exception to the Excludes1 definition is the circumstance when the two conditions are unrelated to each other. If it is not clear whether the two conditions involving an Excludes1 note are related or not, query the provider. For example, code F45.8, Other somatoform disorders, has an Excludes1 note for "sleep related teeth grinding (G47.63)," because "teeth grinding" is an inclusion term under F45.8. Only one of these two codes should be assigned for teeth grinding. However psychogenic dysmenorrhea is also an inclusion term under F45.8, and a patient could have both this condition and sleep related teeth grinding. In this case, the two conditions are clearly unrelated to each other, and so it would be appropriate to report F45.8 and G47.63 together.

Excludes 2

An EXCLUDES 2 note means "NOT INCLUDED HERE." An Excludes 2 note indicates that although the excluded condition is not part of the condition it is excluded from, a patient may have both conditions at the same time. Therefore, when an Excludes 2 note appears under a code, it may be acceptable to use both the code and the excluded code together if supported by the medical documentation.

Note

NOTE The term "NOTE" appears as an icon and precedes the instructional information. These notes function as alerts to highlight coding instructions within the text.

Default Codes

In the Index, the default code is the code listed next to the main term. The default code represents the condition most commonly associated with the main term. This code may be assigned when documentation does not facilitate reporting a more specific code. Alternatively, it may provide an unspecified code for the condition.

Syndromes

Follow the Alphabetic Index guidance when coding syndromes. In the absence of index guidance, assign codes for the documented manifestations of the syndrome.

And

When the term "and" is used in a narrative statement or code title, it may be interpreted as "and/or."

With

The word "with" or "in" should be interpreted to mean "associated with" or "due to" when it appears in a code title, the Alphabetic Index, or an instructional note in the Tabular List. The classification presumes a causal relationship between the two conditions linked by these terms in the Alphabetic Index or Tabular List. These conditions should be coded as related even in the absence of provider documentation explicitly linking them, unless the documentation clearly states the conditions are unrelated or when another guideline exists that specifically requires a documented linkage between two conditions (e.g., sepsis guideline for "acute organ dysfunction that is not clearly associated with the sepsis"). For conditions not specifically linked by these relational terms in the classification or when a guideline requires that a linkage between two conditions be explicitly documented, provider documentation must link the conditions in order to code them as related.

The word "with" in the Alphabetic Index is sequenced immediately following the main term, not in alphabetical order.

See and See Also

The instruction "See" following a main term in the alphabetic index indicates that another term must be referenced in order to locate the correct code. The instructional note "See also" simply provides alternative terms that may be useful in determining the correct code but are not necessary to look up if the main term supplies the appropriate code.

Instructional Notes Used in the Tabular List

In the tabular section, the following instructional notes appear in red type for emphasis:

Code First/Use additional/In diseases classified elsewhere code:

These instructional notes provide sequencing instruction. They may appear independently of each other or to designate certain etiology/manifestation paired codes. These instructions signal the coder that an additional code should be reported to provide a more complete picture of that diagnosis.

In etiology/manifestation coding, ICD-10-CM requires the underlying condition to be sequenced first, followed by the manifestation. In these situations, codes with "In diseases classified elsewhere" in the code description are never permitted as a first-listed or principal diagnosis code and must be sequenced following the underlying condition code.

Code Also:

A "code also" note alerts the coder that more than one code may be required to fully describe the condition. The sequencing depends on the circumstances of the encounter. Factors that may determine sequencing include severity and reason for the encounter.

Code Assignment and Clinical Criteria

Diagnosis code assignment must be based on the provider's diagnostic statement that the condition exists and is not based on clinical criteria used by the provider to establish the diagnosis. Conflicting documentation must be queried.

Additional Annotations

Code-Level Notations

The tabular section of ICD-10-CM has various colors, symbol, and other tabular annotations that may help in code selection, provide clinical or coding information, or alert the coder to reimbursement issues affected by the diagnosis code assignment. Some codes may have more than one annotation. For quick reference to the meanings of the colors and symbols, look at the color/symbol legend at the bottom of each page in the tabular list.

Italics

Italicized type is used for all exclusion notes and to identify manifestation codes, those codes that should not be reported as first-listed (principal) diagnoses.

Color Coding/Symbols

New Code

This ● icon identifies the codes that are new to the classification system for the current year. The new code icon is to the left of the code.

Revised Code Title

This ▲ icon to the left of a code alerts the user to a change in that code's title. This change may be as simple as adding or removing punctuation, which may or may not change the intent of the code, to adding or removing specific terms from a code description that completely alter the circumstances in which the code would be used.

Revised Text

The revised text ▶◀ "bow ties" alert the user to changes in parenthetical notes for the current year. Revised text may include the following:

- A change in a current parenthetical description

- A change in the code(s) associated with a current parenthetical note

- A change in how a current parenthetical note is classified (e.g., an Excludes 1 note that changed to an Excludes 2 note)

- Addition of a new parenthetical note(s) to a code

Deleted Text

Strikethrough on code description(s) and/or code note(s) indicates a deletion from the classification for the current year. For example:

✓4ᵗʰ N25 Disorders resulting from impaired renal tubular function
    EXCLUDES 1 ~~metabolic disorders classifiable to E70-E88~~

The strikethrough over the Excludes 1 note indicates that this note was deleted from the classification and is no longer applicable to codes in category N25.

    ✓7ᵗʰ ~~S63.131 Subluxation of proximal interphalangeal joint of right thumb~~

The strikethrough over the code and the code description indicates that all codes in subcategory S63.131 (S63.131A, S63.131D, and S63.131S) have been deleted from the classification.

Additional Characters Required

✓4ᵗʰ This symbol indicates that the code requires a 4th character.

✓5ᵗʰ This symbol indicates that the code requires a 5th character.

✓6ᵗʰ This symbol indicates that the code requires a 6th character.

✓7ᵗʰ This symbol indicates that the code requires a 7th character.

✓x7ᵗʰ This symbol indicates that the code requires a 7th character following the placeholder "X". Codes with fewer than six characters that require a 7th character must contain placeholder "X" to fill in the empty character(s).

Key Word

Green font is used throughout the Tabular List of Diseases to differentiate the key words that appear in similar code descriptions in a given category or subcategory.

For example, refer to the list of codes below from category C7A:

C7A.020	Malignant carcinoid tumor of the **appendix**
C7A.021	Malignant carcinoid tumor of the **cecum**
C7A.022	Malignant carcinoid tumor of the **ascending colon**
C7A.023	Malignant carcinoid tumor of the **transverse colon**
C7A.024	Malignant carcinoid tumor of the **descending colon**
C7A.025	Malignant carcinoid tumor of the **sigmoid colon**
C7A.026	Malignant carcinoid tumor of the **rectum**
C7A.029	Malignant carcinoid tumor of the large intestine, **unspecified portion**

The portion of the code description that appears in **green font** in the tabular list helps the coder quickly identify the key terms and the correct code. This convention is especially useful when the codes describe laterality, such as the following codes from subcategory H40.22:

H40.221	Chronic angle-closure glaucoma, **right** eye
H40.222	Chronic angle-closure glaucoma, **left** eye
H40.223	Chronic angle-closure glaucoma, **bilateral**
H40.229	Chronic angle-closure glaucoma, **unspecified** eye

The key word convention is used only in those categories in which there are multiple codes with very similar descriptions with only a few words that differentiate them.

Medicare Code Edits

Medicare Administrative Contractors (MACs) and many payers use Medicare code edits to check the coding accuracy on claims. The coding edit information in this manual is used for acute care hospital inpatient admissions and has been updated to reflect v34 changes to the Medicare Code Editor (MCE) and ICD-10 MS-DRG Definitions Manual as well as changes identified in *Federal Register,* volume 82, number 81, April 28, 2017 ("Hospital Inpatient Prospective Payment Systems for Acute Care Hospitals and the Long-Term Care Hospital Prospective Payment System and Proposed Policy Changes and Fiscal Year 2018 Rates; Proposed Rule").

The Medicare code edits for diagnoses are listed below:

- Invalid diagnosis or procedure code

- External causes of morbidity codes as principal diagnosis

- Duplicate of PDx

- *Age conflict

- *Sex conflict

- *Manifestation code as principal diagnosis

- *Questionable principal diagnosis

- *Unacceptable principal diagnosis

- Invalid age

- Invalid sex

- *Wrong procedure performed

Starred edits above are identified in this manual by color bars, symbols, or footnotes as described below.

Age and Sex Edit
The age and sex edits below are used to detect inconsistencies between the patient's age and/or sex and the patient's diagnosis. The following edit symbols appear in the tabular list to the right of the code description.

Newborn Age: 0   **N**
These diagnoses are intended for newborns and neonates and the patient's age must be 0 years.

Pediatric Age: 0-17   **P**
These diagnoses are intended for children and the patient's age must between 0 and 17 years.

Maternity Age: 12-55   **M**
These diagnoses are intended for childbearing patients between the age of 12 and 55 years.

Adult Age: 15-124   **A**
These diagnoses are intended for patients between the age of 15 and 124 years.

Male diagnosis only   ♂

Female diagnosis only   ♀

Manifestation Code
These codes appear in italic type, with a **blue color bar** over the title. A manifestation code cannot be reported as a first-listed or principal diagnosis. By definition, a manifestation code represents a demonstration of some aspect of an underlying disease, which is separately classifiable. In the alphabetic index, these codes are listed as the secondary code in brackets. The underlying disease code is listed first.

Unacceptable PDx/Questionable Admission Dx
Unacceptable principal diagnoses will appear with a **gray color bar** over the code title. These codes do not describe a current illness or injury, but a circumstance which influences a patient's health status. They are considered an unacceptable principal diagnosis for *inpatient* admission.

Questionable admission diagnoses will also appear with a **gray color bar** over the code title along with a reference to footnote 4. These codes, although not unacceptable as a PDx, may be considered a "questionable admission" when used as PDx in an acute care hospital.

Wrong Procedure Performed Edit
The Wrong Procedure Performed edit was created to identify cases in which wrong surgeries occurred. Any claim with a code from the Y65.51-Y65.53 will be denied and returned to the provider. A surgical or other invasive procedure is considered to be a wrong procedure if:

- The procedure was performed on the wrong site
- The procedure was performed on the wrong patient, or
- The incorrect procedure was performed on a patient.

ICD-10 MS-DRG Definitions Manual Edits
An MS-DRG is assigned based on specific patient attributes, such as principal diagnosis, secondary diagnoses, procedures, and discharge status. The attributes (edits) provided in this manual are only those directly related to ICD-10-CM diagnoses and are used for acute care hospital inpatient admissions.

Hospital Acquired Condition (HAC)   **H1 — H14**
These codes identify conditions that are high cost or high volume or both, are either a complication or comorbidity (CC) or major complication or comorbidity (MCC) that as a secondary diagnosis results in assignment of a case to a higher-paying MS-DRG. These conditions are reasonably preventable through the application of evidence-based guidelines. If the condition is not present on admission (meaning it developed during the hospital admission), the case will not group to the higher-paying MS-DRG

based solely upon the reporting of the HAC code. Many of these HACs are conditional, and are based on reporting the specific diagnosis code(s) in combination with certain procedure codes, notated in footnotes.

The HAC icon with the specific HAC table number in which this code is classified appears to the right of the code description. The comprehensive list of HAC tables that coincide with these icon numbers appears in appendix I of this book.

CC Condition   **CC**
This symbol designates a complication or comorbidity diagnosis that may affect DRG assignment. A complication or comorbidity diagnosis, CC condition, is defined as a significant acute disease, a significant acute manifestation of a chronic disease, an advanced or end-stage chronic disease, or a chronic disease associated with systemic physiological decompensation and debility that have consistently greater impact on hospital resources.

A CC icon appears to the right of the code description.

MCC Condition   **MCC**
This symbol designates a major complication or comorbidity diagnosis that may affect DRG assignment. An MCC condition meets the same criteria as a CC condition but is associated with a higher acuity level and hospital resource consumption is expected to be higher than that for a CC condition. There are fewer conditions that meet the criteria as an MCC than those for a CC condition.

An MCC icon appears to the right of the code description.

CC Excludes Notations
The assignment of an MS-DRG often depends on the presence or absence of a secondary diagnosis code that is designated as an MCC or CC. However, in some instances the MCC or CC designation for that secondary diagnosis code is negated due to its relationship with the principal diagnosis.

To save space in this coding manual and provide a more comprehensive reference for the user, the CC Exclusion notations have been restructured. Instead of the individual codes being listed in the reference, which can in many cases be extensive, only the principal diagnosis collection (PDX collection) number is provided. A PDX collection contains a specific list of ICD-10-CM codes and their official descriptions that when used as principal diagnosis would render the MCC/CC designation ineffective. Each PDX collection is provided in an easily searchable data file which can be accessed at the following:

> https://www.optum360coding.com/ProductUpdates/
>
> Title: "2018 ICD-10-CM for Hospitals CC Excludes Data File"
>
> Password: OptumCCExcl18

Similar to the parenthetical notes, the CC Exclusion notations are provided at the category, subcategory, and/or code level. If a CC Exclusion notation is found at the category or subcategory level, all the CC and/or MCC codes in that category or subcategory share the same PDX collection listed in that notation. For example:

G43.6   Persistent migraine aura with cerebral infarction

> **CC Excl: For CC codes in subcategory G43.6, unless otherwise noted:** PDX collection 584

There are four codes with a CC designation in subcategory G43.6; the CC Excludes notation applies to all four codes.

Often a CC exclusion reference is specific to laterality for CC/MCC codes in a category or subcategory. Where possible, a CC exclusion reference is placed at the category or subcategory level with the PDX collection identified for the right, left, or unspecified side. For example:

S58   Traumatic amputation of elbow and forearm

> **CC Excl: For CC codes in category S58:**
> **Right side:** PDX collection 1266
> **Left side:** PDX collection 1267
> **Unspecified side:** PDX collection 1268

All CC codes that are specific to the right side in category S58 are excluded from being a CC for any principal diagnosis found in PDX collection 1266.

Where possible a "see" reference may also be used, referring the user to a previously designated CC excludes notation. For example:

S72.Ø   Fracture of head and neck of femur

> **CC Excl: For CC/MCC codes in subcategory S72.Ø:**
> **Right side:** See code S72.ØØ1
> **Left side:** See code S72.ØØ2
> **Unspecified side:** See code S72.ØØ9

If users want to know the principal diagnoses to which code S72.Ø22 Displaced fracture of epiphysis (separation) (upper) of left femur, may not function as a CC or MCC, they would be referred to the CC excludes notation under code S72.ØØ2.

Certain codes may also have no principal diagnosis codes to which they would be excluded from functioning as a CC or MCC. These are identified as follows:

A17.83   Tuberculosis neuritis

> **CC Excl:** No Excl

By definition of being a condition that acts as its own CC or MCC, the CC exclusion concept (two conditions being too interrelated) does not apply to PDxCC or PDxMCC (see "PDxCC or PDxMCC Condition"). However, if a condition carries separate PDxCC/PDxMCC and MCC/CC designations, a CC Excludes notation does appear for the CC and/or MCC designations.

PDxCC or PDxMCC Condition   `PDx CC` `PDx MCC`

Many ICD-10-CM codes identify multiple clinical concepts, typically describing an underlying condition and its associated acute manifestation; these are often referred to as combination codes. To continue to appropriately capture the complication/comorbidity (CC) or major complication/comorbidity (MCC) included in these combination codes, CMS introduced the concept of a diagnosis combination code acting as its own CC or MCC. For example, code I26.Ø9 Other pulmonary embolism with acute cor pulmonale, is designated as a principal diagnosis that can act as its own MCC to capture the severity and resource consumption related to a pulmonary embolism that is exacerbated by acute cor pulmonale but is represented by one ICD-10-CM code.

The PDxCC and PDxMCC icons appear to the right of the code description.

HIV   `HIV`

This symbol indicates that the condition is considered a major HIV-related diagnosis. When the condition is coded in combination with a diagnosis of human immunodeficiency virus (HIV), code B2Ø, the case will move from MS-DRG 977 to MS-DRGs 974-976.

The HIV icon appears to the right of the code description.

Medicare Advantage Risk Adjustment Edits

Medicare Advantage plans provided as part of the Medicare Part C program uses a risk-adjustment model to plan for future healthcare costs to Medicare Part C participants. The risk-adjustment model measures disease burden by designating certain ICD-10-CM diagnosis codes as falling into hierarchical condition categories (HCC). The HCC information in this manual has been updated to reflect the CMS-HCC model category for v22 of the CMS-HCC risk-adjustment software.

HCC   `HCC`

This symbol indicates that the condition is considered a CMS-HCC diagnosis. All HCC conditions that are appropriately documented are used in the risk-adjustment model for Medicare Advantage to provide a means of comparing quality of care across Medicare Part C participants as well as predict future healthcare costs.

The HCC icon appears to the right of the code description.

Other Code-Level Notations

AHA:

This symbol precedes official citations from AHA's *Coding Clinic for ICD-10-CM/PCS*. Similar to the parenthetical notes, AHA references are placed in a hierarchical pattern at the chapter, code block, category, subcategory, or valid code level. This means that the information found in the reference applies to one or more codes depending on where the citation is placed.

The citations appear in purple type and are listed with the most current citation first. *Coding Clinic* citations included in this edition have been updated through second quarter 2017.

DEF:

This symbol precedes a definition of a condition or disease.

The definition appears in purple type directly under the code.

TIP:

This symbol precedes coding advice that is not readily available within the ICD-10-CM classification. It may relate official coding guidelines, indexing nuances, or advice from *AHA's Coding Clinic for ICD-10-CM/PCS*.

The tip appears in purple type directly under the code.

Footnotes

All footnotes are identified by a numerical superscript that appears to the upper left of the code. For example:

[1] **I49.Ø1   Ventricular fibrillation**   `MCC`

The footnote 1 indicates "MCC = Only if patient is discharged alive." This means that ventricular fibrillation is considered a major complication or comorbidity that may affect DRG assignment only if the patient is discharged alive. Otherwise ventricular fibrillation is assigned as a non-MCC condition.

The following list identifies the meaning of each footnote number in the Tabular List of diseases:

1   These codes are considered major complication/comorbidity (MCC) conditions and may affect MS-DRG assignment only if the patient is discharged alive.

2   These codes indicate that the wrong procedure was performed on the patient and reimbursement may be affected.

3   This condition represents an unacceptable PDx for all encounters – initial, subsequent, and sequela (7th character A, D or S).

4   These codes, although not unacceptable as PDx, would be considered questionable as a PDx for acute care hospital admissions.

5   This code is considered an unacceptable PDx unless a relevant secondary diagnosis is also reported.

6   This condition is considered an MCC only when reported as an initial encounter for an open fracture (7th character B or C specific to category).

7   This condition is considered a CC only when reported as an initial encounter for a fracture (7th character A, B, or C specific to category) or a subsequent encounter for nonunion or malunion fracture (7th character K, M, N, P, Q, or R specific to category).

8   This condition is considered a CC only when reported as a subsequent encounter for a nonunion or malunion fracture (7th character K, M, N, P, Q, or R specific to category).

9   This condition is considered a CC only when reported as an initial encounter or subsequent encounter (7th character A or D).

10   This condition is considered an HCC when reported as initial encounter (7th character A, B, or C specific to category).

11   This condition is considered an HCC when reported as initial encounter (7th character A or B specific to category) or as a sequela.

12   This condition is considered an HCC when reported as a sequela.

Chapter-Level Notations

Chapter-Specific Guidelines with Coding Examples

Each chapter begins with the Official Guidelines for Coding and Reporting specific to that chapter, where provided. Coding examples specific to inpatient care settings have been provided to illustrate the coding and/or sequencing guidance in these guidelines.

Muscle and Tendon Table

ICD-10-CM categorizes certain muscles and tendons in the upper and lower extremities by their action (e.g., extension or flexion) as well as their anatomical location. The Muscle/Tendon table is provided at the beginning of chapter 13 and chapter 19 to help users when code selection depends on the action of the muscle and/or tendon.

Note: This table is not all-inclusive, and proper code assignment should be based on the provider's documentation.

Index Notations

▽ Subterms under main terms may continue to next column or page. This warning statement is a reminder to always check for additional subterms and information that may continue onto the next page or column before making a final selection.

Following References

The Index includes following references to assist in locating "out-of-sequence" codes in the tabular list. "Out-of-sequence" codes contain an alphabetic character (letter) in the 3rd or 4th character position. These codes are placed according to the classification rules — the placement of the codes according to condition — not according to alphabetic or numeric sequencing rules.

Examples:

Carcinoma (malignant) (*see also* Neoplasm, by site, malignant)
neuroendocrine (*see also* Tumor, neuroendocrine)
    high grade, any site C7A.1 (*following* C75)
    poorly differentiated, any site C7A.1 (*following* C75)

In the tabular rubric, C7A is included after rubric C75 and before C76.

Gout, chronic (*see also* Gout, gouty) M1A.9
    drug-induced M1A.2Ø (*following* MØ8)
        ankle M1A.27-(*following* MØ8)
        elbow M1A.22-(*following* MØ8)

In the tabular rubric, M1A is included after rubric MØ8 and before M1Ø.

ICD-10-CM Official Guidelines for Coding and Reporting

Narrative changes appear in **bold** text

Items underlined have been moved within the guidelines since the FY 2017 version

Italics are used to indicate revisions to heading changes

The Centers for Medicare and Medicaid Services (CMS) and the National Center for Health Statistics (NCHS), two departments within the U.S. Federal Government's Department of Health and Human Services (DHHS) provide the following guidelines for coding and reporting using the International Classification of Diseases, 10th Revision, Clinical Modification (ICD-10-CM). These guidelines should be used as a companion document to the official version of the ICD-10-CM as published on the NCHS website. The ICD-10-CM is a morbidity classification published by the United States for classifying diagnoses and reason for visits in all health care settings. The ICD-10-CM is based on the ICD-10, the statistical classification of disease published by the World Health Organization (WHO).

These guidelines have been approved by the four organizations that make up the Cooperating Parties for the ICD-10-CM: the American Hospital Association (AHA), the American Health Information Management Association (AHIMA), CMS, and NCHS.

These guidelines are a set of rules that have been developed to accompany and complement the official conventions and instructions provided within the ICD-10-CM itself. The instructions and conventions of the classification take precedence over guidelines. These guidelines are based on the coding and sequencing instructions in the Tabular List and Alphabetic Index of ICD-10-CM, but provide additional instruction. Adherence to these guidelines when assigning ICD-10-CM diagnosis codes is required under the Health Insurance Portability and Accountability Act (HIPAA). The diagnosis codes (Tabular List and Alphabetic Index) have been adopted under HIPAA for all healthcare settings. A joint effort between the healthcare provider and the coder is essential to achieve complete and accurate documentation, code assignment, and reporting of diagnoses and procedures. These guidelines have been developed to assist both the healthcare provider and the coder in identifying those diagnoses that are to be reported. The importance of consistent, complete documentation in the medical record cannot be overemphasized. Without such documentation accurate coding cannot be achieved. The entire record should be reviewed to determine the specific reason for the encounter and the conditions treated.

The term encounter is used for all settings, including hospital admissions. In the context of these guidelines, the term provider is used throughout the guidelines to mean physician or any qualified health care practitioner who is legally accountable for establishing the patient's diagnosis. Only this set of guidelines, approved by the Cooperating Parties, is official.

The guidelines are organized into sections. Section I includes the structure and conventions of the classification and general guidelines that apply to the entire classification, and chapter-specific guidelines that correspond to the chapters as they are arranged in the classification. Section II includes guidelines for selection of principal diagnosis for non-outpatient settings. Section III includes guidelines for reporting additional diagnoses in non-outpatient settings. Section IV is for outpatient coding and reporting. It is necessary to review all sections of the guidelines to fully understand all of the rules and instructions needed to code properly.

Section I. Conventions, general coding guidelines and chapter specific guidelines

The conventions, general guidelines and chapter-specific guidelines are applicable to all health care settings unless otherwise indicated. The conventions and instructions of the classification take precedence over guidelines.

A. Conventions for the ICD-10-CM

The conventions for the ICD-10-CM are the general rules for use of the classification independent of the guidelines. These conventions are incorporated within the Alphabetic Index and Tabular List of the ICD-10-CM as instructional notes.

1. The Alphabetic Index and Tabular List
The ICD-10-CM is divided into the Alphabetic Index, an alphabetical list of terms and their corresponding code, and the Tabular List, a structured list of codes divided into chapters based on body system or condition. The Alphabetic Index consists of the following parts: the Index of Diseases and Injury, the Index of External Causes of Injury, the Table of Neoplasms and the Table of Drugs and Chemicals.

See Section I.C2. General guidelines

See Section I.C.19. Adverse effects, poisoning, underdosing and toxic effects

2. Format and Structure:
The ICD-10-CM Tabular List contains categories, subcategories and codes. Characters for categories, subcategories and codes may be either a letter or a number. All categories are 3 characters. A three-character category that has no further subdivision is equivalent to a code. Subcategories are either 4 or 5 characters. Codes may be 3, 4, 5, 6 or 7 characters. That is, each level of subdivision after a category is a subcategory. The final level of subdivision is a code. Codes that have applicable 7th characters are still referred to as codes, not subcategories. A code that has an applicable 7th character is considered invalid without the 7th character.

The ICD-10-CM uses an indented format for ease in reference.

3. Use of codes for reporting purposes
For reporting purposes only codes are permissible, not categories or subcategories, and any applicable 7th character is required.

4. Placeholder character
The ICD-10-CM utilizes a placeholder character "X". The "X" is used as a placeholder at certain codes to allow for future expansion. An example of this is at the poisoning, adverse effect and underdosing codes, categories T36-T50.

Where a placeholder exists, the X must be used in order for the code to be considered a valid code.

5. 7th Characters
Certain ICD-10-CM categories have applicable 7th characters. The applicable 7th character is required for all codes within the category, or as the notes in the Tabular List instruct. The 7th character must always be the 7th character in the data field. If a code that requires a 7th character is not 6 characters, a placeholder X must be used to fill in the empty characters.

6. Abbreviations
a. Alphabetic Index abbreviations
NEC "Not elsewhere classifiable"

This abbreviation in the Alphabetic Index represents "other specified." When a specific code is not available for a condition, the Alphabetic Index directs the coder to the "other specified" code in the Tabular List.

NOS "Not otherwise specified"

This abbreviation is the equivalent of unspecified.

b. Tabular List abbreviations
NEC "Not elsewhere classifiable"

This abbreviation in the Tabular List represents "other specified". When a specific code is not available for a condition, the Tabular List includes an NEC entry under a code to identify the code as the "other specified" code.

NOS "Not otherwise specified"

This abbreviation is the equivalent of unspecified.

7. Punctuation
[ ] Brackets are used in the Tabular List to enclose synonyms, alternative wording or explanatory phrases. Brackets are used in the Alphabetic Index to identify manifestation codes.

( ) Parentheses are used in both the Alphabetic Index and Tabular List to enclose supplementary words that may be present or absent in the statement of a disease or procedure without affecting the code number to which it is assigned. The terms within the parentheses are referred to as nonessential modifiers. The nonessential modifiers in the Alphabetic Index to Diseases apply to subterms following a main term except when a nonessential modifier and a subentry are mutually exclusive, the subentry takes precedence. For example, in the ICD-10-CM Alphabetic Index under the main term Enteritis, "acute" is a nonessential modifier and "chronic" is a subentry. In this case, the nonessential modifier "acute" does not apply to the subentry "chronic".

: Colons are used in the Tabular List after an incomplete term which needs one or more of the modifiers following the colon to make it assignable to a given category.

8. Use of "and".
See Section I.A.14. Use of the term "And"

9. Other and Unspecified codes
a. "Other" codes
Codes titled "other" or "other specified" are for use when the information in the medical record provides detail for which a specific code does not exist. Alphabetic Index entries with NEC in the line designate "other" codes in the Tabular List. These Alphabetic Index entries represent specific disease entities for which no specific code exists so the term is included within an "other" code.

b. "Unspecified" codes
Codes titled "unspecified" are for use when the information in the medical record is insufficient to assign a more specific code. For those categories for which an unspecified code is not provided, the "other specified" code may represent both other and unspecified.

See Section I.B.18 Use of Signs/Symptom/Unspecified Codes

10. Includes Notes
This note appears immediately under a three character code title to further define, or give examples of, the content of the category.

11. Inclusion terms
List of terms is included under some codes. These terms are the conditions for which that code is to be used. The terms may be synonyms of the code title, or, in the case of "other specified" codes, the terms are a list of the various conditions assigned to that code. The inclusion terms are not necessarily exhaustive. Additional terms found only in the Alphabetic Index may also be assigned to a code.

12. Excludes Notes
The ICD-10-CM has two types of excludes notes. Each type of note has a different definition for use but they are all similar in that they indicate that codes excluded from each other are independent of each other.

a. Excludes1
A type 1 Excludes note is a pure excludes note. It means "NOT CODED HERE!" An Excludes1 note indicates that the code excluded should never be used at the same time as the code above the Excludes1 note. An Excludes1 is used when two conditions cannot occur together, such as a congenital form versus an acquired form of the same condition.

An exception to the Excludes1 definition is the circumstance when the two conditions are unrelated to each other. If it is not clear whether the two conditions involving an Excludes1 note are related or not, query the provider. For example, code F45.8, Other somatoform disorders, has an Excludes1 note for "sleep related teeth grinding (G47.63)," because "teeth grinding" is an inclusion term under F45.8. Only one of these two codes should be assigned for teeth grinding. However psychogenic dysmenorrhea is also an inclusion term under F45.8, and a patient could have both this condition and sleep related teeth grinding. In this case, the two conditions are clearly unrelated to each other, and so it would be appropriate to report F45.8 and G47.63 together.

b. **Excludes2**

A type 2 Excludes note represents "Not included here." An excludes2 note indicates that the condition excluded is not part of the condition represented by the code, but a patient may have both conditions at the same time. When an Excludes2 note appears under a code, it is acceptable to use both the code and the excluded code together, when appropriate.

13. **Etiology/manifestation convention ("code first", "use additional code" and "in diseases classified elsewhere" notes)**

Certain conditions have both an underlying etiology and multiple body system manifestations due to the underlying etiology. For such conditions, the ICD-10-CM has a coding convention that requires the underlying condition be sequenced first, if applicable, followed by the manifestation. Wherever such a combination exists, there is a "use additional code" note at the etiology code, and a "code first" note at the manifestation code. These instructional notes indicate the proper sequencing order of the codes, etiology followed by manifestation.

In most cases the manifestation codes will have in the code title, "in diseases classified elsewhere." Codes with this title are a component of the etiology/ manifestation convention. The code title indicates that it is a manifestation code. "In diseases classified elsewhere" codes are never permitted to be used as first-listed or principal diagnosis codes. They must be used in conjunction with an underlying condition code and they must be listed following the underlying condition. See category F02, Dementia in other diseases classified elsewhere, for an example of this convention.

There are manifestation codes that do not have "in diseases classified elsewhere" in the title. For such codes, there is a "use additional code" note at the etiology code and a "code first" note at the manifestation code, and the rules for sequencing apply.

In addition to the notes in the Tabular List, these conditions also have a specific Alphabetic Index entry structure. In the Alphabetic Index both conditions are listed together with the etiology code first followed by the manifestation codes in brackets. The code in brackets is always to be sequenced second.

An example of the etiology/manifestation convention is dementia in Parkinson's disease. In the Alphabetic Index, code G20 is listed first, followed by code F02.80 or F02.81 in brackets. Code G20 represents the underlying etiology, Parkinson's disease, and must be sequenced first, whereas code F02.80 and F02.81 represent the manifestation of dementia in diseases classified elsewhere, with or without behavioral disturbance.

"Code first" and "Use additional code" notes are also used as sequencing rules in the classification for certain codes that are not part of an etiology/ manifestation combination.

See Section I.B.7. Multiple coding for a single condition.

14. **"And"**

The word "and" should be interpreted to mean either "and" or "or" when it appears in a title.

For example, cases of "tuberculosis of bones", "tuberculosis of joints" and "tuberculosis of bones and joints" are classified to subcategory A18.0, Tuberculosis of bones and joints.

15. **"With"**

The word "with" **or "in"** should be interpreted to mean "associated with" or "due to" when it appears in a code title, the Alphabetic Index, or an instructional note in the Tabular List. The classification presumes a causal relationship between the two conditions linked by these terms in the Alphabetic Index or Tabular List. These conditions should be coded as related even in the absence of provider documentation explicitly linking them, unless the documentation clearly states the conditions are unrelated **or when another guideline exists that specifically requires a documented linkage between two conditions (e.g., sepsis guideline for "acute organ dysfunction that is not clearly associated with the sepsis").**

For conditions not specifically linked by these relational terms in the classification **or when a guideline requires that a linkage between two conditions be explicitly documented,** provider documentation must link the conditions in order to code them as related.

The word "with" in the Alphabetic Index is sequenced immediately following the main term, not in alphabetical order.

16. **"See" and "See Also"**

The "see" instruction following a main term in the Alphabetic Index indicates that another term should be referenced. It is necessary to go to the main term referenced with the "see" note to locate the correct code.

A "see also" instruction following a main term in the Alphabetic Index instructs that there is another main term that may also be referenced that may provide additional Alphabetic Index entries that may be useful. It is not necessary to follow the "see also" note when the original main term provides the necessary code.

17. **"Code also" note**

A "code also" note instructs that two codes may be required to fully describe a condition, but this note does not provide sequencing direction. **The sequencing depends on the circumstances of the encounter.**

18. **Default codes**

A code listed next to a main term in the ICD-10-CM Alphabetic Index is referred to as a default code. The default code represents that condition that is most commonly associated with the main term, or is the unspecified code for the condition. If a condition is documented in a medical record (for example, appendicitis) without any additional information, such as acute or chronic, the default code should be assigned.

19. **Code assignment and Clinical Criteria**

The assignment of a diagnosis code is based on the provider's diagnostic statement that the condition exists. The provider's statement that the patient has a particular condition is sufficient. Code assignment is not based on clinical criteria used by the provider to establish the diagnosis.

B. General Coding Guidelines

1. **Locating a code in the ICD-10-CM**

To select a code in the classification that corresponds to a diagnosis or reason for visit documented in a medical record, first locate the term in the Alphabetic Index, and then verify the code in the Tabular List. Read and be guided by instructional notations that appear in both the Alphabetic Index and the Tabular List.

It is essential to use both the Alphabetic Index and Tabular List when locating and assigning a code. The Alphabetic Index does not always provide the full code. Selection of the full code, including laterality and any applicable 7th character can only be done in the Tabular List. A dash (-) at the end of an Alphabetic Index entry indicates that additional characters are required. Even if a dash is not included at the Alphabetic Index entry, it is necessary to refer to the Tabular List to verify that no 7th character is required.

2. **Level of Detail in Coding**

Diagnosis codes are to be used and reported at their highest number of characters available.

ICD-10-CM diagnosis codes are composed of codes with 3, 4, 5, 6 or 7 characters. Codes with three characters are included in ICD-10-CM as the heading of a category of codes that may be further subdivided by the use of fourth and/or fifth characters and/or sixth characters, which provide greater detail.

A three-character code is to be used only if it is not further subdivided. A code is invalid if it has not been coded to the full number of characters required for that code, including the 7th character, if applicable.

3. **Code or codes from A00.0 through T88.9, Z00-Z99.8**

The appropriate code or codes from A00.0 through T88.9, Z00-Z99.8 must be used to identify diagnoses, symptoms, conditions, problems, complaints or other reason(s) for the encounter/visit.

4. **Signs and symptoms**

Codes that describe symptoms and signs, as opposed to diagnoses, are acceptable for reporting purposes when a related definitive diagnosis has not been established (confirmed) by the provider. Chapter 18 of ICD-10-CM, Symptoms, Signs, and Abnormal Clinical and Laboratory Findings, Not Elsewhere Classified (codes R00.0 - R99) contains many, but not all, codes for symptoms.

See Section I.B.18 Use of Signs/Symptom/Unspecified Codes

5. **Conditions that are an integral part of a disease process**

Signs and symptoms that are associated routinely with a disease process should not be assigned as additional codes, unless otherwise instructed by the classification.

6. **Conditions that are not an integral part of a disease process**

   Additional signs and symptoms that may not be associated routinely with a disease process should be coded when present.

7. **Multiple coding for a single condition**

   In addition to the etiology/manifestation convention that requires two codes to fully describe a single condition that affects multiple body systems, there are other single conditions that also require more than one code. "Use additional code" notes are found in the Tabular List at codes that are not part of an etiology/manifestation pair where a secondary code is useful to fully describe a condition. The sequencing rule is the same as the etiology/manifestation pair, "use additional code" indicates that a secondary code should be added, **if known.**

   For example, for bacterial infections that are not included in chapter 1, a secondary code from category B95, Streptococcus, Staphylococcus, and Enterococcus, as the cause of diseases classified elsewhere, or B96, Other bacterial agents as the cause of diseases classified elsewhere, may be required to identify the bacterial organism causing the infection. A "use additional code" note will normally be found at the infectious disease code, indicating a need for the organism code to be added as a secondary code.

   "Code first" notes are also under certain codes that are not specifically manifestation codes but may be due to an underlying cause. When there is a "code first" note and an underlying condition is present, the underlying condition should be sequenced first, **if known.**

   "Code, if applicable, any causal condition first" notes indicate that this code may be assigned as a principal diagnosis when the causal condition is unknown or not applicable. If a causal condition is known, then the code for that condition should be sequenced as the principal or first-listed diagnosis.

   Multiple codes may be needed for sequela, complication codes and obstetric codes to more fully describe a condition. See the specific guidelines for these conditions for further instruction.

8. **Acute and Chronic Conditions**

   If the same condition is described as both acute (subacute) and chronic, and separate subentries exist in the Alphabetic Index at the same indentation level, code both and sequence the acute (subacute) code first.

9. **Combination Code**

   A combination code is a single code used to classify:

   > Two diagnoses, or

   > A diagnosis with an associated secondary process (manifestation)

   > A diagnosis with an associated complication

   Combination codes are identified by referring to subterm entries in the Alphabetic Index and by reading the inclusion and exclusion notes in the Tabular List.

   Assign only the combination code when that code fully identifies the diagnostic conditions involved or when the Alphabetic Index so directs. Multiple coding should not be used when the classification provides a combination code that clearly identifies all of the elements documented in the diagnosis. When the combination code lacks necessary specificity in describing the manifestation or complication, an additional code should be used as a secondary code.

10. **Sequela (Late Effects)**

   A sequela is the residual effect (condition produced) after the acute phase of an illness or injury has terminated. There is no time limit on when a sequela code can be used. The residual may be apparent early, such as in cerebral infarction, or it may occur months or years later, such as that due to a previous injury. Examples of sequela include: scar formation resulting from a burn, deviated septum due to a nasal fracture, and infertility due to tubal occlusion from old tuberculosis. Coding of sequela generally requires two codes sequenced in the following order: the condition or nature of the sequela is sequenced first. The sequela code is sequenced second.

   An exception to the above guidelines are those instances where the code for the sequela is followed by a manifestation code identified in the Tabular List and title, or the sequela code has been expanded (at the fourth, fifth or sixth character levels) to include the manifestation(s). The code for the acute phase of an illness or injury that led to the sequela is never used with a code for the late effect.

   See Section I.C.9. Sequelae of cerebrovascular disease

   See Section I.C.15. Sequelae of complication of pregnancy, childbirth and the puerperium

See Section I.C.19. Application of 7th characters for Chapter 19

11. **Impending or Threatened Condition**

   Code any condition described at the time of discharge as "impending" or "threatened" as follows:

   > If it did occur, code as confirmed diagnosis.

   > If it did not occur, reference the Alphabetic Index to determine if the condition has a subentry term for "impending" or "threatened" and also reference main term entries for "Impending" and for "Threatened."

   > If the subterms are listed, assign the given code.

   > If the subterms are not listed, code the existing underlying condition(s) and not the condition described as impending or threatened.

12. **Reporting Same Diagnosis Code More than Once**

   Each unique ICD-10-CM diagnosis code may be reported only once for an encounter. This applies to bilateral conditions when there are no distinct codes identifying laterality or two different conditions classified to the same ICD-10-CM diagnosis code.

13. **Laterality**

   Some ICD-10-CM codes indicate laterality, specifying whether the condition occurs on the left, right or is bilateral. If no bilateral code is provided and the condition is bilateral, assign separate codes for both the left and right side. If the side is not identified in the medical record, assign the code for the unspecified side.

   When a patient has a bilateral condition and each side is treated during separate encounters, assign the "bilateral" code (as the condition still exists on both sides), including for the encounter to treat the first side. For the second encounter for treatment after one side has previously been treated and the condition no longer exists on that side, assign the appropriate unilateral code for the side where the condition still exists (e.g., cataract surgery performed on each eye in separate encounters). The bilateral code would not be assigned for the subsequent encounter, as the patient no longer has the condition in the previously-treated site. If the treatment on the first side did not completely resolve the condition, then the bilateral code would still be appropriate.

14. **Documentation for BMI, Depth of Non-pressure ulcers, Pressure Ulcer Stages, Coma Scale, and NIH Stroke Scale**

   For the Body Mass Index (BMI), depth of non-pressure chronic ulcers, pressure ulcer stage, coma scale, and NIH stroke scale (NIHSS) codes, code assignment may be based on medical record documentation from clinicians who are not the patient's provider (i.e., physician or other qualified healthcare practitioner legally accountable for establishing the patient's diagnosis), since this information is typically documented by other clinicians involved in the care of the patient (e.g., a dietitian often documents the BMI, a nurse often documents the pressure ulcer stages, and an emergency medical technician often documents the coma scale). However, the associated diagnosis (such as overweight, obesity, acute stroke, or pressure ulcer) must be documented by the patient's provider. If there is conflicting medical record documentation, either from the same clinician or different clinicians, the patient's attending provider should be queried for clarification.

   The BMI, coma scale, and NIHSS codes should only be reported as secondary diagnoses.

15. **Syndromes**

   Follow the Alphabetic Index guidance when coding syndromes. In the absence of Alphabetic Index guidance, assign codes for the documented manifestations of the syndrome. Additional codes for manifestations that are not an integral part of the disease process may also be assigned when the condition does not have a unique code.

16. **Documentation of Complications of Care**

   Code assignment is based on the provider's documentation of the relationship between the condition and the care or procedure, unless otherwise instructed by the classification. The guideline extends to any complications of care, regardless of the chapter the code is located in. It is important to note that not all conditions that occur during or following medical care or surgery are classified as complications. There must be a cause-and-effect relationship between the care provided and the condition, and an indication in the documentation that it is a complication. Query the provider for clarification, if the complication is not clearly documented.

17. **Borderline Diagnosis**
If the provider documents a "borderline" diagnosis at the time of discharge, the diagnosis is coded as confirmed, unless the classification provides a specific entry (e.g., borderline diabetes). If a borderline condition has a specific index entry in ICD-10-CM, it should be coded as such. Since borderline conditions are not uncertain diagnoses, no distinction is made between the care setting (inpatient versus outpatient). Whenever the documentation is unclear regarding a borderline condition, coders are encouraged to query for clarification.

18. **Use of Sign/Symptom/Unspecified Codes**
Sign/symptom and "unspecified" codes have acceptable, even necessary, uses. While specific diagnosis codes should be reported when they are supported by the available medical record documentation and clinical knowledge of the patient's health condition, there are instances when signs/symptoms or unspecified codes are the best choices for accurately reflecting the healthcare encounter. Each healthcare encounter should be coded to the level of certainty known for that encounter.

If a definitive diagnosis has not been established by the end of the encounter, it is appropriate to report codes for sign(s) and/or symptom(s) in lieu of a definitive diagnosis. When sufficient clinical information isn't known or available about a particular health condition to assign a more specific code, it is acceptable to report the appropriate "unspecified" code (e.g., a diagnosis of pneumonia has been determined, but not the specific type). Unspecified codes should be reported when they are the codes that most accurately reflect what is known about the patient's condition at the time of that particular encounter. It would be inappropriate to select a specific code that is not supported by the medical record documentation or conduct medically unnecessary diagnostic testing in order to determine a more specific code.

C. Chapter-Specific Coding Guidelines
In addition to general coding guidelines, there are guidelines for specific diagnoses and/or conditions in the classification. Unless otherwise indicated, these guidelines apply to all health care settings. Please refer to Section II for guidelines on the selection of principal diagnosis.

1. **Chapter 1: Certain Infectious and Parasitic Diseases (A00-B99)**
   a. **Human Immunodeficiency Virus (HIV) Infections**
      1) **Code only confirmed cases**
         Code only confirmed cases of HIV infection/illness. This is an exception to the hospital inpatient guideline Section II, H.

         In this context, "confirmation" does not require documentation of positive serology or culture for HIV; the provider's diagnostic statement that the patient is HIV positive, or has an HIV-related illness is sufficient.

      2) **Selection and sequencing of HIV codes**
         (a) **Patient admitted for HIV-related condition**
            If a patient is admitted for an HIV-related condition, the principal diagnosis should be B20, Human immunodeficiency virus [HIV] disease followed by additional diagnosis codes for all reported HIV-related conditions.

         (b) **Patient with HIV disease admitted for unrelated condition**
            If a patient with HIV disease is admitted for an unrelated condition (such as a traumatic injury), the code for the unrelated condition (e.g., the nature of injury code) should be the principal diagnosis. Other diagnoses would be B20 followed by additional diagnosis codes for all reported HIV-related conditions.

         (c) **Whether the patient is newly diagnosed**
            Whether the patient is newly diagnosed or has had previous admissions/encounters for HIV conditions is irrelevant to the sequencing decision.

         (d) **Asymptomatic human immunodeficiency virus**
            Z21, Asymptomatic human immunodeficiency virus [HIV] infection status, is to be applied when the patient without any documentation of symptoms is listed as being "HIV positive," "known HIV," "HIV test positive," or similar terminology. Do not use this code if the term "AIDS" is used

or if the patient is treated for any HIV-related illness or is described as having any condition(s) resulting from his/her HIV positive status; use B20 in these cases.

(e) **Patients with inconclusive HIV serology**
Patients with inconclusive HIV serology, but no definitive diagnosis or manifestations of the illness, may be assigned code R75, Inconclusive laboratory evidence of human immunodeficiency virus [HIV].

(f) **Previously diagnosed HIV-related illness**
Patients with any known prior diagnosis of an HIV-related illness should be coded to B20. Once a patient has developed an HIV-related illness, the patient should always be assigned code B20 on every subsequent admission/encounter. Patients previously diagnosed with any HIV illness (B20) should never be assigned to R75 or Z21, Asymptomatic human immunodeficiency virus [HIV] infection status.

(g) **HIV Infection in Pregnancy, Childbirth and the Puerperium**
During pregnancy, childbirth or the puerperium, a patient admitted (or presenting for a health care encounter) because of an HIV-related illness should receive a principal diagnosis code of O98.7-, Human immunodeficiency [HIV] disease complicating pregnancy, childbirth and the puerperium, followed by B20 and the code(s) for the HIV-related illness(es). Codes from Chapter 15 always take sequencing priority.

Patients with asymptomatic HIV infection status admitted (or presenting for a health care encounter) during pregnancy, childbirth, or the puerperium should receive codes of O98.7- and Z21.

(h) **Encounters for testing for HIV**
If a patient is being seen to determine his/her HIV status, use code Z11.4, Encounter for screening for human immunodeficiency virus [HIV]. Use additional codes for any associated high risk behavior.

If a patient with signs or symptoms is being seen for HIV testing, code the signs and symptoms. An additional counseling code Z71.7, Human immunodeficiency virus [HIV] counseling, may be used if counseling is provided during the encounter for the test.

When a patient returns to be informed of his/her HIV test results and the test result is negative, use code Z71.7, Human immunodeficiency virus [HIV] counseling.

If the results are positive, see previous guidelines and assign codes as appropriate.

b. **Infectious agents as the cause of diseases classified to other chapters**
Certain infections are classified in chapters other than Chapter 1 and no organism is identified as part of the infection code. In these instances, it is necessary to use an additional code from Chapter 1 to identify the organism. A code from category B95, Streptococcus, Staphylococcus, and Enterococcus as the cause of diseases classified to other chapters, B96, Other bacterial agents as the cause of diseases classified to other chapters, or B97, Viral agents as the cause of diseases classified to other chapters, is to be used as an additional code to identify the organism. An instructional note will be found at the infection code advising that an additional organism code is required.

c. **Infections resistant to antibiotics**
Many bacterial infections are resistant to current antibiotics. It is necessary to identify all infections documented as antibiotic resistant. Assign a code from category Z16, Resistance to antimicrobial drugs, following the infection code only if the infection code does not identify drug resistance.

d. **Sepsis, Severe Sepsis, and Septic Shock**
   1) **Coding of Sepsis and Severe Sepsis**
      (a) **Sepsis**
         For a diagnosis of sepsis, assign the appropriate code for the underlying systemic infection. If the type of infection or causal organism is not further specified, assign code A41.9, Sepsis, unspecified organism.

A code from subcategory R65.2, Severe sepsis, should not be assigned unless severe sepsis or an associated acute organ dysfunction is documented.

(i) Negative or inconclusive blood cultures and sepsis

Negative or inconclusive blood cultures do not preclude a diagnosis of sepsis in patients with clinical evidence of the condition; however, the provider should be queried.

(ii) Urosepsis

The term urosepsis is a nonspecific term. It is not to be considered synonymous with sepsis. It has no default code in the Alphabetic Index. Should a provider use this term, he/she must be queried for clarification.

(iii) Sepsis with organ dysfunction

If a patient has sepsis and associated acute organ dysfunction or multiple organ dysfunction (MOD), follow the instructions for coding severe sepsis.

(iv) Acute organ dysfunction that is not clearly associated with the sepsis

If a patient has sepsis and an acute organ dysfunction, but the medical record documentation indicates that the acute organ dysfunction is related to a medical condition other than the sepsis, do not assign a code from subcategory R65.2, Severe sepsis. An acute organ dysfunction must be associated with the sepsis in order to assign the severe sepsis code. If the documentation is not clear as to whether an acute organ dysfunction is related to the sepsis or another medical condition, query the provider.

(b) Severe sepsis

The coding of severe sepsis requires a minimum of 2 codes: first a code for the underlying systemic infection, followed by a code from subcategory R65.2, Severe sepsis. If the causal organism is not documented, assign code A41.9, Sepsis, unspecified organism, for the infection. Additional code(s) for the associated acute organ dysfunction are also required.

Due to the complex nature of severe sepsis, some cases may require querying the provider prior to assignment of the codes.

2) Septic shock

(a) Septic shock generally refers to circulatory failure associated with severe sepsis, and therefore, it represents a type of acute organ dysfunction.

For cases of septic shock, the code for the systemic infection should be sequenced first, followed by code R65.21, Severe sepsis with septic shock or code T81.12, Postprocedural septic shock. Any additional codes for the other acute organ dysfunctions should also be assigned. As noted in the sequencing instructions in the Tabular List, the code for septic shock cannot be assigned as a principal diagnosis.

3) Sequencing of severe sepsis

If severe sepsis is present on admission, and meets the definition of principal diagnosis, the underlying systemic infection should be assigned as principal diagnosis followed by the appropriate code from subcategory R65.2 as required by the sequencing rules in the Tabular List. A code from subcategory R65.2 can never be assigned as a principal diagnosis.

When severe sepsis develops during an encounter (it was not present on admission), the underlying systemic infection and the appropriate code from subcategory R65.2 should be assigned as secondary diagnoses.

Severe sepsis may be present on admission, but the diagnosis may not be confirmed until sometime after admission. If the documentation is not clear whether severe sepsis was present on admission, the provider should be queried.

4) Sepsis and severe sepsis with a localized infection

If the reason for admission is both sepsis or severe sepsis and a localized infection, such as pneumonia or cellulitis, a code(s) for the underlying systemic infection should be assigned first and the code for the localized infection should be assigned as a secondary diagnosis. If the patient has severe sepsis, a code from subcategory R65.2 should also be assigned as a secondary diagnosis. If the patient is admitted with a localized infection, such as pneumonia, and sepsis/severe sepsis doesn't develop until after admission, the localized infection should be assigned first, followed by the appropriate sepsis/severe sepsis codes.

5) Sepsis due to a postprocedural infection

(a) Documentation of causal relationship

As with all postprocedural complications, code assignment is based on the provider's documentation of the relationship between the infection and the procedure.

(b) Sepsis due to a postprocedural infection

For such cases, the postprocedural infection code, such as T80.2, Infections following infusion, transfusion, and therapeutic injection, T81.4, Infection following a procedure, T88.0, Infection following immunization, or O86.0, Infection of obstetric surgical wound, should be coded first, followed by the code for the specific infection. If the patient has severe sepsis, the appropriate code from subcategory R65.2 should also be assigned with the additional code(s) for any acute organ dysfunction.

(c) Postprocedural infection and postprocedural septic shock

In cases where a postprocedural infection has occurred and has resulted in severe sepsis the code for the precipitating complication such as code T81.4, Infection following a procedure, or O86.0, Infection of obstetrical surgical wound should be coded first followed by code R65.20, Severe sepsis without septic shock. A code for the systemic infection should also be assigned.

If a postprocedural infection has resulted in postprocedural septic shock, the code for the precipitating complication such as code T81.4, Infection following a procedure, or O86.0, Infection of obstetrical surgical wound should be coded first followed by code T81.12-, Postprocedural septic shock. A code for the systemic infection should also be assigned.

6) Sepsis and severe sepsis associated with a noninfectious process (condition)

In some cases a noninfectious process (condition), such as trauma, may lead to an infection which can result in sepsis or severe sepsis. If sepsis or severe sepsis is documented as associated with a noninfectious condition, such as a burn or serious injury, and this condition meets the definition for principal diagnosis, the code for the noninfectious condition should be sequenced first, followed by the code for the resulting infection. If severe sepsis is present, a code from subcategory R65.2 should also be assigned with any associated organ dysfunction(s) codes. It is not necessary to assign a code from subcategory R65.1, Systemic inflammatory response syndrome (SIRS) of non-infectious origin, for these cases.

If the infection meets the definition of principal diagnosis, it should be sequenced before the non-infectious condition. When both the associated non-infectious condition and the infection meet the definition of principal diagnosis, either may be assigned as principal diagnosis.

Only one code from category R65, Symptoms and signs specifically associated with systemic inflammation and infection, should be assigned. Therefore, when a non-infectious condition leads to an infection resulting in severe sepsis, assign the appropriate code from subcategory R65.2, Severe sepsis. Do not additionally assign a code from subcategory R65.1, Systemic inflammatory response syndrome (SIRS) of non-infectious origin.

See Section I.C.18. SIRS due to non-infectious process

7) Sepsis and septic shock complicating abortion, pregnancy, childbirth, and the puerperium

See Section I.C.15. Sepsis and septic shock complicating abortion, pregnancy, childbirth and the puerperium

8) Newborn sepsis

See Section I.C.16. f. Bacterial sepsis of Newborn

e. Methicillin Resistant Staphylococcus aureus (MRSA) Conditions

1) Selection and sequencing of MRSA codes

(a) Combination codes for MRSA infection

When a patient is diagnosed with an infection that is due to methicillin resistant *Staphylococcus aureus* (MRSA), and that infection has a combination code that includes the causal organism (e.g., sepsis, pneumonia) assign the appropriate combination code for the condition (e.g., code A41.02, Sepsis due to Methicillin resistant Staphylococcus aureus or code J15.212, Pneumonia due to Methicillin resistant Staphylococcus aureus). Do not assign code B95.62, Methicillin resistant Staphylococcus aureus infection as the cause of diseases classified elsewhere, as an additional code, because the combination code includes the type of infection and the MRSA organism. Do not assign a code from subcategory Z16.11, Resistance to penicillins, as an additional diagnosis.

See Section C.1. for instructions on coding and sequencing of sepsis and severe sepsis.

(b) Other codes for MRSA infection

When there is documentation of a current infection (e.g., wound infection, stitch abscess, urinary tract infection) due to MRSA, and that infection does not have a combination code that includes the causal organism, assign the appropriate code to identify the condition along with code B95.62, Methicillin resistant Staphylococcus aureus infection as the cause of diseases classified elsewhere for the MRSA infection. Do not assign a code from subcategory Z16.11, Resistance to penicillins.

(c) Methicillin susceptible Staphylococcus aureus (MSSA) and MRSA colonization

The condition or state of being colonized or carrying MSSA or MRSA is called colonization or carriage, while an individual person is described as being colonized or being a carrier. Colonization means that MSSA or MSRA is present on or in the body without necessarily causing illness. A positive MRSA colonization test might be documented by the provider as "MRSA screen positive" or "MRSA nasal swab positive".

Assign code Z22.322, Carrier or suspected carrier of Methicillin resistant Staphylococcus aureus, for patients documented as having MRSA colonization. Assign code Z22.321, Carrier or suspected carrier of Methicillin susceptible Staphylococcus aureus, for patient documented as having MSSA colonization. Colonization is not necessarily indicative of a disease process or as the cause of a specific condition the patient may have unless documented as such by the provider.

(d) MRSA colonization and infection

If a patient is documented as having both MRSA colonization and infection during a hospital admission, code Z22.322, Carrier or suspected carrier of Methicillin resistant Staphylococcus aureus, and a code for the MRSA infection may both be assigned.

f. Zika virus infections

1) Code only confirmed cases

Code only a confirmed diagnosis of Zika virus (A92.5, Zika virus disease) as documented by the provider. This is an exception to the hospital inpatient guideline Section II, H. In this context, "confirmation" does not require documentation of the type of test performed; the physician's diagnostic statement that the condition is confirmed is sufficient. This code should be assigned regardless of the stated mode of transmission.

If the provider documents "suspected", "possible" or "probable" Zika, do not assign code A92.5. Assign a code(s) explaining the reason for encounter (such as fever, rash, or joint pain) or Z20.828, Contact with and (suspected) exposure to other viral communicable diseases.

2. Chapter 2: Neoplasms (C00-D49)
General guidelines

Chapter 2 of the ICD-10-CM contains the codes for most benign and all malignant neoplasms. Certain benign neoplasms, such as prostatic adenomas, may be found in the specific body system chapters. To properly code a neoplasm it is necessary to determine from the record if

the neoplasm is benign, in-situ, malignant, or of uncertain histologic behavior. If malignant, any secondary (metastatic) sites should also be determined.

Primary malignant neoplasms overlapping site boundaries

A primary malignant neoplasm that overlaps two or more contiguous (next to each other) sites should be classified to the subcategory/code .8 ('overlapping lesion'), unless the combination is specifically indexed elsewhere. For multiple neoplasms of the same site that are not contiguous such as tumors in different quadrants of the same breast, codes for each site should be assigned.

Malignant neoplasm of ectopic tissue

Malignant neoplasms of ectopic tissue are to be coded to the site of origin mentioned, e.g., ectopic pancreatic malignant neoplasms involving the stomach are coded to **malignant neoplasm of** pancreas, unspecified (C25.9).

The neoplasm table in the Alphabetic Index should be referenced first. However, if the histological term is documented, that term should be referenced first, rather than going immediately to the Neoplasm Table, in order to determine which column in the Neoplasm Table is appropriate. For example, if the documentation indicates "adenoma," refer to the term in the Alphabetic Index to review the entries under this term and the instructional note to "see also neoplasm, by site, benign." The table provides the proper code based on the type of neoplasm and the site. It is important to select the proper column in the table that corresponds to the type of neoplasm. The Tabular List should then be referenced to verify that the correct code has been selected from the table and that a more specific site code does not exist.

See Section I.C.21. Factors influencing health status and contact with health services, Status, for information regarding Z15.0, codes for genetic susceptibility to cancer.

a. Treatment directed at the malignancy

If the treatment is directed at the malignancy, designate the malignancy as the principal diagnosis.

The only exception to this guideline is if a patient admission/encounter is solely for the administration of chemotherapy, immunotherapy or **external beam** radiation therapy, assign the appropriate Z51.-- code as the first-listed or principal diagnosis, and the diagnosis or problem for which the service is being performed as a secondary diagnosis.

b. Treatment of secondary site

When a patient is admitted because of a primary neoplasm with metastasis and treatment is directed toward the secondary site only, the secondary neoplasm is designated as the principal diagnosis even though the primary malignancy is still present.

c. Coding and sequencing of complications

Coding and sequencing of complications associated with the malignancies or with the therapy thereof are subject to the following guidelines:

1) Anemia associated with malignancy

When admission/encounter is for management of an anemia associated with the malignancy, and the treatment is only for anemia, the appropriate code for the malignancy is sequenced as the principal or first-listed diagnosis followed by the appropriate code for the anemia (such as code D63.0, Anemia in neoplastic disease**).**

2) Anemia associated with chemotherapy, immunotherapy and radiation therapy

When the admission/encounter is for management of an anemia associated with an adverse effect of the administration of chemotherapy or immunotherapy and the only treatment is for the anemia, the anemia code is sequenced first followed by the appropriate codes for the neoplasm and the adverse effect (T45.1X5-, Adverse effect of antineoplastic and immunosuppressive drugs).

When the admission/encounter is for management of an anemia associated with an adverse effect of radiotherapy, the anemia code should be sequenced first, followed by the appropriate neoplasm code and code Y84.2, Radiological procedure and radiotherapy as the cause of abnormal reaction of the patient, or of later complication, without mention of misadventure at the time of the procedure.

  3) **Management of dehydration due to the malignancy**
When the admission/encounter is for management of dehydration due to the malignancy and only the dehydration is being treated (intravenous rehydration), the dehydration is sequenced first, followed by the code(s) for the malignancy.

  4) **Treatment of a complication resulting from a surgical procedure**
When the admission/encounter is for treatment of a complication resulting from a surgical procedure, designate the complication as the principal or first-listed diagnosis if treatment is directed at resolving the complication.

d. Primary malignancy previously excised
When a primary malignancy has been previously excised or eradicated from its site and there is no further treatment directed to that site and there is no evidence of any existing primary malignancy, a code from category Z85, Personal history of malignant neoplasm, should be used to indicate the former site of the malignancy. Any mention of extension, invasion, or metastasis to another site is coded as a secondary malignant neoplasm to that site. The secondary site may be the principal or first-listed with the Z85 code used as a secondary code.

e. Admissions/Encounters involving chemotherapy, immunotherapy and radiation therapy

  1) **Episode of care involves surgical removal of neoplasm**
When an episode of care involves the surgical removal of a neoplasm, primary or secondary site, followed by adjunct chemotherapy or radiation treatment during the same episode of care, the code for the neoplasm should be assigned as principal or first-listed diagnosis.

  2) **Patient admission/encounter solely for administration of chemotherapy, immunotherapy and radiation therapy**
If a patient admission/encounter is solely for the administration of chemotherapy, immunotherapy or **external beam** radiation therapy assign code Z51.0, Encounter for antineoplastic radiation therapy, or Z51.11, Encounter for antineoplastic chemotherapy, or Z51.12, Encounter for antineoplastic immunotherapy as the first-listed or principal diagnosis. If a patient receives more than one of these therapies during the same admission more than one of these codes may be assigned, in any sequence.

The malignancy for which the therapy is being administered should be assigned as a secondary diagnosis.

If a patient admission/encounter is for the insertion or implantation of radioactive elements (e.g., brachytherapy) the appropriate code for the malignancy is sequenced as the principal or first-listed diagnosis. Code Z51.0 should not be assigned.

  3) **Patient admitted for radiation therapy, chemotherapy or immunotherapy and develops complications**
When a patient is admitted for the purpose of **external beam** radiotherapy, immunotherapy or chemotherapy and develops complications such as uncontrolled nausea and vomiting or dehydration, the principal or first-listed diagnosis is Z51.0, Encounter for antineoplastic radiation therapy, or Z51.11, Encounter for antineoplastic chemotherapy, or Z51.12, Encounter for antineoplastic immunotherapy followed by any codes for the complications.

When a patient is admitted for the purpose of insertion or implantation of radioactive elements (e.g., brachytherapy) and develops complications such as uncontrolled nausea and vomiting or dehydration, the principal or first-listed diagnosis is the appropriate code for the malignancy followed by any codes for the complications.

f. Admission/encounter to determine extent of malignancy
When the reason for admission/encounter is to determine the extent of the malignancy, or for a procedure such as paracentesis or thoracentesis, the primary malignancy or appropriate metastatic site is designated as the principal or first-listed diagnosis, even though chemotherapy or radiotherapy is administered.

g. Symptoms, signs, and abnormal findings listed in Chapter 18 associated with neoplasms
Symptoms, signs, and ill-defined conditions listed in Chapter 18 characteristic of, or associated with, an existing primary or

secondary site malignancy cannot be used to replace the malignancy as principal or first-listed diagnosis, regardless of the number of admissions or encounters for treatment and care of the neoplasm.
See section I.C.21. Factors influencing health status and contact with health services, Encounter for prophylactic organ removal.

h. Admission/encounter for pain control/management
See Section I.C.6. for information on coding admission/encounter for pain control/management.

i. Malignancy in two or more noncontiguous sites
A patient may have more than one malignant tumor in the same organ. These tumors may represent different primaries or metastatic disease, depending on the site. Should the documentation be unclear, the provider should be queried as to the status of each tumor so that the correct codes can be assigned.

j. Disseminated malignant neoplasm, unspecified
Code C80.0, Disseminated malignant neoplasm, unspecified, is for use only in those cases where the patient has advanced metastatic disease and no known primary or secondary sites are specified. It should not be used in place of assigning codes for the primary site and all known secondary sites.

k. Malignant neoplasm without specification of site
Code C80.1, Malignant (primary) neoplasm, unspecified, equates to Cancer, unspecified. This code should only be used when no determination can be made as to the primary site of a malignancy. This code should rarely be used in the inpatient setting.

l. Sequencing of neoplasm codes

  1) **Encounter for treatment of primary malignancy**
If the reason for the encounter is for treatment of a primary malignancy, assign the malignancy as the principal/first-listed diagnosis. The primary site is to be sequenced first, followed by any metastatic sites.

  2) **Encounter for treatment of secondary malignancy**
When an encounter is for a primary malignancy with metastasis and treatment is directed toward the metastatic (secondary) site(s) only, the metastatic site(s) is designated as the principal/first-listed diagnosis. The primary malignancy is coded as an additional code.

  3) **Malignant neoplasm in a pregnant patient**
When a pregnant woman has a malignant neoplasm, a code from subcategory O9A.1-, Malignant neoplasm complicating pregnancy, childbirth, and the puerperium, should be sequenced first, followed by the appropriate code from Chapter 2 to indicate the type of neoplasm.

  4) **Encounter for complication associated with a neoplasm**
When an encounter is for management of a complication associated with a neoplasm, such as dehydration, and the treatment is only for the complication, the complication is coded first, followed by the appropriate code(s) for the neoplasm.

The exception to this guideline is anemia. When the admission/encounter is for management of an anemia associated with the malignancy, and the treatment is only for anemia, the appropriate code for the malignancy is sequenced as the principal or first-listed diagnosis followed by code D63.0, Anemia in neoplastic disease.

  5) **Complication from surgical procedure for treatment of a neoplasm**
When an encounter is for treatment of a complication resulting from a surgical procedure performed for the treatment of the neoplasm, designate the complication as the principal/first-listed diagnosis. See guideline regarding the coding of a current malignancy versus personal history to determine if the code for the neoplasm should also be assigned.

  6) **Pathologic fracture due to a neoplasm**
When an encounter is for a pathological fracture due to a neoplasm, and the focus of treatment is the fracture, a code from subcategory M84.5, Pathological fracture in neoplastic disease, should be sequenced first, followed by the code for the neoplasm.

If the focus of treatment is the neoplasm with an associated pathological fracture, the neoplasm code should be sequenced first, followed by a code from M84.5 for the pathological fracture.

m. Current malignancy versus personal history of malignancy
When a primary malignancy has been excised but further treatment, such as an additional surgery for the malignancy, radiation therapy or chemotherapy is directed to that site, the primary malignancy code should be used until treatment is completed.

When a primary malignancy has been previously excised or eradicated from its site, there is no further treatment (of the malignancy) directed to that site, and there is no evidence of any existing primary malignancy, a code from category Z85, Personal history of malignant neoplasm, should be used to indicate the former site of the malignancy.

See Section I.C.21. Factors influencing health status and contact with health services, History (of)

n. Leukemia, Multiple Myeloma, and Malignant Plasma Cell Neoplasms in remission versus personal history
The categories for leukemia, and category C90, Multiple myeloma and malignant plasma cell neoplasms, have codes indicating whether or not the leukemia has achieved remission. There are also codes Z85.6, Personal history of leukemia, and Z85.79, Personal history of other malignant neoplasms of lymphoid, hematopoietic and related tissues. If the documentation is unclear as to whether the leukemia has achieved remission, the provider should be queried.

See Section I.C.21. Factors influencing health status and contact with health services, History (of)

o. Aftercare following surgery for neoplasm
See Section I.C.21. Factors influencing health status and contact with health services, Aftercare

p. Follow-up care for completed treatment of a malignancy
See Section I.C.21. Factors influencing health status and contact with health services, Follow-up

q. Prophylactic organ removal for prevention of malignancy
See Section I.C. 21, Factors influencing health status and contact with health services, Prophylactic organ removal

r. Malignant neoplasm associated with transplanted organ
A malignant neoplasm of a transplanted organ should be coded as a transplant complication. Assign first the appropriate code from category T86.-, Complications of transplanted organs and tissue, followed by code C80.2, Malignant neoplasm associated with transplanted organ. Use an additional code for the specific malignancy.

3. Chapter 3: Disease of the blood and blood-forming organs and certain disorders involving the immune mechanism (D50-D89)
Reserved for future guideline expansion

4. Chapter 4: Endocrine, Nutritional, and Metabolic Diseases (E00-E89)

a. Diabetes mellitus
The diabetes mellitus codes are combination codes that include the type of diabetes mellitus, the body system affected, and the complications affecting that body system. As many codes within a particular category as are necessary to describe all of the complications of the disease may be used. They should be sequenced based on the reason for a particular encounter. Assign as many codes from categories E08 – E13 as needed to identify all of the associated conditions that the patient has.

1) Type of diabetes
The age of a patient is not the sole determining factor, though most type 1 diabetics develop the condition before reaching puberty. For this reason type 1 diabetes mellitus is also referred to as juvenile diabetes.

2) Type of diabetes mellitus not documented
If the type of diabetes mellitus is not documented in the medical record the default is E11.-, Type 2 diabetes mellitus.

3) Diabetes mellitus and the use of insulin and oral hypoglycemics
If the documentation in a medical record does not indicate the type of diabetes but does indicate that the patient uses insulin, code E11-, Type 2 diabetes mellitus, should be assigned. **An additional code should be assigned from category Z79 to**

identify the long-term (current) use of insulin or oral hypoglycemic drugs. If the patient is treated with both oral medications and insulin, only the code for long-term (current) use of insulin should be assigned. Code Z79.4 should not be assigned if insulin is given temporarily to bring a type 2 patient's blood sugar under control during an encounter.

4) Diabetes mellitus in pregnancy and gestational diabetes
See Section I.C.15. Diabetes mellitus in pregnancy.

See Section I.C.15. Gestational (pregnancy induced) diabetes

5) Complications due to insulin pump malfunction

(a) Underdose of insulin due to insulin pump failure
An underdose of insulin due to an insulin pump failure should be assigned to a code from subcategory T85.6, Mechanical complication of other specified internal and external prosthetic devices, implants and grafts, that specifies the type of pump malfunction, as the principal or first-listed code, followed by code T38.3X6-, Underdosing of insulin and oral hypoglycemic [antidiabetic] drugs. Additional codes for the type of diabetes mellitus and any associated complications due to the underdosing should also be assigned.

(b) Overdose of insulin due to insulin pump failure
The principal or first-listed code for an encounter due to an insulin pump malfunction resulting in an overdose of insulin, should also be T85.6-, Mechanical complication of other specified internal and external prosthetic devices, implants and grafts, followed by code T38.3X1-, Poisoning by insulin and oral hypoglycemic [antidiabetic] drugs, accidental (unintentional).

6) Secondary diabetes mellitus
Codes under categories E08, Diabetes mellitus due to underlying condition, E09, Drug or chemical induced diabetes mellitus, and E13, Other specified diabetes mellitus, identify complications/manifestations associated with secondary diabetes mellitus. Secondary diabetes is always caused by another condition or event (e.g., cystic fibrosis, malignant neoplasm of pancreas, pancreatectomy, adverse effect of drug, or poisoning).

(a) Secondary diabetes mellitus and the use of insulin or *oral* hypoglycemic drugs
For patients with secondary diabetes mellitus who routinely use insulin or oral hypoglycemic drugs, an additional code from category Z79 should be assigned to identify the long-term (current) use of insulin or oral hypoglycemic drugs. If the patient is treated with both oral medications and insulin, only the code for long-term (current) use of insulin should be assigned. Code Z79.4 should not be assigned if insulin is given temporarily to bring a type 2 patient's blood sugar under control during an encounter.

(b) Assigning and sequencing secondary diabetes codes and its causes
The sequencing of the secondary diabetes codes in relationship to codes for the cause of the diabetes is based on the Tabular List instructions for categories E08, E09 and E13.

(i) Secondary diabetes mellitus due to pancreatectomy
For postpancreatectomy diabetes mellitus (lack of insulin due to the surgical removal of all or part of the pancreas), assign code E89.1, Postprocedural hypoinsulinemia. Assign a code from category E13 and a code from subcategory Z90.41, Acquired absence of pancreas, as additional codes.

(ii) Secondary diabetes due to drugs
Secondary diabetes may be caused by an adverse effect of correctly administered medications, poisoning or sequela of poisoning.
See section I.C.19.e for coding of adverse effects and poisoning, and section I.C.20 for external cause code reporting.

5. **Chapter 5: Mental, Behavioral and Neurodevelopmental disorders (F01 – F99)**

   a. **Pain disorders related to psychological factors**

   Assign code F45.41, for pain that is exclusively related to psychological disorders. As indicated by the Excludes 1 note under category G89, a code from category G89 should not be assigned with code F45.41.

   Code F45.42, Pain disorders with related psychological factors, should be used with a code from category G89, Pain, not elsewhere classified, if there is documentation of a psychological component for a patient with acute or chronic pain.

   See Section I.C.6. Pain

   b. **Mental and behavioral disorders due to psychoactive substance use**

   1) **In Remission**

   Selection of codes for "in remission" for categories F10-F19, Mental and behavioral disorders due to psychoactive substance use (categories F10-F19 with **-11,** -.21) requires the provider's clinical judgment. The appropriate codes for "in remission" are assigned only on the basis of provider documentation (as defined in the Official Guidelines for Coding and Reporting), **unless otherwise instructed by the classification.**

   Mild substance use disorders in early or sustained remission are classified to the appropriate codes for substance abuse in remission, and moderate or severe substance use disorders in early or sustained remission are classified to the appropriate codes for substance dependence in remission.

   2) **Psychoactive Substance Use, Abuse and Dependence**

   When the provider documentation refers to use, abuse and dependence of the same substance (e.g. alcohol, opioid, cannabis, etc.), only one code should be assigned to identify the pattern of use based on the following hierarchy:

   - If both use and abuse are documented, assign only the code for abuse
   - If both abuse and dependence are documented, assign only the code for dependence
   - If use, abuse and dependence are all documented, assign only the code for dependence
   - If both use and dependence are documented, assign only the code for dependence.

   3) **Psychoactive Substance Use** *Disorders*

   As with all other diagnoses, the codes for psychoactive substance use **disorders** (F10.9-, F11.9-, F12.9-, F13.9-, F14.9-, F15.9-, F16.9-) should only be assigned based on provider documentation and when they meet the definition of a reportable diagnosis (see Section III, Reporting Additional Diagnoses). The codes are to be used only when the psychoactive substance use is associated with a **physical,** mental or behavioral disorder, and such a relationship is documented by the provider.

6. **Chapter 6: Diseases of the Nervous System (G00-G99)**

   a. **Dominant/nondominant side**

   Codes from category G81, Hemiplegia and hemiparesis, and subcategories G83.1, Monoplegia of lower limb, G83.2, Monoplegia of upper limb, and G83.3, Monoplegia, unspecified, identify whether the dominant or nondominant side is affected. Should the affected side be documented, but not specified as dominant or nondominant, and the classification system does not indicate a default, code selection is as follows:

   - For ambidextrous patients, the default should be dominant.
   - If the left side is affected, the default is non-dominant.
   - If the right side is affected, the default is dominant.

   b. **Pain - Category G89**

   1) **General coding information**

   Codes in category G89, Pain, not elsewhere classified, may be used in conjunction with codes from other categories and chapters to provide more detail about acute or chronic pain and neoplasm-related pain, unless otherwise indicated below.

   If the pain is not specified as acute or chronic, post-thoracotomy, postprocedural, or neoplasm-related, do not assign codes from category G89.

A code from category G89 should not be assigned if the underlying (definitive) diagnosis is known, unless the reason for the encounter is pain control/ management and not management of the underlying condition.

When an admission or encounter is for a procedure aimed at treating the underlying condition (e.g., spinal fusion, kyphoplasty), a code for the underlying condition (e.g., vertebral fracture, spinal stenosis) should be assigned as the principal diagnosis. No code from category G89 should be assigned.

(a) **Category G89 Codes as Principal or First-Listed Diagnosis**

Category G89 codes are acceptable as principal diagnosis or the first-listed code:

- When pain control or pain management is the reason for the admission/encounter (e.g., a patient with displaced intervertebral disc, nerve impingement and severe back pain presents for injection of steroid into the spinal canal). The underlying cause of the pain should be reported as an additional diagnosis, if known.

- When a patient is admitted for the insertion of a neurostimulator for pain control, assign the appropriate pain code as the principal or first-listed diagnosis. When an admission or encounter is for a procedure aimed at treating the underlying condition and a neurostimulator is inserted for pain control during the same admission/encounter, a code for the underlying condition should be assigned as the principal diagnosis and the appropriate pain code should be assigned as a secondary diagnosis.

(b) **Use of Category G89 Codes in Conjunction with Site Specific Pain Codes**

(i) **Assigning Category G89 and Site-Specific Pain Codes**

Codes from category G89 may be used in conjunction with codes that identify the site of pain (including codes from chapter 18) if the category G89 code provides additional information. For example, if the code describes the site of the pain, but does not fully describe whether the pain is acute or chronic, then both codes should be assigned.

(ii) **Sequencing of Category G89 Codes with Site-Specific Pain Codes**

The sequencing of category G89 codes with site-specific pain codes (including chapter 18 codes), is dependent on the circumstances of the encounter/admission as follows:

- If the encounter is for pain control or pain management, assign the code from category G89 followed by the code identifying the specific site of pain (e.g., encounter for pain management for acute neck pain from trauma is assigned code G89.11, Acute pain due to trauma, followed by code M54.2, Cervicalgia, to identify the site of pain).

- If the encounter is for any other reason except pain control or pain management, and a related definitive diagnosis has not been established (confirmed) by the provider, assign the code for the specific site of pain first, followed by the appropriate code from category G89.

2) **Pain due to devices, implants and grafts**
   See Section I.C.19. Pain due to medical devices

3) **Postoperative Pain**

The provider's documentation should be used to guide the coding of postoperative pain, as well as *Section III. Reporting Additional Diagnoses and Section IV. Diagnostic Coding and Reporting in the Outpatient Setting.*

The default for post-thoracotomy and other postoperative pain not specified as acute or chronic is the code for the acute form.

Routine or expected postoperative pain immediately after surgery should not be coded.

(a) Postoperative pain not associated with specific postoperative complication

Postoperative pain not associated with a specific postoperative complication is assigned to the appropriate postoperative pain code in category G89.

(b) Postoperative pain associated with specific postoperative complication

Postoperative pain associated with a specific postoperative complication (such as painful wire sutures) is assigned to the appropriate code(s) found in Chapter 19, Injury, poisoning, and certain other consequences of external causes. If appropriate, use additional code(s) from category G89 to identify acute or chronic pain (G89.18 or G89.28).

4) Chronic pain

Chronic pain is classified to subcategory G89.2. There is no time frame defining when pain becomes chronic pain. The provider's documentation should be used to guide use of these codes.

5) Neoplasm Related Pain

Code G89.3 is assigned to pain documented as being related, associated or due to cancer, primary or secondary malignancy, or tumor. This code is assigned regardless of whether the pain is acute or chronic.

This code may be assigned as the principal or first-listed code when the stated reason for the admission/encounter is documented as pain control/pain management. The underlying neoplasm should be reported as an additional diagnosis.

When the reason for the admission/encounter is management of the neoplasm and the pain associated with the neoplasm is also documented, code G89.3 may be assigned as an additional diagnosis. It is not necessary to assign an additional code for the site of the pain.

See Section I.C.2 for instructions on the sequencing of neoplasms for all other stated reasons for the admission/encounter (except for pain control/pain management).

6) Chronic pain syndrome

Central pain syndrome (G89.0) and chronic pain syndrome (G89.4) are different than the term "chronic pain," and therefore codes should only be used when the provider has specifically documented this condition.

See Section I.C.5. Pain disorders related to psychological factors

7. Chapter 7: Diseases of the Eye and Adnexa (H00-H59)
a. Glaucoma

1) Assigning Glaucoma Codes

Assign as many codes from category H40, Glaucoma, as needed to identify the type of glaucoma, the affected eye, and the glaucoma stage.

2) Bilateral glaucoma with same type and stage

When a patient has bilateral glaucoma and both eyes are documented as being the same type and stage, and there is a code for bilateral glaucoma, report only the code for the type of glaucoma, bilateral, with the seventh character for the stage.

When a patient has bilateral glaucoma and both eyes are documented as being the same type and stage, and the classification does not provide a code for bilateral glaucoma (i.e. subcategories H40.10, H40.11 and H40.20) report only one code for the type of glaucoma with the appropriate seventh character for the stage.

3) Bilateral glaucoma stage with different types or stages

When a patient has bilateral glaucoma and each eye is documented as having a different type or stage, and the classification distinguishes laterality, assign the appropriate code for each eye rather than the code for bilateral glaucoma.

When a patient has bilateral glaucoma and each eye is documented as having a different type, and the classification does not distinguish laterality (i.e. subcategories H40.10, H40.11 and H40.20), assign one code for each type of glaucoma with the appropriate seventh character for the stage.

When a patient has bilateral glaucoma and each eye is documented as having the same type, but different stage, and the classification does not distinguish laterality (i.e. subcategories H40.10, H40.11 and H40.20), assign a code for

the type of glaucoma for each eye with the seventh character for the specific glaucoma stage documented for each eye.

4) Patient admitted with glaucoma and stage evolves during the admission

If a patient is admitted with glaucoma and the stage progresses during the admission, assign the code for highest stage documented.

5) Indeterminate stage glaucoma

Assignment of the seventh character "4" for "indeterminate stage" should be based on the clinical documentation. The seventh character "4" is used for glaucomas whose stage cannot be clinically determined. This seventh character should not be confused with the seventh character "0", unspecified, which should be assigned when there is no documentation regarding the stage of the glaucoma.

b. Blindness

If "blindness" or "low vision" of both eyes is documented but the visual impairment category is not documented, assign code H54.3, Unqualified visual loss, both eyes. If "blindness" or "low vision" in one eye is documented but the visual impairment category is not documented, assign a code from H54.6-, Unqualified visual loss, one eye. If "blindness" or "visual loss" is documented without any information about whether one or both eyes are affected, assign code H54.7, Unspecified visual loss.

8. Chapter 8: Diseases of the Ear and Mastoid Process (H60-H95)
Reserved for future guideline expansion

9. Chapter 9: Diseases of the Circulatory System (I00-I99)
a. Hypertension

The classification presumes a causal relationship between hypertension and heart involvement and between hypertension and kidney involvement, as the two conditions are linked by the term "with" in the Alphabetic Index. These conditions should be coded as related even in the absence of provider documentation explicitly linking them, unless the documentation clearly states the conditions are unrelated.

For hypertension and conditions not specifically linked by relational terms such as "with," "associated with" or "due to" in the classification, provider documentation must link the conditions in order to code them as related.

1) Hypertension with Heart Disease

Hypertension with heart conditions classified to I50.- or I51.4-I51.9, are assigned to a code from category I11, Hypertensive heart disease. Use additional code(s) from category I50, Heart failure, to identify the type(s) of heart failure in those patients with heart failure.

The same heart conditions (I50.-, I51.4-I51.9) with hypertension are coded separately if the provider has specifically documented a different cause. Sequence according to the circumstances of the admission/encounter.

2) Hypertensive Chronic Kidney Disease

Assign codes from category I12, Hypertensive chronic kidney disease, when both hypertension and a condition classifiable to category N18, Chronic kidney disease (CKD), are present. CKD should not be coded as hypertensive if the physician has specifically documented a different cause.

The appropriate code from category N18 should be used as a secondary code with a code from category I12 to identify the stage of chronic kidney disease.

See Section I.C.14. Chronic kidney disease.

If a patient has hypertensive chronic kidney disease and acute renal failure, an additional code for the acute renal failure is required.

3) Hypertensive Heart and Chronic Kidney Disease

Assign codes from combination category I13, Hypertensive heart and chronic kidney disease, when there is hypertension with both heart and kidney involvement. If heart failure is present, assign an additional code from category I50 to identify the type of heart failure.

The appropriate code from category N18, Chronic kidney disease, should be used as a secondary code with a code from category I13 to identify the stage of chronic kidney disease.

See Section I.C.14. Chronic kidney disease.

The codes in category I13, Hypertensive heart and chronic kidney disease, are combination codes that include hypertension, heart disease and chronic kidney disease. The Includes note at I13 specifies that the conditions included at I11 and I12 are included together in I13. If a patient has hypertension, heart disease and chronic kidney disease, then a code from I13 should be used, not individual codes for hypertension, heart disease and chronic kidney disease, or codes from I11 or I12.

For patients with both acute renal failure and chronic kidney disease, an additional code for acute renal failure is required.

4) Hypertensive Cerebrovascular Disease
For hypertensive cerebrovascular disease, first assign the appropriate code from categories I60-I69, followed by the appropriate hypertension code.

5) Hypertensive Retinopathy
Subcategory H35.0, Background retinopathy and retinal vascular changes, should be used with a code from category I10- I15, Hypertensive disease to include the systemic hypertension. The sequencing is based on the reason for the encounter.

6) Hypertension, Secondary
Secondary hypertension is due to an underlying condition. Two codes are required: one to identify the underlying etiology and one from category I15 to identify the hypertension. Sequencing of codes is determined by the reason for admission/encounter.

7) Hypertension, Transient
Assign code R03.0, Elevated blood pressure reading without diagnosis of hypertension, unless patient has an established diagnosis of hypertension. Assign code O13.-, Gestational [pregnancy-induced] hypertension without significant proteinuria, or O14.-, Pre-eclampsia, for transient hypertension of pregnancy.

8) Hypertension, Controlled
This diagnostic statement usually refers to an existing state of hypertension under control by therapy. Assign the appropriate code from categories I10-I15, Hypertensive diseases.

9) Hypertension, Uncontrolled
Uncontrolled hypertension may refer to untreated hypertension or hypertension not responding to current therapeutic regimen. In either case, assign the appropriate code from categories I10-I15, Hypertensive diseases.

10) Hypertensive Crisis
Assign a code from category I16, Hypertensive crisis, for documented hypertensive urgency, hypertensive emergency or unspecified hypertensive crisis. Code also any identified hypertensive disease (I10-I15). The sequencing is based on the reason for the encounter.

10) Pulmonary Hypertension
Pulmonary hypertension is classified to category I27, Other pulmonary heart diseases. For secondary pulmonary hypertension (I27.1, I27.2-), code also any associated conditions or adverse effects of drugs or toxins. The sequencing is based on the reason for the encounter.

b. Atherosclerotic Coronary Artery Disease and Angina
ICD-10-CM has combination codes for atherosclerotic heart disease with angina pectoris. The subcategories for these codes are I25.11, Atherosclerotic heart disease of native coronary artery with angina pectoris and I25.7, Atherosclerosis of coronary artery bypass graft(s) and coronary artery of transplanted heart with angina pectoris.

When using one of these combination codes it is not necessary to use an additional code for angina pectoris. A causal relationship can be assumed in a patient with both atherosclerosis and angina pectoris, unless the documentation indicates the angina is due to something other than the atherosclerosis.

If a patient with coronary artery disease is admitted due to an acute myocardial infarction (AMI), the AMI should be sequenced before the coronary artery disease.

See Section I.C.9. Acute myocardial infarction (AMI)

c. Intraoperative and Postprocedural Cerebrovascular Accident
Medical record documentation should clearly specify the cause-and-effect relationship between the medical intervention and the cerebrovascular accident in order to assign a code for intraoperative or postprocedural cerebrovascular accident.

Proper code assignment depends on whether it was an infarction or hemorrhage and whether it occurred intraoperatively or postoperatively. If it was a cerebral hemorrhage, code assignment depends on the type of procedure performed.

d. Sequelae of Cerebrovascular Disease

1) Category I69, Sequelae of Cerebrovascular disease
Category I69 is used to indicate conditions classifiable to categories I60-I67 as the causes of sequela (neurologic deficits), themselves classified elsewhere. These "late effects" include neurologic deficits that persist after initial onset of conditions classifiable to categories I60-I67. The neurologic deficits caused by cerebrovascular disease may be present from the onset or may arise at any time after the onset of the condition classifiable to categories I60-I67.

Codes from category I69, Sequelae of cerebrovascular disease, that specify hemiplegia, hemiparesis and monoplegia identify whether the dominant or nondominant side is affected. Should the affected side be documented, but not specified as dominant or nondominant, and the classification system does not indicate a default, code selection is as follows:

- For ambidextrous patients, the default should be dominant.
- If the left side is affected, the default is non-dominant.
- If the right side is affected, the default is dominant.

2) Codes from category I69 with codes from I60-I67
Codes from category I69 may be assigned on a health care record with codes from I60-I67, if the patient has a current cerebrovascular disease and deficits from an old cerebrovascular disease.

3) Codes from category I69 and Personal history of transient ischemic attack (TIA) and cerebral infarction (Z86.73)
Codes from category I69 should not be assigned if the patient does not have neurologic deficits.

See Section I.C.21. 4. History (of) for use of personal history codes

e. Acute myocardial infarction (AMI)

1) Type 1 ST elevation myocardial infarction (STEMI) and non-ST elevation myocardial infarction (NSTEMI)
The ICD-10-CM codes for **type 1** acute myocardial infarction (AMI) identify the site, such as anterolateral wall or true posterior wall. Subcategories I21.0-I21.2 and code I21.3 are used for **type 1** ST elevation myocardial infarction (STEMI). Code I21.4, Non-ST elevation (NSTEMI) myocardial infarction, is used for **type 1** non ST elevation myocardial infarction (NSTEMI) and nontransmural MIs.

If **a type 1** NSTEMI evolves to STEMI, assign the STEMI code. If **a type 1** STEMI converts to NSTEMI due to thrombolytic therapy, it is still coded as STEMI.

For encounters occurring while the myocardial infarction is equal to, or less than, four weeks old, including transfers to another acute setting or a postacute setting, and the myocardial infarction meets the definition for "other diagnoses" (see Section III, Reporting Additional Diagnoses), codes from category I21 may continue to be reported. For encounters after the 4 week time frame and the patient is still receiving care related to the myocardial infarction, the appropriate aftercare code should be assigned, rather than a code from category I21. For old or healed myocardial infarctions not requiring further care, code I25.2, Old myocardial infarction, may be assigned.

2) Acute myocardial infarction, unspecified
Code **I21.9, Acute myocardial infarction, unspecified,** is the default for unspecified acute myocardial infarction **or unspecified type**. If only **type 1** STEMI or transmural MI without the site is documented, assign code I21.3, **ST elevation (STEMI) myocardial infarction of unspecified site**.

3) AMI documented as nontransmural or subendocardial but site provided
If an AMI is documented as nontransmural or subendocardial, but the site is provided, it is still coded as a subendocardial AMI.

See Section I.C.21.3 for information on coding status post administration of tPA in a different facility within the last 24 hours.

4) Subsequent acute myocardial infarction
A code from category I22, Subsequent ST elevation (STEMI) and non-ST elevation (NSTEMI) myocardial infarction, is to be used when a patient who has suffered **a type 1 or unspecified** AMI has a new AMI within the 4 week time frame of the initial AMI. A code from category I22 must be used in conjunction with a code from category I21. The sequencing of the I22 and I21 codes depends on the circumstances of the encounter.

Do not assign code I22 for subsequent myocardial infarctions other than type 1 or unspecified. For subsequent type 2 AMI assign only code I21.A1. For subsequent type 4 or type 5 AMI, assign only code I21.A9.

5) Other Types of Myocardial Infarction
The ICD-10-CM provides codes for different types of myocardial infarction. Type 1 myocardial infarctions are assigned to codes I21.0-I21.4.

Type 2 myocardial infarction, and myocardial infarction due to demand ischemia or secondary to ischemic balance, is assigned to code I21.A1, Myocardial infarction type 2 with a code for the underlying cause. Do not assign code I24.8, Other forms of acute ischemic heart disease for the demand ischemia. Sequencing of type 2 AMI or the underlying cause is dependent on the circumstances of admission. When a type 2 AMI code is described as NSTEMI or STEMI, only assign code I21.A1. Codes I21.01-I21.4 should only be assigned for type 1 AMIs.

Acute myocardial infarctions type 3, 4a, 4b, 4c and 5 are assigned to code I21.A9, Other myocardial infarction type.

The "Code also" and "Code first" notes should be followed related to complications, and for coding of postprocedural myocardial infarctions during or following cardiac surgery.

10. Chapter 10: Diseases of the Respiratory System (J00-J99)
   a. Chronic Obstructive Pulmonary Disease [COPD] and Asthma
      1) Acute exacerbation of chronic obstructive bronchitis and asthma
      The codes in categories J44 and J45 distinguish between uncomplicated cases and those in acute exacerbation. An acute exacerbation is a worsening or a decompensation of a chronic condition. An acute exacerbation is not equivalent to an infection superimposed on a chronic condition, though an exacerbation may be triggered by an infection.

   b. Acute Respiratory Failure
      1) Acute respiratory failure as principal diagnosis
      A code from subcategory J96.0, Acute respiratory failure, or subcategory J96.2, Acute and chronic respiratory failure, may be assigned as a principal diagnosis when it is the condition established after study to be chiefly responsible for occasioning the admission to the hospital, and the selection is supported by the Alphabetic Index and Tabular List. However, chapter-specific coding guidelines (such as obstetrics, poisoning, HIV, newborn) that provide sequencing direction take precedence.

      2) Acute respiratory failure as secondary diagnosis
      Respiratory failure may be listed as a secondary diagnosis if it occurs after admission, or if it is present on admission, but does not meet the definition of principal diagnosis.

      3) Sequencing of acute respiratory failure and another acute condition
      When a patient is admitted with respiratory failure and another acute condition, (e.g., myocardial infarction, cerebrovascular accident, aspiration pneumonia), the principal diagnosis will not be the same in every situation. This applies whether the other acute condition is a respiratory or nonrespiratory condition. Selection of the principal diagnosis will be dependent on the circumstances of admission. If both the respiratory failure and the other acute condition are equally responsible for occasioning the admission to the hospital, and there are no chapter-specific sequencing rules, the guideline regarding two or more diagnoses that equally meet the definition for principal diagnosis *(Section II, C.)* may be applied in these situations.

If the documentation is not clear as to whether acute respiratory failure and another condition are equally responsible for occasioning the admission, query the provider for clarification.

   c. Influenza due to certain identified influenza viruses
   Code only confirmed cases of influenza due to certain identified influenza viruses (category J09), and due to other identified influenza virus (category J10). This is an exception to the hospital inpatient guideline Section II, H. (Uncertain Diagnosis).

   In this context, "confirmation" does not require documentation of positive laboratory testing specific for avian or other novel influenza A or other identified influenza virus. However, coding should be based on the provider's diagnostic statement that the patient has avian influenza, or other novel influenza A, for category J09, or has another particular identified strain of influenza, such as H1N1 or H3N2, but not identified as novel or variant, for category J10.

   If the provider records "suspected" or "possible" or "probable" avian influenza, or novel influenza, or other identified influenza, then the appropriate influenza code from category J11, Influenza due to unidentified influenza virus, should be assigned. A code from category J09, Influenza due to certain identified influenza viruses, should not be assigned nor should a code from category J10, Influenza due to other identified influenza virus.

   d. Ventilator associated Pneumonia
      1) Documentation of Ventilator associated Pneumonia
      As with all procedural or postprocedural complications, code assignment is based on the provider's documentation of the relationship between the condition and the procedure.

      Code J95.851, Ventilator associated pneumonia, should be assigned only when the provider has documented ventilator associated pneumonia (VAP). An additional code to identify the organism (e.g., Pseudomonas aeruginosa, code B96.5) should also be assigned. Do not assign an additional code from categories J12-J18 to identify the type of pneumonia.

      Code J95.851 should not be assigned for cases where the patient has pneumonia and is on a mechanical ventilator and the provider has not specifically stated that the pneumonia is ventilator-associated pneumonia. If the documentation is unclear as to whether the patient has a pneumonia that is a complication attributable to the mechanical ventilator, query the provider.

      2) Ventilator associated Pneumonia Develops after Admission
      A patient may be admitted with one type of pneumonia (e.g., code J13, Pneumonia due to Streptococcus pneumonia) and subsequently develop VAP. In this instance, the principal diagnosis would be the appropriate code from categories J12-J18 for the pneumonia diagnosed at the time of admission. Code J95.851, Ventilator associated pneumonia, would be assigned as an additional diagnosis when the provider has also documented the presence of ventilator associated pneumonia.

11. Chapter 11: Diseases of the Digestive System (K00-K95)
Reserved for future guideline expansion

12. Chapter 12: Diseases of the Skin and Subcutaneous Tissue (L00-L99)
   a. Pressure ulcer stage codes
      1) Pressure ulcer stages
      Codes from category L89, Pressure ulcer, identify the site of the pressure ulcer as well as the stage of the ulcer.

      The ICD-10-CM classifies pressure ulcer stages based on severity, which is designated by stages 1-4, unspecified stage and unstageable.

      Assign as many codes from category L89 as needed to identify all the pressure ulcers the patient has, if applicable.

      2) Unstageable pressure ulcers
      Assignment of the code for unstageable pressure ulcer (L89.--0) should be based on the clinical documentation. These codes are used for pressure ulcers whose stage cannot be clinically determined (e.g., the ulcer is covered by eschar or has been treated with a skin or muscle graft) and pressure ulcers that are documented as deep tissue injury but not documented as due to trauma. This code should not be confused with the codes for unspecified stage (L89.--9). When there is no documentation

regarding the stage of the pressure ulcer, assign the appropriate code for unspecified stage (L89.--9).

3) Documented pressure ulcer stage
Assignment of the pressure ulcer stage code should be guided by clinical documentation of the stage or documentation of the terms found in the Alphabetic Index. For clinical terms describing the stage that are not found in the Alphabetic Index, and there is no documentation of the stage, the provider should be queried.

4) Patients admitted with pressure ulcers documented as healed
No code is assigned if the documentation states that the pressure ulcer is completely healed.

5) Patients admitted with pressure ulcers documented as healing
Pressure ulcers described as healing should be assigned the appropriate pressure ulcer stage code based on the documentation in the medical record. If the documentation does not provide information about the stage of the healing pressure ulcer, assign the appropriate code for unspecified stage.

If the documentation is unclear as to whether the patient has a current (new) pressure ulcer or if the patient is being treated for a healing pressure ulcer, query the provider.

For ulcers that were present on admission but healed at the time of discharge, assign the code for the site and stage of the pressure ulcer at the time of admission.

6) Patient admitted with pressure ulcer evolving into another stage during the admission
If a patient is admitted **to an inpatient hospital** with a pressure ulcer at one stage and it progresses to a higher stage, two separate codes should be assigned: one code for the site and stage of the ulcer on admission and a second code for the same ulcer site and the highest stage reported during the stay.

b. Non-Pressure Chronic Ulcers

1) Patients admitted with non-pressure ulcers documented as healed
No code is assigned if the documentation states that the non-pressure ulcer is completely healed.

2) Patients admitted with non-pressure ulcers documented as healing
Non-pressure ulcers described as healing should be assigned the appropriate non-pressure ulcer code based on the documentation in the medical record. If the documentation does not provide information about the severity of the healing non-pressure ulcer, assign the appropriate code for unspecified severity.

If the documentation is unclear as to whether the patient has a current (new) non-pressure ulcer or if the patient is being treated for a healing non-pressure ulcer, query the provider.

For ulcers that were present on admission but healed at the time of discharge, assign the code for the site and severity of the non-pressure ulcer at the time of admission.

3) Patient admitted with non-pressure ulcer that progresses to another severity level during the admission
If a patient is admitted to an inpatient hospital with a non-pressure ulcer at one severity level and it progresses to a higher severity level, two separate codes should be assigned: one code for the site and severity level of the ulcer on admission and a second code for the same ulcer site and the highest severity level reported during the stay.

13. Chapter 13: Diseases of the Musculoskeletal System and Connective Tissue (M00-M99)

a. Site and laterality
Most of the codes within Chapter 13 have site and laterality designations. The site represents the bone, joint or the muscle involved. For some conditions where more than one bone, joint or muscle is usually involved, such as osteoarthritis, there is a "multiple sites" code available. For categories where no multiple site code is provided and more than one bone, joint or muscle is involved,

multiple codes should be used to indicate the different sites involved.

1) Bone versus joint
For certain conditions, the bone may be affected at the upper or lower end, (e.g., avascular necrosis of bone, M87, Osteoporosis, M80, M81). Though the portion of the bone affected may be at the joint, the site designation will be the bone, not the joint.

b. Acute traumatic versus chronic or recurrent musculoskeletal conditions
Many musculoskeletal conditions are a result of previous injury or trauma to a site, or are recurrent conditions. Bone, joint or muscle conditions that are the result of a healed injury are usually found in chapter 13. Recurrent bone, joint or muscle conditions are also usually found in chapter 13. Any current, acute injury should be coded to the appropriate injury code from chapter 19. Chronic or recurrent conditions should generally be coded with a code from chapter 13. If it is difficult to determine from the documentation in the record which code is best to describe a condition, query the provider.

c. Coding of Pathologic Fractures
7th character A is for use as long as the patient is receiving active treatment for the fracture. While the patient may be seen by a new or different provider over the course of treatment for a pathological fracture, assignment of the 7th character is based on whether the patient is undergoing active treatment and not whether the provider is seeing the patient for the first time.

7th character D is to be used for encounters after the patient has completed active treatment **for the fracture and is receiving routine care for the fracture during the healing or recovery phase.** The other 7th characters, listed under each subcategory in the Tabular List, are to be used for subsequent encounters for treatment of problems associated with the healing, such as malunions, nonunions, and sequelae.

Care for complications of surgical treatment for fracture repairs during the healing or recovery phase should be coded with the appropriate complication codes.

See Section I.C.19. Coding of traumatic fractures.

d. Osteoporosis
Osteoporosis is a systemic condition, meaning that all bones of the musculoskeletal system are affected. Therefore, site is not a component of the codes under category M81, Osteoporosis without current pathological fracture. The site codes under category M80, Osteoporosis with current pathological fracture, identify the site of the fracture, not the osteoporosis.

1) Osteoporosis without pathological fracture
Category M81, Osteoporosis without current pathological fracture, is for use for patients with osteoporosis who do not currently have a pathologic fracture due to the osteoporosis, even if they have had a fracture in the past. For patients with a history of osteoporosis fractures, status code Z87.310, Personal history of (healed) osteoporosis fracture, should follow the code from M81.

2) Osteoporosis with current pathological fracture
Category M80, Osteoporosis with current pathological fracture, is for patients who have a current pathologic fracture at the time of an encounter. The codes under M80 identify the site of the fracture. A code from category M80, not a traumatic fracture code, should be used for any patient with known osteoporosis who suffers a fracture, even if the patient had a minor fall or trauma, if that fall or trauma would not usually break a normal, healthy bone.

14. Chapter 14: Diseases of Genitourinary System (N00-N99)

a. Chronic kidney disease

1) Stages of chronic kidney disease (CKD)
The ICD-10-CM classifies CKD based on severity. The severity of CKD is designated by stages 1-5. Stage 2, code N18.2, equates to mild CKD; stage 3, code N18.3, equates to moderate CKD; and stage 4, code N18.4, equates to severe CKD. Code N18.6, End stage renal disease (ESRD), is assigned when the provider has documented end-stage-renal disease (ESRD).

If both a stage of CKD and ESRD are documented, assign code N18.6 only.

2) **Chronic kidney disease and kidney transplant status**
Patients who have undergone kidney transplant may still have some form of chronic kidney disease (CKD) because the kidney transplant may not fully restore kidney function. Therefore, the presence of CKD alone does not constitute a transplant complication. Assign the appropriate N18 code for the patient's stage of CKD and code Z94.0, Kidney transplant status. If a transplant complication such as failure or rejection or other transplant complication is documented, see section I.C.19.g for information on coding complications of a kidney transplant. If the documentation is unclear as to whether the patient has a complication of the transplant, query the provider.

3) **Chronic kidney disease with other conditions**
Patients with CKD may also suffer from other serious conditions, most commonly diabetes mellitus and hypertension. The sequencing of the CKD code in relationship to codes for other contributing conditions is based on the conventions in the Tabular List.

See I.C.9. Hypertensive chronic kidney disease.

See I.C.19. Chronic kidney disease and kidney transplant complications.

15. **Chapter 15: Pregnancy, Childbirth, and the Puerperium (O00-O9A)**
a. **General Rules for Obstetric Cases**
1) **Codes from chapter 15 and sequencing priority**
Obstetric cases require codes from chapter 15, codes in the range O00-O9A, Pregnancy, Childbirth, and the Puerperium. Chapter 15 codes have sequencing priority over codes from other chapters. Additional codes from other chapters may be used in conjunction with chapter 15 codes to further specify conditions. Should the provider document that the pregnancy is incidental to the encounter, then code Z33.1, Pregnant state, incidental, should be used in place of any chapter 15 codes. It is the provider's responsibility to state that the condition being treated is not affecting the pregnancy.

2) **Chapter 15 codes used only on the maternal record**
Chapter 15 codes are to be used only on the maternal record, never on the record of the newborn.

3) **Final character for trimester**
The majority of codes in Chapter 15 have a final character indicating the trimester of pregnancy. The timeframes for the trimesters are indicated at the beginning of the chapter. If trimester is not a component of a code, it is because the condition always occurs in a specific trimester, or the concept of trimester of pregnancy is not applicable. Certain codes have characters for only certain trimesters because the condition does not occur in all trimesters, but it may occur in more than just one.

Assignment of the final character for trimester should be based on the provider's documentation of the trimester (or number of weeks) for the current admission/encounter. This applies to the assignment of trimester for pre-existing conditions as well as those that develop during or are due to the pregnancy. The provider's documentation of the number of weeks may be used to assign the appropriate code identifying the trimester.

Whenever delivery occurs during the current admission, and there is an "in childbirth" option for the obstetric complication being coded, the "in childbirth" code should be assigned.

4) **Selection of trimester for inpatient admissions that encompass more than one trimester**
In instances when a patient is admitted to a hospital for complications of pregnancy during one trimester and remains in the hospital into a subsequent trimester, the trimester character for the antepartum complication code should be assigned on the basis of the trimester when the complication developed, not the trimester of the discharge. If the condition developed prior to the current admission/encounter or represents a pre-existing condition, the trimester character for the trimester at the time of the admission/encounter should be assigned.

5) **Unspecified trimester**
Each category that includes codes for trimester has a code for "unspecified trimester." The "unspecified trimester" code should rarely be used, such as when the documentation in the record is insufficient to determine the trimester and it is not possible to obtain clarification.

6) **7th character for Fetus Identification**
Where applicable, a 7th character is to be assigned for certain categories (O31, O32, O33.3 - O33.6, O35, O36, O40, O41, O60.1, O60.2, O64, and O69) to identify the fetus for which the complication code applies.

Assign 7th character "0":
- For single gestations
- When the documentation in the record is insufficient to determine the fetus affected and it is not possible to obtain clarification.
- When it is not possible to clinically determine which fetus is affected.

b. **Selection of OB Principal or First-listed Diagnosis**
1) **Routine outpatient prenatal visits**
For routine outpatient prenatal visits when no complications are present, a code from category Z34, Encounter for supervision of normal pregnancy, should be used as the first-listed diagnosis. These codes should not be used in conjunction with chapter 15 codes.

2) **Supervision of High-Risk Pregnancy**
Codes from category O09, Supervision of high-risk pregnancy, are intended for use only during the prenatal period. For complications during the labor or delivery episode as a result of a high-risk pregnancy, assign the applicable complication codes from Chapter 15. If there are no complications during the labor or delivery episode, assign code O80, Encounter for full-term uncomplicated delivery.

For routine prenatal outpatient visits for patients with high-risk pregnancies, a code from category O09, Supervision of high-risk pregnancy, should be used as the first-listed diagnosis. Secondary chapter 15 codes may be used in conjunction with these codes if appropriate.

3) **Episodes when no delivery occurs**
In episodes when no delivery occurs, the principal diagnosis should correspond to the principal complication of the pregnancy which necessitated the encounter. Should more than one complication exist, all of which are treated or monitored, any of the complications codes may be sequenced first.

4) **When a delivery occurs**
When an obstetric patient is admitted and delivers during that admission, the condition that prompted the admission should be sequenced as the principal diagnosis. If multiple conditions prompted the admission, sequence the one most related to the delivery as the principal diagnosis. A code for any complication of the delivery should be assigned as an additional diagnosis. In cases of cesarean delivery, if the patient was admitted with a condition that resulted in the performance of a cesarean procedure, that condition should be selected as the principal diagnosis. If the reason for the admission was unrelated to the condition resulting in the cesarean delivery, the condition related to the reason for the admission should be selected as the principal diagnosis.

5) **Outcome of delivery**
A code from category Z37, Outcome of delivery, should be included on every maternal record when a delivery has occurred. These codes are not to be used on subsequent records or on the newborn record.

c. **Pre-existing conditions versus conditions due to the pregnancy**
Certain categories in Chapter 15 distinguish between conditions of the mother that existed prior to pregnancy (pre-existing) and those that are a direct result of pregnancy. When assigning codes from Chapter 15, it is important to assess if a condition was pre-existing prior to pregnancy or developed during or due to the pregnancy in order to assign the correct code.

Categories that do not distinguish between pre-existing and pregnancy-related conditions may be used for either. It is acceptable to use codes specifically for the puerperium with codes complicating pregnancy and childbirth if a condition arises postpartum during the delivery encounter.

d. Pre-existing hypertension in pregnancy

Category O10, Pre-existing hypertension complicating pregnancy, childbirth and the puerperium, includes codes for hypertensive heart and hypertensive chronic kidney disease. When assigning one of the O10 codes that includes hypertensive heart disease or hypertensive chronic kidney disease, it is necessary to add a secondary code from the appropriate hypertension category to specify the type of heart failure or chronic kidney disease.

See Section I.C.9. Hypertension.

e. Fetal Conditions Affecting the Management of the Mother

1) Codes from categories O35 and O36

Codes from categories O35, Maternal care for known or suspected fetal abnormality and damage, and O36, Maternal care for other fetal problems, are assigned only when the fetal condition is actually responsible for modifying the management of the mother, i.e., by requiring diagnostic studies, additional observation, special care, or termination of pregnancy. The fact that the fetal condition exists does not justify assigning a code from this series to the mother's record.

2) In utero surgery

In cases when surgery is performed on the fetus, a diagnosis code from category O35, Maternal care for known or suspected fetal abnormality and damage, should be assigned identifying the fetal condition. Assign the appropriate procedure code for the procedure performed.

No code from Chapter 16, the perinatal codes, should be used on the mother's record to identify fetal conditions. Surgery performed in utero on a fetus is still to be coded as an obstetric encounter.

f. HIV Infection in Pregnancy, Childbirth and the Puerperium

During pregnancy, childbirth or the puerperium, a patient admitted because of an HIV-related illness should receive a principal diagnosis from subcategory O98.7-, Human immunodeficiency [HIV] disease complicating pregnancy, childbirth and the puerperium, followed by the code(s) for the HIV-related illness(es).

Patients with asymptomatic HIV infection status admitted during pregnancy, childbirth, or the puerperium should receive codes of O98.7- and Z21, Asymptomatic human immunodeficiency virus [HIV] infection status.

g. Diabetes mellitus in pregnancy

Diabetes mellitus is a significant complicating factor in pregnancy. Pregnant women who are diabetic should be assigned a code from category O24, Diabetes mellitus in pregnancy, childbirth, and the puerperium, first, followed by the appropriate diabetes code(s) (E08-E13) from Chapter 4.

h. Long term use of insulin and oral hypoglycemics

See section I.C.4.a.3 for information on the long term use of insulin and oral hypoglycemic.

i. Gestational (pregnancy induced) diabetes

Gestational (pregnancy induced) diabetes can occur during the second and third trimester of pregnancy in women who were not diabetic prior to pregnancy. Gestational diabetes can cause complications in the pregnancy similar to those of pre-existing diabetes mellitus. It also puts the woman at greater risk of developing diabetes after the pregnancy. Codes for gestational diabetes are in subcategory O24.4, Gestational diabetes mellitus. No other code from category O24, Diabetes mellitus in pregnancy, childbirth, and the puerperium, should be used with a code from O24.4.

The codes under subcategory O24.4 include diet controlled, insulin controlled, and controlled by oral hypoglycemic drugs. If a patient with gestational diabetes is treated with both diet and insulin, only the code for insulin-controlled is required. If a patient with gestational diabetes is treated with both diet and oral hypoglycemic medications, only the code for "controlled by oral hypoglycemic drugs" is required. Code Z79.4, Long-term (current) use of insulin or code Z79.84, Long-term (current) use of oral hypoglycemic drugs, should not be assigned with codes from subcategory O24.4.

An abnormal glucose tolerance in pregnancy is assigned a code from subcategory O99.81, Abnormal glucose complicating pregnancy, childbirth, and the puerperium.

j. Sepsis and septic shock complicating abortion, pregnancy, childbirth and the puerperium

When assigning a chapter 15 code for sepsis complicating abortion, pregnancy, childbirth, and the puerperium, a code for the specific type of infection should be assigned as an additional diagnosis. If severe sepsis is present, a code from subcategory R65.2, Severe sepsis, and code(s) for associated organ dysfunction(s) should also be assigned as additional diagnoses.

k. Puerperal sepsis

Code O85, Puerperal sepsis, should be assigned with a secondary code to identify the causal organism (e.g., for a bacterial infection, assign a code from category B95-B96, Bacterial infections in conditions classified elsewhere). A code from category A40, Streptococcal sepsis, or A41, Other sepsis, should not be used for puerperal sepsis. If applicable, use additional codes to identify severe sepsis (R65.2-) and any associated acute organ dysfunction.

l. Alcohol and tobacco use during pregnancy, childbirth and the puerperium

1) Alcohol use during pregnancy, childbirth and the puerperium

Codes under subcategory O99.31, Alcohol use complicating pregnancy, childbirth, and the puerperium, should be assigned for any pregnancy case when a mother uses alcohol during the pregnancy or postpartum. A secondary code from category F10, Alcohol related disorders, should also be assigned to identify manifestations of the alcohol use.

2) Tobacco use during pregnancy, childbirth and the puerperium

Codes under subcategory O99.33, Smoking (tobacco) complicating pregnancy, childbirth, and the puerperium, should be assigned for any pregnancy case when a mother uses any type of tobacco product during the pregnancy or postpartum. A secondary code from category F17, Nicotine dependence, should also be assigned to identify the type of nicotine dependence.

m. Poisoning, toxic effects, adverse effects and underdosing in a pregnant patient

A code from subcategory O9A.2, Injury, poisoning and certain other consequences of external causes complicating pregnancy, childbirth, and the puerperium, should be sequenced first, followed by the appropriate injury, poisoning, toxic effect, adverse effect or underdosing code, and then the additional code(s) that specifies the condition caused by the poisoning, toxic effect, adverse effect or underdosing.

See Section I.C.19. Adverse effects, poisoning, underdosing and toxic effects.

n. Normal Delivery, Code O80

1) Encounter for full term uncomplicated delivery

Code O80 should be assigned when a woman is admitted for a full-term normal delivery and delivers a single, healthy infant without any complications antepartum, during the delivery, or postpartum during the delivery episode. Code O80 is always a principal diagnosis. It is not to be used if any other code from chapter 15 is needed to describe a current complication of the antenatal, delivery, or perinatal period. Additional codes from other chapters may be used with code O80 if they are not related to or are in any way complicating the pregnancy.

2) Uncomplicated delivery with resolved antepartum complication

Code O80 may be used if the patient had a complication at some point during the pregnancy, but the complication is not present at the time of the admission for delivery.

3) Outcome of delivery for O80

Z37.0, Single live birth, is the only outcome of delivery code appropriate for use with O80.

o. The Peripartum and Postpartum Periods

1) Peripartum and Postpartum periods

The postpartum period begins immediately after delivery and continues for six weeks following delivery. The peripartum period is defined as the last month of pregnancy to five months postpartum.

2) Peripartum and postpartum complication

A postpartum complication is any complication occurring within the six-week period.

3) Pregnancy-related complications after 6 week period

Chapter 15 codes may also be used to describe pregnancy-related complications after the peripartum or postpartum period if the provider documents that a condition is pregnancy related.

4) Admission for routine postpartum care following delivery outside hospital

When the mother delivers outside the hospital prior to admission and is admitted for routine postpartum care and no complications are noted, code Z39.0, Encounter for care and examination of mother immediately after delivery, should be assigned as the principal diagnosis.

5) Pregnancy associated cardiomyopathy

Pregnancy associated cardiomyopathy, code O90.3, is unique in that it may be diagnosed in the third trimester of pregnancy but may continue to progress months after delivery. For this reason, it is referred to as peripartum cardiomyopathy. Code O90.3 is only for use when the cardiomyopathy develops as a result of pregnancy in a woman who did not have pre-existing heart disease.

p. Code O94, Sequelae of complication of pregnancy, childbirth, and the puerperium

1) Code O94

Code O94, Sequelae of complication of pregnancy, childbirth, and the puerperium, is for use in those cases when an initial complication of a pregnancy develops a sequelae requiring care or treatment at a future date.

2) After the initial postpartum period

This code may be used at any time after the initial postpartum period.

3) Sequencing of Code O94

- This code, like all sequela codes, is to be sequenced following the code describing the sequelae of the complication.

q. Termination of Pregnancy and Spontaneous abortions

1) Abortion with Liveborn Fetus

When an attempted termination of pregnancy results in a liveborn fetus, assign code Z33.2, Encounter for elective termination of pregnancy and a code from category Z37, Outcome of Delivery.

2) Retained Products of Conception following an abortion

Subsequent encounters for retained products of conception following a spontaneous abortion or elective termination of pregnancy, **without complications** are assigned O03.**4, Incomplete spontaneous,** abortion **without complication**, or codes O07.4, Failed attempted termination of pregnancy without complication. This advice is appropriate even when the patient was discharged previously with a discharge diagnosis of complete abortion. **If the patient has a specific complication associated with the spontaneous abortion or elective termination of pregnancy in addition to retained products of conception, assign the appropriate complication in category O03 or O07 instead of code O03.4 or O07.4**

3) Complications leading to abortion

Codes from Chapter 15 may be used as additional codes to identify any documented complications of the pregnancy in conjunction with codes in categories in **O04**, O07 and O08.

r. Abuse in a pregnant patient

For suspected or confirmed cases of abuse of a pregnant patient, a code(s) from subcategories O9A.3, Physical abuse complicating pregnancy, childbirth, and the puerperium, O9A.4, Sexual abuse complicating pregnancy, childbirth, and the puerperium, and O9A.5, Psychological abuse complicating pregnancy, childbirth, and the puerperium, should be sequenced first, followed by the appropriate codes (if applicable) to identify any associated current injury due to physical abuse, sexual abuse, and the perpetrator of abuse.

See Section I.C.19. Adult and child abuse, neglect and other maltreatment.

16. Chapter 16: Certain Conditions Originating in the Perinatal Period (P00-P96)

For coding and reporting purposes the perinatal period is defined as before birth through the 28th day following birth. The following guidelines are provided for reporting purposes.

a. General Perinatal Rules

1) Use of Chapter 16 Codes

Codes in this chapter are never for use on the maternal record. Codes from Chapter 15, the obstetric chapter, are never permitted on the newborn record. Chapter 16 codes may be used throughout the life of the patient if the condition is still present.

2) Principal Diagnosis for Birth Record

When coding the birth episode in a newborn record, assign a code from category Z38, Liveborn infants according to place of birth and type of delivery, as the principal diagnosis. A code from category Z38 is assigned only once, to a newborn at the time of birth. If a newborn is transferred to another institution, a code from category Z38 should not be used at the receiving hospital.

A code from category Z38 is used only on the newborn record, not on the mother's record.

3) Use of Codes from other Chapters with Codes from Chapter 16

Codes from other chapters may be used with codes from chapter 16 if the codes from the other chapters provide more specific detail. Codes for signs and symptoms may be assigned when a definitive diagnosis has not been established. If the reason for the encounter is a perinatal condition, the code from chapter 16 should be sequenced first.

4) Use of Chapter 16 Codes after the Perinatal Period

Should a condition originate in the perinatal period, and continue throughout the life of the patient, the perinatal code should continue to be used regardless of the patient's age.

5) Birth process or community acquired conditions

If a newborn has a condition that may be either due to the birth process or community acquired and the documentation does not indicate which it is, the default is due to the birth process and the code from Chapter 16 should be used. If the condition is community-acquired, a code from Chapter 16 should not be assigned.

6) Code all clinically significant conditions

All clinically significant conditions noted on routine newborn examination should be coded. A condition is clinically significant if it requires:

- clinical evaluation; or
- therapeutic treatment; or
- diagnostic procedures; or
- extended length of hospital stay; or
- increased nursing care and/or monitoring; or
- has implications for future health care needs

Note: The perinatal guidelines listed above are the same as the general coding guidelines for "additional diagnoses", except for the final point regarding implications for future health care needs. Codes should be assigned for conditions that have been specified by the provider as having implications for future health care needs.

b. Observation and Evaluation of Newborns for Suspected Conditions not Found

1) Use of Z05 codes

Assign a code from category Z05, Observation and evaluation of newborns and infants for suspected conditions ruled out, to identify those instances when a healthy newborn is evaluated for a suspected condition that is determined after study not to be present. Do not use a code from category Z05 when the patient has identified signs or symptoms of a suspected problem; in such cases code the sign or symptom.

2) Z05 on Other than the Birth Record

A code from category Z05 may also be assigned as a principal or first-listed code for readmissions or encounters when the code from category Z38 code no longer applies. Codes from category

Z05 are for use only for healthy newborns and infants for which no condition after study is found to be present.

3) Z05 on a birth record

A code from category Z05 is to be used as a secondary code after the code from category Z38, Liveborn infants according to place of birth and type of delivery.

c. Coding Additional Perinatal Diagnoses

1) Assigning codes for conditions that require treatment

Assign codes for conditions that require treatment or further investigation, prolong the length of stay, or require resource utilization.

2) Codes for conditions specified as having implications for future health care needs

Assign codes for conditions that have been specified by the provider as having implications for future health care needs.

Note: This guideline should not be used for adult patients.

d. Prematurity and Fetal Growth Retardation

Providers utilize different criteria in determining prematurity. A code for prematurity should not be assigned unless it is documented. Assignment of codes in categories P05, Disorders of newborn related to slow fetal growth and fetal malnutrition, and P07, Disorders of newborn related to short gestation and low birth weight, not elsewhere classified, should be based on the recorded birth weight and estimated gestational age.

When both birth weight and gestational age are available, two codes from category P07 should be assigned, with the code for birth weight sequenced before the code for gestational age.

e. Low birth weight and immaturity status

Codes from category P07, Disorders of newborn related to short gestation and low birth weight, not elsewhere classified, are for use for a child or adult who was premature or had a low birth weight as a newborn and this is affecting the patient's current health status.

See Section I.C.21. Factors influencing health status and contact with health services, Status.

f. Bacterial Sepsis of Newborn

Category P36, Bacterial sepsis of newborn, includes congenital sepsis. If a perinate is documented as having sepsis without documentation of congenital or community acquired, the default is congenital and a code from category P36 should be assigned. If the P36 code includes the causal organism, an additional code from category B95, Streptococcus, Staphylococcus, and Enterococcus as the cause of diseases classified elsewhere, or B96, Other bacterial agents as the cause of diseases classified elsewhere, should not be assigned. If the P36 code does not include the causal organism, assign an additional code from category B96. If applicable, use additional codes to identify severe sepsis (R65.2-) and any associated acute organ dysfunction.

g. Stillbirth

Code P95, Stillbirth, is only for use in institutions that maintain separate records for stillbirths. No other code should be used with P95. Code P95 should not be used on the mother's record.

17. Chapter 17: Congenital malformations, deformations, and chromosomal abnormalities (Q00-Q99)

Assign an appropriate code(s) from categories Q00-Q99, Congenital malformations, deformations, and chromosomal abnormalities when a malformation/deformation or chromosomal abnormality is documented. A malformation/deformation/or chromosomal abnormality may be the principal/first-listed diagnosis on a record or a secondary diagnosis.

When a malformation/deformation or chromosomal abnormality does not have a unique code assignment, assign additional code(s) for any manifestations that may be present.

When the code assignment specifically identifies the malformation/deformation or chromosomal abnormality, manifestations that are an inherent component of the anomaly should not be coded separately. Additional codes should be assigned for manifestations that are not an inherent component.

Codes from Chapter 17 may be used throughout the life of the patient. If a congenital malformation or deformity has been corrected, a personal history code should be used to identify the history of the malformation or deformity. Although present at birth, malformation/deformation/or chromosomal abnormality may not be identified until later in life.

Whenever the condition is diagnosed by the physician, it is appropriate to assign a code from codes Q00-Q99.For the birth admission, the appropriate code from category Z38, Liveborn infants, according to place of birth and type of delivery, should be sequenced as the principal diagnosis, followed by any congenital anomaly codes, Q00- Q99.

18. Chapter 18: Symptoms, signs, and abnormal clinical and laboratory findings, not elsewhere classified (R00-R99)

Chapter 18 includes symptoms, signs, abnormal results of clinical or other investigative procedures, and ill-defined conditions regarding which no diagnosis classifiable elsewhere is recorded. Signs and symptoms that point to a specific diagnosis have been assigned to a category in other chapters of the classification.

a. Use of symptom codes

Codes that describe symptoms and signs are acceptable for reporting purposes when a related definitive diagnosis has not been established (confirmed) by the provider.

b. Use of a symptom code with a definitive diagnosis code

Codes for signs and symptoms may be reported in addition to a related definitive diagnosis when the sign or symptom is not routinely associated with that diagnosis, such as the various signs and symptoms associated with complex syndromes. The definitive diagnosis code should be sequenced before the symptom code.

Signs or symptoms that are associated routinely with a disease process should not be assigned as additional codes, unless otherwise instructed by the classification.

c. Combination codes that include symptoms

ICD-10-CM contains a number of combination codes that identify both the definitive diagnosis and common symptoms of that diagnosis.

When using one of these combination codes, an additional code should not be assigned for the symptom.

d. Repeated falls

Code R29.6, Repeated falls, is for use for encounters when a patient has recently fallen and the reason for the fall is being investigated.

Code Z91.81, History of falling, is for use when a patient has fallen in the past and is at risk for future falls. When appropriate, both codes R29.6 and Z91.81 may be assigned together.

e. Coma scale

The coma scale codes (R40.2-) can be used in conjunction with traumatic brain injury codes, acute cerebrovascular disease or sequelae of cerebrovascular disease codes. These codes are primarily for use by trauma registries, but they may be used in any setting where this information is collected. The coma scale may also be used to assess the status of the central nervous system for other non-trauma conditions, such as monitoring patients in the intensive care unit regardless of medical condition. The coma scale codes should be sequenced after the diagnosis code(s).

These codes, one from each subcategory, are needed to complete the scale. The 7th character indicates when the scale was recorded. The 7th character should match for all three codes.

At a minimum, report the initial score documented on presentation at your facility. This may be a score from the emergency medicine technician (EMT) or in the emergency department. If desired, a facility may choose to capture multiple coma scale scores.

Assign code R40.24, Glasgow coma scale, total score, when only the total score is documented in the medical record and not the individual score(s).

f. Functional quadriplegia

GUIDELINE HAS BEEN DELETED EFFECTIVE OCTOBER 1, 2017

g. SIRS due to Non-Infectious Process

The systemic inflammatory response syndrome (SIRS) can develop as a result of certain non-infectious disease processes, such as trauma, malignant neoplasm, or pancreatitis. When SIRS is documented with a noninfectious condition, and no subsequent infection is documented, the code for the underlying condition, such as an injury, should be assigned, followed by code R65.10, Systemic inflammatory response syndrome (SIRS) of non-infectious origin without acute organ dysfunction, or code R65.11, Systemic inflammatory response syndrome (SIRS) of non-infectious origin with acute organ dysfunction. If an associated acute organ dysfunction is documented, the appropriate code(s) for the specific type of organ dysfunction(s) should be assigned in addition to code

R65.11. If acute organ dysfunction is documented, but it cannot be determined if the acute organ dysfunction is associated with SIRS or due to another condition (e.g., directly due to the trauma), the provider should be queried.

h. Death NOS

Code R99, Ill-defined and unknown cause of mortality, is only for use in the very limited circumstance when a patient who has already died is brought into an emergency department or other healthcare facility and is pronounced dead upon arrival. It does not represent the discharge disposition of death.

i. NIHSS Stroke Scale

The NIH stroke scale (NIHSS) codes (R29.7- -) can be used in conjunction with acute stroke codes (I63) to identify the patient's neurological status and the severity of the stroke. The stroke scale codes should be sequenced after the acute stroke diagnosis code(s).

At a minimum, report the initial score documented. If desired, a facility may choose to capture multiple stroke scale scores.

See Section I.B.14. for information concerning the medical record documentation that may be used for assignment of the NIHSS codes.

19. Chapter 19: Injury, poisoning, and certain other consequences of external causes (S00-T88)

a. Application of 7th Characters in Chapter 19

Most categories in chapter 19 have a 7th character requirement for each applicable code. Most categories in this chapter have three 7th character values (with the exception of fractures): A, initial encounter, D, subsequent encounter and S, sequela. Categories for traumatic fractures have additional 7th character values. While the patient may be seen by a new or different provider over the course of treatment for an injury, assignment of the 7th character is based on whether the patient is undergoing active treatment and not whether the provider is seeing the patient for the first time.

For complication codes, active treatment refers to treatment for the condition described by the code, even though it may be related to an earlier precipitating problem. For example, code T84.50XA, Infection and inflammatory reaction due to unspecified internal joint prosthesis, initial encounter, is used when active treatment is provided for the infection, even though the condition relates to the prosthetic device, implant or graft that was placed at a previous encounter.

7th character "A", initial encounter is used for each encounter where the patient is receiving active treatment for the condition.

7th character "D" subsequent encounter is used for encounters after the patient has completed active treatment of the condition and is receiving routine care for the condition during the healing or recovery phase.

The aftercare Z codes should not be used for aftercare for conditions such as injuries or poisonings, where 7th characters are provided to identify subsequent care. For example, for aftercare of an injury, assign the acute injury code with the 7th character "D" (subsequent encounter).

7th character "S", sequela, is for use for complications or conditions that arise as a direct result of a condition, such as scar formation after a burn. The scars are sequelae of the burn. When using 7th character "S", it is necessary to use both the injury code that precipitated the sequela and the code for the sequela itself. The "S" is added only to the injury code, not the sequela code. The 7th character "S" identifies the injury responsible for the sequela. The specific type of sequela (e.g. scar) is sequenced first, followed by the injury code.

See Section I.B.10 Sequelae, (Late Effects)

b. Coding of Injuries

When coding injuries, assign separate codes for each injury unless a combination code is provided, in which case the combination code is assigned. **Codes from category T07**, Unspecified multiple injuries should not be assigned in the inpatient setting unless information for a more specific code is not available. Traumatic injury codes (S00-T14.9) are not to be used for normal, healing surgical wounds or to identify complications of surgical wounds.

The code for the most serious injury, as determined by the provider and the focus of treatment, is sequenced first.

1) Superficial injuries

Superficial injuries such as abrasions or contusions are not coded when associated with more severe injuries of the same site.

2) Primary injury with damage to nerves/blood vessels

When a primary injury results in minor damage to peripheral nerves or blood vessels, the primary injury is sequenced first with additional code(s) for injuries to nerves and spinal cord (such as category S04), and/or injury to blood vessels (such as category S15). When the primary injury is to the blood vessels or nerves, that injury should be sequenced first.

c. Coding of Traumatic Fractures

The principles of multiple coding of injuries should be followed in coding fractures. Fractures of specified sites are coded individually by site in accordance with both the provisions within categories S02, S12, S22, S32, S42, S49, S52, S59, S62, S72, S79, S82, S89, S92 and the level of detail furnished by medical record content.

A fracture not indicated as open or closed should be coded to closed. A fracture not indicated whether displaced or not displaced should be coded to displaced.

More specific guidelines are as follows:

1) Initial vs. Subsequent Encounter for Fractures

Traumatic fractures are coded using the appropriate 7th character for initial encounter (A, B, C) for each encounter where the patient is receiving active treatment for the fracture. The appropriate 7th character for initial encounter should also be assigned for a patient who delayed seeking treatment for the fracture or nonunion.

Fractures are coded using the appropriate 7th character for subsequent care for encounters after the patient has completed active treatment of the fracture and is receiving routine care for the fracture during the healing or recovery phase.

Care for complications of surgical treatment for fracture repairs during the healing or recovery phase should be coded with the appropriate complication codes.

Care of complications of fractures, such as malunion and nonunion, should be reported with the appropriate 7th character for subsequent care with nonunion (K, M, N,) or subsequent care with malunion (P, Q, R).

Malunion/nonunion: The appropriate 7th character for initial encounter should also be assigned for a patient who delayed seeking treatment for the fracture or nonunion.

The open fracture designations in the assignment of the 7th character for fractures of the forearm, femur and lower leg, including ankle are based on the Gustilo open fracture classification. When the Gustilo classification type is not specified for an open fracture, the 7th character for open fracture type I or II should be assigned (B, E, H, M, Q).

A code from category M80, not a traumatic fracture code, should be used for any patient with known osteoporosis who suffers a fracture, even if the patient had a minor fall or trauma, if that fall or trauma would not usually break a normal, healthy bone.

See Section I.C.13. Osteoporosis.

The aftercare Z codes should not be used for aftercare for traumatic fractures. For aftercare of a traumatic fracture, assign the acute fracture code with the appropriate 7th character.

2) Multiple fractures sequencing

Multiple fractures are sequenced in accordance with the severity of the fracture.

d. Coding of Burns and Corrosions

The ICD-10-CM makes a distinction between burns and corrosions. The burn codes are for thermal burns, except sunburns, that come from a heat source, such as a fire or hot appliance. The burn codes are also for burns resulting from electricity and radiation. Corrosions are burns due to chemicals. The guidelines are the same for burns and corrosions.

Current burns (T20-T25) are classified by depth, extent and by agent (X code). Burns are classified by depth as first degree (erythema), second degree (blistering), and third degree (full-thickness involvement). Burns of the eye and internal organs (T26-T28) are classified by site, but not by degree.

1) **Sequencing of burn and related condition codes**
   Sequence first the code that reflects the highest degree of burn when more than one burn is present.

   a. When the reason for the admission or encounter is for treatment of external multiple burns, sequence first the code that reflects the burn of the highest degree.

   b. When a patient has both internal and external burns, the circumstances of admission govern the selection of the principal diagnosis or first-listed diagnosis.

   c. When a patient is admitted for burn injuries and other related conditions such as smoke inhalation and/or respiratory failure, the circumstances of admission govern the selection of the principal or first-listed diagnosis.

2) **Burns of the same local site**
   Classify burns of the same local site (three-character category level, T20-T28) but of different degrees to the subcategory identifying the highest degree recorded in the diagnosis.

3) **Non-healing burns**
   Non-healing burns are coded as acute burns.

   Necrosis of burned skin should be coded as a non-healed burn.

4) **Infected Burn**
   For any documented infected burn site, use an additional code for the infection.

5) **Assign separate codes for each burn site**
   When coding burns, assign separate codes for each burn site. Category T30, Burn and corrosion, body region unspecified is extremely vague and should rarely be used.

6) **Burns and Corrosions Classified According to Extent of Body Surface Involved**
   Assign codes from category T31, Burns classified according to extent of body surface involved, or T32, Corrosions classified according to extent of body surface involved, when the site of the burn is not specified or when there is a need for additional data. It is advisable to use category T31 as additional coding when needed to provide data for evaluating burn mortality, such as that needed by burn units. It is also advisable to use category T31 as an additional code for reporting purposes when there is mention of a third-degree burn involving 20 percent or more of the body surface.

   Categories T31 and T32 are based on the classic "rule of nines" in estimating body surface involved: head and neck are assigned nine percent, each arm nine percent, each leg 18 percent, the anterior trunk 18 percent, posterior trunk 18 percent, and genitalia one percent. Providers may change these percentage assignments where necessary to accommodate infants and children who have proportionately larger heads than adults, and patients who have large buttocks, thighs, or abdomen that involve burns.

7) **Encounters for treatment of sequela of burns**
   Encounters for the treatment of the late effects of burns or corrosions (i.e., scars or joint contractures) should be coded with a burn or corrosion code with the 7th character "S" for sequela.

8) **Sequelae with a late effect code and current burn**
   When appropriate, both a code for a current burn or corrosion with 7th character "A" or "D" and a burn or corrosion code with 7th character "S" may be assigned on the same record (when both a current burn and sequelae of an old burn exist). Burns and corrosions do not heal at the same rate and a current healing wound may still exist with sequela of a healed burn or corrosion.

   See Section I.B.10 Sequela (Late Effects)

9) **Use of an external cause code with burns and corrosions**
   An external cause code should be used with burns and corrosions to identify the source and intent of the burn, as well as the place where it occurred.

e. **Adverse Effects, Poisoning, Underdosing and Toxic Effects**
   Codes in categories T36-T65 are combination codes that include the substance that was taken as well as the intent. No additional external cause code is required for poisonings, toxic effects, adverse effects and underdosing codes.

1) **Do not code directly from the Table of Drugs**
   Do not code directly from the Table of Drugs and Chemicals. Always refer back to the Tabular List.

2) **Use as many codes as necessary to describe**
   Use as many codes as necessary to describe completely all drugs, medicinal or biological substances.

3) **If the same code would describe the causative agent**
   If the same code would describe the causative agent for more than one adverse reaction, poisoning, toxic effect or underdosing, assign the code only once.

4) **If two or more drugs, medicinal or biological substances**
   If two or more drugs, medicinal or biological substances are reported, code each individually unless a combination code is listed in the Table of Drugs and Chemicals.

5) **The occurrence of drug toxicity is classified in ICD-10-CM as follows:**

   (a) **Adverse Effect**
   When coding an adverse effect of a drug that has been correctly prescribed and properly administered, assign the appropriate code for the nature of the adverse effect followed by the appropriate code for the adverse effect of the drug (T36-T50). The code for the drug should have a 5th or 6th character "5" (for example T36.0X5-) Examples of the nature of an adverse effect are tachycardia, delirium, gastrointestinal hemorrhaging, vomiting, hypokalemia, hepatitis, renal failure, or respiratory failure.

   (b) **Poisoning**
   When coding a poisoning or reaction to the improper use of a medication (e.g., overdose, wrong substance given or taken in error, wrong route of administration), first assign the appropriate code from categories T36-T50. The poisoning codes have an associated intent as their 5th or 6th character (accidental, intentional self-harm, assault and undetermined. If the intent of the poisoning is unknown or unspecified, code the intent as accidental intent. The undetermined intent is only for use if the documentation in the record specifies that the intent cannot be determined. Use additional code(s) for all manifestations of poisonings.

   If there is also a diagnosis of abuse or dependence of the substance, the abuse or dependence is assigned as an additional code.

   Examples of poisoning include:

   (i) Error was made in drug prescription
   Errors made in drug prescription or in the administration of the drug by provider, nurse, patient, or other person.

   (ii) Overdose of a drug intentionally taken
   If an overdose of a drug was intentionally taken or administered and resulted in drug toxicity, it would be coded as a poisoning.

   (iii) Nonprescribed drug taken with correctly prescribed and properly administered drug
   If a nonprescribed drug or medicinal agent was taken in combination with a correctly prescribed and properly administered drug, any drug toxicity or other reaction resulting from the interaction of the two drugs would be classified as a poisoning.

   (iv) Interaction of drug(s) and alcohol
   When a reaction results from the interaction of a drug(s) and alcohol, this would be classified as poisoning.

   See Section I.C.4. if poisoning is the result of insulin pump malfunctions.

   (c) **Underdosing**
   Underdosing refers to taking less of a medication than is prescribed by a provider or a manufacturer's instruction. For underdosing, assign the code from categories T36-T50 (fifth or sixth character "6").

   Codes for underdosing should never be assigned as principal or first-listed codes. If a patient has a relapse or exacerbation of the medical condition for which the drug is prescribed because of the reduction in dose, then the medical condition itself should be coded.

Noncompliance (Z91.12-, Z91.13-) or complication of care (Y63.6-Y63.9) codes are to be used with an underdosing code to indicate intent, if known.

(d) Toxic Effects

When a harmful substance is ingested or comes in contact with a person, this is classified as a toxic effect. The toxic effect codes are in categories T51-T65.

Toxic effect codes have an associated intent: accidental, intentional self-harm, assault and undetermined.

f. Adult and child abuse, neglect and other maltreatment

Sequence first the appropriate code from categories T74, Adult and child abuse, neglect and other maltreatment, confirmed) or T76, Adult and child abuse, neglect and other maltreatment, suspected) for abuse, neglect and other maltreatment, followed by any accompanying mental health or injury code(s).

If the documentation in the medical record states abuse or neglect it is coded as confirmed (T74.-). It is coded as suspected if it is documented as suspected (T76.-).

For cases of confirmed abuse or neglect an external cause code from the assault section (X92-Y09) should be added to identify the cause of any physical injuries. A perpetrator code (Y07) should be added when the perpetrator of the abuse is known. For suspected cases of abuse or neglect, do not report external cause or perpetrator code.

If a suspected case of abuse, neglect or mistreatment is ruled out during an encounter code Z04.71, Encounter for examination and observation following alleged physical adult abuse, ruled out, or code Z04.72, Encounter for examination and observation following alleged child physical abuse, ruled out, should be used, not a code from T76.

If a suspected case of alleged rape or sexual abuse is ruled out during an encounter code Z04.41, Encounter for examination and observation following alleged adult rape or code Z04.42, Encounter for examination and observation following alleged child rape, should be used, not a code from T76.

See Section I.C.15. Abuse in a pregnant patient.

g. Complications of care

1) General guidelines for complications of care

(a) Documentation of complications of care

See Section I.B.16. for information on documentation of complications of care.

2) Pain due to medical devices

Pain associated with devices, implants or grafts left in a surgical site (for example painful hip prosthesis) is assigned to the appropriate code(s) found in Chapter 19, Injury, poisoning, and certain other consequences of external causes. Specific codes for pain due to medical devices are found in the T code section of the ICD-10-CM. Use additional code(s) from category G89 to identify acute or chronic pain due to presence of the device, implant or graft (G89.18 or G89.28).

3) Transplant complications

(a) Transplant complications other than kidney

Codes under category T86, Complications of transplanted organs and tissues, are for use for both complications and rejection of transplanted organs. A transplant complication code is only assigned if the complication affects the function of the transplanted organ. Two codes are required to fully describe a transplant complication: the appropriate code from category T86 and a secondary code that identifies the complication.

Pre-existing conditions or conditions that develop after the transplant are not coded as complications unless they affect the function of the transplanted organs.

See I.C.21. for transplant organ removal status

See I.C.2. for malignant neoplasm associated with transplanted organ.

(b) Kidney transplant complications

Patients who have undergone kidney transplant may still have some form of chronic kidney disease (CKD) because the kidney transplant may not fully restore kidney function.

Code T86.1- should be assigned for documented complications of a kidney transplant, such as transplant failure or rejection or other transplant complication. Code T86.1- should not be assigned for post kidney transplant patients who have chronic kidney (CKD) unless a transplant complication such as transplant failure or rejection is documented. If the documentation is unclear as to whether the patient has a complication of the transplant, query the provider.

Conditions that affect the function of the transplanted kidney, other than CKD, should be assigned a code from subcategory T86.1, Complications of transplanted organ, Kidney, and a secondary code that identifies the complication.

For patients with CKD following a kidney transplant, but who do not have a complication such as failure or rejection, *see section I.C.14. Chronic kidney disease and kidney transplant status.*

4) Complication codes that include the external cause

As with certain other T codes, some of the complications of care codes have the external cause included in the code. The code includes the nature of the complication as well as the type of procedure that caused the complication. No external cause code indicating the type of procedure is necessary for these codes.

5) Complications of care codes within the body system chapters

Intraoperative and postprocedural complication codes are found within the body system chapters with codes specific to the organs and structures of that body system. These codes should be sequenced first, followed by a code(s) for the specific complication, if applicable.

20. Chapter 20: External Causes of Morbidity (V00-Y99)

The external causes of morbidity codes should never be sequenced as the first-listed or principal diagnosis.

External cause codes are intended to provide data for injury research and evaluation of injury prevention strategies. These codes capture how the injury or health condition happened (cause), the intent (unintentional or accidental; or intentional, such as suicide or assault), the place where the event occurred the activity of the patient at the time of the event, and the person's status (e.g., civilian, military).

There is no national requirement for mandatory ICD-10-CM external cause code reporting. Unless a provider is subject to a state-based external cause code reporting mandate or these codes are required by a particular payer, reporting of ICD-10-CM codes in Chapter 20, External Causes of Morbidity, is not required. In the absence of a mandatory reporting requirement, providers are encouraged to voluntarily report external cause codes, as they provide valuable data for injury research and evaluation of injury prevention strategies.

a. General External Cause Coding Guidelines

1) Used with any code in the range of A00.0-T88.9 Z00-Z99

An external cause code may be used with any code in the range of A00.0-T88.9, Z00-Z99, classification that **represent**s a health condition due to an external cause. Though they are most applicable to injuries, they are also valid for use with such things as infections or diseases due to an external source, and other health conditions, such as a heart attack that occurs during strenuous physical activity.

2) External cause code used for length of treatment

Assign the external cause code, with the appropriate 7th character (initial encounter, subsequent encounter or sequela) for each encounter for which the injury or condition is being treated.

Most categories in chapter 20 have a 7th character requirement for each applicable code. Most categories in this chapter have three 7th character values: A, initial encounter, D, subsequent encounter and S, sequela. While the patient may be seen by a new or different provider over the course of treatment for an injury or condition, assignment of the 7th character for external cause should match the 7th character of the code assigned for the associated injury or condition for the encounter.

3) **Use the full range of external cause codes**
Use the full range of external cause codes to completely describe the cause, the intent, the place of occurrence, and if applicable, the activity of the patient at the time of the event, and the patient's status, for all injuries, and other health conditions due to an external cause.

4) **Assign as many external cause codes as necessary**
Assign as many external cause codes as necessary to fully explain each cause. If only one external code can be recorded, assign the code most related to the principal diagnosis.

5) **The selection of the appropriate external cause code**
The selection of the appropriate external cause code is guided by the Alphabetic Index of External Causes and by Inclusion and Exclusion notes in the Tabular List.

6) **External cause code can never be a principal diagnosis**
An external cause code can never be a principal (first-listed) diagnosis.

7) **Combination external cause codes**
Certain of the external cause codes are combination codes that identify sequential events that result in an injury, such as a fall which results in striking against an object. The injury may be due to either event or both. The combination external cause code used should correspond to the sequence of events regardless of which caused the most serious injury.

8) **No external cause code needed in certain circumstances**
No external cause code from Chapter 20 is needed if the external cause and intent are included in a code from another chapter (e.g. T36.0X1- Poisoning by penicillins, accidental (unintentional)).

b. **Place of Occurrence Guideline**
Codes from category Y92, Place of occurrence of the external cause, are secondary codes for use after other external cause codes to identify the location of the patient at the time of injury or other condition.

Generally, a place of occurrence code is assigned only once, at the initial encounter for treatment. However, in the rare instance that a new injury occurs during hospitalization, an additional place of occurrence code may be assigned. No 7th characters are used for Y92.

Do not use place of occurrence code Y92.9 if the place is not stated or is not applicable.

c. **Activity Code**
Assign a code from category Y93, Activity code, to describe the activity of the patient at the time the injury or other health condition occurred.

An activity code is used only once, at the initial encounter for treatment. Only one code from Y93 should be recorded on a medical record.

The activity codes are not applicable to poisonings, adverse effects, misadventures or sequela.

Do not assign Y93.9, Unspecified activity, if the activity is not stated.

A code from category Y93 is appropriate for use with external cause and intent codes if identifying the activity provides additional information about the event.

d. **Place of Occurrence, Activity, and Status Codes Used with other External Cause Code**
When applicable, place of occurrence, activity, and external cause status codes are sequenced after the main external cause code(s). Regardless of the number of external cause codes assigned, generally there should be only one place of occurrence code, one activity code, and one external cause status code assigned to an encounter. However, in the rare instance that a new injury occurs during hospitalization, an additional place of occurrence code may be assigned.

e. **If the Reporting Format Limits the Number of External Cause Codes**
If the reporting format limits the number of external cause codes that can be used in reporting clinical data, report the code for the cause/intent most related to the principal diagnosis. If the format permits capture of additional external cause codes, the cause/intent, including medical misadventures, of the additional

events should be reported rather than the codes for place, activity, or external status.

f. **Multiple External Cause Coding Guidelines**
More than one external cause code is required to fully describe the external cause of an illness or injury. The assignment of external cause codes should be sequenced in the following priority:

If two or more events cause separate injuries, an external cause code should be assigned for each cause. The first-listed external cause code will be selected in the following order:

External codes for child and adult abuse take priority over all other external cause codes.

See Section I.C.19., Child and Adult abuse guidelines.

External cause codes for terrorism events take priority over all other external cause codes except child and adult abuse.

External cause codes for cataclysmic events take priority over all other external cause codes except child and adult abuse and terrorism.

External cause codes for transport accidents take priority over all other external cause codes except cataclysmic events, child and adult abuse and terrorism.

Activity and external cause status codes are assigned following all causal (intent) external cause codes.

The first-listed external cause code should correspond to the cause of the most serious diagnosis due to an assault, accident, or self-harm, following the order of hierarchy listed above.

g. **Child and Adult Abuse Guideline**
Adult and child abuse, neglect and maltreatment are classified as assault. Any of the assault codes may be used to indicate the external cause of any injury resulting from the confirmed abuse.

For confirmed cases of abuse, neglect and maltreatment, when the perpetrator is known, a code from Y07, Perpetrator of maltreatment and neglect, should accompany any other assault codes.

See Section I.C.19. Adult and child abuse, neglect and other maltreatment

h. **Unknown or Undetermined Intent Guideline**
If the intent (accident, self-harm, assault) of the cause of an injury or other condition is unknown or unspecified, code the intent as accidental intent. All transport accident categories assume accidental intent.

1) **Use of undetermined intent**
External cause codes for events of undetermined intent are only for use if the documentation in the record specifies that the intent cannot be determined.

i. **Sequelae (Late Effects) of External Cause Guidelines**
1) **Sequelae external cause codes**
Sequela are reported using the external cause code with the 7th character "S" for sequela. These codes should be used with any report of a late effect or sequela resulting from a previous injury.

See Section I.B.10 Sequela (Late Effects)

2) **Sequela external cause code with a related current injury**
A sequela external cause code should never be used with a related current nature of injury code.

3) **Use of sequela external cause codes for subsequent visits**
Use a late effect external cause code for subsequent visits when a late effect of the initial injury is being treated. Do not use a late effect external cause code for subsequent visits for follow-up care (e.g., to assess healing, to receive rehabilitative therapy) of the injury when no late effect of the injury has been documented.

j. **Terrorism Guidelines**
1) **Cause of injury identified by the Federal Government (FBI) as terrorism**
When the cause of an injury is identified by the Federal Government (FBI) as terrorism, the first-listed external cause code should be a code from category Y38, Terrorism. The definition of terrorism employed by the FBI is found at the inclusion note at the beginning of category Y38. Use additional code for place of occurrence (Y92.-). More than one Y38 code

may be assigned if the injury is the result of more than one mechanism of terrorism.

2) **Cause of an injury is suspected to be the result of terrorism**
When the cause of an injury is suspected to be the result of terrorism a code from category Y38 should not be assigned. Suspected cases should be classified as assault.

3) **Code Y38.9, Terrorism, secondary effects**
Assign code Y38.9, Terrorism, secondary effects, for conditions occurring subsequent to the terrorist event. This code should not be assigned for conditions that are due to the initial terrorist act.

It is acceptable to assign code Y38.9 with another code from Y38 if there is an injury due to the initial terrorist event and an injury that is a subsequent result of the terrorist event.

k. External cause status
A code from category Y99, External cause status, should be assigned whenever any other external cause code is assigned for an encounter, including an Activity code, except for the events noted below. Assign a code from category Y99, External cause status, to indicate the work status of the person at the time the event occurred. The status code indicates whether the event occurred during military activity, whether a non-military person was at work, whether an individual including a student or volunteer was involved in a non-work activity at the time of the causal event.

A code from Y99, External cause status, should be assigned, when applicable, with other external cause codes, such as transport accidents and falls. The external cause status codes are not applicable to poisonings, adverse effects, misadventures or late effects.

Do not assign a code from category Y99 if no other external cause codes (cause, activity) are applicable for the encounter.

An external cause status code is used only once, at the initial encounter for treatment. Only one code from Y99 should be recorded on a medical record.

Do not assign code Y99.9, Unspecified external cause status, if the status is not stated.

21. Chapter 21: Factors influencing health status and contact with health services (Z00-Z99)
Note: The chapter specific guidelines provide additional information about the use of Z codes for specified encounters.

a. Use of Z codes in any healthcare setting
Z codes are for use in any healthcare setting. Z codes may be used as either a first-listed (principal diagnosis code in the inpatient setting) or secondary code, depending on the circumstances of the encounter. Certain Z codes may only be used as first-listed or principal diagnosis.

b. Z Codes indicate a reason for an encounter
Z codes are not procedure codes. A corresponding procedure code must accompany a Z code to describe any procedure performed.

c. Categories of Z Codes

1) Contact/Exposure
Category Z20 indicates contact with, and suspected exposure to, communicable diseases. These codes are for patients who do not show any sign or symptom of a disease but are suspected to have been exposed to it by close personal contact with an infected individual or are in an area where a disease is epidemic.

Category Z77, Other contact with and (suspected) exposures hazardous to health, indicates contact with and suspected exposures hazardous to health.

Contact/exposure codes may be used as a first-listed code to explain an encounter for testing, or, more commonly, as a secondary code to identify a potential risk.

2) Inoculations and vaccinations
Code Z23 is for encounters for inoculations and vaccinations. It indicates that a patient is being seen to receive a prophylactic inoculation against a disease. Procedure codes are required to identify the actual administration of the injection and the type(s) of immunizations given. Code Z23 may be used as a secondary code if the inoculation is given as a routine part of preventive health care, such as a well-baby visit.

3) Status
Status codes indicate that a patient is either a carrier of a disease or has the sequelae or residual of a past disease or condition. This includes such things as the presence of prosthetic or mechanical devices resulting from past treatment. A status code is informative, because the status may affect the course of treatment and its outcome. A status code is distinct from a history code. The history code indicates that the patient no longer has the condition.

A status code should not be used with a diagnosis code from one of the body system chapters, if the diagnosis code includes the information provided by the status code. For example, code Z94.1, Heart transplant status, should not be used with a code from subcategory T86.2, Complications of heart transplant. The status code does not provide additional information. The complication code indicates that the patient is a heart transplant patient.

For encounters for weaning from a mechanical ventilator, assign a code from subcategory J96.1, Chronic respiratory failure, followed by code Z99.11, Dependence on respirator [ventilator] status.

The status Z codes/categories are:

Z14 Genetic carrier

Genetic carrier status indicates that a person carries a gene, associated with a particular disease, which may be passed to offspring who may develop that disease. The person does not have the disease and is not at risk of developing the disease.

Z15 Genetic susceptibility to disease

Genetic susceptibility indicates that a person has a gene that increases the risk of that person developing the disease.

Codes from category Z15 should not be used as principal or first-listed codes. If the patient has the condition to which he/she is susceptible, and that condition is the reason for the encounter, the code for the current condition should be sequenced first. If the patient is being seen for follow-up after completed treatment for this condition, and the condition no longer exists, a follow-up code should be sequenced first, followed by the appropriate personal history and genetic susceptibility codes. If the purpose of the encounter is genetic counseling associated with procreative management, code Z31.5, Encounter for genetic counseling, should be assigned as the first-listed code, followed by a code from category Z15. Additional codes should be assigned for any applicable family or personal history.

Z16 Resistance to antimicrobial drugs

This code indicates that a patient has a condition that is resistant to antimicrobial drug treatment. Sequence the infection code first.

Z17 Estrogen receptor status

Z18 Retained foreign body fragments

Z19 Hormone sensitivity malignancy status

Z21 Asymptomatic HIV infection status

This code indicates that a patient has tested positive for HIV but has manifested no signs or symptoms of the disease.

Z22 Carrier of infectious disease

Carrier status indicates that a person harbors the specific organisms of a disease without manifest symptoms and is capable of transmitting the infection.

Z28.3 Underimmunization status

Z33.1 Pregnant state, incidental

This code is a secondary code only for use when the pregnancy is in no way complicating the reason for visit. Otherwise, a code from the obstetric chapter is required.

Z66 Do not resuscitate

This code may be used when it is documented by the provider that a patient is on do not resuscitate status at any time during the stay.

Z67   Blood type

Z68   Body mass index (BMI)

As with all other secondary diagnosis codes, the BMI codes should only be assigned when they meet the definition of a reportable diagnosis (see Section III, Reporting Additional Diagnoses).

Z74.01 Bed confinement status

Z76.82 Awaiting organ transplant status

Z78   Other specified health status

Code Z78.1, Physical restraint status, may be used when it is documented by the provider that a patient has been put in restraints during the current encounter. Please note that this code should not be reported when it is documented by the provider that a patient is temporarily restrained during a procedure.

Z79   Long-term (current) drug therapy

Codes from this category indicate a patient's continuous use of a prescribed drug (including such things as aspirin therapy) for the long-term treatment of a condition or for prophylactic use. It is not for use for patients who have addictions to drugs. This subcategory is not for use of medications for detoxification or maintenance programs to prevent withdrawal symptoms in patients with drug dependence (e.g., methadone maintenance for opiate dependence). Assign the appropriate code for the drug dependence instead.

Assign a code from Z79 if the patient is receiving a medication for an extended period as a prophylactic measure (such as for the prevention of deep vein thrombosis) or as treatment of a chronic condition (such as arthritis) or a disease requiring a lengthy course of treatment (such as cancer). Do not assign a code from category Z79 for medication being administered for a brief period of time to treat an acute illness or injury (such as a course of antibiotics to treat acute bronchitis).

Z88   Allergy status to drugs, medicaments and biological substances

Except: Z88.9, Allergy status to unspecified drugs, medicaments and biological substances status

Z89   Acquired absence of limb

Z90   Acquired absence of organs, not elsewhere classified

Z91.0- Allergy status, other than to drugs and biological substances

Z92.82 Status post administration of tPA (rtPA) in a different facility within the last 24 hours prior to admission to a current facility

Assign code Z92.82, Status post administration of tPA (rtPA) in a different facility within the last 24 hours prior to admission to current facility, as a secondary diagnosis when a patient is received by transfer into a facility and documentation indicates they were administered tissue plasminogen activator (tPA) within the last 24 hours prior to admission to the current facility.

This guideline applies even if the patient is still receiving the tPA at the time they are received into the current facility.

The appropriate code for the condition for which the tPA was administered (such as cerebrovascular disease or myocardial infarction) should be assigned first.

Code Z92.82 is only applicable to the receiving facility record and not to the transferring facility record.

Z93   Artificial opening status

Z94   Transplanted organ and tissue status

Z95   Presence of cardiac and vascular implants and grafts

Z96   Presence of other functional implants

Z97   Presence of other devices

Z98   Other postprocedural states

Assign code Z98.85, Transplanted organ removal status, to indicate that a transplanted organ has been previously removed. This code should not be assigned for the encounter in which the transplanted organ is removed. The complication necessitating removal of the transplant organ should be assigned for that encounter.

See section I.C19. for information on the coding of organ transplant complications.

Z99   Dependence on enabling machines and devices, not elsewhere classified

Note: Categories Z89-Z90 and Z93-Z99 are for use only if there are no complications or malfunctions of the organ or tissue replaced, the amputation site or the equipment on which the patient is dependent.

4) **History (of)**

There are two types of history Z codes, personal and family. Personal history codes explain a patient's past medical condition that no longer exists and is not receiving any treatment, but that has the potential for recurrence, and therefore may require continued monitoring.

Family history codes are for use when a patient has a family member(s) who has had a particular disease that causes the patient to be at higher risk of also contracting the disease.

Personal history codes may be used in conjunction with follow-up codes and family history codes may be used in conjunction with screening codes to explain the need for a test or procedure. History codes are also acceptable on any medical record regardless of the reason for visit. A history of an illness, even if no longer present, is important information that may alter the type of treatment ordered.

The history Z code categories are:

Z80   Family history of primary malignant neoplasm

Z81   Family history of mental and behavioral disorders

Z82   Family history of certain disabilities and chronic diseases (leading to disablement)

Z83   Family history of other specific disorders

Z84   Family history of other conditions

Z85   Personal history of malignant neoplasm

Z86   Personal history of certain other diseases

Z87   Personal history of other diseases and conditions

Z91.4- Personal history of psychological trauma, not elsewhere classified

Z91.5   Personal history of self-harm

Z91.81 History of falling

Z91.82 Personal history of military deployment

Z92   Personal history of medical treatment

Except: Z92.0, Personal history of contraception

Except: Z92.82, Status post administration of tPA (rtPA) in a different facility within the last 24 hours prior to admission to a current facility

5) **Screening**

Screening is the testing for disease or disease precursors in seemingly well individuals so that early detection and treatment can be provided for those who test positive for the disease (e.g., screening mammogram).

The testing of a person to rule out or confirm a suspected diagnosis because the patient has some sign or symptom is a diagnostic examination, not a screening. In these cases, the sign or symptom is used to explain the reason for the test.

A screening code may be a first-listed code if the reason for the visit is specifically the screening exam. It may also be used as an additional code if the screening is done during an office visit for other health problems. A screening code is not necessary if the screening is inherent to a routine examination, such as a pap smear done during a routine pelvic examination.

Should a condition be discovered during the screening then the code for the condition may be assigned as an additional diagnosis.

The Z code indicates that a screening exam is planned. A procedure code is required to confirm that the screening was performed.

The screening Z codes/categories:

Z11   Encounter for screening for infectious and parasitic diseases

Z12   Encounter for screening for malignant neoplasms

Z13   Encounter for screening for other diseases and disorders

       Except: Z13.9, Encounter for screening, unspecified

Z36   Encounter for antenatal screening for mother

6) Observation

There are three observation Z code categories. They are for use in very limited circumstances when a person is being observed for a suspected condition that is ruled out. The observation codes are not for use if an injury or illness or any signs or symptoms related to the suspected condition are present. In such cases the diagnosis/symptom code is used with the corresponding external cause code.

The observation codes are to be used as principal diagnosis only. The only exception to this is when the principal diagnosis is required to be a code from category Z38, Liveborn infants according to place of birth and type of delivery. Then a code from category Z05, Encounter for observation and evaluation of newborn for suspected diseases and conditions ruled out, is sequenced after the Z38 code. Additional codes may be used in addition to the observation code, but only if they are unrelated to the suspected condition being observed.

Codes from subcategory Z03.7, Encounter for suspected maternal and fetal conditions ruled out, may either be used as a first-listed or as an additional code assignment depending on the case. They are for use in very limited circumstances on a maternal record when an encounter is for a suspected maternal or fetal condition that is ruled out during that encounter (for example, a maternal or fetal condition may be suspected due to an abnormal test result). These codes should not be used when the condition is confirmed. In those cases, the confirmed condition should be coded. In addition, these codes are not for use if an illness or any signs or symptoms related to the suspected condition or problem are present. In such cases the diagnosis/symptom code is used.

Additional codes may be used in addition to the code from subcategory Z03.7, but only if they are unrelated to the suspected condition being evaluated.

Codes from subcategory Z03.7 may not be used for encounters for antenatal screening of mother. *See Section I.C.21. Screening.*

For encounters for suspected fetal condition that are inconclusive following testing and evaluation, assign the appropriate code from category O35, O36, O40 or O41.

The observation Z code categories:

Z03   Encounter for medical observation for suspected diseases and conditions ruled out

Z04   Encounter for examination and observation for other reasons

       Except: Z04.9, Encounter for examination and observation for unspecified reason

Z05   Encounter for observation and evaluation of newborn for suspected diseases and conditions ruled out

7) Aftercare

Aftercare visit codes cover situations when the initial treatment of a disease has been performed and the patient requires continued care during the healing or recovery phase, or for the long-term consequences of the disease. The aftercare Z code should not be used if treatment is directed at a current, acute disease. The diagnosis code is to be used in these cases. Exceptions to this rule are codes Z51.0, Encounter for antineoplastic radiation therapy, and codes from subcategory Z51.1, Encounter for antineoplastic chemotherapy and

immunotherapy. These codes are to be first-listed, followed by the diagnosis code when a patient's encounter is solely to receive radiation therapy, chemotherapy, or immunotherapy for the treatment of a neoplasm. If the reason for the encounter is more than one type of antineoplastic therapy, code Z51.0 and a code from subcategory Z51.1 may be assigned together, in which case one of these codes would be reported as a secondary diagnosis.

The aftercare Z codes should also not be used for aftercare for injuries. For aftercare of an injury, assign the acute injury code with the appropriate 7th character (for subsequent encounter).

The aftercare codes are generally first-listed to explain the specific reason for the encounter. An aftercare code may be used as an additional code when some type of aftercare is provided in addition to the reason for admission and no diagnosis code is applicable. An example of this would be the closure of a colostomy during an encounter for treatment of another condition.

Aftercare codes should be used in conjunction with other aftercare codes or diagnosis codes to provide better detail on the specifics of an aftercare encounter visit, unless otherwise directed by the classification. Should a patient receive multiple types of antineoplastic therapy during the same encounter, code Z51.0, Encounter for antineoplastic radiation therapy, and codes from subcategory Z51.1, Encounter for antineoplastic chemotherapy and immunotherapy, may be used together on a record. The sequencing of multiple aftercare codes depends on the circumstances of the encounter.

Certain aftercare Z code categories need a secondary diagnosis code to describe the resolving condition or sequelae. For others, the condition is included in the code title.

Additional Z code aftercare category terms include fitting and adjustment, and attention to artificial openings.

Status Z codes may be used with aftercare Z codes to indicate the nature of the aftercare. For example code Z95.1, Presence of aortocoronary bypass graft, may be used with code Z48.812, Encounter for surgical aftercare following surgery on the circulatory system, to indicate the surgery for which the aftercare is being performed. A status code should not be used when the aftercare code indicates the type of status, such as using Z43.0, Encounter for attention to tracheostomy, with Z93.0, Tracheostomy status.

The aftercare Z category/codes:

Z42   Encounter for plastic and reconstructive surgery following medical procedure or healed injury

Z43   Encounter for attention to artificial openings

Z44   Encounter for fitting and adjustment of external prosthetic device

Z45   Encounter for adjustment and management of implanted device

Z46   Encounter for fitting and adjustment of other devices

Z47   Orthopedic aftercare

Z48   Encounter for other postprocedural aftercare

Z49   Encounter for care involving renal dialysis

Z51   Encounter for other aftercare and medical care

8) Follow-up

The follow-up codes are used to explain continuing surveillance following completed treatment of a disease, condition, or injury. They imply that the condition has been fully treated and no longer exists. They should not be confused with aftercare codes, or injury codes with a 7th character for subsequent encounter, that explain ongoing care of a healing condition or its sequelae. Follow-up codes may be used in conjunction with history codes to provide the full picture of the healed condition and its treatment. The follow-up code is sequenced first, followed by the history code.

A follow-up code may be used to explain multiple visits. Should a condition be found to have recurred on the follow-up visit, then the diagnosis code for the condition should be assigned in place of the follow-up code.

The follow-up Z code categories:

Z08   Encounter for follow-up examination after completed treatment for malignant neoplasm

Z09   Encounter for follow-up examination after completed treatment for conditions other than malignant neoplasm

Z39   Encounter for maternal postpartum care and examination

9) Donor

Codes in category Z52, Donors of organs and tissues, are used for living individuals who are donating blood or other body tissue. These codes are only for individuals donating for others, not for self-donations. They are not used to identify cadaveric donations.

10) Counseling

Counseling Z codes are used when a patient or family member receives assistance in the aftermath of an illness or injury, or when support is required in coping with family or social problems.

The counseling Z codes/categories:

Z30.0-   Encounter for general counseling and advice on contraception

Z31.5   Encounter for **procreative** genetic counseling

Z31.6-   Encounter for general counseling and advice on procreation

Z32.2   Encounter for childbirth instruction

Z32.3   Encounter for childcare instruction

Z69   Encounter for mental health services for victim and perpetrator of abuse

Z70   Counseling related to sexual attitude, behavior and orientation

Z71   Persons encountering health services for other counseling and medical advice, not elsewhere classified

Z76.81 Expectant mother prebirth pediatrician visit

· 11) Encounters for Obstetrical and Reproductive Services

See Section I.C.15. Pregnancy, Childbirth, and the Puerperium, for further instruction on the use of these codes.

Z codes for pregnancy are for use in those circumstances when none of the problems or complications included in the codes from the Obstetrics chapter exist (a routine prenatal visit or postpartum care). Codes in category Z34, Encounter for supervision of normal pregnancy, are always first-listed and are not to be used with any other code from the OB chapter.

Codes in category Z3A, Weeks of gestation, may be assigned to provide additional information about the pregnancy. Category Z3A codes should not be assigned for pregnancies with abortive outcomes (categories O00-O08), elective termination of pregnancy (code **Z33.2**), nor for postpartum conditions, as category Z3A is not applicable to these conditions. The date of the admission should be used to determine weeks of gestation for inpatient admissions that encompass more than one gestational week.

The outcome of delivery, category Z37, should be included on all maternal delivery records. It is always a secondary code. Codes in category Z37 should not be used on the newborn record.

Z codes for family planning (contraceptive) or procreative management and counseling should be included on an obstetric record either during the pregnancy or the postpartum stage, if applicable.

Z codes/categories for obstetrical and reproductive services:

Z30   Encounter for contraceptive management

Z31   Encounter for procreative management

Z32.2   Encounter for childbirth instruction

Z32.3   Encounter for childcare instruction

Z33   Pregnant state

Z34   Encounter for supervision of normal pregnancy

Z36   Encounter for antenatal screening of mother

Z3A   Weeks of gestation

Z37   Outcome of delivery

Z39   Encounter for maternal postpartum care and examination

Z76.81 Expectant mother prebirth pediatrician visit

12) Newborns and Infants

See Section I.C.16. Newborn (Perinatal) Guidelines, for further instruction on the use of these codes.

Newborn Z codes/categories:

Z76.1   Encounter for health supervision and care of foundling

Z00.1-   Encounter for routine child health examination

Z38'   Liveborn infants according to place of birth and type of delivery

13) Routine and administrative examinations

The Z codes allow for the description of encounters for routine examinations, such as, a general check-up, or, examinations for administrative purposes, such as, a pre-employment physical. The codes are not to be used if the examination is for diagnosis of a suspected condition or for treatment purposes. In such cases the diagnosis code is used. During a routine exam, should a diagnosis or condition be discovered, it should be coded as an additional code. Pre-existing and chronic conditions and history codes may also be included as additional codes as long as the examination is for administrative purposes and not focused on any particular condition.

Some of the codes for routine health examinations distinguish between "with" and "without" abnormal findings. Code assignment depends on the information that is known at the time the encounter is being coded. For example, if no abnormal findings were found during the examination, but the encounter is being coded before test results are back, it is acceptable to assign the code for "without abnormal findings." When assigning a code for "with abnormal findings," additional code(s) should be assigned to identify the specific abnormal finding(s).

Pre-operative examination and pre-procedural laboratory examination Z codes are for use only in those situations when a patient is being cleared for a procedure or surgery and no treatment is given.

The Z codes/categories for routine and administrative examinations:

Z00   Encounter for general examination without complaint, suspected or reported diagnosis

Z01   Encounter for other special examination without complaint, suspected or reported diagnosis

Z02   Encounter for administrative examination

Except: Z02.9, Encounter for administrative examinations, unspecified

Z32.0-   Encounter for pregnancy test

14) Miscellaneous Z codes

The miscellaneous Z codes capture a number of other health care encounters that do not fall into one of the other categories.

Certain of these codes identify the reason for the encounter; others are for use as additional codes that provide useful information on circumstances that may affect a patient's care and treatment.

Prophylactic Organ Removal

For encounters specifically for prophylactic removal of an organ (such as prophylactic removal of breasts due to a genetic susceptibility to cancer or a family history of cancer), the principal or first-listed code should be a code from category Z40, Encounter for prophylactic surgery, followed by the appropriate codes to identify the associated risk factor (such as genetic susceptibility or family history).

If the patient has a malignancy of one site and is having prophylactic removal at another site to prevent either a new primary malignancy or metastatic disease, a code for the malignancy should also be assigned in addition to a code from subcategory Z40.0, Encounter for prophylactic surgery for risk factors related to malignant neoplasms. A Z40.0 code should not be assigned if the patient is having organ removal for treatment of a malignancy, such as the removal of the testes for the treatment of prostate cancer.

Miscellaneous Z codes/categories:

Z28   Immunization not carried out

      Except: Z28.3, Underimmunization status

Z29   Encounter for other prophylactic measures

Z40   Encounter for prophylactic surgery

Z41   Encounter for procedures for purposes other than remedying health state

      Except: Z41.9, Encounter for procedure for purposes other than remedying health state, unspecified

Z53   Persons encountering health services for specific procedures and treatment, not carried out

Z55   Problems related to education and literacy

Z56   Problems related to employment and unemployment

Z57   Occupational exposure to risk factors

Z58   Problems related to physical environment

Z59   Problems related to housing and economic circumstances

Z60   Problems related to social environment

Z62   Problems related to upbringing

Z63   Other problems related to primary support group, including family circumstances

Z64   Problems related to certain psychosocial circumstances

Z65   Problems related to other psychosocial circumstances

Z72   Problems related to lifestyle

      Note: These codes should be assigned only when the documentation specifies that the patient has an associated problem

Z73   Problems related to life management difficulty

Z74   Problems related to care provider dependency

      Except: Z74.01, Bed confinement status

Z75   Problems related to medical facilities and other health care

Z76.0   Encounter for issue of repeat prescription

Z76.3   Healthy person accompanying sick person

Z76.4   Other boarder to healthcare facility

Z76.5   Malingerer [conscious simulation]

Z91.1-   Patient's noncompliance with medical treatment and regimen

Z91.83   Wandering in diseases classified elsewhere

Z91.84-Oral health risk factors

Z91.89   Other specified personal risk factors, not elsewhere classified

15) Nonspecific Z codes

Certain Z codes are so non-specific, or potentially redundant with other codes in the classification, that there can be little justification for their use in the inpatient setting. Their use in the outpatient setting should be limited to those instances when there is no further documentation to permit more precise coding. Otherwise, any sign or symptom or any other reason for visit that is captured in another code should be used.

Nonspecific Z codes/categories:

Z02.9   Encounter for administrative examinations, unspecified

Z04.9   Encounter for examination and observation for unspecified reason

Z13.9   Encounter for screening, unspecified

Z41.9   Encounter for procedure for purposes other than remedying health state, unspecified

Z52.9   Donor of unspecified organ or tissue

Z86.59   Personal history of other mental and behavioral disorders

Z88.9   Allergy status to unspecified drugs, medicaments and biological substances status

Z92.0   Personal history of contraception

16) Z Codes That May Only be Principal/First-Listed Diagnosis

The following Z codes/categories may only be reported as the principal/first-listed diagnosis, except when there are multiple encounters on the same day and the medical records for the encounters are combined:

Z00   Encounter for general examination without complaint, suspected or reported diagnosis

      Except: Z00.6

Z01   Encounter for other special examination without complaint, suspected or reported diagnosis

Z02   Encounter for administrative examination

Z03   Encounter for medical observation for suspected diseases and conditions ruled out

Z04   Encounter for examination and observation for other reasons

Z33.2   Encounter for elective termination of pregnancy

Z31.81   Encounter for male factor infertility in female patient

Z31.83   Encounter for assisted reproductive fertility procedure cycle

Z31.84   Encounter for fertility preservation procedure

Z34   Encounter for supervision of normal pregnancy

Z39   Encounter for maternal postpartum care and examination

Z38   Liveborn infants according to place of birth and type of delivery

Z40   Encounter for prophylactic surgery

Z42   Encounter for plastic and reconstructive surgery following medical procedure or healed injury

Z51.0   Encounter for antineoplastic radiation therapy

Z51.1-   Encounter for antineoplastic chemotherapy and immunotherapy

Z52   Donors of organs and tissues

      Except: Z52.9, Donor of unspecified organ or tissue

Z76.1   Encounter for health supervision and care of foundling

Z76.2   Encounter for health supervision and care of other healthy infant and child

Z99.12   Encounter for respirator [ventilator] dependence during power failure

Section II. Selection of Principal Diagnosis

The circumstances of inpatient admission always govern the selection of principal diagnosis. The principal diagnosis is defined in the Uniform Hospital Discharge Data Set (UHDDS) as "that condition established after study to be chiefly responsible for occasioning the admission of the patient to the hospital for care."

The UHDDS definitions are used by hospitals to report inpatient data elements in a standardized manner. These data elements and their definitions can be found in the July 31, 1985, Federal Register (Vol. 50, No, 147), pp. 31038-40.

Since that time the application of the UHDDS definitions has been expanded to include all non-outpatient settings (acute care, short term, long term care and psychiatric hospitals; home health agencies; rehab facilities; nursing homes, etc). The UHDDS definitions also apply to hospice services (all levels of care).

In determining principal diagnosis, coding conventions in the ICD-10-CM, the Tabular List and Alphabetic Index take precedence over these official coding guidelines.

(See Section I.A., Conventions for the ICD-10-CM)

The importance of consistent, complete documentation in the medical record cannot be overemphasized. Without such documentation the application of all coding guidelines is a difficult, if not impossible, task.

A. Codes for symptoms, signs, and ill-defined conditions
Codes for symptoms, signs, and ill-defined conditions from Chapter 18 are not to be used as principal diagnosis when a related definitive diagnosis has been established.

B. Two or more interrelated conditions, each potentially meeting the definition for principal diagnosis.
When there are two or more interrelated conditions (such as diseases in the same ICD-10-CM chapter or manifestations characteristically associated with a certain disease) potentially meeting the definition of principal diagnosis, either condition may be sequenced first, unless the circumstances of the admission, the therapy provided, the Tabular List, or the Alphabetic Index indicate otherwise.

C. Two or more diagnoses that equally meet the definition for principal diagnosis
In the unusual instance when two or more diagnoses equally meet the criteria for principal diagnosis as determined by the circumstances of admission, diagnostic workup and/or therapy provided, and the Alphabetic Index, Tabular List, or another coding guidelines does not provide sequencing direction, any one of the diagnoses may be sequenced first.

D. Two or more comparative or contrasting conditions
In those rare instances when two or more contrasting or comparative diagnoses are documented as "either/or" (or similar terminology), they are coded as if the diagnoses were confirmed and the diagnoses are sequenced according to the circumstances of the admission. If no further determination can be made as to which diagnosis should be principal, either diagnosis may be sequenced first.

E. A symptom(s) followed by contrasting/comparative diagnoses
GUIDELINE HAS BEEN DELETED EFFECTIVE OCTOBER 1, 2014

F. Original treatment plan not carried out
Sequence as the principal diagnosis the condition, which after study occasioned the admission to the hospital, even though treatment may not have been carried out due to unforeseen circumstances.

G. Complications of surgery and other medical care
When the admission is for treatment of a complication resulting from surgery or other medical care, the complication code is sequenced as the principal diagnosis. If the complication is classified to the T80-T88 series and the code lacks the necessary specificity in describing the complication, an additional code for the specific complication should be assigned.

H. Uncertain Diagnosis
If the diagnosis documented at the time of discharge is qualified as "probable", "suspected", "likely", "questionable", "possible", or "still to be ruled out", or other similar terms indicating uncertainty, code the condition as if it existed or was established. The bases for these guidelines are the diagnostic workup, arrangements for further workup or observation, and initial therapeutic approach that correspond most closely with the established diagnosis.

Note: This guideline is applicable only to inpatient admissions to short-term, acute, long-term care and psychiatric hospitals.

I. Admission from Observation Unit
1. Admission Following Medical Observation
When a patient is admitted to an observation unit for a medical condition, which either worsens or does not improve, and is subsequently admitted as an inpatient of the same hospital for this same medical condition, the principal diagnosis would be the medical condition which led to the hospital admission.

2. Admission Following Post-Operative Observation
When a patient is admitted to an observation unit to monitor a condition (or complication) that develops following outpatient surgery, and then is subsequently admitted as an inpatient of the same hospital, hospitals should apply the Uniform Hospital Discharge Data Set (UHDDS) definition of principal diagnosis as "that condition established after study to be chiefly responsible for occasioning the admission of the patient to the hospital for care."

J. Admission from Outpatient Surgery
When a patient receives surgery in the hospital's outpatient surgery department and is subsequently admitted for continuing inpatient care at the same hospital, the following guidelines should be followed in selecting the principal diagnosis for the inpatient admission:

- If the reason for the inpatient admission is a complication, assign the complication as the principal diagnosis.

- If no complication, or other condition, is documented as the reason for the inpatient admission, assign the reason for the outpatient surgery as the principal diagnosis.

- If the reason for the inpatient admission is another condition unrelated to the surgery, assign the unrelated condition as the principal diagnosis.

K. Admissions/Encounters for Rehabilitation
When the purpose for the admission/encounter is rehabilitation, sequence first the code for the condition for which the service is being performed. For example, for an admission/encounter for rehabilitation for right-sided dominant hemiplegia following a cerebrovascular infarction, report code I69.351, Hemiplegia and hemiparesis following cerebral infarction affecting right dominant side, as the first-listed or principal diagnosis.

If the condition for which the rehabilitation service is no longer present, report the appropriate aftercare code **as the first-listed or principal diagnosis, unless the rehabilitation service is being provided following an injury. For rehabilitation services following active treatment of an injury, assign the injury code with the appropriate seventh character for subsequent encounter** as the first-listed or principal diagnosis. For example, if a patient with severe degenerative osteoarthritis of the hip, underwent hip replacement and the current encounter/admission is for rehabilitation, report code Z47.1, Aftercare following joint replacement surgery, as the first-listed or principal diagnosis. **If the patient requires rehabilitation post hip replacement for right intertrochanteric femur fracture, report code S72.141D, Displaced intertrochanteric fracture of right femur, subsequent encounter for closed fracture with routine healing, as the first-listed or principal diagnosis.**

See Section I.C.21.c.7, Factors influencing health states and contact with health services, Aftercare.

See Section I.C.19.a for additional information about the use of 7th characters for injury codes.

Section III. Reporting Additional Diagnoses

GENERAL RULES FOR OTHER (ADDITIONAL) DIAGNOSES

For reporting purposes the definition for "other diagnoses" is interpreted as additional conditions that affect patient care in terms of requiring:

> clinical evaluation; or
> therapeutic treatment; or
> diagnostic procedures; or
> extended length of hospital stay; or
> increased nursing care and/or monitoring.

The UHDDS item #11-b defines Other Diagnoses as "all conditions that coexist at the time of admission, that develop subsequently, or that affect the treatment received and/or the length of stay. Diagnoses that relate to an earlier episode which have no bearing on the current hospital stay are to be excluded." UHDDS definitions apply to inpatients in acute care, short-term, long term care and psychiatric hospital setting. The UHDDS definitions are used by acute care short-term hospitals to report inpatient data elements in a standardized manner. These data elements and their definitions can be found in the July 31, 1985, Federal Register (Vol. 50, No, 147), pp. 31038-40.

Since that time the application of the UHDDS definitions has been expanded to include all non-outpatient settings (acute care, short term, long term care and psychiatric hospitals; home health agencies; rehab facilities; nursing homes, etc). The UHDDS definitions also apply to hospice services (all levels of care).

The following guidelines are to be applied in designating "other diagnoses" when neither the Alphabetic Index nor the Tabular List in ICD-10-CM provide direction. The listing of the diagnoses in the patient record is the responsibility of the attending provider.

A. Previous conditions
If the provider has included a diagnosis in the final diagnostic statement, such as the discharge summary or the face sheet, it should ordinarily be coded. Some providers include in the diagnostic statement resolved conditions or diagnoses and status-post procedures from previous admission that have no bearing on the current stay. Such conditions are not to be reported and are coded only if required by hospital policy.

However, history codes (categories Z80-Z87) may be used as secondary codes if the historical condition or family history has an impact on current care or influences treatment.

B. Abnormal findings

Abnormal findings (laboratory, x-ray, pathologic, and other diagnostic results) are not coded and reported unless the provider indicates their clinical significance. If the findings are outside the normal range and the attending provider has ordered other tests to evaluate the condition or prescribed treatment, it is appropriate to ask the provider whether the abnormal finding should be added.

Please note: This differs from the coding practices in the outpatient setting for coding encounters for diagnostic tests that have been interpreted by a provider.

C. Uncertain Diagnosis

If the diagnosis documented at the time of discharge is qualified as "probable", "suspected", "likely", "questionable", "possible", or "still to be ruled out" or other similar terms indicating uncertainty, code the condition as if it existed or was established. The bases for these guidelines are the diagnostic workup, arrangements for further workup or observation, and initial therapeutic approach that correspond most closely with the established diagnosis.

Note: This guideline is applicable only to inpatient admissions to short-term, acute, long-term care and psychiatric hospitals.

Section IV. Diagnostic Coding and Reporting Guidelines for Outpatient Services

These coding guidelines for outpatient diagnoses have been approved for use by hospitals/ providers in coding and reporting hospital-based outpatient services and provider-based office visits. Guidelines in Section I, Conventions, general coding guidelines and chapter-specific guidelines, should also be applied for outpatient services and office visits.

Information about the use of certain abbreviations, punctuation, symbols, and other conventions used in the ICD-10-CM Tabular List (code numbers and titles), can be found in Section IA of these guidelines, under "Conventions Used in the Tabular List." Section I.B. contains general guidelines that apply to the entire classification. Section I.C. contains chapter-specific guidelines that correspond to the chapters as they are arranged in the classification. Information about the correct sequence to use in finding a code is also described in Section I.

The terms encounter and visit are often used interchangeably in describing outpatient service contacts and, therefore, appear together in these guidelines without distinguishing one from the other.

Though the conventions and general guidelines apply to all settings, coding guidelines for outpatient and provider reporting of diagnoses will vary in a number of instances from those for inpatient diagnoses, recognizing that:

The Uniform Hospital Discharge Data Set (UHDDS) definition of principal diagnosis does not apply to hospital-based outpatient services and provider-based office visits.

Coding guidelines for inconclusive diagnoses (probable, suspected, rule out, etc.) were developed for inpatient reporting and do not apply to outpatients.

A. Selection of first-listed condition

In the outpatient setting, the term first-listed diagnosis is used in lieu of principal diagnosis.

In determining the first-listed diagnosis the coding conventions of ICD-10-CM, as well as the general and disease specific guidelines take precedence over the outpatient guidelines.

Diagnoses often are not established at the time of the initial encounter/visit. It may take two or more visits before the diagnosis is confirmed.

The most critical rule involves beginning the search for the correct code assignment through the Alphabetic Index. Never begin searching initially in the Tabular List as this will lead to coding errors.

1. Outpatient Surgery

When a patient presents for outpatient surgery (same day surgery), code the reason for the surgery as the first-listed diagnosis (reason for the encounter), even if the surgery is not performed due to a contraindication.

2. Observation Stay

When a patient is admitted for observation for a medical condition, assign a code for the medical condition as the first-listed diagnosis.

When a patient presents for outpatient surgery and develops complications requiring admission to observation, code the reason for the surgery as the first reported diagnosis (reason for the encounter), followed by codes for the complications as secondary diagnoses.

B. Codes from A00.0 through T88.9, Z00-Z99

The appropriate code(s) from A00.0 through T88.9, Z00-Z99 must be used to identify diagnoses, symptoms, conditions, problems, complaints, or other reason(s) for the encounter/visit.

C. Accurate reporting of ICD-10-CM diagnosis codes

For accurate reporting of ICD-10-CM diagnosis codes, the documentation should describe the patient's condition, using terminology which includes specific diagnoses as well as symptoms, problems, or reasons for the encounter. There are ICD-10-CM codes to describe all of these.

D. Codes that describe symptoms and signs

Codes that describe symptoms and signs, as opposed to diagnoses, are acceptable for reporting purposes when a diagnosis has not been established (confirmed) by the provider. Chapter 18 of ICD-10-CM, Symptoms, Signs, and Abnormal Clinical and Laboratory Findings Not Elsewhere Classified (codes R00-R99) contain many, but not all codes for symptoms.

E. Encounters for circumstances other than a disease or injury

ICD-10-CM provides codes to deal with encounters for circumstances other than a disease or injury. The Factors Influencing Health Status and Contact with Health Services codes (Z00-Z99) are provided to deal with occasions when circumstances other than a disease or injury are recorded as diagnosis or problems.

See Section I.C.21. Factors influencing health status and contact with health services.

F. Level of Detail in Coding

1. ICD-10-CM codes with 3, 4, 5, 6 or 7 characters

ICD-10-CM is composed of codes with 3, 4, 5, 6 or 7 characters. Codes with three characters are included in ICD-10-CM as the heading of a category of codes that may be further subdivided by the use of fourth, fifth, sixth or seventh characters to provide greater specificity.

2. Use of full number of characters required for a code

A three-character code is to be used only if it is not further subdivided. A code is invalid if it has not been coded to the full number of characters required for that code, including the 7th character, if applicable.

G. ICD-10-CM code for the diagnosis, condition, problem, or other reason for encounter/visit

List first the ICD-10-CM code for the diagnosis, condition, problem, or other reason for encounter/visit shown in the medical record to be chiefly responsible for the services provided. List additional codes that describe any coexisting conditions. In some cases the first-listed diagnosis may be a symptom when a diagnosis has not been established (confirmed) by the physician.

H. Uncertain diagnosis

Do not code diagnoses documented as "probable", "suspected," "questionable," "rule out," or "working diagnosis" or other similar terms indicating uncertainty. Rather, code the condition(s) to the highest degree of certainty for that encounter/visit, such as symptoms, signs, abnormal test results, or other reason for the visit.

Please note: This differs from the coding practices used by short-term, acute care, long-term care and psychiatric hospitals.

I. Chronic diseases

Chronic diseases treated on an ongoing basis may be coded and reported as many times as the patient receives treatment and care for the condition(s)

J. Code all documented conditions that coexist

Code all documented conditions that coexist at the time of the encounter/visit, and require or affect patient care treatment or management. Do not code conditions that were previously treated and no longer exist. However, history codes (categories Z80-Z87) may be used as secondary codes if the historical condition or family history has an impact on current care or influences treatment.

K. Patients receiving diagnostic services only

For patients receiving diagnostic services only during an encounter/visit, sequence first the diagnosis, condition, problem, or other reason for encounter/visit shown in the medical record to be chiefly responsible for the outpatient services provided during the encounter/visit. Codes for other diagnoses (e.g., chronic conditions) may be sequenced as additional diagnoses.

For encounters for routine laboratory/radiology testing in the absence of any signs, symptoms, or associated diagnosis, assign Z01.89, Encounter for other specified special examinations. If routine testing is performed during the same encounter as a test to evaluate a sign, symptom, or diagnosis, it is appropriate to assign both the Z code and the code describing the reason for the non-routine test.

For outpatient encounters for diagnostic tests that have been interpreted by a physician, and the final report is available at the time of coding, code any confirmed or definitive diagnosis(es) documented in the interpretation. Do not code related signs and symptoms as additional diagnoses.

Please note: This differs from the coding practice in the hospital inpatient setting regarding abnormal findings on test results.

L. Patients receiving therapeutic services only

For patients receiving therapeutic services only during an encounter/visit, sequence first the diagnosis, condition, problem, or other reason for encounter/visit shown in the medical record to be chiefly responsible for the outpatient services provided during the encounter/visit. Codes for other diagnoses (e.g., chronic conditions) may be sequenced as additional diagnoses.

The only exception to this rule is that when the primary reason for the admission/encounter is chemotherapy or radiation therapy, the appropriate Z code for the service is listed first, and the diagnosis or problem for which the service is being performed listed second.

M. Patients receiving preoperative evaluations only

For patients receiving preoperative evaluations only, sequence first a code from subcategory Z01.81, Encounter for pre-procedural examinations, to describe the pre-op consultations. Assign a code for the condition to describe the reason for the surgery as an additional diagnosis. Code also any findings related to the pre-op evaluation.

N. Ambulatory surgery

For ambulatory surgery, code the diagnosis for which the surgery was performed. If the postoperative diagnosis is known to be different from the preoperative diagnosis at the time the diagnosis is confirmed, select the postoperative diagnosis for coding, since it is the most definitive.

O. Routine outpatient prenatal visits

See Section I.C.15. Routine outpatient prenatal visits.

P. Encounters for general medical examinations with abnormal findings

The subcategories for encounters for general medical examinations, **Z00.0-** and encounter for routine child health examination, **Z00.12-**, provide codes for with and without abnormal findings. Should a general medical examination result in an abnormal finding, the code for general medical examination with abnormal finding should be assigned as the first-listed diagnosis. An examination with abnormal findings refers to a condition/diagnosis that is newly identified or a change in severity of a chronic condition (such as uncontrolled hypertension, or an acute exacerbation of chronic obstructive pulmonary disease) during a routine physical examination. A secondary code for the abnormal finding should also be coded.

Q. Encounters for routine health screenings

See Section I.C.21. Factors influencing health status and contact with health services, Screening

Appendix I. Present on Admission Reporting Guidelines

Introduction

These guidelines are to be used as a supplement to the *ICD-10-CM Official Guidelines for Coding and Reporting* to facilitate the assignment of the Present on Admission (POA) indicator for each diagnosis and external cause of injury code reported on claim forms (UB-04 and 837 Institutional).

These guidelines are not intended to replace any guidelines in the main body of the *ICD-10-CM Official Guidelines for Coding and Reporting*. The POA guidelines are not intended to provide guidance on when a condition should

be coded, but rather, how to apply the POA indicator to the final set of diagnosis codes that have been assigned in accordance with Sections I, II, and III of the official coding guidelines. Subsequent to the assignment of the ICD-10-CM codes, the POA indicator should then be assigned to those conditions that have been coded.

As stated in the Introduction to the ICD-10-CM Official Guidelines for Coding and Reporting, a joint effort between the healthcare provider and the coder is essential to achieve complete and accurate documentation, code assignment, and reporting of diagnoses and procedures. The importance of consistent, complete documentation in the medical record cannot be overemphasized. Medical record documentation from any provider involved in the care and treatment of the patient may be used to support the determination of whether a condition was present on admission or not. In the context of the official coding guidelines, the term "provider" means a physician or any qualified healthcare practitioner who is legally accountable for establishing the patient's diagnosis.

These guidelines are not a substitute for the provider's clinical judgment as to the determination of whether a condition was/was not present on admission. The provider should be queried regarding issues related to the linking of signs/symptoms, timing of test results, and the timing of findings.

Please see the CDC website for the detailed list of ICD-10-CM codes that do not require the use of a POA indicator (https://www.cdc.gov/nchs/icd/icd10cm.htm) (https://www.cms.gov/Medicare/Coding/ICD10/2018-ICD-10-CM-and-GEMs.html). The **codes and categories** on this exempt list **are** for circumstances regarding the healthcare encounter or factors influencing health status that do not represent a current disease or injury or **that describe conditions that** are always present on admission.

General Reporting Requirements

All claims involving inpatient admissions to general acute care hospitals or other facilities that are subject to a law or regulation mandating collection of present on admission information.

Present on admission is defined as present at the time the order for inpatient admission occurs -- conditions that develop during an outpatient encounter, including emergency department, observation, or outpatient surgery, are considered as present on admission.

POA indicator is assigned to principal and secondary diagnoses (as defined in Section II of the Official Guidelines for Coding and Reporting) and the external cause of injury codes.

Issues related to inconsistent, missing, conflicting or unclear documentation must still be resolved by the provider.

If a condition would not be coded and reported based on UHDDS definitions and current official coding guidelines, then the POA indicator would not be reported.

Reporting Options

　Y - Yes

　N - No

　U - Unknown

　W – Clinically undetermined

Unreported/Not used – (Exempt from POA reporting)

Reporting Definitions

　Y = present at the time of inpatient admission

　N = not present at the time of inpatient admission

　U = documentation is insufficient to determine if condition is present on admission

　W = provider is unable to clinically determine whether condition was present on admission or not

Timeframe for POA Identification and Documentation

There is no required timeframe as to when a provider (per the definition of "provider" used in these guidelines) must identify or document a condition to be present on admission. In some clinical situations, it may not be possible for a provider to make a definitive diagnosis (or a condition may not be recognized or reported by the patient) for a period of time after admission. In some cases it may be several days before the provider arrives at a definitive diagnosis. This does not mean that the condition was not present on admission. Determination of whether the condition was present on admission or not will be based on the applicable POA guideline as identified in this document, or on the provider's best clinical judgment.

If at the time of code assignment the documentation is unclear as to whether a condition was present on admission or not, it is appropriate to query the provider for clarification.

Assigning the POA Indicator

Condition is on the "Exempt from Reporting" list

Leave the "present on admission" field blank if the condition is on the list of ICD-10-CM codes for which this field is not applicable. This is the only circumstance in which the field may be left blank.

POA Explicitly Documented

Assign Y for any condition the provider explicitly documents as being present on admission.

Assign N for any condition the provider explicitly documents as not present at the time of admission.

Conditions diagnosed prior to inpatient admission

Assign "Y" for conditions that were diagnosed prior to admission (example: hypertension, diabetes mellitus, asthma)

Conditions diagnosed during the admission but clearly present before admission

Assign "Y" for conditions diagnosed during the admission that were clearly present but not diagnosed until after admission occurred.

Diagnoses subsequently confirmed after admission are considered present on admission if at the time of admission they are documented as suspected, possible, rule out, differential diagnosis, or constitute an underlying cause of a symptom that is present at the time of admission.

Condition develops during outpatient encounter prior to inpatient admission

Assign Y for any condition that develops during an outpatient encounter prior to a written order for inpatient admission.

Documentation does not indicate whether condition was present on admission

Assign "U" when the medical record documentation is unclear as to whether the condition was present on admission. "U" should not be routinely assigned and used only in very limited circumstances. Coders are encouraged to query the providers when the documentation is unclear.

Documentation states that it cannot be determined whether the condition was or was not present on admission

Assign "W" when the medical record documentation indicates that it cannot be clinically determined whether or not the condition was present on admission.

Chronic condition with acute exacerbation during the admission

If a single code identifies both the chronic condition and the acute exacerbation, see POA guidelines pertaining to codes that contain multiple clinical concepts.

If a single code only identifies the chronic condition and not the acute exacerbation (e.g., acute exacerbation of chronic leukemia), assign "Y."

Conditions documented as possible, probable, suspected, or rule out at the time of discharge

If the final diagnosis contains a possible, probable, suspected, or rule out diagnosis, and this diagnosis was based on signs, symptoms or clinical findings suspected at the time of inpatient admission, assign "Y."

If the final diagnosis contains a possible, probable, suspected, or rule out diagnosis, and this diagnosis was based on signs, symptoms or clinical findings that were not present on admission, assign "N".

Conditions documented as impending or threatened at the time of discharge

If the final diagnosis contains an impending or threatened diagnosis, and this diagnosis is based on symptoms or clinical findings that were present on admission, assign "Y".

If the final diagnosis contains an impending or threatened diagnosis, and this diagnosis is based on symptoms or clinical findings that were not present on admission, assign "N".

Acute and Chronic Conditions

Assign "Y" for acute conditions that are present at time of admission and N for acute conditions that are not present at time of admission.

Assign "Y" for chronic conditions, even though the condition may not be diagnosed until after admission.

If a single code identifies both an acute and chronic condition, see the POA guidelines for codes that contain multiple clinical concepts.

Codes That Contain Multiple Clinical Concepts

Assign "N" if at least one of the clinical concepts included in the code was not present on admission (e.g., COPD with acute exacerbation and the exacerbation was not present on admission; gastric ulcer that does not start bleeding until after admission; asthma patient develops status asthmaticus after admission).

Assign "Y" if all of the clinical concepts included in the code were present on admission (e.g., duodenal ulcer that perforates prior to admission).

For infection codes that include the causal organism, assign "Y" if the infection (or signs of the infection) were present on admission, even though the culture results may not be known until after admission (e.g., patient is admitted with pneumonia and the provider documents Pseudomonas as the causal organism a few days later).

Same Diagnosis Code for Two or More Conditions

When the same ICD-10-CM diagnosis code applies to two or more conditions during the same encounter (e.g. two separate conditions classified to the same ICD-10-CM diagnosis code):

Assign "Y" if all conditions represented by the single ICD-10-CM code were present on admission (e.g. bilateral unspecified age-related cataracts).

Assign "N" if any of the conditions represented by the single ICD-10-CM code was not present on admission (e.g. traumatic secondary and recurrent hemorrhage and seroma is assigned to a single code T79.2, but only one of the conditions was present on admission).

Obstetrical conditions

Whether or not the patient delivers during the current hospitalization does not affect assignment of the POA indicator. The determining factor for POA assignment is whether the pregnancy complication or obstetrical condition described by the code was present at the time of admission or not.

If the pregnancy complication or obstetrical condition was present on admission (e.g., patient admitted in preterm labor), assign "Y".

If the pregnancy complication or obstetrical condition was not present on admission (e.g., 2nd degree laceration during delivery, postpartum hemorrhage that occurred during current hospitalization, fetal distress develops after admission), assign "N".

If the obstetrical code includes more than one diagnosis and any of the diagnoses identified by the code were not present on admission assign "N". (e.g., Category O11, Pre-existing hypertension with pre-eclampsia)

Perinatal conditions

Newborns are not considered to be admitted until after birth. Therefore, any condition present at birth or that developed in utero is considered present at admission and should be assigned "Y". This includes conditions that occur during delivery (e.g., injury during delivery, meconium aspiration, exposure to streptococcus B in the vaginal canal).

Congenital conditions and anomalies

Assign "Y" for congenital conditions and anomalies except for categories Q00-Q99, Congenital anomalies, which are on the exempt list. Congenital conditions are always considered present on admission.

External cause of injury codes

Assign "Y" for any external cause code representing an external cause of morbidity that occurred prior to inpatient admission (e.g., patient fell out of bed at home, patient fell out of bed in emergency room prior to admission)

Assign "N" for any external cause code representing an external cause of morbidity that occurred during inpatient hospitalization (e.g., patient fell out of hospital bed during hospital stay, patient experienced an adverse reaction to a medication administered after inpatient admission)

ICD-10-CM Index to Diseases and Injuries

A

Aarskog's syndrome Q87.1
Abandonment — *see* Maltreatment
Abasia (-astasia) (hysterical) F44.4
Abderhalden-Kaufmann-Lignac syndrome (cystinosis) E72.04
Abdomen, abdominal (*see also* condition)
 acute R10.0
 angina K55.1
 muscle deficiency syndrome Q79.4
Abdominalgia — *see* Pain, abdominal
Abduction contracture, hip or other joint — *see* Contraction, joint
Aberrant (congenital) (*see also* Malposition, congenital)
 adrenal gland Q89.1
 artery (peripheral) Q27.8
  basilar NEC Q28.1
  cerebral Q28.3
  coronary Q24.5
  digestive system Q27.8
  eye Q15.8
  lower limb Q27.8
  precerebral Q28.1
  pulmonary Q25.79
  renal Q27.2
  retina Q14.1
  specified site NEC Q27.8
  subclavian Q27.8
  upper limb Q27.8
  vertebral Q28.1
 breast Q83.8
 endocrine gland NEC Q89.2
 hepatic duct Q44.5
 pancreas Q45.3
 parathyroid gland Q89.2
 pituitary gland Q89.2
 sebaceous glands, mucous membrane, mouth, congenital Q38.6
 spleen Q89.09
 subclavian artery Q27.8
 thymus (gland) Q89.2
 thyroid gland Q89.2
 vein (peripheral) NEC Q27.8
  cerebral Q28.3
  digestive system Q27.8
  lower limb Q27.8
  precerebral Q28.1
  specified site NEC Q27.8
  upper limb Q27.8
Aberration
 distantial — *see* Disturbance, visual
 mental F99
Abetalipoproteinemia E78.6
Abiotrophy R68.89
Ablatio, ablation
 retinae — *see* Detachment, retina
Ablepharia, ablepharon Q10.3
Abnormal, abnormality, abnormalities (*see also* Anomaly)
 acid-base balance (mixed) E87.4
 albumin R77.0
 alphafetoprotein R77.2
 alveolar ridge K08.9
 anatomical relationship Q89.9
 apertures, congenital, diaphragm Q79.1
 auditory perception H93.29- ☑
  diplacusis — *see* Diplacusis
  hyperacusis — *see* Hyperacusis
  recruitment — *see* Recruitment, auditory
  threshold shift — *see* Shift, auditory threshold
 autosomes Q99.9
  fragile site Q95.5
 basal metabolic rate R94.8
 biosynthesis, testicular androgen E29.1
 bleeding time R79.1
 blood level (of)
  cobalt R79.0
  copper R79.0
  iron R79.0
  lithium R78.89
  magnesium R79.0

Abnormal, abnormality, abnormalities — *continued*
 blood level — *continued*
  mineral NEC R79.0
  zinc R79.0
 blood pressure
  elevated R03.0
  low reading (nonspecific) R03.1
 blood sugar R73.09
 blood-gas level R79.81
 bowel sounds R19.15
  absent R19.11
  hyperactive R19.12
 brain scan R94.02
 breathing R06.9
 caloric test R94.138
 cerebrospinal fluid R83.9
  cytology R83.6
  drug level R83.2
  enzyme level R83.0
  hormones R83.1
  immunology R83.4
  microbiology R83.5
  nonmedicinal level R83.3
  specified type NEC R83.8
 chemistry, blood R79.9
  C-reactive protein R79.82
  drugs — *see* Findings, abnormal, in blood
  gas level R79.81
  minerals R79.0
  pancytopenia D61.818
  PTT R79.1
  specified NEC R79.89
  toxins — *see* Findings, abnormal, in blood
 chest sounds (friction) (rales) R09.89
 chromosome, chromosomal Q99.9
  with more than three X chromosomes, female Q97.1
  analysis result R89.8
   bronchial washings R84.8
   cerebrospinal fluid R83.8
   cervix uteri NEC R87.89
   nasal secretions R84.8
   nipple discharge R89.8
   peritoneal fluid R85.89
   pleural fluid R84.8
   prostatic secretions R86.8
   saliva R85.89
   seminal fluid R86.8
   sputum R84.8
   synovial fluid R89.8
   throat scrapings R84.8
   vagina R87.89
   vulva R87.89
   wound secretions R89.8
  dicentric replacement Q93.2
  ring replacement Q93.2
  sex Q99.8
   female phenotype Q97.9
    specified NEC Q97.8
   male phenotype Q98.9
    specified NEC Q98.8
   structural male Q98.6
  specified NEC Q99.8
 clinical findings NEC R68.89
 coagulation D68.9
  newborn, transient P61.6
  profile R79.1
  time R79.1
 communication — *see* Fistula
 conjunctiva, vascular H11.41- ☑
 coronary artery Q24.5
 cortisol-binding globulin E27.8
 course, eustachian tube Q17.8
 creatinine clearance R94.4
 cytology
  anus R85.619
   atypical squamous cells cannot exclude high grade squamous intraepithelial lesion (ASC-H) R85.611
   atypical squamous cells of undetermined significance (ASC-US) R85.610
   cytologic evidence of malignancy R85.614

Abnormal, abnormality, abnormalities — *continued*
 cytology — *continued*
  anus — *continued*
   high grade squamous intraepithelial lesion (HGSIL) R85.613
   human papillomavirus (HPV) DNA test
    high risk positive R85.81
    low risk postive R85.82
   inadequate smear R85.615
   low grade squamous intraepithelial lesion (LGSIL) R85.612
   satisfactory anal smear but lacking transformation zone R85.616
   specified NEC R85.618
   unsatisfactory smear R85.615
  female genital organs — *see* Abnormal, Papanicolaou (smear)
 dark adaptation curve H53.61
 dentofacial NEC — *see* Anomaly, dentofacial
 development, developmental Q89.9
  central nervous system Q07.9
 diagnostic imaging
  abdomen, abdominal region NEC R93.5
  biliary tract R93.2
  bladder R93.41
  breast R92.8
  central nervous system NEC R90.89
  cerebrovascular NEC R90.89
  coronary circulation R93.1
  digestive tract NEC R93.3
  gastrointestinal (tract) R93.3
  genitourinary organs R93.8
  head R93.0
  heart R93.1
  intrathoracic organ NEC R93.8
  kidney R93.42- ☑
  limbs R93.6
  liver R93.2
  lung (field) R91.8
  musculoskeletal system NEC R93.7
  renal pelvis R93.41
  retroperitoneum R93.5
  site specified NEC R93.8
  skin and subcutaneous tissue R93.8
  skull R93.0
  ureter R93.41
  urinary organs specified NEC R93.49
 direction, teeth, fully erupted M26.30
 ear ossicles, acquired NEC H74.39- ☑
  ankylosis — *see* Ankylosis, ear ossicles
  discontinuity — *see* Discontinuity, ossicles, ear
  partial loss — *see* Loss, ossicles, ear (partial)
 Ebstein Q22.5
 echocardiogram R93.1
 echoencephalogram R90.81
 echogram — *see* Abnormal, diagnostic imaging
 electrocardiogram [ECG] [EKG] R94.31
 electroencephalogram [EEG] R94.01
 electrolyte — *see* Imbalance, electrolyte
 electromyogram [EMG] R94.131
 electro-oculogram [EOG] R94.110
 electrophysiological intracardiac studies R94.39
 electroretinogram [ERG] R94.111
 erythrocytes
  congenital, with perinatal jaundice D58.9
 feces (color) (contents) (mucus) R19.5
 finding — *see* Findings, abnormal, without diagnosis
 fluid
  amniotic — *see* Abnormal, specimen, specified
  cerebrospinal — *see* Abnormal, cerebrospinal fluid
  peritoneal — *see* Abnormal, specimen, digestive organs
  pleural — *see* Abnormal, specimen, respiratory organs
  synovial — *see* Abnormal, specimen, specified
  thorax (bronchial washings) (pleural fluid) — *see* Abnormal, specimen, respiratory organs
  vaginal — *see* Abnormal, specimen, female genital organs
 form
  teeth K00.2
  uterus — *see* Anomaly, uterus

Abnormal, abnormality, abnormalities — *continued*
function studies
auditory R94.120
bladder R94.8
brain R94.09
cardiovascular R94.30
ear R94.128
endocrine NEC R94.7
eye NEC R94.118
kidney R94.4
liver R94.5
nervous system
central NEC R94.09
peripheral NEC R94.138
pancreas R94.8
placenta R94.8
pulmonary R94.2
special senses NEC R94.128
spleen R94.8
thyroid R94.6
vestibular R94.121
gait — *see* Gait
hysterical F44.4
gastrin secretion E16.4
globulin R77.1
cortisol-binding E27.8
thyroid-binding E07.89
glomerular, minor (*see also* N00-N07 with fourth
character .0) N05.0
glucagon secretion E16.3
glucose tolerance (test) (non-fasting) R73.09
gravitational (G) forces or states (effect of) T75.81 ☑
hair (color) (shaft) L67.9
specified NEC L67.8
hard tissue formation in pulp (dental) K04.3
head movement R25.0
heart
rate R00.9
specified NEC R00.8
shadow R93.1
sounds NEC R01.2
hemoglobin (disease) (*see also* Disease, hemoglobin)
D58.2
trait — *see* Trait, hemoglobin, abnormal
histology NEC R89.7
immunological findings R89.4
in serum R76.9
specified NEC R76.8
increase in appetite R63.2
involuntary movement — *see* Abnormal, movement,
involuntary
jaw closure M26.51
karyotype R89.8
kidney function test R94.4
knee jerk R29.2
leukocyte (cell) (differential) NEC D72.9
liver function test R94.5
loss of
height R29.890
weight R63.4
mammogram NEC R92.8
calcification (calculus) R92.1
microcalcification R92.0
Mantoux test R76.11
movement (disorder) (*see also* Disorder, movement)
head R25.0
involuntary R25.9
fasciculation R25.3
of head R25.0
spasm R25.2
specified type NEC R25.8
tremor R25.1
myoglobin (Aberdeen) (Annapolis) R89.7
neonatal screening P09
oculomotor study R94.113
palmar creases Q82.8
Papanicolaou (smear)
anus R85.619
atypical squamous cells cannot exclude high
grade squamous intraepithelial lesion
(ASC-H) R85.611
atypical squamous cells of undetermined significance (ASC-US) R85.610
cytologic evidence of malignancy R85.614
high grade squamous intraepithelial lesion
(HGSIL) R85.613
human papillomavirus (HPV) DNA test
high risk positive R85.81

Abnormal, abnormality, abnormalities — *continued*
Papanicolaou — *continued*
anus — *continued*
human papillomavirus DNA test — *continued*
low risk positive R85.82
inadequate smear R85.615
low grade squamous intraepithelial lesion
(LGSIL) R85.612
satisfactory anal smear but lacking transformation zone R85.616
specified NEC R85.618
unsatisfactory smear R85.615
bronchial washings R84.6
cerebrospinal fluid R83.6
cervix R87.619
atypical squamous cells cannot exclude high
grade squamous intraepithelial lesion
(ASC-H) R87.611
atypical squamous cells of undetermined significance (ASC-US) R87.610
cytologic evidence of malignancy R87.614
high grade squamous intraepithelial lesion
(HGSIL) R87.613
inadequate smear R87.615
low grade squamous intraepithelial lesion
(LGSIL) R87.612
non-atypical endometrial cells R87.618
satisfactory cervical smear but lacking transformation zone R87.616
specified NEC R87.618
thin preparaton R87.619
unsatisfactory smear R87.615
nasal secretions R84.6
nipple discharge R89.6
peritoneal fluid R85.69
pleural fluid R84.6
prostatic secretions R86.6
saliva R85.69
seminal fluid R86.6
sites NEC R89.6
sputum R84.6
synovial fluid R89.6
throat scrapings R84.6
vagina R87.629
atypical squamous cells cannot exclude high
grade squamous intraepithelial lesion
(ASC-H) R87.621
atypical squamous cells of undetermined significance (ASC-US) R87.620
cytologic evidence of malignancy R87.624
high grade squamous intraepithelial lesion
(HGSIL) R87.623
inadequate smear R87.625
low grade squamous intraepithelial lesion
(LGSIL) R87.622
specified NEC R87.628
thin preparation R87.629
unsatisfactory smear R87.625
vulva R87.69
wound secretions R89.6
partial thromboplastin time (PTT) R79.1
pelvis (bony) — *see* Deformity, pelvis
percussion, chest (tympany) R09.89
periods (grossly) — *see* Menstruation
phonocardiogram R94.39
plantar reflex R29.2
plasma
protein R77.9
specified NEC R77.8
viscosity R70.1
pleural (folds) Q34.0
posture R29.3
product of conception O02.9
specified type NEC O02.89
prothrombin time (PT) R79.1
pulmonary
artery, congenital Q25.79
function, newborn P28.89
test results R94.2
pulsations in neck R00.2
pupillary H21.56- ☑
function (reaction) (reflex) — *see* Anomaly, pupil,
function
radiological examination — *see* Abnormal, diagnostic
imaging
red blood cell(s) (morphology) (volume) R71.8
reflex — *see* Reflex

Abnormal, abnormality, abnormalities — *continued*
renal function test R94.4
response to nerve stimulation R94.130
retinal correspondence H53.31
retinal function study R94.111
rhythm, heart (*see also* Arrhythmia)
saliva — *see* Abnormal, specimen, digestive organs
scan
kidney R94.4
liver R93.2
thyroid R94.6
secretion
gastrin E16.4
glucagon E16.3
semen, seminal fluid — *see* Abnormal, specimen, male
genital organs
serum level (of)
acid phosphatase R74.8
alkaline phosphatase R74.8
amylase R74.8
enzymes R74.9
specified NEC R74.8
lipase R74.8
triacylglycerol lipase R74.8
shape
gravid uterus — *see* Anomaly, uterus
sinus venosus Q21.1
size, tooth, teeth K00.2
spacing, tooth, teeth, fully erupted M26.30
specimen
digestive organs (peritoneal fluid) (saliva) R85.9
cytology R85.69
drug level R85.2
enzyme level R85.0
histology R85.7
hormones R85.1
immunology R85.4
microbiology R85.5
nonmedicinal level R85.3
specified type NEC R85.89
female genital organs (secretions) (smears) R87.9
cytology R87.69
cervix R87.619
human papillomavirus (HPV) DNA test
high risk positive R87.810
low risk positive R87.820
inadequate (unsatisfactory) smear
R87.615
non-atypical endometrial cells R87.618
specified NEC R87.618
vagina R87.629
human papillomavirus (HPV) DNA test
high risk positive R87.811
low risk positive R87.821
inadequate (unsatisfactory) smear
R87.625
vulva R87.69
drug level R87.2
enzyme level R87.0
histological R87.7
hormones R87.1
immunology R87.4
microbiology R87.5
nonmedicinal level R87.3
specified type NEC R87.89
male genital organs (prostatic secretions) (semen)
R86.9
cytology R86.6
drug level R86.2
enzyme level R86.0
histological R86.7
hormones R86.1
immunology R86.4
microbiology R86.5
nonmedicinal level R86.3
specified type NEC R86.8
nipple discharge — *see* Abnormal, specimen,
specified
respiratory organs (bronchial washings) (nasal secretions) (pleural fluid) (sputum) R84.9
cytology R84.6
drug level R84.2
enzyme level R84.0
histology R84.7
hormones R84.1
immunology R84.4
microbiology R84.5
nonmedicinal level R84.3

Abnormal, abnormality, abnormalities — *continued*
specimen — *continued*
  respiratory organs — *continued*
    specified type NEC R84.8
  specified organ, system and tissue NOS R89.9
    cytology R89.6
    drug level R89.2
    enzyme level R89.0
    histology R89.7
    hormones R89.1
    immunology R89.4
    microbiology R89.5
    nonmedicinal level R89.3
    specified type NEC R89.8
  synovial fluid — *see* Abnormal, specimen, specified
  thorax (bronchial washings) (pleural fluids) — *see* Abnormal, specimen, respiratory organs
  vagina (secretion) (smear) R87.629
  vulva (secretion) (smear) R87.69
  wound secretion — *see* Abnormal, specimen, specified
spermatozoa — *see* Abnormal, specimen, male genital organs
sputum (amount) (color) (odor) R09.3
stool (color) (contents) (mucus) R19.5
  bloody K92.1
  guaiac positive R19.5
synchondrosis Q78.8
thermography (*see also* Abnormal, diagnostic imaging) R93.8
thyroid-binding globulin E07.89
tooth, teeth (form) (size) K00.2
toxicology (findings) R78.9
transport protein E88.09
tumor marker NEC R97.8
ultrasound results — *see* Abnormal, diagnostic imaging
umbilical cord complicating delivery O69.9 ☑
urination NEC R39.198
urine (constituents) R82.90
  bile R82.2
  cytological examination R82.8
  drugs R82.5
  fat R82.0
  glucose R81
  heavy metals R82.6
  hemoglobin R82.3
  histological examination R82.8
  ketones R82.4
  microbiological examination (culture) R82.79
  myoglobin R82.1
  positive culture R82.79
  protein — *see* Proteinuria
  specified substance NEC R82.99
    chromoabnormality NEC R82.91
  substances nonmedical R82.6
uterine hemorrhage — *see* Hemorrhage, uterus
vectorcardiogram R94.39
visually evoked potential (VEP) R94.112
white blood cells D72.9
  specified NEC D72.89
X-ray examination — *see* Abnormal, diagnostic imaging
Abnormity (any organ or part) — *see* Anomaly
Abocclusion M26.29
hemolytic disease (newborn) P55.1
incompatibility reaction ABO — *see* Complication(s), transfusion, incompatibility reaction, ABO
Abolition, language R48.8
Aborter, habitual or recurrent — *see* Loss (of), pregnancy, recurrent
Abortion (complete) (spontaneous) O03.9
with
  retained products of conception — *see* Abortion, incomplete
attempted (elective) (failed) O07.4
  complicated by O07.30
    afibrinogenemia O07.1
    cardiac arrest O07.36
    chemical damage of pelvic organ(s) O07.34
    circulatory collapse O07.31
    cystitis O07.38
    defibrination syndrome O07.1
    electrolyte imbalance O07.33
    embolism (air) (amniotic fluid) (blood clot) (fat) (pulmonary) (septic) (soap) O07.2
    endometritis O07.0

Abortion — *continued*
attempted — *continued*
  complicated by — *continued*
    genital tract and pelvic infection O07.0
    hemolysis O07.1
    hemorrhage (delayed) (excessive) O07.1
    infection
      genital tract or pelvic O07.0
      urinary tract tract O07.38
    intravascular coagulation O07.1
    laceration of pelvic organ(s) O07.34
    metabolic disorder O07.33
    oliguria O07.32
    oophoritis O07.0
    parametritis O07.0
    pelvic peritonitis O07.0
    perforation of pelvic organ(s) O07.34
    renal failure or shutdown O07.32
    salpingitis or salpingo-oophoritis O07.0
    sepsis O07.37
    shock O07.31
    specified condition NEC O07.39
    tubular necrosis (renal) O07.32
    uremia O07.32
    urinary tract infection O07.38
    venous complication NEC O07.35
      embolism (air) (amniotic fluid) (blood clot) (fat) (pulmonary) (septic) (soap) O07.2
complicated (by) (following) O03.80
  afibrinogenemia O03.6
  cardiac arrest O03.86
  chemical damage of pelvic organ(s) O03.84
  circulatory collapse O03.81
  cystitis O03.88
  defibrination syndrome O03.6
  electrolyte imbalance O03.83
  embolism (air) (amniotic fluid) (blood clot) (fat) (pulmonary) (septic) (soap) O03.7
  endometritis O03.5
  genital tract and pelvic infection O03.5
  hemolysis O03.6
  hemorrhage (delayed) (excessive) O03.6
  infection
    genital tract or pelvic O03.5
    urinary tract O03.88
  intravascular coagulation O03.6
  laceration of pelvic organ(s) O03.84
  metabolic disorder O03.83
  oliguria O03.82
  oophoritis O03.5
  parametritis O03.5
  pelvic peritonitis O03.5
  perforation of pelvic organ(s) O03.84
  renal failure or shutdown O03.82
  salpingitis or salpingo-oophoritis O03.5
  sepsis O03.87
  shock O03.81
  specified condition NEC O03.89
  tubular necrosis (renal) O03.82
  uremia O03.82
  urinary tract infection O03.88
  venous complication NEC O03.85
    embolism (air) (amniotic fluid) (blood clot) (fat) (pulmonary) (septic) (soap) O03.7
failed — *see* Abortion, attempted
habitual or recurrent N96
  with current abortion — *see* categories O03-O04
  without current pregnancy N96
  care in current pregnancy O26.2- ☑
incomplete (spontaneous) O03.4
  complicated (by) (following) O03.30
    afibrinogenemia O03.1
    cardiac arrest O03.36
    chemical damage of pelvic organ(s) O03.34
    circulatory collapse O03.31
    cystitis O03.38
    defibrination syndrome O03.1
    electrolyte imbalance O03.33
    embolism (air) (amniotic fluid) (blood clot) (fat) (pulmonary) (septic) (soap) O03.2
    endometritis O03.0
    genital tract and pelvic infection O03.0
    hemolysis O03.1
    hemorrhage (delayed) (excessive) O03.1
    infection
      genital tract or pelvic O03.0
      urinary tract O03.38
    intravascular coagulation O03.1
    laceration of pelvic organ(s) O03.34

Abortion — *continued*
incomplete — *continued*
  complicated — *continued*
    metabolic disorder O03.33
    oliguria O03.32
    oophoritis O03.0
    parametritis O03.0
    pelvic peritonitis O03.0
    perforation of pelvic organ(s) O03.34
    renal failure or shutdown O03.32
    salpingitis or salpingo-oophoritis O03.0
    sepsis O03.37
    shock O03.31
    specified condition NEC O03.39
    tubular necrosis (renal) O03.32
    uremia O03.32
    urinary infection O03.38
    venous complication NEC O03.35
      embolism (air) (amniotic fluid) (blood clot) (fat) (pulmonary) (soap) O03.2
induced (encounter for) Z33.2
  complicated by O04.80
    afibrinogenemia O04.6
    cardiac arrest O04.86
    chemical damage of pelvic organ(s) O04.84
    circulatory collapse O04.81
    cystitis O04.88
    defibrination syndrome O04.6
    electrolyte imbalance O04.83
    embolism (air) (amniotic fluid) (blood clot) (fat) (pulmonary) (septic) (soap) O04.7
    endometritis O04.5
    genital tract and pelvic infection O04.5
    hemolysis O04.6
    hemorrhage (delayed) (excessive) O04.6
    infection
      genital tract or pelvic O04.5
      urinary tract O04.88
    intravascular coagulation O04.6
    laceration of pelvic organ(s) O04.84
    metabolic disorder O04.83
    oliguria O04.82
    oophoritis O04.5
    parametritis O04.5
    pelvic peritonitis O04.5
    perforation of pelvic organ(s) O04.84
    renal failure or shutdown O04.82
    salpingitis or salpingo-oophoritis O04.5
    sepsis O04.87
    shock O04.81
    specified condition NEC O04.89
    tubular necrosis (renal) O04.82
    uremia O04.82
    urinary tract infection O04.88
    venous complication NEC O04.85
      embolism (air) (amniotic fluid) (blood clot) (fat) (pulmonary) (septic) (soap) O04.7
missed O02.1
spontaneous — *see* Abortion (complete) (spontaneous)
  threatened O20.0
threatened (spontaneous) O20.0
tubal O00.10- ☑
  with intrauterine pregnancy O00.11- ☑
Abortus fever A23.1
Aboulomania F60.7
Abrami's disease D59.8
Abramov-Fiedler myocarditis (acute isolated myocarditis) I40.1
Abrasion T14.8 ☑
abdomen, abdominal (wall) S30.811 ☑
alveolar process S00.512 ☑
ankle S90.51- ☑
antecubital space — *see* Abrasion, elbow
anus S30.817 ☑
arm (upper) S40.81- ☑
auditory canal — *see* Abrasion, ear
auricle — *see* Abrasion, ear
axilla — *see* Abrasion, arm
back, lower S30.810 ☑
breast S20.11- ☑
brow S00.81 ☑
buttock S30.810 ☑
calf — *see* Abrasion, leg
canthus — *see* Abrasion, eyelid
cheek S00.81 ☑
  internal S00.512 ☑
chest wall — *see* Abrasion, thorax

Abrasion — *continued*
chin S00.81 ☑
clitoris S30.814 ☑
cornea S05.0- ☑
costal region — *see* Abrasion, thorax
dental K03.1
digit(s)
   foot — *see* Abrasion, toe
   hand — *see* Abrasion, finger
ear S00.41- ☑
elbow S50.31- ☑
epididymis S30.813 ☑
epigastric region S30.811 ☑
epiglottis S10.11 ☑
esophagus (thoracic) S27.818 ☑
   cervical S10.11 ☑
eyebrow — *see* Abrasion, eyelid
eyelid S00.21- ☑
face S00.81 ☑
finger(s) S60.41- ☑
   index S60.41- ☑
   little S60.41- ☑
   middle S60.41- ☑
   ring S60.41- ☑
flank S30.811 ☑
foot (except toe(s) alone) S90.81- ☑
   toe — *see* Abrasion, toe
forearm S50.81- ☑
   elbow only — *see* Abrasion, elbow
forehead S00.81 ☑
genital organs, external
   female S30.816 ☑
   male S30.815 ☑
groin S30.811 ☑
gum S00.512 ☑
hand S60.51- ☑
head S00.91 ☑
   ear — *see* Abrasion, ear
   eyelid — *see* Abrasion, eyelid
   lip S00.511 ☑
   nose S00.31 ☑
   oral cavity S00.512 ☑
   scalp S00.01 ☑
   specified site NEC S00.81 ☑
heel — *see* Abrasion, foot
hip S70.21- ☑
inguinal region S30.811 ☑
interscapular region S20.419 ☑
jaw S00.81 ☑
knee S80.21- ☑
labium (majus) (minus) S30.814 ☑
larynx S10.11 ☑
leg (lower) S80.81- ☑
   knee — *see* Abrasion, knee
   upper — *see* Abrasion, thigh
lip S00.511 ☑
lower back S30.810 ☑
lumbar region S30.810 ☑
malar region S00.81 ☑
mammary — *see* Abrasion, breast
mastoid region S00.81 ☑
mouth S00.512 ☑
nail
   finger — *see* Abrasion, finger
   toe — *see* Abrasion, toe
nape S10.81 ☑
nasal S00.31 ☑
neck S10.91 ☑
   specified site NEC S10.81 ☑
   throat S10.11 ☑
nose S00.31 ☑
occipital region S00.01 ☑
oral cavity S00.512 ☑
orbital region — *see* Abrasion, eyelid
palate S00.512 ☑
palm — *see* Abrasion, hand
parietal region S00.01 ☑
pelvis S30.810 ☑
penis S30.812 ☑
perineum
   female S30.814 ☑
   male S30.810 ☑
periocular area — *see* Abrasion, eyelid
phalanges
   finger — *see* Abrasion, finger
   toe — *see* Abrasion, toe

Abrasion — *continued*
pharynx S10.11 ☑
pinna — *see* Abrasion, ear
popliteal space — *see* Abrasion, knee
prepuce S30.812 ☑
pubic region S30.810 ☑
pudendum
   female S30.816 ☑
   male S30.815 ☑
sacral region S30.810 ☑
scalp S00.01 ☑
scapular region — *see* Abrasion, shoulder
scrotum S30.813 ☑
shin — *see* Abrasion, leg
shoulder S40.21- ☑
skin NEC T14.8
sternal region S20.319 ☑
submaxillary region S00.81 ☑
submental region S00.81 ☑
subungual
   finger(s) — *see* Abrasion, finger
   toe(s) — *see* Abrasion, toe
supraclavicular fossa S10.81 ☑
supraorbital S00.81 ☑
temple S00.81 ☑
temporal region S00.81 ☑
testis S30.813 ☑
thigh S70.31- ☑
thorax, thoracic (wall) S20.91 ☑
   back S20.41- ☑
   front S20.31- ☑
throat S10.11 ☑
thumb S60.31- ☑
toe(s) (lesser) S90.416 ☑
   great S90.41- ☑
tongue S00.512 ☑
tooth, teeth (dentifrice) (habitual) (hard tissues) (occupational) (ritual) (traditional) K03.1
trachea S10.11 ☑
tunica vaginalis S30.813 ☑
tympanum, tympanic membrane — *see* Abrasion, ear
uvula S00.512 ☑
vagina S30.814 ☑
vocal cords S10.11 ☑
vulva S30.814 ☑
wrist S60.81- ☑
Abrism — *see* Poisoning, food, noxious, plant
Abruptio placentae O45.9- ☑
   with
      afibrinogenemia O45.01- ☑
      coagulation defect O45.00- ☑
         specified NEC O45.09- ☑
      disseminated intravascular coagulation O45.02- ☑
      hypofibrinogenemia O45.01- ☑
   specified NEC O45.8- ☑
Abruption, placenta — *see* Abruptio placentae
Abscess (connective tissue) (embolic) (fistulous) (infective) (metastatic) (multiple) (pernicious) (pyogenic) (septic) L02.91
   with
      diverticular disease (intestine) K57.80
         with bleeding K57.81
         large intestine K57.20
            with
               bleeding K57.21
               small intestine K57.40
                  with bleeding K57.41
         small intestine K57.00
            with
               bleeding K57.01
               large intestine K57.40
                  with bleeding K57.41
      lymphangitis — *code by* site under Abscess
   abdomen, abdominal
      cavity K65.1
      wall L02.211
   abdominopelvic K65.1
   accessory sinus — *see* Sinusitis
   adrenal (capsule) (gland) E27.8
   alveolar K04.7
      with sinus K04.6
   amebic A06.4
      brain (and liver or lung abscess) A06.6
      genitourinary tract A06.82
      liver (without mention of brain or lung abscess) A06.4

Abscess — *continued*
   amebic — *continued*
      lung (and liver) (without mention of brain abscess) A06.5
      specified site NEC A06.89
      spleen A06.89
   anerobic A48.0
   ankle — *see* Abscess, lower limb
   anorectal K61.2
   antecubital space — *see* Abscess, upper limb
   antrum (chronic) (Highmore) — *see* Sinusitis, maxillary
   anus K61.0
   apical (tooth) K04.7
      with sinus (alveolar) K04.6
   appendix K35.3
   areola (acute) (chronic) (nonpuerperal) N61.1
      puerperal, postpartum or gestational — *see* Infection, nipple
   arm (any part) — *see* Abscess, upper limb
   artery (wall) I77.89
   atheromatous I77.2
   auricle, ear — *see* Abscess, ear, external
   axilla (region) L02.41- ☑
      lymph gland or node L04.2
   back (any part, except buttock) L02.212
   Bartholin's gland N75.1
      with
         abortion — *see* Abortion, by type complicated by, sepsis
         ectopic or molar pregnancy O08.0
      following ectopic or molar pregnancy O08.0
   Bezold's — *see* Mastoiditis, acute
   bilharziasis B65.1
   bladder (wall) — *see* Cystitis, specified type NEC
   bone (subperiosteal) (*see also* Osteomyelitis, specified type NEC)
      accessory sinus (chronic) — *see* Sinusitis
      chronic or old — *see* Osteomyelitis, chronic
      jaw (lower) (upper) M27.2
      mastoid — *see* Mastoiditis, acute, subperiosteal
      petrous — *see* Petrositis
      spinal (tuberculous) A18.01
         nontuberculous — *see* Osteomyelitis, vertebra
   bowel K63.0
   brain (any part) (cystic) (otogenic) G06.0
      amebic (with abscess of any other site) A06.6
      gonococcal A54.82
      pheomycotic (chromomycotic) B43.1
      tuberculous A17.81
   breast (acute) (chronic) (nonpuerperal) N61.1
      newborn P39.0
      puerperal, postpartum, gestational — *see* Mastitis, obstetric, purulent
   broad ligament N73.2
      acute N73.0
      chronic N73.1
   Brodie's (localized) (chronic) M86.8X- ☑
   bronchi J98.09
   buccal cavity K12.2
   bulbourethral gland N34.0
   bursa M71.00
      ankle M71.07- ☑
      elbow M71.02- ☑
      foot M71.07- ☑
      hand M71.04- ☑
      hip M71.05- ☑
      knee M71.06- ☑
      multiple sites M71.09
      pharyngeal J39.1
      shoulder M71.01- ☑
      specified site NEC M71.08
      wrist M71.03- ☑
   buttock L02.31
   canthus — *see* Blepharoconjunctivitis
   cartilage — *see* Disorder, cartilage, specified type NEC
   cecum K35.3
   cerebellum, cerebellar G06.0
      sequelae G09
   cerebral (embolic) G06.0
      sequelae G09
   cervical (meaning neck) L02.11
      lymph gland or node L04.0
   cervix (stump) (uteri) — *see* Cervicitis
   cheek (external) L02.01
      inner K12.2
   chest J86.9
      with fistula J86.0
      wall L02.213

Abscess — continued
  chin L02.01
  choroid — see Inflammation, chorioretinal
  circumtonsillar J36
  cold (lung) (tuberculous) (see also Tuberculosis, abscess, lung)
    articular — see Tuberculosis, joint
  colon (wall) K63.0
  colostomy K94.02
  conjunctiva — see Conjunctivitis, acute
  cornea H16.31- ☑
  corpus
    cavernosum N48.21
    luteum — see Oophoritis
  Cowper's gland N34.0
  cranium G06.0
  cul-de-sac (Douglas') (posterior) — see Peritonitis, pelvic, female
  cutaneous — see Abscess, by site
  dental K04.7
    with sinus (alveolar) K04.6
  dentoalveolar K04.7
    with sinus K04.6
  diaphragm, diaphragmatic K65.1
  Douglas' cul-de-sac or pouch — see Peritonitis, pelvic, female
  Dubois A50.59
  ear (middle) (see also Otitis, media, suppurative)
    acute — see Otitis, media, suppurative, acute
    external H60.0- ☑
  entamebic — see Abscess, amebic
  enterostomy K94.12
  epididymis N45.4
  epidural G06.2
    brain G06.0
    spinal cord G06.1
  epiglottis J38.7
  epiploon, epiploic K65.1
  erysipelatous — see Erysipelas
  esophagus K20.8
  ethmoid (bone) (chronic) (sinus) J32.2
  external auditory canal — see Abscess, ear, external
  extradural G06.2
    brain G06.0
      sequelae G09
    spinal cord G06.1
  extraperitoneal K68.19
  eye — see Endophthalmitis, purulent
  eyelid H00.03- ☑
  face (any part, except ear, eye and nose) L02.01
  fallopian tube — see Salpingitis
  fascia M72.8
  fauces J39.1
  fecal K63.0
  femoral (region) — see Abscess, lower limb
  filaria, filarial — see Infestation, filarial
  finger (any) (see also Abscess, hand)
    nail — see Cellulitis, finger
  foot L02.61- ☑
  forehead L02.01
  frontal sinus (chronic) J32.1
  gallbladder K81.0
  genital organ or tract
    female (external) N76.4
    male N49.9
      multiple sites N49.8
      specified NEC N49.8
  gestational mammary O91.11- ☑
  gestational subareolar O91.11- ☑
  gingival — see Peridontitis, aggressive, localized
  gland, glandular (lymph) (acute) — see Lymphadenitis, acute
  gluteal (region) L02.31
  gonorrheal — see Gonococcus
  groin L02.214
  gum — see Peridontitis, aggressive, localized
  hand L02.51- ☑
  head NEC L02.811
    face (any part, except ear, eye and nose) L02.01
  heart — see Carditis
  heel — see Abscess, foot
  helminthic — see Infestation, helminth
  hepatic (cholangitic) (hematogenic) (lymphogenic) (pylephlebitic) K75.0
    amebic A06.4
  hip (region) — see Abscess, lower limb
  ileocecal K35.3
  ileostomy (bud) K94.12

Abscess — continued
  iliac (region) L02.214
    fossa K35.3
  infraclavicular (fossa) — see Abscess, upper limb
  inguinal (region) L02.214
    lymph gland or node L04.1
  intestine, intestinal NEC K63.0
    rectal K61.1
  intra-abdominal (see also Abscess, peritoneum) K65.1
    postprocedural T81.4 ☑
      retroperitoneal K68.11
  intracranial G06.0
  intramammary — see Abscess, breast
  intraorbital — see Abscess, orbit
  intraperitoneal K65.1
  intrasphincteric (anus) K61.4
  intraspinal G06.1
  intratonsillar J36
  ischiorectal (fossa) K61.3
  jaw (bone) (lower) (upper) M27.2
  joint — see Arthritis, pyogenic or pyemic
    spine (tuberculous) A18.01
      nontuberculous — see Spondylopathy, infective
  kidney N15.1
    with calculus N20.0
      with hydronephrosis N13.6
    puerperal (postpartum) O86.21
  knee (see also Abscess, lower limb)
    joint M00.9
  labium (majus) (minus) N76.4
  lacrimal
    caruncle — see Inflammation, lacrimal, passages, acute
    gland — see Dacryoadenitis
    passages (duct) (sac) — see Inflammation, lacrimal, passages, acute
  lacunar N34.0
  larynx J38.7
  lateral (alveolar) K04.7
    with sinus K04.6
  leg (any part) — see Abscess, lower limb
  lens H27.8
  lingual K14.0
    tonsil J36
  lip K13.0
  Littre's gland N34.0
  liver (cholangitic) (hematogenic) (lymphogenic) (pylephlebitic) (pyogenic) K75.0
    amebic (due to Entamoeba histolytica) (dysenteric) (tropical) A06.4
      with
        brain abscess (and liver or lung abscess) A06.6
        lung abscess A06.5
  loin (region) L02.211
  lower limb L02.41- ☑
  lumbar (tuberculous) A18.01
    nontuberculous L02.212
  lung (miliary) (putrid) J85.2
    with pneumonia J85.1
      due to specified organism (see Pneumonia, in (due to))
    amebic (with liver abscess) A06.5
      with
        brain abscess A06.6
        pneumonia A06.5
  lymph, lymphatic, gland or node (acute) (see also Lymphadenitis, acute)
    mesentery I88.0
  malar M27.2
  mammary gland — see Abscess, breast
  marginal, anus K61.0
  mastoid — see Mastoiditis, acute
  maxilla, maxillary M27.2
    molar (tooth) K04.7
      with sinus K04.6
    premolar K04.7
    sinus (chronic) J32.0
  mediastinum J85.3
  meibomian gland — see Hordeolum
  meninges G06.2
  mesentery, mesenteric K65.1
  mesosalpinx — see Salpingitis
  mons pubis L02.215
  mouth (floor) K12.2
  muscle — see Myositis, infective
  myocardium I40.0

Abscess — continued
  nabothian (follicle) — see Cervicitis
  nasal J32.9
  nasopharyngeal J39.1
  navel L02.216
    newborn P38.9
      with mild hemorrhage P38.1
      without hemorrhage P38.9
  neck (region) L02.11
    lymph gland or node L04.0
  nephritic — see Abscess, kidney
  nipple N61.1
    associated with
      lactation — see Pregnancy, complicated by
      pregnancy — see Pregnancy, complicated by
  nose (external) (fossa) (septum) J34.0
    sinus (chronic) — see Sinusitis
  omentum K65.1
  operative wound T81.4 ☑
  orbit, orbital — see Cellulitis, orbit
  otogenic G06.0
  ovary, ovarian (corpus luteum) — see Oophoritis
  oviduct — see Oophoritis
  palate (soft) K12.2
    hard M27.2
  palmar (space) — see Abscess, hand
  pancreas (duct) — see Pancreatitis, acute
  parafrenal N48.21
  parametric, parametrium N73.2
    acute N73.0
    chronic N73.1
  paranephric N15.1
  parapancreatic — see Pancreatitis, acute
  parapharyngeal J39.0
  pararectal K61.1
  parasinus — see Sinusitis
  parauterine (see also Disease, pelvis, inflammatory) N73.2
  paravaginal — see Vaginitis
  parietal region (scalp) L02.811
  parodontal — see Peridontitis, aggressive, localized
  parotid (duct) (gland) K11.3
    region K12.2
  pectoral (region) L02.213
  pelvis, pelvic
    female — see Disease, pelvis, inflammatory
    male, peritoneal K65.1
  penis N48.21
    gonococcal (accessory gland) (periurethral) A54.1
  perianal K61.0
  periapical K04.7
    with sinus (alveolar) K04.6
  periappendicular K35.3
  pericardial I30.1
  pericecal K35.3
  pericemental — see Peridontitis, aggressive, localized
  pericholecystic — see Cholecystitis, acute
  pericoronal — see Peridontitis, aggressive, localized
  peridental — see Peridontitis, aggressive, localized
  perimetric (see also Disease, pelvis, inflammatory) N73.2
  perinephric, perinephritic — see Abscess, kidney
  perineum, perineal (superficial) L02.215
    urethra N34.0
  periodontal (parietal) — see Peridontitis, aggressive, localized
    apical K04.7
  periosteum, periosteal (see also Osteomyelitis, specified type NEC)
    with osteomyelitis (see also Osteomyelitis, specified type NEC)
      acute — see Osteomyelitis, acute
      chronic — see Osteomyelitis, chronic
  peripharyngeal J39.0
  peripleuritic J86.9
    with fistula J86.0
  periprostatic N41.2
  perirectal K61.1
  perirenal (tissue) — see Abscess, kidney
  perisinuous (nose) — see Sinusitis
  peritoneum, peritoneal (perforated) (ruptured) K65.1
    with appendicitis K35.3
    pelvic
      female — see Peritonitis, pelvic, female
      male K65.1
    postoperative T81.4 ☑
    puerperal, postpartum, childbirth O85
    tuberculous A18.31

Abscess — *continued*
peritonsillar J36
perityphlic K35.3
periureteral N28.89
periurethral N34.0
   gonococcal (accessory gland) (periurethral) A54.1
periuterine (*see also* Disease, pelvis, inflammatory) N73.2
perivesical — *see* Cystitis, specified type NEC
petrous bone — *see* Petrositis
phagedenic NOS L02.91
   chancroid A57
pharynx, pharyngeal (lateral) J39.1
pilonidal L05.01
pituitary (gland) E23.6
pleura J86.9
   with fistula J86.0
popliteal — *see* Abscess, lower limb
postcecal K35.3
postlaryngeal J38.7
postnasal J34.0
postoperative (any site) T81.4 ☑
   retroperitoneal K68.11
postpharyngeal J39.0
posttonsillar J36
post-typhoid A01.09
pouch of Douglas — *see* Peritonitis, pelvic, female
premammary — *see* Abscess, breast
prepatellar — *see* Abscess, lower limb
prostate N41.2
   gonococcal (acute) (chronic) A54.22
psoas muscle K68.12
puerperal — *code by* site under Puerperal, abscess
pulmonary — *see* Abscess, lung
pulp, pulpal (dental) K04.01
   irreversible K04.02
   reversible K04.01
rectovaginal septum K63.0
rectovesical — *see* Cystitis, specified type NEC
rectum K61.1
renal — *see* Abscess, kidney
retina — *see* Inflammation, chorioretinal
retrobulbar — *see* Abscess, orbit
retrocecal K65.1
retrolaryngeal J38.7
retromammary — *see* Abscess, breast
retroperitoneal NEC K68.19
   postprocedural K68.11
retropharyngeal J39.0
retrouterine — *see* Peritonitis, pelvic, female
retrovesical — *see* Cystitis, specified type NEC
root, tooth K04.7
   with sinus (alveolar) K04.6
round ligament (*see also* Disease, pelvis, inflammatory) N73.2
rupture (spontaneous) NOS L02.91
sacrum (tuberculous) A18.01
   nontuberculous M46.28
salivary (duct) (gland) K11.3
scalp (any part) L02.811
scapular — *see* Osteomyelitis, specified type NEC
sclera — *see* Scleritis
scrofulous (tuberculous) A18.2
scrotum N49.2
seminal vesicle N49.0
septal, dental K04.7
   with sinus (alveolar) K04.6
serous — *see* Periostitis
shoulder (region) — *see* Abscess, upper limb
sigmoid K63.0
sinus (accessory) (chronic) (nasal) (*see also* Sinusitis)
   intracranial venous (any) G06.0
Skene's duct or gland N34.0
skin — *see* Abscess, by site
specified site NEC L02.818
spermatic cord N49.1
sphenoidal (sinus) (chronic) J32.3
spinal cord (any part) (staphylococcal) G06.1
   tuberculous A17.81
spine (column) (tuberculous) A18.01
   epidural G06.1
   nontuberculous — *see* Osteomyelitis, vertebra
spleen D73.3
   amebic A06.89
stitch T81.4 ☑
subarachnoid G06.2
   brain G06.0
   spinal cord G06.1

Abscess — *continued*
subareolar — *see* Abscess, breast
subcecal K35.3
subcutaneous (*see also* Abscess, by site)
   pheomycotic (chromomycotic) B43.2
subdiaphragmatic K65.1
subdural G06.2
   brain G06.0
     sequelae G09
   spinal cord G06.1
subgaleal L02.811
subhepatic K65.1
sublingual K12.2
   gland K11.3
submammary — *see* Abscess, breast
submandibular (region) (space) (triangle) K12.2
   gland K11.3
submaxillary (region) L02.01
   gland K11.3
submental L02.01
   gland K11.3
subperiosteal — *see* Osteomyelitis, specified type NEC
subphrenic K65.1
   postoperative T81.4 ☑
suburethral N34.0
sudoriparous L75.8
supraclavicular (fossa) — *see* Abscess, upper limb
suprapelvic, acute N73.0
suprarenal (capsule) (gland) E27.8
sweat gland L74.8
tear duct — *see* Inflammation, lacrimal, passages, acute
temple L02.01
temporal region L02.01
temporosphenoidal G06.0
tendon (sheath) M65.00
   ankle M65.07- ☑
   foot M65.07- ☑
   forearm M65.03- ☑
   hand M65.04- ☑
   lower leg M65.06- ☑
   pelvic region M65.05- ☑
   shoulder region M65.01- ☑
   specified site NEC M65.08
   thigh M65.05- ☑
   upper arm M65.02- ☑
testis N45.4
thigh — *see* Abscess, lower limb
thorax J86.9
   with fistula J86.0
throat J39.1
thumb (*see also* Abscess, hand)
   nail — *see* Cellulitis, finger
thymus (gland) E32.1
thyroid (gland) E06.0
toe (any) (*see also* Abscess, foot)
   nail — *see* Cellulitis, toe
tongue (staphylococcal) K14.0
tonsil(s) (lingual) J36
tonsillopharyngeal J36
tooth, teeth (root) K04.7
   with sinus (alveolar) K04.6
   supporting structures NEC — *see* Peridontitis, aggressive, localized
trachea J39.8
trunk L02.219
   abdominal wall L02.211
   back L02.212
   chest wall L02.213
   groin L02.214
   perineum L02.215
   umbilicus L02.216
tubal — *see* Salpingitis
tuberculous — *see* Tuberculosis, abscess
tubo-ovarian — *see* Salpingo-oophoritis
tunica vaginalis N49.1
umbilicus L02.216
upper
   limb L02.41- ☑
   respiratory J39.8
urethral (gland) N34.0
urinary N34.0
uterus, uterine (wall) (*see also* Endometritis)
   ligament (*see also* Disease, pelvis, inflammatory) N73.2
   neck — *see* Cervicitis
uvula K12.2
vagina (wall) — *see* Vaginitis

Abscess — *continued*
vaginorectal — *see* Vaginitis
vas deferens N49.1
vermiform appendix K35.3
vertebra (column) (tuberculous) A18.01
   nontuberculous — *see* Osteomyelitis, vertebra
vesical — *see* Cystitis, specified type NEC
vesico-uterine pouch — *see* Peritonitis, pelvic, female
vitreous (humor) — *see* Endophthalmitis, purulent
vocal cord J38.3
von Bezold's — *see* Mastoiditis, acute
vulva N76.4
vulvovaginal gland N75.1
web space — *see* Abscess, hand
wound T81.4 ☑
wrist — *see* Abscess, upper limb
Absence (of) (organ or part) (complete or partial)
adrenal (gland) (congenital) Q89.1
   acquired E89.6
albumin in blood E88.09
alimentary tract (congenital) Q45.8
   upper Q40.8
alveolar process (acquired) — *see* Anomaly, alveolar
ankle (acquired) Z89.44- ☑
anus (congenital) Q42.3
   with fistula Q42.2
aorta (congenital) Q25.41
appendix, congenital Q42.8
arm (acquired) Z89.20- ☑
   above elbow Z89.22- ☑
     congenital (with hand present) — *see* Agenesis, arm, with hand present
     and hand — *see* Agenesis, forearm, and hand
   below elbow Z89.21- ☑
     congenital (with hand present) — *see* Agenesis, arm, with hand present
     and hand — *see* Agenesis, forearm, and hand
   congenital — *see* Defect, reduction, upper limb
   shoulder (following explantation of shoulder joint prosthesis) (joint) (with or without presence of antibiotic-impregnated cement spacer) Z89.23- ☑
     congenital (with hand present) — *see* Agenesis, arm, with hand present
artery (congenital) (peripheral) Q27.8
   brain Q28.3
   coronary Q24.5
   pulmonary Q25.79
   specified NEC Q27.8
   umbilical Q27.0
atrial septum (congenital) Q21.1
auditory canal (congenital) (external) Q16.1
auricle (ear), congenital Q16.0
bile, biliary duct, congenital Q44.5
bladder (acquired) Z90.6
   congenital Q64.5
bowel sounds R19.11
brain Q00.0
   part of Q04.3
breast(s) (and nipple(s)) (acquired) Z90.1- ☑
   congenital Q83.8
broad ligament Q50.6
bronchus (congenital) Q32.4
canaliculus lacrimalis, congenital Q10.4
cerebellum (vermis) Q04.3
cervix (acquired) (with uterus) Z90.710
   with remaining uterus Z90.712
   congenital Q51.5
chin, congenital Q18.8
cilia (congenital) Q10.3
   acquired — *see* Madarosis
clitoris (congenital) Q52.6
coccyx, congenital Q76.49
cold sense R20.8
congenital
   lumen — *see* Atresia
   organ or site NEC — *see* Agenesis
   septum — *see* Imperfect, closure
corpus callosum Q04.0
cricoid cartilage, congenital Q31.8
diaphragm (with hernia), congenital Q79.1
digestive organ(s) or tract, congenital Q45.8
   acquired NEC Z90.49
   upper Q40.8
ductus arteriosus Q28.8
duodenum (acquired) Z90.49

Absence — *continued*
  duodenum — *continued*
    congenital Q41.0
  ear, congenital Q16.9
    acquired H93.8- ☑
    auricle Q16.0
    external Q16.0
    inner Q16.5
    lobe, lobule Q17.8
    middle, except ossicles Q16.4
      ossicles Q16.3
    ossicles Q16.3
  ejaculatory duct (congenital) Q55.4
  endocrine gland (congenital) NEC Q89.2
    acquired E89.89
  epididymis (congenital) Q55.4
    acquired Z90.79
  epiglottis, congenital Q31.8
  esophagus (congenital) Q39.8
    acquired (partial) Z90.49
  eustachian tube (congenital) Q16.2
  extremity (acquired) Z89.9
    congenital Q73.0
    knee (following explantation of knee joint prosthe-
        sis) (joint) (with or without presence of an-
        tibiotic-impregnated cement spacer)
        Z89.52- ☑
    lower (above knee) Z89.619
      below knee Z89.51- ☑
    upper — *see* Absence, arm
  eye (acquired) Z90.01
    congenital Q11.1
    muscle (congenital) Q10.3
  eyeball (acquired) Z90.01
  eyelid (fold) (congenital) Q10.3
    acquired Z90.01
  face, specified part NEC Q18.8
  fallopian tube(s) (acquired) Z90.79
    congenital Q50.6
  family member (causing problem in home) NEC (*see
    also* Disruption, family) Z63.32
  femur, congenital — *see* Defect, reduction, lower limb,
    longitudinal, femur
  fibrinogen (congenital) D68.2
    acquired D65
  finger(s) (acquired) Z89.02- ☑
    congenital — *see* Agenesis, hand
  foot (acquired) Z89.43- ☑
    congenital — *see* Agenesis, foot
  forearm (acquired) — *see* Absence, arm, below elbow
  gallbladder (acquired) Z90.49
    congenital Q44.0
  gamma globulin in blood D80.1
    hereditary D80.0
  genital organs
    acquired (female) (male) Z90.79
    female, congenital Q52.8
      external Q52.71
      internal NEC Q52.8
    male, congenital Q55.8
  genitourinary organs, congenital NEC
    female Q52.8
    male Q55.8
  globe (acquired) Z90.01
    congenital Q11.1
  glottis, congenital Q31.8
  hand and wrist (acquired) Z89.11- ☑
    congenital — *see* Agenesis, hand
  head, part (acquired) NEC Z90.09
  heat sense R20.8
  hip (following explantation of hip joint prosthesis)
      (joint) (with or without presence of antibiotic-
      impregnated cement spacer) Z89.62- ☑
  hymen (congenital) Q52.4
  ileum (acquired) Z90.49
    congenital Q41.2
  immunoglobulin, isolated NEC D80.3
    IgA D80.2
    IgG D80.3
    IgM D80.4
  incus (acquired) — *see* Loss, ossicles, ear
    congenital Q16.3
  inner ear, congenital Q16.5
  intestine (acquired) (small) Z90.49
    congenital Q41.9
      specified NEC Q41.8
    large Z90.49
      congenital Q42.9

Absence — *continued*
  intestine — *continued*
    large — *continued*
      congenital — *continued*
        specified NEC Q42.8
  iris, congenital Q13.1
  jejunum (acquired) Z90.49
    congenital Q41.1
  joint
    acquired
      hip (following explantation of hip joint prosthe-
          sis) (with or without presence of antibiot-
          ic-impregnated cement spacer)
          Z89.62- ☑
      knee (following explantation of knee joint
          prosthesis) (with or without presence of
          antibiotic-impregnated cement spacer)
          Z89.52- ☑
      shoulder (following explantation of shoulder
          joint prosthesis) (with or without pres-
          ence of antibiotic-impregnated cement
          spacer) Z89.23- ☑
    congenital NEC Q74.8
  kidney(s) (acquired) Z90.5
    congenital Q60.2
      bilateral Q60.1
      unilateral Q60.0
  knee (following explantation of knee joint prosthesis)
      (joint) (with or without presence of antibiotic-
      impregnated cement spacer) Z89.52- ☑
  labyrinth, membranous Q16.5
  larynx (congenital) Q31.8
    acquired Z90.02
  leg (acquired) (above knee) Z89.61- ☑
    below knee (acquired) Z89.51- ☑
    congenital — *see* Defect, reduction, lower limb
  lens (acquired) (*see also* Aphakia)
    congenital Q12.3
    post cataract extraction Z98.4- ☑
  limb (acquired) — *see* Absence, extremity
  lip Q38.6
  liver (congenital) Q44.7
  lung (fissure) (lobe) (bilateral) (unilateral) (congenital)
      Q33.3
    acquired (any part) Z90.2
  menstruation — *see* Amenorrhea
  muscle (congenital) (pectoral) Q79.8
    ocular Q10.3
  neck, part Q18.8
  neutrophil — *see* Agranulocytosis
  nipple(s) (with breast(s)) (acquired) Z90.1- ☑
    congenital Q83.2
  nose (congenital) Q30.1
    acquired Z90.09
  organ
    of Corti, congenital Q16.5
    or site, congenital NEC Q89.8
      acquired NEC Z90.89
  osseous meatus (ear) Q16.4
  ovary (acquired)
    bilateral Z90.722
    congenital
      bilateral Q50.02
      unilateral Q50.01
    unilateral Z90.721
  oviduct (acquired)
    bilateral Z90.722
    congenital Q50.6
    unilateral Z90.721
  pancreas (congenital) Q45.0
    acquired Z90.410
      complete Z90.410
      partial Z90.411
      total Z90.410
  parathyroid gland (acquired) E89.2
    congenital Q89.2
  patella, congenital Q74.1
  penis (congenital) Q55.5
    acquired Z90.79
  pericardium (congenital) Q24.8
  pituitary gland (congenital) Q89.2
    acquired E89.3
  prostate (acquired) Z90.79
    congenital Q55.4
  pulmonary valve Q22.0
  punctum lacrimale (congenital) Q10.4
  radius, congenital — *see* Defect, reduction, upper limb,
    longitudinal, radius

Absence — *continued*
  rectum (congenital) Q42.1
    with fistula Q42.0
    acquired Z90.49
  respiratory organ NOS Q34.9
  rib (acquired) Z90.89
    congenital Q76.6
  sacrum, congenital Q76.49
  salivary gland(s), congenital Q38.4
  scrotum, congenital Q55.29
  seminal vesicles (congenital) Q55.4
    acquired Z90.79
  septum
    atrial (congenital) Q21.1
    between aorta and pulmonary artery Q21.4
    ventricular (congenital) Q20.4
  sex chromosome
    female phenotype Q97.8
    male phenotype Q98.8
  skull bone (congenital) Q75.8
    with
      anencephaly Q00.0
      encephalocele — *see* Encephalocele
      hydrocephalus Q03.9
        with spina bifida — *see* Spina bifida, by site,
          with hydrocephalus
      microcephaly Q02
  spermatic cord, congenital Q55.4
  spine, congenital Q76.49
  spleen (congenital) Q89.01
    acquired Z90.81
  sternum, congenital Q76.7
  stomach (acquired) (partial) Z90.3
    congenital Q40.2
  superior vena cava, congenital Q26.8
  teeth, tooth (congenital) K00.0
    acquired (complete) K08.109
      class I K08.101
      class II K08.102
      class III K08.103
      class IV K08.104
      due to
        caries K08.139
          class I K08.131
          class II K08.132
          class III K08.133
          class IV K08.134
        periodontal disease K08.129
          class I K08.121
          class II K08.122
          class III K08.123
          class IV K08.124
        specified NEC K08.199
          class I K08.191
          class II K08.192
          class III K08.193
          class IV K08.194
        trauma K08.119
          class I K08.111
          class II K08.112
          class III K08.113
          class IV K08.114
      partial K08.409
        class I K08.401
        class II K08.402
        class III K08.403
        class IV K08.404
        due to
          caries K08.439
            class I K08.431
            class II K08.432
            class III K08.433
            class IV K08.434
          periodontal disease K08.429
            class I K08.421
            class II K08.422
            class III K08.423
            class IV K08.424
          specified NEC K08.499
            class I K08.491
            class II K08.492
            class III K08.493
            class IV K08.494
          trauma K08.419
            class I K08.411
            class II K08.412
            class III K08.413
            class IV K08.414
  tendon (congenital) Q79.8

Absence — *continued*
  testis (congenital) Q55.0
    acquired Z90.79
  thumb (acquired) Z89.01- ☑
    congenital — *see* Agenesis, hand
  thymus gland Q89.2
  thyroid (gland) (acquired) E89.0
    cartilage, congenital Q31.8
    congenital E03.1
  toe(s) (acquired) Z89.42- ☑
    with foot — *see* Absence, foot and ankle
    congenital — *see* Agenesis, foot
    great Z89.41- ☑
  tongue, congenital Q38.3
  trachea (cartilage), congenital Q32.1
  transverse aortic arch, congenital Q25.49
  tricuspid valve Q22.4
  umbilical artery, congenital Q27.0
  upper arm and forearm with hand present, congenital — *see* Agenesis, arm, with hand present
  ureter (congenital) Q62.4
    acquired Z90.6
  urethra, congenital Q64.5
  uterus (acquired) Z90.710
    with cervix Z90.710
    with remaining cervical stump Z90.711
    congenital Q51.0
  uvula, congenital Q38.5
  vagina, congenital Q52.0
  vas deferens (congenital) Q55.4
    acquired Z90.79
  vein (peripheral) congenital NEC Q27.8
    cerebral Q28.3
    digestive system Q27.8
    great Q26.8
    lower limb Q27.8
    portal Q26.5
    precerebral Q28.1
    specified site NEC Q27.8
    upper limb Q27.8
  vena cava (inferior) (superior), congenital Q26.8
  ventricular septum Q20.4
  vertebra, congenital Q76.49
  vulva, congenital Q52.71
  wrist (acquired) Z89.12- ☑

Absorbent system disease I87.8

Absorption
  carbohydrate, disturbance K90.49
  chemical — *see* Table of Drugs and Chemicals
    through placenta (newborn) P04.9
      environmental substance P04.6
      nutritional substance P04.5
      obstetric anesthetic or analgesic drug P04.0
  drug NEC — *see* Table of Drugs and Chemicals
    addictive
      through placenta (newborn) P04.49
        cocaine P04.41
    medicinal
      through placenta (newborn) P04.1
    through placenta (newborn) P04.1
      obstetric anesthetic or analgesic drug P04.0
  fat, disturbance K90.49
    pancreatic K90.3
  noxious substance — *see* Table of Drugs and Chemicals
  protein, disturbance K90.49
  starch, disturbance K90.49
  toxic substance — *see* Table of Drugs and Chemicals
  uremic — *see* Uremia

Abstinence symptoms, syndrome
  alcohol F10.239
    with delirium F10.231
  cocaine F14.23
  neonatal P96.1
  nicotine — *see* Dependence, drug, nicotine, with, withdrawal
  opioid F11.93
    with dependence F11.23
  psychoactive NEC F19.939
    with
      delirium F19.931
      dependence F19.239
        with
          delirium F19.231
          perceptual disturbance F19.232
        uncomplicated F19.230
      perceptual disturbance F19.932
      uncomplicated F19.930

Abstinence symptoms, syndrome — *continued*
  sedative F13.939
    with
      delirium F13.931
      dependence F13.239
        with
          delirium F13.231
          perceptual disturbance F13.232
        uncomplicated F13.230
      perceptual disturbance F13.932
      uncomplicated F13.930
  stimulant NEC F15.93
    with dependence F15.23

Abulia R68.89

Abulomania F60.7

Abuse
  adult — *see* Maltreatment, adult
    as reason for
      couple seeking advice (including offender) Z63.0
  alcohol (non-dependent) F10.10
    with
      anxiety disorder F10.180
      intoxication F10.129
        with delirium F10.121
        uncomplicated F10.120
      mood disorder F10.14
      other specified disorder F10.188
      psychosis F10.159
        delusions F10.150
        hallucinations F10.151
      sexual dysfunction F10.181
      sleep disorder F10.182
      unspecified disorder F10.19
    counseling and surveillance Z71.41
    in remission (early) (sustained) F10.11
  amphetamine (or related substance) — *see* Abuse, drug, stimulant NEC
  analgesics (non-prescribed) (over the counter) F55.8
  antacids F55.0
  antidepressants — *see* Abuse, drug, psychoactive NEC
  anxiolytic — *see* Abuse, drug, sedative
  barbiturates — *see* Abuse, drug, sedative
  caffeine — *see* Abuse, drug, stimulant NEC
  cannabis, cannabinoids — *see* Abuse, drug, cannabis
  child — *see* Maltreatment, child
  cocaine — *see* Abuse, drug, cocaine
  drug NEC (non-dependent) F19.10
    with sleep disorder F19.182
    amphetamine type — *see* Abuse, drug, stimulant NEC
    analgesics (non-prescribed) (over the counter) F55.8
    antacids F55.0
    antidepressants — *see* Abuse, drug, psychoactive NEC
    anxiolytics — *see* Abuse, drug, sedative
    barbiturates — *see* Abuse, drug, sedative
    caffeine — *see* Abuse, drug, stimulant NEC
    cannabis F12.10
      with
        anxiety disorder F12.180
        intoxication F12.129
          with
            delirium F12.121
            perceptual disturbance F12.122
          uncomplicated F12.120
        other specified disorder F12.188
        psychosis F12.159
          delusions F12.150
          hallucinations F12.151
        unspecified disorder F12.19
      in remission (early) (sustained) F12.11
    cocaine F14.10
      with
        anxiety disorder F14.180
        intoxication F14.129
          with
            delirium F14.121
            perceptual disturbance F14.122
          uncomplicated F14.120
        mood disorder F14.14
        other specified disorder F14.188
        psychosis F14.159
          delusions F14.150
          hallucinations F14.151
        sexual dysfunction F14.181
        sleep disorder F14.182

Abuse — *continued*
  drug — *continued*
    cocaine — *continued*
      with — *continued*
        unspecified disorder F14.19
      in remission (early) (sustained) F14.11
    counseling and surveillance Z71.51
    hallucinogen F16.10
      with
        anxiety disorder F16.180
        flashbacks F16.183
        intoxication F16.129
          with
            delirium F16.121
            perceptual disturbance F16.122
          uncomplicated F16.120
        mood disorder F16.14
        other specified disorder F16.188
        perception disorder, persisting F16.183
        psychosis F16.159
          delusions F16.150
          hallucinations F16.151
        unspecified disorder F16.19
      in remission (early) (sustained) F16.11
    hashish — *see* Abuse, drug, cannabis
    herbal or folk remedies F55.1
    hormones F55.3
    hypnotics — *see* Abuse, drug, sedative
    in remission (early) (sustained) F19.11
    inhalant F18.10
      with
        anxiety disorder F18.180
        dementia, persisting F18.17
        intoxication F18.129
          with delirium F18.121
          uncomplicated F18.120
        mood disorder F18.14
        other specified disorder F18.188
        psychosis F18.159
          delusions F18.150
          hallucinations F18.151
        unspecified disorder F18.19
      in remission (early) (sustained) F18.11
    laxatives F55.2
    LSD — *see* Abuse, drug, hallucinogen
    marihuana — *see* Abuse, drug, cannabis
    morphine type (opioids) — *see* Abuse, drug, opioid
    opioid F11.10
      with
        intoxication F11.129
          with
            delirium F11.121
            perceptual disturbance F11.122
          uncomplicated F11.120
        mood disorder F11.14
        other specified disorder F11.188
        psychosis F11.159
          delusions F11.150
          hallucinations F11.151
        sexual dysfunction F11.181
        sleep disorder F11.182
        unspecified disorder F11.19
      in remission (early) (sustained) F11.11
    PCP (phencyclidine) (or related substance) — *see* Abuse, drug, hallucinogen
    psychoactive NEC F19.10
      with
        amnestic disorder F19.16
        anxiety disorder F19.180
        dementia F19.17
        intoxication F19.129
          with
            delirium F19.121
            perceptual disturbance F19.122
          uncomplicated F19.120
        mood disorder F19.14
        other specified disorder F19.188
        psychosis F19.159
          delusions F19.150
          hallucinations F19.151
        sexual dysfunction F19.181
        sleep disorder F19.182
        unspecified disorder F19.19
    sedative, hypnotic or anxiolytic F13.10
      with
        anxiety disorder F13.180
        intoxication F13.129
          with delirium F13.121
          uncomplicated F13.120

Abuse — *continued*
  drug — *continued*
    sedative, hypnotic or anxiolytic — *continued*
      with — *continued*
        mood disorder F13.14
        other specified disorder F13.188
        psychosis F13.159
          delusions F13.150
          hallucinations F13.151
        sexual dysfunction F13.181
        sleep disorder F13.182
        unspecified disorder F13.19
      in remission (early) (sustained) F13.11
    solvent — *see* Abuse, drug, inhalant
    steroids F55.3
    stimulant NEC F15.10
      with
        anxiety disorder F15.180
        intoxication F15.129
          with
            delirium F15.121
            perceptual disturbance F15.122
          uncomplicated F15.120
        mood disorder F15.14
        other specified disorder F15.188
        psychosis F15.159
          delusions F15.150
          hallucinations F15.151
        sexual dysfunction F15.181
        sleep disorder F15.182
        unspecified disorder F15.19
      in remission (early) (sustained) F15.11
    tranquilizers — *see* Abuse, drug, sedative
    vitamins F55.4
  hallucinogens — *see* Abuse, drug, hallucinogen
  hashish — *see* Abuse, drug, cannabis
  herbal or folk remedies F55.1
  hormones F55.3
  hypnotic — *see* Abuse, drug, sedative
  inhalant — *see* Abuse, drug, inhalant
  laxatives F55.2
  LSD — *see* Abuse, drug, hallucinogen
  marihuana — *see* Abuse, drug, cannabis
  morphine type (opioids) — *see* Abuse, drug, opioid
  non-psychoactive substance NEC F55.8
    antacids F55.0
    folk remedies F55.1
    herbal remedies F55.1
    hormones F55.3
    laxatives F55.2
    steroids F55.3
    vitamins F55.4
  opioids — *see* Abuse, drug, opioid
  PCP (phencyclidine) (or related substance) — *see* Abuse, drug, hallucinogen
  physical (adult) (child) — *see* Maltreatment
  psychoactive substance — *see* Abuse, drug, psychoactive NEC
  psychological (adult) (child) — *see* Maltreatment
  sedative — *see* Abuse, drug, sedative
  sexual — *see* Maltreatment
  solvent — *see* Abuse, drug, inhalant
  steroids F55.3
  vitamins F55.4
Acalculia R48.8
  developmental F81.2
Acanthamebiasis (with) B60.10
  conjunctiva B60.12
  keratoconjunctivitis B60.13
  meningoencephalitis B60.11
  other specified B60.19
Acanthocephaliasis B83.8
Acanthocheilonemiasis B74.4
Acanthocytosis E78.6
Acantholysis L11.9
Acanthosis (acquired) (nigricans) L83
  benign Q82.8
  congenital Q82.8
  seborrheic L82.1
    inflamed L82.0
  tongue K14.3
Acapnia E87.3
Acarbia E87.2
Acardia, acardius Q89.8
Acardiacus amorphus Q89.8
Acardiotrophia I51.4
Acariasis B88.0
  scabies B86

Acarodermatitis (urticarioides) B88.0
Acarophobia F40.218
Acatalasemia, acatalasia E80.3
Acathisia (drug induced) G25.71
Accelerated atrioventricular conduction I45.6
Accentuation of personality traits (type A) Z73.1
Accessory (congenital)
  adrenal gland Q89.1
  anus Q43.4
  appendix Q43.4
  atrioventricular conduction I45.6
  auditory ossicles Q16.3
  auricle (ear) Q17.0
  biliary duct or passage Q44.5
  bladder Q64.79
  blood vessels NEC Q27.9
    coronary Q24.5
  bone NEC Q79.8
  breast tissue, axilla Q83.1
  carpal bones Q74.0
  cecum Q43.4
  chromosome(s) NEC (nonsex) Q92.9
    with complex rearrangements NEC Q92.5
      seen only at prometaphase Q92.8
    13 — *see* Trisomy, 13
    18 — *see* Trisomy, 18
    21 — *see* Trisomy, 21
    partial Q92.9
    sex
      female phenotype Q97.8
  coronary artery Q24.5
  cusp(s), heart valve NEC Q24.8
    pulmonary Q22.3
  cystic duct Q44.5
  digit(s) Q69.9
  ear (auricle) (lobe) Q17.0
  endocrine gland NEC Q89.2
  eye muscle Q10.3
  eyelid Q10.3
  face bone(s) Q75.8
  fallopian tube (fimbria) (ostium) Q50.6
  finger(s) Q69.0
  foreskin N47.8
  frontonasal process Q75.8
  gallbladder Q44.1
  genital organ(s)
    female Q52.8
      external Q52.79
      internal NEC Q52.8
    male Q55.8
  genitourinary organs NEC Q89.8
    female Q52.8
    male Q55.8
  hallux Q69.2
  heart Q24.8
    valve NEC Q24.8
      pulmonary Q22.3
  hepatic ducts Q44.5
  hymen Q52.4
  intestine (large) (small) Q43.4
  kidney Q63.0
  lacrimal canal Q10.6
  leaflet, heart valve NEC Q24.8
  ligament, broad Q50.6
  liver Q44.7
    duct Q44.5
  lobule (ear) Q17.0
  lung (lobe) Q33.1
  muscle Q79.8
  navicular of carpus Q74.0
  nervous system, part NEC Q07.8
  nipple Q83.3
  nose Q30.8
  organ or site not listed — *see* Anomaly, by site
  ovary Q50.31
  oviduct Q50.6
  pancreas Q45.3
  parathyroid gland Q89.2
  parotid gland (and duct) Q38.4
  pituitary gland Q89.2
  preauricular appendage Q17.0
  prepuce N47.8
  renal arteries (multiple) Q27.2
  rib Q76.6
    cervical Q76.5
  roots (teeth) K00.2
  salivary gland Q38.4
  sesamoid bones Q74.8

Accessory — *continued*
  sesamoid bones — *continued*
    foot Q74.2
    hand Q74.0
  skin tags Q82.8
  spleen Q89.09
  sternum Q76.7
  submaxillary gland Q38.4
  tarsal bones Q74.2
  teeth, tooth K00.1
  tendon Q79.8
  thumb Q69.1
  thymus gland Q89.2
  thyroid gland Q89.2
  toes Q69.2
  tongue Q38.3
  tooth, teeth K00.1
  tragus Q17.0
  ureter Q62.5
  urethra Q64.79
  urinary organ or tract NEC Q64.8
  uterus Q51.2
  vagina Q52.10
  valve, heart NEC Q24.8
    pulmonary Q22.3
  vertebra Q76.49
  vocal cords Q31.8
  vulva Q52.79
Accident
  birth — *see* Birth, injury
  cardiac — *see* Infarct, myocardium
  cerebral I63.9
  cerebrovascular (embolic) (ischemic) (thrombotic) I63.9
    aborted I63.9
    hemorrhagic — *see* Hemorrhage, intracranial, intracerebral
    old (without sequelae) Z86.73
      with sequelae (of) — *see* Sequelae, infarction, cerebral
  coronary — *see* Infarct, myocardium
  craniovascular I63.9
  vascular, brain I63.9
Accidental — *see* condition
Accommodation (disorder) (*see also* condition)
  hysterical paralysis of F44.89
  insufficiency of H52.4
  paresis — *see* Paresis, of accommodation
  spasm — *see* Spasm, of accommodation
Accouchement — *see* Delivery
Accreta placenta O43.21- ☑
Accretio cordis (nonrheumatic) I31.0
Accretions, tooth, teeth K03.6
Acculturation difficulty Z60.3
Accumulation secretion, prostate N42.89
Acephalia, acephalism, acephalus, acephaly Q00.0
Acephalobrachia monster Q89.8
Acephalochirus monster Q89.8
Acephalogaster Q89.8
Acephalostomus monster Q89.8
Acephalothorax Q89.8
Acerophobia F40.298
Acetonemia R79.89
  in Type 1 diabetes E10.10
    with coma E10.11
Acetonuria R82.4
Achalasia (cardia) (esophagus) K22.0
  congenital Q39.5
  pylorus Q40.0
  sphincteral NEC K59.8
Ache(s) — *see* Pain
Acheilia Q38.6
Achillobursitis — *see* Tendinitis, Achilles
Achillodynia — *see* Tendinitis, Achilles
Achlorhydria, achlorhydric (neurogenic) K31.83
  anemia D50.8
  diarrhea K31.83
  psychogenic F45.8
  secondary to vagotomy K91.1
Achluophobia F40.228
Acholia K82.8
Acholuric jaundice (familial) (splenomegalic) (*see also* Spherocytosis)
  acquired D59.8
Achondrogenesis Q77.0
Achondroplasia (osteosclerosis congenita) Q77.4
Achroma, cutis L80

Achromat (ism), achromatopsia (acquired) (congenital) H53.51
Achromia, congenital — *see* Albinism
Achromia parasitica B36.0
Achylia gastrica K31.89
  psychogenic F45.8
Acid
  burn — *see* Corrosion
  deficiency
    amide nicotinic E52
    ascorbic E54
    folic E53.8
    nicotinic E52
    pantothenic E53.8
  intoxication E87.2
  peptic disease K30
  phosphatase deficiency E83.39
  stomach K30
    psychogenic F45.8
Acidemia E87.2
  argininosuccinic E72.22
  isovaleric E71.110
  metabolic (newborn) P19.9
    first noted before onset of labor P19.0
    first noted during labor P19.1
    noted at birth P19.2
  methylmalonic E71.120
  pipecolic E72.3
  propionic E71.121
Acidity, gastric (high) K30
  psychogenic F45.8
Acidocytopenia — *see* Agranulocytosis
Acidocytosis D72.1
Acidopenia — *see* Agranulocytosis
Acidosis (lactic) (respiratory) E87.2
  in Type 1 diabetes E10.10
    with coma E10.11
  kidney, tubular N25.89
  lactic E87.2
  metabolic NEC E87.2
    with respiratory acidosis E87.4
    late, of newborn P74.0
  mixed metabolic and respiratory, newborn P84
  newborn P84
  renal (hyperchloremic) (tubular) N25.89
  respiratory E87.2
    complicated by
      metabolic
        acidosis E87.4
        alkalosis E87.4
Aciduria
  argininosuccinic E72.22
  glutaric (type I) E72.3
    type II E71.313 ☑
    type III E71.5- ☑
  orotic (congenital) (hereditary) (pyrimidine deficiency) E79.8
    anemia D53.0
Acladiosis (skin) B36.0
Aclasis, diaphyseal Q78.6
Acleistocardia Q21.1
Aclusion — *see* Anomaly, dentofacial, malocclusion
Acne L70.9
  artificialis L70.8
  atrophica L70.2
  cachecticorum (Hebra) L70.8
  conglobata L70.1
  cystic L70.0
  decalvans L66.2
  excoriée (des jeunes filles) L70.5
  frontalis L70.2
  indurata L70.0
  infantile L70.4
  keloid L73.0
  lupoid L70.2
  necrotic, necrotica (miliaris) L70.2
  neonatal L70.4
  nodular L70.0
  occupational L70.8
  picker's L70.5
  pustular L70.0
  rodens L70.2
  rosacea L71.9
  specified NEC L70.8
  tropica L70.3
  varioliformis L70.2
  vulgaris L70.0
Acnitis (primary) A18.4

Acosta's disease T70.29 ☑
Acoustic — *see* condition
Acousticophobia F40.298
Acquired (*see also* condition)
  immunodeficiency syndrome (AIDS) B20
Acrania Q00.0
Acroangiodermatitis I78.9
Acroasphyxia, chronic I73.89
Acrobystitis N47.7
Acrocephalopolysyndactyly Q87.0
Acrocephalosyndactyly Q87.0
Acrocephaly Q75.0
Acrochondrohyperplasia — *see* Syndrome, Marfan's
Acrocyanosis I73.8 ☑
  newborn P28.2
    meaning transient blue hands and feet — *omit code*
Acrodermatitis L30.8
  atrophicans (chronica) L90.4
  continua (Hallopeau) L40.2
  enteropathica (hereditary) E83.2
  Hallopeau's L40.2
  infantile papular L44.4
  perstans L40.2
  pustulosa continua L40.2
  recalcitrant pustular L40.2
Acrodynia — *see* Poisoning, mercury
Acromegaly, acromegalia E22.0
Acromelalgia I73.81
Acromicria, acromikria Q79.8
Acronyx L60.0
Acropachy, thyroid — *see* Thyrotoxicosis
Acroparesthesia (simple) (vasomotor) I73.89
Acropathy, thyroid — *see* Thyrotoxicosis
Acrophobia F40.241
Acroposthitis N47.7
Acroscleriasis, acroscleroderma, acrosclerosis — *see* Sclerosis, systemic
Acrosphacelus I96
Acrospiroma, eccrine — *see* Neoplasm, skin, benign
Acrostealgia — *see* Osteochondropathy
Acrotrophodynia — *see* Immersion
ACTH ectopic syndrome E24.3
Actinic — *see* condition
Actinobacillosis, actinobacillus A28.8
  mallei A24.0
  muris A25.1
Actinomyces israelii (infection) — *see* Actinomycosis
Actinomycetoma (foot) B47.1
Actinomycosis, actinomycotic A42.9
  with pneumonia A42.0
  abdominal A42.1
  cervicofacial A42.2
  cutaneous A42.89
  gastrointestinal A42.1
  pulmonary A42.0
  sepsis A42.7
  specified site NEC A42.89
Actinoneuritis G62.82
Action, heart
  disorder I49.9
  irregular I49.9
    psychogenic F45.8
Activated protein C resistance D68.51
Activation
  mast cell (disorder) (syndrome) D89.40
    idiopathic D89.42
    monoclonal D89.41
    secondary D89.43
    specified type NEC D89.49
Active — *see* condition
Acute (*see also* condition)
  abdomen R10.0
  gallbladder — *see* Cholecystitis, acute
Acyanotic heart disease (congenital) Q24.9
Acystia Q64.5
Adair-Dighton syndrome (brittle bones and blue sclera, deafness) Q78.0
Adamantinoblastoma — *see* Ameloblastoma
Adamantinoma (*see also* Cyst, calcifying odontogenic)
  long bones C40.90
    lower limb C40.2- ☑
    upper limb C40.0- ☑
  malignant C41.1
    jaw (bone) (lower) C41.1
      upper C41.0
  tibial C40.2- ☑

Adamantoblastoma — *see* Ameloblastoma
Adams-Stokes (-Morgagni) disease or syndrome I45.9
Adaption reaction — *see* Disorder, adjustment
Addiction (*see also* Dependence) F19.20
  alcohol, alcoholic (ethyl) (methyl) (wood) (without remission) F10.20
    with remission F10.21
  drug — *see* Dependence, drug
  ethyl alcohol (without remission) F10.20
    with remission F10.21
  heroin — *see* Dependence, drug, opioid
  methyl alcohol (without remission) F10.20
    with remission F10.21
  methylated spirit (without remission) F10.20
    with remission F10.21
  morphine (-like substances) — *see* Dependence, drug, opioid
  nicotine — *see* Dependence, drug, nicotine
  opium and opioids — *see* Dependence, drug, opioid
  tobacco — *see* Dependence, drug, nicotine
Addison-Biermer anemia (pernicious) D51.0
Addisonian crisis E27.2
Addison's
  anemia (pernicious) D51.0
  disease (bronze) or syndrome E27.1
    tuberculous A18.7
  keloid L94.0
Addison-Schilder complex E71.528
Additional (*see also* Accessory)
  chromosome(s) Q99.8
    21 — *see* Trisomy, 21
    sex — *see* Abnormal, chromosome, sex
Adduction contracture, hip or other joint — *see* Contraction, joint
Adenitis (*see also* Lymphadenitis)
  acute, unspecified site L04.9
  axillary I88.9
    acute L04.2
    chronic or subacute I88.1
  Bartholin's gland N75.8
  bulbourethral gland — *see* Urethritis
  cervical I88.9
    acute L04.0
    chronic or subacute I88.1
  chancroid (Hemophilus ducreyi) A57
  chronic, unspecified site I88.1
  Cowper's gland — *see* Urethritis
  due to Pasteurella multocida (P. septica) A28.0
  epidemic, acute B27.09
  gangrenous L04.9
  gonorrheal NEC A54.89
  groin I88.9
    acute L04.1
    chronic or subacute I88.1
  infectious (acute) (epidemic) B27.09
  inguinal I88.9
    acute L04.1
    chronic or subacute I88.1
  lymph gland or node, except mesenteric I88.9
    acute — *see* Lymphadenitis, acute
    chronic or subacute I88.1
  mesenteric (acute) (chronic) (nonspecific) (subacute) I88.0
  parotid gland (suppurative) — *see* Sialoadenitis
  salivary gland (any) (suppurative) — *see* Sialoadenitis
  scrofulous (tuberculous) A18.2
  Skene's duct or gland — *see* Urethritis
  strumous, tuberculous A18.2
  subacute, unspecified site I88.1
  sublingual gland (suppurative) — *see* Sialoadenitis
  submandibular gland (suppurative) — *see* Sialoadenitis
  submaxillary gland (suppurative) — *see* Sialoadenitis
  tuberculous — *see* Tuberculosis, lymph gland
  urethral gland — *see* Urethritis
  Wharton's duct (suppurative) — *see* Sialoadenitis
Adenoacanthoma — *see* Neoplasm, malignant, by site
Adenoameloblastoma — *see* Cyst, calcifying odontogenic
Adenocarcinoid (tumor) — *see* Neoplasm, malignant, by site
Adenocarcinoma (*see also* Neoplasm, malignant, by site)
  acidophil
    specified site — *see* Neoplasm, malignant, by site
    unspecified site C75.1
  adrenal cortical C74.0- ☑
  alveolar — *see* Neoplasm, lung, malignant

☑ **Additional Character Required** — Refer to the Tabular List for Character Selection ▽ Subterms under main terms may continue to next column or page

Adenocarcinoma — *continued*
  apocrine
    breast — *see* Neoplasm, breast, malignant
    in situ
      breast D05.8- ☑
      specified site NEC — *see* Neoplasm, skin, in situ
      unspecified site D04.9
    specified site NEC — *see* Neoplasm, skin, malignant
    unspecified site C44.99
  basal cell
    specified site — *see* Neoplasm, skin, malignant
    unspecified site C08.9
  basophil
    specified site — *see* Neoplasm, malignant, by site
    unspecified site C75.1
  bile duct type C22.1
    liver C22.1
    specified site NEC — *see* Neoplasm, malignant, by site
    unspecified site C22.1
  bronchiolar — *see* Neoplasm, lung, malignant
  bronchioloalveolar — *see* Neoplasm, lung, malignant
  ceruminous C44.29- ☑
  cervix, in situ (*see also* Carcinoma, cervix uteri, in situ) D06.9
  chromophobe
    specified site — *see* Neoplasm, malignant, by site
    unspecified site C75.1
  diffuse type
    specified site — *see* Neoplasm, malignant, by site
    unspecified site C16.9
  duct
    infiltrating
      with Paget's disease — *see* Neoplasm, breast, malignant
      specified site — *see* Neoplasm, malignant, by site
      unspecified site (female) C50.91- ☑
        male C50.92- ☑
    specified site — *see* Neoplasm, malignant, by site
    unspecified site
      female C56.9
      male C61
  eosinophil
    specified site — *see* Neoplasm, malignant, by site
    unspecified site C75.1
  follicular
    with papillary C73
    moderately differentiated C73
    specified site — *see* Neoplasm, malignant, by site
    trabecular C73
    unspecified site C73
    well differentiated C73
  Hurthle cell C73
  in
    adenomatous
      polyposis coli C18.9
  infiltrating duct
    with Paget's disease — *see* Neoplasm, breast, malignant
    specified site — *see* Neoplasm, by site, malignant
    unspecified site (female) C50.91- ☑
      male C50.92- ☑
  inflammatory
    specified site — *see* Neoplasm, by site, malignant
    unspecified site (female) C50.91- ☑
      male C50.92- ☑
  intestinal type
    specified site — *see* Neoplasm, by site, malignant
    unspecified site C16.9
  intracystic papillary
  intraductal
    breast D05.1- ☑
    noninfiltrating
      breast D05.1- ☑
      papillary
        with invasion
          specified site — *see* Neoplasm, by site, malignant
          unspecified site (female) C50.91- ☑
            male C50.92- ☑
        breast D05.1- ☑
        specified site NEC — *see* Neoplasm, in situ, by site
        unspecified site D05.1- ☑
      specified site NEC — *see* Neoplasm, in situ, by site

Adenocarcinoma — *continued*
  intraductal — *continued*
    noninfiltrating — *continued*
      unspecified site D05.1- ☑
      papillary
        with invasion
          specified site — *see* Neoplasm, malignant, by site
          unspecified site (female) C50.91- ☑
            male C50.92- ☑
        breast D05.1- ☑
        specified site — *see* Neoplasm, in situ, by site
        unspecified site D05.1- ☑
      specified site NEC — *see* Neoplasm, in situ, by site
      unspecified site D05.1- ☑
  islet cell
    with exocrine, mixed
      specified site — *see* Neoplasm, malignant, by site
      unspecified site C25.9
    pancreas C25.4
    specified site NEC — *see* Neoplasm, malignant, by site
    unspecified site C25.4
  lobular
    in situ
      breast D05.0- ☑
      specified site NEC — *see* Neoplasm, in situ, by site
      unspecified site D05.0- ☑
    specified site — *see* Neoplasm, malignant, by site
    unspecified site (female) C50.91- ☑
      male C50.92- ☑
  mucoid (*see also* Neoplasm, malignant, by site)
    cell
      specified site — *see* Neoplasm, malignant, by site
      unspecified site C75.1
  nonencapsulated sclerosing C73
  papillary
    with follicular C73
    follicular variant C73
    intraductal (noninfiltrating)
      with invasion
        specified site — *see* Neoplasm, malignant, by site
        unspecified site (female) C50.91- ☑
          male C50.92- ☑
      breast D05.1- ☑
      specified site NEC — *see* Neoplasm, in situ, by site
      unspecified site D05.1- ☑
    serous
      specified site — *see* Neoplasm, malignant, by site
      unspecified site C56.9
  papillocystic
    specified site — *see* Neoplasm, malignant, by site
    unspecified site C56.9
  pseudomucinous
    specified site — *see* Neoplasm, malignant, by site
    unspecified site C56.9
  renal cell C64- ☑
  sebaceous — *see* Neoplasm, skin, malignant
  serous (*see also* Neoplasm, malignant, by site)
    papillary
      specified site — *see* Neoplasm, malignant, by site
      unspecified site C56.9
  sweat gland — *see* Neoplasm, skin, malignant
  water-clear cell C75.0

Adenocarcinoma-in-situ (*see also* Neoplasm, in situ, by site)
  breast D05.9- ☑

Adenofibroma
  clear cell — *see* Neoplasm, benign, by site
  endometrioid D27.9
    borderline malignancy D39.10
    malignant C56- ☑
  mucinous
    specified site — *see* Neoplasm, benign, by site
    unspecified site D27.9
  papillary
    specified site — *see* Neoplasm, benign, by site
    unspecified site D27.9
  prostate — *see* Enlargement, enlarged, prostate

Adenofibroma — *continued*
  serous
    specified site — *see* Neoplasm, benign, by site
    unspecified site D27.9
  specified site — *see* Neoplasm, benign, by site
  unspecified site D27.9
Adenofibrosis
  breast — *see* Fibroadenosis, breast
  endometrioid N80.0
Adenoiditis (chronic) J35.02
  with tonsillitis J35.03
  acute J03.90
    recurrent J03.91
    specified organism NEC J03.80
      recurrent J03.81
    staphylococcal J03.80
      recurrent J03.81
    streptococcal J03.00
      recurrent J03.01
Adenoids — *see* condition
Adenolipoma — *see* Neoplasm, benign, by site
Adenolipomatosis, Launois-Bensaude E88.89
Adenolymphoma
  specified site — *see* Neoplasm, benign, by site
  unspecified site D11.9
Adenoma (*see also* Neoplasm, benign, by site)
  acidophil
    specified site — *see* Neoplasm, benign, by site
    unspecified site D35.2
  acidophil-basophil, mixed
    specified site — *see* Neoplasm, benign, by site
    unspecified site D35.2
  adrenal (cortical) D35.00
    clear cell D35.00
    compact cell D35.00
    glomerulosa cell D35.00
    heavily pigmented variant D35.00
    mixed cell D35.00
  alpha-cell
    pancreas D13.7
    specified site NEC — *see* Neoplasm, benign, by site
    unspecified site D13.7
  alveolar D14.30
  apocrine
    breast D24- ☑
    specified site NEC — *see* Neoplasm, skin, benign, by site
    unspecified site D23.9
  basal cell D11.9
  basophil
    specified site — *see* Neoplasm, benign, by site
    unspecified site D35.2
  basophil-acidophil, mixed
    specified site — *see* Neoplasm, benign, by site
    unspecified site D35.2
  beta-cell
    pancreas D13.7
    specified site NEC — *see* Neoplasm, benign, by site
    unspecified site D13.7
  bile duct D13.4
    common D13.5
    extrahepatic D13.5
    intrahepatic D13.4
    specified site NEC — *see* Neoplasm, benign, by site
    unspecified site D13.4
  black D35.00
  bronchial D38.1
    cylindroid type — *see* Neoplasm, lung, malignant
  ceruminous D23.2- ☑
  chief cell D35.1
  chromophobe
    specified site — *see* Neoplasm, benign, by site
    unspecified site D35.2
  colloid
    specified site — *see* Neoplasm, benign, by site
    unspecified site D34
  duct
  eccrine, papillary — *see* Neoplasm, skin, benign
  endocrine, multiple
    single specified site — *see* Neoplasm, uncertain behavior, by site
    two or more specified sites D44- ☑
    unspecified site D44.9
  endometrioid (*see also* Neoplasm, benign)
    borderline malignancy — *see* Neoplasm, uncertain behavior, by site
  eosinophil
    specified site — *see* Neoplasm, benign, by site

Subterms under main terms may continue to next column or page   ☑ Additional Character Required — Refer to the Tabular List for Character Selection   11

Adenocarcinoma — Adenoma

Adenoma — *continued*
  eosinophil — *continued*
    unspecified site D35.2
  fetal
    specified site — *see* Neoplasm, benign, by site
    unspecified site D34
  follicular
    specified site — *see* Neoplasm, benign, by site
    unspecified site D34
  hepatocellular D13.4
  Hurthle cell D34
  islet cell
    pancreas D13.7
    specified site NEC — *see* Neoplasm, benign, by site
    unspecified site D13.7
  liver cell D13.4
  macrofollicular
    specified site — *see* Neoplasm, benign, by site
    unspecified site D34
  malignant, malignum — *see* Neoplasm, malignant, by site
  microcystic
    pancreas D13.6
    specified site NEC — *see* Neoplasm, benign, by site
    unspecified site D13.6
  microfollicular
    specified site — *see* Neoplasm, benign, by site
    unspecified site D34
  mucoid cell
    specified site — *see* Neoplasm, benign, by site
    unspecified site D35.2
  multiple endocrine
    single specified site — *see* Neoplasm, uncertain behavior, by site
    two or more specified sites D44- ☑
    unspecified site D44.9
  nipple D24- ☑
  papillary (*see also* Neoplasm, benign, by site)
    eccrine — *see* Neoplasm, skin, benign, by site
  Pick's tubular
    specified site — *see* Neoplasm, benign, by site
    unspecified site
      female D27.9
      male D29.20
  pleomorphic
    carcinoma in — *see* Neoplasm, salivary gland, malignant
    specified site — *see* Neoplasm, malignant, by site
    unspecified site C08.9
  polypoid (*see also* Neoplasm, benign)
    adenocarcinoma in — *see* Neoplasm, malignant, by site
    adenocarcinoma in situ — *see* Neoplasm, in situ, by site
  prostate — *see* Neoplasm, benign, prostate
  rete cell D29.20
  sebaceous — *see* Neoplasm, skin, benign
  Sertoli cell
    specified site — *see* Neoplasm, benign, by site
    unspecified site
      female D27.9
      male D29.20
  skin appendage — *see* Neoplasm, skin, benign
  sudoriferous gland — *see* Neoplasm, skin, benign
  sweat gland — *see* Neoplasm, skin, benign
  testicular
    specified site — *see* Neoplasm, benign, by site
    unspecified site
      female D27.9
      male D29.20
  tubular (*see also* Neoplasm, benign, by site)
    adenocarcinoma in — *see* Neoplasm, malignant, by site
    adenocarcinoma in situ — *see* Neoplasm, in situ, by site
    Pick's
      specified site — *see* Neoplasm, benign, by site
      unspecified site
        female D27.9
        male D29.20
  tubulovillous (*see also* Neoplasm, benign, by site)
    adenocarcinoma in — *see* Neoplasm, malignant, by site
    adenocarcinoma in situ — *see* Neoplasm, in situ, by site
  villous — *see* Neoplasm, uncertain behavior, by site

Adenoma — *continued*
  villous — *see* Neoplasm, uncertain behavior, by site — *continued*
    adenocarcinoma in — *see* Neoplasm, malignant, by site
    adenocarcinoma in situ — *see* Neoplasm, in situ, by site
  water-clear cell D35.1
Adenomatosis
  endocrine (multiple) E31.20
    single specified site — *see* Neoplasm, uncertain behavior, by site
  erosive of nipple D24- ☑
  pluriendocrine — *see* Adenomatosis, endocrine
  pulmonary D38.1
    malignant — *see* Neoplasm, lung, malignant
  specified site — *see* Neoplasm, benign, by site
  unspecified site D12.6
Adenomatous
  goiter (nontoxic) E04.9
    with hyperthyroidism — *see* Hyperthyroidism, with, goiter, nodular
    toxic — *see* Hyperthyroidism, with, goiter, nodular
Adenomyoma (*see also* Neoplasm, benign, by site)
  prostate — *see* Enlarged, prostate
Adenomyometritis N80.0
Adenomyosis N80.0
Adenopathy (lymph gland) R59.9
  generalized R59.1
  inguinal R59.0
  localized R59.0
  mediastinal R59.0
  mesentery R59.0
  syphilitic (secondary) A51.49
  tracheobronchial R59.0
    tuberculous A15.4
      primary (progressive) A15.7
  tuberculous (*see also* Tuberculosis, lymph gland)
    tracheobronchial A15.4
      primary (progressive) A15.7
Adenosalpingitis — *see* Salpingitis
Adenosarcoma — *see* Neoplasm, malignant, by site
Adenosclerosis I88.8
Adenosis (sclerosing) breast — *see* Fibroadenosis, breast
Adenovirus, as cause of disease classified elsewhere B97.0
Adentia (complete) (partial) — *see* Absence, teeth
Adherent (*see also* Adhesions)
  labia (minora) N90.89
  pericardium (nonrheumatic) I31.0
    rheumatic I09.2
  placenta (with hemorrhage) O72.0
    without hemorrhage O73.0
  prepuce, newborn N47.0
  scar (skin) L90.5
  tendon in scar L90.5
Adhesions, adhesive (postinfective) K66.0
  with intestinal obstruction K56.50
    complete K56.52
    incomplete K56.51
    partial K56.51
  abdominal (wall) — *see* Adhesions, peritoneum
  appendix K38.8
  bile duct (common) (hepatic) K83.8
  bladder (sphincter) N32.89
  bowel — *see* Adhesions, peritoneum
  cardiac I31.0
    rheumatic I09.2
  cecum — *see* Adhesions, peritoneum
  cervicovaginal N88.1
    congenital Q52.8
    postpartal O90.89
      old N88.1
  cervix N88.1
  ciliary body NEC — *see* Adhesions, iris
  clitoris N90.89
  colon — *see* Adhesions, peritoneum
  common duct K83.8
  congenital (*see also* Anomaly, by site)
    fingers — *see* Syndactylism, complex, fingers
    omental, anomalous Q43.3
    peritoneal Q43.3
    tongue (to gum or roof of mouth) Q38.3
  conjunctiva (acquired) H11.21- ☑
    congenital Q15.8
  cystic duct K82.8
  diaphragm — *see* Adhesions, peritoneum
  due to foreign body — *see* Foreign body

Adhesions, adhesive — *continued*
  duodenum — *see* Adhesions, peritoneum
  ear
    middle H74.1- ☑
  epididymis N50.89
  epidural — *see* Adhesions, meninges
  epiglottis J38.7
  eyelid H02.59
  female pelvis N73.6
  gallbladder K82.8
  globe H44.89
  heart I31.0
    rheumatic I09.2
  ileocecal (coil) — *see* Adhesions, peritoneum
  ileum — *see* Adhesions, peritoneum
  intestine (*see also* Adhesions, peritoneum)
    with obstruction K56.50
      complete K56.52
      incomplete K56.51
      partial K56.51
  intra-abdominal — *see* Adhesions, peritoneum
  iris H21.50- ☑
    anterior H21.51- ☑
    goniosynechiae H21.52- ☑
    posterior H21.54- ☑
    to corneal graft T85.898 ☑
  joint — *see* Ankylosis
    knee M23.8X ☑
    temporomandibular M26.61- ☑
  labium (majus) (minus), congenital Q52.5
  liver — *see* Adhesions, peritoneum
  lung J98.4
  mediastinum J98.59
  meninges (cerebral) (spinal) G96.12
    congenital Q07.8
    tuberculous (cerebral) (spinal) A17.0
  mesenteric — *see* Adhesions, peritoneum
  nasal (septum) (to turbinates) J34.89
  ocular muscle — *see* Strabismus, mechanical
  omentum — *see* Adhesions, peritoneum
  ovary N73.6
    congenital (to cecum, kidney or omentum) Q50.39
  paraovarian N73.6
  pelvic (peritoneal)
    female N73.6
      postprocedural N99.4
    male — *see* Adhesions, peritoneum
    postpartal (old) N73.6
    tuberculous A18.17
  penis to scrotum (congenital) Q55.8
  periappendiceal (*see also* Adhesions, peritoneum)
  pericardium (nonrheumatic) I31.0
    focal I31.8
    rheumatic I09.2
    tuberculous A18.84
  pericholecystic K82.8
  perigastric — *see* Adhesions, peritoneum
  periovarian N73.6
  periprostatic N42.89
  perirectal — *see* Adhesions, peritoneum
  perirenal N28.89
  peritoneum, peritoneal (postinfective)
    with obstruction (intestinal) K56.50
      complete K56.52
      incomplete K56.51
      partial K56.51
    congenital Q43.3
    pelvic, female N73.6
      postprocedural N99.4
    postpartal, pelvic N73.6
    postprocedural K66.0
    to uterus N73.6
  peritubal N73.6
  periureteral N28.89
  periuterine N73.6
  perivesical N32.89
  perivesicular (seminal vesicle) N50.89
  pleura, pleuritic J94.8
    tuberculous NEC A15.6
  pleuropericardial J94.8
  postoperative (gastrointestinal tract) K66.0
    with obstruction (*see also* Obstruction, intestine, postoperative) K91.30
    due to foreign body accidentally left in wound — *see* Foreign body, accidentally left during a procedure
    pelvic peritoneal N99.4
  urethra — *see* Stricture, urethra, postprocedural

☑ Additional Character Required — Refer to the Tabular List for Character Selection   ▽ Subterms under main terms may continue to next column or page

Adhesions, adhesive — *continued*
  postoperative — *continued*
    vagina N99.2
  postpartal, old (vulva or perineum) N90.89
  preputial, prepuce N47.5
  pulmonary J98.4
  pylorus — *see* Adhesions, peritoneum
  sciatic nerve — *see* Lesion, nerve, sciatic
  seminal vesicle N50.89
  shoulder (joint) — *see* Capsulitis, adhesive
  sigmoid flexure — *see* Adhesions, peritoneum
  spermatic cord (acquired) N50.89
    congenital Q55.4
  spinal canal G96.12
  stomach — *see* Adhesions, peritoneum
  subscapular — *see* Capsulitis, adhesive
  temporomandibular M26.61- ☑
  tendinitis (*see also* Tenosynovitis, specified type NEC)
    shoulder — *see* Capsulitis, adhesive
  testis N44.8
  tongue, congenital (to gum or roof of mouth) Q38.3
    acquired K14.8
  trachea J39.8
  tubo-ovarian N73.6
  tunica vaginalis N44.8
  uterus N73.6
    internal N85.6
    to abdominal wall N73.6
  vagina (chronic) N89.5
    postoperative N99.2
  vitreomacular H43.82- ☑
  vitreous H43.89
  vulva N90.89
Adiaspiromycosis B48.8
Adie (-Holmes) **pupil or syndrome** — *see* Anomaly, pupil, function, tonic pupil
Adiponecrosis neonatorum P83.88
Adiposis (*see also* Obesity)
  cerebralis E23.6
  dolorosa E88.2
Adiposity (*see also* Obesity)
  heart — *see* Degeneration, myocardial
  localized E65
Adiposogenital dystrophy E23.6
Adjustment
  disorder — *see* Disorder, adjustment
  implanted device — *see* Encounter (for), adjustment (of)
  prosthesis, external — *see* Fitting
  reaction — *see* Disorder, adjustment
Administration of tPA (rtPA) in a different facility within the last 24 hours prior to admission to current facility Z92.82
Admission (for) (*see also* Encounter (for))
  adjustment (of)
    artificial
      arm Z44.00- ☑
        complete Z44.01- ☑
        partial Z44.02- ☑
      eye Z44.2 ☑
      leg Z44.10- ☑
        complete Z44.11- ☑
        partial Z44.12- ☑
    brain neuropacemaker Z46.2
      implanted Z45.42
    breast
      implant Z45.81 ☑
      prosthesis (external) Z44.3 ☑
    colostomy belt Z46.89
    contact lenses Z46.0
    cystostomy device Z46.6
    dental prosthesis Z46.3
    device NEC
      abdominal Z46.89
      implanted Z45.89
        cardiac Z45.09
          defibrillator (with synchronous cardiace pacemaker) Z45.02
          pacemaker (cardiac resynchronization therapy (CRT-P)) Z45.018
            pulse generator Z45.010
          resynchronization therapy defibrillator (CRT-D) Z45.02
        hearing device Z45.328
          bone conduction Z45.320
          cochlear Z45.321
        infusion pump Z45.1
        nervous system Z45.49

Admission — *continued*
  adjustment — *continued*
    device — *continued*
      implanted — *continued*
        nervous system — *continued*
          CSF drainage Z45.41
          hearing device — *see* Admission, adjustment, device, implanted, hearing device
          neuropacemaker Z45.42
          visual substitution Z45.31
        specified NEC Z45.89
        vascular access Z45.2
        visual substitution Z45.31
      nervous system Z46.2
        implanted — *see* Admission, adjustment, device, implanted, nervous system
      orthodontic Z46.4
      prosthetic Z44.9
        arm — *see* Admission, adjustment, artificial, arm
        breast Z44.3 ☑
        dental Z46.3
        eye Z44.2 ☑
        leg — *see* Admission, adjustment, artificial, leg
        specified type NEC Z44.8
      substitution
        auditory Z46.2
          implanted — *see* Admission, adjustment, device, implanted, hearing device
        nervous system Z46.2
          implanted — *see* Admission, adjustment, device, implanted, nervous system
        visual Z46.2
          implanted Z45.31
      urinary Z46.6
    hearing aid Z46.1
      implanted — *see* Admission, adjustment, device, implanted, hearing device
    ileostomy device Z46.89
    intestinal appliance or device NEC Z46.89
    neuropacemaker (brain) (peripheral nerve) (spinal cord) Z46.2
      implanted Z45.42
    orthodontic device Z46.4
    orthopedic (brace) (cast) (device) (shoes) Z46.89
    pacemaker (cardiac resynchronization therapy (CRT-P))
      cardiac Z45.018
        pulse generator Z45.010
      nervous system Z46.2
        implanted Z45.42
    portacath (port-a-cath) Z45.2
    prosthesis Z44.9
      arm — *see* Admission, adjustment, artificial, arm
      breast Z44.3 ☑
      dental Z46.3
      eye Z44.2 ☑
      leg — *see* Admission, adjustment, artificial, leg
      specified NEC Z44.8
    spectacles Z46.0
  aftercare (*see also* Aftercare) Z51.89
    postpartum
      immediately after delivery Z39.0
      routine follow-up Z39.2
    radiation therapy (antineoplastic) Z51.0
  attention to artificial opening (of) Z43.9
    artificial vagina Z43.7
    colostomy Z43.3
    cystostomy Z43.5
    enterostomy Z43.4
    gastrostomy Z43.1
    ileostomy Z43.2
    jejunostomy Z43.4
    nephrostomy Z43.6
    specified site NEC Z43.8
      intestinal tract Z43.4
      urinary tract Z43.6
    tracheostomy Z43.0
    ureterostomy Z43.6
    urethrostomy Z43.6
  breast augmentation or reduction Z41.1
  breast reconstruction following mastectomy Z42.1

Admission — *continued*
  change of
    dressing (nonsurgical) Z48.00
    neuropacemaker device (brain) (peripheral nerve) (spinal cord) Z46.2
      implanted Z45.42
    surgical dressing Z48.01
  circumcision, ritual or routine (in absence of diagnosis) Z41.2
  clinical research investigation (control) (normal comparison) (participant) Z00.6
  contraceptive management Z30.9
  cosmetic surgery NEC Z41.1
  counseling (*see also* Counseling)
    dietary Z71.3
    gestational carrier Z31.7
    HIV Z71.7
    human immunodeficiency virus Z71.7
    nonattending third party Z71.0
    procreative management NEC Z31.69
  delivery, full-term, uncomplicated O80
    cesarean, without indication O82
  desensitization to allergens Z51.6
  dietary surveillance and counseling Z71.3
  ear piercing Z41.3
  examination at health care facility (adult) (*see also* Examination) Z00.00
    with abnormal findings Z00.01
    clinical research investigation (control) (normal comparison) (participant) Z00.6
    dental Z01.20
      with abnormal findings Z01.21
    donor (potential) Z00.5
    ear Z01.10
      with abnormal findings NEC Z01.118
    eye Z01.00
      with abnormal findings Z01.01
    general, specified reason NEC Z00.8
    hearing Z01.10
      with abnormal findings NEC Z01.118
    postpartum checkup Z39.2
    psychiatric (general) Z00.8
      requested by authority Z04.6
    vision Z01.00
      with abnormal findings Z01.01
  fitting (of)
    artificial
      arm — *see* Admission, adjustment, artificial, arm
      eye Z44.2 ☑
      leg — *see* Admission, adjustment, artificial, leg
    brain neuropacemaker Z46.2
      implanted Z45.42
    breast prosthesis (external) Z44.3 ☑
    colostomy belt Z46.89
    contact lenses Z46.0
    cystostomy device Z46.6
    dental prosthesis Z46.3
    dentures Z46.3
    device NEC
      abdominal Z46.89
      nervous system Z46.2
        implanted — *see* Admission, adjustment, device, implanted, nervous system
      orthodontic Z46.4
      prosthetic Z44.9
        breast Z44.3 ☑
        dental Z46.3
        eye Z44.2 ☑
      substitution
        auditory Z46.2
          implanted — *see* Admission, adjustment, device, implanted, hearing device
        nervous system Z46.2
          implanted — *see* Admission, adjustment, device, implanted, nervous system
        visual Z46.2
          implanted Z45.31
    hearing aid Z46.1
    ileostomy device Z46.89
    intestinal appliance or device NEC Z46.89
    neuropacemaker (brain) (peripheral nerve) (spinal cord) Z46.2
      implanted Z45.42
    orthodontic device Z46.4
    orthopedic device (brace) (cast) (shoes) Z46.89

Adhesions, adhesive — Admission

☜ Subterms under main terms may continue to next column or page   ☑ Additional Character Required — Refer to the Tabular List for Character Selection   13

Admission — *continued*
  fitting — *continued*
    prosthesis Z44.9
      arm — *see* Admission, adjustment, artificial, arm
      breast Z44.3 ☑
      dental Z46.3
      eye Z44.2 ☑
      leg — *see* Admission, adjustment, artificial, leg
      specified type NEC Z44.8
      spectacles Z46.0
  follow-up examination Z09
  intrauterine device management Z30.431
    initial prescription Z30.014
  mental health evaluation Z00.8
    requested by authority Z04.6
  observation — *see* Observation
  Papanicolaou smear, cervix Z12.4
    for suspected malignant neoplasm Z12.4
  plastic and reconstructive surgery following medical procedure or healed injury NEC Z42.8
  plastic surgery, cosmetic NEC Z41.1
  postpartum observation
    immediately after delivery Z39.0
    routine follow-up Z39.2
  poststerilization (for restoration) Z31.0
    aftercare Z31.42
  procreative management Z31.9
  prophylactic (measure) — (*see also* Encounter, prophylactic measures)
    organ removal Z40.00
      breast Z40.01
      fallopian tube(s) Z40.03
        with ovary(s) Z40.02
      ovary(s) Z40.02
      specified organ NEC Z40.09
      testes Z40.09
    vaccination Z23
  psychiatric examination (general) Z00.8
    requested by authority Z04.6
  radiation therapy (antineoplastic) Z51.0
  reconstructive surgery following medical procedure or healed injury NEC Z42.8
  removal of
    cystostomy catheter Z43.5
    drains Z48.03
    dressing (nonsurgical) Z48.00
    implantable subdermal contraceptive Z30.46
    intrauterine contraceptive device Z30.432
    neuropacemaker (brain) (peripheral nerve) (spinal cord) Z46.2
      implanted Z45.42
    staples Z48.02
    surgical dressing Z48.01
    sutures Z48.02
    ureteral stent Z46.6
  respirator [ventilator] use during power failure Z99.12
  restoration of organ continuity (poststerilization) Z31.0
    aftercare Z31.42
  sensitivity test (*see also* Test, skin)
    allergy NEC Z01.82
    Mantoux Z11.1
  tuboplasty following previous sterilization Z31.0
    aftercare Z31.42
  vasoplasty following previous sterilization Z31.0
    aftercare Z31.42
  vision examination Z01.00
    with abnormal findings Z01.01
  waiting period for admission to other facility Z75.1
Adnexitis (suppurative) — *see* Salpingo-oophoritis
Adolescent X-linked adrenoleukodystrophy E71.521
Adrenal (gland) — *see* condition
Adrenalism, tuberculous A18.7
Adrenalitis, adrenitis E27.8
  autoimmune E27.1
  meningococcal, hemorrhagic A39.1
Adrenarche, premature E27.0
Adrenocortical syndrome — *see* Cushing's, syndrome
Adrenogenital syndrome E25.9
  acquired E25.8
  congenital E25.0
  salt loss E25.0
Adrenogenitalism, congenital E25.0
Adrenoleukodystrophy E71.529
  neonatal E71.511
  X-linked E71.529
    Addison only phenotype E71.528
    Addison-Schilder E71.528

Adrenoleukodystrophy — *continued*
  X-linked — *continued*
    adolescent E71.521
    adrenomyeloneuropathy E71.522
    childhood cerebral E71.520
    other specified E71.528
Adrenomyeloneuropathy E71.522
Adventitious bursa — *see* Bursopathy, specified type NEC
Adverse effect — *see* Table of Drugs and Chemicals, categories T36-T50, with 6th character 5
Advice — *see* Counseling
Adynamia (episodica) (hereditary) (periodic) G72.3
Aeration lung imperfect, newborn — *see* Atelectasis
Aerobullosis T70.3 ☑
Aerocele — *see* Embolism, air
Aerodermectasia
  subcutaneous (traumatic) T79.7 ☑
Aerodontalgia T70.29 ☑
Aeroembolism T70.3 ☑
Aerogenes capsulatus infection A48.0
Aero-otitis media T70.0 ☑
Aerophagy, aerophagia (psychogenic) F45.8
Aerophobia F40.228
Aerosinusitis T70.1 ☑
Aerotitis T70.0 ☑
Affection — *see* Disease
Afibrinogenemia (*see also* Defect, coagulation) D68.8
  acquired D65
  congenital D68.2
  following ectopic or molar pregnancy O08.1
  in abortion — *see* Abortion, by type, complicated by, afibrinogenemia
  puerperal O72.3
African
  sleeping sickness B56.9
  tick fever A68.1
  trypanosomiasis B56.9
    gambian B56.0
    rhodesian B56.1
Aftercare (*see also* Care) Z51.89
  following surgery (for) (on)
    amputation Z47.81
    attention to
      drains Z48.03
      dressings (nonsurgical) Z48.00
        surgical Z48.01
      sutures Z48.02
    circulatory system Z48.812
    delayed (planned) wound closure Z48.1
    digestive system Z48.815
    explantation of joint prosthesis (staged procedure)
      hip Z47.32
      knee Z47.33
      shoulder Z47.31
    genitourinary system Z48.816
    joint replacement Z47.1
    neoplasm Z48.3
    nervous system Z48.811
    oral cavity Z48.814
    organ transplant
      bone marrow Z48.290
      heart Z48.21
      heart-lung Z48.280
      kidney Z48.22
      liver Z48.23
      lung Z48.24
      multiple organs NEC Z48.288
      specified NEC Z48.298
    orthopedic NEC Z47.89
    planned wound closure Z48.1
    removal of internal fixation device Z47.2
    respiratory system Z48.813
    scoliosis Z47.82
    sense organs Z48.810
    skin and subcutaneous tissue Z48.817
    specified body system
      circulatory Z48.812
      digestive Z48.815
      genitourinary Z48.816
      nervous Z48.811
      oral cavity Z48.814
      respiratory Z48.813
      sense organs Z48.810
      skin and subcutaneous tissue Z48.817
      teeth Z48.814
    specified NEC Z48.89
    spinal Z47.89

Aftercare — *continued*
  following surgery — *continued*
    teeth Z48.814
  fracture — *code to* fracture with seventh character D
  involving
    removal of
      drains Z48.03
      dressings (nonsurgical) Z48.00
      staples Z48.02
      surgical dressings Z48.01
      sutures Z48.02
    neuropacemaker (brain) (peripheral nerve) (spinal cord) Z46.2
      implanted Z45.42
    orthopedic NEC Z47.89
  postprocedural — *see* Aftercare, following surgery
After-cataract — *see* Cataract, secondary
Agalactia (primary) O92.3
  elective, secondary or therapeutic O92.5
Agammaglobulinemia (acquired) (secondary) (nonfamilial) D80.1
  with
    immunoglobulin-bearing B-lymphocytes D80.1
    lymphopenia D81.9
  autosomal recessive (Swiss type) D80.0
  Bruton's X-linked D80.0
  common variable (CVAgamma) D80.1
  congenital sex-linked D80.0
  hereditary D80.0
  lymphopenic D81.9
  Swiss type (autosomal recessive) D80.0
  X-linked (with growth hormone deficiency) (Bruton) D80.0
Aganglionosis (bowel) (colon) Q43.1
Age (old) — *see* Senility
Agenesis
  adrenal (gland) Q89.1
  alimentary tract (complete) (partial) NEC Q45.8
    upper Q40.8
  anus, anal (canal) Q42.3
    with fistula Q42.2
  aorta Q25.41
  appendix Q42.8
  arm (complete) Q71.0- ☑
    with hand present Q71.1- ☑
  artery (peripheral) Q27.9
    brain Q28.3
    coronary Q24.5
    pulmonary Q25.79
    specified NEC Q27.8
    umbilical Q27.0
  auditory (canal) (external) Q16.1
  auricle (ear) Q16.0
  bile duct or passage Q44.5
  bladder Q64.5
  bone Q79.9
  brain Q00.0
    part of Q04.3
  breast (with nipple present) Q83.8
    with absent nipple Q83.0
  bronchus Q32.4
  canaliculus lacrimalis Q10.4
  carpus — *see* Agenesis, hand
  cartilage Q79.9
  cecum Q42.8
  cerebellum Q04.3
  cervix Q51.5
  chin Q18.8
  cilia Q10.3
  circulatory system, part NOS Q28.9
  clavicle Q74.0
  clitoris Q52.6
  coccyx Q76.49
  colon Q42.9
    specified NEC Q42.8
  corpus callosum Q04.0
  cricoid cartilage Q31.8
  diaphragm (with hernia) Q79.1
  digestive organ(s) or tract (complete) (partial) NEC Q45.8
    upper Q40.8
  ductus arteriosus Q28.8
  duodenum Q41.0
  ear Q16.9
    auricle Q16.0
    lobe Q17.8
  ejaculatory duct Q55.4
  endocrine (gland) NEC Q89.2

Agenesis — *continued*
epiglottis Q31.8
esophagus Q39.8
eustachian tube Q16.2
eye Q11.1
adnexa Q15.8
eyelid (fold) Q10.3
face
bones NEC Q75.8
specified part NEC Q18.8
fallopian tube Q50.6
femur — *see* Defect, reduction, lower limb, longitudinal, femur
fibula — *see* Defect, reduction, lower limb, longitudinal, fibula
finger (complete) (partial) — *see* Agenesis, hand
foot (and toes) (complete) (partial) Q72.3- ☑
forearm (with hand present) — *see* Agenesis, arm, with hand present
and hand Q71.2- ☑
gallbladder Q44.0
gastric Q40.2
genitalia, genital (organ(s))
female Q52.8
external Q52.71
internal NEC Q52.8
male Q55.8
glottis Q31.8
hair Q84.0
hand (and fingers) (complete) (partial) Q71.3- ☑
heart Q24.8
valve NEC Q24.8
pulmonary Q22.0
hepatic Q44.7
humerus — *see* Defect, reduction, upper limb
hymen Q52.4
ileum Q41.2
incus Q16.3
intestine (small) Q41.9
large Q42.9
specified NEC Q42.8
iris (dilator fibers) Q13.1
jaw M26.09
jejunum Q41.1
kidney(s) (partial) Q60.2
bilateral Q60.1
unilateral Q60.0
labium (majus) (minus) Q52.71
labyrinth, membranous Q16.5
lacrimal apparatus Q10.4
larynx Q31.8
leg (complete) Q72.0- ☑
with foot present Q72.1- ☑
lower leg (with foot present) — *see* Agenesis, leg, with foot present
and foot Q72.2- ☑
lens Q12.3
limb (complete) Q73.0
lower — *see* Agenesis, leg
upper — *see* Agenesis, arm
lip Q38.0
liver Q44.7
lung (fissure) (lobe) (bilateral) (unilateral) Q33.3
mandible, maxilla M26.09
metacarpus — *see* Agenesis, hand
metatarsus — *see* Agenesis, foot
muscle Q79.8
eyelid Q10.3
ocular Q15.8
musculoskeletal system NEC Q79.8
nail(s) Q84.3
neck, part Q18.8
nerve Q07.8
nervous system, part NEC Q07.8
nipple Q83.2
nose Q30.1
nuclear Q07.8
organ
of Corti Q16.5
or site not listed — *see* Anomaly, by site
osseous meatus (ear) Q16.1
ovary
bilateral Q50.02
unilateral Q50.01
oviduct Q50.6
pancreas Q45.0
parathyroid (gland) Q89.2
parotid gland(s) Q38.4

Agenesis — *continued*
patella Q74.1
pelvic girdle (complete) (partial) Q74.2
penis Q55.5
pericardium Q24.8
pituitary (gland) Q89.2
prostate Q55.4
punctum lacrimale Q10.4
radioulnar — *see* Defect, reduction, upper limb
radius — *see* Defect, reduction, upper limb, longitudinal, radius
rectum Q42.1
with fistula Q42.0
renal Q60.2
bilateral Q60.1
unilateral Q60.0
respiratory organ NEC Q34.8
rib Q76.6
roof of orbit Q75.8
round ligament Q52.8
sacrum Q76.49
salivary gland Q38.4
scapula Q74.0
scrotum Q55.29
seminal vesicles Q55.4
septum
atrial Q21.1
between aorta and pulmonary artery Q21.4
ventricular Q20.4
shoulder girdle (complete) (partial) Q74.0
skull (bone) Q75.8
with
anencephaly Q00.0
encephalocele — *see* Encephalocele
hydrocephalus Q03.9
with spina bifida — *see* Spina bifida, by site, with hydrocephalus
microcephaly Q02
spermatic cord Q55.4
spinal cord Q06.0
spine Q76.49
spleen Q89.01
sternum Q76.7
stomach Q40.2
submaxillary gland(s) (congenital) Q38.4
tarsus — *see* Agenesis, foot
tendon Q79.8
testicle Q55.0
thymus (gland) Q89.2
thyroid (gland) E03.1
cartilage Q31.8
tibia — *see* Defect, reduction, lower limb, longitudinal, tibia
tibiofibular — *see* Defect, reduction, lower limb, specified type NEC
toe (and foot) (complete) (partial) — *see* Agenesis, foot
tongue Q38.3
trachea (cartilage) Q32.1
ulna — *see* Defect, reduction, upper limb, longitudinal, ulna
upper limb — *see* Agenesis, arm
ureter Q62.4
urethra Q64.5
urinary tract NEC Q64.8
uterus Q51.0
uvula Q38.5
vagina Q52.0
vas deferens Q55.4
vein(s) (peripheral) Q27.9
brain Q28.3
great NEC Q26.8
portal Q26.5
vena cava (inferior) (superior) Q26.8
vermis of cerebellum Q04.3
vertebra Q76.49
vulva Q52.71
Ageusia R43.2
Agitated — *see* condition
Agitation R45.1
Aglossia (congenital) Q38.3
Aglossia-adactylia syndrome Q87.0
Aglycogenosis E74.00
Agnosia (body image) (other senses) (tactile) R48.1
developmental F88
verbal R48.1
auditory R48.1
developmental F80.2

Agnosia — *continued*
verbal — *continued*
developmental F80.2
visual (object) R48.3
Agoraphobia F40.00
with panic disorder F40.01
without panic disorder F40.02
Agrammatism R48.8
Agranulocytopenia — *see* Agranulocytosis
Agranulocytosis (chronic) (cyclical) (genetic) (infantile) (periodic) (pernicious) (*see also* Neutropenia) D70.9
congenital D70.0
cytoreductive cancer chemotherapy sequela D70.1
drug-induced D70.2
due to cytoreductive cancer chemotherapy D70.1
due to infection D70.3
secondary D70.4
drug-induced D70.2
due to cytoreductive cancer chemotherapy D70.1
Agraphia (absolute) R48.8
with alexia R48.0
developmental F81.81
Ague (dumb) — *see* Malaria
Agyria Q04.3
Ahumada-del Castillo syndrome E23.0
Aichomophobia F40.298
AIDS (related complex) B20
Ailment heart — *see* Disease, heart
Ailurophobia F40.218
AIN — *see* Neoplasia, intraepithelial, anal
Ainhum (disease) L94.6
AIPHI (acute idiopathic pulmonary hemorrhage in infants (over 28 days old)) R04.81
Air
anterior mediastinum J98.2
compressed, disease T70.3 ☑
conditioner lung or pneumonitis J67.7
embolism (artery) (cerebral) (any site) T79.0 ☑
with ectopic or molar pregnancy O08.2
due to implanted device NEC — *see* Complications, by site and type, specified NEC
following
abortion — *see* Abortion by type, complicated by, embolism
ectopic or molar pregnancy O08.2
infusion, therapeutic injection or transfusion T80.0 ☑
in pregnancy, childbirth or puerperium — *see* Embolism, obstetric
traumatic T79.0 ☑
hunger, psychogenic F45.8
rarefied, effects of — *see* Effect, adverse, high altitude
sickness T75.3 ☑
Airplane sickness T75.3 ☑
Akathisia (drug-induced) (treatment-induced) G25.71
neuroleptic induced (acute) G25.71
tardive G25.71
Akinesia R29.898
Akinetic mutism R41.89
Akureyri's disease G93.3
Alactasia, congenital E73.0
Alagille's syndrome Q44.7
Alastrim B03
Albers-Schönberg syndrome Q78.2
Albert's syndrome — *see* Tendinitis, Achilles
Albinism, albino E70.30
with hematologic abnormality E70.339
Chédiak-Higashi syndrome E70.330
Hermansky-Pudlak syndrome E70.331
other specified E70.338
I E70.320
II E70.321
ocular E70.319
autosomal recessive E70.311
other specified E70.318
X-linked E70.310
oculocutaneous E70.329
other specified E70.328
tyrosinase (ty) negative E70.320
tyrosinase (ty) positive E70.321
other specified E70.39
Albinismus E70.30
Albright (-McCune)(-Sternberg) syndrome Q78.1
Albuminous — *see* condition
Albuminuria, albuminuric (acute) (chronic) (subacute) (*see also* Proteinuria) R80.9

Subterms under main terms may continue to next column or page   ☑ Additional Character Required — Refer to the Tabular List for Character Selection   **15**

Agenesis — Albuminuria, albuminuric

Albuminuria, albuminuric — continued
- complicating pregnancy — see Proteinuria, gestational
  - with
    - gestational hypertension — see Pre-eclampsia
    - pre-existing hypertension — see Hypertension, complicating pregnancy, pre-existing, with, pre-eclampsia
  - gestational — see Proteinuria, gestational
    - with
      - gestational hypertension — see Pre-eclampsia
      - pre-existing hypertension — see Hypertension, complicating pregnancy, pre-existing, with, pre-eclampsia
- orthostatic R80.2
- postural R80.2
- pre-eclamptic — see Pre-eclampsia
- scarlatinal A38.8

Albuminurophobia F40.298
Alcaptonuria E70.29
Alcohol, alcoholic, alcohol-induced
- addiction (without remission) F10.20
  - with remission F10.21
- amnestic disorder, persisting F10.96
  - with dependence F10.26
- anxiety disorder F10.980
- bipolar and related disorder F10.94
- brain syndrome, chronic F10.97
  - with dependence F10.27
- cardiopathy I42.6
- counseling and surveillance Z71.41
  - family member Z71.42
- delirium (acute) (tremens) (withdrawal) F10.231
  - with intoxication F10.921
    - in
      - abuse F10.121
      - dependence F10.221
- dementia F10.97
  - with dependence F10.27
- depressive disorder F10.94
- deterioration F10.97
  - with dependence F10.27
- hallucinosis (acute) F10.951
  - in
    - abuse F10.151
    - dependence F10.251
- insanity F10.959
- intoxication (acute) (without dependence) F10.129
  - with
    - delirium F10.121
    - dependence F10.229
      - with delirium F10.221
      - uncomplicated F10.220
    - uncomplicated F10.120
- jealousy F10.988
- Korsakoff's, Korsakov's, Korsakow's F10.26
- liver K70.9
  - acute — see Disease, liver, alcoholic, hepatitis
- major neurocognitive disorder, amnestic-confabulatory type F10.96
- major neurocognitive disorder, nonamnestic-confabulatory type F10.97
- mania (acute) (chronic) F10.959
- mild neurocognitive disorder F10.988
- paranoia, paranoid (type) psychosis F10.950
- pellagra E52
- poisoning, accidental (acute) NEC — see Table of Drugs and Chemicals, alcohol, poisoning
- psychosis — see Psychosis, alcoholic
- psychotic disorder F10.959
- sexual dysfunction F10.981
- sleep disorder F10.982
- withdrawal (without convulsions) F10.239
  - with delirium F10.231
Alcoholism (chronic) (without remission) F10.20
- with
  - psychosis — see Psychosis, alcoholic
  - remission F10.21
  - Korsakov's F10.96
    - with dependence F10.26
Alder (-Reilly) **anomaly or syndrome** (leukocyte granulation) D72.0
Aldosteronism E26.9
- familial (type I) E26.02
- glucocorticoid-remediable E26.02
- primary (due to (bilateral) adrenal hyperplasia) E26.09
- primary NEC E26.09
- secondary E26.1
- specified NEC E26.89

Aldosteronoma D44.10
Aldrich (-Wiskott) **syndrome** (eczema-thrombocytopenia) D82.0
Alektorophobia F40.218
Aleppo boil B55.1
Aleukemic — see condition
Aleukia
- congenital D70.0
- hemorrhagica D61.9
  - congenital D61.09
- splenica D73.1
Alexia R48.0
- developmental F81.0
- secondary to organic lesion R48.0
Algoneurodystrophy M89.00
- ankle M89.07- ☑
- foot M89.07- ☑
- forearm M89.03- ☑
- hand M89.04- ☑
- lower leg M89.06- ☑
- multiple sites M89.0- ☑
- shoulder M89.01- ☑
- specified site NEC M89.08
- thigh M89.05- ☑
- upper arm M89.02- ☑
Algophobia F40.298
Alienation, mental — see Psychosis
Alkalemia E87.3
Alkalosis E87.3
- metabolic E87.3
  - with respiratory acidosis E87.4
- respiratory E87.3
Alkaptonuria E70.29
Allen-Masters syndrome N83.8
Allergy, allergic (reaction) (to) T78.40 ☑
- air-borne substance NEC (rhinitis) J30.89
- alveolitis (extrinsic) J67.9
  - due to
    - Aspergillus clavatus J67.4
    - Cryptostroma corticale J67.6
    - organisms (fungal, thermophilic actinomycete) growing in ventilation (air conditioning) systems J67.7
  - specified type NEC J67.8
- anaphylactic reaction or shock T78.2 ☑
- angioneurotic edema T78.3 ☑
- animal (dander) (epidermal) (hair) (rhinitis) J30.81
- bee sting (anaphylactic shock) — see Toxicity, venom, arthropod, bee
- biological — see Allergy, drug
- colitis (see also Colitis, allergic) K52.29
- dander (animal) (rhinitis) J30.81
- dandruff (rhinitis) J30.81
- dental restorative material (existing) K08.55
- dermatitis — see Dermatitis, contact, allergic
- diathesis — see History, allergy
- drug, medicament & biological (any) (external) (internal) T78.40 ☑
  - correct substance properly administered — see Table of Drugs and Chemicals, by drug, adverse effect
  - wrong substance given or taken NEC (by accident) — see Table of Drugs and Chemicals, by drug, poisoning
- due to pollen J30.1
- dust (house) (stock) (rhinitis) J30.89
  - with asthma — see Asthma, allergic extrinsic
- eczema — see Dermatitis, contact, allergic
- epidermal (animal) (rhinitis) J30.81
- feathers (rhinitis) J30.89
- food (any) (ingested) NEC T78.1 ☑
  - anaphylactic shock — see Shock, anaphylactic, due to food
  - dermatitis — see Dermatitis, due to, food
  - dietary counseling and surveillance Z71.3
  - in contact with skin L23.6
  - rhinitis J30.5
  - status (without reaction) Z91.018
    - eggs Z91.012
    - milk products Z91.011
    - peanuts Z91.010
    - seafood Z91.013
    - specified NEC Z91.018
- gastrointestinal — see also specific type of allergic reaction
  - meaning colitis (see also Colitis, allergic) K52.29

Allergy, allergic — continued
- gastrointestinal — see also specific type of allergic reaction — continued
  - meaning gastroenteritis (see also Gastroenteritis, allergic) K52.29
  - meaning other adverse food reaction not elsewhere classified T78.1 ☑
- grain J30.1
- grass (hay fever) (pollen) J30.1
  - asthma — see Asthma, allergic extrinsic
- hair (animal) (rhinitis) J30.81
- history (of) — see History, allergy
- horse serum — see Allergy, serum
- inhalant (rhinitis) J30.89
  - pollen J30.1
- kapok (rhinitis) J30.89
- medicine — see Allergy, drug
- milk protein (see also Allergy, food) Z91.011
  - anaphylactic reaction T78.07 ☑
  - dermatitis L27.2
  - enterocolitis syndrome K52.21
  - enteropathy K52.22
  - gastroenteritis K52.29
  - gastroesophageal reflux (see also Reaction, adverse, food) K21.9
    - with esophagitis K21.0
  - proctocolitis K52.82
- nasal, seasonal due to pollen J30.1
- pneumonia J82
- pollen (any) (hay fever) J30.1
  - asthma — see Asthma, allergic extrinsic
- primrose J30.1
- primula J30.1
- proctocolitis K52.82
- purpura D69.0
- ragweed (hay fever) (pollen) J30.1
  - asthma — see Asthma, allergic extrinsic
- rose (pollen) J30.1
- seasonal NEC J30.2
- Senecio jacobae (pollen) J30.1
- serum (see also Reaction, serum) T80.69 ☑
  - anaphylactic shock T80.59 ☑
- shock (anaphylactic) T78.2 ☑
  - due to
    - administration of blood and blood products T80.51 ☑
    - adverse effect of correct medicinal substance properly administered T88.6 ☑
    - immunization T80.52 ☑
    - serum NEC T80.59 ☑
    - vaccination T80.52 ☑
- specific NEC T78.49 ☑
- tree (any) (hay fever) (pollen) J30.1
  - asthma — see Asthma, allergic extrinsic
- upper respiratory J30.9
- urticaria L50.0
- vaccine — see Allergy, serum
- wheat — see Allergy, food
Allescheriasis B48.2
Alligator skin disease Q80.9
Allocheiria, allochiria R20.8
Almeida's disease — see Paracoccidioidomycosis
Alopecia (hereditaria) (seborrheica) L65.9
- androgenic L64.9
  - drug-induced L64.0
  - specified NEC L64.8
- areata L63.9
  - ophiasis L63.2
  - specified NEC L63.8
  - totalis L63.0
  - universalis L63.1
- cicatricial L66.9
  - specified NEC L66.8
- circumscripta L63.9
- congenital, congenitalis Q84.0
- due to cytotoxic drugs NEC L65.8
- mucinosa L65.2
- postinfective NEC L65.8
- postpartum L65.0
- premature L64.8
- specific (syphilitic) A51.32
- specified NEC L65.8
- syphilitic (secondary) A51.32
- totalis (capitis) L63.0
- universalis (entire body) L63.1
- X-ray L58.1
Alpers' disease G31.81
Alpine sickness T70.29 ☑

Alport syndrome Q87.81
ALTE (apparent life threatening event) **in newborn and infant** R68.13
Alteration (of), **Altered**
  awareness
    transient R40.4
    unintended under general anesthesia, during procedure T88.53 ☑
  mental status R41.82
  pattern of family relationships affecting child Z62.898
  sensation
    following
      cerebrovascular disease I69.998
        cerebral infarction I69.398
        intracerebral hemorrhage I69.198
        nontraumatic intracranial hemorrhage NEC I69.298
        specified disease NEC I69.898
        subarachnoid hemorrhage I69.098
Alternating — *see* condition
Altitude, high (effects) — *see* Effect, adverse, high altitude
Aluminosis (of lung) J63.0
Alveolitis
  allergic (extrinsic) — *see* Pneumonitis, hypersensitivity
  due to
    Aspergillus clavatus J67.4
    Cryptostroma corticale J67.6
  fibrosing (cryptogenic) (idiopathic) J84.112
  jaw M27.3
  sicca dolorosa M27.3
Alveolus, alveolar — *see* condition
Alymphocytosis D72.810
  thymic (with immunodeficiency) D82.1
Alymphoplasia, thymic D82.1
Alzheimer's disease or sclerosis — *see* Disease, Alzheimer's
Amastia (with nipple present) Q83.8
  with absent nipple Q83.0
Amathophobia F40.228
Amaurosis (acquired) (congenital) (*see also* Blindness)
  fugax G45.3
  hysterical F44.6
  Leber's congenital H35.50
  uremic — *see* Uremia
Amaurotic idiocy (infantile) (juvenile) (late) E75.4
Amaxophobia F40.248
Ambiguous genitalia Q56.4
Amblyopia (congenital) (ex anopsia) (partial) (suppression) H53.00- ☑
  anisometropic — *see* Amblyopia, refractive
  deprivation H53.01- ☑
  hysterical F44.6
  nocturnal (*see also* Blindness, night)
    vitamin A deficiency E50.5
  refractive H53.02- ☑
  strabismic H53.03- ☑
  suspect H53.04- ☑
  tobacco H53.8
  toxic NEC H53.8
  uremic — *see* Uremia
Ameba, amebic (histolytica) (*see also* Amebiasis)
  abscess (liver) A06.4
Amebiasis A06.9
  with abscess — *see* Abscess, amebic
  acute A06.0
  chronic (intestine) A06.1
    with abscess — *see* Abscess, amebic
  cutaneous A06.7
  cutis A06.7
  cystitis A06.81
  genitourinary tract NEC A06.82
  hepatic — *see* Abscess, liver, amebic
  intestine A06.0
  nondysenteric colitis A06.2
  skin A06.7
  specified site NEC A06.89
Ameboma (of intestine) A06.3
Amelia Q73.0
  lower limb — *see* Agenesis, leg
  upper limb — *see* Agenesis, arm
Ameloblastoma (*see also* Cyst, calcifying odontogenic)
  long bones C40.9- ☑
    lower limb C40.2- ☑
    upper limb C40.0- ☑
  malignant C41.1
    jaw (bone) (lower) C41.1

Ameloblastoma — *continued*
  malignant — *continued*
    jaw — *continued*
      upper C41.0
  tibial C40.2- ☑
Amelogenesis imperfecta K00.5
  nonhereditaria (segmentalis) K00.4
Amenorrhea N91.2
  hyperhormonal E28.8
  primary N91.0
  secondary N91.1
Amentia — *see* Disability, intellectual
  Meynert's (nonalcoholic) F04
American
  leishmaniasis B55.2
  mountain tick fever A93.2
Ametropia — *see* Disorder, refraction
AMH (asymptomatic microscopic hematuria) R31.21
Amianthosis J61
Amimia R48.8
Amino-acid disorder E72.9
  anemia D53.0
Aminoacidopathy E72.9
Aminoaciduria E72.9
Amnesia R41.3
  anterograde R41.1
  auditory R48.8
  dissociative F44.0
    with dissociative fugue F44.1
  hysterical F44.0
  postictal in epilepsy — *see* Epilepsy
  psychogenic F44.0
  retrograde R41.2
  transient global G45.4
Amnes(t)ic syndrome (post-traumatic) F04
  induced by
    alcohol F10.96
      with dependence F10.26
    psychoactive NEC F19.96
      with
        abuse F19.16
        dependence F19.26
    sedative F13.96
      with dependence F13.26
Amnion, amniotic — *see* condition
Amnionitis — *see* Pregnancy, complicated by
Amok F68.8
Amoral traits F60.89
Amphetamine (or other stimulant) **-induced**
  anxiety disorder F15.980
  bipolar and related disorder F15.94
  delirium F15.921
  depressive disorder F15.94
  obsessive-compulsive and related disorder F15.988
  psychotic disorder F15.959
  sexual dysfunction F15.981
  sleep disorder F15.982
  stimulant withdrawal F15.23
Ampulla
  lower esophagus K22.8
  phrenic K22.8
Amputation (*see also* Absence, by site, acquired)
  neuroma (postoperative) (traumatic) — *see* Complications, amputation stump, neuroma
  stump (surgical)
    abnormal, painful, or with complication (late) — *see* Complications, amputation stump
    healed or old NOS Z89.9
  traumatic (complete) (partial)
    arm (upper) (complete) S48.91- ☑
      at
        elbow S58.01- ☑
          partial S58.02- ☑
        shoulder joint (complete) S48.01- ☑
          partial S48.02- ☑
      between
        elbow and wrist (complete) S58.11- ☑
          partial S58.12- ☑
        shoulder and elbow (complete) S48.11- ☑
          partial S48.12- ☑
      partial S48.92- ☑
    breast (complete) S28.21- ☑
      partial S28.22- ☑
    clitoris (complete) S38.211
      partial S38.212
    ear (complete) S08.11- ☑
      partial S08.12- ☑

Amputation — *continued*
  traumatic — *continued*
    finger (complete) (metacarpophalangeal) S68.11- ☑
      index S68.11- ☑
      little S68.11- ☑
      middle S68.11- ☑
      partial S68.12- ☑
        index S68.12- ☑
        little S68.12- ☑
        middle S68.12- ☑
        ring S68.12- ☑
      ring S68.11- ☑
      thumb — *see* Amputation, traumatic, thumb
      transphalangeal (complete) S68.61- ☑
        index S68.61- ☑
        little S68.61- ☑
        middle S68.61- ☑
        partial S68.62- ☑
          index S68.62- ☑
          little S68.62- ☑
          middle S68.62- ☑
          ring S68.62- ☑
        ring S68.61- ☑
    foot (complete) S98.91- ☑
      at ankle level S98.01- ☑
        partial S98.02- ☑
      midfoot S98.31- ☑
        partial S98.32- ☑
      partial S98.92- ☑
    forearm (complete) S58.91- ☑
      at elbow level (complete) S58.01- ☑
        partial S58.02- ☑
      between elbow and wrist (complete) S58.11- ☑
        partial S58.12- ☑
      partial S58.92- ☑
    genital organ(s) (external)
      female (complete) S38.211 ☑
        partial S38.212 ☑
      male
        penis (complete) S38.221 ☑
          partial S38.222 ☑
        scrotum (complete) S38.231 ☑
          partial S38.232 ☑
        testes (complete) S38.231 ☑
          partial S38.232 ☑
    hand (complete) (wrist level) S68.41- ☑
      finger(s) alone — *see* Amputation, traumatic, finger
      partial S68.42- ☑
      thumb alone — *see* Amputation, traumatic, thumb
      transmetacarpal (complete) S68.71- ☑
        partial S68.72- ☑
    head
      ear — *see* Amputation, traumatic, ear
      nose (partial) S08.812 ☑
        complete S08.811 ☑
      part S08.89 ☑
      scalp S08.0 ☑
    hip (and thigh) (complete) S78.91- ☑
      at hip joint (complete) S78.01- ☑
        partial S78.02- ☑
      between hip and knee (complete) S78.11- ☑
        partial S78.12- ☑
      partial S78.92- ☑
    labium (majus) (minus) (complete) S38.21- ☑
      partial S38.21- ☑
    leg (lower) S88.91- ☑
      at knee level S88.01- ☑
        partial S88.02- ☑
      between knee and ankle S88.11- ☑
        partial S88.12- ☑
      partial S88.92- ☑
    nose (partial) S08.812 ☑
      complete S08.811 ☑
    penis (complete) S38.221 ☑
      partial S38.222 ☑
    scrotum (complete) S38.231 ☑
      partial S38.232 ☑
    shoulder — *see* Amputation, traumatic, arm
      at shoulder joint — *see* Amputation, traumatic, arm, at shoulder joint
    testes (complete) S38.231 ☑
      partial S38.232 ☑
    thigh — *see* Amputation, traumatic, hip

⬟ Subterms under main terms may continue to next column or page   ☑ Additional Character Required — Refer to the Tabular List for Character Selection   **17**

Alport syndrome — Amputation

Amputation — *continued*
  traumatic — *continued*
    thorax, part of S28.1 ☑
      breast — *see* Amputation, traumatic, breast
    thumb (complete) (metacarpophalangeal) S68.01- ☑
      partial S68.02- ☑
      transphalangeal (complete) S68.51- ☑
        partial S68.52- ☑
    toe (lesser) S98.13- ☑
      great S98.11- ☑
        partial S98.12- ☑
      more than one S98.21- ☑
        partial S98.22- ☑
      partial S98.14- ☑
    vulva (complete) S38.211 ☑
      partial S38.212 ☑
Amputee (bilateral) (old) Z89.9
Amsterdam dwarfism Q87.1
Amusia R48.8
  developmental F80.89
Amyelencephalus, amyelencephaly Q00.0
Amyelia Q06.0
Amygdalitis — *see* Tonsillitis
Amygdalolith J35.8
Amyloid heart (disease) E85.4 [I43]
Amyloidosis (generalized) (primary) E85.9
  with lung involvement E85.4 [J99]
  familial E85.2
  genetic E85.2
  heart E85.4 [I43]
  hemodialysis-associated E85.3
  light chain (AL) E85.81
  liver E85.4 [K77]
  localized E85.4
  neuropathic heredofamilial E85.1
  non-neuropathic heredofamilial E85.0
  organ limited E85.4
  Portuguese E85.1
  pulmonary E85.4 [J99]
  secondary systemic E85.3
  senile systemic (SSA) E85.82
  skin (lichen) (macular) E85.4 [L99]
  specified NEC E85.89
  subglottic E85.4 [J99]
  wild-type transthyretin-related (ATTR) E85.82
Amylopectinosis (brancher enzyme deficiency) E74.03
Amylophagia — *see* Pica
Amyoplasia congenita Q79.8
Amyotonia M62.89
  congenita G70.2
Amyotrophia, amyotrophy, amyotrophic G71.8
  congenita Q79.8
  diabetic — *see* Diabetes, amyotrophy
  lateral sclerosis G12.21
  neuralgic G54.5
  spinal progressive G12.25
Anacidity, gastric K31.83
  psychogenic F45.8
Anaerosis of newborn P28.89
Analbuminemia E88.09
Analgesia — *see* Anesthesia
Analphalipoproteinemia E78.6
Anaphylactic
  purpura D69.0
  shock or reaction — *see* Shock, anaphylactic
Anaphylactoid shock or reaction — *see* Shock, anaphylactic
Anaphylactoid syndrome of pregnancy O88.01- ☑
Anaphylaxis — *see* Shock, anaphylactic
Anaplasia cervix (*see also* Dysplasia, cervix) N87.9
Anaplasmosis, human A77.49
Anarthria R47.1
Anasarca R60.1
  cardiac — *see* Failure, heart, congestive
  lung J18.2
  newborn P83.2
  nutritional E43
  pulmonary J18.2
  renal N04.9
Anastomosis
  aneurysmal — *see* Aneurysm
  arteriovenous ruptured brain I60.8
  intestinal K63.89
    complicated NEC K91.89
      involving urinary tract N99.89
  retinal and choroidal vessels (congenital) Q14.8

Anatomical narrow angle H40.03- ☑
Ancylostoma, ancylostomiasis (braziliense) (caninum) (ceylanicum) (duodenale) B76.0
  Necator americanus B76.1
Andersen's disease (glycogen storage) E74.09
Anderson-Fabry disease E75.21
Andes disease T70.29 ☑
Andrews' disease (bacterid) L08.89
Androblastoma
  benign
    specified site — *see* Neoplasm, benign, by site
    unspecified site
      female D27.9
      male D29.20
  malignant
    specified site — *see* Neoplasm, malignant, by site
    unspecified site
      female C56.9
      male C62.90
  specified site — *see* Neoplasm, uncertain behavior, by site
  tubular
    with lipid storage
      specified site — *see* Neoplasm, benign, by site
      unspecified site
        female D27.9
        male D29.20
    specified site — *see* Neoplasm, benign, by site
    unspecified site
      female D27.9
      male D29.20
  unspecified site
    female D39.10
    male D40.10
Androgen insensitivity syndrome (*see also* Syndrome, androgen insensitivity) E34.50
Androgen resistance syndrome (*see also* Syndrome, androgen insensitivity) E34.50
Android pelvis Q74.2
  with disproportion (fetopelvic) O33.3 ☑
    causing obstructed labor O65.3
Androphobia F40.290
Anectasis, pulmonary (newborn) — *see* Atelectasis
Anemia (essential) (general) (hemoglobin deficiency) (infantile) (primary) (profound) D64.9
  with (due to) (in)
    disorder of
      anaerobic glycolysis D55.2
      pentose phosphate pathway D55.1
    koilonychia D50.9
  achlorhydric D50.8
  achrestic D53.1
  Addison (-Biermer) (pernicious) D51.0
  agranulocytic — *see* Agranulocytosis
  amino-acid-deficiency D53.0
  aplastic D61.9
    congenital D61.09
    drug-induced D61.1
    due to
      drugs D61.1
      external agents NEC D61.2
      infection D61.2
      radiation D61.2
    idiopathic D61.3
    red cell (pure) D60.9
      chronic D60.0
      congenital D61.01
      specified type NEC D60.8
      transient D60.1
    specified type NEC D61.89
    toxic D61.2
  aregenerative
    congenital D61.09
  asiderotic D50.9
  atypical (primary) D64.9
  Baghdad spring D55.0
  Balantidium coli A07.0
  Biermer's (pernicious) D51.0
  blood loss (chronic) D50.0
    acute D62
  bothriocephalus B70.0 [D63.8]
  brickmaker's B76.9 [D63.8]
  cerebral I67.89
  childhood D58.9
  chlorotic D50.8
  chronic
    blood loss D50.0
    hemolytic D58.9

Anemia — *continued*
  chronic — *continued*
    hemolytic — *continued*
      idiopathic D59.9
    simple D53.9
  chronica congenita aregenerativa D61.09
  combined system disease NEC D51.0 [G32.0]
    due to dietary vitamin B12 deficiency D51.3 [G32.0]
  complicating pregnancy, childbirth or puerperium — *see* Pregnancy, complicated by (management affected by), anemia
  congenital P61.4
    aplastic D61.09
    due to isoimmunization NOS P55.9
    dyserythropoietic, dyshematopoietic D64.4
    following fetal blood loss P61.3
    Heinz body D58.2
    hereditary hemolytic NOS D58.9
    pernicious D51.0
    spherocytic D58.0
  Cooley's (erythroblastic) D56.1
  cytogenic D51.0
  deficiency D53.9
    6-PGD D55.1
    2, 3 diphosphoglycurate mutase D55.2
    2, 3 PG D55.2
    6 phosphogluconate dehydrogenase D55.1
    amino-acid D53.0
    combined B12 and folate D53.1
    enzyme D55.9
      drug-induced (hemolytic) D59.2
      glucose-6-phosphate dehydrogenase (G6PD) D55.0
      glycolytic D55.2
      nucleotide metabolism D55.3
      related to hexose monophosphate (HMP) shunt pathway NEC D55.1
      specified type NEC D55.8
    erythrocytic glutathione D55.1
    folate D52.9
      dietary D52.0
      drug-induced D52.1
    folic acid D52.9
      dietary D52.0
      drug-induced D52.1
    G SH D55.1
    G6PD D55.0
    GGS-R D55.1
    glucose-6-phosphate dehydrogenase D55.0
    glutathione reductase D55.1
    glyceraldehyde phosphate dehydrogenase D55.2
    hexokinase D55.2
    iron D50.9
      secondary to blood loss (chronic) D50.0
    nutritional D53.9
      with
        poor iron absorption D50.8
        specified deficiency NEC D53.8
    phosphofructo-aldolase D55.2
    phosphoglycerate kinase D55.2
    PK D55.2
    protein D53.0
    pyruvate kinase D55.2
    transcobalamin II D51.2
    triose-phosphate isomerase D55.2
    vitamin B12 NOS D51.9
      dietary D51.3
      due to
        intrinsic factor deficiency D51.0
        selective vitamin B12 malabsorption with proteinuria D51.1
      pernicious D51.0
      specified type NEC D51.8
  Diamond-Blackfan (congenital hypoplastic) D61.01
  dibothriocephalus B70.0 [D63.8]
  dimorphic D53.1
  diphasic D53.1
  Diphyllobothrium (Dibothriocephalus) B70.0 [D63.8]
  due to (in) (with)
    antineoplastic chemotherapy D64.81
    blood loss (chronic) D50.0
      acute D62
    chemotherapy, antineoplastic D64.81
    chronic disease classified elsewhere NEC D63.8
    chronic kidney disease D63.1
    deficiency
      amino-acid D53.0
      copper D53.8
      folate (folic acid) D52.9

Anemia — *continued*
  due to — *continued*
    deficiency — *continued*
      folate — *continued*
        dietary D52.0
        drug-induced D52.1
      molybdenum D53.8
      protein D53.0
      zinc D53.8
    dietary vitamin B12 deficiency D51.3
    disorder of
      glutathione metabolism D55.1
      nucleotide metabolism D55.3
    drug — *see* Anemia, by type (*see also* Table of
        Drugs and Chemicals)
    end stage renal disease D63.1
    enzyme disorder D55.9
    fetal blood loss P61.3
    fish tapeworm (D.latum) infestation B70.0 [D63.8]
    hemorrhage (chronic) D50.0
      acute D62
    impaired absorption D50.9
    loss of blood (chronic) D50.0
      acute D62
    myxedema E03.9 [D63.8]
    Necator americanus B76.1 [D63.8]
    prematurity P61.2
    selective vitamin B12 malabsorption with protein-
        uria D51.1
    transcobalamin II deficiency D51.2
  Dyke-Young type (secondary) (symptomatic) D59.1
  dyserythropoietic (congenital) D64.4
  dyshematopoietic (congenital) D64.4
  Egyptian B76.9 [D63.8]
  elliptocytosis — *see* Elliptocytosis
  enzyme-deficiency, drug-induced D59.2
  epidemic (*see also* Ancylostomiasis) B76.9 [D63.8]
  erythroblastic
    familial D56.1
    newborn (*see also* Disease, hemolytic) P55.9
    of childhood D56.1
  erythrocytic glutathione deficiency D55.1
  erythropoietin-resistant anemia (EPO resistant anemia)
      D63.1
  Faber's (achlorhydric anemia) D50.9
  factitious (self-induced blood letting) D50.0
  familial erythroblastic D56.1
  Fanconi's (congenital pancytopenia) D61.09
  favism D55.0
  fish tapeworm (D. latum) infestation B70.0 [D63.8]
  folate (folic acid) deficiency D52.9
  glucose-6-phosphate dehydrogenase (G6PD) deficien-
      cy D55.0
  glutathione-reductase deficiency D55.1
  goat's milk D52.0
  granulocytic — *see* Agranulocytosis
  Heinz body, congenital D58.2
  hemolytic D58.9
    acquired D59.9
      with hemoglobinuria NEC D59.6
      autoimmune NEC D59.1
      infectious D59.4
      specified type NEC D59.8
      toxic D59.4
    acute D59.9
      due to enzyme deficiency specified type NEC
          D55.8
      Lederer's D59.1
    autoimmune D59.1
      drug-induced D59.0
    chronic D58.9
      idiopathic D59.9
    cold type (secondary) (symptomatic) D59.1
    congenital (spherocytic) — *see* Spherocytosis
    due to
      cardiac conditions D59.4
      drugs (nonautoimmune) D59.2
        autoimmune D59.0
      enzyme disorder D55.9
        drug-induced D59.2
      presence of shunt or other internal prosthetic
          device D59.4
    familial D58.9
    hereditary D58.9
      due to enzyme disorder D55.9
        specified type NEC D55.8
      specified type NEC D58.8
    idiopathic (chronic) D59.9
    mechanical D59.4

Anemia — *continued*
  hemolytic — *continued*
    microangiopathic D59.4
    nonautoimmune D59.4
      drug-induced D59.2
    nonspherocytic
      congenital or hereditary NEC D55.8
        glucose-6-phosphate dehydrogenase defi-
            ciency D55.0
        pyruvate kinase deficiency D55.2
      type
        I D55.1
        II D55.2
      type
        I D55.1
        II D55.2
    secondary D59.4
      autoimmune D59.1
    specified (hereditary) type NEC D58.8
    Stransky-Regala type (*see also* Hemoglobinopathy)
        D58.8
    symptomatic D59.4
      autoimmune D59.1
    toxic D59.4
    warm type (secondary) (symptomatic) D59.1
  hemorrhagic (chronic) D50.0
    acute D62
  Herrick's D57.1
  hexokinase deficiency D55.2
  hookworm B76.9 [D63.8]
  hypochromic (idiopathic) (microcytic) (normoblastic)
      D50.9
    due to blood loss (chronic) D50.0
      acute D62
    familial sex-linked D64.0
    pyridoxine-responsive D64.3
    sideroblastic, sex-linked D64.0
  hypoplasia, red blood cells D61.9
    congenital or familial D61.01
  hypoplastic (idiopathic) D61.9
    congenital or familial (of childhood) D61.01
  hypoproliferative (refractive) D61.9
  idiopathic D64.9
    aplastic D61.3
    hemolytic, chronic D59.9
  in (due to) (with)
    chronic kidney disease D63.1
    end stage renal disease D63.1
    failure, kidney (renal) D63.1
    neoplastic disease (*see also* Neoplasm) D63.0
  intertropical (*see also* Ancylostomiasis) D63.8
  iron deficiency D50.9
    secondary to blood loss (chronic) D50.0
      acute D62
    specified type NEC D50.8
  Joseph-Diamond-Blackfan (congenital hypoplastic)
      D61.01
  Lederer's (hemolytic) D59.1
  leukoerythroblastic D61.82
  macrocytic D53.9
    nutritional D52.0
    tropical D52.8
  malarial (*see also* Malaria) B54 [D63.8]
  malignant (progressive) D51.0
  malnutrition D53.9
  marsh (*see also* Malaria) B54 [D63.8]
  Mediterranean (with other hemoglobinopathy) D56.9
  megaloblastic D53.1
    combined B12 and folate deficiency D53.1
    hereditary D51.1
    nutritional D52.0
    orotic aciduria D53.0
    refractory D53.1
    specified type NEC D53.1
  megalocytic D53.1
  microcytic (hypochromic) D50.9
    due to blood loss (chronic) D50.0
      acute D62
    familial D56.8
  microdrepanocytosis D57.40
  microelliptopoikilocytic (Rietti-Greppi- Micheli) D56.9
  miner's B76.9 [D63.8]
  myelodysplastic D46.9
  myelofibrosis D75.81
  myelogenous D64.89
  myelopathic D64.89
  myelophthisic D61.82
  myeloproliferative D47.Z9 (*following* D47.4)
  newborn P61.4

Anemia — *continued*
  newborn — *continued*
    due to
      ABO (antibodies, isoimmunization, maternal/fe-
          tal incompatibility) P55.1
      Rh (antibodies, isoimmunization, maternal/fetal
          incompatibility) P55.0
    following fetal blood loss P61.3
    posthemorrhagic (fetal) P61.3
  nonspherocytic hemolytic — *see* Anemia, hemolytic,
      nonspherocytic
  normocytic (infectional) D64.9
    due to blood loss (chronic) D50.0
      acute D62
    myelophthisic D61.82
  nutritional (deficiency) D53.9
    with
      poor iron absorption D50.8
      specified deficiency NEC D53.8
    megaloblastic D52.0
  of prematurity P61.2
  orotaciduric (congenital) (hereditary) D53.0
  osteosclerotic D64.89
  ovalocytosis (hereditary) — *see* Elliptocytosis
  paludal (*see also* Malaria) B54 [D63.8]
  pernicious (congenital) (malignant) (progressive) D51.0
  pleochromic D64.89
    of sprue D52.8
  posthemorrhagic (chronic) D50.0
    acute D62
    newborn P61.3
  postoperative (postprocedural)
    due to (acute) blood loss D62
      chronic blood loss D50.0
    specified NEC D64.9
  postpartum O90.81
  pressure D64.89
  progressive D64.9
    malignant D51.0
    pernicious D51.0
  protein-deficiency D53.0
  pseudoleukemica infantum D64.89
  pure red cell D60.9
    congenital D61.01
  pyridoxine-responsive D64.3
  pyruvate kinase deficiency D55.2
  refractory D46.4
    with
      excess of blasts D46.20
        1 (RAEB 1) D46.21
        2 (RAEB 2) D46.22
        in transformation (RAEB T) — *see* Leukemia,
            acute myeloblastic
      hemochromatosis D46.1
      sideroblasts (ring) (RARS) D46.1
    without ring sideroblasts, so stated D46.0
    without sideroblasts without excess of blasts D46.0
    megaloblastic D53.1
    sideroblastic D46.1
    sideropenic D50.9
  Rietti-Greppi-Micheli D56.9
  scorbutic D53.2
  secondary to
    blood loss (chronic) D50.0
      acute D62
    hemorrhage (chronic) D50.0
      acute D62
  semiplastic D61.89
  sickle-cell — *see* Disease, sickle-cell
  sideroblastic D64.3
    hereditary D64.0
    hypochromic, sex-linked D64.0
    pyridoxine-responsive NEC D64.3
    refractory D46.1
    secondary (due to)
      disease D64.1
      drugs and toxins D64.2
    specified type NEC D64.3
  sideropenic (refractory) D50.9
    due to blood loss (chronic) D50.0
      acute D62
  simple chronic D53.9
  specified type NEC D64.89
  spherocytic (hereditary) — *see* Spherocytosis
  splenic D64.89
  splenomegalic D64.89
  stomatocytosis D58.8
  syphilitic (acquired) (late) A52.79 [D63.8]
  target cell D64.89

Anemia — *continued*
  thalassemia D56.9
  thrombocytopenic — *see* Thrombocytopenia
  toxic D61.2
  tropical B76.9 [D63.8]
    macrocytic D52.8
  tuberculous A18.89 [D63.8]
  vegan D51.3
  vitamin
    B6-responsive D64.3
    B12 deficiency (dietary) pernicious D51.0
  von Jaksch's D64.89
  Witts' (achlorhydric anemia) D50.8
Anemophobia F40.228
Anencephalus, anencephaly Q00.0
Anergasia — *see* Psychosis, organic
Anesthesia, anesthetic R20.0
  complication or reaction NEC (*see also* Complications, anesthesia) T88.59 ☑
    due to
      correct substance properly administered — *see* Table of Drugs and Chemicals, by drug, adverse effect
      overdose or wrong substance given — *see* Table of Drugs and Chemicals, by drug, poisoning
      unintended awareness under general anesthesia during procedure T88.53 ☑
        personal history of Z92.84
  cornea H18.81- ☑
  dissociative F44.6
  functional (hysterical) F44.6
  hyperesthetic, thalamic G89.0
  hysterical F44.6
  local skin lesion R20.0
  sexual (psychogenic) F52.1
  shock (due to) T88.2 ☑
  skin R20.0
  testicular N50.9
Anetoderma (maculosum) (of) L90.8
  Jadassohn-Pellizzari L90.2
  Schweniger-Buzzi L90.1
Aneurin deficiency E51.9
Aneurysm (anastomotic) (artery) (cirsoid) (diffuse) (false) (fusiform) (multiple) (saccular) I72.9
  abdominal (aorta) I71.4
    ruptured I71.3
    syphilitic A52.01
  aorta, aortic (nonsyphilitic) I71.9
    abdominal I71.4
      ruptured I71.3
    arch I71.2
      ruptured I71.1
    arteriosclerotic I71.9
      ruptured I71.8
    ascending I71.2
      ruptured I71.1
    congenital Q25.43
    descending I71.9
      abdominal I71.4
        ruptured I71.3
      ruptured I71.8
      thoracic I71.2
        ruptured I71.1
    root Q25.43
    ruptured I71.8
    sinus, congenital Q25.43
    syphilitic A52.01
    thoracic I71.2
      ruptured I71.1
    thoracoabdominal I71.6
      ruptured I71.5
    thorax, thoracic (arch) I71.2
      ruptured I71.1
    transverse I71.2
      ruptured I71.1
    valve (heart) (*see also* Endocarditis, aortic) I35.8
  arteriosclerotic I72.9
    cerebral I67.1
      ruptured — *see* Hemorrhage, intracranial, subarachnoid
    arteriovenous (congenital) (*see also* Malformation, arteriovenous)
      acquired I77.0
        brain I67.1
        coronary I25.41
        pulmonary I28.0
      brain Q28.2

Aneurysm — *continued*
  arteriovenous (*see also* Malformation, arteriovenous) — *continued*
    brain — *continued*
      ruptured I60.8
    peripheral — *see* Malformation, arteriovenous, peripheral
    precerebral vessels Q28.0
    specified site NEC (*see also* Malformation, arteriovenous)
      acquired I77.0
  basal — *see* Aneurysm, brain
  basilar (trunk) I72.5
  berry (congenital) (nonruptured) I67.1
    ruptured I60.7
  brain I67.1
    arteriosclerotic I67.1
      ruptured — *see* Hemorrhage, intracranial, subarachnoid
    arteriovenous (congenital) (nonruptured) Q28.2
      acquired I67.1
        ruptured I60.8
      ruptured I60.8
    berry (congenital) (nonruptured) I67.1
      ruptured (*see also* Hemorrhage, intracranial, subarachnoid) I60.7
    congenital Q28.3
      ruptured I60.8
    meninges I67.1
      ruptured I60.8
    miliary (congenital) (nonruptured) I67.1
      ruptured (*see also* Hemorrhage, intracranial, subarachnoid) I60.7
    mycotic I33.0
    ruptured — *see* Hemorrhage, intracranial, subarachnoid
    syphilitic (hemorrhage) A52.05
  cardiac (false) (*see also* Aneurysm, heart) I25.3
  carotid artery (common) (external) I72.0
    internal (intracranial) I67.1
      extracranial portion I72.0
      ruptured into brain I60.0- ☑
    syphilitic A52.09
      intracranial A52.05
  cavernous sinus I67.1
    arteriovenous (congenital) (nonruptured) Q28.3
      ruptured I60.8
  celiac I72.8
  central nervous system, syphilitic A52.05
  cerebral — *see* Aneurysm, brain
  chest — *see* Aneurysm, thorax
  circle of Willis I67.1
    congenital Q28.3
      ruptured I60.6
    ruptured I60.6
  common iliac artery I72.3
  congenital (peripheral) Q27.8
    aorta (root) (sinus) Q25.43
    brain Q28.3
      ruptured I60.7
    coronary Q24.5
    digestive system Q27.8
    lower limb Q27.8
    pulmonary Q25.79
    retina Q14.1
    specified site NEC Q27.8
    upper limb Q27.8
  conjunctiva — *see* Abnormality, conjunctiva, vascular
  conus arteriosus — *see* Aneurysm, heart
  coronary (arteriosclerotic) (artery) I25.41
    arteriovenous, congenital Q24.5
    congenital Q24.5
    ruptured — *see* Infarct, myocardium
    syphilitic A52.06
    vein I25.89
  cylindroid (aorta) I71.9
    ruptured I71.8
    syphilitic A52.01
  ductus arteriosus Q25.0
  endocardial, infective (any valve) I33.0
  femoral (artery) (ruptured) I72.4
  gastroduodenal I72.8
  gastroepiploic I72.8
  heart (wall) (chronic or with a stated duration of over 4 weeks) I25.3
    valve — *see* Endocarditis
  hepatic I72.8
  iliac (common) (artery) (ruptured) I72.3

Aneurysm — *continued*
  infective I72.9
    endocardial (any valve) I33.0
  innominate (nonsyphilitic) I72.8
    syphilitic A52.09
  interauricular septum — *see* Aneurysm, heart
  interventricular septum — *see* Aneurysm, heart
  intrathoracic (nonsyphilitic) I71.2
    ruptured I71.1
    syphilitic A52.01
  lower limb I72.4
  lung (pulmonary artery) I28.1
  mediastinal (nonsyphilitic) I72.8
    syphilitic A52.09
  miliary (congenital) I67.1
    ruptured — *see* Hemorrhage, intracerebral, subarachnoid, intracranial
  mitral (heart) (valve) I34.8
  mural — *see* Aneurysm, heart
  mycotic I72.9
    endocardial (any valve) I33.0
    ruptured, brain — *see* Hemorrhage, intracerebral, subarachnoid
  myocardium — *see* Aneurysm, heart
  neck I72.0
  pancreaticoduodenal I72.8
  patent ductus arteriosus Q25.0
  peripheral NEC I72.8
    congenital Q27.8
      digestive system Q27.8
      lower limb Q27.8
      specified site NEC Q27.8
      upper limb Q27.8
  popliteal (artery) (ruptured) I72.4
  precerebral
    congenital (nonruptured) Q28.1
    specified site, NEC I72.5
  pulmonary I28.1
    arteriovenous Q25.72
      acquired I28.0
    syphilitic A52.09
    valve (heart) — *see* Endocarditis, pulmonary
  racemose (peripheral) I72.9
    congenital — *see* Aneurysm, congenital
  radial I72.1
  Rasmussen NEC A15.0
  renal (artery) I72.2
  retina (*see also* Disorder, retina, microaneurysms)
    congenital Q14.1
    diabetic — *see* Diabetes, microaneurysms, retinal
  sinus of Valsalva Q25.49
  specified NEC I72.8
  spinal (cord) I72.8
    syphilitic (hemorrhage) A52.09
  splenic I72.8
  subclavian (artery) (ruptured) I72.8
    syphilitic A52.09
  superior mesenteric I72.8
  syphilitic (aorta) A52.01
    central nervous system A52.05
    congenital (late) A50.54 [I79.0]
    spine, spinal A52.09
  thoracoabdominal (aorta) I71.6
    ruptured I71.5
    syphilitic A52.01
  thorax, thoracic (aorta) (arch) (nonsyphilitic) I71.2
    ruptured I71.1
    syphilitic A52.01
  traumatic (complication) (early), specified site — *see* Injury, blood vessel
  tricuspid (heart) (valve) I07.8
  ulnar I72.1
  upper limb (ruptured) I72.1
  valve, valvular — *see* Endocarditis
  venous (*see also* Varix) I86.8
    congenital Q27.8
      digestive system Q27.8
      lower limb Q27.8
      specified site NEC Q27.8
      upper limb Q27.8
  ventricle — *see* Aneurysm, heart
  vertebral artery I72.6
  visceral NEC I72.8
Angelman syndrome Q93.5
Anger R45.4
Angiectasis, angiectopia I99.8
Angiitis I77.6
  allergic granulomatous M30.1

☑ **Additional Character Required** — **Refer to the Tabular List for Character Selection**   ▽ **Subterms under main terms may continue to next column or page**

Angiitis — *continued*
hypersensitivity M31.0
necrotizing M31.9
specified NEC M31.8
nervous system, granulomatous I67.7
Angina (attack) (cardiac) (chest) (heart) (pectoris) (syndrome) (vasomotor) I20.9
with
atherosclerotic heart disease — *see* Arteriosclerosis, coronary (artery),
documented spasm I20.1
abdominal K55.1
accelerated — *see* Angina, unstable
agranulocytic — *see* Agranulocytosis
angiospastic — *see* Angina, with documented spasm
aphthous B08.5
crescendo — *see* Angina, unstable
croupous J05.0
cruris I73.9
de novo effort — *see* Angina, unstable
diphtheritic, membranous A36.0
equivalent I20.8
exudative, chronic J37.0
following acute myocardial infarction I23.7
gangrenous diphtheritic A36.0
intestinal K55.1
Ludovici K12.2
Ludwig's K12.2
malignant diphtheritic A36.0
membranous J05.0
diphtheritic A36.0
Vincent's A69.1
mesenteric K55.1
monocytic — *see* Mononucleosis, infectious
of effort — *see* Angina, specified NEC
phlegmonous J36
diphtheritic A36.0
post-infarctional I23.7
pre-infarctional — *see* Angina, unstable
Prinzmetal — *see* Angina, with documented spasm
progressive — *see* Angina, unstable
pseudomembranous A69.1
pultaceous, diphtheritic A36.0
spasm-induced — *see* Angina, with documented spasm
specified NEC I20.8
stable I20.8
stenocardia — *see* Angina, specified NEC
stridulous, diphtheritic A36.2
tonsil J36
trachealis J05.0
unstable I20.0
variant — *see* Angina, with documented spasm
Vincent's A69.1
worsening effort — *see* Angina, unstable
Angioblastoma — *see* Neoplasm, connective tissue, uncertain behavior
Angiocholecystitis — *see* Cholecystitis, acute
Angiocholitis (*see also* Cholecystitis, acute) K83.0
Angiodysgenesis spinalis G95.19
Angiodysplasia (cecum) (colon) K55.20
with bleeding K55.21
duodenum (and stomach) K31.819
with bleeding K31.811
stomach (and duodenum) K31.819
with bleeding K31.811
Angioedema (allergic) (any site) (with urticaria) T78.3 ☑
hereditary D84.1
Angioendothelioma — *see* Neoplasm, uncertain behavior, by site
benign D18.00
intra-abdominal D18.03
intracranial D18.02
skin D18.01
specified site NEC D18.09
bone — *see* Neoplasm, bone, malignant
Ewing's — *see* Neoplasm, bone, malignant
Angioendotheliomatosis C85.8- ☑
Angiofibroma (*see also* Neoplasm, benign, by site)
juvenile
specified site — *see* Neoplasm, benign, by site
unspecified site D10.6
Angiohemophilia (A) (B) D68.0
Angioid streaks (choroid) (macula) (retina) H35.33
Angiokeratoma — *see* Neoplasm, skin, benign
corporis diffusum E75.21
Angioleiomyoma — *see* Neoplasm, connective tissue, benign

Angiolipoma (*see also* Lipoma)
infiltrating — *see* Lipoma
Angioma (*see also* Hemangioma, by site)
capillary I78.1
hemorrhagicum hereditaria I78.0
intra-abdominal D18.03
intracranial D18.02
malignant — *see* Neoplasm, connective tissue, malignant
plexiform D18.00
intra-abdominal D18.03
intracranial D18.02
skin D18.01
specified site NEC D18.09
senile I78.1
serpiginosum L81.7
skin D18.01
specified site NEC D18.09
spider I78.1
stellate I78.1
venous Q28.3
Angiomatosis Q82.8
bacillary A79.89
encephalotrigeminal Q85.8
hemorrhagic familial I78.0
hereditary familial I78.0
liver K76.4
Angiomyolipoma — *see* Lipoma
Angiomyoliposarcoma — *see* Neoplasm, connective tissue, malignant
Angiomyoma — *see* Neoplasm, connective tissue, benign
Angiomyosarcoma — *see* Neoplasm, connective tissue, malignant
Angiomyxoma — *see* Neoplasm, connective tissue, uncertain behavior
Angioneurosis F45.8
Angioneurotic edema (allergic) (any site) (with urticaria) T78.3 ☑
hereditary D84.1
Angiopathia, angiopathy I99.9
cerebral I67.9
amyloid E85.4 [I68.0]
diabetic (peripheral) — *see* Diabetes, angiopathy
peripheral I73.9
diabetic — *see* Diabetes, angiopathy
specified type NEC I73.89
retinae syphilitica A52.05
retinalis (juvenilis)
diabetic — *see* Diabetes, retinopathy
proliferative — *see* Retinopathy, proliferative
Angiosarcoma (*see also* Neoplasm, connective tissue, malignant)
liver C22.3
Angiosclerosis — *see* Arteriosclerosis
Angiospasm (peripheral) (traumatic) (vessel) I73.9
brachial plexus G54.0
cerebral G45.9
cervical plexus G54.2
nerve
arm — *see* Mononeuropathy, upper limb
axillary G54.0
median — *see* Lesion, nerve, median
ulnar — *see* Lesion, nerve, ulnar
axillary G54.0
leg — *see* Mononeuropathy, lower limb
median — *see* Lesion, nerve, median
plantar — *see* Lesion, nerve, plantar
ulnar — *see* Lesion, nerve, ulnar
Angiospastic disease or edema I73.9
Angiostrongyliasis
due to
Parastrongylus
cantonensis B83.2
costaricensis B81.3
intestinal B81.3
Anguillulosis — *see* Strongyloidiasis
Angulation
cecum — *see* Obstruction, intestine
coccyx (acquired) (*see also* subcategory) M43.8 ☑
congenital NEC Q76.49
femur (acquired) (*see also* Deformity, limb, specified type NEC, thigh)
congenital Q74.2
intestine (large) (small) — *see* Obstruction, intestine
sacrum (acquired) (*see also* subcategory) M43.8 ☑
congenital NEC Q76.49
sigmoid (flexure) — *see* Obstruction, intestine

Angulation — *continued*
spine — *see* Dorsopathy, deforming, specified NEC
tibia (acquired) (*see also* Deformity, limb, specified type NEC, lower leg)
congenital Q74.2
ureter N13.5
with infection N13.6
wrist (acquired) (*see also* Deformity, limb, specified type NEC, forearm)
congenital Q74.0
Angulus infectiosus (lips) K13.0
Anhedonia R45.84
sexual F52.0
Anhidrosis L74.4
Anhydration E86.0
Anhydremia E86.0
Anidrosis L74.4
Aniridia (congenital) Q13.1
Anisakiasis (infection) (infestation) B81.0
Anisakis larvae infestation B81.0
Aniseikonia H52.32
Anisocoria (pupil) H57.02
congenital Q13.2
Anisocytosis R71.8
Anisometropia (congenital) H52.31
Ankle — *see* condition
Ankyloblepharon (eyelid) (acquired) (*see also* Blepharophimosis)
filiforme (adnatum) (congenital) Q10.3
total Q10.3
Ankyloglossia Q38.1
Ankylosis (fibrous) (osseous) (joint) M24.60
ankle M24.67- ☑
arthrodesis status Z98.1
cricoarytenoid (cartilage) (joint) (larynx) J38.7
dental K03.5
ear ossicles H74.31- ☑
elbow M24.62- ☑
foot M24.67- ☑
hand M24.64- ☑
hip M24.65- ☑
incostapedial joint (infectional) — *see* Ankylosis, ear ossicles
jaw (temporomandibular) M26.61- ☑
knee M24.66- ☑
lumbosacral (joint) M43.27
postoperative (status) Z98.1
produced by surgical fusion, status Z98.1
sacro-iliac (joint) M43.28
shoulder M24.61- ☑
spine (joint) (*see also* Fusion, spine)
spondylitic — *see* Spondylitis, ankylosing
surgical Z98.1
temporomandibular M26.61- ☑
tooth, teeth (hard tissues) K03.5
wrist M24.63- ☑
Ankylostoma — *see* Ancylostoma
Ankylostomiasis — *see* Ancylostomiasis
Ankylurethria — *see* Stricture, urethra
Annular (*see also* condition)
detachment, cervix N88.8
organ or site, congenital NEC — *see* Distortion
pancreas (congenital) Q45.1
Anodontia (complete) (partial) (vera) K00.0
acquired K08.10 ☑
Anomaly, anomalous (congenital) (unspecified type) Q89.9
abdominal wall NEC Q79.59
acoustic nerve Q07.8
adrenal (gland) Q89.1
Alder (-Reilly) (leukocyte granulation) D72.0
alimentary tract Q45.9
upper Q40.9
alveolar M26.70
hyperplasia M26.79
mandibular M26.72
maxillary M26.71
hypoplasia M26.79
mandibular M26.74
maxillary M26.73
ridge (process) M26.79
specified NEC M26.79
ankle (joint) Q74.2
anus Q43.9
aorta (arch) NEC Q25.40
coarctation (preductal) (postductal) Q25.1
aortic cusp or valve Q23.9

Index

Anomaly, anomalous — Anomaly, anomalous

Anomaly, anomalous — *continued*
   appendix Q43.8
   apple peel syndrome Q41.1
   aqueduct of Sylvius Q03.0
      with spina bifida — *see* Spina bifida, with hydro-
         cephalus
   arm Q74.0
   arteriovenous NEC
      coronary Q24.5
      gastrointestinal Q27.33
         acquired — *see* Angiodysplasia
   artery (peripheral) Q27.9
      basilar NEC Q28.1
      cerebral Q28.3
      coronary Q24.5
      digestive system Q27.8
      eye Q15.8
      great Q25.9
         specified NEC Q25.8
      lower limb Q27.8
      peripheral Q27.9
         specified NEC Q27.8
      pulmonary NEC Q25.79
      renal Q27.2
      retina Q14.1
      specified site NEC Q27.8
      subclavian Q27.8
         origin Q25.48
      umbilical Q27.0
      upper limb Q27.8
      vertebral NEC Q28.1
   aryteno-epiglottic folds Q31.8
   atrial
      bands or folds Q20.8
      septa Q21.1
   atrioventricular
      excitation I45.6
      septum Q21.0
   auditory canal Q17.8
   auricle
      ear Q17.8
         causing impairment of hearing Q16.9
      heart Q20.8
   Axenfeld's Q15.0
   back Q89.9
   band
      atrial Q20.8
      heart Q24.8
      ventricular Q24.8
   Bartholin's duct Q38.4
   biliary duct or passage Q44.5
   bladder Q64.70
      absence Q64.5
      diverticulum Q64.6
      exstrophy Q64.10
         cloacal Q64.12
         extroversion Q64.19
         specified type NEC Q64.19
         supravesical fissure Q64.11
      neck obstruction Q64.31
      specified type NEC Q64.79
   bone Q79.9
      arm Q74.0
      face Q75.9
      leg Q74.2
      pelvic girdle Q74.2
      shoulder girdle Q74.0
      skull Q75.9
         with
            anencephaly Q00.0
            encephalocele — *see* Encephalocele
            hydrocephalus Q03.9
               with spina bifida — *see* Spina bifida, by
                  site, with hydrocephalus
            microcephaly Q02
   brain (multiple) Q04.9
      vessel Q28.3
   breast Q83.9
   broad ligament Q50.6
   bronchus Q32.4
   bulbus cordis Q21.9
   bursa Q79.9
   canal of Nuck Q52.4
   canthus Q10.3
   capillary Q27.9
   cardiac Q24.9
      chambers Q20.9
         specified NEC Q20.8
      septal closure Q21.9

Anomaly, anomalous — *continued*
   cardiac — *continued*
      septal closure — *continued*
         specified NEC Q21.8
      valve NEC Q24.8
         pulmonary Q22.3
   cardiovascular system Q28.8
   carpus Q74.0
   caruncle, lacrimal Q10.6
   cascade stomach Q40.2
   cauda equina Q06.3
   cecum Q43.9
   cerebral Q04.9
      vessels Q28.3
   cervix Q51.9
   Chédiak-Higashi (-Steinbrinck) (congenital gigantism
      of peroxidase granules) E70.330
   cheek Q18.9
   chest wall Q67.8
      bones Q76.9
   chin Q18.9
   chordae tendineae Q24.8
   choroid Q14.3
      plexus Q07.8
   chromosomes, chromosomal Q99.9
      D (1) — *see* condition, chromosome 13
      E (3) — *see* condition, chromosome 18
      G — *see* condition, chromosome 21
      sex
         female phenotype Q97.8
         gonadal dysgenesis (pure) Q99.1
         Klinefelter's Q98.4
         male phenotype Q98.9
         Turner's Q96.9
      specified NEC Q99.8
   cilia Q10.3
   circulatory system Q28.9
   clavicle Q74.0
   clitoris Q52.6
   coccyx Q76.49
   colon Q43.9
   common duct Q44.5
   communication
      coronary artery Q24.5
      left ventricle with right atrium Q21.0
   concha (ear) Q17.3
   connection
      portal vein Q26.5
      pulmonary venous Q26.4
         partial Q26.3
         total Q26.2
      renal artery with kidney Q27.2
   cornea (shape) Q13.4
   coronary artery or vein Q24.5
   cranium — *see* Anomaly, skull
   cricoid cartilage Q31.8
   cystic duct Q44.5
   dental
      alveolar — *see* Anomaly, alveolar
      arch relationship M26.20
         specified NEC M26.29
   dentofacial M26.9
      alveolar — *see* Anomaly, alveolar
      dental arch relationship M26.20
         specified NEC M26.29
      functional M26.50
         specified NEC M26.59
      jaw size M26.00
         macrogenia M26.05
         mandibular
            hyperplasia M26.03
            hypoplasia M26.04
         maxillary
            hyperplasia M26.01
            hypoplasia M26.02
         microgenia M26.06
         specified type NEC M26.09
      jaw-cranial base relationship M26.10
         asymmetry M26.12
            maxillary M26.11
         specified type NEC M26.19
      malocclusion M26.4
         dental arch relationship NEC M26.29
         jaw size — *see* Anomaly, dentofacial, jaw size
         jaw-cranial base relationship — *see* Anomaly,
            dentofacial, jaw-cranial base relationship
      specified type NEC M26.89
      temporomandibular joint M26.60- ☑

Anomaly, anomalous — *continued*
   dentofacial — *continued*
      temporomandibular joint — *continued*
         adhesions M26.61- ☑
         ankylosis M26.61- ☑
         arthralgia M26.62- ☑
         articular disc M26.63- ☑
         specified type NEC M26.69
      tooth position, fully erupted M26.30
         specified NEC M26.39
   dermatoglyphic Q82.8
   diaphragm (apertures) NEC Q79.1
   digestive organ(s) or tract Q45.9
      lower Q43.9
      upper Q40.9
   distance, interarch (excessive) (inadequate) M26.25
   distribution, coronary artery Q24.5
   ductus
      arteriosus Q25.0
      botalli Q25.0
   duodenum Q43.9
   dura (brain) Q04.9
      spinal cord Q06.9
   ear (external) Q17.9
      causing impairment of hearing Q16.9
      inner Q16.5
      middle (causing impairment of hearing) Q16.4
         ossicles Q16.3
   Ebstein's (heart) (tricuspid valve) Q22.5
   ectodermal Q82.9
   Eisenmenger's (ventricular septal defect) Q21.8
   ejaculatory duct Q55.4
   elbow Q74.0
   endocrine gland NEC Q89.2
   epididymis Q55.4
   epiglottis Q31.8
   esophagus Q39.9
   eustachian tube Q17.8
   eye Q15.9
      anterior segment Q13.9
         specified NEC Q13.89
      posterior segment Q14.9
         specified NEC Q14.8
      ptosis (eyelid) Q10.0
      specified NEC Q15.8
   eyebrow Q18.8
   eyelid Q10.3
      ptosis Q10.0
   face Q18.9
      bone(s) Q75.9
   fallopian tube Q50.6
   fascia Q79.9
   femur NEC Q74.2
   fibula NEC Q74.2
   finger Q74.0
   fixation, intestine Q43.3
   flexion (joint) NOS Q74.9
      hip or thigh Q65.89
   foot NEC Q74.2
      varus (congenital) Q66.3
   foramen
      Botalli Q21.1
      ovale Q21.1
   forearm Q74.0
   forehead Q75.8
   form, teeth K00.2
   fovea centralis Q14.1
   frontal bone — *see* Anomaly, skull
   gallbladder (position) (shape) (size) Q44.1
   Gartner's duct Q52.4
   gastrointestinal tract Q45.9
   genitalia, genital organ(s) or system
      female Q52.9
         external Q52.70
         internal NOS Q52.9
      male Q55.9
         hydrocele P83.5
         specified NEC Q55.8
   genitourinary NEC
      female Q52.9
      male Q55.9
   Gerbode Q21.0
   glottis Q31.8
   granulation or granulocyte, genetic (constitutional)
      (leukocyte) D72.0
   gum Q38.6
   gyri Q07.9
   hair Q84.2
   hand Q74.0

Anomaly, anomalous — *continued*
  hard tissue formation in pulp K04.3
  head — *see* Anomaly, skull
  heart Q24.9
    auricle Q20.8
    bands or folds Q24.8
    fibroelastosis cordis I42.4
    obstructive NEC Q22.6
    patent ductus arteriosus (Botalli) Q25.0
    septum Q21.9
      auricular Q21.1
      interatrial Q21.1
      interventricular Q21.0
        with pulmonary stenosis or atresia, dextra-
          position of aorta and hypertrophy of
          right ventricle Q21.3
      specified NEC Q21.8
      ventricular Q21.0
        with pulmonary stenosis or atresia, dextra-
          position of aorta and hypertrophy of
          right ventricle Q21.3
    tetralogy of Fallot Q21.3
    valve NEC Q24.8
      aortic
        bicuspid valve Q23.1
        insufficiency Q23.1
        stenosis Q23.0
          subaortic Q24.4
      mitral
        insufficiency Q23.3
        stenosis Q23.2
      pulmonary Q22.3
        atresia Q22.0
        insufficiency Q22.2
        stenosis Q22.1
          infundibular Q24.3
          subvalvular Q24.3
      tricuspid
        atresia Q22.4
        stenosis Q22.4
    ventricle Q20.8
  heel NEC Q74.2
  Hegglin's D72.0
  hemianencephaly Q00.0
  hemicephaly Q00.0
  hemicrania Q00.0
  hepatic duct Q44.5
  hip NEC Q74.2
  hourglass stomach Q40.2
  humerus Q74.0
  hydatid of Morgagni
    female Q50.5
    male (epididymal) Q55.4
      testicular Q55.29
  hymen Q52.4
  hypersegmentation of neutrophils, hereditary D72.0
  hypophyseal Q89.2
  ileocecal (coil) (valve) Q43.9
  ileum Q43.9
  ilium NEC Q74.2
  integument Q84.9
    specified NEC Q84.8
  interarch distance (excessive) (inadequate) M26.25
  intervertebral cartilage or disc Q76.49
  intestine (large) (small) Q43.9
    with anomalous adhesions, fixation or malrotation
      Q43.3
  iris Q13.2
  ischium NEC Q74.2
  jaw — *see* Anomaly, dentofacial
    alveolar — *see* Anomaly, alveolar
  jaw-cranial base relationship — *see* Anomaly, dento-
    facial, jaw-cranial base relationship
  jejunum Q43.8
  joint Q74.9
    specified NEC Q74.8
  Jordan's D72.0
  kidney(s) (calyx) (pelvis) Q63.9
    artery Q27.2
    specified NEC Q63.8
  Klippel-Feil (brevicollis) Q76.1
  knee Q74.1
  labium (majus) (minus) Q52.70
  labyrinth, membranous Q16.5
  lacrimal apparatus or duct Q10.6
  larynx, laryngeal (muscle) Q31.9
    web (bed) Q31.0
  lens Q12.9
  leukocytes, genetic D72.0

Anomaly, anomalous — *continued*
  leukocytes, genetic — *continued*
    granulation (constitutional) D72.0
  lid (fold) Q10.3
  ligament Q79.9
    broad Q50.6
    round Q52.8
  limb Q74.9
    lower NEC Q74.2
      reduction deformity — *see* Defect, reduction,
        lower limb
    upper Q74.0
  lip Q38.0
  liver Q44.7
    duct Q44.5
  lower limb NEC Q74.2
  lumbosacral (joint) (region) Q76.49
    kyphosis — *see* Kyphosis, congenital
    lordosis — *see* Lordosis, congenital
  lung (fissure) (lobe) Q33.9
  mandible — *see* Anomaly, dentofacial
  maxilla — *see* Anomaly, dentofacial
  May (-Hegglin) D72.0
  meatus urinarius NEC Q64.79
  meningeal bands or folds Q07.9
    constriction of Q07.8
    spinal Q06.9
  meninges Q07.9
    cerebral Q04.8
    spinal Q06.9
  meningocele Q05.9
  mesentery Q45.9
  metacarpus Q74.0
  metatarsus NEC Q74.2
  middle ear Q16.4
    ossicles Q16.3
  mitral (leaflets) (valve) Q23.9
    insufficiency Q23.3
    specified NEC Q23.8
    stenosis Q23.2
  mouth Q38.6
  Müllerian (*see also* Anomaly, by site)
    uterus NEC Q51.818
  multiple NEC Q89.7
  muscle Q79.9
    eyelid Q10.3
  musculoskeletal system, except limbs Q79.9
  myocardium Q24.8
  nail Q84.6
  narrowness, eyelid Q10.3
  nasal sinus (wall) Q30.8
  neck (any part) Q18.9
  nerve Q07.9
    acoustic Q07.8
    optic Q07.8
  nervous system (central) Q07.9
  nipple Q83.9
  nose, nasal (bones) (cartilage) (septum) (sinus) Q30.9
    specified NEC Q30.8
  ocular muscle Q15.8
  omphalomesenteric duct Q43.0
  opening, pulmonary veins Q26.4
  optic
    disc Q14.2
    nerve Q07.8
  opticociliary vessels Q13.2
  orbit (eye) Q10.7
  organ Q89.9
    of Corti Q16.5
  origin
    artery
      innominate Q25.8
      pulmonary Q25.79
      renal Q27.2
      subclavian Q25.48
  osseous meatus (ear) Q16.1
  ovary Q50.39
  oviduct Q50.6
  palate (hard) (soft) NEC Q38.5
  pancreas or pancreatic duct Q45.3
  papillary muscles Q24.8
  parathyroid gland Q89.2
  paraurethral ducts Q64.79
  parotid (gland) Q38.4
  patella Q74.1
  Pelger-Huët (hereditary hyposegmentation) D72.0
  pelvic girdle NEC Q74.2
  pelvis (bony) NEC Q74.2
    rachitic E64.3

Anomaly, anomalous — *continued*
  penis (glans) Q55.69
  pericardium Q24.8
  peripheral vascular system Q27.9
  Peter's Q13.4
  pharynx Q38.8
  pigmentation L81.9
    congenital Q82.8
  pituitary (gland) Q89.2
  pleural (folds) Q34.0
  portal vein Q26.5
    connection Q26.5
  position, tooth, teeth, fully erupted M26.30
    specified NEC M26.39
  precerebral vessel Q28.1
  prepuce Q55.69
  prostate Q55.4
  pulmonary Q33.9
    artery NEC Q25.79
    valve Q22.3
      atresia Q22.0
      insufficiency Q22.2
      specified type NEC Q22.3
      stenosis Q22.1
        infundibular Q24.3
        subvalvular Q24.3
    venous connection Q26.4
      partial Q26.3
      total Q26.2
  pupil Q13.2
    function H57.00
      anisocoria H57.02
      Argyll Robertson pupil H57.01
      miosis H57.03
      mydriasis H57.04
      specified type NEC H57.09
      tonic pupil H57.05- ☑
  pylorus Q40.3
  radius Q74.0
  rectum Q43.9
  reduction (extremity) (limb)
    femur (longitudinal) — *see* Defect, reduction,
      lower limb, longitudinal, femur
    fibula (longitudinal) — *see* Defect, reduction, lower
      limb, longitudinal, fibula
    lower limb — *see* Defect, reduction, lower limb
    radius (longitudinal) — *see* Defect, reduction, up-
      per limb, longitudinal, radius
    tibia (longitudinal) — *see* Defect, reduction, lower
      limb, longitudinal, tibia
    ulna (longitudinal) — *see* Defect, reduction, upper
      limb, longitudinal, ulna
    upper limb — *see* Defect, reduction, upper limb
  refraction — *see* Disorder, refraction
  renal Q63.9
    artery Q27.2
    pelvis Q63.9
      specified NEC Q63.8
  respiratory system Q34.9
    specified NEC Q34.8
  retina Q14.1
  rib Q76.6
    cervical Q76.5
  Rieger's Q13.81
  rotation — *see* Malrotation
    hip or thigh Q65.89
  round ligament Q52.8
  sacroiliac (joint) NEC Q74.2
  sacrum NEC Q76.49
    kyphosis — *see* Kyphosis, congenital
    lordosis — *see* Lordosis, congenital
  saddle nose, syphilitic A50.57
  salivary duct or gland Q38.4
  scapula Q74.0
  scrotum — *see* Malformation, testis and scrotum
  sebaceous gland Q82.9
  seminal vesicles Q55.4
  sense organs NEC Q07.8
  sex chromosomes NEC (*see also* Anomaly, chromo-
    somes)
    female phenotype Q97.8
    male phenotype Q98.9
  shoulder (girdle) (joint) Q74.0
  sigmoid (flexure) Q43.9
  simian crease Q82.8
  sinus of Valsalva Q25.49
  skeleton generalized Q78.9
  skin (appendage) Q82.9

Index

Anomaly, anomalous — Anxiety

Anomaly, anomalous — continued
  skull Q75.9
    with
      anencephaly Q00.0
      encephalocele — see Encephalocele
      hydrocephalus Q03.9
        with spina bifida — see Spina bifida, by site,
          with hydrocephalus
      microcephaly Q02
  specified organ or site NEC Q89.8
  spermatic cord Q55.4
  spine, spinal NEC Q76.49
    column NEC Q76.49
      kyphosis — see Kyphosis, congenital
      lordosis — see Lordosis, congenital
    cord Q06.9
    nerve root Q07.8
  spleen Q89.09
    agenesis Q89.01
  stenonian duct Q38.4
  sternum NEC Q76.7
  stomach Q40.3
  submaxillary gland Q38.4
  tarsus NEC Q74.2
  tendon Q79.9
  testis — see Malformation, testis and scrotum
  thigh NEC Q74.2
  thorax (wall) Q67.8
    bony Q76.9
  throat Q38.8
  thumb Q74.0
  thymus gland Q89.2
  thyroid (gland) Q89.2
    cartilage Q31.8
  tibia NEC Q74.2
    saber A50.56
  toe Q74.2
  tongue Q38.3
  tooth, teeth K00.9
    eruption K00.6
    position, fully erupted M26.30
    spacing, fully erupted M26.30
  trachea (cartilage) Q32.1
  tragus Q17.9
  tricuspid (leaflet) (valve) Q22.9
    atresia or stenosis Q22.4
    Ebstein's Q22.5
  Uhl's (hypoplasia of myocardium, right ventricle) Q24.8
  ulna Q74.0
  umbilical artery Q27.0
  union
    cricoid cartilage and thyroid cartilage Q31.8
    thyroid cartilage and hyoid bone Q31.8
    trachea with larynx Q31.8
  upper limb Q74.0
  urachus Q64.4
  ureter Q62.8
    obstructive NEC Q62.39
      cecoureterocele Q62.32
      orthotopic ureterocele Q62.31
  urethra Q64.70
    absence Q64.5
    double Q64.74
    fistula to rectum Q64.73
    obstructive Q64.39
      stricture Q64.32
    prolapse Q64.71
    specified type NEC Q64.79
  urinary tract Q64.9
  uterus Q51.9
    with only one functioning horn Q51.4
  uvula Q38.5
  vagina Q52.4
  valleculae Q31.8
  valve (heart) NEC Q24.8
    coronary sinus Q24.5
    inferior vena cava Q24.8
    pulmonary Q22.3
    sinus coronario Q24.5
    venae cavae inferioris Q24.8
  vas deferens Q55.4
  vascular Q27.9
    brain Q28.3
    ring Q25.45
  vein(s) (peripheral) Q27.9
    brain Q28.3
    cerebral Q28.3
    coronary Q24.5
    developmental Q28.3

Anomaly, anomalous — continued
  vein(s) — continued
    great Q26.9
      specified NEC Q26.8
  vena cava (inferior) (superior) Q26.9
  venous — see Anomaly, vein(s)
  venous return Q26.8
  ventricular
    bands or folds Q24.8
    septa Q21.0
  vertebra Q76.49
    kyphosis — see Kyphosis, congenital
    lordosis — see Lordosis, congenital
  vesicourethral orifice Q64.79
  vessel(s) Q27.9
    optic papilla Q14.2
    precerebral Q28.1
  vitelline duct Q43.0
  vitreous body or humor Q14.0
  vulva Q52.70
  wrist (joint) Q74.0
Anomia R48.8
Anonychia (congenital) Q84.3
  acquired L60.8
Anophthalmos, anophthalmus (congenital) (globe)
    Q11.1
  acquired Z90.01
Anopia, anopsia H53.46- ☑
  quadrant H53.46- ☑
Anorchia, anorchism, anorchidism Q55.0
Anorexia R63.0
  hysterical F44.89
  nervosa F50.00
    atypical F50.9
    binge-eating type F50.2
      with purging F50.02
    restricting type F50.01
Anorgasmy, psychogenic (female) F52.31
  male F52.32
Anosmia R43.0
  hysterical F44.6
  postinfectional J39.8
Anosognosia R41.89
Anosteoplasia Q78.9
Anovulatory cycle N97.0
Anoxemia R09.02
  newborn P84
Anoxia (pathological) R09.02
  altitude T70.29 ☑
  cerebral G93.1
    complicating
      anesthesia (general) (local) or other sedation
        T88.59 ☑
        in labor and delivery O74.3
        in pregnancy O29.21- ☑
        postpartum, puerperal O89.2
      delivery (cesarean) (instrumental) O75.4
    during a procedure G97.81
    newborn P84
    resulting from a procedure G97.82
  due to
    drowning T75.1 ☑
    high altitude T70.29 ☑
  heart — see Insufficiency, coronary
  intrauterine P84
  myocardial — see Insufficiency, coronary
  newborn P84
  spinal cord G95.11
  systemic (by suffocation) (low content in atmosphere)
    — see Asphyxia, traumatic
Anteflexion — see Anteversion
Antenatal
  care (normal pregnancy) Z34.90
  screening (encounter for) of mother (see also En-
    counter, antenatal screening) Z36.9
Antepartum — see condition
Anterior — see condition
Antero-occlusion M26.220
Anteversion
  cervix — see Anteversion, uterus
  femur (neck), congenital Q65.89
  uterus, uterine (cervix) (postinfectional) (postpartal,
    old) N85.4
    congenital Q51.818
    in pregnancy or childbirth — see Pregnancy,
      complicated by
Anthophobia F40.228
Anthracosilicosis J60

Anthracosis (lung) (occupational) J60
  lingua K14.3
Anthrax A22.9
  with pneumonia A22.1
  cerebral A22.8
  colitis A22.2
  cutaneous A22.0
  gastrointestinal A22.2
  inhalation A22.1
  intestinal A22.2
  meningitis A22.8
  pulmonary A22.1
  respiratory A22.1
  sepsis A22.7
  specified manifestation NEC A22.8
Anthropoid pelvis Q74.2
  with disproportion (fetopelvic) O33.0
Anthropophobia F40.10
  generalized F40.11
Antibodies, maternal (blood group) — see Isoimmu-
    nization, affecting management of pregnancy
  anti-D — see Isoimmunization, affecting management
    of pregnancy, Rh
  newborn P55.0
Antibody
  anticardiolipin R76.0
    with
      hemorrhagic disorder D68.312
      hypercoagulable state D68.61
  antiphosphatidylglycerol R76.0
    with
      hemorrhagic disorder D68.312
      hypercoagulable state D68.61
  antiphosphatidylinositol R76.0
    with
      hemorrhagic disorder D68.312
      hypercoagulable state D68.61
  antiphosphatidylserine R76.0
    with
      hemorrhagic disorder D68.312
      hypercoagulable state D68.61
  antiphospholipid R76.0
    with
      hemorrhagic disorder D68.312
      hypercoagulable state D68.61
Anticardiolipin syndrome D68.61
Anticoagulant, circulating (intrinsic) (see also Disorder,
    hemorrhagic) D68.318
  drug-induced (extrinsic) (see also Disorder, hemorrhag-
    ic) D68.32
  iatrogenic D68.32
Antidiuretic hormone syndrome E22.2
Antimonial cholera — see Poisoning, antimony
Antiphospholipid
  antibody
    with hemorrhagic disorder D68.312
  syndrome D68.61
Antisocial personality F60.2
Antithrombinemia — see Circulating anticoagulants
Antithromboplastinemia D68.318
Antithromboplastinogenemia D68.318
Antitoxin complication or reaction — see Complica-
    tions, vaccination
Antlophobia F40.228
Antritis J32.0
  maxilla J32.0
    acute J01.00
      recurrent J01.01
  stomach K29.60
    with bleeding K29.61
Antrum, antral — see condition
Anuria R34
  calculous (impacted) (recurrent) (see also Calculus,
    urinary) N20.9
  following
    abortion — see Abortion by type complicated by,
      renal failure
    ectopic or molar pregnancy O08.4
  newborn P96.0
  postprocedural N99.0
  postrenal N13.8
  traumatic (following crushing) T79.5 ☑
Anus, anal — see condition
Anusitis K62.89
Anxiety F41.9
  depression F41.8
  episodic paroxysmal F41.0
  generalized F41.1

☑ Subterms under main terms may continue to next column or page   ☑ Additional Character Required — Refer to the Tabular List for Character Selection   25

Anxiety — Argyria, argyriasis

Index

Argyria, argyriasis — Arteriosclerosis, arteriosclerotic

Argyria, argyriasis — *continued*
  from drug or medicament — *see* Table of Drugs and
    Chemicals, by substance
Argyrosis, conjunctival H11.13- ☑
Arhinencephaly Q04.1
Ariboflavinosis E53.0
Arm — *see* condition
Arnold-Chiari disease, obstruction or syndrome (type
    II) Q07.00
  with
    hydrocephalus Q07.02
      with spina bifida Q07.03
    spina bifida Q07.01
      with hydrocephalus Q07.03
  type III — *see* Encephalocele
  type IV Q04.8
Aromatic amino-acid metabolism disorder E70.9
  specified NEC E70.8
Arousals, confusional G47.51
Arrest, arrested
  cardiac I46.9
    complicating
      abortion — *see* Abortion, by type, complicated
        by, cardiac arrest
      anesthesia (general) (local) or other sedation
        — *see* Table of Drugs and Chemicals, by
        drug
        in labor and delivery O74.2
        in pregnancy O29.11- ☑
        postpartum, puerperal O89.1
      delivery (cesarean) (instrumental) O75.4
    due to
      cardiac condition I46.2
      specified condition NEC I46.8
    intraoperative I97.71- ☑
    newborn P29.81
    personal history, successfully resuscitated Z86.74
    postprocedural I97.12- ☑
      obstetric procedure O75.4
  cardiorespiratory — *see* Arrest, cardiac
  circulatory — *see* Arrest, cardiac
  deep transverse O64.0 ☑
  development or growth
    bone — *see* Disorder, bone, development or
      growth
    child R62.50
    tracheal rings Q32.1
  epiphyseal
    complete
      femur M89.15- ☑
      humerus M89.12- ☑
      tibia M89.16- ☑
      ulna M89.13- ☑
      forearm M89.13- ☑
        specified NEC M89.13- ☑
      ulna — *see* Arrest, epiphyseal, by type, ulna
    lower leg M89.16- ☑
      specified NEC M89.168
      tibia — *see* Arrest, epiphyseal, by type, tibia
    partial
      femur M89.15- ☑
      humerus M89.12- ☑
      tibia M89.16- ☑
      ulna M89.13- ☑
      specified NEC M89.18
  granulopoiesis — *see* Agranulocytosis
  growth plate — *see* Arrest, epiphyseal
  heart — *see* Arrest, cardiac
  legal, anxiety concerning Z65.3
  physeal — *see* Arrest, epiphyseal
  respiratory R09.2
    newborn P28.81
  sinus I45.5
  spermatogenesis (complete) — *see* Azoospermia
    incomplete — *see* Oligospermia
  transverse (deep) O64.0 ☑
Arrhenoblastoma
  benign
    specified site — *see* Neoplasm, benign, by site
    unspecified site
      female D27.9
      male D29.20
  malignant
    specified site — *see* Neoplasm, malignant, by site
    unspecified site
      female C56.9
      male C62.90

Arrhenoblastoma — *continued*
  specified site — *see* Neoplasm, uncertain behavior,
    by site
  unspecified site
    female D39.10
    male D40.10
Arrhythmia (auricle) (cardiac) (juvenile) (nodal) (reflex)
    (sinus) (supraventricular) (transitory) (ventricle) I49.9
  block I45.9
  extrasystolic I49.49
  newborn
    bradycardia P29.12
    occurring before birth P03.819
      before onset of labor P03.810
      during labor P03.811
    tachycardia P29.11
  psychogenic F45.8
  specified NEC I49.8
  vagal R55
  ventricular re-entry I47.0
Arrillaga-Ayerza syndrome (pulmonary sclerosis with
    pulmonary hypertension) I27.0
Arsenical pigmentation L81.8
  from drug or medicament — *see* Table of Drugs and
    Chemicals
Arsenism — *see* Poisoning, arsenic
Arterial — *see* condition
Arteriofibrosis — *see* Arteriosclerosis
Arteriolar sclerosis — *see* Arteriosclerosis
Arteriolith — *see* Arteriosclerosis
Arteriolitis I77.6
  necrotizing, kidney I77.5
  renal — *see* Hypertension, kidney
Arteriolosclerosis — *see* Arteriosclerosis
Arterionephrosclerosis — *see* Hypertension, kidney
Arteriopathy I77.9
Arteriosclerosis, arteriosclerotic (diffuse) (obliterans)
    (of) (senile) (with calcification) I70.90
  aorta I70.0
  arteries of extremities — *see* Arteriosclerosis, extrem-
    ities
  brain I67.2
  bypass graft
    coronary — *see* Arteriosclerosis, coronary, bypass
      graft
    extremities — *see* Arteriosclerosis, extremities,
      bypass graft
  cardiac — *see* Disease, heart, ischemic, atherosclerotic
  cardiopathy — *see* Disease, heart, ischemic,
    atherosclerotic
  cardiorenal — *see* Hypertension, cardiorenal
  cardiovascular — *see* Disease, heart, ischemic,
    atherosclerotic
  carotid (*see also* Occlusion, artery, carotid) I65.2- ☑
  central nervous system I67.2
  cerebral I67.2
  cerebrovascular I67.2
  coronary (artery) I25.10
    bypass graft I25.810
      with
        angina pectoris I25.709
          with documented spasm I25.701
          specified type NEC I25.708
          unstable I25.700
        ischemic chest pain I25.709
      autologous artery I25.810
        with
          angina pectoris I25.729
            with documented spasm I25.721
            specified type I25.728
            unstable I25.720
          ischemic chest pain I25.729
      autologous vein I25.810
        with
          angina pectoris I25.719
            with documented spasm I25.711
            specified type I25.718
            unstable I25.710
          ischemic chest pain I25.719
      nonautologous biological I25.810
        with
          angina pectoris I25.739
            with documented spasm I25.731
            specified type I25.738
            unstable I25.730
          ischemic chest pain I25.739
      specified type NEC I25.810

Arteriosclerosis, arteriosclerotic — *continued*
  coronary — *continued*
    bypass graft — *continued*
      specified type — *continued*
        with
          angina pectoris I25.799
            with documented spasm I25.791
            specified type I25.798
            unstable I25.790
          ischemic chest pain I25.799
    due to
      calcified coronary lesion (severely) I25.84
      lipid rich plaque I25.83
    native vessel
      with
        angina pectoris I25.119
          with documented spasm I25.111
          specified type NEC I25.118
          unstable I25.110
        ischemic chest pain I25.119
    transplanted heart I25.811
      bypass graft I25.812
        with
          angina pectoris I25.769
            with documented spasm I25.761
            specified type I25.768
            unstable I25.760
          ischemic chest pain I25.769
      native coronary artery I25.811
        with
          angina pectoris I25.759
            with documented spasm I25.751
            specified type I25.758
            unstable I25.750
          ischemic chest pain I25.759
  extremities (native arteries) I70.209
    bypass graft I70.309
      autologous vein graft I70.409
        leg I70.409
          with
            gangrene (and intermittent claudica-
              tion, rest pain and ulcer)
              I70.469
            intermittent claudication I70.419
            rest pain (and intermittent claudica-
              tion) I70.429
        bilateral I70.403
          with
            gangrene (and intermittent clau-
              dication, rest pain and ul-
              cer) I70.463
            intermittent claudication I70.463
            rest pain (and intermittent claudi-
              cation) I70.423
            specified type NEC I70.493
        left I70.402
          with
            gangrene (and intermittent clau-
              dication, rest pain and ul-
              cer) I70.462
            intermittent claudication I70.412
            rest pain (and intermittent claudi-
              cation) I70.422
            ulceration (and intermittent
              claudication and rest pain)
              I70.449
              ankle I70.443
              calf I70.442
              foot site NEC I70.445
              heel I70.444
              lower leg NEC I70.448
              midfoot I70.444
              thigh I70.441
            specified type NEC I70.492
        right I70.401
          with
            gangrene (and intermittent clau-
              dication, rest pain and ul-
              cer) I70.461
            intermittent claudication I70.411
            rest pain (and intermittent claudi-
              cation) I70.421
            ulceration (and intermittent
              claudication and rest pain)
              I70.439
              ankle I70.433
              calf I70.432
              foot site NEC I70.435
              heel I70.434

☑ **Additional Character Required** — **Refer to the Tabular List for Character Selection** ▽ **Subterms under main terms may continue to next column or page**

Arteriosclerosis, arteriosclerotic — *continued*
  extremities — *continued*
    bypass graft — *continued*
      autologous vein graft — *continued*
        leg — *continued*
          right — *continued*
            with — *continued*
              ulceration — *continued*
                lower leg NEC I70.438
                midfoot I70.434
                thigh I70.431
              specified type NEC I70.491
            specified type NEC I70.499
          specified NEC I70.408
            with
              gangrene (and intermittent claudication, rest pain and ulcer) I70.468
              intermittent claudication I70.418
              rest pain (and intermittent claudication) I70.428
              ulceration (and intermittent claudication and rest pain) I70.45
            specified type NEC I70.498
        leg I70.309
          with
            gangrene (and intermittent claudication, rest pain and ulcer) I70.369
            intermittent claudication I70.319
            rest pain (and intermittent claudication) I70.329
          bilateral I70.303
            with
              gangrene (and intermittent claudication, rest pain and ulcer) I70.363
              intermittent claudication I70.313
              rest pain (and intermittent claudication) I70.323
            specified type NEC I70.393
          left I70.302
            with
              gangrene (and intermittent claudication, rest pain and ulcer) I70.362
              intermittent claudication I70.312
              rest pain (and intermittent claudication) I70.322
              ulceration (and intermittent claudication and rest pain) I70.349
                ankle I70.343
                calf I70.342
                foot site NEC I70.345
                heel I70.344
                lower leg NEC I70.348
                midfoot I70.344
                thigh I70.341
            specified type NEC I70.392
          right I70.301
            with
              gangrene (and intermittent claudication, rest pain and ulcer) I70.361
              intermittent claudication I70.311
              rest pain (and intermittent claudication) I70.321
              ulceration (and intermittent claudication and rest pain I70.339
                ankle I70.333
                calf I70.332
                foot site NEC I70.335
                heel I70.334
                lower leg NEC I70.338
                midfoot I70.334
                thigh I70.331
            specified type NEC I70.391
        specified type NEC I70.399
      nonautologous biological graft I70.509
        leg I70.509
          with
            gangrene (and intermittent claudication, rest pain and ulcer) I70.569
            intermittent claudication I70.519
            rest pain (and intermittent claudication) I70.529
          bilateral I70.503

Arteriosclerosis, arteriosclerotic — *continued*
  extremities — *continued*
    bypass graft — *continued*
      nonautologous biological graft — *continued*
        leg — *continued*
          bilateral — *continued*
            with
              gangrene (and intermittent claudication, rest pain and ulcer) I70.563
              intermittent claudication I70.513
              rest pain (and intermittent claudication) I70.523
            specified type NEC I70.593
          left I70.502
            with
              gangrene (and intermittent claudication, rest pain and ulcer) I70.562
              intermittent claudication I70.512
              rest pain (and intermittent claudication) I70.522
              ulceration (and intermittent claudication and rest pain) I70.549
                ankle I70.543
                calf I70.542
                foot site NEC I70.545
                heel I70.544
                lower leg NEC I70.548
                midfoot I70.544
                thigh I70.541
            specified type NEC I70.592
          right I70.501
            with
              gangrene (and intermittent claudication, rest pain and ulcer) I70.561
              intermittent claudication I70.511
              rest pain (and intermittent claudication) I70.521
              ulceration (and intermittent claudication and rest pain) I70.539
                ankle I70.533
                calf I70.532
                foot site NEC I70.535
                heel I70.534
                lower leg NEC I70.538
                midfoot I70.534
                thigh I70.531
            specified type NEC I70.591
        specified type NEC I70.599
        specified NEC I70.508
          with
            gangrene (and intermittent claudication, rest pain and ulcer) I70.568
            intermittent claudication I70.518
            rest pain (and intermittent claudication) I70.528
            ulceration (and intermittent claudication and rest pain) I70.55
          specified type NEC I70.598
      nonbiological graft I70.609
        leg I70.609
          with
            gangrene (and intermittent claudication, rest pain and ulcer) I70.669
            intermittent claudication I70.619
            rest pain (and intermittent claudication) I70.629
          bilateral I70.603
            with
              gangrene (and intermittent claudication, rest pain and ulcer) I70.663
              intermittent claudication I70.613
              rest pain (and intermittent claudication) I70.623
            specified type NEC I70.693
          left I70.602
            with
              gangrene (and intermittent claudication, rest pain and ulcer) I70.662
              intermittent claudication I70.612

Arteriosclerosis, arteriosclerotic — *continued*
  extremities — *continued*
    bypass graft — *continued*
      nonbiological graft — *continued*
        leg — *continued*
          left — *continued*
            with — *continued*
              rest pain (and intermittent claudication) I70.622
              ulceration (and intermittent claudication and rest pain) I70.649
                ankle I70.643
                calf I70.642
                foot site NEC I70.645
                heel I70.644
                lower leg NEC I70.648
                midfoot I70.644
                thigh I70.641
            specified type NEC I70.692
          right I70.601
            with
              gangrene (and intermittent claudication, rest pain and ulcer) I70.661
              intermittent claudication I70.611
              rest pain (and intermittent claudication) I70.621
              ulceration (and intermittent claudication and rest pain) I70.639
                ankle I70.633
                calf I70.632
                foot site NEC I70.635
                heel I70.634
                lower leg NEC I70.638
                midfoot I70.634
                thigh I70.631
            specified type NEC I70.691
        specified type NEC I70.699
        specified NEC I70.608
          with
            gangrene (and intermittent claudication, rest pain and ulcer) I70.668
            intermittent claudication I70.618
            rest pain (and intermittent claudication) I70.628
            ulceration (and intermittent claudication and rest pain) I70.65
          specified type NEC I70.698
      specified graft NEC I70.709
        leg I70.709
          with
            gangrene (and intermittent claudication, rest pain and ulcer) I70.769
            intermittent claudication I70.719
            rest pain (and intermittent claudication) I70.729
          bilateral I70.703
            with
              gangrene (and intermittent claudication, rest pain and ulcer) I70.763
              intermittent claudication I70.713
              rest pain (and intermittent claudication) I70.723
            specified type NEC I70.793
          left I70.702
            with
              gangrene (and intermittent claudication, rest pain and ulcer) I70.762
              intermittent claudication I70.712
              rest pain (and intermittent claudication) I70.722
              ulceration (and intermittent claudication and rest pain) I70.749
                ankle I70.743
                calf I70.742
                foot site NEC I70.745
                heel I70.744
                lower leg NEC I70.748
                midfoot I70.744
                thigh I70.741
            specified type NEC I70.792
          right I70.701

Arteriosclerosis, arteriosclerotic — continued
extremities — continued
- bypass graft — continued
  - specified graft — continued
    - leg — continued
      - right — continued
        - with
          - gangrene (and intermittent claudication, rest pain and ulcer) I70.761
          - intermittent claudication I70.711
          - rest pain (and intermittent claudication) I70.721
          - ulceration (and intermittent claudication and rest pain) I70.739
            - ankle I70.733
            - calf I70.732
            - foot site NEC I70.735
            - heel I70.734
            - lower leg NEC I70.738
            - midfoot I70.734
            - thigh I70.731
          - specified type NEC I70.791
      - specified type NEC I70.799
    - specified NEC I70.708
      - with
        - gangrene (and intermittent claudication, rest pain and ulcer) I70.768
        - intermittent claudication I70.718
        - rest pain (and intermittent claudication) I70.728
        - ulceration (and intermittent claudication and rest pain) I70.75
        - specified type NEC I70.798
  - specified NEC I70.308
    - with
      - gangrene (and intermittent claudication, rest pain and ulcer) I70.368
      - intermittent claudication I70.318
      - rest pain (and intermittent claudication) I70.328
      - ulceration (and intermittent claudication and rest pain) I70.35
      - specifiec type NEC I70.398
  - leg I70.209
    - with
      - gangrene (and intermittent claudication, rest pain and ulcer) I70.269
      - intermittent claudication I70.219
      - rest pain (and intermittent claudication) I70.229
    - bilateral I70.203
      - with
        - gangrene (and intermittent claudication, rest pain and ulcer) I70.263
        - intermittent claudication I70.213
        - rest pain (and intermittent claudication) I70.223
        - specified type NEC I70.293
    - left I70.202
      - with
        - gangrene (and intermittent claudication, rest pain and ulcer) I70.262
        - intermittent claudication I70.212
        - rest pain (and intermittent claudication) I70.222
        - ulceration (and intermittent claudication and rest pain) I70.249
          - ankle I70.243
          - calf I70.242
          - foot site NEC I70.245
          - heel I70.244
          - lower leg NEC I70.248
          - midfoot I70.244
          - thigh I70.241
        - specified type NEC I70.292
    - right I70.201
      - with
        - gangrene (and intermittent claudication, rest pain and ulcer) I70.261
        - intermittent claudication I70.211
        - rest pain (and intermittent claudication) I70.221
        - ulceration (and intermittent claudication and rest pain) I70.239
          - ankle I70.233
          - calf I70.232

Arteriosclerosis, arteriosclerotic — continued
extremities — continued
- leg — continued
  - right — continued
    - with — continued
      - ulceration — continued
        - foot site NEC I70.235
        - heel I70.234
        - lower leg NEC I70.238
        - midfoot I70.234
        - thigh I70.231
      - specified type NEC I70.291
    - specified type NEC I70.299
  - specified site NEC I70.208
    - with
      - gangrene (and intermittent claudication, rest pain and ulcer) I70.268
      - intermittent claudication I70.218
      - rest pain (and intermittent claudication) I70.228
      - ulceration (and intermittent claudication and rest pain) I70.25
      - specified type NEC I70.298
- generalized I70.91
- heart (disease) — see Arteriosclerosis, coronary (artery),
- kidney — see Hypertension, kidney
- medial — see Arteriosclerosis, extremities
- mesenteric (artery) K55.1
- Mönckeberg's — see Arteriosclerosis, extremities
- myocarditis I51.4
- peripheral (of extremities) — see Arteriosclerosis, extremities
- pulmonary (idiopathic) I27.0
- renal (arterioles) (see also Hypertension, kidney)
  - artery I70.1
- retina (vascular) I70.8 [H35.0-] ☑
- specified artery NEC I70.8
- spinal (cord) G95.19
- vertebral (artery) I67.2

Arteriospasm I73.9

Arteriovenous — see condition

Arteritis I77.6
- allergic M31.0
- aorta (nonsyphilitic) I77.6
  - syphilitic A52.02
- aortic arch M31.4
- brachiocephalic M31.4
- brain I67.7
  - syphilitic A52.04
- cerebral I67.7
  - in systemic lupus erythematosus M32.19
  - listerial A32.89
  - syphilitic A52.04
  - tuberculous A18.89
- coronary (artery) I25.89
  - rheumatic I01.8
    - chronic I09.89
  - syphilitic A52.06
- cranial (left) (right), giant cell M31.6
- deformans — see Arteriosclerosis
- giant cell NEC M31.6
  - with polymyalgia rheumatica M31.5
- necrosing or necrotizing M31.9
  - specified NEC M31.8
- nodosa M30.0
- obliterans — see Arteriosclerosis
- pulmonary I28.8
- rheumatic — see Fever, rheumatic
- senile — see Arteriosclerosis
- suppurative I77.2
- syphilitic (general) A52.09
  - brain A52.04
  - coronary A52.06
  - spinal A52.09
- temporal, giant cell M31.6
- young female aortic arch syndrome M31.4

Artery, arterial (see also condition)
- abscess I77.89
- single umbilical Q27.0

Arthralgia (allergic) (see also Pain, joint) M19.90
- in caisson disease T70.3 ☑
- temporomandibular M26.62- ☑

Arthritis, arthritic (acute) (chronic) (nonpyogenic) (subacute) M19.90
- allergic — see Arthritis, specified form NEC
- ankylosing (crippling) (spine) (see also Spondylitis, ankylosing)

Arthritis, arthritic — continued
- ankylosing (see also Spondylitis, ankylosing) — continued
  - sites other than spine — see Arthritis, specified form NEC
- atrophic — see Osteoarthritis
  - spine — see Spondylitis, ankylosing
- back — see Spondylopathy, inflammatory
- blennorrhagic (gonococcal) A54.42
- Charcot's — see Arthropathy, neuropathic
  - diabetic — see Diabetes, arthropathy, neuropathic
  - syringomyelic G95.0
- chylous (filarial) (see also category M01) B74.9
- climacteric (any site) NEC — see Arthritis, specified form NEC
- crystal (-induced) — see Arthritis, in, crystals
- deformans — see Osteoarthritis
- degenerative — see Osteoarthritis
- due to or associated with
  - acromegaly E22.0
  - brucellosis — see Brucellosis
  - caisson disease T70.3 ☑
  - diabetes — see Diabetes, arthropathy
  - dracontiasis (see also category M01) B72
  - enteritis NEC
    - regional — see Enteritis, regional
  - erysipelas (see also category M01) A46
  - erythema
    - epidemic A25.1
    - nodosum L52
  - filariasis NOS B74.9
  - glanders A24.0
  - helminthiasis (see also category M01) B83.9
  - hemophilia D66 [M36.2]
  - Henoch- (Schönlein) purpura D69.0 [M36.4]
  - human parvovirus (see also category M01) B97.6
  - infectious disease NEC M01 ☑
  - leprosy (see also category M01) (see also Leprosy) A30.9
  - Lyme disease A69.23
  - mycobacteria (see also category M01) A31.8
  - parasitic disease NEC (see also category M01) B89
  - paratyphoid fever (see also category M01) (see also Fever, paratyphoid) A01.4
  - rat bite fever (see also category M01) A25.1
  - regional enteritis — see Enteritis, regional
  - respiratory disorder NOS J98.9
  - serum sickness (see also Reaction, serum) T80.69 ☑
  - syringomyelia G95.0
  - typhoid fever A01.04
- epidemic erythema A25.1
- febrile — see Fever, rheumatic
- gonococcal A54.42
- gouty (acute) — see Gout
- in (due to)
  - acromegaly (see also subcategory M14.8-) E22.0
  - amyloidosis (see also subcategory M14.8-) E85.4
  - bacterial disease (see also subcategory M01) A49.9
  - Behçet's syndrome M35.2
  - caisson disease (see also subcategory M14.8-) T70.3 ☑
  - coliform bacilli (Escherichia coli) — see Arthritis, in, pyogenic organism NEC
  - crystals M11.9
    - dicalcium phosphate — see Arthritis, in, crystals, specified type NEC
    - hydroxyapatite M11.0- ☑
    - pyrophosphate — see Arthritis, in, crystals, specified type NEC
    - specified type NEC M11.80
      - ankle M11.87- ☑
      - elbow M11.82- ☑
      - foot joint M11.87- ☑
      - hand joint M11.84- ☑
      - hip M11.85- ☑
      - knee M11.86- ☑
      - multiple sites M11.8- ☑
      - shoulder M11.81- ☑
      - vertebrae M11.88
      - wrist M11.83- ☑
  - dermatoarthritis, lipoid E78.81
  - dracontiasis (dracunculiasis) (see also category M01) B72
  - endocrine disorder NEC (see also subcategory M14.8-) E34.9
  - enteritis, infectious NEC (see also category M01) A09

☑ Additional Character Required — Refer to the Tabular List for Character Selection   ▽ Subterms under main terms may continue to next column or page

Arthritis, arthritic — *continued*
  in — *continued*
    enteritis, infectious (*see also* category M01) —
      continued
      specified organism NEC (*see also* category M01)
        A08.8
    erythema
      multiforme (*see also* subcategory M14.8-) L51.9
      nodosum (*see also* subcategory M14.8-) L52
    gout — *see* Gout
    helminthiasis NEC (*see also* category M01) B83.9
    hemochromatosis (*see also* subcategory M14.8-)
      E83.118
    hemoglobinopathy NEC D58.2 [M36.3]
    hemophilia NEC D66 [M36.2]
    Hemophilus influenzae M00.8- ☑ [B96.3]
    Henoch (-Schönlein) purpura D69.0 [M36.4]
    hyperparathyroidism NEC (*see also* subcategory
      M14.8-) E21.3
    hypersensitivity reaction NEC T78.49 ☑ [M36.4]
    hypogammaglobulinemia (*see also* subcategory
      M14.8-) D80.1
    hypothyroidism NEC (*see also* subcategory M14.8-)
      E03.9
    infection — *see* Arthritis, pyogenic or pyemic
      spine — *see* Spondylopathy, infective
    infectious disease NEC M01 ☑
    leprosy (*see also* category M01) A30.9
    leukemia NEC C95.9- ☑ [M36.1]
    lipoid dermatoarthritis E78.81
    Lyme disease A69.23
    Mediterranean fever, familial (*see also* subcategory
      M14.8-) M04.1
    Meningococcus A39.83
    metabolic disorder NEC (*see also* subcategory
      M14.8-) E88.9
    multiple myelomatosis C90.0- ☑ [M36.1]
    mumps B26.85
    mycosis NEC (*see also* category M01) B49
    myelomatosis (multiple) C90.0- ☑ [M36.1]
    neurological disorder NEC G98.0
    ochronosis (*see also* subcategory M14.8-) E70.29
    O'nyong-nyong (*see also* category M01) A92.1
    parasitic disease NEC (*see also* category M01) B89
    paratyphoid fever (*see also* category M01) A01.4
    Pseudomonas — *see* Arthritis, pyogenic, bacterial
      NEC
    psoriasis L40.50
    pyogenic organism NEC — *see* Arthritis, pyogenic,
      bacterial NEC
    Reiter's disease — *see* Reiter's disease
    respiratory disorder NEC (*see also* subcategory
      M14.8-) J98.9
    reticulosis, malignant (*see also* subcategory M14.8-
) C86.0
    rubella B06.82
    Salmonella (arizonae) (cholerae-suis) (enteritidis)
      (typhimurium) A02.23
    sarcoidosis D86.86
    specified bacteria NEC — *see* Arthritis, pyogenic,
      bacterial NEC
    sporotrichosis B42.82
    syringomyelia G95.0
    thalassemia NEC D56.9 [M36.3]
    tuberculosis — *see* Tuberculosis, arthritis
    typhoid fever A01.04
    urethritis, Reiter's — *see* Reiter's disease
    viral disease NEC (*see also* category M01) B34.9
  infectious or infective (*see also* Arthritis, pyogenic or
    pyemic)
    spine — *see* Spondylopathy, infective
  juvenile M08.90
    with systemic onset — *see* Still's disease
    ankle M08.97- ☑
    elbow M08.92- ☑
    foot joint M08.97- ☑
    hand joint M08.94- ☑
    hip M08.95- ☑
    knee M08.96- ☑
    multiple site M08.99
    pauciarticular M08.40
      ankle M08.47- ☑
      elbow M08.42- ☑
      foot joint M08.47- ☑
      hand joint M08.44- ☑
      hip M08.45- ☑
      knee M08.46- ☑

Arthritis, arthritic — *continued*
  juvenile — *continued*
    pauciarticular — *continued*
      shoulder M08.41- ☑
      vertebrae M08.48
      wrist M08.43- ☑
    psoriatic L40.54
    rheumatoid — *see* Arthritis, rheumatoid, juvenile
    shoulder M08.91- ☑
    specified type NEC M08.80
      ankle M08.87- ☑
      elbow M08.82- ☑
      foot joint M08.87- ☑
      hand joint M08.84- ☑
      hip M08.85- ☑
      knee M08.86- ☑
      multiple site M08.89
      shoulder M08.81- ☑
      specified joint NEC M08.88
      vertebrae M08.88
      wrist M08.83- ☑
    wrist M08.93- ☑
  meaning osteoarthritis — *see* Osteoarthritis
  meningococcal A39.83
  menopausal (any site) NEC — *see* Arthritis, specified
    form NEC
  mutilans (psoriatic) L40.52
  mycotic NEC (*see also* category M01) B49
  neuropathic (Charcot) — *see* Arthropathy, neuropathic
    diabetic — *see* Diabetes, arthropathy, neuropathic
    nonsyphilitic NEC G98.0
    syringomyelic G95.0
  ochronotic (*see also* subcategory M14.8-) E70.29
  palindromic (any site) — *see* Rheumatism, palindromic
  pneumococcal M00.10
    ankle M00.17- ☑
    elbow M00.12- ☑
    foot joint — *see* Arthritis, pneumococcal, ankle
    hand joint M00.14- ☑
    hip M00.15- ☑
    knee M00.16- ☑
    multiple site M00.19
    shoulder M00.11- ☑
    vertebra M00.18
    wrist M00.13- ☑
  postdysenteric — *see* Arthropathy, postdysenteric
  postmeningococcal A39.84
  postrheumatic, chronic — *see* Arthropathy,
    postrheumatic, chronic
  primary progressive (*see also* Arthritis, specified form
    NEC)
    spine — *see* Spondylitis, ankylosing
  psoriatic L40.50
  purulent (any site except spine) — *see* Arthritis, pyo-
    genic or pyemic
    spine — *see* Spondylopathy, infective
  pyogenic or pyemic (any site except spine) M00.9
    bacterial NEC M00.80
      ankle M00.87- ☑
      elbow M00.82- ☑
      foot joint — *see* Arthritis, pyogenic, bacterial
        NEC, ankle
      hand joint M00.84- ☑
      hip M00.85- ☑
      knee M00.86- ☑
      multiple site M00.89
      shoulder M00.81- ☑
      vertebra M00.88
      wrist M00.83- ☑
    pneumococcal — *see* Arthritis, pneumococcal
    spine — *see* Spondylopathy, infective
    staphylococcal — *see* Arthritis, staphylococcal
    streptococcal — *see* Arthritis, streptococcal NEC
      pneumococcal — *see* Arthritis, pneumococcal
  reactive — *see* Reiter's disease
  rheumatic (*see also* Arthritis, rheumatoid)
    acute or subacute — *see* Fever, rheumatic
  rheumatoid M06.9
    with
      carditis — *see* Rheumatoid, carditis
      endocarditis — *see* Rheumatoid, carditis
      heart involvement NEC — *see* Rheumatoid,
        carditis
      lung involvement — *see* Rheumatoid, lung
      myocarditis — *see* Rheumatoid, carditis
      myopathy — *see* Rheumatoid, myopathy
      pericarditis — *see* Rheumatoid, carditis

Arthritis, arthritic — *continued*
  rheumatoid — *continued*
    with — *continued*
      polyneuropathy — *see* Rheumatoid, polyneu-
        ropathy
      rheumatoid factor — *see* Arthritis, rheumatoid,
        seropositive
      splenoadenomegaly and leukopenia — *see*
        Felty's syndrome
      vasculitis — *see* Rheumatoid, vasculitis
      visceral involvement NEC — *see* Rheumatoid,
        arthritis, with involvement of organs NEC
    juvenile (with or without rheumatoid factor)
      M08.00
      ankle M08.07- ☑
      elbow M08.02- ☑
      foot joint M08.07- ☑
      hand joint M08.04- ☑
      hip M08.05- ☑
      knee M08.06- ☑
      multiple site M08.09
      shoulder M08.01- ☑
      vertebra M08.08
      wrist M08.03- ☑
    seronegative M06.00
      ankle M06.07- ☑
      elbow M06.02- ☑
      foot joint M06.07- ☑
      hand joint M06.04- ☑
      hip M06.05- ☑
      knee M06.06- ☑
      multiple site M06.09
      shoulder M06.01- ☑
      vertebra M06.08
      wrist M06.03- ☑
    seropositive M05.9
      without organ involvement M05.70
        ankle M05.77- ☑
        elbow M05.72- ☑
        foot joint M05.77- ☑
        hand joint M05.74- ☑
        hip M05.75- ☑
        knee M05.76- ☑
        multiple sites M05.79
        shoulder M05.71- ☑
        vertebra — *see* Spondylitis, ankylosing
        wrist M05.73- ☑
      specified NEC M05.80
        ankle M05.87- ☑
        elbow M05.82- ☑
        foot joint M05.87- ☑
        hand joint M05.84- ☑
        hip M05.85- ☑
        knee M05.86- ☑
        multiple sites M05.89
        shoulder M05.81- ☑
        vertebra — *see* Spondylitis, ankylosing
        wrist M05.83- ☑
    specified type NEC M06.80
      ankle M06.87- ☑
      elbow M06.82- ☑
      foot joint M06.87- ☑
      hand joint M06.84- ☑
      hip M06.85- ☑
      knee M06.86- ☑
      multiple site M06.89
      shoulder M06.81- ☑
      vertebra M06.88
      wrist M06.83- ☑
    spine — *see* Spondylitis, ankylosing
  rubella B06.82
  scorbutic (*see also* subcategory M14.8-) E54
  senile or senescent — *see* Osteoarthritis
  septic (any site except spine) — *see* Arthritis, pyogenic
    or pyemic
    spine — *see* Spondylopathy, infective
  serum (nontherapeutic) (therapeutic) — *see*
    Arthropathy, postimmunization
  specified form NEC M13.80
    ankle M13.87- ☑
    elbow M13.82- ☑
    foot joint M13.87- ☑
    hand joint M13.84- ☑
    hip M13.85- ☑
    knee M13.86- ☑
    multiple site M13.89

Arthritis, arthritic — *continued*
  specified form — *continued*
    shoulder M13.81-☑
    specified joint NEC M13.88
    wrist M13.83-☑
  spine (*see also* Spondylopathy, inflammatory)
    infectious or infective NEC — *see* Spondylopathy, infective
    Marie-Strümpell — *see* Spondylitis, ankylosing
    pyogenic — *see* Spondylopathy, infective
    rheumatoid — *see* Spondylitis, ankylosing
    traumatic (old) — *see* Spondylopathy, traumatic
    tuberculous A18.01
  staphylococcal M00.00
    ankle M00.07-☑
    elbow M00.02-☑
    foot joint — *see* Arthritis, staphylococcal, ankle
    hand joint M00.04-☑
    hip M00.05-☑
    knee M00.06-☑
    multiple site M00.09
    shoulder M00.01-☑
    vertebra M00.08
    wrist M00.03-☑
  streptococcal NEC M00.20
    ankle M00.27-☑
    elbow M00.22-☑
    foot joint — *see* Arthritis, streptococcal, ankle
    hand joint M00.24-☑
    hip M00.25-☑
    knee M00.26-☑
    multiple site M00.29
    shoulder M00.21-☑
    vertebra M00.28
    wrist M00.23-☑
  suppurative — *see* Arthritis, pyogenic or pyemic
  syphilitic (late) A52.16
    congenital A50.55 [M12.80]
  syphilitica deformans (Charcot) A52.16
  temporomandibular M26.69
  toxic of menopause (any site) — *see* Arthritis, specified form NEC
  transient — *see* Arthropathy, specified form NEC
  traumatic (chronic) — *see* Arthropathy, traumatic
  tuberculous A18.02
    spine A18.01
  uratic — *see* Gout
  urethritica (Reiter's) — *see* Reiter's disease
  vertebral — *see* Spondylopathy, inflammatory
  villous (any site) — *see* Arthropathy, specified form NEC
Arthrocele — *see* Effusion, joint
Arthrodesis status Z98.1
Arthrodynia (*see also* Pain, joint)
Arthrodysplasia Q74.9
Arthrofibrosis, joint — *see* Ankylosis
Arthrogryposis (congenital) Q68.8
  multiplex congenita Q74.3
Arthrokatadysis M24.7
Arthropathy (*see also* Arthritis) M12.9
  Charcot's — *see* Arthropathy, neuropathic
    diabetic — *see* Diabetes, arthropathy, neuropathic
    syringomyelic G95.0
  cricoarytenoid J38.7
  crystal (-induced) — *see* Arthritis, in, crystals
  diabetic NEC — *see* Diabetes, arthropathy
  distal interphalangeal, psoriatic L40.51
  enteropathic M07.60
    ankle M07.67-☑
    elbow M07.62-☑
    foot joint M07.67-☑
    hand joint M07.64-☑
    hip M07.65-☑
    knee M07.66-☑
    multiple site M07.69
    shoulder M07.61-☑
    vertebra M07.68
    wrist M07.63-☑
  following intestinal bypass M02.00
    ankle M02.07-☑
    elbow M02.02-☑
    foot joint M02.07-☑
    hand joint M02.04-☑
    hip M02.05-☑
    knee M02.06-☑
    multiple site M02.09
    shoulder M02.01-☑

Arthropathy — *continued*
  following intestinal bypass — *continued*
    vertebra M02.08
    wrist M02.03-☑
  gouty (*see also* Gout)
    in (due to)
      Lesch-Nyhan syndrome E79.1 [M14.8-] ☑
      sickle-cell disorders D57- ☑ [M14.8-] ☑
  hemophilic NEC D66 [M36.2]
    in (due to)
      hyperparathyroidism NEC E21.3 [M14.8-] ☑
      metabolic disease NOS E88.9 [M14.8-] ☑
  in (due to)
    acromegaly E22.0 [M14.8-] ☑
    amyloidosis E85.4 [M14.8-] ☑
    blood disorder NOS D75.9 [M36.3]
    diabetes — *see* Diabetes, arthropathy
    endocrine disease NOS E34.9 [M14.8-] ☑
    erythema
      multiforme L51.9 [M14.8-] ☑
      nodosum L52 [M14.8-] ☑
    hemochromatosis E83.118 [M14.8-] ☑
    hemoglobinopathy NEC D58.2 [M36.3]
    hemophilia NEC D66 [M36.2]
    Henoch-Schönlein purpura D69.0 [M36.4]
    hyperthyroidism E05.90 [M14.8-] ☑
    hypothyroidism E03.9 [M14.8-] ☑
    infective endocarditis I33.0 [M12.80]
    leukemia NEC C95.9- ☑ [M36.1]
    malignant histiocytosis C96.A [M36.1]
    metabolic disease NOS E88.9 [M14.8-] ☑
    multiple myeloma C90.0- ☑ [M36.1]
    neoplastic disease NOS (*see also* Neoplasm) D49.9 [M36.1]
    nutritional deficiency (*see also* subcategory M14.8-) E63.9
    psoriasis NOS L40.50
    sarcoidosis D86.86
    syphilis (late) A52.77
      congenital A50.55 [M12.80]
    thyrotoxicosis (*see also* subcategory M14.8-) E05.90
    ulcerative colitis K51.90 [M07.60]
    viral hepatitis (postinfectious) NEC B19.9 [M12.80]
    Whipple's disease (*see also* subcategory M14.8-) K90.81
  Jaccoud — *see* Arthropathy, postrheumatic, chronic
  juvenile — *see* Arthritis, juvenile
    psoriatic L40.54
  mutilans (psoriatic) L40.52
  neuropathic (Charcot) M14.60
    ankle M14.67-☑
    diabetic — *see* Diabetes, arthropathy, neuropathic
    elbow M14.62-☑
    foot joint M14.67-☑
    hand joint M14.64-☑
    hip M14.65-☑
    knee M14.66-☑
    multiple site M14.69
    nonsyphilitic NEC G98.0
    shoulder M14.61-☑
    syringomyelic G95.0
    vertebra M14.68
    wrist M14.63-☑
  osteopulmonary — *see* Osteoarthropathy, hypertrophic, specified NEC
  postdysenteric M02.10
    ankle M02.17-☑
    elbow M02.12-☑
    foot joint M02.17-☑
    hand joint M02.14-☑
    hip M02.15-☑
    knee M02.16-☑
    multiple site M02.19
    shoulder M02.11-☑
    vertebra M02.18
    wrist M02.13-☑
  postimmunization M02.20
    ankle M02.27-☑
    elbow M02.22-☑
    foot joint M02.27-☑
    hand joint M02.24-☑
    hip M02.25-☑
    knee M02.26-☑
    multiple site M02.29
    shoulder M02.21-☑
    vertebra M02.28
    wrist M02.23-☑

Arthropathy — *continued*
  postinfectious NEC B99 ☑ [M12.80]
    in (due to)
      enteritis due to Yersinia enterocolitica A04.6 [M12.80]
      syphilis A52.77
      viral hepatitis NEC B19.9 [M12.80]
  postrheumatic, chronic (Jaccoud) M12.00
    ankle M12.07-☑
    elbow M12.02-☑
    foot joint M12.07-☑
    hand joint M12.04-☑
    hip M12.05-☑
    knee M12.06-☑
    multiple site M12.09
    shoulder M12.01-☑
    specified joint NEC M12.08
    vertebrae M12.08
    wrist M12.03-☑
  psoriatic NEC L40.59
    interphalangeal, distal L40.51
  reactive M02.9
    in (due to)
      infective endocarditis I33.0 [M02.9]
    specified type NEC M02.80
      ankle M02.87-☑
      elbow M02.82-☑
      foot joint M02.87-☑
      hand joint M02.84-☑
      hip M02.85-☑
      knee M02.86-☑
      multiple site M02.89
      shoulder M02.81-☑
      vertebra M02.88
      wrist M02.83-☑
  specified form NEC M12.80
    ankle M12.87-☑
    elbow M12.82-☑
    foot joint M12.87-☑
    hand joint M12.84-☑
    hip M12.85-☑
    knee M12.86-☑
    multiple site M12.89
    shoulder M12.81-☑
    specified joint NEC M12.88
    vertebrae M12.88
    wrist M12.83-☑
  syringomyelic G95.0
  tabes dorsalis A52.16
  tabetic A52.16
  transient — *see* Arthropathy, specified form NEC
  traumatic M12.50
    ankle M12.57-☑
    elbow M12.52-☑
    foot joint M12.57-☑
    hand joint M12.54-☑
    hip M12.55-☑
    knee M12.56-☑
    multiple site M12.59
    shoulder M12.51-☑
    specified joint NEC M12.58
    vertebrae M12.58
    wrist M12.53-☑
Arthropyosis — *see* Arthritis, pyogenic or pyemic
Arthrosis (deformans) (degenerative) (localized) (*see also* Osteoarthritis) M19.90
  spine — *see* Spondylosis
Arthus' phenomenon or reaction T78.41 ☑
  due to
    drug — *see* Table of Drugs and Chemicals, by drug
Articular — *see* condition
Articulation, reverse (teeth) M26.24
Artificial
  insemination complication — *see* Complications, artificial, fertilization
  opening status (functioning) (without complication) Z93.9
    anus (colostomy) Z93.3
    colostomy Z93.3
    cystostomy Z93.50
      appendico-vesicostomy Z93.52
      cutaneous Z93.51
      specified NEC Z93.59
    enterostomy Z93.4
    gastrostomy Z93.1
    ileostomy Z93.2
    intestinal tract NEC Z93.4

Artificial — *continued*
opening status — *continued*
jejunostomy Z93.4
nephrostomy Z93.6
specified site NEC Z93.8
tracheostomy Z93.0
ureterostomy Z93.6
urethrostomy Z93.6
urinary tract NEC Z93.6
vagina Z93.8
vagina status Z93.8
Arytenoid — *see* condition
Asbestosis (occupational) J61
Ascariasis B77.9
with
complications NEC B77.89
intestinal complications B77.0
pneumonia, pneumonitis B77.81
Ascaridosis, ascariasis — *see* Ascariasis
Ascaris (infection) (infestation) (lumbricoides) — *see*
Ascariasis
Ascending — *see* condition
ASC-H (atypical squamous cells cannot exclude high
grade squamous intraepithelial lesion on cytologic
smear)
anus R85.611
cervix R87.611
vagina R87.621
Aschoff's bodies — *see* Myocarditis, rheumatic
Ascites (abdominal) R18.8
cardiac (*see also* Failure, heart, right) I50.810
chylous (nonfilarial) I89.8
filarial — *see* Infestation, filarial
due to
cirrhosis, alcoholic K70.31
hepatitis
alcoholic K70.11
chronic active K71.51
S. japonicum B65.2
heart (*see also* Failure, heart, right) I50.810
malignant R18.0
pseudochylous R18.8
syphilitic A52.74
tuberculous A18.31
ASC-US (atypical squamous cells of undetermined significance on cytologic smear)
anus R85.610
cervix R87.610
vagina R87.620
Aseptic — *see* condition
Asherman's syndrome N85.6
Asialia K11.7
Asiatic cholera — *see* Cholera
Asimultagnosia (simultanagnosia) R48.3
Askin's tumor — *see* Neoplasm, connective tissue, malignant
Asocial personality F60.2
Asomatognosia R41.4
Aspartylglucosaminuria E77.1
Asperger's disease or syndrome F84.5
Aspergilloma — *see* Aspergillosis
Aspergillosis (with pneumonia) B44.9
bronchopulmonary, allergic B44.81
disseminated B44.7
generalized B44.7
pulmonary NEC B44.1
allergic B44.81
invasive B44.0
specified NEC B44.89
tonsillar B44.2
Aspergillus (flavus) (fumigatus) (infection) (terreus) —
see Aspergillosis
Aspermatogenesis — *see* Azoospermia
Aspermia (testis) — *see* Azoospermia
Asphyxia, asphyxiation (by) R09.01
antenatal P84
birth P84
bunny bag — *see* Asphyxia, due to, mechanical threat
to breathing, trapped in bed clothes
crushing S28.0 ☑
drowning T75.1 ☑
gas, fumes, or vapor — *see* Table of Drugs and Chemicals
inhalation — *see* Inhalation
intrauterine P84
local I73.00
with gangrene I73.01

Asphyxia, asphyxiation — *continued*
mucus (*see also* Foreign body, respiratory tract, causing
asphyxia)
newborn P84
pathological R09.01
postnatal P84
mechanical — *see* Asphyxia, due to, mechanical
threat to breathing
prenatal P84
reticularis R23.1
strangulation — *see* Asphyxia, due to, mechanical
threat to breathing
submersion T75.1
traumatic T71.9 ☑
due to
crushed chest S28.0 ☑
foreign body (in) — *see* Foreign body, respiratory tract, causing asphyxia
low oxygen content of ambient air T71.20 ☑
due to
being trapped in
low oxygen environment T71.29 ☑
in car trunk T71.221 ☑
circumstances undetermined
T71.224 ☑
done with intent to harm by
another person T71.223 ☑
self T71.222 ☑
in refrigerator T71.231 ☑
circumstances undetermined
T71.234 ☑
done with intent to harm by
another person T71.233 ☑
self T71.232 ☑
cave-in T71.21 ☑
mechanical threat to breathing (accidental)
T71.191 ☑
circumstances undetermined T71.194 ☑
done with intent to harm by
another person T71.193 ☑
self T71.192 ☑
hanging T71.161 ☑
circumstances undetermined T71.164 ☑
done with intent to harm by
another person T71.163 ☑
self T71.162 ☑
plastic bag T71.121 ☑
circumstances undetermined T71.124 ☑
done with intent to harm by
another person T71.123 ☑
self T71.122 ☑
smothering
in furniture T71.151 ☑
circumstances undetermined
T71.154 ☑
done with intent to harm by
another person T71.153 ☑
self T71.152 ☑
under
another person's body T71.141 ☑
circumstances undetermined
T71.144 ☑
done with intent to harm
T71.143 ☑
pillow T71.111 ☑
circumstances undetermined
T71.114 ☑
done with intent to harm by
another person T71.113 ☑
self T71.112 ☑
trapped in bed clothes T71.131 ☑
circumstances undetermined T71.134 ☑
done with intent to harm by
another person T71.133 ☑
self T71.132 ☑
vomiting, vomitus — *see* Foreign body, respiratory
tract, causing asphyxia
Aspiration
amniotic (clear) fluid (newborn) P24.10
with
pneumonia (pneumonitis) P24.11
respiratory symptoms P24.11
blood
newborn (without respiratory symptoms) P24.20
with
pneumonia (pneumonitis) P24.21
respiratory symptoms P24.21

Aspiration — *continued*
blood — *continued*
specified age NEC — *see* Foreign body, respiratory
tract
bronchitis J69.0
food or foreign body (with asphyxiation) — *see* Asphyxia, food
liquor (amnii) (newborn) P24.10
with
pneumonia (pneumonitis) P24.11
respiratory symptoms P24.11
meconium (newborn) (without respiratory symptoms)
P24.00
with
pneumonitis (pneumonitis) P24.01
respiratory symptoms P24.01
milk (newborn) (without respiratory symptoms) P24.30
with
pneumonia (pneumonitis) P24.31
respiratory symptoms P24.31
specified age NEC — *see* Foreign body, respiratory
tract
mucus (*see also* Foreign body, by site, causing asphyxia)
newborn P24.10
with
pneumonia (pneumonitis) P24.11
respiratory symptoms P24.11
neonatal P24.9
specific NEC (without respiratory symptoms) P24.80
with
pneumonia (pneumonitis) P24.81
respiratory symptoms P24.81
newborn P24.9
specific NEC (without respiratory symptoms) P24.80
with
pneumonia (pneumonitis) P24.81
respiratory symptoms P24.81
pneumonia J69.0
pneumonitis J69.0
syndrome of newborn — *see* Aspiration, by substance,
with pneumonia
vernix caseosa (newborn) P24.80
with
pneumonia (pneumonitis) P24.81
respiratory symptoms P24.81
vomitus (*see also* Foreign body, respiratory tract)
newborn (without respiratory symptoms) P24.30
with
pneumonia (pneumonitis) P24.31
respiratory symptoms P24.31
Asplenia (congenital) Q89.01
postsurgical Z90.81
Assam fever B55.0
Assault, sexual — *see* Maltreatment
Assmann's focus NEC A15.0
Astasia (-abasia) (hysterical) F44.4
Asteatosis cutis L85.3
Astereognosia, astereognosis R48.1
Asterixis R27.8
in liver disease K71.3
Asteroid hyalitis — *see* Deposit, crystalline
Asthenia, asthenic R53.1
cardiac (*see also* Failure, heart) I50.9
psychogenic F45.8
cardiovascular (*see also* Failure, heart) I50.9
psychogenic F45.8
heart (*see also* Failure, heart) I50.9
psychogenic F45.8
hysterical F44.4
myocardial (*see also* Failure, heart) I50.9
psychogenic F45.8
nervous F48.8
neurocirculatory F45.8
neurotic F48.8
psychogenic F48.8
psychoneurotic F48.8
psychophysiologic F48.8
reaction (psychophysiologic) F48.8
senile R54
Asthenopia (*see also* Discomfort, visual)
hysterical F44.6
psychogenic F44.6
Asthenospermia — *see* Abnormal, specimen, male
genital organs
Asthma, asthmatic (bronchial) (catarrh) (spasmodic)
J45.909

Artificial — Asthma, asthmatic

Index

Asthma, asthmatic — Atheroma, atheromatous

Asthma, asthmatic — *continued*
with
chronic obstructive bronchitis J44.9
with
acute lower respiratory infection J44.0
exacerbation (acute) J44.1
chronic obstructive pulmonary disease J44.9
with
acute lower respiratory infection J44.0
exacerbation (acute) J44.1
exacerbation (acute) J45.901
hay fever — *see* Asthma, allergic extrinsic
rhinitis, allergic — *see* Asthma, allergic extrinsic
status asthmaticus J45.902
allergic extrinsic J45.909
with
exacerbation (acute) J45.901
status asthmaticus J45.902
atopic — *see* Asthma, allergic extrinsic
cardiac — *see* Failure, ventricular, left
cardiobronchial I50.1
childhood J45.909
with
exacerbation (acute) J45.901
status asthmaticus J45.902
chronic obstructive J44.9
with
acute lower respiratory infection J44.0
exacerbation (acute) J44.1
collier's J60
cough variant J45.991
detergent J69.8
due to
detergent J69.8
inhalation of fumes J68.3
eosinophilic J82
extrinsic, allergic — *see* Asthma, allergic extrinsic
grinder's J62.8
hay — *see* Asthma, allergic extrinsic
heart I50.1
idiosyncratic — *see* Asthma, nonallergic
intermittent (mild) J45.20
with
exacerbation (acute) J45.21
status asthmaticus J45.22
intrinsic, nonallergic — *see* Asthma, nonallergic
Kopp's E32.8
late-onset J45.909
with
exacerbation (acute) J45.901
status asthmaticus J45.902
mild intermittent J45.20
with
exacerbation (acute) J45.21
status asthmaticus J45.22
mild persistent J45.30
with
exacerbation (acute) J45.31
status asthmaticus J45.32
Millar's (laryngismus stridulus) J38.5
miner's J60
mixed J45.909
with
exacerbation (acute) J45.901
status asthmaticus J45.902
moderate persistent J45.40
with
exacerbation (acute) J45.41
status asthmaticus J45.42
nervous — *see* Asthma, nonallergic
nonallergic (intrinsic) J45.909
with
exacerbation (acute) J45.901
status asthmaticus J45.902
persistent
mild J45.30
with
exacerbation (acute) J45.31
status asthmaticus J45.32
moderate J45.40
with
exacerbation (acute) J45.41
status asthmaticus J45.42
severe J45.50
with
exacerbation (acute) J45.51
status asthmaticus J45.52
platinum J45.998

Asthma, asthmatic — *continued*
pneumoconiotic NEC J64
potter's J62.8
predominantly allergic J45.909
psychogenic F54
pulmonary eosinophilic J82
red cedar J67.8
Rostan's I50.1
sandblaster's J62.8
sequoiosis J67.8
severe persistent J45.50
with
exacerbation (acute) J45.51
status asthmaticus J45.52
specified NEC J45.998
stonemason's J62.8
thymic E32.8
tuberculous — *see* Tuberculosis, pulmonary
Wichmann's (laryngismus stridulus) J38.5
wood J67.8
Astigmatism (compound) (congenital) H52.20- ☑
irregular H52.21- ☑
regular H52.22- ☑
Astraphobia F40.220
Astroblastoma
specified site — *see* Neoplasm, malignant, by site
unspecified site C71.9
Astrocytoma (cystic)
anaplastic
specified site — *see* Neoplasm, malignant, by site
unspecified site C71.9
fibrillary
specified site — *see* Neoplasm, malignant, by site
unspecified site C71.9
fibrous
specified site — *see* Neoplasm, malignant, by site
unspecified site C71.9
gemistocytic
specified site — *see* Neoplasm, malignant, by site
unspecified site C71.9
juvenile
specified site — *see* Neoplasm, malignant, by site
unspecified site C71.9
pilocytic
specified site — *see* Neoplasm, malignant, by site
unspecified site C71.9
piloid
specified site — *see* Neoplasm, malignant, by site
unspecified site C71.9
protoplasmic
specified site — *see* Neoplasm, malignant, by site
unspecified site C71.9
specified site NEC — *see* Neoplasm, malignant, by site
subependymal D43.2
giant cell
specified site — *see* Neoplasm, uncertain behavior, by site
unspecified site D43.2
specified site — *see* Neoplasm, uncertain behavior,
by site
unspecified site D43.2
unspecified site C71.9
Astroglioma
specified site — *see* Neoplasm, malignant, by site
unspecified site C71.9
Asymbolia R48.8
Asymmetry (*see also* Distortion)
between native and reconstructed breast N65.1
face Q67.0
jaw (lower) — *see* Anomaly, dentofacial, jaw-cranial
base relationship, asymmetry
Asynergia, asynergy R27.8
ventricular I51.89
Asystole (heart) — *see* Arrest, cardiac
At risk
for
dental caries Z91.849
high Z91.843
low Z91.841
moderate Z91.842
falling Z91.81
Ataxia, ataxy, ataxic R27.0
acute R27.8
brain (hereditary) G11.9
cerebellar (hereditary) G11.9
with defective DNA repair G11.3
alcoholic G31.2
early-onset G11.1

Ataxia, ataxy, ataxic — *continued*
cerebellar — *continued*
in
alcoholism G31.2
myxedema E03.9 [G13.2]
neoplastic disease (*see also* Neoplasm)
D49.9 [G32.81]
specified disease NEC G32.81
late-onset (Marie's) G11.2
cerebral (hereditary) G11.9
congenital nonprogressive G11.0
family, familial — *see* Ataxia, hereditary
following
cerebrovascular disease I69.993
cerebral infarction I69.393
intracerebral hemorrhage I69.193
nontraumatic intracranial hemorrhage NEC
I69.293
specified disease NEC I69.893
subarachnoid hemorrhage I69.093
Friedreich's (heredofamilial) (cerebellar) (spinal) G11.1
gait R26.0
hysterical F44.4
general R27.8
gluten M35.9 [G32.81]
with celiac disease K90.0 [G32.81]
hereditary G11.9
with neuropathy G60.2
cerebellar — *see* Ataxia, cerebellar
spastic G11.4
specified NEC G11.8
spinal (Friedreich's) G11.1
heredofamilial — *see* Ataxia, hereditary
Hunt's G11.1
hysterical F44.4
locomotor (progressive) (syphilitic) (partial) (spastic)
A52.11
diabetic — *see* Diabetes, ataxia
Marie's (cerebellar) (heredofamilial) (late-onset) G11.2
nonorganic origin F44.4
nonprogressive, congenital G11.0
psychogenic F44.4
Roussy-Lévy G60.0
Sanger-Brown's (hereditary) G11.2
spastic hereditary G11.4
spinal
hereditary (Friedreich's) G11.1
progressive (syphilitic) A52.11
spinocerebellar, X-linked recessive G11.1
telangiectasia (Louis-Bar) G11.3
Ataxia-telangiectasia (Louis-Bar) G11.3
Atelectasis (massive) (partial) (pressure) (pulmonary)
J98.11
newborn P28.10
due to resorption P28.11
partial P28.19
primary P28.0
secondary P28.19
primary (newborn) P28.0
tuberculous — *see* Tuberculosis, pulmonary
Atelocardia Q24.9
Atelomyelia Q06.1
Atheroembolism
of
extremities
lower I75.02- ☑
upper I75.01- ☑
kidney I75.81
specified NEC I75.89
Atheroma, atheromatous (*see also* Arteriosclerosis)
I70.90
aorta, aortic I70.0
valve (*see also* Endocarditis, aortic) I35.8
aorto-iliac I70.0
artery — *see* Arteriosclerosis
basilar (artery) I67.2
carotid (artery) (common) (internal) I67.2
cerebral (arteries) I67.2
coronary (artery) I25.10
with angina pectoris — *see* Arteriosclerosis, coronary (artery),
degeneration — *see* Arteriosclerosis
heart, cardiac — *see* Disease, heart, ischemic,
atherosclerotic
mitral (valve) I34.8
myocardium, myocardial — *see* Disease, heart, ischemic, atherosclerotic

☑ Additional Character Required — Refer to the Tabular List for Character Selection   ▽ Subterms under main terms may continue to next column or page

Atheroma, atheromatous — *continued*
  pulmonary valve (heart) (*see also* Endocarditis, pulmonary) I37.8
  tricuspid (heart) (valve) I36.8
  valve, valvular — *see* Endocarditis
  vertebral (artery) I67.2
Atheromatosis — *see* Arteriosclerosis
Atherosclerosis (*see also* Arteriosclerosis)
  coronary
    artery I25.10
      with angina pectoris — *see* Arteriosclerosis, coronary (artery),
      due to
        calcified coronary lesion (severely) I25.84
        lipid rich plaque I25.83
    transplanted heart I25.811
      bypass graft I25.812
        with angina pectoris — *see* Arteriosclerosis, coronary (artery),
      native coronary artery I25.811
        with angina pectoris — *see* Arteriosclerosis, coronary (artery),
Athetosis (acquired) R25.8
  bilateral (congenital) G80.3
  congenital (bilateral) (double) G80.3
  double (congenital) G80.3
  unilateral R25.8
Athlete's
  foot B35.3
  heart I51.7
Athrepsia E41
Athyrea (acquired) (*see also* Hypothyroidism)
  congenital E03.1
Atonia, atony, atonic
  bladder (sphincter) (neurogenic) N31.2
  capillary I78.8
  cecum K59.8
    psychogenic F45.8
  colon — *see* Atony, intestine
  congenital P94.2
  esophagus K22.8
  intestine K59.8
    psychogenic F45.8
  stomach K31.89
    neurotic or psychogenic F45.8
  uterus (during labor) O62.2
    with hemorrhage (postpartum) O72.1
    postpartum (with hemorrhage) O72.1
      without hemorrhage O75.89
Atopy — *see* History, allergy
Atransferrinemia, congenital E88.09
Atresia, atretic
  alimentary organ or tract NEC Q45.8
    upper Q40.8
  ani, anus, anal (canal) Q42.3
    with fistula Q42.2
  aorta (ring) Q25.29
  aortic (orifice) (valve) Q23.0
    arch Q25.21
    congenital with hypoplasia of ascending aorta and defective development of left ventricle (with mitral stenosis) Q23.4
    in hypoplastic left heart syndrome Q23.4
  aqueduct of Sylvius Q03.0
    with spina bifida — *see* Spina bifida, with hydrocephalus
  artery NEC Q27.8
    cerebral Q28.3
    coronary Q24.5
    digestive system Q27.8
    eye Q15.8
    lower limb Q27.8
    pulmonary Q25.5
    specified site NEC Q27.8
    umbilical Q27.0
    upper limb Q27.8
  auditory canal (external) Q16.1
  bile duct (common) (congenital) (hepatic) Q44.2
    acquired — *see* Obstruction, bile duct
  bladder (neck) Q64.39
    obstruction Q64.31
  bronchus Q32.4
  cecum Q42.8
  cervix (acquired) N88.2
    congenital Q51.828
    in pregnancy or childbirth — *see* Anomaly, cervix, in pregnancy or childbirth
      causing obstructed labor O65.5

Atresia, atretic — *continued*
  choana Q30.0
  colon Q42.9
    specified NEC Q42.8
  common duct Q44.2
  cricoid cartilage Q31.8
  cystic duct Q44.2
    acquired K82.8
      with obstruction K82.0
  digestive organs NEC Q45.8
  duodenum Q41.0
  ear canal Q16.1
  ejaculatory duct Q55.4
  epiglottis Q31.8
  esophagus Q39.0
    with tracheoesophageal fistula Q39.1
  eustachian tube Q17.8
  fallopian tube (congenital) Q50.6
    acquired N97.1
  follicular cyst N83.0- ☑
  foramen of
    Luschka Q03.1
      with spina bifida — *see* Spina bifida, with hydrocephalus
    Magendie Q03.1
      with spina bifida — *see* Spina bifida, with hydrocephalus
  gallbladder Q44.1
  genital organ
    external
      female Q52.79
      male Q55.8
    internal
      female Q52.8
      male Q55.8
  glottis Q31.8
  gullet Q39.0
    with tracheoesophageal fistula Q39.1
  heart valve NEC Q24.8
    pulmonary Q22.0
    tricuspid Q22.4
  hymen Q52.3
    acquired (postinfective) N89.6
  ileum Q41.2
  intestine (small) Q41.9
    large Q42.9
      specified NEC Q42.8
  iris, filtration angle Q15.0
  jejunum Q41.1
  lacrimal apparatus Q10.4
  larynx Q31.8
  meatus urinarius Q64.33
  mitral valve Q23.2
    in hypoplastic left heart syndrome Q23.4
  nares (anterior) (posterior) Q30.0
  nasopharynx Q34.8
  nose, nostril Q30.0
    acquired J34.89
  organ or site NEC Q89.8
  osseous meatus (ear) Q16.1
  oviduct (congenital) Q50.6
    acquired N97.1
  parotid duct Q38.4
    acquired K11.8
  pulmonary (artery) Q25.5
    valve Q22.0
  pulmonic Q22.0
  pupil Q13.2
  rectum Q42.1
    with fistula Q42.0
  salivary duct Q38.4
    acquired K11.8
  sublingual duct Q38.4
    acquired K11.8
  submandibular duct Q38.4
    acquired K11.8
  submaxillary duct Q38.4
    acquired K11.8
  thyroid cartilage Q31.8
  trachea Q32.1
  tricuspid valve Q22.4
  ureter Q62.10
    pelvic junction Q62.11
    vesical orifice Q62.12
  ureteropelvic junction Q62.11
  ureterovesical orifice Q62.12
  urethra (valvular) Q64.39
    stricture Q64.32
  urinary tract NEC Q64.8

Atresia, atretic — *continued*
  uterus Q51.818
    acquired N85.8
  vagina (congenital) Q52.4
    acquired (postinfectional) (senile) N89.5
  vas deferens Q55.3
  vascular NEC Q27.8
    cerebral Q28.3
    digestive system Q27.8
    lower limb Q27.8
    specified site NEC Q27.8
    upper limb Q27.8
  vein NEC Q27.8
    digestive system Q27.8
    great Q26.8
    lower limb Q27.8
    portal Q26.5
    pulmonary Q26.4
      partial Q26.3
      total Q26.2
    specified site NEC Q27.8
    upper limb Q27.8
  vena cava (inferior) (superior) Q26.8
  vesicourethral orifice Q64.31
  vulva Q52.79
    acquired N90.5
Atrichia, atrichosis — *see* Alopecia
Atrophia (*see also* Atrophy)
  cutis senilis L90.8
    due to radiation L57.8
  gyrata of choroid and retina H31.23
  senilis R54
    dermatological L90.8
      due to radiation (nonionizing) (solar) L57.8
  unguium L60.3
    congenita Q84.6
Atrophie blanche (en plaque) (de Milian) L95.0
Atrophoderma, atrophodermia (of) L90.9
  diffusum (idiopathic) L90.4
  maculatum L90.8
    et striatum L90.8
      due to syphilis A52.79
    syphilitic A51.39
  neuriticum L90.8
  Pasini and Pierini L90.3
  pigmentosum Q82.1
  reticulatum symmetricum faciei L66.4
  senile L90.8
    due to radiation (nonionizing) (solar) L57.8
  vermiculata (cheeks) L66.4
Atrophy, atrophic (of)
  adrenal (capsule) (gland) E27.49
    primary (autoimmune) E27.1
  alveolar process or ridge (edentulous) K08.20
  anal sphincter (disuse) N81.84
  appendix K38.8
  arteriosclerotic — *see* Arteriosclerosis
  bile duct (common) (hepatic) K83.8
  bladder N32.89
    neurogenic N31.8
  blanche (en plaque) (of Milian) L95.0
  bone (senile) NEC (*see also* Disorder, bone, specified type NEC)
    due to
      tabes dorsalis (neurogenic) A52.11
  brain (cortex) (progressive) G31.9
    frontotemporal circumscribed G31.01 [F02.80]
      with behavioral disturbance G31.01 [F02.81]
    senile NEC G31.1
  breast N64.2
    obstetric — *see* Disorder, breast, specified type NEC
  buccal cavity K13.79
  cardiac — *see* Degeneration, myocardial
  cartilage (infectional) (joint) — *see* Disorder, cartilage, specified NEC
  cerebellar — *see* Atrophy, brain
  cerebral — *see* Atrophy, brain
  cervix (mucosa) (senile) (uteri) N88.8
    menopausal N95.8
  Charcot-Marie-Tooth G60.0
  choroid (central) (macular) (myopic) (retina) H31.10- ☑
    diffuse secondary H31.12- ☑
    gyrate H31.23
    senile H31.11- ☑
  ciliary body — *see* Atrophy, iris
  conjunctiva (senile) H11.89
  corpus cavernosum N48.89

Index

Atrophy, atrophic — Attack, attacks

Atrophy, atrophic — *continued*
cortical — *see* Atrophy, brain
cystic duct K82.8
Déjérine-Thomas G23.8
disuse NEC — *see* Atrophy, muscle
Duchenne-Aran G12.21
ear H93.8- ☑
edentulous alveolar ridge K08.20
endometrium (senile) N85.8
   cervix N88.8
enteric K63.89
epididymis N50.89
eyeball — *see* Disorder, globe, degenerated condition, atrophy
eyelid (senile) — *see* Disorder, eyelid, degenerative
facial (skin) L90.9
fallopian tube (senile) N83.32- ☑
   with ovary N83.33- ☑
fascioscapulohumeral (Landouzy- Déjérine) G71.0
fatty, thymus (gland) E32.8
gallbladder K82.8
gastric K29.40
   with bleeding K29.41
gastrointestinal K63.89
glandular I89.8
globe H44.52- ☑
gum — *see* Recession, gingival
hair L67.8
heart (brown) — *see* Degeneration, myocardial
hemifacial Q67.4
   Romberg G51.8
infantile E41
   paralysis, acute — *see* Poliomyelitis, paralytic
intestine K63.89
iris (essential) (progressive) H21.26- ☑
   specified NEC H21.29
kidney (senile) (terminal) (*see also* Sclerosis, renal) N26.1
   congenital or infantile Q60.5
      bilateral Q60.4
      unilateral Q60.3
   hydronephrotic — *see* Hydronephrosis
lacrimal gland (primary) H04.14- ☑
   secondary H04.15- ☑
Landouzy-Déjérine G71.0
laryngitis, infective J37.0
larynx J38.7
Leber's optic (hereditary) H47.22
lip K13.0
liver (yellow) K72.90
   with coma K72.91
   acute, subacute K72.00
      with coma K72.01
   chronic K72.10
      with coma K72.11
lung (senile) J98.4
macular (dermatological) L90.8
   syphilitic, skin A51.39
      striated A52.79
mandible (edentulous) K08.20
   minimal K08.21
   moderate K08.22
   severe K08.23
maxilla K08.20
   minimal K08.24
   moderate K08.25
   severe K08.26
muscle, muscular (diffuse) (general) (idiopathic) (primary) M62.50
   ankle M62.57- ☑
   Duchenne-Aran G12.21
   foot M62.57- ☑
   forearm M62.53- ☑
   hand M62.54- ☑
   infantile spinal G12.0
   lower leg M62.56- ☑
   multiple sites M62.59
   myelopathic — *see* Atrophy, muscle, spinal
   myotonic G71.11
   neuritic G58.9
   neuropathic (peroneal) (progressive) G60.0
   pelvic (disuse) N81.84
   peroneal G60.0
   progressive (bulbar) G12.21
      adult G12.1
      infantile (spinal) G12.0
      spinal G12.25
         adult G12.1

Atrophy, atrophic — *continued*
muscle, muscular — *continued*
   progressive — *continued*
      spinal — *continued*
         infantile G12.0
   pseudohypertrophic G71.0
   shoulder region M62.51- ☑
   specified site NEC M62.58
   spinal G12.9
      adult form G12.1
      Aran-Duchenne G12.21
      childhood form, type II G12.1
      distal G12.1
      hereditary NEC G12.1
      infantile, type I (Werdnig-Hoffmann) G12.0
      juvenile form, type III (Kugelberg- Welander) G12.1
      progressive G12.25
      scapuloperoneal form G12.1
      specified NEC G12.8
   syphilitic A52.78
   thigh M62.55- ☑
   upper arm M62.52- ☑
myocardium — *see* Degeneration, myocardial
myometrium (senile) N85.8
   cervix N88.8
myopathic NEC — *see* Atrophy, muscle
myotonia G71.11
nail L60.3
nasopharynx J31.1
nerve (*see also* Disorder, nerve)
   abducens — *see* Strabismus, paralytic, sixth nerve
   accessory G52.8
   acoustic or auditory H93.3 ☑
   cranial G52.9
      eighth (auditory) H93.3 ☑
      eleventh (accessory) G52.8
      fifth (trigeminal) G50.8
      first (olfactory) G52.0
      fourth (trochlear) — *see* Strabismus, paralytic, fourth nerve
      second (optic) H47.20
      sixth (abducens) — *see* Strabismus, paralytic, sixth nerve
      tenth (pneumogastric) (vagus) G52.2
      third (oculomotor) — *see* Strabismus, paralytic, third nerve
      twelfth (hypoglossal) G52.3
   hypoglossal G52.3
   oculomotor — *see* Strabismus, paralytic, third nerve
   olfactory G52.0
   optic (papillomacular bundle)
      syphilitic (late) A52.15
         congenital A50.44
   pneumogastric G52.2
   trigeminal G50.8
   trochlear — *see* Strabismus, paralytic, fourth nerve
   vagus (pneumogastric) G52.2
neurogenic, bone, tabetic A52.11
nutritional E41
old age R54
olivopontocerebellar G23.8
optic (nerve) H47.20
   glaucomatous H47.23- ☑
   hereditary H47.22
   primary H47.21- ☑
   specified type NEC H47.29- ☑
   syphilitic (late) A52.15
      congenital A50.44
orbit H05.31- ☑
ovary (senile) N83.31- ☑
   with fallopian tube N83.33- ☑
oviduct (senile) — *see* Atrophy, fallopian tube
palsy, diffuse (progressive) G12.22
pancreas (duct) (senile) K86.89
parotid gland K11.0
pelvic muscle N81.84
penis N48.89
pharynx J39.2
pluriglandular E31.8
   autoimmune E31.0
polyarthritis M15.9
prostate N42.89
pseudohypertrophic (muscle) G71.0
renal (*see also* Sclerosis, renal) N26.1
retina, retinal (postinfectional) H35.89
rhinitis J31.0

Atrophy, atrophic — *continued*
salivary gland K11.0
scar L90.5
sclerosis, lobar (of brain) G31.09 [F02.80]
   with behavioral disturbance G31.09 [F02.81]
scrotum N50.89
seminal vesicle N50.89
senile R54
   due to radiation (nonionizing) (solar) L57.8
skin (patches) (spots) L90.9
   degenerative (senile) L90.8
   due to radiation (nonionizing) (solar) L57.8
   senile L90.8
spermatic cord N50.89
spinal (acute) (cord) G95.89
   muscular — *see* Atrophy, muscle, spinal
   paralysis G12.20
      acute — *see* Poliomyelitis, paralytic
      meaning progressive muscular atrophy G12.21
spine (column) — *see* Spondylopathy, specified NEC
spleen (senile) D73.0
stomach K29.40
   with bleeding K29.41
striate (skin) L90.6
   syphilitic A52.79
subcutaneous L90.9
sublingual gland K11.0
submandibular gland K11.0
submaxillary gland K11.0
Sudeck's — *see* Algoneurodystrophy
suprarenal (capsule) (gland) E27.49
   primary E27.1
systemic affecting central nervous system in
      myxedema E03.9 [G13.2]
      neoplastic disease (*see also* Neoplasm) D49.9 [G13.1]
      specified disease NEC G13.8
tarso-orbital fascia, congenital Q10.3
testis N50.0
thenar, partial — *see* Syndrome, carpal tunnel
thymus (fatty) E32.8
thyroid (gland) (acquired) E03.4
   with cretinism E03.1
   congenital (with myxedema) E03.1
tongue (senile) K14.8
   papillae K14.4
trachea J39.8
tunica vaginalis N50.89
turbinate J34.89
tympanic membrane (nonflaccid) H73.82- ☑
   flaccid H73.81- ☑
upper respiratory tract J39.8
uterus, uterine (senile) N85.8
   cervix N88.8
   due to radiation (intended effect) N85.8
      adverse effect or misadventure N99.89
vagina (senile) N95.2
vas deferens N50.89
vascular I99.8
vertebra (senile) — *see* Spondylopathy, specified NEC
vulva (senile) N90.5
Werdnig-Hoffmann G12.0
yellow — *see* Failure, hepatic

Attack, attacks
   with alteration of consciousness (with automatisms) — *see* Epilepsy, localization-related, symptomatic, with complex partial seizures
   without alteration of consciousness — *see* Epilepsy, localization-related, symptomatic, with simple partial seizures
   Adams-Stokes I45.9
   akinetic — *see* Epilepsy, generalized, specified NEC
   angina — *see* Angina
   atonic — *see* Epilepsy, generalized, specified NEC
   benign shuddering G25.83
   cataleptic — *see* Catalepsy
   coronary — *see* Infarct, myocardium
   cyanotic, newborn P28.2
   drop NEC R55
   epileptic — *see* Epilepsy
   heart — *see* infarct, myocardium
   hysterical F44.9
   jacksonian — *see* Epilepsy, localization-related, symptomatic, with simple partial seizures
   myocardium, myocardial — *see* Infarct, myocardium
   myoclonic — *see* Epilepsy, generalized, specified NEC
   panic F41.0

☑ Additional Character Required — Refer to the Tabular List for Character Selection   ▽ Subterms under main terms may continue to next column or page

Attack, attacks — *continued*
  psychomotor — *see* Epilepsy, localization-related, symptomatic, with complex partial seizures
  salaam — *see* Epilepsy, spasms
  schizophreniform, brief F23
  shuddering, benign G25.83
  Stokes-Adams I45.9
  syncope R55
  transient ischemic (TIA) G45.9
    specified NEC G45.8
  unconsciousness R55
    hysterical F44.89
  vasomotor R55
  vasovagal (paroxysmal) (idiopathic) R55
Attention (to)
  artificial
    opening (of) Z43.9
      digestive tract NEC Z43.4
        colon Z43.3
        ilium Z43.2
        stomach Z43.1
      specified NEC Z43.8
      trachea Z43.0
      urinary tract NEC Z43.6
        cystostomy Z43.5
        nephrostomy Z43.6
        ureterostomy Z43.6
        urethrostomy Z43.6
      vagina Z43.7
    colostomy Z43.3
    cystostomy Z43.5
    deficit disorder or syndrome F98.8
      with hyperactivity — *see* Disorder, attention-deficit hyperactivity
    gastrostomy Z43.1
    ileostomy Z43.2
    jejunostomy Z43.4
    nephrostomy Z43.6
    surgical dressings Z48.01
    sutures Z48.02
    tracheostomy Z43.0
    ureterostomy Z43.6
    urethrostomy Z43.6
Attrition
  gum — *see* Recession, gingival
  tooth, teeth (excessive) (hard tissues) K03.0
Atypical, atypism (*see also* condition)
  cells (on cytolgocial smear) (endocervical) (endometrial) (glandular)
    cervix R87.619
    vagina R87.629
  cervical N87.9
  endometrium N85.9
    hyperplasia N85.00
  parenting situation Z62.9
Auditory — *see* condition
Aujeszky's disease B33.8
Aurantiasis, cutis E67.1
Auricle, auricular (*see also* condition)
  cervical Q18.2
Auriculotemporal syndrome G50.8
Austin Flint murmur (aortic insufficiency) I35.1
Australian
  Q fever A78
  X disease A83.4
Autism, autistic (childhood) (infantile) F84.0
  atypical F84.9
  spectrum disorder F84.0
Autodigestion R68.89
Autoerythrocyte sensitization (syndrome) D69.2
Autographism L50.3
Autoimmune
  disease (systemic) M35.9
  inhibitors to clotting factors D68.311
  lymphoproliferative syndrome [ALPS] D89.82
  thyroiditis E06.3
Autointoxication R68.89
Automatism G93.89
  with temporal sclerosis G93.81
  epileptic — *see* Epilepsy, localization-related, symptomatic, with complex partial seizures
  paroxysmal, idiopathic — *see* Epilepsy, localization-related, symptomatic, with complex partial seizures
Autonomic, autonomous
  bladder (neurogenic) N31.2
  hysteria seizure F44.5
Autosensitivity, erythrocyte D69.2

Autosensitization, cutaneous L30.2
Autosome — *see* condition by chromosome involved
Autotopagnosia R48.1
Autotoxemia R68.89
Autumn — *see* condition
Avellis' syndrome G46.8
Aversion
  oral R63.3
    newborn P92.- ☑
    nonorganic origin F98.2 ☑
  sexual F52.1
Aviator's
  disease or sickness — *see* Effect, adverse, high altitude
  ear T70.0 ☑
Avitaminosis (multiple) (*see also* Deficiency, vitamin) E56.9
  B E53.9
    with
      beriberi E51.11
      pellagra E52
  B2 E53.0
  B6 E53.1
  B12 E53.8
  D E55.9
    with rickets E55.0
  G E53.0
  K E56.1
  nicotinic acid E52
AVNRT (atrioventricular nodal re-entrant tachycardia) I47.1
AVRT (atrioventricular nodal re-entrant tachycardia) I47.1
Avulsion (traumatic)
  blood vessel — *see* Injury, blood vessel
  bone — *see* Fracture, by site
  cartilage (*see also* Dislocation, by site)
    symphyseal (inner), complicating delivery O71.6
  external site other than limb — *see* Wound, open, by site
  eye S05.7- ☑
  head (intracranial)
    external site NEC S08.89 ☑
    scalp S08.0 ☑
  internal organ or site — *see* Injury, by site
  joint (*see also* Dislocation, by site)
    capsule — *see* Sprain, by site
  kidney S37.06- ☑
  ligament — *see* Sprain, by site
  limb (*see also* Amputation, traumatic, by site)
    skin and subcutaneous tissue — *see* Wound, open, by site
  muscle — *see* Injury, muscle
  nerve (root) — *see* Injury, nerve
  scalp S08.0 ☑
  skin and subcutaneous tissue — *see* Wound, open, by site
  spleen S36.032 ☑
  symphyseal cartilage (inner), complicating delivery O71.6
  tendon — *see* Injury, muscle
  tooth S03.2 ☑
Awareness of heart beat R00.2
Axenfeld's
  anomaly or syndrome Q15.0
  degeneration (calcareous) Q13.4
Axilla, axillary (*see also* condition)
  breast Q83.1
Axonotmesis — *see* Injury, nerve
Ayerza's disease or syndrome (pulmonary artery sclerosis with pulmonary hypertension) I27.0
Azoospermia (organic) N46.01
  due to
    drug therapy N46.021
    efferent duct obstruction N46.023
    infection N46.022
    radiation N46.024
    specified cause NEC N46.029
    systemic disease N46.025
Azotemia R79.89
  meaning uremia N19
Aztec ear Q17.3
Azygos
  continuation inferior vena cava Q26.8
  lobe (lung) Q33.1

B

Baastrup's disease — *see* Kissing spine

Babesiosis B60.0
Babington's disease (familial hemorrhagic telangiectasia) I78.0
Babinski's syndrome A52.79
Baby
  crying constantly R68.11
  floppy (syndrome) P94.2
Bacillary — *see* condition
Bacilluria R82.71
Bacillus (*see also* Infection, bacillus)
  abortus infection A23.1
  anthracis infection A22.9
  coli infection (*see also* Escherichia coli) B96.20
  Flexner's A03.1
  mallei infection A24.0
  Shiga's A03.0
  suipestifer infection — *see* Infection, salmonella
Back — *see* condition
Backache (postural) M54.9
  sacroiliac M53.3
  specified NEC M54.89
Backflow — *see* Reflux
Backward reading (dyslexia) F81.0
Bacteremia R78.81
  with sepsis — *see* Sepsis
Bactericholia — *see* Cholecystitis, acute
Bacterid, bacteride (pustular) L40.3
Bacterium, bacteria, bacterial
  agent NEC, as cause of disease classified elsewhere B96.89
  in blood — *see* Bacteremia
  in urine — *see* Bacteriuria
Bacteriuria, bacteruria R82.71
  asymptomatic R82.71
Bacteroides
  fragilis, as cause of disease classified elsewhere B96.6
Bad
  heart — *see* Disease, heart
  trip
    due to drug abuse — *see* Abuse, drug, hallucinogen
    due to drug dependence — *see* Dependence, drug, hallucinogen
Baelz's disease (cheilitis glandularis apostematosa) K13.0
Baerensprung's disease (eczema marginatum) B35.6
Bagasse disease or pneumonitis J67.1
Bagassosis J67.1
Baker's cyst — *see* Cyst, Baker's
Bakwin-Krida syndrome (metaphyseal dysplasia) Q78.5
Balancing side interference M26.56
Balanitis (circinata) (erosiva) (gangrenosa) (phagedenic) (vulgaris) N48.1
  amebic A06.82
  candidal B37.42
  due to Haemophilus ducreyi A57
  gonococcal (acute) (chronic) A54.09
  xerotica obliterans N48.0
Balanoposthitis N47.6
  gonococcal (acute) (chronic) A54.09
  ulcerative (specific) A63.8
Balanorrhagia — *see* Balanitis
Balantidiasis, balantidiosis A07.0
Bald tongue K14.4
Baldness (*see also* Alopecia)
  male-pattern — *see* Alopecia, androgenic
Balkan grippe A78
Balloon disease — *see* Effect, adverse, high altitude
Balo's disease (concentric sclerosis) G37.5
Bamberger-Marie disease — *see* Osteoarthropathy, hypertrophic, specified type NEC
Bancroft's filariasis B74.0
Band(s)
  adhesive — *see* Adhesions, peritoneum
  anomalous or congenital (*see also* Anomaly, by site)
    heart (atrial) (ventricular) Q24.8
    intestine Q43.3
    omentum Q43.3
  cervix N88.1
  constricting, congenital Q79.8
  gallbladder (congenital) Q44.1
  intestinal (adhesive) — *see* Adhesions, peritoneum
  obstructive
    intestine K56.50
      complete K56.52
      incomplete K56.51
      partial K56.51
    peritoneum K56.50

Band(s) — *continued*
  obstructive — *continued*
    peritoneum — *continued*
      complete K56.52
      incomplete K56.51
      partial K56.51
  periappendiceal, congenital Q43.3
  peritoneal (adhesive) — *see* Adhesions, peritoneum
    uterus N73.6
      internal N85.6
    vagina N89.5
Bandemia D72.825
Bandl's ring (contraction), complicating delivery O62.4
Bangkok hemorrhagic fever A91
Bang's disease (brucella abortus) A23.1
Bankruptcy, anxiety concerning Z59.8
Bannister's disease T78.3 ☑
  hereditary D84.1
Banti's disease or syndrome (with cirrhosis) (with portal hypertension) K76.6
Bar, median, prostate — *see* Enlargement, enlarged, prostate
Barcoo disease or rot — *see* Ulcer, skin
Barlow's disease E54
Barodontalgia T70.29 ☑
Baron Münchausen syndrome — *see* Disorder, factitious
Barosinusitis T70.1 ☑
Barotitis T70.0 ☑
Barotrauma T70.29 ☑
  odontalgia T70.29 ☑
  otitic T70.0 ☑
  sinus T70.1 ☑
Barraquer (-Simons) **disease or syndrome** (progressive lipodystrophy) E88.1
Barré-Guillain disease or syndrome G61.0
Barrel chest M95.4
Barré-Liéou syndrome (posterior cervical sympathetic) M53.0
Barrett's
  disease — *see* Barrett's, esophagus
  esophagus K22.70
    with dysplasia K22.719
      high grade K22.711
      low grade K22.710
    without dysplasia K22.70
  syndrome — *see* Barrett's, esophagus
  ulcer K22.10
    with bleeding K22.11
    without bleeding K22.10
Bársony (-Polgár) (-Teschendorf) **syndrome** (corkscrew esophagus) K22.4
Barth syndrome E78.71
Bartholinitis (suppurating) N75.8
  gonococcal (acute) (chronic) (with abscess) A54.1
Bartonellosis A44.9
  cutaneous A44.1
  mucocutaneous A44.1
  specified NEC A44.8
  systemic A44.0
Barton's fracture S52.56- ☑
Bartter's syndrome E26.81
Basal — *see* condition
Basan's (hidrotic) ectodermal dysplasia Q82.4
Baseball finger — *see* Dislocation, finger
Basedow's disease (exophthalmic goiter) — *see* Hyperthyroidism, with, goiter
Basic — *see* condition
Basilar — *see* condition
Bason's (hidrotic) ectodermal dysplasia Q82.4
Basopenia — *see* Agranulocytosis
Basophilia D72.824
Basophilism (cortico-adrenal) (Cushing's) (pituitary) E24.0
Bassen-Kornzweig disease or syndrome E78.6
Bat ear Q17.5
Bateman's
  disease B08.1
  purpura (senile) D69.2
Bathing cramp T75.1 ☑
Bathophobia F40.248
Batten (-Mayou) **disease** E75.4
  retina E75.4 [H36]
Batten-Steinert syndrome G71.11
Battered — *see* Maltreatment
Battey Mycobacterium infection A31.0
Battle exhaustion F43.0

Battledore placenta O43.19- ☑
Baumgarten-Cruveilhier cirrhosis, disease or syndrome K74.69
Bauxite fibrosis (of lung) J63.1
Bayle's disease (general paresis) A52.17
Bazin's disease (primary) (tuberculous) A18.4
Beach ear — *see* Swimmer's, ear
Beaded hair (congenital) Q84.1
Béal conjunctivitis or syndrome B30.2
Beard's disease (neurasthenia) F48.8
Beat(s)
  atrial, premature I49.1
  ectopic I49.49
  elbow — *see* Bursitis, elbow
  escaped, heart I49.49
  hand — *see* Bursitis, hand
  knee — *see* Bursitis, knee
  premature I49.40
    atrial I49.1
    auricular I49.1
    supraventricular I49.1
Beau's
  disease or syndrome — *see* Degeneration, myocardial
  lines (transverse furrows on fingernails) L60.4
Bechterev's syndrome — *see* Spondylitis, ankylosing
Becker's
  cardiomyopathy I42.8
  disease
    idiopathic mural endomyocardial disease I42.3
    myotonia congenita, recessive form G71.12
  dystrophy G71.0
  pigmented hairy nevus D22.5
Beck's syndrome (anterior spinal artery occlusion) I65.8
Beckwith-Wiedemann syndrome Q87.3
Bed confinement status Z74.01
Bed sore — *see* Ulcer, pressure, by site
Bedbug bite(s) — *see* Bite(s), by site, superficial, insect
Bedclothes, asphyxiation or suffocation by — *see* Asphyxia, traumatic, due to, mechanical, trapped
Bednar's
  aphthae K12.0
  tumor — *see* Neoplasm, malignant, by site
Bedridden Z74.01
Bedsore — *see* Ulcer, pressure, by site
Bedwetting — *see* Enuresis
Bee sting (with allergic or anaphylactic shock) — *see* Toxicity, venom, arthropod, bee
Beer drinker's heart (disease) I42.6
Begbie's disease (exophthalmic goiter) — *see* Hyperthyroidism, with, goiter
Behavior
  antisocial
    adult Z72.811
    child or adolescent Z72.810
  disorder, disturbance — *see* Disorder, conduct
  disruptive — *see* Disorder, conduct
  drug seeking Z76.5
  inexplicable R46.2
  marked evasiveness R46.5
  obsessive-compulsive R46.81
  overactivity R46.3
  poor responsiveness R46.4
  self-damaging (life-style) Z72.89
  sleep-incompatible Z72.821
  slowness R46.4
  specified NEC R46.89
  strange (and inexplicable) R46.2
  suspiciousness R46.5
  type A pattern Z73.1
  undue concern or preoccupation with stressful events R46.6
  verbosity and circumstantial detail obscuring reason for contact R46.7
Behçet's disease or syndrome M35.2
Behr's disease — *see* Degeneration, macula
Beigel's disease or morbus (white piedra) B36.2
Bejel A65
Bekhterev's syndrome — *see* Spondylitis, ankylosing
Belching — *see* Eructation
Bell's
  mania F30.8
  palsy, paralysis G51.0
    infant or newborn P11.3
  spasm G51.3
Bence Jones albuminuria or proteinuria NEC R80.3
Bends T70.3 ☑
Benedikt's paralysis or syndrome G46.3

Benign (*see also* condition)
  prostatic hyperplasia — *see* Hyperplasia, prostate
Bennett's fracture (displaced) S62.21- ☑
Benson's disease — *see* Deposit, crystalline
Bent
  back (hysterical) F44.4
  nose M95.0
    congenital Q67.4
Bereavement (uncomplicated) Z63.4
Bergeron's disease (hysterical chorea) F44.4
Berger's disease — *see* Nephropathy, IgA
Beriberi (dry) E51.11
  heart (disease) E51.12
  polyneuropathy E51.11
  wet E51.12
    involving circulatory system E51.11
Berlin's disease or edema (traumatic) S05.8X- ☑
Berlock (berloque) **dermatitis** L56.2
Bernard-Horner syndrome G90.2
Bernard-Soulier disease or thrombopathia D69.1
Bernhardt (-Roth) **disease** — *see* Mononeuropathy, lower limb, meralgia paresthetica
Bernheim's syndrome — *see* Failure, heart, right
Bertielliasis B71.8
Berylliosis (lung) J63.2
Besnier-Boeck (-Schaumann) **disease** — *see* Sarcoidosis
Besnier's
  lupus pernio D86.3
  prurigo L20.0
Bestiality F65.89
Best's disease H35.50
Betalipoproteinemia, broad or floating E78.2
Beta-mercaptolactate-cysteine disulfiduria E72.09
Betting and gambling Z72.6
  pathological (compulsive) F63.0
Bezoar T18.9 ☑
  intestine T18.3 ☑
  stomach T18.2 ☑
Bezold's abscess — *see* Mastoiditis, acute
Bianchi's syndrome R48.8
Bicornate or bicornis uterus Q51.3
  in pregnancy or childbirth O34.00
    causing obstructed labor O65.5
Bicuspid aortic valve Q23.1
Biedl-Bardet syndrome Q87.89
Bielschowsky (-Jansky) **disease** E75.4
Biermer's (pernicious) **anemia or disease** D51.0
Biett's disease L93.0
Bifid (congenital)
  apex, heart Q24.8
  clitoris Q52.6
  kidney Q63.8
  nose Q30.2
  patella Q74.1
  scrotum Q55.29
  toe NEC Q74.2
  tongue Q38.3
  ureter Q62.8
  uterus Q51.3
  uvula Q35.7
Biforis uterus (suprasimplex) Q51.3
Bifurcation (congenital)
  gallbladder Q44.1
  kidney pelvis Q63.8
  renal pelvis Q63.8
  rib Q76.6
  tongue, congenital Q38.3
  trachea Q32.1
  ureter Q62.8
  urethra Q64.74
  vertebra Q76.49
Big spleen syndrome D73.1
Bigeminal pulse R00.8
Bilateral — *see* condition
Bile
  duct — *see* condition
  pigments in urine R82.2
Bilharziasis (*see also* Schistosomiasis)
  chyluria B65.0
  cutaneous B65.3
  galacturia B65.0
  hematochyluria B65.0
  intestinal B65.1
  lipemia B65.9
  lipuria B65.0
  oriental B65.2
  piarhemia B65.9

Bilharziasis — *continued*
pulmonary NOS B65.9 [J99]
  pneumonia B65.9 [J17]
tropical hematuria B65.0
vesical B65.0
Biliary — *see* condition
Bilirubin metabolism disorder E80.7
specified NEC E80.6
Bilirubinemia, familial nonhemolytic E80.4
Bilirubinuria R82.2
Biliuria R82.2
Bilocular stomach K31.2
Binswanger's disease I67.3
Biparta, bipartite
carpal scaphoid Q74.0
patella Q74.1
vagina Q52.10
Bird
face Q75.8
fancier's disease or lung J67.2
Birth
complications in mother — *see* Delivery, complicated
compression during NOS P15.9
defect — *see* Anomaly
immature (less than 37 completed weeks) — *see* Preterm, newborn
  extremely (less than 28 completed weeks) — *see* Immaturity, extreme
inattention, at or after — *see* Maltreatment, child, neglect
injury NOS P15.9
basal ganglia P11.1
brachial plexus NEC P14.3
brain (compression) (pressure) P11.2
central nervous system NOS P11.9
cerebellum P11.1
cerebral hemorrhage P10.1
external genitalia P15.5
eye P15.3
face P15.4
fracture
  bone P13.9
    specified NEC P13.8
  clavicle P13.4
  femur P13.2
  humerus P13.3
  long bone, except femur P13.3
  radius and ulna P13.3
  skull P13.0
  spine P11.5
  tibia and fibula P13.3
intracranial P11.2
  laceration or hemorrhage P10.9
    specified NEC P10.8
intraventricular hemorrhage P10.2
laceration
  brain P10.1
  by scalpel P15.8
  peripheral nerve P14.9
liver P15.0
meninges
  brain P11.1
  spinal cord P11.5
nerve
  brachial plexus P14.3
  cranial NEC (except facial) P11.4
  facial P11.3
  peripheral P14.9
  phrenic (paralysis) P14.2
paralysis
  facial nerve P11.3
  spinal P11.5
penis P15.5
rupture
  spinal cord P11.5
scalp P12.9
scalpel wound P15.8
scrotum P15.5
skull NEC P13.1
  fracture P13.0
specified type NEC P15.8
spinal cord P11.5
spine P11.5
spleen P15.1
sternomastoid (hematoma) P15.2
subarachnoid hemorrhage P10.3
subcutaneous fat necrosis P15.6
subdural hemorrhage P10.0

Birth — *continued*
injury — *continued*
  tentorial tear P10.4
  testes P15.5
  vulva P15.5
lack of care, at or after — *see* Maltreatment, child, neglect
neglect, at or after — *see* Maltreatment, child, neglect
palsy or paralysis, newborn, NOS (birth injury) P14.9
premature (infant) — *see* Preterm, newborn
shock, newborn P96.89
trauma — *see* Birth, injury
weight
  4000 grams to 4499 grams P08.1
  4500 grams or more P08.0
  low (2499 grams or less) — *see* Low, birthweight
    extremely (999 grams or less) — *see* Low, birthweight, extreme
Birthmark Q82.5
Birt-Hogg-Dube syndrome Q87.89
Bisalbuminemia E88.09
Biskra's button B55.1
Bite(s) (animal) (human)
abdomen, abdominal
wall S31.159 ☑
  with penetration into peritoneal cavity S31.659 ☑
  epigastric region S31.152 ☑
    with penetration into peritoneal cavity S31.652 ☑
  left
    lower quadrant S31.154 ☑
      with penetration into peritoneal cavity S31.654 ☑
    upper quadrant S31.151 ☑
      with penetration into peritoneal cavity S31.651 ☑
  periumbilic region S31.155 ☑
    with penetration into peritoneal cavity S31.655 ☑
  right
    lower quadrant S31.153 ☑
      with penetration into peritoneal cavity S31.653 ☑
    upper quadrant S31.150 ☑
      with penetration into peritoneal cavity S31.650 ☑
  superficial NEC S30.871 ☑
    insect S30.861 ☑
alveolar (process) — *see* Bite, oral cavity
amphibian (venomous) — *see* Venom, bite, amphibian
animal (*see also* Bite, by site)
  venomous — *see* Venom
ankle S91.05- ☑
  superficial NEC S90.57- ☑
    insect S90.56- ☑
antecubital space — *see* Bite, elbow
anus S31.835 ☑
  superficial NEC S30.877 ☑
    insect S30.867 ☑
arm (upper) S41.15- ☑
  lower — *see* Bite, forearm
  superficial NEC S40.87- ☑
    insect S40.86- ☑
arthropod NEC — *see* Venom, bite, arthropod
auditory canal (external) (meatus) — *see* Bite, ear
auricle, ear — *see* Bite, ear
axilla — *see* Bite, arm
back (*see also* Bite, thorax, back)
  lower S31.050 ☑
    with penetration into retroperitoneal space S31.051 ☑
  superficial NEC S30.870 ☑
    insect S30.860 ☑
bedbug — *see* Bite(s), by site, superficial, insect
breast S21.05- ☑
  superficial NEC S20.17- ☑
    insect S20.16- ☑
brow — *see* Bite, head, specified site NEC
buttock S31.805 ☑
  left S31.825 ☑
  right S31.815 ☑
  superficial NEC S30.870 ☑
    insect S30.860 ☑
calf — *see* Bite, leg
canaliculus lacrimalis — *see* Bite, eyelid

Bite(s) — *continued*
canthus, eye — *see* Bite, eyelid
centipede — *see* Toxicity, venom, arthropod, centipede
cheek (external) S01.45- ☑
  internal — *see* Bite, oral cavity
  superficial NEC S00.87 ☑
    insect S00.86 ☑
chest wall — *see* Bite, thorax
chigger B88.0
chin — *see* Bite, head, specified site NEC
clitoris — *see* Bite, vulva
costal region — *see* Bite, thorax
digit(s)
  hand — *see* Bite, finger
  toe — *see* Bite, toe
ear (canal) (external) S01.35- ☑
  superficial NEC S00.47- ☑
    insect S00.46- ☑
elbow S51.05- ☑
  superficial NEC S50.37- ☑
    insect S50.36- ☑
epididymis — *see* Bite, testis
epigastric region — *see* Bite, abdomen
epiglottis — *see* Bite, neck, specified site NEC
esophagus, cervical S11.25 ☑
  superficial NEC S10.17 ☑
    insect S10.16 ☑
eyebrow — *see* Bite, eyelid
eyelid S01.15- ☑
  superficial NEC S00.27- ☑
    insect S00.26- ☑
face NEC — *see* Bite, head, specified site NEC
finger(s) S61.259 ☑
  with
    damage to nail S61.359 ☑
  index S61.258 ☑
    with
      damage to nail S61.358 ☑
    left S61.251 ☑
      with
        damage to nail S61.351 ☑
    right S61.250 ☑
      with
        damage to nail S61.350 ☑
    superficial NEC S60.478 ☑
      insect S60.46- ☑
  little S61.25- ☑
    with
      damage to nail S61.35- ☑
    superficial NEC S60.47- ☑
      insect S60.46- ☑
  middle S61.25- ☑
    with
      damage to nail S61.35- ☑
    superficial NEC S60.47- ☑
      insect S60.46- ☑
  ring S61.25- ☑
    with
      damage to nail S61.35- ☑
    superficial NEC S60.47- ☑
      insect S60.46- ☑
  superficial NEC S60.479 ☑
    insect S60.469 ☑
  thumb — *see* Bite, thumb
flank — *see* Bite, abdomen, wall
flea — *see* Bite, by site, superficial, Insect
foot (except toe(s) alone) S91.35- ☑
  superficial NEC S90.87- ☑
    insect S90.86- ☑
  toe — *see* Bite, toe
forearm S51.85- ☑
  elbow only — *see* Bite, elbow
  superficial NEC S50.87- ☑
    insect S50.86- ☑
forehead — *see* Bite, head, specified site NEC
genital organs, external
  female S31.552 ☑
    superficial NEC S30.876 ☑
      insect S30.866 ☑
    vagina and vulva — *see* Bite, vulva
  male S31.551 ☑
    penis — *see* Bite, penis
    scrotum — *see* Bite, scrotum
    superficial NEC S30.875 ☑
      insect S30.865 ☑

Index (side) — **Bite — Blastomycosis, blastomycotic**

Bite(s) — *continued*
genital organs, external — *continued*
  male — *continued*
   testes — *see* Bite, testis
 groin — *see* Bite, abdomen, wall
 gum — *see* Bite, oral cavity
 hand S61.45- ☑
  finger — *see* Bite, finger
  superficial NEC S60.57- ☑
   insect S60.56- ☑
  thumb — *see* Bite, thumb
 head S01.95 ☑
  cheek — *see* Bite, cheek
  ear — *see* Bite, ear
  eyelid — *see* Bite, eyelid
  lip — *see* Bite, lip
  nose — *see* Bite, nose
  oral cavity — *see* Bite, oral cavity
  scalp — *see* Bite, scalp
  specified site NEC S01.85 ☑
   superficial NEC S00.87 ☑
    insect S00.86 ☑
  superficial NEC S00.97 ☑
   insect S00.96 ☑
  temporomandibular area — *see* Bite, cheek
 heel — *see* Bite, foot
 hip S71.05- ☑
  superficial NEC S70.27- ☑
   insect S70.26- ☑
 hymen S31.45 ☑
 hypochondrium — *see* Bite, abdomen, wall
 hypogastric region — *see* Bite, abdomen, wall
 inguinal region — *see* Bite, abdomen, wall
 insect — *see* Bite, by site, superficial, insect
 instep — *see* Bite, foot
 interscapular region — *see* Bite, thorax, back
 jaw — *see* Bite, head, specified site NEC
 knee S81.05- ☑
  superficial NEC S80.27- ☑
   insect S80.26- ☑
 labium (majus) (minus) — *see* Bite, vulva
 lacrimal duct — *see* Bite, eyelid
 larynx S11.015 ☑
  superficial NEC S10.17 ☑
   insect S10.16 ☑
 leg (lower) S81.85- ☑
  ankle — *see* Bite, ankle
  foot — *see* Bite, foot
  knee — *see* Bite, knee
  superficial NEC S80.87- ☑
   insect S80.86- ☑
  toe — *see* Bite, toe
  upper — *see* Bite, thigh
 lip S01.551 ☑
  superficial NEC S00.571 ☑
   insect S00.561 ☑
 lizard (venomous) — *see* Venom, bite, reptile
 loin — *see* Bite, abdomen, wall
 lower back — *see* Bite, back, lower
 lumbar region — *see* Bite, back, lower
 malar region — *see* Bite, head, specified site NEC
 mammary — *see* Bite, breast
 marine animals (venomous) — *see* Toxicity, venom, marine animal
 mastoid region — *see* Bite, head, specified site NEC
 mouth — *see* Bite, oral cavity
 nail
  finger — *see* Bite, finger
  toe — *see* Bite, toe
 nape — *see* Bite, neck, specified site NEC
 nasal (septum) (sinus) — *see* Bite, nose
 nasopharynx — *see* Bite, head, specified site NEC
 neck S11.95 ☑
  involving
   cervical esophagus — *see* Bite, esophagus, cervical
   larynx — *see* Bite, larynx
   pharynx — *see* Bite, pharynx
   thyroid gland S11.15 ☑
   trachea — *see* Bite, trachea
  specified site NEC S11.85 ☑
   superficial NEC S10.87 ☑
    insect S10.86 ☑
  superficial NEC S10.97 ☑
   insect S10.96 ☑
  throat S11.85 ☑

Bite(s) — *continued*
 neck — *continued*
  throat — *continued*
   superficial NEC S10.17 ☑
    insect S10.16 ☑
 nose (septum) (sinus) S01.25 ☑
  superficial NEC S00.37 ☑
   insect S00.36 ☑
 occipital region — *see* Bite, scalp
 oral cavity S01.552 ☑
  superficial NEC S00.572 ☑
   insect S00.562 ☑
 orbital region — *see* Bite, eyelid
 palate — *see* Bite, oral cavity
 palm — *see* Bite, hand
 parietal region — *see* Bite, scalp
 pelvis S31.050 ☑
  with penetration into retroperitoneal space S31.051 ☑
  superficial NEC S30.870 ☑
   insect S30.860 ☑
 penis S31.25 ☑
  superficial NEC S30.872 ☑
   insect S30.862 ☑
 perineum
  female — *see* Bite, vulva
  male — *see* Bite, pelvis
 periocular area (with or without lacrimal passages) — *see* Bite, eyelid
 phalanges
  finger — *see* Bite, finger
  toe — *see* Bite, toe
 pharynx S11.25 ☑
  superficial NEC S10.17 ☑
   insect S10.16 ☑
 pinna — *see* Bite, ear
 poisonous — *see* Venom
 popliteal space — *see* Bite, knee
 prepuce — *see* Bite, penis
 pubic region — *see* Bite, abdomen, wall
 rectovaginal septum — *see* Bite, vulva
 red bug B88.0
 reptile NEC (*see also* Venom, bite, reptile)
  nonvenomous — *see* Bite, by site
  snake — *see* Venom, bite, snake
 sacral region — *see* Bite, back, lower
 sacroiliac region — *see* Bite, back, lower
 salivary gland — *see* Bite, oral cavity
 scalp S01.05 ☑
  superficial NEC S00.07 ☑
   insect S00.06 ☑
 scapular region — *see* Bite, shoulder
 scrotum S31.35 ☑
  superficial NEC S30.873 ☑
   insect S30.863 ☑
 sea-snake (venomous) — *see* Toxicity, venom, snake, sea snake
 shin — *see* Bite, leg
 shoulder S41.05- ☑
  superficial NEC S40.27- ☑
   insect S40.26- ☑
 snake (*see also* Venom, bite, snake)
  nonvenomous — *see* Bite, by site
 spermatic cord — *see* Bite, testis
 spider (venomous) — *see* Toxicity, venom, spider
  nonvenomous — *see* Bite, by site, superficial, insect
 sternal region — *see* Bite, thorax, front
 submaxillary region — *see* Bite, head, specified site NEC
 submental region — *see* Bite, head, specified site NEC
 subungual
  finger(s) — *see* Bite, finger
  toe — *see* Bite, toe
 superficial — *see* Bite, by site, superficial
 supraclavicular fossa S11.85 ☑
 supraorbital — *see* Bite, head, specified site NEC
 temple, temporal region — *see* Bite, head, specified site NEC
 temporomandibular area — *see* Bite, cheek
 testis S31.35 ☑
  superficial NEC S30.873 ☑
   insect S30.863 ☑
 thigh S71.15- ☑
  superficial NEC S70.37- ☑
   insect S70.36- ☑
 thorax, thoracic (wall) S21.95 ☑

Bite(s) — *continued*
 thorax, thoracic — *continued*
  back S21.25- ☑
   with penetration into thoracic cavity S21.45- ☑
  breast — *see* Bite, breast
  front S21.15- ☑
   with penetration into thoracic cavity S21.35- ☑
  superficial NEC S20.97 ☑
   back S20.47- ☑
   front S20.37- ☑
   insect S20.96 ☑
    back S20.46- ☑
    front S20.36- ☑
 throat — *see* Bite, neck, throat
 thumb S61.05- ☑
  with
   damage to nail S61.15- ☑
  superficial NEC S60.37- ☑
   insect S60.36- ☑
 thyroid S11.15 ☑
  superficial NEC S10.87 ☑
   insect S10.86 ☑
 toe(s) S91.15- ☑
  with
   damage to nail S91.25- ☑
  great S91.15- ☑
   with
    damage to nail S91.25- ☑
  lesser S91.15- ☑
   with
    damage to nail S91.25- ☑
  superficial NEC S90.47- ☑
   great S90.47- ☑
   insect S90.46- ☑
    great S90.46- ☑
 tongue S01.552 ☑
 trachea S11.025 ☑
  superficial NEC S10.17 ☑
   insect S10.16 ☑
 tunica vaginalis — *see* Bite, testis
 tympanum, tympanic membrane — *see* Bite, ear
 umbilical region S31.155 ☑
 uvula — *see* Bite, oral cavity
 vagina — *see* Bite, vulva
 venomous — *see* Venom
 vocal cords S11.035 ☑
  superficial NEC S10.17 ☑
   insect S10.16 ☑
 vulva S31.45 ☑
  superficial NEC S30.874 ☑
   insect S30.864 ☑
 wrist S61.55- ☑
  superficial NEC S60.87- ☑
   insect S60.86- ☑
Biting, cheek or lip K13.1
Biventricular failure (heart) I50.82
Björck (-Thorson) **syndrome** (malignant carcinoid) E34.0
Black
 death A20.9
 eye S00.1- ☑
 hairy tongue K14.3
 heel (foot) S90.3- ☑
 lung (disease) J60
 palm (hand) S60.22- ☑
Blackfan-Diamond anemia or syndrome (congenital hypoplastic anemia) D61.01
Blackhead L70.0
Blackout R55
Bladder — *see* condition
Blast (air) (hydraulic) (immersion) (underwater)
 blindness S05.8X- ☑
 injury
  abdomen or thorax — *see* Injury, by site
  ear (acoustic nerve trauma) — *see* Injury, nerve, acoustic, specified type NEC
  syndrome NEC T70.8 ☑
Blastoma — *see* Neoplasm, malignant, by site
 pulmonary — *see* Neoplasm, lung, malignant
Blastomycosis, blastomycotic B40.9
 Brazilian — *see* Paracoccidioidomycosis
 cutaneous B40.3
 disseminated B40.7
 European — *see* Cryptococcosis
 generalized B40.7
 keloidal B48.0
 North American B40.9

Blastomycosis, blastomycotic — *continued*
  primary pulmonary B40.0
  pulmonary B40.2
    acute B40.0
    chronic B40.1
  skin B40.3
  South American — *see* Paracoccidioidomycosis
  specified NEC B40.89
Bleb(s) R23.8
  emphysematous (lung) (solitary) J43.9
  endophthalmitis H59.43
  filtering (vitreous), after glaucoma surgery Z98.83
  inflammed (infected), postprocedural H59.40
    stage 1 H59.41
    stage 2 H59.42
    stage 3 H59.43
  lung (ruptured) J43.9
    congenital — *see* Atelectasis
    newborn P25.8
  subpleural (emphysematous) J43.9
Blebitis, postprocedural H59.40
  stage 1 H59.41
  stage 2 H59.42
  stage 3 H59.43
Bleeder (familial) (hereditary) — *see* Hemophilia
Bleeding (*see also* Hemorrhage)
  anal K62.5
  anovulatory N97.0
  atonic, following delivery O72.1
  capillary I78.8
    puerperal O72.2
  contact (postcoital) N93.0
  due to uterine subinvolution N85.3
  ear — *see* Otorrhagia
  excessive, associated with menopausal onset N92.4
  familial — *see* Defect, coagulation
  following intercourse N93.0
  gastrointestinal K92.2
  hemorrhoids — *see* Hemorrhoids
  intermenstrual (regular) N92.3
    irregular N92.1
  intraoperative — *see* Complication, intraoperative, hemorrhage
  irregular N92.6
  menopausal N92.4
  newborn, intraventricular — *see* Newborn, affected by, hemorrhage, intraventricular
  nipple N64.59
  nose R04.0
  ovulation N92.3
  postclimacteric N95.0
  postcoital N93.0
  postmenopausal N95.0
  postoperative — *see* Complication, postprocedural, hemorrhage
  preclimacteric N92.4
  pre-pubertal vaginal N93.1
  puberty (excessive, with onset of menstrual periods) N92.2
  rectum, rectal K62.5
    newborn P54.2
  tendencies — *see* Defect, coagulation
  throat R04.1
  tooth socket (post-extraction) K91.840
  umbilical stump P51.9
  uterus, uterine NEC N93.9
    climacteric N92.4
    dysfunctional or functional N93.8
    menopausal N92.4
    preclimacteric or premenopausal N92.4
    unrelated to menstrual cycle N93.9
  vagina, vaginal (abnormal) N93.9
    dysfunctional or functional N93.8
    newborn P54.6
    pre-pubertal N93.1
  vicarious N94.89
Blennorrhagia, blennorrhagic — *see* Gonorrhea
Blennorrhea (acute) (chronic) (*see also* Gonorrhea)
  inclusion (neonatal) (newborn) P39.1
  lower genitourinary tract (gonococcal) A54.00
  neonatorum (gonococcal ophthalmia) A54.31
Blepharelosis — *see* Entropion
Blepharitis (angularis) (ciliaris) (eyelid) (marginal) (nonulcerative) H01.009
  herpes zoster B02.39
  left H01.006
    lower H01.005
    upper H01.004

Blepharitis — *continued*
  right H01.003
    lower H01.002
    upper H01.001
  squamous H01.029
    left H01.026
      lower H01.025
      upper H01.024
    right H01.023
      lower H01.022
      upper H01.021
  ulcerative H01.019
    left H01.016
      lower H01.015
      upper H01.014
    right H01.013
      lower H01.012
      upper H01.011
Blepharochalasis H02.30
  congenital Q10.0
  left H02.36
    lower H02.35
    upper H02.34
  right H02.33
    lower H02.32
    upper H02.31
Blepharoclonus H02.59
Blepharoconjunctivitis H10.50- ☑
  angular H10.52- ☑
  contact H10.53- ☑
  ligneous H10.51- ☑
Blepharophimosis (eyelid) H02.529
  congenital Q10.3
  left H02.526
    lower H02.525
    upper H02.524
  right H02.523
    lower H02.522
    upper H02.521
Blepharoptosis H02.40- ☑
  congenital Q10.0
  mechanical H02.41- ☑
  myogenic H02.42- ☑
  neurogenic H02.43- ☑
  paralytic H02.43- ☑
Blepharopyorrhea, gonococcal A54.39
Blepharospasm G24.5
  drug induced G24.01
Blighted ovum O02.0
Blind (*see also* Blindness)
  bronchus (congenital) Q32.4
  loop syndrome K90.2
    congenital Q43.8
  sac, fallopian tube (congenital) Q50.6
  spot, enlarged — *see* Defect, visual field, localized, scotoma, blind spot area
  tract or tube, congenital NEC — *see* Atresia, by site
Blindness (acquired) (congenital) (both eyes) H54.0X- ☑
  blast S05.8X- ☑
  color — *see* Deficiency, color vision
  concussion S05.8X- ☑
  cortical H47.619
    left brain H47.612
    right brain H47.611
  day H53.11
  due to injury (current episode) S05.9- ☑
    sequelae — *code to* injury with seventh character S
  eclipse (total) — *see* Retinopathy, solar
  emotional (hysterical) F44.6
  face H53.16
  hysterical F44.6
  legal (both eyes) (USA definition) H54.8
  mind R48.8
  night H53.60
    abnormal dark adaptation curve H53.61
    acquired H53.62
    congenital H53.63
    specified type NEC H53.69
    vitamin A deficiency E50.5
  one eye (other eye normal) H54.40
    left (normal vision on right) H54.42- ☑
      low vision on right H54.12- ☑
    low vision, other eye H54.10
    right (normal vision on left) H54.41- ☑
      low vision on left H54.11- ☑
  psychic R48.8
  river B73.01

Blindness — *continued*
  snow — *see* Photokeratitis
  sun, solar — *see* Retinopathy, solar
  transient — *see* Disturbance, vision, subjective, loss, transient
  traumatic (current episode) S05.9- ☑
  word (developmental) F81.0
    acquired R48.0
    secondary to organic lesion R48.0
Blister (nonthermal)
  abdominal wall S30.821 ☑
  alveolar process S00.522 ☑
  ankle S90.52- ☑
  antecubital space — *see* Blister, elbow
  anus S30.827 ☑
  arm (upper) S40.82- ☑
  auditory canal — *see* Blister, ear
  auricle — *see* Blister, ear
  axilla — *see* Blister, arm
  back, lower S30.820 ☑
  beetle dermatitis L24.89
  breast S20.12- ☑
  brow S00.82 ☑
  calf — *see* Blister, leg
  canthus — *see* Blister, eyelid
  cheek S00.82 ☑
    internal S00.522 ☑
  chest wall — *see* Blister, thorax
  chin S00.82 ☑
  costal region — *see* Blister, thorax
  digit(s)
    foot — *see* Blister, toe
    hand — *see* Blister, finger
  due to burn — *see* Burn, by site, second degree
  ear S00.42- ☑
  elbow S50.32- ☑
  epiglottis S10.12 ☑
  esophagus, cervical S10.12 ☑
  eyebrow — *see* Blister, eyelid
  eyelid S00.22- ☑
  face S00.82 ☑
  fever B00.1
  finger(s) S60.429 ☑
    index S60.42- ☑
    little S60.42- ☑
    middle S60.42- ☑
    ring S60.42- ☑
  foot (except toe(s) alone) S90.82- ☑
    toe — *see* Blister, toe
  forearm S50.82- ☑
    elbow only — *see* Blister, elbow
  forehead S00.82 ☑
  fracture — *omit code*
  genital organ
    female S30.826 ☑
    male S30.825 ☑
  gum S00.522 ☑
  hand S60.52- ☑
  head S00.92 ☑
    ear — *see* Blister, ear
    eyelid — *see* Blister, eyelid
    lip S00.521 ☑
    nose S00.32 ☑
    oral cavity S00.522 ☑
    scalp S00.02 ☑
    specified site NEC S00.82 ☑
  heel — *see* Blister, foot
  hip S70.22- ☑
  interscapular region S20.429 ☑
  jaw S00.82 ☑
  knee S80.22- ☑
  larynx S10.12 ☑
  leg (lower) S80.82- ☑
    knee — *see* Blister, knee
    upper — *see* Blister, thigh
  lip S00.521 ☑
  malar region S00.82 ☑
  mammary — *see* Blister, breast
  mastoid region S00.82 ☑
  mouth S00.522 ☑
  multiple, skin, nontraumatic R23.8
  nail
    finger — *see* Blister, finger
    toe — *see* Blister, toe
  nasal S00.32 ☑
  neck S10.92 ☑

Blastomycosis, blastomycotic — Blister

Subterms under main terms may continue to next column or page   ☑ Additional Character Required — Refer to the Tabular List for Character Selection   39

Blister — *continued*
 neck — *continued*
  specified site NEC S10.82 ☑
   throat S10.12 ☑
 nose S00.32 ☑
 occipital region S00.02 ☑
 oral cavity S00.522 ☑
 orbital region — *see* Blister, eyelid
 palate S00.522 ☑
 palm — *see* Blister, hand
 parietal region S00.02 ☑
 pelvis S30.820 ☑
 penis S30.822 ☑
 periocular area — *see* Blister, eyelid
 phalanges
  finger — *see* Blister, finger
  toe — *see* Blister, toe
 pharynx S10.12 ☑
 pinna — *see* Blister, ear
 popliteal space — *see* Blister, knee
 scalp S00.02 ☑
 scapular region — *see* Blister, shoulder
 scrotum S30.823 ☑
 shin — *see* Blister, leg
 shoulder S40.22- ☑
 sternal region S20.329 ☑
 submaxillary region S00.82 ☑
 submental region S00.82 ☑
 subungual
  finger(s) — *see* Blister, finger
  toe(s) — *see* Blister, toe
 supraclavicular fossa S10.82 ☑
 supraorbital S00.82 ☑
 temple S00.82 ☑
 temporal region S00.82 ☑
 testis S30.823 ☑
 thermal — *see* Burn, second degree, by site
 thigh S70.32- ☑
 thorax, thoracic (wall) S20.92 ☑
  back S20.42- ☑
  front S20.32- ☑
 throat S10.12 ☑
 thumb S60.32- ☑
 toe(s) S90.42- ☑
  great S90.42- ☑
 tongue S00.522 ☑
 trachea S10.12 ☑
 tympanum, tympanic membrane — *see* Blister, ear
 upper arm — *see* Blister, arm (upper)
 uvula S00.522 ☑
 vagina S30.824 ☑
 vocal cords S10.12 ☑
 vulva S30.824 ☑
 wrist S60.82- ☑
Bloating R14.0
Bloch-Sulzberger disease or syndrome Q82.3
Block, blocked
 alveolocapillary J84.10
 arborization (heart) I45.5
 arrhythmic I45.9
 atrioventricular (incomplete) (partial) I44.30
  with atrioventricular dissociation I44.2
  complete I44.2
   congenital Q24.6
  congenital Q24.6
  first degree I44.0
  second degree (types I and II) I44.1
  specified NEC I44.39
  third degree I44.2
  types I and II I44.1
 auriculoventricular — *see* Block, atrioventricular
 bifascicular (cardiac) I45.2
 bundle-branch (complete) (false) (incomplete) I45.4
  bilateral I45.2
  left I44.7
   with right bundle branch block I45.2
   hemiblock I44.60
    anterior I44.4
    posterior I44.5
   incomplete I44.7
    with right bundle branch block I45.2
  right I45.10
   with
    left bundle branch block I45.2
    left fascicular block I45.2
   specified NEC I45.19
  Wilson's type I45.19

Block, blocked — *continued*
 cardiac I45.9
 conduction I45.9
  complete I44.2
 fascicular (left) I44.60
  anterior I44.4
  posterior I44.5
  right I45.0
  specified NEC I44.69
 foramen Magendie (acquired) G91.1
  congenital Q03.1
   with spina bifida — *see* Spina bifida, by site, with hydrocephalus
 heart I45.9
  bundle branch I45.4
   bilateral I45.2
  complete (atrioventricular) I44.2
  congenital Q24.6
  first degree (atrioventricular) I44.0
  second degree (atrioventricular) I44.1
  specified type NEC I45.5
  third degree (atrioventricular) I44.2
 hepatic vein I82.0
 intraventricular (nonspecific) I45.4
  bundle branch
   bilateral I45.2
 kidney N28.9
  postcystoscopic or postprocedural N99.0
 Mobitz (types I and II) I44.1
 myocardial — *see* Block, heart
 nodal I45.5
 organ or site, congenital NEC — *see* Atresia, by site
 portal (vein) I81
 second degree (types I and II) I44.1
 sinoatrial I45.5
 sinoauricular I45.5
 third degree I44.2
 trifascicular I45.3
 tubal N97.1
 vein NOS I82.90
 Wenckebach (types I and II) I44.1
Blockage — *see* Obstruction
Blocq's disease F44.4
Blood
 constituents, abnormal R78.9
 disease D75.9
 donor — *see* Donor, blood
 dyscrasia D75.9
  with
   abortion — *see* Abortion, by type, complicated by, hemorrhage
   ectopic pregnancy O08.1
   molar pregnancy O08.1
  following ectopic or molar pregnancy O08.1
  newborn P61.9
  puerperal, postpartum O72.3
 flukes NEC — *see* Schistosomiasis
 in
  feces K92.1
   occult R19.5
  urine — *see* Hematuria
 mole O02.0
 occult in feces R19.5
 pressure
  decreased, due to shock following injury T79.4 ☑
  examination only Z01.30
  fluctuating I99.8
  high — *see* Hypertension
   borderline R03.0
   incidental reading, without diagnosis of hypertension R03.0
  low (*see also* Hypotension)
   incidental reading, without diagnosis of hypotension R03.1
 spitting — *see* Hemoptysis
 staining cornea — *see* Pigmentation, cornea, stromal
 transfusion
  reaction or complication — *see* Complications, transfusion
 type
  A (Rh positive) Z67.10
   Rh negative Z67.11
  AB (Rh positive) Z67.30
   Rh negative Z67.31
  B (Rh positive) Z67.20
   Rh negative Z67.21
  O (Rh positive) Z67.40
   Rh negative Z67.41

Blood — *continued*
 type — *continued*
  Rh (positive) Z67.90
   negative Z67.91
 vessel rupture — *see* Hemorrhage
 vomiting — *see* Hematemesis
Blood-forming organs, disease D75.9
Bloodgood's disease — *see* Mastopathy, cystic
Bloom (-Machacek)(-Torre) **syndrome** Q82.8
Blount's disease or osteochondrosis — *see* Osteochondrosis, juvenile, tibia
Blue
 baby Q24.9
 diaper syndrome E72.09
 dome cyst (breast) — *see* Cyst, breast
 dot cataract Q12.0
 nevus D22.9
 sclera Q13.5
  with fragility of bone and deafness Q78.0
 toe syndrome I75.02- ☑
Blueness — *see* Cyanosis
Blues, postpartal O90.6
 baby O90.6
Blurring, visual H53.8
Blushing (abnormal) (excessive) R23.2
BMI — *see* Body, mass index
Boarder, hospital NEC Z76.4
 accompanying sick person Z76.3
 healthy infant or child Z76.2
  foundling Z76.1
Bockhart's impetigo L01.02
Bodechtel-Guttman disease (subacute sclerosing panencephalitis) A81.1
Boder-Sedgwick syndrome (ataxia-telangiectasia) G11.3
Body, bodies
 Aschoff's — *see* Myocarditis, rheumatic
 asteroid, vitreous — *see* Deposit, crystalline
 cytoid (retina) — *see* Occlusion, artery, retina
 drusen (degenerative) (macula) (retinal) (*see also* Degeneration, macula, drusen)
  optic disc — *see* Drusen, optic disc
 foreign — *see* Foreign body
 loose
  joint, except knee — *see* Loose, body, joint
   knee M23.4- ☑
  sheath, tendon — *see* Disorder, tendon, specified type NEC
 mass index (BMI)
  adult
   19.9 or less Z68.1
   20.0-20.9 Z68.20
   21.0-21.9 Z68.21
   22.0-22.9 Z68.22
   23.0-23.9 Z68.23
   24.0-24.9 Z68.24
   25.0-25.9 Z68.25
   26.0-26.9 Z68.26
   27.0-27.9 Z68.27
   28.0-28.9 Z68.28
   29.0-29.9 Z68.29
   30.0-30.9 Z68.30
   31.0-31.9 Z68.31
   32.0-32.9 Z68.32
   33.0-33.9 Z68.33
   34.0-34.9 Z68.34
   35.0-35.9 Z68.35
   36.0-36.9 Z68.36
   37.0-37.9 Z68.37
   38.0-38.9 Z68.38
   39.0-39.9 Z68.39
   40.0-44.9 Z68.41
   45.0-49.9 Z68.42
   50.0-59.9 Z68.43
   60.0-69.9 Z68.44
   70 and over Z68.45
  pediatric
   5th percentile to less than 85th percentile for age Z68.52
   85th percentile to less than 95th percentile for age Z68.53
   less than fifth percentile for age Z68.51
   greater than or equal to ninety-fifth percentile for age Z68.54
 Mooser's A75.2
 rice (*see also* Loose, body, joint)
  knee M23.4- ☑
 rocking F98.4

☑ **Additional Character Required — Refer to the Tabular List for Character Selection**   ▽ Subterms under main terms may continue to next column or page

Boeck's
　disease or sarcoid — see Sarcoidosis
　lupoid (miliary) D86.3
Boerhaave's syndrome (spontaneous esophageal rupture) K22.3
Boggy
　cervix N88.8
　uterus N85.8
Boil (see also Furuncle, by site)
　Aleppo B55.1
　Baghdad B55.1
　Delhi B55.1
　lacrimal
　　gland — see Dacryoadenitis
　　passages (duct) (sac) — see Inflammation, lacrimal, passages, acute
　Natal B55.1
　orbit, orbital — see Abscess, orbit
　tropical B55.1
Bold hives — see Urticaria
Bombé, iris — see Membrane, pupillary
Bone — see condition
Bonnevie-Ullrich syndrome (see also Turner's syndrome) Q87.1
Bonnier's syndrome H81.8 ☑
Bonvale dam fever T73.3 ☑
Bony block of joint — see Ankylosis
BOOP (bronchiolitis obliterans organized pneumonia) J84.89
Borderline
　diabetes mellitus R73.03
　hypertension R03.0
　osteopenia M85.8- ☑
　pelvis, with obstruction during labor O65.1
　personality F60.3
Borna disease A83.9
Bornholm disease B33.0
Boston exanthem A88.0
Botalli, ductus (patent) (persistent) Q25.0
Bothriocephalus latus infestation B70.0
Botulism (foodborne intoxication) A05.1
　infant A48.51
　non-foodborne A48.52
　wound A48.52
Bouba — see Yaws
Bouchard's nodes (with arthropathy) M15.2
Bouffée délirante F23
Bouillaud's disease or syndrome (rheumatic heart disease) I01.9
Bourneville's disease Q85.1
Boutonniere deformity (finger) — see Deformity, finger, boutonniere
Bouveret (-Hoffmann) **syndrome** (paroxysmal tachycardia) I47.9
Bovine heart — see Hypertrophy, cardiac
Bowel — see condition
Bowen's
　dermatosis (precancerous) — see Neoplasm, skin, in situ
　disease — see Neoplasm, skin, in situ
　epithelioma — see Neoplasm, skin, in situ
　type
　　epidermoid carcinoma-in-situ — see Neoplasm, skin, in situ
　　intraepidermal squamous cell carcinoma — see Neoplasm, skin, in situ
Bowing
　femur (see also Deformity, limb, specified type NEC, thigh)
　　congenital Q68.3
　fibula (see also Deformity, limb, specified type NEC, lower leg)
　　congenital Q68.4
　forearm — see Deformity, limb, specified type NEC, forearm
　leg(s), long bones, congenital Q68.5
　radius — see Deformity, limb, specified type NEC, forearm
　tibia (see also Deformity, limb, specified type NEC, lower leg)
　　congenital Q68.4
Bowleg(s) (acquired) M21.16- ☑
　congenital Q68.5
　rachitic E64.3
Boyd's dysentery A03.2
Brachial — see condition
Brachycardia R00.1

Brachycephaly Q75.0
Bradley's disease A08.19
Bradyarrhythmia, cardiac I49.8
Bradycardia (sinoatrial) (sinus) (vagal) R00.1
　neonatal P29.12
　reflex G90.09
　tachycardia syndrome I49.5
Bradykinesia R25.8
Bradypnea R06.89
Bradytachycardia I49.5
Brailsford's disease or osteochondrosis — see Osteochondrosis, juvenile, radius
Brain (see also condition)
　death G93.82
　syndrome — see Syndrome, brain
Branched-chain amino-acid disorder E71.2
Branchial — see condition
　cartilage, congenital Q18.2
Branchiogenic remnant (in neck) Q18.0
Brandt's syndrome (acrodermatitis enteropathica) E83.2
Brash (water) R12
Bravais-jacksonian epilepsy — see Epilepsy, localization-related, symptomatic, with simple partial seizures
Braxton Hicks contractions — see False, labor
Brazilian leishmaniasis B55.2
BRBPR K62.5
Break, retina (without detachment) H33.30- ☑
　with retinal detachment — see Detachment, retina
　horseshoe tear H33.31- ☑
　multiple H33.33- ☑
　round hole H33.32- ☑
Breakdown
　device, graft or implant (see also Complications, by site and type, mechanical) T85.618 ☑
　　arterial graft NEC — see Complication, cardiovascular device, mechanical, vascular
　　breast (implant) T85.41 ☑
　　catheter NEC T85.618 ☑
　　　cystostomy T83.010 ☑
　　　dialysis (renal) T82.41 ☑
　　　　intraperitoneal T85.611 ☑
　　　Hopkins T83.018 ☑
　　　ileostomy T83.018 ☑
　　　infusion NEC T82.514 ☑
　　　　cranial T85.610- ☑
　　　　epidural T85.610 ☑
　　　　intrathecal T85.610 ☑
　　　　spinal T85.610 ☑
　　　　subarachnoid T85.610 ☑
　　　　subdural T85.610 ☑
　　　nephrostomy T83.012 ☑
　　　urethral indwelling T83.011 ☑
　　　urinary NEC T83.018 ☑
　　　urostomy T83.018 ☑
　　electronic (electrode) (pulse generator) (stimulator)
　　　bone T84.310 ☑
　　　cardiac T82.119 ☑
　　　　electrode T82.110 ☑
　　　　pulse generator T82.111 ☑
　　　　specified type NEC T82.118 ☑
　　　nervous system — see Complication, prosthetic device, mechanical, electronic nervous system stimulator
　　　urinary — see Complication, genitourinary, device, urinary, mechanical
　　fixation, internal (orthopedic) NEC — see Complication, fixation device, mechanical
　　gastrointestinal — see Complications, prosthetic device, mechanical, gastrointestinal device
　　genital NEC T83.418 ☑
　　　intrauterine contraceptive device T83.31 ☑
　　　penile prosthesis (cylinder) (implanted) (pump) (resevoir) T83.410 ☑
　　　testicular prosthesis T83.411 ☑
　　heart NEC — see Complication, cardiovascular device, mechanical
　　intrathecal infusion pump T85.615 ☑
　　joint prosthesis — see Complications..., joint prosthesis, internal, mechanical, by site
　　nervous system, specified device NEC T85.615 ☑
　　ocular NEC — see Complications, prosthetic device, mechanical, ocular device
　　orthopedic NEC — see Complication, orthopedic, device, mechanical
　　specified NEC T85.618 ☑

Breakdown — continued
　device, graft or implant (see also Complications, by site and type, mechanical) — continued
　　subcutaneous device pocket
　　　nervous system prosthetic device, implant, or graft T85.890 ☑
　　　other internal prosthetic device, implant, or graft T85.898 ☑
　　sutures, permanent T85.612 ☑
　　　used in bone repair — see Complications, fixation device, internal (orthopedic), mechanical
　　urinary NEC T83.118 ☑
　　　graft T83.21 ☑
　　　sphincter, implanted T83.111 ☑
　　　stent (ileal conduit) (nephroureteral) T83.113 ☑
　　　　ureteral indwelling T83.112 ☑
　　　vascular NEC — see Complication, cardiovascular device, mechanical
　　ventricular intracranial shunt T85.01 ☑
　nervous F48.8
　perineum O90.1
　respirator J95.850
　　specified NEC J95.859
　ventilator J95.850
　　specified NEC J95.859
Breast (see also condition)
　buds E30.1
　　in newborn P96.89
　dense R92.2
　nodule (see also Lump, breast) N63.0
Breath
　foul R19.6
　holder, child R06.89
　holding spell R06.89
　shortness R06.02
Breathing
　labored — see Hyperventilation
　mouth R06.5
　　causing malocclusion M26.5 ☑
　periodic R06.3
　　high altitude G47.32
Breathlessness R06.81
Breda's disease — see Yaws
Breech presentation (mother) O32.1 ☑
　causing obstructed labor O64.1 ☑
　footling O32.8 ☑
　　causing obstructed labor O64.8 ☑
　incomplete O32.8 ☑
　　causing obstructed labor O64.8 ☑
Breisky's disease N90.4
Brennemann's syndrome I88.0
Brenner
　tumor (benign) D27.9
　　borderline malignancy D39.1- ☑
　　malignant C56 ☑
　　proliferating D39.1- ☑
Bretonneau's disease or angina A36.0
Breus' mole O02.0
Brevicollis Q76.49
Brickmakers' anemia B76.9 [D63.8]
Bridge, myocardial Q24.5
Bright red blood per rectum (BRBPR) K62.5
Bright's disease (see also Nephritis)
　arteriosclerotic — see Hypertension, kidney
Brill (-Zinsser) **disease** (recrudescent typhus) A75.1
　flea-borne A75.2
　louse-borne A75.1
Brill-Symmers' disease C82.90
Brion-Kayser disease — see Fever, parathyroid
Briquet's disorder or syndrome F45.0
Brissaud's
　infantilism or dwarfism E23.0
　motor-verbal tic F95.2
Brittle
　bones disease Q78.0
　nails L60.3
　　congenital Q84.6
Broad (see also condition)
　beta disease E78.2
　ligament laceration syndrome N83.8
Broad- or floating-betalipoproteinemia E78.2
Brock's syndrome (atelectasis due to enlarged lymph nodes) J98.19
Brocq-Duhring disease (dermatitis herpetiformis) L13.0
Brodie's abscess or disease M86.8X- ☑

Broken
arches (see also Deformity, limb, flat foot)
arm (meaning upper limb) — see Fracture, arm
back — see Fracture, vertebra
bone — see Fracture
implant or internal device — see Complications, by site and type, mechanical
leg (meaning lower limb) — see Fracture, leg
nose S02.2 ☑
tooth, teeth — see Fracture, tooth
Bromhidrosis, bromidrosis L75.0
Bromidism, bromism G92
chronic (dependence) F13.20
due to
correct substance properly administered — see Table of Drugs and Chemicals, by drug, adverse effect
overdose or wrong substance given or taken — see Table of Drugs and Chemicals, by drug, poisoning
Bromidrosiphobia F40.298
Bronchi, bronchial — see condition
Bronchiectasis (cylindrical) (diffuse) (fusiform) (localized) (saccular) J47.9
with
acute
bronchitis J47.0
lower respiratory infection J47.0
exacerbation (acute) J47.1
congenital Q33.4
tuberculous NEC — see Tuberculosis, pulmonary
Bronchiolectasis — see Bronchiectasis
Bronchiolitis (acute) (infective) (subacute) J21.9
with
bronchospasm or obstruction J21.9
influenza, flu or grippe — see Influenza, with, respiratory manifestations NEC
chemical (chronic) J68.4
acute J68.0
chronic (fibrosing) (obliterative) J44.9
due to
external agent — see Bronchitis, acute, due to
human metapneumovirus J21.1
respiratory syncytial virus J21.0
specified organism NEC J21.8
fibrosa obliterans J44.9
influenzal — see Influenza, with, respiratory manifestations NEC
obliterans J42
with organizing pneumonia (BOOP) J84.89
obliterative (chronic) (subacute) J44.9
due to chemicals, gases, fumes or vapors (inhalation) J68.4
due to fumes or vapors J68.4
respiratory, interstitial lung disease J84.115
Bronchitis (diffuse) (fibrinous) (hypostatic) (infective) (membranous) J40
with
influenza, flu or grippe — see Influenza, with, respiratory manifestations NEC
obstruction (airway) (lung) J44.9
tracheitis (15 years of age and above) J40
acute or subacute J20.9
chronic J42
under 15 years of age J20.9
acute or subacute (with bronchospasm or obstruction) J20.9
with
bronchiectasis J47.0
chronic obstructive pulmonary disease J44.0
chemical (due to gases, fumes or vapors) J68.0
due to
fumes or vapors J68.0
Haemophilus influenzae J20.1
Mycoplasma pneumoniae J20.0
radiation J70.0
specified organism NEC J20.8
Streptococcus J20.2
virus
coxsackie J20.3
echovirus J20.7
parainfluenzae J20.4
respiratory syncytial J20.5
rhinovirus J20.6
viral NEC J20.8
allergic (acute) J45.909
with
exacerbation (acute) J45.901

Bronchitis — continued
allergic — continued
with — continued
status asthmaticus J45.902
arachidic T17.528 ☑
aspiration (due to fumes or vapors) J68.0
asthmatic J45.9 ☑
chronic J44.9
with
acute lower respiratory infection J44.0
exacerbation (acute) J44.1
capillary — see Pneumonia, broncho
caseous (tuberculous) A15.5
Castellani's A69.8
catarrhal (15 years of age and above) J40
acute — see Bronchitis, acute
chronic J41.0
under 15 years of age J20.9
chemical (acute) (subacute) J68.0
chronic J68.4
due to fumes or vapors J68.0
chronic J68.4
chronic J42
with
airways obstruction J44.9
tracheitis (chronic) J42
asthmatic (obstructive) J44.9
catarrhal J41.0
chemical (due to fumes or vapors) J68.4
due to
chemicals, gases, fumes or vapors (inhalation) J68.4
radiation J70.1
tobacco smoking J41.0
emphysematous J44.9
mucopurulent J41.1
non-obstructive J41.0
obliterans J44.9
obstructive J44.9
purulent J41.1
simple J41.0
croupous — see Bronchitis, acute
due to gases, fumes or vapors (chemical) J68.0
emphysematous (obstructive) J44.9
exudative — see Bronchitis, acute
fetid J41.1
grippal — see Influenza, with, respiratory manifestations NEC
in those under 15 years age — see Bronchitis, acute
chronic — see Bronchitis, chronic
influenzal — see Influenza, with, respiratory manifestations NEC
mixed simple and mucopurulent J41.8
moulder's J62.8
mucopurulent (chronic) (recurrent) J41.1
acute or subacute J20.9
simple (mixed) J41.8
obliterans (chronic) J44.9
obstructive (chronic) (diffuse) J44.9
pituitous J41.1
pneumococcal, acute or subacute J20.2
pseudomembranous, acute or subacute — see Bronchitis, acute
purulent (chronic) (recurrent) J41.1
acute or subacute — see Bronchitis, acute
putrid J41.1
senile (chronic) J42
simple and mucopurulent (mixed) J41.8
smokers' J41.0
spirochetal NEC A69.8
subacute — see Bronchitis, acute
suppurative (chronic) J41.1
acute or subacute — see Bronchitis, acute
tuberculous A15.5
under 15 years of age — see Bronchitis, acute
chronic — see Bronchitis, chronic
viral NEC, acute or subacute (see also Bronchitis, acute) J20.8
Bronchoalveolitis J18.0
Bronchoaspergillosis B44.1
Bronchocele meaning goiter E04.0
Broncholithiasis J98.09
tuberculous NEC A15.5
Bronchomalacia J98.09
congenital Q32.2
Bronchomycosis NOS B49 [J99]
candidal B37.1
Bronchopleuropneumonia — see Pneumonia, broncho

Bronchopneumonia — see Pneumonia, broncho
Bronchopneumonitis — see Pneumonia, broncho
Bronchopulmonary — see condition
Bronchopulmonitis — see Pneumonia, broncho
Bronchorrhagia (see Hemoptysis)
Bronchorrhea J98.09
acute J20.9
chronic (infective) (purulent) J42
Bronchospasm (acute) J98.01
with
bronchiolitis, acute J21.9
bronchitis, acute (conditions in J20) — see Bronchitis, acute
due to external agent — see condition, respiratory, acute, due to
exercise induced J45.990
Bronchospirochetosis A69.8
Castellani A69.8
Bronchostenosis J98.09
Bronchus — see condition
Brontophobia F40.220
Bronze baby syndrome P83.88
Brooke's tumor — see Neoplasm, skin, benign
Brown enamel of teeth (hereditary) K00.5
Brown's sheath syndrome H50.61- ☑
Brown-Séquard disease, paralysis or syndrome G83.81
Bruce sepsis A23.0
Brucellosis (infection) A23.9
abortus A23.1
canis A23.3
dermatitis A23.9
melitensis A23.0
mixed A23.8
sepsis A23.9
melitensis A23.0
specified NEC A23.8
suis A23.2
Bruck-de Lange disease Q87.1
Bruck's disease — see Deformity, limb
BRUE (brief resolved unexplained event) R68.13
Brugsch's syndrome Q82.8
Bruise (skin surface intact) (see also Contusion)
with
open wound — see Wound, open
internal organ — see Injury, by site
newborn P54.5
scalp, due to birth injury, newborn P12.3
umbilical cord O69.5 ☑
Bruit (arterial) R09.89
cardiac R01.1
Brush burn — see Abrasion, by site
Bruton's X-linked agammaglobulinemia D80.0
Bruxism
psychogenic F45.8
sleep related G47.63
Bubbly lung syndrome P27.0
Bubo I88.8
blennorrhagic (gonococcal) A54.89
chancroidal A57
climatic A55
due to Haemophilus ducreyi A57
gonococcal A54.89
indolent (nonspecific) I88.8
inguinal (nonspecific) I88.8
chancroidal A57
climatic A55
due to H. ducreyi A57
infective I88.8
scrofulous (tuberculous) A18.2
soft chancre A57
suppurating — see Lymphadenitis, acute
syphilitic (primary) A51.0
congenital A50.07
tropical A55
virulent (chancroidal) A57
Bubonic plague A20.0
Bubonocele — see Hernia, inguinal
Buccal — see condition
Buchanan's disease or osteochondrosis M91.0
Buchem's syndrome (hyperostosis corticalis) M85.2
Bucket-handle fracture or tear (semilunar cartilage) — see Tear, meniscus
Budd-Chiari syndrome (hepatic vein thrombosis) I82.0
Budgerigar fancier's disease or lung J67.2
Buds
breast E30.1

☑ Additional Character Required — Refer to the Tabular List for Character Selection ▽ Subterms under main terms may continue to next column or page

Buds — *continued*
  breast — *continued*
    in newborn P96.89
Buerger's disease (thromboangiitis obliterans) I73.1
Bulbar — *see* condition
Bulbus cordis (left ventricle) (persistent) Q21.8
Bulimia (nervosa) F50.2
  atypical F50.9
  normal weight F50.9
Bulky
  stools R19.5
  uterus N85.2
Bulla (e) R23.8
  lung (emphysematous) (solitary) J43.9
    newborn P25.8
Bullet wound (*see also* Wound, open)
  fracture — *code as* Fracture, by site
  internal organ — *see* Injury, by site
Bundle
  branch block (complete) (false) (incomplete) — *see*
    Block, bundle-branch
  of His — *see* condition
Bunion M21.61- ☑
  tailor's M21.62- ☑
Bunionette M21.62- ☑
Buphthalmia, buphthalmos (congenital) Q15.0
Burdwan fever B55.0
Bürger-Grütz disease or syndrome E78.3
Buried
  penis (congenital) Q55.64
    acquired N48.83
  roots K08.3
Burke's syndrome K86.89
Burkitt
  cell leukemia C91.0- ☑
  lymphoma (malignant) C83.7- ☑
    small noncleaved, diffuse C83.7- ☑
    spleen C83.77
    undifferentiated C83.7- ☑
  tumor C83.7- ☑
  type
    acute lymphoblastic leukemia C91.0- ☑
    undifferentiated C83.7- ☑
Burn (electricity) (flame) (hot gas, liquid or hot object) (radiation) (steam) (thermal) T30.0
  abdomen, abdominal (muscle) (wall) T21.02 ☑
    first degree T21.12 ☑
    second degree T21.22 ☑
    third degree T21.32 ☑
  above elbow T22.039 ☑
    first degree T22.139 ☑
    left T22.032 ☑
      first degree T22.132 ☑
      second degree T22.232 ☑
      third degree T22.332 ☑
    right T22.031 ☑
      first degree T22.131 ☑
      second degree T22.231 ☑
      third degree T22.331 ☑
    second degree T22.239 ☑
    third degree T22.339 ☑
  acid (caustic) (external) (internal) — *see* Corrosion, by site
  alimentary tract NEC T28.2 ☑
    esophagus T28.1 ☑
    mouth T28.0 ☑
    pharynx T28.0 ☑
  alkaline (caustic) (external) (internal) — *see* Corrosion, by site
  ankle T25.019 ☑
    first degree T25.119 ☑
    left T25.012 ☑
      first degree T25.112 ☑
      second degree T25.212 ☑
      third degree T25.312 ☑
    multiple with foot — *see* Burn, lower, limb, multiple, ankle and foot
    right T25.011 ☑
      first degree T25.111 ☑
      second degree T25.211 ☑
      third degree T25.311 ☑
    second degree T25.219 ☑
    third degree T25.319 ☑
  anus — *see* Burn, buttock
  arm (lower) (upper) — *see* Burn, upper, limb
  axilla T22.049 ☑

Burn — *continued*
  axilla — *continued*
    first degree T22.149 ☑
    left T22.042 ☑
      first degree T22.142 ☑
      second degree T22.242 ☑
      third degree T22.342 ☑
    right T22.041 ☑
      first degree T22.141 ☑
      second degree T22.241 ☑
      third degree T22.341 ☑
    second degree T22.249 ☑
    third degree T22.349 ☑
  back (lower) T21.04 ☑
    first degree T21.14 ☑
    second degree T21.24 ☑
    third degree T21.34 ☑
    upper T21.03 ☑
      first degree T21.13 ☑
      second degree T21.23 ☑
      third degree T21.33 ☑
  blisters — *code as* Burn, second degree, by site
  breast(s) — *see* Burn, chest wall
  buttock(s) T21.05 ☑
    first degree T21.15 ☑
    second degree T21.25 ☑
    third degree T21.35 ☑
  calf T24.039 ☑
    first degree T24.139 ☑
    left T24.032 ☑
      first degree T24.132 ☑
      second degree T24.232 ☑
      third degree T24.332 ☑
    right T24.031 ☑
      first degree T24.131 ☑
      second degree T24.231 ☑
      third degree T24.331 ☑
    second degree T24.239 ☑
    third degree T24.339 ☑
  canthus (eye) — *see* Burn, eyelid
  caustic acid or alkaline — *see* Corrosion, by site
  cervix T28.3 ☑
  cheek T20.06 ☑
    first degree T20.16 ☑
    second degree T20.26 ☑
    third degree T20.36 ☑
  chemical (acids) (alkalines) (caustics) (external) (internal) — *see* Corrosion, by site
  chest wall T21.01 ☑
    first degree T21.11 ☑
    second degree T21.21 ☑
    third degree T21.31 ☑
  chin T20.03 ☑
    first degree T20.13 ☑
    second degree T20.23 ☑
    third degree T20.33 ☑
  colon T28.2 ☑
  conjunctiva (and cornea) — *see* Burn, cornea
  cornea (and conjunctiva) T26.1- ☑
    chemical — *see* Corrosion, cornea
  corrosion (external) (internal) — *see* Corrosion, by site
  deep necrosis of underlying tissue — *code as* Burn, third degree, by site
  dorsum of hand T23.069 ☑
    first degree T23.169 ☑
    left T23.062 ☑
      first degree T23.162 ☑
      second degree T23.262 ☑
      third degree T23.362 ☑
    right T23.061 ☑
      first degree T23.161 ☑
      second degree T23.261 ☑
      third degree T23.361 ☑
    second degree T23.269 ☑
    third degree T23.369 ☑
  due to ingested chemical agent — *see* Corrosion, by site
  ear (auricle) (external) (canal) T20.01 ☑
    first degree T20.11 ☑
    second degree T20.21 ☑
    third degree T20.31 ☑
  elbow T22.029 ☑
    first degree T22.129 ☑
    left T22.022 ☑
      first degree T22.122 ☑
      second degree T22.222 ☑

Burn — *continued*
  elbow — *continued*
    left — *continued*
      third degree T22.322 ☑
    right T22.021 ☑
      first degree T22.121 ☑
      second degree T22.221 ☑
      third degree T22.321 ☑
    second degree T22.229 ☑
    third degree T22.329 ☑
  epidermal loss — *code as* Burn, second degree, by site
  erythema, erythematous — *code as* Burn, first degree, by site
  esophagus T28.1 ☑
  extent (percentage of body surface)
    less than 10 percent T31.0
    10-19 percent T31.10
      with 0-9 percent third degree burns T31.10
      with 10-19 percent third degree burns T31.11
    20-29 percent T31.20
      with 0-9 percent third degree burns T31.20
      with 10-19 percent third degree burns T31.21
      with 20-29 percent third degree burns T31.22
    30-39 percent T31.30
      with 0-9 percent third degree burns T31.30
      with 10-19 percent third degree burns T31.31
      with 20-29 percent third degree burns T31.32
      with 30-39 percent third degree burns T31.33
    40-49 percent T31.40
      with 0-9 percent third degree burns T31.40
      with 10-19 percent third degree burns T31.41
      with 20-29 percent third degree burns T31.42
      with 30-39 percent third degree burns T31.43
      with 40-49 percent third degree burns T31.44
    50-59 percent T31.50
      with 0-9 percent third degree burns T31.50
      with 10-19 percent third degree burns T31.51
      with 20-29 percent third degree burns T31.52
      with 30-39 percent third degree burns T31.53
      with 40-49 percent third degree burns T31.54
      with 50-59 percent third degree burns T31.55
    60-69 percent T31.60
      with 0-9 percent third degree burns T31.60
      with 10-19 percent third degree burns T31.61
      with 20-29 percent third degree burns T31.62
      with 30-39 percent third degree burns T31.63
      with 40-49 percent third degree burns T31.64
      with 50-59 percent third degree burns T31.65
      with 60-69 percent third degree burns T31.66
    70-79 percent T31.70
      with 0-9 percent third degree burns T31.70
      with 10-19 percent third degree burns T31.71
      with 20-29 percent third degree burns T31.72
      with 30-39 percent third degree burns T31.73
      with 40-49 percent third degree burns T31.74
      with 50-59 percent third degree burns T31.75
      with 60-69 percent third degree burns T31.76
      with 70-79 percent third degree burns T31.77
    80-89 percent T31.80
      with 0-9 percent third degree burns T31.80
      with 10-19 percent third degree burns T31.81
      with 20-29 percent third degree burns T31.82
      with 30-39 percent third degree burns T31.83
      with 40-49 percent third degree burns T31.84
      with 50-59 percent third degree burns T31.85
      with 60-69 percent third degree burns T31.86
      with 70-79 percent third degree burns T31.87
      with 80-89 percent third degree burns T31.88
    90 percent or more T31.90
      with 0-9 percent third degree burns T31.90
      with 10-19 percent third degree burns T31.91
      with 20-29 percent third degree burns T31.92
      with 30-39 percent third degree burns T31.93
      with 40-49 percent third degree burns T31.94
      with 50-59 percent third degree burns T31.95
      with 60-69 percent third degree burns T31.96
      with 70-79 percent third degree burns T31.97
      with 80-89 percent third degree burns T31.98
      with 90 percent or more third degree burns T31.99
  extremity — *see* Burn, limb
  eye(s) and adnexa T26.4- ☑
    with resulting rupture and destruction of eyeball T26.2- ☑
    conjunctival sac — *see* Burn, cornea
    cornea — *see* Burn, cornea
    lid — *see* Burn, eyelid
    periocular area — *see* Burn, eyelid

Burn — *continued*
  eye(s) and adnexa — *continued*
    specified site NEC T26.3- ☑
  eyeball — *see* Burn, eye
  eyelid(s) T26.0- ☑
    chemical — *see* Corrosion, eyelid
  face — *see* Burn, head
  finger T23.029 ☑
    first degree T23.129 ☑
    left T23.022 ☑
      first degree T23.122 ☑
      second degree T23.222 ☑
      third degree T23.322 ☑
    multiple sites (without thumb) T23.039 ☑
      with thumb T23.049 ☑
        first degree T23.149 ☑
        left T23.042 ☑
          first degree T23.142 ☑
          second degree T23.242 ☑
          third degree T23.342 ☑
        right T23.041 ☑
          first degree T23.141 ☑
          second degree T23.241 ☑
          third degree T23.341 ☑
      second degree T23.249 ☑
      third degree T23.349 ☑
    first degree T23.139 ☑
    left T23.032 ☑
      first degree T23.132 ☑
      second degree T23.232 ☑
      third degree T23.332 ☑
    right T23.031 ☑
      first degree T23.131 ☑
      second degree T23.231 ☑
      third degree T23.331 ☑
    second degree T23.239 ☑
    third degree T23.339 ☑
    right T23.021 ☑
      first degree T23.121 ☑
      second degree T23.221 ☑
      third degree T23.321 ☑
    second degree T23.229 ☑
    third degree T23.329 ☑
  flank — *see* Burn, abdominal wall
  foot T25.029 ☑
    first degree T25.129 ☑
    left T25.022 ☑
      first degree T25.122 ☑
      second degree T25.222 ☑
      third degree T25.322 ☑
    multiple with ankle — *see* Burn, lower, limb, multiple, ankle and foot
    right T25.021 ☑
      first degree T25.121 ☑
      second degree T25.221 ☑
      third degree T25.321 ☑
    second degree T25.229 ☑
    third degree T25.329 ☑
  forearm T22.019 ☑
    first degree T22.119 ☑
    left T22.012 ☑
      first degree T22.112 ☑
      second degree T22.212 ☑
      third degree T22.312 ☑
    right T22.011 ☑
      first degree T22.111 ☑
      second degree T22.211 ☑
      third degree T22.311 ☑
    second degree T22.219 ☑
    third degree T22.319 ☑
  forehead T20.06 ☑
    first degree T20.16 ☑
    second degree T20.26 ☑
    third degree T20.36 ☑
  fourth degree — *code as* Burn, third degree, by site
  friction — *see* Burn, by site
  from swallowing caustic or corrosive substance NEC — *see* Corrosion, by site
  full thickness skin loss — *code as* Burn, third degree, by site
  gastrointestinal tract NEC T28.2 ☑
    from swallowing caustic or corrosive substance T28.7 ☑
  genital organs
    external
      female T21.07 ☑

Burn — *continued*
  genital organs — *continued*
    external — *continued*
      female — *continued*
        first degree T21.17 ☑
        second degree T21.27 ☑
        third degree T21.37 ☑
      male T21.06 ☑
        first degree T21.16 ☑
        second degree T21.26 ☑
        third degree T21.36 ☑
    internal T28.3 ☑
      from caustic or corrosive substance T28.8 ☑
  groin — *see* Burn, abdominal wall
  hand(s) T23.009 ☑
    back — *see* Burn, dorsum of hand
    finger — *see* Burn, finger
    first degree T23.109 ☑
    left T23.002 ☑
      first degree T23.102 ☑
      second degree T23.202 ☑
      third degree T23.302 ☑
    multiple sites with wrist T23.099 ☑
      first degree T23.199 ☑
      left T23.092 ☑
        first degree T23.192 ☑
        second degree T23.292 ☑
        third degree T23.392 ☑
      right T23.091 ☑
        first degree T23.191 ☑
        second degree T23.291 ☑
        third degree T23.391 ☑
      second degree T23.299 ☑
      third degree T23.399 ☑
    palm — *see* Burn, palm
    right T23.001 ☑
      first degree T23.101 ☑
      second degree T23.201 ☑
      third degree T23.301 ☑
    second degree T23.209 ☑
    third degree T23.309 ☑
    thumb — *see* Burn, thumb
  head (and face) (and neck) T20.00 ☑
    cheek — *see* Burn, cheek
    chin — *see* Burn, chin
    ear — *see* Burn, ear
    eye(s) only — *see* Burn, eye
    first degree T20.10 ☑
    forehead — *see* Burn, forehead
    lip — *see* Burn, lip
    multiple sites T20.09 ☑
      first degree T20.19 ☑
      second degree T20.29 ☑
      third degree T20.39 ☑
    neck — *see* Burn, neck
    nose — *see* Burn, nose
    scalp — *see* Burn, scalp
    second degree T20.20 ☑
    third degree T20.30 ☑
  hip(s) — *see* Burn, thigh
  inhalation — *see* Burn, respiratory tract
    caustic or corrosive substance (fumes) — *see* Corrosion, respiratory tract
  internal organ(s) T28.40 ☑
    alimentary tract T28.2 ☑
      esophagus T28.1 ☑
    eardrum T28.41 ☑
    esophagus T28.1 ☑
    from caustic or corrosive substance (swallowing) NEC — *see* Corrosion, by site
    genitourinary T28.3 ☑
    mouth T28.0 ☑
    pharynx T28.0 ☑
    respiratory tract — *see* Burn, respiratory tract
    specified organ NEC T28.49 ☑
  interscapular region — *see* Burn, back, upper
  intestine (large) (small) T28.2 ☑
  knee T24.029 ☑
    first degree T24.129 ☑
    left T24.022 ☑
      first degree T24.122 ☑
      second degree T24.222 ☑
      third degree T24.322 ☑
    right T24.021 ☑
      first degree T24.121 ☑
      second degree T24.221 ☑

Burn — *continued*
  knee — *continued*
    right — *continued*
      third degree T24.321 ☑
    second degree T24.229 ☑
    third degree T24.329 ☑
  labium (majus) (minus) — *see* Burn, genital organs, external, female
  lacrimal apparatus, duct, gland or sac — *see* Burn, eye, specified site NEC
  larynx T27.0 ☑
    with lung T27.1 ☑
  leg(s) (lower) (upper) — *see* Burn, lower, limb
  lightning — *see* Burn, by site
  limb(s)
    lower (except ankle or foot alone) — *see* Burn, lower, limb
    upper — *see* Burn, upper limb
  lip(s) T20.02 ☑
    first degree T20.12 ☑
    second degree T20.22 ☑
    third degree T20.32 ☑
  lower
    back — *see* Burn, back
    limb T24.009 ☑
      ankle — *see* Burn, ankle
      calf — *see* Burn, calf
      first degree T24.109 ☑
      foot — *see* Burn, foot
      hip — *see* Burn, thigh
      knee — *see* Burn, knee
      left T24.002 ☑
        first degree T24.102 ☑
        second degree T24.202 ☑
        third degree T24.302 ☑
      multiple sites, except ankle and foot T24.099 ☑
        ankle and foot T25.099 ☑
          first degree T25.199 ☑
          left T25.092 ☑
            first degree T25.192 ☑
            second degree T25.292 ☑
            third degree T25.392 ☑
          right T25.091 ☑
            first degree T25.191 ☑
            second degree T25.291 ☑
            third degree T25.391 ☑
          second degree T25.299 ☑
          third degree T25.399 ☑
        first degree T24.199 ☑
        left T24.092 ☑
          first degree T24.192 ☑
          second degree T24.292 ☑
          third degree T24.392 ☑
        right T24.091 ☑
          first degree T24.191 ☑
          second degree T24.291 ☑
          third degree T24.391 ☑
        second degree T24.299 ☑
        third degree T24.399 ☑
      right T24.001 ☑
        first degree T24.101 ☑
        second degree T24.201 ☑
        third degree T24.301 ☑
      second degree T24.209 ☑
      thigh — *see* Burn, thigh
      third degree T24.309 ☑
      toe — *see* Burn, toe
  lung (with larynx and trachea) T27.1 ☑
  mouth T28.0 ☑
  neck T20.07 ☑
    first degree T20.17 ☑
    second degree T20.27 ☑
    third degree T20.37 ☑
  nose (septum) T20.04 ☑
    first degree T20.14 ☑
    second degree T20.24 ☑
    third degree T20.34 ☑
  ocular adnexa — *see* Burn, eye
  orbit region — *see* Burn, eyelid
  palm T23.059 ☑
    first degree T23.159 ☑
    left T23.052 ☑
      first degree T23.152 ☑
      second degree T23.252 ☑
      third degree T23.352 ☑
    right T23.051 ☑

☑ **Additional Character Required — Refer to the Tabular List for Character Selection**   ▽ **Subterms under main terms may continue to next column or page**

Burn — *continued*
  wrist — *continued*
    multiple sites with hand — *continued*
      right — *continued*
        second degree T23.291 ☑
         third degree T23.391 ☑
      second degree T23.299 ☑
      third degree T23.399 ☑
    right T23.071 ☑
      first degree T23.171 ☑
      second degree T23.271 ☑
      third degree T23.371 ☑
    second degree T23.279 ☑
    third degree T23.379 ☑
Burnett's syndrome E83.52
Burning
  feet syndrome E53.9
  sensation R20.8
  tongue K14.6
Burn-out (state) Z73.0
Burns' disease or osteochondrosis — *see* Osteochondrosis, juvenile, ulna
Bursa — *see* condition
Bursitis M71.9
  Achilles — *see* Tendinitis, Achilles
  adhesive — *see* Bursitis, specified NEC
  ankle — *see* Enthesopathy, lower limb, ankle, specified type NEC
  calcaneal — *see* Enthesopathy, foot, specified type NEC
  collateral ligament, tibial — *see* Bursitis, tibial collateral
  due to use, overuse, pressure (*see also* Disorder, soft tissue, due to use, specified type NEC)
    specified NEC — *see* Disorder, soft tissue, due to use, specified NEC
  Duplay's M75.0 ☑
  elbow NEC M70.3- ☑
    olecranon M70.2- ☑
  finger — *see* Disorder, soft tissue, due to use, specified type NEC, hand
  foot — *see* Enthesopathy, foot, specified type NEC
  gonococcal A54.49
  gouty — *see* Gout
  hand M70.1- ☑
  hip NEC M70.7- ☑
    trochanteric M70.6- ☑
  infective NEC M71.10
    abscess — *see* Abscess, bursa
    ankle M71.17- ☑
    elbow M71.12- ☑
    foot M71.17- ☑
    hand M71.14- ☑
    hip M71.15- ☑
    knee M71.16- ☑
    multiple sites M71.19
    shoulder M71.11- ☑
    specified site NEC M71.18
    wrist M71.13- ☑
  ischial — *see* Bursitis, hip
  knee NEC M70.5- ☑
    prepatellar M70.4- ☑
  occupational NEC (*see also* Disorder, soft tissue, due to, use)
  olecranon — *see* Bursitis, elbow, olecranon
  pharyngeal J39.1
  popliteal — *see* Bursitis, knee
  prepatellar M70.4- ☑
  radiohumeral M77.8
  rheumatoid M06.20
    ankle M06.27- ☑
    elbow M06.22- ☑
    foot joint M06.27- ☑
    hand joint M06.24- ☑
    hip M06.25- ☑
    knee M06.26- ☑
    multiple site M06.29
    shoulder M06.21- ☑
    vertebra M06.28
    wrist M06.23- ☑
  scapulohumeral — *see* Bursitis, shoulder
  semimembranous muscle (knee) — *see* Bursitis, knee
  shoulder M75.5- ☑
    adhesive — *see* Capsulitis, adhesive
  specified NEC M71.50
    ankle M71.57- ☑

Bursitis — *continued*
  specified — *continued*
    due to use, overuse or pressure — *see* Disorder, soft tissue, due to, use
    elbow M71.52- ☑
    foot M71.57- ☑
    hand M71.54- ☑
    hip M71.55- ☑
    knee M71.56- ☑
    shoulder — *see* Bursitis, shoulder
    specified site NEC M71.58
    tibial collateral M76.4- ☑
    wrist M71.53- ☑
  subacromial — *see* Bursitis, shoulder
  subcoracoid — *see* Bursitis, shoulder
  subdeltoid — *see* Bursitis, shoulder
  syphilitic A52.78
  Thornwaldt, Tornwaldt J39.2
  tibial collateral M76.4- ☑
  toe — *see* Enthesopathy, foot, specified type NEC
  trochanteric (area) — *see* Bursitis, hip, trochanteric
  wrist — *see* Bursitis, hand
Bursopathy M71.9
  specified type NEC M71.80
    ankle M71.87- ☑
    elbow M71.82- ☑
    foot M71.87- ☑
    hand M71.84- ☑
    hip M71.85- ☑
    knee M71.86- ☑
    multiple sites M71.89
    shoulder M71.81- ☑
    specified site NEC M71.88
    wrist M71.83- ☑
Burst stitches or sutures (complication of surgery) T81.31
  external operation wound T81.31
  internal operation wound T81.32
Buruli ulcer A31.1
Bury's disease L95.1
Buschke's
  disease B45.3
  scleredema — *see* Sclerosis, systemic
Busse-Buschke disease B45.3
Buttock — *see* condition
Button
  Biskra B55.1
  Delhi B55.1
  oriental B55.1
Buttonhole deformity (finger) — *see* Deformity, finger, boutonniere
Bwamba fever A92.8
Byssinosis J66.0
Bywaters' syndrome T79.5 ☑

C

Cachexia R64
  cancerous R64
  cardiac — *see* Disease, heart
  dehydration E86.0
  due to malnutrition R64
  exophthalmic — *see* Hyperthyroidism
  heart — *see* Disease, heart
  hypophyseal E23.0
  hypopituitary E23.0
  lead — *see* Poisoning, lead
  malignant R64
  marsh — *see* Malaria
  nervous F48.8
  old age R54
  paludal — *see* Malaria
  pituitary E23.0
  renal N28.9
  saturnine — *see* Poisoning, lead
  senile R54
  Simmonds' E23.0
  splenica D73.0
  strumipriva E03.4
  tuberculous NEC — *see* Tuberculosis
Café, au lait spots L81.3
Caffeine-induced
  anxiety disorder F15.980
  sleep disorder F15.982
Caffey's syndrome Q78.8
Caisson disease T70.3 ☑
Cake kidney Q63.1

Caked breast (puerperal, postpartum) O92.79
Calabar swelling B74.3
Calcaneal spur — *see* Spur, bone, calcaneal
Calcaneo-apophysitis M92.8
Calcareous — *see* condition
Calcicosis J62.8
Calciferol (vitamin D) deficiency E55.9
  with rickets E55.0
Calcification
  adrenal (capsule) (gland) E27.49
    tuberculous E35 [B90.8]
  aorta I70.0
  artery (annular) — *see* Arteriosclerosis
  auricle (ear) — *see* Disorder, pinna, specified type NEC
  basal ganglia G23.8
  bladder N32.89
    due to Schistosoma hematobium B65.0
  brain (cortex) — *see* Calcification, cerebral
  bronchus J98.09
  bursa M71.40
    ankle M71.47- ☑
    elbow M71.42- ☑
    foot M71.47- ☑
    hand M71.44- ☑
    hip M71.45- ☑
    knee M71.46- ☑
    multiple sites M71.49
    shoulder M75.3- ☑
    specified site NEC M71.48
    wrist M71.43- ☑
  cardiac — *see* Degeneration, myocardial
  cerebral (cortex) G93.89
    artery I67.2
  cervix (uteri) N88.8
  choroid plexus G93.89
  conjunctiva — *see* Concretion, conjunctiva
  corpora cavernosa (penis) N48.89
  cortex (brain) — *see* Calcification, cerebral
  dental pulp (nodular) K04.2
  dentinal papilla K00.4
  fallopian tube N83.8
  falx cerebri G96.19
  gallbladder K82.8
  general E83.59
  heart (*see also* Degeneration, myocardial)
    valve — *see* Endocarditis
  idiopathic infantile arterial (IIAC) Q28.8
  intervertebral cartilage or disc (postinfective) — *see* Disorder, disc, specified NEC
  intracranial — *see* Calcification, cerebral
  joint — *see* Disorder, joint, specified type NEC
  kidney N28.89
    tuberculous N29 [B90.1]
  larynx (senile) J38.7
  lens — *see* Cataract, specified NEC
  lung (active) (postinfectional) J98.4
    tuberculous B90.9
  lymph gland or node (postinfectional) I89.8
    tuberculous (*see also* Tuberculosis, lymph gland) B90.8
  mammographic R92.1
  massive (paraplegic) — *see* Myositis, ossificans, in, quadriplegia
  medial — *see* Arteriosclerosis, extremities
  meninges (cerebral) (spinal) G96.19
  metastatic E83.59
  Mönckeberg's — *see* Arteriosclerosis, extremities
  muscle M61.9
    due to burns — *see* Myositis, ossificans, in, burns
    paralytic — *see* Myositis, ossificans, in, quadriplegia
    specified type NEC M61.40
      ankle M61.47- ☑
      foot M61.47- ☑
      forearm M61.43- ☑
      hand M61.44- ☑
      lower leg M61.46- ☑
      multiple sites M61.49
      pelvic region M61.45- ☑
      shoulder region M61.41- ☑
      specified site NEC M61.48
      thigh M61.45- ☑
      upper arm M61.42- ☑
  myocardium, myocardial — *see* Degeneration, myocardial
  ovary N83.8
  pancreas K86.89
  penis N48.89

☑ **Additional Character Required** — **Refer to the Tabular List for Character Selection**   ▽ **Subterms under main terms may continue to next column or page**

Calcification — *continued*
  periarticular — *see* Disorder, joint, specified type NEC
  pericardium (*see also* Pericarditis) I31.1
  pineal gland E34.8
  pleura J94.8
    postinfectional J94.8
    tuberculous NEC B90.9
  pulpal (dental) (nodular) K04.2
  sclera H15.89
  spleen D73.89
  subcutaneous L94.2
  suprarenal (capsule) (gland) E27.49
  tendon (sheath) (*see also* Tenosynovitis, specified type NEC)
    with bursitis, synovitis or tenosynovitis — *see* Tendinitis, calcific
  trachea J39.8
  ureter N28.89
  uterus N85.8
  vitreous — *see* Deposit, crystalline
Calcified — *see* Calcification
Calcinosis (interstitial) (tumoral) (universalis) E83.59
  with Raynaud's phenomenon, esophageal dysfunction, sclerodactyly, telangiectasia (CREST syndrome) M34.1
  circumscripta (skin) L94.2
  cutis L94.2
Calciphylaxis (*see also* Calcification, by site) E83.59
Calcium
  deposits — *see* Calcification, by site
  metabolism disorder E83.50
  salts or soaps in vitreous — *see* Deposit, crystalline
Calciuria R82.99
Calculi — *see* Calculus
Calculosis, intrahepatic — *see* Calculus, bile duct
Calculus, calculi, calculous
  ampulla of Vater — *see* Calculus, bile duct
  anuria (impacted) (recurrent) (*see also* Calculus, urinary) N20.9
  appendix K38.1
  bile duct (common) (hepatic) K80.50
    with
      calculus of gallbladder — *see* Calculus, gallbladder and bile duct
      cholangitis K80.30
        with
          cholecystitis — *see* Calculus, bile duct, with cholecystitis
          obstruction K80.31
        acute K80.32
          with
            chronic cholangitis K80.36
              with obstruction K80.37
            obstruction K80.33
        chronic K80.34
          with
            acute cholangitis K80.36
              with obstruction K80.37
            obstruction K80.35
      cholecystitis (with cholangitis) K80.40
        with obstruction K80.41
        acute K80.42
          with
            chronic cholecystitis K80.46
              with obstruction K80.47
            obstruction K80.43
        chronic K80.44
          with
            acute cholecystitis K80.46
              with obstruction K80.47
            obstruction K80.45
  biliary (*see also* Calculus, gallbladder)
    specified NEC K80.80
      with obstruction K80.81
  bilirubin, multiple — *see* Calculus, gallbladder
  bladder (encysted) (impacted) (urinary) (diverticulum) N21.0
  bronchus J98.09
  calyx (kidney) (renal) — *see* Calculus, kidney
  cholesterol (pure) (solitary) — *see* Calculus, gallbladder
  common duct (bile) — *see* Calculus, bile duct
  conjunctiva — *see* Concretion, conjunctiva
  cystic N21.0
    duct — *see* Calculus, gallbladder
  dental (subgingival) (supragingival) K03.6
  diverticulum
    bladder N21.0
    kidney N20.0

Calculus, calculi, calculous — *continued*
  epididymis N50.89
  gallbladder K80.20
    with
      bile duct calculus — *see* Calculus, gallbladder and bile duct
      cholecystitis K80.10
        with obstruction K80.11
        acute K80.00
          with
            chronic cholecystitis K80.12
              with obstruction K80.13
            obstruction K80.01
        chronic K80.10
          with
            acute cholecystitis K80.12
              with obstruction K80.13
            obstruction K80.11
        specified NEC K80.18
          with obstruction K80.19
      obstruction K80.21
  gallbladder and bile duct K80.70
    with
      cholecystitis K80.60
        with obstruction K80.61
        acute K80.62
          with
            chronic cholecystitis K80.66
              with obstruction K80.67
            obstruction K80.63
        chronic K80.64
          with
            acute cholecystitis K80.66
              with obstruction K80.67
            obstruction K80.65
      obstruction K80.71
  hepatic (duct) — *see* Calculus, bile duct
  ileal conduit N21.8
  intestinal (impaction) (obstruction) K56.49
  kidney (impacted) (multiple) (pelvis) (recurrent) (staghorn) N20.0
    with calculus, ureter N20.2
    congenital Q63.8
  lacrimal passages — *see* Dacryolith
  liver (impacted) — *see* Calculus, bile duct
  lung J98.4
  mammographic R92.1
  nephritic (impacted) (recurrent) — *see* Calculus, kidney
  nose J34.89
  pancreas (duct) K86.89
  parotid duct or gland K11.5
  pelvis, encysted — *see* Calculus, kidney
  prostate N42.0
  pulmonary J98.4
  pyelitis (impacted) (recurrent) N20.0
    with hydronephrosis N13.2
  pyelonephritis (impacted) (recurrent) N20 ☑
    with hydronephrosis N13.2
  renal (impacted) (recurrent) — *see* Calculus, kidney
  salivary (duct) (gland) K11.5
  seminal vesicle N50.89
  staghorn — *see* Calculus, kidney
  Stensen's duct K11.5
  stomach K31.89
  sublingual duct or gland K11.5
    congenital Q38.4
  submandibular duct, gland or region K11.5
  submaxillary duct, gland or region K11.5
  suburethral N21.8
  tonsil J35.8
  tooth, teeth (subgingival) (supragingival) K03.6
  tunica vaginalis N50.89
  ureter (impacted) (recurrent) N20.1
    with calculus, kidney N20.2
      with hydronephrosis N13.2
        with infection N13.6
  urethra (impacted) N21.1
  urinary (duct) (impacted) (passage) (tract) N20.9
    with hydronephrosis N13.2
      with infection N13.6
    in (due to)
      lower N21.9
        specified NEC N21.8
  vagina N89.8
  vesical (impacted) N21.0
  Wharton's duct K11.5
  xanthine E79.8 [N22]
Caliectasis N28.89

Caliectasis N28.89
California
  disease B38.9
  encephalitis A83.5
Caligo cornea — *see* Opacity, cornea, central
Callositas, callosity (infected) L84
Callus (infected) L84
  bone — *see* Osteophyte
    excessive, following fracture — *code as* Sequelae of fracture
CALME (childhood asymmetric labium majus enlargement) N90.61
Calorie deficiency or malnutrition (*see also* Malnutrition) E46
Calvé-Perthes disease — *see* Legg-Calvé-Perthes disease
Calvé's disease — *see* Osteochondrosis, juvenile, spine
Calvities — *see* Alopecia, androgenic
Cameroon fever — *see* Malaria
Camptocormia (hysterical) F44.4
Camurati-Engelmann syndrome Q78.3
Canal (*see also* condition)
  atrioventricular common Q21.2
Canaliculitis (lacrimal) (acute) (subacute) H04.33- ☑
  Actinomyces A42.89
  chronic H04.42- ☑
Canavan's disease E75.29
Canceled procedure (surgical) Z53.9
  because of
    contraindication Z53.09
      smoking Z53.01
    left against medical advice (AMA) Z53.21
    patient's decision Z53.20
      for reasons of belief or group pressure Z53.1
        specified reason NEC Z53.29
    specified reason NEC Z53.8
Cancer (*see also* Neoplasm, by site, malignant)
  bile duct type liver C22.1
  blood — *see* Leukemia
  breast (*see also* Neoplasm, breast, malignant) C50.91- ☑
  hepatocellular C22.0
  lung (*see also* Neoplasm, lung, malignant) C34.90
  ovarian (*see also* Neoplasm ovary, malignant) C56.9
  unspecified site (primary) C80.1
Cancer (o)phobia F45.29
Cancerous — *see* Neoplasm, malignant, by site
Cancrum oris A69.0
Candidiasis, candidal B37.9
  balanitis B37.42
  bronchitis B37.1
  cheilitis B37.83
  congenital P37.5
  cystitis B37.41
  disseminated B37.7
  endocarditis B37.6
  enteritis B37.82
  esophagitis B37.81
  intertrigo B37.2
  lung B37.1
  meningitis B37.5
  mouth B37.0
  nails B37.2
  neonatal P37.5
  onychia B37.2
  oral B37.0
  osteomyelitis B37.89
  otitis externa B37.84
  paronychia B37.2
  perionyxis B37.2
  pneumonia B37.1
  proctitis B37.82
  pulmonary B37.1
  pyelonephritis B37.49
  sepsis B37.7
  skin B37.2
  specified site NEC B37.89
  stomatitis B37.0
  systemic B37.7
  urethritis B37.41
  urogenital site NEC B37.49
  vagina B37.3
  vulva B37.3
  vulvovaginitis B37.3
Candidid L30.2
Candidosis — *see* Candidiasis
Candiru infection or infestation B88.8
Canities (premature) L67.1

▽ Subterms under main terms may continue to next column or page   ☑ Additional Character Required — Refer to the Tabular List for Character Selection   **47**

Calcification — Canities

Canities — *continued*
  congenital Q84.2
Canker (mouth) (sore) K12.0
  rash A38.9
Cannabinosis J66.2
Cannabis induced
  anxiety disorder F12.980
  psychotic disorder F12.959
  sleep disorder F12.988
Canton fever A75.9
Cantrell's syndrome Q87.89
Capillariasis (intestinal) B81.1
  hepatic B83.8
Capillary — *see* condition
Caplan's syndrome — *see* Rheumatoid, lung
Capsule — *see* condition
Capsulitis (joint) (*see also* Enthesopathy)
  adhesive (shoulder) M75.0- ☑
  hepatic K65.8
  labyrinthine — *see* Otosclerosis, specified NEC
  thyroid E06.9
Caput
  crepitus Q75.8
  medusae I86.8
  succedaneum P12.81
Car sickness T75.3 ☑
Carapata (disease) A68.0
Carate — *see* Pinta
Carbon lung J60
Carbuncle L02.93
  abdominal wall L02.231
  anus K61.0
  auditory canal, external — *see* Abscess, ear, external
  auricle ear — *see* Abscess, ear, external
  axilla L02.43- ☑
  back (any part) L02.232
  breast N61.1
  buttock L02.33
  cheek (external) L02.03
  chest wall L02.233
  chin L02.03
  corpus cavernosum N48.21
  ear (any part) (external) (middle) — *see* Abscess, ear, external
  external auditory canal — *see* Abscess, ear, external
  eyelid — *see* Abscess, eyelid
  face NEC L02.03
  femoral (region) — *see* Carbuncle, lower limb
  finger — *see* Carbuncle, hand
  flank L02.231
  foot L02.63- ☑
  forehead L02.03
  genital — *see* Abscess, genital
  gluteal (region) L02.33
  groin L02.234
  hand L02.53- ☑
  head NEC L02.831
  heel — *see* Carbuncle, foot
  hip — *see* Carbuncle, lower limb
  kidney — *see* Abscess, kidney
  knee — *see* Carbuncle, lower limb
  labium (majus) (minus) N76.4
  lacrimal
    gland — *see* Dacryoadenitis
    passages (duct) (sac) — *see* Inflammation, lacrimal, passages, acute
  leg — *see* Carbuncle, lower limb
  lower limb L02.43- ☑
  malignant A22.0
  navel L02.236
  neck L02.13
  nose (external) (septum) J34.0
  orbit, orbital — *see* Abscess, orbit
  palmar (space) — *see* Carbuncle, hand
  partes posteriores L02.33
  pectoral region L02.233
  penis N48.21
  perineum L02.235
  pinna — *see* Abscess, ear, external
  popliteal — *see* Carbuncle, lower limb
  scalp L02.831
  seminal vesicle N49.0
  shoulder — *see* Carbuncle, upper limb
  specified site NEC L02.838
  temple (region) L02.03
  thumb — *see* Carbuncle, hand
  toe — *see* Carbuncle, foot

Carbuncle — *continued*
  trunk L02.239
    abdominal wall L02.231
    back L02.232
    chest wall L02.233
    groin L02.234
    perineum L02.235
    umbilicus L02.236
  umbilicus L02.236
  upper limb L02.43- ☑
  urethra N34.0
  vulva N76.4
Carbunculus — *see* Carbuncle
Carcinoid (tumor) — *see* Tumor, carcinoid
Carcinoidosis E34.0
Carcinoma (malignant) (*see also* Neoplasm, by site, malignant)
  acidophil
    specified site — *see* Neoplasm, malignant, by site
    unspecified site C75.1
  acidophil-basophil, mixed
    specified site — *see* Neoplasm, malignant, by site
    unspecified site C75.1
  adnexal (skin) — *see* Neoplasm, skin, malignant
  adrenal cortical C74.0- ☑
  alveolar — *see* Neoplasm, lung, malignant
    cell — *see* Neoplasm, lung, malignant
  ameloblastic C41.1
    upper jaw (bone) C41.0
  apocrine
    breast — *see* Neoplasm, breast, malignant
    specified site NEC — *see* Neoplasm, skin, malignant
    unspecified site C44.99
  basal cell (pigmented) (*see also* Neoplasm, skin, malignant) C44.91
    fibro-epithelial — *see* Neoplasm, skin, malignant
    morphea — *see* Neoplasm, skin, malignant
    multicentric — *see* Neoplasm, skin, malignant
  basaloid
  basal-squamous cell, mixed — *see* Neoplasm, skin, malignant
  basophil
    specified site — *see* Neoplasm, malignant, by site
    unspecified site C75.1
  basophil-acidophil, mixed
    specified site — *see* Neoplasm, malignant, by site
    unspecified site C75.1
  basosquamous — *see* Neoplasm, skin, malignant
  bile duct
    with hepatocellular, mixed C22.0
    liver C22.1
    specified site NEC — *see* Neoplasm, malignant, by site
    unspecified site C22.1
  branchial or branchiogenic C10.4
  bronchial or bronchogenic — *see* Neoplasm, lung, malignant
  bronchiolar — *see* Neoplasm, lung, malignant
  bronchioloalveolar — *see* Neoplasm, lung, malignant
  C cell
    specified site — *see* Neoplasm, malignant, by site
    unspecified site C73
  ceruminous C44.29- ☑
  cervix uteri
    in situ D06.9
      endocervix D06.0
      exocervix D06.1
      specified site NEC D06.7
  chorionic
    specified site — *see* Neoplasm, malignant, by site
    unspecified site
      female C58
      male C62.90
  chromophobe
    specified site — *see* Neoplasm, malignant, by site
    unspecified site C75.1
  cloacogenic
    specified site — *see* Neoplasm, malignant, by site
    unspecified site C21.2
  diffuse type
    specified site — *see* Neoplasm, malignant, by site
    unspecified site C16.9
  duct (cell)
    with Paget's disease — *see* Neoplasm, breast, malignant

Carcinoma — *continued*
  duct — *continued*
    infiltrating
      with lobular carcinoma (in situ)
        specified site — *see* Neoplasm, malignant, by site
        unspecified site (female) C50.91- ☑
          male C50.92- ☑
      specified site — *see* Neoplasm, malignant, by site
      unspecified site (female) C50.91- ☑
        male C50.92- ☑
  ductal
    with lobular
      specified site — *see* Neoplasm, malignant, by site
      unspecified site (female) C50.91- ☑
        male C50.92- ☑
  ductular, infiltrating
    specified site — *see* Neoplasm, malignant, by site
    unspecified site (female) C50.91- ☑
      male C50.92- ☑
  embryonal
    liver C22.7
  endometrioid
    specified site — *see* Neoplasm, malignant, by site
    unspecified site
      female C56.9
      male C61
  eosinophil
    specified site — *see* Neoplasm, malignant, by site
    unspecified site C75.1
  epidermoid (*see also* Neoplasm, skin, malignant)
    in situ, Bowen's type — *see* Neoplasm, skin, in situ
  fibroepithelial, basal cell — *see* Neoplasm, skin, malignant
  follicular
    with papillary (mixed) C73
    moderately differentiated C73
    pure follicle C73
    specified site — *see* Neoplasm, malignant, by site
    trabecular C73
    unspecified site C73
    well differentiated C73
  generalized, with unspecified primary site C80.0
  glycogen-rich — *see* Neoplasm, breast, malignant
  granulosa cell C56- ☑
  hepatic cell C22.0
  hepatocellular C22.0
    with bile duct, mixed C22.0
    fibrolamellar C22.0
  hepatocholangiolitic C22.0
  Hurthle cell C73
  in
    adenomatous
      polyposis coli C18.9
    pleomorphic adenoma — *see* Neoplasm, salivary glands, malignant
    situ — *see* Carcinoma-in-situ
  infiltrating
    duct
      with lobular
        specified site — *see* Neoplasm, malignant, by site
        unspecified site (female) C50.91- ☑
          male C50.92- ☑
      with Paget's disease — *see* Neoplasm, breast, malignant
      specified site — *see* Neoplasm, malignant
      unspecified site (female) C50.91- ☑
        male C50.92- ☑
    ductular
      specified site — *see* Neoplasm, malignant
      unspecified site (female) C50.91- ☑
        male C50.92- ☑
    lobular
      specified site — *see* Neoplasm, malignant
      unspecified site (female) C50.91- ☑
        male C50.92- ☑
  inflammatory
    specified site — *see* Neoplasm, malignant
    unspecified site (female) C50.91- ☑
      male C50.92- ☑
  intestinal type
    specified site — *see* Neoplasm, malignant, by site
    unspecified site C16.9

☑ Additional Character Required — Refer to the Tabular List for Character Selection   ▽ Subterms under main terms may continue to next column or page

Carcinoma — *continued*
  intracystic
    noninfiltrating — *see* Neoplasm, in situ, by site
  intraductal (noninfiltrating)
    with Paget's disease — *see* Neoplasm, breast, malignant
    breast D05.1- ☑
    papillary
      with invasion
        specified site — *see* Neoplasm, malignant, by site
        unspecified site (female) C50.91- ☑
          male C50.92- ☑
      breast D05.1- ☑
      specified site NEC — *see* Neoplasm, in situ, by site
      unspecified site (female) D05.1- ☑
    specified site NEC — *see* Neoplasm, in situ, by site
    unspecified site (female) D05.1- ☑
  intraepidermal — *see* Neoplasm, in situ
    squamous cell, Bowen's type — *see* Neoplasm, skin, in situ
  intraepithelial — *see* Neoplasm, in situ, by site
    squamous cell — *see* Neoplasm, in situ, by site
  intraosseous C41.1
    upper jaw (bone) C41.0
  islet cell
    with exocrine, mixed
      specified site — *see* Neoplasm, malignant, by site
      unspecified site C25.9
    pancreas C25.4
    specified site NEC — *see* Neoplasm, malignant, by site
    unspecified site C25.4
  juvenile, breast — *see* Neoplasm, breast, malignant
  large cell
    small cell
      specified site — *see* Neoplasm, malignant, by site
      unspecified site C34.90
  Leydig cell (testis)
    specified site — *see* Neoplasm, malignant, by site
    unspecified site
      female C56.9
      male C62.90
  lipid-rich (female) C50.91- ☑
    male C50.92- ☑
  liver cell C22.0
  liver NEC C22.7
  lobular (infiltrating)
    with intraductal
      specified site — *see* Neoplasm, malignant, by site
      unspecified site (female) C50.91- ☑
        male C50.92- ☑
    noninfiltrating
      breast D05.0- ☑
      specified site NEC — *see* Neoplasm, in situ, by site
      unspecified site D05.0- ☑
    specified site — *see* Neoplasm, malignant, by site
    unspecified site (female) C50.91- ☑
      male C50.92- ☑
  medullary
    with
      amyloid stroma
        specified site — *see* Neoplasm, malignant, by site
        unspecified site C73
      lymphoid stroma
        specified site — *see* Neoplasm, malignant, by site
        unspecified site (female) C50.91- ☑
          male C50.92- ☑
  Merkel cell C4A.9 (*following* C43)
    anal margin C4A.51 (*following* C43)
    anal skin C4A.51 (*following* C43)
    canthus C4A.1- ☑ (*following* C43)
    ear and external auricular canal C4A.2- ☑ (*following* C43)
    external auricular canal C4A.2- ☑ (*following* C43)
    eyelid, including canthus C4A.1- ☑ (*following* C43)
    face C4A.30 (*following* C43)
      specified NEC C4A.39 (*following* C43)
    hip C4A.7- ☑ (*following* C43)
    lip C4A.0 (*following* C43)

Carcinoma — *continued*
  Merkel cell — *continued*
    lower limb, including hip C4A.7- ☑ (*following* C43)
    neck C4A.4 (*following* C43)
    nodal presentation C7B.1 (*following* C75)
    nose C4A.31 (*following* C43)
    overlapping sites C4A.8 (*following* C43)
    perianal skin C4A.51 (*following* C43)
    scalp C4A.4 (*following* C43)
    secondary C7B.1 (*following* C75)
    shoulder C4A.6- ☑ (*following* C43)
    skin of breast C4A.52 (*following* C43)
    trunk NEC C4A.59 (*following* C43)
    upper limb, including shoulder C4A.6- ☑ (*following* C43)
    visceral metastatic C7B.1 (*following* C75)
  metastatic — *see* Neoplasm, secondary, by site
  metatypical — *see* Neoplasm, skin, malignant
  morphea, basal cell — *see* Neoplasm, skin, malignant
  mucoid
    cell
      specified site — *see* Neoplasm, malignant, by site
      unspecified site C75.1
  neuroendocrine (*see also* Tumor, neuroendocrine)
    high grade, any site C7A.1 (*following* C75)
    poorly differentiated, any site C7A.1 (*following* C75)
  nonencapsulated sclerosing C73
  noninfiltrating
    intracystic — *see* Neoplasm, in situ, by site
    intraductal
      breast D05.1- ☑
      papillary
        breast D05.1- ☑
        specified site NEC — *see* Neoplasm, in situ, by site
        unspecified site D05.1- ☑
      specified site — *see* Neoplasm, in situ, by site
      unspecified site D05.1- ☑
    lobular
      breast D05.0- ☑
      specified site NEC — *see* Neoplasm, in situ, by site
      unspecified site (female) D05.0- ☑
  oat cell
    specified site — *see* Neoplasm, malignant, by site
    unspecified site C34.90
  odontogenic C41.1
    upper jaw (bone) C41.0
  papillary
    with follicular (mixed) C73
    follicular variant C73
    intraductal (noninfiltrating)
      with invasion
        specified site — *see* Neoplasm, malignant, by site
        unspecified site (female) C50.91- ☑
          male C50.92- ☑
      breast D05.1- ☑
      specified site NEC — *see* Neoplasm, in situ, by site
      unspecified site D05.1- ☑
    serous
      specified site — *see* Neoplasm, malignant, by site
    surface
      specified site — *see* Neoplasm, malignant, by site
      unspecified site C56.9
    unspecified site C56.9
  papillocystic
    specified site — *see* Neoplasm, malignant, by site
    unspecified site C56.9
  parafollicular cell
    specified site — *see* Neoplasm, malignant, by site
    unspecified site C73
  pilomatrix — *see* Neoplasm, skin, malignant
  pseudomucinous
    specified site — *see* Neoplasm, malignant, by site
    unspecified site C56.9
  renal cell C64- ☑
  Schmincke — *see* Neoplasm, nasopharynx, malignant
  Schneiderian
    specified site — *see* Neoplasm, malignant, by site
    unspecified site C30.0
  sebaceous — *see* Neoplasm, skin, malignant

Carcinoma — *continued*
  secondary (*see also* Neoplasm, secondary, by site)
    Merkel cell C7B.1 (*following* C75)
  secretory, breast — *see* Neoplasm, breast, malignant
  serous
    papillary
      specified site — *see* Neoplasm, malignant, by site
      unspecified site C56.9
    surface, papillary
      specified site — *see* Neoplasm, malignant, by site
      unspecified site C56.9
  Sertoli cell
    specified site — *see* Neoplasm, malignant, by site
    unspecified site C62.90
      female C56.9
      male C62.90
  skin appendage — *see* Neoplasm, skin, malignant
  small cell
    fusiform cell
      specified site — *see* Neoplasm, malignant, by site
      unspecified site C34.90
    intermediate cell
      specified site — *see* Neoplasm, malignant, by site
      unspecified site C34.90
    large cell
      specified site — *see* Neoplasm, malignant, by site
      unspecified site C34.90
  solid
    with amyloid stroma
      specified site — *see* Neoplasm, malignant, by site
      unspecified site C73
    microinvasive
      specified site — *see* Neoplasm, malignant, by site
      unspecified site C53.9
  sweat gland — *see* Neoplasm, skin, malignant
  theca cell C56.- ☑
  thymic C37
  unspecified site (primary) C80.1
  water-clear cell C75.0
Carcinoma-in-situ (*see also* Neoplasm, in situ, by site)
  breast NOS D05.9- ☑
    specified type NEC D05.8- ☑
  epidermoid (*see also* Neoplasm, in situ, by site)
    with questionable stromal invasion
      cervix D06.9
      specified site NEC — *see* Neoplasm, in situ, by site
      unspecified site D06.9
    Bowen's type — *see* Neoplasm, skin, in situ
  intraductal
    breast D05.1- ☑
    specified site NEC — *see* Neoplasm, in situ, by site
    unspecified site D05.1- ☑
  lobular
    with
      infiltrating duct
        breast (female) C50.91- ☑
          male C50.92- ☑
        specified site NEC — *see* Neoplasm, malignant
        unspecified site (female) C50.91- ☑
          male C50.92- ☑
      intraductal
        breast D05.8- ☑
        specified site NEC — *see* Neoplasm, in situ, by site
        unspecified site (female) D05.8- ☑
    breast D05.0- ☑
    specified site NEC — *see* Neoplasm, in situ, by site
    unspecified site D05.0- ☑
  squamous cell (*see also* Neoplasm, in situ, by site)
    with questionable stromal invasion
      cervix D06.9
      specified site NEC — *see* Neoplasm, in situ, by site
      unspecified site D06.9
Carcinomaphobia F45.29
Carcinomatosis C80.0
  peritonei C78.6

Carcinomatosis — *continued*
  unspecified site (primary) (secondary) C80.0
Carcinosarcoma — *see* Neoplasm, malignant, by site
  embryonal — *see* Neoplasm, malignant, by site
Cardia, cardial — *see* condition
Cardiac (*see also* condition)
  death, sudden — *see* Arrest, cardiac
  pacemaker
    in situ Z95.0
      management or adjustment Z45.018
  tamponade I31.4
Cardialgia — *see* Pain, precordial
Cardiectasis — *see* Hypertrophy, cardiac
Cardiochalasia K21.9
Cardiomalacia I51.5
Cardiomegalia glycogenica diffusa E74.02 [I43]
Cardiomegaly (*see also* Hypertrophy, cardiac)
  congenital Q24.8
  glycogen E74.02 [I43]
  idiopathic I51.7
Cardiomyoliposis I51.5
Cardiomyopathy (familial) (idiopathic) I42.9
  alcoholic I42.6
  amyloid E85.4 [I43]
    transthyretin-related (ATTR) familial E85.4
  arteriosclerotic — *see* Disease, heart, ischemic,
    atherosclerotic
  beriberi E51.12
  cobalt-beer I42.6
  congenital I42.4
  congestive I42.0
  constrictive NOS I42.5
  dilated I42.0
  due to
    alcohol I42.6
    beriberi E51.12
    cardiac glycogenosis E74.02 [I43]
    drugs I42.7
    external agents NEC I42.7
    Friedreich's ataxia G11.1
    myotonia atrophica G71.11 [I43]
    progressive muscular dystrophy G71.0 [I43]
  glycogen storage E74.02 [I43]
  hypertensive — *see* Hypertension, heart
  hypertrophic (nonobstructive) I42.2
    obstructive I42.1
      congenital Q24.8
  in
    Chagas' disease (chronic) B57.2
      acute B57.0
    sarcoidosis D86.85
  ischemic I25.5
  metabolic E88.9 [I43]
    thyrotoxic E05.90 [I43]
      with thyroid storm E05.91 [I43]
  newborn I42.8
    congenital I42.4
  nutritional E63.9 [I43]
    beriberi E51.12
  obscure of Africa I42.8
  peripartum O90.3
  postpartum O90.3
  restrictive NEC I42.5
  rheumatic I09.0
  secondary I42.9
  stress induced I51.81
  takotsubo I51.81
  thyrotoxic E05.90 [I43]
    with thyroid storm E05.91 [I43]
  toxic NEC I42.7
  transthyretin-related (ATTR) familial amyloid E85.4
  tuberculous A18.84
  viral B33.24
Cardionephritis — *see* Hypertension, cardiorenal
Cardionephropathy — *see* Hypertension, cardiorenal
Cardionephrosis — *see* Hypertension, cardiorenal
Cardiopathia nigra I27.0
Cardiopathy (*see also* Disease, heart) I51.9
  idiopathic I42.9
  mucopolysaccharidosis E76.3 [I52]
Cardiopericarditis — *see* Pericarditis
Cardiophobia F45.29
Cardiorenal — *see* condition
Cardiorrhexis — *see* Infarct, myocardium
Cardiosclerosis — *see* Disease, heart, ischemic,
    atherosclerotic
Cardiosis — *see* Disease, heart
Cardiospasm (esophagus) (reflex) (stomach) K22.0

Cardiospasm — *continued*
  congenital Q39.5
    with megaesophagus Q39.5
Cardiostenosis — *see* Disease, heart
Cardiosymphysis I31.0
Cardiovascular — *see* condition
Carditis (acute) (bacterial) (chronic) (subacute) I51.89
  meningococcal A39.50
  rheumatic — *see* Disease, heart, rheumatic
  rheumatoid — *see* Rheumatoid, carditis
  viral B33.20
Care (of) (for) (following)
  child (routine) Z76.2
  family member (handicapped) (sick)
    creating problem for family Z63.6
    provided away from home for holiday relief Z75.5
    unavailable, due to
      absence (person rendering care) (sufferer) Z74.2
      inability (any reason) of person rendering care
        Z74.2
  foundling Z76.1
  holiday relief Z75.5
  improper — *see* Maltreatment
  lack of (at or after birth) (infant) — *see* Maltreatment,
    child, neglect
  lactating mother Z39.1
  palliative Z51.5
  postpartum
    immediately after delivery Z39.0
    routine follow-up Z39.2
  respite Z75.5
  unavailable, due to
    absence of person rendering care Z74.2
    inability (any reason) of person rendering care
      Z74.2
  well-baby Z76.2
Caries
  bone NEC A18.03
  dental (dentino enamel junction) (early childhood) (of
      dentine) (pre-eruptive) (recurrent) (to the pulp)
      K02.9
    arrested (coronal) (root) K02.3
    chewing surface
      limited to enamel K02.51
      penetrating into dentin K02.52
      penetrating into pulp K02.53
    coronal surface
      chewing surface
        limited to enamel K02.51
        penetrating into dentin K02.52
        penetrating into pulp K02.53
      pit and fissure surface
        limited to enamel K02.51
        penetrating into dentin K02.52
        penetrating into pulp K02.53
      smooth surface
        limited to enamel K02.61
        penetrating into dentin K02.62
        penetrating into pulp K02.63
    pit and fissure surface
      limited to enamel K02.51
      penetrating into dentin K02.52
      penetrating into pulp K02.53
    primary, cervical origin K02.52
    root K02.7
    smooth surface
      limited to enamel K02.61
      penetrating into dentin K02.62
      penetrating into pulp K02.63
  external meatus — *see* Disorder, ear, external, speci-
    fied type NEC
  hip (tuberculous) A18.02
  initial (tooth)
    chewing surface K02.51
    pit and fissure surface K02.51
    smooth surface K02.61
  knee (tuberculous) A18.02
  labyrinth H83.8 ☑
  limb NEC (tuberculous) A18.03
  mastoid process (chronic) — *see* Mastoiditis, chronic
    tuberculous A18.03
  middle ear H74.8 ☑
  nose (tuberculous) A18.03
  orbit (tuberculous) A18.03
  ossicles, ear — *see* Abnormal, ear ossicles
  petrous bone — *see* Petrositis
  root (dental) (tooth) K02.7
  sacrum (tuberculous) A18.01

Caries — *continued*
  spine, spinal (column) (tuberculous) A18.01
  syphilitic A52.77
    congenital (early) A50.02 [M90.80]
  tooth, teeth — *see* Caries, dental
  tuberculous A18.03
  vertebra (column) (tuberculous) A18.01
Carious teeth — *see* Caries, dental
Carneous mole O02.0
Carnitine insufficiency E71.40
Carotid body or sinus syndrome G90.01
Carotidynia G90.01
Carotinemia (dietary) E67.1
Carotinosis (cutis) (skin) E67.1
Carpal tunnel syndrome — *see* Syndrome, carpal tunnel
Carpenter's syndrome Q87.0
Carpopedal spasm — *see* Tetany
Carr-Barr-Plunkett syndrome Q97.1
Carrier (suspected) of
  amebiasis Z22.1
  bacterial disease NEC Z22.39
    diphtheria Z22.2
    intestinal infectious NEC Z22.1
      typhoid Z22.0
    meningococcal Z22.31
    sexually transmitted Z22.4
    specified NEC Z22.39
    staphylococcal (Methicillin susceptible) Z22.321
      Methicillin resistant Z22.322
    streptococcal Z22.338
      group B Z22.330
        complicating pregnancy or delivery
          O99.82- ☑
    typhoid Z22.0
  cholera Z22.1
  diphtheria Z22.2
  gastrointestinal pathogens NEC Z22.1
  genetic Z14.8
    cystic fibrosis Z14.1
    hemophilia A (asymptomatic) Z14.01
      symptomatic Z14.02
  gestational, pregnant Z33.1
  gonorrhea Z22.4
  HAA (hepatitis Australian-antigen) B18.8
  HB (c)(s)-AG B18.1
  hepatitis (viral) B18.9
    Australia-antigen (HAA) B18.8
    B surface antigen (HBsAg) B18.1
      with acute delta- (super)infection B17.0
    C B18.2
    specified NEC B18.8
  human T-cell lymphotropic virus type-1 (HTLV-1) infec-
    tion Z22.6
  infectious organism Z22.9
    specified NEC Z22.8
  meningococci Z22.31
  Salmonella typhosa Z22.0
  serum hepatitis — *see* Carrier, hepatitis
  staphylococci (Methicillin susceptible) Z22.321
    Methicillin resistant Z22.322
  streptococci Z22.338
    group B Z22.330
      complicating pregnancy or delivery O99.82- ☑
  syphilis Z22.4
  typhoid Z22.0
  venereal disease NEC Z22.4
Carrion's disease A44.0
Carter's relapsing fever (Asiatic) A68.1
Cartilage — *see* condition
Caruncle (inflamed)
  conjunctiva (acute) — *see* Conjunctivitis, acute
  labium (majus) (minus) N90.89
  lacrimal — *see* Inflammation, lacrimal, passages
  myrtiform N89.8
  urethral (benign) N36.2
Cascade stomach K31.2
Caseation lymphatic gland (tuberculous) A18.2
Cassidy (-Scholte) syndrome (malignant carcinoid) E34.0
Castellani's disease A69.8
Castration, traumatic, male S38.231 ☑
Casts in urine R82.99
Cat
  cry syndrome Q93.4
  ear Q17.3
  eye syndrome Q92.8
Catabolism, senile R54
Catalepsy (hysterical) F44.2
  schizophrenic F20.2

☑ Additional Character Required — Refer to the Tabular List for Character Selection   ▽ Subterms under main terms may continue to next column or page

Cataplexy (idiopathic) — see Narcolepsy
Cataract (cortical) (immature) (incipient) H26.9
  with
    neovascularization — see Cataract, complicated
  age-related — see Cataract, senile
  anterior
    and posterior axial embryonal Q12.0
    pyramidal Q12.0
  associated with
    galactosemia E74.21 [H28]
    myotonic disorders G71.19 [H28]
  blue Q12.0
  central Q12.0
  cerulean Q12.0
  complicated H26.20
    with
      neovascularization H26.21- ☑
      ocular disorder H26.22- ☑
      glaucomatous flecks H26.23- ☑
  congenital Q12.0
  coraliform Q12.0
  coronary Q12.0
  crystalline Q12.0
  diabetic — see Diabetes, cataract
  drug-induced H26.3- ☑
  due to
    ocular disorder — see Cataract, complicated
    radiation H26.8
  electric H26.8
  extraction status Z98.4- ☑
  glass-blower's H26.8
  heat ray H26.8
  heterochromic — see Cataract, complicated
  hypermature — see Cataract, senile, morgagnian type
  in (due to)
    chronic iridocyclitis — see Cataract, complicated
    diabetes — see Diabetes, cataract
    endocrine disease E34.9 [H28]
    eye disease — see Cataract, complicated
    hypoparathyroidism E20.9 [H28]
    malnutrition-dehydration E46 [H28]
    metabolic disease E88.9 [H28]
    myotonic disorders G71.19 [H28]
    nutritional disease E63.9 [H28]
  infantile — see Cataract, presenile
  irradiational — see Cataract, specified NEC
  juvenile — see Cataract, presenile
  malnutrition-dehydration E46 [H28]
  morgagnian — see Cataract, senile, morgagnian type
  myotonic G71.19 [H28]
  myxedema E03.9 [H28]
  nuclear
    embryonal Q12.0
    sclerosis — see Cataract, senile, nuclear
  presenile H26.00- ☑
    combined forms H26.06- ☑
    cortical H26.01- ☑
    lamellar — see Cataract, presenile, cortical
    nuclear H26.03- ☑
    specified NEC H26.09
    subcapsular polar (anterior) H26.04- ☑
      posterior H26.05- ☑
    zonular — see Cataract, presenile, cortical
  secondary H26.40
    Soemmering's ring H26.41- ☑
    specified NEC H26.49- ☑
    to eye disease — see Cataract, complicated
  senile H25.9
    brunescens — see Cataract, senile, nuclear
    combined forms H25.81- ☑
    coronary — see Cataract, senile, incipient
    cortical H25.01- ☑
    hypermature — see Cataract, senile, morgagnian type
    incipient (mature) (total) H25.09- ☑
      cortical — see Cataract, senile, cortical
      subcapsular — see Cataract, senile, subcapsular
    morgagnian type (hypermature) H25.2- ☑
    nuclear (sclerosis) H25.1- ☑
    polar subcapsular (anterior) (posterior) — see Cataract, senile, incipient
    punctate — see Cataract, senile, incipient
    specified NEC H25.89
    subcapsular polar (anterior) H25.03- ☑
      posterior H25.04- ☑
  snowflake — see Diabetes, cataract
  specified NEC H26.8

Cataract — continued
  toxic — see Cataract, drug-induced
  traumatic H26.10- ☑
    localized H26.11- ☑
    partially resolved H26.12- ☑
    total H26.13- ☑
  zonular (perinuclear) Q12.0
Cataracta (see also Cataract)
  brunescens — see Cataract, senile, nuclear
  centralis pulverulenta Q12.0
  cerulea Q12.0
  complicata — see Cataract, complicated
  congenita Q12.0
  coralliformis Q12.0
  coronaria Q12.0
  diabetic — see Diabetes, cataract
  membranacea
    accreta — see Cataract, secondary
    congenita Q12.0
  nigra — see Cataract, senile, nuclear
  sunflower — see Cataract, complicated
Catarrh, catarrhal (acute) (febrile) (infectious) (inflammation) (see also condition) J00
  bronchial — see Bronchitis
  chest — see Bronchitis
  chronic J31.0
  due to congenital syphilis A50.03
  enteric — see Enteritis
  eustachian H68.009
  fauces — see Pharyngitis
  gastrointestinal — see Enteritis
  gingivitis K05.00
    nonplaque induced K05.01
    plaque induced K05.00
  hay — see Fever, hay
  intestinal — see Enteritis
  larynx, chronic J37.0
  liver B15.9
    with hepatic coma B15.0
  lung — see Bronchitis
  middle ear, chronic — see Otitis, media, nonsuppurative, chronic, serous
  mouth K12.1
  nasal (chronic) — see Rhinitis
  nasobronchial J31.1
  nasopharyngeal (chronic) J31.1
    acute J00
  pulmonary — see Bronchitis
  spring (eye) (vernal) — see Conjunctivitis, acute, atopic
  summer (hay) — see Fever, hay
  throat J31.2
  tubotympanal (see also Otitis, media, nonsuppurative)
    chronic — see Otitis, media, nonsuppurative, chronic, serous
Catatonia (schizophrenic) F20.2
Catatonic
  disorder due to known physiologic condition F06.1
  schizophrenia F20.2
  stupor R40.1
Cat-scratch (see also Abrasion)
  disease or fever A28.1
Cauda equina — see condition
Cauliflower ear M95.1- ☑
Causalgia (upper limb) G56.4- ☑
  lower limb G57.7- ☑
Cause
  external, general effects T75.89 ☑
Caustic burn — see Corrosion, by site
Cavare's disease (familial periodic paralysis) G72.3
Cave-in, injury
  crushing (severe) — see Crush
  suffocation — see Asphyxia, traumatic, due to low oxygen, due to cave-in
Cavernitis (penis) N48.29
Cavernositis N48.29
Cavernous — see condition
Cavitation of lung (see also Tuberculosis, pulmonary)
  nontuberculous J98.4
Cavities, dental — see Caries, dental
Cavity
  lung — see Cavitation of lung
  optic papilla Q14.2
  pulmonary — see Cavitation of lung
Cavovarus foot, congenital Q66.1
Cavus foot (congenital) Q66.7
  acquired — see Deformity, limb, foot, specified NEC
Cazenave's disease L10.2

Cecitis K52.9
  with perforation, peritonitis, or rupture K65.8
Cecum — see condition
Celiac
  artery compression syndrome I77.4
  disease (with steatorrhea) K90.0
  infantilism K90.0
Cell(s), **cellular** (see also condition)
  in urine R82.99
Cellulitis (diffuse) (phlegmonous) (septic) (suppurative) L03.90
  abdominal wall L03.311
  anaerobic A48.0
  ankle — see Cellulitis, lower limb
  anus K61.0
  arm — see Cellulitis, upper limb
  auricle (ear) — see Cellulitis, ear
  axilla L03.11- ☑
  back (any part) L03.312
  breast (acute) (nonpuerperal) (subacute) N61.0
    nipple N61.0
  broad ligament
    acute N73.0
  buttock L03.317
  cervical (meaning neck) L03.221
  cervix (uteri) — see Cervicitis
  cheek (external) L03.211
    internal K12.2
  chest wall L03.313
  chronic L03.90
  clostridial A48.0
  corpus cavernosum N48.22
  digit
    finger — see Cellulitis, finger
    toe — see Cellulitis, toe
  Douglas' cul-de-sac or pouch
    acute N73.0
  drainage site (following operation) T81.4 ☑
  ear (external) H60.1- ☑
  eosinophilic (granulomatous) L98.3
  erysipelatous — see Erysipelas
  external auditory canal — see Cellulitis, ear
  eyelid — see Abscess, eyelid
  face NEC L03.211
  finger (intrathecal) (periosteal) (subcutaneous) (subcuticular) L03.01- ☑
  foot — see Cellulitis, lower limb
  gangrenous — see Gangrene
  genital organ NEC
    female (external) N76.4
    male N49.9
      multiple sites N49.8
      specified NEC N49.8
  gluteal (region) L03.317
  gonococcal A54.89
  groin L03.314
  hand — see Cellulitis, upper limb
  head NEC L03.811
    face (any part, except ear, eye and nose) L03.211
  heel — see Cellulitis, lower limb
  hip — see Cellulitis, lower limb
  jaw (region) L03.211
  knee — see Cellulitis, lower limb
  labium (majus) (minus) — see Vulvitis
  lacrimal passages — see Inflammation, lacrimal, passages
  larynx J38.7
  leg — see Cellulitis, lower limb
  lip K13.0
  lower limb L03.11- ☑
    toe — see Cellulitis, toe
  mouth (floor) K12.2
  multiple sites, so stated L03.90
  nasopharynx J39.1
  navel L03.316
    newborn P38.9
      with mild hemorrhage P38.1
      without hemorrhage P38.9
  neck (region) L03.221
  nipple (acute) (nonpuerperal) (subacute) N61.0
  nose (septum) (external) J34.0
  orbit, orbital H05.01- ☑
  palate (soft) K12.2
  pectoral (region) L03.313
  pelvis, pelvic (chronic)
    female (see also Disease, pelvis, inflammatory) N73.2
      acute N73.0

Index

Cellulitis — Change

Cellulitis — *continued*
  pelvis, pelvic — *continued*
    following ectopic or molar pregnancy O08.0
    male K65.0
  penis N48.22
  perineal, perineum L03.315
  periorbital L03.213
  perirectal K61.1
  peritonsillar J36
  periurethral N34.0
  periuterine (*see also* Disease, pelvis, inflammatory) N73.2
    acute N73.0
  pharynx J39.1
  preseptal L03.213
  rectum K61.1
  retroperitoneal K68.9
  round ligament
    acute N73.0
  scalp (any part) L03.811
  scrotum N49.2
  seminal vesicle N49.0
  shoulder — *see* Cellulitis, upper limb
  specified site NEC L03.818
  submandibular (region) (space) (triangle) K12.2
    gland K11.3
  submaxillary (region) K12.2
    gland K11.3
  thigh — *see* Cellulitis, lower limb
  thumb (intrathecal) (periosteal) (subcutaneous) (subcuticular) — *see* Cellulitis, finger
  toe (intrathecal) (periosteal) (subcutaneous) (subcuticular) L03.03- ☑
  tonsil J36
  trunk L03.319
    abdominal wall L03.311
    back (any part) L03.312
    buttock L03.317
    chest wall L03.313
    groin L03.314
    perineal, perineum L03.315
    umbilicus L03.316
  tuberculous (primary) A18.4
  umbilicus L03.316
  upper limb L03.11- ☑
    axilla — *see* Cellulitis, axilla
    finger — *see* Cellulitis, finger
    thumb — *see* Cellulitis, finger
  vaccinal T88.0 ☑
  vocal cord J38.3
  vulva — *see* Vulvitis
  wrist — *see* Cellulitis, upper limb
Cementoblastoma, benign — *see* Cyst, calcifying odontogenic
Cementoma — *see* Cyst, calcifying odontogenic
Cementoperiostitis — *see* Periodontitis
Cementosis K03.4
Central auditory processing disorder H93.25
Central pain syndrome G89.0
Cephalematocele, cephal (o)hematocele
  newborn P52.8
    birth injury P10.8
  traumatic — *see* Hematoma, brain
Cephalematoma, cephalhematoma (calcified)
  newborn (birth injury) P12.0
  traumatic — *see* Hematoma, brain
Cephalgia, cephalalgia (*see also* Headache)
  histamine G44.009
    intractable G44.001
    not intractable G44.009
  trigeminal autonomic (TAC) NEC G44.099
    intractable G44.091
    not intractable G44.099
Cephalic — *see* condition
Cephalitis — *see* Encephalitis
Cephalocele — *see* Encephalocele
Cephalomenia N94.89
Cephalopelvic — *see* condition
Cerclage (with cervical incompetence) in pregnancy — *see* Incompetence, cervix, in pregnancy
Cerebellitis — *see* Encephalitis
Cerebellum, cerebellar — *see* condition
Cerebral — *see* condition
Cerebritis — *see* Encephalitis
Cerebro-hepato-renal syndrome Q87.89
Cerebromalacia — *see* Softening, brain
  sequelae of cerebrovascular disease I69.398
Cerebroside lipidosis E75.22

Cerebrospasticity (congenital) G80.1
Cerebrospinal — *see* condition
Cerebrum — *see* condition
Ceroid-lipofuscinosis, neuronal E75.4
Cerumen (accumulation) (impacted) H61.2- ☑
Cervical (*see also* condition)
  auricle Q18.2
  dysplasia in pregnancy — *see* Abnormal, cervix, in pregnancy or childbirth
  erosion in pregnancy — *see* Abnormal, cervix, in pregnancy or childbirth
  fibrosis in pregnancy — *see* Abnormal, cervix, in pregnancy or childbirth
  fusion syndrome Q76.1
  rib Q76.5
  shortening (complicating pregnancy) O26.87- ☑
Cervicalgia M54.2
Cervicitis (acute) (chronic) (nonvenereal) (senile (atrophic)) (subacute) (with ulceration) N72
  with
    abortion — *see* Abortion, by type complicated by genital tract and pelvic infection
    ectopic pregnancy O08.0
    molar pregnancy O08.0
  chlamydial A56.09
  gonococcal A54.03
  herpesviral A60.03
  puerperal (postpartum) O86.11
  syphilitic A52.76
  trichomonal A59.09
  tuberculous A18.16
Cervicocolpitis (emphysematosa) (*see also* Cervicitis) N72
Cervix — *see* condition
Cesarean delivery, previous, affecting management of pregnancy O34.219
  classical (vertical) scar O34.212
  low transverse scar O34.211
Céstan (-Chenais) paralysis or syndrome G46.3
Céstan-Raymond syndrome I65.8
Cestode infestation B71.9
  specified type NEC B71.8
Cestodiasis B71.9
Chabert's disease A22.9
Chacaleh E53.8
Chafing L30.4
Chagas' (-Mazza) disease (chronic) B57.2
  with
    cardiovascular involvement NEC B57.2
    digestive system involvement B57.30
      megacolon B57.32
      megaesophagus B57.31
      other specified B57.39
    megacolon B57.32
    megaesophagus B57.31
    myocarditis B57.2
    nervous system involvement B57.40
      meningitis B57.41
      meningoencephalitis B57.42
      other specified B57.49
    specified organ involvement NEC B57.5
  acute (with) B57.1
    cardiovascular NEC B57.0
    myocarditis B57.0
Chagres fever B50.9
Chairridden Z74.09
Chalasia (cardiac sphincter) K21.9
Chalazion H00.19
  left H00.16
    lower H00.15
    upper H00.14
  right H00.13
    lower H00.12
    upper H00.11
Chalcosis (*see also* Disorder, globe, degenerative, chalcosis)
  cornea — *see* Deposit, cornea
  crystalline lens — *see* Cataract, complicated
  retina H35.89
Chalicosis (pulmonum) J62.8
Chancre (any genital site) (hard) (hunterian) (mixed) (primary) (seronegative) (seropositive) (syphilitic) A51.0
  congenital A50.07
  conjunctiva NEC A51.2
  Ducrey's A57
  extragenital A51.2
  eyelid A51.2

Chancre — *continued*
  lip A51.2
  nipple A51.2
  Nisbet's A57
  of
    carate A67.0
    pinta A67.0
    yaws A66.0
  palate, soft A51.2
  phagedenic A57
  simple A57
  soft A57
    bubo A57
    palate A51.2
  urethra A51.0
  yaws A66.0
Chancroid (anus) (genital) (penis) (perineum) (rectum) (urethra) (vulva) A57
Chandler's disease (osteochondritis dissecans, hip) — *see* Osteochondritis, dissecans, hip
Change(s) (in) (of) (*see also* Removal)
  arteriosclerotic — *see* Arteriosclerosis
  bone (*see also* Disorder, bone)
    diabetic — *see* Diabetes, bone change
  bowel habit R19.4
  cardiorenal (vascular) — *see* Hypertension, cardiorenal
  cardiovascular — *see* Disease, cardiovascular
  circulatory I99.9
  cognitive (mild) (organic) R41.89
  color, tooth, teeth
    during formation K00.8
    posteruptive K03.7
  contraceptive device Z30.433
  corneal membrane H18.30
    Bowman's membrane fold or rupture H18.31- ☑
    Descemet's membrane
      fold H18.32- ☑
      rupture H18.33- ☑
  coronary — *see* Disease, heart, ischemic
  degenerative, spine or vertebra — *see* Spondylosis
  dental pulp, regressive K04.2
  dressing (nonsurgical) Z48.00
    surgical Z48.01
  heart — *see* Disease, heart
  hip joint — *see* Derangement, joint, hip
  hyperplastic larynx J38.7
  hypertrophic
    nasal sinus J34.89
    turbinate, nasal J34.3
    upper respiratory tract J39.8
  indwelling catheter Z46.6
  inflammatory (*see also* Inflammation)
    sacroiliac M46.1
  job, anxiety concerning Z56.1
  joint — *see* Derangement, joint
  life — *see* Menopause
  mental status R41.82
  minimal (glomerular) (*see also* N00-N07 with fourth character .0) N05.0
  myocardium, myocardial — *see* Degeneration, myocardial
  of life — *see* Menopause
  pacemaker Z45.018
    pulse generator Z45.010
  personality (enduring) F68.8
    due to (secondary to)
      general medical condition F07.0
      secondary (nonspecific) F60.89
  regressive, dental pulp K04.2
  renal — *see* Disease, renal
  retina H35.9
    myopic (*see also* Myopia, degenerative) H44.2- ☑
  sacroiliac joint M53.3
  senile (*see also* condition) R54
  sensory R20.8
  skin R23.9
    acute, due to ultraviolet radiation L56.9
      specified NEC L56.8
    chronic, due to nonionizing radiation L57.9
      specified NEC L57.8
    cyanosis R23.0
    flushing R23.2
    pallor R23.1
    petechiae R23.3
    specified change NEC R23.8
    swelling — *see* Mass, localized
    texture R23.4

☑ Additional Character Required — Refer to the Tabular List for Character Selection   Subterms under main terms may continue to next column or page

Change(s) — continued
  trophic
    arm — see Mononeuropathy, upper limb
    leg — see Mononeuropathy, lower limb
  vascular I99.9
  vasomotor I73.9
  voice R49.9
    psychogenic F44.4
    specified NEC R49.8
Changing sleep-work schedule, affecting sleep G47.26
Changuinola fever A93.1
Chapping skin T69.8 ☑
Charcot-Marie-Tooth disease, paralysis or syndrome G60.0
Charcot's
  arthropathy — see Arthropathy, neuropathic
  cirrhosis K74.3
  disease (tabetic arthropathy) A52.16
  joint (disease) (tabetic) A52.16
    diabetic — see Diabetes, with, arthropathy
    syringomyelic G95.0
  syndrome (intermittent claudication) I73.9
CHARGE association Q89.8
Charley-horse (quadriceps) M62.831
  traumatic (quadriceps) S76.11- ☑
Charlouis' disease — see Yaws
Cheadle's disease E54
Checking (of)
  cardiac pacemaker (battery) (electrode(s)) Z45.018
    pulse generator Z45.010
  implantable subdermal contraceptive Z30.46
  intrauterine contraceptive device Z30.431
  wound Z48.0- ☑
    due to injury — code to Injury, by site, using appropriate seventh character for subsequent encounter
Check-up — see Examination
Chédiak-Higashi (-Steinbrinck) **syndrome** (congenital gigantism of peroxidase granules) E70.330
Cheek — see condition
Cheese itch B88.0
Cheese-washer's lung J67.8
Cheese-worker's lung J67.8
Cheilitis (acute) (angular) (catarrhal) (chronic) (exfoliative) (gangrenous) (glandular) (infectional) (suppurative) (ulcerative) (vesicular) K13.0
  actinic (due to sun) L56.8
    other than from sun L59.8
  candidal B37.83
Cheilodynia K13.0
Cheiloschisis — see Cleft, lip
Cheilosis (angular) K13.0
  with pellagra E52
  due to
    vitamin B2 (riboflavin) deficiency E53.0
Cheiromegaly M79.89
Cheiropompholyx L30.1
Cheloid — see Keloid
Chemical burn — see Corrosion, by site
Chemodectoma — see Paraganglioma, nonchromaffin
Chemosis, conjunctiva — see Edema, conjunctiva
Chemotherapy (session) (for)
  cancer Z51.11
  neoplasm Z51.11
Cherubism M27.8
Chest — see condition
Cheyne-Stokes breathing (respiration) R06.3
Chiari's
  disease or syndrome (hepatic vein thrombosis) I82.0
  malformation
    type I G93.5
    type II — see Spina bifida
  net Q24.8
Chicago disease B40.9
Chickenpox — see Varicella
Chiclero ulcer or sore B55.1
Chigger (infestation) B88.0
Chignon (disease) B36.8
  newborn (from vacuum extraction) (birth injury) P12.1
Chilaiditi's syndrome (subphrenic displacement, colon) Q43.3
Chilblain(s) (lupus) T69.1 ☑
Child
  custody dispute Z65.3
Childbirth — see Delivery

Childhood
  cerebral X-linked adrenoleukodystrophy E71.520
  period of rapid growth Z00.2
Chill(s) R68.83
  with fever R50.9
  without fever R68.83
  congestive in malarial regions B54
Chilomastigiasis A07.8
Chimera 46,XX/46,XY Q99.0
Chin — see condition
Chinese dysentery A03.9
Chionophobia F40.228
Chitral fever A93.1
Chlamydia, chlamydial A74.9
  cervicitis A56.09
  conjunctivitis A74.0
  cystitis A56.01
  endometritis A56.11
  epididymitis A56.19
  female
    pelvic inflammatory disease A56.11
    pelviperitonitis A56.11
  orchitis A56.19
  peritonitis A74.81
  pharyngitis A56.4
  proctitis A56.3
  psittaci (infection) A70
  salpingitis A56.11
  sexually-transmitted infection NEC A56.8
  specified NEC A74.89
  urethritis A56.01
  vulvovaginitis A56.02
Chlamydiosis — see Chlamydia
Chloasma (skin) (idiopathic) (symptomatic) L81.1
  eyelid H02.719
    hyperthyroid E05.90 [H02.719]
      with thyroid storm E05.91 [H02.719]
    left H02.716
      lower H02.715
      upper H02.714
    right H02.713
      lower H02.712
      upper H02.711
Chloroma C92.3- ☑
Chlorosis D50.9
  Egyptian B76.9 [D63.8]
  miner's B76.9 [D63.8]
Chlorotic anemia D50.8
Chocolate cyst (ovary) N80.1
Choked
  disc or disk — see Papilledema
  on food, phlegm, or vomitus NOS — see Foreign body, by site
  while vomiting NOS — see Foreign body, by site
Chokes (resulting from bends) T70.3 ☑
Choking sensation R09.89
Cholangiectasis K83.8
Cholangiocarcinoma
  with hepatocellular carcinoma, combined C22.0
  liver C22.1
  specified site NEC — see Neoplasm, malignant, by site
  unspecified site C22.1
Cholangiohepatitis K83.8
  due to fluke infestation B66.1
Cholangiohepatoma C22.0
Cholangiolitis (acute) (chronic) (extrahepatic) (gangrenous) (intrahepatic) K83.0
  paratyphoidal — see Fever, paratyphoid
  typhoidal A01.09
Cholangioma D13.4
  malignant — see Cholangiocarcinoma
Cholangitis (ascending) (primary) (recurrent) (sclerosing) (secondary) (stenosing) (suppurative) K83.0
  with calculus, bile duct — see Calculus, bile duct, with cholangitis
  chronic nonsuppurative destructive K74.3
Cholecystectasia K82.8
Cholecystitis K81.9
  with
    calculus, stones in
      bile duct (common) (hepatic) — see Calculus, bile duct, with cholecystitis
      cystic duct — see Calculus, gallbladder, with cholecystitis
      gallbladder — see Calculus, gallbladder, with cholecystitis
      choledocholithiasis — see Calculus, bile duct, with cholecystitis

Cholecystitis — continued
  with — continued
    cholelithiasis — see Calculus, gallbladder, with cholecystitis
  acute (emphysematous) (gangrenous) (suppurative) K81.0
    with
      calculus, stones in
        cystic duct — see Calculus, gallbladder, with cholecystitis, acute
        gallbladder — see Calculus, gallbladder, with cholecystitis, acute
        choledocholithiasis — see Calculus, bile duct, with cholecystitis, acute
        cholelithiasis — see Calculus, gallbladder, with cholecystitis, acute
      chronic cholecystitis K81.2
        with gallbladder calculus K80.12
          with obstruction K80.13
  chronic K81.1
    with acute cholecystitis K81.2
      with gallbladder calculus K80.12
        with obstruction K80.13
  emphysematous (acute) — see Cholecystitis, acute
  gangrenous — see Cholecystitis, acute
  paratyphoidal, current A01.4
  suppurative — see Cholecystitis, acute
  typhoidal A01.09
Cholecystolithiasis — see Calculus, gallbladder
Choledochitis (suppurative) K83.0
Choledocholith — see Calculus, bile duct
Choledocholithiasis (common duct) (hepatic duct) — see Calculus, bile duct
  cystic — see Calculus, gallbladder
  typhoidal A01.09
Cholelithiasis (cystic duct) (gallbladder) (impacted) (multiple) — see Calculus, gallbladder
  bile duct (common) (hepatic) — see Calculus, bile duct
  hepatic duct — see Calculus, bile duct
  specified NEC K80.80
    with obstruction K80.81
Cholemia (see also Jaundice)
  familial (simple) (congenital) E80.4
  Gilbert's E80.4
Choleperitoneum, choleperitonitis K65.3
Cholera (Asiatic) (epidemic) (malignant) A00.9
  antimonial — see Poisoning, antimony
  classical A00.0
  due to Vibrio cholerae 01 A00.9
    biovar cholerae A00.0
    biovar eltor A00.1
    el tor A00.1
  el tor A00.1
Cholerine — see Cholera
Cholestasis NEC K83.1
  with hepatocyte injury K71.0
  due to total parenteral nutrition (TPN) K76.89
  pure K71.0
Cholesteatoma (ear) (middle) (with reaction) H71.9- ☑
  attic H71.0- ☑
  external ear (canal) H60.4- ☑
  mastoid H71.2- ☑
  postmastoidectomy cavity (recurrent) — see Complications, postmastoidectomy, recurrent cholesteatoma
  recurrent (postmastoidectomy) — see Complications, postmastoidectomy, recurrent cholesteatoma
  tympanum H71.1- ☑
Cholesteatosis, diffuse H71.3- ☑
Cholesteremia E78.00
Cholesterin in vitreous — see Deposit, crystalline
Cholesterol
  deposit
    retina H35.89
    vitreous — see Deposit, crystalline
  elevated (high) E78.00
    with elevated (high) triglycerides E78.2
    screening for Z13.220
  imbibition of gallbladder K82.4
Cholesterolemia (essential) (pure) E78.00
  familial E78.01
  hereditary E78.01
Cholesterolosis, cholesterosis (gallbladder) K82.4
  cerebrotendinous E75.5
Cholocolic fistula K82.3
Choluria R82.2
Chondritis M94.8X9

Ⓥ **Subterms under main terms may continue to next column or page**   ☑ **Additional Character Required** — Refer to the Tabular List for Character Selection   **53**

Change — Chondritis

Chondritis — *continued*
aurical H61.03- ☑
costal (Tietze's) M94.0
external ear H61.03- ☑
patella, posttraumatic — *see* Chondromalacia, patella
pinna H61.03- ☑
purulent M94.8X- ☑
tuberculous NEC A18.02
intervertebral A18.01
Chondroblastoma (*see also* Neoplasm, bone, benign)
malignant — *see* Neoplasm, bone, malignant
Chondrocalcinosis M11.20
ankle M11.27- ☑
elbow M11.22- ☑
familial M11.10
ankle M11.17- ☑
elbow M11.12- ☑
foot joint M11.17- ☑
hand joint M11.14- ☑
hip M11.15- ☑
knee M11.16- ☑
multiple site M11.19
shoulder M11.11- ☑
vertebrae M11.18
wrist M11.13- ☑
foot joint M11.27- ☑
hand joint M11.24- ☑
hip M11.25- ☑
knee M11.26- ☑
multiple site M11.29
shoulder M11.21- ☑
specified type NEC M11.20
ankle M11.27- ☑
elbow M11.22- ☑
foot joint M11.27- ☑
hand joint M11.24- ☑
hip M11.25- ☑
knee M11.26- ☑
multiple site M11.29
shoulder M11.21- ☑
vertebrae M11.28
wrist M11.23- ☑
vertebrae M11.28
wrist M11.23- ☑
Chondrodermatitis nodularis helicis or anthelicis
— *see* Perichondritis, ear
Chondrodysplasia Q78.9
with hemangioma Q78.4
calcificans congenita Q77.3
fetalis Q77.4
metaphyseal (Jansen's) (McKusick's) (Schmid's) Q78.8
punctata Q77.3
Chondrodystrophy, chondrodystrophia (familial)
(fetalis) (hypoplastic) Q78.9
calcificans congenita Q77.3
myotonic (congenital) G71.13
punctata Q77.3
Chondroectodermal dysplasia Q77.6
Chondrogenesis imperfecta Q77.4
Chondrolysis M94.35- ☑
Chondroma (*see also* Neoplasm, cartilage, benign)
juxtacortical — *see* Neoplasm, bone, benign
periosteal — *see* Neoplasm, bone, benign
Chondromalacia (systemic) M94.20
acromioclavicular joint M94.21- ☑
ankle M94.27- ☑
elbow M94.22- ☑
foot joint M94.27- ☑
glenohumeral joint M94.21- ☑
hand joint M94.24- ☑
hip M94.25- ☑
knee M94.26- ☑
patella M22.4- ☑
multiple sites M94.29
patella M22.4- ☑
rib M94.28
sacroiliac joint M94.259
shoulder M94.21- ☑
sternoclavicular joint M94.21- ☑
vertebral joint M94.28
wrist M94.23- ☑
Chondromatosis (*see also* Neoplasm, cartilage, uncertain behavior)
internal Q78.4
Chondromyxosarcoma — *see* Neoplasm, cartilage, malignant

Chondro-osteodysplasia (Morquio-Brailsford type) E76.219
Chondro-osteodystrophy E76.29
Chondro-osteoma — *see* Neoplasm, bone, benign
Chondropathia tuberosa M94.0
Chondrosarcoma — *see* Neoplasm, cartilage, malignant
juxtacortical — *see* Neoplasm, bone, malignant
mesenchymal — *see* Neoplasm, connective tissue, malignant
myxoid — *see* Neoplasm, cartilage, malignant
Chordee (nonvenereal) N48.89
congenital Q54.4
gonococcal A54.09
Chorditis (fibrinous) (nodosa) (tuberosa) J38.2
Chordoma — *see* Neoplasm, vertebral (column), malignant
Chorea (chronic) (gravis) (posthemiplegic) (senile) (spasmodic) G25.5
with
heart involvement I02.0
active or acute (conditions in I01-) I02.0
rheumatic I02.9
with valvular disorder I02.0
rheumatic heart disease (chronic) (inactive)(quiescent) — *code to* rheumatic heart condition involved
drug-induced G25.4
habit F95.8
hereditary G10
Huntington's G10
hysterical F44.4
minor I02.9
with heart involvement I02.0
progressive G25.5
hereditary G10
rheumatic (chronic) I02.9
with heart involvement I02.0
Sydenham's I02.9
with heart involvement — *see* Chorea, with rheumatic heart disease
nonrheumatic G25.5
Choreoathetosis (paroxysmal) G25.5
Chorioadenoma (destruens) D39.2
Chorioamnionitis O41.12- ☑
Chorioangioma D26.7
Choriocarcinoma — *see* Neoplasm, malignant, by site
combined with
embryonal carcinoma — *see* Neoplasm, malignant, by site
other germ cell elements — *see* Neoplasm, malignant, by site
teratoma — *see* Neoplasm, malignant, by site
specified site — *see* Neoplasm, malignant, by site
unspecified site
female C58
male C62.90
Chorioencephalitis (acute) (lymphocytic) (serous) A87.2
Chorioepithelioma — *see* Choriocarcinoma
Choriomeningitis (acute) (lymphocytic) (serous) A87.2
Chorionepithelioma — *see* Choriocarcinoma
Chorioretinitis (*see also* Inflammation, chorioretinal)
disseminated (*see also* Inflammation, chorioretinal, disseminated)
in neurosyphilis A52.19
Egyptian B76.9 [D63.8]
focal (*see also* Inflammation, chorioretinal, focal)
histoplasmic B39.9 [H32]
in (due to)
histoplasmosis B39.9 [H32]
syphilis (secondary) A51.43
late A52.71
toxoplasmosis (acquired) B58.01
congenital (active) P37.1 [H32]
tuberculosis A18.53
juxtapapillary, juxtapapillaris — *see* Inflammation, chorioretinal, focal, juxtapapillary
leprous A30.9 [H32]
miner's B76.9 [D63.8]
progressive myopia (degeneration) (*see also* Myopia, degenerative) H44.2- ☑
syphilitic (secondary) A51.43
congenital (early) A50.01 [H32]
late A50.32
late A52.71
tuberculous A18.53
Chorioretinopathy, central serous H35.71- ☑
Choroid — *see* condition
Choroideremia H31.21

Choroiditis — *see* Chorioretinitis
Choroidopathy — *see* Disorder, choroid
Choroidoretinitis — *see* Chorioretinitis
Choroidoretinopathy, central serous — *see* Chorioretinopathy, central serous
Christian-Weber disease M35.6
Christmas disease D67
Chromaffinoma (*see also* Neoplasm, benign, by site)
malignant — *see* Neoplasm, malignant, by site
Chromatopsia — *see* Deficiency, color vision
Chromhidrosis, chromidrosis L75.1
Chromoblastomycosis — *see* Chromomycosis
Chromoconversion R82.91
Chromomycosis B43.9
brain abscess B43.1
cerebral B43.1
cutaneous B43.0
skin B43.0
specified NEC B43.8
subcutaneous abscess or cyst B43.2
Chromophytosis B36.0
Chromosome — *see* Anomaly, by chromosome involved
D (1) — *see* Anomaly, chromosome 13
E (3) — *see* Anomaly, chromosome 18
G — *see* Anomaly, chromosome 21
Chromotrichomycosis B36.8
Chronic — *see* condition
fracture — *see* Fracture, pathological
Churg-Strauss syndrome M30.1
Chyle cyst, mesentery I89.8
Chylocele (nonfilarial) I89.8
filarial (*see also* Infestation, filarial) B74.9 [N51]
tunica vaginalis N50.89
filarial (*see also* Infestation, filarial) B74.9 [N51]
Chylomicronemia (fasting) (with hyperprebetalipoproteinemia) E78.3
Chylopericardium I31.3
acute I30.9
Chylothorax (nonfilarial) I89.8
filarial (*see also* Infestation, filarial) B74.9 [J91.8]
Chylous — *see* condition
Chyluria (nonfilarial) R82.0
due to
bilharziasis B65.0
Brugia (malayi) B74.1
timori B74.2
schistosomiasis (bilharziasis) B65.0
Wuchereria (bancrofti) B74.0
filarial — *see* Infestation, filarial
Cicatricial (deformity) — *see* Cicatrix
Cicatrix (adherent) (contracted) (painful) (vicious) (*see also* Scar) L90.5
adenoid (and tonsil) J35.8
alveolar process M26.79
anus K62.89
auricle — *see* Disorder, pinna, specified type NEC
bile duct (common) (hepatic) K83.8
bladder N32.89
bone — *see* Disorder, bone, specified type NEC
brain G93.89
cervix (postoperative) (postpartal) N88.1
common duct K83.8
cornea H17.9
tuberculous A18.59
duodenum (bulb), obstructive K31.5
esophagus K22.2
eyelid — *see* Disorder, eyelid function
hypopharynx J39.2
lacrimal passages — *see* Obstruction, lacrimal
larynx J38.7
lung J98.4
middle ear H74.8 ☑
mouth K13.79
muscle M62.89
with contracture — *see* Contraction, muscle NEC
nasopharynx J39.2
palate (soft) K13.79
penis N48.89
pharynx J39.2
prostate N42.89
rectum K62.89
retina — *see* Scar, chorioretinal
semilunar cartilage — *see* Derangement, meniscus
seminal vesicle N50.89
skin L90.5
infected L08.89
postinfective L90.5

☑ **Additional Character Required** — Refer to the Tabular List for Character Selection   ▽ Subterms under main terms may continue to next column or page

Cicatrix — *continued*
  skin — *continued*
    tuberculous B90.8
    specified site NEC L90.5
  throat J39.2
  tongue K14.8
  tonsil (and adenoid) J35.8
  trachea J39.8
  tuberculous NEC B90.9
  urethra N36.8
  uterus N85.8
  vagina N89.8
    postoperative N99.2
  vocal cord J38.3
  wrist, constricting (annular) L90.5
CIDP (chronic inflammatory demyelinating polyneuropathy) G61.81
CIN — *see* Neoplasia, intraepithelial, cervix
CINCA (chronic infantile neurological, cutaneous and articular syndrome) M04.2
Cinchonism — *see* Deafness, ototoxic
  correct substance properly administered — *see* Table of Drugs and Chemicals, by drug, adverse effect
  overdose or wrong substance given or taken — *see* Table of Drugs and Chemicals, by drug, poisoning
Circle of Willis — *see* condition
Circular — *see* condition
Circulating anticoagulants (*see also* Disorder, hemorrhagic) D68.318
  due to drugs (*see also* Disorder, hemorrhagic) D68.32
  following childbirth O72.3
Circulation
  collateral, any site I99.8
  defective (lower extremity) I99.9
    congenital Q28.9
  embryonic Q28.9
  failure (peripheral) R57.9
    newborn P29.89
  fetal, persistent P29.38
  heart, incomplete Q28.9
Circulatory system — *see* condition
Circulus senilis (cornea) — *see* Degeneration, cornea, senile
Circumcision (in absence of medical indication) (ritual) (routine) Z41.2
Circumscribed — *see* condition
Circumvallate placenta O43.11- ☑
Cirrhosis, cirrhotic (hepatic) (liver) K74.60
  alcoholic K70.30
    with ascites K70.31
  atrophic — *see* Cirrhosis, liver
  Baumgarten-Cruveilhier K74.69
  biliary (cholangiolitic) (cholangitic) (hypertrophic) (obstructive) (pericholangiolitic) K74.5
    due to
      Clonorchiasis B66.1
      flukes B66.3
    primary K74.3
    secondary K74.4
  cardiac (of liver) K76.1
  Charcot's K74.3
  cholangiolitic, cholangitic, cholostatic (primary) K74.3
  congestive K76.1
  Cruveilhier-Baumgarten K74.69
  cryptogenic (liver) K74.69
  due to
    hepatolenticular degeneration E83.01
    Wilson's disease E83.01
    xanthomatosis E78.2
  fatty K76.0
    alcoholic K70.0
  Hanot's (hypertrophic) K74.3
  hepatic — *see* Cirrhosis, liver
  hypertrophic K74.3
  Indian childhood K74.69
  kidney — *see* Sclerosis, renal
  Laennec's K70.30
    with ascites K70.31
    alcoholic K70.30
      with ascites K70.31
    nonalcoholic K74.69
  liver K74.60
    alcoholic K70.30
      with ascites K70.31
      fatty K70.0
    congenital P78.81
    syphilitic A52.74

Cirrhosis, cirrhotic — *continued*
  lung (chronic) J84.10
  macronodular K74.69
    alcoholic K70.30
      with ascites K70.31
  micronodular K74.69
    alcoholic K70.30
      with ascites K70.31
  mixed type K74.69
  monolobular K74.3
  nephritis — *see* Sclerosis, renal
  nutritional K74.69
    alcoholic K70.30
      with ascites K70.31
  obstructive — *see* Cirrhosis, biliary
  ovarian N83.8
  pancreas (duct) K86.89
  pigmentary E83.110
  portal K74.69
    alcoholic K70.30
      with ascites K70.31
  postnecrotic K74.69
    alcoholic K70.30
      with ascites K70.31
  pulmonary J84.10
  renal — *see* Sclerosis, renal
  spleen D73.2
  stasis K76.1
  Todd's K74.3
  unilobar K74.3
  xanthomatous (biliary) K74.5
    due to xanthomatosis (familial) (metabolic) (primary) E78.2
Cistern, subarachnoid R93.0
Citrullinemia E72.23
Citrullinuria E72.23
Civatte's disease or poikiloderma L57.3
Clam digger's itch B65.3
Clammy skin R23.1
Clap — *see* Gonorrhea
Clarke-Hadfield syndrome (pancreatic infantilism) K86.89
Clark's paralysis G80.9
Clastothrix L67.8
Claude Bernard-Horner syndrome G90.2
  traumatic — *see* Injury, nerve, cervical sympathetic
Claude's disease or syndrome G46.3
Claudicatio venosa intermittens I87.8
Claudication (intermittent) I73.9
  cerebral (artery) G45.9
  spinal cord (arteriosclerotic) G95.19
    syphilitic A52.09
  venous (axillary) I87.8
Claustrophobia F40.240
Clavus (infected) L84
Clawfoot (congenital) Q66.89
  acquired — *see* Deformity, limb, clawfoot
Clawhand (acquired) (*see also* Deformity, limb, clawhand)
  congenital Q68.1
Clawtoe (congenital) Q66.89
  acquired — *see* Deformity, toe, specified NEC
Clay eating — *see* Pica
Cleansing of artificial opening — *see* Attention to, artificial, opening
Cleft (congenital) — *see also* Imperfect, closure
  alveolar process M26.79
  branchial (persistent) Q18.2
    cyst Q18.0
      fistula Q18.0
      sinus Q18.0
  cricoid cartilage, posterior Q31.8
  cyst Q18.0
    fistula Q18.0
    sinus Q18.0
  foot Q72.7 ☑
  hand Q71.6 ☑
  lip (unilateral) Q36.9
    with cleft palate Q37.9
      hard Q37.1
        with soft Q37.5
      soft Q37.3
        with hard Q37.5
    bilateral Q36.0
      with cleft palate Q37.8
        hard Q37.0
          with soft Q37.4
        soft Q37.2
          with hard Q37.4

Cleft — *continued*
  lip — *continued*
    median Q36.1
  nose Q30.2
  palate Q35.9
    with cleft lip (unilateral) Q37.9
      bilateral Q37.8
    hard Q35.1
      with
        cleft lip (unilateral) Q37.1
          bilateral Q37.0
        soft Q35.5
          with cleft lip (unilateral) Q37.5
            bilateral Q37.4
    medial Q35.5
    soft Q35.3
      with
        cleft lip (unilateral) Q37.3
          bilateral Q37.2
        hard Q35.5
          with cleft lip (unilateral) Q37.5
            bilateral Q37.4
  penis Q55.69
  scrotum Q55.29
  thyroid cartilage Q31.8
  uvula Q35.7
Cleidocranial dysostosis Q74.0
Cleptomania F63.2
Clicking hip (newborn) R29.4
Climacteric (female) (*see also* Menopause)
  arthritis (any site) NEC — *see* Arthritis, specified form NEC
  depression (single episode) F32.89
    recurrent episode F33.8
  male (symptoms) (syndrome) NEC N50.89
  melancholia (single episode) F32.89
    recurrent episode F33.8
  paranoid state F22
  polyarthritis NEC — *see* Arthritis, specified form NEC
  symptoms (female) N95.1
Clinical research investigation (clinical trial) (control subject) (normal comparison) (participant) Z00.6
Clitoris — *see* condition
Cloaca (persistent) Q43.7
Clonorchiasis, clonorchis infection (liver) B66.1
Clonus R25.8
Closed bite M26.29
Clostridium (C.) **perfringens, as cause of disease classified elsewhere** B96.7
Closure
  congenital, nose Q30.0
  cranial sutures, premature Q75.0
  defective or imperfect NEC — *see* Imperfect, closure
  fistula, delayed — *see* Fistula
  foramen ovale, imperfect Q21.1
  hymen N89.6
  interauricular septum, defective Q21.1
  interventricular septum, defective Q21.0
  lacrimal duct (*see also* Stenosis, lacrimal, duct)
    congenital Q10.5
  nose (congenital) Q30.0
    acquired M95.0
  of artificial opening — *see* Attention to, artificial, opening
  vagina N89.5
  valve — *see* Endocarditis
  vulva N90.5
Clot (blood) (*see also* Embolism)
  artery (obstruction) (occlusion) — *see* Embolism
  bladder N32.89
  brain (intradural or extradural) — *see* Occlusion, artery, cerebral
  circulation I74.9
  heart (*see also* Infarct, myocardium)
    not resulting in infarction I51.3
  vein — *see* Thrombosis
Clouded state R40.1
  epileptic — *see* Epilepsy, specified NEC
  paroxysmal — *see* Epilepsy, specified NEC
Cloudy antrum, antra J32.0
Clouston's (hidrotic) **ectodermal dysplasia** Q82.4
Clubbed nail pachydermoperiostosis M89.40 [L62]
Clubbing of finger(s) (nails) R68.3
Clubfinger R68.3
  congenital Q68.1
Clubfoot (congenital) Q66.89
  acquired — *see* Deformity, limb, clubfoot
  equinovarus Q66.0

⬆ **Subterms under main terms may continue to next column or page**   ☑ **Additional Character Required** — **Refer to the Tabular List for Character Selection**   **55**

Cicatrix — Clubfoot

Clubfoot — *continued*
paralytic — *see* Deformity, limb, clubfoot
Clubhand (congenital) (radial) Q71.4- ☑
acquired — *see* Deformity, limb, clubhand
Clubnail R68.3
congenital Q84.6
Clump, kidney Q63.1
Clumsiness, clumsy child syndrome F82
Cluttering F80.81
Clutton's joints A50.51 [M12.80]
Coagulation, intravascular (diffuse) (disseminated)
(*see also* Defibrination syndrome)
complicating abortion — *see* Abortion, by type, complicated by, intravascular coagulation
following ectopic or molar pregnancy O08.1
Coagulopathy (*see also* Defect, coagulation)
consumption D65
intravascular D65
newborn P60
Coalition
calcaneo-scaphoid Q66.89
tarsal Q66.89
Coalminer's
elbow — *see* Bursitis, elbow, olecranon
lung or pneumoconiosis J60
Coalworker's lung or pneumoconiosis J60
Coarctation
aorta (preductal) (postductal) Q25.1
pulmonary artery Q25.71
Coated tongue K14.3
Coats' disease (exudative retinopathy) — *see*
Retinopathy, exudative
Cocaine-induced
anxiety disorder F14.980
bipolar and related disorder F14.94
depressive disorder F14.94
obsessive-compulsive and related disorder F14.988
psychotic disorder F14.959
sexual dysfunction F14.981
sleep disorder F14.982
Cocainism — *see* Disorder, cocaine use
Coccidioidomycosis B38.9
cutaneous B38.3
disseminated B38.7
generalized B38.7
meninges B38.4
prostate B38.81
pulmonary B38.2
acute B38.0
chronic B38.1
skin B38.3
specified NEC B38.89
Coccidioidosis — *see* Coccidioidomycosis
Coccidiosis (intestinal) A07.3
Coccydynia, coccygodynia M53.3
Coccyx — *see* condition
Cochin-China diarrhea K90.1
Cockayne's syndrome Q87.1
Cocked up toe — *see* Deformity, toe, specified NEC
Cock's peculiar tumor L72.3
Codman's tumor — *see* Neoplasm, bone, benign
Coenurosis B71.8
Coffee-worker's lung J67.8
Cogan's syndrome H16.32- ☑
oculomotor apraxia H51.8
Coitus, painful (female) N94.10
male N53.12
psychogenic F52.6
Cold J00
with influenza, flu, or grippe — *see* Influenza, with, respiratory manifestations NEC
agglutinin disease or hemoglobinuria (chronic) D59.1
bronchial — *see* Bronchitis
chest — *see* Bronchitis
common (head) J00
effects of T69.9 ☑
specified effect NEC T69.8 ☑
excessive, effects of T69.9 ☑
specified effect NEC T69.8 ☑
exhaustion from T69.8 ☑
exposure to T69.9 ☑
specified effect NEC T69.8 ☑
head J00
injury syndrome (newborn) P80.0
on lung — *see* Bronchitis
rose J30.1
sensitivity, auto-immune D59.1

Cold — *continued*
symptoms J00
virus J00
Coldsore B00.1
Colibacillosis A49.8
as the cause of other disease (*see also* Escherichia coli)
B96.20
generalized A41.50
Colic (bilious) (infantile) (intestinal) (recurrent) (spasmodic) R10.83
abdomen R10.83
psychogenic F45.8
appendix, appendicular K38.8
bile duct — *see* Calculus, bile duct
biliary — *see* Calculus, bile duct
common duct — *see* Calculus, bile duct
cystic duct — *see* Calculus, gallbladder
Devonshire NEC — *see* Poisoning, lead
gallbladder — *see* Calculus, gallbladder
gallstone — *see* Calculus, gallbladder
gallbladder or cystic duct — *see* Calculus, gallbladder
hepatic (duct) — *see* Calculus, bile duct
hysterical F45.8
kidney N23
lead NEC — *see* Poisoning, lead
mucous K58.9
with diarrhea K58.0
psychogenic F54
nephritic N23
painter's NEC — *see* Poisoning, lead
pancreas K86.89
psychogenic F45.8
renal N23
saturnine NEC — *see* Poisoning, lead
ureter N23
urethral N36.8
due to calculus N21.1
uterus NEC N94.89
menstrual — *see* Dysmenorrhea
worm NOS B83.9
Colicystitis — *see* Cystitis
Colitis (acute) (catarrhal) (chronic) (noninfective) (hemorrhagic) (*see also* Enteritis) K52.9
allergic K52.29
with
food protein-induced enterocolitis syndrome K52.21
proctocolitis K52.82
amebic (acute) (*see also* Amebiasis) A06.0
nondysenteric A06.2
anthrax A22.2
bacillary — *see* Infection, Shigella
balantidial A07.0
Clostridium difficile
not specified as recurrent A04.72
recurrent A04.71
coccidial A07.3
collagenous K52.831
cystica superficialis K52.89
dietary counseling and surveillance (for) Z71.3
dietetic (*see also* Colitis, allergic) K52.29
drug-induced K52.1
due to radiation K52.0
eosinophilic K52.82
food hypersensitivity (*see also* Colitis, allergic) K52.29
giardial A07.1
granulomatous — *see* Enteritis, regional, large intestine
indeterminate, so stated K52.3
infectious — *see* Enteritis, infectious
ischemic K55.9
acute (subacute) (*see also* Ischemia, intestine, acute) K55.039
chronic K55.1
due to mesenteric artery insufficiency K55.1
fulminant (acute) (*see also* Ischemia, intestine, acute) K55.039
left sided K51.50
with
abscess K51.514
complication K51.519
specified NEC K51.518
fistula K51.513
obstruction K51.512
rectal bleeding K51.511
lymphocytic K52.832

Colitis — *continued*
membranous
psychogenic F54
microscopic K52.839
specified NEC K52.838
mucous — *see* Syndrome, irritable, bowel
psychogenic F54
noninfective K52.9
specified NEC K52.89
polyposa — *see* Polyp, colon, inflammatory
protozoal A07.9
pseudomembranous
not specified as recurrent A04.72
recurrent A04.71
pseudomucinous — *see* Syndrome, irritable, bowel
regional — *see* Enteritis, regional, large intestine
infectious A09
segmental — *see* Enteritis, regional, large intestine
septic — *see* Enteritis, infectious
spastic K58.9
with diarrhea K58.0
psychogenic F54
staphylococcal A04.8
foodborne A05.0
subacute ischemic (*see also* Ischemia, intestine, acute)
K55.039
thromboulcerative (*see also* Ischemia, intestine, acute)
K55.039
toxic NEC K52.1
due to Clostridium difficile
not specified as recurrent A04.72
recurrent A04.71
transmural — *see* Enteritis, regional, large intestine
trichomonal A07.8
tuberculous (ulcerative) A18.32
ulcerative (chronic) K51.90
with
complication K51.919
abscess K51.914
fistula K51.913
obstruction K51.912
rectal bleeding K51.911
specified complication NEC K51.918
enterocolitis — *see* Enterocolitis, ulcerative
ileocolitis — *see* Ileocolitis, ulcerative
mucosal proctocolitis — *see* Proctocolitis, mucosal
proctitis — *see* Proctitis, ulcerative
pseudopolyposis — *see* Polyp, colon, inflammatory
psychogenic F54
rectosigmoiditis — *see* Rectosigmoiditis, ulcerative
specified type NEC K51.80
with
complication K51.819
abscess K51.814
fistula K51.813
obstruction K51.812
rectal bleeding K51.811
specified complication NEC K51.818
Collagenosis, collagen disease (nonvascular) (vascular)
M35.9
cardiovascular I42.8
reactive perforating L87.1
specified NEC M35.8
Collapse R55
adrenal E27.2
cardiorespiratory R57.0
cardiovascular R57.0
newborn P29.89
circulatory (peripheral) R57.9
during or after labor and delivery O75.1
following ectopic or molar pregnancy O08.3
newborn P29.89
during or
after labor and delivery O75.1
resulting from a procedure, not elsewhere classified T81.10 ☑
external ear canal — *see* Stenosis, external ear canal
general R55
heart — *see* Disease, heart
heat T67.1 ☑
hysterical F44.89
labyrinth, membranous (congenital) Q16.5
lung (massive) (*see also* Atelectasis) J98.19
pressure due to anesthesia (general) (local) or other sedation T88.2
during labor and delivery O74.1
in pregnancy O29.02- ☑
postpartum, puerperal O89.09

Collapse — continued
  myocardial — see Disease, heart
  nervous F48.8
  neurocirculatory F45.8
  nose M95.0
  postoperative T81.10 ☑
  pulmonary (see also Atelectasis) J98.19
    newborn — see Atelectasis
  trachea J39.8
  tracheobronchial J98.09
  valvular — see Endocarditis
  vascular (peripheral) R57.9
    during or after labor and delivery O75.1
    following ectopic or molar pregnancy O08.3
    newborn P29.89
  vertebra M48.50- ☑
    cervical region M48.52- ☑
    cervicothoracic region M48.53- ☑
    in (due to)
        metastasis — see Collapse, vertebra, in, speci-
          fied disease NEC
        osteoporosis (see also Osteoporosis) M80.88 ☑
          cervical region M80.88 ☑
          cervicothoracic region M80.88 ☑
          lumbar region M80.88 ☑
          lumbosacral region M80.88 ☑
          multiple sites M80.88 ☑
          occipito-atlanto-axial region M80.88 ☑
          sacrococcygeal region M80.88 ☑
          thoracic region M80.88 ☑
          thoracolumbar region M80.88 ☑
        specified disease NEC M48.50- ☑
          cervical region M48.52- ☑
          cervicothoracic region M48.53- ☑
          lumbar region M48.56- ☑
          lumbosacral region M48.57- ☑
          occipito-atlanto-axial region M48.51- ☑
          sacrococcygeal region M48.58- ☑
          thoracic region M48.54- ☑
          thoracolumbar region M48.55- ☑
    lumbar region M48.56- ☑
    lumbosacral region M48.57- ☑
    occipito-atlanto-axial region M48.51- ☑
    sacrococcygeal region M48.58- ☑
    thoracic region M48.54- ☑
    thoracolumbar region M48.55- ☑
Collateral (see also condition)
  circulation (venous) I87.8
  dilation, veins I87.8
Colles' fracture S52.53- ☑
Collet (-Sicard) syndrome G52.7
Collier's asthma or lung J60
Collodion baby Q80.2
Colloid nodule (of thyroid) (cystic) E04.1
Coloboma (iris) Q13.0
  eyelid Q10.3
  fundus Q14.8
  lens Q12.2
  optic disc (congenital) Q14.2
    acquired H47.31- ☑
Coloenteritis — see Enteritis
Colon — see condition
Colonization
  MRSA (Methicillin resistant Staphylococcus aureus)
    Z22.322
  MSSA (Methicillin susceptible Staphylococcus aureus)
    Z22.321
  status — see Carrier (suspected) of
Coloptosis K63.4
Color blindness — see Deficiency, color vision
Colostomy
  attention to Z43.3
  fitting or adjustment Z46.89
  malfunctioning K94.03
  status Z93.3
Colpitis (acute) — see Vaginitis
Colpocele N81.5
Colpocystitis — see Vaginitis
Colpospasm N94.2
Column, spinal, vertebral — see condition
Coma R40.20
  with
    motor response (none) R40.231 ☑
      abnormal extensor posturing to pain or noxious
        stimuli (< 2 years of age) R40.232 ☑
      abnormal flexure posturing to pain or noxious
        stimuli (0-5 years of age) R40.233 ☑

Coma — continued
  with — continued
    motor response — continued
      extensor posturing to pain or noxious stimuli
        (2-5 years of age) R40.232 ☑
      flexion/decorticate posturing (< 2 years of age)
        R40.233 ☑
      localizes pain (2-5 years of age) R40.235 ☑
      normal or spontaneous movement (< 2 years
        of age) R40.236 ☑
      obeys commands (2-5 years of age) R40.236 ☑
      withdraws from pain or noxious stimuli (0-5
        years of age) R40.234 ☑
      withdraws to touch (< 2 years of age)
        R40.235 ☑
    opening of eyes (never) R40.211 ☑
      in response to
        pain R40.212 ☑
        sound R40.213 ☑
      spontaneous R40.214 ☑
    verbal response (none) R40.221 ☑
      confused conversation R40.224 ☑
      cooing or babbling or crying appropriately
        (< 2 years of age) R40.225 ☑
      inappropriate crying or screaming (< 2 years of
        age) R40.223 ☑
      inappropriate words (2-5 years of age)
        R40.224 ☑
      incomprehensible sounds (2-5 years of age)
        R40.222 ☑
      incomprehensible words R40.222 ☑
      irritable cries (< 2 years of age) R40.224 ☑
      moans/grunts to pain; restless (< 2 years old)
        R40.222 ☑
      oriented R40.225 ☑
      screaming (2-5 years of age) R40.223 ☑
      uses appropriate words (2-5 years of age)
        R40.225 ☑
  eclamptic — see Eclampsia
  epileptic — see Epilepsy
  Glasgow, scale score — see Glasgow coma scale
  hepatic — see Failure, hepatic, by type, with coma
  hyperglycemic (diabetic) — see Diabetes, by type,
    with hyperosmolarity, with coma
  hyperosmolar (diabetic) — see Diabetes, by type, with
    hyperosmolarity, with coma
  hypoglycemic (diabetic) — see Diabetes, by type, with
    hypoglycemia, with coma
    nondiabetic E15
  in diabetes — see Diabetes, coma
  insulin-induced — see Coma, hypoglycemic
  ketoacidotic (diabetic) — see Diabetes, by type, with
    ketoacidosis, with coma
  myxedematous E03.5
  newborn P91.5
  persistent vegetative state R40.3
  specified NEC, without documented Glasgow coma
    scale score, or with partial Glasgow coma scale
    score reported R40.244 ☑
Comatose — see Coma
Combat fatigue F43.0
Combined — see condition
Comedo, comedones (giant) L70.0
Comedocarcinoma (see also Neoplasm, breast, malignant)
  noninfiltrating
    breast D05.8- ☑
    specified site — see Neoplasm, in situ, by site
    unspecified site D05.8- ☑
Comedomastitis — see Ectasia, mammary duct
Comminuted fracture — code as Fracture, closed
Common
  arterial trunk Q20.0
  atrioventricular canal Q21.2
  atrium Q21.1
  cold (head) J00
  truncus (arteriosus) Q20.0
  variable immunodeficiency — see Immunodeficiency,
    common variable
  ventricle Q20.4
Commotio, commotion (current)
  brain — see Injury, intracranial, concussion
  cerebri — see Injury, intracranial, concussion
  retinae S05.8X- ☑
  spinal cord — see Injury, spinal cord, by region
  spinalis — see Injury, spinal cord, by region

Communication
  between
    base of aorta and pulmonary artery Q21.4
    left ventricle and right atrium Q20.5
    pericardial sac and pleural sac Q34.8
    pulmonary artery and pulmonary vein, congenital
      Q25.72
  congenital between uterus and digestive or urinary
    tract Q51.7
Compartment syndrome (deep) (posterior) (traumatic)
  T79.A0 ☑ (following T79.7)
  abdomen T79.A3 ☑ (following T79.7)
  lower extremity (hip, buttock, thigh, leg, foot, toes)
    T79.A2 ☑ (following T79.7)
  nontraumatic
    abdomen M79.A3 (following M79.7)
    lower extremity (hip, buttock, thigh, leg, foot, toes)
      M79.A2- ☑ (following M79.7)
    specified site NEC M79.A9 (following M79.7)
    upper extremity (shoulder, arm, forearm, wrist,
      hand, fingers) M79.A1- ☑ (following M79.7)
  specified site NEC T79.A9 ☑ (following T79.7)
  upper extremity (shoulder, arm, forearm, wrist, hand,
    fingers) T79.A1- ☑ (following T79.7)
Compensation
  failure — see Disease, heart
  neurosis, psychoneurosis — see Disorder, factitious
Complaint (see also Disease)
  bowel, functional K59.9
    psychogenic F45.8
  intestine, functional K59.9
    psychogenic F45.8
  kidney — see Disease, renal
  miners' J60
Complete — see condition
Complex
  Addison-Schilder E71.528
  cardiorenal — see Hypertension, cardiorenal
  Costen's M26.69
  disseminated mycobacterium avium- intracellulare
    (DMAC) A31.2
  Eisenmenger's (ventricular septal defect) I27.83
  hypersexual F52.8
  jumped process, spine — see Dislocation, vertebra
  primary, tuberculous A15.7
  Schilder-Addison E71.528
  subluxation (vertebral) M99.19
    abdomen M99.19
    acromioclavicular M99.17
    cervical region M99.11
    cervicothoracic M99.11
    costochondral M99.18
    costovertebral M99.18
    head region M99.10
    hip M99.15
    lower extremity M99.16
    lumbar region M99.13
    lumbosacral M99.13
    occipitocervical M99.10
    pelvic region M99.15
    pubic M99.15
    rib cage M99.18
    sacral region M99.14
    sacrococcygeal M99.14
    sacroiliac M99.14
    specified NEC M99.19
    sternochondral M99.18
    sternoclavicular M99.17
    thoracic region M99.12
    thoracolumbar M99.12
    upper extremity M99.17
  Taussig-Bing (transposition, aorta and overriding pul-
    monary artery) Q20.1
Complication(s) (from) (of)
  accidental puncture or laceration during a procedure
    (of) — see Complications, intraoperative (in-
    traprocedural), puncture or laceration
  amputation stump (surgical) (late) NEC T87.9
    dehiscence T87.81
    infection or inflammation T87.40
      lower limb T87.4- ☑
      upper limb T87.4- ☑
    necrosis T87.50
      lower limb T87.5- ☑
      upper limb T87.5- ☑
    neuroma T87.30
      lower limb T87.3- ☑
      upper limb T87.3- ☑

Complication(s) — *continued*
- amputation stump — *continued*
  - specified type NEC T87.89
- anastomosis (and bypass) (*see also* Complications, prosthetic device or implant)
  - intestinal (internal) NEC K91.89
    - involving urinary tract N99.89
  - urinary tract (involving intestinal tract) N99.89
  - vascular — *see* Complications, cardiovascular device or implant
- anesthesia, anesthetic (*see also* Anesthesia, complication) T88.59 ☑
  - brain, postpartum, puerperal O89.2
  - cardiac
    - in
      - labor and delivery O74.2
      - pregnancy O29.19- ☑
    - postpartum, puerperal O89.1
  - central nervous system
    - in
      - labor and delivery O74.3
      - pregnancy O29.29- ☑
    - postpartum, puerperal O89.2
  - difficult or failed intubation T88.4 ☑
    - in pregnancy O29.6- ☑
  - failed sedation (conscious) (moderate) during procedure T88.52 ☑
  - general, unintended awareness during procedure T88.53 ☑
  - hyperthermia, malignant T88.3 ☑
  - hypothermia T88.51 ☑
  - intubation failure T88.4 ☑
  - malignant hyperthermia T88.3 ☑
  - pulmonary
    - in
      - labor and delivery O74.1
      - pregnancy NEC O29.09- ☑
    - postpartum, puerperal O89.09
  - shock T88.2 ☑
  - spinal and epidural
    - in
      - labor and delivery NEC O74.6
        - headache O74.5
      - pregnancy NEC O29.5X- ☑
    - postpartum, puerperal NEC O89.5
      - headache O89.4
  - unintended awareness under general anesthesia during procedure T88.53 ☑
- anti-reflux device — *see* Complications, esophageal anti-reflux device
- aortic (bifurcation) graft — *see* Complications, graft, vascular
- aortocoronary (bypass) graft — *see* Complications, coronary artery (bypass) graft
- aortofemoral (bypass) graft — *see* Complications, extremity artery (bypass) graft
- arteriovenous
  - fistula, surgically created T82.9 ☑
    - embolism T82.818 ☑
    - fibrosis T82.828 ☑
    - hemorrhage T82.838 ☑
    - infection or inflammation T82.7 ☑
    - mechanical
      - breakdown T82.510 ☑
      - displacement T82.520 ☑
      - leakage T82.530 ☑
      - malposition T82.520 ☑
      - obstruction T82.590 ☑
      - perforation T82.590 ☑
      - protrusion T82.590 ☑
    - pain T82.848 ☑
    - specified type NEC T82.898 ☑
    - stenosis T82.858 ☑
    - thrombosis T82.868 ☑
  - shunt, surgically created T82.9 ☑
    - embolism T82.818 ☑
    - fibrosis T82.828 ☑
    - hemorrhage T82.838 ☑
    - infection or inflammation T82.7 ☑
    - mechanical
      - breakdown T82.511 ☑
      - displacement T82.521 ☑
      - leakage T82.531 ☑
      - malposition T82.521 ☑
      - obstruction T82.591 ☑
      - perforation T82.591 ☑
      - protrusion T82.591 ☑

Complication(s) — *continued*
- arteriovenous — *continued*
  - shunt, surgically created — *continued*
    - pain T82.848 ☑
    - specified type NEC T82.898 ☑
    - stenosis T82.858 ☑
    - thrombosis T82.868 ☑
- arthroplasty — *see* Complications, joint prosthesis
- artificial
  - fertilization or insemination N98.9
    - attempted introduction (of)
      - embryo in embryo transfer N98.3
      - ovum following in vitro fertilization N98.2
    - hyperstimulation of ovaries N98.1
    - infection N98.0
    - specified NEC N98.8
  - heart T82.9 ☑
    - embolism T82.817 ☑
    - fibrosis T82.827 ☑
    - hemorrhage T82.837 ☑
    - infection or inflammation T82.7 ☑
    - mechanical
      - breakdown T82.512 ☑
      - displacement T82.522 ☑
      - leakage T82.532 ☑
      - malposition T82.522 ☑
      - obstruction T82.592 ☑
      - perforation T82.592 ☑
      - protrusion T82.592 ☑
    - pain T82.847 ☑
    - specified type NEC T82.897 ☑
    - stenosis T82.857 ☑
    - thrombosis T82.867 ☑
  - opening
    - cecostomy — *see* Complications, colostomy
    - colostomy — *see* Complications, colostomy
    - cystostomy — *see* Complications, cystostomy
    - enterostomy — *see* Complications, enterostomy
    - gastrostomy — *see* Complications, gastrostomy
    - ileostomy — *see* Complications, enterostomy
    - jejunostomy — *see* Complications, enterostomy
    - nephrostomy — *see* Complications, stoma, urinary tract
    - tracheostomy — *see* Complications, tracheostomy
    - ureterostomy — *see* Complications, stoma, urinary tract
    - urethrostomy — *see* Complications, stoma, urinary tract
- balloon implant or device
  - gastrointestinal T85.9 ☑
    - embolism T85.818 ☑
    - fibrosis T85.828 ☑
    - hemorrhage T85.838 ☑
    - infection and inflammation T85.79 ☑
    - pain T85.848 ☑
    - specified type NEC T85.898 ☑
    - stenosis T85.858 ☑
    - thrombosis T85.868 ☑
  - vascular (counterpulsation) T82.9 ☑
    - embolism T82.818 ☑
    - fibrosis T82.828 ☑
    - hemorrhage T82.838 ☑
    - infection or inflammation T82.7 ☑
    - mechanical
      - breakdown T82.513 ☑
      - displacement T82.523 ☑
      - leakage T82.533 ☑
      - malposition T82.523 ☑
      - obstruction T82.593 ☑
      - perforation T82.593 ☑
      - protrusion T82.593 ☑
    - pain T82.848 ☑
    - specified type NEC T82.898 ☑
    - stenosis T82.858 ☑
    - thrombosis T82.868 ☑
- bariatric procedure
  - gastric band procedure K95.09
    - infection K95.01
  - specified procedure NEC K95.89
    - infection K95.81
- bile duct implant (prosthetic) T85.9 ☑
  - embolism T85.818 ☑
  - fibrosis T85.828 ☑
  - hemorrhage T85.838 ☑

Complication(s) — *continued*
- bile duct implant — *continued*
  - infection and inflammation T85.79 ☑
  - mechanical
    - breakdown T85.510 ☑
    - displacement T85.520 ☑
    - malfunction T85.510 ☑
    - malposition T85.520 ☑
    - obstruction T85.590 ☑
    - perforation T85.590 ☑
    - protrusion T85.590 ☑
    - specified NEC T85.590 ☑
  - pain T85.848 ☑
  - specified type NEC T85.898 ☑
  - stenosis T85.858 ☑
  - thrombosis T85.868 ☑
- bladder device (auxiliary) — *see* Complications, genitourinary, device or implant, urinary system
- bleeding (postoperative) — *see* Complication, postoperative, hemorrhage
  - intraoperative — *see* Complication, intraoperative, hemorrhage
- blood vessel graft — *see* Complications, graft, vascular
- bone
  - device NEC T84.9 ☑
    - embolism T84.81 ☑
    - fibrosis T84.82 ☑
    - hemorrhage T84.83 ☑
    - infection or inflammation T84.7 ☑
    - mechanical
      - breakdown T84.318 ☑
      - displacement T84.328 ☑
      - malposition T84.328 ☑
      - obstruction T84.398 ☑
      - perforation T84.398 ☑
      - protrusion T84.398 ☑
    - pain T84.84 ☑
    - specified type NEC T84.89 ☑
    - stenosis T84.85 ☑
    - thrombosis T84.86 ☑
  - graft — *see* Complications, graft, bone
  - growth stimulator (electrode) — *see* Complications, electronic stimulator device, bone
  - marrow transplant — *see* Complications, transplant, bone, marrow
- brain neurostimulator (electrode) — *see* Complications, electronic stimulator device, brain
- breast implant (prosthetic) T85.9 ☑
  - capsular contracture T85.44 ☑
  - embolism T85.818 ☑
  - fibrosis T85.828 ☑
  - hemorrhage T85.838 ☑
  - infection and inflammation T85.79 ☑
  - mechanical
    - breakdown T85.41 ☑
    - displacement T85.42 ☑
    - leakage T85.43 ☑
    - malposition T85.42 ☑
    - obstruction T85.49 ☑
    - perforation T85.49 ☑
    - protrusion T85.49 ☑
    - specified NEC T85.49 ☑
  - pain T85.848 ☑
  - specified type NEC T85.898 ☑
  - stenosis T85.858 ☑
  - thrombosis T85.868 ☑
- bypass (*see also* Complications, prosthetic device or implant)
  - aortocoronary — *see* Complications, coronary artery (bypass) graft
  - arterial (*see also* Complications, graft, vascular)
    - extremity — *see* Complications, extremity artery (bypass) graft
- cardiac (*see also* Disease, heart)
  - device, implant or graft T82.9 ☑
    - embolism T82.817 ☑
    - fibrosis T82.827 ☑
    - hemorrhage T82.837 ☑
    - infection or inflammation T82.7 ☑
      - valve prosthesis T82.6 ☑
    - mechanical
      - breakdown T82.519 ☑
        - specified device NEC T82.518 ☑
      - displacement T82.529 ☑
        - specified device NEC T82.528 ☑
      - leakage T82.539 ☑

☑ **Additional Character Required** — **Refer to the Tabular List for Character Selection**   ▽ **Subterms under main terms may continue to next column or page**

Complication — Complication

Complication(s) — *continued*
  cardiac (*see also* Disease, heart) — *continued*
    device, implant or graft — *continued*
      mechanical — *continued*
        leakage — *continued*
          specified device NEC T82.538 ☑
        malposition T82.529 ☑
          specified device NEC T82.528 ☑
        obstruction T82.599 ☑
          specified device NEC T82.598 ☑
        perforation T82.599 ☑
          specified device NEC T82.598 ☑
        protrusion T82.599 ☑
          specified device NEC T82.598 ☑
      pain T82.847 ☑
      specified type NEC T82.897 ☑
      stenosis T82.857 ☑
      thrombosis T82.867 ☑
  cardiovascular device, graft or implant T82.9
    aortic graft — *see* Complications, graft, vascular
    arteriovenous
      fistula, artificial — *see* Complication, arteriovenous, fistula, surgically created
      shunt — *see* Complication, arteriovenous, shunt, surgically created
    artificial heart — *see* Complication, artificial, heart
    balloon (counterpulsation) device — *see* Complication, balloon implant, vascular
    carotid artery graft — *see* Complications, graft, vascular
    coronary bypass graft — *see* Complication, coronary artery (bypass) graft
    dialysis catheter (vascular) — *see* Complication, catheter, dialysis
    electronic T82.9 ☑
      electrode T82.9 ☑
        embolism T82.817 ☑
        fibrosis T82.827 ☑
        hemorrhage T82.837 ☑
        infection T82.7 ☑
        mechanical
          breakdown T82.110 ☑
          displacement T82.120 ☑
          leakage T82.190 ☑
          obstruction T82.190 ☑
          perforation T82.190 ☑
          protrusion T82.190 ☑
          specified type NEC T82.190 ☑
        pain T82.847 ☑
        specified NEC T82.897 ☑
        stenosis T82.857 ☑
        thrombosis T82.867 ☑
      embolism T82.817 ☑
      fibrosis T82.827 ☑
      hemorrhage T82.837 ☑
      infection T82.7 ☑
      mechanical
        breakdown T82.119 ☑
        displacement T82.129 ☑
        leakage T82.199 ☑
        obstruction T82.199 ☑
        perforation T82.199 ☑
        protrusion T82.199 ☑
        specified type NEC T82.199 ☑
      pain T82.847 ☑
      pulse generator T82.9 ☑
        embolism T82.817 ☑
        fibrosis T82.827 ☑
        hemorrhage T82.837 ☑
        infection T82.7 ☑
        mechanical
          breakdown T82.111 ☑
          displacement T82.121 ☑
          leakage T82.191 ☑
          obstruction T82.191 ☑
          perforation T82.191 ☑
          protrusion T82.191 ☑
          specified type NEC T82.191 ☑
        pain T82.847 ☑
        specified NEC T82.897 ☑
        stenosis T82.857 ☑
        thrombosis T82.867 ☑
      specified condition NEC T82.897 ☑
      specified device NEC T82.9 ☑
        embolism T82.817 ☑
        fibrosis T82.827 ☑

Complication(s) — *continued*
  cardiovascular device, graft or implant — *continued*
    electronic — *continued*
      specified device — *continued*
        hemorrhage T82.837 ☑
        infection T82.7 ☑
        mechanical
          breakdown T82.118 ☑
          displacement T82.128 ☑
          leakage T82.198 ☑
          obstruction T82.198 ☑
          perforation T82.198 ☑
          protrusion T82.198 ☑
          specified type NEC T82.198 ☑
        pain T82.847 ☑
        specified NEC T82.897 ☑
        stenosis T82.857 ☑
        thrombosis T82.867 ☑
      stenosis T82.857 ☑
      thrombosis T82.867 ☑
    extremity artery graft — *see* Complication, extremity artery (bypass) graft
    femoral artery graft — *see* Complication, extremity artery (bypass) graft
    heart
      transplant — *see* Complication, transplant, heart
      valve — *see* Complication, prosthetic device, heart valve
      graft — *see* Complication, heart, valve, graft
    heart-lung transplant — *see* Complication, transplant, heart, with lung
    infection or inflammation T82.7 ☑
    umbrella device — *see* Complication, umbrella device, vascular
    vascular graft (or anastomosis) — *see* Complication, graft, vascular
  carotid artery (bypass) graft — *see* Complications, graft, vascular
  catheter (device) NEC (*see also* Complications, prosthetic device or implant)
    cranial infusion
      infection and inflammation T85.735 ☑
      mechanical
        breakdown T85.610 ☑
        displacement T85.620 ☑
        leakage T85.630 ☑
        malfunction T85.690 ☑
        malposition T85.620 ☑
        obstruction T85.690 ☑
        perforation T85.690 ☑
        protrusion T85.690 ☑
        specified NEC T85.690 ☑
    cystostomy T83.9 ☑
      embolism T83.81 ☑
      fibrosis T83.82 ☑
      hemorrhage T83.83 ☑
      infection and inflammation T83.510 ☑
      mechanical
        breakdown T83.010 ☑
        displacement T83.020 ☑
        leakage T83.030 ☑
        malposition T83.020 ☑
        obstruction T83.090 ☑
        perforation T83.090 ☑
        protrusion T83.090 ☑
        specified NEC T83.090 ☑
      pain T83.84 ☑
      specified type NEC T83.89 ☑
      stenosis T83.85 ☑
      thrombosis T83.86 ☑
    dialysis (vascular) T82.9 ☑
      embolism T82.818 ☑
      fibrosis T82.828 ☑
      hemorrhage T82.838 ☑
      infection and inflammation T82.7 ☑
      intraperitoneal — *see* Complications, catheter, intraperitoneal
      mechanical
        breakdown T82.41 ☑
        displacement T82.42 ☑
        leakage T82.43 ☑
        malposition T82.42 ☑
        obstruction T82.49 ☑
        perforation T82.49 ☑

Complication(s) — *continued*
  catheter (*see also* Complications, prosthetic device or implant) — *continued*
    dialysis — *continued*
      mechanical — *continued*
        protrusion T82.49 ☑
      pain T82.848 ☑
      specified type NEC T82.898 ☑
      stenosis T82.858 ☑
      thrombosis T82.868 ☑
    epidural infusion T85.9
      embolism T85.810 ☑
      fibrosis T85.820 ☑
      hemorrhage T85.830 ☑
      infection and inflammation T85.735 ☑
      mechanical
        breakdown T85.610 ☑
        displacement T85.620 ☑
        leakage T85.630 ☑
        malfunction T85.610 ☑
        malposition T85.620 ☑
        obstruction T85.690 ☑
        perforation T85.690 ☑
        protrusion T85.690 ☑
        specified NEC T85.690 ☑
      pain T85.840 ☑
      specified type NEC T85.890 ☑
      stenosis T85.850 ☑
      thrombosis T85.860 ☑
    intraperitoneal dialysis T85.9 ☑
      embolism T85.818 ☑
      fibrosis T85.828 ☑
      hemorrhage T85.838 ☑
      infection and inflammation T85.71 ☑
      mechanical
        breakdown T85.611 ☑
        displacement T85.621 ☑
        leakage T85.631 ☑
        malfunction T85.611 ☑
        malposition T85.621 ☑
        obstruction T85.691 ☑
        perforation T85.691 ☑
        protrusion T85.691 ☑
        specified NEC T85.691 ☑
      pain T85.848 ☑
      specified type NEC T85.898 ☑
      stenosis T85.858 ☑
      thrombosis T85.868 ☑
    intrathecal infusion
      infection and inflammation T85.735 ☑
      mechanical
        breakdown T85.610 ☑
        displacement T85.620 ☑
        leakage T85.630 ☑
        malfunction T85.690 ☑
        malposition T85.620 ☑
        obstruction T85.690 ☑
        perforation T85.690 ☑
        protrusion T85.690 ☑
        specified NEC T85.690 ☑
    intravenous infusion T82.9 ☑
      embolism T82.818 ☑
      fibrosis T82.828 ☑
      hemorrhage T82.838 ☑
      infection or inflammation T82.7 ☑
      mechanical
        breakdown T82.514 ☑
        displacement T82.524 ☑
        leakage T82.534 ☑
        malposition T82.524 ☑
        obstruction T82.594 ☑
        perforation T82.594 ☑
        protrusion T82.594 ☑
      pain T82.848 ☑
      specified type NEC T82.898 ☑
      stenosis T82.858 ☑
      thrombosis T82.868 ☑
    spinal infusion
      infection and inflammation T85.735 ☑
      mechanical
        breakdown T85.610 ☑
        displacement T85.620 ☑
        leakage T85.630 ☑
        malfunction T85.690 ☑
        malposition T85.620 ☑
        obstruction T85.690 ☑

▽ Subterms under main terms may continue to next column or page   ☑ Additional Character Required — Refer to the Tabular List for Character Selection   59

Complication — Complication

Complication(s) — *continued*
  catheter (*see also* Complications, prosthetic device or implant) — *continued*
    spinal infusion — *continued*
      mechanical — *continued*
        perforation T85.690 ☑
        protrusion T85.690 ☑
        specified NEC T85.690 ☑
    subarachnoid infusion
      infection and inflammation T85.735 ☑
      mechanical
        breakdown T85.610 ☑
        displacement T85.620 ☑
        leakage T85.630 ☑
        malfunction T85.690 ☑
        malposition T85.620 ☑
        obstruction T85.690 ☑
        perforation T85.690 ☑
        protrusion T85.690 ☑
        specified NEC T85.690 ☑
    subdural infusion T85.9 ☑
      embolism T85.810 ☑
      fibrosis T85.820 ☑
      hemorrhage T85.830 ☑
      infection and inflammation T85.735 ☑
      mechanical
        breakdown T85.610 ☑
        displacement T85.620 ☑
        leakage T85.630 ☑
        malfunction T85.610 ☑
        malposition T85.620 ☑
        obstruction T85.690 ☑
        perforation T85.690 ☑
        protrusion T85.690 ☑
        specified NEC T85.690 ☑
      pain T85.840 ☑
      specified type NEC T85.890 ☑
      stenosis T85.850 ☑
      thrombosis T85.860 ☑
    urethral T83.9 ☑
      displacement T83.028 ☑
      embolism T83.81 ☑
      fibrosis T83.82 ☑
      hemorrhage T83.83 ☑
      indwelling
        breakdown T83.011 ☑
        displacement T83.021 ☑
        infection and inflammation T83.511 ☑
        leakage T83.031 ☑
        specified complication NEC T83.091 ☑
      infection and inflammation T83.511 ☑
      leakage T83.038 ☑
      malposition T83.028 ☑
      mechanical
        breakdown T83.011 ☑
      obstruction (mechanical) T83.091 ☑
      pain T83.84 ☑
      perforation T83.091 ☑
      protrusion T83.091 ☑
      specified type NEC T83.091 ☑
      stenosis T83.85 ☑
      thrombosis T83.86 ☑
    urinary NEC
      breakdown T83.018 ☑
      displacement T83.028 ☑
      infection and inflammation T83.518 ☑
      leakage T83.038 ☑
      specified complication NEC T83.098 ☑
  cecostomy (stoma) — *see* Complications, colostomy
  cesarean delivery wound NEC O90.89
    disruption O90.0
    hematoma O90.2
    infection (following delivery) O86.0
  chemotherapy (antineoplastic) NEC T88.7 ☑
  chin implant (prosthetic) — *see* Complication, prosthetic device or implant, specified NEC
  circulatory system I99.8
    intraoperative I97.88
    postprocedural I97.89
      following cardiac surgery (*see also* Infarct, myocardium, associated with revascularization procedure) I97.19-
        postcardiotomy syndrome I97.0
      hypertension I97.3
      lymphedema after mastectomy I97.2
      postcardiotomy syndrome I97.0

Complication(s) — *continued*
  circulatory system — *continued*
    postprocedural — *continued*
      specified NEC I97.89
  colostomy (stoma) K94.00
    hemorrhage K94.01
    infection K94.02
    malfunction K94.03
    mechanical K94.03
    specified complication NEC K94.09
  contraceptive device, intrauterine — *see* Complications, intrauterine, contraceptive device
  cord (umbilical) — *see* Complications, umbilical cord
  corneal graft — *see* Complications, graft, cornea
  coronary artery (bypass) graft T82.9
    atherosclerosis — *see* Arteriosclerosis, coronary (artery),
    embolism T82.818 ☑
    fibrosis T82.828 ☑
    hemorrhage T82.838 ☑
    infection and inflammation T82.7 ☑
    mechanical
      breakdown T82.211 ☑
      displacement T82.212 ☑
      leakage T82.213 ☑
      malposition T82.212 ☑
      obstruction T82.218 ☑
      perforation T82.218 ☑
      protrusion T82.218 ☑
      specified NEC T82.218 ☑
    pain T82.848 ☑
    specified type NEC T82.898 ☑
    stenosis T82.858 ☑
    thrombosis T82.868 ☑
  counterpulsation device (balloon), intra- aortic — *see* Complications, balloon implant, vascular
  cystostomy (stoma) N99.518
    catheter — *see* Complications, catheter, cystostomy
    hemorrhage N99.510
    infection N99.511
    malfunction N99.512
    specified type NEC N99.518
  delivery (*see also* Complications, obstetric) O75.9
    procedure (instrumental) (manual) (surgical) O75.4
    specified NEC O75.89
  dialysis (peritoneal) (renal) (*see also* Complications, infusion)
    catheter (vascular) — *see* Complication, catheter, dialysis
      peritoneal, intraperitoneal — *see* Complications, catheter, intraperitoneal
  dorsal column (spinal) neurostimulator — *see* Complications, electronic stimulator device, spinal cord
  drug NEC T88.7 ☑
  ear procedure (*see also* Disorder, ear)
    intraoperative H95.88
      hematoma — *see* Complications, intraoperative, hemorrhage (hematoma) (of), ear
      hemorrhage — *see* Complications, intraoperative, hemorrhage (hematoma) (of), ear
      laceration — *see* Complications, intraoperative, puncture or laceration..., ear
      specified NEC H95.88
    postoperative H95.89
      external ear canal stenosis H95.81- ☑
      hematoma — *see* Complications, postprocedural, hematoma (of), ear
      hemorrhage — *see* Complications, postprocedural, hemorrhage (of), ear
      postmastoidectomy — *see* Complications, postmastoidectomy
      seroma — *see* Complications, postprocedural, seroma (of), mastoid process
      specified NEC H95.89
  ectopic pregnancy O08.9
    damage to pelvic organs O08.6
    embolism O08.2
    genital infection O08.0
    hemorrhage (delayed) (excessive) O08.1
    metabolic disorder O08.5
    renal failure O08.4
    shock O08.3
    specified type NEC O08.0
    venous complication NEC O08.7

Complication(s) — *continued*
  electronic stimulator device
    bladder (urinary) — *see* Complications, electronic stimulator device, urinary
    bone T84.9 ☑
      breakdown T84.310 ☑
      displacement T84.320 ☑
      embolism T84.81 ☑
      fibrosis T84.82 ☑
      hemorrhage T84.83 ☑
      infection or inflammation T84.7 ☑
      malfunction T84.310 ☑
      malposition T84.320 ☑
      mechanical NEC T84.390 ☑
      obstruction T84.390 ☑
      pain T84.84 ☑
      perforation T84.390 ☑
      protrusion T84.390 ☑
      specified type NEC T84.89 ☑
      stenosis T84.85 ☑
      thrombosis T84.86 ☑
    brain T85.9 ☑
      embolism T85.810 ☑
      fibrosis T85.820 ☑
      hemorrhage T85.830 ☑
      infection and inflammation T85.731 ☑
      mechanical
        breakdown T85.110 ☑
        displacement T85.120 ☑
        leakage T85.190 ☑
        malposition T85.120 ☑
        obstruction T85.190 ☑
        perforation T85.190 ☑
        protrusion T85.190 ☑
        specified NEC T85.190 ☑
      pain T85.840 ☑
      specified type NEC T85.890 ☑
      stenosis T85.850 ☑
      thrombosis T85.860 ☑
    cardiac (defibrillator) (pacemaker) — *see* Complications, cardiovascular device or implant, electronic
    generator (brain) (gastric) (peripheral) (sacral) (spinal)
      breakdown T85.113 ☑
      displacement T85.123 ☑
      leakage T85.193 ☑
      malposition T85.123 ☑
      obstruction T85.193 ☑
      perforation T85.193 ☑
      protrusion T85.193 ☑
      specified type NEC T85.193 ☑
    muscle T84.9 ☑
      breakdown T84.418 ☑
      displacement T84.428 ☑
      embolism T84.81 ☑
      fibrosis T84.82 ☑
      hemorrhage T84.83 ☑
      infection or inflammation T84.7 ☑
      mechanical NEC T84.498 ☑
      pain T84.84 ☑
      specified type NEC T84.89 ☑
      stenosis T84.85 ☑
      thrombosis T84.86 ☑
    nervous system T85.9 ☑
      brain — *see* Complications, electronic stimulator device, brain
      cranial nerve — *see* Complications, electronic stimulator device, peripheral nerve
      embolism T85.810 ☑
      fibrosis T85.820 ☑
      gastric nerve — *see* Complications, electronic stimulator device, peripheral nerve
      hemorrhage T85.830 ☑
      infection and inflammation T85.738 ☑
      mechanical
        breakdown T85.118 ☑
        displacement T85.128 ☑
        leakage T85.199 ☑
        malposition T85.128 ☑
        obstruction T85.199 ☑
        perforation T85.199 ☑
        protrusion T85.199 ☑
        specified NEC T85.199 ☑
      pain T85.840 ☑

Index

plication — Complication

Complication(s) — *continued*
- electronic stimulator device — *continued*
  - nervous system — *continued*
    - peripheral nerve — *see* Complications, electronic stimulator device, peripheral nerve
    - sacral nerve — *see* Complications, electronic stimulator device, peripheral nerve
    - specified type NEC T85.890 ☑
    - spinal cord — *see* Complications, electronic stimulator device, spinal cord
    - stenosis T85.850 ☑
    - thrombosis T85.860 ☑
    - vagal nerve — *see* Complications, electronic stimulator device, peripheral nerve
  - peripheral nerve T85.9 ☑
    - embolism T85.810 ☑
    - fibrosis T85.820 ☑
    - hemorrhage T85.830 ☑
    - infection and inflammation T85.732 ☑
    - mechanical
      - breakdown T85.111 ☑
      - displacement T85.121 ☑
      - leakage T85.191 ☑
      - malposition T85.121 ☑
      - obstruction T85.191 ☑
      - perforation T85.191 ☑
      - protrusion T85.191 ☑
      - specified NEC T85.191 ☑
    - pain T85.840 ☑
    - specified type NEC T85.890 ☑
    - stenosis T85.850 ☑
    - thrombosis T85.860 ☑
  - spinal cord T85.9 ☑
    - embolism T85.810 ☑
    - fibrosis T85.820 ☑
    - hemorrhage T85.830 ☑
    - infection and inflammation T85.733 ☑
    - mechanical
      - breakdown T85.112 ☑
      - displacement T85.122 ☑
      - leakage T85.192 ☑
      - malposition T85.122 ☑
      - obstruction T85.192 ☑
      - perforation T85.192 ☑
      - protrusion T85.192 ☑
      - specified NEC T85.192 ☑
    - pain T85.840 ☑
    - specified type NEC T85.890 ☑
    - stenosis T85.850 ☑
    - thrombosis T85.860 ☑
  - urinary T83.9 ☑
    - embolism T83.81 ☑
    - fibrosis T83.82 ☑
    - hemorrhage T83.83 ☑
    - infection and inflammation T83.598 ☑
    - mechanical
      - breakdown T83.110 ☑
      - displacement T83.120 ☑
      - malposition T83.120 ☑
      - perforation T83.190 ☑
      - protrusion T83.190 ☑
      - specified NEC T83.190 ☑
    - pain T83.84 ☑
    - specified type NEC T83.89 ☑
    - stenosis T83.85 ☑
    - thrombosis T83.86 ☑
- electroshock therapy T88.9 ☑
  - specified NEC T88.8 ☑
- endocrine E34.9
  - postprocedural
    - adrenal hypofunction E89.6
    - hypoinsulinemia E89.1
    - hypoparathyroidism E89.2
    - hypopituitarism E89.3
    - hypothyroidism E89.0
    - ovarian failure E89.40
      - asymptomatic E89.40
      - symptomatic E89.41
    - specified NEC E89.89
    - testicular hypofunction E89.5
- endodontic treatment NEC M27.59
- enterostomy (stoma) K94.10 ☑
  - hemorrhage K94.11
  - infection K94.12
  - malfunction K94.13
  - mechanical K94.13

Complication(s) — *continued*
- enterostomy — *continued*
  - specified complication NEC K94.19
- episiotomy, disruption O90.1
- esophageal anti-reflux device T85.9 ☑
  - embolism T85.818 ☑
  - fibrosis T85.828 ☑
  - hemorrhage T85.838 ☑
  - infection and inflammation T85.79 ☑
  - mechanical
    - breakdown T85.511 ☑
    - displacement T85.521 ☑
    - malfunction T85.511 ☑
    - malposition T85.521 ☑
    - obstruction T85.591 ☑
    - perforation T85.591 ☑
    - protrusion T85.591 ☑
    - specified NEC T85.591 ☑
  - pain T85.848 ☑
  - specified type NEC T85.898 ☑
  - stenosis T85.858 ☑
  - thrombosis T85.868 ☑
- esophagostomy K94.30
  - hemorrhage K94.31
  - infection K94.32
  - malfunction K94.33
  - mechanical K94.33
  - specified complication NEC K94.39
- extracorporeal circulation T80.90 ☑
- extremity artery (bypass) graft T82.9 ☑
  - arteriosclerosis — *see* Arteriosclerosis, extremities, bypass graft
  - embolism T82.818 ☑
  - fibrosis T82.828 ☑
  - hemorrhage T82.838 ☑
  - infection and inflammation T82.7 ☑
  - mechanical
    - breakdown T82.318 ☑
      - femoral artery T82.312 ☑
    - displacement T82.328 ☑
      - femoral artery T82.322 ☑
    - leakage T82.338 ☑
      - femoral artery T82.332 ☑
    - malposition T82.328 ☑
      - femoral artery T82.322 ☑
    - obstruction T82.398 ☑
      - femoral artery T82.392 ☑
    - perforation T82.398 ☑
      - femoral artery T82.392 ☑
    - protrusion T82.398 ☑
      - femoral artery T82.392 ☑
  - pain T82.848 ☑
  - specified type NEC T82.898 ☑
  - stenosis T82.858 ☑
  - thrombosis T82.868 ☑
- eye H57.9
  - corneal graft — *see* Complications, graft, cornea
  - implant (prosthetic) T85.9 ☑
    - embolism T85.818 ☑
    - fibrosis T85.828 ☑
    - hemorrhage T85.838 ☑
    - infection and inflammation T85.79 ☑
    - mechanical
      - breakdown T85.318 ☑
      - displacement T85.328 ☑
      - leakage T85.398 ☑
      - malposition T85.328 ☑
      - obstruction T85.398 ☑
      - perforation T85.398 ☑
      - protrusion T85.398 ☑
      - specified NEC T85.398 ☑
    - pain T85.848 ☑
    - specified type NEC T85.898 ☑
    - stenosis T85.858 ☑
    - thrombosis T85.868 ☑
  - intraocular lens — *see* Complications, intraocular lens
  - orbital prosthesis — *see* Complications, orbital prosthesis
- female genital N94.9
  - device, implant or graft NEC — *see* Complications, genitourinary, device or implant, genital tract
- femoral artery (bypass) graft — *see* Complication, extremity artery (bypass) graft
- fixation device, internal (orthopedic) T84.9 ☑
  - infection and inflammation T84.60 ☑

Complication(s) — *continued*
- fixation device, internal — *continued*
  - infection and inflammation — *continued*
    - arm T84.61- ☑
      - humerus T84.61- ☑
      - radius T84.61- ☑
      - ulna T84.61- ☑
    - leg T84.629 ☑
      - femur T84.62- ☑
      - fibula T84.62- ☑
      - tibia T84.62- ☑
    - specified site NEC T84.89 ☑
    - spine T84.63 ☑
  - mechanical
    - breakdown
      - limb T84.119 ☑
        - carpal T84.210 ☑
        - femur T84.11- ☑
        - fibula T84.11- ☑
        - humerus T84.11- ☑
        - metacarpal T84.210 ☑
        - metatarsal T84.213 ☑
        - phalanx
          - foot T84.213 ☑
          - hand T84.210 ☑
        - radius T84.11- ☑
        - tarsal T84.213 ☑
        - tibia T84.11- ☑
        - ulna T84.11- ☑
      - specified bone NEC T84.218 ☑
      - spine T84.216 ☑
    - displacement
      - limb T84.129 ☑
        - carpal T84.220 ☑
        - femur T84.12- ☑
        - fibula T84.12- ☑
        - humerus T84.12- ☑
        - metacarpal T84.220 ☑
        - metatarsal T84.223 ☑
        - phalanx
          - foot T84.223 ☑
          - hand T84.220 ☑
        - radius T84.12- ☑
        - tarsal T84.223 ☑
        - tibia T84.12- ☑
        - ulna T84.12- ☑
      - specified bone NEC T84.228 ☑
      - spine T84.226 ☑
    - malposition — *see* Complications, fixation device, internal, mechanical, displacement
    - obstruction — *see* Complications, fixation device, internal, mechanical, specified type NEC
    - perforation — *see* Complications, fixation device, internal, mechanical, specified type NEC
    - protrusion — *see* Complications, fixation device, internal, mechanical, specified type NEC
    - specified type NEC
      - limb T84.199 ☑
        - carpal T84.290 ☑
        - femur T84.19- ☑
        - fibula T84.19- ☑
        - humerus T84.19- ☑
        - metacarpal T84.290 ☑
        - metatarsal T84.293 ☑
        - phalanx
          - foot T84.293 ☑
          - hand T84.290 ☑
        - radius T84.19- ☑
        - tarsal T84.293 ☑
        - tibia T84.19- ☑
        - ulna T84.19- ☑
      - specified bone NEC T84.298 ☑
      - vertebra T84.296 ☑
  - specified type NEC T84.89 ☑
    - embolism T84.81 ☑
    - fibrosis T84.82 ☑
    - hemorrhage T84.83 ☑
    - pain T84.84 ☑
    - specified complication NEC T84.89 ☑
    - stenosis T84.85 ☑
    - thrombosis T84.86 ☑
- following
  - acute myocardial infarction NEC I23.8

Complication(s) — *continued*
　following — *continued*
　　acute myocardial infarction — *continued*
　　　aneurysm (false) (of cardiac wall) (of heart wall) (ruptured) I23.3
　　　angina I23.7
　　　atrial
　　　　septal defect I23.1
　　　　thrombosis I23.6
　　　cardiac wall rupture I23.3
　　　chordae tendinae rupture I23.4
　　　defect
　　　　septal
　　　　　atrial (heart) I23.1
　　　　　ventricular (heart) I23.2
　　　hemopericardium I23.0
　　　papillary muscle rupture I23.5
　　　rupture
　　　　cardiac wall I23.3
　　　　　with hemopericardium I23.0
　　　　chordae tendineae I23.4
　　　　papillary muscle I23.5
　　　specified NEC I23.8
　　　thrombosis
　　　　atrium I23.6
　　　　auricular appendage I23.6
　　　　ventricle (heart) I23.6
　　　ventricular
　　　　septal defect I23.2
　　　　thrombosis I23.6
　　ectopic or molar pregnancy O08.9
　　　cardiac arrest O08.81
　　　sepsis O08.82
　　　specified type NEC O08.89
　　　urinary tract infection O08.83
　　termination of pregnancy — *see* Abortion
　gastrointestinal K92.9
　　bile duct prosthesis — *see* Complications, bile duct implant
　　esophageal anti-reflux device — *see* Complications, esophageal anti-reflux device
　　postoperative
　　　colostomy — *see* Complications, colostomy
　　　dumping syndrome K91.1
　　　enterostomy — *see* Complications, enterostomy
　　　gastrostomy — *see* Complications, gastrostomy
　　　malabsorption NEC K91.2
　　　obstruction (*see also* Obstruction, intestine, postoperative) K91.30
　　　postcholecystectomy syndrome K91.5
　　　specified NEC K91.89
　　　vomiting after GI surgery K91.0
　　prosthetic device or implant
　　　bile duct prosthesis — *see* Complications, bile duct implant
　　　esophageal anti-reflux device — *see* Complications, esophageal anti-reflux device
　　　specified type NEC
　　　　embolism T85.818 ☑
　　　　fibrosis T85.828 ☑
　　　　hemorrhage T85.838 ☑
　　　　mechanical
　　　　　breakdown T85.518 ☑
　　　　　displacement T85.528 ☑
　　　　　malfunction T85.518 ☑
　　　　　malposition T85.528 ☑
　　　　　obstruction T85.598 ☑
　　　　　perforation T85.598 ☑
　　　　　protrusion T85.598 ☑
　　　　　specified NEC T85.598 ☑
　　　　pain T85.848 ☑
　　　　specified complication NEC T85.898 ☑
　　　　stenosis T85.858 ☑
　　　　thrombosis T85.868 ☑
　gastrostomy (stoma) K94.20
　　hemorrhage K94.21
　　infection K94.22
　　malfunction K94.23
　　mechanical K94.23
　　specified complication NEC K94.29
　genitourinary
　　device or implant T83.9 ☑
　　　genital tract T83.9 ☑
　　　　infection or inflammation T83.69 ☑
　　　　intrauterine contraceptive device — *see* Complications, intrauterine, contraceptive device

Complication(s) — *continued*
　genitourinary — *continued*
　　device or implant — *continued*
　　　genital tract — *continued*
　　　　mechanical — *see* Complications, by device, mechanical
　　　　mesh — *see* Complications, mesh
　　　　penile prosthesis — *see* Complications, prosthetic device, penile
　　　　specified type NEC T83.89 ☑
　　　　　embolism T83.81 ☑
　　　　　fibrosis T83.82 ☑
　　　　　hemorrhage T83.83 ☑
　　　　　pain T83.84 ☑
　　　　　specified complication NEC T83.89 ☑
　　　　　stenosis T83.85 ☑
　　　　　thrombosis T83.86 ☑
　　　　vaginal mesh — *see* Complications, mesh
　　　urinary system T83.9 ☑
　　　　cystostomy catheter — *see* Complication, catheter, cystostomy
　　　　electronic stimulator — *see* Complications, electronic stimulator device, urinary
　　　　indwelling urethral catheter — *see* Complications, catheter, urethral, indwelling
　　　　infection or inflammation T83.598 ☑
　　　　　indwelling urethral catheter T83.511 ☑
　　　　kidney transplant — *see* Complication, transplant, kidney
　　　　organ graft — *see* Complication, graft, urinary organ
　　　　specified type NEC T83.89 ☑
　　　　　embolism T83.81 ☑
　　　　　fibrosis T83.82 ☑
　　　　　hemorrhage T83.83 ☑
　　　　　mechanical T83.198 ☑
　　　　　　breakdown T83.118 ☑
　　　　　　displacement T83.128 ☑
　　　　　　malfunction T83.118 ☑
　　　　　　malposition T83.128 ☑
　　　　　　obstruction T83.198 ☑
　　　　　　perforation T83.198 ☑
　　　　　　protrusion T83.198 ☑
　　　　　　specified NEC T83.198 ☑
　　　　sphincter implant — *see* Complications, implant, urinary sphincter
　　　　sphincter, implanted T83.191 ☑
　　　　stent (ileal conduit) (nephroureteral) T83.193 ☑
　　　　　pain T83.84 ☑
　　　　　specified complication NEC T83.89 ☑
　　　　　stenosis T83.85 ☑
　　　　　thrombosis T83.86 ☑
　　　　　ureteral indwelling T83.192 ☑
　　postprocedural
　　　pelvic peritoneal adhesions N99.4
　　　renal failure N99.0
　　　specified NEC N99.89
　　　stoma — *see* Complications, stoma, urinary tract
　　　urethral stricture — *see* Stricture, urethra, postprocedural
　　　vaginal
　　　　adhesions N99.2
　　　　vault prolapse N99.3
　graft (bypass) (patch) (*see also* Complications, prosthetic device or implant)
　　aorta — *see* Complications, graft, vascular
　　arterial — *see* Complication, graft, vascular
　　bone T86.839
　　　failure T86.831
　　　infection T86.832
　　　mechanical T84.318 ☑
　　　　breakdown T84.318 ☑
　　　　displacement T84.328 ☑
　　　　protrusion T84.398 ☑
　　　　specified type NEC T84.398 ☑
　　　rejection T86.830
　　　specified type NEC T86.838
　　carotid artery — *see* Complications, graft, vascular
　　cornea T86.849
　　　failure T86.841
　　　infection T86.842
　　　mechanical T85.398 ☑
　　　　breakdown T85.318 ☑
　　　　displacement T85.328 ☑
　　　　protrusion T85.398 ☑

Complication(s) — *continued*
　graft (*see also* Complications, prosthetic device or implant) — *continued*
　　cornea — *continued*
　　　mechanical — *continued*
　　　　specified type NEC T85.398 ☑
　　　rejection T86.840
　　　retroprosthetic membrane T85.398 ☑
　　　specified type NEC T86.848
　　femoral artery (bypass) — *see* Complication, extremity artery (bypass) graft
　　genital organ or tract — *see* Complications, genitourinary, device or implant, genital tract
　　muscle T84.9 ☑
　　　breakdown T84.410 ☑
　　　displacement T84.420 ☑
　　　embolism T84.81 ☑
　　　fibrosis T84.82 ☑
　　　hemorrhage T84.83 ☑
　　　infection and inflammation T84.7 ☑
　　　mechanical NEC T84.490 ☑
　　　pain T84.84 ☑
　　　specified type NEC T84.89 ☑
　　　stenosis T84.85 ☑
　　　thrombosis T84.86 ☑
　　nerve — *see* Complication, prosthetic device or implant, specified NEC
　　skin — *see* Complications, prosthetic device or implant, skin graft
　　tendon T84.9 ☑
　　　breakdown T84.410 ☑
　　　displacement T84.420 ☑
　　　embolism T84.81 ☑
　　　fibrosis T84.82 ☑
　　　hemorrhage T84.83 ☑
　　　infection and inflammation T84.7 ☑
　　　mechanical NEC T84.490 ☑
　　　pain T84.84 ☑
　　　specified type NEC T84.89 ☑
　　　stenosis T84.85 ☑
　　　thrombosis T84.86 ☑
　　urinary organ T83.9 ☑
　　　embolism T83.81 ☑
　　　fibrosis T83.82 ☑
　　　hemorrhage T83.83 ☑
　　　infection and inflammation T83.598 ☑
　　　　indwelling urethral catheter T83.511 ☑
　　　mechanical
　　　　breakdown T83.21 ☑
　　　　displacement T83.22 ☑
　　　　erosion T83.24 ☑
　　　　exposure T83.25 ☑
　　　　leakage T83.23 ☑
　　　　malposition T83.22 ☑
　　　　obstruction T83.29 ☑
　　　　perforation T83.29 ☑
　　　　protrusion T83.29 ☑
　　　　specified NEC T83.29 ☑
　　　pain T83.84 ☑
　　　specified type NEC T83.89 ☑
　　　stenosis T83.85 ☑
　　　thrombosis T83.86 ☑
　　vascular T82.9 ☑
　　　embolism T82.818 ☑
　　　femoral artery — *see* Complication, extremity artery (bypass) graft
　　　fibrosis T82.828 ☑
　　　hemorrhage T82.838 ☑
　　　mechanical
　　　　breakdown T82.319 ☑
　　　　　aorta (bifurcation) T82.310 ☑
　　　　　carotid artery T82.311 ☑
　　　　　specified vessel NEC T82.318 ☑
　　　　displacement T82.329 ☑
　　　　　aorta (bifurcation) T82.320 ☑
　　　　　carotid artery T82.321 ☑
　　　　　specified vessel NEC T82.328 ☑
　　　　leakage T82.339 ☑
　　　　　aorta (bifurcation) T82.330 ☑
　　　　　carotid artery T82.331 ☑
　　　　　specified vessel NEC T82.338 ☑
　　　　malposition T82.329 ☑
　　　　　aorta (bifurcation) T82.320 ☑
　　　　　carotid artery T82.321 ☑
　　　　　specified vessel NEC T82.328 ☑
　　　　obstruction T82.399 ☑

☑ **Additional Character Required — Refer to the Tabular List for Character Selection**　　🔽 **Subterms under main terms may continue to next column or page**

Index

Complication(s) — *continued*
graft (*see also* Complications, prosthetic device or implant) — *continued*
  vascular — *continued*
    mechanical — *continued*
      obstruction — *continued*
        aorta (bifurcation) T82.390 ☑
        carotid artery T82.391 ☑
        specified vessel NEC T82.398 ☑
      perforation T82.399 ☑
        aorta (bifurcation) T82.390 ☑
        carotid artery T82.391 ☑
        specified vessel NEC T82.398 ☑
      protrusion T82.399 ☑
        aorta (bifurcation) T82.390 ☑
        carotid artery T82.391 ☑
        specified vessel NEC T82.398 ☑
    pain T82.848 ☑
    specified complication NEC T82.898 ☑
    stenosis T82.858 ☑
    thrombosis T82.868 ☑
heart I51.9
  assist device
    infection and inflammation T82.7 ☑
  following acute myocardial infarction — *see* Complications, following, acute myocardial infarction
  postoperative — *see* Complications, circulatory system
  transplant — *see* Complication, transplant, heart and lung(s) — *see* Complications, transplant, heart, with lung
  valve
    graft (biological) T82.9 ☑
      embolism T82.817 ☑
      fibrosis T82.827 ☑
      hemorrhage T82.837 ☑
      infection and inflammation T82.7 ☑
      mechanical T82.228 ☑
        breakdown T82.221 ☑
        displacement T82.222 ☑
        leakage T82.223 ☑
        malposition T82.222 ☑
        obstruction T82.228 ☑
        perforation T82.228 ☑
        protrusion T82.228 ☑
      pain T82.847 ☑
      specified type NEC T82.897 ☑
      stenosis T82.857 ☑
      thrombosis T82.867 ☑
    prosthesis T82.9 ☑
      embolism T82.817 ☑
      fibrosis T82.827 ☑
      hemorrhage T82.837 ☑
      infection or inflammation T82.6 ☑
      mechanical T82.09 ☑
        breakdown T82.01 ☑
        displacement T82.02 ☑
        leakage T82.03 ☑
        malposition T82.02 ☑
        obstruction T82.09 ☑
        perforation T82.09 ☑
        protrusion T82.09 ☑
      pain T82.847 ☑
      specified type NEC T82.897 ☑
        mechanical T82.09 ☑
      stenosis T82.857 ☑
      thrombosis T82.867 ☑
hematoma
  intraoperative — *see* Complication, intraoperative, hemorrhage
  postprocedural — *see* Complication, postprocedural, hematoma
hemodialysis — *see* Complications, dialysis
hemorrhage
  intraoperative — *see* Complication, intraoperative, hemorrhage
  postprocedural — *see* Complication, postprocedural, hemorrhage
ileostomy (stoma) — *see* Complications, enterostomy
immunization (procedure) — *see* Complications, vaccination
implant (*see also* Complications, by site and type)
  urinary sphincter T83.9 ☑
    embolism T83.81 ☑
    fibrosis T83.82 ☑

Complication(s) — *continued*
implant (*see also* Complications, by site and type) — *continued*
  urinary sphincter — *continued*
    hemorrhage T83.83 ☑
    infection and inflammation T83.591 ☑
    mechanical
      breakdown T83.111 ☑
      displacement T83.121 ☑
      leakage T83.191 ☑
      malposition T83.121 ☑
      obstruction T83.191 ☑
      perforation T83.191 ☑
      protrusion T83.191 ☑
      specified NEC T83.191 ☑
    pain T83.84 ☑
    specified type NEC T83.89 ☑
    stenosis T83.85 ☑
    thrombosis T83.86 ☑
infusion (procedure) T80.90 ☑
  air embolism T80.0 ☑
  blood — *see* Complications, transfusion
  catheter — *see* Complications, catheter
  infection T80.29 ☑
  pump — *see* Complications, cardiovascular, device or implant
  sepsis T80.29 ☑
  serum reaction (*see also* Reaction, serum) T80.69 ☑
    anaphylactic shock (*see also* Shock, anaphylactic) T80.59 ☑
  specified type NEC T80.89 ☑
inhalation therapy NEC T81.81 ☑
injection (procedure) T80.90 ☑
  drug reaction — *see* Reaction, drug
  infection T80.29 ☑
  sepsis T80.29 ☑
  serum (prophylactic) (therapeutic) — *see* Complications, vaccination
  specified type NEC T80.89 ☑
  vaccine (any) — *see* Complications, vaccination
inoculation (any) — *see* Complications, vaccination
insulin pump
  infection and inflammation T85.72 ☑
  mechanical
    breakdown T85.614 ☑
    displacement T85.624 ☑
    leakage T85.633 ☑
    malposition T85.624 ☑
    obstruction T85.694 ☑
    perforation T85.694 ☑
    protrusion T85.694 ☑
    specified NEC T85.694 ☑
intestinal pouch NEC K91.858
intraocular lens (prosthetic) T85.9 ☑
  embolism T85.818 ☑
  fibrosis T85.828 ☑
  hemorrhage T85.838 ☑
  infection and inflammation T85.79 ☑
  mechanical
    breakdown T85.21 ☑
    displacement T85.22 ☑
    malposition T85.22 ☑
    obstruction T85.29 ☑
    perforation T85.29 ☑
    protrusion T85.29 ☑
    specified NEC T85.29 ☑
  pain T85.848 ☑
  specified type NEC T85.898 ☑
  stenosis T85.858 ☑
  thrombosis T85.868 ☑
intraoperative (intraprocedural)
  cardiac arrest (*see also* Infarct, myocardium, associated with revascularization procedure)
    during cardiac surgery I97.710 ☑
    during other surgery I97.711
  cardiac functional disturbance NEC (*see also* Infarct, myocardium, associated with revascularization procedure)
    during cardiac surgery I97.790
    during other surgery I97.791
  hemorrhage (hematoma) (of)
    circulatory system organ or structure
      during cardiac bypass I97.411
      during cardiac catheterization I97.410
      during other circulatory system procedure I97.418

Complication(s) — *continued*
intraoperative — *continued*
  hemorrhage — *continued*
    circulatory system organ or structure — *continued*
      during other procedure I97.42
    digestive system organ
      during procedure on digestive system K91.61
      during procedure on other organ K91.62
    ear
      during procedure on ear and mastoid process H95.21
      during procedure on other organ H95.22
    endocrine system organ or structure
      during procedure on endocrine system organ or structure E36.01
      during procedure on other organ E36.02
    eye and adnexa
      during ophthalmic procedure H59.11- ☑
      during other procedure H59.12- ☑
    genitourinary organ or structure
      during procedure on genitourinary organ or structure N99.61
      during procedure on other organ N99.62
    mastoid process
      during procedure on ear and mastoid process H95.21
      during procedure on other organ H95.22
    musculoskeletal structure
      during musculoskeletal surgery M96.810
      during non-orthopedic surgery M96.811
      during orthopedic surgery M96.810
    nervous system
      during a nervous system procedure G97.31
      during other procedure G97.32
    respiratory system
      during other procedure J95.62
      during procedure on respiratory system organ or structure J95.61
    skin and subcutaneous tissue
      during a dermatologic procedure L76.01
      during a procedure on other organ L76.02
    spleen
      during a procedure on other organ D78.02
      during a procedure on the spleen D78.01
  puncture or laceration (accidental) (unintentional) (of)
    brain
      during a nervous system procedure G97.48
      during other procedure G97.49
    circulatory system organ or structure
      during circulatory system procedure I97.51
      during other procedure I97.52
    digestive system
      during procedure on digestive system K91.71
      during procedure on other organ K91.72
    ear
      during procedure on ear and mastoid process H95.31
      during procedure on other organ H95.32
    endocrine system organ or structure
      during procedure on endocrine system organ or structure E36.11
      during procedure on other organ E36.12
    eye and adnexa
      during ophthalmic procedure H59.21- ☑
      during other procedure H59.22- ☑
    genitourinary organ or structure
      during procedure on genitourinary organ or structure N99.71
      during procedure on other organ N99.72
    mastoid process
      during procedure on ear and mastoid process H95.31
      during procedure on other organ H95.32
    musculoskeletal structure
      during musculoskeletal surgery M96.820
      during non-orthopedic surgery M96.821
      during orthopedic surgery M96.820
    nervous system
      during a nervous system procedure G97.48
      during other procedure G97.49
    respiratory system
      during other procedure J95.72
      during procedure on respiratory system organ or structure J95.71

Complication — Complication

Complication(s) — *continued*
  intraoperative — *continued*
    puncture or laceration — *continued*
      skin and subcutaneous tissue
        during a dermatologic procedure L76.11
        during a procedure on other organ L76.12
      spleen
        during a procedure on other organ D78.12
        during a procedure on the spleen D78.11
    specified NEC
      circulatory system I97.88
      digestive system K91.81
      ear H95.88
      endocrine system E36.8
      eye and adnexa H59.88
      genitourinary system N99.81
      mastoid process H95.88
      musculoskeletal structure M96.89
      nervous system G97.81
      respiratory system J95.88
      skin and subcutaneous tissue L76.81
      spleen D78.81
  intraperitoneal catheter (dialysis) (infusion) — *see* Complications, catheter, intraperitoneal
  intrathecal infusion pump
    infection and inflammation T85.738 ☑
    mechanical
      breakdown T85.615 ☑
      displacement T85.625 ☑
      leakage T85.635 ☑
      malfunction T85.695 ☑
      malposition T85.625 ☑
      obstruction T85.695 ☑
      perforation T85.695 ☑
      protrusion T85.695 ☑
      specified NEC T85.695 ☑
  intrauterine
    contraceptive device
      embolism T83.81 ☑
      fibrosis T83.82 ☑
      hemorrhage T83.83 ☑
      infection and inflammation T83.69 ☑
      mechanical
        breakdown T83.31 ☑
        displacement T83.32 ☑
        malposition T83.32 ☑
        obstruction T83.39 ☑
        perforation T83.39 ☑
        protrusion T83.39 ☑
        specified NEC T83.39 ☑
      pain T83.84 ☑
      specified type NEC T83.89 ☑
      stenosis T83.85 ☑
      thrombosis T83.86 ☑
    procedure (fetal), to newborn P96.5
  jejunostomy (stoma) — *see* Complications, enterostomy
  joint prosthesis, internal T84.9 ☑
    breakage (fracture) T84.01- ☑
    dislocation T84.02- ☑
    fracture T84.01- ☑
    infection or inflammation T84.50 ☑
      hip T84.5- ☑
      knee T84.5- ☑
      specified joint NEC T84.59 ☑
    instability T84.02- ☑
    malposition — *see* Complications, joint prosthesis, mechanical, displacement
    mechanical
      breakage, broken T84.01- ☑
      dislocation T84.02- ☑
      fracture T84.01- ☑
      instability T84.02- ☑
      leakage — *see* Complications, joint prosthesis, mechanical, specified NEC
      loosening T84.039 ☑
        hip T84.03- ☑
        knee T84.03- ☑
        specified joint NEC T84.038 ☑
      obstruction — *see* Complications, joint prosthesis, mechanical, specified NEC
      perforation — *see* Complications, joint prosthesis, mechanical, specified NEC
      osteolysis T84.059 ☑
        hip T84.05- ☑
        knee T84.05- ☑
        other specified joint T84.058 ☑

Complication(s) — *continued*
  joint prosthesis, internal — *continued*
    mechanical — *continued*
      protrusion — *see* Complications, joint prosthesis, mechanical, specified NEC
      specified complication NEC T84.099 ☑
        hip T84.09- ☑
        knee T84.09- ☑
        other specified joint T84.098 ☑
      subluxation T84.02- ☑
      wear of articular bearing surface T84.069 ☑
        hip T84.06- ☑
        knee T84.06- ☑
        other specified joint T84.068 ☑
    specified joint NEC T84.89 ☑
    embolism T84.81 ☑
    fibrosis T84.82 ☑
    hemorrhage T84.83 ☑
    pain T84.84 ☑
    specified complication NEC T84.89 ☑
    stenosis T84.85 ☑
    thrombosis T84.86 ☑
    subluxation T84.02- ☑
  kidney transplant — *see* Complications, transplant, kidney
  labor O75.9
    specified NEC O75.89
  liver transplant (immune or nonimmune) — *see* Complications, transplant, liver
  lumbar puncture G97.1
    cerebrospinal fluid leak G97.0
    headache or reaction G97.1
  lung transplant — *see* Complications, transplant, lung
    and heart — *see* Complications, transplant, lung, with heart
  male genital N50.9
    device, implant or graft — *see* Complications, genitourinary, device or implant, genital tract
    postprocedural or postoperative — *see* Complications, genitourinary, postprocedural
    specified NEC N99.89
  mastoid (process) procedure
    intraoperative H95.88
      hematoma — *see* Complications, intraoperative, hemorrhage (hematoma) (of), mastoid process
      hemorrhage — *see* Complications, intraoperative, hemorrhage (hematoma) (of), mastoid process
      laceration — *see* Complications, intraoperative, puncture or laceration, mastoid process
      specified NEC H95.88
    postmastoidectomy — *see* Complications, postmastoidectomy
    postoperative H95.89
      external ear canal stenosis H95.81
      hematoma — *see* Complications, postprocedural, hematoma (of), mastoid process
      hemorrhage — *see* Complications, postprocedural, hemorrhage (of), mastoid process
      postmastoidectomy — *see* Complications, postmastoidectomy
      seroma — *see* Complications, postprocedural, seroma (of), mastoid process
      specified NEC H95.89
  mastoidectomy cavity — *see* Complications, postmastoidectomy
  mechanical — *see* Complications, by site and type, mechanical
  medical procedures (*see also* Complication(s), intraoperative) T88.9
  metabolic E88.9
    postoperative E89.89
    specified NEC E89.89
  molar pregnancy NOS O08.9
    damage to pelvic organs O08.6
    embolism O08.2
    genital infection O08.0
    hemorrhage (delayed) (excessive) O08.1
    metabolic disorder O08.5
    renal failure O08.4
    shock O08.3
    specified type NEC O08.0
    venous complication NEC O08.7

Complication(s) — *continued*
  musculoskeletal system (*see also* Complication, intraoperative (intraprocedural), by site)
    device, implant or graft NEC — *see* Complications, orthopedic, device or implant
    internal fixation (nail) (plate) (rod) — *see* Complications, fixation device, internal
    joint prosthesis — *see* Complications, joint prosthesis
    post radiation M96.89
      kyphosis M96.2
      scoliosis M96.5
      specified complication NEC M96.89
    postoperative (postprocedural) M96.89
      with osteoporosis — *see* Osteoporosis
      fracture following insertion of device — *see* Fracture, following insertion of orthopedic implant, joint prosthesis or bone plate
      joint instability after prosthesis removal M96.89
      lordosis M96.4
      postlaminectomy syndrome NEC M96.1
        kyphosis M96.3
      pseudarthrosis M96.0
      specified complication NEC M96.89
  nephrostomy (stoma) — *see* Complications, stoma, urinary tract, external NEC
  nervous system G98.8
    central G96.9
    device, implant or graft (*see also* Complication, prosthetic device or implant, specified NEC)
      electronic stimulator (electrode(s)) — *see* Complications, electronic stimulator device
      specified NEC
        infection and inflammation T85.738 ☑
        mechanical T85.695 ☑
          breakdown T85.615 ☑
          displacement T85.625 ☑
          leakage T85.635 ☑
          malfunction T85.695 ☑
          malposition T85.625 ☑
          obstruction T85.695 ☑
          perforation T85.695 ☑
          protrusion T85.695 ☑
          specified NEC T85.695 ☑
      ventricular shunt — *see* Complications, ventricular shunt
    electronic stimulator (electrode(s)) — *see* Complications, electronic stimulator device
    postprocedural G97.82
      intracranial hypotension G97.2
      specified NEC G97.82
      spinal fluid leak G97.0
  newborn, due to intrauterine (fetal) procedure P96.5
  nonabsorbable (permanent) sutures — *see* Complication, sutures, permanent
  obstetric O75.9
    procedure (instrumental) (manual) (surgical) specified NEC O75.4
    specified NEC O75.89
    surgical wound NEC O90.89
      hematoma O90.2
      infection O86.0
  ocular lens implant — *see* Complications, intraocular lens
  ophthalmologic
    postprocedural bleb — *see* Blebitis
  orbital prosthesis T85.9 ☑
    embolism T85.818 ☑
    fibrosis T85.828 ☑
    hemorrhage T85.838 ☑
    infection and inflammation T85.79 ☑
    mechanical
      breakdown T85.31- ☑
      displacement T85.32- ☑
      malposition T85.32- ☑
      obstruction T85.39- ☑
      perforation T85.39- ☑
      protrusion T85.39- ☑
      specified NEC T85.39- ☑
    pain T85.848 ☑
    specified type NEC T85.898 ☑
    stenosis T85.858 ☑
    thrombosis T85.868 ☑
  organ or tissue transplant (partial) (total) — *see* Complications, transplant

☑ Additional Character Required — Refer to the Tabular List for Character Selection   ▽ Subterms under main terms may continue to next column or page

Complication(s) — *continued*
orthopedic (*see also* Disorder, soft tissue)
device or implant T84.9 ☑
bone
device or implant — *see* Complication, bone, device NEC
graft — *see* Complication, graft, bone
breakdown T84.418 ☑
displacement T84.428 ☑
electronic bone stimulator — *see* Complications, electronic stimulator device, bone
embolism T84.81 ☑
fibrosis T84.82 ☑
fixation device — *see* Complication, fixation device, internal
hemorrhage T84.83 ☑
infection or inflammation T84.7 ☑
joint prosthesis — *see* Complication, joint prosthesis, internal
malfunction T84.418 ☑
malposition T84.428 ☑
mechanical NEC T84.498 ☑
muscle graft — *see* Complications, graft, muscle
obstruction T84.498 ☑
pain T84.84 ☑
perforation T84.498 ☑
protrusion T84.498 ☑
specified complication NEC T84.89 ☑
stenosis T84.85 ☑
tendon graft — *see* Complications, graft, tendon
thrombosis T84.86 ☑
fracture (following insertion of device) — *see* Fracture, following insertion of orthopedic implant, joint prosthesis or bone plate
postprocedural M96.89
fracture — *see* Fracture, following insertion of orthopedic implant, joint prosthesis or bone plate
postlaminectomy syndrome NEC M96.1
kyphosis M96.3
lordosis M96.4
postradiation
kyphosis M96.2
scoliosis M96.5
pseudarthrosis post-fusion M96.0
specified type NEC M96.89
pacemaker (cardiac) — *see* Complications, cardiovascular device or implant, electronic
pancreas transplant — *see* Complications, transplant, pancreas
penile prosthesis (implant) — *see* Complications, prosthetic device, penile
perfusion NEC T80.90 ☑
perineal repair (obstetrical) NEC O90.89
disruption O90.1
hematoma O90.2
infection (following delivery) O86.0
phototherapy T88.9 ☑
specified NEC T88.8 ☑
postmastoidectomy NEC H95.19- ☑
cyst, mucosal H95.13- ☑
granulation H95.12- ☑
inflammation, chronic H95.11- ☑
recurrent cholesteatoma H95.0- ☑
postoperative — *see* Complications, postprocedural
circulatory — *see* Complications, circulatory system
ear — *see* Complications, ear
endocrine — *see* Complications, endocrine
eye — *see* Complications, eye
lumbar puncture G97.1
cerebrospinal fluid leak G97.0
nervous system (central) (peripheral) — *see* Complications, nervous system
respiratory system — *see* Complications, respiratory system
postprocedural (*see also* Complications, surgical procedure)
cardiac arrest (*see also* Infarct, myocardium, associated with revascularization procedure)
following cardiac surgery I97.120
following other surgery I97.121
cardiac functional disturbance NEC (*see also* Infarct, myocardium, associated with revascularization procedure)
following cardiac surgery I97.190

Complication(s) — *continued*
postprocedural (*see also* Complications, surgical procedure) — *continued*
cardiac functional disturbance (*see also* Infarct, myocardium, associated with revascularization procedure) — *continued*
following other surgery I97.191
cardiac insufficiency
following cardiac surgery I97.110
following other surgery I97.111
chorioretinal scars following retinal surgery H59.81- ☑
following cataract surgery
cataract (lens) fragments H59.02- ☑
cystoid macular edema H59.03- ☑
specified NEC H59.09- ☑
vitreous (touch) syndrome H59.01- ☑
heart failure
following cardiac surgery I97.130
following other surgery I97.131
hematoma (of)
circulatory system organ or structure
following cardiac bypass I97.631
following cardiac catheterization I97.630
following other circulatory system procedure I97.638
following other procedure I97.621
digestive system
following procedure on digestive system K91.870
following procedure on other organ K91.871
ear
following other procedure H95.52
following procedure on ear and mastoid process H95.51
endocrine system
following endocrine system procedure E89.820
following other procedure E89.821
eye and adnexa
following ophthalmic procedure H59.33- ☑
following other procedure H59.34- ☑
genitourinary organ or structure
following procedure on genitourinary organ or structure N99.840
following procedure on other organ N99.841
mastoid process
following other procedure H95.52
following procedure on ear and mastoid process H95.51
musculoskeletal structure
following musculoskeletal surgery M96.840
following non-orthopedic surgery M96.841
following orthopedic surgery M96.840
nervous system
following nervous system procedure G97.61
following other procedure G97.62
respiratory system
following other procedure J95.861
following procedure on respiratory system organ or structure J95.860
skin and subcutaneous tissue
following dermatologic procedure L76.31
following procedure on other organ L76.32
spleen
following procedure on other organ D78.32
following procedure on the spleen D78.31
hemorrhage (of)
circulatory system organ or structure
following cardiac bypass I97.611
following cardiac catheterization I97.610
following other circulatory system procedure I97.618
following other procedure I97.620
digestive system
following procedure on digestive system K91.840
following procedure on other organ K91.841
ear
following other procedure H95.42
following procedure on ear and mastoid process H95.41
endocrine system
following endocrine system procedure E89.810
following other procedure E89.811

Complication(s) — *continued*
postprocedural (*see also* Complications, surgical procedure) — *continued*
hemorrhage — *continued*
eye and adnexa
following ophthalmic procedure H59.31- ☑
following other procedure H59.32- ☑
genitourinary organ or structure
following procedure on genitourinary organ or structure N99.820
following procedure on other organ N99.821
mastoid process
following other procedure H95.42
following procedure on ear and mastoid process H95.41
musculoskeletal structure
following musculoskeletal surgery M96.830
following non-orthopedic surgery M96.831
following orthopedic surgery M96.830
nervous system
following nervous system procedure G97.51
following other procedure G97.52
respiratory system
following a respiratory system procedure J95.830
following other procedure J95.831
skin and subcutaneous tissue
following a procedure on other organ L76.22
following dermatologic procedure L76.21
spleen
following procedure on other organ D78.22
following procedure on the spleen D78.21
seroma (of)
circulatory system organ or structure
following cardiac bypass I97.641
following cardiac catheterization I97.640
following other circulatory system procedure I97.648
following other procedure I97.622
digestive system
following procedure on digestive system K91.872
following procedure on other organ K91.873
ear
following other procedure H95.54
following procedure on ear and mastoid process H95.53
endocrine system
following endocrine system procedure E89.822
following other procedure E89.823
eye and adnexa
following ophthalmic procedure H59.35- ☑
following other procedure H59.36- ☑
genitourinary organ or structure
following procedure on genitourinary organ or structure N99.842
following procedure on other organ N99.843
mastoid process
following other procedure H95.54
following procedure on ear and mastoid process H95.53
musculoskeletal structure
following musculoskeletal surgery M96.842
following non-orthopedic surgery M96.843
following orthopedic surgery M96.842
nervous system
following nervous system procedure G97.63
following other procedure G97.64
respiratory system
following other procedure J95.863
following procedure on respiratory system organ or structure J95.862
skin and subcutaneous tissue
following dermatologic procedure L76.33
following procedure on other organ L76.34
spleen
following procedure on other organ D78.34
following procedure on the spleen D78.33
specified NEC
circulatory system I97.89
digestive K91.89
ear H95.89
endocrine E89.89
eye and adnexa H59.89
genitourinary N99.89

☑ **Additional Character Required — Refer to the Tabular List for Character Selection**   ▼ **Subterms under main terms may continue to next column or page**

Complication(s) — continued
- stent — continued
  - urinary — continued
    - infection and inflammation T83.593 ☑
    - mechanical
      - breakdown T83.113 ☑
      - displacement T83.123 ☑
      - leakage T83.193 ☑
      - malposition T83.123 ☑
      - obstruction T83.193 ☑
      - perforation T83.193 ☑
      - protrusion T83.193 ☑
      - specified NEC T83.193 ☑
    - pain T83.84 ☑
    - specified type NEC T83.89 ☑
    - stenosis T83.85 ☑
    - thrombosis T83.86 ☑
  - vascular
    - end stent stenosis — see Restenosis, stent
    - in stent stenosis — see Restenosis, stent
- stoma
  - digestive tract
    - colostomy — see Complications, colostomy
    - enterostomy — see Complications, enterostomy
    - esophagostomy — see Complications, esophagostomy
    - gastrostomy — see Complications, gastrostomy
  - urinary tract N99.528
    - continent N99.538
      - hemorrhage N99.530
      - herniation N99.533
      - infection N99.531
      - malfunction N99.532
      - specified type NEC N99.538
      - stenosis N99.534
    - cystostomy — see Complications, cystostomy
    - external NOS N99.528
    - hemorrhage N99.520
    - herniation N99.523
    - incontinent N99.528
      - hemorrhage N99.520
      - herniation N99.523
      - infection N99.521
      - malfunction N99.522
      - specified type NEC N99.528
      - stenosis N99.524
    - infection N99.521
    - malfunction N99.522
    - specified type NEC N99.528
    - stenosis N99.524
- stomach banding — see Complication(s), bariatric procedure
- stomach stapling — see Complication(s), bariatric procedure
- surgical material, nonabsorbable — see Complication, suture, permanent
- surgical procedure (on) T81.9 ☑
  - amputation stump (late) — see Complications, amputation stump
  - cardiac — see Complications, circulatory system
  - cholesteatoma, recurrent — see Complications, postmastoidectomy, recurrent cholesteatoma
  - circulatory (early) — see Complications, circulatory system
  - digestive system — see Complications, gastrointestinal
  - dumping syndrome (postgastrectomy) K91.1
  - ear — see Complications, ear
  - elephantiasis or lymphedema I97.89
    - postmastectomy I97.2
  - emphysema (surgical) T81.82 ☑
  - endocrine — see Complications, endocrine
  - eye — see Complications, eye
  - fistula (persistent postoperative) T81.83 ☑
  - foreign body inadvertently left in wound (sponge) (suture) (swab) — see Foreign body, accidentally left during a procedure
  - gastrointestinal — see Complications, gastrointestinal
  - genitourinary NEC N99.89
  - hematoma
    - intraoperative — see Complication, intraoperative, hemorrhage
    - postprocedural — see Complication, postprocedural, hematoma

Complication(s) — continued
- surgical procedure — continued
  - hemorrhage
    - intraoperative — see Complication, intraoperative, hemorrhage
    - postprocedural — see Complication, postprocedural, hemorrhage
  - hepatic failure K91.82
  - hyperglycemia (postpancreatectomy) E89.1
  - hypoinsulinemia (postpancreatectomy) E89.1
  - hypoparathyroidism (postparathyroidectomy) E89.2
  - hypopituitarism (posthypophysectomy) E89.3
  - hypothyroidism (post-thyroidectomy) E89.0
  - intestinal obstruction (see also Obstruction, intestine, postoperative) K91.30
  - intracranial hypotension following ventricular shunting (ventriculostomy) G97.2
  - lymphedema I97.89
    - postmastectomy I97.2
  - malabsorption (postsurgical) NEC K91.2
    - osteoporosis — see Osteoporosis, postsurgical malabsorption
  - mastoidectomy cavity NEC — see Complications, postmastoidectomy
  - metabolic E89.89
    - specified NEC E89.89
  - musculoskeletal — see Complications, musculoskeletal system
  - nervous system (central) (peripheral) — see Complications, nervous system
  - ovarian failure E89.40
    - asymptomatic E89.40
    - symptomatic E89.41
  - peripheral vascular — see Complications, surgical procedure, vascular
  - postcardiotomy syndrome I97.0
  - postcholecystectomy syndrome K91.5
  - postcommissurotomy syndrome I97.0
  - postgastrectomy dumping syndrome K91.1
  - postlaminectomy syndrome NEC M96.1
    - kyphosis M96.3
  - postmastectomy lymphedema syndrome I97.2
  - postmastoidectomy cholesteatoma — see Complications, postmastoidectomy, recurrent cholesteatoma
  - postvagotomy syndrome K91.1
  - postvalvulotomy syndrome I97.0
  - pulmonary insufficiency (acute) J95.2
    - chronic J95.3
    - following thoracic surgery J95.1
  - reattached body part — see Complications, reattached
  - respiratory — see Complications, respiratory system
  - shock (hypovolemic) T81.19 ☑
  - spleen (postoperative) D78.89
    - intraoperative D78.81
  - stitch abscess T81.4 ☑
  - subglottic stenosis (postsurgical) J95.5
  - testicular hypofunction E89.5
  - transplant — see Complications, organ or tissue transplant
  - urinary NEC N99.89
  - vaginal vault prolapse (posthysterectomy) N99.3
  - vascular (peripheral)
    - artery T81.719 ☑
      - mesenteric T81.710 ☑
      - renal T81.711 ☑
      - specified NEC T81.718 ☑
    - vein T81.72 ☑
  - wound infection T81.4 ☑
- suture, permanent (wire) NEC T85.9 ☑
  - with repair of bone — see Complications, fixation device, internal
  - embolism T85.818 ☑
  - fibrosis T85.828 ☑
  - hemorrhage T85.838 ☑
  - infection and inflammation T85.79 ☑
  - mechanical
    - breakdown T85.612 ☑
    - displacement T85.622 ☑
    - malfunction T85.612 ☑
    - malposition T85.622 ☑
    - obstruction T85.692 ☑
    - perforation T85.692 ☑
    - protrusion T85.692 ☑

Complication(s) — continued
- suture, permanent — continued
  - mechanical — continued
    - specified NEC T85.692 ☑
  - pain T85.848 ☑
  - specified type NEC T85.898 ☑
  - stenosis T85.858 ☑
  - thrombosis T85.868 ☑
- tracheostomy J95.00
  - granuloma J95.09
  - hemorrhage J95.01
  - infection J95.02
  - malfunction J95.03
  - mechanical J95.03
  - obstruction J95.03
  - specified type NEC J95.09
  - tracheo-esophageal fistula J95.04
- transfusion (blood) (lymphocytes) (plasma) T80.92 ☑
  - air embolism T80.0 ☑
  - circulatory overload E87.71
  - febrile nonhemolytic transfusion reaction R50.84
  - hemochromatosis E83.111
  - hemolysis T80.89 ☑
  - hemolytic reaction (antigen unspecified) T80.919 ☑
  - incompatibility reaction (antigen unspecified) T80.919 ☑
    - ABO T80.30 ☑
      - delayed serologic (DSTR) T80.39 ☑
      - hemolytic transfusion reaction (HTR) (unspecified time after transfusion) T80.319 ☑
        - acute (AHTR) (less than 24 hours after transfusion) T80.310 ☑
        - delayed (DHTR) (24 hours or more after transfusion) T80.311 ☑
      - specified NEC T80.39 ☑
    - acute (antigen unspecified) T80.910 ☑
    - delayed (antigen unspecified) T80.911 ☑
    - delayed serologic (DSTR) T80.89 ☑
    - non-ABO (minor antigens (Duffy) (Kell) (Kidd) (Lewis) (M) (N) (P) (S)) T80.A0 ☑ (following T80.4)
      - delayed serologic (DSTR) T80.A9 ☑ (following T80.4)
      - hemolytic transfusion reaction (HTR) (unspecified time after transfusion) T80.A19 ☑ (following T80.4)
        - acute (AHTR) (less than 24 hours after transfusion) T80.A10 ☑ (following T80.4)
        - delayed (DHTR) (24 hours or more after transfusion) T80.A11 ☑ (following T80.4)
      - specified NEC T80.A9 ☑ (following T80.4)
    - Rh (antigens (C) (c) (D) (E) (e)) (factor) T80.40 ☑
      - delayed serologic (DSTR) T80.49 ☑
      - hemolytic transfusion reaction (HTR) (unspecified time after transfusion) T80.419 ☑
        - acute (AHTR) (less than 24 hours after transfusion) T80.410 ☑
        - delayed (DHTR) (24 hours or more after transfusion) T80.411 ☑
      - specified NEC T80.49 ☑
  - infection T80.29 ☑
    - acute T80.22- ☑
  - reaction NEC T80.89 ☑
  - sepsis T80.29 ☑
  - shock T80.89 ☑
- transplant T86.90
  - bone T86.839
    - failure T86.831
    - infection T86.832
    - rejection T86.830
    - specified type NEC T86.838
  - bone marrow T86.00
    - failure T86.02
    - infection T86.03
    - rejection T86.01
    - specified type NEC T86.09
  - cornea T86.849
    - failure T86.841
    - infection T86.842
    - rejection T86.840
    - specified type NEC T86.848
  - failure T86.92

Index

Complication(s) — *continued*
  transplant — *continued*
    heart T86.20
      with lung T86.30
        cardiac allograft vasculopathy T86.290
          failure T86.32
          infection T86.33
          rejection T86.31
          specified type NEC T86.39
      failure T86.22
      infection T86.23
      rejection T86.21
      specified type NEC T86.298
    infection T86.93
    intestine T86.859
      failure T86.851
      infection T86.852
      rejection T86.850
      specified type NEC T86.858
    kidney T86.10
      failure T86.12
      infection T86.13
      rejection T86.11
      specified type NEC T86.19
    liver T86.40
      failure T86.42
      infection T86.43
      rejection T86.41
      specified type NEC T86.49
    lung T86.819
      with heart T86.30
        failure T86.32
        infection T86.33
        rejection T86.31
        specified type NEC T86.39
      failure T86.811
      infection T86.812
      rejection T86.810
      specified type NEC T86.818
    malignant neoplasm C80.2
    pancreas T86.899
      failure T86.891
      infection T86.892
      rejection T86.890
      specified type NEC T86.898
    peripheral blood stem cells T86.5
    post-transplant lymphoproliferative disorder (PTLD) D47.Z1 (*following* D47.4)
    rejection T86.91
    skin T86.829
      failure T86.821
      infection T86.822
      rejection T86.820
      specified type NEC T86.828
    specified
      tissue T86.899
        failure T86.891
        infection T86.892
        rejection T86.890
        specified type NEC T86.898
      type NEC T86.99
    stem cell (from peripheral blood) (from umbilical cord) T86.5
    umbilical cord stem cells T86.5
  trauma (early) T79.9 ☑
    specified NEC T79.8 ☑
  ultrasound therapy NEC T88.9 ☑
  umbilical cord NEC
    complicating delivery O69.9 ☑
      specified NEC O69.89 ☑
  umbrella device, vascular T82.9 ☑
    embolism T82.818 ☑
    fibrosis T82.828 ☑
    hemorrhage T82.838 ☑
    infection or inflammation T82.7 ☑
    mechanical
      breakdown T82.515 ☑
      displacement T82.525 ☑
      leakage T82.535 ☑
      malposition T82.525 ☑
      obstruction T82.595 ☑
      perforation T82.595 ☑
      protrusion T82.595 ☑
    pain T82.848 ☑
    specified type NEC T82.898 ☑
    stenosis T82.858 ☑
    thrombosis T82.868 ☑

Complication(s) — *continued*
  urethral catheter — *see* Complications, catheter, urethral, indwelling
  vaccination T88.1 ☑
    anaphylaxis NEC T80.52 ☑
    arthropathy — *see* Arthropathy, postimmunization
    cellulitis T88.0 ☑
    encephalitis or encephalomyelitis G04.02
    infection (general) (local) NEC T88.0 ☑
    meningitis G03.8
    myelitis G04.02
    protein sickness T80.62 ☑
    rash T88.1 ☑
    reaction (allergic) T88.1 ☑
      serum T80.62 ☑
    sepsis T88.0 ☑
    serum intoxication, sickness, rash, or other serum reaction NEC T80.62 ☑
      anaphylactic shock T80.52 ☑
    shock (allergic) (anaphylactic) T80.52 ☑
    vaccinia (generalized) (localized) T88.1 ☑
  vas deferens device or implant — *see* Complications, genitourinary, device or implant, genital tract
  vascular I99.9
    device or implant T82.9 ☑
      embolism T82.818 ☑
      fibrosis T82.828 ☑
      hemorrhage T82.838 ☑
      infection or inflammation T82.7 ☑
      mechanical
        breakdown T82.519 ☑
          specified device NEC T82.518 ☑
        displacement T82.529 ☑
          specified device NEC T82.528 ☑
        leakage T82.539 ☑
          specified device NEC T82.538 ☑
        malposition T82.529 ☑
          specified device NEC T82.528 ☑
        obstruction T82.599 ☑
          specified device NEC T82.598 ☑
        perforation T82.599 ☑
          specified device NEC T82.598 ☑
        protrusion T82.599 ☑
          specified device NEC T82.598 ☑
      pain T82.848 ☑
      specified type NEC T82.898 ☑
      stenosis T82.858 ☑
      thrombosis T82.868 ☑
    dialysis catheter — *see* Complication, catheter, dialysis
    following infusion, therapeutic injection or transfusion T80.1 ☑
    graft T82.9 ☑
      embolism T82.818 ☑
      fibrosis T82.828 ☑
      hemorrhage T82.838 ☑
      mechanical
        breakdown T82.319 ☑
          aorta (bifurcation) T82.310 ☑
          carotid artery T82.311 ☑
          specified vessel NEC T82.318 ☑
        displacement T82.329 ☑
          aorta (bifurcation) T82.320 ☑
          carotid artery T82.321 ☑
          specified vessel NEC T82.328 ☑
        leakage T82.339 ☑
          aorta (bifurcation) T82.330 ☑
          carotid artery T82.331 ☑
          specified vessel NEC T82.338 ☑
        malposition T82.329 ☑
          aorta (bifurcation) T82.320 ☑
          carotid artery T82.321 ☑
          specified vessel NEC T82.328 ☑
        obstruction T82.399 ☑
          aorta (bifurcation) T82.390 ☑
          carotid artery T82.391 ☑
          specified vessel NEC T82.398 ☑
        perforation T82.399 ☑
          aorta (bifurcation) T82.390 ☑
          carotid artery T82.391 ☑
          specified vessel NEC T82.398 ☑
        protrusion T82.399 ☑
          aorta (bifurcation) T82.390 ☑
          carotid artery T82.391 ☑
          specified vessel NEC T82.398 ☑
      pain T82.848 ☑

Complication(s) — *continued*
  vascular — *continued*
    graft — *continued*
      specified complication NEC T82.898 ☑
      stenosis T82.858 ☑
      thrombosis T82.868 ☑
    postoperative — *see* Complications, postoperative, circulatory
  vena cava device (filter) (sieve) (umbrella) — *see* Complications, umbrella device, vascular
  ventilation therapy NEC T81.81 ☑
  ventilator
    mechanical J95.850
      specified NEC J95.859
  ventricular (communicating) shunt (device) T85.9 ☑
    embolism T85.810 ☑
    fibrosis T85.820 ☑
    hemorrhage T85.830 ☑
    infection and inflammation T85.730 ☑
    mechanical
      breakdown T85.01 ☑
      displacement T85.02 ☑
      leakage T85.03 ☑
      malposition T85.02 ☑
      obstruction T85.09 ☑
      perforation T85.09 ☑
      protrusion T85.09 ☑
      specified NEC T85.09 ☑
    pain T85.840 ☑
    specified type NEC T85.890 ☑
    stenosis T85.850 ☑
    thrombosis T85.860 ☑
  wire suture, permanent (implanted) — *see* Complications, suture, permanent
Compressed air disease T70.3 ☑
Compression
  with injury — *code by* Nature of injury
  artery I77.1
    celiac, syndrome I77.4
  brachial plexus G54.0
  brain (stem) G93.5
    due to
      contusion (diffuse) — *see* Injury, intracranial, diffuse
        focal — *see* Injury, intracranial, focal
      injury NEC — *see* Injury, intracranial, diffuse
      traumatic — *see* Injury, intracranial, diffuse
  bronchus J98.09
  cauda equina G83.4
  celiac (artery) (axis) I77.4
  cerebral — *see* Compression, brain
  cervical plexus G54.2
  cord
    spinal — *see* Compression, spinal
    umbilical — *see* Compression, umbilical cord
  cranial nerve G52.9
    eighth H93.3 ☑
    eleventh G52.8
    fifth G50.8
    first G52.0
    fourth — *see* Strabismus, paralytic, fourth nerve
    ninth G52.1
    second — *see* Disorder, nerve, optic
    seventh G51.8
    sixth — *see* Strabismus, paralytic, sixth nerve
    tenth G52.2
    third — *see* Strabismus, paralytic, third nerve
    twelfth G52.3
  diver's squeeze T70.3 ☑
  during birth (newborn) P15.9
  esophagus K22.2
  eustachian tube — *see* Obstruction, eustachian tube, cartilaginous
  facies Q67.1
  fracture
    nontraumatic NOS — *see* Collapse, vertebra
    pathological — *see* Fracture, pathological
    traumatic — *see* Fracture, traumatic
  heart — *see* Disease, heart
  intestine — *see* Obstruction, intestine
  laryngeal nerve, recurrent G52.2
    with paralysis of vocal cords and larynx J38.00
      bilateral J38.02
      unilateral J38.01
  lumbosacral plexus G54.1
  lung J98.4
  lymphatic vessel I89.0

Complication — Compression

Compression — *continued*
  medulla — *see* Compression, brain
  nerve (*see also* Disorder, nerve) G58.9
    arm NEC — *see* Mononeuropathy, upper limb
    axillary G54.0
    cranial — *see* Compression, cranial nerve
    leg NEC — *see* Mononeuropathy, lower limb
    median (in carpal tunnel) — *see* Syndrome, carpal tunnel
    optic — *see* Disorder, nerve, optic
    plantar — *see* Lesion, nerve, plantar
    posterior tibial (in tarsal tunnel) — *see* Syndrome, tarsal tunnel
    root or plexus NOS (in) G54.9
      intervertebral disc disorder NEC — *see* Disorder, disc, with, radiculopathy
      with myelopathy — *see* Disorder, disc, with, myelopathy
      neoplastic disease (*see also* Neoplasm) D49.9 [G55]
      spondylosis — *see* Spondylosis, with radiculopathy
    sciatic (acute) — *see* Lesion, nerve, sciatic
    sympathetic G90.8
    traumatic — *see* Injury, nerve
    ulnar — *see* Lesion, nerve, ulnar
    upper extremity NEC — *see* Mononeuropathy, upper limb
  spinal (cord) G95.20
    by displacement of intervertebral disc NEC (*see also* Disorder, disc, with, myelopathy)
    nerve root NOS G54.9
      due to displacement of intervertebral disc NEC — *see* Disorder, disc, with, radiculopathy
      with myelopathy — *see* Disorder, disc, with, myelopathy
    specified NEC G95.29
    spondylogenic (cervical) (lumbar, lumbosacral) (thoracic) — *see* Spondylosis, with myelopathy NEC
      anterior — *see* Syndrome, anterior, spinal artery, compression
    traumatic — *see* Injury, spinal cord, by region
  subcostal nerve (syndrome) — *see* Mononeuropathy, upper limb, specified NEC
  sympathetic nerve NEC G90.8
  syndrome T79.5 ☑
  trachea J39.8
  ulnar nerve (by scar tissue) — *see* Lesion, nerve, ulnar
  umbilical cord
    complicating delivery O69.2 ☑
      cord around neck O69.1 ☑
      prolapse O69.0 ☑
      specified NEC O69.2 ☑
  ureter N13.5
  vein I87.1
  vena cava (inferior) (superior) I87.1
Compulsion, compulsive
  gambling F63.0
  neurosis F42.8
  personality F60.5
  states F42.8
  swearing F42.8
    in Gilles de la Tourette's syndrome F95.2
  tics and spasms F95.9
Concato's disease (pericardial polyserositis) A19.9
  nontubercular I31.1
  pleural — *see* Pleurisy, with effusion
Concavity chest wall M95.4
Concealed penis Q55.69
Concern (normal) **about sick person in family** Z63.6
Concrescence (teeth) K00.2
Concretio cordis I31.1
  rheumatic I09.2
Concretion (*see also* Calculus)
  appendicular K38.1
  canaliculus — *see* Dacryolith
  clitoris N90.89
  conjunctiva H11.12- ☑
  eyelid — *see* Disorder, eyelid, specified type NEC
  lacrimal passages — *see* Dacryolith
  prepuce (male) N47.8
  salivary gland (any) K11.5
  seminal vesicle N50.89
  tonsil J35.8
Concussion (brain) (cerebral) (current) S06.0X9 ☑

Concussion — *continued*
  with
    loss of consciousness of 30 minutes or less S06.0X1 ☑
    loss of consciousness of unspecified duration S06.0X9 ☑
    without loss of consciousness S06.0X0 ☑
  blast (air) (hydraulic) (immersion) (underwater)
    abdomen or thorax — *see* Injury, blast, by site
    ear with acoustic nerve injury — *see* Injury, nerve, acoustic, specified type NEC
  cauda equina S34.3 ☑
  conus medullaris S34.02 ☑
  ocular S05.8X- ☑
  spinal (cord)
    cervical S14.0 ☑
    lumbar S34.01 ☑
    sacral S34.02 ☑
    thoracic S24.0 ☑
  syndrome F07.81
Condition — *see* Disease
Conditions arising in the perinatal period — *see* Newborn, affected by
Conduct disorder — *see* Disorder, conduct
Condyloma A63.0
  acuminatum A63.0
  gonorrheal A54.09
  latum A51.31
  syphilitic A51.31
    congenital A50.07
  venereal, syphilitic A51.31
Conflagration (*see also* Burn)
  asphyxia (by inhalation of gases, fumes or vapors) (*see also* Table of Drugs and Chemicals) T59.9- ☑
Conflict (with) (*see also* Discord)
  family Z73.9
  marital Z63.0
    involving divorce or estrangement Z63.5
  parent-child Z62.820
    parent-adopted child Z62.821
    parent-biological child Z62.820
    parent-foster child Z62.822
  social role NEC Z73.5
Confluent — *see* condition
Confusion, confused R41.0
  epileptic F05
  mental state (psychogenic) F44.89
  psychogenic F44.89
  reactive (from emotional stress, psychological trauma) F44.89
Confusional arousals G47.51
Congelation T69.9 ☑
Congenital (*see also* condition)
  aortic septum Q25.49
  intrinsic factor deficiency D51.0
  malformation — *see* Anomaly
Congestion, congestive
  bladder N32.89
  bowel K63.89
  brain G93.89
  breast N64.59
  bronchial J98.09
  catarrhal J31.0
  chest R09.89
  chill, malarial — *see* Malaria
  circulatory NEC I99.8
  duodenum K31.89
  eye — *see* Hyperemia, conjunctiva
  facial, due to birth injury P15.4
  general R68.89
  glottis J37.0
  heart — *see* Failure, heart, congestive
  hepatic K76.1
  hypostatic (lung) — *see* Edema, lung
  intestine K63.89
  kidney N28.89
  labyrinth H83.8 ☑
  larynx J37.0
  liver K76.1
  lung R09.89
    active or acute — *see* Pneumonia
  malaria, malarial — *see* Malaria
  nasal R09.81
  nose R09.81
  orbit, orbital (*see also* Exophthalmos)
    inflammatory (chronic) — *see* Inflammation, orbit
  ovary N83.8

Congestion, congestive — *continued*
  pancreas K86.89
  pelvic, female N94.89
  pleural J94.8
  prostate (active) N42.1
  pulmonary — *see* Congestion, lung
  renal N28.89
  retina H35.81
  seminal vesicle N50.1
  spinal cord G95.19
  spleen (chronic) D73.2
  stomach K31.89
  trachea — *see* Tracheitis
  urethra N36.8
  uterus N85.8
    with subinvolution N85.3
  venous (passive) I87.8
  viscera R68.89
Congestive — *see* Congestion
Conical
  cervix (hypertrophic elongation) N88.4
  cornea — *see* Keratoconus
  teeth K00.2
Conjoined twins Q89.4
Conjugal maladjustment Z63.0
  involving divorce or estrangement Z63.5
Conjunctiva — *see* condition
Conjunctivitis (staphylococcal) (streptococcal) NOS H10.9
  Acanthamoeba B60.12
  acute H10.3- ☑
    atopic H10.1- ☑
    chemical (*see also* Corrosion, cornea) H10.21- ☑
    mucopurulent H10.02- ☑
      follicular H10.01- ☑
    pseudomembranous H10.22- ☑
    serous except viral H10.23- ☑
      viral — *see* Conjunctivitis, viral
    toxic H10.21- ☑
  adenoviral (acute) (follicular) B30.1
  allergic (acute) — *see* Conjunctivitis, acute, atopic
    chronic H10.45
      vernal H10.44
  anaphylactic — *see* Conjunctivitis, acute, atopic
  Apollo B30.3
  atopic (acute) — *see* Conjunctivitis, acute, atopic
  Béal's B30.2
  blennorrhagic (gonococcal) (neonatorum) A54.31
  chemical (acute) (*see also* Corrosion, cornea) H10.21- ☑
  chlamydial A74.0
    due to trachoma A71.1
    neonatal P39.1
  chronic (nodosa) (petrificans) (phlyctenular) H10.40- ☑
    allergic H10.45
      vernal H10.44
    follicular H10.43- ☑
    giant papillary H10.41- ☑
    simple H10.42- ☑
    vernal H10.44
  coxsackievirus 24 B30.3
  diphtheritic A36.86
  due to
    dust — *see* Conjunctivitis, acute, atopic
    filariasis B74.9
    mucocutaneous leishmaniasis B55.2
  enterovirus type 70 (hemorrhagic) B30.3
  epidemic (viral) B30.9
    hemorrhagic B30.3
  gonococcal (neonatorum) A54.31
  granular (trachomatous) A71.1
    sequelae (late effect) B94.0
  hemorrhagic (acute) (epidemic) B30.3
  herpes zoster B02.31
  in (due to)
    Acanthamoeba B60.12
    adenovirus (acute) (follicular) B30.1
    Chlamydia A74.0
    coxsackievirus 24 B30.3
    diphtheria A36.86
    enterovirus type 70 (hemorrhagic) B30.3
    filariasis B74.9
    gonococci A54.31
    herpes (simplex) virus B00.53
      zoster B02.31
    infectious disease NEC B99 ☑
    meningococci A39.89
    mucocutaneous leishmaniasis B55.2

⚑ Subterms under main terms may continue to next column or page   ☑ Additional Character Required — Refer to the Tabular List for Character Selection   69

Compression — Conjunctivitis

Conjunctivitis — *continued*
- in — *continued*
  - rosacea L71.9
  - syphilis (late) A52.71
  - zoster B02.31
- inclusion A74.0
- infantile P39.1
  - gonococcal A54.31
- Koch-Weeks' — *see* Conjunctivitis, acute, mucopurulent
- light — *see* Conjunctivitis, acute, atopic
- ligneous — *see* Blepharoconjunctivitis, ligneous
- meningococcal A39.89
- mucopurulent — *see* Conjunctivitis, acute, mucopurulent
- neonatal P39.1
  - gonococcal A54.31
- Newcastle B30.8
- of Béal B30.2
- parasitic
  - filariasis B74.9
  - mucocutaneous leishmaniasis B55.2
- Parinaud's H10.89
- petrificans H10.89
- rosacea L71.9
- specified NEC H10.89
- swimming-pool B30.1
- trachomatous A71.1
  - acute A71.0
  - sequelae (late effect) B94.0
- traumatic NEC H10.89
- tuberculous A18.59
- tularemic A21.1
- tularensis A21.1
- viral B30.9
  - due to
    - adenovirus B30.1
    - enterovirus B30.3
  - specified NEC B30.8

Conjunctivochalasis H11.82- ☑
Connective tissue — *see* condition
Conn's syndrome E26.01
Conradi (-Hunermann) **disease** Q77.3
Consanguinity Z84.3
- counseling Z71.89

Conscious simulation (of illness) Z76.5
Consecutive — *see* condition
Consolidation lung (base) — *see* Pneumonia, lobar
Constipation (atonic) (neurogenic) (simple) (spastic) K59.00
- chronic K59.09
  - idiopathic K59.04
- drug-induced K59.03
- functional K59.04
- outlet dysfunction K59.02
- psychogenic F45.8
- slow transit K59.01
- specified NEC K59.09

Constitutional (*see also* condition)
- substandard F60.7
Constitutionally substandard F60.7
Constriction (*see also* Stricture)
- auditory canal — *see* Stenosis, external ear canal
- bronchial J98.09
- duodenum K31.5
- esophagus K22.2
- external
  - abdomen, abdominal (wall) S30.841 ☑
  - alveolar process S00.542 ☑
  - ankle S90.54- ☑
  - antecubital space — *see* Constriction, external, forearm
  - arm (upper) S40.84- ☑
  - auricle — *see* Constriction, external, ear
  - axilla — *see* Constriction, external, arm
  - back, lower S30.840 ☑
  - breast S20.14- ☑
  - brow S00.84 ☑
  - buttock S30.840 ☑
  - calf — *see* Constriction, external, leg
  - canthus — *see* Constriction, external, eyelid
  - cheek S00.84 ☑
    - internal S00.542 ☑
  - chest wall — *see* Constriction, external, thorax
  - chin S00.84 ☑
  - clitoris S30.844 ☑
  - costal region — *see* Constriction, external, thorax

Constriction — *continued*
- external — *continued*
  - digit(s)
    - foot — *see* Constriction, external, toe
    - hand — *see* Constriction, external, finger
  - ear S00.44- ☑
  - elbow S50.34- ☑
  - epididymis S30.843 ☑
  - epigastric region S30.841 ☑
  - esophagus, cervical S10.14 ☑
  - eyebrow — *see* Constriction, external, eyelid
  - eyelid S00.24- ☑
  - face S00.84 ☑
  - finger(s) S60.44- ☑
    - index S60.44- ☑
    - little S60.44- ☑
    - middle S60.44- ☑
    - ring S60.44- ☑
  - flank S30.841 ☑
  - foot (except toe(s) alone) S90.84- ☑
    - toe — *see* Constriction, external, toe
  - forearm S50.84- ☑
    - elbow only — *see* Constriction, external, elbow
  - forehead S00.84 ☑
  - genital organs, external
    - female S30.846 ☑
    - male S30.845 ☑
  - groin S30.841 ☑
  - gum S00.542 ☑
  - hand S60.54- ☑
  - head S00.94 ☑
    - ear — *see* Constriction, external, ear
    - eyelid — *see* Constriction, external, eyelid
    - lip S00.541 ☑
    - nose S00.34 ☑
    - oral cavity S00.542 ☑
    - scalp S00.04 ☑
    - specified site NEC S00.84 ☑
  - heel — *see* Constriction, external, foot
  - hip S70.24- ☑
  - inguinal region S30.841 ☑
  - interscapular region S20.449 ☑
  - jaw S00.84 ☑
  - knee S80.24- ☑
  - labium (majus) (minus) S30.844 ☑
  - larynx S10.14 ☑
  - leg (lower) S80.84- ☑
    - knee — *see* Constriction, external, knee
    - upper — *see* Constriction, external, thigh
  - lip S00.541 ☑
  - lower back S30.840 ☑
  - lumbar region S30.840 ☑
  - malar region S00.84 ☑
  - mammary — *see* Constriction, external, breast
  - mastoid region S00.84 ☑
  - mouth S00.542 ☑
  - nail
    - finger — *see* Constriction, external, finger
    - toe — *see* Constriction, external, toe
  - nasal S00.34 ☑
  - neck S10.94 ☑
    - specified site NEC S10.84 ☑
    - throat S10.14 ☑
  - nose S00.34 ☑
  - occipital region S00.04 ☑
  - oral cavity S00.542 ☑
  - orbital region — *see* Constriction, external, eyelid
  - palate S00.542 ☑
  - palm — *see* Constriction, external, hand
  - parietal region S00.04 ☑
  - pelvis S30.840 ☑
  - penis S30.842 ☑
  - perineum
    - female S30.844 ☑
    - male S30.840 ☑
  - periocular area — *see* Constriction, external, eyelid
  - phalanges
    - finger — *see* Constriction, external, finger
    - toe — *see* Constriction, external, toe
  - pharynx S10.14 ☑
  - pinna — *see* Constriction, external, ear
  - popliteal space — *see* Constriction, external, knee
  - prepuce S30.842 ☑
  - pubic region S30.840 ☑
  - pudendum
    - female S30.846 ☑

Constriction — *continued*
- external — *continued*
  - pudendum — *continued*
    - male S30.845 ☑
  - sacral region S30.840 ☑
  - scalp S00.04 ☑
  - scapular region — *see* Constriction, external, shoulder
  - scrotum S30.843 ☑
  - shin — *see* Constriction, external, leg
  - shoulder S40.24- ☑
  - sternal region S20.349 ☑
  - submaxillary region S00.84 ☑
  - submental region S00.84 ☑
  - subungual
    - finger(s) — *see* Constriction, external, finger
    - toe(s) — *see* Constriction, external, toe
  - supraclavicular fossa S10.84 ☑
  - supraorbital S00.84 ☑
  - temple S00.84 ☑
  - temporal region S00.84 ☑
  - testis S30.843 ☑
  - thigh S70.34- ☑
  - thorax, thoracic (wall) S20.94 ☑
    - back S20.44- ☑
    - front S20.34- ☑
  - throat S10.14 ☑
  - thumb S60.34- ☑
  - toe(s) (lesser) S90.44- ☑
    - great S90.44- ☑
  - tongue S00.542 ☑
  - trachea S10.14 ☑
  - tunica vaginalis S30.843 ☑
  - uvula S00.542 ☑
  - vagina S30.844 ☑
  - vulva S30.844 ☑
  - wrist S60.84- ☑
- gallbladder — *see* Obstruction, gallbladder
- intestine — *see* Obstruction, intestine
- larynx J38.6
  - congenital Q31.8
    - specified NEC Q31.8
    - subglottic Q31.1
- organ or site, congenital NEC — *see* Atresia, by site
- prepuce (acquired) (congenital) N47.1
- pylorus (adult hypertrophic) K31.1
  - congenital or infantile Q40.0
  - newborn Q40.0
- ring dystocia (uterus) O62.4
- spastic (*see also* Spasm)
  - ureter N13.5
- ureter N13.5
  - with infection N13.6
- urethra — *see* Stricture, urethra
- visual field (peripheral) (functional) — *see* Defect, visual field

Constrictive — *see* condition
Consultation
- without complaint or sickness Z71.9
  - feared complaint unfounded Z71.1
  - specified reason NEC Z71.89
- medical — *see* Counseling, medical
- religious Z71.81
- specified reason NEC Z71.89
- spiritual Z71.81

Consumption — *see* Tuberculosis
Contact (with) (*see also* Exposure (to))
- acariasis Z20.7
- AIDS virus Z20.6
- air pollution Z77.110
- algae and algae toxins Z77.121
- algae bloom Z77.121
- anthrax Z20.810
- aromatic amines Z77.020
- aromatic (hazardous) compounds NEC Z77.028
- aromatic dyes NOS Z77.028
- arsenic Z77.010
- asbestos Z77.090
- bacterial disease NEC Z20.818
- benzene Z77.021
- blue-green algae bloom Z77.121
- body fluids (potentially hazardous) Z77.21
- brown tide Z77.121
- chemicals (chiefly nonmedicinal) (hazardous) NEC Z77.098
- cholera Z20.09
- chromium compounds Z77.018

Index

Contraction(s), contracture, contracted — Contusion

Contraction(s), contracture, contracted — *continued*
- vesical — *continued*
  - neck or urethral orifice N32.0
- visual field — *see* Defect, visual field, generalized
- Volkmann's (ischemic) T79.6 ☑

Contusion (skin surface intact) T14.8 ☑
- abdomen, abdominal (muscle) (wall) S30.1
- adnexa, eye NEC S05.8X- ☑
- adrenal gland S37.812 ☑
- alveolar process S00.532 ☑
- ankle S90.0- ☑
- antecubital space — *see* Contusion, forearm
- anus S30.3 ☑
- arm (upper) S40.02- ☑
  - lower (with elbow) — *see* Contusion, forearm
- auditory canal — *see* Contusion, ear
- auricle — *see* Contusion, ear
- axilla — *see* Contusion, arm, upper
- back (*see also* Contusion, thorax, back)
  - lower S30.0 ☑
- bile duct S36.13 ☑
- bladder S37.22 ☑
- bone NEC T14.8 ☑
- brain (diffuse) — *see* Injury, intracranial, diffuse
  - focal — *see* Injury, intracranial, focal
- brainstem S06.38- ☑
- breast S20.0- ☑
- broad ligament S37.892 ☑
- brow S00.83 ☑
- buttock S30.0 ☑
- canthus, eye S00.1- ☑
- cauda equina S34.3 ☑
- cerebellar, traumatic S06.37- ☑
- cerebral S06.33- ☑
  - left side S06.32- ☑
  - right side S06.31- ☑
- cheek S00.83 ☑
  - internal S00.532 ☑
- chest (wall) — *see* Contusion, thorax
- chin S00.83 ☑
- clitoris S30.23 ☑
- colon — *see* Injury, intestine, large, contusion
- common bile duct S36.13 ☑
- conjunctiva S05.1- ☑
  - with foreign body (in conjunctival sac) — *see* Foreign body, conjunctival sac
- conus medullaris (spine) S34.139 ☑
- cornea — *see* Contusion, eyeball
  - with foreign body — *see* Foreign body, cornea
- corpus cavernosum S30.21 ☑
- cortex (brain) (cerebral) — *see* Injury, intracranial, diffuse
  - focal — *see* Injury, intracranial, focal
- costal region — *see* Contusion, thorax
- cystic duct S36.13 ☑
- diaphragm S27.802 ☑
- duodenum S36.420 ☑
- ear S00.43- ☑
- elbow S50.0- ☑
  - with forearm — *see* Contusion, forearm
- epididymis S30.22 ☑
- epigastric region S30.1 ☑
- epiglottis S10.0 ☑
- esophagus (thoracic) S27.812 ☑
  - cervical S10.0 ☑
- eyeball S05.1- ☑
- eyebrow S00.1- ☑
- eyelid (and periocular area) S00.1- ☑
- face NEC S00.83 ☑
- fallopian tube S37.529 ☑
  - bilateral S37.522 ☑
  - unilateral S37.521 ☑
- femoral triangle S30.1 ☑
- finger(s) S60.00 ☑
  - with damage to nail (matrix) S60.10 ☑
  - index S60.02- ☑
    - with damage to nail S60.12- ☑
  - little S60.05- ☑
    - with damage to nail S60.15- ☑
  - middle S60.03- ☑
    - with damage to nail S60.13- ☑
  - ring S60.04- ☑
    - with damage to nail S60.14- ☑
  - thumb — *see* Contusion, thumb
- flank S30.1 ☑

Contusion — *continued*
- foot (except toe(s) alone) S90.3- ☑
  - toe — *see* Contusion, toe
- forearm S50.1- ☑
  - elbow only — *see* Contusion, elbow
- forehead S00.83 ☑
- gallbladder S36.122 ☑
- genital organs, external
  - female S30.202 ☑
  - male S30.201 ☑
- globe (eye) — *see* Contusion, eyeball
- groin S30.1 ☑
- gum S00.532 ☑
- hand S60.22- ☑
  - finger(s) — *see* Contusion, finger
  - wrist — *see* Contusion, wrist
- head S00.93 ☑
  - ear — *see* Contusion, ear
  - eyelid — *see* Contusion, eyelid
  - lip S00.531 ☑
  - nose S00.33 ☑
  - oral cavity S00.532 ☑
  - scalp S00.03 ☑
  - specified part NEC S00.83 ☑
- heart (*see also* Injury, heart) S26.91 ☑
- heel — *see* Contusion, foot
- hepatic duct S36.13 ☑
- hip S70.0- ☑
- ileum S36.428 ☑
- iliac region S30.1 ☑
- inguinal region S30.1 ☑
- interscapular region S20.229 ☑
- intra-abdominal organ S36.92 ☑
  - colon — *see* Injury, intestine, large, contusion
  - liver S36.112 ☑
  - pancreas — *see* Contusion, pancreas
  - rectum S36.62 ☑
  - small intestine — *see* Injury, intestine, small, contusion
  - specified organ NEC S36.892 ☑
  - spleen — *see* Contusion, spleen
  - stomach S36.32 ☑
- iris (eye) — *see* Contusion, eyeball
- jaw S00.83 ☑
- jejunum S36.428 ☑
- kidney S37.01- ☑
  - major (greater than 2 cm) S37.02- ☑
  - minor (less than 2 cm) S37.01- ☑
- knee S80.0- ☑
- labium (majus) (minus) S30.23 ☑
- lacrimal apparatus, gland or sac S05.8X- ☑
- larynx S10.0 ☑
- leg (lower) S80.1- ☑
  - knee — *see* Contusion, knee
- lens — *see* Contusion, eyeball
- lip S00.531 ☑
- liver S36.112 ☑
- lower back S30.0 ☑
- lumbar region S30.0 ☑
- lung S27.329 ☑
  - bilateral S27.322 ☑
  - unilateral S27.321 ☑
- malar region S00.83 ☑
- mastoid region S00.83 ☑
- membrane, brain — *see* Injury, intracranial, diffuse
  - focal — *see* Injury, intracranial, focal
- mesentery S36.892 ☑
- mesosalpinx S37.892 ☑
- mouth S00.532 ☑
- muscle — *see* Contusion, by site
- nail
  - finger — *see* Contusion, finger, with damage to nail
  - toe — *see* Contusion, toe, with damage to nail
- nasal S00.33 ☑
- neck S10.93 ☑
  - specified site NEC S10.83 ☑
  - throat S10.0 ☑
- nerve — *see* Injury, nerve
- newborn P54.5
- nose S00.33 ☑
- occipital
  - lobe (brain) — *see* Injury, intracranial, diffuse
    - focal — *see* Injury, intracranial, focal
  - region (scalp) S00.03 ☑
- orbit (region) (tissues) S05.1- ☑

Contusion — *continued*
- ovary S37.429 ☑
  - bilateral S37.422 ☑
  - unilateral S37.421 ☑
- palate S00.532 ☑
- pancreas S36.229 ☑
  - body S36.221 ☑
  - head S36.220 ☑
  - tail S36.222 ☑
- parietal
  - lobe (brain) — *see* Injury, intracranial, diffuse
    - focal — *see* Injury, intracranial, focal
  - region (scalp) S00.03 ☑
- pelvic organ S37.92 ☑
  - adrenal gland S37.812 ☑
  - bladder S37.22 ☑
  - fallopian tube — *see* Contusion, fallopian tube
  - kidney — *see* Contusion, kidney
  - ovary — *see* Contusion, ovary
  - prostate S37.822 ☑
  - specified organ NEC S37.892 ☑
  - ureter S37.12 ☑
  - urethra S37.32 ☑
  - uterus S37.62 ☑
- pelvis S30.0 ☑
- penis S30.21 ☑
- perineum
  - female S30.23 ☑
  - male S30.0 ☑
- periocular area S00.1- ☑
- peritoneum S36.81 ☑
- periurethral tissue — *see* Contusion, urethra
- pharynx S10.0 ☑
- pinna — *see* Contusion, ear
- popliteal space — *see* Contusion, knee
- prepuce S30.21 ☑
- prostate S37.822 ☑
- pubic region S30.1 ☑
- pudendum
  - female S30.202 ☑
  - male S30.201 ☑
- quadriceps femoris — *see* Contusion, thigh
- rectum S36.62 ☑
- retroperitoneum S36.892 ☑
- round ligament S37.892 ☑
- sacral region S30.0 ☑
- scalp S00.03 ☑
  - due to birth injury P12.3
- scapular region — *see* Contusion, shoulder
- sclera — *see* Contusion, eyeball
- scrotum S30.22 ☑
- seminal vesicle S37.892 ☑
- shoulder S40.01- ☑
- skin NEC T14.8 ☑
- small intestine — *see* Injury, intestine, small, contusion
- spermatic cord S30.22 ☑
- spinal cord — *see* Injury, spinal cord, by region
  - cauda equina S34.3 ☑
  - conus medullaris S34.139 ☑
- spleen S36.029 ☑
  - major S36.021 ☑
  - minor S36.020 ☑
- sternal region S20.219 ☑
- stomach S36.32 ☑
- subconjunctival S05.1- ☑
- subcutaneous NEC T14.8 ☑
- submaxillary region S00.83 ☑
- submental region S00.83 ☑
- subperiosteal NEC T14.8 ☑
- subungual
  - finger — *see* Contusion, finger, with damage to nail
  - toe — *see* Contusion, toe, with damage to nail
- supraclavicular fossa S10.83 ☑
- supraorbital S00.83 ☑
- suprarenal gland S37.812 ☑
- temple (region) S00.83 ☑
- temporal
  - lobe (brain) — *see* Injury, intracranial, diffuse
    - focal — *see* Injury, intracranial, focal
  - region S00.83 ☑
- testis S30.22 ☑
- thigh S70.1- ☑
- thorax (wall) S20.20 ☑
  - back S20.22- ☑
  - front S20.21- ☑

Contusion — *continued*
- throat S10.0 ☑
- thumb S60.01 ☑
  - with damage to nail S60.11- ☑
- toe(s) (lesser) S90.12- ☑
  - with damage to nail S90.22- ☑
  - great S90.11-
    - with damage to nail S90.21- ☑
- tongue S00.532 ☑
- trachea (cervical) S10.0 ☑
  - thoracic S27.52 ☑
- tunica vaginalis S30.22 ☑
- tympanum, tympanic membrane — *see* Contusion, ear
- ureter S37.12 ☑
- urethra S37.32 ☑
- urinary organ NEC S37.892 ☑
- uterus S37.62 ☑
- uvula S00.532 ☑
- vagina S30.23 ☑
- vas deferens S37.892 ☑
- vesical S37.22 ☑
- vocal cord(s) S10.0 ☑
- vulva S30.23 ☑
- wrist S60.21-

Conus (congenital) (any type) Q14.8
- cornea — *see* Keratoconus
- medullaris syndrome G95.81

Conversion hysteria, neurosis or reaction F44.9
Converter, tuberculosis (test reaction) R76.11
Conviction (legal), **anxiety concerning** Z65.0
- with imprisonment Z65.1

Convulsions (idiopathic) (*see also* Seizure(s)) R56.9
- apoplectiform (cerebral ischemia) I67.82
- dissociative F44.5
- epileptic — *see* Epilepsy
- epileptiform, epileptoid — *see* Seizure, epileptiform
- ether (anesthetic) — *see* Table of Drugs and Chemicals, by drug
- febrile R56.00
  - with status epilepticus G40.901
  - complex R56.01
    - with status epilepticus G40.901
  - simple R56.00
- hysterical F44.5
- infantile P90
  - epilepsy — *see* Epilepsy
- jacksonian — *see* Epilepsy, localization-related, symptomatic, with simple partial seizures
- myoclonic G25.3
- newborn P90
- obstetrical (nephritic) (uremic) — *see* Eclampsia
- paretic A52.17
- post traumatic R56.1
- psychomotor — *see* Epilepsy, localization-related, symptomatic, with complex partial seizures
- recurrent R56.9
- reflex R25.8
- scarlatinal A38.8
- tetanus, tetanic — *see* Tetanus
- thymic E32.8

Convulsive (*see also* Convulsions)
Cooley's anemia D56.1
Coolie itch B76.9
Cooper's
- disease — *see* Mastopathy, cystic
- hernia — *see* Hernia, abdomen, specified site NEC

Copra itch B88.0
Coprophagy F50.89
Coprophobia F40.298
Coproporphyria, hereditary E80.29
Cor
- biloculare Q20.8
- bovis, bovinum — *see* Hypertrophy, cardiac
- pulmonale (chronic) I27.81
  - acute I26.09
- triatriatum, triatrium Q24.2
- triloculare Q20.8
  - biatrium Q20.4
  - biventriculare Q21.1

Corbus' disease (gangrenous balanitis) N48.1
Cord (*see also* condition)
- around neck
  - complicating delivery O69.81 ☑
    - with compression O69.1 ☑
- bladder G95.89
  - tabetic A52.19

Cordis ectopia Q24.8
Corditis (spermatic) N49.1
Corectopia Q13.2
Cori's disease (glycogen storage) E74.03
Corkhandler's disease or lung J67.3
Corkscrew esophagus K22.4
Corkworker's disease or lung J67.3
Corn (infected) L84
Cornea (*see also* condition)
- donor Z52.5
- plana Q13.4

Cornelia de Lange syndrome Q87.1
Cornu cutaneum L85.8
Cornual gestation or pregnancy O00.80
- with intrauterine pregnancy O00.81

Coronary (artery) — *see* condition
Coronavirus, as cause of disease classified elsewhere B97.29
- SARS-associated B97.21

Corpora (*see also* condition)
- amylacea, prostate N42.89
- cavernosa — *see* condition

Corpulence — *see* Obesity
Corpus — *see* condition
Corrected transposition Q20.5
Corrosion (injury) (acid) (caustic) (chemical) (lime) (external) (internal) T30.4
- abdomen, abdominal (muscle) (wall) T21.42 ☑
  - first degree T21.52 ☑
  - second degree T21.62 ☑
  - third degree T21.72 ☑
- above elbow T22.439 ☑
  - first degree T22.539 ☑
  - left T22.432 ☑
    - first degree T22.532 ☑
    - second degree T22.632 ☑
    - third degree T22.732 ☑
  - right T22.431 ☑
    - first degree T22.531 ☑
    - second degree T22.631 ☑
    - third degree T22.731 ☑
  - second degree T22.639 ☑
  - third degree T22.739 ☑
- alimentary tract NEC T28.7 ☑
- ankle T25.419 ☑
  - first degree T25.519 ☑
  - left T25.412 ☑
    - first degree T25.512 ☑
    - second degree T25.612 ☑
    - third degree T25.712 ☑
  - multiple with foot — *see* Corrosion, lower, limb, multiple, ankle and foot
  - right T25.411 ☑
    - first degree T25.511 ☑
    - second degree T25.611 ☑
    - third degree T25.711 ☑
  - second degree T25.619 ☑
  - third degree T25.719 ☑
- anus — *see* Corrosion, buttock
- arm(s) (meaning upper limb(s)) — *see* Corrosion, upper limb
- axilla T22.449 ☑
  - first degree T22.549 ☑
  - left T22.442 ☑
    - first degree T22.542 ☑
    - second degree T22.642 ☑
    - third degree T22.742 ☑
  - right T22.441 ☑
    - first degree T22.541 ☑
    - second degree T22.641 ☑
    - third degree T22.741 ☑
  - second degree T22.649 ☑
  - third degree T22.749 ☑
- back (lower) T21.44 ☑
  - first degree T21.54 ☑
  - second degree T21.64 ☑
  - third degree T21.74 ☑
  - upper T21.43 ☑
    - first degree T21.53 ☑
    - second degree T21.63 ☑
    - third degree T21.73 ☑
- blisters — *code as* Corrosion, second degree, by site
- breast — *see* Corrosion, chest wall
- buttock(s) T21.45 ☑
  - first degree T21.55 ☑
  - second degree T21.65 ☑

Corrosion — *continued*
- buttock(s) — *continued*
  - third degree T21.75 ☑
- calf T24.439 ☑
  - first degree T24.539 ☑
  - left T24.432 ☑
    - first degree T24.532 ☑
    - second degree T24.632 ☑
    - third degree T24.732 ☑
  - right T24.431 ☑
    - first degree T24.531 ☑
    - second degree T24.631 ☑
    - third degree T24.731 ☑
  - second degree T24.639 ☑
  - third degree T24.739 ☑
- canthus (eye) — *see* Corrosion, eyelid
- cervix T28.8 ☑
- cheek T20.46 ☑
  - first degree T20.56 ☑
  - second degree T20.66 ☑
  - third degree T20.76 ☑
- chest wall T21.41 ☑
  - first degree T21.51 ☑
  - second degree T21.61 ☑
  - third degree T21.71 ☑
- chin T20.43 ☑
  - first degree T20.53 ☑
  - second degree T20.63 ☑
  - third degree T20.73 ☑
- colon T28.7 ☑
- conjunctiva (and cornea) — *see* Corrosion, cornea
- cornea (and conjunctiva) T26.6- ☑
- deep necrosis of underlying tissue — *code as* Corrosion, third degree, by site
- dorsum of hand T23.469 ☑
  - first degree T23.569 ☑
  - left T23.462 ☑
    - first degree T23.562 ☑
    - second degree T23.662 ☑
    - third degree T23.762 ☑
  - right T23.461 ☑
    - first degree T23.561 ☑
    - second degree T23.661 ☑
    - third degree T23.761 ☑
  - second degree T23.669 ☑
  - third degree T23.769 ☑
- ear (auricle) (external) (canal) T20.41 ☑
  - drum T28.91 ☑
  - first degree T20.51 ☑
  - second degree T20.61 ☑
  - third degree T20.71 ☑
- elbow T22.429 ☑
  - first degree T22.529 ☑
  - left T22.422 ☑
    - first degree T22.522 ☑
    - second degree T22.622 ☑
    - third degree T22.722 ☑
  - right T22.421 ☑
    - first degree T22.521 ☑
    - second degree T22.621 ☑
    - third degree T22.721 ☑
  - second degree T22.629 ☑
  - third degree T22.729 ☑
- entire body — *see* Corrosion, multiple body regions
- epidermal loss — *code as* Corrosion, second degree, by site
- epiglottis T27.4 ☑
- erythema, erythematous — *code as* Corrosion, first degree, by site
- esophagus T28.6 ☑
- extent (percentage of body surface)
  - less than 10 percent T32.0
  - 10-19 percent (0-9 percent third degree) T32.10
    - with 10-19 percent third degree T32.11
  - 20-29 percent (0-9 percent third degree) T32.20
    - with
      - 10-19 percent third degree T32.21
      - 20-29 percent third degree T32.22
  - 30-39 percent (0-9 percent third degree) T32.30
    - with
      - 10-19 percent third degree T32.31
      - 20-29 percent third degree T32.32
      - 30-39 percent third degree T32.33
  - 40-49 percent (0-9 percent third degree) T32.40
    - with
      - 10-19 percent third degree T32.41

⚐ Subterms under main terms may continue to next column or page   ☑ Additional Character Required — Refer to the Tabular List for Character Selection   73

Contusion — Corrosion

Corrosion — *continued*
  extent — *continued*
    40-49 percent — *continued*
     with — *continued*
      20-29 percent third degree T32.42
      30-39 percent third degree T32.43
      40-49 percent third degree T32.44
    50-59 percent (0-9 percent third degree) T32.50
     with
      10-19 percent third degree T32.51
      20-29 percent third degree T32.52
      30-39 percent third degree T32.53
      40-49 percent third degree T32.54
      50-59 percent third degree T32.55
    60-69 percent (0-9 percent third degree) T32.60
     with
      10-19 percent third degree T32.61
      20-29 percent third degree T32.62
      30-39 percent third degree T32.63
      40-49 percent third degree T32.64
      50-59 percent third degree T32.65
      60-69 percent third degree T32.66
    70-79 percent (0-9 percent third degree) T32.70
     with
      10-19 percent third degree T32.71
      20-29 percent third degree T32.72
      30-39 percent third degree T32.73
      40-49 percent third degree T32.74
      50-59 percent third degree T32.75
      60-69 percent third degree T32.76
      70-79 percent third degree T32.77
    80-89 percent (0-9 percent third degree) T32.80
     with
      10-19 percent third degree T32.81
      20-29 percent third degree T32.82
      30-39 percent third degree T32.83
      40-49 percent third degree T32.84
      50-59 percent third degree T32.85
      60-69 percent third degree T32.86
      70-79 percent third degree T32.87
      80-89 percent third degree T32.88
    90 percent or more (0-9 percent third degree) T32.90
     with
      10-19 percent third degree T32.91
      20-29 percent third degree T32.92
      30-39 percent third degree T32.93
      40-49 percent third degree T32.94
      50-59 percent third degree T32.95
      60-69 percent third degree T32.96
      70-79 percent third degree T32.97
      80-89 percent third degree T32.98
      90-99 percent third degree T32.99
  extremity — *see* Corrosion, limb
  eye(s) and adnexa T26.9- ☑
    with resulting rupture and destruction of eyeball T26.7- ☑
    conjunctival sac — *see* Corrosion, cornea
    cornea — *see* Corrosion, cornea
    lid — *see* Corrosion, eyelid
    periocular area — *see* Corrosion eyelid
    specified site NEC T26.8- ☑
  eyeball — *see* Corrosion, eye
  eyelid(s) T26.5- ☑
  face — *see* Corrosion, head
  finger T23.429 ☑
    first degree T23.529 ☑
    left T23.422 ☑
     first degree T23.522 ☑
     second degree T23.622 ☑
     third degree T23.722 ☑
    multiple sites (without thumb) T23.439 ☑
     with thumb T23.449 ☑
      first degree T23.549 ☑
      left T23.442 ☑
       first degree T23.542 ☑
       second degree T23.642 ☑
       third degree T23.742 ☑
      right T23.441 ☑
       first degree T23.541 ☑
       second degree T23.641 ☑
       third degree T23.741 ☑
      second degree T23.649 ☑
      third degree T23.749 ☑
     first degree T23.539 ☑
     left T23.432 ☑
      first degree T23.532 ☑

Corrosion — *continued*
  finger — *continued*
    multiple sites — *continued*
     left — *continued*
      second degree T23.632 ☑
      third degree T23.732 ☑
     right T23.431 ☑
      first degree T23.531 ☑
      second degree T23.631 ☑
      third degree T23.731 ☑
     second degree T23.639 ☑
     third degree T23.739 ☑
    right T23.421 ☑
     first degree T23.521 ☑
     second degree T23.621 ☑
     third degree T23.721 ☑
    second degree T23.629 ☑
    third degree T23.729 ☑
  flank — *see* Corrosion, abdomen
  foot T25.429 ☑
    first degree T25.529 ☑
    left T25.422 ☑
     first degree T25.522 ☑
     second degree T25.622 ☑
     third degree T25.722 ☑
    multiple with ankle — *see* Corrosion, lower, limb, multiple, ankle and foot
    right T25.421 ☑
     first degree T25.521 ☑
     second degree T25.621 ☑
     third degree T25.721 ☑
    second degree T25.629 ☑
    third degree T25.729 ☑
  forearm T22.419 ☑
    first degree T22.519 ☑
    left T22.412 ☑
     first degree T22.512 ☑
     second degree T22.612 ☑
     third degree T22.712 ☑
    right T22.411 ☑
     first degree T22.511 ☑
     second degree T22.611 ☑
     third degree T22.711 ☑
    second degree T22.619 ☑
    third degree T22.719 ☑
  forehead T20.46 ☑
    first degree T20.56 ☑
    second degree T20.66 ☑
    third degree T20.76 ☑
  fourth degree — *code as* Corrosion, third degree, by site
  full thickness skin loss — *code as* Corrosion, third degree, by site
  gastrointestinal tract NEC T28.7 ☑
  genital organs
    external
     female T21.47 ☑
      first degree T21.57 ☑
      second degree T21.67 ☑
      third degree T21.77 ☑
     male T21.46 ☑
      first degree T21.56 ☑
      second degree T21.66 ☑
      third degree T21.76 ☑
    internal T28.8 ☑
  groin — *see* Corrosion, abdominal wall
  hand(s) T23.409 ☑
    back — *see* Corrosion, dorsum of hand
    finger — *see* Corrosion, finger
    first degree T23.509 ☑
    left T23.402 ☑
     first degree T23.502 ☑
     second degree T23.602 ☑
     third degree T23.702 ☑
    multiple sites with wrist T23.499 ☑
     first degree T23.599 ☑
     left T23.492 ☑
      first degree T23.592 ☑
      second degree T23.692 ☑
      third degree T23.792 ☑
     right T23.491 ☑
      first degree T23.591 ☑
      second degree T23.691 ☑
      third degree T23.791 ☑
     second degree T23.699 ☑
     third degree T23.799 ☑

Corrosion — *continued*
  hand(s) — *continued*
    palm — *see* Corrosion, palm
    right T23.401 ☑
     first degree T23.501 ☑
     second degree T23.601 ☑
     third degree T23.701 ☑
    second degree T23.609 ☑
    third degree T23.709 ☑
    thumb — *see* Corrosion, thumb
  head (and face) (and neck) T20.40 ☑
    cheek — *see* Corrosion, cheek
    chin — *see* Corrosion, chin
    ear — *see* Corrosion, ear
    eye(s) only — *see* Corrosion, eye
    first degree T20.50 ☑
    forehead — *see* Corrosion, forehead
    lip — *see* Corrosion, lip
    multiple sites T20.49 ☑
     first degree T20.59 ☑
     second degree T20.69 ☑
     third degree T20.79 ☑
    neck — *see* Corrosion, neck
    nose — *see* Corrosion, nose
    scalp — *see* Corrosion, scalp
    second degree T20.60 ☑
    third degree T20.70 ☑
  hip(s) — *see* Corrosion, lower, limb
  inhalation — *see* Corrosion, respiratory tract
  internal organ(s) (*see also* Corrosion, by site) T28.90 ☑
    alimentary tract T28.7 ☑
     esophagus T28.6 ☑
    esophagus T28.6 ☑
    genitourinary T28.8 ☑
    mouth T28.5 ☑
    pharynx T28.5 ☑
    specified organ NEC T28.99 ☑
  interscapular region — *see* Corrosion, back, upper
  intestine (large) (small) T28.7 ☑
  knee T24.429 ☑
    first degree T24.529 ☑
    left T24.422 ☑
     first degree T24.522 ☑
     second degree T24.622 ☑
     third degree T24.722 ☑
    right T24.421 ☑
     first degree T24.521 ☑
     second degree T24.621 ☑
     third degree T24.721 ☑
    second degree T24.629 ☑
    third degree T24.729 ☑
  labium (majus) (minus) — *see* Corrosion, genital organs, external, female
  lacrimal apparatus, duct, gland or sac — *see* Corrosion, eye, specified site NEC
  larynx T27.4 ☑
    with lung T27.5 ☑
  leg(s) (meaning lower limb(s)) — *see* Corrosion, lower limb
  limb(s)
    lower — *see* Corrosion, lower, limb
    upper — *see* Corrosion, upper limb
  lip(s) T20.42 ☑
    first degree T20.52 ☑
    second degree T20.62 ☑
    third degree T20.72 ☑
  lower
    back — *see* Corrosion, back
    limb T24.409 ☑
     ankle — *see* Corrosion, ankle
     calf — *see* Corrosion, calf
     first degree T24.509 ☑
     foot — *see* Corrosion, foot
     knee — *see* Corrosion, knee
     left T24.402 ☑
      first degree T24.502 ☑
      second degree T24.602 ☑
      third degree T24.702 ☑
     multiple sites, except ankle and foot T24.499 ☑
      ankle and foot T25.499 ☑
       first degree T25.599 ☑
       left T25.492 ☑
        first degree T25.592 ☑
        second degree T25.692 ☑
        third degree T25.792 ☑
       right T25.491 ☑

☑ Additional Character Required — Refer to the Tabular List for Character Selection   ▽ Subterms under main terms may continue to next column or page

Corrosion — *continued*
  lower — *continued*
    limb — *continued*
      multiple sites, except ankle and foot — *continued*
        ankle and foot — *continued*
          right — *continued*
            first degree T25.591 ☑
            second degree T25.691 ☑
            third degree T25.791 ☑
          second degree T25.699 ☑
          third degree T25.799 ☑
      first degree T24.599 ☑
      left T24.492 ☑
        first degree T24.592 ☑
        second degree T24.692 ☑
        third degree T24.792 ☑
      right T24.491 ☑
        first degree T24.591 ☑
        second degree T24.691 ☑
        third degree T24.791 ☑
      second degree T24.699 ☑
      right T24.401 ☑
        first degree T24.501 ☑
        second degree T24.601 ☑
        third degree T24.701 ☑
      second degree T24.609 ☑
      thigh — *see* Corrosion, thigh
      third degree T24.709 ☑
  lung (with larynx and trachea) T27.5 ☑
  mouth T28.5 ☑
  neck T20.47 ☑
    first degree T20.57 ☑
    second degree T20.67 ☑
    third degree T20.77 ☑
  nose (septum) T20.44 ☑
    first degree T20.54 ☑
    second degree T20.64 ☑
    third degree T20.74 ☑
  ocular adnexa — *see* Corrosion, eye
  orbit region — *see* Corrosion, eyelid
  palm T23.459 ☑
    first degree T23.559 ☑
    left T23.452 ☑
      first degree T23.552 ☑
      second degree T23.652 ☑
      third degree T23.752 ☑
    right T23.451 ☑
      first degree T23.551 ☑
      second degree T23.651 ☑
      third degree T23.751 ☑
    second degree T23.659 ☑
    third degree T23.759 ☑
  partial thickness — *code as* Corrosion, unspecified degree, by site
  pelvis — *see* Corrosion, trunk
  penis — *see* Corrosion, genital organs, external, male
  perineum
    female — *see* Corrosion, genital organs, external, female
    male — *see* Corrosion, genital organs, external, male
  periocular area — *see* Corrosion, eyelid
  pharynx T28.5 ☑
  rectum T28.7 ☑
  respiratory tract T27.7 ☑
    larynx — *see* Corrosion, larynx
    specified part NEC T27.6 ☑
    trachea — *see* Corrosion, larynx
  sac, lacrimal — *see* Corrosion, eye, specified site NEC
  scalp T20.45 ☑
    first degree T20.55 ☑
    second degree T20.65 ☑
    third degree T20.75 ☑
  scapular region T22.469 ☑
    first degree T22.569 ☑
    left T22.462 ☑
      first degree T22.562 ☑
      second degree T22.662 ☑
      third degree T22.762 ☑
    right T22.461 ☑
      first degree T22.561 ☑
      second degree T22.661 ☑
      third degree T22.761 ☑
    second degree T22.669 ☑

Corrosion — *continued*
  scapular region — *continued*
    third degree T22.769 ☑
  sclera — *see* Corrosion, eye, specified site NEC
  scrotum — *see* Corrosion, genital organs, external, male
  shoulder T22.459 ☑
    first degree T22.559 ☑
    left T22.452 ☑
      first degree T22.552 ☑
      second degree T22.652 ☑
      third degree T22.752 ☑
    right T22.451 ☑
      first degree T22.551 ☑
      second degree T22.651 ☑
      third degree T22.751 ☑
    second degree T22.659 ☑
    third degree T22.759 ☑
  stomach T28.7 ☑
  temple — *see* Corrosion, head
  testis — *see* Corrosion, genital organs, external, male
  thigh T24.419 ☑
    first degree T24.519 ☑
    left T24.412 ☑
      first degree T24.512 ☑
      second degree T24.612 ☑
      third degree T24.712 ☑
    right T24.411 ☑
      first degree T24.511 ☑
      second degree T24.611 ☑
      third degree T24.711 ☑
    second degree T24.619 ☑
    third degree T24.719 ☑
  thorax (external) — *see* Corrosion, trunk
  throat (meaning pharynx) T28.5 ☑
  thumb(s) T23.419 ☑
    first degree T23.519 ☑
    left T23.412 ☑
      first degree T23.512 ☑
      second degree T23.612 ☑
      third degree T23.712 ☑
    multiple sites with fingers T23.449 ☑
      first degree T23.549 ☑
      left T23.442 ☑
        first degree T23.542 ☑
        second degree T23.642 ☑
        third degree T23.742 ☑
      right T23.441 ☑
        first degree T23.541 ☑
        second degree T23.641 ☑
        third degree T23.741 ☑
      second degree T23.649 ☑
      third degree T23.749 ☑
    right T23.411 ☑
      first degree T23.511 ☑
      second degree T23.611 ☑
      third degree T23.711 ☑
    second degree T23.619 ☑
    third degree T23.719 ☑
  toe T25.439 ☑
    first degree T25.539 ☑
    left T25.432 ☑
      first degree T25.532 ☑
      second degree T25.632 ☑
      third degree T25.732 ☑
    right T25.431 ☑
      first degree T25.531 ☑
      second degree T25.631 ☑
      third degree T25.731 ☑
    second degree T25.639 ☑
    third degree T25.739 ☑
  tongue T28.5 ☑
  tonsil(s) T28.5 ☑
  total body — *see* Corrosion, multiple body regions
  trachea T27.4 ☑
    with lung T27.5 ☑
  trunk T21.40 ☑
    abdominal wall — *see* Corrosion, abdominal wall
    anus — *see* Corrosion, buttock
    axilla — *see* Corrosion, upper limb
    back — *see* Corrosion, back
    breast — *see* Corrosion, chest wall
    buttock — *see* Corrosion, buttock
    chest wall — *see* Corrosion, chest wall
    first degree T21.50 ☑
    flank — *see* Corrosion, abdominal wall

Corrosion — *continued*
  trunk — *continued*
    genital
      female — *see* Corrosion, genital organs, external, female
      male — *see* Corrosion, genital organs, external, male
    groin — *see* Corrosion, abdominal wall
    interscapular region — *see* Corrosion, back, upper
    labia — *see* Corrosion, genital organs, external, female
    lower back — *see* Corrosion, back
    penis — *see* Corrosion, genital organs, external, male
    perineum
      female — *see* Corrosion, genital organs, external, female
      male — *see* Corrosion, genital organs, external, male
    scapular region — *see* Corrosion, upper limb
    scrotum — *see* Corrosion, genital organs, external, male
    second degree T21.60 ☑
    shoulder — *see* Corrosion, upper limb
    specified site NEC T21.49 ☑
      first degree T21.59 ☑
      second degree T21.69 ☑
      third degree T21.79 ☑
    testes — *see* Corrosion, genital organs, external, male
    third degree T21.70 ☑
    upper back — *see* Corrosion, back, upper
    vagina T28.8 ☑
    vulva — *see* Corrosion, genital organs, external, female
  unspecified site with extent of body surface involved specified
    less than 10 percent T32.0
    10-19 percent (0-9 percent third degree) T32.10
      with 10-19 percent third degree T32.11
    20-29 percent (0-9 percent third degree) T32.20
      with
        10-19 percent third degree T32.21
        20-29 percent third degree T32.22
    30-39 percent (0-9 percent third degree) T32.30
      with
        10-19 percent third degree T32.31
        20-29 percent third degree T32.32
        30-39 percent third degree T32.33
    40-49 percent (0-9 percent third degree) T32.40
      with
        10-19 percent third degree T32.41
        20-29 percent third degree T32.42
        30-39 percent third degree T32.43
        40-49 percent third degree T32.44
    50-59 percent (0-9 percent third degree) T32.50
      with
        10-19 percent third degree T32.51
        20-29 percent third degree T32.52
        30-39 percent third degree T32.53
        40-49 percent third degree T32.54
        50-59 percent third degree T32.55
    60-69 percent (0-9 percent third degree) T32.60
      with
        10-19 percent third degree T32.61
        20-29 percent third degree T32.62
        30-39 percent third degree T32.63
        40-49 percent third degree T32.64
        50-59 percent third degree T32.65
        60-69 percent third degree T32.66
    70-79 percent (0-9 percent third degree) T32.70
      with
        10-19 percent third degree T32.71
        20-29 percent third degree T32.72
        30-39 percent third degree T32.73
        40-49 percent third degree T32.74
        50-59 percent third degree T32.75
        60-69 percent third degree T32.76
        70-79 percent third degree T32.77
    80-89 percent (0-9 percent third degree) T32.80
      with
        10-19 percent third degree T32.81
        20-29 percent third degree T32.82
        30-39 percent third degree T32.83
        40-49 percent third degree T32.84
        50-59 percent third degree T32.85
        60-69 percent third degree T32.86
        70-79 percent third degree T32.87

Corrosion — *continued*
  unspecified site with extent of body surface involved
    specified — *continued*
    80-89 percent — *continued*
      with — *continued*
        80-89 percent third degree T32.88
    90 percent or more (0-9 percent third degree)
      T32.90
      with
        10-19 percent third degree T32.91
        20-29 percent third degree T32.92
        30-39 percent third degree T32.93
        40-49 percent third degree T32.94
        50-59 percent third degree T32.95
        60-69 percent third degree T32.96
        70-79 percent third degree T32.97
        80-89 percent third degree T32.98
        90-99 percent third degree T32.99
  upper limb (axilla) (scapular region) T22.40 ☑
    above elbow — *see* Corrosion, above elbow
    axilla — *see* Corrosion, axilla
    elbow — *see* Corrosion, elbow
    first degree T22.50 ☑
    forearm — *see* Corrosion, forearm
    hand — *see* Corrosion, hand
    interscapular region — *see* Corrosion, back, upper
    multiple sites T22.499 ☑
      first degree T22.599 ☑
      left T22.492 ☑
        first degree T22.592 ☑
        second degree T22.692 ☑
        third degree T22.792 ☑
      right T22.491 ☑
        first degree T22.591 ☑
        second degree T22.691 ☑
        third degree T22.791 ☑
      second degree T22.699 ☑
      third degree T22.799 ☑
    scapular region — *see* Corrosion, scapular region
    second degree T22.60 ☑
    shoulder — *see* Corrosion, shoulder
    third degree T22.70 ☑
    wrist — *see* Corrosion, hand
  uterus T28.8 ☑
  vagina T28.8 ☑
  vulva — *see* Corrosion, genital organs, external, female
  wrist T23.479 ☑
    first degree T23.579 ☑
    left T23.472 ☑
      first degree T23.572 ☑
      second degree T23.672 ☑
      third degree T23.772 ☑
    multiple sites with hand T23.499 ☑
      first degree T23.599 ☑
      left T23.492 ☑
        first degree T23.592 ☑
        second degree T23.692 ☑
        third degree T23.792 ☑
      right T23.491 ☑
        first degree T23.591 ☑
        second degree T23.691 ☑
        third degree T23.791 ☑
      second degree T23.699 ☑
      third degree T23.799 ☑
    right T23.471 ☑
      first degree T23.571 ☑
      second degree T23.671 ☑
      third degree T23.771 ☑
    second degree T23.679 ☑
    third degree T23.779 ☑
Corrosive burn — *see* Corrosion
Corsican fever — *see* Malaria
Cortical — *see* condition
Cortico-adrenal — *see* condition
Coryza (acute) J00
  with grippe or influenza — *see* Influenza, with, respiratory manifestations NEC
  syphilitic
    congenital (chronic) A50.05
Costen's syndrome or complex M26.69
Costiveness — *see* Constipation
Costochondritis M94.0
Cot death R99
Cotard's syndrome F22
Cotia virus B08.8
Cotton wool spots (retinal) H35.81

Cotungo's disease — *see* Sciatica
Cough (affected) (chronic) (epidemic) (nervous) R05
  with hemorrhage — *see* Hemoptysis
  bronchial R05
    with grippe or influenza — *see* Influenza, with, respiratory manifestations NEC
  functional F45.8
  hysterical F45.8
  laryngeal, spasmodic R05
  psychogenic F45.8
  smokers' J41.0
  tea taster's B49
Counseling (for) Z71.9
  abuse NEC
    perpetrator Z69.82
    victim Z69.81
  alcohol abuser Z71.41
    family Z71.42
  child abuse
    nonparental
      perpetrator Z69.021
      victim Z69.020
    parental
      perpetrator Z69.011
      victim Z69.010
  consanguinity Z71.89
  contraceptive Z30.09
  dietary Z71.3
  drug abuser Z71.51
    family member Z71.52
  exercise Z71.82
  family Z71.89
  fertility preservation (prior to cancer therapy) (prior to removal of gonads) Z31.62
  for non-attending third party Z71.0
    related to sexual behavior or orientation Z70.2
  genetic
    nonprocreative Z71.83
    procreative NEC Z31.5
  gestational carrier Z31.7
  health (advice) (education) (instruction) — *see* Counseling, medical
  human immunodeficiency virus (HIV) Z71.7
  impotence Z70.1
  insulin pump use Z46.81
  medical (for) Z71.9
    boarding school resident Z59.3
    consanguinity Z71.89
    feared complaint and no disease found Z71.1
    human immunodeficiency virus (HIV) Z71.7
    institutional resident Z59.3
    on behalf of another Z71.0
      related to sexual behavior or orientation Z70.2
    person living alone Z60.2
    specified reason NEC Z71.89
  natural family planning
    procreative Z31.61
    to avoid pregnancy Z30.02
  perpetrator (of)
    abuse NEC Z69.82
    child abuse
      non-parental Z69.021
      parental Z69.011
    rape NEC Z69.82
    spousal abuse Z69.12
  procreative NEC Z31.69
    fertility preservation (prior to cancer therapy) (prior to removal of gonads) Z31.62
    using natural family planning Z31.61
  promiscuity Z70.1
  rape victim Z69.81
  religious Z71.81
  sex, sexual (related to) Z70.9
    attitude(s) Z70.0
    behavior or orientation Z70.1
    combined concerns Z70.3
    non-responsiveness Z70.1
    on behalf of third party Z70.2
    specified reason NEC Z70.8
  specified reason NEC Z71.89
  spiritual Z71.81
  spousal abuse (perpetrator) Z69.12
    victim Z69.11
  substance abuse Z71.89
    alcohol Z71.41
    drug Z71.51
    tobacco Z71.6
  tobacco use Z71.6

Counseling — *continued*
  use (of)
    insulin pump Z46.81
  victim (of)
    abuse Z69.81
    child abuse
      by parent Z69.010
      non-parental Z69.020
    rape NEC Z69.81
Coupled rhythm R00.8
Couvelaire syndrome or uterus (complicating delivery) O45.8X- ☑
Cowperitis — *see* Urethritis
Cowper's gland — *see* condition
Cowpox B08.010
  due to vaccination T88.1 ☑
Coxa
  magna M91.4- ☑
  plana M91.2- ☑
  valga (acquired) (*see also* Deformity, limb, specified type NEC, thigh)
    congenital Q65.81
    sequelae (late effect) of rickets E64.3
  vara (acquired) (*see also* Deformity, limb, specified type NEC, thigh)
    congenital Q65.82
    sequelae (late effect) of rickets E64.3
Coxalgia, coxalgic (nontuberculous) (*see also* Pain, joint, hip)
  tuberculous A18.02
Coxitis — *see* Monoarthritis, hip
Coxsackie (virus) (infection) B34.1
  as cause of disease classified elsewhere B97.11
  carditis B33.20
  central nervous system NEC A88.8
  endocarditis B33.21
  enteritis A08.39
  meningitis (aseptic) A87.0
  myocarditis B33.22
  pericarditis B33.23
  pharyngitis B08.5
  pleurodynia B33.0
  specific disease NEC B33.8
Crabs, meaning pubic lice B85.3
Crack baby P04.41
Cracked nipple N64.0
  associated with
    lactation O92.13
    pregnancy O92.11- ☑
    puerperium O92.12
Cracked tooth K03.81
Cradle cap L21.0
Craft neurosis F48.8
Cramp(s) R25.2
  abdominal — *see* Pain, abdominal
  bathing T75.1 ☑
  colic R10.83
    psychogenic F45.8
  due to immersion T75.1 ☑
  fireman T67.2 ☑
  heat T67.2 ☑
  immersion T75.1 ☑
  intestinal — *see* Pain, abdominal
    psychogenic F45.8
  leg, sleep related G47.62
  limb (lower) (upper) NEC R25.2
    sleep related G47.62
  linotypist's F48.8
    organic G25.89
  muscle (limb) (general) R25.2
    due to immersion T75.1 ☑
    psychogenic F45.8
  occupational (hand) F48.8
    organic G25.89
  salt-depletion E87.1
  sleep related, leg G47.62
  stoker's T67.2 ☑
  swimmer's T75.1 ☑
  telegrapher's F48.8
    organic G25.89
  typist's F48.8
    organic G25.89
  uterus N94.89
    menstrual — *see* Dysmenorrhea
  writer's F48.8
    organic G25.89
Cranial — *see* condition

Index

Curvature — Cyst

Curvature
organ or site, congenital NEC — see Distortion
penis (lateral) Q55.61
Pott's (spinal) A18.01
radius, idiopathic, progressive (congenital) Q74.0
spine (acquired) (angular) (idiopathic) (incorrect)
(postural) — see Dorsopathy, deforming
congenital Q67.5
due to or associated with
Charcot-Marie-Tooth disease (see also subcategory M49.8) G60.0
osteitis
deformans M88.88
fibrosa cystica (see also subcategory M49.8)
E21.0
tuberculosis (Pott's curvature) A18.01
sequelae (late effect) of rickets E64.3
tuberculous A18.01
Cushingoid due to steroid therapy E24.2
correct substance properly administered — see Table
of Drugs and Chemicals, by drug, adverse effect
overdose or wrong substance given or taken — see
Table of Drugs and Chemicals, by drug, poisoning
Cushing's
syndrome or disease E24.9
drug-induced E24.2
iatrogenic E24.2
pituitary-dependent E24.0
specified NEC E24.8
ulcer — see Ulcer, peptic, acute
Cusp, Carabelli — omit code
Cut (external) (see also Laceration)
muscle — see Injury, muscle
Cutaneous (see also condition)
hemorrhage R23.3
larva migrans B76.9
Cutis (see also condition)
hyperelastica Q82.8
acquired L57.4
laxa (hyperelastica) — see Dermatolysis
marmorata R23.8
osteosis L94.2
pendula — see Dermatolysis
rhomboidalis nuchae L57.2
verticis gyrata Q82.8
acquired L91.8
Cyanosis R23.0
due to
patent foramen botalli Q21.1
persistent foramen ovale Q21.1
enterogenous D74.8
paroxysmal digital — see Raynaud's disease
with gangrene I73.01
retina, retinal H35.89
Cyanotic heart disease I24.9
congenital Q24.9
Cycle
anovulatory N97.0
menstrual, irregular N92.6
Cyclencephaly Q04.9
Cyclical vomiting (see also Vomiting, cyclical) G43.A0
(following G43.7)
psychogenic F50.89
Cyclitis (see also Iridocyclitis) H20.9
chronic — see Iridocyclitis, chronic
Fuchs' heterochromic H20.81- ☑
granulomatous — see Iridocyclitis, chronic
lens-induced — see Iridocyclitis, lens-induced
posterior H30.2- ☑
Cycloid personality F34.0
Cyclophoria H50.54
Cyclopia, cyclops Q87.0
Cyclopism Q87.0
Cyclosporiasis A07.4
Cyclothymia F34.0
Cyclothymic personality F34.0
Cyclotropia H50.41- ☑
Cylindroma (see also Neoplasm, malignant, by site)
eccrine dermal — see Neoplasm, skin, benign
skin — see Neoplasm, skin, benign
Cylindruria R82.99
Cynanche
diphtheritic A36.2
tonsillaris J36
Cynophobia F40.218
Cynorexia R63.2

Cyphosis — see Kyphosis
Cyprus fever — see Brucellosis
Cyst (colloid) (mucous) (simple) (retention)
adenoid (infected) J35.8
adrenal gland E27.8
congenital Q89.1
air, lung J98.4
allantoic Q64.4
alveolar process (jaw bone) M27.40
amnion, amniotic O41.8X- ☑
aneurysmal M27.49
anterior
chamber (eye) — see Cyst, iris
nasopalatine K09.1
antrum J34.1
anus K62.89
apical (tooth) (periodontal) K04.8
appendix K38.8
arachnoid, brain (acquired) G93.0
congenital Q04.6
arytenoid J38.7
Baker's M71.2- ☑
ruptured M66.0
tuberculous A18.02
Bartholin's gland N75.0
bile duct (common) (hepatic) K83.5
bladder (multiple) (trigone) N32.89
blue dome (breast) — see Cyst, breast
bone (local) NEC M85.60
aneurysmal M85.50
ankle M85.57- ☑
foot M85.57- ☑
forearm M85.53- ☑
hand M85.54- ☑
jaw M27.49
lower leg M85.56- ☑
multiple site M85.59
neck M85.58
rib M85.58
shoulder M85.51- ☑
skull M85.58
specified site NEC M85.58
thigh M85.55- ☑
toe M85.57- ☑
upper arm M85.52- ☑
vertebra M85.58
solitary M85.40
ankle M85.47- ☑
fibula M85.46- ☑
foot M85.47- ☑
hand M85.44- ☑
humerus M85.42- ☑
jaw M27.49
neck M85.48
pelvis M85.45- ☑
radius M85.43- ☑
rib M85.48
shoulder M85.41- ☑
skull M85.48
specified site NEC M85.48
tibia M85.46- ☑
toe M85.47- ☑
ulna M85.43- ☑
vertebra M85.48
specified type NEC M85.60
ankle M85.67- ☑
foot M85.67- ☑
forearm M85.63- ☑
hand M85.64- ☑
jaw M27.40
developmental (nonodontogenic) K09.1
odontogenic K09.0
latent M27.0
lower leg M85.66- ☑
multiple site M85.69
neck M85.68
rib M85.68
shoulder M85.61- ☑
skull M85.68
specified site NEC M85.68
thigh M85.65- ☑
toe M85.67- ☑
upper arm M85.62- ☑
vertebra M85.68
brain (acquired) G93.0
congenital Q04.6
hydatid B67.99 [G94]

Cyst — continued
brain — continued
third ventricle (colloid), congenital Q04.6
branchial (cleft) Q18.0
branchiogenic Q18.0
breast (benign) (blue dome) (pedunculated) (solitary)
N60.0- ☑
involution — see Dysplasia, mammary, specified
type NEC
sebaceous — see Dysplasia, mammary, specified
type NEC
broad ligament (benign) N83.8
bronchogenic (mediastinal) (sequestration) J98.4
congenital Q33.0
buccal K09.8
bulbourethral gland N36.8
bursa, bursal NEC M71.30
with rupture — see Rupture, synovium
ankle M71.37- ☑
elbow M71.32- ☑
foot M71.37- ☑
hand M71.34- ☑
hip M71.35- ☑
multiple sites M71.39
pharyngeal J39.2
popliteal space — see Cyst, Baker's
shoulder M71.31- ☑
specified site NEC M71.38
wrist M71.33- ☑
calcifying odontogenic D16.5
upper jaw (bone) (maxilla) D16.4
canal of Nuck (female) N94.89
congenital Q52.4
canthus — see Cyst, conjunctiva
carcinomatous — see Neoplasm, malignant, by site
cauda equina G95.89
cavum septi pellucidi — see Cyst, brain
celomic (pericardium) Q24.8
cerebellopontine (angle) — see Cyst, brain
cerebellum — see Cyst, brain
cerebral — see Cyst, brain
cervical lateral Q18.0
cervix NEC N88.8
embryonic Q51.6
nabothian N88.8
chiasmal optic NEC — see Disorder, optic, chiasm
chocolate (ovary) N80.1
choledochus, congenital Q44.4
chorion O41.8X- ☑
choroid plexus G93.0
ciliary body — see Cyst, iris
clitoris N90.7
colon K63.89
common (bile) duct K83.5
congenital NEC Q89.8
adrenal gland Q89.1
epiglottis Q31.8
esophagus Q39.8
fallopian tube Q50.4
kidney Q61.00
more than one (multiple) Q61.02
specified as polycystic Q61.3
adult type Q61.2
infantile type NEC Q61.19
collecting duct dilation Q61.11
solitary Q61.01
larynx Q31.8
liver Q44.6
lung Q33.0
mediastinum Q34.1
ovary Q50.1
oviduct Q50.4
periurethral (tissue) Q64.79
prepuce Q55.69
salivary gland (any) Q38.4
sublingual Q38.6
submaxillary gland Q38.6
thymus (gland) Q89.2
tongue Q38.3
ureterovesical orifice Q62.8
vulva Q52.79
conjunctiva H11.44- ☑
cornea H18.89- ☑
corpora quadrigemina G93.0
corpus
albicans N83.29- ☑
luteum (hemorrhagic) (ruptured) N83.1- ☑
Cowper's gland (benign) (infected) N36.8

☑ Additional Character Required — Refer to the Tabular List for Character Selection   ▽ Subterms under main terms may continue to next column or page

Cyst — *continued*
  cranial meninges G93.0
  craniobuccal pouch E23.6
  craniopharyngeal pouch E23.6
  cystic duct K82.8
  Cysticercus — *see* Cysticercosis
  Dandy-Walker Q03.1
    with spina bifida — *see* Spina bifida
  dental (root) K04.8
    developmental K09.0
    eruption K09.0
    primordial K09.0
  dentigerous (mandible) (maxilla) K09.0
  dermoid — *see* Neoplasm, benign, by site
    with malignant transformation C56.- ☑
    implantation
      external area or site (skin) NEC L72.0
      iris — *see* Cyst, iris, implantation
      vagina N89.8
      vulva N90.7
    mouth K09.8
    oral soft tissue K09.8
    sacrococcygeal — *see* Cyst, pilonidal
  developmental K09.1
    odontogenic K09.0
    oral region (nonodontogenic) K09.1
    ovary, ovarian Q50.1
  dura (cerebral) G93.0
    spinal G96.19
  ear (external) Q18.1
  echinococcal — *see* Echinococcus
  embryonic
    cervix uteri Q51.6
    fallopian tube Q50.4
    vagina Q52.4
  endometrium, endometrial (uterus) N85.8
    ectopic — *see* Endometriosis
  enterogenous Q43.8
  epidermal, epidermoid (inclusion) (*see also* Cyst, skin)
    L72.0
    mouth K09.8
    oral soft tissue K09.8
  epididymis N50.3
  epiglottis J38.7
  epiphysis cerebri E34.8
  epithelial (inclusion) L72.0
  epoophoron Q50.5
  eruption K09.0
  esophagus K22.8
  ethmoid sinus J34.1
  external female genital organs NEC N90.7
  eyelid (sebaceous) H02.829
    infected — *see* Hordeolum
    left H02.826
      lower H02.825
      upper H02.824
    right H02.823
      lower H02.822
      upper H02.821
  eye NEC H57.8
    congenital Q15.8
  fallopian tube N83.8
    congenital Q50.4
  fimbrial (twisted) Q50.4
  fissural (oral region) K09.1
  follicle (graafian) (hemorrhagic) N83.0- ☑
    nabothian N88.8
  follicular (atretic) (hemorrhagic) (ovarian) N83.0- ☑
    dentigerous K09.0
    odontogenic K09.0
    skin L72.9
      specified NEC L72.8
  frontal sinus J34.1
  gallbladder K82.8
  ganglion — *see* Ganglion
  Gartner's duct Q52.4
  gingiva K09.0
  gland of Moll — *see* Cyst, eyelid
  globulomaxillary K09.1
  graafian follicle (hemorrhagic) N83.0- ☑
  granulosal lutein (hemorrhagic) N83.1- ☑
  hemangiomatous D18.00
    intra-abdominal D18.03
    intracranial D18.02
    skin D18.01
    specified site NEC D18.09
  hemorrhagic M27.49
  hydatid (*see also* Echinococcus) B67.90

Cyst — *continued*
  hydatid (*see also* Echinococcus) — *continued*
    brain B67.99 [G94]
    liver (*see also* Cyst, liver, hydatid) B67.8
    lung NEC B67.99 [J99]
    Morgagni
      female Q50.5
      male (epididymal) Q55.4
        testicular Q55.29
    specified site NEC B67.99
  hymen N89.8
    embryonic Q52.4
  hypopharynx J39.2
  hypophysis, hypophyseal (duct) (recurrent) E23.6
    cerebri E23.6
  implantation (dermoid)
    external area or site (skin) NEC L72.0
    iris — *see* Cyst, iris, implantation
    vagina N89.8
    vulva N90.7
  incisive canal K09.1
  inclusion (epidermal) (epithelial) (epidermoid) (squa-
    mous) L72.0
    not of skin — *code under* Cyst, by site
  intestine (large) (small) K63.89
  intracranial — *see* Cyst, brain
  intraligamentous (*see also* Disorder, ligament)
    knee — *see* Derangement, knee
  intrasellar E23.6
  iris H21.309
    exudative H21.31- ☑
    idiopathic H21.30- ☑
    implantation H21.32- ☑
    parasitic H21.33- ☑
    pars plana (primary) H21.34- ☑
      exudative H21.35- ☑
  jaw (bone) M27.40
    aneurysmal M27.49
    developmental (odontogenic) K09.0
    fissural K09.1
    hemorrhagic M27.49
    traumatic M27.49
  joint NEC — *see* Disorder, joint, specified type NEC
  kidney (acquired) N28.1
    calyceal — *see* Hydronephrosis
    congenital Q61.00
    more than one (multiple) Q61.02
      specified as polycystic Q61.3
        adult type (autosomal dominant) Q61.2
        infantile type (autosomal recessive) NEC
          Q61.19
          collecting duct dilation Q61.11
    pyelogenic — *see* Hydronephrosis
    simple N28.1
    solitary (single) Q61.01
      acquired N28.1
  labium (majus) (minus) N90.7
    sebaceous N90.7
  lacrimal (*see also* Disorder, lacrimal system, specified
    NEC)
    gland H04.13- ☑
    passages or sac — *see* Disorder, lacrimal system,
      specified NEC
  larynx J38.7
  lateral periodontal K09.0
  lens H27.8
    congenital Q12.8
  lip (gland) K13.0
  liver (idiopathic) (simple) K76.89
    congenital Q44.6
    hydatid B67.8
      granulosus B67.0
      multilocularis B67.5
  lung J98.4
    congenital Q33.0
    giant bullous J43.9
  lutein N83.1- ☑
  lymphangiomatous D18.1
  lymphoepithelial, oral soft tissue K09.8
  macula — *see* Degeneration, macula, hole
  malignant — *see* Neoplasm, malignant, by site
  mammary gland — *see* Cyst, breast
  mandible M27.40
    dentigerous K09.0
    radicular K04.8
  maxilla M27.40
    dentigerous K09.0
    radicular K04.8

Cyst — *continued*
  medial, face and neck Q18.8
  median
    anterior maxillary K09.1
    palatal K09.1
  mediastinum, congenital Q34.1
  meibomian (gland) — *see* Chalazion
    infected — *see* Hordeolum
  membrane, brain G93.0
  meninges (cerebral) G93.0
    spinal G96.19
  meniscus, knee — *see* Derangement, knee, meniscus,
    cystic
  mesentery, mesenteric K66.8
    chyle I89.8
  mesonephric duct
    female Q50.5
    male Q55.4
  milk N64.89
  Morgagni (hydatid)
    female Q50.5
    male (epididymal) Q55.4
      testicular Q55.29
  mouth K09.8
  Müllerian duct Q50.4
    appendix testis Q55.29
    cervix Q51.6
    fallopian tube Q50.4
    female Q50.4
    male Q55.29
    prostatic utricle Q55.4
    vagina (embryonal) Q52.4
  multilocular (ovary) D39.10
    benign — *see* Neoplasm, benign, by site
  myometrium N85.8
  nabothian (follicle) (ruptured) N88.8
  nasoalveolar K09.1
  nasolabial K09.1
  nasopalatine (anterior) (duct) K09.1
  nasopharynx J39.2
  neoplastic — *see* Neoplasm, uncertain behavior, by
    site
    benign — *see* Neoplasm, benign, by site
  nervous system NEC G96.8
  neuroenteric (congenital) Q06.8
  nipple — *see* Cyst, breast
  nose (turbinates) J34.1
    sinus J34.1
  odontogenic, developmental K09.0
  omentum (lesser) K66.8
    congenital Q45.8
  ora serrata — *see* Cyst, retina, ora serrata
  oral
    region K09.9
      developmental (nonodontogenic) K09.1
      specified NEC K09.8
    soft tissue K09.9
      specified NEC K09.8
  orbit H05.81- ☑
  ovary, ovarian (twisted) N83.20- ☑
    adherent N83.20- ☑
    chocolate N80.1
    corpus
      albicans N83.29- ☑
      luteum (hemorrhagic) N83.1- ☑
    dermoid D27.9
    developmental Q50.1
    due to failure of involution NEC N83.20- ☑
    endometrial N80.1
    follicular (graafian) (hemorrhagic) N83.0- ☑
    hemorrhagic N83.20- ☑
    in pregnancy or childbirth O34.8- ☑
      with obstructed labor O65.5
    multilocular D39.10
    pseudomucinous D27.9
    retention N83.29- ☑
    serous N83.20- ☑
    specified NEC N83.29- ☑
    theca lutein (hemorrhagic) N83.1- ☑
    tuberculous A18.18
  oviduct N83.8
  palate (median) (fissural) K09.1
  palatine papilla (jaw) K09.1
  pancreas, pancreatic (hemorrhagic) (true) K86.2
    congenital Q45.2
    false K86.3
  paralabral
    hip M24.85- ☑

Cyst — *continued*

paralabral — *continued*
  shoulder S43.43- ☑
paramesonephric duct Q50.4
  female Q50.4
  male Q55.29
paranephric N28.1
paraphysis, cerebri, congenital Q04.6
parasitic B89
parathyroid (gland) E21.4
paratubal N83.8
paraurethral duct N36.8
paroophoron Q50.5
parotid gland K11.6
parovarian Q50.5
pelvis, female N94.89
  in pregnancy or childbirth O34.8- ☑
    causing obstructed labor O65.5
penis (sebaceous) N48.89
periapical K04.8
pericardial (congenital) Q24.8
  acquired (secondary) I31.8
pericoronal K09.0
periodontal K04.8
  lateral K09.0
peripelvic (lymphatic) N28.1
peritoneum K66.8
  chylous I89.8
periventricular, acquired, newborn P91.1
pharynx (wall) J39.2
pilar L72.11
pilonidal (infected) (rectum) L05.91
  with abscess L05.01
  malignant C44.59- ☑
pituitary (duct) (gland) E23.6
placenta O43.19- ☑
pleura J94.8
popliteal — *see* Cyst, Baker's
porencephalic Q04.6
  acquired G93.0
postanal (infected) — *see* Cyst, pilonidal
postmastoidectomy cavity (mucosal) — *see* Complications, postmastoidectomy, cyst
preauricular Q18.1
prepuce N47.4
  congenital Q55.69
primordial (jaw) K09.0
prostate N42.83
pseudomucinous (ovary) D27.9
pupillary, miotic H21.27- ☑
radicular (residual) K04.8
radiculodental K04.8
ranular K11.8
Rathke's pouch E23.6
rectum (epithelium) (mucous) K62.89
renal — *see* Cyst, kidney
residual (radicular) K04.8
retention (ovary) N83.29- ☑
  salivary gland K11.6
retina H33.19- ☑
  ora serrata H33.11- ☑
  parasitic H33.12- ☑
retroperitoneal K68.9
sacrococcygeal (dermoid) — *see* Cyst, pilonidal
salivary gland or duct (mucous extravasation or retention) K11.6
Sampson's N80.1
sclera H15.89
scrotum L72.9
  sebaceous L72.3
sebaceous (duct) (gland) L72.3
  breast — *see* Dysplasia, mammary, specified type NEC
  eyelid — *see* Cyst, eyelid
  genital organ NEC
    female N94.89
    male N50.89
  scrotum L72.3
semilunar cartilage (knee) (multiple) — *see* Derangement, knee, meniscus, cystic
seminal vesicle N50.89
serous (ovary) N83.20- ☑
sinus (accessory) (nasal) J34.1
Skene's gland N36.8
skin L72.9
  breast — *see* Dysplasia, mammary, specified type NEC
  epidermal, epidermoid L72.0

Cyst — *continued*

skin — *continued*
  epithelial L72.0
  eyelid — *see* Cyst, eyelid
  genital organ NEC
    female N90.7
    male N50.89
  inclusion L72.0
  scrotum L72.9
  sebaceous L72.3
  sweat gland or duct L74.8
solitary
  bone — *see* Cyst, bone, solitary
  jaw M27.40
  kidney N28.1
spermatic cord N50.89
sphenoid sinus J34.1
spinal meninges G96.19
spleen NEC D73.4
  congenital Q89.09
  hydatid (*see also* Echinococcus) B67.99 [D77]
Stafne's M27.0
subarachnoid intrasellar R93.0
subcutaneous, pheomycotic (chromomycotic) B43.2
subdural (cerebral) G93.0
  spinal cord G96.19
sublingual gland K11.6
submandibular gland K11.6
submaxillary gland K11.6
suburethral N36.8
suprarenal gland E27.8
suprasellar — *see* Cyst, brain
sweat gland or duct L74.8
synovial (*see also* Cyst, bursa)
  ruptured — *see* Rupture, synovium
tarsal — *see* Chalazion
tendon (sheath) — *see* Disorder, tendon, specified type NEC
testis N44.2
  tunica albuginea N44.1
theca lutein (ovary) N83.1- ☑
Thornwaldt's J39.2
thymus (gland) E32.8
thyroglossal duct (infected) (persistent) Q89.2
thyroid (gland) E04.1
thyrolingual duct (infected) (persistent) Q89.2
tongue K14.8
tonsil J35.8
tooth — *see* Cyst, dental
Tornwaldt's J39.2
trichilemmal (proliferating) L72.12
trichodermal L72.12
tubal (fallopian) N83.8
  inflammatory — *see* Salpingitis, chronic
tubo-ovarian N83.8
  inflammatory N70.13
tunica
  albuginea testis N44.1
  vaginalis N50.89
turbinate (nose) J34.1
Tyson's gland N48.89
urachus, congenital Q64.4
ureter N28.89
ureterovesical orifice N28.89
urethra, urethral (gland) N36.8
uterine ligament N83.8
uterus (body) (corpus) (recurrent) N85.8
  embryonic Q51.818
    cervix Q51.6
vagina, vaginal (implantation) (inclusion) (squamous cell) (wall) N89.8
  embryonic Q52.4
vallecula, vallecular (epiglottis) J38.7
vesical (orifice) N32.89
vitreous body H43.89
vulva (implantation) (inclusion) N90.7
  congenital Q52.79
  sebaceous gland N90.7
vulvovaginal gland N90.7
wolffian
  female Q50.5
  male Q55.4

Cystadenocarcinoma — *see* Neoplasm, malignant, by site

bile duct C22.1
endometrioid — *see* Neoplasm, malignant, by site
  specified site — *see* Neoplasm, malignant, by site

Cystadenocarcinoma — *continued*

endometrioid — *see* Neoplasm, malignant, by site — *continued*
  unspecified site
    female C56.9
    male C61
mucinous
  papillary
    specified site — *see* Neoplasm, malignant, by site
    unspecified site C56.9
  specified site — *see* Neoplasm, malignant, by site
  unspecified site C56.9
papillary
  mucinous
    specified site — *see* Neoplasm, malignant, by site
    unspecified site C56.9
  pseudomucinous
    specified site — *see* Neoplasm, malignant, by site
    unspecified site C56.9
  serous
    specified site — *see* Neoplasm, malignant, by site
    unspecified site C56.9
  specified site — *see* Neoplasm, malignant, by site
  unspecified site C56.9
pseudomucinous
  papillary
    specified site — *see* Neoplasm, malignant, by site
    unspecified site C56.9
  specified site — *see* Neoplasm, malignant, by site
  unspecified site C56.9
serous
  papillary
    specified site — *see* Neoplasm, malignant, by site
    unspecified site C56.9
  specified site — *see* Neoplasm, malignant, by site
  unspecified site C56.9

Cystadenofibroma

clear cell — *see* Neoplasm, benign, by site
endometrioid D27.9
  borderline malignancy D39.1- ☑
  malignant C56.- ☑
mucinous
  specified site — *see* Neoplasm, benign, by site
  unspecified site D27.9
serous
  specified site — *see* Neoplasm, benign, by site
  unspecified site D27.9
specified site — *see* Neoplasm, benign, by site
unspecified site D27.9

Cystadenoma (*see also* Neoplasm, benign, by site)

bile duct D13.4
endometrioid — *see* Neoplasm, benign, by site
  borderline malignancy — *see* Neoplasm, uncertain behavior, by site
malignant — *see* Neoplasm, malignant, by site
mucinous
  borderline malignancy
    ovary C56.- ☑
    specified site NEC — *see* Neoplasm, uncertain behavior, by site
    unspecified site C56.9
  papillary
    borderline malignancy
      ovary C56.- ☑
      specified site NEC — *see* Neoplasm, uncertain behavior, by site
      unspecified site C56.9
    specified site — *see* Neoplasm, benign, by site
    unspecified site D27.9
  specified site — *see* Neoplasm, benign, by site
  unspecified site D27.9
papillary
  borderline malignancy
    ovary C56.- ☑
    specified site NEC — *see* Neoplasm, uncertain behavior, by site
    unspecified site C56.9
  lymphomatosum
    specified site — *see* Neoplasm, benign, by site
    unspecified site D11.9

Cystadenoma — *continued*
  papillary — *continued*
    mucinous
      borderline malignancy
        ovary C56.- ☑
        specified site NEC — *see* Neoplasm, uncertain behavior, by site
        unspecified site C56.9
      specified site — *see* Neoplasm, benign, by site
      unspecified site D27.9
    pseudomucinous
      borderline malignancy
        ovary C56.- ☑
        specified site NEC — *see* Neoplasm, uncertain behavior, by site
        unspecified site C56.9
      specified site — *see* Neoplasm, benign, by site
      unspecified site D27.9
    serous
      borderline malignancy
        ovary C56.- ☑
        specified site NEC — *see* Neoplasm, uncertain behavior, by site
        unspecified site C56.9
      specified site — *see* Neoplasm, benign, by site
      unspecified site D27.9
  pseudomucinous
    borderline malignancy
      ovary C56.- ☑
      specified site NEC — *see* Neoplasm, uncertain behavior, by site
      unspecified site C56.9
    papillary
      borderline malignancy
        ovary C56.- ☑
        specified site NEC — *see* Neoplasm, uncertain behavior, by site
        unspecified site C56.9
      specified site — *see* Neoplasm, benign, by site
      unspecified site D27.9
    specified site — *see* Neoplasm, benign, by site
    unspecified site D27.9
  serous
    borderline malignancy
      ovary C56.- ☑
      specified site NEC — *see* Neoplasm, uncertain behavior, by site
      unspecified site C56.9
    papillary
      borderline malignancy
        ovary C56.- ☑
        specified site NEC — *see* Neoplasm, uncertain behavior, by site
        unspecified site C56.9
      specified site — *see* Neoplasm, benign, by site
      unspecified site D27.9
    specified site — *see* Neoplasm, benign, by site
    unspecified site D27.9
Cystathionine synthase deficiency E72.11
Cystathioninemia E72.19
Cystathioninuria E72.19
Cystic (*see also* condition)
  breast (chronic) — *see* Mastopathy, cystic
  corpora lutea (hemorrhagic) N83.1- ☑
  duct — *see* condition
  eyeball (congenital) Q11.0
  fibrosis — *see* Fibrosis, cystic
  kidney (congenital) Q61.9

Cystic — *continued*
  kidney — *continued*
    adult type Q61.2
    infantile type NEC Q61.19
      collecting duct dilatation Q61.11
    medullary Q61.5
  liver, congenital Q44.6
  lung disease J98.4
    congenital Q33.0
  mastitis, chronic — *see* Mastopathy, cystic
  medullary, kidney Q61.5
  meniscus — *see* Derangement, knee, meniscus, cystic
  ovary N83.20- ☑
Cysticercosis, cysticerciasis B69.9
  with
    epileptiform fits B69.0
    myositis B69.81
  brain B69.0
  central nervous system B69.0
  cerebral B69.0
  ocular B69.1
  specified NEC B69.89
Cysticercus cellulose infestation — *see* Cysticercosis
Cystinosis (malignant) E72.04
Cystinuria E72.01
Cystitis (exudative) (hemorrhagic) (septic) (suppurative) N30.90
  with
    fibrosis — *see* Cystitis, chronic, interstitial
    hematuria N30.91
    leukoplakia — *see* Cystitis, chronic, interstitial
    malakoplakia — *see* Cystitis, chronic, interstitial
    metaplasia — *see* Cystitis, chronic, interstitial
    prostatitis N41.3
  acute N30.00
    with hematuria N30.01
    of trigone N30.30
      with hematuria N30.31
  allergic — *see* Cystitis, specified type NEC
  amebic A06.81
  bilharzial B65.9 [N33]
  blennorrhagic (gonococcal) A54.01
  bullous — *see* Cystitis, specified type NEC
  calculous N21.0
  chlamydial A56.01
  chronic N30.20
    with hematuria N30.21
    interstitial N30.10
      with hematuria N30.11
    of trigone N30.30
      with hematuria N30.31
    specified NEC N30.20
      with hematuria N30.21
  cystic (a) — *see* Cystitis, specified type NEC
  diphtheritic A36.85
  echinococcal
    granulosus B67.39
    multilocularis B67.69
  emphysematous — *see* Cystitis, specified type NEC
  encysted — *see* Cystitis, specified type NEC
  eosinophilic — *see* Cystitis, specified type NEC
  follicular — *see* Cystitis, of trigone
  gangrenous — *see* Cystitis, specified type NEC
  glandularis — *see* Cystitis, specified type NEC
  gonococcal A54.01
  incrusted — *see* Cystitis, specified type NEC
  interstitial (chronic) — *see* Cystitis, chronic, interstitial
  irradiation N30.40
    with hematuria N30.41
  irritation — *see* Cystitis, specified type NEC

Cystitis — *continued*
  malignant — *see* Cystitis, specified type NEC
  of trigone N30.30
    with hematuria N30.31
  panmural — *see* Cystitis, chronic, interstitial
  polyposa — *see* Cystitis, specified type NEC
  prostatic N41.3
  puerperal (postpartum) O86.22
  radiation — *see* Cystitis, irradiation
  specified type NEC N30.80
    with hematuria N30.81
  subacute — *see* Cystitis, chronic
  submucous — *see* Cystitis, chronic, interstitial
  syphilitic (late) A52.76
  trichomonal A59.03
  tuberculous A18.12
  ulcerative — *see* Cystitis, chronic, interstitial
Cystocele (-urethrocele)
  female N81.10
    with prolapse of uterus — *see* Prolapse, uterus
    lateral N81.12
    midline N81.11
    paravaginal N81.12
  in pregnancy or childbirth O34.8- ☑
    causing obstructed labor O65.5
  male N32.89
Cystolithiasis N21.0
Cystoma (*see also* Neoplasm, benign, by site)
  endometrial, ovary N80.1
  mucinous
    specified site — *see* Neoplasm, benign, by site
    unspecified site D27.9
  serous
    specified site — *see* Neoplasm, benign, by site
    unspecified site D27.9
  simple (ovary) N83.29- ☑
Cystoplegia N31.2
Cystoptosis N32.89
Cystopyelitis — *see* Pyelonephritis
Cystorrhagia N32.89
Cystosarcoma phyllodes D48.6- ☑
  benign D24- ☑
  malignant — *see* Neoplasm, breast, malignant
Cystostomy
  attention to Z43.5
  complication — *see* Complications, cystostomy
  status Z93.50
    appendico-vesicostomy Z93.52
    cutaneous Z93.51
    specified NEC Z93.59
Cystourethritis — *see* Urethritis
Cystourethrocele (*see also* Cystocele)
  female N81.10
    with uterine prolapse — *see* Prolapse, uterus
    lateral N81.12
    midline N81.11
    paravaginal N81.12
  male N32.89
Cytomegalic inclusion disease
  congenital P35.1
Cytomegalovirus infection B25.9
Cytomycosis (reticuloendothelial) B39.4
Cytopenia D75.9
  refractory
    with multilineage dysplasia D46.A (*following* D46.2)
      and ring sideroblasts (RCMD RS) D46.B (*following* D46.2)
Czerny's disease (periodic hydrarthrosis of the knee) — *see* Effusion, joint, knee

D

Da Costa's syndrome F45.8
Daae (-Finsen) **disease** (epidemic pleurodynia) B33.0
Dabney's grip B33.0
Dacryoadenitis, dacryadenitis H04.00- ☑
  acute H04.01- ☑
  chronic H04.02- ☑
Dacryocystitis H04.30- ☑
  acute H04.32- ☑
  chronic H04.41- ☑
  neonatal P39.1
  phlegmonous H04.31- ☑
  syphilitic A52.71
    congenital (early) A50.01
  trachomatous, active A71.1
    sequelae (late effect) B94.0
Dacryocystoblenorrhea — *see* Inflammation, lacrimal, passages, chronic
Dacryocystocele — *see* Disorder, lacrimal system, changes
Dacryolith, dacryolithiasis H04.51- ☑
Dacryoma — *see* Disorder, lacrimal system, changes
Dacryopericystitis — *see* Dacryocystitis
Dacryops H04.11- ☑
Dacryostenosis (*see also* Stenosis, lacrimal)
  congenital Q10.5
Dactylitis
  bone — *see* Osteomyelitis
  sickle-cell D57.00
    Hb C D57.219
    Hb SS D57.00
    specified NEC D57.819
  skin L08.9
  syphilitic A52.77
  tuberculous A18.03
Dactylolysis spontanea (ainhum) L94.6
Dactylosymphysis Q70.9
  fingers — *see* Syndactylism, complex, fingers
  toes — *see* Syndactylism, complex, toes
Damage
  arteriosclerotic — *see* Arteriosclerosis
  brain (nontraumatic) G93.9
    anoxic, hypoxic G93.1
      resulting from a procedure G97.82
    child NEC G80.9
    due to birth injury P11.2
  cardiorenal (vascular) — *see* Hypertension, cardiorenal
  cerebral NEC — *see* Damage, brain
  coccyx, complicating delivery O71.6
  coronary — *see* Disease, heart, ischemic
  eye, birth injury P15.3
  liver (nontraumatic) K76.9
    alcoholic K70.9
    due to drugs — *see* Disease, liver, toxic
    toxic — *see* Disease, liver, toxic
  medication T88.7 ☑
  pelvic
    joint or ligament, during delivery O71.6
    organ NEC
      during delivery O71.5
      following ectopic or molar pregnancy O08.6
  renal — *see* Disease, renal
  subendocardium, subendocardial — *see* Degeneration, myocardial
  vascular I99.9
Dana-Putnam syndrome (subacute combined sclerosis with pernicious anemia) — *see* Degeneration, combined
Danbolt (-Cross) **syndrome** (acrodermatitis enteropathica) E83.2
Dandruff L21.0
Dandy-Walker syndrome Q03.1
  with spina bifida — *see* Spina bifida
Danlos' syndrome Q79.6
Darier (-White) **disease** (congenital) Q82.8
  meaning erythema annulare centrifugum L53.1
Darier-Roussy sarcoid D86.3
Darling's disease or histoplasmosis B39.4
Darwin's tubercle Q17.8
Dawson's (inclusion body) **encephalitis** A81.1

De Beurmann (-Gougerot) **disease** B42.1
De la Tourette's syndrome F95.2
De Lange's syndrome Q87.1
De Morgan's spots (senile angiomas) I78.1
De Quervain's
  disease (tendon sheath) M65.4
  syndrome E34.51
  thyroiditis (subacute granulomatous thyroiditis) E06.1
De Toni-Fanconi (-Debré) **syndrome** E72.09
  with cystinosis E72.04
Dead
  fetus, retained (mother) O36.4 ☑
    early pregnancy O02.1
  labyrinth H83.2 ☑
  ovum, retained O02.0
Deaf nonspeaking NEC H91.3
Deafmutism (acquired) (congenital) NEC H91.3
  hysterical F44.6
  syphilitic, congenital (*see also* subcategory) H94.8 A50.09
Deafness (acquired) (complete) (hereditary) (partial) H91.9- ☑
  with blue sclera and fragility of bone Q78.0
  auditory fatigue — *see* Deafness, specified type NEC
  aviation T70.0 ☑
    nerve injury — *see* Injury, nerve, acoustic, specified type NEC
  boilermaker's H83.3 ☑
  central — *see* Deafness, sensorineural
  conductive H90.2
    and sensorineural
      mixed H90.8
        bilateral H90.6
    bilateral H90.0
    unilateral H90.1- ☑
      with restricted hearing on the contralateral side H90.A- ☑
  congenital H90.5
    with blue sclera and fragility of bone Q78.0
  due to toxic agents — *see* Deafness, ototoxic
  emotional (hysterical) F44.6
  functional (hysterical) F44.6
  high frequency H91.9- ☑
  hysterical F44.6
  low frequency H91.9- ☑
  mental R48.8
  mixed conductive and sensorineural H90.8
    bilateral H90.6
    unilateral H90.7- ☑
  nerve — *see* Deafness, sensorineural
  neural — *see* Deafness, sensorineural
  noise-induced (*see also* subcategory) H83.3 ☑
    nerve injury — *see* Injury, nerve, acoustic, specified type NEC
  nonspeaking H91.3
  ototoxic H91.0 ☑
  perceptive — *see* Deafness, sensorineural
  psychogenic (hysterical) F44.6
  sensorineural H90.5
    and conductive
      bilateral H90.6
      mixed H90.8
        bilateral H90.6
    bilateral H90.3
    unilateral H90.4- ☑
      with restricted hearing on the contralateral side H90.A- ☑
  sensory — *see* Deafness, sensorineural
  specified type NEC H91.8 ☑
  sudden (idiopathic) H91.2- ☑
  syphilitic A52.15
  transient ischemic H93.01- ☑
  traumatic — *see* Injury, nerve, acoustic, specified type NEC
  word (developmental) H93.25
Death (cause unknown) (of) (unexplained) (unspecified cause) R99
  brain G93.82
  cardiac (sudden) (with successful resuscitation) — *code to* underlying disease
    family history of Z82.41
    personal history of Z86.74

Death — *continued*
  family member (assumed) Z63.4
Debility (chronic) (general) (nervous) R53.81
  congenital or neonatal NOS P96.9
  nervous R53.81
  old age R54
  senile R54
Débove's disease (splenomegaly) R16.1
Decalcification
  bone — *see* Osteoporosis
  teeth K03.89
Decapsulation, kidney N28.89
Decay
  dental — *see* Caries, dental
  senile R54
  tooth, teeth — *see* Caries, dental
Deciduitis (acute)
  following ectopic or molar pregnancy O08.0
Decline (general) — *see* Debility
  cognitive, age-associated R41.81
Decompensation
  cardiac (acute) (chronic) — *see* Disease, heart
  cardiovascular — *see* Disease, cardiovascular
  heart — *see* Disease, heart
  hepatic — *see* Failure, hepatic
  myocardial (acute) (chronic) — *see* Disease, heart
  respiratory J98.8
Decompression sickness T70.3 ☑
Decrease (d)
  absolute neutrophile count — *see* Neutropenia
  blood
    platelets — *see* Thrombocytopenia
    pressure R03.1
      due to shock following
        injury T79.4 ☑
        operation T81.19 ☑
  estrogen E28.39
    postablative E89.40
      asymptomatic E89.40
      symptomatic E89.41
  fragility of erythrocytes D58.8
  function
    lipase (pancreatic) K90.3
    ovary in hypopituitarism E23.0
    parenchyma of pancreas K86.89
    pituitary (gland) (anterior) (lobe) E23.0
      posterior (lobe) E23.0
  functional activity R68.89
  glucose R73.09
  hematocrit R71.0
  hemoglobin R71.0
  leukocytes D72.819
    specified NEC D72.818
  libido R68.82
  lymphocytes D72.810
  platelets D69.6
  respiration, due to shock following injury T79.4 ☑
  sexual desire R68.82
  tear secretion NEC — *see* Syndrome, dry eye
  tolerance
    fat K90.49
    glucose R73.09
    pancreatic K90.3
    salt and water E87.8
  vision NEC H54.7
  white blood cell count D72.819
    specified NEC D72.818
Decubitus (ulcer) — *see* Ulcer, pressure, by site
  cervix N86
Deepening acetabulum — *see* Derangement, joint, specified type NEC, hip
Defect, defective Q89.9
  3-beta-hydroxysteroid dehydrogenase E25.0
  11-hydroxylase E25.0
  21-hydroxylase E25.0
  abdominal wall, congenital Q79.59
  antibody immunodeficiency D80.9
  aorticopulmonary septum Q21.4
  atrial septal (ostium secundum type) Q21.1
    following acute myocardial infarction (current complication) I23.1
    ostium primum type Q21.2

Defect, defective — *continued*
  atrioventricular
    canal Q21.2
    septum Q21.2
  auricular septal Q21.1
  bilirubin excretion NEC E80.6
  biosynthesis, androgen (testicular) E29.1
  bulbar septum Q21.0
  catalase E80.3
  cell membrane receptor complex (CR3) D71
  circulation I99.9
    congenital Q28.9
    newborn Q28.9
  coagulation (factor) (*see also* Deficiency, factor) D68.9
    with
      ectopic pregnancy O08.1
      molar pregnancy O08.1
    acquired D68.4
    antepartum with hemorrhage — *see* Hemorrhage, antepartum, with coagulation defect
    due to
      liver disease D68.4
      vitamin K deficiency D68.4
    hereditary NEC D68.2
    intrapartum O67.0
    newborn, transient P61.6
    postpartum O99.13
      with hemorrhage O72.3
    specified type NEC D68.8
  complement system D84.1
  conduction (heart) I45.9
    bone — *see* Deafness, conductive
  congenital, organ or site not listed — *see* Anomaly, by site
  coronary sinus Q21.1
  cushion, endocardial Q21.2
  degradation, glycoprotein E77.1
  dental bridge, crown, fillings — *see* Defect, dental restoration
  dental restoration K08.50
    specified NEC K08.59
  dentin (hereditary) K00.5
  Descemet's membrane, congenital Q13.89
  developmental (*see also* Anomaly)
    cauda equina Q06.3
  diaphragm
    with elevation, eventration or hernia — *see* Hernia, diaphragm
    congenital Q79.1
      with hernia Q79.0
      gross (with hernia) Q79.0
  ectodermal, congenital Q82.9
  Eisenmenger's Q21.8
  enzyme
    catalase E80.3
    peroxidase E80.3
  esophagus, congenital Q39.9
  extensor retinaculum M62.89
  fibrin polymerization D68.2
  filling
    bladder R93.41
    kidney R93.42- ☑
    renal pelvis R93.41
    stomach R93.3
    ureter R93.41
    urinary organs, specified NEC R93.49
  Gerbode Q21.0
  glycoprotein degradation E77.1
  Hageman (factor) D68.2
  hearing — *see* Deafness
  high grade F70
  interatrial septal Q21.1
  interauricular septal Q21.1
  interventricular septal Q21.0
    with dextroposition of aorta, pulmonary stenosis and hypertrophy of right ventricle Q21.3
    in tetralogy of Fallot Q21.3
  learning (specific) — *see* Disorder, learning
  lymphocyte function antigen-1 (LFA-1) D84.0
  lysosomal enzyme, post-translational modification E77.0
  major osseous M89.70
    ankle M89.77- ☑
    carpus M89.74- ☑
    clavicle M89.71- ☑
    femur M89.75- ☑
    fibula M89.76- ☑
    fingers M89.74- ☑

Defect, defective — *continued*
  major osseous — *continued*
    foot M89.77- ☑
    forearm M89.73- ☑
    hand M89.74- ☑
    humerus M89.72- ☑
    lower leg M89.76- ☑
    metacarpus M89.74- ☑
    metatarsus M89.77- ☑
    multiple sites M89.79
    pelvic region M89.75- ☑
    pelvis M89.75- ☑
    radius M89.73- ☑
    scapula M89.71- ☑
    shoulder region M89.71- ☑
    specified NEC M89.78
    tarsus M89.77- ☑
    thigh M89.75- ☑
    tibia M89.76- ☑
    toes M89.77- ☑
    ulna M89.73- ☑
  mental — *see* Disability, intellectual
  modification, lysosomal enzymes, post-translational E77.0
  obstructive, congenital
    renal pelvis Q62.39
    ureter Q62.39
      atresia — *see* Atresia, ureter
      cecoureterocele Q62.32
      megaureter Q62.2
      orthotopic ureterocele Q62.31
  osseous, major M89.70
    ankle M89.77- ☑
    carpus M89.74- ☑
    clavicle M89.71- ☑
    femur M89.75- ☑
    fibula M89.76- ☑
    fingers M89.74- ☑
    foot M89.77- ☑
    forearm M89.73- ☑
    hand M89.74- ☑
    humerus M89.72- ☑
    lower leg M89.76- ☑
    metacarpus M89.74- ☑
    metatarsus M89.77- ☑
    multiple sites M89.9
    pelvic region M89.75- ☑
    pelvis M89.75- ☑
    radius M89.73- ☑
    scapula M89.71- ☑
    shoulder region M89.71- ☑
    specified NEC M89.78
    tarsus M89.77- ☑
    thigh M89.75- ☑
    tibia M89.76- ☑
    toes M89.77- ☑
    ulna M89.73- ☑
  osteochondral NEC (*see also* Deformity) M95.8
  ostium
    primum Q21.2
    secundum Q21.1
  peroxidase E80.3
  placental blood supply — *see* Insufficiency, placental
  platelets, qualitative D69.1
    constitutional D68.0
  postural NEC, spine — *see* Dorsopathy, deforming
  reduction
    limb Q73.8
      lower Q72.9- ☑
        absence — *see* Agenesis, leg
          foot — *see* Agenesis, foot
        longitudinal
          femur Q72.4- ☑
          fibula Q72.6- ☑
          tibia Q72.5- ☑
        specified type NEC Q72.89- ☑
        split foot Q72.7- ☑
      specified type NEC Q73.8
      upper Q71.9- ☑
        absence — *see* Agenesis, arm
          forearm — *see* Agenesis, forearm
          hand — *see* Agenesis, hand
        lobster-claw hand Q71.6- ☑
        longitudinal
          radius Q71.4- ☑
          ulna Q71.5- ☑

Defect, defective — *continued*
  reduction — *continued*
    limb — *continued*
      upper — *continued*
        specified type NEC Q71.89- ☑
  renal pelvis Q63.8
    obstructive Q62.39
  respiratory system, congenital Q34.9
  restoration, dental K08.50
    specified NEC K08.59
  retinal nerve bundle fibers H35.89
  septal (heart) NOS Q21.9
    acquired (atrial) (auricular) (ventricular) (old) I51.0
    atrial Q21.1
      concurrent with acute myocardial infarction — *see* Infarct, myocardium
      following acute myocardial infarction (current complication) I23.1
    ventricular (*see also* Defect, ventricular septal) Q21.0
  sinus venosus Q21.1
  speech R47.9
    developmental F80.9
    specified NEC R47.89
  Taussig-Bing (aortic transposition and overriding pulmonary artery) Q20.1
  teeth, wedge K03.1
  vascular (local) I99.9
    congenital Q27.9
  ventricular septal Q21.0
    concurrent with acute myocardial infarction — *see* Infarct, myocardium
    following acute myocardial infarction (current complication) I23.2
    in tetralogy of Fallot Q21.3
  vision NEC H54.7
  visual field H53.40
    bilateral
      heteronymous H53.47
      homonymous H53.46- ☑
    generalized contraction H53.48- ☑
    localized
      arcuate H53.43- ☑
      scotoma (central area) H53.41- ☑
        blind spot area H53.42- ☑
      sector H53.43- ☑
      specified type NEC H53.45- ☑
  voice R49.9
    specified NEC R49.8
  wedge, tooth, teeth (abrasion) K03.1
Deferentitis N49.1
  gonorrheal (acute) (chronic) A54.23
Defibrination (syndrome) D65
  antepartum — *see* Hemorrhage, antepartum, with coagulation defect, disseminated intravascular coagulation
  following ectopic or molar pregnancy O08.1
  intrapartum O67.0
  newborn P60
  postpartum O72.3
Deficiency, deficient
  3-beta hydroxysteroid dehydrogenase E25.0
  5-alpha reductase (with male pseudo-hermaphroditism) E29.1
  11-hydroxylase E25.0
  21-hydroxylase E25.0
  abdominal muscle syndrome Q79.4
  AC globulin (congenital) (hereditary) D68.2
    acquired D68.4
  accelerator globulin (Ac G) (blood) D68.2
  acid phosphatase E83.39
  activating factor (blood) D68.2
  adenosine deaminase (ADA) D81.3
  aldolase (hereditary) E74.19
  alpha-1-antitrypsin E88.01
  amino-acids E72.9
  anemia — *see* Anemia
  aneurin E51.9
  antibody with
    hyperimmunoglobulinemia D80.6
    near-normal immunoglobins D80.6
  antidiuretic hormone E23.2
  anti-hemophilic
    factor (A) D66
      B D67
      C D68.1
    globulin (AHG) NEC D66
  antithrombin (antithrombin III) D68.59

Index

Deficiency, deficient — Deficiency, deficient

Deficiency, deficient — *continued*
ascorbic acid E54
attention (disorder) (syndrome) F98.8
  with hyperactivity — *see* Disorder, attention-deficit
    hyperactivity
autoprothrombin
  C D68.2
  I D68.2
  II D67
beta-glucuronidase E76.29
biotin E53.8
biotin-dependent carboxylase D81.819
biotinidase D81.810
brancher enzyme (amylopectinosis) E74.03
C1 esterase inhibitor (C1-INH) D84.1
calciferol E55.9
  with
    adult osteomalacia M83.8
    rickets — *see* Rickets
calcium (dietary) E58
calorie, severe E43
  with marasmus E41
    and kwashiorkor E42
cardiac — *see* Insufficiency, myocardial
carnitine E71.40
  due to
    hemodialysis E71.43
    inborn errors of metabolism E71.42
    Valproic acid therapy E71.43
  iatrogenic E71.43
  muscle palmityltransferase E71.314
  primary E71.41
  secondary E71.448
carotene E50.9
central nervous system G96.8
ceruloplasmin (Wilson) E83.01
choline E53.8
Christmas factor D67
chromium E61.4
clotting (blood) (*see also* Deficiency, coagulation factor) D68.9
clotting factor NEC (hereditary) (*see also* Deficiency, factor) D68.2
coagulation NOS D68.9
  with
    ectopic pregnancy O08.1
    molar pregnancy O08.1
  acquired (any) D68.4
  antepartum hemorrhage — *see* Hemorrhage, antepartum, with coagulation defect
  clotting factor NEC (*see also* Deficiency, factor) D68.2
  due to
    hyperprothrombinemia D68.4
    liver disease D68.4
    vitamin K deficiency D68.4
  newborn, transient P61.6
  postpartum O72.3
  specified NEC D68.8
cognitive F09
color vision H53.50
  achromatopsia H53.51
  acquired H53.52
  deuteranomaly H53.53
  protanomaly H53.54
  specified type NEC H53.59
  tritanomaly H53.55
combined glucocorticoid and mineralocorticoid E27.49
contact factor D68.2
copper (nutritional) E61.0
corticoadrenal E27.40
  primary E27.1
craniofacial axis Q75.0
cyanocobalamin E53.8
debrancher enzyme (limit dextrinosis) E74.03
dehydrogenase
  long chain/very long chain acyl CoA E71.310
  medium chain acyl CoA E71.311
  short chain acyl CoA E71.312
diet E63.9
dihydropyrimidine dehydrogenase (DPD) E88.89
disaccharidase E73.9
edema — *see* Malnutrition, severe
endocrine E34.9
energy-supply — *see* Malnutrition
enzymes, circulating NEC E88.09
ergosterol E55.9

Deficiency, deficient — *continued*
ergosterol — *continued*
  with
    adult osteomalacia M83.8
    rickets — *see* Rickets
essential fatty acid (EFA) E63.0
factor (*see also* Deficiency, coagulation)
  Hageman D68.2
  I (congenital) (hereditary) D68.2
  II (congenital) (hereditary) D68.2
  IX (congenital) (functional) (hereditary) (with functional defect) D67
  multiple (congenital) D68.8
    acquired D68.4
  V (congenital) (hereditary) D68.2
  VII (congenital) (hereditary) D68.2
  VIII (congenital) (functional) (hereditary) (with functional defect) D66
    with vascular defect D68.0
  X (congenital) (hereditary) D68.2
  XI (congenital) (hereditary) D68.1
  XII (congenital) (hereditary) D68.2
  XIII (congenital) (hereditary) D68.2
femoral, proximal focal (congenital) — *see* Defect, reduction, lower limb, longitudinal, femur
fibrinase D68.2
fibrinogen (congenital) (hereditary) D68.2
  acquired D65
fibrin-stabilizing factor (congenital) (hereditary) D68.2
  acquired D68.4
folate E53.8
folic acid E53.8
foreskin N47.3
fructokinase E74.11
fructose 1,6-diphosphatase E74.19
fructose-1-phosphate aldolase E74.19
galactokinase E74.29
galactose-1-phosphate uridyl transferase E74.29
gammaglobulin in blood D80.1
  hereditary D80.0
glass factor D68.2
glucocorticoid E27.49
  mineralocorticoid E27.49
glucose-6-phosphatase E74.01
glucose-6-phosphate dehydrogenase anemia D55.0
glucuronyl transferase E80.5
glycogen synthetase E74.09
gonadotropin (isolated) E23.0
growth hormone (idiopathic) (isolated) E23.0
Hageman factor D68.2
hemoglobin D64.9
hepatophosphorylase E74.09
homogentisate 1,2-dioxygenase E70.29
hormone
  anterior pituitary (partial) NEC E23.0
    growth E23.0
  growth (isolated) E23.0
  pituitary E23.0
  testicular E29.1
hypoxanthine- (guanine)-phosphoribosyltransferase (HG- PRT) (total H-PRT) E79.1
immunity D84.9
  cell-mediated D84.8
    with thrombocytopenia and eczema D82.0
  combined D81.9
  humoral D80.9
  IgA (secretory) D80.2
  IgG D80.3
  IgM D80.4
immuno — *see* Immunodeficiency
immunoglobulin, selective
  A (IgA) D80.2
  G (IgG) (subclasses) D80.3
  M (IgM) D80.4
inositol (B complex) E53.8
intrinsic
  factor (congenital) D51.0
  sphincter N36.42
    with urethral hypermobility N36.43
iodine E61.8
  congenital syndrome — *see* Syndrome, iodine-deficiency, congenital
iron E61.1
  anemia D50.9
kalium E87.6
kappa-light chain D80.8
labile factor (congenital) (hereditary) D68.2
  acquired D68.4

Deficiency, deficient — *continued*
lacrimal fluid (acquired) (*see also* Syndrome, dry eye)
  congenital Q10.6
lactase
  congenital E73.0
  secondary E73.1
Laki-Lorand factor D68.2
lecithin cholesterol acyltransferase E78.6
lipocaic K86.89
lipoprotein (familial) (high density) E78.6
liver phosphorylase E74.09
lysosomal alpha-1, 4 glucosidase E74.02
magnesium E61.2
major histocompatibility complex
  class I D81.6
  class II D81.7
manganese E61.3
menadione (vitamin K) E56.1
  newborn P53
mental (familial) (hereditary) — *see* Disability, intellectual
methylenetetrahydrofolate reductase (MTHFR) E72.12
mevalonate kinase M04.1
mineralocorticoid E27.49
  with glucocorticoid E27.49
mineral NEC E61.8
molybdenum (nutritional) E61.5
moral F60.2
multiple nutrient elements E61.7
muscle
  carnitine (palmityltransferase) E71.314
  phosphofructokinase E74.09
myoadenylate deaminase E79.2
myocardial — *see* Insufficiency, myocardial
myophosphorylase E74.04
NADH diaphorase or reductase (congenital) D74.0
NADH-methemoglobin reductase (congenital) D74.0
natrium E87.1
niacin (amide) (-tryptophan) E52
nicotinamide E52
nicotinic acid E52
number of teeth — *see* Anodontia
nutrient element E61.9
  multiple E61.7
  specified NEC E61.8
nutrition, nutritional E63.9
  sequelae — *see* Sequelae, nutritional deficiency
  specified NEC E63.8
of interleukin 1 receptor antagonist [DIRA] M04.8
ornithine transcarbamylase E72.4
ovarian E28.39
oxygen — *see* Anoxia
pantothenic acid E53.8
parathyroid (gland) E20.9
perineum (female) N81.89
phenylalanine hydroxylase E70.1
phosphoenolpyruvate carboxykinase E74.4
phosphofructokinase E74.19
phosphomannomutase E74.8
phosphomannose isomerase E74.8
phosphomannosyl mutase E74.8
phosphorylase kinase, liver E74.09
pituitary hormone (isolated) E23.0
plasma thromboplastin
  antecedent (PTA) D68.1
  component (PTC) D67
platelet NEC D69.1
  constitutional D68.0
polyglandular E31.8
  autoimmune E31.0
potassium (K) E87.6
prepuce N47.3
proaccelerin (congenital) (hereditary) D68.2
  acquired D68.4
proconvertin factor (congenital) (hereditary) D68.2
  acquired D68.4
protein (*see also* Malnutrition) E46
  anemia D53.0
  C D68.59
  S D68.59
prothrombin (congenital) (hereditary) D68.2
  acquired D68.4
Prower factor D68.2
pseudocholinesterase E88.09
PTA (plasma thromboplastin antecedent) D68.1
PTC (plasma thromboplastin component) D67
purine nucleoside phosphorylase (PNP) D81.5

☑ Additional Character Required — Refer to the Tabular List for Character Selection   ▽ Subterms under main terms may continue to next column or page

Deficiency, deficient — *continued*
  pyracin (alpha) (beta) E53.1
  pyridoxal E53.1
  pyridoxamine E53.1
  pyridoxine (derivatives) E53.1
  pyruvate
    carboxylase E74.4
    dehydrogenase E74.4
  riboflavin (vitamin B2) E53.0
  salt E87.1
  secretion
    ovary E28.39
    salivary gland (any) K11.7
    urine R34
  selenium (dietary) E59
  serum antitrypsin, familial E88.01
  short stature homeobox gene (SHOX)
    with
      dyschondrosteosis Q78.8
      short stature (idiopathic) E34.3
      Turner's syndrome Q96.9
  sodium (Na) E87.1
  SPCA (factor VII) D68.2
  sphincter, intrinsic N36.42
    with urethral hypermobility N36.43
  stable factor (congenital) (hereditary) D68.2
    acquired D68.4
  Stuart-Prower (factor X) D68.2
  sucrase E74.39
  sulfatase E75.29
  sulfite oxidase E72.19
  thiamin, thiaminic (chloride) E51.9
    beriberi (dry) E51.11
      wet E51.12
  thrombokinase D68.2
    newborn P53
  thyroid (gland) — *see* Hypothyroidism
  tocopherol E56.0
  tooth bud K00.0
  transcobalamine II (anemia) D51.2
  vanadium E61.6
  vascular I99.9
  vasopressin E23.2
  vertical ridge K06.8
  viosterol — *see* Deficiency, calciferol
  vitamin (multiple) NOS E56.9
    A E50.9
      with
        Bitot's spot (corneal) E50.1
        follicular keratosis E50.8
        keratomalacia E50.4
        manifestations NEC E50.8
        night blindness E50.5
        scar of cornea, xerophthalmic E50.6
        xeroderma E50.8
        xerophthalmia E50.7
        xerosis
          conjunctival E50.0
            and Bitot's spot E50.1
          cornea E50.2
            and ulceration E50.3
      sequelae E64.1
    B (complex) NOS E53.9
      with
        beriberi (dry) E51.11
          wet E51.12
        pellagra E52
    B1 NOS E51.9
      beriberi (dry) E51.11
        with circulatory system manifestations
          E51.11
        wet E51.12
    B2 (riboflavin) E53.0
    B6 E53.1
    B12 E53.8
    C E54
      sequelae E64.2
    D E55.9
      with
        adult osteomalacia M83.8
        rickets — *see* Rickets
        25-hydroxylase E83.32
    E E56.0
    folic acid E53.8
    G E53.0
    group B E53.9
      specified NEC E53.8
    H (biotin) E53.8
    K E56.1

Deficiency, deficient — *continued*
  vitamin — *continued*
    K — *continued*
      of newborn P53
    nicotinic E52
    P E56.8
    PP (pellagra-preventing) E52
    specified NEC E56.8
    thiamin E51.9
      beriberi — *see* Beriberi
  zinc, dietary E60
Deficit (*see also* Deficiency)
  attention and concentration R41.840
    disorder — *see* Attention, deficit
    following
      cerebral infarction I69.310
      cerebrovascular disease I69.910
        specified disease NEC I69.810
      nontraumatic
        intracerebral hemorrhage I69.110
        specified intracranial hemorrhage NEC
          I69.210
        subarachnoid hemorrhage I69.010
  cognitive
    communication R41.841
    emotional
      following
        cerebral infarction I69.315
        cerebrovascular disease I69.915
          specified disease NEC I69.815
        nontraumatic
          intracerebral hemorrhage I69.115
          specified intracranial hemorrhage NEC
            I69.215
          subarachnoid hemorrhage I69.015
    following
      cerebral infarction I69.319
      cerebrovascular disease I69.919
        specified disease NEC I69.819
      nontraumatic
        intracerebral hemorrhage I69.119
        specified intracranial hemorrhage NEC
          I69.219
        subarachnoid hemorrhage I69.019
    social
      following
        cerebral infarction I69.315
        cerebrovascular disease I69.915
          specified disease NEC I69.815
        nontraumatic
          intracerebral hemorrhage I69.115
          specified intracranial hemorrhage NEC
            I69.215
          subarachnoid hemorrhage I69.015
  cognitive NEC R41.89
    following
      cerebral infarction I69.318
      cerebrovascular disease I69.918
        specified disease NEC I69.818
      nontraumatic
        intracerebral hemorrhage I69.118
        specified intracranial hemorrhage NEC
          I69.218
        subarachnoid hemorrhage I69.018
  concentration R41.840
  executive function R41.844
    following
      cerebral infarction I69.314
      cerebrovascular disease I69.914
        specified disease NEC I69.814
      nontraumatic
        intracerebral hemorrhage I69.114
        specified intracranial hemorrhage NEC
          I69.214
        subarachnoid hemorrhage I69.014
  frontal lobe R41.844
    following
      cerebral infarction I69.314
      cerebrovascular disease I69.914
        specified disease NEC I69.814
      nontraumatic
        intracerebral hemorrhage I69.114
        specified intracranial hemorrhage NEC
          I69.214
        subarachnoid hemorrhage I69.014
  memory
    following
      cerebral infarction I69.311
      cerebrovascular disease I69.911

Deficit — *continued*
  memory — *continued*
    following — *continued*
      cerebrovascular disease — *continued*
        specified disease NEC I69.811
      nontraumatic
        intracerebral hemorrhage I69.111
        specified intracranial hemorrhage NEC
          I69.211
        subarachnoid hemorrhage I69.011
  neurologic NEC R29.818
    ischemic
      reversible (RIND) I63.9
      prolonged (PRIND) I63.9
  oxygen R09.02
  prolonged reversible ischemic neurologic (PRIND) I63.9
  psychomotor R41.843
    following
      cerebral infarction I69.313
      cerebrovascular disease I69.913
        specified disease NEC I69.813
      nontraumatic
        intracerebral hemorrhage I69.113
        specified intracranial hemorrhage NEC
          I69.213
        subarachnoid hemorrhage I69.013
  visuospatial R41.842
    following
      cerebral infarction I69.312
      cerebrovascular disease I69.912
        specified disease NEC I69.812
      nontraumatic
        intracerebral hemorrhage I69.112
        specified intracranial hemorrhage NEC
          I69.212
        subarachnoid hemorrhage I69.012
Deflection
  radius — *see* Deformity, limb, specified type NEC,
    forearm
  septum (acquired) (nasal) (nose) J34.2
  spine — *see* Curvature, spine
  turbinate (nose) J34.2
Defluvium
  capillorum — *see* Alopecia
  ciliorum — *see* Madarosis
  unguium L60.8
Deformity Q89.9
  abdomen, congenital Q89.9
  abdominal wall
    acquired M95.8
    congenital Q79.59
  acquired (unspecified site) M95.9
  adrenal gland Q89.1
  alimentary tract, congenital Q45.9
    upper Q40.9
  ankle (joint) (acquired) (*see also* Deformity, limb, lower
    leg)
    abduction — *see* Contraction, joint, ankle
    congenital Q68.8
    contraction — *see* Contraction, joint, ankle
    specified type NEC — *see* Deformity, limb, foot,
      specified NEC
  anus (acquired) K62.89
    congenital Q43.9
  aorta (arch) (congenital) Q25.40
    acquired I77.89
  aortic
    arch, acquired I77.89
    cusp or valve (congenital) Q23.8
      acquired (*see also* Endocarditis, aortic) I35.8
  arm (acquired) (upper) (*see also* Deformity, limb, upper
    arm)
    congenital Q68.8
    forearm — *see* Deformity, limb, forearm
  artery (congenital) (peripheral) NOS Q27.9
    acquired I77.89
    coronary (acquired) I25.9
      congenital Q24.5
    umbilical Q27.0
  atrial septal Q21.1
  auditory canal (external) (congenital) (*see also* Malfor-
    mation, ear, external)
    acquired — *see* Disorder, ear, external, specified
      type NEC
  auricle
    ear (congenital) (*see also* Malformation, ear, exter-
      nal)
      acquired — *see* Disorder, pinna, deformity

☑ **Additional Character Required** — **Refer to the Tabular List for Character Selection**   **Subterms under main terms may continue to next column or page**

Index

Deformity — Deformity

Deformity — *continued*
- limb — *continued*
  - specified type NEC M21.80
    - forearm M21.83- ☑
    - lower leg M21.86- ☑
    - thigh M21.85- ☑
    - upper arm M21.82- ☑
  - thigh M21.95- ☑
  - unequal length M21.70
    - short site is
      - femur M21.75- ☑
      - fibula M21.76- ☑
      - humerus M21.72- ☑
      - radius M21.73- ☑
      - tibia M21.76- ☑
      - ulna M21.73- ☑
    - upper arm M21.92- ☑
  - valgus — *see* Deformity, valgus
  - varus — *see* Deformity, varus
  - wrist drop M21.33- ☑
- lip (acquired) NEC K13.0
  - congenital Q38.0
- liver (congenital) Q44.7
  - acquired K76.89
- lumbosacral (congenital) (joint) (region) Q76.49
  - acquired — *see* subcategory M43.8 ☑
  - kyphosis — *see* Kyphosis, congenital
  - lordosis — *see* Lordosis, congenital
- lung (congenital) Q33.9
  - acquired J98.4
- lymphatic system, congenital Q89.9
- Madelung's (radius) Q74.0
- mandible (acquired) (congenital) M26.9
- maxilla (acquired) (congenital) M26.9
- meninges or membrane (congenital) Q07.9
  - cerebral Q04.8
    - acquired G96.19
  - spinal cord (congenital) G96.19
    - acquired G96.19
- metacarpus (acquired) — *see* Deformity, limb, forearm
  - congenital Q74.0
- metatarsus (acquired) — *see* Deformity, foot
  - congenital Q66.9
- middle ear (congenital) Q16.4
  - ossicles Q16.3
- mitral (leaflets) (valve) I05.8
  - parachute Q23.2
  - stenosis, congenital Q23.2
- mouth (acquired) K13.79
  - congenital Q38.6
- multiple, congenital NEC Q89.7
- muscle (acquired) M62.89
  - congenital Q79.9
    - sternocleidomastoid Q68.0
- musculoskeletal system (acquired) M95.9
  - congenital Q79.9
  - specified NEC M95.8
- nail (acquired) L60.8
  - congenital Q84.6
- nasal — *see* Deformity, nose
- neck (acquired) M95.3
  - congenital Q18.9
    - sternocleidomastoid Q68.0
- nervous system (congenital) Q07.9
- nipple (congenital) Q83.9
  - acquired N64.89
- nose (acquired) (cartilage) M95.0
  - bone (turbinate) M95.0
  - congenital Q30.9
    - bent or squashed Q67.4
  - saddle M95.0
    - syphilitic A50.57
  - septum (acquired) J34.2
    - congenital Q30.8
  - sinus (wall) (congenital) Q30.8
    - acquired M95.0
  - syphilitic (congenital) A50.57
    - late A52.73
- ocular muscle (congenital) Q10.3
  - acquired — *see* Strabismus, mechanical
- opticociliary vessels (congenital) Q13.2
- orbit (eye) (acquired) H05.30
  - atrophy — *see* Atrophy, orbit
  - congenital Q10.7
  - due to
    - bone disease NEC H05.32- ☑
    - trauma or surgery H05.33- ☑
  - enlargement — *see* Enlargement, orbit

Deformity — *continued*
- orbit — *continued*
  - exostosis — *see* Exostosis, orbit
- organ of Corti (congenital) Q16.5
- ovary (congenital) Q50.39
  - acquired N83.8
- oviduct, acquired N83.8
- palate (congenital) Q38.5
  - acquired M27.8
  - cleft (congenital) — *see* Cleft, palate
- pancreas (congenital) Q45.3
  - acquired K86.89
- parathyroid (gland) Q89.2
- parotid (gland) (congenital) Q38.4
  - acquired K11.8
- patella (acquired) — *see* Disorder, patella, specified NEC
- pelvis, pelvic (acquired) (bony) M95.5
  - with disproportion (fetopelvic) O33.0
    - causing obstructed labor O65.0
  - congenital Q74.2
  - rachitic sequelae (late effect) E64.3
- penis (glans) (congenital) Q55.69
  - acquired N48.89
- pericardium (congenital) Q24.8
  - acquired — *see* Pericarditis
- pharynx (congenital) Q38.8
  - acquired J39.2
- pinna, acquired (*see also* Disorder, pinna, deformity)
  - congenital Q17.9
- pituitary (congenital) Q89.2
- posture — *see* Dorsopathy, deforming
- prepuce (congenital) Q55.69
  - acquired N47.8
- prostate (congenital) Q55.4
  - acquired N42.89
- pupil (congenital) Q13.2
  - acquired — *see* Abnormality, pupillary
- pylorus (congenital) Q40.3
  - acquired K31.89
- rachitic (acquired), old or healed E64.3
- radius (acquired) (*see also* Deformity, limb, forearm)
  - congenital Q68.8
- rectum (congenital) Q43.9
  - acquired K62.89
- reduction (extremity) (limb), congenital (*see also* condition and site) Q73.8
  - brain Q04.3
  - lower — *see* Defect, reduction, lower limb
  - upper — *see* Defect, reduction, upper limb
- renal — *see* Deformity, kidney
- respiratory system (congenital) Q34.9
- rib (acquired) M95.4
  - congenital Q76.6
    - cervical Q76.5
- rotation (joint) (acquired) — *see* Deformity, limb, specified site NEC
  - congenital Q74.9
  - hip — *see* Deformity, limb, specified type NEC, thigh
    - congenital Q65.89
- sacroiliac joint (congenital) — *see* subcategory Q74.2
  - acquired — *see* subcategory M43.8 ☑
- sacrum (acquired) — *see* subcategory M43.8 ☑
- saddle
  - back — *see* Lordosis
  - nose M95.0
    - syphilitic A50.57
- salivary gland or duct (congenital) Q38.4
  - acquired K11.8
- scapula (acquired) M95.8
  - congenital Q68.8
- scrotum (congenital) (*see also* Malformation, testis and scrotum)
  - acquired N50.89
- seminal vesicles (congenital) Q55.4
  - acquired N50.89
- septum, nasal (acquired) J34.2
- shoulder (joint) (acquired) — *see* Deformity, limb, upper arm
  - congenital Q74.0
  - contraction — *see* Contraction, joint, shoulder
- sigmoid (flexure) (congenital) Q43.9
  - acquired K63.89
- skin (congenital) Q82.9
- skull (acquired) M95.2
  - congenital Q75.8

Deformity — *continued*
- skull — *continued*
  - congenital — *continued*
    - with
      - anencephaly Q00.0
      - encephalocele — *see* Encephalocele
      - hydrocephalus Q03.9
        - with spina bifida — *see* Spina bifida, by site, with hydrocephalus
      - microcephaly Q02
- soft parts, organs or tissues (of pelvis)
  - in pregnancy or childbirth NEC O34.8- ☑
    - causing obstructed labor O65.5
- spermatic cord (congenital) Q55.4
  - acquired N50.89
  - torsion — *see* Torsion, spermatic cord
- spinal — *see* Dorsopathy, deforming
  - column (acquired) — *see* Dorsopathy, deforming
  - congenital Q67.5
  - cord (congenital) Q06.9
    - acquired G95.89
  - nerve root (congenital) Q07.9
- spine (acquired) (*see also* Dorsopathy, deforming)
  - congenital Q67.5
  - rachitic E64.3
  - specified NEC — *see* Dorsopathy, deforming, specified NEC
- spleen
  - acquired D73.89
  - congenital Q89.09
- Sprengel's (congenital) Q74.0
- sternocleidomastoid (muscle), congenital Q68.0
- sternum (acquired) M95.4
  - congenital NEC Q76.7
- stomach (congenital) Q40.3
  - acquired K31.89
- submandibular gland (congenital) Q38.4
- submaxillary gland (congenital) Q38.4
  - acquired K11.8
- talipes — *see* Talipes
- testis (congenital) (*see also* Malformation, testis and scrotum)
  - acquired N44.8
  - torsion — *see* Torsion, testis
- thigh (acquired) (*see also* Deformity, limb, thigh)
  - congenital NEC Q68.8
- thorax (acquired) (wall) M95.4
  - congenital Q67.8
  - sequelae of rickets E64.3
- thumb (acquired) (*see also* Deformity, finger)
  - congenital NEC Q68.1
- thymus (tissue) (congenital) Q89.2
- thyroid (gland) (congenital) Q89.2
  - cartilage Q31.8
    - acquired J38.7
- tibia (acquired) (*see also* Deformity, limb, specified type NEC, lower leg)
  - congenital NEC Q68.8
  - saber (syphilitic) A50.56
- toe (acquired) M20.6- ☑
  - congenital Q66.9
  - hallux rigidus M20.2- ☑
  - hallux valgus M20.1- ☑
  - hallux varus M20.3- ☑
  - hammer toe M20.4- ☑
  - specified NEC M20.5X- ☑
- tongue (congenital) Q38.3
  - acquired K14.8
- tooth, teeth K00.2
- trachea (rings) (congenital) Q32.1
  - acquired J39.8
- transverse aortic arch (congenital) Q25.49
- tricuspid (leaflets) (valve) I07.8
  - atresia or stenosis Q22.4
  - Ebstein's Q22.5
- trunk (acquired) M95.8
  - congenital Q89.9
- ulna (acquired) (*see also* Deformity, limb, forearm)
  - congenital NEC Q68.8
- urachus, congenital Q64.4
- ureter (opening) (congenital) Q62.8
  - acquired N28.89
- urethra (congenital) Q64.79
  - acquired N36.8
- urinary tract (congenital) Q64.9
  - urachus Q64.4
- uterus (congenital) Q51.9
  - acquired N85.8

Index

Deformity — Degeneration, degenerative

Deformity — *continued*
uvula (congenital) Q38.5
vagina (acquired) N89.8
  congenital Q52.4
valgus NEC M21.00
  ankle M21.07- ☑
  elbow M21.02- ☑
  hip M21.05- ☑
  knee M21.06- ☑
valve, valvular (congenital) (heart) Q24.8
  acquired — *see* Endocarditis
varus NEC M21.10
  ankle M21.17- ☑
  elbow M21.12- ☑
  hip M21.15 ☑
  knee M21.16- ☑
  tibia — *see* Osteochondrosis, juvenile, tibia
vas deferens (congenital) Q55.4
  acquired N50.89
vein (congenital) Q27.9
  great Q26.9
vertebra — *see* Dorsopathy, deforming
vertical talus (congenital) Q66.80
  left foot Q66.82
  right foot Q66.81
vesicourethral orifice (acquired) N32.89
  congenital NEC Q64.79
vessels of optic papilla (congenital) Q14.2
visual field (contraction) — *see* Defect, visual field
vitreous body, acquired H43.89
vulva (congenital) Q52.79
  acquired N90.89
wrist (joint) (acquired) (*see also* Deformity, limb, forearm)
  congenital Q68.8
  contraction — *see* Contraction, joint, wrist

Degeneration, degenerative
adrenal (capsule) (fatty) (gland) (hyaline) (infectional) E27.8
amyloid (*see also* Amyloidosis) E85.9
anterior cornua, spinal cord G12.29
anterior labral S43.49- ☑
aorta, aortic I70.0
  fatty I77.89
aortic valve (heart) — *see* Endocarditis, aortic
arteriovascular — *see* Arteriosclerosis
artery, arterial (atheromatous) (calcareous) (*see also* Arteriosclerosis)
  cerebral, amyloid E85.4 [I68.0]
  medial — *see* Arteriosclerosis, extremities
articular cartilage NEC — *see* Derangement, joint, articular cartilage, by site
atheromatous — *see* Arteriosclerosis
basal nuclei or ganglia G23.9
  specified NEC G23.8
bone NEC — *see* Disorder, bone, specified type NEC
brachial plexus G54.0
brain (cortical) (progressive) G31.9
  alcoholic G31.2
  arteriosclerotic I67.2
  childhood G31.9
    specified NEC G31.89
  cystic G31.89
    congenital Q04.6
  in
    alcoholism G31.2
    beriberi E51.2
    cerebrovascular disease I67.9
    congenital hydrocephalus Q03.9
      with spina bifida (*see also* Spina bifida)
    Fabry-Anderson disease E75.21
    Gaucher's disease E75.22
    Hunter's syndrome E76.1
    lipidosis
      cerebral E75.4
      generalized E75.6
    mucopolysaccharidosis — *see* Mucopolysaccharidosis
    myxedema E03.9 [G32.89]
    neoplastic disease (*see also* Neoplasm) D49.6 [G32.89]
    Niemann-Pick disease E75.249 [G32.89]
    sphingolipidosis E75.3 [G32.89]
    vitamin B12 deficiency E53.8 [G32.89]
  senile NEC G31.1
breast N64.89
Bruch's membrane — *see* Degeneration, choroid
capillaries (fatty) I78.8

Degeneration, degenerative — *continued*
capillaries — *continued*
  amyloid E85.89 [I79.8]
cardiac (*see also* Degeneration, myocardial)
  valve, valvular — *see* Endocarditis
cardiorenal — *see* Hypertension, cardiorenal
cardiovascular (*see also* Disease, cardiovascular)
  renal — *see* Hypertension, cardiorenal
cerebellar NOS G31.9
  alcoholic G31.2
  primary (hereditary) (sporadic) G11.9
cerebral — *see* Degeneration, brain
cerebrovascular I67.9
  due to hypertension I67.4
cervical plexus G54.2
cervix N88.8
  due to radiation (intended effect) N88.8
    adverse effect or misadventure N99.89
chamber angle H21.21- ☑
changes, spine or vertebra — *see* Spondylosis
chorioretinal (*see also* Degeneration, choroid)
  hereditary H31.20
choroid (colloid) (drusen) H31.10- ☑
  atrophy — *see* Atrophy, choroidal
  hereditary — *see* Dystrophy, choroidal, hereditary
ciliary body H21.22- ☑
cochlear — *see* subcategory H83.8 ☑
combined (spinal cord) (subacute) E53.8 [G32.0]
  with anemia (pernicious) D51.0 [G32.0]
    due to dietary vitamin B12 deficiency D51.3 [G32.0]
  in (due to)
    vitamin B12 deficiency E53.8 [G32.0]
    anemia D51.9 [G32.0]
conjunctiva H11.10
  concretions — *see* Concretion, conjunctiva
  deposits — *see* Deposit, conjunctiva
  pigmentations — *see* Pigmentation, conjunctiva
  pinguecula — *see* Pinguecula
  xerosis — *see* Xerosis, conjunctiva
cornea H18.40
  calcerous H18.43
    band keratopathy H18.42- ☑
  familial, hereditary — *see* Dystrophy, cornea
  hyaline (of old scars) H18.49
  keratomalacia — *see* Keratomalacia
  nodular H18.45- ☑
  peripheral H18.46- ☑
  senile H18.41- ☑
  specified type NEC H18.49
cortical (cerebellar) (parenchymatous) G31.89
  alcoholic G31.2
  diffuse, due to arteriopathy I67.2
corticobasal G31.85
cutis L98.8
  amyloid E85.4 [L99]
dental pulp K04.2
disc disease — *see* Degeneration, intervertebral disc NEC
dorsolateral (spinal cord) — *see* Degeneration, combined
extrapyramidal G25.9
eye, macular (*see also* Degeneration, macula)
  congenital or hereditary — *see* Dystrophy, retina
facet joints — *see* Spondylosis
fatty
  liver NEC K76.0
    alcoholic K70.0
grey matter (brain) (Alpers') G31.81
heart (*see also* Degeneration, myocardial)
  amyloid E85.4 [I43]
  atheromatous — *see* Disease, heart, ischemic, atherosclerotic
  ischemic — *see* Disease, heart, ischemic
hepatolenticular (Wilson's) E83.01
hepatorenal K76.7
hyaline (diffuse) (generalized)
  localized — *see* Degeneration, by site
infrapatellar fat pad M79.4
intervertebral disc NOS
  with
    myelopathy — *see* Disorder, disc, with, myelopathy
    radiculitis or radiculopathy — *see* Disorder, disc, with, radiculopathy
  cervical, cervicothoracic — *see* Disorder, disc, cervical, degeneration

Degeneration, degenerative — *continued*
intervertebral disc — *continued*
  cervical, cervicothoracic — *see* Disorder, disc, cervical, degeneration — *continued*
    with
      myelopathy — *see* Disorder, disc, cervical, with myelopathy
      neuritis, radiculitis or radiculopathy — *see* Disorder, disc, cervical, with neuritis
  lumbar region M51.36
    with
      myelopathy M51.06
      neuritis, radiculitis, radiculopathy or sciatica M51.16
  lumbosacral region M51.37
    with
      neuritis, radiculitis, radiculopathy or sciatica M51.17
  sacrococcygeal region M53.3
  thoracic region M51.34
    with
      myelopathy M51.04
      neuritis, radiculitis, radiculopathy M51.14
  thoracolumbar region M51.35
    with
      myelopathy M51.05
      neuritis, radiculitis, radiculopathy M51.15
intestine, amyloid E85.4
iris (pigmentary) H21.23- ☑
ischemic — *see* Ischemia
joint disease — *see* Osteoarthritis
kidney N28.89
  amyloid E85.4 [N29]
  cystic, congenital Q61.9
  fatty N28.89
  polycystic Q61.3
    adult type (autosomal dominant) Q61.2
    infantile type (autosomal recessive) NEC Q61.19
      collecting duct dilatation Q61.11
Kuhnt-Junius (*see also* Degeneration, macula) H35.32- ☑
lens — *see* Cataract
lenticular (familial) (progressive) (Wilson's) (with cirrhosis of liver) E83.01
liver (diffuse) NEC K76.89
  amyloid E85.4 [K77]
  cystic K76.89
    congenital Q44.6
  fatty NEC K76.0
    alcoholic K70.0
  hypertrophic K76.89
  parenchymatous, acute or subacute K72.00
    with coma K72.01
  pigmentary K76.89
  toxic (acute) K71.9
lung J98.4
lymph gland I89.8
  hyaline I89.8
macula, macular (acquired) (age-related) (senile) H35.30
  angioid streaks H35.33
  atrophic age-related H35.31- ☑
  congenital or hereditary — *see* Dystrophy, retina
  cystoid H35.35- ☑
  drusen H35.36- ☑
  dry age-related H35.31- ☑
  exudative H35.32- ☑
  hole H35.34- ☑
  nonexudative H35.31- ☑
  puckering H35.37- ☑
  toxic H35.38- ☑
  wet age-related H35.32- ☑
membranous labyrinth, congenital (causing impairment of hearing) Q16.5
meniscus — *see* Derangement, meniscus
mitral — *see* Insufficiency, mitral
Mönckeberg's — *see* Arteriosclerosis, extremities
motor centers, senile G31.1
multi-system G90.3
mural — *see* Degeneration, myocardial
muscle (fatty) (fibrous) (hyaline) (progressive) M62.89
  heart — *see* Degeneration, myocardial
myelin, central nervous system G37.9
myocardial, myocardium (fatty) (hyaline) (senile) I51.5
  with rheumatic fever (conditions in I00) I09.9
    active, acute or subacute I01.2
      with chorea I02.0
    inactive or quiescent (with chorea) I09.0

Degeneration, degenerative — *continued*
  myocardial, myocardium — *continued*
    hypertensive — *see* Hypertension, heart
    rheumatic — *see* Degeneration, myocardial, with
      rheumatic fever
    syphilitic A52.06
  nasal sinus (mucosa) J32.9
    frontal J32.1
    maxillary J32.0
  nerve — *see* Disorder, nerve
  nervous system G31.9
    alcoholic G31.2
    amyloid E85.4 [G99.8]
    autonomic G90.9
    fatty G31.89
    specified NEC G31.89
  nipple N64.89
  olivopontocerebellar (hereditary) (familial) G23.8
  osseous labyrinth — *see* subcategory H83.8 ☑
  ovary N83.8
    cystic N83.20- ☑
    microcystic N83.20- ☑
  pallidal pigmentary (progressive) G23.0
  pancreas K86.89
    tuberculous A18.83
  penis N48.89
  pigmentary (diffuse) (general)
    localized — *see* Degeneration, by site
    pallidal (progressive) G23.0
  pineal gland E34.8
  pituitary (gland) E23.6
  popliteal fat pad M79.4
  posterolateral (spinal cord) — *see* Degeneration,
    combined
  pulmonary valve (heart) I37.8
  pulp (tooth) K04.2
  pupillary margin H21.24- ☑
  renal — *see* Degeneration, kidney
  retina H35.9
    hereditary (cerebroretinal) (congenital) (juvenile)
      (macula) (peripheral) (pigmentary) — *see*
      Dystrophy, retina
    Kuhnt-Junius (*see also* Degeneration, macula)
      H35.32- ☑
    macula (cystic) (exudative) (hole) (nonexudative)
      (pseudohole) (senile) (toxic) — *see* Degener-
      ation, macula
    peripheral H35.40
      lattice H35.41- ☑
      microcystoid H35.42- ☑
      paving stone H35.43- ☑
      secondary
        pigmentary H35.45- ☑
        vitreoretinal H35.46- ☑
      senile reticular H35.44- ☑
    pigmentary (primary) (*see also* Dystrophy, retina)
      secondary — *see* Degeneration, retina, periph-
      eral, secondary
    posterior pole — *see* Degeneration, macula
  saccule, congenital (causing impairment of hearing)
    Q16.5
  senile R54
    brain G31.1
    cardiac, heart or myocardium — *see* Degeneration,
      myocardial
    motor centers G31.1
    vascular — *see* Arteriosclerosis
  sinus (cystic) (*see also* Sinusitis)
    polypoid J33.1
  skin L98.8
    amyloid E85.4 [L99]
    colloid L98.8
  spinal (cord) G31.89
    amyloid E85.4 [G32.89]
    combined (subacute) — *see* Degeneration, com-
      bined
    dorsolateral — *see* Degeneration, combined
    familial NEC G31.89
    fatty G31.89
    funicular — *see* Degeneration, combined
    posterolateral — *see* Degeneration, combined
    subacute combined — *see* Degeneration, com-
      bined
    tuberculous A17.81
  spleen D73.0
    amyloid E85.4 [D77]
  stomach K31.89
  striatonigral G23.2

Degeneration, degenerative — *continued*
  suprarenal (capsule) (gland) E27.8
  synovial membrane (pulpy) — *see* Disorder, synovium,
    specified type NEC
  tapetoretinal — *see* Dystrophy, retina
  thymus (gland) E32.8
    fatty E32.8
  thyroid (gland) E07.89
  tricuspid (heart) (valve) I07.9
  tuberculous NEC — *see* Tuberculosis
  turbinate J34.89
  uterus (cystic) N85.8
  vascular (senile) — *see* Arteriosclerosis
    hypertensive — *see* Hypertension
  vitreoretinal, secondary — *see* Degeneration, retina,
    peripheral, secondary, vitreoretinal
  vitreous (body) H43.81- ☑
  Wallerian — *see* Disorder, nerve
  Wilson's hepatolenticular E83.01
Deglutition
  paralysis R13.0
    hysterical F44.4
  pneumonia J69.0
Degos' disease I77.89
Dehiscence (of)
  amputation stump T87.81
  cesarean wound O90.0
  closure of
    cornea T81.31 ☑
    craniotomy T81.32 ☑
    fascia (muscular) (superficial) T81.32 ☑
    internal organ or tissue T81.32 ☑
    laceration (external) (internal) T81.33 ☑
    ligament T81.32 ☑
    mucosa T81.31 ☑
    muscle or muscle flap T81.32 ☑
    ribs or rib cage T81.32 ☑
    skin and subcutaneous tissue (full-thickness) (su-
      perficial) T81.31 ☑
    skull T81.32 ☑
    sternum (sternotomy) T81.32 ☑
    tendon T81.32 ☑
    traumatic laceration (external) (internal) T81.33 ☑
  episiotomy O90.1
  operation wound NEC T81.31 ☑
    external operation wound (superficial) T81.31 ☑
    internal operation wound (deep) T81.32 ☑
  perineal wound (postpartum) O90.1
  traumatic injury wound repair T81.33 ☑
  wound T81.30 ☑
    traumatic repair T81.33 ☑
Dehydration E86.0
  newborn P74.1
Déjérine-Roussy syndrome G89.0
Déjérine-Sottas disease or neuropathy (hypertrophic)
  G60.0
Déjérine-Thomas atrophy G23.8
Delay, delayed
  any plane in pelvis
    complicating delivery O66.9
  birth or delivery NOS O63.9
  closure, ductus arteriosus (Botalli) P29.38
  coagulation — *see* Defect, coagulation
  conduction (cardiac) (ventricular) I45.9
  delivery, second twin, triplet, etc O63.2
  development R62.50
    global F88
    intellectual (specific) F81.9
    language F80.9
      due to hearing loss F80.4
    learning F81.9
    pervasive F84.9
    physiological R62.50
      specified stage NEC R62.0
    reading F81.0
    sexual E30.0
    speech F80.9
      due to hearing loss F80.4
    spelling F81.81
  ejaculation F52.32
  gastric emptying K30
  menarche E30.0
  menstruation (cause unknown) N91.0
  milestone R62.0
  passage of meconium (newborn) P76.0
  primary respiration P28.9
  puberty (constitutional) E30.0

Delay, delayed — *continued*
  separation of umbilical cord P96.82
  sexual maturation, female E30.0
  sleep phase syndrome G47.21
  union, fracture — *see* Fracture, by site
  vaccination Z28.9
Deletion(s)
  autosome Q93.9
    identified by fluorescence in situ hybridization
      (FISH) Q93.89
    identified by in situ hybridization (ISH) Q93.89
  chromosome
    with complex rearrangements NEC Q93.7
    part of NEC Q93.5
    seen only at prometaphase Q93.89
    short arm
      22q11.2 Q93.81
      4 Q93.3
      5p Q93.4
    specified NEC Q93.89
  long arm chromosome 18 or 21 Q93.89
    with complex rearrangements NEC Q93.7
  microdeletions NEC Q93.88
Delhi boil or button B55.1
Delinquency (juvenile) (neurotic) F91.8
  group Z72.810
Delinquent immunization status Z28.3
Delirium, delirious (acute or subacute) (not alcohol- or
  drug-induced) (with dementia) R41.0
  alcoholic (acute) (tremens) (withdrawal) F10.921
    with intoxication F10.921
      in
        abuse F10.121
        dependence F10.221
  due to (secondary to)
    alcohol
      intoxication F10.921
        in
          abuse F10.121
          dependence F10.221
      withdrawal F10.231
    amphetamine intoxication F15.921
      in
        abuse F15.121
        dependence F15.221
    anxiolytic
      intoxication F13.921
        in
          abuse F13.121
          dependence F13.221
      withdrawal F13.231
    cannabis intoxication (acute) F12.921
      in
        abuse F12.121
        dependence F12.221
    cocaine intoxication (acute) F14.921
      in
        abuse F14.121
        dependence F14.221
    general medical condition F05
    hallucinogen intoxication F16.921
      in
        abuse F16.121
        dependence F16.221
    hypnotic
      intoxication F13.921
        in
          abuse F13.121
          dependence F13.221
      withdrawal F13.231
    inhalant intoxication (acute) F18.921
      in
        abuse F18.121
        dependence F18.221
    multiple etiologies F05
    opioid intoxication (acute) F11.921
      in
        abuse F11.121
        dependence F11.221
    other (or unknown) substance F19.921
    phencyclidine intoxication (acute) F16.921
      in
        abuse F16.121
        dependence F16.221
    psychoactive substance NEC intoxication (acute)
      F19.921
      in
        abuse F19.121
        dependence F19.221

Delirium, delirious — *continued*
　due to — *continued*
　　sedative
　　　intoxication F13.921
　　　　in
　　　　　abuse F13.121
　　　　　dependence F13.221
　　　withdrawal F13.231
　　unknown etiology F05
　exhaustion F43.0
　hysterical F44.89
　postprocedural (postoperative) F05
　puerperal F05
　thyroid — *see* Thyrotoxicosis with thyroid storm
　traumatic — *see* Injury, intracranial
　tremens (alcohol-induced) F10.231
　　sedative-induced F13.231
Delivery (childbirth) (labor)
　arrested active phase O62.1
　cesarean (for)
　　without indication O82
　　abnormal
　　　pelvis (bony) (deformity) (major) NEC with disproportion (fetopelvic) O33.0
　　　　with obstructed labor O65.0
　　　presentation or position O32.9 ☑
　　abruptio placentae (*see also* Abruptio placentae) O45.9-
　　acromion presentation O32.2
　　atony, uterus O62.2
　　breech presentation O32.1 ☑
　　　incomplete O32.8
　　brow presentation O32.3 ☑
　　cephalopelvic disproportion O33.9
　　cerclage O34.3- ☑
　　chin presentation O32.3 ☑
　　cicatrix of cervix O34.4- ☑
　　contracted pelvis (general)
　　　inlet O33.2
　　　outlet O33.3 ☑
　　cord presentation or prolapse O69.0 ☑
　　cystocele O34.8- ☑
　　deformity (acquired) (congenital)
　　　pelvic organs or tissues NEC O34.8- ☑
　　　pelvis (bony) NEC O33.0
　　disproportion NOS O33.9
　　eclampsia — *see* Eclampsia
　　face presentation O32.3 ☑
　　failed
　　　forceps O66.5
　　　induction of labor O61.9
　　　　instrumental O61.1
　　　　mechanical O61.1
　　　　medical O61.0
　　　　specified NEC O61.8
　　　　surgical O61.1
　　　trial of labor NOS O66.40
　　　　following previous cesarean delivery O66.41
　　　vacuum extraction O66.5
　　　ventouse O66.5
　　fetal-maternal hemorrhage O43.01- ☑
　　hemorrhage (intrapartum) O67.9
　　　with coagulation defect O67.0
　　　specified cause NEC O67.8
　　high head at term O32.4 ☑
　　hydrocephalic fetus O33.6 ☑
　　incarceration of uterus O34.51- ☑
　　incoordinate uterine action O62.4
　　increased size, fetus O33.5 ☑
　　inertia, uterus O62.2
　　　primary O62.0
　　　secondary O62.1
　　lateroversion, uterus O34.59- ☑
　　mal lie O32.9 ☑
　　malposition
　　　fetus O32.9 ☑
　　　pelvic organs or tissues NEC O34.8- ☑
　　　uterus NEC O34.59- ☑
　　malpresentation NOS O32.9 ☑
　　oblique presentation O32.2 ☑
　　occurring after 37 completed weeks of gestation but before 39 completed weeks gestation due to (spontaneous) onset of labor O75.82
　　oversize fetus O33.5 ☑
　　pelvic tumor NEC O34.8- ☑
　　placenta previa O44.0- ☑
　　　complete O44.0- ☑

Delivery — *continued*
　cesarean — *continued*
　　placenta previa — *continued*
　　　complete — *continued*
　　　　with hemorrhage O44.1- ☑
　　placental insufficiency O36.51- ☑
　　planned, occurring after 37 completed weeks of gestation but before 39 completed weeks gestation due to (spontaneous) onset of labor O75.82
　　polyp, cervix O34.4- ☑
　　　causing obstructed labor O65.5
　　poor dilatation, cervix O62.0
　　pre-eclampsia O14.94
　　　mild O14.04
　　　moderate O14.04
　　　severe O14.14
　　　　with hemolysis, elevated liver enzymes and low platelet count (HELLP) O14.24
　　previous
　　　cesarean delivery O34.219
　　　　classical (vertical) scar O34.212
　　　　low transverse scar O34.211
　　　surgery (to)
　　　　cervix O34.4- ☑
　　　　gynecological NEC O34.8- ☑
　　　　rectum O34.7- ☑
　　　　uterus O34.29
　　　　vagina O34.6- ☑
　　prolapse
　　　arm or hand O32.2 ☑
　　　uterus O34.52- ☑
　　prolonged labor NOS O63.9
　　rectocele O34.8- ☑
　　retroversion
　　　uterus O34.53- ☑
　　rigid
　　　cervix O34.4- ☑
　　　pelvic floor O34.8- ☑
　　　perineum O34.7- ☑
　　　vagina O34.6- ☑
　　　vulva O34.7- ☑
　　sacculation, pregnant uterus O34.59- ☑
　　scar(s)
　　　cervix O34.4- ☑
　　　cesarean delivery O34.219
　　　　classical (vertical) O34.212
　　　　low transverse O34.211
　　　transmural uterine O34.29
　　　uterus O34.29
　　Shirodkar suture in situ O34.3- ☑
　　shoulder presentation O32.2 ☑
　　stenosis or stricture, cervix O34.4- ☑
　　streptococcus group B (GBS) carrier state O99.824
　　transmural uterine scar O34.29
　　transverse presentation or lie O32.2 ☑
　　tumor, pelvic organs or tissues NEC O34.8- ☑
　　　cervix O34.4- ☑
　　umbilical cord presentation or prolapse O69.0 ☑
　completely normal case O80
　complicated O75.9
　　by
　　　abnormal, abnormality (of)
　　　　forces of labor O62.9
　　　　　specified type NEC O62.8
　　　　glucose O99.814
　　　　uterine contractions NOS O62.9
　　　abruptio placentae (*see also* Abruptio placentae) O45.9- ☑
　　　abuse
　　　　physical O9A.32 (*following* O99)
　　　　psychological O9A.52 (*following* O99)
　　　　sexual O9A.42 (*following* O99)
　　　adherent placenta O72.0
　　　　without hemorrhage O73.0
　　　alcohol use O99.314
　　　anemia (pre-existing) O99.02
　　　anesthetic death O74.8
　　　annular detachment of cervix O71.3
　　　atony, uterus O62.2
　　　attempted vacuum extraction and forceps O66.5
　　　Bandl's ring O62.4
　　　bariatric surgery status O99.844
　　　biliary tract disorder O26.62
　　　bleeding — *see* Delivery, complicated by, hemorrhage
　　　blood disorder NEC O99.12

Delivery — *continued*
　complicated — *continued*
　　by — *continued*
　　　cervical dystocia (hypotonic) O62.2
　　　　primary O62.0
　　　　secondary O62.1
　　　circulatory system disorder O99.42
　　　compression of cord (umbilical) NEC O69.2 ☑
　　　condition NEC O99.89
　　　contraction, contracted ring O62.4
　　　cord (umbilical)
　　　　around neck
　　　　　with compression O69.1 ☑
　　　　　without compression O69.81 ☑
　　　　bruising O69.5 ☑
　　　　complication O69.9 ☑
　　　　　specified NEC O69.89 ☑
　　　　compression NEC O69.2 ☑
　　　　entanglement O69.2 ☑
　　　　　without compression O69.82 ☑
　　　　hematoma O69.5 ☑
　　　　presentation O69.0 ☑
　　　　prolapse O69.0 ☑
　　　　short O69.3 ☑
　　　　thrombosis (vessels) O69.5 ☑
　　　　vascular lesion O69.5 ☑
　　　Couvelaire uterus O45.8X- ☑
　　　damage to (injury to) NEC
　　　　perineum O71.82
　　　　periurethral tissue O71.82
　　　　vulva O71.82
　　　delay following rupture of membranes (spontaneous) — *see* Pregnancy, complicated by, premature rupture of membranes
　　　depressed fetal heart tones O76
　　　diabetes O24.92
　　　　gestational O24.429
　　　　　diet controlled O24.420
　　　　　insulin controlled O24.424
　　　　　oral drug controlled (antidiabetic) (hypoglycemic) O24.425
　　　　pre-existing O24.32
　　　　　specified NEC O24.82
　　　　　type 1 O24.02
　　　　　type 2 O24.12
　　　diastasis recti (abdominis) O71.89
　　　dilatation
　　　　bladder O66.8
　　　　cervix incomplete, poor or slow O62.0
　　　disease NEC O99.89
　　　disruptio uteri — *see* Delivery, complicated by, rupture, uterus
　　　drug use O99.324
　　　dysfunction, uterus NOS O62.9
　　　　hypertonic O62.4
　　　　hypotonic O62.2
　　　　　primary O62.0
　　　　　secondary O62.1
　　　　incoordinate O62.4
　　　eclampsia O15.1
　　　embolism (pulmonary) — *see* Embolism, obstetric
　　　endocrine, nutritional or metabolic disease NEC O99.284
　　　failed
　　　　attempted vaginal birth after previous cesarean delivery O66.41
　　　　induction of labor O61.9
　　　　　instrumental O61.1
　　　　　mechanical O61.1
　　　　　medical O61.0
　　　　　specified NEC O61.8
　　　　　surgical O61.1
　　　　trial of labor O66.40
　　　female genital mutilation O65.5
　　　fetal
　　　　abnormal acid-base balance O68
　　　　acidemia O68
　　　　acidosis O68
　　　　alkalosis O68
　　　　death, early O02.1
　　　　deformity O66.3
　　　　heart rate or rhythm (abnormal) (non-reassuring) O76
　　　　hypoxia O77.8
　　　　stress O77.9
　　　　　due to drug administration O77.1
　　　　　electrocardiographic evidence of O77.8

☑ **Additional Character Required — Refer to the Tabular List for Character Selection** 　 Subterms under main terms may continue to next column or page

Delivery — *continued*
  complicated — *continued*
    by — *continued*
      fetal — *continued*
        stress — *continued*
          specified NEC O77.8
          ultrasound evidence of O77.8
      fever during labor O75.2
      gastric banding status O99.844
      gastric bypass status O99.844
      gastrointestinal disease NEC O99.62
      gestational
        diabetes O24.429
          diet controlled O24.420
          insulin (and diet) controlled O24.424
          oral drug controlled (antidiabetic) (hypo-glycemic) O24.425
        edema O12.04
          with proteinuria O12.24
        proteinuria O12.14
      gonorrhea O98.22
      hematoma O71.7
        ischial spine O71.7
        pelvic O71.7
        vagina O71.7
        vulva or perineum O71.7
      hemorrhage (uterine) O67.9
        associated with
          afibrinogenemia O67.0
          coagulation defect O67.0
          hyperfibrinolysis O67.0
          hypofibrinogenemia O67.0
        due to
          low implantation of placenta O44.5- ☑
          low-lying placenta O44.5- ☑
          placenta previa O44.1- ☑
            marginal O44.3- ☑
            partial O44.3- ☑
          premature separation of placenta (nor-mally implanted) (*see also* Abrup-tio placentae) O45.9- ☑
          retained placenta O72.0
          uterine leiomyoma O67.8
        placenta NEC O67.8
        postpartum NEC (atonic) (immediate) O72.1
          with retained or trapped placenta O72.0
          delayed O72.2
          secondary O72.2
          third stage O72.0
      hourglass contraction, uterus O62.4
      hypertension, hypertensive (pre-existing) — *see* Hypertension, complicated by, child-birth (labor)
      hypotension O26.5- ☑
      incomplete dilatation (cervix) O62.0
      incoordinate uterus contractions O62.4
      inertia, uterus O62.2
        during latent phase of labor O62.0
        primary O62.0
        secondary O62.1
      infection (maternal) O98.92
        carrier state NEC O99.834
        gonorrhea O98.22
        human immunodeficiency virus (HIV) O98.72
        sexually transmitted NEC O98.32
        specified NEC O98.82
        syphilis O98.12
        tuberculosis O98.02
        viral hepatitis O98.42
        viral NEC O98.52
      injury (to mother) (*see also* Delivery, complicat-ed, by, damage to) O71.9
        nonobstetric O9A.22 (*following* O99)
          caused by abuse — *see* Delivery, compli-cated by, abuse
      intrauterine fetal death, early O02.1
      inversion, uterus O71.2
      laceration (perineal) O70.9
        anus (sphincter) O70.4
          with third degree laceration (*see also* Delivery, complicated, by, lacera-tion, perineum, third degree) O70.20
            with mucosa O70.3
          without third degree laceration O70.2 ☑
        bladder (urinary) O71.5
        bowel O71.5

      laceration — *continued*
        cervix (uteri) O71.3
        fourchette O70.0
        hymen O70.0
        labia O70.0
        pelvic
          floor O70.1
          organ NEC O71.5
        perineum, perineal O70.9
          first degree O70.0
          fourth degree O70.3
          muscles O70.1
          second degree O70.1
          skin O70.0
          slight O70.0
          third degree O70.20
            with
              less than 50% of external anal sphincter (EAS) thickness torn (IIIa) O70.21
              both external anal sphincter (EAS) and internal anal sphincter (IAS) torn (IIIc) O70.23
              more than 50% external anal sphincter (EAS) thickness torn (IIIb) O70.22
            IIIa O70.21
            IIIb O70.22
            IIIc O70.23
        peritoneum (pelvic) O71.5
        rectovaginal (septum) (without perineal laceration) O71.4
          with perineum (*see also* Delivery, compli-cated, by, laceration, perineum, third degree) O70.20
            with anal or rectal mucosa O70.3
        specified NEC O71.89
        sphincter ani — *see* Delivery, complicated, by, laceration, anus (sphincter)
        urethra O71.5
        uterus O71.81
          before labor O71.81
        vagina, vaginal (deep) (high) (without per-ineal laceration) O71.4
          with perineum O70.0
          muscles, with perineum O70.1
        vulva O70.0
      liver disorder O26.62
      malignancy O9A.12 (*following* O99)
      malnutrition O25.2
      malposition, malpresentation
        without obstruction (*see also* Delivery, complicated by, obstruction) O32.9 ☑
          breech O32.1 ☑
          compound O32.6 ☑
          face (brow) (chin) O32.3 ☑
          footling O32.8 ☑
          high head O32.4 ☑
          oblique O32.2 ☑
          specified NEC O32.8 ☑
          transverse O32.2 ☑
          unstable lie O32.0 ☑
        placenta O44.0- ☑
          with hemorrhage O44.1- ☑
        uterus or cervix O65.5
      meconium in amniotic fluid O77.0
      mental disorder NEC O99.344
      metrorrhexis — *see* Delivery, complicated by, rupture, uterus
      nervous system disorder O99.354
      obesity (pre-existing) O99.214
      obesity surgery status O99.844
      obstetric trauma O71.9
        specified NEC O71.89
      obstructed labor
        due to
          breech (complete) (frank) presentation O64.1 ☑
            incomplete O64.8 ☑
          brow presenation O64.3 ☑
          buttock presentation O64.1 ☑
          chin presentation O64.2 ☑
          compound presentation O64.5 ☑
          contracted pelvis O65.1
          deep transverse arrest O64.0 ☑

      obstructed labor — *continued*
        due to — *continued*
          deformed pelvis O65.0
          dystocia (fetal) O66.9
            due to
              conjoined twins O66.3
              fetal
                abnormality NEC O66.3
                ascites O66.3
                hydrops O66.3
                meningomyelocele O66.3
                sacral teratoma O66.3
                tumor O66.3
              hydrocephalic fetus O66.3
              shoulder O66.0
          face presentation O64.2 ☑
          fetopelvic disproportion O65.4
          footling presentation O64.8 ☑
          impacted shoulders O66.0
          incomplete rotation of fetal head O64.0 ☑
          large fetus O66.2
          locked twins O66.1
          malposition O64.9 ☑
            specified NEC O64.8 ☑
          malpresentation O64.9 ☑
            specified NEC O64.8 ☑
          multiple fetuses NEC O66.6
          pelvic
            abnormality (maternal) O65.9
              organ O65.5
              specified NEC O65.8
            contraction
              inlet O65.2
              mid-cavity O65.3
              outlet O65.3
          persistent (position)
            occipitoiliac O64.0 ☑
            occipitoposterior O64.0 ☑
            occipitosacral O64.0 ☑
            occipitotransverse O64.0 ☑
          prolapsed arm O64.4 ☑
          shoulder presentation O64.4 ☑
        specified NEC O66.8
      pathological retraction ring, uterus O62.4
      penetration, pregnant uterus by instrument O71.1
      perforation — *see* Delivery, complicated by, laceration
      placenta, placental
        ablatio (*see also* Abruptio placentae) O45.9- ☑
        abnormality O43.9- ☑
          specified NEC O43.89- ☑
        abruptio (*see also* Abruptio placentae) O45.9- ☑
        accreta O43.21- ☑
        adherent (with hemorrhage) O72.0
          without hemorrhage O73.0
        detachment (premature) (*see also* Abruptio placentae) O45.9- ☑
        disorder O43.9- ☑
          specified NEC O43.89- ☑
        hemorrhage NEC O67.8
        increta O43.22- ☑
        low (implantation) (lying) O44.4- ☑
          with hemorrhage O44.5- ☑
        malformation O43.10- ☑
        malposition O44.0- ☑
          without hemorrhage O44.1- ☑
        percreta O43.23- ☑
        previa (central) (complete) (lateral) (total) O44.0- ☑
          with hemorrhage O44.1- ☑
          marginal O44.2- ☑
            with hemorrhage O44.3- ☑
          partial O44.2- ☑
            with hemorrhage O44.3- ☑
        retained (with hemorrhage) O72.0
          without hemorrhage O73.0
        separation (premature) O45.9- ☑
          specified NEC O45.8X- ☑
        vicious insertion O44.1- ☑
      precipitate labor O62.3

Subterms under main terms may continue to next column or page   ☑ Additional Character Required — Refer to the Tabular List for Character Selection   91

Delivery — Delivery

Delivery — *continued*
  complicated — *continued*
    by — *continued*
      premature rupture, membranes (*see also* Pregnancy, complicated by, premature rupture of membranes) O42.90
      prolapse
        arm or hand O32.2 ☑
        cord (umbilical) O69.0 ☑
        foot or leg O32.8 ☑
        uterus O34.52- ☑
      prolonged labor O63.9
        first stage O63.0
        second stage O63.1
      protozoal disease (maternal) O98.62
      respiratory disease NEC O99.52
      retained membranes or portions of placenta O72.2
        without hemorrhage O73.1
      retarded birth O63.9
      retention of secundines (with hemorrhage) O72.0
        without hemorrhage O73.0
        partial O72.2
          without hemorrhage O73.1
      rupture
        bladder (urinary) O71.5
        cervix O71.3
        pelvic organ NEC O71.5
        urethra O71.5
        uterus (during or after labor) O71.1
          before labor O71.0- ☑
      separation, pubic bone (symphysis pubis) O71.6
      shock O75.1
      shoulder presentation O64.4 ☑
      skin disorder NEC O99.72
      spasm, cervix O62.4
      stenosis or stricture, cervix O65.5
      streptococcus group B (GBS) carrier state O99.824
      subluxation of symphysis (pubis) O26.72
      syphilis (maternal) O98.12
      tear — *see* Delivery, complicated by, laceration
      tetanic uterus O62.4
      trauma (obstetrical) (*see also* Delivery, complicated, by, damage to) O71.9
        non-obstetric O9A.22 (*following* O99)
        periurethral O71.82
        specified NEC O71.89
      tuberculosis (maternal) O98.02
      tumor, pelvic organs or tissues NEC O65.5
      umbilical cord around neck
        with compression O69.1 ☑
        without compression O69.81 ☑
      uterine inertia O62.2
        during latent phase of labor O62.0
        primary O62.0
        secondary O62.1
      vasa previa O69.4 ☑
      velamentous insertion of cord O43.12- ☑
    specified complication NEC O75.89
  delayed NOS O63.9
    following rupture of membranes
      artificial O75.5
    second twin, triplet, etc. O63.2
  forceps, low following failed vacuum extraction O66.5
  missed (at or near term) O36.4 ☑
  normal O80
  obstructed — *see* Delivery, complicated by, obstructed labor
  precipitate O62.3
  preterm (*see also* Pregnancy, complicated by, preterm labor) O60.10 ☑
  spontaneous O80
  term pregnancy NOS O80
  uncomplicated O80
  vaginal, following previous cesarean delivery O34.219
    classical (vertical) scar O34.212
    low transverse scar O34.211
Delusions (paranoid) — *see* Disorder, delusional
Dementia (degenerative (primary)) (old age) (persisting) F03.90
  with
    aggressive behavior F03.91
    behavioral disturbance F03.91
    combative behavior F03.91
    Lewy bodies G31.83 [F02.80]
      with behavioral disturbance G31.83 [F02.81]

Dementia — *continued*
  with — *continued*
    Parkinsonism G31.83 [F02.80]
      with behavioral disturbance G31.83 [F02.81]
    Parkinson's disease G20 [F02.80]
      with behavioral disturbance G20 [F02.81]
    violent behavior F03.91
  alcoholic F10.97
    with dependence F10.27
  Alzheimer's type — *see* Disease, Alzheimer's
  arteriosclerotic — *see* Dementia, vascular
  atypical, Alzheimer's type — *see* Disease, Alzheimer's, specified NEC
  congenital — *see* Disability, intellectual
  frontal (lobe) G31.09 [F02.80]
    with behavioral disturbance G31.09 [F02.81]
  frontotemporal G31.09 [F02.80]
    with behavioral disturbance G31.09 [F02.81]
    specified NEC G31.09 [F02.80]
      with behavioral disturbance G31.09 [F02.81]
  Huntington's disease or chorea G10
    with dementia G10 [F02.80]
  in (due to)
    with behavioral disturbance G31.83 [F02.81]
    alcohol F10.97
      with dependence F10.27
    Alzheimer's disease — *see* Disease, Alzheimer's
    arteriosclerotic brain disease — *see* Dementia, vascular
    cerebral lipidoses E75.- ☑ [F02.80]
      with behavioral disturbance E75.- ☑ [F02.81]
    Creutzfeldt-Jakob disease (*see also* Creutzfeldt-Jakob disease or syndrome (with dementia)) A81.00
    epilepsy G40.- ☑ [F02.80]
      with behavioral disturbance G40.- ☑ [F02.81]
    hepatolenticular degeneration E83.01 [F02.80]
      with behavioral disturbance E83.01 [F02.81]
    human immunodeficiency virus (HIV) disease B20 [F02.80]
      with behavioral disturbance B20 [F02.81]
    Huntington's disease or chorea G10 [F02.80]
      with behavioral disturbance G10 [F02.81]
    hypercalcemia E83.52 [F02.80]
      with behavioral disturbance E83.52 [F02.81]
    hypothyroidism, acquired E03.9 [F02.80]
      with behavioral disturbance E03.9 [F02.81]
      due to iodine deficiency E01.8 [F02.80]
        with behavioral disturbance E01.8 [F02.81]
    inhalants F18.97
      with dependence F18.27
    multiple
      etiologies F03 ☑
      sclerosis G35 [F02.80]
        with behavioral disturbance G35 [F02.81]
    neurosyphilis A52.17 [F02.80]
      with behavioral disturbance A52.17 [F02.81]
      juvenile A50.49 [F02.80]
        with behavioral disturbance A50.49 [F02.81]
    niacin deficiency E52 [F02.80]
      with behavioral disturbance E52 [F02.81]
    paralysis agitans G20 [F02.80]
      with behavioral disturbance G20 [F02.81]
    Parkinson's disease G20 [F02.80]
    pellagra E52 [F02.80]
      with behavioral disturbance E52 [F02.81]
    Pick's G31.01 [F02.80]
      with behavioral disturbance G31.01 [F02.81]
    polyarteritis nodosa M30.0 [F02.80]
      with behavioral disturbance M30.0 [F02.81]
    psychoactive drug F19.97
      with dependence F19.27
      inhalants F18.97
        with dependence F18.27
      sedatives, hypnotics or anxiolytics F13.97
        with dependence F13.27
    sedatives, hypnotics or anxiolytics F13.97
      with dependence F13.27
    systemic lupus erythematosus M32.- ☑ [F02.80]
      with behavioral disturbance M32.- ☑ [F02.81]
    trypanosomiasis
      African B56.9 [F02.80]
        with behavioral disturbance B56.9 [F02.81]
    unknown etiology F03 ☑
    vitamin B12 deficiency E53.8 [F02.80]
      with behavioral disturbance E53.8 [F02.81]
    volatile solvents F18.97
      with dependence F18.27

Dementia — *continued*
  infantile, infantilis F84.3
  Lewy body G31.83 [F02.80]
    with behavioral disturbance G31.83 [F02.81]
  multi-infarct — *see* Dementia, vascular
  paralytica, paralytic (syphilitic) A52.17 [F02.80]
    with behavioral disturbance A52.17 [F02.81]
    juvenilis A50.45
  paretic A52.17
  praecox — *see* Schizophrenia
  presenile F03 ☑
    Alzheimer's type — *see* Disease, Alzheimer's, early onset
  primary degenerative F03 ☑
  progressive, syphilitic A52.17
  senile F03 ☑
    with acute confusional state F05
    Alzheimer's type — *see* Disease, Alzheimer's, late onset
    depressed or paranoid type F03 ☑
  vascular (acute onset) (mixed) (multi-infarct) (subcortical) F01.50
    with behavioral disturbance F01.51
Demineralization, bone — *see* Osteoporosis
Demodex folliculorum (infestation) B88.0
Demophobia F40.248
Demoralization R45.3
Demyelination, demyelinization
  central nervous system G37.9
    specified NEC G37.8
  corpus callosum (central) G37.1
  disseminated, acute G36.9
    specified NEC G36.8
  global G35
  in optic neuritis G36.0
Dengue (classical) (fever) A90
  hemorrhagic A91
  sandfly A93.1
Dennie-Marfan syphilitic syndrome A50.45
Dens evaginatus, in dente or invaginatus K00.2
Dense breasts R92.2
Density
  increased, bone (disseminated) (generalized) (spotted) — *see* Disorder, bone, density and structure, specified type NEC
  lung (nodular) J98.4
Dental (*see also* condition)
  examination Z01.20
    with abnormal findings Z01.21
  restoration
    aesthetically inadequate or displeasing K08.56
    defective K08.50
      specified NEC K08.59
    failure of marginal integrity K08.51
    failure of periodontal anatomical integrity K08.54
Dentia praecox K00.6
Denticles (pulp) K04.2
Dentigerous cyst K09.0
Dentin
  irregular (in pulp) K04.3
  opalescent K00.5
  secondary (in pulp) K04.3
  sensitive K03.89
Dentinogenesis imperfecta K00.5
Dentinoma — *see* Cyst, calcifying odontogenic
Dentition (syndrome) K00.7
  delayed K00.6
  difficult K00.7
  precocious K00.6
  premature K00.6
  retarded K00.6
Dependence (on) (syndrome) F19.20
  with remission F19.21
  alcohol (ethyl) (methyl) (without remission) F10.20
    with
      amnestic disorder, persisting F10.26
      anxiety disorder F10.280
      dementia, persisting F10.27
      intoxication F10.229
        with delirium F10.221
        uncomplicated F10.220
      mood disorder F10.24
      psychotic disorder F10.259
        with
          delusions F10.250
          hallucinations F10.251
      remission F10.21
      sexual dysfunction F10.281

Delivery — Dependence

Dependence — *continued*
  alcohol — *continued*
    with — *continued*
      sleep disorder F10.282
      specified disorder NEC F10.288
      withdrawal F10.239
        with
          delirium F10.231
          perceptual disturbance F10.232
        uncomplicated F10.230
    counseling and surveillance Z71.41
  amobarbital — *see* Dependence, drug, sedative
  amphetamine(s) (type) — *see* Dependence, drug, stimulant NEC
  amytal (sodium) — *see* Dependence, drug, sedative
  analgesic NEC F55.8
  anesthetic (agent) (gas) (general) (local) NEC — *see* Dependence, drug, psychoactive NEC
  anxiolytic NEC — *see* Dependence, drug, sedative
  barbital(s) — *see* Dependence, drug, sedative
  barbiturate(s) (compounds) (drugs classifiable to T42) — *see* Dependence, drug, sedative
  benzedrine — *see* Dependence, drug, stimulant NEC
  bhang — *see* Dependence, drug, cannabis
  bromide(s) NEC — *see* Dependence, drug, sedative
  caffeine — *see* Dependence, drug, stimulant NEC
  cannabis (sativa) (indica) (resin) (derivatives) (type) — *see* Dependence, drug, cannabis
  chloral (betaine) (hydrate) — *see* Dependence, drug, sedative
  chlordiazepoxide — *see* Dependence, drug, sedative
  coca (leaf) (derivatives) — *see* Dependence, drug, cocaine
  cocaine — *see* Dependence, drug, cocaine
  codeine — *see* Dependence, drug, opioid
  combinations of drugs F19.20
  dagga — *see* Dependence, drug, cannabis
  demerol — *see* Dependence, drug, opioid
  dexamphetamine — *see* Dependence, drug, stimulant NEC
  dexedrine — *see* Dependence, drug, stimulant NEC
  dextromethorphan — *see* Dependence, drug, opioid
  dextromoramide — *see* Dependence, drug, opioid
  dextro-nor-pseudo-ephedrine — *see* Dependence, drug, stimulant NEC
  dextrorphan — *see* Dependence, drug, opioid
  diazepam — *see* Dependence, drug, sedative
  dilaudid — *see* Dependence, drug, opioid
  D-lysergic acid diethylamide — *see* Dependence, drug, hallucinogen
  drug NEC F19.20
    with sleep disorder F19.282
    cannabis F12.20
      with
        anxiety disorder F12.280
        intoxication F12.229
          with
            delirium F12.221
            perceptual disturbance F12.222
          uncomplicated F12.220
        other specified disorder F12.288
        psychosis F12.259
          delusions F12.250
          hallucinations F12.251
        unspecified disorder F12.29
      in remission F12.21
    cocaine F14.20
      with
        anxiety disorder F14.280
        intoxication F14.229
          with
            delirium F14.221
            perceptual disturbance F14.222
          uncomplicated F14.220
        mood disorder F14.24
        other specified disorder F14.288
        psychosis F14.259
          delusions F14.250
          hallucinations F14.251
        sexual dysfunction F14.281
        sleep disorder F14.282
        unspecified disorder F14.29
        withdrawal F14.23
      in remission F14.21
      withdrawal symptoms in newborn P96.1
  counseling and surveillance Z71.51
  hallucinogen F16.20

Dependence — *continued*
  drug — *continued*
    hallucinogen — *continued*
      with
        anxiety disorder F16.280
        flashbacks F16.283
        intoxication F16.229
          with delirium F16.221
          uncomplicated F16.220
        mood disorder F16.24
        other specified disorder F16.288
        perception disorder, persisting F16.283
        psychosis F16.259
          delusions F16.250
          hallucinations F16.251
        unspecified disorder F16.29
      in remission F16.21
    in remission F19.21
    inhalant F18.20
      with
        anxiety disorder F18.280
        dementia, persisting F18.27
        intoxication F18.229
          with delirium F18.221
          uncomplicated F18.220
        mood disorder F18.24
        other specified disorder F18.288
        psychosis F18.259
          delusions F18.250
          hallucinations F18.251
        unspecified disorder F18.29
      in remission F18.21
    nicotine F17.200
      with disorder F17.209
        in remission F17.201
        specified disorder NEC F17.208
        withdrawal F17.203
      chewing tobacco F17.220
        with disorder F17.229
          in remission F17.221
          specified disorder NEC F17.228
          withdrawal F17.223
      cigarettes F17.210
        with disorder F17.219
          in remission F17.211
          specified disorder NEC F17.218
          withdrawal F17.213
      specified product NEC F17.290
        with disorder F17.299
          remission F17.291
          specified disorder NEC F17.298
          withdrawal F17.293
    opioid F11.20
      with
        intoxication F11.229
          with
            delirium F11.221
            perceptual disturbance F11.222
          uncomplicated F11.220
        mood disorder F11.24
        other specified disorder F11.288
        psychosis F11.259
          delusions F11.250
          hallucinations F11.251
        sexual dysfunction F11.281
        sleep disorder F11.282
        unspecified disorder F11.29
        withdrawal F11.23
      in remission F11.21
    psychoactive NEC F19.20
      with
        amnestic disorder F19.26
        anxiety disorder F19.280
        dementia F19.27
        intoxication F19.229
          with
            delirium F19.221
            perceptual disturbance F19.222
          uncomplicated F19.220
        mood disorder F19.24
        other specified disorder F19.288
        psychosis F19.259
          delusions F19.250
          hallucinations F19.251
        sexual dysfunction F19.281
        sleep disorder F19.282
        unspecified disorder F19.29
        withdrawal F19.239

Dependence — *continued*
  drug — *continued*
    psychoactive — *continued*
      with — *continued*
        withdrawal — *continued*
          with
            delirium F19.231
            perceptual disturbance F19.232
          uncomplicated F19.230
    sedative, hypnotic or anxiolytic F13.20
      with
        amnestic disorder F13.26
        anxiety disorder F13.280
        dementia, persisting F13.27
        intoxication F13.229
          with delirium F13.221
          uncomplicated F13.220
        mood disorder F13.24
        other specified disorder F13.288
        psychosis F13.259
          delusions F13.250
          hallucinations F13.251
        sexual dysfunction F13.281
        sleep disorder F13.282
        unspecified disorder F13.29
        withdrawal F13.239
          with
            delirium F13.231
            perceptual disturbance F13.232
          uncomplicated F13.230
      in remission F13.21
    stimulant NEC F15.20
      with
        anxiety disorder F15.280
        intoxication F15.229
          with
            delirium F15.221
            perceptual disturbance F15.222
          uncomplicated F15.220
        mood disorder F15.24
        other specified disorder F15.288
        psychosis F15.259
          delusions F15.250
          hallucinations F15.251
        sexual dysfunction F15.281
        sleep disorder F15.282
        unspecified disorder F15.29
        withdrawal F15.23
      in remission F15.21
  ethyl
    alcohol (without remission) F10.20
      with remission F10.21
    bromide — *see* Dependence, drug, sedative
    carbamate F19.20
    chloride F19.20
    morphine — *see* Dependence, drug, opioid
  ganja — *see* Dependence, drug, cannabis
  glue (airplane) (sniffing) — *see* Dependence, drug, inhalant
  glutethimide — *see* Dependence, drug, sedative
  hallucinogenics — *see* Dependence, drug, hallucinogen
  hashish — *see* Dependence, drug, cannabis
  hemp — *see* Dependence, drug, cannabis
  heroin (salt) (any) — *see* Dependence, drug, opioid
  hypnotic NEC — *see* Dependence, drug, sedative
  Indian hemp — *see* Dependence, drug, cannabis
  inhalants — *see* Dependence, drug, inhalant
  khat — *see* Dependence, drug, stimulant NEC
  laudanum — *see* Dependence, drug, opioid
  LSD (-25) (derivatives) — *see* Dependence, drug, hallucinogen
  luminal — *see* Dependence, drug, sedative
  lysergic acid — *see* Dependence, drug, hallucinogen
  maconha — *see* Dependence, drug, cannabis
  marihuana — *see* Dependence, drug, cannabis
  meprobamate — *see* Dependence, drug, sedative
  mescaline — *see* Dependence, drug, hallucinogen
  methadone — *see* Dependence, drug, opioid
  methamphetamine(s) — *see* Dependence, drug, stimulant NEC
  methaqualone — *see* Dependence, drug, sedative
  methyl
    alcohol (without remission) F10.20
      with remission F10.21
    bromide — *see* Dependence, drug, sedative
    morphine — *see* Dependence, drug, opioid

Index

Dependence — Derangement

Dependence — *continued*
  methyl — *continued*
    phenidate — *see* Dependence, drug, stimulant NEC
    sulfonal — *see* Dependence, drug, sedative
  morphine (sulfate) (sulfite) (type) — *see* Dependence, drug, opioid
  narcotic (drug) NEC — *see* Dependence, drug, opioid
  nembutal — *see* Dependence, drug, sedative
  neraval — *see* Dependence, drug, sedative
  neravan — *see* Dependence, drug, sedative
  neurobarb — *see* Dependence, drug, sedative
  nicotine — *see* Dependence, drug, nicotine
  nitrous oxide F19.2Ø
  nonbarbiturate sedatives and tranquilizers with similar effect — *see* Dependence, drug, sedative
  on
    artificial heart (fully implantable) (mechanical) Z95.812
    aspirator Z99.Ø
    care provider (because of) Z74.9
      impaired mobility Z74.Ø9
      need for
        assistance with personal care Z74.1
        continuous supervision Z74.3
        no other household member able to render care Z74.2
      specified reason NEC Z74.8
    machine Z99.89
      enabling NEC Z99.89
      specified type NEC Z99.89
    renal dialysis (hemodialysis) (peritoneal) Z99.2
    respirator Z99.11
    ventilator Z99.11
    wheelchair Z99.3
  opiate — *see* Dependence, drug, opioid
  opioids — *see* Dependence, drug, opioid
  opium (alkaloids) (derivatives) (tincture) — *see* Dependence, drug, opioid
  oxygen (long-term) (supplemental) Z99.81
  paraldehyde — *see* Dependence, drug, sedative
  paregoric — *see* Dependence, drug, opioid
  PCP (phencyclidine) (or related substance) — *see* Dependence, drug, hallucinogen
  pentobarbital — *see* Dependence, drug, sedative
  pentobarbitone (sodium) — *see* Dependence, drug, sedative
  pentothal — *see* Dependence, drug, sedative
  peyote — *see* Dependence, drug, hallucinogen
  phencyclidine (PCP) (or related substance) — *see* Dependence, drug, hallucinogen
  phenmetrazine — *see* Dependence, drug, stimulant NEC
  phenobarbital — *see* Dependence, drug, sedative
  polysubstance F19.2Ø
  psilocibin, psilocin, psilocyn, psilocyline — *see* Dependence, drug, hallucinogen
  psychostimulant NEC — *see* Dependence, drug, stimulant NEC
  secobarbital — *see* Dependence, drug, sedative
  seconal — *see* Dependence, drug, sedative
  sedative NEC — *see* Dependence, drug, sedative
  specified drug NEC — *see* Dependence, drug
  stimulant NEC — *see* Dependence, drug, stimulant NEC
  substance NEC — *see* Dependence, drug
  supplemental oxygen Z99.81
  tobacco — *see* Dependence, drug, nicotine
    counseling and surveillance Z71.6
  tranquilizer NEC — *see* Dependence, drug, sedative
  vitamin B6 E53.1
  volatile solvents — *see* Dependence, drug, inhalant
Dependency
  care-provider Z74.9
  passive F6Ø.7
  reactions (persistent) F6Ø.7
Depersonalization (in neurotic state) (neurotic) (syndrome) F48.1
Depletion
  extracellular fluid E86.9
  plasma E86.1
  potassium E87.6
    nephropathy N25.89
  salt or sodium E87.1
    causing heat exhaustion or prostration T67.4 ☑
    nephropathy N28.9
  volume NOS E86.9

Deployment (current) (military) status Z56.82
  in theater or in support of military war, peacekeeping and humanitarian operations Z56.82
  personal history of Z91.82
    military war, peacekeeping and humanitarian deployment (current or past conflict) Z91.82
  returned from Z91.82
Depolarization, premature I49.4Ø
  atrial I49.1
  junctional I49.2
  specified NEC I49.49
  ventricular I49.3
Deposit
  bone in Boeck's sarcoid D86.89
  calcareous, calcium — *see* Calcification
  cholesterol
    retina H35.89
    vitreous (body) (humor) — *see* Deposit, crystalline
  conjunctiva H11.11- ☑
  cornea H18.ØØ- ☑
    argentous H18.Ø2- ☑
    due to metabolic disorder H18.Ø3- ☑
    Kayser-Fleischer ring H18.Ø4- ☑
    pigmentation — *see* Pigmentation, cornea
  crystalline, vitreous (body) (humor) H43.2- ☑
  hemosiderin in old scars of cornea — *see* Pigmentation, cornea, stromal
  metallic in lens — *see* Cataract, specified NEC
  skin R23.8
  tooth, teeth (betel) (black) (green) (materia alba) (orange) (tobacco) KØ3.6
  urate, kidney — *see* Calculus, kidney
Depraved appetite — *see* Pica
Depressed
  HDL cholesterol E78.6
Depression (acute) (mental) F32.9
  agitated (single episode) F32.2
  anaclitic — *see* Disorder, adjustment
  anxiety F41.8
    persistent F34.1
  arches (*see also* Deformity, limb, flat foot)
  atypical (single episode) F32.89
    recurrent episode F33.8
  basal metabolic rate R94.8
  bone marrow D75.89
  central nervous system RØ9.2
  cerebral R29.818
    newborn P91.4
  cerebrovascular I67.9
  chest wall M95.4
  climacteric (single episode) F32.89
    recurrent episode F33.8
  endogenous (without psychotic symptoms) F33.2
    with psychotic symptoms F33.3
  functional activity R68.89
  hysterical F44.89
  involutional (single episode) F32.89
    recurrent episode F33.8
  major F32.9
    with psychotic symptoms F32.3
    recurrent — *see* Disorder, depressive, recurrent
  manic-depressive — *see* Disorder, depressive, recurrent
  masked (single episode) F32.89
  medullary G93.89
  menopausal (single episode) F32.89
    recurrent episode F33.8
  metatarsus — *see* Depression, arches
  monopolar F33.9
  nervous F34.1
  neurotic F34.1
  nose M95.Ø
  postnatal F53
  postpartum F53
  post-psychotic of schizophrenia F32.89
  post-schizophrenic F32.89
  psychogenic (reactive) (single episode) F32.9
  psychoneurotic F34.1
  psychotic (single episode) F32.3
    recurrent F33.3
  reactive (psychogenic) (single episode) F32.9
    psychotic (single episode) F32.3
  recurrent — *see* Disorder, depressive, recurrent
  respiratory center G93.89
  seasonal — *see* Disorder, depressive, recurrent
  senile FØ3 ☑
  severe, single episode F32.2
  situational F43.21

Depression — *continued*
  skull Q67.4
  specified NEC (single episode) F32.89
  sternum M95.4
  visual field — *see* Defect, visual field
  vital (recurrent) (without psychotic symptoms) F33.2
    with psychotic symptoms F33.3
    single episode F32.2
Deprivation
  cultural Z6Ø.3
  effects NOS T73.9 ☑
    specified NEC T73.8 ☑
  emotional NEC Z65.8
    affecting infant or child — *see* Maltreatment, child, psychological
  food T73.Ø ☑
  protein — *see* Malnutrition
  sleep Z72.82Ø
  social Z6Ø.4
    affecting infant or child — *see* Maltreatment, child, psychological
  specified NEC T73.8 ☑
  vitamins — *see* Deficiency, vitamin
  water T73.1 ☑
Derangement
  ankle (internal) — *see* Derangement, joint, ankle
  cartilage (articular) NEC — *see* Derangement, joint, articular cartilage, by site
    recurrent — *see* Dislocation, recurrent
  cruciate ligament, anterior, current injury — *see* Sprain, knee, cruciate, anterior
  elbow (internal) — *see* Derangement, joint, elbow
  hip (joint) (internal) (old) — *see* Derangement, joint, hip
  joint (internal) M24.9
    ankylosis — *see* Ankylosis
    articular cartilage M24.1Ø
      ankle M24.17- ☑
      elbow M24.12- ☑
      foot M24.17- ☑
      hand M24.14- ☑
      hip M24.15- ☑
      knee NEC M23.9- ☑
      loose body — *see* Loose, body
      shoulder M24.11- ☑
      wrist M24.13- ☑
    contracture — *see* Contraction, joint
    current injury (*see also* Dislocation)
      knee, meniscus or cartilage — *see* Tear, meniscus
    dislocation
      pathological — *see* Dislocation, pathological
      recurrent — *see* Dislocation, recurrent
    knee — *see* Derangement, knee
    ligament — *see* Disorder, ligament
    loose body — *see* Loose, body
    recurrent — *see* Dislocation, recurrent
    specified type NEC M24.8Ø
      ankle M24.87- ☑
      elbow M24.82- ☑
      foot joint M24.87- ☑
      hand joint M24.84- ☑
      hip M24.85- ☑
      shoulder M24.81- ☑
      wrist M24.83- ☑
    temporomandibular M26.69
  knee (recurrent) M23.9- ☑
    ligament disruption, spontaneous M23.6Ø- ☑
      anterior cruciate M23.61- ☑
      capsular M23.67- ☑
      instability, chronic M23.5- ☑
      lateral collateral M23.64- ☑
      medial collateral M23.63- ☑
      posterior cruciate M23.62- ☑
    loose body M23.4- ☑
    meniscus M23.3Ø- ☑
      cystic M23.ØØ- ☑
        lateral M23.ØØ2
          anterior horn M23.Ø4- ☑
          posterior horn M23.Ø5- ☑
          specified NEC M23.Ø6- ☑
        medial M23.ØØ5
          anterior horn M23.Ø1- ☑
          posterior horn M23.Ø2- ☑
          specified NEC M23.Ø3- ☑

☑ **Additional Character Required** — Refer to the Tabular List for Character Selection   ⍦ **Subterms under main terms may continue to next column or page**

Derangement — *continued*
  knee — *continued*
    meniscus — *continued*
      degenerate — *see* Derangement, knee, menis-
        cus, specified NEC
      detached — *see* Derangement, knee, meniscus,
        specified NEC
      due to old tear or injury M23.20- ☑
        lateral M23.20- ☑
          anterior horn M23.24- ☑
          posterior horn M23.25- ☑
          specified NEC M23.26- ☑
        medial M23.20- ☑
          anterior horn M23.21- ☑
          posterior horn M23.22- ☑
          specified NEC M23.23- ☑
      retained — *see* Derangement, knee, meniscus,
        specified NEC
      specified NEC M23.30- ☑
        lateral M23.30- ☑
          anterior horn M23.34- ☑
          posterior horn M23.35- ☑
          specified NEC M23.36- ☑
        medial M23.30- ☑
          anterior horn M23.31- ☑
          posterior horn M23.32- ☑
          specified NEC M23.33- ☑
      old M23.8X- ☑
      specified NEC — *see* subcategory M23.8 ☑
  low back NEC — *see* Dorsopathy, specified NEC
  meniscus — *see* Derangement, knee, meniscus
  mental — *see* Psychosis
  patella, specified NEC — *see* Disorder, patella, derange-
    ment NEC
  semilunar cartilage (knee) — *see* Derangement, knee,
    meniscus, specified NEC
  shoulder (internal) — *see* Derangement, joint, shoul-
    der
Dercum's disease E88.2
Derealization (neurotic) F48.1
Dermal — *see* condition
Dermaphytid — *see* Dermatophytosis
Dermatitis (eczematous) L30.9
  ab igne L59.0
  acarine B88.0
  actinic (due to sun) L57.8
    other than from sun L59.8
  allergic — *see* Dermatitis, contact, allergic
  ambustionis, due to burn or scald — *see* Burn
  amebic A06.7
  ammonia L22
  arsenical (ingested) L27.8
  artefacta L98.1
    psychogenic F54
  atopic L20.9
    psychogenic F54
    specified NEC L20.89
  autoimmune progesterone L30.8
  berlock, berloque L56.2
  blastomycotic B40.3
  blister beetle L24.89
  bullous, bullosa L13.9
    mucosynechial, atrophic L12.1
    seasonal L30.8
    specified NEC L13.8
  calorica L59.0
    due to burn or scald — *see* Burn
  caterpillar L24.89
  cercarial B65.3
  combustionis L59.0
    due to burn or scald — *see* Burn
  congelationis T69.1 ☑
  contact (occupational) L25.9
    allergic L23.9
      due to
        adhesives L23.1
        cement L23.5
        chemical products NEC L23.5
        chromium L23.0
        cosmetics L23.2
        dander (cat) (dog) L23.81
        drugs in contact with skin L23.3
        dyes L23.4
        food in contact with skin L23.6
        hair (cat) (dog) L23.81
        insecticide L23.5
        metals L23.0

Dermatitis — *continued*
  contact — *continued*
    allergic — *continued*
      due to — *continued*
        nickel L23.0
        plants, non-food L23.7
        plastic L23.5
        rubber L23.5
        specified agent NEC L23.89
      due to
        cement L25.3
        chemical products NEC L25.3
        cosmetics L25.0
        dander (cat) (dog) L23.81
        drugs in contact with skin L25.1
        dyes L25.2
        food in contact with skin L25.4
        hair (cat) (dog) L23.81
        plants, non-food L25.5
        specified agent NEC L25.8
    irritant L24.9
      due to
        cement L24.5
        chemical products NEC L24.5
        cosmetics L24.3
        detergents L24.0
        drugs in contact with skin L24.4
        food in contact with skin L24.6
        oils and greases L24.1
        plants, non-food L24.7
        solvents L24.2
        specified agent NEC L24.89
  contusiformis L52
  diabetic — *see* E08-E13 with .620
  diaper L22
  diphtheritica A36.3
  dry skin L85.3
  due to
    acetone (contact) (irritant) L24.2
    acids (contact) (irritant) L24.5
    adhesive(s) (allergic) (contact) (plaster) L23.1
      irritant L24.5
    alcohol (irritant) (skin contact) (substances in cate-
      gory T51) L24.2
      taken internally L27.8
    alkalis (contact) (irritant) L24.5
    arsenic (ingested) L27.8
    carbon disulfide (contact) (irritant) L24.2
    caustics (contact) (irritant) L24.5
    cement (contact) L25.3
    cereal (ingested) L27.2
    chemical(s) NEC L25.3
      taken internally L27.8
    chlorocompounds L24.2
    chromium (contact) (irritant) L24.81
    coffee (ingested) L27.2
    cold weather L30.8
    cosmetics (contact) L25.0
      allergic L23.2
      irritant L24.3
    cyclohexanes L24.2
    dander (cat) (dog) L23.81
    Demodex species B88.0
    Dermanyssus gallinae B88.0
    detergents (contact) (irritant) L24.0
    dichromate L24.81
    drugs and medicaments (generalized) (internal
      use) L27.0
      external — *see* Dermatitis, due to, drugs, in
        contact with skin
      in contact with skin L25.1
        allergic L23.3
        irritant L24.4
      localized skin eruption L27.1
      specified substance — *see* Table of Drugs and
        Chemicals
    dyes (contact) L25.2
      allergic L23.4
      irritant L24.89
    epidermophytosis — *see* Dermatophytosis
    esters L24.2
    external irritant NEC L24.9
    fish (ingested) L27.2
    flour (ingested) L27.2
    food (ingested) L27.2
      in contact with skin L25.4
    fruit (ingested) L27.2
    furs (allergic) (contact) L23.81
    glues — *see* Dermatitis, due to, adhesives

Dermatitis — *continued*
  due to — *continued*
    glycols L24.2
    greases NEC (contact) (irritant) L24.1
    hair (cat) (dog) L23.81
    hot
      objects and materials — *see* Burn
      weather or places L59.0
    hydrocarbons L24.2
    infrared rays L59.8
    ingestion, ingested substance L27.9
      chemical NEC L27.8
      drugs and medicaments — *see* Dermatitis, due
        to, drugs
      food L27.2
      specified NEC L27.8
    insecticide in contact with skin L24.5
    internal agent L27.9
      drugs and medicaments (generalized) — *see*
        Dermatitis, due to, drugs
      food L27.2
    irradiation — *see* Dermatitis, due to, radioactive
      substance
    ketones L24.2
    lacquer tree (allergic) (contact) L23.7
    light (sun) NEC L57.8
      acute L56.8
      other L59.8
    Liponyssoides sanguineus B88.0
    low temperature L30.8
    meat (ingested) L27.2
    metals, metal salts (contact) (irritant) L24.81
    milk (ingested) L27.2
    nickel (contact) (irritant) L24.81
    nylon (contact) (irritant) L24.5
    oils NEC (contact) (irritant) L24.1
    paint solvent (contact) (irritant) L24.2
    petroleum products (contact) (irritant) (substances
      in T52.0) L24.2
    plants NEC (contact) L25.5
      allergic L23.7
      irritant L24.7
    plasters (adhesive) (any) (allergic) (contact) L23.1
      irritant L24.5
    plastic L25.3
    preservatives (contact) — *see* Dermatitis, due to,
      chemical, in contact with skin
    primrose (allergic) (contact) L23.7
    primula (allergic) (contact) L23.7
    radiation L59.8
      nonionizing (chronic exposure) L57.8
      sun NEC L57.8
        acute L56.8
    radioactive substance L58.9
      acute L58.0
      chronic L58.1
    radium L58.9
      acute L58.0
      chronic L58.1
    ragweed (allergic) (contact) L23.7
    Rhus (allergic) (contact) (diversiloba) (radicans)
      (toxicodendron) (venenata) (verniciflua)
      L23.7
    rubber (contact) L24.5
    Senecio jacobaea (allergic) (contact) L23.7
    solvents (contact) (irritant) (substances in category
      T52) L24.2
    specified agent NEC (contact) L25.8
      allergic L23.89
      irritant L24.89
    sunshine NEC L57.8
      acute L56.8
    tetrachlorethylene (contact) (irritant) L24.2
    toluene (contact) (irritant) L24.2
    turpentine (contact) L24.2
    ultraviolet rays (sun NEC) (chronic exposure) L57.8
      acute L56.8
    vaccine or vaccination L27.0
      specified substance — *see* Table of Drugs and
        Chemicals
    varicose veins — *see* Varix, leg, with, inflammation
    X-rays L58.9
      acute L58.0
      chronic L58.1
  dyshydrotic L30.1
  dysmenorrheica N94.6
  escharotica — *see* Burn
  exfoliative, exfoliativa (generalized) L26

Dermatitis — *continued*
exfoliative, exfoliativa — *continued*
neonatorum L00
eyelid (*see also* Dermatosis, eyelid)
allergic H01.119
left H01.116
lower H01.115
upper H01.114
right H01.113
lower H01.112
upper H01.111
contact — *see* Dermatitis, eyelid, allergic
due to
Demodex species B88.0
herpes (zoster) B02.39
simplex B00.59
eczematous H01.139
left H01.136
lower H01.135
upper H01.134
right H01.133
lower H01.132
upper H01.131
facta, factitia, factitial L98.1
psychogenic F54
flexural NEC L20.82
friction L30.4
fungus B36.9
specified type NEC B36.8
gangrenosa, gangrenous infantum L08.0
harvest mite B88.0
heat L59.0
herpesviral, vesicular (ear) (lip) B00.1
herpetiformis (bullous) (erythematous) (pustular)
(vesicular) L13.0
juvenile L12.2
senile L12.0
hiemalis L30.8
hypostatic, hypostatica — *see* Varix, leg, with, inflammation
infectious eczematoid L30.3
infective L30.3
irritant — *see* Dermatitis, contact, irritant
Jacquet's (diaper dermatitis) L22
Leptus B88.0
lichenified NEC L28.0
medicamentosa (generalized) (internal use) — *see*
Dermatitis, due to drugs
mite B88.0
multiformis L13.0
juvenile L12.2
napkin L22
neurotica L13.0
nummular L30.0
papillaris capillitii L73.0
pellagrous E52
perioral L71.0
photocontact L56.2
polymorpha dolorosa L13.0
pruriginosa L13.0
pruritic NEC L30.8
psychogenic F54
purulent L08.0
pustular
contagious B08.02
subcorneal L13.1
pyococcal L08.0
pyogenica L08.0
repens L40.2
Ritter's (exfoliativa) L00
Schamberg's L81.7
schistosome B65.3
seasonal bullous L30.8
seborrheic L21.9
infantile L21.1
specified NEC L21.8
sensitization NOS L23.9
septic L08.0
solare L57.8
specified NEC L30.8
stasis I87.2
with
varicose ulcer — *see* Varix, leg, with ulcer, with
inflammation
varicose veins — *see* Varix, leg, with, inflammation
due to postthrombotic syndrome — *see* Syndrome,
postthrombotic

Dermatitis — *continued*
suppurative L08.0
traumatic NEC L30.4
trophoneurotica L13.0
ultraviolet (sun) (chronic exposure) L57.8
acute L56.8
varicose — *see* Varix, leg, with, inflammation
vegetans L10.1
verrucosa B43.0
vesicular, herpesviral B00.1
Dermatoarthritis, lipoid E78.81
Dermatochalasis, eyelid H02.839
left H02.836
lower H02.835
upper H02.834
right H02.833
lower H02.832
upper H02.831
Dermatofibroma (lenticulare) — *see* Neoplasm, skin,
benign
protuberans — *see* Neoplasm, skin, uncertain behavior
Dermatofibrosarcoma (pigmented) (protuberans) —
see Neoplasm, skin, malignant
Dermatographia L50.3
Dermatolysis (exfoliativa) (congenital) Q82.8
acquired L57.4
eyelids — *see* Blepharochalasis
palpebrarum — *see* Blepharochalasis
senile L57.4
Dermatomegaly NEC Q82.8
Dermatomucosomyositis M33.10
with
myopathy M33.12
respiratory involvement M33.11
specified organ involvement NEC M33.19
Dermatomycosis B36.9
furfuracea B36.0
specified type NEC B36.8
Dermatomyositis (acute) (chronic) (*see also* Dermatopolymyositis)
adult (*see also* Dermatomyositis, specified NEC) M33.10
in (due to) neoplastic disease (*see also* Neoplasm)
D49.9 [M36.0]
juvenile M33.00
with
myopathy M33.02
respiratory involvement M33.01
specified organ involvement NEC M33.09
without myopathy M33.03
specified NEC M33.10
with
myopathy M33.12
respiratory involvement M33.11
specified organ involvement NEC M33.19
without myopathy M33.13
Dermatoneuritis of children — *see* Poisoning, mercury
Dermatophilosis A48.8
Dermatophytid L30.2
Dermatophytide — *see* Dermatophytosis
Dermatophytosis (epidermophyton) (infection) (Microsporum) (tinea) (Trichophyton) B35.9
beard B35.0
body B35.4
capitis B35.0
corporis B35.4
deep-seated B35.8
disseminated B35.8
foot B35.3
granulomatous B35.8
groin B35.6
hand B35.2
nail B35.1
perianal (area) B35.6
scalp B35.0
specified NEC B35.8
Dermatopolymyositis M33.90
with
myopathy M33.92
respiratory involvement M33.91
specified organ involvement NEC M33.99
without myopathy M33.93
in neoplastic disease (*see also* Neoplasm)
D49.9 [M36.0]
juvenile M33.00
with
myopathy M33.02
respiratory involvement M33.01
specified organ involvement NEC M33.09

Dermatopolymyositis — *continued*
specified NEC M33.10
myopathy M33.12
respiratory involvement M33.11
specified organ involvement NEC M33.19
Dermatopolyneuritis — *see* Poisoning, mercury
Dermatorrhexis Q79.6
acquired L57.4
Dermatosclerosis (*see also* Scleroderma)
localized L94.0
Dermatosis L98.9
Andrews' L08.89
Bowen's — *see* Neoplasm, skin, in situ
bullous L13.9
specified NEC L13.8
exfoliativa L26
eyelid (noninfectious)
dermatitis — *see* Dermatitis, eyelid
discoid lupus erythematosus — *see* Lupus, erythematosus, eyelid
xeroderma — *see* Xeroderma, acquired, eyelid
factitial L98.1
febrile neutrophilic L98.2
gonococcal A54.89
herpetiformis L13.0
juvenile L12.2
linear IgA L13.8
menstrual NEC L98.8
neutrophilic, febrile L98.2
occupational — *see* Dermatitis, contact
papulosa nigra L82.1
pigmentary L81.9
progressive L81.7
Schamberg's L81.7
psychogenic F54
purpuric, pigmented L81.7
pustular, subcorneal L13.1
transient acantholytic L11.1
Dermographia, dermographism L50.3
Dermoid (cyst) (*see also* Neoplasm, benign, by site)
with malignant transformation C56- ☑
due to radiation (nonionizing) L57.8
Dermopathy
infiltrative with thyrotoxicosis — *see* Thyrotoxicosis
nephrogenic fibrosing L90.8
Dermophytosis — *see* Dermatophytosis
Descemetocele H18.73- ☑
Descemet's membrane — *see* condition
Descending — *see* condition
Descensus uteri — *see* Prolapse, uterus
Desert
rheumatism B38.0
sore — *see* Ulcer, skin
Desertion (newborn) — *see* Maltreatment
Desmoid (extra-abdominal) (tumor) — *see* Neoplasm,
connective tissue, uncertain behavior
abdominal D48.1
Despondency F32.9
Desquamation, skin R23.4
Destruction, destructive (*see also* Damage)
articular facet (*see also* Derangement, joint, specified
type NEC)
knee M23.8X- ☑
vertebra — *see* Spondylosis
bone (*see also* Disorder, bone, specified type NEC)
syphilitic A52.77
joint (*see also* Derangement, joint, specified type NEC)
sacroiliac M53.3
rectal sphincter K62.89
septum (nasal) J34.89
tuberculous NEC — *see* Tuberculosis
tympanum, tympanic membrane (nontraumatic) —
see Disorder, tympanic membrane, specified
NEC
vertebral disc — *see* Degeneration, intervertebral disc
Destructiveness (*see also* Disorder, conduct)
adjustment reaction — *see* Disorder, adjustment
Desultory labor O62.2
Detachment
cartilage — *see* Sprain
cervix, annular N88.8
complicating delivery O71.3
choroid (old) (postinfectional) (simple) (spontaneous)
H31.40- ☑
hemorrhagic H31.41- ☑
serous H31.42- ☑
ligament — *see* Sprain

Detachment — *continued*
  meniscus (knee) (*see also* Derangement, knee, meniscus, specified NEC)
    current injury — *see* Tear, meniscus
    due to old tear or injury — *see* Derangement, knee, meniscus, due to old tear
  retina (without retinal break) (serous) H33.2- ☑
    with retinal:
      break H33.00- ☑
        giant H33.03- ☑
        multiple H33.02- ☑
        single H33.01- ☑
      dialysis H33.04- ☑
    pigment epithelium — *see* Degeneration, retina, separation of layers, pigment epithelium detachment
    rhegmatogenous — *see* Detachment, retina, with retinal, break
    specified NEC H33.8
    total H33.05- ☑
    traction H33.4- ☑
  vitreous (body) H43.81 ☑
Detergent asthma J69.8
Deterioration
  epileptic F06.8
  general physical R53.81
  heart, cardiac — *see* Degeneration, myocardial
  mental — *see* Psychosis
  myocardial, myocardium — *see* Degeneration, myocardial
  senile (simple) R54
Deuteranomaly (anomalous trichromat) H53.53
Deuteranopia (complete) (incomplete) H53.53
Development
  abnormal, bone Q79.9
  arrested R62.50
    bone — *see* Arrest, development or growth, bone
    child R62.50
    due to malnutrition E45
  defective, congenital (*see also* Anomaly, by site)
    cauda equina Q06.3
    left ventricle Q24.8
      in hypoplastic left heart syndrome Q23.4
    valve Q24.8
      pulmonary Q22.3
  delayed (*see also* Delay, development) R62.50
    arithmetical skills F81.2
    language (skills) (expressive) F80.1
    learning skill F81.9
    mixed skills F88
    motor coordination F82
    reading F81.0
    specified learning skill NEC F81.89
    speech F80.9
    spelling F81.81
    written expression F81.81
  imperfect, congenital (*see also* Anomaly, by site)
    heart Q24.9
    lungs Q33.6
  incomplete
    bronchial tree Q32.4
    organ or site not listed — *see* Hypoplasia, by site
    respiratory system Q34.9
  sexual, precocious NEC E30.1
  tardy, mental (*see also* Disability, intellectual) F79
Developmental — *see* condition
  testing, infant or child — *see* Examination, child
Devergie's disease (pityriasis rubra pilaris) L44.0
Deviation (in)
  conjugate palsy (eye) (spastic) H51.0
  esophagus (acquired) K22.8
  eye, skew H51.8
  midline (jaw) (teeth) (dental arch) M26.29
    specified site NEC — *see* Malposition
  nasal septum J34.2
    congenital Q67.4
  opening and closing of the mandible M26.53
  organ or site, congenital NEC — *see* Malposition, congenital
  septum (nasal) (acquired) J34.2
    congenital Q67.4
  sexual F65.9
    bestiality F65.89
    erotomania F52.8
    exhibitionism F65.2
    fetishism, fetishistic F65.0
      transvestism F65.1
    frotteurism F65.81

Deviation — *continued*
  sexual — *continued*
    masochism F65.51
    multiple F65.89
    necrophilia F65.89
    nymphomania F52.8
    pederosis F65.4
    pedophilia F65.4
    sadism, sadomasochism F65.52
    satyriasis F52.8
    specified type NEC F65.89
    transvestism F64.1
    voyeurism F65.3
  teeth, midline M26.29
  trachea J39.8
  ureter, congenital Q62.61
Device
  cerebral ventricle (communicating) in situ Z98.2
  contraceptive — *see* Contraceptive, device
  drainage, cerebrospinal fluid, in situ Z98.2
Devic's disease G36.0
Devil's
  grip B33.0
  pinches (purpura simplex) D69.2
Devitalized tooth K04.99
Devonshire colic — *see* Poisoning, lead
Dextraposition, aorta Q20.3
  in tetralogy of Fallot Q21.3
Dextrinosis, limit (debrancher enzyme deficiency) E74.03
Dextrocardia (true) Q24.0
  with
    complete transposition of viscera Q89.3
    situs inversus Q89.3
Dextrotransposition, aorta Q20.3
d-glycericacidemia E72.59
Dhat syndrome F48.8
Dhobi itch B35.6
Di George's syndrome D82.1
Di Guglielmo's disease C94.0- ☑
Diabetes, diabetic (mellitus) (sugar) E11.9
  with
    amyotrophy E11.44
    arthropathy NEC E11.618
    autonomic (poly)neuropathy E11.43
    cataract E11.36
    Charcot's joints E11.610
    chronic kidney disease E11.22
    circulatory complication NEC E11.59
    complication E11.8
      specified NEC E11.69
    dermatitis E11.620
    foot ulcer E11.621
    gangrene E11.52
    gastroparalysis E11.43
    gastroparesis E11.43
    glomerulonephrosis, intracapillary E11.21
    glomerulosclerosis, intercapillary E11.21
    hyperglycemia E11.65
    hyperosmolarity E11.00
      with coma E11.01
    hypoglycemia E11.649
      with coma E11.641
    ketoacidosis E11.10
      with coma E11.11
    kidney complications NEC E11.29
    Kimmelstiel-Wilson disease E11.21
    loss of protective sensation (LOPS) — *see* Diabetes, by type, with neuropathy
    mononeuropathy E11.41
    myasthenia E11.44
    necrobiosis lipoidica E11.620
    nephropathy E11.21
    neuralgia E11.42
    neurologic complication NEC E11.49
    neuropathic arthropathy E11.610
    neuropathy E11.40
    ophthalmic complication NEC E11.39
    oral complication NEC E11.638
    osteomyelitis E11.69
    periodontal disease E11.630
    peripheral angiopathy E11.51
      with gangrene E11.52
    polyneuropathy E11.42
    renal complication NEC E11.29
    renal tubular degeneration E11.29
    retinopathy E11.319
      with macular edema E11.311

Diabetes, diabetic — *continued*
  with — *continued*
    retinopathy — *continued*
      with macular edema — *continued*
        resolved following treatment E11.37 ☑
      nonproliferative E11.329 ☑
        with macular edema E11.321 ☑
        mild E11.329 ☑
          with macular edema E11.321 ☑
        moderate E11.339 ☑
          with macular edema E11.331 ☑
        severe E11.349 ☑
          with macular edema E11.341 ☑
      proliferative E11.359 ☑
        with
          combined traction retinal detachment and rhegmatogenous retinal detachment E11.354 ☑
          macular edema E11.351 ☑
          stable proliferative diabetic retinopathy E11.355 ☑
          traction retinal detachment involving the macula E11.352 ☑
          traction retinal detachment not involving the macula E11.353 ☑
    skin complication NEC E11.628
    skin ulcer NEC E11.622
  brittle — *see* Diabetes, type 1
  bronzed E83.110
  complicating pregnancy — *see* Pregnancy, complicated by, diabetes
  dietary counseling and surveillance Z71.3
  due to
    autoimmune process — *see* Diabetes, type 1
    immune mediated pancreatic islet beta-cell destruction — *see* Diabetes, type 1
  due to drug or chemical E09.9
    with
      amyotrophy E09.44
      arthropathy NEC E09.618
      autonomic (poly)neuropathy E09.43
      cataract E09.36
      Charcot's joints E09.610
      chronic kidney disease E09.22
      circulatory complication NEC E09.59
      complication E09.8
        specified NEC E09.69
      dermatitis E09.620
      foot ulcer E09.621
      gangrene E09.52
      gastroparalysis E09.43
      gastroparesis E09.43
      glomerulonephrosis, intracapillary E09.21
      glomerulosclerosis, intercapillary E09.21
      hyperglycemia E09.65
      hyperosmolarity E09.00
        with coma E09.01
      hypoglycemia E09.649
        with coma E09.641
      ketoacidosis E09.10
        with coma E09.11
      kidney complications NEC E09.29
      Kimmelstiel-Wilson disease E09.21
      mononeuropathy E09.41
      myasthenia E09.44
      necrobiosis lipoidica E09.620
      nephropathy E09.21
      neuralgia E09.42
      neurologic complication NEC E09.49
      neuropathic arthropathy E09.610
      neuropathy E09.40
      ophthalmic complication NEC E09.39
      oral complication NEC E09.638
      periodontal disease E09.630
      peripheral angiopathy E09.51
        with gangrene E09.52
      polyneuropathy E09.42
      renal complication NEC E09.29
      renal tubular degeneration E09.29
      retinopathy E09.319
        with macular edema E09.311
        nonproliferative E09.329 ☑
          with macular edema E09.321 ☑
          mild E09.329 ☑
            with macular edema E09.321 ☑
          moderate E09.339 ☑
            with macular edema E09.331 ☑
          severe E09.349 ☑

Diabetes, diabetic — *continued*
  due to drug or chemical — *continued*
    with — *continued*
      retinopathy — *continued*
        nonproliferative — *continued*
          severe — *continued*
            with macular edema E09.341 ☑
          proliferative E09.359 ☑
            with
              combined traction retinal detach-
                ment and rhegmatogenous
                retinal detachment E09.354 ☑
              macular edema E09.351 ☑
              stable proliferative diabetic
                retinopathy E09.355 ☑
              traction retinal detachment involving
                the macula E09.352 ☑
              traction retinal detachment not in-
                volving the macula E09.353 ☑
          resolved following treatment E09.37 ☑
      skin complication NEC E09.628
      skin ulcer NEC E09.622
  due to underlying condition E08.9
    with
      amyotrophy E08.44
      arthropathy NEC E08.618
      autonomic (poly)neuropathy E08.43
      cataract E08.36
      Charcot's joints E08.610
      chronic kidney disease E08.22
      circulatory complication NEC E08.59
      complication E08.8
        specified NEC E08.69
      dermatitis E08.620
      foot ulcer E08.621
      gangrene E08.52
      gastroparalysis E08.43
      gastroparesis E08.43
      glomerulonephrosis, intracapillary E08.21
      glomerulosclerosis, intercapillary E08.21
      hyperglycemia E08.65
      hyperosmolarity E08.00
        with coma E08.01
      hypoglycemia E08.649
        with coma E08.641
      ketoacidosis E08.10
        with coma E08.11
      kidney complications NEC E08.29
      Kimmelsteil-WIlson disease E08.21
      mononeuropathy E08.41
      myasthenia E08.44
      necrobiosis lipoidica E08.620
      nephropathy E08.21
      neuralgia E08.42
      neurologic complication NEC E08.49
      neuropathic arthropathy E08.610
      neuropathy E08.40
      ophthalmic complication NEC E08.39
      oral complication NEC E08.638
      periodontal disease E08.630
      peripheral angiopathy E08.51
        with gangrene E08.52
      polyneuropathy E08.42
      renal complication NEC E08.29
      renal tubular degeneration E08.29
      retinopathy E08.319
        with macular edema E08.311
        nonproliferative E08.329 ☑
          with macular edema E08.321 ☑
          mild E08.329 ☑
            with macular edema E08.321 ☑
          moderate E08.339 ☑
            with macular edema E08.331 ☑
          severe E08.349 ☑
            with macular edema E08.341 ☑
        proliferative E08.359 ☑
          with
            combined traction retinal detach-
              ment and rhegmatogenous
              retinal detachment E08.354 ☑
            macular edema E08.351 ☑
            stable proliferative diabetic
              retinopathy E08.355 ☑
            traction retinal detachment involving
              the macula E08.352 ☑
            traction retinal detachment not in-
              volving the macula E08.353 ☑
        resolved following treatment E08.37 ☑

Diabetes, diabetic — *continued*
  due to underlying condition — *continued*
    with — *continued*
      skin complication NEC E08.628
      skin ulcer NEC E08.622
  gestational (in pregnancy) O24.419
    affecting newborn P70.0
    diet controlled O24.410
    in childbirth O24.429
      diet controlled O24.420
      insulin (and diet) controlled O24.424
      oral drug controlled (antidiabetic) (hypo-
        glycemic) O24.425
    insulin (and diet) controlled O24.414
    oral drug controlled (antidiabetic) (hypoglycemic)
      O24.415
    puerperal O24.439
      diet controlled O24.430
      insulin (and diet) controlled O24.434
      oral drug controlled (antidiabetic) (hypo-
        glycemic) O24.435
  hepatogenous E13.9
  idiopathic — *see* Diabetes, type 1
  inadequately controlled — *code to* Diabetes, by type,
      with hyperglycemia
  insipidus E23.2
    nephrogenic N25.1
    pituitary E23.2
    vasopressin resistant N25.1
  insulin dependent — *code to* type of diabetes
  juvenile-onset — *see* Diabetes, type 1
  ketosis-prone — *see* Diabetes, type 1
  latent R73.03
  neonatal (transient) P70.2
  non-insulin dependent — *code to* type of diabetes
  out of control — *code to* Diabetes, by type, with hyper-
      glycemia
  phosphate E83.39
  poorly controlled — *code to* Diabetes, by type, with
      hyperglycemia
  postpancreatectomy — *see* Diabetes, specified type
      NEC
  postprocedural — *see* Diabetes, specified type NEC
  secondary diabetes mellitus NEC — *see* Diabetes,
      specified type NEC
  specified type NEC E13.9
    with
      amyotrophy E13.44
      arthropathy NEC E13.618
      autonomic (poly)neuropathy E13.43
      cataract E13.36
      Charcot's joints E13.610
      chronic kidney disease E13.22
      circulatory complication NEC E13.59
      complication E13.8
        specified NEC E13.69
      dermatitis E13.620
      foot ulcer E13.621
      gangrene E13.52
      gastroparalysis E13.43
      gastroparesis E13.43
      glomerulonephrosis, intracapillary E13.21
      glomerulosclerosis, intercapillary E13.21
      hyperglycemia E13.65
      hyperosmolarity E13.00
        with coma E13.01
      hypoglycemia E13.649
        with coma E13.641
      ketoacidosis E13.10
        with coma E13.11
      kidney complications NEC E13.29
      Kimmelsteil-Wilson disease E13.21
      mononeuropathy E13.41
      myasthenia E13.44
      necrobiosis lipoidica E13.620
      nephropathy E13.21
      neuralgia E13.42
      neurologic complication NEC E13.49
      neuropathic arthropathy E13.610
      neuropathy E13.40
      ophthalmic complication NEC E13.39
      oral complication NEC E13.638
      periodontal disease E13.630
      peripheral angiopathy E13.51
        with gangrene E13.52
      polyneuropathy E13.42
      renal complication NEC E13.29
      renal tubular degeneration E13.29

Diabetes, diabetic — *continued*
  specified type — *continued*
    with — *continued*
      retinopathy E13.319
        with macular edema E13.311
        nonproliferative E13.329 ☑
          with macular edema E13.321 ☑
          mild E13.329 ☑
            with macular edema E13.321 ☑
          moderate E13.339 ☑
            with macular edema E13.331 ☑
          severe E13.349 ☑
            with macular edema E13.341 ☑
        proliferative E13.359 ☑
          with
            combined traction retinal detach-
              ment and rhegmatogenous
              retinal detachment E13.354 ☑
            macular edema E13.351 ☑
            stable proliferative diabetic
              retinopathy E13.355 ☑
            traction retinal detachment involving
              the macula E13.352 ☑
            traction retinal detachment not in-
              volving the macula E13.353 ☑
        resolved following treatment E13.37 ☑
      skin complication NEC E13.628
      skin ulcer NEC E13.622
  steroid-induced — *see* Diabetes, due to, drug or
      chemical
  type 1 E10.9
    with
      amyotrophy E10.44
      arthropathy NEC E10.618
      autonomic (poly)neuropathy E10.43
      cataract E10.36
      Charcot's joints E10.610
      chronic kidney disease E10.22
      circulatory complication NEC E10.59
      complication E10.8
        specified NEC E10.69
      dermatitis E10.620
      foot ulcer E10.621
      gangrene E10.52
      gastroparalysis E10.43
      gastroparesis E10.43
      glomerulonephrosis, intracapillary E10.21
      glomerulosclerosis, intercapillary E10.21
      hyperglycemia E10.65
      hypoglycemia E10.649
        with coma E10.641
      ketoacidosis E10.10
        with coma E10.11
      kidney complications NEC E10.29
      Kimmelsteil-Wilson disease E10.21
      mononeuropathy E10.41
      myasthenia E10.44
      necrobiosis lipoidica E10.620
      nephropathy E10.21
      neuralgia E10.42
      neurologic complication NEC E10.49
      neuropathic arthropathy E10.610
      neuropathy E10.40
      ophthalmic complication NEC E10.39
      oral complication NEC E10.638
      osteomyelitis E10.69
      periodontal disease E10.630
      peripheral angiopathy E10.51
        with gangrene E10.52
      polyneuropathy E10.42
      renal complication NEC E10.29
      renal tubular degeneration E10.29
      retinopathy E10.319
        with macular edema E10.311
        nonproliferative E10.329 ☑
          with macular edema E10.321 ☑
          mild E10.329 ☑
            with macular edema E10.321 ☑
          moderate E10.339 ☑
            with macular edema E10.331 ☑
          severe E10.349 ☑
            with macular edema E10.341 ☑
        proliferative E10.359 ☑
          with
            combined traction retinal detach-
              ment and rhegmatogenous
              retinal detachment E10.354 ☑
            macular edema E10.351 ☑

☑ **Additional Character Required** — **Refer to the Tabular List for Character Selection**   ▽ **Subterms under main terms may continue to next column or page**

Diabetes, diabetic — *continued*
  type 1 — *continued*
    with — *continued*
      retinopathy — *continued*
        proliferative — *continued*
          with — *continued*
            stable proliferative diabetic
              retinopathy E10.355 ☑
            traction retinal detachment involving
              the macula E10.352 ☑
            traction retinal detachment not in-
              volving the macula E10.353 ☑
          resolved following treatment E10.37 ☑
      skin complication NEC E10.628
      skin ulcer NEC E10.622
  type 2 E11.9
    with
      amyotrophy E11.44
      arthropathy NEC E11.618
      autonomic (poly)neuropathy E11.43
      cataract E11.36
      Charcot's joints E11.610
      chronic kidney disease E11.22
      circulatory complication NEC E11.59
      complication E11.8
        specified NEC E11.69
      dermatitis E11.620
      foot ulcer E11.621
      gangrene E11.52
      gastroparalysis E11.43
      gastroparesis E11.43
      glomerulonephrosis, intracapillary E11.21
      glomerulosclerosis, intercapillary E11.21
      hyperglycemia E11.65
      hyperosmolarity E11.00
        with coma E11.01
      hypoglycemia E11.649
        with coma E11.641
      ketoacidosis E11.10
        with coma E11.11
      kidney complications NEC E11.29
      Kimmelstiel-Wilson disease E11.21
      mononeuropathy E11.41
      myasthenia E11.44
      necrobiosis lipoidica E11.620
      nephropathy E11.21
      neuralgia E11.42
      neurologic complication NEC E11.49
      neuropathic arthropathy E11.610
      neuropathy E11.40
      ophthalmic complication NEC E11.39
      oral complication NEC E11.638
      osteomyelitis E11.69
      periodontal disease E11.630
      peripheral angiopathy E11.51
        with gangrene E11.52
      polyneuropathy E11.42
      renal complication NEC E11.29
      renal tubular degeneration E11.29
      retinopathy E11.319
        with macular edema E11.311
        nonproliferative E11.329 ☑
          with macular edema E11.321 ☑
          mild E11.329 ☑
            with macular edema E11.321 ☑
          moderate E11.339 ☑
            with macular edema E11.331 ☑
          severe E11.349 ☑
            with macular edema E11.341 ☑
        proliferative E11.359 ☑
          with
            combined traction retinal detach-
              ment and rhegmatogenous
              retinal detachment E11.354 ☑
            macular edema E11.351 ☑
            stable proliferative diabetic
              retinopathy E11.355 ☑
            traction retinal detachment involving
              the macula E11.352 ☑
            traction retinal detachment not in-
              volving the macula E11.353 ☑
        resolved following treatment E11.37 ☑
      skin complication NEC E11.628
      skin ulcer NEC E11.622
  uncontrolled
    meaning
      hyperglycemia — *see* Diabetes, by type, with,
        hyperglycemia

Diabetes, diabetic — *continued*
  uncontrolled — *continued*
    meaning — *continued*
      hypoglycemia — *see* Diabetes, by type, with,
        hypoglycemia
Diacyclothrombopathia D69.1
Diagnosis deferred R69
Dialysis (intermittent) (treatment)
  noncompliance (with) Z91.15
  renal (hemodialysis) (peritoneal), status Z99.2
  retina, retinal — *see* Detachment, retina, with retinal,
    dialysis
Diamond-Blackfan anemia (congenital hypoplastic)
  D61.01
Diamond-Gardener syndrome (autoerythrocyte sensi-
  tization) D69.2
Diaper rash L22
Diaphoresis (excessive) R61
Diaphragm — *see* condition
Diaphragmalgia R07.1
Diaphragmatitis, diaphragmitis J98.6
Diaphysial aclasis Q78.6
Diaphysitis — *see* Osteomyelitis, specified type NEC
Diarrhea, diarrheal (disease) (infantile) (inflammatory)
  R19.7
  achlorhydric K31.83
  allergic K52.29
    due to
      colitis — *see* Colitis, allergic
      enteritis — *see* Enteritis, allergic
  amebic (*see also* Amebiasis) A06.0
    with abscess — *see* Abscess, amebic
    acute A06.0
    chronic A06.1
    nondysenteric A06.2
  bacillary — *see* Dysentery, bacillary
  balantidial A07.0
  cachectic NEC K52.89
  Chilomastix A07.8
  choleriformis A00.1
  chronic (noninfectious) K52.9
  coccidial A07.3
  Cochin-China K90.1
    strongyloidiasis B78.0
  Dientamoeba A07.8
  dietetic (*see also* Diarrhea, allergic) K52.29
  drug-induced K52.1
  due to
    bacteria A04.9
      specified NEC A04.8
    Campylobacter A04.5
    Capillaria philippinensis B81.1
    Clostridium difficile
      not specified as recurrent A04.72
      recurrent A04.71
    Clostridium perfringens (C) (F) A04.8
    Cryptosporidium A07.2
    drugs K52.1
    Escherichia coli A04.4
      enteroaggregative A04.4
      enterohemorrhagic A04.3
      enteroinvasive A04.2
      enteropathogenic A04.0
      enterotoxigenic A04.1
      specified NEC A04.4
    food hypersensitivity (*see also* Diarrhea, allergic)
      K52.29
    Necator americanus B76.1
    S. japonicum B65.2
    specified organism NEC A08.8
      bacterial A04.8
      viral A08.39
    Staphylococcus A04.8
    Trichuris trichiuria B79
    virus — *see* Enteritis, viral
    Yersinia enterocolitica A04.6
  dysenteric A09
  endemic A09
  epidemic A09
  flagellate A07.9
  Flexner's (ulcerative) A03.1
  functional K59.1
    following gastrointestinal surgery K91.89
    psychogenic F45.8
  Giardia lamblia A07.1
  giardial A07.1
  hill K90.1
  infectious A09

Diarrhea, diarrheal — *continued*
  malarial — *see* Malaria
  mite B88.0
  mycotic NEC B49
  neonatal (noninfectious) P78.3
  nervous F45.8
  neurogenic K59.1
  noninfectious K52.9
  postgastrectomy K91.1
  postvagotomy K91.1
  protozoal A07.9
    specified NEC A07.8
  psychogenic F45.8
  specified
    bacterium NEC A04.8
    virus NEC A08.39
  strongyloidiasis B78.0
  toxic K52.1
  trichomonal A07.8
  tropical K90.1
  tuberculous A18.32
  viral — *see* Enteritis, viral
Diastasis
  cranial bones M84.88
    congenital NEC Q75.8
  joint (traumatic) — *see* Dislocation
  muscle M62.00
    ankle M62.07- ☑
    congenital Q79.8
    foot M62.07- ☑
    forearm M62.03- ☑
    hand M62.04- ☑
    lower leg M62.06- ☑
    pelvic region M62.05- ☑
    shoulder region M62.01- ☑
    specified site NEC M62.08
    thigh M62.05- ☑
    upper arm M62.02- ☑
  recti (abdomen)
    complicating delivery O71.89
    congenital Q79.59
Diastema, tooth, teeth, fully erupted M26.32
Diastematomyelia Q06.2
Diataxia, cerebral G80.4
Diathesis
  allergic — *see* History, allergy
  bleeding (familial) D69.9
  cystine (familial) E72.00
  gouty — *see* Gout
  hemorrhagic (familial) D69.9
    newborn NEC P53
  spasmophilic R29.0
Diaz's disease or osteochondrosis (juvenile) (talus) —
  see Osteochondrosis, juvenile, tarsus
Dibothriocephalus, dibothriocephaliasis (latus) (infection) (infestation) B70.0
  larval B70.1
Dicephalus, dicephaly Q89.4
Dichotomy, teeth K00.2
Dichromat, dichromatopsia (congenital) — *see* Deficiency, color vision
Dichuchwa A65
Dicroceliasis B66.2
Didelphia, didelphys — *see* Double uterus
Didymytis N45.1
  with orchitis N45.3
Dietary
  inadequacy or deficiency E63.9
  surveillance and counseling Z71.3
Dietl's crisis N13.8
Dieulafoy lesion (hemorrhagic)
  duodenum K31.82
  esophagus K22.8
  intestine (colon) K63.81
  stomach K31.82
Difficult, difficulty (in)
  acculturation Z60.3
  feeding R63.3
    newborn P92.9
      breast P92.5
      specified NEC P92.8
    nonorganic (infant or child) F98.29
  intubation, in anesthesia T88.4 ☑
  mechanical, gastroduodenal stoma K91.89
    causing obstruction (*see also* Obstruction, intestine,
      postoperative) K91.30
  micturition
    need to immediately re-void R39.191

☑ Subterms under main terms may continue to next column or page   ☑ Additional Character Required — Refer to the Tabular List for Character Selection   99

Diabetes, diabetic — Difficult, difficulty

Difficult, difficulty — continued
  micturition — continued
    position dependent R39.192
    specified NEC R39.198
  reading (developmental) F81.0
    secondary to emotional disorders F93.9
  spelling (specific) F81.81
    with reading disorder F81.89
    due to inadequate teaching Z55.8
  swallowing — see Dysphagia
  walking R26.2
  work
    conditions NEC Z56.5
    schedule Z56.3
Diffuse — see condition
Digestive — see condition
Dihydropyrimidine dehydrogenase disease (DPD) E88.89
Diktyoma — see Neoplasm, malignant, by site
Dilaceration, tooth K00.4
Dilatation
  anus K59.8
    venule — see Hemorrhoids
  aorta (focal) (general) — see Ectasia, aorta
    with aneuysm — see Aneurysm, aorta
    congenital Q25.44
  artery — see Aneurysm
  bladder (sphincter) N32.89
    congenital Q64.79
  blood vessel I99.8
  bronchial J47.9
    with
      exacerbation (acute) J47.1
      lower respiratory infection J47.0
  calyx (due to obstruction) — see Hydronephrosis
  capillaries I78.8
  cardiac (acute) (chronic) (see also Hypertrophy, cardiac)
    congenital Q24.8
      valve NEC Q24.8
        pulmonary Q22.3
    valve — see Endocarditis
  cavum septi pellucidi Q06.8
  cervix (uteri) (see also Incompetency, cervix)
    incomplete, poor, slow complicating delivery O62.0
  colon K59.39
    congenital Q43.1
    psychogenic F45.8
    toxic K59.31
  common duct (acquired) K83.8
    congenital Q44.5
  cystic duct (acquired) K82.8
    congenital Q44.5
  duct, mammary — see Ectasia, mammary duct
  duodenum K59.8
  esophagus K22.8
    congenital Q39.5
    due to achalasia K22.0
  eustachian tube, congenital Q17.8
  gallbladder K82.8
  gastric — see Dilatation, stomach
  heart (acute) (chronic) (see also Hypertrophy, cardiac)
    congenital Q24.8
    valve — see Endocarditis
  ileum K59.8
    psychogenic F45.8
  jejunum K59.8
    psychogenic F45.8
  kidney (calyx) (collecting structures) (cystic) (parenchyma) (pelvis) (idiopathic) N28.89
  lacrimal passages or duct — see Disorder, lacrimal system, changes
  lymphatic vessel I89.0
  mammary duct — see Ectasia, mammary duct
  Meckel's diverticulum (congenital) Q43.0
    malignant — see Table of Neoplasms, small intestine, malignant
  myocardium (acute) (chronic) — see Hypertrophy, cardiac
  organ or site, congenital NEC — see Distortion
  pancreatic duct K86.89
  pericardium — see Pericarditis
  pharynx J39.2
  prostate N42.89
  pulmonary
    artery (idiopathic) I28.8
    valve, congenital Q22.3
  pupil H57.04
  rectum K59.39

Dilatation — continued
  saccule, congenital Q16.5
  salivary gland (duct) K11.8
  sphincter ani K62.89
  stomach K31.89
    acute K31.0
    psychogenic F45.8
  submaxillary duct K11.8
  trachea, congenital Q32.1
  ureter (idiopathic) N28.82
    congenital Q62.2
    due to obstruction N13.4
  urethra (acquired) N36.8
  vasomotor I73.9
  vein I86.8
  ventricular, ventricle (acute) (chronic) (see also Hypertrophy, cardiac)
    cerebral, congenital Q04.8
  venule NEC I86.8
  vesical orifice N32.89
Dilated, dilation — see Dilatation
Diminished, diminution
  hearing (acuity) — see Deafness
  sense or sensation (cold) (heat) (tactile) (vibratory) R20.8
  vision NEC H54.7
  vital capacity R94.2
Diminuta taenia B71.0
Dimitri-Sturge-Weber disease Q85.8
Dimple
  congenital sacral Q82.6
  parasacral Q82.6
  pilonidal or postanal — see Cyst, pilonidal
Dioctophyme renalis (infection) (infestation) B83.8
Dipetalonemiasis B74.4
Diphallus Q55.69
Diphtheria, diphtheritic (gangrenous) (hemorrhagic) A36.9
  carrier (suspected) Z22.2
  cutaneous A36.3
  faucial A36.0
  infection of wound A36.3
  laryngeal A36.2
  myocarditis A36.81
  nasal, anterior A36.89
  nasopharyngeal A36.1
  neurological complication A36.89
  pharyngeal A36.0
  specified site NEC A36.89
  tonsillar A36.0
Diphyllobothriasis (intestine) B70.0
  larval B70.1
Diplacusis H93.22- ☑
Diplegia (upper limbs) G83.0
  congenital (cerebral) G80.8
  facial G51.0
  lower limbs G82.20
  spastic G80.1
Diplococcus, diplococcal — see condition
Diplopia H53.2
Dipsomania F10.20
  with
    psychosis — see Psychosis, alcoholic
    remission F10.21
Dipylidiasis B71.1
DIRA (deficiency of interleukin 1 receptor antagonist) M04.8
Direction, teeth, abnormal, fully erupted M26.30
Dirofilariasis B74.8
Dirt-eating child F98.3
Disability, disabilities
  heart — see Disease, heart
  intellectual F79
    with
      autistic features F84.9
      mild (I.Q. 50-69) F70
      moderate (I.Q. 35-49) F71
      profound (I.Q. under 20) F73
      severe (I.Q. 20-34) F72
      specified level NEC F78
  knowledge acquisition F81.9
  learning F81.9
  limiting activities Z73.6
  spelling, specific F81.81
Disappearance of family member Z63.4
Disarticulation — see Amputation
  meaning traumatic amputation — see Amputation, traumatic

Discharge (from)
  abnormal finding in — see Abnormal, specimen
  breast (female) (male) N64.52
  diencephalic autonomic idiopathic — see Epilepsy, specified NEC
  ear (see also Otorrhea)
    blood — see Otorrhagia
  excessive urine R35.8
  nipple N64.52
  penile R36.9
  postnasal R09.82
  prison, anxiety concerning Z65.2
  urethral R36.9
    without blood R36.0
    hematospermia R36.1
  vaginal N89.8
Discitis, diskitis M46.40
  cervical region M46.42
  cervicothoracic region M46.43
  lumbar region M46.46
  lumbosacral region M46.47
  multiple sites M46.49
  occipito-atlanto-axial region M46.41
  pyogenic — see Infection, intervertebral disc, pyogenic
  sacrococcygeal region M46.48
  thoracic region M46.44
  thoracolumbar region M46.45
Discoid
  meniscus (congenital) Q68.6
  semilunar cartilage (congenital) — see Derangement, knee, meniscus, specified NEC
Discoloration
  nails L60.8
  teeth (posteruptive) K03.7
    during formation K00.8
Discomfort
  chest R07.89
  visual H53.14- ☑
Discontinuity, ossicles, ear H74.2- ☑
Discord (with)
  boss Z56.4
  classmates Z55.4
  counselor Z64.4
  employer Z56.4
  family Z63.8
  fellow employees Z56.4
  in-laws Z63.1
  landlord Z59.2
  lodgers Z59.2
  neighbors Z59.2
  probation officer Z64.4
  social worker Z64.4
  teachers Z55.4
  workmates Z56.4
Discordant connection
  atrioventricular (congenital) Q20.5
  ventriculoarterial Q20.3
Discrepancy
  centric occlusion maximum intercuspation M26.55
  leg length (acquired) — see Deformity, limb, unequal length
    congenital — see Defect, reduction, lower limb
  uterine size date O26.84- ☑
Discrimination
  ethnic Z60.5
  political Z60.5
  racial Z60.5
  religious Z60.5
  sex Z60.5
Disease, diseased (see also Syndrome)
  absorbent system I87.8
  acid-peptic K30
  Acosta's T70.29 ☑
  Adams-Stokes (-Morgagni) (syncope with heart block) I45.9
  Addison's anemia (pernicious) D51.0
  adenoids (and tonsils) J35.9
  adrenal (capsule) (cortex) (gland) (medullary) E27.9
    hyperfunction E27.0
    specified NEC E27.8
  ainhum L94.6
  airway
    obstructive, chronic J44.9
      due to
        cotton dust J66.0
        specific organic dusts NEC J66.8
      reactive — see Asthma
  akamushi (scrub typhus) A75.3

☑ **Additional Character Required** — **Refer to the Tabular List for Character Selection**   ▽ **Subterms under main terms may continue to next column or page**

Disease, diseased — *continued*
- Albers-Schönberg (marble bones) Q78.2
- Albert's — *see* Tendinitis, Achilles
- alimentary canal K63.9
- alligator-skin Q80.9
  - acquired L85.0
- alpha heavy chain C88.3
- alpine T70.29 ☑
- altitude T70.20 ☑
- alveolar ridge
  - edentulous K06.9
    - specified NEC K06.8
- alveoli, teeth K08.9
- Alzheimer's G30.9 [F02.80]
  - with behavioral disturbance G30.9 [F02.81]
  - early onset G30.0 [F02.80]
    - with behavioral disturbance G30.0 [F02.81]
  - late onset G30.1 [F02.80]
    - with behavioral disturbance G30.1 [F02.81]
  - specified NEC G30.8 [F02.80]
    - with behavioral disturbance G30.8 [F02.81]
- amyloid — *see* Amyloidosis
- Andersen's (glycogenosis IV) E74.09
- Andes T70.29 ☑
- Andrews' (bacterid) L08.89
- angiospastic I73.9
  - cerebral G45.9
  - vein I87.8
- anterior
  - chamber H21.9
  - horn cell G12.29
- antiglomerular basement membrane (anti- GBM) antibody M31.0
  - tubulo-interstitial nephritis N12
- antral — *see* Sinusitis, maxillary
- anus K62.9
  - specified NEC K62.89
- aorta (nonsyphilitic) I77.9
  - syphilitic NEC A52.02
- aortic (heart) (valve) I35.9
  - rheumatic I06.9
- Apollo B30.3
- aponeuroses — *see* Enthesopathy
- appendix K38.9
  - specified NEC K38.8
- aqueous (chamber) H21.9
- Arnold-Chiari — *see* Arnold-Chiari disease
- arterial I77.9
  - occlusive — *see* Occlusion, by site
  - due to stricture or stenosis I77.1
- arteriocardiorenal — *see* Hypertension, cardiorenal
- arteriolar (generalized) (obliterative) I77.9
- arteriorenal — *see* Hypertension, kidney
- arteriosclerotic (*see also* Arteriosclerosis)
  - cardiovascular — *see* Disease, heart, ischemic, atherosclerotic
  - coronary (artery) — *see* Disease, heart, ischemic, atherosclerotic
  - heart — *see* Disease, heart, ischemic, atherosclerotic
- artery I77.9
  - cerebral I67.9
  - coronary I25.10
    - with angina pectoris — *see* Arteriosclerosis, coronary (artery)
- arthropod-borne NOS (viral) A94
  - specified type NEC A93.8
- atticoantral, chronic H66.20
  - left H66.22
    - with right H66.23
  - right H66.21
    - with left H66.23
- auditory canal — *see* Disorder, ear, external
- auricle, ear NEC — *see* Disorder, pinna
- Australian X A83.4
- autoimmune (systemic) NOS M35.9
  - hemolytic (cold type) (warm type) D59.1
    - drug-induced D59.0
  - thyroid E06.3
- aviator's — *see* Effect, adverse, high altitude
- Ayerza's (pulmonary artery sclerosis with pulmonary hypertension) I27.0
- Babington's (familial hemorrhagic telangiectasia) I78.0
- bacterial A49.9
  - specified NEC A48.8
  - zoonotic A28.9
    - specified type NEC A28.8
- Baelz's (cheilitis glandularis apostematosa) K13.0

Disease, diseased — *continued*
- bagasse J67.1
- balloon — *see* Effect, adverse, high altitude
- Bang's (brucella abortus) A23.1
- Bannister's T78.3 ☑
- barometer makers' — *see* Poisoning, mercury
- Barraquer (-Simons') (progressive lipodystrophy) E88.1
- Barrett's — *see* Barrett's, esophagus
- Bartholin's gland N75.9
- basal ganglia G25.9
  - degenerative G23.9
    - specified NEC G23.8
  - specified NEC G25.89
- Basedow's (exophthalmic goiter) — *see* Hyperthyroidism, with, goiter (diffuse)
- Bateman's B08.1
- Batten-Steinert G71.11
- Battey A31.0
- Beard's (neurasthenia) F48.8
- Becker
  - idiopathic mural endomyocardial I42.3
  - myotonia congenita G71.12
- Begbie's (exophthalmic goiter) — *see* Hyperthyroidism, with, goiter (diffuse)
- behavioral, organic F07.9
- Beigel's (white piedra) B36.2
- Benson's — *see* Deposit, crystalline
- Bernard-Soulier (thrombopathy) D69.1
- Bernhardt (-Roth) — *see* Mononeuropathy, lower limb, meralgia paresthetica
- Biermer's (pernicious anemia) D51.0
- bile duct (common) (hepatic) K83.9
  - with calculus, stones — *see* Calculus, bile duct
  - specified NEC K83.8
- biliary (tract) K83.9
  - specified NEC K83.8
- Billroth's — *see* Spina bifida
- bird fancier's J67.2
- black lung J60
- bladder N32.9
  - in (due to)
    - schistosomiasis (bilharziasis) B65.0 [N33]
  - specified NEC N32.89
- bleeder's D66
- blood D75.9
  - forming organs D75.9
  - vessel I99.9
- Bloodgood's — *see* Mastopathy, cystic
- Bodechtel-Guttmann (subacute sclerosing panencephalitis) A81.1
- bone (*see also* Disorder, bone)
  - aluminum M83.4
  - fibrocystic NEC
    - jaw M27.49
  - bone-marrow D75.9
- Borna A83.9
- Bornholm (epidemic pleurodynia) B33.0
- Bouchard's (myopathic dilatation of the stomach) K31.0
- Bouillaud's (rheumatic heart disease) I01.9
- Bourneville (-Brissaud) (tuberous sclerosis) Q85.1
- Bouveret (-Hoffmann) (paroxysmal tachycardia) I47.9
- bowel K63.9
  - functional K59.9
    - psychogenic F45.8
- brain G93.9
  - arterial, artery I67.9
  - arteriosclerotic I67.2
  - congenital Q04.9
  - degenerative — *see* Degeneration, brain
  - inflammatory — *see* Encephalitis
  - organic G93.9
    - arteriosclerotic I67.2
  - parasitic NEC B71.9 [G94]
  - senile NEC G31.1
  - specified NEC G93.89
- breast (*see also* Disorder, breast) N64.9
  - cystic (chronic) — *see* Mastopathy, cystic
  - fibrocystic — *see* Mastopathy, cystic
  - Paget's
    - female, unspecified side C50.91- ☑
    - male, unspecified side C50.92- ☑
  - specified NEC N64.89
- Breda's — *see* Yaws
- Bretonneau's (diphtheritic malignant angina) A36.0
- Bright's — *see* Nephritis
  - arteriosclerotic — *see* Hypertension, kidney
- Brill's (recrudescent typhus) A75.1

Disease, diseased — *continued*
- Brill-Zinsser (recrudescent typhus) A75.1
- Brion-Kayser — *see* Fever, paratyphoid
- broad
  - beta E78.2
  - ligament (noninflammatory) N83.9
    - inflammatory — *see* Disease, pelvis, inflammatory
    - specified NEC N83.8
- Brocq-Duhring (dermatitis herpetiformis) L13.0
- Brocq's
  - meaning
    - dermatitis herpetiformis L13.0
    - prurigo L28.2
- bronchopulmonary J98.4
- bronchus NEC J98.09
- bronze Addison's E27.1
  - tuberculous A18.7
- budgerigar fancier's J67.2
- Buerger's (thromboangiitis obliterans) I73.1
- bullous L13.9
  - chronic of childhood L12.2
  - specified NEC L13.8
- Bürger-Grütz (essential familial hyperlipemia) E78.3
- bursa — *see* Bursopathy
- caisson T70.3 ☑
- California — *see* Coccidioidomycosis
- capillaries I78.9
  - specified NEC I78.8
- Carapata A68.0
- cardiac — *see* Disease, heart
- cardiopulmonary, chronic I27.9
- cardiorenal (hepatic) (hypertensive) (vascular) — *see* Hypertension, cardiorenal
- cardiovascular (atherosclerotic) I25.10
  - with angina pectoris — *see* Arteriosclerosis, coronary (artery),
  - congenital Q28.9
  - hypertensive — *see* Hypertension, heart
  - newborn P29.9
    - specified NEC P29.89
  - renal (hypertensive) — *see* Hypertension, cardiorenal
  - syphilitic (asymptomatic) A52.00
- cartilage — *see* Disorder, cartilage
- Castellani's A69.8
- Castleman (unicentric) (multicentric) D47.Z2
  - HHV-8-associated (*see also* Herpesvirus, human, 8) D47.Z2
- cat-scratch A28.1
- Cavare's (familial periodic paralysis) G72.3
- cecum K63.9
- celiac (adult) (infantile) (with steatorrhea) K90.0
- cellular tissue L98.9
- central core G71.2
- cerebellar, cerebellum — *see* Disease, brain
- cerebral (*see also* Disease, brain)
  - degenerative — *see* Degeneration, brain
- cerebrospinal G96.9
- cerebrovascular I67.9
  - acute I67.89
    - embolic I63.4- ☑
    - thrombotic I63.3- ☑
  - arteriosclerotic I67.2
  - specified NEC I67.89
- cervix (uteri) (noninflammatory) N88.9
  - inflammatory — *see* Cervicitis
  - specified NEC N88.8
- Chabert's A22.9
- Chandler's (osteochondritis dissecans, hip) — *see* Osteochondritis, dissecans, hip
- Charlouis — *see* Yaws
- Chédiak-Steinbrinck (-Higashi) (congenital gigantism of peroxidase granules) E70.330
- chest J98.9
- Chiari's (hepatic vein thrombosis) I82.0
- Chicago B40.9
- Chignon B36.8
- chigo, chigoe B88.1
- childhood granulomatous D71
- Chinese liver fluke B66.1
- chlamydial A74.9
  - specified NEC A74.89
- cholecystic K82.9
- choroid H31.9
  - specified NEC H31.8
- Christmas D67
- chronic bullous of childhood L12.2

Disease, diseased — *continued*
chylomicron retention E78.3
ciliary body H21.9
  specified NEC H21.89
circulatory (system) NEC I99.8
  newborn P29.9
  syphilitic A52.00
    congenital A50.54
coagulation factor deficiency (congenital) — *see* Defect, coagulation
coccidioidal — *see* Coccidioidomycosis
cold
  agglutinin or hemoglobinuria D59.1
    paroxysmal D59.6
  hemagglutinin (chronic) D59.1
collagen NOS (nonvascular) (vascular) M35.9
  specified NEC M35.8
colon K63.9
  functional K59.9
    congenital Q43.2
  ischemic (*see also* Ischemia, intestine, acute) K55.039
colonic inflammatory bowel, unclassified (IBDU) K52.3
combined system — *see* Degeneration, combined
compressed air T70.3 ☑
Concato's (pericardial polyserositis) A19.9
  nontubercular I31.1
  pleural — *see* Pleurisy, with effusion
conjunctiva H11.9
  chlamydial A74.0
  specified NEC H11.89
  viral B30.9
    specified NEC B30.8
connective tissue, systemic (diffuse) M35.9
  in (due to)
    hypogammaglobulinemia D80.1 [M36.8]
    ochronosis E70.29 [M36.8]
  specified NEC M35.8
Conor and Bruch's (boutonneuse fever) A77.1
Cooper's — *see* Mastopathy, cystic
Cori's (glycogenosis III) E74.03
corkhandler's or corkworker's J67.3
cornea H18.9
  specified NEC H18.89- ☑
coronary (artery) — *see* Disease, heart, ischemic, atherosclerotic
  congenital Q24.5
  ostial, syphilitic (aortic) (mitral) (pulmonary) A52.03
corpus cavernosum N48.9
  specified NEC N48.89
Cotugno's — *see* Sciatica
coxsackie (virus) NEC B34.1
cranial nerve NOS G52.9
Creutzfeldt-Jakob — *see* Creutzfeldt-Jakob disease or syndrome
Crocq's (acrocyanosis) I73.89
Crohn's — *see* Enteritis, regional
Curschmann G71.11
cystic
  breast (chronic) — *see* Mastopathy, cystic
  kidney, congenital Q61.9
  liver, congenital Q44.6
  lung J98.4
    congenital Q33.0
cytomegalic inclusion (generalized) B25.9
  with pneumonia B25.0
  congenital P35.1
cytomegaloviral B25.9
  specified NEC B25.8
Czerny's (periodic hydrarthrosis of the knee) — *see* Effusion, joint, knee
Daae (-Finsen) (epidemic pleurodynia) B33.0
Darling's — *see* Histoplasmosis capsulati
de Quervain's (tendon sheath) M65.4
  thyroid (subacute granulomatous thyroiditis) E06.1
Débove's (splenomegaly) R16.1
deer fly — *see* Tularemia
Degos' I77.89
demyelinating, demyelinizating (nervous system) G37.9
  multiple sclerosis G35
  specified NEC G37.8
dense deposit (*see also* N00-N07 with fourth character .6) N05.6
deposition, hydroxyapatite — *see* Disease, hydroxyapatite deposition
Devergie's (pityriasis rubra pilaris) L44.0
Devic's G36.0

Disease, diseased — *continued*
diaphorase deficiency D74.0
diaphragm J98.6
diarrheal, infectious NEC A09
digestive system K92.9
  specified NEC K92.89
disc, degenerative — *see* Degeneration, intervertebral disc
discogenic (*see also* Displacement, intervertebral disc NEC)
  with myelopathy — *see* Disorder, disc, with, myelopathy
diverticular — *see* Diverticula
Dubois (thymus) A50.59 [E35]
Duchenne-Griesinger G71.0
Duchenne's
  muscular dystrophy G71.0
  pseudohypertrophy, muscles G71.0
ductless glands E34.9
Duhring's (dermatitis herpetiformis) L13.0
duodenum K31.9
  specified NEC K31.89
Dupré's (meningism) R29.1
Dupuytren's (muscle contracture) M72.0
Durand-Nicholas-Favre (climatic bubo) A55
Duroziez's (congenital mitral stenosis) Q23.2
ear — *see* Disorder, ear
Eberth's — *see* Fever, typhoid
Ebola (virus) A98.4
Ebstein's heart Q22.5
Echinococcus — *see* Echinococcus
echovirus NEC B34.1
Eddowes' (brittle bones and blue sclera) Q78.0
edentulous (alveolar) ridge K06.9
  specified NEC K06.8
Edsall's T67.2 ☑
Eichstedt's (pityriasis versicolor) B36.0
Eisenmenger's (irreversible) I27.83
Ellis-van Creveld (chondroectodermal dysplasia) Q77.6
end stage renal (ESRD) N18.6
  due to hypertension I12.0
endocrine glands or system NEC E34.9
endomyocardial (eosinophilic) I42.3
English (rickets) E55.0
enteroviral, enterovirus NEC B34.1
  central nervous system NEC A88.8
epidemic B99.9
  specified NEC B99.8
epididymis N50.9
Erb (-Landouzy) G71.0
Erdheim-Chester (ECD) E88.89
esophagus K22.9
  functional K22.4
  psychogenic F45.8
  specified NEC K22.8
Eulenburg's (congenital paramyotonia) G71.19
eustachian tube — *see* Disorder, eustachian tube
external
  auditory canal — *see* Disorder, ear, external
  ear — *see* Disorder, ear, external
extrapyramidal G25.9
  specified NEC G25.89
eye H57.9
  anterior chamber H21.9
  inflammatory NEC H57.8
  muscle (external) — *see* Strabismus
  specified NEC H57.8
  syphilitic — *see* Oculopathy, syphilitic
eyeball H44.9
  specified NEC H44.89
eyelid — *see* Disorder, eyelid
  specified NEC — *see* Disorder, eyelid, specified type NEC
eyeworm of Africa B74.3
facial nerve (seventh) G51.9
  newborn (birth injury) P11.3
Fahr (of brain) G23.8
Fahr Volhard (of kidney) I12.- ☑
fallopian tube (noninflammatory) N83.9
  inflammatory — *see* Salpingo-oophoritis
  specified NEC N83.8
familial periodic paralysis G72.3
Fanconi's (congenital pancytopenia) D61.09
fascia NEC (*see also* Disorder, muscle)
  inflammatory — *see* Myositis
  specified NEC M62.89
Fauchard's (periodontitis) — *see* Periodontitis
Favre-Durand-Nicolas (climatic bubo) A55

Disease, diseased — *continued*
Fede's K14.0
Feer's — *see* Poisoning, mercury
female pelvic inflammatory (*see also* Disease, pelvis, inflammatory) N73.9
  syphilitic (secondary) A51.42
  tuberculous A18.17
Fernels' (aortic aneurysm) I71.9
fibrocaseous of lung — *see* Tuberculosis, pulmonary
fibrocystic — *see* Fibrocystic disease
Fiedler's (leptospiral jaundice) A27.0
fifth B08.3
file-cutter's — *see* Poisoning, lead
fish-skin Q80.9
  acquired L85.0
Flajani (-Basedow) (exophthalmic goiter) — *see* Hyperthyroidism, with, goiter (diffuse)
flax-dresser's J66.1
fluke — *see* Infestation, fluke
foot and mouth B08.8
foot process N04.9
Forbes' (glycogenosis III) E74.03
Fordyce-Fox (apocrine miliaria) L75.2
Fordyce's (ectopic sebaceous glands) (mouth) Q38.6
Forestier's (rhizomelic pseudopolyarthritis) M35.3
  meaning ankylosing hyperostosis — *see* Hyperostosis, ankylosing
Fothergill's
  neuralgia — *see* Neuralgia, trigeminal
  scarlatina anginosa A38.9
Fournier (gangrene) N49.3
  female N76.89
fourth B08.8
Fox (-Fordyce) (apocrine miliaria) L75.2
Francis' — *see* Tularemia
Franklin C88.2
Frei's (climatic bubo) A55
Friedreich's
  combined systemic or ataxia G11.1
  myoclonia G25.3
frontal sinus — *see* Sinusitis, frontal
fungus NEC B49
Gaisböck's (polycythemia hypertonica) D75.1
gallbladder K82.9
  calculus — *see* Calculus, gallbladder
  cholecystitis — *see* Cholecystitis
  cholesterolosis K82.4
  fistula — *see* Fistula, gallbladder
  hydrops K82.1
  obstruction — *see* Obstruction, gallbladder
  perforation K82.2
  specified NEC K82.8
gamma heavy chain C88.2
Gamna's (siderotic splenomegaly) D73.2
Gamstorp's (adynamia episodica hereditaria) G72.3
Gandy-Nanta (siderotic splenomegaly) D73.2
ganister J62.8
gastric — *see* Disease, stomach
gastroesophageal reflux (GERD) K21.9
  with esophagitis K21.0
gastrointestinal (tract) K92.9
  amyloid E85.4
  functional K59.9
    psychogenic F45.8
  specified NEC K92.89
Gee (-Herter) (-Heubner) (-Thaysen) (nontropical sprue) K90.0
genital organs
  female N94.9
  male N50.9
Gerhardt's (erythromelalgia) I73.81
Gibert's (pityriasis rosea) L42
Gierke's (glycogenosis I) E74.01
Gilles de la Tourette's (motor-verbal tic) F95.2
gingiva K06.9
  plaque induced K05.00
  specified NEC K06.8
gland (lymph) I89.9
Glanzmann's (hereditary hemorrhagic thrombasthenia) D69.1
glass-blower's (cataract) — *see* Cataract, specified NEC
  salivary gland hypertrophy K11.1
Glisson's — *see* Rickets
globe H44.9
  specified NEC H44.89
glomerular (*see also* Glomerulonephritis)
  with edema — *see* Nephrosis
  acute — *see* Nephritis, acute

   ☑ **Additional Character Required** — **Refer to the Tabular List for Character Selection**   🔽 **Subterms under main terms may continue to next column or page**

Disease, diseased — *continued*
- glomerular (*see also* Glomerulonephritis) — *continued*
  - chronic — *see* Nephritis, chronic
  - minimal change N05.0
  - rapidly progressive N01.9
- glycogen storage E74.00
  - Andersen's E74.09
  - Cori's E74.03
  - Forbes' E74.03
  - generalized E74.00
  - glucose-6-phosphatase deficiency E74.01
  - heart E74.02 [I43]
  - hepatorenal E74.09
  - Hers' E74.09
  - liver and kidney E74.09
  - McArdle's E74.04
  - muscle phosphofructokinase E74.09
  - myocardium E74.02 [I43]
  - Pompe's E74.02
  - Tauri's E74.09
  - type 0 E74.09
  - type I E74.01
  - type II E74.02
  - type III E74.03
  - type IV E74.09
  - type V E74.04
  - type VI-XI E74.09
  - Von Gierke's E74.01
- Goldstein's (familial hemorrhagic telangiectasia) I78.0
- gonococcal NOS A54.9
- graft-versus-host (GVH) D89.813
  - acute D89.810
  - acute on chronic D89.812
  - chronic D89.811
- grainhandler's J67.8
- granulomatous (childhood) (chronic) D71
- Graves' (exophthalmic goiter) — *see* Hyperthyroidism, with, goiter (diffuse)
- Griesinger's — *see* Ancylostomiasis
- Grisel's M43.6
- Gruby's (tinea tonsurans) B35.0
- Guillain-Barré G61.0
- Guinon's (motor-verbal tic) F95.2
- gum K06.9
- gynecological N94.9
- H (Hartnup's) E72.02
- Haff — *see* Poisoning, mercury
- Hageman (congenital factor XII deficiency) D68.2
- hair (color) (shaft) L67.9
  - follicles L73.9
    - specified NEC L73.8
- Hamman's (spontaneous mediastinal emphysema) J98.2
- hand, foot and mouth B08.4
- Hansen's — *see* Leprosy
- Hantavirus, with pulmonary manifestations B33.4
  - with renal manifestations A98.5
- Harada's H30.81- ☑
- Hartnup (pellagra-cerebellar ataxia-renal aminoaciduria) E72.02
- Hart's (pellagra-cerebellar ataxia-renal aminoaciduria) E72.02
- Hashimoto's (struma lymphomatosa) E06.3
- Hb — *see* Disease, hemoglobin
- heart (organic) I51.9
  - with
    - pulmonary edema (acute) (*see also* Failure, ventricular, left) I50.1
    - rheumatic fever (conditions in I00)
      - active I01.9
        - with chorea I02.0
        - specified NEC I01.8
      - inactive or quiescent (with chorea) I09.9
        - specified NEC I09.89
  - amyloid E85.4 [I43]
  - aortic (valve) I35.9
  - arteriosclerotic or sclerotic (senile) — *see* Disease, heart, ischemic, atherosclerotic
  - artery, arterial — *see* Disease, heart, ischemic, atherosclerotic
  - beer drinkers' I42.6
  - beriberi (wet) E51.12
  - black I27.0
  - congenital Q24.9
    - cyanotic Q24.9
    - specified NEC Q24.8
  - coronary — *see* Disease, heart, ischemic

Disease, diseased — *continued*
- heart — *continued*
  - cryptogenic I51.9
  - fibroid — *see* Myocarditis
  - functional I51.89
    - psychogenic F45.8
  - glycogen storage E74.02 [I43]
  - gonococcal A54.83
  - hypertensive — *see* Hypertension, heart
  - hyperthyroid (*see also* Hyperthyroidism) E05.90 [I43]
    - with thyroid storm E05.91 [I43]
  - ischemic (chronic or with a stated duration of over 4 weeks) I25.9
    - atherosclerotic (of) I25.10
      - with angina pectoris — *see* Arteriosclerosis, coronary (artery)
      - coronary artery bypass graft — *see* Arteriosclerosis, coronary (artery), cardiomyopathy I25.5
    - diagnosed on ECG or other special investigation, but currently presenting no symptoms I25.6
    - silent I25.6
    - specified form NEC I25.89
  - kyphoscoliotic I27.1
  - meningococcal A39.50
    - endocarditis A39.51
    - myocarditis A39.52
    - pericarditis A39.53
  - mitral I05.9
    - specified NEC I05.8
  - muscular — *see* Degeneration, myocardial
  - psychogenic (functional) F45.8
  - pulmonary (chronic) I27.9
    - in schistosomiasis B65.9 [I52]
    - specified NEC I27.89
  - rheumatic (chronic) (inactive) (old) (quiescent) (with chorea) I09.9
    - active or acute I01.9
      - with chorea (acute) (rheumatic) (Sydenham's) I02.9
    - specified NEC I09.89
  - senile — *see* Myocarditis
  - syphilitic A52.06
    - aortic A52.03
      - aneurysm A52.01
    - congenital A50.54 [I52]
  - thyrotoxic (*see also* Thyrotoxicosis) E05.90 [I43]
    - with thyroid storm E05.91 [I43]
  - valve, valvular (obstructive) (regurgitant) (*see also* Endocarditis)
    - congenital NEC Q24.8
      - pulmonary Q22.3
  - vascular — *see* Disease, cardiovascular
- heavy chain NEC C88.2
  - alpha C88.3
  - gamma C88.2
  - mu C88.2
- Hebra's
  - pityriasis
    - maculata et circinata L42
    - rubra pilaris L44.0
  - prurigo L28.2
- hematopoietic organs D75.9
- hemoglobin or Hb
  - abnormal (mixed) NEC D58.2
    - with thalassemia D56.9
  - AS genotype D57.3
  - Bart's D56.0
  - C (Hb-C) D58.2
    - with other abnormal hemoglobin NEC D58.2
    - elliptocytosis D58.1
    - Hb-S D57.2- ☑
    - sickle-cell D57.2- ☑
    - thalassemia D56.8
  - Constant Spring D58.2
  - D (Hb-D) D58.2
  - E (Hb-E) D58.2
  - E-beta thalassemia D56.5
  - elliptocytosis D58.1
  - H (Hb-H) (thalassemia) D56.0
    - with other abnormal hemoglobin NEC D56.9
    - Constant Spring D56.0
  - I thalassemia D56.9
  - M D74.0
  - S or SS D57.1
  - SC D57.2- ☑

Disease, diseased — *continued*
- hemoglobin or Hb — *continued*
  - SD D57.8- ☑
  - SE D57.8- ☑
  - spherocytosis D58.0
  - unstable, hemolytic D58.2
- hemolytic (newborn) P55.9
  - autoimmune (cold type) (warm type) D59.1
  - drug-induced D59.0
  - due to or with
    - incompatibility
      - ABO (blood group) P55.1
      - blood (group) (Duffy) (K(ell)) (Kidd) (Lewis) (M) (S) NEC P55.8
      - Rh (blood group) (factor) P55.0
    - Rh negative mother P55.0
  - specified type NEC P55.8
  - unstable hemoglobin D58.2
- hemorrhagic D69.9
  - newborn P53
- Henoch (-Schönlein) (purpura nervosa) D69.0
- hepatic — *see* Disease, liver
- hepatolenticular E83.01
- heredodegenerative NEC
  - spinal cord G95.89
- herpesviral, disseminated B00.7
- Hers' (glycogenosis VI) E74.09
- Herter (-Gee) (-Heubner) (nontropical sprue) K90.0
- Heubner-Herter (nontropical sprue) K90.0
- high fetal gene or hemoglobin thalassemia D56.9
- Hildenbrand's — *see* Typhus
- hip (joint) M25.9
  - congenital Q65.89
  - suppurative M00.9
  - tuberculous A18.02
- His (-Werner) (trench fever) A79.0
- Hodgson's I71.2
  - ruptured I71.1
- Holla — *see* Spherocytosis
- hookworm B76.9
  - specified NEC B76.8
- host-versus-graft D89.813
  - acute D89.810
  - acute on chronic D89.812
  - chronic D89.811
- human immunodeficiency virus (HIV) B20
- Huntington's G10
  - with dementia G10 [F02.80]
- Hutchinson's (cheiropompholyx) — *see* Hutchinson's disease
- hyaline (diffuse) (generalized)
  - membrane (lung) (newborn) P22.0
    - adult J80
- hydatid — *see* Echinococcus
- hydroxyapatite deposition M11.00
  - ankle M11.07- ☑
  - elbow M11.02- ☑
  - foot joint M11.07- ☑
  - hand joint M11.04- ☑
  - hip M11.05- ☑
  - knee M11.06- ☑
  - multiple site M11.09
  - shoulder M11.01- ☑
  - vertebra M11.08
  - wrist M11.03- ☑
- hyperkinetic — *see* Hyperkinesia
- hypertensive — *see* Hypertension
- hypophysis E23.7
- Iceland G93.3
- I-cell E77.0
- immune D89.9
- immunoproliferative (malignant) C88.9
  - small intestinal C88.3
  - specified NEC C88.8
- inclusion B25.9
  - salivary gland B25.9
- infectious, infective B99.9
  - congenital P37.9
    - specified NEC P37.8
  - viral P35.9
    - specified type NEC P35.8
  - specified NEC B99.8
- inflammatory
  - penis N48.29
    - abscess N48.21
    - cellulitis N48.22
  - prepuce N47.7
    - balanoposthitis N47.6

Index

Disease, diseased — Disease, diseased

Disease, diseased — *continued*
inflammatory — *continued*
tubo-ovarian — *see* Salpingo-oophoritis
intervertebral disc (*see also* Disorder, disc)
with myelopathy — *see* Disorder, disc, with, myelopathy
cervical, cervicothoracic — *see* Disorder, disc, cervical
with
myelopathy — *see* Disorder, disc, cervical, with myelopathy
neuritis, radiculitis or radiculopathy — *see* Disorder, disc, cervical, with neuritis
specified NEC — *see* Disorder, disc, cervical, specified type NEC
lumbar (with)
myelopathy M51.06
neuritis, radiculitis, radiculopathy or sciatica M51.16
specified NEC M51.86
lumbosacral (with)
neuritis, radiculitis, radiculopathy or sciatica M51.17
specified NEC M51.87
specified NEC — *see* Disorder, disc, specified NEC
thoracic (with)
myelopathy M51.04
neuritis, radiculitis or radiculopathy M51.14
specified NEC M51.84
thoracolumbar (with)
myelopathy M51.05
neuritis, radiculitis or radiculopathy M51.15
specified NEC M51.85
intestine K63.9
functional K59.9
psychogenic F45.8
specified NEC K59.8
organic K63.9
protozoal A07.9
specified NEC K63.89
iris H21.9
specified NEC H21.89
iron metabolism or storage E83.10
island (scrub typhus) A75.3
itai-itai — *see* Poisoning, cadmium
Jakob-Creutzfeldt — *see* Creutzfeldt-Jakob disease or syndrome
jaw M27.9
fibrocystic M27.49
specified NEC M27.8
jigger B88.1
joint (*see also* Disorder, joint)
Charcot's — *see* Arthropathy, neuropathic (Charcot)
degenerative — *see* Osteoarthritis
multiple M15.9
spine — *see* Spondylosis
hypertrophic — *see* Osteoarthritis
sacroiliac M53.3
specified NEC — *see* Disorder, joint, specified type NEC
spine NEC — *see* Dorsopathy
suppurative — *see* Arthritis, pyogenic or pyemic
Jourdain's (acute gingivitis) K05.00
nonplaque induced K05.01
plaque induced K05.00
Kaschin-Beck (endemic polyarthritis) M12.10
ankle M12.17- ☑
elbow M12.12- ☑
foot joint M12.17- ☑
hand joint M12.14- ☑
hip M12.15- ☑
knee M12.16- ☑
multiple site M12.19
shoulder M12.11- ☑
vertebra M12.18
wrist M12.13- ☑
Katayama B65.2
Kedani (scrub typhus) A75.3
Keshan E59
kidney (functional) (pelvis) N28.9
chronic N18.9
hypertensive — *see* Hypertension, kidney
stage 1 N18.1
stage 2 (mild) N18.2
stage 3 (moderate) N18.3
stage 4 (severe) N18.4
stage 5 N18.5

Disease, diseased — *continued*
kidney — *continued*
complicating pregnancy — *see* Pregnancy, complicated by, renal disease
cystic (congenital) Q61.9
fibrocystic (congenital) Q61.8
hypertensive — *see* Hypertension, kidney
in (due to)
schistosomiasis (bilharziasis) B65.9 [N29]
multicystic Q61.4
polycystic Q61.3
adult type Q61.2
childhood type NEC Q61.19
collecting duct dilatation Q61.11
Kimmelstiel (-Wilson) (intercapillary polycystic (congenital) glomerulosclerosis) — *see* E08-E13 with .21
Kinnier Wilson's (hepatolenticular degeneration) E83.01
kissing — *see* Mononucleosis, infectious
Klebs' (*see also* Glomerulonephritis) N05- ☑
Klippel-Feil (brevicollis) Q76.1
Köhler-Pellegrini-Stieda (calcification, knee joint) — *see* Bursitis, tibial collateral
Kok Q89.8
König's (osteochondritis dissecans) — *see* Osteochondritis, dissecans
Korsakoff's (nonalcoholic) F04
alcoholic F10.96
with dependence F10.26
Kostmann's (infantile genetic agranulocytosis) D70.0
kuru A81.81
Kyasanur Forest A98.2
labyrinth, ear — *see* Disorder, ear, inner
lacrimal system — *see* Disorder, lacrimal system
Lafora's — *see* Epilepsy, generalized, idiopathic
Lancereaux-Mathieu (leptospiral jaundice) A27.0
Landry's G61.0
Larrey-Weil (leptospiral jaundice) A27.0
larynx J38.7
legionnaires' A48.1
nonpneumonic A48.2
Lenegre's I44.2
lens H27.9
specified NEC H27.8
Lev's (acquired complete heart block) I44.2
Lewy body (dementia) G31.83 [F02.80]
with behavioral disturbance G31.83 [F02.81]
Lichtheim's (subacute combined sclerosis with pernicious anemia) D51.0
Lightwood's (renal tubular acidosis) N25.89
Lignac's (cystinosis) E72.04
lip K13.0
lipid-storage E75.6
specified NEC E75.5
Lipschütz's N76.6
liver (chronic) (organic) K76.9
alcoholic (chronic) K70.9
acute — *see* Disease, liver, alcoholic, hepatitis
cirrhosis K70.30
with ascites K70.31
failure K70.40
with coma K70.41
fatty liver K70.0
fibrosis K70.2
hepatitis K70.10
with ascites K70.11
sclerosis K70.2
cystic, congenital Q44.6
drug-induced (idiosyncratic) (toxic) (predictable) (unpredictable) — *see* Disease, liver, toxic
end stage K72.90
due to hepatitis — *see* Hepatitis
fatty, nonalcoholic (NAFLD) K76.0
alcoholic K70.0
fibrocystic (congenital) Q44.6
fluke
Chinese B66.1
oriental B66.1
sheep B66.3
gestational alloimmune (GALD) P78.84
glycogen storage E74.09 [K77]
in (due to)
schistosomiasis (bilharziasis) B65.9 [K77]
inflammatory K75.9
alcoholic K70.1 ☑
specified NEC K75.89
polycystic (congenital) Q44.6

Disease, diseased — *continued*
liver — *continued*
toxic K71.9
with
cholestasis K71.0
cirrhosis (liver) K71.7
fibrosis (liver) K71.7
focal nodular hyperplasia K71.8
hepatic granuloma K71.8
hepatic necrosis K71.10
with coma K71.11
hepatitis NEC K71.6
acute K71.2
chronic
active K71.50
with ascites K71.51
lobular K71.4
persistent K71.3
lupoid K71.50
with ascites K71.51
peliosis hepatis K71.8
veno-occlusive disease (VOD) of liver K71.8
veno-occlusive K76.5
Lobo's (keloid blastomycosis) B48.0
Lobstein's (brittle bones and blue sclera) Q78.0
Ludwig's (submaxillary cellulitis) K12.2
lumbosacral region M53.87
lung J98.4
black J60
congenital Q33.9
cystic J98.4
congenital Q33.0
fibroid (chronic) — *see* Fibrosis, lung
fluke B66.4
oriental B66.4
in
amyloidosis E85.4 [J99]
sarcoidosis D86.0
Sjögren's syndrome M35.02
systemic
lupus erythematosus M32.13
sclerosis M34.81
interstitial J84.9
of childhood, specified NEC J84.848
respiratory bronchiolitis J84.115
specified NEC J84.89
obstructive (chronic) J44.9
with
acute
bronchitis J44.0
exacerbation NEC J44.1
lower respiratory infection J44.0
alveolitis, allergic J67.9
asthma J44.9
bronchiectasis J47.9
with
exacerbation (acute) J47.1
lower respiratory infection J47.0
bronchitis J44.9
with
exacerbation (acute) J44.1
lower respiratory infection J44.0
emphysema J43.9
hypersensitivity pneumonitis J67.9
decompensated J44.1
with
exacerbation (acute) J44.1
polycystic J98.4
congenital Q33.0
rheumatoid (diffuse) (interstitial) — *see* Rheumatoid, lung
Lutembacher's (atrial septal defect with mitral stenosis) Q21.1
Lyme A69.20
lymphatic (gland) (system) (channel) (vessel) I89.9
lymphoproliferative D47.9
specified NEC D47.Z9 (*following* D47.4)
T-gamma D47.Z9 (*following* D47.4)
X-linked D82.3
Magitot's M27.2
malarial — *see* Malaria
malignant (*see also* Neoplasm, malignant, by site)
Manson's B65.1
maple bark J67.6
maple-syrup-urine E71.0
Marburg (virus) A98.3
Marion's (bladder neck obstruction) N32.0
Marsh's (exophthalmic goiter) — *see* Hyperthyroidism, with, goiter (diffuse)

☑ **Additional Character Required** — Refer to the Tabular List for Character Selection   ▽ Subterms under main terms may continue to next column or page

Disease, diseased — *continued*
- mastoid (process) — *see* Disorder, ear, middle
- Mathieu's (leptospiral jaundice) A27.Ø
- Maxcy's A75.2
- McArdle (-Schmid-Pearson) (glycogenosis V) E74.Ø4
- mediastinum J98.59
- medullary center (idiopathic) (respiratory) G93.89
- Meige's (chronic hereditary edema) Q82.Ø
- meningococcal — *see* Infection, meningococcal
- mental F99
  - organic FØ9
- mesenchymal M35.9
- mesenteric embolic (*see also* Ischemia, intestine, acute) K55.Ø39
- metabolic, metabolism E88.9
  - bilirubin E8Ø.7
- metal-polisher's J62.8
- metastatic (*see also* Neoplasm, secondary, by site) C79.9
- microvascular - code to condition
- microvillus
  - atrophy Q43.8
  - inclusion (MVD) Q43.8
- middle ear — *see* Disorder, ear, middle
- Mikulicz' (dryness of mouth, absent or decreased lacrimation) K11.8
- Milroy's (chronic hereditary edema) Q82.Ø
- Minamata — *see* Poisoning, mercury
- minicore G71.2
- Minor's G95.19
- Minot's (hemorrhagic disease, newborn) P53
- Minot-von Willebrand-Jürgens (angiohemophilia) D68.Ø
- Mitchell's (erythromelalgia) I73.81
- mitral (valve) IØ5.9
  - nonrheumatic I34.9
- mixed connective tissue M35.1
- moldy hay J67.Ø
- Monge's T7Ø.29 ☑
- Morgagni-Adams-Stokes (syncope with heart block) I45.9
- Morgagni's (syndrome) (hyperostosis frontalis interna) M85.2
- Morton's (with metatarsalgia) — *see* Lesion, nerve, plantar
- Morvan's G6Ø.8
- motor neuron (bulbar) (mixed type) (spinal) G12.2Ø
  - amyotrophic lateral sclerosis G12.21
  - familial G12.24
  - progressive bulbar palsy G12.22
  - specified NEC G12.29
- moyamoya I67.5
- mu heavy chain disease C88.2
- multicore G71.2
- muscle (*see also* Disorder, muscle)
  - inflammatory — *see* Myositis
  - ocular (external) — *see* Strabismus
- musculoskeletal system, soft tissue — *see also* Disorder, soft tissue
  - specified NEC — *see* Disorder, soft tissue, specified type NEC
- mushroom workers' J67.5
- mycotic B49
- myelodysplastic, not classified C94.6
- myeloproliferative, not classified C94.6
  - chronic D47.1
- myocardium, myocardial (*see also* Degeneration, myocardial) I51.5
  - primary (idiopathic) I42.9
- myoneural G7Ø.9
- Naegeli's D69.1
- nails L6Ø.9
  - specified NEC L6Ø.8
- Nairobi (sheep virus) A93.8
- nasal J34.9
- nemaline body G71.2
- nerve — *see* Disorder, nerve
- nervous system G98.8
  - autonomic G9Ø.9
  - central G96.9
    - specified NEC G96.8
  - congenital QØ7.9
  - parasympathetic G9Ø.9
  - specified NEC G98.8
  - sympathetic G9Ø.9
  - vegetative G9Ø.9
- neuromuscular system G7Ø.9
- Newcastle B3Ø.8

Disease, diseased — *continued*
- Nicolas (-Durand)-Favre (climatic bubo) A55
- nipple N64.9
  - Paget's C5Ø.9- ☑
    - female C5Ø.Ø1- ☑
    - male C5Ø.Ø2- ☑
- Nishimoto (-Takeuchi) I67.5
- nonarthropod-borne NOS (viral) B34.9
  - enterovirus NEC B34.1
- nonautoimmune hemolytic D59.4
  - drug-induced D59.2
- Nonne-Milroy-Meige (chronic hereditary edema) Q82.Ø
- nose J34.9
- nucleus pulposus — *see* Disorder, disc
- nutritional E63.9
- oast-house-urine E72.19
  - ocular
    - herpesviral BØØ.5Ø
    - zoster BØ2.3Ø
- obliterative vascular I77.1
- Ohara's — *see* Tularemia
- Opitz's (congestive splenomegaly) D73.2
- Oppenheim-Urbach (necrobiosis lipoidica diabeticorum) — *see* EØ8-E13 with .62Ø
- optic nerve NEC — *see* Disorder, nerve, optic
- orbit — *see* Disorder, orbit
- Oriental liver fluke B66.1
- Oriental lung fluke B66.4
- Ormond's N13.5
- Oropouche virus A93.Ø
- Osler-Rendu (familial hemorrhagic telangiectasia) I78.Ø
- osteofibrocystic E21.Ø
- Otto's M24.7
- outer ear — *see* Disorder, ear, external
- ovary (noninflammatory) N83.9
  - cystic N83.2Ø- ☑
  - inflammatory — *see* Salpingo-oophoritis
  - polycystic E28.2
  - specified NEC N83.8
- Owren's (congenital) — *see* Defect, coagulation
- pancreas K86.9
  - cystic K86.2
  - fibrocystic E84.9
  - specified NEC K86.89
- panvalvular IØ8.9
  - specified NEC IØ8.8
- parametrium (noninflammatory) N83.9
- parasitic B89
  - cerebral NEC B71.9 [G94]
  - intestinal NOS B82.9
  - mouth B37.Ø
  - skin NOS B88.9
  - specified type — *see* Infestation
  - tongue B37.Ø
- parathyroid (gland) E21.5
  - specified NEC E21.4
- Parkinson's G2Ø
- parodontal KØ5.6
- Parrot's (syphilitic osteochondritis) A5Ø.Ø2
- Parry's (exophthalmic goiter) — *see* Hyperthyroidism, with, goiter (diffuse)
- Parson's (exophthalmic goiter) — *see* Hyperthyroidism, with, goiter (diffuse)
- Paxton's (white piedra) B36.2
- pearl-worker's — *see* Osteomyelitis, specified type NEC
- Pellegrini-Stieda (calcification, knee joint) — *see* Bursitis, tibial collateral
- pelvis, pelvic
  - female NOS N94.9
    - specified NEC N94.89
  - gonococcal (acute) (chronic) A54.24
  - inflammatory (female) N73.9
    - acute N73.Ø
    - chlamydial A56.11
    - chronic N73.1
    - specified NEC N73.8
    - syphilitic (secondary) A51.42
      - late A52.76
    - tuberculous A18.17
  - organ, female N94.9
  - peritoneum, female NEC N94.89
- penis N48.9
  - inflammatory N48.29
    - abscess N48.21
    - cellulitis N48.22
  - specified NEC N48.89
- periapical tissues NOS KØ4.9Ø

Disease, diseased — *continued*
- periodontal KØ5.6
  - specified NEC KØ5.5
- periosteum — *see* Disorder, bone, specified type NEC
- peripheral
  - arterial I73.9
  - autonomic nervous system G9Ø.9
  - nerves — *see* Polyneuropathy
  - vascular NOS I73.9
- peritoneum K66.9
  - pelvic, female NEC N94.89
  - specified NEC K66.8
- persistent mucosal (middle ear) H66.2Ø
  - left H66.22
    - with right H66.23
  - right H66.21
    - with left H66.23
- Petit's — *see* Hernia, abdomen, specified site NEC
- pharynx J39.2
  - specified NEC J39.2
- Phocas' — *see* Mastopathy, cystic
- photochromogenic (acid-fast bacilli) (pulmonary) A31.Ø
  - nonpulmonary A31.9
- Pick's G31.Ø1 [FØ2.8Ø]
  - with behavioral disturbance G31.Ø1 [FØ2.81]
  - brain G31.Ø1 [FØ2.8Ø]
    - with behavioral disturbance G31.Ø1 [FØ2.81]
  - of pericardium (pericardial pseudocirrhosis of liver) I31.1
- pigeon fancier's J67.2
- pineal gland E34.8
- pink — *see* Poisoning, mercury
- Pinkus' (lichen nitidus) L44.1
- pinworm B8Ø
- Piry virus A93.8
- pituitary (gland) E23.7
- pituitary-snuff-taker's J67.8
- pleura (cavity) J94.9
  - specified NEC J94.8
- pneumatic drill (hammer) T75.21 ☑
- Pollitzer's (hidradenitis suppurativa) L73.2
- polycystic
  - kidney or renal Q61.3
    - adult type Q61.2
    - childhood type NEC Q61.19
      - collecting duct dilatation Q61.11
  - liver or hepatic Q44.6
  - lung or pulmonary J98.4
    - congenital Q33.Ø
  - ovary, ovaries E28.2
  - spleen Q89.Ø9
- polyethylene T84.Ø5- ☑
- Pompe's (glycogenosis II) E74.Ø2
- Posadas-Wernicke B38.9
- Potain's (pulmonary edema) — *see* Edema, lung
- prepuce N47.8
  - inflammatory N47.7
    - balanoposthitis N47.6
- Pringle's (tuberous sclerosis) Q85.1
- prion, central nervous system A81.9
  - specified NEC A81.89
- prostate N42.9
  - specified NEC N42.89
- protozoal B64
  - acanthamebiasis — *see* Acanthamebiasis
  - African trypanosomiasis — *see* African trypanosomiasis
  - babesiosis B6Ø.Ø
  - Chagas disease — *see* Chagas disease
  - intestine, intestinal AØ7.9
  - leishmaniasis — *see* Leishmaniasis
  - malaria — *see* Malaria
  - naegleriasis B6Ø.2
  - pneumocystosis B59
  - specified organism NEC B6Ø.8
  - toxoplasmosis — *see* Toxoplasmosis
- pseudo-Hurler's E77.Ø
- psychiatric F99
- psychotic — *see* Psychosis
- Puente's (simple glandular cheilitis) K13.Ø
- puerperal (*see also* Puerperal) O9Ø.89
- pulmonary (*see also* Disease, lung)
  - artery I28.9
  - chronic obstructive J44.9
    - with
      - acute bronchitis J44.Ø
      - exacerbation (acute) J44.1

Disease, diseased — *continued*
  pulmonary (*see also* Disease, lung) — *continued*
    chronic obstructive — *continued*
      with — *continued*
        lower respiratory infection (acute) J44.0
      decompensated J44.1
        with
          exacerbation (acute) J44.1
    heart I27.9
      specified NEC I27.89
    hypertensive (vascular) (*see also* Hypertension, pulmonary) I27.20
      primary (idiopathic) I27.0
      NEC I27.2 ☑
    valve I37.9
      rheumatic I09.89
  pulp (dental) NOS K04.90
  pulseless M31.4
  Putnam's (subacute combined sclerosis with pernicious anemia) D51.0
  Pyle (-Cohn) (metaphyseal dysplasia) Q78.5
  ragpicker's or ragsorter's A22.1
  Raynaud's — *see* Raynaud's disease
  reactive airway — *see* Asthma
  Reclus' (cystic) — *see* Mastopathy, cystic
  rectum K62.9
    specified NEC K62.89
  Refsum's (heredopathia atactica polyneuritiformis) G60.1
  renal (functional) (pelvis) (*see also* Disease, kidney) N28.9
    with
      edema — *see* Nephrosis
      glomerular lesion — *see* Glomerulonephritis
        with edema — *see* Nephrosis
      interstitial nephritis N12
    acute N28.9
    chronic (*see also* Disease, kidney, chronic) N18.9
    cystic, congenital Q61.9
    diabetic — *see* E08-E13 with .22
    end-stage (failure) N18.6
      due to hypertension I12.0
    fibrocystic (congenital) Q61.8
    hypertensive — *see* Hypertension, kidney
    lupus M32.14
    phosphate-losing (tubular) N25.0
    polycystic (congenital) Q61.3
      adult type Q61.2
      childhood type NEC Q61.19
        collecting duct dilatation Q61.11
    rapidly progressive N01.9
    subacute N01.9
  Rendu-Osler-Weber (familial hemorrhagic telangiectasia) I78.0
  renovascular (arteriosclerotic) — *see* Hypertension, kidney
  respiratory (tract) J98.9
    acute or subacute NOS J06.9
      due to
        chemicals, gases, fumes or vapors (inhalation) J68.3
        external agent J70.9
          specified NEC J70.8
        radiation J70.0
        smoke inhalation J70.5
      noninfectious J39.8
    chronic NOS J98.9
      due to
        chemicals, gases, fumes or vapors J68.4
        external agent J70.9
          specified NEC J70.8
        radiation J70.1
      newborn P27.9
        specified NEC P27.8
    due to
      chemicals, gases, fumes or vapors J68.9
        acute or subacute NEC J68.3
        chronic J68.4
      external agent J70.9
        specified NEC J70.8
    newborn P28.9
      specified type NEC P28.89
    upper J39.9
      acute or subacute J06.9
      noninfectious NEC J39.8
      specified NEC J39.8
      streptococcal J06.9
  retina, retinal H35.9

Disease, diseased — *continued*
  retina, retinal — *continued*
    Batten's or Batten-Mayou E75.4 [H36]
    specified NEC H35.89
  rheumatoid — *see* Arthritis, rheumatoid
  rickettsial NOS A79.9
    specified type NEC A79.89
  Riga (-Fede) (cachectic aphthae) K14.0
  Riggs' (compound periodontitis) — *see* Periodontitis
  Ritter's L00
  Rivalta's (cervicofacial actinomycosis) A42.2
  Robles' (onchocerciasis) B73.01
  Roger's (congenital interventricular septal defect) Q21.0
  Rosenthal's (factor XI deficiency) D68.1
  Ross River B33.1
  Rossbach's (hyperchlorhydria) K30
  Rotes Quérol — *see* Hyperostosis, ankylosing
  Roth (-Bernhardt) — *see* Mononeuropathy, lower limb, meralgia paresthetica
  Runeberg's (progressive pernicious anemia) D51.0
  sacroiliac NEC M53.3
  salivary gland or duct K11.9
    inclusion B25.9
    specified NEC K11.8
    virus B25.9
  sandworm B76.9
  Schimmelbusch's — *see* Mastopathy, cystic
  Schmorl's — *see* Schmorl's disease or nodes
  Schönlein (-Henoch) (purpura rheumatica) D69.0
  Schottmüller's — *see* Fever, paratyphoid
  Schultz's (agranulocytosis) — *see* Agranulocytosis
  Schwalbe-Ziehen-Oppenheim G24.1
  Schwartz-Jampel G71.13
  sclera H15.9
    specified NEC H15.89
  scrofulous (tuberculous) A18.2
  scrotum N50.9
  sebaceous glands L73.9
  semilunar cartilage, cystic (*see also* Derangement, knee, meniscus, cystic)
  seminal vesicle N50.9
  serum NEC (*see also* Reaction, serum) T80.69 ☑
  sexually transmitted A64
    anogenital
      herpesviral infection — *see* Herpes, anogenital
      warts A63.0
    chancroid A57
    chlamydial infection — *see* Chlamydia
    gonorrhea — *see* Gonorrhea
    granuloma inguinale A58
    specified organism NEC A63.8
    syphilis — *see* Syphilis
    trichomoniasis — *see* Trichomoniasis
  Sézary C84.1- ☑
  shimamushi (scrub typhus) A75.3
  shipyard B30.0
  sickle-cell D57.1
    with crisis (vasoocclusive pain) D57.00
      with
        acute chest syndrome D57.01
        splenic sequestration D57.02
    elliptocytosis D57.8- ☑
    Hb-C D57.20
      with crisis (vasoocclusive pain) D57.219
        with
          acute chest syndrome D57.211
          splenic sequestration D57.212
      without crisis D57.20
    Hb-SD D57.80
      with crisis D57.819
        with
          acute chest syndrome D57.811
          splenic sequestration D57.812
    Hb-SE D57.80
      with crisis D57.819
        with
          acute chest syndrome D57.811
          splenic sequestration D57.812
    specified NEC D57.80
      with crisis D57.819
        with
          acute chest syndrome D57.811
          splenic sequestration D57.812
    spherocytosis D57.80
      with crisis D57.819
        with
          acute chest syndrome D57.811

Disease, diseased — *continued*
  sickle-cell — *continued*
    spherocytosis — *continued*
      with crisis — *continued*
        with — *continued*
          splenic sequestration D57.812
    thalassemia D57.40
      with crisis (vasoocclusive pain) D57.419
        with
          acute chest syndrome D57.411
          splenic sequestration D57.412
      without crisis D57.40
  silo-filler's J68.8
    bronchitis J68.0
    pneumonitis J68.0
    pulmonary edema J68.1
  simian B B00.4
  Simons' (progressive lipodystrophy) E88.1
  sin nombre virus B33.4
  sinus — *see* Sinusitis
  Sirkari's B55.0
  sixth B08.20
    due to human herpesvirus 6 B08.21
    due to human herpesvirus 7 B08.22
  skin L98.9
    due to metabolic disorder NEC E88.9 [L99]
    specified NEC L98.8
  slim (HIV) B20
  small vessel I73.9
  Sneddon-Wilkinson (subcorneal pustular dermatosis) L13.1
  South African creeping B88.0
  spinal (cord) G95.9
    congenital Q06.9
    specified NEC G95.89
  spine (*see also* Spondylopathy)
    joint — *see* Dorsopathy
    tuberculous A18.01
  spinocerebellar (hereditary) G11.9
    specified NEC G11.8
  spleen D73.9
    amyloid E85.4 [D77]
    organic D73.9
    polycystic Q89.09
    postinfectional D73.89
  sponge-diver's — *see* Toxicity, venom, marine animal, sea anemone
  Startle Q89.8
  Steinert's G71.11
  Sticker's (erythema infectiosum) B08.3
  Stieda's (calcification, knee joint) — *see* Bursitis, tibial collateral
  Stokes' (exophthalmic goiter) — *see* Hyperthyroidism, with, goiter (diffuse)
  Stokes-Adams (syncope with heart block) I45.9
  stomach K31.9
    functional, psychogenic F45.8
    specified NEC K31.89
  stonemason's J62.8
  storage
    glycogen — *see* Disease, glycogen storage
    mucopolysaccharide — *see* Mucopolysaccharidosis
  striatopallidal system NEC G25.89
  Stuart-Prower (congenital factor X deficiency) D68.2
  Stuart's (congenital factor X deficiency) D68.2
  subcutaneous tissue — *see* Disease, skin
  supporting structures of teeth K08.9
    specified NEC K08.89
  suprarenal (capsule) (gland) E27.9
    hyperfunction E27.0
    specified NEC E27.8
  sweat glands L74.9
    specified NEC L74.8
  Sweeley-Klionsky E75.21
  Swift (-Feer) — *see* Poisoning, mercury
  swimming-pool granuloma A31.1
  Sylvest's (epidemic pleurodynia) B33.0
  sympathetic nervous system G90.9
  synovium — *see* Disorder, synovium
  syphilitic — *see* Syphilis
  systemic tissue mast cell C96.20
  tanapox (virus) B08.71
  Tangier E78.6
  Tarral-Besnier (pityriasis rubra pilaris) L44.0
  Tauri's E74.09
  tear duct — *see* Disorder, lacrimal system
  tendon, tendinous (*see also* Disorder, tendon)
    nodular — *see* Trigger finger

☑ Additional Character Required — Refer to the Tabular List for Character Selection   ▽ Subterms under main terms may continue to next column or page

Disease, diseased — *continued*
- terminal vessel I73.9
- testis N50.9
- thalassemia Hb-S — *see* Disease, sickle-cell, thalassemia
- Thaysen-Gee (nontropical sprue) K90.0
- Thomsen G71.12
- throat J39.2
  - septic J02.0
- thromboembolic — *see* Embolism
- thymus (gland) E32.9
  - specified NEC E32.8
- thyroid (gland) E07.9
  - heart (*see also* Hyperthyroidism) E05.90 [I43]
    - with thyroid storm E05.91 [I43]
  - specified NEC E07.89
- Tietze's M94.0
- tongue K14.9
  - specified NEC K14.8
- tonsils, tonsillar (and adenoids) J35.9
- tooth, teeth K08.9
  - hard tissues K03.9
    - specified NEC K03.89
  - pulp NEC K04.99
  - specified NEC K08.89
- Tourette's F95.2
- trachea NEC J39.8
- tricuspid I07.9
  - nonrheumatic I36.9
- triglyceride-storage E75.5
- trophoblastic — *see* Mole, hydatidiform
- tsutsugamushi A75.3
- tube (fallopian) (noninflammatory) N83.9
  - inflammatory — *see* Salpingitis
  - specified NEC N83.8
- tuberculous NEC — *see* Tuberculosis
- tubo-ovarian (noninflammatory) N83.9
  - inflammatory — *see* Salpingo-oophoritis
  - specified NEC N83.8
- tubotympanic, chronic — *see* Otitis, media, suppurative, chronic, tubotympanic
- tubulo-interstitial N15.9
  - specified NEC N15.8
- tympanum — *see* Disorder, tympanic membrane
- Uhl's Q24.8
- Underwood's (sclerema neonatorum) P83.0
- Unverricht (-Lundborg) — *see* Epilepsy, generalized, idiopathic
- Urbach-Oppenheim (necrobiosis lipoidica diabeticorum) — *see* E08-E13 with .620
- ureter N28.9
  - in (due to)
    - schistosomiasis (bilharziasis) B65.0 [N29]
- urethra N36.9
  - specified NEC N36.8
- urinary (tract) N39.9
  - bladder N32.9
    - specified NEC N32.89
  - specified NEC N39.8
- uterus (noninflammatory) N85.9
  - infective — *see* Endometritis
  - inflammatory — *see* Endometritis
  - specified NEC N85.8
- uveal tract (anterior) H21.9
  - posterior H31.9
- vagabond's B85.1
- vagina, vaginal (noninflammatory) N89.9
  - inflammatory NEC N76.89
  - specified NEC N89.8
- valve, valvular I38
  - multiple I08.9
    - specified NEC I08.8
- van Creveld-von Gierke (glycogenosis I) E74.01
- vas deferens N50.9
- vascular I99.9
  - arteriosclerotic — *see* Arteriosclerosis
  - ciliary body NEC — *see* Disorder, iris, vascular
  - hypertensive — *see* Hypertension
  - iris NEC — *see* Disorder, iris, vascular
  - obliterative I77.1
    - peripheral I73.9
  - occlusive I99.8
  - peripheral (occlusive) I73.9
    - in diabetes mellitus — *see* E08-E13 with .51
  - vasomotor I73.9
- vasospastic I73.9
- vein I87.9
- venereal (*see also* Disease, sexually transmitted) A64

Disease, diseased — *continued*
- venereal (*see also* Disease, sexually transmitted) — *continued*
  - chlamydial NEC A56.8
    - anus A56.3
    - genitourinary NOS A56.2
    - pharynx A56.4
    - rectum A56.3
  - fifth A55
  - sixth A55
  - specified nature or type NEC A63.8
- vertebra, vertebral (*see also* Spondylopathy)
  - disc — *see* Disorder, disc
- vibration — *see* Vibration, adverse effects
- viral, virus (*see also* Disease, by type of virus) B34.9
  - arbovirus NOS A94
  - arthropod-borne NOS A94
  - congenital P35.9
    - specified NEC P35.8
  - Hanta (with renal manifestations) (Dobrava) (Puumala) (Seoul) A98.5
    - with pulmonary manifestations (Andes) (Bayou) (Bermejo) (Black Creek Canal) (Choclo) (Juquitiba) (Laguna negra) (Lechiguanas) (New York) (Oran) (Sin nombre) B33.4
  - Hantaan (Korean hemorrhagic fever) A98.5
  - human immunodeficiency (HIV) B20
  - Kunjin A83.4
  - nonarthropod-borne NOS B34.9
  - Powassan A84.8
  - Rocio (encephalitis) A83.6
  - Sin nombre (Hantavirus) (cardio)-pulmonary syndrome) B33.4
  - Tahyna B33.8
  - vesicular stomatitis A93.8
- vitreous H43.9
  - specified NEC H43.89
- vocal cord J38.3
- Volkmann's, acquired T79.6 ☑
- von Eulenburg's (congenital paramyotonia) G71.19
- von Gierke's (glycogenosis I) E74.01
- von Graefe's — *see* Strabismus, paralytic, ophthalmoplegia, progressive
- von Willebrand (-Jürgens) (angiohemophilia) D68.0
- Vrolik's (osteogenesis imperfecta) Q78.0
- vulva (noninflammatory) N90.9
  - inflammatory NEC N76.89
  - specified NEC N90.89
- Wallgren's (obstruction of splenic vein with collateral circulation) I87.8
- Wassilieff's (leptospiral jaundice) A27.0
- wasting NEC R64
  - due to malnutrition E41
- Waterhouse-Friderichsen A39.1
- Wegner's (syphilitic osteochondritis) A50.02
- Weil's (leptospiral jaundice of lung) A27.0
- Weir Mitchell's (erythromelalgia) I73.81
- Werdnig-Hoffmann G12.0
- Wermer's E31.21
- Werner-His (trench fever) A79.0
- Werner-Schultz (neutropenic splenomegaly) D73.81
- Wernicke-Posadas B38.9
- whipworm B79
- white blood cells D72.9
  - specified NEC D72.89
- white matter R90.82
- white-spot, meaning lichen sclerosus et atrophicus L90.0
  - penis N48.0
  - vulva N90.4
- Wilkie's K55.1
- Wilkinson-Sneddon (subcorneal pustular dermatosis) L13.1
- Willis' — *see* Diabetes
- Wilson's (hepatolenticular degeneration) E83.01
- woolsorter's A22.1
- yaba monkey tumor B08.72
- yaba pox (virus) B08.72
- Zika virus A92.5
- zoonotic, bacterial A28.9
  - specified type NEC A28.8

Disfigurement (due to scar) L90.5
Disgerminoma — *see* Dysgerminoma
DISH (diffuse idiopathic skeletal hyperostosis) — *see* Hyperostosis, ankylosing
Disinsertion, retina — *see* Detachment, retina
Dislocatable hip, congenital Q65.6

Dislocation (articular)
- with fracture — *see* Fracture
- acromioclavicular (joint) S43.10- ☑
  - with displacement
    - 100%-200% S43.12- ☑
    - more than 200% S43.13- ☑
  - inferior S43.14- ☑
  - posterior S43.15- ☑
- ankle S93.0- ☑
- astragalus — *see* Dislocation, ankle
- atlantoaxial S13.121 ☑
- atlantooccipital S13.111 ☑
- atloidooccipital S13.111 ☑
- breast bone S23.29
- capsule, joint — *code by* site under Dislocation
- carpal (bone) — *see* Dislocation, wrist
- carpometacarpal (joint) NEC S63.05- ☑
  - thumb S63.04- ☑
- cartilage (joint) — *code by* site under Dislocation
- cervical spine (vertebra) — *see* Dislocation, vertebra, cervical
- chronic — *see* Dislocation, recurrent
- clavicle — *see* Dislocation, acromioclavicular joint
- coccyx S33.2 ☑
- congenital NEC Q68.8
- coracoid — *see* Dislocation, shoulder
- costal cartilage S23.29 ☑
- costochondral S23.29 ☑
- cricoarytenoid articulation S13.29 ☑
- cricothyroid articulation S13.29 ☑
- dorsal vertebra — *see* Dislocation, vertebra, thoracic
- ear ossicle — *see* Discontinuity, ossicles, ear
- elbow S53.10- ☑
  - congenital Q68.8
  - pathological — *see* Dislocation, pathological NEC, elbow
  - radial head alone — *see* Dislocation, radial head
  - recurrent — *see* Dislocation, recurrent, elbow
  - traumatic S53.10- ☑
    - anterior S53.11- ☑
    - lateral S53.14- ☑
    - medial S53.13- ☑
    - posterior S53.12- ☑
    - specified type NEC S53.19- ☑
- eye, nontraumatic — *see* Luxation, globe
- eyeball, nontraumatic — *see* Luxation, globe
- femur
  - distal end — *see* Dislocation, knee
  - proximal end — *see* Dislocation, hip
- fibula
  - distal end — *see* Dislocation, ankle
  - proximal end — *see* Dislocation, knee
- finger S63.25- ☑
  - index S63.25- ☑
  - interphalangeal S63.27- ☑
    - distal S63.29- ☑
      - index S63.29- ☑
      - little S63.29- ☑
      - middle S63.29- ☑
      - ring S63.29- ☑
    - index S63.27- ☑
    - little S63.27- ☑
    - middle S63.27- ☑
    - proximal S63.28- ☑
      - index S63.28- ☑
      - little S63.28- ☑
      - middle S63.28- ☑
      - ring S63.28- ☑
    - ring S63.27- ☑
  - little S63.25- ☑
  - metacarpophalangeal S63.26- ☑
    - index S63.26- ☑
    - little S63.26- ☑
    - middle S63.26- ☑
    - ring S63.26- ☑
  - middle S63.25- ☑
  - recurrent — *see* Dislocation, recurrent, finger
  - ring S63.25- ☑
  - thumb — *see* Dislocation, thumb
- foot S93.30- ☑
  - recurrent — *see* Dislocation, recurrent, foot
  - specified site NEC S93.33- ☑
  - tarsal joint S93.31- ☑
  - tarsometatarsal joint S93.32- ☑
  - toe — *see* Dislocation, toe
- fracture — *see* Fracture

Dislocation — *continued*
glenohumeral (joint) — *see* Dislocation, shoulder
glenoid — *see* Dislocation, shoulder
habitual — *see* Dislocation, recurrent
hip S73.00- ☑
 anterior S73.03- ☑
  obturator S73.02- ☑
 central S73.04- ☑
 congenital (total) Q65.2
  bilateral Q65.1
  partial Q65.5
   bilateral Q65.4
   unilateral Q65.3- ☑
  unilateral Q65.0- ☑
 developmental M24.85- ☑
 pathological — *see* Dislocation, pathological NEC,
  hip
 posterior S73.01- ☑
 recurrent — *see* Dislocation, recurrent, hip
humerus, proximal end — *see* Dislocation, shoulder
incomplete — *see* Subluxation, by site
incus — *see* Discontinuity, ossicles, ear
infracoracoid — *see* Dislocation, shoulder
innominate (pubic junction) (sacral junction) S33.39 ☑
 acetabulum — *see* Dislocation, hip
interphalangeal (joint(s))
 finger S63.279 ☑
  distal S63.29- ☑
   index S63.29- ☑
   little S63.29- ☑
   middle S63.29- ☑
   ring S63.29- ☑
  index S63.27- ☑
  little S63.27- ☑
  middle S63.27- ☑
  proximal S63.28- ☑
   index S63.28- ☑
   little S63.28- ☑
   middle S63.28- ☑
   ring S63.28- ☑
  ring S63.27- ☑
 foot or toe — *see* Dislocation, toe
 thumb S63.12- ☑
  distal joint S63.14- ☑
  proximal joint S63.13- ☑
jaw (cartilage) (meniscus) S03.0- ☑
joint prosthesis — *see* Complications, joint prosthesis,
 mechanical, displacement, by site
knee S83.106 ☑
 cap — *see* Dislocation, patella
 congenital Q68.2
 old M23.8X- ☑
 patella — *see* Dislocation, patella
 pathological — *see* Dislocation, pathological NEC,
  knee
 proximal tibia
  anteriorly S83.11- ☑
  laterally S83.14- ☑
  medially S83.13- ☑
  posteriorly S83.12- ☑
 recurrent (*see also* Derangement, knee, specified
  NEC)
 specified type NEC S83.19- ☑
lacrimal gland H04.16- ☑
lens (complete) H27.10
 anterior H27.12- ☑
 congenital Q12.1
 ocular implant — *see* Complications, intraocular
  lens
 partial H27.11- ☑
 posterior H27.13- ☑
 traumatic S05.8X- ☑
ligament — *code by* site under Dislocation
lumbar (vertebra) — *see* Dislocation, vertebra, lumbar
lumbosacral (vertebra) (*see also* Dislocation, vertebra,
 lumbar)
 congenital Q76.49
mandible S03.0- ☑
meniscus (knee) — *see* Tear, meniscus
 other sites - code by site under Dislocation
metacarpal (bone)
 distal end — *see* Dislocation, finger
 proximal end S63.06- ☑
metacarpophalangeal (joint)
 finger S63.26- ☑
  index S63.26- ☑

Dislocation — *continued*
metacarpophalangeal — *continued*
 finger — *continued*
  little S63.26- ☑
  middle S63.26- ☑
  ring S63.26- ☑
  thumb S63.11- ☑
metatarsal (bone) — *see* Dislocation, foot
metatarsophalangeal (joint(s)) — *see* Dislocation, toe
midcarpal (joint) S63.03- ☑
midtarsal (joint) — *see* Dislocation, foot
neck S13.20 ☑
 specified site NEC S13.29 ☑
 vertebra — *see* Dislocation, vertebra, cervical
nose (septal cartilage) S03.1 ☑
occipitoatloid S13.111 ☑
old — *see* Derangement, joint, specified type NEC
ossicles, ear — *see* Discontinuity, ossicles, ear
partial — *see* Subluxation, by site
patella S83.006 ☑
 congenital Q74.1
 lateral S83.01- ☑
 recurrent (nontraumatic) M22.0- ☑
  incomplete M22.1- ☑
 specified type NEC S83.09- ☑
pathological NEC M24.30
 ankle M24.37- ☑
 elbow M24.32- ☑
 foot joint M24.37- ☑
 hand joint M24.34- ☑
 hip M24.35- ☑
 knee M24.36- ☑
 lumbosacral joint — *see* subcategory M53.2
 pelvic region — *see* Dislocation, pathological, hip
 sacroiliac — *see* subcategory M53.2 ☑
 shoulder M24.31- ☑
 wrist M24.33- ☑
pelvis NEC S33.30 ☑
 specified NEC S33.39 ☑
phalanx
 finger or hand — *see* Dislocation, finger
 foot or toe — *see* Dislocation, toe
prosthesis, internal — *see* Complications, prosthetic
 device, by site, mechanical
radial head S53.006 ☑
 anterior S53.01- ☑
 posterior S53.02- ☑
 specified type NEC S53.09- ☑
radiocarpal (joint) S63.02- ☑
radiohumeral (joint) — *see* Dislocation, radial head
radioulnar (joint)
 distal S63.01- ☑
 proximal — *see* Dislocation, elbow
radius
 distal end — *see* Dislocation, wrist
 proximal end — *see* Dislocation, radial head
recurrent M24.40
 ankle M24.47- ☑
 elbow M24.42- ☑
 finger M24.44- ☑
 foot joint M24.47- ☑
 hand joint M24.44- ☑
 hip M24.45- ☑
 knee M24.46- ☑
  patella — *see* Dislocation, patella, recurrent
 patella — *see* Dislocation, patella, recurrent
 sacroiliac — *see* subcategory M53.2 ☑
 shoulder M24.41- ☑
 toe M24.47- ☑
 vertebra (*see also* subcategory) M43.5 ☑
  atlantoaxial M43.4
   with myelopathy M43.3
 wrist M24.43- ☑
rib (cartilage) S23.29 ☑
sacrococcygeal S33.2 ☑
sacroiliac (joint) (ligament) S33.2 ☑
 congenital Q74.2
 recurrent — *see* subcategory M53.2 ☑
sacrum S33.2 ☑
scaphoid (bone) (hand) (wrist) — *see* Dislocation, wrist
 foot — *see* Dislocation, foot
scapula — *see* Dislocation, shoulder, girdle, scapula
semilunar cartilage, knee — *see* Tear, meniscus
septal cartilage (nose) S03.1 ☑
septum (nasal) (old) J34.2

Dislocation — *continued*
sesamoid bone — *code by* site under Dislocation
shoulder (blade) (ligament) (joint) (traumatic)
 S43.006 ☑
 acromioclavicular — *see* Dislocation, acromioclavicular
 chronic — *see* Dislocation, recurrent, shoulder
 congenital Q68.8
 girdle S43.30- ☑
  scapula S43.31- ☑
  specified site NEC S43.39- ☑
 humerus S43.00- ☑
  anterior S43.01- ☑
  inferior S43.03- ☑
  posterior S43.02- ☑
 pathological — *see* Dislocation, pathological NEC,
  shoulder
 recurrent — *see* Dislocation, recurrent, shoulder
 specified type NEC S43.08- ☑
spine
 cervical — *see* Dislocation, vertebra, cervical
 congenital Q76.49
 due to birth trauma P11.5
 lumbar — *see* Dislocation, vertebra, lumbar
 thoracic — *see* Dislocation, vertebra, thoracic
spontaneous — *see* Dislocation, pathological
sternoclavicular (joint) S43.206 ☑
 anterior S43.21- ☑
 posterior S43.22- ☑
sternum S23.29 ☑
subglenoid — *see* Dislocation, shoulder
symphysis pubis S33.4 ☑
talus — *see* Dislocation, ankle
tarsal (bone(s)) (joint(s)) — *see* Dislocation, foot
tarsometatarsal (joint(s)) — *see* Dislocation, foot
temporomandibular (joint) S03.0- ☑
thigh, proximal end — *see* Dislocation, hip
thorax S23.20 ☑
 specified site NEC S23.29 ☑
 vertebra — *see* Dislocation, vertebra
thumb S63.10- ☑
 interphalangeal joint — *see* Dislocation, interphalangeal (joint), thumb
 metacarpophalangeal joint — *see* Dislocation,
  metacarpophalangeal (joint), thumb
thyroid cartilage S13.29 ☑
tibia
 distal end — *see* Dislocation, ankle
 proximal end — *see* Dislocation, knee
tibiofibular (joint)
 distal — *see* Dislocation, ankle
 superior — *see* Dislocation, knee
toe(s) S93.106 ☑
 great S93.10- ☑
  interphalangeal joint S93.11- ☑
  metatarsophalangeal joint S93.12- ☑
 interphalangeal joint S93.119 ☑
 lesser S93.106 ☑
  interphalangeal joint S93.11- ☑
  metatarsophalangeal joint S93.12- ☑
 metatarsophalangeal joint S93.12- ☑
tooth S03.2 ☑
trachea S23.29 ☑
ulna
 distal end S63.07- ☑
 proximal end — *see* Dislocation, elbow
ulnohumeral (joint) — *see* Dislocation, elbow
vertebra (articular process) (body) (traumatic)
 cervical S13.101 ☑
  atlantoaxial joint S13.121 ☑
  atlantooccipital joint S13.111 ☑
  atloidooccipital joint S13.111 ☑
  joint between
   C0 and C1 S13.111 ☑
   C1 and C2 S13.121 ☑
   C2 and C3 S13.131 ☑
   C3 and C4 S13.141 ☑
   C4 and C5 S13.151 ☑
   C5 and C6 S13.161 ☑
   C6 and C7 S13.171 ☑
   C7 and T1 S13.181 ☑
  occipitoatloid joint S13.111 ☑
 congenital Q76.49
 lumbar S33.101 ☑
  joint between
   L1 and L2 S33.111 ☑

Dislocation — continued
  vertebra — continued
    lumbar — continued
      joint between — continued
        L2 and L3 S33.121 ☑
        L3 and L4 S33.131 ☑
        L4 and L5 S33.141 ☑
    nontraumatic — see Displacement, intervertebral disc
    partial — see Subluxation, by site
    recurrent NEC — see subcategory M43.5 ☑
    thoracic S23.101 ☑
      joint between
        T1 and T2 S23.111 ☑
        T2 and T3 S23.121 ☑
        T3 and T4 S23.123 ☑
        T4 and T5 S23.131 ☑
        T5 and T6 S23.133 ☑
        T6 and T7 S23.141 ☑
        T7 and T8 S23.143 ☑
        T8 and T9 S23.151 ☑
        T9 and T10 S23.153 ☑
        T10 and T11 S23.161 ☑
        T11 and T12 S23.163 ☑
        T12 and L1 S23.171 ☑
  wrist (carpal bone) S63.006 ☑
    carpometacarpal joint — see Dislocation, carpometacarpal (joint)
    distal radioulnar joint — see Dislocation, radioulnar (joint), distal
    metacarpal bone, proximal — see Dislocation, metacarpal (bone), proximal end
    midcarpal — see Dislocation, midcarpal (joint)
    radiocarpal joint — see Dislocation, radiocarpal (joint)
    recurrent — see Dislocation, recurrent, wrist
    specified site NEC S63.09- ☑
    ulna — see Dislocation, ulna, distal end
  xiphoid cartilage S23.29 ☑
Disorder (of) (see also Disease)
  acantholytic L11.9
    specified NEC L11.8
  acute
    psychotic — see Psychosis, acute
    stress F43.0
  adjustment (grief) F43.20
    with
      anxiety F43.22
        with depressed mood F43.23
      conduct disturbance F43.24
        with emotional disturbance F43.25
      depressed mood F43.21
        with anxiety F43.23
      other specified symptom F43.29
  adrenal (capsule) (gland) (medullary) E27.9
    specified NEC E27.8
  adrenogenital E25.9
    drug-induced E25.8
    iatrogenic E25.8
    idiopathic E25.8
  adult personality (and behavior) F69
    specified NEC F68.8
  affective (mood) — see Disorder, mood
  aggressive, unsocialized F91.1
  alcohol use
    mild F10.10
      with
        alcohol intoxication F10.129
          delirium F10.121
        alcohol-induced
          anxiety disorder F10.180
          bipolar and related disorder F10.14
          depressive disorder F10.14
          psychotic disorder F10.159
          sexual dysfunction F10.181
          sleep disorder F10.182
      in remission (early) (sustained) F10.11
    moderate or severe F10.20
      with
        alcohol intoxication F10.229
          delirium F10.221
        alcohol-induced
          anxiety disorder F10.280
          bipolar and related disorder F10.24
          depressive disorder F10.24
          major neurocognitive disorder, amnestic-confabulatory type F10.26

Disorder — continued
  alcohol use — continued
    moderate or severe — continued
      with — continued
        alcohol-induced — continued
          major neurocognitive disorder, non-amnestic-confabulatory type F10.27
          mild neurocognitive disorder F10.288
          psychotic disorder F10.259
          sexual dysfunction F10.281
          sleep disorder F10.282
      in remission (early) (sustained) F10.21
  alcohol-related F10.99
    with
      amnestic disorder, persisting F10.96
      anxiety disorder F10.980
      dementia, persisting F10.97
      intoxication F10.929
        with delirium F10.921
        uncomplicated F10.920
      mood disorder F10.94
      other specified F10.988
      psychotic disorder F10.959
        with
          delusions F10.950
          hallucinations F10.951
      sexual dysfunction F10.981
      sleep disorder F10.982
  allergic — see Allergy
  alveolar NEC J84.09
  amino-acid
    cystathioninuria E72.19
    cystinosis E72.04
    cystinuria E72.01
    glycinuria E72.09
    homocystinuria E72.11
    metabolism — see Disturbance, metabolism, amino-acid
    specified NEC E72.8
  neonatal, transitory P74.8
  renal transport NEC E72.09
  transport NEC E72.09
  amnesic, amnestic
    alcohol-induced F10.96
      with dependence F10.26
    due to (secondary to) general medical condition F04
    psychoactive NEC-induced F19.96
      with
        abuse F19.16
        dependence F19.26
    sedative, hypnotic or anxiolytic-induced F13.96
      with dependence F13.26
  amphetamine (or other stimulant) use
    mild
      with
        amphetamine, cocaine, or other stimulant intoxication
          with perceptual disturbances F15.122
          without perceptual disturbances F15.129
        amphetamine (or other stimulant) -induced
          anxiety disorder F15.180
          bipolar and related disorder F15.14
          depressive disorder F15.14
          obsessive-compulsive and related disorder F15.188
          psychotic disorder F15.159
          sexual dysfunction F15.181
        intoxication delirium F15.121
    moderate or severe
      with
        amphetamine, cocaine, or other stimulant intoxication
          with perceptual disturbances F15.222
          without perceptual disturbances F15.229
        amphetamine (or other stimulant) -induced
          anxiety disorder F15.280
          bipolar and related disorder F15.24
          depressive disorder F15.24
          obsessive-compulsive and related disorder F15.288
          psychotic disorder F15.259
          sexual dysfunction F15.281
        intoxication delirium F15.221
  amphetamine-type substance use
    mild F15.10
      in remission (early) (sustained) F15.11
    moderate F15.20

Disorder — continued
  amphetamine-type substance use — continued
    moderate — continued
      in remission (early) (sustained) F15.21
    severe F15.20
      in remission (early) (sustained) F15.21
  anaerobic glycolysis with anemia D55.2
  anxiety F41.9
    due to (secondary to)
      alcohol F10.980
        in
          abuse F10.180
          dependence F10.280
      amphetamine F15.980
        in
          abuse F15.180
          dependence F15.280
      anxiolytic F13.980
        in
          abuse F13.180
          dependence F13.280
      caffeine F15.980
        in
          abuse F15.180
          dependence F15.280
      cannabis F12.980
        in
          abuse F12.180
          dependence F12.280
      cocaine F14.980
        in
          abuse F14.180
          dependence F14.180
      general medical condition F06.4
      hallucinogen F16.980
        in
          abuse F16.180
          dependence F16.280
      hypnotic F13.980
        in
          abuse F13.180
          dependence F13.280
      inhalant F18.980
        in
          abuse F18.180
          dependence F18.280
      phencyclidine F16.980
        in
          abuse F16.180
          dependence F16.280
      psychoactive substance NEC F19.980
        in
          abuse F19.180
          dependence F19.280
      sedative F13.980
        in
          abuse F13.180
          dependence F13.280
      volatile solvents F18.980
        in
          abuse F18.180
          dependence F18.280
    generalized F41.1
    illness F45.21
    mixed
      with depression (mild) F41.8
      specified NEC F41.3
    organic F06.4
    phobic F40.9
      of childhood F40.8
    specified NEC F41.8
  aortic valve — see Endocarditis, aortic
  aromatic amino-acid metabolism E70.9
    specified NEC E70.8
  arteriole NEC I77.89
  artery NEC I77.89
  articulation — see Disorder, joint
  attachment (childhood)
    disinhibited F94.2
    reactive F94.1
  attention-deficit hyperactivity (adolescent) (adult) (child) F90.9
    combined
      presentation F90.2
      type F90.2
    hyperactive
      impulsive presentation F90.1
      type F90.1

▽ Subterms under main terms may continue to next column or page   ☑ Additional Character Required — Refer to the Tabular List for Character Selection   109

Dislocation — Disorder

Disorder — *continued*
  attention-deficit hyperactivity — *continued*
    inattentive
      presentation F90.0
      type F90.0
    specified type NEC F90.8
  attention-deficit without hyperactivity (adolescent) (adult) (child) F98.8
  auditory processing (central) H93.25
  autism spectrum F84.0
  autistic F84.0
  autoimmune D89.89
  autonomic nervous system G90.9
    specified NEC G90.8
  avoidant
    child or adolescent F40.10
    restrictive food intake F50.82
  balance
    acid-base E87.8
      mixed E87.4
    electrolyte E87.8
    fluid NEC E87.8
  behavioral (disruptive) — *see* Disorder, conduct
  beta-amino-acid metabolism E72.8
  bile acid and cholesterol metabolism E78.70
    Barth syndrome E78.71
    other specified E78.79
    Smith-Lemli-Opitz syndrome E78.72
  bilirubin excretion E80.6
  binge eating F50.81
  binocular
    movement H51.9
      convergence
        excess H51.12
        insufficiency H51.11
      internuclear ophthalmoplegia — *see* Ophthalmoplegia, internuclear
      palsy of conjugate gaze H51.0
      specified type NEC H51.8
    vision NEC — *see* Disorder, vision, binocular
  bipolar (I) (type I) F31.9
    and related due to a known physiological condition
      with
        manic features F06.33
        manic- or hypomanic-like episodes F06.33
        mixed features F06.34
    current (or most recent) episode
      depressed F31.9
        with psychotic features F31.5
        without psychotic features F31.30
          mild F31.31
          moderate F31.32
          severe (without psychotic features) F31.4
            with psychotic features F31.5
      hypomanic F31.0
      manic F31.9
        with psychotic features F31.2
        without psychotic features F31.10
          mild F31.11
          moderate F31.12
          severe (without psychotic features) F31.13
            with psychotic features F31.2
      mixed F31.60
        mild F31.61
        moderate F31.62
        severe (without psychotic features) F31.63
          with psychotic features F31.64
      severe depression (without psychotic features) F31.4
        with psychotic features F31.5
    in remission (currently) F31.70
      in full remission
        most recent episode
          depressed F31.76
          hypomanic F31.72
          manic F31.74
          mixed F31.78
      in partial remission
        most recent episode
          depressed F31.75
          hypomanic F31.71
          manic F31.73
          mixed F31.77
    organic F06.30
    single manic episode F30.9
      mild F30.11
      moderate F30.12
      severe (without psychotic symptoms) F30.13

Disorder — *continued*
  bipolar — *continued*
    single manic episode — *continued*
      severe — *continued*
        with psychotic symptoms F30.2
      specified NEC F31.89
  bipolar II (type 2) F31.81
  bladder N32.9
    functional NEC N31.9
    in schistosomiasis B65.0 [N33]
    specified NEC N32.89
  bleeding D68.9
  blood D75.9
    in congenital early syphilis A50.09 [D77]
  body dysmorphic F45.22
  bone M89.9
    continuity M84.9
      specified type NEC M84.80
        ankle M84.87- ☑
        fibula M84.86- ☑
        foot M84.87- ☑
        hand M84.84- ☑
        humerus M84.82- ☑
        neck M84.88
        pelvis M84.859
        radius M84.83- ☑
        rib M84.88
        shoulder M84.81- ☑
        skull M84.88
        thigh M84.85- ☑
        tibia M84.86- ☑
        ulna M84.83- ☑
        vertebra M84.88
    density and structure M85.9
      cyst (*see also* Cyst, bone, specified type NEC)
        aneurysmal — *see* Cyst, bone, aneurysmal
        solitary — *see* Cyst, bone, solitary
      diffuse idiopathic skeletal hyperostosis — *see* Hyperostosis, ankylosing
      fibrous dysplasia (monostotic) — *see* Dysplasia, fibrous, bone
      fluorosis — *see* Fluorosis, skeletal
      hyperostosis of skull M85.2
      osteitis condensans — *see* Osteitis, condensans
      specified type NEC M85.8- ☑
        ankle M85.87- ☑
        foot M85.87- ☑
        forearm M85.83- ☑
        hand M85.84- ☑
        lower leg M85.86- ☑
        multiple sites M85.89
        neck M85.88
        rib M85.88
        shoulder M85.81- ☑
        skull M85.88
        thigh M85.85- ☑
        upper arm M85.82- ☑
        vertebra M85.88
    development and growth NEC M89.20
      carpus M89.24- ☑
      clavicle M89.21- ☑
      femur M89.25- ☑
      fibula M89.26- ☑
      finger M89.24- ☑
      humerus M89.22- ☑
      ilium M89.259
      ischium M89.259
      metacarpus M89.24- ☑
      metatarsus M89.27- ☑
      multiple sites M89.29
      neck M89.28
      radius M89.23- ☑
      rib M89.28
      scapula M89.21- ☑
      skull M89.28
      tarsus M89.27- ☑
      tibia M89.26- ☑
      toe M89.27- ☑
      ulna M89.23- ☑
      vertebra M89.28
    specified type NEC M89.8X- ☑
  brachial plexus G54.0
  branched-chain amino-acid metabolism E71.2
    specified NEC E71.19
  breast N64.9
    agalactia — *see* Agalactia

Disorder — *continued*
  breast — *continued*
    associated with
      lactation O92.70
        specified NEC O92.79
      pregnancy O92.20
        specified NEC O92.29
      puerperium O92.20
        specified NEC O92.29
    cracked nipple — *see* Cracked nipple
    galactorrhea — *see* Galactorrhea
    hypogalactia O92.4
    lactation disorder NEC O92.79
    mastitis — *see* Mastitis
    nipple infection — *see* Infection, nipple
    retracted nipple — *see* Retraction, nipple
    specified type NEC N64.89
  Briquet's F45.0
  bullous, in diseases classified elsewhere L14
  caffeine use
    mild
      with
        caffeine-induced
          anxiety disorder F15.180
          sleep disorder F15.182
    moderate or severe
      with
        caffeine-induced
          anxiety disorder F15.280
          sleep disorder F15.282
  cannabis use
    mild F12.10
      with
        cannabis intoxication delirium F12.121
          with perceptual disturbances F12.122
          without perceptual disturbances F12.129
        cannabis-induced
          anxiety disorder F12.180
          psychotic disorder F12.159
          sleep disorder F12.188
      in remission (early) (sustained) F12.11
    moderate or severe F12.20
      with
        cannabis intoxication
          with perceptual disturbances F12.222
          without perceptual disturbances F12.229
        cannabis-induced
          anxiety disorder F12.280
          psychotic disorder F12.259
          sleep disorder F12.288
        delirium F12.221
      in remission (early) (sustained) F12.21
  carbohydrate
    absorption, intestinal NEC E74.39
    metabolism (congenital) E74.9
      specified NEC E74.8
  cardiac, functional I51.89
  carnitine metabolism E71.40
  cartilage M94.9
    articular NEC — *see* Derangement, joint, articular cartilage
    chondrocalcinosis — *see* Chondrocalcinosis
    specified type NEC M94.8X- ☑
      articular — *see* Derangement, joint, articular cartilage
      multiple sites M94.8X0
  catatonia (due to known physiological condition) (with another mental disorder) F06.1
  catatonic
    due to (secondary to) known physiological condition F06.1
    organic F06.1
  central auditory processing H93.25
  cervical
    region NEC M53.82
    root (nerve) NEC G54.2
  character NOS F60.9
  childhood disintegrative NEC F84.3
  cholesterol and bile acid metabolism E78.70
    Barth syndrome E78.71
    other specified E78.79
    Smith-Lemli-Opitz syndrome E78.72
  choroid H31.9
    atrophy — *see* Atrophy, choroid
    degeneration — *see* Degeneration, choroid
    detachment — *see* Detachment, choroid
    dystrophy — *see* Dystrophy, choroid
    hemorrhage — *see* Hemorrhage, choroid

☑ Additional Character Required — Refer to the Tabular List for Character Selection   ▽ Subterms under main terms may continue to next column or page

Disorder — continued
  choroid — continued
    rupture — see Rupture, choroid
    scar — see Scar, chorioretinal
    solar retinopathy — see Retinopathy, solar
    specified type NEC H31.8
  ciliary body — see Disorder, iris
    degeneration — see Degeneration, ciliary body
  coagulation (factor) (see also Defect, coagulation)
    D68.9
    newborn, transient P61.6
  cocaine use
    mild F14.10
      with
        amphetamine, cocaine, or other stimulant
          intoxication
            with perceptual disturbances F14.122
            without perceptual disturbances F14.129
        cocaine intoxication delirium F14.121
        cocaine-induced
          anxiety disorder F14.180
          bipolar and related disorder F14.14
          depressive disorder F14.14
          obsessive-compulsive and related disor-
            der F14.188
          psychotic disorder F14.159
          sexual dysfunction F14.181
          sleep disorder F14.182
      in remission (early) (sustained) F14.11
    moderate or severe F14.20
      with
        amphetamine, cocaine, or other stimulant
          intoxication
            with perceptual disturbances F14.222
            without perceptual disturbances F14.229
        cocaine intoxication delirium F14.221
        cocaine-induced
          anxiety disorder F14.280
          bipolar and related disorder F14.24
          depressive disorder F14.24
          obsessive-compulsive and related disor-
            der F14.288
          psychotic disorder F14.259
          sexual dysfunction F14.281
          sleep disorder F14.282
      in remission (early) (sustained) F14.21
  coccyx NEC M53.3
  cognitive F09
    due to (secondary to) general medical condition
      F09
    persisting R41.89
      due to
        alcohol F10.97
          with dependence F10.27
        anxiolytics F13.97
          with dependence F13.27
        hypnotics F13.97
          with dependence F13.27
        sedatives F13.97
          with dependence F13.27
        specified substance NEC F19.97
          with
            abuse F19.17
            dependence F19.27
  communication F80.9
    social pragmatic F80.82
  conduct (childhood) F91.9
    adjustment reaction — see Disorder, adjustment
    adolescent onset type F91.2
    childhood onset type F91.1
    compulsive F63.9
    confined to family context F91.0
    depressive F91.8
    group type F91.2
    hyperkinetic — see Disorder, attention-deficit hy-
      peractivity
    oppositional defiance F91.3
    socialized F91.2
    solitary aggressive type F91.1
    specified NEC F91.8
    unsocialized (aggressive) F91.1
  conduction, heart I45.9
  congenital glycosylation (CDG) E74.8
  conjunctiva H11.9
    infection — see Conjunctivitis
  connective tissue, localized L94.9
    specified NEC L94.8

Disorder — continued
  conversion (functional neurological symptom disorder)
    with
      abnormal movement F44.4
      anesthesia or sensory loss F44.6
      attacks or seizures F44.5
      mixed symptoms F44.7
      special sensory symptoms F44.6
      speech symptoms F44.4
      swallowing symptoms F44.4
      weakness or paralysis F44.4
  convulsive (secondary) — see Convulsions
  cornea H18.9
    deformity — see Deformity, cornea
    degeneration — see Degeneration, cornea
    deposits — see Deposit, cornea
    due to contact lens H18.82- ☑
      specified as edema — see Edema, cornea
    edema — see Edema, cornea
    keratitis — see Keratitis
    keratoconjunctivitis — see Keratoconjunctivitis
    membrane change — see Change, corneal mem-
      brane
    neovascularization — see Neovascularization,
      cornea
    scar — see Opacity, cornea ☑
    specified type NEC H18.89- ☑
    ulcer — see Ulcer, cornea
  corpus cavernosum N48.9
  cranial nerve — see Disorder, nerve, cranial
  cyclothymic F34.0
  defiant oppositional F91.3
  delusional (persistent) (systematized) F22
    induced F24
  depersonalization F48.1
  depressive F32.9
    due to known physiological condition
      with
        depressive features F06.31
        major depressive-like episode F06.32
        mixed features F06.34
    major F32.9
      with psychotic symptoms F32.3
      in remission (full) F32.5
        partial F32.4
      recurrent F33.9
        with psychotic features F33.3
      single episode F32.9
        mild F32.0
        moderate F32.1
        severe (without psychotic symptoms) F32.2
          with psychotic symptoms F32.3
    organic F06.31
    persistent F34.1
    recurrent F33.9
      current episode
        mild F33.0
        moderate F33.1
        severe (without psychotic symptoms) F33.2
          with psychotic symptoms F33.3
      in remission F33.40
        full F33.42
        partial F33.41
      specified NEC F33.8
    single episode — see Episode, depressive
    specified NEC F32.89
  developmental F89
    arithmetical skills F81.2
    coordination (motor) F82
    expressive writing F81.81
    language F80.9
      expressive F80.1
      mixed receptive and expressive F80.2
      receptive type F80.2
      specified NEC F80.89
    learning F81.9
      arithmetical F81.2
      reading F81.0
    mixed F88
    motor coordination or function F82
    pervasive F84.9
      specified NEC F84.8
    phonological F80.0
    reading F81.0
    scholastic skills (see also Disorder, learning)
      mixed F81.89
    specified NEC F88
    speech F80.9

Disorder — continued
  developmental — continued
    speech — continued
      articulation F80.0
      specified NEC F80.89
    written expression F81.81
  diaphragm J98.6
  digestive (system) K92.9
    newborn P78.9
      specified NEC P78.89
    postprocedural — see Complication, gastrointesti-
      nal
    psychogenic F45.8
  disc (intervertebral) M51.9
    with
      myelopathy
        cervical region M50.00
        cervicothoracic region M50.03
        high cervical region M50.01
        lumbar region M51.06
        mid-cervical region M50.020
        sacrococcygeal region M53.3
        thoracic region M51.04
        thoracolumbar region M51.05
      radiculopathy
        cervical region M50.10
        cervicothoracic region M50.13
        high cervical region M50.11
        lumbar region M51.16
        lumbosacral region M51.17
        mid-cervical region M50.120
        sacrococcygeal region M53.3
        thoracic region M51.14
        thoracolumbar region M51.15
  cervical M50.90
    with
      myelopathy M50.00
        C2-C3 M50.01
        C3-C4 M50.01
        C4-C5 M50.021
        C5-C6 M50.022
        C6-C7 M50.023
        C7-T1 M50.03
        cervicothoracic region M50.03
        high cervical region M50.01
        mid-cervical region M50.020
      neuritis, radiculitis or radiculopathy M50.10
        C2-C3 M50.11
        C3-C4 M50.11
        C4-C5 M50.121
        C5-C6 M50.122
        C6-C7 M50.123
        C7-T1 M50.13
        cervicothoracic region M50.13
        high cervical region M50.11
        mid-cervical region M50.120
    C2-C3 M50.91
    C3-C4 M50.91
    C4-C5 M50.921
    C5-C6 M50.922
    C6-C7 M50.923
    C7-T1 M50.93
    cervicothoracic region M50.93
    degeneration M50.30
      C2-C3 M50.31
      C3-C4 M50.31
      C4-C5 M50.321
      C5-C6 M50.322
      C6-C7 M50.323
      C7-T1 M50.33
      cervicothoracic region M50.33
      high cervical region M50.31
      mid-cervical region M50.320
    displacement M50.20
      C2-C3 M50.21
      C3-C4 M50.21
      C4-C5 M50.221
      C5-C6 M50.222
      C6-C7 M50.223
      C7-T1 M50.23
      cervicothoracic region M50.23
      high cervical region M50.21
      mid-cervical region M50.220
    high cervical region M50.91
    mid-cervical region M50.920
    specified type NEC M50.80
      C2-C3 M50.81
      C3-C4 M50.81
      C4-C5 M50.821

Disorder — continued
  disc — continued
    cervical — continued
      specified type — continued
        C5-C6 M50.822
        C6-C7 M50.823
        C7-T1 M50.83
        cervicothoracic region M50.83
        high cervical region M50.81
        mid-cervical region M50.820
      specified NEC
        lumbar region M51.86
        lumbosacral region M51.87
        sacrococcygeal region M53.3
        thoracic region M51.84
        thoracolumbar region M51.85
  disinhibited attachment (childhood) F94.2
  disintegrative, childhood NEC F84.3
  disruptive F91.9
    mood dysregulation F34.81
    specified NEC F91.8
  disruptive behavior — see Disorder, conduct
  dissocial personality F60.2
  dissociative F44.9
    affecting
      motor function F44.4
        and sensation F44.7
      sensation F44.6
        and motor function F44.7
    brief reactive F43.0
    due to (secondary to) general medical condition F06.8
    mixed F44.7
    organic F06.8
    other specified NEC F44.89
  double heterozygous sickling — see Disease, sickle-cell
  dream anxiety F51.5
  drug induced hemorrhagic D68.32
  drug related F19.99
    abuse — see Abuse, drug
    dependence — see Dependence, drug
  dysmorphic body F45.22
  dysthymic F34.1
  ear H93.9- ☑
    bleeding — see Otorrhagia
    deafness — see Deafness
    degenerative H93.09- ☑
    discharge — see Otorrhea
    external H61.9- ☑
      auditory canal stenosis — see Stenosis, external ear canal
      exostosis — see Exostosis, external ear canal
      impacted cerumen — see Impaction, cerumen
      otitis — see Otitis, externa
      perichondritis — see Perichondritis, ear
      pinna — see Disorder, pinna
      specified type NEC H61.89- ☑
    inner H83.9- ☑
      vestibular dysfunction — see Disorder, vestibular function
    middle H74.9- ☑
      adhesive H74.1- ☑
      ossicle — see Abnormal, ear ossicles
      polyp — see Polyp, ear (middle)
      specified NEC, in diseases classified elsewhere H75.8- ☑
    postprocedural — see Complications, ear, procedure
    specified NEC, in diseases classified elsewhere H94.8- ☑
  eating (adult) (psychogenic) F50.9
    anorexia — see Anorexia
    binge F50.81
    bulimia F50.2
    child F98.29
      pica F98.3
      rumination disorder F98.21
    pica F50.89
      childhood F98.3
  electrolyte (balance) NEC E87.8
    with
      abortion — see Abortion by type complicated by specified condition NEC
      ectopic pregnancy O08.5
      molar pregnancy O08.5
    acidosis (metabolic) (respiratory) E87.2
    alkalosis (metabolic) (respiratory) E87.3

Disorder — continued
  elimination, transepidermal L87.9
    specified NEC L87.8
  emotional (persistent) F34.9
    of childhood F93.9
      specified NEC F93.8
  endocrine E34.9
    postprocedural E89.89
      specified NEC E89.89
  erectile (male) (organic) (see also Dysfunction, sexual, male, erectile) N52.9
    nonorganic F52.21
  erythematous — see Erythema
  esophagus K22.9
    functional K22.4
    psychogenic F45.8
  eustachian tube H69.9- ☑
    infection — see Salpingitis, eustachian
    obstruction — see Obstruction, eustachian tube
    patulous — see Patulous, eustachian tube
    specified NEC H69.8- ☑
  exhibitionistic F65.2
  extrapyramidal G25.9
    in deseases classified elsewhere — see category G26
    specified type NEC G25.89
  eye H57.9
    postprocedural — see Complication, postprocedural, eye
  eyelid H02.9
    cyst — see Cyst, eyelid
    degenerative H02.70
      chloasma — see Chloasma, eyelid
      madarosis — see Madarosis
      specified type NEC H02.79
      vitiligo — see Vitiligo, eyelid
      xanthelasma — see Xanthelasma
    dermatochalasis — see Dermatochalasis
    edema — see Edema, eyelid
    elephantiasis — see Elephantiasis, eyelid
    foreign body, retained — see Foreign body, retained, eyelid
    function H02.59
      abnormal innervation syndrome — see Syndrome, abnormal innervation
      blepharochalasis — see Blepharochalasis
      blepharoclonus — see Blepharoclonus
      blepharophimosis — see Blepharophimosis
      blepharoptosis — see Blepharoptosis
      lagophthalmos — see Lagophthalmos
      lid retraction — see Retraction, lid
    hypertrichosis — see Hypertrichosis, eyelid
    specified type NEC H02.89
    vascular H02.879
      left H02.876
        lower H02.875
        upper H02.874
      right H02.873
        lower H02.872
        upper H02.871
  factitious F68.10
    with predominantly
      physical symptoms F68.12
        with psychological symptoms F68.13
      psychological symptoms F68.11
        with physical symptoms F68.13
  factor, coagulation — see Defect, coagulation
  fatty acid
    metabolism E71.30
      specified NEC E71.39
    oxidation
      LCAD E71.310
      MCAD E71.311
      SCAD E71.312
      specified deficiency NEC E71.318
  feeding (infant or child) (see also Disorder, eating) R63.3
    or eating disorder F50.9
    specified NEC F50.9
  feigned (with obvious motivation) Z76.5
    without obvious motivation — see Disorder, factitious
  female
    hypoactive sexual desire F52.0
    orgasmic F52.31
    sexual interest/arousal F52.22
  fetishistic F65.0
  fibroblastic M72.9

Disorder — continued
  fibroblastic — continued
    specified NEC M72.8
  fluency
    adult onset F98.5
    childhood onset F80.81
    following
      cerebral infarction I69.323
      cerebrovascular disease I69.923
        specified disease NEC I69.823
      intracerebral hemorrhage I69.123
      nontraumatic intracranial hemorrhage NEC I69.223
      subarachnoid hemorrhage I69.023
    in conditions classified elsewhere R47.82
  fluid balance E87.8
  follicular (skin) L73.9
    specified NEC L73.8
  frotteuristic F65.81
  fructose metabolism E74.10
    essential fructosuria E74.11
    fructokinase deficiency E74.11
    fructose-1, 6-diphosphatase deficiency E74.19
    hereditary fructose intolerance E74.12
    other specified E74.19
  functional polymorphonuclear neutrophils D71
  gallbladder, biliary tract and pancreas in diseases classified elsewhere K87
  gambling F63.0
  gamma-glutamyl cycle E72.8
  gastric (functional) K31.9
    motility K30
    psychogenic F45.8
    secretion K30
  gastrointestinal (functional) NOS K92.9
    newborn P78.9
    psychogenic F45.8
  gender-identity or -role F64.9
    childhood F64.2
    effect on relationship F66
    of adolescence or adulthood F64.0
      nontranssexual F64.8
    specified NEC F64.8
    uncertainty F66
  genito-pelvic pain penetration F52.6
  genitourinary system
    female N94.9
    male N50.9
    psychogenic F45.8
  globe H44.9
    degenerated condition H44.50
      absolute glaucoma H44.51- ☑
      atrophy H44.52- ☑
      leucocoria H44.53- ☑
    degenerative H44.30
      chalcosis H44.31- ☑
      myopia (see also Myopia, degenerative) H44.2- ☑
      siderosis H44.32- ☑
      specified type NEC H44.39- ☑
    endophthalmitis — see Endophthalmitis
    foreign body, retained — see Foreign body, intraocular, old, retained
    hemophthalmos — see Hemophthalmos
    hypotony H44.40
      due to
        ocular fistula H44.42- ☑
        specified disorder NEC H44.43- ☑
      flat anterior chamber H44.41- ☑
      primary H44.44- ☑
    luxation — see Luxation, globe
    specified type NEC H44.89
  glomerular (in) N05.9
    amyloidosis E85.4 [N08]
    cryoglobulinemia D89.1 [N08]
    disseminated intravascular coagulation D65 [N08]
    Fabry's disease E75.21 [N08]
    familial lecithin cholesterol acyltransferase deficiency E78.6 [N08]
    Goodpasture's syndrome M31.0
    hemolytic-uremic syndrome D59.3
    Henoch (-Schönlein) purpura D69.0 [N08]
    malariae malaria B52.0
    microscopic polyangiitis M31.7 [N08]
    multiple myeloma C90.0- ☑ [N08]
    mumps B26.83
    schistosomiasis B65.9 [N08]
    sepsis NEC A41.- ☑ [N08]

Disorder — *continued*
  glomerular — *continued*
    sepsis — *continued*
      streptococcal A40.- ☑ [N08]
    sickle-cell disorders D57.- ☑ [N08]
    strongyloidiasis B78.9 [N08]
    subacute bacterial endocarditis I33.0 [N08]
    syphilis A52.75
    systemic lupus erythematosus M32.14
    thrombotic thrombocytopenic purpura
      M31.1 [N08]
    Waldenström macroglobulinemia C88.0 [N08]
    Wegener's granulomatosis M31.31
  gluconeogenesis E74.4
  glucosaminoglycan metabolism — *see* Disorder,
    metabolism, glucosaminoglycan
  glycine metabolism E72.50
    d-glycericacidemia E72.59
    hyperhydroxyprolinemia E72.59
    hyperoxaluria E72.53
    hyperprolinemia E72.59
    non-ketotic hyperglycinemia E72.51
    oxalosis E72.53
    oxaluria E72.53
    sarcosinemia E72.59
    trimethylaminuria E72.52
  glycoprotein metabolism E77.9
    specified NEC E77.8
  habit (and impulse) F63.9
    involving sexual behavior NEC F65.9
    specified NEC F63.89
  hallucinogen use
    mild F16.10
      with
        hallucinogen intoxication delirium F16.121
        hallucinogen-induced
          anxiety disorder F16.180
          bipolar and related disorder F16.14
          depressive disorder F16.14
          psychotic disorder F16.159
        other hallucinogen intoxication F16.129
      in remission (early) (sustained) F16.11
    moderate or severe F16.20
      with
        hallucinogen intoxication delirium F16.221
        hallucinogen-induced
          anxiety disorder F16.280
          bipolar and related disorder F16.24
          depressive disorder F16.24
          psychotic disorder F16.259
        other hallucinogen intoxication F16.229
      in remission (early) (sustained) F16.21
  heart action I49.9
  hematological D75.9
    newborn (transient) P61.9
      specified NEC P61.8
  hematopoietic organs D75.9
  hemorrhagic NEC D69.9
    drug-induced D68.32
    due to
      extrinsic circulating anticoagulants D68.32
      increase in
        anti-IIa D68.32
        anti-Xa D68.32
      intrinsic
        circulating anticoagulants D68.318
        increase in
          anti-IXa D68.318
          antithrombin D68.318
          anti-VIIIa D68.318
          anti-XIa D68.318
    following childbirth O72.3
  hemostasis — *see* Defect, coagulation
  histidine metabolism E70.40
    histidinemia E70.41
    other specified E70.49
  hoarding F42.3
  hyperkinetic — *see* Disorder, attention-deficit hyper-
    activity
  hyperleucine-isoleucinemia E71.19
  hypervalinemia E71.19
  hypoactive sexual desire F52.0
  hypochondriacal F45.20
    body dysmorphic F45.22
    neurosis F45.21
    other specified F45.29
  identity
    dissociative F44.81
    illness anxiety F45.21

Disorder — *continued*
  identity — *continued*
    of childhood F93.8
  immune mechanism (immunity) D89.9
    specified type NEC D89.89
  impaired renal tubular function N25.9
    specified NEC N25.89
  impulse (control) F63.9
  inflammatory
    pelvic, in diseases classified elsewhere — *see* cate-
      gory N74
    penis N48.29
      abscess N48.21
      cellulitis N48.22
  inhalant use
    mild F18.10
      with
        inhalant intoxication F18.129
        inhalant intoxication delirium F18.121
        inhalant-induced
          anxiety disorder F18.180
          depressive disorder F18.14
          major neurocognitive disorder F18.17
          mild neurocognitive disorder F18.188
          psychotic disorder F18.159
      in remission (early) (sustained) F18.11
    moderate or severe F18.20
      with
        inhalant intoxication F18.229
        inhalant intoxication delirium F18.221
        inhalant-induced
          anxiety disorder F18.280
          depressive disorder F18.24
          major neurocognitive disorder F18.27
          mild neurocognitive disorder F18.288
          psychotic disorder F18.259
      in remission (early) (sustained) F18.21
  integument, newborn P83.9
    specified NEC P83.88
  intermittent explosive F63.81
  internal secretion pancreas — *see* Increased, secretion,
    pancreas, endocrine
  intestine, intestinal
    carbohydrate absorption NEC E74.39
      postoperative K91.2
    functional NEC K59.9
      postoperative K91.89
    psychogenic F45.8
    vascular K55.9
      chronic K55.1
      specified NEC K55.8
  intraoperative (intraprocedural) — *see* Complications,
    intraoperative
  involuntary emotional expression (IEED) F07.89
  iris H21.9
    adhesions — *see* Adhesions, iris
    atrophy — *see* Atrophy, iris
    chamber angle recession — *see* Recession, cham-
      ber angle
    cyst — *see* Cyst, iris
    degeneration — *see* Degeneration, iris
    in diseases classified elsewhere H22
    iridodialysis — *see* Iridodialysis
    iridoschisis — *see* Iridoschisis
    miotic pupillary cyst — *see* Cyst, pupillary
    pupillary
      abnormality — *see* Abnormality, pupillary
      membrane — *see* Membrane, pupillary
    specified type NEC H21.89
    vascular NEC H21.1X- ☑
  iron metabolism E83.10
    specified NEC E83.19
  isovaleric acidemia E71.110
  jaw, developmental M27.0
    temporomandibular (*see also* Anomaly, dentofacial,
      temporomandibular joint) M26.60- ☑
  joint M25.9
    derangement — *see* Derangement, joint
    effusion — *see* Effusion, joint
    fistula — *see* Fistula, joint
    hemarthrosis — *see* Hemarthrosis
    instability — *see* Instability, joint
    osteophyte — *see* Osteophyte
    pain — *see* Pain, joint
    psychogenic F45.8
    specified type NEC M25.80
      ankle M25.87- ☑
      elbow M25.82- ☑

Disorder — *continued*
  joint — *continued*
    specified type — *continued*
      foot joint M25.87- ☑
      hand joint M25.84- ☑
      hip M25.85- ☑
      knee M25.86- ☑
      shoulder M25.81- ☑
      wrist M25.83- ☑
    stiffness — *see* Stiffness, joint
  ketone metabolism E71.32
  kidney N28.9
    functional (tubular) N25.9
    in
      schistosomiasis B65.9 [N29]
    tubular function N25.9
      specified NEC N25.89
  lacrimal system H04.9
    changes H04.69
      fistula — *see* Fistula, lacrimal
    gland H04.19
      atrophy — *see* Atrophy, lacrimal gland
      cyst — *see* Cyst, lacrimal, gland
      dacryops — *see* Dacryops
      dislocation — *see* Dislocation, lacrimal gland
      dry eye syndrome — *see* Syndrome, dry eye
      infection — *see* Dacryoadenitis
      granuloma — *see* Granuloma, lacrimal
      inflammation — *see* Inflammation, lacrimal
      obstruction — *see* Obstruction, lacrimal
      specified NEC H04.89
  lactation NEC O92.79
  language (developmental) F80.9
    expressive F80.1
    mixed receptive and expressive F80.2
    receptive F80.2
  late luteal phase dysphoric N94.89
  learning (specific) F81.9
    acalculia R48.8
    alexia R48.0
    mathematics F81.2
    reading F81.0
    specified
      with impairment in
        mathematics F81.2
        reading F81.0
        written expression F81.81
    specified NEC F81.89
    spelling F81.81
    written expression F81.81
  lens H27.9
    aphakia — *see* Aphakia
    cataract — *see* Cataract
    dislocation — *see* Dislocation, lens
    specified type NEC H27.8
  ligament M24.20
    ankle M24.27- ☑
    attachment, spine — *see* Enthesopathy, spinal
    elbow M24.22- ☑
    foot joint M24.27- ☑
    hand joint M24.24- ☑
    hip M24.25- ☑
    knee — *see* Derangement, knee, specified NEC
    shoulder M24.21- ☑
    vertebra M24.28
    wrist M24.23- ☑
  ligamentous attachments (*see also* Enthesopathy)
    spine — *see* Enthesopathy, spinal
  lipid
    metabolism, congenital E78.9
    storage E75.6
      specified NEC E75.5
  lipoprotein
    deficiency (familial) E78.6
    metabolism E78.9
      specified NEC E78.89
  liver K76.9
    malarial B54 [K77]
  low back (*see also* Dorsopathy, specified NEC)
  lumbosacral
    plexus G54.1
    root (nerve) NEC G54.4
  lung, interstitial, drug-induced J70.4
    acute J70.2
    chronic J70.3
  lymphoproliferative, post-transplant (PTLD) D47.Z1
    (*following* D47.4)
  lysine and hydroxylysine metabolism E72.3

△ Subterms under main terms may continue to next column or page   ☑ Additional Character Required — Refer to the Tabular List for Character Selection   113

Disorder — Disorder

Disorder — *continued*
- major neurocognitive — *see* Dementia, in (due to)
- male
  - erectile (organic) (*see also* Dysfunction, sexual, male, erectile) N52.9
    - nonorganic F52.21
  - hypoactive sexual desire F52.0
  - orgasmic F52.32
- manic F30.9
  - organic F06.33
- mast cell activation — *see* Activation, mast cell
- mastoid (*see also* Disorder, ear, middle)
  - postprocedural — *see* Complications, ear, procedure
- meniscus — *see* Derangement, knee, meniscus
- menopausal N95.9
  - specified NEC N95.8
- menstrual N92.6
  - psychogenic F45.8
  - specified NEC N92.5
- mental (or behavioral) (nonpsychotic) F99
  - due to (secondary to)
    - amphetamine
      - due to drug abuse — *see* Abuse, drug, stimulant
      - due to drug dependence — *see* Dependence, drug, stimulant
    - brain disease, damage and dysfunction F09
    - caffeine use
      - due to drug abuse — *see* Abuse, drug, stimulant
      - due to drug dependence — *see* Dependence, drug, stimulant
    - cannabis use
      - due to drug abuse — *see* Abuse, drug, cannabis
      - due to drug dependence — *see* Dependence, drug, cannabis
    - general medical condition F09
    - sedative or hypnotic use
      - due to drug abuse — *see* Abuse, drug, sedative
      - due to drug dependence — *see* Dependence, drug, sedative
    - tobacco (nicotine) use — *see* Dependence, drug, nicotine
  - following organic brain damage F07.9
    - frontal lobe syndrome F07.0
    - personality change F07.0
    - postconcussional syndrome F07.81
    - specified NEC F07.89
  - infancy, childhood or adolescence F98.9
  - neurotic — *see* Neurosis
  - organic or symptomatic F09
  - presenile, psychotic F03 ☑
  - problem NEC
  - psychoneurotic — *see* Neurosis
  - psychotic — *see* Psychosis
  - puerperal F53
  - senile, psychotic NEC F03 ☑
- metabolic, amino acid, transitory, newborn P74.8
- metabolism NOS E88.9
  - amino-acid E72.9
    - aromatic E70.9
      - albinism — *see* Albinism
      - histidine E70.40
        - histidinemia E70.41
        - other specified E70.49
      - hyperphenylalaninemia E70.1
        - classical phenylketonuria E70.0
      - other specified E70.8
      - tryptophan E70.5
      - tyrosine E70.20
        - hypertyrosinemia E70.21
        - other specified E70.29
    - branched chain E71.2
      - 3-methylglutaconic aciduria E71.111
      - hyperleucine-isoleucinemia E71.19
      - hypervalinemia E71.19
      - isovaleric acidemia E71.110
      - maple syrup urine disease E71.0
      - methylmalonic acidemia E71.120
      - organic aciduria NEC E71.118
      - other specified E71.19
      - proprionate NEC E71.128
      - proprionic acidemia E71.121
    - glycine E72.50
      - d-glycericacidemia E72.59

Disorder — *continued*
- metabolism — *continued*
  - amino-acid — *continued*
    - glycine — *continued*
      - hyperhydroxyprolinemia E72.59
      - hyperoxaluria E72.53
      - hyperprolinemia E72.59
      - non-ketotic hyperglycinemia E72.51
      - other specified E72.59
      - sarcosinemia E72.59
      - trimethylaminuria E72.52
    - hydroxylysine E72.3
    - lysine E72.3
    - ornithine E72.4
    - other specified E72.8
      - beta-amino acid E72.8
      - gamma-glutamyl cycle E72.8
      - straight-chain E72.8
    - sulfur-bearing E72.10
      - homocystinuria E72.11
      - methylenetetrahydrofolate reductase deficiency E72.12
      - other specified E72.19
  - bile acid and cholesterol metabolism E78.70
  - bilirubin E80.7
    - specified NEC E80.6
  - calcium E83.50
    - hypercalcemia E83.52
    - hypocalcemia E83.51
    - other specified E83.59
  - carbohydrate E74.9
    - specified NEC E74.8
  - cholesterol and bile acid metabolism E78.70
  - congenital E88.9
  - copper E83.00
    - specified type NEC E83.09
    - Wilson's disease E83.01
  - cystinuria E72.01
  - fructose E74.10
  - galactose E74.20
  - glucosaminoglycan E76.9
    - mucopolysaccharidosis — *see* Mucopolysaccharidosis
    - specified NEC E76.8
  - glutamine E72.8
  - glycine E72.50
  - glycogen storage (hepatorenal) E74.09
  - glycoprotein E77.9
    - specified NEC E77.8
  - glycosaminoglycan E76.9
    - specified NEC E76.8
  - in labor and delivery O75.89
  - iron E83.10
  - isoleucine E71.19
  - leucine E71.19
  - lipoid E78.9
  - lipoprotein E78.9
    - specified NEC E78.89
  - magnesium E83.40
    - hypermagnesemia E83.41
    - hypomagnesemia E83.42
    - other specified E83.49
  - mineral E83.9
    - specified NEC E83.89
  - mitochondrial E88.40
    - MELAS syndrome E88.41
    - MERRF syndrome (myoclonic epilepsy associated with ragged-red fibers) E88.42
    - other specified E88.49
  - ornithine E72.4
  - phosphatases E83.30
  - phosphorus E83.30
    - acid phosphatase deficiency E83.39
    - hypophosphatasia E83.39
    - hypophosphatemia E83.39
      - familial E83.31
    - other specified E83.39
    - pseudovitamin D deficiency E83.32
  - plasma protein NEC E88.09
  - porphyrin — *see* Porphyria
  - postprocedural E89.89
    - specified NEC E89.89
  - purine E79.9
    - specified NEC E79.8
  - pyrimidine E79.9
    - specified NEC E79.8
  - pyruvate E74.4
  - serine E72.8
  - sodium E87.8

Disorder — *continued*
- metabolism — *continued*
  - specified NEC E88.89
  - threonine E72.8
  - valine E71.19
  - zinc E83.2
- methylmalonic acidemia E71.120
- micturition NEC (*see also* Difficulty, micturition) R39.198
  - feeling of incomplete emptying R39.14
  - hesitancy R39.11
  - poor stream R39.12
  - psychogenic F45.8
  - split stream R39.13
  - straining R39.16
  - urgency R39.15
- mild neurocognitive G31.84
- mitochondrial metabolism E88.40
- mitral (valve) — *see* Endocarditis, mitral
- mixed
  - anxiety and depressive F41.8
  - of scholastic skills (developmental) F81.89
  - receptive expressive language F80.2
- mood F39
  - bipolar — *see* Disorder, bipolar
  - depressive — *see* Disorder, depressive
  - due to (secondary to)
    - alcohol F10.94
    - amphetamine F15.94
      - in
        - abuse F15.14
        - dependence F15.24
    - anxiolytic F13.94
      - in
        - abuse F13.14
        - dependence F13.24
    - cocaine F14.94
      - in
        - abuse F14.14
        - dependence F14.24
    - general medical condition F06.30
    - hallucinogen F16.94
      - in
        - abuse F16.14
        - dependence F16.24
    - hypnotic F13.94
      - in
        - abuse F13.14
        - dependence F13.24
    - inhalant F18.94
      - in
        - abuse F18.14
        - dependence F18.24
    - opioid F11.94
      - in
        - abuse F11.14
        - dependence F11.24
    - phencyclidine (PCP) F16.94
      - in
        - abuse F16.14
        - dependence F16.24
    - physiological condition F06.30
      - with
        - depressive features F06.31
        - major depressive-like episode F06.32
        - manic features F06.33
        - mixed features F06.34
    - psychoactive substance NEC F19.94
      - in
        - abuse F19.14
        - dependence F19.24
    - sedative F13.94
      - in
        - abuse F13.14
        - dependence F13.24
    - volatile solvents F18.94
      - in
        - abuse F18.14
        - dependence F18.24
  - manic episode F30.9
    - with psychotic symptoms F30.2
    - without psychotic symptoms F30.10
      - mild F30.11
      - moderate F30.12
      - severe F30.13
    - in remission (full) F30.4
      - partial F30.3
    - specified type NEC F30.8
  - organic F06.30

Disorder — continued
  mood — continued
    organic — continued
      right hemisphere F07.89
    persistent F34.9
      cyclothymia F34.0
      dysthymia F34.1
      specified type NEC F34.89
    recurrent F39
    right hemisphere organic F07.89
  movement G25.9
    drug-induced G25.70
      akathisia G25.71
      specified NEC G25.79
    hysterical F44.4
    in diseases classified elsewhere — see category G26
    periodic limb G47.61
      sleep related G47.61
    sleep related NEC G47.69
    specified NEC G25.89
    stereotyped F98.4
    treatment-induced G25.9
  multiple personality F44.81
  muscle M62.9
    attachment, spine — see Enthesopathy, spinal
    in trichinellosis — see Trichinellosis, with muscle disorder
    psychogenic F45.8
    specified type NEC M62.89
    tone, newborn P94.9
      specified NEC P94.8
  muscular
    attachments (see also Enthesopathy)
      spine — see Enthesopathy, spinal
    urethra N36.44
  musculoskeletal system, soft tissue — see Disorder, soft tissue
    postprocedural M96.89
    psychogenic F45.8
  myoneural G70.9
    due to lead G70.1
    specified NEC G70.89
    toxic G70.1
  myotonic NEC G71.19
  nail, in diseases classified elsewhere L62
  neck region NEC — see Dorsopathy, specified NEC
  neonatal onset multisystemic inflammatory (NOMID) M04.2
  nerve G58.9
    abducent NEC — see Strabismus, paralytic, sixth nerve
    accessory G52.8
    acoustic — see subcategory H93.3 ☑
    auditory — see subcategory H93.3 ☑
    auriculotemporal G50.8
    axillary G54.0
    cerebral — see Disorder, nerve, cranial
    cranial G52.9
      eighth — see subcategory H93.3 ☑
      eleventh G52.8
      fifth G50.9
      first G52.0
      fourth NEC — see Strabismus, paralytic, fourth nerve
      multiple G52.7
      ninth G52.1
      second NEC — see Disorder, nerve, optic
      seventh NEC G51.8
      sixth NEC — see Strabismus, paralytic, sixth nerve
      specified NEC G52.8
      tenth G52.2
      third NEC — see Strabismus, paralytic, third nerve
      twelfth G52.3
    entrapment — see Neuropathy, entrapment
    facial G51.9
      specified NEC G51.8
    femoral — see Lesion, nerve, femoral
    glossopharyngeal NEC G52.1
    hypoglossal G52.3
    intercostal G58.0
    lateral
      cutaneous of thigh — see Mononeuropathy, lower limb, meralgia paresthetica
      popliteal — see Lesion, nerve, popliteal
    lower limb — see Mononeuropathy, lower limb

Disorder — continued
  nerve — continued
    medial popliteal — see Lesion, nerve, popliteal, medial
    median NEC — see Lesion, nerve, median
    multiple G58.7
    oculomotor NEC — see Strabismus, paralytic, third nerve
    olfactory G52.0
    optic NEC H47.09- ☑
      hemorrhage into sheath — see Hemorrhage, optic nerve
      ischemic H47.01- ☑
    peroneal — see Lesion, nerve, popliteal
    phrenic G58.8
    plantar — see Lesion, nerve, plantar
    pneumogastric G52.2
    posterior tibial — see Syndrome, tarsal tunnel
    radial — see Lesion, nerve, radial
    recurrent laryngeal G52.2
    root G54.9
      cervical G54.2
      lumbosacral G54.1
      specified NEC G54.8
      thoracic G54.3
    sciatic NEC — see Lesion, nerve, sciatic
    specified NEC G58.8
      lower limb — see Mononeuropathy, lower limb, specified NEC
      upper limb — see Mononeuropathy, upper limb, specified NEC
    sympathetic G90.9
    tibial — see Lesion, nerve, popliteal, medial
    trigeminal G50.9
      specified NEC G50.8
    trochlear NEC — see Strabismus, paralytic, fourth nerve
    ulnar — see Lesion, nerve, ulnar
    upper limb — see Mononeuropathy, upper limb
    vagus G52.2
  nervous system G98.8
    autonomic (peripheral) G90.9
      specified NEC G90.8
    central G96.9
      specified NEC G96.8
    parasympathetic G90.9
    specified NEC G98.8
    sympathetic G90.9
    vegetative G90.9
  neurocognitive R41.9
    major
      with
        aggressive behavior F01.51
        combative behavior F01.51
        violent behavior F01.51
      without behavioral disturbance F01.50
      due to vascular disease, with behavioral disturbance F01.51
      in (due to) (other diseases classified elsewhere) (see also Dementia, in (due to)) F02.80
        with
          aggressive behavior F02.81
          combative behavior F02.81
          violent behavior F02.81
    mild G31.84
  neurodevelopmental F89
    specified NEC F88
  neurohypophysis NEC E23.3
  neurological NEC R29.818
  neuromuscular G70.9
    hereditary NEC G71.9
    specified NEC G70.89
    toxic G70.1
  neurotic F48.9
    specified NEC F48.8
  neutrophil, polymorphonuclear D71
  nicotine use — see Dependence, drug, nicotine
  nightmare F51.5
  non-rapid eye movement sleep arousal
    sleep terror type F51.4
    sleepwalking type F51.3
  nose J34.9
    specified NEC J34.89
  obsessive-compulsive F42.9
    and related disorder due to a known physiological condition F06.8
  odontogenesis NOS K00.9

Disorder — continued
  opioid use
    with
      opioid-induced psychotic disorder F11.959
        with
          delusions F11.950
          hallucinations F11.951
    due to drug abuse — see Abuse, drug, opioid
    due to drug dependence — see Dependence, drug, opioid
    mild F11.10
      with
        opioid intoxication
          with perceptual disturbances F11.122
          without perceptual disturbances F11.129
          delirium F11.121
        opioid-induced
          anxiety disorder F11.188
          depressive disorder F11.14
          sexual dysfunction F11.181
      in remission (early) (sustained) F11.11
    moderate or severe F11.20
      with
        opioid intoxication
          with perceptual disturbances F11.222
          without perceptual disturbances F11.229
          delirium F11.221
        opioid-induced
          anxiety disorder F11.288
          anxiety disorder F11.988
          depressive disorder F11.24
          depressive disorder F11.94
          sexual dysfunction F11.281
          sexual dysfunction F11.981
      in remission (early) (sustained) F11.21
  oppositional defiant F91.3
  optic
    chiasm H47.49
      due to
        inflammatory disorder H47.41
        neoplasm H47.42
        vascular disorder H47.43
    disc H47.39- ☑
      coloboma — see Coloboma, optic disc
      drusen — see Drusen, optic disc
      pseudopapilledema — see Pseudopapilledema
    radiations — see Disorder, visual, pathway
    tracts — see Disorder, visual, pathway
  orbit H05.9
    cyst — see Cyst, orbit
    deformity — see Deformity, orbit
    edema — see Edema, orbit
    enophthalmos — see Enophthalmos
    exophthalmos — see Exophthalmos
    hemorrhage — see Hemorrhage, orbit
    inflammation — see Inflammation, orbit
    myopathy — see Myopathy, extraocular muscles
    retained foreign body — see Foreign body, orbit, old
    specified type NEC H05.89
  organic
    anxiety F06.4
    catatonic F06.1
    delusional F06.2
    dissociative F06.8
    emotionally labile (asthenic) F06.8
    mood (affective) F06.30
    schizophrenia-like F06.2
  orgasmic (female) F52.31
    male F52.32
  ornithine metabolism E72.4
  overanxious F41.1
    of childhood F93.8
  pain
    with related psychological factors F45.42
    exclusively related to psychological factors F45.41
    genito-pelvic penetration disorder F52.6
  pancreatic internal secretion E16.9
    specified NEC E16.8
  panic F41.0
    with agoraphobia F40.01
  papulosquamous L44.9
    in diseases classified elsewhere L45
    specified NEC L44.8
  paranoid F22
    induced F24
    shared F24
  paraphilic F65.9

Index

Disorder — Disorder

Disorder — *continued*
  paraphilic — *continued*
    specified NEC F65.89
  parathyroid (gland) E21.5
    specified NEC E21.4
  parietoalveolar NEC J84.09
  paroxysmal, mixed R56.9
  patella M22.9- ☑
    chondromalacia — *see* Chondromalacia, patella
    derangement NEC M22.3X- ☑
    recurrent
      dislocation — *see* Dislocation, patella, recurrent
      subluxation — *see* Dislocation, patella, recurrent, incomplete
    specified NEC M22.8X- ☑
  patellofemoral M22.2X- ☑
  pedophilic F65.4
  pentose phosphate pathway with anemia D55.1
  perception, due to hallucinogens F16.983
    in
      abuse F16.183
      dependence F16.283
  peripheral nervous system NEC G64
  peroxisomal E71.50
    biogenesis
      neonatal adrenoleukodystrophy E71.511
      specified disorder NEC E71.518
      Zellweger syndrome E71.510
    rhizomelic chondrodysplasia punctata E71.540
    specified form NEC E71.548
      group 1 E71.518
      group 2 E71.53
      group 3 E71.542
    X-linked adrenoleukodystrophy E71.529
      adolescent E71.521
      adrenomyeloneuropathy E71.522
      childhood E71.520
      specified form NEC E71.528
    Zellweger-like syndrome E71.541
  persistent
    (somatoform) pain F45.41
    affective (mood) F34.9
  personality (*see also* Personality) F60.9
    affective F34.0
    aggressive F60.3
    amoral F60.2
    anankastic F60.5
    antisocial F60.2
    anxious F60.6
    asocial F60.2
    asthenic F60.7
    avoidant F60.6
    borderline F60.3
    change (secondary) due to general medical condition F07.0
    compulsive F60.5
    cyclothymic F34.0
    dependent (passive) F60.7
    depressive F34.1
    dissocial F60.2
    emotional instability F60.3
    expansive paranoid F60.0
    explosive F60.3
    following organic brain damage F07.9
    histrionic F60.4
    hyperthymic F34.0
    hypothymic F34.1
    hysterical F60.4
    immature F60.89
    inadequate F60.7
    labile F60.3
    mixed (nonspecific) F60.89
    moral deficiency F60.2
    narcissistic F60.81
    negativistic F60.89
    obsessional F60.5
    obsessive (-compulsive) F60.5
    organic F07.9
    overconscientious F60.5
    paranoid F60.0
    passive (-dependent) F60.7
    passive-aggressive F60.89
    pathological NEC F60.9
    pseudosocial F60.2
    psychopathic F60.2
    schizoid F60.1
    schizotypal F21
    self-defeating F60.7

Disorder — *continued*
  personality (*see also* Personality) — *continued*
    specified NEC F60.89
    type A F60.5
    unstable (emotional) F60.3
  pervasive, developmental F84.9
  phencyclidine use
    mild F16.10
      with
        phencyclidine intoxication F16.129
        phencyclidine intoxication delirium F16.121
        phencyclidine-induced
          anxiety disorder F16.180
          bipolar and related disorder F16.14
          depressive disorder F16.14
          psychotic disorder F16.159
      in remission (early) (sustained) F16.11
    moderate or severe F16.20
      with
        phencyclidine intoxication F16.229
        phencyclidine intoxication delirium F16.221
        phencyclidine-induced
          anxiety disorder F16.280
          bipolar and related disorder F16.14
          depressive disorder F16.24
          psychotic disorder F16.259
      in remission (early) (sustained) F16.21
  phobic anxiety, childhood F40.8
  phosphate-losing tubular N25.0
  pigmentation L81.9
    choroid, congenital Q14.3
    diminished melanin formation L81.6
    iron L81.8
    specified NEC L81.8
  pinna (noninfective) H61.10- ☑
    deformity, acquired H61.11- ☑
    hematoma H61.12- ☑
    perichondritis — *see* Perichondritis, ear
    specified type NEC H61.19- ☑
  pituitary gland E23.7
    iatrogenic (postprocedural) E89.3
    specified NEC E23.6
  platelets D69.1
  plexus G54.9
    specified NEC G54.8
  polymorphonuclear neutrophils D71
  porphyrin metabolism — *see* Porphyria
  postconcussional F07.81
  posthallucinogen perception F16.983
    in
      abuse F16.183
      dependence F16.283
  postmenopausal N95.9
    specified NEC N95.8
  postprocedural (postoperative) — *see* Complications, postprocedural
  post-transplant lymphoproliferative D47.Z1 (*following* D47.4)
  post-traumatic stress (PTSD) F43.10
    acute F43.11
    chronic F43.12
  premenstrual dysphoric (PMDD) F32.81
  prepuce N47.8
  propionic acidemia E71.121
  prostate N42.9
    specified NEC N42.89
  psychogenic NOS (*see also* condition) F45.9
    anxiety F41.8
    appetite F50.9
    asthenic F48.8
    cardiovascular (system) F45.8
    compulsive F42.8
    cutaneous F54
    depressive F32.9
    digestive (system) F45.8
    dysmenorrheic F45.8
    dyspneic F45.8
    endocrine (system) F54
    eye NEC F45.8
    feeding — *see* Disorder, eating
    functional NEC F45.8
    gastric F45.8
    gastrointestinal (system) F45.8
    genitourinary (system) F45.8
    heart (function) (rhythm) F45.8
    hyperventilatory F45.8
    hypochondriacal — *see* Disorder, hypochondriacal
    intestinal F45.8

Disorder — *continued*
  psychogenic (*see also* condition) — *continued*
    joint F45.8
    learning F81.9
    limb F45.8
    lymphatic (system) F45.8
    menstrual F45.8
    micturition F45.8
    monoplegic NEC F44.4
    motor F44.4
    muscle F45.8
    musculoskeletal F45.8
    neurocirculatory F45.8
    obsessive F42.8
    occupational F48.8
    organ or part of body NEC F45.8
    paralytic NEC F44.4
    phobic F40.9
    physical NEC F45.8
    rectal F45.8
    respiratory (system) F45.8
    rheumatic F45.8
    sexual (function) F52.9
    skin (allergic) (eczematous) F54
    sleep F51.9
    specified part of body NEC F45.8
    stomach F45.8
  psychological F99
    associated with
      disease classified elsewhere F54
      sexual
        development F66
        relationship F66
      uncertainty about gender identity F64.9
  psychomotor NEC F44.4
    hysterical F44.4
  psychoneurotic (*see also* Neurosis)
    mixed NEC F48.8
  psychophysiologic — *see* Disorder, somatoform
  psychosexual F65.9
    development F66
    identity of childhood F64.2
  psychosomatic NOS — *see* Disorder, somatoform
    multiple F45.0
    undifferentiated F45.1
  psychotic — *see* Psychosis
    transient (acute) F23
  puberty E30.9
    specified NEC E30.8
  pulmonary (valve) — *see* Endocarditis, pulmonary
  purine metabolism E79.9
  pyrimidine metabolism E79.9
  pyruvate metabolism E74.4
  reactive attachment (childhood) F94.1
  reading R48.0
    developmental (specific) F81.0
  receptive language F80.2
  receptor, hormonal, peripheral (*see also* Syndrome, androgen insensitivity) E34.50
  recurrent brief depressive F33.8
  reflex R29.2
  refraction H52.7
    aniseikonia H52.32
    anisometropia H52.31
    astigmatism — *see* Astigmatism
    hypermetropia — *see* Hypermetropia
    myopia — *see* Myopia
    presbyopia H52.4
    specified NEC H52.6
  relationship F68.8
    due to sexual orientation F66
  REM sleep behavior G47.52
  renal function, impaired (tubular) N25.9
  resonance R49.9
    specified NEC R49.8
  respiratory function, impaired (*see also* Failure, respiration)
    postprocedural — *see* Complication, postoperative, respiratory system
    psychogenic F45.8
  retina H35.9
    angioid streaks H35.33
    changes in vascular appearance H35.01- ☑
    degeneration — *see* Degeneration, retina
    dystrophy (hereditary) — *see* Dystrophy, retina
    edema H35.81
    hemorrhage — *see* Hemorrhage, retina
    ischemia H35.82

☑ Additional Character Required — Refer to the Tabular List for Character Selection   ▽ Subterms under main terms may continue to next column or page

Disorder — continued
  retina — continued
    macular degeneration — see Degeneration, macula
    microaneurysms H35.04- ☑
    microvascular abnormality NEC H35.09
    neovascularization — see Neovascularization, retina
    retinopathy — see Retinopathy
    separation of layers H35.70
      central serous chorioretinopathy H35.71- ☑
      pigment epithelium detachment (serous) H35.72- ☑
        hemorrhagic H35.73- ☑
    specified type NEC H35.89
    telangiectasis — see Telangiectasis, retina
    vasculitis — see Vasculitis, retina
  retroperitoneal K68.9
  right hemisphere organic affective F07.89
  rumination (infant or child) F98.21
  sacrum, sacrococcygeal NEC M53.3
  schizoaffective F25.9
    bipolar type F25.0
    depressive type F25.1
    manic type F25.0
    mixed type F25.0
    specified NEC F25.8
  schizoid of childhood F84.5
  schizophrenia spectrum and other psychotic disorder F29
    specified NEC F28
  schizophreniform F20.81
    brief F23
  schizotypal (personality) F21
  secretion, thyrocalcitonin E07.0
  sedative, hypnotic, or anxiolytic use
    mild F13.10
      with
        sedative, hypnotic, or anxiolytic intoxication F13.129
        sedative, hypnotic, or anxiolytic intoxication delirium F13.121
        sedative, hypnotic, or anxiolytic-induced
          anxiety disorder F13.180
          bipolar and related disorder F13.14
          depressive disorder F13.14
          psychotic disorder F13.159
          sexual dysfunction F13.181
      in remission (early) (sustained) F13.11
    moderate or severe F13.20
      with
        sedative, hypnotic, or anxiolytic intoxication F13.229
        sedative, hypnotic, or anxiolytic intoxication delirium F13.221
        sedative, hypnotic, or anxiolytic-induced
          anxiety disorder F13.280
          bipolar and related disorder F13.24
          depressive disorder F13.24
          major neurocognitive disorder F13.27
          mild neurocognitive disorder F13.288
          psychotic disorder F13.259
          sexual dysfunction F13.281
      in remission (early) (sustained) F13.21
  seizure (see also Epilepsy) G40.909
    intractable G40.919
      with status epilepticus G40.911
  semantic pragmatic F80.89
    with autism F84.0
  sense of smell R43.1
    psychogenic F45.8
  separation anxiety, of childhood F93.0
  sexual
    aversion F52.1
    function, psychogenic F52.9
    interest/arousal, female F52.22
    masochism F65.51
    maturation F66
    nonorganic F52.9
    preference (see also Deviation, sexual) F65.9
      fetishistic transvestism F65.1
    relationship F66
    sadism F65.52
  shyness, of childhood and adolescence F40.10
  sibling rivalry F93.8
  sickle-cell (sickling) (homozygous) — see Disease, sickle-cell
    heterozygous D57.3
    specified type NEC D57.8- ☑

Disorder — continued
  sickle-cell — see Disease, sickle-cell — continued
    trait D57.3
  sinus (nasal) J34.9
    specified NEC J34.89
  skin L98.9
    atrophic L90.9
      specified NEC L90.8
    granulomatous L92.9
      specified NEC L92.8
    hypertrophic L91.9
      specified NEC L91.8
    infiltrative NEC L98.6
    newborn P83.9
      specified NEC P83.88
    picking F42.4
    psychogenic (allergic) (eczematous) F54
  sleep G47.9
    breathing-related — see Apnea, sleep
    circadian rhythm G47.20
      advance sleep phase type G47.22
      delayed sleep phase type G47.21
      due to
        alcohol
          abuse F10.182
          dependence F10.282
          use F10.982
        amphetamines
          abuse F15.182
          dependence F15.282
          use F15.982
        caffeine
          abuse F15.182
          dependence F15.282
          use F15.982
        cocaine
          abuse F14.182
          dependence F14.282
          use F14.982
        drug NEC
          abuse F19.182
          dependence F19.282
          use F19.982
        opioid
          abuse F11.182
          dependence F11.282
          use F11.982
        psychoactive substance NEC
          abuse F19.182
          dependence F19.282
          use F19.982
        sedative, hypnotic, or anxiolytic
          abuse F13.182
          dependence F13.282
          use F13.982
        stimulant NEC
          abuse F15.182
          dependence F15.282
          use F15.982
      free running type G47.24
      in conditions classified elsewhere G47.27
      irregular sleep wake type G47.23
      jet lag type G47.25
      non-24-hour sleep-wake type G47.24
      shift work type G47.26
      specified NEC G47.29
    due to
      alcohol
        abuse F10.182
        dependence F10.282
        use F10.982
      amphetamine
        abuse F15.182
        dependence F15.282
        use F15.982
      anxiolytic
        abuse F13.182
        dependence F13.282
        use F13.982
      caffeine
        abuse F15.182
        dependence F15.282
        use F15.982
      cocaine
        abuse F14.182
        dependence F14.282
        use F14.982
      drug NEC
        abuse F19.182

Disorder — continued
  sleep — continued
    due to — continued
      drug — continued
        dependence F19.282
        use F19.982
      hypnotic
        abuse F13.182
        dependence F13.282
        use F13.982
      opioid
        abuse F11.182
        dependence F11.282
        use F11.982
      psychoactive substance NEC
        abuse F19.182
        dependence F19.282
        use F19.982
      sedative
        abuse F13.182
        dependence F13.282
        use F13.982
      stimulant NEC
        abuse F15.182
        dependence F15.282
        use F15.982
    emotional F51.9
    excessive somnolence — see Hypersomnia
    hypersomnia type — see Hypersomnia
    initiating or maintaining — see Insomnia
    nightmares F51.5
    nonorganic F51.9
      specified NEC F51.8
    parasomnia type G47.50
    specified NEC G47.8
    terrors F51.4
    walking F51.3
  sleep-wake pattern or schedule (see also Disorder, sleep, circadian rhythm) G47.9
    specified NEC G47.8
  social
    anxiety (of childhood) F40.10
      generalized F40.11
    functioning in childhood F94.9
      specified NEC F94.8
    pragmatic F80.82
  soft tissue M79.9
    ankle M79.9
    due to use, overuse and pressure M70.90
      ankle M70.97- ☑
      bursitis — see Bursitis
      foot M70.97- ☑
      forearm M70.93- ☑
      hand M70.94- ☑
      lower leg M70.96- ☑
      multiple sites M70.99
      pelvic region M70.95- ☑
      shoulder region M70.91- ☑
      specified site NEC M70.98
      specified type NEC M70.80
        ankle M70.87- ☑
        foot M70.87- ☑
        forearm M70.83- ☑
        hand M70.84- ☑
        lower leg M70.86- ☑
        multiple sites M70.89
        pelvic region M70.85- ☑
        shoulder region M70.81- ☑
        specified site NEC M70.88
        thigh M70.85- ☑
        upper arm M70.82- ☑
      thigh M70.95- ☑
      upper arm M70.92- ☑
    foot M79.9
    forearm M79.9
    hand M79.9
    lower leg M79.9
    multiple sites M79.9
    occupational — see Disorder, soft tissue, due to use, overuse and pressure
    pelvic region M79.9
    shoulder region M79.9
    specified type NEC M79.89
    thigh M79.9
    upper arm M79.9
  somatic symptom F45.1
  somatization F45.0
  somatoform F45.9

Disorder — *continued*
  somatoform — *continued*
    pain (persistent) F45.41
    somatization (multiple) (long-lasting) F45.0
    specified NEC F45.8
    undifferentiated F45.1
  somnolence, excessive — *see* Hypersomnia
  specific
    arithmetical F81.2
    developmental, of motor F82
    reading F81.0
    speech and language F80.9
    spelling F81.81
    written expression F81.81
  speech R47.9
    articulation (functional) (specific) F80.0
    developmental F80.9
    specified NEC R47.89
  speech-sound F80.0
  spelling (specific) F81.81
  spine (*see also* Dorsopathy)
    ligamentous or muscular attachments, peripheral
      — *see* Enthesopathy, spinal
    specified NEC — *see* Dorsopathy, specified NEC
  stereotyped, habit or movement F98.4
  stimulant use (other) (unspecified)
    mild F15.10
      in remission (early) (sustained) F15.11
    moderate or severe F15.20
      in remission (early) (sustained) F15.21
  stomach (functional) — *see* Disorder, gastric
  stress F43.9
    acute F43.0
    post-traumatic F43.10
      acute F43.11
      chronic F43.12
  substance use (other) (unknown)
    mild F19.10
      with substance-induced
        anxiety disorder F19.180
        bipolar and related disorder F19.14
        depressive disorder F19.14
        major neurocognitive disorder F19.17
        mild neurocognitive disorder F19.188
        obsessive-compulsive and related disorder F19.188
        sexual dysfunction F19.181
      substance intoxication F19.129
      substance intoxication delirium F19.121
    moderate or severe F19.20
      with substance-induced
        anxiety disorder F19.280
        bipolar and related disorder F19.24
        depressive disorder F19.24
        major neurocognitive disorder F19.27
        mild neurocognitive disorder F19.288
        obsessive-compulsive and related disorder F19.288
        sexual dysfunction F19.281
      in remission (early) (sustained) F19.21
      substance intoxication F19.229
      substance intoxication delirium F19.221
  sulfur-bearing amino-acid metabolism E72.10
  sweat gland (eccrine) L74.9
    apocrine L75.9
      specified NEC L75.8
    specified NEC L74.8
  synovium M67.90
    acromioclavicular M67.91- ☑
    ankle M67.97- ☑
    elbow M67.92- ☑
    foot M67.97- ☑
    forearm M67.93- ☑
    hand M67.94- ☑
    hip M67.95- ☑
    knee M67.96- ☑
    multiple sites M67.99
    rupture — *see* Rupture, synovium
    shoulder M67.91- ☑
    specified type NEC M67.80
      acromioclavicular M67.81- ☑
      ankle M67.87- ☑
      elbow M67.82- ☑
      foot M67.87- ☑
      hand M67.84- ☑
      hip M67.85- ☑
      knee M67.86- ☑
      multiple sites M67.89

Disorder — *continued*
  synovium — *continued*
    specified type — *continued*
      wrist M67.83- ☑
    synovitis — *see* Synovitis
    upper arm M67.92- ☑
    wrist M67.93- ☑
  temperature regulation, newborn P81.9
    specified NEC P81.8
  temporomandibular joint M26.60- ☑
  tendon M67.90
    acromioclavicular M67.91- ☑
    ankle M67.97- ☑
    contracture — *see* Contracture, tendon
    elbow M67.92- ☑
    foot M67.97- ☑
    forearm M67.93- ☑
    hand M67.94- ☑
    hip M67.95- ☑
    knee M67.96- ☑
    multiple sites M67.99
    rupture — *see* Rupture, tendon
    shoulder M67.91- ☑
    specified type NEC M67.80
      acromioclavicular M67.81- ☑
      ankle M67.87- ☑
      elbow M67.82- ☑
      foot M67.87- ☑
      hand M67.84- ☑
      hip M67.85- ☑
      knee M67.86- ☑
      multiple sites M67.89
      trunk M67.88
      wrist M67.83- ☑
    synovitis — *see* Synovitis
    tendinitis — *see* Tendinitis
    tenosynovitis — *see* Tenosynovitis
    trunk M67.98
    upper arm M67.92- ☑
    wrist M67.93- ☑
  thoracic root (nerve) NEC G54.3
  thyrocalcitonin hypersecretion E07.0
  thyroid (gland) E07.9
    function NEC, neonatal, transitory P72.2
    iodine-deficiency related E01.8
    specified NEC E07.89
  tic — *see* Tic
  tobacco use
    chewing tobacco (mild) (moderate) (severe)
      in remission (early) (sustained) F17.221
    cigarettes (mild) (moderate) (severe)
      in remission (early) (sustained) F17.211
    mild Z72.0
      in remission (early) (sustained) F17.201
    moderate F17.200
      in remission (early) (sustained) F17.201
    severe F17.200
      in remission (early) (sustained) F17.201
    specified product NEC (mild) (moderate) (severe)
      in remission (early) (sustained) F17.291
  tooth K08.9
    development K00.9
      specified NEC K00.8
    eruption K00.6
  Tourette's F95.2
  trance and possession F44.89
  transvestic F65.1
  trauma and stressor-related F43.9
    other specified F43.8
  tricuspid (valve) — *see* Endocarditis, tricuspid
  tryptophan metabolism E70.5
  tubular, phosphate-losing N25.0
  tubulo-interstitial (in)
    brucellosis A23.9 [N16]
    cystinosis E72.04
    diphtheria A36.84
    glycogen storage disease E74.00 [N16]
    leukemia NEC C95.9- ☑ [N16]
    lymphoma NEC C85.9- ☑ [N16]
    mixed cryoglobulinemia D89.1 [N16]
    multiple myeloma C90.0- ☑ [N16]
    Salmonella infection A02.25
    sarcoidosis D86.84
    sepsis A41.9 [N16]
      streptococcal A40.9 [N16]
    systemic lupus erythematosus M32.15
    toxoplasmosis B58.83

Disorder — *continued*
  tubulo-interstitial — *continued*
    transplant rejection T86.91 [N16]
    Wilson's disease E83.01 [N16]
  tubulo-renal function, impaired N25.9
    specified NEC N25.89
  tympanic membrane H73.9- ☑
    atrophy — *see* Atrophy, tympanic membrane
    infection — *see* Myringitis
    perforation — *see* Perforation, tympanum
    specified NEC H73.89- ☑
  unsocialized aggressive F91.1
  urea cycle metabolism E72.20
    argininemia E72.21
    arginosuccinic aciduria E72.22
    citrullinemia E72.23
    ornithine transcarbamylase deficiency E72.4
    other specified E72.29
  ureter (in) N28.9
    schistosomiasis B65.0 [N29]
    tuberculosis A18.11
  urethra N36.9
    specified NEC N36.8
  urinary system N39.9
    specified NEC N39.8
  valve, heart
    aortic — *see* Endocarditis, aortic
    mitral — *see* Endocarditis, mitral
    pulmonary — *see* Endocarditis, pulmonary
    rheumatic
      aortic — *see* Endocarditis, aortic, rheumatic
      mitral — *see* Endocarditis, mitral
      pulmonary — *see* Endocarditis, pulmonary, rheumatic
      tricuspid — *see* Endocarditis, tricuspid
    tricuspid — *see* Endocarditis, tricuspid
  vestibular function H81.9- ☑
    specified NEC — *see* subcategory H81.8 ☑
      in diseases classified elsewhere H82.- ☑
    vertigo — *see* Vertigo
  vision, binocular H53.30
    abnormal retinal correspondence H53.31
    diplopia H53.2
    fusion with defective stereopsis H53.32
    simultaneous perception H53.33
    suppression H53.34
  visual
    cortex
      blindness H47.619
        left brain H47.612
        right brain H47.611
      due to
        inflammatory disorder H47.629
          left brain H47.622
          right brain H47.621
        neoplasm H47.639
          left brain H47.632
          right brain H47.631
        vascular disorder H47.649
          left brain H47.642
          right brain H47.641
    pathway H47.9
      due to
        inflammatory disorder H47.51- ☑
        neoplasm H47.52- ☑
        vascular disorder H47.53- ☑
      optic chiasm — *see* Disorder, optic, chiasm
  vitreous body H43.9
    crystalline deposits — *see* Deposit, crystalline
    degeneration — *see* Degeneration, vitreous
    hemorrhage — *see* Hemorrhage, vitreous
    opacities — *see* Opacity, vitreous
    prolapse — *see* Prolapse, vitreous
    specified type NEC H43.89
  voice R49.9
    specified type NEC R49.8
  volatile solvent use
    due to drug abuse — *see* Abuse, drug, inhalant
    due to drug dependence — *see* Dependence, drug, inhalant
  voyeuristic F65.3
  white blood cells D72.9
    specified NEC D72.89
  withdrawing, child or adolescent F40.10
Disorientation R41.0
Displacement, displaced
  acquired traumatic of bone, cartilage, joint, tendon
    NEC — *see* Dislocation

☑ **Additional Character Required** — **Refer to the Tabular List for Character Selection**

▽ **Subterms under main terms may continue to next column or page**

Index

Displacement, displaced — *continued*
  adrenal gland (congenital) Q89.1
  appendix, retrocecal (congenital) Q43.8
  auricle (congenital) Q17.4
  bladder (acquired) N32.89
    congenital Q64.19
  brachial plexus (congenital) Q07.8
  brain stem, caudal (congenital) Q04.8
  canaliculus (lacrimalis), congenital Q10.6
  cardia through esophageal hiatus (congenital) Q40.1
  cerebellum, caudal (congenital) Q04.8
  cervix — *see* Malposition, uterus
  colon (congenital) Q43.3
  device, implant or graft (*see also* Complications, by
      site and type, mechanical) T85.628 ☑
    arterial graft NEC — *see* Complication, cardiovas-
        cular device, mechanical, vascular
    breast (implant) T85.42 ☑
    catheter NEC T85.628 ☑
      dialysis (renal) T82.42 ☑
        intraperitoneal T85.621 ☑
      infusion NEC T82.524 ☑
        spinal (epidural) (subdural) T85.620 ☑
      urinary
        cystostomy T83.020 ☑
        Hopkins T83.028 ☑
        ileostomy T83.028 ☑
        indwelling T83.021 ☑
        nephrostomy T83.022 ☑
        specified NEC T83.028 ☑
        urostomy T83.028 ☑
    electronic (electrode) (pulse generator) (stimulator)
        — *see* Complication, electronic stimulator
    fixation, internal (orthopedic) NEC — *see* Compli-
        cation, fixation device, mechanical
    gastrointestinal — *see* Complications, prosthetic
        device, mechanical, gastrointestinal device
    genital NEC T83.428 ☑
      intrauterine contraceptive device (string)
          T83.32 ☑
      penile prosthesis (cylinder) (implanted) (pump)
          (reservoir) T83.420 ☑
      testicular prosthesis T83.421 ☑
    heart NEC — *see* Complication, cardiovascular de-
        vice, mechanical
    joint prosthesis — *see* Complications, joint prosthe-
        sis, mechanical
    ocular — *see* Complications, prosthetic device,
        mechanical, ocular device
    orthopedic NEC — *see* Complication, orthopedic,
        device or graft, mechanical
    specified NEC T85.628 ☑
    urinary NEC T83.128 ☑
      graft T83.22 ☑
      sphincter, implanted T83.121 ☑
      stent (ileal conduit) (nephroureteral) T83.123 ☑
        ureteral indwelling T83.122 ☑
    vascular NEC — *see* Complication, cardiovascular
        device, mechanical
    ventricular intracranial shunt T85.02 ☑
  electronic stimulator
    bone T84.320 ☑
    cardiac — *see* Complications, cardiac device, elec-
        tronic
    nervous system — *see* Complication, prosthetic
        device, mechanical, electronic nervous sys-
        tem stimulator
    urinary — *see* Complications, electronic stimulator,
        urinary
  esophageal mucosa into cardia of stomach, congenital
      Q39.8
  esophagus (acquired) K22.8
    congenital Q39.8
  eyeball (acquired) (lateral) (old) — *see* Displacement,
      globe
    congenital Q15.8
    current — *see* Avulsion, eye
  fallopian tube (acquired) N83.4- ☑
    congenital Q50.6
    opening (congenital) Q50.6
  gallbladder (congenital) Q44.1
  gastric mucosa (congenital) Q40.2
  globe (acquired) (old) (lateral) H05.21- ☑
    current — *see* Avulsion, eye
  heart (congenital) Q24.8
    acquired I51.89
  hymen (upward) (congenital) Q52.4

Displacement, displaced — *continued*
  intervertebral disc NEC
    with myelopathy — *see* Disorder, disc, with,
        myelopathy
    cervical, cervicothoracic (with) M50.20
      myelopathy — *see* Disorder, disc, cervical, with
          myelopathy
      neuritis, radiculitis or radiculopathy — *see* Dis-
          order, disc, cervical, with neuritis
    due to trauma — *see* Dislocation, vertebra
    lumbar region M51.26
      with
        myelopathy M51.06
        neuritis, radiculitis, radiculopathy or sciatica
            M51.16
    lumbosacral region M51.27
      with
        neuritis, radiculitis, radiculopathy or sciatica
            M51.17
    sacrococcygeal region M53.3
    thoracic region M51.24
      with
        myelopathy M51.04
        neuritis, radiculitis, radiculopathy M51.14
    thoracolumbar region M51.25
      with
        myelopathy M51.05
        neuritis, radiculitis, radiculopathy M51.15
  intrauterine device (string) T83.32 ☑
  kidney (acquired) N28.83
    congenital Q63.2
  lachrymal, lacrimal apparatus or duct (congenital)
      Q10.6
  lens, congenital Q12.1
  macula (congenital) Q14.1
  Meckel's diverticulum Q43.0
    malignant — *see* Table of Neoplasms, small intes-
        tine, malignant
  nail (congenital) Q84.6
    acquired L60.8
  opening of Wharton's duct in mouth Q38.4
  organ or site, congenital NEC — *see* Malposition,
      congenital
  ovary (acquired) N83.4- ☑
    congenital Q50.39
    free in peritoneal cavity (congenital) Q50.39
    into hernial sac N83.4- ☑
  oviduct (acquired) N83.4- ☑
    congenital Q50.6
  parathyroid (gland) E21.4
  parotid gland (congenital) Q38.4
  punctum lacrimale (congenital) Q10.6
  sacro-iliac (joint) (congenital) Q74.2
    current injury S33.2 ☑
    old — *see* subcategory M53.2 ☑
  salivary gland (any) (congenital) Q38.4
  spleen (congenital) Q89.09
  stomach, congenital Q40.2
  sublingual duct Q38.4
  tongue (downward) (congenital) Q38.3
  tooth, teeth, fully erupted M26.30
    horizontal M26.33
    vertical M26.34
  trachea (congenital) Q32.1
  ureter or ureteric opening or orifice (congenital)
      Q62.62
  uterine opening of oviducts or fallopian tubes Q50.6
  uterus, uterine — *see* Malposition, uterus
  ventricular septum Q21.0
    with rudimentary ventricle Q20.4

Disproportion
  between native and reconstructed breast N65.1
  fiber-type G71.2
Disruptio uteri — *see* Rupture, uterus
Disruption (of)
  ciliary body NEC H21.89
  closure of
    cornea T81.31 ☑
    craniotomy T81.32 ☑
    fascia (muscular) (superficial) T81.32 ☑
    internal organ or tissue T81.32 ☑
    laceration (external) (internal) T81.33 ☑
    ligament T81.32 ☑
    mucosa T81.31 ☑
    muscle or muscle flap T81.32 ☑
    ribs or rib cage T81.32 ☑
    skin and subcutaneous tissue (full-thickness) (su-
        perficial) T81.31 ☑

Disruption — *continued*
  closure of — *continued*
    skull T81.32 ☑
    sternum (sternotomy) T81.32 ☑
    tendon T81.32 ☑
    traumatic laceration (external) (internal) T81.33 ☑
  family Z63.8
    due to
      absence of family member due to military de-
          ployment Z63.31
      absence of family member NEC Z63.32
      alcoholism and drug addiction in family Z63.72
      bereavement Z63.4
      death (assumed) or disappearance of family
          member Z63.4
      divorce or separation Z63.5
      drug addiction in family Z63.72
      return of family member from military deploy-
          ment (current or past conflict) Z63.71
      stressful life events NEC Z63.79
  iris NEC H21.89
  ligament(s) (*see also* Sprain)
    knee
      current injury — *see* Dislocation, knee
      old (chronic) — *see* Derangement, knee, insta-
          bility
      spontaneous NEC — *see* Derangement, knee,
          disruption ligament
  ossicular chain — *see* Discontinuity, ossicles, ear
  pelvic ring (stable) S32.810 ☑
    unstable S32.811 ☑
  traumatic injury wound repair T81.33 ☑
  wound T81.30 ☑
    episiotomy O90.1
    operation T81.31 ☑
      cesarean O90.0
      external operation wound (superficial)
          T81.31 ☑
      internal operation wound (deep) T81.32 ☑
    perineal (obstetric) O90.1
    traumatic injury repair T81.33 ☑
Dissatisfaction with
  employment Z56.9
  school environment Z55.4
Dissecting — *see* condition
Dissection
  aorta I71.00
    abdominal I71.02
    thoracic I71.01
    thoracoabdominal I71.03
  artery I77.70
    basilar (trunk) I77.75
    carotid I77.71
    cerebral (nonruptured) I67.0
      ruptured — *see* Hemorrhage, intracranial,
          subarachnoid
    coronary I25.42
    extremity
      lower I77.77
      upper I77.76
    iliac I77.72
    precerebral
      congenital (nonruptured) Q28.1
      specified site NEC I77.75
    renal I77.73
    specified NEC I77.79
    vertebral I77.74
  precerbral artery, congenital (nonruptured) Q28.1
      Heartland A93.8
  traumatic — *see* Wound, open, by site
  vascular I99.8
  wound — *see* Wound, open
Disseminated — *see* condition
Dissociation
  auriculoventricular or atrioventricular (AV) (any de-
      gree) (isorhythmic) I45.89
    with heart block I44.2
  interference I45.89
Dissociative reaction, state F44.9
Dissolution, vertebra — *see* Osteoporosis
Distension, distention
  abdomen R14.0
  bladder N32.89
  cecum K63.89
  colon K63.89
  gallbladder K82.8
  intestine K63.89
  kidney N28.89

Displacement, displaced — Distension, distention

Distension, distention — *continued*
- liver K76.89
- seminal vesicle N50.89
- stomach K31.89
    - acute K31.0
    - psychogenic F45.8
- ureter — *see* Dilatation, ureter
- uterus N85.8

Distoma hepaticum infestation B66.3

Distomiasis B66.9
- bile passages B66.3
- hemic B65.9
- hepatic B66.3
    - due to Clonorchis sinensis B66.1
- intestinal B66.5
- liver B66.3
    - due to Clonorchis sinensis B66.1
- lung B66.4
- pulmonary B66.4

Distomolar (fourth molar) K00.1

Disto-occlusion (Division I) (Division II) M26.212

Distortion(s) (congenital)
- adrenal (gland) Q89.1
- arm NEC Q68.8
- bile duct or passage Q44.5
- bladder Q64.79
- brain Q04.9
- cervix (uteri) Q51.9
- chest (wall) Q67.8
    - bones Q76.8
- clavicle Q74.0
- clitoris Q52.6
- coccyx Q76.49
- common duct Q44.5
- coronary Q24.5
- cystic duct Q44.5
- ear (auricle) (external) Q17.3
    - inner Q16.5
    - middle Q16.4
        - ossicles Q16.3
- endocrine NEC Q89.2
- eustachian tube Q17.8
- eye (adnexa) Q15.8
- face bone(s) NEC Q75.8
- fallopian tube Q50.6
- femur NEC Q68.8
- fibula NEC Q68.8
- finger(s) Q68.1
- foot Q66.9
- genitalia, genital organ(s)
    - female Q52.8
        - external Q52.79
        - internal NEC Q52.8
- gyri Q04.8
- hand bone(s) Q68.1
- heart (auricle) (ventricle) Q24.8
    - valve (cusp) Q24.8
- hepatic duct Q44.5
- humerus NEC Q68.8
- hymen Q52.4
- intrafamilial communications Z63.8
- jaw NEC M26.89
- labium (majus) (minus) Q52.79
- leg NEC Q68.8
- lens Q12.8
- liver Q44.7
- lumbar spine Q76.49
    - with disproportion O33.8
        - causing obstructed labor O65.0
- lumbosacral (joint) (region) Q76.49
    - kyphosis — *see* Kyphosis, congenital
    - lordosis — *see* Lordosis, congenital
- nerve Q07.8
- nose Q30.8
- organ
    - of Corti Q16.5
    - or site not listed — *see* Anomaly, by site
- ossicles, ear Q16.3
- oviduct Q50.6
- pancreas Q45.3
- parathyroid (gland) Q89.2
- pituitary (gland) Q89.2
- radius NEC Q68.8
- sacroiliac joint Q74.2
- sacrum Q76.49
- scapula Q74.0
- shoulder girdle Q74.0
- skull bone(s) NEC Q75.8

Distortion(s) — *continued*
- skull bone(s) — *continued*
    - with
        - anencephalus Q00.0
        - encephalocele — *see* Encephalocele
        - hydrocephalus Q03.9
            - with spina bifida — *see* Spina bifida, with hydrocephalus
        - microcephaly Q02
- spinal cord Q06.8
- spine Q76.49
    - kyphosis — *see* Kyphosis, congenital
    - lordosis — *see* Lordosis, congenital
- spleen Q89.09
- sternum NEC Q76.7
- thorax (wall) Q67.8
    - bony Q76.8
- thymus (gland) Q89.2
- thyroid (gland) Q89.2
- tibia NEC Q68.8
- toe(s) Q66.9
- tongue Q38.3
- trachea (cartilage) Q32.1
- ulna NEC Q68.8
- ureter Q62.8
- urethra Q64.79
    - causing obstruction Q64.39
- uterus Q51.9
- vagina Q52.4
- vertebra Q76.49
    - kyphosis — *see* Kyphosis, congenital
    - lordosis — *see* Lordosis, congenital
- visual (*see also* Disturbance, vision)
    - shape and size H53.15
- vulva Q52.79
- wrist (bones) (joint) Q68.8

Distress
- abdomen — *see* Pain, abdominal
- acute respiratory R06.03
    - syndrome (adult) (child) J80
- epigastric R10.13
- fetal P84
    - complicating pregnancy — *see* Stress, fetal
- gastrointestinal (functional) K30
    - psychogenic F45.8
- intestinal (functional) NOS K59.9
    - psychogenic F45.8
- maternal, during labor and delivery O75.0
- relationship, with spouse or intimate partner Z63.0
- respiratory (adult) (child) R06.03
    - newborn P22.9
        - specified NEC P22.8
    - orthopnea R06.01
    - psychogenic F45.8
    - shortness of breath R06.02
    - specified type NEC R06.09

Distribution vessel, atypical Q27.9
- coronary artery Q24.5
- precerebral Q28.1

Districhiasis L68.8

Disturbance(s) (*see also* Disease)
- absorption K90.9
    - calcium E58
    - carbohydrate K90.49
    - fat K90.49
        - pancreatic K90.3
    - protein K90.49
    - starch K90.49
    - vitamin — *see* Deficiency, vitamin
- acid-base equilibrium E87.8
    - mixed E87.4
- activity and attention (with hyperkinesis) — *see* Disorder, attention-deficit hyperactivity
- amino acid transport E72.00
- assimilation, food K90.9
- auditory nerve, except deafness — *see* subcategory H93.3 ☑
- behavior — *see* Disorder, conduct
- blood clotting (mechanism) (*see also* Defect, coagulation) D68.9
- cerebral
    - nerve — *see* Disorder, nerve, cranial
    - status, newborn P91.9
        - specified NEC P91.88
- circulatory I99.9
- conduct (*see also* Disorder, conduct) F91.9
    - adjustment reaction — *see* Disorder, adjustment
    - compulsive F63.9

Disturbance(s) — *continued*
- conduct (*see also* Disorder, conduct) — *continued*
    - disruptive F91.9
    - hyperkinetic — *see* Disorder, attention-deficit hyperactivity
    - socialized F91.2
    - specified NEC F91.8
    - unsocialized F91.1
- coordination R27.8
- cranial nerve — *see* Disorder, nerve, cranial
- deep sensibility — *see* Disturbance, sensation
- digestive K30
    - psychogenic F45.8
- electrolyte (*see also* Imbalance, electrolyte)
    - newborn, transitory P74.4
        - hyperammonemia P74.6
        - potassium balance P74.3
        - sodium balance P74.2
        - specified type NEC P74.4
- emotions specific to childhood and adolescence F93.9
    - with
        - anxiety and fearfulness NEC F93.8
        - elective mutism F94.0
        - oppositional disorder F91.3
        - sensitivity (withdrawal) F40.10
        - shyness F40.10
        - social withdrawal F40.10
    - involving relationship problems F93.8
    - mixed F93.8
    - specified NEC F93.8
- endocrine (gland) E34.9
    - neonatal, transitory P72.9
        - specified NEC P72.8
- equilibrium R42
- fructose metabolism E74.10
- gait — *see* Gait
    - hysterical F44.4
    - psychogenic F44.4
- gastrointestinal (functional) K30
    - psychogenic F45.8
- habit, child F98.9
- hearing, except deafness and tinnitus — *see* Abnormal, auditory perception
- heart, functional (conditions in I44-I50)
    - due to presence of (cardiac) prosthesis I97.19- ☑
    - postoperative I97.89
        - cardiac surgery (*see also* Infarct, myocardium, associated with revascularization procedure) I97.19- ☑
- hormones E34.9
- innervation uterus (parasympathetic) (sympathetic) N85.8
- keratinization NEC
    - gingiva K05.10
        - nonplaque induced K05.11
        - plaque induced K05.10
    - lip K13.0
    - oral (mucosa) (soft tissue) K13.29
    - tongue K13.29
- learning (specific) — *see* Disorder, learning
- memory — *see* Amnesia
    - mild, following organic brain damage F06.8
- mental F99
    - associated with diseases classified elsewhere F54
- metabolism E88.9
    - with
        - abortion — *see* Abortion, by type with other specified complication
        - ectopic pregnancy O08.5
        - molar pregnancy O08.5
    - amino-acid E72.9
        - aromatic E70.9
        - branched-chain E71.2
            - straight-chain E72.8
            - sulfur-bearing E72.10
        - ammonia E72.20
        - arginine E72.21
        - argininosuccinic acid E72.22
        - carbohydrate E74.9
        - cholesterol E78.9
        - citrulline E72.23
        - cystathionine E72.19
        - general E88.9
        - glutamine E72.8
        - histidine E70.40
        - homocystine E72.19
        - hydroxylysine E72.3
    - in labor or delivery O75.89

Disturbance(s) — *continued*
  metabolism — *continued*
    iron E83.10
    lipoid E78.9
    lysine E72.3
    methionine E72.19
    neonatal, transitory P74.9
      calcium and magnesium P71.9
        specified type NEC P71.8
      carbohydrate metabolism P70.9
        specified type NEC P70.8
      specified NEC P74.8
    ornithine E72.4
    phosphate E83.39
    sodium NEC E87.8
    threonine E72.8
    tryptophan E70.5
    tyrosine E70.20
    urea cycle E72.20
  motor R29.2
  nervous, functional R45.0
  neuromuscular mechanism (eye), due to syphilis
    A52.15
  nutritional E63.9
    nail L60.3
  ocular motion H51.9
    psychogenic F45.8
  oculogyric H51.8
    psychogenic F45.8
  oculomotor H51.9
    psychogenic F45.8
  olfactory nerve R43.1
  optic nerve NEC — *see* Disorder, nerve, optic
  oral epithelium, including tongue NEC K13.29
  perceptual due to
    alcohol withdrawal F10.232
    amphetamine intoxication F15.922
      in
        abuse F15.122
        dependence F15.222
    anxiolytic withdrawal F13.232
    cannabis intoxication (acute) F12.922
      in
        abuse F12.122
        dependence F12.222
    cocaine intoxication (acute) F14.922
      in
        abuse F14.122
        dependence F14.222
    hypnotic withdrawal F13.232
    opioid intoxication (acute) F11.922
      in
        abuse F11.122
        dependence F11.222
    phencyclidine intoxication (acute) F16.122
    sedative withdrawal F13.232
  personality (pattern) (trait) (*see also* Disorder, person-
    ality) F60.9
    following organic brain damage F07.9
  polyglandular E31.9
    specified NEC E31.8
  potassium balance, newborn P74.3
  psychogenic F45.9
  psychomotor F44.4
  psychophysical visual H53.16
  pupillary — *see* Anomaly, pupil, function
  reflex R29.2
  rhythm, heart I49.9
  salivary secretion K11.7
  sensation (cold) (heat) (localization) (tactile discrimi-
    nation) (texture) (vibratory) NEC R20.9
    hysterical F44.6
    skin R20.9
      anesthesia R20.0
      hyperesthesia R20.3
      hypoesthesia R20.1
      paresthesia R20.2
      specified type NEC R20.8
    smell R43.9
      and taste (mixed) R43.8
      anosmia R43.0
      parosmia R43.1
      specified NEC R43.8
    taste R43.9
      and smell (mixed) R43.8
      parageusia R43.2
      specified NEC R43.8
  sensory — *see* Disturbance, sensation

Disturbance(s) — *continued*
  situational (transient) (*see also* Disorder,
    adjustment)
    acute F43.0
  sleep G47.9
    nonorganic origin F51.9
  smell — *see* Disturbance, sensation, smell
  sociopathic F60.2
  sodium balance, newborn P74.2
  speech R47.9
    developmental F80.9
    specified NEC R47.89
  stomach (functional) K31.9
  sympathetic (nerve) G90.9
  taste — *see* Disturbance, sensation, taste
  temperature
    regulation, newborn P81.9
      specified NEC P81.8
    sense R20.8
      hysterical F44.6
  tooth
    eruption K00.6
    formation K00.4
    structure, hereditary NEC K00.5
  touch — *see* Disturbance, sensation
  vascular I99.9
    arteriosclerotic — *see* Arteriosclerosis
  vasomotor I73.9
  vasospastic I73.9
  vision, visual H53.9
    following
      cerebral infarction I69.398
      cerebrovascular disease I69.998
        specified NEC I69.898
      intracerebral hemorrhage I69.198
      nontraumatic intracranial hemorrhage NEC
        I69.298
      specified disease NEC I69.898
      subarachnoid hemorrhage I69.098
    psychophysical H53.16
    specified NEC H53.8
    subjective H53.10
      day blindness H53.11
      discomfort H53.14- ☑
      distortions of shape and size H53.15
      loss
        sudden H53.13- ☑
        transient H53.12- ☑
      specified type NEC H53.19
  voice R49.9
    psychogenic F44.4
    specified NEC R49.8
Diuresis R35.8
Diver's palsy, paralysis or squeeze T70.3 ☑
Diverticulitis (acute) K57.92
  bladder — *see* Cystitis
  ileum — *see* Diverticulitis, intestine, small
  intestine K57.92
    with
      abscess, perforation or peritonitis K57.80
        with bleeding K57.81
      bleeding K57.93
    congenital Q43.8
    large K57.32
      with
        abscess, perforation or peritonitis K57.20
          with bleeding K57.21
        bleeding K57.33
        small intestine K57.52
          with
            abscess, perforation or peritonitis
              K57.40
              with bleeding K57.41
            bleeding K57.53
    small K57.12
      with
        abscess, perforation or peritonitis K57.00
          with bleeding K57.01
        bleeding K57.13
        large intestine K57.52
          with
            abscess, perforation or peritonitis
              K57.40
              with bleeding K57.41
            bleeding K57.53
Diverticulosis K57.90
  with bleeding K57.91
  large intestine K57.30

Diverticulosis — *continued*
  large intestine — *continued*
    with
      bleeding K57.31
      small intestine K57.50
        with bleeding K57.51
    small intestine K57.10
    with
      bleeding K57.11
      large intestine K57.50
        with bleeding K57.51
Diverticulum, diverticula (multiple) K57.90
  appendix (noninflammatory) K38.2
  bladder (sphincter) N32.3
    congenital Q64.6
  bronchus (congenital) Q32.4
    acquired J98.09
  calyx, calyceal (kidney) N28.89
  cardia (stomach) K31.4
  cecum — *see* Diverticulosis, intestine, large
    congenital Q43.8
  colon — *see* Diverticulosis, intestine, large
    congenital Q43.8
  duodenum — *see* Diverticulosis, intestine, small
    congenital Q43.8
  epiphrenic (esophagus) K22.5
  esophagus (congenital) Q39.6
    acquired (epiphrenic) (pulsion) (traction) K22.5
  eustachian tube — *see* Disorder, eustachian tube,
    specified NEC
  fallopian tube N83.8
  gastric K31.4
  heart (congenital) Q24.8
  ileum — *see* Diverticulosis, intestine, small
  jejunum — *see* Diverticulosis, intestine, small
  kidney (pelvis) (calyces) N28.89
    with calculus — *see* Calculus, kidney
  Meckel's (displaced) (hypertrophic) Q43.0
    malignant — *see* Table of Neoplasms, small intes-
      tine, malignant
  midthoracic K22.5
  organ or site, congenital NEC — *see* Distortion
  pericardium (congenital) (cyst) Q24.8
    acquired I31.8
  pharyngoesophageal (congenital) Q39.6
    acquired K22.5
  pharynx (congenital) Q38.7
  rectosigmoid — *see* Diverticulosis, intestine, large
    congenital Q43.8
  rectum — *see* Diverticulosis, intestine, large
  Rokitansky's K22.5
  seminal vesicle N50.89
  sigmoid — *see* Diverticulosis, intestine, large
    congenital Q43.8
  stomach (acquired) K31.4
    congenital Q40.2
  trachea (acquired) J39.8
  ureter (acquired) N28.89
    congenital Q62.8
  ureterovesical orifice N28.89
  urethra (acquired) N36.1
    congenital Q64.79
  ventricle, left (congenital) Q24.8
  vesical N32.3
    congenital Q64.6
  Zenker's (esophagus) K22.5
Division
  cervix uteri (acquired) N88.8
  glans penis Q55.69
  labia minora (congenital) Q52.79
  ligament (partial or complete) (current) (*see also*
    Sprain)
    with open wound — *see* Wound, open
  muscle (partial or complete) (current) (*see also* Injury,
    muscle)
    with open wound — *see* Wound, open
  nerve (traumatic) — *see* Injury, nerve
  spinal cord — *see* Injury, spinal cord, by region
  vein I87.8
Divorce, causing family disruption Z63.5
Dix-Hallpike neurolabyrinthitis — *see* Neuronitis,
  vestibular
Dizziness R42
  hysterical F44.89
  psychogenic F45.8
DMAC (disseminated mycobacterium avium- intracellulare complex) A31.2
DNR (do not resuscitate) Z66

Index

Doan-Wiseman syndrome — Dwarfism

Doan-Wiseman syndrome (primary splenic neutropenia) — *see* Agranulocytosis
Doehle-Heller aortitis A52.02
Dog bite — *see* Bite
Dohle body panmyelopathic syndrome D72.0
Dolichocephaly Q67.2
Dolichocolon Q43.8
Dolichostenomelia — *see* Syndrome, Marfan's
Donohue's syndrome E34.8
Donor (organ or tissue) Z52.9
　blood (whole) Z52.000
　　autologous Z52.010
　　specified component (lymphocytes) (platelets) NEC Z52.008
　　　autologous Z52.018
　　　specified donor NEC Z52.098
　　specified donor NEC Z52.090
　　stem cells Z52.001
　　　autologous Z52.011
　　　specified donor NEC Z52.091
　bone Z52.20
　　autologous Z52.21
　　marrow Z52.3
　　specified type NEC Z52.29
　cornea Z52.5
　egg (Oocyte) Z52.819
　　age 35 and over Z52.812
　　　anonymous recipient Z52.812
　　　designated recipient Z52.813
　　under age 35 Z52.810
　　　anonymous recipient Z52.810
　　　designated recipient Z52.811
　kidney Z52.4
　liver Z52.6
　lung Z52.89
　lymphocyte — *see* Donor, blood, specified components NEC
　Oocyte — *see* Donor, egg
　platelets Z52.008
　potential, examination of Z00.5
　semen Z52.89
　skin Z52.10
　　autologous Z52.11
　　specified type NEC Z52.19
　specified organ or tissue NEC Z52.89
　sperm Z52.89
Donovanosis A58
Dorsalgia M54.9
　psychogenic F45.41
　specified NEC M54.89
Dorsopathy M53.9
　deforming M43.9
　　specified NEC — *see* subcategory M43.8 ☑
　specified NEC M53.80
　　cervical region M53.82
　　cervicothoracic region M53.83
　　lumbar region M53.86
　　lumbosacral region M53.87
　　occipito-atlanto-axial region M53.81
　　sacrococcygeal region M53.88
　　thoracic region M53.84
　　thoracolumbar region M53.85
Double
　albumin E88.09
　aortic arch Q25.45
　auditory canal Q17.8
　auricle (heart) Q20.8
　bladder Q64.79
　cervix Q51.820
　　with doubling of uterus (and vagina) Q51.10
　　　with obstruction Q51.11
　inlet ventricle Q20.4
　kidney with double pelvis (renal) Q63.0
　meatus urinarius Q64.75
　monster Q89.4
　outlet
　　left ventricle Q20.2
　　right ventricle Q20.1
　pelvis (renal) with double ureter Q62.5
　tongue Q38.3
　ureter (one or both sides) Q62.5
　　with double pelvis (renal) Q62.5
　urethra Q64.74
　urinary meatus Q64.75
　uterus Q51.2
　　with
　　　doubling of cervix (and vagina) Q51.10
　　　　with obstruction Q51.11

Double — *continued*
　uterus — *continued*
　　in pregnancy or childbirth O34.59- ☑
　　　causing obstructed labor O65.5
　　vagina Q52.10
　　　with doubling of uterus (and cervix) Q51.10
　　　　with obstruction Q51.11
　　vision H53.2
　　vulva Q52.79
Douglas' pouch, cul-de-sac — *see* condition
Down syndrome Q90.9
　meiotic nondisjunction Q90.0
　mitotic nondisjunction Q90.1
　mosaicism Q90.1
　translocation Q90.2
DPD (dihydropyrimidine dehydrogenase deficiency) E88.89
Dracontiasis B72
Dracunculiasis, dracunculosis B72
Dream state, hysterical F44.89
Drepanocytic anemia — *see* Disease, sickle-cell
Dresbach's syndrome (elliptocytosis) D58.1
Dreschlera (hawaiiensis) (infection) B43.8
Dressler's syndrome I24.1
Drift, ulnar — *see* Deformity, limb, specified type NEC, forearm
Drinking (alcohol)
　excessive, to excess NEC (without dependence) F10.10
　　habitual (continual) (without remission) F10.20
　　　with remission F10.21
Drip, postnasal (chronic) R09.82
　due to
　　allergic rhinitis — *see* Rhinitis, allergic
　　common cold J00
　　gastroesophageal reflux — *see* Reflux, gastroesophageal
　　nasopharyngitis — *see* Nasopharyngitis
　　other known condition — *code to* condition
　　sinusitis — *see* Sinusitis
Droop
　facial R29.810
　　cerebrovascular disease I69.992
　　　cerebral infarction I69.392
　　　intracerebral hemorrhage I69.192
　　　nontraumatic intracranial hemorrhage NEC I69.292
　　　specified disease NEC I69.892
　　　subarachnoid hemorrhage I69.092
Drop (in)
　attack NEC R55
　finger — *see* Deformity, finger
　foot — *see* Deformity, limb, foot, drop
　hematocrit (precipitous) R71.0
　hemoglobin R71.0
　toe — *see* Deformity, toe, specified NEC
　wrist — *see* Deformity, limb, wrist drop
Dropped heart beats I45.9
Dropsy, dropsical (*see also* Hydrops)
　abdomen R18.8
　brain — *see* Hydrocephalus
　cardiac, heart — *see* Failure, heart, congestive
　gangrenous — *see* Gangrene
　heart — *see* Failure, heart, congestive
　kidney — *see* Nephrosis
　lung — *see* Edema, lung
　newborn due to isoimmunization P56.0
　pericardium — *see* Pericarditis
Drowned, drowning (near) T75.1 ☑
Drowsiness R40.0
Drug
　abuse counseling and surveillance Z71.51
　addiction — *see* Dependence
　dependence — *see* Dependence
　habit — *see* Dependence
　harmful use — *see* Abuse, drug
　induced fever R50.2
　overdose — *see* Table of Drugs and Chemicals, by drug, poisoning
　poisoning — *see* Table of Drugs and Chemicals, by drug, poisoning
　resistant organism infection (*see also* Resistant, organism, to, drug) Z16.30
　therapy
　　long term (current) (prophylactic) — *see* Therapy, drug long-term (current) (prophylactic)

Drug — *continued*
　therapy — *continued*
　　short term — *omit code*
　　wrong substance given or taken in error — *see* Table of Drugs and Chemicals, by drug, poisoning
Drunkenness (without dependence) F10.129
　acute in alcoholism F10.229
　chronic (without remission) F10.20
　　with remission F10.21
　pathological (without dependence) F10.129
　　with dependence F10.229
　sleep F51.9
Drusen
　macula (degenerative) (retina) — *see* Degeneration, macula, drusen
　optic disc H47.32- ☑
Dry, dryness (*see also* condition)
　larynx J38.7
　mouth R68.2
　　due to dehydration E86.0
　nose J34.89
　socket (teeth) M27.3
　throat J39.2
DSAP L56.5
Duane's syndrome H50.81- ☑
Dubin-Johnson disease or syndrome E80.6
Dubois' disease (thymus gland) A50.59 [E35]
Dubowitz' syndrome Q87.1
Duchenne-Aran muscular atrophy G12.21
Duchenne-Griesinger disease G71.0
Duchenne's
　disease or syndrome
　　motor neuron disease G12.22
　　muscular dystrophy G71.0
　locomotor ataxia (syphilitic) A52.11
　paralysis
　　birth injury P14.0
　　due to or associated with
　　　motor neuron disease G12.22
　　　muscular dystrophy G71.0
Ducrey's chancre A57
Duct, ductus — *see* condition
Duhring's disease (dermatitis herpetiformis) L13.0
Dullness, cardiac (decreased) (increased) R01.2
Dumb ague — *see* Malaria
Dumbness — *see* Aphasia
Dumdum fever B55.0
Dumping syndrome (postgastrectomy) K91.1
Duodenitis (nonspecific) (peptic) K29.80
　with bleeding K29.81
Duodenocholangitis — *see* Cholangitis
Duodenum, duodenal — *see* condition
Duplay's bursitis or periarthritis — *see* Tendinitis, calcific, shoulder
Duplication, duplex (*see also* Accessory)
　alimentary tract Q45.8
　anus Q43.4
　appendix (and cecum) Q43.4
　biliary duct (any) Q44.5
　bladder Q64.79
　cecum (and appendix) Q43.4
　cervix Q51.820
　chromosome NEC
　　with complex rearrangements NEC Q92.5
　　seen only at prometaphase Q92.8
　cystic duct Q44.5
　digestive organs Q45.8
　esophagus Q39.8
　frontonasal process Q75.8
　intestine (large) (small) Q43.4
　kidney Q63.0
　liver Q44.7
　pancreas Q45.3
　penis Q55.69
　respiratory organs NEC Q34.8
　salivary duct Q38.4
　spinal cord (incomplete) Q06.2
　stomach Q40.2
Dupré's disease (meningism) R29.1
Dupuytren's contraction or disease M72.0
Durand-Nicolas-Favre disease A55
Durotomy (inadvertent) (incidental) G97.41
Duroziez's disease (congenital mitral stenosis) Q23.2
Dutton's relapsing fever (West African) A68.1
Dwarfism E34.3
　achondroplastic Q77.4
　congenital E34.3
　constitutional E34.3

Dwarfism — *continued*
  hypochondroplastic Q77.4
  hypophyseal E23.0
  infantile E34.3
  Laron-type E34.3
  Lorain (-Levi) type E23.0
  metatropic Q77.8
  nephrotic-glycosuric (with hypophosphatemic rickets) E72.09
  nutritional E45
  pancreatic K86.89
  pituitary E23.0
  renal N25.0
  thanatophoric Q77.1
Dyke-Young anemia (secondary) (symptomatic) D59.1
Dysacusis — *see* Abnormal, auditory perception
Dysadrenocortism E27.9
  hyperfunction E27.0
Dysarthria R47.1
  following
    cerebral infarction I69.322
    cerebrovascular disease I69.922
      specified disease NEC I69.822
    intracerebral hemorrhage I69.122
    nontraumatic intracranial hemorrhage NEC I69.222
    subarachnoid hemorrhage I69.022
Dysautonomia (familial) G90.1
Dysbarism T70.3 ☑
Dysbasia R26.2
  angiosclerotica intermittens I73.9
  hysterical F44.4
  lordotica (progressiva) G24.1
  nonorganic origin F44.4
  psychogenic F44.4
Dysbetalipoproteinemia (familial) E78.2
Dyscalculia R48.8
  developmental F81.2
Dyschezia K59.00
Dyschondroplasia (with hemangiomata) Q78.4
Dyschromia (skin) L81.9
Dyscollagenosis M35.9
Dyscranio-pygo-phalangy Q87.0
Dyscrasia
  blood (with) D75.9
    antepartum hemorrhage — *see* Hemorrhage, antepartum, with coagulation defect
    intrapartum hemorrhage O67.0
    newborn P61.9
      specified type NEC P61.8
    puerperal, postpartum O72.3
    polyglandular, pluriglandular E31.9
Dysendocrinism E34.9
Dysentery, dysenteric (catarrhal) (diarrhea) (epidemic) (hemorrhagic) (infectious) (sporadic) (tropical) A09
  abscess, liver A06.4
  amebic (*see also* Amebiasis) A06.0
    with abscess — *see* Abscess, amebic
    acute A06.0
    chronic A06.1
  arthritis (*see also* category M01) A09
    bacillary (*see also* category M01) A03.9
  bacillary A03.9
    arthritis (*see also* category M01) A03.9
    Boyd A03.2
    Flexner A03.1
    Schmitz (-Stutzer) A03.0
    Shiga (-Kruse) A03.0
    Shigella A03.9
      boydii A03.2
      dysenteriae A03.0
      flexneri A03.1
      group A A03.0
      group B A03.1
      group C A03.2
      group D A03.3
      sonnei A03.3
      specified type NEC A03.8
    Sonne A03.3
    specified type NEC A03.8
  balantidial A07.0
  Balantidium coli A07.0
  Boyd's A03.2
  candidal B37.82
  Chilomastix A07.8
  Chinese A03.9
  coccidial A07.3
  Dientamoeba (fragilis) A07.8
  Embadomonas A07.8

Dysentery, dysenteric — *continued*
  Entamoeba, entamebic — *see* Dysentery, amebic
  Flexner-Boyd A03.2
  Flexner's A03.1
  Giardia lamblia A07.1
  Hiss-Russell A03.1
  Lamblia A07.1
  leishmanial B55.0
  malarial — *see* Malaria
  metazoal B82.0
  monilial B37.82
  protozoal A07.9
  Salmonella A02.0
  schistosomal B65.1
  Schmitz (-Stutzer) A03.0
  Shiga (-Kruse) A03.0
  Shigella NOS — *see* Dysentery, bacillary
  Sonne A03.3
  strongyloidiasis B78.0
  trichomonal A07.8
  viral (*see also* Enteritis, viral) A08.4
Dysequilibrium R42
Dysesthesia R20.8
  hysterical F44.6
Dysfibrinogenemia (congenital) D68.2
Dysfunction
  adrenal E27.9
    hyperfunction E27.0
  autonomic
    due to alcohol G31.2
    somatoform F45.8
  bladder N31.9
    neurogenic NOS — *see* Dysfunction, bladder, neuromuscular
    neuromuscular NOS N31.9
      atonic (motor) (sensory) N31.2
      autonomous N31.2
      flaccid N31.2
      nonreflex N31.2
      reflex N31.1
      specified NEC N31.8
      uninhibited N31.0
  bleeding, uterus N93.8
  cerebral G93.89
  colon K59.9
    psychogenic F45.8
  colostomy K94.03
  cystic duct K82.8
  cystostomy (stoma) — *see* Complications, cystostomy
  ejaculatory N53.19
    anejaculatory orgasm N53.13
    painful N53.12
    premature F52.4
    retarded N53.11
  endocrine NOS E34.9
  endometrium N85.8
  enterostomy K94.13
  erectile — *see* Dysfunction, sexual, male, erectile
  gallbladder K82.8
  gastrostomy (stoma) K94.23
  gland, glandular NOS E34.9
  heart I51.89
  hemoglobin D75.89
  hepatic K76.89
  hypophysis E23.7
  hypothalamic NEC E23.3
  ileostomy (stoma) K94.13
  jejunostomy (stoma) K94.13
  kidney — *see* Disease, renal
  labyrinthine — *see* subcategory H83.2 ☑
  left ventricular, following sudden emotional stress I51.81
  liver K76.89
  male — *see* Dysfunction, sexual, male
  orgasmic (female) F52.31
    male F52.32
  ovary E28.9
    specified NEC E28.8
  papillary muscle I51.89
  parathyroid E21.4
  physiological NEC R68.89
    psychogenic F59
  pineal gland E34.8
  pituitary (gland) E23.3
  platelets D69.1
  polyglandular E31.9
    specified NEC E31.8
  psychophysiologic F59

Dysfunction — *continued*
  psychosexual F52.9
    with
      dyspareunia F52.6
      premature ejaculation F52.4
      vaginismus F52.5
  pylorus K31.9
  rectum K59.9
    psychogenic F45.8
  reflex (sympathetic) — *see* Syndrome, pain, complex regional I
  segmental — *see* Dysfunction, somatic
  senile R54
  sexual (due to) R37
    alcohol F10.981
    amphetamine F15.981
      in
        abuse F15.181
        dependence F15.281
    anxiolytic F13.981
      in
        abuse F13.181
        dependence F13.281
    cocaine F14.981
      in
        abuse F14.181
        dependence F14.281
    excessive sexual drive F52.8
    failure of genital response (male) F52.21
      female F52.22
    female N94.9
      aversion F52.1
      dyspareunia N94.10
        psychogenic F52.6
      frigidity F52.22
      nymphomania F52.8
      orgasmic F52.31
      psychogenic F52.9
        aversion F52.1
        dyspareunia F52.6
        frigidity F52.22
        nymphomania F52.8
        orgasmic F52.31
        vaginismus F52.5
      vaginismus N94.2
        psychogenic F52.5
    hypnotic F13.981
      in
        abuse F13.181
        dependence F13.281
    inhibited orgasm (female) F52.31
      male F52.32
    lack
      of sexual enjoyment F52.1
      or loss of sexual desire F52.0
    male N53.9
      anejaculatory orgasm N53.13
      ejaculatory N53.19
        painful N53.12
        premature F52.4
        retarded N53.11
      erectile N52.9
        drug induced N52.2
        due to
          disease classified elsewhere N52.1
          drug N52.2
        postoperative (postprocedural) N52.39
          following
            cryotherapy N52.37
            interstitial seed therapy N52.36
            prostate ablative therapy N52.37
            prostatectomy N52.34
              radical N52.31
            radiation therapy N52.35
            radical cystectomy N52.32
            ultrasound ablative therapy N52.37
            urethral surgery N52.33
        psychogenic F52.21
        specified cause NEC N52.8
        vasculogenic
          arterial insufficiency N52.01
            with corporo-venous occlusive N52.03
          corporo-venous occlusive N52.02
            with arterial insufficiency N52.03
      impotence — *see* Dysfunction, sexual, male, erectile
      psychogenic F52.9
        aversion F52.1

Dysfunction — *continued*
  sexual — *continued*
    male — *continued*
      psychogenic — *continued*
        erectile F52.21
        orgasmic F52.32
        premature ejaculation F52.4
        satyriasis F52.8
        specified type NEC F52.8
      specified type NEC N53.8
    nonorganic F52.9
    specified NEC F52.8
    opioid F11.981
      in
        abuse F11.181
        dependence F11.281
    orgasmic dysfunction (female) F52.31
      male F52.32
    premature ejaculation F52.4
    psychoactive substances NEC F19.981
      in
        abuse F19.181
        dependence F19.281
    psychogenic F52.9
    sedative F13.981
      in
        abuse F13.181
        dependence F13.281
  sexual aversion F52.1
  vaginismus (nonorganic) (psychogenic) F52.5
  sinoatrial node I49.5
  somatic M99.09
    abdomen M99.09
    acromioclavicular M99.07
    cervical region M99.01
    cervicothoracic M99.01
    costochondral M99.08
    costovertebral M99.08
    head region M99.00
    hip M99.05
    lower extremity M99.06
    lumbar region M99.03
    lumbosacral M99.03
    occipitocervical M99.00
    pelvic region M99.05
    pubic M99.05
    rib cage M99.08
    sacral region M99.04
    sacrococcygeal M99.04
    sacroiliac M99.04
    specified NEC M99.09
    sternochondral M99.08
    sternoclavicular M99.07
    thoracic region M99.02
    thoracolumbar M99.02
    upper extremity M99.07
  somatoform autonomic F45.8
  stomach K31.89
    psychogenic F45.8
  suprarenal E27.9
    hyperfunction E27.0
  symbolic R48.9
    specified type NEC R48.8
  temporomandibular (joint) M26.69
    joint-pain syndrome M26.62- ☑
  testicular (endocrine) E29.9
    specified NEC E29.8
  thymus E32.9
  thyroid E07.9
  ureterostomy (stoma) — *see* Complications, stoma, urinary tract
  urethrostomy (stoma) — *see* Complications, stoma, urinary tract
  uterus, complicating delivery O62.9
    hypertonic O62.4
    hypotonic O62.2
      primary O62.0
      secondary O62.1
  ventricular I51.9
    with congestive heart failure (*see also* Failure, heart) I50.9
    left, reversible, following sudden emotional stress I51.81

Dysgenesis
  gonadal (due to chromosomal anomaly) Q96.9
    pure Q99.1
  renal Q60.5
    bilateral Q60.4
    unilateral Q60.3

Dysgenesis — *continued*
  reticular D72.0
  tidal platelet D69.3
Dysgerminoma
  specified site — *see* Neoplasm, malignant, by site
  unspecified site
    female C56.9
    male C62.90
Dysgeusia R43.2
Dysgraphia R27.8
Dyshidrosis, dysidrosis L30.1
Dyskaryotic cervical smear R87.619
Dyskeratosis L85.8
  cervix — *see* Dysplasia, cervix
  congenital Q82.8
  uterus NEC N85.8
Dyskinesia G24.9
  biliary (cystic duct or gallbladder) K82.8
  drug induced
    orofacial G24.01
  esophagus K22.4
  hysterical F44.4
  intestinal K59.8
  nonorganic origin F44.4
  orofacial (idiopathic) G24.4
    drug induced G24.01
  psychogenic F44.4
  subacute, drug induced G24.01
  tardive G24.01
    neuroleptic induced G24.01
  trachea J39.8
  tracheobronchial J98.09
Dyslalia (developmental) F80.0
Dyslexia R48.0
  developmental F81.0
Dyslipidemia E78.5
  depressed HDL cholesterol E78.6
  elevated fasting triglycerides E78.1
Dysmaturity (*see also* Light for dates)
  pulmonary (newborn) (Wilson-Mikity) P27.0
Dysmenorrhea (essential) (exfoliative) N94.6
  congestive (syndrome) N94.6
  primary N94.4
  psychogenic F45.8
  secondary N94.5
Dysmetabolic syndrome X E88.81
Dysmetria R27.8
Dysmorphism (due to)
  alcohol Q86.0
  exogenous cause NEC Q86.8
  hydantoin Q86.1
  warfarin Q86.2
Dysmorphophobia (nondelusional) F45.22
  delusional F22
Dysnomia R47.01
Dysorexia R63.0
  psychogenic F50.89
Dysostosis
  cleidocranial, cleidocranialis Q74.0
  craniofacial Q75.1
  Fairbank's (idiopathic familial generalized osteophytosis) Q78.9
  mandibulofacial (incomplete) Q75.4
  multiplex E76.01
  oculomandibular Q75.5
Dyspareunia (female) N94.10
  deep N94.12
  male N53.12
  nonorganic F52.6
  psychogenic F52.6
  secondary N94.19
  specified NEC N94.19
  superficial (introital) N94.11
Dyspepsia R10.13
  atonic K30
  functional (allergic) (congenital) (gastrointestinal) (occupational) (reflex) K30
  intestinal K59.8
  nervous F45.8
  neurotic F45.8
  psychogenic F45.8
Dysphagia R13.10
  cervical R13.19
  following
    cerebral infarction I69.391
    cerebrovascular disease I69.991
      specified NEC I69.891
    intracerebral hemorrhage I69.191

Dysphagia — *continued*
  following — *continued*
    nontraumatic intracranial hemorrhage NEC I69.291
    specified disease NEC I69.891
    subarachnoid hemorrhage I69.091
  functional (hysterical) F45.8
  hysterical F45.8
  nervous (hysterical) F45.8
  neurogenic R13.19
  oral phase R13.11
  oropharyngeal phase R13.12
  pharyngeal phase R13.13
  pharyngoesophageal phase R13.14
  psychogenic F45.8
  sideropenic D50.1
  spastica K22.4
  specified NEC R13.19
Dysphagocytosis, congenital D71
Dysphasia R47.02
  developmental
    expressive type F80.1
    receptive type F80.2
  following
    cerebrovascular disease I69.921
      cerebral infarction I69.321
      intracerebral hemorrhage I69.121
      nontraumatic intracranial hemorrhage NEC I69.221
      specified disease NEC I69.821
      subarachnoid hemorrhage I69.021
Dysphonia R49.0
  functional F44.4
  hysterical F44.4
  psychogenic F44.4
  spastica J38.3
Dysphoria
  gender F64.9
    in
      adolescence and adulthood F64.0
      children F64.2
    specified NEC F64.8
  postpartal O90.6
Dyspituitarism E23.3
Dysplasia (*see also* Anomaly)
  acetabular, congenital Q65.89
  alveolar capillary, with vein misalignment J84.843
  anus (histologically confirmed) (mild) (moderate) K62.82
    severe D01.3
  arrhythmogenic right ventricular I42.8
  arterial, fibromuscular I77.3
  asphyxiating thoracic (congenital) Q77.2
  brain Q07.9
  bronchopulmonary, perinatal P27.1
  cervix (uteri) N87.9
    mild N87.0
    moderate N87.1
    severe D06.9
  chondroectodermal Q77.6
  colon D12.6
  craniometaphyseal Q78.8
  dentinal K00.5
  diaphyseal, progressive Q78.3
  dystrophic Q77.5
  ectodermal (anhidrotic) (congenital) (hereditary) Q82.4
    hydrotic Q82.8
  epithelial, uterine cervix — *see* Dysplasia, cervix
  eye (congenital) Q11.2
  fibrous
    bone NEC (monostotic) M85.00
      ankle M85.07- ☑
      foot M85.07- ☑
      forearm M85.03- ☑
      hand M85.04- ☑
      lower leg M85.06- ☑
      multiple site M85.09
      neck M85.08
      rib M85.08
      shoulder M85.01- ☑
      skull M85.08
      specified site NEC M85.08
      thigh M85.05- ☑
      toe M85.07- ☑
      upper arm M85.02- ☑
      vertebra M85.08
  diaphyseal, progressive Q78.3
  jaw M27.8
  polyostotic Q78.1

Dysplasia — *continued*
  florid osseous (*see also* Cyst, calcifying odontogenic)
  high grade, focal D12.6
  hip, congenital Q65.89
  joint, congenital Q74.8
  kidney Q61.4
    multicystic Q61.4
  leg Q74.2
  lung, congenital (not associated with short gestation) Q33.6
  mammary (gland) (benign) N60.9- ☑
    cyst (solitary) — *see* Cyst, breast
    cystic — *see* Mastopathy, cystic
    duct ectasia — *see* Ectasia, mammary duct
    fibroadenosis — *see* Fibroadenosis, breast
    fibrosclerosis — *see* Fibrosclerosis, breast
    specified type NEC N60.8- ☑
  metaphyseal Q78.5
  muscle Q79.8
  oculodentodigital Q87.0
  periapical (cemental) (cemento-osseous) — *see* Cyst, calcifying odontogenic
  periosteum — *see* Disorder, bone, specified type NEC
  polyostotic fibrous Q78.1
  prostate (*see also* Neoplasia, intraepithelial, prostate) N42.30
    severe D07.5
    specified NEC N42.39
  renal Q61.4
    multicystic Q61.4
  retinal, congenital Q14.1
  right ventricular, arrhythmogenic I42.8
  septo-optic Q04.4
  skin L98.8
  spinal cord Q06.1
  spondyloepiphyseal Q77.7
  thymic, with immunodeficiency D82.1
  vagina N89.3
    mild N89.0
    moderate N89.1
    severe NEC D07.2
  vulva N90.3
    mild N90.0
    moderate N90.1
    severe NEC D07.1
Dyspnea (nocturnal) (paroxysmal) R06.00
  asthmatic (bronchial) J45.909
    with
      bronchitis J45.909
        with
          exacerbation (acute) J45.901
          status asthmaticus J45.902
        chronic J44.9
      exacerbation (acute) J45.901
      status asthmaticus J45.902
  cardiac — *see* Failure, ventricular, left
  cardiac — *see* Failure, ventricular, left
  functional F45.8
  hyperventilation R06.4
  hysterical F45.8
  newborn P28.89
  orthopnea R06.01
  psychogenic F45.8
  shortness of breath R06.02
  specified type NEC R06.09
Dyspraxia R27.8
  developmental (syndrome) F82
Dysproteinemia E88.09
Dysreflexia, autonomic G90.4
Dysrhythmia
  cardiac I49.9
    newborn
      bradycardia P29.12
        occurring before birth P03.819
          before onset of labor P03.810
          during labor P03.811
      tachycardia P29.11
    postoperative I97.89
  cerebral or cortical — *see* Epilepsy
Dyssomnia — *see* Disorder, sleep
Dyssynergia
  biliary K83.8
  bladder sphincter N36.44
  cerebellaris myoclonica (Hunt's ataxia) G11.1
Dysthymia F34.1
Dysthyroidism E07.9
Dystocia O66.9
  affecting newborn P03.1

Dystocia — *continued*
  cervical (hypotonic) O62.2
    affecting newborn P03.6
    primary O62.0
    secondary O62.1
  contraction ring O62.4
  fetal O66.9
    abnormality NEC O66.3
    conjoined twins O66.3
    oversize O66.2
  maternal O66.9
  positional O64.9 ☑
  shoulder (girdle) O66.0
    causing obstructed labor O66.0
  uterine NEC O62.4
Dystonia G24.9
  deformans progressiva G24.1
  drug induced NEC G24.09
    acute G24.02
    specified NEC G24.09
  familial G24.1
  idiopathic G24.1
    familial G24.1
    nonfamilial G24.2
    orofacial G24.4
  lenticularis G24.8
  musculorum deformans G24.1
  neuroleptic induced (acute) G24.02
  orofacial (idiopathic) G24.4
  oromandibular G24.4
    due to drug G24.01
  specified NEC G24.8
  torsion (familial) (idiopathic) G24.1
    acquired G24.8
    genetic G24.1
    symptomatic (nonfamilial) G24.2
Dystonic movements R25.8
Dystrophy, dystrophia
  adiposogenital E23.6
  Becker's type G71.0
  cervical sympathetic G90.2
  choroid (hereditary) H31.20
    central areolar H31.22
    choroideremia H31.21
    gyrate atrophy H31.23
    specified type NEC H31.29
  cornea (hereditary) H18.50
    endothelial H18.51
    epithelial H18.52
    granular H18.53
    lattice H18.54
    macular H18.55
    specified type NEC H18.59
  Duchenne's type G71.0
  due to malnutrition E45
  Erb's G71.0
  Fuchs' H18.51
  Gower's muscular G71.0
  hair L67.8
  infantile neuraxonal G31.89
  Landouzy-Déjérine G71.0
  Leyden-Möbius G71.0
  muscular G71.0
    benign (Becker type) G71.0
    congenital (hereditary) (progressive) (with specific morphological abnormalities of the muscle fiber) G71.0
      myotonic G71.11
    distal G71.0
    Duchenne type G71.0
    Emery-Dreifuss G71.0
    Erb type G71.0
    facioscapulohumeral G71.0
    Gower's G71.0
    hereditary (progressive) G71.0
    Landouzy-Déjérine type G71.0
    limb-girdle G71.0
    myotonic G71.11
    progressive (hereditary) G71.0
      Charcot-Marie (-Tooth) type G60.0
    pseudohypertrophic (infantile) G71.0
    severe (Duchenne type) G71.0
  myocardium, myocardial — *see* Degeneration, myocardial
  nail L60.3
    congenital Q84.6
  nutritional E45
  ocular G71.0
  oculocerebrorenal E72.03

Dystrophy, dystrophia — *continued*
  oculopharyngeal G71.0
  ovarian N83.8
  polyglandular E31.8
  reflex (neuromuscular) (sympathetic) — *see* Syndrome, pain, complex regional I
  retinal (hereditary) H35.50
    in
      lipid storage disorders E75.6 [H36]
      systemic lipidoses E75.6 [H36]
    involving
      pigment epithelium H35.54
      sensory area H35.53
    pigmentary H35.52
    vitreoretinal H35.51
  Salzmann's nodular — *see* Degeneration, cornea, nodular
  scapuloperoneal G71.0
  skin NEC L98.8
  sympathetic (reflex) — *see* Syndrome, pain, complex regional I
    cervical G90.2
  tapetoretinal H35.54
  thoracic, asphyxiating Q77.2
  unguium L60.3
    congenital Q84.6
  vitreoretinal H35.51
  vulva N90.4
  yellow (liver) — *see* Failure, hepatic
Dysuria R30.0
  psychogenic F45.8

E

Eales' disease H35.06- ☑
Ear (*see also* condition)
  piercing Z41.3
  tropical NEC B36.9 [H62.40]
    in
      aspergillosis B44.89
      candidiasis B37.84
      moniliasis B37.84
  wax (impacted) H61.20
    left H61.22
      with right H61.23
    right H61.21
      with left H61.23
Earache — *see* subcategory H92.0 ☑
Early satiety R68.81
Eaton-Lambert syndrome — *see* Syndrome, Lambert-Eaton
Eberth's disease (typhoid fever) A01.00
Ebola virus disease A98.4
Ebstein's anomaly or syndrome (heart) Q22.5
Eccentro-osteochondrodysplasia E76.29
Ecchondroma — *see* Neoplasm, bone, benign
Ecchondrosis D48.0
Ecchymosis R58
  conjunctiva — *see* Hemorrhage, conjunctiva
  eye (traumatic) — *see* Contusion, eyeball
  eyelid (traumatic) — *see* Contusion, eyelid
  newborn P54.5
  spontaneous R23.3
  traumatic — *see* Contusion
Echinococciasis — *see* Echinococcus
Echinococcosis — *see* Echinococcus
Echinococcus (infection) B67.90
  granulosus B67.4
    bone B67.2
    liver B67.0
    lung B67.1
    multiple sites B67.32
    specified site NEC B67.39
    thyroid B67.31
  liver NOS B67.8
    granulosus B67.0
    multilocularis B67.5
  lung NEC B67.99
    granulosus B67.1
    multilocularis B67.69
  multilocularis B67.7
    liver B67.5
    multiple sites B67.61
    specified site NEC B67.69
  specified site NEC B67.99
    granulosus B67.39
    multilocularis B67.69
  thyroid NEC B67.99

▽ Subterms under main terms may continue to next column or page   ☑ Additional Character Required — Refer to the Tabular List for Character Selection   **125**

Dysplasia — Echinococcus

Echinococcus — continued
  thyroid — continued
    granulosus B67.31
    multilocularis B67.69 [E35]
Echinorhynchiasis B83.8
Echinostomiasis B66.8
Echolalia R48.8
Echovirus, as cause of disease classified elsewhere
  B97.12
Eclampsia, eclamptic (coma) (convulsions) (delirium)
  (with hypertension) NEC O15.9
  complicating
    labor and delivery O15.1
    postpartum O15.2
    pregnancy O15.0- ☑
    puerperium O15.2
Economic circumstances affecting care Z59.9
Economo's disease A85.8
Ectasia, ectasis
  annuloaortic I35.8
  aorta I77.819
    with aneurysm — see Aneurysm, aorta
    abdominal I77.811
    thoracic I77.810
    thoracoabdominal I77.812
  breast — see Ectasia, mammary duct
  capillary I78.8
  cornea H18.71- ☑
  gastric antral vascular (GAVE) K31.819
    with hemorrhage K31.811
    without hemorrhage K31.819
  mammary duct N60.4- ☑
  salivary gland (duct) K11.8
  sclera — see Sclerectasia
Ecthyma L08.0
  contagiosum B08.02
  gangrenosum L08.0
  infectiosum B08.02
Ectocardia Q24.8
Ectodermal dysplasia (anhidrotic) Q82.4
Ectodermosis erosiva pluriorificialis L51.1
Ectopic, ectopia (congenital)
  abdominal viscera Q45.8
    due to defect in anterior abdominal wall Q79.59
  ACTH syndrome E24.3
  adrenal gland Q89.1
  anus Q43.5
  atrial beats I49.1
  beats I49.49
    atrial I49.1
    ventricular I49.3
  bladder Q64.10
  bone and cartilage in lung Q33.5
  brain Q04.8
  breast tissue Q83.8
  cardiac Q24.8
  cerebral Q04.8
  cordis Q24.8
  endometrium — see Endometriosis
  gastric mucosa Q40.2
  gestation — see Pregnancy, by site
  heart Q24.8
  hormone secretion NEC E34.2
  kidney (crossed) (pelvis) Q63.2
  lens, lentis Q12.1
  mole — see Pregnancy, by site
  organ or site NEC — see Malposition, congenital
  pancreas Q45.3
  pregnancy — see Pregnancy, ectopic
  pupil — see Abnormality, pupillary
  renal Q63.2
  sebaceous glands of mouth Q38.6
  spleen Q89.09
  testis Q53.00
    bilateral Q53.02
    unilateral Q53.01
  thyroid Q89.2
  tissue in lung Q33.5
  ureter Q62.63
  ventricular beats I49.3
  vesicae Q64.10
Ectromelia Q73.8
  lower limb — see Defect, reduction, limb, lower,
    specified type NEC
  upper limb — see Defect, reduction, limb, upper,
    specified type NEC
Ectropion H02.109
  cervix N86

Ectropion — continued
  cervix — continued
    with cervicitis N72
  congenital Q10.1
  eyelid (paralytic) H02.109
    cicatricial H02.119
      left H02.116
        lower H02.115
        upper H02.114
      right H02.113
        lower H02.112
        upper H02.111
    congenital Q10.1
    left H02.106
      lower H02.105
      upper H02.104
    mechanical H02.129
      left H02.126
        lower H02.125
        upper H02.124
      right H02.123
        lower H02.122
        upper H02.121
    right H02.103
      lower H02.102
      upper H02.101
    senile H02.139
      left H02.136
        lower H02.135
        upper H02.134
      right H02.133
        lower H02.132
        upper H02.131
    spastic H02.149
      left H02.146
        lower H02.145
        upper H02.144
      right H02.143
        lower H02.142
        upper H02.141
  iris H21.89
  lip (acquired) K13.0
    congenital Q38.0
  urethra N36.8
  uvea H21.89
Eczema (acute) (chronic) (erythematous) (fissum)
  (rubrum) (squamous) (see also Dermatitis) L30.9
  contact — see Dermatitis, contact
  dyshydrotic L30.1
  external ear — see Otitis, externa, acute, eczematoid
  flexural L20.82
  herpeticum B00.0
  hypertrophicum L28.0
  hypostatic — see Varix, leg, with, inflammation
  impetiginous L01.1
  infantile (due to any substance) L20.83
    intertriginous L21.1
    seborrheic L21.1
  intertriginous NEC L30.4
    infantile L21.1
  intrinsic (allergic) L20.84
  lichenified NEC L28.0
  marginatum (hebrae) B35.6
  pustular L30.3
  stasis I87.2
    with varicose veins — see Varix, leg, with, inflam-
      mation
  vaccination, vaccinatum T88.1 ☑
  varicose — see Varix, leg, with, inflammation
Eczematid L30.2
Eddowes (-Spurway) **syndrome** Q78.0
Edema, edematous (infectious) (pitting) (toxic) R60.9
  with nephritis — see Nephrosis
  allergic T78.3 ☑
  amputation stump (surgical) (sequelae) (late effect))
    T87.89
  angioneurotic (allergic) (any site) (with urticaria)
    T78.3 ☑
    hereditary D84.1
  angiospastic I73.9
  Berlin's (traumatic) S05.8X- ☑
  brain (cytotoxic) (vasogenic) G93.6
    due to birth injury P11.0
    newborn (anoxia or hypoxia) P52.4
      birth injury P11.0
    traumatic — see Injury, intracranial, cerebral edema
  cardiac — see Failure, heart, congestive
  cardiovascular — see Failure, heart, congestive

Edema, edematous — continued
  cerebral — see Edema, brain
  cerebrospinal — see Edema, brain
  cervix (uteri) (acute) N88.8
    puerperal, postpartum O90.89
  chronic hereditary Q82.0
  circumscribed, acute T78.3 ☑
    hereditary D84.1
  conjunctiva H11.42- ☑
  cornea H18.2- ☑
    idiopathic H18.22- ☑
    secondary H18.23- ☑
      due to contact lens H18.21- ☑
  due to
    lymphatic obstruction I89.0
    salt retention E87.0
  epiglottis — see Edema, glottis
  essential, acute T78.3 ☑
    hereditary D84.1
  extremities, lower — see Edema, legs
  eyelid NEC H02.849
    left H02.846
      lower H02.845
      upper H02.844
    right H02.843
      lower H02.842
      upper H02.841
  familial, hereditary Q82.0
  famine — see Malnutrition, severe
  generalized R60.1
  glottis, glottic, glottidis (obstructive) (passive) J38.4
    allergic T78.3 ☑
      hereditary D84.1
  heart — see Failure, heart, congestive
  heat T67.7 ☑
  hereditary Q82.0
  inanition — see Malnutrition, severe
  intracranial G93.6
  iris H21.89
  joint — see Effusion, joint
  larynx — see Edema, glottis
  legs R60.0
    due to venous obstruction I87.1
    hereditary Q82.0
  localized R60.0
    due to venous obstruction I87.1
  lower limbs — see Edema, legs
  lung J81.1
    with heart condition or failure — see Failure, ven-
      tricular, left
    acute J81.0
      chemical (acute) J68.1
        chronic J68.1
      chronic J81.1
        due to
          chemicals, gases, fumes or vapors (inhala-
            tion) J68.1
          external agent J70.9
            specified NEC J70.8
          radiation J70.1
    due to
      chemicals, fumes or vapors (inhalation) J68.1
      external agent J70.9
        specified NEC J70.8
      high altitude T70.29 ☑
      near drowning T75.1 ☑
      radiation J70.0
    meaning failure, left ventricle I50.1
  lymphatic I89.0
    due to mastectomy I97.2
  macula H35.81
    cystoid, following cataract surgery — see Compli-
      cations, postprocedural, following cataract
      surgery
    diabetic — see Diabetes, by type, with, retinopathy,
      with macular edema
  malignant — see Gangrene, gas
  Milroy's Q82.0
  nasopharynx J39.2
  newborn P83.30
    hydrops fetalis — see Hydrops, fetalis
    specified NEC P83.39
  nutritional (see also Malnutrition, severe)
    with dyspigmentation, skin and hair E40
  optic disc or nerve — see Papilledema
  orbit H05.22- ☑
  pancreas K86.89
  papilla, optic — see Papilledema

Edema, edematous — *continued*
- penis N48.89
- periodic T78.3 ☑
  - hereditary D84.1
- pharynx J39.2
- pulmonary — *see* Edema, lung
- Quincke's T78.3 ☑
  - hereditary D84.1
- renal — *see* Nephrosis
- retina H35.81
  - diabetic — *see* Diabetes, by type, with, retinopathy, with macular edema
- salt E87.0
- scrotum N50.89
- seminal vesicle N50.89
- spermatic cord N50.89
- spinal (cord) (vascular) (nontraumatic) G95.19
- starvation — *see* Malnutrition, severe
- stasis — *see* Hypertension, venous, (chronic)
- subglottic — *see* Edema, glottis
- supraglottic — *see* Edema, glottis
- testis N44.8
- tunica vaginalis N50.89
- vas deferens N50.89
- vulva (acute) N90.89

Edentulism — *see* Absence, teeth, acquired

Edsall's disease T67.2 ☑

Educational handicap Z55.9
- specified NEC Z55.8

Edward's syndrome — *see* Trisomy, 18

Effect(s) (of) (from) — *see* Effect, adverse NEC

Effect, adverse
- abnormal gravitational (G) forces or states T75.81 ☑
- abuse — *see* Maltreatment
- air pressure T70.9 ☑
  - specified NEC T70.8 ☑
- altitude (high) — *see* Effect, adverse, high altitude
- anesthesia (*see also* Anesthesia) T88.59 ☑
  - in labor and delivery O74.9
  - local, toxic
    - in labor and delivery O74.4
    - in pregnancy NEC O29.3- ☑
    - postpartum, puerperal O89.3
  - postpartum, puerperal O89.9
  - specified NEC T88.59 ☑
    - in labor and delivery O74.8
    - postpartum, puerperal O89.8
  - spinal and epidural T88.59 ☑
    - headache T88.59 ☑
      - in labor and delivery O74.5
      - postpartum, puerperal O89.4
    - specified NEC
      - in labor and delivery O74.6
      - postpartum, puerperal O89.5
- antitoxin — *see* Complications, vaccination
- atmospheric pressure T70.9 ☑
  - due to explosion T70.8 ☑
  - high T70.3 ☑
  - low — *see* Effect, adverse, high altitude
  - specified effect NEC T70.8 ☑
- biological, correct substance properly administered — *see* Effect, adverse, drug
- blood (derivatives) (serum) (transfusion) — *see* Complications, transfusion
- chemical substance — *see* Table of Drugs and Chemicals
- cold (temperature) (weather) T69.9 ☑
  - chilblains T69.1 ☑
  - frostbite — *see* Frostbite
  - specified effect NEC T69.8 ☑
- drugs and medicaments T88.7 ☑
  - specified drug — *see* Table of Drugs and Chemicals, by drug, adverse effect
  - specified effect — *code to* condition
- electric current, electricity (shock) T75.4 ☑
  - burn — *see* Burn
- exertion (excessive) T73.3 ☑
- exposure — *see* Exposure
- external cause NEC T75.89 ☑
- foodstuffs T78.1 ☑
  - allergic reaction — *see* Allergy, food
    - causing anaphylaxis — *see* Shock, anaphylactic, due to food
  - noxious — *see* Poisoning, food, noxious
- gases, fumes, or vapors T59.9- ☑
  - specified agent — *see* Table of Drugs and Chemicals

Effect, adverse — *continued*
- glue (airplane) sniffing
  - due to drug abuse — *see* Abuse, drug, inhalant
  - due to drug dependence — *see* Dependence, drug, inhalant
- heat — *see* Heat
- high altitude NEC T70.29 ☑
  - anoxia T70.29 ☑
  - on
    - ears T70.0 ☑
    - sinuses T70.1 ☑
  - polycythemia D75.1
- high pressure fluids T70.4 ☑
- hot weather — *see* Heat
- hunger T73.0 ☑
- immersion, foot — *see* Immersion
- immunization — *see* Complications, vaccination
- immunological agents — *see* Complications, vaccination
- infrared (radiation) (rays) NOS T66 ☑
  - dermatitis or eczema L59.8
- infusion — *see* Complications, infusion
- lack of care of infants — *see* Maltreatment, child
- lightning — *see* Lightning
- medical care T88.9 ☑
  - specified NEC T88.8 ☑
- medicinal substance, correct, properly administered — *see* Effect, adverse, drug
- motion T75.3 ☑
- noise, on inner ear — *see* subcategory H83.3 ☑
- overheated places — *see* Heat
- psychosocial, of work environment Z56.5
- radiation (diagnostic) (infrared) (natural source) (therapeutic) (ultraviolet) (X-ray) NOS T66 ☑
  - dermatitis or eczema — *see* Dermatitis, due to, radiation
  - fibrosis of lung J70.1
  - pneumonitis J70.0
  - pulmonary manifestations
    - acute J70.0
    - chronic J70.1
  - skin L59.9
- radioactive substance NOS
  - dermatitis or eczema — *see* Radiodermatitis
- reduced temperature T69.9 ☑
  - immersion foot or hand — *see* Immersion
  - specified effect NEC T69.8 ☑
- serum NEC (*see also* Reaction, serum) T80.69 ☑
- specified NEC T78.8 ☑
  - external cause NEC T75.89 ☑
- strangulation — *see* Asphyxia, traumatic
- submersion T75.1 ☑
- thirst T73.1 ☑
- toxic — *see* Toxicity
- transfusion — *see* Complications, transfusion
- ultraviolet (radiation) (rays) NOS T66 ☑
  - burn — *see* Burn
  - dermatitis or eczema — *see* Dermatitis, due to, ultraviolet rays
    - acute L56.8
- vaccine (any) — *see* Complications, vaccination
- vibration — *see* Vibration, adverse effects
- water pressure NEC T70.9 ☑
  - specified NEC T70.8 ☑
- weightlessness T75.82 ☑
- whole blood — *see* Complications, transfusion
- work environment Z56.5

Effects, late — *see* Sequelae

Effluvium
- anagen L65.1
- telogen L65.0

Effort syndrome (psychogenic) F45.8

Effusion
- amniotic fluid — *see* Pregnancy, complicated by, premature rupture of membranes
- brain (serous) G93.6
- bronchial — *see* Bronchitis
- cerebral G93.6
- cerebrospinal (*see also* Meningitis)
  - vessel G93.6
- chest — *see* Effusion, pleura
- chylous, chyliform (pleura) J94.0
- intracranial G93.6
- joint M25.40
  - ankle M25.47- ☑
  - elbow M25.42- ☑
  - foot joint M25.47- ☑

Effusion — *continued*
- joint — *continued*
  - hand joint M25.44- ☑
  - hip M25.45- ☑
  - knee M25.46- ☑
  - shoulder M25.41- ☑
  - specified joint NEC M25.48
  - wrist M25.43- ☑
- malignant pleural J91.0
- meninges — *see* Meningitis
- pericardium, pericardial (noninflammatory) I31.3
  - acute — *see* Pericarditis, acute
- peritoneal (chronic) R18.8
- pleura, pleurisy, pleuritic, pleuropericardial J90
  - chylous, chyliform J94.0
  - due to systemic lupus erythematosis M32.13
  - in conditions classified elsewhere J91.8
  - influenzal — *see* Influenza, with, respiratory manifestations NEC
  - malignant J91.0
  - newborn P28.89
  - tuberculous NEC A15.6
    - primary (progressive) A15.7
- spinal — *see* Meningitis
- thorax, thoracic — *see* Effusion, pleura

Egg shell nails L60.3
- congenital Q84.6

Egyptian splenomegaly B65.1

Ehlers-Danlos syndrome Q79.6

Ehrlichiosis A77.40
- due to
  - E. chafeensis A77.41
  - E. sennetsu A79.81
  - specified organism NEC A77.49

Eichstedt's disease B36.0

Eisenmenger's
- complex or syndrome I27.83
- defect Q21.8

Ejaculation
- delayed F52.32
- painful N53.12
- premature F52.4
- retarded N53.11
- retrograde N53.14
- semen, painful N53.12
  - psychogenic F52.6

Ekbom's syndrome (restless legs) G25.81

Ekman's syndrome (brittle bones and blue sclera) Q78.0

Elastic skin Q82.8
- acquired L57.4

Elastofibroma — *see* Neoplasm, connective tissue, benign

Elastoma (juvenile) Q82.8
- Miescher's L87.2

Elastomyofibrosis I42.4

Elastosis
- actinic, solar L57.8
- atrophicans (senile) L57.4
- perforans serpiginosa L87.2
- senilis L57.4

Elbow — *see* condition

Electric current, electricity, effects (concussion) (fatal) (nonfatal) (shock) T75.4 ☑
- burn — *see* Burn

Electric feet syndrome E53.8

Electrocution T75.4 ☑
- from electroshock gun (taser) T75.4 ☑

Electrolyte imbalance E87.8
- with
  - abortion — *see* Abortion by type, complicated by, electrolyte imbalance
  - ectopic pregnancy O08.5
  - molar pregnancy O08.5

Elephantiasis (nonfilarial) I89.0
- arabicum — *see* Infestation, filarial
- bancroftian B74.0
- congenital (any site) (hereditary) Q82.0
- due to
  - Brugia (malayi) B74.1
    - timori B74.2
  - mastectomy I97.2
  - Wuchereria (bancrofti) B74.0
- eyelid H02.859
  - left H02.856
    - lower H02.855
    - upper H02.854
  - right H02.853
    - lower H02.852

Index

Elephantiasis — Embolism

Elephantiasis — continued
  eyelid — continued
    right — continued
      upper H02.851
  filarial, filariensis — see Infestation, filarial
  glandular I89.0
  graecorum A30.9
  lymphangiectatic I89.0
  lymphatic vessel I89.0
    due to mastectomy I97.2
  scrotum (nonfilarial) I89.0
  streptococcal I89.0
  surgical I97.89
    postmastectomy I97.2
  telangiectodes I89.0
  vulva (nonfilarial) N90.89

Elevated, elevation
  antibody titer R76.0
  basal metabolic rate R94.8
  blood pressure (see also Hypertension)
    reading (incidental) (isolated) (nonspecific), no diagnosis of hypertension R03.0
  blood sugar R73.9
  body temperature (of unknown origin) R50.9
  cancer antigen 125 [CA 125] R97.1
  carcinoembryonic antigen [CEA] R97.0
  cholesterol E78.00
    with high triglycerides E78.2
  conjugate, eye H51.0
  C-reactive protein (CRP) R79.82
  diaphragm, congenital Q79.1
  erythrocyte sedimentation rate R70.0
  fasting glucose R73.01
  fasting triglycerides E78.1
  finding on laboratory examination — see Findings, abnormal, inconclusive, without diagnosis, by type of exam
  GFR (glomerular filtration rate) — see Findings, abnormal, inconclusive, without diagnosis, by type of exam
  glucose tolerance (oral) R73.02
  immunoglobulin level R76.8
  indoleacetic acid R82.5
  lactic acid dehydrogenase (LDH) level R74.0
  leukocytes D72.829
  lipoprotein a level E78.8 ☑
  liver function
    study R94.5
    test R79.89
      alkaline phosphatase R74.8
      aminotransferase R74.0
      bilirubin R17
      hepatic enzyme R74.8
      lactate dehydrogenase R74.0
  lymphocytes D72.820
  prostate specific antigen [PSA] R97.20
  Rh titer — see Complication(s), transfusion, incompatibility reaction, Rh (factor)
  scapula, congenital Q74.0
  sedimentation rate R70.0
  SGOT R74.0
  SGPT R74.0
  transaminase level R74.0
  triglycerides E78.1
    with high cholesterol E78.2
  tumor associated antigens [TAA] NEC R97.8
  tumor specific antigens [TSA] NEC R97.8
  urine level of
    17-ketosteroids R82.5
    catecholamine R82.5
    indoleacetic acid R82.5
    steroids R82.5
    vanillylmandelic acid (VMA) R82.5
  venous pressure I87.8
  white blood cell count D72.829
    specified NEC D72.828

Elliptocytosis (congenital) (hereditary) D58.1
  Hb C (disease) D58.1
  hemoglobin disease D58.1
  sickle-cell (disease) D57.8- ☑
    trait D57.3

Ellison-Zollinger syndrome E16.4
Ellis-van Creveld syndrome (chondroectodermal dysplasia) Q77.6
Elongated, elongation (congenital) (see also Distortion)
  bone Q79.9
  cervix (uteri) Q51.828
    acquired N88.4

Elongated, elongation — continued
  cervix — continued
    hypertrophic N88.4
  colon Q43.8
  common bile duct Q44.5
  cystic duct Q44.5
  frenulum, penis Q55.69
  labia minora (acquired) N90.69
  ligamentum patellae Q74.1
  petiolus (epiglottidis) Q31.8
  tooth, teeth K00.2
  uvula Q38.6

Eltor cholera A00.1
Emaciation (due to malnutrition) E41
Embadomoniasis A07.8
Embedded tooth, teeth K01.0
  root only K08.3
Embolic — see condition
Embolism (multiple) (paradoxical) I74.9
  air (any site) (traumatic) T79.0 ☑
    following
      abortion — see Abortion by type complicated by embolism
      ectopic pregnancy O08.2
    infusion, therapeutic injection or transfusion T80.0 ☑
    molar pregnancy O08.2
    procedure NEC
      artery T81.719 ☑
        mesenteric T81.710 ☑
        renal T81.711 ☑
        specified NEC T81.718 ☑
      vein T81.72 ☑
  in pregnancy, childbirth or puerperium — see Embolism, obstetric
  amniotic fluid (pulmonary) (see also Embolism, obstetric)
    following
      abortion — see Abortion by type complicated by embolism
      ectopic pregnancy O08.2
      molar pregnancy O08.2
  aorta, aortic I74.10
    abdominal I74.09
      saddle I74.01
    bifurcation I74.09
    saddle I74.01
    thoracic I74.11
  artery I74.9
    auditory, internal I65.8
    basilar — see Occlusion, artery, basilar
    carotid (common) (internal) — see Occlusion, artery, carotid
    cerebellar (anterior inferior) (posterior inferior) (superior) I66.3
    cerebral — see Occlusion, artery, cerebral
    choroidal (anterior) I65.8
    communicating posterior I65.8
    coronary (see also Infarct, myocardium)
      not resulting in infarction I24.0
    extremity I74.4
      lower I74.3
      upper I74.2
    hypophyseal I65.8
    iliac I74.5
    limb I74.4
      lower I74.3
      upper I74.2
    mesenteric (with gangrene) (see also Ischemia, intestine, acute) K55.059
    ophthalmic — see Occlusion, artery, retina
    peripheral I74.4
    pontine I65.8
    precerebral — see Occlusion, artery, precerebral
    pulmonary — see Embolism, pulmonary
    renal N28.0
    retinal — see Occlusion, artery, retina
    septic I76
    specified NEC I74.8
    vertebral — see Occlusion, artery, vertebral
  basilar (artery) I65.1
  blood clot
    following
      abortion — see Abortion by type complicated by embolism
      ectopic or molar pregnancy O08.2
    in pregnancy, childbirth or puerperium — see Embolism, obstetric

Embolism — continued
  brain (see also Occlusion, artery, cerebral)
    following
      abortion — see Abortion by type complicated by embolism
      ectopic or molar pregnancy O08.2
    puerperal, postpartum, childbirth — see Embolism, obstetric
  capillary I78.8
  cardiac (see also Infarct, myocardium)
    not resulting in infarction I51.3
  carotid (artery) (common) (internal) — see Occlusion, artery, carotid
  cavernous sinus (venous) — see Embolism, intracranial venous sinus
  cerebral — see Occlusion, artery, cerebral
  cholesterol — see Atheroembolism
  coronary (artery or vein) (systemic) — see Occlusion, coronary
  due to device, implant or graft (see also Complications, by site and type, specified NEC)
    arterial graft NEC T82.818 ☑
    breast (implant) T85.818 ☑
    catheter NEC T85.818 ☑
      dialysis (renal) T82.818 ☑
        intraperitoneal T85.818 ☑
      infusion NEC T82.818 ☑
        spinal (epidural) (subdural) T85.810 ☑
      urinary (indwelling) T83.81 ☑
    electronic (electrode) (pulse generator) (stimulator)
      bone T84.81 ☑
      cardiac T82.817 ☑
      nervous system (brain) (peripheral nerve) (spinal) T85.810 ☑
      urinary T83.81 ☑
    fixation, internal (orthopedic) NEC T84.81 ☑
    gastrointestinal (bile duct) (esophagus) T85.818 ☑
    genital NEC T83.81 ☑
    heart (graft) (valve) T82.817 ☑
    joint prosthesis T84.81 ☑
    ocular (corneal graft) (orbital implant) T85.818 ☑
    orthopedic (bone graft) NEC T86.838
    specified NEC T85.818 ☑
    urinary (graft) NEC T83.81 ☑
    vascular NEC T82.818 ☑
    ventricular intracranial shunt T85.810 ☑
  extremities
    lower — see Embolism, vein, lower extremity
      arterial I74.3
    upper I74.2
  eye H34.9
  fat (cerebral) (pulmonary) (systemic) T79.1 ☑
    complicating delivery — see Embolism, obstetric
    following
      abortion — see Abortion by type complicated by embolism
      ectopic or molar pregnancy O08.2
  following
    abortion — see Abortion by type complicated by embolism
    ectopic or molar pregnancy O08.2
    infusion, therapeutic injection or transfusion
      air T80.0 ☑
  heart (fatty) (see also Infarct, myocardium)
    not resulting in infarction I51.3
  hepatic (vein) I82.0
  in pregnancy, childbirth or puerperium — see Embolism, obstetric
  intestine (artery) (vein) (with gangrene) (see also Ischemia, intestine, acute) K55.039
  intracranial (see also Occlusion, artery, cerebral)
    venous sinus (any) G08
      nonpyogenic I67.6
  intraspinal venous sinuses or veins G08
    nonpyogenic G95.19
  kidney (artery) N28.0
  lateral sinus (venous) — see Embolism, intracranial, venous sinus
  leg — see Embolism, vein, lower extremity
    arterial I74.3
  longitudinal sinus (venous) — see Embolism, intracranial, venous sinus
  lung (massive) — see Embolism, pulmonary
  meninges I66.8
  mesenteric (artery) (vein) (with gangrene) (see also Ischemia, intestine, acute) K55.059

☑ Additional Character Required — Refer to the Tabular List for Character Selection ▽ Subterms under main terms may continue to next column or page

Embolism — *continued*
  obstetric (in) (pulmonary)
    childbirth O88.22
      air O88.02
      amniotic fluid O88.12
      blood clot O88.22
      fat O88.82
      pyemic O88.32
      septic O88.32
      specified type NEC O88.82
    pregnancy O88.21- ☑
      air O88.01- ☑
      amniotic fluid O88.11- ☑
      blood clot O88.21- ☑
      fat O88.81- ☑
      pyemic O88.31- ☑
      septic O88.31- ☑
      specified type NEC O88.81- ☑
    puerperal O88.23
      air O88.03
      amniotic fluid O88.13
      blood clot O88.23
      fat O88.83
      pyemic O88.33
      septic O88.33
      specified type NEC O88.83
  ophthalmic — *see* Occlusion, artery, retina
  penis N48.81
  peripheral artery NOS I74.4
  pituitary E23.6
  popliteal (artery) I74.3
  portal (vein) I81
  postoperative, postprocedural
    artery T81.719 ☑
      mesenteric T81.710 ☑
      renal T81.711 ☑
      specified NEC T81.718 ☑
    vein T81.72 ☑
  precerebral artery — *see* Occlusion, artery, precerebral
  puerperal — *see* Embolism, obstetric
  pulmonary (acute) (artery) (vein) I26.99
    with acute cor pulmonale I26.09
    chronic I27.82
    following
      abortion — *see* Abortion by type complicated
        by embolism
      ectopic or molar pregnancy O08.2
    healed or old Z86.711
    in pregnancy, childbirth or puerperium — *see*
      Embolism, obstetric
    personal history of Z86.711
    saddle I26.92
      with acute cor pulmonale I26.02
    septic I26.90
      with acute cor pulmonale I26.01
  pyemic (multiple) I76
    following
      abortion — *see* Abortion by type complicated
        by embolism
      ectopic or molar pregnancy O08.2
    Hemophilus influenzae A41.3
    pneumococcal A40.3
      with pneumonia J13
    puerperal, postpartum, childbirth (any organism)
      — *see* Embolism, obstetric
    specified organism NEC A41.89
    staphylococcal A41.2
    streptococcal A40.9
  renal (artery) N28.0
    vein I82.3
  retina, retinal — *see* Occlusion, artery, retina
  saddle
    abdominal aorta I74.01
    pulmonary artery I26.92
      with acute cor pulmonale I26.02
  septic (arterial) I76
    complicating abortion — *see* Abortion, by type,
      complicated by, embolism
  sinus — *see* Embolism, intracranial, venous sinus
  soap complicating abortion — *see* Abortion, by type,
    complicated by, embolism
  spinal cord G95.19
    pyogenic origin G06.1
  spleen, splenic (artery) I74.8
  upper extremity I74.2
  vein (acute) I82.90
    antecubital I82.61- ☑
      chronic I82.71- ☑

Embolism — *continued*
  vein — *continued*
    axillary I82.A1- ☑ (*following* I82.7)
      chronic I82.A2- ☑ (*following* I82.7)
    basilic I82.61- ☑
      chronic I82.71- ☑
    brachial I82.62- ☑
      chronic I82.72- ☑
    brachiocephalic (innominate) I82.290
      chronic I82.291
    cephalic I82.61- ☑
      chronic I82.71- ☑
    chronic I82.91
    deep (DVT) I82.40- ☑
      calf I82.4Z- ☑
        chronic I82.5Z- ☑
      lower leg I82.4Z- ☑
        chronic I82.5Z- ☑
      thigh I82.4Y- ☑
        chronic I82.5Y- ☑
      upper leg I82.4Y ☑
        chronic I82.5Y-
    femoral I82.41- ☑
      chronic I82.51- ☑
    iliac (iliofemoral) I82.42- ☑
      chronic I82.52- ☑
    innominate I82.290
      chronic I82.291
    internal jugular I82.C1- ☑ (*following* I82.7)
      chronic I82.C2- ☑ (*following* I82.7)
    lower extremity
      deep I82.40- ☑
        chronic I82.50- ☑
        specified NEC I82.49- ☑
          chronic NEC I82.59- ☑
      distal
        deep I82.4Z- ☑
      proximal
        deep I82.4Y- ☑
          chronic I82.5Y- ☑
      superficial I82.81- ☑
    popliteal I82.43- ☑
      chronic I82.53- ☑
    radial I82.62- ☑
      chronic I82.72- ☑
    renal I82.3
    saphenous (greater) (lesser) I82.81- ☑
    specified NEC I82.890
      chronic NEC I82.891
    subclavian I82.B1- ☑ (*following* I82.7)
      chronic I82.B2- ☑ (*following* I82.7)
    thoracic NEC I82.290
      chronic I82.291
    tibial I82.44- ☑
      chronic I82.54- ☑
    ulnar I82.62- ☑
      chronic I82.72- ☑
    upper extremity I82.60- ☑
      chronic I82.70- ☑
      deep I82.62- ☑
        chronic I82.72- ☑
      superficial I82.61- ☑
        chronic I82.71- ☑
  vena cava
    inferior (acute) I82.220
      chronic I82.221
    superior (acute) I82.210
      chronic I82.211
  venous sinus G08
  vessels of brain — *see* Occlusion, artery, cerebral
Embolus — *see* Embolism
Embryoma (*see also* Neoplasm, uncertain behavior, by
  site)
  benign — *see* Neoplasm, benign, by site
  kidney C64.- ☑
  liver C22.0
  malignant (*see also* Neoplasm, malignant, by site)
    kidney C64.- ☑
    liver C22.0
    testis C62.9- ☑
      descended (scrotal) C62.1- ☑
      undescended C62.0- ☑
  testis C62.9- ☑
    descended (scrotal) C62.1- ☑
    undescended C62.0- ☑

Embryonic
  circulation Q28.9
  heart Q28.9
  vas deferens Q55.4
Embryopathia NOS Q89.9
Embryotoxon Q13.4
Emesis — *see* Vomiting
Emotional lability R45.86
Emotionality, pathological F60.3
Emotogenic disease — *see* Disorder, psychogenic
Emphysema (atrophic) (bullous) (chronic) (interlobular)
    (lung) (obstructive) (pulmonary) (senile) (vesicular)
    J43.9
  cellular tissue (traumatic) T79.7 ☑
    surgical T81.82 ☑
  centrilobular J43.2
  compensatory J98.3
  congenital (interstitial) P25.0
  conjunctiva H11.89
  connective tissue (traumatic) T79.7 ☑
    surgical T81.82 ☑
  due to chemicals, gases, fumes or vapors J68.4
  eyelid(s) — *see* Disorder, eyelid, specified type NEC
    surgical T81.82 ☑
    traumatic T79.7 ☑
  interstitial J98.2
    congenital P25.0
    perinatal period P25.0
  laminated tissue T79.7 ☑
    surgical T81.82 ☑
  mediastinal J98.2
    newborn P25.2
  orbit, orbital — *see* Disorder, orbit, specified type NEC
  panacinar J43.1
  panlobular J43.1
  specified NEC J43.8
  subcutaneous (traumatic) T79.7 ☑
    nontraumatic J98.2
    postprocedural T81.82 ☑
    surgical T81.82 ☑
  surgical T81.82 ☑
  thymus (gland) (congenital) E32.8
  traumatic (subcutaneous) T79.7 ☑
  unilateral J43.0
Empty nest syndrome Z60.0
Empyema (acute) (chest) (double) (pleura) (supradi-
    aphragmatic) (thorax) J86.9
  with fistula J86.0
  accessory sinus (chronic) — *see* Sinusitis
  antrum (chronic) — *see* Sinusitis, maxillary
  brain (any part) — *see* Abscess, brain
  ethmoidal (chronic) (sinus) — *see* Sinusitis, ethmoidal
  extradural — *see* Abscess, extradural
  frontal (chronic) (sinus) — *see* Sinusitis, frontal
  gallbladder K81.0
  mastoid (process) (acute) — *see* Mastoiditis, acute
  maxilla, maxillary M27.2
    sinus (chronic) — *see* Sinusitis, maxillary
  nasal sinus (chronic) — *see* Sinusitis
  sinus (accessory) (chronic) (nasal) — *see* Sinusitis
  sphenoidal (sinus) (chronic) — *see* Sinusitis, sphe-
    noidal
  subarachnoid — *see* Abscess, extradural
  subdural — *see* Abscess, subdural
  tuberculous A15.6
  ureter — *see* Ureteritis
  ventricular — *see* Abscess, brain
En coup de sabre lesion L94.1
Enamel pearls K00.2
Enameloma K00.2
Enanthema, viral B09
Encephalitis (chronic) (hemorrhagic) (idiopathic)
    (nonepidemic) (spurious) (subacute) G04.90
  acute (*see also* Encephalitis, viral) A86
    disseminated G04.00
      infectious G04.01
      noninfectious G04.81
      postimmunization (postvaccination) G04.02
      postinfectious G04.01
    inclusion body A85.8
    necrotizing hemorrhagic G04.30
      postimmunization G04.32
      postinfectious G04.31
      specified NEC G04.39
  arboviral, arbovirus NEC A85.2
  arthropod-borne NEC (viral) A85.2
  Australian A83.4

Encephalitis — *continued*
  California (virus) A83.5
  Central European (tick-borne) A84.1
  Czechoslovakian A84.1
  Dawson's (inclusion body) A81.1
  diffuse sclerosing A81.1
  disseminated, acute G04.00
  due to
    cat scratch disease A28.1
    human immunodeficiency virus (HIV) disease
      B20 [G05.3]
    malaria — *see* Malaria
    rickettsiosis — *see* Rickettsiosis
    smallpox inoculation G04.02
    typhus — *see* Typhus
  Eastern equine A83.2
  endemic (viral) A86
  epidemic NEC (viral) A86
  equine (acute) (infectious) (viral) A83.9
    Eastern A83.2
    Venezuelan A92.2
    Western A83.1
  Far Eastern (tick-borne) A84.0
  following vaccination or other immunization proce-
    dure G04.02
  herpes zoster B02.0
  herpesviral B00.4
    due to herpesvirus 6 B10.01
    due to herpesvirus 7 B10.09
    specified NEC B10.09
  Ilheus (virus) A83.8
  in (due to)
    actinomycosis A42.82
    adenovirus A85.1
    African trypanosomiasis B56.9 [G05.3]
    Chagas' disease (chronic) B57.42
    cytomegalovirus B25.8
    enterovirus A85.0
    herpes (simplex) virus B00.4
      due to herpesvirus 6 B10.01
      due to herpesvirus 7 B10.09
      specified NEC B10.09
    infectious disease NEC B99 ✓ [G05.3]
    influenza — *see* Influenza, with, encephalopathy
    listeriosis A32.12
    measles B05.0
    mumps B26.2
    naegleriasis B60.2
    parasitic disease NEC B89 [G05.3]
    poliovirus A80.9 [G05.3]
    rubella B06.01
    syphilis
      congenital A50.42
      late A52.14
    systemic lupus erythematosus M32.19
    toxoplasmosis (acquired) B58.2
      congenital P37.1
    tuberculosis A17.82
    zoster B02.0
  inclusion body A81.1
  infectious (acute) (virus) NEC A86
  Japanese (B type) A83.0
  La Crosse A83.5
  lead — *see* Poisoning, lead
  lethargica (acute) (infectious) A85.8
  louping ill A84.8
  lupus erythematosus, systemic M32.19
  lymphatica A87.2
  Mengo A85.8
  meningococcal A39.81
  Murray Valley A83.4
  otitic NEC H66.40 [G05.3]
  parasitic NOS B71.9
  periaxial G37.0
  periaxialis (concentrica) (diffuse) G37.5
  postchickenpox B01.11
  postexanthematous NEC B09
  postimmunization G04.02
  postinfectious NEC G04.01
  postmeasles B05.0
  postvaccinal G04.02
  postvaricella B01.11
  postviral NEC A86
  Powassan A84.8
  Rasmussen G04.81
  Rio Bravo A85.8
  Russian
    autumnal A83.0
    spring-summer (taiga) A84.0

Encephalitis — *continued*
  saturnine — *see* Poisoning, lead
  specified NEC G04.81
  St. Louis A83.3
  subacute sclerosing A81.1
  summer A83.0
  suppurative G04.81
  tick-borne A84.9
  Torula, torular (cryptococcal) B45.1
  toxic NEC G92
  trichinosis B75 [G05.3]
  type
    B A83.0
    C A83.3
  van Bogaert's A81.1
  Venezuelan equine A92.2
  Vienna A85.8
  viral, virus A86
    arthropod-borne NEC A85.2
      mosquito-borne A83.9
        Australian X disease A83.4
        California virus A83.5
        Eastern equine A83.2
        Japanese (B type) A83.0
        Murray Valley A83.4
        specified NEC A83.8
        St. Louis A83.3
        type B A83.0
        type C A83.3
        Western equine A83.1
      tick-borne A84.9
        biundulant A84.1
        central European A84.1
        Czechoslovakian A84.1
        diphasic meningoencephalitis A84.1
        Far Eastern A84.0
        Russian spring-summer (taiga) A84.0
        specified NEC A84.8
    specified type NEC A85.8
  Western equine A83.1
Encephalocele Q01.9
  frontal Q01.0
  nasofrontal Q01.1
  occipital Q01.2
  specified NEC Q01.8
Encephalocystocele — *see* Encephalocele
Encephaloduroarteriomyosynangiosis (EDAMS) I67.5
Encephalomalacia (brain) (cerebellar) (cerebral) — *see*
  Softening, brain
Encephalomeningitis — *see* Meningoencephalitis
Encephalomeningocele — *see* Encephalocele
Encephalomeningomyelitis — *see* Meningoencephalitis
Encephalomyelitis (*see also* Encephalitis) G04.90
  acute disseminated G04.00
    infectious G04.01
    noninfectious G04.81
    postimmunization G04.02
    postinfectious G04.01
  acute necrotizing hemorrhagic G04.30
    postimmunization G04.32
    postinfectious G04.31
    specified NEC G04.39
  benign myalgic G93.3
  equine A83.9
    Eastern A83.2
    Venezuelan A92.2
    Western A83.1
  in diseases classified elsewhere G05.3
  myalgic, benign G93.3
  postchickenpox B01.11
  postinfectious NEC G04.01
  postmeasles B05.0
  postvaccinal G04.02
  postvaricella B01.11
  rubella B06.01
  specified NEC G04.81
  Venezuelan equine A92.2
Encephalomyelocele — *see* Encephalocele
Encephalomyelomeningitis — *see* Meningoencephalitis
Encephalomyelopathy G96.9
Encephalomyeloradiculitis (acute) G61.0
Encephalomyeloradiculoneuritis (acute) (Guillain-
  Barré) G61.0
Encephalomyeloradiculopathy G96.9
Encephalopathia hyperbilirubinemica, newborn
  P57.9

Encephalopathia hyperbilirubinemica, newborn —
  continued
  due to isoimmunization (conditions in P55) P57.0
Encephalopathy (acute) G93.40
  acute necrotizing hemorrhagic G04.30
    postimmunization G04.32
    postinfectious G04.31
    specified NEC G04.39
  alcoholic G31.2
  anoxic — *see* Damage, brain, anoxic
  arteriosclerotic I67.2
  centrolobar progressive (Schilder) G37.0
  congenital Q07.9
  degenerative, in specified disease NEC G32.89
  demyelinating callosal G37.1
  due to
    drugs (*see also* Table of Drugs and Chemicals) G92
  hepatic — *see* Failure, hepatic
  hyperbilirubinemic, newborn P57.9
    due to isoimmunization (conditions in P55) P57.0
  hypertensive I67.4
  hypoglycemic E16.2
  hypoxic — *see* Damage, brain, anoxic
  hypoxic ischemic P91.60
    mild P91.61
    moderate P91.62
    severe P91.63
  in (due to) (with)
    birth injury P11.1
    hyperinsulinism E16.1 [G94]
    influenza — *see* Influenza, with, encephalopathy
    lack of vitamin (*see also* Deficiency, vitamin)
      E56.9 [G32.89]
    neoplastic disease (*see also* Neoplasm)
      D49.9 [G13.1]
    serum (*see also* Reaction, serum) T80.69 ✓
    syphilis A52.17
    trauma (postconcussional) F07.81
      current injury — *see* Injury, intracranial
    vaccination G04.02
  lead — *see* Poisoning, lead
  metabolic G93.41
    drug induced G92
    toxic G92
  myoclonic, early, symptomatic — *see* Epilepsy, gener-
    alized, specified NEC
  necrotizing, subacute (Leigh) G31.82
  neonatal P91.819
    in diseases classified elsewhere P91.811
  pellagrous E52 [G32.89]
  portosystemic — *see* Failure, hepatic
  postcontusional F07.81
    current injury — *see* Injury, intracranial, diffuse
  posthypoglycemic (coma) E16.1 [G94]
  postradiation G93.89
  saturnine — *see* Poisoning, lead
  septic G93.41
  specified NEC G93.49
  spongioform, subacute (viral) A81.09
  toxic G92
    metabolic G92
  traumatic (postconcussional) F07.81
    current injury — *see* Injury, intracranial
  vitamin B deficiency NEC E53.9 [G32.89]
    vitamin B1 E51.2
  Wernicke's E51.2
Encephalorrhagia — *see* Hemorrhage, intracranial, intracerebral
Encephalosis, posttraumatic F07.81
Enchondroma (*see also* Neoplasm, bone, benign)
Enchondromatosis (cartilaginous) (multiple) Q78.4
Encopresis R15.9
  functional F98.1
  nonorganic origin F98.1
  psychogenic F98.1
Encounter (with health service) (for) Z76.89
  adjustment and management (of)
    breast implant Z45.81 ✓
    implanted device NEC Z45.89
    myringotomy device (stent) (tube) Z45.82
  administrative purpose only Z02.9
    examination for
      adoption Z02.82
      armed forces Z02.3
      disability determination Z02.71
      driving license Z02.4
      employment Z02.1
      insurance Z02.6

✓ **Additional Character Required** — Refer to the Tabular List for Character Selection   ▽ **Subterms under main terms may continue to next column or page**

Encounter — *continued*
  administrative purpose only — *continued*
    examination for — *continued*
      medical certificate NEC Z02.79
      paternity testing Z02.81
      residential institution admission Z02.2
      school admission Z02.0
      sports Z02.5
      specified reason NEC Z02.89
  aftercare — *see* Aftercare
  antenatal screening Z36.9
    cervical length Z36.86
    chromosomal anomalies Z36.0
    congenital cardiac abnormalities Z36.83
    elevated maternal serum alphafetoprotein Z36.1
    fetal growth retardation Z36.4
    fetal lung maturity Z36.84
    fetal macrosomia Z36.88
    hydrops fetalis Z36.81
    intrauterine growth restriction (IUGR) /small-for-
        dates Z36.4
    isoimmunization Z36.5
    large-for-dates Z36.88
    malformations Z36.3
    non-visualized anatomy on a previous scan Z36.2
    nuchal translucency Z36.82
    raised alphafetoprotein level Z36.1
    risk of pre-term labor Z36.86
    specified follow-up NEC Z36.2
    specified genetic defects NEC Z36.8A
    specified type NEC Z36.89
    Streptococcus B Z36.85
    suspected anomaly Z36.3
    uncertain dates Z36.87
  assisted reproductive fertility procedure cycle Z31.83
  blood typing Z01.83
    Rh typing Z01.83
  breast augmentation or reduction Z41.1
  breast implant exchange (different material) (different
      size) Z45.81 ☑
  breast reconstruction following mastectomy Z42.1
  check-up — *see* Examination
  chemotherapy for neoplasm Z51.11
  colonoscopy, screening Z12.11
  counseling — *see* Counseling
  delivery, full-term, uncomplicated O80
    cesarean, without indication O82
  desensitization to allergens Z51.6
  ear piercing Z41.3
  examination — *see* Examination
  expectant parent(s) (adoptive) pre-birth pediatrician
      visit Z76.81
  fertility preservation procedure (prior to cancer thera-
      py) (prior to removal of gonads) Z31.84
  fitting (of) — *see* Fitting (and adjustment) (of)
  genetic
    counseling
      nonprocreative Z71.83
      procreative Z31.5
    testing — *see* Test, genetic
  hearing conservation and treatment Z01.12
  immunotherapy for neoplasm Z51.12
  in vitro fertilization cycle Z31.83
  instruction (in)
    child care (postpartal) (prenatal) Z32.3
    childbirth Z32.2
    natural family planning
      procreative Z31.61
      to avoid pregnancy Z30.02
  insulin pump titration Z46.81
  joint prosthesis insertion following prior explantation
      of joint prosthesis (staged procedure)
    hip Z47.32
    knee Z47.33
    shoulder Z47.31
  laboratory (as part of a general medical examination)
      Z00.00
    with abnormal findings Z00.01
  mental health services (for)
    abuse NEC
      perpetrator Z69.82
      victim Z69.81
    child abuse
      nonparental
        perpetrator Z69.021
        victim Z69.020
      parental
        perpetrator Z69.011

Encounter — *continued*
  mental health services — *continued*
    child abuse — *continued*
      parental — *continued*
        victim Z69.010
    child neglect
      nonparental
        perpetrator Z69.021
        victim Z69.020
      parental
        perpetrator Z69.011
    child psychological abuse
      nonparental
        perpetrator Z69.021
        victim Z69.020
      parental
        perpetrator Z69.011
        victim Z69.010
    child sexual abuse
      nonparental
        perpetrator Z69.021
        victim Z69.020
      parental
        perpetrator Z69.011
        victim Z69.010
    non-spousal adult abuse (perpetrator) (victim)
        Z69.81
    spousal or partner
      abuse
        perpetrator Z69.12
        victim Z69.11
      neglect
        perpetrator Z69.12
        victim Z69.11
      psychological abuse
        perpetrator Z69.12
        victim Z69.11
      violence
        perpetrator (physical) (sexual) Z69.12
        victim (physical) Z69.11
          sexual Z69.81
  observation (for) (ruled out)
    exposure to (suspected)
      anthrax Z03.810
      biological agent NEC Z03.818
  pediatrician visit, by expectant parent(s) (adoptive)
      Z76.81
  placental sample (taken vaginally) (*see also* Encounter,
      antenatal screening) Z36.9
  plastic and reconstructive surgery following medical
      procedure or healed injury NEC Z42.8
  pregnancy
    supervision of — *see* Pregnancy, supervision of
    test Z32.00
      result negative Z32.02
      result positive Z32.01
  procreative management and counseling for gestation-
      al carrier Z31.7
  prophylactic measures Z29.9
    antivenin Z29.12
    fluoride administration Z29.3
    immunotherapy for respiratory syncytial virus (RSV)
        Z29.11
    rabies immune globin Z29.14
    Rho (D) immune globulin Z29.13
    specified NEC Z29.8
  radiation therapy (antineoplastic) Z51.0
  radiological (as part of a general medical examination)
      Z00.00
    with abnormal findings Z00.01
  reconstructive surgery following medical procedure
      or healed injury NEC Z42.8
  removal (of) (*see also* Removal)
    artificial
      arm Z44.00- ☑
        complete Z44.01- ☑
        partial Z44.02- ☑
      eye Z44.2- ☑
      leg Z44.10- ☑
        complete Z44.11- ☑
        partial Z44.12- ☑
    breast implant Z45.81 ☑
      tissue expander (without synchronous insertion
          of permanent implant) Z45.81 ☑
    device Z46.9
      specified NEC Z46.89

Encounter — *continued*
  removal (*see also* Removal) — *continued*
    external
      fixation device — *code to* fracture with seventh
          character D
      prosthesis, prosthetic device Z44.9
        breast Z44.3- ☑
        specified NEC Z44.8
    implanted device NEC Z45.89
    insulin pump Z46.81
    internal fixation device Z47.2
    myringotomy device (stent) (tube) Z45.82
    nervous system device NEC Z46.2
      brain neuropacemaker Z46.2
      visual substitution device Z46.2
        implanted Z45.31
    non-vascular catheter Z46.82
    orthodontic device Z46.4
    stent
      ureteral Z46.6
    urinary device Z46.6
  repeat cervical smear to confirm findings of recent
      normal smear following initial abnormal smear
      Z01.42
  respirator [ventilator] use during power failure Z99.12
  Rh typing Z01.83
  screening — *see* Screening
  specified NEC Z76.89
  sterilization Z30.2
  suspected condition, ruled out
    amniotic cavity and membrane Z03.71
    cervical shortening Z03.75
    fetal anomaly Z03.73
    fetal growth Z03.74
    maternal and fetal conditions NEC Z03.79
    oligohydramnios Z03.71
    placental problem Z03.72
    polyhydramnios Z03.71
  suspected exposure (to), ruled out
    anthrax Z03.810
    biological agents NEC Z03.818
  termination of pregnancy, elective Z33.2
  testing — *see* Test
  therapeutic drug level monitoring Z51.81
  titration, insulin pump Z46.81
  to determine fetal viability of pregnancy O36.80 ☑
  training
    insulin pump Z46.81
  X-ray of chest (as part of a general medical examina-
      tion) Z00.00
    with abnormal findings Z00.01
Encystment — *see* Cyst
Endarteritis (bacterial, subacute) (infective) I77.6
  brain I67.7
  cerebral or cerebrospinal I67.7
  deformans — *see* Arteriosclerosis
  embolic — *see* Embolism
  obliterans (*see also* Arteriosclerosis)
    pulmonary I28.8
  pulmonary I28.8
  retina — *see* Vasculitis, retina
  senile — *see* Arteriosclerosis
  syphilitic A52.09
    brain or cerebral A52.04
    congenital A50.54 [I79.8]
  tuberculous A18.89
Endemic — *see* condition
Endocarditis (chronic) (marantic) (nonbacterial)
    (thrombotic) (valvular) I38
  with rheumatic fever (conditions in I00)
    active — *see* Endocarditis, acute, rheumatic
    inactive or quiescent (with chorea) I09.1
  acute or subacute I33.9
    infective I33.0
    rheumatic (aortic) (mitral) (pulmonary) (tricuspid)
        I01.1
      with chorea (acute) (rheumatic) (Sydenham's)
          I02.0
  aortic (heart) (nonrheumatic) (valve) I35.8
    with
      mitral disease I08.0
        with tricuspid (valve) disease I08.3
        active or acute I01.1
          with chorea (acute) (rheumatic) (Syden-
              ham's) I02.0
      rheumatic fever (conditions in I00)
        active — *see* Endocarditis, acute, rheumatic
        inactive or quiescent (with chorea) I06.9

Index

Endocarditis — Enlargement, enlarged

Endocarditis — continued
aortic — continued
  with — continued
    tricuspid (valve) disease I08.2
      with mitral (valve) disease I08.3
  acute or subacute I33.9
  arteriosclerotic I35.8
  rheumatic I06.9
    with mitral disease I08.0
      with tricuspid (valve) disease I08.3
        active or acute I01.1
          with chorea (acute) (rheumatic) (Sydenham's) I02.0
      active or acute I01.1
        with chorea (acute) (rheumatic) (Sydenham's) I02.0
    specified NEC I06.8
  specified cause NEC I35.8
  syphilitic A52.03
arteriosclerotic I38
atypical verrucous (Libman-Sacks) M32.11
bacterial (acute) (any valve) (subacute) I33.0
candidal B37.6
congenital Q24.8
constrictive I33.0
Coxiella burnetii A78 [I39]
Coxsackie B33.21
due to
  prosthetic cardiac valve T82.6 ☑
  Q fever A78 [I39]
  Serratia marcescens I33.0
  typhoid (fever) A01.02
gonococcal A54.83
infectious or infective (acute) (any valve) (subacute) I33.0
lenta (acute) (any valve) (subacute) I33.0
Libman-Sacks M32.11
listerial A32.82
Löffler's I42.3
malignant (acute) (any valve) (subacute) I33.0
meningococcal A39.51
mitral (chronic) (double) (fibroid) (heart) (inactive) (valve) (with chorea) I05.9
  with
    aortic (valve) disease I08.0
      with tricuspid (valve) disease I08.3
        active or acute I01.1
          with chorea (acute) (rheumatic) (Sydenham's) I02.0
    rheumatic fever (conditions in I00)
      active — see Endocarditis, acute, rheumatic
      inactive or quiescent (with chorea) I05.9
    tricuspid (valve) disease I08.1
      with aortic (valve) disease I08.3
  active or acute I01.1
    with chorea (acute) (rheumatic) (Sydenham's) I02.0
    bacterial I33.0
  arteriosclerotic I34.8
  nonrheumatic I34.8
    acute or subacute I33.9
  specified NEC I05.8
monilial B37.6
multiple valves I08.9
  specified disorders I08.8
mycotic (acute) (any valve) (subacute) I33.0
pneumococcal (acute) (any valve) (subacute) I33.0
pulmonary (chronic) (heart) (valve) I37.8
  with rheumatic fever (conditions in I00)
    active — see Endocarditis, acute, rheumatic
    inactive or quiescent (with chorea) I09.89
      with aortic, mitral or tricuspid disease I08.8
  acute or subacute I33.9
    rheumatic I01.1
      with chorea (acute) (rheumatic) (Sydenham's) I02.0
  arteriosclerotic I37.8
  congenital Q22.2
  rheumatic (chronic) (inactive) (with chorea) I09.89
    active or acute I01.1
      with chorea (acute) (rheumatic) (Sydenham's) I02.0
  syphilitic A52.03
purulent (acute) (any valve) (subacute) I33.0
Q fever A78 [I39]
rheumatic (chronic) (inactive) (with chorea) I09.1
  active or acute (aortic) (mitral) (pulmonary) (tricuspid) I01.1

Endocarditis — continued
rheumatic — continued
  active or acute — continued
    with chorea (acute) (rheumatic) (Sydenham's) I02.0
rheumatoid — see Rheumatoid, carditis
septic (acute) (any valve) (subacute) I33.0
streptococcal (acute) (any valve) (subacute) I33.0
subacute — see Endocarditis, acute
suppurative (acute) (any valve) (subacute) I33.0
syphilitic A52.03
toxic I33.9
tricuspid (chronic) (heart) (inactive) (rheumatic) (valve) (with chorea) I07.9
  with
    aortic (valve) disease I08.2
      mitral (valve) disease I08.3
    mitral (valve) disease I08.1
      aortic (valve) disease I08.3
    rheumatic fever (conditions in I00)
      active — see Endocarditis, acute, rheumatic
      inactive or quiescent (with chorea) I07.8
  active or acute I01.1
    with chorea (acute) (rheumatic) (Sydenham's) I02.0
  arteriosclerotic I36.8
  nonrheumatic I36.8
    acute or subacute I33.9
  specified cause, except rheumatic I36.8
tuberculous — see Tuberculosis, endocarditis
typhoid A01.02
ulcerative (acute) (any valve) (subacute) I33.0
vegetative (acute) (any valve) (subacute) I33.0
verrucous (atypical) (nonbacterial) (nonrheumatic) M32.11

Endocardium, endocardial (see also condition)
  cushion defect Q21.2
Endocervicitis (see also Cervicitis)
  due to intrauterine (contraceptive) device T83.69 ☑
  hyperplastic N72
Endocrine — see condition
Endocrinopathy, pluriglandular E31.9
Endodontic
  overfill M27.52
  underfill M27.53
Endodontitis K04.01
  irreversible K04.02
  reversible K04.01
Endomastoiditis — see Mastoiditis
Endometrioma N80.9
Endometriosis N80.9
  appendix N80.5
  bladder N80.8
  bowel N80.5
  broad ligament N80.3
  cervix N80.0
  colon N80.5
  cul-de-sac (Douglas') N80.3
  exocervix N80.0
  fallopian tube N80.2
  female genital organ NEC N80.8
  gallbladder N80.8
  in scar of skin N80.6
  internal N80.0
  intestine N80.5
  lung N80.8
  myometrium N80.0
  ovary N80.1
  parametrium N80.3
  pelvic peritoneum N80.3
  peritoneal (pelvic) N80.3
  rectovaginal septum N80.4
  rectum N80.5
  round ligament N80.3
  skin (scar) N80.6
  specified site NEC N80.8
  stromal D39.0
  thorax N80.8
  umbilicus N80.8
  uterus (internal) N80.0
  vagina N80.4
  vulva N80.8
Endometritis (decidual) (nonspecific) (purulent) (senile) (atrophic) (suppurative) N71.9
  with ectopic pregnancy O08.0
  acute N71.0
  blenorrhagic (gonococcal) (acute) (chronic) A54.24

Endometritis — continued
  cervix, cervical (with erosion or ectropion) (see also Cervicitis)
    hyperplastic N72
  chlamydial A56.11
  chronic N71.1
  following
    abortion — see Abortion by type complicated by genital infection
    ectopic or molar pregnancy O08.0
  gonococcal, gonorrheal (acute) (chronic) A54.24
  hyperplastic (see also Hyperplasia, endometrial) N85.00
    cervix N72
  puerperal, postpartum, childbirth O86.12
  subacute N71.0
  tuberculous A18.17
Endometrium — see condition
Endomyocardiopathy, South African I42.3
Endomyocarditis — see Endocarditis
Endomyofibrosis I42.3
Endomyometritis — see Endometritis
Endopericarditis — see Endocarditis
Endoperineuritis — see Disorder, nerve
Endophlebitis — see Phlebitis
Endophthalmia — see Endophthalmitis, purulent
Endophthalmitis (acute) (infective) (metastatic) (subacute) H44.009
  bleb associated (see also Bleb, inflammed (infected), postprocedural H59.4 ☑
  gonorrheal A54.39
  in (due to)
    cysticercosis B69.1
    onchocerciasis B73.01
    toxocariasis B83.0
  panuveitis — see Panuveitis
  parasitic H44.12- ☑
  purulent H44.00- ☑
    panophthalmitis — see Panophthalmitis
    vitreous abscess H44.02- ☑
  specified NEC H44.19
  sympathetic — see Uveitis, sympathetic
Endosalpingioma D28.2
Endosalpingiosis N94.89
Endosteitis — see Osteomyelitis
Endothelioma, bone — see Neoplasm, bone, malignant
Endotheliosis (hemorrhagic infectional) D69.8
Endotoxemia — code to condition
Endotrachelitis — see Cervicitis
Engelmann (-Camurati) **syndrome** Q78.3
English disease — see Rickets
Engman's disease L30.3
Engorgement
  breast N64.59
    newborn P83.4
    puerperal, postpartum O92.79
  lung (passive) — see Edema, lung
  pulmonary (passive) — see Edema, lung
  stomach K31.89
  venous, retina — see Occlusion, retina, vein, engorgement
Enlargement, enlarged (see also Hypertrophy)
  adenoids J35.2
    with tonsils J35.3
  alveolar ridge K08.89
    congenital — see Anomaly, alveolar
  apertures of diaphragm (congenital) Q79.1
  gingival K06.1
  heart, cardiac — see Hypertrophy, cardiac
  labium majus, childhood asymmetric (CALME) N90.61
  lacrimal gland, chronic H04.03- ☑
  liver — see Hypertrophy, liver
  lymph gland or node R59.9
    generalized R59.1
    localized R59.0
  orbit H05.34- ☑
  organ or site, congenital NEC — see Anomaly, by site
  parathyroid (gland) E21.0
  pituitary fossa R93.0
  prostate N40.0
    with lower urinary tract symptoms (LUTS) N40.1
    without lower urinary tract symtpoms (LUTS) N40.0
  sella turcica R93.0
  spleen — see Splenomegaly
  thymus (gland) (congenital) E32.0
  thyroid (gland) — see Goiter
  tongue K14.8
  tonsils J35.1

Enlargement, enlarged — *continued*
  tonsils — *continued*
    with adenoids J35.3
  uterus N85.2
  vestibular aqueduct Q16.5
Enophthalmos H05.40- ☑
  due to
    orbital tissue atrophy H05.41- ☑
    trauma or surgery H05.42- ☑
Enostosis M27.8
Entamebic, entamebiasis — *see* Amebiasis
Entanglement
  umbilical cord(s) O69.82 ☑
    with compression O69.2 ☑
    without compression O69.82 ☑
    around neck (with compression) O69.81 ☑
      with compression O69.1 ☑
      without compression O69.81 ☑
    of twins in monoamniotic sac O69.2 ☑
Enteralgia — *see* Pain, abdominal
Enteric — *see* condition
Enteritis (acute) (diarrheal) (hemorrhagic) (noninfective)
  K52.9
  adenovirus A08.2
  aertrycke infection A02.0
  allergic K52.29
    with
      eosinophilic gastritis or gastroenteritis K52.81
      food protein-induced enterocolitis syndrome
        K52.21
      food protein-induced enteropathy K52.22
  amebic (acute) A06.0
    with abscess — *see* Abscess, amebic
    chronic A06.1
      with abscess — *see* Abscess, amebic
      nondysenteric A06.2
    nondysenteric A06.2
  astrovirus A08.32
  bacillary NOS A03.9
  bacterial A04.9
    specified NEC A04.8
  calicivirus A08.31
  candidal B37.82
  Chilomastix A07.8
  choleriformis A00.1
  chronic (noninfectious) K52.9
    ulcerative — *see* Colitis, ulcerative
  cicatrizing (chronic) — *see* Enteritis, regional, small
    intestine
  Clostridium
    botulinum (food poisoning) A05.1
    difficile
      not specified as recurrent A04.72
      recurrent A04.71
  coccidial A07.3
  coxsackie virus A08.39
  dietetic (*see also* Enteritis, allergic) K52.29
  drug-induced K52.1
  due to
    astrovirus A08.32
    calicivirus A08.31
    coxsackie virus A08.39
    drugs K52.1
    echovirus A08.39
    enterovirus NEC A08.39
    food hypersensitivity (*see also* Enteritis, allergic)
      K52.29
    infectious organism (bacterial) (viral) — *see* Enteri-
      tis, infectious
    torovirus A08.39
    Yersinia enterocolitica A04.6
  echovirus A08.39
  eltor A00.1
  enterovirus NEC A08.39
  eosinophilic K52.81
  epidemic (infectious) A09
  fulminant (*see also* Ischemia, intestine, acute) K55.019
  gangrenous — *see* Enteritis, infectious
  giardial A07.1
  infectious NOS A09
    due to
      adenovirus A08.2
      Aerobacter aerogenes A04.8
      Arizona (bacillus) A02.0
      bacteria NOS A04.9
        specified NEC A04.8
      Campylobacter A04.5

Enteritis — *continued*
  infectious — *continued*
    due to — *continued*
      Clostridium difficile
        not specified as recurrent A04.72
        recurrent A04.71
      Clostridium perfringens A04.8
      Enterobacter aerogenes A04.8
      enterovirus A08.39
      Escherichia coli A04.4
        enteroaggregative A04.4
        enterohemorrhagic A04.3
        enteroinvasive A04.2
        enteropathogenic A04.0
        enterotoxigenic A04.1
        specified NEC A04.4
      specified
        bacteria NEC A04.8
        virus NEC A08.39
      Staphylococcus A04.8
      virus NEC A08.4
        specified type NEC A08.39
      Yersinia enterocolitica A04.6
    specified organism NEC A08.8
  influenzal — *see* Influenza, with, digestive manifesta-
    tions
  ischemic K55.9
    acute (*see also* Ischemia, intestine, acute) K55.019
    chronic K55.1
  microsporidial A07.8
  mucomembranous, myxomembranous — *see* Syn-
    drome, irritable bowel
  mucous — *see* Syndrome, irritable bowel
  necroticans A05.2
  necrotizing of newborn — *see* Enterocolitis, necrotiz-
    ing, in newborn
  neurogenic — *see* Syndrome, irritable bowel
  newborn necrotizing — *see* Enterocolitis, necrotizing,
    in newborn
  noninfectious K52.9
  norovirus A08.11
  parasitic NEC B82.9
  paratyphoid (fever) — *see* Fever, paratyphoid
  protozoal A07.9
    specified NEC A07.8
  radiation K52.0
  regional (of) K50.90
    with
      complication K50.919
        abscess K50.914
        fistula K50.913
        intestinal obstruction K50.912
        rectal bleeding K50.911
        specified complication NEC K50.918
    colon — *see* Enteritis, regional, large intestine
    duodenum — *see* Enteritis, regional, small intestine
    ileum — *see* Enteritis, regional, small intestine
    jejunum — *see* Enteritis, regional, small intestine
    large bowel — *see* Enteritis, regional, large intes-
      tine
    large intestine (colon) (rectum) K50.10
      with
        complication K50.119
          abscess K50.114
          fistula K50.113
          intestinal obstruction K50.112
          rectal bleeding K50.111
          small intestine (duodenum) (ileum) (je-
            junum) involvement K50.80
            with
              complication K50.819
                abscess K50.814
                fistula K50.813
                intestinal obstruction K50.812
                rectal bleeding K50.811
                specified complication NEC
                  K50.818
        specified complication NEC K50.118
    rectum — *see* Enteritis, regional, large intestine
    small intestine (duodenum) (ileum) (jejunum)
      K50.00
      with
        complication K50.019
          abscess K50.014
          fistula K50.013
          intestinal obstruction K50.012
          large intestine (colon) (rectum) involve-
            ment K50.80

Enteritis — *continued*
  regional — *continued*
    small intestine — *continued*
      with — *continued*
        complication — *continued*
          large intestine involvement — *contin-*
            ued
            with
              complication K50.819
                abscess K50.814
                fistula K50.813
                intestinal obstruction K50.812
                rectal bleeding K50.811
                specified complication NEC
                  K50.818
          rectal bleeding K50.011
          specified complication NEC K50.018
    rotaviral A08.0
    Salmonella, salmonellosis (arizonae) (cholerae-suis)
      (enteritidis) (typhimurium) A02.0
    segmental — *see* Enteritis, regional
    septic A09
    Shigella — *see* Infection, Shigella
    small round structured NEC A08.19
    spasmodic, spastic — *see* Syndrome, irritable bowel
    staphylococcal A04.8
      due to food A05.0
    torovirus A08.39
    toxic NEC K52.1
      due to Clostridium difficile
        not specified as recurrent A04.72
        recurrent A04.71
    trichomonal A07.8
    tuberculous A18.32
    typhosa A01.00
    ulcerative (chronic) — *see* Colitis, ulcerative
    viral A08.4
      adenovirus A08.2
      enterovirus A08.39
      Rotavirus A08.0
      small round structured NEC A08.19
      specified NEC A08.39
      virus specified NEC A08.39
Enterobiasis B80
Enterobius vermicularis (infection) (infestation) B80
Enterocele (*see also* Hernia, abdomen)
  pelvic, pelvis (acquired) (congenital) N81.5
  vagina, vaginal (acquired) (congenital) NEC N81.5
Enterocolitis (*see also* Enteritis) K52.9
  due to Clostridium difficile
    not specified as recurrent A04.72
    recurrent A04.71
  fulminant ischemic (*see also* Ischemia, intestine, acute)
    K55.059
  granulomatous — *see* Enteritis, regional
  hemorrhagic (acute) (*see also* Ischemia, intestine,
    acute) K55.059
    chronic K55.1
  infectious NEC A09
  ischemic K55.9
  necrotizing K55.30
    with
      perforation K55.33
      pneumatosis K55.32
        and perforation K55.33
    without pneumatosis or perforation K55.31
    due to Clostridium difficile
      not specified as recurrent A04.72
      recurrent A04.71
    in newborn P77.9
      stage 1 (without pneumatosis, without perfora-
        tion) P77.1
      stage 2 (with pneumatosis, without perforation)
        P77.2
      stage 3 (with pneumatosis, with perforation)
        P77.3
    in non-newborn K55.30
      stage 1 (without pneumatosis, without perfora-
        tion) K55.31
      stage 2 (with pneumatosis, without perforation)
        K55.32
      stage 3 (with pneumatosis, with perforation)
        K55.33
  noninfectious K52.9
    newborn — *see* Enterocolitis, necrotizing, in new-
      born
  pseudomembranous (newborn)
    not specified as recurrent A04.72

Enterocolitis — continued
  pseudomembranous — continued
    recurrent A04.71
  radiation K52.0
    newborn — see Enterocolitis, necrotizing, in newborn
  ulcerative (chronic) — see Pancolitis, ulcerative (chronic)
Enterogastritis — see Enteritis
Enteropathy K63.9
  celiac-gluten-sensitive K90.0
    non-celiac K90.41
  food protein-induced enterocolitis K52.22
  hemorrhagic, terminal (see also Ischemia, intestine, acute) K55.059
  protein-losing K90.49
Enteroperitonitis — see Peritonitis
Enteroptosis K63.4
Enterorrhagia K92.2
Enterospasm (see also Syndrome, irritable, bowel)
  psychogenic F45.8
Enterostenosis (see also Obstruction, intestine, specified NEC) K56.699
Enterostomy
  complication — see Complication, enterostomy
  status Z93.4
Enterovirus, as cause of disease classified elsewhere B97.10
  coxsackievirus B97.11
  echovirus B97.12
  other specified B97.19
Enthesopathy (peripheral) M77.9
  Achilles tendinitis — see Tendinitis, Achilles
  ankle and tarsus M77.9
    specified type NEC — see Enthesopathy, foot, specified type NEC
  anterior tibial syndrome M76.81- ☑
  calcaneal spur — see Spur, bone, calcaneal
  elbow region M77.8
    lateral epicondylitis — see Epicondylitis, lateral
    medial epicondylitis — see Epicondylitis, medial
  foot NEC M77.9
    metatarsalgia — see Metatarsalgia
    specified type NEC M77.5- ☑
  forearm M77.9
  gluteal tendinitis — see Tendinitis, gluteal
  hand M77.9
  hip — see Enthesopathy, lower limb, specified type NEC
  iliac crest spur — see Spur, bone, iliac crest
  iliotibial band syndrome — see Syndrome, iliotibial band
  knee — see Enthesopathy, lower limb, lower leg, specified type NEC
  lateral epicondylitis — see Epicondylitis, lateral
  lower limb (excluding foot) M76.9
    Achilles tendinitis — see Tendinitis, Achilles
    anterior tibial syndrome M76.81- ☑
    gluteal tendinitis — see Tendinitis, gluteal
    iliac crest spur — see Spur, bone, iliac crest
    iliotibial band syndrome — see Syndrome, iliotibial band
    patellar tendinitis — see Tendinitis, patellar
    pelvic region — see Enthesopathy, lower limb, specified type NEC
    peroneal tendinitis — see Tendinitis, peroneal
    posterior tibial syndrome M76.82- ☑
    psoas tendinitis — see Tendinitis, psoas
    shoulder M77.9
    specified type NEC M76.89- ☑
    tibial collateral bursitis — see Bursitis, tibial collateral
  medial epicondylitis — see Epicondylitis, medial
  metatarsalgia — see Metatarsalgia
  multiple sites M77.9
  patellar tendinitis — see Tendinitis, patellar
  pelvis M77.9
  periarthritis of wrist — see Periarthritis, wrist
  peroneal tendinitis — see Tendinitis, peroneal
  posterior tibial syndrome M76.82- ☑
  psoas tendinitis — see Tendinitis, psoas
  shoulder region — see Lesion, shoulder
  specified site NEC M77.9
  specified type NEC M77.8
  spinal M46.00
    cervical region M46.02
      cervicothoracic region M46.03

Enthesopathy — continued
  spinal — continued
    lumbar region M46.06
    lumbosacral region M46.07
    multiple sites M46.09
    occipito-atlanto-axial region M46.01
    sacrococcygeal region M46.08
    thoracic region M46.04
    thoracolumbar region M46.05
  tibial collateral bursitis — see Bursitis, tibial collateral
  upper arm M77.9
  wrist and carpus NEC M77.8
    calcaneal spur — see Spur, bone, calcaneal
    periarthritis of wrist — see Periarthritis, wrist
Entomophobia F40.218
Entomophthoromycosis B46.8
Entrance, air into vein — see Embolism, air
Entrapment, nerve — see Neuropathy, entrapment
Entropion (eyelid) (paralytic) H02.009
  cicatricial H02.019
    left H02.016
      lower H02.015
      upper H02.014
    right H02.013
      lower H02.012
      upper H02.011
  congenital Q10.2
  left H02.006
    lower H02.005
    upper H02.004
  mechanical H02.029
    left H02.026
      lower H02.025
      upper H02.024
    right H02.023
      lower H02.022
      upper H02.021
  right H02.003
    lower H02.002
    upper H02.001
  senile H02.039
    left H02.036
      lower H02.035
      upper H02.034
    right H02.033
      lower H02.032
      upper H02.031
  spastic H02.049
    left H02.046
      lower H02.045
      upper H02.044
    right H02.043
      lower H02.042
      upper H02.041
Enucleated eye (traumatic, current) S05.7- ☑
Enuresis R32
  functional F98.0
  habit disturbance F98.0
  nocturnal N39.44
    psychogenic F98.0
  nonorganic origin F98.0
  psychogenic F98.0
Eosinopenia — see Agranulocytosis
Eosinophilia (allergic) (hereditary) (idiopathic) (secondary) D72.1
  with
    angiolymphoid hyperplasia (ALHE) D18.01
  infiltrative J82
  Löffler's J82
  peritoneal — see Peritonitis, eosinophilic
  pulmonary NEC J82
  tropical (pulmonary) J82
Eosinophilia-myalgia syndrome M35.8
Ependymitis (acute) (cerebral) (chronic) (granular) — see Encephalomyelitis
Ependymoblastoma
  specified site — see Neoplasm, malignant, by site
  unspecified site C71.9
Ependymoma (epithelial) (malignant)
  anaplastic
    specified site — see Neoplasm, malignant, by site
    unspecified site C71.9
  benign
    specified site — see Neoplasm, benign, by site
    unspecified site D33.2
  myxopapillary D43.2
    specified site — see Neoplasm, uncertain behavior, by site

Ependymoma — continued
  myxopapillary — continued
    unspecified site D43.2
  papillary D43.2
    specified site — see Neoplasm, uncertain behavior, by site
    unspecified site D43.2
  specified site — see Neoplasm, malignant, by site
  unspecified site C71.9
Ependymopathy G93.89
Ephelis, ephelides L81.2
Epiblepharon (congenital) Q10.3
Epicanthus, epicanthic fold (eyelid) (congenital) Q10.3
Epicondylitis (elbow)
  lateral M77.1- ☑
  medial M77.0- ☑
Epicystitis — see Cystitis
Epidemic — see condition
Epidermidalization, cervix — see Dysplasia, cervix
Epidermis, epidermal — see condition
Epidermodysplasia verruciformis B07.8
Epidermolysis
  bullosa (congenital) Q81.9
    acquired L12.30
      drug-induced L12.31
      specified cause NEC L12.35
    dystrophica Q81.2
    letalis Q81.1
    simplex Q81.0
    specified NEC Q81.8
  necroticans combustiformis L51.2
    due to drug — see Table of Drugs and Chemicals, by drug
Epidermophytid — see Dermatophytosis
Epidermophytosis (infected) — see Dermatophytosis
Epididymis — see condition
Epididymitis (acute) (nonvenereal) (recurrent) (residual) N45.1
  with orchitis N45.3
  blennorrhagic (gonococcal) A54.23
  caseous (tuberculous) A18.15
  chlamydial A56.19
  filarial (see also Infestation, filarial) B74.9 [N51]
  gonococcal A54.23
  syphilitic A52.76
  tuberculous A18.15
Epididymo-orchitis (see also Epididymitis) N45.3
Epidural — see condition
Epigastrium, epigastric — see condition
Epigastrocele — see Hernia, ventral
Epiglottis — see condition
Epiglottitis, epiglottiditis (acute) J05.10
  with obstruction J05.11
  chronic J37.0
Epignathus Q89.4
Epilepsia partialis continua (see also Kozhevnikof's epilepsy) G40.1- ☑
Epilepsy, epileptic, epilepsia (attack) (cerebral) (convulsion) (fit) (seizure) G40.909

> Note: the following terms are to be considered equivalent to intractable: pharmacoresistant (pharmacologically resistant), treatment resistant, refractory (medically) and poorly controlled

  with
    complex partial seizures — see Epilepsy, localization-related, symptomatic, with complex partial seizures
    grand mal seizures on awakening — see Epilepsy, generalized, specified NEC
    myoclonic absences — see Epilepsy, generalized, specified NEC
    myoclonic-astatic seizures — see Epilepsy, generalized, specified NEC
    simple partial seizures — see Epilepsy, localization-related, symptomatic, with simple partial seizures
  akinetic — see Epilepsy, generalized, specified NEC
  benign childhood with centrotemporal EEG spikes — see Epilepsy, localization-related, idiopathic
  benign myoclonic in infancy G40.80- ☑
  Bravais-jacksonian — see Epilepsy, localization-related, symptomatic, with simple partial seizures
  childhood
    with occipital EEG paroxysms — see Epilepsy, localization-related, idiopathic
    absence G40.A09 (following G40.3)

☑ **Additional Character Required** — Refer to the Tabular List for Character Selection   ▽ **Subterms under main terms may continue to next column or page**

Epilepsy, epileptic, epilepsia — *continued*
  childhood — *continued*
    absence — *continued*
      intractable G40.A19 (*following* G40.3)
        with status epilepticus G40.A11 (*following* G40.3)
        without status epilepticus G40.A19 (*following* G40.3)
      not intractable G40.A09 (*following* G40.3)
        with status epilepticus G40.A01 (*following* G40.3)
        without status epilepticus G40.A09 (*following* G40.3)
  climacteric — *see* Epilepsy, specified NEC
  cysticercosis B69.0
  deterioration (mental) F06.8
  due to syphilis A52.19
  focal — *see* Epilepsy, localization-related, symptomatic, with simple partial seizures
  generalized
    idiopathic G40.309
      intractable G40.319
        with status epilepticus G40.311
        without status epilepticus G40.319
      not intractable G40.309
        with status epilepticus G40.301
        without status epilepticus G40.309
    specified NEC G40.409
      intractable G40.419
        with status epilepticus G40.411
        without status epilepticus G40.419
      not intractable G40.409
        with status epilepticus G40.401
        without status epilepticus G40.409
  impulsive petit mal — *see* Epilepsy, juvenile myoclonic
  intractable G40.919
    with status epilepticus G40.911
    without status epilepticus G40.919
  juvenile absence G40.A09 (*following* G40.3)
    intractable G40.A19 (*following* G40.3)
      with status epilepticus G40.A11 (*following* G40.3)
      without status epilepticus G40.A19 (*following* G40.3)
    not intractable G40.A09 (*following* G40.3)
      with status epilepticus G40.A01 (*following* G40.3)
      without status epilepticus G40.A09 (*following* G40.3)
  juvenile myoclonic G40.B09 (*following* G40.3)
    intractable G40.B19 (*following* G40.3)
      with status epilepticus G40.B11 (*following* G40.3)
      without status epilepticus G40.B19 (*following* G40.3)
    not intractable G40.B09 (*following* G40.3)
      with status epilepticus G40.B01 (*following* G40.3)
      without status epilepticus G40.B09 (*following* G40.3)
  localization-related (focal) (partial)
    idiopathic G40.009
      with seizures of localized onset G40.009
        intractable G40.019
          with status epilepticus G40.011
          without status epilepticus G40.019
        not intractable G40.009
          with status epilepticus G40.001
          without status epilepticus G40.009
    symptomatic
      with complex partial seizures G40.209
        intractable G40.219
          with status epilepticus G40.211
          without status epilepticus G40.219
        not intractable G40.209
          with status epilepticus G40.201
          without status epilepticus G40.209
      with simple partial seizures G40.109
        intractable G40.119
          with status epilepticus G40.111
          without status epilepticus G40.119
        not intractable G40.109
          with status epilepticus G40.101
          without status epilepticus G40.109
  myoclonus, myoclonic — *see* Epilepsy, generalized, specified NEC
    progressive — *see* Epilepsy, generalized, idiopathic
  not intractable G40.909
    with status epilepticus G40.901

Epilepsy, epileptic, epilepsia — *continued*
  not intractable — *continued*
    without status epilepticus G40.909
  on awakening — *see* Epilepsy, generalized, specified NEC
  parasitic NOS B71.9 [G94]
  partialis continua (*see also* Kozhevnikof's epilepsy) G40.1- ☑
  peripheral — *see* Epilepsy, specified NEC
  procursiva — *see* Epilepsy, localization-related, symptomatic, with simple partial seizures
  progressive (familial) myoclonic — *see* Epilepsy, generalized, idiopathic
  reflex — *see* Epilepsy, specified NEC
  related to
    alcohol G40.509
      not intractable G40.509
        with status epilepticus G40.501
        without status epilepticus G40.509
    drugs G40.509
      not intractable G40.509
        with status epilepticus G40.501
        without status epilepticus G40.509
    external causes G40.509
      not intractable G40.509
        with status epilepticus G40.501
        without status epilepticus G40.509
    hormonal changes G40.509
      not intractable G40.509
        with status epilepticus G40.501
        without status epilepticus G40.509
    sleep deprivation G40.509
      not intractable G40.509
        with status epilepticus G40.501
        without status epilepticus G40.509
    stress G40.509
      not intractable G40.509
        with status epilepticus G40.501
        without status epilepticus G40.509
  somatomotor — *see* Epilepsy, localization-related, symptomatic, with simple partial seizures
  somatosensory — *see* Epilepsy, localization-related, symptomatic, with simple partial seizures
  spasms G40.822
    intractable G40.824
      with status epilepticus G40.823
      without status epilepticus G40.824
    not intractable G40.822
      with status epilepticus G40.821
      without status epilepticus G40.822
  specified NEC G40.802
    intractable G40.804
      with status epilepticus G40.803
      without status epilepticus G40.804
    not intractable G40.802
      with status epilepticus G40.801
      without status epilepticus G40.802
  syndromes
    generalized
      idiopathic G40.309
        intractable G40.319
          with status epilepticus G40.311
          without status epilepticus G40.319
        not intractable G40.309
          with status epilepticus G40.301
          without status epilepticus G40.309
      specified NEC G40.409
        intractable G40.419
          with status epilepticus G40.411
          without status epilepticus G40.419
        not intractable G40.409
          with status epilepticus G40.401
          without status epilepticus G40.409
    localization-related (focal) (partial)
      idiopathic G40.009
        with seizures of localized onset G40.009
          intractable G40.019
            with status epilepticus G40.011
            without status epilepticus G40.019
          not intractable G40.009
            with status epilepticus G40.001
            without status epilepticus G40.009
      symptomatic
        with complex partial seizures G40.209
          intractable G40.219
            with status epilepticus G40.211
            without status epilepticus G40.219
          not intractable G40.209

Epilepsy, epileptic, epilepsia — *continued*
  syndromes — *continued*
    localization-related — *continued*
      symptomatic — *continued*
        with complex partial seizures — *continued*
          not intractable — *continued*
            with status epilepticus G40.201
            without status epilepticus G40.209
        with simple partial seizures G40.109
          intractable G40.119
            with status epilepticus G40.111
            without status epilepticus G40.119
          not intractable G40.109
            with status epilepticus G40.101
            without status epilepticus G40.109
      specified NEC G40.802
        intractable G40.804
          with status epilepticus G40.803
          without status epilepticus G40.804
        not intractable G40.802
          with status epilepticus G40.801
          without status epilepticus G40.802
  tonic (-clonic) — *see* Epilepsy, generalized, specified NEC
  twilight F05
  uncinate (gyrus) — *see* Epilepsy, localization-related, symptomatic, with complex partial seizures
  Unverricht (-Lundborg) (familial myoclonic) — *see* Epilepsy, generalized, idiopathic
  visceral — *see* Epilepsy, specified NEC
  visual — *see* Epilepsy, specified NEC
Epiloia Q85.1
Epimenorrhea N92.0
Epipharyngitis — *see* Nasopharyngitis
Epiphora H04.20- ☑
  due to
    excess lacrimation H04.21- ☑
    insufficient drainage H04.22- ☑
Epiphyseal arrest — *see* Arrest, epiphyseal
Epiphyseolysis, epiphysiolysis — *see* Osteochondropathy
Epiphysitis (*see also* Osteochondropathy)
  juvenile M92.9
  syphilitic (congenital) A50.02
Epiplocele — *see* Hernia, abdomen
Epiploitis — *see* Peritonitis
Epiplosarcomphalocele — *see* Hernia, umbilicus
Episcleritis (suppurative) H15.10- ☑
  in (due to)
    syphilis A52.71
    tuberculosis A18.51
  nodular H15.12- ☑
  periodica fugax H15.11- ☑
    angioneurotic — *see* Edema, angioneurotic
  syphilitic (late) A52.71
  tuberculous A18.51
Episode
  affective, mixed F39
  depersonalization (in neurotic state) F48.1
  depressive F32.9
    major F32.9
      mild F32.0
      moderate F32.1
      severe (without psychotic symptoms) F32.2
        with psychotic symptoms F32.3
    recurrent F33.9
      brief F33.8
    specified NEC F32.89
  hypomanic F30.8
  manic F30.9
    with
      psychotic symptoms F30.2
      remission (full) F30.4
        partial F30.3
    without psychotic symptoms F30.10
      mild F30.11
      moderate F30.12
      severe (without psychotic symptoms) F30.13
        with psychotic symptoms F30.2
    other specified F30.8
    recurrent F31.89
  psychotic F23
    organic F06.8
  schizophrenic (acute) NEC, brief F23
Epispadias (female) (male) Q64.0
Episplenitis D73.89
Epistaxis (multiple) R04.0

Epistaxis — continued
  hereditary I78.0
  vicarious menstruation N94.89
Epithelioma (malignant) (see also Neoplasm, malignant, by site)
  adenoides cysticum — see Neoplasm, skin, benign
  basal cell — see Neoplasm, skin, malignant
  benign — see Neoplasm, benign, by site
  Bowen's — see Neoplasm, skin, in situ
  calcifying, of Malherbe — see Neoplasm, skin, benign
  external site — see Neoplasm, skin, malignant
  intraepidermal, Jadassohn — see Neoplasm, skin, benign
  squamous cell — see Neoplasm, malignant, by site
Epitheliomatosis pigmented Q82.1
Epitheliopathy, multifocal placoid pigment H30.14- ☑
Epithelium, epithelial — see condition
Epituberculosis (with atelectasis) (allergic) A15.7
Eponychia Q84.6
Epstein's
  nephrosis or syndrome — see Nephrosis
  pearl K09.8
Epulis (gingiva) (fibrous) (giant cell) K06.8
Equinia A24.0
Equinovarus (congenital) (talipes) Q66.0
  acquired — see Deformity, limb, clubfoot
Equivalent
  convulsive (abdominal) — see Epilepsy, specified NEC
  epileptic (psychic) — see Epilepsy, localization-related, symptomatic, with complex partial seizures
Erb (-Duchenne) **paralysis** (birth injury) (newborn) P14.0
Erb-Goldflam disease or syndrome G70.00
  with exacerbation (acute) G70.01
  in crisis G70.01
Erb's
  disease G71.0
  palsy, paralysis (brachial) (birth) (newborn) P14.0
    spinal (spastic) syphilitic A52.17
  pseudohypertrophic muscular dystrophy G71.0
Erdheim's syndrome (acromegalic macrospondylitis) E22.0
Erection, painful (persistent) — see Priapism
Ergosterol deficiency (vitamin D) E55.9
  with
    adult osteomalacia M83.8
    rickets — see Rickets
Ergotism (see also Poisoning, food, noxious, plant)
  from ergot used as drug (migraine therapy) — see Table of Drugs and Chemicals
Erosio interdigitalis blastomycetica B37.2
Erosion
  artery I77.2
    without rupture I77.89
  bone — see Disorder, bone, density and structure, specified NEC
  bronchus J98.09
  cartilage (joint) — see Disorder, cartilage, specified type NEC
  cervix (uteri) (acquired) (chronic) (congenital) N86
    with cervicitis N72
  cornea (nontraumatic) — see Ulcer, cornea
    recurrent H18.83- ☑
    traumatic — see Abrasion, cornea
  dental (idiopathic) (occupational) (due to diet, drugs or vomiting) K03.2
  duodenum, postpyloric — see Ulcer, duodenum
  esophagus K22.10
    with bleeding K22.11
  gastric — see Ulcer, stomach
  gastrojejunal — see Ulcer, gastrojejunal
  implanted mesh — see Complications, mesh
  intestine K63.3
  lymphatic vessel I89.8
  pylorus, pyloric (ulcer) — see Ulcer, stomach
  spine, aneurysmal A52.09
  stomach — see Ulcer, stomach
  subcutaneous device pocket
    nervous system prosthetic device, implant, or graft T85.890 ☑
    other internal prosthetic device, implant, or graft T85.898 ☑
  teeth (idiopathic) (occupational) (due to diet, drugs or vomiting) K03.2
  urethra N36.8
  uterus N85.8
Erotomania F52.8

Error
  metabolism, inborn — see Disorder, metabolism
  refractive — see Disorder, refraction
Eructation R14.2
  nervous or psychogenic F45.8
Eruption
  creeping B76.9
  drug (generalized) (taken internally) L27.0
    fixed L27.1
    in contact with skin — see Dermatitis, due to drugs
    localized L27.1
  Hutchinson, summer L56.4
  Kaposi's varicelliform B00.0
  napkin L22
  polymorphous light (sun) L56.4
  recalcitrant pustular L13.8
  ringed R23.8
  skin (nonspecific) R21
    creeping (meaning hookworm) B76.9
    due to inoculation/vaccination (generalized) (see also Dermatitis, due to, vaccine) L27.0
      localized L27.1
    erysipeloid A26.0
    feigned L98.1
    Kaposi's varicelliform B00.0
    lichenoid L28.0
    meaning dermatitis — see Dermatitis
    toxic NEC L53.0
  tooth, teeth, abnormal (incomplete) (late) (premature) (sequence) K00.6
  vesicular R23.8
Erysipelas (gangrenous) (infantile) (newborn) (phlegmonous) (suppurative) A46
  external ear A46 [H62.40]
  puerperal, postpartum O86.89
Erysipeloid A26.9
  cutaneous (Rosenbach's) A26.0
  disseminated A26.8
  sepsis A26.7
  specified NEC A26.8
Erythema, erythematous (infectional) (inflammation) L53.9
  ab igne L59.0
  annulare (centrifugum) (rheumaticum) L53.1
  arthriticum epidemicum A25.1
  brucellum — see Brucellosis
  chronic figurate NEC L53.3
  chronicum migrans (Borrelia burgdorferi) A69.20
  diaper L22
  due to
    chemical NEC L53.0
      in contact with skin L24.5
    drug (internal use) — see Dermatitis, due to, drugs
  elevatum diutinum L95.1
  endemic E52
  epidemic, arthritic A25.1
  figuratum perstans L53.3
  gluteal L22
  heat — code by site under Burn, first degree
  ichthyosiforme congenitum bullous Q80.3
  in diseases classified elsewhere L54
  induratum (nontuberculous) L52
    tuberculous A18.4
  infectiosum B08.3
  intertrigo L30.4
  iris L51.9
  marginatum L53.2
    in (due to) acute rheumatic fever I00
  medicamentosum — see Dermatitis, due to, drugs
  migrans A26.0
    chronicum A69.20
    tongue K14.1
  multiforme (major) (minor) L51.9
    bullous, bullosum L51.1
    conjunctiva L51.1
    nonbullous L51.0
    pemphigoides L12.0
    specified NEC L51.8
  napkin L22
  neonatorum P83.88
    toxic P83.1
  nodosum L52
    tuberculous A18.4
  palmar L53.8
  pernio T69.1 ☑
  rash, newborn P83.88
  scarlatiniform (recurrent) (exfoliative) L53.8
  solare L55.0

Erythema, erythematous — continued
  specified NEC L53.8
  toxic, toxicum NEC L53.0
    newborn P83.1
  tuberculous (primary) A18.4
Erythematous, erythematosus — see condition
Erythermalgia (primary) I73.81
Erythralgia I73.81
Erythrasma L08.1
Erythredema (polyneuropathy) — see Poisoning, mercury
Erythremia (acute) C94.0- ☑
  chronic D45
  secondary D75.1
Erythroblastopenia (see also Aplasia, red cell) D60.9
  congenital D61.01
Erythroblastophthisis D61.09
Erythroblastosis (fetalis) (newborn) P55.9
  due to
    ABO (antibodies) (incompatibility) (isoimmunization) P55.1
    Rh (antibodies) (incompatibility) (isoimmunization) P55.0
Erythrocyanosis (crurum) I73.89
Erythrocythemia — see Erythremia
Erythrocytosis (megalosplenic) (secondary) D75.1
  familial D75.0
  oval, hereditary — see Elliptocytosis
  secondary D75.1
  stress D75.1
Erythroderma (secondary) (see also Erythema) L53.9
  bullous ichthyosiform, congenital Q80.3
  desquamativum L21.1
  ichthyosiform, congenital (bullous) Q80.3
  neonatorum P83.88
  psoriaticum L40.8
Erythrodysesthesia, palmar plantar (PPE) L27.1
Erythrogenesis imperfecta D61.09
Erythroleukemia C94.0- ☑
Erythromelalgia I73.81
Erythrophagocytosis D75.89
Erythrophobia F40.298
Erythroplakia, oral epithelium, and tongue K13.29
Erythroplasia (Queyrat) D07.4
  specified site — see Neoplasm, skin, in situ
  unspecified site D07.4
Escherichia coli (E. coli), **as cause of disease classified elsewhere** B96.20
  non-O157 Shiga toxin-producing (with known O group) B96.22
  non-Shiga toxin-producing B96.29
  O157 B96.21
  O157 with confirmation of Shiga toxin when H antigen is unknown, or is not H7 B96.21
  O157:H- (nonmotile) with confirmation of Shiga toxin B96.21
  O157:H7 with or without confirmation of Shiga toxin-production B96.21
  Shiga toxin-producing (with unspecified O group) (STEC) B96.23
  specified NEC B96.29
Esophagismus K22.4
Esophagitis (acute) (alkaline) (chemical) (chronic) (infectional) (necrotic) (peptic) (postoperative) K20.9
  candidal B37.81
  due to gastrointestinal reflux disease K21.0
  eosinophilic K20.0
  reflux K21.0
  specified NEC K20.8
  tuberculous A18.83
  ulcerative K22.10
    with bleeding K22.11
Esophagocele K22.5
Esophagomalacia K22.8
Esophagospasm K22.4
Esophagostenosis K22.2
Esophagostomiasis B81.8
Esophagotracheal — see condition
Esophagus — see condition
Esophoria H50.51
  convergence, excess H51.12
  divergence, insufficiency H51.8
Esotropia — see Strabismus, convergent concomitant
Espundia B55.2
Essential — see condition
Esthesioneuroblastoma C30.0
Esthesioneurocytoma C30.0

Esthesioneuroepithelioma C30.0
Esthiomene A55
Estivo-autumnal malaria (fever) B50.9
Estrangement (marital) Z63.5
　parent-child NEC Z62.890
Estriasis — *see* Myiasis
Ethanolism — *see* Alcoholism
Etherism — *see* Dependence, drug, inhalant
Ethmoid, ethmoidal — *see* condition
Ethmoiditis (chronic) (nonpurulent) (purulent) (*see also*
　Sinusitis, ethmoidal)
　influenzal — *see* Influenza, with, respiratory manifes-
　　tations NEC
　Woakes' J33.1
Ethylism — *see* Alcoholism
Eulenburg's disease (congenital paramyotonia) G71.19
Eumycetoma B47.0
Eunuchoidism E29.1
　hypogonadotropic E23.0
European blastomycosis — *see* Cryptococcosis
Eustachian — *see* condition
Evaluation (for) (of)
　development state
　　adolescent Z00.3
　　period of
　　　delayed growth in childhood Z00.70
　　　　with abnormal findings Z00.71
　　　rapid growth in childhood Z00.2
　　　puberty Z00.3
　growth and developmental state (period of rapid
　　growth) Z00.2
　　delayed growth Z00.70
　　　with abnormal findings Z00.71
　mental health (status) Z00.8
　　requested by authority Z04.6
　period of
　　delayed growth in childhood Z00.70
　　　with abnormal findings Z00.71
　　rapid growth in childhood Z00.2
　suspected condition — *see* Observation
Evans syndrome D69.41
Event
　apparent life threatening in newborn and infant (ALTE)
　　R68.13
　brief resolved unexplained event (BRUE) R68.13
Eventration (*see also* Hernia, ventral)
　colon into chest — *see* Hernia, diaphragm
　diaphragm (congenital) Q79.1
Eversion
　bladder N32.89
　cervix (uteri) N86
　　with cervicitis N72
　foot NEC (*see also* Deformity, valgus, ankle)
　　congenital Q66.6
　punctum lacrimale (postinfectional) (senile) H04.52- ☑
　ureter (meatus) N28.89
　urethra (meatus) N36.8
　uterus N81.4
Evidence
　cytologic
　　of malignancy on anal smear R85.614
　　of malignancy on cervical smear R87.614
　　of malignancy on vaginal smear R87.624
Evisceration
　birth injury P15.8
　traumatic NEC
　　eye — *see* Enucleated eye
Evulsion — *see* Avulsion
Ewing's sarcoma or tumor — *see* Neoplasm, bone,
　malignant
Examination (for) (following) (general) (of) (routine)
　Z00.00
　with abnormal findings Z00.01
　abuse, physical (alleged), ruled out
　　adult Z04.71
　　child Z04.72
　adolescent (development state) Z00.3
　alleged rape or sexual assault (victim), ruled out
　　adult Z04.41
　　child Z04.42
　allergy Z01.82
　annual (adult) (periodic) (physical) Z00.00
　　with abnormal findings Z00.01
　　gynecological Z01.419
　　　with abnormal findings Z01.411
　antibody response Z01.84
　blood — *see* Examination, laboratory
　blood pressure Z01.30

Examination — *continued*
　blood pressure — *continued*
　　with abnormal findings Z01.31
　cancer staging — *see* Neoplasm, malignant, by site
　cervical Papanicolaou smear Z12.4
　　as part of routine gynecological examination
　　　Z01.419
　　with abnormal findings Z01.411
　child (over 28 days old) Z00.129
　　with abnormal findings Z00.121
　　under 28 days old — *see* Newborn, examination
　clinical research control or normal comparison (con-
　　trol) (participant) Z00.6
　contraceptive (drug) maintenance (routine) Z30.8
　　device (intrauterine) Z30.431
　dental Z01.20
　　with abnormal findings Z01.21
　developmental — *see* Examination, child
　donor (potential) Z00.5
　ear Z01.10
　　with abnormal findings NEC Z01.118
　eye Z01.00
　　with abnormal findings Z01.01
　following
　　accident NEC Z04.3
　　　transport Z04.1
　　　work Z04.2
　　assault, alleged, ruled out
　　　adult Z04.71
　　　child Z04.72
　　motor vehicle accident Z04.1
　　treatment (for) Z09
　　　combined NEC Z09
　　　　fracture Z09
　　　　malignant neoplasm Z08
　　　malignant neoplasm Z08
　　　mental disorder Z09
　　　specified condition NEC Z09
　follow-up (routine) (following) Z09
　　chemotherapy NEC Z09
　　　malignant neoplasm Z08
　　fracture Z09
　　malignant neoplasm Z08
　　postpartum Z39.2
　　psychotherapy Z09
　　radiotherapy NEC Z09
　　　malignant neoplasm Z08
　　surgery NEC Z09
　　　malignant neoplasm Z08
　gynecological Z01.419
　　with abnormal findings Z01.411
　　for contraceptive maintenance Z30.8
　health — *see* Examination, medical
　hearing Z01.10
　　with abnormal findings NEC Z01.118
　　following failed hearing screening Z01.110
　immunity status testing Z01.84
　laboratory (as part of a general medical examination)
　　Z00.00
　　with abnormal findings Z00.01
　　preprocedural Z01.812
　lactating mother Z39.1
　medical (adult) (for) (of) Z00.00
　　with abnormal findings Z00.01
　　administrative purpose only Z02.9
　　　specified NEC Z02.89
　　admission to
　　　armed forces Z02.3
　　　old age home Z02.2
　　　prison Z02.89
　　　residential institution Z02.2
　　　school Z02.0
　　　　following illness or medical treatment Z02.0
　　　summer camp Z02.89
　　adoption Z02.82
　　blood alcohol or drug level Z02.83
　　camp (summer) Z02.89
　　clinical research, normal subject (control) (partici-
　　　pant) Z00.6
　　control subject in clinical research (normal compar-
　　　ison) (participant) Z00.6
　　donor (potential) Z00.5
　　driving license Z02.4
　　general (adult) Z00.00
　　　with abnormal findings Z00.01
　　immigration Z02.89
　　insurance purposes Z02.6
　　marriage Z02.89
　　medicolegal reasons NEC Z04.8

Examination — *continued*
　medical — *continued*
　　naturalization Z02.89
　　participation in sport Z02.5
　　paternity testing Z02.81
　　population survey Z00.8
　　pre-employment Z02.1
　　pre-operative — *see* Examination, pre-procedural
　　pre-procedural
　　　cardiovascular Z01.810
　　　respiratory Z01.811
　　　specified NEC Z01.818
　　preschool children
　　　for admission to school Z02.0
　　prisoners
　　　for entrance into prison Z02.89
　　recruitment for armed forces Z02.3
　　specified NEC Z00.8
　　sport competition Z02.5
　medicolegal reason NEC Z04.8
　newborn — *see* Newborn, examination
　pelvic (annual) (periodic) Z01.419
　　with abnormal findings Z01.411
　period of rapid growth in childhood Z00.2
　periodic (adult) (annual) (routine) Z00.00
　　with abnormal findings Z00.01
　physical (adult) (*see also* Examination, medical) Z00.00
　　sports Z02.5
　postpartum
　　immediately after delivery Z39.0
　　routine follow-up Z39.2
　pre-chemotherapy (antineoplastic) Z01.818
　prenatal (normal pregnancy) (*see also* Pregnancy,
　　normal) Z34.9- ☑
　pre-procedural (pre-operative)
　　cardiovascular Z01.810
　　laboratory Z01.812
　　respiratory Z01.811
　　specified NEC Z01.818
　prior to chemotherapy (antineoplastic) Z01.818
　psychiatric NEC Z00.8
　　follow-up not needing further care Z09
　　requested by authority Z04.6
　radiological (as part of a general medical examination)
　　Z00.00
　　with abnormal findings Z00.01
　repeat cervical smear to confirm findings of recent
　　normal smear following initial abnormal smear
　　Z01.42
　skin (hypersensitivity) Z01.82
　special (*see also* Examination, by type) Z01.89
　　specified type NEC Z01.89
　specified type or reason NEC Z04.8
　teeth Z01.20
　　with abnormal findings Z01.21
　urine — *see* Examination, laboratory
　vision Z01.00
　　with abnormal findings Z01.01
Exanthem, exanthema (*see also* Rash)
　with enteroviral vesicular stomatitis B08.4
　Boston A88.0
　epidemic with meningitis A88.0 [G02]
　subitum B08.20
　　due to human herpesvirus 6 B08.21
　　due to human herpesvirus 7 B08.22
　viral, virus B09
　　specified type NEC B08.8
Excess, excessive, excessively
　alcohol level in blood R78.0
　androgen (ovarian) E28.1
　attrition, tooth, teeth K03.0
　carotene, carotin (dietary) E67.1
　cold, effects of T69.9 ☑
　　specified effect NEC T69.8 ☑
　convergence H51.12
　crying
　　in child, adolescent, or adult R45.83
　　in infant R68.11
　development, breast N62
　divergence H51.8
　drinking (alcohol) NEC (without dependence) F10.10
　　habitual (continual) (without remission) F10.20
　eating R63.2
　estrogen E28.0
　fat (*see also* Obesity)
　　in heart — *see* Degeneration, myocardial
　　localized E65
　foreskin N47.8

Excess, excessive, excessively — *continued*
  gas R14.0
  glucagon E16.3
  heat — *see* Heat
  intermaxillary vertical dimension of fully erupted teeth M26.37
  interocclusal distance of fully erupted teeth M26.37
  kalium E87.5
  large
    colon K59.39
      congenital Q43.8
    infant P08.0
    organ or site, congenital NEC — *see* Anomaly, by site
  long
    organ or site, congenital NEC — *see* Anomaly, by site
  menstruation (with regular cycle) N92.0
    with irregular cycle N92.1
  napping Z72.821
  natrium E87.0
  number of teeth K00.1
  nutrient (dietary) NEC R63.2
  potassium (K) E87.5
  salivation K11.7
  secretion (*see also* Hypersecretion)
    milk O92.6
    sputum R09.3
    sweat R61
  sexual drive F52.8
  short
    organ or site, congenital NEC — *see* Anomaly, by site
    umbilical cord in labor or delivery O69.3 ☑
  skin L98.7
    and subcutaneous tissue L98.7
    eyelid (acquired) — *see* Blepharochalasis
      congenital Q10.3
  sodium (Na) E87.0
  spacing of fully erupted teeth M26.32
  sputum R09.3
  sweating R61
  thirst R63.1
    due to deprivation of water T73.1 ☑
  tuberosity of jaw M26.07
  vitamin
    A (dietary) E67.0
      administered as drug (prolonged intake) — *see* Table of Drugs and Chemicals, vitamins, adverse effect
      overdose or wrong substance given or taken — *see* Table of Drugs and Chemicals, vitamins, poisoning
    D (dietary) E67.3
      administered as drug (prolonged intake) — *see* Table of Drugs and Chemicals, vitamins, adverse effect
      overdose or wrong substance given or taken — *see* Table of Drugs and Chemicals, vitamins, poisoning
  weight
    gain R63.5
    loss R63.4
Excitability, abnormal, under minor stress (personality disorder) F60.3
Excitation
  anomalous atrioventricular I45.6
  psychogenic F30.8
  reactive (from emotional stress, psychological trauma) F30.8
Excitement
  hypomanic F30.8
  manic F30.9
  mental, reactive (from emotional stress, psychological trauma) F30.8
  state, reactive (from emotional stress, psychological trauma) F30.8
Excoriation (traumatic) (*see also* Abrasion)
  neurotic L98.1
  skin picking disorder F42.4
Exfoliation
  due to erythematous conditions according to extent of body surface involved L49.0
    less than 10 percent of body surface L49.0
    10-19 percent of body surface L49.1
    20-29 percent of body surface L49.2
    30-39 percent of body surface L49.3
    40-49 percent of body surface L49.4

Exfoliation — *continued*
  due to erythematous conditions according to extent of body surface involved — *continued*
    50-59 percent of body surface L49.5
    60-69 percent of body surface L49.6
    70-79 percent of body surface L49.7
    80-89 percent of body surface L49.8
    90-99 percent of body surface L49.9
  teeth, due to systemic causes K08.0
Exfoliative — *see* condition
Exhaustion, exhaustive (physical NEC) R53.83
  battle F43.0
  cardiac — *see* Failure, heart
  delirium F43.0
  due to
    cold T69.8 ☑
    excessive exertion T73.3 ☑
    exposure T73.2 ☑
    neurasthenia F48.8
  heart — *see* Failure, heart
  heat (*see also* Heat, exhaustion) T67.5 ☑
    due to
      salt depletion T67.4 ☑
      water depletion T67.3 ☑
  maternal, complicating delivery O75.81
  mental F48.8
  myocardium, myocardial — *see* Failure, heart
  nervous F48.8
  old age R54
  psychogenic F48.8
  psychosis F43.0
  senile R54
  vital NEC Z73.0
Exhibitionism F65.2
Exocervicitis — *see* Cervicitis
Exomphalos Q79.2
  meaning hernia — *see* Hernia, umbilicus
Exophoria H50.52
  convergence, insufficiency H51.11
  divergence, excess H51.8
Exophthalmos H05.2- ☑
  congenital Q15.8
  constant NEC H05.24- ☑
  displacement, globe — *see* Displacement, globe
  due to thyrotoxicosis (hyperthyroidism) — *see* Hyperthyroidism, with, goiter (diffuse)
  dysthyroid — *see* Hyperthyroidism, with, goiter (diffuse)
  goiter — *see* Hyperthyroidism, with, goiter (diffuse)
  intermittent NEC H05.25- ☑
  malignant — *see* Hyperthyroidism, with, goiter (diffuse)
  orbital
    edema — *see* Edema, orbit
    hemorrhage — *see* Hemorrhage, orbit
  pulsating NEC H05.26- ☑
  thyrotoxic, thyrotropic — *see* Hyperthyroidism, with, goiter (diffuse)
Exostosis (*see also* Disorder, bone)
  cartilaginous — *see* Neoplasm, bone, benign
  congenital (multiple) Q78.6
  external ear canal H61.81- ☑
  gonococcal A54.49
  jaw (bone) M27.8
  multiple, congenital Q78.6
  orbit H05.35- ☑
  osteocartilaginous — *see* Neoplasm, bone, benign
  syphilitic A52.77
Exotropia — *see* Strabismus, divergent concomitant
Explanation of
  investigation finding Z71.2
  medication Z71.89
Exposure (to) (*see also* Contact, with) T75.89 ☑
  acariasis Z20.7
  AIDS virus Z20.6
  air pollution Z77.110
  algae and algae toxins Z77.121
  algae bloom Z77.121
  anthrax Z20.810
  aromatic amines Z77.020
  aromatic (hazardous) compounds NEC Z77.028
  aromatic dyes NOS Z77.028
  arsenic Z77.010
  asbestos Z77.090
  bacterial disease NEC Z20.818
  benzene Z77.021
  blue-green algae bloom Z77.121

Exposure — *continued*
  body fluids (potentially hazardous) Z77.21
  brown tide Z77.121
  chemicals (chiefly nonmedicinal) (hazardous) NEC Z77.098
  cholera Z20.09
  chromium compounds Z77.018
  cold, effects of T69.9 ☑
    specified effect NEC T69.8 ☑
  communicable disease Z20.9
    bacterial NEC Z20.818
    specified NEC Z20.89
    viral NEC Z20.828
  cyanobacteria bloom Z77.121
  disaster Z65.5
  discrimination Z60.5
  dyes Z77.098
  effects of T73.9 ☑
  environmental tobacco smoke (acute) (chronic) Z77.22
  Escherichia coli (E. coli) Z20.01
  exhaustion due to T73.2 ☑
  fiberglass — *see* Table of Drugs and Chemicals, fiberglass
  German measles Z20.4
  gonorrhea Z20.2
  hazardous metals NEC Z77.018
  hazardous substances NEC Z77.29
  hazards in the physical environment NEC Z77.128
  hazards to health NEC Z77.9
  human immunodeficiency virus (HIV) Z20.6
  human T-lymphotropic virus type-1 (HTLV-1) Z20.89
  implanted
    mesh — *see* Complications, mesh
    prosthetic materials NEC — *see* Complications, prosthetic materials NEC
  infestation (parasitic) NEC Z20.7
  intestinal infectious disease NEC Z20.09
    Escherichia coli (E. coli) Z20.01
  lead Z77.011
  meningococcus Z20.811
  mold (toxic) Z77.120
  nickel dust Z77.018
  noise Z77.122
  occupational
    air contaminants NEC Z57.39
    dust Z57.2
    environmental tobacco smoke Z57.31
    extreme temperature Z57.6
    noise Z57.0
    radiation Z57.1
    risk factors Z57.9
      specified NEC Z57.8
    toxic agents (gases) (liquids) (solids) (vapors) in agriculture Z57.4
    toxic agents (gases) (liquids) (solids) (vapors) in industry NEC Z57.5
    vibration Z57.7
  parasitic disease NEC Z20.7
  pediculosis Z20.7
  persecution Z60.5
  pfiesteria piscicida Z77.121
  poliomyelitis Z20.89
  pollution
    air Z77.110
    environmental NEC Z77.118
    soil Z77.112
    water Z77.111
  polycyclic aromatic hydrocarbons Z77.028
  prenatal (drugs) (toxic chemicals) — *see* Newborn, affected by, noxious substances transmitted via placenta or breast milk
  rabies Z20.3
  radiation, naturally occurring NEC Z77.123
  radon Z77.123
  red tide (Florida) Z77.121
  rubella Z20.4
  second hand tobacco smoke (acute) (chronic) Z77.22
    in the perinatal period P96.81
  sexually-transmitted disease Z20.2
  smallpox (laboratory) Z20.89
  syphilis Z20.2
  terrorism Z65.4
  torture Z65.4
  tuberculosis Z20.1
  uranium Z77.012
  varicella Z20.820
  venereal disease Z20.2
  viral disease NEC Z20.828

☑ Additional Character Required — Refer to the Tabular List for Character Selection   ▽ Subterms under main terms may continue to next column or page

Exposure — *continued*
  war Z65.5
  water pollution Z77.111
Exsanguination — *see* Hemorrhage
Exstrophy
  abdominal contents Q45.8
  bladder Q64.10
    cloacal Q64.12
    specified type NEC Q64.19
    supravesical fissure Q64.11
Extensive — *see* condition
Extra (*see also* Accessory)
  marker chromosomes (normal individual) Q92.61
    in abnormal individual Q92.62
  rib Q76.6
    cervical Q76.5
Extrasystoles (supraventricular) I49.49
  atrial I49.1
  auricular I49.1
  junctional I49.2
  ventricular I49.3
Extrauterine gestation or pregnancy — *see* Pregnancy, by site
Extravasation
  blood R58
  chyle into mesentery I89.8
  pelvicalyceal N13.8
  pyelosinus N13.8
  urine (from ureter) R39.0
  vesicant agent
    antineoplastic chemotherapy T80.810 ☑
    other agent NEC T80.818 ☑
Extremity — *see* condition, limb
Extrophy — *see* Exstrophy
Extroversion
  bladder Q64.19
  uterus N81.4
    complicating delivery O71.2
    postpartal (old) N81.4
Extruded tooth (teeth) M26.34
Extrusion
  breast implant (prosthetic) T85.42 ☑
  eye implant (globe) (ball) T85.328 ☑
  intervertebral disc — *see* Displacement, intervertebral disc
  ocular lens implant (prosthetic) — *see* Complications, intraocular lens
  vitreous — *see* Prolapse, vitreous
Exudate
  pleural — *see* Effusion, pleura
  retina H35.89
Exudative — *see* condition
Eye, eyeball, eyelid — *see* condition
Eyestrain — *see* Disturbance, vision, subjective
Eyeworm disease of Africa B74.3

F

Faber's syndrome (achlorhydric anemia) D50.9
Fabry (-Anderson) **disease** E75.21
Faciocephalalgia, autonomic (*see also* Neuropathy, peripheral, autonomic) G90.09
Factor(s)
  psychic, associated with diseases classified elsewhere F54
  psychological
    affecting physical conditions F54
    or behavioral
      affecting general medical condition F54
      associated with disorders or diseases classified elsewhere F54
Fahr disease (of brain) G23.8
Fahr Volhard disease (of kidney) I12.- ☑
Failure, failed
  abortion — *see* Abortion, attempted
  aortic (valve) I35.8
    rheumatic I06.8
  attempted abortion — *see* Abortion, attempted
  biventricular I50.82
    due to left heart failure I50.814
  bone marrow — *see* Anemia, aplastic
  cardiac — *see* Failure, heart
  cardiorenal (chronic) (*see also* Failure, renal, and Failure, heart) I50.9
    hypertensive I13.2
  cardiorespiratory (*see also* Failure, heart) R09.2
  cardiovascular (chronic) — *see* Failure, heart

Failure, failed — *continued*
  cerebrovascular I67.9
  cervical dilatation in labor O62.0
  circulation, circulatory (peripheral) R57.9
    newborn P29.89
  compensation — *see* Disease, heart
  compliance with medical treatment or regimen — *see* Noncompliance
  congestive — *see* Failure, heart, congestive
  dental implant (endosseous) M27.69
    due to
      failure of dental prosthesis M27.63
      lack of attached gingiva M27.62
      occlusal trauma (poor prosthetic design) M27.62
      parafunctional habits M27.62
      periodontal infection (peri-implantitis) M27.62
      poor oral hygiene M27.62
    osseointegration M27.61
      due to
        complications of systemic disease M27.61
        poor bone quality M27.61
      iatrogenic M27.61
    post-osseointegration
      biological M27.62
      due to complications of systemic disease M27.62
      iatrogenic M27.62
      mechanical M27.63
    pre-integration M27.61
    pre-osseointegration M27.61
    specified NEC M27.69
  descent of head (at term) of pregnancy (mother) O32.4 ☑
  endosseous dental implant — *see* Failure, dental implant
  engagement of head (term of pregnancy) (mother) O32.4 ☑
  erection (penile) (*see also* Dysfunction, sexual, male, erectile) N52.9
    nonorganic F52.21
  examination(s), anxiety concerning Z55.2
  expansion terminal respiratory units (newborn) (primary) P28.0
  forceps NOS (with subsequent cesarean delivery) O66.5
  gain weight (child over 28 days old) R62.51
    adult R62.7
    newborn P92.6
  genital response (male) F52.21
    female F52.22
  heart (acute) (senile) (sudden) I50.9
    with
      acute pulmonary edema — *see* Failure, ventricular, left
      decompensation (*see also* Failure, heart, by type as diastolic or systolic, acute and chronic) I50.9
      dilatation — *see* Disease, heart
      normal ejection fraction — *see* Failure, heart, diastolic
      preserved ejection fraction — *see* Failure, heart, diastolic
      reduced ejection fraction — *see* Failure, heart, systolic
    arteriosclerotic I70.90
    biventricular I50.82
      due to left heart failure I50.814
    combined left-right sided I50.82
      due to left heart failure I50.814
    compensated (*see also* Failure, heart, by type as diastolic or systolic, chronic) I50.9
    complicating
      anesthesia (general) (local) or other sedation
        in labor and delivery O74.2
        in pregnancy O29.12- ☑
        postpartum, puerperal O89.1
      delivery (cesarean) (instrumental) O75.4
    congestive I50.9
      with rheumatic fever (conditions in I00)
        active I01.8
        inactive or quiescent (with chorea) I09.81
      newborn P29.0
      rheumatic (chronic) (inactive) (with chorea) I09.81
        active or acute I01.8
          with chorea I02.0
    decompensated (*see also* Failure, heart, by type as diastolic or systolic, acute and chronic) I50.9

Failure, failed — *continued*
  heart — *continued*
    degenerative — *see* Degeneration, myocardial
    diastolic (congestive) (left ventricular) I50.30
      acute (congestive) I50.31
        and (on) chronic (congestive) I50.33
      chronic (congestive) I50.32
        and (on) acute (congestive) I50.33
      combined with systolic (congestive) I50.40
        acute (congestive) I50.41
          and (on) chronic (congestive) I50.43
        chronic (congestive) I50.42
          and (on) acute (congestive) I50.43
    due to presence of cardiac prosthesis I97.13- ☑
    end stage (*see also* Failure, heart, by type as diastolic or systolic, chronic) I50.84
    following cardiac surgery I97.13- ☑
    high output NOS I50.83
    hypertensive — *see* Hypertension, heart
    left (ventricular) (*see also* Failure, ventricular, left)
      combined diastolic and systolic — *see* Failure, heart, diastolic, combined with systolic
      diastolic — *see* Failure, heart, diastolic
      systolic — *see* Failure, heart, systolic
    low output (syndrome) NOS I50.9
    newborn P29.0
    organic — *see* Disease, heart
    peripartum O90.3
    postprocedural I97.13- ☑
    rheumatic (chronic) (inactive) I09.9
    right (isolated) (ventricular) I50.810
      acute I50.811
        and (on) chronic I50.813
      chronic I50.812
        and acute I50.813
      secondary to left heart failure I50.814
    specified NEC I50.89

> Note: heart failure stages A, B, C, and D are based on the American College of Cardiology and American Heart Association stages of heart failure, which complement and should not be confused with the New York Heart Association Classification of Heart Failure, into Class I, Class II, Class III, and Class IV

    stage A Z91.89
    stage B (*see also* Failure, heart, by type as diastolic or systolic) I50.9
    stage C (*see also* Failure, heart, by type as diastolic or systolic) I50.9
    stage D (*see also* Failure, heart, by type as diastolic or systolic, chronic) I50.84
    systolic (congestive) (left ventricular) I50.20
      acute (congestive) I50.21
        and (on) chronic (congestive) I50.23
      chronic (congestive) I50.22
        and (on) acute (congestive) I50.23
      combined with diastolic (congestive) I50.40
        acute (congestive) I50.41
          and (on) chronic (congestive) I50.43
        chronic (congestive) I50.42
          and (on) acute (congestive) I50.43
    thyrotoxic (*see also* Thyrotoxicosis) E05.90 [I43]
      with
        high output (*see also* Thyrotoxicosis) I50.83
        thyroid storm E05.91 [I43]
          high output (*see also* Thyrotoxicosis) I50.83
    valvular — *see* Endocarditis
  hepatic K72.90
    with coma K72.91
    acute or subacute K72.00
      with coma K72.01
      due to drugs K71.10
        with coma K71.11
    alcoholic (acute) (chronic) (subacute) K70.40
      with coma K70.41
    chronic K72.10
      with coma K72.11
      due to drugs (acute) (subacute) (chronic) K71.10
        with coma K71.11
    due to drugs (acute) (subacute) (chronic) K71.10
      with coma K71.11
    postprocedural K91.82
  hepatorenal K76.7
  induction (of labor) O61.9
    abortion — *see* Abortion, attempted
    by
      oxytocic drugs O61.0

Failure, failed — continued
  induction — continued
    by — continued
      prostaglandins O61.0
    instrumental O61.1
    mechanical O61.1
    medical O61.0
    specified NEC O61.8
    surgical O61.1
  intubation during anesthesia T88.4 ☑
    in pregnancy O29.6- ☑
    labor and delivery O74.7
    postpartum, puerperal O89.6
  involution, thymus (gland) E32.0
  kidney (see also Disease, kidney, chronic) N19
    acute (see also Failure, renal, acute) N17.9
  lactation (complete) O92.3
    partial O92.4
  Leydig's cell, adult E29.1
  liver — see Failure, hepatic
  menstruation at puberty N91.0
  mitral I05.8
  myocardial, myocardium (see also Failure, heart) I50.9
    chronic (see also Failure, heart, congestive) I50.9
    congestive (see also Failure, heart, congestive) I50.9
  orgasm (female) (psychogenic) F52.31
    male F52.32
  ovarian (primary) E28.39
    iatrogenic E89.40
      asymptomatic E89.40
      symptomatic E89.41
    postprocedural (postablative) (postirradiation)
      (postsurgical) E89.40
      asymptomatic E89.40
      symptomatic E89.41
  ovulation causing infertility N97.0
  polyglandular, autoimmune E31.0
  prosthetic joint implant — see Complications, joint
    prosthesis, mechanical, breakdown, by site
  renal N19
    with
      tubular necrosis (acute) N17.0
    acute N17.9
      with
        cortical necrosis N17.1
        medullary necrosis N17.2
        tubular necrosis N17.0
      specified NEC N17.8
    chronic N18.9
      hypertensive — see Hypertension, kidney
    congenital P96.0
    end stage (chronic) N18.6
      due to hypertension I12.0
    following
      abortion — see Abortion by type complicated
        by specified condition NEC
      crushing T79.5 ☑
      ectopic or molar pregnancy O08.4
      labor and delivery (acute) O90.4
    hypertensive — see Hypertension, kidney
    postprocedural N99.0
  respiration, respiratory J96.90
    with
      hypercapnia J96.92
      hypercarbia J96.02
      hypoxia J96.91
    acute J96.00
      with
        hypercapnia J96.02
        hypercarbia J96.02
        hypoxia J96.01
    acute and (on) chronic J96.20
      with
        hypercapnia J96.22
        hypercarbia J96.22
        hypoxia J96.21
    center G93.89
    chronic J96.10
      with
        hypercapnia J96.12
        hypercarbia J96.12
        hypoxia J96.11
    newborn P28.5
    postprocedural (acute) J95.821
      acute and chronic J95.822
  rotation
    cecum Q43.3
    colon Q43.3

Failure, failed — continued
  rotation — continued
    intestine Q43.3
    kidney Q63.2
  sedation (conscious) (moderate) during procedure
    T88.52 ☑
    history of Z92.83
  segmentation (see also Fusion)
    fingers — see Syndactylism, complex, fingers
    vertebra Q76.49
      with scoliosis Q76.3
  seminiferous tubule, adult E29.1
  senile (general) R54
  sexual arousal (male) F52.21
    female F52.22
  testicular endocrine function E29.1
  to thrive (child over 28 days old) R62.51
    adult R62.7
    newborn P92.6
  transplant T86.92
    bone T86.831
      marrow T86.02
    cornea T86.841
    heart T86.22
      with lung(s) T86.32
    intestine T86.851
    kidney T86.12
    liver T86.42
    lung(s) T86.811
      with heart T86.32
    pancreas T86.891
    skin (allograft) (autograft) T86.821
    specified organ or tissue NEC T86.891
    stem cell (peripheral blood) (umbilical cord) T86.5
  trial of labor (with subsequent cesarean delivery)
    O66.40
    following previous cesarean delivery O66.41
  tubal ligation N99.89
  urinary — see Disease, kidney, chronic
  vacuum extraction NOS (with subsequent cesarean
    delivery) O66.5
  vasectomy N99.89
  ventouse NOS (with subsequent cesarean delivery)
    O66.5
  ventricular (see also Failure, heart) I50.9
    left (see also Failure, heart, left) I50.1
      with rheumatic fever (conditions in I00)
        active I01.8
          with chorea I02.0
        inactive or quiescent (with chorea) I09.81
        rheumatic (chronic) (inactive) (with chorea)
          I09.81
          active or acute I01.8
            with chorea I02.0
    right — see Failure, heart, right
  vital centers, newborn P91.88
Fainting (fit) R55
Fallen arches — see Deformity, limb, flat foot
Falling, falls (repeated) R29.6
  any organ or part — see Prolapse
Fallopian
  insufflation Z31.41
  tube — see condition
Fallot's
  pentalogy Q21.8
  tetrad or tetralogy Q21.3
  triad or trilogy Q22.3
False (see also condition)
  croup J38.5
  joint — see Nonunion, fracture
  labor (pains) O47.9
    at or after 37 completed weeks of gestation O47.1
    before 37 completed weeks of gestation O47.0- ☑
  passage, urethra (prostatic) N36.5
  pregnancy F45.8
Family, familial (see also condition)
  disruption Z63.8
    involving divorce or separation Z63.5
  Li-Fraumeni (syndrome) Z15.01
  planning advice Z30.09
  problem Z63.9
    specified NEC Z63.8
  retinoblastoma C69.2- ☑
Famine (effects of) T73.0 ☑
  edema — see Malnutrition, severe
Fanconi (-de Toni)(-Debré) **syndrome** E72.09
  with cystinosis E72.04
Fanconi's anemia (congenital pancytopenia) D61.09

Farber's disease or syndrome E75.29
Farcy A24.0
Farmer's
  lung J67.0
  skin L57.8
Farsightedness — see Hypermetropia
Fascia — see condition
Fasciculation R25.3
Fasciitis M72.9
  diffuse (eosinophilic) M35.4
  infective M72.8
    necrotizing M72.6
  necrotizing M72.6
  nodular M72.4
  perirenal (with ureteral obstruction) N13.5
    with infection N13.6
  plantar M72.2
  specified NEC M72.8
  traumatic (old) M72.8
    current — code by site under Sprain
Fascioliasis B66.3
Fasciolopsis, fasciolopsiasis (intestinal) B66.5
Fascioscapulohumeral myopathy G71.0
Fast pulse R00.0
Fat
  embolism — see Embolism, fat
  excessive (see also Obesity)
    in heart — see Degeneration, myocardial
  in stool R19.5
  localized (pad) E65
    heart — see Degeneration, myocardial
    knee M79.4
    retropatellar M79.4
  necrosis
    breast N64.1
    mesentery K65.4
    omentum K65.4
  pad E65
    knee M79.4
Fatigue R53.83
  auditory deafness — see Deafness
  chronic R53.82
  combat F43.0
  general R53.83
    psychogenic F48.8
  heat (transient) T67.6 ☑
  muscle M62.89
  myocardium — see Failure, heart
  neoplasm-related R53.0
  nervous, neurosis F48.8
  operational F48.8
  psychogenic (general) F48.8
  senile R54
  voice R49.8
Fatness — see Obesity
Fatty (see also condition)
  apron E65
  degeneration — see Degeneration, fatty
  heart (enlarged) — see Degeneration, myocardial
  liver NEC K76.0
    alcoholic K70.0
    nonalcoholic K76.0
  necrosis — see Degeneration, fatty
Fauces — see condition
Fauchard's disease (periodontitis) — see Periodontitis
Faucitis J02.9
Favism (anemia) D55.0
Favus — see Dermatophytosis
Fazio-Londe disease or syndrome G12.1
Fear complex or reaction F40.9
Fear of — see Phobia
Feared complaint unfounded Z71.1
Febris, febrile (see also Fever)
  flava (see also Fever, yellow) A95.9
  melitensis A23.0
  pestis — see Plague
  recurrens — see Fever, relapsing
  rubra A38.9
Fecal
  incontinence R15.9
  smearing R15.1
  soiling R15.1
  urgency R15.2
Fecalith (impaction) K56.41
  appendix K38.1
  congenital P76.8
Fede's disease K14.0

Feeble rapid pulse due to shock following injury
  T79.4 ☑
Feeble-minded F70
Feeding
  difficulties R63.3
  problem R63.3
    newborn P92.9
      specified NEC P92.8
    nonorganic (adult) — *see* Disorder, eating
Feeling (of)
  foreign body in throat R09.89
Feer's disease — *see* Poisoning, mercury
Feet — *see* condition
Feigned illness Z76.5
Feil-Klippel syndrome (brevicollis) Q76.1
Feinmesser's (hidrotic) **ectodermal dysplasia** Q82.4
Felinophobia F40.218
Felon (*see also* Cellulitis, digit)
  with lymphangitis — *see* Lymphangitis, acute, digit
Felty's syndrome M05.00
  ankle M05.07- ☑
  elbow M05.02- ☑
  foot joint M05.07- ☑
  hand joint M05.04- ☑
  hip M05.05- ☑
  knee M05.06- ☑
  multiple site M05.09
  shoulder M05.01- ☑
  vertebra — *see* Spondylitis, ankylosing
  wrist M05.03- ☑
Female genital cutting status — *see* Female genital
  mutilation status (FGM)
Female genital mutilation status (FGM) N90.810
  specified NEC N90.818
  type I (clitorectomy status) N90.811
  type II (clitorectomy with excision of labia minora status) N90.812
  type III (infibulation status) N90.813
  type IV N90.818
Femur, femoral — *see* condition
Fenestration, fenestrated (*see also* Imperfect, closure)
  aortico-pulmonary Q21.4
  cusps, heart valve NEC Q24.8
    pulmonary Q22.3
  pulmonic cusps Q22.3
Fernell's disease (aortic aneurysm) I71.9
Fertile eunuch syndrome E23.0
Fetid
  breath R19.6
  sweat L75.0
Fetishism F65.0
  transvestic F65.1
Fetus, fetal (*see also* condition)
  alcohol syndrome (dysmorphic) Q86.0
  compressus O31.0- ☑
  hydantoin syndrome Q86.1
  lung tissue P28.0
  papyraceous O31.0- ☑
Fever (inanition) (of unknown origin) (persistent) (with chills) (with rigor) R50.9
  abortus A23.1
  Aden (dengue) A90
  African tick-borne A68.1
  American
    mountain (tick) A93.2
    spotted A77.0
  aphthous B08.8
  arbovirus, arboviral A94
    hemorrhagic A94
    specified NEC A93.8
  Argentinian hemorrhagic A96.0
  Assam B55.0
  Australian Q A78
  Bangkok hemorrhagic A91
  Barmah forest A92.8
  Bartonella A44.0
  bilious, hemoglobinuric B50.8
  blackwater B50.8
  blister B00.1
  Bolivian hemorrhagic A96.1
  Bonvale dam T73.3 ☑
  boutonneuse A77.1
  brain — *see* Encephalitis
  Brazilian purpuric A48.4
  breakbone A90
  Bullis A77.0
  Bunyamwera A92.8

Fever — *continued*
  Burdwan B55.0
  Bwamba A92.8
  Cameroon — *see* Malaria
  Canton A75.9
  catarrhal (acute) J00
    chronic J31.0
  cat-scratch A28.1
  Central Asian hemorrhagic A98.0
  cerebral — *see* Encephalitis
  cerebrospinal meningococcal A39.0
  Chagres B50.9
  Chandipura A92.8
  Changuinola A93.1
  Charcot's (biliary) (hepatic) (intermittent) — *see* Calculus, bile duct
  Chikungunya (viral) (hemorrhagic) A92.0
  Chitral A93.1
  Colombo — *see* Fever, paratyphoid
  Colorado tick (virus) A93.2
  congestive (remittent) — *see* Malaria
  Congo virus A98.0
  continued malarial B50.9
  Corsican — *see* Malaria
  Crimean-Congo hemorrhagic A98.0
  Cyprus — *see* Brucellosis
  dandy A90
  deer fly — *see* Tularemia
  dengue (virus) A90
    hemorrhagic A91
    sandfly A93.1
  desert B38.0
  drug induced R50.2
  due to
    conditions classified elsewhere R50.81
    heat T67.0 ☑
  enteric A01.00
  enteroviral exanthematous (Boston exanthem) A88.0
  ephemeral (of unknown origin) R50.9
  epidemic hemorrhagic A98.5
  erysipelatous — *see* Erysipelas
  estivo-autumnal (malarial) B50.9
  famine A75.0
  five day A79.0
  following delivery O86.4
  Fort Bragg A27.89
  gastroenteric A01.00
  gastromalarial — *see* Malaria
  Gibraltar — *see* Brucellosis
  glandular — *see* Mononucleosis, infectious
  Guama (viral) A92.8
  Haverhill A25.1
  hay (allergic) J30.1
    with asthma (bronchial) J45.909
      with
        exacerbation (acute) J45.901
        status asthmaticus J45.902
      due to
        allergen other than pollen J30.89
        pollen, any plant or tree J30.1
  heat (effects) T67.0 ☑
  hematuric, bilious B50.8
  hemoglobinuric (malarial) (bilious) B50.8
  hemorrhagic (arthropod-borne) NOS A94
    with renal syndrome A98.5
    arenaviral A96.9
      specified NEC A96.8
    Argentinian A96.0
    Bangkok A91
    Bolivian A96.1
    Central Asian A98.0
    Chikungunya A92.0
    Crimean-Congo A98.0
    dengue (virus) A91
    epidemic A98.5
    Junin (virus) A96.0
    Korean A98.5
    Kyasanur forest A98.2
    Machupo (virus) A96.1
    mite-borne A93.8
    mosquito-borne A92.8
    Omsk A98.1
    Philippine A91
    Russian A98.5
    Singapore A91
    Southeast Asia A91
    Thailand A91
    tick-borne NEC A93.8

Fever — *continued*
  hemorrhagic — *continued*
    viral A99
      specified NEC A98.8
  hepatic — *see* Cholecystitis
  herpetic — *see* Herpes
  icterohemorrhagic A27.0
  Indiana A93.8
  infective B99.9
    specified NEC B99.8
  intermittent (bilious) (*see also* Malaria)
    of unknown origin R50.9
    pernicious B50.9
  iodide R50.2
  Japanese river A75.3
  jungle (*see also* Malaria)
    yellow A95.0
  Junin (virus) hemorrhagic A96.0
  Katayama B65.2
  kedani A75.3
  Kenya (tick) A77.1
  Kew Garden A79.1
  Korean hemorrhagic A98.5
  Lassa A96.2
  Lone Star A77.0
  Machupo (virus) hemorrhagic A96.1
  malaria, malarial — *see* Malaria
  Malta A23.9
  Marseilles A77.1
  marsh — *see* Malaria
  Mayaro (viral) A92.8
  Mediterranean (*see also* Brucellosis) A23.9
    familial M04.1
    tick A77.1
  meningeal — *see* Meningitis
  Meuse A79.0
  Mexican A75.2
  mianeh A68.1
  miasmatic — *see* Malaria
  mosquito-borne (viral) A92.9
    hemorrhagic A92.8
  mountain (*see also* Brucellosis)
    meaning Rocky Mountain spotted fever A77.0
    tick (American) (Colorado) (viral) A93.2
  Mucambo (viral) A92.8
  mud A27.89
  Neapolitan — *see* Brucellosis
  neutropenic D70.9
  newborn P81.9
    environmental P81.0
  Nine-Mile A78
  non-exanthematous tick A93.2
  North Asian tick-borne A77.2
  Omsk hemorrhagic A98.1
  O'nyong-nyong (viral) A92.1
  Oropouche (viral) A93.0
  Oroya A44.0
  paludal — *see* Malaria
  Panama (malarial) B50.9
  Pappataci A93.1
  paratyphoid A01.4
    A A01.1
    B A01.2
    C A01.3
  parrot A70
  periodic (Mediterranean) M04.1
  persistent (of unknown origin) R50.9
  petechial A39.0
  pharyngoconjunctival B30.2
  Philippine hemorrhagic A91
  phlebotomus A93.1
  Piry (virus) A93.8
  Pixuna (viral) A92.8
  Plasmodium ovale B53.0
  polioviral (nonparalytic) A80.4
  Pontiac A48.2
  postimmunization R50.83
  postoperative R50.82
    due to infection T81.4 ☑
  posttransfusion R50.84
  postvaccination R50.83
  presenting with conditions classified elsewhere R50.81
  pretibial A27.89
  puerperal O86.4
  Q A78
  quadrilateral A78
  quartan (malaria) B52.9
  Queensland (coastal) (tick) A77.3

Fever — *continued*
quintan A79.0
rabbit — *see* Tularemia
rat-bite A25.9
    due to
        Spirillum A25.0
        Streptobacillus moniliformis A25.1
recurrent — *see* Fever, relapsing
relapsing (Borrelia) A68.9
    Carter's (Asiatic) A68.1
    Dutton's (West African) A68.1
    Koch's A68.9
    louse-borne A68.0
    Novy's
        louse-borne A68.0
        tick-borne A68.1
    Obermeyer's (European) A68.0
    tick-borne A68.1
remittent (bilious) (congestive) (gastric) — *see* Malaria
rheumatic (active) (acute) (chronic) (subacute) I00
    with central nervous system involvement I02.9
    active with heart involvement — *see* category
        I01 ☑
    inactive or quiescent with
        cardiac hypertrophy I09.89
        carditis I09.9
        endocarditis I09.1
            aortic (valve) I06.9
                with mitral (valve) disease I08.0
            mitral (valve) I05.9
                with aortic (valve) disease I08.0
            pulmonary (valve) I09.89
            tricuspid (valve) I07.8
        heart disease NEC I09.89
        heart failure (congestive) (conditions in I50.)
            I09.81
        left ventricular failure (conditions in I50.1- I50.4-)
            I09.81
        myocarditis, myocardial degeneration (condi-
            tions in I51.4) I09.0
        pancarditis I09.9
        pericarditis I09.2
Rift Valley (viral) A92.4
Rocky Mountain spotted A77.0
rose J30.1
Ross River B33.1
Russian hemorrhagic A98.5
San Joaquin (Valley) B38.0
sandfly A93.1
Sao Paulo A77.0
scarlet A38.9
seven day (leptospirosis) (autumnal) (Japanese) A27.89
    dengue A90
shin-bone A79.0
Singapore hemorrhagic A91
solar A90
Songo A98.5
sore B00.1
South African tick-bite A68.1
Southeast Asia hemorrhagic A91
spinal — *see* Meningitis
spirillary A25.0
splenic — *see* Anthrax
spotted A77.9
    American A77.0
    Brazilian A77.0
    cerebrospinal meningitis A39.0
    Colombian A77.0
    due to Rickettsia
        australis A77.3
        conorii A77.1
        rickettsii A77.0
        sibirica A77.2
        specified type NEC A77.8
    Ehrlichiosis A77.40
        due to
            E. chafeensis A77.41
            specified organism NEC A77.49
    Rocky Mountain A77.0
steroid R50.2
streptobacillary A25.1
subtertian B50.9
Sumatran mite A75.3
sun A90
swamp A27.9
swine A02.8
sylvatic, yellow A95.0
Tahyna B33.8

Fever — *continued*
tertian — *see* Malaria, tertian
Thailand hemorrhagic A91
thermic T67.0 ☑
three-day A93.1
tick
    American mountain A93.2
    Colorado A93.2
    Kemerovo A93.8
    Mediterranean A77.1
    mountain A93.2
    nonexanthematous A93.2
    Quaranfil A93.8
tick-bite NEC A93.8
tick-borne (hemorrhagic) NEC A93.8
trench A79.0
tsutsugamushi A75.3
typhogastric A01.00
typhoid (abortive) (hemorrhagic) (intermittent) (ma-
    lignant) A01.00
    complicated by
        arthritis A01.04
        heart involvement A01.02
        meningitis A01.01
        osteomyelitis A01.05
        pneumonia A01.03
        specified NEC A01.09
typhomalarial — *see* Malaria
typhus — *see* Typhus (fever)
undulant — *see* Brucellosis
unknown origin R50.9
uveoparotid D86.89
valley B38.0
Venezuelan equine A92.2
vesicular stomatitis A93.8
viral hemorrhagic — *see* Fever, hemorrhagic, by type
    of virus
Volhynian A79.0
Wesselsbron (viral) A92.8
West
    African B50.8
    Nile (viral) A92.30
        with
            complications NEC A92.39
            cranial nerve disorders A92.32
            encephalitis A92.31
            encephalomyelitis A92.31
            neurologic manifestation NEC A92.32
            optic neuritis A92.32
            polyradiculitis A92.32
Whitmore's — *see* Melioidosis
Wolhynian A79.0
worm B83.9
yellow A95.9
    jungle A95.0
    sylvatic A95.0
    urban A95.1
Zika virus A92.5
Fibrillation
atrial or auricular (established) I48.91
    chronic I48.2
    paroxysmal I48.0
    permanent I48.2
    persistent I48.1
cardiac I49.8
heart I49.8
muscular M62.89
ventricular I49.01
Fibrin
ball or bodies, pleural (sac) J94.1
chamber, anterior (eye) (gelatinous exudate) — *see*
    Iridocyclitis, acute
Fibrinogenolysis — *see* Fibrinolysis
Fibrinogenopenia D68.8
acquired D65
congenital D68.2
Fibrinolysis (hemorrhagic) (acquired) D65
antepartum hemorrhage — *see* Hemorrhage, antepar-
    tum, with coagulation defect
following
    abortion — *see* Abortion by type complicated by
        hemorrhage
    ectopic or molar pregnancy O08.1
intrapartum O67.0
newborn, transient P60
postpartum O72.3
Fibrinopenia (hereditary) D68.2
acquired D68.4

Fibrinopurulent — *see* condition
Fibrinous — *see* condition
Fibroadenoma
cellular intracanalicular D24- ☑
giant D24- ☑
intracanalicular
    cellular D24- ☑
    giant D24- ☑
    specified site — *see* Neoplasm, benign, by site
    unspecified site D24- ☑
juvenile D24- ☑
pericanalicular
    specified site — *see* Neoplasm, benign, by site
    unspecified site D24- ☑
phyllodes D24- ☑
prostate D29.1
specified site NEC — *see* Neoplasm, benign, by site
unspecified site D24- ☑
Fibroadenosis, breast (chronic) (cystic) (diffuse) (peri-
    odic) (segmental) N60.2- ☑
Fibroangioma (see also Neoplasm, benign, by site)
juvenile
    specified site — *see* Neoplasm, benign, by site
    unspecified site D10.6
Fibrochondrosarcoma — *see* Neoplasm, cartilage,
    malignant
Fibrocystic
disease (see also Fibrosis, cystic)
    breast — *see* Mastopathy, cystic
    jaw M27.49
    kidney (congenital) Q61.8
    liver Q44.6
    pancreas E84.9
kidney (congenital) Q61.8
Fibrodysplasia ossificans progressiva — *see* Myositis,
    ossificans, progressiva
Fibroelastosis (cordis) (endocardial) (endomyocardial)
    I42.4
Fibroid (tumor) (see also Neoplasm, connective tissue,
    benign)
disease, lung (chronic) — *see* Fibrosis, lung
heart (disease) — *see* Myocarditis
in pregnancy or childbirth O34.1- ☑
    causing obstructed labor O65.5
induration, lung (chronic) — *see* Fibrosis, lung
lung — *see* Fibrosis, lung
pneumonia (chronic) — *see* Fibrosis, lung
uterus (see also Leiomyoma, uterus) D25.9
Fibrolipoma — *see* Lipoma
Fibroliposarcoma — *see* Neoplasm, connective tissue,
    malignant
Fibroma (see also Neoplasm, connective tissue, benign)
ameloblastic — *see* Cyst, calcifying odontogenic
bone (nonossifying) — *see* Disorder, bone, specified
    type NEC
    ossifying — *see* Neoplasm, bone, benign
cementifying — *see* Neoplasm, bone, benign
chondromyxoid — *see* Neoplasm, bone, benign
desmoplastic — *see* Neoplasm, connective tissue,
    uncertain behavior
durum — *see* Neoplasm, connective tissue, benign
fascial — *see* Neoplasm, connective tissue, benign
invasive — *see* Neoplasm, connective tissue, uncertain
    behavior
molle — *see* Lipoma
myxoid — *see* Neoplasm, connective tissue, benign
nasopharynx, nasopharyngeal (juvenile) D10.6
nonosteogenic (nonossifying) — *see* Dysplasia, fibrous
odontogenic (central) — *see* Cyst, calcifying odonto-
    genic
ossifying — *see* Neoplasm, bone, benign
periosteal — *see* Neoplasm, bone, benign
soft — *see* Lipoma
Fibromatosis M72.9
abdominal — *see* Neoplasm, connective tissue, uncer-
    tain behavior
aggressive — *see* Neoplasm, connective tissue, uncer-
    tain behavior
congenital generalized — *see* Neoplasm, connective
    tissue, uncertain behavior
Dupuytren's M72.0
gingival K06.1
palmar (fascial) M72.0
plantar (fascial) M72.2
pseudosarcomatous (proliferative) (subcutaneous)
    M72.4
retroperitoneal D48.3

Fibromatosis — *continued*
  specified NEC M72.8
Fibromyalgia M79.7
Fibromyoma (*see also* Neoplasm, connective tissue, benign)
  uterus (corpus) (*see also* Leiomyoma, uterus)
    in pregnancy or childbirth — *see* Fibroid, in pregnancy or childbirth
      causing obstructed labor O65.5
Fibromyositis M79.7
Fibromyxolipoma D17.9
Fibromyxoma — *see* Neoplasm, connective tissue, benign
Fibromyxosarcoma — *see* Neoplasm, connective tissue, malignant
Fibro-odontoma, ameloblastic — *see* Cyst, calcifying odontogenic
Fibro-osteoma — *see* Neoplasm, bone, benign
Fibroplasia, retrolental H35.17- ☑
Fibropurulent — *see* condition
Fibrosarcoma (*see also* Neoplasm, connective tissue, malignant)
  ameloblastic C41.1
    upper jaw (bone) C41.0
  congenital — *see* Neoplasm, connective tissue, malignant
  fascial — *see* Neoplasm, connective tissue, malignant
  infantile — *see* Neoplasm, connective tissue, malignant
  odontogenic C41.1
    upper jaw (bone) C41.0
  periosteal — *see* Neoplasm, bone, malignant
Fibrosclerosis
  breast N60.3- ☑
  multifocal M35.5
  penis (corpora cavernosa) N48.6
Fibrosis, fibrotic
  adrenal (gland) E27.8
  amnion O41.8X- ☑
  anal papillae K62.89
  arteriocapillary — *see* Arteriosclerosis
  bladder N32.89
    interstitial — *see* Cystitis, chronic, interstitial
    localized submucosal — *see* Cystitis, chronic, interstitial
    panmural — *see* Cystitis, chronic, interstitial
  breast — *see* Fibrosclerosis, breast
  capillary (*see also* Arteriosclerosis) I70.90
    lung (chronic) — *see* Fibrosis, lung
  cardiac — *see* Myocarditis
  cervix N88.8
  chorion O41.8X- ☑
  corpus cavernosum (sclerosing) N48.6
  cystic (of pancreas) E84.9
    with
      distal intestinal obstruction syndrome E84.19
      fecal impaction E84.19
      intestinal manifestations NEC E84.19
      pulmonary manifestations E84.0
      specified manifestations NEC E84.8
  due to device, implant or graft (*see also* Complications, by site and type, specified NEC) T85.828 ☑
    arterial graft NEC T82.828 ☑
    breast (implant) T85.828 ☑
    catheter NEC T85.828 ☑
      dialysis (renal) T82.828 ☑
        intraperitoneal T85.828 ☑
      infusion NEC T82.828 ☑
        spinal (epidural) (subdural) T85.820 ☑
      urinary (indwelling) T83.82 ☑
    electronic (electrode) (pulse generator) (stimulator)
      bone T84.82 ☑
      cardiac T82.827 ☑
      nervous system (brain) (peripheral nerve) (spinal) T85.820 ☑
      urinary T83.82 ☑
    fixation, internal (orthopedic) NEC T84.82 ☑
    gastrointestinal (bile duct) (esophagus) T85.828 ☑
    genital NEC T83.82 ☑
    heart NEC T82.827 ☑
    joint prosthesis T84.82 ☑
    ocular (corneal graft) (orbital implant) NEC T85.828 ☑
    orthopedic NEC T84.82 ☑
    specified NEC T85.828 ☑
    urinary NEC T83.82 ☑
    vascular NEC T82.828 ☑

Fibrosis, fibrotic — *continued*
  due to device, implant or graft (*see also* Complications, by site and type, specified) — *continued*
    ventricular intracranial shunt T85.820 ☑
  ejaculatory duct N50.89
  endocardium — *see* Endocarditis
  endomyocardial (tropical) I42.3
  epididymis N50.89
  eye muscle — *see* Strabismus, mechanical
  heart — *see* Myocarditis
  hepatic — *see* Fibrosis, liver
  hepatolienal (portal hypertension) K76.6
  hepatosplenic (portal hypertension) K76.6
  infrapatellar fat pad M79.4
  intrascrotal N50.89
  kidney N26.9
  liver K74.0
    with sclerosis K74.2
    alcoholic K70.2
  lung (atrophic) (chronic) (confluent) (massive) (perialveolar) (peribronchial) J84.10
    with
      anthracosilicosis J60
      anthracosis J60
      asbestosis J61
      bagassosis J67.1
      bauxite J63.1
      berylliosis J63.2
      byssinosis J66.0
      calcicosis J62.8
      chalicosis J62.8
      dust reticulation J64
      farmer's lung J67.0
      ganister disease J62.8
      graphite J63.3
      pneumoconiosis NOS J64
      siderosis J63.4
      silicosis J62.8
  capillary J84.10
  congenital P27.8
  diffuse (idiopathic) J84.10
    chemicals, gases, fumes or vapors (inhalation) J68.4
    interstitial J84.10
      acute J84.114
    talc J62.0
  following radiation J70.1
  idiopathic J84.112
  postinflammatory J84.10
  silicotic J62.8
  tuberculous — *see* Tuberculosis, pulmonary
  lymphatic gland I89.8
  median bar — *see* Hyperplasia, prostate
  mediastinum (idiopathic) J98.59
  meninges G96.19
  myocardium, myocardial — *see* Myocarditis
  ovary N83.8
  oviduct N83.8
  pancreas K86.89
  penis NEC N48.6
  pericardium I31.0
  perineum, in pregnancy or childbirth O34.7- ☑
    causing obstructed labor O65.5
  pleura J94.1
  popliteal fat pad M79.4
  prostate (chronic) — *see* Hyperplasia, prostate
  pulmonary (*see also* Fibrosis, lung) J84.10
    congenital P27.8
    idiopathic J84.112
  rectal sphincter K62.89
  retroperitoneal, idiopathic (with ureteral obstruction) N13.5
    with infection N13.6
  sclerosing mesenteric (idiopathic) K65.4
  scrotum N50.89
  seminal vesicle N50.89
  senile R54
  skin L90.5
  spermatic cord N50.89
  spleen D73.89
    in schistosomiasis (bilharziasis) B65.9 [D77]
  subepidermal nodular — *see* Neoplasm, skin, benign
  submucous (oral) (tongue) K13.5
  testis N44.8
    chronic, due to syphilis A52.76
  thymus (gland) E32.8
  tongue, submucous K13.5
  tunica vaginalis N50.89

Fibrosis, fibrotic — *continued*
  uterus (non-neoplastic) N85.8
  vagina N89.8
  valve, heart — *see* Endocarditis
  vas deferens N50.89
  vein I87.8
Fibrositis (periarticular) M79.7
  nodular, chronic (Jaccoud's) (rheumatoid) — *see* Arthropathy, postrheumatic, chronic
Fibrothorax J94.1
Fibrotic — *see* Fibrosis
Fibrous — *see* condition
Fibroxanthoma (*see also* Neoplasm, connective tissue, benign)
  atypical — *see* Neoplasm, connective tissue, uncertain behavior
  malignant — *see* Neoplasm, connective tissue, malignant
Fibroxanthosarcoma — *see* Neoplasm, connective tissue, malignant
Fiedler's
  disease (icterohemorrhagic leptospirosis) A27.0
  myocarditis (acute) I40.1
Fifth disease B08.3
  venereal A55
Filaria, filarial, filariasis — *see* Infestation, filarial
Filatov's disease — *see* Mononucleosis, infectious
File-cutter's disease — *see* Poisoning, lead
Filling defect
  biliary tract R93.2
  bladder R93.41
  duodenum R93.3
  gallbladder R93.2
  gastrointestinal tract R93.3
  intestine R93.3
  kidney R93.42- ☑
  stomach R93.3
  ureter R93.41
  urinary organs, specified NEC R93.49
Fimbrial cyst Q50.4
Financial problem affecting care NOS Z59.9
  bankruptcy Z59.8
  foreclosure on loan Z59.8
Findings, abnormal, inconclusive, without diagnosis
  (*see also* Abnormal)
  17-ketosteroids, elevated R82.5
  acetonuria R82.4
  alcohol in blood R78.0
  anisocytosis R71.8
  antenatal screening of mother O28.9
    biochemical O28.1
    chromosomal O28.5
    cytological O28.2
    genetic O28.5
    hematological O28.0
    radiological O28.4
    specified NEC O28.8
    ultrasonic O28.3
  antibody titer, elevated R76.0
  anticardiolipin antibody R76.0
  antiphosphatidylglycerol antibody R76.0
  antiphosphatidylinositol antibody R76.0
  antiphosphatidylserine antibody R76.0
  antiphospholipid antibody R76.0
  bacteriuria R82.71
  bicarbonate E87.8
  bile in urine R82.2
  blood sugar R73.09
    high R73.9
    low (transient) E16.2
  body fluid or substance, specified NEC R88.8
  casts, urine R82.99
  catecholamines R82.5
  cells, urine R82.99
  chloride E87.8
  cholesterol E78.9
    high E78.00
      with high triglycerides E78.2
  chyluria R82.0
  cloudy
    dialysis effluent R88.0
    urine R82.90
  creatinine clearance R94.4
  crystals, urine R82.99
  culture
    blood R78.81
    positive — *see* Positive, culture
  echocardiogram R93.1

Findings, abnormal, inconclusive, without diagnosis
— *continued*
electrolyte level, urinary R82.99
function study NEC R94.8
  bladder R94.8
  endocrine NEC R94.7
    thyroid R94.6
  kidney R94.4
  liver R94.5
  pancreas R94.8
  placenta R94.8
  pulmonary R94.2
  spleen R94.8
gallbladder, nonvisualization R93.2
glucose (tolerance test) (non-fasting) R73.09
glycosuria R81
heart
  shadow R93.1
  sounds R01.2
hematinuria R82.3
hematocrit drop (precipitous) R71.0
hemoglobinuria R82.3
human papillomavirus (HPV) DNA test positive
  cervix
    high risk R87.810
    low risk R87.820
  vagina
    high risk R87.811
    low risk R87.821
in blood (of substance not normally found in blood)
    R78.9
  addictive drug NEC R78.4
  alcohol (excessive level) R78.0
  cocaine R78.2
  hallucinogen R78.3
  heavy metals (abnormal level) R78.79
  lead R78.71
  lithium (abnormal level) R78.89
  opiate drug R78.1
  psychotropic drug R78.5
  specified substance NEC R78.89
  steroid agent R78.6
indoleacetic acid, elevated R82.5
ketonuria R82.4
lactic acid dehydrogenase (LDH) R74.0
liver function test R79.89
mammogram NEC R92.8
  calcification (calculus) R92.1
  inconclusive result (due to dense breasts) R92.2
  microcalcification R92.0
mediastinal shift R93.8
melanin, urine R82.99
myoglobinuria R82.1
neonatal screening P09
nonvisualization of gallbladder R93.2
odor of urine NOS R82.90
Papanicolaou cervix R87.619
  non-atypical endometrial cells R87.618
pneumoencephalogram R93.0
poikilocytosis R71.8
potassium (deficiency) E87.6
  excess E87.5
PPD R76.11
radiologic (X-ray) R93.8
  abdomen R93.5
  biliary tract R93.2
  breast R92.8
  gastrointestinal tract R93.3
  genitourinary organs R93.8
  head R93.0
  inconclusive due to excess body fat of patient R93.9
  intrathoracic organs NEC R93.1
  placenta R93.8
  retroperitoneum R93.5
  skin R93.8
  skull R93.0
  subcutaneous tissue R93.8
red blood cell (count) (morphology) (sickling) (volume)
    R71.8
scan NEC R94.8
  bladder R94.8
  bone R94.8
  kidney R94.4
  liver R93.2
  lung R94.2
  pancreas R94.8
  placental R94.8
  spleen R94.8
  thyroid R94.6

Findings, abnormal, inconclusive, without diagnosis
— *continued*
sedimentation rate, elevated R70.0
SGOT R74.0
SGPT R74.0
sodium (deficiency) E87.1
  excess E87.0
specified body fluid NEC R88.8
stress test R94.39
thyroid (function) (metabolic rate) (scan) (uptake)
    R94.6
transaminase (level) R74.0
triglycerides E78.9
  high E78.1
    with high cholesterol E78.2
tuberculin skin test (without active tuberculosis)
    R76.11
urine R82.90
  acetone R82.4
  bacteria R82.71
  bile R82.2
  casts or cells R82.99
  chyle R82.0
  culture positive R82.79
  glucose R81
  hemoglobin R82.3
  ketone R82.4
  sugar R81
vanillylmandelic acid (VMA), elevated R82.5
vectorcardiogram (VCG) R94.39
ventriculogram R93.0
white blood cell (count) (differential) (morphology)
    D72.9
xerography R92.8
Finger — *see* condition
Fire, Saint Anthony's — *see* Erysipelas
Fire-setting
  pathological (compulsive) F63.1
Fish hook stomach K31.89
Fishmeal-worker's lung J67.8
Fissure, fissured
  anus, anal K60.2
    acute K60.0
    chronic K60.1
    congenital Q43.8
  ear, lobule, congenital Q17.8
  epiglottis (congenital) Q31.8
  larynx J38.7
    congenital Q31.8
  lip K13.0
    congenital — *see* Cleft, lip
  nipple N64.0
    associated with
      lactation O92.13
      pregnancy O92.11- ☑
      puerperium O92.12
  nose Q30.2
  palate (congenital) — *see* Cleft, palate
  skin R23.4
  spine (congenital) (*see also* Spina bifida)
    with hydrocephalus — *see* Spina bifida, by site,
      with hydrocephalus
  tongue (acquired) K14.5
    congenital Q38.3
Fistula (cutaneous) L98.8
  abdomen (wall) K63.2
    bladder N32.2
    intestine NEC K63.2
    ureter N28.89
    uterus N82.5
  abdominorectal K63.2
  abdominosigmoidal K63.2
  abdominothoracic J86.0
  abdominouterine N82.5
    congenital Q51.7
  abdominovesical N32.2
  accessory sinuses — *see* Sinusitis
  actinomycotic — *see* Actinomycosis
  alveolar antrum — *see* Sinusitis, maxillary
  alveolar process K04.6
  anorectal K60.5
  antrobuccal — *see* Sinusitis, maxillary
  antrum — *see* Sinusitis, maxillary
  anus, anal (recurrent) (infectional) K60.3
    congenital Q43.6
      with absence, atresia and stenosis Q42.2
    tuberculous A18.32
  aorta-duodenal I77.2

Fistula — *continued*
  appendix, appendicular K38.3
  arteriovenous (acquired) (nonruptured) I77.0
    brain I67.1
      congenital Q28.2
        ruptured I60.8
      ruptured I60.8
    cerebral — *see* Fistula, arteriovenous, brain
    congenital (peripheral) (*see also* Malformation, ar-
      teriovenous)
      brain Q28.2
        ruptured I60.8
      coronary Q24.5
      pulmonary Q25.72
    coronary I25.41
      congenital Q24.5
    pulmonary I28.0
      congenital Q25.72
    surgically created (for dialysis) Z99.2
      complication — *see* Complication, arteriove-
        nous, fistula, surgically created
    traumatic — *see* Injury, blood vessel
  artery I77.2
  aural (mastoid) — *see* Mastoiditis, chronic
  auricle (*see also* Disorder, pinna, specified type NEC)
    congenital Q18.1
  Bartholin's gland N82.8
  bile duct (common) (hepatic) K83.3
    with calculus, stones — *see* Calculus, bile duct
  biliary (tract) — *see* Fistula, bile duct
  bladder (sphincter) NEC (*see also* Fistula, vesico-) N32.2
    into seminal vesicle N32.2
  bone (*see also* Disorder, bone, specified type NEC)
    with osteomyelitis, chronic — *see* Osteomyelitis,
      chronic, with draining sinus
  brain G93.89
    arteriovenous (acquired) I67.1
      congenital Q28.2
  branchial (cleft) Q18.0
  branchiogenous Q18.0
  breast N61.0
    puerperal, postpartum or gestational, due to mas-
      titis (purulent) — *see* Mastitis, obstetric, pu-
      rulent
  bronchial J86.0
  bronchocutaneous, bronchomediastinal, bronchopleu-
    ral, bronchopleuromediastinal (infective) J86.0
    tuberculous NEC A15.5
  bronchoesophageal J86.0
    congenital Q39.2
      with atresia of esophagus Q39.1
  bronchovisceral J86.0
  buccal cavity (infective) K12.2
  cecosigmoidal K63.2
  cecum K63.2
  cerebrospinal (fluid) G96.0
  cervical, lateral Q18.1
  cervicoaural Q18.1
  cervicosigmoidal N82.4
  cervicovesical N82.1
  cervix N82.8
  chest (wall) J86.0
  cholecystenteric — *see* Fistula, gallbladder
  cholecystocolic — *see* Fistula, gallbladder
  cholecystocolonic — *see* Fistula, gallbladder
  cholecystoduodenal — *see* Fistula, gallbladder
  cholecystogastric — *see* Fistula, gallbladder
  cholecystointestinal — *see* Fistula, gallbladder
  choledochoduodenal — *see* Fistula, bile duct
  cholocolic K82.3
  coccyx — *see* Sinus, pilonidal
  colon K63.2
  colostomy K94.09
  common duct — *see* Fistula, bile duct
  congenital, site not listed — *see* Anomaly, by site
  coronary, arteriovenous I25.41
    congenital Q24.5
  costal region J86.0
  cul-de-sac, Douglas' N82.8
  cystic duct (*see also* Fistula, gallbladder)
    congenital Q44.5
  dental K04.6
  diaphragm J86.0
  duodenum K31.6
  ear (external) (canal) — *see* Disorder, ear, external,
    specified type NEC
  enterocolic K63.2
  enterocutaneous K63.2

Fistula — *continued*
enterouterine N82.4
  congenital Q51.7
enterovaginal N82.4
  congenital Q52.2
  large intestine N82.3
  small intestine N82.2
enterovesical N32.1
epididymis N50.89
  tuberculous A18.15
esophagobronchial J86.0
  congenital Q39.2
    with atresia of esophagus Q39.1
esophagocutaneous K22.8
esophagopleural-cutaneous J86.0
esophagotracheal J86.0
  congenital Q39.2
    with atresia of esophagus Q39.1
esophagus K22.8
  congenital Q39.2
    with atresia of esophagus Q39.1
ethmoid — *see* Sinusitis, ethmoidal
eyeball (cornea) (sclera) — *see* Disorder, globe, hypotony
eyelid H01.8
fallopian tube, external N82.5
fecal K63.2
  congenital Q43.6
from periapical abscess K04.6
frontal sinus — *see* Sinusitis, frontal
gallbladder K82.3
  with calculus, cholelithiasis, stones — *see* Calculus, gallbladder
gastric K31.6
gastrocolic K31.6
  congenital Q40.2
  tuberculous A18.32
gastroenterocolic K31.6
gastroesophageal K31.6
gastrojejunal K31.6
gastrojejunocolic K31.6
genital tract (female) N82.9
  specified NEC N82.8
  to intestine NEC N82.4
  to skin N82.5
hepatic artery-portal vein, congenital Q26.6
hepatopleural J86.0
hepatopulmonary J86.0
ileorectal or ileosigmoidal K63.2
ileovaginal N82.2
ileovesical N32.1
ileum K63.2
in ano K60.3
  tuberculous A18.32
inner ear (labyrinth) — *see* subcategory H83.1 ☑
intestine NEC K63.2
intestinocolonic (abdominal) K63.2
intestinoureteral N28.89
intestinouterine N82.4
intestinovaginal N82.4
  large intestine N82.3
  small intestine N82.2
intestinovesical N32.1
ischiorectal (fossa) K61.3
jejunum K63.2
joint M25.10
  ankle M25.17- ☑
  elbow M25.12- ☑
  foot joint M25.17- ☑
  hand joint M25.14- ☑
  hip M25.15- ☑
  knee M25.16- ☑
  shoulder M25.11- ☑
  specified joint NEC M25.18
  tuberculous — *see* Tuberculosis, joint
  vertebrae M25.18
  wrist M25.13- ☑
kidney N28.89
labium (majus) (minus) N82.8
labyrinth — *see* subcategory H83.1 ☑
lacrimal (gland) (sac) H04.61- ☑
lacrimonasal duct — *see* Fistula, lacrimal
laryngotracheal, congenital Q34.8
larynx J38.7
lip K13.0
  congenital Q38.0
lumbar, tuberculous A18.01
lung J86.0

Fistula — *continued*
lymphatic I89.8
mammary (gland) N61.0
mastoid (process) (region) — *see* Mastoiditis, chronic
maxillary J32.0
medial, face and neck Q18.8
mediastinal J86.0
mediastinobronchial J86.0
mediastinocutaneous J86.0
middle ear — *see* subcategory H74.8 ☑
mouth K12.2
nasal J34.89
  sinus — *see* Sinusitis
nasopharynx J39.2
nipple N64.0
nose J34.89
oral (cutaneous) K12.2
  maxillary J32.0
  nasal (with cleft palate) — *see* Cleft, palate
orbit, orbital — *see* Disorder, orbit, specified type NEC
oroantral J32.0
oviduct, external N82.5
palate (hard) M27.8
pancreatic K86.89
pancreaticoduodenal K86.89
parotid (gland) K11.4
  region K12.2
penis N48.89
perianal K60.3
pericardium (pleura) (sac) — *see* Pericarditis
pericecal K63.2
perineorectal K60.4
perineosigmoidal K63.2
perineum, perineal (with urethral involvement) NEC N36.0
  tuberculous A18.13
  ureter N28.89
perirectal K60.4
  tuberculous A18.32
peritoneum K65.9
pharyngoesophageal J39.2
pharynx J39.2
  branchial cleft (congenital) Q18.0
pilonidal (infected) (rectum) — *see* Sinus, pilonidal
pleura, pleural, pleurocutaneous, pleuroperitoneal J86.0
  tuberculous NEC A15.6
pleuropericardial I31.8
portal vein-hepatic artery, congenital Q26.6
postauricular H70.81- ☑
postoperative, persistent T81.83 ☑
  specified site — *see* Fistula, by site
preauricular (congenital) Q18.1
prostate N42.89
pulmonary J86.0
  arteriovenous I28.0
    congenital Q25.72
  tuberculous — *see* Tuberculosis, pulmonary
pulmonoperitoneal J86.0
rectolabial N82.4
rectosigmoid (intercommunicating) K63.2
rectoureteral N28.89
rectourethral N36.0
  congenital Q64.73
rectouterine N82.4
  congenital Q51.7
rectovaginal N82.3
  congenital Q52.2
  tuberculous A18.18
rectovesical N32.1
  congenital Q64.79
rectovesicovaginal N82.3
rectovulval N82.4
  congenital Q52.79
rectum (to skin) K60.4
  congenital Q43.6
    with absence, atresia and stenosis Q42.0
  tuberculous A18.32
renal N28.89
retroauricular — *see* Fistula, postauricular
salivary duct or gland (any) K11.4
  congenital Q38.4
scrotum (urinary) N50.89
  tuberculous A18.15
semicircular canals — *see* subcategory H83.1 ☑
sigmoid K63.2
  to bladder N32.1
sinus — *see* Sinusitis

Fistula — *continued*
skin L98.8
  to genital tract (female) N82.5
splenocolic D73.89
stercoral K63.2
stomach K31.6
sublingual gland K11.4
submandibular gland K11.4
submaxillary (gland) K11.4
  region K12.2
thoracic J86.0
  duct I89.8
thoracoabdominal J86.0
thoracogastric J86.0
thoracointestinal J86.0
thorax J86.0
thyroglossal duct Q89.2
thyroid E07.89
trachea, congenital (external) (internal) Q32.1
tracheoesophageal J86.0
  congenital Q39.2
    with atresia of esophagus Q39.1
  following tracheostomy J95.04
traumatic arteriovenous — *see* Injury, blood vessel, by site
tuberculous — *code by* site under Tuberculosis
typhoid A01.09
umbilicourinary Q64.8
urachus, congenital Q64.4
ureter (persistent) N28.89
ureteroabdominal N28.89
ureterorectal N28.89
ureterosigmoido-abdominal N28.89
ureterovaginal N82.1
ureterovesical N32.2
urethra N36.0
  congenital Q64.79
  tuberculous A18.13
urethroperineal N36.0
urethroperineovesical N32.2
urethrorectal N36.0
  congenital Q64.73
urethroscrotal N50.89
urethrovaginal N82.1
urethrovesical N32.2
urinary (tract) (persistent) (recurrent) N36.0
uteroabdominal N82.5
  congenital Q51.7
uteroenteric, uterointestinal N82.4
  congenital Q51.7
uterorectal N82.4
  congenital Q51.7
uteroureteric N82.1
uterourethral Q51.7
uterovaginal N82.8
uterovesical N82.1
  congenital Q51.7
uterus N82.8
vagina (postpartal) (wall) N82.8
vaginocutaneous (postpartal) N82.5
vaginointestinal NEC N82.4
  large intestine N82.3
  small intestine N82.2
vaginoperineal N82.5
vasocutaneous, congenital Q55.7
vesical NEC N32.2
vesicoabdominal N32.2
vesicocervicovaginal N82.1
vesicocolic N32.1
vesicocutaneous N32.2
vesicoenteric N32.1
vesicointestinal N32.1
vesicometrorectal N82.4
vesicoperineal N32.2
vesicorectal N32.1
  congenital Q64.79
vesicosigmoidal N32.1
vesicosigmoidovaginal N82.3
vesicoureteral N32.2
vesicoureterovaginal N82.1
vesicourethral N32.2
vesicourethrorectal N32.1
vesicouterine N82.1
  congenital Q51.7
vesicovaginal N82.0
vulvorectal N82.4
  congenital Q52.79
Fit R56.9
  epileptic — *see* Epilepsy

Fit — *continued*
  fainting R55
  hysterical F44.5
  newborn P9Ø
Fitting (and adjustment) (of)
  artificial
    arm — *see* Admission, adjustment, artificial, arm
    breast Z44.3 ☑
    eye Z44.2 ☑
    leg — *see* Admission, adjustment, artificial, leg
  automatic implantable cardiac defibrillator (with synchronous cardiac pacemaker) Z45.02
  brain neuropacemaker Z46.2
    implanted Z45.42
  cardiac defibrillator — *see* Fitting (and adjustment) (of), automatic implantable cardiac defibrillator
  catheter, non-vascular Z46.82
  colostomy belt Z46.89
  contact lenses Z46.Ø
  CRT-D (resynchronization therapy defibrillator) Z45.02
  CRT-P (cardiac resynchronization therapy pacemaker) Z45.Ø18
    pulse generator Z45.Ø1Ø
  cystostomy device Z46.6
  defibrillator, cardiac — *see* Fitting (and adjustment) (of), automatic implantable cardiac defibrillator
  dentures Z46.3
  device NOS Z46.9
    abdominal Z46.89
    gastrointestinal NEC Z46.59
    implanted NEC Z45.89
    nervous system Z46.2
      implanted — *see* Admission, adjustment, device, implanted, nervous system
    orthodontic Z46.4
    orthoptic Z46.Ø
    orthotic Z46.89
    prosthetic (external) Z44.9
      breast Z44.3 ☑
      dental Z46.3
      eye Z44.2 ☑
      specified NEC Z44.8
    specified NEC Z46.89
  substitution
    auditory Z46.2
      implanted — *see* Admission, adjustment, device, implanted, hearing device
    nervous system Z46.2
      implanted — *see* Admission, adjustment, device, implanted, nervous system
    visual Z46.2
      implanted Z45.31
    urinary Z46.6
  gastric lap band Z46.51
  gastrointestinal appliance NEC Z46.59
  glasses (reading) Z46.Ø
  hearing aid Z46.1
  ileostomy device Z46.89
  insulin pump Z46.81
  intestinal appliance NEC Z46.89
  myringotomy device (stent) (tube) Z45.82
  neuropacemaker Z46.2
    implanted Z45.42
  non-vascular catheter Z46.82
  orthodontic device Z46.4
  orthopedic device (brace) (cast) (corset) (shoes) Z46.89
  pacemaker (cardiac) (cardiac resynchronization therapy (CRT-P)) Z45.Ø18
    nervous system (brain) (peripheral nerve) (spinal cord) Z46.2
      implanted Z45.42
    pulse generator Z45.Ø1Ø
  portacath (port-a-cath) Z45.2
  prosthesis (external) Z44.9
    arm — *see* Admission, adjustment, artificial, arm
    breast Z44.3 ☑
    dental Z46.3
    eye Z44.2 ☑
    leg — *see* Admission, adjustment, artificial, leg
    specified NEC Z44.8
  spectacles Z46.Ø
  wheelchair Z46.89
Fitzhugh-Curtis syndrome
  due to
    Chlamydia trachomatis A74.81
    Neisseria gonorrhorea (gonococcal peritonitis) A54.85

Fitz's syndrome (acute hemorrhagic pancreatitis) (*see also* Pancreatitis, acute) K85.8Ø
Fixation
  joint — *see* Ankylosis
  larynx J38.7
  stapes — *see* Ankylosis, ear ossicles
    deafness — *see* Deafness, conductive
  uterus (acquired) — *see* Malposition, uterus
  vocal cord J38.3
Flabby ridge KØ6.8
Flaccid (*see also* condition)
  palate, congenital Q38.5
Flail
  chest S22.5 ☑
    newborn (birth injury) P13.8
  joint (paralytic) M25.2Ø
    ankle M25.27- ☑
    elbow M25.22- ☑
    foot joint M25.27- ☑
    hand joint M25.24- ☑
    hip M25.25- ☑
    knee M25.26- ☑
    shoulder M25.21- ☑
    specified joint NEC M25.28
    wrist M25.23- ☑
Flajani's disease — *see* Hyperthyroidism, with, goiter (diffuse)
Flap, liver K71.3
Flashbacks (residual to hallucinogen use) F16.283
Flat
  chamber (eye) — *see* Disorder, globe, hypotony, flat anterior chamber
  chest, congenital Q67.8
  foot (acquired) (fixed type) (painful) (postural) (*see also* Deformity, limb, flat foot)
    congenital (rigid) (spastic) (everted) Q66.5- ☑
    rachitic sequelae (late effect) E64.3
  organ or site, congenital NEC — *see* Anomaly, by site
  pelvis M95.5
    with disproportion (fetopelvic) O33.Ø
      causing obstructed labor O65.Ø
    congenital Q74.2
Flatau-Schilder disease G37.Ø
Flatback syndrome M4Ø.3Ø
  lumbar region M4Ø.36
  lumbosacral region M4Ø.37
  thoracolumbar region M4Ø.35
Flattening
  head, femur M89.8X5
  hip — *see* Coxa, plana
  lip (congenital) Q18.8
  nose (congenital) Q67.4
    acquired M95.Ø
Flatulence R14.3
  psychogenic F45.8
Flatus R14.3
  vaginalis N89.8
Flax-dresser's disease J66.1
Flea bite — *see* Injury, bite, by site, superficial, insect
Flecks, glaucomatous (subcapsular) — *see* Cataract, complicated
Fleischer (-Kayser) **ring** (cornea) H18.Ø4- ☑
Fleshy mole OØ2.Ø
Flexibilitas cerea — *see* Catalepsy
Flexion
  amputation stump (surgical) T87.89
  cervix — *see* Malposition, uterus
  contracture, joint — *see* Contraction, joint
  deformity, joint (*see also* Deformity, limb, flexion) M21.2Ø
    hip, congenital Q65.89
  uterus (*see also* Malposition, uterus)
    lateral — *see* Lateroversion, uterus
Flexner-Boyd dysentery AØ3.2
Flexner's dysentery AØ3.1
Flexure — *see* Flexion
Flint murmur (aortic insufficiency) I35.1
Floater, vitreous — *see* Opacity, vitreous
Floating
  cartilage (joint) (*see also* Loose, body, joint)
    knee — *see* Derangement, knee, loose body
  gallbladder, congenital Q44.1
  kidney N28.89
    congenital Q63.8
  spleen D73.89
Flooding N92.Ø
Floor — *see* condition

Floppy
  baby syndrome (nonspecific) P94.2
  iris syndrome (intraoperative) (IFIS) H21.81
  nonrheumatic mitral valve syndrome I34.1
Flu (*see also* Influenza)
  avian (*see also* Influenza, due to, identified novel influenza A virus) JØ9.X2
  bird (*see also* Influenza, due to, identified novel influenza A virus) JØ9.X2
  intestinal NEC AØ8.4
  swine (viruses that normally cause infections in pigs) (*see also* Influenza, due to, identified novel influenza A virus) JØ9.X2
Fluctuating blood pressure I99.8
Fluid
  abdomen R18.8
  chest J94.8
  heart — *see* Failure, heart, congestive
  joint — *see* Effusion, joint
  loss (acute) E86.9
  lung — *see* Edema, lung
  overload E87.7Ø
    specified NEC E87.79
  peritoneal cavity R18.8
  pleural cavity J94.8
  retention R6Ø.9
Flukes NEC (*see also* Infestation, fluke)
  blood NEC — *See* Schistosomiasis
  liver B66.3
Fluor (vaginalis) N89.8
  trichomonal or due to Trichomonas (vaginalis) A59.ØØ
Fluorosis
  dental KØØ.3
  skeletal M85.1Ø
    ankle M85.17- ☑
    foot M85.17- ☑
    forearm M85.13- ☑
    hand M85.14- ☑
    lower leg M85.16- ☑
    multiple site M85.19
    neck M85.18
    rib M85.18
    shoulder M85.11- ☑
    skull M85.18
    specified site NEC M85.18
    thigh M85.15- ☑
    toe M85.17- ☑
    upper arm M85.12- ☑
    vertebra M85.18
Flush syndrome E34.Ø
Flushing R23.2
  menopausal N95.1
Flutter
  atrial or auricular I48.92
    atypical I48.4
    type I I48.3
    type II I48.4
    typical I48.3
  heart I49.8
    atrial or auricular I48.92
      atypical I48.4
      type I I48.3
      type II I48.4
      typical I48.3
    ventricular I49.Ø2
  ventricular I49.Ø2
FNHTR (febrile nonhemolytic transfusion reaction) R5Ø.84
Fochier's abscess — *code by* site under Abscess
Focus, Assmann's — *see* Tuberculosis, pulmonary
Fogo selvagem L1Ø.3
Foix-Alajouanine syndrome G95.19
Fold, folds (anomalous) (*see also* Anomaly, by site)
  Descemet's membrane — *see* Change, corneal membrane, Descemet's, fold
  epicanthic Q1Ø.3
  heart Q24.8
Folie à deux F24
Follicle
  cervix (nabothian) (ruptured) N88.8
  graafian, ruptured, with hemorrhage N83.Ø- ☑
  nabothian N88.8
Follicular — *see* condition
Folliculitis (superficial) L73.9
  abscedens et suffodiens L66.3
  cyst N83.Ø- ☑
  decalvans L66.2
  deep — *see* Furuncle, by site

☑ **Additional Character Required** — **Refer to the Tabular List for Character Selection**   ⊽ **Subterms under main terms may continue to next column or page**

Folliculitis — *continued*
  gonococcal (acute) (chronic) A54.01
  keloid, keloidalis L73.0
  pustular L01.02
  ulerythematosa reticulata L66.4
Folliculome lipidique
  specified site — *see* Neoplasm, benign, by site
  unspecified site
    female D27.9
    male D29.20
Følling's disease E70.0
Follow-up — *see* Examination, follow-up
Fong's syndrome (hereditary osteo-onychodysplasia) Q87.2
Food
  allergy L27.2
  asphyxia (from aspiration or inhalation) — *see* Foreign body, by site
  choked on — *see* Foreign body, by site
  deprivation T73.0 ☑
    specified kind of food NEC E63.8
  intoxication — *see* Poisoning, food
  lack of T73.0 ☑
  poisoning — *see* Poisoning, food
  rejection NEC — *see* Disorder, eating
  strangulation or suffocation — *see* Foreign body, by site
  toxemia — *see* Poisoning, food
Foot — *see* condition
Foramen ovale (nonclosure) (patent) (persistent) Q21.1
Forbes' glycogen storage disease E74.03
Fordyce-Fox disease L75.2
Fordyce's disease (mouth) Q38.6
Forearm — *see* condition
Foreign body
  with
    laceration — *see* Laceration, by site, with foreign body
    puncture wound — *see* Puncture, by site, with foreign body
  accidentally left following a procedure T81.509 ☑
    aspiration T81.506 ☑
      resulting in
        adhesions T81.516 ☑
        obstruction T81.526 ☑
        perforation T81.536 ☑
        specified complication NEC T81.596 ☑
    cardiac catheterization T81.505 ☑
      resulting in
        acute reaction T81.60 ☑
          aseptic peritonitis T81.61 ☑
            specified NEC T81.69 ☑
        adhesions T81.515 ☑
        obstruction T81.525 ☑
        perforation T81.535 ☑
        specified complication NEC T81.595 ☑
    causing
      acute reaction T81.60 ☑
        aseptic peritonitis T81.61 ☑
          specified complication NEC T81.69 ☑
      adhesions T81.519 ☑
      aseptic peritonitis T81.61 ☑
      obstruction T81.529 ☑
      perforation T81.539 ☑
      specified complication NEC T81.599 ☑
    endoscopy T81.504 ☑
      resulting in
        adhesions T81.514 ☑
        obstruction T81.524 ☑
        perforation T81.534 ☑
        specified complication NEC T81.594 ☑
    immunization T81.503 ☑
      resulting in
        adhesions T81.513 ☑
        obstruction T81.523 ☑
        perforation T81.533 ☑
        specified complication NEC T81.593 ☑
    infusion T81.501 ☑
      resulting in
        adhesions T81.511 ☑
        obstruction T81.521 ☑
        perforation T81.531 ☑
        specified complication NEC T81.591 ☑
    injection T81.503 ☑
      resulting in
        adhesions T81.513 ☑

Foreign body — *continued*
  accidentally left following a procedure — *continued*
    injection — *continued*
      resulting in — *continued*
        obstruction T81.523 ☑
        perforation T81.533 ☑
        specified complication NEC T81.593 ☑
    kidney dialysis T81.502 ☑
      resulting in
        adhesions T81.512 ☑
        obstruction T81.522 ☑
        perforation T81.532 ☑
        specified complication NEC T81.592 ☑
    packing removal T81.507 ☑
      resulting in
        acute reaction T81.60 ☑
          aseptic peritonitis T81.61 ☑
            specified NEC T81.69 ☑
        adhesions T81.517 ☑
        obstruction T81.527 ☑
        perforation T81.537 ☑
        specified complication NEC T81.597 ☑
    puncture T81.506 ☑
      resulting in
        adhesions T81.516 ☑
        obstruction T81.526 ☑
        perforation T81.536 ☑
        specified complication NEC T81.596 ☑
    specified procedure NEC T81.508 ☑
      resulting in
        acute reaction T81.60 ☑
          aseptic peritonitis T81.61 ☑
            specified NEC T81.69 ☑
        adhesions T81.518 ☑
        obstruction T81.528 ☑
        perforation T81.538 ☑
        specified complication NEC T81.598 ☑
    surgical operation T81.500 ☑
      resulting in
        acute reaction T81.60 ☑
          aseptic peritonitis T81.61 ☑
            specified NEC T81.69 ☑
        adhesions T81.510 ☑
        obstruction T81.520 ☑
        perforation T81.530 ☑
        specified complication NEC T81.590 ☑
    transfusion T81.501 ☑
      resulting in
        adhesions T81.511 ☑
        obstruction T81.521 ☑
        perforation T81.531 ☑
        specified complication NEC T81.591 ☑
  alimentary tract T18.9 ☑
    anus T18.5 ☑
    colon T18.4 ☑
    esophagus — *see* Foreign body, esophagus
    mouth T18.0 ☑
    multiple sites T18.8 ☑
    rectosigmoid (junction) T18.5 ☑
    rectum T18.5 ☑
    small intestine T18.3 ☑
    specified site NEC T18.8 ☑
    stomach T18.2 ☑
  anterior chamber (eye) S05.5- ☑
  auditory canal — *see* Foreign body, entering through orifice, ear
  bronchus T17.508 ☑
    causing
      asphyxiation T17.500 ☑
        food (bone) (seed) T17.520 ☑
        gastric contents (vomitus) T17.510 ☑
        specified type NEC T17.590 ☑
      injury NEC T17.508 ☑
        food (bone) (seed) T17.528 ☑
        gastric contents (vomitus) T17.518 ☑
        specified type NEC T17.598 ☑
  canthus — *see* Foreign body, conjunctival sac
  ciliary body (eye) S05.5- ☑
  conjunctival sac T15.1- ☑
  cornea T15.0- ☑
  entering through orifice
    accessory sinus T17.0 ☑
    alimentary canal T18.9 ☑
      multiple parts T18.8 ☑
      specified part NEC T18.8 ☑

Foreign body — *continued*
  entering through orifice — *continued*
    alveolar process T18.0 ☑
    antrum (Highmore's) T17.0 ☑
    anus T18.5 ☑
    appendix T18.4 ☑
    auditory canal — *see* Foreign body, entering through orifice, ear
    auricle — *see* Foreign body, entering through orifice, ear
    bladder T19.1 ☑
    bronchioles — *see* Foreign body, respiratory tract, specified site NEC
    bronchus (main) — *see* Foreign body, bronchus
    buccal cavity T18.0 ☑
    canthus (inner) — *see* Foreign body, conjunctival sac
    cecum T18.4 ☑
    cervix (canal) (uteri) T19.3 ☑
    colon T18.4 ☑
    conjunctival sac — *see* Foreign body, conjunctival sac
    cornea — *see* Foreign body, cornea
    digestive organ or tract NOS T18.9 ☑
      multiple parts T18.8 ☑
      specified part NEC T18.8 ☑
    duodenum T18.3 ☑
    ear (external) T16.- ☑
    esophagus — *see* Foreign body, esophagus
    eye (external) NOS T15.9- ☑
      conjunctival sac — *see* Foreign body, conjunctival sac
      cornea — *see* Foreign body, cornea
      specified part NEC T15.8- ☑
    eyeball (*see also* Foreign body, entering through orifice, eye, specified part NEC)
      with penetrating wound — *see* Puncture, eyeball
    eyelid (*see also* Foreign body, conjunctival sac)
      with
        laceration — *see* Laceration, eyelid, with foreign body
        puncture — *see* Puncture, eyelid, with foreign body
        superficial injury — *see* Foreign body, superficial, eyelid
    gastrointestinal tract T18.9 ☑
      multiple parts T18.8 ☑
      specified part NEC T18.8 ☑
    genitourinary tract T19.9 ☑
      multiple parts T19.8 ☑
      specified part NEC T19.8 ☑
    globe — *see* Foreign body, entering through orifice, eyeball
    gum T18.0 ☑
    Highmore's antrum T17.0 ☑
    hypopharynx — *see* Foreign body, pharynx
    ileum T18.3 ☑
    intestine (small) T18.3 ☑
      large T18.4 ☑
    lacrimal apparatus (punctum) — *see* Foreign body, entering through orifice, eye, specified part NEC
    large intestine T18.4 ☑
    larynx — *see* Foreign body, larynx
    lung — *see* Foreign body, respiratory tract, specified site NEC
    maxillary sinus T17.0 ☑
    mouth T18.0 ☑
    nasal sinus T17.0 ☑
    nasopharynx — *see* Foreign body, pharynx
    nose (passage) T17.1 ☑
    nostril T17.1 ☑
    oral cavity T18.0 ☑
    palate T18.0 ☑
    penis T19.4 ☑
    pharynx — *see* Foreign body, pharynx
    piriform sinus — *see* Foreign body, pharynx
    rectosigmoid (junction) T18.5 ☑
    rectum T18.5 ☑
    respiratory tract — *see* Foreign body, respiratory tract
    sinus (accessory) (frontal) (maxillary) (nasal) T17.0 ☑
      piriform — *see* Foreign body, pharynx
    small intestine T18.3 ☑

Foreign body — *continued*
  entering through orifice — *continued*
    stomach T18.2 ☑
    suffocation by — *see* Foreign body, by site
    tear ducts or glands — *see* Foreign body, entering through orifice, eye, specified part NEC
    throat — *see* Foreign body, pharynx
    tongue T18.0 ☑
    tonsil, tonsillar (fossa) — *see* Foreign body, pharynx
    trachea — *see* Foreign body, trachea
    ureter T19.8 ☑
    urethra T19.0 ☑
    uterus (any part) T19.3 ☑
    vagina T19.2 ☑
    vulva T19.2 ☑
  esophagus T18.108 ☑
    causing
      injury NEC T18.108 ☑
        food (bone) (seed) T18.128 ☑
        gastric contents (vomitus) T18.118 ☑
        specified type NEC T18.198 ☑
      tracheal compression T18.100 ☑
        food (bone) (seed) T18.120 ☑
        gastric contents (vomitus) T18.110 ☑
        specified type NEC T18.190 ☑
  feeling of, in throat R09.89
  fragment — *see* Retained, foreign body fragments (type of)
  genitourinary tract T19.9 ☑
    bladder T19.1 ☑
    multiple parts T19.8 ☑
    penis T19.4 ☑
    specified site NEC T19.8 ☑
    urethra T19.0 ☑
    uterus T19.3 ☑
      IUD Z97.5
    vagina T19.2 ☑
      contraceptive device Z97.5
    vulva T19.2 ☑
  granuloma (old) (soft tissue) (*see also* Granuloma, foreign body)
    skin L92.3
  in
    laceration — *see* Laceration, by site, with foreign body
    puncture wound — *see* Puncture, by site, with foreign body
    soft tissue (residual) M79.5
  inadvertently left in operation wound — *see* Foreign body, accidentally left during a procedure
  ingestion, ingested NOS T18.9 ☑
  inhalation or inspiration — *see* Foreign body, by site
  internal organ, not entering through a natural orifice — code as specific injury with foreign body
  intraocular S05.5- ☑
    old, retained (nonmagnetic) H44.70- ☑
      anterior chamber H44.71- ☑
      ciliary body H44.72- ☑
      iris H44.72- ☑
      lens H44.73- ☑
      magnetic H44.60- ☑
        anterior chamber H44.61- ☑
        ciliary body H44.62- ☑
        iris H44.62- ☑
        lens H44.63- ☑
        posterior wall H44.64- ☑
        specified site NEC H44.69- ☑
        vitreous body H44.65- ☑
      posterior wall H44.74- ☑
      specified site NEC H44.79- ☑
      vitreous body H44.75- ☑
  iris — *see* Foreign body, intraocular
  lacrimal punctum — *see* Foreign body, entering through orifice, eye, specified part NEC
  larynx T17.308 ☑
    causing
      asphyxiation T17.300 ☑
        food (bone) (seed) T17.320 ☑
        gastric contents (vomitus) T17.310 ☑
        specified type NEC T17.390 ☑
      injury NEC T17.308 ☑
        food (bone) (seed) T17.328 ☑
        gastric contents (vomitus) T17.318 ☑
        specified type NEC T17.398 ☑
  lens — *see* Foreign body, intraocular
  ocular muscle S05.4- ☑

Foreign body — *continued*
  ocular muscle — *continued*
    old, retained — *see* Foreign body, orbit, old
  old or residual
    soft tissue (residual) M79.5
  operation wound, left accidentally — *see* Foreign body, accidentally left during a procedure
  orbit S05.4- ☑
    old, retained H05.5- ☑
  pharynx T17.208 ☑
    causing
      asphyxiation T17.200 ☑
        food (bone) (seed) T17.220 ☑
        gastric contents (vomitus) T17.210 ☑
        specified type NEC T17.290 ☑
      injury NEC T17.208 ☑
        food (bone) (seed) T17.228 ☑
        gastric contents (vomitus) T17.218 ☑
        specified type NEC T17.298 ☑
  respiratory tract T17.908 ☑
    bronchioles — *see* Foreign body, respiratory tract, specified site NEC
    bronchus — *see* Foreign body, bronchus
    causing
      asphyxiation T17.900 ☑
        food (bone) (seed) T17.920 ☑
        gastric contents (vomitus) T17.910 ☑
        specified type NEC T17.990 ☑
      injury NEC T17.908 ☑
        food (bone) (seed) T17.928 ☑
        gastric contents (vomitus) T17.918 ☑
        specified type NEC T17.998 ☑
    larynx — *see* Foreign body, larynx
    lung — *see* Foreign body, respiratory tract, specified site NEC
    multiple parts — *see* Foreign body, respiratory tract, specified site NEC
    nasal sinus T17.0 ☑
    nasopharynx — *see* Foreign body, pharynx
    nose T17.1 ☑
    nostril T17.1 ☑
    pharynx — *see* Foreign body, pharynx
    specified site NEC T17.808 ☑
      causing
        asphyxiation T17.800 ☑
          food (bone) (seed) T17.820 ☑
          gastric contents (vomitus) T17.810 ☑
          specified type NEC T17.890 ☑
        injury NEC T17.808 ☑
          food (bone) (seed) T17.828 ☑
          gastric contents (vomitus) T17.818 ☑
          specified type NEC T17.898 ☑
    throat — *see* Foreign body, pharynx
    trachea — *see* Foreign body, trachea
  retained (old) (nonmagnetic) (in)
    anterior chamber (eye) — *see* Foreign body, intraocular, old, retained, anterior chamber
      magnetic — *see* Foreign body, intraocular, old, retained, magnetic, anterior chamber
    ciliary body — *see* Foreign body, intraocular, old, retained, ciliary body
      magnetic — *see* Foreign body, intraocular, old, retained, magnetic, ciliary body
    eyelid H02.819
      left H02.816
        lower H02.815
        upper H02.814
      right H02.813
        lower H02.812
        upper H02.811
    fragments — *see* Retained, foreign body fragments (type of)
    globe — *see* Foreign body, intraocular, old, retained
      magnetic — *see* Foreign body, intraocular, old, retained, magnetic
    intraocular — *see* Foreign body, intraocular, old, retained
      magnetic — *see* Foreign body, intraocular, old, retained, magnetic
    iris — *see* Foreign body, intraocular, old, retained, iris
      magnetic — *see* Foreign body, intraocular, old, retained, magnetic, iris
    lens — *see* Foreign body, intraocular, old, retained, lens

Foreign body — *continued*
  retained — *continued*
    lens — *see* Foreign body, intraocular, old, retained, lens — *continued*
      magnetic — *see* Foreign body, intraocular, old, retained, magnetic, lens
    muscle — *see* Foreign body, retained, soft tissue
    orbit — *see* Foreign body, orbit, old
    posterior wall of globe — *see* Foreign body, intraocular, old, retained, posterior wall
      magnetic — *see* Foreign body, intraocular, old, retained, magnetic, posterior wall
    retrobulbar — *see* Foreign body, orbit, old, retrobulbar
    soft tissue M79.5
    vitreous — *see* Foreign body, intraocular, old, retained, vitreous body
      magnetic — *see* Foreign body, intraocular, old, retained, magnetic, vitreous body
  retina S05.5- ☑
  superficial, without open wound
    abdomen, abdominal (wall) S30.851 ☑
    alveolar process S00.552 ☑
    ankle S90.55- ☑
    antecubital space — *see* Foreign body, superficial, forearm
    anus S30.857 ☑
    arm (upper) S40.85- ☑
    auditory canal — *see* Foreign body, superficial, ear
    auricle — *see* Foreign body, superficial, ear
    axilla — *see* Foreign body, superficial, arm
    back, lower S30.850 ☑
    breast S20.15- ☑
    brow S00.85 ☑
    buttock S30.850 ☑
    calf — *see* Foreign body, superficial, leg
    canthus — *see* Foreign body, superficial, eyelid
    cheek S00.85 ☑
      internal S00.552 ☑
    chest wall — *see* Foreign body, superficial, thorax
    chin S00.85 ☑
    clitoris S30.854 ☑
    costal region — *see* Foreign body, superficial, thorax
    digit(s)
      foot — *see* Foreign body, superficial, toe
      hand — *see* Foreign body, superficial, finger
    ear S00.45- ☑
    elbow S50.35- ☑
    epididymis S30.853 ☑
    epigastric region S30.851 ☑
    epiglottis S10.15 ☑
    esophagus, cervical S10.15 ☑
    eyebrow — *see* Foreign body, superficial, eyelid
    eyelid S00.25- ☑
    face S00.85 ☑
    finger(s) S60.459 ☑
      index S60.45- ☑
      little S60.45- ☑
      middle S60.45- ☑
      ring S60.45- ☑
    flank S30.851 ☑
    foot (except toe(s) alone) S90.85- ☑
      toe — *see* Foreign body, superficial, toe
    forearm S50.85- ☑
      elbow only — *see* Foreign body, superficial, elbow
    forehead S00.85 ☑
    genital organs, external
      female S30.856 ☑
      male S30.855 ☑
    groin S30.851 ☑
    gum S00.552 ☑
    hand S60.55- ☑
    head S00.95 ☑
      ear — *see* Foreign body, superficial, ear
      eyelid — *see* Foreign body, superficial, eyelid
      lip S00.551 ☑
      nose S00.35 ☑
      oral cavity S00.552 ☑
      scalp S00.05 ☑
      specified site NEC S00.85 ☑
    heel — *see* Foreign body, superficial, foot
    hip S70.25- ☑
    inguinal region S30.851 ☑
    interscapular region S20.459 ☑

☑ **Additional Character Required** — **Refer to the Tabular List for Character Selection**   ▽ Subterms under main terms may continue to next column or page

Foreign body — *continued*
  superficial, without open wound — *continued*
    jaw S00.85 ☑
    knee S80.25- ☑
    labium (majus) (minus) S30.854 ☑
    larynx S10.15 ☑
    leg (lower) S80.85- ☑
      knee — *see* Foreign body, superficial, knee
      upper — *see* Foreign body, superficial, thigh
    lip S00.551 ☑
    lower back S30.850 ☑
    lumbar region S30.850 ☑
    malar region S00.85 ☑
    mammary — *see* Foreign body, superficial, breast
    mastoid region S00.85 ☑
    mouth S00.552 ☑
    nail
      finger — *see* Foreign body, superficial, finger
      toe — *see* Foreign body, superficial, toe
    nape S10.85 ☑
    nasal S00.35 ☑
    neck S10.95 ☑
      specified site NEC S10.85 ☑
      throat S10.15 ☑
    nose S00.35 ☑
    occipital region S00.05 ☑
    oral cavity S00.552 ☑
    orbital region — *see* Foreign body, superficial, eyelid
    palate S00.552 ☑
    palm — *see* Foreign body, superficial, hand
    parietal region S00.05 ☑
    pelvis S30.850 ☑
    penis S30.852 ☑
    perineum
      female S30.854 ☑
      male S30.850 ☑
    periocular area — *see* Foreign body, superficial, eyelid
    phalanges
      finger — *see* Foreign body, superficial, finger
      toe — *see* Foreign body, superficial, toe
    pharynx S10.15 ☑
    pinna — *see* Foreign body, superficial, ear
    popliteal space — *see* Foreign body, superficial, knee
    prepuce S30.852 ☑
    pubic region S30.850 ☑
    pudendum
      female S30.856 ☑
      male S30.855 ☑
    sacral region S30.850 ☑
    scalp S00.05 ☑
    scapular region — *see* Foreign body, superficial, shoulder
    scrotum S30.853 ☑
    shin — *see* Foreign body, superficial, leg
    shoulder S40.25- ☑
    sternal region S20.359 ☑
    submaxillary region S00.85 ☑
    submental region S00.85 ☑
    subungual
      finger(s) — *see* Foreign body, superficial, finger
      toe(s) — *see* Foreign body, superficial, toe
    supraclavicular fossa S10.85 ☑
    supraorbital S00.85 ☑
    temple S00.85 ☑
    temporal region S00.85 ☑
    testis S30.853 ☑
    thigh S70.35- ☑
    thorax, thoracic (wall) S20.95 ☑
      back S20.45- ☑
      front S20.35- ☑
    throat S10.15 ☑
    thumb S60.35- ☑
    toe(s) (lesser) S90.456 ☑
      great S90.45- ☑
    tongue S00.552 ☑
    trachea S10.15 ☑
    tunica vaginalis S30.853 ☑
    tympanum, tympanic membrane — *see* Foreign body, superficial, ear
    uvula S00.552 ☑
    vagina S30.854 ☑
    vocal cords S10.15 ☑
    vulva S30.854 ☑

Foreign body — *continued*
  superficial, without open wound — *continued*
    wrist S60.85- ☑
  swallowed T18.9 ☑
  trachea T17.408 ☑
    causing
      asphyxiation T17.400 ☑
        food (bone) (seed) T17.420 ☑
        gastric contents (vomitus) T17.410 ☑
        specified type NEC T17.490 ☑
      injury NEC T17.408 ☑
        food (bone) (seed) T17.428 ☑
        gastric contents (vomitus) T17.418 ☑
        specified type NEC T17.498 ☑
  type of fragment — *see* Retained, foreign body fragments (type of)
  vitreous (humor) S05.5- ☑

Forestier's disease (rhizomelic pseudopolyarthritis) M35.3
  meaning ankylosing hyperostosis — *see* Hyperostosis, ankylosing

Formation
  hyalin in cornea — *see* Degeneration, cornea
  sequestrum in bone (due to infection) — *see* Osteomyelitis, chronic
  valve
    colon, congenital Q43.8
    ureter (congenital) Q62.39

Formication R20.2
Fort Bragg fever A27.89
Fossa (*see also* condition)
  pyriform — *see* condition
Foster-Kennedy syndrome H47.14- ☑
Fothergill's
  disease (trigeminal neuralgia) (*see also* Neuralgia, trigeminal)
  scarlatina anginosa A38.9
Foul breath R19.6
Foundling Z76.1
Fournier disease or gangrene N49.3
  female N76.89
Fourth
  cranial nerve — *see* condition
  molar K00.1
Foville's (peduncular) **disease or syndrome** G46.3
Fox (-Fordyce) disease (apocrine miliaria) L75.2
Fracture, burst — *see* Fracture, traumatic, by site
Fracture, chronic — *see* Fracture, pathological, by site
Fracture, insufficiency — *see* Fracture, pathological, by site
Fracture, nontraumatic, NEC
  atypical
    femur M84.750- ☑
      complete
        oblique M84.759 ☑
          left side M84.758 ☑
          right side M84.757 ☑
        transverse M84.756 ☑
          left side M84.755 ☑
          right side M84.754 ☑
      incomplete M84.753 ☑
        left side M84.752 ☑
        right side M84.751 ☑
Fracture, pathological (pathologic) (*see also* Fracture, traumatic) M84.40 ☑
  ankle M84.47- ☑
  carpus M84.44- ☑
  clavicle M84.41- ☑
  compression (not due to trauma) (*see also* Collapse, vertebra) M48.50- ☑
  dental implant M27.63
  dental restorative material K08.539
    with loss of material K08.531
    without loss of material K08.530
  due to
    neoplastic disease NEC (*see also* Neoplasm) M84.50 ☑
      ankle M84.57- ☑
      carpus M84.54- ☑
      clavicle M84.51- ☑
      femur M84.55- ☑
      fibula M84.56- ☑
      finger M84.54- ☑
      hip M84.559 ☑
      humerus M84.52- ☑
      ilium M84.550 ☑

Fracture, pathological — *continued*
  due to — *continued*
    neoplastic disease (*see also* Neoplasm) — *continued*
      ischium M84.550 ☑
      metacarpus M84.54- ☑
      metatarsus M84.57- ☑
      neck M84.58 ☑
      pelvis M84.550 ☑
      radius M84.53- ☑
      rib M84.58 ☑
      scapula M84.51- ☑
      skull M84.58 ☑
      specified site NEC M84.58 ☑
      tarsus M84.57- ☑
      tibia M84.56- ☑
      toe M84.57- ☑
      ulna M84.53- ☑
      vertebra M84.58 ☑
    osteoporosis M80.00 ☑
      disuse — *see* Osteoporosis, specified type NEC, with pathological fracture
      drug-induced — *see* Osteoporosis, drug induced, with pathological fracture
      idiopathic — *see* Osteoporosis, specified type NEC, with pathological fracture
      postmenopausal — *see* Osteoporosis, postmenopausal, with pathological fracture
      postoophorectomy — *see* Osteoporosis, postoophorectomy, with pathological fracture
      postsurgical malabsorption — *see* Osteoporosis, specified type NEC, with pathological fracture
      specified cause NEC — *see* Osteoporosis, specified type NEC, with pathological fracture
    specified disease NEC M84.60 ☑
      ankle M84.67- ☑
      carpus M84.64- ☑
      clavicle M84.61- ☑
      femur M84.65- ☑
      fibula M84.66- ☑
      finger M84.64- ☑
      hip M84.65- ☑
      humerus M84.62- ☑
      ilium M84.650 ☑
      ischium M84.650 ☑
      metacarpus M84.64- ☑
      metatarsus M84.67- ☑
      neck M84.68 ☑
      radius M84.63- ☑
      rib M84.68 ☑
      scapula M84.61- ☑
      skull M84.68 ☑
      tarsus M84.67- ☑
      tibia M84.66- ☑
      toe M84.67- ☑
      ulna M84.63- ☑
      vertebra M84.68 ☑
  femur M84.45- ☑
  fibula M84.46- ☑
  finger M84.44- ☑
  hip M84.459 ☑
  humerus M84.42- ☑
  ilium M84.454 ☑
  ischium M84.454 ☑
  joint prosthesis — *see* Complications, joint prosthesis, mechanical, breakdown, by site
    periprosthetic — *see* Fracture, pathological, periprosthetic
  metacarpus M84.44- ☑
  metatarsus M84.47- ☑
  neck M84.48 ☑
  pelvis M84.454 ☑
  periprosthetic M97.9 ☑
    ankle M97.2- ☑
    elbow M97.4- ☑
    finger M97.8 ☑
    hip M97.0- ☑
    knee M97.1- ☑
    other specified joint M97.8 ☑
    shoulder M97.3- ☑
    spinal joint M97.8 ☑
    toe joint M97.8 ☑
    wrist joint M97.8 ☑
  radius M84.43- ☑

▼ Subterms under main terms may continue to next column or page   ☑ Additional Character Required — Refer to the Tabular List for Character Selection   149

Index

Foreign body — Fracture, pathological

Fracture, pathological — *continued*
  restorative material (dental) K08.539
    with loss of material K08.531
    without loss of material K08.530
  rib M84.48 ☑
  scapula M84.41- ☑
  skull M84.48 ☑
  tarsus M84.47- ☑
  tibia M84.46- ☑
  toe M84.47- ☑
  ulna M84.43- ☑
  vertebra M84.48 ☑
Fracture, traumatic (abduction) (adduction) (separation)
  (*see also* Fracture, pathological) T14.8 ☑
  acetabulum S32.40- ☑
    column
      anterior (displaced) (iliopubic) S32.43- ☑
        nondisplaced S32.436
      posterior (displaced) (ilioischial) S32.443 ☑
        nondisplaced S32.44- ☑
    dome (displaced) S32.48- ☑
      nondisplaced S32.48 ☑
    specified NEC S32.49- ☑
    transverse (displaced) S32.45- ☑
      with associated posterior wall fracture (displaced) S32.46- ☑
        nondisplaced S32.46- ☑
      nondisplaced S32.45- ☑
    wall
      anterior (displaced) S32.41- ☑
        nondisplaced S32.41- ☑
      medial (displaced) S32.47- ☑
        nondisplaced S32.47- ☑
      posterior (displaced) S32.42- ☑
        with associated transverse fracture (displaced) S32.46- ☑
        nondisplaced S32.46- ☑
        nondisplaced S32.42- ☑
  acromion — *see* Fracture, scapula, acromial process
  ankle S82.899 ☑
    bimalleolar (displaced) S82.84- ☑
      nondisplaced S82.84- ☑
    lateral malleolus only (displaced) S82.6- ☑
      nondisplaced S82.6- ☑
    medial malleolus (displaced) S82.5- ☑
      associated with Maisonneuve's fracture — *see* Fracture, Maisonneuve's
      nondisplaced S82.5- ☑
    talus — *see* Fracture, tarsal, talus
    trimalleolar (displaced) S82.85- ☑
      nondisplaced S82.85- ☑
  arm (upper) (*see also* Fracture, humerus, shaft)
    humerus — *see* Fracture, humerus
    radius — *see* Fracture, radius
    ulna — *see* Fracture, ulna
  astragalus — *see* Fracture, tarsal, talus
  atlas — *see* Fracture, neck, cervical vertebra, first
  axis — *see* Fracture, neck, cervical vertebra, second
  back — *see* Fracture, vertebra
  Barton's — *see* Barton's fracture
  base of skull — *see* Fracture, skull, base
  basicervical (basal) (femoral) S72.0 ☑
  Bennett's — *see* Bennett's fracture
  bimalleolar — *see* Fracture, ankle, bimalleolar
  blow-out S02.3- ☑
  bone NEC T14.8 ☑
    birth injury P13.9
    following insertion of orthopedic implant, joint prosthesis or bone plate — *see* Fracture, following insertion of orthopedic implant, joint prosthesis or bone plate
    in (due to) neoplastic disease NEC — *see* Fracture, pathological, due to, neoplastic disease
    pathological (cause unknown) — *see* Fracture, pathological
  breast bone — *see* Fracture, sternum
  bucket handle (semilunar cartilage) — *see* Tear, meniscus
  burst — *see* Fracture, traumatic, by site
  calcaneus — *see* Fracture, tarsal, calcaneus
  carpal bone(s) S62.10- ☑
    capitate (displaced) S62.13- ☑
      nondisplaced S62.13- ☑
    cuneiform — *see* Fracture, carpal bone, triquetrum
    hamate (body) (displaced) S62.143 ☑
      hook process (displaced) S62.15- ☑

Fracture, traumatic — *continued*
  carpal bone(s) — *continued*
    hamate — *continued*
      hook process — *continued*
        nondisplaced S62.15- ☑
        nondisplaced S62.14- ☑
    larger multangular — *see* Fracture, carpal bones, trapezium
    lunate (displaced) S62.12- ☑
      nondisplaced S62.12- ☑
    navicular S62.00- ☑
      distal pole (displaced) S62.01- ☑
        nondisplaced S62.01- ☑
      middle third (displaced) S62.02- ☑
        nondisplaced S62.02- ☑
      proximal third (displaced) S62.03- ☑
        nondisplaced S62.03- ☑
      volar tuberosity — *see* Fracture, carpal bones, navicular, distal pole
    os magnum — *see* Fracture, carpal bones, capitate
    pisiform (displaced) S62.16- ☑
      nondisplaced S62.16- ☑
    semilunar — *see* Fracture, carpal bones, lunate
    smaller multangular — *see* Fracture, carpal bones, trapezoid
    trapezium (displaced) S62.17- ☑
      nondisplaced S62.17- ☑
    trapezoid (displaced) S62.18- ☑
      nondisplaced S62.18- ☑
    triquetrum (displaced) S62.11- ☑
      nondisplaced S62.11- ☑
    unciform — *see* Fracture, carpal bones, hamate
  cervical — *see* Fracture, vertebra, cervical
  clavicle S42.00- ☑
    acromial end (displaced) S42.03- ☑
      nondisplaced S42.03- ☑
    birth injury P13.4
    lateral end — *see* Fracture, clavicle, acromial end
    shaft (displaced) S42.02- ☑
      nondisplaced S42.02- ☑
    sternal end (anterior) (displaced) S42.01- ☑
      nondisplaced S42.01- ☑
      posterior S42.01- ☑
  coccyx S32.2 ☑
  collapsed — *see* Collapse, vertebra
  collar bone — *see* Fracture, clavicle
  Colles' — *see* Colles' fracture
  coronoid process — *see* Fracture, ulna, upper end, coronoid process
  corpus cavernosum penis S39.840 ☑
  costochondral cartilage S23.41 ☑
  costochondral, costosternal junction — *see* Fracture, rib
  cranium — *see* Fracture, skull
  cricoid cartilage S12.8 ☑
  cuboid (ankle) — *see* Fracture, tarsal, cuboid
  cuneiform
    foot — *see* Fracture, tarsal, cuneiform
    wrist — *see* Fracture, carpal, triquetrum
  delayed union — *see* Delay, union, fracture
  dental restorative material K08.539
    with loss of material K08.531
    without loss of material K08.530
  due to
    birth injury — *see* Birth, injury, fracture
    osteoporosis — *see* Osteoporosis, with fracture
  Dupuytren's — *see* Fracture, ankle, lateral malleolus
  elbow S42.40- ☑
  ethmoid (bone) (sinus) — *see* Fracture, skull, base
  face bone S02.92 ☑
  fatigue (*see also* Fracture, stress)
    vertebra M48.40 ☑
      cervical region M48.42 ☑
      cervicothoracic region M48.43 ☑
      lumbar region M48.46 ☑
      lumbosacral region M48.47 ☑
      occipito-atlanto-axial region M48.41 ☑
      sacrococcygeal region M48.48 ☑
      thoracic region M48.44 ☑
      thoracolumbar region M48.45 ☑
  femur, femoral S72.9- ☑
    basicervical (basal) S72.0 ☑
    birth injury P13.2
    capital epiphysial S79.01- ☑
    condyles, epicondyles — *see* Fracture, femur, lower end

Fracture, traumatic — *continued*
  femur, femoral — *continued*
    distal end — *see* Fracture, femur, lower end
    epiphysis
      head — *see* Fracture, femur, upper end, epiphysis
      lower — *see* Fracture, femur, lower end, epiphysis
      upper — *see* Fracture, femur, upper end, epiphysis
    following insertion of implant, prosthesis or plate M96.66- ☑
    head — *see* Fracture, femur, upper end, head
    intertrochanteric — *see* Fracture, femur, trochanteric
    intratrochanteric — *see* Fracture, femur, trochanteric
    lower end S72.40- ☑
      condyle (displaced) S72.41- ☑
        lateral (displaced) S72.42- ☑
          nondisplaced S72.42- ☑
        medial (displaced) S72.43- ☑
          nondisplaced S72.43- ☑
        nondisplaced S72.41- ☑
      epiphysis (displaced) S72.44- ☑
        nondisplaced S72.44- ☑
      physeal S79.10- ☑
        Salter-Harris
          Type I S79.11- ☑
          Type II S79.12- ☑
          Type III S79.13- ☑
          Type IV S79.14- ☑
        specified NEC S79.19- ☑
      specified NEC S72.49- ☑
      supracondylar (displaced) S72.45- ☑
        with intracondylar extension (displaced) S72.46- ☑
          nondisplaced S72.46- ☑
        nondisplaced S72.45- ☑
      torus S72.47- ☑
    neck — *see* Fracture, femur, upper end, neck
    pertrochanteric — *see* Fracture, femur, trochanteric
    shaft (lower third) (middle third) (upper third) S72.30- ☑
      comminuted (displaced) S72.35- ☑
        nondisplaced S72.35- ☑
      oblique (displaced) S72.33- ☑
        nondisplaced S72.33- ☑
      segmental (displaced) S72.36- ☑
        nondisplaced S72.36- ☑
      specified NEC S72.39- ☑
      spiral (displaced) S72.34- ☑
        nondisplaced S72.34- ☑
      transverse (displaced) S72.32- ☑
        nondisplaced S72.32- ☑
    specified site NEC — *see* subcategory S72.8 ☑
    subcapital (displaced) S72.01- ☑
    subtrochanteric (region) (section) (displaced) S72.2- ☑
      nondisplaced S72.2- ☑
    transcervical — *see* Fracture, femur, upper end, neck
    transtrochanteric — *see* Fracture, femur, trochanteric
    trochanteric S72.10- ☑
      apophyseal (displaced) S72.13- ☑
        nondisplaced S72.13- ☑
      greater trochanter (displaced) S72.11- ☑
        nondisplaced S72.11- ☑
      intertrochanteric (displaced) S72.14- ☑
        nondisplaced S72.14- ☑
      lesser trochanter (displaced) S72.12- ☑
        nondisplaced S72.12- ☑
    upper end S72.00- ☑
      apophyseal (displaced) S72.13- ☑
        nondisplaced S72.13- ☑
      cervicotrochanteric — *see* Fracture, femur, upper end, neck, base
      epiphysis (displaced) S72.02- ☑
        nondisplaced S72.02- ☑
      head S72.05- ☑
        articular (displaced) S72.06- ☑
          nondisplaced S72.06- ☑
        specified NEC S72.09- ☑
      intertrochanteric (displaced) S72.14- ☑

Fracture, traumatic — *continued*
- femur, femoral — *continued*
  - upper end — *continued*
    - intertrochanteric — *continued*
      - nondisplaced S72.14- ☑
    - intracapsular S72.01- ☑
    - midcervical (displaced) S72.03- ☑
      - nondisplaced S72.03- ☑
    - neck S72.00- ☑
      - base (displaced) S72.04- ☑
        - nondisplaced S72.04- ☑
      - specified NEC S72.09- ☑
    - pertrochanteric — *see* Fracture, femur, upper end, trochanteric
    - physeal S79.00- ☑
      - Salter-Harris type I S79.01- ☑
      - specified NEC S79.09- ☑
    - subcapital (displaced) S72.01- ☑
    - subtrochanteric (displaced) S72.2- ☑
      - nondisplaced S72.2- ☑
    - transcervical — *see* Fracture, femur, upper end, midcervical
    - trochanteric S72.10- ☑
      - greater (displaced) S72.11- ☑
        - nondisplaced S72.11- ☑
      - lesser (displaced) S72.12- ☑
        - nondisplaced S72.12- ☑
- fibula (shaft) (styloid) S82.40- ☑
  - comminuted (displaced) S82.45- ☑
    - nondisplaced S82.45- ☑
  - following insertion of implant, prosthesis or plate M96.67- ☑
  - involving ankle or malleolus — *see* Fracture, fibula, lateral malleolus
  - lateral malleolus (displaced) S82.6- ☑
    - nondisplaced S82.6- ☑
  - lower end
    - physeal S89.30- ☑
      - Salter-Harris
        - Type I S89.31- ☑
        - Type II S89.32- ☑
        - specified NEC S89.39- ☑
      - specified NEC S82.83- ☑
    - torus S82.82- ☑
  - oblique (displaced) S82.43- ☑
    - nondisplaced S82.43- ☑
  - segmental (displaced) S82.46- ☑
    - nondisplaced S82.46- ☑
  - specified NEC S82.49- ☑
  - spiral (displaced) S82.44- ☑
    - nondisplaced S82.44- ☑
  - transverse (displaced) S82.42- ☑
    - nondisplaced S82.42- ☑
  - upper end
    - physeal S89.20- ☑
      - Salter-Harris
        - Type I S89.21- ☑
        - Type II S89.22- ☑
        - specified NEC S89.29- ☑
      - specified NEC S82.83- ☑
    - torus S82.81- ☑
- finger (except thumb) S62.60- ☑
  - distal phalanx (displaced) S62.63- ☑
    - nondisplaced S62.66- ☑
  - index S62.60- ☑
    - distal phalanx (displaced) S62.63- ☑
      - nondisplaced S62.66- ☑
    - medial phalanx (displaced) S62.62- ☑
      - nondisplaced S62.65- ☑
    - proximal phalanx (displaced) S62.61- ☑
      - nondisplaced S62.64- ☑
  - little S62.60- ☑
    - distal phalanx (displaced) S62.63- ☑
      - nondisplaced S62.66- ☑
    - medial phalanx (displaced) S62.62- ☑
      - nondisplaced S62.65- ☑
    - proximal phalanx (displaced) S62.61- ☑
      - nondisplaced S62.64- ☑
  - medial phalanx (displaced) S62.62- ☑
    - nondisplaced S62.65- ☑
  - middle S62.60- ☑
    - distal phalanx (displaced) S62.63- ☑
      - nondisplaced S62.66- ☑
    - medial phalanx (displaced) S62.62- ☑
      - nondisplaced S62.65- ☑
    - proximal phalanx (displaced) S62.61- ☑

Fracture, traumatic — *continued*
- finger — *continued*
  - middle — *continued*
    - proximal phalanx — *continued*
      - nondisplaced S62.64- ☑
    - proximal phalanx (displaced) S62.61- ☑
      - nondisplaced S62.64- ☑
  - ring S62.60- ☑
    - distal phalanx (displaced) S62.63- ☑
      - nondisplaced S62.66- ☑
    - medial phalanx (displaced) S62.62- ☑
      - nondisplaced S62.65- ☑
    - proximal phalanx (displaced) S62.61- ☑
      - nondisplaced S62.64- ☑
  - thumb — *see* Fracture, thumb
- following insertion (intraoperative) (postoperative) of orthopedic implant, joint prosthesis or bone plate M96.69
  - femur M96.66- ☑
  - fibula M96.67- ☑
  - humerus M96.62- ☑
  - pelvis M96.65
  - radius M96.63- ☑
  - specified bone NEC M96.69
  - tibia M96.67- ☑
  - ulna M96.63- ☑
- foot S92.90- ☑
  - astragalus — *see* Fracture, tarsal, talus
  - calcaneus — *see* Fracture, tarsal, calcaneus
  - cuboid — *see* Fracture, tarsal, cuboid
  - cuneiform — *see* Fracture, tarsal, cuneiform
  - metatarsal — *see* Fracture, metatarsal
  - navicular — *see* Fracture, tarsal, navicular
  - sesamoid S92.81- ☑
  - specified NEC S92.81- ☑
  - talus — *see* Fracture, tarsal, talus
  - tarsal — *see* Fracture, tarsal
  - toe — *see* Fracture, toe
- forearm S52.9- ☑
  - radius — *see* Fracture, radius
  - ulna — *see* Fracture, ulna
- fossa (anterior) (middle) (posterior) S02.19 ☑
- frontal (bone) (skull) S02.0 ☑
  - sinus S02.19
- glenoid (cavity) (scapula) — *see* Fracture, scapula, glenoid cavity
- greenstick — *see* Fracture, by site
- hallux — *see* Fracture, toe, great
- hand S62.9- ☑
  - carpal — *see* Fracture, carpal bone
  - finger (except thumb) — *see* Fracture, finger
  - metacarpal — *see* Fracture, metacarpal
  - navicular (scaphoid) (hand) — *see* Fracture, carpal bone, navicular
  - thumb — *see* Fracture, thumb
- healed or old
  - with complications — *code by* Nature of the complication
- heel bone — *see* Fracture, tarsal, calcaneus
- Hill-Sachs S42.29- ☑
- hip — *see* Fracture, femur, neck
- humerus S42.30- ☑
  - anatomical neck — *see* Fracture, humerus, upper end
  - articular process — *see* Fracture, humerus, lower end
  - capitellum — *see* Fracture, humerus, lower end, condyle, lateral
  - distal end — *see* Fracture, humerus, lower end
  - epiphysis
    - lower — *see* Fracture, humerus, lower end, physeal
    - upper — *see* Fracture, humerus, upper end, physeal
  - external condyle — *see* Fracture, humerus, lower end, condyle, lateral
  - following insertion of implant, prosthesis or plate M96.62- ☑
  - great tuberosity — *see* Fracture, humerus, upper end, greater tuberosity
  - intercondylar — *see* Fracture, humerus, lower end
  - internal epicondyle — *see* Fracture, humerus, lower end, epicondyle, medial
  - lesser tuberosity — *see* Fracture, humerus, upper end, lesser tuberosity
  - lower end S42.40- ☑

Fracture, traumatic — *continued*
- humerus — *continued*
  - lower end — *continued*
    - condyle
      - lateral (displaced) S42.45- ☑
        - nondisplaced S42.45- ☑
      - medial (displaced) S42.46- ☑
        - nondisplaced S42.46- ☑
    - epicondyle
      - lateral (displaced) S42.43- ☑
        - nondisplaced S42.43- ☑
      - medial (displaced) S42.44- ☑
        - incarcerated S42.44- ☑
        - nondisplaced S42.44- ☑
    - physeal S49.10- ☑
      - Salter-Harris
        - Type I S49.11- ☑
        - Type II S49.12- ☑
        - Type III S49.13- ☑
        - Type IV S49.14- ☑
        - specified NEC S49.19- ☑
    - specified NEC (displaced) S42.49- ☑
      - nondisplaced S42.49- ☑
    - supracondylar (simple) (displaced) S42.41- ☑
      - with intercondylar fracture — *see* Fracture, humerus, lower end
      - comminuted (displaced) S42.42- ☑
        - nondisplaced S42.42- ☑
      - nondisplaced S42.41- ☑
    - torus S42.48- ☑
    - transcondylar (displaced) S42.47- ☑
      - nondisplaced S42.47- ☑
  - proximal end — *see* Fracture, humerus, upper end
  - shaft S42.30- ☑
    - comminuted (displaced) S42.35- ☑
      - nondisplaced S42.35- ☑
    - greenstick S42.31- ☑
    - oblique (displaced) S42.33- ☑
      - nondisplaced S42.33- ☑
    - segmental (displaced) S42.36- ☑
      - nondisplaced S42.36- ☑
    - specified NEC S42.39- ☑
    - spiral (displaced) S42.34- ☑
      - nondisplaced S42.34- ☑
    - transverse (displaced) S42.32- ☑
      - nondisplaced S42.32- ☑
  - supracondylar — *see* Fracture, humerus, lower end
  - surgical neck — *see* Fracture, humerus, upper end, surgical neck
  - trochlea — *see* Fracture, humerus, lower end, condyle, medial
  - tuberosity — *see* Fracture, humerus, upper end
  - upper end S42.20- ☑
    - anatomical neck — *see* Fracture, humerus, upper end, specified NEC
    - articular head — *see* Fracture, humerus, upper end, specified NEC
    - epiphysis — *see* Fracture, humerus, upper end, physeal
    - greater tuberosity (displaced) S42.25- ☑
      - nondisplaced S42.25- ☑
    - lesser tuberosity (displaced) S42.26- ☑
      - nondisplaced S42.26- ☑
    - physeal S49.00- ☑
      - Salter-Harris
        - Type I S49.01- ☑
        - Type II S49.02- ☑
        - Type III S49.03- ☑
        - Type IV S49.04- ☑
        - specified NEC S49.09- ☑
    - specified NEC (displaced) S42.29- ☑
      - nondisplaced S42.29- ☑
    - surgical neck (displaced) S42.21- ☑
      - four-part S42.24- ☑
      - nondisplaced S42.21- ☑
      - three-part S42.23- ☑
      - two-part (displaced) S42.22- ☑
        - nondisplaced S42.22- ☑
    - torus S42.27- ☑
    - transepiphyseal — *see* Fracture, humerus, upper end, physeal
- hyoid bone S12.8 ☑
- ilium S32.30- ☑
  - with disruption of pelvic ring — *see* Disruption, pelvic ring
  - avulsion (displaced) S32.31- ☑

▼ **Subterms under main terms may continue to next column or page**   ☑ **Additional Character Required — Refer to the Tabular List for Character Selection**   **151**

Fracture, traumatic — Fracture, traumatic

Fracture, traumatic — *continued*
ilium — *continued*
  avulsion — *continued*
    nondisplaced S32.31- ☑
    specified NEC S32.39- ☑
  impaction, impacted — *code as* Fracture, by site
innominate bone — *see* Fracture, ilium
instep — *see* Fracture, foot
ischium S32.60- ☑
  with disruption of pelvic ring — *see* Disruption,
    pelvic ring
  avulsion (displaced) S32.61- ☑
    nondisplaced S32.61- ☑
  specified NEC S32.69- ☑
jaw (bone) (lower) — *see* Fracture, mandible
  upper — *see* Fracture, maxilla
joint prosthesis — *see* Complications, joint prosthesis,
  mechanical, breakdown, by site
  periprosthetic — *see* Fracture, traumatic,
    periprosthetic
knee cap — *see* Fracture, patella
larynx S12.8 ☑
late effects — *see* Sequelae, fracture
leg (lower) S82.9- ☑
  ankle — *see* Fracture, ankle
  femur — *see* Fracture, femur
  fibula — *see* Fracture, fibula
  malleolus — *see* Fracture, ankle
  patella — *see* Fracture, patella
  specified site NEC S82.89- ☑
  tibia — *see* Fracture, tibia
lumbar spine — *see* Fracture, vertebra, lumbar
lumbosacral spine S32.9 ☑
Maisonneuve's (displaced) S82.86- ☑
  nondisplaced S82.86- ☑
malar bone (*see also* Fracture, maxilla) S02.40Ø ☑
  left side S02.40B ☑
  right side S02.40A ☑
malleolus — *see* Fracture, ankle
malunion — *see* Fracture, by site
mandible (lower jaw (bone)) S02.609 ☑
  alveolus S02.67- ☑
  angle (of jaw) S02.65- ☑
  body, unspecified S02.600 ☑
    left side S02.602 ☑
    right side S02.601 ☑
  condylar process S02.61- ☑
  coronoid process S02.63- ☑
  ramus, unspecified S02.64- ☑
  specified site NEC S02.69 ☑
  subcondylar process S02.62- ☑
  symphysis S02.66 ☑
manubrium (sterni) S22.21 ☑
  dissociation from sternum S22.23 ☑
march — *see* Fracture, traumatic, stress, by site
maxilla, maxillary (bone) (sinus) (superior) (upper jaw)
    S02.401 ☑
  alveolus S02.42 ☑
  inferior — *see* Fracture, mandible
  LeFort I S02.411 ☑
  LeFort II S02.412 ☑
  LeFort III S02.413 ☑
  left side S02.40D ☑
  right side S02.40C ☑
metacarpal S62.309 ☑
  base (displaced) S62.319 ☑
    nondisplaced S62.349 ☑
  fifth S62.30- ☑
    base (displaced) S62.31- ☑
      nondisplaced S62.34- ☑
    neck (displaced) S62.33- ☑
      nondisplaced S62.36- ☑
    shaft (displaced) S62.32- ☑
      nondisplaced S62.35- ☑
    specified NEC S62.398 ☑
  first S62.20- ☑
    base NEC (displaced) S62.23- ☑
      nondisplaced S62.23- ☑
    Bennett's — *see* Bennett's fracture
    neck (displaced) S62.25- ☑
      nondisplaced S62.25- ☑
    shaft (displaced) S62.24- ☑
      nondisplaced S62.24- ☑
    specified NEC S62.29- ☑
  fourth S62.30- ☑
    base (displaced) S62.31- ☑

Fracture, traumatic — *continued*
metacarpal — *continued*
  fourth — *continued*
    base — *continued*
      nondisplaced S62.34- ☑
    neck (displaced) S62.33- ☑
      nondisplaced S62.36- ☑
    shaft (displaced) S62.32- ☑
      nondisplaced S62.35- ☑
    specified NEC S62.39- ☑
  neck (displaced) S62.33- ☑
    nondisplaced S62.36- ☑
  Rolando's — *see* Rolando's fracture
  second S62.30- ☑
    base (displaced) S62.31- ☑
      nondisplaced S62.34- ☑
    neck (displaced) S62.33- ☑
      nondisplaced S62.36- ☑
    shaft (displaced) S62.32- ☑
      nondisplaced S62.35- ☑
    specified NEC S62.39- ☑
  shaft (displaced) S62.32- ☑
    nondisplaced S62.35- ☑
  specified NEC S62.399 ☑
  third S62.30- ☑
    base (displaced) S62.31- ☑
      nondisplaced S62.34- ☑
    neck (displaced) S62.33- ☑
      nondisplaced S62.36- ☑
    shaft (displaced) S62.32- ☑
      nondisplaced S62.35- ☑
    specified NEC S62.39- ☑
metastatic — *see* Fracture, pathological, due to, neoplastic disease (*see also* Neoplasm)
metatarsal bone S92.30- ☑
  fifth (displaced) S92.35- ☑
    nondisplaced S92.35- ☑
  first (displaced) S92.31- ☑
    nondisplaced S92.31- ☑
  fourth (displaced) S92.34- ☑
    nondisplaced S92.34- ☑
  physeal S99.10- ☑
    Salter-Harris
      Type I S99.11- ☑
      Type II S99.12- ☑
      Type III S99.13- ☑
      Type IV S99.14- ☑
    specified NEC S99.19- ☑
  second (displaced) S92.32- ☑
    nondisplaced S92.32- ☑
  third (displaced) S92.33- ☑
    nondisplaced S92.33- ☑
Monteggia's — *see* Monteggia's fracture
multiple
  hand (and wrist) NEC — *see* Fracture, by site
  ribs — *see* Fracture, rib, multiple
nasal (bone(s)) S02.2 ☑
navicular (scaphoid) (foot) (*see also* Fracture, tarsal,
  navicular)
  hand — *see* Fracture, carpal, navicular
neck S12.9 ☑
  cervical vertebra S12.9 ☑
    fifth (displaced) S12.400 ☑
      nondisplaced S12.401 ☑
      specified type NEC (displaced) S12.490 ☑
        nondisplaced S12.491 ☑
    first (displaced) S12.000 ☑
      burst (stable) S12.01 ☑
        unstable S12.02 ☑
      lateral mass (displaced) S12.040 ☑
        nondisplaced S12.041 ☑
      nondisplaced S12.001 ☑
      posterior arch (displaced) S12.030 ☑
        nondisplaced S12.031 ☑
      specified type NEC (displaced) S12.090 ☑
        nondisplaced S12.091 ☑
    fourth (displaced) S12.300 ☑
      nondisplaced S12.301 ☑
      specified type NEC (displaced) S12.390 ☑
        nondisplaced S12.391 ☑
    second (displaced) S12.100 ☑
      dens (anterior) (displaced) (type II)
        S12.110 ☑
        nondisplaced S12.112 ☑
        posterior S12.111 ☑

Fracture, traumatic — *continued*
neck — *continued*
  cervical vertebra — *continued*
    second — *continued*
      dens — *continued*
        specified type NEC (displaced)
          S12.120 ☑
          nondisplaced S12.121 ☑
      nondisplaced S12.101 ☑
      specified type NEC (displaced) S12.190 ☑
        nondisplaced S12.191 ☑
    seventh (displaced) S12.600 ☑
      nondisplaced S12.601 ☑
      specified type NEC (displaced) S12.690 ☑
        nondisplaced S12.691 ☑
    sixth (displaced) S12.500 ☑
      nondisplaced S12.501 ☑
      specified type NEC (displaced) S12.590 ☑
        nondisplaced S12.591 ☑
    third (displaced) S12.200 ☑
      nondisplaced S12.201 ☑
      specified type NEC (displaced) S12.290 ☑
        nondisplaced S12.291 ☑
  hyoid bone S12.8 ☑
  larynx S12.8 ☑
  specified site NEC S12.8 ☑
  thyroid cartilage S12.8 ☑
  trachea S12.8 ☑
neoplastic NEC — *see* Fracture, pathological, due to,
  neoplastic disease
neural arch — *see* Fracture, vertebra
newborn — *see* Birth, injury, fracture
nontraumatic — *see* Fracture, pathological
nonunion — *see* Nonunion, fracture
nose, nasal (bone) (septum) S02.2 ☑
occiput — *see* Fracture, skull, base, occiput
odontoid process — *see* Fracture, neck, cervical vertebra, second
olecranon (process) (ulna) — *see* Fracture, ulna, upper
  end, olecranon process
orbit, orbital (bone) (region) S02.8- ☑
  floor (blow-out) S02.3- ☑
  roof S02.19 ☑
os
  calcis — *see* Fracture, tarsal, calcaneus
  magnum — *see* Fracture, carpal, capitate
  pubis — *see* Fracture, pubis
palate S02.8- ☑
parietal bone (skull) S02.0 ☑
patella S82.00- ☑
  comminuted (displaced) S82.04- ☑
    nondisplaced S82.04- ☑
  longitudinal (displaced) S82.02- ☑
    nondisplaced S82.02- ☑
  osteochondral (displaced) S82.01- ☑
    nondisplaced S82.01- ☑
  specified NEC S82.09- ☑
  transverse (displaced) S82.03- ☑
    nondisplaced S82.03- ☑
pedicle (of vertebral arch) — *see* Fracture, vertebra
pelvis, pelvic (bone) S32.9 ☑
  acetabulum — *see* Fracture, acetabulum
  circle — *see* Disruption, pelvic ring
  following insertion of implant, prosthesis or plate
    M96.65
  ilium — *see* Fracture, ilium
  ischium — *see* Fracture, ischium
  multiple
    with disruption of pelvic ring (circle) — *see*
      Disruption, pelvic ring
    without disruption of pelvic ring (circle)
      S32.82 ☑
  pubis — *see* Fracture, pubis
  sacrum — *see* Fracture, sacrum
  specified site NEC S32.89 ☑
periprosthetic, around internal prosthetic joint
  M97.9
  ankle M97.2- ☑
  elbow M97.4- ☑
  finger M97.8 ☑
  hip M97.0- ☑
  knee M97.1- ☑
  shoulder M97.3- ☑
  specified joint NEC M97.8 ☑
  spine M97.8 ☑
  toe M97.8 ☑

Fracture, traumatic — *continued*
- periprosthetic, around internal prosthetic joint — *continued*
  - wrist M97.8 ☑
- phalanx
  - foot — *see* Fracture, toe
  - hand — *see* Fracture, finger
- pisiform — *see* Fracture, carpal, pisiform
- pond — *see* Fracture, skull
- prosthetic device, internal — *see* Complications, prosthetic device, by site, mechanical
- pubis S32.50- ☑
  - with disruption of pelvic ring — *see* Disruption, pelvic ring
  - specified site NEC S32.59- ☑
  - superior rim S32.51- ☑
- radius S52.9- ☑
  - distal end — *see* Fracture, radius, lower end
  - following insertion of implant, prosthesis or plate M96.63- ☑
  - head — *see* Fracture, radius, upper end, head
  - lower end S52.50- ☑
    - Barton's — *see* Barton's fracture
    - Colles' — *see* Colles' fracture
    - extraarticular NEC S52.55- ☑
    - intraarticular NEC S52.57- ☑
    - physeal S59.20- ☑
      - Salter-Harris
        - Type I S59.21- ☑
        - Type II S59.22- ☑
        - Type III S59.23- ☑
        - Type IV S59.24- ☑
        - specified NEC S59.29- ☑
    - Smith's — *see* Smith's fracture
    - specified NEC S52.59- ☑
    - styloid process (displaced) S52.51- ☑
      - nondisplaced S52.51- ☑
    - torus S52.52- ☑
  - neck — *see* Fracture, radius, upper end
  - proximal end — *see* Fracture, radius, upper end
  - shaft S52.30- ☑
    - bent bone S52.38- ☑
    - comminuted (displaced) S52.35- ☑
      - nondisplaced S52.35- ☑
    - Galeazzi's — *see* Galeazzi's fracture
    - greenstick S52.31- ☑
    - oblique (displaced) S52.33- ☑
      - nondisplaced S52.33- ☑
    - segmental (displaced) S52.36- ☑
      - nondisplaced S52.36- ☑
    - specified NEC S52.39- ☑
    - spiral (displaced) S52.34- ☑
      - nondisplaced S52.34- ☑
    - transverse (displaced) S52.32- ☑
      - nondisplaced S52.32- ☑
  - upper end S52.10- ☑
    - head (displaced) S52.12- ☑
      - nondisplaced S52.12- ☑
    - neck (displaced) S52.13- ☑
      - nondisplaced S52.13- ☑
    - physeal S59.10- ☑
      - Salter-Harris
        - Type I S59.11- ☑
        - Type II S59.12- ☑
        - Type III S59.13- ☑
        - Type IV S59.14- ☑
        - specified NEC S59.19- ☑
    - specified NEC S52.18- ☑
    - torus S52.11- ☑
- ramus
  - inferior or superior, pubis — *see* Fracture, pubis
  - mandible — *see* Fracture, mandible
- restorative material (dental) K08.539
  - with loss of material K08.531
  - without loss of material K08.530
- rib S22.3- ☑
  - with flail chest — *see* Flail, chest
  - multiple S22.4- ☑
    - with flail chest — *see* Flail, chest
- root, tooth — *see* Fracture, tooth
- sacrum S32.10- ☑
  - specified NEC S32.19 ☑
  - Type
    - 1 S32.14 ☑
    - 2 S32.15 ☑
    - 3 S32.16 ☑

Fracture, traumatic — *continued*
- sacrum — *continued*
  - Type — *continued*
    - 4 S32.17 ☑
  - Zone
    - I S32.119 ☑
      - displaced (minimally) S32.111 ☑
        - severely S32.112 ☑
      - nondisplaced S32.110 ☑
    - II S32.129 ☑
      - displaced (minimally) S32.121 ☑
        - severely S32.122 ☑
      - nondisplaced S32.120 ☑
    - III S32.139 ☑
      - displaced (minimally) S32.131 ☑
        - severely S32.132 ☑
      - nondisplaced S32.130 ☑
- scaphoid (hand) (*see also* Fracture, carpal, navicular)
  - foot — *see* Fracture, tarsal, navicular
- scapula S42.10- ☑
  - acromial process (displaced) S42.12- ☑
    - nondisplaced S42.12- ☑
  - body (displaced) S42.11- ☑
    - nondisplaced S42.11- ☑
  - coracoid process (displaced) S42.13- ☑
    - nondisplaced S42.13- ☑
  - glenoid cavity (displaced) S42.14- ☑
    - nondisplaced S42.14- ☑
  - neck (displaced) S42.15- ☑
    - nondisplaced S42.15- ☑
  - specified NEC S42.19- ☑
- semilunar bone, wrist — *see* Fracture, carpal, lunate
- sequelae — *see* Sequelae, fracture
- sesamoid bone
  - foot S92.81- ☑
  - hand — *see* Fracture, carpal
  - other — *see* Fracture, traumatic, by site
- shepherd's — *see* Fracture, tarsal, talus
- shoulder (girdle) S42.9- ☑
  - blade — *see* Fracture, scapula
- sinus (ethmoid) (frontal) S02.19 ☑
- skull S02.91 ☑
  - base S02.10- ☑
    - occiput S02.119 ☑
      - condyle S02.113 ☑
        - specified NEC S02.118 ☑
          - left side S02.11H ☑
          - right side S02.11G ☑
        - type I S02.110 ☑
          - left side S02.11B ☑
          - right side S02.11A ☑
        - type II S02.111 ☑
          - left side S02.11D ☑
          - right side S02.11C ☑
        - type III S02.112 ☑
          - left side S02.11F ☑
          - right side S02.11E ☑
      - specified NEC S02.19 ☑
  - birth injury P13.0
  - frontal bone S02.0 ☑
  - parietal bone S02.0 ☑
  - specified site NEC S02.8- ☑
  - temporal bone S02.19 ☑
  - vault S02.0 ☑
- Smith's — *see* Smith's fracture
- sphenoid (bone) (sinus) S02.19 ☑
- spine — *see* Fracture, vertebra
- spinous process — *see* Fracture, vertebra
- spontaneous (cause unknown) — *see* Fracture, pathological
- stave (of thumb) — *see* Fracture, metacarpal, first
- sternum S22.20 ☑
  - with flail chest — *see* Flail, chest
  - body S22.22 ☑
  - manubrium S22.21 ☑
  - xiphoid (process) S22.24 ☑
- stress M84.30 ☑
  - ankle M84.37- ☑
  - carpus M84.34- ☑
  - clavicle M84.31- ☑
  - femoral neck M84.359 ☑
  - femur M84.35- ☑
  - fibula M84.36- ☑
  - finger M84.34- ☑
  - hip M84.359 ☑
  - humerus M84.32- ☑

Fracture, traumatic — *continued*
- stress — *continued*
  - ilium M84.350 ☑
  - ischium M84.350 ☑
  - metacarpus M84.34- ☑
  - metatarsus M84.37- ☑
  - neck — *see* Fracture, fatigue, vertebra
  - pelvis M84.350 ☑
  - radius M84.33- ☑
  - rib M84.38 ☑
  - scapula M84.31- ☑
  - skull M84.38 ☑
  - tarsus M84.37- ☑
  - tibia M84.36- ☑
  - toe M84.37- ☑
  - ulna M84.33- ☑
  - vertebra — *see* Fracture, fatigue, vertebra
- supracondylar, elbow — *see* Fracture, humerus, lower end, supracondylar
- symphysis pubis — *see* Fracture, pubis
- talus (ankle bone) — *see* Fracture, tarsal, talus
- tarsal bone(s) S92.20- ☑
  - astragalus — *see* Fracture, tarsal, talus
  - calcaneus S92.00- ☑
    - anterior process (displaced) S92.02- ☑
      - nondisplaced S92.02- ☑
    - body (displaced) S92.01- ☑
      - nondisplaced S92.01- ☑
    - extraarticular NEC (displaced) S92.05- ☑
      - nondisplaced S92.05- ☑
    - intraarticular (displaced) S92.06- ☑
      - nondisplaced S92.06- ☑
    - physeal S99.00- ☑
      - Salter-Harris
        - Type I S99.01- ☑
        - Type II S99.02- ☑
        - Type III S99.03- ☑
        - Type IV S99.04- ☑
        - specified NEC S99.09- ☑
    - tuberosity (displaced) S92.04- ☑
      - avulsion (displaced) S92.03- ☑
        - nondisplaced S92.03- ☑
      - nondisplaced S92.04- ☑
  - cuboid (displaced) S92.21- ☑
    - nondisplaced S92.21- ☑
  - cuneiform
    - intermediate (displaced) S92.23- ☑
      - nondisplaced S92.23- ☑
    - lateral (displaced) S92.22- ☑
      - nondisplaced S92.22- ☑
    - medial (displaced) S92.24- ☑
      - nondisplaced S92.24- ☑
  - navicular (displaced) S92.25- ☑
    - nondisplaced S92.25- ☑
  - scaphoid — *see* Fracture, tarsal, navicular
  - talus S92.10- ☑
    - avulsion (displaced) S92.15- ☑
      - nondisplaced S92.15- ☑
    - body (displaced) S92.12- ☑
      - nondisplaced S92.12- ☑
    - dome (displaced) S92.14- ☑
      - nondisplaced S92.14- ☑
    - head (displaced) S92.12- ☑
      - nondisplaced S92.12- ☑
    - lateral process (displaced) S92.14- ☑
      - nondisplaced S92.14- ☑
    - neck (displaced) S92.11- ☑
      - nondisplaced S92.11- ☑
    - posterior process (displaced) S92.13- ☑
      - nondisplaced S92.13- ☑
    - specified NEC S92.19- ☑
- temporal bone (styloid) S02.19 ☑
- thorax (bony) S22.9 ☑
  - with flail chest — *see* Flail, chest
  - rib S22.3- ☑
    - multiple S22.4- ☑
      - with flail chest — *see* Flail, chest
  - sternum S22.20 ☑
    - body S22.22 ☑
    - manubrium S22.21 ☑
    - xiphoid process S22.24 ☑
  - vertebra (displaced) S22.009 ☑
    - burst (stable) S22.001
      - unstable S22.002 ☑
    - eighth S22.069 ☑
      - burst (stable) S22.061

▽ Subterms under main terms may continue to next column or page   ☑ Additional Character Required — Refer to the Tabular List for Character Selection   153

Fracture, traumatic — Fracture, traumatic

Fracture, traumatic — *continued*
thorax — *continued*
  vertebra — *continued*
    eighth — *continued*
      burst — *continued*
        unstable S22.062 ✓
      specified type NEC S22.068 ✓
      wedge compression S22.060 ✓
    eleventh S22.089 ✓
      burst (stable) S22.081 ✓
        unstable S22.082 ✓
      specified type NEC S22.088 ✓
      wedge compression S22.080 ✓
    fifth S22.059 ✓
      burst (stable) S22.051 ✓
        unstable S22.052 ✓
      specified type NEC S22.058 ✓
      wedge compression S22.050 ✓
    first S22.019 ✓
      burst (stable) S22.011 ✓
        unstable S22.012 ✓
      specified type NEC S22.018 ✓
      wedge compression S22.010 ✓
    fourth S22.049 ✓
      burst (stable) S22.041 ✓
        unstable S22.042 ✓
      specified type NEC S22.048 ✓
      wedge compression S22.040 ✓
    ninth S22.079 ✓
      burst (stable) S22.071 ✓
        unstable S22.072 ✓
      specified type NEC S22.078 ✓
      wedge compression S22.070 ✓
    nondisplaced S22.001 ✓
    second S22.029 ✓
      burst (stable) S22.021 ✓
        unstable S22.022 ✓
      specified type NEC S22.028 ✓
      wedge compression S22.020 ✓
    seventh S22.069 ✓
      burst (stable) S22.061 ✓
        unstable S22.062 ✓
      specified type NEC S22.068 ✓
      wedge compression S22.060 ✓
    sixth S22.059 ✓
      burst (stable) S22.051 ✓
        unstable S22.052 ✓
      specified type NEC S22.058 ✓
      wedge compression S22.050 ✓
    specified type NEC S22.008 ✓
    tenth S22.079 ✓
      burst (stable) S22.071 ✓
        unstable S22.072 ✓
      specified type NEC S22.078 ✓
      wedge compression S22.070 ✓
    third S22.039 ✓
      burst (stable) S22.031 ✓
        unstable S22.032 ✓
      specified type NEC S22.038 ✓
      wedge compression S22.030 ✓
    twelfth S22.089 ✓
      burst (stable) S22.081 ✓
        unstable S22.082 ✓
      specified type NEC S22.088 ✓
      wedge compression S22.080 ✓
    wedge compression S22.000 ✓
  thumb S62.50- ✓
    distal phalanx (displaced) S62.52- ✓
    nondisplaced S62.52- ✓
    proximal phalanx (displaced) S62.51- ✓
    nondisplaced S62.51- ✓
  thyroid cartilage S12.8 ✓
  tibia (shaft) S82.20- ✓
    comminuted (displaced) S82.25- ✓
    nondisplaced S82.25- ✓
    condyles — *see* Fracture, tibia, upper end
    distal end — *see* Fracture, tibia, lower end
    epiphysis
      lower — *see* Fracture, tibia, lower end
      upper — *see* Fracture, tibia, upper end
    following insertion of implant, prosthesis or plate
      M96.67- ✓
    head (involving knee joint) — *see* Fracture, tibia,
      upper end
    intercondyloid eminence — *see* Fracture, tibia,
      upper end

Fracture, traumatic — *continued*
tibia — *continued*
  involving ankle or malleolus — *see* Fracture, ankle,
    medial malleolus
  lower end S82.30- ✓
    physeal S89.10- ✓
      Salter-Harris
        Type I S89.11- ✓
        Type II S89.12- ✓
        Type III S89.13- ✓
        Type IV S89.14- ✓
      specified NEC S89.19- ✓
    pilon (displaced) S82.87- ✓
      nondisplaced S82.87- ✓
    specified NEC S82.39- ✓
    torus S82.31- ✓
  malleolus — *see* Fracture, ankle, medial malleolus
  oblique (displaced) S82.23- ✓
    nondisplaced S82.23- ✓
  pilon — *see* Fracture, tibia, lower end, pilon
  proximal end — *see* Fracture, tibia, upper end
  segmental (displaced) S82.26- ✓
    nondisplaced S82.26- ✓
  specified NEC S82.29- ✓
  spine — *see* Fracture, tibia, upper end, spine
  spiral (displaced) S82.24- ✓
    nondisplaced S82.24- ✓
  transverse (displaced) S82.22- ✓
    nondisplaced S82.22- ✓
  tuberosity — *see* Fracture, tibia, upper end,
    tuberosity
  upper end S82.10- ✓
    bicondylar (displaced) S82.14- ✓
      nondisplaced S82.14- ✓
    lateral condyle (displaced) S82.12- ✓
      nondisplaced S82.12- ✓
    medial condyle (displaced) S82.13- ✓
      nondisplaced S82.13- ✓
    physeal S89.00- ✓
      Salter-Harris
        Type I S89.01- ✓
        Type II S89.02- ✓
        Type III S89.03- ✓
        Type IV S89.04- ✓
      specified NEC S89.09- ✓
    plateau — *see* Fracture, tibia, upper end, bi-
      condylar
    specified NEC S82.19- ✓
    spine (displaced) S82.11- ✓
      nondisplaced S82.11- ✓
    torus S82.16- ✓
    tuberosity (displaced) S82.15- ✓
      nondisplaced S82.15- ✓
  toe S92.91- ✓
    great (displaced) S92.40- ✓
      distal phalanx (displaced) S92.42- ✓
        nondisplaced S92.42- ✓
      nondisplaced S92.40- ✓
      proximal phalanx (displaced) S92.41- ✓
        nondisplaced S92.41- ✓
      specified NEC S92.49- ✓
    lesser (displaced) S92.50- ✓
      distal phalanx (displaced) S92.53- ✓
        nondisplaced S92.53- ✓
      medial phalanx (displaced) S92.52- ✓
        nondisplaced S92.52- ✓
      nondisplaced S92.50- ✓
      proximal phalanx (displaced) S92.51- ✓
        nondisplaced S92.51- ✓
      specified NEC S92.59- ✓
    physeal
      phalanx S99.20- ✓
        Salter-Harris
          Type I S99.21- ✓
          Type II S99.22- ✓
          Type III S99.23- ✓
          Type IV S99.24- ✓
        specified NEC S99.29- ✓
  tooth (root) S02.5 ✓
  trachea (cartilage) S12.8 ✓
  transverse process — *see* Fracture, vertebra
  trapezium or trapezoid bone — *see* Fracture, carpal
  trimalleolar — *see* Fracture, ankle, trimalleolar
  triquetrum (cuneiform of carpus) — *see* Fracture,
    carpal, triquetrum
  trochanter — *see* Fracture, femur, trochanteric

Fracture, traumatic — *continued*
tuberosity (external) — *see* Fracture, traumatic, by site
ulna (shaft) S52.20- ✓
  bent bone S52.28- ✓
  coronoid process — *see* Fracture, ulna, upper end,
    coronoid process
  distal end — *see* Fracture, ulna, lower end
  following insertion of implant, prosthesis or plate
    M96.63- ✓
  head S52.60- ✓
  lower end S52.60- ✓
    physeal S59.00- ✓
      Salter-Harris
        Type I S59.01- ✓
        Type II S59.02- ✓
        Type III S59.03- ✓
        Type IV S59.04- ✓
      specified NEC S59.09- ✓
    specified NEC S52.69- ✓
    styloid process (displaced) S52.61- ✓
      nondisplaced S52.61- ✓
    torus S52.62- ✓
  proximal end — *see* Fracture, ulna, upper end
  shaft S52.20- ✓
    comminuted (displaced) S52.25- ✓
      nondisplaced S52.25- ✓
    greenstick S52.21- ✓
    Monteggia's — *see* Monteggia's fracture
    oblique (displaced) S52.23- ✓
      nondisplaced S52.23- ✓
    segmental (displaced) S52.26- ✓
      nondisplaced S52.26- ✓
    specified NEC S52.29- ✓
    spiral (displaced) S52.24- ✓
      nondisplaced S52.24- ✓
    transverse (displaced) S52.22- ✓
      nondisplaced S52.22- ✓
  upper end S52.00- ✓
    coronoid process (displaced) S52.04- ✓
      nondisplaced S52.04- ✓
    olecranon process (displaced) S52.02- ✓
      with intraarticular extension S52.03- ✓
      nondisplaced S52.02- ✓
        with intraarticular extension S52.03- ✓
    specified NEC S52.09- ✓
    torus S52.01- ✓
unciform — *see* Fracture, carpal, hamate
vault of skull S02.0 ✓
vertebra, vertebral (arch) (body) (column) (neural arch)
  (pedicle) (spinous process) (transverse process)
  atlas — *see* Fracture, neck, cervical vertebra, first
  axis — *see* Fracture, neck, cervical vertebra, second
  cervical (teardrop) S12.9 ✓
    axis — *see* Fracture, neck, cervical vertebra,
      second
    first (atlas) — *see* Fracture, neck, cervical verte-
      bra, first
    second (axis) — *see* Fracture, neck, cervical
      vertebra, second
  chronic M84.48 ✓
  coccyx S32.2 ✓
  dorsal — *see* Fracture, thorax, vertebra
  lumbar S32.009 ✓
    burst (stable) S32.001 ✓
      unstable S32.002 ✓
    fifth S32.059 ✓
      burst (stable) S32.051 ✓
        unstable S32.052 ✓
      specified type NEC S32.058 ✓
      wedge compression S32.050 ✓
    first S32.019 ✓
      burst (stable) S32.011 ✓
        unstable S32.012 ✓
      specified type NEC S32.018 ✓
      wedge compression S32.010 ✓
    fourth S32.049 ✓
      burst (stable) S32.041 ✓
        unstable S32.042 ✓
      specified type NEC S32.048 ✓
      wedge compression S32.040 ✓
    second S32.029 ✓
      burst (stable) S32.021 ✓
        unstable S32.022 ✓
      specified type NEC S32.028 ✓
      wedge compression S32.020 ✓
    specified type NEC S32.008 ✓

✓ Additional Character Required — Refer to the Tabular List for Character Selection   ▽ Subterms under main terms may continue to next column or page

Fracture, traumatic — *continued*
  vertebra, vertebral — *continued*
    lumbar — *continued*
      third S32.039 ☑
        burst (stable) S32.031 ☑
          unstable S32.032 ☑
        specified type NEC S32.038 ☑
        wedge compression S32.030 ☑
        wedge compression S32.000 ☑
    metastatic — *see* Collapse, vertebra, in, specified disease NEC (*see also* Neoplasm)
    newborn (birth injury) P11.5
    sacrum S32.10 ☑
      specified NEC S32.19 ☑
      Type
        1 S32.14 ☑
        2 S32.15 ☑
        3 S32.16 ☑
        4 S32.17 ☑
      Zone
        I S32.119 ☑
          displaced (minimally) S32.111 ☑
            severely S32.112 ☑
          nondisplaced S32.110 ☑
        II S32.129 ☑
          displaced (minimally) S32.121 ☑
            severely S32.122 ☑
          nondisplaced S32.120 ☑
        III S32.139 ☑
          displaced (minimally) S32.131 ☑
            severely S32.132 ☑
          nondisplaced S32.130 ☑
    thoracic — *see* Fracture, thorax, vertebra
  vertex S02.0 ☑
  vomer (bone) S02.2 ☑
  wrist S62.10- ☑
    carpal — *see* Fracture, carpal bone
    navicular (scaphoid) (hand) — *see* Fracture, carpal, navicular
  xiphisternum, xiphoid (process) S22.24 ☑
  zygoma S02.402 ☑
    left side S02.40F ☑
    right side S02.40E ☑
Fragile, fragility
  autosomal site Q95.5
  bone, congenital (with blue sclera) Q78.0
  capillary (hereditary) D69.8
  hair L67.8
  nails L60.3
  non-sex chromosome site Q95.5
  X chromosome Q99.2
Fragilitas
  crinium L67.8
  ossium (with blue sclerae) (hereditary) Q78.0
  unguium L60.3
    congenital Q84.6
Fragments, cataract (lens), **following cataract surgery** H59.02- ☑
  retained foreign body — *see* Retained, foreign body fragments (type of)
Frailty (frail) R54
  mental R41.81
Frambesia, frambesial (tropica) (*see also* Yaws)
  initial lesion or ulcer A66.0
  primary A66.0
Frambeside
  gummatous A66.4
  of early yaws A66.2
Frambesioma A66.1
Franceschetti-Klein (-Wildervanck) **disease or syndrome** Q75.4
Francis' disease — *see* Tularemia
Franklin disease C88.2
Frank's essential thrombocytopenia D69.3
Fraser's syndrome Q87.0
Freckle(s) L81.2
  malignant melanoma in — *see* Melanoma
  melanotic (Hutchinson's) — *see* Melanoma, in situ
  retinal D49.81
Frederickson's hyperlipoproteinemia, type
  I and V E78.3
  IIA E78.00
  IIB and III E78.2
  IV E78.1
Freeman Sheldon syndrome Q87.0
Freezing (*see also* Effect, adverse, cold) T69.9 ☑

Freiberg's disease (infraction of metatarsal head or osteochondrosis) — *see* Osteochondrosis, juvenile, metatarsus
Frei's disease A55
Fremitus, friction, cardiac R01.2
Frenum, frenulum
  external os Q51.828
  tongue (shortening) (congenital) Q38.1
Frequency micturition (nocturnal) R35.0
  psychogenic F45.8
Frey's syndrome
  auriculotemporal G50.8
  hyperhidrosis L74.52
Friction
  burn — *see* Burn, by site
  fremitus, cardiac R01.2
  precordial R01.2
  sounds, chest R09.89
Friderichsen-Waterhouse syndrome or disease A39.1
Friedländer's B (bacillus) **NEC** (*see also* condition) A49.8
Friedreich's
  ataxia G11.1
  combined systemic disease G11.1
  facial hemihypertrophy Q67.4
  sclerosis (cerebellum) (spinal cord) G11.1
Frigidity F52.22
Fröhlich's syndrome E23.6
Frontal (*see also* condition)
  lobe syndrome F07.0
Frostbite (superficial) T33.90 ☑
  with
    partial thickness skin loss — *see* Frostbite (superficial), by site
    tissue necrosis T34.90 ☑
  abdominal wall T33.3 ☑
    with tissue necrosis T34.3 ☑
  ankle T33.81- ☑
    with tissue necrosis T34.81- ☑
  arm T33.4- ☑
    with tissue necrosis T34.4- ☑
    finger(s) — *see* Frostbite, finger
    hand — *see* Frostbite, hand
    wrist — *see* Frostbite, wrist
  ear T33.01- ☑
    with tissue necrosis T34.01- ☑
  face T33.09 ☑
    with tissue necrosis T34.09 ☑
  finger T33.53- ☑
    with tissue necrosis T34.53- ☑
  foot T33.82- ☑
    with tissue necrosis T34.82- ☑
  hand T33.52- ☑
    with tissue necrosis T34.52- ☑
  head T33.09 ☑
    with tissue necrosis T34.09 ☑
    ear — *see* Frostbite, ear
    nose — *see* Frostbite, nose
  hip (and thigh) T33.6- ☑
    with tissue necrosis T34.6- ☑
  knee T33.7- ☑
    with tissue necrosis T34.7- ☑
  leg T33.9- ☑
    with tissue necrosis T34.9- ☑
    ankle — *see* Frostbite, ankle
    foot — *see* Frostbite, foot
    knee — *see* Frostbite, knee
    lower T33.7- ☑
      with tissue necrosis T34.7- ☑
    thigh — *see* Frostbite, hip
    toe — *see* Frostbite, toe
  limb
    lower T33.99 ☑
      with tissue necrosis T34.99 ☑
    upper — *see* Frostbite, arm
  neck T33.1 ☑
    with tissue necrosis T34.1 ☑
  nose T33.02 ☑
    with tissue necrosis T34.02 ☑
  pelvis T33.3 ☑
    with tissue necrosis T34.3 ☑
  specified site NEC T33.99 ☑
    with tissue necrosis T34.99 ☑
  thigh — *see* Frostbite, hip
  thorax T33.2 ☑
    with tissue necrosis T34.2 ☑
  toes T33.83- ☑

Frostbite — *continued*
  toes — *continued*
    with tissue necrosis T34.83- ☑
  trunk T33.99 ☑
    with tissue necrosis T34.99 ☑
  wrist T33.51- ☑
    with tissue necrosis T34.51- ☑
Frotteurism F65.81
Frozen (*see also* Effect, adverse, cold) T69.9 ☑
  pelvis (female) N94.89
    male K66.8
  shoulder — *see* Capsulitis, adhesive
Fructokinase deficiency E74.11
Fructose 1,6 diphosphatase deficiency E74.19
Fructosemia (benign) (essential) E74.12
Fructosuria (benign) (essential) E74.11
Fuchs'
  black spot (myopic) (*see also* Myopia, degenerative) H44.2- ☑
  dystrophy (corneal endothelium) H18.51
  heterochromic cyclitis — *see* Cyclitis, Fuchs' heterochromic
Fucosidosis E77.1
Fugue R68.89
  dissociative F44.1
  hysterical (dissociative) F44.1
  postictal in epilepsy — *see* Epilepsy
  reaction to exceptional stress (transient) F43.0
Fulminant, fulminating — *see* condition
Functional (*see also* condition)
  bleeding (uterus) N93.8
Functioning, intellectual, borderline R41.83
Fundus — *see* condition
Fungemia NOS B49
Fungus, fungous
  cerebral G93.89
  disease NOS B49
  infection — *see* Infection, fungus
Funiculitis (acute) (chronic) (endemic) N49.1
  gonococcal (acute) (chronic) A54.23
  tuberculous A18.15
Funnel
  breast (acquired) M95.4
    congenital Q67.6
    sequelae (late effect) of rickets E64.3
  chest (acquired) M95.4
    congenital Q67.6
    sequelae (late effect) of rickets E64.3
  pelvis (acquired) M95.5
    with disproportion (fetopelvic) O33.3 ☑
      causing obstructed labor O65.3
    congenital Q74.2
FUO (fever of unknown origin) R50.9
Furfur L21.0
  microsporon B36.0
Furrier's lung J67.8
Furrowed K14.5
  nail(s) (transverse) L60.4
    congenital Q84.6
  tongue K14.5
    congenital Q38.3
Furuncle L02.92
  abdominal wall L02.221
  ankle — *see* Furuncle, lower limb
  antecubital space — *see* Furuncle, upper limb
  anus K61.0
  arm — *see* Furuncle, upper limb
  auditory canal, external — *see* Abscess, ear, external
  auricle (ear) — *see* Abscess, ear, external
  axilla (region) L02.42- ☑
  back (any part) L02.222
  breast N61.1
  buttock L02.32
  cheek (external) L02.02
  chest wall L02.223
  chin L02.02
  corpus cavernosum N48.21
  ear, external — *see* Abscess, ear, external
  external auditory canal — *see* Abscess, ear, external
  eyelid — *see* Abscess, eyelid
  face L02.02
  femoral (region) — *see* Furuncle, lower limb
  finger — *see* Furuncle, hand
  flank L02.221
  foot L02.62- ☑
  forehead L02.02
  gluteal (region) L02.32

Furuncle — continued
  groin L02.224
  hand L02.52- ☑
  head L02.821
    face L02.02
  hip — see Furuncle, lower limb
  kidney — see Abscess, kidney
  knee — see Furuncle, lower limb
  labium (majus) (minus) N76.4
  lacrimal
    gland — see Dacryoadenitis
    passages (duct) (sac) — see Inflammation, lacrimal,
      passages, acute
  leg (any part) — see Furuncle, lower limb
  lower limb L02.42- ☑
  malignant A22.0
  mouth K12.2
  navel L02.226
  neck L02.12
  nose J34.0
  orbit, orbital — see Abscess, orbit
  palmar (space) — see Furuncle, hand
  partes posteriores L02.32
  pectoral region L02.223
  penis N48.21
  perineum L02.225
  pinna — see Abscess, ear, external
  popliteal — see Furuncle, lower limb
  prepatellar — see Furuncle, lower limb
  scalp L02.821
  seminal vesicle N49.0
  shoulder — see Furuncle, upper limb
  specified site NEC L02.828
  submandibular K12.2
  temple (region) L02.02
  thumb — see Furuncle, hand
  toe — see Furuncle, foot
  trunk L02.229
    abdominal wall L02.221
    back L02.222

Furuncle — continued
  trunk — continued
    chest wall L02.223
    groin L02.224
    perineum L02.225
    umbilicus L02.226
  umbilicus L02.226
  upper limb L02.42- ☑
  vulva N76.4
Furunculosis — see Furuncle
Fused — see Fusion, fused
Fusion, fused (congenital)
  astragaloscaphoid Q74.2
  atria Q21.1
  auditory canal Q16.1
  auricles, heart Q21.1
  binocular with defective stereopsis H53.32
  bone Q79.8
  cervical spine M43.22
  choanal Q30.0
  commissure, mitral valve Q23.2
  cusps, heart valve NEC Q24.8
    mitral Q23.2
    pulmonary Q22.1
    tricuspid Q22.4
  ear ossicles Q16.3
  fingers Q70.0 ☑
  hymen Q52.3
  joint (acquired) (see also Ankylosis)
    congenital Q74.8
  kidneys (incomplete) Q63.1
  labium (majus) (minus) Q52.5
  larynx and trachea Q34.8
  limb, congenital Q74.8
    lower Q74.2
    upper Q74.0
  lobes, lung Q33.8
  lumbosacral (acquired) M43.27
    arthrodesis status Z98.1
    congenital Q76.49

Fusion, fused — continued
  lumbosacral — continued
    postprocedural status Z98.1
  nares, nose, nasal, nostril(s) Q30.0
  organ or site not listed — see Anomaly, by site
  ossicles Q79.9
    auditory Q16.3
  pulmonic cusps Q22.1
  ribs Q76.6
  sacroiliac (joint) (acquired) M43.28
    arthrodesis status Z98.1
    congenital Q74.2
    postprocedural status Z98.1
  spine (acquired) NEC M43.20
    arthrodesis status Z98.1
    cervical region M43.22
    cervicothoracic region M43.23
    congenital Q76.49
    lumbar M43.26
    lumbosacral region M43.27
    occipito-atlanto-axial region M43.21
    postoperative status Z98.1
    sacrococcygeal region M43.28
    thoracic region M43.24
    thoracolumbar region M43.25
  sublingual duct with submaxillary duct at opening in
    mouth Q38.4
  testes Q55.1
  toes Q70.2- ☑
  tooth, teeth K00.2
  trachea and esophagus Q39.8
  twins Q89.4
  vagina Q52.4
  ventricles, heart Q21.0
  vertebra (arch) — see Fusion, spine
  vulva Q52.5
Fusospirillosis (mouth) (tongue) (tonsil) A69.1
Fussy baby R68.12

G

Gain in weight (abnormal) (excessive) (see also Weight, gain)
Gaisböck's disease (polycythemia hypertonica) D75.1
Gait abnormality R26.9
  ataxic R26.0
  falling R29.6
  hysterical (ataxic) (staggering) F44.4
  paralytic R26.1
  spastic R26.1
  specified type NEC R26.89
  staggering R26.0
  unsteadiness R26.81
  walking difficulty NEC R26.2
Galactocele (breast) N64.89
  puerperal, postpartum O92.79
Galactokinase deficiency E74.29
Galactophoritis N61.0
  gestational, puerperal, postpartum O91.2- ☑
Galactorrhea O92.6
  not associated with childbirth N64.3
Galactosemia (classic) (congenital) E74.21
Galactosuria E74.29
Galacturia R82.0
  schistosomiasis (bilharziasis) B65.0
GALD (gestational alloimmune liver disease) P78.84
Galeazzi's fracture S52.37- ☑
Galen's vein — see condition
Galeophobia F40.218
Gall duct — see condition
Gallbladder (see also condition)
  acute K81.0
Gallop rhythm R00.8
Gallstone (colic) (cystic duct) (gallbladder) (impacted) (multiple) (see also Calculus, gallbladder)
  with
    cholecystitis — see Calculus, gallbladder, with cholecystitis
  bile duct (common) (hepatic) — see Calculus, bile duct
  causing intestinal obstruction K56.3
  specified NEC K80.80
    with obstruction K80.81
Gambling Z72.6
  pathological (compulsive) F63.0
Gammopathy (of undetermined significance [MGUS]) D47.2
  associated with lymphoplasmacytic dyscrasia D47.2
  monoclonal D47.2
  polyclonal D89.0
Gamna's disease (siderotic splenomegaly) D73.1
Gamophobia F40.298
Gampsodactylia (congenital) Q66.7
Gamstorp's disease (adynamia episodica hereditaria) G72.3
Gandy-Nanta disease (siderotic splenomegaly) D73.1
Gang
  membership offenses Z72.810
Gangliocytoma D36.10
Ganglioglioma — see Neoplasm, uncertain behavior, by site
Ganglion (compound) (diffuse) (joint) (tendon (sheath)) M67.40
  ankle M67.47- ☑
  foot M67.47- ☑
  forearm M67.43- ☑
  hand M67.44- ☑
  lower leg M67.46- ☑
  multiple sites M67.49
  of yaws (early) (late) A66.6
  pelvic region M67.45- ☑
  periosteal — see Periostitis
  shoulder region M67.41- ☑
  specified site NEC M67.48
  thigh region M67.45- ☑
  tuberculous A18.09
  upper arm M67.42- ☑
  wrist M67.43- ☑
Ganglioneuroblastoma — see Neoplasm, nerve, malignant
Ganglioneuroma D36.10
  malignant — see Neoplasm, nerve, malignant
Ganglioneuromatosis D36.10
Ganglionitis
  fifth nerve — see Neuralgia, trigeminal
  gasserian (postherpetic) (postzoster) B02.21

Ganglionitis — continued
  geniculate G51.1
    newborn (birth injury) P11.3
    postherpetic, postzoster B02.21
  herpes zoster B02.21
  postherpetic geniculate B02.21
Gangliosidosis E75.10
  GM1 E75.19
  GM2 E75.00
    other specified E75.09
    Sandhoff disease E75.01
    Tay-Sachs disease E75.02
  GM3 E75.19
  mucolipidosis IV E75.11
Gangosa A66.5
Gangrene, gangrenous (connective tissue) (dropsical) (dry) (moist) (skin) (ulcer) (see also Necrosis) I96
  with diabetes (mellitus) — see Diabetes, gangrene
  abdomen (wall) I96
  alveolar M27.3
  appendix K35.80
    with
      perforation or rupture K35.2
      peritoneal abscess K35.3
      peritonitis NEC K35.3
        generalized (with perforation or rupture) K35.2
        localized (with perforation or rupture) K35.3
  arteriosclerotic (general) (senile) — see Arteriosclerosis, extremities, with, gangrene
  auricle I96
  Bacillus welchii A48.0
  bladder (infectious) — see Cystitis, specified type NEC
  bowel, cecum, or colon — see Gangrene, intestine
  Clostridium perfringens or welchii A48.0
  cornea H18.89- ☑
  corpora cavernosa N48.29
    noninfective N48.89
  cutaneous, spreading I96
  decubital — see Ulcer, pressure, by site
  diabetic (any site) — see Diabetes, gangrene
  emphysematous — see Gangrene, gas
  epidemic — see Poisoning, food, noxious, plant
  epididymis (infectional) N45.1
  erysipelas — see Erysipelas
  extremity (lower) (upper) I96
  Fournier N49.3
    female N76.89
  fusospirochetal A69.0
  gallbladder — see Cholecystitis, acute
  gas (bacillus) A48.0
    following
      abortion — see Abortion by type complicated by infection
      ectopic or molar pregnancy O08.0
  glossitis K14.0
  hernia — see Hernia, by site, with gangrene
  intestine, intestinal (hemorrhagic) (massive) (see also Infarct, intestine) K55.069
    with
      mesenteric embolism (see also Infarct, intestine) K55.069
      obstruction — see Obstruction, intestine
  laryngitis J04.0
  limb (lower) (upper) I96
  lung J85.0
    spirochetal A69.8
  lymphangitis I89.1
  Meleney's (synergistic) — see Ulcer, skin
  mesentery (see also Infarct, intestine) K55.069
    with
      embolism (see also Infarct, intestine) K55.069
      intestinal obstruction — see Obstruction, intestine
  mouth A69.0
  ovary — see Oophoritis
  pancreas — see Pancreatitis, acute
  penis N48.29
    noninfective N48.89
  perineum I96
  pharynx (see also Pharyngitis)
    Vincent's A69.1
  presenile I73.1
  progressive synergistic — see Ulcer, skin
  pulmonary J85.0
  pulpal (dental) K04.1
  quinsy J36
  Raynaud's (symmetric gangrene) I73.01

Gangrene, gangrenous — continued
  retropharyngeal J39.2
  scrotum N49.3
    noninfective N50.89
  senile (atherosclerotic) — see Arteriosclerosis, extremities, with, gangrene
  spermatic cord N49.1
    noninfective N50.89
  spine I96
  spirochetal NEC A69.8
  spreading cutaneous I96
  stomatitis A69.0
  symmetrical I73.01
  testis (infectional) N45.2
    noninfective N44.8
  throat (see also Pharyngitis)
    diphtheritic A36.0
    Vincent's A69.1
  thyroid (gland) E07.89
  tooth (pulp) K04.1
  tuberculous NEC — see Tuberculosis
  tunica vaginalis N49.1
    noninfective N50.89
  umbilicus I96
  uterus — see Endometritis
  uvulitis K12.2
  vas deferens N49.1
    noninfective N50.89
  vulva N76.89
Ganister disease J62.8
Ganser's syndrome (hysterical) F44.89
Gardner-Diamond syndrome (autoerythrocyte sensitization) D69.2
Gargoylism E76.01
Garré's disease, osteitis (sclerosing), osteomyelitis — see Osteomyelitis, specified type NEC
Garrod's pad, knuckle M72.1
Gartner's duct
  cyst Q52.4
  persistent Q50.6
Gas R14.3
  asphyxiation, inhalation, poisoning, suffocation NEC — see Table of Drugs and Chemicals
  excessive R14.0
  gangrene A48.0
    following
      abortion — see Abortion by type complicated by infection
      ectopic or molar pregnancy O08.0
  on stomach R14.0
  pains R14.1
Gastralgia (see also Pain, abdominal)
Gastrectasis K31.0
  psychogenic F45.8
Gastric — see condition
Gastrinoma
  malignant
    pancreas C25.4
    specified site NEC — see Neoplasm, malignant, by site
    unspecified site C25.4
  specified site — see Neoplasm, uncertain behavior
  unspecified site D37.9
Gastritis (simple) K29.70
  with bleeding K29.71
  acute (erosive) K29.00
    with bleeding K29.01
  alcoholic K29.20
    with bleeding K29.21
  allergic K29.60
    with bleeding K29.61
  atrophic (chronic) K29.40
    with bleeding K29.41
  chronic (antral) (fundal) K29.50
    with bleeding K29.51
    atrophic K29.40
      with bleeding K29.41
    superficial K29.30
      with bleeding K29.31
  dietary counseling and surveillance Z71.3
  due to diet deficiency E63.9
  eosinophilic K52.81
  giant hypertrophic K29.60
    with bleeding K29.61
  granulomatous K29.60
    with bleeding K29.61
  hypertrophic (mucosa) K29.60
    with bleeding K29.61

⬛ Subterms under main terms may continue to next column or page   ☑ Additional Character Required — Refer to the Tabular List for Character Selection   157

Gain in weight — Gastritis

Gastritis — continued
  nervous F54
  spastic K29.60
    with bleeding K29.61
  specified NEC K29.60
    with bleeding K29.61
  superficial chronic K29.30
    with bleeding K29.31
  tuberculous A18.83
  viral NEC A08.4
Gastrocarcinoma — see Neoplasm, malignant, stomach
Gastrocolic — see condition
Gastrodisciasis, gastrodiscoidiasis B66.8
Gastroduodenitis K29.90
  with bleeding K29.91
  virus, viral A08.4
    specified type NEC A08.39
Gastrodynia — see Pain, abdominal
Gastroenteritis (acute) (chronic) (noninfectious) (see
    also Enteritis) K52.9
  allergic K52.29
    with
      eosinophilic gastritis or gastroenteritis K52.81
      food protein-induced enterocolitis syndrome
        K52.21
      food protein-induced enteropathy K52.22
  dietetic (see also Gastroenteritis, allergic) K52.29
  drug-induced K52.1
  due to
    Cryptosporidium A07.2
    drugs K52.1
    food poisoning — see Intoxication, foodborne
    radiation K52.0
  eosinophilic K52.81
  epidemic (infectious) A09
  food hypersensitivity (see also Gastroenteritis, allergic)
    K52.29
  infectious — see Enteritis, infectious
  influenzal — see Influenza, with gastroenteritis
  noninfectious K52.9
    specified NEC K52.89
  rotaviral A08.0
  Salmonella A02.0
  toxic K52.1
  viral NEC A08.4
    acute infectious A08.39
      type Norwalk A08.11
    infantile (acute) A08.39
    Norwalk agent A08.11
    rotaviral A08.0
    severe of infants A08.39
    specified type NEC A08.39
Gastroenteropathy (see also Gastroenteritis) K52.9
  acute, due to Norovirus A08.11
  acute, due to Norwalk agent A08.11
  infectious A09
Gastroenteroptosis K63.4
**Gastroesophageal laceration- hemorrhage syn-
    drome** K22.6
Gastrointestinal — see condition
Gastrojejunal — see condition
Gastrojejunitis (see also Enteritis) K52.9
Gastrojejunocolic — see condition
Gastroliths K31.89
Gastromalacia K31.89
Gastroparalysis K31.84
  diabetic — see Diabetes, gastroparalysis
Gastroparesis K31.84
  diabetic — see Diabetes, by type, with gastroparesis
Gastropathy K31.9
  congestive portal K31.89
  erythematous K29.70
  exudative K90.89
  portal hypertensive K31.89
Gastroptosis K31.89
Gastrorrhagia K92.2
  psychogenic F45.8
Gastroschisis (congenital) Q79.3
Gastrospasm (neurogenic) (reflex) K31.89
  neurotic F45.8
  psychogenic F45.8
Gastrostaxis — see Gastritis, with bleeding
Gastrostenosis K31.89
Gastrostomy
  attention to Z43.1
  status Z93.1
Gastrosuccorrhea (continuous) (intermittent) K31.89
  neurotic F45.8

Gastrosuccorrhea — continued
  psychogenic F45.8
Gatophobia F40.218
Gaucher's disease or splenomegaly (adult) (infantile)
    E75.22
Gee (-Herter)(-Thaysen) **disease** (nontropical sprue) K90.0
Gélineau's syndrome G47.419
  with cataplexy G47.411
Gemination, tooth, teeth K00.2
Gemistocytoma
  specified site — see Neoplasm, malignant, by site
  unspecified site C71.9
General, generalized — see condition
Genetic
  carrier (status)
    cystic fibrosis Z14.1
    hemophilia A (asymptomatic) Z14.01
      symptomatic Z14.02
    specified NEC Z14.8
  susceptibility to disease NEC Z15.89
    malignant neoplasm Z15.09
      breast Z15.01
      endometrium Z15.04
      ovary Z15.02
      prostate Z15.03
      specified NEC Z15.09
    multiple endocrine neoplasia Z15.81
Genital — see condition
Genito-anorectal syndrome A55
Genitourinary system — see condition
Genu
  congenital Q74.1
  extrorsum (acquired) (see also Deformity, varus, knee)
    congenital Q74.1
    sequelae (late effect) of rickets E64.3
  introrsum (acquired) (see also Deformity, valgus, knee)
    congenital Q74.1
    sequelae (late effect) of rickets E64.3
  rachitic (old) E64.3
  recurvatum (acquired) (see also Deformity, limb,
      specified type NEC, lower leg)
    congenital Q68.2
    sequelae (late effect) of rickets E64.3
  valgum (acquired) (knock-knee) M21.06- ☑
    congenital Q74.1
    sequelae (late effect) of rickets E64.3
  varum (acquired) (bowleg) M21.16- ☑
    congenital Q74.1
    sequelae (late effect) of rickets E64.3
Geographic tongue K14.1
Geophagia — see Pica
Geotrichosis B48.3
  stomatitis B48.3
Gephyrophobia F40.242
Gerbode defect Q21.0
GERD (gastroesophageal reflux disease) K21.9
Gerhardt's
  disease (erythromelalgia) I73.81
  syndrome (vocal cord paralysis) J38.00
    bilateral J38.02
    unilateral J38.01
German measles (see also Rubella)
  exposure to Z20.4
Germinoblastoma (diffuse) C85.9- ☑
  follicular C82.9- ☑
Germinoma — see Neoplasm, malignant, by site
Gerontoxon — see Degeneration, cornea, senile
Gerstmann's syndrome R48.8
  developmental F81.2
Gerstmann-Sträussler-Scheinker syndrome (GSS)
    A81.82
Gestation (period) (see also Pregnancy)
  ectopic — see Pregnancy, by site
  multiple O30.9- ☑
    greater than quadruplets — see Pregnancy, multi-
      ple (gestation), specified NEC
    specified NEC — see Pregnancy, multiple (gesta-
      tion), specified NEC
Gestational
  mammary abscess O91.11- ☑
  purulent mastitis O91.11- ☑
  subareolar abscess O91.11- ☑
Ghon tubercle, primary infection A15.7
Ghost
  teeth K00.4
  vessels (cornea) H16.41- ☑
Ghoul hand A66.3

Gianotti-Crosti disease L44.4
Giant
  cell
    epulis K06.8
    peripheral granuloma K06.8
  esophagus, congenital Q39.5
  kidney, congenital Q63.3
  urticaria T78.3 ☑
    hereditary D84.1
Giardiasis A07.1
Gibert's disease or pityriasis L42
Giddiness R42
  hysterical F44.89
  psychogenic F45.8
Gierke's disease (glycogenosis I) E74.01
Gigantism (cerebral) (hypophyseal) (pituitary) E22.0
  constitutional E34.4
Gilbert's disease or syndrome E80.4
Gilchrist's disease B40.9
Gilford-Hutchinson disease E34.8
Gilles de la Tourette's disease or syndrome (motor-
    verbal tic) F95.2
Gingivitis K05.10
  acute (catarrhal) K05.00
    necrotizing A69.1
    nonplaque induced K05.01
    plaque induced K05.00
  chronic (desquamative) (hyperplastic) (simple
      marginal) (pregnancy associated) (ulcerative)
      K05.10
    nonplaque induced K05.11
    plaque induced K05.10
  expulsiva — see Periodontitis
  necrotizing ulcerative (acute) A69.1
  pellagrous E52
    acute necrotizing A69.1
  Vincent's A69.1
Gingivoglossitis K14.0
Gingivopericementitis — see Periodontitis
Gingivosis — see Gingivitis, chronic
Gingivostomatitis K05.10
  herpesviral B00.2
  necrotizing ulcerative (acute) A69.1
Gland, glandular — see condition
Glanders A24.0
Glanzmann (-Naegeli) **disease or thrombasthenia**
    D69.1
Glasgow coma scale
  total score
    3-8 R40.243 ☑
    9-12 R40.242 ☑
    13-15 R40.241 ☑
Glass-blower's disease (cataract) — see Cataract,
    specified NEC
Glaucoma H40.9
  with
    increased episcleral venous pressure H40.81- ☑
    pseudoexfoliation of lens — see Glaucoma, open
      angle, primary, capsular
  absolute H44.51- ☑
  angle-closure (primary) H40.20- ☑
    acute (attack) (crisis) H40.21- ☑
    chronic H40.22- ☑
    intermittent H40.23- ☑
    residual stage H40.24- ☑
  borderline H40.00- ☑
  capsular (with pseudoexfoliation of lens) — see Glau-
    coma, open angle, primary, capsular
  childhood Q15.0
  closed angle — see Glaucoma, angle-closure
  congenital Q15.0
  corticosteroid-induced — see Glaucoma, secondary,
    drugs
  hypersecretion H40.82- ☑
  in (due to)
    amyloidosis E85.4 [H42]
    aniridia Q13.1 [H42]
    concussion of globe — see Glaucoma, secondary,
      trauma
    dislocation of lens — see Glaucoma, secondary
    disorder of lens NEC — see Glaucoma, secondary
    drugs — see Glaucoma, secondary, drugs
    endocrine disease NOS E34.9 [H42]
    eye
      inflammation — see Glaucoma, secondary, in-
        flammation
      trauma — see Glaucoma, secondary, trauma

Glaucoma — continued
  in — continued
    hypermature cataract — see Glaucoma, secondary
    iridocyclitis — see Glaucoma, secondary, inflammation
    lens disorder — see Glaucoma, secondary
    Lowe's syndrome E72.03 [H42]
    metabolic disease NOS E88.9 [H42]
    ocular disorders NEC — see Glaucoma, secondary
    onchocerciasis B73.02
    pupillary block — see Glaucoma, secondary
    retinal vein occlusion — see Glaucoma, secondary
    Rieger's anomaly Q13.81 [H42]
    rubeosis of iris — see Glaucoma, secondary
    tumor of globe — see Glaucoma, secondary
  infantile Q15.0
  low tension — see Glaucoma, open angle, primary, low-tension
  malignant H40.83- ☑
  narrow angle — see Glaucoma, angle-closure
  newborn Q15.0
  noncongestive (chronic) — see Glaucoma, open angle
  nonobstructive — see Glaucoma, open angle
  obstructive (see also Glaucoma, angle-closure)
    due to lens changes — see Glaucoma, secondary
  open angle H40.10- ☑
    primary H40.11- ☑
      capsular (with pseudoexfoliation of lens) H40.14- ☑
      low-tension H40.12- ☑
      pigmentary H40.13- ☑
      residual stage H40.15- ☑
  phacolytic — see Glaucoma, secondary
  pigmentary — see Glaucoma, open angle, primary, pigmentary
  postinfectious — see Glaucoma, secondary, inflammation
  secondary (to) H40.5- ☑
    drugs H40.6- ☑
    inflammation H40.4- ☑
    trauma H40.3- ☑
  simple (chronic) H40.11- ☑
  simplex H40.11- ☑
  specified type NEC H40.89
  suspect H40.00- ☑
  syphilitic A52.71
  traumatic (see also Glaucoma, secondary, trauma)
    newborn (birth injury) P15.3
  tuberculous A18.59
Glaucomatous flecks (subcapsular) — see Cataract, complicated
Glazed tongue K14.4
Gleet (gonococcal) A54.01
Glénard's disease K63.4
Glioblastoma (multiforme)
  with sarcomatous component
    specified site — see Neoplasm, malignant, by site
    unspecified site C71.9
  giant cell
    specified site — see Neoplasm, malignant, by site
    unspecified site C71.9
  specified site — see Neoplasm, malignant, by site
  unspecified site C71.9
Glioma (malignant)
  astrocytic
    specified site — see Neoplasm, malignant, by site
    unspecified site C71.9
  mixed
    specified site — see Neoplasm, malignant, by site
    unspecified site C71.9
  nose Q30.8
  specified site NEC — see Neoplasm, malignant, by site
  subependymal D43.2
    specified site — see Neoplasm, uncertain behavior, by site
    unspecified site D43.2
  unspecified site C71.9
Gliomatosis cerebri C71.0
Glioneuroma — see Neoplasm, uncertain behavior, by site
Gliosarcoma
  specified site — see Neoplasm, malignant, by site
  unspecified site C71.9
Gliosis (cerebral) G93.89
  spinal G95.89
Glisson's disease — see Rickets
Globinuria R82.3

Globus (hystericus) F45.8
Glomangioma D18.00
  intra-abdominal D18.03
  intracranial D18.02
  skin D18.01
  specified site NEC D18.09
Glomangiomyoma D18.00
  intra-abdominal D18.03
  intracranial D18.02
  skin D18.01
  specified site NEC D18.09
Glomangiosarcoma — see Neoplasm, connective tissue, malignant
Glomerular
  disease in syphilis A52.75
  nephritis — see Glomerulonephritis
Glomerulitis — see Glomerulonephritis
Glomerulonephritis (see also Nephritis) N05.9
  with
    edema — see Nephrosis
    minimal change N05.0
    minor glomerular abnormality N05.0
  acute N00.9
  chronic N03.9
  crescentic (diffuse) NEC (see also N00-N07 with fourth character .7) N05.7
  dense deposit (see also N00-N07 with fourth character .6) N05.6
  diffuse
    crescentic (see also N00-N07 with fourth character .7) N05.7
    endocapillary proliferative (see also N00-N07 with fourth character .4) N05.4
    membranous (see also N00-N07 with fourth character .2) N05.2
    mesangial proliferative (see also N00-N07 with fourth character .3) N05.3
    mesangiocapillary (see also N00-N07 with fourth character .5) N05.5
    sclerosing N18.9
  endocapillary proliferative (diffuse) NEC (see also N00-N07 with fourth character .4) N05.4
  extracapillary NEC (see also N00-N07 with fourth character .7) N05.7
  focal (and segmental) (see also N00-N07 with fourth character .1) N05.1
  hypocomplementemic — see Glomerulonephritis, membranoproliferative
  IgA — see Nephropathy, IgA
  immune complex (circulating) NEC N05.8
  in (due to)
    amyloidosis E85.4 [N08]
    bilharziasis B65.9 [N08]
    cryoglobulinemia D89.1 [N08]
    defibrination syndrome D65 [N08]
    diabetes mellitus — see Diabetes, glomerulosclerosis
    disseminated intravascular coagulation D65 [N08]
    Fabry (-Anderson) disease E75.21 [N08]
    Goodpasture's syndrome M31.0
    hemolytic-uremic syndrome D59.3
    Henoch (-Schönlein) purpura D69.0 [N08]
    lecithin cholesterol acyltransferase deficiency E78.6 [N08]
    microscopic polyangiitis M31.7 [N08]
    multiple myeloma C90.0- ☑ [N08]
    Plasmodium malariae B52.0
    schistosomiasis B65.9 [N08]
    sepsis A41.9 [N08]
      streptococcal A40- ☑ [N08]
    sickle-cell disorders D57.- ☑ [N08]
    strongyloidiasis B78.9 [N08]
    subacute bacterial endocarditis I33.0 [N08]
    syphilis (late) congenital A50.59 [N08]
    systemic lupus erythematosus M32.14
    thrombotic thrombocytopenic purpura M31.1 [N08]
    typhoid fever A01.09
    Waldenström macroglobulinemia C88.0 [N08]
    Wegener's granulomatosis M31.31
  latent or quiescent N03.9
  lobular, lobulonodular — see Glomerulonephritis, membranoproliferative
  membranoproliferative (diffuse)(type 1 or 3) (see also N00-N07 with fourth character .5) N05.5
    dense deposit (type 2) NEC (see also N00-N07 with fourth character .6) N05.6

Glomerulonephritis — continued
  membranous (diffuse) NEC (see also N00-N07 with fourth character .2) N05.2
  mesangial
    IgA/IgG — see Nephropathy, IgA
    proliferative (diffuse) NEC (see also N00-N07 with fourth character .3) N05.3
  mesangiocapillary (diffuse) NEC (see also N00-N07 with fourth character .5) N05.5
  necrotic, necrotizing NEC (see also N00- N07 with fourth character .8) N05.8
  nodular — see Glomerulonephritis, membranoproliferative
  poststreptococcal NEC N05.9
    acute N00.9
    chronic N03.9
    rapidly progressive N01.9
  proliferative NEC (see also N00-N07 with fourth character .8) N05.8
    diffuse (lupus) M32.14
  rapidly progressive N01.9
  sclerosing, diffuse N18.9
  specified pathology NEC (see also N00- N07 with fourth character .8) N05.8
  subacute N01.9
Glomerulopathy — see Glomerulonephritis
Glomerulosclerosis (see also Sclerosis, renal)
  intercapillary (nodular) (with diabetes) — see Diabetes, glomerulosclerosis
  intracapillary — see Diabetes, glomerulosclerosis
Glossagra K14.6
Glossalgia K14.6
Glossitis (chronic superficial) (gangrenous) (Moeller's) K14.0
  areata exfoliativa K14.1
  atrophic K14.4
  benign migratory K14.1
  cortical superficial, sclerotic K14.0
  Hunter's D51.0
  interstitial, sclerous K14.0
  median rhomboid K14.2
  pellagrous E52
  superficial, chronic K14.0
Glossocele K14.8
Glossodynia K14.6
  exfoliativa K14.4
Glossoncus K14.8
Glossopathy K14.9
Glossophytia K14.3
Glossoplegia K14.8
Glossoptosis K14.8
Glossopyrosis K14.6
Glossotrichia K14.3
Glossy skin L90.8
Glottis — see condition
Glottitis (see also Laryngitis) J04.0
Glucagonoma
  pancreas
    benign D13.7
    malignant C25.4
    uncertain behavior D37.8
  specified site NEC
    benign — see Neoplasm, benign, by site
    malignant — see Neoplasm, malignant, by site
    uncertain behavior — see Neoplasm, uncertain behavior, by site
  unspecified site
    benign D13.7
    malignant C25.4
    uncertain behavior D37.8
Glucoglycinuria E72.51
Glucose-galactose malabsorption E74.39
Glue
  ear — see Otitis, media, nonsuppurative, chronic, mucoid
  sniffing (airplane) — see Abuse, drug, inhalant dependence — see Dependence, drug, inhalant
Glutaric aciduria E72.3
Glycinemia E72.51
Glycinuria (renal) (with ketosis) E72.09
Glycogen
  infiltration — see Disease, glycogen storage
  storage disease — see Disease, glycogen storage
Glycogenosis (diffuse) (generalized) (see also Disease, glycogen storage)
  cardiac E74.02 [I43]

Index

Glycogenosis — Gout, gouty

Glycogenosis — continued
  diabetic, secondary — see Diabetes, glycogenosis, secondary
  pulmonary interstitial J84.842
Glycopenia E16.2
Glycosuria R81
  renal E74.8
Gnathostoma spinigerum (infection) (infestation), **gnathostomiasis** (wandering swelling) B83.1
Goiter (plunging) (substernal) E04.9
  with
    hyperthyroidism (recurrent) — see Hyperthyroidism, with, goiter
    thyrotoxicosis — see Hyperthyroidism, with, goiter
  adenomatous — see Goiter, nodular
  cancerous C73
  congenital (nontoxic) E03.0
    diffuse E03.0
    parenchymatous E03.0
    transitory, with normal functioning P72.0
  cystic E04.2
    due to iodine-deficiency E01.1
  due to
    enzyme defect in synthesis of thyroid hormone E07.1
    iodine-deficiency (endemic) E01.2
  dyshormonogenetic (familial) E07.1
  endemic (iodine-deficiency) E01.2
    diffuse E01.0
    multinodular E01.1
  exophthalmic — see Hyperthyroidism, with, goiter
  iodine-deficiency (endemic) E01.2
    diffuse E01.0
    multinodular E01.1
    nodular E01.1
  lingual Q89.2
  lymphadenoid E06.3
  malignant C73
  multinodular (cystic) (nontoxic) E04.2
    toxic or with hyperthyroidism E05.20
      with thyroid storm E05.21
  neonatal NEC P72.0
  nodular (nontoxic) (due to) E04.9
    with
      hyperthyroidism E05.20
        with thyroid storm E05.21
      thyrotoxicosis E05.20
        with thyroid storm E05.21
    endemic E01.1
    iodine-deficiency E01.1
    sporadic E04.9
    toxic E05.20
      with thyroid storm E05.21
  nontoxic E04.9
    diffuse (colloid) E04.0
    multinodular E04.2
    simple E04.0
    specified NEC E04.8
    uninodular E04.1
  simple E04.0
  toxic — see Hyperthyroidism, with, goiter
  uninodular (nontoxic) E04.1
    toxic or with hyperthyroidism E05.10
      with thyroid storm E05.11
Goiter-deafness syndrome E07.1
Goldberg syndrome Q89.8
Goldberg-Maxwell syndrome E34.51
Goldblatt's hypertension or kidney I70.1
Goldenhar (-Gorlin) **syndrome** Q87.0
Goldflam-Erb disease or syndrome G70.00
  with exacerbation (acute) G70.01
  in crisis G70.01
Goldscheider's disease Q81.8
Goldstein's disease (familial hemorrhagic telangiectasia) I78.0
Golfer's elbow — see Epicondylitis, medial
Gonadoblastoma
  specified site — see Neoplasm, uncertain behavior, by site
  unspecified site
    female D39.10
    male D40.10
Gonecystitis — see Vesiculitis
Gongylonemiasis B83.8
Goniosynechiae — see Adhesions, iris, goniosynechiae
Gonococcemia A54.86
Gonococcus, gonococcal (disease) (infection) (see also condition) A54.9

Gonococcus, gonococcal — continued
  anus A54.6
  bursa, bursitis A54.49
  conjunctiva, conjunctivitis (neonatorum) A54.31
  endocardium A54.83
  eye A54.30
    conjunctivitis A54.31
    iridocyclitis A54.32
    keratitis A54.33
    newborn A54.31
    other specified A54.39
  fallopian tubes (acute) (chronic) A54.24
  genitourinary (organ) (system) (tract) (acute)
    lower A54.00
      with abscess (accessory gland) (periurethral) A54.1
    upper (see also condition) A54.29
  heart A54.83
  iridocyclitis A54.32
  joint A54.42
  lymphatic (gland) (node) A54.89
  meninges, meningitis A54.81
  musculoskeletal A54.40
    arthritis A54.42
    osteomyelitis A54.43
    other specified A54.49
    spondylopathy A54.41
  pelviperitonitis A54.24
  pelvis (acute) (chronic) A54.24
  pharynx A54.5
  proctitis A54.6
  pyosalpinx (acute) (chronic) A54.24
  rectum A54.6
  skin A54.89
  specified site NEC A54.89
  tendon sheath A54.49
  throat A54.5
  urethra (acute) (chronic) A54.01
    with abscess (accessory gland) (periurethral) A54.1
  vulva (acute) (chronic) A54.02
Gonocytoma
  specified site — see Neoplasm, uncertain behavior, by site
  unspecified site
    female D39.10
    male D40.10
Gonorrhea (acute) (chronic) A54.9
  Bartholin's gland (acute) (chronic) (purulent) A54.02
    with abscess (accessory gland) (periurethral) A54.1
  bladder A54.01
  cervix A54.03
  conjunctiva, conjunctivitis (neonatorum) A54.31
  contact Z20.2
  Cowper's gland (with abscess) A54.1
  exposure to Z20.2
  fallopian tube (acute) (chronic) A54.24
  kidney (acute) (chronic) A54.21
  lower genitourinary tract A54.00
    with abscess (accessory gland) (periurethral) A54.1
  ovary (acute) (chronic) A54.24
  pelvis (acute) (chronic) A54.24
    female pelvic inflammatory disease A54.24
  penis A54.09
  prostate (acute) (chronic) A54.22
  seminal vesicle (acute) (chronic) A54.23
  specified site not listed (see also Gonococcus) A54.89
  spermatic cord (acute) (chronic) A54.23
  urethra A54.01
    with abscess (accessory gland) (periurethral) A54.1
  vagina A54.02
  vas deferens (acute) (chronic) A54.23
  vulva A54.02
Goodall's disease A08.19
Goodpasture's syndrome M31.0
Gopalan's syndrome (burning feet) E53.0
Gorlin-Chaudry-Moss syndrome Q87.0
Gottron's papules L94.4
Gougerot-Blum syndrome (pigmented purpuric lichenoid dermatitis) L81.7
Gougerot-Carteaud disease or syndrome (confluent reticulate papillomatosis) L83
Gougerot's syndrome (trisymptomatic) L81.7
Gouley's syndrome (constrictive pericarditis) I31.1
Goundou A66.6
Gout, chronic (see also Gout, gouty) M1A.9 ☑ (following M08)
  drug-induced M1A.20 ☑ (following M08)
    ankle M1A.27- ☑ (following M08)

Gout, chronic — continued
  drug-induced — continued
    elbow M1A.22- ☑ (following M08)
    foot joint M1A.27- ☑ (following M08)
    hand joint M1A.24- ☑ (following M08)
    hip M1A.25- ☑ (following M08)
    knee M1A.26- ☑ (following M08)
    multiple site M1A.29- ☑ (following M08)
    shoulder M1A.21- ☑ (following M08)
    vertebrae M1A.28 ☑ (following M08)
    wrist M1A.23- ☑ (following M08)
  idiopathic M1A.00 ☑ (following M08)
    ankle M1A.07- ☑ (following M08)
    elbow M1A.02- ☑ (following M08)
    foot joint M1A.07- ☑ (following M08)
    hand joint M1A.04- ☑ (following M08)
    hip M1A.05- ☑ (following M08)
    knee M1A.06- ☑ (following M08)
    multiple site M1A.09 ☑ (following M08)
    shoulder M1A.01- ☑ (following M08)
    vertebrae M1A.08 ☑ (following M08)
    wrist M1A.03- ☑ (following M08)
  in (due to) renal impairment M1A.30 ☑ (following M08)
    ankle M1A.37- ☑ (following M08)
    elbow M1A.32- ☑ (following M08)
    foot joint M1A.37- ☑ (following M08)
    hand joint M1A.34- ☑ (following M08)
    hip M1A.35- ☑ (following M08)
    knee M1A.36- ☑ (following M08)
    multiple site M1A.39 ☑ (following M08)
    shoulder M1A.31- ☑ (following M08)
    vertebrae M1A.38 ☑ (following M08)
    wrist M1A.33- ☑ (following M08)
  lead-induced M1A.10 ☑ (following M08)
    ankle M1A.17- ☑ (following M08)
    elbow M1A.12- ☑ (following M08)
    foot joint M1A.17- ☑ (following M08)
    hand joint M1A.14- ☑ (following M08)
    hip M1A.15- ☑ (following M08)
    knee M1A.16- ☑ (following M08)
    multiple site M1A.19 ☑ (following M08)
    shoulder M1A.11- ☑ (following M08)
    vertebrae M1A.18 ☑ (following M08)
    wrist M1A.13- ☑ (following M08)
  primary — see Gout, chronic, idiopathic
  saturnine — see Gout, chronic, lead-induced
  secondary NEC M1A.40 ☑ (following M08)
    ankle M1A.47- ☑ (following M08)
    elbow M1A.42- ☑ (following M08)
    foot joint M1A.47- ☑ (following M08)
    hand joint M1A.44- ☑ (following M08)
    hip M1A.45- ☑ (following M08)
    knee M1A.46- ☑ (following M08)
    multiple site M1A.49 ☑ (following M08)
    shoulder M1A.41- ☑ (following M08)
    vertebrae M1A.48 ☑ (following M08)
    wrist M1A.43- ☑ (following M08)
  syphilitic (see also subcategory M14.8-) A52.77
  tophi M1A.9 ☑ (following M08)
Gout, gouty (acute) (attack) (flare) (see also Gout, chronic) M10.9
  drug-induced M10.20
    ankle M10.27- ☑
    elbow M10.22- ☑
    foot joint M10.27- ☑
    hand joint M10.24- ☑
    hip M10.25- ☑
    knee M10.26- ☑
    multiple site M10.29
    shoulder M10.21- ☑
    vertebrae M10.28
    wrist M10.23- ☑
  idiopathic M10.00
    ankle M10.07- ☑
    elbow M10.02- ☑
    foot joint M10.07- ☑
    hand joint M10.04- ☑
    hip M10.05- ☑
    knee M10.06- ☑
    multiple site M10.09
    shoulder M10.01- ☑
    vertebrae M10.08
    wrist M10.03- ☑
  in (due to) renal impairment M10.30
    ankle M10.37- ☑

☑ Additional Character Required — Refer to the Tabular List for Character Selection   ▿ Subterms under main terms may continue to next column or page

Gout, gouty — *continued*
  in renal impairment — *continued*
    elbow M10.32- ☑
    foot joint M10.37- ☑
    hand joint M10.34- ☑
    hip M10.35- ☑
    knee M10.36- ☑
    multiple site M10.39
    shoulder M10.31- ☑
    vertebrae M10.38
    wrist M10.33- ☑
  lead-induced M10.10
    ankle M10.17- ☑
    elbow M10.12- ☑
    foot joint M10.17- ☑
    hand joint M10.14- ☑
    hip M10.15- ☑
    knee M10.16- ☑
    multiple site M10.19
    shoulder M10.11- ☑
    vertebrae M10.18
    wrist M10.13- ☑
  primary — *see* Gout, idiopathic
  saturnine — *see* Gout, lead-induced
  secondary NEC M10.40
    ankle M10.47- ☑
    elbow M10.42- ☑
    foot joint M10.47- ☑
    hand joint M10.44- ☑
    hip M10.45- ☑
    knee M10.46- ☑
    multiple site M10.49
    shoulder M10.41- ☑
    vertebrae M10.48
    wrist M10.43- ☑
  syphilitic (*see also* subcategory M14.8-) A52.77
  tophi — *see* Gout, chronic
Gower's
  muscular dystrophy G71.0
  syndrome (vasovagal attack) R55
Gradenigo's syndrome — *see* Otitis, media, suppurative, acute
Graefe's disease — *see* Strabismus, paralytic, ophthalmoplegia, progressive
Graft-versus-host disease D89.813
  acute D89.810
  acute on chronic D89.812
  chronic D89.811
Grain mite (itch) B88.0
Grainhandler's disease or lung J67.8
Grand mal — *see* Epilepsy, generalized, specified NEC
Grand multipara status only (not pregnant) Z64.1
  pregnant — *see* Pregnancy, complicated by, grand multiparity
Granite worker's lung J62.8
Granular (*see also* condition)
  inflammation, pharynx J31.2
  kidney (contracting) — *see* Sclerosis, renal
  liver K74.69
Granulation tissue (abnormal) (excessive) L92.9
  postmastoidectomy cavity — *see* Complications, postmastoidectomy, granulation
Granulocytopenia (primary) (malignant) — *see* Agranulocytosis
Granuloma L92.9
  abdomen K66.8
    from residual foreign body L92.3
    pyogenicum L98.0
  actinic L57.5
  annulare (perforating) L92.0
  apical K04.5
  aural — *see* Otitis, externa, specified NEC
  beryllium (skin) L92.3
  bone
    eosinophilic C96.6
    from residual foreign body — *see* Osteomyelitis, specified type NEC
    lung C96.6
  brain (any site) G06.0
    schistosomiasis B65.9 [G07]
  canaliculus lacrimalis — *see* Granuloma, lacrimal
  candidal (cutaneous) B37.2
  cerebral (any site) G06.0
  coccidioidal (primary) (progressive) B38.7
    lung B38.1
    meninges B38.4
  colon K63.89

Granuloma — *continued*
  conjunctiva H11.22- ☑
  dental K04.5
  ear, middle — *see* Cholesteatoma
  eosinophilic C96.6
    bone C96.6
    lung C96.6
    oral mucosa K13.4
    skin L92.2
  eyelid H01.8
  facial (e) L92.2
  foreign body (in soft tissue) NEC M60.20
    ankle M60.27- ☑
    foot M60.27- ☑
    forearm M60.23- ☑
    hand M60.24- ☑
    in operation wound — *see* Foreign body, accidentally left during a procedure
    lower leg M60.26- ☑
    pelvic region M60.25- ☑
    shoulder region M60.21- ☑
    skin L92.3
    specified site NEC M60.28
    subcutaneous tissue L92.3
    thigh M60.25- ☑
    upper arm M60.22- ☑
  gangraenescens M31.2
  genito-inguinale A58
  giant cell (central) (reparative) (jaw) M27.1
    gingiva (peripheral) K06.8
  gland (lymph) I88.8
  hepatic NEC K75.3
    in (due to)
      berylliosis J63.2 [K77]
      sarcoidosis D86.89
  Hodgkin C81.9 ☑
  ileum K63.89
  infectious B99.9
    specified NEC B99.8
  inguinale (Donovan) (venereal) A58
  intestine NEC K63.89
  intracranial (any site) G06.0
  intraspinal (any part) G06.1
  iridocyclitis — *see* Iridocyclitis, chronic
  jaw (bone) (central) M27.1
    reparative giant cell M27.1
  kidney (*see also* Infection, kidney) N15.8
  lacrimal H04.81- ☑
  larynx J38.7
  lethal midline (faciale(e)) M31.2
  liver NEC — *see* Granuloma, hepatic
  lung (infectious) (*see also* Fibrosis, lung)
    coccidioidal B38.1
    eosinophilic C96.6
  Majocchi's B35.8
  malignant (facial(e)) M31.2
  mandible (central) M27.1
  midline (lethal) M31.2
  monilial (cutaneous) B37.2
  nasal sinus — *see* Sinusitis
  operation wound T81.89 ☑
    foreign body — *see* Foreign body, accidentally left during a procedure
    stitch T81.89 ☑
    talc — *see* Foreign body, accidentally left during a procedure
  oral mucosa K13.4
  orbit, orbital H05.11- ☑
  paracoccidioidal B41.8
  penis, venereal A58
  periapical K04.5
  peritoneum K66.8
    due to ova of helminths NOS (*see also* Helminthiasis) B83.9 [K67]
  postmastoidectomy cavity — *see* Complications, postmastoidectomy, recurrent cholesteatoma
  prostate N42.89
  pudendi (ulcerating) A58
  pulp, internal (tooth) K03.3
  pyogenic, pyogenicum (of) (skin) L98.0
    gingiva K06.8
    maxillary alveolar ridge K04.5
    oral mucosa K13.4
  rectum K62.89
  reticulohistiocytic D76.3
  rubrum nasi L74.8
  Schistosoma — *see* Schistosomiasis
  septic (skin) L98.0

Granuloma — *continued*
  silica (skin) L92.3
  sinus (accessory) (infective) (nasal) — *see* Sinusitis
  skin L92.9
    from residual foreign body L92.3
    pyogenicum L98.0
  spine
    syphilitic (epidural) A52.19
    tuberculous A18.01
  stitch (postoperative) T81.89 ☑
  suppurative (skin) L98.0
  swimming pool A31.1
  talc (*see also* Granuloma, foreign body)
    in operation wound — *see* Foreign body, accidentally left during a procedure
  telangiectaticum (skin) L98.0
  tracheostomy J95.09
  trichophyticum B35.8
  tropicum A66.4
  umbilical P83.81
  umbilicus P83.81
  urethra N36.8
  uveitis — *see* Iridocyclitis, chronic
  vagina A58
  venereum A58
  vocal cord J38.3
Granulomatosis L92.9
  lymphoid C83.8- ☑
  miliary (listerial) A32.89
  necrotizing, respiratory M31.30
  progressive septic D71
  specified NEC L92.8
  Wegener's M31.30
    with renal involvement M31.31
Granulomatous tissue (abnormal) (excessive) L92.9
Granulosis rubra nasi L74.8
Graphite fibrosis (of lung) J63.3
Graphospasm F48.8
  organic G25.89
Grating scapula M89.8X1
Gravel (urinary) — *see* Calculus, urinary
Graves' disease — *see* Hyperthyroidism, with, goiter
Gravis — *see* condition
Grawitz tumor C64.- ☑
Gray syndrome (newborn) P93.0
Grayness, hair (premature) L67.1
  congenital Q84.2
Green sickness D50.8
Greenfield's disease
  meaning
    concentric sclerosis (encephalitis periaxialis concentrica) G37.5
    metachromatic leukodystrophy E75.25
Greenstick fracture — *code as* Fracture, by site
Grey syndrome (newborn) P93.0
Grief F43.21
  prolonged F43.29
  reaction (*see also* Disorder, adjustment) F43.20
Griesinger's disease B76.9
Grinder's lung or pneumoconiosis J62.8
Grinding, teeth
  psychogenic F45.8
  sleep related G47.63
Grip
  Dabney's B33.0
  devil's B33.0
Grippe, grippal (*see also* Influenza)
  Balkan A78
  summer, of Italy A93.1
Grisel's disease M43.6
Groin — *see* condition
Grooved tongue K14.5
Ground itch B76.9
Grover's disease or syndrome L11.1
Growing pains, children R29.898
Growth (fungoid) (neoplastic) (new) (*see also* Neoplasm)
  adenoid (vegetative) J35.8
  benign — *see* Neoplasm, benign, by site
  malignant — *see* Neoplasm, malignant, by site
  rapid, childhood Z00.2
  secondary — *see* Neoplasm, secondary, by site
Gruby's disease B35.0
Gubler-Millard paralysis or syndrome G46.3
Guerin-Stern syndrome Q74.3
Guidance, insufficient anterior (occlusal) M26.54
Guillain-Barré disease or syndrome G61.0
  sequelae G65.0

Guinea worms (infection) (infestation) B72
Guinon's disease (motor-verbal tic) F95.2
Gull's disease E03.4
Gum — see condition
Gumboil K04.7
  with sinus K04.6
Gumma (syphilitic) A52.79
  artery A52.09
    cerebral A52.04
  bone A52.77
    of yaws (late) A66.6
  brain A52.19
  cauda equina A52.19
  central nervous system A52.3
  ciliary body A52.71
  congenital A50.59
  eyelid A52.71
  heart A52.06
  intracranial A52.19
  iris A52.71
  kidney A52.75
  larynx A52.73
  leptomeninges A52.19
  liver A52.74
  meninges A52.19
  myocardium A52.06
  nasopharynx A52.73
  neurosyphilitic A52.3
  nose A52.73
  orbit A52.71
  palate (soft) A52.79
  penis A52.76
  pericardium A52.06
  pharynx A52.73
  pituitary A52.79
  scrofulous (tuberculous) A18.4
  skin A52.79
  specified site NEC A52.79
  spinal cord A52.19
  tongue A52.79
  tonsil A52.73
  trachea A52.73
  tuberculous A18.4
  ulcerative due to yaws A66.4
  ureter A52.75
  yaws A66.4
    bone A66.6
Gunn's syndrome Q07.8
Gunshot wound (see also Wound, open)
  fracture — code as Fracture, by site
  internal organs — see Injury, by site
Gynandrism Q56.0
Gynandroblastoma
  specified site — see Neoplasm, uncertain behavior,
    by site
  unspecified site
    female D39.10
    male D40.10
Gynecological examination (periodic) (routine) Z01.419
  with abnormal findings Z01.411
Gynecomastia N62
Gynephobia F40.291
Gyrate scalp Q82.8

H

H (Hartnup's) **disease** E72.02
Haas' disease or osteochondrosis (juvenile) (head of
  humerus) — see Osteochondrosis, juvenile,
  humerus
Habit, habituation
  bad sleep Z72.821
  chorea F95.8
  disturbance, child F98.9
  drug — see Dependence, drug
  irregular sleep Z72.821
  laxative F55.2
  spasm — see Tic
  tic — see Tic
Haemophilus (H.) **influenzae, as cause of disease
  classified elsewhere** B96.3
Haff disease — see Poisoning, mercury
Hageman's factor defect, deficiency or disease D68.2
Haglund's disease or osteochondrosis (juvenile) (os
  tibiale externum) — see Osteochondrosis, juvenile,
  tarsus
Hailey-Hailey disease Q82.8

Hair (see also condition)
  plucking F63.3
    in stereotyped movement disorder F98.4
  tourniquet syndrome (see also Constriction, external,
    by site)
    finger S60.44- ☑
    penis S30.842 ☑
    thumb S60.34- ☑
    toe S90.44- ☑
Hairball in stomach T18.2 ☑
Hair-pulling, pathological (compulsive) F63.3
Hairy black tongue K14.3
Half vertebra Q76.49
Halitosis R19.6
Hallerman-Streiff syndrome Q87.0
Hallervorden-Spatz disease G23.0
Hallopeau's acrodermatitis or disease L40.2
Hallucination R44.3
  auditory R44.0
  gustatory R44.2
  olfactory R44.2
  specified NEC R44.2
  tactile R44.2
  visual R44.1
Hallucinosis (chronic) F28
  alcoholic (acute) F10.951
    in
      abuse F10.151
      dependence F10.251
  drug-induced F19.951
    cannabis F12.951
    cocaine F14.951
    hallucinogen F16.151
    in
      abuse F19.151
        cannabis F12.151
        cocaine F14.151
        hallucinogen F16.151
        inhalant F18.151
        opioid F11.151
        sedative, anxiolytic or hypnotic F13.151
        stimulant NEC F15.151
      dependence F19.251
        cannabis F12.251
        cocaine F14.251
        hallucinogen F16.251
        inhalant F18.251
        opioid F11.251
        sedative, anxiolytic or hypnotic F13.251
        stimulant NEC F15.251
    inhalant F18.951
    opioid F11.951
    sedative, anxiolytic or hypnotic F13.951
    stimulant NEC F15.951
  organic F06.0
Hallux
  deformity (acquired) NEC M20.5X- ☑
  limitus M20.5X-
  malleus (acquired) NEC M20.3- ☑
  rigidus (acquired) M20.2- ☑
    congenital Q74.2
    sequelae (late effect) of rickets E64.3
  valgus (acquired) M20.1- ☑
    congenital Q66.6
  varus (acquired) M20.3- ☑
    congenital Q66.3
Halo, visual H53.19
Hamartoma, hamartoblastoma Q85.9
  epithelial (gingival), odontogenic, central or peripheral
    — see Cyst, calcifying odontogenic
Hamartosis Q85.9
Hamman-Rich syndrome J84.114
Hammer toe (acquired) NEC (see also Deformity, toe,
  hammer toe)
  congenital Q66.89
  sequelae (late effect) of rickets E64.3
Hand — see condition
Hand-foot syndrome L27.1
Handicap, handicapped
  educational Z55.9
  specified NEC Z55.8
Hand-Schüller-Christian disease or syndrome C96.5
Hanging (asphyxia) (strangulation) (suffocation) — see
  Asphyxia, traumatic, due to mechanical threat
Hangnail (see also Cellulitis, digit)
  with lymphangitis — see Lymphangitis, acute, digit
Hangover (alcohol) F10.129

Hanhart's syndrome Q87.0
Hanot-Chauffard (-Troisier) **syndrome** E83.19
Hanot's cirrhosis or disease K74.3
Hansen's disease — see Leprosy
Hantaan virus disease (Korean hemorrhagic fever) A98.5
Hantavirus disease (with renal manifestations) (Dobra-
  va) (Puumala) (Seoul) A98.5
  with pulmonary manifestations (Andes) (Bayou)
    (Bermejo) (Black Creek Canal) (Choclo) (Juquiti-
    ba) (Laguna negra) (Lechiguanas) (New York)
    (Oran) (Sin nombre) B33.4
Happy puppet syndrome Q93.5
Harada's disease or syndrome H30.81- ☑
Hardening
  artery — See Arteriosclerosis
  brain G93.89
Harelip (complete) (incomplete) — see Cleft, lip
Harlequin (newborn) Q80.4
Harley's disease D59.6
Harmful use (of)
  alcohol F10.10
  anxiolytics — see Abuse, drug, sedative
  cannabinoids — see Abuse, drug, cannabis
  cocaine — see Abuse, drug, cocaine
  drug — see Abuse, drug
  hallucinogens — see Abuse, drug, hallucinogen
  hypnotics — see Abuse, drug, sedative
  opioids — see Abuse, drug, opioid
  PCP (phencyclidine) — see Abuse, drug, hallucinogen
  sedatives — see Abuse, drug, sedative
  stimulants NEC — see Abuse, drug, stimulant
Harris' lines — see Arrest, epiphyseal
Hartnup's disease E72.02
Harvester's lung J67.0
Harvesting ovum for in vitro fertilization Z31.83
Hashimoto's disease or thyroiditis E06.3
Hashitoxicosis (transient) E06.3
Hassal-Henle bodies or warts (cornea) H18.49
Haut mal — see Epilepsy, generalized, specified NEC
Haverhill fever A25.1
Hay fever (see also Fever, hay) J30.1
Hayem-Widal syndrome D59.8
Haygarth's nodes M15.8
Haymaker's lung J67.0
Hb (abnormal)
  Bart's disease D56.0
  disease — see Disease, hemoglobin
  trait — see Trait
Head — see condition
Headache R51
  allergic NEC G44.89
  associated with sexual activity G44.82
  chronic daily R51
  cluster G44.009
    chronic G44.029
      intractable G44.021
      not intractable G44.029
    episodic G44.019
      intractable G44.011
      not intractable G44.019
    intractable G44.001
    not intractable G44.009
  cough (primary) G44.83
  daily chronic R51
  drug-induced NEC G44.40
    intractable G44.41
    not intractable G44.40
  exertional (primary) G44.84
  histamine G44.009
    intractable G44.001
    not intractable G44.009
  hypnic G44.81
  lumbar puncture G97.1
  medication overuse G44.40
    intractable G44.41
    not intractable G44.40
  menstrual — see Migraine, menstrual
  migraine (type) (see also Migraine) G43.909
  nasal septum R51
  neuralgiform, short lasting unilateral, with conjunctival
    injection and tearing (SUNCT) G44.059
    intractable G44.051
    not intractable G44.059
  new daily persistent (NDPH) G44.52
  orgasmic G44.82
  periodic syndromes in adults and children G43.C0
    (following G43.7)

☑ **Additional Character Required** — Refer to the Tabular List for Character Selection
▽ **Subterms under main terms may continue to next column or page**

Headache — *continued*
  periodic syndromes in adults and children — *continued*
    with refractory migraine G43.C1 (*following* G43.7)
    without refractory migraine G43.C0 (*following* G43.7)
    intractable G43.C1 (*following* G43.7)
    not intractable G43.C0 (*following* G43.7)
  postspinal puncture G97.1
  post-traumatic G44.309
    acute G44.319
      intractable G44.311
      not intractable G44.319
    chronic G44.329
      intractable G44.321
      not intractable G44.329
    intractable G44.301
    not intractable G44.309
  pre-menstrual — *see* Migraine, menstrual
  preorgasmic G44.82
  primary
    cough G44.83
    exertional G44.84
    stabbing G44.85
    thunderclap G44.53
  rebound G44.40
    intractable G44.41
    not intractable G44.40
  short lasting unilateral neuralgiform, with conjunctival injection and tearing (SUNCT) G44.059
    intractable G44.051
    not intractable G44.059
  specified syndrome NEC G44.89
  spinal and epidural anesthesia - induced T88.59 ☑
    in labor and delivery O74.5
    in pregnancy O29.4- ☑
    postpartum, puerperal O89.4
  spinal fluid loss (from puncture) G97.1
  stabbing (primary) G44.85
  tension (-type) G44.209
    chronic G44.229
      intractable G44.221
      not intractable G44.229
    episodic G44.219
      intractable G44.211
      not intractable G44.219
    intractable G44.201
    not intractable G44.209
  thunderclap (primary) G44.53
  vascular NEC G44.1
Healthy
  infant
    accompanying sick mother Z76.3
    receiving care Z76.2
  person accompanying sick person Z76.3
Hearing examination Z01.10
  with abnormal findings NEC Z01.118
  following failed hearing screening Z01.110
  for hearing conservation and treatment Z01.12
Heart — *see* condition
Heart beat
  abnormality R00.9
    specified NEC R00.8
  awareness R00.2
  rapid R00.0
  slow R00.1
Heartburn R12
  psychogenic F45.8
Heartland virus disease A93.8
Heat (effects) T67.9 ☑
  apoplexy T67.0 ☑
  burn (*see also* Burn) L55.9
  collapse T67.1 ☑
  cramps T67.2 ☑
  dermatitis or eczema L59.0
  edema T67.7 ☑
  erythema — *code by site under* Burn, first degree
  excessive T67.9 ☑
    specified effect NEC T67.8 ☑
  exhaustion T67.5 ☑
    anhydrotic T67.3 ☑
    due to
      salt (and water) depletion T67.4 ☑
      water depletion T67.3 ☑
        with salt depletion T67.4 ☑
  fatigue (transient) T67.6 ☑
  fever T67.0 ☑
  hyperpyrexia T67.0 ☑

Heat — *continued*
  prickly L74.0
  prostration — *see* Heat, exhaustion
  pyrexia T67.0 ☑
  rash L74.0
  specified effect NEC T67.8 ☑
  stroke T67.0 ☑
  sunburn — *see* Sunburn
  syncope T67.1 ☑
Heavy-for-dates NEC (infant) (4000g to 4499g) P08.1
  exceptionally (4500g or more) P08.0
Hebephrenia, hebephrenic (schizophrenia) F20.1
Heberden's disease or nodes (with arthropathy) M15.1
Hebra's
  pityriasis L26
  prurigo L28.2
Heel — *see* condition
Heerfordt's disease D86.89
Hegglin's anomaly or syndrome D72.0
Heilmeyer-Schoner disease D45
Heine-Medin disease A80.9
Heinz body anemia, congenital D58.2
Heliophobia F40.228
Heller's disease or syndrome F84.3
HELLP syndrome (hemolysis, elevated liver enzymes and low platelet count) O14.2- ☑
  complicating
    childbirth O14.24
    puerperium O14.25
Helminthiasis (*see also* Infestation, helminth)
  Ancylostoma B76.0
  intestinal B82.0
    mixed types (types classifiable to more than one of the titles B65.0-B81.3 and B81.8) B81.4
    specified type NEC B81.8
  mixed types (intestinal) (types classifiable to more than one of the titles B65.0-B81.3 and B81.8) B81.4
  Necator (americanus) B76.1
  specified type NEC B83.8
Heloma L84
Hemangioblastoma — *see* Neoplasm, connective tissue, uncertain behavior
  malignant — *see* Neoplasm, connective tissue, malignant
Hemangioendothelioma (*see also* Neoplasm, uncertain behavior, by site)
  benign D18.00
    intra-abdominal D18.03
    intracranial D18.02
    skin D18.01
    specified site NEC D18.09
  bone (diffuse) — *see* Neoplasm, bone, malignant
  epithelioid (*see also* Neoplasm, uncertain behavior, by site)
    malignant — *see* Neoplasm, malignant, by site
  malignant — *see* Neoplasm, connective tissue, malignant
Hemangiofibroma — *see* Neoplasm, benign, by site
Hemangiolipoma — *see* Lipoma
Hemangioma D18.00
  arteriovenous D18.00
    intra-abdominal D18.03
    intracranial D18.02
    skin D18.01
    specified site NEC D18.09
  capillary D18.00
    intra-abdominal D18.03
    intracranial D18.02
    skin D18.01
    specified site NEC D18.09
  cavernous D18.00
    intra-abdominal D18.03
    intracranial D18.02
    skin D18.01
    specified site NEC D18.09
  epithelioid D18.00
    intra-abdominal D18.03
    intracranial D18.02
    skin D18.01
    specified site NEC D18.09
  histiocytoid D18.00
    intra-abdominal D18.03
    intracranial D18.02
    skin D18.01
    specified site NEC D18.09
  infantile D18.00
    intra-abdominal D18.03

Hemangioma — *continued*
  infantile — *continued*
    intracranial D18.02
    skin D18.01
    specified site NEC D18.09
  intra-abdominal D18.03
  intracranial D18.02
  intramuscular D18.00
    intra-abdominal D18.03
    intracranial D18.02
    skin D18.01
    specified site NEC D18.09
  intrathoracic structures D18.09
  juvenile D18.00
  malignant — *see* Neoplasm, connective tissue, malignant
  plexiform D18.00
    intra-abdominal D18.03
    intracranial D18.02
    skin D18.01
    specified site NEC D18.09
  racemose D18.00
    intra-abdominal D18.03
    intracranial D18.02
    skin D18.01
    specified site NEC D18.09
  sclerosing — *see* Neoplasm, skin, benign
  simplex D18.00
    intra-abdominal D18.03
    intracranial D18.02
    skin D18.01
    specified site NEC D18.09
  skin D18.01
  specified site NEC D18.09
  venous D18.00
    intra-abdominal D18.03
    intracranial D18.02
    skin D18.01
    specified site NEC D18.09
  verrucous keratotic D18.00
    intra-abdominal D18.03
    intracranial D18.02
    skin D18.01
    specified site NEC D18.09
Hemangiomatosis (systemic) I78.8
  involving single site — *see* Hemangioma
Hemangiopericytoma (*see also* Neoplasm, connective tissue, uncertain behavior)
  benign — *see* Neoplasm, connective tissue, benign
  malignant — *see* Neoplasm, connective tissue, malignant
Hemangiosarcoma — *see* Neoplasm, connective tissue, malignant
Hemarthrosis (nontraumatic) M25.00
  ankle M25.07- ☑
  elbow M25.02- ☑
  foot joint M25.07- ☑
  hand joint M25.04- ☑
  hip M25.05- ☑
  in hemophilic arthropathy — *see* Arthropathy, hemophilic
  knee M25.06- ☑
  shoulder M25.01- ☑
  specified joint NEC M25.08
  traumatic — *see* Sprain, by site
  vertebrae M25.08
  wrist M25.03- ☑
Hematemesis K92.0
  with ulcer — *code by site under* Ulcer, with hemorrhage K27.4
  newborn, neonatal P54.0
    due to swallowed maternal blood P78.2
Hematidrosis L74.8
Hematinuria (*see also* Hemoglobinuria)
  malarial B50.8
Hematobilia K83.8
Hematocele
  female NEC N94.89
    with ectopic pregnancy O00.90
      with intrauterine pregnancy O00.91
    ovary N83.8
  male N50.1
Hematochezia (*see also* Melena) K92.1
Hematochyluria (*see also* Infestation, filarial)
  schistosomiasis (bilharziasis) B65.0
Hematocolpos (with hematometra or hematosalpinx) N89.7
Hematocornea — *see* Pigmentation, cornea, stromal

Index

Hematogenous — Hemiplegia

Hematogenous — *see* condition
Hematoma (traumatic) (skin surface intact) (*see also* Contusion)
  with
    injury of internal organs — *see* Injury, by site
    open wound — *see* Wound, open
  amputation stump (surgical) (late) T87.89
  aorta, dissecting I71.00
    abdominal I71.02
    thoracic I71.01
    thoracoabdominal I71.03
  aortic intramural — *see* Dissection, aorta
  arterial (complicating trauma) — *see* Injury, blood vessel, by site
  auricle — *see* Contusion, ear
    nontraumatic — *see* Disorder, pinna, hematoma
  birth injury NEC P15.8
  brain (traumatic)
    with
      cerebral laceration or contusion (diffuse) — *see* Injury, intracranial, diffuse
        focal — *see* Injury, intracranial, focal
    cerebellar, traumatic S06.37- ☑
    intracerebral, traumatic — *see* Injury, intracranial, intracerebral hemorrhage
    newborn NEC P52.4
      birth injury P10.1
    nontraumatic — *see* Hemorrhage, intracranial
    subarachnoid, arachnoid, traumatic — *see* Injury, intracranial, subarachnoid hemorrhage
    subdural, traumatic — *see* Injury, intracranial, subdural hemorrhage
  breast (nontraumatic) N64.89
  broad ligament (nontraumatic) N83.7
    traumatic S37.892 ☑
  cerebellar, traumatic S06.37- ☑
  cerebral — *see* Hematoma, brain
  cerebrum S06.36- ☑
    left S06.35- ☑
    right S06.34- ☑
  cesarean delivery wound O90.2
  complicating delivery (perineal) (pelvic) (vagina) (vulva) O71.7
  corpus cavernosum (nontraumatic) N48.89
  epididymis (nontraumatic) N50.1
  epidural (traumatic) — *see* Injury, intracranial, epidural hemorrhage
    spinal — *see* Injury, spinal cord, by region
  episiotomy O90.2
  face, birth injury P15.4
  genital organ NEC (nontraumatic)
    female (nonobstetric) N94.89
      traumatic S30.202 ☑
    male N50.1
      traumatic S30.201 ☑
  internal organs — *see* Injury, by site
  intracerebral, traumatic — *see* Injury, intracranial, intracerebral hemorrhage
  intraoperative — *see* Complications, intraoperative, hemorrhage
  labia (nontraumatic) (nonobstetric) N90.89
  liver (subcapsular) (nontraumatic) K76.89
    birth injury P15.0
  mediastinum — *see* Injury, intrathoracic
  mesosalpinx (nontraumatic) N83.7
    traumatic S37.898 ☑
  muscle — code by site under Contusion
  nontraumatic
    muscle M79.81
    soft tissue M79.81
  obstetrical surgical wound O90.2
  orbit, orbital (nontraumatic) (*see also* Hemorrhage, orbit)
    traumatic — *see* Contusion, orbit
  pelvis (female) (nontraumatic) (nonobstetric) N94.89
    obstetric O71.7
    traumatic — *see* Injury, by site
  penis (nontraumatic) N48.89
    birth injury P15.5
  perianal (nontraumatic) K64.5
  perineal S30.23 ☑
    complicating delivery O71.7
  perirenal — *see* Injury, kidney
  pinna — *see* Contusion, ear
    nontraumatic — *see* Disorder, pinna, hematoma
  placenta O43.89- ☑

Hematoma — *continued*
  postoperative (postprocedural) — *see* Complication, postprocedural, hematoma
  retroperitoneal (nontraumatic) K66.1
    traumatic S36.892 ☑
  scrotum, superficial S30.22 ☑
    birth injury P15.5
  seminal vesicle (nontraumatic) N50.1
    traumatic S37.892 ☑
  spermatic cord (traumatic) S37.892 ☑
    nontraumatic N50.1
  spinal (cord) (meninges) (*see also* Injury, spinal cord, by region)
    newborn (birth injury) P11.5
  spleen D73.5
    intraoperative — *see* Complications, intraoperative, hemorrhage, spleen
    postprocedural (postoperative) — *see* Complications, postprocedural, hemorrhage, spleen
  sternocleidomastoid, birth injury P15.2
  sternomastoid, birth injury P15.2
  subarachnoid (traumatic) — *see* Injury, intracranial, subarachnoid hemorrhage
    newborn (nontraumatic) P52.5
      due to birth injury P10.3
    nontraumatic — *see* Hemorrhage, intracranial, subarachnoid
  subdural (traumatic) — *see* Injury, intracranial, subdural hemorrhage
    newborn (localized) P52.8
      birth injury P10.0
    nontraumatic — *see* Hemorrhage, intracranial, subdural
  superficial, newborn P54.5
  testis (nontraumatic) N50.1
    birth injury P15.5
  tunica vaginalis (nontraumatic) N50.1
  umbilical cord, complicating delivery O69.5 ☑
  uterine ligament (broad) (nontraumatic) N83.7
    traumatic S37.892 ☑
  vagina (ruptured) (nontraumatic) N89.8
    complicating delivery O71.7
  vas deferens (nontraumatic) N50.1
    traumatic S37.892 ☑
  vitreous — *see* Hemorrhage, vitreous
  vulva (nontraumatic) (nonobstetric) N90.89
    complicating delivery O71.7
    newborn (birth injury) P15.5
Hematometra N85.7
  with hematocolpos N89.7
Hematomyelia (central) G95.19
  newborn (birth injury) P11.5
  traumatic T14.8 ☑
Hematomyelitis G04.90
Hematoperitoneum — *see* Hemoperitoneum
Hematophobia F40.230
Hematopneumothorax (see Hemothorax)
Hematopoiesis, cyclic D70.4
Hematoporphyria — *see* Porphyria
Hematorachis, hematorrhachis G95.19
  newborn (birth injury) P11.5
Hematosalpinx N83.6
  with
    hematocolpos N89.7
    hematometra N85.7
      with hematocolpos N89.7
  infectional — *see* Salpingitis
Hematospermia R36.1
Hematothorax (see Hemothorax)
Hematuria R31.9
  benign (familial) (of childhood) (*see also* Hematuria, idiopathic)
    essential microscopic R31.1
  due to sulphonamide, sulfonamide — *see* Table of Drugs and Chemicals, by drug
  endemic (*see also* Schistosomiasis) B65.0
  gross R31.0
  idiopathic N02.9
    with glomerular lesion
      crescentic (diffuse) glomerulonephritis N02.7
      dense deposit disease N02.6
      endocapillary proliferative glomerulonephritis N02.4
      focal and segmental hyalinosis or sclerosis N02.1
      membranoproliferative (diffuse) N02.5
      membranous (diffuse) N02.2
      mesangial proliferative (diffuse) N02.3

Hematuria — *continued*
  idiopathic — *continued*
    with glomerular lesion — *continued*
      mesangiocapillary (diffuse) N02.5
      minor abnormality N02.0
      proliferative NEC N02.8
      specified pathology NEC N02.8
  intermittent — *see* Hematuria, idiopathic
  malarial B50.8
  microscopic NEC (with symptoms) R31.29
    asymptomatic R31.21
    benign essential R31.1
  paroxysmal (*see also* Hematuria, idiopathic)
    nocturnal D59.5
  persistent — *see* Hematuria, idiopathic
  recurrent — *see* Hematuria, idiopathic
  tropical (*see also* Schistosomiasis) B65.0
  tuberculous A18.13
Hemeralopia (day blindness) H53.11
  vitamin A deficiency E50.5
Hemi-akinesia R41.4
Hemianalgesia R20.0
Hemianencephaly Q00.0
Hemianesthesia R20.0
Hemianopia, hemianopsia (heteronymous) H53.47
  homonymous H53.46- ☑
  syphilitic A52.71
Hemiathetosis R25.8
Hemiatrophy R68.89
  cerebellar G31.9
  face, facial, progressive (Romberg) G51.8
  tongue K14.8
Hemiballism (us) G25.5
Hemicardia Q24.8
Hemicephalus, hemicephaly Q00.0
Hemichorea G25.5
Hemicolitis, left — *see* Colitis, left sided
Hemicrania
  congenital malformation Q00.0
  continua G44.51
  meaning migraine (*see also* Migraine) G43.909
  paroxysmal G44.039
    chronic G44.049
      intractable G44.041
      not intractable G44.049
    episodic G44.039
      intractable G44.031
      not intractable G44.039
    intractable G44.031
    not intractable G44.039
Hemidystrophy — *see* Hemiatrophy
Hemiectromelia Q73.8
Hemihypalgesia R20.8
Hemihypesthesia R20.1
Hemi-inattention R41.4
Hemimelia Q73.8
  lower limb — *see* Defect, reduction, lower limb, specified type NEC
  upper limb — *see* Defect, reduction, upper limb, specified type NEC
Hemiparalysis — *see* Hemiplegia
Hemiparesis — *see* Hemiplegia
Hemiparesthesia R20.2
Hemiparkinsonism G20
Hemiplegia G81.9- ☑
  alternans facialis G83.89
  ascending NEC G81.90
    spinal G95.89
  congenital (cerebral) G80.8
    spastic G80.2
  embolic (current episode) I63.4- ☑
  flaccid G81.0- ☑
  following
    cerebrovascular disease I69.959
      cerebral infarction I69.35- ☑
      intracerebral hemorrhage I69.15- ☑
      nontraumatic intracranial hemorrhage NEC I69.25- ☑
      specified disease NEC I69.85- ☑
      stroke NOS I69.35- ☑
      subarachnoid hemorrhage I69.05- ☑
  hysterical F44.4
  newborn NEC P91.88
    birth injury P11.9
  spastic G81.1- ☑
    congenital G80.2
  thrombotic (current episode) I63.3- ☑

☑ Additional Character Required — Refer to the Tabular List for Character Selection   🔺 Subterms under main terms may continue to next column or page

Hemisection, spinal cord — *see* Injury, spinal cord, by region
Hemispasm (facial) R25.2
Hemisporosis B48.8
Hemitremor R25.1
Hemivertebra Q76.49
  failure of segmentation with scoliosis Q76.3
  fusion with scoliosis Q76.3
Hemochromatosis E83.119
  with refractory anemia D46.1
  due to repeated red blood cell transfusion E83.111
  hereditary (primary) E83.110
  neonatal P78.84
  primary E83.110
  specified NEC E83.118
Hemoglobin (*see also* condition)
  abnormal (disease) — *see* Disease, hemoglobin
  AS genotype D57.3
  Constant Spring D58.2
  E-beta thalassemia D56.5
  fetal, hereditary persistence (HPFH) D56.4
  H Constant Spring D56.0
  low NOS D64.9
  S (Hb S), heterozygous D57.3
Hemoglobinemia D59.9
  due to blood transfusion T80.89 ☑
  paroxysmal D59.6
    nocturnal D59.5
Hemoglobinopathy (mixed) D58.2
  with thalassemia D56.8
  sickle-cell D57.1
    with thalassemia D57.40
      with crisis (vasoocclusive pain) D57.419
        with
          acute chest syndrome D57.411
          splenic sequestration D57.412
      without crisis D57.40
Hemoglobinuria R82.3
  with anemia, hemolytic, acquired (chronic) NEC D59.6
  cold (agglutinin) (paroxysmal) (with Raynaud's syndrome) D59.6
  due to exertion or hemolysis NEC D59.6
  intermittent D59.6
  malarial B50.8
  march D59.6
  nocturnal (paroxysmal) D59.5
  paroxysmal (cold) D59.6
    nocturnal D59.5
Hemolymphangioma D18.1
Hemolysis
  intravascular
    with
      abortion — *see* Abortion, by type, complicated by, hemorrhage
      ectopic or molar pregnancy O08.1
      hemorrhage
        antepartum — *see* Hemorrhage, antepartum, with coagulation defect
        intrapartum (*see also* Hemorrhage, complicating, delivery) O67.0
      postpartum O72.3
  neonatal (excessive) P58.9
    specified NEC P58.8
Hemolytic — *see* condition
Hemopericardium I31.2
  following acute myocardial infarction (current complication) I23.0
  newborn P54.8
  traumatic — *see* Injury, heart, with hemopericardium
Hemoperitoneum K66.1
  infectional K65.9
  traumatic S36.899 ☑
    with open wound — *see* Wound, open, with penetration into peritoneal cavity
Hemophilia (classical) (familial) (hereditary) D66
  A D66
  acquired D68.311
  autoimmune D68.311
  B D67
  C D68.1
  calcipriva (*see also* Defect, coagulation) D68.4
  nonfamilial (*see also* Defect, coagulation) D68.4
  secondary D68.311
  vascular D68.0
Hemophthalmos H44.81- ☑
Hemopneumothorax (*see also* Hemothorax)
  traumatic S27.2 ☑
Hemoptysis R04.2

Hemoptysis — *continued*
  newborn P26.9
  tuberculous — *see* Tuberculosis, pulmonary
Hemorrhage, hemorrhagic (concealed) R58
  abdomen R58
  accidental antepartum — *see* Hemorrhage, antepartum
  acute idiopathic pulmonary, in infants R04.81
  adenoid J35.8
  adrenal (capsule) (gland) E27.49
    medulla E27.8
    newborn P54.4
  after delivery — *see* Hemorrhage, postpartum
  alveolar
    lung, newborn P26.8
    process K08.89
  alveolus K08.89
  amputation stump (surgical) T87.89
  anemia (chronic) D50.0
    acute D62
  antepartum (with) O46.90
    with coagulation defect O46.00- ☑
      afibrinogenemia O46.01- ☑
      disseminated intravascular coagulation O46.02- ☑
      hypofibrinogenemia O46.01- ☑
      specified defect NEC O46.09- ☑
    before 20 weeks gestation O20.9
      specified type NEC O20.8
      threatened abortion O20.0
    due to
      abruptio placenta (*see also* Abruptio placentae) O45.9- ☑
      leiomyoma, uterus — *see* Hemorrhage, antepartum, specified cause NEC
      placenta previa O44.1- ☑
    specified cause NEC — *see* subcategory O46.8X- ☑
  anus (sphincter) K62.5
  apoplexy (stroke) — *see* Hemorrhage, intracranial, intracerebral
  arachnoid — *see* Hemorrhage, intracranial, subarachnoid
  artery R58
    brain — *see* Hemorrhage, intracranial, intracerebral
  basilar (ganglion) I61.0
  bladder N32.89
  bowel K92.2
    newborn P54.3
  brain (miliary) (nontraumatic) — *see* Hemorrhage, intracranial, intracerebral
    due to
      birth injury P10.1
      syphilis A52.05
    epidural or extradural (traumatic) — *see* Injury, intracranial, epidural hemorrhage
    newborn P52.4
      birth injury P10.1
    subarachnoid — *see* Hemorrhage, intracranial, subarachnoid
    subdural — *see* Hemorrhage, intracranial, subdural
  brainstem (nontraumatic) I61.3
    traumatic S06.38- ☑
  breast N64.59
  bronchial tube — *see* Hemorrhage, lung
  bronchopulmonary — *see* Hemorrhage, lung
  bronchus — *see* Hemorrhage, lung
  bulbar I61.5
  capillary I78.8
    primary D69.8
  cecum K92.2
  cerebellar, cerebellum (nontraumatic) I61.4
    newborn P52.6
    traumatic S06.37- ☑
  cerebral, cerebrum (*see also* Hemorrhage, intracranial, intracerebral)
    lobe I61.1
    newborn (anoxic) P52.4
      birth injury P10.1
  cerebromeningeal I61.8
  cerebrospinal — *see* Hemorrhage, intracranial, intracerebral
  cervix (uteri) (stump) NEC N88.8
  chamber, anterior (eye) — *see* Hyphema
  childbirth — *see* Hemorrhage, complicating, delivery
  choroid H31.30- ☑
    expulsive H31.31- ☑
  ciliary body — *see* Hyphema
  cochlea — *see* subcategory H83.8 ☑

Hemorrhage, hemorrhagic — *continued*
  colon K92.2
  complicating
    abortion — *see* Abortion, by type, complicated by, hemorrhage
    delivery O67.9
      associated with coagulation defect (afibrinogenemia) (DIC) (hyperfibrinolysis) O67.0
      specified cause NEC O67.8
    surgical procedure — *see* Hemorrhage, intraoperative
  conjunctiva H11.3- ☑
    newborn P54.8
  cord, newborn (stump) P51.9
  corpus luteum (ruptured) cyst N83.1- ☑
  cortical (brain) I61.1
  cranial — *see* Hemorrhage, intracranial
  cutaneous R23.3
    due to autosensitivity, erythrocyte D69.2
    newborn P54.5
  delayed
    following ectopic or molar pregnancy O08.1
    postpartum O72.2
  diathesis (familial) D69.9
  disease D69.9
    newborn P53
    specified type NEC D69.8
  due to or associated with
    afibrinogenemia or other coagulation defect (conditions in categories D65- D69)
      antepartum — *see* Hemorrhage, antepartum, with coagulation defect
      intrapartum O67.0
    dental implant M27.61
    device, implant or graft (*see also* Complications, by site and type, specified NEC) T85.838 ☑
      arterial graft NEC T82.838 ☑
      breast T85.838 ☑
      catheter NEC T85.838 ☑
        dialysis (renal) T82.838 ☑
          intraperitoneal T85.838 ☑
        infusion NEC T82.838 ☑
          spinal (epidural) (subdural) T85.830 ☑
        urinary (indwelling) T83.83 ☑
      electronic (electrode) (pulse generator) (stimulator)
        bone T84.83 ☑
        cardiac T82.837 ☑
        nervous system (brain) (peripheral nerve) (spinal) T85.830 ☑
        urinary T83.83 ☑
      fixation, internal (orthopedic) NEC T84.83 ☑
      gastrointestinal (bile duct) (esophagus) T85.838 ☑
      genital NEC T83.83 ☑
      heart NEC T82.837 ☑
      joint prosthesis T84.83 ☑
      ocular (corneal graft) (orbital implant) NEC T85.838 ☑
      orthopedic NEC T84.83 ☑
        bone graft T86.838 ☑
      specified NEC T85.838 ☑
      urinary NEC T83.83 ☑
      vascular NEC T82.838 ☑
      ventricular intracranial shunt T85.830 ☑
  duodenum, duodenal K92.2
    ulcer — *see* Ulcer, duodenum, with hemorrhage
  dura mater — *see* Hemorrhage, intracranial, subdural
  endotracheal — *see* Hemorrhage, lung
  epicranial subaponeurotic (massive), birth injury P12.2
  epidural (traumatic) (*see also* Injury, intracranial, epidural hemorrhage)
    nontraumatic I62.1
  esophagus K22.8
    varix I85.01
      secondary I85.11
  excessive, following ectopic gestation (subsequent episode) O08.1
  extradural (traumatic) — *see* Injury, intracranial, epidural hemorrhage
    birth injury P10.8
    newborn (anoxic) (nontraumatic) P52.8
    nontraumatic I62.1
  eye NEC H57.8
    fundus — *see* Hemorrhage, retina
    lid — *see* Disorder, eyelid, specified type NEC
  fallopian tube N83.6

Hemorrhage, hemorrhagic — *continued*
fibrinogenolysis — *see* Fibrinolysis
fibrinolytic (acquired) — *see* Fibrinolysis
from
  ear (nontraumatic) — *see* Otorrhagia
  tracheostomy stoma J95.01
fundus, eye — *see* Hemorrhage, retina
funis — *see* Hemorrhage, umbilicus, cord
gastric — *see* Hemorrhage, stomach
gastroenteric K92.2
  newborn P54.3
gastrointestinal (tract) K92.2
  newborn P54.3
genital organ, male N50.1
genitourinary (tract) NOS R31.9
gingiva K06.8
globe (eye) — *see* Hemophthalmos
graafian follicle cyst (ruptured) N83.0- ☑
gum K06.8
heart I51.89
hypopharyngeal (throat) R04.1
intermenstrual (regular) N92.3
  irregular N92.1
internal (organs) NEC R58
  capsule I61.0
  ear — *see* subcategory H83.8 ☑
  newborn P54.8
intestine K92.2
  newborn P54.3
intra-abdominal R58
intra-alveolar (lung), newborn P26.8
intracerebral (nontraumatic) — *see* Hemorrhage, intracranial, intracerebral
intracranial (nontraumatic) I62.9
  birth injury P10.9
  epidural, nontraumatic I62.1
  extradural, nontraumatic I62.1
  intracerebral (nontraumatic) (in) I61.9
    brain stem I61.3
    cerebellum I61.4
    hemisphere I61.2
      cortical (superficial) I61.1
      subcortical (deep) I61.0
    intraoperative
      during a nervous system procedure G97.31
      during other procedure G97.32
    intraventricular I61.5
    multiple localized I61.6
    newborn P52.4
      birth injury P10.1
    postprocedural
      following a nervous system procedure G97.51
      following other procedure G97.52
    specified NEC I61.8
    superficial I61.1
    traumatic (diffuse) — *see* Injury, intracranial, diffuse
      focal — *see* Injury, intracranial, focal
  newborn P52.9
    specified NEC P52.8
  subarachnoid (nontraumatic) (from) I60.9
    intracranial (cerebral) artery I60.7
      anterior communicating I60.2
      basilar I60.4
      carotid siphon and bifurcation I60.0- ☑
      communicating I60.7
        anterior I60.2
        posterior I60.3- ☑
      middle cerebral I60.1- ☑
      posterior communicating I60.3- ☑
      specified artery NEC I60.6
      vertebral I60.5- ☑
    newborn P52.5
      birth injury P10.3
    specified NEC I60.8
    traumatic S06.6X- ☑
  subdural (nontraumatic) I62.00
    acute I62.01
    birth injury P10.0
    chronic I62.03
    newborn (anoxic) (hypoxic) P52.8
      birth injury P10.0
    spinal G95.19
    subacute I62.02
    traumatic — *see* Injury, intracranial, subdural hemorrhage

Hemorrhage, hemorrhagic — *continued*
intracranial — *continued*
  traumatic — *see* Injury, intracranial, focal brain injury
intramedullary NEC G95.19
intraocular — *see* Hemophthalmos
intraoperative, intraprocedural — *see* Complication, hemorrhage (hematoma), intraoperative (intraprocedural), by site
intrapartum — *see* Hemorrhage, complicating, delivery
intrapelvic
  female N94.89
  male K66.1
intraperitoneal K66.1
intrapontine I61.3
intraprocedural — *see* Complication, hemorrhage (hematoma), intraoperative (intraprocedural), by site
intrauterine N85.7
  complicating delivery (*see also* Hemorrhage, complicating, delivery) O67.9
  postpartum — *see* Hemorrhage, postpartum
intraventricular I61.5
  newborn (nontraumatic) (*see also* Newborn, affected by, hemorrhage) P52.3
    due to birth injury P10.2
    grade
      1 P52.0
      2 P52.1
      3 P52.21
      4 P52.22
intravesical N32.89
iris (postinfectional) (postinflammatory) (toxic) — *see* Hyphema
joint (nontraumatic) — *see* Hemarthrosis
kidney N28.89
knee (joint) (nontraumatic) — *see* Hemarthrosis, knee
labyrinth — *see* subcategory H83.8 ☑
lenticular striate artery I61.0
ligature, vessel — *see* Hemorrhage, postoperative
liver K76.89
lung R04.89
  newborn P26.9
    massive P26.1
    specified NEC P26.8
  tuberculous — *see* Tuberculosis, pulmonary
massive umbilical, newborn P51.0
mediastinum — *see* Hemorrhage, lung
medulla I61.3
membrane (brain) I60.8
  spinal cord — *see* Hemorrhage, spinal cord
meninges, meningeal (brain) (middle) I60.8
  spinal cord — *see* Hemorrhage, spinal cord
mesentery K66.1
metritis — *see* Endometritis
mouth K13.79
mucous membrane NEC R58
  newborn P54.8
muscle M62.89
nail (subungual) L60.8
nasal turbinate R04.0
  newborn P54.8
navel, newborn P51.9
newborn P54.9
  specified NEC P54.8
nipple N64.59
nose R04.0
  newborn P54.8
omentum K66.1
optic nerve (sheath) H47.02- ☑
orbit, orbital H05.23- ☑
ovary NEC N83.8
oviduct N83.6
pancreas K86.89
parathyroid (gland) (spontaneous) E21.4
parturition — *see* Hemorrhage, complicating, delivery
penis N48.89
pericardium, pericarditis I31.2
peritoneum, peritoneal K66.1
peritonsillar tissue J35.8
  due to infection J36
petechial R23.3
  due to autosensitivity, erythrocyte D69.2
pituitary (gland) E23.6
pleura — *see* Hemorrhage, lung
polioencephalitis, superior E51.2
polymyositis — *see* Polymyositis

Hemorrhage, hemorrhagic — *continued*
pons, pontine I61.3
posterior fossa (nontraumatic) I61.8
  newborn P52.6
postmenopausal N95.0
postnasal R04.0
postoperative — *see* Complications, postprocedural, hemorrhage, by site
postpartum NEC (following delivery of placenta) O72.1
  delayed or secondary O72.2
  retained placenta O72.0
  third stage O72.0
pregnancy — *see* Hemorrhage, antepartum
preretinal — *see* Hemorrhage, retina
prostate N42.1
puerperal — *see* Hemorrhage, postpartum
  delayed or secondary O72.2
pulmonary R04.89
  newborn P26.9
    massive P26.1
    specified NEC P26.8
  tuberculous — *see* Tuberculosis, pulmonary
purpura (primary) D69.3
rectum (sphincter) K62.5
  newborn P54.2
recurring, following initial hemorrhage at time of injury T79.2 ☑
renal N28.89
respiratory passage or tract R04.9
  specified NEC R04.89
retina, retinal (vessels) H35.6- ☑
  diabetic — *see* Diabetes, retinal, hemorrhage
retroperitoneal R58
scalp R58
scrotum N50.1
secondary (nontraumatic) R58
  following initial hemorrhage at time of injury T79.2 ☑
seminal vesicle N50.1
skin R23.3
  newborn P54.5
slipped umbilical ligature P51.8
spermatic cord N50.1
spinal (cord) G95.19
  newborn (birth injury) P11.5
spleen D73.5
  intraoperative — *see* Complications, intraoperative, hemorrhage, spleen
  postprocedural — *see* Complications, postprocedural, hemorrhage, spleen
stomach K92.2
  newborn P54.3
  ulcer — *see* Ulcer, stomach, with hemorrhage
subarachnoid (nontraumatic) — *see* Hemorrhage, intracranial, subarachnoid
subconjunctival (*see also* Hemorrhage, conjunctiva)
  birth injury P15.3
subcortical (brain) I61.0
subcutaneous R23.3
subdiaphragmatic R58
subdural (acute) (nontraumatic) — *see* Hemorrhage, intracranial, subdural
subependymal
  newborn P52.0
    with intraventricular extension P52.1
      and intracerebral extension P52.22
subgaleal P12.2
subhyaloid — *see* Hemorrhage, retina
subperiosteal — *see* Disorder, bone, specified type NEC
subretinal — *see* Hemorrhage, retina
subtentorial — *see* Hemorrhage, intracranial, subdural
subungual L60.8
suprarenal (capsule) (gland) E27.49
  newborn P54.4
tentorium (traumatic) NEC — *see* Hemorrhage, brain
  newborn (birth injury) P10.4
testis N50.1
third stage (postpartum) O72.0
thorax — *see* Hemorrhage, lung
throat R04.1
thymus (gland) E32.8
thyroid (cyst) (gland) E07.89
tongue K14.8
tonsil J35.8
trachea — *see* Hemorrhage, lung
tracheobronchial R04.89
  newborn P26.0

☑ **Additional Character Required** — **Refer to the Tabular List for Character Selection**

🔻 **Subterms under main terms may continue to next column or page**

Hemorrhage, hemorrhagic — *continued*
  traumatic — *code to specific injury*
    cerebellar — *see* Hemorrhage, brain
    intracranial — *see* Hemorrhage, brain
    recurring or secondary (following initial hemor-
      rhage at time of injury) T79.2 ☑
  tuberculous NEC (*see also* Tuberculosis, pulmonary)
    A15.0
  tunica vaginalis N50.1
  ulcer — *code by* site under Ulcer, with hemorrhage
    K27.4
  umbilicus, umbilical
    cord
      after birth, newborn P51.9
      complicating delivery O69.5 ☑
    newborn P51.9
      massive P51.0
      slipped ligature P51.8
    stump P51.9
  urethra (idiopathic) N36.8
  uterus, uterine (abnormal) N93.9
    climacteric N92.4
    complicating delivery — *see* Hemorrhage, compli-
      cating, delivery
    dysfunctional or functional N93.8
    intermenstrual (regular) N92.3
      irregular N92.1
    postmenopausal N95.0
    postpartum — *see* Hemorrhage, postpartum
    preclimacteric or premenopausal N92.4
    prepubertal N93.8
    pubertal N92.2
  vagina (abnormal) N93.9
    newborn P54.6
  vas deferens N50.1
  vasa previa O69.4 ☑
  ventricular I61.5
  vesical N32.89
  viscera NEC R58
    newborn P54.8
  vitreous (humor) (intraocular) H43.1- ☑
  vulva N90.89
Hemorrhoids (bleeding) (without mention of degree)
    K64.9
  1st degree (grade/stage I) (without prolapse outside
    of anal canal) K64.0
  2nd degree (grade/stage II) (that prolapse with
    straining but retract spontaneously) K64.1
  3rd degree (grade/stage III) (that prolapse with
    straining and require manual replacement back
    inside anal canal) K64.2
  4th degree (grade/stage IV) (with prolapsed tissue that
    cannot be manually replaced) K64.3
  complicating
    pregnancy O22.4 ☑
    puerperium O87.2
  external K64.4
    with
      thrombosis K64.5
  internal (without mention of degree) K64.8
  prolapsed K64.8
  skin tags
    anus K64.4
    residual K64.4
  specified NEC K64.8
  strangulated (*see also* Hemorrhoids, by degree) K64.8
  thrombosed (*see also* Hemorrhoids, by degree) K64.5
  ulcerated (*see also* Hemorrhoids, by degree) K64.8
Hemosalpinx N83.6
  with
    hematocolpos N89.7
    hematometra N85.7
      with hematocolpos N89.7
Hemosiderosis (dietary) E83.19
  pulmonary, idiopathic E83.1- ☑ [J84.03]
  transfusion T80.89 ☑
Hemothorax (bacterial) (nontuberculous) J94.2
  newborn P54.8
  traumatic S27.1 ☑
    with pneumothorax S27.2 ☑
  tuberculous NEC A15.6
Henoch (-Schönlein) **disease or syndrome** (purpura)
    D69.0
Henpue, henpuye A66.6
Hepar lobatum (syphilitic) A52.74
Hepatalgia K76.89
Hepatitis K75.9
  acute B17.9

Hepatitis — *continued*
  acute — *continued*
    with coma K72.01
    with hepatic failure — *see* Failure, hepatic
    alcoholic — *see* Hepatitis, alcoholic
    infectious B17.9
    non-viral K72.0 ☑
    viral B17.9
  alcoholic (acute) (chronic) K70.10
    with ascites K70.11
  amebic — *see* Abscess, liver, amebic
  anicteric, (viral) — *see* Hepatitis, viral
  antigen-associated (HAA) — *see* Hepatitis, B
  Australia-antigen (positive) — *see* Hepatitis, B
  autoimmune K75.4
  B B19.10
    with hepatic coma B19.11
    acute B16.9
      with
        delta-agent (coinfection) (without hepatic
          coma) B16.1
          with hepatic coma B16.0
        hepatic coma (without delta-agent coinfec-
          tion) B16.2
    chronic B18.1
      with delta-agent B18.0
  bacterial NEC K75.89
  C (viral) B19.20
    with hepatic coma B19.21
    acute B17.10
      with hepatic coma B17.11
    chronic B18.2
  catarrhal (acute) B15.9
    with hepatic coma B15.0
  cholangiolitic K75.89
  cholestatic K75.89
  chronic K73.9
    active NEC K73.2
    lobular NEC K73.1
    persistent NEC K73.0
    specified NEC K73.8
  cytomegaloviral B25.1
  due to ethanol (acute) (chronic) — *see* Hepatitis, alco-
    holic
  epidemic B15.9
    with hepatic coma B15.0
  fulminant NEC (viral) — *see* Hepatitis, viral
  granulomatous NEC K75.3
  herpesviral B00.81
  history of
    B Z86.19
    C Z86.19
  homologous serum — *see* Hepatitis, viral, type B
  in (due to)
    mumps B26.81
    toxoplasmosis (acquired) B58.1
      congenital (active) P37.1 [K77]
  infectious, infective B15.9
    acute (subacute) B17.9
    chronic B18.9
  inoculation — *see* Hepatitis, viral, type B
  interstitial (chronic) K74.69
  lupoid NEC K75.4
  malignant NEC (with hepatic failure) K72.90
    with coma K72.91
  neonatal (idiopathic) (toxic) P59.29
  neonatal giant cell P59.29
  newborn P59.29
  non-viral K72.0 ☑
  postimmunization — *see* Hepatitis, viral, type B
  post-transfusion — *see* Hepatitis, viral, type B
  reactive, nonspecific K75.2
  serum — *see* Hepatitis, viral, type B
  specified type NEC
    with hepatic failure — *see* Failure, hepatic
  syphilitic (late) A52.74
    congenital (early) A50.08 [K77]
    late A50.59 [K77]
    secondary A51.45
  toxic (*see also* Disease, liver, toxic) K71.6
  tuberculous A18.83
  viral, virus B19.9
    with hepatic coma B19.0
    acute B17.9
    chronic B18.9
      specified NEC B18.8
      type
        B B18.1

Hepatitis — *continued*
  viral, virus — *continued*
    chronic — *continued*
      type — *continued*
        B — *continued*
          with delta-agent B18.0
        C B18.2
    congenital P35.3
    coxsackie B33.8 [K77]
    cytomegalic inclusion B25.1
    in remission, any type — *code to* Hepatitis, chronic,
      by type
    non-A, non-B B17.8
    specified type NEC (with or without coma) B17.8
    type
      A B15.9
        with hepatic coma B15.0
      B B19.10
        with hepatic coma B19.11
        acute B16.9
          with
            delta-agent (coinfection) (without
              hepatic coma) B16.1
              with hepatic coma B16.0
            hepatic coma (without delta-agent
              coinfection) B16.2
        chronic B18.1
          with delta-agent B18.0
      C B19.20
        with hepatic coma B19.21
        acute B17.10
          with hepatic coma B17.11
        chronic B18.2
      E B17.2
      non-A, non-B B17.8
Hepatization lung (acute) — *see* Pneumonia, lobar
Hepatoblastoma C22.2
Hepatocarcinoma C22.0
Hepatocholangiocarcinoma C22.0
Hepatocholangioma, benign D13.4
Hepatocholangitis K75.89
Hepatolenticular degeneration E83.01
Hepatoma (malignant) C22.0
  benign D13.4
  embryonal C22.0
Hepatomegaly (*see also* Hypertrophy, liver)
  with splenomegaly R16.2
  congenital Q44.7
  in mononucleosis
    gammaherpesviral B27.09
    infectious specified NEC B27.89
Hepatoptosis K76.89
Hepatorenal syndrome following labor and delivery
    O90.4
Hepatosis K76.89
Hepatosplenomegaly R16.2
  hyperlipemic (Bürger-Grütz type) E78.3 [K77]
Hereditary — *see* condition
Heredodegeneration, macular — *see* Dystrophy, retina
Heredopathia atactica polyneuritiformis G60.1
Heredosyphilis — *see* Syphilis, congenital
Herlitz' syndrome Q81.1
Hermansky-Pudlak syndrome E70.331
Hermaphrodite, hermaphroditism (true) Q56.0
  46,XX with streak gonads Q99.1
  46,XX/46,XY Q99.0
  46,XY with streak gonads Q99.1
  chimera 46,XX/46,XY Q99.0
Hernia, hernial (acquired) (recurrent) K46.9
  with
    gangrene — *see* Hernia, by site, with, gangrene
    incarceration — *see* Hernia, by site, with, obstruc-
      tion
    irreducible — *see* Hernia, by site, with, obstruction
    obstruction — *see* Hernia, by site, with, obstruction
    strangulation — *see* Hernia, by site, with, obstruc-
      tion
  abdomen, abdominal K46.9
    with
      gangrene (and obstruction) K46.1
      obstruction K46.0
    femoral — *see* Hernia, femoral
    incisional — *see* Hernia, incisional
    inguinal — *see* Hernia, inguinal
    specified site NEC K45.8
      with
        gangrene (and obstruction) K45.1
        obstruction K45.0

Hernia, hernial — *continued*
   abdomen, abdominal — *continued*
      umbilical — *see* Hernia, umbilical
      wall — *see* Hernia, ventral
   appendix — *see* Hernia, abdomen
   bladder (mucosa) (sphincter)
      congenital (female) (male) Q79.51
      female — *see* Cystocele
      male N32.89
   brain, congenital — *see* Encephalocele
   cartilage, vertebra — *see* Displacement, intervertebral
      disc
   cerebral, congenital (*see also* Encephalocele)
      endaural Q01.8
   ciliary body (traumatic) S05.2- ☑
   colon — *see* Hernia, abdomen
   Cooper's — *see* Hernia, abdomen, specified site NEC
   crural — *see* Hernia, femoral
   diaphragm, diaphragmatic K44.9
      with
         gangrene (and obstruction) K44.1
         obstruction K44.0
      congenital Q79.0
   direct (inguinal) — *see* Hernia, inguinal
   diverticulum, intestine — *see* Hernia, abdomen
   double (inguinal) — *see* Hernia, inguinal, bilateral
   due to adhesions (with obstruction) K56.50
   epigastric (*see also* Hernia, ventral) K43.9
   esophageal hiatus — *see* Hernia, hiatal
   external (inguinal) — *see* Hernia, inguinal
   fallopian tube N83.4- ☑
   fascia M62.89
   femoral K41.90
      with
         gangrene (and obstruction) K41.40
            not specified as recurrent K41.40
            recurrent K41.41
         obstruction K41.30
            not specified as recurrent K41.30
            recurrent K41.31
      bilateral K41.20
         with
            gangrene (and obstruction) K41.10
               not specified as recurrent K41.10
               recurrent K41.11
            obstruction K41.00
               not specified as recurrent K41.00
               recurrent K41.01
         not specified as recurrent K41.20
         recurrent K41.21
      not specified as recurrent K41.90
      recurrent K41.91
      unilateral K41.90
         with
            gangrene (and obstruction) K41.40
               not specified as recurrent K41.40
               recurrent K41.41
            obstruction K41.30
               not specified as recurrent K41.30
               recurrent K41.31
         not specified as recurrent K41.90
         recurrent K41.91
   foramen magnum G93.5
      congenital Q01.8
   funicular (umbilical) (*see also* Hernia, umbilicus)
      spermatic (cord) — *see* Hernia, inguinal
   gastrointestinal tract — *see* Hernia, abdomen
   Hesselbach's — *see* Hernia, femoral, specified site NEC
   hiatal (esophageal) (sliding) K44.9
      with
         gangrene (and obstruction) K44.1
         obstruction K44.0
      congenital Q40.1
   hypogastric — *see* Hernia, ventral
   incarcerated (*see also* Hernia, by site, with obstruction)
      with gangrene — *see* Hernia, by site, with gan-
         grene
   incisional K43.2
      with
         gangrene (and obstruction) K43.1
         obstruction K43.0
   indirect (inguinal) — *see* Hernia, inguinal
   inguinal (direct) (external) (funicular) (indirect) (inter-
      nal) (oblique) (scrotal) (sliding) K40.90
      with
         gangrene (and obstruction) K40.40
            not specified as recurrent K40.40
            recurrent K40.41

inguinal — *continued*
   with — *continued*
      obstruction K40.30
         not specified as recurrent K40.30
         recurrent K40.31
      bilateral K40.20
         with
            gangrene (and obstruction) K40.10
               not specified as recurrent K40.10
               recurrent K40.11
            obstruction K40.00
               not specified as recurrent K40.00
               recurrent K40.01
         not specified as recurrent K40.20
         recurrent K40.21
      not specified as recurrent K40.90
      recurrent K40.91
      unilateral K40.90
         with
            gangrene (and obstruction) K40.40
               not specified as recurrent K40.40
               recurrent K40.41
            obstruction K40.30
               not specified as recurrent K40.30
               recurrent K40.31
         not specified as recurrent K40.90
         recurrent K40.91
   internal (*see also* Hernia, abdomen)
      inguinal — *see* Hernia, inguinal
   interstitial — *see* Hernia, abdomen
   intervertebral cartilage or disc — *see* Displacement,
      intervertebral disc
   intestine, intestinal — *see* Hernia, by site
   intra-abdominal — *see* Hernia, abdomen
   iris (traumatic) S05.2- ☑
   irreducible (*see also* Hernia, by site, with obstruction)
      with gangrene — *see* Hernia, by site, with gan-
         grene
   ischiatic — *see* Hernia, abdomen, specified site NEC
   ischiorectal — *see* Hernia, abdomen, specified site
      NEC
   lens (traumatic) S05.2- ☑
   linea (alba) (semilunaris) — *see* Hernia, ventral
   Littre's — *see* Hernia, abdomen
   lumbar — *see* Hernia, abdomen, specified site NEC
   lung (subcutaneous) J98.4
   mediastinum J98.59
   mesenteric (internal) — *see* Hernia, abdomen
   midline — *see* Hernia, ventral
   muscle (sheath) M62.89
   nucleus pulposus — *see* Displacement, intervertebral
      disc
   oblique (inguinal) — *see* Hernia, inguinal
   obstructive (*see also* Hernia, by site, with obstruction)
      with gangrene — *see* Hernia, by site, with gan-
         grene
   obturator — *see* Hernia, abdomen, specified site NEC
   omental — *see* Hernia, abdomen
   ovary N83.4- ☑
   oviduct N83.4- ☑
   paraesophageal (*see also* Hernia, diaphragm)
      congenital Q40.1
   parastomal K43.5
      with
         gangrene (and obstruction) K43.4
         obstruction K43.3
   paraumbilical — *see* Hernia, umbilicus
   perineal — *see* Hernia, abdomen, specified site NEC
   Petit's — *see* Hernia, abdomen, specified site NEC
   postoperative — *see* Hernia, incisional
   pregnant uterus — *see* Abnormal, uterus in pregnancy
      or childbirth
   prevesical N32.89
   properitoneal — *see* Hernia, abdomen, specified site
      NEC
   pudendal — *see* Hernia, abdomen, specified site NEC
   rectovaginal N81.6
   retroperitoneal — *see* Hernia, abdomen, specified site
      NEC
   Richter's — *see* Hernia, abdomen, with obstruction
   Rieux's, Riex's — *see* Hernia, abdomen, specified site
      NEC
   sac condition (adhesion) (dropsy) (inflammation)
      (laceration) (suppuration) — *code by site under*
      Hernia
   sciatic — *see* Hernia, abdomen, specified site NEC

scrotum, scrotal — *see* Hernia, inguinal
   sliding (inguinal) (*see also* Hernia, inguinal)
      hiatus — *see* Hernia, hiatal
   spigelian — *see* Hernia, ventral
   spinal — *see* Spina bifida
   strangulated (*see also* Hernia, by site, with obstruction)
      with gangrene — *see* Hernia, by site, with gan-
         grene
   subxiphoid — *see* Hernia, ventral
   supra-umbilicus — *see* Hernia, ventral
   tendon — *see* Disorder, tendon, specified type NEC
   Treitz's (fossa) — *see* Hernia, abdomen, specified site
      NEC
   tunica vaginalis Q55.29
   umbilicus, umbilical K42.9
      with
         gangrene (and obstruction) K42.1
         obstruction K42.0
   ureter N28.89
   urethra, congenital Q64.79
   urinary meatus, congenital Q64.79
   uterus N81.4
      pregnant — *see* Abnormal, uterus in pregnancy or
         childbirth
   vaginal (anterior) (wall) — *see* Cystocele
   Velpeau's — *see* Hernia, femoral
   ventral K43.9
      with
         gangrene (and obstruction) K43.7
         obstruction K43.6
      incisional K43.2
         with
            gangrene (and obstruction) K43.1
            obstruction K43.0
         recurrent — *see* Hernia, incisional
      specified NEC K43.9
         with
            gangrene (and obstruction) K43.7
            obstruction K43.6
   vesical
      congenital (female) (male) Q79.51
      female — *see* Cystocele
      male N32.89
   vitreous (into wound) S05.2- ☑
      into anterior chamber — *see* Prolapse, vitreous
Herniation (*see also* Hernia)
   brain (stem) G93.5
   cerebral G93.5
   mediastinum J98.59
   nucleus pulposus — *see* Displacement, intervertebral
      disc
Herpangina B08.5
Herpes, herpesvirus, herpetic B00.9
   anogenital A60.9
      perianal skin A60.1
      rectum A60.1
      urogenital tract A60.00
         cervix A60.03
         male genital organ NEC A60.02
         penis A60.01
         specified site NEC A60.09
         vagina A60.04
         vulva A60.04
   blepharitis (zoster) B02.39
      simplex B00.59
   circinatus B35.4
      bullosus L12.0
   conjunctivitis (simplex) B00.53
      zoster B02.31
   cornea B02.33
   encephalitis B00.4
      due to herpesvirus 6 B10.01
      due to herpesvirus 7 B10.09
      specified NEC B10.09
   eye (zoster) B02.30
      simplex B00.50
   eyelid (zoster) B02.39
      simplex B00.59
   facialis B00.1
   febrilis B00.1
   geniculate ganglionitis B02.21
   genital, genitalis A60.00
      female A60.09
      male A60.02
   gestational, gestationis O26.4- ☑
   gingivostomatitis B00.2
   human B00.9

☑ **Additional Character Required** — Refer to the Tabular List for Character Selection   ▽ **Subterms under main terms may continue to next column or page**

Herpes, herpesvirus, herpetic — *continued*
- human — *continued*
  - 1 — *see* Herpes, simplex
  - 2 — *see* Herpes, simplex
  - 3 — *see* Varicella
  - 4 — *see* Mononucleosis, Epstein-Barr (virus)
  - 5 — *see* Disease, cytomegalic inclusion (generalized)
  - 6
    - encephalitis B10.01
    - specified NEC B10.81
  - 7
    - encephalitis B10.09
    - specified NEC B10.82
  - 8 B10.89
- infection NEC B10.89
  - Kaposi's sarcoma associated B10.89
- iridocyclitis (simplex) B00.51
  - zoster B02.32
- iris (vesicular erythema multiforme) L51.9
- iritis (simplex) B00.51
- Kaposi's sarcoma associated B10.89
- keratitis (simplex) (dendritic) (disciform) (interstitial) B00.52
  - zoster (interstitial) B02.33
- keratoconjunctivitis (simplex) B00.52
  - zoster B02.33
- labialis B00.1
- lip B00.1
- meningitis (simplex) B00.3
  - zoster B02.1
- ophthalmicus (zoster) NEC B02.30
  - simplex B00.50
- penis A60.01
- perianal skin A60.1
- pharyngitis, pharyngotonsillitis B00.2
- rectum A60.1
- scrotum A60.02
- sepsis B00.7
- simplex B00.9
  - complicated NEC B00.89
  - congenital P35.2
  - conjunctivitis B00.53
  - external ear B00.1
  - eyelid B00.59
  - hepatitis B00.81
  - keratitis (interstitial) B00.52
  - myeilitis B00.82
  - specified complication NEC B00.89
  - visceral B00.89
- stomatitis B00.2
- tonsurans B35.0
- visceral B00.89
- vulva A60.04
- whitlow B00.89
- zoster (*see also* condition) B02.9
  - auricularis B02.21
  - complicated NEC B02.8
  - conjunctivitis B02.31
  - disseminated B02.7
  - encephalitis B02.0
  - eye (lid) B02.39
  - geniculate ganglionitis B02.21
  - keratitis (interstitial) B02.33
  - meningitis B02.1
  - myelitis B02.24
  - neuritis, neuralgia B02.29
  - ophthalmicus NEC B02.30
  - oticus B02.21
  - polyneuropathy B02.23
  - specified complication NEC B02.8
  - trigeminal neuralgia B02.22

Herpesvirus (human) — *see* Herpes
Herpetophobia F40.218
Herrick's anemia — *see* Disease, sickle-cell
Hers' disease E74.09
Herter-Gee syndrome K90.0
Herxheimer's reaction R68.89
Hesitancy
- of micturition R39.11
- urinary R39.11

Hesselbach's hernia — *see* Hernia, femoral, specified site NEC
Heterochromia (congenital) Q13.2
- cataract — *see* Cataract, complicated
- cyclitis (Fuchs) — *see* Cyclitis, Fuchs' heterochromic
- hair L67.1
- iritis — *see* Cyclitis, Fuchs' heterochromic

Heterochromia — *continued*
- retained metallic foreign body (nonmagnetic) — *see* Foreign body, intraocular, old, retained
  - magnetic — *see* Foreign body, intraocular, old, retained, magnetic
- uveitis — *see* Cyclitis, Fuchs' heterochromic
Heterophoria — *see* Strabismus, heterophoria
Heterophyes, heterophyiasis (small intestine) B66.8
Heterotopia, heterotopic (*see also* Malposition, congenital)
- cerebralis Q04.8
Heterotropia — *see* Strabismus
Heubner-Herter disease K90.0
Hexadactylism Q69.9
HGSIL (cytology finding) (high grade squamous intraepithelial lesion on cytologic smear) (Pap smear finding)
- anus R85.613
- cervix R87.613
  - biopsy (histology) finding — *see* Neoplasia, intraepithelial, cervix, grade II or grade III
- vagina R87.623
  - biopsy (histology) finding — *see* Neoplasia, intraepithelial, cervix, grade II or grade III
Hibernoma — *see* Lipoma
Hiccup, hiccough R06.6
- epidemic B33.0
- psychogenic F45.8
Hidden penis (congenital) Q55.64
- acquired N48.83
Hidradenitis (axillaris) (suppurative) L73.2
Hidradenoma (nodular) (*see also* Neoplasm, skin, benign)
- clear cell — *see* Neoplasm, skin, benign
- papillary — *see* Neoplasm, skin, benign
Hidrocystoma — *see* Neoplasm, skin, benign
High
- altitude effects T70.20 ✓
  - anoxia T70.29 ✓
  - on
    - ears T70.0 ✓
    - sinuses T70.1 ✓
  - polycythemia D75.1
- arch
  - foot Q66.7
  - palate, congenital Q38.5
- arterial tension — *see* Hypertension
- basal metabolic rate R94.8
- blood pressure (*see also* Hypertension)
  - borderline R03.0
  - reading (incidental) (isolated) (nonspecific), without diagnosis of hypertension R03.0
- cholesterol E78.00
  - with high triglycerides E78.2
- diaphragm (congenital) Q79.1
- expressed emotional level within family Z63.8
- head at term O32.4 ✓
- palate, congenital Q38.5
- risk
  - infant NEC Z76.2
  - sexual behavior (heterosexual) Z72.51
    - bisexual Z72.53
    - homosexual Z72.52
- scrotal testis, testes
  - bilateral Q53.23
  - unilateral Q53.13
- temperature (of unknown origin) R50.9
- thoracic rib Q76.6
- triglycerides E78.1
  - with high cholesterol E78.2
Hildenbrand's disease A75.0
Hilum — *see* condition
Hip — *see* condition
Hippel's disease Q85.8
Hippophobia F40.218
Hippus H57.09
Hirschsprung's disease or megacolon Q43.1
Hirsutism, hirsuties L68.0
Hirudiniasis
- external B88.3
- internal B83.4
Hiss-Russell dysentery A03.1
Histidinemia, histidinuria E70.41
Histiocytoma (*see also* Neoplasm, skin, benign)
- fibrous (*see also* Neoplasm, skin, benign)
  - atypical — *see* Neoplasm, connective tissue, uncertain behavior

Histiocytoma — *continued*
- fibrous (*see also* Neoplasm, skin, benign) — *continued*
  - malignant — *see* Neoplasm, connective tissue, malignant
Histiocytosis D76.3
- acute differentiated progressive C96.0
- Langerhans' cell NEC C96.6
  - multifocal X
    - multisystemic (disseminated) C96.0
    - unisystemic C96.5
  - pulmonary, adult (adult PLCH) J84.82
  - unifocal (X) C96.6
- lipid, lipoid D76.3
  - essential E75.29
- malignant C96.A (*following* C96.6)
- mononuclear phagocytes NEC D76.1
  - Langerhans' cells C96.6
- non-Langerhans cell D76.3
- polyostotic sclerosing D76.3
- sinus, with massive lymphadenopathy D76.3
- syndrome NEC D76.3
- X NEC C96.6
  - acute (progressive) C96.0
  - chronic C96.6
  - multifocal C96.5
  - multisystemic C96.0
  - unifocal C96.6
Histoplasmosis B39.9
- with pneumonia NEC B39.2
- African B39.5
- American — *see* Histoplasmosis, capsulati
- capsulati B39.4
  - disseminated B39.3
  - generalized B39.3
  - pulmonary B39.2
    - acute B39.0
    - chronic B39.1
- Darling's B39.4
- duboisii B39.5
- lung NEC B39.2
History
- family (of) (*see also* History, personal (of))
  - alcohol abuse Z81.1
  - allergy NEC Z84.89
  - anemia Z83.2
  - arthritis Z82.61
  - asthma Z82.5
  - blindness Z82.1
  - cardiac death (sudden) Z82.41
  - carrier of genetic disease Z84.81
  - chromosomal anomaly Z82.79
  - chronic
    - disabling disease NEC Z82.8
    - lower respiratory disease Z82.5
  - colonic polyps Z83.71
  - congenital malformations and deformations Z82.79
    - polycystic kidney Z82.71
  - consanguinity Z84.3
  - deafness Z82.2
  - diabetes mellitus Z83.3
  - disability NEC Z82.8
  - disease or disorder (of)
    - allergic NEC Z84.89
    - behavioral NEC Z81.8
    - blood and blood-forming organs Z83.2
    - cardiovascular NEC Z82.49
    - chronic disabling NEC Z82.8
    - digestive Z83.79
    - ear NEC Z83.52
    - endocrine NEC Z83.49
    - eye NEC Z83.518
      - glaucoma Z83.511
    - familial hypercholesterolemia Z83.42
    - genitourinary NEC Z84.2
    - glaucoma Z83.511
    - hematological Z83.2
    - immune mechanism Z83.2
    - infectious NEC Z83.1
    - ischemic heart Z82.49
    - kidney Z84.1
    - mental NEC Z81.8
    - metabolic Z83.49
    - musculoskeletal NEC Z82.69
    - neurological NEC Z82.0
    - nutritional Z83.49
    - parasitic NEC Z83.1
    - psychiatric NEC Z81.8
    - respiratory NEC Z83.6

History — *continued*
family (*see also* History, personal) — *continued*
  disease or disorder — *continued*
    skin and subcutaneous tissue NEC Z84.0
      specified NEC Z84.89
  drug abuse NEC Z81.3
  epilepsy Z82.0
  familial hypercholesterolemia Z83.42
  genetic disease carrier Z84.81
  glaucoma Z83.511
  hearing loss Z82.2
  human immunodeficiency virus (HIV) infection Z83.0
  Huntington's chorea Z82.0
  intellectual disability Z81.0
  leukemia Z80.6
  malignant neoplasm (of) NOS Z80.9
    bladder Z80.52
    breast Z80.3
    bronchus Z80.1
    digestive organ Z80.0
    gastrointestinal tract Z80.0
    genital organ Z80.49
      ovary Z80.41
      prostate Z80.42
      specified organ NEC Z80.49
      testis Z80.43
    hematopoietic NEC Z80.7
    intrathoracic organ NEC Z80.2
    kidney Z80.51
    lung Z80.1
    lymphatic NEC Z80.7
    ovary Z80.41
    prostate Z80.42
    respiratory organ NEC Z80.2
    specified site NEC Z80.8
    testis Z80.43
    trachea Z80.1
    urinary organ or tract Z80.59
      bladder Z80.52
      kidney Z80.51
  mental
    disorder NEC Z81.8
  multiple endocrine neoplasia (MEN) syndrome Z83.41
  osteoporosis Z82.62
  polycystic kidney Z82.71
  polyps (colon) Z83.71
  psychiatric disorder Z81.8
  psychoactive substance abuse NEC Z81.3
  respiratory condition NEC Z83.6
    asthma and other lower respiratory conditions Z82.5
  self-harmful behavior Z81.8
  SIDS (sudden infant death syndrome) Z84.82
  skin condition Z84.0
  specified condition NEC Z84.89
  stroke (cerebrovascular) Z82.3
  substance abuse NEC Z81.4
    alcohol Z81.1
    drug NEC Z81.3
    psychoactive NEC Z81.3
    tobacco Z81.2
  sudden
    cardiac death Z82.41
    infant death syndrome (SIDS) Z84.82
  tobacco abuse Z81.2
  violence, violent behavior Z81.8
  visual loss Z82.1
personal (of) (*see also* History, family (of))
  abuse
    adult Z91.419
      physical and sexual Z91.410
      psychological Z91.411
    childhood Z62.819
      physical Z62.810
      psychological Z62.811
      sexual Z62.810
  alcohol dependence F10.21
  allergy (to) Z88.9
    analgesic agent NEC Z88.6
    anesthetic Z88.4
    antibiotic agent NEC Z88.1
    anti-infective agent NEC Z88.3
    contrast media Z91.041
    drugs, medicaments and biological substances Z88.9
      specified NEC Z88.8
    food Z91.018

History — *continued*
personal (*see also* History, family) — *continued*
  allergy — *continued*
    food — *continued*
      additives Z91.02
      eggs Z91.012
      milk products Z91.011
      peanuts Z91.010
      seafood Z91.013
      specified food NEC Z91.018
    insect Z91.038
      bee Z91.030
    latex Z91.040
    medicinal agents Z88.9
      specified NEC Z88.8
    narcotic agent NEC Z88.5
    nonmedicinal agents Z91.048
    penicillin Z88.0
    serum Z88.7
    specified NEC Z91.09
    sulfonamides Z88.2
    vaccine Z88.7
  anaphylactic shock Z87.892
  anaphylaxis Z87.892
  behavioral disorders Z86.59
  benign carcinoid tumor Z86.012
  benign neoplasm Z86.018
    brain Z86.011
    carcinoid Z86.012
    colonic polyps Z86.010
  brain injury (traumatic) Z87.820
  breast implant removal Z98.86
  calculi, renal Z87.442
  cancer — *see* History, personal (of), malignant neoplasm (of)
  cardiac arrest (death), successfully resuscitated Z86.74
  cerebral infarction without residual deficit Z86.73
  cervical dysplasia Z87.410
  chemotherapy for neoplastic condition Z92.21
  childhood abuse — *see* History, personal (of), abuse
  cleft lip (corrected) Z87.730
  cleft palate (corrected) Z87.730
  collapsed vertebra (healed) Z87.311
    due to osteoporosis Z87.310
  combat and operational stress reaction Z86.51
  congenital malformation (corrected) Z87.798
    circulatory system (corrected) Z87.74
    digestive system (corrected) NEC Z87.738
    ear (corrected) Z87.721
    eye (corrected) Z87.720
    face and neck (corrected) Z87.790
    genitourinary system (corrected) NEC Z87.718
    heart (corrected) Z87.74
    integument (corrected) Z87.76
    limb(s) (corrected) Z87.76
    musculoskeletal system (corrected) Z87.76
    neck (corrected) Z87.790
    nervous system (corrected) NEC Z87.728
    respiratory system (corrected) Z87.75
    sense organs (corrected) NEC Z87.728
    specified NEC Z87.798
  contraception Z92.0
  deployment (military) Z91.82
  diabetic foot ulcer Z86.31
  disease or disorder (of) Z87.898
    anaphylaxis Z87.892
    blood and blood-forming organs Z86.2
    circulatory system Z86.79
      specified condition NEC Z86.79
    connective tissue Z87.39
    digestive system Z87.19
      colonic polyp Z86.010
      peptic ulcer disease Z87.11
      specified condition NEC Z87.19
    ear Z86.69
    endocrine Z86.39
      diabetic foot ulcer Z86.31
      gestational diabetes Z86.32
      specified type NEC Z86.39
    eye Z86.69
    genital (track) system NEC
      female Z87.42
      male Z87.438
    hematological Z86.2
    Hodgkin Z85.71
    immune mechanism Z86.2
    infectious Z86.19

History — *continued*
personal (*see also* History, family) — *continued*
  disease or disorder — *continued*
    infectious — *continued*
      malaria Z86.13
      Methicillin resistant Staphylococcus aureus (MRSA) Z86.14
      poliomyelitis Z86.12
      specified NEC Z86.19
      tuberculosis Z86.11
    mental NEC Z86.59
    metabolic Z86.39
      diabetic foot ulcer Z86.31
      gestational diabetes Z86.32
      specified type NEC Z86.39
    musculoskeletal NEC Z87.39
    nervous system Z86.69
    nutritional Z86.39
    parasitic Z86.19
    respiratory system NEC Z87.09
    sense organs Z86.69
    skin Z87.2
    specified site or type NEC Z87.898
    subcutaneous tissue Z87.2
    trophoblastic Z87.59
    urinary system NEC Z87.448
  drug dependence — *see* Dependence, drug, by type, in remission
  drug therapy
    antineoplastic chemotherapy Z92.21
    estrogen Z92.23
    immunosupression Z92.25
    inhaled steroids Z92.240
    monoclonal drug Z92.22
    specified NEC Z92.29
    steroid Z92.241
    systemic steroids Z92.241
  dysplasia
    cervical (mild) (moderate) Z87.410
      severe (grade III) Z86.001
    prostatic Z87.430
    vaginal (mild) (moderate) Z87.411
      severe (grade III) Z86.008
    vulvar (mild) (moderate) Z87.412
      severe (grade III) Z86.008
  embolism (venous) Z86.718
    pulmonary Z86.711
  encephalitis Z86.61
  estrogen therapy Z92.23
  extracorporeal membrane oxygenation (ECMO) Z92.81
  failed conscious sedation Z92.83
  failed moderate sedation Z92.83
  fall, falling Z91.81
  fracture (healed)
    fatigue Z87.312
    fragility Z87.310
    osteoporosis Z87.310
    pathological NEC Z87.311
    stress Z87.312
    traumatic Z87.81
  gestational diabetes Z86.32
  hepatitis
    B Z86.19
    C Z86.19
  Hodgkin disease Z85.71
  hyperthermia, malignant Z88.4
  hypospadias (corrected) Z87.710
  hysterectomy Z90.710
  immunosupression therapy Z92.25
  in situ neoplasm
    breast Z86.000
    cervix uteri Z86.001
    specified NEC Z86.008
  in utero procedure during pregnancy Z98.870
  in utero procedure while a fetus Z98.871
  infection NEC Z86.19
    central nervous system Z86.61
    Methicillin resistant Staphylococcus aureus (MRSA) Z86.14
    urinary (recurrent) (tract) Z87.440
  injury NEC Z87.828
  irradiation Z92.3
  kidney stones Z87.442
  leukemia Z85.6
  lymphoma (non-Hodgkin) Z85.72
  malignant melanoma (skin) Z85.820
  malignant neoplasm (of) Z85.9
    accessory sinuses Z85.22

☑ Additional Character Required — Refer to the Tabular List for Character Selection　　▼ Subterms under main terms may continue to next column or page

History — *continued*
  personal (*see also* History, family) — *continued*
    malignant neoplasm — *continued*
      anus NEC Z85.048
        carcinoid Z85.040
      bladder Z85.51
      bone Z85.830
      brain Z85.841
      breast Z85.3
      bronchus NEC Z85.118
        carcinoid Z85.110
      carcinoid — *see* History, personal (of), malig-
        nant neoplasm, by site, carcinioid
      cervix Z85.41
      colon NEC Z85.038
        carcinoid Z85.030
      digestive organ Z85.00
        specified NEC Z85.09
      endocrine gland NEC Z85.858
      epididymis Z85.48
      esophagus Z85.01
      eye Z85.840
      gastrointestinal tract — *see* History, malignant
        neoplasm, digestive organ
      genital organ
        female Z85.40
          specified NEC Z85.44
        male Z85.45
          specified NEC Z85.49
      hematopoietic NEC Z85.79
      intrathoracic organ Z85.20
      kidney NEC Z85.528
        carcinoid Z85.520
      large intestine NEC Z85.038
        carcinoid Z85.030
      larynx Z85.21
      liver Z85.05
      lung NEC Z85.118
        carcinoid Z85.110
      mediastinum Z85.29
      Merkel cell Z85.821
      middle ear Z85.22
      nasal cavities Z85.22
      nervous system NEC Z85.848
      oral cavity Z85.819
        specified site NEC Z85.818
      ovary Z85.43
      pancreas Z85.07
      pelvis Z85.53
      pharynx Z85.819
        specified site NEC Z85.818
      pleura Z85.29
      prostate Z85.46
      rectosigmoid junction NEC Z85.048
        carcinoid Z85.040
      rectum NEC Z85.048
        carcinoid Z85.040
      respiratory organ Z85.20
      sinuses, accessory Z85.22
      skin NEC Z85.828
        melanoma Z85.820
        Merkel cell Z85.821
      small intestine NEC Z85.068
        carcinoid Z85.060
      soft tissue Z85.831
      specified site NEC Z85.89
      stomach NEC Z85.028
        carcinoid Z85.020
      testis Z85.47
      thymus NEC Z85.238
        carcinoid Z85.230
      thyroid Z85.850
      tongue Z85.810
      trachea Z85.12
      urinary organ or tract Z85.50
        specified NEC Z85.59
      uterus Z85.42
    maltreatment Z91.89
    medical treatment NEC Z92.89
    melanoma (malignant) (skin) Z85.820
    meningitis Z86.61
    mental disorder Z86.59
    Merkel cell carcinoma (skin) Z85.821
    Methicillin resistant Staphylococcus aureus (MRSA)
      Z86.14
    military deployment Z91.82
    military war, peacekeeping and humanitarian de-
      ployment (current or past conflict) Z91.82
    myocardial infarction (old) I25.2

History — *continued*
  personal (*see also* History, family) — *continued*
    neglect (in)
      adult Z91.412
      childhood Z62.812
    neoplasm
      benign Z86.018
        brain Z86.011
        colon polyp Z86.010
      in situ
        breast Z86.000
        cervix uteri Z86.001
        specified NEC Z86.008
      malignant — *see* History of, malignant neo-
        plasm
      uncertain behavior Z86.03
    nephrotic syndrome Z87.441
    nicotine dependence Z87.891
    noncompliance with medical treatment or regimen
      — *see* Noncompliance
    nutritional deficiency Z86.39
    obstetric complications Z87.59
      childbirth Z87.59
      pregnancy Z87.59
      pre-term labor Z87.51
      puerperium Z87.59
    osteoporosis fractures Z87.31 ☑
    parasuicide (attempt) Z91.5
    physical trauma NEC Z87.828
      self-harm or suicide attempt Z91.5
    pneumonia (recurrent) Z87.01
    poisoning NEC Z91.89
      self-harm or suicide attempt Z91.5
    poor personal hygiene Z91.89
    preterm labor Z87.51
    procedure during pregnancy Z98.870
    procedure while a fetus Z98.871
    prolonged reversible ischemic neurologic deficit
      (PRIND) Z86.73
    prostatic dysplasia Z87.430
    psychological
      abuse
        adult Z91.411
        child Z62.811
      trauma, specified NEC Z91.49
    radiation therapy Z92.3
    removal
      implant
        breast Z98.86
    renal calculi Z87.442
    respiratory condition NEC Z87.09
    retained foreign body fully removed Z87.821
    risk factors NEC Z91.89
    self-harm Z91.5
    self-poisoning attempt Z91.5
    sex reassignment Z87.890
    sleep-wake cycle problem Z72.821
    specified NEC Z87.898
    steroid therapy (systemic) Z92.241
      inhaled Z92.240
    stroke without residual deficits Z86.73
    substance abuse NEC F10-F19
    sudden cardiac arrest Z86.74
    sudden cardiac death successfully resuscitated
      Z86.74
    suicide attempt Z91.5
    surgery NEC Z98.890
      with uterine scar Z98.891
      sex reassignment Z87.890
      transplant — *see* Transplant
    thrombophlebitis Z86.72
    thrombosis (venous) Z86.718
      pulmonary Z86.711
    tobacco dependence Z87.891
    transient ischemic attack (TIA) without residual
      deficits Z86.73
    trauma (physical) NEC Z87.828
      psychological NEC Z91.49
      self-harm Z91.5
    traumatic brain injury Z87.820
    unhealthy sleep-wake cycle Z72.821
    unintended awareness under general anesthesia
      Z92.84
    urinary calculi Z87.442
    urinary (recurrent) (tract) infection(s) Z87.440
    uterine scar from previous surgery Z98.891
    vaginal dysplasia Z87.411
    venous thrombosis or embolism Z86.718
      pulmonary Z86.711

History — *continued*
  personal (*see also* History, family) — *continued*
    vulvar dysplasia Z87.412
His-Werner disease A79.0
HIV (*see also* Human, immunodeficiency virus) B20
  laboratory evidence (nonconclusive) R75
  nonconclusive test (in infants) R75
  positive, seropositive Z21
Hives (bold) — *see* Urticaria
Hoarseness R49.0
Hobo Z59.0
Hodgkin disease — *see* Lymphoma, Hodgkin
Hodgson's disease I71.2
  ruptured I71.1
Hoffa-Kastert disease E88.89
Hoffa's disease E88.89
Hoffmann-Bouveret syndrome I47.9
Hoffmann's syndrome E03.9 [G73.7]
Hole (round)
  macula H35.34- ☑
  retina (without detachment) — *see* Break, retina,
    round hole
    with detachment — *see* Detachment, retina, with
      retinal, break
Holiday relief care Z75.5
Hollenhorst's plaque — *see* Occlusion, artery, retina
Hollow foot (congenital) Q66.7
  acquired — *see* Deformity, limb, foot, specified NEC
Holoprosencephaly Q04.2
Holt-Oram syndrome Q87.2
Homelessness Z59.0
Homesickness — *see* Disorder, adjustment
Homocystinemia, homocystinuria E72.11
Homogentisate 1,2-dioxygenase deficiency E70.29
Homologous serum hepatitis (prophylactic) (therapeu-
  tic) — *see* Hepatitis, viral, type B
Honeycomb lung J98.4
  congenital Q33.0
Hooded
  clitoris Q52.6
  penis Q55.69
Hookworm (anemia) (disease) (infection) (infestation)
  B76.9
  specified NEC B76.8
Hordeolum (eyelid) (externum) (recurrent) H00.019
  internum H00.029
    left H00.026
      lower H00.025
      upper H00.024
    right H00.023
      lower H00.022
      upper H00.021
  left H00.016
    lower H00.015
    upper H00.014
  right H00.013
    lower H00.012
    upper H00.011
Horn
  cutaneous L85.8
  nail L60.2
    congenital Q84.6
Horner (-Claude Bernard) **syndrome** G90.2
  traumatic — *see* Injury, nerve, cervical sympathetic
Horseshoe kidney (congenital) Q63.1
Horton's headache or neuralgia G44.099
  intractable G44.091
  not intractable G44.099
Hospital hopper syndrome — *see* Disorder, factitious
Hospitalism in children — *see* Disorder, adjustment
Hostility R45.5
  towards child Z62.3
Hot flashes
  menopausal N95.1
Hourglass (contracture) (*see also* Contraction, hourglass)
  stomach K31.89
    congenital Q40.2
    stricture K31.2
Household, housing circumstance affecting care
  Z59.9
  specified NEC Z59.8
Housemaid's knee — *see* Bursitis, prepatellar
Hudson (-Stähli) **line** (cornea) — *see* Pigmentation,
  cornea, anterior
Human
  bite (open wound) (*see also* Bite)
    intact skin surface — *see* Bite, superficial

ᴺᴱᵂ Subterms under main terms may continue to next column or page   ☑ Additional Character Required — Refer to the Tabular List for Character Selection   **171**

History — Human

Human — *continued*
  herpesvirus — *see* Herpes
  immunodeficiency virus (HIV) disease (infection) B20
    asymptomatic status Z21
    contact Z20.6
    counseling Z71.7
    dementia B20 [F02.80]
      with behavioral disturbance B20 [F02.81]
    exposure to Z20.6
    laboratory evidence R75
    type-2 (HIV 2) as cause of disease classified else-
        where B97.35
  papillomavirus (HPV)
    DNA test positive
      high risk
        cervix R87.810
        vagina R87.811
      low risk
        cervix R87.820
        vagina R87.821
    screening for Z11.51
  T-cell lymphotropic virus
    type-1 (HTLV-I) infection B33.3
      as cause of disease classified elsewhere B97.33
      carrier Z22.6
    type-2 (HTLV-II) as cause of disease classified else-
        where B97.34
Humidifier lung or pneumonitis J67.7
Humiliation (experience) **in childhood** Z62.898
Humpback (acquired) — *see* Kyphosis
Hunchback (acquired) — *see* Kyphosis
Hunger T73.0 ☑
  air, psychogenic F45.8
Hungry bone syndrome E83.81
Hunner's ulcer — *see* Cystitis, chronic, interstitial
Hunter's
  glossitis D51.0
  syndrome E76.1
Huntington's disease or chorea G10
  with dementia G10 [F02.80]
    with behavioral disturbance G10 [F02.81]
Hunt's
  disease or syndrome (herpetic geniculate ganglionitis)
      B02.21
    dyssynergia cerebellaris myoclonica G11.1
  neuralgia B02.21
Hurler (-Scheie) **disease or syndrome** E76.02
Hurst's disease G36.1
Hurthle cell
  adenocarcinoma C73
  adenoma D34
  carcinoma C73
  tumor D34
Hutchinson-Boeck disease or syndrome — *see* Sar-
    coidosis
Hutchinson-Gilford disease or syndrome E34.8
Hutchinson's
  disease, meaning
    angioma serpiginosum L81.7
    pompholyx (cheiropompholyx) L30.1
    prurigo estivalis L56.4
    summer eruption or summer prurigo L56.4
  melanotic freckle — *see* Melanoma, in situ
    malignant melanoma in — *see* Melanoma
  teeth or incisors (congenital syphilis) A50.52
  triad (congenital syphilis) A50.53
Hyalin plaque, sclera, senile H15.89
Hyaline membrane (disease) (lung) (pulmonary) (new-
    born) P22.0
Hyalinosis
  cutis (et mucosae) E78.89
  focal and segmental (glomerular) (*see also* N00-N07
      with fourth character .1) N05.1
Hyalitis, hyalosis, asteroid (*see also* Deposit, crystalline)
  syphilitic (late) A52.71
Hydatid
  cyst or tumor — *see* Echinococcus
  mole — *see* Hydatidiform mole
  Morgagni
    female Q50.5
    male (epididymal) Q55.4
      testicular Q55.29
Hydatidiform mole (benign) (complicating pregnancy)
    (delivered) (undelivered) O01.9
  classical O01.0
  complete O01.0
  incomplete O01.1
  invasive D39.2

Hydatidiform mole — *continued*
  malignant D39.2
  partial O01.1
Hydatidosis — *see* Echinococcus
Hydradenitis (axillaris) (suppurative) L73.2
Hydradenoma — *see* Hidradenoma
Hydramnios O40.- ☑
Hydrancephaly, hydranencephaly Q04.3
  with spina bifida — *see* Spina bifida, with hydro-
      cephalus
Hydrargyrism NEC — *see* Poisoning, mercury
Hydrarthrosis (*see also* Effusion, joint)
  gonococcal A54.42
  intermittent M12.40
    ankle M12.47- ☑
    elbow M12.42- ☑
    foot joint M12.47- ☑
    hand joint M12.44- ☑
    hip M12.45- ☑
    knee M12.46- ☑
    multiple site M12.49
    shoulder M12.41- ☑
    specified joint NEC M12.48
    wrist M12.43- ☑
  of yaws (early) (late) (*see also* subcategory M14.8-)
      A66.6
  syphilitic (late) A52.77
    congenital A50.55 [M12.80]
Hydremia D64.89
Hydrencephalocele (congenital) — *see* Encephalocele
Hydrencephalomeningocele (congenital) — *see* En-
    cephalocele
Hydroa R23.8
  aestivale L56.4
  vacciniforme L56.4
Hydroadenitis (axillaris) (suppurative) L73.2
Hydrocalycosis — *see* Hydronephrosis
Hydrocele (spermatic cord) (testis) (tunica vaginalis)
    N43.3
  canal of Nuck N94.89
  communicating N43.2
  congenital P83.5
  encysted N43.0
  female NEC N94.89
  infected N43.1
  newborn P83.5
  round ligament N94.89
  specified NEC N43.2
  spinalis — *see* Spina bifida
  vulva N90.89
Hydrocephalus (acquired) (external) (internal) (malig-
    nant) (recurrent) G91.9
  aqueduct Sylvius stricture Q03.0
  causing disproportion O33.6 ☑
    with obstructed labor O66.3
  communicating G91.0
  congenital (external) (internal) Q03.9
    with spina bifida Q05.4
      cervical Q05.0
      dorsal Q05.1
      lumbar Q05.2
      lumbosacral Q05.2
      sacral Q05.3
      thoracic Q05.1
      thoracolumbar Q05.1
    specified NEC Q03.8
  due to toxoplasmosis (congenital) P37.1
  foramen Magendie block (acquired) G91.1
    congenital (*see also* Hydrocephalus, congenital)
        Q03.1
  in (due to)
    infectious disease NEC B89 [G91.4]
    neoplastic disease NEC (*see also* Neoplasm) G91.4
    parasitic disease B89 [G91.4]
  newborn Q03.9
    with spina bifida — *see* Spina bifida, with hydro-
        cephalus
  noncommunicating G91.1
  normal pressure G91.2
    secondary G91.0
  obstructive G91.1
  otitic G93.2
  post-traumatic NEC G91.3
  secondary G91.4
    post-traumatic G91.3
  specified NEC G91.8
  syphilitic, congenital A50.49

Hydrocolpos (congenital) N89.8
Hydrocystoma — *see* Neoplasm, skin, benign
Hydroencephalocele (congenital) — *see* Encephalocele
Hydroencephalomeningocele (congenital) — *see* En-
    cephalocele
Hydrohematopneumothorax — *see* Hemothorax
Hydromeningitis — *see* Meningitis
Hydromeningocele (spinal) (*see also* Spina bifida)
  cranial — *see* Encephalocele
Hydrometra N85.8
Hydrometrocolpos N89.8
Hydromicrocephaly Q02
Hydromphalos (since birth) Q45.8
Hydromyelia Q06.4
Hydromyelocele — *see* Spina bifida
Hydronephrosis (atrophic) (early) (functionless) (inter-
    mittent) (primary) (secondary) NEC N13.30
  with
    infection N13.6
    obstruction (by) (of)
      renal calculus N13.2
        with infection N13.6
      ureteral NEC N13.1
        with infection N13.6
        calculus N13.2
          with infection N13.6
      ureteropelvic junction (congenital) Q62.11
        acquired N13.0
          with infection N13.6
      ureteral stricture NEC N13.1
        with infection N13.6
  congenital Q62.0
  due to acquired occlusion of ureteropelvic junction
      N13.0
  specified type NEC N13.39
  tuberculous A18.11
Hydropericarditis — *see* Pericarditis
Hydropericardium — *see* Pericarditis
Hydroperitoneum R18.8
Hydrophobia — *see* Rabies
Hydrophthalmos Q15.0
Hydropneumohemothorax — *see* Hemothorax
Hydropneumopericarditis — *see* Pericarditis
Hydropneumopericardium — *see* Pericarditis
Hydropneumothorax J94.8
  traumatic — *see* Injury, intrathoracic, lung
  tuberculous NEC A15.6
Hydrops R60.9
  abdominis R18.8
  articulorum intermittens — *see* Hydrarthrosis, inter-
      mittent
  cardiac — *see* Failure, heart, congestive
  causing obstructed labor (mother) O66.3
  endolymphatic H81.0- ☑
  fetal — *see* Pregnancy, complicated by, hydrops, fetalis
  fetalis P83.2
    due to
      ABO isoimmunization P56.0
      alpha thalassemia D56.0
      hemolytic disease P56.90
        specified NEC P56.99
      isoimmunization (ABO) (Rh) P56.0
      other specified nonhemolytic disease NEC P83.2
      Rh incompatibility P56.0
    during pregnancy — *see* Pregnancy, complicated
        by, hydrops, fetalis
  gallbladder K82.1
  joint — *see* Effusion, joint
  labyrinth H81.0- ☑
  newborn (idiopathic) P83.2
    due to
      ABO isoimmunization P56.0
      alpha thalassemia D56.0
      hemolytic disease P56.90
        specified NEC P56.99
      isoimmunization (ABO) (Rh) P56.0
      Rh incompatibility P56.0
  nutritional — *see* Malnutrition, severe
  pericardium — *see* Pericarditis
  pleura — *see* Hydrothorax
  spermatic cord — *see* Hydrocele
Hydropyonephrosis N13.6
Hydrorachis Q06.4
Hydrorrhea (nasal) J34.89
  pregnancy — *see* Rupture, membranes, premature
Hydrosadenitis (axillaris) (suppurative) L73.2
Hydrosalpinx (fallopian tube) (follicularis) N70.11

172

☑ **Additional Character Required** — **Refer to the Tabular List for Character Selection**   ⤷ **Subterms under main terms may continue to next column or page**

Hydrothorax (double) (pleura) J94.8
  chylous (nonfilarial) I89.8
    filarial (*see also* Infestation, filarial) B74.9 [J91.8]
  traumatic — *see* Injury, intrathoracic
  tuberculous NEC (non primary) A15.6
Hydroureter (*see also* Hydronephrosis) N13.4
  with infection N13.6
  congenital Q62.39
Hydroureteronephrosis — *see* Hydronephrosis
Hydrourethra N36.8
Hydroxykynureninuria E70.8
Hydroxylysinemia E72.3
Hydroxyprolinemia E72.59
Hygiene, sleep
  abuse Z72.821
  inadequate Z72.821
  poor Z72.821
Hygroma (congenital) (cystic) D18.1
  praepatellare, prepatellar — *see* Bursitis, prepatellar
  subdural I62.03
Hymen — *see* condition
Hymenolepis, hymenolepiasis (diminuta) (infection) (infestation) (nana) B71.0
Hypalgesia R20.8
Hyperacidity (gastric) K31.89
  psychogenic F45.8
Hyperactive, hyperactivity F90.9
  basal cell, uterine cervix — *see* Dysplasia, cervix
  bowel sounds R19.12
  cervix epithelial (basal) — *see* Dysplasia, cervix
  child F90.9
    attention deficit — *see* Disorder, attention-deficit hyperactivity
  detrusor muscle N32.81
  gastrointestinal K31.89
    psychogenic F45.8
  nasal mucous membrane J34.3
  stomach K31.89
  thyroid (gland) — *see* Hyperthyroidism
Hyperacusis H93.23- ☑
Hyperadrenalism E27.5
Hyperadrenocorticism E24.9
  congenital E25.0
  iatrogenic E24.2
    correct substance properly administered — *see* Table of Drugs and Chemicals, by drug, adverse effect
    overdose or wrong substance given or taken — *see* Table of Drugs and Chemicals, by drug, poisoning
  not associated with Cushing's syndrome E27.0
  pituitary-dependent E24.0
Hyperaldosteronism E26.9
  familial (type I) E26.02
  glucocorticoid-remediable E26.02
  primary (due to (bilateral) adrenal hyperplasia) E26.09
  primary NEC E26.09
  secondary E26.1
  specified NEC E26.89
Hyperalgesia R20.8
Hyperalimentation R63.2
  carotene, carotin E67.1
  specified NEC E67.8
  vitamin
    A E67.0
    D E67.3
Hyperaminoaciduria
  arginine E72.21
  cystine E72.01
  lysine E72.3
  ornithine E72.4
Hyperammonemia (congenital) E72.20
Hyperazotemia — *see* Uremia
Hyperbetalipoproteinemia (familial) E78.00
  with prebetalipoproteinemia E78.2
Hyperbilirubinemia
  constitutional E80.6
  familial conjugated E80.6
  neonatal (transient) — *see* Jaundice, newborn
Hypercalcemia, hypocalciuric, familial E83.52
Hypercalciuria, idiopathic E83.52
Hypercapnia R06.89
  newborn P84
Hypercarotenemia, hypercarotinemia (dietary) E67.1
Hypercementosis K03.4
Hyperchloremia E87.8
Hyperchlorhydria K31.89

Hyperchlorhydria — *continued*
  neurotic F45.8
  psychogenic F45.8
Hypercholesterinemia — *see* Hypercholesterolemia
Hypercholesterolemia (essential) (primary) (pure) E78.00
  with hyperglyceridemia, endogenous E78.2
  dietary counseling and surveillance Z71.3
  familial E78.01
  hereditary E78.01
Hyperchylia gastrica, psychogenic F45.8
Hyperchylomicronemia (familial) (primary) E78.3
  with hyperbetalipoproteinemia E78.3
Hypercoagulable (state) D68.59
  activated protein C resistance D68.51
  antithrombin (III) deficiency D68.59
  factor V Leiden mutation D68.51
  primary NEC D68.59
  protein C deficiency D68.59
  protein S deficiency D68.59
  prothrombin gene mutation D68.52
  secondary D68.69
  specified NEC D68.69
Hypercoagulation (state) D68.59
Hypercorticalism, pituitary-dependent E24.0
Hypercorticosolism — *see* Cushing's, syndrome
Hypercorticosteronism E24.2
  correct substance properly administered — *see* Table of Drugs and Chemicals, by drug, adverse effect
  overdose or wrong substance given or taken — *see* Table of Drugs and Chemicals, by drug, poisoning
Hypercortisonism E24.2
  correct substance properly administered — *see* Table of Drugs and Chemicals, by drug, adverse effect
  overdose or wrong substance given or taken — *see* Table of Drugs and Chemicals, by drug, poisoning
Hyperekplexia Q89.8
Hyperelectrolytemia E87.8
Hyperemesis R11.10
  with nausea R11.2
  gravidarum (mild) O21.0
    with
      carbohydrate depletion O21.1
      dehydration O21.1
      electrolyte imbalance O21.1
      metabolic disturbance O21.1
      severe (with metabolic disturbance) O21.1
  projectile R11.12
  psychogenic F45.8
Hyperemia (acute) (passive) R68.89
  anal mucosa K62.89
  bladder N32.89
  cerebral I67.89
  conjunctiva H11.43- ☑
  ear internal, acute — *see* subcategory H83.0 ☑
  enteric K59.8
  eye — *see* Hyperemia, conjunctiva
  eyelid (active) (passive) — *see* Disorder, eyelid, specified type NEC
  intestine K59.8
  iris — *see* Disorder, iris, vascular
  kidney N28.89
  labyrinth — *see* subcategory H83.0 ☑
  liver (active) K76.89
  lung (passive) — *see* Edema, lung
  pulmonary (passive) — *see* Edema, lung
  renal N28.89
  retina H35.89
  stomach K31.89
Hyperesthesia (body surface) R20.3
  larynx (reflex) J38.7
    hysterical F44.89
  pharynx (reflex) J39.2
    hysterical F44.89
Hyperestrogenism (drug-induced) (iatrogenic) E28.0
Hyperexplexia Q89.8
Hyperfibrinolysis — *see* Fibrinolysis
Hyperfructosemia E74.19
Hyperfunction
  adrenal cortex, not associated with Cushing's syndrome E27.0
  medulla E27.5
    adrenomedullary E27.5
  virilism E25.9
    congenital E25.0
  ovarian E28.8

Hyperfunction — *continued*
  pancreas K86.89
  parathyroid (gland) E21.3
  pituitary (gland) (anterior) E22.9
    specified NEC E22.8
  polyglandular E31.1
  testicular E29.0
Hypergammaglobulinemia D89.2
  polyclonal D89.0
  Waldenström D89.0
Hypergastrinemia E16.4
Hyperglobulinemia R77.1
Hyperglycemia, hyperglycemic (transient) R73.9
  coma — *see* Diabetes, by type, with coma
  postpancreatectomy E89.1
Hyperglyceridemia (endogenous) (essential) (familial) (hereditary) (pure) E78.1
  mixed E78.3
Hyperglycinemia (non-ketotic) E72.51
Hypergonadism
  ovarian E28.8
  testicular (primary) (infantile) E29.0
Hyperheparinemia D68.32
Hyperhidrosis, hyperidrosis R61
  focal
    primary L74.519
      axilla L74.510
      face L74.511
      palms L74.512
      soles L74.513
    secondary L74.52
  generalized R61
  localized
    primary L74.519
      axilla L74.510
      face L74.511
      palms L74.512
      soles L74.513
    secondary L74.52
  psychogenic F45.8
  secondary R61
    focal L74.52
Hyperhistidinemia E70.41
Hyperhomocysteinemia E72.11
Hyperhydroxyprolinemia E72.59
Hyperinsulinism (functional) E16.1
  with
    coma (hypoglycemic) E15
    encephalopathy E16.1 [G94]
  ectopic E16.1
  therapeutic misadventure (from administration of insulin) — *see* subcategory T38.3 ☑
Hyperkalemia E87.5
Hyperkeratosis (*see also* Keratosis) L85.9
  cervix N88.0
  due to yaws (early) (late) (palmar or plantar) A66.3
  follicularis Q82.8
    penetrans (in cutem) L87.0
  palmoplantaris climacterica L85.1
  pinta A67.1
  senile (with pruritus) L57.0
  universalis congenita Q80.8
  vocal cord J38.3
  vulva N90.4
Hyperkinesia, hyperkinetic (disease) (reaction) (syndrome) (childhood) (adolescence) (*see also* Disorder, attention-deficit hyperactivity)
  heart I51.89
Hyperleucine-isoleucinemia E71.19
Hyperlipemia, hyperlipidemia E78.5
  combined E78.2
    familial E78.4
  group
    A E78.00
    B E78.1
    C E78.2
    D E78.3
  mixed E78.2
  specified NEC E78.4
Hyperlipidosis E75.6
  hereditary NEC E75.5
Hyperlipoproteinemia E78.5
  Fredrickson's type
    I E78.3
    IIa E78.00
    IIb E78.2
    III E78.2
    IV E78.1

Hyperlipoproteinemia — *continued*
  Fredrickson's type — *continued*
    V E78.3
    low-density-lipoprotein-type (LDL) E78.00
    very-low-density-lipoprotein-type (VLDL) E78.1
Hyperlucent lung, unilateral J43.0
Hyperlysinemia E72.3
Hypermagnesemia E83.41
  neonatal P71.8
Hypermenorrhea N92.0
Hypermethioninemia E72.19
Hypermetropia (congenital) H52.0- ☑
Hypermobility, hypermotility
  cecum — *see* Syndrome, irritable bowel
  coccyx — *see* subcategory M53.2 ☑
  colon — *see* Syndrome, irritable bowel
    psychogenic F45.8
  ileum K58.9
  intestine (*see also* Syndrome, irritable bowel) K58.9
    psychogenic F45.8
  meniscus (knee) — *see* Derangement, knee, meniscus
  scapula — *see* Instability, joint, shoulder
  stomach K31.89
    psychogenic F45.8
  syndrome M35.7
  urethra N36.41
    with intrinsic sphincter deficiency N36.43
Hypernasality R49.21
Hypernatremia E87.0
Hypernephroma C64.- ☑
Hyperopia — *see* Hypermetropia
Hyperorexia nervosa F50.2
Hyperornithinemia E72.4
Hyperosmia R43.1
Hyperosmolality E87.0
Hyperostosis (monomelic) (*see also* Disorder, bone, density and structure, specified NEC)
  ankylosing (spine) M48.10
    cervical region M48.12
    cervicothoracic region M48.13
    lumbar region M48.16
    lumbosacral region M48.17
    multiple sites M48.19
    occipito-atlanto-axial region M48.11
    sacrococcygeal region M48.18
    thoracic region M48.14
    thoracolumbar region M48.15
  cortical (skull) M85.2
    infantile M89.8X- ☑
  frontal, internal of skull M85.2
  interna frontalis M85.2
  skeletal, diffuse idiopathic — *see* Hyperostosis, ankylosing
  skull M85.2
    congenital Q75.8
  vertebral, ankylosing — *see* Hyperostosis, ankylosing
Hyperovarism E28.8
Hyperoxaluria (primary) E72.53
Hyperparathyroidism E21.3
  primary E21.0
  secondary (renal) N25.81
    non-renal E21.1
  specified NEC E21.2
  tertiary E21.2
Hyperpathia R20.8
Hyperperistalsis R19.2
  psychogenic F45.8
Hyperpermeability, capillary I78.8
Hyperphagia R63.2
Hyperphenylalaninemia NEC E70.1
Hyperphoria (alternating) H50.53
Hyperphosphatemia E83.39
Hyperpiesis, hyperpiesia — *see* Hypertension
Hyperpigmentation (*see also* Pigmentation)
  melanin NEC L81.4
  postinflammatory L81.0
Hyperpinealism E34.8
Hyperpituitarism E22.9
Hyperplasia, hyperplastic
  adenoids J35.2
  adrenal (capsule) (cortex) (gland) E27.8
    with
      sexual precocity (male) E25.9
        congenital E25.0
      virilism, adrenal E25.9
        congenital E25.0
      virilization (female) E25.9

Hyperplasia, hyperplastic — *continued*
  adrenal — *continued*
    with — *continued*
      virilization — *continued*
        congenital E25.0
    congenital E25.0
      salt-losing E25.0
  adrenomedullary E27.5
  angiolymphoid, eosinophilia (ALHE) D18.01
  appendix (lymphoid) K38.0
  artery, fibromuscular I77.3
  bone (*see also* Hypertrophy, bone)
    marrow D75.89
  breast (*see also* Hypertrophy, breast)
    ductal (atypical) N60.9- ☑
  C-cell, thyroid E07.0
  cementation (tooth) (teeth) K03.4
  cervical gland R59.0
  cervix (uteri) (basal cell) (endometrium) (polypoid) (*see also* Dysplasia, cervix)
    congenital Q51.828
  clitoris, congenital Q52.6
  denture K06.2
  endocervicitis N72
  endometrium, endometrial (adenomatous) (benign) (cystic) (glandular) (glandular-cystic) (polypoid) N85.00
    with atypia N85.02
    cervix — *see* Dysplasia, cervix
    complex (without atypia) N85.01
    simple (without atypia) N85.01
  epithelial L85.9
    focal, oral, including tongue K13.29
    nipple N62
    skin L85.9
    tongue K13.29
    vaginal wall N89.3
  erythroid D75.89
  fibromuscular of artery (carotid) (renal) I77.3
  genital
    female NEC N94.89
    male N50.89
  gingiva K06.1
  glandularis cystica uteri (interstitialis) (*see also* Hyperplasia, endometrial) N85.00
  gum K06.1
  hymen, congenital Q52.4
  irritative, edentulous (alveolar) K06.2
  jaw M26.09
    alveolar M26.79
    lower M26.03
      alveolar M26.72
    upper M26.01
      alveolar M26.71
  kidney (congenital) Q63.3
  labia N90.69
    epithelial N90.3
  liver (congenital) Q44.7
    nodular, focal K76.89
  lymph gland or node R59.9
  mandible, mandibular M26.03
    alveolar M26.72
    unilateral condylar M27.8
  maxilla, maxillary M26.01
    alveolar M26.71
  myometrium, myometrial N85.2
  neuroendocrine cell, of infancy J84.841
  nose
    lymphoid J34.89
    polypoid J33.9
  oral mucosa (irritative) K13.6
  organ or site, congenital NEC — *see* Anomaly, by site
  ovary N83.8
  palate, papillary (irritative) K13.6
  pancreatic islet cells E16.9
    alpha E16.8
      with excess
        gastrin E16.4
        glucagon E16.3
    beta E16.1
  parathyroid (gland) E21.0
  pharynx (lymphoid) J39.2
  prostate (adenofibromatous) (nodular) N40.0
    with lower urinary tract symptoms (LUTS) N40.1
    without lower urinary tract symptoms (LUTS) N40.0
  renal artery I77.89
  reticulo-endothelial (cell) D75.89
  salivary gland (any) K11.1

Hyperplasia, hyperplastic — *continued*
  Schimmelbusch's — *see* Mastopathy, cystic
  suprarenal capsule (gland) E27.8
  thymus (gland) (persistent) E32.0
  thyroid (gland) — *see* Goiter
  tonsils (faucial) (infective) (lingual) (lymphoid) J35.1
    with adenoids J35.3
  unilateral condylar M27.8
  uterus, uterine N85.2
    endometrium (glandular) (*see also* Hyperplasia, endometrial) N85.00
  vulva N90.69
    epithelial N90.3
Hyperpnea — *see* Hyperventilation
Hyperpotassemia E87.5
Hyperprebetalipoproteinemia (familial) E78.1
Hyperprolactinemia E22.1
Hyperprolinemia (type I) (type II) E72.59
Hyperproteinemia E88.09
Hyperprothrombinemia, causing coagulation factor deficiency D68.4
Hyperpyrexia R50.9
  heat (effects) T67.0 ☑
  malignant, due to anesthetic T88.3 ☑
  rheumatic — *see* Fever, rheumatic
  unknown origin R50.9
Hyper-reflexia R29.2
Hypersalivation K11.7
Hypersecretion
  ACTH (not associated with Cushing's syndrome) E27.0
    pituitary E24.0
  adrenaline E27.5
  adrenomedullary E27.5
  androgen (testicular) E29.0
    ovarian (drug-induced) (iatrogenic) E28.1
  calcitonin E07.0
  catecholamine E27.5
  corticoadrenal E24.9
  cortisol E24.9
  epinephrine E27.5
  estrogen E28.0
  gastric K31.89
    psychogenic F45.8
  gastrin E16.4
  glucagon E16.3
  hormone(s)
    ACTH (not associated with Cushing's syndrome) E27.0
      pituitary E24.0
    antidiuretic E22.2
    growth E22.0
    intestinal NEC E34.1
    ovarian androgen E28.1
    pituitary E22.9
    testicular E29.0
    thyroid stimulating E05.80
      with thyroid storm E05.81
  insulin — *see* Hyperinsulinism
  lacrimal glands — *see* Epiphora
  medulloadrenal E27.5
  milk O92.6
  ovarian androgens E28.1
  salivary gland (any) K11.7
  thyrocalcitonin E07.0
  upper respiratory J39.8
Hypersegmentation, leukocytic, hereditary D72.0
Hypersensitive, hypersensitiveness, hypersensitivity (*see also* Allergy)
  carotid sinus G90.01
  colon — *see* Irritable, colon
  drug T88.7 ☑
  gastrointestinal K52.29
    immediate K52.29
    psychogenic F45.8
  labyrinth — *see* subcategory H83.2 ☑
  pain R20.8
  pneumonitis — *see* Pneumonitis, allergic
  reaction T78.40 ☑
    upper respiratory tract NEC J39.3
Hypersomnia (organic) G47.10
  due to
    alcohol
      abuse F10.182
      dependence F10.282
      use F10.982
    amphetamines
      abuse F15.182
      dependence F15.282

☑ Additional Character Required — Refer to the Tabular List for Character Selection   ▽ Subterms under main terms may continue to next column or page

Hypersomnia — *continued*
- due to — *continued*
  - amphetamines — *continued*
    - use F15.982
  - caffeine
    - abuse F15.182
    - dependence F15.282
    - use F15.982
  - cocaine
    - abuse F14.182
    - dependence F14.282
    - use F14.982
  - drug NEC
    - abuse F19.182
    - dependence F19.282
    - use F19.982
  - medical condition G47.14
  - mental disorder F51.13
  - opioid
    - abuse F11.182
    - dependence F11.282
    - use F11.982
  - psychoactive substance NEC
    - abuse F19.182
    - dependence F19.282
    - use F19.982
  - sedative, hypnotic, or anxiolytic
    - abuse F13.182
    - dependence F13.282
    - use F13.982
  - stimulant NEC
    - abuse F15.182
    - dependence F15.282
    - use F15.982
- idiopathic G47.11
  - with long sleep time G47.11
  - without long sleep time G47.12
- menstrual related G47.13
- nonorganic origin F51.11
  - specified NEC F51.19
- not due to a substance or known physiological condition F51.11
  - specified NEC F51.19
- primary F51.11
- recurrent G47.13
- specified NEC G47.19

Hypersplenia, hypersplenism D73.1
Hyperstimulation, ovaries (associated with induced ovulation) N98.1
Hypersusceptibility — *see* Allergy
Hypertelorism (ocular) (orbital) Q75.2
Hypertension, hypertensive (accelerated) (benign) (essential) (idiopathic) (malignant) (systemic) I10
- with
  - heart failure (congestive) I11.0
  - heart involvement (conditions in I50.-, I51.4-I51.9 due to hypertension) — *see* Hypertension, heart
  - kidney involvement — *see* Hypertension, kidney
- benign, intracranial G93.2
- borderline R03.0
- cardiorenal (disease) I13.10
  - with heart failure I13.0
    - with stage 1 through stage 4 chronic kidney disease I13.0
    - with stage 5 or end stage renal disease I13.2
  - without heart failure I13.10
    - with stage 1 through stage 4 chronic kidney disease I13.10
    - with stage 5 or end stage renal disease I13.11
- cardiovascular
  - disease (arteriosclerotic) (sclerotic) — *see* Hypertension, heart
  - renal (disease) — *see* Hypertension, cardiorenal
- chronic venous — *see* Hypertension, venous (chronic)
- complicating
  - childbirth (labor) O16.4
    - pre-existing O10.92
      - with
        - heart disease O10.12
          - with renal disease O10.32
        - pre-eclampsia O11.4
        - renal disease O10.22
          - with heart disease O10.32
        - essential O10.02
      - secondary O10.42
  - pregnancy O16.-
    - with edema (*see also* Pre-eclampsia) O14.9- ☑

Hypertension, hypertensive — *continued*
- complicating — *continued*
  - pregnancy — *continued*
    - gestational (pregnancy induced) (without proteinuria) O13.- ☑
      - with proteinuria O14.9- ☑
        - mild pre-eclampsia O14.0- ☑
        - moderate pre-eclampsia O14.0- ☑
        - severe pre-eclampsia O14.1- ☑
          - with hemolysis, elevated liver enzymes and low platelet count (HELLP) O14.2- ☑
    - pre-existing O10.91- ☑
      - with
        - heart disease O10.11- ☑
          - with renal disease O10.31- ☑
        - pre-eclampsia — *see* category O11
        - renal disease O10.21- ☑
          - with heart disease O10.31- ☑
        - essential O10.01- ☑
      - secondary O10.41- ☑
    - transient O13- ☑
  - puerperium, pre-existing O16.5
    - pre-existing
      - with
        - heart disease O10.13
          - with renal disease O10.33
        - pre-eclampsia O11.5
        - renal disease O10.23
          - with heart disease O10.33
        - essential O10.03
    - pregnancy-induced O13.9
    - secondary O10.43
- crisis I16.9
- due to
  - endocrine disorders I15.2
  - pheochromocytoma I15.2
  - renal disorders NEC I15.1
    - arterial I15.0
  - renovascular disorders I15.0
  - specified disease NEC I15.8
- emergency I16.1
- encephalopathy I67.4
- gestational (without significant proteinuria) (pregnancy-induced) (transient) O13.- ☑
  - with significant proteinuria — *see* Pre-eclampsia
  - complicating
    - delivery O13.4
    - puerperium O13.5
- Goldblatt's I70.1
- heart (disease) (conditions in I51.4-I51.9 due to hypertension) I11.9
  - with
    - heart failure (congestive) I11.0
    - kidney disease (chronic) — *see* Hypertension, cardiorenal
- intracranial (benign) G93.2
- kidney I12.9
  - with
    - heart disease — *see* Hypertension, cardiorenal
    - stage 1 through stage 4 chronic kidney disease I12.9
    - stage 5 chronic kidney disease (CKD) or end stage renal disease (ESRD) I12.0
- lesser circulation I27.0
- maternal O16- ☑
- newborn P29.2
  - pulmonary (persistent) P29.30
- ocular H40.05- ☑
- pancreatic duct — *code to* underlying condition
  - with chronic pancreatitis K86.1
- portal (due to chronic liver disease) (idiopathic) K76.6
  - gastropathy K31.89
  - in (due to) schistosomiasis (bilharziasis) B65.9 [K77]
- postoperative I97.3
- psychogenic F45.8
- pulmonary I27.20
  - with
    - cor pulmonale (chronic) I27.29
      - acute I26.09
    - right heart ventricular strain/failure I27.29
      - acute I26.09
    - right to left shunt related to congenital heart disease I27.83
    - unclear multifactorial mechanisms I27.29
  - arterial (associated) (drug-induced) (toxin-induced) I27.21
  - chronic thromboembolic I27.24

Hypertension, hypertensive — *continued*
- pulmonary — *continued*
  - due to
    - hematologic disorders I27.29
    - left heart disease I27.22
    - lung diseases and hypoxia I27.23
    - metabolic disorders I27.29
    - specified systemic disorders I27.29
  - group 1 (associated) (drug-induced) (toxin-induced) I27.21
  - group 2 I27.22
  - group 3 I27.23
  - group 4 I27.24
  - group 5 I27.29
  - of newborn (persistent) P29.30
  - primary (idiopathic) I27.0
  - secondary
    - arterial I27.21
    - specified NEC I27.29
- renal — *see* Hypertension, kidney
- renovascular I15.0
- secondary NEC I15.9
  - due to
    - endocrine disorders I15.2
    - pheochromocytoma I15.2
    - renal disorders NEC I15.1
      - arterial I15.0
    - renovascular disorders I15.0
  - specified NEC I15.8
- transient, of pregnancy O13- ☑
- urgency I16.0
- venous (chronic)
  - due to
    - deep vein thrombosis — *see* Syndrome, post-thrombotic
    - idiopathic I87.309
      - with
        - inflammation I87.32- ☑
          - with ulcer I87.33- ☑
        - specified complication NEC I87.39- ☑
        - ulcer I87.31- ☑
          - with inflammation I87.33- ☑
        - asymptomatic I87.30- ☑

Hypertensive urgency — *see* Hypertension
Hyperthecosis ovary E28.8
Hyperthermia (of unknown origin) (*see also* Hyperpyrexia)
- malignant, due to anesthesia T88.3 ☑
- newborn P81.9
  - environmental P81.0
Hyperthyroid (recurrent) — *see* Hyperthyroidism
Hyperthyroidism (latent) (pre-adult) (recurrent) E05.90
- with
  - goiter (diffuse) E05.00
    - with thyroid storm E05.01
    - nodular (multinodular) E05.20
      - with thyroid storm E05.21
      - uninodular E05.10
        - with thyroid storm E05.11
  - storm E05.91
- due to ectopic thyroid tissue E05.30
  - with thyroid storm E05.31
- neonatal, transitory P72.1
- specified NEC E05.80
  - with thyroid storm E05.81
Hypertony, hypertonia, hypertonicity
- bladder N31.8
- congenital P94.1
- stomach K31.89
  - psychogenic F45.8
- uterus, uterine (contractions) (complicating delivery) O62.4
Hypertrichosis L68.9
- congenital Q84.2
- eyelid H02.869
  - left H02.869
    - lower H02.865
    - upper H02.864
  - right H02.863
    - lower H02.862
    - upper H02.861
- lanuginosa Q84.2
  - acquired L68.1
- localized L68.2
- specified NEC L68.8
Hypertriglyceridemia, essential E78.1

Hypertrophy, hypertrophic
adenofibromatous, prostate — *see* Enlargement, enlarged, prostate
adenoids (infective) J35.2
　with tonsils J35.3
adrenal cortex E27.8
alveolar process or ridge — *see* Anomaly, alveolar
anal papillae K62.89
artery I77.89
　congenital NEC Q27.8
　　digestive system Q27.8
　　lower limb Q27.8
　　specified site NEC Q27.8
　　upper limb Q27.8
auricular — *see* Hypertrophy, cardiac
Bartholin's gland N75.8
bile duct (common) (hepatic) K83.8
bladder (sphincter) (trigone) N32.89
bone M89.30
　carpus M89.34- ☑
　clavicle M89.31- ☑
　femur M89.35- ☑
　fibula M89.36- ☑
　finger M89.34- ☑
　humerus M89.32- ☑
　ilium M89.359
　ischium M89.359
　metacarpus M89.34- ☑
　metatarsus M89.37- ☑
　multiple sites M89.39
　neck M89.38
　radius M89.33- ☑
　rib M89.38
　scapula M89.31- ☑
　skull M89.38
　tarsus M89.37- ☑
　tibia M89.36- ☑
　toe M89.37- ☑
　ulna M89.33- ☑
　vertebra M89.38
brain G93.89
breast N62
　cystic — *see* Mastopathy, cystic
　newborn P83.4
　pubertal, massive N62
　puerperal, postpartum — *see* Disorder, breast, specified type NEC
　senile (parenchymatous) N62
cardiac (chronic) (idiopathic) I51.7
　with rheumatic fever (conditions in I00)
　　active I01.8
　　inactive or quiescent (with chorea) I09.89
　congenital NEC Q24.8
　fatty — *see* Degeneration, myocardial
　hypertensive — *see* Hypertension, heart
　rheumatic (with chorea) I09.89
　　active or acute I01.8
　　　with chorea I02.0
　valve — *see* Endocarditis
cartilage — *see* Disorder, cartilage, specified type NEC
cecum — *see* Megacolon
cervix (uteri) N88.8
　congenital Q51.828
　elongation N88.4
clitoris (cirrhotic) N90.89
　congenital Q52.6
colon (*see also* Megacolon)
　congenital Q43.2
conjunctiva, lymphoid H11.89
corpora cavernosa N48.89
cystic duct K82.8
duodenum K31.89
endometrium (glandular) (*see also* Hyperplasia, endometrial) N85.00
　cervix N88.8
epididymis N50.89
esophageal hiatus (congenital) Q79.1
　with hernia — *see* Hernia, hiatal
eyelid — *see* Disorder, eyelid, specified type NEC
fat pad E65
　knee (infrapatellar) (popliteal) (prepatellar) (retropatellar) M79.4
foot (congenital) Q74.2
frenulum, frenum (tongue) K14.8
　lip K13.0
gallbladder K82.8
gastric mucosa K29.60
　with bleeding K29.61

Hypertrophy, hypertrophic — *continued*
gland, glandular R59.9
　generalized R59.1
　localized R59.0
gum (mucous membrane) K06.1
heart (idiopathic) (*see also* Hypertrophy, cardiac)
　valve (*see also* Endocarditis) I38
hemifacial Q67.4
hepatic — *see* Hypertrophy, liver
hiatus (esophageal) Q79.1
hilus gland R59.0
hymen, congenital Q52.4
ileum K63.89
intestine NEC K63.89
jejunum K63.89
kidney (compensatory) N28.81
　congenital Q63.3
labium (majus) (minus) N90.60
ligament — *see* Disorder, ligament
lingual tonsil (infective) J35.1
　with adenoids J35.3
lip K13.0
　congenital Q18.6
liver R16.0
　acute K76.89
　cirrhotic — *see* Cirrhosis, liver
　congenital Q44.7
　fatty — *see* Fatty, liver
lymph, lymphatic gland R59.9
　generalized R59.1
　localized R59.0
　tuberculous — *see* Tuberculosis, lymph gland
mammary gland — *see* Hypertrophy, breast
Meckel's diverticulum (congenital) Q43.0
　malignant — *see* Table of Neoplasms, small intestine, malignant
median bar — *see* Hyperplasia, prostate
meibomian gland — *see* Chalazion
meniscus, knee, congenital Q74.1
metatarsal head — *see* Hypertrophy, bone, metatarsus
metatarsus — *see* Hypertrophy, bone, metatarsus
mucous membrane
　alveolar ridge K06.2
　gum K06.1
　nose (turbinate) J34.3
muscle M62.89
muscular coat, artery I77.89
myocardium (*see also* Hypertrophy, cardiac)
　idiopathic I42.2
myometrium N85.2
nail L60.2
　congenital Q84.5
nasal J34.89
　alae J34.89
　bone J34.89
　cartilage J34.89
　mucous membrane (septum) J34.3
　sinus J34.89
　turbinate J34.3
nasopharynx, lymphoid (infectional) (tissue) (wall) J35.2
nipple N62
organ or site, congenital NEC — *see* Anomaly, by site
ovary N83.8
palate (hard) M27.8
　soft K13.79
pancreas, congenital Q45.3
parathyroid (gland) E21.0
parotid gland K11.1
penis N48.89
pharyngeal tonsil J35.2
pharynx J39.2
　lymphoid (infectional) (tissue) (wall) J35.2
pituitary (anterior) (fossa) (gland) E23.6
prepuce (congenital) N47.8
　female N90.89
prostate — *see* Enlargement, enlarged, prostate
　congenital Q55.4
pseudomuscular G71.0
pylorus (adult) (muscle) (sphincter) K31.1
　congenital or infantile Q40.0
rectal, rectum (sphincter) K62.89
rhinitis (turbinate) J31.0
salivary gland (any) K11.1
　congenital Q38.4
scaphoid (tarsal) — *see* Hypertrophy, bone, tarsus
scar L91.0
scrotum N50.89

Hypertrophy, hypertrophic — *continued*
seminal vesicle N50.89
sigmoid — *see* Megacolon
skin L91.9
　specified NEC L91.8
spermatic cord N50.89
spleen — *see* Splenomegaly
spondylitis — *see* Spondylosis
stomach K31.89
sublingual gland K11.1
submandibular gland K11.1
suprarenal cortex (gland) E27.8
synovial NEC M67.20
　acromioclavicular M67.21- ☑
　ankle M67.27- ☑
　elbow M67.22- ☑
　foot M67.27- ☑
　hand M67.24- ☑
　hip M67.25- ☑
　knee M67.26- ☑
　multiple sites M67.29
　specified site NEC M67.28
　wrist M67.23- ☑
tendon — *see* Disorder, tendon, specified type NEC
testis N44.8
　congenital Q55.29
thymic, thymus (gland) (congenital) E32.0
thyroid (gland) — *see* Goiter
toe (congenital) Q74.2
　acquired (*see also* Deformity, toe, specified NEC)
tongue K14.8
　congenital Q38.2
　papillae (foliate) K14.3
tonsils (faucial) (infective) (lingual) (lymphoid) J35.1
　with adenoids J35.3
tunica vaginalis N50.89
ureter N28.89
urethra N36.8
uterus N85.2
　neck (with elongation) N88.4
　puerperal O90.89
uvula K13.79
vagina N89.8
vas deferens N50.89
vein I87.8
ventricle, ventricular (heart) (*see also* Hypertrophy, cardiac)
　congenital Q24.8
　in tetralogy of Fallot Q21.3
verumontanum N36.8
vocal cord J38.3
vulva N90.60
　stasis (nonfilarial) N90.69
Hypertropia H50.2- ☑
Hypertyrosinemia E70.21
Hyperuricemia (asymptomatic) E79.0
Hypervalinemia E71.19
Hyperventilation (tetany) R06.4
　hysterical F45.8
　psychogenic F45.8
　syndrome F45.8
Hypervitaminosis (dietary) NEC E67.8
　A E67.0
　　administered as drug (prolonged intake) — *see* Table of Drugs and Chemicals, vitamins, adverse effect
　　overdose or wrong substance given or taken — *see* Table of Drugs and Chemicals, vitamins, poisoning
　B6 E67.2
　D E67.3
　　administered as drug (prolonged intake) — *see* Table of Drugs and Chemicals, vitamins, adverse effect
　　overdose or wrong substance given or taken — *see* Table of Drugs and Chemicals, vitamins, poisoning
　K E67.8
　　administered as drug (prolonged intake) — *see* Table of Drugs and Chemicals, vitamins, adverse effect
　　overdose or wrong substance given or taken — *see* Table of Drugs and Chemicals, vitamins, poisoning
Hypervolemia E87.70
　specified NEC E87.79
Hypesthesia R20.1
　cornea — *see* Anesthesia, cornea

Hyphema H21.0- ☑
  traumatic S05.1- ☑
Hypoacidity, gastric K31.89
  psychogenic F45.8
Hypoadrenalism, hypoadrenia E27.40
  primary E27.1
  tuberculous A18.7
Hypoadrenocorticism E27.40
  pituitary E23.0
  primary E27.1
Hypoalbuminemia E88.09
Hypoaldosteronism E27.40
Hypoalphalipoproteinemia E78.6
Hypobarism T70.29 ☑
Hypobaropathy T70.29 ☑
Hypobetalipoproteinemia (familial) E78.6
Hypocalcemia E83.51
  dietary E58
  neonatal P71.1
    due to cow's milk P71.0
  phosphate-loading (newborn) P71.1
Hypochloremia E87.8
Hypochlorhydria K31.89
  neurotic F45.8
  psychogenic F45.8
Hypochondria, hypochondriac, hypochondriasis
  (reaction) F45.21
  sleep F51.03
Hypochondrogenesis Q77.0
Hypochondroplasia Q77.4
Hypochromasia, blood cells D50.8
Hypodontia — see Anodontia
Hypoeosinophilia D72.89
Hypoesthesia R20.1
Hypofibrinogenemia D68.8
  acquired D65
  congenital (hereditary) D68.2
Hypofunction
  adrenocortical E27.40
    drug-induced E27.3
    postprocedural E89.6
    primary E27.1
  adrenomedullary, postprocedural E89.6
  cerebral R29.818
  corticoadrenal NEC E27.40
  intestinal K59.8
  labyrinth — see subcategory H83.2 ☑
  ovary E28.39
  pituitary (gland) (anterior) E23.0
  testicular E29.1
    postprocedural (postsurgical) (postirradiation) (iatrogenic) E89.5
Hypogalactia O92.4
Hypogammaglobulinemia (see also Agammaglobulinemia) D80.1
  hereditary D80.0
  nonfamilial D80.1
  transient, of infancy D80.7
Hypogenitalism (congenital) — see Hypogonadism
Hypoglossia Q38.3
Hypoglycemia (spontaneous) E16.2
  coma E15
    diabetic — see Diabetes, by type, with hypoglycemia, with coma
  diabetic — see Diabetes, hypoglycemia
  dietary counseling and surveillance Z71.3
  drug-induced E16.0
    with coma (nondiabetic) E15
  due to insulin E16.0
    with coma (nondiabetic) E15
    therapeutic misadventure — see subcategory T38.3 ☑
  functional, nonhyperinsulinemic E16.1
  iatrogenic E16.0
    with coma (nondiabetic) E15
  in infant of diabetic mother P70.1
    gestational diabetes P70.0
  infantile E16.1
  leucine-induced E71.19
  neonatal (transitory) P70.4
    iatrogenic P70.3
  reactive (not drug-induced) E16.1
  transitory neonatal P70.4
Hypogonadism
  female E28.39
  hypogonadotropic E23.0
  male E29.1
  ovarian (primary) E28.39

Hypogonadism — continued
  pituitary E23.0
  testicular (primary) E29.1
Hypohidrosis, hypoidrosis L74.4
Hypoinsulinemia, postprocedural E89.1
Hypokalemia E87.6
Hypoleukocytosis — see Agranulocytosis
Hypolipoproteinemia (alpha) (beta) E78.6
Hypomagnesemia E83.42
  neonatal P71.2
Hypomania, hypomanic reaction F30.8
Hypomenorrhea — see Oligomenorrhea
Hypometabolism R63.8
Hypomotility
  gastrointestinal (tract) K31.89
    psychogenic F45.8
  intestine K59.8
    psychogenic F45.8
  stomach K31.89
    psychogenic F45.8
Hyponasality R49.22
Hyponatremia E87.1
Hypo-osmolality E87.1
Hypo-ovarianism, hypo-ovarism E28.39
Hypoparathyroidism E20.9
  familial E20.8
  idiopathic E20.0
  neonatal, transitory P71.4
  postprocedural E89.2
  specified NEC E20.8
Hypoperfusion (in)
  newborn P96.89
Hypopharyngitis — see Laryngopharyngitis
Hypophoria H50.53
Hypophosphatemia, hypophosphatasia (acquired) (congenital) (renal) E83.39
  familial E83.31
Hypophyseal, hypophysis (see also condition)
  dwarfism E23.0
  gigantism E22.0
Hypopiesis — see Hypotension
Hypopinealism E34.8
Hypopituitarism (juvenile) E23.0
  drug-induced E23.1
  due to
    hypophysectomy E89.3
    radiotherapy E89.3
  iatrogenic NEC E23.1
  postirradiation E89.3
  postpartum O99.285
  postprocedural E89.3
Hypoplasia, hypoplastic
  adrenal (gland), congenital Q89.1
  alimentary tract, congenital Q45.8
    upper Q40.8
  anus, anal (canal) Q42.3
    with fistula Q42.2
  aorta, aortic Q25.42
    ascending, in hypoplastic left heart syndrome Q23.4
    valve Q23.1
      in hypoplastic left heart syndrome Q23.4
  areola, congenital Q83.8
  arm (congenital) — see Defect, reduction, upper limb
  artery (peripheral) Q27.8
    brain (congenital) Q28.3
    coronary Q24.5
    digestive system Q27.8
    lower limb Q27.8
    pulmonary Q25.79
      functional, unilateral J43.0
    retinal (congenital) Q14.1
    specified site NEC Q27.8
    umbilical Q27.0
    upper limb Q27.8
  auditory canal Q17.8
    causing impairment of hearing Q16.9
  biliary duct or passage Q44.5
  bone NOS Q79.9
    face Q75.8
    marrow D61.9
      megakaryocytic D69.49
    skull — see Hypoplasia, skull
  brain Q02
    gyri Q04.3
    part of Q04.3
  breast (areola) N64.82
  bronchus Q32.4

Hypoplasia, hypoplastic — continued
  cardiac Q24.8
  carpus — see Defect, reduction, upper limb, specified type NEC
  cartilage hair Q78.8
  cecum Q42.8
  cementum K00.4
  cephalic Q02
  cerebellum Q04.3
  cervix (uteri), congenital Q51.821
  clavicle (congenital) Q74.0
  coccyx Q76.49
  colon Q42.9
    specified NEC Q42.8
  corpus callosum Q04.0
  cricoid cartilage Q31.2
  digestive organ(s) or tract NEC Q45.8
    upper (congenital) Q40.8
  ear (auricle) (lobe) Q17.2
    middle Q16.4
  enamel of teeth (neonatal) (postnatal) (prenatal) K00.4
  endocrine (gland) NEC Q89.2
  endometrium N85.8
  epididymis (congenital) Q55.4
  epiglottis Q31.2
  erythroid, congenital D61.01
  esophagus (congenital) Q39.8
  eustachian tube Q17.8
  eye Q11.2
  eyelid (congenital) Q10.3
  face Q18.8
    bone(s) Q75.8
  femur (congenital) — see Defect, reduction, lower limb, specified type NEC
  fibula (congenital) — see Defect, reduction, lower limb, specified type NEC
  finger (congenital) — see Defect, reduction, upper limb, specified type NEC
  focal dermal Q82.8
  foot — see Defect, reduction, lower limb, specified type NEC
  gallbladder Q44.0
  genitalia, genital organ(s)
    female, congenital Q52.8
      external Q52.79
      internal NEC Q52.8
    in adiposogenital dystrophy E23.6
  glottis Q31.2
  hair Q84.2
  hand (congenital) — see Defect, reduction, upper limb, specified type NEC
  heart Q24.8
  humerus (congenital) — see Defect, reduction, upper limb, specified type NEC
  intestine (small) Q41.9
    large Q42.9
      specified NEC Q42.8
  jaw M26.09
    alveolar M26.79
    lower M26.04
      alveolar M26.74
    upper M26.02
      alveolar M26.73
  kidney(s) Q60.5
    bilateral Q60.4
    unilateral Q60.3
  labium (majus) (minus), congenital Q52.79
  larynx Q31.2
  left heart syndrome Q23.4
  leg (congenital) — see Defect, reduction, lower limb
  limb Q73.8
    lower (congenital) — see Defect, reduction, lower limb
    upper (congenital) — see Defect, reduction, upper limb
  liver Q44.7
  lung (lobe) (not associated with short gestation) Q33.6
    associated with immaturity, low birth weight, prematurity, or short gestation P28.0
  mammary (areola), congenital Q83.8
  mandible, mandibular M26.04
    alveolar M26.74
    unilateral condylar M27.8
  maxillary M26.02
    alveolar M26.73
  medullary D61.9
  megakaryocytic D69.49

Hypoplasia, hypoplastic — continued
metacarpus — see Defect, reduction, upper limb, specified type NEC
metatarsus — see Defect, reduction, lower limb, specified type NEC
muscle Q79.8
nail(s) Q84.6
nose, nasal Q30.1-
optic nerve H47.03- ☑
osseous meatus (ear) Q17.8
ovary, congenital Q50.39
pancreas Q45.0
parathyroid (gland) Q89.2
parotid gland Q38.4
patella Q74.1
pelvis, pelvic girdle Q74.2
penis (congenital) Q55.62
peripheral vascular system Q27.8
  digestive system Q27.8
  lower limb Q27.8
  specified site NEC Q27.8
  upper limb Q27.8
pituitary (gland) (congenital) Q89.2
pulmonary (not associated with short gestation) Q33.6
  artery, functional J43.0
  associated with short gestation P28.0
radioulnar — see Defect, reduction, upper limb, specified type NEC
radius — see Defect, reduction, upper limb
rectum Q42.1
  with fistula Q42.0
respiratory system NEC Q34.8
rib Q76.6
right heart syndrome Q22.6
sacrum Q76.49
scapula Q74.0
scrotum Q55.1
shoulder girdle Q74.0
skin Q82.8
skull (bone) Q75.8
  with
    anencephaly Q00.0
    encephalocele — see Encephalocele
    hydrocephalus Q03.9
      with spina bifida — see Spina bifida, by site, with hydrocephalus
    microcephaly Q02
spinal (cord) (ventral horn cell) Q06.1
spine Q76.49
sternum Q76.7
tarsus — see Defect, reduction, lower limb, specified type NEC
testis Q55.1
thymic, with immunodeficiency D82.1
thymus (gland) Q89.2
  with immunodeficiency D82.1
thyroid (gland) E03.1
  cartilage Q31.2
tibiofibular (congenital) — see Defect, reduction, lower limb, specified type NEC
toe — see Defect, reduction, lower limb, specified type NEC
tongue Q38.3
Turner's K00.4
ulna (congenital) — see Defect, reduction, upper limb
umbilical artery Q27.0
unilateral condylar M27.8
ureter Q62.8
uterus, congenital Q51.811
vagina Q52.4
vascular NEC peripheral Q27.8
  brain Q28.3
  digestive system Q27.8
  lower limb Q27.8
  specified site NEC Q27.8
  upper limb Q27.8
vein(s) (peripheral) Q27.8
  brain Q28.3
  digestive system Q27.8
  great Q26.8
  lower limb Q27.8
  specified site NEC Q27.8
  upper limb Q27.8
vena cava (inferior) (superior) Q26.8
vertebra Q76.49
vulva, congenital Q52.79
zonule (ciliary) Q12.8
Hypopnea, obstructive sleep apnea G47.33

Hypopotassemia E87.6
Hypoproconvertinemia, congenital (hereditary) D68.2
Hypoproteinemia E77.8
Hypoprothrombinemia (congenital) (hereditary) (idiopathic) D68.2
  acquired D68.4
  newborn, transient P61.6
Hypoptyalism K11.7
Hypopyon (eye) (anterior chamber) — see Iridocyclitis, acute, hypopyon
Hypopyrexia R68.0
Hyporeflexia R29.2
Hyposecretion
  ACTH E23.0
  antidiuretic hormone E23.2
  ovary E28.39
  salivary gland (any) K11.7
  vasopressin E23.2
Hyposegmentation, leukocytic, hereditary D72.0
Hyposiderinemia D50.9
Hypospadias Q54.9
  balanic Q54.0
  coronal Q54.0
  glandular Q54.0
  penile Q54.1
  penoscrotal Q54.2
  perineal Q54.3
  specified NEC Q54.8
Hypospermatogenesis — see Oligospermia
Hyposplenism D73.0
Hypostasis pulmonary, passive — see Edema, lung
Hypostatic — see condition
Hyposthenuria N28.89
Hypotension (arterial) (constitutional) I95.9
  chronic I95.89
  drug-induced I95.2
  due to (of) hemodialysis I95.3
  iatrogenic I95.89
  idiopathic (permanent) I95.0
  intracranial, following ventricular shunting (ventriculostomy) G97.2
  intra-dialytic I95.3
  maternal, syndrome (following labor and delivery) O26.5- ☑
  neurogenic, orthostatic G90.3
  orthostatic (chronic) I95.1
    due to drugs I95.2
    neurogenic G90.3
  postoperative I95.81
  postural I95.1
  specified NEC I95.89
Hypothermia (accidental) T68 ☑
  due to anesthesia, anesthetic T88.51 ☑
  low environmental temperature T68 ☑
  neonatal P80.9
    environmental (mild) NEC P80.8
    mild P80.8
    severe (chronic) (cold injury syndrome) P80.0
    specified NEC P80.8
  not associated with low environmental temperature R68.0
Hypothyroidism (acquired) E03.9
  autoimmune — see Thyroiditis, autoimmune
  congenital (without goiter) E03.1
    with goiter (diffuse) E03.0
  due to
    exogenous substance NEC E03.2
    iodine-deficiency, acquired E01.8
      subclinical E02
    irradiation therapy E89.0
    medicament NEC E03.2
    P-aminosalicylic acid (PAS) E03.2
    phenylbutazone E03.2
    resorcinol E03.2
    sulfonamide E03.2
    surgery E89.0
    thiourea group drugs E03.2
  iatrogenic NEC E03.2
  iodine-deficiency (acquired) E01.8
    congenital — see Syndrome, iodine- deficiency, congenital
    subclinical E02
  neonatal, transitory P72.2
  postinfectious E03.3
  postirradiation E89.0
  postprocedural E89.0
  postsurgical E89.0
  specified NEC E03.8

Hypothyroidism — continued
  subclinical, iodine-deficiency related E02
Hypotonia, hypotonicity, hypotony
  bladder N31.2
  congenital (benign) P94.2
  eye — see Disorder, globe, hypotony
Hypotrichosis — see Alopecia
Hypotropia H50.2- ☑
Hypoventilation R06.89
  congenital central alveolar G47.35
  sleep related
    idiopathic nonobstructive alveolar G47.34
    in conditions classified elsewhere G47.36
Hypovitaminosis — see Deficiency, vitamin
Hypovolemia E86.1
  surgical shock T81.19 ☑
  traumatic (shock) T79.4 ☑
Hypoxemia R09.02
  newborn P84
  sleep related, in conditions classified elsewhere G47.36
Hypoxia (see also Anoxia) R09.02
  cerebral, during a procedure NEC G97.81
    postprocedural NEC G97.82
  intrauterine P84
  myocardial — see Insufficiency, coronary
  newborn P84
  sleep-related G47.34
Hypsarrhythmia — see Epilepsy, generalized, specified NEC
Hysteralgia, pregnant uterus O26.89- ☑
Hysteria, hysterical (conversion) (dissociative state) F44.9
  anxiety F41.8
  convulsions F44.5
  psychosis, acute F44.9
Hysteroepilepsy F44.5

I

IBDU (colonic inflammatory bowel dissease unclassified) K52.3
Ichthyoparasitism due to Vandellia cirrhosa B88.8
Ichthyosis (congenital) Q80.9
  acquired L85.0
  fetalis Q80.4
  hystrix Q80.8
  lamellar Q80.2
  lingual K13.29
  palmaris and plantaris Q82.8
  simplex Q80.0
  vera Q80.8
  vulgaris Q80.0
  X-linked Q80.1
Ichthyotoxism — see Poisoning, fish
  bacterial — see Intoxication, foodborne
Icteroanemia, hemolytic (acquired) D59.9
  congenital — see Spherocytosis
Icterus (see also Jaundice)
  conjunctiva R17
  gravis, newborn P55.0
  hematogenous (acquired) D59.9
  hemolytic (acquired) D59.9
    congenital — see Spherocytosis
  hemorrhagic (acute) (leptospiral) (spirochetal) A27.0
    newborn P53
  infectious B15.9
    with hepatic coma B15.0
    leptospiral A27.0
    spirochetal A27.0
  neonatorum — see Jaundice, newborn
  newborn P59.9
  spirochetal A27.0
Ictus solaris, solis T67.0 ☑
Id reaction (due to bacteria) L30.2
Ideation
  homicidal R45.850
  suicidal R45.851
Identity disorder (child) F64.9
  gender role F64.2
  psychosexual F64.2
Idioglossia F80.0
Idiopathic — see condition
Idiot, idiocy (congenital) F73
  amaurotic (Bielschowsky(-Jansky)) (family) (infantile (late)) (juvenile (late)) (Vogt-Spielmeyer) E75.4
  microcephalic Q02
IgE asthma J45.909

IIAC (idiopathic infantile arterial calcification) Q28.8
Ileitis (chronic) (noninfectious) (*see also* Enteritis) K52.9
  backwash — *see* Pancolitis, ulcerative (chronic)
  infectious A09
  regional (ulcerative) — *see* Enteritis, regional, small
    intestine
  segmental — *see* Enteritis, regional
  terminal (ulcerative) — *see* Enteritis, regional, small
    intestine
Ileocolitis (*see also* Enteritis) K52.9
  infectious A09
  regional — *see* Enteritis, regional
  ulcerative K51.0- ☑
Ileostomy
  attention to Z43.2
  malfunctioning K94.13
  status Z93.2
    with complication — *see* Complications, enterostomy
Ileotyphus — *see* Typhoid
Ileum — *see* condition
Ileus (bowel) (colon) (inhibitory) (intestine) K56.7
  adynamic K56.0
  due to gallstone (in intestine) K56.3
  duodenal (chronic) K31.5
  gallstone K56.3
  mechanical NEC (*see also* Obstruction, intestine, specified NEC) K56.699
  meconium P76.0
    in cystic fibrosis E84.11
    meaning meconium plug (without cystic fibrosis) P76.0
  myxedema K59.8
  neurogenic K56.0
    Hirschsprung's disease or megacolon Q43.1
  newborn
    due to meconium P76.0
      in cystic fibrosis E84.11
      meaning meconium plug (without cystic fibrosis) P76.0
    transitory P76.1
  obstructive (*see also* Obstruction, intestine, specified NEC) K56.699
  paralytic K56.0
  postoperative K91.89
Iliac — *see* condition
Iliotibial band syndrome M76.3- ☑
Illiteracy Z55.0
Illness (*see also* Disease) R69
  manic-depressive — *see* Disorder, bipolar
Imbalance R26.89
  autonomic G90.8
  constituents of food intake E63.1
  electrolyte E87.8
    with
      abortion — *see* Abortion by type, complicated by, electrolyte imbalance
      molar pregnancy O08.5
    due to hyperemesis gravidarum O21.1
    following ectopic or molar pregnancy O08.5
    neonatal, transitory NEC P74.4
      potassium P74.3
      sodium P74.2
  endocrine E34.9
  eye muscle NOS H50.9
  hormone E34.9
  hysterical F44.4
  labyrinth — *see* subcategory H83.2 ☑
  posture R29.3
  protein-energy — *see* Malnutrition
  sympathetic G90.8
Imbecile, imbecility (I.Q. 35-49) F71
Imbedding, intrauterine device T83.39 ☑
Imbibition, cholesterol (gallbladder) K82.4
Imbrication, teeth,, fully erupted M26.30
Imerslund (-Gräsbeck) **syndrome** D51.1
Immature (*see also* Immaturity)
  birth (less than 37 completed weeks) — *see* Preterm, newborn
    extremely (less than 28 completed weeks) — *see* Immaturity, extreme
  personality F60.89
Immaturity (less than 37 completed weeks) (*see also* Preterm, newborn)
  extreme of newborn (less than 28 completed weeks of gestation) (less than 196 completed days of gestation) (unspecified weeks of gestation) P07.20

Immaturity — *continued*
  extreme of newborn — *continued*
    gestational age
      less than 23 completed weeks P07.21
      23 completed weeks (23 weeks, 0 days through 23 weeks, 6 days) P07.22
      24 completed weeks (24 weeks, 0 days through 24 weeks, 6 days) P07.23
      25 completed weeks (25 weeks, 0 days through 25 weeks, 6 days) P07.24
      26 completed weeks (26 weeks, 0 days through 26 weeks, 6 days) P07.25
      27 completed weeks (27 weeks, 0 days through 27 weeks, 6 days) P07.26
  fetus or infant light-for-dates — *see* Light-for-dates
  lung, newborn P28.0
  organ or site NEC — *see* Hypoplasia
  pulmonary, newborn P28.0
  reaction F60.89
  sexual (female) (male), after puberty E30.0
Immersion T75.1 ☑
  foot T69.02- ☑
  hand T69.01- ☑
Immobile, immobility
  complete, due to severe physical disability or frailty R53.2
  intestine K59.8
  syndrome (paraplegic) M62.3
Immune reconstitution (inflammatory) syndrome [IRIS] D89.3
Immunization (*see also* Vaccination)
  ABO — *see* Incompatibility, ABO
    in newborn P55.1
  complication — *see* Complications, vaccination
  encounter for Z23
  not done (not carried out) Z28.9
    because (of)
      acute illness of patient Z28.01
      allergy to vaccine (or component) Z28.04
      caregiver refusal Z28.82
      chronic illness of patient Z28.02
      contraindication NEC Z28.09
      group pressure Z28.1
      guardian refusal Z28.82
      immune compromised state of patient Z28.03
      parent refusal Z28.82
      patient had disease being vaccinated against Z28.81
      patient refusal Z28.21
      patient's belief Z28.1
      religious beliefs of patient Z28.1
      specified reason NEC Z28.89
        of patient Z28.29
      unspecified patient reason Z28.20
  Rh factor
    affecting management of pregnancy NEC O36.09- ☑
      anti-D antibody O36.01- ☑
    from transfusion — *see* Complication(s), transfusion, incompatibility reaction, Rh (factor)
Immunocytoma C83.0- ☑
Immunodeficiency D84.9
  with
    adenosine-deaminase deficiency D81.3
    antibody defects D80.9
      specified type NEC D80.8
    hyperimmunoglobulinemia D80.6
    increased immunoglobulin M (IgM) D80.5
    major defect D82.9
      specified type NEC D82.8
    partial albinism D82.8
    short-limbed stature D82.2
    thrombocytopenia and eczema D82.0
  antibody with
    hyperimmunoglobulinemia D80.6
    near-normal immunoglobulins D80.6
  autosomal recessive, Swiss type D80.0
  combined D81.9
    biotin-dependent carboxylase D81.819
      biotinidase D81.810
      holocarboxylase synthetase D81.818
      specified type NEC D81.818
    severe (SCID) D81.9
      with
        low or normal B-cell numbers D81.2
        low T- and B-cell numbers D81.1
        reticular dysgenesis D81.0
    specified type NEC D81.89

Immunodeficiency — *continued*
  common variable D83.9
    with
      abnormalities of B-cell numbers and function D83.0
      autoantibodies to B- or T-cells D83.2
      immunoregulatory T-cell disorders D83.1
    specified type NEC D83.8
  following hereditary defective response to Epstein-Barr virus (EBV) D82.3
  selective, immunoglobulin
    A (IgA) D80.2
    G (IgG) (subclasses) D80.3
    M (IgM) D80.4
  severe combined (SCID) D81.9
  specified type NEC D84.8
  X-linked, with increased IgM D80.5
Immunotherapy (encounter for)
  antineoplastic Z51.12
Impaction, impacted
  bowel, colon, rectum (*see also* Impaction, fecal) K56.49
    by gallstone K56.3
  calculus — *see* Calculus
  cerumen (ear) (external) H61.2- ☑
  cuspid — *see* Impaction, tooth
  dental (same or adjacent tooth) K01.1
  fecal, feces K56.41
  fracture — *see* Fracture, by site
  gallbladder — *see* Calculus, gallbladder
  gallstone(s) — *see* Calculus, gallbladder
    bile duct (common) (hepatic) — *see* Calculus, bile duct
    cystic duct — *see* Calculus, gallbladder
    in intestine, with obstruction (any part) K56.3
  intestine (calculous) NEC (*see also* Impaction, fecal) K56.49
    gallstone, with ileus K56.3
  intrauterine device (IUD) T83.39 ☑
  molar — *see* Impaction, tooth
  shoulder, causing obstructed labor O66.0
  tooth, teeth K01.1
  turbinate J34.89
Impaired, impairment (function)
  auditory discrimination — *see* Abnormal, auditory perception
  cognitive, mild, so stated G31.84
  dual sensory Z73.82
  fasting glucose R73.01
  glucose tolerance (oral) R73.02
  hearing — *see* Deafness
  heart — *see* Disease, heart
  kidney N28.9
    disorder resulting from N25.9
    specified NEC N25.89
  liver K72.90
    with coma K72.91
  mastication K08.89
  mild cognitive, so stated G31.84
  mobility
    ear ossicles — *see* Ankylosis, ear ossicles
    requiring care provider Z74.09
  myocardium, myocardial — *see* Insufficiency, myocardial
  rectal sphincter R19.8
  renal (acute) (chronic) N28.9
    disorder resulting from N25.9
    specified NEC N25.89
  vision NEC H54.7
    both eyes H54.3
Impediment, speech R47.9
  psychogenic (childhood) F98.8
  slurring R47.81
  specified NEC R47.89
Impending
  coronary syndrome I20.0
  delirium tremens F10.239
  myocardial infarction I20.0
Imperception auditory (acquired) (*see also* Deafness)
  congenital H93.25
Imperfect
  aeration, lung (newborn) NEC — *see* Atelectasis
  closure (congenital)
    alimentary tract NEC Q45.8
      lower Q43.8
      upper Q40.8
    atrioventricular ostium Q21.2
    atrium (secundum) Q21.1
    branchial cleft NOS Q18.2

▽ Subterms under main terms may continue to next column or page   ☑ Additional Character Required — Refer to the Tabular List for Character Selection   179

IIAC — Imperfect

Imperfect — *continued*
closure — *continued*
  branchial cleft — *continued*
    cyst Q18.0
    fistula Q18.0
    sinus Q18.0
  choroid Q14.3
  cricoid cartilage Q31.8
  cusps, heart valve NEC Q24.8
    pulmonary Q22.3
  ductus
    arteriosus Q25.0
    Botalli Q25.0
  ear drum (causing impairment of hearing) Q16.4
  esophagus with communication to bronchus or trachea Q39.1
  eyelid Q10.3
  foramen
    botalli Q21.1
    ovale Q21.1
  genitalia, genital organ(s) or system
    female Q52.8
      external Q52.79
      internal NEC Q52.8
    male Q55.8
  glottis Q31.8
  interatrial ostium or septum Q21.1
  interauricular ostium or septum Q21.1
  interventricular ostium or septum Q21.0
  larynx Q31.8
  lip — *see* Cleft, lip
  nasal septum Q30.3
  nose Q30.2
  omphalomesenteric duct Q43.0
  optic nerve entry Q14.2
  organ or site not listed — *see* Anomaly, by site
  ostium
    interatrial Q21.1
    interauricular Q21.1
    interventricular Q21.0
  palate — *see* Cleft, palate
  preauricular sinus Q18.1
  retina Q14.1
  roof of orbit Q75.8
  sclera Q13.5
  septum
    aorticopulmonary Q21.4
    atrial (secundum) Q21.1
    between aorta and pulmonary artery Q21.4
    heart Q21.9
    interatrial (secundum) Q21.1
    interauricular (secundum) Q21.1
    interventricular Q21.0
      in tetralogy of Fallot Q21.3
    nasal Q30.3
    ventricular Q21.0
      with pulmonary stenosis or atresia, dextraposition of aorta, and hypertrophy of right ventricle Q21.3
      in tetralogy of Fallot Q21.3
  skull Q75.0
    with
      anencephaly Q00.0
      encephalocele — *see* Encephalocele
      hydrocephalus Q03.9
        with spina bifida — *see* Spina bifida, by site, with hydrocephalus
      microcephaly Q02
  spine (with meningocele) — *see* Spina bifida
  trachea Q32.1
  tympanic membrane (causing impairment of hearing) Q16.4
  uterus Q51.818
  vitelline duct Q43.0
 erection — *see* Dysfunction, sexual, male, erectile
 fusion — *see* Imperfect, closure
 inflation, lung (newborn) — *see* Atelectasis
 posture R29.3
 rotation, intestine Q43.3
 septum, ventricular Q21.0
Imperfectly descended testis — *see* Cryptorchid
Imperforate (congenital) (*see also* Atresia)
 anus Q42.3
  with fistula Q42.2
 cervix (uteri) Q51.828
 esophagus Q39.0
  with tracheoesophageal fistula Q39.1
 hymen Q52.3

Imperforate — *continued*
 jejunum Q41.1
 pharynx Q38.8
 rectum Q42.1
  with fistula Q42.0
 urethra Q64.39
 vagina Q52.4
Impervious (congenital) (*see also* Atresia)
 anus Q42.3
  with fistula Q42.2
 bile duct Q44.2
 esophagus Q39.0
  with tracheoesophageal fistula Q39.1
 intestine (small) Q41.9
  large Q42.9
    specified NEC Q42.8
 rectum Q42.1
  with fistula Q42.0
 ureter — *see* Atresia, ureter
 urethra Q64.39
Impetiginization of dermatoses L01.1
Impetigo (any organism) (any site) (circinate) (contagiosa) (simplex) (vulgaris) L01.00
 Bockhart's L01.02
 bullous, bullosa L01.03
 external ear L01.00 [H62.40]
 follicularis L01.02
 furfuracea L30.5
 herpetiformis L40.1
  nonobstetrical L40.1
 neonatorum L01.03
 nonbullous L01.01
 specified type NEC L01.09
 ulcerative L01.09
Impingement (on teeth)
 soft tissue
  anterior M26.81
  posterior M26.82
Implant, endometrial N80.9
Implantation
 anomalous — *see* Anomaly, by site
  ureter Q62.63
 cyst
  external area or site (skin) NEC L72.0
  iris — *see* Cyst, iris, implantation
  vagina N89.8
  vulva N90.7
 dermoid (cyst) — *see* Implantation, cyst
Impotence (sexual) N52.9
 counseling Z70.1
 organic origin (*see also* Dysfunction, sexual, male, erectile) N52.9
 psychogenic F52.21
Impression, basilar Q75.8
Imprisonment, anxiety concerning Z65.1
Improper care (child) (newborn) — *see* Maltreatment
Improperly tied umbilical cord (causing hemorrhage) P51.8
Impulsiveness (impulsive) R45.87
Inability to swallow — *see* Aphagia
Inaccessible, inaccessibility
 health care NEC Z75.3
  due to
    waiting period Z75.2
      for admission to facility elsewhere Z75.1
  other helping agencies Z75.4
Inactive — *see* condition
Inadequate, inadequacy
 aesthetics of dental restoration K08.56
 biologic, constitutional, functional, or social F60.7
 development
  child R62.50
  genitalia
    after puberty NEC E30.0
    congenital
      female Q52.8
        external Q52.79
        internal Q52.8
      male Q55.8
  lungs Q33.6
    associated with short gestation P28.0
  organ or site not listed — *see* Anomaly, by site
 diet (causing nutritional deficiency) E63.9
 eating habits Z72.4
 environment, household Z59.1
 family support Z63.8
 food (supply) NEC Z59.4
  hunger effects T73.0 ☑

Inadequate, inadequacy — *continued*
 functional F60.7
 household care, due to
  family member
    handicapped or ill Z74.2
    on vacation Z75.5
    temporarily away from home Z74.2
  technical defects in home Z59.1
  temporary absence from home of person rendering care Z74.2
 housing (heating) (space) Z59.1
 income (financial) Z59.6
 intrafamilial communication Z63.8
 material resources Z59.9
 mental — *see* Disability, intellectual
 parental supervision or control of child Z62.0
 personality F60.7
 pulmonary
  function R06.89
    newborn P28.5
  ventilation, newborn P28.5
 sample of cytologic smear
  anus R85.615
  cervix R87.615
  vagina R87.625
 social F60.7
  insurance Z59.7
  skills NEC Z73.4
 supervision of child by parent Z62.0
 teaching affecting education Z55.8
 welfare support Z59.7
Inanition R64
 with edema — *see* Malnutrition, severe
 due to
  deprivation of food T73.0 ☑
  malnutrition — *see* Malnutrition
 fever R50.9
Inappropriate
 change in quantitative human chorionic gonadotropin (hCG) in early pregnancy O02.81
 diet or eating habits Z72.4
 level of quantitative human chorionic gonadotropin (hCG) for gestational age in early pregnancy O02.81
 secretion
  antidiuretic hormone (ADH) (excessive) E22.2
    deficiency E23.2
  pituitary (posterior) E22.2
Inattention at or after birth — *see* Neglect
Incarceration, incarcerated
 enterocele K46.0
  gangrenous K46.1
 epiplocele K46.0
  gangrenous K46.1
 exomphalos K42.0
  gangrenous K42.1
 hernia (*see also* Hernia, by site, with obstruction)
  with gangrene — *see* Hernia, by site, with gangrene
 iris, in wound — *see* Injury, eye, laceration, with prolapse
 lens, in wound — *see* Injury, eye, laceration, with prolapse
 omphalocele K42.0
 prison, anxiety concerning Z65.1
 rupture — *see* Hernia, by site
 sarcoepiplocele K46.0
  gangrenous K46.1
 sarcoepiplomphalocele K42.0
  with gangrene K42.1
 uterus N85.8
  gravid O34.51- ☑
    causing obstructed labor O65.5
Incised wound
 external — *see* Laceration
 internal organs — *see* Injury, by site
Incision, incisional
 hernia K43.2
  with
    gangrene (and obstruction) K43.1
    obstruction K43.0
  surgical, complication — *see* Complications, surgical procedure
 traumatic
  external — *see* Laceration
  internal organs — *see* Injury, by site
Inclusion
 azurophilic leukocytic D72.0

☑ **Additional Character Required — Refer to the Tabular List for Character Selection**   ▥ **Subterms under main terms may continue to next column or page**

Inclusion — *continued*
  blennorrhea (neonatal) (newborn) P39.1
  gallbladder in liver (congenital) Q44.1
Incompatibility
  ABO
    affecting management of pregnancy O36.11- ☑
      anti-A sensitization O36.11- ☑
      anti-B sensitization O36.19- ☑
      specified NEC O36.19- ☑
    infusion or transfusion reaction — *see* Complication(s), transfusion, incompatibility reaction, ABO
    newborn P55.1
  blood (group) (Duffy) (K(ell)) (Kidd) (Lewis) (M) (S) NEC
    affecting management of pregnancy O36.11- ☑
      anti-A sensitization O36.11- ☑
      anti-B sensitization O36.19- ☑
    infusion or transfusion reaction T80.89 ☑
    newborn P55.8
  divorce or estrangement Z63.5
  Rh (blood group) (factor) Z31.82
    affecting management of pregnancy NEC O36.09- ☑
      anti-D antibody O36.01- ☑
    infusion or transfusion reaction — *see* Complication(s), transfusion, incompatibility reaction, Rh (factor)
    newborn P55.0
  rhesus — *see* Incompatibility, Rh
Incompetency, incompetent, incompetence
  annular
    aortic (valve) — *see* Insufficiency, aortic
    mitral (valve) I34.0
    pulmonary valve (heart) I37.1
  aortic (valve) — *see* Insufficiency, aortic
  cardiac valve — *see* Endocarditis
  cervix, cervical (os) N88.3
    in pregnancy O34.3- ☑
  chronotropic I45.89
    with
      autonomic dysfunction G90.8
      ischemic heart disease I25.89
      left ventricular dysfunction I51.89
      sinus node dysfunction I49.8
  esophagogastric (junction) (sphincter) K22.0
  mitral (valve) — *see* Insufficiency, mitral
  pelvic fundus N81.89
  pubocervical tissue N81.82
  pulmonary valve (heart) I37.1
    congenital Q22.3
  rectovaginal tissue N81.83
  tricuspid (annular) (valve) — *see* Insufficiency, tricuspid
  valvular — *see* Endocarditis
    congenital Q24.8
  vein, venous (saphenous) (varicose) — *see* Varix, leg
Incomplete (*see also* condition)
  bladder, emptying R33.9
  defecation R15.0
  expansion lungs (newborn) NEC — *see* Atelectasis
  rotation, intestine Q43.3
Inconclusive
  diagnostic imaging due to excess body fat of patient R93.9
  findings on diagnostic imaging of breast NEC R92.8
  mammogram (due to dense breasts) R92.2
Incontinence R32
  anal sphincter R15.9
  coital N39.491
  feces R15.9
    nonorganic origin F98.1
  insensible (urinary) N39.42
  overflow N39.490
  postural (urinary) N39.492
  psychogenic F45.8
  rectal R15.9
  reflex N39.498
  stress (female) (male) N39.3
    and urge N39.46
  urethral sphincter R32
  urge N39.41
    and stress (female) (male) N39.46
  urine (urinary) R32
    continuous N39.45
    due to cognitive impairment, or severe physical disability or immobility R39.81
    functional R39.81
    insensible N39.42
    mixed (stress and urge) N39.46

Incontinence — *continued*
  urine — *continued*
    nocturnal N39.44
    nonorganic origin F98.0
    overflow N39.490
    post dribbling N39.43
    postural N39.492
    reflex N39.498
    specified NEC N39.498
    stress (female) (male) N39.3
      and urge N39.46
    total N39.498
    unaware N39.42
    urge N39.41
      and stress (female) (male) N39.46
Incontinentia pigmenti Q82.3
Incoordinate, incoordination
  esophageal-pharyngeal (newborn) — *see* Dysphagia
  muscular R27.8
  uterus (action) (contractions) (complicating delivery) O62.4
Increase, increased
  abnormal, in development R63.8
  androgens (ovarian) E28.1
  anticoagulants (antithrombin) (anti-VIIIa) (anti-IXa) (anti-Xa) (anti-XIa) — *see* Circulating anticoagulants
  cold sense R20.8
  estrogen E28.0
  function
    adrenal
      cortex — *see* Cushing's, syndrome
      medulla E27.5
    pituitary (gland) (anterior) (lobe) E22.9
      posterior E22.2
  heat sense R20.8
  intracranial pressure (benign) G93.2
  permeability, capillaries I78.8
  pressure, intracranial G93.2
  secretion
    gastrin E16.4
    glucagon E16.3
    pancreas, endocrine E16.9
      growth hormone-releasing hormone E16.8
      pancreatic polypeptide E16.8
      somatostatin E16.8
      vasoactive-intestinal polypeptide E16.8
  sphericity, lens Q12.4
  splenic activity D73.1
  venous pressure I87.8
    portal K76.6
Increta placenta O43.22- ☑
Incrustation, cornea, foreign body (lead)(zinc) — *see* Foreign body, cornea
Incyclophoria H50.54
Incyclotropia — *see* Cyclotropia
Indeterminate sex Q56.4
India rubber skin Q82.8
Indigestion (acid) (bilious) (functional) K30
  catarrhal K31.89
  due to decomposed food NOS A05.9
  nervous F45.8
  psychogenic F45.8
Indirect — *see* condition
Induratio penis plastica N48.6
Induration, indurated
  brain G93.89
  breast (fibrous) N64.51
    puerperal, postpartum O92.29
  broad ligament N83.8
  chancre
    anus A51.1
    congenital A50.07
    extragenital NEC A51.2
  corpora cavernosa (penis) (plastic) N48.6
  liver (chronic) K76.89
  lung (black) (chronic) (fibroid) (*see also* Fibrosis, lung) J84.10
    essential brown J84.03
  penile (plastic) N48.6
  phlebitic — *see* Phlebitis
  skin R23.4
Inebriety (without dependence) — *see* Alcohol, intoxication
Inefficiency, kidney N28.9
Inelasticity, skin R23.4
Inequality, leg (length) (acquired) (*see also* Deformity, limb, unequal length)
  congenital — *see* Defect, reduction, lower limb

Inequality, leg — *continued*
  lower leg — *see* Deformity, limb, unequal length
Inertia
  bladder (neurogenic) N31.2
  stomach K31.89
    psychogenic F45.8
  uterus, uterine during labor O62.2
    during latent phase of labor O62.0
    primary O62.0
    secondary O62.1
  vesical (neurogenic) N31.2
Infancy, infantile, infantilism (*see also* condition)
  celiac K90.0
  genitalia, genitals (after puberty) E30.0
  Herter's (nontropical sprue) K90.0
  intestinal K90.0
  Lorain E23.0
  pancreatic K86.89
  pelvis M95.5
    with disproportion (fetopelvic) O33.1
      causing obstructed labor O65.1
  pituitary E23.0
  renal N25.0
  uterus — *see* Infantile, genitalia
Infant(s) (*see also* Infancy)
  excessive crying R68.11
  irritable child R68.12
  lack of care — *see* Neglect
  liveborn (singleton) Z38.2
    born in hospital Z38.00
      by cesarean Z38.01
    born outside hospital Z38.1
    multiple NEC Z38.8
      born in hospital Z38.68
        by cesarean Z38.69
      born outside hospital Z38.7
    quadruplet Z38.8
      born in hospital Z38.63
        by cesarean Z38.64
      born outside hospital Z38.7
    quintuplet Z38.8
      born in hospital Z38.65
        by cesarean Z38.66
      born outside hospital Z38.7
    triplet Z38.8
      born in hospital Z38.61
        by cesarean Z38.62
      born outside hospital Z38.7
    twin Z38.5
      born in hospital Z38.30
        by cesarean Z38.31
      born outside hospital Z38.4
  of diabetic mother (syndrome of) P70.1
    gestational diabetes P70.0
Infantile (*see also* condition)
  genitalia, genitals E30.0
  os, uterine E30.0
  penis E30.0
  testis E29.1
  uterus E30.0
Infantilism — *see* Infancy
Infarct, infarction
  adrenal (capsule) (gland) E27.49
  appendices epiploicae (*see also* Infarct, intestine) K55.069
  bowel (*see also* Infarct, intestine) K55.069
  brain (stem) — *see* Infarct, cerebral
  breast N64.89
  brewer's (kidney) N28.0
  cardiac — *see* Infarct, myocardium
  cerebellar — *see* Infarct, cerebral
  cerebral (*see also* Occlusion, artery cerebral or precerebral, with infarction) I63.9
    aborted I63.9
    cortical I63.9
    due to
      cerebral venous thrombosis, nonpyogenic I63.6
      embolism
        cerebral arteries I63.4- ☑
        precerebral arteries I63.1- ☑
      occlusion NEC
        cerebral arteries I63.5- ☑
        precerebral arteries I63.2- ☑
      stenosis NEC
        cerebral arteries I63.5- ☑
        precerebral arteries I63.2- ☑

Infarct, infarction — *continued*
cerebral (*see also* Occlusion, artery cerebral or precerebral, with infarction) — *continued*
due to — *continued*
thrombosis
cerebral artery I63.3- ☑
precerebral artery I63.0- ☑
intraoperative
during cardiac surgery I97.810
during other surgery I97.811
postprocedural
following cardiac surgery I97.820
following other surgery I97.821
specified NEC I63.8
colon (acute) (agnogenic) (embolic) (hemorrhagic)
(nonocclusive) (nonthrombotic) (occlusive)
(segmental) (thrombotic) (with gangrene) (*see
also* Infarct, intestine) K55.049
coronary artery — *see* Infarct, myocardium
embolic — *see* Embolism
fallopian tube N83.8
gallbladder K82.8
heart — *see* Infarct, myocardium
hepatic K76.3
hypophysis (anterior lobe) E23.6
impending (myocardium) I20.0
intestine (acute) (agnogenic) (embolic) (hemorrhagic)
(nonocclusive) (nonthrombotic) (occlusive)
(thrombotic) (with gangrene) K55.069
diffuse K55.062
focal K55.061
large K55.049
diffuse K55.042
focal K55.041
small K55.029
diffuse K55.022
focal K55.021
kidney N28.0
liver K76.3
lung (embolic) (thrombotic) — *see* Embolism, pulmonary
lymph node I89.8
mesentery, mesenteric (embolic) (thrombotic) (with
gangrene) (*see also* Infarct, intestine) K55.069
muscle (ischemic) M62.20
ankle M62.27- ☑
foot M62.27- ☑
forearm M62.23- ☑
hand M62.24- ☑
lower leg M62.26- ☑
pelvic region M62.25- ☑
shoulder region M62.21- ☑
specified site NEC M62.28
thigh M62.25- ☑
upper arm M62.22- ☑
myocardium, myocardial (acute) (with stated duration
of 4 weeks or less) I21.9
associated with revascularization procedure I21.A9
diagnosed on ECG, but presenting no symptoms
I25.2
due to
demand ischemia I21.A1
ischemic imbalance I21.A1
healed or old I25.2
intraoperative (*see also* Infarct, myocardium, associated with revascularization procedure)
during cardiac surgery I97.790
during other surgery I97.791
non-Q wave I21.4
non-ST elevation (NSTEMI) I21.4
subsequent I22.2
nontransmural I21.4
past (diagnosed on ECG or other investigation, but
currently presenting no symptoms) I25.2
postprocedural (*see also* Infarct, myocardium, associated with revascularization procedure)
following cardiac surgery (*see also* Infarct, myocardium, type 4 or type 5) I97.190
following other surgery I97.191
Q wave (see also, Infarct, myocardium, by site) I21.3
secondary to
demand ischemia I21.A1
ischemic imbalance I21.A1
ST elevation (STEMI) I21.3
anterior (anteroapical) (anterolateral) (anteroseptal) (Q wave) (wall) I21.09
subsequent I22.0

Infarct, infarction — *continued*
myocardium, myocardial — *continued*
ST elevation — *continued*
inferior (diaphragmatic) (inferolateral) (inferoposterior) (wall) NEC I21.19
subsequent I22.1
inferoposterior transmural (Q wave) I21.11
involving
coronary artery of anterior wall NEC I21.09
coronary artery of inferior wall NEC I21.19
diagonal coronary artery I21.02
left anterior descending coronary artery
I21.02
left circumflex coronary artery I21.21
left main coronary artery I21.01
oblique marginal coronary artery I21.21
right coronary artery I21.11
lateral (apical-lateral) (basal-lateral) (high)
I21.29
subsequent I22.8
posterior (posterobasal) (posterolateral) (posteroseptal) (true) I21.29
subsequent I22.8
septal I21.29
subsequent I22.8
specified NEC I21.29
subsequent I22.8
subsequent I22.9
subsequent (recurrent) (reinfarction) I22.9
anterior (anteroapical) (anterolateral) (anteroseptal) (wall) I22.0
diaphragmatic (wall) I22.1
inferior (diaphragmatic) (inferolateral) (inferoposterior) (wall) I22.1
lateral (apical-lateral) (basal-lateral) (high) I22.8
non-ST elevation (NSTEMI) I22.2
posterior (posterobasal) (posterolateral) (posteroseptal) (true) I22.8
septal I22.8
specified NEC I22.8
ST elevation I22.9
anterior (anteroapical) (anterolateral) (anteroseptal) (wall) I22.0
inferior (diaphragmatic) (inferolateral) (inferoposterior) (wall) I22.1
specified NEC I22.8
subendocardial I22.2
transmural I22.9
anterior (anteroapical) (anterolateral) (anteroseptal) (wall) I22.0
diaphragmatic (wall) I22.1
inferior (diaphragmatic) (inferolateral) (inferoposterior) (wall) I22.1
lateral (apical-lateral) (basal-lateral) (high)
I22.8
posterior (posterobasal) (posterolateral)
(posteroseptal) (true) I22.8
specified NEC I22.8
type 1 (*see also* Infarction, myocardial, subsequent, by site, or by ST elevation or non-
ST elevation) I22.9
type 2 I21.A1
type 3 I21.A9
type 4 I21.A9
type 5 I21.A9
syphilitic A52.06
transmural I21.9
anterior (anteroapical) (anterolateral) (anteroseptal) (Q wave) (wall) NEC I21.09
inferior (diaphragmatic) (inferolateral) (inferoposterior) (Q wave) (wall) NEC I21.19
inferoposterior (Q wave) I21.11
lateral (apical-lateral) (basal-lateral) (high) NEC
I21.29
posterior (posterobasal) (posterolateral) (posteroseptal) (true) NEC I21.29
septal NEC I21.29
specified NEC I21.29
type 1 (*see also* Infarction, myocardial, by site, or
by ST elevation or non-ST elevation) I21.9
type 2 I21.A1
type 3 I21.A9
type 4 (a) (b) (c) I21.A9
type 5 I21.A9
nontransmural I21.4
omentum (*see also* Infarct, intestine) K55.069
ovary N83.8
pancreas K86.89
papillary muscle — *see* Infarct, myocardium

Infarct, infarction — *continued*
parathyroid gland E21.4
pituitary (gland) E23.6
placenta O43.81- ☑
prostate N42.89
pulmonary (artery) (vein) (hemorrhagic) — *see* Embolism, pulmonary
renal (embolic) (thrombotic) N28.0
retina, retinal (artery) — *see* Occlusion, artery, retina
spinal (cord) (acute) (embolic) (nonembolic) G95.11
spleen D73.5
embolic or thrombotic I74.8
subendocardial (acute) (nontransmural) I21.4
suprarenal (capsule) (gland) E27.49
testis N50.1
thrombotic (*see also* Thrombosis)
artery, arterial — *see* Embolism
thyroid (gland) E07.89
ventricle (heart) — *see* Infarct, myocardium
Infecting — *see* condition
Infection, infected, infective (opportunistic) B99.9
with
drug resistant organism — *see* Resistance (to), drug
(*see also* specific organism)
lymphangitis — *see* Lymphangitis
organ dysfunction (acute) R65.20
with septic shock R65.21
abscess (skin) — *code by* site under Abscess
Absidia — *see* Mucormycosis
Acanthamoeba — *see* Acanthamebiasis
Acanthocheilonema (perstans) (streptocerca) B74.4
accessory sinus (chronic) — *see* Sinusitis
achorion — *see* Dermatophytosis
acromioclavicular M00.9
Acremonium falciforme B47.0
Actinobacillus (actinomycetem-comitans) A28.8
mallei A24.0
muris A25.1
Actinomadura B47.1
Actinomyces (israelii) (*see also* Actinomycosis) A42.9
Actinomycetales — *see* Actinomycosis
actinomycotic NOS — *see* Actinomycosis
adenoid (and tonsil) J03.90
chronic J35.02
adenovirus NEC
as cause of disease classified elsewhere B97.0
unspecified nature or site B34.0
aerogenes capsulatus A48.0
aertrycke — *see* Infection, salmonella
alimentary canal NOS — *see* Enteritis, infectious
Allescheria boydii B48.2
Alternaria B48.8
alveolus, alveolar (process) K04.7
Ameba, amebic (histolytica) — *see* Amebiasis
amniotic fluid, sac or cavity O41.10- ☑
chorioamnionitis O41.12- ☑
placentitis O41.14- ☑
amputation stump (surgical) — *see* Complication,
amputation stump, infection
Ancylostoma (duodenalis) B76.0
Anisakiasis, Anisakis larvae B81.0
anthrax — *see* Anthrax
antrum (chronic) — *see* Sinusitis, maxillary
anus, anal (papillae) (sphincter) K62.89
arbovirus (arbor virus) A94
specified type NEC A93.8
artificial insemination N98.0
Ascaris lumbricoides — *see* Ascariasis
Ascomycetes B47.0
Aspergillus (flavus) (fumigatus) (terreus) — *see* Aspergillosis
atypical
acid-fast (bacilli) — *see* Mycobacterium, atypical
mycobacteria — *see* Mycobacterium, atypical
virus A81.9
specified type NEC A81.89
auditory meatus (external) — *see* Otitis, externa, infective
auricle (ear) — *see* Otitis, externa, infective
axillary gland (lymph) L04.2
Bacillus A49.9
abortus A23.1
anthracis — *see* Anthrax
Ducrey's (any location) A57
Flexner's A03.1
Friedländer's NEC A49.8
gas (gangrene) A48.0
mallei A24.0

☑ Additional Character Required — Refer to the Tabular List for Character Selection   ⟱ Subterms under main terms may continue to next column or page

Infection, infected, infective — *continued*
Bacillus — *continued*
  melitensis A23.0
  paratyphoid, paratyphosus A01.4
    A A01.1
    B A01.2
    C A01.3
  Shiga (-Kruse) A03.0
  suipestifer — *see* Infection, salmonella
  swimming pool A31.1
  typhosa A01.00
  welchii — *see* Gangrene, gas
bacterial NOS A49.9
  as cause of disease classified elsewhere B96.89
    Bacteroides fragilis [B. fragilis] B96.6
    Clostridium perfringens [C. perfringens] B96.7
    Enterobacter sakazakii B96.89
    Enterococcus B95.2
    Escherichia coli [E. coli] (*see also* Escherichia
      coli) B96.20
    Helicobacter pylori [H.pylori] B96.81
    Hemophilus influenzae [H. influenzae] B96.3
    Klebsiella pneumoniae [K. pneumoniae] B96.1
    Mycoplasma pneumoniae [M. pneumoniae]
      B96.0
    Proteus (mirabilis) (morganii) B96.4
    Pseudomonas (aeruginosa) (mallei) (pseudoma-
      llei) B96.5
    Staphylococcus B95.8
      aureus (methicillin susceptible) (MSSA)
        B95.61
        methicillin resistant (MRSA) B95.62
      specified NEC B95.7
    Streptococcus B95.5
      group A B95.0
      group B B95.1
      pneumoniae B95.3
      specified NEC B95.4
    Vibrio vulnificus B96.82
  specified NEC A48.8
Bacterium
  paratyphosum A01.4
    A A01.1
    B A01.2
    C A01.3
  typhosum A01.00
Bacteroides NEC A49.8
  fragilis, as cause of disease classified elsewhere
    B96.6
Balantidium coli A07.0
Bartholin's gland N75.8
Basidiobolus B46.8
bile duct (common) (hepatic) — *see* Cholangitis
bladder — *see* Cystitis
Blastomyces, blastomycotic (*see also* Blastomycosis)
  brasiliensis — *see* Paracoccidioidomycosis
  dermatitidis — *see* Blastomycosis
  European — *see* Cryptococcosis
  Loboi B48.0
  North American B40.9
  South American — *see* Paracoccidioidomycosis
bleb, postprocedure — *see* Blebitis
bone — *see* Osteomyelitis
Bordetella — *see* Whooping cough
Borrelia bergdorfi A69.20
brain (*see also* Encephalitis) G04.90
  membranes — *see* Meningitis
  septic G06.0
    meninges — *see* Meningitis, bacterial
branchial cyst Q18.0
breast — *see* Mastitis
bronchus — *see* Bronchitis
Brucella A23.9
  abortus A23.1
  canis A23.3
  melitensis A23.0
  mixed A23.8
  specified NEC A23.8
  suis A23.2
Brugia (malayi) B74.1
  timori B74.2
bursa — *see* Bursitis, infective
buttocks (skin) L08.9
Campylobacter, intestinal A04.5
  as cause of disease classified elsewhere B96.81
Candida (albicans) (tropicalis) — *see* Candidiasis
candiru B88.8
Capillaria (intestinal) B81.1

Infection, infected, infective — *continued*
Capillaria — *continued*
  hepatica B83.8
  philippinensis B81.1
cartilage — *see* Disorder, cartilage, specified type NEC
cat liver fluke B66.0
catheter-related bloodstream (CRBSI) T80.211 ☑
cellulitis — *code by* site under Cellulitis
central line-associated T80.219 ☑
  bloodstream (CLABSI) T80.211 ☑
  specified NEC T80.218 ☑
Cephalosporium falciforme B47.0
cerebrospinal — *see* Meningitis
cervical gland (lymph) L04.0
cervix — *see* Cervicitis
cesarean delivery wound (puerperal) O86.0
cestodes — *see* Infestation, cestodes
chest J22
Chilomastix (intestinal) A07.8
Chlamydia, chlamydial A74.9
  anus A56.3
  genitourinary tract A56.2
    lower A56.00
    specified NEC A56.19
  lymphogranuloma A55
  pharynx A56.4
  psittaci A70
  rectum A56.3
  sexually transmitted NEC A56.8
cholera — *see* Cholera
Cladosporium
  bantianum (brain abscess) B43.1
  carrionii B43.0
  castellanii B36.1
  trichoides (brain abscess) B43.1
  werneckii B36.1
Clonorchis (sinensis) (liver) B66.1
Clostridium NEC
  bifermentans A48.0
  botulinum (food poisoning) A05.1
    infant A48.51
    wound A48.52
  difficile
    as cause of disease classified elsewhere B96.89
    foodborne (disease)
      not specified as recurrent A04.72
      recurrent A04.71
    gas gangrene A48.0
    necrotizing enterocolitis
      not specified as recurrent A04.72
      recurrent A04.71
    sepsis A41.4
  gas-forming NEC A48.0
  histolyticum A48.0
  novyi, causing gas gangrene A48.0
  oedematiens A48.0
  perfringens
    as cause of disease classified elsewhere B96.7
    due to food A05.2
    foodborne (disease) A05.2
    gas gangrene A48.0
    sepsis A41.4
  septicum, causing gas gangrene A48.0
  sordellii, causing gas gangrene A48.0
  welchii
    as cause of disease classified elsewhere B96.7
    foodborne (disease) A05.2
    gas gangrene A48.0
    necrotizing enteritis A05.2
    sepsis A41.4
Coccidioides (immitis) — *see* Coccidioidomycosis
colon — *see* Enteritis, infectious
colostomy K94.02
common duct — *see* Cholangitis
congenital P39.9
  Candida (albicans) P37.5
  cytomegalovirus P35.1
  hepatitis, viral P35.3
  herpes simplex P35.2
  infectious or parasitic disease P37.9
    specified NEC P37.8
  listeriosis (disseminated) P37.2
  malaria NEC P37.4
    falciparum P37.3
  Plasmodium falciparum P37.3
  poliomyelitis P35.8
  rubella P35.0
  skin P39.4

Infection, infected, infective — *continued*
congenital — *continued*
  toxoplasmosis (acute) (subacute) (chronic) P37.1
  tuberculosis P37.0
  urinary (tract) P39.3
  vaccinia P35.8
  virus P35.9
    specified type NEC P35.8
Conidiobolus B46.8
coronavirus B34.2
  as cause of disease classified elsewhere B97.29
  severe acute respiratory syndrome (SARS associat-
    ed) B97.21
corpus luteum — *see* Salpingo-oophoritis
Corynebacterium diphtheriae — *see* Diphtheria
cotia virus B08.8
Coxiella burnetii A78
coxsackie — *see* Coxsackie
Cryptococcus neoformans — *see* Cryptococcosis
Cryptosporidium A07.2
Cunninghamella — *see* Mucormycosis
cyst — *see* Cyst
cystic duct (*see also* Cholecystitis) K81.9
Cysticercus cellulosae — *see* Cysticercosis
cytomegalovirus, cytomegaloviral B25.9
  congenital P35.1
  maternal, maternal care for (suspected) damage
    to fetus O35.3 ☑
  mononucleosis B27.10
    with
      complication NEC B27.19
      meningitis B27.12
      polyneuropathy B27.11
delta-agent (acute), in hepatitis B carrier B17.0
dental (pulpal origin) K04.7
Deuteromycetes B47.0
Dicrocoelium dendriticum B66.2
Dipetalonema (perstans) (streptocerca) B74.4
diphtherial — *see* Diphtheria
Diphyllobothrium (adult) (latum) (pacificum) B70.0
  larval B70.1
Diplogonoporus (grandis) B71.8
Dipylidium caninum B67.4
Dirofilaria B74.8
Dracunculus medinensis B72
Drechslera (hawaiiensis) B43.8
Ducrey Haemophilus (any location) A57
due to or resulting from
  artificial insemination N98.0
  central venous catheter T80.219 ☑
    bloodstream T80.211 ☑
    exit or insertion site T80.212 ☑
    localized T80.212 ☑
    port or reservoir T80.212 ☑
    specified NEC T80.218 ☑
    tunnel T80.212 ☑
  device, implant or graft (*see also* Complications,
    by site and type, infection or inflammation)
    T85.79 ☑
    arterial graft NEC T82.7 ☑
    breast (implant) T85.79 ☑
    catheter NEC T85.79 ☑
      dialysis (renal) T82.7 ☑
        intraperitoneal T85.71 ☑
      infusion NEC T82.7 ☑
        cranial T85.735 ☑
        intrathecal T85.735 ☑
        spinal (epidural) (subdural) T85.735 ☑
        subarachnoid T85.735 ☑
      urinary T83.518 ☑
        cystostomy T83.510 ☑
        Hopkins T83.518 ☑
        ileostomy T83.518 ☑
        nephrostomy T83.512 ☑
        specified NEC T83.518 ☑
        urethral indwelling T83.511 ☑
        urostomy T83.518 ☑
    electronic (electrode) (pulse generator) (stimu-
      lator)
      bone T84.7 ☑
      cardiac T82.7 ☑
      nervous system T85.738 ☑
        brain T85.731 ☑
        cranial nerve T85.732 ☑
        gastric nerve T85.732 ☑
        generator pocket T85.734 ☑
        neurostimulator generator T85.734 ☑

Index

Infection, infected, infective — *continued*
  due to or resulting from — *continued*
    device, implant or graft (*see also* Complications, by site and type, infection or inflammation) — *continued*
      electronic — *continued*
        nervous system — *continued*
          peripheral nerve T85.732 ☑
          sacral nerve T85.732 ☑
          spinal cord T85.733 ☑
          vagal nerve T85.732 ☑
          urinary (indwelling) T83.51 ☑
      fixation, internal (orthopedic) NEC — *see* Complication, fixation device, infection
      gastrointestinal (bile duct) (esophagus) T85.79
        neurostimulator electrode (lead) T85.732 ☑
      genital NEC T83.69 ☑
      heart NEC T82.7
        valve (prosthesis) T82.6 ☑
          graft T82.7 ☑
      joint prosthesis — *see* Complication, joint prosthesis, infection
      ocular (corneal graft) (orbital implant) NEC T85.79
      orthopedic NEC T84.7 ☑
      penile (cylinder) (pump) (resevoir) T83.61 ☑
      specified NEC T85.79 ☑
      testicular T83.62 ☑
      urinary NEC T83.598 ☑
        ileal conduit stent T83.593 ☑
        implanted neurostimulation T83.590 ☑
        implanted sphincter T83.591 ☑
        indwelling ureteral stent T83.592 ☑
        nephroureteral stent T83.593 ☑
        specified stent NEC T83.593 ☑
      vascular NEC T82.7 ☑
      ventricular intracranial (communicating) shunt T85.730 ☑
    Hickman catheter T80.219 ☑
      bloodstream T80.211 ☑
      localized T80.212 ☑
      specified NEC T80.218 ☑
    immunization or vaccination T88.0 ☑
    infusion, injection or transfusion NEC T80.29 ☑
    injury NEC — *code by* site under Wound, open
    peripherally inserted central catheter (PICC) T80.219 ☑
      bloodstream T80.211 ☑
      localized T80.212 ☑
      specified NEC T80.218 ☑
    portacath (port-a-cath) T80.219 ☑
      bloodstream T80.211 ☑
      localized T80.212 ☑
      specified NEC T80.218 ☑
    pulmonary artery catheter — *see* Infection, due to or resulting from, central venous catheter
    surgery T81.4 ☑
    Swan Ganz catheter — *see* Infection, due to or resulting from, central venous catheter
    triple lumen catheter T80.219 ☑
      bloodstream T80.211 ☑
      localized T80.212 ☑
      specified NEC T80.218 ☑
    umbilical venous catheter T80.219 ☑
      bloodstream T80.211 ☑
      localized T80.212 ☑
      specified NEC T80.218 ☑
  during labor NEC O75.3
  ear (middle) (*see also* Otitis media)
    external — *see* Otitis, externa, infective
    inner — *see* subcategory H83.0 ☑
  Eberthella typhosa A01.00
  Echinococcus — *see* Echinococcus
  echovirus
    as cause of disease classified elsewhere B97.12
    unspecified nature or site B34.1
  endocardium I33.0
  endocervix — *see* Cervicitis
  Entamoeba — *see* Amebiasis
  enteric — *see* Enteritis, infectious
  Enterobacter sakazakii B96.89
  Enterobius vermicularis B80
  enterostomy K94.12
  enterovirus B34.1
    as cause of disease classified elsewhere B97.10

enterovirus — *continued*
  as cause of disease classified elsewhere — *continued*
    coxsackievirus B97.11
    echovirus B97.12
    specified NEC B97.19
Entomophthora B46.8
Epidermophyton — *see* Dermatophytosis
epididymis — *see* Epididymitis
episiotomy (puerperal) O86.0
Erysipelothrix (insidiosa) (rhusiopathiae) — *see* Erysipeloid
erythema infectiosum B08.3
Escherichia (E.) coli NEC A49.8
  as cause of disease classified elsewhere (*see also* Escherichia coli) B96.20
  congenital P39.8
    sepsis P36.4
  generalized A41.51
  intestinal — *see* Enteritis, infectious, due to, Escherichia coli
ethmoidal (chronic) (sinus) — *see* Sinusitis, ethmoidal
eustachian tube (ear) — *see* Salpingitis, eustachian
external auditory canal (meatus) NEC — *see* Otitis, externa, infective
eye (purulent) — *see* Endophthalmitis, purulent
eyelid — *see* Inflammation, eyelid
fallopian tube — *see* Salpingo-oophoritis
Fasciola (gigantica) (hepatica) (indica) B66.3
Fasciolopsis (buski) B66.5
filarial — *see* Infestation, filarial
finger (skin) L08.9
  nail L03.01- ☑
    fungus B35.1
fish tapeworm B70.0
  larval B70.1
flagellate, intestinal A07.9
fluke — *see* Infestation, fluke
focal
  teeth (pulpal origin) K04.7
  tonsils J35.01
Fonsecaea (compactum) (pedrosoi) B43.0
food — *see* Intoxication, foodborne
foot (skin) L08.9
  dermatophytic fungus B35.3
Francisella tularensis — *see* Tularemia
frontal (sinus) (chronic) — *see* Sinusitis, frontal
fungus NOS B49
  beard B35.0
  dermatophytic — *see* Dermatophytosis
  foot B35.3
  groin B35.6
  hand B35.2
  nail B35.1
  pathogenic to compromised host only B48.8
  perianal (area) B35.6
  scalp B35.0
  skin B36.9
    foot B35.3
    hand B35.2
    toenails B35.1
Fusarium B48.8
gallbladder — *see* Cholecystitis
gas bacillus — *see* Gangrene, gas
gastrointestinal — *see* Enteritis, infectious
generalized NEC — *see* Sepsis
generator pocket, implanted electronic neurostimulator T85.734 ☑
genital organ or tract
  female — *see* Disease, pelvis, inflammatory
  male N49.9
    multiple sites N49.8
    specified NEC N49.8
Ghon tubercle, primary A15.7
Giardia lamblia A07.1
gingiva (chronic) K05.10
  acute K05.00
    nonplaque induced K05.01
    plaque induced K05.00
  nonplaque induced K05.11
  plaque induced K05.10
glanders A24.0
glenosporopsis B48.0
Gnathostoma (spinigerum) B83.1
Gongylonema B83.8
gonococcal — *see* Gonococcus
gram-negative bacilli NOS A49.9

Infection, infected, infective — *continued*
guinea worm B72
gum (chronic) K05.10
  acute K05.00
    nonplaque induced K05.01
    plaque induced K05.00
  nonplaque induced K05.11
  plaque induced K05.10
Haemophilus — *see* Infection, Hemophilus
heart — *see* Carditis
Helicobacter pylori A04.8
  as cause of disease classified elsewhere B96.81
helminths B83.9
  intestinal B82.0
    mixed (types classifiable to more than one of the titles B65.0-B81.3 and B81.8) B81.4
    specified type NEC B81.8
  specified type NEC B83.8
Hemophilus
  aegyptius, systemic A48.4
  ducrey (any location) A57
  generalized A41.3
  influenzae NEC A49.2
    as cause of disease classified elsewhere B96.3
herpes (simplex) (*see also* Herpes)
  congenital P35.2
  disseminated B00.7
  zoster B02.9
herpesvirus, herpesviral — *see* Herpes
Heterophyes (heterophyes) B66.8
hip (joint) NEC M00.9
  due to internal joint prosthesis
    left T84.52 ☑
    right T84.51 ☑
  skin NEC L08.9
Histoplasma — *see* Histoplasmosis
  American B39.4
  capsulatum B39.4
hookworm B76.9
human
  papilloma virus A63.0
  T-cell lymphotropic virus type-1 (HTLV-1) B33.3
hydrocele N43.0
Hymenolepis B71.0
hypopharynx — *see* Pharyngitis
inguinal (lymph) glands L04.1
  due to soft chancre A57
intervertebral disc, pyogenic M46.30
  cervical region M46.32
  cervicothoracic region M46.33
  lumbar region M46.36
  lumbosacral region M46.37
  multiple sites M46.39
  occipito-atlanto-axial region M46.31
  sacrococcygeal region M46.38
  thoracic region M46.34
  thoracolumbar region M46.35
intestine, intestinal — *see* Enteritis, infectious
  specified NEC A08.8
intra-amniotic affecting newborn NEC P39.2
Isospora belli or hominis A07.3
Japanese B encephalitis A83.0
jaw (bone) (lower) (upper) M27.2
joint NEC M00.9
  due to internal joint prosthesis T84.50 ☑
kidney (cortex) (hematogenous) N15.9
  with calculus N20.0
    with hydronephrosis N13.6
  following ectopic gestation O08.83
  pelvis and ureter (cystic) N28.85
  puerperal (postpartum) O86.21
  specified NEC N15.8
Klebsiella (K.) pneumoniae NEC A49.8
  as cause of disease classified elsewhere B96.1
knee (joint) NEC M00.9
  due to internal joint prosthesis
    left T84.54 ☑
    right T84.53 ☑
  joint M00.9
  skin L08.9
Koch's — *see* Tuberculosis
labia (majora) (minora) (acute) — *see* Vulvitis
lacrimal
  gland — *see* Dacryoadenitis
  passages (duct) (sac) — *see* Inflammation, lacrimal, passages
lancet fluke B66.2
larynx NEC J38.7

☑ Additional Character Required — Refer to the Tabular List for Character Selection   ▽ Subterms under main terms may continue to next column or page

Infection, infected, infective — Infection, infected, infective

Infection, infected, infective — *continued*
- leg (skin) NOS L08.9
- Legionella pneumophila A48.1
  - nonpneumonic A48.2
- Leishmania (*see also* Leishmaniasis)
  - aethiopica B55.1
  - braziliensis B55.2
  - chagasi B55.0
  - donovani B55.0
  - infantum B55.0
  - major B55.1
  - mexicana B55.1
  - tropica B55.1
- lentivirus, as cause of disease classified elsewhere B97.31
- Leptosphaeria senegalensis B47.0
- Leptospira interrogans A27.9
  - autumnalis A27.89
  - canicola A27.89
  - hebdomadis A27.89
  - icterohaemorrhagiae A27.0
  - pomona A27.89
  - specified type NEC A27.89
- leptospirochetal NEC — *see* Leptospirosis
- Listeria monocytogenes (*see also* Listeriosis)
  - congenital P37.2
- Loa loa B74.3
  - with conjunctival infestation B74.3
  - eyelid B74.3
- Loboa loboi B48.0
- local, skin (staphylococcal) (streptococcal) L08.9
  - abscess — *code by* site under Abscess
  - cellulitis — *code by* site under Cellulitis
  - specified NEC L08.89
  - ulcer — *see* Ulcer, skin
- Loefflerella mallei A24.0
- lung (*see also* Pneumonia) J18.9
  - atypical Mycobacterium A31.0
  - spirochetal A69.8
  - tuberculous — *see* Tuberculosis, pulmonary
  - virus — *see* Pneumonia, viral
- lymph gland (*see also* Lymphadenitis, acute)
  - mesenteric I88.0
- lymphoid tissue, base of tongue or posterior pharynx, NEC (chronic) J35.03
- Madurella (grisea) (mycetomii) B47.0
- major
  - following ectopic or molar pregnancy O08.0
  - puerperal, postpartum, childbirth O85
- Malassezia furfur B36.0
- Malleomyces
  - mallei A24.0
  - pseudomallei (whitmori) — *see* Melioidosis
- mammary gland N61.0
- Mansonella (ozzardi) (perstans) (streptocerca) B74.4
- mastoid — *see* Mastoiditis
- maxilla, maxillary M27.2
  - sinus (chronic) — *see* Sinusitis, maxillary
- mediastinum J98.51
- Medina (worm) B72
- meibomian cyst or gland — *see* Hordeolum
- meninges — *see* Meningitis, bacterial
- meningococcal (*see also* condition) A39.9
  - adrenals A39.1
  - brain A39.81
  - cerebrospinal A39.0
  - conjunctiva A39.89
  - endocardium A39.51
  - heart A39.50
    - endocardium A39.51
    - myocardium A39.52
    - pericardium A39.53
  - joint A39.83
  - meninges A39.0
  - meningococcemia A39.4
    - acute A39.2
    - chronic A39.3
  - myocardium A39.52
  - pericardium A39.53
  - retrobulbar neuritis A39.82
  - specified site NEC A39.89
- mesenteric lymph nodes or glands NEC I88.0
- Metagonimus B66.8
- metatarsophalangeal M00.9
- methicillin
  - resistant Staphylococcus aureus (MRSA) A49.02
  - susceptible Staphylococcus aureus (MSSA) A49.01
- Microsporum, microsporic — *see* Dermatophytosis

Infection, infected, infective — *continued*
- mixed flora (bacterial) NEC A49.8
- Monilia — *see* Candidiasis
- Monosporium apiospermum B48.2
- mouth, parasitic B37.0
- Mucor — *see* Mucormycosis
- muscle NEC — *see* Myositis, infective
- mycelium NOS B49
- mycetoma B47.9
  - actinomycotic NEC B47.1
  - mycotic NEC B47.0
- Mycobacterium, mycobacterial — *see* Mycobacterium
- Mycoplasma NEC A49.3
  - pneumoniae, as cause of disease classified elsewhere B96.0
- mycotic NOS B49
  - pathogenic to compromised host only B48.8
  - skin NOS B36.9
- myocardium NEC I40.0
- nail (chronic)
  - with lymphangitis — *see* Lymphangitis, acute, digit
  - finger L03.01- ☑
    - fungus B35.1
  - ingrowing L60.0
  - toe L03.03- ☑
    - fungus B35.1
- nasal sinus (chronic) — *see* Sinusitis
- nasopharynx — *see* Nasopharyngitis
- navel L08.82
- Necator americanus B76.1
- Neisseria — *see* Gonococcus
- Neotestudina rosatii B47.0
- newborn P39.9
  - intra-amniotic NEC P39.2
  - skin P39.4
  - specified type NEC P39.8
- nipple N61.0
  - associated with
    - lactation O91.03
    - pregnancy O91.01- ☑
    - puerperium O91.02
- Nocardia — *see* Nocardiosis
- obstetrical surgical wound (puerperal) O86.0
- Oesophagostomum (apiostomum) B81.8
- Oestrus ovis — *see* Myiasis
- Oidium albicans B37.9
- Onchocerca (volvulus) — *see* Onchocerciasis
- oncovirus, as cause of disease classified elsewhere B97.32
- operation wound T81.4 ☑
- Opisthorchis (felineus) (viverrini) B66.0
- orbit, orbital — *see* Inflammation, orbit
- orthopoxvirus NEC B08.09
- ovary — *see* Salpingo-oophoritis
- Oxyuris vermicularis B80
- pancreas (acute) — *see* Pancreatitis, acute
  - abscess — *see* Pancreatitis, acute
  - specified NEC (*see also* Pancreatitis, acute) K85.80
- papillomavirus, as cause of disease classified elsewhere B97.7
- papovavirus NEC B34.4
- Paracoccidioides brasiliensis — *see* Paracoccidioidomycosis
- Paragonimus (westermani) B66.4
- parainfluenza virus B34.8
- parameningococcus NOS A39.9
- parapoxvirus B08.60
  - specified NEC B08.69
- parasitic B89
- Parastrongylus
  - cantonensis B83.2
  - costaricensis B81.3
  - paratyphoid A01.4
    - Type A A01.1
    - Type B A01.2
    - Type C A01.3
- paraurethral ducts N34.2
- parotid gland — *see* Sialoadenitis
- parvovirus NEC B34.3
  - as cause of disease classified elsewhere B97.6
- Pasteurella NEC A28.0
  - multocida A28.0
  - pestis — *see* Plague
  - pseudotuberculosis A28.2
  - septica (cat bite) (dog bite) A28.0
  - tularensis — *see* Tularemia
- pelvic, female — *see* Disease, pelvis, inflammatory

Infection, infected, infective — *continued*
- Penicillium (marneffei) B48.4
- penis (glans) (retention) NEC N48.29
- periapical K04.5
- peridental, periodontal K05.20
  - generalized — *see* Peridontitis, aggressive, generalized
  - localized — *see* Peridontitis, aggressive, localized
- perinatal period P39.9
  - specified type NEC P39.8
- perineal repair (puerperal) O86.0
- periorbital — *see* Inflammation, orbit
- perirectal K62.89
- perirenal — *see* Infection, kidney
- peritoneal — *see* Peritonitis
- periureteral N28.89
- Petriellidium boydii B48.2
- pharynx (*see also* Pharyngitis)
  - coxsackievirus B08.5
  - posterior, lymphoid (chronic) J35.03
- Phialophora
  - gougerotii (subcutaneous abscess or cyst) B43.2
  - jeanselmei (subcutaneous abscess or cyst) B43.2
  - verrucosa (skin) B43.0
- Piedraia hortae B36.3
- pinta A67.9
  - intermediate A67.1
  - late A67.2
  - mixed A67.3
  - primary A67.0
- pinworm B80
- pityrosporum furfur B36.0
- pleuro-pneumonia-like organism (PPLO) NEC A49.3
  - as cause of disease classified elsewhere B96.0
- pneumococcus, pneumococcal NEC A49.1
  - as cause of disease classified elsewhere B95.3
  - generalized (purulent) A40.3
    - with pneumonia J13
- Pneumocystis carinii (pneumonia) B59
- Pneumocystis jiroveci (pneumonia) B59
- port or reservoir T80.212 ☑
- postoperative T81.4 ☑
- postoperative wound T81.4 ☑
- postprocedural T81.4 ☑
- postvaccinal T88.0 ☑
- prepuce NEC N47.7
  - with penile inflammation N47.6
- prion — *see* Disease, prion, central nervous system
- prostate (capsule) — *see* Prostatitis
- Proteus (mirabilis) (morganii) (vulgaris) NEC A49.8
  - as cause of disease classified elsewhere B96.4
- protozoal NEC B64
  - intestinal A07.9
    - specified NEC A07.8
  - specified NEC B60.8
- Pseudoallescheria boydii B48.2
- Pseudomonas NEC A49.8
  - as cause of disease classified elsewhere B96.5
  - mallei A24.0
  - pneumonia J15.1
  - pseudomallei — *see* Melioidosis
- puerperal O86.4
  - genitourinary tract NEC O86.89
  - major or generalized O85
  - minor O86.4
  - specified NEC O86.89
- pulmonary — *see* Infection, lung
- purulent — *see* Abscess
- Pyrenochaeta romeroi B47.0
- Q fever A78
- rectum (sphincter) K62.89
- renal (*see also* Infection, kidney)
  - pelvis and ureter (cystic) N28.85
- reovirus, as cause of disease classified elsewhere B97.5
- respiratory (tract) NEC J98.8
  - acute J22
  - chronic J98.8
  - influenzal (upper) (acute) — *see* Influenza, with, respiratory manifestations NEC
  - lower (acute) J22
    - chronic — *see* Bronchitis, chronic
  - rhinovirus J00
  - syncytial virus, as cause of disease classified elsewhere B97.4
  - upper (acute) NOS J06.9
    - chronic J39.8
    - streptococcal J06.9
    - viral NOS J06.9

Infection, infected, infective — *continued*
  resulting from
    presence of internal prosthesis, implant, graft —
      see Complications, by site and type, infection
  retortamoniasis A07.8
  retroperitoneal NEC K68.9
  retrovirus B33.3
    as cause of disease classified elsewhere B97.30
      human
        immunodeficiency, type 2 (HIV 2) B97.35
        T-cell lymphotropic
          type I (HTLV-I) B97.33
          type II (HTLV-II) B97.34
      lentivirus B97.31
      oncovirus B97.32
      specified NEC B97.39
  Rhinosporidium (seeberi) B48.1
  rhinovirus
    as cause of disease classified elsewhere B97.89
    unspecified nature or site B34.8
  Rhizopus — *see* Mucormycosis
  rickettsial NOS A79.9
  roundworm (large) NEC B82.0
    Ascariasis (*see also* Ascariasis) B77.9
  rubella — *see* Rubella
  Saccharomyces — *see* Candidiasis
  salivary duct or gland (any) — *see* Sialoadenitis
  Salmonella (aertrycke) (arizonae) (callinarum)
      (cholerae-suis) (enteritidis) (suipestifer) (ty-
      phimurium) A02.9
    with
      (gastro)enteritis A02.0
      sepsis A02.1
      specified manifestation NEC A02.8
    due to food (poisoning) A02.9
    hirschfeldii A01.3
    localized A02.20
      arthritis A02.23
      meningitis A02.21
      osteomyelitis A02.24
      pneumonia A02.22
      pyelonephritis A02.25
      specified NEC A02.29
    paratyphi A01.4
      A A01.1
      B A01.2
      C A01.3
    schottmuelleri A01.2
    typhi, typhosa — *see* Typhoid
  Sarcocystis A07.8
  scabies B86
  Schistosoma — *see* Infestation, Schistosoma
  scrotum (acute) NEC N49.2
  seminal vesicle — *see* Vesiculitis
  septic
    localized, skin — *see* Abscess
  sheep liver fluke B66.3
  Shigella A03.9
    boydii A03.2
    dysenteriae A03.0
    flexneri A03.1
    group
      A A03.0
      B A03.1
      C A03.2
      D A03.3
    Schmitz (-Stutzer) A03.0
    schmitzii A03.0
    shigae A03.0
    sonnei A03.3
    specified NEC A03.8
  shoulder (joint) NEC M00.9
    due to internal joint prosthesis T84.59 ☑
    skin NEC L08.9
  sinus (accessory) (chronic) (nasal) (*see also* Sinusitis)
    pilonidal — *see* Sinus, pilonidal
    skin NEC L08.89
  Skene's duct or gland — *see* Urethritis
  skin (local) (staphylococcal) (streptococcal) L08.9
    abscess — *code by* site under Abscess
    cellulitis — *code by* site under Cellulitis
    due to fungus B36.9
      specified type NEC B36.8
    mycotic B36.9
      specified type NEC B36.8
    newborn P39.4
    ulcer — *see* Ulcer, skin
  slow virus A81.9

Infection, infected, infective — *continued*
  slow virus — *continued*
    specified NEC A81.89
  Sparganum (mansoni) (proliferum) (baxteri) B70.1
  specific (*see also* Syphilis)
    to perinatal period — *see* Infection, congenital
  specified NEC B99.8
  spermatic cord NEC N49.1
  sphenoidal (sinus) — *see* Sinusitis, sphenoidal
  spinal cord NOS (*see also* Myelitis) G04.91
    abscess G06.1
    meninges — *see* Meningitis
    streptococcal G04.89
  Spirillum A25.0
  spirochetal NOS A69.9
    lung A69.8
    specified NEC A69.8
  Spirometra larvae B70.1
  spleen D73.89
  Sporotrichum, Sporothrix (schenckii) — *see* Sporotri-
    chosis
  staphylococcal, unspecified site
    as cause of disease classified elsewhere B95.8
      aureus (methicillin susceptible) (MSSA) B95.61
        methicillin resistant (MRSA) B95.62
      specified NEC B95.7
    aureus (methicillin susceptible) (MSSA) A49.01
      methicillin resistant (MRSA) A49.02
    food poisoning A05.0
    generalized (purulent) A41.2
    pneumonia — *see* Pneumonia, staphylococcal
  Stellantchasmus falcatus B66.8
  streptobacillus moniliformis A25.1
  streptococcal NEC A49.1
    as cause of disease classified elsewhere B95.5
    B genitourinary complicating
      childbirth O98.82
      pregnancy O98.81- ☑
      puerperium O98.83
    congenital
      sepsis P36.10
        group B P36.0
        specified NEC P36.19
    generalized (purulent) A40.9
  Streptomyces B47.1
  Strongyloides (stercoralis) — *see* Strongyloidiasis
  stump (amputation) (surgical) — *see* Complication,
    amputation stump, infection
  subcutaneous tissue, local L08.9
  suipestifer — *see* Infection, salmonella
  swimming pool bacillus A31.1
  Taenia — *see* Infestation, Taenia
  Taeniarhynchus saginatus B68.1
  tapeworm — *see* Infestation, tapeworm
  tendon (sheath) — *see* Tenosynovitis, infective NEC
  Ternidens diminutus B81.8
  testis — *see* Orchitis
  threadworm B80
  throat — *see* Pharyngitis
  thyroglossal duct K14.8
  toe (skin) L08.9
    cellulitis L03.03- ☑
      fungus B35.1
    nail L03.03- ☑
      fungus B35.1
  tongue NEC K14.0
    parasitic B37.0
  tonsil (and adenoid) (faucial) (lingual) (pharyngeal) —
    see Tonsillitis
  tooth, teeth K04.7
    periapical K04.7
    peridental, periodontal K05.20
      generalized — *see* Peridontitis, aggressive,
        generalized
      localized — *see* Peridontitis, aggressive, local-
        ized
    pulp K04.01
      irreversible K04.02
      reversible K04.01
    socket M27.3
  TORCH — *see* Infection, congenital
    without active infection P00.2
  Torula histolytica — *see* Cryptococcosis
  Toxocara (canis) (cati) (felis) B83.0
  Toxoplasma gondii — *see* Toxoplasma
  trachea, chronic J42
  trematode NEC — *see* Infestation, fluke
  trench fever A79.0

Infection, infected, infective — *continued*
  Treponema pallidum — *see* Syphilis
  Trichinella (spiralis) B75
  Trichomonas A59.9
    cervix A59.09
    intestine A07.8
    prostate A59.02
    specified site NEC A59.8
    urethra A59.03
    urogenitalis A59.00
    vagina A59.01
    vulva A59.01
  Trichophyton, trichophytic — *see* Dermatophytosis
  Trichosporon (beigelii) cutaneum B36.2
  Trichostrongylus B81.2
  Trichuris (trichiura) B79
  Trombicula (irritans) B88.0
  Trypanosoma
    brucei
      gambiense B56.0
      rhodesiense B56.1
    cruzi — *see* Chagas' disease
  tubal — *see* Salpingo-oophoritis
  tuberculous NEC — *see* Tuberculosis
  tubo-ovarian — *see* Salpingo-oophoritis
  tunica vaginalis N49.1
  tunnel T80.212 ☑
  tympanic membrane NEC — *see* Myringitis
  typhoid (abortive) (ambulant) (bacillus) — *see* Typhoid
  typhus A75.9
    flea-borne A75.2
    mite-borne A75.3
    recrudescent A75.1
    tick-borne A77.9
      African A77.1
      North Asian A77.2
  umbilicus L08.82
  ureter N28.86
  urethra — *see* Urethritis
  urinary (tract) N39.0
    bladder — *see* Cystitis
    complicating
      pregnancy O23.4- ☑
        specified type NEC O23.3- ☑
    kidney — *see* Infection, kidney
    newborn P39.3
    puerperal (postpartum) O86.20
    tuberculous A18.13
    urethra — *see* Urethritis
  uterus, uterine — *see* Endometritis
  vaccination T88.0 ☑
  vaccinia not from vaccination B08.011
  vagina (acute) — *see* Vaginitis
  varicella B01.9
  varicose veins — *see* Varix
  vas deferens NEC N49.1
  vesical — *see* Cystitis
  Vibrio
    cholerae A00.0
      El Tor A00.1
    parahaemolyticus (food poisoning) A05.3
    vulnificus
      as cause of disease classified elsewhere B96.82
      foodborne intoxication A05.5
  Vincent's (gum) (mouth) (tonsil) A69.1
  virus, viral NOS B34.9
    adenovirus
      as cause of disease classified elsewhere B97.0
      unspecified nature or site B34.0
    arborvirus, arbovirus arthropod-borne A94
    as cause of disease classified elsewhere B97.89
      adenovirus B97.0
      coronavirus B97.29
        SARS-associated B97.21
      coxsackievirus B97.11
      echovirus B97.12
      enterovirus B97.10
        coxsackievirus B97.11
        echovirus B97.12
        specified NEC B97.19
      human
        immunodeficiency, type 2 (HIV 2) B97.35
        metapneumovirus B97.81
        T-cell lymphotropic,
          type I (HTLV-I) B97.33
          type II (HTLV-II) B97.34
      papillomavirus B97.7
      parvovirus B97.6

Infection, infected, infective — *continued*
  virus, viral — *continued*
    as cause of disease classified elsewhere — *continued*
      reovirus B97.5
      respiratory syncytial B97.4
      retrovirus B97.30
        human
          immunodeficiency, type 2 (HIV 2) B97.35
          T-cell lymphotropic,
            type I (HTLV-I) B97.33
            type II (HTLV-II) B97.34
        lentivirus B97.31
        oncovirus B97.32
        specified NEC B97.39
      specified NEC B97.89
    central nervous system A89
      atypical A81.9
        specified NEC A81.89
      enterovirus NEC A88.8
        meningitis A87.0
      slow virus A81.9
        specified NEC A81.89
      specified NEC A88.8
    chest J98.8
    cotia B08.8
    coxsackie (*see also* Infection, coxsackie) B34.1
      as cause of disease classified elsewhere B97.11
    ECHO
      as cause of disease classified elsewhere B97.12
      unspecified nature or site B34.1
    encephalitis, tick-borne A84.9
    enterovirus, as cause of disease classified elsewhere B97.10
      coxsackievirus B97.11
      echovirus B97.12
      specified NEC B97.19
    exanthem NOS B09
    human metapneumovirus as cause of disease classified elsewhere B97.81
    human papilloma as cause of disease classified elsewhere B97.7
    intestine — *see* Enteritis, viral
    respiratory syncytial
      as cause of disease classified elsewhere B97.4
      bronchopneumonia J12.1
      common cold syndrome J00
      nasopharyngitis (acute) J00
    rhinovirus
      as cause of disease classified elsewhere B97.89
      unspecified nature or site B34.8
    slow A81.9
      specified NEC A81.89
    specified type NEC B33.8
      as cause of disease classified elsewhere B97.89
      unspecified nature or site B34.8
    unspecified nature or site B34.9
    West Nile — *see* Virus, West Nile
  vulva (acute) — *see* Vulvitis
  West Nile — *see* Virus, West Nile
  whipworm B79
  worms B83.9
    specified type NEC B83.8
  Wuchereria (bancrofti) B74.0
    malayi B74.1
  yatapoxvirus B08.70
    specified NEC B08.79
  yeast (*see also* Candidiasis) B37.9
  yellow fever — *see* Fever, yellow
  Yersinia
    enterocolitica (intestinal) A04.6
    pestis — *see* Plague
    pseudotuberculosis A28.2
  Zeis' gland — *see* Hordeolum
  Zika virus A92.5
  zoonotic bacterial NOS A28.9
  Zopfia senegalensis B47.0
Infective, infectious — *see* condition
Infertility
  female N97.9
    age-related N97.8
    associated with
      anovulation N97.0
      cervical (mucus) disease or anomaly N88.3
      congenital anomaly
        cervix N88.3
        fallopian tube N97.1
        uterus N97.2

Infertility — *continued*
  female — *continued*
    associated with — *continued*
      congenital anomaly — *continued*
        vagina N97.8
      dysmucorrhea N88.3
      fallopian tube disease or anomaly N97.1
      pituitary-hypothalamic origin E23.0
      specified origin NEC N97.8
      Stein-Leventhal syndrome E28.2
      uterine disease or anomaly N97.2
      vaginal disease or anomaly N97.8
    due to
      cervical anomaly N88.3
      fallopian tube anomaly N97.1
      ovarian failure E28.39
      Stein-Leventhal syndrome E28.2
      uterine anomaly N97.2
      vaginal anomaly N97.8
    nonimplantation N97.2
    origin
      cervical N88.3
      tubal (block) (occlusion) (stenosis) N97.1
      uterine N97.2
      vaginal N97.8
  male N46.9
    azoospermia N46.01
      extratesticular cause N46.029
        drug therapy N46.021
        efferent duct obstruction N46.023
        infection N46.022
        radiation N46.024
        specified cause NEC N46.029
        systemic disease N46.025
    oligospermia N46.11
      extratesticular cause N46.129
        drug therapy N46.121
        efferent duct obstruction N46.123
        infection N46.122
        radiation N46.124
        specified cause NEC N46.129
        systemic disease N46.125
    specified type NEC N46.8
Infestation B88.9
  Acanthocheilonema (perstans) (streptocerca) B74.4
  Acariasis B88.0
    demodex folliculorum B88.0
    sarcoptes scabiei B86
    trombiculae B88.0
  Agamofilaria streptocerca B74.4
  Ancylostoma, ankylostoma (braziliense) (caninum) (ceylanicum) (duodenale) B76.0
    americanum B76.1
    new world B76.1
  Anisakis larvae, anisakiasis B81.0
  arthropod NEC B88.2
  Ascaris lumbricoides — *see* Ascariasis
  Balantidium coli A07.0
  beef tapeworm B68.1
  Bothriocephalus (latus) B70.0
    larval B70.1
  broad tapeworm B70.0
    larval B70.1
  Brugia (malayi) B74.1
    timori B74.2
  candiru B88.8
  Capillaria
    hepatica B83.8
    philippinensis B81.1
  cat liver fluke B66.0
  cestodes B71.9
    diphyllobothrium — *see* Infestation, diphyllobothrium
    dipylidiasis B71.1
    hymenolepiasis B71.0
    specified type NEC B71.8
  chigger B88.0
  chigo, chigoe B88.1
  Clonorchis (sinensis) (liver) B66.1
  coccidial A07.3
  crab-lice B85.3
  Cysticercus cellulosae — *see* Cysticercosis
  Demodex (folliculorum) B88.0
  Dermanyssus gallinae B88.0
  Dermatobia (hominis) — *see* Myiasis
  Dibothriocephalus (latus) B70.0
    larval B70.1
  Dicrocoelium dendriticum B66.2

Infestation — *continued*
  Diphyllobothrium (adult) (latum) (intestinal) (pacificum) B70.0
    larval B70.1
  Diplogonoporus (grandis) B71.8
  Dipylidium caninum B67.4
  Distoma hepaticum B66.3
  dog tapeworm B67.4
  Dracunculus medinensis B72
  dragon worm B72
  dwarf tapeworm B71.0
  Echinococcus — *see* Echinococcus
  Echinostomum ilocanum B66.8
  Entamoeba (histolytica) — *see* Infection, Ameba
  Enterobius vermicularis B80
  eyelid
    in (due to)
      leishmaniasis B55.1
      loiasis B74.3
      onchocerciasis B73.09
      phthiriasis B85.3
      parasitic NOS B89
  eyeworm B74.3
  Fasciola (gigantica) (hepatica) (indica) B66.3
  Fasciolopsis (buski) (intestine) B66.5
  filarial B74.9
    bancroftian B74.0
    conjunctiva B74.9
    due to
      Acanthocheilonema (perstans) (streptocerca) B74.4
      Brugia (malayi) B74.1
        timori B74.2
      Dracunculus medinensis B72
      guinea worm B72
      loa loa B74.3
      Mansonella (ozzardi) (perstans) (streptocerca) B74.4
      Onchocerca volvulus B73.00
        eye B73.00
        eyelid B73.09
      Wuchereria (bancrofti) B74.0
    Malayan B74.1
    ozzardi B74.4
    specified type NEC B74.8
  fish tapeworm B70.0
    larval B70.1
  fluke B66.9
    blood NOS — *see* Schistosomiasis
    cat liver B66.0
    intestinal B66.5
    lancet B66.2
    liver (sheep) B66.3
      cat B66.0
      Chinese B66.1
      due to clonorchiasis B66.1
      oriental B66.1
    lung (oriental) B66.4
    sheep liver B66.3
    specified type NEC B66.8
  fly larvae — *see* Myiasis
  Gasterophilus (intestinalis) — *see* Myiasis
  Gastrodiscoides hominis B66.8
  Giardia lamblia A07.1
  Gnathostoma (spinigerum) B83.1
  Gongylonema B83.8
  guinea worm B72
  helminth B83.9
    angiostrongyliasis B83.2
      intestinal B81.3
    gnathostomiasis B83.1
    hirudiniasis, internal B83.4
    intestinal B82.0
      angiostrongyliasis B81.3
      anisakiasis B81.0
      ascariasis — *see* Ascariasis
      capillariasis B81.1
      cysticercosis — *see* Cysticercosis
      diphyllobothriasis — *see* Infestation, diphyllobothriasis
      dracunculiasis B72
      echinococcus — *see* Echinococcosis
      enterobiasis B80
      filariasis — *see* Infestation, filarial
      fluke — *see* Infestation, fluke
      hookworm — *see* Infestation, hookworm
      mixed (types classifiable to more than one of the titles B65.0-B81.3 and B81.8) B81.4

▼ **Subterms under main terms may continue to next column or page**   ☑ **Additional Character Required — Refer to the Tabular List for Character Selection**   **187**

Infection, infected, infective — Infestation

Index — Infestation — Inflammation, inflamed, inflammatory

Infestation — *continued*
  helminth — *continued*
    intestinal — *continued*
      onchocerciasis — *see* Onchocerciasis
      schistosomiasis — *see* Infestation, schistosoma
      specified
        cestode NEC — *see* Infestation, cestode
        type NEC B81.8
      strongyloidiasis — *see* Strongyloidiasis
      taenia — *see* Infestation, taenia
      trichinellosis B75
      trichostrongyliasis B81.2
      trichuriasis B79
    specified type NEC B83.8
    syngamiasis B83.3
    visceral larva migrans B83.0
  Heterophyes (heterophyes) B66.8
  hookworm B76.9
    ancylostomiasis B76.0
    necatoriasis B76.1
    specified type NEC B76.8
  Hymenolepis (diminuta) (nana) B71.0
  intestinal NEC B82.9
  leeches (aquatic) (land) — *see* Hirudiniasis
  Leishmania — *see* Leishmaniasis
  lice, louse — *see* Infestation, Pediculus
  Linguatula B88.8
  Liponyssoides sanguineus B88.0
  Loa loa B74.3
    conjunctival B74.3
    eyelid B74.3
  louse — *see* Infestation, Pediculus
  maggots — *see* Myiasis
  Mansonella (ozzardi) (perstans) (streptocerca) B74.4
  Medina (worm) B72
  Metagonimus (yokogawai) B66.8
  microfilaria streptocerca — *see* Onchocerciasis
    eye B73.00
    eyelid B73.09
  mites B88.9
    scabic B86
  Monilia (albicans) — *see* Candidiasis
  mouth B37.0
  Necator americanus B76.1
  nematode NEC (intestinal) B82.0
    Ancylostoma B76.0
    conjunctiva NEC B83.9
    Enterobius vermicularis B80
    Gnathostoma spinigerum B83.1
    physaloptera B80
    specified NEC B81.8
    trichostrongylus B81.2
    trichuris (trichuria) B79
  Oesophagostomum (apiostomum) B81.8
  Oestrus ovis (*see also* Myiasis) B87.9
  Onchocerca (volvulus) — *see* Onchocerciasis
  Opisthorchis (felineus) (viverrini) B66.0
  orbit, parasitic NOS B89
  Oxyuris vermicularis B80
  Paragonimus (westermani) B66.4
  parasite, parasitic B89
    eyelid B89
    intestinal NOS B82.9
    mouth B37.0
    skin B88.9
    tongue B37.0
  Parastrongylus
    cantonensis B83.2
    costaricensis B81.3
  Pediculus B85.2
    body B85.1
    capitis (humanus) (any site) B85.0
    corporis (humanus) (any site) B85.1
    head B85.0
    mixed (classifiable to more than one of the titles B85.0 - B85.3) B85.4
    pubis (any site) B85.3
  Pentastoma B88.8
  Phthirus (pubis) (any site) B85.3
    with any infestation classifiable to B85.0 - B85.2 B85.4
  pinworm B80
  pork tapeworm (adult) B68.0
  protozoal NEC B64
    intestinal A07.9
      specified NEC A07.8
    specified NEC B60.8
  pubic, louse B85.3

Infestation — *continued*
  rat tapeworm B71.0
  red bug B88.0
  roundworm (large) NEC B82.0
    Ascariasis (*see also* Ascariasis) B77.9
  sandflea B88.1
  Sarcoptes scabiei B86
  scabies B86
  Schistosoma B65.9
    bovis B65.8
    cercariae B65.3
    haematobium B65.0
    intercalatum B65.8
    japonicum B65.2
    mansoni B65.1
    mattheei B65.8
    mekongi B65.8
    specified type NEC B65.8
    spindale B65.8
  screw worms — *see* Myiasis
  skin NOS B88.9
  Sparganum (mansoni) (proliferum) (baxteri) B70.1
    larval B70.1
  specified type NEC B88.8
  Spirometra larvae B70.1
  Stellantchasmus falcatus B66.8
  Strongyloides stercoralis — *see* Strongyloidiasis
  Taenia B68.9
    diminuta B71.0
    echinococcus — *see* Echinococcus
    mediocanellata B68.1
    nana B71.0
    saginata B68.1
    solium (intestinal form) B68.0
      larval form — *see* Cysticercosis
  Taeniarhynchus saginatus B68.1
  tapeworm B71.9
    beef B68.1
    broad B70.0
      larval B70.1
    dog B67.4
    dwarf B71.0
    fish B70.0
      larval B70.1
    pork B68.0
    rat B71.0
  Ternidens diminutus B81.8
  Tetranychus molestissimus B88.0
  threadworm B80
  tongue B37.0
  Toxocara (canis) (cati) (felis) B83.0
  trematode(s) NEC — *see* Infestation, fluke
  Trichinella (spiralis) B75
  Trichocephalus B79
  Trichomonas — *see* Trichomoniasis
  Trichostrongylus B81.2
  Trichuris (trichiura) B79
  Trombicula (irritans) B88.0
  Tunga penetrans B88.1
  Uncinaria americana B76.1
  Vandellia cirrhosa B88.8
  whipworm B79
  worms B83.9
    intestinal B82.0
  Wuchereria (bancrofti) B74.0

Infiltrate, infiltration
  amyloid (generalized) (localized) — *see* Amyloidosis
  calcareous NEC R89.7
    localized — *see* Degeneration, by site
  calcium salt R89.7
  cardiac
    fatty — *see* Degeneration, myocardial
    glycogenic E74.02 [I43]
  corneal — *see* Edema, cornea
  eyelid — *see* Inflammation, eyelid
  glycogen, glycogenic — *see* Disease, glycogen storage
  heart, cardiac
    fatty — *see* Degeneration, myocardial
    glycogenic E74.02 [I43]
  inflammatory in vitreous H43.89
  kidney N28.89
  leukemic — *see* Leukemia
  liver K76.89
    fatty — *see* Fatty, liver NEC
    glycogen (*see also* Disease, glycogen storage) E74.03 [K77]
  lung R91.8
    eosinophilic J82

Infiltrate, infiltration — *continued*
  lymphatic (*see also* Leukemia, lymphatic) C91.9- ☑
    gland I88.9
  muscle, fatty M62.89
  myocardium, myocardial
    fatty — *see* Degeneration, myocardial
    glycogenic E74.02 [I43]
  on chest x-ray R91.8
  pulmonary R91.8
    with eosinophilia J82
  skin (lymphocytic) L98.6
  thymus (gland) (fatty) E32.8
  urine R39.0
  vesicant agent
    antineoplastic chemotherapy T80.810 ☑
    other agent NEC T80.818 ☑
  vitreous body H43.89

Infirmity R68.89
  senile R54

Inflammation, inflamed, inflammatory (with exudation)
  abducent (nerve) — *see* Strabismus, paralytic, sixth nerve
  accessory sinus (chronic) — *see* Sinusitis
  adrenal (gland) E27.8
  alveoli, teeth M27.3
    scorbutic E54
  anal canal, anus K62.89
  antrum (chronic) — *see* Sinusitis, maxillary
  appendix — *see* Appendicitis
  arachnoid — *see* Meningitis
  areola N61.0
    puerperal, postpartum or gestational — *see* Infection, nipple
  areolar tissue NOS L08.9
  artery — *see* Arteritis
  auditory meatus (external) — *see* Otitis, externa
  Bartholin's gland N75.8
  bile duct (common) (hepatic) or passage — *see* Cholangitis
  bladder — *see* Cystitis
  bone — *see* Osteomyelitis
  brain (*see also* Encephalitis)
    membrane — *see* Meningitis
  breast N61.0
    puerperal, postpartum, gestational — *see* Mastitis, obstetric
  broad ligament — *see* Disease, pelvis, inflammatory
  bronchi — *see* Bronchitis
  catarrhal J00
  cecum — *see* Appendicitis
  cerebral (*see also* Encephalitis)
    membrane — *see* Meningitis
  cerebrospinal
    meningococcal A39.0
  cervix (uteri) — *see* Cervicitis
  chest J98.8
  chorioretinal H30.9- ☑
    cyclitis — *see* Cyclitis
    disseminated H30.10- ☑
      generalized H30.13- ☑
      peripheral H30.12- ☑
      posterior pole H30.11- ☑
    epitheliopathy — *see* Epitheliopathy
    focal H30.00- ☑
      juxtapapillary H30.01- ☑
      macular H30.04- ☑
      paramacular — *see* Inflammation, chorioretinal, focal, macular
      peripheral H30.03- ☑
      posterior pole H30.02- ☑
    specified type NEC H30.89- ☑
  choroid — *see* Inflammation, chorioretinal
  chronic, postmastoidectomy cavity — *see* Complications, postmastoidectomy, inflammation
  colon — *see* Enteritis
  connective tissue (diffuse) NEC — *see* Disorder, soft tissue, specified type NEC
  cornea — *see* Keratitis
  corpora cavernosa N48.29
  cranial nerve — *see* Disorder, nerve, cranial
  Douglas' cul-de-sac or pouch (chronic) N73.0
  due to device, implant or graft (*see also* Complications, by site and type, infection or inflammation)
    arterial graft T82.7 ☑
    breast (implant) T85.79 ☑
    catheter T85.79 ☑

☑ Additional Character Required — Refer to the Tabular List for Character Selection   Subterms under main terms may continue to next column or page

Index

Inflammation, inflamed, inflammatory —
  continued
  due to device, implant or graft (*see also* Complications, by site and type, infection or inflammation) — *continued*
    catheter — *continued*
      dialysis (renal) T82.7 ☑
        intraperitoneal T85.71 ☑
      infusion T82.7 ☑
        cranial T85.735 ☑
        intrathecal T85.735 ☑
        spinal (epidural) (subdural) T85.735 ☑
        subarachnoid T85.735 ☑
      urinary T83.518 ☑
        cystostomy T83.510 ☑
        Hopkins T83.518 ☑
        ileostomy T83.518 ☑
        nephrostomy T83.512 ☑
        specified NEC T83.518 ☑
        urethral indwelling T83.511 ☑
        urostomy T83.518 ☑
    electronic (electrode) (pulse generator) (stimulator)
      bone T84.7 ☑
      cardiac T82.7 ☑
      nervous system T85.738 ☑
        brain T85.731 ☑
        cranial nerve T85.732 ☑
        gastric nerve T85.732 ☑
        neurostimulator generator T85.734 ☑
        peripheral nerve T85.732 ☑
        sacral nerve T85.732 ☑
        spinal cord T85.733 ☑
        vagal nerve T85.732 ☑
      urinary T83.590 ☑
    fixation, internal (orthopedic) NEC — *see* Complication, fixation device, infection
    gastrointestinal (bile duct) (esophagus) T85.79 ☑
      neurostimulator electrode (lead) T85.732 ☑
    genital NEC T83.69 ☑
    heart NEC T82.7 ☑
      valve (prosthesis) T82.6 ☑
        graft T82.7 ☑
    joint prosthesis — *see* Complication, joint prosthesis, infection
    ocular (corneal graft) (orbital implant) NEC T85.79 ☑
    orthopedic NEC T84.7 ☑
    penile (cylinder) (pump) (resevoir) T83.61 ☑
    specified NEC T85.79 ☑
    testicular T83.62 ☑
    urinary NEC T83.598 ☑
      ileal conduit stent T83.593 ☑
      implanted neurostimulation T83.590 ☑
      implanted sphincter T83.591 ☑
      indwelling ureteral stent T83.592 ☑
      nephroureteral stent T83.593 ☑
      specified stent NEC T83.593 ☑
    vascular NEC T82.7 ☑
    ventricular intracranial (communicating) shunt T85.730 ☑
  duodenum K29.80
    with bleeding K29.81
  dura mater — *see* Meningitis
  ear (middle) (*see also* Otitis, media)
    external — *see* Otitis, externa
    inner — *see* subcategory H83.0 ☑
  epididymis — *see* Epididymitis
  esophagus K20.9
  ethmoidal (sinus) (chronic) — *see* Sinusitis, ethmoidal
  eustachian tube (catarrhal) — *see* Salpingitis, eustachian
  eyelid H01.9
    abscess — *see* Abscess, eyelid
    blepharitis — *see* Blepharitis
    chalazion — *see* Chalazion
    dermatosis (noninfectious) — *see* Dermatosis, eyelid
    hordeolum — *see* Hordeolum
    specified NEC H01.8
  fallopian tube — *see* Salpingo-oophoritis
  fascia — *see* Myositis
  follicular, pharynx J31.2
  frontal (sinus) (chronic) — *see* Sinusitis, frontal
  gallbladder — *see* Cholecystitis
  gastric — *see* Gastritis
  gastrointestinal — *see* Enteritis

Inflammation, inflamed, inflammatory —
  continued
  genital organ (internal) (diffuse)
    female — *see* Disease, pelvis, inflammatory
    male N49.9
      multiple sites N49.8
      specified NEC N49.8
  gland (lymph) — *see* Lymphadenitis
  glottis — *see* Laryngitis
  granular, pharynx J31.2
  gum K05.10
    nonplaque induced K05.11
    plaque induced K05.10
  heart — *see* Carditis
  hepatic duct — *see* Cholangitis
  ileoanal (internal) pouch K91.850
  ileum (*see also* Enteritis)
    regional or terminal — *see* Enteritis, regional
  intestinal pouch K91.850
  intestine (any part) — *see* Enteritis
  jaw (acute) (bone) (chronic) (lower) (suppurative) (upper) M27.2
  joint NEC — *see* Arthritis
    sacroiliac M46.1
  kidney — *see* Nephritis
  knee (joint) M13.169
    tuberculous A18.02
  labium (majus) (minus) — *see* Vulvitis
  lacrimal
    gland — *see* Dacryoadenitis
    passages (duct) (sac) (*see also* Dacryocystitis)
      canaliculitis — *see* Canaliculitis, lacrimal
  larynx — *see* Laryngitis
  leg NOS L08.9
  lip K13.0
  liver (capsule) (*see also* Hepatitis)
    chronic K73.9
    suppurative K75.0
  lung (acute) (*see also* Pneumonia)
    chronic J98.4
  lymph gland or node — *see* Lymphadenitis
  lymphatic vessel — *see* Lymphangitis
  maxilla, maxillary M27.2
    sinus (chronic) — *see* Sinusitis, maxillary
  membranes of brain or spinal cord — *see* Meningitis
  meninges — *see* Meningitis
  mouth K12.1
  muscle — *see* Myositis
  myocardium — *see* Myocarditis
  nasal sinus (chronic) — *see* Sinusitis
  nasopharynx — *see* Nasopharyngitis
  navel L08.82
  nerve NEC — *see* Neuralgia
  nipple N61.0
    puerperal, postpartum or gestational — *see* Infection, nipple
  nose — *see* Rhinitis
  oculomotor (nerve) — *see* Strabismus, paralytic, third nerve
  optic nerve — *see* Neuritis, optic
  orbit (chronic) H05.10
    acute H05.00
      abscess — *see* Abscess, orbit
      cellulitis — *see* Cellulitis, orbit
      osteomyelitis — *see* Osteomyelitis, orbit
      periostitis — *see* Periostitis, orbital
      tenonitis — *see* Tenonitis, eye
    granuloma — *see* Granuloma, orbit
    myositis — *see* Myositis, orbital
  ovary — *see* Salpingo-oophoritis
  oviduct — *see* Salpingo-oophoritis
  pancreas (acute) — *see* Pancreatitis
  parametrium N73.0
  parotid region L08.9
  pelvis, female — *see* Disease, pelvis, inflammatory
  penis (corpora cavernosa) N48.29
  perianal K62.89
  pericardium — *see* Pericarditis
  perineum (female) (male) L08.9
  perirectal K62.89
  peritoneum — *see* Peritonitis
  periuterine — *see* Disease, pelvis, inflammatory
  perivesical — *see* Cystitis
  petrous bone (acute) (chronic) — *see* Petrositis
  pharynx (acute) — *see* Pharyngitis
  pia mater — *see* Meningitis
  pleura — *see* Pleurisy

Inflammation, inflamed, inflammatory —
  continued
  polyp, colon (*see also* Polyp, colon, inflammatory) K51.40
  prostate (*see also* Prostatitis)
    specified type NEC N41.8
  rectosigmoid — *see* Rectosigmoiditis
  rectum (*see also* Proctitis) K62.89
  respiratory, upper (*see also* Infection, respiratory, upper) J06.9
    acute, due to radiation J70.0
    chronic, due to external agent — *see* condition, respiratory, chronic, due to
    due to
      chemicals, gases, fumes or vapors (inhalation) J68.2
      radiation J70.1
  retina — *see* Chorioretinitis
  retrocecal — *see* Appendicitis
  retroperitoneal — *see* Peritonitis
  salivary duct or gland (any) (suppurative) — *see* Sialoadenitis
  scorbutic, alveoli, teeth E54
  scrotum N49.2
  seminal vesicle — *see* Vesiculitis
  sigmoid — *see* Enteritis
  sinus — *see* Sinusitis
  Skene's duct or gland — *see* Urethritis
  skin L08.9
  spermatic cord N49.1
  sphenoidal (sinus) — *see* Sinusitis, sphenoidal
  spinal
    cord — *see* Encephalitis
    membrane — *see* Meningitis
    nerve — *see* Disorder, nerve
  spine — *see* Spondylopathy, inflammatory
  spleen (capsule) D73.89
  stomach — *see* Gastritis
  subcutaneous tissue L08.9
  suprarenal (gland) E27.8
  synovial — *see* Tenosynovitis
  tendon (sheath) NEC — *see* Tenosynovitis
  testis — *see* Orchitis
  throat (acute) — *see* Pharyngitis
  thymus (gland) E32.8
  thyroid (gland) — *see* Thyroiditis
  tongue K14.0
  tonsil — *see* Tonsillitis
  trachea — *see* Tracheitis
  trochlear (nerve) — *see* Strabismus, paralytic, fourth nerve
  tubal — *see* Salpingo-oophoritis
  tuberculous NEC — *see* Tuberculosis
  tubo-ovarian — *see* Salpingo-oophoritis
  tunica vaginalis N49.1
  tympanic membrane — *see* Tympanitis
  umbilicus, umbilical L08.82
  uterine ligament — *see* Disease, pelvis, inflammatory
  uterus (catarrhal) — *see* Endometritis
  uveal tract (anterior) NOS (*see also* Iridocyclitis)
    posterior — *see* Chorioretinitis
  vagina — *see* Vaginitis
  vas deferens N49.1
  vein (*see also* Phlebitis)
    intracranial or intraspinal (septic) G08
    thrombotic I80.9
      leg — *see* Phlebitis, leg
      lower extremity — *see* Phlebitis, leg
  vocal cord J38.3
  vulva — *see* Vulvitis
  Wharton's duct (suppurative) — *see* Sialoadenitis
Inflation, lung, imperfect (newborn) — *see* Atelectasis
Influenza (bronchial) (epidemic) (respiratory (upper)) (unidentified influenza virus) J11.1
  with
    digestive manifestations J11.2
    encephalopathy J11.81
    enteritis J11.2
    gastroenteritis J11.2
    gastrointestinal manifestations J11.2
    laryngitis J11.1
    myocarditis J11.82
    otitis media J11.83
    pharyngitis J11.1
    pneumonia J11.00
      specified type J11.08
    respiratory manifestations NEC J11.1

▽ Subterms under main terms may continue to next column or page   ☑ **Additional Character Required** — Refer to the Tabular List for Character Selection   **189**

Inflammation, inflamed, inflammatory — Influenza

Influenza — *continued*
with — *continued*
  specified manifestation NEC J11.89
A/H5N1 (*see also* Influenza, due to, identified novel
    influenza A virus) J09.X2
avian (*see also* Influenza, due to, identified novel in-
    fluenza A virus) J09.X2
bird (*see also* Influenza, due to, identified novel influen-
    za A virus) J09.X2
due to
  avian (*see also* Influenza, due to, identified novel
      influenza A virus) J09.X2
  identified influenza virus NEC J10.1
    with
      digestive manifestations J10.2
      encephalopathy J10.81
      enteritis J10.2
      gastroenteritis J10.2
      gastrointestinal manifestations J10.2
      laryngitis J10.1
      myocarditis J10.82
      otitis media J10.83
      pharyngitis J10.1
      pneumonia (unspecified type) J10.00
        with same identified influenza virus
          J10.01
        specified type NEC J10.08
      respiratory manifestations NEC J10.1
      specified manifestation NEC J10.89
  identified novel influenza A virus J09.X2
    with
      digestive manifestations J09.X3
      encephalopathy J09.X9
      enteritis J09.X3
      gastroenteritis J09.X3
      gastrointestinal manifestations J09.X3
      laryngitis J09.X2
      myocarditis J09.X9
      otitis media J09.X9
      pharyngitis J09.X2
      pneumonia J09.X1
      respiratory manifestations NEC J09.X2
      specified manifestation NEC J09.X9
      upper respiratory symptoms J09.X2
  novel (2009) H1N1 influenza (*see also* Influenza, due
      to, identified influenza virus NEC) J10.1
  novel influenza A/H1N1 (*see also* Influenza, due to,
      identified influenza virus NEC) J10.1
  of other animal origin, not bird or swine (*see also* In-
      fluenza, due to, identified novel influenza A
      virus) J09.X2
  swine (viruses that normally cause infections in pigs)
      (*see also* Influenza, due to, identified novel in-
      fluenza A virus) J09.X2
Influenzal — *see* Influenza
Influenza-like disease — *see* Influenza
Infraction, Freiberg's (metatarsal head) — *see* Osteo-
    chondrosis, juvenile, metatarsus
Infraeruption of tooth (teeth) M26.34
Infusion complication, misadventure, or reaction
    — *see* Complications, infusion
Ingestion
  chemical — *see* Table of Drugs and Chemicals, by
      substance, poisoning
  drug or medicament
    correct substance properly administered — *see*
        Table of Drugs and Chemicals, by drug, ad-
        verse effect
    overdose or wrong substance given or taken —
        see Table of Drugs and Chemicals, by drug,
        poisoning
  foreign body — *see* Foreign body, alimentary tract
  tularemia A21.3
Ingrowing
  hair (beard) L73.1
  nail (finger) (toe) L60.0
Inguinal (*see also* condition)
  testicle Q53.9
    bilateral Q53.212
    unilateral Q53.112
Inhalant-induced
  anxiety disorder F18.980
  depressive disorder F18.94
  major neurocognitive disorder F18.97
  mild neurocognitive disorder F18.988
  psychotic disorder F18.959
Inhalation
  anthrax A22.1

Inhalation — *continued*
  flame T27.3 ☑
  food or foreign body — *see* Foreign body, by site
  gases, fumes, or vapors NEC T59.9- ☑
    specified agent — *see* Table of Drugs and Chemi-
        cals, by substance
  liquid or vomitus — *see* Asphyxia
  meconium (newborn) P24.00
    with
      with respiratory symptoms P24.01
      pneumonia (pneumonitis) P24.01
  mucus — *see* Asphyxia, mucus
  oil or gasoline (causing suffocation) — *see* Foreign
      body, by site
  smoke J70.5
    due to chemicals, gases, fumes and vapors J68.9
  steam — *see* Toxicity, vapors
  stomach contents or secretions — *see* Foreign body,
      by site
    due to anesthesia (general) (local) or other sedation
        T88.59 ☑
      in labor and delivery O74.0
      in pregnancy O29.01- ☑
      postpartum, puerperal O89.01
Inhibition, orgasm
  female F52.31
  male F52.32
Inhibitor, systemic lupus erythematosus (presence
    of) D68.62
Iniencephalus, iniencephaly Q00.2
Injection, traumatic jet (air) (industrial) (water) (paint
    or dye) T70.4 ☑
Injury (*see also* specified injury type) T14.90 ☑
  abdomen, abdominal S39.91 ☑
    blood vessel — *see* Injury, blood vessel, abdomen
    cavity — *see* Injury, intra-abdominal
    contusion S30.1 ☑
    internal — *see* Injury, intra-abdominal
    intra-abdominal organ — *see* Injury, intra-abdom-
        inal
    nerve — *see* Injury, nerve, abdomen
    open — *see* Wound, open, abdomen
    specified NEC S39.81 ☑
    superficial — *see* Injury, superficial, abdomen
  Achilles tendon S86.00- ☑
    laceration S86.02- ☑
    specified type NEC S86.09- ☑
    strain S86.01- ☑
  acoustic, resulting in deafness — *see* Injury, nerve,
      acoustic
  adrenal (gland) S37.819 ☑
    contusion S37.812 ☑
    laceration S37.813 ☑
    specified type NEC S37.818 ☑
  alveolar (process) S09.93 ☑
  ankle S99.91- ☑
    contusion — *see* Contusion, ankle
    dislocation — *see* Dislocation, ankle
    fracture — *see* Fracture, ankle
    nerve — *see* Injury, nerve, ankle
    open — *see* Wound, open, ankle
    specified type NEC S99.81- ☑
    sprain — *see* Sprain, ankle
    superficial — *see* Injury, superficial, ankle
  anterior chamber, eye — *see* Injury, eye, specified site
      NEC
  anus — *see* Injury, abdomen
  aorta (thoracic) S25.00 ☑
    abdominal S35.00 ☑
      laceration (minor) (superficial) S35.01 ☑
        major S35.02 ☑
      specified type NEC S35.09 ☑
    laceration (minor) (superficial) S25.01 ☑
      major S25.02 ☑
    specified type NEC S25.09 ☑
  arm (upper) S49.9- ☑
    blood vessel — *see* Injury, blood vessel, arm
    contusion — *see* Contusion, arm, upper
    fracture — *see* Fracture, humerus
    lower — *see* Injury, forearm
    muscle — *see* Injury, muscle, shoulder
    nerve — *see* Injury, nerve, arm
    open — *see* Wound, open, arm
    specified type NEC S49.8- ☑
    superficial — *see* Injury, superficial, arm

Injury — *continued*
  artery (complicating trauma) (*see also* Injury, blood
      vessel, by site)
    cerebral or meningeal — *see* Injury, intracranial
  auditory canal (external) (meatus) S09.91 ☑
  auricle, auris, ear S09.91 ☑
  axilla — *see* Injury, shoulder
  back — *see* Injury, back, lower
  bile duct S36.13 ☑
  birth (*see also* Birth, injury) P15.9
  bladder (sphincter) S37.20 ☑
    at delivery O71.5
    contusion S37.22 ☑
    laceration S37.23 ☑
    obstetrical trauma O71.5
    specified type NEC S37.29 ☑
  blast (air) (hydraulic) (immersion) (underwater) NEC
      T14.8 ☑
    acoustic nerve trauma — *see* Injury, nerve, acoustic
    bladder — *see* Injury, bladder
    brain — *see* Concussion
    colon — *see* Injury, intestine, large
    ear (primary) S09.31- ☑
      secondary S09.39- ☑
    generalized T70.8 ☑
    lung — *see* Injury, intrathoracic, lung
    multiple body organs T70.8 ☑
    peritoneum S36.81 ☑
    rectum S36.61 ☑
    retroperitoneum S36.898 ☑
    small intestine S36.419 ☑
      duodenum S36.410 ☑
      specified site NEC S36.418 ☑
    specified
      intra-abdominal organ NEC S36.898 ☑
      pelvic organ NEC S37.899 ☑
  blood vessel NEC T14.8 ☑
    abdomen S35.9 ☑
      aorta — *see* Injury, aorta, abdominal
      celiac artery — *see* Injury, blood vessel, celiac
          artery
      iliac vessel — *see* Injury, blood vessel, iliac
      laceration S35.91 ☑
      mesenteric vessel — *see* Injury, mesenteric
      portal vein — *see* Injury, blood vessel, portal
          vein
      renal vessel — *see* Injury, blood vessel, renal
      specified vessel NEC S35.8X- ☑
      splenic vessel — *see* Injury, blood vessel,
          splenic
      vena cava — *see* Injury, vena cava, inferior
    ankle — *see* Injury, blood vessel, foot
    aorta (abdominal) (thoracic) — *see* Injury, aorta
    arm (upper) NEC S45.90- ☑
      forearm — *see* Injury, blood vessel, forearm
      laceration S45.91- ☑
      specified
        site NEC S45.80- ☑
          laceration S45.81- ☑
          specified type NEC S45.89- ☑
        type NEC S45.99- ☑
      superficial vein S45.30- ☑
        laceration S45.31- ☑
        specified type NEC S45.39- ☑
    axillary
      artery S45.00- ☑
        laceration S45.01- ☑
        specified type NEC S45.09- ☑
      vein S45.20- ☑
        laceration S45.21- ☑
        specified type NEC S45.29- ☑
    azygos vein — *see* Injury, blood vessel, thoracic,
        specified site NEC
    brachial
      artery S45.10- ☑
        laceration S45.11- ☑
        specified type NEC S45.19- ☑
      vein S45.20- ☑
        laceration S45.219 ☑
        specified type NEC S45.29- ☑
    carotid artery (common) (external) (internal, ex-
        tracranial) S15.00- ☑
      internal, intracranial S06.8- ☑
      laceration (minor) (superficial) S15.01- ☑
        major S15.02- ☑
      specified type NEC S15.09- ☑

☑ **Additional Character Required — Refer to the Tabular List for Character Selection**   ⟳ **Subterms under main terms may continue to next column or page**

Injury — *continued*
  blood vessel — *continued*
    celiac artery S35.219 ☑
      branch S35.299 ☑
        laceration (minor) (superficial) S35.291 ☑
          major S35.292 ☑
        specified NEC S35.298 ☑
      laceration (minor) (superficial) S35.211 ☑
        major S35.212 ☑
      specified type NEC S35.218 ☑
    cerebral — *see* Injury, intracranial
    deep plantar — *see* Injury, blood vessel, plantar artery
    digital (hand) — *see* Injury, blood vessel, finger
    dorsal
      artery (foot) S95.00- ☑
        laceration S95.01- ☑
        specified type NEC S95.09- ☑
      vein (foot) S95.20- ☑
        laceration S95.21- ☑
        specified type NEC S95.29- ☑
    due to accidental laceration during procedure — *see* Laceration, accidental complicating surgery
    extremity — *see* Injury, blood vessel, limb
    femoral
      artery (common) (superficial) S75.00- ☑
        laceration (minor) (superficial) S75.01- ☑
          major S75.02- ☑
        specified type NEC S75.09- ☑
      vein (hip level) (thigh level) S75.10- ☑
        laceration (minor) (superficial) S75.11- ☑
          major S75.12- ☑
        specified type NEC S75.19- ☑
    finger S65.50- ☑
      index S65.50- ☑
        laceration S65.51- ☑
        specified type NEC S65.59- ☑
      laceration S65.51- ☑
      little S65.50- ☑
        laceration S65.51- ☑
        specified type NEC S65.59- ☑
      middle S65.50- ☑
        laceration S65.51- ☑
        specified type NEC S65.59- ☑
      specified type NEC S65.59- ☑
      thumb — *see* Injury, blood vessel, thumb
    foot S95.90- ☑
      dorsal
        artery — *see* Injury, blood vessel, dorsal, artery
        vein — *see* Injury, blood vessel, dorsal, vein
      laceration S95.91- ☑
      plantar artery — *see* Injury, blood vessel, plantar artery
      specified
        site NEC S95.80- ☑
          laceration S95.81- ☑
          specified type NEC S95.89- ☑
        specified type NEC S95.99- ☑
    forearm S55.90- ☑
      laceration S55.91- ☑
      radial artery — *see* Injury, blood vessel, radial artery
      specified
        site NEC S55.80- ☑
          laceration S55.81- ☑
          specified type NEC S55.89- ☑
        type NEC S55.99- ☑
      ulnar artery — *see* Injury, blood vessel, ulnar artery
      vein S55.20- ☑
        laceration S55.21- ☑
        specified type NEC S55.29- ☑
    gastric
      artery — *see* Injury, mesenteric, artery, branch
      vein — *see* Injury, blood vessel, abdomen
    gastroduodenal artery — *see* Injury, mesenteric, artery, branch
    greater saphenous vein (lower leg level) S85.30- ☑
      hip (and thigh) level S75.20- ☑
        laceration (minor) (superficial) S75.21- ☑
          major S75.22- ☑
        specified type NEC S75.29- ☑
      laceration S85.31- ☑
      specified type NEC S85.39- ☑

Injury — *continued*
  blood vessel — *continued*
    hand (level) S65.90- ☑
      finger — *see* Injury, blood vessel, finger
      laceration S65.91- ☑
      palmar arch — *see* Injury, blood vessel, palmar arch
      radial artery — *see* Injury, blood vessel, radial artery, hand
      specified
        site NEC S65.80- ☑
          laceration S65.81- ☑
          specified type NEC S65.89- ☑
        type NEC S65.99- ☑
      thumb — *see* Injury, blood vessel, thumb
      ulnar artery — *see* Injury, blood vessel, ulnar artery, hand
    head S09.0 ☑
      intracranial — *see* Injury, intracranial
      multiple S09.0 ☑
    hepatic
      artery — *see* Injury, mesenteric, artery
      vein — *see* Injury, vena cava, inferior
    hip S75.90- ☑
      femoral artery — *see* Injury, blood vessel, femoral, artery
      femoral vein — *see* Injury, blood vessel, femoral, vein
      greater saphenous vein — *see* Injury, blood vessel, greater saphenous, hip level
      laceration S75.91- ☑
      specified
        site NEC S75.80- ☑
          laceration S75.81- ☑
          specified type NEC S75.89- ☑
        type NEC S75.99- ☑
    hypogastric (artery) (vein) — *see* Injury, blood vessel, iliac
    iliac S35.5- ☑
      artery S35.51- ☑
      specified vessel NEC S35.5- ☑
      uterine vessel — *see* Injury, blood vessel, uterine
      vein S35.51- ☑
    innominate — *see* Injury, blood vessel, thoracic, innominate
    intercostal (artery) (vein) — *see* Injury, blood vessel, thoracic, intercostal
    jugular vein (external) S15.20- ☑
      internal S15.30- ☑
        laceration (minor) (superficial) S15.31- ☑
          major S15.32- ☑
        specified type NEC S15.39- ☑
      laceration (minor) (superficial) S15.21- ☑
        major S15.22- ☑
      specified type NEC S15.29- ☑
    leg (level) (lower) S85.90- ☑
      greater saphenous — *see* Injury, blood vessel, greater saphenous
      laceration S85.91- ☑
      lesser saphenous — *see* Injury, blood vessel, lesser saphenous
      peroneal artery — *see* Injury, blood vessel, peroneal artery
      popliteal
        artery — *see* Injury, blood vessel, popliteal, artery
        vein — *see* Injury, blood vessel, popliteal, vein
      specified
        site NEC S85.80- ☑
          laceration S85.81- ☑
          specified type NEC S85.89- ☑
        type NEC S85.99- ☑
      thigh — *see* Injury, blood vessel, hip
      tibial artery — *see* Injury, blood vessel, tibial artery
    lesser saphenous vein (lower leg level) S85.40- ☑
      laceration S85.41- ☑
      specified type NEC S85.49- ☑
    limb
      lower — *see* Injury, blood vessel, leg
      upper — *see* Injury, blood vessel, arm
    lower back — *see* Injury, blood vessel, abdomen
      specified NEC — *see* Injury, blood vessel, abdomen, specified, site NEC

Injury — *continued*
  blood vessel — *continued*
    mammary (artery) (vein) — *see* Injury, blood vessel, thoracic, specified site NEC
    mesenteric (inferior) (superior)
      artery — *see* Injury, mesenteric, artery
      vein — *see* Injury, blood vessel, mesenteric, vein
    neck S15.9
      specified site NEC S15.8 ☑
    ovarian (artery) (vein) — *see* subcategory S35.8 ☑
    palmar arch (superficial) S65.20- ☑
      deep S65.30- ☑
        laceration S65.31- ☑
        specified type NEC S65.39- ☑
      laceration S65.21- ☑
      specified type NEC S65.29- ☑
    pelvis — *see* Injury, blood vessel, abdomen
      specified NEC — *see* Injury, blood vessel, abdomen, specified, site NEC
    peroneal artery S85.20- ☑
      laceration S85.21- ☑
      specified type NEC S85.29- ☑
    plantar artery (deep) (foot) S95.10- ☑
      laceration S95.11- ☑
      specified type NEC S95.19- ☑
    popliteal
      artery S85.00- ☑
        laceration S85.01- ☑
        specified type NEC S85.09- ☑
      vein S85.50- ☑
        laceration S85.51- ☑
        specified type NEC S85.59- ☑
    portal vein S35.319 ☑
      laceration S35.311 ☑
      specified type NEC S35.318 ☑
    precerebral — *see* Injury, blood vessel, neck
    pulmonary (artery) (vein) — *see* Injury, blood vessel, thoracic, pulmonary
    radial artery (forearm level) S55.10- ☑
      hand and wrist (level) S65.10- ☑
        laceration S65.11- ☑
        specified type NEC S65.19- ☑
      laceration S55.11- ☑
      specified type NEC S55.19- ☑
    renal
      artery S35.40- ☑
        laceration S35.41- ☑
        specified NEC S35.49- ☑
      vein S35.40- ☑
        laceration S35.41- ☑
        specified NEC S35.49- ☑
    saphenous vein (greater) (lower leg level) — *see* Injury, blood vessel, greater saphenous
      hip and thigh level — *see* Injury, blood vessel, greater saphenous, hip level
      lesser — *see* Injury, blood vessel, lesser saphenous
    shoulder
      specified NEC — *see* Injury, blood vessel, arm, specified site NEC
      superficial vein — *see* Injury, blood vessel, arm, superficial vein
    specified NEC T14.8 ☑
    splenic
      artery — *see* Injury, blood vessel, celiac artery, branch
      vein S35.329 ☑
        laceration S35.321 ☑
        specified NEC S35.328 ☑
    subclavian — *see* Injury, blood vessel, thoracic, innominate
    thigh — *see* Injury, blood vessel, hip
    thoracic S25.90 ☑
      aorta S25.00 ☑
        laceration (minor) (superficial) S25.01 ☑
          major S25.02 ☑
        specified type NEC S25.09 ☑
      azygos vein — *see* Injury, blood vessel, thoracic, specified, site NEC
      innominate
        artery S25.10- ☑
          laceration (minor) (superficial) S25.11- ☑
            major S25.12- ☑
          specified type NEC S25.19- ☑

Injury — *continued*
blood vessel — *continued*
thoracic — *continued*
innominate — *continued*
vein S25.30- ☑
laceration (minor) (superficial)
S25.31- ☑
major S25.32- ☑
specified type NEC S25.39- ☑
intercostal S25.50- ☑
laceration S25.51- ☑
specified type NEC S25.59- ☑
laceration S25.91 ☑
mammary vessel — *see* Injury, blood vessel, thoracic, specified, site NEC
pulmonary S25.40- ☑
laceration (minor) (superficial) S25.41- ☑
major S25.42- ☑
specified type NEC S25.49- ☑
specified
site NEC S25.80- ☑
laceration S25.81 ☑
specified type NEC S25.89 ☑
type NEC S25.99 ☑
subclavian — *see* Injury, blood vessel, thoracic, innominate
vena cava (superior) S25.20 ☑
laceration (minor) (superficial) S25.21 ☑
major S25.22 ☑
specified type NEC S25.29 ☑
thumb S65.40- ☑
laceration S65.41- ☑
specified type NEC S65.49- ☑
tibial artery S85.10- ☑
anterior S85.13- ☑
laceration S85.14- ☑
specified injury NEC S85.15- ☑
laceration S85.11- ☑
posterior S85.16- ☑
laceration S85.17- ☑
specified injury NEC S85.18- ☑
specified injury NEC S85.12- ☑
ulnar artery (forearm level) S55.00- ☑
hand and wrist (level) S65.00- ☑
laceration S65.01- ☑
specified type NEC S65.09- ☑
laceration S55.01- ☑
specified type NEC S55.09- ☑
upper arm (level) — *see* Injury, blood vessel, arm
superficial vein — *see* Injury, blood vessel, arm, superficial vein
uterine S35.5- ☑
artery S35.53- ☑
vein S35.53- ☑
vena cava — *see* Injury, vena cava
vertebral artery S15.10- ☑
laceration (minor) (superficial) S15.11- ☑
major S15.12- ☑
specified type NEC S15.19- ☑
wrist (level) — *see* Injury, blood vessel, hand
brachial plexus S14.3 ☑
newborn P14.3
brain (traumatic) S06.9- ☑
diffuse (axonal) S06.2X- ☑
focal S06.30- ☑
brainstem S06.38- ☑
breast NOS S29.9 ☑
broad ligament — *see* Injury, pelvic organ, specified site NEC
bronchus, bronchi — *see* Injury, intrathoracic, bronchus
brow S09.90 ☑
buttock S39.92 ☑
canthus, eye S05.90 ☑
cardiac plexus — *see* Injury, nerve, thorax, sympathetic
cauda equina S34.3 ☑
cavernous sinus — *see* Injury, intracranial
cecum — *see* Injury, colon
celiac ganglion or plexus — *see* Injury, nerve, lumbosacral, sympathetic
cerebellum — *see* Injury, intracranial
cerebral — *see* Injury, intracranial
cervix (uteri) — *see* Injury, uterus
cheek (wall) S09.93 ☑
chest — *see* Injury, thorax

Injury — *continued*
childbirth (newborn) (*see also* Birth, injury)
maternal NEC O71.9
chin S09.93 ☑
choroid (eye) — *see* Injury, eye, specified site NEC
clitoris S39.94 ☑
coccyx (*see also* Injury, back, lower)
complicating delivery O71.6
colon — *see* Injury, intestine, large
common bile duct — *see* Injury, liver
conjunctiva (superficial) — *see* Injury, eye, conjunctiva
conus medullaris — *see* Injury, spinal, sacral
cord
spermatic (pelvic region) S37.898 ☑
scrotal region S39.848 ☑
spinal — *see* Injury, spinal cord, by region
cornea — *see* Injury, eye, specified site NEC
abrasion — *see* Injury, eye, cornea, abrasion
cortex (cerebral) (*see also* Injury, intracranial)
visual — *see* Injury, nerve, optic
costal region NEC S29.9 ☑
costochondral NEC S29.9 ☑
cranial
cavity — *see* Injury, intracranial
nerve — *see* Injury, nerve, cranial
crushing — *see* Crush
cutaneous sensory nerve
cystic duct — *see* Injury, liver
deep tissue — *see* Contusion, by site
meaning pressure ulcer — *see* Ulcer, pressure, unstageable, by site
delivery (newborn) P15.9
maternal NEC O71.9
Descemet's membrane — *see* Injury, eyeball, penetrating
diaphragm — *see* Injury, intracranial, diaphragm
duodenum — *see* Injury, intestine, small, duodenum
ear (auricle) (external) (canal) S09.91 ☑
abrasion — *see* Abrasion, ear
bite — *see* Bite, ear
blister — *see* Blister, ear
bruise — *see* Contusion, ear
contusion — *see* Contusion, ear
external constriction — *see* Constriction, external, ear
hematoma — *see* Hematoma, ear
inner — *see* Injury, ear, middle
laceration — *see* Laceration, ear
middle S09.30- ☑
blast — *see* Injury, blast, ear
specified NEC S09.39- ☑
puncture — *see* Puncture, ear
superficial — *see* Injury, superficial, ear
eighth cranial nerve (acoustic or auditory) — *see* Injury, nerve, acoustic
elbow S59.90- ☑
contusion — *see* Contusion, elbow
dislocation — *see* Dislocation, elbow
fracture — *see* Fracture, ulna, upper end
open — *see* Wound, open, elbow
specified NEC S59.80- ☑
sprain — *see* Sprain, elbow
superficial — *see* Injury, superficial, elbow
eleventh cranial nerve (accessory) — *see* Injury, nerve, accessory
epididymis S39.94 ☑
epigastric region S39.91 ☑
epiglottis NEC S19.89 ☑
esophageal plexus — *see* Injury, nerve, thorax, sympathetic
esophagus (thoracic part) (*see also* Injury, intrathoracic, esophagus)
cervical NEC S19.85 ☑
eustachian tube S09.30 ☑
eye S05.9- ☑
avulsion S05.7- ☑
ball — *see* Injury, eyeball
conjunctiva S05.0- ☑
cornea
abrasion S05.0- ☑
laceration S05.3- ☑
with prolapse S05.2- ☑
lacrimal apparatus S05.8X- ☑
orbit penetration S05.4- ☑
specified site NEC S05.8X- ☑
eyeball S05.8X- ☑

Injury — *continued*
eyeball — *continued*
contusion S05.1- ☑
penetrating S05.6- ☑
with
foreign body S05.5- ☑
prolapse or loss of intraocular tissue S05.2- ☑
without prolapse or loss of intraocular tissue S05.3- ☑
specified type NEC S05.8- ☑
eyebrow S09.93 ☑
eyelid S09.93 ☑
abrasion — *see* Abrasion, eyelid
contusion — *see* Contusion, eyelid
open — *see* Wound, open, eyelid
face S09.93 ☑
fallopian tube S37.509 ☑
bilateral S37.502 ☑
blast injury S37.512 ☑
contusion S37.522 ☑
laceration S37.532 ☑
specified type NEC S37.592 ☑
blast injury (primary) S37.519 ☑
bilateral S37.512 ☑
secondary — *see* Injury, fallopian tube, specified type NEC
unilateral S37.511 ☑
contusion S37.529 ☑
bilateral S37.522 ☑
unilateral S37.521 ☑
laceration S37.539 ☑
bilateral S37.532 ☑
unilateral S37.531 ☑
specified type NEC S37.599 ☑
bilateral S37.592 ☑
unilateral S37.591 ☑
unilateral S37.501 ☑
blast injury S37.511 ☑
contusion S37.521 ☑
laceration S37.531 ☑
specified type NEC S37.591 ☑
fascia — *see* Injury, muscle
fifth cranial nerve (trigeminal) — *see* Injury, nerve, trigeminal
finger (nail) S69.9- ☑
blood vessel — *see* Injury, blood vessel, finger
contusion — *see* Contusion, finger
dislocation — *see* Dislocation, finger
fracture — *see* Fracture, finger
muscle — *see* Injury, muscle, finger
nerve — *see* Injury, nerve, digital, finger
open — *see* Wound, open, finger
specified NEC S69.8- ☑
sprain — *see* Sprain, finger
superficial — *see* Injury, superficial, finger
first cranial nerve (olfactory) — *see* Injury, nerve, olfactory
flank — *see* Injury, abdomen
foot S99.92- ☑
blood vessel — *see* Injury, blood vessel, foot
contusion — *see* Contusion, foot
dislocation — *see* Dislocation, foot
fracture — *see* Fracture, foot
muscle — *see* Injury, muscle, foot
open — *see* Wound, open, foot
specified type NEC S99.82- ☑
sprain — *see* Sprain, foot
superficial — *see* Injury, superficial, foot
forceps NOS P15.9
forearm S59.91- ☑
blood vessel — *see* Injury, blood vessel, forearm
contusion — *see* Contusion, forearm
fracture — *see* Fracture, forearm
muscle — *see* Injury, muscle, forearm
nerve — *see* Injury, nerve, forearm
open — *see* Wound, open, forearm
specified NEC S59.81- ☑
superficial — *see* Injury, superficial, forearm
forehead S09.90 ☑
fourth cranial nerve (trochlear) — *see* Injury, nerve, trochlear
gallbladder S36.129 ☑
contusion S36.122 ☑
laceration S36.123 ☑
specified NEC S36.128 ☑

☑ **Additional Character Required** — Refer to the Tabular List for Character Selection   ▽ **Subterms under main terms may continue to next column or page**

Injury — *continued*
  ganglion
    celiac, coeliac — *see* Injury, nerve, lumbosacral, sympathetic
    gasserian — *see* Injury, nerve, trigeminal
    stellate — *see* Injury, nerve, thorax, sympathetic
    thoracic sympathetic — *see* Injury, nerve, thorax, sympathetic
  gasserian ganglion — *see* Injury, nerve, trigeminal
  gastric artery — *see* Injury, blood vessel, celiac artery, branch
  gastroduodenal artery — *see* Injury, blood vessel, celiac artery, branch
  gastrointestinal tract — *see* Injury, intra-abdominal
    with open wound into abdominal cavity — *see* Wound, open, with penetration into peritoneal cavity
    colon — *see* Injury, intestine, large
    rectum — *see* Injury, intestine, large, rectum
      with open wound into abdominal cavity S36.61 ☑
    small intestine — *see* Injury, intestine, small
    specified site NEC — *see* Injury, intra-abdominal, specified, site NEC
    stomach — *see* Injury, stomach
  genital organ(s)
    external S39.94 ☑
      specified NEC S39.848 ☑
    internal S37.90 ☑
      fallopian tube — *see* Injury, fallopian tube
      ovary — *see* Injury, ovary
      prostate — *see* Injury, prostate
      seminal vesicle — *see* Injury, pelvis, organ, specified site NEC
      uterus — *see* Injury, uterus
      vas deferens — *see* Injury, pelvis, organ, specified site NEC
    obstetrical trauma O71.9
  gland
    lacrimal laceration — *see* Injury, eye, specified site NEC
    salivary S09.93 ☑
    thyroid NEC S19.84 ☑
  globe (eye) S05.90 ☑
    specified NEC S05.8X- ☑
  groin — *see* Injury, abdomen
  gum S09.90 ☑
  hand S69.9- ☑
    blood vessel — *see* Injury, blood vessel, hand
    contusion — *see* Contusion, hand
    fracture — *see* Fracture, hand
    muscle — *see* Injury, muscle, hand
    nerve — *see* Injury, nerve, hand
    open — *see* Wound, open, hand
    specified NEC S69.8- ☑
    sprain — *see* Sprain, hand
    superficial — *see* Injury, superficial, hand
  head S09.90 ☑
    with loss of consciousness S06.9- ☑
    specified NEC S09.8 ☑
  heart S26.90 ☑
    with hemopericardium S26.00 ☑
      contusion S26.01 ☑
      laceration (mild) S26.020 ☑
        major S26.022 ☑
        moderate S26.021 ☑
      specified type NEC S26.09 ☑
    without hemopericardium S26.10 ☑
      contusion S26.11 ☑
      laceration S26.12 ☑
      specified type NEC S26.19 ☑
    contusion S26.91 ☑
    laceration S26.92 ☑
    specified type NEC S26.99 ☑
  heel — *see* Injury, foot
  hepatic
    artery — *see* Injury, blood vessel, celiac artery, branch
    duct — *see* Injury, liver
    vein — *see* Injury, vena cava, inferior
  hip S79.91- ☑
    blood vessel — *see* Injury, blood vessel, hip
    contusion — *see* Contusion, hip
    dislocation — *see* Dislocation, hip
    fracture — *see* Fracture, femur, neck
    muscle — *see* Injury, muscle, hip

Injury — *continued*
  hip — *continued*
    nerve — *see* Injury, nerve, hip
    open — *see* Wound, open, hip
    specified NEC S79.81- ☑
    sprain — *see* Sprain, hip
    superficial — *see* Injury, superficial, hip
  hymen S39.94 ☑
  hypogastric
    blood vessel — *see* Injury, blood vessel, iliac
    plexus — *see* Injury, nerve, lumbosacral, sympathetic
  ileum — *see* Injury, intestine, small
  iliac region S39.91 ☑
  instrumental (during surgery) — *see* Laceration, accidental complicating surgery
    birth injury — *see* Birth, injury
    nonsurgical — *see* Injury, by site
    obstetrical O71.9
      bladder O71.5
      cervix O71.3
      high vaginal O71.4
      perineal NOS O70.9
      urethra O71.5
      uterus O71.5
        with rupture or perforation O71.1
  internal T14.8 ☑
    aorta — *see* Injury, aorta
    bladder (sphincter) — *see* Injury, bladder
      with
        ectopic or molar pregnancy O08.6
        following ectopic or molar pregnancy O08.6
        obstetrical trauma O71.5
    bronchus, bronchi — *see* Injury, intrathoracic, bronchus
    cecum — *see* Injury, intestine, large
    cervix (uteri) (*see also* Injury, uterus)
      with ectopic or molar pregnancy O08.6
      following ectopic or molar pregnancy O08.6
      obstetrical trauma O71.3
    chest — *see* Injury, intrathoracic
    gastrointestinal tract — *see* Injury, intra-abdominal
    heart — *see* Injury, heart
    intestine NEC — *see* Injury, intestine
    intrauterine — *see* Injury, uterus
    mesentery — *see* Injury, intra-abdominal, specified, site NEC
    pelvis, pelvic (organ) S37.90 ☑
      following ectopic or molar pregnancy (subsequent episode) O08.6
      obstetrical trauma NEC O71.5
        rupture or perforation O71.1
      specified NEC S39.83 ☑
    rectum — *see* Injury, intestine, large, rectum
    stomach — *see* Injury, stomach
    ureter — *see* Injury, ureter
    urethra (sphincter) following ectopic or molar pregnancy O08.6
    uterus — *see* Injury, uterus
  interscapular area — *see* Injury, thorax
  intestine
    large S36.509 ☑
      ascending (right) S36.500 ☑
        blast injury (primary) S36.510 ☑
          secondary S36.590 ☑
        contusion S36.520 ☑
        laceration S36.530 ☑
        specified type NEC S36.590 ☑
      blast injury (primary) S36.519 ☑
        ascending (right) S36.510 ☑
        descending (left) S36.512 ☑
        rectum S36.61 ☑
        sigmoid S36.513 ☑
        specified site NEC S36.518 ☑
        transverse S36.511 ☑
      contusion S36.529 ☑
        ascending (right) S36.520 ☑
        descending (left) S36.522 ☑
        rectum S36.62 ☑
        sigmoid S36.523 ☑
        specified site NEC S36.528 ☑
        transverse S36.521 ☑
      descending (left) S36.502 ☑
        blast injury (primary) S36.512 ☑
          secondary S36.592 ☑
        contusion S36.522 ☑
        laceration S36.532 ☑

Injury — *continued*
  intestine — *continued*
    large — *continued*
      descending — *continued*
        specified type NEC S36.592 ☑
      laceration S36.539 ☑
        ascending (right) S36.530 ☑
        descending (left) S36.532 ☑
        rectum S36.63 ☑
        sigmoid S36.533 ☑
        specified site NEC S36.538 ☑
        transverse S36.531 ☑
      rectum S36.60 ☑
        blast injury (primary) S36.61 ☑
          secondary S36.69 ☑
        contusion S36.62 ☑
        laceration S36.63 ☑
        specified type NEC S36.69 ☑
      sigmoid S36.503 ☑
        blast injury (primary) S36.513 ☑
          secondary S36.593 ☑
        contusion S36.523 ☑
        laceration S36.533 ☑
        specified type NEC S36.593 ☑
      specified
        site NEC S36.508 ☑
          blast injury (primary) S36.518 ☑
            secondary S36.598 ☑
          contusion S36.528 ☑
          laceration S36.538 ☑
          specified type NEC S36.598 ☑
        type NEC S36.599 ☑
          ascending (right) S36.590 ☑
          descending (left) S36.592 ☑
          rectum S36.69 ☑
          sigmoid S36.593 ☑
          specified site NEC S36.598 ☑
          transverse S36.591 ☑
      transverse S36.501 ☑
        blast injury (primary) S36.511 ☑
          secondary S36.591 ☑
        contusion S36.521 ☑
        laceration S36.531 ☑
        specified type NEC S36.591 ☑
    small S36.409 ☑
      blast injury (primary) S36.419 ☑
        duodenum S36.410 ☑
        secondary S36.499 ☑
          duodenum S36.490 ☑
          specified site NEC S36.498 ☑
        specified site NEC S36.418 ☑
      contusion S36.429 ☑
        duodenum S36.420 ☑
        specified site NEC S36.428 ☑
      duodenum S36.400 ☑
        blast injury (primary) S36.410 ☑
          secondary S36.490 ☑
        contusion S36.420 ☑
        laceration S36.430 ☑
        specified NEC S36.490 ☑
      laceration S36.439 ☑
        duodenum S36.430 ☑
        specified site NEC S36.438 ☑
      specified
        site NEC S36.408 ☑
        type NEC S36.499 ☑
          duodenum S36.490 ☑
          specified site NEC S36.498 ☑
  intra-abdominal S36.90 ☑
    adrenal gland — *see* Injury, adrenal gland
    bladder — *see* Injury, bladder
    colon — *see* Injury, intestine, large
    contusion S36.92 ☑
    fallopian tube — *see* Injury, fallopian tube
    gallbladder — *see* Injury, gallbladder
    intestine — *see* Injury, intestine
    kidney — *see* Injury, kidney
    laceration S36.93 ☑
    liver — *see* Injury, liver
    ovary — *see* Injury, ovary
    pancreas — *see* Injury, pancreas
    pelvic NOS S37.90 ☑
    peritoneum — *see* Injury, intra-abdominal, specified, site NEC
    prostate — *see* Injury, prostate
    rectum — *see* Injury, intestine, large, rectum

Index

Injury — Injury

Injury — *continued*
  intra-abdominal — *continued*
    retroperitoneum — *see* Injury, intra-abdominal, specified, site NEC
    seminal vesicle — *see* Injury, pelvis, organ, specified site NEC
    small intestine — *see* Injury, intestine, small
    specified
      pelvic S37.90 ☑
        specified
          site NEC S37.899 ☑
            specified type NEC S37.898 ☑
          type NEC S37.99 ☑
      site NEC S36.899 ☑
        contusion S36.892 ☑
        laceration S36.893 ☑
        specified type NEC S36.898 ☑
      type NEC S36.99 ☑
    spleen — *see* Injury, spleen
    stomach — *see* Injury, stomach
    ureter — *see* Injury, ureter
    urethra — *see* Injury, urethra
    uterus — *see* Injury, uterus
    vas deferens — *see* Injury, pelvis, organ, specified site NEC
  intracranial (traumatic) S06.9- ☑
    cerebellar hemorrhage, traumatic — *see* Injury, intracranial, focal
    cerebral edema, traumatic S06.1X- ☑
      diffuse S06.1X- ☑
      focal S06.1X- ☑
    diffuse (axonal) S06.2X- ☑
    epidural hemorrhage (traumatic) S06.4X- ☑
    focal brain injury S06.30- ☑
      contusion — *see* Contusion, cerebral
      laceration — *see* Laceration, cerebral
    intracerebral hemorrhage, traumatic S06.36- ☑
      left side S06.35- ☑
      right side S06.34- ☑
    subarachnoid hemorrhage, traumatic S06.6X- ☑
    subdural hemorrhage, traumatic S06.5X- ☑
  intraocular — *see* Injury, eyeball, penetrating
  intrathoracic S27.9 ☑
    bronchus S27.409 ☑
      bilateral S27.402 ☑
      blast injury (primary) S27.419 ☑
        bilateral S27.412 ☑
        secondary — *see* Injury, intrathoracic, bronchus, specified type NEC
        unilateral S27.411 ☑
      contusion S27.429 ☑
        bilateral S27.422 ☑
        unilateral S27.421 ☑
      laceration S27.439 ☑
        bilateral S27.432 ☑
        unilateral S27.431 ☑
      specified type NEC S27.499 ☑
        bilateral S27.492 ☑
        unilateral S27.491 ☑
      unilateral S27.401 ☑
    diaphragm S27.809 ☑
      contusion S27.802 ☑
      laceration S27.803 ☑
      specified type NEC S27.808 ☑
    esophagus (thoracic) S27.819 ☑
      contusion S27.812 ☑
      laceration S27.813 ☑
      specified type NEC S27.818 ☑
    heart — *see* Injury, heart
    hemopneumothorax S27.2 ☑
    hemothorax S27.1 ☑
    lung S27.309 ☑
      aspiration J69.0
      bilateral S27.302 ☑
      blast injury (primary) S27.319 ☑
        bilateral S27.312 ☑
        secondary — *see* Injury, intrathoracic, lung, specified type NEC
        unilateral S27.311 ☑
      contusion S27.329 ☑
        bilateral S27.322 ☑
        unilateral S27.321 ☑
      laceration S27.339 ☑
        bilateral S27.332 ☑
        unilateral S27.331 ☑
      specified type NEC S27.399 ☑

Injury — *continued*
  intrathoracic — *continued*
    lung — *continued*
      specified type — *continued*
        bilateral S27.392 ☑
        unilateral S27.391 ☑
      unilateral S27.301 ☑
    pleura S27.60 ☑
      laceration S27.63 ☑
      specified type NEC S27.69 ☑
    pneumothorax S27.0 ☑
    specified organ NEC S27.899 ☑
      contusion S27.892 ☑
      laceration S27.893 ☑
      specified type NEC S27.898 ☑
    thoracic duct — *see* Injury, intrathoracic, specified organ NEC
    thymus gland — *see* Injury, intrathoracic, specified organ NEC
    trachea, thoracic S27.50 ☑
      blast (primary) S27.51 ☑
      contusion S27.52 ☑
      laceration S27.53 ☑
      specified type NEC S27.59 ☑
  iris — *see* Injury, eye, specified site NEC
    penetrating — *see* Injury, eyeball, penetrating
  jaw S09.93 ☑
  jejunum — *see* Injury, intestine, small
  joint NOS T14.8 ☑
    old or residual — *see* Disorder, joint, specified type NEC
  kidney S37.00- ☑
    acute (nontraumatic) N17.9
    contusion — *see* Contusion, kidney
    laceration — *see* Laceration, kidney
    specified NEC S37.09- ☑
  knee S89.9- ☑
    contusion — *see* Contusion, knee
    dislocation — *see* Dislocation, knee
    meniscus (lateral) (medial) — *see* Sprain, knee, specified site NEC
      old injury or tear — *see* Derangement, knee, meniscus, due to old injury
    open — *see* Wound, open, knee
    specified NEC S89.8- ☑
    sprain — *see* Sprain, knee
    superficial — *see* Injury, superficial, knee
  labium (majus) (minus) S39.94 ☑
  labyrinth, ear S09.30- ☑
  lacrimal apparatus, duct, gland, or sac — *see* Injury, eye, specified site NEC
  larynx NEC S19.81 ☑
  leg (lower) S89.9- ☑
    blood vessel — *see* Injury, blood vessel, leg
    contusion — *see* Contusion, leg
    fracture — *see* Fracture, leg
    muscle — *see* Injury, muscle, leg
    nerve — *see* Injury, nerve, leg
    open — *see* Wound, open, leg
    specified NEC S89.8- ☑
    superficial — *see* Injury, superficial, leg
  lens, eye — *see* Injury, eye, specified site NEC
    penetrating — *see* Injury, eyeball, penetrating
  limb NEC T14.8 ☑
  lip S09.93 ☑
  liver S36.119 ☑
    contusion S36.112 ☑
    laceration S36.113 ☑
      major (stellate) S36.116 ☑
      minor S36.114 ☑
      moderate S36.115 ☑
    specified NEC S36.118 ☑
  lower back S39.92 ☑
    specified NEC S39.82 ☑
  lumbar, lumbosacral (region) S39.92 ☑
    plexus — *see* Injury, lumbosacral plexus
  lumbosacral plexus S34.4 ☑
  lung (*see also* Injury, intrathoracic, lung)
    aspiration J69.0
    transfusion-related (TRALI) J95.84
  lymphatic thoracic duct — *see* Injury, intrathoracic, specified organ NEC
  malar region S09.93 ☑
  mastoid region S09.90 ☑
  maxilla S09.93 ☑

Injury — *continued*
  mediastinum — *see* Injury, intrathoracic, specified organ NEC
  membrane, brain — *see* Injury, intracranial
  meningeal artery — *see* Injury, intracranial, subdural hemorrhage
  meninges (cerebral) — *see* Injury, intracranial
  mesenteric
    artery
      branch S35.299 ☑
        laceration (minor) (superficial) S35.291 ☑
          major S35.292 ☑
        specified NEC S35.298 ☑
      inferior S35.239 ☑
        laceration (minor) (superficial) S35.231 ☑
          major S35.232 ☑
        specified NEC S35.238 ☑
      superior S35.229 ☑
        laceration (minor) (superficial) S35.221 ☑
          major S35.222 ☑
        specified NEC S35.228 ☑
    plexus (inferior) (superior) — *see* Injury, nerve, lumbosacral, sympathetic
    vein
      inferior S35.349 ☑
        laceration S35.341 ☑
        specified NEC S35.348 ☑
      superior S35.339 ☑
        laceration S35.331 ☑
        specified NEC S35.338 ☑
  mesentery — *see* Injury, intra-abdominal, specified site NEC
  mesosalpinx — *see* Injury, pelvic organ, specified site NEC
  middle ear S09.30- ☑
  midthoracic region NOS S29.9 ☑
  mouth S09.93 ☑
  multiple NOS T07 ☑
  muscle (and fascia) (and tendon)
    abdomen S39.001 ☑
      laceration S39.021 ☑
      specified type NEC S39.091 ☑
      strain S39.011 ☑
    abductor
      thumb, forearm level — *see* Injury, muscle, thumb, abductor
    adductor
      thigh S76.20- ☑
        laceration S76.22- ☑
        specified type NEC S76.29- ☑
        strain S76.21- ☑
    ankle — *see* Injury, muscle, foot
    anterior muscle group, at leg level (lower) S86.20- ☑
      laceration S86.22- ☑
      specified type NEC S86.29- ☑
      strain S86.21- ☑
    arm (upper) — *see* Injury, muscle, shoulder
    biceps (parts NEC) S46.20- ☑
      laceration S46.22- ☑
      long head S46.10- ☑
        laceration S46.12- ☑
        specified type NEC S46.19- ☑
        strain S46.11- ☑
      specified type NEC S46.29- ☑
      strain S46.21- ☑
    extensor
      finger(s) (other than thumb) — *see* Injury, muscle, finger by site, extensor
      forearm level, specified NEC — *see* Injury, muscle, forearm, extensor
      thumb — *see* Injury, muscle, thumb, extensor
      toe (large) (ankle level) (foot level) — *see* Injury, muscle, toe, extensor
    finger
      extensor (forearm level) S56.40- ☑
        hand level S66.309 ☑
          laceration S66.329 ☑
          specified type NEC S66.399 ☑
          strain S66.319 ☑
        laceration S56.429 ☑
        specified type NEC S56.499 ☑
        strain S56.419 ☑
      flexor (forearm level) S56.10- ☑
        hand level S66.109 ☑
          laceration S66.129 ☑

☑ **Additional Character Required — Refer to the Tabular List for Character Selection**   ▽ **Subterms under main terms may continue to next column or page**

Injury — *continued*
  muscle — *continued*
    finger — *continued*
      flexor — *continued*
        hand level — *continued*
          specified type NEC S66.199 ☑
          strain S66.119 ☑
        laceration S56.129 ☑
        specified type NEC S56.199 ☑
        strain S56.119 ☑
      index
        extensor (forearm level)
          hand level S66.308 ☑
            laceration S66.32- ☑
            specified type NEC S66.39- ☑
            strain S66.31- ☑
          specified type NEC S56.492 ☑
        flexor (forearm level)
          hand level S66.108 ☑
            laceration S66.12- ☑
            specified type NEC S66.19- ☑
            strain S66.11- ☑
          specified type NEC S56.19- ☑
          strain S56.11- ☑
        intrinsic S66.50- ☑
          laceration S66.52- ☑
          specified type NEC S66.59- ☑
          strain S66.51- ☑
      intrinsic S66.509
        laceration S66.529 ☑
        specified type NEC S66.599 ☑
        strain S66.519 ☑
      little
        extensor (forearm level)
          hand level S66.30- ☑
            laceration S66.32- ☑
            specified type NEC S66.39- ☑
            strain S66.31- ☑
          laceration S56.42- ☑
          specified type NEC S56.49- ☑
          strain S56.41- ☑
        flexor (forearm level)
          hand level S66.10- ☑
            laceration S66.12- ☑
            specified type NEC S66.19- ☑
            strain S66.11- ☑
          laceration S56.12- ☑
          specified type NEC S56.19- ☑
          strain S56.11- ☑
        intrinsic S66.50- ☑
          laceration S66.52- ☑
          specified type NEC S66.59- ☑
          strain S66.51- ☑
      middle
        extensor (forearm level)
          hand level S66.30- ☑
            laceration S66.32- ☑
            specified type NEC S66.39- ☑
            strain S66.31- ☑
          laceration S56.42- ☑
          specified type NEC S56.49- ☑
          strain S56.41- ☑
        flexor (forearm level)
          hand level S66.10- ☑
            laceration S66.12- ☑
            specified type NEC S66.19- ☑
            strain S66.11- ☑
          laceration S56.12- ☑
          specified type NEC S56.19- ☑
          strain S56.11- ☑
        intrinsic S66.50- ☑
          laceration S66.52- ☑
          specified type NEC S66.59- ☑
          strain S66.51- ☑
      ring
        extensor (forearm level)
          hand level S66.30- ☑
            laceration S66.32- ☑
            specified type NEC S66.39- ☑
            strain S66.31- ☑
          laceration S56.42- ☑
          specified type NEC S56.49- ☑
          strain S56.41- ☑
        flexor (forearm level)
          hand level S66.10- ☑
            laceration S66.12- ☑

Injury — *continued*
  muscle — *continued*
    finger — *continued*
      ring — *continued*
        flexor — *continued*
          hand level — *continued*
            specified type NEC S66.19- ☑
            strain S66.11- ☑
          laceration S56.12- ☑
          specified type NEC S56.19- ☑
          strain S56.11- ☑
        intrinsic S66.50- ☑
          laceration S66.52- ☑
          specified type NEC S66.59- ☑
          strain S66.51- ☑
    flexor
      finger(s) (other than thumb) — *see* Injury, muscle, finger
      forearm level, specified NEC — *see* Injury, muscle, forearm, flexor
      thumb — *see* Injury, muscle, thumb, flexor
      toe (long) (ankle level) (foot level) — *see* Injury, muscle, toe, flexor
    foot S96.90- ☑
      intrinsic S96.20- ☑
        laceration S96.22- ☑
        specified type NEC S96.29- ☑
        strain S96.21- ☑
      laceration S96.92- ☑
      long extensor, toe — *see* Injury, muscle, toe, extensor
      long flexor, toe — *see* Injury, muscle, toe, flexor
      specified
        site NEC S96.80- ☑
          laceration S96.82- ☑
          specified type NEC S96.89- ☑
          strain S96.81- ☑
        type S96.99- ☑
      strain S96.91- ☑
    forearm (level) S56.90- ☑
      extensor S56.50- ☑
        laceration S56.52- ☑
        specified type NEC S56.59- ☑
        strain S56.51- ☑
      flexor S56.20- ☑
        laceration S56.22- ☑
        specified type NEC S56.29- ☑
        strain S56.21- ☑
      laceration S56.92- ☑
      specified S56.99- ☑
        site NEC S56.80- ☑
          laceration S56.82- ☑
          strain S56.81- ☑
          type NEC S56.89- ☑
      strain S56.91- ☑
    hand (level) S66.90- ☑
      laceration S66.92- ☑
      specified
        site NEC S66.80- ☑
          laceration S66.82- ☑
          specified type NEC S66.89- ☑
          strain S66.81- ☑
          type NEC S66.99- ☑
      strain S66.91- ☑
    head S09.10 ☑
      laceration S09.12 ☑
      specified type NEC S09.19 ☑
      strain S09.11 ☑
    hip NEC S76.00- ☑
      laceration S76.02- ☑
      specified type NEC S76.09- ☑
      strain S76.01- ☑
    intrinsic
      ankle and foot level — *see* Injury, muscle, foot, intrinsic
      finger (other than thumb) — *see* Injury, muscle, finger by site, intrinsic
      foot (level) — *see* Injury, muscle, foot, intrinsic
      thumb — *see* Injury, muscle, thumb, intrinsic
    leg (level) (lower) S86.90- ☑
      Achilles tendon — *see* Injury, Achilles tendon
      anterior muscle group — *see* Injury, muscle, anterior muscle group
      laceration S86.92- ☑
      peroneal muscle group — *see* Injury, muscle, peroneal muscle group

Injury — *continued*
  muscle — *continued*
    leg — *continued*
      posterior muscle group — *see* Injury, muscle, posterior muscle group, leg level
      specified
        site NEC S86.80- ☑
          laceration S86.82- ☑
          specified type NEC S86.89- ☑
          strain S86.81- ☑
        type NEC S86.99- ☑
      strain S86.91- ☑
    long
      extensor toe, at ankle and foot level — *see* Injury, muscle, toe, extensor
      flexor, toe, at ankle and foot level — *see* Injury, muscle, toe, flexor
      head, biceps — *see* Injury, muscle, biceps, long head
    lower back S39.002 ☑
      laceration S39.022 ☑
      specified type NEC S39.092 ☑
      strain S39.012 ☑
    neck (level) S16.9 ☑
      laceration S16.2 ☑
      specified type NEC S16.8 ☑
      strain S16.1 ☑
    pelvis S39.003 ☑
      laceration S39.023 ☑
      specified type NEC S39.093 ☑
      strain S39.013 ☑
    peroneal muscle group, at leg level (lower) S86.30- ☑
      laceration S86.32- ☑
      specified type NEC S86.39- ☑
      strain S86.31- ☑
    posterior muscle (group)
      leg level (lower) S86.10- ☑
        laceration S86.12- ☑
        specified type NEC S86.19- ☑
        strain S86.11- ☑
      thigh level S76.30- ☑
        laceration S76.32- ☑
        specified type NEC S76.39- ☑
        strain S76.31- ☑
    quadriceps (thigh) S76.10- ☑
      laceration S76.12- ☑
      specified type NEC S76.19- ☑
      strain S76.11- ☑
    shoulder S46.90- ☑
      laceration S46.92- ☑
      rotator cuff — *see* Injury, rotator cuff
      specified site NEC S46.80- ☑
        laceration S46.82- ☑
        specified type NEC S46.89- ☑
        strain S46.81- ☑
      specified type NEC S46.99- ☑
      strain S46.91- ☑
    thigh NEC (level) S76.90- ☑
      adductor — *see* Injury, muscle, adductor, thigh
      laceration S76.92- ☑
      posterior muscle (group) — *see* Injury, muscle, posterior muscle, thigh level
      quadriceps — *see* Injury, muscle, quadriceps
      specified
        site NEC S76.80- ☑
          laceration S76.82- ☑
          specified type NEC S76.89- ☑
          strain S76.81- ☑
        type NEC S76.99- ☑
      strain S76.91- ☑
    thorax (level) S29.009 ☑
      back wall S29.002 ☑
      front wall S29.001 ☑
      laceration S29.029 ☑
        back wall S29.022 ☑
        front wall S29.021 ☑
      specified type NEC S29.099 ☑
        back wall S29.092 ☑
        front wall S29.091 ☑
      strain S29.019 ☑
        back wall S29.012 ☑
        front wall S29.011 ☑
    thumb
      abductor (forearm level) S56.30- ☑
        laceration S56.32- ☑

▽ Subterms under main terms may continue to next column or page   ☑ Additional Character Required — Refer to the Tabular List for Character Selection   **195**

Injury — Injury

Injury — *continued*
  muscle — *continued*
    thumb — *continued*
      abductor — *continued*
        specified type NEC S56.39- ☑
        strain S56.31- ☑
      extensor (forearm level) S56.30- ☑
        hand level S66.20- ☑
          laceration S66.22- ☑
          specified type NEC S66.29- ☑
          strain S66.21- ☑
        laceration S56.32- ☑
        specified type NEC S56.39- ☑
        strain S56.31- ☑
      flexor (forearm level) S56.00- ☑
        hand level S66.00- ☑
          laceration S66.02- ☑
          specified type NEC S66.09- ☑
          strain S66.01- ☑
        laceration S56.02- ☑
        specified type NEC S56.09- ☑
        strain S56.01- ☑
      wrist level — *see* Injury, muscle, thumb,
          flexor, hand level
    intrinsic S66.40- ☑
      laceration S66.42- ☑
      specified type NEC S66.49- ☑
      strain S66.41- ☑
    toe (*see also* Injury, muscle, foot)
      extensor, long S96.10- ☑
        laceration S96.12- ☑
        specified type NEC S96.19- ☑
        strain S96.11- ☑
      flexor, long S96.00- ☑
        laceration S96.02- ☑
        specified type NEC S96.09- ☑
        strain S96.01- ☑
    triceps S46.30- ☑
      laceration S46.32- ☑
      specified type NEC S46.39- ☑
      strain S46.31- ☑
    wrist (and hand) level — *see* Injury, muscle, hand
  musculocutaneous nerve — *see* Injury, nerve, muscu-
      locutaneous
  myocardium — *see* Injury, heart
  nape — *see* Injury, neck
  nasal (septum) (sinus) S09.92 ☑
  nasopharynx S09.92 ☑
  neck S19.9 ☑
    specified NEC S19.80 ☑
      specified site NEC S19.89 ☑
  nerve NEC T14.8 ☑
    abdomen S34.9 ☑
      peripheral S34.6 ☑
      specified site NEC S34.8 ☑
    abducens S04.4- ☑
      contusion S04.4- ☑
      laceration S04.4- ☑
      specified type NEC S04.4- ☑
    abducent — *see* Injury, nerve, abducens
    accessory S04.7- ☑
      contusion S04.7- ☑
      laceration S04.7- ☑
      specified type NEC S04.7- ☑
    acoustic S04.6- ☑
      contusion S04.6- ☑
      laceration S04.6- ☑
      specified type NEC S04.6- ☑
    ankle S94.9- ☑
      cutaneous sensory S94.3- ☑
      specified site NEC — *see* subcategory S94.8 ☑
    anterior crural, femoral — *see* Injury, nerve, femoral
    arm (upper) S44.9- ☑
      axillary — *see* Injury, nerve, axillary
      cutaneous — *see* Injury, nerve, cutaneous, arm
      median — *see* Injury, nerve, median, upper arm
      musculocutaneous — *see* Injury, nerve, muscu-
          locutaneous
      radial — *see* Injury, nerve, radial, upper arm
      specified site NEC — *see* subcategory S44.8 ☑
      ulnar — *see* Injury, nerve, ulnar, arm
    auditory — *see* Injury, nerve, acoustic
    axillary S44.3- ☑
    brachial plexus — *see* Injury, brachial plexus
    cervical sympathetic S14.5 ☑
    cranial S04.9 ☑

Injury — *continued*
  nerve — *continued*
    cranial — *continued*
      contusion S04.9 ☑
      eighth (acoustic or auditory) — *see* Injury,
          nerve, acoustic
      eleventh (accessory) — *see* Injury, nerve, acces-
          sory
      fifth (trigeminal) — *see* Injury, nerve, trigeminal
      first (olfactory) — *see* Injury, nerve, olfactory
      fourth (trochlear) — *see* Injury, nerve, trochlear
      laceration S04.9 ☑
      ninth (glossopharyngeal) — *see* Injury, nerve,
          glossopharyngeal
      second (optic) — *see* Injury, nerve, optic
      seventh (facial) — *see* Injury, nerve, facial
      sixth (abducent) — *see* Injury, nerve, abducens
      specified
        nerve NEC S04.89- ☑
          contusion S04.89- ☑
          laceration S04.89- ☑
          specified type NEC S04.89- ☑
        type NEC S04.9 ☑
      tenth (pneumogastric or vagus) — *see* Injury,
          nerve, vagus
      third (oculomotor) — *see* Injury, nerve, oculo-
          motor
      twelfth (hypoglossal) — *see* Injury, nerve, hy-
          poglossal
    cutaneous sensory
      ankle (level) S94.3- ☑
      arm (upper) (level) S44.5- ☑
      foot (level) — *see* Injury, nerve, cutaneous
          sensory, ankle
      forearm (level) S54.3- ☑
      hip (level) S74.2- ☑
      leg (lower level) S84.2- ☑
      shoulder (level) — *see* Injury, nerve, cutaneous
          sensory, arm
      thigh (level) — *see* Injury, nerve, cutaneous
          sensory, hip
    deep peroneal — *see* Injury, nerve, peroneal, foot
    digital
      finger S64.4- ☑
        index S64.49- ☑
        little S64.49- ☑
        middle S64.49- ☑
        ring S64.49- ☑
      thumb S64.3- ☑
      toe — *see* Injury, nerve, ankle, specified site
          NEC
    eighth cranial (acoustic or auditory) — *see* Injury,
        nerve, acoustic
    eleventh cranial (accessory) — *see* Injury, nerve,
        accessory
    facial S04.5- ☑
      contusion S04.5- ☑
      laceration S04.5- ☑
      newborn P11.3
      specified type NEC S04.5- ☑
    femoral (hip level) (thigh level) S74.1- ☑
    fifth cranial (trigeminal) — *see* Injury, nerve,
        trigeminal
    finger (digital) — *see* Injury, nerve, digital, finger
    first cranial (olfactory) — *see* Injury, nerve, olfactory
    foot S94.9- ☑
      cutaneous sensory S94.3- ☑
      deep peroneal S94.2- ☑
      lateral plantar S94.0- ☑
      medial plantar S94.1- ☑
      specified site NEC — *see* subcategory S94.8 ☑
    forearm (level) S54.9- ☑
      cutaneous sensory — *see* Injury, nerve, cuta-
          neous sensory, forearm
      median — *see* Injury, nerve, median
      radial — *see* Injury, nerve, radial
      specified site NEC — *see* subcategory S54.8 ☑
      ulnar — *see* Injury, nerve, ulnar
    fourth cranial (trochlear) — *see* Injury, nerve,
        trochlear
    glossopharyngeal S04.89- ☑
      specified type NEC S04.89- ☑
    hand S64.9- ☑
      median — *see* Injury, nerve, median, hand
      radial — *see* Injury, nerve, radial, hand
      specified NEC — *see* subcategory S64.8 ☑

Injury — *continued*
  nerve — *continued*
    hand — *continued*
      ulnar — *see* Injury, nerve, ulnar, hand
    hip (level) S74.9- ☑
      cutaneous sensory — *see* Injury, nerve, cuta-
          neous sensory, hip
      femoral — *see* Injury, nerve, femoral
      sciatic — *see* Injury, nerve, sciatic
      specified site NEC — *see* subcategory S74.8 ☑
    hypoglossal S04.89- ☑
      specified type NEC S04.89- ☑
    lateral plantar S94.0- ☑
    leg (lower) S84.9- ☑
      cutaneous sensory — *see* Injury, nerve, cuta-
          neous sensory, leg
      peroneal — *see* Injury, nerve, peroneal
      specified site NEC — *see* subcategory S84.8 ☑
      tibial — *see* Injury, nerve, tibial
      upper — *see* Injury, nerve, thigh
    lower
      back — *see* Injury, nerve, abdomen, specified
          site NEC
        peripheral — *see* Injury, nerve, abdomen,
            peripheral
      limb — *see* Injury, nerve, leg
    lumbar plexus — *see* Injury, nerve, lumbosacral,
        sympathetic
    lumbar spinal — *see* Injury, nerve, spinal, lumbar
    lumbosacral
      plexus — *see* Injury, nerve, lumbosacral, sym-
          pathetic
      sympathetic S34.5 ☑
    medial plantar S94.1- ☑
    median (forearm level) S54.1- ☑
      hand (level) S64.1- ☑
      upper arm (level) S44.1- ☑
      wrist (level) — *see* Injury, nerve, median, hand
    musculocutaneous S44.4- ☑
    musculospiral (upper arm level) — *see* Injury,
        nerve, radial, upper arm
    neck S14.9 ☑
      peripheral S14.4 ☑
      specified site NEC S14.8 ☑
      sympathetic S14.5 ☑
    ninth cranial (glossopharyngeal) — *see* Injury,
        nerve, glossopharyngeal
    oculomotor S04.1- ☑
      contusion S04.1- ☑
      laceration S04.1- ☑
      specified type NEC S04.1- ☑
    olfactory S04.81- ☑
      specified type NEC S04.81- ☑
    optic S04.01- ☑
      contusion S04.01- ☑
      laceration S04.01- ☑
      specified type NEC S04.01- ☑
    pelvic girdle — *see* Injury, nerve, hip
    pelvis — *see* Injury, nerve, abdomen, specified site
        NEC
      peripheral — *see* Injury, nerve, abdomen, pe-
          ripheral
    peripheral NEC T14.8 ☑
      abdomen — *see* Injury, nerve, abdomen, periph-
          eral
      lower back — *see* Injury, nerve, abdomen, pe-
          ripheral
      neck — *see* Injury, nerve, neck, peripheral
      pelvis — *see* Injury, nerve, abdomen, peripheral
      specified NEC T14.8 ☑
    peroneal (lower leg level) S84.1- ☑
      foot S94.2- ☑
    plexus
      brachial — *see* Injury, brachial plexus
      celiac, coeliac — *see* Injury, nerve, lumbosacral,
          sympathetic
      mesenteric, inferior — *see* Injury, nerve, lum-
          bosacral, sympathetic
      sacral — *see* Injury, lumbosacral plexus
      spinal
        brachial — *see* Injury, brachial plexus
        lumbosacral — *see* Injury, lumbosacral
            plexus
    pneumogastric — *see* Injury, nerve, vagus
    radial (forearm level) S54.2- ☑
      hand (level) S64.2- ☑

☑ **Additional Character Required** — **Refer to the Tabular List for Character Selection**   ▽ **Subterms under main terms may continue to next column or page**

Injury — continued
nerve — continued
  radial — continued
    upper arm (level) S44.2- ☑
    wrist (level) — see Injury, nerve, radial, hand
  root — see Injury, nerve, spinal, root
  sacral plexus — see Injury, lumbosacral plexus
  sacral spinal — see Injury, nerve, spinal, sacral
  sciatic (hip level) (thigh level) S74.0- ☑
  second cranial (optic) — see Injury, nerve, optic
  seventh cranial (facial) — see Injury, nerve, facial
  shoulder — see Injury, nerve, arm
  sixth cranial (abducent) — see Injury, nerve, abducens
  spinal
    plexus — see Injury, nerve, plexus, spinal
    root
      cervical S14.2 ☑
      dorsal S24.2 ☑
      lumbar S34.21 ☑
      sacral S34.22 ☑
      thoracic — see Injury, nerve, spinal, root, dorsal
  splanchnic — see Injury, nerve, lumbosacral, sympathetic
  sympathetic NEC — see Injury, nerve, lumbosacral, sympathetic
    cervical — see Injury, nerve, cervical sympathetic
  tenth cranial (pneumogastric or vagus) — see Injury, nerve, vagus
  thigh (level) — see Injury, nerve, hip
    cutaneous sensory — see Injury, nerve, cutaneous sensory, hip
    femoral — see Injury, nerve, femoral
    sciatic — see Injury, nerve, sciatic
    specified NEC — see Injury, nerve, hip
  third cranial (oculomotor) — see Injury, nerve, oculomotor
  thorax S24.9 ☑
    peripheral S24.3 ☑
    specified site NEC S24.8 ☑
    sympathetic S24.4 ☑
  thumb, digital — see Injury, nerve, digital, thumb
  tibial (lower leg level) (posterior) S84.0- ☑
  toe — see Injury, nerve, ankle
  trigeminal S04.3- ☑
    contusion S04.3- ☑
    laceration S04.3- ☑
    specified type NEC S04.3- ☑
  trochlear S04.2- ☑
    contusion S04.2- ☑
    laceration S04.2- ☑
    specified type NEC S04.2- ☑
  twelfth cranial (hypoglossal) — see Injury, nerve, hypoglossal
  ulnar (forearm level) S54.0- ☑
    arm (upper) (level) S44.0- ☑
    hand (level) S64.0- ☑
    wrist (level) — see Injury, nerve, ulnar, hand
  vagus S04.89- ☑
    specified type NEC S04.89- ☑
  wrist (level) — see Injury, nerve, hand
  ninth cranial nerve (glossopharyngeal) — see Injury, nerve, glossopharyngeal
nose (septum) S09.92 ☑
obstetrical O71.9
  specified NEC O71.89
occipital (region) (scalp) S09.90 ☑
  lobe — see Injury, intracranial
optic chiasm S04.02 ☑
optic radiation S04.03- ☑
optic tract and pathways S04.03- ☑
orbit, orbital (region) — see Injury, eye
  penetrating (with foreign body) — see Injury, eye, orbit, penetrating
  specified NEC — see Injury, eye, specified site NEC
ovary, ovarian S37.409 ☑
  bilateral S37.402 ☑
    contusion S37.422 ☑
    laceration S37.432 ☑
    specified type NEC S37.492 ☑
  blood vessel — see Injury, blood vessel, ovarian
  contusion S37.429 ☑
    bilateral S37.422 ☑
    unilateral S37.421 ☑

ovary, ovarian — continued
  laceration S37.439 ☑
    bilateral S37.432 ☑
    unilateral S37.431 ☑
  specified type NEC S37.499 ☑
    bilateral S37.492 ☑
    unilateral S37.491 ☑
  unilateral S37.401 ☑
    contusion S37.421 ☑
    laceration S37.431 ☑
    specified type NEC S37.491 ☑
palate (hard) (soft) S09.93 ☑
pancreas S36.209 ☑
  body S36.201 ☑
    contusion S36.221 ☑
    laceration S36.231 ☑
      major S36.261 ☑
      minor S36.241 ☑
      moderate S36.251 ☑
    specified type NEC S36.291 ☑
  contusion S36.229 ☑
  head S36.200 ☑
    contusion S36.220 ☑
    laceration S36.230 ☑
      major S36.260 ☑
      minor S36.240 ☑
      moderate S36.250 ☑
    specified type NEC S36.290 ☑
  laceration S36.239 ☑
    major S36.269 ☑
    minor S36.249 ☑
    moderate S36.259 ☑
  specified type NEC S36.299 ☑
  tail S36.202 ☑
    contusion S36.222 ☑
    laceration S36.232 ☑
      major S36.262 ☑
      minor S36.242 ☑
      moderate S36.252 ☑
    specified type NEC S36.292 ☑
parietal (region) (scalp) S09.90 ☑
  lobe — see Injury, intracranial
patellar ligament (tendon) S76.10- ☑
  laceration S76.12- ☑
  specified NEC S76.19- ☑
  strain S76.11- ☑
pelvis, pelvic (floor) S39.93 ☑
  complicating delivery O70.1
  joint or ligament, complicating delivery O71.6
  organ S37.90 ☑
    with ectopic or molar pregnancy O08.6
    complication of abortion — see Abortion
    contusion S37.92 ☑
    following ectopic or molar pregnancy O08.6
    laceration S37.93 ☑
    obstetrical trauma NEC O71.5
    specified
      site NEC S37.899 ☑
        contusion S37.892 ☑
        laceration S37.893 ☑
        specified type NEC S37.898 ☑
      type NEC S37.99 ☑
  specified NEC S39.83 ☑
penis S39.94 ☑
perineum S39.94 ☑
peritoneum S36.81 ☑
  laceration S36.893 ☑
periurethral tissue — see Injury, urethra
  complicating delivery O71.82
phalanges
  foot — see Injury, foot
  hand — see Injury, hand
pharynx NEC S19.85 ☑
pleura — see Injury, intrathoracic, pleura
plexus
  brachial — see Injury, brachial plexus
  cardiac — see Injury, nerve, thorax, sympathetic
  celiac, coeliac — see Injury, nerve, lumbosacral, sympathetic
  esophageal — see Injury, nerve, thorax, sympathetic
  hypogastric — see Injury, nerve, lumbosacral, sympathetic
  lumbar, lumbosacral — see Injury, lumbosacral plexus

plexus — continued
  mesenteric — see Injury, nerve, lumbosacral, sympathetic
  pulmonary — see Injury, nerve, thorax, sympathetic
postcardiac surgery (syndrome) I97.0
prepuce S39.94 ☑
prostate S37.829 ☑
  contusion S37.822 ☑
  laceration S37.823 ☑
  specified type NEC S37.828 ☑
pubic region S39.94 ☑
pudendum S39.94 ☑
pulmonary plexus — see Injury, nerve, thorax, sympathetic
rectovaginal septum NEC S39.83 ☑
rectum — see Injury, intestine, large, rectum
retina — see Injury, eye, specified site NEC
  penetrating — see Injury, eyeball, penetrating
retroperitoneal — see Injury, intra-abdominal, specified site NEC
rotator cuff (muscle(s)) (tendon(s)) S46.00- ☑
  laceration S46.02- ☑
  specified type NEC S46.09- ☑
  strain S46.01- ☑
round ligament — see Injury, pelvic organ, specified site NEC
sacral plexus — see Injury, lumbosacral plexus
salivary duct or gland S09.93 ☑
scalp S09.90 ☑
  newborn (birth injury) P12.9
    due to monitoring (electrode) (sampling incision) P12.4
    specified NEC P12.89
      caput succedaneum P12.81
scapular region — see Injury, shoulder
sclera — see Injury, eye, specified site NEC
  penetrating — see Injury, eyeball, penetrating
scrotum S39.94 ☑
second cranial nerve (optic) — see Injury, nerve, optic
seminal vesicle — see Injury, pelvic organ, specified site NEC
seventh cranial nerve (facial) — see Injury, nerve, facial
shoulder S49.9- ☑
  blood vessel — see Injury, blood vessel, arm
  contusion — see Contusion, shoulder
  dislocation — see Dislocation, shoulder
  fracture — see Fracture, shoulder
  muscle — see Injury, muscle, shoulder
  nerve — see Injury, nerve, shoulder
  open — see Wound, open, shoulder
  specified type NEC S49.8- ☑
  sprain — see Sprain, shoulder girdle
  superficial — see Injury, superficial, shoulder
sinus
  cavernous — see Injury, intracranial
  nasal S09.92 ☑
sixth cranial nerve (abducent) — see Injury, nerve, abducens
skeleton, birth injury P13.9
  specified part NEC P13.8
skin NEC T14.8 ☑
  surface intact — see Injury, superficial
skull NEC S09.90 ☑
specified NEC T14.8 ☑
spermatic cord (pelvic region) S37.898 ☑
  scrotal region S39.848 ☑
spinal (cord)
  cervical (neck) S14.109 ☑
    anterior cord syndrome S14.139 ☑
      C1 level S14.131 ☑
      C2 level S14.132 ☑
      C3 level S14.133 ☑
      C4 level S14.134 ☑
      C5 level S14.135 ☑
      C6 level S14.136 ☑
      C7 level S14.137 ☑
      C8 level S14.138 ☑
    Brown-Séquard syndrome S14.149 ☑
      C1 level S14.141 ☑
      C2 level S14.142 ☑
      C3 level S14.143 ☑
      C4 level S14.144 ☑
      C5 level S14.145 ☑
      C6 level S14.146 ☑

Injury — *continued*
  spinal — *continued*
    cervical — *continued*
      Brown-Séquard syndrome — *continued*
        C7 level S14.147 ☑
        C8 level S14.148 ☑
      C1 level S14.101 ☑
      C2 level S14.102 ☑
      C3 level S14.103 ☑
      C4 level S14.104 ☑
      C5 level S14.105 ☑
      C6 level S14.106 ☑
      C7 level S14.107 ☑
      C8 level S14.108 ☑
      central cord syndrome S14.129 ☑
        C1 level S14.121 ☑
        C2 level S14.122 ☑
        C3 level S14.123 ☑
        C4 level S14.124 ☑
        C5 level S14.125 ☑
        C6 level S14.126 ☑
        C7 level S14.127 ☑
        C8 level S14.128 ☑
      complete lesion S14.119 ☑
        C1 level S14.111 ☑
        C2 level S14.112 ☑
        C3 level S14.113 ☑
        C4 level S14.114 ☑
        C5 level S14.115 ☑
        C6 level S14.116 ☑
        C7 level S14.117 ☑
        C8 level S14.118 ☑
      concussion S14.0 ☑
      edema S14.0 ☑
      incomplete lesion specified NEC S14.159 ☑
        C1 level S14.151 ☑
        C2 level S14.152 ☑
        C3 level S14.153 ☑
        C4 level S14.154 ☑
        C5 level S14.155 ☑
        C6 level S14.156 ☑
        C7 level S14.157 ☑
        C8 level S14.158 ☑
      posterior cord syndrome S14.159 ☑
        C1 level S14.151 ☑
        C2 level S14.152 ☑
        C3 level S14.153 ☑
        C4 level S14.154 ☑
        C5 level S14.155 ☑
        C6 level S14.156 ☑
        C7 level S14.157 ☑
        C8 level S14.158 ☑
    dorsal — *see* Injury, spinal, thoracic
    lumbar S34.109 ☑
      complete lesion S34.119 ☑
        L1 level S34.111 ☑
        L2 level S34.112 ☑
        L3 level S34.113 ☑
        L4 level S34.114 ☑
        L5 level S34.115 ☑
      concussion S34.01 ☑
      edema S34.01 ☑
      incomplete lesion S34.129 ☑
        L1 level S34.121 ☑
        L2 level S34.122 ☑
        L3 level S34.123 ☑
        L4 level S34.124 ☑
        L5 level S34.125 ☑
      L1 level S34.101 ☑
      L2 level S34.102 ☑
      L3 level S34.103 ☑
      L4 level S34.104 ☑
      L5 level S34.105 ☑
    nerve root NEC
      cervical — *see* Injury, nerve, spinal, root, cervical
      dorsal — *see* Injury, nerve, spinal, root, dorsal
      lumbar S34.21 ☑
      sacral S34.22 ☑
      thoracic — *see* Injury, nerve, spinal, root, dorsal
    plexus
      brachial — *see* Injury, brachial plexus
      lumbosacral — *see* Injury, lumbosacral plexus
    sacral S34.139 ☑
      complete lesion S34.131 ☑
      incomplete lesion S34.132 ☑

Injury — *continued*
  spinal — *continued*
    thoracic S24.109 ☑
      anterior cord syndrome S24.139 ☑
        T1 level S24.131 ☑
        T2-T6 level S24.132 ☑
        T7-T10 level S24.133 ☑
        T11-T12 level S24.134 ☑
      Brown-Séquard syndrome S24.149 ☑
        T1 level S24.141 ☑
        T2-T6 level S24.142 ☑
        T7-T10 level S24.143 ☑
        T11-T12 level S24.144 ☑
      complete lesion S24.119 ☑
        T1 level S24.111 ☑
        T2-T6 level S24.112 ☑
        T7-T10 level S24.113 ☑
        T11-T12 level S24.114 ☑
      concussion S24.0 ☑
      edema S24.0 ☑
      incomplete lesion specified NEC S24.159 ☑
        T1 level S24.151 ☑
        T2-T6 level S24.152 ☑
        T7-T10 level S24.153 ☑
        T11-T12 level S24.154 ☑
      posterior cord syndrome S24.159 ☑
        T1 level S24.151 ☑
        T2-T6 level S24.152 ☑
        T7-T10 level S24.153 ☑
        T11-T12 level S24.154 ☑
      T1 level S24.101 ☑
      T2-T6 level S24.102 ☑
      T7-T10 level S24.103 ☑
      T11-T12 level S24.104 ☑
    splanchnic nerve — *see* Injury, nerve, lumbosacral, sympathetic
  spleen S36.00 ☑
    contusion S36.029 ☑
      major S36.021 ☑
      minor S36.020 ☑
    laceration S36.039 ☑
      major (massive) (stellate) S36.032 ☑
      moderate S36.031 ☑
      superficial (capsular) (minor) S36.030 ☑
    specified type NEC S36.09 ☑
  splenic artery — *see* Injury, blood vessel, celiac artery, branch
  stellate ganglion — *see* Injury, nerve, thorax, sympathetic
  sternal region S29.9 ☑
  stomach S36.30 ☑
    contusion S36.32 ☑
    laceration S36.33 ☑
    specified type NEC S36.39 ☑
  subconjunctival — *see* Injury, eye, conjunctiva
  subcutaneous NEC T14.8 ☑
  submaxillary region S09.93 ☑
  submental region S09.93 ☑
  subungual
    fingers — *see* Injury, hand
    toes — *see* Injury, foot
  superficial NEC T14.8 ☑
    abdomen, abdominal (wall) S30.92 ☑
      abrasion S30.811 ☑
      bite S30.871 ☑
        insect S30.861 ☑
      contusion S30.1 ☑
      external constriction S30.841 ☑
      foreign body S30.851 ☑
    abrasion — *see* Abrasion, by site
    adnexa, eye NEC — *see* Injury, eye, specified site NEC
    alveolar process — *see* Injury, superficial, oral cavity
    ankle S90.91- ☑
      abrasion — *see* Abrasion, ankle
      bite — *see* Bite, ankle
      blister — *see* Blister, ankle
      contusion — *see* Contusion, ankle
      external constriction — *see* Constriction, external, ankle
      foreign body — *see* Foreign body, superficial, ankle
    anus S30.98 ☑
    arm (upper) S40.92- ☑
      abrasion — *see* Abrasion, arm

Injury — *continued*
  superficial — *continued*
    arm — *continued*
      bite — *see* Bite, superficial, arm
      blister — *see* Blister, arm (upper)
      contusion — *see* Contusion, arm
      external constriction — *see* Constriction, external, arm
      foreign body — *see* Foreign body, superficial, arm
    auditory canal (external) (meatus) — *see* Injury, superficial, ear
    auricle — *see* Injury, superficial, ear
    axilla — *see* Injury, superficial, arm
    back (*see also* Injury, superficial, thorax, back)
      lower S30.91 ☑
        abrasion S30.810 ☑
        contusion S30.0 ☑
        external constriction S30.840 ☑
        superficial
          bite NEC S30.870 ☑
            insect S30.860 ☑
          foreign body S30.850 ☑
    bite NEC — *see* Bite, superficial NEC, by site
    blister — *see* Blister, by site
    breast S20.10- ☑
      abrasion — *see* Abrasion, breast
      bite — *see* Bite, superficial, breast
      contusion — *see* Contusion, breast
      external constriction — *see* Constriction, external, breast
      foreign body — *see* Foreign body, superficial, breast
    brow — *see* Injury, superficial, head, specified NEC
    buttock S30.91 ☑
    calf — *see* Injury, superficial, leg
    canthus, eye — *see* Injury, superficial, periocular area
    cheek (external) — *see* Injury, superficial, head, specified NEC
      internal — *see* Injury, superficial, oral cavity
    chest wall — *see* Injury, superficial, thorax
    chin — *see* Injury, superficial, head NEC
    clitoris S30.95 ☑
    conjunctiva — *see* Injury, eye, conjunctiva
      with foreign body (in conjunctival sac) — *see* Foreign body, conjunctival sac
    contusion — *see* Contusion, by site
    costal region — *see* Injury, superficial, thorax
    digit(s)
      hand — *see* Injury, superficial, finger
    ear (auricle) (canal) (external) S00.40- ☑
      abrasion — *see* Abrasion, ear
      bite — *see* Bite, superficial, ear
      contusion — *see* Contusion, ear
      external constriction — *see* Constriction, external, ear
      foreign body — *see* Foreign body, superficial, ear
    elbow S50.90- ☑
      abrasion — *see* Abrasion, elbow
      bite — *see* Bite, superficial, elbow
      blister — *see* Blister, elbow
      contusion — *see* Contusion, elbow
      external constriction — *see* Constriction, external, elbow
      foreign body — *see* Foreign body, superficial, elbow
    epididymis S30.94 ☑
    epigastric region S30.92 ☑
    epiglottis — *see* Injury, superficial, throat
    esophagus
      cervical — *see* Injury, superficial, throat
    external constriction — *see* Constriction, external, by site
    extremity NEC T14.8 ☑
    eyeball NEC — *see* Injury, eye, specified site NEC
    eyebrow — *see* Injury, superficial, periocular area
    eyelid S00.20- ☑
      abrasion — *see* Abrasion, eyelid
      bite — *see* Bite, superficial, eyelid
      contusion — *see* Contusion, eyelid
      external constriction — *see* Constriction, external, eyelid
      foreign body — *see* Foreign body, superficial, eyelid

Injury — continued
  superficial — continued
    face NEC — see Injury, superficial, head, specified NEC
    finger(s) S60.949 ☑
      abrasion — see Abrasion, finger
      bite — see Bite, superficial, finger
      blister — see Blister, finger
      contusion — see Contusion, finger
      external constriction — see Constriction, external, finger
      foreign body — see Foreign body, superficial, finger
      index S60.94- ☑
      insect bite — see Bite, by site, superficial, insect
      little S60.94- ☑
      middle S60.94- ☑
      ring S60.94- ☑
    flank S30.92 ☑
    foot S90.92- ☑
      abrasion — see Abrasion, foot
      bite — see Bite, foot
      blister — see Blister, foot
      contusion — see Contusion, foot
      external constriction — see Constriction, external, foot
      foreign body — see Foreign body, superficial, foot
    forearm S50.91- ☑
      abrasion — see Abrasion, forearm
      bite — see Bite, forearm, superficial
      blister — see Blister, forearm
      contusion — see Contusion, forearm
      elbow only — see Injury, superficial, elbow
      external constriction — see Constriction, external, forearm
      foreign body — see Foreign body, superficial, forearm
    forehead — see Injury, superficial, head NEC
    foreign body — see Foreign body, superficial
    genital organs, external
      female S30.97 ☑
      male S30.96 ☑
    globe (eye) — see Injury, eye, specified site NEC
    groin S30.92 ☑
    gum — see Injury, superficial, oral cavity
    hand S60.92- ☑
      abrasion — see Abrasion, hand
      bite — see Bite, superficial, hand
      contusion — see Contusion, hand
      external constriction — see Constriction, external, hand
      foreign body — see Foreign body, superficial, hand
    head S00.90 ☑
      ear — see Injury, superficial, ear
      eyelid — see Injury, superficial, eyelid
      nose S00.30 ☑
      oral cavity S00.502 ☑
      scalp S00.00 ☑
      specified site NEC S00.80 ☑
    heel — see Injury, superficial, foot
    hip S70.91- ☑
      abrasion — see Abrasion, hip
      bite — see Bite, superficial, hip
      blister — see Blister, hip
      contusion — see Contusion, hip
      external constriction — see Constriction, external, hip
      foreign body — see Foreign body, superficial, hip
    iliac region — see Injury, superficial, abdomen
    inguinal region — see Injury, superficial, abdomen
    insect bite — see Bite, by site, superficial, insect
    interscapular region — see Injury, superficial, thorax, back
    jaw — see Injury, superficial, head, specified NEC
    knee S80.91- ☑
      abrasion — see Abrasion, knee
      bite — see Bite, superficial, knee
      blister — see Blister, knee
      contusion — see Contusion, knee
      external constriction — see Constriction, external, knee
      foreign body — see Foreign body, superficial, knee

Injury — continued
  superficial — continued
    labium (majus) (minus) S30.95 ☑
    lacrimal (apparatus) (gland) (sac) — see Injury, eye, specified site NEC
    larynx — see Injury, superficial, throat
    leg (lower) S80.92- ☑
      abrasion — see Abrasion, leg
      bite — see Bite, superficial, leg
      contusion — see Contusion, leg
      external constriction — see Constriction, external, leg
      foreign body — see Foreign body, superficial, leg
      knee — see Injury, superficial, knee
    limb NEC T14.8 ☑
    lip S00.501 ☑
    lower back S30.91 ☑
    lumbar region S30.91 ☑
    malar region — see Injury, superficial, head, specified NEC
    mammary — see Injury, superficial, breast
    mastoid region — see Injury, superficial, head, specified NEC
    mouth — see Injury, superficial, oral cavity
    muscle NEC T14.8 ☑
    nail NEC T14.8 ☑
      finger — see Injury, superficial, finger
      toe — see Injury, superficial, toe
    nasal (septum) — see Injury, superficial, nose
    neck S10.90 ☑
      specified site NEC S10.80 ☑
    nose (septum) S00.30 ☑
    occipital region — see Injury, superficial, scalp
    oral cavity S00.502 ☑
    orbital region — see Injury, superficial, periocular area
    palate — see Injury, superficial, oral cavity
    palm — see Injury, superficial, hand
    parietal region — see Injury, superficial, scalp
    pelvis S30.91 ☑
      girdle — see Injury, superficial, hip
    penis S30.93 ☑
    perineum
      female S30.95 ☑
      male S30.91 ☑
    periocular area S00.20- ☑
      abrasion — see Abrasion, eyelid
      bite — see Bite, superficial, eyelid
      contusion — see Contusion, eyelid
      external constriction — see Constriction, external, eyelid
      foreign body — see Foreign body, superficial, eyelid
    phalanges
      finger — see Injury, superficial, finger
      toe — see Injury, superficial, toe
    pharynx — see Injury, superficial, throat
    pinna — see Injury, superficial, ear
    popliteal space — see Injury, superficial, knee
    prepuce S30.93 ☑
    pubic region S30.91 ☑
    pudendum
      female S30.97 ☑
      male S30.96 ☑
    sacral region S30.91 ☑
    scalp S00.00 ☑
    scapular region — see Injury, superficial, shoulder
    sclera — see Injury, eye, specified site NEC
    scrotum S30.94 ☑
    shin — see Injury, superficial, leg
    shoulder S40.91- ☑
      abrasion — see Abrasion, shoulder
      bite — see Bite, superficial, shoulder
      blister — see Blister, shoulder
      contusion — see Contusion, shoulder
      external constriction — see Constriction, external, shoulder
      foreign body — see Foreign body, superficial, shoulder
    skin NEC T14.8 ☑
    sternal region — see Injury, superficial, thorax, front
    subconjunctival — see Injury, eye, specified site NEC
    subcutaneous NEC T14.8 ☑

Injury — continued
  superficial — continued
    submaxillary region — see Injury, superficial, head, specified NEC
    submental region — see Injury, superficial, head, specified NEC
    subungual
      finger(s) — see Injury, superficial, finger
      toe(s) — see Injury, superficial, toe
    supraclavicular fossa — see Injury, superficial, neck
    supraorbital — see Injury, superficial, head, specified NEC
    temple — see Injury, superficial, head, specified NEC
    temporal region — see Injury, superficial, head, specified NEC
    testis S30.94 ☑
    thigh S70.92- ☑
      abrasion — see Abrasion, thigh
      bite — see Bite, superficial, thigh
      blister — see Blister, thigh
      contusion — see Contusion, thigh
      external constriction — see Constriction, external, thigh
      foreign body — see Foreign body, superficial, thigh
    thorax, thoracic (wall) S20.90 ☑
      abrasion — see Abrasion, thorax
      back S20.40- ☑
      bite — see Bite, thorax, superficial
      blister — see Blister, thorax
      contusion — see Contusion, thorax
      external constriction — see Constriction, external, thorax
      foreign body — see Foreign body, superficial, thorax
      front S20.30- ☑
    throat S10.10 ☑
      abrasion S10.11 ☑
      bite S10.17 ☑
        insect S10.16 ☑
      blister S10.12 ☑
      contusion S10.0 ☑
      external constriction S10.14 ☑
      foreign body S10.15 ☑
    thumb S60.93- ☑
      abrasion — see Abrasion, thumb
      bite — see Bite, superficial, thumb
      blister — see Blister, thumb
      contusion — see Contusion, thumb
      external constriction — see Constriction, external, thumb
      foreign body — see Foreign body, superficial, thumb
      insect bite — see Bite, by site, superficial, insect
      specified type NEC S60.39 ☑
    toe(s) S90.93- ☑
      abrasion — see Abrasion, toe
      bite — see Bite, toe
      blister — see Blister, toe
      contusion — see Contusion, toe
      external constriction — see Constriction, external, toe
      foreign body — see Foreign body, superficial, toe
      great S90.93- ☑
    tongue — see Injury, superficial, oral cavity
    tooth, teeth — see Injury, superficial, oral cavity
    trachea S10.10 ☑
    tunica vaginalis S30.94 ☑
    tympanum, tympanic membrane — see Injury, superficial, ear
    uvula — see Injury, superficial, oral cavity
    vagina S30.95 ☑
    vocal cords — see Injury, superficial, throat
    vulva S30.95 ☑
    wrist S60.91- ☑
  supraclavicular region — see Injury, neck
  supraorbital S09.93 ☑
  suprarenal gland (multiple) — see Injury, adrenal
  surgical complication (external or internal site) — see Laceration, accidental complicating surgery
  temple S09.90 ☑
  temporal region S09.90 ☑
  tendon (see also Injury, muscle, by site)
    abdomen — see Injury, muscle, abdomen

Injury — *continued*
 tendon (*see also* Injury, muscle, by site) — *continued*
  Achilles — *see* Injury, Achilles tendon
  lower back — *see* Injury, muscle, lower back
  pelvic organs — *see* Injury, muscle, pelvis
 tenth cranial nerve (pneumogastric or vagus) — *see* Injury, nerve, vagus
 testis S39.94 ☑
 thigh S79.92-☑
  blood vessel — *see* Injury, blood vessel, hip
  contusion — *see* Contusion, thigh
  fracture — *see* Fracture, femur
  muscle — *see* Injury, muscle, thigh
  nerve — *see* Injury, nerve, thigh
  open — *see* Wound, open, thigh
  specified NEC S79.82-☑
  superficial — *see* Injury, superficial, thigh
 third cranial nerve (oculomotor) — *see* Injury, nerve, oculomotor
 thorax, thoracic S29.9 ☑
  blood vessel — *see* Injury, blood vessel, thorax
  cavity — *see* Injury, intrathoracic
  dislocation — *see* Dislocation, thorax
  external (wall) S29.9 ☑
   contusion — *see* Contusion, thorax
   nerve — *see* Injury, nerve, thorax
   open — *see* Wound, open, thorax
   specified NEC S29.8 ☑
   sprain — *see* Sprain, thorax
   superficial — *see* Injury, superficial, thorax
  fracture — *see* Fracture, thorax
  internal — *see* Injury, intrathoracic
  intrathoracic organ — *see* Injury, intrathoracic
  sympathetic ganglion — *see* Injury, nerve, thorax, sympathetic
 throat (*see also* Injury, neck) S19.9 ☑
 thumb S69.9-☑
  blood vessel — *see* Injury, blood vessel, thumb
  contusion — *see* Contusion, thumb
  dislocation — *see* Dislocation, thumb
  fracture — *see* Fracture, thumb
  muscle — *see* Injury, muscle, thumb
  nerve — *see* Injury, nerve, digital, thumb
  open — *see* Wound, open, thumb
  specified NEC S69.8-☑
  sprain — *see* Sprain, thumb
  superficial — *see* Injury, superficial, thumb
 thymus (gland) — *see* Injury, intrathoracic, specified organ NEC
 thyroid (gland) NEC S19.84 ☑
 toe S99.92-☑
  contusion — *see* Contusion, toe
  dislocation — *see* Dislocation, toe
  fracture — *see* Fracture, toe
  muscle — *see* Injury, muscle, toe
  open — *see* Wound, open, toe
  specified type NEC S99.82-☑
  sprain — *see* Sprain, toe
  superficial — *see* Injury, superficial, toe
 tongue S09.93 ☑
 tonsil S09.93 ☑
 tooth S09.93 ☑
 trachea (cervical) NEC S19.82 ☑
  thoracic — *see* Injury, intrathoracic, trachea, thoracic
 transfusion-related acute lung (TRALI) J95.84
 tunica vaginalis S39.94 ☑
 twelfth cranial nerve (hypoglossal) — *see* Injury, nerve, hypoglossal
 ureter S37.10 ☑
  contusion S37.12 ☑
  laceration S37.13 ☑
  specified type NEC S37.19 ☑
 urethra (sphincter) S37.30 ☑
  at delivery O71.5
  contusion S37.32 ☑
  laceration S37.33 ☑
  specified type NEC S37.39 ☑
 urinary organ S37.90 ☑
  contusion S37.92 ☑
  laceration S37.93 ☑
  specified
   site NEC S37.899 ☑
    contusion S37.892 ☑
    laceration S37.893 ☑

Injury — *continued*
 urinary organ — *continued*
  specified — *continued*
   site — *continued*
    specified type NEC S37.898 ☑
    type NEC S37.99 ☑
 uterus, uterine S37.60 ☑
  with ectopic or molar pregnancy O08.6
  blood vessel — *see* Injury, blood vessel, iliac
  contusion S37.62 ☑
  laceration S37.63 ☑
   cervix at delivery O71.3
  rupture associated with obstetrics — *see* Rupture, uterus
  specified type NEC S37.69 ☑
 uvula S09.93 ☑
 vagina S39.93 ☑
  abrasion S30.814 ☑
  bite S31.45 ☑
   insect S30.864 ☑
   superficial NEC S30.874 ☑
  contusion S30.23 ☑
  crush S38.03 ☑
  during delivery — *see* Laceration, vagina, during delivery
  external constriction S30.844 ☑
  insect bite S30.864 ☑
  laceration S31.41 ☑
   with foreign body S31.42 ☑
  open wound S31.40 ☑
  puncture S31.43 ☑
   with foreign body S31.44 ☑
  superficial S30.95 ☑
   foreign body S30.854 ☑
 vas deferens — *see* Injury, pelvic organ, specified site NEC
 vascular NEC T14.8 ☑
 vein — *see* Injury, blood vessel
 vena cava (superior) S25.20 ☑
  inferior S35.10 ☑
   laceration (minor) (superficial) S35.11 ☑
    major S35.12 ☑
   specified type NEC S35.19 ☑
  laceration (minor) (superficial) S25.21 ☑
   major S25.22 ☑
  specified type NEC S25.29 ☑
 vesical (sphincter) — *see* Injury, bladder
 visual cortex S04.04-☑
 vitreous (humor) S05.90 ☑
  specified NEC S05.8X-☑
 vocal cord NEC S19.83 ☑
 vulva S39.94 ☑
  abrasion S30.814 ☑
  bite S31.45 ☑
   insect S30.864 ☑
   superficial NEC S30.874 ☑
  contusion S30.23 ☑
  crush S38.03 ☑
  during delivery — *see* Laceration, perineum, female, during delivery
  external constriction S30.844 ☑
  insect bite S30.864 ☑
  laceration S31.41 ☑
   with foreign body S31.42 ☑
  open wound S31.40 ☑
  puncture S31.43 ☑
   with foreign body S31.44 ☑
  superficial S30.95 ☑
   foreign body S30.854 ☑
 whiplash (cervical spine) S13.4 ☑
 wrist S69.9-☑
  blood vessel — *see* Injury, blood vessel, hand
  contusion — *see* Contusion, wrist
  dislocation — *see* Dislocation, wrist
  fracture — *see* Fracture, wrist
  muscle — *see* Injury, muscle, hand
  nerve — *see* Injury, nerve, hand
  open — *see* Wound, open, wrist
  specified NEC S69.8-☑
  sprain — *see* Sprain, wrist
  superficial — *see* Injury, superficial, wrist
Inoculation (*see also* Vaccination)
 complication or reaction — *see* Complications, vaccination
Insanity, insane (*see also* Psychosis)
 adolescent — *see* Schizophrenia

Insanity, insane — *continued*
 confusional F28
  acute or subacute F05
 delusional F22
 senile F03 ☑
Insect
 bite — *see* Bite, by site, superficial, insect
 venomous, poisoning NEC (by) — *see* Venom, arthropod
Insensitivity
 adrenocorticotropin hormone (ACTH) E27.49
 androgen E34.50
  complete E34.51
  partial E34.52
Insertion
 cord (umbilical) lateral or velamentous O43.12-☑
 intrauterine contraceptive device (encounter for) — *see* Intrauterine contraceptive device
Insolation (sunstroke) T67.0 ☑
Insomnia (organic) G47.00
 without objective findings F51.02
 adjustment F51.02
 adjustment disorder F51.02
 behavioral, of childhood Z73.819
  combined type Z73.812
  limit setting type Z73.811
  sleep-onset association type Z73.810
 childhood Z73.819
 chronic F51.04
  somatized tension F51.04
 conditioned F51.04
 due to
  alcohol
   abuse F10.182
   dependence F10.282
   use F10.982
  amphetamines
   abuse F15.182
   dependence F15.282
   use F15.982
  anxiety disorder F51.05
  caffeine
   abuse F15.182
   dependence F15.282
   use F15.982
  cocaine
   abuse F14.182
   dependence F14.282
   use F14.982
  depression F51.05
  drug NEC
   abuse F19.182
   dependence F19.282
   use F19.982
  medical condition G47.01
  mental disorder NEC F51.05
  opioid
   abuse F11.182
   dependence F11.282
   use F11.982
  psychoactive substance NEC
   abuse F19.182
   dependence F19.182
   use F19.982
  sedative, hypnotic, or anxiolytic
   abuse F13.182
   dependence F13.282
   use F13.982
  stimulant NEC
   abuse F15.182
   dependence F15.282
   use F15.982
 fatal familial (FFI) A81.83
 idiopathic F51.01
 learned F51.3
 nonorganic origin F51.01
 not due to a substance or known physiological condition F51.01
 specified NEC F51.09
 paradoxical F51.03
 primary F51.01
 psychiatric F51.05
 psychophysiologic F51.04
 related to psychopathology F51.05
 short-term F51.02
 specified NEC G47.09
 stress-related F51.02
 transient F51.02

☑ Additional Character Required — Refer to the Tabular List for Character Selection   Subterms under main terms may continue to next column or page

Inspiration
food or foreign body — *see* Foreign body, by site
mucus — *see* Asphyxia, mucus
Inspissated bile syndrome (newborn) P59.1
Instability
emotional (excessive) F60.3
joint (post-traumatic) M25.30
ankle M25.37- ☑
due to old ligament injury — *see* Disorder, ligament
elbow M25.32- ☑
flail — *see* Flail, joint
foot M25.37- ☑
hand M25.34- ☑
hip M25.35- ☑
knee M25.36- ☑
lumbosacral — *see* subcategory M53.2 ☑
prosthesis — *see* Complications, joint prosthesis, mechanical, displacement, by site
sacroiliac — *see* subcategory M53.2 ☑
secondary to
old ligament injury — *see* Disorder, ligament
removal of joint prosthesis M96.89
shoulder (region) M25.31- ☑
spine — *see* subcategory M53.2 ☑
wrist M25.33- ☑
knee (chronic) M23.5- ☑
lumbosacral — *see* subcategory M53.2 ☑
nervous F48.8
personality (emotional) F60.3
spine — *see* Instability, joint, spine
vasomotor R55
Institutional syndrome (childhood) F94.2
Institutionalization, affecting child Z62.22
disinhibited attachment F94.2
Insufficiency, insufficient
accommodation, old age H52.4
adrenal (gland) E27.40
primary E27.1
adrenocortical E27.40
drug-induced E27.3
iatrogenic E27.3
primary E27.1
anatomic crown height K08.89
anterior (occlusal) guidance M26.54
anus K62.89
aortic (valve) I35.1
with
mitral (valve) disease I08.0
with tricuspid (valve) disease I08.3
stenosis I35.2
tricuspid (valve) disease I08.2
with mitral (valve) disease I08.3
congenital Q23.1
rheumatic I06.1
with
mitral (valve) disease I08.0
with tricuspid (valve) disease I08.3
stenosis I06.2
with mitral (valve) disease I08.0
with tricuspid (valve) disease I08.3
tricuspid (valve) disease I08.2
with mitral (valve) disease I08.3
specified cause NEC I35.1
syphilitic A52.03
arterial I77.1
basilar G45.0
carotid (hemispheric) G45.1
cerebral I67.81
coronary (acute or subacute) I24.8
mesenteric K55.1
peripheral I73.9
precerebral (multiple) (bilateral) G45.2
vertebral G45.0
arteriovenous I99.8
biliary K83.8
cardiac (*see also* Insufficiency, myocardial)
due to presence of (cardiac) prosthesis I97.11- ☑
postprocedural I97.11- ☑
cardiorenal, hypertensive I13.2
cardiovascular — *see* Disease, cardiovascular
cerebrovascular (acute) I67.81
with transient focal neurological signs and symptoms G45.8
circulatory NEC I99.8
newborn P29.89
clinical crown length K08.89
convergence H51.11

Insufficiency, insufficient — *continued*
coronary (acute or subacute) I24.8
chronic or with a stated duration of over 4 weeks I25.89
corticoadrenal E27.40
primary E27.1
dietary E63.9
divergence H51.8
food T73.0 ☑
gastroesophageal K22.8
gonadal
ovary E28.39
testis E29.1
heart (*see also* Insufficiency, myocardial)
newborn P29.0
valve — *see* Endocarditis
hepatic — *see* Failure, hepatic
idiopathic autonomic G90.09
interocclusal distance of fully erupted teeth (ridge) M26.36
kidney N28.9
acute N28.9
chronic N18.9
lacrimal (secretion) H04.12- ☑
passages — *see* Stenosis, lacrimal
liver — *see* Failure, hepatic
lung — *see* Insufficiency, pulmonary
mental (congenital) — *see* Disability, intellectual
mesenteric K55.1
mitral (valve) I34.0
with
aortic valve disease I08.0
with tricuspid (valve) disease I08.3
obstruction or stenosis I05.2
with aortic valve disease I08.0
tricuspid (valve) disease I08.1
with aortic (valve) disease I08.3
congenital Q23.3
rheumatic I05.1
with
aortic valve disease I08.0
with tricuspid (valve) disease I08.3
obstruction or stenosis I05.2
with aortic valve disease I08.0
with tricuspid (valve) disease I08.3
tricuspid (valve) disease I08.1
with aortic (valve) disease I08.3
active or acute I01.1
with chorea, rheumatic (Sydenham's) I02.0
specified cause, except rheumatic I34.0
muscle (*see also* Disease, muscle)
heart — *see* Insufficiency, myocardial
ocular NEC H50.9
myocardial, myocardium (with arteriosclerosis) (*see also* Failure, heart) I50.9
with
rheumatic fever (conditions in I00) I09.0
active, acute or subacute I01.2
with chorea I02.0
inactive or quiescent (with chorea) I09.0
congenital Q24.8
hypertensive — *see* Hypertension, heart
newborn P29.0
rheumatic I09.0
active, acute, or subacute I01.2
syphilitic A52.06
nourishment T73.0 ☑
pancreatic K86.89
exocrine K86.81
parathyroid (gland) E20.9
peripheral vascular (arterial) I73.9
pituitary E23.0
placental (mother) O36.51- ☑
platelets D69.6
prenatal care affecting management of pregnancy O09.3- ☑
progressive pluriglandular E31.0
pulmonary J98.4
acute, following surgery (nonthoracic) J95.2
thoracic J95.1
chronic, following surgery J95.3
following
shock J98.4
trauma J98.4
newborn P28.5
valve I37.1
with stenosis I37.2
congenital Q22.2

Insufficiency, insufficient — *continued*
pulmonary — *continued*
valve — *continued*
rheumatic I09.89
with aortic, mitral or tricuspid (valve) disease I08.8
pyloric K31.89
renal (acute) N28.9
chronic N18.9
respiratory R06.89
newborn P28.5
rotation — *see* Malrotation
sleep syndrome F51.12
social insurance Z59.7
suprarenal E27.40
primary E27.1
tarso-orbital fascia, congenital Q10.3
testis E29.1
thyroid (gland) (acquired) E03.9
congenital E03.1
tricuspid (valve) (rheumatic) I07.1
with
aortic (valve) disease I08.2
with mitral (valve) disease I08.3
mitral (valve) disease I08.1
with aortic (valve) disease I08.3
obstruction or stenosis I07.2
with aortic (valve) disease I08.2
with mitral (valve) disease I08.3
congenital Q22.8
nonrheumatic I36.1
with stenosis I36.2
urethral sphincter R32
valve, valvular (heart) I38
aortic — *see* Insufficiency, aortic (valve)
congenital Q24.8
mitral — *see* Insufficiency, mitral (valve)
pulmonary — *see* Insufficiency, pulmonary, valve
tricuspid — *see* Insufficiency, tricuspid (valve)
vascular I99.8
intestine K55.9
acute (*see also* Ischemia, intestine, acute) K55.059
mesenteric K55.1
peripheral I73.9
renal — *see* Hypertension, kidney
velopharyngeal
acquired K13.79
congenital Q38.8
venous (chronic) (peripheral) I87.2
ventricular — *see* Insufficiency, myocardial
welfare support Z59.7
Insufflation, fallopian Z31.41
Insular — *see* condition
Insulinoma
pancreas
benign D13.7
malignant C25.4
uncertain behavior D37.8
specified site
benign — *see* Neoplasm, by site, benign
malignant — *see* Neoplasm, by site, malignant
uncertain behavior — *see* Neoplasm, by site, uncertain behavior
unspecified site
benign D13.7
malignant C25.4
uncertain behavior D37.8
Insuloma — *see* Insulinoma
Interference
balancing side M26.56
non-working side M26.56
Intermenstrual — *see* condition
Intermittent — *see* condition
Internal — *see* condition
Interrogation
cardiac defibrillator (automatic) (implantable) Z45.02
cardiac pacemaker Z45.018
cardiac (event) (loop) recorder Z45.09
infusion pump (implanted) (intrathecal) Z45.1
neurostimulator Z46.2
Interruption
aortic arch Q25.21
bundle of His I44.30
phase-shift, sleep cycle — *see* Disorder, sleep, circadian rhythm
sleep phase-shift, or 24 hour sleep-wake cycle — *see* Disorder, sleep, circadian rhythm

Interstitial — see condition
Intertrigo L30.4
  labialis K13.0
Intervertebral disc — see condition
Intestine, intestinal — see condition
Intolerance
  carbohydrate K90.49
  disaccharide, hereditary E73.0
  fat NEC K90.49
    pancreatic K90.3
  food K90.49
    dietary counseling and surveillance Z71.3
  fructose E74.10
    hereditary E74.12
  glucose (-galactose) E74.39
  gluten K90.41
  lactose E73.9
    specified NEC E73.8
  lysine E72.3
  milk NEC K90.49
    lactose E73.9
  protein K90.49
  starch NEC K90.49
  sucrose (-isomaltose) E74.31
Intoxicated NEC (without dependence) — see Alcohol, intoxication
Intoxication
  acid E87.2
  alcoholic (acute) (without dependence) — see Alcohol, intoxication
  alimentary canal K52.1
  amphetamine (without dependence) — see Abuse, drug, stimulant, with intoxication
    with dependence — see Dependence, drug, stimulant, with intoxication
  anxiolytic (acute) (without dependence) — see Abuse, drug, sedative, with intoxication
    with dependence — see Dependence, drug, sedative, with intoxication
  caffeine F15.929
    with dependence — see Dependence, drug, stimulant, with intoxication
  cannabinoids (acute) (without dependence) — see Use, cannabis, with intoxication
    with
      abuse — see Abuse, drug, cannabis, with intoxication
      dependence — see Dependence, drug, cannabis, with intoxication
  chemical — see Table of Drugs and Chemicals
    via placenta or breast milk — see - Absorption, chemical, through placenta
  cocaine (acute) (without dependence) — see Abuse, drug, cocaine, with intoxication
    with dependence — see Dependence, drug, cocaine, with intoxication
  drug
    acute (without dependence) — see Abuse, drug, by type with intoxication
      with dependence — see Dependence, drug, by type with intoxication
    addictive
      via placenta or breast milk — see Absorption, drug, addictive, through placenta
    newborn P93.8
      gray baby syndrome P93.0
    overdose or wrong substance given or taken — see Table of Drugs and Chemicals, by drug, poisoning
  enteric K52.1
  foodborne A05.9
    bacterial A05.9
    classical (Clostridium botulinum) A05.1
    due to
      Bacillus cereus A05.4
      bacterium A05.9
        specified NEC A05.8
      Clostridium
        botulinum A05.1
        perfringens A05.2
        welchii A05.2
      Salmonella A02.9
        with
          (gastro)enteritis A02.0
          localized infection(s) A02.20
            arthritis A02.23
            meningitis A02.21
            osteomyelitis A02.24

Intoxication — continued
  foodborne — continued
    due to — continued
      Salmonella — continued
        with — continued
          localized infection(s) — continued
            pneumonia A02.22
            pyelonephritis A02.25
            specified NEC A02.29
          sepsis A02.1
          specified manifestation NEC A02.8
      Staphylococcus A05.0
      Vibrio
        parahaemolyticus A05.3
        vulnificus A05.5
    enterotoxin, staphylococcal A05.0
    noxious — see Poisoning, food, noxious
  gastrointestinal K52.1
  hallucinogenic (without dependence) — see Abuse, drug, hallucinogen, with intoxication
    with dependence — see Dependence, drug, hallucinogen, with intoxication
  hypnotic (acute) (without dependence) — see Abuse, drug, sedative, with intoxication
    with dependence — see Dependence, drug, sedative, with intoxication
  inhalant (acute) (without dependence) — see Abuse, drug, inhalant, with intoxication
    with dependence — see Dependence, drug, inhalant, with intoxication
  meaning
    inebriation — see category F10 ☑
    poisoning — see Table of Drugs and Chemicals
  methyl alcohol (acute) (without dependence) — see Alcohol, intoxication
  opioid (acute) (without dependence) — see Abuse, drug, opioid, with intoxication
    with dependence — see Dependence, drug, opioid, with intoxication
  pathologic NEC (without dependence) — see Alcohol, intoxication
  phencyclidine (without dependence) — see Abuse, drug, hallucinogen, with intoxication
    with dependence — see Dependence, drug, hallucinogen, with intoxication
  potassium (K) E87.5
  psychoactive substance NEC (without dependence) — see Abuse, drug, psychoactive NEC, with intoxication
    with dependence — see Dependence, drug, psychoactive NEC, with intoxication
  sedative (acute) (without dependence) — see Abuse, drug, sedative, with intoxication
    with dependence — see Dependence, drug, sedative, with intoxication
  serum (see also Reaction, serum) T80.69 ☑
  uremic — see Uremia
  volatile solvents (acute) (without dependence) — see Abuse, drug, inhalant, with intoxication
    with dependence — see Dependence, drug, inhalant, with intoxication
  water E87.79
Intraabdominal testis, testes
  bilateral Q53.211
  unilateral Q53.111
Intracranial — see condition
Intrahepatic gallbladder Q44.1
Intraligamentous — see condition
Intrathoracic (see also condition)
  kidney Q63.2
Intrauterine contraceptive device
  checking Z30.431
  in situ Z97.5
  insertion Z30.430
    immediately following removal Z30.433
  management Z30.431
  reinsertion Z30.433
  removal Z30.432
  replacement Z30.433
  retention in pregnancy O26.3- ☑
Intraventricular — see condition
Intrinsic deformity — see Deformity
Intubation, difficult or failed T88.4 ☑
Intumescence, lens (eye) (cataract) — see Cataract
Intussusception (bowel) (colon) (enteric) (ileocecal) (ileocolic) (intestine) (rectum) K56.1
  appendix K38.8
  congenital Q43.8

Intussusception — continued
  ureter (with obstruction) N13.5
Invagination (bowel, colon, intestine or rectum) K56.1
Inversion
  albumin-globulin (A-G) ratio E88.09
  bladder N32.89
  cecum — see Intussusception
  cervix N88.8
  chromosome in normal individual Q95.1
  circadian rhythm — see Disorder, sleep, circadian rhythm
  nipple N64.59
    congenital Q83.8
    gestational — see Retraction, nipple
    puerperal, postpartum — see Retraction, nipple
  nyctohemeral rhythm — see Disorder, sleep, circadian rhythm
  optic papilla Q14.2
  organ or site, congenital NEC — see Anomaly, by site
  sleep rhythm — see Disorder, sleep, circadian rhythm
  testis (congenital) Q55.29
  uterus (chronic) (postinfectional) (postpartal, old) N85.5
    postpartum O71.2
  vagina (posthysterectomy) N99.3
  ventricular Q20.5
Investigation (see also Examination) Z04.9
  clinical research subject (control) (normal comparison) (participant) Z00.6
Involuntary movement, abnormal R25.9
Involution, involutional (see also condition)
  breast, cystic — see Dysplasia, mammary, specified type NEC
  depression (single episode) F32.89
    recurrent episode F33.9
  melancholia (single episode) F32.89
    recurrent episode F33.8
  ovary, senile — see Atrophy, ovary
  thymus failure E32.8
I.Q.
  under 20 F73
  20-34 F72
  35-49 F71
  50-69 F70
IRDS (type I) P22.0
  type II P22.1
Irideremia Q13.1
Iridis rubeosis — see Disorder, iris, vascular
Iridochoroiditis (panuveitis) — see Panuveitis
Iridocyclitis H20.9
  acute H20.0- ☑
    hypopyon H20.05- ☑
    primary H20.01- ☑
    recurrent H20.02- ☑
    secondary (noninfectious) H20.04- ☑
      infectious H20.03- ☑
  chronic H20.1- ☑
  due to allergy — see Iridocyclitis, acute, secondary
  endogenous — see Iridocyclitis, acute, primary
  Fuchs' — see Cyclitis, Fuchs' heterochromic
  gonococcal A54.32
  granulomatous — see Iridocyclitis, chronic
  herpes, herpetic (simplex) B00.51
    zoster B02.32
  hypopyon — see Iridocyclitis, acute, hypopyon
  in (due to)
    ankylosing spondylitis M45.9
    gonococcal infection A54.32
    herpes (simplex) virus B00.51
      zoster B02.32
    infectious disease NOS B99 ☑
    parasitic disease NOS B89 [H22]
    sarcoidosis D86.83
    syphilis A51.43
    tuberculosis A18.54
    zoster B02.32
  lens-induced H20.2- ☑
  nongranulomatous — see Iridocyclitis, acute
  recurrent — see Iridocyclitis, acute, recurrent
  rheumatic — see Iridocyclitis, chronic
  subacute — see Iridocyclitis, acute
  sympathetic — see Uveitis, sympathetic
  syphilitic (secondary) A51.43
  tuberculous (chronic) A18.54
  Vogt-Koyanagi H20.82- ☑
Iridocyclochoroiditis (panuveitis) — see Panuveitis
Iridodialysis H21.53- ☑

☑ Additional Character Required — Refer to the Tabular List for Character Selection   ▽ Subterms under main terms may continue to next column or page

Iridodonesis H21.89
Iridoplegia (complete) (partial) (reflex) H57.09
Iridoschisis H21.25- ☑
Iris (see also condition)
  bombé — see Membrane, pupillary
Iritis (see also Iridocyclitis)
  chronic — see Iridocyclitis, chronic
  diabetic — see E08-E13 with .39
  due to
    herpes simplex B00.51
    leprosy A30.9 [H22]
  gonococcal A54.32
  gouty (see also Gout, by type) M10.9 [H22]
  granulomatous — see Iridocyclitis, chronic
  lens induced — see Iridocyclitis, lens-induced
  papulosa (syphilitic) A52.71
  rheumatic — see Iridocyclitis, chronic
  syphilitic (secondary) A51.43
    congenital (early) A50.01
    late A52.71
  tuberculous A18.54
Iron — see condition
Iron-miner's lung J63.4
Irradiated enamel (tooth, teeth) K03.89
Irradiation effects, adverse T66 ☑
Irreducible, irreducibility — see condition
Irregular, irregularity
  action, heart I49.9
  alveolar process K08.89
  bleeding N92.6
  breathing R06.89
  contour of cornea (acquired) — see Deformity, cornea
    congenital Q13.4
  contour, reconstructed breast N65.0
  dentin (in pulp) K04.3
  eye movements H55.89
    nystagmus — see Nystagmus
    saccadic H55.81
  labor O62.2
  menstruation (cause unknown) N92.6
  periods N92.6
  prostate N42.9
  pupil — see Abnormality, pupillary
  reconstructed breast N65.0
  respiratory R06.89
  septum (nasal) J34.2
  shape, organ or site, congenital NEC — see Distortion
  sleep-wake pattern (rhythm) G47.23
Irritable, irritability R45.4
  bladder N32.89
  bowel (syndrome) K58.9
    with
      constipation K58.1
      diarrhea K58.0
    mixed K58.2
    psychogenic F45.8
    specified NEC K58.8
  bronchial — see Bronchitis
  cerebral, in newborn P91.3
  colon (see also Irritable, bowel) K58.9
    with diarrhea K58.0
    psychogenic F45.8
  duodenum K59.8
  heart (psychogenic) F45.8
  hip — see Derangement, joint, specified type NEC, hip
  ileum K59.8
  infant R68.12
  jejunum K59.8
  rectum K59.8
  stomach K31.89
    psychogenic F45.8
  sympathetic G90.8
  urethra N36.8
Irritation
  anus K62.89
  axillary nerve G54.0
  bladder N32.89
  brachial plexus G54.0
  bronchial — see Bronchitis
  cervical plexus G54.2
  cervix — see Cervicitis
  choroid, sympathetic — see Endophthalmitis
  cranial nerve — see Disorder, nerve, cranial
  gastric K31.89
    psychogenic F45.8
  globe, sympathetic — see Uveitis, sympathetic
  labyrinth — see subcategory H83.2 ☑
  lumbosacral plexus G54.1

Irritation — continued
  meninges (traumatic) — see Injury, intracranial
    nontraumatic — see Meningismus
  nerve — see Disorder, nerve
  nervous R45.0
  penis N48.89
  perineum NEC L29.3
  peripheral autonomic nervous system G90.8
  peritoneum — see Peritonitis
  pharynx J39.2
  plantar nerve — see Lesion, nerve, plantar
  spinal (cord) (traumatic) (see also Injury, spinal cord,
    by region)
    nerve G58.9
      root NEC — see Radiculopathy
    nontraumatic — see Myelopathy
  stomach K31.89
    psychogenic F45.8
  sympathetic nerve NEC G90.8
  ulnar nerve — see Lesion, nerve, ulnar
  vagina N89.8
Ischemia, ischemic I99.8
  bowel (transient)
    acute (see also Ischemia, intestine, acute) K55.059
    chronic K55.1
    due to mesenteric artery insufficiency K55.1
  brain — see Ischemia, cerebral
  cardiac (see Disease, heart, ischemic)
  cardiomyopathy I25.5
  cerebral (chronic) (generalized) I67.82
    arteriosclerotic I67.2
    intermittent G45.9
    newborn P91.0
    recurrent focal G45.8
    transient G45.9
  colon chronic (due to mesenteric artery insufficiency)
    K55.1
  coronary — see Disease, heart, ischemic
  demand (coronary) (see also Angina) I24.8
    with myocardial infarction I21.A1
    resulting in myocardial infarction I21.A1
  heart (chronic or with a stated duration of over 4
    weeks) I25.9
    acute or with a stated duration of 4 weeks or less
      I24.9
    subacute I24.9
  infarction, muscle — see Infarct, muscle
  intestine (large) (small) (transient) K55.9
    acute K55.059
      diffuse K55.052
      focal K55.051
      large K55.039
        diffuse K55.032
        focal K55.031
      small K55.019
        diffuse K55.012
        focal K55.011
    chronic K55.1
    due to mesenteric artery insufficiency K55.1
  kidney N28.0
  mesenteric, acute (see also Ischemia, intestine, acute)
    K55.059
  muscle, traumatic T79.6 ☑
  myocardium, myocardial (chronic or with a stated
    duration of over 4 weeks) I25.9
    acute, without myocardial infarction I51.3
    silent (asymptomatic) I25.6
    transient of newborn P29.4
  renal N28.0
  retina, retinal — see Occlusion, artery, retina
  small bowel
    acute K55.019
      diffuse K55.012
      focal K55.011
    chronic K55.1
    due to mesenteric artery insufficiency K55.1
  spinal cord G95.11
  subendocardial — see Insufficiency, coronary
  supply (coronary) (see also Angina) I25.9
    due to vasospasm I20.1
Ischial spine — see condition
Ischialgia — see Sciatica
Ischiopagus Q89.4
Ischium, ischial — see condition
Ischuria R34
Iselin's disease or osteochondrosis — see Osteochon-
  drosis, juvenile, metatarsus

Islands of
  parotid tissue in
    lymph nodes Q38.6
    neck structures Q38.6
  submaxillary glands in
    fascia Q38.6
    lymph nodes Q38.6
    neck muscles Q38.6
Islet cell tumor, pancreas D13.7
Isoimmunization NEC (see also Incompatibility)
  affecting management of pregnancy (ABO) (with hy-
    drops fetalis) O36.11- ☑
    anti-A sensitization O36.11- ☑
    anti-B sensitization O36.19- ☑
    anti-c sensitization O36.09- ☑
    anti-C sensitization O36.09- ☑
    anti-e sensitization O36.09- ☑
    anti-E sensitization O36.09- ☑
    Rh NEC O36.09- ☑
      anti-D antibody O36.01- ☑
    specified NEC O36.19- ☑
  newborn P55.9
    with
      hydrops fetalis P56.0
      kernicterus P57.0
    ABO (blood groups) P55.1
    Rhesus (Rh) factor P55.0
    specified type NEC P55.8
Isolation, isolated
  dwelling Z59.8
  family Z63.79
  social Z60.4
Isoleucinosis E71.19
Isomerism atrial appendages (with asplenia or
  polysplenia) Q20.6
Isosporiasis, isosporosis A07.3
Isovaleric acidemia E71.110
Issue of
  medical certificate Z02.79
    for disability determination Z02.71
  repeat prescription (appliance) (glasses) (medicinal
    substance, medicament, medicine) Z76.0
    contraception — see Contraception
Itch, itching (see also Pruritus)
  baker's L23.6
  barber's B35.0
  bricklayer's L24.5
  cheese B88.0
  clam digger's B65.3
  coolie B76.9
  copra B88.0
  dew B76.9
  dhobi B35.6
  filarial — see Infestation, filarial
  grain B88.0
  grocer's B88.0
  ground B76.9
  harvest B88.0
  jock B35.6
  Malabar B35.5
    beard B35.0
    foot B35.3
    scalp B35.0
  meaning scabies B86
  Norwegian B86
  perianal L29.0
  poultrymen's B88.0
  sarcoptic B86
  scabies B86
  scrub B88.0
  straw B88.0
  swimmer's B65.3
  water B76.9
  winter L29.8
Ivemark's syndrome (asplenia with congenital heart
  disease) Q89.01
Ivory bones Q78.2
Ixodiasis NEC B88.8

J

Jaccoud's syndrome — see Arthropathy, postrheumatic,
  chronic
Jackson's
  membrane Q43.3
  paralysis or syndrome G83.89
  veil Q43.3
Jacquet's dermatitis (diaper dermatitis) L22

Jadassohn-Pellizari's disease or anetoderma L90.2
Jadassohn's
  blue nevus — *see* Nevus
  intraepidermal epithelioma — *see* Neoplasm, skin, benign
Jaffe-Lichtenstein (-Uehlinger) **syndrome** — *see* Dysplasia, fibrous, bone NEC
Jakob-Creutzfeldt disease or syndrome — *see* Creutzfeldt-Jakob disease or syndrome
Jaksch-Luzet disease D64.89
Jamaican
  neuropathy G92
  paraplegic tropical ataxic-spastic syndrome G92
Janet's disease F48.8
Janiceps Q89.4
Jansky-Bielschowsky amaurotic idiocy E75.4
Japanese
  B-type encephalitis A83.0
  river fever A75.3
Jaundice (yellow) R17
  acholuric (familial) (splenomegalic) (*see also* Spherocytosis)
    acquired D59.8
  breast-milk (inhibitor) P59.3
  catarrhal (acute) B15.9
    with hepatic coma B15.0
  cholestatic (benign) R17
  due to or associated with
    delayed conjugation P59.8
      associated with (due to) preterm delivery P59.0
    preterm delivery P59.0
  epidemic (catarrhal) B15.9
    with hepatic coma B15.0
    leptospiral A27.0
    spirochetal A27.0
  familial nonhemolytic (congenital) (Gilbert) E80.4
    Crigler-Najjar E80.5
  febrile (acute) B15.9
    with hepatic coma B15.0
    leptospiral A27.0
    spirochetal A27.0
  hematogenous D59.9
  hemolytic (acquired) D59.9
    congenital — *see* Spherocytosis
  hemorrhagic (acute) (leptospiral) (spirochetal) A27.0
  infectious (acute) (subacute) B15.9
    with hepatic coma B15.0
    leptospiral A27.0
    spirochetal A27.0
  leptospiral (hemorrhagic) A27.0
  malignant (without coma) K72.90
    with coma K72.91
  neonatal — *see* Jaundice, newborn
  newborn P59.9
    due to or associated with
      ABO
        antibodies P55.1
        incompatibility, maternal/fetal P55.1
        isoimmunization P55.1
      absence or deficiency of enzyme system for bilirubin conjugation (congenital) P59.8
      bleeding P58.1
      breast milk inhibitors to conjugation P59.3
        associated with preterm delivery P59.0
      bruising P58.0
      Crigler-Najjar syndrome E80.5
      delayed conjugation P59.8
        associated with preterm delivery P59.0
      drugs or toxins
        given to newborn P58.42
        transmitted from mother P58.41
      excessive hemolysis P58.9
        due to
          bleeding P58.1
          bruising P58.0
          drugs or toxins
            given to newborn P58.42
            transmitted from mother P58.41
          infection P58.2
          polycythemia P58.3
          swallowed maternal blood P58.5
        specified type NEC P58.8
      galactosemia E74.21
      Gilbert syndrome E80.4
      hemolytic disease P55.9
        ABO isoimmunization P55.1
        Rh isoimmunization P55.0
        specified NEC P55.8

Jaundice — *continued*
  newborn — *continued*
    due to or associated with — *continued*
      hepatocellular damage P59.20
        specified NEC P59.29
      hereditary hemolytic anemia P58.8
      hypothyroidism, congenital E03.1
      incompatibility, maternal/fetal NOS P55.9
      infection P58.2
      inspissated bile syndrome P59.1
      isoimmunization NOS P55.9
      mucoviscidosis E84.9
      polycythemia P58.3
      preterm delivery P59.0
      Rh
        antibodies P55.0
        incompatibility, maternal/fetal P55.0
        isoimmunization P55.0
      specified cause NEC P59.8
      swallowed maternal blood P58.5
    spherocytosis (congenital) D58.0
  nonhemolytic congenital familial (Gilbert) E80.4
  nuclear, newborn (*see also* Kernicterus of newborn) P57.9
  obstructive (*see also* Obstruction, bile duct) K83.1
  post-immunization — *see* Hepatitis, viral, type, B
  post-transfusion — *see* Hepatitis, viral, type, B
  regurgitation (*see also* Obstruction, bile duct) K83.1
  serum (homologous) (prophylactic) (therapeutic) — *see* Hepatitis, viral, type, B
  spirochetal (hemorrhagic) A27.0
  symptomatic R17
    newborn P59.9
Jaw — *see* condition
Jaw-winking phenomenon or syndrome Q07.8
Jealousy
  alcoholic F10.988
  childhood F93.8
  sibling F93.8
Jejunitis — *see* Enteritis
Jejunostomy status Z93.4
Jejunum, jejunal — *see* condition
Jensen's disease — *see* Inflammation, chorioretinal, focal, juxtapapillary
Jerks, myoclonic G25.3
Jervell-Lange-Nielsen syndrome I45.81
Jeune's disease Q77.2
Jigger disease B88.1
Job's syndrome (chronic granulomatous disease) D71
Joint (*see also* condition)
  mice — *see* Loose, body, joint
    knee M23.4- ☑
Jordan's anomaly or syndrome D72.0
Joseph-Diamond-Blackfan anemia (congenital hypoplastic) D61.01
Jungle yellow fever A95.0
Jüngling's disease — *see* Sarcoidosis
Juvenile — *see* condition

K

Kahler's disease C90.0- ☑
Kakke E51.11
Kala-azar B55.0
Kallmann's syndrome E23.0
Kanner's syndrome (autism) — *see* Psychosis, childhood
Kaposi's
  dermatosis (xeroderma pigmentosum) Q82.1
  lichen ruber L44.0
    acuminatus L44.0
  sarcoma
    colon C46.4
    connective tissue C46.1
    gastrointestinal organ C46.4
    lung C46.5- ☑
    lymph node (multiple) C46.3
    palate (hard) (soft) C46.2
    rectum C46.4
    skin (multiple sites) C46.0
    specified site NEC C46.7
    stomach C46.4
    unspecified site C46.9
  varicelliform eruption B00.0
    vaccinia T88.1 ☑
Kartagener's syndrome or triad (sinusitis, bronchiectasis, situs inversus) Q89.3

Karyotype
  with abnormality except iso (Xq) Q96.2
  45,X Q96.0
  46,X
    iso (Xq) Q96.1
  46,XX Q98.3
    with streak gonads Q50.32
    hermaphrodite (true) Q99.1
    male Q98.3
  46,XY
    with streak gonads Q56.1
    female Q97.3
    hermaphrodite (true) Q99.1
  47,XXX Q97.0
  47,XXY Q98.0
  47,XYY Q98.5
Kaschin-Beck disease — *see* Disease, Kaschin-Beck
Katayama's disease or fever B65.2
Kawasaki's syndrome M30.3
Kayser-Fleischer ring (cornea) (pseudosclerosis) H18.04- ☑
Kaznelson's syndrome (congenital hypoplastic anemia) D61.01
Kearns-Sayre syndrome H49.81- ☑
Kedani fever A75.3
Kelis L91.0
Kelly (-Patterson) **syndrome** (sideropenic dysphagia) D50.1
Keloid, cheloid L91.0
  acne L73.0
  Addison's L94.0
  cornea — *see* Opacity, cornea
  Hawkin's L91.0
  scar L91.0
Keloma L91.0
Kenya fever A77.1
Keratectasia (*see also* Ectasia, cornea)
  congenital Q13.4
Keratinization of alveolar ridge mucosa
  excessive K13.23
  minimal K13.22
Keratinized residual ridge mucosa
  excessive K13.23
  minimal K13.22
Keratitis (nodular) (nonulcerative) (simple) (zonular) H16.9
  with ulceration (central) (marginal) (perforated) (ring) — *see* Ulcer, cornea
  actinic — *see* Photokeratitis
  arborescens (herpes simplex) B00.52
  areolar H16.11- ☑
  bullosa H16.8
  deep H16.309
    specified type NEC H16.399
  dendritic (a) (herpes simplex) B00.52
  disciform (is) (herpes simplex) B00.52
    varicella B01.81
  filamentary H16.12- ☑
  gonococcal (congenital or prenatal) A54.33
  herpes, herpetic (simplex) B00.52
    zoster B02.33
  in (due to)
    acanthamebiasis B60.13
    adenovirus B30.0
    exanthema (*see also* Exanthem) B09
    herpes (simplex) virus B00.52
    measles B05.81
    syphilis A50.31
    tuberculosis A18.52
    zoster B02.33
  interstitial (nonsyphilitic) H16.30- ☑
    diffuse H16.32- ☑
    herpes, herpetic (simplex) B00.52
      zoster B02.33
    sclerosing H16.33- ☑
    specified type NEC H16.39- ☑
    syphilitic (congenital) (late) A50.31
    tuberculous A18.52
  macular H16.11- ☑
  nummular H16.11- ☑
  oyster shuckers' H16.8
  parenchymatous — *see* Keratitis, interstitial
  petrificans H16.8
  postmeasles B05.81
  punctata
    leprosa A30.9 [H16.14-] ☑
    syphilitic (profunda) A50.31
  punctate H16.14- ☑

☑ Additional Character Required — Refer to the Tabular List for Character Selection   ▽ Subterms under main terms may continue to next column or page

Keratitis — *continued*
 purulent H16.8
 rosacea L71.8
 sclerosing H16.33- ☑
 specified type NEC H16.8
 stellate H16.11- ☑
 striate H16.11- ☑
 superficial H16.10- ☑
  with conjunctivitis — *see* Keratoconjunctivitis
  due to light — *see* Photokeratitis
 suppurative H16.8
 syphilitic (congenital) (prenatal) A50.31
 trachomatous A71.1
  sequelae B94.0
 tuberculous A18.52
 vesicular H16.8
 xerotic (*see also* Keratomalacia) H16.8
  vitamin A deficiency E50.4
Keratoacanthoma L85.8
Keratocele — *see* Descemetocele
Keratoconjunctivitis H16.20- ☑
 Acanthamoeba B60.13
 adenoviral B30.0
 epidemic B30.0
 exposure H16.21- ☑
 herpes, herpetic (simplex) B00.52
  zoster B02.33
 in exanthema (*see also* Exanthem) B09
 infectious B30.0
 lagophthalmic — *see* Keratoconjunctivitis, specified
   type NEC
 neurotrophic H16.23- ☑
 phlyctenular H16.25- ☑
 postmeasles B05.81
 shipyard B30.0
 sicca (Sjogren's) M35.0- ☑
  not Sjogren's H16.22- ☑
 specified type NEC H16.29- ☑
 tuberculous (phlyctenular) A18.52
 vernal H16.26- ☑
Keratoconus H18.60- ☑
 congenital Q13.4
 stable H18.61- ☑
 unstable H18.62- ☑
Keratocyst (dental) (odontogenic) — *see* Cyst, calcifying
   odontogenic
Keratoderma, keratodermia (congenital) (palmaris et
   plantaris) (symmetrical) Q82.8
 acquired L85.1
  in diseases classified elsewhere L86
 climactericum L85.1
 gonococcal A54.89
 gonorrheal A54.89
 punctata L85.2
 Reiter's — *see* Reiter's disease
Keratodermatocele — *see* Descemetocele
Keratoglobus H18.79 ☑
 congenital Q15.8
  with glaucoma Q15.0
Keratohemia — *see* Pigmentation, cornea, stromal
Keratoiritis (*see also* Iridocyclitis)
 syphilitic A50.39
 tuberculous A18.54
Keratoma L57.0
 palmaris and plantaris hereditarium Q82.8
 senile L57.0
Keratomalacia H18.44- ☑
 vitamin A deficiency E50.4
Keratomegaly Q13.4
Keratomycosis B49
 nigrans, nigricans (palmaris) B36.1
Keratopathy H18.9
 band H18.42- ☑
 bullous (aphakic), following cataract surgery
   H59.01- ☑
 bullous H18.1- ☑
Keratoscleritis, tuberculous A18.52
Keratosis L57.0
 actinic L57.0
 arsenical L85.8
 congenital, specified NEC Q80.8
 female genital NEC N94.89
 follicularis Q82.8
  acquired L11.0
  congenita Q82.8
  et parafollicularis in cutem penetrans L87.0
  spinulosa (decalvans) Q82.8

Keratosis — *continued*
 follicularis — *continued*
  vitamin A deficiency E50.8
 gonococcal A54.89
 male genital (external) N50.89
 nigricans L83
 obturans, external ear (canal) — *see* Cholesteatoma,
   external ear
 palmaris et plantaris (inherited) (symmetrical) Q82.8
  acquired L85.1
 penile N48.89
 pharynx J39.2
 pilaris, acquired L85.8
 punctata (palmaris et plantaris) L85.2
 scrotal N50.89
 seborrheic L82.1
  inflamed L82.0
 senile L57.0
 solar L57.0
 tonsillaris J35.8
 vagina N89.4
 vegetans Q82.8
 vitamin A deficiency E50.8
 vocal cord J38.3
Kerato-uveitis — *see* Iridocyclitis
Kerion (celsi) B35.0
Kernicterus of newborn (not due to isoimmunization)
   P57.9
 due to isoimmunization (conditions in P55.0-P55.9)
   P57.0
 specified type NEC P57.8
Kerunoparalysis T75.09 ☑
Keshan disease E59
Ketoacidosis E87.2
 diabetic — *see* Diabetes, by type, with ketoacidosis
Ketonuria R82.4
Ketosis NEC E88.89
 diabetic — *see* Diabetes, by type, with with ketoacidosis
Kew Garden fever A79.1
Kidney — *see* condition
Kienböck's disease (*see also* Osteochondrosis, juvenile,
   hand, carpal lunate)
 adult M93.1
Kimmelstiel (-Wilson) **disease** — *see* Diabetes, Kimmelstiel (-Wilson) disease
Kink, kinking
 artery I77.1
 hair (acquired) L67.8
 ileum or intestine — *see* Obstruction, intestine
 Lane's — *see* Obstruction, intestine
 organ or site, congenital NEC — *see* Anomaly, by site
 ureter (pelvic junction) N13.5
  with
   hydronephrosis N13.1
    with infection N13.6
   pyelonephritis (chronic) N11.1
  congenital Q62.39
 vein(s) I87.8
  caval I87.1
  peripheral I87.1
Kinnier Wilson's disease (hepatolenticular degeneration) E83.01
Kissing spine M48.20
 cervical region M48.22
 cervicothoracic region M48.23
 lumbar region M48.26
 lumbosacral region M48.27
 occipito-atlanto-axial region M48.21
 thoracic region M48.24
 thoracolumbar region M48.25
Klatskin's tumor C22.1
Klauder's disease A26.8
Klebs' disease (*see also* Glomerulonephritis) N05- ☑
Klebsiella (K.) **pneumoniae, as cause of disease
   classified elsewhere** B96.1
Klein (e)-**Levin syndrome** G47.13
Kleptomania F63.2
Klinefelter's syndrome Q98.4
 karyotype 47,XXY Q98.0
 male with more than two X chromosomes Q98.1
Klippel-Feil deficiency, disease, or syndrome (brevi-
   collis) Q76.1
Klippel's disease I67.2
Klippel-Trenaunay (-Weber) **syndrome** Q87.2
Klumpke (-Déjerine) **palsy, paralysis** (birth) (newborn)
   P14.1
Knee — *see* condition

Knock knee (acquired) M21.06- ☑
 congenital Q74.1
Knot(s)
 intestinal, syndrome (volvulus) K56.2
 surfer S89.8- ☑
 umbilical cord (true) O69.2 ☑
Knotting (of)
 hair L67.8
 intestine K56.2
Knuckle pad (Garrod's) M72.1
Koch's
 infection — *see* Tuberculosis
 relapsing fever A68.9
Koch-Weeks' conjunctivitis — *see* Conjunctivitis, acute,
   mucopurulent
Köebner's syndrome Q81.8
Köenig's disease (osteochondritis dissecans) — *see* Osteochondritis, dissecans
Köhler-Pellegrini-Steida disease or syndrome (calcification, knee joint) — *see* Bursitis, tibial collateral
Köhler's disease
 patellar — *see* Osteochondrosis, juvenile, patella
 tarsal navicular — *see* Osteochondrosis, juvenile, tarsus
Koilonychia L60.3
 congenital Q84.6
Kojevnikov's, epilepsy — *see* Kozhevnikof's epilepsy
Koplik's spots B05.9
Kopp's asthma E32.8
Korsakoff's (Wernicke) **disease, psychosis or syndrome** (alcoholic) F10.96
 with dependence F10.26
 drug-induced
  due to drug abuse — *see* Abuse, drug, by type,
    with amnestic disorder
  due to drug dependence — *see* Dependence, drug,
    by type, with amnestic disorder
 nonalcoholic F04
Korsakov's disease, psychosis or syndrome — *see*
   Korsakoff's disease
Korsakow's disease, psychosis or syndrome — *see*
   Korsakoff's disease
Kostmann's disease or syndrome (infantile genetic
   agranulocytosis) — *see* Agranulocytosis
Kozhevnikof's epilepsy G40.109
 intractable G40.119
  with status epilepticus G40.111
  without status epilepticus G40.119
 not intractable G40.109
  with status epilepticus G40.101
  without status epilepticus G40.109
Krabbe's
 disease E75.23
 syndrome, congenital muscle hypoplasia Q79.8
Kraepelin-Morel disease — *see* Schizophrenia
Kraft-Weber-Dimitri disease Q85.8
Kraurosis
 ani K62.89
 penis N48.0
 vagina N89.8
 vulva N90.4
Kreotoxism A05.9
Krukenberg's
 spindle — *see* Pigmentation, cornea, posterior
 tumor C79.6- ☑
Kufs' disease E75.4
Kugelberg-Welander disease G12.1
Kuhnt-Junius degeneration (*see also* Degeneration,
   macula) H35.32- ☑
Kümmell's disease or spondylitis — *see* Spondylopathy, traumatic
Kupffer cell sarcoma C22.3
Kuru A81.81
Kussmaul's
 disease M30.0
 respiration E87.2
  in diabetic acidosis — *see* Diabetes, by type, with
    ketoacidosis
Kwashiorkor E40
 marasmic, marasmus type E42
Kyasanur Forest disease A98.2
Kyphoscoliosis, kyphoscoliotic (acquired) (*see also*
   Scoliosis) M41.9
 congenital Q67.5
 heart (disease) I27.1
 sequelae of rickets E64.3
 tuberculous A18.01
Kyphosis, kyphotic (acquired) M40.209

Kyphosis, kyphotic — *continued*
  cervical region M40.202
  cervicothoracic region M40.203
  congenital Q76.419
    cervical region Q76.412
    cervicothoracic region Q76.413
    occipito-atlanto-axial region Q76.411
    thoracic region Q76.414
    thoracolumbar region Q76.415
  Morquio-Brailsford type (spinal) (*see also* subcategory M49.8) E76.219
  postlaminectomy M96.3
  postradiation therapy M96.2
  postural (adolescent) M40.00
    cervicothoracic region M40.03
    thoracic region M40.04
    thoracolumbar region M40.05
  secondary NEC M40.10
    cervical region M40.12
    cervicothoracic region M40.13
    thoracic region M40.14
    thoracolumbar region M40.15
  sequelae of rickets E64.3
  specified type NEC M40.299
    cervical region M40.292
    cervicothoracic region M40.293
    thoracic region M40.294
    thoracolumbar region M40.295
  syphilitic, congenital A50.56
  thoracic region M40.204
  thoracolumbar region M40.205
  tuberculous A18.01
Kyrle disease L87.0

L

Labia, labium — *see* condition
Labile
  blood pressure R09.89
  vasomotor system I73.9
Labioglossal paralysis G12.29
Labium leporinum — *see* Cleft, lip
Labor — *see* Delivery
Labored breathing — *see* Hyperventilation
Labyrinthitis (circumscribed) (destructive) (diffuse) (inner ear) (latent) (purulent) (suppurative) (*see also* subcategory) H83.0
  syphilitic A52.79
Laceration
  with abortion — *see* Abortion, by type, complicated by laceration of pelvic organs
  abdomen, abdominal
    wall S31.119 ☑
      with
        foreign body S31.129 ☑
        penetration into peritoneal cavity S31.619 ☑
          with foreign body S31.629 ☑
      epigastric region S31.112 ☑
        with
          foreign body S31.122 ☑
          penetration into peritoneal cavity S31.612 ☑
            with foreign body S31.622 ☑
      left
        lower quadrant S31.114 ☑
          with
            foreign body S31.124 ☑
            penetration into peritoneal cavity S31.614 ☑
              with foreign body S31.624 ☑
        upper quadrant S31.111 ☑
          with
            foreign body S31.121 ☑
            penetration into peritoneal cavity S31.611 ☑
              with foreign body S31.621 ☑
      periumbilic region S31.115 ☑
        with
          foreign body S31.125 ☑
          penetration into peritoneal cavity S31.615 ☑
            with foreign body S31.625 ☑
      right
        lower quadrant S31.113 ☑
          with
            foreign body S31.123 ☑

Laceration — *continued*
  abdomen, abdominal — *continued*
    wall — *continued*
      right — *continued*
        lower quadrant — *continued*
          with — *continued*
            penetration into peritoneal cavity S31.613 ☑
              with foreign body S31.623 ☑
          upper quadrant S31.110 ☑
            with
              foreign body S31.120 ☑
              penetration into peritoneal cavity S31.610 ☑
                with foreign body S31.620 ☑
  accidental, complicating surgery — *see* Complications, surgical, accidental puncture or laceration
  Achilles tendon S86.02- ☑
  adrenal gland S37.813 ☑
  alveolar (process) — *see* Laceration, oral cavity
  ankle S91.01- ☑
    with
      foreign body S91.02- ☑
  antecubital space — *see* Laceration, elbow
  anus (sphincter) S31.831 ☑
    with
      ectopic or molar pregnancy O08.6
      foreign body S31.832 ☑
    complicating delivery — *see* Delivery, complicated, by, laceration, anus (sphincter)
    following ectopic or molar pregnancy O08.6
    nontraumatic, nonpuerperal — *see* Fissure, anus
  arm (upper) S41.11- ☑
    with foreign body S41.12- ☑
    lower — *see* Laceration, forearm
  auditory canal (external) (meatus) — *see* Laceration, ear
  auricle, ear — *see* Laceration, ear
  axilla — *see* Laceration, arm
  back (*see also* Laceration, thorax, back)
    lower S31.010 ☑
      with
        foreign body S31.020 ☑
          with penetration into retroperitoneal space S31.021 ☑
        penetration into retroperitoneal space S31.011 ☑
  bile duct S36.13 ☑
  bladder S37.23 ☑
    with ectopic or molar pregnancy O08.6
    following ectopic or molar pregnancy O08.6
    obstetrical trauma O71.5
  blood vessel — *see* Injury, blood vessel
  bowel (*see also* Laceration, intestine)
    with ectopic or molar pregnancy O08.6
    complicating abortion — *see* Abortion, by type, complicated by, specified condition NEC
    following ectopic or molar pregnancy O08.6
    obstetrical trauma O71.5
  brain (any part) (cortex) (diffuse) (membrane) (*see also* Injury, intracranial, diffuse)
    during birth P10.8
      with hemorrhage P10.1
    focal — *see* Injury, intracranial, focal brain injury
  brainstem S06.38- ☑
  breast S21.01- ☑
    with foreign body S21.02- ☑
  broad ligament S37.893 ☑
    with ectopic or molar pregnancy O08.6
    following ectopic or molar pregnancy O08.6
    laceration syndrome N83.8
    obstetrical trauma O71.6
    syndrome (laceration) N83.8
  buttock S31.801 ☑
    with foreign body S31.802 ☑
    left S31.821 ☑
      with foreign body S31.822 ☑
    right S31.811 ☑
      with foreign body S31.812 ☑
  calf — *see* Laceration, leg
  canaliculus lacrimalis — *see* Laceration, eyelid
  canthus, eye — *see* Laceration, eyelid
  capsule, joint — *see* Sprain
  causing eversion of cervix uteri (old) N86
  central (perineal), complicating delivery O70.9
  cerebellum, traumatic S06.37- ☑
  cerebral S06.33- ☑

Laceration — *continued*
  cerebral — *continued*
    during birth P10.8
      with hemorrhage P10.1
    left side S06.32- ☑
    right side S06.31- ☑
  cervix (uteri)
    with ectopic or molar pregnancy O08.6
    following ectopic or molar pregnancy O08.6
    nonpuerperal, nontraumatic N88.1
    obstetrical trauma (current) O71.3
    old (postpartal) N88.1
    traumatic S37.63 ☑
  cheek (external) S01.41- ☑
    with foreign body S01.42- ☑
    internal — *see* Laceration, oral cavity
  chest wall — *see* Laceration, thorax
  chin — *see* Laceration, head, specified site NEC
  chordae tendinae NEC I51.1
    concurrent with acute myocardial infarction — *see* Infarct, myocardium
    following acute myocardial infarction (current complication) I23.4
  clitoris — *see* Laceration, vulva
  colon — *see* Laceration, intestine, large, colon
  common bile duct S36.13 ☑
  cortex (cerebral) — *see* Injury, intracranial, diffuse
  costal region — *see* Laceration, thorax
  cystic duct S36.13 ☑
  diaphragm S27.803 ☑
  digit(s)
    foot — *see* Laceration, toe
    hand — *see* Laceration, finger
  duodenum S36.430 ☑
  ear (canal) (external) S01.31- ☑
    with foreign body S01.32- ☑
    drum S09.2- ☑
  elbow S51.01- ☑
    with
      foreign body S51.02- ☑
  epididymis — *see* Laceration, testis
  epigastric region — *see* Laceration, abdomen, wall, epigastric region
  esophagus K22.8
    traumatic
      cervical S11.21 ☑
        with foreign body S11.22 ☑
      thoracic S27.813 ☑
  eye (ball) S05.3- ☑
    with prolapse or loss of intraocular tissue S05.2- ☑
    penetrating S05.6- ☑
  eyebrow — *see* Laceration, eyelid
  eyelid S01.11- ☑
    with foreign body S01.12- ☑
  face NEC — *see* Laceration, head, specified site NEC
  fallopian tube S37.539 ☑
    bilateral S37.532 ☑
    unilateral S37.531 ☑
  finger(s) S61.219 ☑
    with
      damage to nail S61.319 ☑
        with
          foreign body S61.329 ☑
      foreign body S61.229 ☑
    index S61.218 ☑
      with
        damage to nail S61.318 ☑
          with
            foreign body S61.328 ☑
        foreign body S61.228 ☑
      left S61.211 ☑
        with
          damage to nail S61.311 ☑
            with
              foreign body S61.321 ☑
          foreign body S61.221 ☑
      right S61.210 ☑
        with
          damage to nail S61.310 ☑
            with
              foreign body S61.320 ☑
          foreign body S61.220 ☑
    little S61.218 ☑
      with
        damage to nail S61.318 ☑
          with
            foreign body S61.328 ☑

☑ **Additional Character Required** — Refer to the Tabular List for Character Selection   ▽ **Subterms under main terms may continue to next column or page**

Laceration — *continued*
- finger(s) — *continued*
  - little — *continued*
    - with — *continued*
      - foreign body S61.228 ☑
    - left S61.217 ☑
      - with
        - damage to nail S61.317 ☑
          - with
            - foreign body S61.327 ☑
        - foreign body S61.227 ☑
    - right S61.216 ☑
      - with
        - damage to nail S61.316 ☑
          - with
            - foreign body S61.326 ☑
        - foreign body S61.226 ☑
  - middle S61.218 ☑
    - with
      - damage to nail S61.318 ☑
        - with
          - foreign body S61.328 ☑
      - foreign body S61.228 ☑
    - left S61.213 ☑
      - with
        - damage to nail S61.313 ☑
          - with
            - foreign body S61.323 ☑
        - foreign body S61.223 ☑
    - right S61.212 ☑
      - with
        - damage to nail S61.312 ☑
          - with
            - foreign body S61.322 ☑
        - foreign body S61.222 ☑
  - ring S61.218 ☑
    - with
      - damage to nail S61.318 ☑
        - with
          - foreign body S61.328 ☑
      - foreign body S61.228 ☑
    - left S61.215 ☑
      - with
        - damage to nail S61.315 ☑
          - with
            - foreign body S61.325 ☑
        - foreign body S61.225 ☑
    - right S61.214 ☑
      - with
        - damage to nail S61.314 ☑
          - with
            - foreign body S61.324 ☑
        - foreign body S61.224 ☑
- flank S31.119 ☑
  - with foreign body S31.129 ☑
- foot (except toe(s) alone) S91.319 ☑
  - with foreign body S91.329 ☑
  - left S91.312 ☑
    - with foreign body S91.322 ☑
  - right S91.311 ☑
    - with foreign body S91.321 ☑
  - toe — *see* Laceration, toe
- forearm S51.819 ☑
  - with
    - foreign body S51.829 ☑
  - elbow only — *see* Laceration, elbow
  - left S51.812 ☑
    - with
      - foreign body S51.822 ☑
  - right S51.811 ☑
    - with
      - foreign body S51.821 ☑
- forehead S01.81 ☑
  - with foreign body S01.82 ☑
- fourchette O70.0
  - with ectopic or molar pregnancy O08.6
  - complicating delivery O70.0
  - following ectopic or molar pregnancy O08.6
- gallbladder S36.123 ☑
- genital organs, external
  - female S31.512 ☑
    - with foreign body S31.522 ☑
    - vagina — *see* Laceration, vagina
    - vulva — *see* Laceration, vulva
  - male S31.511 ☑
    - with foreign body S31.521 ☑

Laceration — *continued*
- genital organs, external — *continued*
  - male — *continued*
    - penis — *see* Laceration, penis
    - scrotum — *see* Laceration, scrotum
    - testis — *see* Laceration, testis
  - groin — *see* Laceration, abdomen, wall
  - gum — *see* Laceration, oral cavity
  - hand S61.419 ☑
    - with
      - foreign body S61.429 ☑
    - finger — *see* Laceration, finger
    - left S61.412 ☑
      - with
        - foreign body S61.422 ☑
    - right S61.411 ☑
      - with
        - foreign body S61.421 ☑
    - thumb — *see* Laceration, thumb
  - head S01.91 ☑
    - with foreign body S01.92 ☑
    - cheek — *see* Laceration, cheek
    - ear — *see* Laceration, ear
    - eyelid — *see* Laceration, eyelid
    - lip — *see* Laceration, lip
    - nose — *see* Laceration, nose
    - oral cavity — *see* Laceration, oral cavity
    - scalp S01.01 ☑
      - with foreign body S01.02 ☑
    - specified site NEC S01.81 ☑
      - with foreign body S01.82 ☑
    - temporomandibular area — *see* Laceration, cheek
  - heart — *see* Injury, heart, laceration
  - heel — *see* Laceration, foot
  - hepatic duct S36.13 ☑
  - hip S71.019 ☑
    - with foreign body S71.029 ☑
    - left S71.012 ☑
      - with foreign body S71.022 ☑
    - right S71.011 ☑
      - with foreign body S71.021 ☑
  - hymen — *see* Laceration, vagina
  - hypochondrium — *see* Laceration, abdomen, wall
  - hypogastric region — *see* Laceration, abdomen, wall
  - ileum S36.438 ☑
  - inguinal region — *see* Laceration, abdomen, wall
  - instep — *see* Laceration, foot
  - internal organ — *see* Injury, by site
  - interscapular region — *see* Laceration, thorax, back
  - intestine
    - large
      - colon S36.539 ☑
        - ascending S36.530 ☑
        - descending S36.532 ☑
        - sigmoid S36.533 ☑
        - specified site NEC S36.538 ☑
      - rectum S36.63 ☑
      - transverse S36.531 ☑
    - small S36.439 ☑
      - duodenum S36.430 ☑
      - specified site NEC S36.438 ☑
  - intra-abdominal organ S36.93 ☑
    - intestine — *see* Laceration, intestine
    - liver — *see* Laceration, liver
    - pancreas — *see* Laceration, pancreas
    - peritoneum S36.81 ☑
    - specified site NEC S36.893 ☑
    - spleen — *see* Laceration, spleen
    - stomach — *see* Laceration, stomach
  - intracranial NEC (*see also* Injury, intracranial, diffuse)
    - birth injury P10.9
  - jaw — *see* Laceration, head, specified site NEC
  - jejunum S36.438 ☑
  - joint capsule — *see* Sprain, by site
  - kidney S37.03- ☑
    - major (greater than 3 cm) (massive) (stellate) S37.06- ☑
    - minor (less than 1 cm) S37.04- ☑
    - moderate (1 to 3 cm) S37.05- ☑
    - multiple S37.06- ☑
  - knee S81.01- ☑
    - with foreign body S81.02- ☑
  - labium (majus) (minus) — *see* Laceration, vulva
  - lacrimal duct — *see* Laceration, eyelid
  - large intestine — *see* Laceration, intestine, large
  - larynx S11.011 ☑

Laceration   *continued*
- larynx — *continued*
  - with foreign body S11.012 ☑
  - leg (lower) S81.819 ☑
    - with foreign body S81.829 ☑
    - foot — *see* Laceration, foot
    - knee — *see* Laceration, knee
    - left S81.812 ☑
      - with foreign body S81.822 ☑
    - right S81.811 ☑
      - with foreign body S81.821 ☑
    - upper — *see* Laceration, thigh
  - ligament — *see* Sprain
  - lip S01.511 ☑
    - with foreign body S01.521 ☑
  - liver S36.113 ☑
    - major (stellate) S36.116 ☑
    - minor S36.114 ☑
    - moderate S36.115 ☑
  - loin — *see* Laceration, abdomen, wall
  - lower back — *see* Laceration, back, lower
  - lumbar region — *see* Laceration, back, lower
  - lung S27.339 ☑
    - bilateral S27.332 ☑
    - unilateral S27.331 ☑
  - malar region — *see* Laceration, head, specified site NEC
  - mammary — *see* Laceration, breast
  - mastoid region — *see* Laceration, head, specified site NEC
  - meninges — *see* Injury, intracranial, diffuse
  - meniscus — *see* Tear, meniscus
  - mesentery S36.893 ☑
  - mesosalpinx S37.893 ☑
  - mouth — *see* Laceration, oral cavity
  - muscle — *see* Injury, muscle, by site, laceration
  - nail
    - finger — *see* Laceration, finger, with damage to nail
    - toe — *see* Laceration, toe, with damage to nail
  - nasal (septum) (sinus) — *see* Laceration, nose
  - nasopharynx — *see* Laceration, head, specified site NEC
  - neck S11.91 ☑
    - with foreign body S11.92 ☑
    - involving
      - cervical esophagus S11.21 ☑
        - with foreign body S11.22 ☑
      - larynx — *see* Laceration, larynx
      - pharynx — *see* Laceration, pharynx
      - thyroid gland — *see* Laceration, thyroid gland
      - trachea — *see* Laceration, trachea
    - specified site NEC S11.81 ☑
      - with foreign body S11.82 ☑
  - nerve — *see* Injury, nerve
  - nose (septum) (sinus) S01.21 ☑
    - with foreign body S01.22 ☑
  - ocular NOS S05.3- ☑
    - adnexa NOS S01.11- ☑
  - oral cavity S01.512 ☑
    - with foreign body S01.522 ☑
  - orbit (eye) — *see* Wound, open, ocular, orbit
  - ovary S37.439 ☑
    - bilateral S37.432 ☑
    - unilateral S37.431 ☑
  - palate — *see* Laceration, oral cavity
  - palm — *see* Laceration, hand
  - pancreas S36.239 ☑
  - pelvic S31.010 ☑
    - with
      - foreign body S31.020 ☑
        - penetration into retroperitoneal cavity S31.021 ☑
      - penetration into retroperitoneal cavity S31.011 ☑
    - floor (*see also* Laceration, back, lower)
      - with ectopic or molar pregnancy O08.6
      - complicating delivery O70.1
      - following ectopic or molar pregnancy O08.6
      - old (postpartal) N81.89
    - organ S37.93 ☑
  - penis S31.21 ☑
    - with foreign body S31.22 ☑
  - perineum
    - female S31.41 ☑

⬛ Subterms under main terms may continue to next column or page   ☑ Additional Character Required — Refer to the Tabular List for Character Selection   **207**

Laceration — Laceration

Laceration — continued
  perineum — continued
    female — continued
      with
        ectopic or molar pregnancy O08.6
        foreign body S31.42 ☑
      during delivery O70.9
        first degree O70.0
        fourth degree O70.3
        second degree O70.1
        third degree (see also Delivery, complicated,
          by, laceration, perineum, third de-
          gree) O70.20
      old (postpartal) N81.89
      postpartal N81.89
      secondary (postpartal) O90.1
    male S31.119 ☑
      with foreign body S31.129 ☑
  periocular area (with or without lacrimal passages) —
    see Laceration, eyelid
  peritoneum S36.893 ☑
  periumbilic region — see Laceration, abdomen, wall,
    periumbilic
  periurethral tissue — see Laceration, urethra
  phalanges
    finger — see Laceration, finger
    toe — see Laceration, toe
  pharynx S11.21 ☑
    with foreign body S11.22 ☑
  pinna — see Laceration, ear
  popliteal space — see Laceration, knee
  prepuce — see Laceration, penis
  prostate S37.823 ☑
  pubic region S31.119 ☑
    with foreign body S31.129 ☑
  pudendum — see Laceration, genital organs, external
  rectovaginal septum — see Laceration, vagina
  rectum S36.63 ☑
  retroperitoneum S36.893 ☑
  round ligament S37.893 ☑
  sacral region — see Laceration, back, lower
  sacroiliac region — see Laceration, back, lower
  salivary gland — see Laceration, oral cavity
  scalp S01.01 ☑
    with foreign body S01.02 ☑
  scapular region — see Laceration, shoulder
  scrotum S31.31 ☑
    with foreign body S31.32 ☑
  seminal vesicle S37.893 ☑
  shin — see Laceration, leg
  shoulder S41.019 ☑
    with foreign body S41.029 ☑
    left S41.012 ☑
      with foreign body S41.022 ☑
    right S41.011 ☑
      with foreign body S41.021 ☑
  small intestine — see Laceration, intestine, small
  spermatic cord — see Laceration, testis
  spinal cord (meninges) (see also Injury, spinal cord, by
    region)
    due to injury at birth P11.5
    newborn (birth injury) P11.5
  spleen S36.039 ☑
    major (massive) (stellate) S36.032 ☑
    moderate S36.031 ☑
    superficial (minor) S36.030 ☑
  sternal region — see Laceration, thorax, front
  stomach S36.33 ☑
  submaxillary region — see Laceration, head, specified
    site NEC
  submental region — see Laceration, head, specified
    site NEC
  subungual
    finger(s) — see Laceration, finger, with damage to
      nail
    toe(s) — see Laceration, toe, with damage to nail
  suprarenal gland — see Laceration, adrenal gland
  temple, temporal region — see Laceration, head,
    specified site NEC
  temporomandibular area — see Laceration, cheek
  tendon — see Injury, muscle, by site, laceration
    Achilles S86.02- ☑
  tentorium cerebelli — see Injury, intracranial, diffuse
  testis S31.31 ☑
    with foreign body S31.32 ☑
  thigh S71.11- ☑
    with foreign body S71.12- ☑

Laceration — continued
  thorax, thoracic (wall) S21.91 ☑
    with foreign body S21.92 ☑
    back S21.22- ☑
      with penetration into thoracic cavity
        S21.42- ☑
    front S21.12- ☑
      with penetration into thoracic cavity
        S21.32- ☑
    back S21.21- ☑
      with
        foreign body S21.22- ☑
          with penetration into thoracic cavity
            S21.42- ☑
        penetration into thoracic cavity S21.41- ☑
    breast — see Laceration, breast
    front S21.11- ☑
      with
        foreign body S21.12- ☑
          with penetration into thoracic cavity
            S21.32- ☑
        penetration into thoracic cavity S21.31- ☑
  thumb S61.019 ☑
    with
      damage to nail S61.119 ☑
        with
          foreign body S61.129 ☑
      foreign body S61.029 ☑
    left S61.012 ☑
      with
        damage to nail S61.112 ☑
          with
            foreign body S61.122 ☑
        foreign body S61.022 ☑
    right S61.011 ☑
      with
        damage to nail S61.111 ☑
          with
            foreign body S61.121 ☑
        foreign body S61.021 ☑
  thyroid gland S11.11 ☑
    with foreign body S11.12 ☑
  toe(s) S91.119 ☑
    with
      damage to nail S91.219 ☑
        with
          foreign body S91.229 ☑
      foreign body S91.129 ☑
    great S91.113 ☑
      with
        damage to nail S91.213 ☑
          with
            foreign body S91.223 ☑
        foreign body S91.123 ☑
      left S91.112 ☑
        with
          damage to nail S91.212 ☑
            with
               foreign body S91.222 ☑
          foreign body S91.122 ☑
      right S91.111 ☑
        with
          damage to nail S91.211 ☑
            with
               foreign body S91.221 ☑
          foreign body S91.121 ☑
    lesser S91.116 ☑
      with
        damage to nail S91.216 ☑
          with
            foreign body S91.226 ☑
        foreign body S91.126 ☑
      left S91.115 ☑
        with
          damage to nail S91.215 ☑
            with
               foreign body S91.225 ☑
          foreign body S91.125 ☑
      right S91.114 ☑
        with
          damage to nail S91.214 ☑
            with
               foreign body S91.224 ☑
          foreign body S91.124 ☑
  tongue — see Laceration, oral cavity
  trachea S11.021 ☑

Laceration — continued
  trachea — continued
    with foreign body S11.022 ☑
  tunica vaginalis — see Laceration, testis
  tympanum, tympanic membrane — see Laceration,
    ear, drum
  umbilical region S31.115 ☑
    with foreign body S31.125 ☑
  ureter S37.13 ☑
  urethra S37.33 ☑
    with or following ectopic or molar pregnancy O08.6
    obstetrical trauma O71.5
  urinary organ NEC S37.893 ☑
  uterus S37.63 ☑
    with ectopic or molar pregnancy O08.6
    following ectopic or molar pregnancy O08.6
    nonpuerperal, nontraumatic N85.8
    obstetrical trauma NEC O71.81
    old (postpartal) N85.8
  uvula — see Laceration, oral cavity
  vagina S31.41 ☑
    with
      ectopic or molar pregnancy O08.6
      foreign body S31.42 ☑
    during delivery O71.4
      with perineal laceration — see Laceration, per-
        ineum, female, during delivery
    following ectopic or molar pregnancy O08.6
    nonpuerperal, nontraumatic N89.8
    old (postpartal) N89.8
  vas deferens S37.893 ☑
  vesical — see Laceration, bladder
  vocal cords S11.031 ☑
    with foreign body S11.032 ☑
  vulva S31.41 ☑
    with
      ectopic or molar pregnancy O08.6
      foreign body S31.42 ☑
    complicating delivery O70.0
    following ectopic or molar pregnancy O08.6
    nonpuerperal, nontraumatic N90.89
    old (postpartal) N90.89
  wrist S61.519 ☑
    with
      foreign body S61.529 ☑
    left S61.512 ☑
      with
        foreign body S61.522 ☑
    right S61.511 ☑
      with
        foreign body S61.521 ☑

Lack of
  achievement in school Z55.3
  adequate
    food Z59.4
    intermaxillary vertical dimension of fully erupted
      teeth M26.36
    sleep Z72.820
  appetite (see Anorexia) R63.0
  awareness R41.9
  care
    in home Z74.2
    of infant (at or after birth) T76.02 ☑
      confirmed T74.02 ☑
  cognitive functions R41.9
  coordination R27.9
    ataxia R27.0
    specified type NEC R27.8
  development (physiological) R62.50
    failure to thrive (child over 28 days old) R62.51
      adult R62.7
      newborn P92.6
    short stature R62.52
    specified type NEC R62.59
  energy R53.83
  financial resources Z59.6
  food T73.0 ☑
  growth R62.52
  heating Z59.1
  housing (permanent) (temporary) Z59.0
    adequate Z59.1
  learning experiences in childhood Z62.898
  leisure time (affecting life-style) Z73.2
  material resources Z59.9
  memory (see also Amnesia)
    mild, following organic brain damage F06.8
  ovulation N97.0
  parental supervision or control of child Z62.0

☑ Additional Character Required — Refer to the Tabular List for Character Selection   ▽ Subterms under main terms may continue to next column or page

Lack of — *continued*
 person able to render necessary care Z74.2
 physical exercise Z72.3
 play experience in childhood Z62.898
 posterior occlusal support M26.57
 relaxation (affecting life-style) Z73.2
 sexual
  desire F52.0
  enjoyment F52.1
 shelter Z59.0
 sleep (adequate) Z72.820
 supervision of child by parent Z62.0
 support, posterior occlusal M26.57
 water T73.1 ☑
Lacrimal — *see* condition
Lacrimation, abnormal — *see* Epiphora
Lacrimonasal duct — *see* condition
Lactation, lactating (breast) (puerperal, postpartum)
 associated
  cracked nipple O92.13
  retracted nipple O92.03
 defective O92.4
 disorder NEC O92.79
 excessive O92.6
 failed (complete) O92.3
  partial O92.4
 mastitis NEC — *see* Mastitis, obstetric
 mother (care and/or examination) Z39.1
 nonpuerperal N64.3
Lacticemia, excessive E87.2
Lacunar skull Q75.8
Laennec's cirrhosis K70.30
 with ascites K70.31
 nonalcoholic K74.69
Lafora's disease — *see* Epilepsy, generalized, idiopathic
Lag, lid (nervous) — *see* Retraction, lid
Lagophthalmos (eyelid) (nervous) H02.209
 cicatricial H02.219
  left H02.216
   lower H02.215
   upper H02.214
  right H02.213
   lower H02.212
   upper H02.211
 keratoconjunctivitis — *see* Keratoconjunctivitis
 left H02.206
  lower H02.205
  upper H02.204
 mechanical H02.229
  left H02.226
   lower H02.225
   upper H02.224
  right H02.223
   lower H02.222
   upper H02.221
 paralytic H02.239
  left H02.236
   lower H02.235
   upper H02.234
  right H02.233
   lower H02.232
   upper H02.231
 right H02.203
  lower H02.202
  upper H02.201
Laki-Lorand factor deficiency — *see* Defect, coagulation, specified type NEC
Lalling F80.0
Lambert-Eaton syndrome — *see* Syndrome, Lambert-Eaton
Lambliasis, lambliosis A07.1
Landau-Kleffner syndrome — *see* Epilepsy, specified NEC
Landouzy-Déjérine dystrophy or facioscapulohumeral atrophy G71.0
Landouzy's disease (icterohemorrhagic leptospirosis) A27.0
Landry-Guillain-Barré, syndrome or paralysis G61.0
Landry's disease or paralysis G61.0
Lane's
 band Q43.3
 kink — *see* Obstruction, intestine
 syndrome K90.2
Langdon Down syndrome — *see* Trisomy, 21
Lapsed immunization schedule status Z28.3
Large
 baby (regardless of gestational age) (4000g to 4499g) P08.1

Large — *continued*
 ear, congenital Q17.1
 physiological cup Q14.2
 stature R68.89
Large-for-dates NEC (infant) (4000g to 4499g) P08.1
 affecting management of pregnancy O36.6- ☑
 exceptionally (4500g or more) P08.0
Larsen-Johansson disease orosteochondrosis — *see* Osteochondrosis, juvenile, patella
Larsen's syndrome (flattened facies and multiple congenital dislocations) Q74.8
Larva migrans
 cutaneous B76.9
  Ancylostoma B76.0
 visceral B83.0
Laryngeal — *see* condition
Laryngismus (stridulus) J38.5
 congenital P28.89
 diphtheritic A36.2
Laryngitis (acute) (edematous) (fibrinous) (infective) (infiltrative) (malignant) (membranous) (phlegmonous) (pneumococcal) (pseudomembranous) (septic) (subglottic) (suppurative) (ulcerative) J04.0
 with
  influenza, flu, or grippe — *see* Influenza, with, laryngitis
  tracheitis (acute) — *see* Laryngotracheitis
 atrophic J37.0
 catarrhal J37.0
 chronic J37.0
  with tracheitis (chronic) J37.1
 diphtheritic A36.2
 due to external agent — *see* Inflammation, respiratory, upper, due to
 H. influenzae J04.0
 Hemophilus influenzae J04.0
 hypertrophic J37.0
 influenzal — *see* Influenza, with, respiratory manifestations NEC
 obstructive J05.0
 sicca J37.0
 spasmodic J05.0
  acute J04.0
 streptococcal J04.0
 stridulous J05.0
 syphilitic (late) A52.73
  congenital A50.59 [J99]
   early A50.03 [J99]
 tuberculous A15.5
 Vincent's A69.1
Laryngocele (congenital) (ventricular) Q31.3
Laryngofissure J38.7
 congenital Q31.8
Laryngomalacia (congenital) Q31.5
Laryngopharyngitis (acute) J06.0
 chronic J37.0
 due to external agent — *see* Inflammation, respiratory, upper, due to
Laryngoplegia J38.00
 bilateral J38.02
 unilateral J38.01
Laryngoptosis J38.7
Laryngospasm J38.5
Laryngostenosis J38.6
Laryngotracheitis (acute) (Infectional) (infective) (viral) J04.2
 atrophic J37.1
 catarrhal J37.1
 chronic J37.1
 diphtheritic A36.2
 due to external agent — *see* Inflammation, respiratory, upper, due to
 Hemophilus influenzae J04.2
 hypertrophic J37.1
 influenzal — *see* Influenza, with, respiratory manifestations NEC
 pachydermic J38.7
 sicca J37.1
 spasmodic J38.5
  acute J05.0
 streptococcal J04.2
 stridulous J38.5
 syphilitic (late) A52.73
  congenital A50.59 [J99]
   early A50.03 [J99]
 tuberculous A15.5
 Vincent's A69.1
Laryngotracheobronchitis — *see* Bronchitis

Larynx, laryngeal — *see* condition
Lassa fever A96.2
Lassitude — *see* Weakness
Late
 talker R62.0
 walker R62.0
Late effect(s) — *see* Sequelae
Latent — *see* condition
Laterocession — *see* Lateroversion
Lateroflexion — *see* Lateroversion
Lateroversion
 cervix — *see* Lateroversion, uterus
 uterus, uterine (cervix) (postinfectional) (postpartal, old) N85.4
  congenital Q51.818
  in pregnancy or childbirth O34.59- ☑
Lathyrism — *see* Poisoning, food, noxious, plant
Launois' syndrome (pituitary gigantism) E22.0
Launois-Bensaude adenolipomatosis E88.89
Laurence-Moon (-Bardet)-**Biedl syndrome** Q87.89
Lax, laxity (*see also* Relaxation)
 ligament (ous) (*see also* Disorder, ligament)
  familial M35.7
  knee — *see* Derangement, knee
 skin (acquired) L57.4
  congenital Q82.8
Laxative habit F55.2
Lazy leukocyte syndrome D70.8
Lead miner's lung J63.6
Leak, leakage
 air NEC J93.82
  postprocedural J95.812
 amniotic fluid — *see* Rupture, membranes, premature
 blood (microscopic), fetal, into maternal circulation
  affecting management of pregnancy — *see* Pregnancy, complicated by
 cerebrospinal fluid G96.0
  from spinal (lumbar) puncture G97.0
 device, implant or graft (*see also* Complications, by site and type, mechanical)
  arterial graft NEC — *see* Complication, cardiovascular device, mechanical, vascular
  breast (implant) T85.43 ☑
  catheter NEC T85.638 ☑
   dialysis (renal) T82.43 ☑
    intraperitoneal T85.631 ☑
   infusion NEC T82.534 ☑
    spinal (epidural) (subdural) T85.630 ☑
   urinary T83.038 ☑
    cystostomy T83.030 ☑
    Hopkins T83.038 ☑
    ileostomy T83.038 ☑
    indwelling T83.031 ☑
    nephrostomy T83.032 ☑
    specified T83.038 ☑
    urostomy T83.038 ☑
  gastrointestinal — *see* Complications, prosthetic device, mechanical, gastrointestinal device
  genital NEC T83.498 ☑
   penile prosthesis (cylinder) (implanted) (pump) (reservoir) T83.490 ☑
   testicular prosthesis T83.491 ☑
  heart NEC — *see* Complication, cardiovascular device, mechanical
  joint prosthesis — *see* Complications, joint prosthesis, mechanical, specified NEC, by site
  ocular NEC — *see* Complications, prosthetic device, mechanical, ocular device
  orthopedic NEC — *see* Complication, orthopedic, device, mechanical
  persistent air J93.82
  specified NEC T85.638 ☑
  urinary NEC (*see also* Complication, genitourinary, device, urinary, mechanical)
   graft T83.23 ☑
  vascular NEC — *see* Complication, cardiovascular device, mechanical
  ventricular intracranial shunt T85.03 ☑
 urine — *see* Incontinence
Leaky heart — *see* Endocarditis
Learning defect (specific) F81.9
Leather bottle stomach C16.9
Leber's
 congenital amaurosis H35.50
 optic atrophy (hereditary) H47.22
Lederer's anemia D59.1
Leeches (external) — *see* Hirudiniasis

Index

Leg—Lesion

Leg — *see* condition
Legg (-Calvé)-**Perthes disease, syndrome or osteo-chondrosis** M91.1- ☑
Legionellosis A48.1
　nonpneumonic A48.2
Legionnaires'
　disease A48.1
　　nonpneumonic A48.2
　pneumonia A48.1
Leigh's disease G31.82
Leiner's disease L21.1
Leiofibromyoma — *see* Leiomyoma
Leiomyoblastoma — *see* Neoplasm, connective tissue, benign
Leiomyofibroma (*see also* Neoplasm, connective tissue, benign)
　uterus (cervix) (corpus) D25.9
Leiomyoma (*see also* Neoplasm, connective tissue, benign)
　bizarre — *see* Neoplasm, connective tissue, benign
　cellular — *see* Neoplasm, connective tissue, benign
　epithelioid — *see* Neoplasm, connective tissue, benign
　uterus (cervix) (corpus) D25.9
　　intramural D25.1
　　submucous D25.0
　　subserosal D25.2
　vascular — *see* Neoplasm, connective tissue, benign
Leiomyoma, leiomyomatosis (intravascular) — *see* Neoplasm, connective tissue, uncertain behavior
Leiomyosarcoma (*see also* Neoplasm, connective tissue, malignant)
　epithelioid — *see* Neoplasm, connective tissue, malignant
　myxoid — *see* Neoplasm, connective tissue, malignant
Leishmaniasis B55.9
　American (mucocutaneous) B55.2
　　cutaneous B55.1
　Asian Desert B55.1
　Brazilian B55.2
　cutaneous (any type) B55.1
　dermal (*see also* Leishmaniasis, cutaneous)
　　post-kala-azar B55.0
　eyelid B55.1
　infantile B55.0
　Mediterranean B55.0
　mucocutaneous (American) (New World) B55.2
　naso-oral B55.2
　nasopharyngeal B55.2
　old world B55.1
　tegumentaria diffusa B55.1
　visceral B55.0
Leishmanoid, dermal (*see also* Leishmaniasis, cutaneous)
　post-kala-azar B55.0
Lenegre's disease I44.2
Lengthening, leg — *see* Deformity, limb, unequal length
Lennert's lymphoma — *see* Lymphoma, Lennert's
Lennox-Gastaut syndrome G40.812
　intractable G40.814
　　with status epilepticus G40.813
　　without status epilepticus G40.814
　not intractable G40.812
　　with status epilepticus G40.811
　　without status epilepticus G40.812
Lens — *see* condition
Lenticonus (anterior) (posterior) (congenital) Q12.8
Lenticular degeneration, progressive E83.01
Lentiglobus (posterior) (congenital) Q12.8
Lentigo (congenital) L81.4
　maligna (*see also* Melanoma, in situ)
　　melanoma — *see* Melanoma
Lentivirus, as cause of disease classified elsewhere B97.31
Leontiasis
　ossium M85.2
　syphilitic (late) A52.78
　　congenital A50.59
Lepothrix A48.8
Lepra — *see* Leprosy
Leprechaunism E34.8
Leprosy A30.- ☑
　with muscle disorder A30.9 [M63.80]
　　ankle A30.9 [M63.87-] ☑
　　foot A30.9 [M63.87-] ☑
　　forearm A30.9 [M63.83-] ☑
　　hand A30.9 [M63.84-] ☑
　　lower leg A30.9 [M63.86-] ☑

Leprosy — *continued*
　with muscle disorder — *continued*
　　multiple sites A30.9 [M63.89]
　　pelvic region A30.9 [M63.85-] ☑
　　shoulder region A30.9 [M63.81-] ☑
　　specified site NEC A30.9 [M63.88]
　　thigh A30.9 [M63.85-] ☑
　　upper arm A30.9 [M63.82-] ☑
　anesthetic A30.9
　BB A30.3
　BL A30.4
　borderline (infiltrated) (neuritic) A30.3
　　lepromatous A30.4
　　tuberculoid A30.2
　BT A30.3
　dimorphous (infiltrated) (neuritic) A30.3
　I A30.0
　indeterminate (macular) (neuritic) A30.0
　lepromatous (diffuse) (infiltrated) (macular) (neuritic) (nodular) A30.5
　LL A30.5
　macular (early) (neuritic) (simple) A30.9
　maculoanesthetic A30.9
　mixed A30.3
　neural A30.9
　nodular A30.5
　primary neuritic A30.3
　specified type NEC A30.8
　TT A30.1
　tuberculoid (major) (minor) A30.1
Leptocytosis, hereditary D56.9
Leptomeningitis (chronic) (circumscribed) (hemorrhagic) (nonsuppurative) — *see* Meningitis
Leptomeningopathy G96.19
Leptospiral — *see* condition
Leptospirochetal — *see* condition
Leptospirosis A27.9
　canicola A27.89
　due to Leptospira interrogans serovar icterohaemorrhagiae A27.0
　icterohemorrhagica A27.0
　pomona A27.89
　Weil's disease A27.0
Leptus dermatitis B88.0
Leriche's syndrome (aortic bifurcation occlusion) I74.09
Leri's pleonosteosis Q78.8
Leri-Weill syndrome Q77.8
Lermoyez' syndrome — *see* Vertigo, peripheral NEC
Lesch-Nyhan syndrome E79.1
Leser-Trélat disease L82.1
　inflamed L82.0
Lesion(s) (nontraumatic)
　abducens nerve — *see* Strabismus, paralytic, sixth nerve
　alveolar process K08.9
　angiocentric immunoproliferative D47.Z9 (*following* D47.4)
　anorectal K62.9
　aortic (valve) I35.9
　auditory nerve — *see* subcategory H93.3 ☑
　basal ganglion G25.9
　bile duct — *see* Disease, bile duct
　biomechanical M99.9
　　specified type NEC M99.89
　　　abdomen M99.89
　　　acromioclavicular M99.87
　　　cervical region M99.81
　　　cervicothoracic M99.81
　　　costochondral M99.88
　　　costovertebral M99.88
　　　head region M99.80
　　　hip M99.85
　　　lower extremity M99.86
　　　lumbar region M99.83
　　　lumbosacral M99.83
　　　occipitocervical M99.80
　　　pelvic region M99.85
　　　pubic M99.85
　　　rib cage M99.88
　　　sacral region M99.84
　　　sacrococcygeal M99.84
　　　sacroiliac M99.84
　　　specified NEC M99.89
　　　sternochondral M99.88
　　　sternoclavicular M99.87
　　　thoracic region M99.82
　　　thoracolumbar M99.82
　　　upper extremity M99.87

Lesion(s) — *continued*
　bladder N32.9
　bone — *see* Disorder, bone
　brachial plexus G54.0
　brain G93.9
　　congenital Q04.9
　　vascular I67.9
　　　degenerative I67.9
　　　hypertensive I67.4
　buccal cavity K13.79
　calcified — *see* Calcification
　canthus — *see* Disorder, eyelid
　carate — *see* Pinta, lesions
　cardia K31.9
　cardiac (*see also* Disease, heart) I51.9
　　congenital Q24.9
　　valvular — *see* Endocarditis
　cauda equina G83.4
　cecum K63.9
　cerebral — *see* Lesion, brain
　cerebrovascular I67.9
　　degenerative I67.9
　　hypertensive I67.4
　cervical (nerve) root NEC G54.2
　chiasmal — *see* Disorder, optic, chiasm
　chorda tympani G51.8
　coin, lung R91.1
　colon K63.9
　combined periodontic - endodontic K05.5
　congenital — *see* Anomaly, by site
　conjunctiva H11.9
　conus medullaris — *see* Injury, conus medullaris
　coronary artery — *see* Ischemia, heart
　cranial nerve G52.9
　　eighth — *see* Disorder, ear
　　eleventh G52.9
　　fifth G50.9
　　first G52.0
　　fourth — *see* Strabismus, paralytic, fourth nerve
　　seventh G51.9
　　sixth — *see* Strabismus, paralytic, sixth nerve
　　tenth G52.2
　　twelfth G52.3
　cystic — *see* Cyst
　degenerative — *see* Degeneration
　duodenum K31.9
　edentulous (alveolar) ridge, associated with trauma, due to traumatic occlusion K06.2
　en coup de sabre L94.1
　eyelid — *see* Disorder, eyelid
　gasserian ganglion G50.8
　gastric K31.9
　gastroduodenal K31.9
　gastrointestinal K63.9
　gingiva, associated with trauma K06.2
　glomerular
　　focal and segmental (*see also* N00-N07 with fourth character .1) N05.1
　　minimal change (*see also* N00-N07 with fourth character .0) N05.0
　heart (organic) — *see* Disease, heart
　hyperchromic, due to pinta (carate) A67.1
　hyperkeratotic — *see* Hyperkeratosis
　hypothalamic E23.7
　ileocecal K63.9
　ileum K63.9
　iliohypogastric nerve G57.8- ☑
　inflammatory — *see* Inflammation
　intestine K63.9
　intracerebral — *see* Lesion, brain
　intrachiasmal (optic) — *see* Disorder, optic, chiasm
　intracranial, space-occupying R90.0
　joint — *see* Disorder, joint
　　sacroiliac (old) M53.3
　keratotic — *see* Keratosis
　kidney — *see* Disease, renal
　laryngeal nerve (recurrent) G52.2
　lip K13.0
　liver K76.9
　lumbosacral
　　plexus G54.1
　　root (nerve) NEC G54.4
　lung (coin) R91.1
　maxillary sinus J32.0
　mitral I05.9
　Morel-Lavallée — *see* Hematoma, by site
　motor cortex NEC G93.89
　mouth K13.79

Lesion(s) — continued
  nerve G58.9
    femoral G57.2- ☑
    median G56.1- ☑
      carpal tunnel syndrome — see Syndrome, carpal tunnel
    plantar G57.6- ☑
    popliteal (lateral) G57.3- ☑
      medial G57.4- ☑
    radial G56.3- ☑
    sciatic G57.0- ☑
    spinal — see Injury, nerve, spinal
    ulnar G56.2- ☑
  nervous system, congenital Q07.9
  nonallopathic — see Lesion, biomechanical
  nose (internal) J34.89
  obstructive — see Obstruction
  obturator nerve G57.8- ☑
  oral mucosa K13.70
  organ or site NEC — see Disease, by site
  osteolytic — see Osteolysis
  peptic K27.9
  periodontal, due to traumatic occlusion K05.5
  pharynx J39.2
  pigment, pigmented (skin) L81.9
  pinta — see Pinta, lesions
  polypoid — see Polyp
  prechiasmal (optic) — see Disorder, optic, chiasm
  primary (see also Syphilis, primary) A51.0
    carate A67.0
    pinta A67.0
    yaws A66.0
  pulmonary J98.4
    valve I37.9
  pylorus K31.9
  rectosigmoid K63.9
  retina, retinal H35.9
  sacroiliac (joint) (old) M53.3
  salivary gland K11.9
    benign lymphoepithelial K11.8
  saphenous nerve G57.8- ☑
  sciatic nerve G57.0- ☑
  secondary — see Syphilis, secondary
  shoulder (region) M75.9- ☑
    specified NEC M75.8- ☑
  sigmoid K63.9
  sinus (accessory) (nasal) J34.89
  skin L98.9
    suppurative L08.0
  SLAP S43.43- ☑
  spinal cord G95.9
    congenital Q06.9
  spleen D73.89
  stomach K31.9
  superior glenoid labrum S43.43- ☑
  syphilitic — see Syphilis
  tertiary — see Syphilis, tertiary
  thoracic root (nerve) NEC G54.3
  tonsillar fossa J35.9
  tooth, teeth K08.9
    white spot
      chewing surface K02.51
      pit and fissure surface K02.51
      smooth surface K02.61
  traumatic — see specific type of injury by site
  tricuspid (valve) I07.9
    nonrheumatic I36.9
  trigeminal nerve G50.9
  ulcerated or ulcerative — see Ulcer, skin
  uterus N85.9
  vagus nerve G52.2
  valvular — see Endocarditis
  vascular I99.9
    affecting central nervous system I67.9
    following trauma NEC T14.8 ☑
    umbilical cord, complicating delivery O69.5 ☑
  warty — see Verruca
  white spot (tooth)
    chewing surface K02.51
    pit and fissure surface K02.51
    smooth surface K02.61
Lethargic — see condition
Lethargy R53.83
Letterer-Siwe's disease C96.0
Leukemia, leukemic C95.9- ☑
  acute basophilic C94.8- ☑
  acute bilineal C95.0- ☑

Leukemia, leukemic — continued
  acute erythroid C94.0- ☑
  acute lymphoblastic C91.0- ☑
  acute megakaryoblastic C94.2- ☑
  acute megakaryocytic C94.2- ☑
  acute mixed lineage C95.0- ☑
  acute monoblastic (monoblastic/monocytic) C93.0- ☑
  acute monocytic (monoblastic/monocytic) C93.0- ☑
  acute myeloblastic (minimal differentiation) (with maturation) C92.0- ☑
  acute myeloid
    with
      11q23-abnormality C92.6- ☑
      dysplasia of remaining hematopoesis and/or myelodysplastic disease in its history C92.A- ☑ (following C92.6)
      multilineage dysplasia C92.A- ☑ (following C92.6)
      variation of MLL-gene C92.6- ☑
    M6 (a)(b) C94.0- ☑
    M7 C94.2- ☑
  acute myelomonocytic C92.5- ☑
  acute promyelocytic C92.4- ☑
  adult T-cell (HTLV-1-associated) (acute variant) (chronic variant) (lymphomatoid variant) (smouldering variant) C91.5- ☑
  aggressive NK-cell C94.8- ☑
  AML (1/ETO) (M0) (M1) (M2) (without a FAB classification) C92.0- ☑
  AML M3 C92.4- ☑
  AML M4 (Eo with inv(16) or t(16;16)) C92.5- ☑
  AML M5 C93.0- ☑
  AML M5a C93.0- ☑
  AML M5b C93.0- ☑
  AML Me with t (15;17) and variants C92.4- ☑
  atypical chronic myeloid, BCR/ABL-negative C92.2- ☑
  biphenotypic acute C95.0- ☑
  blast cell C95.0- ☑
  Burkitt-type, mature B-cell C91.A- ☑ (following C91.6)
  chronic lymphocytic, of B-cell type C91.1- ☑
  chronic monocytic C93.1- ☑
  chronic myelogenous (Philadelphia chromosome (Ph1) positive) (t(9;22)) (q34;q11) (with crisis of blast cells) C92.1- ☑
  chronic myeloid, BCR/ABL-positive C92.1- ☑
    atypical, BCR/ABL-negative C92.2- ☑
  chronic myelomonocytic C93.1- ☑
  chronic neutrophilic D47.1
  CMML (-1) (-2) (with eosinophilia) C93.1- ☑
  granulocytic (see also Category C92) C92.9- ☑
  hairy cell C91.4- ☑
  juvenile myelomonocytic C93.3- ☑
  lymphoid C91.9- ☑
    specified NEC C91.Z- ☑ (following C91.6)
  mast cell C94.3- ☑
  mature B-cell, Burkitt-type C91.A- ☑ (following C91.6)
  monocytic (subacute) C93.9- ☑
    specified NEC C93.Z- ☑ (following C93.3)
  myelogenous (see also Category C92) C92.9- ☑
  myeloid C92.9- ☑
    specified NEC C92.Z- ☑ (following C92.6)
  plasma cell C90.1- ☑
  plasmacytic C90.1- ☑
  prolymphocytic
    of B-cell type C91.3- ☑
    of T-cell type C91.6- ☑
  specified NEC C94.8- ☑
  stem cell, of unclear lineage C95.0- ☑
  subacute lymphocytic C91.9- ☑
  T-cell large granular lymphocytic C91.Z- ☑ (following C91.6)
  unspecified cell type C95.9- ☑
    acute C95.0- ☑
    chronic C95.1- ☑
Leukemoid reaction (see also Reaction, leukemoid) D72.823
Leukoaraiosis (hypertensive) I67.81
Leukoariosis — see Leukoaraiosis
Leukocoria — see Disorder, globe, degenerated condition, leucocoria
Leukocytopenia D72.819
Leukocytosis D72.829
  eosinophilic D72.1
Leukoderma, leukodermia NEC L81.5
  syphilitic A51.39
    late A52.79

Leukodystrophy E75.29
Leukoedema, oral epithelium K13.29
Leukoencephalitis G04.81
  acute (subacute) hemorrhagic G36.1
    postimmunization or postvaccinal G04.02
  postinfectious G04.01
  subacute sclerosing A81.1
  van Bogaert's (sclerosing) A81.1
Leukoencephalopathy (see also Encephalopathy) G93.49
  Binswanger's I67.3
  heroin vapor G92
  metachromatic E75.25
  multifocal (progressive) A81.2
  postimmunization and postvaccinal G04.02
  progressive multifocal A81.2
  reversible, posterior G93.6
  van Bogaert's (sclerosing) A81.1
  vascular, progressive I67.3
Leukoerythroblastosis D75.9
Leukokeratosis (see also Leukoplakia)
  mouth K13.21
  nicotina palati K13.24
  oral mucosa K13.21
  tongue K13.21
  vocal cord J38.3
Leukokraurosis vulva (e) N90.4
Leukoma (cornea) (see also Opacity, cornea)
  adherent H17.0- ☑
  interfering with central vision — see Opacity, cornea, central
Leukomalacia, cerebral, newborn P91.2
  periventricular P91.2
Leukomelanopathy, hereditary D72.0
Leukonychia (punctata) (striata) L60.8
  congenital Q84.4
Leukopathia unguium L60.8
  congenital Q84.4
Leukopenia D72.819
  basophilic D72.818
  chemotherapy (cancer) induced D70.1
  congenital D70.0
  cyclic D70.0
  drug induced NEC D70.2
    due to cytoreductive cancer chemotherapy D70.1
  eosinophilic D72.818
  familial D70.0
  infantile genetic D70.0
  malignant D70.9
  periodic D70.0
  transitory neonatal P61.5
Leukopenic — see condition
Leukoplakia
  anus K62.89
  bladder (postinfectional) N32.89
  buccal K13.21
  cervix (uteri) N88.0
  esophagus K22.8
  gingiva K13.21
  hairy (oral mucosa) (tongue) K13.3
  kidney (pelvis) N28.89
  larynx J38.7
  lip K13.21
  mouth K13.21
  oral epithelium, including tongue (mucosa) K13.21
  palate K13.21
  pelvis (kidney) N28.89
  penis (infectional) N48.0
  rectum K62.89
  syphilitic (late) A52.79
  tongue K13.21
  ureter (postinfectional) N28.89
  urethra (postinfectional) N36.8
  uterus N85.8
  vagina N89.4
  vocal cord J38.3
  vulva N90.4
Leukorrhea N89.8
  due to Trichomonas (vaginalis) A59.00
  trichomonal A59.00
Leukosarcoma C85.9- ☑
Levocardia (isolated) Q24.1
  with situs inversus Q89.3
Levotransposition Q20.5
Lev's disease or syndrome (acquired complete heart block) I44.2
Levulosuria — see Fructosuria
Levurid L30.2

Lewy body (ies) (dementia) (disease) G31.83
Leyden-Moebius dystrophy G71.0
Leydig cell
  carcinoma
    specified site — see Neoplasm, malignant, by site
    unspecified site
      female C56.9
      male C62.9- ☑
  tumor
    benign
      specified site — see Neoplasm, benign, by site
      unspecified site
        female D27.- ☑
        male D29.2- ☑
    malignant
      specified site — see Neoplasm, malignant, by site
      unspecified site
        female C56.- ☑
        male C62.9- ☑
    specified site — see Neoplasm, uncertain behavior, by site
    unspecified site
      female D39.1- ☑
      male D40.1- ☑
Leydig-Sertoli cell tumor
  specified site — see Neoplasm, benign, by site
  unspecified site
    female D27.- ☑
    male D29.2- ☑
LGSIL (Low grade squamous intraepithelial lesion on cytologic smear of)
  anus R85.612
  cervix R87.612
  vagina R87.622
Liar, pathologic F60.2
Libido
  decreased R68.82
Libman-Sacks disease M32.11
Lice (infestation) B85.2
  body (Pediculus corporis) B85.1
  crab B85.3
  head (Pediculus capitis) B85.0
  mixed (classifiable to more than one of the titles B85.0-B85.3) B85.4
  pubic (Phthirus pubis) B85.3
Lichen L28.0
  albus L90.0
    penis N48.0
    vulva N90.4
  amyloidosis E85.4 [L99]
  atrophicus L90.0
    penis N48.0
    vulva N90.4
  congenital Q82.8
  myxedematosus L98.5
  nitidus L44.1
  pilaris Q82.8
    acquired L85.8
  planopilaris L66.1
  planus (chronicus) L43.9
    annularis L43.8
    bullous L43.1
    follicular L66.1
    hypertrophic L43.0
    moniliformis L44.3
    of Wilson L43.9
    specified NEC L43.8
    subacute (active) L43.3
    tropicus L43.3
  ruber
    acuminatus L44.0
    moniliformis L44.3
    planus L43.9
  sclerosus (et atrophicus) L90.0
    penis N48.0
    vulva N90.4
  scrofulosus (primary) (tuberculous) A18.4
  simplex (chronicus) (circumscriptus) L28.0
  striatus L44.2
  urticatus L28.2
Lichenification L28.0
Lichenoides tuberculosis (primary) A18.4
Lichtheim's disease or syndrome — see Degeneration, combined
Lien migrans D73.89
Ligament — see condition

Light
  for gestational age — see Light for dates
  headedness R42
Light-for-dates (infant) P05.00
  with weight of
    1000-1249 grams P05.04
    1250-1499 grams P05.05
    1500-1749 grams P05.06
    1750-1999 grams P05.07
    2000-2499 grams P05.08
    2500 grams and over P05.09
    499 grams or less P05.01
    500-749 grams P05.02
    750-999 grams P05.03
  affecting management of pregnancy O36.59- ☑
  and small-for-dates — see Small for dates
  specified NEC P05.09
Lightning (effects) (stroke) (struck by) T75.00 ☑
  burn — see Burn
  foot E53.8
  shock T75.01 ☑
  specified effect NEC T75.09 ☑
Lightwood-Albright syndrome N25.89
Lightwood's disease or syndrome (renal tubular acidosis) N25.89
Lignac (-de Toni) (-Fanconi) (-Debré) **disease or syndrome** E72.09
  with cystinosis E72.04
Ligneous thyroiditis E06.5
Likoff's syndrome I20.8
Limb — see condition
Limbic epilepsy personality syndrome F07.0
Limitation, limited
  activities due to disability Z73.6
  cardiac reserve — see Disease, heart
  eye muscle duction, traumatic — see Strabismus, mechanical
  mandibular range of motion M26.52
Lindau (-von Hippel) **disease** Q85.8
Line(s)
  Beau's L60.4
  Harris' — see Arrest, epiphyseal
  Hudson's (cornea) — see Pigmentation, cornea, anterior
  Stähli's (cornea) — see Pigmentation, cornea, anterior
Linea corneae senilis — see Change, cornea, senile
Lingua
  geographica K14.1
  nigra (villosa) K14.3
  plicata K14.5
  tylosis K13.29
Lingual — see condition
Linguatulosis B88.8
Linitis (gastric) **plastica** C16.9
Lip — see condition
Lipedema — see Edema
Lipemia (see also Hyperlipidemia)
  retina, retinalis E78.3
Lipidosis E75.6
  cerebral (infantile) (juvenile) (late) E75.4
  cerebroretinal E75.4
  cerebroside E75.22
  cholesterol (cerebral) E75.5
  glycolipid E75.21
  hepatosplenomegalic E78.3
  sphingomyelin — see Niemann-Pick disease or syndrome
  sulfatide E75.29
Lipoadenoma — see Neoplasm, benign, by site
Lipoblastoma — see Lipoma
Lipoblastomatosis — see Lipoma
Lipochondrodystrophy E76.01
Lipochrome histiocytosis (familial) D71
Lipodermatosclerosis — see Varix, leg, with, inflammation
  ulcerated — see Varix, leg, with, ulcer, with inflammation by site
Lipodystrophia progressiva E88.1
Lipodystrophy (progressive) E88.1
  insulin E88.1
  intestinal K90.81
  mesenteric K65.4
Lipofibroma — see Lipoma
Lipofuscinosis, neuronal (with ceroidosis) E75.4
Lipogranuloma, sclerosing L92.8
Lipogranulomatosis E78.89
Lipoid (see also condition)

Lipoid — continued
  histiocytosis D76.3
    essential E75.29
  nephrosis N04.9
  proteinosis of Urbach E78.89
Lipoidemia — see Hyperlipidemia
Lipoidosis — see Lipidosis
Lipoma D17.9
  fetal D17.9
    fat cell D17.9
  infiltrating D17.9
  intramuscular D17.9
  pleomorphic D17.9
  site classification
    arms (skin) (subcutaneous) D17.2- ☑
    connective tissue D17.30
      intra-abdominal D17.5
      intrathoracic D17.4
      peritoneum D17.79
      retroperitoneum D17.79
      specified site NEC D17.39
      spermatic cord D17.6
    face (skin) (subcutaneous) D17.0
    genitourinary organ NEC D17.72
    head (skin) (subcutaneous) D17.0
    intra-abdominal D17.5
    intrathoracic D17.4
    kidney D17.71
    legs (skin) (subcutaneous) D17.2- ☑
    neck (skin) (subcutaneous) D17.0
    peritoneum D17.79
    retroperitoneum D17.79
    skin D17.30
      specified site NEC D17.39
    specified site NEC D17.79
    spermatic cord D17.6
    subcutaneous D17.30
      specified site NEC D17.39
    trunk (skin) (subcutaneous) D17.1
    unspecified D17.9
  spindle cell D17.9
Lipomatosis E88.2
  dolorosa (Dercum) E88.2
  fetal — see Lipoma
  Launois-Bensaude E88.89
Lipomyoma — see Lipoma
Lipomyxoma — see Lipoma
Lipomyxosarcoma — see Neoplasm, connective tissue, malignant
Lipoprotein metabolism disorder E78.9
Lipoproteinemia E78.5
  broad-beta E78.2
  floating-beta E78.2
  hyper-pre-beta E78.1
Liposarcoma (see also Neoplasm, connective tissue, malignant)
  dedifferentiated — see Neoplasm, connective tissue, malignant
  differentiated type — see Neoplasm, connective tissue, malignant
  embryonal — see Neoplasm, connective tissue, malignant
  mixed type — see Neoplasm, connective tissue, malignant
  myxoid — see Neoplasm, connective tissue, malignant
  pleomorphic — see Neoplasm, connective tissue, malignant
  round cell — see Neoplasm, connective tissue, malignant
  well differentiated type — see Neoplasm, connective tissue, malignant
Liposynovitis prepatellaris E88.89
Lipping, cervix N86
Lipschütz disease or ulcer N76.6
Lipuria R82.0
  schistosomiasis (bilharziasis) B65.0
Lisping F80.0
Lissauer's paralysis A52.17
Lissencephalia, lissencephaly Q04.3
Listeriosis, listerellosis A32.9
  congenital (disseminated) P37.2
  cutaneous A32.0
  neonatal, newborn (disseminated) P37.2
  oculoglandular A32.81
  specified NEC A32.89
Lithemia E79.0
Lithiasis — see Calculus
Lithosis J62.8

LIthurIa R82.99
Litigation, anxiety concerning Z65.3
Little leaguer's elbow — *see* Epicondylitis, medial
Little's disease G80.9
Littre's
  gland — *see* condition
  hernia — *see* Hernia, abdomen
Littritis — *see* Urethritis
Livedo (annularis) (racemosa) (reticularis) R23.1
Liver — *see* condition
Living alone (problems with) Z60.2
  with handicapped person Z74.2
Lloyd's syndrome — *see* Adenomatosis, endocrine
Loa loa, loaiasis, loasis B74.3
Lobar — *see* condition
Lobomycosis B48.0
Lobo's disease B48.0
Lobotomy syndrome F07.0
Lobstein (-Ekman) **disease or syndrome** Q78.0
Lobster-claw hand Q71.6-
Lobulation (congenital) (*see also* Anomaly, by site)
  kidney, Q63.1
  liver, abnormal Q44.7
  spleen Q89.09
Lobule, lobular — *see* condition
Local, localized — *see* condition
Locked twins causing obstructed labor O66.1
Locked-in state G83.5
Locking
  joint — *see* Derangement, joint, specified type NEC
    knee — *see* Derangement, knee
Lockjaw — *see* Tetanus
Löffler's
  endocarditis I42.3
  eosinophilia J82
  pneumonia J82
  syndrome (eosinophilic pneumonitis) J82
Loiasis (with conjunctival infestation) (eyelid) B74.3
Lone Star fever A77.0
Long
  labor O63.9
    first stage O63.0
    second stage O63.1
  QT syndrome I45.81
Longitudinal stripes or grooves, nails L60.8
  congenital Q84.6
Long-term (current) (prophylactic) **drug therapy** (use of)
  agents affecting estrogen receptors and estrogen levels NEC Z79.818
  anastrozole (Arimidex) Z79.811
  antibiotics Z79.2
    short-term use — *omit code*
  anticoagulants Z79.01
  anti-inflammatory, non-steroidal (NSAID) Z79.1
  antiplatelet Z79.02
  antithrombotics Z79.02
  aromatase inhibitors Z79.811
  aspirin Z79.82
  birth control pill or patch Z79.3
  bisphosphonates Z79.83
  contraceptive, oral Z79.3
  drug, specified NEC Z79.899
  estrogen receptor downregulators Z79.818
  Evista Z79.810
  exemestane (Aromasin) Z79.811
  Fareston Z79.810
  fulvestrant (Faslodex) Z79.818
  gonadotropin-releasing hormone (GnRH) agonist Z79.818
  goserelin acetate (Zoladex) Z79.818
  hormone replacement Z79.890
  insulin Z79.4
  letrozole (Femara) Z79.811
  leuprolide acetate (leuprorelin) (Lupron) Z79.818
  megestrol acetate (Megace) Z79.818
  methadone for pain management Z79.891
  Nolvadex Z79.810
  non-steroidal anti-inflammatories (NSAID) Z79.1
  opiate analgesic Z79.891
  oral
    antidiabetic Z79.84
    contraceptive Z79.3
    hypoglycemic Z79.84
  raloxifene (Evista) Z79.810
  selective estrogen receptor modulators (SERMs) Z79.810

Long-term (current) (prophylactic) **drug therapy** — *continued*
  steroids
    inhaled Z79.51
    systemic Z79.52
  tamoxifen (Nolvadex) Z79.810
  toremifene (Fareston) Z79.810
Loop
  intestine — *see* Volvulus
  vascular on papilla (optic) Q14.2
Loose (*see also* condition)
  body
    joint M24.00
      ankle M24.07- ☑
      elbow M24.02- ☑
      hand M24.04- ☑
      hip M24.05- ☑
      knee M23.4- ☑
      shoulder (region) M24.01- ☑
      specified site NEC M24.08
      toe M24.07- ☑
      vertebra M24.08
      wrist M24.03- ☑
    knee M23.4- ☑
    sheath, tendon — *see* Disorder, tendon, specified type NEC
  cartilage — *see* Loose, body, joint
  skin and subcutaneous tissue (following bariatric surgery weight loss) (following dietary weight loss) L98.7
  tooth, teeth K08.89
Loosening
  aseptic
    joint prosthesis — *see* Complications, joint prosthesis, mechanical, loosening, by site
    epiphysis — *see* Osteochondropathy
  mechanical
    joint prosthesis — *see* Complications, joint prosthesis, mechanical, loosening, by site
Looser-Milkman (-Debray) **syndrome** M83.8
Lop ear (deformity) Q17.3
Lorain (-Levi) **short stature syndrome** E23.0
Lordosis M40.50
  acquired — *see* Lordosis, specified type NEC
  congenital Q76.429
    lumbar region Q76.426
    lumbosacral region Q76.427
    sacral region Q76.428
    sacrococcygeal region Q76.428
    thoracolumbar region Q76.425
  lumbar region M40.56
  lumbosacral region M40.57
  postsurgical M96.4
  postural — *see* Lordosis, specified type NEC
  rachitic (late effect) (sequelae) E64.3
  sequelae of rickets E64.3
  specified type NEC M40.40
    lumbar region M40.46
    lumbosacral region M40.47
    thoracolumbar region M40.45
  thoracolumbar region M40.55
  tuberculous A18.01
Loss (of)
  appetite (*see also* Anorexia) R63.0
    hysterical F50.89
    nonorganic origin F50.89
    psychogenic F50.89
  blood — *see* Hemorrhage
  bone — *see* Loss, substance of, bone
  consciousness, transient R55
    traumatic — *see* Injury, intracranial
  control, sphincter, rectum R15.9
    nonorganic origin F98.1
  elasticity, skin R23.4
  family (member) in childhood Z62.898
  fluid (acute) E86.9
  function of labyrinth — *see* subcategory H83.2 ☑
  hair, nonscarring — *see* Alopecia
  hearing (*see also* Deafness)
    central NOS H90.5
    conductive H90.2
      bilateral H90.0
      unilateral
        with
          restricted hearing on the contralateral side H90.A1- ☑
          unrestricted hearing on the contralateral side H90.1- ☑

Loss — *continued*
  hearing (*see also* Deafness) — *continued*
    mixed conductive and sensorineural hearing loss H90.8
      bilateral H90.6
      unilateral
        with
          restricted hearing on the contralateral side H90.A3- ☑
          unrestricted hearing on the contralateral side H90.7- ☑
    neural NOS H90.5
    perceptive NOS H90.5
    sensorineural NOS H90.5
      bilateral H90.3
      unilateral
        with
          restricted hearing onthe contralateral side H90.A2- ☑
          unrestricted hearing on the contralateral side H90.4- ☑
    sensory NOS H90.5
  height R29.890
  limb or member, traumatic, current — *see* Amputation, traumatic
  love relationship in childhood Z62.898
  memory (*see also* Amnesia)
    mild, following organic brain damage F06.8
  mind — *see* Psychosis
  occlusal vertical dimension of fully erupted teeth M26.37
  organ or part — *see* Absence, by site, acquired
  ossicles, ear (partial) H74.32- ☑
  parent in childhood Z63.4
  pregnancy, recurrent N96
    without current pregnancy N96
    care in current pregnancy O26.2- ☑
  recurrent pregnancy — *see* Loss, pregnancy, recurrent
  self-esteem, in childhood Z62.898
  sense of
    smell — *see* Disturbance, sensation, smell
    taste — *see* Disturbance, sensation, taste
    touch R20.8
  sensory R44.9
    dissociative F44.6
  sexual desire F52.0
  sight (acquired) (complete) (congenital) — *see* Blindness
  substance of
    bone — *see* Disorder, bone, density and structure, specified NEC
      horizontal alveolar K06.3
    cartilage — *see* Disorder, cartilage, specified type NEC
      auricle (ear) — *see* Disorder, pinna, specified type NEC
    vitreous (humor) H15.89
  tooth, teeth — *see* Absence, teeth, acquired
  vision, visual H54.7
    both eyes H54.3
    one eye H54.60
      left (normal vision on right) H54.62
      right (normal vision on left) H54.61
    specified as blindness — *see* Blindness
    subjective
      sudden H53.13- ☑
      transient H53.12- ☑
  vitreous — *see* Prolapse, vitreous
  voice — *see* Aphonia
  weight (abnormal) (cause unknown) R63.4
Louis-Bar syndrome (ataxia-telangiectasia) G11.3
Louping ill (encephalitis) A84.8
Louse, lousiness — *see* Lice
Low
  achiever, school Z55.3
  back syndrome M54.5
  basal metabolic rate R94.8
  birthweight (2499 grams or less) P07.10
    with weight of
      1000-1249 grams P07.14
      1250-1499 grams P07.15
      1500-1749 grams P07.16
      1750-1999 grams P07.17
      2000-2499 grams P07.18
    extreme (999 grams or less) P07.00
      with weight of
        499 grams or less P07.01
        500-749 grams P07.02

Low — continued
  birthweight — continued
    extreme — continued
      with weight of — continued
        750-999 grams P07.03
    for gestational age — see Light for dates
  blood pressure (see also Hypotension)
    reading (incidental) (isolated) (nonspecific) R03.1
  cardiac reserve — see Disease, heart
  function (see also Hypofunction)
    kidney N28.9
  hematocrit D64.9
  hemoglobin D64.9
  income Z59.6
  level of literacy Z55.0
  lying
    kidney N28.89
    organ or site, congenital — see Malposition, congenital
  output syndrome (cardiac) — see Failure, heart
  platelets (blood) — see Thrombocytopenia
  reserve, kidney N28.89
  salt syndrome E87.1
  self esteem R45.81
  set ears Q17.4
  vision H54.2X- ☑
    one eye (other eye normal) H54.50
      left (normal vision on right) H54.52A- ☑
      other eye blind — see Blindness
      right (normal vision on left) H54.511- ☑
Low-density-lipoprotein-type (LDL) **hyperlipoproteinemia** E78.00
Lowe's syndrome E72.03
Lown-Ganong-Levine syndrome I45.6
LSD reaction (acute) (without dependence) F16.90
  with dependence F16.20
L-shaped kidney Q63.8
Ludwig's angina or disease K12.2
Lues (venerea), **luetic** — see Syphilis
Luetscher's syndrome (dehydration) E86.0
Lumbago, lumbalgia M54.5
  with sciatica M54.4- ☑
    due to intervertebral disc disorder M51.17
  due to displacement, intervertebral disc M51.27
    with sciatica M51.17
Lumbar — see condition
Lumbarization, vertebra, congenital Q76.49
Lumbermen's itch B88.0
Lump (see also Mass)
  breast N63.0
    axillary tail
      left N63.32
      right N63.31
    left
      lower inner quadrant N63.24
      lower outer quadrant N63.23
      unspecified quadrant N63.20
      upper inner quadrant N63.22
      upper outer quadrant N63.21
    right
      lower inner quadrant N63.14
      lower outer quadrant N63.13
      unspecified quadrant N63.10
      upper inner quadrant N63.12
      upper outer quadrant N63.11
    subareolar
      left N63.42
      right N63.41
Lunacy — see Psychosis
Lung — see condition
Lupoid (miliary) **of Boeck** D86.3
Lupus
  anticoagulant D68.62
    with
      hemorrhagic disorder D68.312
      hypercoagulable state D68.62
      finding without diagnosis R76.0
  discoid (local) L93.0
  erythematosus (discoid) (local) L93.0
    disseminated — see Lupus, erythematosus, systemic
    eyelid H01.129
      left H01.126
        lower H01.125
        upper H01.124
      right H01.123
        lower H01.122
        upper H01.121

Lupus — continued
  erythematosus — continued
    profundus L93.2
    specified NEC L93.2
    subacute cutaneous L93.1
    systemic M32.9
      with organ or system involvement M32.10
        endocarditis M32.11
        lung M32.13
        pericarditis M32.12
        renal (glomerular) M32.14
          tubulo-interstitial M32.15
        specified organ or system NEC M32.19
      drug-induced M32.0
      inhibitor (presence of) D68.62
        with
          hemorrhagic disorder D68.312
          hypercoagulable state D68.62
        finding without diagnosis R76.0
      specified NEC M32.8
  exedens A18.4
  hydralazine M32.0
    correct substance properly administered — see Table of Drugs and Chemicals, by drug, adverse effect
    overdose or wrong substance given or taken — see Table of Drugs and Chemicals, by drug, poisoning
  nephritis (chronic) M32.14
  nontuberculous, not disseminated L93.0
  panniculitis L93.2
  pernio (Besnier) D86.3
  systemic — see Lupus, erythematosus, systemic
  tuberculous A18.4
    eyelid A18.4
  vulgaris A18.4
    eyelid A18.4
Luteinoma D27.- ☑
Lutembacher's disease or syndrome (atrial septal defect with mitral stenosis) Q21.1
Luteoma D27.- ☑
Lutz (-Splendore-de Almeida) **disease** — see Paracoccidioidomycosis
Luxation (see also Dislocation)
  eyeball (nontraumatic) — see Luxation, globe
    birth injury P15.3
  globe, nontraumatic H44.82- ☑
  lacrimal gland — see Dislocation, lacrimal gland
  lens (old) (partial) (spontaneous)
    congenital Q12.1
      syphilitic A50.39
Lycanthropy F22
Lyell's syndrome L51.2
  due to drug L51.2
    correct substance properly administered — see Table of Drugs and Chemicals, by drug, adverse effect
    overdose or wrong substance given or taken — see Table of Drugs and Chemicals, by drug, poisoning
Lyme disease A69.20
Lymph
  gland or node — see condition
  scrotum — see Infestation, filarial
Lymphadenitis I88.9
  with ectopic or molar pregnancy O08.0
  acute L04.9
    axilla L04.2
    face L04.0
    head L04.0
    hip L04.3
    limb
      lower L04.3
      upper L04.2
    neck L04.0
    shoulder L04.2
    specified site NEC L04.8
    trunk L04.1
  anthracosis (occupational) J60
  any site, except mesenteric I88.9
    chronic I88.1
    subacute I88.1
  breast
    gestational — see Mastitis, obstetric
    puerperal, postpartum (nonpurulent) O91.22
  chancroidal (congenital) A57
  chronic I88.1
    mesenteric I88.0

Lymphadenitis — continued
  due to
    Brugia (malayi) B74.1
      timori B74.2
    chlamydial lymphogranuloma A55
    diphtheria (toxin) A36.89
    lymphogranuloma venereum A55
    Wuchereria bancrofti B74.0
  following ectopic or molar pregnancy O08.0
  gonorrheal A54.89
  infective — see Lymphadenitis, acute
  mesenteric (acute) (chronic) (nonspecific) (subacute) I88.0
    due to Salmonella typhi A01.09
    tuberculous A18.39
  mycobacterial A31.8
  purulent — see Lymphadenitis, acute
  pyogenic — see Lymphadenitis, acute
  regional, nonbacterial I88.8
  septic — see Lymphadenitis, acute
  subacute, unspecified site I88.1
  suppurative — see Lymphadenitis, acute
  syphilitic (early) (secondary) A51.49
    late A52.79
  tuberculous — see Tuberculosis, lymph gland
  venereal (chlamydial) A55
Lymphadenoid goiter E06.3
Lymphadenopathy (generalized) R59.1
  angioimmunoblastic, with dysproteinemia (AILD) C86.5
  due to toxoplasmosis (acquired) B58.89
    congenital (acute) (subacute) (chronic) P37.1
  localized R59.0
  syphilitic (early) (secondary) A51.49
Lymphadenosis R59.1
Lymphangiectasis I89.0
  conjunctiva H11.89
  postinfectional I89.0
  scrotum I89.0
Lymphangiectatic elephantiasis, nonfilarial I89.0
Lymphangioendothelioma D18.1
  malignant — see Neoplasm, connective tissue, malignant
Lymphangioleiomyomatosis J84.81
Lymphangioma D18.1
  capillary D18.1
  cavernous D18.1
  cystic D18.1
  malignant — see Neoplasm, connective tissue, malignant
Lymphangiomyoma D18.1
Lymphangiomyomatosis J84.81
Lymphangiosarcoma — see Neoplasm, connective tissue, malignant
Lymphangitis I89.1
  with
    abscess — code by site under Abscess
    cellulitis — code by site under Cellulitis
    ectopic or molar pregnancy O08.0
  acute L03.91
    abdominal wall L03.321
    ankle — see Lymphangitis, acute, lower limb
    arm — see Lymphangitis, acute, upper limb
    auricle (ear) — see Lymphangitis, acute, ear
    axilla L03.12- ☑
    back (any part) L03.322
    buttock L03.327
    cervical (meaning neck) L03.222
    cheek (external) L03.212
    chest wall L03.323
    digit
      finger — see Lymphangitis, acute, finger
      toe — see Lymphangitis, acute, toe
    ear (external) H60.1- ☑
    external auditory canal — see Lymphangitis, acute, ear
    eyelid — see Abscess, eyelid
    face NEC L03.212
    finger (intrathecal) (periosteal) (subcutaneous) (subcuticular) L03.02- ☑
    foot — see Lymphangitis, acute, lower limb
    gluteal (region) L03.327
    groin L03.324
    hand — see Lymphangitis, acute, upper limb
    head NEC L03.891
      face (any part, except ear, eye and nose) L03.212
    heel — see Lymphangitis, acute, lower limb

☑ Additional Character Required — Refer to the Tabular List for Character Selection   ▽ Subterms under main terms may continue to next column or page

Lymphangitis — *continued*
- acute — *continued*
  - hip — *see* Lymphangitis, acute, lower limb
  - jaw (region) L03.212
  - knee — *see* Lymphangitis, acute, lower limb
  - leg — *see* Lymphangitis, acute, lower limb
  - lower limb L03.12- ☑
    - toe — *see* Lymphangitis, acute, toe
  - navel L03.326
  - neck (region) L03.222
  - orbit, orbital — *see* Cellulitis, orbit
  - pectoral (region) L03.323
  - perineal, perineum L03.325
  - scalp (any part) L03.891
  - shoulder — *see* Lymphangitis, acute, upper limb
  - specified site NEC L03.898
  - thigh — *see* Lymphangitis, acute, lower limb
  - thumb (intrathecal) (periosteal) (subcutaneous) (subcuticular) — *see* Lymphangitis, acute, finger
  - toe (intrathecal) (periosteal) (subcutaneous) (subcuticular) L03.04- ☑
  - trunk L03.329
    - abdominal wall L03.321
    - back (any part) L03.322
    - buttock L03.327
    - chest wall L03.323
    - groin L03.324
    - perineal, perineum L03.325
    - umbilicus L03.326
  - umbilicus L03.326
  - upper limb L03.12- ☑
    - axilla — *see* Lymphangitis, acute, axilla
    - finger — *see* Lymphangitis, acute, finger
    - thumb — *see* Lymphangitis, acute, finger
    - wrist — *see* Lymphangitis, acute, upper limb
- breast
  - gestational — *see* Mastitis, obstetric
- chancroidal A57
- chronic (any site) I89.1
- due to
  - Brugia (malayi) B74.1
    - timori B74.2
  - Wuchereria bancrofti B74.0
- following ectopic or molar pregnancy O08.89
- penis
  - acute N48.29
  - gonococcal (acute) (chronic) A54.09
- puerperal, postpartum, childbirth O86.89
- strumous, tuberculous A18.2
- subacute (any site) I89.1
- tuberculous — *see* Tuberculosis, lymph gland

Lymphatic (vessel) — *see* condition
Lymphatism E32.8
Lymphectasia I89.0
Lymphedema (acquired) (*see also* Elephantiasis)
- congenital Q82.0
- hereditary (chronic) (idiopathic) Q82.0
- postmastectomy I97.2
- praecox I89.0
- secondary I89.0
- surgical NEC I97.89
  - postmastectomy (syndrome) I97.2

Lymphoblastic — *see* condition
Lymphoblastoma (diffuse) — *see* Lymphoma, lymphoblastic (diffuse)
- giant follicular — *see* Lymphoma, lymphoblastic (diffuse)
- macrofollicular — *see* Lymphoma, lymphoblastic (diffuse)

Lymphocele I89.8
Lymphocytic
- chorioencephalitis (acute) (serous) A87.2
- choriomeningitis (acute) (serous) A87.2
- meningoencephalitis A87.2

Lymphocytoma, benign cutis L98.8
Lymphocytopenia D72.810
Lymphocytosis (symptomatic) D72.820
- infectious (acute) B33.8

Lymphoepithelioma — *see* Neoplasm, malignant, by site
Lymphogranuloma (malignant) (*see also* Lymphoma, Hodgkin)
- chlamydial A55
- inguinale A55
- venereum (any site) (chlamydial) (with stricture of rectum) A55

Lymphogranulomatosis (malignant) (*see also* Lymphoma, Hodgkin)
- benign (Boeck's sarcoid) (Schaumann's) D86.1
Lymphohistiocytosis, hemophagocytic (familial) D76.1
Lymphoid — *see* condition
Lymphoma (of) (malignant) C85.90
- adult T-cell (HTLV-1-associated) (acute variant) (chronic variant) (lymphomatoid variant) (smouldering variant) C91.5- ☑
- anaplastic large cell
  - ALK-negative C84.7- ☑
  - ALK-positive C84.6- ☑
  - CD30-positive C84.6- ☑
  - primary cutaneous C86.6
- angioimmunoblastic T-cell C86.5
- BALT C88.4
- B-cell C85.1- ☑
- blastic NK-cell C86.4
- blastic plasmacytoid dendritic cell neoplasm (BPDCN) C86.4
- B-precursor C83.5- ☑
- bronchial-associated lymphoid tissue [BALT-lymphoma] C88.4
- Burkitt (atypical) C83.7- ☑
- Burkitt-like C83.7- ☑
- centrocytic C83.1- ☑
- cutaneous follicle center C82.6- ☑
- cutaneous T-cell C84.A- ☑ (*following* C84.7)
- diffuse follicle center C82.5- ☑
- diffuse large cell C83.3- ☑
  - anaplastic C83.3- ☑
  - B-cell C83.3- ☑
  - CD30-positive C83.3- ☑
  - centroblastic C83.3- ☑
  - immunoblastic C83.3- ☑
  - plasmablastic C83.3- ☑
  - subtype not specified C83.3- ☑
  - T-cell rich C83.3- ☑
- enteropathy-type (associated) (intestinal) T-cell C86.2
- extranodal marginal zone B-cell lymphoma of mucosa-associated lymphoid tissue [MALT-lymphoma] C88.4
- extranodal NK/T-cell, nasal type C86.0
- follicular C82.9- ☑
  - grade
    - I C82.0- ☑
    - II C82.1- ☑
    - III C82.2- ☑
    - IIIa C82.3- ☑
    - IIIb C82.4- ☑
  - specified NEC C82.8- ☑
- hepatosplenic T-cell (alpha-beta) (gamma-delta) C86.1
- histiocytic C85.9- ☑
  - true C96.A (*following* C96.6)
- Hodgkin C81.9 ☑
  - lymphocyte depleted (classical) C81.3- ☑
  - lymphocyte-rich (classical) C81.4- ☑
  - mixed cellularity (classical) C81.2- ☑
  - nodular
    - lymphocyte predominant C81.0- ☑
    - sclerosis (classical) C81.1- ☑
  - nodular sclerosis (classical) C81.1- ☑
  - specified NEC (classical) C81.7- ☑
- intravascular large B-cell C83.8- ☑
- Lennert's C84.4- ☑
- lymphoblastic (diffuse) C83.5- ☑
- lymphoblastic B-cell C83.5- ☑
- lymphoblastic T-cell C83.5- ☑
- lymphoepithelioid C84.4- ☑
- lymphoplasmacytic C83.0- ☑
  - with IgM-production C88.0
- MALT C88.4
- mantle cell C83.1- ☑
- mature T-cell NEC C84.4- ☑
- mature T/NK-cell C84.9- ☑
  - specified NEC C84.Z- ☑ (*following* C84.7)
- mediastinal (thymic) large B-cell C85.2- ☑
- Mediterranean C88.3
- mucosa-associated lymphoid tissue [MALT-lymphoma] C88.4
- NK/T cell C84.9- ☑
- nodal marginal zone C83.0- ☑
- non-follicular (diffuse) C83.9- ☑
  - specified NEC C83.8- ☑
- non-Hodgkin (*see also* Lymphoma, by type) C85.9- ☑
  - specified NEC C85.8- ☑

Lymphoma — *continued*
- non-leukemic variant of B-CLL C83.0- ☑
- peripheral T-cell, not classified C84.4- ☑
- primary cutaneous
  - anaplastic large cell C86.6
  - CD30-positive large T-cell C86.6
- primary effusion B-cell C83.8- ☑
- SALT C88.4
- skin-associated lymphoid tissue [SALT-lymphoma] C88.4
- small cell B-cell C83.0- ☑
- splenic marginal zone C83.0- ☑
- subcutaneous panniculitis-like T-cell C86.3
- T-precursor C83.5- ☑
- true histiocytic C96.A (*following* C96.6)
Lymphomatosis — *see* Lymphoma
Lymphopathia venereum, veneris A55
Lymphopenia D72.810
Lymphoplasmacytic leukemia — *see* Leukemia, chronic lymphocytic, B-cell type
Lymphoproliferation, X-linked disease D82.3
Lymphoreticulosis, benign (of inoculation) A28.1
Lymphorrhea I89.8
Lymphosarcoma (diffuse) (*see also* Lymphoma) C85.9- ☑
Lymphostasis I89.8
Lypemania — *see* Melancholia
Lysine and hydroxylysine metabolism disorder E72.3
Lyssa — *see* Rabies

M

Macacus ear Q17.3
Maceration, wet feet, tropical (syndrome) T69.02- ☑
MacLeod's syndrome J43.0
Macrocephalia, macrocephaly Q75.3
Macrocheilia, macrochilia (congenital) Q18.6
Macrocolon (*see also* Megacolon) Q43.1
Macrocornea Q15.8
- with glaucoma Q15.0
Macrocytic — *see* condition
Macrocytosis D75.89
Macrodactylia, macrodactylism (fingers) (thumbs) Q74.0
- toes Q74.2
Macrodontia K00.2
Macrogenia M26.05
Macrogenitosomia (adrenal) (male) (praecox) E25.9
- congenital E25.0
Macroglobulinemia (idiopathic) (primary) C88.0
- monoclonal (essential) D47.2
- Waldenström C88.0
Macroglossia (congenital) Q38.2
- acquired K14.8
Macrognathia, macrognathism (congenital) (mandibular) (maxillary) M26.09
Macrogyria (congenital) Q04.8
Macrohydrocephalus — *see* Hydrocephalus
Macromastia — *see* Hypertrophy, breast
Macrophthalmos Q11.3
- in congenital glaucoma Q15.0
Macropsia H53.15
Macrosigmoid K59.39
- congenital Q43.2
Macrospondylitis , acromegalic E22.0
Macrostomia (congenital) Q18.4
Macrotia (external ear) (congenital) Q17.1
Macula
- cornea, corneal — *see* Opacity, cornea
- degeneration (atrophic) (exudative) (senile) (*see also* Degeneration, macula)
- hereditary — *see* Dystrophy, retina
Maculae ceruleae B85.1
Maculopathy, toxic — *see* Degeneration, macula, toxic
Madarosis (eyelid) H02.729
- left H02.726
  - lower H02.725
  - upper H02.724
- right H02.723
  - lower H02.722
  - upper H02.721
Madelung's
- deformity (radius) Q74.0
- disease
  - radial deformity Q74.0
  - symmetrical lipomas, neck E88.89
Madness — *see* Psychosis

▼ Subterms under main terms may continue to next column or page   ☑ Additional Character Required — Refer to the Tabular List for Character Selection   **215**

Lymphangitis — Madness

Index

Madura
foot B47.9
actinomycotic B47.1
mycotic B47.0
Maduromycosis B47.0
Maffucci's syndrome Q78.4
Magnesium metabolism disorder — see Disorder, metabolism, magnesium
Main en griffe (acquired) (see also Deformity, limb, clawhand)
congenital Q74.0
Maintenance (encounter for)
antineoplastic chemotherapy Z51.11
antineoplastic radiation therapy Z51.0
methadone F11.20
Majocchi's
disease L81.7
granuloma B35.8
Major — see condition
Mal de los pintos — see Pinta
Mal de mer T75.3 ☑
Malabar itch (any site) B35.5
Malabsorption K90.9
calcium K90.89
carbohydrate K90.49
disaccharide E73.9
fat K90.49
galactose E74.20
glucose (-galactose) E74.39
intestinal K90.9
specified NEC K90.89
isomaltose E74.31
lactose E73.9
methionine E72.19
monosaccharide E74.39
postgastrectomy K91.2
postsurgical K91.2
protein K90.49
starch K90.49
sucrose E74.39
syndrome K90.9
postsurgical K91.2
Malacia, bone (adult) M83.9
juvenile — see Rickets
Malacoplakia
bladder N32.89
pelvis (kidney) N28.89
ureter N28.89
urethra N36.8
Malacosteon, juvenile — see Rickets
Maladaptation — see Maladjustment
Maladie de Roger Q21.0
Maladjustment
conjugal Z63.0
involving divorce or estrangement Z63.5
educational Z55.4
family Z63.9
marital Z63.0
involving divorce or estrangement Z63.5
occupational NEC Z56.89
simple, adult — see Disorder, adjustment
situational — see Disorder, adjustment
social Z60.9
due to
acculturation difficulty Z60.3
discrimination and persecution (perceived) Z60.5
exclusion and isolation Z60.4
life-cycle (phase of life) transition Z60.0
rejection Z60.4
specified reason NEC Z60.8
Malaise R53.81
Malakoplakia — see Malacoplakia
Malaria, malarial (fever) B54
with
blackwater fever B50.8
hemoglobinuric (bilious) B50.8
hemoglobinuria B50.8
accidentally induced (therapeutically) — code by type under Malaria
algid B50.9
cerebral B50.0 [G94]
clinically diagnosed (without parasitological confirmation) B54
congenital NEC P37.4
falciparum P37.3
congestion, congestive B54
continued (fever) B50.9

Malaria, malarial — continued
estivo-autumnal B50.9
falciparum B50.9
with complications NEC B50.8
cerebral B50.0 [G94]
severe B50.8
hemorrhagic B54
malariae B52.9
with
complications NEC B52.8
glomerular disorder B52.0
malignant (tertian) — see Malaria, falciparum
mixed infections — code to first listed type in B50-B53
ovale B53.0
parasitologically confirmed NEC B53.8
pernicious, acute — see Malaria, falciparum
Plasmodium (P.)
falciparum NEC — see Malaria, falciparum
malariae NEC B52.9
with Plasmodium
falciparum (and or vivax) — see Malaria, falciparum
vivax (see also Malaria, vivax)
and falciparum — see Malaria, falciparum
ovale B53.0
with Plasmodium malariae (see also Malaria, malariae)
and vivax (see also Malaria, vivax)
and falciparum — see Malaria, falciparum
simian B53.1
with Plasmodium malariae (see also Malaria, malariae)
and vivax (see also Malaria, vivax)
and falciparum — see Malaria, falciparum
vivax NEC B51.9
with Plasmodium falciparum — see Malaria, falciparum
quartan — see Malaria, malariae
quotidian — see Malaria, falciparum
recurrent B54
remittent B54
specified type NEC (parasitologically confirmed) B53.8
spleen B54
subtertian (fever) — see Malaria, falciparum
tertian (benign) (see also Malaria, vivax)
malignant B50.9
tropical B50.9
typhoid B54
vivax B51.9
with
complications NEC B51.8
ruptured spleen B51.0
Malassez's disease (cystic) N50.89
Malassimilation K90.9
Maldescent, testis Q53.9
bilateral Q53.20
abdominal Q53.211
perineal Q53.22
unilateral Q53.10
abdominal Q53.111
perineal Q53.12
Maldevelopment (see also Anomaly)
brain Q07.9
colon Q43.9
hip Q74.2
congenital dislocation Q65.2
bilateral Q65.1
unilateral Q65.0- ☑
mastoid process Q75.8
middle ear Q16.4
except ossicles Q16.4
ossicles Q16.3
ossicles Q16.3
spine Q76.49
toe Q74.2
Male type pelvis Q74.2
with disproportion (fetopelvic) O33.3 ☑
causing obstructed labor O65.3
Malformation (congenital) (see also Anomaly)
adrenal gland Q89.1
affecting multiple systems with skeletal changes NEC Q87.5
alimentary tract Q45.9
specified type NEC Q45.8
upper Q40.9

Malformation — continued
alimentary tract — continued
upper — continued
specified type NEC Q40.8
aorta Q25.40
absence Q25.41
aneurysm, congenital Q25.43
aplasia Q25.41
atresia Q25.29
aortic arch Q25.21
coarctation (preductal) (postductal) Q25.1
dilatation, congenital Q25.44
hypoplasia Q25.42
patent ductus arteriosus Q25.0
specified type NEC Q25.49
stenosis Q25.1
supravalvular Q25.3
aortic valve Q23.9
specified NEC Q23.8
arteriovenous, aneurysmatic (congenital) Q27.30
brain Q28.2
cerebral Q28.2
peripheral Q27.30
digestive system Q27.33
lower limb Q27.32
other specified site Q27.39
renal vessel Q27.34
upper limb Q27.31
precerebral vessels (nonruptured) Q28.0
auricle
ear (congenital) Q17.3
acquired H61.119
left H61.112
with right H61.113
right H61.111
with left H61.113
bile duct Q44.5
bladder Q64.79
aplasia Q64.5
diverticulum Q64.6
exstrophy — see Exstrophy, bladder
neck obstruction Q64.31
bone Q79.9
face Q75.9
specified type NEC Q75.8
skull Q75.9
specified type NEC Q75.8
brain (multiple) Q04.9
arteriovenous Q28.2
specified type NEC Q04.8
branchial cleft Q18.2
breast Q83.9
specified type NEC Q83.8
broad ligament Q50.6
bronchus Q32.4
bursa Q79.9
cardiac
chambers Q20.9
specified type NEC Q20.8
septum Q21.9
specified type NEC Q21.8
cerebral Q04.9
vessels Q28.3
cervix uteri Q51.9
specified type NEC Q51.828
Chiari
Type I G93.5
Type II Q07.01
choroid (congenital) Q14.3
plexus Q07.8
circulatory system Q28.9
cochlea Q16.5
cornea Q13.4
coronary vessels Q24.5
corpus callosum (congenital) Q04.0
diaphragm Q79.1
digestive system NEC, specified type NEC Q45.8
dura Q07.9
brain Q04.9
spinal Q06.9
ear Q17.9
causing impairment of hearing Q16.9
external Q17.9
accessory auricle Q17.0
causing impairment of hearing Q16.9
absence of
auditory canal Q16.1
auricle Q16.0
macrotia Q17.1

☑ Additional Character Required — Refer to the Tabular List for Character Selection   Subterms under main terms may continue to next column or page

Madura — Malformation

Malformation — *continued*
  ear — *continued*
    external — *continued*
      microtia Q17.2
      misplacement Q17.4
      misshapen NEC Q17.3
      prominence Q17.5
      specified type NEC Q17.8
    inner Q16.5
    middle Q16.4
      absence of eustachian tube Q16.2
      ossicles (fusion) Q16.3
    ossicles Q16.3
    specified type NEC Q17.8
  epididymis Q55.4
  esophagus Q39.9
    specified type NEC Q39.8
  eye Q15.9
    lid Q10.3
    specified NEC Q15.8
  fallopian tube Q50.6
  genital organ — *see* Anomaly, genitalia
  great
    artery Q25.9
      aorta — *see* Malformation, aorta
      pulmonary artery — *see* Malformation, pul-
        monary, artery
      specified type NEC Q25.8
    vein Q26.9
      anomalous
        portal venous connection Q26.5
        pulmonary venous connection Q26.4
          partial Q26.3
          total Q26.2
      persistent left superior vena cava Q26.1
      portal vein-hepatic artery fistula Q26.6
      specified type NEC Q26.8
      vena cava stenosis, congenital Q26.0
  gum Q38.6
  hair Q84.2
  heart Q24.9
    specified type NEC Q24.8
  integument Q84.9
    specified type NEC Q84.8
  internal ear Q16.5
  intestine Q43.9
    specified type NEC Q43.8
  iris Q13.2
  joint Q74.9
    ankle Q74.2
    lumbosacral Q76.49
    sacroiliac Q74.2
    specified type NEC Q74.8
  kidney Q63.9
    accessory Q63.0
    giant Q63.3
    horseshoe Q63.1
    hydronephrosis Q62.0
    malposition Q63.2
    specified type NEC Q63.8
  lacrimal apparatus Q10.6
  lingual Q38.3
  lip Q38.0
  liver Q44.7
  lung Q33.9
  meninges or membrane (congenital) Q07.9
    cerebral Q04.8
    spinal (cord) Q06.9
  middle ear Q16.4
    ossicles Q16.3
  mitral valve Q23.9
    specified NEC Q23.8
  Mondini's (congenital) (malformation, cochlea) Q16.5
  mouth (congenital) Q38.6
  multiple types NEC Q89.7
  musculoskeletal system Q79.9
  myocardium Q24.8
  nail Q84.6
  nervous system (central) Q07.9
  nose Q30.9
    specified type NEC Q30.8
  optic disc Q14.2
  orbit Q10.7
  ovary Q50.39
  palate Q38.5
  parathyroid gland Q89.2
  pelvic organs or tissues NEC
    in pregnancy or childbirth O34.8- ☑
      causing obstructed labor O65.5

Malformation — *continued*
  penis Q55.69
    aplasia Q55.5
    curvature (lateral) Q55.61
    hypoplasia Q55.62
  pericardium Q24.8
  peripheral vascular system Q27.9
    specified type NEC Q27.8
  pharynx Q38.8
  precerebral vessels Q28.1
  prostate Q55.4
  pulmonary
    arteriovenous Q25.72
    artery Q25.9
      atresia Q25.5
      specified type NEC Q25.79
      stenosis Q25.6
    valve Q22.3
  renal artery Q27.2
  respiratory system Q34.9
  retina Q14.1
  scrotum — *see* Malformation, testis and scrotum
  seminal vesicles Q55.4
  sense organs NEC Q07.9
  skin Q82.9
  specified NEC Q89.8
  spinal
    cord Q06.9
    nerve root Q07.8
  spine Q76.49
    kyphosis — *see* Kyphosis, congenital
    lordosis — *see* Lordosis, congenital
  spleen Q89.09
  stomach Q40.3
    specified type NEC Q40.2
  teeth, tooth K00.9
  tendon Q79.9
  testis and scrotum Q55.20
    aplasia Q55.0
    hypoplasia Q55.1
    polyorchism Q55.21
    retractile testis Q55.22
    scrotal transposition Q55.23
    specified NEC Q55.29
  thorax, bony Q76.9
  throat Q38.8
  thyroid gland Q89.2
  tongue (congenital) Q38.3
    hypertrophy Q38.2
    tie Q38.1
  trachea Q32.1
  tricuspid valve Q22.9
    specified type NEC Q22.8
  umbilical cord NEC (complicating delivery) O69.89 ☑
  umbilicus Q89.9
  ureter Q62.8
    agenesis Q62.4
    duplication Q62.5
    malposition — *see* Malposition, congenital, ureter
    obstructive defect — *see* Defect, obstructive, ureter
    vesico-uretero-renal reflux Q62.7
  urethra Q64.79
    aplasia Q64.5
    duplication Q64.74
    posterior valves Q64.2
    prolapse Q64.71
    stricture Q64.32
  urinary system Q64.9
  uterus Q51.9
    specified type NEC Q51.818
  vagina Q52.4
  vas deferens Q55.4
    atresia Q55.3
  vascular system, peripheral Q27.9
  venous — *see* Anomaly, vein(s)
  vulva Q52.70
Malfunction (*see also* Dysfunction)
  cardiac electronic device T82.119 ☑
    electrode T82.110 ☑
    pulse generator T82.111 ☑
    specified type NEC T82.118 ☑
  catheter device NEC T85.618 ☑
    cystostomy T83.010 ☑
    dialysis (renal) (vascular) T82.41 ☑
      intraperitoneal T85.611 ☑
    infusion NEC T82.514 ☑
      cranial T85.610 ☑
      epidural T85.610 ☑

Malfunction — *continued*
  catheter device — *continued*
    infusion — *continued*
      intrathecal T85.610 ☑
      spinal T85.610 ☑
      subarachnoid T85.610 ☑
      subdural T85.610 ☑
    urinary (*see also* Breakdown, device, catheter)
      T83.018 ☑
  colostomy K94.03
    valve K94.03
  cystostomy (stoma) N99.512
    catheter T83.010 ☑
  enteric stoma K94.13
  enterostomy K94.13
  esophagostomy K94.33
  gastroenteric K31.89
  gastrostomy K94.23
  ileostomy K94.13
    valve K94.13
  intrathecal infusion pump T85.615 ☑
  jejunostomy K94.13
  nervous system device, implant or graft, specified NEC
    T85.615 ☑
  pacemaker — *see* Malfunction, cardiac electronic de-
    vice
  prosthetic device, internal — *see* Complications,
    prosthetic device, by site, mechanical
  tracheostomy J95.03
  urinary device NEC — *see* Complication, genitourinary,
    device, urinary, mechanical
  valve
    colostomy K94.03
    heart T82.09 ☑
    ileostomy K94.13
  vascular graft or shunt NEC — *see* Complication, car-
    diovascular device, mechanical, vascular
  ventricular (communicating shunt) T85.01 ☑
Malherbe's tumor — *see* Neoplasm, skin, benign
Malibu disease L98.8
Malignancy (*see also* Neoplasm, malignant, by site)
  unspecified site (primary) C80.1
Malignant — *see* condition
Malingerer, malingering Z76.5
Mallet finger (acquired) — *see* Deformity, finger, mallet
  finger
  congenital Q74.0
  sequelae of rickets E64.3
Malleus A24.0
Mallory's bodies R89.7
Mallory-Weiss syndrome K22.6
Malnutrition E46
  degree
    first E44.1
    mild (protein) E44.1
    moderate (protein) E44.0
    second E44.0
    severe (protein-energy) E43
      intermediate form E42
        with
          kwashiorkor (and marasmus) E42
          marasmus E41
    third E43
  following gastrointestinal surgery K91.2
  intrauterine
    light-for-dates — *see* Light for dates
    small-for-dates — *see* Small for dates
  lack of care, or neglect (child) (infant) T76.02 ☑
    confirmed T74.02 ☑
  malignant E40
  protein E46
    calorie E46
      mild E44.1
      moderate E44.0
      severe E43
        intermediate form E42
          with
            kwashiorkor (and marasmus) E42
            marasmus E41
    energy E46
      mild E44.1
      moderate E44.0
      severe E43
        intermediate form E42
          with
            kwashiorkor (and marasmus) E42
            marasmus E41
  severe (protein-energy) E43

Malnutrition — *continued*
  severe — *continued*
    with
      kwashiorkor (and marasmus) E42
      marasmus E41
Malocclusion (teeth) M26.4
  Angle's M26.219
    class I M26.211
    class II M26.212
    class III M26.213
  due to
    abnormal swallowing M26.59
    mouth breathing M26.59
    tongue, lip or finger habits M26.59
  temporomandibular (joint) M26.69
Malposition
  cervix — *see* Malposition, uterus
  congenital
    adrenal (gland) Q89.1
    alimentary tract Q45.8
      lower Q43.8
      upper Q40.8
    aorta Q25.49
    appendix Q43.8
    arterial trunk Q20.0
    artery (peripheral) Q27.8
      coronary Q24.5
      digestive system Q27.8
      lower limb Q27.8
      pulmonary Q25.79
      specified site NEC Q27.8
      upper limb Q27.8
    auditory canal Q17.8
      causing impairment of hearing Q16.9
    auricle (ear) Q17.4
      causing impairment of hearing Q16.9
      cervical Q18.2
    biliary duct or passage Q44.5
    bladder (mucosa) — *see* Exstrophy, bladder
    brachial plexus Q07.8
    brain tissue Q04.8
    breast Q83.8
    bronchus Q32.4
    cecum Q43.8
    clavicle Q74.0
    colon Q43.8
    digestive organ or tract NEC Q45.8
      lower Q43.8
      upper Q40.8
    ear (auricle) (external) Q17.4
      ossicles Q16.3
    endocrine (gland) NEC Q89.2
    epiglottis Q31.8
    eustachian tube Q17.8
    eye Q15.8
    facial features Q18.8
    fallopian tube Q50.6
    finger(s) Q68.1
      supernumerary Q69.0
    foot Q66.9
    gallbladder Q44.1
    gastrointestinal tract Q45.8
    genitalia, genital organ(s) or tract
      female Q52.8
        external Q52.79
        internal NEC Q52.8
      male Q55.8
    glottis Q31.8
    hand Q68.1
    heart Q24.8
      dextrocardia Q24.0
        with complete transposition of viscera Q89.3
    hepatic duct Q44.5
    hip (joint) Q65.89
    intestine (large) (small) Q43.8
      with anomalous adhesions, fixation or malrotation Q43.3
    joint NEC Q68.8
    kidney Q63.2
    larynx Q31.8
    limb Q68.8
      lower Q68.8
      upper Q68.8
    liver Q44.7
    lung (lobe) Q33.8
    nail(s) Q84.6
    nerve Q07.8
    nervous system NEC Q07.8
    nose, nasal (septum) Q30.8

Malposition — *continued*
  congenital — *continued*
    organ or site not listed — *see* Anomaly, by site
    ovary Q50.39
    pancreas Q45.3
    parathyroid (gland) Q89.2
    patella Q74.1
    peripheral vascular system Q27.8
    pituitary (gland) Q89.2
    respiratory organ or system NEC Q34.8
    rib (cage) Q76.6
      supernumerary in cervical region Q76.5
    scapula Q74.0
    shoulder Q74.0
    spinal cord Q06.8
    spleen Q89.09
    sternum NEC Q76.7
    stomach Q40.2
    symphysis pubis Q74.2
    thymus (gland) Q89.2
    thyroid (gland) (tissue) Q89.2
      cartilage Q31.8
    toe(s) Q66.9
      supernumerary Q69.2
    tongue Q38.3
    trachea Q32.1
    ureter Q62.60
      deviation Q62.61
      displacement Q62.62
      ectopia Q62.63
      specified type NEC Q62.69
    uterus Q51.818
    vein(s) (peripheral) Q27.8
      great Q26.8
    vena cava (inferior) (superior) Q26.8
  device, implant or graft (*see also* Complications, by site and type, mechanical) T85.628 ☑
    arterial graft NEC — *see* Complication, cardiovascular device, mechanical, vascular
    breast (implant) T85.42 ☑
    catheter NEC T85.628 ☑
      cystostomy T83.020 ☑
      dialysis (renal) T82.42 ☑
        intraperitoneal T85.621 ☑
      infusion NEC T82.524 ☑
        spinal (epidural) (subdural) T85.620 ☑
      urinary (*see also* Displacement, device, catheter, urinary) T83.028 ☑
    electronic (electrode) (pulse generator) (stimulator)
      bone T84.320 ☑
      cardiac T82.129 ☑
        electrode T82.120 ☑
        pulse generator T82.121 ☑
        specified type NEC T82.128 ☑
      nervous system — *see* Complication, prosthetic device, mechanical, electronic nervous system stimulator
      urinary — *see* Complication, genitourinary, device, urinary, mechanical
    fixation, internal (orthopedic) NEC — *see* Complication, fixation device, mechanical
    gastrointestinal — *see* Complications, prosthetic device, mechanical, gastrointestinal device
    genital NEC T83.428 ☑
      intrauterine contraceptive device (string) T83.32 ☑
      penile prosthesis (cylinder) (implanted) (pump) (reservoir) T83.420 ☑
      testicular prosthesis T83.421 ☑
    heart NEC — *see* Complication, cardiovascular device, mechanical
    joint prosthesis — *see* Complication, joint prosthesis, mechanical
    ocular NEC — *see* Complications, prosthetic device, mechanical, ocular device
    orthopedic NEC — *see* Complication, orthopedic, device, mechanical
    specified NEC T85.628 ☑
    urinary NEC (*see also* Complication, genitourinary, device, urinary, mechanical)
      graft T83.22 ☑
    vascular NEC — *see* Complication, cardiovascular device, mechanical
    ventricular intracranial shunt T85.02 ☑
  fetus — *see* Pregnancy, complicated by (management affected by), presentation, fetal
  gallbladder K82.8

Malposition — *continued*
  gastrointestinal tract, congenital Q45.8
  heart, congenital NEC Q24.8
  joint prosthesis — *see* Complications, joint prosthesis, mechanical, displacement, by site
  stomach K31.89
    congenital Q40.2
  tooth, teeth, fully erupted M26.30
  uterus (acute) (acquired) (adherent) (asymptomatic) (postinfectional) (postpartal, old) N85.4
    anteflexion or anteversion N85.4
      congenital Q51.818
    flexion N85.4
      lateral — *see* Lateroversion, uterus
    inversion N85.5
    lateral (flexion) (version) — *see* Lateroversion, uterus
    in pregnancy or childbirth — *see* subcategory O34.5 ☑
    retroflexion or retroversion — *see* Retroversion, uterus
Malposture R29.3
Malrotation
  cecum Q43.3
  colon Q43.3
  intestine Q43.3
  kidney Q63.2
Malta fever — *see* Brucellosis
Maltreatment
  adult
    abandonment
      confirmed T74.01 ☑
      suspected T76.01 ☑
    confirmed T74.91 ☑
    history of Z91.419
    neglect
      confirmed T74.01 ☑
      suspected T76.01 ☑
    physical abuse
      confirmed T74.11 ☑
      suspected T76.11 ☑
    psychological abuse
      confirmed T74.31 ☑
      history of Z91.411
      suspected T76.31 ☑
    sexual abuse
      confirmed T74.21 ☑
      suspected T76.21 ☑
    suspected T76.91 ☑
  child
    abandonment
      confirmed T74.02 ☑
      suspected T76.02 ☑
    confirmed T74.92 ☑
    history of — *see* History, personal (of), abuse
    neglect
      confirmed T74.02 ☑
      history of — *see* History, personal (of), abuse
      suspected T76.02 ☑
    physical abuse
      confirmed T74.12 ☑
      history of — *see* History, personal (of), abuse
      suspected T76.12 ☑
    psychological abuse
      confirmed T74.32 ☑
      history of — *see* History, personal (of), abuse
      suspected T76.32 ☑
    sexual abuse
      confirmed T74.22 ☑
      history of — *see* History, personal (of), abuse
      suspected T76.22 ☑
    suspected T76.92 ☑
  personal history of Z91.89
Maltworker's lung J67.4
Malunion, fracture — *see* Fracture, by site
Mammillitis N61.0
  puerperal, postpartum O91.02
Mammitis — *see* Mastitis
Mammogram (examination) Z12.39
  routine Z12.31
Mammoplasia N62
Management (of)
  bone conduction hearing device (implanted) Z45.320
  cardiac pacemaker NEC Z45.018
  cerebrospinal fluid drainage device Z45.41
  cochlear device (implanted) Z45.321
  contraceptive Z30.9

☑ **Additional Character Required — Refer to the Tabular List for Character Selection**   ☝ **Subterms under main terms may continue to next column or page**

Management — *continued*
  contraceptive — *continued*
    specified NEC Z30.8
  implanted device Z45.9
    specified NEC Z45.89
  infusion pump Z45.1
  procreative Z31.9
    male factor infertility in female Z31.81
    specified NEC Z31.89
  prosthesis (external) (*see also* Fitting) Z44.9
    implanted Z45.9
      specified NEC Z45.89
  renal dialysis catheter Z49.01
  vascular access device Z45.2
Mangled — *see* specified injury by site
Mania (monopolar) (*see also* Disorder, mood, manic episode)
  with psychotic symptoms F30.2
  without psychotic symptoms F30.10
    mild F30.11
    moderate F30.12
    severe F30.13
  Bell's F30.8
  chronic (recurrent) F31.89
  hysterical F44.89
  puerperal F30.8
  recurrent F31.89
Manic depression F31.9
Manic-depressive insanity, psychosis, or syndrome — *see* Disorder, bipolar
Mannosidosis E77.1
Mansonelliasis, mansonellosis B74.4
Manson's
  disease B65.1
  schistosomiasis B65.1
Manual — *see* condition
Maple-bark-stripper's lung (disease) J67.6
Maple-syrup-urine disease E71.0
Marable's syndrome (celiac artery compression) I77.4
Marasmus E41
  due to malnutrition E41
  intestinal E41
  nutritional E41
  senile R54
  tuberculous NEC — *see* Tuberculosis
Marble
  bones Q78.2
  skin R23.8
Marburg virus disease A98.3
March
  fracture — *see* Fracture, traumatic, stress, by site
  hemoglobinuria D59.6
Marchesani (-Weill) **syndrome** Q87.0
Marchiafava (-Bignami) **syndrome or disease** G37.1
Marchiafava-Micheli syndrome D59.5
Marcus Gunn's syndrome Q07.8
Marfan's syndrome — *see* Syndrome, Marfan's
Marie-Bamberger disease — *see* Osteoarthropathy, hypertrophic, specified NEC
Marie-Charcot-Tooth neuropathic muscular atrophy G60.0
Marie's
  cerebellar ataxia (late-onset) G11.2
  disease or syndrome (acromegaly) E22.0
Marie-Strümpell arthritis, disease or spondylitis — *see* Spondylitis, ankylosing
Marion's disease (bladder neck obstruction) N32.0
Marital conflict Z63.0
Mark
  port wine Q82.5
  raspberry Q82.5
  strawberry Q82.5
  stretch L90.6
  tattoo L81.8
Marker heterochromatin — *see* Extra, marker chromosomes
Maroteaux-Lamy syndrome (mild) (severe) E76.29
Marrow (bone)
  arrest D61.9
  poor function D75.89
Marseilles fever A77.1
Marsh fever — *see* Malaria
Marshall's (hidrotic) **ectodermal dysplasia** Q82.4
Marsh's disease (exophthalmic goiter) E05.00
  with storm E05.01
Masculinization (female) **with adrenal hyperplasia** E25.9

Masculinization (female) **with adrenal hyperplasia** — *continued*
  congenital E25.0
Masculinovoblastoma D27.- ☑
Masochism (sexual) F65.51
Mason's lung J62.8
Mass
  abdominal R19.00
    epigastric R19.06
    generalized R19.07
    left lower quadrant R19.04
    left upper quadrant R19.02
    periumbilic R19.05
    right lower quadrant R19.03
    right upper quadrant R19.01
    specified site NEC R19.09
  breast (*see also* Lump, breast) N63.0
  chest R22.2
  cystic — *see* Cyst
  ear H93.8- ☑
  head R22.0
  intra-abdominal (diffuse) (generalized) — *see* Mass, abdominal
  kidney N28.89
  liver R16.0
  localized (skin) R22.9
    chest R22.2
    head R22.0
    limb
      lower R22.4- ☑
      upper R22.3- ☑
    neck R22.1
    trunk R22.2
  lung R91.8
  malignant — *see* Neoplasm, malignant, by site
  neck R22.1
  pelvic (diffuse) (generalized) — *see* Mass, abdominal
  specified organ NEC — *see* Disease, by site
  splenic R16.1
  substernal thyroid — *see* Goiter
  superficial (localized) R22.9
  umbilical (diffuse) (generalized) R19.09
Massive — *see* condition
Mast cell
  disease, systemic tissue D47.02
  leukemia C94.3- ☑
  neoplasm
    malignant C96.20
      specified type NEC C96.29
    of uncertain behavior NEC D47.09
  sarcoma C96.22
  tumor D47.09
Mastalgia N64.4
Masters-Allen syndrome N83.8
Mastitis (acute) (diffuse) (nonpuerperal) (subacute) N61.0
  with abscess N61.1
  without abscess N61.0
  chronic (cystic) — *see* Mastopathy, cystic
  cystic (Schimmelbusch's type) — *see* Mastopathy, cystic
  fibrocystic — *see* Mastopathy, cystic
  infective N61.0
    newborn P39.0
  interstitial, gestational or puerperal — *see* Mastitis, obstetric
  neonatal (noninfective) P83.4
    infective P39.0
  obstetric (interstitial) (nonpurulent)
    associated with
      lactation O91.23
      pregnancy O91.21- ☑
      puerperium O91.22
    purulent
      associated with
        lactation O91.13
        pregnancy O91.11- ☑
        puerperium O91.12
  periductal — *see* Ectasia, mammary duct
  phlegmonous — *see* Mastopathy, cystic
  plasma cell — *see* Ectasia, mammary duct
Mastocytoma (extracutaneous) D47.09
  malignant C96.29
  solitary D47.01
Mastocytosis D47.09
  aggressive systemic C96.21
  cutaneous (diffuse) (maculopapular) D47.01
    congenital Q82.2
    of neonatal onset Q82.2

Mastocytosis — *continued*
  cutaneous — *continued*
    of newborn onset Q82.2
  indolent systemic D47.02
  isolated bone marrow D47.02
  malignant C96.29
  systemic (indolent) (smoldering)
    with an associated hematological non-mast cell lineage disease (SM-AHNMD) D47.02
Mastodynia N64.4
Mastoid — *see* condition
Mastoidalgia — *see* subcategory H92.0 ☑
Mastoiditis (coalescent) (hemorrhagic) (suppurative) H70.9-
  acute, subacute H70.00- ☑
    complicated NEC H70.09- ☑
    subperiosteal H70.01- ☑
  chronic (necrotic) (recurrent) H70.1- ☑
  in (due to)
    infectious disease NEC B99 ☑ [H75.0-] ☑
    parasitic disease NEC B89 [H75.0-] ☑
    tuberculosis A18.03
  petrositis — *see* Petrositis
  postauricular fistula — *see* Fistula, postauricular
  specified NEC H70.89- ☑
  tuberculous A18.03
Mastopathy, mastopathia N64.9
  chronica cystica — *see* Mastopathy, cystic
  cystic (chronic) (diffuse) N60.1- ☑
    with epithelial proliferation N60.3- ☑
  diffuse cystic — *see* Mastopathy, cystic
  estrogenic, oestrogenica N64.89
  ovarian origin N64.89
Mastoplasia, mastoplastia N62
Masturbation (excessive) F98.8
Maternal care (for) — *see* Pregnancy (complicated by) (management affected by)
Matheiu's disease (leptospiral jaundice) A27.0
Mauclaire's disease or osteochondrosis — *see* Osteochondrosis, juvenile, hand, metacarpal
Maxcy's disease A75.2
Maxilla, maxillary — *see* condition
May (-Hegglin) **anomaly or syndrome** D72.0
McArdle (-Schmid)(-Pearson) **disease** (glycogen storage) E74.04
McCune-Albright syndrome Q78.1
McQuarrie's syndrome (idiopathic familial hypoglycemia) E16.2
Meadow's syndrome Q86.1
Measles (black) (hemorrhagic) (suppressed) B05.9
  with
    complications NEC B05.89
    encephalitis B05.0
    intestinal complications B05.4
    keratitis (keratoconjunctivitis) B05.81
    meningitis B05.1
    otitis media B05.3
    pneumonia B05.2
  French — *see* Rubella
  German — *see* Rubella
  Liberty — *see* Rubella
Meatitis, urethral — *see* Urethritis
Meatus, meatal — *see* condition
Meat-wrappers' asthma J68.9
Meckel-Gruber syndrome Q61.9
Meckel's diverticulitis, diverticulum (displaced) (hypertrophic) Q43.0
  malignant — *see* Table of Neoplasms, small intestine, malignant
Meconium
  ileus, newborn P76.0
    in cystic fibrosis E84.11
    meaning meconium plug (without cystic fibrosis) P76.0
  obstruction, newborn P76.0
    due to fecaliths P76.0
    in mucoviscidosis E84.11
  peritonitis P78.0
  plug syndrome (newborn) NEC P76.0
Median (*see also* condition)
  arcuate ligament syndrome I77.4
  bar (prostate) (vesical orifice) — *see* Hyperplasia, prostate
  rhomboid glossitis K14.2
Mediastinal shift R93.8
Mediastinitis (acute) (chronic) J98.51
  syphilitic A52.73

▼ Subterms under main terms may continue to next column or page   ☑ Additional Character Required — Refer to the Tabular List for Character Selection   **219**

Management — Mediastinitis

Mediastinitis — *continued*
  tuberculous A15.8
Mediastinopericarditis (*see also* Pericarditis)
  acute I30.9
  adhesive I31.0
  chronic I31.8
    rheumatic I09.2
Mediastinum, mediastinal — *see* condition
Medicine poisoning — *see* Table of Drugs and Chemicals, by drug, poisoning
Mediterranean
  fever — *see* Brucellosis
    familial M04.1
    tick A77.1
  kala-azar B55.0
  leishmaniasis B55.0
  tick fever A77.1
Medulla — *see* condition
Medullary cystic kidney Q61.5
Medullated fibers
  optic (nerve) Q14.8
  retina Q14.1
Medulloblastoma
  desmoplastic C71.6
  specified site — *see* Neoplasm, malignant, by site
  unspecified site C71.6
Medulloepithelioma (*see also* Neoplasm, malignant, by site)
  teratoid — *see* Neoplasm, malignant, by site
Medullomyoblastoma
  specified site — *see* Neoplasm, malignant, by site
  unspecified site C71.6
Meekeren-Ehlers-Danlos syndrome Q79.6
Megacolon (acquired) (functional) (not Hirschsprung's disease) (in) K59.39
  Chagas' disease B57.32
  congenital, congenitum (aganglionic) Q43.1
  Hirschsprung's (disease) Q43.1
  toxic NEC K59.31
    due to Clostridium difficile
      not specified as recurrent A04.72
      recurrent A04.71
Megaesophagus (functional) K22.0
  congenital Q39.5
  in (due to) Chagas' disease B57.31
Megalencephaly Q04.5
Megalerythema (epidemic) B08.3
Megaloappendix Q43.8
Megalocephalus, megalocephaly NEC Q75.3
Megalocornea Q15.8
  with glaucoma Q15.0
Megalocytic anemia D53.1
Megalodactylia (fingers) (thumbs) (congenital) Q74.0
  toes Q74.2
Megaloduodenum Q43.8
Megaloesophagus (functional) K22.0
  congenital Q39.5
Megalogastria (acquired) K31.89
  congenital Q40.2
Megalophthalmos Q11.3
Megalopsia H53.15
Megalosplenia — *see* Splenomegaly
Megaloureter N28.82
  congenital Q62.2
Megarectum K62.89
Megasigmoid K59.39
  congenital Q43.2
Megaureter N28.82
  congenital Q62.2
Megavitamin-B6 syndrome E67.2
Megrim — *see* Migraine
Meibomian
  cyst, infected — *see* Hordeolum
  gland — *see* condition
  sty, stye — *see* Hordeolum
Meibomitis — *see* Hordeolum
Meige-Milroy disease (chronic hereditary edema) Q82.0
Meige's syndrome Q82.0
Melalgia, nutritional E53.8
Melancholia F32.9
  climacteric (single episode) F32.89
    recurrent episode F33.8
  hypochondriac F45.29
  intermittent (single episode) F32.89
    recurrent episode F33.8
  involutional (single episode) F32.89
    recurrent episode F33.8

Melancholia — *continued*
  menopausal (single episode) F32.89
    recurrent episode F33.8
  puerperal F32.89
  reactive (emotional stress or trauma) F32.3
  recurrent F33.9
  senile F03 ☑
  stuporous (single episode) F32.89
    recurrent episode F33.8
Melanemia R79.89
Melanoameloblastoma — *see* Neoplasm, bone, benign
Melanoblastoma — *see* Melanoma
Melanocarcinoma — *see* Melanoma
Melanocytoma, eyeball D31.9-
Melanocytosis, neurocutaneous Q82.8
Melanoderma, melanodermia L81.4
Melanodontia, infantile K03.89
Melanodontoclasia K03.89
Melanoepithelioma — *see* Melanoma
Melanoma (malignant) C43.9
  acral lentiginous, malignant — *see* Melanoma, skin, by site
  amelanotic — *see* Melanoma, skin, by site
  balloon cell — *see* Melanoma, skin, by site
  benign — *see* Nevus
  desmoplastic, malignant — *see* Melanoma, skin, by site
  epithelioid cell — *see* Melanoma, skin, by site
    with spindle cell, mixed — *see* Melanoma, skin, by site
  in
    giant pigmented nevus — *see* Melanoma, skin, by site
    Hutchinson's melanotic freckle — *see* Melanoma, skin, by site
    junctional nevus — *see* Melanoma, skin, by site
    precancerous melanosis — *see* Melanoma, skin, by site
  in situ D03.9
    abdominal wall D03.59
    ala nasi D03.39
    ankle D03.7- ☑
    anus, anal (margin) (skin) D03.51
    arm D03.6- ☑
    auditory canal D03.2- ☑
    auricle (ear) D03.2- ☑
    auricular canal (external) D03.2- ☑
    axilla, axillary fold D03.59
    back D03.59
    breast D03.52
    brow D03.39
    buttock D03.59
    canthus (eye) D03.1- ☑
    cheek (external) D03.39
    chest wall D03.59
    chin D03.39
    choroid D03.8
    conjunctiva D03.8
    ear (external) D03.2- ☑
    external meatus (ear) D03.2- ☑
    eye D03.8
    eyebrow D03.39
    eyelid (lower) (upper) D03.1- ☑
    face D03.30
      specified NEC D03.39
    female genital organ (external) NEC D03.8
    finger D03.6- ☑
    flank D03.59
    foot D03.7- ☑
    forearm D03.6- ☑
    forehead D03.39
    foreskin D03.8
    gluteal region D03.59
    groin D03.59
    hand D03.6- ☑
    heel D03.7- ☑
    helix D03.2- ☑
    hip D03.7- ☑
    interscapular region D03.59
    iris D03.8
    jaw D03.39
    knee D03.7- ☑
    labium (majus) (minus) D03.8
    lacrimal gland D03.8
    leg D03.7- ☑
    lip (lower) (upper) D03.0
    lower limb NEC D03.7- ☑

Melanoma — *continued*
  in situ — *continued*
    male genital organ (external) NEC D03.8
    nail D03.9
      finger D03.6- ☑
      toe D03.7- ☑
    neck D03.4
    nose (external) D03.39
    orbit D03.8
    penis D03.8
    perianal skin D03.51
    perineum D03.51
    pinna D03.2- ☑
    popliteal fossa or space D03.7- ☑
    prepuce D03.8
    pudendum D03.8
    retina D03.8
    retrobulbar D03.8
    scalp D03.4
    scrotum D03.8
    shoulder D03.6- ☑
    specified site NEC D03.8
    submammary fold D03.52
    temple D03.39
    thigh D03.7- ☑
    toe D03.7- ☑
    trunk NEC D03.59
    umbilicus D03.59
    upper limb NEC D03.6- ☑
    vulva D03.8
  juvenile — *see* Nevus
  malignant, of soft parts except skin — *see* Neoplasm, connective tissue, malignant
  metastatic
    breast C79.81
    genital organ C79.82
    specified site NEC C79.89
  neurotropic, malignant — *see* Melanoma, skin, by site
  nodular — *see* Melanoma, skin, by site
  regressing, malignant — *see* Melanoma, skin, by site
  skin C43.9
    abdominal wall C43.59
    ala nasi C43.31
    ankle C43.7- ☑
    anus, anal (skin) C43.51
    arm C43.6- ☑
    auditory canal (external) C43.2- ☑
    auricle (ear) C43.2- ☑
    auricular canal (external) C43.2- ☑
    axilla, axillary fold C43.59
    back C43.59
    breast (female) (male) C43.52
    brow C43.39
    buttock C43.59
    canthus (eye) C43.1- ☑
    cheek (external) C43.39
    chest wall C43.59
    chin C43.39
    ear (external) C43.2- ☑
    elbow C43.6- ☑
    external meatus (ear) C43.2- ☑
    eyebrow C43.39
    eyelid (lower) (upper) C43.1- ☑
    face C43.30
      specified NEC C43.39
    female genital organ (external) NEC C51.9
    finger C43.6- ☑
    flank C43.59
    foot C43.7- ☑
    forearm C43.6- ☑
    forehead C43.39
    foreskin C60.0
    glabella C43.39
    gluteal region C43.59
    groin C43.59
    hand C43.6- ☑
    heel C43.7- ☑
    helix C43.2- ☑
    hip C43.7- ☑
    interscapular region C43.59
    jaw (external) C43.39
    knee C43.7- ☑
    labium C51.9
      majus C51.0
      minus C51.1
    leg C43.7- ☑
    lip (lower) (upper) C43.0

Melanoma — *continued*
- skin — *continued*
  - lower limb NEC C43.7- ☑
  - male genital organ (external) NEC C63.9
  - nail
    - finger C43.6- ☑
    - toe C43.7- ☑
  - nasolabial groove C43.39
  - nates C43.59
  - neck C43.4
  - nose (external) C43.31
  - overlapping site C43.8
  - palpebra C43.1- ☑
  - penis C60.9
  - perianal skin C43.51
  - perineum C43.51
  - pinna C43.2- ☑
  - popliteal fossa or space C43.7- ☑
  - prepuce C60.0
  - pudendum C51.9
  - scalp C43.4
  - scrotum C63.2
  - shoulder C43.6- ☑
  - skin NEC C43.9
  - submammary fold C43.52
  - temple C43.39
  - thigh C43.7- ☑
  - toe C43.7- ☑
  - trunk NEC C43.59
  - umbilicus C43.59
  - upper limb NEC C43.6- ☑
  - vulva C51.9
    - overlapping sites C51.8
- spindle cell
  - with epithelioid, mixed — *see* Melanoma, skin, by site
  - type A C69.4- ☑
  - type B C69.4- ☑
- superficial spreading — *see* Melanoma, skin, by site

Melanosarcoma (*see also* Melanoma)
- epithelioid cell — *see* Melanoma

Melanosis L81.4
- addisonian E27.1
  - tuberculous A18.7
- adrenal E27.1
- colon K63.89
- conjunctiva — *see* Pigmentation, conjunctiva
  - congenital Q13.89
- cornea (presenile) (senile) (*see also* Pigmentation, cornea)
  - congenital Q13.4
- eye NEC H57.8
  - congenital Q15.8
- lenticularis progressiva Q82.1
- liver K76.89
- precancerous (*see also* Melanoma, in situ)
  - malignant melanoma in — *see* Melanoma
- Riehl's L81.4
- sclera H15.89
  - congenital Q13.89
- suprarenal E27.1
- tar L81.4
- toxic L81.4

Melanuria R82.99
MELAS syndrome E88.41
Melasma L81.1
- adrenal (gland) E27.1
- suprarenal (gland) E27.1

Melena K92.1
- with ulcer — *code by* site under Ulcer, with hemorrhage K27.4
- due to swallowed maternal blood P78.2
- newborn, neonatal P54.1
  - due to swallowed maternal blood P78.2

Meleney's
- gangrene (cutaneous) — *see* Ulcer, skin
- ulcer (chronic undermining) — *see* Ulcer, skin

Melioidosis A24.9
- acute A24.1
- chronic A24.2
- fulminating A24.1
- pneumonia A24.1
- pulmonary (chronic) A24.2
  - acute A24.1
  - subacute A24.2
- sepsis A24.1
- specified NEC A24.3
- subacute A24.2

Melitensis, febris A23.0
Melkersson (-Rosenthal) **syndrome** G51.2
Mellitus, diabetes — *see* Diabetes
Melorheostosis (bone) — *see* Disorder, bone, density and structure, specified NEC
Meloschisis Q18.4
Melotia Q17.4
Membrana
- capsularis lentis posterior Q13.89
- epipapillaris Q14.2

Membranacea placenta O43.19- ☑
Membranaceous uterus N85.8
Membrane(s), membranous (*see also* condition)
- cyclitic — *see* Membrane, pupillary
- folds, congenital — *see* Web
- Jackson's Q43.3
- over face of newborn P28.9
- premature rupture — *see* Rupture, membranes, premature
- pupillary H21.4- ☑
  - persistent Q13.89
- retained (with hemorrhage) (complicating delivery) O72.2
  - without hemorrhage O73.1
- secondary cataract — *see* Cataract, secondary
- unruptured (causing asphyxia) — *see* Asphyxia, newborn
- vitreous — *see* Opacity, vitreous, membranes and strands

Membranitis — *see* Chorioamnionitis
Memory disturbance, lack or loss (*see also* Amnesia)
- mild, following organic brain damage F06.8

Menadione deficiency E56.1
Menarche
- delayed E30.0
- precocious E30.1

Mendacity, pathologic F60.2
Mendelson's syndrome (due to anesthesia) J95.4
- in labor and delivery O74.0
- in pregnancy O29.01- ☑
- obstetric O74.0
- postpartum, puerperal O89.01

Ménétrier's disease or syndrome K29.60
- with bleeding K29.61

Ménière's disease, syndrome or vertigo H81.0- ☑
Meninges, meningeal — *see* condition
Meningioma (*see also* Neoplasm, meninges, benign)
- angioblastic — *see* Neoplasm, meninges, benign
- angiomatous — *see* Neoplasm, meninges, benign
- endotheliomatous — *see* Neoplasm, meninges, benign
- fibroblastic — *see* Neoplasm, meninges, benign
- fibrous — *see* Neoplasm, meninges, benign
- hemangioblastic — *see* Neoplasm, meninges, benign
- hemangiopericytic — *see* Neoplasm, meninges, benign
- malignant — *see* Neoplasm, meninges, malignant
- meningiothelial — *see* Neoplasm, meninges, benign
- meningotheliomatous — *see* Neoplasm, meninges, benign
- mixed — *see* Neoplasm, meninges, benign
- multiple — *see* Neoplasm, meninges, uncertain behavior
- papillary — *see* Neoplasm, meninges, uncertain behavior
- psammomatous — *see* Neoplasm, meninges, benign
- syncytial — *see* Neoplasm, meninges, benign
- transitional — *see* Neoplasm, meninges, benign

Meningiomatosis (diffuse) — *see* Neoplasm, meninges, uncertain behavior
Meningism — *see* Meningismus
Meningismus (infectional) (pneumococcal) R29.1
- due to serum or vaccine R29.1
- influenzal — *see* Influenza, with, manifestations NEC

Meningitis (basal) (basic) (brain) (cerebral) (cervical) (congestive) (diffuse) (hemorrhagic) (infantile) (membranous) (metastatic) (nonspecific) (pontine) (progressive) (simple) (spinal) (subacute) (sympathetic) (toxic) G03.9
- abacterial G03.0
- actinomycotic A42.81
- adenoviral A87.1
- arbovirus A87.8
- aseptic (acute) G03.0
- bacterial G00.9
  - Escherichia coli (E. coli) G00.8
  - Friedländer (bacillus) G00.8
  - gram-negative G00.9

Meningitis — *continued*
- bacterial — *continued*
  - H. influenzae G00.0
  - Klebsiella G00.8
  - pneumococcal G00.1
  - specified organism NEC G00.8
  - staphylococcal G00.3
  - streptococcal (acute) G00.2
- benign recurrent (Mollaret) G03.2
- candidal B37.5
- caseous (tuberculous) A17.0
- cerebrospinal A39.0
- chronic NEC G03.1
- clear cerebrospinal fluid NEC G03.0
- coxsackievirus A87.0
- cryptococcal B45.1
- diplococcal (gram positive) A39.0
- echovirus A87.0
- enteroviral A87.0
- eosinophilic B83.2
- epidemic NEC A39.0
- Escherichia coli (E. coli) G00.8
- fibrinopurulent G00.9
  - specified organism NEC G00.8
- Friedländer (bacillus) G00.8
- gonococcal A54.81
- gram-negative cocci G00.9
- gram-positive cocci G00.9
- H. influenzae G00.0
- Haemophilus (influenzae) G00.0
- in (due to)
  - adenovirus A87.1
  - African trypanosomiasis B56.9 [G02]
  - anthrax A22.8
  - bacterial disease NEC A48.8 [G01]
  - Chagas' disease (chronic) B57.41
  - chickenpox B01.0
  - coccidioidomycosis B38.4
  - Diplococcus pneumoniae G00.1
  - enterovirus A87.0
  - herpes (simplex) virus B00.3
    - zoster B02.1
  - infectious mononucleosis B27.92
  - leptospirosis A27.81
  - Listeria monocytogenes A32.11
  - Lyme disease A69.21
  - measles B05.1
  - mumps (virus) B26.1
  - neurosyphilis (late) A52.13
  - parasitic disease NEC B89 [G02]
  - poliovirus A80.9 [G02]
  - preventive immunization, inoculation or vaccination G03.8
  - rubella B06.02
  - Salmonella infection A02.21
  - specified cause NEC G03.8
  - Streptococcal pneumoniae G00.1
  - typhoid fever A01.01
  - varicella B01.0
  - viral disease NEC A87.8
  - whooping cough A37.90
  - zoster B02.1
- infectious G00.9
- influenzal (H. influenzae) G00.0
- Klebsiella G00.8
- leptospiral (aseptic) A27.81
- lymphocytic (acute) (benign) (serous) A87.2
- meningococcal A39.0
- Mima polymorpha G00.8
- Mollaret (benign recurrent) G03.2
- monilial B37.5
- mycotic NEC B49 [G02]
- Neisseria A39.0
- nonbacterial G03.0
- nonpyogenic NEC G03.0
- ossificans G96.19
- pneumococcal streptococcus pneumoniae G00.1
- poliovirus A80.9 [G02]
- postmeasles B05.1
- purulent G00.9
  - specified organism NEC G00.8
- pyogenic G00.9
  - specified organism NEC G00.8
- Salmonella (arizonae) (Cholerae-Suis) (enteritidis) (typhimurium) A02.21
- septic G00.9
  - specified organism NEC G00.8
- serosa circumscripta NEC G03.0
- serous NEC G93.2

Index

Meningitis — Mesothelioma

Meningitis — *continued*
  specified organism NEC G00.8
  sporotrichosis B42.81
  staphylococcal G00.3
  sterile G03.0
  Streptococcal (acute) G00.2
    pneumoniae G00.1
  suppurative G00.9
    specified organism NEC G00.8
  syphilitic (late) (tertiary) A52.13
    acute A51.41
    congenital A50.41
    secondary A51.41
  Torula histolytica (cryptococcal) B45.1
  traumatic (complication of injury) T79.8 ☑
  tuberculous A17.0
  typhoid A01.01
  viral NEC A87.9
  Yersinia pestis A20.3
Meningocele (spinal) (*see also* Spina bifida)
  with hydrocephalus — *see* Spina bifida, by site, with
    hydrocephalus
  acquired (traumatic) G96.19
  cerebral — *see* Encephalocele
Meningocerebritis — *see* Meningoencephalitis
Meningococcemia A39.4
  acute A39.2
  chronic A39.3
Meningococcus, meningococcal (*see also* condition)
  A39.9
  adrenalitis, hemorrhagic A39.1
  carrier (suspected) of Z22.31
  meningitis (cerebrospinal) A39.0
Meningoencephalitis (*see also* Encephalitis) G04.90
  acute NEC (*see also* Encephalitis, viral) A86
  bacterial NEC G04.2
  California A83.5
  diphasic A84.1
  eosinophilic B83.2
  epidemic A39.81
  herpesviral, herpetic B00.4
    due to herpesvirus 6 B10.01
    due to herpesvirus 7 B10.09
    specified NEC B10.09
  in (due to)
    blastomycosis NEC B40.81
    diseases classified elsewhere G05.3
    free-living amebae B60.2
    H. influenzae G00.0
    Hemophilus influenzae (H .influenzae) G00.0
    herpes B00.4
      due to herpesvirus 6 B10.01
      due to herpesvirus 7 B10.09
      specified NEC B10.09
    Lyme disease A69.22
    mercury — *see* subcategory T56.1 ☑
    mumps B26.2
    Naegleria (amebae) (organisms) (fowleri) B60.2
    Parastrongylus cantonensis B83.2
    toxoplasmosis (acquired) B58.2
      congenital P37.1
  infectious (acute) (viral) A86
  influenzal (H. influenzae) G00.0
  Listeria monocytogenes A32.12
  lymphocytic (serous) A87.2
  mumps B26.2
  parasitic NEC B89 [G05.3]
  pneumococcal G04.2
  primary amebic B60.2
  specific (syphilitic) A52.14
  specified organism NEC G04.81
  staphylococcal G04.2
  streptococcal G04.2
  syphilitic A52.14
  toxic NEC G92
    due to mercury — *see* subcategory T56.1 ☑
  tuberculous A17.82
  virus NEC A86
Meningoencephalocele (*see also* Encephalocele)
  syphilitic A52.19
    congenital A50.49
Meningoencephalomyelitis (*see also* Meningoencephalitis)
  acute NEC (viral) A86
    disseminated G04.00
      postimmunization or postvaccination G04.02
      postinfectious G04.01

Meningoencephalomyelitis — *continued*
  due to
    actinomycosis A42.82
    Torula B45.1
    Toxoplasma or toxoplasmosis (acquired) B58.2
      congenital P37.1
  postimmunization or postvaccination G04.02
Meningoencephalomyelopathy G96.9
Meningoencephalopathy G96.9
Meningomyelitis (*see also* Meningoencephalitis)
  bacterial NEC G04.2
  blastomycotic NEC B40.81
  cryptococcal B45.1
  in diseases classified elsewhere G05.4
  meningococcal A39.81
  syphilitic A52.14
  tuberculous A17.82
Meningomyelocele (*see also* Spina bifida)
  syphilitic A52.19
Meningomyeloneuritis — *see* Meningoencephalitis
Meningoradiculitis — *see* Meningitis
Meningovascular — *see* condition
Menkes' disease or syndrome E83.09
  meaning maple-syrup-urine disease E71.0
Menometrorrhagia N92.1
Menopause, menopausal (asymptomatic) (state) Z78.0
  arthritis (any site) NEC — *see* Arthritis, specified form
    NEC
  bleeding N92.4
  depression (single episode) F32.89
    agitated (single episode) F32.2
      recurrent episode F33.9
    psychotic (single episode) F32.89
      recurrent episode F33.9
    recurrent episode F33.8
  melancholia (single episode) F32.89
    recurrent episode F33.8
  paranoid state F22
  premature E28.319
    asymptomatic E28.319
      postirradiation E89.40
      postsurgical E89.40
    symptomatic E28.310
      postirradiation E89.41
      postsurgical E89.41
  psychosis NEC F28
  symptomatic N95.1
  toxic polyarthritis NEC — *see* Arthritis, specified form
    NEC
Menorrhagia (primary) N92.0
  climacteric N92.4
    menopausal N92.4
  menopausal N92.4
  postclimacteric N95.0
  postmenopausal N95.0
  preclimacteric or premenopausal N92.4
  pubertal (menses retained) N92.2
Menostaxis N92.0
Menses, retention N94.89
Menstrual — *see* Menstruation
Menstruation
  absent — *see* Amenorrhea
  anovulatory N97.0
  cycle, irregular N92.6
  delayed N91.0
  disorder N93.9
    psychogenic F45.8
  during pregnancy O20.8
  excessive (with regular cycle) N92.0
    with irregular cycle N92.1
    at puberty N92.2
  frequent N92.0
  infrequent — *see* Oligomenorrhea
  irregular N92.6
    specified NEC N92.5
  latent N92.5
  membranous N92.5
  painful (*see also* Dysmenorrhea) N94.6
    primary N94.4
    psychogenic F45.8
    secondary N94.5
  passage of clots N92.0
  precocious E30.1
  protracted N92.5
  rare — *see* Oligomenorrhea
  retained N94.89
  retrograde N92.5
  scanty — *see* Oligomenorrhea

Menstruation — *continued*
  suppression N94.89
  vicarious (nasal) N94.89
Mental (*see also* condition)
  deficiency — *see* Disability, intellectual
  deterioration — *see* Psychosis
  disorder — *see* Disorder, mental
  exhaustion F48.8
  insufficiency (congenital) — *see* Disability, intellectual
  observation without need for further medical care
    Z03.89
  retardation — *see* Disability, intellectual
  subnormality — *see* Disability, intellectuall
  upset — *see* Disorder, mental
Meralgia paresthetica G57.1- ☑
Mercurial — *see* condition
Mercurialism — *see* subcategory T56.1 ☑
Merkel cell tumor — *see* Carcinoma, Merkel cell
Merocele — *see* Hernia, femoral
Meromelia
  lower limb — *see* Defect, reduction, lower limb
    intercalary
      femur — *see* Defect, reduction, lower limb,
        specified type NEC
        tibiofibular (complete) (incomplete) — *see*
          Defect, reduction, lower limb
  upper limb — *see* Defect, reduction, upper limb
    intercalary, humeral, radioulnar — *see* Agenesis,
      arm, with hand present
MERRF syndrome (myoclonic epilepsy associated with
  ragged-red fiber) E88.42
Merzbacher-Pelizaeus disease E75.29
Mesaortitis — *see* Aortitis
Mesarteritis — *see* Arteritis
Mesencephalitis — *see* Encephalitis
Mesenchymoma (*see also* Neoplasm, connective tissue,
  uncertain behavior)
  benign — *see* Neoplasm, connective tissue, benign
  malignant — *see* Neoplasm, connective tissue, malig-
    nant
Mesenteritis
  retractile K65.4
  sclerosing K65.4
Mesentery, mesenteric — *see* condition
Mesiodens, mesiodentes K00.1
Mesio-occlusion M26.213
Mesocolon — *see* condition
Mesonephroma (malignant) — *see* Neoplasm, malig-
  nant, by site
  benign — *see* Neoplasm, benign, by site
Mesophlebitis — *see* Phlebitis
Mesostromal dysgenesia Q13.89
Mesothelioma (malignant) C45.9
  benign
    mesentery D19.1
    mesocolon D19.1
    omentum D19.1
    peritoneum D19.1
    pleura D19.0
    specified site NEC D19.7
    unspecified site D19.9
  biphasic C45.9
    benign
      mesentery D19.1
      mesocolon D19.1
      omentum D19.1
      peritoneum D19.1
      pleura D19.0
      specified site NEC D19.7
      unspecified site D19.9
  cystic D48.4
  epithelioid C45.9
    benign
      mesentery D19.1
      mesocolon D19.1
      omentum D19.1
      peritoneum D19.1
      pleura D19.0
      specified site NEC D19.7
      unspecified site D19.9
  fibrous C45.9
    benign
      mesentery D19.1
      mesocolon D19.1
      omentum D19.1
      peritoneum D19.1
      pleura D19.0
      specified site NEC D19.7

☑ Additional Character Required — Refer to the Tabular List for Character Selection   ᵂᴱᴮ Subterms under main terms may continue to next column or page

Mesothelioma — *continued*
  fibrous — *continued*
    benign — *continued*
      unspecified site D19.9
    site classification
      liver C45.7
      lung C45.7
      mediastinum C45.7
      mesentery C45.1
      mesocolon C45.1
      omentum C45.1
      pericardium C45.2
      peritoneum C45.1
      pleura C45.0
        parietal C45.0
      retroperitoneum C45.7
      specified site NEC C45.7
      unspecified C45.9
Metabolic syndrome E88.81
Metagonimiasis B66.8
Metagonimus infestation (intestine) B66.8
Metal
  pigmentation L81.8
  polisher's disease J62.8
Metamorphopsia H53.15
Metaplasia
  apocrine (breast) — *see* Dysplasia, mammary, specified type NEC
  cervix (squamous) — *see* Dysplasia, cervix
  endometrium (squamous) (uterus) N85.8
  esophagus K22.7- ☑
  kidney (pelvis) (squamous) N28.89
  myelogenous D73.1
  myeloid (agnogenic) (megakaryocytic) D73.1
  spleen D73.1
  squamous cell, bladder N32.89
Metastasis, metastatic
  abscess — *see* Abscess
  calcification E83.59
  cancer
    from specified site — *see* Neoplasm, malignant, by site
    to specified site — *see* Neoplasm, secondary, by site
  deposits (in) — *see* Neoplasm, secondary, by site
  disease (*see also* Neoplasm, secondary, by site) C79.9
  spread (to) — *see* Neoplasm, secondary, by site
Metastrongyliasis B83.8
Metatarsalgia M77.4- ☑
  anterior G57.6- ☑
  Morton's G57.6- ☑
Metatarsus, metatarsal (*see also* condition)
  adductus, congenital Q66.22
  valgus (abductus), congenital Q66.6
  varus (congenital) Q66.22
    primus Q66.21
Methadone use — *see* Use, opioid
Methemoglobinemia D74.9
  acquired (with sulfhemoglobinemia) D74.8
  congenital D74.0
  enzymatic (congenital) D74.0
  Hb M disease D74.0
  hereditary D74.0
  toxic D74.8
Methemoglobinuria — *see* Hemoglobinuria
Methioninemia E72.19
Methylmalonic acidemia E71.120
Metritis (catarrhal) (hemorrhagic) (septic) (suppurative) (*see also* Endometritis)
  cervical — *see* Cervicitis
Metropathia hemorrhagica N93.8
Metroperitonitis — *see* Peritonitis, pelvic, female
Metrorrhagia N92.1
  climacteric N92.4
  menopausal N92.4
  postpartum NEC (atonic) (following delivery of placenta) O72.1
    delayed or secondary O72.2
  preclimacteric or premenopausal N92.4
  psychogenic F45.8
Metrorrhexis — *see* Rupture, uterus
Metrosalpingitis N70.91
Metrostaxis N93.8
Metrovaginitis — *see* Endometritis
Meyer-Schwickerath and Weyers syndrome Q87.0
Meynert's amentia (nonalcoholic) F04
  alcoholic F10.96

Meynert's amentia — *continued*
  alcoholic — *continued*
    with dependence F10.26
Mibelli's disease (porokeratosis) Q82.8
Mice, joint — *see* Loose, body, joint
  knee M23.4- ☑
Micrencephalon, micrencephaly Q02
Microalbuminuria R80.9
Microaneurysm, retinal (*see also* Disorder, retina, microaneurysms)
  diabetic — *see* E08-E13 with .31
Microangiopathy (peripheral) I73.9
  thrombotic M31.1
Microcalcifications, breast R92.0
Microcephalus, microcephalic, microcephaly Q02
  due to toxoplasmosis (congenital) P37.1
Microcheilia Q18.7
Microcolon (congenital) Q43.8
Microcornea (congenital) Q13.4
Microcytic — *see* condition
Microdeletions NEC Q93.88
Microdontia K00.2
Microdrepanocytosis D57.40
  with crisis (vasoocclusive pain) D57.419
    with
      acute chest syndrome D57.411
      splenic sequestration D57.412
Microembolism
  atherothrombotic — *see* Atheroembolism
  retinal — *see* Occlusion, artery, retina
Microencephalon Q02
Microfilaria streptocerca infestation — *see* Onchocerciasis
Microgastria (congenital) Q40.2
Microgenia M26.06
Microgenitalia, congenital
  female Q52.8
  male Q55.8
Microglioma — *see* Lymphoma, non-Hodgkin, specified NEC
Microglossia (congenital) Q38.3
Micrognathia, micrognathism (congenital) (mandibular) (maxillary) M26.09
Microgyria (congenital) Q04.3
Microinfarct of heart — *see* Insufficiency, coronary
Microlentia (congenital) Q12.8
Microlithiasis, alveolar, pulmonary J84.02
Micromastia N64.82
Micromyelia (congenital) Q06.8
Micropenis Q55.62
Microphakia (congenital) Q12.8
Microphthalmos, microphthalmia (congenital) Q11.2
  due to toxoplasmosis P37.1
Micropsia H53.15
Microscopic polyangiitis (polyarteritis) M31.7
Microsporidiosis B60.8
  intestinal A07.8
Microsporon furfur infestation B36.0
Microsporosis (*see also* Dermatophytosis)
  nigra B36.1
Microstomia (congenital) Q18.5
Microtia (congenital) (external ear) Q17.2
Microtropia H50.40
Microvillus inclusion disease (MVD) (MVID) Q43.8
Micturition
  disorder NEC (*see also* Difficulty, micturition) R39.198
    psychogenic F45.8
  frequency R35.0
    psychogenic F45.8
  hesitancy R39.11
  incomplete emptying R39.14
  nocturnal R35.1
  painful R30.9
    dysuria R30.0
    psychogenic F45.8
    tenesmus R30.1
  poor stream R39.12
  position dependent R39.192
  split stream R39.13
  straining R39.16
  urgency R39.15
Mid plane — *see* condition
Middle
  ear — *see* condition
  lobe (right) syndrome J98.19
Miescher's elastoma L87.2
Mietens' syndrome Q87.2

Migraine (idiopathic) G43.909
  with aura (acute-onset) (prolonged) (typical) (without headache) G43.109
    with refractory migraine G43.119
      with status migrainosus G43.111
      without status migrainosus G43.119
    without mention of refractory migraine G43.109
      with status migrainosus G43.101
      without status migrainosus G43.109
    intractable G43.119
      with status migrainosus G43.111
      without status migrainosus G43.119
    not intractable G43.109
      with status migrainosus G43.101
      without status migrainosus G43.109
    persistent G43.509
      with cerebral infarction G43.609
        with refractory migraine G43.619
          with status migrainosus G43.611
          without status migrainosus G43.619
        without refractory migraine G43.609
          with status migrainosus G43.601
          without status migrainosus G43.609
        intractable G43.619
          with status migrainosus G43.611
          without status migrainosus G43.619
        not intractable G43.609
          with status migrainosus G43.601
          without status migrainosus G43.609
      without cerebral infarction G43.509
        with refractory migraine G43.519
          with status migrainosus G43.511
          without status migrainosus G43.519
        without refractory migraine G43.509
          with status migrainosus G43.501
          without status migrainosus G43.509
        intractable G43.519
          with status migrainosus G43.511
          without status migrainosus G43.519
        not intractable G43.509
          with status migrainosus G43.501
          without status migrainosus G43.509
  with refractory migraine G43.919
    with status migrainosus G43.911
    without status migrainosus G43.919
  without aura G43.009
    with refractory migraine G43.019
      with status migrainosus G43.011
      without status migrainosus G43.019
    without mention of refractory migraine G43.009
      with status migrainosus G43.001
      without status migrainosus G43.009
    chronic G43.709
      with refractory migraine G43.719
        with status migrainosus G43.711
        without status migrainosus G43.719
      without refractory migraine G43.709
        with status migrainosus G43.701
        without status migrainosus G43.709
      intractable
        with status migrainosus G43.711
        without status migrainosus G43.719
      not intractable
        with status migrainosus G43.701
        without status migrainosus G43.709
    intractable
      with status migrainosus G43.011
      without status migrainosus G43.019
    not intractable
      with status migrainosus G43.001
      without status migrainosus G43.009
  without refractory migraine G43.909
    with status migrainosus G43.901
    without status migrainosus G43.919
  abdominal G43.D0 (*following* G43.7)
    with refractory migraine G43.D1 (*following* G43.7)
    without refractory migraine G43.D0 (*following* G43.7)
    intractable G43.D1 (*following* G43.7)
    not intractable G43.D0 (*following* G43.7)
  basilar — *see* Migraine, with aura
  classical — *see* Migraine, with aura
  common — *see* Migraine, without aura
  complicated G43.109
  equivalents — *see* Migraine, with aura
  familiar — *see* Migraine, hemiplegic
  hemiplegic G43.409
    with refractory migraine G43.419
      with status migrainosus G43.411

Migraine — continued
  hemiplegic — continued
    with refractory migraine — continued
      without status migrainosus G43.419
    without refractory migraine G43.409
      with status migrainosus G43.401
      without status migrainosus G43.409
    intractable G43.419
      with status migrainosus G43.411
      without status migrainosus G43.419
    not intractable G43.409
      with status migrainosus G43.401
      without status migrainosus G43.409
  intractable G43.919
    with status migrainosus G43.911
    without status migrainosus G43.919
  menstrual G43.829
    with refractory migraine G43.839
      with status migrainosus G43.831
      without status migrainosus G43.839
    without refractory migraine G43.829
      with status migrainosus G43.821
      without status migrainosus G43.829
    intractable G43.839
      with status migrainosus G43.831
      without status migrainosus G43.839
    not intractable 4G43.829
      with status migrainosus G43.821
      without status migrainosus G43.829
  menstrually related — see Migraine, menstrual
  not intractable G43.909
    with status migrainosus G43.901
    without status migrainosus G43.919
  ophthalmoplegic G43.B0 (following G43.7)
    with refractory migraine G43.B1 (following G43.7)
    without refractory migraine G43.B0 (following G43.7)
    intractable G43.B1 (following G43.7)
    not intractable G43.B0 (following G43.7)
  persistent aura (with, without) cerebral infarction — see Migraine, with aura, persistent
  preceded or accompanied by transient focal neurological phenomena — see Migraine, with aura
  pre-menstrual — see Migraine, menstrual
  pure menstrual — see Migraine, menstrual
  retinal — see Migraine, with aura
  specified NEC G43.809
    intractable G43.819
      with status migrainosus G43.811
      without status migrainosus G43.819
    not intractable G43.809
      with status migrainosus G43.801
      without status migrainosus G43.809
  sporadic — see Migraine, hemiplegic
  transformed — see Migraine, without aura, chronic
  triggered seizures — see Migraine, with aura
Migrant, social Z59.0
Migration, anxiety concerning Z60.3
Migratory, migrating (see also condition)
  person Z59.0
  testis Q55.29
Mikity-Wilson disease or syndrome P27.0
Mikulicz' disease or syndrome K11.8
Miliaria L74.3
  alba L74.1
  apocrine L75.2
  crystallina L74.1
  profunda L74.2
  rubra L74.0
  tropicalis L74.2
Miliary — see condition
Milium L72.0
  colloid L57.8
Milk
  crust L21.0
  excessive secretion O92.6
  poisoning — see Poisoning, food, noxious
  retention O92.79
  sickness — see Poisoning, food, noxious
  spots I31.0
Milk-alkali disease or syndrome E83.52
Milk-leg (deep vessels) (nonpuerperal) — see Embolism, vein, lower extremity
  complicating pregnancy O22.3- ☑
  puerperal, postpartum, childbirth O87.1
Milkman's disease or syndrome M83.8
Milky urine — see Chyluria
Millard-Gubler (-Foville) **paralysis or syndrome** G46.3

Millar's asthma J38.5
Miller Fisher syndrome G61.0
Mills' disease — see Hemiplegia
Millstone maker's pneumoconiosis J62.8
Milroy's disease (chronic hereditary edema) Q82.0
Minamata disease T56.1 ☑
Miners' asthma or lung J60
Minkowski-Chauffard syndrome — see Spherocytosis
Minor — see condition
Minor's disease (hematomyelia) G95.19
Minot's disease (hemorrhagic disease), newborn P53
Minot-von Willebrand-Jurgens disease or syndrome (angiohemophilia) D68.0
Minus (and plus) **hand** (intrinsic) — see Deformity, limb, specified type NEC, forearm
Miosis (pupil) H57.03
Mirizzi's syndrome (hepatic duct stenosis) K83.1
Mirror writing F81.0
Misadventure (of) (prophylactic) (therapeutic) (see also Complications) T88.9 ☑
  administration of insulin (by accident) — see subcategory T38.3 ☑
  infusion — see Complications, infusion
  local applications (of fomentations, plasters, etc.) T88.9 ☑
    burn or scald — see Burn
    specified NEC T88.8 ☑
  medical care (early) (late) T88.9 ☑
    adverse effect of drugs or chemicals — see Table of Drugs and Chemicals
    burn or scald — see Burn
    specified NEC T88.8 ☑
  specified NEC T88.8 ☑
  surgical procedure (early) (late) — see Complications, surgical procedure
  transfusion — see Complications, transfusion
  vaccination or other immunological procedure — see Complications, vaccination
Miscarriage O03.9
Misdirection, aqueous H40.83- ☑
Misperception, sleep state F51.02
Misplaced, misplacement
  ear Q17.4
  kidney (acquired) N28.89
    congenital Q63.2
  organ or site, congenital NEC — see Malposition, congenital
Missed
  abortion O02.1
  delivery O36.4 ☑
Missing (see also Absence)
  string of intrauterine contraceptive device T83.32- ☑
Misuse of drugs F19.99
Mitchell's disease (erythromelalgia) I73.81
Mite(s) (infestation) B88.9
  diarrhea B88.0
  grain (itch) B88.0
  hair follicle (itch) B88.0
  in sputum B88.0
Mitral — see condition
Mittelschmerz N94.0
Mixed — see condition
MMN (multifocal motor neuropathy) G61.82
MNGIE (Mitochondrial Neurogastrointestinal Encephalopathy) **syndrome** E88.49
Mobile, mobility
  cecum Q43.3
  excessive — see Hypermobility
  gallbladder, congenital Q44.1
  kidney N28.89
  organ or site, congenital NEC — see Malposition, congenital
Mobitz heart block (atrioventricular) I44.1
Moebius, Möbius
  disease (ophthalmoplegic migraine) — see Migraine, ophthalmoplegic
  syndrome Q87.0
    congenital oculofacial paralysis (with other anomalies) Q87.0
    ophthalmoplegic migraine — see Migraine, ophthalmoplegic
Moeller's glossitis K14.0
Mohr's syndrome (Types I and II) Q87.0
Mola destruens D39.2
Molar pregnancy O02.0
Molarization of premolars K00.2

Molding, head (during birth) — omit code
Mole (pigmented) (see also Nevus)
  blood O02.0
  Breus' O02.0
  cancerous — see Melanoma
  carneous O02.0
  destructive D39.2
  fleshy O02.0
  hydatid, hydatidiform (benign) (complicating pregnancy) (delivered) (undelivered) O01.9
    classical O01.0
    complete O01.0
    incomplete O01.1
    invasive D39.2
    malignant D39.2
    partial O01.1
  intrauterine O02.0
  invasive (hydatidiform) D39.2
  malignant
    meaning
      malignant hydatidiform mole D39.2
      melanoma — see Melanoma
  nonhydatidiform O02.0
  nonpigmented — see Nevus
  pregnancy NEC O02.0
  skin — see Nevus
  tubal O00.10- ☑
    with intrauterine pregnancy O00.11- ☑
  vesicular — see Mole, hydatidiform
Molimen, molimina (menstrual) N94.3
Molluscum contagiosum (epitheliale) B08.1
Mönckeberg's arteriosclerosis, disease, or sclerosis — see Arteriosclerosis, extremities
Mondini's malformation (cochlea) Q16.5
Mondor's disease I80.8
Monge's disease T70.29 ☑
Monilethrix (congenital) Q84.1
Moniliasis (see also Candidiasis) B37.9
  neonatal P37.5
Monitoring (encounter for)
  therapeutic drug level Z51.81
Monkey malaria B53.1
Monkeypox B04
Monoarthritis M13.10
  ankle M13.17- ☑
  elbow M13.12- ☑
  foot joint M13.17- ☑
  hand joint M13.14- ☑
  hip M13.15- ☑
  knee M13.16- ☑
  shoulder M13.11- ☑
  wrist M13.13- ☑
Monoblastic — see condition
Monochromat (ism), monochromatopsia (acquired) (congenital) H53.51
Monocytic — see condition
Monocytopenia D72.818
Monocytosis (symptomatic) D72.821
Monomania — see Psychosis
Mononeuritis G58.9
  cranial nerve — see Disorder, nerve, cranial
  femoral nerve G57.2- ☑
  lateral
    cutaneous nerve of thigh G57.1- ☑
    popliteal nerve G57.3- ☑
  lower limb G57.9- ☑
    specified nerve NEC G57.8- ☑
  medial popliteal nerve G57.4- ☑
  median nerve G56.1- ☑
  multiplex G58.7
  plantar nerve G57.6- ☑
  posterior tibial nerve G57.5- ☑
  radial nerve G56.3- ☑
  sciatic nerve G57.0- ☑
  specified NEC G58.8
  tibial nerve G57.4- ☑
  ulnar nerve G56.2- ☑
  upper limb G56.9- ☑
    specified nerve NEC G56.8- ☑
  vestibular — see subcategory H93.3 ☑
Mononeuropathy G58.9
  carpal tunnel syndrome — see Syndrome, carpal tunnel
  diabetic NEC — see E08-E13 with .41
  femoral nerve — see Lesion, nerve, femoral
  ilioinguinal nerve G57.8- ☑
  in diseases classified elsewhere — see category G59

☑ Additional Character Required — Refer to the Tabular List for Character Selection   Subterms under main terms may continue to next column or page

Mononeuropathy — *continued*
intercostal G58.0
lower limb G57.9- ☑
causalgia — *see* Causalgia, lower limb
femoral nerve — *see* Lesion, nerve, femoral
meralgia paresthetica G57.1- ☑
plantar nerve — *see* Lesion, nerve, plantar
popliteal nerve — *see* Lesion, nerve, popliteal
sciatic nerve — *see* Lesion, nerve, sciatic
specified NEC G57.8- ☑
tarsal tunnel syndrome — *see* Syndrome, tarsal tunnel
median nerve — *see* Lesion, nerve, median
multiplex G58.7
obturator nerve G57.8- ☑
popliteal nerve — *see* Lesion, nerve, popliteal
radial nerve — *see* Lesion, nerve, radial
saphenous nerve G57.8- ☑
specified NEC G58.8
tarsal tunnel syndrome — *see* Syndrome, tarsal tunnel
tuberculous A17.83
ulnar nerve — *see* Lesion, nerve, ulnar
upper limb G56.9- ☑
carpal tunnel syndrome — *see* Syndrome, carpal tunnel
causalgia — *see* Causalgia
median nerve — *see* Lesion, nerve, median
radial nerve — *see* Lesion, nerve, radial
specified site NEC G56.8- ☑
ulnar nerve — *see* Lesion, nerve, ulnar
Mononucleosis, infectious B27.90
with
complication NEC B27.99
meningitis B27.92
polyneuropathy B27.91
cytomegaloviral B27.10
with
complication NEC B27.19
meningitis B27.12
polyneuropathy B27.11
Epstein-Barr (virus) B27.00
with
complication NEC B27.09
meningitis B27.02
polyneuropathy B27.01
gammaherpesviral B27.00
with
complication NEC B27.09
meningitis B27.02
polyneuropathy B27.01
specified NEC B27.80
with
complication NEC B27.89
meningitis B27.82
polyneuropathy B27.81
Monoplegia G83.3- ☑
congenital (cerebral) G80.8
spastic G80.1
embolic (current episode) I63.4- ☑
following
cerebrovascular disease
cerebral infarction
lower limb I69.34- ☑
upper limb I69.33- ☑
intracerebral hemorrhage
lower limb I69.14- ☑
upper limb I69.13- ☑
lower limb I69.94- ☑
nontraumatic intracranial hemorrhage NEC
lower limb I69.24- ☑
upper limb I69.23- ☑
specified disease NEC
lower limb I69.84- ☑
upper limb I69.83- ☑
stroke NOS
lower limb I69.34- ☑
upper limb I69.33- ☑
subarachnoid hemorrhage
lower limb I69.04- ☑
upper limb I69.03- ☑
upper limb I69.93- ☑
hysterical (transient) F44.4
lower limb G83.1-
psychogenic (conversion reaction) F44.4
thrombotic (current episode) I63.3- ☑
transient R29.818
upper limb G83.2- ☑

Monorchism, monorchidism Q55.0
Monosomy (*see also* Deletion, chromosome) Q93.9
specified NEC Q93.89
whole chromosome
meiotic nondisjunction Q93.0
mitotic nondisjunction Q93.1
mosaicism Q93.1
X Q96.9
Monster, monstrosity (single) Q89.7
acephalic Q00.0
twin Q89.4
Monteggia's fracture (-dislocation) S52.27- ☑
Mooren's ulcer (cornea) — *see* Ulcer, cornea, Mooren's
Moore's syndrome — *see* Epilepsy, specified NEC
Mooser-Neill reaction A75.2
Mooser's bodies A75.2
Morbidity not stated or unknown R69
Morbilli — *see* Measles
Morbus (*see also* Disease)
angelicus, anglorum E55.0
Beigel B36.2
caducus — *see* Epilepsy
celiacus K90.0
comitialis — *see* Epilepsy
cordis (*see also* Disease, heart) I51.9
valvulorum — *see* Endocarditis
coxae senilis M16.9
tuberculous A18.02
hemorrhagicus neonatorum P53
maculosus neonatorum P54.5
Morel (-Stewart)(-Morgagni) **syndrome** M85.2
Morel-Kraepelin disease — *see* Schizophrenia
Morel-Moore syndrome M85.2
Morgagni's
cyst, organ, hydatid, or appendage
female Q50.5
male (epididymal) Q55.4
testicular Q55.29
syndrome M85.2
Morgagni-Stewart-Morel syndrome M85.2
Morgagni-Stokes-Adams syndrome I45.9
Morgagni-Turner (-Albright) **syndrome** Q96.9
Moria F07.0
Moron (I.Q. 50-69) F70
Morphea L94.0
Morphinism (without remission) F11.20
with remission F11.21
Morphinomania (without remission) F11.20
with remission F11.21
Morquio (-Ullrich)(-Brailsford) **disease or syndrome** — *see* Mucopolysaccharidosis
Mortification (dry) (moist) — *see* Gangrene
Morton's metatarsalgia (neuralgia)(neuroma) (syndrome) G57.6- ☑
Morvan's disease or syndrome G60.8
Mosaicism, mosaic (autosomal) (chromosomal)
45,X/46,XX Q96.3
45,X/other cell lines NEC with abnormal sex chromosome Q96.4
sex chromosome
female Q97.8
lines with various numbers of X chromosomes Q97.2
male Q98.7
XY Q96.3
Moschowitz' disease M31.1
Mother yaw A66.0
Motion sickness (from travel, any vehicle) (from roundabouts or swings) T75.3
Mottled, mottling, teeth (enamel) (endemic) (nonendemic) K00.3
Mounier-Kuhn syndrome Q32.4
with bronchiectasis J47.9
exacerbation (acute) J47.1
lower respiratory infection J47.0
acquired J98.09
with bronchiectasis J47.9
with
exacerbation (acute) J47.1
lower respiratory infection J47.0
Mountain
sickness T70.29 ☑
with polycythemia , acquired (acute) D75.1
tick fever A93.2
Mouse, joint — *see* Loose, body, joint
knee M23.4- ☑
Mouth — *see* condition

Movable
coccyx — *see* subcategory M53.2 ☑
kidney N28.89
congenital Q63.8
spleen D73.89
Movements, dystonic R25.8
Moyamoya disease I67.5
MRSA (Methicillin resistant Staphylococcus aureus)
infection A49.02
as the cause of diseases classified elsewhere B95.62
sepsis A41.02
MSSA (Methicillin susceptible Staphylococcus aureus)
infection A49.01
as the cause of diseases classified elsewhere B95.61
sepsis A41.01
Mucha-Habermann disease L41.0
Mucinosis (cutaneous) (focal) (papular) (skin) L98.5
oral K13.79
Mucocele
appendix K38.8
buccal cavity K13.79
gallbladder K82.1
lacrimal sac, chronic H04.43- ☑
nasal sinus J34.1
nose J34.1
salivary gland (any) K11.6
sinus (accessory) (nasal) J34.1
turbinate (bone) (middle) (nasal) J34.1
uterus N85.8
Mucolipidosis
I E77.1
II, III E77.0
IV E75.11
Mucopolysaccharidosis E76.3
beta-gluduronidase deficiency E76.29
cardiopathy E76.3 [I52]
Hunter's syndrome E76.1
Hurler's syndrome E76.01
Hurler-Scheie syndrome E76.02
Maroteaux-Lamy syndrome E76.29
Morquio syndrome E76.219
A E76.210
B E76.211
classic E76.210
Sanfilippo syndrome E76.22
Scheie's syndrome E76.03
specified NEC E76.29
type
I
Hurler's syndrome E76.01
Hurler-Scheie syndrome E76.02
Scheie's syndrome E76.03
II E76.1
III E76.22
IV E76.219
IVA E76.210
IVB E76.211
VI E76.29
VII E76.29
Mucormycosis B46.5
cutaneous B46.3
disseminated B46.4
gastrointestinal B46.2
generalized B46.4
pulmonary B46.0
rhinocerebral B46.1
skin B46.3
subcutaneous B46.3
Mucositis (ulcerative) K12.30
due to drugs NEC K12.32
gastrointestinal K92.81
mouth (oral) (oropharyngeal) K12.30
due to antineoplastic therapy K12.31
due to drugs NEC K12.32
due to radiation K12.33
specified NEC K12.39
viral K12.39
nasal J34.81
oral cavity — *see* Mucositis, mouth
oral soft tissues — *see* Mucositis, mouth
vagina and vulva N76.81
Mucositis necroticans agranulocytica — *see* Agranulocytosis
Mucous (*see also* condition)
patches (syphilitic) A51.39
congenital A50.07
Mucoviscidosis E84.9
with meconium obstruction E84.11

Mucus
- asphyxia or suffocation — see Asphyxia, mucus
- in stool R19.5
- plug — see Asphyxia, mucus

Muguet B37.0
Mulberry molars (congenital syphilis) A50.52
Müllerian mixed tumor
- specified site — see Neoplasm, malignant, by site
- unspecified site C54.9

Multicystic kidney (development) Q61.4
Multiparity (grand) Z64.1
- affecting management of pregnancy, labor and delivery (supervision only) O09.4- ☑
- requiring contraceptive management — see Contraception

Multipartita placenta O43.19- ☑
Multiple, multiplex (see also condition)
- digits (congenital) Q69.9
- endocrine neoplasia — see Neoplasia, endocrine, multiple (MEN)
- personality F44.81

Mumps B26.9
- arthritis B26.85
- complication NEC B26.89
- encephalitis B26.2
- hepatitis B26.81
- meningitis (aseptic) B26.1
- meningoencephalitis B26.2
- myocarditis B26.82
- oophoritis B26.89
- orchitis B26.0
- pancreatitis B26.3
- polyneuropathy B26.84

Mumu (see also Infestation, filarial) B74.9 [N51]
Münchhausen's syndrome — see Disorder, factitious
Münchmeyer's syndrome — see Myositis, ossificans, progressiva
Mural — see condition
Murmur (cardiac) (heart) (organic) R01.1
- abdominal R19.15
- aortic (valve) — see Endocarditis, aortic
- benign R01.0
- diastolic — see Endocarditis
- Flint I35.1
- functional R01.0
- Graham Steell I37.1
- innocent R01.0
- mitral (valve) — see Insufficiency, mitral
- nonorganic R01.0
- presystolic, mitral — see Insufficiency, mitral
- pulmonic (valve) I37.8
- systolic R01.1
- tricuspid (valve) I07.9
- valvular — see Endocarditis

Murri's disease (intermittent hemoglobinuria) D59.6
Muscle, muscular (see also condition)
- carnitine (palmityltransferase) deficiency E71.314

Musculoneuralgia — see Neuralgia
Mushrooming hip — see Derangement, joint, specified NEC, hip
Mushroom-workers' (pickers') **disease or lung** J67.5
Mutation(s)
- factor V Leiden D68.51
- prothrombin gene D68.52
- surfactant, of lung J84.83

Mutism (see also Aphasia)
- deaf (acquired) (congenital) NEC H91.3
- elective (adjustment reaction) (childhood) F94.0
- hysterical F44.4
- selective (childhood) F94.0

MVD (microvillus inclusion disease) Q43.8
MVID (microvillus inclusion disease) Q43.8
Myalgia M79.1
- epidemic (cervical) B33.0
- traumatic NEC T14.8 ☑

Myasthenia G70.9
- congenital G70.2
- cordis — see Failure, heart
- developmental G70.2
- gravis G70.00
  - with exacerbation (acute) G70.01
  - in crisis G70.01
  - neonatal, transient P94.0
  - pseudoparalytica G70.00
    - with exacerbation (acute) G70.01
    - in crisis G70.01
- stomach, psychogenic F45.8

Myasthenia — continued
- syndrome
  - in
    - diabetes mellitus — see E08-E13 with .44
    - neoplastic disease (see also Neoplasm) D49.9 [G73.3]
    - pernicious anemia D51.0 [G73.3]
    - thyrotoxicosis E05.90 [G73.3]
      - with thyroid storm E05.91 [G73.3]

Myasthenic M62.81
Mycelium infection B49
Mycetismus — see Poisoning, food, noxious, mushroom
Mycetoma B47.9
- actinomycotic B47.1
- bone (mycotic) B47.9 [M90.80]
- eumycotic B47.0
- foot B47.9
  - actinomycotic B47.1
  - mycotic B47.0
- madurae NEC B47.9
  - mycotic B47.0
- maduromycotic B47.0
- mycotic B47.0
- nocardial B47.1

Mycobacteriosis — see Mycobacterium
Mycobacterium, mycobacterial (infection) A31.9
- anonymous A31.9
- atypical A31.9
  - cutaneous A31.1
  - pulmonary A31.0
    - tuberculous — see Tuberculosis, pulmonary
  - specified site NEC A31.8
- avium (intracellulare complex) A31.0
- balnei A31.1
- Battey A31.0
- chelonei A31.8
- cutaneous A31.1
- extrapulmonary systemic A31.8
- fortuitum A31.8
- intracellulare (Battey bacillus) A31.0
- kakaferifu A31.8
- kansasii (yellow bacillus) A31.0
- kasongo A31.8
- leprae (see also Leprosy) A30.9
- luciflavum A31.1
- marinum (M. balnei) A31.1
- nonspecific — see Mycobacterium, atypical
- pulmonary (atypical) A31.0
  - tuberculous — see Tuberculosis, pulmonary
- scrofulaceum A31.8
- simiae A31.8
- systemic, extrapulmonary A31.8
- szulgai A31.8
- terrae A31.8
- triviale A31.8
- tuberculosis (human, bovine) — see Tuberculosis
- ulcerans A31.1
- xenopi A31.8

Mycoplasma (M.) **pneumoniae, as cause of disease classified elsewhere** B96.0
Mycosis, mycotic B49
- cutaneous NEC B36.9
- ear B36.9
  - in
    - aspergillosis B44.89
    - candidiasis B37.84
    - moniliasis B37.84
- fungoides (extranodal) (solid organ) C84.0- ☑
- mouth B37.0
- nails B35.1
- opportunistic B48.8
- skin NEC B36.9
- specified NEC B48.8
- stomatitis B37.0
- vagina, vaginitis (candidal) B37.3

Mydriasis (pupil) H57.04
Myelatelia Q06.1
Myelinolysis, pontine, central G37.2
Myelitis (acute) (ascending) (childhood) (chronic) (descending) (diffuse) (disseminated) (idiopathic) (pressure) (progressive) (spinal cord) (subacute) (see also Encephalitis) G04.91
- herpes simplex B00.82
- herpes zoster B02.24
- in diseases classified elsewhere G05.4
- necrotizing, subacute G37.4
- optic neuritis in G36.0
- postchickenpox B01.12

Myelitis — continued
- postherpetic B02.24
- postimmunization G04.02
- postinfectious NEC G04.89
- postvaccinal G04.02
- specified NEC G04.89
- syphilitic (transverse) A52.14
- toxic G92
- transverse (in demyelinating diseases of central nervous system) G37.3
- tuberculous A17.82
- varicella B01.12

Myeloblastic — see condition
Myeloblastoma
- granular cell (see also Neoplasm, connective tissue)
  - malignant — see Neoplasm, connective tissue, malignant
  - tongue D10.1

Myelocele — see Spina bifida
Myelocystocele — see Spina bifida
Myelocytic — see condition
Myelodysplasia D46.9
- specified NEC D46.Z (following D46.4)
- spinal cord (congenital) Q06.1

Myelodysplastic syndrome D46.9
- with
  - 5q deletion D46.C (following D46.2)
  - isolated del (5q) chromosomal abnormality D46.C (following D46.2)
- specified NEC D46.Z (following D46.4)

Myeloencephalitis — see Encephalitis
Myelofibrosis D75.81
- with myeloid metaplasia D47.4
- acute C94.4- ☑
- idiopathic (chronic) D47.4
- primary D47.1
- secondary D75.81
  - in myeloproliferative disease D47.4

Myelogenous — see condition
Myeloid — see condition
Myelokathexis D70.9
Myeloleukodystrophy E75.29
Myelolipoma — see Lipoma
Myeloma (multiple) C90.0- ☑
- monostotic C90.3 ☑
  - plasma cell C90.0- ☑
- plasma cell C90.0- ☑
- solitary (see also Plasmacytoma, solitary) C90.3- ☑

Myelomalacia G95.89
Myelomatosis C90.0- ☑
Myelomeningitis — see Meningoencephalitis
Myelomeningocele (spinal cord) — see Spina bifida
Myelo-osteo-musculodysplasia hereditaria Q79.8
Myelopathic
- anemia D64.89
- muscle atrophy — see Atrophy, muscle, spinal
- pain syndrome G89.0

Myelopathy (spinal cord) G95.9
- drug-induced G95.89
- in (due to)
  - degeneration or displacement, intervertebral disc NEC — see Disorder, disc, with, myelopathy
  - infection — see Encephalitis
  - intervertebral disc disorder (see also Disorder, disc, with, myelopathy)
  - mercury — see subcategory T56.1 ☑
  - neoplastic disease (see also Neoplasm) D49.9 [G99.2]
  - pernicious anemia D51.0 [G99.2]
  - spondylosis — see Spondylosis, with myelopathy NEC
- necrotic (subacute) (vascular) G95.19
- radiation-induced G95.89
- spondylogenic NEC — see Spondylosis, with myelopathy NEC
- toxic G95.89
- transverse, acute G37.3
- vascular G95.19
- vitamin B12 E53.8 [G32.0]

Myelophthisis D61.82
Myeloradiculitis G04.91
Myeloradiculodysplasia (spinal) Q06.1
Myelosarcoma C92.3- ☑
Myelosclerosis D75.89
- with myeloid metaplasia D47.4
- disseminated, of nervous system G35
- megakaryocytic D47.4

Myelosclerosis — *continued*
  megakaryocytic — *continued*
    with myeloid metaplasia D47.4
Myelosis
  acute C92.0- ☑
  aleukemic C92.9- ☑
  chronic D47.1
  erythremic (acute) C94.0- ☑
  megakaryocytic C94.2- ☑
  nonleukemic D72.828
  subacute C92.9- ☑
Myiasis (cavernous) B87.9
  aural B87.4
  creeping B87.0
  cutaneous B87.0
  dermal B87.0
  ear (external) (middle) B87.4
  eye B87.2
  genitourinary B87.81
  intestinal B87.82
  laryngeal B87.3
  nasopharyngeal B87.3
  ocular B87.2
  orbit B87.2
  skin B87.0
  specified site NEC B87.89
  traumatic B87.1
  wound B87.1
Myoadenoma, prostate — *see* Hyperplasia, prostate
Myoblastoma
  granular cell (*see also* Neoplasm, connective tissue, benign)
    malignant — *see* Neoplasm, connective tissue, malignant
  tongue D10.1
Myocardial — *see* condition
Myocardiopathy (congestive) (constrictive) (familial) (hypertrophic nonobstructive) (idiopathic) (infiltrative) (obstructive) (primary) (restrictive) (sporadic) (*see also* Cardiomyopathy) I42.9
  alcoholic I42.6
  cobalt-beer I42.6
  glycogen storage E74.02 [I43]
  hypertrophic obstructive I42.1
  in (due to)
    beriberi E51.12
    cardiac glycogenosis E74.02 [I43]
    Friedreich's ataxia G11.1 [I43]
    myotonia atrophica G71.11 [I43]
    progressive muscular dystrophy G71.0 [I43]
  obscure (African) I42.8
  secondary I42.9
  thyrotoxic E05.90 [I43]
    with storm E05.91 [I43]
  toxic NEC I42.7
Myocarditis (with arteriosclerosis)(chronic)(fibroid) (interstitial) (old) (progressive) (senile) I51.4
  with
    rheumatic fever (conditions in I00) I09.0
      active — *see* Myocarditis, acute, rheumatic
      inactive or quiescent (with chorea) I09.0
  active I40.9
    rheumatic I01.2
      with chorea (acute) (rheumatic) (Sydenham's) I02.0
  acute or subacute (interstitial) I40.9
    due to
      streptococcus (beta-hemolytic) I01.2
    idiopathic I40.1
    rheumatic I01.2
      with chorea (acute) (rheumatic) (Sydenham's) I02.0
    specified NEC I40.8
  aseptic of newborn B33.22
  bacterial (acute) I40.0
  Coxsackie (virus) B33.22
  diphtheritic A36.81
  eosinophilic I40.1
  epidemic of newborn (Coxsackie) B33.22
  Fiedler's (acute) (isolated) I40.1
  giant cell (acute) (subacute) I40.1
  gonococcal A54.83
  granulomatous (idiopathic) (isolated) (nonspecific) I40.1
  hypertensive — *see* Hypertension, heart
  idiopathic (granulomatous) I40.1
  in (due to)
    diphtheria A36.81

Myocarditis — *continued*
  in — *continued*
    epidemic louse-borne typhus A75.0 [I41]
    Lyme disease A69.29
    sarcoidosis D86.85
    scarlet fever A38.1
    toxoplasmosis (acquired) B58.81
    typhoid A01.02
    typhus NEC A75.9 [I41]
  infective I40.0
  influenzal — *see* Influenza, with, myocarditis
  isolated (acute) I40.1
  meningococcal A39.52
  mumps B26.82
  nonrheumatic, active I40.9
  parenchymatous I40.9
  pneumococcal I40.0
  rheumatic (chronic) (inactive) (with chorea) I09.0
    active or acute I01.2
      with chorea (acute) (rheumatic) (Sydenham's) I02.0
  rheumatoid — *see* Rheumatoid, carditis
  septic I40.0
  staphylococcal I40.0
  suppurative I40.0
  syphilitic (chronic) A52.06
  toxic I40.8
    rheumatic — *see* Myocarditis, acute, rheumatic
  tuberculous A18.84
  typhoid A01.02
  valvular — *see* Endocarditis
  virus, viral I40.0
    of newborn (Coxsackie) B33.22
Myocardium, myocardial — *see* condition
Myocardosis — *see* Cardiomyopathy
Myoclonus, myoclonic, myoclonia (familial) (essential) (multifocal) (simplex) G25.3
  drug-induced G25.3
  epilepsy (*see also* Epilepsy, generalized, specified NEC) G40.4- ☑
    familial (progressive) G25.3
  epileptica G40.409
    with status epilepticus G40.401
  facial G51.3
  familial progressive G25.3
  Friedreich's G25.3
  jerks G25.3
  massive G25.3
  palatal G25.3
  pharyngeal G25.3
Myocytolysis I51.5
Myodiastasis — *see* Diastasis, muscle
Myoendocarditis — *see* Endocarditis
Myoepithelioma — *see* Neoplasm, benign, by site
Myofasciitis (acute) — *see* Myositis
Myofibroma (*see also* Neoplasm, connective tissue, benign)
  uterus (cervix) (corpus) — *see* Leiomyoma
Myofibromatosis D48.1
  infantile Q89.8
Myofibrosis M62.89
  heart — *see* Myocarditis
  scapulohumeral — *see* Lesion, shoulder, specified NEC
Myofibrositis M79.7
  scapulohumeral — *see* Lesion, shoulder, specified NEC
Myoglobulinuria, myoglobinuria (primary) R82.1
Myokymia, facial G51.4
Myolipoma — *see* Lipoma
Myoma (*see also* Neoplasm, connective tissue, benign)
  malignant — *see* Neoplasm, connective tissue, malignant
  prostate D29.1
  uterus (cervix) (corpus) — *see* Leiomyoma
Myomalacia M62.89
Myometritis — *see* Endometritis
Myometrium — *see* condition
Myonecrosis, clostridial A48.0
Myopathy G72.9
  acute
    necrotizing G72.81
    quadriplegic G72.81
  alcoholic G72.1
  benign congenital G71.2
  central core G71.2
  centronuclear G71.2
  congenital (benign) G71.2
  critical illness G72.81
  distal G71.0

Myopathy — *continued*
  drug-induced G72.0
  endocrine NEC E34.9 [G73.7]
  extraocular muscles H05.82- ☑
  facioscapulohumeral G71.0
  hereditary G71.9
    specified NEC G71.8
  immune NEC G72.49
  in (due to)
    Addison's disease E27.1 [G73.7]
    alcohol G72.1
    amyloidosis E85.0 [G73.7]
    cretinism E00.9 [G73.7]
    Cushing's syndrome E24.9 [G73.7]
    drugs G72.0
    endocrine disease NEC E34.9 [G73.7]
    giant cell arteritis M31.6 [G73.7]
    glycogen storage disease E74.00 [G73.7]
    hyperadrenocorticism E24.9 [G73.7]
    hyperparathyroidism NEC E21.3 [G73.7]
    hypoparathyroidism E20.9 [G73.7]
    hypopituitarism E23.0 [G73.7]
    hypothyroidism E03.9 [G73.7]
    infectious disease NEC B99 ☑ [G73.7]
    lipid storage disease E75.6 [G73.7]
    metabolic disease NEC E88.9 [G73.7]
    myxedema E03.9 [G73.7]
    parasitic disease NEC B89 [G73.7]
    polyarteritis nodosa M30.0 [G73.7]
    rheumatoid arthritis — *see* Rheumatoid, myopathy
    sarcoidosis D86.87
    scleroderma M34.82
    sicca syndrome M35.03
    Sjögren's syndrome M35.03
    systemic lupus erythematosus M32.19
    thyrotoxicosis (hyperthyroidism) E05.90 [G73.7]
      with thyroid storm E05.91 [G73.7]
    toxic agent NEC G72.2
  inflammatory NEC G72.49
  intensive care (ICU) G72.81
  limb-girdle G71.0
  mitochondrial NEC G71.3
  myotubular G71.2
  mytonic, proximal (PROMM) G71.11
  nemaline G71.2
  ocular G71.0
  oculopharyngeal G71.0
  of critical illness G72.81
  primary G71.9
    specified NEC G71.8
  progressive NEC G72.89
  proximal myotonic (PROMM) G71.11
  rod G71.2
  scapulohumeral G71.0
  specified NEC G72.89
  toxic G72.2
Myopericarditis (*see also* Pericarditis)
  chronic rheumatic I09.2
Myopia (axial) (congenital) H52.1- ☑
  degenerative (malignant) H44.20
    with
      choroidal neovascularization H44.2A- ☑
      foveoschisis H44.2D- ☑
      macular hole H44.2B- ☑
      retinal detachment H44.2C- ☑
      specified maculopathy NEC H44.2E- ☑
    bilateral H44.23
    left eye H44.22
    right eye H44.21
  malignant (*see also* Myopia, degenerative) H44.2- ☑
  pernicious (*see also* Myopia, degenerative) H44.2- ☑
  progressive high (degenerative) (*see also* Myopia, degenerative) H44.2- ☑
Myosarcoma — *see* Neoplasm, connective tissue, malignant
Myosis (pupil) H57.03
  stromal (endolymphatic) D39.0
Myositis M60.9
  clostridial A48.0
  due to posture — *see* Myositis, specified type NEC
  epidemic B33.0
  fibrosa or fibrous (chronic), Volkmann's T79.6 ☑
  foreign body granuloma — *see* Granuloma, foreign body
  in (due to)
    bilharziasis B65.9 [M63.8-] ☑
    cysticercosis B69.81
    leprosy A30.9 [M63.8-] ☑

▼ Subterms under main terms may continue to next column or page   ☑ Additional Character Required — Refer to the Tabular List for Character Selection   **227**

Myelosclerosis — Myositis

Myositis — *continued*
  in — *continued*
    mycosis B49 [M63.8-] ☑
    sarcoidosis D86.87
    schistosomiasis B65.9 [M63.8-] ☑
    syphilis
      late A52.78
      secondary A51.49
    toxoplasmosis (acquired) B58.82
    trichinellosis B75 [M63.8-] ☑
    tuberculosis A18.09
  inclusion body [IBM] G72.41
  infective M60.009
    arm M60.002
      left M60.001
      right M60.000
    leg M60.005
      left M60.004
      right M60.003
    lower limb M60.005
      ankle M60.07- ☑
      foot M60.07- ☑
      lower leg M60.06- ☑
      thigh M60.05- ☑
      toe M60.07- ☑
    multiple sites M60.09
    specified site NEC M60.08
    upper limb M60.002
      finger M60.04- ☑
      forearm M60.03- ☑
      hand M60.04- ☑
      shoulder region M60.01- ☑
      upper arm M60.02- ☑
  interstitial M60.10
    ankle M60.17- ☑
    foot M60.17- ☑
    forearm M60.13- ☑
    hand M60.14- ☑
    lower leg M60.16- ☑
    multiple sites M60.19
    shoulder region M60.11- ☑
    specified site NEC M60.18
    thigh M60.15- ☑
    upper arm M60.12- ☑
  mycotic B49 [M63.8-] ☑
  orbital, chronic H05.12- ☑
  ossificans or ossifying (circumscripta) (*see also* Ossifi-
    cation, muscle, specified NEC)
    in (due to)
      burns M61.30
        ankle M61.37- ☑
        foot M61.37- ☑
        forearm M61.33- ☑
        hand M61.34- ☑
        lower leg M61.36- ☑
        multiple sites M61.39
        pelvic region M61.35- ☑

Myositis — *continued*
  ossificans or ossifying (*see also* Ossification, muscle,
    specified) — *continued*
    in — *continued*
      burns — *continued*
        shoulder region M61.31- ☑
        specified site NEC M61.38
        thigh M61.35- ☑
        upper arm M61.32- ☑
      quadriplegia or paraplegia M61.20
        ankle M61.27- ☑
        foot M61.27- ☑
        forearm M61.23- ☑
        hand M61.24- ☑
        lower leg M61.26- ☑
        multiple sites M61.29
        pelvic region M61.25- ☑
        shoulder region M61.21- ☑
        specified site NEC M61.28
        thigh M61.25- ☑
        upper arm M61.22- ☑
    progressiva M61.10
      ankle M61.17- ☑
      finger M61.14- ☑
      foot M61.17- ☑
      forearm M61.13- ☑
      hand M61.14- ☑
      lower leg M61.16- ☑
      multiple sites M61.19
      pelvic region M61.15- ☑
      shoulder region M61.11- ☑
      specified site NEC M61.18
      thigh M61.15- ☑
      toe M61.17- ☑
      upper arm M61.12- ☑
    traumatica M61.00
      ankle M61.07- ☑
      foot M61.07- ☑
      forearm M61.03- ☑
      hand M61.04- ☑
      lower leg M61.06- ☑
      multiple sites M61.09
      pelvic region M61.05- ☑
      shoulder region M61.01- ☑
      specified site NEC M61.08
      thigh M61.05- ☑
      upper arm M61.02- ☑
  purulent — *see* Myositis, infective
  specified type NEC M60.80
    ankle M60.87- ☑
    foot M60.87- ☑
    forearm M60.83- ☑
    hand M60.84- ☑
    lower leg M60.86- ☑
    multiple sites M60.89
    pelvic region M60.85- ☑
    shoulder region M60.81- ☑

Myositis — *continued*
  specified type — *continued*
    specified site NEC M60.88
    thigh M60.85- ☑
    upper arm M60.82- ☑
  suppurative — *see* Myositis, infective
  traumatic (old) — *see* Myositis, specified type NEC
Myospasia impulsiva F95.2
Myotonia (acquisita) (intermittens) M62.89
  atrophica G71.11
  chondrodystrophic G71.13
  congenita (acetazolamide responsive) (dominant)
    (recessive) G71.12
  drug-induced G71.14
  dystrophica G71.11
  fluctuans G71.19
  levior G71.12
  permanens G71.19
  symptomatic G71.19
Myotonic pupil — *see* Anomaly, pupil, function, tonic
  pupil
Myriapodiasis B88.2
Myringitis H73.2- ☑
  with otitis media — *see* Otitis, media
  acute H73.00- ☑
    bullous H73.01- ☑
    specified NEC H73.09- ☑
  bullous — *see* Myringitis, acute, bullous
  chronic H73.1- ☑
Mysophobia F40.228
Mytilotoxism — *see* Poisoning, fish
Myxadenitis labialis K13.0
Myxedema (adult) (idiocy) (infantile) (juvenile) (*see also*
  Hypothyroidism) E03.9
  circumscribed E05.90
    with storm E05.91
  coma E03.5
  congenital E00.1
  cutis L98.5
  localized (pretibial) E05.90
    with storm E05.91
  papular L98.5
Myxochondrosarcoma — *see* Neoplasm, cartilage,
  malignant
Myxofibroma — *see* Neoplasm, connective tissue, benign
  odontogenic — *see* Cyst, calcifying odontogenic
Myxofibrosarcoma — *see* Neoplasm, connective tissue,
  malignant
Myxolipoma D17.9
Myxoliposarcoma — *see* Neoplasm, connective tissue,
  malignant
Myxoma (*see also* Neoplasm, connective tissue, benign)
  nerve sheath — *see* Neoplasm, nerve, benign
  odontogenic — *see* Cyst, calcifying odontogenic
Myxosarcoma — *see* Neoplasm, connective tissue, malignant

228
☑ **Additional Character Required — Refer to the Tabular List for Character Selection**
⬝ **Subterms under main terms may continue to next column or page**

Myositis — Myxosarcoma

N

Naegeli's
  disease Q82.8
  leukemia, monocytic C93.1- ☑
Naegleriasis (with meningoencephalitis) B60.2
Naffziger's syndrome G54.0
Naga sore — *see* Ulcer, skin
Nägele's pelvis M95.5
  with disproportion (fetopelvic) O33.0
    causing obstructed labor O65.0
Nail (*see also* condition)
  biting F98.8
  patella syndrome Q87.2
Nanism, nanosomia — *see* Dwarfism
Nanophyetiasis B66.8
Nanukayami A27.89
Napkin rash L22
Narcolepsy G47.419
  with cataplexy G47.411
  in conditions classified elsewhere G47.429
    with cataplexy G47.421
Narcosis R06.89
Narcotism — *see* Dependence
NARP (Neuropathy, Ataxia and Retinitis pigmentosa)
  syndrome E88.49
Narrow
  anterior chamber angle H40.03- ☑
  gingival width (of periodontal soft tissue) K05.5
  pelvis — *see* Contraction, pelvis
Narrowing (*see also* Stenosis)
  artery I77.1
    auditory, internal I65.8
    basilar — *see* Occlusion, artery, basilar
    carotid — *see* Occlusion, artery, carotid
    cerebellar — *see* Occlusion, artery, cerebellar
    cerebral — *see* Occlusion artery, cerebral
    choroidal — *see* Occlusion, artery, cerebral, specified NEC
    communicating posterior — *see* Occlusion, artery, cerebral, specified NEC
    coronary (*see also* Disease, heart, ischemic, atherosclerotic)
      congenital Q24.5
      syphilitic A50.54 [I52]
      due to syphilis NEC A52.06
    hypophyseal — *see* Occlusion, artery, cerebral, specified NEC
    pontine — *see* Occlusion, artery, cerebral, specified NEC
    precerebral — *see* Occlusion, artery, precerebral
    vertebral — *see* Occlusion, artery, vertebral
  auditory canal (external) — *see* Stenosis, external ear canal
  eustachian tube — *see* Obstruction, eustachian tube
  eyelid — *see* Disorder, eyelid function
  larynx J38.6
  mesenteric artery (*see also* Ischemia, intestine, acute) K55.059
  palate M26.89
  palpebral fissure — *see* Disorder, eyelid function
  ureter N13.5
    with infection N13.6
  urethra — *see* Stricture, urethra
Narrowness, abnormal, eyelid Q10.3
Nasal — *see* condition
Nasolachrymal, nasolacrimal — *see* condition
Nasopharyngeal (*see also* condition)
  pituitary gland Q89.2
  torticollis M43.6
Nasopharyngitis (acute) (infective) (streptococcal) (subacute) J00
  chronic (suppurative) (ulcerative) J31.1
Nasopharynx, nasopharyngeal — *see* condition
Natal tooth, teeth K00.6
Nausea (without vomiting) R11.0
  with vomiting R11.2
  gravidarum — *see* Hyperemesis, gravidarum
  marina T75.3 ☑
  navalis T75.3 ☑
Navel — *see* condition
Neapolitan fever — *see* Brucellosis
Near drowning T75.1 ☑
Nearsightedness — *see* Myopia
Near-syncope R55
Nebula, cornea — *see* Opacity, cornea

Necator americanus infestation B76.1
Necatoriasis B76.1
Neck — *see* condition
Necrobiosis R68.89
  lipoidica NEC L92.1
    with diabetes — *see* E08-E13 with .620
Necrolysis, toxic epidermal L51.2
  due to drug
    correct substance properly administered — *see* Table of Drugs and Chemicals, by drug, adverse effect
    overdose or wrong substance given or taken — *see* Table of Drugs and Chemicals, by drug, poisoning
Necrophilia F65.89
Necrosis, necrotic (ischemic) (*see also* Gangrene)
  adrenal (capsule) (gland) E27.49
  amputation stump (surgical) (late) T87.50
    arm T87.5- ☑
    leg T87.5- ☑
  antrum J32.0
  aorta (hyaline) (*see also* Aneurysm, aorta)
    cystic medial — *see* Dissection, aorta
  artery I77.5
  bladder (aseptic) (sphincter) N32.89
  bone (*see also* Osteonecrosis) M87.9
    aseptic or avascular — *see* Osteonecrosis
      idiopathic M87.00
    ethmoid J32.2
    jaw M27.2
    tuberculous — *see* Tuberculosis, bone
  brain I67.89
  breast (aseptic) (fat) (segmental) N64.1
  bronchus J98.09
  central nervous system NEC I67.89
  cerebellar I67.89
  cerebral I67.89
  colon (*see also* Infarct, intestine) K55.049
  cornea H18.89- ☑
  cortical (acute) (renal) N17.1
  cystic medial (aorta) — *see* Dissection, aorta
  dental pulp K04.1
  esophagus K22.8
  ethmoid (bone) J32.2
  eyelid — *see* Disorder, eyelid, degenerative
  fat, fatty (generalized) (*see also* Disorder, soft tissue, specified type NEC)
    abdominal wall K65.4
    breast (aseptic) (segmental) N64.1
    localized — *see* Degeneration, by site, fatty
    mesentery K65.4
    omentum K65.4
    pancreas K86.89
    peritoneum K65.4
    skin (subcutaneous), newborn P83.0
    subcutaneous, due to birth injury P15.6
  gallbladder — *see* Cholecystitis, acute
  heart — *see* Infarct, myocardium
  hip, aseptic or avascular — *see* Osteonecrosis, by type, femur
  intestine (acute) (hemorrhagic) (massive) (*see also* Infarct, intestine) K55.069
  jaw M27.2
  kidney (bilateral) N28.0
    acute N17.9
    cortical (acute) (bilateral) N17.1
      with ectopic or molar pregnancy O08.4
    medullary (bilateral) (in acute renal failure) (papillary) N17.2
    papillary (bilateral) (in acute renal failure) N17.2
    tubular N17.0
      with ectopic or molar pregnancy O08.4
      complicating
        abortion — *see* Abortion, by type, complicated by, tubular necrosis
        ectopic or molar pregnancy O08.4
        pregnancy — *see* Pregnancy, complicated by, diseases of, specified type or system NEC
      following ectopic or molar pregnancy O08.4
      traumatic T79.5 ☑
  larynx J38.7
  liver (with hepatic failure) (cell) — *see* Failure, hepatic
    hemorrhagic, central K76.2
  lung J85.0
  lymphatic gland — *see* Lymphadenitis, acute
  mammary gland (fat) (segmental) N64.1
  mastoid (chronic) — *see* Mastoiditis, chronic

Necrosis, necrotic — *continued*
  medullary (acute) (renal) N17.2
  mesentery (*see also* Infarct, intestine) K55.069
    fat K65.4
  mitral valve — *see* Insufficiency, mitral
  myocardium, myocardial — *see* Infarct, myocardium
  nose J34.0
  omentum (with mesenteric infarction) (*see also* Infarct, intestine) K55.069
    fat K65.4
  orbit, orbital — *see* Osteomyelitis, orbit
  ossicles, ear — *see* Abnormal, ear ossicles
  ovary N70.92
  pancreas (aseptic) (duct) (fat) K86.89
    acute (infective) — *see* Pancreatitis, acute
    infective — *see* Pancreatitis, acute
  papillary (acute) (renal) N17.2
  perineum N90.89
  peritoneum (with mesenteric infarction) (*see also* Infarct, intestine) K55.069
    fat K65.4
  pharynx J02.9
    in granulocytopenia — *see* Neutropenia
    Vincent's A69.1
  phosphorus — *see* subcategory T54.2 ☑
  pituitary (gland) E23.0
    postpartum O99.285
    Sheehan O99.285
  pressure — *see* Ulcer, pressure, by site
  pulmonary J85.0
  pulp (dental) K04.1
  radiation — *see* Necrosis, by site
  radium — *see* Necrosis, by site
  renal — *see* Necrosis, kidney
  sclera H15.89
  scrotum N50.89
  skin or subcutaneous tissue NEC I96
  spine, spinal (column) (*see also* Osteonecrosis, by type, vertebra)
    cord G95.19
  spleen D73.5
  stomach K31.89
  stomatitis (ulcerative) A69.0
  subcutaneous fat, newborn P83.88
  subendocardial (acute) I21.4
    chronic I25.89
  suprarenal (capsule) (gland) E27.49
  testis N50.89
  thymus (gland) E32.8
  tonsil J35.8
  trachea J39.8
  tuberculous NEC — *see* Tuberculosis
  tubular (acute) (anoxic) (renal) (toxic) N17.0
    postprocedural N99.0
  vagina N89.8
  vertebra (*see also* Osteonecrosis, by type, vertebra)
    tuberculous A18.01
  vulva N90.89
  X-ray — *see* Necrosis, by site
Necrospermia — *see* Infertility, male
Need (for)
  care provider because of (of)
    assistance with personal care Z74.1
    continuous supervision required Z74.3
    impaired mobility Z74.09
    no other household member able to render care Z74.2
    specified reason NEC Z74.8
  immunization — *see* Vaccination
  vaccination — *see* Vaccination
Neglect
  adult
    confirmed T74.01 ☑
    history of Z91.412
    suspected T76.01 ☑
  child (childhood)
    confirmed T74.02 ☑
    history of Z62.812
    suspected T76.02 ☑
  emotional, in childhood Z62.898
  hemispatial R41.4
  left-sided R41.4
  sensory R41.4
  visuospatial R41.4
Neisserian infection NEC — *see* Gonococcus
Nelaton's syndrome G60.8
Nelson's syndrome E24.1
Nematodiasis (intestinal) B82.0

Nematodiasis — *continued*
Ancylostoma B76.0
Neonatal (*see also* Newborn)
acne L70.4
bradycardia P29.12
screening, abnormal findings on P09
tachycardia P29.11
tooth, teeth K00.6
Neonatorum — *see* condition
Neoplasia
endocrine, multiple (MEN) E31.20
type I E31.21
type IIA E31.22
type IIB E31.23
intraepithelial (histologically confirmed)
anal (AIN) (histologically confirmed) K62.82
grade I K62.82
grade II K62.82
severe D01.3
cervical glandular (histologically confirmed) D06.9
cervix (uteri) (CIN) (histologically confirmed) N87.9
glandular D06.9
grade I N87.0
grade II N87.1
grade III (severe dysplasia) (*see also* Carcinoma, cervix uteri, in situ) D06.9
prostate (histologically confirmed) (PIN) N42.31
grade I N42.31
grade II N42.31
grade III (severe dysplasia) D07.5
vagina (histologically confirmed) (VAIN) N89.3
grade I N89.0
grade II N89.1
grade III (severe dysplasia) D07.2
vulva (histologically confirmed) (VIN) N90.3
grade I N90.0
grade II N90.1
grade III (severe dysplasia) D07.1
Neoplasm, neoplastic (*see also* Table of Neoplasms)
lipomatous, benign — *see* Lipoma
malignant mast cell C96.20
specified type NEC C96.29
mast cell, of uncertain behavior NEC D47.09
Neovascularization
ciliary body — *see* Disorder, iris, vascular
cornea H16.40- ☑
deep H16.44- ☑
ghost vessels — *see* Ghost, vessels
localized H16.43- ☑
pannus — *see* Pannus
iris — *see* Disorder, iris, vascular
retina H35.05- ☑
Nephralgia N23
Nephritis, nephritic (albuminuric) (azotemic) (congenital) (disseminated) (epithelial) (familial) (focal) (granulomatous) (hemorrhagic) (infantile) (nonsuppurative, excretory) (uremic) N05.9
with
dense deposit disease N05.6
diffuse
crescentic glomerulonephritis N05.7
endocapillary proliferative glomerulonephritis N05.4
membranous glomerulonephritis N05.2
mesangial proliferative glomerulonephritis N05.3
mesangiocapillary glomerulonephritis N05.5
edema — *see* Nephrosis
focal and segmental glomerular lesions N05.1
foot process disease N04.9
glomerular lesion
diffuse sclerosing N05.8
hypocomplementemic — *see* Nephritis, membranoproliferative
IgA — *see* Nephropathy, IgA
lobular, lobulonodular — *see* Nephritis, membranoproliferative
nodular — *see* Nephritis, membranoproliferative
lesion of
glomerulonephritis, proliferative N05.8
renal necrosis N05.9
minor glomerular abnormality N05.0
specified morphological changes NEC N05.8
acute N00.9
with
dense deposit disease N00.6

Nephritis, nephritic — *continued*
acute — *continued*
with — *continued*
diffuse
crescentic glomerulonephritis N00.7
endocapillary proliferative glomerulonephritis N00.4
membranous glomerulonephritis N00.2
mesangial proliferative glomerulonephritis N00.3
mesangiocapillary glomerulonephritis N00.5
focal and segmental glomerular lesions N00.1
minor glomerular abnormality N00.0
specified morphological changes NEC N00.8
amyloid E85.4 [N08]
antiglomerular basement membrane (anti-GBM) antibody NEC
in Goodpasture's syndrome M31.0
antitubular basement membrane (tubulo-interstitial) NEC N12
toxic — *see* Nephropathy, toxic
arteriolar — *see* Hypertension, kidney
arteriosclerotic — *see* Hypertension, kidney
ascending — *see* Nephritis, tubulo-interstitial
atrophic N03.9
Balkan (endemic) N15.0
calculous, calculus — *see* Calculus, kidney
cardiac — *see* Hypertension, kidney
cardiovascular — *see* Hypertension, kidney
chronic N03.9
with
dense deposit disease N03.6
diffuse
crescentic glomerulonephritis N03.7
endocapillary proliferative glomerulonephritis N03.4
membranous glomerulonephritis N03.2
mesangial proliferative glomerulonephritis N03.3
mesangiocapillary glomerulonephritis N03.5
focal and segmental glomerular lesions N03.1
minor glomerular abnormality N03.0
specified morphological changes NEC N03.8
arteriosclerotic — *see* Hypertension, kidney
cirrhotic N26.9
complicating pregnancy O26.83- ☑
croupous N00.9
degenerative — *see* Nephrosis
diffuse sclerosing N05.8
due to
diabetes mellitus — *see* E08-E13 with .21
subacute bacterial endocarditis I33.0
systemic lupus erythematosus (chronic) M32.14
typhoid fever A01.09
gonococcal (acute) (chronic) A54.21
hypocomplementemic — *see* Nephritis, membranoproliferative
IgA — *see* Nephropathy, IgA
immune complex (circulating) NEC N05.8
infective — *see* Nephritis, tubulo-interstitial
interstitial — *see* Nephritis, tubulo-interstitial
lead N14.3
membranoproliferative (diffuse) (type 1 or 3) (*see also* N00-N07 with fourth character .5) N05.5
type 2 (*see also* N00-N07 with fourth character .6) N05.6
minimal change N05.0
necrotic, necrotizing NEC (*see also* N00-N07 with fourth character .8) N05.8
nephrotic — *see* Nephrosis
nodular — *see* Nephritis, membranoproliferative
polycystic Q61.3
adult type Q61.2
autosomal
dominant Q61.2
recessive NEC Q61.19
childhood type NEC Q61.19
infantile type NEC Q61.19
poststreptococcal N05.9
acute N00.0
chronic N03.9
rapidly progressive N01.9
proliferative NEC (*see also* N00-N07 with fourth character .8) N05.8
purulent — *see* Nephritis, tubulo-interstitial
rapidly progressive N01.9
with
dense deposit disease N01.6

Nephritis, nephritic — *continued*
rapidly progressive — *continued*
with — *continued*
diffuse
crescentic glomerulonephritis N01.7
endocapillary proliferative glomerulonephritis N01.4
membranous glomerulonephritis N01.2
mesangial proliferative glomerulonephritis N01.3
mesangiocapillary glomerulonephritis N01.5
focal and segmental glomerular lesions N01.1
minor glomerular abnormality N01.0
specified morphological changes NEC N01.8
salt losing or wasting NEC N28.89
saturnine N14.3
sclerosing, diffuse N05.8
septic — *see* Nephritis, tubulo-interstitial
specified pathology NEC (*see also* N00-N07 with fourth character .8) N05.8
subacute N01.9
suppurative — *see* Nephritis, tubulo-interstitial
syphilitic (late) A52.75
congenital A50.59 [N08]
early (secondary) A51.44
toxic — *see* Nephropathy, toxic
tubal, tubular — *see* Nephritis, tubulo-interstitial
tuberculous A18.11
tubulo-interstitial (in) N12
acute (infectious) N10
chronic (infectious) N11.9
nonobstructive N11.8
reflux-associated N11.0
obstructive N11.1
specified NEC N11.8
due to
brucellosis A23.9 [N16]
cryoglobulinemia D89.1 [N16]
glycogen storage disease E74.00 [N16]
Sjögren's syndrome M35.04
vascular — *see* Hypertension, kidney
war N00.9
Nephroblastoma (epithelial) (mesenchymal) C64- ☑
Nephrocalcinosis E83.59 [N29]
Nephrocystitis, pustular — *see* Nephritis, tubulo-interstitial
Nephrolithiasis (congenital) (pelvis) (recurrent) (*see also* Calculus, kidney)
Nephroma C64- ☑
mesoblastic D41.0- ☑
Nephronephritis — *see* Nephrosis
Nephronophthisis Q61.5
Nephropathia epidemica A98.5
Nephropathy (*see also* Nephritis) N28.9
with
edema — *see* Nephrosis
glomerular lesion — *see* Glomerulonephritis
amyloid, hereditary E85.0
analgesic N14.0
with medullary necrosis, acute N17.2
Balkan (endemic) N15.0
chemical — *see* Nephropathy, toxic
diabetic — *see* E08-E13 with .21
drug-induced N14.2
specified NEC N14.1
focal and segmental hyalinosis or sclerosis N02.1
heavy metal-induced N14.3
hereditary NEC N07.9
with
dense deposit disease N07.6
diffuse
crescentic glomerulonephritis N07.7
endocapillary proliferative glomerulonephritis N07.4
membranous glomerulonephritis N07.2
mesangial proliferative glomerulonephritis N07.3
mesangiocapillary glomerulonephritis N07.5
focal and segmental glomerular lesions N07.1
minor glomerular abnormality N07.0
specified morphological changes NEC N07.8
hypercalcemic N25.89
hypertensive — *see* Hypertension, kidney
hypokalemic (vacuolar) N25.89
IgA N02.8
with glomerular lesion N02.9
focal and segmental hyalinosis or sclerosis N02.1

☑ Additional Character Required — Refer to the Tabular List for Character Selection   ▼ Subterms under main terms may continue to next column or page

Nephropathy — *continued*
  IgA — *continued*
    with glomerular lesion — *continued*
      membranoproliferative (diffuse) N02.5
      membranous (diffuse) N02.2
      mesangial proliferative (diffuse) N02.3
      mesangiocapillary (diffuse) N02.5
      proliferative NEC N02.8
      specified pathology NEC N02.8
  lead N14.3
  membranoproliferative (diffuse) N02.5
  membranous (diffuse) N02.2
  mesangial (IgA/IgG) — *see* Nephropathy, IgA
    proliferative (diffuse) N02.3
  mesangiocapillary (diffuse) N02.5
  obstructive N13.8
  phenacetin N17.2
  phosphate-losing N25.0
  potassium depletion N25.89
  pregnancy-related O26.83- ☑
  proliferative NEC (*see also* N00-N07 with fourth character .8) N05.8
  protein-losing N25.89
  saturnine N14.3
  sickle-cell D57.- ☑ [N08]
  toxic NEC N14.4
    due to
      drugs N14.2
        analgesic N14.0
        specified NEC N14.1
      heavy metals N14.3
  vasomotor N17.0
  water-losing N25.89
Nephroptosis N28.83
Nephropyosis — *see* Abscess, kidney
Nephrorrhagia N28.89
Nephrosclerosis (arteriolar)(arteriosclerotic) (chronic) (hyaline) (*see also* Hypertension, kidney)
  hyperplastic — *see* Hypertension, kidney
  senile N26.9
Nephrosis, nephrotic (Epstein's) (syndrome) (congenital) N04.9
  with
    foot process disease N04.9
    glomerular lesion N04.1
    hypocomplementemic N04.5
  acute N04.9
  anoxic — *see* Nephrosis, tubular
  chemical — *see* Nephrosis, tubular
  cholemic K76.7
  diabetic — *see* E08-E13 with .21
  Finnish type (congenital) Q89.8
  hemoglobin N10
  hemoglobinuric — *see* Nephrosis, tubular
  in
    amyloidosis E85.4 [N08]
    diabetes mellitus — *see* E08-E13 with .21
    epidemic hemorrhagic fever A98.5
    malaria (malariae) B52.0
  ischemic — *see* Nephrosis, tubular
  lipoid N04.9
  lower nephron — *see* Nephrosis, tubular
  malarial (malariae) B52.0
  minimal change N04.0
  myoglobin N10
  necrotizing — *see* Nephrosis, tubular
  osmotic (sucrose) N25.89
  radiation N04.9
  syphilitic (late) A52.75
  toxic — *see* Nephrosis, tubular
  tubular (acute) N17.0
    postprocedural N99.0
    radiation N04.9
Nephrosonephritis, hemorrhagic (endemic) A98.5
Nephrostomy
  attention to Z43.6
  status Z93.6
Nerve (*see also* condition)
  injury — *see* Injury, nerve, by body site
Nerves R45.0
Nervous (*see also* condition) R45.0
  heart F45.8
  stomach F45.8
  tension R45.0
Nervousness R45.0
Nesidioblastoma
  pancreas D13.7
  specified site NEC — *see* Neoplasm, benign, by site

Nesidioblastoma — *continued*
  unspecified site D13.7
Nettleship's syndrome — *see* Urticaria pigmentosa
Neumann's disease or syndrome L10.1
Neuralgia, neuralgic (acute) M79.2
  accessory (nerve) G52.8
  acoustic (nerve) — *see* subcategory H93.3 ☑
  auditory (nerve) — *see* subcategory H93.3 ☑
  ciliary G44.009
    intractable G44.001
    not intractable G44.009
  cranial
    nerve (*see also* Disorder, nerve, cranial)
      fifth or trigeminal — *see* Neuralgia, trigeminal
    postherpetic, postzoster B02.29
  ear — *see* subcategory H92.0 ☑
  facialis vera G51.1
  Fothergill's — *see* Neuralgia, trigeminal
  glossopharyngeal (nerve) G52.1
  Horton's G44.099
    intractable G44.091
    not intractable G44.099
  Hunt's B02.21
  hypoglossal (nerve) G52.3
  infraorbital — *see* Neuralgia, trigeminal
  malarial — *see* Malaria
  migrainous G44.009
    intractable G44.001
    not intractable G44.009
  Morton's G57.6- ☑
  nerve, cranial — *see* Disorder, nerve, cranial
  nose G52.0
  occipital M54.81
  olfactory G52.0
  penis N48.9
  perineum R10.2
  postherpetic NEC B02.29
    trigeminal B02.22
  pubic region R10.2
  scrotum R10.2
  Sluder's G44.89
  specified nerve NEC G58.8
  spermatic cord R10.2
  sphenopalatine (ganglion) G90.09
  trifacial — *see* Neuralgia, trigeminal
  trigeminal G50.0
    postherpetic, postzoster B02.22
  vagus (nerve) G52.2
  writer's F48.8
    organic G25.89
Neurapraxia — *see* Injury, nerve
Neurasthenia F48.8
  cardiac F45.8
  gastric F45.8
  heart F45.8
Neurilemmoma (*see also* Neoplasm, nerve, benign)
  acoustic (nerve) D33.3
  malignant (*see also* Neoplasm, nerve, malignant)
    acoustic (nerve) C72.4- ☑
Neurilemmosarcoma — *see* Neoplasm, nerve, malignant
Neurinoma — *see* Neoplasm, nerve, benign
Neurinomatosis — *see* Neoplasm, nerve, uncertain behavior
Neuritis (rheumatoid) M79.2
  abducens (nerve) — *see* Strabismus, paralytic, sixth nerve
  accessory (nerve) G52.8
  acoustic (nerve) (*see also* subcategory) H93.3 ☑
    in (due to)
      infectious disease NEC B99 ☑ [H94.0-] ☑
      parasitic disease NEC B89 [H94.0-] ☑
    syphilitic A52.15
  alcoholic G62.1
    with psychosis — *see* Psychosis, alcoholic
  amyloid, any site E85.4 [G63]
  auditory (nerve) — *see* subcategory H93.3 ☑
  brachial — *see* Radiculopathy
    due to displacement, intervertebral disc — *see* Disorder, disc, cervical, with neuritis
  cranial nerve
    due to Lyme disease A69.22
    eighth or acoustic or auditory — *see* subcategory H93.3 ☑
    eleventh or accessory G52.8
    fifth or trigeminal G51.0
    first or olfactory G52.0

Neuritis   *continued*
  cranial nerve — *continued*
    fourth or trochlear — *see* Strabismus, paralytic, fourth nerve
    second or optic — *see* Neuritis, optic
    seventh or facial G51.8
      newborn (birth injury) P11.3
    sixth or abducent — *see* Strabismus, paralytic, sixth nerve
    tenth or vagus G52.2
    third or oculomotor — *see* Strabismus, paralytic, third nerve
    twelfth or hypoglossal G52.3
  Déjérine-Sottas G60.0
  diabetic (mononeuropathy) — *see* E08-E13 with .41
    polyneuropathy — *see* E08-E13 with .42
  due to
    beriberi E51.11
    displacement, prolapse or rupture, intervertebral disc — *see* Disorder, disc, with, radiculopathy
    herniation, nucleus pulposus M51.9 [G55]
  endemic E51.11
  facial G51.8
    newborn (birth injury) P11.3
  general — *see* Polyneuropathy
  geniculate ganglion G51.1
    due to herpes (zoster) B02.21
  gouty (*see also* Gout, by type) M10.9 [G63]
  hypoglossal (nerve) G52.3
  ilioinguinal (nerve) G57.9- ☑
  infectious (multiple) NEC G61.0
  interstitial hypertrophic progressive G60.0
  lumbar M54.16
  lumbosacral M54.17
  multiple (*see also* Polyneuropathy)
    endemic E51.11
    infective, acute G61.0
  multiplex endemica E51.11
  nerve root — *see* Radiculopathy
  oculomotor (nerve) — *see* Strabismus, paralytic, third nerve
  olfactory nerve G52.0
  optic (nerve) (hereditary) (sympathetic) H46.9
    with demyelination G36.0
    in myelitis G36.0
    nutritional H46.2
    papillitis — *see* Papillitis, optic
    retrobulbar H46.1- ☑
    specified type NEC H46.8
    toxic H46.3
  peripheral (nerve) G62.9
    multiple — *see* Polyneuropathy
    single — *see* Mononeuritis
  pneumogastric (nerve) G52.2
  postherpetic, postzoster B02.29
  progressive hypertrophic interstitial G60.0
  retrobulbar (*see also* Neuritis, optic, retrobulbar)
    in (due to)
      late syphilis A52.15
      meningococcal infection A39.82
    meningococcal A39.82
    syphilitic A52.15
  sciatic (nerve) (*see also* Sciatica)
    due to displacement of intervertebral disc — *see* Disorder, disc, with, radiculopathy
  serum (*see also* Reaction, serum) T80.69 ☑
  shoulder-girdle G54.5
  specified nerve NEC G58.8
  spinal (nerve) root — *see* Radiculopathy
  syphilitic A52.15
  thenar (median) G56.1- ☑
  thoracic M54.14
  toxic NEC G62.2
  trochlear (nerve) — *see* Strabismus, paralytic, fourth nerve
  vagus (nerve) G52.2
Neuroastrocytoma — *see* Neoplasm, uncertain behavior, by site
Neuroavitaminosis E56.9 [G99.8]
Neuroblastoma
  olfactory C30.0
  specified site — *see* Neoplasm, malignant, by site
  unspecified site C74.90
Neurochorioretinitis — *see* Chorioretinitis
Neurocirculatory asthenia F45.8
Neurocysticercosis B69.0
Neurocytoma — *see* Neoplasm, benign, by site

Neurodermatitis (circumscribed) (circumscripta) (local) L28.0
  atopic L20.81
  diffuse (Brocq) L20.81
  disseminated L20.81
Neuroencephalomyelopathy, optic G36.0
Neuroepithelioma (see also Neoplasm, malignant, by site)
  olfactory C30.0
Neurofibroma (see also Neoplasm, nerve, benign)
  melanotic — see Neoplasm, nerve, benign
  multiple — see Neurofibromatosis
  plexiform — see Neoplasm, nerve, benign
Neurofibromatosis (multiple) (nonmalignant) Q85.00
  acoustic Q85.02
  malignant — see Neoplasm, nerve, malignant
  specified NEC Q85.09
  type 1 (von Recklinghausen) Q85.01
  type 2 Q85.02
Neurofibrosarcoma — see Neoplasm, nerve, malignant
Neurogenic (see also condition)
  bladder (see also Dysfunction, bladder, neuromuscular) N31.9
    cauda equina syndrome G83.4
  bowel NEC K59.2
  heart F45.8
Neuroglioma — see Neoplasm, uncertain behavior, by site
Neurolabyrinthitis (of Dix and Hallpike) — see Neuronitis, vestibular
Neurolathyrism — see Poisoning, food, noxious, plant
Neuroleprosy A30.9
Neuroma (see also Neoplasm, nerve, benign)
  acoustic (nerve) D33.3
  amputation (stump) (traumatic) (surgical complication) (late) T87.3- ☑
    arm T87.3- ☑
    leg T87.3- ☑
  digital (toe) G57.6- ☑
  interdigital G58.8
    lower limb (toe) G57.8- ☑
    upper limb G56.8- ☑
  intermetatarsal G57.8- ☑
  Morton's G57.6- ☑
  nonneoplastic
    arm G56.9- ☑
    leg G57.9- ☑
    lower extremity G57.9- ☑
    upper extremity G56.9- ☑
  optic (nerve) D33.3
  plantar G57.6- ☑
  plexiform — see Neoplasm, nerve, benign
  surgical (nonneoplastic)
    arm G56.9- ☑
    leg G57.9- ☑
    lower extremity G57.9- ☑
    upper extremity G56.9- ☑
Neuromyalgia — see Neuralgia
Neuromyasthenia (epidemic) (postinfectious) G93.3
Neuromyelitis G36.9
  ascending G61.0
  optica G36.0
Neuromyopathy G70.9
  paraneoplastic D49.9 [G13.0]
Neuromyotonia (Isaacs) G71.19
Neuronevus — see Nevus
Neuronitis G58.9
  ascending (acute) G57.2- ☑
  vestibular H81.2- ☑
Neuroparalytic — see condition
Neuropathy, neuropathic G62.9
  acute motor G62.81
  alcoholic G62.1
    with psychosis — see Psychosis, alcoholic
  arm G56.9- ☑
  autonomic, peripheral — see Neuropathy, peripheral, autonomic
  axillary G56.9- ☑
  bladder N31.9
    atonic (motor) (sensory) N31.2
    autonomous N31.2
    flaccid N31.2
    nonreflex N31.2
    reflex N31.1
    uninhibited N31.0
  brachial plexus G54.0
  cervical plexus G54.2

Neuropathy, neuropathic — continued
  chronic
    progressive segmentally demyelinating G62.89
    relapsing demyelinating G62.89
  Déjérine-Sottas G60.0
  diabetic — see E08-E13 with .40
    mononeuropathy — see E08-E13 with .41
    polyneuropathy — see E08-E13 with .42
  entrapment G58.9
    iliohypogastric nerve G57.8- ☑
    ilioinguinal nerve G57.8- ☑
    lateral cutaneous nerve of thigh G57.1- ☑
    median nerve G56.0- ☑
    obturator nerve G57.8- ☑
    peroneal nerve G57.3- ☑
    posterior tibial nerve G57.5- ☑
    saphenous nerve G57.8- ☑
    ulnar nerve G56.2- ☑
  facial nerve G51.9
  hereditary G60.9
    motor and sensory (types I-IV) G60.0
    sensory G60.8
    specified NEC G60.8
  hypertrophic G60.0
    Charcot-Marie-Tooth G60.0
    Déjérine-Sottas G60.0
    interstitial progressive G60.0
    of infancy G60.0
    Refsum G60.1
  idiopathic G60.9
    progressive G60.3
    specified NEC G60.8
  in association with hereditary ataxia G60.2
  intercostal G58.0
  ischemic — see Disorder, nerve
  Jamaica (ginger) G62.2
  leg NEC G57.9- ☑
  lower extremity G57.9- ☑
  lumbar plexus G54.1
  median nerve G56.1- ☑
  motor and sensory (see also Polyneuropathy)
    hereditary (types I-IV) G60.0
  multifocal motor (MMN) G61.82
  multiple (acute) (chronic) — see Polyneuropathy
  optic (nerve) (see also Neuritis, optic)
    ischemic H47.01- ☑
  paraneoplastic (sensorial) (Denny Brown) D49.9 [G13.0]
  peripheral (nerve) (see also Polyneuropathy) G62.9
    autonomic G90.9
      idiopathic G90.09
      in (due to)
        amyloidosis E85.4 [G99.0]
        diabetes mellitus — see E08-E13 with .43
        endocrine disease NEC E34.9 [G99.0]
        gout M10.00 [G99.0]
        hyperthyroidism E05.90 [G99.0]
          with thyroid storm E05.91 [G99.0]
        metabolic disease NEC E88.9 [G99.0]
    idiopathic G60.9
      progressive G60.3
    in (due to)
      antitetanus serum G62.0
      arsenic G62.2
      drugs NEC G62.0
      lead G62.2
      organophosphate compounds G62.2
      toxic agent NEC G62.2
  plantar nerves G57.6- ☑
  progressive
    hypertrophic interstitial G60.0
    inflammatory G62.81
  radicular NEC — see Radiculopathy
  sacral plexus G54.1
  sciatic G57.0- ☑
  serum G61.1
  toxic NEC G62.2
  trigeminal sensory G50.8
  ulnar nerve G56.2- ☑
  uremic N18.9 [G63]
  vitamin B12 E53.8 [G63]
    with anemia (pernicious) D51.0 [G63]
      due to dietary deficiency D51.3 [G63]
Neurophthisis (see also Disorder, nerve)
  peripheral, diabetic — see E08-E13 with .42
Neuroretinitis — see Chorioretinitis
Neuroretinopathy, hereditary optic H47.22
Neurosarcoma — see Neoplasm, nerve, malignant
Neurosclerosis — see Disorder, nerve

Neurosis, neurotic F48.9
  anankastic F42.8
  anxiety (state) F41.1
    panic type F41.0
  asthenic F48.8
  bladder F45.8
  cardiac (reflex) F45.8
  cardiovascular F45.8
  character F60.9
  colon F45.8
  compensation F68.1 ☑
  compulsive, compulsion F42.8
  conversion F44.9
  craft F48.8
  cutaneous F45.8
  depersonalization F48.1
  depressive (reaction) (type) F34.1
  environmental F48.8
  excoriation L98.1
  fatigue F48.8
  functional — see Disorder, somatoform
  gastric F45.8
  gastrointestinal F45.8
  heart F45.8
  hypochondriacal F45.21
  hysterical F44.9
  incoordination F45.8
    larynx F45.8
    vocal cord F45.8
  intestine F45.8
  larynx (sensory) F45.8
    hysterical F44.4
  mixed NEC F48.8
  musculoskeletal F45.8
  obsessional F42.8
  obsessive-compulsive F42.8
  occupational F48.8
  ocular NEC F45.8
  organ — see Disorder, somatoform
  pharynx F45.8
  phobic F40.9
  posttraumatic (situational) F43.10
    acute F43.11
    chronic F43.12
  psychasthenic (type) F48.8
  railroad F48.8
  rectum F45.8
  respiratory F45.8
  rumination F45.8
  sexual F65.9
  situational F48.8
  social F40.10
    generalized F40.11
  specified type NEC F48.8
  state F48.9
    with depersonalization episode F48.1
  stomach F45.8
  traumatic F43.10
    acute F43.11
    chronic F43.12
  vasomotor F45.8
  visceral F45.8
  war F48.8
Neurospongioblastosis diffusa Q85.1
Neurosyphilis (arrested) (early) (gumma) (late) (latent) (recurrent) (relapse) A52.3
  with ataxia (cerebellar) (locomotor) (spastic) (spinal) A52.19
  aneurysm (cerebral) A52.05
  arachnoid (adhesive) A52.13
  arteritis (any artery) (cerebral) A52.04
  asymptomatic A52.2
  congenital A50.40
  dura (mater) A52.13
  general paresis A52.17
  hemorrhagic A52.05
  juvenile (asymptomatic) (meningeal) A50.40
  leptomeninges (aseptic) A52.13
  meningeal, meninges (adhesive) A52.13
  meningitis A52.13
  meningovascular (diffuse) A52.13
  optic atrophy A52.15
  parenchymatous (degenerative) A52.19
  paresis, paretic A52.17
    juvenile A50.45
  remission in (sustained) A52.3
  serological (without symptoms) A52.2
  specified nature or site NEC A52.19
  tabes, tabetic (dorsalis) A52.11

☑ **Additional Character Required** — **Refer to the Tabular List for Character Selection**   ▽ **Subterms under main terms may continue to next column or page**

Neurosyphilis — *continued*
  tabes, tabetic — *continued*
    juvenile A50.45
  taboparesis A52.17
    juvenile A50.45
  thrombosis (cerebral) A52.05
  vascular (cerebral) NEC A52.05
Neurothekeoma — *see* Neoplasm, nerve, benign
Neurotic — *see* Neurosis
Neurotoxemia — *see* Toxemia
Neuroclusion M26.211
Neutropenia, neutropenic (chronic) (genetic) (idiopathic) (immune) (infantile) (malignant) (pernicious) (splenic) D70.9
  congenital (primary) D70.0
  cyclic D70.4
  cytoreductive cancer chemotherapy sequela D70.1
  drug-induced D70.2
    due to cytoreductive cancer chemotherapy D70.1
  due to infection D70.3
  fever D70.9
  neonatal, transitory (isoimmune) (maternal transfer) P61.5
  periodic D70.4
  secondary (cyclic) (periodic) (splenic) D70.4
    drug-induced D70.2
      due to cytoreductive cancer chemotherapy D70.1
  toxic D70.8
Neutrophilia, hereditary giant D72.0
Nevocarcinoma — *see* Melanoma
Nevus D22.9
  achromic — *see* Neoplasm, skin, benign
  amelanotic — *see* Neoplasm, skin, benign
  angiomatous D18.00
    intra-abdominal D18.03
    intracranial D18.02
    skin D18.01
    specified site NEC D18.09
  araneus I78.1
  balloon cell — *see* Neoplasm, skin, benign
  bathing trunk D48.5
  blue — *see* Neoplasm, skin, benign
    cellular — *see* Neoplasm, skin, benign
    giant — *see* Neoplasm, skin, benign
    Jadassohn's — *see* Neoplasm, skin, benign
    malignant — *see* Melanoma
  capillary D18.00
    intra-abdominal D18.03
    intracranial D18.02
    skin D18.01
    specified site NEC D18.09
  cavernous D18.00
    intra-abdominal D18.03
    intracranial D18.02
    skin D18.01
    specified site NEC D18.09
  cellular — *see* Neoplasm, skin, benign
    blue — *see* Neoplasm, skin, benign
  choroid D31.3- ☑
  comedonicus Q82.5
  conjunctiva D31.0- ☑
  dermal — *see* Neoplasm, skin, benign
    with epidermal nevus — *see* Neoplasm, skin, benign
  dysplastic — *see* Neoplasm, skin, benign
  eye D31.9- ☑
  flammeus Q82.5
  hemangiomatous D18.00
    intra-abdominal D18.03
    intracranial D18.02
    skin D18.01
    specified site NEC D18.09
  iris D31.4- ☑
  lacrimal gland D31.5- ☑
  lymphatic D18.1
  magnocellular
    specified site — *see* Neoplasm, benign, by site
    unspecified site D31.40
  malignant — *see* Melanoma
  meaning hemangioma D18.00
    intra-abdominal D18.03
    intracranial D18.02
    skin D18.01
    specified site NEC D18.09
  mouth (mucosa) D10.30
    specified site NEC D10.39
    white sponge Q38.6

Nevus — *continued*
  multiplex Q85.1
  non-neoplastic I78.1
  oral mucosa D10.30
    specified site NEC D10.39
    white sponge Q38.6
  orbit D31.6- ☑
  pigmented
    giant (*see also* Neoplasm, skin, uncertain behavior) D48.5
      malignant melanoma in — *see* Melanoma
  portwine Q82.5
  retina D31.2- ☑
  retrobulbar D31.6- ☑
  sanguineous Q82.5
  senile I78.1
  skin D22.9
    abdominal wall D22.5
    ala nasi D22.39
    ankle D22.7- ☑
    anus, anal D22.5
    arm D22.6- ☑
    auditory canal (external) D22.2- ☑
    auricle (ear) D22.2- ☑
    auricular canal (external) D22.2- ☑
    axilla, axillary fold D22.5
    back D22.5
    breast D22.5
    brow D22.39
    buttock D22.5
    canthus (eye) D22.1- ☑
    cheek (external) D22.39
    chest wall D22.5
    chin D22.39
    ear (external) D22.2- ☑
    external meatus (ear) D22.2- ☑
    eyebrow D22.39
    eyelid (lower) (upper) D22.1- ☑
    face D22.30
      specified NEC D22.39
    female genital organ (external) NEC D28.0
    finger D22.6- ☑
    flank D22.5
    foot D22.7- ☑
    forearm D22.6- ☑
    forehead D22.39
    foreskin D29.0
    genital organ (external) NEC
      female D28.0
      male D29.9
    gluteal region D22.5
    groin D22.5
    hand D22.6- ☑
    heel D22.7- ☑
    helix D22.2- ☑
    hip D22.7- ☑
    interscapular region D22.5
    jaw D22.39
    knee D22.7- ☑
    labium (majus) (minus) D28.0
    leg D22.7- ☑
    lip (lower) (upper) D22.0
    lower limb D22.7- ☑
    male genital organ (external) D29.9
    nail D22.9
      finger D22.6- ☑
      toe D22.7- ☑
    nasolabial groove D22.39
    nates D22.5
    neck D22.4
    nose (external) D22.39
    palpebra D22.1- ☑
    penis D29.0
    perianal skin D22.5
    perineum D22.5
    pinna D22.2- ☑
    popliteal fossa or space D22.7- ☑
    prepuce D29.0
    pudendum D28.0
    scalp D22.4
    scrotum D29.4
    shoulder D22.6- ☑
    submammary fold D22.5
    temple D22.39
    thigh D22.7- ☑
    toe D22.7- ☑
    trunk NEC D22.5

Nevus — *continued*
  skin — *continued*
    umbilicus D22.5
    upper limb D22.6- ☑
    vulva D28.0
  specified site NEC — *see* Neoplasm, by site, benign
  spider I78.1
  stellar I78.1
  strawberry Q82.5
  Sutton's benign D22.9
  unius lateris Q82.5
  Unna's Q82.5
  vascular Q82.5
  verrucous Q82.5
Newborn (infant) (liveborn) (singleton) Z38.2
  abstinence syndrome P96.1
  acne L70.4
  affected by
    abnormalities of membranes P02.9
      specified NEC P02.8
    abruptio placenta P02.1
    amino-acid metabolic disorder, transitory P74.8
    amniocentesis (while in utero) P00.6
    amnionitis P02.7
    apparent life threatening event (ALTE) R68.13
    bleeding (into)
      cerebral cortex P52.22
      germinal matrix P52.0
      ventricles P52.1
    breech delivery P03.0
    cardiac arrest P29.81
    cardiomyopathy I42.8
      congenital I42.4
    cerebral ischemia P91.0
    Cesarean delivery P03.4
    chemotherapy agents P04.1
    chorioamnionitis P02.7
    cocaine (crack) P04.41
    complications of labor and delivery P03.9
      specified NEC P03.89
    compression of umbilical cord NEC P02.5
    contracted pelvis P03.1
    delivery P03.9
      Cesarean P03.4
      forceps P03.2
      vacuum extractor P03.3
    entanglement (knot) in umbilical cord P02.5
    environmental chemicals P04.6
    fetal (intrauterine)
      growth retardation P05.9
      malnutrition not light or small for gestational age P05.2
    forceps delivery P03.2
    heart rate abnormalities
      bradycardia P29.12
      intrauterine P03.819
        before onset of labor P03.810
        during labor P03.811
      tachycardia P29.11
    hemorrhage (antepartum) P02.1
      cerebellar (nontraumatic) P52.6
      intracerebral (nontraumatic) P52.4
      intracranial (nontraumatic) P52.9
        specified NEC P52.8
      intraventricular (nontraumatic) P52.3
        grade 1 P52.0
        grade 2 P52.1
        grade 3 P52.21
        grade 4 P52.22
      posterior fossa (nontraumatic) P52.6
      subarachnoid (nontraumatic) P52.5
      subependymal P52.0
        with intracerebral extension P52.22
        with intraventricular extension P52.1
          with enlargment of ventricles P52.21
        without intraventricular extension P52.0
    hypoxic ischemic encephalopathy [HIE] P91.60
      mild P91.61
      moderate P91.62
      severe P91.63
    induction of labor P03.89
    intestinal perforation P78.0
    intrauterine (fetal) blood loss P50.9
      due to (from)
        cut end of co-twin cord P50.5
        hemorrhage into
          co-twin P50.3
          maternal circulation P50.4
        placenta P50.2

Newborn — *continued*
  affected by — *continued*
    intrauterine blood loss — *continued*
      due to — *continued*
        ruptured cord blood P50.1
        vasa previa P50.0
      specified NEC P50.8
    intrauterine (fetal) hemorrhage P50.9
    intrauterine (in utero) procedure P96.5
    malpresentation (malposition) NEC P03.1
    maternal (complication of) (use of)
      alcohol P04.3
      analgesia (maternal) P04.0
      anesthesia (maternal) P04.0
      blood loss P02.1
      circulatory disease P00.3
      condition P00.9
        specified NEC P00.89
      delivery P03.9
        Cesarean P03.4
        forceps P03.2
        vacuum extractor P03.3
      diabetes mellitus (pre-existing) P70.1
      disorder P00.9
        specified NEC P00.89
      drugs (addictive) (illegal) NEC P04.49
      ectopic pregnancy P01.4
      gestational diabetes P70.0
      hemorrhage P02.1
      hypertensive disorder P00.0
      incompetent cervix P01.0
      infectious disease P00.2
      injury P00.5
      labor and delivery P03.9
      malpresentation before labor P01.7
      maternal death P01.6
      medical procedure P00.7
      medication P04.1
      multiple pregnancy P01.5
      nutritional disorder P00.4
      oligohydramnios P01.2
      parasitic disease P00.2
      periodontal disease P00.81
      placenta previa P02.0
      polyhydramnios P01.3
      precipitate delivery P03.5
      pregnancy P01.9
        specified P01.8
      premature rupture of membranes P01.1
      renal disease P00.1
      respiratory disease P00.3
      surgical procedure P00.6
      urinary tract disease P00.1
      uterine contraction (abnormal) P03.6
    meconium peritonitis P78.0
    medication (legal) (maternal use) (prescribed) P04.1
    membrane abnormalities P02.9
      specified NEC P02.8
    membranitis P02.7
    methamphetamine(s) P04.49
    mixed metabolic and respiratory acidosis P84
    neonatal abstinence syndrome P96.1
    noxious substances transmitted via placenta or
      breast milk P04.9
      specified NEC P04.8
    nutritional supplements P04.5
    placenta previa P02.0
    placental
      abnormality (functional) (morphological)
        P02.20
        specified NEC P02.29
      dysfunction P02.29
      infarction P02.29
      insufficiency P02.29
      separation NEC P02.1
      transfusion syndromes P02.3
    placentitis P02.7
    precipitate delivery P03.5
    prolapsed cord P02.4
    respiratory arrest P28.81
    slow intrauterine growth P05.9
    tobacco P04.2
    twin to twin transplacental transfusion P02.3
    umbilical cord (tightly) around neck P02.5
    umbilical cord condition P02.60
      short cord P02.69
      specified NEC P02.69
    uterine contractions (abnormal) P03.6
    vasa previa P02.69

Newborn — *continued*
  affected by — *continued*
    vasa previa — *continued*
      from intrauterine blood loss P50.0
    apnea P28.4
      obstructive P28.4
      primary P28.3
      sleep (central) (obstructive) (primary) P28.3
    born in hospital Z38.00
      by cesarean Z38.01
    born outside hospital Z38.1
    breast buds P96.89
    breast engorgement P83.4
    check-up — *see* Newborn, examination
    convulsion P90
    dehydration P74.1
    examination
      8 to 28 days old Z00.111
      under 8 days old Z00.110
    fever P81.9
      environmentally-induced P81.0
    hyperbilirubinemia P59.9
      of prematurity P59.0
    hypernatremia P74.2
    hyponatremia P74.2
    infection P39.9
      candidal P37.5
      specified NEC P39.8
      urinary tract P39.3
    jaundice P59.9
      due to
        breast milk inhibitor P59.3
        hepatocellular damage P59.20
          specified NEC P59.29
        preterm delivery P59.0
      of prematurity P59.0
      specified NEC P59.8
    late metabolic acidosis P74.0
    mastitis P39.0
      infective P39.0
      noninfective P83.4
    multiple born NEC Z38.8
      born in hospital Z38.68
        by cesarean Z38.69
      born outside hospital Z38.7
    omphalitis P38.9
      with mild hemorrhage P38.1
      without hemorrhage P38.9
    post-term P08.21
    prolonged gestation (over 42 completed weeks)
      P08.22
    quadruplet Z38.8
      born in hospital Z38.63
        by cesarean Z38.64
      born outside hospital Z38.7
    quintuplet Z38.8
      born in hospital Z38.65
        by cesarean Z38.66
      born outside hospital Z38.7
    seizure P90
    sepsis (congenital) P36.9
      due to
        anaerobes NEC P36.5
        Escherichia coli P36.4
        Staphylococcus P36.30
          aureus P36.2
          specified NEC P36.39
        Streptococcus P36.10
          group B P36.0
          specified NEC P36.19
      specified NEC P36.8
    triplet Z38.8
      born in hospital Z38.61
        by cesarean Z38.62
      born outside hospital Z38.7
    twin Z38.5
      born in hospital Z38.30
        by cesarean Z38.31
      born outside hospital Z38.4
    vomiting P92.09
      bilious P92.01
    weight check Z00.111
Newcastle conjunctivitis or disease B30.8
Nezelof's syndrome (pure alymphocytosis) D81.4
Niacin (amide) **deficiency** E52
Nicolas (-Durand)-**Favre disease** A55
Nicotine — *see* Tobacco
Nicotinic acid deficiency E52

Niemann-Pick disease or syndrome E75.249
  specified NEC E75.248
  type
    A E75.240
    B E75.241
    C E75.242
    D E75.243
Night
  blindness — *see* Blindness, night
  sweats R61
  terrors (child) F51.4
Nightmares (REM sleep type) F51.5
NIHSS (National Institutes of Health Stroke Scale) **score**
  R29.7- ☑
Nipple — *see* condition
Nisbet's chancre A57
Nishimoto (-Takeuchi) **disease** I67.5
Nitritoid crisis or reaction — *see* Crisis, nitritoid
Nitrosohemoglobinemia D74.8
Njovera A65
Nocardiosis, nocardiasis A43.9
  cutaneous A43.1
  lung A43.0
  pneumonia A43.0
  pulmonary A43.0
  specified site NEC A43.8
Nocturia R35.1
  psychogenic F45.8
Nocturnal — *see* condition
Nodal rhythm I49.8
Node(s) (*see also* Nodule)
  Bouchard's (with arthropathy) M15.2
  Haygarth's M15.8
  Heberden's (with arthropathy) M15.1
  larynx J38.7
  lymph — *see* condition
  milker's B08.03
  Osler's I33.0
  Schmorl's — *see* Schmorl's disease
  singer's J38.2
  teacher's J38.2
  tuberculous — *see* Tuberculosis, lymph gland
  vocal cord J38.2
Nodule(s), nodular
  actinomycotic — *see* Actinomycosis
  breast NEC (*see also* Lump, breast) N63.0
  colloid (cystic), thyroid E04.1
  cutaneous — *see* Swelling, localized
  endometrial (stromal) D26.1
  Haygarth's M15.8
  inflammatory — *see* Inflammation
  juxta-articular
    syphilitic A52.77
    yaws A66.7
  larynx J38.7
  lung, solitary (subsegmental branch of the bronchial
    tree) R91.1
    multiple R91.8
  milker's B08.03
  prostate N40.2
    with lower urinary tract symptoms (LUTS) N40.3
    without lower urinary tract symptpoms (LUTS) N40.2
  pulmonary, solitary (subsegmental branch of the
    bronchial tree) R91.1
  retrocardiac R09.89
  rheumatoid M06.30
    ankle M06.37- ☑
    elbow M06.32- ☑
    foot joint M06.37- ☑
    hand joint M06.34- ☑
    hip M06.35- ☑
    knee M06.36- ☑
    multiple site M06.39
    shoulder M06.31- ☑
    vertebra M06.38
    wrist M06.33- ☑
  scrotum (inflammatory) N49.2
  singer's J38.2
  solitary, lung (subsegmental branch of the bronchial
    tree) R91.1
    multiple R91.8
  subcutaneous — *see* Swelling, localized
  teacher's J38.2
  thyroid (cold) (gland) (nontoxic) E04.1
    with thyrotoxicosis E05.20
      with thyroid storm E05.21
    toxic or with hyperthyroidism E05.20
      with thyroid storm E05.21

Nodule(s), **nodular** — *continued*
  vocal cord J38.2
Noma (gangrenous) (hospital) (infective) A69.0
  auricle I96
  mouth A69.0
  pudendi N76.89
  vulvae N76.89
Nomad, nomadism Z59.0
NOMID (neonatal onset multisystemic inflammatory disorder) M04.2
Nonadherence to medical treatment Z91.19
Nonautoimmune hemolytic anemia D59.4
  drug-induced D59.2
Nonclosure (*see also* Imperfect, closure)
  ductus arteriosus (Botallo's) Q25.0
  foramen
    botalli Q21.1
    ovale Q21.1
Noncompliance Z91.19
  with
    dialysis Z91.15
    dietary regimen Z91.11
    medical treatment Z91.19
    medication regimen NEC Z91.14
      underdosing (*see also* Table of Drugs and Chemicals, categories T36-T50, with final character 6) Z91.14
      intentional NEC Z91.128
        due to financial hardship of patient Z91.120
      unintentional NEC Z91.138
        due to patient's age related debility Z91.130
    renal dialysis Z91.15
Nondescent (congenital) (*see also* Malposition, congenital)
  cecum Q43.3
  colon Q43.3
  testicle Q53.9
    bilateral Q53.20
      abdominal Q53.211
      perineal Q53.22
    unilateral Q53.10
      abdominal Q53.111
      perineal Q53.12
Nondevelopment
  brain Q02
    part of Q04.3
  heart Q24.8
  organ or site, congenital NEC — *see* Hypoplasia
Nonengagement
  head NEC O32.4 ☑
    in labor, causing obstructed labor O64.8 ☑
Nonexanthematous tick fever A93.2
Nonexpansion, lung (newborn) P28.0
Nonfunctioning
  cystic duct (*see also* Disease, gallbladder) K82.8
  gallbladder (*see also* Disease, gallbladder) K82.8
  kidney N28.9
  labyrinth — *see* subcategory H83.2 ☑
Non-Hodgkin lymphoma NEC — *see* Lymphoma, non-Hodgkin
Nonimplantation, ovum N97.2
Noninsufflation, fallopian tube N97.1
Non-ketotic hyperglycinemia E72.51
Nonne-Milroy syndrome Q82.0
Nonovulation N97.0
Non-palpable testicle(s)
  bilateral R39.84
  unilateral R39.83
Nonpatent fallopian tube N97.1
Nonpneumatization, lung NEC P28.0
Nonrotation — *see* Malrotation
Nonsecretion, urine — *see* Anuria
Nonunion
  fracture — *see* Fracture, by site
  joint, following fusion or arthrodesis M96.0
  organ or site, congenital NEC — *see* Imperfect, closure
  symphysis pubis, congenital Q74.2
Nonvisualization, gallbladder R93.2
Nonvital, nonvitalized tooth K04.99
Non-working side interference M26.56
Noonan's syndrome Q87.1
Normocytic anemia (infectional) due to blood loss (chronic) D50.0
  acute D62
Norrie's disease (congenital) Q15.8

North American blastomycosis B40.9
Norwegian itch B86
Nose, nasal — *see* condition
Nosebleed R04.0
Nose-picking F98.8
Nosomania F45.21
Nosophobia F45.22
Nostalgia F43.20
Notch of iris Q13.2
Notching nose, congenital (tip) Q30.2
Nothnagel's
  syndrome — *see* Strabismus, paralytic, third nerve
  vasomotor acroparesthesia I73.89
Novy's relapsing fever A68.9
  louse-borne A68.0
  tick-borne A68.1
Noxious
  foodstuffs, poisoning by — *see* Poisoning, food, noxious, plant
  substances transmitted through placenta or breast milk P04.9
Nucleus pulposus — *see* condition
Numbness R20.0
Nuns' knee — *see* Bursitis, prepatellar
Nursemaid's elbow S53.03- ☑
Nutcracker esophagus K22.4
Nutmeg liver K76.1
Nutrient element deficiency E61.9
  specified NEC E61.8
Nutrition deficient or insufficient (*see also* Malnutrition) E46
  due to
    insufficient food T73.0 ☑
    lack of
      care (child) T76.02 ☑
        adult T76.01 ☑
      food T73.0 ☑
Nutritional stunting E45
Nyctalopia (night blindness) — *see* Blindness, night
Nycturia R35.1
  psychogenic F45.8
Nymphomania F52.8
Nystagmus H55.00
  benign paroxysmal — *see* Vertigo, benign paroxysmal
  central positional H81.4- ☑
  congenital H55.01
  dissociated H55.04
  latent H55.02
  miners' H55.09
  positional
    benign paroxysmal H81.4- ☑
    central H81.4- ☑
  specified form NEC H55.09
  visual deprivation H55.03

O

Obermeyer's relapsing fever (European) A68.0
Obesity E66.9
  with alveolar hypoventilation E66.2
  adrenal E27.8
  complicating
    childbirth O99.214
    pregnancy O99.21- ☑
    puerperium O99.215
  constitutional E66.8
  dietary counseling and surveillance Z71.3
  drug-induced E66.1
  due to
    drug E66.1
    excess calories E66.09
      morbid E66.01
      severe E66.01
  endocrine E66.8
  endogenous E66.8
  exogenous E66.09
  familial E66.8
  glandular E66.8
  hypothyroid — *see* Hypothyroidism
  hypoventilation syndrome (OHS) E66.2
  morbid E66.01
    with
      alveolar hypoventilation E66.2
      obesity hypoventilation syndrome (OHS) E66.2
    due to excess calories E66.01
  nutritional E66.09
  pituitary E23.6

Obesity — *continued*
  severe E66.01
  specified type NEC E66.8
Oblique — *see* condition
Obliteration
  appendix (lumen) K38.8
  artery I77.1
  bile duct (noncalculous) K83.1
  common duct (noncalculous) K83.1
  cystic duct — *see* Obstruction, gallbladder
  disease, arteriolar I77.1
  endometrium N85.8
  eye, anterior chamber — *see* Disorder, globe, hypotony
  fallopian tube N97.1
  lymphatic vessel I89.0
    due to mastectomy I97.2
  organ or site, congenital NEC — *see* Atresia, by site
  ureter N13.5
    with infection N13.6
  urethra — *see* Stricture, urethra
  vein I87.8
  vestibule (oral) K08.89
Observation (following) (for) (without need for further medical care) Z04.9
  accident NEC Z04.3
    at work Z04.2
    transport Z04.1
  adverse effect of drug Z03.6
  alleged rape or sexual assault (victim), ruled out
    adult Z04.41
    child Z04.42
  criminal assault Z04.8
  development state
    adolescent Z00.3
    period of rapid growth in childhood Z00.2
    puberty Z00.3
  disease, specified NEC Z03.89
  following work accident Z04.2
  growth and development state — *see* Observation, development state
  injuries (accidental) NEC (*see also* Observation, accident)
  newborn (for)
    suspected condition, related to exposure from the mother or birth process — *see* Newborn, affected by, maternal
    ruled out Z05.9
      cardiac Z05.0
      connective tissue Z05.73
      gastrointestinal Z05.5
      genetic Z05.41
      genitourinary Z05.6
      immunologic Z05.43
      infectious Z05.1
      metabolic Z05.42
      musculoskeletal Z05.72
      neurological Z05.2
      respiratory Z05.3
      skin and subcutaneous tissue Z05.71
      specified condition NEC Z05.8
  postpartum
    immediately after delivery Z39.0
    routine follow-up Z39.2
  pregnancy (normal) (without complication) Z34.9- ☑
    high risk O09.9- ☑
  suicide attempt, alleged NEC Z03.89
    self-poisoning Z03.6
  suspected, ruled out (*see also* Suspected condition, ruled out)
    abuse, physical
      adult Z04.71
      child Z04.72
    accident at work Z04.2
    adult battering victim Z04.71
    child battering victim Z04.72
    condition NEC Z03.89
      newborn (*see also* Observation, newborn (for), suspected condition, ruled out) Z05.9
    drug poisoning or adverse effect Z03.6
    exposure (to)
      anthrax Z03.810
      biological agent NEC Z03.818
    inflicted injury NEC Z04.8
    suicide attempt, alleged Z03.89
      self-poisoning Z03.6
    toxic effects from ingested substance (drug) (poison) Z03.6

Observation — *continued*
  toxic effects from ingested substance (drug) (poison)
    Z03.6
Obsession, obsessional state F42.8
  mixed thoughts and acts F42.2
Obsessive-compulsive neurosis or reaction F42.8
Obstetric embolism, septic — *see* Embolism, obstetric,
  septic
Obstetrical trauma (complicating delivery) O71.9
  with or following ectopic or molar pregnancy O08.6
  specified type NEC O71.89
Obstipation — *see* Constipation
Obstruction, obstructed, obstructive
  airway J98.8
    with
      allergic alveolitis J67.9
      asthma J45.909
        with
          exacerbation (acute) J45.901
          status asthmaticus J45.902
      bronchiectasis J47.9
        with
          exacerbation (acute) J47.1
          lower respiratory infection J47.0
      bronchitis (chronic) J44.9
      emphysema J43.9
    chronic J44.9
      with
        allergic alveolitis — *see* Pneumonitis, hyper-
          sensitivity
        bronchiectasis J47.9
          with
            exacerbation (acute) J47.1
            lower respiratory infection J47.0
    due to
      foreign body — *see* Foreign body, by site,
        causing asphyxia
      inhalation of fumes or vapors J68.9
      laryngospasm J38.5
  ampulla of Vater K83.1
  aortic (heart) (valve) — *see* Stenosis, aortic
  aortoiliac I74.09
  aqueduct of Sylvius G91.1
    congenital Q03.0
      with spina bifida — *see* Spina bifida, by site,
        with hydrocephalus
  Arnold-Chiari — *see* Arnold-Chiari disease
  artery (*see also* Atherosclerosis, artery) I70.9 ☑
    basilar (complete) (partial) — *see* Occlusion, artery,
      basilar
    carotid (complete) (partial) — *see* Occlusion, artery,
      carotid
    cerebellar — *see* Occlusion, artery, cerebellar
    cerebral (anterior) (middle) (posterior) — *see* Oc-
      clusion, artery, cerebral
    precerebral — *see* Occlusion, artery, precerebral
    renal N28.0
    retinal NEC — *see* Occlusion, artery, retina
    stent — *see* Restenosis, stent
    vertebral (complete) (partial) — *see* Occlusion,
      artery, vertebral
  band (intestinal) (*see also* Obstruction, intestine,
    specified NEC) K56.699
  bile duct or passage (common) (hepatic) (noncalcu-
    lous) K83.1
    with calculus K80.51
    congenital (causing jaundice) Q44.3
  biliary (duct) (tract) K83.1
    gallbladder K82.0
  bladder-neck (acquired) N32.0
    congenital Q64.31
    due to hyperplasia (hypertrophy) of prostate —
      see Hyperplasia, prostate
  bowel — *see* Obstruction, intestine
  bronchus J98.09
  canal, ear — *see* Stenosis, external ear canal
  cardia K22.2
  caval veins (inferior) (superior) I87.1
  cecum — *see* Obstruction, intestine
  circulatory I99.8
  colon — *see* Obstruction, intestine
  common duct (noncalculous) K83.1
  coronary (artery) — *see* Occlusion, coronary
  cystic duct (*see also* Obstruction, gallbladder)
    with calculus K80.21
  device, implant or graft (*see also* Complications, by
    site and type, mechanical) T85.698 ☑

Obstruction, obstructed, obstructive — *continued*
  device, implant or graft (*see also* Complications, by site
    and type, mechanical) — *continued*
    arterial graft NEC — *see* Complication, cardiovas-
      cular device, mechanical, vascular
    catheter NEC T85.628 ☑
      cystostomy T83.090 ☑
      dialysis (renal) T82.49 ☑
        intraperitoneal T85.691 ☑
      Hopkins T83.098 ☑
      ileostomy T83.098 ☑
      infusion NEC T82.594 ☑
        spinal (epidural) (subdural) T85.690 ☑
      nephrostomy T83.092 ☑
      urethral indwelling T83.091 ☑
      urinary T83.098 ☑
      urostomy T83.098 ☑
    due to infection T85.79 ☑
    gastrointestinal — *see* Complications, prosthetic
      device, mechanical, gastrointestinal device
    genital NEC T83.498 ☑
      intrauterine contraceptive device T83.39 ☑
      penile prosthesis (cylinder) (implanted) (pump)
        (resevoir) T83.490 ☑
      testicular prosthesis T83.491 ☑
    heart NEC — *see* Complication, cardiovascular de-
      vice, mechanical
    joint prosthesis — *see* Complications, joint prosthe-
      sis, mechanical, specified NEC, by site
    orthopedic NEC — *see* Complication, orthopedic,
      device, mechanical
    specified NEC T85.628 ☑
    urinary NEC (*see also* Complication, genitourinary,
      device, urinary, mechanical)
      graft T83.29 ☑
    vascular NEC — *see* Complication, cardiovascular
      device, mechanical
    ventricular intracranial shunt T85.09 ☑
  due to foreign body accidentally left in operative
    wound T81.529 ☑
  duodenum K31.5
  ejaculatory duct N50.89
  esophagus K22.2
  eustachian tube (complete) (partial) H68.10- ☑
    cartilagenous (extrinsic) H68.13- ☑
      intrinsic H68.12- ☑
      osseous H68.11- ☑
  fallopian tube (bilateral) N97.1
  fecal K56.41
    with hernia — *see* Hernia, by site, with obstruction
  foramen of Monro (congenital) Q03.8
    with spina bifida — *see* Spina bifida, by site, with
      hydrocephalus
  foreign body — *see* Foreign body
  gallbladder K82.0
    with calculus, stones K80.21
    congenital Q44.1
  gastric outlet K31.1
  gastrointestinal — *see* Obstruction, intestine
  hepatic K76.89
    duct (noncalculous) K83.1
  ileum — *see* Obstruction, intestine
  iliofemoral (artery) I74.5
  intestine K56.609
    with
      adhesions (intestinal) (peritoneal) K56.50
        complete K56.52
        incomplete K56.51
        partial K56.51
    adynamic K56.0
    by gallstone K56.3
    complete K56.601
    congenital (small) Q41.9
      large Q42.9
        specified part NEC Q42.8
    incomplete K56.600
    neurogenic K56.0
      Hirschsprung's disease or megacolon Q43.1
    newborn P76.9
      due to
        fecaliths P76.8
        inspissated milk P76.2
        meconium (plug) P76.0
          in mucoviscidosis E84.11
      specified NEC P76.8
    partial K56.600
    postoperative K91.30

Obstruction, obstructed, obstructive — *continued*
  intestine — *continued*
    postoperative — *continued*
      complete K91.32
      incomplete K91.31
      partial K91.31
    reflex K56.0
    specified NEC K56.699
      complete K56.691
      incomplete K56.690
      partial K56.690
    volvulus K56.2
  intracardiac ball valve prosthesis T82.09 ☑
  jejunum — *see* Obstruction, intestine
  joint prosthesis — *see* Complications, joint prosthesis,
    mechanical, specified NEC, by site
  kidney (calices) N28.89
  labor — *see* Delivery
  lacrimal (passages) (duct)
    by
      dacryolith — *see* Dacryolith
      stenosis — *see* Stenosis, lacrimal
    congenital Q10.5
    neonatal H04.53- ☑
  lacrimonasal duct — *see* Obstruction, lacrimal
  lacteal, with steatorrhea K90.2
  laryngitis — *see* Laryngitis
  larynx NEC J38.6
    congenital Q31.8
  lung J98.4
    disease, chronic J44.9
  lymphatic I89.0
  meconium (plug)
    newborn P76.0
      due to fecaliths P76.0
      in mucoviscidosis E84.11
  mitral — *see* Stenosis, mitral
  nasal J34.89
  nasolacrimal duct (*see also* Obstruction, lacrimal)
    congenital Q10.5
  nasopharynx J39.2
  nose J34.89
  organ or site, congenital NEC — *see* Atresia, by site
  pancreatic duct K86.89
  parotid duct or gland K11.8
  pelviureteral junction N13.5
    with hydronephrosis N13.0
    congenital Q62.39
  pharynx J39.2
  portal (circulation) (vein) I81
  prostate (*see also* Hyperplasia, prostate)
    valve (urinary) N32.0
  pulmonary valve (heart) I37.0
  pyelonephritis (chronic) N11.1
  pylorus
    adult K31.1
    congenital or infantile Q40.0
  rectosigmoid — *see* Obstruction, intestine
  rectum K62.4
  renal N28.89
    outflow N13.8
    pelvis, congenital Q62.39
  respiratory J98.8
    chronic J44.9
  retinal (vessels) H34.9
  salivary duct (any) K11.8
    with calculus K11.5
  sigmoid — *see* Obstruction, intestine
  sinus (accessory) (nasal) J34.89
  Stensen's duct K11.8
  stomach NEC K31.89
    acute K31.0
    congenital Q40.2
    due to pylorospasm K31.3
  submandibular duct K11.8
  submaxillary gland K11.8
    with calculus K11.5
  thoracic duct I89.0
  thrombotic — *see* Thrombosis
  trachea J39.8
  tracheostomy airway J95.03
  tricuspid (valve) — *see* Stenosis, tricuspid
  upper respiratory, congenital Q34.8
  ureter (functional) (pelvic junction) NEC N13.5
    with
      hydronephrosis N13.1
        with infection N13.6
      pyelonephritis (chronic) N11.1

☑ **Additional Character Required** — Refer to the Tabular List for Character Selection   ▽ **Subterms under main terms may continue to next column or page**

Obstruction, obstructed, obstructive — *continued*
  ureter — *continued*
    congenital Q62.39
      due to calculus — *see* Calculus, ureter
  urethra NEC N36.8
    congenital Q64.39
  urinary (moderate) N13.9
    due to hyperplasia (hypertrophy) of prostate —
      see Hyperplasia, prostate
    organ or tract (lower) N13.9
    prostatic valve N32.0
    specified NEC N13.8
  uropathy N13.9
  uterus N85.8
  vagina N89.5
  valvular — *see* Endocarditis
  vein, venous I87.1
    caval (inferior) (superior) I87.1
    thrombotic — *see* Thrombosis
  vena cava (inferior) (superior) I87.1
  vesical NEC N32.0
  vesicourethral orifice N32.0
    congenital Q64.31
  vessel NEC I99.8
    stent — *see* Restenosis, stent
Obturator — *see* condition
Occlusal wear, teeth K03.0
Occlusio pupillae — *see* Membrane, pupillary
Occlusion, occluded
  anus K62.4
    congenital Q42.3
      with fistula Q42.2
  aortoiliac (chronic) I74.09
  aqueduct of Sylvius G91.1
    congenital Q03.0
      with spina bifida — *see* Spina bifida, by site,
        with hydrocephalus
  artery (*see also* Atherosclerosis, artery) I70.9 ☑
    auditory, internal I65.8
    basilar I65.1
      with
        infarction I63.22
          due to
            embolism I63.12
            thrombosis I63.02
    brain or cerebral I66.9
      with infarction (due to) I63.5- ☑
        embolism I63.4- ☑
        thrombosis I63.3- ☑
    carotid I65.2- ☑
      with
        infarction I63.23- ☑
          due to
            embolism I63.13- ☑
            thrombosis I63.03- ☑
    cerebellar (anterior inferior) (posterior inferior)
      (superior) I66.3
      with infarction I63.54- ☑
        due to
          embolism I63.44- ☑
          thrombosis I63.34- ☑
    cerebral I66.9
      with infarction I63.50
        due to
          embolism I63.40
            specified NEC I63.49
          thrombosis I63.30
            specified NEC I63.39
      anterior I66.1- ☑
        with infarction I63.52- ☑
          due to
            embolism I63.42- ☑
            thrombosis I63.32- ☑
      middle I66.0- ☑
        with infarction I63.51- ☑
          due to
            embolism I63.41- ☑
            thrombosis I63.31- ☑
      posterior I66.2- ☑
        with infarction I63.53- ☑
          due to
            embolism I63.43- ☑
            thrombosis I63.33- ☑
      specified NEC I66.8
        with infarction I63.59
          due to
            embolism I63.4- ☑

Occlusion, occluded — *continued*
  artery (*see also* Atherosclerosis, artery) — *continued*
    cerebral — *continued*
      specified — *continued*
        with infarction — *continued*
          due to — *continued*
            thrombosis I63.3- ☑
    choroidal (anterior) — *see* Occlusion, artery, pre-
      cerebral, specified NEC
    communicating posterior — *see* Occlusion, artery,
      precerebral, specified NEC
    complete
      coronary I25.82
      extremities I70.92
    coronary (acute) (thrombotic) (without myocardial
      infarction) I24.0
      with myocardial infarction — *see* Infarction,
        myocardium
      chronic total I25.82
      complete I25.82
      healed or old I25.2
      total (chronic) I25.82
    hypophyseal — *see* Occlusion, artery, precerebral,
      specified NEC
    iliac I74.5
    lower extremities due to stenosis or stricture I77.1
    mesenteric (embolic) (thrombotic) (*see also* Infarct,
      intestine) K55.069
    perforating — *see* Occlusion, artery, cerebral,
      specified NEC
    peripheral I77.9
      thrombotic or embolic I74.4
    pontine — *see* Occlusion, artery, precerebral,
      specified NEC
    precerebral I65.9
      with infarction I63.20
        due to
          embolism I63.10
            specified NEC I63.19
          thrombosis I63.00
            specified NEC I63.09
        specified NEC I63.29
      basilar — *see* Occlusion, artery, basilar
      carotid — *see* Occlusion, artery, carotid
      puerperal O88.23
      specified NEC I65.8
        with infarction I63.29
          due to
            embolism I63.19
            thrombosis I63.09
      vertebral — *see* Occlusion, artery, vertebral
    renal N28.0
    retinal
      branch H34.23- ☑
      central H34.1- ☑
      partial H34.21- ☑
      transient H34.0- ☑
    spinal — *see* Occlusion, artery, precerebral, verte-
      bral
    total (chronic)
      coronary I25.82
      extremities I70.92
    vertebral I65.0- ☑
      with
        infarction I63.21- ☑
          due to
            embolism I63.11- ☑
            thrombosis I63.01- ☑
  basilar artery — *see* Occlusion, artery, basilar
  bile duct (common) (hepatic) (noncalculous) K83.1
  bowel — *see* Obstruction, intestine
  carotid (artery) (common) (internal) — *see* Occlusion,
    artery, carotid
  centric (of teeth) M26.59
    maximum intercuspation discrepancy M26.55
  cerebellar (artery) — *see* Occlusion, artery, cerebellar
  cerebral (artery) — *see* Occlusion, artery, cerebral
  cerebrovascular (*see also* Occlusion, artery, cerebral)
    with infarction I63.5- ☑
  cervical canal — *see* Stricture, cervix
  cervix (uteri) — *see* Stricture, cervix
  choanal Q30.0
  choroidal (artery) — *see* Occlusion, artery, precerebral,
    specified NEC
  colon — *see* Obstruction, intestine
  communicating posterior artery — *see* Occlusion,
    artery, precerebral, specified NEC

Occlusion, occluded — *continued*
  coronary (artery) (vein) (thrombotic) (*see also* Infarct,
    myocardium)
    chronic total I25.82
    healed or old I25.2
    not resulting in infarction I24.0
    total (chronic) I25.82
  cystic duct — *see* Obstruction, gallbladder
  embolic — *see* Embolism
  fallopian tube N97.1
    congenital Q50.6
  gallbladder (*see also* Obstruction, gallbladder)
    congenital (causing jaundice) Q44.1
  gingiva, traumatic K06.2
  hymen N89.6
    congenital Q52.3
  hypophyseal (artery) — *see* Occlusion, artery, precere-
    bral, specified NEC
  iliac artery I74.5
  intestine — *see* Obstruction, intestine
  lacrimal passages — *see* Obstruction, lacrimal
  lung J98.4
  lymph or lymphatic channel I89.0
  mammary duct N64.89
  mesenteric artery (embolic) (thrombotic) (*see also* In-
    farct, intestine) K55.069
  nose J34.89
    congenital Q30.0
  organ or site, congenital NEC — *see* Atresia, by site
  oviduct N97.1
    congenital Q50.6
  peripheral arteries
    due to stricture or stenosis I77.1
    upper extremity I74.2
  pontine (artery) — *see* Occlusion, artery, precerebral,
    specified NEC
  posterior lingual, of mandibular teeth M26.29
  precerebral artery — *see* Occlusion, artery, precerebral
  punctum lacrimale — *see* Obstruction, lacrimal
  pupil — *see* Membrane, pupillary
  pylorus, adult (*see also* Stricture, pylorus) K31.1
  renal artery N28.0
  retina, retinal
    artery — *see* Occlusion, artery, retinal
    vein (central) H34.81- ☑
      engorgement H34.82- ☑
      tributary H34.83- ☑
    vessels H34.9
  spinal artery — *see* Occlusion, artery, precerebral,
    vertebral
  teeth (mandibular) (posterior lingual) M26.29
  thoracic duct I89.0
  thrombotic — *see* Thrombosis, artery
  traumatic
    edentulous (alveolar) ridge K06.2
    gingiva K06.2
    periodontal K05.5
  tubal N97.1
  ureter (complete) (partial) N13.5
    congenital Q62.10
  ureteropelvic junction N13.5
    congenital Q62.11
  ureterovesical orifice N13.5
    congenital Q62.12
  urethra — *see* Stricture, urethra
  uterus N85.8
  vagina N89.5
  vascular NEC I99.8
  vein — *see* Thrombosis
    retinal — *see* Occlusion, retinal, vein
  vena cava (inferior) (superior) — *see* Embolism, vena
    cava
  ventricle (brain) NEC G91.1
  vertebral (artery) — *see* Occlusion, artery, vertebral
  vessel (blood) I99.8
  vulva N90.5
Occult
  blood in feces (stools) R19.5
Occupational
  problems NEC Z56.89
Ochlophobia — *see* Agoraphobia
Ochronosis (endogenous) E70.29
Ocular muscle — *see* condition
Oculogyric crisis or disturbance H51.8
  psychogenic F45.8
Oculomotor syndrome H51.9
Oculopathy
  syphilitic NEC A52.71

Oculopathy — *continued*
  syphilitic — *continued*
    congenital
      early A50.01
        late A50.30
    early (secondary) A51.43
    late A52.71
Oddi's sphincter spasm K83.4
Odontalgia K08.89
Odontoameloblastoma — *see* Cyst, calcifying odontogenic
Odontoclasia K03.89
Odontodysplasia, regional K00.4
Odontogenesis imperfecta K00.5
Odontoma (ameloblastic) (complex) (compound) (fibroameloblastic) — *see* Cyst, calcifying odontogenic
Odontomyelitis (closed) (open) K04.01
  irreversible K04.02
  reversible K04.01
Odontorrhagia K08.89
Odontosarcoma, ameloblastic C41.1
  upper jaw (bone) C41.0
Oestriasis — *see* Myiasis
Oguchi's disease H53.63
Ohara's disease — *see* Tularemia
OHS (obesity hypoventilation syndrome) E66.2
Oidiomycosis — *see* Candidiasis
Oidium albicans infection — *see* Candidiasis
Old age (without mention of debility) R54
  dementia F03 ☑
Old (previous) **myocardial infarction** I25.2
Olfactory — *see* condition
Oligemia — *see* Anemia
Oligoastrocytoma
  specified site — *see* Neoplasm, malignant, by site
  unspecified site C71.9
Oligocythemia D64.9
Oligodendroblastoma
  specified site — *see* Neoplasm, malignant
  unspecified site C71.9
Oligodendroglioma
  anaplastic type
    specified site — *see* Neoplasm, malignant, by site
    unspecified site C71.9
  specified site — *see* Neoplasm, malignant, by site
  unspecified site C71.9
Oligodontia — *see* Anodontia
Oligoencephalon Q02
Oligohidrosis L74.4
Oligohydramnios O41.0- ☑
Oligohydrosis L74.4
Oligomenorrhea N91.5
  primary N91.3
  secondary N91.4
Oligophrenia (*see also* Disability, intellectual)
  phenylpyruvic E70.0
Oligospermia N46.11
  due to
    drug therapy N46.121
    efferent duct obstruction N46.123
    infection N46.122
    radiation N46.124
    specified cause NEC N46.129
    systemic disease N46.125
Oligotrichia — *see* Alopecia
Oliguria R34
  postprocedural N99.0
  with, complicating or following ectopic or molar pregnancy O08.4
Ollier's disease Q78.4
Omenotocele — *see* Hernia, abdomen, specified site NEC
Omentitis — *see* Peritonitis
Omentum, omental — *see* condition
Omphalitis (congenital) (newborn) P38.9
  with mild hemorrhage P38.1
  without hemorrhage P38.9
  not of newborn L08.82
  tetanus A33
Omphalocele Q79.2
Omphalomesenteric duct, persistent Q43.0
Omphalorrhagia, newborn P51.9
Omsk hemorrhagic fever A98.1
Onanism (excessive) F98.8
Onchocerciasis, onchocercosis B73.1
  with
    eye disease B73.00

Onchocerciasis, onchocercosis — *continued*
  with — *continued*
    eye disease — *continued*
      endophthalmitis B73.01
      eyelid B73.09
      glaucoma B73.02
      specified NEC B73.09
    eyelid B73.09
    eye NEC B73.00
Oncocytoma — *see* Neoplasm, benign, by site
Oncovirus, as cause of disease classified elsewhere B97.32
Ondine's curse — *see* Apnea, sleep
Oneirophrenia F23
Onychauxis L60.2
  congenital Q84.5
Onychia (*see also* Cellulitis, digit)
  with lymphangitis — *see* Lymphangitis, acute, digit
  candidal B37.2
  dermatophytic B35.1
Onychitis (*see also* Cellulitis, digit)
  with lymphangitis — *see* Lymphangitis, acute, digit
Onychocryptosis L60.0
Onychodystrophy L60.3
  congenital Q84.6
Onychogryphosis, onychogryposis L60.2
Onycholysis L60.1
Onychomadesis L60.8
Onychomalacia L60.3
Onychomycosis (finger) (toe) B35.1
Onycho-osteodysplasia Q87.2
Onychophagia F98.8
Onychophosis L60.8
Onychoptosis L60.8
Onychorrhexis L60.3
  congenital Q84.6
Onychoschizia L60.3
Onyxis (finger) (toe) L60.0
Onyxitis (*see also* Cellulitis, digit)
  with lymphangitis — *see* Lymphangitis, acute, digit
Oophoritis (cystic) (infectional) (interstitial) N70.92
  with salpingitis N70.93
  acute N70.02
    with salpingitis N70.03
  chronic N70.12
    with salpingitis N70.13
  complicating abortion — *see* Abortion, by type, complicated by, oophoritis
Oophorocele N83.4- ☑
Opacity, opacities
  cornea H17.- ☑
    central H17.1- ☑
    congenital Q13.3
    degenerative — *see* Degeneration, cornea
    hereditary — *see* Dystrophy, cornea
    inflammatory — *see* Keratitis
    minor H17.81- ☑
    peripheral H17.82- ☑
    sequelae of trachoma (healed) B94.0
    specified NEC H17.89
  enamel (teeth) (fluoride) (nonfluoride) K00.3
  lens — *see* Cataract
  snowball — *see* Deposit, crystalline
  vitreous (humor) NEC H43.39- ☑
    congenital Q14.0
    membranes and strands H43.31- ☑
Opalescent dentin (hereditary) K00.5
Open, opening
  abnormal, organ or site, congenital — *see* Imperfect, closure
  angle with
    borderline
      findings
        high risk H40.02- ☑
        low risk H40.01- ☑
      intraocular pressure H40.00- ☑
    cupping of discs H40.01- ☑
    glaucoma (primary) — *see* Glaucoma, open angle
  bite
    anterior M26.220
    posterior M26.221
  false — *see* Imperfect, closure
  margin on tooth restoration K08.51
  restoration margins of tooth K08.51
  wound — *see* Wound, open
Operational fatigue F48.8
Operative — *see* condition

Operculitis — *see* Periodontitis
Operculum — *see* Break, retina
Ophiasis L63.2
Ophthalmia (*see also* Conjunctivitis) H10.9
  actinic rays — *see* Photokeratitis
  allergic (acute) — *see* Conjunctivitis, acute, atopic
  blennorrhagic (gonococcal) (neonatorum) A54.31
  diphtheritic A36.86
  Egyptian A71.1
  electrica — *see* Photokeratitis
  gonococcal (neonatorum) A54.31
  metastatic — *see* Endophthalmitis, purulent
  migraine — *see* Migraine, ophthalmoplegic
  neonatorum, newborn P39.1
    gonococcal A54.31
  nodosa H16.24- ☑
  purulent — *see* Conjunctivitis, acute, mucopurulent
  spring — *see* Conjunctivitis, acute, atopic
  sympathetic — *see* Uveitis, sympathetic
Ophthalmitis — *see* Ophthalmia
Ophthalmocele (congenital) Q15.8
Ophthalmoneuromyelitis G36.0
Ophthalmoplegia (*see also* Strabismus, paralytic)
  anterior internuclear — *see* Ophthalmoplegia, internuclear
  ataxia-areflexia G61.0
  diabetic — *see* E08-E13 with .39
  exophthalmic E05.00
    with thyroid storm E05.01
  external H49.88- ☑
    progressive H49.4- ☑
      with pigmentary retinopathy — *see* Kearns-Sayre syndrome
    total H49.3- ☑
  internal (complete) (total) H52.51- ☑
  internuclear H51.2- ☑
  migraine — *see* Migraine, ophthalmoplegic
  Parinaud's H49.88- ☑
  progressive external — *see* Ophthalmoplegia, external, progressive
  supranuclear, progressive G23.1
  total (external) — *see* Ophthalmoplegia, external, total
Opioid(s)
  abuse — *see* Abuse, drug, opioids
  dependence — *see* Dependence, drug, opioids
  induced, without use disorder
    anxiety disorder F11.988
    delirium F11.921
    depressive disorder F11.94
    sexual dysfunction F11.981
    sleep disorder F11.982
Opisthognathism M26.09
Opisthorchiasis (felineus) (viverrini) B66.0
Opitz' disease D73.2
Opiumism — *see* Dependence, drug, opioid
Oppenheim's disease G70.2
Oppenheim-Urbach disease (necrobiosis lipoidica diabeticorum) — *see* E08-E13 with .620
Optic nerve — *see* condition
Orbit — *see* condition
Orchioblastoma C62.9- ☑
Orchitis (gangrenous) (nonspecific) (septic) (suppurative) N45.2
  blennorrhagic (gonococcal) (acute) (chronic) A54.23
  chlamydial A56.19
  filarial (*see also* Infestation, filarial) B74.9 [N51]
  gonococcal (acute) (chronic) A54.23
  mumps B26.0
  syphilitic A52.76
  tuberculous A18.15
Orf (virus disease) B08.02
Organic (*see also* condition)
  brain syndrome F09
  heart — *see* Disease, heart
  mental disorder F09
  psychosis F09
Orgasm
  anejaculatory N53.13
Oriental
  bilharziasis B65.2
  schistosomiasis B65.2
Orifice — *see* condition
Origin of both great vessels from right ventricle Q20.1
Ormond's disease (with ureteral obstruction) N13.5
  with infection N13.6
Ornithine metabolism disorder E72.4

☑ Additional Character Required — Refer to the Tabular List for Character Selection   ▽ Subterms under main terms may continue to next column or page

Ornithinemia (Type I) (Type II) E72.4
Ornithosis A70
Orotaciduria, oroticaciduria (congenital) (hereditary) (pyrimidine deficiency) E79.8
   anemia D53.0
Orthodontics
   adjustment Z46.4
   fitting Z46.4
Orthopnea R06.01
Orthopoxvirus B08.09
   specified NEC B08.09
Os, uterus — *see* condition
Osgood-Schlatter disease or osteochondrosis — *see* Osteochondrosis, juvenile, tibia
Osler (-Weber)-**Rendu disease** I78.0
Osler's nodes I33.0
Osmidrosis L75.0
Osseous — *see* condition
Ossification
   artery — *see* Arteriosclerosis
   auricle (ear) — *see* Disorder, pinna, specified type NEC
   bronchial J98.09
   cardiac — *see* Degeneration, myocardial
   cartilage (senile) — *see* Disorder, cartilage, specified type NEC
   coronary (artery) — *see* Disease, heart, ischemic, atherosclerotic
   diaphragm J98.6
   ear, middle — *see* Otosclerosis
   falx cerebri G96.19
   fontanel, premature Q75.0
   heart (*see also* Degeneration, myocardial)
      valve — *see* Endocarditis
   larynx J38.7
   ligament — *see* Disorder, tendon, specified type NEC
      posterior longitudinal — *see* Spondylopathy, specified NEC
   meninges (cerebral) (spinal) G96.19
   multiple, eccentric centers — *see* Disorder, bone, development or growth
   muscle (*see also* Calcification, muscle)
      due to burns — *see* Myositis, ossificans, in, burns
      paralytic — *see* Myositis, ossificans, in, quadriplegia
      progressive — *see* Myositis, ossificans, progressiva
      specified NEC M61.50
         ankle M61.57- ☑
         foot M61.57- ☑
         forearm M61.53- ☑
         hand M61.54- ☑
         lower leg M61.56- ☑
         multiple sites M61.59
         pelvic region M61.55- ☑
         shoulder region M61.51- ☑
         specified site NEC M61.58
         thigh M61.55- ☑
         upper arm M61.52- ☑
      traumatic — *see* Myositis, ossificans, traumatica
   myocardium, myocardial — *see* Degeneration, myocardial
   penis N48.89
   periarticular — *see* Disorder, joint, specified type NEC
   pinna — *see* Disorder, pinna, specified type NEC
   rider's bone — *see* Ossification, muscle, specified NEC
   sclera H15.89
   subperiosteal, post-traumatic M89.8X- ☑
   tendon — *see* Disorder, tendon, specified type NEC
   trachea J39.8
   tympanic membrane — *see* Disorder, tympanic membrane, specified NEC
   vitreous (humor) — *see* Deposit, crystalline
Osteitis (*see also* Osteomyelitis)
   alveolar M27.3
   condensans M85.30
      ankle M85.37- ☑
      foot M85.37- ☑
      forearm M85.33- ☑
      hand M85.34- ☑
      lower leg M85.36- ☑
      multiple site M85.39
      neck M85.38
      rib M85.38
      shoulder M85.31- ☑
      skull M85.38
      specified site NEC M85.38
      thigh M85.35- ☑
      toe M85.37- ☑
      upper arm M85.32- ☑

Osteitis — *continued*
   condensans — *continued*
      vertebra M85.38
   deformans M88.9
      in (due to)
         malignant neoplasm of bone C41.9 [M90.60]
         neoplastic disease (*see also* Neoplasm) D49.9 [M90.60]
            carpus D49.9 [M90.64-] ☑
            clavicle D49.9 [M90.61-] ☑
            femur D49.9 [M90.65-] ☑
            fibula D49.9 [M90.66-] ☑
            finger D49.9 [M90.64-] ☑
            humerus D49.9 [M90.62-] ☑
            ilium D49.9 [M90.65-] ☑
            ischium D49.9 [M90.65-] ☑
            metacarpus D49.9 [M90.64-] ☑
            metatarsus D49.9 [M90.67-] ☑
            multiple sites D49.9 [M90.69]
            neck D49.9 [M90.68]
            radius D49.9 [M90.63-] ☑
            rib D49.9 [M90.68]
            scapula D49.9 [M90.61-] ☑
            skull D49.9 [M90.68]
            tarsus D49.9 [M90.67-] ☑
            tibia D49.9 [M90.66-] ☑
            toe D49.9 [M90.67-] ☑
            ulna D49.9 [M90.63-] ☑
            vertebra D49.9 [M90.68]
      skull M88.0
      specified NEC — *see* Paget's disease, bone, by site
      vertebra M88.1
   due to yaws A66.6
   fibrosa NEC — *see* Cyst, bone, by site
      circumscripta — *see* Dysplasia, fibrous, bone NEC
      cystica (generalisata) E21.0
      disseminata Q78.1
      osteoplastica E21.0
   fragilitans Q78.0
   Garr's (sclerosing) — *see* Osteomyelitis, specified type NEC
   jaw (acute) (chronic) (lower) (suppurative) (upper) M27.2
   parathyroid E21.0
   petrous bone (acute) (chronic) — *see* Petrositis
   sclerotic, nonsuppurative — *see* Osteomyelitis, specified type NEC
   tuberculosa A18.09
      cystica D86.89
      multiplex cystoides D86.89
Osteoarthritis M19.90
   ankle M19.07- ☑
   elbow M19.02- ☑
   foot joint M19.07- ☑
   generalized M15.9
      erosive M15.4
      primary M15.0
      specified NEC M15.8
   hand joint M19.04- ☑
      first carpometacarpal joint M18.9
   hip M16.1- ☑
      bilateral M16.0
      due to hip dysplasia (unilateral) M16.3- ☑
         bilateral M16.2
   interphalangeal
      distal (Heberden) M15.1
      proximal (Bouchard) M15.2
   knee M17.1- ☑
      bilateral M17.0
   post-traumatic NEC M19.92
      ankle M19.17- ☑
      elbow M19.12- ☑
      foot joint M19.17- ☑
      hand joint M19.14- ☑
         first carpometacarpal joint M18.3- ☑
            bilateral M18.2
      hip M16.5- ☑
         bilateral M16.4
      knee M17.3- ☑
         bilateral M17.2
      shoulder M19.11- ☑
      wrist M19.13- ☑
   primary M19.91
      ankle M19.07- ☑
      elbow M19.02- ☑
      foot joint M19.07- ☑
      hand joint M19.04- ☑

Osteoarthritis — *continued*
   primary — *continued*
      hand joint — *continued*
         first carpometacarpal joint M18.1- ☑
            bilateral M18.0
      hip M16.1- ☑
         bilateral M16.0
      knee M17.1- ☑
         bilateral M17.0
      shoulder M19.01- ☑
      spine — *see* Spondylosis
      wrist M19.03- ☑
   secondary M19.93
      ankle M19.27- ☑
      elbow M19.22- ☑
      foot joint M19.27- ☑
      hand joint M19.24- ☑
         first carpometacarpal joint M18.5- ☑
            bilateral M18.4
      hip M16.7
         bilateral M16.6
      knee M17.5
         bilateral M17.4
      multiple M15.3
      shoulder M19.21- ☑
      spine — *see* Spondylosis
      wrist M19.23- ☑
   shoulder M19.01- ☑
   spine — *see* Spondylosis
   wrist M19.03- ☑
Osteoarthropathy (hypertrophic) M19.90
   ankle — *see* Osteoarthritis, primary, ankle
   elbow — *see* Osteoarthritis, primary, elbow
   foot joint — *see* Osteoarthritis, primary, foot
   hand joint — *see* Osteoarthritis, primary, hand joint
   knee joint — *see* Osteoarthritis, primary, knee
   multiple site — *see* Osteoarthritis, primary, multiple joint
   pulmonary (*see also* Osteoarthropathy, specified type NEC)
      hypertrophic — *see* Osteoarthropathy, hypertrophic, specified type NEC
   secondary — *see* Osteoarthropathy, specified type NEC
   secondary hypertrophic — *see* Osteoarthropathy, specified type NEC
   shoulder — *see* Osteoarthritis, primary, shoulder
   specified joint NEC — *see* Osteoarthritis, primary, specified joint NEC
   specified type NEC M89.40
      carpus M89.44- ☑
      clavicle M89.41- ☑
      femur M89.45- ☑
      fibula M89.46- ☑
      finger M89.44- ☑
      humerus M89.42- ☑
      ilium M89.459
      ischium M89.459
      metacarpus M89.44- ☑
      metatarsus M89.47- ☑
      multiple sites M89.49
      neck M89.48
      radius M89.43- ☑
      rib M89.48
      scapula M89.41- ☑
      skull M89.48
      tarsus M89.47- ☑
      tibia M89.46- ☑
      toe M89.47- ☑
      ulna M89.43- ☑
      vertebra M89.48
   spine — *see* Spondylosis
   wrist — *see* Osteoarthritis, primary, wrist
Osteoarthrosis (degenerative) (hypertrophic) (joint) (*see also* Osteoarthritis)
   deformans alkaptonurica E70.29 [M36.8]
   erosive M15.4
   generalized M15.9
      primary M15.0
   polyarticular M15.9
   spine — *see* Spondylosis
Osteoblastoma — *see* Neoplasm, bone, benign
   aggressive — *see* Neoplasm, bone, uncertain behavior
Osteochondritis (*see also* Osteochondropathy, by site)
   Brailsford's — *see* Osteochondrosis, juvenile, radius
   dissecans M93.20
      ankle M93.27- ☑

Osteochondritis — *continued*
 dissecans — *continued*
  elbow M93.22- ☑
  foot M93.27- ☑
  hand M93.24- ☑
  hip M93.25- ☑
  knee M93.26- ☑
  multiple sites M93.29
  shoulder joint M93.21- ☑
  specified site NEC M93.28
  wrist M93.23- ☑
 juvenile M92.9
  patellar — *see* Osteochondrosis, juvenile, patella
 syphilitic (congenital) (early) A50.02 [M90.80]
  ankle A50.02 [M90.87-] ☑
  elbow A50.02 [M90.82-] ☑
  foot A50.02 [M90.87-] ☑
  forearm A50.02 [M90.83-] ☑
  hand A50.02 [M90.84-] ☑
  hip A50.02 [M90.85-] ☑
  knee A50.02 [M90.86-] ☑
  multiple sites A50.02 [M90.89]
  shoulder joint A50.02 [M90.81-] ☑
  specified site NEC A50.02 [M90.88]
Osteochondroarthrosis deformans endemica — *see* Disease, Kaschin-Beck
Osteochondrodysplasia Q78.9
 with defects of growth of tubular bones and spine Q77.9
  specified NEC Q77.8
 specified NEC Q78.8
Osteochondrodystrophy E78.9
Osteochondrolysis — *see* Osteochondritis, dissecans
Osteochondroma — *see* Neoplasm, bone, benign
Osteochondromatosis D48.0
 syndrome Q78.4
Osteochondromyxosarcoma — *see* Neoplasm, bone, malignant
Osteochondropathy M93.90
 ankle M93.97- ☑
 elbow M93.92- ☑
 foot M93.97- ☑
 hand M93.94- ☑
 hip M93.95- ☑
 Kienböck's disease of adults M93.1
 knee M93.96- ☑
 multiple joints M93.99
 osteochondritis dissecans — *see* Osteochondritis, dissecans
 osteochondrosis — *see* Osteochondrosis
 shoulder region M93.91- ☑
 slipped upper femoral epiphysis — *see* Slipped, epiphysis, upper femoral
 specified joint NEC M93.98
 specified type NEC M93.80
  ankle M93.87- ☑
  elbow M93.82- ☑
  foot M93.87- ☑
  hand M93.84- ☑
  hip M93.85- ☑
  knee M93.86- ☑
  multiple joints M93.89
  shoulder region M93.81- ☑
  specified joint NEC M93.88
  wrist M93.83- ☑
 syphilitic, congenital
  early A50.02 [M90.80]
  late A50.56 [M90.80]
 wrist M93.93- ☑
Osteochondrosarcoma — *see* Neoplasm, bone, malignant
Osteochondrosis (*see also* Osteochondropathy, by site)
 acetabulum (juvenile) M91.0
 adult — *see* Osteochondropathy, specified type NEC, by site
 astragalus (juvenile) — *see* Osteochondrosis, juvenile, tarsus
 Blount's — *see* Osteochondrosis, juvenile, tibia
 Buchanan's M91.0
 Burns' — *see* Osteochondrosis, juvenile, ulna
 calcaneus (juvenile) — *see* Osteochondrosis, juvenile, tarsus
 capitular epiphysis (femur) (juvenile) — *see* Legg-Calvé-Perthes disease
 carpal (juvenile) (lunate) (scaphoid) — *see* Osteochondrosis, juvenile, hand, carpal lunate
  adult M93.1

Osteochondrosis — *continued*
 coxae juvenilis — *see* Legg-Calvé-Perthes disease
 deformans juvenilis, coxae — *see* Legg-Calvé-Perthes disease
 Diaz's — *see* Osteochondrosis, juvenile, tarsus
 dissecans (knee) (shoulder) — *see* Osteochondritis, dissecans
 femoral capital epiphysis (juvenile) — *see* Legg-Calvé-Perthes disease
 femur (head), juvenile — *see* Legg-Calvé-Perthes disease
 fibula (juvenile) — *see* Osteochondrosis, juvenile, fibula
 foot NEC (juvenile) M92.8
 Freiberg's — *see* Osteochondrosis, juvenile, metatarsus
 Haas' (juvenile) — *see* Osteochondrosis, juvenile, humerus
 Haglund's — *see* Osteochondrosis, juvenile, tarsus
 hip — *see* Legg-Calvé-Perthes disease
 humerus (capitulum) (head) (juvenile) — *see* Osteochondrosis, juvenile, humerus
 ilium, iliac crest (juvenile) M91.0
 ischiopubic synchondrosis M91.0
 Iselin's — *see* Osteochondrosis, juvenile, metatarsus
 juvenile, juvenilis M92.9
  after congenital dislocation of hip reduction — *see* Osteochondrosis, juvenile, hip, specified NEC
  arm — *see* Osteochondrosis, juvenile, upper limb NEC
  capitular epiphysis (femur) — *see* Legg-Calvé-Perthes disease
  clavicle, sternal epiphysis — *see* Osteochondrosis, juvenile, upper limb NEC
  coxae — *see* Legg-Calvé-Perthes disease
  deformans M92.9
  fibula M92.5- ☑
  foot NEC M92.8
  hand M92.20- ☑
   carpal lunate M92.21- ☑
   metacarpal head M92.22- ☑
   specified site NEC M92.29- ☑
  head of femur — *see* Legg-Calvé-Perthes disease
  hip and pelvis M91.9- ☑
   coxa plana — *see* Coxa, plana
   femoral head — *see* Legg-Calvé-Perthes disease
   pelvis M91.0
   pseudocoxalgia — *see* Pseudocoxalgia
   specified NEC M91.8- ☑
  humerus M92.0- ☑
  limb
   lower NEC M92.8
   upper NEC — *see* Osteochondrosis, juvenile, upper limb NEC
  medial cuneiform bone — *see* Osteochondrosis, juvenile, tarsus
  metatarsus M92.7- ☑
  patella M92.4- ☑
  radius M92.1- ☑
  specified site NEC M92.8
  spine M42.00
   cervical region M42.02
   cervicothoracic region M42.03
   lumbar region M42.06
   lumbosacral region M42.07
   multiple sites M42.09
   occipito-atlanto-axial region M42.01
   sacrococcygeal region M42.08
   thoracic region M42.04
   thoracolumbar region M42.05
  tarsus M92.6- ☑
  tibia M92.5- ☑
  ulna M92.1- ☑
  upper limb NEC M92.3- ☑
  vertebra (body) (epiphyseal plates) (Calvé's) (Scheuermann's) — *see* Osteochondrosis, juvenile, spine
 Kienböck's — *see* Osteochondrosis, juvenile, hand, carpal lunate
  adult M93.1
 Köhler's
  patellar — *see* Osteochondrosis, juvenile, patella
  tarsal navicular — *see* Osteochondrosis, juvenile, tarsus
 Legg-Perthes (-Calvé)(-Waldenström) — *see* Legg-Calvé-Perthes disease
 limb
  lower NEC (juvenile) M92.8

Osteochondrosis — *continued*
 limb — *continued*
  upper NEC (juvenile) — *see* Osteochondrosis, juvenile, upper limb NEC
 lunate bone (carpal) (juvenile) (*see also* Osteochondrosis, juvenile, hand, carpal lunate)
  adult M93.1
 Mauclaire's — *see* Osteochondrosis, juvenile, hand, metacarpal
 metacarpal (head) (juvenile) — *see* Osteochondrosis, juvenile, hand, metacarpal
 metatarsus (fifth) (head) (juvenile) (second) — *see* Osteochondrosis, juvenile, metatarsus
 navicular (juvenile) — *see* Osteochondrosis, juvenile, tarsus
 os
  calcis (juvenile) — *see* Osteochondrosis, juvenile, tarsus
  tibiale externum (juvenile) — *see* Osteochondrosis, juvenile, tarsus
 Osgood-Schlatter — *see* Osteochondrosis, juvenile, tibia
 Panner's — *see* Osteochondrosis, juvenile, humerus
 patellar center (juvenile) (primary) (secondary) — *see* Osteochondrosis, juvenile, patella
 pelvis (juvenile) M91.0
 Pierson's M91.0
 radius (head) (juvenile) — *see* Osteochondrosis, juvenile, radius
 Scheuermann's — *see* Osteochondrosis, juvenile, spine
 Sever's — *see* Osteochondrosis, juvenile, tarsus
 Sinding-Larsen — *see* Osteochondrosis, juvenile, patella
 spine M42.9
  adult M42.10
   cervical region M42.12
   cervicothoracic region M42.13
   lumbar region M42.16
   lumbosacral region M42.17
   multiple sites M42.19
   occipito-atlanto-axial region M42.11
   sacrococcygeal region M42.18
   thoracic region M42.14
   thoracolumbar region M42.15
  juvenile — *see* Osteochondrosis, juvenile, spine
 symphysis pubis (juvenile) M91.0
 syphilitic (congenital) A50.02
 talus (juvenile) — *see* Osteochondrosis, juvenile, tarsus
 tarsus (navicular) (juvenile) — *see* Osteochondrosis, juvenile, tarsus
 tibia (proximal) (tubercle) (juvenile) — *see* Osteochondrosis, juvenile, tibia
 tuberculous — *see* Tuberculosis, bone
 ulna (lower) (juvenile) — *see* Osteochondrosis, juvenile, ulna
 van Neck's M91.0
 vertebral — *see* Osteochondrosis, spine
Osteoclastoma D48.0
 malignant — *see* Neoplasm, bone, malignant
Osteodynia — *see* Disorder, bone, specified type NEC
Osteodystrophy Q78.9
 azotemic N25.0
 congenital Q78.9
 parathyroid, secondary E21.1
 renal N25.0
Osteofibroma — *see* Neoplasm, bone, benign
Osteofibrosarcoma — *see* Neoplasm, bone, malignant
Osteogenesis imperfecta Q78.0
Osteogenic — *see* condition
Osteolysis M89.50
 carpus M89.54- ☑
 clavicle M89.51- ☑
 femur M89.55- ☑
 fibula M89.56- ☑
 finger M89.54- ☑
 humerus M89.52- ☑
 ilium M89.559
 ischium M89.559
 joint prosthesis (periprosthetic) — *see* Complications, joint prosthesis, mechanical, periprosthetic, osteolysis, by site
 metacarpus M89.54- ☑
 metatarsus M89.57- ☑
 multiple sites M89.59
 neck M89.58
 periprosthetic — *see* Complications, joint prosthesis, mechanical, periprosthetic, osteolysis, by site

☑ **Additional Character Required — Refer to the Tabular List for Character Selection**   ▼ **Subterms under main terms may continue to next column or page**

Osteolysis — continued
  radius M89.53- ☑
  rib M89.58
  scapula M89.51- ☑
  skull M89.58
  tarsus M89.57- ☑
  tibia M89.56- ☑
  toe M89.57- ☑
  ulna M89.53- ☑
  vertebra M89.58
Osteoma (see also Neoplasm, bone, benign)
  osteoid (see also Neoplasm, bone, benign)
    giant — see Neoplasm, bone, benign
Osteomalacia M83.9
  adult M83.9
    drug-induced NEC M83.5
    due to
      malabsorption (postsurgical) M83.2
      malnutrition M83.3
    specified NEC M83.8
  aluminium-induced M83.4
  infantile — see Rickets
  juvenile — see Rickets
  oncogenic E83.89
  pelvis M83.8
  puerperal M83.0
  senile M83.1
  vitamin-D-resistant in adults E83.31 [M90.8-] ☑
    carpus E83.31 [M90.84-] ☑
    clavicle E83.31 [M90.81-] ☑
    femur E83.31 [M90.85-] ☑
    fibula E83.31 [M90.86-] ☑
    finger E83.31 [M90.84-] ☑
    humerus E83.31 [M90.82-] ☑
    ilium E83.31 [M90.859]
    ischium E83.31 [M90.859]
    metacarpus E83.31 [M90.84-] ☑
    metatarsus E83.31 [M90.87-] ☑
    multiple sites E83.31 [M90.89]
    neck E83.31 [M90.88]
    radius E83.31 [M90.83-] ☑
    rib E83.31 [M90.88]
    scapula E83.31 [M90.819]
    skull E83.31 [M90.88]
    tarsus E83.31 [M90.879]
    tibia E83.31 [M90.869]
    toe E83.31 [M90.879]
    ulna E83.31 [M90.839]
    vertebra E83.31 [M90.88]
Osteomyelitis (general) (infective) (localized) (neonatal)
  (purulent) (septic) (staphylococcal) (streptococcal)
  (suppurative) (with periostitis) M86.9
  acute M86.10
    carpus M86.14- ☑
    clavicle M86.11- ☑
    femur M86.15- ☑
    fibula M86.16- ☑
    finger M86.14- ☑
    hematogenous M86.00
      carpus M86.04- ☑
      clavicle M86.01- ☑
      femur M86.05- ☑
      fibula M86.06- ☑
      finger M86.04- ☑
      humerus M86.02- ☑
      ilium M86.059
      ischium M86.059
      mandible M27.2
      metacarpus M86.04- ☑
      metatarsus M86.07- ☑
      multiple sites M86.09
      neck M86.08
      orbit H05.02- ☑
      petrous bone — see Petrositis
      radius M86.03- ☑
      rib M86.08
      scapula M86.01- ☑
      skull M86.08
      tarsus M86.07- ☑
      tibia M86.06- ☑
      toe M86.07- ☑
      ulna M86.03- ☑
      vertebra — see Osteomyelitis, vertebra
    humerus M86.12- ☑
    ilium M86.159
    ischium M86.159
    mandible M27.2

Osteomyelitis — continued
  acute — continued
    metacarpus M86.14- ☑
    metatarsus M86.17- ☑
    multiple sites M86.19
    neck M86.18
    orbit H05.02- ☑
    petrous bone — see Petrositis
    radius M86.13- ☑
    rib M86.18
    scapula M86.11- ☑
    skull M86.18
    tarsus M86.17- ☑
    tibia M86.16- ☑
    toe M86.17- ☑
    ulna M86.13- ☑
    vertebra — see Osteomyelitis, vertebra
  chronic (or old) M86.60
    with draining sinus M86.40
      carpus M86.44- ☑
      clavicle M86.41- ☑
      femur M86.45- ☑
      fibula M86.46- ☑
      finger M86.44- ☑
      humerus M86.42- ☑
      ilium M86.459
      ischium M86.459
      mandible M27.2
      metacarpus M86.44- ☑
      metatarsus M86.47- ☑
      multiple sites M86.49
      neck M86.48
      orbit H05.02- ☑
      petrous bone — see Petrositis
      radius M86.43- ☑
      rib M86.48
      scapula M86.41- ☑
      skull M86.48
      tarsus M86.47- ☑
      tibia M86.46- ☑
      toe M86.47- ☑
      ulna M86.43- ☑
      vertebra — see Osteomyelitis, vertebra
    carpus M86.64- ☑
    clavicle M86.61- ☑
    femur M86.65- ☑
    fibula M86.66- ☑
    finger M86.64- ☑
    hematogenous NEC M86.50
      carpus M86.54- ☑
      clavicle M86.51- ☑
      femur M86.55- ☑
      fibula M86.56- ☑
      finger M86.54- ☑
      humerus M86.52- ☑
      ilium M86.559
      ischium M86.559
      mandible M27.2
      metacarpus M86.54- ☑
      metatarsus M86.57- ☑
      multifocal M86.30
        carpus M86.34- ☑
        clavicle M86.31- ☑
        femur M86.35- ☑
        fibula M86.36- ☑
        finger M86.34- ☑
        humerus M86.32- ☑
        ilium M86.359
        ischium M86.359
        metacarpus M86.34- ☑
        metatarsus M86.37- ☑
        multiple sites M86.39
        neck M86.38
        radius M86.33- ☑
        rib M86.38
        scapula M86.31- ☑
        skull M86.38
        tarsus M86.37- ☑
        tibia M86.36- ☑
        toe M86.37- ☑
        ulna M86.33- ☑
        vertebra — see Osteomyelitis, vertebra
      multiple sites M86.59
      neck M86.58
      orbit H05.02- ☑
      petrous bone — see Petrositis

Osteomyelitis — continued
  chronic — continued
    hematogenous — continued
      radius M86.53- ☑
      rib M86.58
      scapula M86.51- ☑
      skull M86.58
      tarsus M86.57- ☑
      tibia M86.56- ☑
      toe M86.57- ☑
      ulna M86.53- ☑
      vertebra — see Osteomyelitis, vertebra
    humerus M86.62- ☑
    ilium M86.659
    ischium M86.659
    mandible M27.2
    metacarpus M86.64- ☑
    metatarsus M86.67- ☑
    multifocal — see Osteomyelitis, chronic,
      hematogenous, multifocal
    multiple sites M86.69
    neck M86.68
    orbit H05.02- ☑
    petrous bone — see Petrositis
    radius M86.63- ☑
    rib M86.68
    scapula M86.61- ☑
    skull M86.68
    tarsus M86.67- ☑
    tibia M86.66- ☑
    toe M86.67- ☑
    ulna M86.63- ☑
    vertebra — see Osteomyelitis, vertebra
  echinococcal B67.2
  Garr's — see Osteomyelitis, specified type NEC
  in diabetes mellitus — see E08-E13 with .69
  jaw (acute) (chronic) (lower) (neonatal) (suppurative)
    (upper) M27.2
  nonsuppurating — see Osteomyelitis, specified type
    NEC
  orbit H05.02- ☑
  petrous bone — see Petrositis
  Salmonella (arizonae) (cholerae-suis) (enteritidis) (ty-
    phimurium) A02.24
  sclerosing, nonsuppurative — see Osteomyelitis,
    specified type NEC
  specified type NEC (see also subcategory) M86.8X- ☑
    mandible M27.2
    orbit H05.02- ☑
    petrous bone — see Petrositis
    vertebra — see Osteomyelitis, vertebra
  subacute M86.20
    carpus M86.24- ☑
    clavicle M86.21- ☑
    femur M86.25- ☑
    fibula M86.26- ☑
    finger M86.24- ☑
    humerus M86.22- ☑
    mandible M27.2
    metacarpus M86.24- ☑
    metatarsus M86.27- ☑
    multiple sites M86.29
    neck M86.28
    orbit H05.02- ☑
    petrous bone — see Petrositis
    radius M86.23- ☑
    rib M86.28
    scapula M86.21- ☑
    skull M86.28
    tarsus M86.27- ☑
    tibia M86.26- ☑
    toe M86.27- ☑
    ulna M86.23- ☑
    vertebra — see Osteomyelitis, vertebra
  syphilitic A52.77
    congenital (early) A50.02 [M90.80]
  tuberculous — see Tuberculosis, bone
  typhoid A01.05
  vertebra M46.20
    cervical region M46.22
    cervicothoracic region M46.23
    lumbar region M46.26
    lumbosacral region M46.27
    occipito-atlanto-axial region M46.21
    sacrococcygeal region M46.28
    thoracic region M46.24
    thoracolumbar region M46.25

Index

Osteomyelofibrosis — Osteoporosis

Osteomyelofibrosis D47.4
Osteomyelosclerosis D75.89
Osteonecrosis M87.9
  due to
    drugs — *see* Osteonecrosis, secondary, due to, drugs
    trauma — *see* Osteonecrosis, secondary, due to, trauma
  idiopathic aseptic M87.00
    ankle M87.07- ☑
    carpus M87.03- ☑
    clavicle M87.01- ☑
    femur M87.05- ☑
    fibula M87.06- ☑
    finger M87.04- ☑
    humerus M87.02- ☑
    ilium M87.050
    ischium M87.050
    metacarpus M87.04- ☑
    metatarsus M87.07- ☑
    multiple sites M87.09
    neck M87.08
    pelvis M87.050
    radius M87.03- ☑
    rib M87.08
    scapula M87.01- ☑
    skull M87.08
    tarsus M87.07- ☑
    tibia M87.06- ☑
    toe M87.07- ☑
    ulna M87.03- ☑
    vertebra M87.08
  secondary NEC M87.30
    carpus M87.33- ☑
    clavicle M87.31- ☑
    due to
      drugs M87.10
        carpus M87.13- ☑
        clavicle M87.11- ☑
        femur M87.15- ☑
        fibula M87.16- ☑
        finger M87.14- ☑
        humerus M87.12- ☑
        ilium M87.159
        ischium M87.159
        jaw M87.180
        metacarpus M87.14- ☑
        metatarsus M87.17- ☑
        multiple sites M87.19
        neck M87.18 ☑
        radius M87.13- ☑
        rib M87.18 ☑
        scapula M87.11- ☑
        skull M87.18 ☑
        tarsus M87.17- ☑
        tibia M87.16- ☑
        toe M87.17- ☑
        ulna M87.13- ☑
        vertebra M87.18 ☑
      hemoglobinopathy NEC D58.2 [M90.50]
        carpus D58.2 [M90.54-] ☑
        clavicle D58.2 [M90.51-] ☑
        femur D58.2 [M90.55-] ☑
        fibula D58.2 [M90.56-] ☑
        finger D58.2 [M90.54-] ☑
        humerus D58.2 [M90.52-] ☑
        ilium D58.2 [M90.55-] ☑
        ischium D58.2 [M90.55-] ☑
        metacarpus D58.2 [M90.54-] ☑
        metatarsus D58.2 [M90.57-] ☑
        multiple sites D58.2 [M90.58]
        neck D58.2 [M90.58]
        radius D58.2 [M90.53-] ☑
        rib D58.2 [M90.58]
        scapula D58.2 [M90.51-] ☑
        skull D58.2 [M90.58]
        tarsus D58.2 [M90.57-] ☑
        tibia D58.2 [M90.56-] ☑
        toe D58.2 [M90.57-] ☑
        ulna D58.2 [M90.53-] ☑
        vertebra D58.2 [M90.58]
      trauma (previous) M87.20
        carpus M87.23- ☑
        clavicle M87.21- ☑
        femur M87.25- ☑
        fibula M87.26- ☑

Osteonecrosis — *continued*
  secondary — *continued*
    due to — *continued*
      trauma — *continued*
        finger M87.24- ☑
        humerus M87.22- ☑
        ilium M87.25- ☑
        ischium M87.25- ☑
        metacarpus M87.24- ☑
        metatarsus M87.27- ☑
        multiple sites M87.29
        neck M87.28
        radius M87.23- ☑
        rib M87.28
        scapula M87.21- ☑
        skull M87.28
        tarsus M87.27- ☑
        tibia M87.26- ☑
        toe M87.27- ☑
        ulna M87.23- ☑
        vertebra M87.28
    femur M87.35- ☑
    fibula M87.36- ☑
    finger M87.34- ☑
    humerus M87.32- ☑
    ilium M87.350
    in
      caisson disease T70.3 ☑ [M90.50]
        carpus T70.3 ☑ [M90.54-] ☑
        clavicle T70.3 ☑ [M90.51-] ☑
        femur T70.3 ☑ [M90.55-] ☑
        fibula T70.3 ☑ [M90.56-] ☑
        finger T70.3 ☑ [M90.54-] ☑
        humerus T70.3 ☑ [M90.52-] ☑
        ilium T70.3 ☑ [M90.55-] ☑
        ischium T70.3 ☑ [M90.55-] ☑
        metacarpus T70.3 ☑ [M90.54-] ☑
        metatarsus T70.3 ☑ [M90.57-] ☑
        multiple sites T70.3 ☑ [M90.59]
        neck T70.3 ☑ [M90.58]
        radius T70.3 ☑ [M90.53-] ☑
        rib T70.3 ☑ [M90.58]
        scapula T70.3 ☑ [M90.51-] ☑
        skull T70.3 ☑ [M90.58]
        tarsus T70.3 ☑ [M90.57-] ☑
        tibia T70.3 ☑ [M90.56-] ☑
        toe T70.3 ☑ [M90.57-] ☑
        ulna T70.3 ☑ [M90.53-] ☑
        vertebra T70.3 ☑ [M90.58]
    ischium M87.350
    metacarpus M87.34- ☑
    metatarsus M87.37- ☑
    multiple site M87.39
    neck M87.38
    radius M87.33- ☑
    rib M87.38
    scapula M87.319
    skull M87.38
    tarsus M87.379
    tibia M87.366
    toe M87.379
    ulna M87.33- ☑
    vertebra M87.38
  specified type NEC M87.80
    carpus M87.83- ☑
    clavicle M87.81- ☑
    femur M87.85- ☑
    fibula M87.86- ☑
    finger M87.84- ☑
    humerus M87.82- ☑
    ilium M87.85- ☑
    ischium M87.85- ☑
    metacarpus M87.84- ☑
    metatarsus M87.87- ☑
    multiple sites M87.89
    neck M87.88
    radius M87.83- ☑
    rib M87.88
    scapula M87.81- ☑
    skull M87.88
    tarsus M87.87- ☑
    tibia M87.86- ☑
    toe M87.87- ☑
    ulna M87.83- ☑
    vertebra M87.88
Osteo-onycho-arthro-dysplasia Q87.2

Osteo-onychodysplasia, hereditary Q87.2
Osteopathia condensans disseminata Q78.8
Osteopathy (*see also* Osteomyelitis, Osteonecrosis, Osteoporosis)
  after poliomyelitis M89.60
    carpus M89.64- ☑
    clavicle M89.61- ☑
    femur M89.65- ☑
    fibula M89.66- ☑
    finger M89.64- ☑
    humerus M89.62- ☑
    ilium M89.659
    ischium M89.659
    metacarpus M89.64- ☑
    metatarsus M89.67- ☑
    multiple sites M89.69
    neck M89.68
    radius M89.63- ☑
    rib M89.68
    scapula M89.61- ☑
    skull M89.68
    tarsus M89.67- ☑
    tibia M89.66- ☑
    toe M89.67- ☑
    ulna M89.63- ☑
    vertebra M89.68
  in (due to)
    renal osteodystrophy N25.0
    specified diseases classified elsewhere — *see* subcategory M90.8 ☑
Osteopenia M85.8- ☑
  borderline M85.8- ☑
Osteoperiostitis — *see* Osteomyelitis, specified type NEC
Osteopetrosis (familial) Q78.2
Osteophyte M25.70
  ankle M25.77- ☑
  elbow M25.72- ☑
  foot joint M25.77- ☑
  hand joint M25.74- ☑
  hip M25.75- ☑
  knee M25.76- ☑
  shoulder M25.71- ☑
  spine M25.78
  vertebrae M25.78
  wrist M25.73- ☑
Osteopoikilosis Q78.8
Osteoporosis (female) (male) M81.0
  with current pathological fracture M80.00 ☑
  age-related M81.0
    with current pathologic fracture M80.00 ☑
      carpus M80.04- ☑
      clavicle M80.01- ☑
      fibula M80.06- ☑
      finger M80.04- ☑
      humerus M80.02- ☑
      ilium M80.05- ☑
      ischium M80.05- ☑
      metacarpus M80.04- ☑
      metatarsus M80.07- ☑
      pelvis M80.05- ☑
      radius M80.03- ☑
      scapula M80.01- ☑
      tarsus M80.07- ☑
      tibia M80.06- ☑
      toe M80.07- ☑
      ulna M80.03- ☑
      vertebra M80.08 ☑
  disuse M81.8
    with current pathological fracture M80.80 ☑
      carpus M80.84- ☑
      clavicle M80.81- ☑
      fibula M80.86- ☑
      finger M80.84- ☑
      humerus M80.82- ☑
      ilium M80.85- ☑
      ischium M80.85- ☑
      metacarpus M80.84- ☑
      metatarsus M80.87- ☑
      pelvis M80.85- ☑
      radius M80.83- ☑
      scapula M80.81- ☑
      tarsus M80.87- ☑
      tibia M80.86- ☑
      toe M80.87- ☑
      ulna M80.83- ☑

☑ Additional Character Required — Refer to the Tabular List for Character Selection   ▽ Subterms under main terms may continue to next column or page

Osteoporosis — *continued*
  disuse — *continued*
    with current pathological fracture — *continued*
      vertebra M80.88 ☑
  drug-induced — *see* Osteoporosis, specified type NEC
  idiopathic — *see* Osteoporosis, specified type NEC
  involutional — *see* Osteoporosis, age-related
  Lequesne M81.6
  localized M81.6
  postmenopausal M81.0
    with pathological fracture M80.00 ☑
      carpus M80.04- ☑
      clavicle M80.01- ☑
      fibula M80.06- ☑
      finger M80.04- ☑
      humerus M80.02- ☑
      ilium M80.05- ☑
      ischium M80.05- ☑
      metacarpus M80.04- ☑
      metatarsus M80.07- ☑
      pelvis M80.05- ☑
      radius M80.03- ☑
      scapula M80.01- ☑
      tarsus M80.07- ☑
      tibia M80.06- ☑
      toe M80.07- ☑
      ulna M80.03- ☑
      vertebra M80.08 ☑
  postoophorectomy — *see* Osteoporosis, specified type NEC
  postsurgical malabsorption — *see* Osteoporosis, specified type NEC
  post-traumatic — *see* Osteoporosis, specified type NEC
  senile — *see* Osteoporosis, age-related
  specified type NEC M81.8
    with pathological fracture M80.80 ☑
      carpus M80.84- ☑
      clavicle M80.81- ☑
      fibula M80.86- ☑
      finger M80.84- ☑
      humerus M80.82- ☑
      ilium M80.85- ☑
      ischium M80.85- ☑
      metacarpus M80.84- ☑
      metatarsus M80.87- ☑
      pelvis M80.85- ☑
      radius M80.83- ☑
      scapula M80.81- ☑
      tarsus M80.87- ☑
      tibia M80.86- ☑
      toe M80.87- ☑
      ulna M80.83- ☑
      vertebra M80.88 ☑
Osteopsathyrosis (idiopathica) Q78.0
Osteoradionecrosis, jaw (acute) (chronic) (lower) (suppurative) (upper) M27.2
Osteosarcoma (any form) — *see* Neoplasm, bone, malignant
Osteosclerosis Q78.2
  acquired M85.8- ☑
  congenita Q77.4
  fragilitas (generalisata) Q78.2
  myelofibrosis D75.81
Osteosclerotic anemia D64.89
Osteosis
  cutis L94.2
  renal fibrocystic N25.0
Österreicher-Turner syndrome Q87.2
Ostium
  atrioventriculare commune Q21.2
  primum (arteriosum) (defect) (persistent) Q21.2
  secundum (arteriosum) (defect) (patent) (persistent) Q21.1
Ostrum-Furst syndrome Q75.8
Otalgia H92.0 ☑
Otitis (acute) H66.90
  with effusion (*see also* Otitis, media, nonsuppurative)
    purulent — *see* Otitis, media, suppurative
  adhesive — *see* subcategory H74.1
  chronic (*see also* Otitis, media, chronic)
    with effusion (*see also* Otitis, media, nonsuppurative, chronic)
  externa H60.9- ☑
    abscess — *see* Abscess, ear, external
    acute (noninfective) H60.50- ☑

Otitis — *continued*
  externa — *continued*
    acute — *continued*
      actinic H60.51- ☑
      chemical H60.52- ☑
      contact H60.53- ☑
      eczematoid H60.54- ☑
      infective — *see* Otitis, externa, infective
      reactive H60.55- ☑
      specified NEC H60.59- ☑
    cellulitis — *see* Cellulitis, ear
    chronic H60.6-
    diffuse — *see* Otitis, externa, infective, diffuse
    hemorrhagic — *see* Otitis, externa, infective, hemorrhagic
    in (due to)
      aspergillosis B44.89
      candidiasis B37.84
      erysipelas A46 [H62.40]
      herpes (simplex) virus infection B00.1
        zoster B02.8
      impetigo L01.00 [H62.40]
      infectious disease NEC B99 ☑ [H62.4-] ☑
      mycosis NEC B36.9 [H62.40]
      parasitic disease NEC B89 [H62.40]
      viral disease NEC B34.9 [H62.40]
      zoster B02.8
    infective NEC H60.39- ☑
      abscess — *see* Abscess, ear, external
      cellulitis — *see* Cellulitis, ear
      diffuse H60.31- ☑
      hemorrhagic H60.32- ☑
      swimmer's ear — *see* Swimmer's, ear
    malignant H60.2- ☑
    mycotic NEC B36.9 [H62.40]
      in
        aspergillosis B44.89
        candidiasis B37.84
        moniliasis B37.84
    necrotizing — *see* Otitis, externa, malignant
    Pseudomonas aeruginosa — *see* Otitis, externa, malignant
    reactive — *see* Otitis, externa, acute, reactive
    specified NEC — *see* subcategory H60.8 ☑
    tropical NEC B36.9 [H62.40]
      in
        aspergillosis B44.89
        candidiasis B37.84
        moniliasis B37.84
  insidiosa — *see* Otosclerosis
  interna H83.0 ☑
  media (hemorrhagic) (staphylococcal) (streptococcal) H66.9- ☑
    with effusion (nonpurulent) — *see* Otitis, media, nonsuppurative
    acute, subacute H66.90
      allergic — *see* Otitis, media, nonsuppurative, acute, allergic
      exudative — *see* Otitis, media, suppurative, acute
      mucoid — *see* Otitis, media, nonsuppurative, acute
      necrotizing (*see also* Otitis, media, suppurative, acute)
        in
          measles B05.3
          scarlet fever A38.0
      nonsuppurative NEC — *see* Otitis, media, nonsuppurative, acute
      purulent — *see* Otitis, media, suppurative, acute
      sanguinous — *see* Otitis, media, nonsuppurative, acute
      secretory — *see* Otitis, media, nonsuppurative, acute, serous
      seromucinous — *see* Otitis, media, nonsuppurative, acute
      serous — *see* Otitis, media, nonsuppurative, acute, serous
      suppurative — *see* Otitis, media, suppurative, acute
    allergic — *see* Otitis, media, nonsuppurative
    catarrhal — *see* Otitis, media, nonsuppurative
    chronic H66.90
      with effusion (nonpurulent) — *see* Otitis, media, nonsuppurative, chronic

Otitis — *continued*
  media — *continued*
    chronic — *continued*
      allergic — *see* Otitis, media, nonsuppurative, chronic, allergic
      benign suppurative — *see* Otitis, media, suppurative, chronic, tubotympanic
      catarrhal — *see* Otitis, media, nonsuppurative, chronic, serous
      exudative — *see* Otitis, media, nonsuppurative, chronic
      mucinous — *see* Otitis, media, nonsuppurative, chronic, mucoid
      mucoid — *see* Otitis, media, nonsuppurative, chronic, mucoid
      nonsuppurative NEC — *see* Otitis, media, nonsuppurative, chronic
      purulent — *see* Otitis, media, suppurative, chronic
      secretory — *see* Otitis, media, nonsuppurative, chronic, mucoid
      seromucinous — *see* Otitis, media, nonsuppurative, chronic
      serous — *see* Otitis, media, nonsuppurative, chronic, serous
      suppurative — *see* Otitis, media, suppurative, chronic
      transudative — *see* Otitis, media, nonsuppurative, chronic, mucoid
    exudative — *see* Otitis, media, suppurative
    in (due to) (with)
      influenza — *see* Influenza, with, otitis media
      measles B05.3
      scarlet fever A38.0
      tuberculosis A18.6
      viral disease NEC B34.- ☑ [H67.-] ☑
    mucoid — *see* Otitis, media, nonsuppurative
    nonsuppurative H65.9- ☑
      acute or subacute NEC H65.19- ☑
        allergic H65.11- ☑
          recurrent H65.11- ☑
        recurrent H65.19- ☑
        secretory — *see* Otitis, media, nonsuppurative, serous
        serous H65.0- ☑
          recurrent H65.0- ☑
      chronic H65.49- ☑
        allergic H65.41- ☑
        mucoid H65.3- ☑
        serous H65.2- ☑
    postmeasles B05.3
    purulent — *see* Otitis, media, suppurative
    secretory — *see* Otitis, media, nonsuppurative
    seromucinous — *see* Otitis, media, nonsuppurative
    serous — *see* Otitis, media, nonsuppurative
    suppurative H66.4- ☑
      acute H66.00- ☑
        with rupture of ear drum H66.01- ☑
        recurrent H66.00- ☑
          with rupture of ear drum H66.01- ☑
      chronic (*see also* subcategory) H66.3 ☑
        atticoantral H66.2- ☑
        benign — *see* Otitis, media, suppurative, chronic, tubotympanic
        tubotympanic H66.1- ☑
    transudative — *see* Otitis, media, nonsuppurative
    tuberculous A18.6
Otocephaly Q18.2
Otolith syndrome — *see* subcategory H81.8 ☑
Otomycosis (diffuse) NEC B36.9 [H62.40]
  in
    aspergillosis B44.89
    candidiasis B37.84
    moniliasis B37.84
Otoporosis — *see* Otosclerosis
Otorrhagia (nontraumatic) H92.2- ☑
  traumatic — *code by* Type of injury
Otorrhea H92.1- ☑
  cerebrospinal G96.0
Otosclerosis (general) H80.9- ☑
  cochlear (endosteal) H80.2- ☑
  involving
    otic capsule — *see* Otosclerosis, cochlear
    oval window
      nonobliterative H80.0- ☑
      obliterative H80.1- ☑
    round window — *see* Otosclerosis, cochlear

Otosclerosis — *continued*
  nonobliterative — *see* Otosclerosis, involving, oval window, nonobliterative
  obliterative — *see* Otosclerosis, involving, oval window, obliterative
  specified NEC H80.8- ☑
Otospongiosis — *see* Otosclerosis
Otto's disease or pelvis M24.7
Outcome of delivery Z37.9
  multiple births Z37.9
    all liveborn Z37.50
      quadruplets Z37.52
      quintuplets Z37.53
      sextuplets Z37.54
      specified number NEC Z37.59
      triplets Z37.51
    all stillborn Z37.7
    some liveborn Z37.60
      quadruplets Z37.62
      quintuplets Z37.63
      sextuplets Z37.64
      specified number NEC Z37.69
      triplets Z37.61
  single NEC Z37.9
    liveborn Z37.0
    stillborn Z37.1
  twins NEC Z37.9
    both liveborn Z37.2
    both stillborn Z37.4
    one liveborn, one stillborn Z37.3
Outlet — *see* condition
Ovalocytosis (congenital) (hereditary) — *see* Elliptocytosis
Ovarian — *see* Condition
Ovariocele N83.4- ☑
Ovaritis (cystic) — *see* Oophoritis
Ovary, ovarian (*see also* condition)
  resistant syndrome E28.39
  vein syndrome N13.8
Overactive (*see also* Hyperfunction)
  adrenal cortex NEC E27.0
  bladder N32.81
  hypothalamus E23.3
  thyroid — *see* Hyperthyroidism
Overactivity R46.3
  child — *see* Disorder, attention-deficit hyperactivity
Overbite (deep) (excessive) (horizontal) (vertical) M26.29
Overbreathing — *see* Hyperventilation
Overconscientious personality F60.5
Overdevelopment — *see* Hypertrophy
Overdistension — *see* Distension
Overdose, overdosage (drug) — *see* Table of Drugs and Chemicals, by drug, poisoning
Overeating R63.2
  nonorganic origin F50.89
  psychogenic F50.89
Overexertion (effects) (exhaustion) T73.3 ☑
Overexposure (effects) T73.9 ☑
  exhaustion T73.2 ☑
Overfeeding — *see* Overeating
  newborn P92.4
Overfill, endodontic M27.52
Overgrowth, bone — *see* Hypertrophy, bone
Overhanging of dental restorative material (unrepairable) K08.52
Overheated (places) (effects) — *see* Heat
Overjet (excessive horizontal) M26.23
Overlaid, overlying (suffocation) — *see* Asphyxia, traumatic, due to mechanical threat
Overlap, excessive horizontal (teeth) M26.23
Overlapping toe (acquired) (*see also* Deformity, toe, specified NEC)
  congenital (fifth toe) Q66.89
Overload
  circulatory, due to transfusion (blood) (blood components) (TACO) E87.71
  fluid E87.70
    due to transfusion (blood) (blood components) E87.71
    specified NEC E87.79
  iron, due to repeated red blood cell transfusions E83.111
  potassium (K) E87.5
  sodium (Na) E87.0
Overnutrition — *see* Hyperalimentation
Overproduction (*see also* Hypersecretion)
  ACTH E27.0

Overproduction — *continued*
  catecholamine E27.5
  growth hormone E22.0
Overprotection, child by parent Z62.1
Overriding
  aorta Q25.49
  finger (acquired) — *see* Deformity, finger
    congenital Q68.1
  toe (acquired) (*see also* Deformity, toe, specified NEC)
    congenital Q66.89
Overstrained R53.83
  heart — *see* Hypertrophy, cardiac
Overuse, muscle NEC M70.8- ☑
Overweight E66.3
Overworked R53.83
Oviduct — *see* condition
Ovotestis Q56.0
Ovulation (cycle)
  failure or lack of N97.0
  pain N94.0
Ovum — *see* condition
Owren's disease or syndrome (parahemophilia) D68.2
Ox heart — *see* Hypertrophy, cardiac
Oxalosis E72.53
Oxaluria E72.53
Oxycephaly, oxycephalic Q75.0
  syphilitic, congenital A50.02
Oxyuriasis B80
Oxyuris vermicularis (infestation) B80
Ozena J31.0

P

Pachyderma, pachydermia L85.9
  larynx (verrucosa) J38.7
Pachydermatocele (congenital) Q82.8
Pachydermoperiostosis (*see also* Osteoarthropathy, hypertrophic, specified type NEC)
  clubbed nail M89.40 [L62]
Pachygyria Q04.3
Pachymeningitis (adhesive) (basal) (brain) (cervical) (chronic)(circumscribed) (external) (fibrous) (hemorrhagic) (hypertrophic) (internal) (purulent) (spinal) (suppurative) — *see* Meningitis
Pachyonychia (congenital) Q84.5
Pacinian tumor — *see* Neoplasm, skin, benign
Pad, knuckle or Garrod's M72.1
Paget's disease
  with infiltrating duct carcinoma — *see* Neoplasm, breast, malignant
  bone M88.9
    carpus M88.84- ☑
    clavicle M88.81- ☑
    femur M88.85- ☑
    fibula M88.86- ☑
    finger M88.84- ☑
    humerus M88.82- ☑
    ilium M88.85- ☑
    in neoplastic disease — *see* Osteitis, deformans, in neoplastic disease
    ischium M88.85- ☑
    metacarpus M88.84- ☑
    metatarsus M88.87- ☑
    multiple sites M88.89
    neck M88.88
    radius M88.83- ☑
    rib M88.88
    scapula M88.81- ☑
    skull M88.0
    tarsus M88.87- ☑
    tibia M88.86- ☑
    toe M88.87- ☑
    ulna M88.83- ☑
    vertebra M88.88
  breast (female) C50.01- ☑
    male C50.02- ☑
  extramammary (*see also* Neoplasm, skin, malignant)
    anus C21.0
      margin C44.590
      skin C44.590
  intraductal carcinoma — *see* Neoplasm, breast, malignant
  malignant — *see* Neoplasm, skin, malignant
    breast (female) C50.01- ☑
      male C50.02- ☑
    unspecified site (female) C50.01- ☑
      male C50.02- ☑

Paget's disease — *continued*
  mammary — *see* Paget's disease, breast
  nipple — *see* Paget's disease, breast
  osteitis deformans — *see* Paget's disease, bone
Paget-Schroetter syndrome I82.890
Pain(s) (*see also* Painful) R52
  abdominal R10.9
    colic R10.83
    generalized R10.84
      with acute abdomen R10.0
    lower R10.30
      left quadrant R10.32
      pelvic or perineal R10.2
      periumbilical R10.33
      right quadrant R10.31
    rebound — *see* Tenderness, abdominal, rebound
    severe with abdominal rigidity R10.0
    tenderness — *see* Tenderness, abdominal
    upper R10.10
      epigastric R10.13
      left quadrant R10.12
      right quadrant R10.11
  acute R52
    due to trauma G89.11
    neoplasm related G89.3
    postprocedural NEC G89.18
    post-thoracotomy G89.12
    specified by site — *code to* Pain, by site
  adnexa (uteri) R10.2
  anginoid — *see* Pain, precordial
  anus K62.89
  arm — *see* Pain, limb, upper
  axillary (axilla) M79.62- ☑
  back (postural) M54.9
  bladder R39.89
    associated with micturition — *see* Micturition, painful
    chronic R39.82
  bone — *see* Disorder, bone, specified type NEC
  breast N64.4
  broad ligament R10.2
  cancer associated (acute) (chronic) G89.3
  cecum — *see* Pain, abdominal
  cervicobrachial M53.1
  chest (central) R07.9
    anterior wall R07.89
    atypical R07.89
    ischemic I20.9
    musculoskeletal R07.89
    non-cardiac R07.89
    on breathing R07.1
    pleurodynia R07.81
    precordial R07.2
    wall (anterior) R07.89
  chronic G89.29
    associated with significant psychosocial dysfunction G89.4
    due to trauma G89.21
    neoplasm related G89.3
    postoperative NEC G89.28
    postprocedural NEC G89.28
    post-thoracotomy G89.22
    specified NEC G89.29
  coccyx M53.3
  colon — *see* Pain, abdominal
  coronary — *see* Angina
  costochondral R07.1
  diaphragm R07.1
  due to cancer G89.3
  due to device, implant or graft (*see also* Complications, by site and type, specified NEC) T85.848 ☑
    arterial graft NEC T82.848 ☑
    breast (implant) T85.848 ☑
    catheter NEC T85.848 ☑
      dialysis (renal) T82.848 ☑
        intraperitoneal T85.848 ☑
      infusion NEC T82.848 ☑
        spinal (epidural) (subdural) T85.840 ☑
      urinary (indwelling) T83.84 ☑
    electronic (electrode) (pulse generator) (stimulator)
      bone T85.840 ☑
      cardiac T82.847 ☑
      nervous system (brain) (peripheral nerve) (spinal) T85.84 ☑
      urinary T83.84 ☑
    fixation, internal (orthopedic) NEC T84.84 ☑
    gastrointestinal (bile duct) (esophagus) T85.848 ☑
    genital NEC T83.84 ☑

Pain(s) — *continued*
due to device, implant or graft (*see also* Complications, by site and type, specified) — *continued*
  heart NEC T82.847 ☑
  infusion NEC T85.848 ☑
  joint prosthesis T84.84 ☑
  ocular (corneal graft) (orbital implant) NEC T85.848 ☑
  orthopedic NEC T84.84 ☑
  specified NEC T85.848 ☑
  urinary NEC T83.84 ☑
  vascular NEC T82.848 ☑
  ventricular intracranial shunt T85.840 ☑
due to malignancy (primary) (secondary) G89.3
ear — *see* subcategory H92.0 ☑
epigastric, epigastrium R10.13
eye — *see* Pain, ocular
face, facial R51
  atypical G50.1
female genital organs NEC N94.89
finger — *see* Pain, limb, upper
flank — *see* Pain, abdominal
foot — *see* Pain, limb, lower
gallbladder K82.9
gas (intestinal) R14.1
gastric — *see* Pain, abdominal
generalized NOS R52
genital organ
  female N94.89
  male N50.89
groin — *see* Pain, abdominal, lower
hand — *see* Pain, limb, upper
head — *see* Headache
heart — *see* Pain, precordial
infra-orbital — *see* Neuralgia, trigeminal
intercostal R07.82
intermenstrual N94.0
jaw R68.84
joint M25.50
  ankle M25.57- ☑
  elbow M25.52- ☑
  finger M25.54- ☑
  foot M25.57- ☑
  hand M25.54- ☑
  hip M25.55- ☑
  knee M25.56- ☑
  shoulder M25.51- ☑
  toe M25.57- ☑
  wrist M25.53- ☑
kidney N23
laryngeal R07.0
leg — *see* Pain, limb, lower
limb M79.609
  lower M79.60- ☑
   foot M79.67- ☑
   lower leg M79.66- ☑
   thigh M79.65- ☑
   toe M79.67- ☑
  upper M79.60- ☑
   axilla M79.62- ☑
   finger M79.64- ☑
   forearm M79.63- ☑
   hand M79.64- ☑
   upper arm M79.62- ☑
loin M54.5
low back M54.5
lumbar region M54.5
mandibular R68.84
mastoid — *see* subcategory H92.0 ☑
maxilla R68.84
menstrual (*see also* Dysmenorrhea) N94.6
metacarpophalangeal (joint) — *see* Pain, joint, hand
metatarsophalangeal (joint) — *see* Pain, joint, foot
mouth K13.79
muscle — *see* Myalgia
musculoskeletal (*see also* Pain, by site) M79.1
myofascial M79.1
nasal J34.89
nasopharynx J39.2
neck NEC M54.2
nerve NEC — *see* Neuralgia
neuromuscular — *see* Neuralgia
nose J34.89
ocular H57.1- ☑
ophthalmic — *see* Pain, ocular
orbital region — *see* Pain, ocular
ovary N94.89

Pain(s) — *continued*
over heart — *see* Pain, precordial
ovulation N94.0
pelvic (female) R10.2
penis N48.89
pericardial — *see* Pain, precordial
perineal, perineum R10.2
pharynx J39.2
pleura, pleural, pleuritic R07.81
postoperative NOS G89.18
postprocedural NOS G89.18
post-thoracotomy G89.12
precordial (region) R07.2
premenstrual N94.3
psychogenic (persistent) (any site) F45.41
radicular (spinal) — *see* Radiculopathy
rectum K62.89
respiration R07.1
retrosternal R07.2
rheumatoid, muscular — *see* Myalgia
rib R07.81
root (spinal) — *see* Radiculopathy
round ligament (stretch) R10.2
sacroiliac M53.3
sciatic — *see* Sciatica
scrotum N50.82
seminal vesicle N50.89
shoulder M25.51- ☑
spermatic cord N50.89
spinal root — *see* Radiculopathy
spine M54.9
  cervical M54.2
  low back M54.5
   with sciatica M54.4- ☑
  thoracic M54.6
stomach — *see* Pain, abdominal
substernal R07.2
temporomandibular (joint) M26.62- ☑
testis N50.81- ☑
thoracic spine M54.6
  with radicular and visceral pain M54.14
throat R07.0
tibia — *see* Pain, limb, lower
toe — *see* Pain, limb, lower
tongue K14.6
tooth K08.89
trigeminal — *see* Neuralgia, trigeminal
tumor associated G89.3
ureter N23
urinary (organ) (system) N23
uterus NEC N94.89
vagina R10.2
vertebrogenic (syndrome) M54.89
vesical R39.89
  associated with micturition — *see* Micturition, painful
vulva R10.2
Painful (*see also* Pain)
coitus
  female N94.10
  male N53.12
  psychogenic F52.6
ejaculation (semen) N53.12
  psychogenic F52.6
erection — *see* Priapism
feet syndrome E53.8
joint replacement (hip) (knee) T84.84 ☑
menstruation — *see* Dysmenorrhea
  psychogenic F45.8
micturition — *see* Micturition, painful
respiration R07.1
scar NEC L90.5
wire sutures T81.89 ☑
Painter's colic — *see* subcategory T56.0 ☑
Palate — *see* condition
Palatoplegia K13.79
Palatoschisis — *see* Cleft, palate
Palilalia R48.8
Palliative care Z51.5
Pallor R23.1
optic disc, temporal — *see* Atrophy, optic
Palmar (*see also* condition)
fascia — *see* condition
Palpable
cecum K63.89
kidney N28.89
ovary N83.8
prostate N42.9

Palpable — *continued*
spleen — *see* Splenomegaly
Palpitations (heart) R00.2
psychogenic F45.8
Palsy (*see also* Paralysis) G83.9
atrophic diffuse (progressive) G12.22
Bell's (*see also* Palsy, facial)
  newborn P11.3
brachial plexus NEC G54.0
  newborn (birth injury) P14.3
brain — *see* Palsy, cerebral
bulbar (progressive) (chronic) G12.22
  of childhood (Fazio-Londe) G12.1
  pseudo NEC G12.29
  supranuclear (progressive) G23.1
cerebral (congenital) G80.9
  ataxic G80.4
  athetoid G80.3
  choreathetoid G80.3
  diplegic G80.8
   spastic G80.1
  dyskinetic G80.3
   athetoid G80.3
   choreathetoid G80.3
   distonic G80.3
  dystonic G80.3
  hemiplegic G80.8
   spastic G80.2
  mixed G80.8
  monoplegic G80.8
   spastic G80.1
  paraplegic G80.8
   spastic G80.1
  quadriplegic G80.8
   spastic G80.0
  spastic G80.1
   diplegic G80.1
   hemiplegic G80.2
   monoplegic G80.1
   quadriplegic G80.0
   specified NEC G80.1
   tetrapelgic G80.0
  specified NEC G80.8
  syphilitic A52.12
   congenital A50.49
  tetraplegic G80.8
   spastic G80.0
cranial nerve (*see also* Disorder, nerve, cranial)
  multiple G52.7
   in
    infectious disease B99 ☑ [G53]
    neoplastic disease (*see also* Neoplasm) D49.9 [G53]
    parasitic disease B89 [G53]
    sarcoidosis D86.82
creeping G12.22
diver's T70.3 ☑
Erb's P14.0
facial G51.0
  newborn (birth injury) P11.3
glossopharyngeal G52.1
Klumpke (-Déjérine) P14.1
lead — *see* subcategory T56.0 ☑
median nerve (tardy) G56.1- ☑
nerve G58.9
  specified NEC G58.8
peroneal nerve (acute) G57.3- ☑
progressive supranuclear G23.1
pseudobulbar NEC G12.29
radial nerve (acute) G56.3- ☑
seventh nerve (*see also* Palsy, facial)
  newborn P11.3
shaking — *see* Parkinsonism
spastic (cerebral) (spinal) G80.1
ulnar nerve (tardy) G56.2- ☑
wasting G12.29
Paludism — *see* Malaria
Panangiitis M30.0
Panaris, panaritium (*see also* Cellulitis, digit)
with lymphangitis — *see* Lymphangitis, acute, digit
Panarteritis nodosa M30.0
brain or cerebral I67.7
Pancake heart R93.1
with cor pulmonale (chronic) I27.81
Pancarditis (acute) (chronic) I51.89
rheumatic I09.89
  active or acute I01.8
Pancoast's syndrome or tumor C34.1- ☑

Pancolitis, ulcerative (chronic) K51.00
  with
    abscess K51.014
    complication K51.019
    fistula K51.013
    obstruction K51.012
    rectal bleeding K51.011
    specified complication NEC K51.018
Pancreas, pancreatic — see condition
Pancreatitis (annular) (apoplectic) (calcareous) (edematous) (hemorrhagic) (malignant) (recurrent) (subacute) (suppurative) K85.90
  with necrosis (uninfected) K85.91
    infected K85.92
  acute (without necrosis or infection) K85.90
    with necrosis (uninfected) K85.91
      infected K85.92
    alcohol induced (without necrosis or infection) K85.20
      with necrosis (uninfected) K85.21
        infected K85.22
    biliary (without necrosis or infection) K85.10
      with necrosis (uninfected) K85.11
        infected K85.12
    drug induced (without necrosis or infection) K85.30
      with necrosis (uninfected) K85.31
        infected K85.32
    gallstone (without necrosis or infection) K85.10
      with necrosis (uninfected) K85.11
        infected K85.12
    idiopathic (without necrosis or infection) K85.00
      with necrosis (uninfected) K85.01
        infected K85.02
    specified NEC (without necrosis or infection) K85.80
      with necrosis (uninfected) K85.81
        infected K85.82
  chronic (infectious) K86.1
    alcohol-induced K86.0
    recurrent K86.1
    relapsing K86.1
  cystic (chronic) K86.1
  cytomegaloviral B25.2
  fibrous (chronic) K86.1
  gallstone (without necrosis or infection) K85.10
    with necrosis (uninfected) K85.11
      infected K85.12
  gangrenous — see Pancreatitis, acute
  interstitial (chronic) K86.1
    acute (see also Pancreatitis, acute) K85.80
  mumps B26.3
  recurrent (chronic) K86.1
  relapsing, chronic K86.1
  syphilitic A52.74
Pancreatoblastoma — see Neoplasm, pancreas, malignant
Pancreolithiasis K86.89
Pancytolysis D75.89
Pancytopenia (acquired) D61.818
  with
    malformations D61.09
    myelodysplastic syndrome — see Syndrome, myelodysplastic
  antineoplastic chemotherapy induced D61.810
  congenital D61.09
  drug-induced NEC D61.811
PANDAS (pediatric autoimmune neuropsychiatric disorders associated with streptococcal infections syndrome) D89.89
Panencephalitis, subacute, sclerosing A81.1
Panhematopenia D61.9
  congenital D61.09
  constitutional D61.09
  splenic, primary D73.1
Panhemocytopenia D61.9
  congenital D61.09
  constitutional D61.09
Panhypogonadism E29.1
Panhypopituitarism E23.0
  prepubertal E23.0
Panic (attack) (state) F41.0
  reaction to exceptional stress (transient) F43.0
Panmyelopathy, familial, constitutional D61.09
Panmyelophthisis D61.82
  congenital D61.09
Panmyelosis (acute) (with myelofibrosis) C94.4- ☑
Panner's disease — see Osteochondrosis, juvenile, humerus
Panneuritis endemica E51.11

Panniculitis (nodular) (nonsuppurative) M79.3
  back M54.00
    cervical region M54.02
    cervicothoracic region M54.03
    lumbar region M54.06
    lumbosacral region M54.07
    multiple sites M54.09
    occipito-atlanto-axial region M54.01
    sacrococcygeal region M54.08
    thoracic region M54.04
    thoracolumbar region M54.05
  lupus L93.2
  mesenteric K65.4
  neck M54.02
    cervicothoracic region M54.03
    occipito-atlanto-axial region M54.01
  relapsing M35.6
Panniculus adiposus (abdominal) E65
Pannus (allergic) (cornea) (degenerativus) (keratic) H16.42- ☑
  abdominal (symptomatic) E65
  trachomatosus, trachomatous (active) A71.1
Panophthalmitis H44.01- ☑
Pansinusitis (chronic) (hyperplastic) (nonpurulent) (purulent) J32.4
  acute J01.40
    recurrent J01.41
  tuberculous A15.8
Panuveitis (sympathetic) H44.11- ☑
Panvalvular disease I08.9
  specified NEC I08.8
PAPA (pyogenic arthritis, pyoderma gangrenosum, and acne syndrome) M04.8
Papanicolaou smear, cervix Z12.4
  as part of routine gynecological examination Z01.419
    with abnormal findings Z01.411
  for suspected neoplasm Z12.4
  nonspecific abnormal finding R87.619
  routine Z01.419
    with abnormal findings Z01.411
Papilledema (choked disc) H47.10
  associated with
    decreased ocular pressure H47.12
    increased intracranial pressure H47.11
    retinal disorder H47.13
  Foster-Kennedy syndrome H47.14- ☑
Papillitis H46.00
  anus K62.89
  chronic lingual K14.4
  necrotizing, kidney N17.2
  optic H46.0- ☑
  rectum K62.89
  renal, necrotizing N17.2
  tongue K14.0
Papilloma (see also Neoplasm, benign, by site)
  acuminatum (female) (male) (anogenital) A63.0
  basal cell L82.1
    inflamed L82.0
  benign pinta (primary) A67.0
  bladder (urinary) (transitional cell) D41.4
  choroid plexus (lateral ventricle) (third ventricle) D33.0
    anaplastic C71.5
    fourth ventricle D33.1
    malignant C71.5
  renal pelvis (transitional cell) D41.1- ☑
    benign D30.1- ☑
  Schneiderian
    specified site — see Neoplasm, benign, by site
    unspecified site D14.0
  serous surface
    borderline malignancy
      specified site — see Neoplasm, uncertain behavior, by site
      unspecified site D39.10
    specified site — see Neoplasm, benign, by site
    unspecified site D27.9
  transitional (cell)
    bladder (urinary) D41.4
    inverted type — see Neoplasm, uncertain behavior, by site
    renal pelvis D41.1- ☑
    ureter D41.2- ☑
  ureter (transitional cell) D41.2- ☑
    benign D30.2- ☑
  urothelial — see Neoplasm, uncertain behavior, by site
  villous — see Neoplasm, uncertain behavior, by site

Papilloma — continued
  villous — see Neoplasm, uncertain behavior, by site — continued
    adenocarcinoma in — see Neoplasm, malignant, by site
    in situ — see Neoplasm, in situ
  yaws, plantar or palmar A66.1
Papillomata, multiple, of yaws A66.1
Papillomatosis (see also Neoplasm, benign, by site)
  confluent and reticulated L83
  cystic, breast — see Mastopathy, cystic
  ductal, breast — see Mastopathy, cystic
  intraductal (diffuse) — see Neoplasm, benign, by site
  subareolar duct D24- ☑
Papillomavirus, as cause of disease classified elsewhere B97.7
Papillon-Léage and Psaume syndrome Q87.0
Papule(s) R23.8
  carate (primary) A67.0
  fibrous, of nose D22.39
  Gottron's L94.4
  pinta (primary) A67.0
Papulosis
  lymphomatoid C86.6
  malignant I77.89
Papyraceous fetus O31.0- ☑
Para-albuminemia E88.09
Paracephalus Q89.7
Parachute mitral valve Q23.2
Paracoccidioidomycosis B41.9
  disseminated B41.7
  generalized B41.7
  mucocutaneous-lymphangitic B41.8
  pulmonary B41.0
  specified NEC B41.8
  visceral B41.8
Paradentosis K05.4
Paraffinoma T88.8 ☑
Paraganglioma D44.7
  adrenal D35.0- ☑
    malignant C74.1- ☑
  aortic body D44.7
    malignant C75.5
  carotid body D44.6
    malignant C75.4
  chromaffin (see also Neoplasm, benign, by site)
    malignant — see Neoplasm, malignant, by site
  extra-adrenal D44.7
    malignant C75.5
      specified site — see Neoplasm, malignant, by site
      unspecified site C75.5
    specified site — see Neoplasm, uncertain behavior, by site
    unspecified site D44.7
  gangliocytic D13.2
    specified site — see Neoplasm, benign, by site
    unspecified site D13.2
  glomus jugulare D44.7
    malignant C75.5
  jugular D44.7
  malignant C75.5
    specified site — see Neoplasm, malignant, by site
    unspecified site C75.5
  nonchromaffin D44.7
    malignant C75.5
      specified site — see Neoplasm, malignant, by site
      unspecified site C75.5
    specified site — see Neoplasm, uncertain behavior, by site
    unspecified site D44.7
  parasympathetic D44.7
    specified site — see Neoplasm, uncertain behavior, by site
    unspecified site D44.7
  specified site — see Neoplasm, uncertain behavior, by site
  sympathetic D44.7
    specified site — see Neoplasm, uncertain behavior, by site
    unspecified site D44.7
  unspecified site D44.7
Parageusia R43.2
  psychogenic F45.8
Paragonimiasis B66.4

☑ Additional Character Required — Refer to the Tabular List for Character Selection ▽ Subterms under main terms may continue to next column or page

Paragranuloma, Hodgkin — *see* Lymphoma, Hodgkin, specified NEC
Parahemophilia (*see also* Defect, coagulation) D68.2
Parakeratosis R23.4
  variegata L41.0
Paralysis, paralytic (complete) (incomplete) G83.9
  with
    syphilis A52.17
  abducens, abducent (nerve) — *see* Strabismus, paralytic, sixth nerve
  abductor, lower extremity G57.9- ☑
  accessory nerve G52.8
  accommodation (*see also* Paresis, of accommodation)
    hysterical F44.89
  acoustic nerve (except Deafness) H93.3 ☑
  agitans (*see also* Parkinsonism) G20
    arteriosclerotic G21.4
  alternating (oculomotor) G83.89
  amyotrophic G12.21
  ankle G57.9- ☑
  anus (sphincter) K62.89
  arm — *see* Monoplegia, upper limb
  ascending (spinal), acute G61.0
  association G12.29
  asthenic bulbar G70.00
    with exacerbation (acute) G70.01
    in crisis G70.01
  ataxic (hereditary) G11.9
    general (syphilitic) A52.17
  atrophic G58.9
    infantile, acute — *see* Poliomyelitis, paralytic
    progressive G12.22
    spinal (acute) — *see* Poliomyelitis, paralytic
  axillary G54.0
  Babinski-Nageotte's G83.89
  Bell's G51.0
    newborn P11.3
  Benedikt's G46.3
  birth injury P14.9
    spinal cord P11.5
  bladder (neurogenic) (sphincter) N31.2
  bowel, colon or intestine K56.0
  brachial plexus G54.0
    birth injury P14.3
    newborn (birth injury) P14.3
  brain G83.9
    diplegia G83.0
    triplegia G83.89
  bronchial J98.09
  Brown-Séquard G83.81
  bulbar (chronic) (progressive) G12.22
    infantile — *see* Poliomyelitis, paralytic
    poliomyelitic — *see* Poliomyelitis, paralytic
    pseudo G12.29
  bulbospinal G70.00
    with exacerbation (acute) G70.01
    in crisis G70.01
  cardiac (*see also* Failure, heart) I50.9
  cerebrocerebellar, diplegic G80.1
  cervical
    plexus G54.2
    sympathetic G90.09
  Céstan-Chenais G46.3
  Charcot-Marie-Tooth type G60.0
  Clark's G80.9
  colon K56.0
  compressed air T70.3 ☑
  compression
    arm G56.9- ☑
    leg G57.9- ☑
    lower extremity G57.9- ☑
    upper extremity G56.9- ☑
  congenital (cerebral) — *see* Palsy, cerebral
  conjugate movement (gaze) (of eye) H51.0
    cortical (nuclear) (supranuclear) H51.0
  cordis — *see* Failure, heart
  cranial or cerebral nerve G52.9
  creeping G12.22
  crossed leg G83.89
  crutch — *see* Injury, brachial plexus
  deglutition R13.0
    hysterical F44.4
  dementia A52.17
  descending (spinal) NEC G12.29
  diaphragm (flaccid) J98.6
    due to accidental dissection of phrenic nerve during procedure — *see* Puncture, accidental complicating surgery

Paralysis, paralytic — *continued*
  digestive organs NEC K59.8
  diplegic — *see* Diplegia
  divergence (nuclear) H51.8
  diver's T70.3 ☑
  Duchenne's
    birth injury P14.0
    due to or associated with
      motor neuron disease G12.22
      muscular dystrophy G71.0
  due to intracranial or spinal birth injury — *see* Palsy, cerebral
  embolic (current episode) I63.4- ☑
  Erb (-Duchenne) (birth) (newborn) P14.0
  Erb's syphilitic spastic spinal A52.17
  esophagus K22.8
  eye muscle (extrinsic) H49.9
    intrinsic (*see also* Paresis, of accommodation)
  facial (nerve) G51.0
    birth injury P11.3
    congenital P11.3
    following operation NEC — *see* Puncture, accidental complicating surgery
    newborn (birth injury) P11.3
  familial (recurrent) (periodic) G72.3
    spastic G11.4
  fauces J39.2
  finger G56.9- ☑
  gait R26.1
  gastric nerve (nondiabetic) G52.2
  gaze, conjugate H51.0
  general (progressive) (syphilitic) A52.17
    juvenile A50.45
  glottis J38.00
    bilateral J38.02
    unilateral J38.01
  gluteal G54.1
  Gubler (-Millard) G46.3
  hand — *see* Monoplegia, upper limb
  heart — *see* Arrest, cardiac
  hemiplegic — *see* Hemiplegia
  hyperkalemic periodic (familial) G72.3
  hypoglossal (nerve) G52.3
  hypokalemic periodic G72.3
  hysterical F44.4
  ileus K56.0
  infantile (*see also* Poliomyelitis, paralytic) A80.30
    bulbar — *see* Poliomyelitis, paralytic
    cerebral — *see* Palsy, cerebral
    spastic — *see* Palsy, cerebral, spastic
  infective — *see* Poliomyelitis, paralytic
  inferior nuclear G83.9
  internuclear — *see* Ophthalmoplegia, internuclear
  intestine K56.0
  iris H57.09
    due to diphtheria (toxin) A36.89
  ischemic, Volkmann's (complicating trauma) T79.6 ☑
  Jackson's G83.89
  jake — *see* Poisoning, food, noxious, plant
  Jamaica ginger (jake) G62.2
  juvenile general A50.45
  Klumpke (-Déjérine) (birth) (newborn) P14.1
  labioglossal (laryngeal) (pharyngeal) G12.29
  Landry's G61.0
  laryngeal nerve (recurrent) (superior) (unilateral) J38.00
    bilateral J38.02
    unilateral J38.01
  larynx J38.00
    bilateral J38.02
    due to diphtheria (toxin) A36.2
    unilateral J38.01
  lateral G12.23
  lead T56.0 ☑
  left side — *see* Hemiplegia
  leg G83.1- ☑
    both — *see* Paraplegia
    crossed G83.89
    hysterical F44.4
    psychogenic F44.4
    transient or transitory R29.818
    traumatic NEC — *see* Injury, nerve, leg
  levator palpebrae superioris — *see* Blepharoptosis, paralytic
  limb — *see* Monoplegia
  lip K13.39
  Lissauer's A52.17
  lower limb — *see* Monoplegia, lower limb
    both — *see* Paraplegia

Paralysis, paralytic — *continued*
  lung J98.4
  median nerve G56.1- ☑
  medullary (tegmental) G83.89
  mesencephalic NEC G83.89
    tegmental G83.89
  middle alternating G83.89
  Millard-Gubler-Foville G46.3
  monoplegic — *see* Monoplegia
  motor G83.9
  muscle, muscular NEC G72.89
    due to nerve lesion G58.9
    eye (extrinsic) H49.9
      intrinsic — *see* Paresis, of accommodation
      oblique — *see* Strabismus, paralytic, fourth nerve
    iris sphincter H21.9
    ischemic (Volkmann's) (complicating trauma) T79.6
    progressive G12.21
    pseudohypertrophic G71.0
  musculocutaneous nerve G56.9- ☑
  musculospiral G56.9- ☑
  nerve (*see also* Disorder, nerve)
    abducent — *see* Strabismus, paralytic, sixth nerve
    accessory G52.8
    auditory (except Deafness) H93.3 ☑
    birth injury P14.9
    cranial or cerebral G52.9
    facial G51.0
      birth injury P11.3
      congenital P11.3
      newborn (birth injury) P11.3
    fourth or trochlear — *see* Strabismus, paralytic, fourth nerve
    newborn (birth injury) P14.9
    oculomotor — *see* Strabismus, paralytic, third nerve
    phrenic (birth injury) P14.2
    radial G56.3- ☑
    seventh or facial G51.0
      newborn (birth injury) P11.3
    sixth or abducent — *see* Strabismus, paralytic, sixth nerve
    syphilitic A52.15
    third or oculomotor — *see* Strabismus, paralytic, third nerve
    trigeminal G50.9
    trochlear — *see* Strabismus, paralytic, fourth nerve
    ulnar G56.2- ☑
  normokalemic periodic G72.3
  ocular H49.9
    alternating G83.89
  oculofacial, congenital (Moebius) Q87.0
  oculomotor (external bilateral) (nerve) — *see* Strabismus, paralytic, third nerve
  palate (soft) K13.79
  paratrigeminal G50.9
  periodic (familial) (hyperkalemic) (hypokalemic) (myotonic) (normokalemic) (potassium sensitive) (secondary) G72.3
  peripheral autonomic nervous system — *see* Neuropathy, peripheral, autonomic
  peroneal (nerve) G57.3- ☑
  pharynx J39.2
  phrenic nerve G56.8- ☑
  plantar nerve(s) G57.6- ☑
  pneumogastric nerve G52.2
  poliomyelitis (current) — *see* Poliomyelitis, paralytic
  popliteal nerve G57.3- ☑
  postepileptic transitory G83.84
  progressive (atrophic) (bulbar) (spinal) G12.22
    general A52.17
    infantile acute — *see* Poliomyelitis, paralytic
    supranuclear G23.1
  pseudobulbar G12.29
  pseudohypertrophic (muscle) G71.0
  psychogenic F44.4
  quadriceps G57.9- ☑
  quadriplegic — *see* Tetraplegia
  radial nerve G56.3- ☑
  rectus muscle (eye) H49.9
  recurrent isolated sleep G47.53
  respiratory (muscle) (system) (tract) R06.81
    center NEC G93.89
    congenital P28.89
    newborn P28.89
  right side — *see* Hemiplegia

Paralysis, paralytic — *continued*
  saturnine T56.0 ☑
  sciatic nerve G57.0- ☑
  senile G83.9
  shaking — *see* Parkinsonism
  shoulder G56.9- ☑
  sleep, recurrent isolated G47.53
  spastic G83.9
    cerebral — *see* Palsy, cerebral, spastic
    congenital (cerebral) — *see* Palsy, cerebral, spastic
    familial G11.4
    hereditary G11.4
    quadriplegic G80.0
    syphilitic (spinal) A52.17
  sphincter, bladder — *see* Paralysis, bladder
  spinal (cord) G83.9
    accessory nerve G52.8
    acute — *see* Poliomyelitis, paralytic
    ascending acute G61.0
    atrophic (acute) (*see also* Poliomyelitis, paralytic)
      spastic, syphilitic A52.17
    congenital NEC — *see* Palsy, cerebral
    hereditary G95.89
    infantile — *see* Poliomyelitis, paralytic
    progressive G12.21
    sequelae NEC G83.89
  sternomastoid G52.8
  stomach K31.84
    diabetic — *see* Diabetes, by type, with gastroparesis
    nerve G52.2
      diabetic — *see* Diabetes, by type, with gastroparesis
  stroke — *see* Infarct, brain
  subcapsularis G56.8- ☑
  supranuclear (progressive) G23.1
  sympathetic G90.8
    cervical G90.09
    nervous system — *see* Neuropathy, peripheral, autonomic
  syndrome G83.9
    specified NEC G83.89
  syphilitic spastic spinal (Erb's) A52.17
  thigh G57.9- ☑
  throat J39.2
    diphtheritic A36.0
    muscle J39.2
  thrombotic (current episode) I63.3- ☑
  thumb G56.9- ☑
  tick — *see* Toxicity, venom, arthropod, specified NEC
  Todd's (postepileptic transitory paralysis) G83.84
  toe G57.6- ☑
  tongue K14.8
  transient R29.5
    arm or leg NEC R29.818
    traumatic NEC — *see* Injury, nerve
  trapezius G52.8
  traumatic, transient NEC — *see* Injury, nerve
  trembling — *see* Parkinsonism
  triceps brachii G56.9- ☑
  trigeminal nerve G50.9
  trochlear (nerve) — *see* Strabismus, paralytic, fourth nerve
  ulnar nerve G56.2- ☑
  upper limb — *see* Monoplegia, upper limb
  uremic N18.9 [G99.8]
  uveoparotitic D86.89
  uvula K13.79
    postdiphtheritic A36.0
  vagus nerve G52.2
  vasomotor NEC G90.8
  velum palati K13.79
  vesical — *see* Paralysis, bladder
  vestibular nerve (except Vertigo) H93.3 ☑
  vocal cords J38.00
    bilateral J38.02
    unilateral J38.01
  Volkmann's (complicating trauma) T79.6 ☑
  wasting G12.29
  Weber's G46.3
  wrist G56.9- ☑
Paramedial urethrovesical orifice Q64.79
Paramenia N92.6
Parametritis (*see also* Disease, pelvis, inflammatory) N73.2
  acute N73.0

Parametritis — *continued*
  complicating abortion — *see* Abortion, by type, complicated by, parametritis
Parametrium, parametric — *see* condition
Paramnesia — *see* Amnesia
Paramolar K00.1
Paramyloidosis E85.89
Paramyoclonus multiplex G25.3
Paramyotonia (congenita) G71.19
Parangi — *see* Yaws
Paranoia (querulans) F22
  senile F03 ☑
Paranoid
  dementia (senile) F03 ☑
    praecox — *see* Schizophrenia
  personality F60.0
  psychosis (climacteric) (involutional) (menopausal) F22
    psychogenic (acute) F23
    senile F03 ☑
  reaction (acute) F23
    chronic F22
  schizophrenia F20.0
  state (climacteric) (involutional) (menopausal) (simple) F22
    senile F03 ☑
  tendencies F60.0
  traits F60.0
  trends F60.0
  type, psychopathic personality F60.0
Paraparesis — *see* Paraplegia
Paraphasia R47.02
Paraphilia F65.9
Paraphimosis (congenital) N47.2
  chancroidal A57
Paraphrenia, paraphrenic (late) F22
  schizophrenia F20.0
Paraplegia (lower) G82.20
  ataxic — *see* Degeneration, combined, spinal cord
  complete G82.21
  congenital (cerebral) G80.8
    spastic G80.1
  familial spastic G11.4
  functional (hysterical) F44.4
  hereditary, spastic G11.4
  hysterical F44.4
  incomplete G82.22
  Pott's A18.01
  psychogenic F44.4
  spastic
    Erb's spinal, syphilitic A52.17
    hereditary G11.4
    tropical G04.1
  syphilitic (spastic) A52.17
  tropical spastic G04.1
Parapoxvirus B08.60
  specified NEC B08.69
Paraproteinemia D89.2
  benign (familial) D89.2
  monoclonal D47.2
  secondary to malignant disease D47.2
Parapsoriasis L41.9
  en plaques L41.4
  guttata L41.1
  large plaque L41.4
  retiform, retiformis L41.5
  small plaque L41.3
  specified NEC L41.8
  varioliformis (acuta) L41.0
Parasitic (*see also* condition)
  disease NEC B89
  stomatitis B37.0
  sycosis (beard) (scalp) B35.0
  twin Q89.4
Parasitism B89
  intestinal B82.9
  skin B88.9
  specified — *see* Infestation
Parasitophobia F40.218
Parasomnia G47.50
  due to
    alcohol
      abuse F10.182
      dependence F10.282
      use F10.982
    amphetamines
      abuse F15.182
      dependence F15.282

Parasomnia — *continued*
  due to — *continued*
    amphetamines — *continued*
      use F15.982
    caffeine
      abuse F15.182
      dependence F15.282
      use F15.982
    cocaine
      abuse F14.182
      dependence F14.282
      use F14.982
    drug NEC
      abuse F19.182
      dependence F19.282
      use F19.982
    opioid
      abuse F11.182
      dependence F11.282
      use F11.982
    psychoactive substance NEC
      abuse F19.182
      dependence F19.282
      use F19.982
    sedative, hypnotic, or anxiolytic
      abuse F13.182
      dependence F13.282
      use F13.982
    stimulant NEC
      abuse F15.182
      dependence F15.282
      use F15.982
  in conditions classified elsewhere G47.54
  nonorganic origin F51.8
  organic G47.50
  specified NEC G47.59
Paraspadias Q54.9
Paraspasmus facialis G51.8
Parasuicide (attempt)
  history of (personal) Z91.5
    in family Z81.8
Parathyroid gland — *see* condition
Parathyroid tetany E20.9
Paratrachoma A74.0
Parathyphilitis — *see* Appendicitis
Paratyphoid (fever) — *see* Fever, paratyphoid
Paratyphus — *see* Fever, paratyphoid
Paraurethral duct Q64.79
  nonorganic origin F51.5
Paraurethritis (*see also* Urethritis)
  gonococcal (acute) (chronic) (with abscess) A54.1
Paravaccinia NEC B08.04
Paravaginitis — *see* Vaginitis
Parencephalitis (*see also* Encephalitis)
  sequelae G09
Parent-child conflict — *see* Conflict, parent-child
  estrangement NEC Z62.890
Paresis (*see also* Paralysis)
  accommodation — *see* Paresis, of accommodation
  Bernhardt's G57.1- ☑
  bladder (sphincter) (*see also* Paralysis, bladder)
    tabetic A52.17
  bowel, colon or intestine K56.0
  extrinsic muscle, eye H49.9
  general (progressive) (syphilitic) A52.17
    juvenile A50.45
  heart — *see* Failure, heart
  insane (syphilitic) A52.17
  juvenile (general) A50.45
  of accommodation H52.52- ☑
  peripheral progressive (idiopathic) G60.3
  pseudohypertrophic G71.0
  senile G83.9
  syphilitic (general) A52.17
    congenital A50.45
  vesical NEC N31.2
Paresthesia (*see also* Disturbance, sensation, skin) R20.2
  Bernhardt G57.1- ☑
Paretic — *see* condition
Parinaud's
  conjunctivitis H10.89
  oculoglandular syndrome H10.89
  ophthalmoplegia H49.88- ☑
Parkinsonism (idiopathic) (primary) G20
  with neurogenic orthostatic hypotension (symptomatic) G90.3
  arteriosclerotic G21.4
  dementia G31.83 [F02.80]

Parkinsonism — *continued*
  dementia — *continued*
    with behavioral disturbance G31.83 [F02.81]
  due to
    drugs NEC G21.19
      neuroleptic G21.11
    medication-induced NEC G21.19
    neuroleptic induced G21.11
    postencephalitic G21.3
    secondary G21.9
      due to
        arteriosclerosis G21.4
        drugs NEC G21.19
          neuroleptic G21.11
        encephalitis G21.3
        external agents NEC G21.2
        syphilis A52.19
      specified NEC G21.8
    syphilitic A52.19
    treatment-induced NEC G21.19
    vascular G21.4
Parkinson's disease, syndrome or tremor — *see* Parkinsonism
Parodontitis — *see* Periodontitis
Parodontosis K05.4
Paronychia (*see also* Cellulitis, digit)
  with lymphangitis — *see* Lymphangitis, acute, digit
  candidal (chronic) B37.2
  tuberculous (primary) A18.4
Parorexia (psychogenic) F50.89
Parosmia R43.1
  psychogenic F45.8
Parotid gland — *see* condition
Parotitis, parotiditis (allergic)(nonspecific toxic) (purulent) (septic) (suppurative) (*see also* Sialoadenitis)
  epidemic — *see* Mumps
  infectious — *see* Mumps
  postoperative K91.89
  surgical K91.89
Parrot fever A70
Parrot's disease (early congenital syphilitic pseudoparalysis) A50.02
Parry-Romberg syndrome G51.8
Parry's disease or syndrome E05.00
  with thyroid storm E05.01
Pars planitis — *see* Cyclitis
Parsonage (-Aldren)-**Turner syndrome** G54.5
Parson's disease (exophthalmic goiter) E05.00
  with thyroid storm E05.01
Particolored infant Q82.8
Parturition — *see* Delivery
Parulis K04.7
  with sinus K04.6
Parvovirus, as cause of disease classified elsewhere B97.6
Pasini and Pierini's atrophoderma L90.3
Passage
  false, urethra N36.5
  meconium (newborn) during delivery P03.82
  of sounds or bougies — *see* Attention to, artificial, opening
Passive — *see* condition
  smoking Z77.22
Pasteurella septica A28.0
Pasteurellosis — *see* Infection, Pasteurella
PAT (paroxysmal atrial tachycardia) I47.1
Patau's syndrome — *see* Trisomy, 13
Patches
  mucous (syphilitic) A51.39
    congenital A50.07
  smokers' (mouth) K13.24
Patellar — *see* condition
Patent (*see also* Imperfect, closure)
  canal of Nuck Q52.4
  cervix N88.3
  ductus arteriosus or Botallo's Q25.0
  foramen
    botalli Q21.1
    ovale Q21.1
  interauricular septum Q21.1
  interventricular septum Q21.0
  omphalomesenteric duct Q43.0
  os (uteri) — *see* Patent, cervix
  ostium secundum Q21.1
  urachus Q64.4
  vitelline duct Q43.0
Paterson (-Brown)(-Kelly) **syndrome or web** D50.1

Pathologic, pathological (*see also* condition)
  asphyxia R09.01
  fire-setting F63.1
  gambling F63.0
  ovum O02.0
  resorption, tooth K03.3
  stealing F63.2
Pathology (of) — *see* Disease
  periradicular, associated with previous endodontic treatment NEC M27.59
Pattern, sleep-wake, irregular G47.23
Patulous (*see also* Imperfect, closure (congenital))
  alimentary tract Q45.8
    lower Q43.8
    upper Q40.8
  eustachian tube H69.0- ☑
Pause, sinoatrial I49.5
Paxton's disease B36.2
Pearl(s)
  enamel K00.2
  Epstein's K09.8
Pearl-worker's disease — *see* Osteomyelitis, specified type NEC
Pectenosis K62.4
Pectoral — *see* condition
Pectus
  carinatum (congenital) Q67.7
    acquired M95.4
    rachitic sequelae (late effect) E64.3
  excavatum (congenital) Q67.6
    acquired M95.4
    rachitic sequelae (late effect) E64.3
  recurvatum (congenital) Q67.6
Pedatrophia E41
Pederosis F65.4
Pediculosis (infestation) B85.2
  capitis (head-louse) (any site) B85.0
  corporis (body-louse) (any site) B85.1
  eyelid B85.0
  mixed (classifiable to more than one of the titles B85.0-B85.3) B85.4
  pubis (pubic louse) (any site) B85.3
  vestimenti B85.1
  vulvae B85.3
Pediculus (infestation) — *see* Pediculosis
Pedophilia F65.4
Peg-shaped teeth K00.2
Pelade — *see* Alopecia, areata
Pelger-Huët anomaly or syndrome D72.0
Peliosis (rheumatica) D69.0
  hepatis K76.4
    with toxic liver disease K71.8
Pelizaeus-Merzbacher disease E75.29
Pellagra (alcoholic) (with polyneuropathy) E52
Pellagra-cerebellar-ataxia-renal aminoaciduria syndrome E72.02
Pellegrini (-Stieda) **disease or syndrome** — *see* Bursitis, tibial collateral
Pellizzi's syndrome E34.8
Pel's crisis A52.11
Pelvic (*see also* condition)
  examination (periodic) (routine) Z01.419
    with abnormal findings Z01.411
  kidney, congenital Q63.2
Pelviolithiasis — *see* Calculus, kidney
Pelviperitonitis (*see also* Peritonitis, pelvic)
  gonococcal A54.24
  puerperal O85
Pelvis — *see* condition or type
Pemphigoid L12.9
  benign, mucous membrane L12.1
  bullous L12.0
  cicatricial L12.1
  juvenile L12.2
  ocular L12.1
  specified NEC L12.8
Pemphigus L10.9
  benign familial (chronic) Q82.8
  Brazilian L10.3
  circinatus L13.0
  conjunctiva L12.1
  drug-induced L10.5
  erythematosus L10.4
  foliaceus L10.2
  gangrenous — *see* Gangrene
  neonatorum L01.03
  ocular L12.1
  paraneoplastic L10.81

Pemphigus — *continued*
  specified NEC L10.89
  syphilitic (congenital) A50.06
  vegetans L10.1
  vulgaris L10.0
  wildfire L10.3
Pendred's syndrome E07.1
Pendulous
  abdomen, in pregnancy — *see* Pregnancy, complicated by, abnormal, pelvic organs or tissues NEC
  breast N64.89
Penetrating wound (*see also* Puncture)
  with internal injury — *see* Injury, by site
  eyeball — *see* Puncture, eyeball
  orbit (with or without foreign body) — *see* Puncture, orbit
  uterus by instrument with or following ectopic or molar pregnancy O08.6
Penicillosis B48.4
Penis — *see* condition
Penitis N48.29
Pentalogy of Fallot Q21.8
Pentasomy X syndrome Q97.1
Pentosuria (essential) E74.8
Percreta placenta - O43.23 ☑
Peregrinating patient — *see* Disorder, factitious
Perforation, perforated (nontraumatic) (of)
  accidental during procedure (blood vessel) (nerve) (organ) — *see* Complication, accidental puncture or laceration
  antrum — *see* Sinusitis, maxillary
  appendix K35.2
    with localized peritonitis K35.3
  atrial septum, multiple Q21.1
  attic, ear — *see* Perforation, tympanum, attic
  bile duct (common) (hepatic) K83.2
    cystic K82.2
  bladder (urinary)
    with or following ectopic or molar pregnancy O08.6
    obstetrical trauma O71.5
    traumatic S37.29 ☑
      at delivery O71.5
  bowel K63.1
    with or following ectopic or molar pregnancy O08.6
    newborn P78.0
    obstetrical trauma O71.5
    traumatic — *see* Laceration, intestine
  broad ligament N83.8
    with or following ectopic or molar pregnancy O08.6
    obstetrical trauma O71.6
  by
    device, implant or graft (*see also* Complications, by site and type, mechanical) T85.628 ☑
      arterial graft NEC — *see* Complication, cardiovascular device, mechanical, vascular
      breast (implant) T85.49 ☑
      catheter NEC T85.698 ☑
        cystostomy T83.090 ☑
        dialysis (renal) T82.49 ☑
          intraperitoneal T85.691 ☑
        infusion NEC T82.594 ☑
          spinal (epidural) (subdural) T85.690 ☑
        urinary (*see also* Complications, catheter, urinary T83.098 ☑
      electronic (electrode) (pulse generator) (stimulator)
        bone T84.390 ☑
        cardiac T82.199 ☑
          electrode T82.190 ☑
          pulse generator T82.191 ☑
          specified type NEC T82.198 ☑
        nervous system — *see* Complication, prosthetic device, mechanical, electronic nervous system stimulator
        urinary — *see* Complication, genitourinary, device, urinary, mechanical
      fixation, internal (orthopedic) NEC — *see* Complication, fixation device, mechanical
      gastrointestinal — *see* Complications, prosthetic device, mechanical, gastrointestinal device
      genital NEC T83.498 ☑
        intrauterine contraceptive device T83.39 ☑
        penile prosthesis T83.490 ☑
      heart NEC — *see* Complication, cardiovascular device, mechanical

Index

Perforation, perforated — Perichondritis

Perforation, perforated — *continued*
by — *continued*
 device, implant or graft (*see also* Complications, by site and type, mechanical) — *continued*
  joint prosthesis — *see* Complications, joint prosthesis, mechanical, specified NEC, by site
  ocular NEC — *see* Complications, prosthetic device, mechanical, ocular device
  orthopedic NEC — *see* Complication, orthopedic, device, mechanical
  specified NEC T85.628 ☑
  urinary NEC (*see also* Complication, genitourinary, device, urinary, mechanical)
   graft T83.29 ☑
  vascular NEC — *see* Complication, cardiovascular device, mechanical
  ventricular intracranial shunt T85.09 ☑
 foreign body left accidentally in operative wound T81.539 ☑
 instrument (any) during a procedure, accidental — *see* Puncture, accidental complicating surgery
cecum K35.2
 with localized peritonitis K35.3
cervix (uteri) N88.8
 with or following ectopic or molar pregnancy O08.6
 obstetrical trauma O71.3
colon K63.1
 newborn P78.0
 obstetrical trauma O71.5
 traumatic — *see* Laceration, intestine, large
common duct (bile) K83.2
cornea (due to ulceration) — *see* Ulcer, cornea, perforated
cystic duct K82.2
diverticulum (intestine) K57.80
 with bleeding K57.81
 large intestine K57.20
  with
   bleeding K57.21
   small intestine K57.40
    with bleeding K57.41
 small intestine K57.00
  with
   bleeding K57.01
   large intestine K57.40
    with bleeding K57.41
ear drum — *see* Perforation, tympanum
esophagus K22.3
ethmoidal sinus — *see* Sinusitis, ethmoidal
frontal sinus — *see* Sinusitis, frontal
gallbladder K82.2
heart valve — *see* Endocarditis
ileum K63.1
 newborn P78.0
 obstetrical trauma O71.5
 traumatic — *see* Laceration, intestine, small
instrumental, surgical (accidental) (blood vessel) (nerve) (organ) — *see* Puncture, accidental complicating surgery
intestine NEC K63.1
 with ectopic or molar pregnancy O08.6
 newborn P78.0
 obstetrical trauma O71.5
 traumatic — *see* Laceration, intestine
 ulcerative NEC K63.1
  newborn P78.0
jejunum, jejunal K63.1
 obstetrical trauma O71.5
 traumatic — *see* Laceration, intestine, small
 ulcer — *see* Ulcer, gastrojejunal, with perforation
joint prosthesis — *see* Complications, joint prosthesis, mechanical, specified NEC, by site
mastoid (antrum) (cell) — *see* Disorder, mastoid, specified NEC
maxillary sinus — *see* Sinusitis, maxillary
membrana tympani — *see* Perforation, tympanum
nasal
 septum J34.89
  congenital Q30.3
  syphilitic A52.73
 sinus J34.89
  congenital Q30.8
  due to sinusitis — *see* Sinusitis
palate (*see also* Cleft, palate) Q35.9
 syphilitic A52.79
palatine vault (*see also* Cleft, palate, hard) Q35.1

Perforation, perforated — *continued*
palatine vault (*see also* Cleft, palate, hard) — *continued*
 syphilitic A52.79
 congenital A50.59
pars flaccida (ear drum) — *see* Perforation, tympanum, attic
pelvic
 floor S31.030 ☑
  with
   ectopic or molar pregnancy O08.6
   penetration into retroperitoneal space S31.031 ☑
   retained foreign body S31.040 ☑
    with penetration into retroperitoneal space S31.041 ☑
  following ectopic or molar pregnancy O08.6
  obstetrical trauma O70.1
 organ S37.99
  adrenal gland S37.818 ☑
  bladder — *see* Perforation, bladder
  fallopian tube S37.599 ☑
   bilateral S37.592 ☑
   unilateral S37.591 ☑
  kidney S37.09- ☑
  obstetrical trauma O71.5
  ovary S37.499 ☑
   bilateral S37.492 ☑
   unilateral S37.491 ☑
  prostate S37.828 ☑
  specified organ NEC S37.898 ☑
  ureter — *see* Perforation, ureter
  urethra — *see* Perforation, urethra
  uterus — *see* Perforation, uterus
perineum — *see* Laceration, perineum
pharynx J39.2
rectum K63.1
 newborn P78.0
 obstetrical trauma O71.5
 traumatic S36.63 ☑
root canal space due to endodontic treatment M27.51
sigmoid K63.1
 newborn P78.0
 obstetrical trauma O71.5
 traumatic S36.533 ☑
sinus (accessory) (chronic) (nasal) J34.89
sphenoidal sinus — *see* Sinusitis, sphenoidal
surgical (accidental) (by instrument) (blood vessel) (nerve) (organ) — *see* Puncture, accidental complicating surgery
traumatic
 external — *see* Puncture
 eye — *see* Puncture, eyeball
 internal organ — *see* Injury, by site
tympanum, tympanic (membrane) (persistent post-traumatic) (postinflammatory) H72.9- ☑
 attic H72.1- ☑
  multiple — *see* Perforation, tympanum, multiple
  total — *see* Perforation, tympanum, total
 central H72.0- ☑
  multiple — *see* Perforation, tympanum, multiple
  total — *see* Perforation, tympanum, total
 marginal NEC — *see* subcategory H72.2 ☑
 multiple H72.81- ☑
 pars flaccida — *see* Perforation, tympanum, attic
 total H72.82- ☑
 traumatic, current episode S09.2- ☑
typhoid, gastrointestinal — *see* Typhoid
ulcer — *see* Ulcer, by site, with perforation
ureter N28.89
 traumatic S37.19 ☑
urethra N36.8
 with ectopic or molar pregnancy O08.6
 following ectopic or molar pregnancy O08.6
 obstetrical trauma O71.5
 traumatic S37.39 ☑
  at delivery O71.5
uterus
 with ectopic or molar pregnancy O08.6
 by intrauterine contraceptive device T83.39 ☑
 following ectopic or molar pregnancy O08.6
 obstetrical trauma O71.1
 traumatic S37.69 ☑
  obstetric O71.1
uvula K13.79

Perforation, perforated — *continued*
uvula — *continued*
 syphilitic A52.79
vagina O71.4
 obstetrical trauma O71.4
 other trauma — *see* Puncture, vagina
Periadenitis mucosa necrotica recurrens K12.0
Periappendicitis (acute) — *see* Appendicitis
Periarteritis nodosa (disseminated) (infectious) (necrotizing) M30.0
Periarthritis (joint) (*see also* Enthesopathy)
 Duplay's M75.0- ☑
 gonococcal A54.42
 humeroscapularis — *see* Capsulitis, adhesive
 scapulohumeral — *see* Capsulitis, adhesive
 shoulder — *see* Capsulitis, adhesive
 wrist M77.2- ☑
Periarthrosis (angioneural) — *see* Enthesopathy
Pericapsulitis, adhesive (shoulder) — *see* Capsulitis, adhesive
Pericarditis (with decompensation) (with effusion) I31.9
 with rheumatic fever (conditions in I00)
  active — *see* Pericarditis, rheumatic
  inactive or quiescent I09.2
 acute (hemorrhagic) (nonrheumatic) (Sicca) I30.9
  with chorea (acute) (rheumatic) (Sydenham's) I02.0
  benign I30.8
  nonspecific I30.0
  rheumatic I01.0
   with chorea (acute) (Sydenham's) I02.0
 adhesive or adherent (chronic) (external) (internal) I31.0
  acute — *see* Pericarditis, acute
  rheumatic I09.2
 bacterial (acute) (subacute) (with serous or seropurulent effusion) I30.1
 calcareous I31.1
 cholesterol (chronic) I31.8
  acute I30.9
 chronic (nonrheumatic) I31.9
  rheumatic I09.2
 constrictive (chronic) I31.1
 coxsackie B33.23
 fibrinocaseous (tuberculous) A18.84
 fibrinopurulent I30.1
 fibrinous I30.8
 fibrous I31.0
 gonococcal A54.83
 idiopathic I30.0
 in systemic lupus erythematosus M32.12
 infective I30.1
 meningococcal A39.53
 neoplastic (chronic) I31.8
  acute I30.9
 obliterans, obliterating I31.0
 plastic I31.0
 pneumococcal I30.1
 postinfarction I24.1
 purulent I30.1
 rheumatic (active) (acute) (with effusion) (with pneumonia) I01.0
  with chorea (acute) (rheumatic) (Sydenham's) I02.0
  chronic or inactive (with chorea) I09.2
 rheumatoid — *see* Rheumatoid, carditis
 septic I30.1
 serofibrinous I30.8
 staphylococcal I30.1
 streptococcal I30.1
 suppurative I30.1
 syphilitic A52.06
 tuberculous A18.84
 uremic N18.9 [I32]
 viral I30.1
Pericardium, pericardial — *see* condition
Pericellulitis — *see* Cellulitis
Pericementitis (chronic) (suppurative) (*see also* Periodontitis)
 acute K05.20
  generalized — *see* Peridontitis, aggressive, generalized
  localized — *see* Peridontitis, aggressive, localized
Perichondritis
 auricle — *see* Perichondritis, ear
 bronchus J98.09
 ear (external) H61.00- ☑
  acute H61.01- ☑
  chronic H61.02- ☑
  external auditory canal — *see* Perichondritis, ear

Perichondritis — *continued*
  larynx J38.7
    syphilitic A52.73
    typhoid A01.09
  nose J34.89
  pinna — *see* Perichondritis, ear
  trachea J39.8
Periclasia K05.4
Pericoronitis — *see* Periodontitis
Pericystitis N30.90
  with hematuria N30.91
Peridiverticulitis (intestine) K57.92
  cecum — *see* Diverticulitis, intestine, large
  colon — *see* Diverticulitis, intestine, large
  duodenum — *see* Diverticulitis, intestine, small
  intestine — *see* Diverticulitis, intestine
  jejunum — *see* Diverticulitis, intestine, small
  rectosigmoid — *see* Diverticulitis, intestine, large
  rectum — *see* Diverticulitis, intestine, large
  sigmoid — *see* Diverticulitis, intestine, large
Periendocarditis — *see* Endocarditis
Periepididymitis N45.1
Perifolliculitis L01.02
  abscedens, caput, scalp L66.3
  capitis, abscedens (et suffodiens) L66.3
  superficial pustular L01.02
Perihepatitis K65.8
Perilabyrinthitis (acute) — *see* subcategory H83.0 ☑
Perimeningitis — *see* Meningitis
Perimetritis — *see* Endometritis
Perimetrosalpingitis — *see* Salpingo-oophoritis
Perineocele N81.81
Perinephric, perinephritic — *see* condition
Perinephritis (*see also* Infection, kidney)
  purulent — *see* Abscess, kidney
Perineum, perineal — *see* condition
Perineuritis NEC — *see* Neuralgia
Periodic — *see* condition
Periodontitis (chronic) (complex) (compound) (local)
  (simplex) K05.30
  acute K05.20
    generalized K05.229
      moderate K05.222
      severe K05.223
      slight K05.221
    localized K05.219
      moderate K05.212
      severe K05.213
      slight K05.211
  apical K04.5
    acute (pulpal origin) K04.4
  generalized K05.329
    moderate K05.322
    severe K05.323
    slight K05.321
  localized K05.319
    moderate K05.312
    severe K05.313
    slight K05.311
Periodontoclasia K05.4
Periodontosis (juvenile) K05.4
Periods (*see also* Menstruation)
  heavy N92.0
  irregular N92.6
  shortened intervals (irregular) N92.1
Perionychia (*see also* Cellulitis, digit)
  with lymphangitis — *see* Lymphangitis, acute, digit
Perioophoritis — *see* Salpingo-oophoritis
Periorchitis N45.2
Periosteum, periosteal — *see* condition
Periostitis (albuminosa) (circumscribed) (diffuse) (infective) (monomelic) (*see also* Osteomyelitis)
  alveolar M27.3
  alveolodental M27.3
  dental M27.3
  gonorrheal A54.43
  jaw (lower) (upper) M27.2
  orbit H05.03- ☑
  syphilitic A52.77
    congenital (early) A50.02 [M90.80]
    secondary A51.46
  tuberculous — *see* Tuberculosis, bone
  yaws (hypertrophic) (early) (late) A66.6 [M90.80]
Periostosis (hyperplastic) (*see also* Disorder, bone, specified type NEC)
  with osteomyelitis — *see* Osteomyelitis, specified type NEC

Peripartum
  cardiomyopathy O90.3
Periphlebitis — *see* Phlebitis
Periproctitis K62.89
Periprostatitis — *see* Prostatitis
Perirectal — *see* condition
Perirenal — *see* condition
Perisalpingitis — *see* Salpingo-oophoritis
Perisplenitis (infectional) D73.89
Peristalsis, visible or reversed R19.2
Peritendinitis — *see* Enthesopathy
Peritoneum, peritoneal — *see* condition
Peritonitis (adhesive) (bacterial) (fibrinous) (hemorrhagic) (idiopathic) (localized) (perforative) (primary) (with adhesions) (with effusion) K65.9
  with or following
    abscess K65.1
    appendicitis K35.3
      with perforation or rupture K35.2
      generalized K35.2
      localized K35.3
    diverticular disease (intestine) K57.80
      with bleeding K57.81
      ectopic or molar pregnancy O08.0
      large intestine K57.20
        with
          bleeding K57.21
          small intestine K57.40
            with bleeding K57.41
      small intestine K57.00
        with
          bleeding K57.01
          large intestine K57.40
            with bleeding K57.41
  acute (generalized) K65.0
  aseptic T81.61 ☑
  bile, biliary K65.3
  chemical T81.61 ☑
  chlamydial A74.81
  chronic proliferative K65.8
  complicating abortion — *see* Abortion, by type, complicated by, pelvic peritonitis
  congenital P78.1
  diaphragmatic K65.0
  diffuse K65.0
  diphtheritic A36.89
  disseminated K65.0
  due to
    bile K65.3
    foreign
      body or object accidentally left during a procedure (instrument) (sponge) (swab) T81.599 ☑
      substance accidentally left during a procedure (chemical) (powder) (talc) T81.61 ☑
    talc T81.61 ☑
    urine K65.8
  eosinophilic K65.8
    acute K65.0
  fibrocaseous (tuberculous) A18.31
  fibropurulent K65.0
  following ectopic or molar pregnancy O08.0
  general (ized) K65.0
  gonococcal A54.85
  meconium (newborn) P78.0
  neonatal P78.1
    meconium P78.0
  pancreatic K65.0
  paroxysmal, familial E85.0
    benign E85.0
  pelvic
    female N73.5
      acute N73.3
      chronic N73.4
        with adhesions N73.6
    male K65.0
  periodic, familial E85.0
  proliferative, chronic K65.8
  puerperal, postpartum, childbirth O85
  purulent K65.0
  septic K65.0
  specified NEC K65.8
  spontaneous bacterial K65.2
  subdiaphragmatic K65.0
  subphrenic K65.0
  suppurative K65.0
  syphilitic A52.74
    congenital (early) A50.08 [K67]

Peritonitis — *continued*
  talc T81.61 ☑
  tuberculous A18.31
  urine K65.8
Peritonsillar — *see* condition
Peritonsillitis J36
Perityphlitis K37
Periureteritis N28.89
Periurethral — *see* condition
Periurethritis (gangrenous) — *see* Urethritis
Periuterine — *see* condition
Perivaginitis — *see* Vaginitis
Perivasculitis, retinal H35.06- ☑
Perivasitis (chronic) N49.1
Perivesiculitis (seminal) — *see* Vesiculitis
Perlèche NEC K13.0
  due to
    candidiasis B37.83
    moniliasis B37.83
    riboflavin deficiency E53.0
    vitamin B2 (riboflavin) deficiency E53.0
Pernicious — *see* condition
Pernio, perniosis T69.1 ☑
Perpetrator (of abuse) — *see* Index to External Causes of Injury, Perpetrator
Persecution
  delusion F22
  social Z60.5
Perseveration (tonic) R48.8
Persistence, persistent (congenital)
  anal membrane Q42.3
    with fistula Q42.2
  arteria stapedia Q16.3
  atrioventricular canal Q21.2
  branchial cleft NOS Q18.2
    cyst Q18.0
    fistula Q18.0
    sinus Q18.0
  bulbus cordis in left ventricle Q21.8
  canal of Cloquet Q14.0
  capsule (opaque) Q12.8
  cilioretinal artery or vein Q14.8
  cloaca Q43.7
  communication — *see* Fistula, congenital
  convolutions
    aortic arch Q25.46
    fallopian tube Q50.6
    oviduct Q50.6
    uterine tube Q50.6
  double aortic arch Q25.45
  ductus arteriosus (Botalli) Q25.0
  fetal
    circulation P29.38
    form of cervix (uteri) Q51.828
    hemoglobin, hereditary (HPFH) D56.4
  foramen
    Botalli Q21.1
    ovale Q21.1
  Gartner's duct Q52.4
  hemoglobin, fetal (hereditary) (HPFH) D56.4
  hyaloid
    artery (generally incomplete) Q14.0
    system Q14.8
  hymen, in pregnancy or childbirth — *see* Pregnancy, complicated by, abnormal, vulva
  lanugo Q84.2
  left
    posterior cardinal vein Q26.8
    root with right arch of aorta Q25.49
    superior vena cava Q26.1
  Meckel's diverticulum Q43.0
    malignant — *see* Table of Neoplasms, small intestine, malignant
  mucosal disease (middle ear) — *see* Otitis, media, suppurative, chronic, tubotympanic
  nail(s), anomalous Q84.6
  omphalomesenteric duct Q43.0
  organ or site not listed — *see* Anomaly, by site
  ostium
    atrioventriculare commune Q21.2
    primum Q21.2
    secundum Q21.1
  ovarian rests in fallopian tube Q50.6
  pancreatic tissue in intestinal tract Q43.8
  primary (deciduous)
    teeth K00.6
    vitreous hyperplasia Q14.0
  pupillary membrane Q13.89

Index

Persistence, persistent — *continued*
  rhesus (Rh) titer — *see* Complication(s), transfusion, incompatibility reaction, Rh (factor)
  right aortic arch Q25.47
  sinus
    urogenitalis
      female Q52.8
      male Q55.8
    venosus with imperfect incorporation in right auricle Q26.8
  thymus (gland) (hyperplasia) E32.0
  thyroglossal duct Q89.2
  thyrolingual duct Q89.2
  truncus arteriosus or communis Q20.0
  tunica vasculosa lentis Q12.2
  umbilical sinus Q64.4
  urachus Q64.4
  vitelline duct Q43.0
Person (with)
  admitted for clinical research, as a control subject (normal comparison) (participant) Z00.6
  awaiting admission to adequate facility elsewhere Z75.1
  concern (normal) about sick person in family Z63.6
  consulting on behalf of another Z71.0
  feigning illness Z76.5
  living (in)
    without
      adequate housing (heating) (space) Z59.1
      housing (permanent) (temporary) Z59.0
      person able to render necessary care Z74.2
      shelter Z59.0
    alone Z60.2
    boarding school Z59.3
    residential institution Z59.3
  on waiting list Z75.1
  sick or handicapped in family Z63.6
Personality (disorder) F60.9
  accentuation of traits (type A pattern) Z73.1
  affective F34.0
  aggressive F60.3
  amoral F60.2
  anacastic, anankastic F60.5
  antisocial F60.2
  anxious F60.6
  asocial F60.2
  asthenic F60.7
  avoidant F60.6
  borderline F60.3
  change due to organic condition (enduring) F07.0
  compulsive F60.5
  cycloid F34.0
  cyclothymic F34.0
  dependent F60.7
  depressive F34.1
  dissocial F60.2
  dual F44.81
  eccentric F60.89
  emotionally unstable F60.3
  expansive paranoid F60.0
  explosive F60.3
  fanatic F60.0
  haltlose type F60.89
  histrionic F60.4
  hyperthymic F34.0
  hypothymic F34.1
  hysterical F60.4
  immature F60.89
  inadequate F60.7
  labile (emotional) F60.3
  mixed (nonspecific) F60.89
  morally defective F60.2
  multiple F44.81
  narcissistic F60.81
  obsessional F60.5
  obsessive (-compulsive) F60.5
  organic F07.0
  overconscientious F60.5
  paranoid F60.0
  passive (-dependent) F60.7
  passive-aggressive F60.89
  pathologic F60.9
  pattern defect or disturbance F60.9
  pseudopsychopathic (organic) F07.0
  pseudoretarded (organic) F07.0
  psychoinfantile F60.4
  psychoneurotic NEC F60.89
  psychopathic F60.2
  querulant F60.0

Personality — *continued*
  sadistic F60.89
  schizoid F60.1
  self-defeating F60.7
  sensitive paranoid F60.0
  sociopathic (amoral) (antisocial) (asocial) (dissocial) F60.2
  specified NEC F60.89
  type A Z73.1
  unstable (emotional) F60.3
Perthes' disease — *see* Legg-Calvé-Perthes disease
Pertussis (*see also* Whooping cough) A37.90
Perversion, perverted
  appetite F50.89
    psychogenic F50.89
  function
    pituitary gland E23.2
      posterior lobe E22.2
  sense of smell and taste R43.8
    psychogenic F45.8
  sexual — *see* Deviation, sexual
Pervious, congenital (*see also* Imperfect, closure)
  ductus arteriosus Q25.0
Pes (congenital) (*see also* Talipes)
  acquired (*see also* Deformity, limb, foot, specified NEC)
    planus — *see* Deformity, limb, flat foot
  adductus Q66.89
  cavus Q66.7
  deformity NEC, acquired — *see* Deformity, limb, foot, specified NEC
  planus (acquired) (any degree) (*see also* Deformity, limb, flat foot)
    rachitic sequelae (late effect) E64.3
  valgus Q66.6
Pest, pestis — *see* Plague
Petechia, petechiae R23.3
  newborn P54.5
Petechial typhus A75.9
Peter's anomaly Q13.4
Petit mal seizure — *see* Epilepsy, generalized, specified NEC
Petit's hernia — *see* Hernia, abdomen, specified site NEC
Petrellidosis B48.2
Petrositis H70.20- ☑
  acute H70.21- ☑
  chronic H70.22- ☑
Peutz-Jeghers disease or syndrome Q85.8
Peyronie's disease N48.6
PFAPA (periodic fever, aphthous stomatitis, pharyngitis, and adenopathy syndrome) M04.8
Pfeiffer's disease — *see* Mononucleosis, infectious
Phagedena (dry) (moist) (sloughing) (*see also* Gangrene)
  geometric L88
  penis N48.29
  tropical — *see* Ulcer, skin
  vulva N76.6
Phagedenic — *see* condition
Phakoma H35.89
Phakomatosis (*see also* specific eponymous syndromes) Q85.9
  Bourneville's Q85.1
  specified NEC Q85.8
Phantom limb syndrome (without pain) G54.7
  with pain G54.6
Pharyngeal pouch syndrome D82.1
Pharyngitis (acute) (catarrhal) (gangrenous) (infective) (malignant) (membranous) (phlegmonous) (pseudomembranous) (simple) (subacute) (suppurative) (ulcerative) (viral) J02.9
  with influenza, flu, or grippe — *see* Influenza, with, pharyngitis
  aphthous B08.5
  atrophic J31.2
  chlamydial A56.4
  chronic (atrophic) (granular) (hypertrophic) J31.2
  coxsackievirus B08.5
  diphtheritic A36.0
  enteroviral vesicular B08.5
  follicular (chronic) J31.2
  fusospirochetal A69.1
  gonococcal A54.5
  granular (chronic) J31.2
  herpesviral B00.2
  hypertrophic J31.2
  infectional, chronic J31.2
  influenzal — *see* Influenza, with, respiratory manifestations NEC

Pharyngitis — *continued*
  lymphonodular, acute (enteroviral) B08.8
  pneumococcal J02.8
  purulent J02.9
  putrid J02.9
  septic J02.0
  sicca J31.2
  specified organism NEC J02.8
  staphylococcal J02.8
  streptococcal J02.0
  syphilitic, congenital (early) A50.03
  tuberculous A15.8
  vesicular, enteroviral B08.5
  viral NEC J02.8
Pharyngoconjunctivitis, viral B30.2
Pharyngolaryngitis (acute) J06.0
  chronic J37.0
Pharyngoplegia J39.2
Pharyngotonsillitis, herpesviral B00.2
Pharyngotracheitis, chronic J42
Pharynx, pharyngeal — *see* condition
Phencyclidine-induced
  anxiety disorder F16.980
  bipolar and related disorder F16.94
  depressive disorder F16.94
  psychotic disorder F16.959
Phenomenon
  Arthus' — *see* Arthus' phenomenon
  jaw-winking Q07.8
  lupus erythematosus (LE) cell M32.9
  Raynaud's (secondary) I73.00
    with gangrene I73.01
  vasomotor R55
  vasospastic I73.9
  vasovagal R55
  Wenckebach's I44.1
Phenylketonuria E70.1
  classical E70.0
  maternal E70.1
Pheochromoblastoma
  specified site — *see* Neoplasm, malignant, by site
  unspecified site C74.10
Pheochromocytoma
  malignant
    specified site — *see* Neoplasm, malignant, by site
    unspecified site C74.10
  specified site — *see* Neoplasm, benign, by site
  unspecified site D35.00
Pheohyphomycosis — *see* Chromomycosis
Pheomycosis — *see* Chromomycosis
Phimosis (congenital) (due to infection) N47.1
  chancroidal A57
Phlebectasia (*see also* Varix)
  congenital Q27.4
Phlebitis (infective) (pyemic) (septic) (suppurative) I80.9
  antepartum — *see* Thrombophlebitis, antepartum
  blue — *see* Phlebitis, leg, deep
  breast, superficial I80.8
  cavernous (venous) sinus — *see* Phlebitis, intracranial (venous) sinus
  cerebral (venous) sinus — *see* Phlebitis, intracranial (venous) sinus
  chest wall, superficial I80.8
  cranial (venous) sinus — *see* Phlebitis, intracranial (venous) sinus
  deep (vessels) — *see* Phlebitis, leg, deep
  due to implanted device — *see* Complications, by site and type, specified NEC
  during or resulting from a procedure T81.72 ☑
  femoral vein (superficial) I80.1- ☑
  femoropopliteal vein I80.0- ☑
  gestational — *see* Phlebopathy, gestational
  hepatic veins I80.8
  iliofemoral — *see* Phlebitis, femoral vein
  intracranial (venous) sinus (any) G08
    nonpyogenic I67.6
  intraspinal venous sinuses and veins G08
    nonpyogenic G95.19
  lateral (venous) sinus — *see* Phlebitis, intracranial (venous) sinus
  leg I80.3
    antepartum — *see* Thrombophlebitis, antepartum
    deep (vessels) NEC I80.20- ☑
      iliac I80.21- ☑
      popliteal vein I80.22- ☑
      specified vessel NEC I80.29- ☑
      tibial vein I80.23- ☑

Persistence, persistent — Phlebitis

Phlebitis — *continued*
  leg — *continued*
    femoral vein (superficial) I80.1- ☑
    superficial (vessels) I80.0- ☑
  longitudinal sinus — *see* Phlebitis, intracranial (venous) sinus
  lower limb — *see* Phlebitis, leg
  migrans, migrating (superficial) I82.1
  pelvic
    with ectopic or molar pregnancy O08.0
    following ectopic or molar pregnancy O08.0
    puerperal, postpartum O87.1
  popliteal vein — *see* Phlebitis, leg, deep, popliteal
  portal (vein) K75.1
  postoperative T81.72 ☑
  pregnancy — *see* Thrombophlebitis, antepartum
  puerperal, postpartum, childbirth O87.0
    deep O87.1
    pelvic O87.1
    superficial O87.0
  retina — *see* Vasculitis, retina
  saphenous (accessory) (great) (long) (small) — *see* Phlebitis, leg, superficial
  sinus (meninges) — *see* Phlebitis, intracranial (venous) sinus
  specified site NEC I80.8
  syphilitic A52.09
  tibial vein — *see* Phlebitis, leg, deep, tibial
  ulcerative I80.9
    leg — *see* Phlebitis, leg
  umbilicus I80.8
  uterus (septic) — *see* Endometritis
  varicose (leg) (lower limb) — *see* Varix, leg, with, inflammation
Phlebofibrosis I87.8
Phleboliths I87.8
Phlebopathy,
  gestational O22.9- ☑
  puerperal O87.9
Phlebosclerosis I87.8
Phlebothrombosis (*see also* Thrombosis)
  antepartum — *see* Thrombophlebitis, antepartum
  pregnancy — *see* Thrombophlebitis, antepartum
  puerperal — *see* Thrombophlebitis, puerperal
Phlebotomus fever A93.1
Phlegmasia
  alba dolens O87.1
    nonpuerperal — *see* Phlebitis, femoral vein
  cerulea dolens — *see* Phlebitis, leg, deep
Phlegmon — *see* Abscess
Phlegmonous — *see* condition
Phlyctenulosis (allergic) (keratoconjunctivitis) (nontuberculous) (*see also* Keratoconjunctivitis)
  cornea — *see* Keratoconjunctivitis
  tuberculous A18.52
Phobia, phobic F40.9
  animal F40.218
    spiders F40.210
  examination F40.298
  reaction F40.9
  simple F40.298
  social F40.10
    generalized F40.11
  specific (isolated) F40.298
    animal F40.218
      spiders F40.210
    blood F40.230
    injection F40.231
    injury F40.233
    men F40.290
    natural environment F40.228
      thunderstorms F40.220
    situational F40.248
      bridges F40.242
      closed in spaces F40.240
      flying F40.243
      heights F40.241
    specified focus NEC F40.298
    transfusion F40.231
    women F40.291
  specified NEC F40.8
    medical care NEC F40.232
  state F40.9
Phocas' disease — *see* Mastopathy, cystic
Phocomelia Q73.1
  lower limb — *see* Agenesis, leg, with foot present
  upper limb — *see* Agenesis, arm, with hand present

Phoria H50.50
Phosphate-losing tubular disorder N25.0
Phosphatemia E83.39
Phosphaturia E83.39
Photodermatitis (sun) L56.8
  chronic L57.8
  due to drug L56.8
  light other than sun L59.8
Photokeratitis H16.13- ☑
Photophobia H53.14- ☑
Photophthalmia — *see* Photokeratitis
Photopsia H53.19
Photoretinitis — *see* Retinopathy, solar
Photosensitivity, photosensitization (sun) skin L56.8
  light other than sun L59.8
Phrenitis — *see* Encephalitis
Phrynoderma (vitamin A deficiency) E50.8
Phthiriasis (pubis) B85.3
  with any infestation classifiable to B85.0-B85.2 B85.4
Phthirus infestation — *see* Phthiriasis
Phthisis (*see also* Tuberculosis)
  bulbi (infectional) — *see* Disorder, globe, degenerated condition, atrophy
  eyeball (due to infection) — *see* Disorder, globe, degenerated condition, atrophy
Phycomycosis — *see* Zygomycosis
Physalopteriasis B81.8
Physical restraint status Z78.1
Phytobezoar T18.9 ☑
  intestine T18.3 ☑
  stomach T18.2 ☑
Pian — *see* Yaws
Pianoma A66.1
Pica F50.89
  in adults F50.89
  infant or child F98.3
Picking, nose F98.8
Pick-Niemann disease — *see* Niemann-Pick disease or syndrome
Pick's
  cerebral atrophy G31.01 [F02.80]
    with behavioral disturbance G31.01 [F02.81]
  disease or syndrome (brain) G31.01 [F02.80]
    with behavioral disturbance G31.01 [F02.81]
    brain G31.01 [F02.80]
      with behavioral disturbance G31.01 [F02.81]
    pericardium (pericardial pseudocirrhosis of liver) I31.1
  syndrome
    brain G31.01 [F02.80]
      with behavioral disturbance G31.01 [F02.81]
    of heart (pericardial pseudocirrhosis of liver) I31.1
Pickwickian syndrome E66.2
Piebaldism E70.39
Piedra (beard) (scalp) B36.8
  black B36.3
  white B36.2
Pierre Robin deformity or syndrome Q87.0
Pierson's disease or osteochondrosis M91.0
Pig-bel A05.2
Pigeon
  breast or chest (acquired) M95.4
    congenital Q67.7
    rachitic sequelae (late effect) E64.3
  breeder's disease or lung J67.2
  fancier's disease or lung J67.2
  toe — *see* Deformity, toe, specified NEC
Pigmentation (abnormal) (anomaly) L81.9
  conjunctiva H11.13- ☑
  cornea (anterior) H18.01- ☑
    posterior H18.05- ☑
    stromal H18.06- ☑
  diminished melanin formation NEC L81.6
  iron L81.8
  lids, congenital Q82.8
  limbus corneae — *see* Pigmentation, cornea
  metals L81.8
  optic papilla, congenital Q14.2
  retina, congenital (grouped) (nevoid) Q14.1
  scrotum, congenital Q82.8
  tattoo L81.8
Piles (*see also* Hemorrhoids) K64.9
Pili
  annulati or torti (congenital) Q84.1
  incarnati L73.1
Pill roller hand (intrinsic) — *see* Parkinsonism
Pilomatrixoma — *see* Neoplasm, skin, benign

Pilomatrixoma — *continued*
  malignant — *see* Neoplasm, skin, malignant
Pilonidal — *see* condition
Pimple R23.8
PIN — *see* Neoplasia, intraepithelial, prostate
Pinched nerve — *see* Neuropathy, entrapment
Pindborg tumor — *see* Cyst, calcifying odontogenic
Pineal body or gland — *see* condition
Pinealoblastoma C75.3
Pinealoma D44.5
  malignant C75.3
Pineoblastoma C75.3
Pineocytoma D44.5
Pinguecula H11.15- ☑
Pingueculitis H10.81- ☑
Pinhole meatus (*see also* Stricture, urethra) N35.9
Pink
  disease — *see* subcategory T56.1 ☑
  eye — *see* Conjunctivitis, acute, mucopurulent
Pinkus' disease (lichen nitidus) L44.1
Pinpoint
  meatus — *see* Stricture, urethra
  os (uteri) — *see* Stricture, cervix
Pins and needles R20.2
Pinta A67.9
  cardiovascular lesions A67.2
  chancre (primary) A67.0
  erythematous plaques A67.1
  hyperchromic lesions A67.1
  hyperkeratosis A67.1
  lesions A67.9
    cardiovascular A67.2
    hyperchromic A67.1
    intermediate A67.1
    late A67.2
    mixed A67.3
    primary A67.0
    skin (achromic) (cicatricial) (dyschromic) A67.2
      hyperchromic A67.1
      mixed (achromic and hyperchromic) A67.3
  papule (primary) A67.0
  skin lesions (achromic) (cicatricial) (dyschromic) A67.2
    hyperchromic A67.1
    mixed (achromic and hyperchromic) A67.3
  vitiligo A67.2
Pintids A67.1
Pinworm (disease) (infection) (infestation) B80
Piroplasmosis B60.0
Pistol wound — *see* Gunshot wound
Pitchers' elbow — *see* Derangement, joint, specified type NEC, elbow
Pithecoid pelvis Q74.2
  with disproportion (fetopelvic) O33.0
    causing obstructed labor O65.0
Pithiatism F48.8
Pitted — *see* Pitting
Pitting (*see also* Edema) R60.9
  lip R60.0
  nail L60.8
  teeth K00.4
Pituitary gland — *see* condition
Pituitary-snuff-taker's disease J67.8
Pityriasis (capitis) L21.0
  alba L30.5
  circinata (et maculata) L42
  furfuracea L21.0
  Hebra's L26
  lichenoides L41.0
    chronica L41.1
    et varioliformis (acuta) L41.0
  maculata (et circinata) L30.5
  nigra B36.1
  pilaris, Hebra's L44.0
  rosea L42
  rotunda L44.8
  rubra (Hebra) pilaris L44.0
  simplex L30.5
  specified type NEC L30.5
  streptogenes L30.5
  versicolor (scrotal) B36.0
Placenta, placental — *see* Pregnancy, complicated by (care of) (management affected by), specified condition
Placentitis O41.14- ☑
Plagiocephaly Q67.3
Plague A20.9
  abortive A20.8

⬇ **Subterms under main terms may continue to next column or page**   ☑ **Additional Character Required — Refer to the Tabular List for Character Selection**   **253**

Phlebitis — Plague

Plague — *continued*
　ambulatory A20.8
　asymptomatic A20.8
　bubonic A20.0
　cellulocutaneous A20.1
　cutaneobubonic A20.1
　lymphatic gland A20.0
　meningitis A20.3
　pharyngeal A20.8
　pneumonic (primary) (secondary) A20.2
　pulmonary, pulmonic A20.2
　septicemic A20.7
　tonsillar A20.8
　　septicemic A20.7
Planning, family
　contraception Z30.9
　procreation Z31.69
Plaque(s)
　artery, arterial — *see* Arteriosclerosis
　calcareous — *see* Calcification
　coronary, lipid rich I25.83
　epicardial I31.8
　erythematous, of pinta A67.1
　Hollenhorst's — *see* Occlusion, artery, retina
　lipid rich, coronary I25.83
　pleural (without asbestos) J92.9
　　with asbestos J92.0
　tongue K13.29
Plasmacytoma C90.3- ☑
　extramedullary C90.2- ☑
　medullary C90.0- ☑
　solitary C90.3- ☑
Plasmacytopenia D72.818
Plasmacytosis D72.822
Plaster ulcer — *see* Ulcer, pressure, by site
Plateau iris syndrome (post-iridectomy) (postprocedural) (without glaucoma) H21.82
　with glaucoma H40.22- ☑
Platybasia Q75.8
Platyonychia (congenital) Q84.6
　acquired L60.8
Platypelloid pelvis M95.5
　with disproportion (fetopelvic) O33.0
　　causing obstructed labor O65.0
　congenital Q74.2
Platyspondylisis Q76.49
Plaut (-Vincent) **disease** (*see also* Vincent's) A69.1
Plethora R23.2
　newborn P61.1
Pleura, pleural — *see* condition
Pleuralgia R07.81
Pleurisy (acute) (adhesive) (chronic) (costal) (diaphragmatic) (double) (dry) (fibrinous) (fibrous) (interlobar) (latent) (plastic) (primary) (residual) (sicca) (sterile) (subacute) (unresolved) R09.1
　with
　　adherent pleura J86.0
　　effusion J90
　　　chylous, chyliform J94.0
　　　tuberculous (non primary) A15.6
　　　　primary (progressive) A15.7
　　　tuberculosis — *see* Pleurisy, tuberculous (non primary)
　encysted — *see* Pleurisy, with effusion
　exudative — *see* Pleurisy, with effusion
　fibrinopurulent, fibropurulent — *see* Pyothorax
　hemorrhagic — *see* Hemothorax
　pneumococcal J90
　purulent — *see* Pyothorax
　septic — *see* Pyothorax
　serofibrinous — *see* Pleurisy, with effusion
　seropurulent — *see* Pyothorax
　serous — *see* Pleurisy, with effusion
　staphylococcal J86.9
　streptococcal J90
　suppurative — *see* Pyothorax
　traumatic (post) (current) — *see* Injury, intrathoracic, pleura
　tuberculous (with effusion) (non primary) A15.6
　　primary (progressive) A15.7
Pleuritis sicca — *see* Pleurisy
Pleurobronchopneumonia — *see* Pneumonia, broncho-
Pleurodynia R07.81
　epidemic B33.0
　viral B33.0
Pleuropericarditis (*see also* Pericarditis)
　acute I30.9

Pleuropneumonia (acute) (bilateral) (double) (septic) (*see also* Pneumonia) J18.8
　chronic — *see* Fibrosis, lung
Pleuro-pneumonia-like-organism (PPLO), as cause of disease classified elsewhere B96.0
Pleurorrhea — *see* Pleurisy, with effusion
Plexitis, brachial G54.0
Plica
　polonica B85.0
　syndrome, knee M67.5- ☑
　tonsil J35.8
Plicated tongue K14.5
Plug
　bronchus NEC J98.09
　meconium (newborn) NEC syndrome P76.0
　mucus — *see* Asphyxia, mucus
Plumbism — *see* subcategory T56.0 ☑
Plummer's disease E05.20
　with thyroid storm E05.21
Plummer-Vinson syndrome D50.1
Pluricarential syndrome of infancy E40
Plus (and minus) **hand** (intrinsic) — *see* Deformity, limb, specified type NEC, forearm
Pneumathemia — *see* Air, embolism
Pneumatic hammer (drill) syndrome T75.21 ☑
Pneumatocele (lung) J98.4
　intracranial G93.89
　tension J44.9
Pneumatosis
　cystoides intestinalis K63.89
　intestinalis K63.89
　peritonei K66.8
Pneumaturia R39.89
Pneumoblastoma — *see* Neoplasm, lung, malignant
Pneumocephalus G93.89
Pneumococcemia A40.3
Pneumococcus, pneumococcal — *see* condition
Pneumoconiosis (due to) (inhalation of) J64
　with tuberculosis (any type in A15) J65
　aluminum J63.0
　asbestos J61
　bagasse, bagassosis J67.1
　bauxite J63.1
　beryllium J63.2
　coal miners' (simple) J60
　coalworkers' (simple) J60
　collier's J60
　cotton dust J66.0
　diatomite (diatomaceous earth) J62.8
　dust
　　inorganic NEC J63.6
　　lime J62.8
　　marble J62.8
　　organic NEC J66.8
　fumes or vapors (from silo) J68.9
　graphite J63.3
　grinder's J62.8
　kaolin J62.8
　mica J62.8
　millstone maker's J62.8
　mineral fibers NEC J61
　miner's J60
　moldy hay J67.0
　potter's J62.8
　rheumatoid — *see* Rheumatoid, lung
　sandblaster's J62.8
　silica, silicate NEC J62.8
　　with carbon J60
　stonemason's J62.8
　talc (dust) J62.0
Pneumocystis carinii pneumonia B59
Pneumocystis jiroveci (pneumonia) B59
Pneumocystosis (with pneumonia) B59
Pneumohemopericardium I31.2
Pneumohemothorax J94.2
　traumatic S27.2 ☑
Pneumohydropericardium — *see* Pericarditis
Pneumohydrothorax — *see* Hydrothorax
Pneumomediastinum J98.2
　congenital or perinatal P25.2
Pneumomycosis B49 [J99]
Pneumonia (acute) (double) (migratory) (purulent) (septic) (unresolved) J18.9
　with
　　influenza — *see* Influenza, with, pneumonia
　　lung abscess J85.1

Pneumonia — *continued*
　with — *continued*
　　lung abscess — *continued*
　　　due to specified organism — *see* Pneumonia, in (due to)
　adenoviral J12.0
　adynamic J18.2
　alba A50.04
　allergic (eosinophilic) J82
　alveolar — *see* Pneumonia, lobar
　anaerobes J15.8
　anthrax A22.1
　apex, apical — *see* Pneumonia, lobar
　Ascaris B77.81
　aspiration J69.0
　　due to
　　　aspiration of microorganisms
　　　　bacterial J15.9
　　　　viral J12.9
　　　food (regurgitated) J69.0
　　　gastric secretions J69.0
　　　milk (regurgitated) J69.0
　　　oils, essences J69.1
　　　solids, liquids NEC J69.8
　　　vomitus J69.0
　　newborn P24.81
　　　amniotic fluid (clear) P24.11
　　　blood P24.21
　　　food (regurgitated) P24.31
　　　liquor (amnii) P24.11
　　　meconium P24.01
　　　milk P24.31
　　　mucus P24.11
　　　specified NEC P24.81
　　　stomach contents P24.31
　　postprocedural J95.4
　atypical NEC J18.9
　bacillus J15.9
　　specified NEC J15.8
　bacterial J15.9
　　specified NEC J15.8
　Bacteroides (fragilis) (oralis) (melaninogenicus) J15.8
　basal, basic, basilar — *see* Pneumonia, by type
　bronchiolitis obliterans organized (BOOP) J84.89
　broncho-, bronchial (confluent) (croupous) (diffuse) (disseminated) (hemorrhagic) (involving lobes) (lobar) (terminal) J18.0
　　allergic (eosinophilic) J82
　　aspiration — *see* Pneumonia, aspiration
　　bacterial J15.9
　　　specified NEC J15.8
　　chronic — *see* Fibrosis, lung
　　diplococcal J13
　　Eaton's agent J15.7
　　Escherichia coli (E. coli) J15.5
　　Friedländer's bacillus J15.0
　　Hemophilus influenzae J14
　　hypostatic J18.2
　　inhalation (*see also* Pneumonia, aspiration)
　　　due to fumes or vapors (chemical) J68.0
　　　of oils or essences J69.1
　　Klebsiella (pneumoniae) J15.0
　　lipid, lipoid J69.1
　　　endogenous J84.89
　　Mycoplasma (pneumoniae) J15.7
　　pleuro-pneumonia-like-organisms (PPLO) J15.7
　　pneumococcal J13
　　Proteus J15.6
　　Pseudomonas J15.1
　　Serratia marcescens J15.6
　　specified organism NEC J16.8
　　staphylococcal — *see* Pneumonia, staphylococcal
　　streptococcal NEC J15.4
　　　group B J15.3
　　　pneumoniae J13
　　viral, virus — *see* Pneumonia, viral
　Butyrivibrio (fibriosolvens) J15.8
　Candida B37.1
　caseous — *see* Tuberculosis, pulmonary
　catarrhal — *see* Pneumonia, broncho
　chlamydial J16.0
　　congenital P23.1
　cholesterol J84.89
　cirrhotic (chronic) — *see* Fibrosis, lung
　Clostridium (haemolyticum) (novyi) J15.8
　confluent — *see* Pneumonia, broncho
　congenital (infective) P23.9

☑ **Additional Character Required** — Refer to the Tabular List for Character Selection　　　▽ **Subterms under main terms may continue to next column or page**

Pneumonia — *continued*
  congenital — *continued*
    due to
      bacterium NEC P23.6
      Chlamydia P23.1
      Escherichia coli P23.4
      Haemophilus influenzae P23.6
      infective organism NEC P23.8
      Klebsiella pneumoniae P23.6
      Mycoplasma P23.6
      Pseudomonas P23.5
      Staphylococcus P23.2
      Streptococcus (except group B) P23.6
        group B P23.3
      viral agent P23.0
    specified NEC P23.8
  croupous — *see* Pneumonia, lobar
  cryptogenic organizing J84.116
  cytomegalic inclusion B25.0
  cytomegaloviral B25.0
  deglutition — *see* Pneumonia, aspiration
  desquamative interstitial J84.117
  diffuse — *see* Pneumonia, broncho
  diplococcal, diplococcus (broncho-) (lobar) J13
  disseminated (focal) — *see* Pneumonia, broncho
  Eaton's agent J15.7
  embolic, embolism — *see* Embolism, pulmonary
  Enterobacter J15.6
  eosinophilic J82
  Escherichia coli (E. coli) J15.5
  Eubacterium J15.8
  fibrinous — *see* Pneumonia, lobar
  fibroid, fibrous (chronic) — *see* Fibrosis, lung
  Friedländer's bacillus J15.0
  Fusobacterium (nucleatum) J15.8
  gangrenous J85.0
  giant cell (measles) B05.2
  gonococcal A54.84
  gram-negative bacteria NEC J15.6
    anaerobic J15.8
  Hemophilus influenzae (broncho) (lobar) J14
  human metapneumovirus J12.3
  hypostatic (broncho) (lobar) J18.2
  in (due to)
    actinomycosis A42.0
    adenovirus J12.0
    anthrax A22.1
    ascariasis B77.81
    aspergillosis B44.9
    Bacillus anthracis A22.1
    Bacterium anitratum J15.6
    candidiasis B37.1
    chickenpox B01.2
    Chlamydia J16.0
      neonatal P23.1
    coccidioidomycosis B38.2
      acute B38.0
      chronic B38.1
    cytomegalovirus disease B25.0
    Eaton's agent J15.7
    Enterobacter J15.6
    Escherichia coli (E. coli) J15.5
    Friedländer's bacillus J15.0
    fumes and vapors (chemical) (inhalation) J68.0
    gonorrhea A54.84
    Hemophilus influenzae (H. influenzae) J14
    Herellea J15.6
    histoplasmosis B39.2
      acute B39.0
      chronic B39.1
    human metapneumovirus J12.3
    Klebsiella (pneumoniae) J15.0
    measles B05.2
    Mycoplasma (pneumoniae) J15.7
    nocardiosis, nocardiasis A43.0
    ornithosis A70
    parainfluenza virus J12.2
    pleuro-pneumonia-like-organism (PPLO) J15.7
    pneumococcus J13
    pneumocystosis (Pneumocystis carinii) (Pneumo-
      cystis jiroveci) B59
    Proteus J15.6
    Pseudomonas NEC J15.1
      pseudomallei A24.1
    psittacosis A70
    Q fever A78
    respiratory syncytial virus J12.1

Pneumonia — *continued*
  in — *continued*
    rheumatic fever I00 [J17]
    rubella B06.81
    Salmonella (infection) A02.22
      typhi A01.03
    schistosomiasis B65.9 [J17]
    Serratia marcescens J15.6
    specified
      bacterium NEC J15.8
      organism NEC J16.8
    spirochetal NEC A69.8
    Staphylococcus J15.20
      aureus (methicillin susceptible) (MSSA) J15.211
        methicillin resistant (MRSA) J15.212
      specified NEC J15.29
    Streptococcus J15.4
      group B J15.3
      pneumoniae J13
      specified NEC J15.4
    toxoplasmosis B58.3
    tularemia A21.2
    typhoid (fever) A01.03
    varicella B01.2
    virus — *see* Pneumonia, viral
    whooping cough A37.91
      due to
        Bordetella parapertussis A37.11
        Bordetella pertussis A37.01
        specified NEC A37.81
    Yersinia pestis A20.2
  inhalation of food or vomit — *see* Pneumonia, aspira-
    tion
  interstitial J84.9
    chronic J84.111
    desquamative J84.117
    due to
      collagen vascular disease J84.17
      known underlying cause J84.17
    idiopathic NOS J84.111
    in disease classified elsewhere J84.17
    lymphocytic (due to collagen vascular disease) (in
      diseases classified elsewhere) J84.17
    lymphoid J84.2
    non-specific J84.89
      due to
        collagen vascular disease J84.17
        known underlying cause J84.17
      idiopathic J84.113
      in diseases classified elsewhere J84.17
    plasma cell B59
    pseudomonas J15.1
    usual J84.112
      due to collagen vascular disease J84.17
      idiopathic J84.112
      in diseases classified elsewhere J84.17
  Klebsiella (pneumoniae) J15.0
  lipid, lipoid (exogenous) J69.1
    endogenous J84.89
  lobar (disseminated) (double) (interstitial) J18.1
    bacterial J15.9
      specified NEC J15.8
    chronic — *see* Fibrosis, lung
    Escherichia coli (E. coli) J15.5
    Friedländer's bacillus J15.0
    Hemophilus influenzae J14
    hypostatic J18.2
    Klebsiella (pneumoniae) J15.0
    pneumococcal J13
    Proteus J15.6
    Pseudomonas J15.1
    specified organism NEC J16.8
    staphylococcal — *see* Pneumonia, staphylococcal
    streptococcal NEC J15.4
    Streptococcus pneumoniae J13
    viral, virus — *see* Pneumonia, viral
  lobular — *see* Pneumonia, broncho
  Löffler's J82
  lymphoid interstitial J84.2
  massive — *see* Pneumonia, lobar
  meconium P24.01
  MRSA (methicillin resistant Staphylococcus aureus)
    J15.212
  MSSA (methicillin susceptible Staphylococcus aureus)
    J15.211
  multilobar — *see* Pneumonia, by type
  Mycoplasma (pneumoniae) J15.7
  necrotic J85.0

Pneumonia — *continued*
  neonatal P23.9
    aspiration — *see* Aspiration, by substance, with
      pneumonia
  nitrogen dioxide J68.0
  organizing J84.89
    due to
      collagen vascular disease J84.17
      known underlying cause J84.17
    in diseases classified elsewhere J84.17
  orthostatic J18.2
  parainfluenza virus J12.2
  parenchymatous — *see* Fibrosis, lung
  passive J18.2
  patchy — *see* Pneumonia, broncho
  Peptococcus J15.8
  Peptostreptococcus J15.8
  plasma cell (of infants) B59
  pleurolobar — *see* Pneumonia, lobar
  pleuro-pneumonia-like organism (PPLO) J15.7
  pneumococcal (broncho) (lobar) J13
  Pneumocystis (carinii) (jiroveci) B59
  postinfectional NEC B99 ☑ [J17]
  postmeasles B05.2
  Proteus J15.6
  Pseudomonas J15.1
  psittacosis A70
  radiation J70.0
  respiratory syncytial virus J12.1
  resulting from a procedure J95.89
  rheumatic I00 [J17]
  Salmonella (arizonae) (cholerae-suis) (enteritidis) (ty-
    phimurium) A02.22
    typhi A01.03
    typhoid fever A01.03
  SARS-associated coronavirus J12.81
  segmented, segmental — *see* Pneumonia, broncho-
  Serratia marcescens J15.6
  specified NEC J18.8
    bacterium NEC J15.8
    organism NEC J16.8
    virus NEC J12.89
  spirochetal NEC A69.8
  staphylococcal (broncho) (lobar) J15.20
    aureus (methicillin susceptible) (MSSA) J15.211
      methicillin resistant (MRSA) J15.212
    specified NEC J15.29
  static, stasis J18.2
  streptococcal NEC (broncho) (lobar) J15.4
    group
      A J15.4
      B J15.3
    specified NEC J15.4
  Streptococcus pneumoniae J13
  syphilitic, congenital (early) A50.04
  traumatic (complication) (early) (secondary) T79.8 ☑
  tuberculous (any) — *see* Tuberculosis, pulmonary
  tularemic A21.2
  varicella B01.2
  Veillonella J15.8
  ventilator associated J95.851
  viral, virus (broncho) (interstitial) (lobar) J12.9
    adenoviral J12.0
    congenital P23.0
    human metapneumovirus J12.3
    parainfluenza J12.2
    respiratory syncytial J12.1
    SARS-associated coronavirus J12.81
    specified NEC J12.89
  white (congenital) A50.04
Pneumonic — *see* condition
Pneumonitis (acute) (primary) (*see also* Pneumonia)
  air-conditioner J67.7
  allergic (due to) J67.9
    organic dust NEC J67.8
    red cedar dust J67.8
    sequoiosis J67.8
    wood dust J67.8
  aspiration J69.0
    due to
      anesthesia J95.4
        during
          labor and delivery O74.0
          pregnancy O29.01- ☑
          puerperium O89.01
      fumes or gases J68.0
    obstetric O74.0

Pneumonitis — *continued*
  chemical (due to gases, fumes or vapors) (inhalation)
      J68.0
    due to anesthesia J95.4
  cholesterol J84.89
  chronic — *see* Fibrosis, lung
  congenital rubella P35.0
  crack (cocaine) J68.0
  due to
    beryllium J68.0
    cadmium J68.0
    crack (cocaine) J68.0
    detergent J69.8
    fluorocarbon-polymer J68.0
    food, vomit (aspiration) J69.0
    fumes or vapors J68.0
    gases, fumes or vapors (inhalation) J68.0
    inhalation
      blood J69.8
      essences J69.1
      food (regurgitated), milk, vomit J69.0
      oils, essences J69.1
      saliva J69.0
      solids, liquids NEC J69.8
    manganese J68.0
    nitrogen dioxide J68.0
    oils, essences J69.1
    solids, liquids NEC J69.8
    toxoplasmosis (acquired) B58.3
      congenital P37.1
    vanadlum J68.0
    ventilator J95.851
  eosinophilic J82
  hypersensitivity J67.9
    air conditioner lung J67.7
    bagassosis J67.1
    bird fancier's lung J67.2
    farmer's lung J67.0
    maltworker's lung J67.4
    maple bark-stripper's lung J67.6
    mushroom worker's lung J67.5
    specified organic dust NEC J67.8
    suberosis J67.3
  interstitial (chronic) J84.89
    acute J84.114
    lymphoid J84.2
    non-specific J84.89
      idiopathic J84.113
  lymphoid, interstitial J84.2
  meconium P24.01
  postanesthetic J95.4
    correct substance properly administered — *see*
        Table of Drugs and Chemicals, by drug, ad-
        verse effect
    in labor and delivery O74.0
    in pregnancy O29.01- ☑
    obstetric O74.0
    overdose or wrong substance given or taken (by
        accident) — *see* Table of Drugs and Chemi-
        cals, by drug, poisoning
    postpartum, puerperal O89.01
  postoperative J95.4
    obstetric O74.0
  radiation J70.0
  rubella, congenital P35.0
  ventilation (air-conditioning) J67.7
  ventilator associated J95.851
  wood-dust J67.8
Pneumonoconiosis — *see* Pneumoconiosis
Pneumoparotid K11.8
Pneumopathy NEC J98.4
  alveolar J84.09
  due to organic dust NEC J66.8
  parietoalveolar J84.09
Pneumopericarditis (*see also* Pericarditis)
  acute I30.9
Pneumopericardium (*see also* Pericarditis)
  congenital P25.3
  newborn P25.3
  traumatic (post) — *see* Injury, heart
Pneumophagia (psychogenic) F45.8
Pneumopleurisy, pneumopleuritis (*see also* Pneumo-
    nia) J18.8
Pneumopyopericardium I30.1
Pneumopyothorax — *see* Pyopneumothorax
  with fistula J86.0
Pneumorrhagia (*see also* Hemorrhage, lung)
  tuberculous — *see* Tuberculosis, pulmonary

Pneumothorax NOS J93.9
  acute J93.83
  chronic J93.81
  congenital P25.1
  perinatal period P25.1
  postprocedural J95.811
  specified NEC J93.83
  spontaneous NOS J93.83
    newborn P25.1
    primary J93.11
    secondary J93.12
    tension J93.0
  tense valvular, infectional J93.0
  tension (spontaneous) J93.0
  traumatic S27.0 ☑
    with hemothorax S27.2 ☑
  tuberculous — *see* Tuberculosis, pulmonary
Podagra (*see also* Gout) M10.9
Podencephalus Q01.9
Poikilocytosis R71.8
Poikiloderma L81.6
  Civatte's L57.3
  congenital Q82.8
  vasculare atrophicans L94.5
Poikilodermatomyositis M33.10
  with
    myopathy M33.12
    respiratory involvement M33.11
    specified organ involvement NEC M33.19
Pointed ear (congenital) Q17.3
Poison ivy, oak, sumac or other plant dermatitis
    (allergic) (contact) L23.7
Poisoning (acute) (*see also* Table of Drugs and Chemicals)
  algae and toxins T65.82- ☑
  Bacillus B (aertrycke) (cholerae (suis)) (paratyphosus)
      (suipestifer) A02.9
    botulinus A05.1
  bacterial toxins A05.9
  berries, noxious — *see* Poisoning, food, noxious,
      berries
  botulism A05.1
  ciguatera fish T61.0- ☑
  Clostridium botulinum A05.1
  death-cap (Amanita phalloides) (Amanita verna) —
      see Poisoning, food, noxious, mushrooms
  drug — *see* Table of Drugs and Chemicals, by drug,
      poisoning
  epidemic, fish (noxious) — *see* Poisoning, seafood
    bacterial A05.9
  fava bean D55.0
  fish (noxious) T61.9- ☑
    bacterial — *see* Intoxication, foodborne, by agent
    ciguatera fish — *see* Poisoning, ciguatera fish
    scombroid fish — *see* Poisoning, scombroid fish
    specified type NEC T61.77- ☑
  food (acute) (diseased) (infected) (noxious) NEC
      T62.9- ☑
    bacterial — *see* Intoxication, foodborne, by agent
    due to
      Bacillus (aertrycke) (choleraesuis) (paratypho-
          sus) (suipestifer) A02.9
        botulinus A05.1
      Clostridium (perfringens) (Welchii) A05.2
      salmonella (aertrycke) (callinarum) (choleraesu-
          is) (enteritidis) (paratyphi) (suipestifer)
          A02.9
        with
          gastroenteritis A02.0
          sepsis A02.1
      staphylococcus A05.0
      Vibrio
        parahaemolyticus A05.3
        vulnificus A05.5
    noxious or naturally toxic T62.9- ☑
      berries — *see* subcategory T62.1 ☑
      fish — *see* Poisoning, seafood
      mushrooms — *see* subcategory T62.0X ☑
      plants NEC — *see* subcategory T62.2X ☑
      seafood — *see* Poisoning, seafood
      specified NEC — *see* subcategory T62.8X ☑
    ichthyotoxism — *see* Poisoning, seafood
    kreotoxism, food A05.9
    latex T65.81- ☑
    lead T56.0- ☑
  mushroom — *see* Poisoning, food, noxious, mushroom
  mussels (*see also* Poisoning, shellfish)
    bacterial — *see* Intoxication, foodborne, by agent

Poisoning — *continued*
  nicotine (tobacco) T65.2- ☑
  noxious foodstuffs — *see* Poisoning, food, noxious
  plants, noxious — *see* Poisoning, food, noxious, plants
      NEC
  ptomaine — *see* Poisoning, food
  radiation J70.0
  Salmonella (arizonae) (cholerae-suis) (enteritidis) (ty-
      phimurium) A02.9
  scombroid fish T61.1- ☑
  seafood (noxious) T61.9- ☑
    bacterial — *see* Intoxication, foodborne, by agent
    fish — *see* Poisoning, fish
    shellfish — *see* Poisoning, shellfish
    specified NEC — *see* subcategory T61.8X ☑
  shellfish (amnesic) (azaspiracid) (diarrheic) (neurotoxic)
      (noxious) (paralytic) T61.78- ☑
    bacterial — *see* Intoxication, foodborne, by agent
    ciguatera mollusk — *see* Poisoning, ciguatera fish
  specified substance NEC T65.891 ☑
  Staphylococcus, food A05.0
  tobacco (nicotine) T65.2- ☑
  water E87.79
Poker spine — *see* Spondylitis, ankylosing
Poland syndrome Q79.8
Polioencephalitis (acute) (bulbar) A80.9
  inferior G12.22
  influenzal — *see* Influenza, with, encephalopathy
  superior hemorrhagic (acute) (Wernicke's) E51.2
  Wernicke's E51.2
Polioencephalomyelitis (acute) (anterior) A80.9
  with beriberi E51.2
Polioencephalopathy, superior hemorrhagic E51.2
  with
    beriberi E51.11
    pellagra E52
Poliomeningoencephalitis — *see* Meningoencephalitis
Poliomyelitis (acute) (anterior) (epidemic) A80.9
  with paralysis (bulbar) — *see* Poliomyelitis, paralytic
  abortive A80.4
  ascending (progressive) — *see* Poliomyelitis, paralytic
  bulbar (paralytic) — *see* Poliomyelitis, paralytic
  congenital P35.8
  nonepidemic A80.9
  nonparalytic A80.4
  paralytic A80.30
    specified NEC A80.39
    vaccine-associated A80.0
    wild virus
      imported A80.1
      indigenous A80.2
  spinal, acute A80.9
Poliosis (eyebrow) (eyelashes) L67.1
  circumscripta, acquired L67.1
Pollakiuria R35.0
  psychogenic F45.8
Pollinosis J30.1
Pollitzer's disease L73.2
Polyadenitis (*see also* Lymphadenitis)
  malignant A20.0
Polyalgia M79.89
Polyangiitis M30.0
  microscopic M31.7
  overlap syndrome M30.8
Polyarteritis
  microscopic M31.7
  nodosa M30.0
    with lung involvement M30.1
    juvenile M30.2
    related condition NEC M30.8
Polyarthralgia — *see* Pain, joint
Polyarthritis, polyarthropathy (*see also* Arthritis) M13.0
  due to or associated with other specified conditions
      — *see* Arthritis
  epidemic (Australian) (with exanthema) B33.1
  infective — *see* Arthritis, pyogenic or pyemic
  inflammatory M06.4
  juvenile (chronic) (seronegative) M08.3
  migratory — *see* Fever, rheumatic
  rheumatic, acute — *see* Fever, rheumatic
Polyarthrosis M15.9
  post-traumatic M15.3
  primary M15.0
  specified NEC M15.8
Polycarential syndrome of infancy E40
Polychondritis (atrophic) (chronic) (*see also* Disorder,
    cartilage, specified type NEC)
  relapsing M94.1

☑ **Additional Character Required** — Refer to the Tabular List for Character Selection   ▽ **Subterms under main terms may continue to next column or page**

Polycoria Q13.2
Polycystic (disease)
  degeneration, kidney Q61.3
    autosomal dominant (adult type) Q61.2
    autosomal recessive (infantile type)
      NEC Q61.19
  kidney Q61.3
    autosomal
      dominant Q61.2
      recessive NEC Q61.19
    autosomal dominant (adult type) Q61.2
    autosomal recessive (childhood type) NEC Q61.19
    infantile type NEC Q61.19
  liver Q44.6
  lung J98.4
    congenital Q33.0
  ovary, ovaries E28.2
  spleen Q89.09
Polycythemia (secondary) D75.1
  acquired D75.1
  benign (familial) D75.0
  due to
    donor twin P61.1
    erythropoietin D75.1
    fall in plasma volume D75.1
    high altitude D75.1
    maternal-fetal transfusion P61.1
    stress D75.1
  emotional D75.1
  erythropoietin D75.1
  familial (benign) D75.0
  Gaisböck's (hypertonica) D75.1
  high altitude D75.1
  hypertonica D75.1
  hypoxemic D75.1
  neonatorum P61.1
  nephrogenous D75.1
  relative D75.1
  secondary D75.1
  spurious D75.1
  stress D75.1
  vera D45
Polycytosis cryptogenica D75.1
Polydactylism, polydactyly Q69.9
  toes Q69.2
Polydipsia R63.1
Polydystrophy, pseudo-Hurler E77.0
Polyembryoma — *see* Neoplasm, malignant, by site
Polyglandular
  deficiency E31.0
  dyscrasia E31.9
  dysfunction E31.9
  syndrome E31.8
Polyhydramnios O40.- ☑
Polymastia Q83.1
Polymenorrhea N92.0
Polymyalgia M35.3
  arteritica, giant cell M31.5
  rheumatica M35.3
    with giant cell arteritis M31.5
Polymyositis (acute) (chronic) (hemorrhagic) M33.20
  with
    myopathy M33.22
    respiratory involvement M33.21
    skin involvement — *see* Dermatopolymyositis
    specified organ involvement NEC M33.29
  ossificans (generalisata) (progressiva) — *see* Myositis, ossificans, progressiva
Polyneuritis, polyneuritic (*see also* Polyneuropathy)
  acute (post-)infective G61.0
  alcoholic G62.1
  cranialis G52.7
  demyelinating, chronic inflammatory (CIDP) G61.81
  diabetic — *see* Diabetes, polyneuropathy
  diphtheritic A36.83
  due to lack of vitamin NEC E56.9 [G63]
  endemic E51.11
  erythredema — *see* subcategory T56.1 ☑
  febrile, acute G61.0
  hereditary ataxic G60.1
  idiopathic, acute G61.0
  infective (acute) G61.0
  inflammatory, chronic demyelinating (CIDP) G61.81
  nutritional E63.9 [G63]
  postinfective (acute) G61.0
  specified NEC G62.89
Polyneuropathy (peripheral) G62.9

Polyneuropathy — *continued*
  alcoholic G62.1
  amyloid (Portuguese) E85.1 [G63]
    transthyretin-related (ATTR) familial E85.1
  arsenical G62.2
  critical illness G62.81
  demyelinating, chronic inflammatory (CIDP) G61.81
  diabetic — *see* Diabetes, polyneuropathy
  drug-induced G62.0
  hereditary G60.9
    specified NEC G60.8
  idiopathic G60.9
    progressive G60.3
  in (due to)
    alcohol G62.1
      sequelae G65.2
    amyloidosis, familial (Portuguese) E85.1 [G63]
    antitetanus serum G61.1
    arsenic G62.2
      sequelae G65.2
    avitaminosis NEC E56.9 [G63]
    beriberi E51.11
    collagen vascular disease NEC M35.9 [G63]
    deficiency (of)
      B (-complex) vitamins E53.9 [G63]
      vitamin B6 E53.1 [G63]
    diabetes — *see* Diabetes, polyneuropathy
    diphtheria A36.83
    drug or medicament G62.0
      correct substance properly administered — *see* Table of Drugs and Chemicals, by drug, adverse effect
      overdose or wrong substance given or taken — *see* Table of Drugs and Chemicals, by drug, poisoning
    endocrine disease NEC E34.9 [G63]
    herpes zoster B02.23
    hypoglycemia E16.2 [G63]
    infectious
      disease NEC B99 ☑ [G63]
      mononucleosis B27.91
    lack of vitamin NEC E56.9 [G63]
    lead G62.2
      sequelae G65.2
    leprosy A30.9 [G63]
    Lyme disease A69.22
    metabolic disease NEC E88.9 [G63]
    microscopic polyangiitis M31.7 [G63]
    mumps B26.84
    neoplastic disease (*see also* Neoplasm) D49.9 [G63]
    nutritional deficiency NEC E63.9 [G63]
    organophosphate compounds G62.2
      sequelae G65.2
    parasitic disease NEC B89 [G63]
    pellagra E52 [G63]
    polyarteritis nodosa M30.0
    porphyria E80.20 [G63]
    radiation G62.82
    rheumatoid arthritis — *see* Rheumatoid, polyneuropathy
    sarcoidosis D86.89
    serum G61.1
    syphilis (late) A52.15
      congenital A50.43
    systemic
      connective tissue disorder M35.9 [G63]
      lupus erythematosus M32.19
    toxic agent NEC G62.2
      sequelae G65.2
  inflammatory G61.9
    chronic demyelinating (CIDP) G61.81
    sequelae G65.1
    specified NEC G61.89
  lead G62.2
    sequelae G65.2
  nutritional NEC E63.9 [G63]
  postherpetic (zoster) B02.23
  progressive G60.3
  radiation-induced G62.82
  sensory (hereditary) (idiopathic) G60.8
  specified NEC G62.89
  syphilitic (late) A52.15
    congenital A50.43
  transthyretin-related (ATTR) familial amyloid E85.1
    triorthocresyl phosphate G62.2
      sequelae G65.2
    tuberculosis A17.89
    uremia N18.9 [G63]

Polyneuropathy — *continued*
  transthyretin-related familial amyloid — *continued*
    vitamin B12 deficiency E53.8 [G63]
      with anemia (pernicious) D51.0 [G63]
        due to dietary deficiency D51.3 [G63]
    zoster B02.23
Polyopia H53.8
Polyorchism, polyorchidism Q55.21
Polyosteoarthritis (*see also* Osteoarthritis, generalized) M15.9
  post-traumatic M15.3
  specified NEC M15.8
Polyostotic fibrous dysplasia Q78.1
Polyotia Q17.0
Polyp, polypus
  accessory sinus J33.8
  adenocarcinoma in — *see* Neoplasm, malignant, by site
  adenocarcinoma in situ in — *see* Neoplasm, in situ, by site
  adenoid tissue J33.0
  adenomatous (*see also* Neoplasm, benign, by site)
    adenocarcinoma in — *see* Neoplasm, malignant, by site
    adenocarcinoma in situ in — *see* Neoplasm, in situ, by site
    carcinoma in — *see* Neoplasm, malignant, by site
    carcinoma in situ in — *see* Neoplasm, in situ, by site
    multiple — *see* Neoplasm, benign
      adenocarcinoma in — *see* Neoplasm, malignant, by site
      adenocarcinoma in situ in — *see* Neoplasm, in situ, by site
  antrum J33.8
  anus, anal (canal) K62.0
  Bartholin's gland N84.3
  bladder D41.4
  carcinoma in — *see* Neoplasm, malignant, by site
  carcinoma in situ in — *see* Neoplasm, in situ, by site
  cecum D12.0
  cervix (uteri) N84.1
    in pregnancy or childbirth — *see* Pregnancy, complicated by, abnormal, cervix
    mucous N84.1
    nonneoplastic N84.1
  choanal J33.0
  cholesterol K82.4
  clitoris N84.3
  colon K63.5
    adenomatous D12.6
    ascending D12.2
    cecum D12.0
    descending D12.4
    inflammatory K51.40
      with
        abscess K51.414
        complication K51.419
          specified NEC K51.418
        fistula K51.413
        intestinal obstruction K51.412
        rectal bleeding K51.411
    sigmoid D12.5
    transverse D12.3
  corpus uteri N84.0
  dental K04.01
    irreversible K04.02
    reversible K04.01
  duodenum K31.7
  ear (middle) H74.4- ☑
  endometrium N84.0
  ethmoidal (sinus) J33.8
  fallopian tube N84.8
  female genital tract N84.9
    specified NEC N84.8
  frontal (sinus) J33.8
  gallbladder K82.4
  gingiva, gum K06.8
  labia, labium (majus) (minus) N84.3
  larynx (mucous) J38.1
    adenomatous D14.1
  malignant — *see* Neoplasm, malignant, by site
  maxillary (sinus) J33.8
  middle ear — *see* Polyp, ear (middle)
  myometrium N84.0
  nares
    anterior J33.9
    posterior J33.0

▼ Subterms under main terms may continue to next column or page   ☑ **Additional Character Required** — **Refer to the Tabular List for Character Selection**   **257**

Polycoria — Polyp, polypus

Polyp, polypus — *continued*
- nasal (mucous) J33.9
  - cavity J33.0
    - septum J33.0
  - nasopharyngeal J33.0
  - nose (mucous) J33.9
  - oviduct N84.8
  - pharynx J39.2
  - placenta O90.89
  - prostate — *see* Enlargement, enlarged, prostate
  - pudenda, pudendum N84.3
  - pulpal (dental) K04.01
    - irreversible K04.02
    - reversible K04.01
  - rectum (nonadenomatous) K62.1
    - adenomatous — *see* Polyp, adenomatous
  - septum (nasal) J33.0
  - sinus (accessory) (ethmoidal) (frontal) (maxillary) (sphenoidal) J33.8
  - sphenoidal (sinus) J33.8
  - stomach K31.7
    - adenomatous D13.1
  - tube, fallopian N84.8
  - turbinate, mucous membrane J33.8
  - umbilical, newborn P83.6
  - ureter N28.89
  - urethra N36.2
  - uterus (body) (corpus) (mucous) N84.0
    - cervix N84.1
    - in pregnancy or childbirth — *see* Pregnancy, complicated by, tumor, uterus
  - vagina N84.2
  - vocal cord (mucous) J38.1
  - vulva N84.3

Polyphagia R63.2
Polyploidy Q92.7
Polypoid — *see* condition
Polyposis (*see also* Polyp)
- coli (adenomatous) D12.6
  - adenocarcinoma in C18.9
  - adenocarcinoma in situ in — *see* Neoplasm, in situ, by site
  - carcinoma in C18.9
- colon (adenomatous) D12.6
- familial D12.6
  - adenocarcinoma in situ in — *see* Neoplasm, in situ, by site
- intestinal (adenomatous) D12.6
- malignant lymphomatous C83.1- ☑
- multiple, adenomatous (*see also* Neoplasm, benign) D36.9

Polyradiculitis — *see* Polyneuropathy
Polyradiculoneuropathy (acute) (postinfective) (segmentally demyelinating) G61.0
Polyserositis
- due to pericarditis I31.1
- pericardial I31.1
- periodic, familial E85.0
- tuberculous A19.9
  - acute A19.1
  - chronic A19.8

Polysplenia syndrome Q89.09
Polysyndactyly (*see also* Syndactylism, syndactyly) Q70.4
Polytrichia L68.3
Polyunguia Q84.6
Polyuria R35.8
- nocturnal R35.1
- psychogenic F45.8

Pompe's disease (glycogen storage) E74.02
Pompholyx L30.1
Poncet's disease (tuberculous rheumatism) A18.09
Pond fracture — *see* Fracture, skull
Ponos B55.0
Pons, pontine — *see* condition
Poor
- aesthetic of existing restoration of tooth K08.56
- contractions, labor O62.2
- gingival margin to tooth restoration K08.51
- personal hygiene R46.0
- prenatal care, affecting management of pregnancy — *see* Pregnancy, complicated by, insufficient, prenatal care
- sucking reflex (newborn) R29.2
- urinary stream R39.12
- vision NEC H54.7

Poradenitis, nostras inguinalis or venerea A55
Porencephaly (congenital) (developmental) (true) Q04.6
- acquired G93.0

Porencephaly — *continued*
- nondevelopmental G93.0
- traumatic (post) F07.89
Porocephaliasis B88.8
Porokeratosis Q82.8
Poroma, eccrine — *see* Neoplasm, skin, benign
Porphyria (South African) E80.20
- acquired E80.20
- acute intermittent (hepatic) (Swedish) E80.21
- cutanea tarda (hereditary) (symptomatic) E80.1
- due to drugs E80.20
  - correct substance properly administered — *see* Table of Drugs and Chemicals, by drug, adverse effect
  - overdose or wrong substance given or taken — *see* Table of Drugs and Chemicals, by drug, poisoning
- erythropoietic (congenital) (hereditary) E80.0
- hepatocutaneous type E80.1
- secondary E80.20
- toxic NEC E80.20
- variegata E80.20
Porphyrinuria — *see* Porphyria
Porphyruria — *see* Porphyria
Port wine nevus, mark, or stain Q82.5
Portal — *see* condition
Posadas-Wernicke disease B38.9
Positive
- culture (nonspecific)
  - blood R78.81
  - bronchial washings R84.5
  - cerebrospinal fluid R83.5
  - cervix uteri R87.5
  - nasal secretions R84.5
  - nipple discharge R89.5
  - nose R84.5
    - staphylococcus (Methicillin susceptible) Z22.321
    - Methicillin resistant Z22.322
  - peritoneal fluid R85.5
  - pleural fluid R84.5
  - prostatic secretions R86.5
  - saliva R85.5
  - seminal fluid R86.5
  - sputum R84.5
  - synovial fluid R89.5
  - throat scrapings R84.5
  - urine R82.79
  - vagina R87.5
  - vulva R87.5
  - wound secretions R89.5
- PPD (skin test) R76.11
- serology for syphilis A53.0
  - with signs or symptoms — *code as* Syphilis, by site and stage
  - false R76.8
- skin test, tuberculin (without active tuberculosis) R76.11
- test, human immunodeficiency virus (HIV) R75
- VDRL A53.0
  - with signs or symptoms — *code by* site and stage under Syphilis A53.9
- Wassermann reaction A53.0
Postcardiotomy syndrome I97.0
Postcaval ureter Q62.62
Postcholecystectomy syndrome K91.5
Postclimacteric bleeding N95.0
Postcommissurotomy syndrome I97.0
Postconcussional syndrome F07.81
Postcontusional syndrome F07.81
Postcricoid region — *see* condition
Post-dates (40-42 weeks) (pregnancy) (mother) O48.0
- more than 42 weeks gestation O48.1
Postencephalitic syndrome F07.89
Posterior — *see* condition
Posterolateral sclerosis (spinal cord) — *see* Degeneration, combined
Postexanthematous — *see* condition
Postfebrile — *see* condition
Postgastrectomy dumping syndrome K91.1
Posthemiplegic chorea — *see* Monoplegia
Posthemorrhagic anemia (chronic) D50.0
- acute D62
- newborn P61.3
Postherpetic neuralgia (zoster) B02.29
- trigeminal B02.22
Posthitis N47.7
Postimmunization complication or reaction — *see* Complications, vaccination

Postinfectious — *see* condition
Postlaminectomy syndrome NEC M96.1
Postleukotomy syndrome F07.0
Postmastectomy lymphedema (syndrome) I97.2
Postmaturity, postmature (over 42 weeks)
- maternal (over 42 weeks gestation) O48.1
- newborn P08.22
Postmeasles complication NEC (*see also* condition) B05.89
Postmenopausal
- endometrium (atrophic) N95.8
  - suppurative (*see also* Endometritis) N71.9
- osteoporosis — *see* Osteoporosis, postmenopausal
Postnasal drip R09.82
- due to
  - allergic rhinitis — *see* Rhinitis, allergic
  - common cold J00
  - gastroesophageal reflux — *see* Reflux, gastroesophageal
  - nasopharyngitis — *see* Nasopharyngitis
  - other known condition — *code to* condition
  - sinusitis — *see* Sinusitis
Postnatal — *see* condition
Postoperative (postprocedural) — *see* Complication, postoperative
- pneumothorax, therapeutic Z98.3
- state NEC Z98.890
Postpancreatectomy hyperglycemia E89.1
Postpartum — *see* Puerperal
Postphlebitic syndrome — *see* Syndrome, postthrombotic
Postpolio (myelitic) **syndrome** G14
Postpoliomyelitic (*see also* condition)
- osteopathy — *see* Osteopathy, after poliomyelitis
Postprocedural (*see also* Postoperative)
- hypoinsulinemia E89.1
Postschizophrenic depression F32.89
Postsurgery status (*see also* Status (post))
- pneumothorax, therapeutic Z98.3
Post-term (40-42 weeks) (pregnancy) (mother) O48.0
- infant P08.21
- more than 42 weeks gestation (mother) O48.1
Post-traumatic brain syndrome, nonpsychotic F07.81
Post-typhoid abscess A01.09
Postures, hysterical F44.2
Postvaccinal reaction or complication — *see* Complications, vaccination
Postvalvulotomy syndrome I97.0
Potain's
- disease (pulmonary edema) — *see* Edema, lung
- syndrome (gastrectasis with dyspepsia) K31.0
Potter's
- asthma J62.8
- facies Q60.6
- lung J62.8
- syndrome (with renal agenesis) Q60.6
Pott's
- curvature (spinal) A18.01
- disease or paraplegia A18.01
- spinal curvature A18.01
- tumor, puffy — *see* Osteomyelitis, specified type NEC
Pouch
- bronchus Q32.4
- Douglas' — *see* condition
- esophagus, esophageal, congenital Q39.6
  - acquired K22.5
- gastric K31.4
- Hartmann's K82.8
- pharynx, pharyngeal (congenital) Q38.7
Pouchitis K91.850
Poultrymen's itch B88.0
Poverty NEC Z59.6
- extreme Z59.5
Poxvirus NEC B08.8
Prader-Willi syndrome Q87.1
Preauricular appendage or tag Q17.0
Prebetalipoproteinemia (acquired) (essential) (familial) (hereditary) (primary) (secondary) E78.1
- with chylomicronemia E78.3
Precipitate labor or delivery O62.3
Preclimacteric bleeding (menorrhagia) N92.4
Precocious
- adrenarche E30.1
- menarche E30.1
- menstruation E30.1
- pubarche E30.1
- puberty E30.1

Precocious — *continued*
  puberty — *continued*
    central E22.8
    sexual development NEC E30.1
    thelarche E30.8
Precocity, sexual (constitutional) (cryptogenic) (female) (idiopathic) (male) E30.1
  with adrenal hyperplasia E25.9
    congenital E25.0
Precordial pain R07.2
Predeciduous teeth K00.2
Prediabetes, prediabetic R73.03
  complicating
    pregnancy — *see* Pregnancy, complicated by, diseases of, specified type or system NEC
    puerperium O99.89
Predislocation status of hip at birth Q65.6
Pre-eclampsia O14.9- ☑
  with pre-existing hypertension — *see* Hypertension, complicating pregnancy, pre-existing, with, pre-eclampsia
  complicating
    childbirth O14.94
    puerperium O14.95
  mild O14.0- ☑
    complicating
      childbirth O14.04
      puerperium O14.05
  moderate O14.0- ☑
    complicating
      childbirth O14.04
      puerperium O14.05
  severe O14.1- ☑
    with hemolysis, elevated liver enzymes and low platelet count (HELLP) O14.2- ☑
      complicating
        childbirth O14.24
        puerperium O14.25
    complicating
      childbirth O14.14
      puerperium O14.15
Pre-eruptive color change, teeth, tooth K00.8
Pre-excitation atrioventricular conduction I45.6
Preglaucoma H40.00- ☑
Pregnancy (single) (uterine) (*see also* Delivery and Puerperal)

Note: The Tabular must be reviewed for assignment of appropriate seventh character for multiple gestation codes in Chapter 15

Note: The Tabular must be reviewed for assignment of the appropriate character indicating the trimester of the pregnancy

  abdominal (ectopic) O00.00
    with intrauterine pregnancy O00.01
    with viable fetus O36.7- ☑
  ampullar O00.10- ☑
    with intrauterine pregnancy O00.11- ☑
  biochemical O02.81
  broad ligament O00.80
    with intrauterine pregnancy O00.81
  cervical O00.8
    with intrauterine pregnancy O00.81
  chemical O02.81
  complicated by (care of) (management affected by)
    abnormal, abnormality
      cervix O34.4- ☑
        causing obstructed labor O65.5
      cord (umbilical) O69.9 ☑
      fetal heart rate or rhythm O36.83- ☑
      findings on antenatal screening of mother O28.9
        biochemical O28.1
        chromosomal O28.5
        cytological O28.2
        genetic O28.5
        hematological O28.0
        radiological O28.4
        specified NEC O28.8
        ultrasonic O28.3
      glucose (tolerance) NEC O99.810
      pelvic organs O34.9- ☑
        specified NEC O34.8- ☑
          causing obstructed labor O65.5
      pelvis (bony) (major) NEC O33.0
      perineum O34.7- ☑

Pregnancy — *continued*
  complicated by — *continued*
    abnormal, abnormality — *continued*
      position
        placenta O44.0- ☑
          with hemorrhage O44.1- ☑
        uterus O34.59- ☑
      uterus O34.59- ☑
        causing obstructed labor O65.5
        congenital O34.0- ☑
      vagina O34.6-
        causing obstructed labor O65.5
      vulva O34.7-
        causing obstructed labor O65.5
    abruptio placentae — *see* Abruptio placentae
    abscess or cellulitis
      bladder O23.1- ☑
      breast O91.11- ☑
      genital organ or tract O23.9- ☑
    abuse
      physical O9A.31 ☑ (*following* O99)
      psychological O9A.51 ☑ (*following* O99)
      sexual O9A.41 ☑ (*following* O99)
    adverse effect anesthesia O29.9- ☑
      aspiration pneumonitis O29.01- ☑
      cardiac arrest O29.11- ☑
      cardiac complication NEC O29.19- ☑
      cardiac failure O29.12- ☑
      central nervous system complication NEC O29.29- ☑
      cerebral anoxia O29.21- ☑
      failed or difficult intubation O29.6- ☑
      inhalation of stomach contents or secretions NOS O29.01- ☑
      local, toxic reaction O29.3X ☑
      Mendelson's syndrome O29.01- ☑
      pressure collapse of lung O29.02- ☑
      pulmonary complications NEC O29.09- ☑
      specified NEC O29.8X- ☑
      spinal and epidural type NEC O29.5X ☑
        induced headache O29.4- ☑
    albuminuria (*see also* Proteinuria, gestational) O12.1- ☑
    alcohol use O99.31- ☑
    amnionitis O41.12- ☑
    anaphylactoid syndrome of pregnancy O88.01- ☑
    anemia (conditions in D50-D64) (pre-existing) O99.01- ☑
      complicating the puerperium O99.03
    antepartum hemorrhage O46.9- ☑
      with coagulation defect — *see* Hemorrhage, antepartum, with coagulation defect
      specified NEC O46.8X- ☑
    appendicitis O99.61- ☑
    atrophy (yellow) (acute) liver (subacute) O26.61- ☑
    bariatric surgery status O99.84- ☑
    bicornis or bicornuate uterus O34.0- ☑
    biliary tract problems O26.61- ☑
    breech presentation O32.1 ☑
    cardiovascular diseases (conditions in I00-I09, I20-I52, I70-I99) O99.41- ☑
    cerebrovascular disorders (conditions in I60-I69) O99.41- ☑
    cervical shortening O26.87- ☑
    cervicitis O23.51- ☑
    chloasma (gravidarum) O26.89- ☑
    cholecystitis O99.61- ☑
    cholestasis (intrahepatic) O26.61- ☑
    chorioamnionitis O41.12- ☑
    circulatory system disorder (conditions in I00-I09, I20-I99, O99.41-)
    compound presentation O32.6 ☑
    conjoined twins O30.02- ☑
    connective system disorders (conditions in M00-M99) O99.89
    contracted pelvis (general) O33.1
      inlet O33.2
      outlet O33.3 ☑
    convulsions (eclamptic) (uremic) (*see also* Eclampsia) O15.9
    cracked nipple O92.11- ☑
    cystitis O23.1- ☑
    cystocele O34.8- ☑
    death of fetus (near term) O36.4 ☑
      early pregnancy O02.1

Pregnancy — *continued*
  complicated by — *continued*
    death of fetus — *continued*
      of one fetus or more in multiple gestation O31.2- ☑
    deciduitis O41.14- ☑
    decreased fetal movement O36.81- ☑
    dental problems O99.61- ☑
    diabetes (mellitus) O24.91- ☑
      gestational (pregnancy induced) — *see* Diabetes, gestational
      pre-existing O24.31- ☑
        specified NEC O24.81- ☑
        type 1 O24.01- ☑
        type 2 O24.11- ☑
    digestive system disorders (conditions in K00-K93) O99.61- ☑
    diseases of — *see* Pregnancy, complicated by, specified body system disease
      biliary tract O26.61- ☑
      blood NEC (conditions in D65-D77) O99.11- ☑
      liver O26.61- ☑
      specified NEC O99.89
    disorders of — *see* Pregnancy, complicated by, specified body system disorder
      amniotic fluid and membranes O41.9- ☑
        specified NEC O41.8X- ☑
      biliary tract O26.61- ☑
      ear and mastoid process (conditions in H60-H95) O99.89
      eye and adnexa (conditions in H00-H59) O99.89
      liver O26.61- ☑
      skin (conditions in L00-L99) O99.71- ☑
      specified NEC O99.89
    displacement, uterus NEC O34.59- ☑
      causing obstructed labor O65.5
    disproportion (due to) O33.9
      fetal (ascites) (hydrops) (meningomyelocele) (sacral teratoma) (tumor) deformities NEC O33.7
      generally contracted pelvis O33.1
      hydrocephalic fetus O33.6 ☑
      inlet contraction of pelvis O33.2
      mixed maternal and fetal origin O33.4 ☑
      specified NEC O33.8
    double uterus O34.0- ☑
      causing obstructed labor O65.5
    drug use (conditions in F11-F19) O99.32- ☑
    eclampsia, eclamptic (coma) (convulsions) (delirium) (nephritis) (uremia) (*see also* Eclampsia) O15.- ☑
    ectopic pregnancy — *see* Pregnancy, ectopic
    edema O12.0- ☑
      with
        gestational hypertension, mild (*see also* Pre-eclampsia) O14.0- ☑
        proteinuria O12.2- ☑
    effusion, amniotic fluid — *see* Pregnancy, complicated by, premature rupture of membranes
    elderly
      multigravida O09.52- ☑
      primigravida O09.51- ☑
    embolism (*see also* Embolism, obstetric, pregnancy) O88.- ☑
    endocrine diseases NEC O99.28- ☑
    endometritis O86.12
    excessive weight gain O26.0- ☑
    exhaustion O26.81- ☑
      during labor and delivery O75.81
    face presentation O32.3 ☑
    failed induction of labor O61.9
      instrumental O61.1
      mechanical O61.1
      medical O61.0
      specified NEC O61.8
      surgical O61.1
    failed or difficult intubation for anesthesia O29.6- ☑
    false labor (pains) O47.9
      at or after 37 completed weeks of pregnancy O47.1
      before 37 completed weeks of pregnancy O47.0- ☑
    fatigue O26.81- ☑
      during labor and delivery O75.81
    fatty metamorphosis of liver O26.61- ☑
    female genital mutilation O34.8- ☑ [N90.81-] ☑

▽ Subterms under main terms may continue to next column or page   ☑ Additional Character Required — Refer to the Tabular List for Character Selection   **259**

Precocious — Pregnancy

Pregnancy — *continued*
  complicated by — *continued*
    fetal (maternal care for)
      abnormality or damage O35.9 ☑
        acid-base balance O68
        specified type NEC O35.8 ☑
      acidemia O68
      acidosis O68
      alkalosis O68
      anemia and thrombocytopenia O36.82- ☑
      anencephaly O35.0 ☑
      chromosomal abnormality (conditions in Q90-Q99) O35.1 ☑
      conjoined twins O30.02- ☑
      damage from
        amniocentesis O35.7 ☑
        biopsy procedures O35.7 ☑
        drug addiction O35.5 ☑
        hematological investigation O35.7 ☑
        intrauterine contraceptive device O35.7 ☑
        maternal
          alcohol addiction O35.4 ☑
          cytomegalovirus infection O35.3 ☑
          disease NEC O35.8 ☑
          drug addiction O35.5 ☑
          listeriosis O35.8 ☑
          rubella O35.3 ☑
          toxoplasmosis O35.8 ☑
          viral infection O35.3 ☑
        medical procedure NEC O35.7 ☑
        radiation O35.6 ☑
      death (near term) O36.4 ☑
        early pregnancy O02.1
      decreased movement O36.81- ☑
      disproportion due to deformity (fetal) O33.7 ☑
      excessive growth (large for dates) O36.6- ☑
      growth retardation O36.59- ☑
        light for dates O36.59- ☑
        small for dates O36.59- ☑
      heart rate irregularity (bradycardia) (decelerations) (tachycardia) O76
      hereditary disease O35.2 ☑
      hydrocephalus O35.0 ☑
      intrauterine death O36.4 ☑
      poor growth O36.59- ☑
        light for dates O36.59- ☑
        small for dates O36.59- ☑
      problem O36.9- ☑
        specified NEC O36.89- ☑
      reduction (elective) O31.3- ☑
      selective termination O31.3- ☑
      spina bifida O35.0 ☑
      thrombocytopenia O36.82- ☑
    fibroid (tumor) (uterus) O34.1- ☑
    fissure of nipple O92.11- ☑
    gallstones O99.61- ☑
    gastric banding status O99.84- ☑
    gastric bypass status O99.84- ☑
    genital herpes (asymptomatic) (history of) (inactive) O98.3- ☑
    genital tract infection O23.9- ☑
    glomerular diseases (conditions in N00-N07) O26.83- ☑
      with hypertension, pre-existing — *see* Hypertension, complicating, pregnancy, pre-existing, with, renal disease
    gonorrhea O98.21- ☑
    grand multiparity O09.4 ☑
    habitual aborter — *see* Pregnancy, complicated by, recurrent pregnancy loss
    HELLP syndrome (hemolysis, elevated liver enzymes and low platelet count) O14.2- ☑
    hemorrhage
      antepartum — *see* Hemorrhage, antepartum
      before 20 completed weeks gestation O20.9
        specified NEC O20.8
      due to premature separation, placenta (*see also* Abruptio placentae) O45.9- ☑
      early O20.9
        specified NEC O20.8
      threatened abortion O20.0
    hemorrhoids O22.4- ☑
    hepatitis (viral) O98.41- ☑
    herniation of uterus O34.59- ☑
    high
      head at term O32.4 ☑

Pregnancy — *continued*
  complicated by — *continued*
    high — *continued*
      risk — *see* Supervision (of) (for), high-risk
    history of in utero procedure during previous pregnancy O09.82- ☑
    HIV O98.71- ☑
    human immunodeficiency virus (HIV) disease O98.71- ☑
    hydatidiform mole (*see also* Mole, hydatidiform) O01.9
    hydramnios O40.- ☑
    hydrocephalic fetus (disproportion) O33.6 ☑
    hydrops
      amnii O40.- ☑
      fetalis O36.2- ☑
        associated with isoimmunization (*see also* Pregnancy, complicated by, isoimmunization) O36.11- ☑
    hydrorrhea O42.90
    hyperemesis (gravidarum) (mild) (*see also* Hyperemesis, gravidarum) O21.0
    hypertension — *see* Hypertension, complicating pregnancy
    hypertensive
      heart and renal disease, pre-existing — *see* Hypertension, complicating, pregnancy, pre-existing, with, heart disease, with renal disease
      heart disease, pre-existing — *see* Hypertension, complicating, pregnancy, pre-existing, with, heart disease
      renal disease, pre-existing — *see* Hypertension, complicating, pregnancy, pre-existing, with, renal disease
    hypotension O26.5- ☑
    immune disorders NEC (conditions in D80-D89) O99.11- ☑
    incarceration, uterus O34.51- ☑
    incompetent cervix O34.3- ☑
    inconclusive fetal viability O36.80 ☑
    infection(s) O98.91- ☑
      amniotic fluid or sac O41.10- ☑
      bladder O23.1- ☑
      carrier state NEC O99.830
        streptococcus B O99.820
      genital organ or tract O23.9- ☑
        specified NEC O23.59- ☑
      genitourinary tract O23.9- ☑
      gonorrhea O98.21- ☑
      hepatitis (viral) O98.41- ☑
      HIV O98.71- ☑
      human immunodeficiency virus (HIV) O98.71- ☑
      kidney O23.0- ☑
      nipple O91.01- ☑
      parasitic disease O98.91- ☑
        specified NEC O98.81- ☑
      protozoal disease O98.61- ☑
      sexually transmitted NEC O98.31- ☑
      specified type NEC O98.81- ☑
      syphilis O98.11- ☑
      tuberculosis O98.01- ☑
      urethra O23.2- ☑
      urinary (tract) O23.4- ☑
        specified NEC O23.3- ☑
      viral disease O98.51- ☑
    injury or poisoning (conditions in S00-T88) O9A.21- ☑ (*following* O99)
      due to abuse
        physical O9A.31- ☑ (*following* O99)
        psychological O9A.51- ☑ (*following* O99)
        sexual O9A.41- ☑ (*following* O99)
    insufficient
      prenatal care O09.3- ☑
      weight gain O26.1- ☑
    insulin resistance O26.89 ☑
    intrauterine fetal death (near term) O36.4 ☑
      early pregnancy O02.1
      multiple gestation (one fetus or more) O31.2- ☑
    isoimmunization O36.11- ☑
      anti-A sensitization O36.11- ☑
      anti-B sensitization O36.19- ☑
      Rh O36.09- ☑
        anti-D antibody O36.01- ☑

Pregnancy — *continued*
  complicated by — *continued*
    isoimmunization — *continued*
      specified NEC O36.19- ☑
    laceration of uterus NEC O71.81
    malformation
      placenta, placental (vessel) O43.10- ☑
        specified NEC O43.19- ☑
      uterus (congenital) O34.0- ☑
    malnutrition (conditions in E40-E46) O25.1- ☑
    maternal hypotension syndrome O26.5- ☑
    mental disorders (conditions in F01-F09, F20-F99) O99.34- ☑
      alcohol use O99.31- ☑
      drug use O99.32- ☑
      smoking O99.33- ☑
    mentum presentation O32.3 ☑
    metabolic disorders O99.28- ☑
    missed
      abortion O02.1
      delivery O36.4 ☑
    multiple gestations O30.9- ☑
      conjoined twins O30.02- ☑
      quadruplet — *see* Pregnancy, quadruplet
      specified complication NEC O31.8X- ☑
      specified number of multiples NEC — *see* Pregnancy, multiple (gestation), specified NEC
      triplet — *see* Pregnancy, triplet
      twin — *see* Pregnancy, twin
    musculoskeletal condition (conditions is M00-M99) O99.89
    necrosis, liver (conditions in K72) O26.61- ☑
    neoplasm
      benign
        cervix O34.4- ☑
        corpus uteri O34.1- ☑
        uterus O34.1- ☑
      malignant O9A.11- ☑ (*following* O99)
    nephropathy NEC O26.83- ☑
    nervous system condition (conditions in G00-G99) O99.35- ☑
    nutritional diseases NEC O99.28- ☑
    obesity (pre-existing) O99.21- ☑
    obesity surgery status O99.84- ☑
    oblique lie or presentation O32.2 ☑
    older mother — *see* Pregnancy, complicated by, elderly
    oligohydramnios O41.0- ☑
      with premature rupture of membranes (*see also* Pregnancy, complicated by, premature rupture of membranes) O42.- ☑
    onset (spontaneous) of labor after 37 completed weeks of gestation but before 39 completed weeks gestation, with delivery by (planned) cesarean section O75.82
    oophoritis O23.52- ☑
    overdose, drug (*see also* Table of Drugs and Chemicals, by drug, poisoning) O9A.21- ☑ (*following* O99)
    oversize fetus O33.5 ☑
    papyraceous fetus O31.0- ☑
    pelvic inflammatory disease O99.89
    periodontal disease O99.61- ☑
    peripheral neuritis O26.82- ☑
    peritoneal (pelvic) adhesions O99.89
    phlebitis O22.9- ☑
    phlebopathy O22.9- ☑
    phlebothrombosis (superficial) O22.2- ☑
      deep O22.3- ☑
    placenta accreta O43.21- ☑
    placenta increta O43.22- ☑
    placenta percreta O43.23- ☑
    placenta previa O44.0- ☑
      complete O44.0- ☑
        with hemorrhage O44.1- ☑
      marginal O44.2- ☑
        with hemorrhage O44.3- ☑
      partial O44.2- ☑
        with hemorrhage O44.3- ☑
    placental disorder O43.9- ☑
      specified NEC O43.89- ☑
    placental dysfunction O43.89- ☑
    placental infarction O43.81- ☑
    placental insufficiency O36.51- ☑

☑ **Additional Character Required** — Refer to the Tabular List for Character Selection
▽ **Subterms under main terms may continue to next column or page**

Pregnancy — *continued*
  complicated by — *continued*
    placental transfusion syndromes
      fetomaternal O43.01- ☑
      fetus to fetus O43.02- ☑
      maternofetal O43.01- ☑
    placentitis O41.14- ☑
    pneumonia O99.51- ☑
    poisoning (*see also* Table of Drugs and Chemicals)
      O9A.21 ☑ (*following* O99)
    polyhydramnios O40- ☑
    polymorphic eruption of pregnancy O26.86
    poor obstetric history NEC O09.29- ☑
    postmaturity (post-term) (40 to 42 weeks) O48.0
      more than 42 completed weeks gestation
        (prolonged) O48.1
    pre-eclampsia O14.9- ☑
      mild O14.0- ☑
      moderate O14.0- ☑
      severe O14.1- ☑
        with hemolysis, elevated liver enzymes and
          low platelet count (HELLP) O14.2- ☑
    premature labor — *see* Pregnancy, complicated
      by, preterm labor
    premature rupture of membranes O42.90
      with onset of labor
        after 24 hours O42.10
          at or after 37 weeks gestation, onset of
            labor more than 24 hours follow-
            ing rupture O42.12
          pre-term (before 37 completed weeks
            of gestation) O42.11- ☑
        within 24 hours O42.00
          at or after 37 weeks gestation, onset of
            labor within 24 hours of rupture
            O42.02
          pre-term (before 37 completed weeks
            of gestation) O42.01- ☑
      at or after 37 weeks gestation, unspecified as
        to length of time between rupture and
        onset of labor O42.92
      full-term, unspecified as to length of time be-
        tween rupture and onset of labor O42.92
      pre-term (before 37 completed weeks of gesta-
        tion) O42.91- ☑
    premature separation of placenta (*see also* Abrup-
      tio placentae) O45.9- ☑
    presentation, fetal — *see* Delivery, complicated
      by, malposition
    preterm delivery O60.10 ☑
    preterm labor
      with delivery O60.10 ☑
        preterm O60.10 ☑
        term O60.20 ☑
      without delivery O60.00
        second trimester O60.02
        third trimester O60.03
      second trimester
        with preterm delivery
          second trimester O60.12 ☑
          third trimester O60.13 ☑
        with term delivery O60.22 ☑
        without delivery O60.02
      third trimester
        with term delivery O60.23 ☑
        with third trimester preterm delivery
          O60.14 ☑
        without delivery O60.03
    previous history of — *see* Pregnancy, supervision
      of, high-risk
    prolapse, uterus O34.52- ☑
    proteinuria (gestational) (*see also* Proteinuria,
      gestational) O12.1- ☑
      with edema O12.2- ☑
    pruritic urticarial papules and plaques of pregnancy
      (PUPPP) O26.86
    pruritus (neurogenic) O26.89- ☑
    psychosis or psychoneurosis (puerperal) F53
    ptyalism O26.89- ☑
    PUPPP (pruritic urticarial papules and plaques of
      pregnancy) O26.86
    pyelitis O23.0- ☑
    recurrent pregnancy loss O26.2- ☑
    renal disease or failure NEC O26.83- ☑
      with secondary hypertension, pre-existing —
        see Hypertension, complicating, pregnan-
        cy, pre-existing, secondary

Pregnancy — *continued*
  complicated by — *continued*
    renal disease or failure — *continued*
      hypertensive, pre-existing — *see* Hypertension,
        complicating, pregnancy, pre-existing,
        with, renal disease
    respiratory condition (conditions in J00-J99)
      O99.51- ☑
    retained, retention
      dead ovum O02.0
      intrauterine contraceptive device O26.3- ☑
    retroversion, uterus O34.53- ☑
    Rh immunization, incompatibility or sensitization
      NEC O36.09- ☑
      anti-D antibody O36.01- ☑
    rupture
      amnion (premature) (*see also* Pregnancy, com-
        plicated by, premature rupture of mem-
        branes) O42- ☑
      membranes (premature) (*see also* Pregnancy,
        complicated by, premature rupture of
        membranes) O42- ☑
      uterus (during labor) O71.1
        before onset of labor O71.0- ☑
    salivation (excessive) O26.89- ☑
    salpingitis O23.52- ☑
    salpingo-oophoritis O23.52- ☑
    sepsis (conditions in A40, A41) O98.81- ☑
    size date discrepancy (uterine) O26.84- ☑
    skin condition (conditions in L00-L99) O99.71- ☑
    smoking (tobacco) O99.33- ☑
    social problem O09.7- ☑
    specified condition NEC O26.89- ☑
    spotting O26.85- ☑
    streptococcus group B (GBS) carrier state O99.820
    subluxation of symphysis (pubis) O26.71- ☑
    syphilis (conditions in A50-A53) O98.11- ☑
    threatened
      abortion O20.0
      labor O47.9
        at or after 37 completed weeks of gestation
          O47.1
        before 37 completed weeks of gestation
          O47.0 ☑
    thrombophlebitis (superficial) O22.2- ☑
    thrombosis O22.9- ☑
      cerebral venous O22.5- ☑
      cerebrovenous sinus O22.5- ☑
      deep O22.3- ☑
    tobacco use disorder (smoking) O99.33- ☑
    torsion of uterus O34.59- ☑
    toxemia O14.9- ☑
    transverse lie or presentation O32.2 ☑
    tuberculosis (conditions in A15-A19) O98.01- ☑
    tumor (benign)
      cervix O34.4- ☑
      malignant O9A.11- ☑ (*following* O99)
      uterus O34.1- ☑
    unstable lie O32.0 ☑
    upper respiratory infection O99.51- ☑
    urethritis O23.2- ☑
    uterine size date discrepancy O26.84- ☑
    vaginitis or vulvitis O23.59- ☑
    varicose veins (lower extremities) O22.0- ☑
      genitals O22.1- ☑
      legs O22.0- ☑
      perineal O22.1- ☑
      vaginal or vulval O22.1- ☑
    venereal disease NEC (conditions in A63.8)
      O98.31- ☑
    venous disorders O22.9- ☑
      specified NEC O22.8X- ☑
    very young mother — *see* Pregnancy, complicated
      by, young mother
    viral diseases (conditions in A80-B09, B25-B34)
      O98.51- ☑
    vomiting O21.9
      due to diseases classified elsewhere O21.8
      hyperemesis gravidarum (mild) (*see also* Hyper-
        emesis, gravidarum) O21.0
      late (occurring after 20 weeks of gestation)
        O21.2
    young mother
      multigravida O09.62- ☑
      primigravida O09.61- ☑
  complicated NOS O26.9- ☑
  concealed O09.3- ☑

Pregnancy — *continued*
  continuing following
    elective fetal reduction of one or more fetus
      O31.3- ☑
    intrauterine death of one or more fetus O31.2- ☑
    spontaneous abortion of one or more fetus
      O31.1- ☑
  cornual O00.80
    with intrauterine pregnancy O00.81
  ectopic (ruptured) O00.90
    with intrauterine pregnancy O00.91
    abdominal O00.00
      with
        intrauterine pregnancy O00.01
        viable fetus O36.7- ☑
    cervical O00.80
      with intrauterine pregnancy O00.81
    complicated (by) O08.9
      afibrinogenemia O08.1
      cardiac arrest O08.81
      chemical damage of pelvic organ(s) O08.6
      circulatory collapse O08.3
      defibrination syndrome O08.1
      electrolyte imbalance O08.5
      embolism (amniotic fluid) (blood clot) (pul-
        monary) (septic) O08.2
      endometritis O08.0
      genital tract and pelvic infection O08.0
      hemorrhage (delayed) (excessive) O08.1
      infection
        genital tract or pelvic O08.0
        kidney O08.83
        urinary tract O08.3
      intravascular coagulation O08.1
      laceration of pelvic organ(s) O08.6
      metabolic disorder O08.5
      oliguria O08.4
      oophoritis O08.0
      parametritis O08.0
      pelvic peritonitis O08.0
      perforation of pelvic organ(s) O08.6
      renal failure or shutdown O08.4
      salpingitis or salpingo-oophoritis O08.0
      sepsis O08.82
      shock O08.83
        septic O08.82
      specified condition NEC O08.89
      tubular necrosis (renal) O08.4
      uremia O08.4
      urinary infection O08.83
      venous complication NEC O08.7
        embolism O08.2
    cornual O00.80
      with intrauterine pregnancy O00.81
    intraligamentous O00.80
      with intrauterine pregnancy O00.81
    mural O00.80
      with intrauterine pregnancy O00.81
    ovarian O00.20- ☑
      with intrauterine pregnancy O00.21- ☑
    specified site NEC O00.80
      with intrauterine pregnancy O00.81
    tubal (ruptured) O00.10- ☑
      with intrauterine pregnancy O00.11- ☑
  examination (normal) Z34.9- ☑
    first Z34.0- ☑
    high-risk — *see* Pregnancy, supervision of, high-
      risk
    specified Z34.8- ☑
  extrauterine — *see* Pregnancy, ectopic
  fallopian O00.10- ☑
    with intrauterine pregnancy O00.11- ☑
  false F45.8
  gestational carrier Z33.3
  hidden O09.3- ☑
  high-risk — *see* Pregnancy, supervision of, high-risk
  incidental finding Z33.1
  interstitial O00.80
    with intrauterine pregnancy O00.81
  intraligamentous O00.80
    with intrauterine pregnancy O00.81
  intramural O00.80
    with intrauterine pregnancy O00.81
  intraperitoneal O00.00
    with intrauterine pregnancy O00.01
  isthmian O00.10- ☑
    with intrauterine pregnancy O00.11- ☑
  mesometric (mural) O00.80

Pregnancy — *continued*
  mesometric — *continued*
    with intrauterine pregnancy O00.81
  molar NEC O02.0
    complicated (by) O08.9
      afibrinogenemia O08.1
      cardiac arrest O08.81
      chemical damage of pelvic organ(s) O08.6
      circulatory collapse O08.3
      defibrination syndrome O08.1
      electrolyte imbalance O08.5
      embolism (amniotic fluid) (blood clot) (pul-
        monary) (septic) O08.2
      endometritis O08.0
      genital tract and pelvic infection O08.0
      hemorrhage (delayed) (excessive) O08.1
      infection
        genital tract or pelvic O08.0
        kidney O08.83
        urinary tract O08.83
      intravascular coagulation O08.1
      laceration of pelvic organ(s) O08.6
      metabolic disorder O08.5
      oliguria O08.4
      oophoritis O08.0
      parametritis O08.0
      pelvic peritonitis O08.0
      perforation of pelvic organ(s) O08.6
      renal failure or shutdown O08.4
      salpingitis or salpingo-oophoritis O08.0
      sepsis O08.82
      shock O08.3
        septic O08.82
      specified condition NEC O08.89
      tubular necrosis (renal) O08.4
      uremia O08.4
      urinary infection O08.83
      venous complication NEC O08.7
        embolism O08.2
    hydatidiform (*see also* Mole, hydatidiform) O01.9
  multiple (gestation) O30.9- ☑
    greater than quadruplets — *see* Pregnancy, multi-
      ple (gestation), specified NEC
    specified NEC O30.80- ☑
      with
        two or more monoamniotic fetuses
          O30.82- ☑
        two or more monochorionic fetuses
          O30.81- ☑
      two or more monoamniotic fetuses O30.82- ☑
      two or more monochorionic fetuses O30.81- ☑
      unable to determine number of placenta and
        number of amniotic sacs O30.89- ☑
      unspecified number of placenta and unspeci-
        fied number of amniotic sacs O30.80- ☑
  mural O00.80
    with intrauterine pregnancy O00.81
  normal (supervision of) Z34.9- ☑
    first Z34.0- ☑
    high-risk — *see* Pregnancy, supervision of, high-
      risk
    specified Z34.8- ☑
  ovarian O00.20- ☑
    with intrauterine pregnancy O00.21- ☑
  postmature (40 to 42 weeks) O48.0
    more than 42 weeks gestation O48.1
  post-term (40 to 42 weeks) O48.0
  prenatal care only Z34.9- ☑
    first Z34.0- ☑
    high-risk — *see* Pregnancy, supervision of, high-
      risk
    specified Z34.8- ☑
  prolonged (more than 42 weeks gestation) O48.1
  quadruplet O30.20- ☑
    with
      two or more monoamniotic fetuses O30.22- ☑
      two or more monochorionic fetuses O30.21- ☑
    two or more monoamniotic fetuses O30.22- ☑
    two or more monochorionic fetuses O30.21- ☑
    unable to determine number of placenta and
      number of amniotic sacs O30.29- ☑
    unspecified number of placenta and unspecified
      number of amniotic sacs O30.20- ☑
  quintuplet — *see* Pregnancy, multiple (gestation),
    specified NEC
  sextuplet — *see* Pregnancy, multiple (gestation),
    specified NEC

Pregnancy — *continued*
  supervision of
    concealed pregnancy O09.3- ☑
    elderly mother
      multigravida O09.52- ☑
      primigravida O09.51- ☑
    hidden pregnancy O09.3- ☑
    high-risk O09.9- ☑
      due to (history of)
        ectopic pregnancy O09.1- ☑
        elderly — *see* Pregnancy, supervision, elder-
          ly mother
        grand multiparity O09.4 ☑
        in utero procedure during previous pregnan-
          cy O09.82- ☑
        in vitro fertilization O09.81- ☑
        infertility O09.0- ☑
        insufficient prenatal care O09.3- ☑
        molar pregnancy O09.A- ☑
        multiple previous pregnancies O09.4- ☑
        older mother — *see* Pregnancy, supervision
          of, elderly mother
        poor reproductive or obstetric history NEC
          O09.29- ☑
        pre-term labor O09.21- ☑
        previous
          neonatal death O09.29- ☑
        social problems O09.7- ☑
        specified NEC O09.89- ☑
        very young mother — *see* Pregnancy, super-
          vision, young mother
      resulting from in vitro fertilization O09.81- ☑
    normal Z34.9- ☑
      first Z34.0- ☑
      specified NEC Z34.8- ☑
    young mother
      multigravida O09.62- ☑
      primigravida O09.61- ☑
  triplet O30.10- ☑
    with
      two or more monoamniotic fetuses O30.12- ☑
      two or more monochorionic fetuses O30.11- ☑
    two or more monoamniotic fetuses O30.12- ☑
    two or more monochorionic fetuses O30.11- ☑
    unable to determine number of placenta and
      number of amniotic sacs O30.19- ☑
    unspecified number of placenta and unspecified
      number of amniotic sacs O30.10- ☑
  tubal (with abortion) (with rupture) O00.10- ☑
    with intrauterine pregnancy O00.11- ☑
  twin O30.00- ☑
    conjoined O30.02- ☑
    dichorionic/diamniotic (two placenta, two amniotic
      sacs) O30.04- ☑
    monochorionic/diamniotic (one placenta, two
      amniotic sacs) O30.03- ☑
    monochorionic/monoamniotic (one placenta, one
      amniotic sac) O30.01- ☑
    unable to determine number of placenta and
      number of amniotic sacs O30.09- ☑
    unspecified number of placenta and unspecified
      number of amniotic sacs O30.00- ☑
  unwanted Z64.0
  weeks of gestation
    less than 8 weeks Z3A.01 (*following* Z36)
    8 weeks Z3A.08 (*following* Z36)
    9 weeks Z3A.09 (*following* Z36)
    10 weeks Z3A.10 (*following* Z36)
    11 weeks Z3A.11 (*following* Z36)
    12 weeks Z3A.12 (*following* Z36)
    13 weeks Z3A.13 (*following* Z36)
    14 weeks Z3A.14 (*following* Z36)
    15 weeks Z3A.15 (*following* Z36)
    16 weeks Z3A.16 (*following* Z36)
    17 weeks Z3A.17 (*following* Z36)
    18 weeks Z3A.18 (*following* Z36)
    19 weeks Z3A.19 (*following* Z36)
    20 weeks Z3A.20 (*following* Z36)
    21 weeks Z3A.21 (*following* Z36)
    22 weeks Z3A.22 (*following* Z36)
    23 weeks Z3A.23 (*following* Z36)
    24 weeks Z3A.24 (*following* Z36)
    25 weeks Z3A.25 (*following* Z36)
    26 weeks Z3A.26 (*following* Z36)
    27 weeks Z3A.27 (*following* Z36)
    28 weeks Z3A.28 (*following* Z36)
    29 weeks Z3A.29 (*following* Z36)

Pregnancy — *continued*
  weeks of gestation — *continued*
    30 weeks Z3A.30 (*following* Z36)
    31 weeks Z3A.31 (*following* Z36)
    32 weeks Z3A.32 (*following* Z36)
    33 weeks Z3A.33 (*following* Z36)
    34 weeks Z3A.34 (*following* Z36)
    35 weeks Z3A.35 (*following* Z36)
    36 weeks Z3A.36 (*following* Z36)
    37 weeks Z3A.37 (*following* Z36)
    38 weeks Z3A.38 (*following* Z36)
    39 weeks Z3A.39 (*following* Z36)
    40 weeks Z3A.40 (*following* Z36)
    41 weeks Z3A.41 (*following* Z36)
    42 weeks Z3A.42 (*following* Z36)
    greater than 42 weeks Z3A.49 (*following* Z36)
    not specified Z3A.00 (*following* Z36)
Preiser's disease — *see* Osteonecrosis, secondary, due
  to, trauma, metacarpus
Pre-kwashiorkor — *see* Malnutrition, severe
Preleukemia (syndrome) D46.9
Preluxation, hip, congenital Q65.6
Premature (*see also* condition)
  adrenarche E27.0
  aging E34.8
  beats I49.40
    atrial I49.1
    auricular I49.1
    supraventricular I49.1
  birth NEC — *see* Preterm, newborn
  closure, foramen ovale Q21.8
  contraction
    atrial I49.1
    atrioventricular I49.2
    auricular I49.1
    auriculoventricular I49.49
    heart (extrasystole) I49.49
    junctional I49.2
    ventricular I49.3
  delivery (*see also* Pregnancy, complicated by, preterm
    labor) O60.10 ☑
  ejaculation F52.4
  infant NEC — *see* Preterm, newborn
    light-for-dates — *see* Light for dates
  labor — *see* Pregnancy, complicated by, preterm labor
  lungs P28.0
  menopause E28.319
    asymptomatic E28.319
    symptomatic E28.310
  newborn
    less than 37 completed weeks — *see* Preterm,
      newborn
    extreme (less than 28 completed weeks) — *see*
      Immaturity, extreme
  puberty E30.1
  rupture membranes or amnion — *see* Pregnancy,
    complicated by, premature rupture of mem-
    branes
  senility E34.8
  thelarche E30.8
  ventricular systole I49.3
Prematurity NEC (less than 37 completed weeks) — *see*
  Preterm, newborn
  extreme (less than 28 completed weeks) — *see* Imma-
    turity, extreme
Premenstrual
  dysphoric disorder (PMDD) F32.81
  tension (syndrome) N94.3
Premolarization, cuspids K00.2
Prenatal
  care, normal pregnancy — *see* Pregnancy, normal
  screening of mother (*see also* Encounter, antenatal
    screening) Z36.9
  teeth K00.6
Preparatory care for subsequent treatment NEC
  for dialysis Z49.01
    peritoneal Z49.02
Prepartum — *see* condition
Preponderance, left or right ventricular I51.7
Prepuce — *see* condition
PRES (posterior reversible encephalopathy syndrome)
  I67.83
Presbycardia R54
Presbycusis, presbyacusia H91.1- ☑
Presbyesophagus K22.8
Presbyophrenia F03 ☑
Presbyopia H52.4
Prescription of contraceptives (initial) Z30.019

☑ Additional Character Required — Refer to the Tabular List for Character Selection ⛛ Subterms under main terms may continue to next column or page

Prescription of contraceptives — *continued*
  barrier Z30.018
  diaphragm Z30.018
  emergency (postcoital) Z30.012
  implantable subdermal Z30.017
  injectable Z30.013
  intrauterine contraceptive device Z30.014
  pills Z30.011
  postcoital (emergency) Z30.012
  repeat Z30.40
    barrier Z30.49
    diaphragm Z30.49
    implantable subdermal Z30.46
    injectable Z30.42
    pills Z30.41
    specified type NEC Z30.49
    transdermal patch hormonal Z30.45
    vaginal ring hormonal Z30.44
  specified type NEC Z30.018
    transdermal patch hormonal Z30.016
    vaginal ring hormonal Z30.015
Presence (of)
  ankle-joint implant (functional) (prosthesis) Z96.66- ☑
  aortocoronary (bypass) graft Z95.1
  arterial-venous shunt (dialysis) Z99.2
  artificial
    eye (globe) Z97.0
    heart (fully implantable) (mechanical) Z95.812
      valve Z95.2
    larynx Z96.3
    lens (intraocular) Z96.1
    limb (complete) (partial) Z97.1- ☑
      arm Z97.1- ☑
        bilateral Z97.15
      leg Z97.1- ☑
        bilateral Z97.16
  audiological implant (functional) Z96.29
  bladder implant (functional) Z96.0
  bone
    conduction hearing device Z96.29
    implant (functional) NEC Z96.7
    joint (prosthesis) — *see* Presence, joint implant
  cardiac
    defibrillator (functional) (with synchronous cardiac pacemaker) Z95.810
    implant or graft Z95.9
      specified type NEC Z95.818
    pacemaker Z95.0
    resynchronization therapy
      defibrillator Z95.810
      pacemaker Z95.0
  cardioverter-defibrillator (ICD) Z95.810
  cerebrospinal fluid drainage device Z98.2
  cochlear implant (functional) Z96.21
  contact lens (es) Z97.3
  coronary artery graft or prosthesis Z95.5
  CRT-D (cardiac resynchronization therapy defibrillator) Z95.810
  CRT-P (cardiac resynchronization therapy pacemaker) Z95.0
  CSF shunt Z98.2
  dental prosthesis device Z97.2
  dentures Z97.2
  device (external) NEC Z97.8
    cardiac NEC Z95.818
    heart assist Z95.811
    implanted (functional) Z96.9
      specified NEC Z96.89
    prosthetic Z97.8
  ear implant Z96.20
    cochlear implant Z96.21
    myringotomy tube Z96.22
    specified type NEC Z96.29
  elbow-joint implant (functional) (prosthesis) Z96.62- ☑
  endocrine implant (functional) NEC Z96.49
  eustachian tube stent or device (functional) Z96.29
  external hearing-aid or device Z97.4
  finger-joint implant (functional) (prosthetic) Z96.69- ☑
  functional implant Z96.9
    specified NEC Z96.89
  graft
    cardiac NEC Z95.818
    vascular NEC Z95.828
  hearing-aid or device (external) Z97.4
    implant (bone) (cochlear) (functional) Z96.21
  heart assist device Z95.811
  heart valve implant (functional) Z95.2

Presence — *continued*
  heart valve implant — *continued*
    prosthetic Z95.2
    specified type NEC Z95.4
    xenogenic Z95.3
  hip-joint implant (functional) (prosthesis) Z96.64- ☑
  ICD (cardioverter-defibrillator) Z95.810
  implanted device (artificial) (functional) (prosthetic) Z96.9
    automatic cardiac defibrillator (with synchronous cardiac pacemaker) Z95.810
    cardiac pacemaker Z95.0
    cochlear Z96.21
    dental Z96.5
    heart Z95.812
    heart valve Z95.2
      prosthetic Z95.2
      specified NEC Z95.4
      xenogenic Z95.3
    insulin pump Z96.41
    intraocular lens Z96.1
    joint Z96.60
      ankle Z96.66- ☑
      elbow Z96.62- ☑
      finger Z96.69- ☑
      hip Z96.64- ☑
      knee Z96.65- ☑
      shoulder Z96.61- ☑
      specified NEC Z96.698
      wrist Z96.63- ☑
    larynx Z96.3
    myringotomy tube Z96.22
    otological Z96.20
      cochlear Z96.21
      eustachian stent Z96.29
      myringotomy Z96.22
      specified NEC Z96.29
      stapes Z96.29
    skin Z96.81
    skull plate Z96.7
    specified NEC Z96.89
    urogenital Z96.0
  insulin pump (functional) Z96.41
  intestinal bypass or anastomosis Z98.0
  intraocular lens (functional) Z96.1
  intrauterine contraceptive device (IUD) Z97.5
  intravascular implant (functional) (prosthetic) NEC Z95.9
    coronary artery Z95.5
    defibrillator (with synchronous cardiac pacemaker) Z95.810
    peripheral vessel (with angioplasty) Z95.820
  joint implant (prosthetic) (any) Z96.60
    ankle — *see* Presence, ankle joint implant
    elbow — *see* Presence, elbow joint implant
    finger — *see* Presence, finger joint implant
    hip — *see* Presence, hip joint implant
    knee — *see* Presence, knee joint implant
    shoulder — *see* Presence, shoulder joint implant
    specified joint NEC Z96.698
    wrist — *see* Presence, wrist joint implant
  knee-joint implant (functional) (prosthesis) Z96.65- ☑
  laryngeal implant (functional) Z96.3
  mandibular implant (dental) Z96.5
  myringotomy tube(s) Z96.22
  orthopedic-joint implant (prosthetic) (any) — *see* Presence, joint implant
  otological implant (functional) Z96.29
  shoulder-joint implant (functional) (prosthesis) Z96.61- ☑
  skull-plate implant Z96.7
  spectacles Z97.3
  stapes implant (functional) Z96.29
  systemic lupus erythematosus [SLE] inhibitor D68.62
  tendon implant (functional) (graft) Z96.7
  tooth root(s) implant Z96.5
  ureteral stent Z96.0
  urethral stent Z96.0
  urogenital implant (functional) Z96.0
  vascular implant or device Z95.9
    access port device Z95.828
    specified type NEC Z95.828
  wrist-joint implant (functional) (prosthesis) Z96.63- ☑
Presenile (*see also* condition)
  dementia F03 ☑
  premature aging E34.8
Presentation, fetal — *see* Delivery, complicated by, malposition

Prespondylolisthesis (congenital) Q76.2
Pressure
  area, skin — *see* Ulcer, pressure, by site
  brachial plexus G54.0
  brain G93.5
    injury at birth NEC P11.1
  cerebral — *see* Pressure, brain
  chest R07.89
  cone, tentorial G93.5
  hyposystolic (*see also* Hypotension)
    incidental reading, without diagnosis of hypotension R03.1
  increased
    intracranial (benign) G93.2
      injury at birth P11.0
    intraocular H40.05- ☑
  lumbosacral plexus G54.1
  mediastinum J98.59
  necrosis (chronic) — *see* Ulcer, pressure, by site
  parental, inappropriate (excessive) Z62.6
  sore (chronic) — *see* Ulcer, pressure, by site
  spinal cord G95.20
  ulcer (chronic) — *see* Ulcer, pressure, by site
  venous, increased I87.8
Pre-syncope R55
Preterm
  delivery (*see also* Pregnancy, complicated by, preterm labor) O60.10 ☑
  labor — *see* Pregnancy, complicated by, preterm labor
  newborn (infant) P07.30
    gestational age
      28 completed weeks (28 weeks, 0 days through 28 weeks, 6 days) P07.31
      29 completed weeks (29 weeks, 0 days through 29 weeks, 6 days) P07.32
      30 completed weeks (30 weeks, 0 days through 30 weeks, 6 days) P07.33
      31 completed weeks (31 weeks, 0 days through 31 weeks, 6 days) P07.34
      32 completed weeks (32 weeks, 0 days through 32 weeks, 6 days) P07.35
      33 completed weeks (33 weeks, 0 days through 33 weeks, 6 days) P07.36
      34 completed weeks (34 weeks, 0 days through 34 weeks, 6 days) P07.37
      35 completed weeks (35 weeks, 0 days through 35 weeks, 6 days) P07.38
      36 completed weeks (36 weeks, 0 days through 36 weeks, 6 days) P07.39
Previa
  placenta (total) (without hemorrhage) O44.0- ☑
    with hemorrhage O44.1- ☑
    complete O44.0- ☑
      with hemorrhage O44.1- ☑
    low (*see also* Delivery, complicated, by, placenta, low) O44.4- ☑
      with hemorrhage O44.5- ☑
    marginal O44.2- ☑
      with hemorrhage O44.3- ☑
    partial O44.2- ☑
      with hemorrhage O44.3- ☑
  vasa O69.4 ☑
Priapism N48.30
  due to
    disease classified elsewhere N48.32
    drug N48.33
    specified cause NEC N48.39
    trauma N48.31
Prickling sensation (skin) R20.2
Prickly heat L74.0
Primary — *see* condition
Primigravida
  elderly, affecting management of pregnancy, labor and delivery (supervision only) — *see* Pregnancy, complicated by, elderly, primigravida
  older, affecting management of pregnancy, labor and delivery (supervision only) — *see* Pregnancy, complicated by, elderly, primigravida
  very young, affecting management of pregnancy, labor and delivery (supervision only) — *see* Pregnancy, complicated by, young mother, primigravida
Primipara
  elderly, affecting management of pregnancy, labor and delivery (supervision only) — *see* Pregnancy, complicated by, elderly, primigravida

Primipara — *continued*
- older, affecting management of pregnancy, labor and delivery (supervision only) — *see* Pregnancy, complicated by, elderly, primigravida
- very young, affecting management of pregnancy, labor and delivery (supervision only) — *see* Pregnancy, complicated by, young mother, primigravida

Primus varus (bilateral) Q66.2 ☑

PRIND (Prolonged reversible ischemic neurologic deficit) I63.9

Pringle's disease (tuberous sclerosis) Q85.1

Prinzmetal angina I20.1

Prizefighter ear — *see* Cauliflower ear

Problem (with) (related to)
- academic Z55.8
- acculturation Z60.3
- adjustment (to)
  - change of job Z56.1
  - life-cycle transition Z60.0
  - pension Z60.0
  - retirement Z60.0
- adopted child Z62.821
- alcoholism in family Z63.72
- atypical parenting situation Z62.9
- bankruptcy Z59.8
- behavioral (adult) F69
  - drug seeking Z76.5
- birth of sibling affecting child Z62.898
- care (of)
  - provider dependency 774.9
    - specified NEC Z74.8
  - sick or handicapped person in family or household Z63.6
- child
  - abuse (affecting the child) — *see* Maltreatment, child
  - custody or support proceedings Z65.3
  - in care of non-parental family member Z62.21
  - in foster care Z62.21
  - in welfare custody Z62.21
  - living in orphanage or group home Z62.22
- child-rearing Z62.9
  - specified NEC Z62.898
- communication (developmental) F80.9
- conflict or discord (with)
  - boss Z56.4
  - classmates Z55.4
  - counselor Z64.4
  - employer Z56.4
  - family Z63.9
    - specified NEC Z63.8
  - probation officer Z64.4
  - social worker Z64.4
  - teachers Z55.4
  - workmates Z56.4
- conviction in legal proceedings Z65.0
  - with imprisonment Z65.1
- counselor Z64.4
- creditors Z59.8
- digestive K92.9
- drug addict in family Z63.72
- ear — *see* Disorder, ear
- economic Z59.9
  - affecting care Z59.9
  - specified NEC Z59.8
- education Z55.9
  - specified NEC Z55.8
- employment Z56.9
  - change of job Z56.1
  - discord Z56.4
  - environment Z56.5
  - sexual harassment Z56.81
  - specified NEC Z56.89
  - stressful schedule Z56.3
  - stress NEC Z56.6
  - threat of job loss Z56.2
  - unemployment Z56.0
- enuresis, child F98.0
- eye H57.9
- failed examinations (school) Z55.2
- falling Z91.81
- family (*see also* Disruption, family) Z63.9
  - specified NEC Z63.8
- feeding (elderly) (infant) R63.3
  - newborn P92.9
    - breast P92.5
    - overfeeding P92.4
    - slow P92.2

Problem — *continued*
- feeding — *continued*
  - newborn — *continued*
    - specified NEC P92.8
    - underfeeding P92.3
  - nonorganic F50.89
- finance Z59.9
  - specified NEC Z59.8
- foreclosure on loan Z59.8
- foster child Z62.822
- frightening experience(s) in childhood Z62.898
- genital NEC
  - female N94.9
  - male N50.9
- health care Z75.9
  - specified NEC Z75.8
- hearing — *see* Deafness
- homelessness Z59.0
- housing Z59.9
  - inadequate Z59.1
  - isolated Z59.8
  - specified NEC Z59.8
- identity (of childhood) F93.8
- illegitimate pregnancy (unwanted) Z64.0
- illiteracy Z55.0
- impaired mobility Z74.09
- imprisonment or incarceration Z65.1
- inadequate teaching affecting education Z55.8
- inappropriate (excessive) parental pressure Z62.6
- influencing health status NEC Z78.9
- in-law Z63.1
- institutionalization, affecting child Z62.22
- intrafamilial communication Z63.8
- jealousy, child F93.8
- landlord Z59.2
- language (developmental) F80.9
- learning (developmental) F81.9
- legal Z65.3
  - conviction without imprisonment Z65.0
  - imprisonment Z65.1
  - release from prison Z65.2
- life-management Z73.9
  - specified NEC Z73.89
- life-style Z72.9
  - gambling Z72.6
  - high-risk sexual behavior (heterosexual) Z72.51
    - bisexual Z72.53
    - homosexual Z72.52
  - inappropriate eating habits Z72.4
  - self-damaging behavior NEC Z72.89
  - specified NEC Z72.89
  - tobacco use Z72.0
- literacy Z55.9
  - low level Z55.0
  - specified NEC Z55.8
- living alone Z60.2
- lodgers Z59.2
- loss of love relationship in childhood Z62.898
- marital Z63.0
  - involving
    - divorce Z63.5
    - estrangement Z63.5
    - gender identity F66
- mastication K08.89
- medical
  - care, within family Z63.6
  - facilities Z75.9
    - specified NEC Z75.8
- mental F48.9
- multiparity Z64.1
- negative life events in childhood Z62.9
  - altered pattern of family relationships Z62.898
  - frightening experience Z62.898
  - loss of
    - love relationship Z62.898
    - self-esteem Z62.898
  - physical abuse (alleged) — *see* Maltreatment, child
  - removal from home Z62.29
  - specified event NEC Z62.898
- neighbor Z59.2
- neurological NEC R29.818
- new step-parent affecting child Z62.898
- none (feared complaint unfounded) Z71.1
- occupational NEC Z56.89
- parent-child — *see* Conflict, parent-child
- personal hygiene Z91.89
- personality F69
- phase-of-life transition, adjustment Z60.0

Problem — *continued*
- presence of sick or disabled person in family or household Z63.79
  - needing care Z63.6
- primary support group (family) Z63.9
  - specified NEC Z63.8
- probation officer Z64.4
- psychiatric F99
- psychosexual (development) F66
- psychosocial Z65.9
  - religious or spiritual Z65.8
  - specified NEC Z65.8
- relationship Z63.9
  - childhood F93.8
- release from prison Z65.2
  - religious or spiritual Z65.8
- removal from home affecting child Z62.29
- seeking and accepting known hazardous and harmful behavioral or psychological interventions Z65.8
  - chemical, nutritional or physical interventions Z65.8
- sexual function (nonorganic) F52.9
- sight H54.7
- sleep disorder, child F51.9
- smell — *see* Disturbance, sensation, smell
- social
  - environment Z60.9
    - specified NEC Z60.8
  - exclusion and rejection Z60.4
  - worker Z64.4
- speech R47.9
  - developmental F80.9
  - specified NEC R47.89
- swallowing — *see* Dysphagia
- taste — *see* Disturbance, sensation, taste
- tic, child F95.0
- underachievement in school Z55.3
- unemployment Z56.0
  - threatened Z56.2
- unwanted pregnancy Z64.0
- upbringing Z62.9
  - specified NEC Z62.898
- urinary N39.9
- voice production R47.89
- work schedule (stressful) Z56.3

Procedure (surgical)
- converted
  - arthroscopic to open Z53.33
  - laparoscopic to open Z53.31
  - specified procedure NEC to open Z53.39
  - thoracoscopic to open Z53.32
- for purpose other than remedying health state Z41.9
  - specified NEC Z41.8
- not done Z53.9
  - because of
    - administrative reasons Z53.8
    - contraindication Z53.09
      - smoking Z53.01
    - patient's decision Z53.20
      - for reasons of belief or group pressure Z53.1
      - left against medical advice (AMA) Z53.21
      - specified reason NEC Z53.29
    - specified reason NEC Z53.8

Procidentia (uteri) N81.3

Proctalgia K62.89
- fugax K59.4
- spasmodic K59.4

Proctitis K62.89
- amebic (acute) A06.0
- chlamydial A56.3
- gonococcal A54.6
- granulomatous — *see* Enteritis, regional, large intestine
- herpetic A60.1
- radiation K62.7
- tuberculous A18.32
- ulcerative (chronic) K51.20
  - with
    - complication K51.219
      - abscess K51.214
      - fistula K51.213
      - obstruction K51.212
      - rectal bleeding K51.211
      - specified NEC K51.218

Proctocele
- female (without uterine prolapse) N81.6
  - with uterine prolapse N81.2
    - complete N81.3
- male K62.3

264   ☑ **Additional Character Required — Refer to the Tabular List for Character Selection**   ⬇ **Subterms under main terms may continue to next column or page**

Primipara — Proctocele

Proctocolitis
food protein-induced K52.82
food-induced eosinophilic K52.82
milk protein-induced K52.82
mucosal — *see* Rectosigmoiditis, ulcerative
Proctoptosis K62.3
Proctorrhagia K62.5
Proctosigmoiditis K63.89
ulcerative (chronic) — *see* Rectosigmoiditis, ulcerative
Proctospasm K59.4
psychogenic F45.8
Profichet's disease — *see* Disorder, soft tissue, specified
type NEC
Progeria E34.8
Prognathism (mandibular) (maxillary) M26.19
Progonoma (melanotic) — *see* Neoplasm, benign, by site
Progressive — *see* condition
Prolactinoma
specified site — *see* Neoplasm, benign, by site
unspecified site D35.2
Prolapse, prolapsed
anus, anal (canal) (sphincter) K62.2
arm or hand O32.2 ☑
causing obstructed labor O64.4 ☑
bladder (mucosa) (sphincter) (acquired)
congenital Q79.4
female — *see* Cystocele
male N32.89
breast implant (prosthetic) T85.49 ☑
cecostomy K94.09
cecum K63.4
cervix, cervical (hypertrophied) N81.2
anterior lip, obstructing labor O65.5
congenital Q51.828
postpartal, old N81.2
stump N81.85
ciliary body (traumatic) — *see* Laceration, eye(ball),
with prolapse or loss of interocular tissue
colon (pedunculated) K63.4
colostomy K94.09
disc (intervertebral) — *see* Displacement, intervertebral disc
eye implant (orbital) T85.398 ☑
lens (ocular) — *see* Complications, intraocular lens
fallopian tube N83.4- ☑
gastric (mucosa) K31.89
genital, female N81.9
specified NEC N81.89
globe, nontraumatic — *see* Luxation, globe
ileostomy bud K94.19
intervertebral disc — *see* Displacement, intervertebral
disc
intestine (small) K63.4
iris (traumatic) — *see* Laceration, eye(ball), with prolapse or loss of interocular tissue
nontraumatic H21.89
kidney N28.83
congenital Q63.2
laryngeal muscles or ventricle J38.7
liver K76.89
meatus urinarius N36.8
mitral (valve) I34.1
ocular lens implant — *see* Complications, intraocular
lens
organ or site, congenital NEC — *see* Malposition,
congenital
ovary N83.4- ☑
pelvic floor, female N81.89
perineum, female N81.89
rectum (mucosa) (sphincter) K62.3
due to trichuris trichuria B79
spleen D73.89
stomach K31.89
umbilical cord
complicating delivery O69.0 ☑
urachus, congenital Q64.4
ureter N28.89
with obstruction N13.5
with infection N13.6
ureterovesical orifice N28.89
urethra (acquired) (infected) (mucosa) N36.8
congenital Q64.71
urinary meatus N36.8
congenital Q64.72
uterovaginal N81.4
complete N81.3
incomplete N81.2

Prolapse, prolapsed — *continued*
uterus (with prolapse of vagina) N81.4
complete N81.3
congenital Q51.818
first degree N81.2
in pregnancy or childbirth — *see* Pregnancy,
complicated by, abnormal, uterus
incomplete N81.2
postpartal (old) N81.4
second degree N81.2
third degree N81.3
uveal (traumatic) — *see* Laceration, eye(ball), with
prolapse or loss of interocular tissue
vagina (anterior) (wall) — *see* Cystocele
with prolapse of uterus N81.4
complete N81.3
incomplete N81.2
posterior wall N81.6
posthysterectomy N99.3
vitreous (humor) H43.0- ☑
in wound — *see* Laceration, eye(ball), with prolapse or loss of interocular tissue
womb — *see* Prolapse, uterus
Prolapsus, female N81.9
specified NEC N81.89
Proliferation(s)
primary cutaneous CD30-positive large T-cell C86.6
prostate, atypical small acinar N42.32
Proliferative — *see* condition
Prolonged, prolongation (of)
bleeding (time) (idiopathic) R79.1
coagulation (time) R79.1
gestation (over 42 completed weeks)
mother O48.1
newborn P08.22
interval I44.0
labor O63.9
first stage O63.0
second stage O63.1
partial thromboplastin time (PTT) R79.1
pregnancy (more than 42 weeks gestation) O48.1
prothrombin time R79.1
QT interval I45.81
uterine contractions in labor O62.4
Prominence, prominent
auricle (congenital) (ear) Q17.5
ischial spine or sacral promontory
with disproportion (fetopelvic) O33.0
causing obstructed labor O65.0
nose (congenital) acquired M95.0
Promiscuity — *see* High, risk, sexual behavior
Pronation
ankle — *see* Deformity, limb, foot, specified NEC
foot (*see also* Deformity, limb, foot, specified NEC)
congenital Q74.2
Prophylactic
administration of
antibiotics, long-term Z79.2
short-term use — *omit code*
drug (*see also* Long-term (current) drug therapy
(use of)) Z79.899
medication Z79.899
organ removal (for neoplasia management) Z40.00
breast Z40.01
fallopian tube(s) Z40.03
with ovary(s) Z40.02
ovary(s) Z40.02
specified site NEC Z40.09
surgery Z40.9
for risk factors related to malignant neoplasm —
see Prophylactic, organ removal
specified NEC Z40.8
vaccination Z23
Propionic acidemia E71.121
Proptosis (ocular) (*see also* Exophthalmos)
thyroid — *see* Hyperthyroidism, with goiter
Prosecution, anxiety concerning Z65.3
Prosopagnosia R48.3
Prostadynia N42.81
Prostate, prostatic — *see* condition
Prostatism — *see* Hyperplasia, prostate
Prostatitis (congestive) (suppurative) (with cystitis) N41.9
acute N41.0
cavitary N41.8
chronic N41.1
diverticular N41.8
due to Trichomonas (vaginalis) A59.02
fibrous N41.1

Prostatitis — *continued*
gonococcal (acute) (chronic) A54.22
granulomatous N41.4
hypertrophic N41.1
subacute N41.1
trichomonal A59.02
tuberculous A18.14
Prostatocystitis N41.3
Prostatorrhea N42.89
Prostatosis N42.82
Prostration R53.83
heat (*see also* Heat, exhaustion)
anhydrotic T67.3 ☑
due to
salt (and water) depletion T67.4 ☑
water depletion T67.3 ☑
nervous F48.8
senile R54
Protanomaly (anomalous trichromat) H53.54
Protanopia (complete) (incomplete) H53.54
Protection (against) (from) — *see* Prophylactic
Protein
deficiency NEC — *see* Malnutrition
malnutrition — *see* Malnutrition
sickness (*see also* Reaction, serum) T80.69 ☑
Proteinemia R77.9
Proteinosis
alveolar (pulmonary) J84.01
lipid or lipoid (of Urbach) E78.89
Proteinuria R80.9
Bence Jones R80.3
complicating pregnancy — *see* Proteinuria, gestational
gestational
complicating
childbirth O12.14
pregnancy O12.1- ☑
with edema O12.2- ☑
puerperium O12.15
idiopathic R80.0
isolated R80.0
with glomerular lesion N06.9
dense deposit disease N06.6
diffuse
crescentic glomerulonephritis N06.7
endocapillary proliferative glomerulonephritis N06.4
mesangiocapillary glomerulonephritis N06.5
focal and segmental hyalinosis or sclerosis
N06.1
membranous (diffuse) N06.2
mesangial proliferative (diffuse) N06.3
minimal change N06.0
specified pathology NEC N06.8
orthostatic R80.2
with glomerular lesion — *see* Proteinuria, isolated,
with glomerular lesion
persistent R80.1
with glomerular lesion — *see* Proteinuria, isolated,
with glomerular lesion
postural R80.2
with glomerular lesion — *see* Proteinuria, isolated,
with glomerular lesion
pre-eclamptic — *see* Pre-eclampsia
puerperal O12.15
specified type NEC R80.8
Proteolysis, pathologic D65
Proteus (mirabilis) (morganii), **as cause of disease
classified elsewhere** B96.4
Prothrombin gene mutation D68.52
Protoporphyria, erythropoietic E80.0
Protozoal (*see also* condition)
disease B64
specified NEC B60.8
Protrusion, protrusio
acetabuli M24.7
acetabulum (into pelvis) M24.7
device, implant or graft (*see also* Complications, by
site and type, mechanical) T85.698 ☑
arterial graft NEC — *see* Complication, cardiovascular device, mechanical, vascular
breast (implant) T85.49 ☑
catheter NEC T85.698 ☑
cystostomy T83.090 ☑
dialysis (renal) T82.49 ☑
intraperitoneal T85.691 ☑
infusion NEC T82.594 ☑
spinal (epidural) (subdural) T85.690 ☑

Protrusion, protrusio — *continued*
device, implant or graft (*see also* Complications, by site and type, mechanical) — *continued*
catheter — *continued*
urinary (*see also* Complications, catheter, urinary) T83.098 ☑
electronic (electrode) (pulse generator) (stimulator)
bone T84.390 ☑
nervous system — *see* Complication, prosthetic device, mechanical, electronic nervous system stimulator
fixation, internal (orthopedic) NEC — *see* Complication, fixation device, mechanical
gastrointestinal — *see* Complications, prosthetic device, mechanical, gastrointestinal device
genital NEC T83.498 ☑
intrauterine contraceptive device T83.39 ☑
penile prosthesis (cylinder) (implanted) (pump) (resevoir) T83.490 ☑
testicular prosthesis T83.491 ☑
heart NEC — *see* Complication, cardiovascular device, mechanical
joint prosthesis — *see* Complications, joint prosthesis, mechanical, specified NEC, by site
ocular NEC — *see* Complications, prosthetic device, mechanical, ocular device
orthopedic NEC — *see* Complication, orthopedic, device, mechanical
specified NEC T85.628 ☑
urinary NEC (*see also* Complication, genitourinary, device, urinary, mechanical)
graft T83.29 ☑
vascular NEC — *see* Complication, cardiovascular device, mechanical
ventricular intracranial shunt T85.09 ☑
intervertebral disc — *see* Displacement, intervertebral disc
joint prosthesis — *see* Complications, joint prosthesis, mechanical, specified NEC, by site
nucleus pulposus — *see* Displacement, intervertebral disc
Prune belly (syndrome) Q79.4
Prurigo (ferox) (gravis) (Hebrae's) (Hebra's) (mitis) (simplex) L28.2
Besnier's L20.0
estivalis L56.4
nodularis L28.1
psychogenic F45.8
Pruritus, pruritic (essential) L29.9
ani, anus L29.0
psychogenic F45.8
anogenital L29.3
psychogenic F45.8
due to onchocerca volvulus B73.1
gravidarum — *see* Pregnancy, complicated by, specified pregnancy-related condition NEC
hiemalis L29.8
neurogenic (any site) F45.8
perianal L29.0
psychogenic (any site) F45.8
scroti, scrotum L29.1
psychogenic F45.8
senile, senilis L29.8
specified NEC L29.8
psychogenic F45.8
Trichomonas A59.9
vulva, vulvae L29.2
psychogenic F45.8
Pseudarthrosis, pseudoarthrosis (bone) — *see* Nonunion, fracture
clavicle, congenital Q74.0
joint, following fusion or arthrodesis M96.0
Pseudoaneurysm — *see* Aneurysm
Pseudoangina (pectoris) — *see* Angina
Pseudoangioma I81
Pseudoarteriosus Q28.8
Pseudoarthrosis — *see* Pseudarthrosis
Pseudobulbar affect (PBA) F48.2
Pseudochromhidrosis L67.8
Pseudocirrhosis, liver, pericardial I31.1
Pseudocowpox B08.03
Pseudocoxalgia M91.3- ☑
Pseudocroup J38.5
Pseudo-Cushing's syndrome, alcohol-induced E24.4
Pseudocyesis F45.8
Pseudocyst
lung J98.4

Pseudocyst — *continued*
pancreas K86.3
retina — *see* Cyst, retina
Pseudoelephantiasis neuroarthritica Q82.0
Pseudoexfoliation, capsule (lens) — *see* Cataract, specified NEC
Pseudofolliculitis barbae L73.1
Pseudoglioma H44.89
Pseudohemophilia (Bernuth's) (hereditary) (type B) D68.0
Type A D69.8
vascular D69.8
Pseudohermaphroditism Q56.3
adrenal E25.8
female Q56.2
with adrenocortical disorder E25.8
without adrenocortical disorder Q56.2
adrenal (congenital) E25.0
unspecified E25.9
male Q56.1
with
5-alpha-reductase deficiency E29.1
adrenocortical disorder E25.8
androgen resistance E34.51
cleft scrotum Q56.1
feminizing testis E34.51
without gonadal disorder Q56.1
adrenal E25.8
unspecified E25.9
Pseudo-Hurler's polydystrophy E77.0
Pseudohydrocephalus G93.2
Pseudohypertrophic muscular dystrophy (Erb's) G71.0
Pseudohypertrophy, muscle G71.0
Pseudohypoparathyroidism E20.1
Pseudoinsomnia F51.03
Pseudoleukemia, infantile D64.89
Pseudomembranous — *see* condition
Pseudomeningocele (cerebral) (infective) (post-traumatic) G96.19
postprocedural (spinal) G97.82
Pseudomenses (newborn) P54.6
Pseudomenstruation (newborn) P54.6
Pseudomonas
aeruginosa, as cause of disease classified elsewhere B96.5
mallei infection A24.0
as cause of disease classified elsewhere B96.5
pseudomallei, as cause of disease classified elsewhere B96.5
Pseudomyotonia G71.19
Pseudomyxoma peritonei C78.6
Pseudoneuritis, optic (nerve) (disc) (papilla), **congenital** Q14.2
Pseudo-obstruction intestine (acute) (chronic) (idiopathic) (intermittent secondary) (primary) K59.8
Pseudopapilledema H47.33- ☑
congenital Q14.2
Pseudoparalysis
arm or leg R29.818
atonic, congenital P94.2
Pseudopelade L66.0
Pseudophakia Z96.1
Pseudopolyarthritis, rhizomelic M35.3
Pseudopolycythemia D75.1
Pseudopseudohypoparathyroidism E20.1
Pseudopterygium H11.81- ☑
Pseudoptosis (eyelid) — *see* Blepharochalasis
Pseudopuberty, precocious
female heterosexual E25.8
male isosexual E25.8
Pseudorickets (renal) N25.0
Pseudorubella B08.20
Pseudosclerema, newborn P83.88
Pseudosclerosis (brain)
Jakob's — *see* Creutzfeldt-Jakob disease or syndrome
of Westphal (Strümpell) E83.01
spastic — *see* Creutzfeldt-Jakob disease or syndrome
Pseudotetanus — *see* Convulsions
Pseudotetany R29.0
hysterical F44.5
Pseudotruncus arteriosus Q25.49
Pseudotuberculosis A28.2
enterocolitis A04.8
pasteurella (infection) A28.0
Pseudotumor
cerebri G93.2
orbital H05.11 ☑

Pseudoxanthoma elasticum Q82.8
Psilosis (sprue) (tropical) K90.1
nontropical K90.0
Psittacosis A70
Psoitis M60.88
Psoriasis L40.9
arthropathic L40.50
arthritis mutilans L40.52
distal interphalangeal L40.51
juvenile L40.54
other specified L40.59
spondylitis L40.53
buccal K13.29
flexural L40.8
guttate L40.4
mouth K13.29
nummular L40.0
plaque L40.0
psychogenic F54
pustular (generalized) L40.1
palmaris et plantaris L40.3
specified NEC L40.8
vulgaris L40.0
Psychasthenia F48.8
Psychiatric disorder or problem F99
Psychogenic (*see also* condition)
factors associated with physical conditions F54
Psychological and behavioral factors affecting medical condition F59
Psychoneurosis, psychoneurotic (*see also* Neurosis)
anxiety (state) F41.1
depersonalization F48.1
hypochondriacal F45.21
hysteria F44.9
neurasthenic F48.8
personality NEC F60.89
Psychopathy, psychopathic
affectionless F94.2
autistic F84.5
constitution, post-traumatic F07.81
personality — *see* Disorder, personality
sexual — *see* Deviation, sexual
state F60.2
Psychosexual identity disorder of childhood F64.2
Psychosis, psychotic F29
acute (transient) F23
hysterical F44.9
affective — *see* Disorder, mood
alcoholic F10.959
with
abuse F10.159
anxiety disorder F10.980
with
abuse F10.180
dependence F10.280
delirium tremens F10.231
delusions F10.950
with
abuse F10.150
dependence F10.250
dementia F10.97
with dependence F10.27
dependence F10.259
hallucinosis F10.951
with
abuse F10.151
dependence F10.251
mood disorder F10.94
with
abuse F10.14
dependence F10.24
paranoia F10.950
with
abuse F10.150
dependence F10.250
persisting amnesia F10.96
with dependence F10.26
amnestic confabulatory F10.96
with dependence F10.26
delirium tremens F10.231
Korsakoff's, Korsakov's, Korsakow's F10.26
paranoid type F10.950
with
abuse F10.150
dependence F10.250
anergastic — *see* Psychosis, organic
arteriosclerotic (simple type) (uncomplicated) F01.50
with behavioral disturbance F01.51

☑ Additional Character Required — Refer to the Tabular List for Character Selection
Subterms under main terms may continue to next column or page

Psychosis, psychotic — *continued*
  childhood F84.0
    atypical F84.8
  climacteric — *see* Psychosis, involutional
  confusional F29
    acute or subacute F05
    reactive F23
  cycloid F23
  depressive — *see* Disorder, depressive
  disintegrative (childhood) F84.3
  drug-induced — *see* F11-F19 with .X59
    paranoid and hallucinatory states — *see* F11-F19
      with .X50 or .X51
  due to or associated with
    addiction, drug — *see* F11-F19 with .X59
    dependence
      alcohol F10.259
      drug — *see* F11-F19 with .X59
    epilepsy F06.8
    Huntington's chorea F06.8
    ischemia, cerebrovascular (generalized) F06.8
    multiple sclerosis F06.8
    physical disease F06.8
    presenile dementia F03 ☑
    senile dementia F03 ☑
    vascular disease (arteriosclerotic) (cerebral) F01.50
      with behavioral disturbance F01.51
  epileptic F06.8
  episode F23
    due to or associated with physical condition F06.8
  exhaustive F43.0
  hallucinatory, chronic F28
  hypomanic F30.8
  hysterical (acute) F44.9
  induced F24
  infantile F84.0
    atypical F84.8
  infective (acute) (subacute) F05
  involutional F28
    depressive — *see* Disorder, depressive
    melancholic — *see* Disorder, depressive
    paranoid (state) F22
  Korsakoff's, Korsakov's, Korsakow's (nonalcoholic) F04
    alcoholic F10.96
      in dependence F10.26
    induced by other psychoactive substance — *see*
      categories F11-F19 with .X5X
  mania, manic (single episode) F30.2
    recurrent type F31.89
  manic-depressive — *see* Disorder, bipolar
  menopausal — *see* Psychosis, involutional
  mixed schizophrenic and affective F25.8
  multi-infarct (cerebrovascular) F01.50
    with behavioral disturbance F01.51
  nonorganic F29
    specified NEC F28
  organic F09
    due to or associated with
      arteriosclerosis (cerebral) — *see* Psychosis, ar-
        teriosclerotic
      cerebrovascular disease, arteriosclerotic — *see*
        Psychosis, arteriosclerotic
      childbirth — *see* Psychosis, puerperal
      Creutzfeldt-Jakob disease or syndrome — *see*
        Creutzfeldt-Jakob disease or syndrome
      dependence, alcohol F10.259
      disease
        alcoholic liver F10.259
        brain, arteriosclerotic — *see* Psychosis, arte-
          riosclerotic
        cerebrovascular F01.50
          with behavioral disturbance F01.51
        Creutzfeldt-Jakob — *see* Creutzfeldt-Jakob
          disease or syndrome
        endocrine or metabolic F06.8
          acute or subacute F05
        liver, alcoholic F10.259
      epilepsy transient (acute) F05
      infection
        brain (intracranial) F06.8
          acute or subacute F05
      intoxication
        alcoholic (acute) F10.259
        drug F11-F19 with .X59
      ischemia, cerebrovascular (generalized) — *see*
        Psychosis, arteriosclerotic
      puerperium — *see* Psychosis, puerperal

Psychosis, psychotic — *continued*
  organic — *continued*
    due to or associated with — *continued*
      trauma, brain (birth) (from electric current)
        (surgical) F06.8
        acute or subacute F05
    infective F06.8
      acute or subacute F05
    post-traumatic F06.8
      acute or subacute F05
  paranoiac F22
  paranoid (climacteric) (involutional) (menopausal) F22
    psychogenic (acute) F23
    schizophrenic F20.0
    senile F03 ☑
  postpartum F53
  presbyophrenic (type) F03 ☑
  presenile F03 ☑
  psychogenic (paranoid) F23
    depressive F32.3
  puerperal F53
    specified type — *see* Psychosis, by type
  reactive (brief) (transient) (emotional stress) (psycho-
    logical trauma) F23
    depressive F32.3
      recurrent F33.3
    excitative type F30.8
  schizoaffective F25.9
    depressive type F25.1
    manic type F25.0
  schizophrenia, schizophrenic — *see* Schizophrenia
  schizophrenia-like, in epilepsy F06.2
  schizophreniform F20.81
    affective type F25.9
    brief F23
    confusional type F23
    mixed type F25.0
  senile NEC F03 ☑
    depressed or paranoid type F03 ☑
    simple deterioration F03 ☑
    specified type — *code to* condition
  shared F24
  situational (reactive) F23
  symbiotic (childhood) F84.3
  symptomatic F09
Psychosomatic — *see* Disorder, psychosomatic
Psychosyndrome, organic F07.9
Psychotic episode due to or associated with physical
    condition F06.8
Pterygium (eye) H11.00- ☑
  amyloid H11.01- ☑
  central H11.02- ☑
  colli Q18.3
  double H11.03- ☑
  peripheral
    progressive H11.05- ☑
    stationary H11.04- ☑
  recurrent H11.06- ☑
Ptilosis (eyelid) — *see* Madarosis
Ptomaine (poisoning) — *see* Poisoning, food
Ptosis (*see also* Blepharoptosis)
  adiposa (false) — *see* Blepharoptosis
  breast N64.81
  cecum K63.4
  colon K63.4
  congenital (eyelid) Q10.0
    specified site NEC — *see* Anomaly, by site
  eyelid — *see* Blepharoptosis
    congenital Q10.0
  gastric K31.89
  intestine K63.4
  kidney N28.83
  liver K76.89
  renal N28.83
  splanchnic K63.4
  spleen D73.89
  stomach K31.89
  viscera K63.4
PTP D69.51
Ptyalism (periodic) K11.7
  hysterical F45.8
  pregnancy — *see* Pregnancy, complicated by, specified
    pregnancy-related condition NEC
  psychogenic F45.8
Ptyalolithiasis K11.5
Pubarche, precocious E30.1
Pubertas praecox E30.1
Puberty (development state) Z00.3

Puberty — *continued*
  bleeding (excessive) N92.2
  delayed E30.0
  precocious (constitutional) (cryptogenic) (idiopathic)
    E30.1
    central E22.8
    due to
      ovarian hyperfunction E28.1
        estrogen E28.0
      testicular hyperfunction E29.0
    premature E30.1
    due to
      adrenal cortical hyperfunction E25.8
      pineal tumor E34.8
      pituitary (anterior) hyperfunction E22.8
Puckering, macula — *see* Degeneration, macula, puckering
Pudenda, pudendum — *see* condition
Puente's disease (simple glandular cheilitis) K13.0
Puerperal, puerperium (complicated by, complications)
  abnormal glucose (tolerance test) O99.815
  abscess
    areola O91.02
      associated with lactation O91.03
    Bartholin's gland O86.19
    breast O91.12
      associated with lactation O91.13
    cervix (uteri) O86.11
    genital organ NEC O86.19
    kidney O86.21
    mammary O91.12
      associated with lactation O91.13
    nipple O91.02
      associated with lactation O91.03
    peritoneum O85
    subareolar O91.12
      associated with lactation O91.13
    urinary tract — *see* Puerperal, infection, urinary
    uterus O86.12
    vagina (wall) O86.13
    vaginorectal O86.13
    vulvovaginal gland O86.13
  adnexitis O86.19
  afibrinogenemia, or other coagulation defect O72.3
  albuminuria (acute) (subacute) — *see* Proteinuria,
    gestational
  alcohol use O99.315
  anemia O99.81
    pre-existing (pre-pregnancy) O99.03
  anesthetic death O89.8
  apoplexy O99.43
  bariatric surgery status O99.845
  blood disorder NEC O99.13
  blood dyscrasia O72.3
  cardiomyopathy O90.3
  cerebrovascular disorder (conditions in I60-I69) O99.43
  cervicitis O86.11
  circulatory system disorder O99.43
  coagulopathy (any) O99.13
    with hemorrhage O72.3
  complications O90.9
    specified NEC O90.89
  convulsions — *see* Eclampsia
  cystitis O86.22
  cystopyelitis O86.29
  delirium NEC F05
  diabetes O24.93
    gestational — *see* Puerperal, gestational diabetes
    pre-existing O24.33
      specified NEC O24.83
      type 1 O24.03
      type 2 O24.13
  digestive system disorder O99.63
  disease O90.9
    breast NEC O92.29
    cerebrovascular (acute) O99.43
    nonobstetric NEC O99.89
    tubo-ovarian O86.19
    Valsuani's O99.03
  disorder O90.9
    biliary tract O26.63
    lactation O92.70
    liver O26.63
    nonobstetric NEC O99.89
  disruption
    cesarean wound O90.0
    episiotomy wound O90.1
    perineal laceration wound O90.1

Index

Puerperal, puerperium — Puncture

Puerperal, puerperium — *continued*
  drug use O99.325
  eclampsia (with pre-existing hypertension) O15.2
  embolism (pulmonary) (blood clot) — *see* Embolism, obstetric, puerperal
  endocrine, nutritional or metabolic disease NEC O99.285
  endophlebitis — *see* Puerperal, phlebitis
  endotrachelitis O86.11
  failure
    lactation (complete) O92.3
      partial O92.4
    renal, acute O90.4
  fever (of unknown origin) O86.4
    septic O85
  fissure, nipple O92.12
    associated with lactation O92.13
  fistula
    breast (due to mastitis) O91.12
      associated with lactation O91.13
    nipple O91.02
      associated with lactation O91.03
  galactophoritis O91.22
    associated with lactation O91.23
  galactorrhea O92.6
  gastric banding status O99.845
  gastric bypass status O99.845
  gastrointestinal disease NEC O99.63
  gestational
    diabetes O24.439
      diet controlled O24.430
      insulin (and diet) controlled O24.434
      oral drug controlled (antidiabetic) (hypoglycemic) O24.435
    edema O12.05
      with proteinuria O12.25
    proteinuria O12.15
  gonorrhea O98.23
  hematoma, subdural O99.43
  hemiplegia, cerebral O99.355
    due to cerbrovascular disorder O99.43
  hemorrhage O72.1
    brain O99.43
    bulbar O99.43
    cerebellar O99.43
    cerebral O99.43
    cortical O99.43
    delayed or secondary O72.2
    extradural O99.43
    internal capsule O99.43
    intracranial O99.43
    intrapontine O99.43
    meningeal O99.43
    pontine O99.43
    retained placenta O72.0
    subarachnoid O99.43
    subcortical O99.43
    subdural O99.43
    third stage O72.0
    uterine, delayed O72.2
    ventricular O99.43
  hemorrhoids O87.2
  hepatorenal syndrome O90.4
  hypertension — *see* Hypertension, complicating, puerperium
  hypertrophy, breast O92.29
  induration breast (fibrous) O92.29
  infection O86.4
    cervix O86.11
    generalized O85
    genital tract NEC O86.19
      obstetric surgical wound O86.0
    kidney (bacillus coli) O86.21
    maternal O98.93
      carrier state NEC O99.835
      gonorrhea O98.23
      human immunodeficiency virus (HIV) O98.73
      protozoal O98.63
      sexually transmitted NEC O98.33
      specified NEC O98.83
      streptococcus group B (GBS) carrier state O99.825
      syphilis O98.13
      tuberculosis O98.03
      viral hepatitis O98.43
      viral NEC O98.53
    nipple O91.02
      associated with lactation O91.03
    peritoneum O85

Puerperal, puerperium — *continued*
  infection — *continued*
    renal O86.21
    specified NEC O86.89
    urinary (asymptomatic) (tract) NEC O86.20
      bladder O86.22
      kidney O86.21
      specified site NEC O86.29
      urethra O86.22
    vagina O86.13
    vein — *see* Puerperal, phlebitis
  ischemia, cerebral O99.43
  lymphangitis O86.89
    breast O91.22
      associated with lactation O91.23
  malignancy O9A.13 (*following* O99)
  malnutrition O25.3
  mammillitis O91.02
    associated with lactation O91.03
  mammitis O91.22
    associated with lactation O91.23
  mania F30.8
  mastitis O91.22
    associated with lactation O91.23
    purulent O91.12
      associated with lactation O91.13
  melancholia — *see* Disorder, depressive
  mental disorder NEC O99.345
  metroperitonitis O85
  metrorrhagia — *see* Hemorrhage, postpartum
  metrosalpingitis O86.19
  metrovaginitis O86.13
  milk leg O87.1
  monoplegia, cerebral O99.43
  mood disturbance O90.6
  necrosis, liver (acute) (subacute) (conditions in subcategory K72.0) O26.63
    with renal failure O90.4
  nervous system disorder O99.355
  obesity (pre-existing prior to pregnancy) O99.215
  obesity surgery status O99.845
  occlusion, precerebral artery O99.43
  paralysis
    bladder (sphincter) O90.89
    cerebral O99.43
  paralytic stroke O99.43
  parametritis O85
  paravaginitis O86.13
  pelviperitonitis O85
  perimetritis O86.12
  perimetrosalpingitis O86.19
  perinephritis O86.21
  periphlebitis — *see* Puerperal phlebitis
  peritoneal infection O85
  peritonitis (pelvic) O85
  perivaginitis O86.13
  phlebitis O87.0
    deep O87.1
    pelvic O87.1
    superficial O87.0
  phlebothrombosis, deep O87.1
  phlegmasia alba dolens O87.1
  placental polyp O90.89
  pneumonia, embolic — *see* Embolism, obstetric, puerperal
  pre-eclampsia — *see* Pre-eclampsia
  psychosis F53
  pyelitis O86.21
  pyelocystitis O86.29
  pyelonephritis O86.21
  pyelonephrosis O86.21
  pyemia O85
  pyocystitis O86.29
  pyohemia O85
  pyometra O86.12
  pyonephritis O86.21
  pyosalpingitis O86.19
  pyrexia (of unknown origin) O86.4
  renal
    disease NEC O90.89
    failure O90.4
  respiratory disease NEC O99.53
  retention
    decidua — *see* Retention, decidua
    placenta O72.0
    secundines — *see* Retention, secundines
  retracted nipple O92.02
  salpingo-ovaritis O86.19

Puerperal, puerperium — *continued*
  salpingoperitonitis O85
  secondary perineal tear O90.1
  sepsis (pelvic) O85
  sepsis O85
  septic thrombophlebitis O86.81
  skin disorder NEC O99.73
  specified condition NEC O99.89
  stroke O99.43
  subinvolution (uterus) O90.89
  subluxation of symphysis (pubis) O26.73
  suppuration — *see* Puerperal, abscess
  tetanus A34
  thelitis O91.02
    associated with lactation O91.03
  thrombocytopenia O72.3
  thrombophlebitis (superficial) O87.0
    deep O87.1
    pelvic O87.1
    septic O86.81
  thrombosis (venous) — *see* Thrombosis, puerperal
  thyroiditis O90.5
  toxemia (eclamptic) (pre-eclamptic) (with convulsions) O15.2
  trauma, non-obstetric O9A.23 (*following* O99)
    caused by abuse (physical) (suspected) O9A.33 (*following* O99)
      confirmed O9A.33 (*following* O99)
      psychological (suspected) O9A.53 (*following* O99)
        confirmed O9A.53 (*following* O99)
      sexual (suspected) O9A.43 (*following* O99)
        confirmed O9A.43 (*following* O99)
  uremia (due to renal failure) O90.4
  urethritis O86.22
  vaginitis O86.13
  varicose veins (legs) O87.4
    vulva or perineum O87.8
  venous O87.9
  vulvitis O86.19
  vulvovaginitis O86.13
  white leg O87.1
Puerperium — *see* Puerperal
Pulmolithiasis J98.4
Pulmonary — *see* condition
Pulpitis (acute) (anachoretic) (chronic) (hyperplastic) (putrescent) (suppurative) (ulcerative) K04.01
  irreversible K04.02
  reversible K04.01
Pulpless tooth K04.99
Pulse
  alternating R00.8
  bigeminal R00.8
  fast R00.0
  feeble, rapid due to shock following injury T79.4 ☑
  rapid R00.0
  weak R09.89
Pulsus alternans or trigeminus R00.8
Punch drunk F07.81
Punctum lacrimale occlusion — *see* Obstruction, lacrimal
Puncture
  abdomen, abdominal
    wall S31.139 ☑
      with
        foreign body S31.149 ☑
        penetration into peritoneal cavity S31.639 ☑
          with foreign body S31.649 ☑
    epigastric region S31.132 ☑
      with
        foreign body S31.142 ☑
        penetration into peritoneal cavity S31.632 ☑
          with foreign body S31.642 ☑
    left
      lower quadrant S31.134 ☑
        with
          foreign body S31.144 ☑
          penetration into peritoneal cavity S31.634 ☑
            with foreign body S31.644 ☑
      upper quadrant S31.131 ☑
        with
          foreign body S31.141 ☑
          penetration into peritoneal cavity S31.631 ☑
            with foreign body S31.641 ☑

☑ Additional Character Required — Refer to the Tabular List for Character Selection   ▽ Subterms under main terms may continue to next column or page

Puncture — *continued*
  abdomen, abdominal — *continued*
    wall — *continued*
      periumbilic region S31.135 ☑
        with
          foreign body S31.145 ☑
          penetration into peritoneal cavity
            S31.635 ☑
            with foreign body S31.645 ☑
      right
        lower quadrant S31.133 ☑
          with
            foreign body S31.143 ☑
            penetration into peritoneal cavity
              S31.633 ☑
              with foreign body S31.643 ☑
        upper quadrant S31.130 ☑
          with
            foreign body S31.140 ☑
            penetration into peritoneal cavity
              S31.630 ☑
              with foreign body S31.640 ☑
  accidental, complicating surgery — *see* Complication,
      accidental puncture or laceration
  alveolar (process) — *see* Puncture, oral cavity
  ankle S91.039 ☑
    with
      foreign body S91.049 ☑
    left S91.032 ☑
      with
        foreign body S91.042 ☑
    right S91.031 ☑
      with
        foreign body S91.041 ☑
  anus S31.833 ☑
    with foreign body S31.834 ☑
  arm (upper) S41.139 ☑
    with foreign body S41.149 ☑
    left S41.132 ☑
      with foreign body S41.142 ☑
    lower — *see* Puncture, forearm
    right S41.131 ☑
      with foreign body S41.141 ☑
  auditory canal (external) (meatus) — *see* Puncture,
      ear
  auricle, ear — *see* Puncture, ear
  axilla — *see* Puncture, arm
  back (*see also* Puncture, thorax, back)
    lower S31.030 ☑
      with
        foreign body S31.040 ☑
          with penetration into retroperitoneal
            space S31.041 ☑
        penetration into retroperitoneal space
          S31.031 ☑
  bladder (traumatic) S37.29 ☑
    nontraumatic N32.89
  breast S21.039 ☑
    with foreign body S21.049 ☑
    left S21.032 ☑
      with foreign body S21.042 ☑
    right S21.031 ☑
      with foreign body S21.041 ☑
  buttock S31.803 ☑
    with foreign body S31.804 ☑
    left S31.823 ☑
      with foreign body S31.824 ☑
    right S31.813 ☑
      with foreign body S31.814 ☑
  by
    device, implant or graft — *see* Complications, by
        site and type, mechanical
    foreign body left accidentally in operative wound
        T81.539 ☑
    instrument (any) during a procedure, accidental
        — *see* Puncture, accidental complicating
        surgery
  calf — *see* Puncture, leg
  canaliculus lacrimalis — *see* Puncture, eyelid
  canthus, eye — *see* Puncture, eyelid
  cervical esophagus S11.23 ☑
    with foreign body S11.24 ☑
  cheek (external) S01.439 ☑
    with foreign body S01.449 ☑
    internal — *see* Puncture, oral cavity
    left S01.432 ☑

Puncture — *continued*
  cheek — *continued*
    left — *continued*
      with foreign body S01.442 ☑
    right S01.431 ☑
      with foreign body S01.441 ☑
  chest wall — *see* Puncture, thorax
  chin — *see* Puncture, head, specified site NEC
  clitoris — *see* Puncture, vulva
  costal region — *see* Puncture, thorax
  digit(s)
    foot — *see* Puncture, toe
    hand — *see* Puncture, finger
  ear (canal) (external) S01.339 ☑
    with foreign body S01.349 ☑
    drum S09.2-
    left S01.332 ☑
      with foreign body S01.342 ☑
    right S01.331 ☑
      with foreign body S01.341 ☑
  elbow S51.039 ☑
    with
      foreign body S51.049 ☑
    left S51.032 ☑
      with
        foreign body S51.042 ☑
    right S51.031 ☑
      with
        foreign body S51.041 ☑
  epididymis — *see* Puncture, testis
  epigastric region — *see* Puncture, abdomen, wall,
      epigastric
  epiglottis S11.83 ☑
    with foreign body S11.84 ☑
  esophagus
    cervical S11.23 ☑
      with foreign body S11.24 ☑
    thoracic S27.818 ☑
  eyeball S05.6-
    with foreign body S05.5-
  eyebrow — *see* Puncture, eyelid
  eyelid S01.13- ☑
    with foreign body S01.14- ☑
    left S01.132 ☑
      with foreign body S01.142 ☑
    right S01.131 ☑
      with foreign body S01.141 ☑
  face NEC — *see* Puncture, head, specified site NEC
  finger(s) S61.239 ☑
    with
      damage to nail S61.339 ☑
        with
          foreign body S61.349 ☑
      foreign body S61.249 ☑
    index S61.238 ☑
      with
        damage to nail S61.338 ☑
          with
            foreign body S61.348 ☑
        foreign body S61.248 ☑
      left S61.231 ☑
        with
          damage to nail S61.331 ☑
            with
              foreign body S61.341 ☑
          foreign body S61.241 ☑
      right S61.230 ☑
        with
          damage to nail S61.330 ☑
            with
              foreign body S61.340 ☑
          foreign body S61.240 ☑
    little S61.238 ☑
      with
        damage to nail S61.338 ☑
          with
            foreign body S61.348 ☑
        foreign body S61.248 ☑
      left S61.237 ☑
        with
          damage to nail S61.337 ☑
            with
              foreign body S61.347 ☑
          foreign body S61.247 ☑
      right S61.236 ☑

Puncture — *continued*
  finger(s) — *continued*
    little — *continued*
      right — *continued*
        with
          damage to nail S61.336 ☑
            with
              foreign body S61.346 ☑
          foreign body S61.246 ☑
    middle S61.238 ☑
      with
        damage to nail S61.338 ☑
          with
            foreign body S61.348 ☑
        foreign body S61.248 ☑
      left S61.233 ☑
        with
          damage to nail S61.333 ☑
            with
              foreign body S61.343 ☑
          foreign body S61.243 ☑
      right S61.232 ☑
        with
          damage to nail S61.332 ☑
            with
              foreign body S61.342 ☑
          foreign body S61.242 ☑
    ring S61.238 ☑
      with
        damage to nail S61.338 ☑
          with
            foreign body S61.348 ☑
        foreign body S61.248 ☑
      left S61.235 ☑
        with
          damage to nail S61.335 ☑
            with
              foreign body S61.345 ☑
          foreign body S61.245 ☑
      right S61.234 ☑
        with
          damage to nail S61.334 ☑
            with
              foreign body S61.344 ☑
          foreign body S61.244 ☑
  flank S31.139 ☑
    with foreign body S31.149 ☑
  foot (except toe(s) alone) S91.339 ☑
    with foreign body S91.349 ☑
    left S91.332 ☑
      with foreign body S91.342 ☑
    right S91.331 ☑
      with foreign body S91.341 ☑
    toe — *see* Puncture, toe
  forearm S51.839 ☑
    with
      foreign body S51.849 ☑
    elbow only — *see* Puncture, elbow
    left S51.832 ☑
      with
        foreign body S51.842 ☑
    right S51.831 ☑
      with
        foreign body S51.841 ☑
  forehead — *see* Puncture, head, specified site NEC
  genital organs, external
    female S31.532 ☑
      with foreign body S31.542 ☑
      vagina — *see* Puncture, vagina
      vulva — *see* Puncture, vulva
    male S31.531 ☑
      with foreign body S31.541 ☑
      penis — *see* Puncture, penis
      scrotum — *see* Puncture, scrotum
      testis — *see* Puncture, testis
  groin — *see* Puncture, abdomen, wall
  gum — *see* Puncture, oral cavity
  hand S61.439 ☑
    with
      foreign body S61.449 ☑
    finger — *see* Puncture, finger
    left S61.432 ☑
      with
        foreign body S61.442 ☑
    right S61.431 ☑

Puncture — *continued*
- hand — *continued*
  - right — *continued*
    - with
      - foreign body S61.441 ☑
    - thumb — *see* Puncture, thumb
- head S01.93 ☑
  - with foreign body S01.94 ☑
  - cheek — *see* Puncture, cheek
  - ear — *see* Puncture, ear
  - eyelid — *see* Puncture, eyelid
  - lip — *see* Puncture, oral cavity
  - nose — *see* Puncture, nose
  - oral cavity — *see* Puncture, oral cavity
  - scalp S01.03 ☑
    - with foreign body S01.04 ☑
  - specified site NEC S01.83 ☑
    - with foreign body S01.84 ☑
  - temporomandibular area — *see* Puncture, cheek
- heart S26.99 ☑
  - with hemopericardium S26.09 ☑
  - without hemopericardium S26.19 ☑
- heel — *see* Puncture, foot
- hip S71.039 ☑
  - with foreign body S71.049 ☑
  - left S71.032 ☑
    - with foreign body S71.042 ☑
  - right S71.031 ☑
    - with foreign body S71.041 ☑
- hymen — *see* Puncture, vagina
- hypochondrium — *see* Puncture, abdomen, wall
- hypogastric region — *see* Puncture, abdomen, wall
- inguinal region — *see* Puncture, abdomen, wall
- instep — *see* Puncture, foot
- internal organs — *see* Injury, by site
- interscapular region — *see* Puncture, thorax, back
- intestine
  - large
    - colon S36.599 ☑
      - ascending S36.590 ☑
      - descending S36.592 ☑
      - sigmoid S36.593 ☑
      - specified site NEC S36.598 ☑
      - transverse S36.591 ☑
    - rectum S36.69 ☑
  - small S36.499 ☑
    - duodenum S36.490 ☑
    - specified site NEC S36.498 ☑
- intra-abdominal organ S36.99 ☑
  - gallbladder S36.128 ☑
  - intestine — *see* Puncture, intestine
  - liver S36.118 ☑
  - pancreas — *see* Puncture, pancreas
  - peritoneum S36.81 ☑
  - specified site NEC S36.898 ☑
  - spleen S36.09 ☑
  - stomach S36.39 ☑
- jaw — *see* Puncture, head, specified site NEC
- knee S81.039 ☑
  - with foreign body S81.049 ☑
  - left S81.032 ☑
    - with foreign body S81.042 ☑
  - right S81.031 ☑
    - with foreign body S81.041 ☑
- labium (majus) (minus) — *see* Puncture, vulva
- lacrimal duct — *see* Puncture, eyelid
- larynx S11.013 ☑
  - with foreign body S11.014 ☑
- leg (lower) S81.839 ☑
  - with foreign body S81.849 ☑
  - foot — *see* Puncture, foot
  - knee — *see* Puncture, knee
  - left S81.832 ☑
    - with foreign body S81.842 ☑
  - right S81.831 ☑
    - with foreign body S81.841 ☑
  - upper — *see* Puncture, thigh
- lip S01.531 ☑
  - with foreign body S01.541 ☑
- loin — *see* Puncture, abdomen, wall
- lower back — *see* Puncture, back, lower
- lumbar region — *see* Puncture, back, lower
- malar region — *see* Puncture, head, specified site NEC
- mammary — *see* Puncture, breast
- mastoid region — *see* Puncture, head, specified site NEC

Puncture — *continued*
- mouth — *see* Puncture, oral cavity
- nail
  - finger — *see* Puncture, finger, with damage to nail
  - toe — *see* Puncture, toe, with damage to nail
- nasal (septum) (sinus) — *see* Puncture, nose
- nasopharynx — *see* Puncture, head, specified site NEC
- neck S11.93 ☑
  - with foreign body S11.94 ☑
  - involving
    - cervical esophagus — *see* Puncture, cervical esophagus
    - larynx — *see* Puncture, larynx
    - pharynx — *see* Puncture, pharynx
    - thyroid gland — *see* Puncture, thyroid gland
    - trachea — *see* Puncture, trachea
  - specified site NEC S11.83 ☑
    - with foreign body S11.84 ☑
- nose (septum) (sinus) S01.23 ☑
  - with foreign body S01.24 ☑
- ocular — *see* Puncture, eyeball
- oral cavity S01.532 ☑
  - with foreign body S01.542 ☑
- orbit S05.4- ☑
- palate — *see* Puncture, oral cavity
- palm — *see* Puncture, hand
- pancreas S36.299 ☑
  - body S36.291 ☑
  - head S36.290 ☑
  - tail S36.292 ☑
- pelvis — *see* Puncture, back, lower
- penis S31.23 ☑
  - with foreign body S31.24 ☑
- perineum
  - female S31.43 ☑
    - with foreign body S31.44 ☑
  - male S31.139 ☑
    - with foreign body S31.149 ☑
- periocular area (with or without lacrimal passages) — *see* Puncture, eyelid
- phalanges
  - finger — *see* Puncture, finger
  - toe — *see* Puncture, toe
- pharynx S11.23 ☑
  - with foreign body S11.24 ☑
- pinna — *see* Puncture, ear
- popliteal space — *see* Puncture, knee
- prepuce — *see* Puncture, penis
- pubic region S31.139 ☑
  - with foreign body S31.149 ☑
- pudendum — *see* Puncture, genital organs, external
- rectovaginal septum — *see* Puncture, vagina
- sacral region — *see* Puncture, back, lower
- sacroiliac region — *see* Puncture, back, lower
- salivary gland — *see* Puncture, oral cavity
- scalp S01.03 ☑
  - with foreign body S01.04 ☑
- scapular region — *see* Puncture, shoulder
- scrotum S31.33 ☑
  - with foreign body S31.34 ☑
- shin — *see* Puncture, leg
- shoulder S41.039 ☑
  - with foreign body S41.049 ☑
  - left S41.032 ☑
    - with foreign body S41.042 ☑
  - right S41.031 ☑
    - with foreign body S41.041 ☑
- spermatic cord — *see* Puncture, testis
- sternal region — *see* Puncture, thorax, front
- submaxillary region — *see* Puncture, head, specified site NEC
- submental region — *see* Puncture, head, specified site NEC
- subungual
  - finger(s) — *see* Puncture, finger, with damage to nail
  - toe — *see* Puncture, toe, with damage to nail
- supraclavicular fossa — *see* Puncture, neck, specified site NEC
- temple, temporal region — *see* Puncture, head, specified site NEC
- temporomandibular area — *see* Puncture, cheek
- testis S31.33 ☑
  - with foreign body S31.34 ☑
- thigh S71.139 ☑
  - with foreign body S71.149 ☑

Puncture — *continued*
- thigh — *continued*
  - left S71.132 ☑
    - with foreign body S71.142 ☑
  - right S71.131 ☑
    - with foreign body S71.141 ☑
- thorax, thoracic (wall) S21.93 ☑
  - with foreign body S21.94 ☑
  - back S21.23- ☑
    - with
      - foreign body S21.24- ☑
        - with penetration S21.44 ☑
      - penetration S21.43 ☑
  - breast — *see* Puncture, breast
  - front S21.13- ☑
    - with
      - foreign body S21.14- ☑
        - with penetration S21.34 ☑
      - penetration S21.33 ☑
- throat — *see* Puncture, neck
- thumb S61.039 ☑
  - with
    - damage to nail S61.139 ☑
      - with
        - foreign body S61.149 ☑
    - foreign body S61.049 ☑
  - left S61.032 ☑
    - with
      - damage to nail S61.132 ☑
        - with
          - foreign body S61.142 ☑
      - foreign body S61.042 ☑
  - right S61.031 ☑
    - with
      - damage to nail S61.131 ☑
        - with
          - foreign body S61.141 ☑
      - foreign body S61.041 ☑
- thyroid gland S11.13 ☑
  - with foreign body S11.14 ☑
- toe(s) S91.139 ☑
  - with
    - damage to nail S91.239 ☑
      - with
        - foreign body S91.249 ☑
    - foreign body S91.149 ☑
  - great S91.133 ☑
    - with
      - damage to nail S91.233 ☑
        - with
          - foreign body S91.243 ☑
      - foreign body S91.143 ☑
    - left S91.132 ☑
      - with
        - damage to nail S91.232 ☑
          - with
            - foreign body S91.242 ☑
        - foreign body S91.142 ☑
    - right S91.131 ☑
      - with
        - damage to nail S91.231 ☑
          - with
            - foreign body S91.241 ☑
        - foreign body S91.141 ☑
  - lesser S91.136 ☑
    - with
      - damage to nail S91.236 ☑
        - with
          - foreign body S91.246 ☑
      - foreign body S91.146 ☑
    - left S91.135 ☑
      - with
        - damage to nail S91.235 ☑
          - with
            - foreign body S91.245 ☑
        - foreign body S91.145 ☑
    - right S91.134 ☑
      - with
        - damage to nail S91.234 ☑
          - with
            - foreign body S91.244 ☑
        - foreign body S91.144 ☑
- tongue — *see* Puncture, oral cavity
- trachea S11.023 ☑
  - with foreign body S11.024 ☑
- tunica vaginalis — *see* Puncture, testis

Puncture — *continued*
　tympanum, tympanic membrane S09.2- ☑
　umbilical region S31.135 ☑
　　with foreign body S31.145 ☑
　uvula — *see* Puncture, oral cavity
　vagina S31.43 ☑
　　with foreign body S31.44 ☑
　vocal cords S11.033 ☑
　　with foreign body S11.034 ☑
　vulva S31.43 ☑
　　with foreign body S31.44 ☑
　wrist S61.539 ☑
　　with
　　　foreign body S61.549 ☑
　　left S61.532 ☑
　　　with
　　　　foreign body S61.542 ☑
　　right S61.531 ☑
　　　with
　　　　foreign body S61.541 ☑
PUO (pyrexia of unknown origin) R50.9
Pupillary membrane (persistent) Q13.89
Pupillotonia — *see* Anomaly, pupil, function, tonic pupil
Purpura D69.2
　abdominal D69.0
　allergic D69.0
　anaphylactoid D69.0
　annularis telangiectodes L81.7
　arthritic D69.0
　autoerythrocyte sensitization D69.2
　autoimmune D69.0
　bacterial D69.0
　Bateman's (senile) D69.2
　capillary fragility (hereditary) (idiopathic) D69.8
　cryoglobulinemic D89.1
　Devil's pinches D69.2
　fibrinolytic — *see* Fibrinolysis
　fulminans, fulminous D65
　gangrenous D65
　hemorrhagic, hemorrhagica D69.3
　　not due to thrombocytopenia D69.0
　Henoch (-Schönlein) (allergic) D69.0
　hypergammaglobulinemic (benign) (Waldenström) D89.0
　idiopathic (thrombocytopenic) D69.3
　　nonthrombocytopenic D69.0
　immune thrombocytopenic D69.3
　infectious D69.0
　malignant D69.0
　neonatorum P54.5
　nervosa D69.0
　newborn P54.5
　nonthrombocytopenic D69.2
　　hemorrhagic D69.0
　　idiopathic D69.0
　nonthrombopenic D69.2
　peliosis rheumatica D69.0
　posttransfusion (post-transfusion) (from (fresh) whole blood or blood products) D69.51
　primary D69.49
　red cell membrane sensitivity D69.2
　rheumatica D69.0
　Schönlein (-Henoch) (allergic) D69.0
　scorbutic E54 [D77]
　senile D69.2
　simplex D69.2
　symptomatica D69.0
　telangiectasia annularis L81.7
　thrombocytopenic D69.49
　　congenital D69.42
　　hemorrhagic D69.3
　　hereditary D69.42
　　idiopathic D69.3
　　immune D69.3
　　neonatal, transitory P61.0
　　thrombotic M31.1
　thrombohemolytic — *see* Fibrinolysis
　thrombolytic — *see* Fibrinolysis
　thrombopenic D69.49
　thrombotic, thrombocytopenic M31.1
　toxic D69.0
　vascular D69.0
　visceral symptoms D69.0
Purpuric spots R23.3
Purulent — *see* condition
Pus
　in
　　stool R19.5

Pus — *continued*
　in — *continued*
　　urine N39.0
　tube (rupture) — *see* Salpingo-oophoritis
Pustular rash L08.0
Pustule (nonmalignant) L08.9
　malignant A22.0
Pustulosis palmaris et plantaris L40.3
Putnam (-Dana) **disease or syndrome** — *see* Degeneration, combined
Putrescent pulp (dental) K04.1
Pyarthritis, pyarthrosis — *see* Arthritis, pyogenic or pyemic
　tuberculous — *see* Tuberculosis, joint
Pyelectasis — *see* Hydronephrosis
Pyelitis (congenital) (uremic) (*see also* Pyelonephritis)
　with
　　calculus — *see* category N20 ☑
　　　with hydronephrosis N13.2
　　　contracted kidney N11.9
　acute N10
　chronic N11.9
　　with calculus — *see* category N20 ☑
　　　with hydronephrosis N13.2
　cystica N28.84
　puerperal (postpartum) O86.21
　tuberculous A18.11
Pyelocystitis — *see* Pyelonephritis
Pyelonephritis (*see also* Nephritis, tubulo-interstitial)
　with
　　calculus — *see* category N20 ☑
　　　with hydronephrosis N13.2
　　　contracted kidney N11.9
　acute N10
　calculus — *see* category N20 ☑
　　with hydronephrosis N13.2
　chronic N11.9
　　with calculus — *see* category N20 ☑
　　　with hydronephrosis N13.2
　　associated with ureteral obstruction or stricture N11.1
　　nonobstructive N11.8
　　　with reflux (vesicoureteral) N11.0
　　obstructive N11.1
　　specified NEC N11.8
　in (due to)
　　brucellosis A23.9 [N16]
　　cryoglobulinemia (mixed) D89.1 [N16]
　　cystinosis E72.04
　　diphtheria A36.84
　　glycogen storage disease E74.09 [N16]
　　leukemia NEC C95.9- ☑ [N16]
　　lymphoma NEC C85.90 [N16]
　　multiple myeloma C90.0- ☑ [N16]
　　obstruction N11.1
　　Salmonella infection A02.25
　　sarcoidosis D86.84
　　sepsis A41.9 [N16]
　　Sjögren's disease M35.04
　　toxoplasmosis B58.83
　　transplant rejection T86.91 [N16]
　　Wilson's disease E83.01 [N16]
　nonobstructive N12
　　with reflux (vesicoureteral) N11.0
　　chronic N11.8
　syphilitic A52.75
Pyelonephrosis (obstructive) N11.1
　chronic N11.9
Pyelophlebitis I80.8
Pyeloureteritis cystica N28.85
Pyemia, pyemic (fever) (infection) (purulent) (*see also* Sepsis)
　joint — *see* Arthritis, pyogenic or pyemic
　liver K75.1
　pneumococcal A40.3
　portal K75.1
　postvaccinal T88.0 ☑
　puerperal, postpartum, childbirth O85
　specified organism NEC A41.89
　tuberculous — *see* Tuberculosis, miliary
Pygopagus Q89.4
Pyknoepilepsy (idiopathic) — *see* Pyknolepsy
Pyknolepsy G40.A09 (*following* G40.3)
　intractable G40.A19 (*following* G40.3)
　　with status epilepticus G40.A11 (*following* G40.3)
　　without status epilepticus G40.A19 (*following* G40.3)
　not intractable G40.A09 (*following* G40.3)

Pyknolepsy — *continued*
　not intractable — *continued*
　　with status epilepticus G40.A01 (*following* G40.3)
　　without status epilepticus G40.A09 (*following* G40.3)
Pylephlebitis K75.1
Pyle's syndrome Q78.5
Pylethrombophlebitis K75.1
Pylethrombosis K75.1
Pyloritis K29.90
　with bleeding K29.91
Pylorospasm (reflex) **NEC** K31.3
　congenital or infantile Q40.0
　neurotic F45.8
　newborn Q40.0
　psychogenic F45.8
Pylorus, pyloric — *see* condition
Pyoarthrosis — *see* Arthritis, pyogenic or pyemic
Pyocele
　mastoid — *see* Mastoiditis, acute
　sinus (accessory) — *see* Sinusitis
　turbinate (bone) J32.9
　urethra (*see also* Urethritis) N34.0
Pyocolpos — *see* Vaginitis
Pyocystitis N30.80
　with hematuria N30.81
Pyoderma, pyodermia L08.0
　gangrenosum L88
　newborn P39.4
　phagedenic L88
　vegetans L08.81
Pyodermatitis L08.0
　vegetans L08.81
Pyogenic — *see* condition
Pyohydronephrosis N13.6
Pyometra, pyometrium, pyometritis — *see* Endometritis
Pyomyositis (tropical) — *see* Myositis, infective
Pyonephritis N12
Pyonephrosis N13.6
　tuberculous A18.11
Pyo-oophoritis — *see* Salpingo-oophoritis
Pyo-ovarium — *see* Salpingo-oophoritis
Pyopericarditis, pyopericardium I30.1
Pyophlebitis — *see* Phlebitis
Pyopneumopericardium I30.1
Pyopneumothorax (infective) J86.9
　with fistula J86.0
　tuberculous NEC A15.6
Pyosalpinx, pyosalpingitis (*see also* Salpingo-oophoritis)
Pyothorax J86.9
　with fistula J86.0
　tuberculous NEC A15.6
Pyoureter N28.89
　tuberculous A18.11
Pyramidopallidonigral syndrome G20
Pyrexia (of unknown origin) R50.9
　atmospheric T67.0 ☑
　during labor NEC O75.2
　heat T67.0 ☑
　newborn P81.9
　　environmentally-induced P81.0
　persistent R50.9
　puerperal O86.4
Pyroglobulinemia NEC E88.09
Pyromania F63.1
Pyrosis R12
Pyuria (bacterial) N39.0

Q

Q fever A78
　with pneumonia A78
Quadricuspid aortic valve Q23.8
Quadrilateral fever A78
Quadriparesis — *see* Quadriplegia
　meaning muscle weakness M62.81
Quadriplegia G82.50
　complete
　　C1-C4 level G82.51
　　C5-C7 level G82.53
　congenital (cerebral) (spinal) G80.8
　　spastic G80.0
　embolic (current episode) I63.4- ☑
　functional R53.2

Quadriplegia — continued
incomplete
C1-C4 level G82.52
C5-C7 level G82.54
thrombotic (current episode) I63.3-
traumatic — code to injury with seventh character S
current episode — see Injury, spinal (cord), cervical
Quadruplet, pregnancy — see Pregnancy, quadruplet
Quarrelsomeness F60.3
Queensland fever A77.3
Quervain's disease M65.4
thyroid E06.1
Queyrat's erythroplasia D07.4
penis D07.4
specified site — see Neoplasm, skin, in situ
unspecified site D07.4
Quincke's disease or edema T78.3 ☑
hereditary D84.1
Quinsy (gangrenous) J36
Quintan fever A79.0
Quintuplet, pregnancy — see Pregnancy, quintuplet

R

Rabbit fever — see Tularemia
Rabies A82.9
contact Z20.3
exposure to Z20.3
inoculation reaction — see Complications, vaccination
sylvatic A82.0
urban A82.1
Rachischisis — see Spina bifida
Rachitic (see also condition)
deformities of spine (late effect) (sequelae) E64.3
pelvis (late effect) (sequelae) E64.3
with disproportion (fetopelvic) O33.0
causing obstructed labor O65.0
Rachitis, rachitism (acute) (tarda) (see also Rickets)
renalis N25.0
sequelae E64.3
Radial nerve — see condition
Radiation
burn — see Burn
effects NOS T66 ☑
sickness NOS T66 ☑
therapy, encounter for Z51.0
Radiculitis (pressure) (vertebrogenic) — see Radiculopathy
Radiculomyelitis (see also Encephalitis)
toxic, due to
Clostridium tetani A35
Corynebacterium diphtheriae A36.82
Radiculopathy M54.10
cervical region M54.12
cervicothoracic region M54.13
due to
disc disorder
C3 M50.11
C4 M50.11
C5 M50.121
C6 M50.122
C7 M50.123
displacement of intervertebral disc — see Disorder, disc, with, radiculopathy
leg M54.1- ☑
lumbar region M54.16
lumbosacral region M54.17
occipito-atlanto-axial region M54.11
postherpetic B02.29
sacrococcygeal region M54.18
syphilitic A52.11
thoracic region (with visceral pain) M54.14
thoracolumbar region M54.15
Radiodermal burns (acute, chronic, or occupational) — see Burn
Radiodermatitis L58.9
acute L58.0
chronic L58.1
Radiotherapy session Z51.0
RAEB (refractory anemia with excess blasts) D46.2- ☑
Rage, meaning rabies — see Rabies
Ragpicker's disease A22.1
Ragsorter's disease A22.1
Raillietiniasis B71.8
Railroad neurosis F48.8
Railway spine F48.8

Raised (see also Elevated)
antibody titer R76.0
Rake teeth, tooth M26.39
Rales R09.89
Ramifying renal pelvis Q63.8
Ramsay-Hunt disease or syndrome (see also Hunt's disease) B02.21
meaning dyssynergia cerebellaris myoclonica G11.1
Ranula K11.6
congenital Q38.4
Rape
adult
confirmed T74.21 ☑
suspected T76.21 ☑
alleged, observation or examination, ruled out
adult Z04.41
child Z04.42
child
confirmed T74.22 ☑
suspected T76.22 ☑
Rapid
feeble pulse, due to shock, following injury T79.4 ☑
heart (beat) R00.0
psychogenic F45.8
second stage (delivery) O62.3
time-zone change syndrome — see Disorder, sleep, circadian rhythm, psychogenic
Rarefaction, bone — see Disorder, bone, density and structure, specified NEC
Rash (toxic) R21
canker A38.9
diaper L22
drug (internal use) L27.0
contact (see also Dermatitis, due to, drugs, external) L25.1
following immunization T88.1 ☑
food — see Dermatitis, due to, food
heat L74.0
napkin (psoriasiform) L22
nettle — see Urticaria
pustular L08.0
rose R21
epidemic B06.9
scarlet A38.9
serum (see also Reaction, serum) T80.69 ☑
wandering tongue K14.1
Rasmussen aneurysm — see Tuberculosis, pulmonary
Rasmussen encephalitis G04.81
Rat-bite fever A25.9
due to Streptobacillus moniliformis A25.1
spirochetal (morsus muris) A25.0
Rathke's pouch tumor D44.3
Raymond (-Céstan) **syndrome** I65.8
Raynaud's disease, phenomenon or syndrome (secondary) I73.00
with gangrene (symmetric) I73.01
RDS (newborn) (type I) P22.0
type II P22.1
Reaction (see also Disorder)
adaptation — see Disorder, adjustment
adjustment (anxiety) (conduct disorder) (depressiveness) (distress) — see Disorder, adjustment
with
mutism, elective (child) (adolescent) F94.0
adverse
food (any) (ingested) NEC T78.1 ☑
anaphylactic — see Shock, anaphylactic, due to food
affective — see Disorder, mood
allergic — see Allergy
anaphylactic — see Shock, anaphylactic
anaphylactoid — see Shock, anaphylactic
anesthesia — see Anesthesia, complication
antitoxin (prophylactic) (therapeutic) — see Complications, vaccination
anxiety F41.1
Arthus — see Arthus' phenomenon
asthenic F48.8
combat and operational stress F43.0
compulsive F42.8
conversion F44.9
crisis, acute F43.0
deoxyribonuclease (DNA) (DNase) hypersensitivity D69.2
depressive (single episode) F32.9
affective (single episode) F31.4
recurrent episode F33.9

Reaction — continued
depressive — continued
neurotic F34.1
psychoneurotic F34.1
psychotic F32.3
recurrent — see Disorder, depressive, recurrent
dissociative F44.9
drug NEC T88.7 ☑
addictive — see Dependence, drug
transmitted via placenta or breast milk — see Absorption, drug, addictive, through placenta
allergic — see Allergy, drug
lichenoid L43.2
newborn P93.8
gray baby syndrome P93.0
overdose or poisoning (by accident) — see Table of Drugs and Chemicals, by drug, poisoning
photoallergic L56.1
phototoxic L56.0
withdrawal — see Dependence, by drug, with, withdrawal
infant of dependent mother P96.1
newborn P96.1
wrong substance given or taken (by accident) — see Table of Drugs and Chemicals, by drug, poisoning
fear F40.9
child (abnormal) F93.8
febrile nonhemolytic transfusion (FNHTR) R50.84
fluid loss, cerebrospinal G97.1
foreign
body NEC — see Granuloma, foreign body
in operative wound (inadvertently left) — see Foreign body, accidentally left during a procedure
substance accidentally left during a procedure (chemical) (powder) (talc) T81.60 ☑
aseptic peritonitis T81.61 ☑
body or object (instrument) (sponge) (swab) — see Foreign body, accidentally left during a procedure
specified reaction NEC T81.69 ☑
grief — see Disorder, adjustment
Herxheimer's R68.89
hyperkinetic — see Hyperkinesia
hypochondriacal F45.20
hypoglycemic, due to insulin E16.0
with coma (diabetic) — see Diabetes, coma
nondiabetic E15
therapeutic misadventure — see subcategory T38.3 ☑
hypomanic F30.8
hysterical F44.9
immunization — see Complications, vaccination
incompatibility
ABO blood group (infusion) (transfusion) — see Complication(s), transfusion, incompatibility reaction, ABO
delayed serologic T80.39 ☑
minor blood group (Duffy) (E) (K(ell)) (Kidd) (Lewis) (M) (N) (P) (S) T80.89 ☑
Rh (factor) (infusion) (transfusion) — see Complication(s), transfusion, incompatibility reaction, Rh (factor)
inflammatory — see Infection
infusion — see Complications, infusion
inoculation (immune serum) — see Complications, vaccination
insulin T38.3- ☑
involutional psychotic — see Disorder, depressive
leukemoid D72.823
basophilic D72.823
lymphocytic D72.823
monocytic D72.823
myelocytic D72.823
neutrophilic D72.823
LSD (acute)
due to drug abuse — see Abuse, drug, hallucinogen
due to drug dependence — see Dependence, drug, hallucinogen
lumbar puncture G97.1
manic-depressive — see Disorder, bipolar
neurasthenic F48.8
neurogenic — see Neurosis
neurotic F48.9
neurotic-depressive F34.1

☑ Additional Character Required — Refer to the Tabular List for Character Selection   ▽ Subterms under main terms may continue to next column or page

Reaction — *continued*
- nitritoid — *see* Crisis, nitritoid
- nonspecific
  - to
    - cell mediated immunity measurement of gamma interferon antigen response without active tuberculosis R76.12
    - QuantiFERON-TB test (QFT) without active tuberculosis R76.12
    - tuberculin test (*see also* Reaction, tuberculin skin test) R76.11
- obsessive-compulsive F42.8
- organic, acute or subacute — *see* Delirium
- paranoid (acute) F23
  - chronic F22
  - senile F03 ☑
- passive dependency F60.7
- phobic F40.9
- post-traumatic stress, uncomplicated Z73.3
- psychogenic F99
- psychoneurotic (*see also* Neurosis)
  - compulsive F42.8
  - depersonalization F48.1
  - depressive F34.1
  - hypochondriacal F45.20
  - neurasthenic F48.8
  - obsessive F42.8
- psychophysiologic — *see* Disorder, somatoform
- psychosomatic — *see* Disorder, somatoform
- psychotic — *see* Psychosis
- scarlet fever toxin — *see* Complications, vaccination
- schizophrenic F23
  - acute (brief) (undifferentiated) F23
  - latent F21
  - undifferentiated (acute) (brief) F23
- serological for syphilis — *see* Serology for syphilis
- serum T80.69 ☑
  - anaphylactic (immediate) (*see also* Shock, anaphylactic) T80.59 ☑
  - specified reaction NEC
    - due to
      - administration of blood and blood products T80.61 ☑
      - immunization T80.62 ☑
      - serum specified NEC T80.69 ☑
      - vaccination T80.62 ☑
- situational — *see* Disorder, adjustment
- somatization — *see* Disorder, somatoform
- spinal puncture G97.1
- stress (severe) F43.9
  - acute (agitation) ("daze") (disorientation) (disturbance of consciousness) (flight reaction) (fugue) F43.0
  - specified NEC F43.8
- surgical procedure — *see* Complications, surgical procedure
- tetanus antitoxin — *see* Complications, vaccination
- toxic, to local anesthesia T88.59 ☑
  - in labor and delivery O74.4
  - in pregnancy O29.3X- ☑
  - postpartum, puerperal O89.3
- toxin-antitoxin — *see* Complications, vaccination
- transfusion (blood) (bone marrow) (lymphocytes) (allergic) — *see* Complications, transfusion
- tuberculin skin test, abnormal R76.11
- vaccination (any) — *see* Complications, vaccination
- withdrawing, child or adolescent F93.8

Reactive airway disease — *see* Asthma
Reactive depression — *see* Reaction, depressive
Rearrangement
- chromosomal
  - balanced (in) Q95.9
    - abnormal individual (autosomal) Q95.2
      - non-sex (autosomal) chromosomes Q95.2
      - sex/non-sex chromosomes Q95.3
    - specified NEC Q95.8
Recalcitrant patient — *see* Noncompliance
Recanalization, thrombus — *see* Thrombosis
Recession, receding
- chamber angle (eye) H21.55- ☑
- chin M26.09
- gingival (postinfective) (postoperative)
  - generalized K06.020
    - minimal K06.021
    - moderate K06.022
    - severe K06.023
  - localized K06.010
    - minimal K06.011

Recession, receding — *continued*
- gingival — *continued*
  - localized — *continued*
    - moderate K06.012
    - severe K06.013
Recklinghausen disease Q85.01
- bones E21.0
Reclus' disease (cystic) — *see* Mastopathy, cystic
Recrudescent typhus (fever) A75.1
Recruitment, auditory H93.21- ☑
Rectalgia K62.89
Rectitis K62.89
Rectocele
- female (without uterine prolapse) N81.6
  - with uterine prolapse N81.4
    - incomplete N81.2
  - in pregnancy — *see* Pregnancy, complicated by, abnormal, pelvic organs or tissues NEC
- male K62.3
Rectosigmoid junction — *see* condition
Rectosigmoiditis K63.89
- ulcerative (chronic) K51.30
  - with
    - complication K51.319
      - abscess K51.314
      - fistula K51.313
      - obstruction K51.312
      - rectal bleeding K51.311
      - specified NEC K51.318
Rectourethral — *see* condition
Rectovaginal — *see* condition
Rectovesical — *see* condition
Rectum, rectal — *see* condition
Recurrent — *see* condition
- pregnancy loss — *see* Loss (of), pregnancy, recurrent
Red bugs B88.0
Red tide (*see also* Table of Drugs and Chemicals) T65.82- ☑
Red-cedar lung or pneumonitis J67.8
Reduced
- mobility Z74.09
- ventilatory or vital capacity R94.2
Redundant, redundancy
- anus (congenital) Q43.8
- clitoris N90.89
- colon (congenital) Q43.8
- foreskin (congenital) N47.8
- intestine (congenital) Q43.8
- labia N90.69
- organ or site, congenital NEC — *see* Accessory
- panniculus (abdominal) E65
- prepuce (congenital) N47.8
- pylorus K31.89
- rectum (congenital) Q43.8
- scrotum N50.89
- sigmoid (congenital) Q43.8
- skin L98.7
  - and subcutaneous tissue L98.7
  - of face L57.4
  - eyelids — *see* Blepharochalasis
- stomach K31.89
Reduplication — *see* Duplication
Reflex R29.2
- hyperactive gag J39.2
- pupillary, abnormal — *see* Anomaly, pupil, function
- vasoconstriction I73.9
- vasovagal R55
Reflux K21.9
- acid K21.9
- esophageal K21.9
  - with esophagitis K21.0
  - newborn P78.83
- gastroesophageal K21.9
  - with esophagitis K21.0
- mitral — *see* Insufficiency, mitral
- ureteral — *see* Reflux, vesicoureteral
- vesicoureteral (with scarring) N13.70
  - with
    - nephropathy N13.729
      - with hydroureter N13.739
        - bilateral N13.732
        - unilateral N13.731
      - without hydroureter N13.729
        - bilateral N13.722
        - unilateral N13.721
    - bilateral N13.722
    - unilateral N13.721
    - pyelonephritis (chronic) N11.0

Reflux — *continued*
- vesicoureteral — *continued*
  - without nephropathy N13.71
  - congenital Q62.7
Reforming, artificial openings — *see* Attention to, artificial, opening
Refractive error — *see* Disorder, refraction
Refsum's disease or syndrome G60.1
Refusal of
- food, psychogenic F50.89
- treatment (because of) Z53.20
  - left against medical advice (AMA) Z53.21
  - patient's decision NEC Z53.29
  - reasons of belief or group pressure Z53.1
Regional — *see* condition
Regurgitation R11.10
- aortic (valve) — *see* Insufficiency, aortic
- food (*see also* Vomiting)
  - with reswallowing — *see* Rumination
  - newborn P92.1
- gastric contents — *see* Vomiting
- heart — *see* Endocarditis
- mitral (valve) — *see* Insufficiency, mitral
  - congenital Q23.3
- myocardial — *see* Endocarditis
- pulmonary (valve) (heart) I37.1
  - congenital Q22.2
  - syphilitic A52.03
- tricuspid — *see* Insufficiency, tricuspid
- valve, valvular — *see* Endocarditis
  - congenital Q24.8
- vesicoureteral — *see* Reflux, vesicoureteral
Reichmann's disease or syndrome K31.89
Reifenstein syndrome E34.52
Reinsertion
- implantable subdermal contraceptive Z30.46
- intrauterine contraceptive device Z30.433
Reiter's disease, syndrome, or urethritis M02.30
- ankle M02.37- ☑
- elbow M02.32- ☑
- foot joint M02.37- ☑
- hand joint M02.34- ☑
- hip M02.35- ☑
- knee M02.36- ☑
- multiple site M02.39
- shoulder M02.31- ☑
- vertebra M02.38
- wrist M02.33- ☑
Rejection
- food, psychogenic F50.89
- transplant T86.91
  - bone T86.830
    - marrow T86.01
  - cornea T86.840
  - heart T86.21
    - with lung(s) T86.31
  - intestine T86.850
  - kidney T86.11
  - liver T86.41
  - lung(s) T86.810
    - with heart T86.31
  - organ (immune or nonimmune cause) T86.91
  - pancreas T86.890
  - skin (allograft) (autograft) T86.820
  - specified NEC T86.890
  - stem cell (peripheral blood) (umbilical cord) T86.5
Relapsing fever A68.9
- Carter's (Asiatic) A68.1
- Dutton's (West African) A68.1
- Koch's A68.9
- louse-borne (epidemic) A68.0
- Novy's (American) A68.1
- Obermeyers's (European) A68.0
- Spirillum A68.9
- tick-borne (endemic) A68.1
Relationship
- occlusal
  - open anterior M26.220
  - open posterior M26.221
Relaxation
- anus (sphincter) K62.89
  - psychogenic F45.8
- arch (foot) (*see also* Deformity, limb, flat foot)
- back ligaments — *see* Instability, joint, spine
- bladder (sphincter) N31.2
- cardioesophageal K21.9
- cervix — *see* Incompetency, cervix
- diaphragm J98.6

Relaxation — *continued*
joint (capsule) (ligament) (paralytic) — *see* Flail, joint
   congenital NEC Q74.8
lumbosacral (joint) — *see* subcategory M53.2 ☑
pelvic floor N81.89
perineum N81.89
posture R29.3
rectum (sphincter) K62.89
sacroiliac (joint) — *see* subcategory M53.2 ☑
scrotum N50.89
urethra (sphincter) N36.44
vesical N31.2
Release from prison, anxiety concerning Z65.2
Remains
canal of Cloquet Q14.0
capsule (opaque) Q14.8
Remittent fever (malarial) B54
Remnant
canal of Cloquet Q14.0
capsule (opaque) Q14.8
cervix, cervical stump (acquired) (postoperative) N88.8
cystic duct, postcholecystectomy K91.5
fingernail L60.8
   congenital Q84.6
meniscus, knee — *see* Derangement, knee, meniscus,
   specified NEC
thyroglossal duct Q89.2
tonsil J35.8
   infected (chronic) J35.01
urachus Q64.4
Removal (from) (of)
artificial
   arm Z44.00- ☑
      complete Z44.01- ☑
      partial Z44.02- ☑
   eye Z44.2- ☑
   leg Z44.10- ☑
      complete Z44.11- ☑
      partial Z44.12- ☑
breast implant Z45.81 ☑
cardiac pulse generator (battery) (end-of-life) Z45.010
catheter (urinary) (indwelling) Z46.6
   from artificial opening — *see* Attention to, artificial,
      opening
   non-vascular Z46.82
   vascular NEC Z45.2
device Z46.9
   contraceptive Z30.432
      implantable subdermal Z30.46
   implanted NEC Z45.89
   specified NEC Z46.89
drains Z48.03
dressing (nonsurgical) Z48.00
   surgical Z48.01
external
   fixation device — *code to* fracture with seventh
      character D
   prosthesis, prosthetic device Z44.9
      breast Z44.3- ☑
      specified NEC Z44.8
home in childhood (to foster home or institution)
   Z62.29
ileostomy Z43.2
insulin pump Z46.81
myringotomy device (stent) (tube) Z45.82
nervous system device NEC Z46.2
   brain neuropacemaker Z46.2
   visual substitution device Z46.2
      implanted Z45.31
non-vascular catheter Z46.82
organ, prophylactic (for neoplasia management) —
   see Prophylactic, organ removal
orthodontic device Z46.4
staples Z48.02
stent
   ureteral Z46.6
suture Z48.02
urinary device Z46.6
vascular access device or catheter Z45.2
Ren
arcuatus Q63.1
mobile, mobilis N28.89
   congenital Q63.8
unguliformis Q63.1
Renal — *see* condition
Rendu-Osler-Weber disease or syndrome I78.0
Reninoma D41.0- ☑
Renon-Delille syndrome E23.3

Reovirus, as cause of disease classified elsewhere
   B97.5
Repeated falls NEC R29.6
Replaced chromosome by dicentric ring Q93.2
Replacement by artificial or mechanical device or
   prosthesis of
bladder Z96.0
blood vessel NEC Z95.828
bone NEC Z96.7
cochlea Z96.21
coronary artery Z95.5
eustachian tube Z96.29
eye globe Z97.0
heart Z95.812
   valve Z95.2
      prosthetic Z95.2
      specified NEC Z95.4
      xenogenic Z95.3
intestine Z96.89
joint Z96.60
   hip — *see* Presence, hip joint implant
   knee — *see* Presence, knee joint implant
   specified site NEC Z96.698
larynx Z96.3
lens Z96.1
limb(s) — *see* Presence, artificial, limb
mandible NEC (for tooth root implant(s)) Z96.5
organ NEC Z96.89
peripheral vessel NEC Z95.828
stapes Z96.29
teeth Z97.2
tendon Z96.7
tissue NEC Z96.89
tooth root(s) Z96.5
vessel NEC Z95.828
   coronary (artery) Z95.5
Request for expert evidence Z04.8
Reserve, decreased or low
cardiac — *see* Disease, heart
kidney N28.89
Residual (*see also* condition)
ovary syndrome N99.83
state, schizophrenic F20.5
urine R39.198
Resistance, resistant (to)
activated protein C D68.51
complicating pregnancy O26.89 ☑
insulin E88.81
organism(s)
   to
      drug Z16.30
         aminoglycosides Z16.29
         amoxicillin Z16.11
         ampicillin Z16.11
         antibiotic(s) Z16.20
            multiple Z16.24
            specified NEC Z16.29
         antifungal Z16.32
         antimicrobial (single) Z16.30
            multiple Z16.35
            specified NEC Z16.39
         antimycobacterial (single) Z16.341
            multiple Z16.342
         antiparasitic Z16.31
         antiviral Z16.33
         beta lactam antibiotics Z16.10
            specified NEC Z16.19
         cephalosporins Z16.19
         extended beta lactamase (ESBL) Z16.12
         fluoroquinolones Z16.23
         macrolides Z16.29
         methicillin — *see* MRSA
         multiple drugs (MDRO)
            antibiotics Z16.24
            antimicrobial Z16.35
            antimycobacterials Z16.342
         penicillins Z16.11
         quinine (and related compounds) Z16.31
         quinolones Z16.23
         sulfonamides Z16.29
         tetracyclines Z16.29
         tuberculostatics (single) Z16.341
            multiple Z16.342
         vancomycin Z16.21
           related antibiotics Z16.22
   thyroid hormone E07.89
Resorption
dental (roots) K03.3

Resorption — *continued*
dental — *continued*
   alveoli M26.79
   teeth (external) (internal) (pathological) (roots) K03.3
Respiration
Cheyne-Stokes R06.3
decreased due to shock, following injury T79.4 ☑
disorder of, psychogenic F45.8
insufficient, or poor R06.89
   newborn P28.5
painful R07.1
sighing, psychogenic F45.8
Respiratory (*see also* condition)
distress syndrome (newborn) (type I) P22.0
   type II P22.1
syncytial virus, as cause of disease classified elsewhere
   B97.4
Respite care Z75.5
Response (drug)
photoallergic L56.1
phototoxic L56.0
Restenosis
stent
   vascular
      end stent
         adjacent to stent — *see* Arteriosclerosis
         within the stent
            coronary T82.855 ☑
            peripheral T82.856 ☑
      in stent
         coronary vessel T82.855 ☑
         peripheral vessel T82.856 ☑
Restless legs (syndrome) G25.81
Restlessness R45.1
Restoration (of)
dental
   aesthetically inadequate or displeasing K08.56
   defective K08.50
      specified NEC K08.59
   failure of marginal integrity K08.51
   failure of periodontal anatomical intergrity K08.54
organ continuity from previous sterilization (tuboplasty) (vasoplasty) Z31.0
   aftercare Z31.42
tooth (existing)
   contours biologically incompatible with oral health
      K08.54
   open margins K08.51
   overhanging K08.52
   poor aesthetic K08.56
   poor gingival margins K08.51
unsatisfactory, of tooth K08.50
   specified NEC K08.59
Restorative material (dental)
allergy to K08.55
fractured K08.539
   with loss of material K08.531
   without loss of material K08.530
unrepairable overhanging of K08.52
Restriction of housing space Z59.1
Rests, ovarian, in fallopian tube Q50.6
Restzustand (schizophrenic) F20.5
Retained (*see also* Retention)
cholelithiasis following cholecystectomy K91.86
foreign body fragments (type of) Z18.9
   acrylics Z18.2
   animal quill(s) or spines Z18.31
   cement Z18.83
   concrete Z18.83
   crystalline Z18.83
   depleted isotope Z18.09
   depleted uranium Z18.01
   diethylhexylphthalates Z18.2
   glass Z18.81
   isocyanate Z18.2
   magnetic metal Z18.11
   metal Z18.10
   nonmagnectic metal Z18.12
   nontherapeutic radioactive Z18.09
   organic NEC Z18.39
   plastic Z18.2
   quill(s) (animal) Z18.31
   radioactive (nontherapeutic) NEC Z18.09
   specified NEC Z18.89
   spine(s) (animal) Z18.31
   stone Z18.83
   tooth (teeth) Z18.32
   wood Z18.33

Retained — *continued*
  fragments (type of) Z18.9
    acrylics Z18.2
    animal quill(s) or spines Z18.31
    cement Z18.83
    concrete Z18.83
    crystalline Z18.83
    depleted isotope Z18.09
    depleted uranium Z18.01
    diethylhexylphthalates Z18.2
    glass Z18.81
    isocyanate Z18.2
    magnetic metal Z18.11
    metal Z18.10
    nonmagnectic metal Z18.12
    nontherapeutic radioactive Z18.09
    organic NEC Z18.39
    plastic Z18.2
    quill(s) (animal) Z18.31
    radioactive (nontherapeutic) NEC Z18.09
    specified NEC Z18.89
    spine(s) (animal) Z18.31
    stone Z18.83
    tooth (teeth) Z18.32
    wood Z18.33
  gallstones, following cholecystectomy K91.86
Retardation
  development, developmental, specific — *see* Disorder, developmental
  endochondral bone growth — *see* Disorder, bone, development or growth
  growth R62.50
    due to malnutrition E45
  mental — *see* Disability, intellectual
  motor function, specific F82
  physical (child) R62.52
    due to malnutrition E45
  reading (specific) F81.0
  spelling (specific) (without reading disorder) F81.81
Retching — *see* Vomiting
Retention (*see also* Retained)
  bladder — *see* Retention, urine
  carbon dioxide E87.2
  cholelithiasis following cholecystectomy K91.86
  cyst — *see* Cyst
  dead
    fetus (at or near term) (mother) O36.4 ☑
      early fetal death O02.1
      ovum O02.0
  decidua (fragments) (following delivery) (with hemorrhage) O72.2
    without hemorrhage O73.1
  deciduous tooth K00.6
  dental root K08.3
  fecal — *see* Constipation
  fetus
    dead O36.4 ☑
      early O02.1
  fluid R60.9
  foreign body (*see also* Foreign body, retained)
    current trauma — *code as* Foreign body, by site or type
  gallstones, following cholecystectomy K91.86
  gastric K31.89
  intrauterine contraceptive device, in pregnancy — *see* Pregnancy, complicated by, retention, intrauterine device
  membranes (complicating delivery) (with hemorrhage) O72.2
    with abortion — *see* Abortion, by type
    without hemorrhage O73.1
  meniscus — *see* Derangement, meniscus
  menses N94.89
  milk (puerperal, postpartum) O92.79
  nitrogen, extrarenal R39.2
  ovary syndrome N99.83
  placenta (total) (with hemorrhage) O72.0
    without hemorrhage O73.0
    portions or fragments (with hemorrhage) O72.2
      without hemorrhage O73.1
  products of conception
    early pregnancy (dead fetus) O02.1
    following
      delivery (with hemorrhage) O72.2
        without hemorrhage O73.1
  secundines (following delivery) (with hemorrhage) O72.0
    without hemorrhage O73.0

Retention — *continued*
  secundines — *continued*
    complicating puerperium (delayed hemorrhage) O72.2
    partial O72.2
      without hemorrhage O73.1
  smegma, clitoris N90.89
  urine R33.9
    drug-induced R33.0
    due to hyperplasia (hypertrophy) of prostate — *see* Hyperplasia, prostate
    organic R33.8
      drug-induced R33.0
    psychogenic F45.8
    specified NEC R33.8
  water (in tissues) — *see* Edema
Reticulation, dust — *see* Pneumoconiosis
Reticulocytosis R70.1
Reticuloendotheliosis
  acute infantile C96.0
  leukemic C91.4- ☑
  nonlipid C96.0
Reticulohistiocytoma (giant-cell) D76.3
Reticuloid, actinic L57.1
Reticulosis (skin)
  acute of infancy C96.0
  hemophagocytic, familial D76.1
  histiocytic medullary C96.A (*following* C96.6)
  lipomelanotic I89.8
  malignant (midline) C86.0
  polymorphic C83.8- ☑
  Sézary — *see* Sézary disease
Retina, retinal (*see also* condition)
  dark area D49.81
Retinitis (*see also* Inflammation, chorioretinal)
  albuminurica N18.9 [H32]
  diabetic — *see* Diabetes, retinitis
  disciformis — *see* Degeneration, macula
  focal — *see* Inflammation, chorioretinal, focal
  gravidarum — *see* Pregnancy, complicated by, specified pregnancy-related condition NEC
  juxtapapillaris — *see* Inflammation, chorioretinal, focal, juxtapapillary
  luetic — *see* Retinitis, syphilitic
  pigmentosa H35.52
  proliferans — *see* Disorder, globe, degenerative, specified type NEC
  proliferating — *see* Disorder, globe, degenerative, specified type NEC
  renal N18.9 [H32]
  syphilitic (early) (secondary) A51.43
    central, recurrent A52.71
    congenital (early) A50.01 [H32]
    late A52.71
  tuberculous A18.53
Retinoblastoma C69.2- ☑
  differentiated C69.2- ☑
  undifferentiated C69.2- ☑
Retinochoroiditis (*see also* Inflammation, chorioretinal)
  disseminated — *see* Inflammation, chorioretinal, disseminated
    syphilitic A52.71
  focal — *see* Inflammation, chorioretinal
  juxtapapillaris — *see* Inflammation, chorioretinal, focal, juxtapapillary
Retinopathy (background) H35.00
  arteriosclerotic I70.8 [H35.0-] ☑
  atherosclerotic I70.8 [H35.0-] ☑
  central serous — *see* Chorioretinopathy, central serous
  Coats H35.02- ☑
  diabetic — *see* Diabetes, retinopathy
  exudative H35.02- ☑
  hypertensive H35.03- ☑
  in (due to)
    diabetes — *see* Diabetes, retinopathy
    sickle-cell disorders D57.- ☑ [H36]
  of prematurity H35.10- ☑
    stage 0 H35.11- ☑
    stage 1 H35.12- ☑
    stage 2 H35.13- ☑
    stage 3 H35.14- ☑
    stage 4 H35.15- ☑
    stage 5 H35.16- ☑
  pigmentary, congenital — *see* Dystrophy, retina
  proliferative NEC H35.2- ☑
    diabetic — *see* Diabetes, retinopathy, proliferative
    sickle-cell D57.- ☑ [H36]

Retinopathy — *continued*
  solar H31.02- ☑
Retinoschisis H33.10- ☑
  congenital Q14.1
  specified type NEC H33.19- ☑
Retortamoniasis A07.8
Retractile testis Q55.22
Retraction
  cervix — *see* Retroversion, uterus
  drum (membrane) — *see* Disorder, tympanic membrane, specified NEC
  finger — *see* Deformity, finger
  lid H02.539
    left H02.536
      lower H02.535
      upper H02.534
    right H02.533
      lower H02.532
      upper H02.531
  lung J98.4
  mediastinum J98.59
  nipple N64.53
    associated with
      lactation O92.03
      pregnancy O92.01- ☑
      puerperium O92.02
    congenital Q83.8
  palmar fascia M72.0
  pleura — *see* Pleurisy
  ring, uterus (Bandl's) (pathological) O62.4
  sternum (congenital) Q76.7
    acquired M95.4
  uterus — *see* Retroversion, uterus
  valve (heart) — *see* Endocarditis
Retrobulbar — *see* condition
Retrocecal — *see* condition
Retrocession — *see* Retroversion
Retrodisplacement — *see* Retroversion
Retroflection, retroflexion — *see* Retroversion
Retrognathia, retrognathism (mandibular) (maxillary) M26.19
Retrograde menstruation N92.5
Retroperineal — *see* condition
Retroperitoneal — *see* condition
Retroperitonitis K68.9
Retropharyngeal — *see* condition
Retroplacental — *see* condition
Retroposition — *see* Retroversion
Retroprosthetic membrane T85.398 ☑
Retrosternal thyroid (congenital) Q89.2
Retroversion, retroverted
  cervix — *see* Retroversion, uterus
  female NEC — *see* Retroversion, uterus
  iris H21.89
  testis (congenital) Q55.29
  uterus (acquired) (acute) (any degree) (asymptomatic) (cervix) (postinfectional) (postpartal, old) N85.4
    congenital Q51.818
    in pregnancy O34.53- ☑
Retrovirus, as cause of disease classified elsewhere B97.30
  human
    immunodeficiency, type 2 (HIV 2) B97.35
    T-cell lymphotropic
      type I (HTLV-I) B97.33
      type II (HTLV-II) B97.34
  lentivirus B97.31
  oncovirus B97.32
  specified NEC B97.39
Retrusion, premaxilla (developmental) M26.09
Rett's disease or syndrome F84.2
Reverse peristalsis R19.2
Reye's syndrome G93.7
Rh (factor)
  hemolytic disease (newborn) P55.5
  incompatibility, immunization or sensitization
    affecting management of pregnancy NEC O36.09- ☑
      anti-D antibody O36.01- ☑
    newborn P55.0
    transfusion reaction — *see* Complication(s), transfusion, incompatibility reaction, Rh (factor)
  negative mother affecting newborn P55.0
  titer elevated — *see* Complication(s), transfusion, incompatibility reaction, Rh (factor)
  transfusion reaction — *see* Complication(s), transfusion, incompatibility reaction, Rh (factor)

▽ Subterms under main terms may continue to next column or page   ☑ Additional Character Required — Refer to the Tabular List for Character Selection   275

Retained — Rh

Index

Rhabdomyolysis (idiopathic) NEC M62.82
traumatic T79.6 ☑
Rhabdomyoma (see also Neoplasm, connective tissue, benign)
adult — see Neoplasm, connective tissue, benign
fetal — see Neoplasm, connective tissue, benign
glycogenic — see Neoplasm, connective tissue, benign
Rhabdomyosarcoma (any type) — see Neoplasm, connective tissue, malignant
Rhabdosarcoma — see Rhabdomyosarcoma
Rhesus (factor) **incompatibility** — see Rh, incompatibility
Rheumatic (acute) (subacute) (chronic)
adherent pericardium I09.2
coronary arteritis I01.9
degeneration, myocardium I09.0
fever (acute) — see Fever, rheumatic
heart — see Disease, heart, rheumatic
myocardial degeneration — see Degeneration, myocardium
myocarditis (chronic) (inactive) (with chorea) I09.0
with chorea (acute) (rheumatic) (Sydenham's) I02.0
active or acute I01.2
pancarditis, acute I01.8
with chorea (acute (rheumatic) Sydenham's) I02.0
pericarditis (active) (acute) (with effusion) (with pneumonia) I01.0
with chorea (acute) (rheumatic) (Sydenham's) I02.0
chronic or inactive I09.2
pneumonia I00 [J17]
torticollis M43.6
typhoid fever A01.09
Rheumatism (articular) (neuralgic) (nonarticular) M79.0
gout — see Arthritis, rheumatoid
intercostal, meaning Tietze's disease M94.0
palindromic (any site) M12.30
ankle M12.37- ☑
elbow M12.32- ☑
foot joint M12.37- ☑
hand joint M12.34- ☑
hip M12.35- ☑
knee M12.36- ☑
multiple site M12.39
shoulder M12.31- ☑
specified joint NEC M12.38
vertebrae M12.38
wrist M12.33- ☑
sciatic M54.4- ☑
Rheumatoid (see also condition)
arthritis (see also Arthritis, rheumatoid)
with involvement of organs NEC M05.60
ankle M05.67- ☑
elbow M05.62- ☑
foot joint M05.67- ☑
hand joint M05.64- ☑
hip M05.65- ☑
knee M05.66- ☑
multiple site M05.69
shoulder M05.61- ☑
vertebra — see Spondylitis, ankylosing
wrist M05.63- ☑
seronegative — see Arthritis, rheumatoid, seronegative
seropositive — see Arthritis, rheumatoid, seropositive
carditis M05.30
ankle M05.37- ☑
elbow M05.32- ☑
foot joint M05.37- ☑
hand joint M05.34- ☑
hip M05.35- ☑
knee M05.36- ☑
multiple site M05.39
shoulder M05.31- ☑
vertebra — see Spondylitis, ankylosing
wrist M05.33- ☑
endocarditis — see Rheumatoid, carditis
lung (disease) M05.10
ankle M05.17- ☑
elbow M05.12- ☑
foot joint M05.17- ☑
hand joint M05.14- ☑
hip M05.15- ☑
knee M05.16- ☑
multiple site M05.19
shoulder M05.11- ☑
vertebra — see Spondylitis, ankylosing

Rheumatoid — continued
lung — continued
wrist M05.13- ☑
myocarditis — see Rheumatoid, carditis
myopathy M05.40
ankle M05.47- ☑
elbow M05.42- ☑
foot joint M05.47- ☑
hand joint M05.44- ☑
hip M05.45- ☑
knee M05.46- ☑
multiple site M05.49
shoulder M05.41- ☑
vertebra — see Spondylitis, ankylosing
wrist M05.43- ☑
pericarditis — see Rheumatoid, carditis
polyarthritis — see Arthritis, rheumatoid
polyneuropathy M05.50
ankle M05.57- ☑
elbow M05.52- ☑
foot joint M05.57- ☑
hand joint M05.54- ☑
hip M05.55- ☑
knee M05.56- ☑
multiple site M05.59
shoulder M05.51- ☑
vertebra — see Spondylitis, ankylosing
wrist M05.53- ☑
vasculitis M05.20
ankle M05.27- ☑
elbow M05.22- ☑
foot joint M05.27- ☑
hand joint M05.24- ☑
hip M05.25- ☑
knee M05.26- ☑
multiple site M05.29
shoulder M05.21- ☑
vertebra — see Spondylitis, ankylosing
wrist M05.23- ☑
Rhinitis (atrophic) (catarrhal) (chronic) (croupous) (fibrinous) (granulomatous) (hyperplastic) (hypertrophic) (membranous) (obstructive) (purulent) (suppurative) (ulcerative) J31.0
with
sore throat — see Nasopharyngitis
acute J00
allergic J30.9
with asthma J45.909
with
exacerbation (acute) J45.901
status asthmaticus J45.902
due to
food J30.5
pollen J30.1
nonseasonal J30.89
perennial J30.89
seasonal NEC J30.2
specified NEC J30.89
infective J00
pneumococcal J00
syphilitic A52.73
congenital A50.05 [J99]
tuberculous A15.8
vasomotor J30.0
Rhinoantritis (chronic) — see Sinusitis, maxillary
Rhinodacryolith — see Dacryolith
Rhinolith (nasal sinus) J34.89
Rhinomegaly J34.89
Rhinopharyngitis (acute) (subacute) (see also Nasopharyngitis)
chronic J31.1
destructive ulcerating A66.5
mutilans A66.5
Rhinophyma L71.1
Rhinorrhea J34.89
cerebrospinal (fluid) G96.0
paroxysmal — see Rhinitis, allergic
spasmodic — see Rhinitis, allergic
Rhinosalpingitis — see Salpingitis, eustachian
Rhinoscleroma A48.8
Rhinosporidiosis B48.1
Rhinovirus infection NEC B34.8
Rhizomelic chondrodysplasia punctata E71.540
Rhythm
atrioventricular nodal I49.8
disorder I49.9
coronary sinus I49.8

Rhythm — continued
disorder — continued
ectopic I49.8
nodal I49.8
escape I49.9
heart, abnormal I49.9
idioventricular I44.2
nodal I49.8
sleep, inversion G47.2- ☑
nonorganic origin — see Disorder, sleep, circadian rhythm, psychogenic
Rhytidosis facialis L98.8
Rib (see also condition)
cervical Q76.5
Riboflavin deficiency E53.0
Rice bodies (see also Loose, body, joint)
knee M23.4- ☑
Richter syndrome — see Leukemia, chronic lymphocytic, B-cell type
Richter's hernia — see Hernia, abdomen, with obstruction
Ricinism — see Poisoning, food, noxious, plant
Rickets (active) (acute) (adolescent) (chest wall) (congenital) (current) (infantile) (intestinal) E55.0
adult — see Osteomalacia
celiac K90.0
hypophosphatemic with nephrotic-glycosuric dwarfism E72.09
inactive E64.3
kidney N25.0
renal N25.0
sequelae, any E64.3
vitamin-D-resistant E83.31 [M90.80]
Rickettsial disease A79.9
specified type NEC A79.89
Rickettsialpox (Rickettsia akari) A79.1
Rickettsiosis A79.9
due to
Ehrlichia sennetsu A79.81
Rickettsia akari (rickettsialpox) A79.1
specified type NEC A79.89
tick-borne A77.9
vesicular A79.1
Rider's bone — see Ossification, muscle, specified NEC
Ridge, alveolus (see also condition)
flabby K06.8
Ridged ear, congenital Q17.3
Riedel's
lobe, liver Q44.7
struma, thyroiditis or disease E06.5
Rieger's anomaly or syndrome Q13.81
Riehl's melanosis L81.4
Rietti-Greppi-Micheli anemia D56.9
Rieux's hernia — see Hernia, abdomen, specified site NEC
Riga (-Fede) **disease** K14.0
Riggs' disease — see Periodontitis
Right aortic arch Q25.47
Right middle lobe syndrome J98.11
Rigid, rigidity (see also condition)
abdominal R19.30
with severe abdominal pain R10.0
epigastric R19.36
generalized R19.37
left lower quadrant R19.34
left upper quadrant R19.32
periumbilic R19.35
right lower quadrant R19.33
right upper quadrant R19.31
articular, multiple, congenital Q68.8
cervix (uteri) in pregnancy — see Pregnancy, complicated by, abnormal, cervix
hymen (acquired) (congenital) N89.6
nuchal R29.1
pelvic floor in pregnancy — see Pregnancy, complicated by, abnormal, pelvic organs or tissues NEC
perineum or vulva in pregnancy — see Pregnancy, complicated by, abnormal, vulva
spine — see Dorsopathy, specified NEC
vagina in pregnancy — see Pregnancy, complicated by, abnormal, vagina
Rigors R68.89
with fever R50.9
Riley-Day syndrome G90.1
RIND (reversible ischemic neurologic deficit) I63.9
Ring(s)
aorta (vascular) Q25.45
Bandl's O62.4

☑ Additional Character Required — Refer to the Tabular List for Character Selection ▽ Subterms under main terms may continue to next column or page

Ring(s) — *continued*
contraction, complicating delivery O62.4
esophageal, lower (muscular) K22.2
Fleischer's (cornea) H18.04- ☑
hymenal, tight (acquired) (congenital) N89.6
Kayser-Fleischer (cornea) H18.04- ☑
retraction, uterus, pathological O62.4
Schatzki's (esophagus) (lower) K22.2
congenital Q39.3
Soemmerring's — *see* Cataract, secondary
vascular (congenital) Q25.8
aorta Q25.45
Ringed hair (congenital) Q84.1
Ringworm B35.9
beard B35.0
black dot B35.0
body B35.4
Burmese B35.5
corporeal B35.4
foot B35.3
groin B35.6
hand B35.2
honeycomb B35.0
nails B35.1
perianal (area) B35.6
scalp B35.0
specified NEC B35.8
Tokelau B35.5
Rise, venous pressure I87.8
Rising, PSA following treatment for malignant neoplasm of prostate R97.21
Risk
for
dental caries Z91.849
high Z91.843
low Z91.841
moderate Z91.842
suicidal
meaning personal history of attempted suicide Z91.5
meaning suicidal ideation — *see* Ideation, suicidal
Ritter's disease L00
Rivalry, sibling Z62.891
Rivalta's disease A42.2
River blindness B73.01
Robert's pelvis Q74.2
with disproportion (fetopelvic) O33.0
causing obstructed labor O65.0
Robin (-Pierre) **syndrome** Q87.0
Robinow-Silvermann-Smith syndrome Q87.1
Robinson's (hidrotic) **ectodermal dysplasia or syndrome** Q82.4
Robles' disease B73.01
Rocky Mountain (spotted) **fever** A77.0
Roetheln — *see* Rubella
Roger's disease Q21.0
Rokitansky-Aschoff sinuses (gallbladder) K82.8
Rolando's fracture (displaced) S62.22- ☑
nondisplaced S62.22- ☑
Romano-Ward (prolonged QT interval) **syndrome** I45.81
Romberg's disease or syndrome G51.8
Roof, mouth — *see* condition
Rosacea L71.9
acne L71.9
keratitis L71.8
specified NEC L71.8
Rosary, rachitic E55.0
Rose
cold J30.1
fever J30.1
rash R21
epidemic B06.9
Rosenbach's erysipeloid A26.0
Rosenthal's disease or syndrome D68.1
Roseola B09
infantum B08.20
due to human herpesvirus 6 B08.21
due to human herpesvirus 7 B08.22
Ross River disease or fever B33.1
Rossbach's disease K31.89
psychogenic F45.8
Rostan's asthma (cardiac) — *see* Failure, ventricular, left
Rotation
anomalous, incomplete or insufficient, intestine Q43.3
cecum (congenital) Q43.3
colon (congenital) Q43.3

Rotation — *continued*
spine, incomplete or insufficient — *see* Dorsopathy, deforming, specified NEC
tooth, teeth, fully erupted M26.35
vertebra, incomplete or insufficient — *see* Dorsopathy, deforming, specified NEC
Rotes Quérol disease or syndrome — *see* Hyperostosis, ankylosing
Roth (-Bernhardt) **disease or syndrome** — *see* Meralgia paraesthetica
Rothmund (-Thomson) **syndrome** Q82.8
Rotor's disease or syndrome E80.6
Round
back (with wedging of vertebrae) — *see* Kyphosis
sequelae (late effect) of rickets E64.3
worms (large) (infestation) NEC B82.0
Ascariasis (*see also* Ascariasis) B77.9
Roussy-Lévy syndrome G60.0
Rubella (German measles) B06.9
complication NEC B06.09
neurological B06.00
congenital P35.0
contact Z20.4
exposure to Z20.4
maternal
care for (suspected) damage to fetus O35.3 ☑
manifest rubella in infant P35.0
suspected damage to fetus affecting management of pregnancy O35.3 ☑
specified complications NEC B06.89
Rubeola (meaning measles) — *see* Measles
meaning rubella — *see* Rubella
Rubeosis, iris — *see* Disorder, iris, vascular
Rubinstein-Taybi syndrome Q87.2
Rudimentary (congenital) (*see also* Agenesis)
arm — *see* Defect, reduction, upper limb
bone Q79.9
cervix uteri Q51.828
eye Q11.2
lobule of ear Q17.3
patella Q74.1
respiratory organs in thoracopagus Q89.4
tracheal bronchus Q32.4
uterus Q51.818
in male Q56.1
vagina Q52.0
Ruled out condition — *see* Observation, suspected
Rumination R11.10
with nausea R11.2
disorder of infancy F98.21
neurotic F42.8
newborn P92.1
obsessional F42.8
psychogenic F42.8
Runeberg's disease D51.0
Runny nose R09.89
Rupia (syphilitic) A51.39
congenital A50.06
tertiary A52.79
Rupture, ruptured
abscess (spontaneous) — *code by* site under Abscess
aneurysm — *see* Aneurysm
anus (sphincter) — *see* Laceration, anus
aorta, aortic I71.8
abdominal I71.3
arch I71.1
ascending I71.1
descending I71.8
abdominal I71.3
thoracic I71.1
syphilitic A52.01
thoracoabdominal I71.5
thorax, thoracic I71.1
transverse I71.1
traumatic — *see* Injury, aorta, laceration, major
valve or cusp (*see also* Endocarditis, aortic) I35.8
appendix (with peritonitis) K35.2
with localized peritonitis K35.3
arteriovenous fistula, brain I60.8
artery I77.2
brain — *see* Hemorrhage, intracranial, intracerebral
coronary — *see* Infarct, myocardium
heart — *see* Infarct, myocardium
pulmonary I28.8
traumatic (complication) — *see* Injury, blood vessel
bile duct (common) (hepatic) K83.2
cystic K82.2

Rupture, ruptured — *continued*
bladder (sphincter) (nontraumatic) (spontaneous) N32.89
following ectopic or molar pregnancy O08.6
obstetrical trauma O71.5
traumatic S37.29 ☑
blood vessel (*see also* Hemorrhage)
brain — *see* Hemorrhage, intracranial, intracerebral
heart — *see* Infarct, myocardium
traumatic (complication) — *see* Injury, blood vessel, laceration, major, by site
bone — *see* Fracture
bowel (nontraumatic) K63.1
brain
aneurysm (congenital) (*see also* Hemorrhage, intracranial, subarachnoid)
syphilitic A52.05
hemorrhagic — *see* Hemorrhage, intracranial, intracerebral
capillaries I78.8
cardiac (auricle) (ventricle) (wall) I23.3
with hemopericardium I23.0
infectional I40.9
traumatic — *see* Injury, heart
cartilage (articular) (current) (*see also* Sprain)
knee S83.3- ☑
semilunar — *see* Tear, meniscus
cecum (with peritonitis) K65.0
with peritoneal abscess K35.3
traumatic S36.598 ☑
celiac artery, traumatic — *see* Injury, blood vessel, celiac artery, laceration, major
cerebral aneurysm (congenital) (*see* Hemorrhage, intracranial, subarachnoid)
cervix (uteri)
with ectopic or molar pregnancy O08.6
following ectopic or molar pregnancy O08.6
obstetrical trauma O71.3
traumatic S37.69 ☑
chordae tendineae NEC I51.1
concurrent with acute myocardial infarction — *see* Infarct, myocardium
following acute myocardial infarction (current complication) I23.4
choroid (direct) (indirect) (traumatic) H31.32- ☑
circle of Willis I60.6
colon (nontraumatic) K63.1
traumatic — *see* Injury, intestine, large
cornea (traumatic) — *see* Injury, eye, laceration
coronary (artery) (thrombotic) — *see* Infarct, myocardium
corpus luteum (infected) (ovary) N83.1- ☑
cyst — *see* Cyst
cystic duct K82.2
Descemet's membrane — *see* Change, corneal membrane, Descemet's, rupture
traumatic — *see* Injury, eye, laceration
diaphragm, traumatic — *see* Injury, intrathoracic, diaphragm
disc — *see* Rupture, intervertebral disc
diverticulum (intestine) K57.80
with bleeding K57.81
bladder N32.3
large intestine K57.20
with
bleeding K57.21
small intestine K57.40
with bleeding K57.41
small intestine K57.00
with
bleeding K57.01
large intestine K57.40
with bleeding K57.41
duodenal stump K31.89
ear drum (nontraumatic) (*see also* Perforation, tympanum)
traumatic S09.2- ☑
due to blast injury — *see* Injury, blast, ear
esophagus K22.3
eye (without prolapse or loss of intraocular tissue) — *see* Injury, eye, laceration
fallopian tube NEC (nonobstetric) (nontraumatic) N83.8
due to pregnancy O00.10- ☑
with intrauterine pregnancy O00.11- ☑
fontanel P13.1
gallbladder K82.2
traumatic S36.128 ☑

Rupture, ruptured — *continued*
gastric (*see also* Rupture, stomach)
  vessel K92.2
globe (eye) (traumatic) — *see* Injury, eye, laceration
graafian follicle (hematoma) N83.0- ☑
heart — *see* Rupture, cardiac
hymen (nontraumatic) (nonintentional) N89.8
internal organ, traumatic — *see* Injury, by site
intervertebral disc — *see* Displacement, intervertebral
  disc
  traumatic — *see* Rupture, traumatic, intervertebral
    disc
intestine NEC (nontraumatic) K63.1
  traumatic — *see* Injury, intestine
iris (*see also* Abnormality, pupillary)
  traumatic — *see* Injury, eye, laceration
joint capsule, traumatic — *see* Sprain
kidney (traumatic) S37.06- ☑
  birth injury P15.8
  nontraumatic N28.89
lacrimal duct (traumatic) — *see* Injury, eye, specified
  site NEC
lens (cataract) (traumatic) — *see* Cataract, traumatic
ligament, traumatic — *see* Rupture, traumatic, ligament, by site
liver S36.116 ☑
  birth injury P15.0
lymphatic vessel I89.8
marginal sinus (placental) (with hemorrhage) — *see*
  Hemorrhage, antepartum, specified cause NEC
membrana tympani (nontraumatic) — *see* Perforation,
  tympanum
membranes (spontaneous)
  artificial
    delayed delivery following O75.5
  delayed delivery following — *see* Pregnancy,
    complicated by, premature rupture of
    membranes
meningeal artery I60.8
meniscus (knee) (*see also* Tear, meniscus)
  old — *see* Derangement, meniscus
  site other than knee — *code as* Sprain
mesenteric artery, traumatic — *see* Injury, mesenteric,
  artery, laceration, major
mesentery (nontraumatic) K66.8
  traumatic — *see* Injury, intra-abdominal, specified,
    site NEC
mitral (valve) I34.8
muscle (traumatic) (*see also* Strain)
  diastasis — *see* Diastasis, muscle
  nontraumatic M62.10
    ankle M62.17- ☑
    foot M62.17- ☑
    forearm M62.13- ☑
    hand M62.14- ☑
    lower leg M62.16- ☑
    pelvic region M62.15- ☑
    shoulder region M62.11- ☑
    specified site NEC M62.18
    thigh M62.15- ☑
    upper arm M62.12- ☑
  traumatic — *see* Strain, by site
musculotendinous junction NEC, nontraumatic — *see*
  Rupture, tendon, spontaneous
mycotic aneurysm causing cerebral hemorrhage —
  see Hemorrhage, intracranial, subarachnoid
myocardium, myocardial — *see* Rupture, cardiac
  traumatic — *see* Injury, heart
nontraumatic, meaning hernia — *see* Hernia
obstructed — *see* Hernia, by site, obstructed
operation wound — *see* Disruption, wound, operation
ovary, ovarian N83.8
  corpus luteum cyst N83.1- ☑
  follicle (graafian) N83.0- ☑
oviduct (nonobstetric) (nontraumatic) N83.8
  due to pregnancy O00.10- ☑
    with intrauterine pregnancy O00.11- ☑
pancreas (nontraumatic) K86.89
  traumatic S36.299 ☑
papillary muscle NEC I51.2
  following acute myocardial infarction (current
    complication) I23.5
pelvic
  floor, complicating delivery O70.1
  organ NEC, obstetrical trauma O71.5
perineum (nonobstetric) (nontraumatic) N90.89

Rupture, ruptured — *continued*
perineum — *continued*
  complicating delivery — *see* Delivery, complicated,
    by, laceration, anus (sphincter)
postoperative wound — *see* Disruption, wound, operation
prostate (traumatic) S37.828 ☑
pulmonary
  artery I28.8
  valve (heart) I37.8
  vein I28.8
  vessel I28.8
pus tube — *see* Salpingitis
pyosalpinx — *see* Salpingitis
rectum (nontraumatic) K63.1
  traumatic S36.69
retina, retinal (traumatic) (without detachment) (*see
  also* Break, retina)
  with detachment — *see* Detachment, retina, with
    retinal, break
rotator cuff (nontraumatic) M75.10- ☑
  complete M75.12- ☑
  incomplete M75.11- ☑
sclera — *see* Injury, eye, laceration
sigmoid (nontraumatic) K63.1
  traumatic S36.593
spinal cord (*see also* Injury, spinal cord, by region)
  due to injury at birth P11.5
  newborn (birth injury) P11.5
spleen (traumatic) S36.09 ☑
  birth injury P15.1
  congenital (birth injury) P15.1
  due to P. vivax malaria B51.0
  nontraumatic D73.5
  spontaneous D73.5
splenic vein R58
  traumatic — *see* Injury, blood vessel, splenic vein
stomach (nontraumatic) (spontaneous) K31.89
  traumatic S36.39
supraspinatus (complete) (incomplete) (nontraumatic)
  — *see* Tear, rotator cuff
symphysis pubis
  obstetric O71.6
  traumatic S33.4 ☑
synovium (cyst) M66.10
  ankle M66.17- ☑
  elbow M66.12- ☑
  finger M66.14- ☑
  foot M66.17- ☑
  forearm M66.13- ☑
  hand M66.14- ☑
  pelvic region M66.15- ☑
  shoulder region M66.11- ☑
  specified site NEC M66.18
  thigh M66.15- ☑
  toe M66.17- ☑
  upper arm M66.12- ☑
  wrist M66.13- ☑
tendon (traumatic) — *see* Strain
  nontraumatic (spontaneous) M66.9
    ankle M66.87- ☑
    extensor M66.20
      ankle M66.27- ☑
      foot M66.27- ☑
      forearm M66.23- ☑
      hand M66.24- ☑
      lower leg M66.26- ☑
      multiple sites M66.29
      pelvic region M66.25- ☑
      shoulder region M66.21- ☑
      specified site NEC M66.28
      thigh M66.25- ☑
      upper arm M66.22- ☑
    flexor M66.30
      ankle M66.37- ☑
      foot M66.37- ☑
      forearm M66.33- ☑
      hand M66.34- ☑
      lower leg M66.36- ☑
      multiple sites M66.39
      pelvic region M66.35- ☑
      shoulder region M66.31- ☑
      specified site NEC M66.38
      thigh M66.35- ☑
      upper arm M66.32- ☑
    foot M66.87- ☑
    forearm M66.83- ☑

Rupture, ruptured — *continued*
tendon — *see* Strain — *continued*
  nontraumatic — *continued*
    hand M66.84- ☑
    lower leg M66.86- ☑
    multiple sites M66.89
    pelvic region M66.85- ☑
    shoulder region M66.81- ☑
    specified
      site NEC M66.88
      tendon M66.80
    thigh M66.85- ☑
    upper arm M66.82- ☑
thoracic duct I89.8
tonsil J35.8
traumatic
  aorta — *see* Injury, aorta, laceration, major
  diaphragm — *see* Injury, intrathoracic, diaphragm
  external site — *see* Wound, open, by site
  eye — *see* Injury, eye, laceration
  internal organ — *see* Injury, by site
  intervertebral disc
    cervical S13.0 ☑
    lumbar S33.0 ☑
    thoracic S23.0 ☑
  kidney S37.06- ☑
  ligament (*see also* Sprain)
    ankle — *see* Sprain, ankle
    carpus — *see* Rupture, traumatic, ligament,
      wrist
    collateral (hand) — *see* Rupture, traumatic,
      ligament, finger, collateral
    finger (metacarpophalangeal) (interphalangeal)
      S63.40- ☑
      collateral S63.41- ☑
        index S63.41- ☑
        little S63.41- ☑
        middle S63.41- ☑
        ring S63.41- ☑
      index S63.40- ☑
      little S63.40- ☑
      middle S63.40- ☑
      palmar S63.42- ☑
        index S63.42- ☑
        little S63.42- ☑
        middle S63.42- ☑
        ring S63.42- ☑
      ring S63.40- ☑
      specified site NEC S63.499 ☑
        index S63.49- ☑
        little S63.49- ☑
        middle S63.49- ☑
        ring S63.49- ☑
      volar plate S63.43- ☑
        index S63.43- ☑
        little S63.43- ☑
        middle S63.43- ☑
        ring S63.43- ☑
    foot — *see* Sprain, foot
    radial collateral S53.2- ☑
    radiocarpal — *see* Rupture, traumatic, ligament,
      wrist, radiocarpal
    ulnar collateral S53.3- ☑
    ulnocarpal — *see* Rupture, traumatic, ligament,
      wrist, ulnocarpal
    wrist S63.30- ☑
      collateral S63.31- ☑
      radiocarpal S63.32- ☑
      specified site NEC S63.39- ☑
      ulnocarpal (palmar) S63.33- ☑
  liver S36.116 ☑
  membrana tympani — *see* Rupture, ear drum,
    traumatic
  muscle or tendon — *see* Strain
  myocardium — *see* Injury, heart
  pancreas S36.299 ☑
  rectum S36.69 ☑
  sigmoid S36.593 ☑
  spleen S36.09 ☑
  stomach S36.39 ☑
  symphysis pubis S33.4 ☑
  tympanum, tympanic (membrane) — *see* Rupture,
    ear drum, traumatic
  ureter S37.19 ☑
  uterus S37.69 ☑
  vagina — *see* Injury, vagina

☑ **Additional Character Required** — **Refer to the Tabular List for Character Selection**   ▽ **Subterms under main terms may continue to next column or page**

Rupture, ruptured — *continued*
  traumatic — *continued*
    vena cava — *see* Injury, vena cava, laceration, major
    tricuspid (heart) (valve) I07.8
    tube, tubal (nonobstetric) (nontraumatic) N83.8
      abscess — *see* Salpingitis
      due to pregnancy O00.10- ☑
        with intrauterine pregnancy O00.11- ☑
    tympanum, tympanic (membrane) (nontraumatic) (*see also* Perforation, tympanic membrane) H72.9- ☑
      traumatic — *see* Rupture, ear drum, traumatic
    umbilical cord, complicating delivery O69.89 ☑
    ureter (traumatic) S37.19 ☑
      nontraumatic N28.89
    urethra (nontraumatic) N36.8
      with ectopic or molar pregnancy O08.6
      following ectopic or molar pregnancy O08.6
      obstetrical trauma O71.5
      traumatic S37.39 ☑
    uterosacral ligament (nonobstetric) (nontraumatic) N83.8
    uterus (traumatic) S37.69 ☑
      before labor O71.0- ☑
      during or after labor O71.1
      nonpuerperal, nontraumatic N85.8
      pregnant (during labor) O71.1
        before labor O71.0- ☑
    vagina — *see* Injury, vagina
    valve, valvular (heart) — *see* Endocarditis
    varicose vein — *see* Varix
    varix — *see* Varix
    vena cava R58
      traumatic — *see* Injury, vena cava, laceration, major
    vesical (urinary) N32.89
    vessel (blood) R58
      pulmonary I28.8
      traumatic — *see* Injury, blood vessel
    viscus R19.8
    vulva complicating delivery O70.0
Russell-Silver syndrome Q87.1
Russian spring-summer type encephalitis A84.0
Rust's disease (tuberculous cervical spondylitis) A18.01
Ruvalcaba-Myhre-Smith syndrome E71.440
Rytand-Lipsitch syndrome I44.2

S

Saber, sabre shin or tibia (syphilitic) A50.56 [M90.8-] ☑
Sac lacrimal — *see* condition
Saccharomyces infection B37.9
Saccharopinuria E72.3
Saccular — *see* condition
Sacculation
  aorta (nonsyphilitic) — *see* Aneurysm, aorta
  bladder N32.3
  intralaryngeal (congenital) (ventricular) Q31.3
  larynx (congenital) (ventricular) Q31.3
  organ or site, congenital — *see* Distortion
  pregnant uterus — *see* Pregnancy, complicated by, abnormal, uterus
  ureter N28.89
  urethra N36.1
  vesical N32.3
Sachs' amaurotic familial idiocy or disease E75.02
Sachs-Tay disease E75.02
Sacks-Libman disease M32.11
Sacralgia M53.3
Sacralization Q76.49
Sacrodynia M53.3
Sacroiliac joint — *see* condition
Sacroiliitis NEC M46.1
Sacrum — *see* condition
Saddle
  back — *see* Lordosis
  embolus
    abdominal aorta I74.01
    pulmonary artery I26.92
      with acute cor pulmonale I26.02
  injury — *code to* condition
  nose M95.0
    due to syphilis A50.57
Sadism (sexual) F65.52
Sadness, postpartal O90.6
Sadomasochism F65.50
Saemisch's ulcer (cornea) — *see* Ulcer, cornea, central

Sagging
  skin and subcutaneous tissue (following bariatric surgery weight loss) (following dietary weight loss) L98.7
Sahib disease B55.0
Sailors' skin L57.8
Saint
  Anthony's fire — *see* Erysipelas
  triad — *see* Hernia, diaphragm
  Vitus' dance — *see* Chorea, Sydenham's
Salaam
  attack(s) — *see* Epilepsy, spasms
  tic R25.8
Salicylism
  abuse F55.8
  overdose or wrong substance given — *see* Table of Drugs and Chemicals, by drug, poisoning
Salivary duct or gland — *see* condition
Salivation, excessive K11.7
Salmonella — *see* Infection, Salmonella
Salmonellosis A02.0
Salpingitis (catarrhal) (fallopian tube) (nodular) (pseudofollicular) (purulent) (septic) N70.91
  with oophoritis N70.93
  acute N70.01
    with oophoritis N70.03
  chlamydial A56.11
  chronic N70.11
    with oophoritis N70.13
  complicating abortion — *see* Abortion, by type, complicated by, salpingitis
  ear — *see* Salpingitis, eustachian
  eustachian (tube) H68.00- ☑
    acute H68.01- ☑
    chronic H68.02- ☑
  follicularis N70.11
    with oophoritis N70.13
  gonococcal (acute) (chronic) A54.24
  interstitial, chronic N70.11
    with oophoritis N70.13
  isthmica nodosa N70.11
    with oophoritis N70.13
  specific (gonococcal) (acute) (chronic) A54.24
  tuberculous (acute) (chronic) A18.17
  venereal (gonococcal) (acute) (chronic) A54.24
Salpingocele N83.4- ☑
Salpingo-oophoritis (catarrhal) (purulent) (ruptured) (septic) (suppurative) N70.93
  acute N70.03
    with ectopic or molar pregnancy O08.0
    following ectopic or molar pregnancy O08.0
    gonococcal A54.24
  chronic N70.13
  following ectopic or molar pregnancy O08.0
  gonococcal (acute) (chronic) A54.24
  puerperal O86.19
  specific (gonococcal) (acute) (chronic) A54.24
  subacute N70.03
  tuberculous (acute) (chronic) A18.17
  venereal (gonococcal) (acute) (chronic) A54.24
Salpingo-ovaritis — *see* Salpingo-oophoritis
Salpingoperitonitis — *see* Salpingo-oophoritis
Salzmann's nodular dystrophy — *see* Degeneration, cornea, nodular
Sampson's cyst or tumor N80.1
San Joaquin (Valley) **fever** B38.0
Sandblaster's asthma, lung or pneumoconiosis J62.8
Sander's disease (paranoia) F22
Sandfly fever A93.1
Sandhoff's disease E75.01
Sanfilippo (Type B) (Type C) (Type D) **syndrome** E76.22
Sanger-Brown ataxia G11.2
Sao Paulo fever or typhus A77.0
Saponification, mesenteric K65.8
Sarcocele (benign)
  syphilitic A52.76
    congenital A50.59
Sarcocystosis A07.8
Sarcoepiplocele — *see* Hernia
Sarcoepiplomphalocele Q79.2
Sarcoid (*see also* Sarcoidosis)
  arthropathy D86.86
  Boeck's D86.9
  Darier-Roussy D86.3
  iridocyclitis D86.83
  meningitis D86.81
  myocarditis D86.85

Sarcoid — *continued*
  myositis D86.87
  pyelonephritis D86.84
  Spiegler-Fendt L08.89
Sarcoidosis D86.9
  with
    cranial nerve palsies D86.82
    hepatic granuloma D86.89
    polyarthritis D86.86
    tubulo-interstitial nephropathy D86.84
  combined sites NEC D86.89
  lung D86.0
    and lymph nodes D86.2
  lymph nodes D86.1
    and lung D86.2
  meninges D86.81
  skin D86.3
  specified type NEC D86.89
Sarcoma (of) (*see also* Neoplasm, connective tissue, malignant)
  alveolar soft part — *see* Neoplasm, connective tissue, malignant
  ameloblastic C41.1
    upper jaw (bone) C41.0
  botryoid — *see* Neoplasm, connective tissue, malignant
  botryoides — *see* Neoplasm, connective tissue, malignant
  cerebellar C71.6
    circumscribed (arachnoidal) C71.6
  circumscribed (arachnoidal) cerebellar C71.6
  clear cell (*see also* Neoplasm, connective tissue, malignant)
    kidney C64.- ☑
  dendritic cells (accessory cells) C96.4
  embryonal — *see* Neoplasm, connective tissue, malignant
  endometrial (stromal) C54.1
    isthmus C54.0
  epithelioid (cell) — *see* Neoplasm, connective tissue, malignant
  Ewing's — *see* Neoplasm, bone, malignant
  follicular dendritic cell C96.4
  germinoblastic (diffuse) — *see* Lymphoma, diffuse large cell
    follicular — *see* Lymphoma, follicular, specified NEC
  giant cell (except of bone) (*see also* Neoplasm, connective tissue, malignant)
    bone — *see* Neoplasm, bone, malignant
  glomoid — *see* Neoplasm, connective tissue, malignant
  granulocytic C92.3- ☑
  hemangioendothelial — *see* Neoplasm, connective tissue, malignant
  hemorrhagic, multiple — *see* Sarcoma, Kaposi's
  histiocytic C96.A (*following* C96.6)
  Hodgkin — *see* Lymphoma, Hodgkin
  immunoblastic (diffuse) — *see* Lymphoma, diffuse large cell
  interdigitating dendritic cell C96.4
  Kaposi's
    colon C46.4
    connective tissue C46.1
    gastrointestinal organ C46.4
    lung C46.5- ☑
    lymph node(s) C46.3
    palate (hard) (soft) C46.2
    rectum C46.4
    skin C46.0
    specified site NEC C46.7
    stomach C46.4
    unspecified site C46.9
  Kupffer cell C22.3
  Langerhans cell C96.4
  leptomeningeal — *see* Neoplasm, meninges, malignant
  liver NEC C22.4
  lymphangioendothelial — *see* Neoplasm, connective tissue, malignant
  lymphoblastic — *see* Lymphoma, lymphoblastic (diffuse)
  lymphocytic — *see* Lymphoma, small cell B-cell
  mast cell C96.22
  melanotic — *see* Melanoma
  meningeal — *see* Neoplasm, meninges, malignant
  meningothelial — *see* Neoplasm, meninges, malignant

☟ Subterms under main terms may continue to next column or page   ☑ Additional Character Required — Refer to the Tabular List for Character Selection   279

Rupture, ruptured — Sarcoma

Sarcoma — *continued*
  mesenchymal (*see also* Neoplasm, connective tissue, malignant)
    mixed — *see* Neoplasm, connective tissue, malignant
  mesothelial — *see* Mesothelioma
  monstrocellular
    specified site — *see* Neoplasm, malignant, by site
    unspecified site C71.9
  myeloid C92.3- ☑
  neurogenic — *see* Neoplasm, nerve, malignant
  odontogenic C41.1
    upper jaw (bone) C41.0
  osteoblastic — *see* Neoplasm, bone, malignant
  osteogenic (*see also* Neoplasm, bone, malignant)
    juxtacortical — *see* Neoplasm, bone, malignant
    periosteal — *see* Neoplasm, bone, malignant
  periosteal (*see also* Neoplasm, bone, malignant)
    osteogenic — *see* Neoplasm, bone, malignant
  pleomorphic cell — *see* Neoplasm, connective tissue, malignant
  reticulum cell (diffuse) — *see* Lymphoma, diffuse large cell
    nodular — *see* Lymphoma, follicular
    pleomorphic cell type — *see* Lymphoma, diffuse large cell
  rhabdoid — *see* Neoplasm, malignant, by site
  round cell — *see* Neoplasm, connective tissue, malignant
  small cell — *see* Neoplasm, connective tissue, malignant
  soft tissue — *see* Neoplasm, connective tissue, malignant
  spindle cell — *see* Neoplasm, connective tissue, malignant
  stromal (endometrial) C54.1
    isthmus C54.0
  synovial (*see also* Neoplasm, connective tissue, malignant)
    biphasic — *see* Neoplasm, connective tissue, malignant
    epithelioid cell — *see* Neoplasm, connective tissue, malignant
    spindle cell — *see* Neoplasm, connective tissue, malignant
Sarcomatosis
  meningeal — *see* Neoplasm, meninges, malignant
  specified site NEC — *see* Neoplasm, connective tissue, malignant
  unspecified site C80.1
Sarcopenia (age-related) M62.84
Sarcosinemia E72.59
Sarcosporidiosis (intestinal) A07.8
Satiety, early R68.81
Saturnine — *see* condition
Saturnism
  overdose or wrong substance given or taken — *see* Table of Drugs and Chemicals, by drug, poisoning
Satyriasis F52.8
Sauriasis — *see* Ichthyosis
SBE (subacute bacterial endocarditis) I33.0
Scabies (any site) B86
Scabs R23.4
Scaglietti-Dagnini syndrome E22.0
Scald — *see* Burn
Scalenus anticus (anterior) **syndrome** G54.0
Scales R23.4
Scaling, skin R23.4
Scalp — *see* condition
Scapegoating affecting child Z62.3
Scaphocephaly Q75.0
Scapulalgia M89.8X1
Scapulohumeral myopathy G71.0
Scar, scarring (*see also* Cicatrix) L90.5
  adherent L90.5
  atrophic L90.5
  cervix
    in pregnancy or childbirth — *see* Pregnancy, complicated by, abnormal cervix
  cheloid L91.0
  chorioretinal H31.00- ☑
    posterior pole macula H31.01- ☑
    postsurgical H59.81-
    solar retinopathy H31.02- ☑
    specified type NEC H31.09- ☑
  choroid — *see* Scar, chorioretinal

Scar, scarring — *continued*
  conjunctiva H11.24- ☑
  cornea H17.9
    xerophthalmic (*see also* Opacity, cornea)
      vitamin A deficiency E50.6
  duodenum, obstructive K31.5
  hypertrophic L91.0
  keloid L91.0
  labia N90.89
  lung (base) J98.4
  macula — *see* Scar, chorioretinal, posterior pole
  muscle M62.89
  myocardium, myocardial I25.2
  painful L90.5
  posterior pole (eye) — *see* Scar, chorioretinal, posterior pole
  retina — *see* Scar, chorioretinal
  trachea J39.8
  transmural uterine, in pregnancy O34.29
  uterus N85.8
    in pregnancy O34.29
  vagina N89.8
    postoperative N99.2
  vulva N90.89
Scarabiasis B88.2
Scarlatina (anginosa) (maligna) A38.9
  myocarditis (acute) A38.1
    old — *see* Myocarditis
  otitis media A38.0
  ulcerosa A38.8
Scarlet fever (albuminuria) (angina) A38.9
Schamberg's disease (progressive pigmentary dermatosis) L81.7
Schatzki's ring (acquired) (esophagus) (lower) K22.2
  congenital Q39.3
Schaufenster krankheit I20.8
Schaumann's
  benign lymphogranulomatosis D86.1
  disease or syndrome — *see* Sarcoidosis
Scheie's syndrome E76.03
Schenck's disease B42.1
Scheuermann's disease or osteochondrosis — *see* Osteochondrosis, juvenile, spine
Schilder (-Flatau) **disease** G37.0
Schilling-type monocytic leukemia C93.0- ☑
Schimmelbusch's disease, cystic mastitis, or hyperplasia — *see* Mastopathy, cystic
Schistosoma infestation — *see* Infestation, Schistosoma
Schistosomiasis B65.9
  with muscle disorder B65.9 [M63.80]
    ankle B65.9 [M63.87-] ☑
    foot B65.9 [M63.87-] ☑
    forearm B65.9 [M63.83-] ☑
    hand B65.9 [M63.84-] ☑
    lower leg B65.9 [M63.86-] ☑
    multiple sites B65.9 [M63.89]
    pelvic region B65.9 [M63.85-] ☑
    shoulder region B65.9 [M63.81-] ☑
    specified site NEC B65.9 [M63.88]
    thigh B65.9 [M63.85-] ☑
    upper arm B65.9 [M63.82-] ☑
  Asiatic B65.2
  bladder B65.0
  chestermani B65.8
  colon B65.1
  cutaneous B65.3
  due to
    S. haematobium B65.0
    S. japonicum B65.2
    S. mansoni B65.1
    S. mattheii B65.8
  Eastern B65.2
  genitourinary tract B65.0
  intestinal B65.1
  lung NEC B65.9 [J99]
    pneumonia B65.9 [J17]
  Manson's (intestinal) B65.1
  oriental B65.2
  pulmonary NEC B65.9 [J99]
    pneumonia B65.9
  Schistosoma
    haematobium B65.0
    japonicum B65.2
    mansoni B65.1
  specified type NEC B65.8
  urinary B65.0
  vesical B65.0
Schizencephaly Q04.6

Schizoaffective psychosis F25.9
Schizodontia K00.2
Schizoid personality F60.1
Schizophrenia, schizophrenic F20.9
  acute (brief) (undifferentiated) F23
  atypical (form) F20.3
  borderline F21
  catalepsy F20.2
  catatonic (type) (excited) (withdrawn) F20.2
  cenesthopathic, cenesthesiopathic F20.89
  childhood type F84.5
  chronic undifferentiated F20.5
  cyclic F25.0
  disorganized (type) F20.1
  flexibilitas cerea F20.2
  hebephrenic (type) F20.1
  incipient F21
  latent F21
  negative type F20.5
  paranoid (type) F20.0
  paraphrenic F20.0
  post-psychotic depression F32.89
  prepsychotic F21
  prodromal F21
  pseudoneurotic F21
  pseudopsychopathic F21
  reaction F23
  residual (state) (type) F20.5
  restzustand F20.5
  schizoaffective (type) — *see* Psychosis, schizoaffective
  simple (type) F20.89
  simplex F20.89
  specified type NEC F20.89
  spectrum and other psychotic disorder F29
    specified NEC F28
  stupor F20.2
  syndrome of childhood F84.5
  undifferentiated (type) F20.3
    chronic F20.5
Schizothymia (persistent) F60.1
Schlatter-Osgood disease or osteochondrosis — *see* Osteochondrosis, juvenile, tibia
Schlatter's tibia — *see* Osteochondrosis, juvenile, tibia
Schmidt's syndrome (polyglandular, autoimmune) E31.0
Schmincke's carcinoma or tumor — *see* Neoplasm, nasopharynx, malignant
Schmitz (-Stutzer) **dysentery** A03.0
Schmorl's disease or nodes
  lumbar region M51.46
  lumbosacral region M51.47
  sacrococcygeal region M53.3
  thoracic region M51.44
  thoracolumbar region M51.45
Schneiderian
  papilloma — *see* Neoplasm, nasopharynx, benign
    specified site — *see* Neoplasm, benign, by site
    unspecified site D14.0
  specified site — *see* Neoplasm, malignant, by site
    unspecified site C30.0
Scholte's syndrome (malignant carcinoid) E34.0
Scholz (-Bielchowsky-Henneberg) **disease or syndrome** E75.25
Schönlein (-Henoch) disease or purpura (primary) (rheumatic) D69.0
Schottmuller's disease A01.4
Schroeder's syndrome (endocrine hypertensive) E27.0
Schüller-Christian disease or syndrome C96.5
Schultze's type acroparesthesia, simple I73.89
Schultz's disease or syndrome — *see* Agranulocytosis
Schwalbe-Ziehen-Oppenheim disease G24.1
Schwannoma (*see also* Neoplasm, nerve, benign)
  malignant (*see also* Neoplasm, nerve, malignant)
    with rhabdomyoblastic differentiation — *see* Neoplasm, nerve, malignant
  melanocytic — *see* Neoplasm, nerve, benign
  pigmented — *see* Neoplasm, nerve, benign
Schwannomatosis Q85.03
Schwartz (-Jampel) **syndrome** G71.13
Schwartz-Bartter syndrome E22.2
Schweniger-Buzzi anetoderma L90.1
Sciatic — *see* condition
Sciatica (infective)
  with lumbago M54.4- ☑
    due to intervertebral disc disorder — *see* Disorder, disc, with, radiculopathy
  due to displacement of intervertebral disc (with lumbago) — *see* Disorder, disc, with, radiculopathy

Sciatica — *continued*
  wallet M54.3- ☑
Scimitar syndrome Q26.8
Sclera — *see* condition
Sclerectasia H15.84- ☑
Scleredema
  adultorum — *see* Sclerosis, systemic
  Buschke's — *see* Sclerosis, systemic
  newborn P83.0
Sclerema (adiposum) (edematosum) (neonatorum)
    (newborn) P83.0
  adultorum — *see* Sclerosis, systemic
Scleriasis — *see* Scleroderma
Scleritis H15.00- ☑
  with corneal involvement H15.04- ☑
  anterior H15.01- ☑
  brawny H15.02- ☑
  in (due to) zoster B02.34
  posterior H15.03- ☑
  specified type NEC H15.09- ☑
  syphilitic A52.71
  tuberculous (nodular) A18.51
Sclerochoroiditis H31.8
Scleroconjunctivitis — *see* Scleritis
Sclerocystic ovary syndrome E28.2
Sclerodactyly, sclerodactylia L94.3
Scleroderma, sclerodermia (acrosclerotic) (diffuse)
    (generalized) (progressive) (pulmonary) (*see also*
    Sclerosis, systemic) M34.9
  circumscribed L94.0
  linear L94.1
  localized L94.0
  newborn P83.88
  systemic M34.9
Sclerokeratitis H16.8
  tuberculous A18.52
Scleroma nasi A48.8
Scleromalacia (perforans) H15.05- ☑
Scleromyxedema L98.5
Sclérose en plaques G35
Sclerosis, sclerotic
  adrenal (gland) E27.8
  Alzheimer's — *see* Disease, Alzheimer's
  amyotrophic (lateral) G12.21
  aorta, aortic I70.0
    valve — *see* Endocarditis, aortic
  artery, arterial, arteriolar, arteriovascular — *see* Arteriosclerosis
  ascending multiple G35
  brain (generalized) (lobular) G37.9
    artery, arterial I67.2
    diffuse G37.0
    disseminated G35
    insular G35
    Krabbe's E75.23
    miliary G35
    multiple G35
    presenile (Alzheimer's) — *see* Disease, Alzheimer's,
      early onset
    senile (arteriosclerotic) I67.2
    stem, multiple G35
    tuberous Q85.1
  bulbar, multiple G35
  bundle of His I44.39
  cardiac — *see* Disease, heart, ischemic, atherosclerotic
  cardiorenal — *see* Hypertension, cardiorenal
  cardiovascular (*see also* Disease, cardiovascular)
    renal — *see* Hypertension, cardiorenal
  cerebellar — *see* Sclerosis, brain
  cerebral — *see* Sclerosis, brain
  cerebrospinal (disseminated) (multiple) G35
  cerebrovascular I67.2
  choroid — *see* Degeneration, choroid
  combined (spinal cord) (*see also* Degeneration, combined)
    multiple G35
  concentric (Balo) G37.5
  cornea — *see* Opacity, cornea
  coronary (artery) I25.10
    with angina pectoris — *see* Arteriosclerosis, coronary (artery),
  corpus cavernosum
    female N90.89
    male N48.6
  diffuse (brain) (spinal cord) G37.0
  disseminated G35
  dorsal G35

Sclerosis, sclerotic — *continued*
  dorsolateral (spinal cord) — *see* Degeneration, combined
  endometrium N85.5
  extrapyramidal G25.9
  eye, nuclear (senile) — *see* Cataract, senile, nuclear
  focal and segmental (glomerular) (*see also* N00-N07
    with fourth character .1) N05.1
  Friedreich's (spinal cord) G11.1
  funicular (spermatic cord) N50.89
  general (vascular) — *see* Arteriosclerosis
  gland (lymphatic) I89.8
  hepatic K74.1
    alcoholic K70.2
  hereditary
    cerebellar G11.9
    spinal (Friedreich's ataxia) G11.1
  hippocampal G93.81
  insular G35
  kidney — *see* Sclerosis, renal
  larynx J38.7
  lateral (amyotrophic) (descending) (spinal) G12.21
    primary G12.23
  lens, senile nuclear — *see* Cataract, senile, nuclear
  liver K74.1
    with fibrosis K74.2
      alcoholic K70.2
    alcoholic K70.2
    cardiac K76.1
  lung — *see* Fibrosis, lung
  mastoid — *see* Mastoiditis, chronic
  mesial temporal G93.81
  mitral I05.8
  Mönckeberg's (medial) — *see* Arteriosclerosis, extremities
  multiple (brain stem) (cerebral) (generalized) (spinal
    cord) G35
  myocardium, myocardial — *see* Disease, heart, ischemic, atherosclerotic
  nuclear (senile), eye — *see* Cataract, senile, nuclear
  ovary N83.8
  pancreas K86.89
  penis N48.6
  peripheral arteries — *see* Arteriosclerosis, extremities
  plaques G35
  pluriglandular E31.8
  polyglandular E31.8
  posterolateral (spinal cord) — *see* Degeneration, combined
  presenile (Alzheimer's) — *see* Disease, Alzheimer's, early onset
  primary, lateral G12.23
  progressive, systemic M34.0
  pulmonary — *see* Fibrosis, lung
    artery I27.0
    valve (heart) — *see* Endocarditis, pulmonary
  renal N26.9
    with
      cystine storage disease E72.09
      hypertensive heart disease (conditions in I11)
        — *see* Hypertension, cardiorenal
      arteriolar (hyaline) (hyperplastic) — *see* Hypertension, kidney
  retina (senile) (vascular) H35.00
  senile (vascular) — *see* Arteriosclerosis
  spinal (cord) (progressive) G95.89
    ascending G61.0
    combined (*see also* Degeneration, combined)
      multiple G35
      syphilitic A52.11
    disseminated G35
    dorsolateral — *see* Degeneration, combined
    hereditary (Friedreich's) (mixed form) G11.1
    lateral (amyotrophic) G12.23
    multiple G35
    posterior (syphilitic) A52.11
  stomach K31.89
  subendocardial, congenital I42.4
  systemic M34.9
    with
      lung involvement M34.81
      myopathy M34.82
      polyneuropathy M34.83
    drug-induced M34.2
    due to chemicals NEC M34.2
    progressive M34.0
    specified NEC M34.89
  temporal (mesial) G93.81

Sclerosis, sclerotic — *continued*
  tricuspid (heart) (valve) I07.8
  tuberous (brain) Q85.1
  tympanic membrane — *see* Disorder, tympanic
    membrane, specified NEC
  valve, valvular (heart) — *see* Endocarditis
  vascular — *see* Arteriosclerosis
  vein I87.8
Scoliosis (acquired) (postural) M41.9
  adolescent (idiopathic) — *see* Scoliosis, idiopathic,
    adolescent
  congenital Q67.5
    due to bony malformation Q76.3
    failure of segmentation (hemivertebra) Q76.3
    hemivertebra fusion Q76.3
    postural Q67.5
  idiopathic M41.20
    adolescent M41.129
      cervical region M41.122
      cervicothoracic region M41.123
      lumbar region M41.126
      lumbosacral region M41.127
      thoracic region M41.124
      thoracolumbar region M41.125
    cervical region M41.22
    cervicothoracic region M41.23
    infantile M41.00
      cervical region M41.02
      cervicothoracic region M41.03
      lumbar region M41.06
      lumbosacral region M41.07
      sacrococcygeal region M41.08
      thoracic region M41.04
      thoracolumbar region M41.05
    juvenile M41.119
      cervical region M41.112
      cervicothoracic region M41.113
      lumbar region M41.116
      lumbosacral region M41.117
      thoracic region M41.114
      thoracolumbar region M41.115
    lumbar region M41.26
    lumbosacral region M41.27
    thoracic region M41.24
    thoracolumbar region M41.25
  infantile — *see* Scoliosis, idiopathic, infantile
  neuromuscular M41.40
    cervical region M41.42
    cervicothoracic region M41.43
    lumbar region M41.46
    lumbosacral region M41.47
    occipito-atlanto-axial region M41.41
    thoracic region M41.44
    thoracolumbar region M41.45
  paralytic — *see* Scoliosis, neuromuscular
  postradiation therapy M96.5
  rachitic (late effect or sequelae) E64.3 [M49.80]
    cervical region E64.3 [M49.82]
    cervicothoracic region E64.3 [M49.83]
    lumbar region E64.3 [M49.86]
    lumbosacral region E64.3 [M49.87]
    multiple sites E64.3 [M49.89]
    occipito-atlanto-axial region E64.3 [M49.81]
    sacrococcygeal region E64.3 [M49.88]
    thoracic region E64.3 [M49.84]
    thoracolumbar region E64.3 [M49.85]
  sciatic M54.4- ☑
  secondary (to) NEC M41.50
    cerebral palsy, Friedreich's ataxia, poliomyelitis,
      neuromuscular disorders — *see* Scoliosis,
      neuromuscular
    cervical region M41.52
    cervicothoracic region M41.53
    lumbar region M41.56
    lumbosacral region M41.57
    thoracic region M41.54
    thoracolumbar region M41.55
  specified form NEC M41.80
    cervical region M41.82
    cervicothoracic region M41.83
    lumbar region M41.86
    lumbosacral region M41.87
    thoracic region M41.84
    thoracolumbar region M41.85
  thoracogenic M41.30
    thoracic region M41.34
    thoracolumbar region M41.35
  tuberculous A18.01

Index

Sciatica — Scoliosis

Scoliotic pelvis
with disproportion (fetopelvic) O33.0
causing obstructed labor O65.0
Scorbutus, scorbutic (see also Scurvy)
anemia D53.2
Score, NIHSS (National Institutes of Health Stroke Scale)
R29.7- ☑
Scotoma (arcuate) (Bjerrum) (central) (ring) (see also
Defect, visual field, localized, scotoma)
scintillating H53.19
Scratch — see Abrasion
Scratchy throat R09.89
Screening (for) Z13.9
alcoholism Z13.89
anemia Z13.0
anomaly, congenital Z13.89
antenatal, of mother (see also Encounter, antenatal
screening) Z36.9
arterial hypertension Z13.6
arthropod-borne viral disease NEC Z11.59
bacteriuria, asymptomatic Z13.89
behavioral disorder Z13.89
brain injury, traumatic Z13.850
bronchitis, chronic Z13.83
brucellosis Z11.2
cardiovascular disorder Z13.6
cataract Z13.5
chlamydial diseases Z11.8
cholera Z11.0
chromosomal abnormalities (nonprocreative) NEC
Z13.79
colonoscopy Z12.11
congenital
dislocation of hip Z13.89
eye disorder Z13.5
malformation or deformation Z13.89
contamination NEC Z13.88
cystic fibrosis Z13.228
dengue fever Z11.59
dental disorder Z13.84
depression Z13.89
developmental handicap Z13.4
in early childhood Z13.4
infant Z13.4
diabetes mellitus Z13.1
diphtheria Z11.2
disability, intellectual Z13.4
infant Z13.4
disease or disorder Z13.9
bacterial NEC Z11.2
intestinal infectious Z11.0
respiratory tuberculosis Z11.1
blood or blood-forming organ Z13.0
cardiovascular Z13.6
Chagas' Z11.6
chlamydial Z11.8
dental Z13.89
developmental Z13.4
in child Z13.4
infant Z13.4
digestive tract NEC Z13.818
lower GI Z13.811
upper GI Z13.810
ear Z13.5
endocrine Z13.29
eye Z13.5
genitourinary Z13.89
heart Z13.6
human immunodeficiency virus (HIV) infection
Z11.4
immunity Z13.0
infection
intestinal Z11.0
specified NEC Z11.6
infectious Z11.9
mental Z13.89
metabolic Z13.228
neurological Z13.89
nutritional Z13.21
metabolic Z13.228
lipoid disorders Z13.220
protozoal Z11.6
intestinal Z11.0
respiratory Z13.83
rheumatic Z13.828
rickettsial Z11.8
sexually-transmitted NEC Z11.3
human immunodeficiency virus (HIV) Z11.4

Screening — continued
disease or disorder — continued
sickle-cell (trait) Z13.0
skin Z13.89
specified NEC Z13.89
spirochetal Z11.8
thyroid Z13.29
vascular Z13.6
venereal Z11.3
viral NEC Z11.59
human immunodeficiency virus (HIV) Z11.4
intestinal Z11.0
elevated titer Z13.89
emphysema Z13.83
encephalitis, viral (mosquito- or tick-borne) Z11.59
exposure to contaminants (toxic) Z13.88
fever
dengue Z11.59
hemorrhagic Z11.59
yellow Z11.59
filariasis Z11.6
galactosemia Z13.228
gastrointestinal condition Z13.818
genetic (nonprocreative) - for procreative management — see Testing, genetic, for procreative
management
disease carrier status (nonprocreative) Z13.71
specified NEC (nonprocreative) Z13.79
genitourinary condition Z13.89
glaucoma Z13.5
gonorrhea Z11.3
gout Z13.89
helminthiasis (intestinal) Z11.6
hematopoietic malignancy Z12.89
hemoglobinopathies NEC Z13.0
hemorrhagic fever Z11.59
Hodgkin disease Z12.89
human immunodeficiency virus (HIV) Z11.4
human papillomavirus Z11.51
hypertension Z13.6
immunity disorders Z13.0
infection
mycotic Z11.8
parasitic Z11.8
ingestion of radioactive substance Z13.88
intellectual disability Z13.4
infant Z13.4
intestinal
helminthiasis Z11.6
infectious disease Z11.0
leishmaniasis Z11.6
leprosy Z11.2
leptospirosis Z11.8
leukemia Z12.89
lymphoma Z12.89
malaria Z11.6
malnutrition Z13.29
metabolic Z13.228
nutritional Z13.21
measles Z11.59
mental disorder Z13.89
metabolic errors, inborn Z13.228
multiphasic Z13.89
musculoskeletal disorder Z13.828
osteoporosis Z13.820
mycoses Z11.8
myocardial infarction (acute) Z13.6
neoplasm (malignant) (of) Z12.9
bladder Z12.6
blood Z12.89
breast Z12.39
routine mammogram Z12.31
cervix Z12.4
colon Z12.11
genitourinary organs NEC Z12.79
bladder Z12.6
cervix Z12.4
ovary Z12.73
prostate Z12.5
testis Z12.71
vagina Z12.72
hematopoietic system Z12.89
intestinal tract Z12.10
colon Z12.11
rectum Z12.12
small intestine Z12.13
lung Z12.2
lymph (glands) Z12.89
nervous system Z12.82

Screening — continued
neoplasm — continued
oral cavity Z12.81
prostate Z12.5
rectum Z12.12
respiratory organs Z12.2
skin Z12.83
small intestine Z12.13
specified site NEC Z12.89
stomach Z12.0
nephropathy Z13.89
nervous system disorders NEC Z13.858
neurological condition Z13.89
osteoporosis Z13.820
parasitic infestation Z11.9
specified NEC Z11.8
phenylketonuria Z13.228
plague Z11.2
poisoning (chemical) (heavy metal) Z13.88
poliomyelitis Z11.59
postnatal, chromosomal abnormalities Z13.89
prenatal, of mother (see also Encounter, antenatal
screening) Z36.9
protozoal disease Z11.6
intestinal Z11.0
pulmonary tuberculosis Z11.1
radiation exposure Z13.88
respiratory condition Z13.83
respiratory tuberculosis Z11.1
rheumatoid arthritis Z13.828
rubella Z11.59
schistosomiasis Z11.6
sexually-transmitted disease NEC Z11.3
human immunodeficiency virus (HIV) Z11.4
sickle-cell disease or trait Z13.0
skin condition Z13.89
sleeping sickness Z11.6
special Z13.9
specified NEC Z13.89
syphilis Z11.3
tetanus Z11.2
trachoma Z11.8
traumatic brain injury Z13.850
trypanosomiasis Z11.6
tuberculosis, respiratory Z11.1
venereal disease Z11.3
viral encephalitis (mosquito- or tick-borne) Z11.59
whooping cough Z11.2
worms, intestinal Z11.6
yaws Z11.8
yellow fever Z11.59
Scrofula, scrofulosis (tuberculosis of cervical lymph
glands) A18.2
Scrofulide (primary) (tuberculous) A18.4
Scrofuloderma, scrofulodermia (any site) (primary)
A18.4
Scrofulosus lichen (primary) (tuberculous) A18.4
Scrofulous — see condition
Scrotal tongue K14.5
Scrotum — see condition
Scurvy, scorbutic E54
anemia D53.2
gum E54
infantile E54
rickets E55.0 [M90.80]
Sealpox B08.62
Seasickness T75.3 ☑
Seatworm (infection) (infestation) B80
Sebaceous (see also condition)
cyst — see Cyst, sebaceous
Seborrhea, seborrheic L21.9
capillitii R23.8
capitis L21.0
dermatitis L21.9
infantile L21.1
eczema L21.9
infantile L21.1
sicca L21.0
Seckel's syndrome Q87.1
Seclusion, pupil — see Membrane, pupillary
Second hand tobacco smoke exposure (acute)
(chronic) Z77.22
in the perinatal period P96.81
Secondary
dentin (in pulp) K04.3
neoplasm, secondaries — see Table of Neoplasms,
secondary

☑ Additional Character Required — Refer to the Tabular List for Character Selection   ▽ Subterms under main terms may continue to next column or page

Secretion
- antidiuretic hormone, inappropriate E22.2
- catecholamine, by pheochromocytoma E27.5
- hormone
  - antidiuretic, inappropriate (syndrome) E22.2
  - by
    - carcinoid tumor E34.0
    - pheochromocytoma E27.5
  - ectopic NEC E34.2
- urinary
  - excessive R35.8
  - suppression R34

Section
- nerve, traumatic — see Injury, nerve

Sedative, hypnotic, or anxiolytic-induced
- anxiety disorder F13.980
- bipolar and related disorder F13.94
- delirium F13.921
- depressive disorder F13.94
- major neurocognitive disorder F13.97
- mild neurocognitive disorder F13.988
- psychotic disorder F13.959
- sexual dysfunction F13.981
- sleep disorder F13.982

Segmentation, incomplete (congenital) (see also Fusion)
- bone NEC Q78.8
- lumbosacral (joint) (vertebra) Q76.49

Seitelberger's syndrome (infantile neuraxonal dystrophy) G31.89

Seizure(s) (see also Convulsions) R56.9
- akinetic — see Epilepsy, generalized, specified NEC
- atonic — see Epilepsy, generalized, specified NEC
- autonomic (hysterical) F44.5
- convulsive — see Convulsions
- cortical (focal) (motor) — see Epilepsy, localization-related, symptomatic, with simple partial seizures
- disorder (see also Epilepsy) G40.909
- due to stroke — see Sequelae (of), disease, cerebrovascular, by type, specified NEC
- epileptic — see Epilepsy
- febrile (simple) R56.00
  - with status epilepticus G40.901
  - complex (atypical) (complicated) R56.01
    - with status epilepticus G40.901
- grand mal G40.409
  - intractable G40.419
    - with status epilepticus G40.411
    - without status epilepticus G40.419
  - not intractable G40.409
    - with status epilepticus G40.401
    - without status epilepticus G40.409
- heart — see Disease, heart
- hysterical F44.5
- intractable G40.919
  - with status epilepticus G40.911
- Jacksonian (focal) (motor type) (sensory type) — see Epilepsy, localization-related, symptomatic, with simple partial seizures
- newborn P90
- nonspecific epileptic
  - atonic — see Epilepsy, generalized, specified NEC
  - clonic — see Epilepsy, generalized, specified NEC
  - myoclonic — see Epilepsy, generalized, specified NEC
  - tonic — see Epilepsy, generalized, specified NEC
  - tonic-clonic — see Epilepsy, generalized, specified NEC
- partial, developing into secondarily generalized seizures
  - complex — see Epilepsy, localization-related, symptomatic, with complex partial seizures
  - simple — see Epilepsy, localization-related, symptomatic, with simple partial seizures
- petit mal G40.409
  - intractable G40.419
    - with status epilepticus G40.411
    - without status epilepticus G40.419
  - not intractable G40.409
    - with status epilepticus G40.401
    - without status epilepticus G40.409
- post traumatic R56.1
- recurrent G40.909
- specified NEC G40.89
- uncinate — see Epilepsy, localization-related, symptomatic, with complex partial seizures

Selenium deficiency, dietary E59

Self-damaging behavior (life-style) Z72.89
Self-harm (attempted)
- history (personal) Z91.5
  - in family Z81.8
Self-mutilation (attempted)
- history (personal) Z91.5
  - in family Z81.8
Self-poisoning
- history (personal) Z91.5
  - in family Z81.8
- observation following (alleged) attempt Z03.6
Semicoma R40.1
Seminal vesiculitis N49.0
Seminoma C62.9- ☑
- specified site — see Neoplasm, malignant, by site
Senear-Usher disease or syndrome L10.4
Senectus R54
Senescence (without mention of psychosis) R54
Senile, senility (see also condition) R41.81
- with
  - acute confusional state F05
  - mental changes NOS F03 ☑
  - psychosis NEC — see Psychosis, senile
- asthenia R54
- cervix (atrophic) N88.8
- debility R54
- endometrium (atrophic) N85.8
- fallopian tube (atrophic) — see Atrophy, fallopian tube
- heart (failure) R54
- ovary (atrophic) — see Atrophy, ovary
- premature E34.8
- vagina, vaginitis (atrophic) N95.2
- wart L82.1
Sensation
- burning (skin) R20.8
  - tongue K14.6
- loss of R20.8
- prickling (skin) R20.2
- tingling (skin) R20.2
Sense loss
- smell — see Disturbance, sensation, smell
- taste — see Disturbance, sensation, taste
- touch R20.8
Sensibility disturbance (cortical) (deep) (vibratory) R20.9
Sensitive, sensitivity (see also Allergy)
- carotid sinus G90.01
- child (excessive) F93.8
- cold, autoimmune D59.1
- dentin K03.89
- gluten (non-celiac) K90.41
- latex Z91.040
- methemoglobin D74.8
- tuberculin, without clinical or radiological symptoms R76.11
- visual
  - glare H53.71
  - impaired contrast H53.72
Sensitiver Beziehungswahn F22
Sensitization, auto-erythrocytic D69.2
Separation
- anxiety, abnormal (of childhood) F93.0
- apophysis, traumatic — code as Fracture, by site
- choroid — see Detachment, choroid
- epiphysis, epiphyseal
  - nontraumatic (see also Osteochondropathy, specified type NEC)
    - upper femoral — see Slipped, epiphysis, upper femoral
  - traumatic — code as Fracture, by site
- fracture — see Fracture
- infundibulum cardiac from right ventricle by a partition Q24.3
- joint (traumatic) (current) — code by site under Dislocation
- pubic bone, obstetrical trauma O71.6
- retina, retinal — see Detachment, retina
- symphysis pubis, obstetrical trauma O71.6
- tracheal ring, incomplete, congenital Q32.1
Sepsis (generalized) (unspecified organism) A41.9
- with
  - organ dysfunction (acute) (multiple) R65.20
    - with septic shock R65.21
- actinomycotic A42.7
- adrenal hemorrhage syndrome (meningococcal) A39.1
- anaerobic A41.4
- Bacillus anthracis A22.7
- Brucella (see also Brucellosis) A23.9

Sepsis — continued
- candidal B37.7
- cryptogenic A41.9
- due to device, implant or graft T85.79 ☑
  - arterial graft NEC T82.7 ☑
  - breast (implant) T85.79 ☑
  - catheter NEC T85.79 ☑
    - dialysis (renal) T82.7 ☑
      - intraperitoneal T85.71 ☑
    - infusion NEC T82.7 ☑
      - spinal (cranial) (epidural) (intrathecal) (spinal) (subarachnoid) (subdural) T85.735 ☑
    - urethral indwelling T83.511 ☑
    - urinary T83.518 ☑
  - ectopic or molar pregnancy O08.82
  - electronic (electrode) (pulse generator) (stimulator)
    - bone T84.7 ☑
    - cardiac T82.7 ☑
    - nervous system T85.738 ☑
      - brain T85.731 ☑
      - neurostimulator generator T85.734 ☑
      - peripheral nerve T85.732 ☑
      - spinal cord T85.733 ☑
    - urinary T83.590 ☑
  - fixation, internal (orthopedic) — see Complication, fixation device, infection
  - gastrointestinal (bile duct) (esophagus) T85.79 ☑
    - neurostimulator electrode (lead) T85.732 ☑
  - genital T83.69 ☑
  - heart NEC T82.7 ☑
    - valve (prosthesis) T82.6 ☑
      - graft T82.7 ☑
  - joint prosthesis — see Complication, joint prosthesis, infection
  - ocular (corneal graft) (orbital implant) T85.79 ☑
  - orthopedic NEC T84.7 ☑
    - fixation device, internal — see Complication, fixation device, infection
  - specified NEC T85.79 ☑
  - vascular T82.7 ☑
  - ventricular intracranial (communicating) shunt T85.730 ☑
- during labor O75.3
- Enterococcus A41.81
- Erysipelothrix (rhusiopathiae) (erysipeloid) A26.7
- Escherichia coli (E. coli) A41.5 ☑
- extraintestinal yersiniosis A28.2
- following
  - abortion (subsequent episode) O08.0
    - current episode — see Abortion
  - ectopic or molar pregnancy O08.82
  - immunization T88.0 ☑
  - infusion, therapeutic injection or transfusion NEC T80.29 ☑
- gangrenous A41.9
- gonococcal A54.86
- Gram-negative (organism) A41.5 ☑
  - anaerobic A41.4
- Haemophilus influenzae A41.3
- herpesviral B00.7
- intra-abdominal K65.1
- intraocular — see Endophthalmitis, purulent
- Listeria monocytogenes A32.7
- localized — code to specific localized infection
  - in operation wound T81.4 ☑
  - skin — see Abscess
- malleus A24.0
- melioidosis A24.1
- meningeal — see Meningitis
- meningococcal A39.4
  - acute A39.2
  - chronic A39.3
- MSSA (Methicillin susceptible Staphylococcus aureus) A41.01
- newborn P36.9
  - due to
    - anaerobes NEC P36.5
    - Escherichia coli P36.4
    - Staphylococcus P36.30
      - aureus P36.2
      - specified NEC P36.39
    - Streptococcus P36.10
      - group B P36.0
      - specified NEC P36.19
  - specified NEC P36.8
- Pasteurella multocida A28.0

Sepsis — continued
- pelvic, puerperal, postpartum, childbirth O85
- pneumococcal A40.3
- postprocedural T81.4 ☑
- puerperal, postpartum, childbirth (pelvic) O85
- Salmonella (arizonae) (cholerae-suis) (enteritidis) (ty-phimurium) A02.1
- severe R65.20
  - with septic shock R65.21
- Shigella (see also Dysentery, bacillary) A03.9
- skin, localized — see Abscess
- specified organism NEC A41.89
- Staphylococcus, staphylococcal A41.2
  - aureus (methicillin susceptible) (MSSA) A41.01
    - methicillin resistant (MRSA) A41.02
  - coagulase-negative A41.1
  - specified NEC A41.1
- Streptococcus, streptococcal A40.9
  - agalactiae A40.1
  - group
    - A A40.0
    - B A40.1
    - D A41.81
  - neonatal P36.10
    - group B P36.0
    - specified NEC P36.19
  - pneumoniae A40.3
  - pyogenes A40.0
  - specified NEC A40.8
- tracheostomy stoma J95.02
- tularemic A21.7
- umbilical, umbilical cord (newborn) — see Sepsis, newborn
- Yersinia pestis A20.7

Septate — see Septum
Septic — see condition
- arm — see Cellulitis, upper limb
  - with lymphangitis — see Lymphangitis, acute, upper limb
- embolus — see Embolism
- finger — see Cellulitis, digit
  - with lymphangitis — see Lymphangitis, acute, digit
- foot — see Cellulitis, lower limb
  - with lymphangitis — see Lymphangitis, acute, lower limb
- gallbladder (acute) K81.0
- hand — see Cellulitis, upper limb
  - with lymphangitis — see Lymphangitis, acute, upper limb
- joint — see Arthritis, pyogenic or pyemic
- leg — see Cellulitis, lower limb
  - with lymphangitis — see Lymphangitis, acute, lower limb
- nail (see also Cellulitis, digit)
  - with lymphangitis — see Lymphangitis, acute, digit
- sore (see also Abscess)
  - throat J02.0
    - streptococcal J02.0
- spleen (acute) D73.89
- teeth, tooth (pulpal origin) K04.4
- throat — see Pharyngitis
- thrombus — see Thrombosis
- toe — see Cellulitis, digit
  - with lymphangitis — see Lymphangitis, acute, digit
- tonsils, chronic J35.01
  - with adenoiditis J35.03
- uterus — see Endometritis

Septicemia A41.9
- meaning sepsis — see Sepsis
Septum, septate (congenital) (see also Anomaly, by site)
- anal Q42.3
  - with fistula Q42.2
- aqueduct of Sylvius Q03.0
  - with spina bifida — see Spina bifida, by site, with hydrocephalus
- uterus (complete) (partial) Q51.2
- vagina Q52.10
  - in pregnancy — see Pregnancy, complicated by, abnormal vagina
    - causing obstructed labor O65.5
  - longitudinal Q52.129
    - microperforate
      - left side Q52.124
      - right side Q52.123
    - nonobstruction Q52.120

Septum, septate — continued
- vagina — continued
  - longitudinal — continued
    - obstructing Q52.129
      - left side Q52.122
      - right side Q52.121
    - transverse Q52.11

Sequelae (of) (see also condition)
- abscess, intracranial or intraspinal (conditions in G06) G09
- amputation — code to injury with seventh character S
- burn and corrosion — code to injury with seventh character S
- calcium deficiency E64.8
- cerebrovascular disease — see Sequelae, disease, cerebrovascular
- childbirth O94
- contusion — code to injury with seventh character S
- corrosion — see Sequelae, burn and corrosion
- crushing injury — code to injury with seventh character S
- disease
  - cerebrovascular I69.90
    - alteration of sensation I69.998
    - aphasia I69.920
    - apraxia I69.990
    - ataxia I69.993
    - cognitive deficits I69.91 ☑
    - disturbance of vision I69.998
    - dysarthria I69.922
    - dysphagia I69.991
    - dysphasia I69.921
    - facial droop I69.992
    - facial weakness I69.992
    - fluency disorder I69.923
    - hemiplegia I69.95- ☑
    - hemorrhage
      - intracerebral — see Sequelae, hemorrhage, intracerebral
      - intracranial, nontraumatic NEC — see Sequelae, hemorrhage, intracranial, nontraumatic
      - subarachnoid — see Sequelae, hemorrhage, subarachnoid
    - language deficit I69.928
    - monoplegia
      - lower limb I69.94- ☑
      - upper limb I69.93- ☑
    - paralytic syndrome I69.96- ☑
    - specified effect NEC I69.998
    - specified type NEC I69.80
      - alteration of sensation I69.898
      - aphasia I69.820
      - apraxia I69.890
      - ataxia I69.893
      - cognitive deficits I69.81 ☑
      - disturbance of vision I69.898
      - dysarthria I69.822
      - dysphagia I69.891
      - dysphasia I69.821
      - facial droop I69.892
      - facial weakness I69.892
      - fluency disorder I69.823
      - hemiplegia I69.85- ☑
      - language deficit I69.828
      - monoplegia
        - lower limb I69.84- ☑
        - upper limb I69.83- ☑
      - paralytic syndrome I69.86- ☑
      - specified effect NEC I69.898
    - speech deficit I69.928
      - speech deficit I69.828
    - stroke NOS — see Sequelae, stroke NOS
- dislocation — code to injury with seventh character S
- encephalitis or encephalomyelitis (conditions in G04) G09
  - in infectious disease NEC B94.8
  - viral B94.1
- external cause — code to injury with seventh character S
- foreign body entering natural orifice — code to injury with seventh character S
- fracture — code to injury with seventh character S
- frostbite — code to injury with seventh character S
- Hansen's disease B92
- hemorrhage
  - intracerebral I69.10

Sequelae — continued
- hemorrhage — continued
  - intracerebral — continued
    - alteration of sensation I69.198
    - aphasia I69.120
    - apraxia I69.190
    - ataxia I69.193
    - cognitive deficits I69.11 ☑
    - disturbance of vision I69.198
    - dysarthria I69.122
    - dysphagia I69.191
    - dysphasia I69.121
    - facial droop I69.192
    - facial weakness I69.192
    - fluency disorder I69.123
    - hemiplegia I69.15- ☑
    - language deficit NEC I69.128
    - monoplegia
      - lower limb I69.14- ☑
      - upper limb I69.13- ☑
    - paralytic syndrome I69.16- ☑
    - specified effect NEC I69.198
    - speech deficit NEC I69.128
  - intracranial, nontraumatic NEC I69.20
    - alteration of sensation I69.298
    - aphasia I69.220
    - apraxia I69.290
    - ataxia I69.293
    - cognitive deficits I69.21 ☑
    - disturbance of vision I69.298
    - dysarthria I69.222
    - dysphagia I69.291
    - dysphasia I69.221
    - facial droop I69.292
    - facial weakness I69.292
    - fluency disorder I69.223
    - hemiplegia I69.25- ☑
    - language deficit NEC I69.228
    - monoplegia
      - lower limb I69.24- ☑
      - upper limb I69.23- ☑
    - paralytic syndrome I69.26- ☑
    - specified effect NEC I69.298
    - speech deficit NEC I69.228
  - subarachnoid I69.00
    - alteration of sensation I69.098
    - aphasia I69.020
    - apraxia I69.090
    - ataxia I69.093
    - cognitive deficits — see subcategory I69.01- ☑
    - disturbance of vision I69.098
    - dysarthria I69.022
    - dysphagia I69.091
    - dysphasia I69.021
    - facial droop I69.092
    - facial weakness I69.092
    - fluency disorder I69.023
    - hemiplegia I69.05- ☑
    - language deficit NEC I69.028
    - monoplegia
      - lower limb I69.04- ☑
      - upper limb I69.03- ☑
    - paralytic syndrome I69.06- ☑
    - specified effect NEC I69.098
    - speech deficit NEC I69.028
- hepatitis, viral B94.2
- hyperalimentation E68
- infarction
  - cerebral I69.30
    - alteration of sensation I69.398
    - aphasia I69.320
    - apraxia I69.390
    - ataxia I69.393
    - cognitive deficits I69.31 ☑
    - disturbance of vision I69.398
    - dysarthria I69.322
    - dysphagia I69.391
    - dysphasia I69.321
    - facial droop I69.392
    - facial weakness I69.392
    - fluency disorder I69.323
    - hemiplegia I69.35- ☑
    - language deficit NEC I69.328
    - monoplegia
      - lower limb I69.34- ☑
      - upper limb I69.33- ☑
    - paralytic syndrome I69.36- ☑
    - specified effect NEC I69.398

☑ **Additional Character Required — Refer to the Tabular List for Character Selection**   🔻 **Subterms under main terms may continue to next column or page**

Sequelae — *continued*
  infarction — *continued*
    cerebral — *continued*
      speech deficit NEC I69.328
  infection, pyogenic, intracranial or intraspinal G09
  infectious disease B94.9
    specified NEC B94.8
  injury — *code to* injury with seventh character S
  leprosy B92
  meningitis
    bacterial (conditions in G00) G09
    other or unspecified cause (conditions in G03) G09
  muscle (and tendon) injury — *code to* injury with seventh character S
  myelitis — *see* Sequelae, encephalitis
  niacin deficiency E64.8
  nutritional deficiency E64.9
    specified NEC E64.8
  obstetrical condition O94
  parasitic disease B94.9
  phlebitis or thrombophlebitis of intracranial or in-traspinal venous sinuses and veins (conditions in G08) G09
  poisoning — *code to* poisoning with seventh character S
    nonmedicinal substance — *see* Sequelae, toxic effect, nonmedicinal substance
  poliomyelitis (acute) B91
  pregnancy O94
  protein-energy malnutrition E64.0
  puerperium O94
  rickets E64.3
  selenium deficiency E64.8
  sprain and strain — *code to* injury with seventh character S
  stroke NOS I69.30
    alteration in sensation I69.398
    aphasia I69.320
    apraxia I69.390
    ataxia I69.393
    cognitive deficits I69.31 ☑
    disturbance of vision I69.398
    dysarthria I69.322
    dysphagia I69.391
    dysphasia I69.321
    facial droop I69.392
    facial weakness I69.392
    hemiplegia I69.35- ☑
    language deficit NEC I69.328
    monoplegia
      lower limb I69.34- ☑
      upper limb I69.33- ☑
    paralytic syndrome I69.36- ☑
    specified effect NEC I69.398
    speech deficit NEC I69.328
  tendon and muscle injury — *code to* injury with seventh character S
  thiamine deficiency E64.8
  trachoma B94.0
  tuberculosis B90.9
    bones and joints B90.2
    central nervous system B90.0
    genitourinary B90.1
    pulmonary (respiratory) B90.9
    specified organs NEC B90.8
  viral
    encephalitis B94.1
    hepatitis B94.2
  vitamin deficiency NEC E64.8
    A E64.1
    B E64.8
    C E64.2
  wound, open — *code to* injury with seventh character S

Sequestration (*see also* Sequestrum)
  disk — *see* Displacement, intervertebral disk
  lung, congenital Q33.2

Sequestrum
  bone — *see* Osteomyelitis, chronic
  dental M27.2
  jaw bone M27.2
  orbit — *see* Osteomyelitis, orbit
  sinus (accessory) (nasal) — *see* Sinusitis

Sequoiosis lung or pneumonitis J67.8

Serology for syphilis
  doubtful
    with signs or symptoms — *code by* site and stage under Syphilis
    follow-up of latent syphilis — *see* Syphilis, latent
  negative, with signs or symptoms — *code by* site and stage under Syphilis
  positive A53.0
    with signs or symptoms — *code by* site and stage under Syphilis
  reactivated A53.0

Seroma (*see also* Hematoma)
  postprocedural — *see* Complication, postprocedural, seroma
  traumatic, secondary and recurrent T79.2 ☑

Seropurulent — *see* condition

Serositis, multiple K65.8
  pericardial I31.1
  peritoneal K65.8

Serous — *see* condition

Sertoli cell
  adenoma
    specified site — *see* Neoplasm, benign, by site
    unspecified site
      female D27.9
      male D29.20
  carcinoma
    specified site — *see* Neoplasm, malignant, by site
    unspecified site (male) C62.9- ☑
      female C56.9
  tumor
    with lipid storage
      specified site — *see* Neoplasm, benign, by site
      unspecified site
        female D27.9
        male D29.20
    specified site — *see* Neoplasm, benign, by site
    unspecified site
      female D27.9
      male D29.20

Sertoli-Leydig cell tumor — *see* Neoplasm, benign, by site
  specified site — *see* Neoplasm, benign, by site
  unspecified site
    female D27.9
    male D29.20

Serum
  allergy, allergic reaction (*see also* Reaction, serum) T80.69 ☑
    shock (*see also* Shock, anaphylactic) T80.59 ☑
  arthritis (*see also* Reaction, serum) T80.69 ☑
  complication or reaction NEC (*see also* Reaction, serum) T80.69 ☑
  disease NEC (*see also* Reaction, serum) T80.69 ☑
  hepatitis (*see also* Hepatitis, viral, type B)
    carrier (suspected) of B18.1
  intoxication (*see also* Reaction, serum) T80.69 ☑
  neuritis (*see also* Reaction, serum) T80.69 ☑
  neuropathy G61.1
  poisoning NEC (*see also* Reaction, serum) T80.69 ☑
  rash NEC (*see also* Reaction, serum) T80.69 ☑
  reaction NEC (*see also* Reaction, serum) T80.69 ☑
  sickness NEC (*see also* Reaction, serum) T80.69 ☑
  urticaria (*see also* Reaction, serum) T80.69 ☑

Sesamoiditis M25.8- ☑

Severe sepsis R65.20
  with septic shock R65.21

Sever's disease or osteochondrosis — *see* Osteochondrosis, juvenile, tarsus

Sex
  chromosome mosaics Q97.8
    lines with various numbers of X chromosomes Q97.2
  education Z70.8
  reassignment surgery status Z87.890

Sextuplet pregnancy — *see* Pregnancy, sextuplet

Sexual
  function, disorder of (psychogenic) F52.9
  immaturity (female) (male) E30.0
  impotence (psychogenic) organic origin NEC — *see* Dysfunction, sexual, male
  precocity (constitutional) (cryptogenic)(female) (idiopathic) (male) E30.1

Sexuality, pathologic — *see* Deviation, sexual

Sézary disease C84.1- ☑

Shadow, lung R91.8

Shaking palsy or paralysis — *see* Parkinsonism

Shallowness, acetabulum — *see* Derangement, joint, specified type NEC, hip

Shaver's disease J63.1

Sheath (tendon) — *see* condition

Sheathing, retinal vessels H35.01- ☑

Shedding
  nail L60.8
  premature, primary (deciduous) teeth K00.6

Sheehan's disease or syndrome E23.0

Shelf, rectal K62.89

Shell teeth K00.5

Shellshock (current) F43.0
  lasting state — *see* Disorder, post-traumatic stress

Shield kidney Q63.1

Shift
  auditory threshold (temporary) H93.24- ☑
  mediastinal R93.8

Shifting sleep-work schedule (affecting sleep) G47.26

Shiga (-Kruse) **dysentery** A03.0

Shiga's bacillus A03.0

Shigella (dysentery) — *see* Dysentery, bacillary

Shigellosis A03.9
  Group A A03.0
  Group B A03.1
  Group C A03.2
  Group D A03.3

Shin splints S86.89- ☑

Shingles — *see* Herpes, zoster

Shipyard disease or eye B30.0

Shirodkar suture, in pregnancy — *see* Pregnancy, complicated by, incompetent cervix

Shock R57.9
  with ectopic or molar pregnancy O08.3
  adrenal (cortical) (Addisonian) E27.2
  adverse food reaction (anaphylactic) — *see* Shock, anaphylactic, due to food
  allergic — *see* Shock, anaphylactic
  anaphylactic T78.2 ☑
    chemical — *see* Table of Drugs and Chemicals
    due to drug or medicinal substance
      correct substance properly administered T88.6 ☑
      overdose or wrong substance given or taken (by accident) — *see* Table of Drugs and Chemicals, by drug, poisoning
    due to food (nonpoisonous) T78.00 ☑
      additives T78.06 ☑
      dairy products T78.07 ☑
      eggs T78.08 ☑
      fish T78.03 ☑
        shellfish T78.02 ☑
      fruit T78.04 ☑
      milk T78.07 ☑
      nuts T78.05 ☑
        multiple types T78.05 ☑
        peanuts T78.01 ☑
      peanuts T78.01 ☑
      seeds T78.05 ☑
      specified type NEC T78.09 ☑
      vegetable T78.04 ☑
    following sting(s) — *see* Venom
    immunization T80.52 ☑
    serum T80.59 ☑
      blood and blood products T80.51 ☑
      immunization T80.52 ☑
      specified NEC T80.59 ☑
      vaccination T80.52 ☑
  anaphylactoid — *see* Shock, anaphylactic
  anesthetic
    correct substance properly administered T88.2 ☑
    overdose or wrong substance given or taken — *see* Table of Drugs and Chemicals, by drug, poisoning
      specified anesthetic — *see* Table of Drugs and Chemicals, by drug, poisoning
  cardiogenic R57.0
  chemical substance — *see* Table of Drugs and Chemicals
  complicating ectopic or molar pregnancy O08.3
  culture — *see* Disorder, adjustment
  drug
    due to correct substance properly administered T88.6 ☑
    overdose or wrong substance given or taken (by accident) — *see* Table of Drugs and Chemicals, by drug, poisoning
  during or after labor and delivery O75.1

Shock — *continued*
electric T75.4 ☑
  (taser) T75.4 ☑
endotoxic R65.21
  postprocedural (resulting from a procedure, not elsewhere classified) T81.12 ☑
following
  ectopic or molar pregnancy O08.3
  injury (immediate) (delayed) T79.4 ☑
  labor and delivery O75.1
food (anaphylactic) — *see* Shock, anaphylactic, due to food
from electroshock gun (taser) T75.4 ☑
gram-negative R65.21
  postprocedural (resulting from a procedure, not elsewhere classified) T81.12 ☑
hematologic R57.8
hemorrhagic R57.8
  surgery (intraoperative) (postoperative) T81.19 ☑
  trauma T79.4 ☑
hypovolemic R57.1
  surgical T81.19 ☑
  traumatic T79.4 ☑
insulin E15
  therapeutic misadventure — *see* subcategory T38.3 ☑
kidney N17.0
  traumatic (following crushing) T79.5 ☑
lightning T75.01 ☑
liver K72.00
lung J80
obstetric O75.1
  with ectopic or molar pregnancy O08.3
  following ectopic or molar pregnancy O08.3
pleural (surgical) T81.19 ☑
  due to trauma T79.4 ☑
postprocedural (postoperative) T81.10 ☑
  with ectopic or molar pregnancy O08.3
  cardiogenic T81.11 ☑
  endotoxic T81.12 ☑
  following ectopic or molar pregnancy O08.3
  gram-negative T81.12 ☑
  hypovolemic T81.19 ☑
  septic T81.12 ☑
  specified type NEC T81.19 ☑
psychic F43.0
septic (due to severe sepsis) R65.21
specified NEC R57.8
surgical T81.10 ☑
taser gun (taser) T75.4 ☑
therapeutic misadventure NEC T81.10 ☑
thyroxin
  overdose or wrong substance given or taken — *see* Table of Drugs and Chemicals, by drug, poisoning
toxic, syndrome A48.3
transfusion — *see* Complications, transfusion
traumatic (immediate) (delayed) T79.4 ☑
Shoemaker's chest M95.4
Short, shortening, shortness
arm (acquired) (*see also* Deformity, limb, unequal length)
  congenital Q71.81- ☑
  forearm — *see* Deformity, limb, unequal length
bowel syndrome K91.2
breath R06.02
cervical (complicating pregnancy) O26.87- ☑
  non-gravid uterus N88.3
common bile duct, congenital Q44.5
cord (umbilical), complicating delivery O69.3 ☑
cystic duct, congenital Q44.5
esophagus (congenital) Q39.8
femur (acquired) — *see* Deformity, limb, unequal length, femur
  congenital — *see* Defect, reduction, lower limb, longitudinal, femur
frenum, frenulum, linguae (congenital) Q38.1
hip (acquired) (*see also* Deformity, limb, unequal length)
  congenital Q65.89
leg (acquired) (*see also* Deformity, limb, unequal length)
  congenital Q72.81- ☑
  lower leg (*see also* Deformity, limb, unequal length)
limbed stature, with immunodeficiency D82.2
lower limb (acquired) (*see also* Deformity, limb, unequal length)

Short, shortening, shortness — *continued*
lower limb (*see also* Deformity, limb, unequal length) — *continued*
  congenital Q72.81- ☑
organ or site, congenital NEC — *see* Distortion
palate, congenital Q38.5
radius (acquired) (*see also* Deformity, limb, unequal length)
  congenital — *see* Defect, reduction, upper limb, longitudinal, radius
rib syndrome Q77.2
stature (child) (hereditary) (idiopathic) NEC R62.52
  constitutional E34.3
  due to endocrine disorder E34.3
  Laron-type E34.3
tendon (*see also* Contraction, tendon)
  with contracture of joint — *see* Contraction, joint
  Achilles (acquired) M67.0- ☑
    congenital Q66.89
  congenital Q79.8
thigh (acquired) (*see also* Deformity, limb, unequal length, femur)
  congenital — *see* Defect, reduction, lower limb, longitudinal, femur
tibialis anterior (tendon) — *see* Contraction, tendon
umbilical cord
  complicating delivery O69.3 ☑
upper limb, congenital — *see* Defect, reduction, upper limb, specified type NEC
urethra N36.8
uvula, congenital Q38.5
vagina (congenital) Q52.4
Shortsightedness — *see* Myopia
Shoshin (acute fulminating beriberi) E51.11
Shoulder — *see* condition
Shovel-shaped incisors K00.2
Shower, thromboembolic — *see* Embolism
Shunt
arterial-venous (dialysis) Z99.2
arteriovenous, pulmonary (acquired) I28.0
  congenital Q25.72
cerebral ventricle (communicating) in situ Z98.2
surgical, prosthetic, with complications — *see* Complications, cardiovascular, device or implant
Shutdown, renal N28.9
Shy-Drager syndrome G90.3
Sialadenitis, sialadenosis (any gland) (chronic) (periodic) (suppurative) — *see* Sialoadenitis
Sialectasia K11.8
Sialidosis E77.1
Sialitis, silitis (any gland) (chronic) (suppurative) — *see* Sialoadenitis
Sialoadenitis (any gland) (periodic) (suppurative) K11.20
acute K11.21
  recurrent K11.22
chronic K11.23
Sialoadenopathy K11.9
Sialoangitis — *see* Sialoadenitis
Sialodochitis (fibrinosa) — *see* Sialoadenitis
Sialodocholithiasis K11.5
Sialolithiasis K11.5
Sialometaplasia, necrotizing K11.8
Sialorrhea (*see also* Ptyalism)
periodic — *see* Sialoadenitis
Sialosis K11.7
Siamese twin Q89.4
Sibling rivalry Z62.891
Sicard's syndrome G52.7
Sicca syndrome M35.00
with
  keratoconjunctivitis M35.01
  lung involvement M35.02
  myopathy M35.03
  renal tubulo-interstitial disorders M35.04
specified organ involvement NEC M35.09
Sick R69
or handicapped person in family Z63.79
  needing care at home Z63.6
sinus (syndrome) I49.5
Sick-euthyroid syndrome E07.81
Sickle-cell
anemia — *see* Disease, sickle-cell
trait D57.3
Sicklemia (*see also* Disease, sickle-cell)
trait D57.3
Sickness
air (travel) T75.3 ☑

Sickness — *continued*
airplane T75.3 ☑
alpine T70.29 ☑
altitude T70.20 ☑
Andes T70.29 ☑
aviator's T70.29 ☑
balloon T70.29 ☑
car T75.3 ☑
compressed air T70.3 ☑
decompression T70.3 ☑
green D50.8
milk — *see* Poisoning, food, noxious
motion T75.3 ☑
mountain T70.29 ☑
  acute D75.1
protein (*see also* Reaction, serum) T80.69 ☑
radiation T66 ☑
roundabout (motion) T75.3 ☑
sea T75.3 ☑
serum NEC (*see also* Reaction, serum) T80.69 ☑
sleeping (African) B56.9
  by Trypanosoma B56.9
    brucei
      gambiense B56.0
      rhodesiense B56.1
  East African B56.1
  Gambian B56.0
  Rhodesian B56.1
  West African B56.0
swing (motion) T75.3 ☑
train (railway) (travel) T75.3 ☑
travel (any vehicle) T75.3 ☑
Sideropenia — *see* Anemia, iron deficiency
Siderosilicosis J62.8
Siderosis (lung) J63.4
eye (globe) — *see* Disorder, globe, degenerative, siderosis
Siemens' syndrome (ectodermal dysplasia) Q82.8
Sighing R06.89
psychogenic F45.8
Sigmoid (*see also* condition)
flexure — *see* condition
kidney Q63.1
Sigmoiditis (*see also* Enteritis) K52.9
infectious A09
noninfectious K52.9
Silfversköld's syndrome Q78.9
Silicosiderosis J62.8
Silicosis, silicotic (simple) (complicated) J62.8
with tuberculosis J65
Silicotuberculosis J65
Silo-fillers' disease J68.8
bronchitis J68.0
pneumonitis J68.0
pulmonary edema J68.1
Silver's syndrome Q87.1
Simian malaria B53.1
Simmonds' cachexia or disease E23.0
Simons' disease or syndrome (progressive lipodystrophy) E88.1
Simple, simplex — *see* condition
Simulation, conscious (of illness) Z76.5
Simultanagnosia (asimultagnosia) R48.3
Sin Nombre virus disease (Hantavirus) (cardio)-pulmonary syndrome) B33.4
Sinding-Larsen disease or osteochondrosis — *see* Osteochondrosis, juvenile, patella
Singapore hemorrhagic fever A91
Singer's node or nodule J38.2
Single
atrium Q21.2
coronary artery Q24.5
umbilical artery Q27.0
ventricle Q20.4
Singultus R06.6
epidemicus B33.0
Sinus (*see also* Fistula)
abdominal K63.89
arrest I45.5
arrhythmia I49.8
bradycardia R00.1
branchial cleft (internal) (external) Q18.0
coccygeal — *see* Sinus, pilonidal
dental K04.6
dermal (congenital) Q06.8
  with abscess Q06.8
coccygeal, pilonidal — *see* Sinus, coccygeal

☑ **Additional Character Required** — Refer to the Tabular List for Character Selection   ⬇ **Subterms under main terms may continue to next column or page**

Sinus — *continued*
  infected, skin NEC L08.89
  marginal, ruptured or bleeding — *see* Hemorrhage, antepartum, specified cause NEC
  medial, face and neck Q18.8
  pause I45.5
  pericranii Q01.9
  pilonidal (infected) (rectum) L05.92
    with abscess L05.02
  preauricular Q18.1
  rectovaginal N82.3
  Rokitansky-Aschoff (gallbladder) K82.8
  sacrococcygeal (dermoid) (infected) — *see* Sinus, pilonidal
  tachycardia R00.0
    paroxysmal I47.1
  tarsi syndrome M25.57- ☑
  testis N50.89
  tract (postinfective) — *see* Fistula
  urachus Q64.4
Sinusitis (accessory) (chronic) (hyperplastic) (nasal) (nonpurulent) (purulent) J32.9
  acute J01.90
    ethmoidal J01.20
      recurrent J01.21
    frontal J01.10
      recurrent J01.11
    involving more than one sinus, other than pansinusitis J01.80
      recurrent J01.81
    maxillary J01.00
      recurrent J01.01
    pansinusitis J01.40
      recurrent J01.41
    recurrent J01.91
    specified NEC J01.80
      recurrent J01.81
    sphenoidal J01.30
      recurrent J01.31
  allergic — *see* Rhinitis, allergic
  due to high altitude T70.1 ☑
  ethmoidal J32.2
    acute J01.20
      recurrent J01.21
  frontal J32.1
    acute J01.10
      recurrent J01.11
  influenzal — *see* Influenza, with, respiratory manifestations NEC
  involving more than one sinus but not pansinusitis J32.8
    acute J01.80
      recurrent J01.81
  maxillary J32.0
    acute J01.00
      recurrent J01.01
  sphenoidal J32.3
    acute J01.30
      recurrent J01.31
  tuberculous, any sinus A15.8
Sinusitis-bronchiectasis-situs inversus (syndrome) (triad) Q89.3
Sipple's syndrome E31.22
Sirenomelia (syndrome) Q87.2
Siriasis T67.0 ☑
Sirkari's disease B55.0
Siti A65
Situation, psychiatric F99
Situational
  disturbance (transient) — *see* Disorder, adjustment
    acute F43.0
  maladjustment — *see* Disorder, adjustment
  reaction — *see* Disorder, adjustment
    acute F43.0
Situs inversus or transversus (abdominalis) (thoracis) Q89.3
Sixth disease B08.20
  due to human herpesvirus 6 B08.21
  due to human herpesvirus 7 B08.22
Sjögren-Larsson syndrome Q87.1
Sjögren's syndrome or disease — *see* Sicca syndrome
Skeletal — *see* condition
Skene's gland — *see* condition
Skenitis — *see* Urethritis
Skerljevo A65
Skevas-Zerfus disease — *see* Toxicity, venom, marine animal, sea anemone
Skin (*see also* condition)

Skin — *continued*
  clammy R23.1
  donor — *see* Donor, skin
  hidebound M35.9
Slate-dressers' or slate-miners' lung J62.8
Sleep
  apnea — *see* Apnea, sleep
  deprivation Z72.820
  disorder or disturbance G47.9
    child F51.9
    nonorganic origin F51.9
    specified NEC G47.8
  disturbance G47.9
    nonorganic origin F51.9
  drunkenness F51.9
  rhythm inversion G47.2- ☑
  terrors F51.4
  walking F51.3
    hysterical F44.89
Sleep hygiene
  abuse Z72.821
  inadequate Z72.821
  poor Z72.821
Sleeping sickness — *see* Sickness, sleeping
Sleeplessness — *see* Insomnia
  menopausal N95.1
Sleep-wake schedule disorder G47.20
Slim disease (in HIV infection) B20
Slipped, slipping
  epiphysis (traumatic) (*see also* Osteochondropathy, specified type NEC)
    capital femoral (traumatic)
      acute (on chronic) S79.01- ☑
    current traumatic — *code as* Fracture, by site
    upper femoral (nontraumatic) M93.00- ☑
      acute M93.01- ☑
        on chronic M93.03- ☑
      chronic M93.02- ☑
  intervertebral disc — *see* Displacement, intervertebral disc
  ligature, umbilical P51.8
  patella — *see* Disorder, patella, derangement NEC
  rib M89.8X8
  sacroiliac joint — *see* subcategory M53.2 ☑
  tendon — *see* Disorder, tendon
  ulnar nerve, nontraumatic — *see* Lesion, nerve, ulnar
  vertebra NEC — *see* Spondylolisthesis
Slocumb's syndrome E27.0
Sloughing (multiple) (phagedena) (skin) (*see also* Gangrene)
  abscess — *see* Abscess
  appendix K38.8
  fascia — *see* Disorder, soft tissue, specified type NEC
  scrotum N50.89
  tendon — *see* Disorder, tendon
  transplanted organ — *see* Rejection, transplant
  ulcer — *see* Ulcer, skin
Slow
  feeding, newborn P92.2
  flow syndrome, coronary I20.8
  heart (beat) R00.1
Slowing, urinary stream R39.198
Sluder's neuralgia (syndrome) G44.89
Slurred, slurring speech R47.81
Small (ness)
  for gestational age — *see* Small for dates
  introitus, vagina N89.6
  kidney (unknown cause) N27.9
    bilateral N27.1
    unilateral N27.0
  ovary (congenital) Q50.39
  pelvis
    with disproportion (fetopelvic) O33.1
      causing obstructed labor O65.1
  uterus N85.8
  white kidney N03.9
Small-and-light-for-dates — *see* Small for dates
Small-for-dates (infant) P05.10
  with weight of
    499 grams or less P05.11
    500-749 grams P05.12
    750-999 grams P05.13
    1000-1249 grams P05.14
    1250-1499 grams P05.15
    1500-1749 grams P05.16
    1750-1999 grams P05.17
    2000-2499 grams P05.18

Small-for-dates — *continued*
  with weight of — *continued*
    2500 grams and over P05.19
    specified NEC P05.19
Smallpox B03
Smearing, fecal R15.1
Smith-Lemli-Opitz syndrome E78.72
Smith's fracture S52.54- ☑
Smoker — *see* Dependence, drug, nicotine
Smoker's
  bronchitis J41.0
  cough J41.0
  palate K13.24
  throat J31.2
  tongue K13.24
Smoking
  passive Z77.22
Smothering spells R06.81
Snaggle teeth, tooth M26.39
Snapping
  finger — *see* Trigger finger
  hip — *see* Derangement, joint, specified type NEC, hip
    involving the iliotiblial band M76.3- ☑
  knee — *see* Derangement, knee
    involving the iliotiblial band M76.3- ☑
Sneddon-Wilkinson disease or syndrome (sub-corneal pustular dermatosis) L13.1
Sneezing (intractable) R06.7
Sniffing
  cocaine
    abuse — *see* Abuse, drug, cocaine
    dependence — *see* Dependence, drug, cocaine
  gasoline
    abuse — *see* Abuse, drug, inhalant
    dependence — *see* Dependence, drug, inhalant
  glue (airplane)
    abuse — *see* Abuse, drug, inhalant
    drug dependence — *see* Dependence, drug, inhalant
Sniffles
  newborn P28.89
Snoring R06.83
Snow blindness — *see* Photokeratitis
Snuffles (non-syphilitic) R06.5
  newborn P28.89
  syphilitic (infant) A50.05 [J99]
Social
  exclusion Z60.4
    due to discrimination or persecution (perceived) Z60.5
  migrant Z59.0
    acculturation difficulty Z60.3
  rejection Z60.4
    due to discrimination or persecution Z60.5
  role conflict NEC Z73.5
  skills inadequacy NEC Z73.4
  transplantation Z60.3
Sodoku A25.0
Soemmerring's ring — *see* Cataract, secondary
Soft (*see also* condition)
  nails L60.3
Softening
  bone — *see* Osteomalacia
  brain (necrotic) (progressive) G93.89
    congenital Q04.8
    embolic I63.4- ☑
    hemorrhagic — *see* Hemorrhage, intracranial, intracerebral
    occlusive I63.5- ☑
      thrombotic I63.3- ☑
  cartilage M94.2- ☑
    patella M22.4- ☑
  cerebellar — *see* Softening, brain
  cerebral — *see* Softening, brain
  cerebrospinal — *see* Softening, brain
  myocardial, heart — *see* Degeneration, myocardial
  spinal cord G95.89
  stomach K31.89
Soldier's
  heart F45.8
  patches I31.0
Solitary
  cyst, kidney N28.1
  kidney, congenital Q60.0
Solvent abuse — *see* Abuse, drug, inhalant
  dependence — *see* Dependence, drug, inhalant

Index

Somatization reaction, somatic reaction — Splenopathy

Somatization reaction, somatic reaction — see Disorder, somatoform
Somnambulism F51.3
  hysterical F44.89
Somnolence R40.0
  nonorganic origin F51.11
Sonne dysentery A03.3
Soor B37.0
Sore
  bed — see Ulcer, pressure, by site
  chiclero B55.1
  Delhi B55.1
  desert — see Ulcer, skin
  eye H57.1- ☑
  Lahore B55.1
  mouth K13.79
    canker K12.0
  muscle M79.1
  Naga — see Ulcer, skin
  of skin — see Ulcer, skin
  oriental B55.1
  pressure — see Ulcer, pressure, by site
  skin L98.9
  soft A57
  throat (acute) (see also Pharyngitis)
    with influenza, flu, or grippe — see Influenza, with, respiratory manifestations NEC
    chronic J31.2
    coxsackie (virus) B08.5
    diphtheritic A36.0
    herpesviral B00.2
    influenzal — see Influenza, with, respiratory manifestations NEC
    septic J02.0
    streptococcal (ulcerative) J02.0
    viral NEC J02.8
      coxsackie B08.5
  tropical — see Ulcer, skin
  veldt — see Ulcer, skin
Soto's syndrome (cerebral gigantism) Q87.3
South African cardiomyopathy syndrome I42.8
Southeast Asian hemorrhagic fever A91
Spacing
  abnormal, tooth, teeth, fully erupted M26.30
  excessive, tooth, fully erupted M26.32
Spade-like hand (congenital) Q68.1
Spading nail L60.8
  congenital Q84.6
Spanish collar N47.1
Sparganosis B70.1
Spasm(s), spastic, spasticity (see also condition) R25.2
  accommodation — see Spasm, of accommodation
  ampulla of Vater K83.4
  anus, ani (sphincter) (reflex) K59.4
    psychogenic F45.8
  artery I73.9
    cerebral G45.9
  Bell's G51.3
  bladder (sphincter, external or internal) N32.89
    psychogenic F45.8
  bronchus, bronchiole J98.01
  cardia K22.0
  cardiac I20.1
  carpopedal — see Tetany
  cerebral (arteries) (vascular) G45.9
  cervix, complicating delivery O62.4
  ciliary body (of accommodation) — see Spasm, of accommodation
  colon (see also Irritable, bowel) K58.9
    with diarrhea K58.0
    psychogenic F45.8
  common duct K83.8
  compulsive — see Tic
  conjugate H51.8
  coronary (artery) I20.1
  diaphragm (reflex) R06.6
    epidemic B33.0
    psychogenic F45.8
  duodenum K59.8
  epidemic diaphragmatic (transient) B33.0
  esophagus (diffuse) K22.4
    psychogenic F45.8
  facial G51.3
  fallopian tube N83.8
  gastrointestinal (tract) K31.89
    psychogenic F45.8
  glottis J38.5
    hysterical F44.4

Spasm(s), spastic, spasticity — continued
  glottis — continued
    psychogenic F45.8
      conversion reaction F44.4
    reflex through recurrent laryngeal nerve J38.5
  habit — see Tic
  heart I20.1
  hemifacial (clonic) G51.3
  hourglass — see Contraction, hourglass
  hysterical F44.4
  infantile — see Epilepsy, spasms
  inferior oblique, eye H51.8
  intestinal (see also Syndrome, irritable bowel) K58.9
    psychogenic F45.8
  larynx, laryngeal J38.5
    hysterical F44.4
    psychogenic F45.8
      conversion reaction F44.4
  levator palpebrae superioris — see Disorder, eyelid function
  muscle NEC M62.838
    back M62.830
  nerve, trigeminal G51.0
  nervous F45.8
  nodding F98.4
  occupational F48.8
  oculogyric H51.8
    psychogenic F45.8
  of accommodation H52.53- ☑
  ophthalmic artery — see Occlusion, artery, retina
  perineal, female N94.89
  peroneo-extensor (see also Deformity, limb, flat foot)
  pharynx (reflex) J39.2
    hysterical F45.8
    psychogenic F45.8
  psychogenic F45.8
  pylorus NEC K31.3
    adult hypertrophic K31.89
    congenital or infantile Q40.0
    psychogenic F45.8
  rectum (sphincter) K59.4
    psychogenic F45.8
  retinal (artery) — see Occlusion, artery, retina
  sigmoid (see also Syndrome, irritable bowel) K58.9
    psychogenic F45.8
  sphincter of Oddi K83.4
  stomach K31.89
    neurotic F45.8
  throat J39.2
    hysterical F45.8
    psychogenic F45.8
  tic F95.9
    chronic F95.1
    transient of childhood F95.0
  tongue K14.8
  torsion (progressive) G24.1
  trigeminal nerve — see Neuralgia, trigeminal
  ureter N13.5
  urethra (sphincter) N35.9
  uterus N85.8
    complicating labor O62.4
  vagina N94.2
    psychogenic F52.5
  vascular I73.9
  vasomotor I73.9
  vein NEC I87.8
  viscera — see Pain, abdominal
Spasmodic — see condition
Spasmophilia — see Tetany
Spasmus nutans F98.4
Spastic, spasticity (see also Spasm)
  child (cerebral) (paralysis) G80.1
Speaker's throat R49.8
Specific, specified — see condition
Speech
  defect, disorder, disturbance, impediment R47.9
    psychogenic, in childhood and adolescence F98.8
    slurring R47.81
    specified NEC R47.89
Spencer's disease A08.19
Spens' syndrome (syncope with heart block) I45.9
Sperm counts (fertility testing) Z31.41
  postvasectomy Z30.8
    reversal Z31.42
Spermatic cord — see condition
Spermatocele N43.40
  congenital Q55.4
  multiple N43.42

Spermatocele — continued
  single N43.41
Spermatocystitis N49.0
Spermatocytoma C62.9- ☑
  specified site — see Neoplasm, malignant, by site
Spermatorrhea N50.89
Sphacelus — see Gangrene
Sphenoidal — see condition
Sphenoiditis (chronic) — see Sinusitis, sphenoidal
Sphenopalatine ganglion neuralgia G90.09
Sphericity, increased, lens (congenital) Q12.4
Spherocytosis (congenital) (familial) (hereditary) D58.0
  hemoglobin disease D58.0
  sickle-cell (disease) D57.8- ☑
Spherophakia Q12.4
Sphincter — see condition
Sphincteritis, sphincter of Oddi — see Cholangitis
Sphingolipidosis E75.3
  specified NEC E75.29
Sphingomyelinosis E75.3
Spicule tooth K00.2
Spider
  bite — see Toxicity, venom, spider
  fingers — see Syndrome, Marfan's
  nevus I78.1
  toes — see Syndrome, Marfan's
  vascular I78.1
Spiegler-Fendt
  benign lymphocytoma L98.8
  sarcoid L08.89
Spielmeyer-Vogt disease E75.4
Spina bifida (aperta) Q05.9
  with hydrocephalus NEC Q05.4
  cervical Q05.5
    with hydrocephalus Q05.0
  dorsal Q05.6
    with hydrocephalus Q05.1
  lumbar Q05.7
    with hydrocephalus Q05.2
  lumbosacral Q05.7
    with hydrocephalus Q05.2
  occulta Q76.0
  sacral Q05.8
    with hydrocephalus Q05.3
  thoracic Q05.6
    with hydrocephalus Q05.1
  thoracolumbar Q05.6
    with hydrocephalus Q05.1
Spindle, Krukenberg's — see Pigmentation, cornea, posterior
Spine, spinal — see condition
Spiradenoma (eccrine) — see Neoplasm, skin, benign
Spirillosis A25.0
Spirillum
  minus A25.0
  obermeieri infection A68.0
Spirochetal — see condition
Spirochetosis A69.9
  arthritic, arthritica A69.9
  bronchopulmonary A69.8
  icterohemorrhagic A27.0
  lung A69.8
Spirometrosis B70.1
Spitting blood — see Hemoptysis
Splanchnoptosis K63.4
Spleen, splenic — see condition
Splenectasis — see Splenomegaly
Splenitis (interstitial) (malignant) (nonspecific) D73.89
  malarial (see also Malaria) B54 [D77]
  tuberculous A18.85
Splenocele D73.89
Splenomegaly, splenomegalia (Bengal) (cryptogenic) (idiopathic) (tropical) R16.1
  with hepatomegaly R16.2
  cirrhotic D73.2
  congenital Q89.09
  congestive, chronic D73.2
  Egyptian B65.1
  Gaucher's E75.22
  malarial (see also Malaria) B54 [D77]
  neutropenic D73.81
  Niemann-Pick — see Niemann-Pick disease or syndrome
  siderotic D73.2
  syphilitic A52.79
    congenital (early) A50.08 [D77]
Splenopathy D73.9

☑ Additional Character Required — Refer to the Tabular List for Character Selection   ▽ Subterms under main terms may continue to next column or page

Splenoptosis D73.89
Splenosis D73.89
Splinter — *see* Foreign body, superficial, by site
Split, splitting
　foot Q72.7- ☑
　hand Q71.6 ☑
　heart sounds R01.2
　lip, congenital — *see* Cleft, lip
　nails L60.3
　urinary stream R39.13
Spondylarthrosis — *see* Spondylosis
Spondylitis (chronic) (*see also* Spondylopathy, inflammatory)
　ankylopoietica — *see* Spondylitis, ankylosing
　ankylosing (chronic) M45.9
　　with lung involvement M45.9 [J99]
　　cervical region M45.2
　　cervicothoracic region M45.3
　　juvenile M08.1
　　lumbar region M45.6
　　lumbosacral region M45.7
　　multiple sites M45.0
　　occipito-atlanto-axial region M45.1
　　sacrococcygeal region M45.8
　　thoracic region M45.4
　　thoracolumbar region M45.5
　atrophic (ligamentous) — *see* Spondylitis, ankylosing
　deformans (chronic) — *see* Spondylosis
　gonococcal A54.41
　gouty (*see also* Gout, by type, vertebrae) M10.08
　in (due to)
　　brucellosis A23.9 [M49.80]
　　　cervical region A23.9 [M49.82]
　　　cervicothoracic region A23.9 [M49.83]
　　　lumbar region A23.9 [M49.86]
　　　lumbosacral region A23.9 [M49.87]
　　　multiple sites A23.9 [M49.89]
　　　occipito-atlanto-axial region A23.9 [M49.81]
　　　sacrococcygeal region A23.9 [M49.88]
　　　thoracic region A23.9 [M49.84]
　　　thoracolumbar region A23.9 [M49.85]
　　enterobacteria (*see also* subcategory M49.8) A04.9
　　tuberculosis A18.01
　infectious NEC — *see* Spondylopathy, infective
　juvenile ankylosing (chronic) M08.1
　Kümmell's — *see* Spondylopathy, traumatic
　Marie-Strümpell — *see* Spondylitis, ankylosing
　muscularis — *see* Spondylopathy, specified NEC
　psoriatic L40.53
　rheumatoid — *see* Spondylitis, ankylosing
　rhizomelica — *see* Spondylitis, ankylosing
　sacroiliac NEC M46.1
　senescent, senile — *see* Spondylosis
　traumatic (chronic) or post-traumatic — *see* Spondylopathy, traumatic
　tuberculous A18.01
　typhosa A01.05
Spondylolisthesis (acquired) (degenerative) M43.10
　with disproportion (fetopelvic) O33.0
　　causing obstructed labor O65.0
　cervical region M43.12
　cervicothoracic region M43.13
　congenital Q76.2
　lumbar region M43.16
　lumbosacral region M43.17
　multiple sites M43.19
　occipito-atlanto-axial region M43.11
　sacrococcygeal region M43.18
　thoracic region M43.14
　thoracolumbar region M43.15
　traumatic (old) M43.10
　　acute
　　　fifth cervical (displaced) S12.430 ☑
　　　　nondisplaced S12.431 ☑
　　　　specified type NEC (displaced) S12.450 ☑
　　　　　nondisplaced S12.451 ☑
　　　　　type III S12.44 ☑
　　　fourth cervical (displaced) S12.330 ☑
　　　　nondisplaced S12.331 ☑
　　　　specified type NEC (displaced) S12.350 ☑
　　　　　nondisplaced S12.351 ☑
　　　　　type III S12.34 ☑
　　　second cervical (displaced) S12.130 ☑
　　　　nondisplaced S12.131 ☑
　　　　specified type NEC (displaced) S12.150 ☑
　　　　　nondisplaced S12.151 ☑
　　　　　type III S12.14 ☑

Spondylolisthesis — *continued*
　traumatic — *continued*
　　acute — *continued*
　　　seventh cervical (displaced) S12.630 ☑
　　　　nondisplaced S12.631 ☑
　　　　specified type NEC (displaced) S12.650 ☑
　　　　　nondisplaced S12.651 ☑
　　　　　type III S12.64 ☑
　　　sixth cervical (displaced) S12.530 ☑
　　　　nondisplaced S12.531 ☑
　　　　specified type NEC (displaced) S12.550 ☑
　　　　　nondisplaced S12.551 ☑
　　　　　type III S12.54 ☑
　　　third cervical (displaced) S12.230 ☑
　　　　nondisplaced S12.231 ☑
　　　　specified type NEC (displaced) S12.250 ☑
　　　　　nondisplaced S12.251 ☑
　　　　　type III S12.24 ☑
Spondylolysis (acquired) M43.00
　cervical region M43.02
　cervicothoracic region M43.03
　congenital Q76.2
　lumbar region M43.06
　lumbosacral region M43.07
　　with disproportion (fetopelvic) O33.0
　　　causing obstructed labor O65.8
　multiple sites M43.09
　occipito-atlanto-axial region M43.01
　sacrococcygeal region M43.08
　thoracic region M43.04
　thoracolumbar region M43.05
Spondylopathy M48.9
　infective NEC M46.50
　　cervical region M46.52
　　cervicothoracic region M46.53
　　lumbar region M46.56
　　lumbosacral region M46.57
　　multiple sites M46.59
　　occipito-atlanto-axial region M46.51
　　sacrococcygeal region M46.58
　　thoracic region M46.54
　　thoracolumbar region M46.55
　inflammatory M46.90
　　cervical region M46.92
　　cervicothoracic region M46.93
　　lumbar region M46.96
　　lumbosacral region M46.97
　　multiple sites M46.99
　　occipito-atlanto-axial region M46.91
　　sacrococcygeal region M46.98
　　specified type NEC M46.80
　　　cervical region M46.82
　　　cervicothoracic region M46.83
　　　lumbar region M46.86
　　　lumbosacral region M46.87
　　　multiple sites M46.89
　　　occipito-atlanto-axial region M46.81
　　　sacrococcygeal region M46.88
　　　thoracic region M46.84
　　　thoracolumbar region M46.85
　　thoracic region M46.94
　　thoracolumbar region M46.95
　neuropathic, in
　　syringomyelia and syringobulbia G95.0
　　tabes dorsalis A52.11
　specified NEC — *see* subcategory M48.8 ☑
　traumatic M48.30
　　cervical region M48.32
　　cervicothoracic region M48.33
　　lumbar region M48.36
　　lumbosacral region M48.37
　　occipito-atlanto-axial region M48.31
　　sacrococcygeal region M48.38
　　thoracic region M48.34
　　thoracolumbar region M48.35
Spondylosis M47.9
　with
　　disproportion (fetopelvic) O33.0
　　　causing obstructed labor O65.0
　　myelopathy NEC M47.10
　　　cervical region M47.12
　　　cervicothoracic region M47.13
　　　lumbar region M47.16
　　　occipito-atlanto-axial region M47.11
　　　thoracic region M47.14
　　　thoracolumbar region M47.15
　　radiculopathy M47.20
　　　cervical region M47.22

Spondylosis — *continued*
　with — *continued*
　　radiculopathy — *continued*
　　　cervicothoracic region M47.23
　　　lumbar region M47.26
　　　lumbosacral region M47.27
　　　occipito-atlanto-axial region M47.21
　　　sacrococcygeal region M47.28
　　　thoracic region M47.24
　　　thoracolumbar region M47.25
　　without myelopathy or radiculopathy M47.819
　　　cervical region M47.812
　　　cervicothoracic region M47.813
　　　lumbar region M47.816
　　　lumbosacral region M47.817
　　　occipito-atlanto-axial region M47.811
　　　sacrococcygeal region M47.818
　　　thoracic region M47.814
　　　thoracolumbar region M47.815
　　specified NEC M47.899
　　　cervical region M47.892
　　　cervicothoracic region M47.893
　　　lumbar region M47.896
　　　lumbosacral region M47.897
　　　occipito-atlanto-axial region M47.891
　　　sacrococcygeal region M47.898
　　　thoracic region M47.894
　　　thoracolumbar region M47.895
　　traumatic — *see* Spondylopathy, traumatic
Sponge
　inadvertently left in operation wound — *see* Foreign body, accidentally left during a procedure
　kidney (medullary) Q61.5
Sponge-diver's disease — *see* Toxicity, venom, marine animal, sea anemone
Spongioblastoma (any type) — *see* Neoplasm, malignant, by site
　specified site — *see* Neoplasm, malignant, by site
　unspecified site C71.9
Spongioneuroblastoma — *see* Neoplasm, malignant, by site
Spontaneous (*see also* condition)
　fracture (cause unknown) — *see* Fracture, pathological
Spoon nail L60.3
　congenital Q84.6
Sporadic — *see* condition
Sporothrix schenckii infection — *see* Sporotrichosis
Sporotrichosis B42.9
　arthritis B42.82
　disseminated B42.7
　generalized B42.7
　lymphocutaneous (fixed) (progressive) B42.1
　pulmonary B42.0
　specified NEC B42.89
Spots, spotting (in) (of)
　Bitot's (*see also* Pigmentation, conjunctiva)
　　in the young child E50.1
　　vitamin A deficiency E50.1
　café, au lait L81.3
　Cayenne pepper I78.1
　cotton wool, retina — *see* Occlusion, artery, retina
　de Morgan's (senile angiomas) I78.1
　Fuchs' black (myopic) (*see also* Myopia, degenerative) H44.2- ☑
　intermenstrual (regular) N92.0
　　irregular N92.1
　Koplik's B05.9
　liver L81.4
　pregnancy O26.85- ☑
　purpuric R23.3
　ruby I78.1
Spotted fever — *see* Fever, spotted N92.3
Sprain (joint) (ligament)
　acromioclavicular joint or ligament S43.5- ☑
　ankle S93.40- ☑
　　calcaneofibular ligament S93.41- ☑
　　deltoid ligament S93.42- ☑
　　internal collateral ligament — *see* Sprain, ankle, specified ligament NEC
　　specified ligament NEC S93.49- ☑
　　talofibular ligament — *see* Sprain, ankle, specified ligament NEC
　　tibiofibular ligament S93.43- ☑
　anterior longitudinal, cervical S13.4
　atlas, atlanto-axial, atlanto-occipital S13.4 ☑
　breast bone — *see* Sprain, sternum
　calcaneofibular — *see* Sprain, ankle
　carpal — *see* Sprain, wrist

Index   **Sprain — Stähli's line**

Sprain — *continued*
  carpometacarpal — *see* Sprain, hand, specified site
    NEC
  cartilage
    costal S23.41 ☑
    semilunar (knee) — *see* Sprain, knee, specified site
      NEC
      with current tear — *see* Tear, meniscus
    thyroid region S13.5 ☑
    xiphoid — *see* Sprain, sternum
  cervical, cervicodorsal, cervicothoracic S13.4 ☑
  chondrosternal S23.421 ☑
  coracoclavicular S43.8- ☑
  coracohumeral S43.41- ☑
  coronary, knee — *see* Sprain, knee, specified site NEC
  costal cartilage S23.41 ☑
  cricoarytenoid articulation or ligament S13.5 ☑
  cricothyroid articulation S13.5 ☑
  cruciate, knee — *see* Sprain, knee, cruciate
  deltoid, ankle — *see* Sprain, ankle
  dorsal (spine) S23.3 ☑
  elbow S53.40- ☑
    radial collateral ligament S53.43- ☑
    radiohumeral S53.41- ☑
    rupture
      radial collateral ligament — *see* Rupture, trau-
        matic, ligament, radial collateral
      ulnar collateral ligament — *see* Rupture, trau-
        matic, ligament, ulnar collateral
    specified type NEC S53.49- ☑
    ulnar collateral ligament S53.44- ☑
    ulnohumeral S53.42- ☑
  femur, head — *see* Sprain, hip
  fibular collateral, knee — *see* Sprain, knee, collateral
  fibulocalcaneal — *see* Sprain, ankle
  finger(s) S63.61- ☑
    index S63.61- ☑
    interphalangeal (joint) S63.63- ☑
      index S63.63- ☑
      little S63.63- ☑
      middle S63.63- ☑
      ring S63.63- ☑
    little S63.61- ☑
    metacarpophalangeal (joint) S63.65- ☑
    middle S63.61- ☑
    ring S63.61- ☑
    specified site NEC S63.69- ☑
      index S63.69- ☑
      little S63.69- ☑
      middle S63.69- ☑
      ring S63.69- ☑
  foot S93.60- ☑
    specified ligament NEC S93.69- ☑
    tarsal ligament S93.61- ☑
    tarsometatarsal ligament S93.62- ☑
    toe — *see* Sprain, toe
  hand S63.9- ☑
    finger — *see* Sprain, finger
    specified site NEC — *see* subcategory S63.8 ☑
    thumb — *see* Sprain, thumb
  head S03.9 ☑
  hip S73.10- ☑
    iliofemoral ligament S73.11- ☑
    ischiocapsular (ligament) S73.12- ☑
    specified NEC S73.19- ☑
  iliofemoral — *see* Sprain, hip
  innominate
    acetabulum — *see* Sprain, hip
    sacral junction S33.6 ☑
  internal
    collateral, ankle — *see* Sprain, ankle
    semilunar cartilage — *see* Sprain, knee, specified
      site NEC
  interphalangeal
    finger — *see* Sprain, finger, interphalangeal (joint)
    toe — *see* Sprain, toe, interphalangeal joint
  ischiocapsular — *see* Sprain, hip
  ischiofemoral — *see* Sprain, hip
  jaw (articular disc) (cartilage) (meniscus) S03.4- ☑
    old M26.69
  knee S83.9- ☑
    collateral ligament S83.40- ☑
      lateral (fibular) S83.42- ☑
      medial (tibial) S83.41- ☑
    cruciate ligament S83.50- ☑
      anterior S83.51- ☑

Sprain — *continued*
  knee — *continued*
    cruciate ligament — *continued*
      posterior S83.52- ☑
    lateral (fibular) collateral ligament S83.42- ☑
    medial (tibial) collateral ligament S83.41- ☑
    patellar ligament S76.11- ☑
    specified site NEC S83.8X- ☑
    superior tibiofibular joint (ligament) S83.6- ☑
  lateral collateral, knee — *see* Sprain, knee, collateral
  lumbar (spine) S33.5 ☑
  lumbosacral S33.9 ☑
  mandible (articular disc) S03.4- ☑
    old M26.69
  medial collateral, knee — *see* Sprain, knee, collateral
  meniscus
    jaw S03.4- ☑
      old M26.69
    knee — *see* Sprain, knee, specified site NEC
      with current tear — *see* Tear, meniscus
        old — *see* Derangement, knee, meniscus,
          due to old tear
    mandible S03.4- ☑
      old M26.69
  metacarpal (distal) (proximal) — *see* Sprain, hand,
    specified site NEC
  metacarpophalangeal — *see* Sprain, finger, metacar-
    pophalangeal (joint)
  metatarsophalangeal — *see* Sprain, toe, metatarsopha-
    langeal joint
  midcarpal — *see* Sprain, hand, specified site NEC
  midtarsal — *see* Sprain, foot, specified site NEC
  neck S13.9 ☑
    anterior longitudinal cervical ligament S13.4 ☑
    atlanto-axial joint S13.4 ☑
    atlanto-occipital joint S13.4 ☑
    cervical spine S13.4 ☑
    cricoarytenoid ligament S13.5 ☑
    cricothyroid ligament S13.5 ☑
    specified site NEC S13.8 ☑
    thyroid region (cartilage) S13.5 ☑
  nose S03.8 ☑
  orbicular, hip — *see* Sprain, hip
  patella — *see* Sprain, knee, specified site NEC
  patellar ligament S76.11- ☑
  pelvis NEC S33.8 ☑
  phalanx
    finger — *see* Sprain, finger
    toe — *see* Sprain, toe
  pubofemoral — *see* Sprain, hip
  radiocarpal — *see* Sprain, wrist
  radiohumeral — *see* Sprain, elbow
  radius, collateral — *see* Rupture, traumatic, ligament,
    radial collateral
  rib (cage) S23.41 ☑
  rotator cuff (capsule) S43.42- ☑
  sacroiliac (region)
    chronic or old — *see* subcategory M53.2 ☑
    joint S33.6 ☑
  scaphoid (hand) — *see* Sprain, hand, specified site
    NEC
  scapula (r) — *see* Sprain, shoulder girdle, specified site
    NEC
  semilunar cartilage (knee) — *see* Sprain, knee, speci-
    fied site NEC
    with current tear — *see* Tear, meniscus
      old — *see* Derangement, knee, meniscus, due
        to old tear
  shoulder joint S43.40- ☑
    acromioclavicular joint (ligament) — *see* Sprain,
      acromioclavicular joint
    blade — *see* Sprain, shoulder, girdle, specified site
      NEC
    coracoclavicular joint (ligament) — *see* Sprain,
      coracoclavicular joint
    coracohumeral ligament — *see* Sprain, coraco-
      humeral joint
    girdle S43.9- ☑
      specified site NEC S43.8- ☑
    rotator cuff — *see* Sprain, rotator cuff
    specified site NEC S43.49- ☑
    sternoclavicular joint (ligament) — *see* Sprain,
      sternoclavicular joint
  spine
    cervical S13.4 ☑
    lumbar S33.5 ☑

Sprain — *continued*
  spine — *continued*
    thoracic S23.3 ☑
  sternoclavicular joint S43.6- ☑
  sternum S23.429 ☑
    chondrosternal joint S23.421 ☑
    specified site NEC S23.428 ☑
    sternoclavicular (joint) (ligament) S23.420 ☑
  symphysis
    jaw S03.4- ☑
      old M26.69
    mandibular S03.4- ☑
      old M26.69
  talofibular — *see* Sprain, ankle
  tarsal — *see* Sprain, foot, specified site NEC
  tarsometatarsal — *see* Sprain, foot, specified site NEC
  temporomandibular S03.4- ☑
    old M26.69
  thorax S23.9 ☑
    ribs S23.41 ☑
    specified site NEC S23.8 ☑
    spine S23.3 ☑
    sternum — *see* Sprain, sternum
  thumb S63.60- ☑
    interphalangeal (joint) S63.62- ☑
    metacarpophalangeal (joint) S63.64- ☑
    specified site NEC S63.68- ☑
  thyroid cartilage or region S13.5 ☑
  tibia (proximal end) — *see* Sprain, knee, specified site
    NEC
  tibial collateral, knee — *see* Sprain, knee, collateral
  tibiofibular
    distal — *see* Sprain, ankle
    superior — *see* Sprain, knee, specified site NEC
  toe(s) S93.50- ☑
    great S93.50- ☑
    interphalangeal joint S93.51- ☑
      great S93.51- ☑
      lesser S93.51- ☑
    lesser S93.50- ☑
    metatarsophalangeal joint S93.52- ☑
      great S93.52- ☑
      lesser S93.52- ☑
  ulna, collateral — *see* Rupture, traumatic, ligament,
    ulnar collateral
  ulnohumeral — *see* Sprain, elbow
  wrist S63.50- ☑
    carpal S63.51- ☑
    radiocarpal S63.52- ☑
    specified site NEC S63.59- ☑
  xiphoid cartilage — *see* Sprain, sternum
Sprengel's deformity (congenital) Q74.0
Sprue (tropical) K90.1
  celiac K90.0
  idiopathic K90.49
  meaning thrush B37.0
  nontropical K90.0
Spur, bone (*see also* Enthesopathy)
  calcaneal M77.3- ☑
  iliac crest M76.2- ☑
  nose (septum) J34.89
Spurway's syndrome Q78.0
Sputum
  abnormal (amount) (color) (odor) (purulent) R09.3
  blood-stained R04.2
  excessive (cause unknown) R09.3
Squamous (*see also* condition)
  epithelium in
    cervical canal (congenital) Q51.828
    uterine mucosa (congenital) Q51.818
Squashed nose M95.0
  congenital Q67.4
Squeeze, diver's T70.3 ☑
Squint (*see also* Strabismus)
  accommodative — *see* Strabismus, convergent con-
    comitant
St. Hubert's disease A82.9
Stab (*see also* Laceration)
  internal organs — *see* Injury, by site
Stafne's cyst or cavity M27.0
Staggering gait R26.0
  hysterical F44.4
Staghorn calculus — *see* Calculus, kidney
Stähli's line (cornea) (pigment) — *see* Pigmentation,
  cornea, anterior

Stain, staining
- meconium (newborn) P96.83
- port wine Q82.5
- tooth, teeth (hard tissues) (extrinsic) K03.6
  - due to
    - accretions K03.6
    - deposits (betel) (black) (green) (materia alba) (orange) (soft) (tobacco) K03.6
    - metals (copper) (silver) K03.7
    - nicotine K03.6
    - pulpal bleeding K03.7
    - tobacco K03.6
  - intrinsic K00.8
Stammering (see also Disorder, fluency) F80.81
Standstill
- auricular I45.5
- cardiac — see Arrest, cardiac
- sinoatrial I45.5
- ventricular — see Arrest, cardiac
Stannosis J63.5
Stanton's disease — see Melioidosis
Staphylitis (acute) (catarrhal) (chronic) (gangrenous) (membranous) (suppurative) (ulcerative) K12.2
Staphylococcal scalded skin syndrome L00
Staphylococcemia A41.2
Staphylococcus, staphylococcal (see also condition)
- as cause of disease classified elsewhere B95.8
  - aureus (methicillin susceptible) (MSSA) B95.61
    - methicillin resistant (MRSA) B95.62
  - specified NEC, as cause of disease classified elsewhere B95.7
Staphyloma (sclera)
- cornea H18.72- ☑
- equatorial H15.81- ☑
- localized (anterior) H15.82- ☑
- posticum H15.83- ☑
- ring H15.85- ☑
Stargardt's disease — see Dystrophy, retina
Starvation (inanition) (due to lack of food) T73.0 ☑
- edema — see Malnutrition, severe
Stasis
- bile (noncalculous) K83.1
- bronchus J98.09
  - with infection — see Bronchitis
- cardiac — see Failure, heart, congestive
- cecum K59.8
- colon K59.8
- dermatitis I87.2
  - with
    - varicose ulcer — see Varix, leg, with ulcer, with inflammation
    - varicose veins — see Varix, leg, with, inflammation
    - due to postthrombotic syndrome — see Syndrome, postthrombotic
- duodenal K31.5
- eczema — see Varix, leg, with, inflammation
- edema — see Hypertension, venous (chronic), idiopathic
- foot T69.0- ☑
- ileocecal coil K59.8
- ileum K59.8
- intestinal K59.8
- jejunum K59.8
- kidney N19
- liver (cirrhotic) K76.1
- lymphatic I89.8
- pneumonia J18.2
- pulmonary — see Edema, lung
- rectal K59.8
- renal N19
  - tubular N17.0
- ulcer — see Varix, leg, with, ulcer
  - without varicose veins I87.2
- urine — see Retention, urine
- venous I87.8
State (of)
- affective and paranoid, mixed, organic psychotic F06.8
- agitated R45.1
  - acute reaction to stress F43.0
- anxiety (neurotic) F41.1
- apprehension F41.1
- burn-out Z73.0
- climacteric, female Z78.0
  - symptomatic N95.1
- compulsive F42.8
  - mixed with obsessional thoughts F42.2
- confusional (psychogenic) F44.89

State — continued
- confusional — continued
  - acute (see also Delirium)
    - with
      - arteriosclerotic dementia F01.50
        - with behavioral disturbance F01.51
      - senility or dementia F05
    - alcoholic F10.231
  - epileptic F05
  - reactive (from emotional stress, psychological trauma) F44.89
  - subacute — see Delirium
- convulsive — see Convulsions
- crisis F43.0
- depressive F32.9
  - neurotic F34.1
- dissociative F44.9
- emotional shock (stress) R45.7
- hypercoagulation — see Hypercoagulable
- locked-in G83.5
- menopausal Z78.0
  - symptomatic N95.1
- neurotic F48.9
  - with depersonalization F48.1
- obsessional F42.8
- oneiroid (schizophrenia-like) F23
- organic
  - hallucinatory (nonalcoholic) F06.0
  - paranoid (-hallucinatory) F06.2
- panic F41.0
- paranoid F22
  - climacteric F22
  - involutional F22
  - menopausal F22
  - organic F06.2
  - senile F03 ☑
  - simple F22
- persistent vegetative R40.3
- phobic F40.9
- postleukotomy F07.0
- pregnant
  - gestational carrier Z33.3
  - incidental Z33.1
- psychogenic, twilight F44.89
- psychopathic (constitutional) F60.2
- psychotic, organic (see also Psychosis, organic)
  - mixed paranoid and affective F06.8
  - senile or presenile F03 ☑
  - transient NEC F06.8
    - with
      - depression F06.31
      - hallucinations F06.0
- residual schizophrenic F20.5
- restlessness R45.1
- stress (emotional) R45.7
- tension (mental) F48.9
  - specified NEC F48.8
- transient organic psychotic NEC F06.8
  - depressive type F06.31
  - hallucinatory type F06.0
- twilight
  - epileptic F05
  - psychogenic F44.89
- vegetative, persistent R40.3
- vital exhaustion Z73.0
- withdrawal, — see Withdrawal, state
Status (post) (see also Presence (of))
- absence, epileptic — see Epilepsy, by type, with status epilepticus
- administration of tPA (rtPA) in a different facility within the last 24 hours prior to admission to current facility Z92.82
- adrenalectomy (unilateral) (bilateral) E89.6
- anastomosis Z98.0
- anginosus I20.9
- angioplasty (peripheral) Z98.62
  - with implant Z95.820
  - coronary artery Z98.61
    - with implant Z95.5
- aortocoronary bypass Z95.1
- arthrodesis Z98.1
- artificial opening (of) Z93.9
  - gastrointestinal tract Z93.4
  - specified NEC Z93.8
  - urinary tract Z93.6
  - vagina Z93.8
- asthmaticus — see Asthma, by type, with status asthmaticus

Status — continued
- awaiting organ transplant Z76.82
- bariatric surgery Z98.84
- bed confinement Z74.01
- bleb, filtering (vitreous), after glaucoma surgery Z98.83
- breast implant Z98.82
  - removal Z98.86
- cataract extraction Z98.4- ☑
- cholecystectomy Z90.49
- clitorectomy N90.811
  - with excision of labia minora N90.812
- colectomy (complete) (partial) Z90.49
- colonization — see Carrier (suspected) of
- colostomy Z93.3
- convulsivus idiopathicus — see Epilepsy, by type, with status epilepticus
- coronary artery angioplasty — see Status, angioplasty, coronary artery
- coronary artery bypass graft Z95.1
- cystectomy (urinary bladder) Z90.6
- cystostomy Z93.50
  - appendico-vesicostomy Z93.52
  - cutaneous Z93.51
  - specified NEC Z93.59
- delinquent immunization Z28.3
- dental Z98.818
  - crown Z98.811
  - fillings Z98.811
  - restoration Z98.811
  - sealant Z98.810
  - specified NEC Z98.818
- deployment (current) (military) Z56.82
- dialysis (hemodialysis) (peritoneal) Z99.2
- do not resuscitate (DNR) Z66
- donor — see Donor
- embedded fragments — see Retained, foreign body fragments (type of)
- embedded splinter — see Retained, foreign body fragments (type of)
- enterostomy Z93.4
- epileptic, epilepticus (see also Epilepsy, by type, with status epilepticus) G40.901
- estrogen receptor
  - negative Z17.1
  - positive Z17.0
- female genital cutting — see Female genital mutilation status
- female genital mutilation — see Female genital mutilation status
- filtering (vitreous) bleb after glaucoma surgery Z98.83
- gastrectomy (complete) (partial) Z90.3
- gastric banding Z98.84
- gastric bypass for obesity Z98.84
- gastrostomy Z93.1
- human immunodeficiency virus (HIV) infection, asymptomatic Z21
- hysterectomy (complete) (total) Z90.710
  - partial (with remaining cervial stump) Z90.711
- ileostomy Z93.2
- implant
  - breast Z98.82
- infibulation N90.813
- intestinal bypass Z98.0
- jejunostomy Z93.4
- lapsed immunization schedule Z28.3
- laryngectomy Z90.02
- lymphaticus E32.8
- malignancy
  - castrate resistant prostate Z19.2
  - hormone resistant Z19.2
  - hormone sensitive Z19.1
- marmoratus G80.3
- mastectomy (unilateral) (bilateral) Z90.1- ☑
- military deployment status (current) Z56.82
  - in theater or in support of military war, peacekeeping and humanitarian operations Z56.82
- nephrectomy (unilateral) (bilateral) Z90.5
- nephrostomy Z93.6
- obesity surgery Z98.84
- oophorectomy
  - bilateral Z90.722
  - unilateral Z90.721
- organ replacement
  - by artificial or mechanical device or prosthesis of
    - artery Z95.828
    - bladder Z96.0
    - blood vessel Z95.828
    - breast Z97.8

Status — *continued*
- organ replacement — *continued*
  - by artificial or mechanical device or prosthesis of — *continued*
    - eye globe Z97.0
    - heart Z95.812
      - valve Z95.2
    - intestine Z97.8
    - joint Z96.60
      - hip — *see* Presence, hip joint implant
      - knee — *see* Presence, knee joint implant
      - specified site NEC Z96.698
    - kidney Z97.8
    - larynx Z96.3
    - lens Z96.1
    - limbs — *see* Presence, artificial, limb
    - liver Z97.8
    - lung Z97.8
    - pancreas Z97.8
  - by organ transplant (heterologous)(homologous) — *see* Transplant
- pacemaker
  - brain Z96.89
  - cardiac Z95.0
  - specified NEC Z96.89
- pancreatectomy Z90.410
  - complete Z90.410
  - partial Z90.411
  - total Z90.410
- physical restraint Z78.1
- pneumonectomy (complete) (partial) Z90.2
- pneumothorax, therapeutic Z98.3
- postcommotio cerebri F07.81
- postoperative (postprocedural) NEC Z98.890
  - breast implant Z98.82
  - dental Z98.818
    - crown Z98.811
    - fillings Z98.811
    - restoration Z98.811
    - sealant Z98.810
    - specified NEC Z98.818
  - pneumothorax, therapeutic Z98.3
  - uterine scar Z98.891
- postpartum (routine follow-up) Z39.2
  - care immediately after delivery Z39.0
- postsurgical (postprocedural) NEC Z98.890
  - pneumothorax, therapeutic Z98.3
- pregnancy, incidental Z33.1
- prosthesis coronary angioplasty Z95.5
- pseudophakia Z96.1
- renal dialysis (hemodialysis) (peritoneal) Z99.2
- retained foreign body — *see* Retained, foreign body fragments (type of)
- reversed jejunal transposition (for bypass) Z98.0
- salpingo-oophorectomy
  - bilateral Z90.722
  - unilateral Z90.721
- sex reassignment surgery status Z87.890
- shunt
  - arteriovenous (for dialysis) Z99.2
  - cerebrospinal fluid Z98.2
  - ventricular (communicating) (for drainage) Z98.2
- splenectomy Z90.81
- thymicolymphaticus E32.8
- thymicus E32.8
- thymolymphaticus E32.8
- thyroidectomy (hypothyroidism) E89.0
- tooth (teeth) extraction (*see also* Absence, teeth, acquired) K08.409
- tPA (rtPA) administration in a different facility within the last 24 hours prior to admission to current facility Z92.82
- tracheostomy Z93.0
- transplant — *see* Transplant
  - organ removed Z98.85
- tubal ligation Z98.51
- underimmunization Z28.3
- ureterostomy Z93.6
- urethrostomy Z93.6
- vagina, artificial Z93.8
- vasectomy Z98.52
- wheelchair confinement Z99.3

Stealing
- child problem F91.8
  - in company with others Z72.810
- pathological (compulsive) F63.2

Steam burn — *see* Burn

Steatocystoma multiplex L72.2

Steatohepatitis (nonalcoholic) (NASH) K75.81

Steatoma L72.3
- eyelid (cystic) — *see* Dermatosis, eyelid
  - infected — *see* Hordeolum

Steatorrhea (chronic) K90.9
- with lacteal obstruction K90.2
- idiopathic (adult) (infantile) K90.9
- pancreatic K90.3
- primary K90.0
- tropical K90.1

Steatosis E88.89
- heart — *see* Degeneration, myocardial
- kidney N28.89
- liver NEC K76.0

Steele-Richardson-Olszewski disease or syndrome G23.1

Steinbrocker's syndrome G90.8

Steinert's disease G71.11

Stein-Leventhal syndrome E28.2

Stein's syndrome E28.2

STEMI (*see also* Infarct, myocardium, ST elevation) I21.3

Stenocardia I20.8

Stenocephaly Q75.8

Stenosis, stenotic (cicatricial) (*see also* Stricture)
- ampulla of Vater K83.1
- anus, anal (canal) (sphincter) K62.4
  - and rectum K62.4
  - congenital Q42.3
    - with fistula Q42.2
- aorta (ascending) (supraventricular) (congenital) Q25.1
  - arteriosclerotic I70.0
  - calcified I70.0
  - supravalvular Q25.3
- aortic (valve) I35.0
  - with insufficiency I35.2
  - congenital Q23.0
  - rheumatic I06.0
    - with
      - incompetency, insufficiency or regurgitation I06.2
        - with mitral (valve) disease I08.0
          - with tricuspid (valve) disease I08.3
      - mitral (valve) disease I08.0
        - with tricuspid (valve) disease I08.3
      - tricuspid (valve) disease I08.2
        - with mitral (valve) disease I08.3
  - specified cause NEC I35.0
  - syphilitic A52.03
- aqueduct of Sylvius (congenital) Q03.0
  - with spina bifida — *see* Spina bifida, by site, with hydrocephalus
  - acquired G91.1
- artery NEC (*see also* Arteriosclerosis) I77.1
  - celiac I77.4
  - cerebral — *see* Occlusion, artery, cerebral
  - extremities — *see* Arteriosclerosis, extremities
  - precerebral — *see* Occlusion, artery, precerebral
  - pulmonary (congenital) Q25.6
    - acquired I28.8
  - renal I70.1
  - stent
    - coronary T82.855 ☑
    - peripheral T82.856 ☑
- bile duct (common) (hepatic) K83.1
  - congenital Q44.3
- bladder-neck (acquired) N32.0
  - congenital Q64.31
- brain G93.89
- bronchus J98.09
  - congenital Q32.3
  - syphilitic A52.72
- cardia (stomach) K22.2
  - congenital Q39.3
- cardiovascular — *see* Disease, cardiovascular
- caudal M48.08
- cervix, cervical (canal) N88.2
  - congenital Q51.828
  - in pregnancy or childbirth — *see* Pregnancy, complicated by, abnormal cervix
- colon (*see also* Obstruction, intestine)
  - congenital Q42.9
    - specified NEC Q42.8
- colostomy K94.03
- common (bile) duct K83.1
  - congenital Q44.3
- coronary (artery) — *see* Disease, heart, ischemic, atherosclerotic
- cystic duct — *see* Obstruction, gallbladder

Stenosis, stenotic — *continued*
- due to presence of device, implant or graft (*see also* Complications, by site and type, specified NEC) T85.858 ☑
  - arterial graft NEC T82.858 ☑
  - breast (implant) T85.858 ☑
  - catheter T85.858 ☑
    - dialysis (renal) T82.858 ☑
      - intraperitoneal T85.858 ☑
    - infusion NEC T82.858 ☑
      - spinal (epidural) (subdural) T85.850 ☑
    - urinary (indwelling) T83.85 ☑
  - fixation, internal (orthopedic) NEC T84.85 ☑
  - gastrointestinal (bile duct) (esophagus) T85.858 ☑
  - genital NEC T83.85 ☑
  - heart NEC T82.857 ☑
  - joint prosthesis T84.85 ☑
  - ocular (corneal graft) (orbital implant) NEC T85.858 ☑
  - orthopedic NEC T84.85 ☑
  - specified NEC T85.858 ☑
  - urinary NEC T83.85 ☑
  - vascular NEC T82.858 ☑
  - ventricular intracranial shunt T85.850 ☑
- duodenum K31.5
  - congenital Q41.0
- ejaculatory duct NEC N50.89
  - stent
    - vascular
      - end stent
        - adjacent to stent — *see* Arteriosclerosis
        - within the stent
          - coronary T82.855 ☑
          - peripheral T82.856 ☑
      - in stent
        - coronary vessel T82.855 ☑
        - peripheral vessel T82.856 ☑
- endocervical os — *see* Stenosis, cervix
- enterostomy K94.13
- esophagus K22.2
  - congenital Q39.3
  - syphilitic A52.79
    - congenital A50.59 [K23]
- eustachian tube — *see* Obstruction, eustachian tube
- external ear canal (acquired) H61.30- ☑
  - congenital Q16.1
  - due to
    - inflammation H61.32- ☑
    - trauma H61.31- ☑
  - postprocedural H95.81- ☑
  - specified cause NEC H61.39- ☑
- gallbladder — *see* Obstruction, gallbladder
- glottis J38.6
- heart valve (congenital) Q24.8
  - aortic Q23.0
  - mitral Q23.2
  - pulmonary Q22.1
  - tricuspid Q22.4
- hepatic duct K83.1
- hymen N89.6
- hypertrophic subaortic (idiopathic) I42.1
- ileum (*see also* Obstruction, intestine, specified NEC) K56.699
  - congenital Q41.2
- infundibulum cardia Q24.3
- intervertebral foramina (*see also* Lesion, biomechanical, specified NEC)
  - connective tissue M99.79
    - abdomen M99.79
    - cervical region M99.71
    - cervicothoracic M99.71
    - head region M99.70
    - lumbar region M99.73
    - lumbosacral M99.73
    - occipitocervical M99.70
    - sacral region M99.74
    - sacrococcygeal M99.74
    - sacroiliac M99.74
    - specified NEC M99.79
    - thoracic region M99.72
    - thoracolumbar M99.72
  - disc M99.79
    - abdomen M99.79
    - cervical region M99.71
    - cervicothoracic M99.71
    - head region M99.70
    - lower extremity M99.76

☑ Additional Character Required — Refer to the Tabular List for Character Selection   ▽ Subterms under main terms may continue to next column or page

Stenosis, stenotic — *continued*
  intervertebral foramina (*see also* Lesion, biomechanical, specified) — *continued*
    disc — *continued*
      lumbar region M99.73
      lumbosacral M99.73
      occipitocervical M99.70
      pelvic M99.75
      rib cage M99.78
      sacral region M99.74
      sacrococcygeal M99.74
      sacroiliac M99.74
      specified NEC M99.79
      thoracic region M99.72
      thoracolumbar M99.72
      upper extremity M99.77
    osseous M99.69
      abdomen M99.69
      cervical region M99.61
      cervicothoracic M99.61
      head region M99.60
      lower extremity M99.66
      lumbar region M99.63
      lumbosacral M99.63
      occipitocervical M99.60
      pelvic M99.65
      rib cage M99.68
      sacral region M99.64
      sacrococcygeal M99.64
      sacroiliac M99.64
      specified NEC M99.69
      thoracic region M99.62
      thoracolumbar M99.62
      upper extremity M99.67
    subluxation — *see* Stenosis, intervertebral foramina, osseous
  intestine (*see also* Obstruction, intestine)
    congenital (small) Q41.9
      large Q42.9
        specified NEC Q42.8
      specified NEC Q41.8
  jejunum (*see also* Obstruction, intestine, specified NEC) K56.699
    congenital Q41.1
  lacrimal (passage)
    canaliculi H04.54- ☑
    congenital Q10.5
    duct H04.55- ☑
    punctum H04.56- ☑
    sac H04.57- ☑
  lacrimonasal duct — *see* Stenosis, lacrimal, duct
    congenital Q10.5
  larynx J38.6
    congenital NEC Q31.8
      subglottic Q31.1
    syphilitic A52.73
      congenital A50.59 [J99]
  mitral (chronic) (inactive) (valve) I05.0
    with
      aortic valve disease I08.0
      incompetency, insufficiency or regurgitation I05.2
    active or acute I01.1
      with rheumatic or Sydenham's chorea I02.0
    congenital Q23.2
    specified cause, except rheumatic I34.2
    syphilitic A52.03
  myocardium, myocardial (*see also* Degeneration, myocardial)
    hypertrophic subaortic (idiopathic) I42.1
  nares (anterior) (posterior) J34.89
    congenital Q30.0
  nasal duct (*see also* Stenosis, lacrimal, duct)
    congenital Q10.5
  nasolacrimal duct (*see also* Stenosis, lacrimal, duct)
    congenital Q10.5
  neural canal (*see also* Lesion, biomechanical, specified NEC)
    connective tissue M99.49
      abdomen M99.49
      cervical region M99.41
      cervicothoracic M99.41
      head region M99.40
      lower extremity M99.46
      lumbar region M99.43
      lumbosacral M99.43
      occipitocervical M99.40
      pelvic M99.45

Stenosis, stenotic — *continued*
  neural canal (*see also* Lesion, biomechanical, specified) — *continued*
    connective tissue — *continued*
      rib cage M99.48
      sacral region M99.44
      sacrococcygeal M99.44
      sacroiliac M99.44
      specified NEC M99.49
      thoracic region M99.42
      thoracolumbar M99.42
      upper extremity M99.47
    intervertebral disc M99.59
      abdomen M99.59
      cervical region M99.51
      cervicothoracic M99.51
      head region M99.50
      lower extremity M99.56
      lumbar region M99.53
      lumbosacral M99.53
      occipitocervical M99.50
      pelvic M99.55
      rib cage M99.58
      sacral region M99.54
      sacrococcygeal M99.54
      sacroiliac M99.54
      specified NEC M99.59
      thoracic region M99.52
      thoracolumbar M99.52
      upper extremity M99.57
    osseous M99.39
      abdomen M99.39
      cervical region M99.31
      cervicothoracic M99.31
      head region M99.30
      lower extremity M99.36
      lumbar region M99.33
      lumbosacral M99.33
      occipitocervical M99.30
      pelvic M99.35
      rib cage M99.38
      sacral region M99.34
      sacrococcygeal M99.34
      sacroiliac M99.34
      specified NEC M99.39
      thoracic region M99.32
      thoracolumbar M99.32
      upper extremity M99.37
    subluxation M99.29
      cervical region M99.21
      cervicothoracic M99.21
      head region M99.20
      lower extremity M99.26
      lumbar region M99.23
      lumbosacral M99.23
      occipitocervical M99.20
      pelvic M99.25
      rib cage M99.28
      sacral region M99.24
      sacrococcygeal M99.24
      sacroiliac M99.24
      specified NEC M99.29
      thoracic region M99.22
      thoracolumbar M99.22
      upper extremity M99.27
  organ or site, congenital NEC — *see* Atresia, by site
  papilla of Vater K83.1
  pulmonary (artery) (congenital) Q25.6
    with ventricular septal defect, transposition of aorta, and hypertrophy of right ventricle Q21.3
    acquired I28.8
    in tetralogy of Fallot Q21.3
    infundibular Q24.3
    subvalvular Q24.3
    supravalvular Q25.6
    valve I37.0
      with insufficiency I37.2
      congenital Q22.1
      rheumatic I09.89
        with aortic, mitral or tricuspid (valve) disease I08.8
    vein, acquired I28.8
    vessel NEC I28.8
  pulmonic (congenital) Q22.1
    infundibular Q24.3
    subvalvular Q24.3
  pylorus (hypertrophic) (acquired) K31.1
    adult K31.1

Stenosis, stenotic — *continued*
  pylorus — *continued*
    congenital Q40.0
    infantile Q40.0
  rectum (sphincter) — *see* Stricture, rectum
  renal artery I70.1
    congenital Q27.1
  salivary duct (any) K11.8
  sphincter of Oddi K83.1
  spinal M48.00
    cervical region M48.02
    cervicothoracic region M48.03
    lumbar region (NOS) (without neurogenic claudication) M48.061
      with neurogenic claudication M48.062
    lumbosacral region M48.07
    occipito-atlanto-axial region M48.01
    sacrococcygeal region M48.08
    thoracic region M48.04
    thoracolumbar region M48.05
  stomach, hourglass K31.2
  subaortic (congenital) Q24.4
    hypertrophic (idiopathic) I42.1
  subglottic J38.6
    congenital Q31.1
    postprocedural J95.5
  trachea J39.8
    congenital Q32.1
    syphilitic A52.73
    tuberculous NEC A15.5
  tracheostomy J95.03
  tricuspid (valve) I07.0
    with
      aortic (valve) disease I08.2
      incompetency, insufficiency or regurgitation I07.2
        with aortic (valve) disease I08.2
          with mitral (valve) disease I08.3
      mitral (valve) disease I08.1
        with aortic (valve) disease I08.3
    congenital Q22.4
    nonrheumatic I36.0
      with insufficiency I36.2
  tubal N97.1
  ureter — *see* Atresia, ureter
  ureteropelvic junction, congenital Q62.11
  ureterovesical orifice, congenital Q62.12
  urethra (valve) (*see also* Stricture, urethra)
    congenital Q64.32
  urinary meatus, congenital Q64.33
  vagina N89.5
    congenital Q52.4
    in pregnancy — *see* Pregnancy, complicated by, abnormal vagina
      causing obstructed labor O65.5
  valve (cardiac) (heart) (*see also* Endocarditis) I38
    congenital Q24.8
      aortic Q23.0
      mitral Q23.2
      pulmonary Q22.1
      tricuspid Q22.4
  vena cava (inferior) (superior) I87.1
    congenital Q26.0
  vesicourethral orifice Q64.31
  vulva N90.5
Stent jail T82.897 ☑
Stercolith (impaction) K56.41
  appendix K38.1
Stercoraceous, stercoral ulcer K63.3
  anus or rectum K62.6
Stereotypies NEC F98.4
Sterility — *see* Infertility
Sterilization — *see* Encounter (for), sterilization
Sternalgia — *see* Angina
Sternopagus Q89.4
Sternum bifidum Q76.7
Steroid
  effects (adverse) (adrenocortical) (iatrogenic)
    cushingoid E24.2
      correct substance properly administered — *see* Table of Drugs and Chemicals, by drug, adverse effect
      overdose or wrong substance given or taken — *see* Table of Drugs and Chemicals, by drug, poisoning
    diabetes — *see* subcategory E09 ☑

▽ Subterms under main terms may continue to next column or page   ☑ Additional Character Required — Refer to the Tabular List for Character Selection   293

Stenosis, stenotic — Steroid

Steroid — *continued*
effects — *continued*
diabetes — *see* subcategory — *continued*
correct substance properly administered — *see* Table of Drugs and Chemicals, by drug, adverse effect
overdose or wrong substance given or taken — *see* Table of Drugs and Chemicals, by drug, poisoning
fever R50.2
insufficiency E27.3
correct substance properly administered — *see* Table of Drugs and Chemicals, by drug, adverse effect
overdose or wrong substance given or taken — *see* Table of Drugs and Chemicals, by drug, poisoning
responder H40.04- ☑
Stevens-Johnson disease or syndrome L51.1
toxic epidermal necrolysis overlap L51.3
Stewart-Morel syndrome M85.2
Sticker's disease B08.3
Sticky eye — *see* Conjunctivitis, acute, mucopurulent
Stieda's disease — *see* Bursitis, tibial collateral
Stiff neck — *see* Torticollis
Stiff-man syndrome G25.82
Stiffness, joint NEC M25.60
ankle M25.67- ☑
ankylosis — *see* Ankylosis, joint
contracture — *see* Contraction, joint
elbow M25.62- ☑
foot M25.67- ☑
hand M25.64- ☑
hip M25.65- ☑
knee M25.66- ☑
shoulder M25.61- ☑
wrist M25.63- ☑
Stigmata congenital syphilis A50.59
Stillbirth P95
Still-Felty syndrome — *see* Felty's syndrome
Still's disease or syndrome (juvenile) M08.20
adult-onset M06.1
ankle M08.27- ☑
elbow M08.22- ☑
foot joint M08.27- ☑
hand joint M08.24- ☑
hip M08.25- ☑
knee M08.26- ☑
multiple site M08.29
shoulder M08.21- ☑
vertebra M08.28
wrist M08.23- ☑
Stimulation, ovary E28.1
Sting (venomous) (with allergic or anaphylactic shock) — *see* Table of Drugs and Chemicals, by animal or substance, poisoning
Stippled epiphyses Q78.8
Stitch
abscess T81.4 ☑
burst (in operation wound) — *see* Disruption, wound, operation
Stokes' disease E05.00
with thyroid storm E05.01
Stokes-Adams disease or syndrome I45.9
Stokvis (-Talma) **disease** D74.8
Stoma malfunction
colostomy K94.03
enterostomy K94.13
gastrostomy K94.23
ileostomy K94.13
tracheostomy J95.03
Stomach — *see* condition
Stomatitis (denture) (ulcerative) K12.1
angular K13.0
due to dietary or vitamin deficiency E53.0
aphthous K12.0
bovine B08.61
candidal B37.0
catarrhal K12.1
diphtheritic A36.89
due to
dietary deficiency E53.0
thrush B37.0
vitamin deficiency
B group NEC E53.9
B2 (riboflavin) E53.0
epidemic B08.8

Stomatitis — *continued*
epizootic B08.8
follicular K12.1
gangrenous A69.0
Geotrichum B48.3
herpesviral, herpetic B00.2
herpetiformis K12.0
malignant K12.1
membranous acute K12.1
monilial B37.0
mycotic B37.0
necrotizing ulcerative A69.0
parasitic B37.0
septic K12.1
spirochetal A69.1
suppurative (acute) K12.2
ulceromembranous A69.1
vesicular K12.1
with exanthem (enteroviral) B08.4
virus disease A93.8
Vincent's A69.1
Stomatocytosis D58.8
Stomatomycosis B37.0
Stomatorrhagia K13.79
Stone(s) (*see also* Calculus)
bladder (diverticulum) N21.0
cystine E72.09
heart syndrome I50.1
kidney N20.0
prostate N42.0
pulpal (dental) K04.2
renal N20.0
salivary gland or duct (any) K11.5
urethra (impacted) N21.1
urinary (duct) (impacted) (passage) N20.9
bladder (diverticulum) N21.0
lower tract N21.9
specified NEC N21.8
xanthine E79.8 [N22]
Stonecutter's lung J62.8
Stonemason's asthma, disease, lung or pneumoconiosis J62.8
Stoppage
heart — *see* Arrest, cardiac
urine — *see* Retention, urine
Storm, thyroid — *see* Thyrotoxicosis
Strabismus (congenital) (nonparalytic) H50.9
concomitant H50.40
convergent — *see* Strabismus, convergent concomitant
divergent — *see* Strabismus, divergent concomitant
convergent concomitant H50.00
accommodative component H50.43
alternating H50.05
with
A pattern H50.06
specified nonconcomitances NEC H50.08
V pattern H50.07
monocular H50.01- ☑
with
A pattern H50.02- ☑
specified nonconcomitances NEC H50.04- ☑
V pattern H50.03- ☑
intermittent H50.31- ☑
alternating H50.32
cyclotropia H50.41 ☑
divergent concomitant H50.10
alternating H50.15
with
A pattern H50.16
specified nonconcomitances NEC H50.18
V pattern H50.17
monocular H50.11- ☑
with
A pattern H50.12- ☑
specified nonconcomitances NEC H50.14- ☑
V pattern H50.13- ☑
intermittent H50.33 ☑
alternating H50.34
Duane's syndrome H50.81- ☑
due to adhesions, scars H50.69
heterophoria H50.50
alternating H50.55
cyclophoria H50.54
esophoria H50.51
exophoria H50.52
vertical H50.53

Strabismus — *continued*
heterotropia H50.40
intermittent H50.30
hypertropia H50.2- ☑
hypotropia — *see* Hypertropia
latent H50.50
mechanical H50.60
Brown's sheath syndrome H50.61- ☑
specified type NEC H50.69
monofixation syndrome H50.42
paralytic H49.9
abducens nerve H49.2- ☑
fourth nerve H49.1- ☑
Kearns-Sayre syndrome H49.81- ☑
ophthalmoplegia (external)
progressive H49.4- ☑
with pigmentary retinopathy H49.81- ☑
total H49.3- ☑
sixth nerve H49.2- ☑
specified type NEC H49.88- ☑
third nerve H49.0- ☑
trochlear nerve H49.1- ☑
specified type NEC H50.89
vertical H50.2- ☑
Strain
back S39.012 ☑
cervical S16.1 ☑
eye NEC — *see* Disturbance, vision, subjective
heart — *see* Disease, heart
low back S39.012 ☑
mental NOS Z73.3
work-related Z56.6
muscle (tendon) — *see* Injury, muscle, by site, strain
neck S16.1 ☑
physical NOS Z73.3
work-related Z56.6
postural (*see also* Disorder, soft tissue, due to use)
psychological NEC Z73.3
tendon — *see* Injury, muscle, by site, strain
Straining, on urination R39.16
Strand, vitreous — *see* Opacity, vitreous, membranes and strands
Strangulation, strangulated (*see also* Asphyxia, traumatic)
appendix K38.8
bladder-neck N32.0
bowel or colon K56.2
food or foreign body — *see* Foreign body, by site
hemorrhoids — *see* Hemorrhoids, with complication
hernia (*see also* Hernia, by site, with obstruction)
with gangrene — *see* Hernia, by site, with gangrene
intestine (large) (small) K56.2
with hernia (*see also* Hernia, by site, with obstruction)
with gangrene — *see* Hernia, by site, with gangrene
mesentery K56.2
mucus — *see* Asphyxia, mucus
omentum K56.2
organ or site, congenital NEC — *see* Atresia, by site
ovary — *see* Torsion, ovary
penis N48.89
foreign body T19.4 ☑
rupture — *see* Hernia, by site, with obstruction
stomach due to hernia (*see also* Hernia, by site, with obstruction)
with gangrene — *see* Hernia, by site, with gangrene
vesicourethral orifice N32.0
Strangury R30.0
Straw itch B88.0
Strawberry
gallbladder K82.4
mark Q82.5
tongue (red) (white) K14.3
Streak(s)
macula, angioid H35.33
ovarian Q50.32
Strephosymbolia F81.0
secondary to organic lesion R48.8
Streptobacillary fever A25.1
Streptobacillosis A25.1
Streptobacillus moniliformis A25.1
Streptococcus, streptococcal (*see also* condition)
as cause of disease classified elsewhere B95.5

☑ Additional Character Required — Refer to the Tabular List for Character Selection ▽ Subterms under main terms may continue to next column or page

Streptococcus, streptococcal — *continued*
  group
    A, as cause of disease classified elsewhere B95.0
    B, as cause of disease classified elsewhere B95.1
    D, as cause of disease classified elsewhere B95.2
  pneumoniae, as cause of disease classified elsewhere
    B95.3
  specified NEC, as cause of disease classified elsewhere
    B95.4
Streptomycosis B47.1
Streptotrichosis A48.8
Stress F43.9
  family — *see* Disruption, family
  fetal P84
    complicating pregnancy O77.9
      due to drug administration O77.1
  mental NEC Z73.3
    work-related Z56.6
  physical NEC Z73.3
    work-related Z56.6
  polycythemia D75.1
  reaction (*see also* Reaction, stress) F43.9
  work schedule Z56.3
Stretching, nerve — *see* Injury, nerve
Striae albicantes, atrophicae or distensae (cutis) L90.6
Stricture (*see also* Stenosis)
  ampulla of Vater K83.1
  anus (sphincter) K62.4
    congenital Q42.3
      with fistula Q42.2
    infantile Q42.3
      with fistula Q42.2
  aorta (ascending) (congenital) Q25.1
    arteriosclerotic I70.0
    calcified I70.0
    supravalvular, congenital Q25.3
  aortic (valve) — *see* Stenosis, aortic
  aqueduct of Sylvius (congenital) Q03.0
    with spina bifida — *see* Spina bifida, by site, with
      hydrocephalus
    acquired G91.1
  artery I77.1
    basilar — *see* Occlusion, artery, basilar
    carotid — *see* Occlusion, artery, carotid
    celiac I77.4
    congenital (peripheral) Q27.8
      cerebral Q28.3
      coronary Q24.5
      digestive system Q27.8
      lower limb Q27.8
      retinal Q14.1
      specified site NEC Q27.8
      umbilical Q27.0
      upper limb Q27.8
    coronary — *see* Disease, heart, ischemic,
      atherosclerotic
      congenital Q24.5
    precerebral — *see* Occlusion, artery, precerebral
    pulmonary (congenital) Q25.6
      acquired I28.8
    renal I70.1
    vertebral — *see* Occlusion, artery, vertebral
  auditory canal (external) (congenital)
    acquired — *see* Stenosis, external ear canal
  bile duct (common) (hepatic) K83.1
    congenital Q44.3
    postoperative K91.89
  bladder N32.89
    neck N32.0
  bowel — *see* Obstruction, intestine
  brain G93.89
  bronchus J98.09
    congenital Q32.3
    syphilitic A52.72
  cardia (stomach) K22.2
    congenital Q39.3
  cardiac (*see also* Disease, heart)
    orifice (stomach) K22.2
  cecum — *see* Obstruction, intestine
  cervix, cervical (canal) N88.2
    congenital Q51.828
    in pregnancy — *see* Pregnancy, complicated by,
      abnormal cervix
        causing obstructed labor O65.5
  colon (*see also* Obstruction, intestine)
    congenital Q42.9
      specified NEC Q42.8
  colostomy K94.03

Stricture — *continued*
  common (bile) duct K83.1
  coronary (artery) — *see* Disease, heart, ischemic,
    atherosclerotic
  cystic duct — *see* Obstruction, gallbladder
  digestive organs NEC, congenital Q45.8
  duodenum K31.5
    congenital Q41.0
  ear canal (external) (congenital) Q16.1
    acquired — *see* Stricture, auditory canal, acquired
  ejaculatory duct N50.89
  enterostomy K94.13
  esophagus K22.2
    congenital Q39.3
    syphilitic A52.79
      congenital A50.59 [K23]
  eustachian tube (*see also* Obstruction, eustachian tube)
    congenital Q17.8
  fallopian tube N97.1
    gonococcal A54.24
    tuberculous A18.17
  gallbladder — *see* Obstruction, gallbladder
  glottis J38.6
  heart (*see also* Disease, heart)
    valve (*see also* Endocarditis) I38
      aortic Q23.0
      mitral Q23.2
      pulmonary Q22.1
      tricuspid Q22.4
  hepatic duct K83.1
  hourglass, of stomach K31.2
  hymen N89.6
  hypopharynx J39.2
  ileum (*see also* Obstruction, intestine, specified NEC)
    K56.699
    congenital Q41.2
  intestine (*see also* Obstruction, intestine)
    congenital (small) Q41.9
      large Q42.9
        specified NEC Q42.8
      specified NEC Q41.8
    ischemic K55.1
  jejunum (*see also* Obstruction, intestine, specified NEC)
    K56.699
    congenital Q41.1
  lacrimal passages (*see also* Stenosis, lacrimal)
    congenital Q10.5
  larynx J38.6
    congenital NEC Q31.8
      subglottic Q31.1
    syphilitic A52.73
      congenital A50.59 [J99]
  meatus
    ear (congenital) Q16.1
      acquired — *see* Stricture, auditory canal, ac-
        quired
    osseous (ear) (congenital) Q16.1
      acquired — *see* Stricture, auditory canal, ac-
        quired
    urinarius (*see also* Stricture, urethra)
      congenital Q64.33
  mitral (valve) — *see* Stenosis, mitral
  myocardium, myocardial I51.5
    hypertrophic subaortic (idiopathic) I42.1
  nares (anterior) (posterior) J34.89
    congenital Q30.0
  nasal duct (*see also* Stenosis, lacrimal, duct)
    congenital Q10.5
  nasolacrimal duct (*see also* Stenosis, lacrimal, duct)
    congenital Q10.5
  nasopharynx J39.2
    syphilitic A52.73
  nose J34.89
    congenital Q30.0
  nostril (anterior) (posterior) J34.89
    congenital Q30.0
    syphilitic A52.73
      congenital A50.59 [J99]
  organ or site, congenital NEC — *see* Atresia, by site
  os uteri — *see* Stricture, cervix
  osseous meatus (ear) (congenital) Q16.1
    acquired — *see* Stricture, auditory canal, acquired
  oviduct — *see* Stricture, fallopian tube
  pelviureteric junction (congenital) Q62.11
    acquired, with hydronephrosis N13.0
  penis, by foreign body T19.4 ☑
  pharynx J39.2
  prostate N42.89

Stricture — *continued*
  pulmonary, pulmonic
    artery (congenital) Q25.6
      acquired I28.8
      noncongenital I28.8
    infundibulum (congenital) Q24.3
    valve I37.0
      congenital Q22.1
    vein, acquired I28.8
    vessel NEC I28.8
  punctum lacrimale (*see also* Stenosis, lacrimal, punc-
    tum)
    congenital Q10.5
  pylorus (hypertrophic) K31.1
    adult K31.1
    congenital Q40.0
    infantile Q40.0
  rectosigmoid (*see also* Obstruction, intestine, specified
    NEC) K56.699
  rectum (sphincter) K62.4
    congenital Q42.1
      with fistula Q42.0
    due to
      chlamydial lymphogranuloma A55
      irradiation K91.89
      lymphogranuloma venereum A55
    gonococcal A54.6
    inflammatory (chlamydial) A55
    syphilitic A52.74
    tuberculous A18.32
  renal artery I70.1
    congenital Q27.1
  salivary duct or gland (any) K11.8
  sigmoid (flexure) — *see* Obstruction, intestine
  spermatic cord N50.89
  stoma (following) (of)
    colostomy K94.03
    enterostomy K94.13
    gastrostomy K94.23
    ileostomy K94.13
    tracheostomy J95.03
  stomach K31.89
    congenital Q40.2
    hourglass K31.2
  subaortic Q24.4
    hypertrophic (acquired) (idiopathic) I42.1
  subglottic J38.6
  syphilitic NEC A52.79
  trachea J39.8
    congenital Q32.1
    syphilitic A52.73
    tuberculous NEC A15.5
  tracheostomy J95.03
  tricuspid (valve) — *see* Stenosis, tricuspid
  tunica vaginalis N50.89
  ureter (postoperative) N13.5
    with
      hydronephrosis N13.1
        with infection N13.6
      pyelonephritis (chronic) N11.1
    congenital — *see* Atresia, ureter
    tuberculous A18.11
  ureteropelvic junction (congenital) Q62.11
    acquired, with hydronephrosis N13.0
  ureterovesical orifice N13.5
    with infection N13.6
  urethra (organic) (spasmodic) N35.9
    associated with schistosomiasis B65.0 [N37]
    congenital Q64.39
      valvular (posterior) Q64.2
    due to
      infection — *see* Stricture, urethra, postinfective
      trauma — *see* Stricture, urethra, post-traumatic
    gonococcal, gonorrheal A54.01
    infective NEC — *see* Stricture, urethra, postinfective
    late effect (sequelae) of injury — *see* Stricture,
      urethra, post-traumatic
    postcatheterization — *see* Stricture, urethra, post-
      procedural
    postinfective NEC
      female N35.12
      male N35.119
        anterior urethra N35.114
        bulbous urethra N35.112
        meatal N35.111
        membranous urethra N35.113
    postobstetric N35.021

Stricture — continued
  urethra — continued
    postoperative — see Stricture, urethra, postprocedural
    postprocedural
      female N99.12
      male N99.114
        anterior bulbous urethra N99.113
        bulbous urethra N99.111
        fossa navicularis N99.115
        meatal N99.110
        membranous urethra N99.112
    post-traumatic
      female N35.028
        due to childbirth N35.021
      male N35.014
        anterior urethra N35.013
        bulbous urethra N35.011
        meatal N35.010
        membranous urethra N35.012
    sequela (late effect) of
      childbirth N35.021
      injury — see Stricture, urethra, post-traumatic
    specified cause NEC N35.8
    syphilitic A52.76
    traumatic — see Stricture, urethra, post-traumatic
    valvular (posterior), congenital Q64.2
  urinary meatus — see Stricture, urethra
  uterus, uterine (synechiae) N85.6
    os (external) (internal) — see Stricture, cervix
  vagina (outlet) — see Stenosis, vagina
  valve (cardiac) (heart) (see also Endocarditis)
    congenital
      aortic Q23.0
      mitral Q23.2
      pulmonary Q22.1
      tricuspid Q22.4
  vas deferens N50.89
    congenital Q55.4
  vein I87.1
  vena cava (inferior) (superior) NEC I87.1
    congenital Q26.0
  vesicourethral orifice N32.0
    congenital Q64.31
  vulva (acquired) N90.5
Stridor R06.1
  congenital (larynx) P28.89
Stridulous — see condition
Stroke (apoplectic) (brain) (embolic) (ischemic) (paralytic) (thrombotic) I63.9
  cryptogenic (see also infarction, cerebral) I63.9
  epileptic — see Epilepsy
  heat T67.0 ☑
  in evolution I63.9
  intraoperative
    during cardiac surgery I97.810
    during other surgery I97.811
  lightning — see Lightning
  meaning
    cerebral hemorrhage — code to Hemorrhage, intracranial
    cerebral infarction — code to Infarction, cerebral
  postprocedural
    following cardiac surgery I97.820
    following other surgery I97.821
  unspecified (NOS) I63.9
Stromatosis, endometrial D39.0
Strongyloidiasis, strongyloidosis B78.9
  cutaneous B78.1
  disseminated B78.7
  intestinal B78.0
Strophulus pruriginosus L28.2
Struck by lightning — see Lightning
Struma (see also Goiter)
  Hashimoto E06.3
  lymphomatosa E06.3
  nodosa (simplex) E04.9
    endemic E01.2
      multinodular E01.1
    multinodular E04.2
      iodine-deficiency related E01.1
    toxic or with hyperthyroidism E05.20
      with thyroid storm E05.21
        multinodular E05.20
          with thyroid storm E05.21
        uninodular E05.10
          with thyroid storm E05.11
    toxicosa E05.20

Struma — continued
  nodosa — continued
    toxicosa — continued
      with thyroid storm E05.21
        multinodular E05.20
          with thyroid storm E05.21
        uninodular E05.10
          with thyroid storm E05.11
    uninodular E04.1
  ovarii D27.-
  Riedel's E06.5
Strumipriva cachexia E03.4
Strümpell-Marie spine — see Spondylitis, ankylosing
Strümpell-Westphal pseudosclerosis E83.01
Stuart deficiency disease (factor X) D68.2
Stuart-Prower factor deficiency (factor X) D68.2
Student's elbow — see Bursitis, elbow, olecranon
Stump — see Amputation
Stunting, nutritional E45
Stupor (catatonic) R40.1
  depressive (single episode) F32.89
    recurrent episode F33.8
  dissociative F44.2
  manic F30.2
  manic-depressive F31.89
  psychogenic (anergic) F44.2
  reaction to exceptional stress (transient) F43.0
Sturge (-Weber) (-Dimitri) (-Kalischer) **disease or syndrome** Q85.8
Stuttering F80.81
  adult onset F98.5
  childhood onset F80.81
  following cerebrovascular disease — see Disorder, fluency. following cerebrovascular disease
  in conditions classified elsewhere R47.82
Sty, stye (external) (internal) (meibomian) (zeisian) — see Hordeolum
Subacidity, gastric K31.89
  psychogenic F45.8
Subacute — see condition
Subarachnoid — see condition
Subcortical — see condition
Subcostal syndrome, nerve compression — see Mononeuropathy, upper limb, specified site NEC
Subcutaneous, subcuticular — see condition
Subdural — see condition
Subendocardium — see condition
Subependymoma
  specified site — see Neoplasm, uncertain behavior, by site
  unspecified site D43.2
Suberosis J67.3
Subglossitis — see Glossitis
Subhemophilia D66
Subinvolution
  breast (postlactational) (postpuerperal) N64.89
  puerperal O90.89
  uterus (chronic) (nonpuerperal) N85.3
    puerperal O90.89
Sublingual — see condition
Sublinguitis — see Sialoadenitis
Subluxatable hip Q65.6
Subluxation (see also Dislocation)
  acromioclavicular S43.11- ☑
  ankle S93.0- ☑
  atlantoaxial, recurrent M43.4
    with myelopathy M43.3
  carpometacarpal (joint) NEC S63.05- ☑
    thumb S63.04- ☑
  complex, vertebral — see Complex, subluxation
  congenital (see also Malposition, congenital)
    hip — see Dislocation, hip, congenital, partial
    joint (excluding hip)
      lower limb Q68.8
      shoulder Q68.8
      upper limb Q68.8
  elbow (traumatic) S53.10- ☑
    anterior S53.11- ☑
    lateral S53.14- ☑
    medial S53.13- ☑
    posterior S53.12- ☑
    specified type NEC S53.19- ☑
  finger S63.20- ☑
    index S63.20- ☑
    interphalangeal S63.22- ☑
      distal S63.24- ☑
        index S63.24- ☑

Subluxation — continued
  finger — continued
    interphalangeal — continued
      distal — continued
        little S63.24- ☑
        middle S63.24- ☑
        ring S63.24- ☑
      index S63.22- ☑
      little S63.22- ☑
      middle S63.22- ☑
      proximal S63.23- ☑
        index S63.23- ☑
        little S63.23- ☑
        middle S63.23- ☑
        ring S63.23- ☑
      ring S63.22- ☑
    little S63.20- ☑
    metacarpophalangeal S63.21- ☑
      index S63.21- ☑
      little S63.21- ☑
      middle S63.21- ☑
      ring S63.21- ☑
    middle S63.20- ☑
    ring S63.20- ☑
  foot S93.30- ☑
    specified site NEC S93.33- ☑
    tarsal joint S93.31- ☑
    tarsometatarsal joint S93.32- ☑
    toe — see Subluxation, toe
  hip S73.00- ☑
    anterior S73.03- ☑
      obturator S73.02- ☑
    central S73.04- ☑
    posterior S73.01- ☑
  interphalangeal (joint)
    finger S63.22- ☑
      distal joint S63.24- ☑
        index S63.24- ☑
        little S63.24- ☑
        middle S63.24- ☑
        ring S63.24- ☑
      index S63.22- ☑
      little S63.22- ☑
      middle S63.22- ☑
      proximal joint S63.23- ☑
        index S63.23- ☑
        little S63.23- ☑
        middle S63.23- ☑
        ring S63.23- ☑
      ring S63.22- ☑
    thumb S63.12- ☑
      distal joint S63.14- ☑
      proximal joint S63.13- ☑
    toe S93.13- ☑
      great S93.13- ☑
      lesser S93.13- ☑
  joint prosthesis — see Complications, joint prosthesis, mechanical, displacement, by site
  knee S83.10- ☑
    cap — see Subluxation, patella
    patella — see Subluxation, patella
    proximal tibia
      anteriorly S83.11- ☑
      laterally S83.14- ☑
      medially S83.13- ☑
      posteriorly S83.12- ☑
      specified type NEC S83.19- ☑
  lens — see Dislocation, lens, partial
  ligament, traumatic — see Sprain, by site
  metacarpal (bone)
    proximal end S63.06- ☑
  metacarpophalangeal (joint)
    finger S63.21- ☑
      index S63.21- ☑
      little S63.21- ☑
      middle S63.21- ☑
      ring S63.21- ☑
    thumb S63.11- ☑
  metatarsophalangeal joint S93.14- ☑
    great toe S93.14- ☑
    lesser toe S93.14- ☑
  midcarpal (joint) S63.03- ☑
  patella S83.00- ☑
    lateral S83.01- ☑
    recurrent (nontraumatic) — see Dislocation, patella, recurrent, incomplete

☑ **Additional Character Required** — Refer to the Tabular List for Character Selection   ▽ **Subterms under main terms may continue to next column or page**

Subluxation — *continued*
  patella — *continued*
    specified type NEC S83.09- ☑
  pathological — *see* Dislocation, pathological
  radial head S53.00- ☑
    anterior S53.01- ☑
    nursemaid's elbow S53.03- ☑
    posterior S53.02- ☑
    specified type NEC S53.09- ☑
  radiocarpal (joint) S63.02- ☑
  radioulnar (joint)
    distal S63.01- ☑
    proximal — *see* Subluxation, elbow
  shoulder
    congenital Q68.8
    girdle S43.30- ☑
      scapula S43.31- ☑
      specified site NEC S43.39- ☑
    traumatic S43.00- ☑
      anterior S43.01- ☑
      inferior S43.03- ☑
      posterior S43.02- ☑
      specified type NEC S43.08- ☑
  sternoclavicular (joint) S43.20- ☑
    anterior S43.21- ☑
    posterior S43.22- ☑
  symphysis (pubis)
  thumb S63.103 ☑
    interphalangeal joint — *see* Subluxation, interphalangeal (joint), thumb
    metacarpophalangeal joint — *see* Subluxation, metacarpophalangeal (joint), thumb
  toe(s) S93.10- ☑
    great S93.10- ☑
      interphalangeal joint S93.13- ☑
      metatarsophalangeal joint S93.14- ☑
    interphalangeal joint S93.13- ☑
    lesser S93.10- ☑
      interphalangeal joint S93.13- ☑
      metatarsophalangeal joint S93.14- ☑
    metatarsophalangeal joint S93.149 ☑
  ulna
    distal end S63.07- ☑
    proximal end — *see* Subluxation, elbow
  ulnohumeral joint — *see* Subluxation, elbow
  vertebral
    recurrent NEC — *see* subcategory M43.5 ☑
    traumatic
      cervical S13.100 ☑
        atlantoaxial joint S13.120 ☑
        atlantooccipital joint S13.110 ☑
        atloidooccipital joint S13.110 ☑
        joint between
          C0 and C1 S13.110 ☑
          C1 and C2 S13.120 ☑
          C2 and C3 S13.130 ☑
          C3 and C4 S13.140 ☑
          C4 and C5 S13.150 ☑
          C5 and C6 S13.160 ☑
          C6 and C7 S13.170 ☑
          C7 and T1 S13.180 ☑
        occipitoatloid joint S13.110 ☑
      lumbar S33.100 ☑
        joint between
          L1 and L2 S33.110 ☑
          L2 and L3 S33.120 ☑
          L3 and L4 S33.130 ☑
          L4 and L5 S33.140 ☑
      thoracic S23.100 ☑
        joint between
          T1 and T2 S23.110 ☑
          T2 and T3 S23.120 ☑
          T3 and T4 S23.122 ☑
          T4 and T5 S23.130 ☑
          T5 and T6 S23.132 ☑
          T6 and T7 S23.140 ☑
          T7 and T8 S23.142 ☑
          T8 and T9 S23.150 ☑
          T9 and T10 S23.152 ☑
          T10 and T11 S23.160 ☑
          T11 and T12 S23.162 ☑
          T12 and L1 S23.170 ☑
  wrist (carpal bone) S63.00- ☑
    carpometacarpal joint — *see* Subluxation, carpometacarpal (joint)

Subluxation — *continued*
  wrist — *continued*
    distal radioulnar joint — *see* Subluxation, radioulnar (joint), distal
    metacarpal bone, proximal — *see* Subluxation, metacarpal (bone), proximal end
    midcarpal — *see* Subluxation, midcarpal (joint)
    radiocarpal joint — *see* Subluxation, radiocarpal (joint)
    recurrent — *see* Dislocation, recurrent, wrist
    specified site NEC S63.09- ☑
    ulna — *see* Subluxation, ulna, distal end
Submaxillary — *see* condition
Submersion (fatal) (nonfatal) T75.1 ☑
Submucous — *see* condition
Subnormal, subnormality
  accommodation (old age) H52.4
  mental — *see* Disability, intellectual
  temperature (accidental) T68 ☑
Subphrenic — *see* condition
Subscapular nerve — *see* condition
Subseptus uterus Q51.2
Subsiding appendicitis K36
Substance (other psychoactive) **-induced**
  anxiety disorder F19.980
  bipolar and related disorder F19.94
  delirium F19.921
  depressive disorder F19.94
  major neurocognitive disorder F19.97
  mild neurocognitive disorder F19.988
  obsessive-compulsive and related disorder F19.988
  psychotic disorder F19.959
  sexual dysfunction F19.981
  sleep disorder F19.982
Substernal thyroid E04.9
  congenital Q89.2
Substitution disorder F44.9
Subtentorial — *see* condition
Subthyroidism (acquired) (*see also* Hypothyroidism)
  congenital E03.1
Succenturiate placenta O43.19- ☑
Sucking thumb, child (excessive) F98.8
Sudamen, sudamina L74.1
Sudanese kala-azar B55.0
Sudden
  hearing loss — *see* Deafness, sudden
  heart failure — *see* Failure, heart
Sudeck's atrophy, disease, or syndrome — *see* Algoneurodystrophy
Suffocation — *see* Asphyxia, traumatic
Sugar
  blood
    high (transient) R73.9
    low (transient) E16.2
  in urine R81
Suicide, suicidal (attempted) T14.91 ☑
  by poisoning — *see* Table of Drugs and Chemicals
  history of (personal) Z91.5
    in family Z81.8
  ideation — *see* Ideation, suicidal
  risk
    meaning personal history of attempted suicide Z91.5
    meaning suicidal ideation — *see* Ideation, suicidal
  tendencies
    meaning personal history of attempted suicide Z91.5
    meaning suicidal ideation — *see* Ideation, suicidal
  trauma — *see* nature of injury by site
Suipestifer infection — *see* Infection, salmonella
Sulfhemoglobinemia, sulphemoglobinemia (acquired) (with methemoglobinemia) D74.8
Sumatran mite fever A75.3
Summer — *see* condition
Sunburn L55.9
  due to
    tanning bed (acute) L56.8
      chronic L57.8
    ultraviolet radiation (acute) L56.8
      chronic L57.8
  first degree L55.0
  second degree L55.1
  third degree L55.2
SUNCT (short lasting unilateral neuralgiform headache with conjunctival injection and tearing) G44.059
  intractable G44.051
  not intractable G44.059

Sundowning F05
Sunken acetabulum — *see* Derangement, joint, specified type NEC, hip
Sunstroke T67.0 ☑
Superfecundation — *see* Pregnancy, multiple
Superfetation — *see* Pregnancy, multiple
Superinvolution (uterus) N85.8
Supernumerary (congenital)
  aortic cusps Q23.8
  auditory ossicles Q16.3
  bone Q79.8
  breast Q83.1
  carpal bones Q74.0
  cusps, heart valve NEC Q24.8
    aortic Q23.8
    mitral Q23.2
    pulmonary Q22.3
  digit(s) Q69.9
  ear (lobule) Q17.0
  fallopian tube Q50.6
  finger Q69.0
  hymen Q52.4
  kidney Q63.0
  lacrimonasal duct Q10.6
  lobule (ear) Q17.0
  mitral cusps Q23.2
  muscle Q79.8
  nipple(s) Q83.3
  organ or site not listed — *see* Accessory
  ossicles, auditory Q16.3
  ovary Q50.31
  oviduct Q50.6
  pulmonary, pulmonic cusps Q22.3
  rib Q76.6
    cervical or first (syndrome) Q76.5
  roots (of teeth) K00.2
  spleen Q89.09
  tarsal bones Q74.2
  teeth K00.1
  testis Q55.29
  thumb Q69.1
  toe Q69.2
  uterus Q51.2
  vagina Q52.1 ☑
  vertebra Q76.49
Supervision (of)
  contraceptive — *see* Prescription, contraceptives
  dietary (for) Z71.3
    allergy (food) Z71.3
    colitis Z71.3
    diabetes mellitus Z71.3
    food allergy or intolerance Z71.3
    gastritis Z71.3
    hypercholesterolemia Z71.3
    hypoglycemia Z71.3
    intolerance (food) Z71.3
    obesity Z71.3
    specified NEC Z71.3
  healthy infant or child Z76.2
    foundling Z76.1
  high-risk pregnancy — *see* Pregnancy, complicated by, high, risk
  lactation Z39.1
  pregnancy — *see* Pregnancy, supervision of
Supplemental teeth K00.1
Suppression
  binocular vision H53.34
  lactation O92.5
  menstruation N94.89
  ovarian secretion E28.39
  renal N28.9
  urine, urinary secretion R34
Suppuration, suppurative (*see also* condition)
  accessory sinus (chronic) — *see* Sinusitis
  adrenal gland
  antrum (chronic) — *see* Sinusitis, maxillary
  bladder — *see* Cystitis
  brain G06.0
    sequelae G09
  breast N61.1
    puerperal, postpartum or gestational — *see* Mastitis, obstetric, purulent
  dental periosteum M27.3
  ear (middle) (*see also* Otitis, media)
    external NEC — *see* Otitis, externa, infective
    internal — *see* subcategory H83.0 ☑
  ethmoidal (chronic) (sinus) — *see* Sinusitis, ethmoidal
  fallopian tube — *see* Salpingo-oophoritis

Suppuration, suppurative — *continued*
  frontal (chronic) (sinus) — *see* Sinusitis, frontal
  gallbladder (acute) K81.0
  gum K05.20
    generalized — *see* Peridontitis, aggressive, generalized
    localized — *see* Peridontitis, aggressive, localized
  intracranial G06.0
  joint — *see* Arthritis, pyogenic or pyemic
  labyrinthine — *see* subcategory H83.0 ☑
  lung — *see* Abscess, lung
  mammary gland N61.1
    puerperal, postpartum O91.12
      associated with lactation O91.13
  maxilla, maxillary M27.2
    sinus (chronic) — *see* Sinusitis, maxillary
  muscle — *see* Myositis, infective
  nasal sinus (chronic) — *see* Sinusitis
  pancreas, acute (*see also* Pancreatitis, acute) K85.80
  parotid gland — *see* Sialoadenitis
  pelvis, pelvic
    female — *see* Disease, pelvis, inflammatory
    male K65.0
  pericranial — *see* Osteomyelitis
  salivary duct or gland (any) — *see* Sialoadenitis
  sinus (accessory) (chronic) (nasal) — *see* Sinusitis
  sphenoidal sinus (chronic) — *see* Sinusitis, sphenoidal
  thymus (gland) E32.1
  thyroid (gland) E06.0
  tonsil — *see* Tonsillitis
  uterus — *see* Endometritis
Supraeruption of tooth (teeth) M26.34
Supraglottitis J04.30
  with obstruction J04.31
Suprarenal (gland) — *see* condition
Suprascapular nerve — *see* condition
Suprasellar — *see* condition
Surfer's knots or nodules S89.8- ☑
Surgical
  emphysema T81.82 ☑
  procedures, complication or misadventure — *see* Complications, surgical procedures
  shock T81.10 ☑
Surveillance (of) (for) (*see also* Observation)
  alcohol abuse Z71.41
  contraceptive — *see* Prescription, contraceptives
  dietary Z71.3
  drug abuse Z71.51
Susceptibility to disease, genetic Z15.89
  malignant neoplasm Z15.09
    breast Z15.01
    endometrium Z15.04
    ovary Z15.02
    prostate Z15.03
    specified NEC Z15.09
  multiple endocrine neoplasia Z15.81
Suspected condition, ruled out (*see also* Observation, suspected)
  amniotic cavity and membrane Z03.71
  cervical shortening Z03.75
  fetal anomaly Z03.73
  fetal growth Z03.74
  maternal and fetal conditions NEC Z03.79
  newborn (*see also* Observation, newborn, suspected condition ruled out) Z05.9
  oligohydramnios Z03.71
  placental problem Z03.72
  polyhydramnios Z03.71
Suspended uterus
  in pregnancy or childbirth — *see* Pregnancy, complicated by, abnormal uterus
Sutton's nevus D22.9
Suture
  burst (in operation wound) T81.31 ☑
    external operation wound T81.31 ☑
    internal operation wound T81.32 ☑
  inadvertently left in operation wound — *see* Foreign body, accidentally left during a procedure
  removal Z48.02
Swab inadvertently left in operation wound — *see* Foreign body, accidentally left during a procedure
Swallowed, swallowing
  difficulty — *see* Dysphagia
  foreign body — *see* Foreign body, alimentary tract
Swan-neck deformity (finger) — *see* Deformity, finger, swan-neck
Swearing, compulsive F42.8

Swearing, compulsive — *continued*
  in Gilles de la Tourette's syndrome F95.2
Sweat, sweats
  fetid L75.0
  night R61
Sweating, excessive R61
Sweeley-Klionsky disease E75.21
Sweet's disease or dermatosis L98.2
Swelling (of) R60.9
  abdomen, abdominal (not referable to any particular organ) — *see* Mass, abdominal
  ankle — *see* Effusion, joint, ankle
  arm M79.89
    forearm M79.89
  breast (*see also* Lump, breast) N63.0
  Calabar B74.3
  cervical gland R59.0
  chest, localized R22.2
  ear H93.8- ☑
  extremity (lower) (upper) — *see* Disorder, soft tissue, specified type NEC
  finger M79.89
  foot M79.89
  glands R59.9
    generalized R59.1
    localized R59.0
  hand M79.89
  head (localized) R22.0
  inflammatory — *see* Inflammation
  intra-abdominal — *see* Mass, abdominal
  joint — *see* Effusion, joint
  leg M79.89
    lower M79.89
  limb — *see* Disorder, soft tissue, specified type NEC
  localized (skin) R22.9
    chest R22.2
    head R22.0
    limb
      lower — *see* Mass, localized, limb, lower
      upper — *see* Mass, localized, limb, upper
    neck R22.1
    trunk R22.2
  neck (localized) R22.1
  pelvic — *see* Mass, abdominal
  scrotum N50.89
  splenic — *see* Splenomegaly
  testis N50.89
  toe M79.89
  umbilical R19.09
  wandering, due to Gnathostoma (spinigerum) B83.1
  white — *see* Tuberculosis, arthritis
Swift (-Feer) **disease**
  overdose or wrong substance given or taken — *see* Table of Drugs and Chemicals, by drug, poisoning
Swimmer's
  cramp T75.1 ☑
  ear H60.33- ☑
  itch B65.3
Swimming in the head R42
Swollen — *see* Swelling
Swyer syndrome Q99.1
Sycosis L73.8
  barbae (not parasitic) L73.8
  contagiosa (mycotic) B35.0
  lupoides L73.8
  mycotic B35.0
  parasitic B35.0
  vulgaris L73.8
Sydenham's chorea — *see* Chorea, Sydenham's
Sylvatic yellow fever A95.0
Sylvest's disease B33.0
Symblepharon H11.23- ☑
  congenital Q10.3
Symond's syndrome G93.2
Sympathetic — *see* condition
Sympatheticotonia G90.8
Sympathicoblastoma
  specified site — *see* Neoplasm, malignant, by site
  unspecified site C74.90
Sympathogonioma — *see* Sympathicoblastoma
Symphalangy (fingers) (toes) Q70.9
Symptoms NEC R68.89
  breast NEC N64.59
  cold J00
  development NEC R63.8
  factitious, self-induced — *see* Disorder, factitious

Symptoms — *continued*
  genital organs, female R10.2
  involving
    abdomen NEC R19.8
    appearance NEC R46.89
    awareness R41.9
      altered mental status R41.82
      amnesia — *see* Amnesia
      borderline intellectual functioning R41.83
      coma — *see* Coma
      disorientation R41.0
      neurologic neglect syndrome R41.4
      senile cognitive decline R41.81
      specified symptom NEC R41.89
    behavior NEC R46.89
    cardiovascular system NEC R09.89
    chest NEC R09.89
    circulatory system NEC R09.89
    cognitive functions R41.9
      altered mental status R41.82
      amnesia — *see* Amnesia
      borderline intellectual functioning R41.83
      coma — *see* Coma
      disorientation R41.0
      neurologic neglect syndrome R41.4
      senile cognitive decline R41.81
      specified symptom NEC R41.89
    development NEC R62.50
    digestive system NEC R19.8
    emotional state NEC R45.89
      emotional lability R45.86
    food and fluid intake R63.8
    general perceptions and sensations R44.9
      specified NEC R44.8
    musculoskeletal system R29.91
      specified NEC R29.898
    nervous system R29.90
      specified NEC R29.818
    pelvis NEC R19.8
    respiratory system NEC R09.89
    skin and integument R23.9
    urinary system R39.9
  menopausal N95.1
  metabolism NEC R63.8
  neurotic F48.8
  of infancy R68.19
  pelvis NEC, female R10.2
  skin and integument NEC R23.9
  subcutaneous tissue NEC R23.9
  viral cold J00
Sympus Q74.2
Syncephalus Q89.4
Synchondrosis
  abnormal (congenital) Q78.8
  ischiopubic M91.0
Synchysis (scintillans) (senile) (vitreous body) H43.89
Syncope (near) (pre-) R55
  anginosa I20.8
  bradycardia R00.1
  cardiac R55
  carotid sinus G90.01
  due to spinal (lumbar) puncture G97.1
  heart R55
  heat T67.1 ☑
  laryngeal R05
  psychogenic F48.8
  tussive R05
  vasoconstriction R55
  vasodepressor R55
  vasomotor R55
  vasovagal R55
Syndactylism, syndactyly Q70.9
  complex (with synostosis)
    fingers Q70.0- ☑
    toes Q70.2- ☑
  simple (without synostosis)
    fingers Q70.1- ☑
    toes Q70.3- ☑
Syndrome (*see also* Disease)
  48,XXXX Q97.1
  49,XXXXX Q97.1
  5q minus NOS D46.C (*following* D46.2)
  abdominal
    acute R10.0
    muscle deficiency Q79.4
  abnormal innervation H02.519
    left H02.516
      lower H02.515

☑ **Additional Character Required** — **Refer to the Tabular List for Character Selection**   ▽ **Subterms under main terms may continue to next column or page**

Syndrome — *continued*
  abnormal innervation — *continued*
    left — *continued*
      upper H02.514
    right H02.513
      lower H02.512
      upper H02.511
  abstinence, neonatal P96.1
  acid pulmonary aspiration, obstetric O74.0
  acquired immunodeficiency — *see* Human, immunodeficiency virus (HIV) disease
  acute abdominal R10.0
  acute respiratory distress (adult) (child) J80
    idiopathic J84.114
  Adair-Dighton Q78.0
  Adams-Stokes (-Morgagni) I45.9
  adiposogenital E23.6
  adrenal
    hemorrhage (meningococcal) A39.1
    meningococcic A39.1
  adrenocortical — *see* Cushing's, syndrome
  adrenogenital E25.9
    congenital, associated with enzyme deficiency E25.0
  afferent loop NEC K91.89
  Alagille's Q44.7
  alcohol withdrawal (without convulsions) — *see* Dependence, alcohol, with, withdrawal
  Alder's D72.0
  Aldrich (-Wiskott) D82.0
  alien hand R41.4
  Alport Q87.81
  alveolar hypoventilation E66.2
  alveolocapillary block J84.10
  amnesic, amnestic (confabulatory) (due to) — *see* Disorder, amnesic
  amyostatic (Wilson's disease) E83.01
  androgen insensitivity E34.50
    complete E34.51
    partial E34.52
  androgen resistance (*see also* Syndrome, androgen insensitivity) E34.50
  Angelman Q93.5
  anginal — *see* Angina
  ankyloglossia superior Q38.1
  anterior
    chest wall R07.89
    cord G83.82
    spinal artery G95.19
      compression M47.019
        cervical region M47.012
        cervicothoracic region M47.013
        lumbar region M47.016
        occipito-atlanto-axial region M47.011
        thoracic region M47.014
        thoracolumbar region M47.015
    tibial M76.81- ☑
  antibody deficiency D80.9
    agammaglobulinemic D80.1
      hereditary D80.0
    congenital D80.0
    hypogammaglobulinemic D80.1
      hereditary D80.0
  anticardiolipin (-antibody) D68.61
  antidepressant discontinuation T43.205 ☑
  antiphospholipid (-antibody) D68.61
  aortic
    arch M31.4
    bifurcation I74.09
  aortomesenteric duodenum occlusion K31.5
  apical ballooning (transient left ventricular) I51.81
  arcuate ligament I77.4
  argentaffin, argintaffinoma E34.0
  Arnold-Chiari — *see* Arnold-Chiari disease
  Arrillaga-Ayerza I27.0
  arterial tortuosity Q87.82
  arteriovenous steal T82.898- ☑
  Asherman's N85.6
  aspiration, of newborn — *see* Aspiration, by substance, with pneumonia
    meconium P24.01
  ataxia-telangiectasia G11.3
  auriculotemporal G50.8
  autoerythrocyte sensitization (Gardner-Diamond) D69.2
  autoimmune lymphoproliferative [ALPS] D89.82
  autoimmune polyglandular E31.0
  autoinflammatory M04.9

Syndrome — *continued*
  autoinflammatory — *continued*
    specified type NEC M04.8
  autosomal — *see* Abnormal, autosomes
  Avellis' G46.8
  Ayerza (-Arrillaga) I27.0
  Babinski-Nageotte G83.89
  Bakwin-Krida Q78.5
  bare lymphocyte D81.6
  Barré-Guillain G61.0
  Barré-Liéou M53.0
  Barrett's — *see* Barrett's, esophagus
  Barsony-Polgar K22.4
  Bársony-Teschendorf K22.4
  Barth E78.71
  Bartter's E26.81
  basal cell nevus Q87.89
  Basedow's E05.00
    with thyroid storm E05.01
  basilar artery G45.0
  Batten-Steinert G71.11
  battered
    baby or child — *see* Maltreatment, child, physical abuse
    spouse — *see* Maltreatment, adult, physical abuse
  Beals Q87.40
  Beau's I51.5
  Beck's I65.8
  Benedikt's G46.3
  Béquez César (-Steinbrinck-Chédiak-Higashi) E70.330
  Bernhardt-Roth — *see* Meralgia paresthetica
  Bernheim's — *see* Failure, heart, right
  big spleen D73.1
  bilateral polycystic ovarian E28.2
  Bing-Horton's — *see* Horton's headache
  Birt-Hogg-Dube syndrome Q87.89
  Björck (-Thorsen) E34.0
  black
    lung J60
    widow spider bite — *see* Toxicity, venom, spider, black widow
  Blackfan-Diamond D61.01
  Blau M04.8
  blind loop K90.2
    congenital Q43.8
    postsurgical K91.2
  blue sclera Q78.0
  blue toe I75.02- ☑
  Boder-Sedgewick G11.3
  Boerhaave's K22.3
  Borjeson Forssman Lehmann Q89.8
  Bouillaud's I01.9
  Bourneville (-Pringle) Q85.1
  Bouveret (-Hoffman) I47.9
  brachial plexus G54.0
  bradycardia-tachycardia I49.5
  brain (nonpsychotic) F09
    with psychosis, psychotic reaction F09
    acute or subacute — *see* Delirium
    congenital — *see* Disability, intellectual
    organic F09
      post-traumatic (nonpsychotic) F07.81
        psychotic F09
      personality change F07.0
      postcontusional F07.81
      post-traumatic, nonpsychotic F07.81
      psycho-organic F09
      psychotic F06.8
  brain stem stroke G46.3
  Brandt's (acrodermatitis enteropathica) E83.2
  broad ligament laceration N83.8
  Brock's J98.11
  bronze baby P83.88
  Brown-Sequard G83.81
  Brugada I49.8
  bubbly lung P27.0
  Buchem's M85.2
  Budd-Chiari I82.0
  Bürger-Grütz E78.3
  Burke's K86.89
  Burnett's (milk-alkali) E83.52
  burning feet E53.9
  Bywaters' T79.5 ☑
  Call-Fleming I67.841
  carbohydrate-deficient glycoprotein (CDGS) E77.8
  carcinogenic thrombophlebitis I82.1
  carcinoid E34.0

Syndrome — *continued*
  cardiac asthma I50.1
  cardiacos negros I27.0
  cardiofaciocutaneous Q87.89
  cardiopulmonary-obesity E66.2
  cardiorenal — *see* Hypertension, cardiorenal
  cardiorespiratory distress (idiopathic), newborn P22.0
  cardiovascular renal — *see* Hypertension, cardiorenal
  carotid
    artery (hemispheric) (internal) G45.1
    body G90.01
    sinus G90.01
  carpal tunnel G56.0- ☑
  Cassidy (-Scholte) E34.0
  cat cry Q93.4
  cat eye Q92.8
  cauda equina G83.4
  causalgia — *see* Causalgia
  celiac K90.0
    artery compression I77.4
    axis I77.4
  central pain G89.0
  cerebellar
    hereditary G11.9
    stroke G46.4
  cerebellomedullary malformation — *see* Spina bifida
  cerebral
    artery
      anterior G46.1
      middle G46.0
      posterior G46.2
    gigantism E22.0
  cervical (root) M53.1
    disc — *see* Disorder, disc, cervical, with neuritis
    fusion Q76.1
    posterior, sympathicus M53.0
    rib Q76.5
    sympathetic paralysis G90.2
  cervicobrachial (diffuse) M53.1
  cervicocranial M53.0
  cervicodorsal outlet G54.2
  cervicothoracic outlet G54.0
  Céstan (-Raymond) I65.8
  Charcot's (angina cruris) (intermittent claudication) I73.9
  Charcot-Weiss-Baker G90.09
  CHARGE Q89.8
  Chédiak-Higashi (-Steinbrinck) E70.330
  chest wall R07.1
  Chiari's (hepatic vein thrombosis) I82.0
  Chilaiditi's Q43.3
  child maltreatment — *see* Maltreatment, child
  chondrocostal junction M94.0
  chondroectodermal dysplasia Q77.6
  chromosome 4 short arm deletion Q93.3
  chromosome 5 short arm deletion Q93.4
  chronic
    infantile neurological, cutaneous and articular (CINCA) M04.2
    pain G89.4
      personality F68.8
  Clarke-Hadfield K86.89
  Clerambault's automatism G93.89
  Clouston's (hidrotic ectodermal dysplasia) Q82.4
  clumsiness, clumsy child F82
  cluster headache G44.009
    intractable G44.001
    not intractable G44.009
  Coffin-Lowry Q89.8
  cold injury (newborn) P80.0
  combined immunity deficiency D81.9
  compartment (deep) (posterior) (traumatic) T79.A0 ☑ (*following* T79.7)
    abdomen T79.A3 ☑ (*following* T79.7)
    lower extremity (hip, buttock, thigh, leg, foot, toes) T79.A2 ☑ (*following* T79.7)
    nontraumatic
      abdomen M79.A3 (*following* M79.7)
      lower extremity (hip, buttock, thigh, leg, foot, toes) M79.A2- ☑ (*following* M79.7)
      specified site NEC M79.A9 (*following* M79.7)
      upper extremity (shoulder, arm, forearm, wrist, hand, fingers) M79.A1- ☑ (*following* M79.7)
    postprocedural — *see* Syndrome, compartment, nontraumatic
    specified site NEC T79.A9 ☑ (*following* T79.7)

Syndrome — *continued*
- compartment — *continued*
  - upper extremity (shoulder, arm, forearm, wrist, hand, fingers) T79.A1 ☑ (*following* T79.7)
  - complex regional pain — *see* Syndrome, pain, complex regional
  - compression T79.5 ☑
    - anterior spinal — *see* Syndrome, anterior, spinal artery, compression
    - cauda equina G83.4
    - celiac artery I77.4
    - vertebral artery M47.029
      - cervical region M47.022
      - occipito-atlanto-axial region M47.021
  - concussion F07.81
  - congenital
    - affecting multiple systems NEC Q87.89
    - central alveolar hypoventilation G47.35
    - facial diplegia Q87.0
    - muscular hypertrophy-cerebral Q87.89
    - oculo-auriculovertebral Q87.0
    - oculofacial diplegia (Moebius) Q87.0
    - rubella (manifest) P35.0
  - congestion-fibrosis (pelvic), female N94.89
  - congestive dysmenorrhea N94.6
  - connective tissue M35.9
    - overlap NEC M35.1
  - Conn's E26.01
  - conus medullaris G95.81
  - cord
    - anterior G83.82
    - posterior G83.83
  - coronary
    - acute NEC I24.9
    - insufficiency or intermediate I20.0
    - slow flow I20.8
  - Costen's (complex) M26.69
  - costochondral junction M94.0
  - costoclavicular G54.0
  - costovertebral E22.0
  - Cowden Q85.8
  - craniovertebral M53.0
  - Creutzfeldt-Jakob — *see* Creutzfeldt-Jakob disease or syndrome
  - crib death R99
  - cricopharyngeal — *see* Dysphagia
  - cri-du-chat Q93.4
  - croup J05.0
  - CRPS I — *see* Syndrome, pain, complex regional I
  - crush T79.5 ☑
  - cryopyrin-associated perodic M04.2
  - cryptophthalmos Q87.0
  - cubital tunnel — *see* Lesion, nerve, ulnar
  - Curschmann (-Batten) (-Steinert) G71.11
  - Cushing's E24.9
    - alcohol-induced E24.4
    - drug-induced E24.2
    - due to
      - alcohol
      - drugs E24.2
      - ectopic ACTH E24.3
      - overproduction of pituitary ACTH E24.0
    - overdose or wrong substance given or taken — *see* Table of Drugs and Chemicals, by drug, poisoning
    - pituitary-dependent E24.0
    - specified type NEC E24.8
  - cystic duct stump K91.5
  - Dana-Putnam D51.0
  - Danbolt (-Cross) (acrodermatitis enteropathica) E83.2
  - Dandy-Walker Q03.1
    - with spina bifida Q07.01
  - Danlos' Q79.6
  - De Quervain E34.51
  - de Toni-Fanconi (-Debré) E72.09
    - with cystinosis E72.04
  - defibrination (*see also* Fibrinolysis)
    - with
      - antepartum hemorrhage — *see* Hemorrhage, antepartum, with coagulation defect
      - intrapartum hemorrhage — *see* Hemorrhage, complicating, delivery
    - newborn P60
    - postpartum O72.3
  - Degos' I77.89
  - Déjérine-Roussy G89.0
  - delayed sleep phase G47.21
  - demyelinating G37.9

Syndrome — *continued*
- dependence — *see* F10-F19 with fourth character .2
- depersonalization (-derealization) F48.1
- di George's D82.1
- diabetes mellitus in newborn infant P70.2
- diabetes mellitus-hypertension-nephrosis — *see* Diabetes, nephrosis
- diabetes-nephrosis — *see* Diabetes, nephrosis
- diabetic amyotrophy — *see* Diabetes, amyotrophy
- dialysis associated steal T82.898- ☑
- Diamond-Blackfan D61.01
- Diamond-Gardener D69.2
- DIC (diffuse or disseminated intravascular coagulopathy) D65
- Dighton's Q78.0
- disequilibrium E87.8
- Döhle body-panmyelopathic D72.0
- dorsolateral medullary G46.4
- double athetosis G80.3
- Down (*see also* Down syndrome) Q90.9
- Dresbach's (elliptocytosis) D58.1
- Dressler's (postmyocardial infarction) I24.1
  - postcardiotomy I97.0
- drug withdrawal, infant of dependent mother P96.1
- dry eye H04.12- ☑
- due to abnormality
  - chromosomal Q99.9
    - sex
      - female phenotype Q97.9
      - male phenotype Q98.9
      - specified NEC Q99.8
- dumping (postgastrectomy) K91.1
  - nonsurgical K31.89
- Dupré's (meningism) R29.1
- dysmetabolic X E88.81
- dyspraxia, developmental F82
- Eagle-Barrett Q79.4
- Eaton-Lambert — *see* Syndrome, Lambert-Eaton
- Ebstein's Q22.5
- ectopic ACTH E24.3
- eczema-thrombocytopenia D82.0
- Eddowes' Q78.0
- effort (psychogenic) F45.8
- Ehlers-Danlos Q79.6
- Eisenmenger's I27.83
- Ekman's Q78.0
- electric feet E53.8
- Ellis-van Creveld Q77.6
- empty nest Z60.0
- endocrine-hypertensive E27.0
- entrapment — *see* Neuropathy, entrapment
- eosinophilia-myalgia M35.8
- epileptic (*see also* Epilepsy, by type)
  - absence G40.A09 (*following* G40.3)
    - intractable G40.A19 (*following* G40.3)
      - with status epilepticus G40.A11 (*following* G40.3)
      - without status epilepticus G40.A19 (*following* G40.3)
    - not intractable G40.A09 (*following* G40.3)
      - with status epilepticus G40.A01 (*following* G40.3)
      - without status epilepticus G40.A09 (*following* G40.3)
- Erdheim-Chester (ECD) E88.89
- Erdheim's E22.0
- erythrocyte fragmentation D59.4
- Evans D69.41
- exhaustion F48.8
- extrapyramidal G25.9
  - specified NEC G25.89
- eye retraction — *see* Strabismus
- eyelid-malar-mandible Q87.0
- Faber's D50.9
- facial nerve, paroxysmal G50.0
- Fallot's Q21.3
- familial cold autoinflammatory M04.2
- familial eczema-thrombocytopenia (Wiskott-Aldrich) D82.0
- Fanconi (-de Toni) (-Debré) E72.09
  - with cystinosis E72.04
- Fanconi's (anemia) (congenital pancytopenia) D61.09
- fatigue
  - chronic R53.82
  - psychogenic F48.8
- faulty bowel habit K59.39
- Feil-Klippel (brevicollis) Q76.1
- Felty's — *see* Felty's syndrome

Syndrome — *continued*
- fertile eunuch E23.0
- fetal
  - alcohol (dysmorphic) Q86.0
  - hydantoin Q86.1
- Fiedler's I40.1
- first arch Q87.0
- fish odor E72.8
- Fisher's G61.0
- Fitzhugh-Curtis
  - due to
    - Chlamydia trachomatis A74.81
    - Neisseria gonorrhorea (gonococcal peritonitis) A54.85
- Fitz's (*see also* Pancreatitis, acute) K85.80
- Flajani (-Basedow) E05.00
  - with thyroid storm E05.01
- flatback — *see* Flatback syndrome
- floppy
  - baby P94.2
  - iris (intraoeprative) (IFIS) H21.81
  - mitral valve I34.1
- flush E34.0
- Foix-Alajouanine G95.19
- Fong's Q87.2
- food protein-induced enterocolitis K52.21
- foramen magnum G93.5
- Foster-Kennedy H47.14- ☑
- Foville's (peduncular) G46.3
- fragile X Q99.2
- Franceschetti Q75.4
- Frey's
  - auriculotemporal G50.8
  - hyperhidrosis L74.52
- Friderichsen-Waterhouse A39.1
- Froin's G95.89
- frontal lobe F07.0
- Fukuhara E88.49
- functional
  - bowel K59.9
  - prepubertal castrate E29.1
- Gaisböck's D75.1
- ganglion (basal ganglia brain) G25.9
  - geniculi G51.1
- Gardner-Diamond D69.2
- gastroesophageal
  - junction K22.0
  - laceration-hemorrhage K22.6
- gastrojejunal loop obstruction K91.89
- Gee-Herter-Heubner K90.0
- Gelineau's G47.419
  - with cataplexy G47.411
- genito-anorectal A55
- Gerstmann-Sträussler-Scheinker (GSS) A81.82
- Gianotti-Crosti L44.4
- giant platelet (Bernard-Soulier) D69.1
- Gilles de la Tourette's F95.2
- goiter-deafness E07.1
- Goldberg Q89.8
- Goldberg-Maxwell E34.51
- Good's D83.8
- Gopalan' (burning feet) E53.8
- Gorlin's Q87.89
- Gougerot-Blum L81.7
- Gouley's I31.1
- Gower's R55
- gray or grey (newborn) P93.0
  - platelet D69.1
- Gubler-Millard G46.3
- Guillain-Barré (-Strohl) G61.0
- gustatory sweating G50.8
- Hadfield-Clarke K86.89
- hair tourniquet — *see* Constriction, external, by site
- Hamman's J98.19
- hand-foot L27.1
- hand-shoulder G90.8
- hantavirus (cardio)-pulmonary (HPS) (HCPS) B33.4
- happy puppet Q93.5
- Harada's H30.81- ☑
- Hayem-Faber D50.9
- headache NEC G44.89
  - complicated NEC G44.59
- Heberden's I20.8
- Hedinger's E34.0
- Hegglin's D72.0
- HELLP (hemolysis, elevated liver enzymes and low platelet count) O14.2- ☑
  - complicating
    - childbirth O14.24

☑ Additional Character Required — Refer to the Tabular List for Character Selection   ▽ Subterms under main terms may continue to next column or page

Syndrome — Syndrome

Index

Syndrome — *continued*
  HELLP — *continued*
    complicating — *continued*
      puerperium O14.25
  hemolytic-uremic D59.3
  hemophagocytic, infection-associated D76.2
  Henoch-Schönlein D69.0
  hepatic flexure K59.8
  hepatopulmonary K76.81
  hepatorenal K76.7
    following delivery O90.4
    postoperative or postprocedural K91.83
    postpartum, puerperal O90.4
  hepatourologic K76.7
  Herter (-Gee) (nontropical sprue) K90.0
  Heubner-Herter K90.0
  Heyd's K76.7
  Hilger's G90.09
  histamine-like (fish poisoning) — *see* Poisoning, fish
  histiocytic D76.3
  histiocytosis NEC D76.3
  HIV infection, acute B20
  Hoffmann-Werdnig G12.0
  Hollander-Simons E88.1
  Hoppe-Goldflam G70.00
    with exacerbation (acute) G70.01
    in crisis G70.01
  Horner's G90.2
  hungry bone E83.81
  hunterian glossitis D51.0
  Hutchinson's triad A50.53
  hyperabduction G54.0
  hyperammonemia-hyperornithinemia-homocitrulline-mia E72.4
  hypereosinophilic (idiopathic) D72.1
  hyperimmunoglobulin D M04.1
  hyperimmunoglobulin E (IgE) D82.4
  hyperkalemic E87.5
  hyperkinetic — *see* Hyperkinesia
  hypermobility M35.7
  hypernatremia E87.0
  hyperosmolarity E87.0
  hyperperfusion G97.82
  hypersplenic D73.1
  hypertransfusion, newborn P61.1
  hyperventilation F45.8
  hyperviscosity (of serum)
    polycythemic D75.1
    sclerothymic D58.8
  hypoglycemic (familial) (neonatal) E16.2
  hypokalemic E87.6
  hyponatremic E87.1
  hypopituitarism E23.0
  hypoplastic left-heart Q23.4
  hypopotassemia E87.6
  hyposmolality E87.1
  hypotension, maternal O26.5- ☑
  hypothenar hammer I73.89
  hypoventilation, obesity (OHS) E66.2
  ICF (intravascular coagulation-fibrinolysis) D65
  idiopathic
    cardiorespiratory distress, newborn P22.0
    nephrotic (infantile) N04.9
  iliotibial band M76.3- ☑
  immobility, immobilization (paraplegic) M62.3
  immune reconstitution D89.3
  immune reconstitution inflammatory [IRIS] D89.3
  immunity deficiency, combined D81.9
  immunodeficiency
    acquired — *see* Human, immunodeficiency virus (HIV) disease
    combined D81.9
  impending coronary I20.0
  impingement, shoulder M75.4- ☑
  inappropriate secretion of antidiuretic hormone E22.2
  infant
    gestational diabetes P70.0
    of diabetic mother P70.1
  infantilism (pituitary) E23.0
  inferior vena cava I87.1
  inspissated bile (newborn) P59.1
  institutional (childhood) F94.2
  insufficient sleep F51.12
  intermediate coronary (artery) I20.0
  interspinous ligament — *see* Spondylopathy, specified NEC
  intestinal
    carcinoid E34.0

Syndrome — *continued*
  intestinal — *continued*
    knot K56.2
  intravascular coagulation-fibrinolysis (ICF) D65
  iodine-deficiency, congenital E00.9
    type
      mixed E00.2
      myxedematous E00.1
      neurological E00.0
  IRDS (Idiopathic respiratory distress, newborn) P22.0
  irritable
    bowel K58.9
      with
        constipation K58.1
        diarrhea K58.0
      mixed K58.2
      psychogenic F45.8
      specified NEC K58.8
    heart (psychogenic) F45.8
    weakness F48.8
  ischemic
    bowel (transient) K55.9
      chronic K55.1
      due to mesenteric artery insufficiency K55.1
    steal T82.898 ☑
  IVC (intravascular coagulopathy) D65
  Ivemark's Q89.01
  Jaccoud's — *see* Arthropathy, postrheumatic, chronic
  Jackson's G83.89
  Jakob-Creutzfeldt — *see* Creutzfeldt-Jakob disease or syndrome
  jaw-winking Q07.8
  Jervell-Lange-Nielsen I45.81
  jet lag G47.25
  Job's D71
  Joseph-Diamond-Blackfan D61.01
  jugular foramen G52.7
  Kabuki Q89.8
  Kanner's (autism) F84.0
  Kartagener's Q89.3
  Kelly's D50.1
  Kimmelsteil-Wilson — *see* Diabetes, specified type, with Kimmelsteil-Wilson disease
  Klein (e)-Levine G47.13
  Klippel-Feil (brevicollis) Q76.1
  Köhler-Pellegrini-Steida — *see* Bursitis, tibial collateral
  König's K59.8
  Korsakoff (-Wernicke) (nonalcoholic) F04
    alcoholic F10.26
  Kostmann's D70.0
  Krabbe's congenital muscle hypoplasia Q79.8
  labyrinthine — *see* subcategory H83.2 ☑
  lacunar NEC G46.7
  Lambert-Eaton G70.80
    in
      neoplastic disease G73.1
      specified disease NEC G70.81
  Landau-Kleffner — *see* Epilepsy, specified NEC
  Larsen's Q74.8
  lateral
    cutaneous nerve of thigh G57.1- ☑
    medullary G46.4
  Launois' E22.0
  lazy
    leukocyte D70.8
    posture M62.3
  Lemiere I80.8
  Lennox-Gastaut G40.812
    intractable G40.814
      with status epilepticus G40.813
      without status epilepticus G40.814
    not intractable G40.812
      with status epilepticus G40.811
      without status epilepticus G40.812
  lenticular, progressive E83.01
  Leopold-Levi's E05.90
  Lev's I44.2
  Lichtheim's D51.0
  Li-Fraumeni Z15.01
  Lightwood's N25.89
  Lignac (de Toni) (-Fanconi) (-Debré) E72.09
    with cystinosis E72.04
  Likoff's I20.8
  limbic epilepsy personality F07.0
  liver-kidney K76.7
  lobotomy F07.0
  Loffler's J82
  long arm 18 or 21 deletion Q93.89

Syndrome — *continued*
  long QT I45.81
  Louis-Barré G11.3
  low
    atmospheric pressure T70.29 ☑
    back M54.5
    output (cardiac) I50.9
  lower radicular, newborn (birth injury) P14.8
  Luetscher's (dehydration) E86.0
  Lupus anticoagulant D68.62
  Lutembacher's Q21.1
  macrophage activation D76.1
    due to infection D76.2
  magnesium-deficiency R29.0
  Majeed M04.8
  Mal de Debarquement R42
  malabsorption K90.9
    postsurgical K91.2
  malformation, congenital, due to
    alcohol Q86.0
    exogenous cause NEC Q86.8
    hydantoin Q86.1
    warfarin Q86.2
  malignant
    carcinoid E34.0
    neuroleptic G21.0
  Mallory-Weiss K22.6
  mandibulofacial dysostosis Q75.4
  manic-depressive — *see* Disorder, bipolar
  maple-syrup-urine E71.0
  Marable's I77.4
  Marfan's Q87.40
    with
      cardiovascular manifestations Q87.418
        aortic dilation Q87.410
      ocular manifestations Q87.42
      skeletal manifestations Q87.43
  Marie's (acromegaly) E22.0
  mast cell activation — *see* Activation, mast cell
  maternal hypotension — *see* Syndrome, hypotension, maternal
  May (-Hegglin) D72.0
  McArdle (-Schmidt) (-Pearson) E74.04
  McQuarrie's E16.2
  meconium plug (newborn) P76.0
  median arcuate ligament I77.4
  Meekeren-Ehlers-Danlos Q79.6
  megavitamin-B6 E67.2
  Meige G24.4
  MELAS E88.41
  Mendelson's O74.0
  MERRF (myoclonic epilepsy associated with ragged-red fibers) E88.42
  mesenteric
    artery (superior) K55.1
    vascular insufficiency K55.1
  metabolic E88.81
  metastatic carcinoid E34.0
  micrognathia-glossoptosis Q87.0
  midbrain NEC G93.89
  middle lobe (lung) J98.19
  middle radicular G54.0
  migraine (*see also* Migraine) G43.909
  Mikulicz' K11.8
  milk-alkali E83.52
  Millard-Gubler G46.3
  Miller-Dieker Q93.88
  Miller-Fisher G61.0
  Minkowski-Chauffard D58.0
  Mirizzi's K83.1
  MNGIE (Mitochondrial Neurogastrointestinal Encephalopathy) E88.49
  Möbius, ophthalmoplegic migraine — *see* Migraine, ophthalmoplegic
  monofixation H50.42
  Morel-Moore M85.2
  Morel-Morgagni M85.2
  Morgagni (-Morel) (-Stewart) M85.2
  Morgagni-Adams-Stokes I45.9
  Mounier-Kuhn Q32.4
    with bronchiectasis J47.9
      with
        exacerbation (acute) J47.1
        lower respiratory infection J47.0
    acquired J98.09
      with bronchiectasis J47.9
        with
          exacerbation (acute) J47.1
          lower respiratory infection J47.0

Syndrome — Syndrome

☑ **Additional Character Required** — Refer to the Tabular List for Character Selection   ▽ **Subterms under main terms may continue to next column or page**

Syndrome — *continued*
  right — *continued*
    ventricular obstruction — *see* Failure, heart, congestive
  Romano-Ward (prolonged QT interval) I45.81
  rotator cuff, shoulder (*see also* Tear, rotator cuff)
    M75.10- ☑
  Rotes Quérol — *see* Hyperostosis, ankylosing
  Roth — *see* Meralgia paresthetica
  rubella (congenital) P35.0
  Ruvalcaba-Myhre-Smith E71.440
  Rytand-Lipsitch I44.2
  salt
    depletion E87.1
      due to heat NEC T67.8 ☑
        causing heat exhaustion or prostration
          T67.4 ☑
    low E87.1
  salt-losing N28.89
  Scaglietti-Dagnini E22.0
  scalenus anticus (anterior) G54.0
  scapulocostal — *see* Mononeuropathy, upper limb, specified site NEC
  scapuloperoneal G71.0
  schizophrenic, of childhood NEC F84.5
  Schnitzler D47.2
  Scholte's E34.0
  Schroeder's E27.0
  Schüller-Christian C96.5
  Schwachman's — *see* Syndrome, Shwachman's
  Schwartz (-Jampel) G71.13
  Schwartz-Bartter E22.2
  scimitar Q26.8
  sclerocystic ovary E28.2
  Seitelberger's G31.89
  septicemic adrenal hemorrhage A39.1
  seroconversion, retroviral (acute) Z21
  serous meningitis G93.2
  severe acute respiratory (SARS) J12.81
  shaken infant T74.4 ☑
  shock (traumatic) T79.4 ☑
    kidney N17.0
      following crush injury T79.5 ☑
    toxic A48.3
  shock-lung J80
  Shone's — *code to* specific anomalies
  short
    bowel K91.2
    rib Q77.2
  shoulder-hand — *see* Algoneurodystrophy
  Shwachman's D70.4
  sicca — *see* Sicca syndrome
  sick
    cell E87.1
    sinus I49.5
  sick-euthyroid E07.81
  sideropenic D50.1
  Siemens' ectodermal dysplasia Q82.4
  Silfversköld's Q78.9
  Simons' E88.1
  sinus tarsi M25.57- ☑
  sinusitis-bronchiectasis-situs inversus Q89.3
  Sipple's E31.22
  sirenomelia Q87.2
  Slocumb's E27.0
  slow flow, coronary I20.8
  Sluder's G44.89
  Smith-Magenis Q93.88
  Sneddon-Wilkinson L13.1
  Sotos' Q87.3
  South African cardiomyopathy I42.8
  spasmodic
    upward movement, eyes H51.8
    winking F95.8
  Spen's I45.9
  splenic
    agenesis Q89.01
    flexure K59.8
    neutropenia D73.81
  Spurway's Q78.0
  staphylococcal scalded skin L00
  steal
    arteriovenous T82.898- ☑
    ischemic T82.898- ☑
    subclavian G45.8
  Stein-Leventhal E28.2
  Stein's E28.2
  Stevens-Johnson syndrome L51.1

Syndrome — *continued*
  Stevens-Johnson syndrome — *continued*
    toxic epidermal necrolysis overlap L51.3
  Stewart-Morel M85.2
  Stickler Q89.8
  stiff baby Q89.8
  stiff man G25.82
  Still-Felty — *see* Felty's syndrome
  Stokes (-Adams) I45.9
  stone heart I50.1
  straight back, congenital Q76.49
  subclavian steal G45.8
  subcoracoid-pectoralis minor G54.0
  subcostal nerve compression I77.89
  subphrenic interposition Q43.3
  superior
    cerebellar artery I63.8
    mesenteric artery K55.1
    semi-circular canal dehiscence H83.8X- ☑
    vena cava I87.1
  supine hypotensive (maternal) — *see* Syndrome, hypotension, maternal
  suprarenal cortical E27.0
  supraspinatus (*see also* Tear, rotator cuff) M75.10- ☑
  Susac G93.49
  swallowed blood P78.2
  sweat retention L74.0
  Swyer Q99.1
  Symond's G93.2
  sympathetic
    cervical paralysis G90.2
    pelvic, female N94.89
  systemic inflammatory response (SIRS), of non-infectious origin (without organ dysfunction) R65.10
    with acute organ dysfunction R65.11
  tachycardia-bradycardia I49.5
  takotsubo I51.81
  TAR (thrombocytopenia with absent radius) Q87.2
  tarsal tunnel G57.5- ☑
  teething K00.7
  tegmental G93.89
  telangiectasic-pigmentation-cataract Q82.8
  temporal pyramidal apex — *see* Otitis, media, suppurative, acute
  temporomandibular joint-pain-dysfunction M26.62- ☑
  Terry's (*see also* Myopia, degenerative) H44.2- ☑
  testicular feminization (*see also* Syndrome, androgen insensitivity) E34.51
  thalamic pain (hyperesthetic) G89.0
  thoracic outlet (compression) G54.0
  Thorson-Björck E34.0
  thrombocytopenia with absent radius (TAR) Q87.2
  thyroid-adrenocortical insufficiency E31.0
  tibial
    anterior M76.81- ☑
    posterior M76.82- ☑
  Tietze's M94.0
  time-zone (rapid) G47.25
  Toni-Fanconi E72.09
    with cystinosis E72.04
  Touraine's Q79.8
  tourniquet — *see* Constriction, external, by site
  toxic shock A48.3
  transient left ventricular apical ballooning I51.81
  traumatic vasospastic T75.22 ☑
  Treacher Collins Q75.4
  triple X, female Q97.0
  trisomy Q92.9
    13 Q91.7
      meiotic nondisjunction Q91.4
      mitotic nondisjunction Q91.5
      mosaicism Q91.5
      translocation Q91.6
    18 Q91.3
      meiotic nondisjunction Q91.0
      mitotic nondisjunction Q91.1
      mosaicism Q91.1
      translocation Q91.2
    20 (q)(p) Q92.8
    21 Q90.9
      meiotic nondisjunction Q90.0
      mitotic nondisjunction Q90.1
      mosaicism Q90.1
      translocation Q90.2
    22 Q92.8
  tropical wet feet T69.0- ☑
  Trousseau's I82.1

Syndrome — *continued*
  tumor lysis (following antineoplastic chemotherapy) (spontaneous) NEC E88.3
  tumor necrosis factor receptor associated periodic (TRAPS) M04.1
  Twiddler's (due to)
    automatic implantable defibrillator T82.198 ☑
    cardiac pacemaker T82.198 ☑
  Unverricht (-Lundborg) — *see* Epilepsy, generalized, idiopathic
  upward gaze H51.8
  uremia, chronic (*see also* Disease, kidney, chronic) N18.9
  urethral N34.3
  urethro-oculo-articular — *see* Reiter's disease
  urohepatic K76.7
  vago-hypoglossal G52.7
  van Buchem's M85.2
  van der Hoeve's Q78.0
  vascular NEC in cerebrovascular disease G46.8
  vasoconstriction, reversible cerebrovascular I67.841
  vasomotor I73.9
  vasospastic (traumatic) T75.22 ☑
  vasovagal R55
  VATER Q87.2
  velo-cardio-facial Q93.81
  vena cava (inferior) (superior) (obstruction) I87.1
  vertebral
    artery G45.0
      compression — *see* Syndrome, anterior, spinal artery, compression
    steal G45.0
  vertebro-basilar artery G45.0
  vertebrogenic (pain) M54.89
  vertiginous — *see* Disorder, vestibular function
  Vinson-Plummer D50.1
  virus B34.9
  visceral larva migrans B83.0
  visual disorientation H53.8
  vitamin B6 deficiency E53.1
  vitreal corneal H59.01- ☑
  vitreous (touch) H59.01- ☑
  Vogt-Koyanagi H20.82- ☑
  Volkmann's T79.6 ☑
  von Schroetter's I82.890
  von Willebrand (-Jürgen) D68.0
  Waldenström-Kjellberg D50.1
  Wallenberg's G46.3
  water retention E87.79
  Waterhouse (-Friderichsen) A39.1
  Weber-Gubler G46.3
  Weber-Leyden G46.3
  Weber's G46.3
  Wegener's M31.30
    with
      kidney involvement M31.31
      lung involvement M31.30
        with kidney involvement M31.31
  Weingarten's (tropical eosinophilia) J82
  Weiss-Baker G90.09
  Werdnig-Hoffman G12.0
  Wermer's E31.21
  Werner's E34.8
  Wernicke-Korsakoff (nonalcoholic) F04
    alcoholic F10.26
  Westphal-Strümpell E83.01
  West's — *see* Epilepsy, spasms
  wet
    feet (maceration) (tropical) T69.0- ☑
    lung, newborn P22.1
  whiplash S13.4 ☑
  whistling face Q87.0
  Wilkie's K55.1
  Wilkinson-Sneddon L13.1
  Willebrand (-Jürgens) D68.0
  Wilson's (hepatolenticular degeneration) E83.01
  Wiskott-Aldrich D82.0
  withdrawal — *see* Withdrawal, state
    drug
      infant of dependent mother P96.1
        therapeutic use, newborn P96.2
  Woakes' (ethmoiditis) J33.1
  Wright's (hyperabduction) G54.0
  X I20.9
  XXXX Q97.1
  XXXXX Q97.1
  XXXXY Q98.1
  XXY Q98.0

Subterms under main terms may continue to next column or page   ☑ Additional Character Required — Refer to the Tabular List for Character Selection   303

Syndrome — Syndrome

Index

Syndrome — *continued*
yellow nail L60.5
Zahorsky's B08.5
Zellweger syndrome E71.510
Zellweger-like syndrome E71.541
Synechia (anterior) (iris) (posterior) (pupil) (*see also* Adhesions, iris)
intra-uterine (traumatic) N85.6
Synesthesia R20.8
Syngamiasis, syngamosis B83.3
Synodontia K00.2
Synorchidism, synorchism Q55.1
Synostosis (congenital) Q78.8
astragalo-scaphoid Q74.2
radioulnar Q74.0
Synovial sarcoma — *see* Neoplasm, connective tissue, malignant
Synovioma (malignant) (*see also* Neoplasm, connective tissue, malignant)
benign — *see* Neoplasm, connective tissue, benign
Synoviosarcoma — *see* Neoplasm, connective tissue, malignant
Synovitis (*see also* Tenosynovitis) M65.9
crepitant
hand M70.0- ☑
wrist M70.03- ☑
gonococcal A54.49
gouty — *see* Gout
in (due to)
crystals M65.8- ☑
gonorrhea A54.49
syphilis (late) A52.78
use, overuse, pressure — *see* Disorder, soft tissue, due to use
infective NEC — *see* Tenosynovitis, infective NEC
specified NEC — *see* Tenosynovitis, specified type NEC
syphilitic A52.78
congenital (early) A50.02
toxic — *see* Synovitis, transient
transient M67.3- ☑
ankle M67.37- ☑
elbow M67.32- ☑
foot joint M67.37- ☑
hand joint M67.34- ☑
hip M67.35- ☑
knee M67.36- ☑
multiple site M67.39
pelvic region M67.35- ☑
shoulder M67.31- ☑
specified joint NEC M67.38
wrist M67.33- ☑
traumatic, current — *see* Sprain
tuberculous — *see* Tuberculosis, synovitis
villonodular (pigmented) M12.2- ☑
ankle M12.27- ☑
elbow M12.22- ☑
foot joint M12.27- ☑
hand joint M12.24- ☑
hip M12.25- ☑
knee M12.26- ☑
multiple site M12.29
pelvic region M12.25- ☑
shoulder M12.21- ☑
specified joint NEC M12.28
vertebrae M12.28
wrist M12.23- ☑
Syphilid A51.39
congenital A50.06
newborn A50.06
tubercular (late) A52.79
Syphilis, syphilitic (acquired) A53.9
abdomen (late) A52.79
acoustic nerve A52.15
adenopathy (secondary) A51.49
adrenal (gland) (with cortical hypofunction) A52.79
age under 2 years NOS (*see also* Syphilis, congenital, early)
acquired A51.9
alopecia (secondary) A51.32
anemia (late) A52.79 [D63.8]
aneurysm (aorta) (ruptured) A52.01
central nervous system A52.05
congenital A50.54 [I79.0]
anus (late) A52.74
primary A51.1
secondary A51.39
aorta (arch) (abdominal) (thoracic) A52.02

Syphilis, syphilitic — *continued*
aorta — *continued*
aneurysm A52.01
aortic (insufficiency) (regurgitation) (stenosis) A52.03
aneurysm A52.01
arachnoid (adhesive) (cerebral) (spinal) A52.13
asymptomatic — *see* Syphilis, latent
ataxia (locomotor) A52.11
atrophoderma maculatum A51.39
auricular fibrillation A52.06
bladder (late) A52.76
bone A52.77
secondary A51.46
brain A52.17
breast (late) A52.79
bronchus (late) A52.72
bubo (primary) A51.0
bulbar palsy A52.19
bursa (late) A52.78
cardiac decompensation A52.06
cardiovascular A52.00
central nervous system (late) (recurrent) (relapse) (tertiary) A52.3
with
ataxia A52.11
general paralysis A52.17
juvenile A50.45
paresis (general) A52.17
juvenile A50.45
tabes (dorsalis) A52.11
juvenile A50.45
taboparesis A52.17
juvenile A50.45
aneurysm A52.05
congenital A50.40
juvenile A50.40
remission in (sustained) A52.3
serology doubtful, negative, or positive A52.3
specified nature or site NEC A52.19
vascular A52.05
cerebral A52.17
meningovascular A52.13
nerves (multiple palsies) A52.15
sclerosis A52.17
thrombosis A52.05
cerebrospinal (tabetic type) A52.12
cerebrovascular A52.05
cervix (late) A52.76
chancre (multiple) A51.0
extragenital A51.2
Rollet's A51.0
Charcot's joint A52.16
chorioretinitis A51.43
congenital A50.01
late A52.71
prenatal A50.01
choroiditis — *see* Syphilitic chorioretinitis
choroidoretinitis — *see* Syphilitic chorioretinitis
ciliary body (secondary) A51.43
late A52.71
colon (late) A52.74
combined spinal sclerosis A52.11
condyloma (latum) A51.31
congenital A50.9
with
paresis (general) A50.45
tabes (dorsalis) A50.45
taboparesis A50.45
early, or less than 2 years after birth NEC A50.2
with manifestations — *see* Syphilis, congenital, early, symptomatic
latent (without manifestations) A50.1
negative spinal fluid test A50.1
serology positive A50.1
symptomatic A50.09
cutaneous A50.06
mucocutaneous A50.07
oculopathy A50.01
osteochondropathy A50.02
pharyngitis A50.03
pneumonia A50.04
rhinitis A50.05
visceral A50.08
chorioretinitis, choroiditis A50.01 [H32]
interstitial keratitis A50.31
juvenile neurosyphilis A50.45
late, or 2 years or more after birth NEC A50.7
chorioretinitis, choroiditis A50.32
interstitial keratitis A50.31

Syphilis, syphilitic — *continued*
congenital — *continued*
late, or 2 years or more after birth — *continued*
juvenile neurosyphilis A50.45
latent (without manifestations) A50.6
negative spinal fluid test A50.6
serology positive A50.6
symptomatic or with manifestations NEC A50.59
arthropathy A50.55
cardiovascular A50.54
Clutton's joints A50.51
Hutchinson's teeth A50.52
Hutchinson's triad A50.53
osteochondropathy A50.56
saddle nose A50.57
conjugal A53.9
tabes A52.11
conjunctiva (late) A52.71
contact Z20.2
cord bladder A52.19
cornea, late A52.71
coronary (artery) (sclerosis) A52.06
coryza, congenital A50.05
cranial nerve A52.15
multiple palsies A52.15
cutaneous — *see* Syphilis, skin
dacryocystitis (late) A52.71
degeneration, spinal cord A52.12
dementia paralytica A52.17
juvenilis A50.45
destruction of bone A52.77
dilatation, aorta A52.01
due to blood transfusion A53.9
dura mater A52.13
ear A52.79
inner A52.79
nerve (eighth) A52.15
neurorecurrence A52.15
early A51.9
cardiovascular A52.00
central nervous system A52.3
latent (without manifestations) (less than 2 years after infection) A51.5
negative spinal fluid test A51.5
serological relapse after treatment A51.5
serology positive A51.5
relapse (treated, untreated) A51.9
skin A51.39
symptomatic A51.9
extragenital chancre A51.2
primary, except extragenital chancre A51.0
secondary (*see also* Syphilis, secondary) A51.39
relapse (treated, untreated) A51.49
ulcer A51.39
eighth nerve (neuritis) A52.15
endemic A65
endocarditis A52.03
aortic A52.03
pulmonary A52.03
epididymis (late) A52.76
epiglottis (late) A52.73
epiphysitis (congenital) (early) A50.02
episcleritis (late) A52.71
esophagus A52.79
eustachian tube A52.73
exposure to Z20.2
eye A52.71
eyelid (late) (with gumma) A52.71
fallopian tube (late) A52.76
fracture A52.77
gallbladder (late) A52.74
gastric (polyposis) (late) A52.74
general A53.9
paralysis A52.17
juvenile A50.45
genital (primary) A51.0
glaucoma A52.71
gumma NEC A52.79
cardiovascular system A52.00
central nervous system A52.3
congenital A50.59
heart (block) (decompensation) (disease) (failure) A52.06 [I52]
valve NEC A52.03
hemianesthesia A52.19
hemianopsia A52.71
hemiparesis A52.17
hemiplegia A52.17

☑ **Additional Character Required** — Refer to the Tabular List for Character Selection   ▽ **Subterms under main terms may continue to next column or page**

Syndrome — Syphilis, syphilitic

Syphilis, syphilitic — *continued*
- hepatic artery A52.09
- hepatis A52.74
- hepatomegaly, congenital A50.08
- hereditaria tarda — *see* Syphilis, congenital, late
- hereditary — *see* Syphilis, congenital
- Hutchinson's teeth A50.52
- hyalitis A52.71
- inactive — *see* Syphilis, latent
- infantum — *see* Syphilis, congenital
- inherited — *see* Syphilis, congenital
- internal ear A52.79
- intestine (late) A52.74
- iris, iritis (secondary) A51.43
  - late A52.71
- joint (late) A52.77
- keratitis (congenital) (interstitial) (late) A50.31
- kidney (late) A52.75
- lacrimal passages (late) A52.71
- larynx (late) A52.73
- late A52.9
  - cardiovascular A52.00
  - central nervous system A52.3
  - kidney A52.75
  - latent or 2 years or more after infection (without manifestations) A52.8
    - negative spinal fluid test A52.8
    - serology positive A52.8
  - paresis A52.17
  - specified site NEC A52.79
  - symptomatic or with manifestations A52.79
  - tabes A52.11
- latent A53.0
  - with signs or symptoms — *code by* site and stage under Syphilis
  - early, or less than 2 years after infection A51.5
  - central nervous system A52.2
  - date of infection unspecified A53.0
  - follow-up of latent syphilis A53.0
    - date of infection unspecified A53.0
    - late, or 2 years or more after infection A52.8
  - late, or 2 years or more after infection A52.8
  - positive serology (only finding) A53.0
    - early, or less than 2 years after infection A51.5
    - date of infection unspecified A53.0
    - late, or 2 years or more after infection A52.8
- lens (late) A52.71
- leukoderma A51.39
  - late A52.79
- lienitis A52.79
- lip A51.39
  - chancre (primary) A51.2
  - late A52.79
- Lissauer's paralysis A52.17
- liver A52.74
- locomotor ataxia A52.11
- lung A52.72
- lymph gland (early) (secondary) A51.49
  - late A52.79
- lymphadenitis (secondary) A51.49
- macular atrophy of skin A51.39
  - striated A52.79
- mediastinum (late) A52.73
- meninges (adhesive) (brain) (spinal cord) A52.13
- meningitis A52.13
  - acute (secondary) A51.41
  - congenital A50.41
- meningoencephalitis A52.14
- meningovascular A52.13
  - congenital A50.41
- mesarteritis A52.09
  - brain A52.04
- middle ear A52.77
- mitral stenosis A52.03
- monoplegia A52.17
- mouth (secondary) A51.39
  - late A52.79
- mucocutaneous (secondary) A51.39
  - late A52.79
- mucous
  - membrane (secondary) A51.39
    - late A52.79
  - patches A51.39
    - congenital A50.07
- mulberry molars A50.52
- muscle A52.78
- myocardium A52.06
- nasal sinus (late) A52.73

Syphilis, syphilitic — *continued*
- neonatorum — *see* Syphilis, congenital
- nephrotic syndrome (secondary) A51.44
- nerve palsy (any cranial nerve) A52.15
  - multiple A52.15
- nervous system, central A52.3
- neuritis A52.15
  - acoustic A52.15
- neurorecidive of retina A52.19
- neuroretinitis A52.19
- newborn — *see* Syphilis, congenital
- nodular superficial (late) A52.79
- nonvenereal A65
- nose (late) A52.73
  - saddle back deformity A50.57
- occlusive arterial disease A52.09
- oculopathy A52.71
- ophthalmic (late) A52.71
- optic nerve (atrophy) (neuritis) (papilla) A52.15
- orbit (late) A52.71
- organic A53.9
- osseous (late) A52.77
- osteochondritis (congenital) (early) A50.02 [M90.80]
- osteoporosis A52.77
- ovary (late) A52.76
- oviduct (late) A52.76
- palate (late) A52.79
- pancreas (late) A52.74
- paralysis A52.17
  - general A52.17
    - juvenile A50.45
- paresis (general) A52.17
  - juvenile A50.45
- paresthesia A52.19
- Parkinson's disease or syndrome A52.19
- paroxysmal tachycardia A52.06
- pemphigus (congenital) A50.06
- penis (chancre) A51.0
  - late A52.76
- pericardium A52.06
- perichondritis, larynx (late) A52.73
- periosteum (late) A52.77
  - congenital (early) A50.02 [M90.80]
  - early (secondary) A51.46
- peripheral nerve A52.79
- petrous bone (late) A52.77
- pharynx (late) A52.73
  - secondary A51.39
- pituitary (gland) A52.79
- pleura (late) A52.73
- pneumonia, white A50.04
- pontine lesion A52.17
- portal vein A52.09
- primary A51.0
  - anal A51.1
  - and secondary — *see* Syphilis, secondary
  - central nervous system A52.3
  - extragenital chancre NEC A51.2
  - fingers A51.2
  - genital A51.0
  - lip A51.2
  - specified site NEC A51.2
  - tonsils A51.2
- prostate (late) A52.76
- ptosis (eyelid) A52.71
- pulmonary (late) A52.72
  - artery A52.09
- pyelonephritis (late) A52.75
- recently acquired, symptomatic A51.9
- rectum (late) A52.74
- respiratory tract (late) A52.73
- retina, late A52.71
- retrobulbar neuritis A52.15
- salpingitis A52.76
- sclera (late) A52.71
- sclerosis
  - cerebral A52.17
  - coronary A52.06
  - multiple A52.11
- scotoma (central) A52.71
- scrotum (late) A52.76
- secondary (and primary) A51.49
  - adenopathy A51.49
  - anus A51.39
  - bone A51.46
  - chorioretinitis, choroiditis A51.43
  - hepatitis A51.45
  - liver A51.45
  - lymphadenitis A51.49

Syphilis, syphilitic — *continued*
- secondary — *continued*
  - meningitis (acute) A51.41
  - mouth A51.39
  - mucous membranes A51.39
  - periosteum, periostitis A51.46
  - pharynx A51.39
  - relapse (treated, untreated) A51.49
  - skin A51.39
  - specified form NEC A51.49
  - tonsil A51.39
  - ulcer A51.39
  - viscera NEC A51.49
  - vulva A51.39
- seminal vesicle (late) A52.76
- seronegative with signs or symptoms — *code by* site and stage under Syphilis
- seropositive
  - with signs or symptoms — *code by* site and stage under Syphilis
  - follow-up of latent syphilis — *see* Syphilis, latent
  - only finding — *see* Syphilis, latent
- seventh nerve (paralysis) A52.15
- sinus, sinusitis (late) A52.73
- skeletal system A52.77
- skin (with ulceration) (early) (secondary) A51.39
  - late or tertiary A52.79
- small intestine A52.74
- spastic spinal paralysis A52.17
- spermatic cord (late) A52.76
- spinal (cord) A52.12
- spleen A52.79
- splenomegaly A52.79
- spondylitis A52.77
- staphyloma A52.71
- stigmata (congenital) A50.59
- stomach A52.74
- synovium A52.78
- tabes dorsalis (late) A52.11
  - juvenile A50.45
- tabetic type A52.11
  - juvenile A50.45
- taboparesis A52.17
  - juvenile A50.45
- tachycardia A52.06
- tendon (late) A52.78
- tertiary A52.9
  - with symptoms NEC A52.79
  - cardiovascular A52.00
  - central nervous system A52.3
  - multiple NEC A52.79
  - specified site NEC A52.79
- testis A52.76
- thorax A52.73
- throat A52.73
- thymus (gland) (late) A52.79
- thyroid (late) A52.79
- tongue (late) A52.79
- tonsil (lingual) (late) A52.73
  - primary A51.2
  - secondary A51.39
- trachea (late) A52.73
- tunica vaginalis (late) A52.76
- ulcer (any site) (early) (secondary) A51.39
  - late A52.79
  - perforating A52.79
    - foot A52.11
- urethra (late) A52.76
- urogenital (late) A52.76
- uterus (late) A52.76
- uveal tract (secondary) A51.43
  - late A52.71
- uveitis (secondary) A51.43
  - late A52.71
- uvula (late) (perforated) A52.79
- vagina A51.0
  - late A52.76
- valvulitis NEC A52.03
- vascular A52.00
  - brain (cerebral) A52.05
- ventriculi A52.74
- vesicae urinariae (late) A52.76
- viscera (abdominal) (late) A52.74
  - secondary A51.49
- vitreous (opacities) (late) A52.71
  - hemorrhage A52.71
- vulva A51.0
  - late A52.76
  - secondary A51.39

☑ Subterms under main terms may continue to next column or page   ☑ **Additional Character Required** — Refer to the Tabular List for Character Selection   **305**

Syphilis, syphilitic — Syphilis, syphilitic

...9
...stem A52.00
...stem A52.3
...A52.00

...5.29
...a (see also Neoplasm, skin, benign)
— see Neoplasm, skin, benign

Syringobulbia G95.0
Syringocystadenoma — *see* Neoplasm, skin, benign
    papillary — *see* Neoplasm, skin, benign
Syringoma (*see also* Neoplasm, skin, benign)
    chondroid — *see* Neoplasm, skin, benign
Syringomyelia G95.0
Syringomyelitis — *see* Encephalitis
Syringomyelocele — *see* Spina bifida

Syringopontia G95.0
System, systemic (*see also* condition)
    disease, combined — *see* Degeneration, combined
    inflammatory response syndrome (SIRS) of non-infec-
      tious origin (without organ dysfunction) R65.10
      with acute organ dysfunction R65.11
    lupus erythematosus M32.9
      inhibitor present D68.62

☑ **Additional Character Required — Refer to the Tabular List for Character Selection**   ▽ **Subterms under main terms may continue to next column or page**

T

Tabacism, tabacosis, tabagism (*see also* Poisoning, tobacco)
  meaning dependence (without remission) F17.200
    with
      disorder F17.299
        in remission F17.211
        specified disorder NEC F17.298
        withdrawal F17.203
Tabardillo A75.9
  flea-borne A75.2
  louse-borne A75.0
Tabes, tabetic A52.10
  with
    central nervous system syphilis A52.10
    Charcot's joint A52.16
    cord bladder A52.19
    crisis, viscera (any) A52.19
    paralysis, general A52.17
    paresis (general) A52.17
    perforating ulcer (foot) A52.19
  arthropathy (Charcot) A52.16
  bladder A52.19
  bone A52.11
  cerebrospinal A52.12
  congenital A50.45
  conjugal A52.10
  dorsalis A52.11
    juvenile A50.49
  juvenile A50.49
  latent A52.19
  mesenterica A18.39
  paralysis, insane, general A52.17
  spasmodic A52.17
  syphilis (cerebrospinal) A52.12
Taboparalysis A52.17
Taboparesis (remission) A52.17
  juvenile A50.45
TAC (trigeminal autonomic cephalgia) NEC G44.099
  intractable G44.091
  not intractable G44.099
Tache noir S60.22- ☑
Tachyalimentation K91.2
Tachyarrhythmia, tachyrhythmia — *see* Tachycardia
Tachycardia R00.0
  atrial (paroxysmal) I47.1
  auricular I47.1
  AV nodal re-entry (re-entrant) I47.1
  junctional (paroxysmal) I47.1
  newborn P29.11
  nodal (paroxysmal) I47.1
  non-paroxysmal AV nodal I45.89
  paroxysmal (sustained) (nonsustained) I47.9
    with sinus bradycardia I49.5
    atrial (PAT) I47.1
    atrioventricular (AV) (re-entrant) I47.1
      psychogenic F54
    junctional I47.1
      ectopic I47.1
    nodal I47.1
    psychogenic (atrial) (supraventricular) (ventricular) F54
    supraventricular (sustained) I47.1
      psychogenic F54
    ventricular I47.2
      psychogenic F54
  psychogenic F45.8
  sick sinus I49.5
  sinoauricular NOS R00.0
    paroxysmal I47.1
  sinus [sinusal] NOS R00.0
    paroxysmal I47.1
  supraventricular I47.1
  ventricular (paroxysmal) (sustained) I47.2
    psychogenic F54
Tachygastria K31.89
Tachypnea R06.82
  hysterical F45.8
  newborn (idiopathic) (transitory) P22.1
  psychogenic F45.8
  transitory, of newborn P22.1
TACO (transfusion associated circulatory overload) E87.71
Taenia (infection) (infestation) B68.9
  diminuta B71.0
  echinococcal infestation B67.90
  mediocanellata B68.1

Taenia — *continued*
  nana B71.0
  saginata B68.1
  solium (intestinal form) B68.0
    larval form — *see* Cysticercosis
Taeniasis (intestine) — *see* Taenia
Tag (hypertrophied skin) (infected) L91.8
  adenoid J35.8
  anus K64.4
  hemorrhoidal K64.4
  hymen N89.8
  perineal N90.89
  preauricular Q17.0
  sentinel K64.4
  skin L91.8
    accessory (congenital) Q82.8
    anus K64.4
    congenital Q82.8
    preauricular Q17.0
  tonsil J35.8
  urethra, urethral N36.8
  vulva N90.89
Tahyna fever B33.8
Takahara's disease E80.3
Takayasu's disease or syndrome M31.4
Talcosis (pulmonary) J62.0
Talipes (congenital) Q66.89
  acquired, planus — *see* Deformity, limb, flat foot
  asymmetric Q66.89
  calcaneovalgus Q66.4
  calcaneovarus Q66.1
  calcaneus Q66.89
  cavus Q66.7
  equinovalgus Q66.6
  equinovarus Q66.0
  equinus Q66.89
  percavus Q66.7
  planovalgus Q66.6
  planus (acquired) (any degree) (*see also* Deformity, limb, flat foot)
    congenital Q66.5- ☑
    due to rickets (sequelae) E64.3
  valgus Q66.6
  varus Q66.3
Tall stature, constitutional E34.4
Talma's disease M62.89
Talon noir S90.3- ☑
  hand S60.22- ☑
  heel S90.3- ☑
  toe S90.1- ☑
Tamponade, heart I31.4
Tanapox (virus disease) B08.71
Tangier disease E78.6
Tantrum, child problem F91.8
Tapeworm (infection) (infestation) — *see* Infestation, tapeworm
Tapia's syndrome G52.7
TAR (thrombocytopenia with absent radius) **syndrome** Q87.2
Tarral-Besnier disease L44.0
Tarsal tunnel syndrome — *see* Syndrome, tarsal tunnel
Tarsalgia — *see* Pain, limb, lower
Tarsitis (eyelid) H01.8
  syphilitic A52.71
  tuberculous A18.4
Tartar (teeth) (dental calculus) K03.6
Tattoo (mark) L81.8
Tauri's disease E74.09
Taurodontism K00.2
Taussig-Bing syndrome Q20.1
Taybi's syndrome Q87.2
Tay-Sachs amaurotic familial idiocy or disease E75.02
TBI (traumatic brain injury) S06.9 ☑
Teacher's node or nodule J38.2
Tear, torn (traumatic) (*see also* Laceration)
  with abortion — *see* Abortion
  annular fibrosis M51.35
  anus, anal (sphincter) S31.831 ☑
    complicating delivery
      with third degree perineal laceration (*see also* Delivery, complicated, by, laceration, perineum, third degree) O70.20
        with mucosa O70.3
      without third degree perineal laceration O70.4
    nontraumatic (healed) (old) K62.81
  articular cartilage, old — *see* Derangement, joint, articular cartilage, by site

Tear, torn — *continued*
  bladder
    with ectopic or molar pregnancy O08.6
    following ectopic or molar pregnancy O08.6
    obstetrical O71.5
    traumatic — *see* Injury, bladder
  bowel
    with ectopic or molar pregnancy O08.6
    following ectopic or molar pregnancy O08.6
    obstetrical trauma O71.5
  broad ligament
    with ectopic or molar pregnancy O08.6
    following ectopic or molar pregnancy O08.6
    obstetrical trauma O71.6
  bucket handle (knee) (meniscus) — *see* Tear, meniscus
  capsule, joint — *see* Sprain
  cartilage (*see also* Sprain)
    articular, old — *see* Derangement, joint, articular cartilage, by slte
  cervix
    with ectopic or molar pregnancy O08.6
    following ectopic or molar pregnancy O08.6
    obstetrical trauma (current) O71.3
    old N88.1
    traumatic — *see* Injury, uterus
  dural G97.41
    nontraumatic G96.11
  internal organ — *see* Injury, by site
  knee cartilage
    articular (current) S83.3- ☑
    old — *see* Derangement, knee, meniscus, due to old tear
  ligament — *see* Sprain
  meniscus (knee) (current injury) S83.209 ☑
    bucket-handle S83.20- ☑
    lateral
      bucket-handle S83.25- ☑
      complex S83.27- ☑
      peripheral S83.26- ☑
      specified type NEC S83.28- ☑
    medial
      bucket-handle S83.21- ☑
      complex S83.23- ☑
      peripheral S83.22- ☑
      specified type NEC S83.24- ☑
    old — *see* Derangement, knee, meniscus, due to old tear
    site other than knee — *code as* Sprain
    specified type NEC S83.20- ☑
  muscle — *see* Strain
  pelvic
    floor, complicating delivery O70.1
    organ NEC, obstetrical trauma O71.5
      with ectopic or molar pregnancy O08.6
      following ectopic or molar pregnancy O08.6
  perineal, secondary O90.1
  periurethral tissue, obstetrical trauma O71.82
    with ectopic or molar pregnancy O08.6
    following ectopic or molar pregnancy O08.6
  rectovaginal septum — *see* Laceration, vagina
  retina, retinal (without detachment) (horseshoe) (*see also* Break, retina, horseshoe)
    with detachment — *see* Detachment, retina, with retinal, break
  rotator cuff (nontraumatic) M75.10- ☑
    complete M75.12- ☑
    incomplete M75.11- ☑
    traumatic S46.01- ☑
      capsule S43.42- ☑
  semilunar cartilage, knee — *see* Tear, meniscus
  supraspinatus (complete) (incomplete) (nontraumatic) (*see also* Tear, rotator cuff) M75.10- ☑
  tendon — *see* Strain
  tentorial, at birth P10.4
  umbilical cord
    complicating delivery O69.89 ☑
  urethra
    with ectopic or molar pregnancy O08.6
    following ectopic or molar pregnancy O08.6
    obstetrical trauma O71.5
  uterus — *see* Injury, uterus
  vagina — *see* Laceration, vagina
  vessel, from catheter — *see* Puncture, accidental complicating surgery
  vulva, complicating delivery O70.0
Tear-stone — *see* Dacryolith

... condition)

... nic F45.8
... ated G47.63
... syndrome) KØØ.7
...ectasia, telangiectasis (verrucous) I78.1
...ic (cerebellar) (Louis-Bar) G11.3
...nilial I78.Ø
hemorrhagic, hereditary (congenital) (senile) I78.Ø
hereditary, hemorrhagic (congenital) (senile) I78.Ø
juxtafoveal H35.Ø7- ☑
macular H35.Ø7- ☑
macularis eruptiva perstans D47.Ø1
parafoveal H35.Ø7- ☑
retinal (idiopathic) (juxtafoveal) (macular) (parafoveal) H35.Ø7- ☑
spider I78.1
Telephone scatologia F65.89
Telescoped bowel or intestine K56.1
congenital Q43.8
Temperature
body, high (of unknown origin) R5Ø.9
cold, trauma from T69.9 ☑
newborn P8Ø.Ø
specified effect NEC T69.8 ☑
Temple — see condition
Temporal — see condition
Temporomandibular joint pain-dysfunction syndrome M26.62- ☑
Temporosphenoidal — see condition
Tendency
bleeding — see Defect, coagulation
suicide
meaning personal history of attempted suicide Z91.5
meaning suicidal ideation — see Ideation, suicidal
to fall R29.6
Tenderness, abdominal R1Ø.819
epigastric R1Ø.816
generalized R1Ø.817
left lower quadrant R1Ø.814
left upper quadrant R1Ø.812
periumbilic R1Ø.815
rebound R1Ø.829
epigastric R1Ø.826
generalized R1Ø.827
left lower quadrant R1Ø.824
left upper quadrant R1Ø.822
periumbilic R1Ø.825
right lower quadrant R1Ø.823
right upper quadrant R1Ø.821
right lower quadrant R1Ø.813
right upper quadrant R1Ø.811
Tendinitis, tendonitis (see also Enthesopathy)
Achilles M76.6- ☑
adhesive — see Tenosynovitis, specified type NEC
shoulder — see Capsulitis, adhesive
bicipital M75.2- ☑
calcific M65.2- ☑
ankle M65.27- ☑
foot M65.27- ☑
forearm M65.23- ☑
hand M65.24- ☑
lower leg M65.26- ☑
multiple sites M65.29
pelvic region M65.25- ☑
shoulder M75.3- ☑
specified site NEC M65.28
thigh M65.25- ☑
upper arm M65.22- ☑
due to use, overuse, pressure (see also Disorder, soft tissue, due to use)
specified NEC — see Disorder, soft tissue, due to use, specified NEC
gluteal M76.Ø- ☑
patellar M76.5- ☑
peroneal M76.7- ☑
psoas M76.1- ☑
tibial (posterior) M76.82- ☑
anterior M76.81- ☑
trochanteric — see Bursitis, hip, trochanteric
Tendon — see condition
Tendosynovitis — see Tenosynovitis
Tenesmus (rectal) R19.8
vesical R3Ø.1
Tennis elbow — see Epicondylitis, lateral

Tenonitis (see also Tenosynovitis)
eye (capsule) HØ5.Ø4- ☑
Tenontosynovitis — see Tenosynovitis
Tenontothecitis — see Tenosynovitis
Tenophyte — see Disorder, synovium, specified type NEC
Tenosynovitis (see also Synovitis) M65.9
adhesive — see Tenosynovitis, specified type NEC
shoulder — see Capsulitis, adhesive
bicipital (calcifying) — see Tendinitis, bicipital
gonococcal A54.49
in (due to)
crystals M65.8- ☑
gonorrhea A54.49
syphilis (late) A52.78
use, overuse, pressure (see also Disorder, soft tissue, due to use)
specified NEC — see Disorder, soft tissue, due to use, specified NEC
infective NEC M65.1- ☑
ankle M65.17- ☑
foot M65.17- ☑
forearm M65.13- ☑
hand M65.14- ☑
lower leg M65.16- ☑
multiple sites M65.19
pelvic region M65.15- ☑
shoulder region M65.11- ☑
specified site NEC M65.18
thigh M65.15- ☑
upper arm M65.12- ☑
radial styloid M65.4
shoulder region M65.81- ☑
adhesive — see Capsulitis, adhesive
specified type NEC M65.88
ankle M65.87- ☑
foot M65.87- ☑
forearm M65.83- ☑
hand M65.84- ☑
lower leg M65.86- ☑
multiple sites M65.89
pelvic region M65.85- ☑
shoulder region M65.81- ☑
specified site NEC M65.88
thigh M65.85- ☑
upper arm M65.82- ☑
tuberculous — see Tuberculosis, tenosynovitis
Tenovaginitis — see Tenosynovitis
Tension
arterial, high (see also Hypertension)
without diagnosis of hypertension RØ3.Ø
headache G44.2Ø9
intractable G44.2Ø1
not intractable G44.2Ø9
nervous R45.Ø
pneumothorax J93.Ø
premenstrual N94.3
state (mental) F48.9
Tentorium — see condition
Teratencephalus Q89.8
Teratism Q89.7
Teratoblastoma (malignant) — see Neoplasm, malignant, by site
Teratocarcinoma (see also Neoplasm, malignant, by site)
liver C22.7
Teratoma (solid) (see also Neoplasm, uncertain behavior, by site)
with embryonal carcinoma, mixed — see Neoplasm, malignant, by site
with malignant transformation — see Neoplasm, malignant, by site
adult (cystic) — see Neoplasm, benign, by site
benign — see Neoplasm, benign, by site
combined with choriocarcinoma — see Neoplasm, malignant, by site
cystic (adult) — see Neoplasm, benign, by site
differentiated — see Neoplasm, benign, by site
embryonal (see also Neoplasm, malignant, by site)
liver C22.7
immature — see Neoplasm, malignant, by site
liver C22.7
adult, benign, cystic, differentiated type or mature D13.4
malignant (see also Neoplasm, malignant, by site)
anaplastic — see Neoplasm, malignant, by site
intermediate — see Neoplasm, malignant, by site

Teratoma — continued
malignant (see also Neoplasm, malignant, by site) — continued
intermediate — see Neoplasm, malignant, by site — continued
specified site — see Neoplasm, malignant, by site
unspecified site C62.9Ø
undifferentiated — see Neoplasm, malignant, by site
mature — see Neoplasm, uncertain behavior, by site
malignant — see Neoplasm, by site, malignant, by site
ovary D27.- ☑
embryonal, immature or malignant C56- ☑
solid — see Neoplasm, uncertain behavior, by site
testis C62.9- ☑
adult, benign, cystic, differentiated type or mature D29.2- ☑
scrotal C62.1- ☑
undescended C62.Ø- ☑
Termination
anomalous (see also Malposition, congenital)
right pulmonary vein Q26.3
pregnancy, elective Z33.2
Ternidens diminutus infestation B81.8
Ternidensiasis B81.8
Terror(s) night (child) F51.4
Terrorism, victim of Z65.4
Terry's syndrome (see also Myopia, degenerative) H44.2- ☑
Tertiary — see condition
Test, tests, testing (for)
adequacy (for dialysis)
hemodialysis Z49.31
peritoneal Z49.32
blood pressure ZØ1.3Ø
abnormal reading — see Blood, pressure
blood typing ZØ1.83
Rh typing ZØ1.83
blood-alcohol ZØ4.8
positive — see Findings, abnormal, in blood
blood-drug ZØ4.8
positive — see Findings, abnormal, in blood
cardiac pulse generator (battery) Z45.Ø1Ø
fertility Z31.41
genetic
disease carrier status for procreative management
female Z31.43Ø
male Z31.44Ø
male partner of patient with recurrent pregnancy loss Z31.441
procreative management NEC
female Z31.438
male Z31.448
hearing ZØ1.1Ø
with abnormal findings NEC ZØ1.118
HIV (human immunodeficiency virus)
nonconclusive (in infants) R75
positive Z21
seropositive Z21
immunity status ZØ1.84
intelligence NEC ZØ1.89
laboratory (as part of a general medical examination) ZØØ.ØØ
with abnormal finding ZØØ.Ø1
for medicolegal reason NEC ZØ4.8
male partner of patient with recurrent pregnancy loss Z31.441
Mantoux (for tuberculosis) Z11.1
abnormal result R76.11
pregnancy, positive first pregnancy — see Pregnancy, normal, first
procreative Z31.49
fertility Z31.41
skin, diagnostic
allergy ZØ1.82
special screening examination — see Screening, by name of disease
Mantoux Z11.1
tuberculin Z11.1
specified NEC ZØ1.89
tuberculin Z11.1
abnormal result R76.11
vision ZØ1.ØØ
with abnormal findings ZØ1.Ø1
Wassermann Z11.3
positive — see Serology for syphilis, positive

☑ Additional Character Required — Refer to the Tabular List for Character Selection ▽ Subterms under main terms may continue to next column or page

Testicle, testicular, testis (*see also* condition)
  feminization syndrome (*see also* Syndrome, androgen
    insensitivity) E34.51
  migrans Q55.29
Tetanus, tetanic (cephalic) (convulsions) A35
  with
    abortion A34
    ectopic or molar pregnancy O08.0
  following ectopic or molar pregnancy O08.0
  inoculation reaction (due to serum) — *see* Complica-
    tions, vaccination
  neonatorum A33
  obstetrical A34
  puerperal, postpartum, childbirth A34
Tetany (due to) R29.0
  alkalosis E87.3
  associated with rickets E55.0
  convulsions R29.0
    hysterical F44.5
  functional (hysterical) F44.5
  hyperkinetic R29.0
    hysterical F44.5
  hyperpnea R06.4
    hysterical F44.5
    psychogenic F45.8
  hyperventilation (*see also* Hyperventilation) R06.4
    hysterical F44.5
  neonatal (without calcium or magnesium deficiency)
    P71.3
  parathyroid (gland) E20.9
  parathyroprival E89.2
  post- (para)thyroidectomy E89.2
  postoperative E89.2
  pseudotetany R29.0
  psychogenic (conversion reaction) F44.5
Tetralogy of Fallot Q21.3
Tetraplegia (chronic) (*see also* Quadriplegia) G82.50
Thailand hemorrhagic fever A91
Thalassanemia — *see* Thalassemia
Thalassemia (anemia) (disease) D56.9
  with other hemoglobinopathy D56.8
  alpha (major) (severe) (triple gene defect) D56.0
    minor D56.3
    silent carrier D56.3
    trait D56.3
  beta (severe) D56.1
    homozygous D56.1
    major D56.1
    minor D56.3
    trait D56.3
  delta-beta (homozygous) D56.2
    minor D56.3
    trait D56.3
  dominant D56.8
  hemoglobin
    C D56.8
    E-beta D56.5
  intermedia D56.1
  major D56.1
  minor D56.3
  mixed D56.8
  sickle-cell — *see* Disease, sickle-cell, thalassemia
  specified type NEC D56.8
  trait D56.3
  variants D56.8
Thanatophoric dwarfism or short stature Q77.1
Thaysen-Gee disease (nontropical sprue) K90.0
Thaysen's disease K90.0
Thecoma D27- ☑
  luteinized D27- ☑
  malignant C56- ☑
Thelarche, premature E30.8
Thelaziasis B83.8
Thelitis N61.0
  puerperal, postpartum or gestational — *see* Infection,
    nipple
Therapeutic — *see* condition
Therapy
  drug, long-term (current) (prophylactic)
    agents affecting estrogen receptors and estrogen
     levels NEC Z79.818
    anastrozole (Arimidex) Z79.811
    antibiotics Z79.2
     short-term use — *omit code*
    anticoagulants Z79.01
    anti-inflammatory Z79.1
    antiplatelet Z79.02
    antithrombotics Z79.02

Therapy — *continued*
  drug, long-term — *continued*
    aromatase inhibitors Z79.811
    aspirin Z79.82
    birth control pill or patch Z79.3
    bisphosphonates Z79.83
    contraceptive, oral Z79.3
    drug, specified NEC Z79.899
    estrogen receptor downregulators Z79.818
    Evista Z79.810
    exemestane (Aromasin) Z79.811
    Fareston Z79.810
    fulvestrant (Faslodex) Z79.818
    gonadotropin-releasing hormone (GnRH) agonist
     Z79.818
    goserelin acetate (Zoladex) Z79.818
    hormone replacement Z79.890
    insulin Z79.4
    letrozole (Femara) Z79.811
    leuprolide acetate (leuprorelin) (Lupron) Z79.818
    megestrol acetate (Megace) Z79.818
    methadone
     for pain management Z79.891
     maintenance therapy F11.20
    Nolvadex Z79.810
    opiate analgesic Z79.891
    oral contraceptive Z79.3
    raloxifene (Evista) Z79.810
    selective estrogen receptor modulators (SERMs)
     Z79.810
    short term — *omit code*
    steroids
     inhaled Z79.51
     systemic Z79.52
    tamoxifen (Nolvadex) Z79.810
    toremifene (Fareston) Z79.810
Thermic — *see* condition
Thermography (abnormal) (*see also* Abnormal, diagnostic imaging) R93.8
  breast R92.8
Thermoplegia T67.0 ☑
Thesaurismosis, glycogen — *see* Disease, glycogen
  storage
Thiamin deficiency E51.9
  specified NEC E51.8
Thiaminic deficiency with beriberi E51.11
Thibierge-Weissenbach syndrome — *see* Sclerosis,
  systemic
Thickening
  bone — *see* Hypertrophy, bone
  breast N64.59
  endometrium R93.8
  epidermal L85.9
    specified NEC L85.8
  hymen N89.6
  larynx J38.7
  nail L60.2
    congenital Q84.5
  periosteal — *see* Hypertrophy, bone
  pleura J92.9
    with asbestos J92.0
  skin R23.4
  subepiglottic J38.7
  tongue K14.8
  valve, heart — *see* Endocarditis
Thigh — *see* condition
Thinning vertebra — *see* Spondylopathy, specified NEC
Thirst, excessive R63.1
  due to deprivation of water T73.1 ☑
Thomsen disease G71.12
Thoracic (*see also* condition)
  kidney Q63.2
  outlet syndrome G54.0
Thoracogastroschisis (congenital) Q79.8
Thoracopagus Q89.4
Thorax — *see* condition
Thorn's syndrome N28.89
Thorson-Björck syndrome E34.0
Threadworm (infection) (infestation) B80
Threatened
  abortion O20.0
    with subsequent abortion O03.9
  job loss, anxiety concerning Z56.2
  labor (without delivery) O47.9
    at or after 37 completed weeks of gestation O47.1
    before 37 completed weeks of gestation O47.0- ☑
  loss of job, anxiety concerning Z56.2
  miscarriage O20.0

Threatened — *continued*
  unemployment, anxiety concerning Z56.2
Three-day fever A93.1
Threshers' lung J67.0
Thrix annulata (congenital) Q84.1
Throat — *see* condition
Thrombasthenia (Glanzmann) (hemorrhagic) (heredi-
  tary) D69.1
Thromboangiitis I73.1
  obliterans (general) I73.1
    cerebral I67.89
    vessels
     brain I67.89
     spinal cord I67.89
Thromboarteritis — *see* Arteritis
Thromboasthenia (Glanzmann) (hemorrhagic) (heredi-
  tary) D69.1
Thrombocytasthenia (Glanzmann) D69.1
Thrombocythemia (essential) (hemorrhagic) (idiopathic)
  (primary) D47.3
Thrombocytopathy (dystrophic) (granulopenic) D69.1
Thrombocytopenia, thrombocytopenic D69.6
  with absent radius (TAR) Q87.2
  congenital D69.42
  dilutional D69.59
  due to
    (massive) blood transfusion D69.59
    drugs D69.59
    extracorporeal circulation of blood D69.59
    platelet alloimmunization D69.59
  essential D69.3
  heparin induced (HIT) D75.82
  hereditary D69.42
  idiopathic D69.3
  neonatal, transitory P61.0
    due to
     exchange transfusion P61.0
     idiopathic maternal thrombocytopenia P61.0
     isoimmunization P61.0
  primary NEC D69.49
    idiopathic D69.3
  puerperal, postpartum O72.3
  secondary D69.59
  transient neonatal P61.0
Thrombocytosis, essential D47.3
  primary D47.3
Thromboembolism — *see* Embolism
Thrombopathy (Bernard-Soulier) D69.1
  constitutional D68.0
  Willebrand-Jurgens D68.0
Thrombopenia — *see* Thrombocytopenia
Thrombophilia D68.59
  primary NEC D68.59
  secondary NEC D68.69
  specified NEC D68.69
Thrombophlebitis I80.9
  antepartum O22.2- ☑
    deep O22.3- ☑
    superficial O22.2- ☑
  cavernous (venous) sinus G08
    complicating pregnancy O22.5- ☑
    nonpyogenic I67.6
  cerebral (sinus) (vein) G08
    nonpyogenic I67.6
    sequelae G09
  due to implanted device — *see* Complications, by site
    and type, specified NEC
  during or resulting from a procedure NEC T81.72 ☑
  femoral vein (superficial) I80.1- ☑
  femoropopliteal vein I80.0- ☑
  hepatic (vein) I80.8
  idiopathic, recurrent I82.1
  iliofemoral I80.1- ☑
  intracranial venous sinus (any) G08
    nonpyogenic I67.6
    sequelae G09
  intraspinal venous sinuses and veins G08
    nonpyogenic G95.19
  lateral (venous) sinus G08
    nonpyogenic I67.6
  leg I80.3
    superficial I80.0- ☑
  longitudinal (venous) sinus G08
    nonpyogenic I67.6
  lower extremity I80.299
  migrans, migrating I82.1
  pelvic
    with ectopic or molar pregnancy O08.0

Thrombophlebitis — *continued*
  pelvic — *continued*
    following ectopic or molar pregnancy O08.0
    puerperal O87.1
  popliteal vein — *see* Phlebitis, leg, deep, popliteal
  portal (vein) K75.1
  postoperative T81.72 ☑
  pregnancy — *see* Thrombophlebitis, antepartum
  puerperal, postpartum, childbirth O87.0
    deep O87.1
    pelvic O87.1
    septic O86.81
    superficial O87.0
  saphenous (greater) (lesser) I80.0- ☑
  sinus (intracranial) G08
    nonpyogenic I67.6
  specified site NEC I80.8
  tibial vein I80.23- ☑

Thrombosis, thrombotic (bland) (multiple) (progressive) (silent) (vessel) I82.90
  anal K64.5
  antepartum — *see* Thrombophlebitis, antepartum
  aorta, aortic I74.10
    abdominal I74.09
      saddle I74.01
    bifurcation I74.09
    saddle I74.01
    specified site NEC I74.19
    terminal I74.09
    thoracic I74.11
    valve — *see* Endocarditis, aortic
  apoplexy I63.3- ☑
  artery, arteries (postinfectional) I74.9
    auditory, internal — *see* Occlusion, artery, precerebral, specified NEC
    basilar — *see* Occlusion, artery, basilar
    carotid (common) (internal) — *see* Occlusion, artery, carotid
    cerebellar (anterior inferior) (posterior inferior) (superior) — *see* Occlusion, artery, cerebellar
    cerebral — *see* Occlusion, artery, cerebral
    choroidal (anterior) — *see* Occlusion, artery, precerebral, specified NEC
    communicating, posterior — *see* Occlusion, artery, precerebral, specified NEC
    coronary (*see also* Infarct, myocardium)
      not resulting in infarction I24.0
    hepatic I74.8
    hypophyseal — *see* Occlusion, artery, precerebral, specified NEC
    iliac I74.5
    limb I74.4
      lower I74.3
      upper I74.2
    meningeal, anterior or posterior — *see* Occlusion, artery, cerebral, specified NEC
    mesenteric (with gangrene) (*see also* Infarct, intestine) K55.069
    ophthalmic — *see* Occlusion, artery, retina
    pontine — *see* Occlusion, artery, precerebral, specified NEC
    precerebral — *see* Occlusion, artery, precerebral
    pulmonary (iatrogenic) — *see* Embolism, pulmonary
    renal N28.0
    retinal — *see* Occlusion, artery, retina
    spinal, anterior or posterior G95.11
    traumatic NEC T14.8 ☑
    vertebral — *see* Occlusion, artery, vertebral
  atrium, auricular (*see also* Infarct, myocardium)
    following acute myocardial infarction (current complication) I23.6
    not resulting in infarction I51.3
    old I51.3
  basilar (artery) — *see* Occlusion, artery, basilar
  brain (artery) (stem) (*see also* Occlusion, artery, cerebral)
    due to syphilis A52.05
    puerperal O99.43
    sinus — *see* Thrombosis, intracranial venous sinus
  capillary I78.8
  cardiac (*see also* Infarct, myocardium)
    not resulting in infarction I51.3
    old I51.3
    valve — *see* Endocarditis
  carotid (artery) (common) (internal) — *see* Occlusion, artery, carotid

Thrombosis, thrombotic — *continued*
  cavernous (venous) sinus — *see* Thrombosis, intracranial venous sinus
  cerebellar artery (anterior inferior) (posterior inferior) (superior) I66.3
  cerebral (artery) — *see* Occlusion, artery, cerebral
  cerebrovenous sinus (*see also* Thrombosis, intracranial venous sinus)
    puerperium O87.3
  chronic I82.91
  coronary (artery) (vein) (*see also* Infarct, myocardium)
    not resulting in infarction I24.0
  corpus cavernosum N48.89
  cortical I66.9
  deep — *see* Embolism, vein, lower extremity
  due to device, implant or graft (*see also* Complications, by site and type, specified NEC) T85.868 ☑
    arterial graft NEC T82.868 ☑
    breast (implant) T85.868 ☑
    catheter NEC T85.868 ☑
      dialysis (renal) T82.868 ☑
        intraperitoneal T85.868 ☑
      infusion NEC T82.868 ☑
        spinal (epidural) (subdural) T85.860 ☑
      urinary (indwelling) T83.86 ☑
    electronic (electrode) (pulse generator) (stimulator)
      bone T84.86 ☑
      cardiac T82.867 ☑
      nervous system (brain) (peripheral nerve) (spinal) T85.860 ☑
      urinary T83.86 ☑
    fixation, internal (orthopedic) NEC T84.86 ☑
    gastrointestinal (bile duct) (esophagus) T85.868 ☑
    genital NEC T83.86 ☑
    heart T82.867 ☑
    joint prosthesis T84.86 ☑
    ocular (corneal graft) (orbital implant) NEC T85.868 ☑
    orthopedic NEC T84.86 ☑
    specified NEC T85.868 ☑
    urinary NEC T83.86 ☑
    vascular NEC T82.868 ☑
    ventricular intracranial shunt T85.860 ☑
  during the puerperium — *see* Thrombosis, puerperal
  endocardial (*see also* Infarct, myocardium)
    not resulting in infarction I51.3
  eye — *see* Occlusion, retina
  genital organ
    female NEC N94.89
      pregnancy — *see* Thrombophlebitis, antepartum
    male N50.1
  gestational — *see* Phlebopathy, gestational
  heart (chamber) (*see also* Infarct, myocardium)
    not resulting in infarction I51.3
    old I51.3
  hepatic (vein) I82.0
    artery I74.8
  history (of) Z86.718
  intestine (with gangrene) (*see also* Infarct, intestine) K55.069
  intracardiac NEC (apical) (atrial) (auricular) (ventricular) (old) I51.3
  intracranial (arterial) I66.9
    venous sinus (any) G08
      nonpyogenic origin I67.6
      puerperium O87.3
  intramural (*see also* Infarct, myocardium)
    not resulting in infarction I51.3
    old I51.3
  intraspinal venous sinuses and veins G08
    nonpyogenic G95.19
  kidney (artery) N28.0
  lateral (venous) sinus — *see* Thrombosis, intracranial venous sinus
  leg — *see* Thrombosis, vein, lower extremity
    arterial I74.3
  liver (venous) I82.0
    artery I74.8
    portal vein I81
  longitudinal (venous) sinus — *see* Thrombosis, intracranial venous sinus
  lower limb — *see* Thrombosis, vein, lower extremity
  lung (iatrogenic) (postoperative) — *see* Embolism, pulmonary
  meninges (brain) (arterial) I66.8

Thrombosis, thrombotic — *continued*
  mesenteric (artery) (with gangrene) (*see also* Infarct, intestine) K55.069
    vein (inferior) (superior) I81
  mitral I34.8
  mural (*see also* Infarct, myocardium)
    due to syphilis A52.06
    not resulting in infarction I51.3
    old I51.3
  omentum (with gangrene) (*see also* Infarct, intestine) K55.069
  ophthalmic — *see* Occlusion, retina
  pampiniform plexus (male) N50.1
  parietal (*see also* Infarct, myocardium)
    not resulting in infarction I24.0
  penis, superficial vein N48.81
  perianal venous K64.5
  peripheral arteries I74.4
    upper I74.2
  personal history (of) Z86.718
  portal I81
    due to syphilis A52.09
  precerebral artery — *see* Occlusion, artery, precerebral
  puerperal, postpartum O87.0
    brain (artery) O99.43
      venous (sinus) O87.3
    cardiac O99.43
    cerebral (artery) O99.43
      venous (sinus) O87.3
    superficial O87.0
  pulmonary (artery) (iatrogenic) (postoperative) (vein) — *see* Embolism, pulmonary
  renal (artery) N28.0
    vein I82.3
  resulting from presence of device, implant or graft — *see* Complications, by site and type, specified NEC
  retina, retinal — *see* Occlusion, retina
  scrotum N50.1
  seminal vesicle N50.1
  sigmoid (venous) sinus — *see* Thrombosis, intracranial venous sinus
  sinus, intracranial (any) — *see* Thrombosis, intracranial venous sinus
  specified site NEC I82.890
    chronic I82.891
  spermatic cord N50.1
  spinal cord (arterial) G95.11
    due to syphilis A52.09
    pyogenic origin G06.1
  spleen, splenic D73.5
    artery I74.8
  testis N50.1
  traumatic NEC T14.8 ☑
  tricuspid I07.8
  tumor — *see* Neoplasm, unspecified behavior, by site
  tunica vaginalis N50.1
  umbilical cord (vessels), complicating delivery O69.5 ☑
  vas deferens N50.1
  vein (acute) I82.90
    antecubital I82.61- ☑
      chronic I82.71- ☑
    axillary I82.A1- ☑ (*following* I82.7)
      chronic I82.A2- ☑ (*following* I82.7)
    basilic I82.61- ☑
      chronic I82.71- ☑
    brachial I82.62- ☑
      chronic I82.72- ☑
    brachiocephalic (innominate) I82.290
      chronic I82.291
    cephalic I82.61- ☑
      chronic I82.71- ☑
    cerebral, nonpyogenic I67.6
    chronic I82.91
    deep (DVT) I82.40- ☑
      calf I82.4Z- ☑
        chronic I82.5Z- ☑
      lower leg I82.4Z- ☑
        chronic I82.5Z- ☑
      thigh I82.4Y- ☑
        chronic I82.5Y- ☑
      upper leg I82.4Y ☑
        chronic I82.5Y- ☑
    femoral I82.41- ☑
      chronic I82.51- ☑
    iliac (iliofemoral) I82.42- ☑
      chronic I82.52- ☑

☑ Additional Character Required — Refer to the Tabular List for Character Selection

▽ Subterms under main terms may continue to next column or page

Index

Thrombosis, thrombotic — *continued*
- vein — *continued*
  - innominate I82.290
    - chronic I82.291
  - internal jugular I82.C1- ☑ (*following* I82.7)
    - chronic I82.C2- ☑ (*following* I82.7)
  - lower extremity
    - deep I82.40- ☑
      - chronic I82.50- ☑
        - specified NEC I82.49- ☑
          - chronic NEC I82.59- ☑
    - distal
      - deep I82.4Z- ☑
    - proximal
      - deep I82.4Y- ☑
        - chronic I82.5Y- ☑
    - superficial I82.81- ☑
  - perianal K64.5
  - popliteal I82.43- ☑
    - chronic I82.53- ☑
  - radial I82.62- ☑
    - chronic I82.72- ☑
  - renal I82.3
  - saphenous (greater) (lesser) I82.81- ☑
  - specified NEC I82.890
    - chronic NEC I82.891
  - subclavian I82.B1- ☑ (*following* I82.7)
    - chronic I82.B2- ☑ (*following* I82.7)
  - thoracic NEC I82.290
    - chronic I82.291
  - tibial I82.44- ☑
    - chronic I82.54- ☑
  - ulnar I82.62- ☑
    - chronic I82.72- ☑
  - upper extremity I82.60- ☑
    - chronic I82.70- ☑
    - deep I82.62- ☑
      - chronic I82.72- ☑
    - superficial I82.61- ☑
      - chronic I82.71- ☑
- vena cava
  - inferior I82.220
    - chronic I82.221
  - superior I82.210
    - chronic I82.211
- venous, perianal K64.5
- ventricle (*see also* Infarct, myocardium)
  - following acute myocardial infarction (current complication) I23.6
  - not resulting in infarction I24.0
  - old I51.3

Thrombus — *see* Thrombosis
Thrush (*see also* Candidiasis)
- newborn P37.5
- oral B37.0
- vaginal B37.3
Thumb (*see also* condition)
- sucking (child problem) F98.8
Thymitis E32.8
Thymoma (benign) D15.0
- malignant C37
Thymus, thymic (gland) — *see* condition
Thyrocele — *see* Goiter
Thyroglossal (*see also* condition)
- cyst Q89.2
- duct, persistent Q89.2
Thyroid (gland) (body) (*see also* condition)
- hormone resistance E07.89
- lingual Q89.2
- nodule (cystic) (nontoxic) (single) E04.1
Thyroiditis E06.9
- acute (nonsuppurative) (pyogenic) (suppurative) E06.0
- autoimmune E06.3
- chronic (nonspecific) (sclerosing) E06.5
  - with thyrotoxicosis, transient E06.2
  - fibrous E06.5
  - lymphadenoid E06.3
  - lymphocytic E06.3
  - lymphoid E06.3
- de Quervain's E06.1
- drug-induced E06.4
- fibrous (chronic) E06.5
- giant-cell (follicular) E06.1
- granulomatous (de Quervain) (subacute) E06.1
- Hashimoto's (struma lymphomatosa) E06.3
- iatrogenic E06.4
- ligneous E06.5

Thyroiditis — *continued*
- lymphocytic (chronic) E06.3
- lymphoid E06.3
- lymphomatous E06.3
- nonsuppurative E06.1
- postpartum, puerperal O90.5
- pseudotuberculous E06.1
- pyogenic E06.0
- radiation E06.4
- Riedel's E06.5
- subacute (granulomatous) E06.1
- suppurative E06.0
- tuberculous A18.81
- viral E06.1
- woody E06.5
Thyrolingual duct, persistent Q89.2
Thyromegaly E01.0
Thyrotoxic
- crisis — *see* Thyrotoxicosis
- heart disease or failure (*see also* Thyrotoxicosis) E05.90 [I43]
  - with thyroid storm E05.91 [I43]
- storm — *see* Thyrotoxicosis
Thyrotoxicosis (recurrent) E05.90
- with
  - goiter (diffuse) E05.00
    - with thyroid storm E05.01
    - adenomatous uninodular E05.10
      - with thyroid storm E05.11
    - multinodular E05.20
      - with thyroid storm E05.21
    - nodular E05.20
      - with thyroid storm E05.21
    - uninodular E05.10
      - with thyroid storm E05.11
  - infiltrative
    - dermopathy E05.00
      - with thyroid storm E05.01
    - ophthalmopathy E05.00
      - with thyroid storm E05.01
  - single thyroid nodule E05.10
    - with thyroid storm E05.11
  - thyroid storm E05.91
- due to
  - ectopic thyroid nodule or tissue E05.30
    - with thyroid storm E05.31
  - ingestion of (excessive) thyroid material E05.40
    - with thyroid storm E05.41
  - overproduction of thyroid-stimulating hormone E05.80
    - with thyroid storm E05.81
  - specified cause NEC E05.80
    - with thyroid storm E05.81
- factitia E05.40
  - with thyroid storm E05.41
- heart (*see also* Failure, heart, high-output) E05.90 [I43]
  - with thyroid storm (*see also* Failure, heart, high-output) E05.91 [I43]
  - failure (*see also* Failure, heart, high-output) E05.90 [I43]
- neonatal (transient) P72.1
- transient with chronic thyroiditis E06.2
Tibia vara — *see* Osteochondrosis, juvenile, tibia
Tic (disorder) F95.9
- breathing F95.8
- child problem F95.0
- compulsive F95.1
- de la Tourette F95.2
- degenerative (generalized) (localized) G25.69
  - facial G25.69
- disorder
  - chronic
    - motor F95.1
    - vocal F95.1
  - combined vocal and multiple motor F95.2
  - transient F95.0
- douloureux G50.0
  - atypical G50.1
  - postherpetic, postzoster B02.22
- drug-induced G25.61
- eyelid F95.9
- habit F95.9
  - chronic F95.1
  - transient of childhood F95.0
- lid, transient of childhood F95.0
- motor-verbal F95.2
- occupational F48.8
- orbicularis F95.8

Tic — *continued*
- orbicularis — *continued*
  - transient of childhood F95.0
- organic origin G25.69
- postchoreic G25.69
- provisional F95.0
- psychogenic, compulsive F95.1
- salaam R25.8
- spasm (motor or vocal) F95.9
  - chronic F95.1
  - transient of childhood F95.0
- specified NEC F95.8
Tick-borne — *see* condition
Tietze's disease or syndrome M94.0
Tight, tightness
- anus K62.89
- chest R07.89
- fascia (lata) M62.89
- foreskin (congenital) N47.1
- hymen, hymenal ring N89.6
- introitus (acquired) (congenital) N89.6
- rectal sphincter K62.89
- tendon — *see* Short, tendon
- urethral sphincter N35.9
Tilting vertebra — *see* Dorsopathy, deforming, specified NEC
Timidity, child F93.8
Tinea (intersecta) (tarsi) B35.9
- amiantacea L44.8
- asbestina B35.0
- barbae B35.0
- beard B35.0
- black dot B35.0
- blanca B36.2
- capitis B35.0
- corporis B35.4
- cruris B35.6
- flava B36.0
- foot B35.3
- furfuracea B36.0
- imbricata (Tokelau) B35.5
- kerion B35.0
- manuum B35.2
- microsporic — *see* Dermatophytosis
- nigra B36.1
- nodosa — *see* Piedra
- pedis B35.3
- scalp B35.0
- specified NEC B35.8
- sycosis B35.0
- tonsurans B35.0
- trichophytic — *see* Dermatophytosis
- unguium B35.1
- versicolor B36.0
Tingling sensation (skin) R20.2
Tin-miner's lung J63.5
Tinnitus NOS H93.1- ☑
- audible H93.1- ☑
- aurium H93.1- ☑
- pulsatile H93.A- ☑
- subjective H93.1- ☑
Tipped tooth (teeth) M26.33
Tipping
- pelvis M95.5
  - with disproportion (fetopelvic) O33.0
    - causing obstructed labor O65.0
- tooth (teeth), fully erupted M26.33
Tiredness R53.83
Tissue — *see* condition
Tobacco (nicotine)
- abuse — *see* Tobacco, use
- dependence — *see* Dependence, drug, nicotine
- harmful use Z72.0
- heart — *see* Tobacco, toxic effect
- maternal use, affecting newborn P04.2
- toxic effect — *see* Table of Drugs and Chemicals, by substance, poisoning
  - chewing tobacco — *see* Table of Drugs and Chemicals, by substance, poisoning
  - cigarettes — *see* Table of Drugs and Chemicals, by substance, poisoning
- use Z72.0
  - complicating
    - childbirth O99.334
    - pregnancy O99.33- ☑
    - puerperium O99.335
  - counseling and surveillance Z71.6
  - history Z87.891

Thrombosis, thrombotic — Tobacco

Tobacco — *continued*
  withdrawal state (*see also* Dependence, drug, nicotine)
    F17.203
Tocopherol deficiency E56.0
Todd's
  cirrhosis K74.3
  paralysis (postepileptic) (transitory) G83.84
Toe — *see* condition
Toilet, artificial opening — *see* Attention to, artificial, opening
Tokelau (ringworm) B35.5
Tollwut — *see* Rabies
Tommaselli's disease R31.9
  correct substance properly administered — *see* Table of Drugs and Chemicals, by drug, adverse effect
  overdose or wrong substance given or taken — *see* Table of Drugs and Chemicals, by drug, poisoning
Tongue (*see also* condition)
  tie Q38.1
Tonic pupil — *see* Anomaly, pupil, function, tonic pupil
Toni-Fanconi syndrome (cystinosis) E72.09
  with cystinosis E72.04
Tonsil — *see* condition
Tonsillitis (acute) (catarrhal) (croupous) (follicular) (gangrenous) (infective) (lacunar) (lingual) (malignant) (membranous) (parenchymatous) (phlegmonous) (pseudomembranous) (purulent) (septic) (subacute) (suppurative) (toxic) (ulcerative) (vesicular) (viral) J03.90
  chronic J35.01
    with adenoiditis J35.03
  diphtheritic A36.0
  hypertrophic J35.01
    with adenoiditis J35.03
  recurrent J03.91
  specified organism NEC J03.80
    recurrent J03.81
  staphylococcal J03.80
    recurrent J03.81
  streptococcal J03.00
    recurrent J03.01
  tuberculous A15.8
  Vincent's A69.1
Tooth, teeth — *see* condition
Toothache K08.89
Topagnosis R20.8
Tophi — *see* Gout, chronic
TORCH infection — *see* Infection, congenital
  without active infection P00.2
Torn — *see* Tear
Tornwaldt's cyst or disease J39.2
Torsion
  accessory tube — *see* Torsion, fallopian tube
  adnexa (female) — *see* Torsion, fallopian tube
  aorta, acquired I77.1
  appendix epididymis N44.04
  appendix testis N44.03
  bile duct (common) (hepatic) K83.8
    congenital Q44.5
  bowel, colon or intestine K56.2
  cervix — *see* Malposition, uterus
  cystic duct K82.8
  dystonia — *see* Dystonia, torsion
  epididymis (appendix) N44.04
  fallopian tube N83.52- ☑
    with ovary N83.53
  gallbladder K82.8
    congenital Q44.1
  hydatid of Morgagni
    female N83.52- ☑
    male N44.03
  kidney (pedicle) (leading to infarction) N28.0
  Meckel's diverticulum (congenital) Q43.0
    malignant — *see* Table of Neoplasms, small intestine, malignant
  mesentery K56.2
  omentum K56.2
  organ or site, congenital NEC — *see* Anomaly, by site
  ovary (pedicle) N83.51- ☑
    with fallopian tube N83.53
    congenital Q50.2
  oviduct — *see* Torsion, fallopian tube
  penis (acquired) N48.82
    congenital Q55.63
  spasm — *see* Dystonia, torsion
  spermatic cord N44.02
    extravaginal N44.01

Torsion — *continued*
  spermatic cord — *continued*
    intravaginal N44.02
  spleen D73.5
  testis, testicle N44.00
    appendix N44.03
  tibia — *see* Deformity, limb, specified type NEC, lower leg
  uterus — *see* Malposition, uterus
Torticollis (intermittent) (spastic) M43.6
  congenital (sternomastoid) Q68.0
  due to birth injury P15.8
  hysterical F44.4
  ocular R29.891
  psychogenic F45.8
    conversion reaction F44.4
  rheumatic M43.6
  rheumatoid M06.88
  spasmodic G24.3
  traumatic, current S13.4 ☑
Tortipelvis G24.1
Tortuous
  aortic arch Q25.46
  artery I77.1
  organ or site, congenital NEC — *see* Distortion
  retinal vessel, congenital Q14.1
  ureter N13.8
  urethra N36.8
  vein — *see* Varix
Torture, victim of Z65.4
Torula, torular (histolytica) (infection) — *see* Cryptococcosis
Torulosis — *see* Cryptococcosis
Torus (mandibularis) (palatinus) M27.0
  fracture — *see* Fracture, by site, torus
Touraine's syndrome Q79.8
Tourette's syndrome F95.2
Tourniquet syndrome — *see* Constriction, external, by site
Tower skull Q75.0
  with exophthalmos Q87.0
Toxemia R68.89
  bacterial — *see* Sepsis
  burn — *see* Burn
  eclamptic (with pre-existing hypertension) — *see* Eclampsia
  erysipelatous — *see* Erysipelas
  fatigue R68.89
  food — *see* Poisoning, food
  gastrointestinal K52.1
  intestinal K52.1
  kidney — *see* Uremia
  malarial — *see* Malaria
  myocardial — *see* Myocarditis, toxic
  of pregnancy — *see* Pre-eclampsia
  pre-eclamptic — *see* Pre-eclampsia
  small intestine K52.1
  staphylococcal, due to food A05.0
  stasis R68.89
  uremic — *see* Uremia
  urinary — *see* Uremia
Toxemica cerebropathia psychica (nonalcoholic) F04
  alcoholic — *see* Alcohol, amnestic disorder ☑
Toxic (poisoning) (*see also* condition) T65.91 ☑
  effect — *see* Table of Drugs and Chemicals, by substance, poisoning
  shock syndrome A48.3
  thyroid (gland) — *see* Thyrotoxicosis
Toxicemia — *see* Toxemia
Toxicity — *see* Table of Drugs and Chemicals, by substance, poisoning
  fava bean D55.0
  food, noxious — *see* Poisoning, food
  from drug or nonmedicinal substance — *see* Table of Drugs and Chemicals, by drug
Toxicosis (*see also* Toxemia)
  capillary, hemorrhagic D69.0
Toxinfection, gastrointestinal K52.1
Toxocariasis B83.0
Toxoplasma, toxoplasmosis (acquired) B58.9
  with
    hepatitis B58.1
    meningoencephalitis B58.2
    ocular involvement B58.00
    other organ involvement B58.89
    pneumonia, pneumonitis B58.3
  congenital (acute) (subacute) (chronic) P37.1

Toxoplasma, toxoplasmosis — *continued*
  maternal, manifest toxoplasmosis in infant (acute) (subacute) (chronic) P37.1
tPA (rtPA) administration in a different facility within the last 24 hours prior to admission to current facility Z92.82
Trabeculation, bladder N32.89
Trachea — *see* condition
Tracheitis (catarrhal) (infantile) (membranous) (plastic) (septal) (suppurative) (viral) J04.10
  with
    bronchitis (15 years of age and above) J40
      acute or subacute — *see* Bronchitis, acute
      chronic J42
      tuberculous NEC A15.5
      under 15 years of age J20.9
    laryngitis (acute) J04.2
      chronic J37.1
      tuberculous NEC A15.5
  acute J04.10
    with obstruction J04.11
  chronic J42
    with
      bronchitis (chronic) J42
      laryngitis (chronic) J37.1
  diphtheritic (membranous) A36.89
  due to external agent — *see* Inflammation, respiratory, upper, due to
  syphilitic A52.73
  tuberculous A15.5
Trachelitis (nonvenereal) — *see* Cervicitis
Tracheobronchial — *see* condition
Tracheobronchitis (15 years of age and above) (*see also* Bronchitis)
  due to
    Bordetella bronchiseptica A37.80
      with pneumonia A37.81
    Francisella tularensis A21.8
Tracheobronchomegaly Q32.4
  with bronchiectasis J47.9
    with
      exacerbation (acute) J47.1
      lower respiratory infection J47.0
  acquired J98.09
    with bronchiectasis J47.9
      with
        exacerbation (acute) J47.1
        lower respiratory infection J47.0
Tracheobronchopneumonitis — *see* Pneumonia, broncho-
Tracheocele (external) (internal) J39.8
  congenital Q32.1
Tracheomalacia J39.8
  congenital Q32.0
Tracheopharyngitis (acute) J06.9
  chronic J42
  due to external agent — *see* Inflammation, respiratory, upper, due to
Tracheostenosis J39.8
Tracheostomy
  complication — *see* Complication, tracheostomy
  status Z93.0
    attention to Z43.0
    malfunctioning J95.03
Trachoma, trachomatous A71.9
  active (stage) A71.1
  contraction of conjunctiva A71.1
  dubium A71.0
  healed or sequelae B94.0
  initial (stage) A71.0
  pannus A71.1
  Türck's J37.0
Traction, vitreomacular H43.82- ☑
Train sickness T75.3 ☑
Trait(s)
  Hb-S D57.3
  hemoglobin
    abnormal NEC D58.2
      with thalassemia D56.3
    C — *see* Disease, hemoglobin C
    S (Hb-S) D57.3
  Lepore D56.3
  personality, accentuated Z73.1
  sickle-cell D57.3
    with elliptocytosis or spherocytosis D57.3
  type A personality Z73.1
Tramp Z59.0
Trance R41.89

Trance — *continued*
 hysterical F44.89
Transaminasemia R74.0
Transection
 abdomen (partial) S38.3 ☑
 aorta (incomplete) (*see also* Injury, aorta)
  complete — *see* Injury, aorta, laceration, major
 carotid artery (incomplete) (*see also* Injury, blood
   vessel, carotid, laceration)
  complete — *see* Injury, blood vessel, carotid, laceration, major
 celiac artery (incomplete) S35.211 ☑
  branch (incomplete) S35.291 ☑
   complete S35.292 ☑
  complete S35.212 ☑
 innominate
  artery (incomplete) (*see also* Injury, blood vessel,
    thoracic, innominate, artery, laceration)
   complete — *see* Injury, blood vessel, thoracic,
    innominate, artery, laceration, major
  vein (incomplete) (*see also* Injury, blood vessel,
    thoracic, innominate, vein, laceration)
   complete — *see* Injury, blood vessel, thoracic,
    innominate, vein, laceration, major
 jugular vein (external) (incomplete) (*see also* Injury,
   blood vessel, jugular vein, laceration)
  complete — *see* Injury, blood vessel, jugular vein,
   laceration, major
  internal (incomplete) (*see also* Injury, blood vessel,
    jugular vein, internal, laceration)
   complete — *see* Injury, blood vessel, jugular
    vein, internal, laceration, major
 mesenteric artery (incomplete) (*see also* Injury,
   mesenteric, artery, laceration)
  complete — *see* Injury, mesenteric artery, laceration, major
 pulmonary vessel (incomplete) (*see also* Injury, blood
   vessel, thoracic, pulmonary, laceration)
  complete — *see* Injury, blood vessel, thoracic,
   pulmonary, laceration, major
 subclavian — *see* Transection, innominate
 vena cava (incomplete) (*see also* Injury, vena cava)
  complete — *see* Injury, vena cava, laceration, major
 vertebral artery (incomplete) (*see also* Injury, blood
   vessel, vertebral, laceration)
  complete — *see* Injury, blood vessel, vertebral,
   laceration, major
Transfusion
 associated (red blood cell) hemochromatosis E83.111
 blood
  ABO incompatible — *see* Complication(s), transfusion, incompatibility reaction, ABO
  minor blood group (Duffy) (E) (K(ell)) (Kidd) (Lewis)
   (M) (N) (P) (S) T80.89 ☑
  reaction or complication — *see* Complications,
   transfusion
 fetomaternal (mother) — *see* Pregnancy, complicated
   by, placenta, transfusion syndrome
 maternofetal (mother) — *see* Pregnancy, complicated
   by, placenta, transfusion syndrome
 placental (syndrome) (mother) — *see* Pregnancy,
   complicated by, placenta, transfusion syndrome
 reaction (adverse) — *see* Complications, transfusion
 related acute lung injury (TRALI) J95.84
 twin-to-twin — *see* Pregnancy, complicated by, placenta, transfusion syndrome, fetus to fetus
Transient (meaning homeless) (*see also* condition) Z59.0
Translocation
 balanced autosomal Q95.9
  in normal individual Q95.0
 chromosomes NEC Q99.8
  balanced and insertion in normal individual Q95.0
 Down syndrome Q90.2
 trisomy
  13 Q91.6
  18 Q91.2
  21 Q90.2
Translucency, iris — *see* Degeneration, iris
Transmission of chemical substances through the
  placenta — *see* Absorption, chemical, through
  placenta
Transparency, lung, unilateral J43.0
Transplant (ed) (status) Z94.9
 awaiting organ Z76.82
 bone Z94.6
  marrow Z94.81
 candidate Z76.82

Transplant — *continued*
 complication — *see* Complication, transplant
 cornea Z94.7
 heart Z94.1
  and lung(s) Z94.3
  valve Z95.2
   prosthetic Z95.2
   specified NEC Z95.4
   xenogenic Z95.3
 intestine Z94.82
 kidney Z94.0
 liver Z94.4
 lung(s) Z94.2
  and heart Z94.3
 organ (failure) (infection) (rejection) Z94.9
  removal status Z98.85
 pancreas Z94.83
 skin Z94.5
 social Z60.3
 specified organ or tissue NEC Z94.89
 stem cells Z94.84
 tissue Z94.9
Transplants, ovarian, endometrial N80.1
Transposed — *see* Transposition
Transposition (congenital) (*see also* Malposition, congenital)
 abdominal viscera Q89.3
 aorta (dextra) Q20.3
 appendix Q43.8
 colon Q43.8
 corrected Q20.5
 great vessels (complete) (partial) Q20.3
 heart Q24.0
  with complete transposition of viscera Q89.3
 intestine (large) (small) Q43.8
 reversed jejunal (for bypass) (status) Z98.0
 scrotum Q55.23
 stomach Q40.2
  with general transposition of viscera Q89.3
 tooth, teeth, fully erupted M26.30
 vessels, great (complete) (partial) Q20.3
 viscera (abdominal) (thoracic) Q89.3
Transsexualism F64.0
Transverse (*see also* condition)
 arrest (deep), in labor O64.0 ☑
 lie (mother) O32.2 ☑
  causing obstructed labor O64.8 ☑
Transvestism, transvestitism (dual-role) F64.1
 fetishistic F65.1
Trapped placenta (with hemorrhage) O72.0
 without hemorrhage O73.0
TRAPS (tumor necrosis factor receptor associated periodic
  syndrome) M04.1
Trauma, traumatism (*see also* Injury)
 acoustic — *see* subcategory H83.3 ☑
 birth — *see* Birth, injury
 complicating ectopic or molar pregnancy O08.6
 during delivery O71.9
 following ectopic or molar pregnancy O08.6
 obstetric O71.9
  specified NEC O71.89
 occusal
  primary K08.81
  secondary K08.82
Traumatic (*see also* condition)
 brain injury S06.9 ☑
Treacher Collins syndrome Q75.4
Treitz's hernia — *see* Hernia, abdomen, specified site
  NEC
Trematode infestation — *see* Infestation, fluke
Trematodiasis — *see* Infestation, fluke
Trembling paralysis — *see* Parkinsonism
Tremor(s) R25.1
 drug induced G25.1
 essential (benign) G25.0
 familial G25.0
 hereditary G25.0
 hysterical F44.4
 intention G25.2
 medication induced postural G25.1
 mercurial — *see* subcategory T56.1 ☑
 Parkinson's — *see* Parkinsonism
 psychogenic (conversion reaction) F44.4
 senilis R54
 specified type NEC G25.2
Trench
 fever A79.0
 foot — *see* Immersion, foot

Trench — *continued*
 mouth A69.1
Treponema pallidum infection — *see* Syphilis
Treponematosis
 due to
  T. pallidum — *see* Syphilis
  T. pertenue — *see* Yaws
Triad
 Hutchinson's (congenital syphilis) A50.53
 Kartagener's Q89.3
 Saint's — *see* Hernia, diaphragm
Trichiasis (eyelid) H02.059
 with entropion — *see* Entropion
 left H02.056
  lower H02.055
  upper H02.054
 right H02.053
  lower H02.052
  upper H02.051
Trichinella spiralis (infection) (infestation) B75
Trichinellosis, trichiniasis, trichinelliasis, trichinosis
  B75
 with muscle disorder B75 [M63.80]
  ankle B75 [M63.87-] ☑
  foot B75 [M63.87-] ☑
  forearm B75 [M63.83-] ☑
  hand B75 [M63.84-] ☑
  lower leg B75 [M63.86-] ☑
  multiple sites B75 [M63.89]
  pelvic region B75 [M63.85-] ☑
  shoulder region B75 [M63.81-] ☑
  specified site NEC B75 [M63.88]
  thigh B75 [M63.85-] ☑
  upper arm B75 [M63.82-] ☑
Trichobezoar T18.9 ☑
 intestine T18.3 ☑
 stomach T18.2 ☑
Trichocephaliasis, trichocephalosis B79
Trichocephalus infestation B79
Trichoclasis L67.8
Trichoepithelioma (*see also* Neoplasm, skin, benign)
 malignant — *see* Neoplasm, skin, malignant
Trichofolliculoma — *see* Neoplasm, skin, benign
Tricholemmoma — *see* Neoplasm, skin, benign
Trichomoniasis A59.9
 bladder A59.03
 cervix A59.09
 intestinal A07.8
 prostate A59.02
 seminal vesicles A59.09
 specified site NEC A59.8
 urethra A59.03
 urogenitalis A59.00
 vagina A59.01
 vulva A59.01
Trichomycosis
 axillaris A48.8
 nodosa, nodularis B36.8
Trichonodosis L67.8
Trichophytid, trichophyton infection — *see* Dermato-
  phytosis
Trichophytobezoar T18.9 ☑
 intestine T18.3 ☑
 stomach T18.2 ☑
Trichophytosis — *see* Dermatophytosis
Trichoptilosis L67.8
Trichorrhexis (nodosa) (invaginata) L67.0
Trichosis axillaris A48.8
Trichosporosis nodosa B36.2
Trichostasis spinulosa (congenital) Q84.1
Trichostrongyliasis, trichostrongylosis (small intes-
  tine) B81.2
Trichostrongylus infection B81.2
Trichotillomania F63.3
Trichromat, trichromatopsia, anomalous (congenital)
  H53.55
Trichuriasis B79
Trichuris trichiura (infection) (infestation) (any site) B79
Tricuspid (valve) — *see* condition
Trifid (*see also* Accessory)
 kidney (pelvis) Q63.8
 tongue Q38.3
Trigeminal neuralgia — *see* Neuralgia, trigeminal
Trigeminy R00.8
Trigger finger (acquired) M65.30
 congenital Q74.0
 index finger M65.32- ☑

Trigger finger — *continued*
little finger M65.35- ☑
middle finger M65.33- ☑
ring finger M65.34- ☑
thumb M65.31- ☑
Trigonitis (bladder) (chronic) (pseudomembranous) N30.30
with hematuria N30.31
Trigonocephaly Q75.0
Trilocular heart — *see* Cor triloculare
Trimethylaminuria E72.52
Tripartite placenta O43.19- ☑
Triphalangeal thumb Q74.0
Triple (*see also* Accessory)
kidneys Q63.0
uteri Q51.818
X, female Q97.0
Triplegia G83.89
congenital G80.8
Triplet (newborn) (*see also* Newborn, triplet)
complicating pregnancy — *see* Pregnancy, triplet
Triplication — *see* Accessory
Triploidy Q92.7
Trismus R25.2
neonatorum A33
newborn A33
Trisomy (syndrome) Q92.9
13 (partial) Q91.7
meiotic nondisjunction Q91.4
mitotic nondisjunction Q91.5
mosaicism Q91.5
translocation Q91.6
18 (partial) Q91.3
meiotic nondisjunction Q91.0
mitotic nondisjunction Q91.1
mosaicism Q91.1
translocation Q91.2
20 Q92.8
21 (partial) Q90.9
meiotic nondisjunction Q90.0
mitotic nondisjunction Q90.1
mosaicism Q90.1
translocation Q90.2
22 Q92.8
autosomes Q92.9
chromosome specified NEC Q92.8
partial Q92.2
due to unbalanced translocation Q92.5
specified NEC Q92.8
whole (nonsex chromosome)
meiotic nondisjunction Q92.0
mitotic nondisjunction Q92.1
mosaicism Q92.1
due to
dicentrics — *see* Extra, marker chromosomes
extra rings — *see* Extra, marker chromosomes
isochromosomes — *see* Extra, marker chromosomes
specified NEC Q92.8
whole chromosome Q92.9
meiotic nondisjunction Q92.0
mitotic nondisjunction Q92.1
mosaicism Q92.1
partial Q92.9
specified NEC Q92.8
Tritanomaly, tritanopia H53.55
Trombiculosis, trombiculiasis, trombidiosis B88.0
Trophedema (congenital) (hereditary) Q82.0
Trophoblastic disease (*see also* Mole, hydatidiform) O01.9
Tropholymphedema Q82.0
Trophoneurosis NEC G96.8
disseminated M34.9
Tropical — *see* condition
Trouble (*see also* Disease)
heart — *see* Disease, heart
kidney — *see* Disease, renal
nervous R45.0
sinus — *see* Sinusitis
Trousseau's syndrome (thrombophlebitis migrans) I82.1
Truancy, childhood
from school Z72.810
Truncus
arteriosus (persistent) Q20.0
communis Q20.0
Trunk — *see* condition

Trypanosomiasis
African B56.9
by Trypanosoma brucei
gambiense B56.0
rhodesiense B56.1
American — *see* Chagas' disease
Brazilian — *see* Chagas' disease
by Trypanosoma
brucei gambiense B56.0
brucei rhodesiense B56.1
cruzi — *see* Chagas' disease
gambiensis, Gambian B56.0
rhodesiensis, Rhodesian B56.1
South American — *see* Chagas' disease
where
African trypanosomiasis is prevalent B56.9
Chagas' disease is prevalent B57.2
T-shaped incisors K00.2
Tsutsugamushi (disease) (fever) A75.3
Tube, tubal, tubular — *see* condition
Tubercle (*see also* Tuberculosis)
brain, solitary A17.81
Darwin's Q17.8
Ghon, primary infection A15.7
Tuberculid, tuberculide (indurating, subcutaneous) (lichenoid) (miliary) (papulonecrotic) (primary) (skin) A18.4
Tuberculoma (*see also* Tuberculosis)
brain A17.81
meninges (cerebral) (spinal) A17.1
spinal cord A17.81
Tuberculosis, tubercular, tuberculous (calcification) (calcified) (caseous) (chromogenic acid-fast bacilli) (degeneration) (fibrocaseous) (fistula) (interstitial) (isolated circumscribed lesions) (necrosis) (parenchymatous) (ulcerative) A15.9
with pneumoconiosis (any condition in J60-J64) J65
abdomen (lymph gland) A18.39
abscess (respiratory) A15.9
bone A18.03
hip A18.02
knee A18.02
sacrum A18.01
specified site NEC A18.03
spinal A18.01
vertebra A18.01
brain A17.81
breast A18.89
Cowper's gland A18.15
dura (mater) (cerebral) (spinal) A17.81
epidural (cerebral) (spinal) A17.81
female pelvis A18.17
frontal sinus A15.8
genital organs NEC A18.10
genitourinary A18.10
gland (lymphatic) — *see* Tuberculosis, lymph gland
hip A18.02
intestine A18.32
ischiorectal A18.32
joint NEC A18.02
hip A18.02
knee A18.02
specified NEC A18.02
vertebral A18.01
kidney A18.11
knee A18.02
latent R76.11
lumbar (spine) A18.01
lung — *see* Tuberculosis, pulmonary
meninges (cerebral) (spinal) A17.0
muscle A18.09
perianal (fistula) A18.32
perinephritic A18.11
perirectal A18.32
rectum A18.32
retropharyngeal A15.8
sacrum A18.01
scrofulous A18.2
scrotum A18.15
skin (primary) A18.4
spinal cord A17.81
spine or vertebra (column) A18.01
subdiaphragmatic A18.31
testis A18.15
urinary A18.13
uterus A18.17
accessory sinus — *see* Tuberculosis, sinus
Addison's disease A18.7

Tuberculosis, tubercular, tuberculous — *continued*
adenitis — *see* Tuberculosis, lymph gland
adenoids A15.8
adenopathy — *see* Tuberculosis, lymph gland
adherent pericardium A18.84
adnexa (uteri) A18.17
adrenal (capsule) (gland) A18.7
alimentary canal A18.32
anemia A18.89
ankle (joint) (bone) A18.02
anus A18.32
apex, apical — *see* Tuberculosis, pulmonary
appendicitis, appendix A18.32
arachnoid A17.0
artery, arteritis A18.89
cerebral A18.89
arthritis (chronic) (synovial) A18.02
spine or vertebra (column) A18.01
articular — *see* Tuberculosis, joint
ascites A18.31
asthma — *see* Tuberculosis, pulmonary
axilla, axillary (gland) A18.2
bladder A18.12
bone A18.03
hip A18.02
knee A18.02
limb NEC A18.03
sacrum A18.01
spine or vertebral column A18.01
bowel (miliary) A18.32
brain A17.81
breast A18.89
broad ligament A18.17
bronchi, bronchial, bronchus A15.5
ectasia, ectasis (bronchiectasis) — *see* Tuberculosis, pulmonary
fistula A15.5
primary (progressive) A15.7
gland or node A15.4
primary (progressive) A15.7
lymph gland or node A15.4
primary (progressive) A15.7
bronchiectasis — *see* Tuberculosis, pulmonary
bronchitis A15.5
bronchopleural A15.6
bronchopneumonia, bronchopneumonic — *see* Tuberculosis, pulmonary
bronchorrhagia A15.5
bronchotracheal A15.5
bronze disease A18.7
buccal cavity A18.83
bulbourethral gland A18.15
bursa A18.09
cachexia A15.9
cardiomyopathy A18.84
caries — *see* Tuberculosis, bone
cartilage A18.02
intervertebral A18.01
catarrhal — *see* Tuberculosis, respiratory
cecum A18.32
cellulitis (primary) A18.4
cerebellum A17.81
cerebral, cerebrum A17.81
cerebrospinal A17.81
meninges A17.0
cervical (lymph gland or node) A18.2
cervicitis, cervix (uteri) A18.16
chest — *see* Tuberculosis, respiratory
chorioretinitis A18.53
choroid, choroiditis A18.53
ciliary body A18.54
colitis A18.32
collier's J65
colliquativa (primary) A18.4
colon A18.32
complex, primary A15.7
congenital P37.0
conjunctiva A18.59
connective tissue (systemic) A18.89
contact Z20.1
cornea (ulcer) A18.52
Cowper's gland A18.15
coxae A18.02
coxalgia A18.02
cul-de-sac of Douglas A18.17
curvature, spine A18.01
cutis (colliquativa) (primary) A18.4
cyst, ovary A18.18

☑ Additional Character Required — Refer to the Tabular List for Character Selection   ▽ Subterms under main terms may continue to next column or page

Tuberculosis, tubercular, tuberculous — *continued*

cystitis A18.12
dactylitis A18.03
diarrhea A18.32
diffuse — *see* Tuberculosis, miliary
digestive tract A18.32
disseminated — *see* Tuberculosis, miliary
duodenum A18.32
dura (mater) (cerebral) (spinal) A17.0
    abscess (cerebral) (spinal) A17.81
dysentery A18.32
ear (inner) (middle) A18.6
    bone A18.03
    external (primary) A18.4
    skin (primary) A18.4
elbow A18.02
emphysema — *see* Tuberculosis, pulmonary
empyema A15.6
encephalitis A17.82
endarteritis A18.89
endocarditis A18.84
    aortic A18.84
    mitral A18.84
    pulmonary A18.84
    tricuspid A18.84
endocrine glands NEC A18.82
endometrium A18.17
enteric, enterica, enteritis A18.32
enterocolitis A18.32
epididymis, epididymitis A18.15
epidural abscess (cerebral) (spinal) A17.81
epiglottis A15.5
episcleritis A18.51
erythema (induratum) (nodosum) (primary) A18.4
esophagus A18.83
eustachian tube A18.6
exposure (to) Z20.1
exudative — *see* Tuberculosis, pulmonary
eye A18.50
eyelid (primary) (lupus) A18.4
fallopian tube (acute) (chronic) A18.17
fascia A18.09
fauces A15.8
female pelvic inflammatory disease A18.17
finger A18.03
first infection A15.7
gallbladder A18.83
ganglion A18.09
gastritis A18.83
gastrocolic fistula A18.32
gastroenteritis A18.32
gastrointestinal tract A18.32
general, generalized — *see* Tuberculosis, miliary
genital organs A18.10
genitourinary A18.10
genu A18.02
glandula suprarenalis A18.7
glandular, general A18.2
glottis A15.5
grinder's J65
gum A18.83
hand A18.03
heart A18.84
hematogenous — *see* Tuberculosis, miliary
hemoptysis — *see* Tuberculosis, pulmonary
hemorrhage NEC — *see* Tuberculosis, pulmonary
hemothorax A15.6
hepatitis A18.83
hilar lymph nodes A15.4
    primary (progressive) A15.7
hip (joint) (disease) (bone) A18.02
hydropneumothorax A15.6
hydrothorax A15.6
hypoadrenalism A18.7
hypopharynx A15.8
ileocecal (hyperplastic) A18.32
ileocolitis A18.32
ileum A18.32
iliac spine (superior) A18.03
immunological findings only A15.7
indurativa (primary) A18.4
infantile A15.7
infection A15.9
    without clinical manifestations A15.7
infraclavicular gland A18.2
inguinal gland A18.2
inguinalis A18.2
intestine (any part) A18.32

Tuberculosis, tubercular, tuberculous — *continued*

iridocyclitis A18.54
iris, iritis A18.54
ischiorectal A18.32
jaw A18.03
jejunum A18.32
joint A18.02
    vertebral A18.01
keratitis (interstitial) A18.52
keratoconjunctivitis A18.52
kidney A18.11
knee (joint) A18.02
kyphosis, kyphoscoliosis A18.01
laryngitis A15.5
larynx A15.5
latent R76.11
leptomeninges, leptomeningitis (cerebral) (spinal) A17.0
lichenoides (primary) A18.4
linguae A18.83
lip A18.83
liver A18.83
lordosis A18.01
lung — *see* Tuberculosis, pulmonary
lupus vulgaris A18.4
lymph gland or node (peripheral) A18.2
    abdomen A18.39
    bronchial A15.4
        primary (progressive) A15.7
    cervical A18.2
    hilar A15.4
        primary (progressive) A15.7
    intrathoracic A15.4
        primary (progressive) A15.7
    mediastinal A15.4
        primary (progressive) A15.7
    mesenteric A18.39
    retroperitoneal A18.39
    tracheobronchial A15.4
        primary (progressive) A15.7
lymphadenitis — *see* Tuberculosis, lymph gland
lymphangitis — *see* Tuberculosis, lymph gland
lymphatic (gland) (vessel) — *see* Tuberculosis, lymph gland
mammary gland A18.89
marasmus A15.9
mastoiditis A18.03
mediastinal lymph gland or node A15.4
    primary (progressive) A15.7
mediastinitis A15.8
    primary (progressive) A15.7
mediastinum A15.8
    primary (progressive) A15.7
medulla A17.81
melanosis, Addisonian A18.7
meninges, meningitis (basilar) (cerebral) (cerebrospinal) (spinal) A17.0
meningoencephalitis A17.82
mesentery, mesenteric (gland or node) A18.39
miliary A19.9
    acute A19.2
        multiple sites A19.1
        single specified site A19.0
    chronic A19.8
    specified NEC A19.8
millstone makers' J65
miner's J65
molder's J65
mouth A18.83
multiple A19.9
    acute A19.1
    chronic A19.8
muscle A18.09
myelitis A17.82
myocardium, myocarditis A18.84
nasal (passage) (sinus) A15.8
nasopharynx A15.8
neck gland A18.2
nephritis A18.11
nerve (mononeuropathy) A17.83
nervous system A17.9
nose (septum) A15.8
ocular A18.50
omentum A18.31
oophoritis (acute) (chronic) A18.17
optic (nerve trunk) (papilla) A18.59
orbit A18.59
orchitis A18.15
organ, specified NEC A18.89

Tuberculosis, tubercular, tuberculous — *continued*

osseous — *see* Tuberculosis, bone
osteitis — *see* Tuberculosis, bone
osteomyelitis — *see* Tuberculosis, bone
otitis media A18.6
ovary, ovaritis (acute) (chronic) A18.17
oviduct (acute) (chronic) A18.17
pachymeningitis A17.0
palate (soft) A18.83
pancreas A18.83
papulonecrotic (a) (primary) A18.4
parathyroid glands A18.82
paronychia (primary) A18.4
parotid gland or region A18.83
pelvis (bony) A18.03
penis A18.15
peribronchitis A15.5
pericardium, pericarditis A18.84
perichondritis, larynx A15.5
periostitis — *see* Tuberculosis, bone
perirectal fistula A18.32
peritoneum NEC A18.31
peritonitis A18.31
pharynx, pharyngitis A15.8
phlyctenulosis (keratoconjunctivitis) A18.52
phthisis NEC — *see* Tuberculosis, pulmonary
pituitary gland A18.82
pleura, pleural, pleurisy, pleuritis (fibrinous) (obliterative) (purulent) (simple plastic) (with effusion) A15.6
    primary (progressive) A15.7
pneumonia, pneumonic — *see* Tuberculosis, pulmonary
pneumothorax (spontaneous) (tense valvular) — *see* Tuberculosis, pulmonary
polyneuropathy A17.89
polyserositis A19.9
    acute A19.1
    chronic A19.8
potter's J65
prepuce A18.15
primary (complex) A15.7
proctitis A18.32
prostate, prostatitis A18.14
pulmonalis — *see* Tuberculosis, pulmonary
pulmonary (cavitated) (fibrotic) (infiltrative) (nodular) A15.0
    childhood type or first infection A15.7
    primary (complex) A15.7
pyelitis A18.11
pyelonephritis A18.11
pyemia — *see* Tuberculosis, miliary
pyonephrosis A18.11
pyopneumothorax A15.6
pyothorax A15.6
rectum (fistula) (with abscess) A18.32
reinfection stage — *see* Tuberculosis, pulmonary
renal A18.11
renis A18.11
respiratory A15.9
    primary A15.7
    specified site NEC A15.8
retina, retinitis A18.53
retroperitoneal (lymph gland or node) A18.39
rheumatism NEC A18.09
rhinitis A15.8
sacroiliac (joint) A18.01
sacrum A18.01
salivary gland A18.83
salpingitis (acute) (chronic) A18.17
sandblaster's J65
sclera A18.51
scoliosis A18.01
scrofulous A18.2
scrotum A18.15
seminal tract or vesicle A18.15
senile A15.9
septic — *see* Tuberculosis, miliary
shoulder (joint) A18.02
    blade A18.03
sigmoid A18.32
sinus (any nasal) A15.8
    bone A18.03
    epididymis A18.15
skeletal NEC A18.03
skin (any site) (primary) A18.4
small intestine A18.32
soft palate A18.83

Tuberculosis, tubercular, tuberculous — *continued*
  spermatic cord A18.15
  spine, spinal (column) A18.01
    cord A17.81
    medulla A17.81
    membrane A17.0
    meninges A17.0
  spleen, splenitis A18.85
  spondylitis A18.01
  sternoclavicular joint A18.02
  stomach A18.83
  stonemason's J65
  subcutaneous tissue (cellular) (primary) A18.4
  subcutis (primary) A18.4
  subdeltoid bursa A18.83
  submaxillary (region) A18.83
  supraclavicular gland A18.2
  suprarenal (capsule) (gland) A18.7
  swelling, joint (*see also* category M01) (*see also* Tuberculosis, joint) A18.02
  symphysis pubis A18.02
  synovitis A18.09
    articular A18.02
    spine or vertebra A18.01
  systemic — *see* Tuberculosis, miliary
  tarsitis A18.4
  tendon (sheath) — *see* Tuberculosis, tenosynovitis
  tenosynovitis A18.09
    spine or vertebra A18.01
  testis A18.15
  throat A15.8
  thymus gland A18.82
  thyroid gland A18.81
  tongue A18.83
  tonsil, tonsillitis A15.8
  trachea, tracheal A15.5
    lymph gland or node A15.4
      primary (progressive) A15.7
  tracheobronchial A15.5
    lymph gland or node A15.4
      primary (progressive) A15.7
  tubal (acute) (chronic) A18.17
  tunica vaginalis A18.15
  ulcer (skin) (primary) A18.4
    bowel or intestine A18.32
    specified NEC — *see* Tuberculosis, by site
  unspecified site A15.9
  ureter A18.11
  urethra, urethral (gland) A18.13
  urinary organ or tract A18.13
  uterus A18.17
  uveal tract A18.54
  uvula A18.83
  vagina A18.18
  vas deferens A18.15
  verruca, verrucosa (cutis) (primary) A18.4
  vertebra (column) A18.01
  vesiculitis A18.15
  vulva A18.18
  wrist (joint) A18.02
Tuberculum
  Carabelli — *see* Excludes Note at K00.2
  occlusal — *see* Excludes Note at K00.2
  paramolare K00.2
Tuberosity, enitre maxillary M26.07
Tuberous sclerosis (brain) Q85.1
Tubo-ovarian — *see* condition
Tuboplasty, after previous sterilization Z31.0
  aftercare Z31.42
Tubotympanitis, catarrhal (chronic) — *see* Otitis, media, nonsuppurative, chronic, serous
Tularemia A21.9
  with
    conjunctivitis A21.1
    pneumonia A21.2
  abdominal A21.3
  bronchopneumonic A21.2
  conjunctivitis A21.1
  cryptogenic A21.3
  enteric A21.3
  gastrointestinal A21.3
  generalized A21.7
  ingestion A21.3
  intestinal A21.3
  oculoglandular A21.1
  ophthalmic A21.1
  pneumonia (any), pneumonic A21.2
  pulmonary A21.2

Tularemia — *continued*
  sepsis A21.7
  specified NEC A21.8
  typhoidal A21.7
  ulceroglandular A21.0
Tularensis conjunctivitis A21.1
Tumefaction (*see also* Swelling)
  liver — *see* Hypertrophy, liver
Tumor (*see also* Neoplasm, unspecified behavior, by site)
  acinar cell — *see* Neoplasm, uncertain behavior, by site
  acinic cell — *see* Neoplasm, uncertain behavior, by site
  adenocarcinoid — *see* Neoplasm, malignant, by site
  adenomatoid (*see also* Neoplasm, benign, by site)
    odontogenic — *see* Cyst, calcifying odontogenic
  adnexal (skin) — *see* Neoplasm, skin, benign, by site
  adrenal
    cortical (benign) D35.0- ☑
      malignant C74.0- ☑
    rest — *see* Neoplasm, benign, by site
  alpha-cell
    malignant
      pancreas C25.4
      specified site NEC — *see* Neoplasm, malignant, by site
      unspecified site C25.4
    pancreas D13.7
    specified site NEC — *see* Neoplasm, benign, by site
    unspecified site D13.7
  aneurysmal — *see* Aneurysm
  aortic body D44.7
    malignant C75.5
  Askin's — *see* Neoplasm, connective tissue, malignant
  basal cell (*see also* Neoplasm, skin, uncertain behavior) D48.5
  Bednar — *see* Neoplasm, skin, malignant
  benign (unclassified) — *see* Neoplasm, benign, by site
  beta-cell
    malignant
      pancreas C25.4
      specified site NEC — *see* Neoplasm, malignant, by site
      unspecified site C25.4
    pancreas D13.7
    specified site NEC — *see* Neoplasm, benign, by site
    unspecified site D13.7
  Brenner D27.9
    borderline malignancy D39.1- ☑
    malignant C56- ☑
    proliferating D39.1- ☑
  bronchial alveolar, intravascular D38.1
  Brooke's — *see* Neoplasm, skin, benign
  brown fat — *see* Lipoma
  Burkitt — *see* Lymphoma, Burkitt
  calcifying epithelial odontogenic — *see* Cyst, calcifying odontogenic
  carcinoid
    benign D3A.00 (*following* D36)
      appendix D3A.020 (*following* D36)
      ascending colon D3A.022 (*following* D36)
      bronchus (lung) D3A.090 (*following* D36)
      cecum D3A.021 (*following* D36)
      colon D3A.029 (*following* D36)
      descending colon D3A.024 (*following* D36)
      duodenum D3A.010 (*following* D36)
      foregut NOS D3A.094 (*following* D36)
      hindgut NOS D3A.096 (*following* D36)
      ileum D3A.012 (*following* D36)
      jejunum D3A.011 (*following* D36)
      kidney D3A.093 (*following* D36)
      large intestine D3A.029 (*following* D36)
      lung (bronchus) D3A.090 (*following* D36)
      midgut NOS D3A.095 (*following* D36)
      rectum D3A.026 (*following* D36)
      sigmoid colon D3A.025 (*following* D36)
      small intestine D3A.019 (*following* D36)
      specified NEC D3A.098 (*following* D36)
      stomach D3A.092 (*following* D36)
      thymus D3A.091 (*following* D36)
      transverse colon D3A.023 (*following* D36)
    malignant C7A.00 (*following* C75)
      appendix C7A.020 (*following* C75)
      ascending colon C7A.022 (*following* C75)
      bronchus (lung) C7A.090 (*following* C75)
      cecum C7A.021 (*following* C75)
      colon C7A.029 (*following* C75)
      descending colon C7A.024 (*following* C75)

Tumor — *continued*
  carcinoid — *continued*
    malignant — *continued*
      duodenum C7A.010 (*following* C75)
      foregut NOS C7A.094 (*following* C75)
      hindgut NOS C7A.096 (*following* C75)
      ileum C7A.012 (*following* C75)
      jejunum C7A.011 (*following* C75)
      kidney C7A.093 (*following* C75)
      large intestine C7A.029 (*following* C75)
      lung (bronchus) C7A.090 (*following* C75)
      midgut NOS C7A.095 (*following* C75)
      rectum C7A.026 (*following* C75)
      sigmoid colon C7A.025 (*following* C75)
      small intestine C7A.019 (*following* C75)
      specified NEC C7A.098 (*following* C75)
      stomach C7A.092 (*following* C75)
      thymus C7A.091 (*following* C75)
      transverse colon C7A.023 (*following* C75)
    mesentary metastasis C7B.04 (*following* C75)
    secondary C7B.00 (*following* C75)
      bone C7B.03 (*following* C75)
      distant lymph nodes C7B.01 (*following* C75)
      liver C7B.02 (*following* C75)
      peritoneum C7B.04 (*following* C75)
      specified NEC C7B.09 (*following* C75)
  carotid body D44.6
    malignant C75.4
  cells (*see also* Neoplasm, unspecified behavior, by site)
    benign — *see* Neoplasm, benign, by site
    malignant — *see* Neoplasm, malignant, by site
    uncertain whether benign or malignant — *see* Neoplasm, uncertain behavior, by site
  cervix, in pregnancy or childbirth — *see* Pregnancy, complicated by, tumor, cervix
  chondromatous giant cell — *see* Neoplasm, bone, benign
  chromaffin (*see also* Neoplasm, benign, by site)
    malignant — *see* Neoplasm, malignant, by site
  Cock's peculiar L72.3
  Codman's — *see* Neoplasm, bone, benign
  dentigerous, mixed — *see* Cyst, calcifying odontogenic
  dermoid — *see* Neoplasm, benign, by site
    with malignant transformation C56- ☑
  desmoid (extra-abdominal) (*see also* Neoplasm, connective tissue, uncertain behavior)
    abdominal — *see* Neoplasm, connective tissue, uncertain behavior
  embolus — *see* Neoplasm, secondary, by site
  embryonal (mixed) (*see also* Neoplasm, uncertain behavior, by site)
    liver C22.7
  endodermal sinus
    specified site — *see* Neoplasm, malignant, by site
    unspecified site
      female C56.- ☑
      male C62.90
  epithelial
    benign — *see* Neoplasm, benign, by site
    malignant — *see* Neoplasm, malignant, by site
  Ewing's — *see* Neoplasm, bone, malignant, by site
  fatty — *see* Lipoma
  fibroid — *see* Leiomyoma
  G cell
    malignant
      pancreas C25.4
      specified site NEC — *see* Neoplasm, malignant, by site
      unspecified site C25.4
    specified site — *see* Neoplasm, uncertain behavior, by site
    unspecified site D37.8
  germ cell (*see also* Neoplasm, malignant, by site)
    mixed — *see* Neoplasm, malignant, by site
  ghost cell, odontogenic — *see* Cyst, calcifying odontogenic
  giant cell (*see also* Neoplasm, uncertain behavior, by site)
    bone D48.0
      malignant — *see* Neoplasm, bone, malignant
      chondromatous — *see* Neoplasm, bone, benign
    malignant — *see* Neoplasm, malignant, by site
    soft parts — *see* Neoplasm, connective tissue, uncertain behavior
      malignant — *see* Neoplasm, connective tissue, malignant
  glomus D18.00
    intra-abdominal D18.03

☑ **Additional Character Required** — **Refer to the Tabular List for Character Selection**
▽ **Subterms under main terms may continue to next column or page**

Tumor — *continued*
glomus — *continued*
  intracranial D18.02
  jugulare D44.7
    malignant C75.5
  skin D18.01
  specified site NEC D18.09
gonadal stromal — *see* Neoplasm, uncertain behavior, by site
granular cell (*see also* Neoplasm, connective tissue, benign)
  malignant — *see* Neoplasm, connective tissue, malignant
granulosa cell D39.1- ☑
  juvenile D39.1- ☑
  malignant C56- ☑
granulosa cell-theca cell D39.1- ☑
  malignant C56- ☑
Grawitz's C64- ☑
hemorrhoidal — *see* Hemorrhoids
hilar cell D27- ☑
hilus cell D27- ☑
Hurthle cell (benign) D34
  malignant C73
hydatid — *see* Echinococcus
hypernephroid (*see also* Neoplasm, uncertain behavior, by site)
interstitial cell (*see also* Neoplasm, uncertain behavior, by site)
  benign — *see* Neoplasm, benign, by site
  malignant — *see* Neoplasm, malignant, by site
intravascular bronchial alveolar D38.1
islet cell — *see* Neoplasm, benign, by site
  malignant — *see* Neoplasm, malignant, by site
    pancreas C25.4
    specified site NEC — *see* Neoplasm, malignant, by site
  pancreas D13.7
  specified site NEC — *see* Neoplasm, benign, by site
  unspecified site D13.7
juxtaglomerular D41.0- ☑
Klatskin's C22.1
Krukenberg's C79.6- ☑
Leydig cell — *see* Neoplasm, uncertain behavior, by site
  benign — *see* Neoplasm, benign, by site
    specified site — *see* Neoplasm, benign, by site
    unspecified site
      female D27.9
      male D29.20
  malignant — *see* Neoplasm, malignant, by site
    specified site — *see* Neoplasm, malignant, by site
    unspecified site
      female C56.9
      male C62.90
  specified site — *see* Neoplasm, uncertain behavior, by site
  unspecified site
    female D39.10
    male D40.10
lipid cell, ovary D27- ☑
lipoid cell, ovary D27- ☑
malignant (*see also* Neoplasm, malignant, by site) C80.1
  fusiform cell (type) C80.1
  giant cell (type) C80.1
  localized, plasma cell — *see* Plasmacytoma, solitary
  mixed NEC C80.1
  small cell (type) C80.1
  spindle cell (type) C80.1
  unclassified C80.1
mast cell D47.09
melanotic, neuroectodermal — *see* Neoplasm, benign, by site
Merkel cell — *see* Carcinoma, Merkel cell
mesenchymal
  malignant — *see* Neoplasm, connective tissue, malignant
  mixed — *see* Neoplasm, connective tissue, uncertain behavior
mesodermal, mixed (*see also* Neoplasm, malignant, by site)
  liver C22.4

Tumor — *continued*
mesonephric (*see also* Neoplasm, uncertain behavior, by site)
  malignant — *see* Neoplasm, malignant, by site
metastatic
  from specified site — *see* Neoplasm, malignant, by site
  of specified site — *see* Neoplasm, malignant, by site
  to specified site — *see* Neoplasm, secondary, by site
mixed NEC (*see also* Neoplasm, benign, by site)
  malignant — *see* Neoplasm, malignant, by site
mucinous of low malignant potential
  specified site — *see* Neoplasm, malignant, by site
  unspecified site C56.9
mucocarcinoid
  specified site — *see* Neoplasm, malignant, by site
  unspecified site C18.1
mucoepidermoid — *see* Neoplasm, uncertain behavior, by site
Müllerian, mixed
  specified site — *see* Neoplasm, malignant, by site
  unspecified site C54.9
myoepithelial — *see* Neoplasm, benign, by site
neuroectodermal (peripheral) — *see* Neoplasm, malignant, by site
  primitive
    specified site — *see* Neoplasm, malignant, by site
    unspecified site C71.9
neuroendocrine D3A.8 (*following* D36)
  malignant poorly differentiated C7A.1 (*following* C75)
  secondary NEC C7B.8 (*following* C75)
  specified NEC C7A.8 (*following* C75)
neurogenic olfactory C30.0
nonencapsulated sclerosing C73
odontogenic (adenomatoid) (benign) (calcifying epithelial) (keratocystic) (squamous) — *see* Cyst, calcifying odontogenic
  malignant C41.1
    upper jaw (bone) C41.0
ovarian stromal D39.1- ☑
ovary, in pregnancy — *see* Pregnancy, complicated by
pacinian — *see* Neoplasm, skin, benign
Pancoast's — *see* Pancoast's syndrome
papillary (*see also* Papilloma)
  cystic D37.9
  mucinous of low malignant potential C56- ☑
    specified site — *see* Neoplasm, malignant, by site
    unspecified site C56.9
  serous of low malignant potential
    specified site — *see* Neoplasm, malignant, by site
    unspecified site C56.9
pelvic, in pregnancy or childbirth — *see* Pregnancy, complicated by
phantom F45.8
phyllodes D48.6- ☑
  benign D24- ☑
  malignant — *see* Neoplasm, breast, malignant
Pindborg — *see* Cyst, calcifying odontogenic
placental site trophoblastic D39.2
plasma cell (malignant) (localized) — *see* Plasmacytoma, solitary
polyvesicular vitelline
  specified site — *see* Neoplasm, malignant, by site
  unspecified site
    female C56.9
    male C62.90
Pott's puffy — *see* Osteomyelitis, specified NEC
Rathke's pouch D44.3
retinal anlage — *see* Neoplasm, benign, by site
salivary gland type, mixed — *see* Neoplasm, salivary gland, benign
  malignant — *see* Neoplasm, salivary gland, malignant
Sampson's N80.1
Schmincke's — *see* Neoplasm, nasopharynx, malignant
sclerosing stromal D27- ☑
sebaceous — *see* Cyst, sebaceous
secondary — *see* Neoplasm, secondary, by site
  carcinoid C7B.00 (*following* C75)
    bone C7B.03 (*following* C75)
    distant lymph nodes C7B.01 (*following* C75)

Tumor — *continued*
secondary — *see* Neoplasm, secondary, by site — *continued*
  carcinoid — *continued*
    liver C7B.02 (*following* C75)
    peritoneum C7B.04 (*following* C75)
    specified NEC C7B.09 (*following* C75)
  neuroendocrine NEC C7B.8 (*following* C75)
serous of low malignant potential
  specified site — *see* Neoplasm, malignant, by site
  unspecified site C56.9
Sertoli cell — *see* Neoplasm, benign, by site
  with lipid storage
    specified site — *see* Neoplasm, benign, by site
    unspecified site
      female D27.9
      male D29.20
  specified site — *see* Neoplasm, benign, by site
  unspecified site
    female D27.9
    male D29.20
Sertoli-Leydig cell — *see* Neoplasm, benign, by site
  specified site — *see* Neoplasm, benign, by site
  unspecified site
    female D27.9
    male D29.20
sex cord (-stromal) — *see* Neoplasm, uncertain behavior, by site
  with annular tubules D39.1- ☑
skin appendage — *see* Neoplasm, skin, benign
smooth muscle — *see* Neoplasm, connective tissue, uncertain behavior
soft tissue
  benign — *see* Neoplasm, connective tissue, benign
  malignant — *see* Neoplasm, connective tissue, malignant
sternomastoid (congenital) Q68.0
stromal
  endometrial D39.0
  gastric D48.1
    benign D21.4
    malignant C16.9
    uncertain behavior D48.1
  gastrointestinal C49.A- ☑
    benign D21.4
    esophagus C49.A1
    malignant C49.A0
      colon C49.A4
      duodenum C49.A3
      esophagus C49.A1
      ileum C49.A3
      jejunum C49.A3
      large intestine C49.A4
      Meckel diverticulum C49.A3
      omentum C49.A9
      peritoneum C49.A9
      rectum C49.A5
      small intestine C49.A3
      specified site NEC C49.A9
      stomach C49.A2
    rectum C49.A5
    small intestine C49.A3
    specified site NEC C49.A9
    stomach C49.A2
    uncertain behavior D48.1
  intestine
    benign D21.4
    malignant
      large C49.A4
      small C49.A3
    uncertain behavior D48.1
  ovarian D39.1- ☑
  stomach C49.A2
    benign D21.4
    malignant C49.A2
    uncertain behavior D48.1
sweat gland (*see also* Neoplasm, skin, uncertain behavior)
  benign — *see* Neoplasm, skin, benign
  malignant — *see* Neoplasm, skin, malignant
syphilitic, brain A52.17
testicular D40.10
testicular stromal D40.1- ☑
theca cell D27.- ☑
theca cell-granulosa cell D39.1- ☑
Triton, malignant — *see* Neoplasm, nerve, malignant
trophoblastic, placental site D39.2
turban D23.4

☑ **Subterms under main terms may continue to next column or page**   ☑ **Additional Character Required — Refer to the Tabular List for Character Selection**

Tumor — continued
  uterus (body), in pregnancy or childbirth — see Pregnancy, complicated by, tumor, uterus
  vagina, in pregnancy or childbirth — see Pregnancy, complicated by
  varicose — see Varix
  von Recklinghausen's — see Neurofibromatosis
  vulva or perineum, in pregnancy or childbirth — see Pregnancy, complicated by
    causing obstructed labor O65.5
  Warthin's — see Neoplasm, salivary gland, benign
  Wilms' C64- ☑
  yolk sac — see Neoplasm, malignant, by site
    specified site — see Neoplasm, malignant, by site
    unspecified site
      female C56.9
      male C62.90
Tumor lysis syndrome (following antineoplastic chemotherapy) (spontaneous) NEC E88.3
Tumorlet — see Neoplasm, uncertain behavior, by site
Tungiasis B88.1
Tunica vasculosa lentis Q12.2
Turban tumor D23.4
Türck's trachoma J37.0
Turner-Kieser syndrome Q87.2
Turner-like syndrome Q87.1
Turner's
  hypoplasia (tooth) K00.4
  syndrome Q96.9
    specified NEC Q96.8
  tooth K00.4
Turner-Ullrich syndrome Q96.9
Tussis convulsiva — see Whooping cough
Twiddler's syndrome (due to)
  automatic implantable defibrillator T82.198
  cardiac pacemaker T82.198 ☑
Twilight state
  epileptic F05
  psychogenic F44.89
Twin (newborn) (see also Newborn, twin)
  conjoined Q89.4
  pregnancy — see Pregnancy, twin
Twinning, teeth K00.2
Twist, twisted
  bowel, colon or intestine K56.2
  hair (congenital) Q84.1
  mesentery K56.2
  omentum K56.2
  organ or site, congenital NEC — see Anomaly, by site
  ovarian pedicle — see Torsion, ovary
Twitching R25.3
Tylosis (acquired) L84
  buccalis K13.29
  linguae K13.29
  palmaris et plantaris (congenital) (inherited) Q82.8
    acquired L85.1
Tympanism R14.0
Tympanites (abdominal) (intestinal) R14.0
Tympanitis — see Myringitis
Tympanosclerosis H74.0 ☑
Tympanum — see condition
Tympany
  abdomen R14.0
  chest R09.89
Type A behavior pattern Z73.1
Typhlitis — see Appendicitis
Typhoenteritis — see Typhoid
Typhoid (abortive) (ambulant) (any site) (clinical) (fever) (hemorrhagic) (infection) (intermittent) (malignant) (rheumatic) (Widal negative) A01.00
  with pneumonia A01.03
  abdominal A01.09
  arthritis A01.04
  carrier (suspected) of Z22.0
  cholecystitis (current) A01.09
  endocarditis A01.02
  heart involvement A01.02
  inoculation reaction — see Complications, vaccination
  meningitis A01.01
  mesenteric lymph nodes A01.09
  myocarditis A01.02
  osteomyelitis A01.05
  perichondritis, larynx A01.09
  pneumonia A01.03
  specified NEC A01.09
  spine A01.05
  ulcer (perforating) A01.09

Typhomalaria (fever) — see Malaria
Typhomania A01.00
Typhoperitonitis A01.09
Typhus (fever) A75.9
  abdominal, abdominalis — see Typhoid
  African tick A77.1
  amarillic A95.9
  brain A75.9 [G94]
  cerebral A75.9 [G94]
  classical A75.0
  due to Rickettsia
    prowazekii A75.0
      recrudescent A75.1
    tsutsugamushi A75.3
    typhi A75.2
  endemic (flea-borne) A75.2
  epidemic (louse-borne) A75.0
  exanthematicus SAI A75.0
    brillii SAI A75.1
    mexicanus SAI A75.2
    typhus murinus A75.2
  exanthematic NEC A75.0
  flea-borne A75.2
  India tick A77.1
  Kenya (tick) A77.1
  louse-borne A75.0
  Mexican A75.2
  mite-borne A75.3
  murine A75.2
  North Asian tick-borne A77.2
  petechial A75.9
  Queensland tick A77.3
  rat A75.2
  recrudescent A75.1
  recurrens — see Fever, relapsing
  Sao Paulo A77.0
  scrub (China) (India) (Malaysia) (New Guinea) A75.3
  shop (of Malaysia) A75.2
  Siberian tick A77.2
  tick-borne A77.9
  tropical (mite-borne) A75.3
Tyrosinemia E70.21
  newborn, transitory P74.5
Tyrosinosis E70.21
Tyrosinuria E70.29

U

Uhl's anomaly or disease Q24.8
Ulcer, ulcerated, ulcerating, ulceration, ulcerative
  alveolar process M27.3
  amebic (intestine) A06.1
    skin A06.7
  anastomotic — see Ulcer, gastrojejunal
  anorectal K62.6
  antral — see Ulcer, stomach
  anus (sphincter) (solitary) K62.6
  aorta — see Aneurysm
  aphthous (oral) (recurrent) K12.0
    genital organ(s)
      female N76.6
      male N50.89
  artery I77.2
  atrophic — see Ulcer, skin
    decubitus — see Ulcer, pressure, by site
  back L98.429
    with
      bone involvement without evidence of necrosis L98.426
      bone necrosis L98.424
      exposed fat layer L98.422
      muscle involvement without evidence of necrosis L98.425
      muscle necrosis L98.423
      skin breakdown only L98.421
      specified severity NEC L98.428
  Barrett's (esophagus) K22.10
    with bleeding K22.11
  bile duct (common) (hepatic) K83.8
  bladder (solitary) (sphincter) NEC N32.89
    bilharzial B65.9 [N33]
    in schistosomiasis (bilharzial) B65.9 [N33]
    submucosal — see Cystitis, interstitial
    tuberculous A18.12
  bleeding K27.4
  bone — see Osteomyelitis, specified type NEC
  bowel — see Ulcer, intestine
  breast N61.1

Ulcer, ulcerated, ulcerating, ulceration, ulcerative — continued
  bronchus J98.09
  buccal (cavity) (traumatic) K12.1
  Buruli A31.1
  buttock L98.419
    with
      bone involvement without evidence of necrosis L98.416
      bone necrosis L98.414
      exposed fat layer L98.412
      muscle involvement without evidence of necrosis L98.415
      muscle necrosis L98.413
      skin breakdown only L98.411
      specified severity NEC L98.418
  cancerous — see Neoplasm, malignant, by site
  cardia K22.10
    with bleeding K22.11
  cardioesophageal (peptic) K22.10
    with bleeding K22.11
  cecum — see Ulcer, intestine
  cervix (uteri) (decubitus) (trophic) N86
    with cervicitis N72
  chancroidal A57
  chiclero B55.1
  chronic (cause unknown) — see Ulcer, skin
  Cochin-China B55.1
  colon — see Ulcer, intestine
  conjunctiva H10.89
  cornea H16.00- ☑
    with hypopyon H16.03- ☑
      central H16.01- ☑
      dendritic (herpes simplex) B00.52
      marginal H16.04- ☑
      Mooren's H16.05- ☑
      mycotic H16.06- ☑
      perforated H16.07- ☑
      ring H16.02- ☑
      tuberculous (phlyctenular) A18.52
  corpus cavernosum (chronic) N48.5
  crural — see Ulcer, lower limb
  Curling's — see Ulcer, peptic, acute
  Cushing's — see Ulcer, peptic, acute
  cystic duct K82.8
  cystitis (interstitial) — see Cystitis, interstitial
  decubitus — see Ulcer, pressure, by site
  dendritic, cornea (herpes simplex) B00.52
  diabetes, diabetic — see Diabetes, ulcer
  Dieulafoy's K25.0
  due to
    infection NEC — see Ulcer, skin
    radiation NEC L59.8
    trophic disturbance (any region) — see Ulcer, skin
    X-ray L58.1
  duodenum, duodenal (eroded) (peptic) K26.9
    with
      hemorrhage K26.4
        and perforation K26.6
      perforation K26.5
    acute K26.3
      with
        hemorrhage K26.0
          and perforation K26.2
        perforation K26.1
    chronic K26.7
      with
        hemorrhage K26.4
          and perforation K26.6
        perforation K26.5
  dysenteric A09
  elusive — see Cystitis, interstitial
  endocarditis (acute) (chronic) (subacute) I28.8
  epiglottis J38.7
  esophagus (peptic) K22.10
    with bleeding K22.11
    due to
      aspirin K22.10
        with bleeding K22.11
      gastrointestinal reflux disease K21.0
      ingestion of chemical or medicament K22.10
        with bleeding K22.11
    fungal K22.10
      with bleeding K22.11
    infective K22.10
      with bleeding K22.11
    varicose — see Varix, esophagus
  eyelid (region) H01.8

Ulcer, ulcerated, ulcerating, ulceration, ulcerative — *continued*

fauces J39.2
Fenwick (-Hunner) (solitary) — *see* Cystitis, interstitial
fistulous — *see* Ulcer, skin
foot (indolent) (trophic) — *see* Ulcer, lower limb
frambesial, initial A66.0
frenum (tongue) K14.0
gallbladder or duct K82.8
gangrenous — *see* Gangrene
gastric — *see* Ulcer, stomach
gastrocolic — *see* Ulcer, gastrojejunal
gastroduodenal — *see* Ulcer, peptic
gastroesophageal — *see* Ulcer, stomach
gastrointestinal — *see* Ulcer, gastrojejunal
gastrojejunal (peptic) K28.9
  with
    hemorrhage K28.4
      and perforation K28.6
    perforation K28.5
  acute K28.3
    with
      hemorrhage K28.0
        and perforation K28.2
      perforation K28.1
  chronic K28.7
    with
      hemorrhage K28.4
        and perforation K28.6
      perforation K28.5
gastrojejunocolic — *see* Ulcer, gastrojejunal
gingiva K06.8
gingivitis K05.10
  nonplaque induced K05.11
  plaque induced K05.10
glottis J38.7
granuloma of pudenda A58
gum K06.8
gumma, due to yaws A66.4
heel — *see* Ulcer, lower limb
hemorrhoid (*see also* Hemorrhoids, by degree) K64.8
Hunner's — *see* Cystitis, interstitial
hypopharynx J39.2
hypopyon (chronic) (subacute) — *see* Ulcer, cornea, with hypopyon
hypostaticum — *see* Ulcer, varicose
ileum — *see* Ulcer, intestine
intestine, intestinal K63.3
  with perforation K63.1
  amebic A06.1
  duodenal — *see* Ulcer, duodenum
  granulocytopenic (with hemorrhage) — *see* Neutropenia
  marginal — *see* Ulcer, gastrojejunal
  perforating K63.1
    newborn P78.0
  primary, small intestine K63.3
  rectum K62.6
  stercoraceous, stercoral K63.3
  tuberculous A18.32
  typhoid (fever) — *see* Typhoid
  varicose I86.8
jejunum, jejunal — *see* Ulcer, gastrojejunal
keratitis — *see* Ulcer, cornea
knee — *see* Ulcer, lower limb
labium (majus) (minus) N76.6
laryngitis — *see* Laryngitis
larynx (aphthous) (contact) J38.7
  diphtheritic A36.2
leg — *see* Ulcer, lower limb
lip K13.0
Lipschütz's N76.6
lower limb (atrophic) (chronic) (neurogenic) (perforating) (pyogenic) (trophic) (tropical) L97.909
  with
    bone involvement without evidence of necrosis L97.906
    bone necrosis L97.904
    exposed fat layer L97.902
    muscle involvement without evidence of necrosis L97.905
    muscle necrosis L97.903
    skin breakdown only L97.901
    specified severity NEC L97.908
  ankle L97.309
    with
      bone involvement without evidence of necrosis L97.306

Ulcer, ulcerated, ulcerating, ulceration, ulcerative — *continued*

lower limb — *continued*
  ankle — *continued*
    with — *continued*
      bone necrosis L97.304
      exposed fat layer L97.302
      muscle involvement without evidence of necrosis L97.305
      muscle necrosis L97.303
      skin breakdown only L97.301
      specified severity NEC L97.308
    left L97.329
      with
        bone involvement without evidence of necrosis L97.326
        bone necrosis L97.324
        exposed fat layer L97.322
        muscle involvement without evidence of necrosis L97.325
        muscle necrosis L97.323
        skin breakdown only L97.321
        specified severity NEC L97.328
    right L97.319
      with
        bone involvement without evidence of necrosis L97.316
        bone necrosis L97.314
        exposed fat layer L97.312
        muscle involvement without evidence of necrosis L97.315
        muscle necrosis L97.313
        skin breakdown only L97.311
        specified severity NEC L97.318
  calf L97.209
    with
      bone involvement without evidence of necrosis L97.206
      bone necrosis L97.204
      exposed fat layer L97.202
      muscle involvement without evidence of necrosis L97.205
      muscle necrosis L97.203
      skin breakdown only L97.201
      specified severity NEC L97.208
    left L97.229
      with
        bone involvement without evidence of necrosis L97.226
        bone necrosis L97.224
        exposed fat layer L97.222
        muscle involvement without evidence of necrosis L97.225
        muscle necrosis L97.223
        skin breakdown only L97.221
        specified severity NEC L97.228
    right L97.219
      with
        bone involvement without evidence of necrosis L97.216
        bone necrosis L97.214
        exposed fat layer L97.212
        muscle involvement without evidence of necrosis L97.215
        muscle necrosis L97.213
        skin breakdown only L97.211
        specified severity NEC L97.218
  decubitus — *see* Ulcer, pressure, by site
  foot specified NEC L97.509
    with
      bone involvement without evidence of necrosis L97.506
      bone necrosis L97.504
      exposed fat layer L97.502
      muscle involvement without evidence of necrosis L97.505
      muscle necrosis L97.503
      skin breakdown only L97.501
      specified severity NEC L97.508
    left L97.529
      with
        bone involvement without evidence of necrosis L97.526
        bone necrosis L97.524
        exposed fat layer L97.522
        muscle involvement without evidence of necrosis L97.525
        muscle necrosis L97.523
        skin breakdown only L97.521

Ulcer, ulcerated, ulcerating, ulceration, ulcerative — *continued*

lower limb — *continued*
  foot specified — *continued*
    left — *continued*
      with — *continued*
        specified severity NEC L97.528
    right L97.519
      with
        bone involvement without evidence of necrosis L97.516
        bone necrosis L97.514
        exposed fat layer L97.512
        muscle involvement without evidence of necrosis L97.515
        muscle necrosis L97.513
        skin breakdown only L97.511
        specified severity NEC L97.518
  heel L97.409
    with
      bone involvement without evidence of necrosis L97.406
      bone necrosis L97.404
      exposed fat layer L97.402
      muscle involvement without evidence of necrosis L97.405
      muscle necrosis L97.403
      skin breakdown only L97.401
      specified severity NEC L97.408
    left L97.429
      with
        bone involvement without evidence of necrosis L97.426
        bone necrosis L97.424
        exposed fat layer L97.422
        muscle involvement without evidence of necrosis L97.425
        muscle necrosis L97.423
        skin breakdown only L97.421
        specified severity NEC L97.428
    right L97.419
      with
        bone involvement without evidence of necrosis L97.416
        bone necrosis L97.414
        exposed fat layer L97.412
        muscle involvement without evidence of necrosis L97.415
        muscle necrosis L97.413
        skin breakdown only L97.411
        specified severity NEC L97.418
  left L97.929
    with
      bone involvement without evidence of necrosis L97.926
      bone necrosis L97.924
      exposed fat layer L97.922
      muscle involvement without evidence of necrosis L97.925
      muscle necrosis L97.923
      skin breakdown only L97.921
      specified severity NEC L97.928
  leprous A30.1
  lower leg NOS L97.909
    with
      bone involvement without evidence of necrosis L97.906
      bone necrosis L97.904
      exposed fat layer L97.902
      muscle involvement without evidence of necrosis L97.905
      muscle necrosis L97.903
      skin breakdown only L97.901
      specified severity NEC L97.908
  left L97.929
    with
      bone involvement without evidence of necrosis L97.926
      bone necrosis L97.924
      exposed fat layer L97.922
      muscle involvement without evidence of necrosis L97.925
      muscle necrosis L97.923
      skin breakdown only L97.921
      specified severity NEC L97.928
  right L97.919
    with
      bone involvement without evidence of necrosis L97.916

Ulcer, ulcerated, ulcerating, ulceration, ulcerative — *continued*
lower limb — *continued*
  lower leg — *continued*
    right — *continued*
      with — *continued*
        bone necrosis L97.914
        exposed fat layer L97.912
        muscle involvement without evidence of necrosis L97.915
        muscle necrosis L97.913
        skin breakdown only L97.911
        specified severity NEC L97.918
  specified site NEC L97.809
    with
      bone involvement without evidence of necrosis L97.806
      bone necrosis L97.804
      exposed fat layer L97.802
      muscle involvement without evidence of necrosis L97.805
      muscle necrosis L97.803
      skin breakdown only L97.801
      specified severity NEC L97.808
    left L97.829
      with
        bone involvement without evidence of necrosis L97.826
        bone necrosis L97.824
        exposed fat layer L97.822
        muscle involvement without evidence of necrosis L97.825
        muscle necrosis L97.823
        skin breakdown only L97.821
        specified severity NEC L97.828
    right L97.819
      with
        bone involvement without evidence of necrosis L97.816
        bone necrosis L97.814
        exposed fat layer L97.812
        muscle involvement without evidence of necrosis L97.815
        muscle necrosis L97.813
        skin breakdown only L97.811
        specified severity NEC L97.818
  midfoot L97.409
    with
      bone involvement without evidence of necrosis L97.406
      bone necrosis L97.404
      exposed fat layer L97.402
      muscle involvement without evidence of necrosis L97.405
      muscle necrosis L97.403
      skin breakdown only L97.401
      specified severity NEC L97.408
    left L97.429
      with
        bone involvement without evidence of necrosis L97.426
        bone necrosis L97.424
        exposed fat layer L97.422
        muscle involvement without evidence of necrosis L97.425
        muscle necrosis L97.423
        skin breakdown only L97.421
        specified severity NEC L97.428
    right L97.419
      with
        bone involvement without evidence of necrosis L97.416
        bone necrosis L97.414
        exposed fat layer L97.412
        muscle involvement without evidence of necrosis L97.415
        muscle necrosis L97.413
        skin breakdown only L97.411
        specified severity NEC L97.418
    right L97.919
      with
        bone involvement without evidence of necrosis L97.916
        bone necrosis L97.914
        exposed fat layer L97.912
        muscle involvement without evidence of necrosis L97.915
        muscle necrosis L97.913
        skin breakdown only L97.911

Ulcer, ulcerated, ulcerating, ulceration, ulcerative — *continued*
lower limb — *continued*
  right — *continued*
    with — *continued*
      specified severity NEC L97.918
  syphilitic A52.19
  thigh L97.109
    with
      bone involvement without evidence of necrosis L97.106
      bone necrosis L97.104
      exposed fat layer L97.102
      muscle involvement without evidence of necrosis L97.105
      muscle necrosis L97.103
      skin breakdown only L97.101
      specified severity NEC L97.108
    left L97.129
      with
        bone involvement without evidence of necrosis L97.126
        bone necrosis L97.124
        exposed fat layer L97.122
        muscle involvement without evidence of necrosis L97.125
        muscle necrosis L97.123
        skin breakdown only L97.121
        specified severity NEC L97.128
    right L97.119
      with
        bone involvement without evidence of necrosis L97.116
        bone necrosis L97.114
        exposed fat layer L97.112
        muscle involvement without evidence of necrosis L97.115
        muscle necrosis L97.113
        skin breakdown only L97.111
        specified severity NEC L97.118
  toe L97.509
    with
      bone involvement without evidence of necrosis L97.506
      bone necrosis L97.504
      exposed fat layer L97.502
      muscle involvement without evidence of necrosis L97.505
      muscle necrosis L97.503
      skin breakdown only L97.501
      specified severity NEC L97.508
    left L97.529
      with
        bone involvement without evidence of necrosis L97.526
        bone necrosis L97.524
        exposed fat layer L97.522
        muscle involvement without evidence of necrosis L97.525
        muscle necrosis L97.523
        skin breakdown only L97.521
        specified severity NEC L97.528
    right L97.519
      with
        bone involvement without evidence of necrosis L97.516
        bone necrosis L97.514
        exposed fat layer L97.512
        muscle involvement without evidence of necrosis L97.515
        muscle necrosis L97.513
        skin breakdown only L97.511
        specified severity NEC L97.518
  varicose — *see* Varix, leg, with, ulcer
luetic — *see* Ulcer, syphilitic
lung J98.4
  tuberculous — *see* Tuberculosis, pulmonary
malignant — *see* Neoplasm, malignant, by site
marginal NEC — *see* Ulcer, gastrojejunal
meatus (urinarius) N34.2
Meckel's diverticulum Q43.0
  malignant — *see* Table of Neoplasms, small intestine, malignant
Meleney's (chronic undermining) — *see* Ulcer, skin
Mooren's (cornea) — *see* Ulcer, cornea, Mooren's
mycobacterial (skin) A31.1
nasopharynx J39.2
neck, uterus N86

Ulcer, ulcerated, ulcerating, ulceration, ulcerative — *continued*
neurogenic NEC — *see* Ulcer, skin
nose, nasal (passage) (infective) (septum) J34.0
  skin — *see* Ulcer, skin
  spirochetal A69.8
  varicose (bleeding) I86.8
oral mucosa (traumatic) K12.1
palate (soft) K12.1
penis (chronic) N48.5
peptic (site unspecified) K27.9
  with
    hemorrhage K27.4
      and perforation K27.6
    perforation K27.5
  acute K27.3
    with
      hemorrhage K27.0
        and perforation K27.2
      perforation K27.1
  chronic K27.7
    with
      hemorrhage K27.4
        and perforation K27.6
      perforation K27.5
  esophagus K22.10
    with bleeding K22.11
  newborn P78.82
perforating K27.5
  skin — *see* Ulcer, skin
peritonsillar J35.8
phagedenic (tropical) — *see* Ulcer, skin
pharynx J39.2
phlebitis — *see* Phlebitis
plaster — *see* Ulcer, pressure, by site
popliteal space — *see* Ulcer, lower limb
postpyloric — *see* Ulcer, duodenum
prepuce N47.7
prepyloric — *see* Ulcer, stomach
pressure (pressure area) L89.9- ☑
  ankle L89.5- ☑
  back L89.1- ☑
  buttock L89.3- ☑
  coccyx L89.15- ☑
  contiguous site of back, buttock, hip L89.4- ☑
  elbow L89.0- ☑
  face L89.81- ☑
  head L89.81- ☑
  heel L89.6- ☑
  hip L89.2- ☑
  sacral region (tailbone) L89.15- ☑
  specified site NEC L89.89- ☑
  stage 1 (healing) (pre-ulcer skin changes limited to persistent focal edema)
    ankle L89.5- ☑
    back L89.1- ☑
    buttock L89.3- ☑
    coccyx L89.15- ☑
    contiguous site of back, buttock, hip L89.4- ☑
    elbow L89.0- ☑
    face L89.81- ☑
    head L89.81- ☑
    heel L89.6- ☑
    hip L89.2- ☑
    sacral region (tailbone) L89.15- ☑
    specified site NEC L89.89- ☑
  stage 2 (healing) (abrasion, blister, partial thickness skin loss involving epidermis and/or dermis)
    ankle L89.5- ☑
    back L89.1- ☑
    buttock L89.3- ☑
    coccyx L89.15- ☑
    contiguous site of back, buttock, hip L89.4- ☑
    elbow L89.0- ☑
    face L89.81- ☑
    head L89.81- ☑
    heel L89.6- ☑
    hip L89.2- ☑
    sacral region (tailbone) L89.15- ☑
    specified site NEC L89.89- ☑
  stage 3 (healing) (full thickness skin loss involving damage or necrosis of subcutaneous tissue)
    ankle L89.5- ☑
    back L89.1- ☑
    buttock L89.3- ☑
    coccyx L89.15- ☑
    contiguous site of back, buttock, hip L89.4- ☑

Ulcer, ulcerated, ulcerating, ulceration, ulcerative
  — *continued*
  pressure — *continued*
    stage 3 — *continued*
      elbow L89.0- ☑
      face L89.81- ☑
      head L89.81- ☑
      heel L89.6- ☑
      hip L89.2- ☑
      sacral region (tailbone) L89.15- ☑
      specified site NEC L89.89- ☑
    stage 4 (healing) (necrosis of soft tissues through
        to underlying muscle, tendon, or bone)
      ankle L89.5- ☑
      back L89.1- ☑
      buttock L89.3- ☑
      coccyx L89.15- ☑
      contiguous site of back, buttock, hip L89.4- ☑
      elbow L89.0- ☑
      face L89.81- ☑
      head L89.81- ☑
      heel L89.6- ☑
      hip L89.2- ☑
      sacral region (tailbone) L89.15- ☑
      specified site NEC L89.89- ☑
    unspecified stage
      ankle L89.5- ☑
      back L89.1- ☑
      buttock L89.3- ☑
      coccyx L89.15- ☑
      contiguous site of back, buttock, hip L89.4- ☑
      elbow L89.0- ☑
      face L89.81- ☑
      head L89.81- ☑
      heel L89.6- ☑
      hip L89.2- ☑
      sacral region (tailbone) L89.15- ☑
      specified site NEC L89.89- ☑
    unstageable
      ankle L89.5- ☑
      back L89.1- ☑
      buttock L89.3- ☑
      coccyx L89.15- ☑
      contiguous site of back, buttock, hip L89.4- ☑
      elbow L89.0- ☑
      face L89.81- ☑
      head L89.81- ☑
      heel L89.6- ☑
      hip L89.2- ☑
      sacral region (tailbone) L89.15- ☑
      specified site NEC L89.89- ☑
  primary of intestine K63.3
    with perforation K63.1
  prostate N41.9
  pyloric — *see* Ulcer, stomach
  rectosigmoid K63.3
    with perforation K63.1
  rectum (sphincter) (solitary) K62.6
    stercoraceous, stercoral K62.6
  retina — *see* Inflammation, chorioretinal
  rodent (*see also* Neoplasm, skin, malignant)
  sclera — *see* Scleritis
  scrofulous (tuberculous) A18.2
  scrotum N50.89
    tuberculous A18.15
    varicose I86.1
  seminal vesicle N50.89
  sigmoid — *see* Ulcer, intestine
  skin (atrophic) (chronic) (neurogenic) (non-healing)
      (perforating) (pyogenic) (trophic) (tropical)
      L98.499
    with gangrene — *see* Gangrene
    amebic A06.7
    back — *see* Ulcer, back
    buttock — *see* Ulcer, buttock
    decubitus — *see* Ulcer, pressure
    lower limb — *see* Ulcer, lower limb
    mycobacterial A31.1
    specified site NEC L98.499
      with
        bone involvement without evidence of
          necrosis L98.496
        bone necrosis L98.494
        exposed fat layer L98.492
        muscle involvement without evidence of
          necrosis L98.495
        muscle necrosis L98.493

Ulcer, ulcerated, ulcerating, ulceration, ulcerative
  — *continued*
  skin — *continued*
    specified site — *continued*
      with — *continued*
        skin breakdown only L98.491
        specified severity NEC L98.498
    tuberculous (primary) A18.4
    varicose — *see* Ulcer, varicose
  sloughing — *see* Ulcer, skin
  solitary, anus or rectum (sphincter) K62.6
  sore throat J02.9
    streptococcal J02.0
  spermatic cord N50.89
  spine (tuberculous) A18.01
  stasis (venous) — *see* Varix, leg, with, ulcer
    without varicose veins I87.2
  stercoraceous, stercoral K63.3
    with perforation K63.1
    anus or rectum K62.6
  stoma, stomal — *see* Ulcer, gastrojejunal
  stomach (eroded) (peptic) (round) K25.9
    with
      hemorrhage K25.4
        and perforation K25.6
      perforation K25.5
    acute K25.3
      with
        hemorrhage K25.0
          and perforation K25.2
        perforation K25.1
    chronic K25.7
      with
        hemorrhage K25.4
          and perforation K25.6
        perforation K25.5
  stomal — *see* Ulcer, gastrojejunal
  stomatitis K12.1
  stress — *see* Ulcer, peptic
  strumous (tuberculous) A18.2
  submucosal, bladder — *see* Cystitis, interstitial
  syphilitic (any site) (early) (secondary) A51.39
    late A52.79
    perforating A52.79
      foot A52.11
  testis N50.89
  thigh — *see* Ulcer, lower limb
  throat J39.2
    diphtheritic A36.0
  toe — *see* Ulcer, lower limb
  tongue (traumatic) K14.0
  tonsil J35.8
    diphtheritic A36.0
  trachea J39.8
  trophic — *see* Ulcer, skin
  tropical — *see* Ulcer, skin
  tuberculous — *see* Tuberculosis, ulcer
  tunica vaginalis N50.89
  turbinate J34.89
  typhoid (perforating) — *see* Typhoid
  unspecified site — *see* Ulcer, skin
  urethra (meatus) — *see* Urethritis
  uterus N85.8
    cervix N86
      with cervicitis N72
    neck N86
      with cervicitis N72
  vagina N76.5
    in Behçet's disease M35.2 [N77.0]
    pessary N89.8
  valve, heart I33.0
  varicose (lower limb, any part) (*see also* Varix, leg, with,
      ulcer)
    broad ligament I86.2
    esophagus — *see* Varix, esophagus
    inflamed or infected — *see* Varix, leg, with ulcer,
      with inflammation
    nasal septum I86.8
    perineum I86.3
    scrotum I86.1
    specified site NEC I86.8
    sublingual I86.0
    vulva I86.3
  vas deferens N50.89
  vulva (acute) (infectional) N76.6
    in (due to)
      Behçet's disease M35.2 [N77.0]
      herpesviral (herpes simplex) infection A60.04

Ulcer, ulcerated, ulcerating, ulceration, ulcerative
  — *continued*
  vulva — *continued*
    in — *continued*
      tuberculosis A18.18
  vulvobuccal, recurring N76.6
  X-ray L58.1
  yaws A66.4
Ulcerosa scarlatina A38.8
Ulcus (*see also* Ulcer)
  cutis tuberculosum A18.4
  duodeni — *see* Ulcer, duodenum
  durum (syphilitic) A51.0
    extragenital A51.2
  gastrojejunale — *see* Ulcer, gastrojejunal
  hypostaticum — *see* Ulcer, varicose
  molle (cutis) (skin) A57
  serpens corneae — *see* Ulcer, cornea, central
  ventriculi — *see* Ulcer, stomach
Ulegyria Q04.8
Ulerythema
  ophryogenes, congenital Q84.2
  sycosiforme L73.8
Ullrich (-Bonnevie)(-Turner) **syndrome** (*see also* Turner's
    syndrome) Q87.1
Ullrich-Feichtiger syndrome Q87.0
Ulnar — *see* condition
Ulorrhagia, ulorrhea K06.8
Umbilicus, umbilical — *see* condition
Unacceptable
  contours of tooth K08.54
  morphology of tooth K08.54
Unavailability (of)
  bed at medical facility Z75.1
  health service-related agencies Z75.4
  medical facilities (at) Z75.3
    due to
      investigation by social service agency Z75.2
      lack of services at home Z75.0
      remoteness from facility Z75.3
      waiting list Z75.1
    home Z75.0
    outpatient clinic Z75.3
  schooling Z55.1
  social service agencies Z75.4
Uncinaria americana infestation B76.1
Uncinariasis B76.9
Uncongenial work Z56.5
Unconscious (ness) — *see* Coma
Under observation — *see* Observation
Underachievement in school Z55.3
Underdevelopment (*see also* Undeveloped)
  nose Q30.1
  sexual E30.0
Underdosing (*see also* Table of Drugs and Chemicals,
    categories T36-T50, with final character 6) Z91.14
  intentional NEC Z91.128
    due to financial hardship of patient Z91.120
  unintentional NEC Z91.138
    due to patient's age related debility Z91.130
Underfeeding, newborn P92.3
Underfill, endodontic M27.53
Underimmunization status Z28.3
Undernourishment — *see* Malnutrition
Undernutrition — *see* Malnutrition
Underweight R63.6
  for gestational age — *see* Light for dates
Underwood's disease P83.0
Undescended (*see also* Malposition, congenital)
  cecum Q43.3
  colon Q43.3
  testicle — *see* Cryptorchid
Undeveloped, undevelopment (*see also* Hypoplasia)
  brain (congenital) Q02
  cerebral (congenital) Q02
  heart Q24.8
  lung Q33.6
  testis E29.1
  uterus E30.0
Undiagnosed (disease) R69
Undulant fever — *see* Brucellosis
Unemployment, anxiety concerning Z56.0
  threatened Z56.2
Unequal length (acquired) (limb) (*see also* Deformity,
    limb, unequal length)
  leg (*see also* Deformity, limb, unequal length)
    congenital Q72.9- ☑

Unextracted dental root KØ8.3
Unguis incarnatus L6Ø.Ø
Unhappiness R45.2
Unicornate uterus Q51.4
  in pregnancy or childbirth O34.ØØ
Unilateral (see also condition)
  development, breast N64.89
  organ or site, congenital NEC — see Agenesis, by site
Unilocular heart Q2Ø.8
Union, abnormal (see also Fusion)
  larynx and trachea Q34.8
Universal mesentery Q43.3
Unrepairable overhanging of dental restorative
  materials KØ8.52
Unsatisfactory
  restoration of tooth KØ8.5Ø
    specified NEC KØ8.59
  sample of cytologic smear
    anus R85.615
    cervix R87.615
    vagina R87.625
  surroundings Z59.1
  work Z56.5
Unsoundness of mind — see Psychosis
Unstable
  back NEC — see Instability, joint, spine
  hip (congenital) Q65.6
    acquired — see Derangement, joint, specified type
      NEC, hip
  joint — see Instability, joint
    secondary to removal of joint prosthesis M96.89
  lie (mother) O32.Ø ☑
  lumbosacral joint (congenital)
    acquired — see subcategory M53.2 ☑
  sacroiliac — see subcategory M53.2 ☑
  spine NEC — see Instability, joint, spine
Unsteadiness on feet R26.81
Untruthfulness, child problem F91.8
Unverricht (-Lundborg) **disease or epilepsy** — see
  Epilepsy, generalized, idiopathic
Unwanted pregnancy Z64.Ø
Upbringing, institutional Z62.22
  away from parents NEC Z62.29
  in care of non-parental family member Z62.21
  in foster care Z62.21
  in orphanage or group home Z62.22
  in welfare custody Z62.21
Upper respiratory — see condition
Upset
  gastric K3Ø
  gastrointestinal K3Ø
    psychogenic F45.8
  intestinal (large) (small) K59.9
    psychogenic F45.8
  menstruation N93.9
  mental F48.9
  stomach K3Ø
    psychogenic F45.8
Urachus (see also condition)
  patent or persistent Q64.4
Urbach-Oppenheim disease (necrobiosis lipoidica diabeticorum) — see E08-E13 with .62Ø
Urbach's lipoid proteinosis E78.89
Urbach-Wiethe disease E78.89
Urban yellow fever A95.1
Urea
  blood, high — see Uremia
  cycle metabolism disorder — see Disorder, urea cycle
    metabolism
Uremia, uremic N19
  with
    ectopic or molar pregnancy O08.4
    polyneuropathy N18.9 [G63]
  chronic NOS (see also Disease, kidney, chronic) N18.9
    due to hypertension — see Hypertensive, kidney
  complicating
    ectopic or molar pregnancy O08.4
  congenital P96.Ø
  extrarenal R39.2
  following ectopic or molar pregnancy O08.4
  newborn P96.Ø
  prerenal R39.2
Ureter, ureteral — see condition
Ureteralgia N23
Ureterectasis — see Hydroureter
Ureteritis N28.89
  cystica N28.86

Ureteritis — continued
  due to calculus N2Ø.1
    with calculus, kidney N2Ø.2
      with hydronephrosis N13.2
  gonococcal (acute) (chronic) A54.21
  nonspecific N28.89
Ureterocele N28.89
  congenital (orthotopic) Q62.31
  ectopic Q62.32
Ureterolith, ureterolithiasis — see Calculus, ureter
Ureterostomy
  attention to Z43.6
  status Z93.6
Urethra, urethral — see condition
Urethralgia R39.89
Urethritis (anterior) (posterior) N34.2
  calculous N21.1
  candidal B37.41
  chlamydial A56.Ø1
  diplococcal (gonococcal) A54.Ø1
    with abscess (accessory gland) (periurethral) A54.1
  gonococcal A54.Ø1
    with abscess (accessory gland) (periurethral) A54.1
  nongonococcal N34.1
    Reiter's — see Reiter's disease
  nonspecific N34.1
  nonvenereal N34.1
  postmenopausal N34.2
  puerperal O86.22
  Reiter's — see Reiter's disease
  specified NEC N34.2
  trichomonal or due to Trichomonas (vaginalis) A59.Ø3
Urethrocele N81.Ø
  with
    cystocele — see Cystocele
    prolapse of uterus — see Prolapse, uterus
Urethrolithiasis (with colic or infection) N21.1
Urethrorectal — see condition
Urethrorrhagia N36.8
Urethrorrhea R36.9
Urethrostomy
  attention to Z43.6
  status Z93.6
Urethrotrigonitis — see Trigonitis
Urethrovaginal — see condition
Urgency
  fecal R15.2
  hypertensive — see Hypertension
  urinary R39.15
Urhidrosis, uridrosis L74.8
Uric acid in blood (increased) E79.Ø
Uricacidemia (asymptomatic) E79.Ø
Uricemia (asymptomatic) E79.Ø
Uricosuria R82.99
Urinary — see condition
Urination
  frequent R35.Ø
  painful R3Ø.9
Urine
  blood in — see Hematuria
  discharge, excessive R35.8
  enuresis, nonorganic origin F98.Ø
  extravasation R39.Ø
  frequency R35.Ø
  incontinence R32
    nonorganic origin F98.Ø
  intermittent stream R39.198
  pus in N39.Ø
  retention or stasis R33.9
    organic R33.8
      drug-induced R33.Ø
    psychogenic F45.8
  secretion
    deficient R34
    excessive R35.8
    frequency R35.Ø
  stream
    intermittent R39.198
    slowing R39.198
    splitting R39.13
    weak R39.12
Urinemia — see Uremia
Urinoma, urethra N36.8
Uroarthritis, infectious (Reiter's) — see Reiter's disease
Urodialysis R34
Urolithiasis — see Calculus, urinary
Uronephrosis — see Hydronephrosis
Uropathy N39.9

Uropathy — continued
  obstructive N13.9
    specified NEC N13.8
  reflux N13.9
    specified NEC N13.8
  vesicoureteral reflux-associated — see Reflux, vesi-
    coureteral
Urosepsis — code to condition
Urticaria L5Ø.9
  with angioneurotic edema T78.3 ☑
    hereditary D84.1
  allergic L5Ø.Ø
  cholinergic L5Ø.5
  chronic L5Ø.8
  cold, familial L5Ø.2
  contact L5Ø.6
  dermatographic L5Ø.3
  due to
    cold or heat L5Ø.2
    drugs L5Ø.Ø
    food L5Ø.Ø
    inhalants L5Ø.Ø
    plants L5Ø.6
    serum (see also Reaction, serum) T80.69 ☑
  factitial L5Ø.3
  familial cold MØ4.2
  giant T78.3 ☑
    hereditary D84.1
  gigantea T78.3 ☑
  idiopathic L5Ø.1
  larynx T78.3 ☑
    hereditary D84.1
  neonatorum P83.88
  nonallergic L5Ø.1
  papulosa (Hebra) L28.2
  pigmentosa D47.Ø1
    congenital Q82.2
    of neonatal onset Q82.2
    of newborn onset Q82.2
  recurrent periodic L5Ø.8
  serum (see also Reaction, serum) T80.69 ☑
  solar L56.3
  specified type NEC L5Ø.8
  thermal (cold) (heat) L5Ø.2
  vibratory L5Ø.4
  xanthelasmoidea — see Urticaria pigmentosa
Use (of)
  alcohol Z72.89
    with
      intoxication F1Ø.929
      sleep disorder F1Ø.982
    harmful — see Abuse, alcohol
  amphetamines — see Use, stimulant NEC
  caffeine — see Use, stimulant NEC
  cannabis F12.9Ø
    with
      anxiety disorder F12.98Ø
      intoxication F12.929
        with
          delirium F12.921
          perceptual disturbance F12.922
        uncomplicated F12.92Ø
      other specified disorder F12.988
      psychosis F12.959
        delusions F12.95Ø
        hallucinations F12.951
      unspecified disorder F12.99
  cocaine F14.9Ø
    with
      anxiety disorder F14.98Ø
      intoxication F14.929
        with
          delirium F14.921
          perceptual disturbance F14.922
        uncomplicated F14.92Ø
      other specified disorder F14.988
      psychosis F14.959
        delusions F14.95Ø
        hallucinations F14.951
      sexual dysfunction F14.981
      sleep disorder F14.982
      unspecified disorder F14.99
    harmful — see Abuse, drug, cocaine
  drug(s) NEC F19.9Ø
    with sleep disorder F19.982
    harmful — see Abuse, drug, by type
  hallucinogen NEC F16.9Ø

☑ **Additional Character Required** — Refer to the Tabular List for Character Selection   ▽ **Subterms under main terms may continue to next column or page**

Unextracted dental root — Use

Use — *continued*
  hallucinogen — *continued*
    with
      anxiety disorder F16.980
      intoxication F16.929
        with
          delirium F16.921
        uncomplicated F16.920
      mood disorder F16.94
      other specified disorder F16.988
      perception disorder (flashbacks) F16.983
      psychosis F16.959
        delusions F16.950
        hallucinations F16.951
      unspecified disorder F16.99
    harmful — *see* Abuse, drug, hallucinogen NEC
  inhalants F18.90
    with
      anxiety disorder F18.980
      intoxication F18.929
        with delirium F18.921
        uncomplicated F18.920
      mood disorder F18.94
      other specified disorder F18.988
      persisting dementia F18.97
      psychosis F18.959
        delusions F18.950
        hallucinations F18.951
      unspecified disorder F18.99
    harmful — *see* Abuse, drug, inhalant
  methadone — *see* Use, opioid
  nonprescribed drugs F19.90
    harmful — *see* Abuse, non-psychoactive substance
  opioid F11.90
    with
      disorder F11.99
        mood F11.94
        sleep F11.982
        specified type NEC F11.988
      intoxication F11.929
        with
          delirium F11.921
          perceptual disturbance F11.922
        uncomplicated F11.920
      withdrawal F11.93
    harmful — *see* Abuse, drug, opioid
  patent medicines F19.90
    harmful — *see* Abuse, non-psychoactive substance
  psychoactive drug NEC F19.90
    with
      anxiety disorder F19.980
      intoxication F19.929
        with
          delirium F19.921
          perceptual disturbance F19.922
        uncomplicated F19.920
      mood disorder F19.94
      other specified disorder F19.988
      persisting
        amnestic disorder F19.96
        dementia F19.97
      psychosis F19.959
        delusions F19.950
        hallucinations F19.951
      sexual dysfunction F19.981
      sleep disorder F19.982
      unspecified disorder F19.99
      withdrawal F19.939
        with
          delirium F19.931
          perceptual disturbance F19.932
        uncomplicated F19.930
    harmful — *see* Abuse, drug NEC, psychoactive NEC
  sedative, hypnotic, or anxiolytic F13.90
    with
      anxiety disorder F13.980
      intoxication F13.929
        with
          delirium F13.921
        uncomplicated F13.920
      other specified disorder F13.988
      persisting
        amnestic disorder F13.96
        dementia F13.97
      psychosis F13.959
        delusions F13.950
        hallucinations F13.951
      sexual dysfunction F13.981

Use — *continued*
  sedative, hypnotic, or anxiolytic — *continued*
    with — *continued*
      sleep disorder F13.982
      unspecified disorder F13.99
    harmful — *see* Abuse, drug, sedative, hypnotic, or anxiolytic
  stimulant NEC F15.90
    with
      anxiety disorder F15.980
      intoxication F15.929
        with
          delirium F15.921
          perceptual disturbance F15.922
        uncomplicated F15.920
      mood disorder F15.94
      other specified disorder F15.988
      psychosis F15.959
        delusions F15.950
        hallucinations F15.951
      sexual dysfunction F15.981
      sleep disorder F15.982
      unspecified disorder F15.99
      withdrawal F15.93
    harmful — *see* Abuse, drug, stimulant NEC
  tobacco Z72.0
    with dependence — *see* Dependence, drug, nicotine
  volatile solvents (*see also* Use, inhalant) F18.90
    harmful — *see* Abuse, drug, inhalant
Usher-Senear disease or syndrome L10.4
Uta B55.1
Uteromegaly N85.2
Uterovaginal — *see* condition
Uterovesical — *see* condition
Uveal — *see* condition
Uveitis (anterior) (*see also* Iridocyclitis)
  acute — *see* Iridocyclitis, acute
  chronic — *see* Iridocyclitis, chronic
  due to toxoplasmosis (acquired) B58.09
    congenital P37.1
  granulomatous — *see* Iridocyclitis, chronic
  heterochromic — *see* Cyclitis, Fuchs' heterochromic
  lens-induced — *see* Iridocyclitis, lens-induced
  posterior — *see* Chorioretinitis
  sympathetic H44.13- ☑
  syphilitic (secondary) A51.43
    congenital (early) A50.01
    late A52.71
  tuberculous A18.54
Uveoencephalitis — *see* Inflammation, chorioretinal
Uveokeratitis — *see* Iridocyclitis
Uveoparotitis D86.89
Uvula — *see* condition
Uvulitis (acute) (catarrhal) (chronic) (membranous) (suppurative) (ulcerative) K12.2

V

Vaccination (prophylactic)
  complication or reaction — *see* Complications, vaccination
  delayed Z28.9
  encounter for Z23
  not done — *see* Immunization, not done, because (of)
Vaccinia (generalized) (localized) T88.1 ☑
  without vaccination B08.011
  congenital P35.8
Vacuum, in sinus (accessory) (nasal) J34.89
Vagabond, vagabondage Z59.0
Vagabond's disease B85.1
Vagina, vaginal — *see* condition
Vaginalitis (tunica) (testis) N49.1
Vaginismus (reflex) N94.2
  functional F52.5
  nonorganic F52.5
  psychogenic F52.5
  secondary N94.2
Vaginitis (acute) (circumscribed) (diffuse) (emphysematous) (nonvenereal) (ulcerative) N76.0
  with ectopic or molar pregnancy O08.0
  amebic A06.82
  atrophic, postmenopausal N95.2
  bacterial N76.0
  blennorrhagic (gonococcal) A54.02
  candidal B37.3
  chlamydial A56.02

Vaginitis — *continued*
  chronic N76.1
  due to Trichomonas (vaginalis) A59.01
  following ectopic or molar pregnancy O08.0
  gonococcal A54.02
    with abscess (accessory gland) (periurethral) A54.1
  granuloma A58
  in (due to)
    candidiasis B37.3
    herpesviral (herpes simplex) infection A60.04
    pinworm infection B80 [N77.1]
  monilial B37.3
  mycotic (candidal) B37.3
  postmenopausal atrophic N95.2
  puerperal (postpartum) O86.13
  senile (atrophic) N95.2
  subacute or chronic N76.1
  syphilitic (early) A51.0
    late A52.76
  trichomonal A59.01
  tuberculous A18.18
Vaginosis — *see* Vaginitis
Vagotonia G52.2
Vagrancy Z59.0
VAIN — *see* Neoplasia, intraepithelial, vagina
Vallecula — *see* condition
Valley fever B38.0
Valsuani's disease — *see* Anemia, obstetric
Valve, valvular (formation) (*see also* condition)
  cerebral ventricle (communicating) in situ Z98.2
  cervix, internal os Q51.828
  congenital NEC — *see* Atresia, by site
  ureter (pelvic junction) (vesical orifice) Q62.39
  urethra (congenital) (posterior) Q64.2
Valvulitis (chronic) — *see* Endocarditis
Valvulopathy — *see* Endocarditis
Van Bogaert's leukoencephalopathy (sclerosing) (subacute) A81.1
Van Bogaert-Scherer-Epstein disease or syndrome E75.5
Van Buchem's syndrome M85.2
Van Creveld-von Gierke disease E74.01
Van der Hoeve (-de Kleyn) **syndrome** Q78.0
Van der Woude's syndrome Q38.0
Van Neck's disease or osteochondrosis M91.0
Vanishing lung J44.9
Vapor asphyxia or suffocation T59.9 ☑
  specified agent — *see* Table of Drugs and Chemicals
Variance, lethal ball, prosthetic heart valve T82.09 ☑
Variants, thalassemic D56.8
Variations in hair color L67.1
Varicella B01.9
  with
    complications NEC B01.89
    encephalitis B01.11
    encephalomyelitis B01.11
    meningitis B01.0
    myelitis B01.12
    pneumonia B01.2
  congenital P35.8
Varices — *see* Varix
Varicocele (scrotum) (thrombosed) I86.1
  ovary I86.2
  perineum I86.3
  spermatic cord (ulcerated) I86.1
Varicose
  aneurysm (ruptured) I77.0
  dermatitis — *see* Varix, leg, with, inflammation
  eczema — *see* Varix, leg, with, inflammation
  phlebitis — *see* Varix, with, inflammation
  tumor — *see* Varix
  ulcer (lower limb, any part) (*see also* Varix, leg, with, ulcer)
    anus (*see also* Hemorrhoids) K64.8
    esophagus — *see* Varix, esophagus
    inflamed or infected — *see* Varix, leg, with ulcer, with inflammation
    nasal septum I86.8
    perineum I86.3
    scrotum I86.1
    specified site NEC I86.8
  vein — *see* Varix
  vessel — *see* Varix, leg
Varicosis, varicosities, varicosity — *see* Varix
Variola (major) (minor) B03
Varioloid B03
Varix (lower limb) (ruptured) I83.90

Varix — continued
  with
    edema I83.899
    inflammation I83.10
      with ulcer (venous) I83.209
    pain I83.819
    specified complication NEC I83.899
    stasis dermatitis I83.10
      with ulcer (venous) I83.209
    swelling I83.899
    ulcer I83.009
      with inflammation I83.209
  aneurysmal I77.0
  asymptomatic I83.9- ☑
  bladder I86.2
  broad ligament I86.2
  complicating
    childbirth (lower extremity) O87.4
      anus or rectum O87.2
      genital (vagina, vulva or perineum) O87.8
    pregnancy (lower extremity) O22.0- ☑
      anus or rectum O22.4- ☑
      genital (vagina, vulva or perineum) O22.1- ☑
    puerperium (lower extremity) O87.4
      anus or rectum O87.2
      genital (vagina, vulva, perineum) O87.8
  congenital (any site) Q27.8
  esophagus (idiopathic) (primary) (ulcerated) I85.00
    bleeding I85.01
    congenital Q27.8
    in (due to)
      alcoholic liver disease I85.10
        bleeding I85.11
      cirrhosis of liver I85.10
        bleeding I85.11
      portal hypertension I85.10
        bleeding I85.11
      schistosomiasis I85.10
        bleeding I85.11
      toxic liver disease I85.10
        bleeding I85.11
    secondary I85.10
      bleeding I85.11
  gastric I86.4
  inflamed or infected I83.10
    ulcerated I83.209
  labia (majora) I86.3
  leg (asymptomatic) I83.90
    with
      edema I83.899
      inflammation I83.10
        with ulcer — see Varix, leg, with, ulcer, with inflammation by site
      pain I83.819
      specified complication NEC I83.899
      swelling I83.899
      ulcer I83.009
        with inflammation I83.209
        ankle I83.003
          with inflammation I83.203
        calf I83.002
          with inflammation I83.202
        foot NEC I83.005
          with inflammation I83.205
        heel I83.004
          with inflammation I83.204
        lower leg NEC I83.008
          with inflammation I83.208
        midfoot I83.004
          with inflammation I83.204
        thigh I83.001
          with inflammation I83.201
    bilateral (asymptomatic) I83.93
      with
        edema I83.893
        pain I83.813
        specified complication NEC I83.893
        swelling I83.893
        ulcer I83.0- ☑
          with inflammation I83.209
    left (asymptomatic) I83.92
      with
        edema I83.892
        inflammation I83.12
          with ulcer — see Varix, leg, with, ulcer, with inflammation by site
        pain I83.812
        specified complication NEC I83.892

Varix — continued
  leg — continued
    left — continued
      with — continued
        swelling I83.892
        ulcer I83.029
          with inflammation I83.229
          ankle I83.023
            with inflammation I83.223
          calf I83.022
            with inflammation I83.222
          foot NEC I83.025
            with inflammation I83.225
          heel I83.024
            with inflammation I83.224
          lower leg NEC I83.028
            with inflammation I83.228
          midfoot I83.024
            with inflammation I83.224
          thigh I83.021
            with inflammation I83.221
    right (asymptomatic) I83.91
      with
        edema I83.891
        inflammation I83.11
          with ulcer — see Varix, leg, with, ulcer, with inflammation by site
        pain I83.811
        specified complication NEC I83.891
        swelling I83.891
        ulcer I83.019
          with inflammation I83.219
          ankle I83.013
            with inflammation I83.213
          calf I83.012
            with inflammation I83.212
          foot NEC I83.015
            with inflammation I83.215
          heel I83.014
            with inflammation I83.214
          lower leg NEC I83.018
            with inflammation I83.218
          midfoot I83.014
            with inflammation I83.214
          thigh I83.011
            with inflammation I83.211
  nasal septum I86.8
  orbit I86.8
    congenital Q27.8
  ovary I86.2
  papillary I78.1
  pelvis I86.2
  perineum I86.3
  pharynx I86.8
  placenta O43.89- ☑
  renal papilla I86.8
  retina H35.09
  scrotum (ulcerated) I86.1
  sigmoid colon I86.8
  specified site NEC I86.8
  spinal (cord) (vessels) I86.8
  spleen, splenic (vein) (with phlebolith) I86.8
  stomach I86.4
  sublingual I86.0
  ulcerated I83.009
    inflamed or infected I83.209
  uterine ligament I86.2
  vagina I86.8
  vocal cord I86.8
  vulva I86.3
Vas deferens — see condition
Vas deferentitis N49.1
Vasa previa O69.4 ☑
  hemorrhage from, affecting newborn P50.0
Vascular (see also condition)
  loop on optic papilla Q14.2
  spasm I73.9
  spider I78.1
Vascularization, cornea — see Neovascularization, cornea
Vasculitis I77.6
  allergic D69.0
  cryoglobulinemic D89.1
  disseminated I77.6
  hypocomplementemic M31.8
  kidney I77.89
  livedoid L95.0
  nodular L95.8

Vasculitis — continued
  retina H35.06- ☑
  rheumatic — see Fever, rheumatic
  rheumatoid — see Rheumatoid, vasculitis
  skin (limited to) L95.9
    specified NEC L95.8
  systemic M31.8
Vasculopathy, necrotizing M31.9
  cardiac allograft T86.290
  specified NEC M31.8
Vasitis (nodosa) N49.1
  tuberculous A18.15
Vasodilation I73.9
Vasomotor — see condition
Vasoplasty, after previous sterilization Z31.0
  aftercare Z31.42
Vasospasm (vasoconstriction) I73.9
  cerebral (cerebrovascular) (artery) I67.848
    reversible I67.841
  coronary I20.1
  nerve
    arm — see Mononeuropathy, upper limb
    brachial plexus G54.0
    cervical plexus G54.2
    leg — see Mononeuropathy, lower limb
  peripheral NOS I73.9
  retina (artery) — see Occlusion, artery, retina
Vasospastic — see condition
Vasovagal attack (paroxysmal) R55
  psychogenic F45.8
VATER syndrome Q87.2
Vater's ampulla — see condition
Vegetation, vegetative
  adenoid (nasal fossa) J35.8
  endocarditis (acute) (any valve) (subacute) I33.0
  heart (mycotic) (valve) I33.0
Veil
  Jackson's Q43.3
Vein, venous — see condition
Veldt sore — see Ulcer, skin
Velpeau's hernia — see Hernia, femoral
Venereal
  bubo A55
  disease A64
  granuloma inguinale A58
  lymphogranuloma (Durand-Nicolas-Favre) A55
Venofibrosis I87.8
Venom, venomous — see Table of Drugs and Chemicals, by animal or substance, poisoning
Venous — see condition
Ventilator lung, newborn P27.8
Ventral — see condition
Ventricle, ventricular (see also condition)
  escape I49.3
  inversion Q20.5
Ventriculitis (cerebral) (see also Encephalitis) G04.90
Ventriculostomy status Z98.2
Vernet's syndrome G52.7
Verneuil's disease (syphilitic bursitis) A52.78
Verruca (due to HPV) (filiformis) (simplex) (viral) (vulgaris) B07.9
  acuminata A63.0
  necrogenica (primary) (tuberculosa) A18.4
  plana B07.8
  plantaris B07.0
  seborrheica L82.1
    inflamed L82.0
  senile (seborrheic) L82.1
    inflamed L82.0
  tuberculosa (primary) A18.4
  venereal A63.0
Verrucosities — see Verruca
Verruga peruana, peruviana A44.1
Version
  with extraction
  cervix — see Malposition, uterus
  uterus (postinfectional) (postpartal, old) — see Malposition, uterus
Vertebra, vertebral — see condition
Vertical talus (congenital) Q66.80
  left foot Q66.82
  right foot Q66.81
Vertigo R42
  auditory — see Vertigo, aural
  aural H81.31- ☑
  benign paroxysmal (positional) H81.1- ☑
  central (origin) H81.4- ☑

☑ Additional Character Required — Refer to the Tabular List for Character Selection   ▽ Subterms under main terms may continue to next column or page

Vertigo — *continued*
  cerebral H81.4- ☑
  Dix and Hallpike (epidemic) — *see* Neuronitis,
    vestibular
  due to infrasound T75.23 ☑
  epidemic A88.1
    Dix and Hallpike — *see* Neuronitis, vestibular
    Pedersen's — *see* Neuronitis, vestibular
    vestibular neuronitis — *see* Neuronitis, vestibular
  hysterical F44.89
  infrasound T75.23 ☑
  labyrinthine — *see* subcategory H81.0 ☑
  laryngeal R05
  malignant positional H81.4- ☑
  Ménière's — *see* subcategory H81.0 ☑
  menopausal N95.1
  otogenic — *see* Vertigo, aural
  paroxysmal positional, benign — *see* Vertigo, benign
    paroxysmal
  Pedersen's (epidemic) — *see* Neuronitis, vestibular
  peripheral NEC H81.39- ☑
  positional
    benign paroxysmal — *see* Vertigo, benign parox-
      ysmal
    malignant H81.4- ☑
Very-low-density-lipoprotein-type (VLDL) **hyper-**
  lipoproteinemia E78.1
Vesania — *see* Psychosis
Vesical — *see* condition
Vesicle
  cutaneous R23.8
  seminal — *see* condition
  skin R23.8
Vesicocolic — *see* condition
Vesicoperineal — *see* condition
Vesicorectal — *see* condition
Vesicourethrorectal — *see* condition
Vesicovaginal — *see* condition
Vesicular — *see* condition
Vesiculitis (seminal) N49.0
  amebic A06.82
  gonorrheal (acute) (chronic) A54.23
  trichomonal A59.09
  tuberculous A18.15
Vestibulitis (ear) (*see also* subcategory) H83.0 ☑ ☑
  nose (external) J34.89
  vulvar N94.810
Vestibulopathy , acute peripheral (recurrent) — *see*
  Neuronitis, vestibular
Vestige, vestigial (*see also* Persistence)
  branchial Q18.0
  structures in vitreous Q14.0
Vibration
  adverse effects T75.20 ☑
    pneumatic hammer syndrome T75.21 ☑
    specified effect NEC T75.29 ☑
    vasospastic syndrome T75.22 ☑
    vertigo from infrasound T75.23 ☑
  exposure (occupational) Z57.7
  vertigo T75.23 ☑
Vibriosis A28.9
Victim (of)
  crime Z65.4
  disaster Z65.5
  terrorism Z65.4
  torture Z65.4
  war Z65.5
Vidal's disease L28.0
Villaret's syndrome G52.7
Villous — *see* condition
VIN — *see* Neoplasia, intraepithelial, vulva
Vincent's infection (angina) (gingivitis) A69.1
  stomatitis NEC A69.1
Vinson-Plummer syndrome D50.1
Violence, physical R45.6
Viosterol deficiency — *see* Deficiency, calciferol
Vipoma — *see* Neoplasm, malignant, by site
Viremia B34.9
Virilism (adrenal) E25.9
  congenital E25.0
Virilization (female) (suprarenal) E25.9
  congenital E25.0
  isosexual E28.2
Virulent bubo A57
Virus, viral (*see also* condition)
  as cause of disease classified elsewhere B97.89
  cytomegalovirus B25.9

Virus, viral — *continued*
  human immunodeficiency (HIV) — *see* Human, immun-
    odeficiency virus (HIV) disease
  infection — *see* Infection, virus
  specified NEC B34.8
  swine influenza (viruses that normally cause infections
    in pigs) (*see also* Influenza, due to, identified
    novel influenza A virus) J09.X2
  West Nile (fever) A92.30
    with
      complications NEC A92.39
      cranial nerve disorders A92.32
      encephalitis A92.31
      encephalomyelitis A92.31
      neurologic manifestation NEC A92.32
      optic neuritis A92.32
      polyradiculitis A92.32
Viscera, visceral — *see* condition
Visceroptosis K63.4
Visible peristalsis R19.2
Vision, visual
  binocular, suppression H53.34
  blurred, blurring H53.8
    hysterical F44.6
  defect, defective NEC H54.7
  disorientation (syndrome) H53.8
  disturbance H53.9
    hysterical F44.6
  double H53.2
  examination Z01.00
    with abnormal findings Z01.01
  field, limitation (defect) — *see* Defect, visual field
  hallucinations R44.1
  halos H53.19
  loss — *see* Loss, vision
    sudden — *see* Disturbance, vision, subjective, loss,
      sudden
  low (both eyes) — *see* Low, vision
  perception, simultaneous without fusion H53.33
Vitality, lack or want of R53.83
  newborn P96.89
Vitamin deficiency — *see* Deficiency, vitamin
Vitelline duct, persistent Q43.0
Vitiligo L80
  eyelid H02.739
    left H02.736
      lower H02.735
      upper H02.734
    right H02.733
      lower H02.732
      upper H02.731
  pinta A67.2
  vulva N90.89
Vitreal corneal syndrome H59.01- ☑
Vitreoretinopathy, proliferative (*see also* Retinopathy,
  proliferative)
  with retinal detachment — *see* Detachment, retina,
    traction
Vitreous (*see also* condition)
  touch syndrome — *see* Complication, postprocedural,
    following cataract surgery
Vocal cord — *see* condition
Vogt-Koyanagi syndrome H20.82- ☑
Vogt's disease or syndrome G80.3
Vogt-Spielmeyer amaurotic idiocy or disease E75.4
Voice
  change R49.9
    specified NEC R49.8
  loss — *see* Aphonia
Volhynian fever A79.0
Volkmann's ischemic contracture or paralysis (complicating trauma) T79.6 ☑
Volvulus (bowel) (colon) (intestine) K56.2
  with perforation K56.2
  congenital Q43.8
  duodenum K31.5
  fallopian tube — *see* Torsion, fallopian tube
  oviduct — *see* Torsion, fallopian tube
  stomach (due to absence of gastrocolic ligament)
    K31.89
Vomiting R11.10
  with nausea R11.2
  without nausea R11.11
  asphyxia — *see* Foreign body, by site, causing asphyx-
    ia, gastric contents
  bilious (cause unknown) R11.14
    following gastro-intestinal surgery K91.0
    in newborn P92.01

Vomiting — *continued*
  blood — *see* Hematemesis
  causing asphyxia, choking, or suffocation — *see* For-
    eign body, by site
  cyclical G43.A0 (*following* G43.7)
    with refractory migraine G43.A1 (*following* G43.7)
    without refractory migraine G43.A0 (*following*
      G43.7)
    intractable G43.A1 (*following* G43.7)
    not intractable G43.A0 (*following* G43.7)
    psychogenic F50.89
  fecal mater R11.13
  following gastrointestinal surgery K91.0
    psychogenic F50.89
  functional K31.89
  hysterical F50.89
  nervous F50.89
  neurotic F50.89
  newborn NEC P92.09
    bilious P92.01
  periodic R11.10
    psychogenic F50.89
  projectile R11.12
  psychogenic F50.89
  uremic — *see* Uremia
Vomito negro — *see* Fever, yellow
Von Bezold's abscess — *see* Mastoiditis, acute
Von Economo-Cruchet disease A85.8
Von Eulenburg's disease G71.19
Von Gierke's disease E74.01
Von Hippel (-Lindau) **disease or syndrome** Q85.8
Von Jaksch's anemia or disease D64.89
Von Recklinghausen
  disease (neurofibromatosis) Q85.01
    bones E21.0
Von Schroetter's syndrome I82.890
Von Willebrand (-Jurgens)(-Minot) **disease or syn-**
  drome D68.0
Von Zumbusch's disease L40.1
Voyeurism F65.3
Vrolik's disease Q78.0
Vulva — *see* condition
Vulvismus N94.2
Vulvitis (acute) (allergic) (atrophic) (hypertrophic) (intertriginous) (senile) N76.2
  with ectopic or molar pregnancy O08.0
  adhesive, congenital Q52.79
  blennorrhagic (gonococcal) A54.02
  candidal B37.3
  chlamydial A56.02
  due to Haemophilus ducreyi A57
  following ectopic or molar pregnancy O08.0
  gonococcal A54.02
    with abscess (accessory gland) (periurethral) A54.1
  herpesviral A60.04
  leukoplakic N90.4
  monilial B37.3
  puerperal (postpartum) O86.19
  subacute or chronic N76.3
  syphilitic (early) A51.0
    late A52.76
  trichomonal A59.01
  tuberculous A18.18
Vulvodynia N94.819
  specified NEC N94.818
Vulvorectal — *see* condition
Vulvovaginitis (acute) — *see* Vaginitis

W

Waiting list, person on Z75.1
  for organ transplant Z76.82
  undergoing social agency investigation Z75.2
Waldenström
  hypergammaglobulinemia D89.0
  syndrome or macroglobulinemia C88.0
Waldenström-Kjellberg syndrome D50.1
Walking
  difficulty R26.2
    psychogenic F44.4
  sleep F51.3
    hysterical F44.89
Wall, abdominal — *see* condition
Wallenberg's disease or syndrome G46.3
Wallgren's disease I87.8
Wandering
  gallbladder, congenital Q44.1
  in diseases classified elsewhere Z91.83

◢ **Subterms under main terms may continue to next column or page**   ☑ **Additional Character Required — Refer to the Tabular List for Character Selection**   **325**

Vertigo — Wandering

Wandering — *continued*
kidney, congenital Q63.8
organ or site, congenital NEC — *see* Malposition, congenital, by site
pacemaker (heart) I49.8
spleen D73.89
War neurosis F48.8
Wart (due to HPV) (filiform) (infectious) (viral) B07.9
anogenital region (venereal) A63.0
common B07.8
external genital organs (venereal) A63.0
flat B07.8
Hassal-Henle's (of cornea) H18.49
Peruvian A44.1
plantar B07.0
prosector (tuberculous) A18.4
seborrheic L82.1
inflamed L82.0
senile (seborrheic) L82.1
inflamed L82.0
tuberculous A18.4
venereal A63.0
Warthin's tumor — *see* Neoplasm, salivary gland, benign
Wassilieff's disease A27.0
Wasting
disease R64
due to malnutrition E41
extreme (due to malnutrition) E41
muscle NEC — *see* Atrophy, muscle
Water
clefts (senile cataract) — *see* Cataract, senile, incipient
deprivation of T73.1 ☑
intoxication E87.79
itch B76.9
lack of T73.1 ☑
loading E87.70
on
brain — *see* Hydrocephalus
chest J94.8
poisoning E87.79
Waterbrash R12
Waterhouse (-Friderichsen) **syndrome or disease** (meningococcal) A39.1
Water-losing nephritis N25.89
Watermelon stomach K31.819
with hemorrhage K31.811
without hemorrhage K31.819
Watsoniasis B66.8
Wax in ear — *see* Impaction, cerumen
Weak, weakening, weakness (generalized) R53.1
arches (acquired) (*see also* Deformity, limb, flat foot)
bladder (sphincter) R32
facial R29.810
following
cerebrovascular disease I69.992
cerebral infarction I69.392
intracerebral hemorrhage I69.192
nontraumatic intracranial hemorrhage NEC I69.292
specified disease NEC I69.892
stroke I69.392
subarachnoid hemorrhage I69.092
foot (double) — *see* Weak, arches
heart, cardiac — *see* Failure, heart
mind F70
muscle M62.81
myocardium — *see* Failure, heart
newborn P96.89
pelvic fundus N81.89
pubocervical tissue N81.82
rectovaginal tissue N81.83
senile R54
urinary stream R39.12
valvular — *see* Endocarditis
Wear, worn (with normal or routine use)
articular bearing surface of internal joint prosthesis — *see* Complications, joint prosthesis, mechanical, wear of articular bearing surfaces, by site
device, implant or graft — *see* Complications, by site, mechanical complication
tooth, teeth (approximal) (hard tissues) (interproximal) (occlusal) K03.0
Weather, weathered
effects of
cold T69.9 ☑
specified effect NEC T69.8 ☑
hot — *see* Heat
skin L57.8

Weaver's syndrome Q87.3
Web, webbed (congenital)
duodenal Q43.8
esophagus Q39.4
fingers Q70.1- ☑
larynx (glottic) (subglottic) Q31.0
neck (pterygium colli) Q18.3
Paterson-Kelly D50.1
popliteal syndrome Q87.89
toes Q70.3- ☑
Weber-Christian disease M35.6
Weber-Cockayne syndrome (epidermolysis bullosa) Q81.8
Weber-Gubler syndrome G46.3
Weber-Leyden syndrome G46.3
Weber-Osler syndrome I78.0
Weber's paralysis or syndrome G46.3
Wedge-shaped or wedging vertebra — *see* Collapse, vertebra NEC
Wegener's granulomatosis or syndrome M31.30
with
kidney involvement M31.31
lung involvement M31.30
with kidney involvement M31.31
Wegner's disease A50.02
Weight
1000-2499 grams at birth (low) — *see* Low, birth-weight
999 grams or less at birth (extremely low) — *see* Low, birthweight, extreme
and length below 10th percentile for gestational age P05.1- ☑
below but length above 10th percentile for gestational age P05.0- ☑
gain (abnormal) (excessive) R63.5
in pregnancy — *see* Pregnancy, complicated by, excessive weight gain
low — *see* Pregnancy, complicated by, insufficient, weight gain
loss (abnormal) (cause unknown) R63.4
Weightlessness (effect of) T75.82 ☑
Weil (l)-**Marchesani syndrome** Q87.1
Weil's disease A27.0
Weingarten's syndrome J82
Weir Mitchell's disease I73.81
Weiss-Baker syndrome G90.09
Wells' disease L98.3
Wen — *see* Cyst, sebaceous
Wenckebach's block or phenomenon I44.1
Werdnig-Hoffmann syndrome (muscular atrophy) G12.0
Werlhof's disease D69.3
Wermer's disease or syndrome E31.21
Werner-His disease A79.0
Werner's disease or syndrome E34.8
Wernicke-Korsakoff's syndrome or psychosis (alcoholic) F10.96
with dependence F10.26
drug-induced
due to drug abuse — *see* Abuse, drug, by type, with amnestic disorder
due to drug dependence — *see* Dependence, drug, by type, with amnestic disorder
nonalcoholic F04
Wernicke-Posadas disease B38.9
Wernicke's
developmental aphasia F80.2
disease or syndrome E51.2
encephalopathy E51.2
polioencephalitis, superior E51.2
West African fever B50.8
Westphal-Strümpell-syndrome E83.01
West's syndrome — *see* Epilepsy, spasms
Wet
feet, tropical (maceration) (syndrome) — *see* Immersion, foot
lung (syndrome), newborn P22.1
Wharton's duct — *see* condition
Wheal — *see* Urticaria
Wheezing R06.2
Whiplash injury S13.4 ☑
Whipple's disease (*see also* subcategory M14.8-) K90.81
Whipworm (disease) (infection) (infestation) B79
Whistling face Q87.0
White (*see also* condition)
kidney, small N03.9
leg, puerperal, postpartum, childbirth O87.1

White — *continued*
mouth B37.0
patches of mouth K13.29
spot lesions, teeth
chewing surface K02.51
pit and fissure surface K02.51
smooth surface K02.61
Whitehead L70.0
Whitlow (*see also* Cellulitis, digit)
with lymphangitis — *see* Lymphangitis, acute, digit
herpesviral B00.89
Whitmore's disease or fever — *see* Melioidosis
Whooping cough A37.90
with pneumonia A37.91
due to Bordetella
bronchiseptica A37.81
parapertussis A37.11
pertussis A37.01
specified organism NEC A37.81
due to
Bordetella
bronchiseptica A37.80
with pneumonia A37.81
parapertussis A37.10
with pneumonia A37.11
pertussis A37.00
with pneumonia A37.01
specified NEC A37.80
with pneumonia A37.81
Wichman's asthma J38.5
Wide cranial sutures, newborn P96.3
Widening aorta — *see* Ectasia, aorta
with aneurysm — *see* Aneurysm, aorta
Wilkie's disease or syndrome K55.1
Wilkinson-Sneddon disease or syndrome L13.1
Willebrand (-Jürgens) **thrombopathy** D68.0
Willige-Hunt disease or syndrome G23.1
Wilms' tumor C64- ☑
Wilson-Mikity syndrome P27.0
Wilson's
disease or syndrome E83.01
hepatolenticular degeneration E83.01
lichen ruber L43.9
Window (*see also* Imperfect, closure)
aorticopulmonary Q21.4
Winter — *see* condition
Wiskott-Aldrich syndrome D82.0
Withdrawal state (*see also* Dependence, drug by type, with withdrawal)
alcohol
with perceptual disturbances F10.232
without perceptual disturbances F10.239
caffeine F15.93
cannabis F12.288
newborn
correct therapeutic substance properly administered P96.2
infant of dependent mother P96.1
therapeutic substance, neonatal P96.2
Witts' anemia D50.8
Witzelsucht F07.0
Woakes' ethmoiditis or syndrome J33.1
Wolff-Hirschorn syndrome Q93.3
Wolff-Parkinson-White syndrome I45.6
Wolhynian fever A79.0
Wolman's disease E75.5
Wood lung or pneumonitis J67.8
Woolly, wooly hair (congenital) (nevus) Q84.1
Woolsorter's disease A22.1
Word
blindness (congenital) (developmental) F81.0
deafness (congenital) (developmental) H93.25
Worm(s) (infection) (infestation) (*see also* Infestation, helminth)
guinea B72
in intestine NEC B82.0
Worm-eaten soles A66.3
Worn out — *see* Exhaustion
cardiac
defibrillator (with synchronous cardiace pacemaker) Z45.02
pacemaker
battery Z45.010
lead Z45.018
device, implant or graft — *see* Complications, by site, mechanical
Worried well Z71.1
Worries R45.82

☑ **Additional Character Required — Refer to the Tabular List for Character Selection**   ▼ **Subterms under main terms may continue to next column or page**

Wound, open — *continued*
 head — *continued*
  eyelid — *see* Wound, open, eyelid
  laceration — *see* Laceration, head
  lip — *see* Wound, open, lip
  nose S01.20 ☑
  oral cavity — *see* Wound, open, oral cavity
  puncture — *see* Puncture, head
  scalp — *see* Wound, open, scalp
  specified site NEC S01.80 ☑
  temporomandibular area — *see* Wound, open, cheek
 heel — *see* Wound, open, foot
 hip S71.00- ☑
  with amputation — *see* Amputation, traumatic, hip
  bite — *see* Bite, hip
  laceration — *see* Laceration, hip
  puncture — *see* Puncture, hip
 hymen S31.40 ☑
  bite — *see* Bite, vulva
  laceration — *see* Laceration, vagina
  puncture — *see* Puncture, vagina
 hypochondrium S31.109 ☑
  bite — *see* Bite, hypochondrium
  laceration — *see* Laceration, hypochondrium
  puncture — *see* Puncture, hypochondrium
 hypogastric region S31.109 ☑
  bite — *see* Bite, hypogastric region
  laceration — *see* Laceration, hypogastric region
  puncture — *see* Puncture, hypogastric region
 iliac (region) — *see* Wound, open, inguinal region
 inguinal region S31.109 ☑
  bite — *see* Bite, abdomen, wall, lower quadrant
  laceration — *see* Laceration, inguinal region
  puncture — *see* Puncture, inguinal region
 instep — *see* Wound, open, foot
 interscapular region — *see* Wound, open, thorax, back
 intraocular — *see* Wound, open, ocular
 iris — *see* Wound, open, ocular
 jaw — *see* Wound, open, head, specified site NEC
 knee S81.00- ☑
  bite — *see* Bite, knee
  laceration — *see* Laceration, knee
  puncture — *see* Puncture, knee
 labium (majus) (minus) — *see* Wound, open, vulva
 laceration — *see* Laceration, by site
 lacrimal duct — *see* Wound, open, eyelid
 larynx S11.019 ☑
  bite — *see* Bite, larynx
  laceration — *see* Laceration, larynx
  puncture — *see* Puncture, larynx
 left
  lower quadrant S31.104 ☑
   with penetration into peritoneal cavity S31.604 ☑
   bite — *see* Bite, abdomen, wall, left, lower quadrant
   laceration — *see* Laceration, abdomen, wall, left, lower quadrant
   puncture — *see* Puncture, abdomen, wall, left, lower quadrant
  upper quadrant S31.101 ☑
   with penetration into peritoneal cavity S31.601 ☑
   bite — *see* Bite, abdomen, wall, left, upper quadrant
   laceration — *see* Laceration, abdomen, wall, left, upper quadrant
   puncture — *see* Puncture, abdomen, wall, left, upper quadrant
 leg (lower) S81.80- ☑
  with amputation — *see* Amputation, traumatic, leg
  ankle — *see* Wound, open, ankle
  bite — *see* Bite, leg
  foot — *see* Wound, open, foot
  knee — *see* Wound, open, knee
  laceration — *see* Laceration, leg
  puncture — *see* Puncture, leg
  toe — *see* Wound, open, toe
  upper — *see* Wound, open, thigh
 lip S01.501 ☑
  bite — *see* Bite, lip
  laceration — *see* Laceration, lip
  puncture — *see* Puncture, lip

Wound, open — *continued*
 loin S31.109 ☑
  bite — *see* Bite, abdomen, wall
  laceration — *see* Laceration, loin
  puncture — *see* Puncture, loin
 lower back — *see* Wound, open, back, lower
 lumbar region — *see* Wound, open, back, lower
 malar region — *see* Wound, open, head, specified site NEC
 mammary — *see* Wound, open, breast
 mastoid region — *see* Wound, open, head, specified site NEC
 mouth — *see* Wound, open, oral cavity
 nail
  finger — *see* Wound, open, finger, with damage to nail
  toe — *see* Wound, open, toe, with damage to nail
 nape (neck) — *see* Wound, open, neck
 nasal (septum) (sinus) — *see* Wound, open, nose
 nasopharynx — *see* Wound, open, head, specified site NEC
 neck S11.90 ☑
  bite — *see* Bite, neck
  involving
   cervical esophagus S11.20 ☑
   larynx — *see* Wound, open, larynx
   pharynx S11.20 ☑
   thyroid S11.10 ☑
   trachea (cervical) S11.029 ☑
    bite — *see* Bite, trachea
    laceration S11.021 ☑
     with foreign body S11.022 ☑
    puncture S11.023 ☑
     with foreign body S11.024 ☑
  laceration — *see* Laceration, neck
  puncture — *see* Puncture, neck
  specified site NEC S11.80 ☑
   specified type NEC S11.89 ☑
 nose (septum) (sinus) S01.20 ☑
  with amputation — *see* Amputation, traumatic, nose
  bite — *see* Bite, nose
  laceration — *see* Laceration, nose
  puncture — *see* Puncture, nose
 ocular S05.90 ☑
  avulsion (traumatic enucleation) S05.7- ☑
  eyeball S05.6- ☑
   with foreign body S05.5- ☑
  eyelid — *see* Wound, open, eyelid
  laceration and rupture S05.3- ☑
   with prolapse or loss of intraocular tissue S05.2- ☑
  orbit (penetrating) (with or without foreign body) S05.4- ☑
  periocular area — *see* Wound, open, eyelid
  specified NEC S05.8X- ☑
 oral cavity S01.502 ☑
  bite S01.552 ☑
  laceration — *see* Laceration, oral cavity
  puncture — *see* Puncture, oral cavity
 orbit — *see* Wound, open, ocular, orbit
 palate — *see* Wound, open, oral cavity
 palm — *see* Wound, open, hand
 pelvis, pelvic (*see also* Wound, open, back, lower)
  girdle — *see* Wound, open, hip
 penetrating — *see* Puncture, by site
 penis S31.20 ☑
  with amputation — *see* Amputation, traumatic, penis
  bite S31.25 ☑
  laceration — *see* Laceration, penis
  puncture — *see* Puncture, penis
 perineum
  bite — *see* Bite, perineum
  female S31.502 ☑
  laceration — *see* Laceration, perineum
  male S31.501 ☑
  puncture — *see* Puncture, perineum
 periocular area (with or without lacrimal passages) — *see* Wound, open, eyelid
 periumbilic region S31.105 ☑
  with penetration into peritoneal cavity S31.605 ☑
  bite — *see* Bite, abdomen, wall, periumbilic region
  laceration — *see* Laceration, abdomen, wall, periumbilic region

Wound, open — *continued*
 periumbilic region — *continued*
  puncture — *see* Puncture, abdomen, wall, periumbilic region
 phalanges
  finger — *see* Wound, open, finger
  toe — *see* Wound, open, toe
 pharynx S11.20 ☑
 pinna — *see* Wound, open, ear
 popliteal space — *see* Wound, open, knee
 prepuce — *see* Wound, open, penis
 pubic region — *see* Wound, open, back, lower
 pudendum — *see* Wound, open, genital organs, external
 puncture wound — *see* Puncture
 rectovaginal septum — *see* Wound, open, vagina
 right
  lower quadrant S31.103 ☑
   with penetration into peritoneal cavity S31.603 ☑
   bite — *see* Bite, abdomen, wall, right, lower quadrant
   laceration — *see* Laceration, abdomen, wall, right, lower quadrant
   puncture — *see* Puncture, abdomen, wall, right, lower quadrant
  upper quadrant S31.100 ☑
   with penetration into peritoneal cavity S31.600 ☑
   bite — *see* Bite, abdomen, wall, right, upper quadrant
   laceration — *see* Laceration, abdomen, wall, right, upper quadrant
   puncture — *see* Puncture, abdomen, wall, right, upper quadrant
 sacral region — *see* Wound, open, back, lower
 sacroiliac region — *see* Wound, open, back, lower
 salivary gland — *see* Wound, open, oral cavity
 scalp S01.00 ☑
  bite S01.05 ☑
  laceration — *see* Laceration, scalp
  puncture — *see* Puncture, scalp
 scalpel, newborn (birth injury) P15.8
 scapular region — *see* Wound, open, shoulder
 sclera — *see* Wound, open, ocular
 scrotum S31.30 ☑
  with amputation — *see* Amputation, traumatic, scrotum
  bite S31.35 ☑
  laceration — *see* Laceration, scrotum
  puncture — *see* Puncture, scrotum
 shin — *see* Wound, open, leg
 shoulder S41.00- ☑
  with amputation — *see* Amputation, traumatic, arm
  bite — *see* Bite, shoulder
  laceration — *see* Laceration, shoulder
  puncture — *see* Puncture, shoulder
 skin NOS T14.8 ☑
 spermatic cord — *see* Wound, open, testis
 sternal region — *see* Wound, open, thorax, front wall
 submaxillary region — *see* Wound, open, head, specified site NEC
 submental region — *see* Wound, open, head, specified site NEC
 subungual
  finger(s) — *see* Wound, open, finger
  toe(s) — *see* Wound, open, toe
 supraclavicular region — *see* Wound, open, neck, specified site NEC
 temple, temporal region — *see* Wound, open, head, specified site NEC
 temporomandibular area — *see* Wound, open, cheek
 testis S31.30 ☑
  with amputation — *see* Amputation, traumatic, testes
  bite S31.35 ☑
  laceration — *see* Laceration, testis
  puncture — *see* Puncture, testis
 thigh S71.10- ☑
  with amputation — *see* Amputation, traumatic, hip
  bite — *see* Bite, thigh
  laceration — *see* Laceration, thigh
  puncture — *see* Puncture, thigh
 thorax, thoracic (wall) S21.90 ☑
  back S21.20- ☑

☑ Additional Character Required — Refer to the Tabular List for Character Selection   ▽ Subterms under main terms may continue to next column or page

Wound, open — *continued*
  thorax, thoracic — *continued*
    back — *continued*
      with penetration S21.40 ☑
    bite — *see* Bite, thorax
    breast — *see* Wound, open, breast
    front S21.10-
      with penetration S21.30 ☑
    laceration — *see* Laceration, thorax
    puncture — *see* Puncture, thorax
  throat — *see* Wound, open, neck
  thumb S61.009 ☑
    with
      amputation — *see* Amputation, traumatic, thumb
      damage to nail S61.109 ☑
    bite — *see* Bite, thumb
    laceration — *see* Laceration, thumb
    left S61.002 ☑
      with
        damage to nail S61.102 ☑
    puncture — *see* Puncture, thumb
    right S61.001 ☑
      with
        damage to nail S61.101 ☑
  thyroid (gland) — *see* Wound, open, neck, thyroid
  toe(s) S91.109 ☑
    with
      amputation — *see* Amputation, traumatic, toe
      damage to nail S91.209 ☑
    bite — *see* Bite, toe
    great S91.103 ☑
      with
        damage to nail S91.203 ☑
      left S91.102 ☑
        with
          damage to nail S91.202 ☑
      right S91.101 ☑
        with
          damage to nail S91.201 ☑
    laceration — *see* Laceration, toe
    lesser S91.106 ☑
      with
        damage to nail S91.206 ☑
      left S91.105 ☑
        with
          damage to nail S91.205 ☑
      right S91.104 ☑
        with
          damage to nail S91.204 ☑
    puncture — *see* Puncture, toe
  tongue — *see* Wound, open, oral cavity
  trachea (cervical region) — *see* Wound, open, neck, trachea
  tunica vaginalis — *see* Wound, open, testis
  tympanum, tympanic membrane S09.2- ☑
    laceration — *see* Laceration, ear, drum
    puncture — *see* Puncture, tympanum
  umbilical region — *see* Wound, open, abdomen, wall, periumbilic region
  uvula — *see* Wound, open, oral cavity
  vagina S31.40 ☑
    bite S31.45 ☑
    laceration — *see* Laceration, vagina
    puncture — *see* Puncture, vagina
  vitreous (humor) — *see* Wound, open, ocular
  vocal cord S11.039 ☑
    bite — *see* Bite, vocal cord
    laceration S11.031 ☑
      with foreign body S11.032 ☑
    puncture S11.033 ☑
      with foreign body S11.034 ☑
  vulva S31.40 ☑
    with amputation — *see* Amputation, traumatic, vulva
    bite S31.45 ☑
    laceration — *see* Laceration, vulva
    puncture — *see* Puncture, vulva
  wrist S61.50- ☑
    bite — *see* Bite, wrist
    laceration — *see* Laceration, wrist
    puncture — *see* Puncture, wrist
Wound, superficial — *see* Injury (*see also* specified injury type)

Wright's syndrome G54.0
Wrist — *see* condition
Wrong drug (by accident) (given in error) — *see* Table of Drugs and Chemicals, by drug, poisoning
Wry neck — *see* Torticollis
Wuchereria (bancrofti) **infestation** B74.0
Wuchereriasis B74.0
Wuchernde Struma Langhans C73

X

Xanthelasma (eyelid) (palpebrarum) H02.60
  left H02.66
    lower H02.65
    upper H02.64
  right H02.63
    lower H02.62
    upper H02.61
Xanthelasmatosis (essential) E78.2
Xanthinuria, hereditary E79.8
Xanthoastrocytoma
  specified site — *see* Neoplasm, malignant, by site
  unspecified site C71.9
Xanthofibroma — *see* Neoplasm, connective tissue, benign
Xanthogranuloma D76.3
Xanthoma(s), xanthomatosis (primary) (familial) (hereditary) E75.5
  with
    hyperlipoproteinemia
      Type I E78.3
      Type III E78.2
      Type IV E78.1
      Type V E78.3
  bone (generalisata) C96.5
  cerebrotendinous E75.5
  cutaneotendinous E75.5
  disseminatum (skin) E78.2
  eruptive E78.2
  hypercholesterinemic E78.00
  hypercholesterolemic E78.00
  hyperlipidemic E78.5
  joint E75.5
  multiple (skin) E78.2
  tendon (sheath) E75.5
  tuberosum E78.2
  tuberous E78.2
  tubo-eruptive E78.2
  verrucous, oral mucosa K13.4
Xanthosis R23.8
Xenophobia F40.10
Xeroderma (*see also* Ichthyosis)
  acquired L85.0
  eyelid H01.149
    left H01.146
      lower H01.145
      upper H01.144
    right H01.143
      lower H01.142
      upper H01.141
  pigmentosum Q82.1
  vitamin A deficiency E50.8
Xerophthalmia (vitamin A deficiency) E50.7
  unrelated to vitamin A deficiency — *see* Keratoconjunctivitis
Xerosis
  conjunctiva H11.14- ☑
    with Bitot's spots (*see also* Pigmentation, conjunctiva)
      vitamin A deficiency E50.1
    vitamin A deficiency E50.0
  cornea H18.89- ☑
    with ulceration — *see* Ulcer, cornea
      vitamin A deficiency E50.3
    vitamin A deficiency E50.2
  cutis L85.3
  skin L85.3
Xerostomia K11.7
Xiphopagus Q89.4
XO syndrome Q96.9
X-ray (of)
  abnormal findings — *see* Abnormal, diagnostic imaging
  breast (mammogram) (routine) Z12.31

X-ray — *continued*
  chest
    routine (as part of a general medical examination) Z00.00
      with abnormal findings Z00.01
  routine (as part of a general medical examination) Z00.00
    with abnormal findings Z00.01
XXXXY syndrome Q98.1
XXY syndrome Q98.0

Y

Yaba pox (virus disease) B08.72
Yatapoxvirus B08.70
  specified NEC B08.79
Yawning R06.89
  psychogenic F45.8
Yaws A66.9
  cutaneous, less than five years after infection A66.2
  bone lesions A66.6
  butter A66.1
  chancre A66.0
  early (cutaneous) (macular) (maculopapular) (micropapular) (papular) A66.2
    frambeside A66.2
    skin lesions NEC A66.2
  eyelid A66.2
  ganglion A66.6
  gangosis, gangosa A66.5
  gumma, gummata A66.4
    bone A66.6
  gummatous
    frambeside A66.4
    osteitis A66.6
    periostitis A66.6
  hydrarthrosis (*see also* subcategory M14.8-) A66.6
  hyperkeratosis (early) (late) A66.3
  initial lesions A66.0
  joint lesions (*see also* subcategory M14.8-) A66.6
  juxta-articular nodules A66.7
  late nodular (ulcerated) A66.4
  latent (without clinical manifestations) (with positive serology) A66.8
  mother A66.0
  mucosal A66.7
  multiple papillomata A66.1
  nodular, late (ulcerated) A66.4
  osteitis A66.6
  papilloma, plantar or palmar A66.1
  periostitis (hypertrophic) A66.6
  specified NEC A66.7
  ulcers A66.4
  wet crab A66.1
Yeast infection (*see also* Candidiasis) B37.9
Yellow
  atrophy (liver) — *see* Failure, hepatic
  fever — *see* Fever, yellow
  jack — *see* Fever, yellow
  jaundice — *see* Jaundice
  nail syndrome L60.5
Yersiniosis (*see also* Infection, Yersinia)
  extraintestinal A28.2
  intestinal A04.6

Z

Zahorsky's syndrome (herpangina) B08.5
Zellweger's syndrome Q87.89
Zenker's diverticulum (esophagus) K22.5
Ziehen-Oppenheim disease G24.1
Zieve's syndrome K70.0
Zika NOS A92.5
Zinc
  deficiency, dietary E60
  metabolism disorder E83.2
Zollinger-Ellison syndrome E16.4
Zona — *see* Herpes, zoster
Zoophobia F40.218
Zoster (herpes) — *see* Herpes, zoster
Zygomycosis B46.9
  specified NEC B46.8
Zymotic — *see* condition

	Malignant Primary	Malignant Secondary	Ca in situ	Benign	Uncertain	Unspecified Behavior

Note: The list below gives the code number for neoplasms by anatomical site. For each site there are six possible code numbers according to whether the neoplasm in question is malignant, benign, in situ, of uncertain behavior, or of unspecified nature. The description of the neoplasm will often indicate which of the six columns is appropriate; e.g., malignant melanoma of skin, benign fibroadenoma of breast, carcinoma in situ of cervix uteri. Where such descriptors are not present, the remainder of the Index should be consulted where guidance is given to the appropriate column for each morphological (histological) variety listed; e.g., Mesonephroma – see Neoplasm, malignant; Embryoma (see also Neoplasm, uncertain behavior); Disease, Bowen's – see Neoplasm, skin, in situ. However, the guidance in the Index can be overridden if one of the descriptors mentioned above is present; e.g., malignant adenoma of colon is coded to C18.9 and not to D12.6 as the adjective "malignant" overrides the Index entry "Adenoma (see also Neoplasm, benign, by site)." Codes listed with a dash -, following the code have a required additional character for laterality. The tabular list must be reviewed for the complete code.

Site	Malignant Primary	Malignant Secondary	Ca in situ	Benign	Uncertain	Unspecified Behavior
Neoplasm, neoplastic	C80.1	C79.9	D09.9	D36.9	D48.9	D49.9
abdomen,						
abdominal	C76.2	C79.8-☑	D09.8	D36.7	D48.7	D49.89
cavity	C76.2	C79.8-☑	D09.8	D36.7	D48.7	D49.89
organ	C76.2	C79.8-☑	D09.8	D36.7	D48.7	D49.89
viscera	C76.2	C79.8-☑	D09.8	D36.7	D48.7	D49.89
wall — see also						
Neoplasm,						
abdomen, wall,						
skin	C44.509	C79.2	D04.5	D23.5	D48.5	D49.2
connective						
tissue	C49.4	C79.8-☑	—	D21.4	D48.1	D49.2
skin	C44.509	—	—	—	—	—
basal cell						
carcinoma	C44.519	—	—	—	—	—
specified type						
NEC	C44.599	—	—	—	—	—
squamous cell						
carcinoma	C44.529	—	—	—	—	—
abdominopelvic	C76.8	C79.8-☑	—	D36.7	D48.7	D49.89
accessory sinus — see						
Neoplasm, sinus						
acoustic nerve	C72.4-☑	C79.49		D33.3	D43.3	D49.7
adenoid (pharynx)						
(tissue)	C11.1	C79.89	D00.08	D10.6	D37.05	D49.0
adipose tissue — see also						
Neoplasm, connective						
tissue	C49.4	C79.89	—	D21.9	D48.1	D49.2
adnexa (uterine)	C57.4	C79.89	D07.39	D28.7	D39.8	D49.59
adrenal	C74.9-☑	C79.7-☑	D09.3	D35.0-☑	D44.1-☑	D49.7
capsule	C74.9-☑	C79.7-☑	D09.3	D35.0-☑	D44.1-☑	D49.7
cortex	C74.0-☑	C79.7-☑	D09.3	D35.0-☑	D44.1-☑	D49.7
gland	C74.9-☑	C79.7-☑	D09.3	D35.0-☑	D44.1-☑	D49.7
medulla	C74.1-☑	C79.7-☑	D09.3	D35.0-☑	D44.1-☑	D49.7
ala nasi (external) — see						
also Neoplasm, skin,						
nose	C44.301	C79.2	D04.39	D23.39	D48.5	D49.2
alimentary canal or tract						
NEC	C26.9	C78.80	D01.9	D13.9	D37.9	D49.0
alveolar	C03.9	C79.89	D00.03	D10.39	D37.09	D49.0
mucosa	C03.9	C79.89	D00.03	D10.39	D37.09	D49.0
lower	C03.1	C79.89	D00.03	D10.39	D37.09	D49.0
upper	C03.0	C79.89	D00.03	D10.39	D37.09	D49.0
ridge or process	C41.1	C79.51	—	D16.5	D48.0	D49.2
carcinoma	C03.9	C79.8-☑	—	—	—	—
lower	C03.1	C79.8-☑	—	—	—	—
upper	C03.0	C79.8-☑	—	—	—	—
lower	C41.1	C79.51	—	D16.5	D48.0	D49.2
mucosa	C03.9	C79.89	D00.03	D10.39	D37.09	D49.0
lower	C03.1	C79.89	D00.03	D10.39	D37.09	D49.0
upper	C03.0	C79.89	D00.03	D10.39	D37.09	D49.0
upper	C41.0	C79.51	—	D16.4	D48.0	D49.2
sulcus	C06.1	C79.89	D00.02	D10.39	D37.09	D49.0
alveolus	C03.9	C79.89	D00.03	D10.39	D37.09	D49.0
lower	C03.1	C79.89	D00.03	D10.39	D37.09	D49.0
upper	C03.0	C79.89	D00.03	D10.39	D37.09	D49.0
ampulla of Vater	C24.1	C78.89	D01.5	D13.5	D37.6	D49.0
ankle NEC	C76.5-☑	C79.89	D04.7-☑	D36.7	D48.7	D49.89
anorectum, anorectal						
(junction)	C21.8	C78.5	D01.3	D12.9	D37.8	D49.0
antecubital fossa or						
space	C76.4-☑	C79.89	D04.6-☑	D36.7	D48.7	D49.89
Neoplasm, neoplastic —						
continued						
antrum (Highmore)						
(maxillary)	C31.0	C78.39	D02.3	D14.0	D38.5	D49.1
pyloric	C16.3	C78.89	D00.2	D13.1	D37.1	D49.0
tympanicum	C30.1	C78.39	D02.3	D14.0	D38.5	D49.1
anus, anal	C21.0	C78.5	D01.3	D12.9	D37.8	D49.0
canal	C21.1	C78.5	D01.3	D12.9	D37.8	D49.0
cloacogenic zone	C21.2	C78.5	D01.3	D12.9	D37.8	D49.0
margin — see also						
Neoplasm, anus,						
skin	C44.500	C79.2	D04.5	D23.5	D48.5	D49.2
overlapping lesion with						
rectosigmoid						
junction or						
rectum	C21.8	—	—	—	—	—
skin	C44.500	C79.2	D04.5	D23.5	D48.5	D49.2
basal cell						
carcinoma	C44.510	—	—	—	—	—
specified type						
NEC	C44.590	—	—	—	—	—
squamous cell						
carcinoma	C44.520	—	—	—	—	—
sphincter	C21.1	C78.5	D01.3	D12.9	D37.8	D49.0
aorta (thoracic)	C49.3	C79.89	—	D21.3	D48.1	D49.2
abdominal	C49.4	C79.89	—	D21.4	D48.1	D49.2
aortic body	C75.5	C79.89	—	D35.6	D44.7	D49.7
aponeurosis	C49.9	C79.89	—	D21.9	D48.1	D49.2
palmar	C49.1-☑	C79.89	—	D21.1-☑	D48.1	D49.2
plantar	C49.2-☑	C79.89	—	D21.2-☑	D48.1	D49.2
appendix	C18.1	C78.5	D01.0	D12.1	D37.3	D49.0
arachnoid	C70.9	C79.49	—	D32.9	D42.9	D49.7
cerebral	C70.0	C79.32	—	D32.0	D42.0	D49.7
spinal	C70.1	C79.49	—	D32.1	D42.1	D49.7
areola	C50.0-☑	C79.81	D05-☑	D24-☑	D48.6-☑	D49.3
arm NEC	C76.4-☑	C79.89	D04.6-☑	D36.7	D48.7	D49.89
artery — see Neoplasm,						
connective tissue						
aryepiglottic fold	C13.1	C79.89	D00.08	D10.7	D37.05	D49.0
hypopharyngeal						
aspect	C13.1	C79.89	D00.08	D10.7	D37.05	D49.0
laryngeal aspect	C32.1	C78.39	D02.0	D14.1	D38.0	D49.1
marginal zone	C13.1	C79.89	D00.08	D10.7	D37.05	D49.0
arytenoid (cartilage)	C32.3	C78.39	D02.0	D14.1	D38.0	D49.1
fold — see Neoplasm,						
aryepiglottic						
associated with						
transplanted						
organ	C80.2	—	—	—	—	—
atlas	C41.2	C79.51	—	D16.6	D48.0	D49.2
atrium, cardiac	C38.0	C79.89	—	D15.1	D48.7	D49.89
auditory						
canal (external)						
(skin)	C44.20-☑	C79.2	D04.2-☑	D23.2-☑	D48.5	D49.2
internal	C30.1	C78.39	D02.3	D14.0	D38.5	D49.1
nerve	C72.4-☑	C79.49	—	D33.3	D43.3	D49.7
tube	C30.1	C78.39	D02.3	D14.0	D38.5	D49.1
opening	C11.2	C79.89	D00.08	D10.6	D37.05	D49.0
auricle, ear — see also						
Neoplasm, skin,						
ear	C44.20-☑	C79.2	D04.2-☑	D23.2-☑	D48.5	D49.2
auricular canal (external)						
— see also Neoplasm,						
skin, ear	C44.20-☑	C79.2	D04.2-☑	D23.2-☑	D48.5	D49.2
internal	C30.1	C78.39	D02.3	D14.0	D38.5	D49.2
autonomic nerve or						
nervous system NEC						
(see Neoplasm, nerve,						
peripheral)						
axilla, axillary	C76.1	C79.89	D09.8	D36.7	D48.7	D49.89
fold — see also						
Neoplasm, skin,						
trunk	C44.509	C79.2	D04.5	D23.5	D48.5	D49.2
back NEC	C76.8	C79.89	D04.5	D36.7	D48.7	D49.89
Bartholin's gland	C51.0	C79.82	D07.1	D28.0	D39.8	D49.59
basal ganglia	C71.0	C79.31	—	D33.0	D43.0	D49.6
basis pedunculi	C71.7	C79.31	—	D33.1	D43.1	D49.6
bile or biliary (tract)	C24.9	C78.89	D01.5	D13.5	D37.6	D49.0
canaliculi (biliferi)						
(intrahepatic)	C22.1	C78.7	D01.5	D13.4	D37.6	D49.0
canals,						
interlobular	C22.1	C78.7	D01.5	D13.4	D37.6	D49.0

Neoplasm, neoplastic — *continued*	Malignant Primary	Malignant Secondary	Ca in situ	Benign	Uncertain	Unspecified Behavior
bile or biliary — continued						
duct or passage (common) (cystic) (extrahepatic)	C24.0	C78.89	D01.5	D13.5	D37.6	D49.0
interlobular	C22.1	C78.89	D01.5	D13.4	D37.6	D49.0
intrahepatic	C22.1	C78.7	D01.5	D13.4	D37.6	D49.0
and extrahepatic	C24.8	C78.89	D01.5	D13.5	D37.6	D49.0
bladder (urinary)	C67.9	C79.11	D09.0	D30.3	D41.4	D49.4
dome	C67.1	C79.11	D09.0	D30.3	D41.4	D49.4
neck	C67.5	C79.11	D09.0	D30.3	D41.4	D49.4
orifice	C67.9	C79.11	D09.0	D30.3	D41.4	D49.4
ureteric	C67.6	C79.11	D09.0	D30.3	D41.4	D49.4
urethral	C67.5	C79.11	D09.0	D30.3	D41.4	D49.4
overlapping lesion	C67.8	—	—	—	—	—
sphincter	C67.8	C79.11	D09.0	D30.3	D41.4	D49.4
trigone	C67.0	C79.11	D09.0	D30.3	D41.4	D49.4
urachus	C67.7	C79.11	D09.0	D30.3	D41.4	D49.4
wall	C67.9	C79.11	D09.0	D30.3	D41.4	D49.4
anterior	C67.3	C79.11	D09.0	D30.3	D41.4	D49.4
lateral	C67.2	C79.11	D09.0	D30.3	D41.4	D49.4
posterior	C67.4	C79.11	D09.0	D30.3	D41.4	D49.4
blood vessel — *see* Neoplasm, connective tissue						
bone (periosteum)	C41.9	C79.51	—	D16.9	D48.0	D49.2
acetabulum	C41.4	C79.51	—	D16.8	D48.0	D49.2
ankle	C40.3-✓	C79.51	—	D16.3-✓	—	—
arm NEC	C40.0-✓	C79.51	—	D16.0-✓	—	—
astragalus	C40.3-✓	C79.51	—	D16.3-✓	—	—
atlas	C41.2	C79.51	—	D16.6	D48.0	D49.2
axis	C41.2	C79.51	—	D16.6	D48.0	D49.2
back NEC	C41.2	C79.51	—	D16.6	D48.0	D49.2
calcaneus	C40.3-✓	C79.51	—	D16.3-✓	—	—
calvarium	C41.0	C79.51	—	D16.4	D48.0	D49.2
carpus (any)	C40.1-✓	C79.51	—	D16.1-✓	—	—
cartilage NEC	C41.9	C79.51	—	D16.9	D48.0	D49.2
clavicle	C41.3	C79.51	—	D16.7	D48.0	D49.2
clivus	C41.0	C79.51	—	D16.4	D48.0	D49.2
coccygeal vertebra	C41.4	C79.51	—	D16.8	D48.0	D49.2
coccyx	C41.4	C79.51	—	D16.8	D48.0	D49.2
costal cartilage	C41.3	C79.51	—	D16.7	D48.0	D49.2
costovertebral joint	C41.3	C79.51	—	D16.7	D48.0	D49.2
cranial	C41.0	C79.51	—	D16.4	D48.0	D49.2
cuboid	C40.3-✓	C79.51	—	D16.3-✓	—	—
cuneiform	C41.9	C79.51	—	D16.9	D48.0	D49.2
elbow	C40.0-✓	C79.51	—	D16.0-✓	—	—
ethmoid (labyrinth)	C41.0	C79.51	—	D16.4	D48.0	D49.2
face	C41.0	C79.51	—	D16.4	D48.0	D49.2
femur (any part)	C40.2-✓	C79.51	—	D16.2-✓	—	—
fibula (any part)	C40.2-✓	C79.51	—	D16.2-✓	—	—
finger (any)	C40.1-✓	C79.51	—	D16.1-✓	—	—
foot	C40.3-✓	C79.51	—	D16.3-✓	—	—
forearm	C40.0-✓	C79.51	—	D16.0-✓	—	—
frontal	C41.0	C79.51	—	D16.4	D48.0	D49.2
hand	C40.1-✓	C79.51	—	D16.1-✓	—	—
heel	C40.3-✓	C79.51	—	D16.3-✓	—	—
hip	C41.4	C79.51	—	D16.8	D48.0	D49.2
humerus (any part)	C40.0-✓	C79.51	—	D16.0-✓	—	—
hyoid	C41.0	C79.51	—	D16.4	D48.0	D49.2
ilium	C41.4	C79.51	—	D16.8	D48.0	D49.2
innominate	C41.4	C79.51	—	D16.8	D48.0	D49.2
intervertebral cartilage or disc	C41.2	C79.51	—	D16.6	D48.0	D49.2
ischium	C41.4	C79.51	—	D16.8	D48.0	D49.2
jaw (lower)	C41.1	C79.51	—	D16.5	D48.0	D49.2
knee	C40.2-✓	C79.51	—	D16.2-✓	—	—
leg NEC	C40.2-✓	C79.51	—	D16.2-✓	—	—
limb NEC	C40.9-✓	C79.51	—	D16.9	—	—
lower (long bones)	C40.2-✓	C79.51	—	D16.2-✓	—	—
short bones	C40.3-✓	C79.51	—	D16.3-✓	—	—
upper (long bones)	C40.0-✓	C79.51	—	D16.0-✓	—	—
short bones	C40.1-✓	C79.51	—	D16.1-✓	—	—
malar	C41.0	C79.51	—	D16.4	D48.0	D49.2

Neoplasm, neoplastic — *continued*	Malignant Primary	Malignant Secondary	Ca in situ	Benign	Uncertain	Unspecified Behavior
bone — continued						
mandible	C41.1	C79.51	—	D16.5	D48.0	D49.2
marrow NEC (any bone)	C96.9	C79.52	—	—	D47.9	D49.89
mastoid	C41.0	C79.51	—	D16.4	D48.0	D49.2
maxilla, maxillary (superior)	C41.0	C79.51	—	D16.4	D48.0	D49.2
inferior	C41.1	C79.51	—	D16.5	D48.0	D49.2
metacarpus (any)	C40.1-✓	C79.51	—	D16.1-✓	—	—
metatarsus (any)	C40.3-✓	C79.51	—	D16.3-✓	—	—
navicular						
ankle	C40.3-✓	C79.51	—	—	—	—
hand	C40.1-✓	C79.51	—	—	—	—
nose, nasal	C41.0	C79.51	—	D16.4	D48.0	D49.2
occipital	C41.0	C79.51	—	D16.4	D48.0	D49.2
orbit	C41.0	C79.51	—	D16.4	D48.0	D49.2
overlapping sites	C40.8-✓	—	—	—	—	—
parietal	C41.0	C79.51	—	D16.4	D48.0	D49.2
patella	C40.2-✓	C79.51	—	—	—	—
pelvic	C41.4	C79.51	—	D16.8	D48.0	D49.2
phalanges						
foot	C40.3-✓	C79.51	—	—	—	—
hand	C40.1-✓	C79.51	—	—	—	—
pubic	C41.4	C79.51	—	D16.8	D48.0	D49.2
radius (any part)	C40.0-✓	C79.51	—	D16.0-✓	—	—
rib	C41.3	C79.51	—	D16.7	D48.0	D49.2
sacral vertebra	C41.4	C79.51	—	D16.8	D48.0	D49.2
sacrum	C41.4	C79.51	—	D16.8	D48.0	D49.2
scaphoid						
of ankle	C40.3-✓	C79.51	—	—	—	—
of hand	C40.1-✓	C79.51	—	—	—	—
scapula (any part)	C40.0-✓	C79.51	—	D16.0-✓	—	—
sella turcica	C41.0	C79.51	—	D16.4	D48.0	D49.2
shoulder	C40.0-✓	C79.51	—	D16.0-✓	—	—
skull	C41.0	C79.51	—	D16.4	D48.0	D49.2
sphenoid	C41.0	C79.51	—	D16.4	D48.0	D49.2
spine, spinal (column)	C41.2	C79.51	—	D16.6	D48.0	D49.2
coccyx	C41.4	C79.51	—	D16.8	D48.0	D49.2
sacrum	C41.4	C79.51	—	D16.8	D48.0	D49.2
sternum	C41.3	C79.51	—	D16.7	D48.0	D49.2
tarsus (any)	C40.3-✓	C79.51	—	—	—	—
temporal	C41.0	C79.51	—	D16.4	D48.0	D49.2
thumb	C40.1-✓	C79.51	—	—	—	—
tibia (any part)	C40.2-✓	C79.51	—	—	—	—
toe (any)	C40.3-✓	C79.51	—	—	—	—
trapezium	C40.1-✓	C79.51	—	—	—	—
trapezoid	C40.1-✓	C79.51	—	—	—	—
turbinate	C41.0	C79.51	—	D16.4	D48.0	D49.2
ulna (any part)	C40.0-✓	C79.51	—	D16.0-✓	—	—
unciform	C40.1-✓	C79.51	—	—	—	—
vertebra (column)	C41.2	C79.51	—	D16.6	D48.0	D49.2
coccyx	C41.4	C79.51	—	D16.8	D48.0	D49.2
sacrum	C41.4	C79.51	—	D16.8	D48.0	D49.2
vomer	C41.0	C79.51	—	D16.4	D48.0	D49.2
wrist	C40.1-✓	C79.51	—	—	—	—
xiphoid process	C41.3	C79.51	—	D16.7	D48.0	D49.2
zygomatic	C41.0	C79.51	—	D16.4	D48.0	D49.2
book-leaf (mouth) — *ventral surface of tongue and floor of mouth*	C06.89	C79.89	D00.00	D10.39	D37.09	D49.0
bowel — *see* Neoplasm, intestine						
brachial plexus	C47.1-✓	C79.89	—	D36.12	D48.2	D49.2
brain NEC	C71.9	C79.31	—	D33.2	D43.2	D49.6
basal ganglia	C71.0	C79.31	—	D33.0	D43.0	D49.6
cerebellopontine angle	C71.6	C79.31	—	D33.1	D43.1	D49.6
cerebellum NOS	C71.6	C79.31	—	D33.1	D43.1	D49.6
cerebrum	C71.0	C79.31	—	D33.0	D43.0	D49.6
choroid plexus	C71.7	C79.31	—	D33.1	D43.1	D49.6
corpus callosum	C71.8	C79.31	—	D33.2	D43.2	D49.6
corpus striatum	C71.0	C79.31	—	D33.0	D43.0	D49.6
cortex (cerebral)	C71.0	C79.31	—	D33.0	D43.0	D49.6
frontal lobe	C71.1	C79.31	—	D33.0	D43.0	D49.6
globus pallidus	C71.0	C79.31	—	D33.0	D43.0	D49.6
hippocampus	C71.2	C79.31	—	D33.0	D43.0	D49.6
hypothalamus	C71.0	C79.31	—	D33.0	D43.0	D49.6
internal capsule	C71.0	C79.31	—	D33.0	D43.0	D49.6

✓ **Additional Character Required** — Refer to the Tabular List for Character Selection   ▽ **Subterms under main terms may continue to next column or page**

Neoplasm, neoplastic — continued

	Malignant Primary	Malignant Secondary	Ca in situ	Benign	Uncertain	Unspecified Behavior
brain — continued						
medulla oblongata	C71.7	C79.31	—	D33.1	D43.1	D49.6
meninges	C70.0	C79.32	—	D32.0	D42.0	D49.7
midbrain	C71.7	C79.31	—	D33.1	D43.1	D49.6
occipital lobe	C71.4	C79.31	—	D33.0	D43.0	D49.6
overlapping lesion	C71.8	C79.31	—	—	—	—
parietal lobe	C71.3	C79.31	—	D33.0	D43.0	D49.6
peduncle	C71.7	C79.31	—	D33.1	D43.1	D49.6
pons	C71.7	C79.31	—	D33.1	D43.1	D49.6
stem	C71.7	C79.31	—	D33.1	D43.1	D49.6
tapetum	C71.8	C79.31	—	D33.2	D43.2	D49.6
temporal lobe	C71.2	C79.31	—	D33.0	D43.0	D49.6
thalamus	C71.0	C79.31	—	D33.0	D43.0	D49.6
uncus	C71.2	C79.31	—	D33.0	D43.0	D49.6
ventricle (floor)	C71.5	C79.31	—	D33.0	D43.0	D49.6
fourth	C71.7	C79.31	—	D33.1	D43.1	D49.6
branchial (cleft) (cyst) (vestiges)	C10.4	C79.89	D00.08	D10.5	D37.05	D49.0
breast (connective tissue) (glandular tissue) (soft parts)	C50.9-☑	C79.81	D05.-☑	D24.-☑	D48.6-☑	D49.3
areola	C50.0-☑	C79.81	D05.-☑	D24.-☑	D48.6-☑	D49.3
axillary tail	C50.6-☑	C79.81	D05.-☑	D24.-☑	D48.6-☑	D49.3
central portion	C50.1-☑	C79.81	D05.-☑	D24.-☑	D48.6-☑	D49.3
inner	C50.8-☑	C79.81	D05.-☑	D24.-☑	D48.6-☑	D49.3
lower	C50.8-☑	C79.81	D05.-☑	D24.-☑	D48.6-☑	D49.3
lower-inner quadrant	C50.3-☑	C79.81	D05.-☑	D24.-☑	D48.6-☑	D49.3
lower-outer quadrant	C50.5-☑	C79.81	D05.-☑	D24.-☑	D48.6-☑	D49.3
mastectomy site (skin) — see also Neoplasm, breast, skin	C44.501	C79.2	—	—	—	—
specified as breast tissue	C50.8-☑	C79.81	—	—	—	—
midline	C50.8-☑	C79.81	D05.-☑	D24.-☑	D48.6-☑	D49.3
nipple	C50.0-☑	C79.81	D05.-☑	D24.-☑	D48.6-☑	D49.3
outer	C50.8-☑	C79.81	D05.-☑	D24.-☑	D48.6-☑	D49.3
overlapping lesion	C50.8-☑	—	—	—	—	—
skin	C44.501	C79.2	D04.5	D23.5	D48.5	D49.2
basal cell carcinoma	C44.511	—	—	—	—	—
specified type NEC	C44.591	—	—	—	—	—
squamous cell carcinoma	C44.521	—	—	—	—	—
tail (axillary)	C50.6-☑	C79.81	D05.-☑	D24.-☑	D48.6-☑	D49.3
upper	C50.8-☑	C79.81	D05.-☑	D24.-☑	D48.6-☑	D49.3
upper-inner quadrant	C50.2-☑	C79.81	D05.-☑	D24.-☑	D48.6-☑	D49.3
upper-outer quadrant	C50.4-☑	C79.81	D05.-☑	D24.-☑	D48.6-☑	D49.3
broad ligament	C57.1-☑	C79.82	D07.39	D28.2	D39.8	D49.59
bronchiogenic, bronchogenic (lung)	C34.9-☑	C78.0-☑	D02.2-☑	D14.3-☑	D38.1	D49.1
bronchiole	C34.9-☑	C78.0-☑	D02.2-☑	D14.3-☑	D38.1	D49.1
bronchus	C34.9-☑	C78.0-☑	D02.2-☑	D14.3-☑	D38.1	D49.1
carina	C34.0-☑	C78.0-☑	D02.2-☑	D14.3-☑	D38.1	D49.1
lower lobe of lung	C34.3-☑	C78.0-☑	D02.2-☑	D14.3-☑	D38.1	D49.1
main	C34.0-☑	C78.0-☑	D02.2-☑	D14.3-☑	D38.1	D49.1
middle lobe of lung	C34.2	C78.0-☑	D02.21	D14.31	D38.1	D49.1
overlapping lesion	C34.8-☑	—	—	—	—	—
upper lobe of lung	C34.1-☑	C78.0-☑	D02.2-☑	D14.3-☑	D38.1	D49.1
brow	C44.309	C79.2	D04.39	D23.39	D48.5	D49.2
basal cell carcinoma	C44.319	—	—	—	—	—
specified type NEC	C44.399	—	—	—	—	—
squamous cell carcinoma	C44.329	—	—	—	—	—
buccal (cavity)	C06.9	C79.89	D00.00	D10.39	D37.09	D49.0
commissure	C06.0	C79.89	D00.02	D10.39	D37.09	D49.0
groove (lower) (upper)	C06.1	C79.89	D00.02	D10.39	D37.09	D49.0
mucosa	C06.0	C79.89	D00.02	D10.39	D37.09	D49.0
sulcus (lower) (upper)	C06.1	C79.89	D00.02	D10.39	D37.09	D49.0

Neoplasm, neoplastic — continued

	Malignant Primary	Malignant Secondary	Ca in situ	Benign	Uncertain	Unspecified Behavior
bulbourethral gland	C68.0	C79.19	D09.19	D30.4	D41.3	D49.59
bursa — see Neoplasm, connective tissue						
buttock NEC	C76.3	C79.89	D04.5	D36.7	D48.7	D49.89
calf	C76.5-☑	C79.89	D04.7-☑	D36.7	D48.7	D49.89
calvarium	C41.0	C79.51	—	D16.4	D48.0	D49.2
calyx, renal	C65.-☑	C79.0-☑	D09.19	D30.1-☑	D41.1-☑	D49.51-☑
canal						
anal	C21.1	C78.5	D01.3	D12.9	D37.8	D49.0
auditory (external) — see also Neoplasm, skin, ear	C44.20-☑	C79.2	D04.2-☑	D23.2-☑	D48.5	D49.2
auricular (external) — see also Neoplasm, skin, ear	C44.20-☑	C79.2	D04.2-☑	D23.2-☑	D48.5	D49.2
canaliculi, biliary (biliferi) (intrahepatic)	C22.1	C78.7	D01.5	D13.4	D37.6	D49.0
canthus (eye) (inner) (outer)	C44.10-☑	C79.2	D04.1-☑	D23.1-☑	D48.5	D49.2
basal cell carcinoma	C44.11-☑	—	—	—	—	—
specified type NEC	C44.19-☑	—	—	—	—	—
squamous cell carcinoma	C44.12-☑	—	—	—	—	—
capillary — see Neoplasm, connective tissue						
caput coli	C18.0	C78.5	D01.0	D12.0	D37.4	D49.0
carcinoid — see Tumor, carcinoid						
cardia (gastric)	C16.0	C78.89	D00.2	D13.1	D37.1	D49.0
cardiac orifice (stomach)	C16.0	C78.89	D00.2	D13.1	D37.1	D49.0
cardio-esophageal junction	C16.0	C78.89	D00.2	D13.1	D37.1	D49.0
cardio-esophagus	C16.0	C78.89	D00.2	D13.1	D37.1	D49.0
carina (bronchus)	C34.0-☑	C78.0-☑	D02.2-☑	D14.3-☑	D38.1	D49.1
carotid (artery)	C49.0	C79.89	—	D21.0	D48.2	D49.2
body	C75.4	C79.89	—	D35.5	D44.6	D49.7
carpus (any bone)	C40.1-☑	C79.51	—	D16.1-☑	—	—
cartilage (articular) (joint) NEC — see also Neoplasm, bone	C41.9	C79.51	—	D16.9	D48.0	D49.2
arytenoid	C32.3	C78.39	D02.0	D14.1	D38.0	D49.1
auricular	C49.0	C79.89	—	D21.0	D48.1	D49.2
bronchi	C34.0-☑	C78.39	—	D14.3-☑	D38.1	D49.1
costal	C41.3	C79.51	—	D16.7	D48.0	D49.2
cricoid	C32.3	C78.39	D02.0	D14.1	D38.0	D49.1
cuneiform	C32.3	C78.39	D02.0	D14.1	D38.0	D49.1
ear (external)	C49.0	C79.89	—	D21.0	D48.1	D49.2
ensiform	C41.3	C79.51	—	D16.7	D48.0	D49.2
epiglottis	C32.1	C78.39	D02.0	D14.1	D38.0	D49.1
anterior surface	C10.1	C79.89	D00.08	D10.5	D37.05	D49.0
eyelid	C49.0	C79.89	—	D21.0	D48.1	D49.2
intervertebral	C41.2	C79.51	—	D16.6	D48.0	D49.2
larynx, laryngeal	C32.3	C78.39	D02.0	D14.1	D38.0	D49.1
nose, nasal	C30.0	C78.39	D02.3	D14.0	D38.5	D49.1
pinna	C49.0	C79.89	—	D21.0	D48.1	D49.2
rib	C41.3	C79.51	—	D16.7	D48.0	D49.2
semilunar (knee)	C40.2-☑	C79.51	—	D16.2-☑	D48.0	D49.2
thyroid	C32.3	C78.39	D02.0	D14.1	D38.0	D49.1
trachea	C33	C78.39	D02.1	D14.2	D38.1	D49.1
cauda equina	C72.1	C79.49	—	D33.4	D43.4	D49.7
cavity						
buccal	C06.9	C79.89	D00.00	D10.30	D37.09	D49.0
nasal	C30.0	C78.39	D02.3	D14.0	D38.5	D49.1
oral	C06.9	C79.89	D00.00	D10.30	D37.09	D49.0
peritoneal	C48.2	C78.6	—	D20.1	D48.4	D49.0
tympanic	C30.1	C78.39	D02.3	D14.0	D38.5	D49.1
cecum	C18.0	C78.5	D01.0	D12.0	D37.4	D49.0
central nervous system	C72.9	C79.40	—	—	—	—
cerebellopontine (angle)	C71.6	C79.31	—	D33.1	D43.1	D49.6
cerebellum, cerebellar	C71.6	C79.31	—	D33.1	D43.1	D49.6
cerebrum, cerebral (cortex) (hemisphere) (white matter)	C71.0	C79.31	—	D33.0	D43.0	D49.6
meninges	C70.0	C79.32	—	D32.0	D42.0	D49.7
peduncle	C71.7	C79.31	—	D33.1	D43.1	D49.6

Neoplasm Table

Neoplasm, cerebrum, cerebral — Neoplasm, connective tissue NEC

	Malignant Primary	Malignant Secondary	Ca in situ	Benign	Uncertain	Unspecified Behavior
Neoplasm, neoplastic — *continued*						
cerebrum, cerebral — *continued*						
ventricle	C71.5	C79.31	—	D33.0	D43.0	D49.6
fourth	C71.7	C79.31	—	D33.1	D43.1	D49.6
cervical region	C76.0	C79.89	D09.8	D36.7	D48.7	D49.89
cervix (cervical) (uteri)						
(uterus)	C53.9	C79.82	D06.9	D26.0	D39.0	D49.59
canal	C53.0	C79.82	D06.0	D26.0	D39.0	D49.59
endocervix (canal)						
(gland)	C53.0	C79.82	D06.0	D26.0	D39.0	D49.59
exocervix	C53.1	C79.82	D06.1	D26.0	D39.0	D49.59
external os	C53.1	C79.82	D06.1	D26.0	D39.0	D49.59
internal os	C53.0	C79.82	D06.0	D26.0	D39.0	D49.59
nabothian gland	C53.0	C79.82	D06.0	D26.0	D39.0	D49.59
overlapping lesion	C53.8	—	—	—	—	—
squamocolumnar junction	C53.8	C79.82	D06.7	D26.0	D39.0	D49.59
stump	C53.8	C79.82	D06.7	D26.0	D39.0	D49.59
cheek	C76.0	C79.89	D09.8	D36.7	D48.7	D49.89
external	C44.309	C79.2	D04.39	D23.39	D48.5	D49.2
basal cell carcinoma	C44.319	—	—	—	—	—
specified type NEC	C44.399	—	—	—	—	—
squamous cell carcinoma	C44.329	—	—	—	—	—
inner aspect	C06.0	C79.89	D00.02	D10.39	D37.09	D49.0
internal	C06.0	C79.89	D00.02	D10.39	D37.09	D49.0
mucosa	C06.0	C79.89	D00.02	D10.39	D37.09	D49.0
chest (wall) NEC	C76.1	C79.89	D09.8	D36.7	D48.7	D49.89
chiasma opticum	C72.3-☑	C79.49	—	D33.3	D43.3	D49.7
chin	C44.309	C79.2	D04.39	D23.39	D48.5	D49.2
basal cell carcinoma	C44.319	—	—	—	—	—
specified type NEC	C44.399	—	—	—	—	—
squamous cell carcinoma	C44.329	—	—	—	—	—
choana	C11.3	C79.89	D00.08	D10.6	D37.05	D49.0
cholangiole	C22.1	C78.89	D01.5	D13.4	D37.6	D49.0
choledochal duct	C24.0	C78.89	D01.5	D13.5	D37.6	D49.0
choroid	C69.3-☑	C79.49	D09.2-☑	D31.3-☑	D48.7	D49.81
plexus	C71.5	C79.31	—	D33.0	D43.0	D49.6
ciliary body	C69.4-☑	C79.49	D09.2-☑	D31.4-☑	D48.7	D49.89
clavicle	C41.3	C79.51	—	D16.7	D48.0	D49.2
clitoris	C51.2	C79.82	D07.1	D28.0	D39.8	D49.59
clivus	C41.0	C79.51	—	D16.4	D48.0	D49.2
cloacogenic zone	C21.2	C78.5	D01.3	D12.9	D37.8	D49.0
coccygeal						
body or glomus	C49.5	C79.89	—	D21.5	D48.1	D49.2
vertebra	C41.4	C79.51	—	D16.8	D48.0	D49.2
coccyx	C41.4	C79.51	—	D16.8	D48.0	D49.2
colon — *see also* Neoplasm, intestine, large	C18.9	C78.5	—	—	—	—
with rectum	C19	C78.5	D01.1	D12.7	D37.5	D49.0
columnella — *see also* Neoplasm, skin, face	C44.390	C79.2	D04.39	D23.39	D48.5	D49.2
column, spinal — *see* Neoplasm, spine						
commissure						
labial, lip	C00.6	C79.89	D00.01	D10.39	D37.01	D49.0
laryngeal	C32.0	C78.39	D02.0	D14.1	D38.0	D49.1
common (bile) duct	C24.0	C78.89	D01.5	D13.5	D37.6	D49.0
concha — *see also* Neoplasm, skin,						
ear	C44.20-☑	C79.2	D04.2-☑	D23.2-☑	D48.5	D49.2
nose	C30.0	C78.39	D02.3	D14.0	D38.5	D49.1
conjunctiva	C69.0-☑	C79.49	D09.2-☑	D31.0-☑	D48.7	D49.89

	Malignant Primary	Malignant Secondary	Ca in situ	Benign	Uncertain	Unspecified Behavior
Neoplasm, neoplastic — *continued*						
connective tissue NEC	C49.9	C79.89	—	D21.9	D48.1	D49.2

Note: For neoplasms of connective tissue (blood vessel, bursa, fascia, ligament, muscle, peripheral nerves, sympathetic and parasympathetic nerves and ganglia, synovia, tendon, etc.) or of morphological types that indicate connective tissue, code according to the list under "Neoplasm, connective tissue". For sites that do not appear in this list, code to neoplasm of that site; e.g., fibrosarcoma, pancreas (C25.9)

Note: Morphological types that indicate connective tissue appear in their proper place in the alphabetic index with the instruction "see Neoplasm, connective tissue ...."

	Malignant Primary	Malignant Secondary	Ca in situ	Benign	Uncertain	Unspecified Behavior
abdomen	C49.4	C79.89	—	D21.4	D48.1	D49.2
abdominal wall	C49.4	C79.89	—	D21.4	D48.1	D49.2
ankle	C49.2-☑	C79.89	—	D21.2-☑	D48.1	D49.2
antecubital fossa or space	C49.1-☑	C79.89	—	D21.1-☑	D48.1	D49.2
arm	C49.1-☑	C79.89	—	D21.1-☑	D48.1	D49.2
auricle (ear)	C49.0	C79.89	—	D21.0	D48.1	D49.2
axilla	C49.3	C79.89	—	D21.3	D48.1	D49.2
back	C49.6	C79.89	—	D21.6	D48.1	D49.2
breast — *see* Neoplasm, breast						
buttock	C49.5	C79.89	—	D21.5	D48.1	D49.2
calf	C49.2-☑	C79.89	—	D21.2-☑	D48.1	D49.2
cervical region	C49.0	C79.89	—	D21.0	D48.1	D49.2
cheek	C49.0	C79.89	—	D21.0	D48.1	D49.2
chest (wall)	C49.3	C79.89	—	D21.3	D48.1	D49.2
chin	C49.0	C79.89	—	D21.0	D48.1	D49.2
diaphragm	C49.3	C79.89	—	D21.3	D48.1	D49.2
ear (external)	C49.0	C79.89	—	D21.0	D48.1	D49.2
elbow	C49.1-☑	C79.89	—	D21.1-☑	D48.1	D49.2
extrarectal	C49.5	C79.89	—	D21.5	D48.1	D49.2
extremity	C49.9	C79.89	—	D21.9	D48.1	D49.2
lower	C49.2-☑	C79.89	—	D21.2-☑	D48.1	D49.2
upper	C49.1-☑	C79.89	—	D21.1-☑	D48.1	D49.2
eyelid	C49.0	C79.89	—	D21.0	D48.1	D49.2
face	C49.0	C79.89	—	D21.0	D48.1	D49.2
finger	C49.1-☑	C79.89	—	D21.1-☑	D48.1	D49.2
flank	C49.6	C79.89	—	D21.6	D48.1	D49.2
foot	C49.2-☑	C79.89	—	D21.2-☑	D48.1	D49.2
forearm	C49.1-☑	C79.89	—	D21.1-☑	D48.1	D49.2
forehead	C49.0	C79.89	—	D21.0	D48.1	D49.2
gastric	C49.4	C79.89	—	D21.4	D48.1	D49.2
gastrointestinal	C49.4	C79.89	—	D21.4	D48.1	D49.2
gluteal region	C49.5	C79.89	—	D21.5	D48.1	D49.2
great vessels NEC	C49.3	C79.89	—	D21.3	D48.1	D49.2
groin	C49.5	C79.89	—	D21.5	D48.1	D49.2
hand	C49.1-☑	C79.89	—	D21.1-☑	D48.1	D49.2
head	C49.0	C79.89	—	D21.0	D48.1	D49.2
heel	C49.2-☑	C79.89	—	D21.2-☑	D48.1	D49.2
hip	C49.2-☑	C79.89	—	D21.2-☑	D48.1	D49.2
hypochondrium	C49.4	C79.89	—	D21.4	D48.1	D49.2
iliopsoas muscle	C49.5	C79.89	—	D21.5	D48.1	D49.2
infraclavicular region	C49.3	C79.89	—	D21.3	D48.1	D49.2
inguinal (canal) (region)	C49.5	C79.89	—	D21.5	D48.1	D49.2
intestinal	C49.4	C79.89	—	D21.4	D48.1	D49.2
intrathoracic	C49.3	C79.89	—	D21.3	D48.1	D49.2
ischiorectal fossa	C49.5	C79.89	—	D21.5	D48.1	D49.2
jaw	C03.9	C79.89	D00.03	D10.39	D48.1	D49.0
knee	C49.2-☑	C79.89	—	D21.2-☑	D48.1	D49.2
leg	C49.2-☑	C79.89	—	D21.2-☑	D48.1	D49.2
limb NEC	C49.9	C79.89	—	D21.9	D48.1	D49.2
lower	C49.2-☑	C79.89	—	D21.2-☑	D48.1	D49.2
upper	C49.1-☑	C79.89	—	D21.1-☑	D48.1	D49.2
nates	C49.5	C79.89	—	D21.5	D48.1	D49.2
neck	C49.0	C79.89	—	D21.0	D48.1	D49.2
orbit	C69.6-☑	C79.49	D09.2-☑	D31.6-☑	D48.1	D49.89
overlapping lesion	C49.8	—	—	—	—	—
pararectal	C49.5	C79.89	—	D21.5	D48.1	D49.2
para-urethral	C49.5	C79.89	—	D21.5	D48.1	D49.2
paravaginal	C49.5	C79.89	—	D21.5	D48.1	D49.2
pelvis (floor)	C49.5	C79.89	—	D21.5	D48.1	D49.2
pelvo-abdominal	C49.8	C79.89	—	D21.6	D48.1	D49.2
perineum	C49.5	C79.89	—	D21.5	D48.1	D49.2
perirectal (tissue)	C49.5	C79.89	—	D21.5	D48.1	D49.2

	Malignant Primary	Malignant Secondary	Ca in situ	Benign	Uncertain	Unspecified Behavior
Neoplasm, neoplastic — *continued*						
connective tissue — *continued*						
periurethral (tissue)	C49.5	C79.89	—	D21.5	D48.1	D49.2
popliteal fossa or space	C49.2-☑	C79.89	—	D21.2-☑	D48.1	D49.2
presacral	C49.5	C79.89	—	D21.5	D48.1	D49.2
psoas muscle	C49.4	C79.89	—	D21.4	D48.1	D49.2
pterygoid fossa	C49.0	C79.89	—	D21.0	D48.1	D49.2
rectovaginal septum or wall	C49.5	C79.89	—	D21.5	D48.1	D49.2
rectovesical	C49.5	C79.89	—	D21.5	D48.1	D49.2
retroperitoneum	C48.0	C78.6	—	D20.0	D48.3	D49.0
sacrococcygeal region	C49.5	C79.89	—	D21.5	D48.1	D49.2
scalp	C49.0	C79.89	—	D21.0	D48.1	D49.2
scapular region	C49.3	C79.89	—	D21.3	D48.1	D49.2
shoulder	C49.1-☑	C79.89	—	D21.1-☑	D48.1	D49.2
skin (dermis) NEC — *see also* Neoplasm, skin, by site	C44.90	C79.2	D04.9	D23.9	D48.5	D49.5
stomach	C49.4	C79.89	—	D21.4	D48.1	D49.2
submental	C49.0	C79.89	—	D21.0	D48.1	D49.2
supraclavicular region	C49.0	C79.89	—	D21.0	D48.1	D49.2
temple	C49.0	C79.89	—	D21.0	D48.1	D49.2
temporal region	C49.0	C79.89	—	D21.0	D48.1	D49.2
thigh	C49.2-☑	C79.89	—	D21.2-☑	D48.1	D49.2
thoracic (duct) (wall)	C49.3	C79.89	—	D21.3	D48.1	D49.2
thorax	C49.3	C79.89	—	D21.3	D48.1	D49.2
thumb	C49.1-☑	C79.89	—	D21.1-☑	D48.1	D49.2
toe	C49.2-☑	C79.89	—	D21.2-☑	D48.1	D49.2
trunk	C49.6	C79.89	—	D21.6	D48.1	D49.2
umbilicus	C49.4	C79.89	—	D21.4	D48.1	D49.2
vesicorectal	C49.5	C79.89	—	D21.5	D48.1	D49.2
wrist	C49.1-☑	C79.89	—	D21.1-☑	D48.1	D49.2
conus medullaris	C72.0	C79.49	—	D33.4	D43.4	D49.7
cord (true) (vocal)	C32.0	C78.39	D02.0	D14.1	D38.0	D49.1
false	C32.1	C78.39	D02.0	D14.1	D38.0	D49.1
spermatic	C63.1-☑	C79.82	D07.69	D29.8	D40.8	D49.59
spinal (cervical) (lumbar) (thoracic)	C72.0	C79.49	—	D33.4	D43.4	D49.7
cornea (limbus)	C69.1-☑	C79.49	D09.2-☑	D31.1-☑	D48.7	D49.89
corpus						
albicans	C56.-☑	C79.6-☑	D07.39	D27.-☑	D39.1-☑	D49.59
callosum, brain	C71.0	C79.31	—	D33.2	D43.2	D49.6
cavernosum	C60.2	C79.82	D07.4	D29.0	D40.8	D49.59
gastric	C16.2	C78.89	D00.2	D13.1	D37.1	D49.0
overlapping sites	C54.8	—	—	—	—	—
penis	C60.2	C79.82	D07.4	D29.0	D40.8	D49.59
striatum, cerebrum	C71.0	C79.31	—	D33.0	D43.0	D49.6
uteri	C54.9	C79.82	D07.0	D26.1	D39.0	D49.59
isthmus	C54.0	C79.82	D07.0	D26.1	D39.0	D49.59
cortex						
adrenal	C74.0-☑	C79.7-☑	D09.3	D35.0-☑	D44.1-☑	D49.7
cerebral	C71.0	C79.31	—	D33.0	D43.0	D49.6
costal cartilage	C41.3	C79.51	—	D16.7	D48.0	D49.2
costovertebral joint	C41.3	C79.51	—	D16.7	D48.0	D49.2
Cowper's gland	C68.0	C79.19	D09.19	D30.4	D41.3	D49.59
cranial (fossa, any)	C71.9	C79.31	—	D33.2	D43.2	D49.6
meninges	C70.0	C79.32	—	D32.0	D42.0	D49.7
nerve	C72.50	C79.49	—	D33.3	D43.3	D49.7
specified NEC	C72.59	C79.49	—	D33.3	D43.3	D49.7
craniobuccal pouch	C75.2	C79.89	D09.3	D35.2	D44.3	D49.7
craniopharyngeal (duct) (pouch)	C75.2	C79.89	D09.3	D35.3	D44.4	D49.7
cricoid	C13.0	C79.89	D00.08	D10.7	D37.05	D49.0
cartilage	C32.3	C78.39	D02.0	D14.1	D38.0	D49.1
cricopharynx	C13.0	C79.89	D00.08	D10.7	D37.05	D49.0
crypt of Morgagni	C21.8	C78.5	D01.3	D12.9	D37.8	D49.0
crystalline lens	C69.4-☑	C79.49	D09.2-☑	D31.4-☑	D48.7	D49.89
cul-de-sac (Douglas')	C48.1	C78.6	—	D20.1	D48.4	D49.0
cuneiform cartilage	C32.3	C78.39	D02.0	D14.1	D38.0	D49.1
cutaneous — *see* Neoplasm, skin						
cutis — *see* Neoplasm, skin						

	Malignant Primary	Malignant Secondary	Ca in situ	Benign	Uncertain	Unspecified Behavior
Neoplasm, neoplastic — *continued*						
cystic (bile) duct (common)	C24.0	C78.89	D01.5	D13.5	D37.6	D49.0
dermis — *see* Neoplasm, skin						
diaphragm	C49.3	C79.89	—	D21.3	D48.1	D49.2
digestive organs, system, tube, or tract						
NEC	C26.9	C78.89	D01.9	D13.9	D37.9	D49.0
disc, intervertebral	C41.2	C79.51	—	D16.6	D48.0	D49.2
disease, generalized	C80.0	—	—	—	—	—
disseminated	C80.0	—	—	—	—	—
Douglas' cul-de-sac or pouch	C48.1	C78.6	—	D20.1	D48.4	D49.0
duodenojejunal junction	C17.8	C78.4	D01.49	D13.39	D37.2	D49.0
duodenum	C17.0	C78.4	D01.49	D13.2	D37.2	D49.0
dura (cranial) (mater)	C70.9	C79.49	—	D32.9	D42.9	D49.7
cerebral	C70.0	C79.32	—	D32.0	D42.0	D49.7
spinal	C70.1	C79.49	—	D32.1	D42.1	D49.7
ear (external) — *see also* Neoplasm, skin, ear	C44.20-☑	C79.2	D04.2-☑	D23.2-☑	D48.5	D49.2
auricle or auris — *see also* Neoplasm, skin, ear	C44.20-☑	C79.2	D04.2-☑	D23.2-☑	D48.5	D49.2
canal, external — *see also* Neoplasm, skin, ear	C44.20-☑	C79.2	D04.2-☑	D23.2-☑	D48.5	D49.2
cartilage	C49.0	C79.89	—	D21.0	D48.1	D49.2
external meatus — *see also* Neoplasm, skin, ear	C44.20-☑	C79.2	D04.2-☑	D23.2-☑	D48.5	D49.2
inner	C30.1	C78.39	D02.3	D14.0	D38.5	D49.1
lobule — *see also* Neoplasm, skin, ear	C44.20-☑	C79.2	D04.2-☑	D23.2-☑	D48.5	D49.2
middle	C30.1	C78.39	D02.3	D14.0	D38.5	D49.1
overlapping lesion with accessory sinuses	C31.8	—	—	—	—	—
skin	C44.20-☑	C79.2	D04.2-☑	D23.2-☑	D48.5	D49.2
basal cell carcinoma	C44.21-☑	—	—	—	—	—
specified type NEC	C44.29-☑	—	—	—	—	—
squamous cell carcinoma	C44.22-☑	—	—	—	—	—
earlobe	C44.20-☑	C79.2	D04.2-☑	D23.2-☑	D48.5	D49.2
basal cell carcinoma	C44.21-☑	—	—	—	—	—
specified type NEC	C44.29-☑	—	—	—	—	—
squamous cell carcinoma	C44.22-☑	—	—	—	—	—
ejaculatory duct	C63.7	C79.82	D07.69	D29.8	D40.8	D49.59
elbow NEC	C76.4-☑	C79.89	D04.6-☑	D36.7	D48.7	D49.89
endocardium	C38.0	C79.89	—	D15.1	D48.7	D49.89
endocervix (canal) (gland)	C53.0	C79.82	D06.0	D26.0	D39.0	D49.59
endocrine gland NEC	C75.9	C79.89	D09.3	D35.9	D44.9	D49.7
pluriglandular	C75.8	C79.89	D09.3	D35.7	D44.9	D49.7
endometrium (gland) (stroma)	C54.1	C79.82	D07.0	D26.1	D39.0	D49.59
ensiform cartilage	C41.3	C79.51	—	D16.7	D48.0	D49.2
enteric — *see* Neoplasm, intestine						
ependyma (brain)	C71.5	C79.31	—	D33.0	D43.0	D49.6
fourth ventricle	C71.7	C79.31	—	D33.1	D43.1	D49.6
epicardium	C38.0	C79.89	—	D15.1	D48.7	D49.89
epididymis	C63.0-☑	C79.82	D07.69	D29.3-☑	D40.8	D49.59
epidural	C72.9	C79.49	—	D33.9	D43.9	D49.7
epiglottis	C32.1	C78.39	D02.0	D14.1	D38.0	D49.1
anterior aspect or surface	C10.1	C79.89	D00.08	D10.5	D37.05	D49.0
cartilage	C32.3	C78.39	D02.0	D14.1	D38.0	D49.1
free border (margin)	C10.1	C79.89	D00.08	D10.5	D37.05	D49.0
junctional region	C10.8	C79.89	D00.08	D10.5	D37.05	D49.0
posterior (laryngeal) surface	C32.1	C78.39	D02.0	D14.1	D38.0	D49.1

Neoplasm Table

Neoplasm, neoplastic —	Malignant Primary	Malignant Secondary	Ca in situ	Benign	Uncertain	Unspecified Behavior
continued						
epiglottis — *continued*						
suprahyoid portion	C32.1	C78.39	D02.0	D14.1	D38.0	D49.1
esophagogastric junction	C16.0	C78.89	D00.2	D13.1	D37.1	D49.0
esophagus	C15.9	C78.89	D00.1	D13.0	D37.8	D49.0
abdominal	C15.5	C78.89	D00.1	D13.0	D37.8	D49.0
cervical	C15.3	C78.89	D00.1	D13.0	D37.8	D49.0
distal (third)	C15.5	C78.89	D00.1	D13.0	D37.8	D49.0
lower (third)	C15.5	C78.89	D00.1	D13.0	D37.8	D49.0
middle (third)	C15.4	C78.89	D00.1	D13.0	D37.8	D49.0
overlapping lesion	C15.8	—	—	—	—	—
proximal (third)	C15.3	C78.89	D00.1	D13.0	D37.8	D49.0
thoracic	C15.4	C78.89	D00.1	D13.0	D37.8	D49.0
upper (third)	C15.3	C78.89	D00.1	D13.0	D37.8	D49.0
ethmoid (sinus)	C31.1	C78.39	D02.3	D14.0	D38.5	D49.1
bone or labyrinth	C41.0	C79.51	—	D16.4	D48.0	D49.2
eustachian tube	C30.1	C78.39	D02.3	D14.0	D38.5	D49.1
exocervix	C53.1	C79.82	D06.1	D26.0	D39.0	D49.59
external						
meatus (ear) — *see also* Neoplasm, skin, ear	C44.20-☑	C79.2	D04.2-☑	D23.2-☑	D48.5	D49.2
os, cervix uteri	C53.1	C79.82	D06.1	D26.0	D39.0	D49.59
extradural	C72.9	C79.49	—	D33.9	D43.9	D49.7
extrahepatic (bile) duct	C24.0	C78.89	D01.5	D13.5	D37.6	D49.0
overlapping lesion with gallbladder	C24.8	—	—	—	—	—
extraocular muscle	C69.6-☑	C79.49	D09.2-☑	D31.6-☑	D48.7	D49.89
extrarectal	C76.3	C79.89	D09.8	D36.7	D48.7	D49.89
extremity	C76.8	C79.89	D04.8	D36.7	D48.7	D49.89
lower	C76.5-☑	C79.89	D04.7-☑	D36.7	D48.7	D49.89
upper	C76.4-☑	C79.89	D04.6-☑	D36.7	D48.7	D49.89
eyeball	C69.9-☑	C79.49	D09.2-☑	D31.9-☑	D48.7	D49.89
eyebrow	C44.309	C79.2	D04.39	D23.39	D48.5	D49.2
basal cell carcinoma	C44.319	—	—	—	—	—
specified type NEC	C44.399	—	—	—	—	—
squamous cell carcinoma	C44.329	—	—	—	—	—
eyelid (lower) (skin) (upper)	C44.10-☑	—	—	—	—	—
basal cell carcinoma	C44.11-☑	—	—	—	—	—
cartilage	C49.0	C79.89	—	D21.0	D48.1	D49.2
specified type NEC	C44.19-☑	—	—	—	—	—
squamous cell carcinoma	C44.12-☑	—	—	—	—	—
eye NEC	C69.9-☑	C79.49	D09.2-☑	D31.9-☑	D48.7	D49.89
overlapping sites	C69.8-☑	—	—	—	—	—
face NEC	C76.0	C79.89	D04.39	D36.7	D48.7	D49.89
fallopian tube (accessory)	C57.0-☑	C79.82	D07.39	D28.2	D39.8	D49.59
falx (cerebella) (cerebri)	C70.0	C79.32	—	D32.0	D42.0	D49.7
fascia — *see also* Neoplasm, connective tissue						
palmar	C49.1-☑	C79.89	—	D21.1-☑	D48.1	D49.2
plantar	C49.2-☑	C79.89	—	D21.2-☑	D48.1	D49.2
fatty tissue — *see* Neoplasm, connective tissue						
fauces, faucial NEC	C10.9	C79.89	D00.08	D10.5	D37.05	D49.0
pillars	C09.1	C79.89	D00.08	D10.5	D37.05	D49.0
tonsil	C09.9	C79.89	D00.08	D10.4	D37.05	D49.0
femur (any part)	C40.2-☑	—	—	D16.2-☑	—	—
fetal membrane	C58	C79.82	D07.0	D26.7	D39.2	D49.59
fibrous tissue — *see* Neoplasm, connective tissue						
fibula (any part)	C40.2-☑	C79.51	—	D16.2-☑	—	—
filum terminale	C72.0	C79.49	—	D33.4	D43.4	D49.7
finger NEC	C76.4-☑	C79.89	D04.6-☑	D36.7	D48.7	D49.89
flank NEC	C76.8	C79.89	D04.5	D36.7	D48.7	D49.89
follicle, nabothian	C53.0	C79.82	D06.0	D26.0	D39.0	D49.59
foot NEC	C76.5-☑	C79.89	D04.7-☑	D36.7	D48.7	D49.89
forearm NEC	C76.4-☑	C79.89	D04.6-☑	D36.7	D48.7	D49.89
forehead (skin)	C44.309	C79.2	D04.39	D23.39	D48.5	D49.2

Neoplasm, neoplastic —	Malignant Primary	Malignant Secondary	Ca in situ	Benign	Uncertain	Unspecified Behavior
continued						
forehead — *continued*						
basal cell carcinoma	C44.319	—	—	—	—	—
specified type NEC	C44.399	—	—	—	—	—
squamous cell carcinoma	C44.329	—	—	—	—	—
foreskin	C60.0	C79.82	D07.4	D29.0	D40.8	D49.59
fornix						
pharyngeal	C11.3	C79.89	D00.08	D10.6	D37.05	D49.0
vagina	C52	C79.82	D07.2	D28.1	D39.8	D49.59
fossa (of)						
anterior (cranial)	C71.9	C79.31	—	D33.2	D43.2	D49.6
cranial	C71.9	C79.31	—	D33.2	D43.2	D49.6
ischiorectal	C76.3	C79.89	D09.8	D36.7	D48.7	D49.89
middle (cranial)	C71.9	C79.31	—	D33.2	D43.2	D49.6
piriform	C12	C79.89	D00.08	D10.7	D37.05	D49.0
pituitary	C75.1	C79.89	D09.3	D35.2	D44.3	D49.7
posterior (cranial)	C71.9	C79.31	—	D33.2	D43.2	D49.6
pterygoid	C49.0	C79.89	—	D21.0	D48.1	D49.2
pyriform	C12	C79.89	D00.08	D10.7	D37.05	D49.0
Rosenmuller	C11.2	C79.89	D00.08	D10.6	D37.05	D49.0
tonsillar	C09.0	C79.89	D00.08	D10.5	D37.05	D49.0
fourchette	C51.9	C79.82	D07.1	D28.0	D39.8	D49.59
frenulum						
labii — *see* Neoplasm, lip, internal						
linguae	C02.2	C79.89	D00.07	D10.1	D37.02	D49.0
frontal						
bone	C41.0	C79.51	—	D16.4	D48.0	D49.2
lobe, brain	C71.1	C79.31	—	D33.0	D43.0	D49.6
pole	C71.1	C79.31	—	D33.0	D43.0	D49.6
sinus	C31.2	C78.39	D02.3	D14.0	D38.5	D49.1
fundus						
stomach	C16.1	C78.89	D00.2	D13.1	D37.1	D49.0
uterus	C54.3	C79.82	D07.0	D26.1	D39.0	D49.59
gallbladder	C23	C78.89	D01.5	D13.5	D37.6	D49.0
overlapping lesion with extrahepatic bile ducts	C24.8	—	—	—	—	—
gall duct						
(extrahepatic)	C24.0	C78.89	D01.5	D13.5	D37.6	D49.0
intrahepatic	C22.1	C78.7	D01.5	D13.4	D37.6	D49.0
ganglia — *see also* Neoplasm, nerve, peripheral	C47.9	C79.89	—	D36.10	D48.2	D49.2
basal	C71.0	C79.31	—	D33.0	D43.0	D49.6
cranial nerve	C72.50	C79.49	—	D33.3	D43.3	D49.7
Gartner's duct	C52	C79.82	D07.2	D28.1	D39.8	D49.59
gastric — *see* Neoplasm, stomach						
gastrocolic	C26.9	C78.89	D01.9	D13.9	D37.9	D49.0
gastroesophageal junction	C16.0	C78.89	D00.2	D13.1	D37.1	D49.0
gastrointestinal (tract) NEC	C26.9	C78.89	D01.9	D13.9	D37.9	D49.0
generalized	C80.0	—	—	—	—	—
genital organ or tract						
female NEC	C57.9	C79.82	D07.30	D28.9	D39.9	D49.59
overlapping lesion	C57.8	—	—	—	—	—
specified site NEC	C57.7	C79.82	D07.39	D28.7	D39.8	D49.59
male NEC	C63.9	C79.82	D07.60	D29.9	D40.9	D49.59
overlapping lesion	C63.8	—	—	—	—	—
specified site NEC	C63.7	C79.82	D07.69	D29.8	D40.8	D49.59
genitourinary tract						
female	C57.9	C79.82	D07.30	D28.9	D39.9	D49.59
male	C63.9	C79.82	D07.60	D29.9	D40.9	D49.59
gingiva (alveolar) (marginal)	C03.9	C79.89	D00.03	D10.39	D37.09	D49.0
lower	C03.1	C79.89	D00.03	D10.39	D37.09	D49.0
mandibular	C03.1	C79.89	D00.03	D10.39	D37.09	D49.0
maxillary	C03.0	C79.89	D00.03	D10.39	D37.09	D49.0
upper	C03.0	C79.89	D00.03	D10.39	D37.09	D49.0
gland, glandular (lymphatic) (system) — *see also* Neoplasm, lymph gland						
endocrine NEC	C75.9	C79.89	D09.3	D35.9	D44.9	D49.7

☑ Additional Character Required — Refer to the Tabular List for Character Selection   ▽ Subterms under main terms may continue to next column or page

Neoplasm, neoplastic — continued	Malignant Primary	Malignant Secondary	Ca in situ	Benign	Uncertain	Unspecified Behavior
gland, glandular — *see also* Neoplasm, lymph gland — *continued*						
salivary — *see* Neoplasm, salivary gland						
glans penis	C60.1	C79.82	D07.4	D29.0	D40.8	D49.59
globus pallidus	C71.0	C79.31	—	D33.0	D43.0	D49.6
glomus						
coccygeal	C49.5	C79.89	—	D21.5	D48.1	D49.2
jugularis	C75.5	C79.89	—	D35.6	D44.7	D49.7
glosso-epiglottic fold(s)	C10.1	C79.89	D00.08	D10.5	D37.05	D49.0
glossopalatine fold	C09.1	C79.89	D00.08	D10.5	D37.05	D49.0
glossopharyngeal sulcus	C09.0	C79.89	D00.08	D10.5	D37.05	D49.0
glottis	C32.0	C78.39	D02.0	D14.1	D38.0	D49.1
gluteal region	C76.3	C79.89	D04.5	D36.7	D48.7	D49.89
great vessels NEC	C49.3	C79.89	—	D21.3	D48.1	D49.2
groin NEC	C76.3	C79.89	D04.5	D36.7	D48.7	D49.89
gum	C03.9	C79.89	D00.03	D10.39	D37.09	D49.0
lower	C03.1	C79.89	D00.03	D10.39	D37.09	D49.0
upper	C03.0	C79.89	D00.03	D10.39	D37.09	D49.0
hand NEC	C76.4-☑	C79.89	D04.6-☑	D36.7	D48.7	D49.89
head NEC	C76.0	C79.89	D04.4	D36.7	D48.7	D49.89
heart	C38.0	C79.89	—	D15.1	D48.7	D49.89
heel NEC	C76.5-☑	C79.89	D04.7-☑	D36.7	D48.7	D49.89
helix — *see also* Neoplasm, skin, ear	C44.20-☑	C79.2	D04.2-☑	D23.2-☑	D48.5	D49.2
hematopoietic, hemopoietic tissue NEC	C96.9	—	—	—	—	—
specified NEC	C96.Z	—	—	—	—	—
hemisphere, cerebral	C71.0	C79.31	—	D33.0	D43.0	D49.6
hemorrhoidal zone	C21.1	C78.5	D01.3	D12.9	D37.8	D49.0
hepatic — *see also* Index to disease, by histology	C22.9	C78.7	D01.5	D13.4	D37.6	D49.0
duct (bile)	C24.0	C78.89	D01.5	D13.5	D37.6	D49.0
flexure (colon)	C18.3	C78.5	D01.0	D12.3	D37.4	D49.0
primary	C22.8	C78.7	D01.5	D13.4	D37.6	D49.0
hepatobiliary	C24.9	C78.89	D01.5	D13.5	D37.6	D49.0
hepatoblastoma	C22.2	C78.7	D01.5	D13.4	D37.6	D49.0
hepatoma	C22.0	C78.7	D01.5	D13.4	D37.6	D49.0
hilus of lung	C34.0-☑	C78.0-☑	D02.2-☑	D14.3-☑	D38.1	D49.1
hippocampus, brain	C71.2	C79.31	—	D33.0	D43.0	D49.6
hip NEC	C76.5-☑	C79.89	D04.7-☑	D36.7	D48.7	D49.89
humerus (any part)	C40.0-☑	C79.51	—	D16.0-☑	—	—
hymen	C52	C79.82	D07.2	D28.1	D39.8	D49.59
hypopharynx, hypopharyngeal NEC	C13.9	C79.89	D00.08	D10.7	D37.05	D49.0
overlapping lesion	C13.8	—	—	—	—	—
postcricoid region	C13.0	C79.89	D00.08	D10.7	D37.05	D49.0
posterior wall	C13.2	C79.89	D00.08	D10.7	D37.05	D49.0
pyriform fossa (sinus)	C12	C79.89	D00.08	D10.7	D37.05	D49.0
hypophysis	C75.1	C79.89	D09.3	D35.2	D44.3	D49.7
hypothalamus	C71.0	C79.31	—	D33.0	D43.0	D49.6
ileocecum, ileocecal (coil) (junction) (valve)	C18.0	C78.5	D01.0	D12.0	D37.4	D49.0
ileum	C17.2	C78.4	D01.49	D13.39	D37.2	D49.0
ilium	C41.4	C79.51	—	D16.8	D48.0	D49.2
immunoproliferative NEC	C88.9	—	—	—	—	—
infraclavicular (region)	C76.1	C79.89	D04.5	D36.7	D48.7	D49.89
inguinal (region)	C76.3	C79.89	D04.5	D36.7	D48.7	D49.89
insula	C71.0	C79.31	—	D33.0	D43.0	D49.6
insular tissue (pancreas)	C25.4	C78.89	D01.7	D13.7	D37.8	D49.0
brain	C71.0	C79.31	—	D33.0	D43.0	D49.6
interarytenoid fold	C13.1	C78.39	D00.08	D10.7	D37.05	D49.0
hypopharyngeal aspect	C13.1	C79.89	D00.08	D10.7	D37.05	D49.0
laryngeal aspect	C32.1	C78.39	D02.0	D14.1	D38.0	D49.1
marginal zone	C13.1	C79.89	D00.08	D10.7	D37.05	D49.0
interdental papillae	C03.9	C79.89	D00.03	D10.39	D37.09	D49.0

Neoplasm, neoplastic — continued	Malignant Primary	Malignant Secondary	Ca in situ	Benign	Uncertain	Unspecified Behavior
interdental papillae — *continued*						
lower	C03.1	C79.89	D00.03	D10.39	D37.09	D49.0
upper	C03.0	C79.89	D00.03	D10.39	D37.09	D49.0
internal						
capsule	C71.0	C79.31	—	D33.0	D43.0	D49.6
os (cervix)	C53.0	C79.82	D06.0	D26.0	D39.0	D49.59
intervertebral cartilage or disc	C41.2	C79.51	—	D16.6	D48.0	D49.2
intestine, intestinal	C26.0	C78.80	D01.40	D13.9	D37.8	D49.0
large	C18.9	C78.5	D01.0	D12.6	D37.4	D49.0
appendix	C18.1	C78.5	D01.0	D12.1	D37.3	D49.0
caput coli	C18.0	C78.5	D01.0	D12.0	D37.4	D49.0
cecum	C18.0	C78.5	D01.0	D12.0	D37.4	D49.0
colon	C18.9	C78.5	D01.0	D12.6	D37.4	D49.0
and rectum	C19	C78.5	D01.1	D12.7	D37.5	D49.0
ascending	C18.2	C78.5	D01.0	D12.2	D37.4	D49.0
caput	C18.0	C78.5	D01.0	D12.0	D37.4	D49.0
descending	C18.6	C78.5	D01.0	D12.4	D37.4	D49.0
distal	C18.6	C78.5	D01.0	D12.4	D37.4	D49.0
left	C18.6	C78.5	D01.0	D12.4	D37.4	D49.0
overlapping lesion	C18.8	—	—	—	—	—
pelvic	C18.7	C78.5	D01.0	D12.5	D37.4	D49.0
right	C18.2	C78.5	D01.0	D12.2	D37.4	D49.0
sigmoid (flexure)	C18.7	C78.5	D01.0	D12.5	D37.4	D49.0
transverse	C18.4	C78.5	D01.0	D12.3	D37.4	D49.0
hepatic flexure	C18.3	C78.5	D01.0	D12.3	D37.4	D49.0
ileocecum, ileocecal (coil) (valve)	C18.0	C78.5	D01.0	D12.0	D37.4	D49.0
overlapping lesion	C18.8	—	—	—	—	—
sigmoid flexure (lower) (upper)	C18.7	C78.5	D01.0	D12.5	D37.4	D49.0
splenic flexure	C18.5	C78.5	D01.0	D12.3	D37.4	D49.0
small	C17.9	C78.4	D01.40	D13.30	D37.2	D49.0
duodenum	C17.0	C78.4	D01.49	D13.2	D37.2	D49.0
ileum	C17.2	C78.4	D01.49	D13.39	D37.2	D49.0
jejunum	C17.1	C78.4	D01.49	D13.39	D37.2	D49.0
overlapping lesion	C17.8	—	—	—	—	—
tract NEC	C26.0	C78.89	D01.40	D13.9	D37.8	D49.0
intra-abdominal	C76.2	C79.89	D09.8	D36.7	D48.7	D49.89
intracranial NEC	C71.9	C79.31	—	D33.2	D43.2	D49.6
intrahepatic (bile) duct	C22.1	C78.7	D01.5	D13.4	D37.6	D49.0
intraocular	C69.9-☑	C79.49	D09.2-☑	D31.9-☑	D48.7	D49.89
intraorbital	C69.6-☑	C79.49	D09.2-☑	D31.6-☑	D48.7	D49.89
intrasellar	C75.1	C79.89	D09.3	D35.2	D44.3	D49.7
intrathoracic (cavity) (organs)	C76.1	C79.89	D09.8	D15.9	D48.7	D49.89
specified NEC	C76.1	C79.89	D09.8	D15.7	—	—
iris	C69.4-☑	C79.49	D09.2-☑	D31.4-☑	D48.7	D49.89
ischiorectal (fossa)	C76.3	C79.89	D09.8	D36.7	D48.7	D49.89
ischium	C41.4	C79.51	—	D16.8	D48.0	D49.2
island of Reil	C71.0	C79.31	—	D33.0	D43.0	D49.6
islands or islets of Langerhans	C25.4	C78.89	D01.7	D13.7	D37.8	D49.0
isthmus uteri	C54.0	C79.82	D07.0	D26.1	D39.0	D49.59
jaw	C76.0	C79.89	D09.8	D36.7	D48.7	D49.89
bone	C41.1	C79.51	—	D16.5	D48.0	D49.2
lower	C41.1	C79.51	—	D16.5	—	—
upper	C41.0	C79.51	—	D16.4	—	—
carcinoma (any type) (lower) (upper)	C76.0	C79.89	—	—	—	—
skin — *see also* Neoplasm, skin, face	C44.309	C79.2	D04.39	D23.39	D48.5	D49.2
soft tissues	C03.9	C79.89	D00.03	D10.39	D37.09	D49.0
lower	C03.1	C79.89	D00.03	D10.39	D37.09	D49.0
upper	C03.0	C79.89	D00.03	D10.39	D37.09	D49.0
jejunum	C17.1	C78.4	D01.49	D13.39	D37.2	D49.0
joint NEC — *see also* Neoplasm, bone	C41.9	C79.51	—	D16.9	D48.0	D49.2
acromioclavicular	C40.0-☑	C79.51	—	D16.0-☑	—	—

☟ Subterms under main terms may continue to next column or page   ☑ Additional Character Required — Refer to the Tabular List for Character Selection

Neoplasm, neoplastic — continued

	Malignant Primary	Malignant Secondary	Ca in situ	Benign	Uncertain	Unspecified Behavior
joint — see also Neoplasm, bone — continued						
bursa or synovial membrane — see Neoplasm, connective tissue						
costovertebral	C41.3	C79.51	—	D16.7	D48.0	D49.2
sternocostal	C41.3	C79.51	—	D16.7	D48.0	D49.2
temporomandibular	C41.1	C79.51	—	D16.5	D48.0	D49.2
junction						
anorectal	C21.8	C78.5	D01.3	D12.9	D37.8	D49.0
cardioesophageal	C16.0	C78.89	D00.2	D13.1	D37.1	D49.0
esophagogastric	C16.0	C78.89	D00.2	D13.1	D37.1	D49.0
gastroesophageal	C16.0	C78.89	D00.2	D13.1	D37.1	D49.0
hard and soft palate	C05.9	C79.89	D00.00	D10.39	D37.09	D49.0
ileocecal	C18.0	C78.5	D01.0	D12.0	D37.4	D49.0
pelvirectal	C19	C78.5	D01.1	D12.7	D37.5	D49.0
pelviureteric	C65.-✓	C79.0-✓	D09.19	D30.1-✓	D41.1-✓	D49.59
rectosigmoid	C19	C78.5	D01.1	D12.7	D37.5	D49.0
squamocolumnar, of cervix	C53.8	C79.82	D06.7	D26.0	D39.0	D49.59
Kaposi's sarcoma — see Kaposi's, sarcoma						
kidney (parenchymal)	C64.-✓	C79.0-✓	D09.19	D30.0-✓	D41.0-✓	D49.51-✓
calyx	C65.-✓	C79.0-✓	D09.19	D30.1-✓	D41.1-✓	D49.51-✓
hilus	C65.-✓	C79.0-✓	D09.19	D30.1-✓	D41.1-✓	D49.51-✓
pelvis	C65.-✓	C79.0-✓	D09.19	D30.1-✓	D41.1-✓	D49.51-✓
knee NEC	C76.5-✓	C79.89	D04.7-✓	D36.7	D48.7	D49.89
labia (skin)	C51.9	C79.82	D07.1	D28.0	D39.8	D49.59
majora	C51.0	C79.82	D07.1	D28.0	D39.8	D49.59
minora	C51.1	C79.82	D07.1	D28.0	D39.8	D49.59
labial — see also Neoplasm, lip	C00.9	C79.89	D00.01	D10.0	D37.01	D49.0
sulcus (lower) (upper)	C06.1	C79.89	D00.02	D10.39	D37.09	D49.0
labium (skin)	C51.9	C79.82	D07.1	D28.0	D39.8	D49.59
majus	C51.0	C79.82	D07.1	D28.0	D39.8	D49.59
minus	C51.1	C79.82	D07.1	D28.0	D39.8	D49.59
lacrimal						
canaliculi	C69.5-✓	C79.49	D09.2-✓	D31.5-✓	D48.7	D49.89
duct (nasal)	C69.5-✓	C79.49	D09.2-✓	D31.5-✓	D48.7	D49.89
gland	C69.5-✓	C79.49	D09.2-✓	D31.5-✓	D48.7	D49.89
punctum	C69.5-✓	C79.49	D09.2-✓	D31.5-✓	D48.7	D49.89
sac	C69.5-✓	C79.49	D09.2-✓	D31.5-✓	D48.7	D49.89
Langerhans, islands or islets	C25.4	C78.89	D01.7	D13.7	D37.8	D49.0
laryngopharynx	C13.9	C79.89	D00.08	D10.7	D37.05	D49.0
larynx, laryngeal NEC	C32.9	C78.39	D02.0	D14.1	D38.0	D49.1
aryepiglottic fold	C32.1	C78.39	D02.0	D14.1	D38.0	D49.1
cartilage (arytenoid) (cricoid) (cuneiform) (thyroid)	C32.3	C78.39	D02.0	D14.1	D38.0	D49.1
commissure (anterior) (posterior)	C32.0	C78.39	D02.0	D14.1	D38.0	D49.1
extrinsic NEC	C32.1	C78.39	D02.0	D14.1	D38.0	D49.1
meaning hypopharynx	C13.9	C79.89	D00.08	D10.7	D37.05	D49.0
interarytenoid fold	C32.1	C78.39	D02.0	D14.1	D38.0	D49.1
intrinsic	C32.0	C78.39	D02.0	D14.1	D38.0	D49.1
overlapping lesion	C32.8	—	—	—	—	—
ventricular band	C32.1	C78.39	D02.0	D14.1	D38.0	D49.1
leg NEC	C76.5-✓	C79.89	D04.7-✓	D36.7	D48.7	D49.89
lens, crystalline	C69.4-✓	C79.49	D09.2-✓	D31.4-✓	D48.7	D49.89
lid (lower) (upper)	C44.10-✓	C79.2	D04.1-✓	D23.1-✓	D48.5	D49.2
basal cell carcinoma	C44.11-✓	—	—	—	—	—
specified type NEC	C44.19-✓	—	—	—	—	—
squamous cell carcinoma	C44.12-✓	—	—	—	—	—

Neoplasm, neoplastic — continued

	Malignant Primary	Malignant Secondary	Ca in situ	Benign	Uncertain	Unspecified Behavior
ligament — see also Neoplasm, connective tissue						
broad	C57.1-✓	C79.82	D07.39	D28.2	D39.8	D49.59
Mackenrodt's	C57.7	C79.82	D07.39	D28.7	D39.8	D49.59
non-uterine — see Neoplasm, connective tissue						
round	C57.2-✓	C79.82	—	D28.2	D39.8	D49.59
sacro-uterine	C57.3	C79.82	—	D28.2	D39.8	D49.59
uterine	C57.3	C79.82	—	D28.2	D39.8	D49.59
utero-ovarian	C57.7	C79.82	D07.39	D28.2	D39.8	D49.59
uterosacral	C57.3	C79.82	—	D28.2	D39.8	D49.59
limb	C76.8	C79.89	D04.8	D36.7	D48.7	D49.89
lower	C76.5-✓	C79.89	D04.7-✓	D36.7	D48.7	D49.89
upper	C76.4-✓	C79.89	D04.6-✓	D36.7	D48.7	D49.89
limbus of cornea	C69.1-✓	C79.49	D09.2-✓	D31.1-✓	D48.7	D49.89
lingual NEC — see also Neoplasm, tongue	C02.9	C79.89	D00.07	D10.1	D37.02	D49.0
lingula, lung	C34.1-✓	C78.0-✓	D02.2-✓	D14.3-✓	D38.1	D49.1
lip	C00.9	C79.89	D00.01	D10.0	D37.01	D49.0
buccal aspect — see Neoplasm, lip, internal						
commissure	C00.6	C79.89	D00.01	D10.0	D37.01	D49.0
external	C00.2	C79.89	D00.01	D10.0	D37.01	D49.0
lower	C00.1	C79.89	D00.01	D10.0	D37.01	D49.0
upper	C00.0	C79.89	D00.01	D10.0	D37.01	D49.0
frenulum — see Neoplasm, lip, internal						
inner aspect — see Neoplasm, lip, internal						
internal	C00.5	C79.89	D00.01	D10.0	D37.01	D49.0
lower	C00.4	C79.89	D00.01	D10.0	D37.01	D49.0
upper	C00.3	C79.89	D00.01	D10.0	D37.01	D49.0
lipstick area	C00.2	C79.89	D00.01	D10.0	D37.01	D49.0
lower	C00.1	C79.89	D00.01	D10.0	D37.01	D49.0
upper	C00.0	C79.89	D00.01	D10.0	D37.01	D49.0
lower	C00.1	C79.89	D00.01	D10.0	D37.01	D49.0
internal	C00.4	C79.89	D00.01	D10.0	D37.01	D49.0
mucosa — see Neoplasm, lip, internal						
oral aspect — see Neoplasm, lip, internal						
overlapping lesion	C00.8	—	—	—	—	—
with oral cavity or pharynx	C14.8	—	—	—	—	—
skin (commissure) (lower) (upper)	C44.00	C79.2	D04.0	D23.0	D48.5	D49.2
basal cell carcinoma	C44.01	—	—	—	—	—
specified type NEC	C44.09	—	—	—	—	—
squamous cell carcinoma	C44.02	—	—	—	—	—
upper	C00.0	C79.89	D00.01	D10.0	D37.01	D49.0
internal	C00.3	C79.89	D00.01	D10.0	D37.01	D49.0
vermilion border	C00.2	C79.89	D00.01	D10.0	D37.01	D49.0
lower	C00.1	C79.89	D00.01	D10.0	D37.01	D49.0
upper	C00.0	C79.89	D00.01	D10.0	D37.01	D49.0
lipomatous — see Lipoma, by site						
liver — see also Index to disease, by histology	C22.9	C78.7	D01.5	D13.4	D37.6	D49.0
primary	C22.8	C78.7	D01.5	D13.4	D37.6	D49.0
lumbosacral plexus	C47.5	C79.89		D36.16	D48.2	D49.2
lung	C34.9-✓	C78.0-✓	D02.2-✓	D14.3-✓	D38.1	D49.1
azygos lobe	C34.1-✓	C78.0-✓	D02.2-✓	D14.3-✓	D38.1	D49.1
carina	C34.0-✓	C78.0-✓	D02.2-✓	D14.3-✓	D38.1	D49.1
hilus	C34.0-✓	C78.0-✓	D02.2-✓	D14.3-✓	D38.1	D49.1
lingula	C34.1-✓	C78.0-✓	D02.2-✓	D14.3-✓	D38.1	D49.1
lobe NEC	C34.9-✓	C78.0-✓	D02.2-✓	D14.3-✓	D38.1	D49.1
lower lobe	C34.3-✓	C78.0-✓	D02.2-✓	D14.3-✓	D38.1	D49.1

✓ Additional Character Required — Refer to the Tabular List for Character Selection

▽ Subterms under main terms may continue to next column or page

Neoplasm, neoplastic — continued

	Malignant Primary	Malignant Secondary	Ca in situ	Benign	Uncertain	Unspecified Behavior
lung — continued						
main bronchus	C34.0-☑	C78.0-☑	D02.2-☑	D14.3-☑	D38.1	D49.1
mesothelioma — *see* Mesothelioma						
middle lobe	C34.2	C78.0-☑	D02.21	D14.31	D38.1	D49.1
overlapping lesion	C34.8-☑	—	—	—	—	—
upper lobe	C34.1-☑	C78.0-☑	D02.2-☑	D14.3-☑	D38.1	D49.1
lymph, lymphatic channel						
NEC	C49.9	C79.89	—	D21.9	D48.1	D49.2
gland (secondary)	—	C77.9	—	D36.0	D48.7	D49.89
abdominal	—	C77.2	—	D36.0	D48.7	D49.89
aortic	—	C77.2	—	D36.0	D48.7	D49.89
arm	—	C77.3	—	D36.0	D48.7	D49.89
auricular (anterior) (posterior)	—	C77.0	—	D36.0	D48.7	D49.89
axilla, axillary	—	C77.3	—	D36.0	D48.7	D49.89
brachial	—	C77.3	—	D36.0	D48.7	D49.89
bronchial	—	C77.1	—	D36.0	D48.7	D49.89
bronchopulmonary	—	C77.1	—	D36.0	D48.7	D49.89
celiac	—	C77.2	—	D36.0	D48.7	D49.89
cervical	—	C77.0	—	D36.0	D48.7	D49.89
cervicofacial	—	C77.0	—	D36.0	D48.7	D49.89
Cloquet	—	C77.4	—	D36.0	D48.7	D49.89
colic	—	C77.2	—	D36.0	D48.7	D49.89
common duct	—	C77.2	—	D36.0	D48.7	D49.89
cubital	—	C77.3	—	D36.0	D48.7	D49.89
diaphragmatic	—	C77.1	—	D36.0	D48.7	D49.89
epigastric, inferior	—	C77.1	—	D36.0	D48.7	D49.89
epitrochlear	—	C77.3	—	D36.0	D48.7	D49.89
esophageal	—	C77.1	—	D36.0	D48.7	D49.89
face	—	C77.0	—	D36.0	D48.7	D49.89
femoral	—	C77.4	—	D36.0	D48.7	D49.89
gastric	—	C77.2	—	D36.0	D48.7	D49.89
groin	—	C77.4	—	D36.0	D48.7	D49.89
head	—	C77.0	—	D36.0	D48.7	D49.89
hepatic	—	C77.2	—	D36.0	D48.7	D49.89
hilar (pulmonary)	—	C77.1	—	D36.0	D48.7	D49.89
splenic	—	C77.2	—	D36.0	D48.7	D49.89
hypogastric	—	C77.5	—	D36.0	D48.7	D49.89
ileocolic	—	C77.2	—	D36.0	D48.7	D49.89
iliac	—	C77.5	—	D36.0	D48.7	D49.89
infraclavicular	—	C77.3	—	D36.0	D48.7	D49.89
inguina, inguinal	—	C77.4	—	D36.0	D48.7	D49.89
innominate	—	C77.1	—	D36.0	D48.7	D49.89
intercostal	—	C77.1	—	D36.0	D48.7	D49.89
intestinal	—	C77.2	—	D36.0	D48.7	D49.89
intrabdominal	—	C77.2	—	D36.0	D48.7	D49.89
intrapelvic	—	C77.5	—	D36.0	D48.7	D49.89
intrathoracic	—	C77.1	—	D36.0	D48.7	D49.89
jugular	—	C77.0	—	D36.0	D48.7	D49.89
leg	—	C77.4	—	D36.0	D48.7	D49.89
limb, lower	—	C77.4	—	D36.0	D48.7	D49.89
upper	—	C77.3	—	D36.0	D48.7	D49.89
lower limb	—	C77.4	—	D36.0	D48.7	D49.89
lumbar	—	C77.2	—	D36.0	D48.7	D49.89
mandibular	—	C77.0	—	D36.0	D48.7	D49.89
mediastinal	—	C77.1	—	D36.0	D48.7	D49.89
mesenteric (inferior) (superior)	—	C77.2	—	D36.0	D48.7	D49.89
midcolic	—	C77.2	—	D36.0	D48.7	D49.89
multiple sites in categories C77.0-C77.5	—	C77.8	—	D36.0	D48.7	D49.89
neck	—	C77.0	—	D36.0	D48.7	D49.89
obturator	—	C77.5	—	D36.0	D48.7	D49.89
occipital	—	C77.0	—	D36.0	D48.7	D49.89
pancreatic	—	C77.2	—	D36.0	D48.7	D49.89
para-aortic	—	C77.2	—	D36.0	D48.7	D49.89
paracervical	—	C77.5	—	D36.0	D48.7	D49.89
parametrial	—	C77.5	—	D36.0	D48.7	D49.89
parasternal	—	C77.1	—	D36.0	D48.7	D49.89
parotid	—	C77.0	—	D36.0	D48.7	D49.89
pectoral	—	C77.3	—	D36.0	D48.7	D49.89
pelvic	—	C77.5	—	D36.0	D48.7	D49.89
peri-aortic	—	C77.2	—	D36.0	D48.7	D49.89
peripancreatic	—	C77.2	—	D36.0	D48.7	D49.89
popliteal	—	C77.4	—	D36.0	D48.7	D49.89
porta hepatis	—	C77.2	—	D36.0	D48.7	D49.89

Neoplasm, neoplastic — continued

	Malignant Primary	Malignant Secondary	Ca in situ	Benign	Uncertain	Unspecified Behavior
lymph, lymphatic channel — continued						
gland — continued						
portal	—	C77.2	—	D36.0	D48.7	D49.89
preauricular	—	C77.0	—	D36.0	D48.7	D49.89
prelaryngeal	—	C77.0	—	D36.0	D48.7	D49.89
presymphysial	—	C77.5	—	D36.0	D48.7	D49.89
pretracheal	—	C77.0	—	D36.0	D48.7	D49.89
primary (any site) NEC	C96.9	—	—	—	—	—
pulmonary (hiler)	—	C77.1	—	D36.0	D48.7	D49.89
pyloric	—	C77.2	—	D36.0	D48.7	D49.89
retroperitoneal	—	C77.2	—	D36.0	D48.7	D49.89
retropharyngeal	—	C77.0	—	D36.0	D48.7	D49.89
Rosenmuller's	—	C77.4	—	D36.0	D48.7	D49.89
sacral	—	C77.5	—	D36.0	D48.7	D49.89
scalene	—	C77.0	—	D36.0	D48.7	D49.89
site NEC	—	C77.9	—	D36.0	D48.7	D49.89
splenic (hilar)	—	C77.2	—	D36.0	D48.7	D49.89
subclavicular	—	C77.3	—	D36.0	D48.7	D49.89
subinguinal	—	C77.4	—	D36.0	D48.7	D49.89
sublingual	—	C77.0	—	D36.0	D48.7	D49.89
submandibular	—	C77.0	—	D36.0	D48.7	D49.89
submaxillary	—	C77.0	—	D36.0	D48.7	D49.89
submental	—	C77.0	—	D36.0	D48.7	D49.89
subscapular	—	C77.3	—	D36.0	D48.7	D49.89
supraclavicular	—	C77.0	—	D36.0	D48.7	D49.89
thoracic	—	C77.1	—	D36.0	D48.7	D49.89
tibial	—	C77.4	—	D36.0	D48.7	D49.89
tracheal	—	C77.1	—	D36.0	D48.7	D49.89
tracheobronchial	—	C77.1	—	D36.0	D48.7	D49.89
upper limb	—	C77.3	—	D36.0	D48.7	D49.89
Virchow's	—	C77.0	—	D36.0	D48.7	D49.89
node — *see also* Neoplasm, lymph gland						
primary NEC	C96.9	—	—	—	—	—
vessel — *see also* Neoplasm, connective tissue	C49.9	C79.89	—	D21.9	D48.1	D49.2
Mackenrodt's ligament	C57.7	C79.82	D07.39	D28.7	D39.8	D49.59
malar	C41.0	C79.51	—	D16.4	D48.0	D49.2
region — *see* Neoplasm, cheek						
mammary gland — *see* Neoplasm, breast						
mandible	C41.1	C79.51	—	D16.5	D48.0	D49.2
alveolar mucosa (carcinoma)	C03.1	C79.89	D00.03	D10.39	D37.09	D49.0
ridge or process	C41.1	C79.51	—	D16.5	D48.0	D49.2
marrow (bone) NEC	C96.9	C79.52	—	—	D47.9	D49.89
mastectomy site (skin) — *see also* Neoplasm, breast, skin	C44.501	C79.2	—	—	—	—
specified as breast tissue	C50.8-☑	C79.81	—	—	—	—
mastoid (air cells) (antrum) (cavity)	C30.1	C78.39	D02.3	D14.0	D38.5	D49.1
bone or process	C41.0	C79.51	—	D16.4	D48.0	D49.2
maxilla, maxillary (superior)	C41.0	C79.51	—	D16.4	D48.0	D49.2
alveolar mucosa	C03.0	C79.89	D00.03	D10.39	D37.09	D49.0
ridge or process (carcinoma)	C41.0	C79.51	—	D16.4	D48.0	D49.2
antrum	C31.0	C78.39	D02.3	D14.0	D38.5	D49.1
carcinoma	C03.0	C79.51	—	—	—	—
inferior — *see* Neoplasm, mandible						
sinus	C31.0	C78.39	D02.3	D14.0	D38.5	D49.1
meatus external (ear) — *see also* Neoplasm, skin, ear	C44.20-☑	C79.2	D04.2-☑	D23.2-☑	D48.5	D49.2
Meckel diverticulum, malignant	C17.3	C78.4	D01.49	D13.39	D37.2	D49.0
mediastinum, mediastinal	C38.3	C78.1	—	D15.2	D38.3	D49.89

Neoplasm, neoplastic — continued

	Malignant Primary	Malignant Secondary	Ca in situ	Benign	Uncertain	Unspecified Behavior
mediastinum, mediastinal — continued						
anterior	C38.1	C78.1	—	D15.2	D38.3	D49.89
posterior	C38.2	C78.1	—	D15.2	D38.3	D49.89
medulla						
adrenal	C74.1-☑	C79.7-☑	D09.3	D35.0-☑	D44.1-☑	D49.7
oblongata	C71.7	C79.31		D33.1	D43.1	D49.6
meibomian gland	C44.10-☑	C79.2	D04.1-☑	D23.1-☑	D48.5	D49.2
basal cell carcinoma	C44.11-☑	—	—	—	—	—
specified type NEC	C44.19-☑	—	—	—	—	—
squamous cell carcinoma	C44.12-☑	—	—	—	—	—
melanoma — see Melanoma						
meninges	C70.9	C79.49	—	D32.9	D42.9	D49.7
brain	C70.0	C79.32	—	D32.0	D42.0	D49.7
cerebral	C70.0	C79.32	—	D32.0	D42.0	D49.7
crainial	C70.0	C79.32	—	D32.0	D42.0	D49.7
intracranial	C70.0	C79.32	—	D32.0	D42.0	D49.7
spinal (cord)	C70.1	C79.49	—	D32.1	D42.1	D49.7
meniscus, knee joint (lateral) (medial)	C40.2-☑	C79.51	—	D16.2-☑	D48.0	D49.2
Merkel cell — see Carcinoma, Merkel cell						
mesentery, mesenteric	C48.1	C78.6	—	D20.1	D48.4	D49.0
mesoappendix	C48.1	C78.6	—	D20.1	D48.4	D49.0
mesocolon	C48.1	C78.6	—	D20.1	D48.4	D49.0
mesopharynx — see Neoplasm, oropharynx						
mesosalpinx	C57.1-☑	C79.82	D07.39	D28.2	D39.8	D49.59
mesothelial tissue — see Mesothelioma						
mesothelioma — see Mesothelioma						
mesovarium	C57.1-☑	C79.82	D07.39	D28.2	D39.8	D49.59
metacarpus (any bone)	C40.1-☑	C79.51	—	D16.1-☑	—	—
metastatic NEC — see also Neoplasm, by site, secondary	—	C79.9	—	—	—	—
metatarsus (any bone)	C40.3-☑	C79.51	—	D16.3-☑	—	—
midbrain	C71.7	C79.31		D33.1	D43.1	D49.6
milk duct — see Neoplasm, breast						
mons						
pubis	C51.9	C79.82	D07.1	D28.0	D39.8	D49.59
veneris	C51.9	C79.82	D07.1	D28.0	D39.8	D49.59
motor tract	C72.9	C79.49	—	D33.9	D43.9	D49.7
brain	C71.9	C79.31	—	D33.2	D43.2	D49.6
cauda equina	C72.1	C79.49	—	D33.4	D43.4	D49.7
spinal	C72.0	C79.49	—	D33.4	D43.4	D49.7
mouth	C06.9	C79.89	D00.00	D10.30	D37.09	D49.0
book-leaf	C06.89	C79.89	—	—	—	—
floor	C04.9	C79.89	D00.06	D10.2	D37.09	D49.0
anterior portion	C04.0	C79.89	D00.06	D10.2	D37.09	D49.0
lateral portion	C04.1	C79.89	D00.06	D10.2	D37.09	D49.0
overlapping lesion	C04.8	—	—	—	—	—
overlapping NEC	C06.80	—	—	—	—	—
roof	C05.9	C79.89	D00.00	D10.39	D37.09	D49.0
specified part NEC	C06.89	C79.89	D00.00	D10.39	D37.09	D49.0
vestibule	C06.1	C79.89	D00.00	D10.39	D37.09	D49.0
mucosa						
alveolar (ridge or process)	C03.9	C79.89	D00.03	D10.39	D37.09	D49.0
lower	C03.1	C79.89	D00.03	D10.39	D37.09	D49.0
upper	C03.0	C79.89	D00.03	D10.39	D37.09	D49.0
buccal	C06.0	C79.89	D00.02	D10.39	D37.09	D49.0
cheek	C06.0	C79.89	D00.02	D10.39	D37.09	D49.0
lip — see Neoplasm, lip, internal						
nasal	C30.0	C78.39	D02.3	D14.0	D38.5	D49.1
oral	C06.0	C79.89	D00.02	D10.39	D37.09	D49.0
Mullerian duct						
female	C57.7	C79.82	D07.39	D28.7	D39.8	D49.59
male	C63.7	C79.82	D07.69	D29.8	D40.8	D49.59

Neoplasm, neoplastic — continued

	Malignant Primary	Malignant Secondary	Ca in situ	Benign	Uncertain	Unspecified Behavior
muscle — see also Neoplasm, connective tissue						
extraocular	C69.6-☑	C79.49	D09.2-☑	D31.6-☑	D48.7	D49.89
myocardium	C38.0	C79.89	—	D15.1	D48.7	D49.89
myometrium	C54.2	C79.82	D07.0	D26.1	D39.0	D49.59
myopericardium	C38.0	C79.89	—	D15.1	D48.7	D49.89
nabothian gland (follicle)	C53.0	C79.82	D06.0	D26.0	D39.0	D49.59
nail — see also Neoplasm, skin, limb	C44.90	C79.2	D04.9	D23.9	D48.5	D49.2
finger — see also Neoplasm, skin, limb, upper	C44.60-☑	C79.2	D04.6-☑	D23.6-☑	D48.5	D49.2
toe — see also Neoplasm, skin, limb, lower	C44.70-☑	C79.2	D04.7-☑	D23.7-☑	D48.5	D49.2
nares, naris (anterior) (posterior)	C30.0	C78.39	D02.3	D14.0	D38.5	D49.1
nasal — see Neoplasm, nose						
nasolabial groove — see also Neoplasm, skin, face	C44.309	C79.2	D04.39	D23.39	D48.5	D49.2
nasolacrimal duct	C69.5-☑	C79.49	D09.2-☑	D31.5-☑	D48.7	D49.89
nasopharynx, nasopharyngeal	C11.9	C79.89	D00.08	D10.6	D37.05	D49.0
floor	C11.3	C79.89	D00.08	D10.6	D37.05	D49.0
overlapping lesion	C11.8	—	—	—	—	—
roof	C11.0	C79.89	D00.08	D10.6	D37.05	D49.0
wall	C11.9	C79.89	D00.08	D10.6	D37.05	D49.0
anterior	C11.3	C79.89	D00.08	D10.6	D37.05	D49.0
lateral	C11.2	C79.89	D00.08	D10.6	D37.05	D49.0
posterior	C11.1	C79.89	D00.08	D10.6	D37.05	D49.0
superior	C11.0	C79.89	D00.08	D10.6	D37.05	D49.0
nates — see also Neoplasm, skin, trunk	C44.509	C79.2	D04.5	D23.5	D48.5	D49.2
neck NEC	C76.0	C79.89	D09.8	D36.7	D48.7	D49.89
skin	C44.40	—	—	—	—	—
basal cell carcinoma	C44.41	—	—	—	—	—
specified type NEC	C44.49	—	—	—	—	—
squamous cell carcinoma	C44.42	—	—	—	—	—
nerve (ganglion)	C47.9	C79.89	—	D36.10	D48.2	D49.2
abducens	C72.59	C79.49	—	D33.3	D43.3	D49.7
accessory (spinal)	C72.59	C79.49	—	D33.3	D43.3	D49.7
acoustic	C72.4-☑	C79.49	—	D33.3	D43.3	D49.7
auditory	C72.4-☑	C79.49	—	D33.3	D43.3	D49.7
autonomic NEC — see also Neoplasm, nerve, peripheral	C47.9	C79.89	—	D36.10	D48.2	D49.2
brachial	C47.1-☑	C79.89	—	D36.12	D48.2	D49.2
cranial	C72.50	C79.49	—	D33.3	D43.3	D49.7
specified NEC	C72.59	C79.49	—	D33.3	D43.3	D49.7
facial	C72.59	C79.49	—	D33.3	D43.3	D49.7
femoral	C47.2-☑	C79.89	—	D36.13	D48.2	D49.2
ganglion NEC — see also Neoplasm, nerve, peripheral	C47.9	C79.89	—	D36.10	D48.2	D49.2
glossopharyngeal	C72.59	C79.49	—	D33.3	D43.3	D49.7
hypoglossal	C72.59	C79.49	—	D33.3	D43.3	D49.7
intercostal	C47.3	C79.89	—	D36.14	D48.2	D49.2
lumbar	C47.6	C79.89	—	D36.17	D48.2	D49.2
median	C47.1-☑	C79.89	—	D36.12	D48.2	D49.2
obturator	C47.2-☑	C79.89	—	D36.13	D48.2	D49.2
oculomotor	C72.59	C79.49	—	D33.3	D43.3	D49.7
olfactory	C47.2-☑	C79.49	—	D33.3	D43.3	D49.7
optic	C72.3-☑	C79.49	—	D33.3	D43.3	D49.7
parasympathetic NEC	C47.9	C79.89	—	D36.10	D48.2	D49.2
peripheral NEC	C47.9	C79.89	—	D36.10	D48.2	D49.2
abdomen	C47.4	C79.89	—	D36.15	D48.2	D49.2
abdominal wall	C47.4	C79.89	—	D36.15	D48.2	D49.2
ankle	C47.2-☑	C79.89	—	D36.13	D48.2	D49.2
antecubital fossa or space	C47.1-☑	C79.89	—	D36.12	D48.2	D49.2

☑ Additional Character Required — Refer to the Tabular List for Character Selection   ▽ Subterms under main terms may continue to next column or page

Neoplasm, neoplastic —	Malignant Primary	Malignant Secondary	Ca in situ	Benign	Uncertain	Unspecified Behavior
continued						
nerve — *continued*						
peripheral — *continued*						
arm	C47.1-☑	C79.89	—	D36.12	D48.2	D49.2
auricle (ear)	C47.0	C79.89	—	D36.11	D48.2	D49.2
axilla	C47.3	C79.89	—	D36.12	D48.2	D49.2
back	C47.6	C79.89	—	D36.17	D48.2	D49.2
buttock	C47.5	C79.89	—	D36.16	D48.2	D49.2
calf	C47.2-☑	C79.89	—	D36.13	D48.2	D49.2
cervical region	C47.0	C79.89	—	D36.11	D48.2	D49.2
cheek	C47.0	C79.89	—	D36.11	D48.2	D49.2
chest (wall)	C47.3	C79.89	—	D36.14	D48.2	D49.2
chin	C47.0	C79.89	—	D36.11	D48.2	D49.2
ear (external)	C47.0	C79.89	—	D36.11	D48.2	D49.2
elbow	C47.1-☑	C79.89	—	D36.12	D48.2	D49.2
extrarectal	C47.5	C79.89	—	D36.16	D48.2	D49.2
extremity	C47.9	C79.89	—	D36.10	D48.2	D49.2
lower	C47.2-☑	C79.89	—	D36.13	D48.2	D49.2
upper	C47.1-☑	C79.89	—	D36.12	D48.2	D49.2
eyelid	C47.0	C79.89	—	D36.11	D48.2	D49.2
face	C47.0	C79.89	—	D36.11	D48.2	D49.2
finger	C47.1-☑	C79.89	—	D36.12	D48.2	D49.2
flank	C47.6	C79.89	—	D36.17	D48.2	D49.2
foot	C47.2-☑	C79.89	—	D36.13	D48.2	D49.2
forearm	C47.1-☑	C79.89	—	D36.12	D48.2	D49.2
forehead	C47.0	C79.89	—	D36.11	D48.2	D49.2
gluteal region	C47.5	C79.89	—	D36.16	D48.2	D49.2
groin	C47.5	C79.89	—	D36.16	D48.2	D49.2
hand	C47.1-☑	C79.89	—	D36.12	D48.2	D49.2
head	C47.0	C79.89	—	D36.11	D48.2	D49.2
heel	C47.2-☑	C79.89	—	D36.13	D48.2	D49.2
hip	C47.2-☑	C79.89	—	D36.13	D48.2	D49.2
infraclavicular region	C47.3	C79.89	—	D36.14	D48.2	D49.2
inguinal (canal) (region)	C47.5	C79.89	—	D36.16	D48.2	D49.2
intrathoracic	C47.3	C79.89	—	D36.14	D48.2	D49.2
ischiorectal fossa	C47.5	C79.89	—	D36.16	D48.2	D49.2
knee	C47.2-☑	C79.89	—	D36.13	D48.2	D49.2
leg	C47.2-☑	C79.89	—	D36.13	D48.2	D49.2
limb NEC	C47.9	C79.89	—	D36.10	D48.2	D49.2
lower	C47.2-☑	C79.89	—	D36.13	D48.2	D49.2
upper	C47.1-☑	C79.89	—	D36.12	D48.2	D49.2
nates	C47.5	C79.89	—	D36.16	D48.2	D49.2
neck	C47.0	C79.89	—	D36.11	D48.2	D49.2
orbit	C69.6-☑	C79.49	—	D31.6-☑	D48.7	D49.2
pararectal	C47.5	C79.89	—	D36.16	D48.2	D49.2
paraurethral	C47.5	C79.89	—	D36.16	D48.2	D49.2
paravaginal	C47.5	C79.89	—	D36.16	D48.2	D49.2
pelvis (floor)	C47.5	C79.89	—	D36.16	D48.2	D49.2
pelvoabdominal	C47.8	C79.89	—	D36.17	D48.2	D49.2
perineum	C47.5	C79.89	—	D36.16	D48.2	D49.2
perirectal (tissue)	C47.5	C79.89	—	D36.16	D48.2	D49.2
periurethral (tissue)	C47.5	C79.89	—	D36.16	D48.2	D49.2
popliteal fossa or space	C47.2-☑	C79.89	—	D36.13	D48.2	D49.2
presacral	C47.5	C79.89	—	D36.16	D48.2	D49.2
pterygoid fossa	C47.0	C79.89	—	D36.11	D48.2	D49.2
rectovaginal septum or wall	C47.5	C79.89	—	D36.16	D48.2	D49.2
rectovesical	C47.5	C79.89	—	D36.16	D48.2	D49.2
sacrococcygeal region	C47.5	C79.89	—	D36.16	D48.2	D49.2
scalp	C47.0	C79.89	—	D36.11	D48.2	D49.2
scapular region	C47.3	C79.89	—	D36.14	D48.2	D49.2
shoulder	C47.1-☑	C79.89	—	D36.12	D48.2	D49.2
submental	C47.0	C79.89	—	D36.11	D48.2	D49.2
supraclavicular region	C47.0	C79.89	—	D36.11	D48.2	D49.2
temple	C47.0	C79.89	—	D36.11	D48.2	D49.2
temporal region	C47.0	C79.89	—	D36.11	D48.2	D49.2
thigh	C47.2-☑	C79.89	—	D36.13	D48.2	D49.2
thoracic (duct) (wall)	C47.3	C79.89	—	D36.14	D48.2	D49.2
thorax	C47.3	C79.89	—	D36.14	D48.2	D49.2
thumb	C47.1-☑	C79.89	—	D36.12	D48.2	D49.2
toe	C47.2-☑	C79.89	—	D36.13	D48.2	D49.2
trunk	C47.6	C79.89	—	D36.17	D48.2	D49.2

Neoplasm, neoplastic —	Malignant Primary	Malignant Secondary	Ca in situ	Benign	Uncertain	Unspecified Behavior
continued						
nerve — *continued*						
peripheral — *continued*						
umbilicus	C47.4	C79.89	—	D36.15	D48.2	D49.2
vesicorectal	C47.5	C79.89	—	D36.16	D48.2	D49.2
wrist	C47.1-☑	C79.89	—	D36.12	D48.2	D49.2
radial	C47.1-☑	C79.89	—	D36.12	D48.2	D49.2
sacral	C47.5	C79.89	—	D36.16	D48.2	D49.2
sciatic	C47.2-☑	C79.89	—	D36.13	D48.2	D49.2
spinal NEC	C47.9	C79.89	—	D36.10	D48.2	D49.2
accessory	C72.59	C79.49	—	D33.3	D43.3	D49.7
sympathetic NEC — *see also* Neoplasm, nerve, peripheral	C47.9	C79.89	—	D36.10	D48.2	D49.2
trigeminal	C72.59	C79.49	—	D33.3	D43.3	D49.7
trochlear	C72.59	C79.49	—	D33.3	D43.3	D49.7
ulnar	C47.1-☑	C79.89	—	D36.12	D48.2	D49.2
vagus	C72.59	C79.49	—	D33.3	D43.3	D49.7
nervous system (central)	C72.9	C79.40	—	D33.9	D43.9	D49.7
autonomic — *see* Neoplasm, nerve, peripheral						
parasympathetic — *see* Neoplasm, nerve, peripheral						
specified site NEC	—	C79.49	—	D33.7	D43.8	—
sympathetic — *see* Neoplasm, nerve, peripheral						
nevus — *see* Nevus						
nipple	C50.0-☑	C79.81	D05.-☑	D24.-☑	—	—
nose, nasal	C76.0	C79.89	D09.8	D36.7	D48.7	D49.89
ala (external) (nasi) — *see also* Neoplasm, nose, skin	C44.301	C79.2	D04.39	D23.39	D48.5	D49.2
bone	C41.0	C79.51	—	D16.4	D48.0	D49.2
cartilage	C30.0	C78.39	D02.3	D14.0	D38.5	D49.1
cavity	C30.0	C78.39	D02.3	D14.0	D38.5	D49.1
choana	C11.3	C79.89	D00.08	D10.6	D37.05	D49.0
external (skin) — *see also* Neoplasm, nose, skin	C44.301	C79.2	D04.39	D23.39	D48.5	D49.2
fossa	C30.0	C78.39	D02.3	D14.0	D38.5	D49.1
internal	C30.0	C78.39	D02.3	D14.0	D38.5	D49.1
mucosa	C30.0	C78.39	D02.3	D14.0	D38.5	D49.1
septum	C30.0	C78.39	D02.3	D14.0	D38.5	D49.1
posterior margin	C11.3	C79.89	D00.08	D10.6	D37.05	D49.0
sinus — *see* Neoplasm, sinus						
skin	C44.301	C79.2	D04.39	D23.39	D48.5	D49.2
basal cell carcinoma	C44.311	—	—	—	—	—
specified type NEC	C44.391	—	—	—	—	—
squamous cell carcinoma	C44.321	—	—	—	—	—
turbinate (mucosa)	C30.0	C78.39	D02.3	D14.0	D38.5	D49.1
bone	C41.0	C79.51	—	D16.4	D48.0	D49.2
vestibule	C30.0	C78.39	D02.3	D14.0	D38.5	D49.1
nostril	C30.0	C78.39	D02.3	D14.0	D38.5	D49.1
nucleus pulposus	C41.2	C79.51	—	D16.6	D48.0	D49.2
occipital						
bone	C41.0	C79.51	—	D16.4	D48.0	D49.2
lobe or pole, brain	C71.4	C79.31	—	D33.0	D43.0	D49.6
odontogenic — *see* Neoplasm, jaw bone						
olfactory nerve or bulb	C72.2-☑	C79.49	—	D33.3	D43.3	D49.7
olive (brain)	C71.7	C79.31	—	D33.1	D43.1	D49.6
omentum	C48.1	C78.6	—	D20.1	D48.4	D49.0
operculum (brain)	C71.0	C79.31	—	D33.0	D43.0	D49.6
optic nerve, chiasm, or tract	C72.3-☑	C79.49	—	D33.3	D43.3	D49.7
oral (cavity)	C06.9	C79.89	D00.00	D10.30	D37.09	D49.0
ill-defined	C14.8	C79.89	D00.00	D10.30	D37.09	D49.0
mucosa	C06.0	C79.89	D00.02	D10.39	D37.09	D49.0
orbit	C69.6-☑	C79.49	D09.2-☑	D31.6-☑	D48.7	D49.89
autonomic nerve	C69.6-☑	C79.49	—	D31.6-☑	D48.7	D49.2
bone	C41.0	C79.51	—	D16.4	D48.0	D49.2

☑ Subterms under main terms may continue to next column or page   ☑ Additional Character Required — Refer to the Tabular List for Character Selection   341

Neoplasm, nerve — Neoplasm, orbit

Neoplasm, neoplastic — continued	Malignant Primary	Malignant Secondary	Ca in situ	Benign	Uncertain	Unspecified Behavior
orbit — continued						
eye	C69.6-✓	C79.49	D09.2-✓	D31.6-✓	D48.7	D49.89
peripheral nerves	C69.6-✓	C79.49	—	D31.6-✓	D48.7	D49.2
soft parts	C69.6-✓	C79.49	D09.2-✓	D31.6-✓	D48.7	D49.89
organ of Zuckerkandl	C75.5	C79.89	—	D35.6	D44.7	D49.7
oropharynx	C10.9	C79.89	D00.08	D10.5	D37.05	D49.0
branchial cleft (vestige)	C10.4	C79.89	D00.08	D10.5	D37.05	D49.0
junctional region	C10.8	C79.89	D00.08	D10.5	D37.05	D49.0
lateral wall	C10.2	C79.89	D00.08	D10.5	D37.05	D49.0
overlapping lesion	C10.8	—	—	—	—	—
pillars or fauces	C09.1	C79.89	D00.08	D10.5	D37.05	D49.0
posterior wall	C10.3	C79.89	D00.08	D10.5	D37.05	D49.0
vallecula	C10.0	C79.89	D00.08	D10.5	D37.05	D49.0
os						
external	C53.1	C79.82	D06.1	D26.0	D39.0	D49.59
internal	C53.0	C79.82	D06.0	D26.0	D39.0	D49.59
ovary	C56.-✓	C79.6-✓	D07.39	D27.-✓	D39.1-✓	D49.59
oviduct	C57.0-✓	C79.82	D07.39	D28.2	D39.8	D49.59
palate	C05.9	C79.89	D00.00	D10.39	D37.09	D49.0
hard	C05.0	C79.89	D00.05	D10.39	D37.09	D49.0
junction of hard and soft palate	C05.9	C79.89	D00.00	D10.39	D37.09	D49.0
overlapping lesions	C05.8	—	—	—	—	—
soft	C05.1	C79.89	D00.04	D10.39	D37.09	D49.0
nasopharyngeal surface	C11.3	C79.89	D00.08	D10.6	D37.05	D49.0
posterior surface	C11.3	C79.89	D00.08	D10.6	D37.05	D49.0
superior surface	C11.3	C79.89	D00.08	D10.6	D37.05	D49.0
palatoglossal arch	C09.1	C79.89	D00.00	D10.5	D37.09	D49.0
palatopharyngeal arch	C09.1	C79.89	D00.00	D10.5	D37.09	D49.0
pallium	C71.0	C79.31	—	D33.0	D43.0	D49.6
palpebra	C44.10-✓	C79.2	D04.1-✓	D23.1-✓	D48.5	D49.2
basal cell carcinoma	C44.11-✓	—	—	—	—	—
specified type NEC	C44.19-✓	—	—	—	—	—
squamous cell carcinoma	C44.12-✓	—	—	—	—	—
pancreas	C25.9	C78.89	D01.7	D13.6	D37.8	D49.0
body	C25.1	C78.89	D01.7	D13.6	D37.8	D49.0
duct (of Santorini) (of Wirsung)	C25.3	C78.89	D01.7	D13.6	D37.8	D49.0
ectopic tissue	C25.7	C78.89	—	D13.6	D37.8	D49.0
head	C25.0	C78.89	D01.7	D13.6	D37.8	D49.0
islet cells	C25.4	C78.89	D01.7	D13.7	D37.8	D49.0
neck	C25.7	C78.89	D01.7	D13.6	D37.8	D49.0
overlapping lesion	C25.8	—	—	—	—	—
tail	C25.2	C78.89	D01.7	D13.6	D37.8	D49.0
para-aortic body	C75.5	C79.89	—	D35.6	D44.7	D49.7
paraganglion NEC	C75.5	C79.89	—	D35.6	D44.7	D49.7
parametrium	C57.3	C79.82	—	D28.2	D39.8	D49.59
paranephric	C48.0	C78.6	—	D20.0	D48.3	D49.0
pararectal	C76.3	C79.89	—	D36.7	D48.7	D49.89
parasagittal (region)	C76.0	C79.89	D09.8	D36.7	D48.7	D49.89
parasellar	C72.9	C79.49	—	D33.9	D43.8	D49.7
parathyroid (gland)	C75.0	C79.89	D09.3	D35.1	D44.2	D49.7
paraurethral	C76.3	C79.89	—	D36.7	D48.7	D49.89
gland	C68.1	C79.19	D09.19	D30.8	D41.8	D49.59
paravaginal	C76.3	C79.89	—	D36.7	D48.7	D49.89
parenchyma, kidney	C64.-✓	C79.0-✓	D09.19	D30.0-✓	D41.0-✓	D49.51-✓
parietal						
bone	C41.0	C79.51	—	D16.4	D48.0	D49.2
lobe, brain	C71.3	C79.31	—	D33.0	D43.0	D49.6
paroophoron	C57.1-✓	C79.82	D07.39	D28.2	D39.8	D49.59
parotid (duct) (gland)	C07	C79.89	D00.00	D11.0	D37.030	D49.0
parovarium	C57.1-✓	C79.82	D07.39	D28.2	D39.8	D49.59
patella	C40.20	C79.51	—	—	—	—
peduncle, cerebral	C71.7	C79.31	—	D33.1	D43.1	D49.6
pelvirectal junction	C19	C78.5	D01.1	D12.7	D37.5	D49.0
pelvis, pelvic	C76.3	C79.89	D09.8	D36.7	D48.7	D49.89
bone	C41.4	C79.51	—	D16.8	D48.0	D49.2
floor	C76.3	C79.89	D09.8	D36.7	D48.7	D49.89
renal	C65.-✓	C79.0-✓	D09.19	D30.1-✓	D41.1-✓	D49.51-✓
viscera	C76.3	C79.89	D09.8	D36.7	D48.7	D49.89
wall	C76.3	C79.89	D09.8	D36.7	D48.7	D49.89
pelvo-abdominal	C76.8	C79.89	D09.8	D36.7	D48.7	D49.89
penis	C60.9	C79.82	D07.4	D29.0	D40.8	D49.59

Neoplasm, neoplastic — continued	Malignant Primary	Malignant Secondary	Ca in situ	Benign	Uncertain	Unspecified Behavior
penis — continued						
body	C60.2	C79.82	D07.4	D29.0	D40.8	D49.59
corpus (cavernosum)	C60.2	C79.82	D07.4	D29.0	D40.8	D49.59
glans	C60.1	C79.82	D07.4	D29.0	D40.8	D49.59
overlapping sites	C60.8	—	—	—	—	—
skin NEC	C60.9	C79.82	D07.4	D29.0	D40.8	D49.59
periadrenal (tissue)	C48.0	C78.6	—	D20.0	D48.3	D49.0
perianal (skin) — see also Neoplasm, anus, skin	C44.500	C79.2	D04.5	D23.5	D48.5	D49.2
pericardium	C38.0	C79.89	—	D15.1	D48.7	D49.89
perinephric	C48.0	C78.6	—	D20.0	D48.3	D49.0
perineum	C76.3	C79.89	D09.8	D36.7	D48.7	D49.89
periodontal tissue NEC	C03.9	C79.89	D00.03	D10.39	D37.09	D49.0
periosteum — see Neoplasm, bone						
peripancreatic	C48.0	C78.6	—	D20.0	D48.3	D49.0
peripheral nerve NEC	C47.9	C79.89	—	D36.10	D48.2	D49.2
perirectal (tissue)	C76.3	C79.89	—	D36.7	D48.7	D49.89
perirenal (tissue)	C48.0	C78.6	—	D20.0	D48.3	D49.0
peritoneum, peritoneal (cavity)	C48.2	C78.6	—	D20.1	D48.4	D49.0
benign mesothelial tissue — see Mesothelioma, benign						
overlapping lesion	C48.8	—	—	—	—	—
with digestive organs	C26.9					
parietal	C48.1	C78.6	—	D20.1	D48.4	D49.0
pelvic	C48.1	C78.6	—	D20.1	D48.4	D49.0
specified part NEC	C48.1	C78.6	—	D20.1	D48.4	D49.0
peritonsillar (tissue)	C76.0	C79.89	D09.8	D36.7	D48.7	D49.89
periurethral tissue	C76.3	C79.89	—	D36.7	D48.7	D49.89
phalanges						
foot	C40.3-✓	C79.51	—	D16.3-✓	—	—
hand	C40.1-✓	C79.51	—	D16.1-✓	—	—
pharynx, pharyngeal	C14.0	C79.89	D00.08	D10.9	D37.05	D49.0
bursa	C11.1	C79.89	D00.08	D10.6	D37.05	D49.0
fornix	C11.3	C79.89	D00.08	D10.6	D37.05	D49.0
recess	C11.2	C79.89	D00.08	D10.6	D37.05	D49.0
region	C14.0	C79.89	D00.08	D10.9	D37.05	D49.0
tonsil	C11.1	C79.89	D00.08	D10.6	D37.05	D49.0
wall (lateral) (posterior)	C14.0	C79.89	D00.08	D10.9	D37.05	D49.0
pia mater	C70.9	C79.40	—	D32.9	D42.9	D49.7
cerebral	C70.0	C79.32	—	D32.0	D42.0	D49.7
cranial	C70.0	C79.32	—	D32.0	D42.0	D49.7
spinal	C70.1	C79.49	—	D32.1	D42.1	D49.7
pillars of fauces	C09.1	C79.89	D00.08	D10.5	D37.05	D49.0
pineal (body) (gland)	C75.3	C79.89	D09.3	D35.4	D44.5	D49.7
pinna (ear) NEC — see also Neoplasm, skin, ear	C44.20-✓	C79.2	D04.2-✓	D23.2-✓	D48.5	D49.2
piriform fossa or sinus	C12	C79.89	D00.08	D10.7	D37.05	D49.0
pituitary (body) (fossa) (gland) (lobe)	C75.1	C79.89	D09.3	D35.2	D44.3	D49.7
placenta	C58	C79.82	D07.0	D26.7	D39.2	D49.59
pleura, pleural (cavity)	C38.4	C78.2	—	D19.0	D38.2	D49.1
overlapping lesion with heart or mediastinum	C38.8	—	—	—	—	—
parietal	C38.4	C78.2	—	D19.0	D38.2	D49.1
visceral	C38.4	C78.2	—	D19.0	D38.2	D49.1
plexus						
brachial	C47.1-✓	C79.89	—	D36.12	D48.2	D49.2
cervical	C47.0	C79.89	—	D36.11	D48.2	D49.2
choroid	C71.5	C79.31	—	D33.0	D43.0	D49.6
lumbosacral	C47.5	C79.89	—	D36.16	D48.2	D49.2
sacral	C47.5	C79.89	—	D36.16	D48.2	D49.2
pluriendocrine	C75.8	C79.89	D09.3	D35.7	D44.9	D49.7
pole						
frontal	C71.1	C79.31	—	D33.0	D43.0	D49.6
occipital	C71.4	C79.31	—	D33.0	D43.0	D49.6
pons (varolii)	C71.7	C79.31	—	D33.1	D43.1	D49.6

✓ Additional Character Required — Refer to the Tabular List for Character Selection   Subterms under main terms may continue to next column or page

Neoplasm, neoplastic — *continued*	Malignant Primary	Malignant Secondary	Ca in situ	Benign	Uncertain	Unspecified Behavior
popliteal fossa or space	C76.5-☑	C79.89	D04.7-☑	D36.7	D48.7	D49.89
postcricoid (region)	C13.0	C79.89	D00.08	D10.7	D37.05	D49.0
posterior fossa (cranial)	C71.9	C79.31	—	D33.2	D43.2	D49.6
postnasal space	C11.9	C79.89	D00.08	D10.6	D37.05	D49.0
prepuce	C60.0	C79.82	D07.4	D29.0	D40.8	D49.59
prepylorus	C16.4	C78.89	D00.2	D13.1	D37.1	D49.0
presacral (region)	C76.3	C79.89	—	D36.7	D48.7	D49.89
prostate (gland)	C61	C79.82	D07.5	D29.1	D40.0	D49.59
utricle	C68.0	C79.19	D09.19	D30.4	D41.3	D49.59
pterygoid fossa	C49.0	C79.89	—	D21.0	D48.1	D49.2
pubic bone	C41.4	C79.51	—	D16.8	D48.0	D49.2
pudenda, pudendum (female)	C51.9	C79.82	D07.1	D28.0	D39.8	D49.59
pulmonary — *see also* Neoplasm, lung	C34.9-☑	C78.0-☑	D02.2-☑	D14.3-☑	D38.1	D49.1
putamen	C71.0	C79.31	—	D33.0	D43.0	D49.6
pyloric						
antrum	C16.3	C78.89	D00.2	D13.1	D37.1	D49.0
canal	C16.4	C78.89	D00.2	D13.1	D37.1	D49.0
pylorus	C16.4	C78.89	D00.2	D13.1	D37.1	D49.0
pyramid (brain)	C71.7	C79.31	—	D33.1	D43.1	D49.6
pyriform fossa or sinus	C12	C79.89	D00.08	D10.7	D37.05	D49.0
radius (any part)	C40.0-☑	C79.51	—	D16.0-☑	—	—
Rathke's pouch	C75.1	C79.89	D09.3	D35.2	D44.3	D49.7
rectosigmoid (junction)	C19	C78.5	D01.1	D12.7	D37.5	D49.0
overlapping lesion with anus or rectum	C21.8	—	—	—	—	—
rectouterine pouch	C48.1	C78.6	—	D20.1	D48.4	D49.0
rectovaginal septum or wall	C76.3	C79.89	D09.8	D36.7	D48.7	D49.89
rectovesical septum	C76.3	C79.89	D09.8	D36.7	D48.7	D49.89
rectum (ampulla)	C20	C78.5	D01.2	D12.8	D37.5	D49.0
and colon	C19	C78.5	D01.1	D12.7	D37.5	D49.0
overlapping lesion with anus or rectosigmoid junction	C21.8	—	—	—	—	—
renal	C64.-☑	C79.0-☑	D09.19	D30.0-☑	D41.0-☑	D49.51-☑
calyx	C65.-☑	C79.0-☑	D09.19	D30.1-☑	D41.1-☑	D49.51-☑
hilus	C65.-☑	C79.0-☑	D09.19	D30.1-☑	D41.1-☑	D49.51-☑
parenchyma	C64.-☑	C79.0-☑	D09.19	D30.0-☑	D41.0-☑	D49.51-☑
pelvis	C65.-☑	C79.0-☑	D09.19	D30.1-☑	D41.1-☑	D49.51-☑
respiratory organs or system NEC	C39.9	C78.30	D02.4	D14.4	D38.6	D49.1
tract NEC	C39.9	C78.30	D02.4	D14.4	D38.5	D49.1
upper	C39.0	C78.30	D02.4	D14.4	D38.5	D49.1
retina	C69.2-☑	C79.49	D09.2-☑	D31.2-☑	D48.7	D49.81
retrobulbar	C69.6-☑	C79.49	—	D31.6-☑	D48.7	D49.89
retrocecal	C48.0	C78.6	—	D20.0	D48.3	D49.0
retromolar (area) (triangle) (trigone)	C06.2	C79.89	D00.00	D10.39	D37.09	D49.0
retro-orbital	C76.0	C79.89	D09.8	D36.7	D48.7	D49.89
retroperitoneal (space) (tissue)	C48.0	C78.6	—	D20.0	D48.3	D49.0
retroperitoneum	C48.0	C78.6	—	D20.0	D48.3	D49.0
retropharyngeal	C14.0	C79.89	D00.08	D10.9	D37.05	D49.0
retrovesical (septum)	C76.3	C79.89	D09.8	D36.7	D48.7	D49.89
rhinencephalon	C71.0	C79.31	—	D33.0	D43.0	D49.6
rib	C41.3	C79.51	—	D16.7	D48.0	D49.2
Rosenmuller's fossa	C11.2	C79.89	D00.08	D10.6	D37.05	D49.0
round ligament	C57.2-☑	C79.82	—	D28.2	D39.8	D49.59
sacrococcyx, sacrococcygeal	C41.4	C79.51	—	D16.8	D48.0	D49.2
region	C76.3	C79.89	D09.8	D36.7	D48.7	D49.89
sacrouterine ligament	C57.3	C79.82	—	D28.2	D39.8	D49.59
sacrum, sacral (vertebra)	C41.4	C79.51	—	D16.8	D48.0	D49.2
salivary gland or duct (major)	C08.9	C79.89	D00.00	D11.9	D37.039	D49.0
minor NEC	C06.9	C79.89	D00.00	D10.39	D37.04	D49.0
overlapping lesion	C08.9	—	—	—	—	—
parotid	C07	C79.89	D00.00	D11.0	D37.030	D49.0

Neoplasm, neoplastic — *continued*	Malignant Primary	Malignant Secondary	Ca in situ	Benign	Uncertain	Unspecified Behavior
salivary gland or duct — *continued*						
pluriglandular	C08.9	C79.89	D00.00	D11.9	D37.039	D49.0
sublingual	C08.1	C79.89	D00.00	D11.7	D37.031	D49.0
submandibular	C08.0	C79.89	D00.00	D11.7	D37.032	D49.0
submaxillary	C08.0	C79.89	D00.00	D11.7	D37.032	D49.0
salpinx (uterine)	C57.0-☑	C79.82	D07.39	D28.2	D39.8	D49.59
Santorini's duct	C25.3	C78.89	D01.7	D13.6	D37.8	D49.0
scalp	C44.40	C79.2	D04.4	D23.4	D48.5	D49.2
basal cell carcinoma	C44.41	—	—	—	—	—
specified type NEC	C44.49	—	—	—	—	—
squamous cell carcinoma	C44.42	—	—	—	—	—
scapula (any part)	C40.0-☑	C79.51	—	D16.0-☑	—	—
scapular region	C76.1	C79.89	D09.8	D36.7	D48.7	D49.89
scar NEC — *see also* Neoplasm, skin, by site	C44.90	C79.2	D04.9	D23.9	D48.5	D49.2
sciatic nerve	C47.2-☑	C79.89	—	D36.13	D48.2	D49.2
sclera	C69.4-☑	C79.49	D09.2-☑	D31.4-☑	D48.7	D49.89
scrotum (skin)	C63.2	C79.82	D07.61	D29.4	D40.8	D49.59
sebaceous gland — *see* Neoplasm, skin						
sella turcica	C75.1	C79.89	D09.3	D35.2	D44.3	D49.7
bone	C41.0	C79.51	—	D16.4	D48.0	D49.2
semilunar cartilage (knee)	C40.2-☑	C79.51	—	D16.2-☑	D48.0	D49.2
seminal vesicle	C63.7	C79.82	D07.69	D29.8	D40.8	D49.59
septum						
nasal	C30.0	C78.39	D02.3	D14.0	D38.5	D49.1
posterior margin	C11.3	C79.89	D00.08	D10.6	D37.05	D49.0
rectovaginal	C76.3	C79.89	D09.8	D36.7	D48.7	D49.89
rectovesical	C76.3	C79.89	D09.8	D36.7	D48.7	D49.89
urethrovaginal	C57.9	C79.82	D07.30	D28.9	D39.9	D49.59
vesicovaginal	C57.9	C79.82	D07.30	D28.9	D39.9	D49.59
shoulder NEC	C76.4-☑	C79.89	D04.6-☑	D36.7	D48.7	D49.89
sigmoid flexure (lower) (upper)	C18.7	C78.5	D01.0	D12.5	D37.4	D49.0
sinus (accessory)	C31.9	C78.39	D02.3	D14.0	D38.5	D49.1
bone (any)	C41.0	C79.51	—	D16.4	D48.0	D49.2
ethmoidal	C31.1	C78.39	D02.3	D14.0	D38.5	D49.1
frontal	C31.2	C78.39	D02.3	D14.0	D38.5	D49.1
maxillary	C31.0	C78.39	D02.3	D14.0	D38.5	D49.1
nasal, paranasal NEC	C31.9	C78.39	D02.3	D14.0	D38.5	D49.1
overlapping lesion	C31.8	—	—	—	—	—
pyriform	C12	C79.89	D00.08	D10.7	D37.05	D49.0
sphenoid	C31.3	C78.39	D02.3	D14.0	D38.5	D49.1
skeleton, skeletal NEC	C41.9	C79.51	—	D16.9	D48.0	D49.2
Skene's gland	C68.1	C79.19	D09.19	D30.8	D41.8	D49.59
skin NOS	C44.90	C79.2	D04.9	D23.9	D48.5	D49.2
abdominal wall	C44.509	C79.2	D04.5	D23.5	D48.5	D49.2
basal cell carcinoma	C44.519	—	—	—	—	—
specified type NEC	C44.599	—	—	—	—	—
squamous cell carcinoma	C44.529	—	—	—	—	—
ala nasi — *see also* Neoplasm, nose, skin	C44.301	C79.2	D04.39	D23.39	D48.5	D49.2
ankle — *see also* Neoplasm, skin, limb, lower	C44.70-☑	C79.2	D04.7-☑	D23.7-☑	D48.5	D49.2
antecubital space — *see also* Neoplasm, skin, limb, upper	C44.60-☑	C79.2	D04.6-☑	D23.6-☑	D48.5	D49.2
anus	C44.500	C79.2	D04.5	D23.5	D48.5	D49.2
basal cell carcinoma	C44.510	—	—	—	—	—
specified type NEC	C44.590	—	—	—	—	—
squamous cell carcinoma	C44.520	—	—	—	—	—
arm — *see also* Neoplasm, skin, limb, upper	C44.60-☑	C79.2	D04.6-☑	D23.6-☑	D48.5	D49.2

Neoplasm, neoplastic — continued	Malignant Primary	Malignant Secondary	Ca in situ	Benign	Uncertain	Unspecified Behavior
skin — continued						
auditory canal (external) — *see also* Neoplasm, skin, ear	C44.2Ø-☑	C79.2	DØ4.2-☑	D23.2-☑	D48.5	D49.2
auricle (ear) — *see also* Neoplasm, skin, ear	C44.2Ø-☑	C79.2	DØ4.2-☑	D23.2-☑	D48.5	D49.2
auricular canal (external) — *see also* Neoplasm, skin, ear	C44.2Ø-☑	C79.2	DØ4.2-☑	D23.2-☑	D48.5	D49.2
axilla, axillary fold — *see also* Neoplasm, skin, trunk	C44.5Ø9	C79.2	DØ4.5	D23.5	D48.5	D49.2
back — *see also* Neoplasm, skin, trunk	C44.5Ø9	C79.2	DØ4.5	D23.5	D48.5	D49.2
basal cell carcinoma	C44.91	—	—	—	—	—
breast	C44.5Ø1	C79.2	DØ4.5	D23.5	D48.5	D49.2
basal cell carcinoma	C44.511	—	—	—	—	—
specified type NEC	C44.591	—	—	—	—	—
squamous cell carcinoma	C44.521	—	—	—	—	—
brow — *see also* Neoplasm, skin, face	C44.3Ø9	C79.2	DØ4.39	D23.39	D48.5	D49.2
buttock — *see also* Neoplasm, skin, trunk	C44.5Ø9	C79.2	DØ4.5	D23.5	D48.5	D49.2
calf — *see also* Neoplasm, skin, limb, lower	C44.7Ø-☑	C79.2	DØ4.7-☑	D23.7-☑	D48.5	D49.2
canthus (eye) (inner) (outer)	C44.1Ø-☑	C79.2	DØ4.1-☑	D23.1-☑	D48.5	D49.2
basal cell carcinoma	C44.11-☑	—	—	—	—	—
specified type NEC	C44.19-☑	—	—	—	—	—
squamous cell carcinoma	C44.12-☑	—	—	—	—	—
cervical region — *see also* Neoplasm, skin, neck	C44.4Ø	C79.2	DØ4.4	D23.4	D48.5	D49.2
cheek (external) — *see also* Neoplasm, skin, face	C44.3Ø9	C79.2	DØ4.39	D23.39	D48.5	D49.2
chest (wall) — *see also* Neoplasm, skin, trunk	C44.5Ø9	C79.2	DØ4.5	D23.5	D48.5	D49.2
chin — *see also* Neoplasm, skin, face	C44.3Ø9	C79.2	DØ4.39	D23.39	D48.5	D49.2
clavicular area — *see also* Neoplasm, skin, trunk	C44.5Ø9	C79.2	DØ4.5	D23.5	D48.5	D49.2
clitoris	C51.2	C79.82	DØ7.1	D28.Ø	D39.8	D49.59
columnella — *see also* Neoplasm, skin, face	C44.3Ø9	C79.2	DØ4.39	D23.39	D48.5	D49.2
concha — *see also* Neoplasm, skin, ear	C44.2Ø-☑	C79.2	DØ4.2-☑	D23.2-☑	D48.5	D49.2
ear (external)	C44.2Ø-☑	C79.2	DØ4.2-☑	D23.2-☑	D48.5	D49.2
basal cell carcinoma	C44.21-☑	—	—	—	—	—
specified type NEC	C44.29-☑	—	—	—	—	—
squamous cell carcinoma	C44.22-☑	—	—	—	—	—
elbow — *see also* Neoplasm, skin, limb, upper	C44.6Ø-☑	C79.2	DØ4.6-☑	D23.6-☑	D48.5	D49.2
eyebrow — *see also* Neoplasm, skin, face	C44.3Ø9	C79.2	DØ4.39	D23.39	D48.5	D49.2
eyelid	C44.1Ø-☑	C79.2	DØ4.1-☑	D23.1-☑	D48.5	D49.2
Neoplasm, neoplastic — continued						
skin — continued						
eyelid — *continued*						
basal cell carcinoma	C44.11-☑	—	—	—	—	—
specified type NEC	C44.19-☑	—	—	—	—	—
squamous cell carcinoma	C44.12-☑	—	—	—	—	—
face NOS	C44.3ØØ	C79.2	DØ4.3Ø	D23.3Ø	D48.5	D49.2
basal cell carcinoma	C44.31Ø	—	—	—	—	—
specified type NEC	C44.39Ø	—	—	—	—	—
squamous cell carcinoma	C44.32Ø	—	—	—	—	—
female genital organs (external)	C51.9	C79.82	DØ7.1	D28.Ø	D39.8	D49.59
clitoris	C51.2	C79.82	DØ7.1	D28.Ø	D39.8	D49.59
labium NEC	C51.9	C79.82	DØ7.1	D28.Ø	D39.8	D49.59
majus	C51.Ø	C79.82	DØ7.1	D28.Ø	D39.8	D49.59
minus	C51.1	C79.82	DØ7.1	D28.Ø	D39.8	D49.59
pudendum	C51.9	C79.82	DØ7.1	D28.Ø	D39.8	D49.59
vulva	C51.9	C79.82	DØ7.1	D28.Ø	D39.8	D49.59
finger — *see also* Neoplasm, skin, limb, upper	C44.6Ø-☑	C79.2	DØ4.6-☑	D23.6-☑	D48.5	D49.2
flank — *see also* Neoplasm, skin, trunk	C44.5Ø9	C79.2	DØ4.5	D23.5	D48.5	D49.2
foot — *see also* Neoplasm, skin, limb, lower	C44.7Ø-☑	C79.2	DØ4.7-☑	D23.7-☑	D48.5	D49.2
forearm — *see also* Neoplasm, skin, limb, upper	C44.6Ø-☑	C79.2	DØ4.6-☑	D23.6-☑	D48.5	D49.2
forehead — *see also* Neoplasm, skin, face	C44.3Ø9	C79.2	DØ4.39	D23.39	D48.5	D49.2
glabella — *see also* Neoplasm, skin, face	C44.3Ø9	C79.2	DØ4.39	D23.39	D48.5	D49.2
gluteal region — *see also* Neoplasm, skin, trunk	C44.5Ø9	C79.2	DØ4.5	D23.5	D48.5	D49.2
groin — *see also* Neoplasm, skin, trunk	C44.5Ø9	C79.2	DØ4.5	D23.5	D48.5	D49.2
hand — *see also* Neoplasm, skin, limb, upper	C44.6Ø-☑	C79.2	DØ4.6-☑	D23.6-☑	D48.5	D49.2
head NEC — *see also* Neoplasm, skin, scalp	C44.4Ø	C79.2	DØ4.4	D23.4	D48.5	D49.2
heel — *see also* Neoplasm, skin, limb, lower	C44.7Ø-☑	C79.2	DØ4.7-☑	D23.7-☑	D48.5	D49.2
helix — *see also* Neoplasm, skin, ear	C44.2Ø-☑	C79.2	DØ4.2-☑	D23.2-☑	D48.5	D49.2
hip — *see also* Neoplasm, skin, limb, lower	C44.7Ø-☑	C79.2	DØ4.7-☑	D23.7-☑	D48.5	D49.2
infraclavicular region — *see also* Neoplasm, skin, trunk	C44.5Ø9	C79.2	DØ4.5	D23.5	D48.5	D49.2
inguinal region — *see also* Neoplasm, skin, trunk	C44.5Ø9	C79.2	DØ4.5	D23.5	D48.5	D49.2
jaw — *see also* Neoplasm, skin, face	C44.3Ø9	C79.2	DØ4.39	D23.39	D48.5	D49.2
Kaposi's sarcoma — *see* Kaposi's, sarcoma, skin						
knee — *see also* Neoplasm, skin, limb, lower	C44.7Ø-☑	C79.2	DØ4.7-☑	D23.7-☑	D48.5	D49.2
labia						
majora	C51.Ø	C79.82	DØ7.1	D28.Ø	D39.8	D49.59
minora	C51.1	C79.82	DØ7.1	D28.Ø	D39.8	D49.59

☑ Additional Character Required — Refer to the Tabular List for Character Selection   ▽ Subterms under main terms may continue to next column or page

Neoplasm, neoplastic — continued	Malignant Primary	Malignant Secondary	Ca in situ	Benign	Uncertain	Unspecified Behavior
skin — continued						
leg — see also Neoplasm, skin, limb, lower	C44.70-☑	C79.2	D04.7-☑	D23.7-☑	D48.5	D49.2
lid (lower) (upper)	C44.10-☑	C79.2	D04.1-☑	D23.1-☑	D48.5	D49.2
basal cell carcinoma	C44.11-☑	—	—	—	—	—
specified type NEC	C44.19-☑	—	—	—	—	—
squamous cell carcinoma	C44.12-☑	—	—	—	—	—
limb NEC	C44.90	C79.2	D04.9	D23.9	D48.5	D49.2
basal cell carcinoma	C44.91	—	—	—	—	—
lower	C44.70-☑	C79.2	D04.7-☑	D23.7-☑	D48.5	D49.2
basal cell carcinoma	C44.71-☑	—	—	—	—	—
specified type NEC	C44.79-☑	—	—	—	—	—
squamous cell carcinoma	C44.72-☑	—	—	—	—	—
upper	C44.60-☑	C79.2	D04.6-☑	D23.6-☑	D48.5	D49.2
basal cell carcinoma	C44.61-☑	—	—	—	—	—
specified type NEC	C44.69-☑	—	—	—	—	—
squamous cell carcinoma	C44.62-☑	—	—	—	—	—
lip (lower) (upper)	C44.00	C79.2	D04.0	D23.0	D48.5	D49.2
basal cell carcinoma	C44.01	—	—	—	—	—
specified type NEC	C44.09	—	—	—	—	—
squamous cell carcinoma	C44.02	—	—	—	—	—
male genital						
organs	C63.9	C79.82	D07.60	D29.9	D40.8	D49.59
penis	C60.9	C79.82	D07.4	D29.0	D40.8	D49.59
prepuce	C60.0	C79.82	D07.4	D29.0	D40.8	D49.59
scrotum	C63.2	C79.82	D07.61	D29.4	D40.8	D49.59
mastectomy site (skin) — see also Neoplasm, skin, breast	C44.501	C79.2	—	—	—	—
specified as breast tissue	C50.8-☑	C79.81	—	—	—	—
meatus, acoustic (external) — see also Neoplasm, skin, ear	C44.20-☑	C79.2	D04.2-☑	D23.2-☑	D48.5	D49.2
melanotic — see Melanoma						
Merkel cell — see Carcinoma, Merkel cell						
nates — see also Neoplasm, skin, trunk	C44.509	C79.2	D04.5	D23.5	D48.5	D49.2
neck	C44.40	C79.2	D04.4	D23.4	D48.5	D49.2
basal cell carcinoma	C44.41	—	—	—	—	—
specified type NEC	C44.49	—	—	—	—	—
squamous cell carcinoma	C44.42	—	—	—	—	—
nevus — see Nevus, skin						
nose (external) — see also Neoplasm, nose, skin	C44.301	C79.2	D04.39	D23.39	D48.5	D49.2
overlapping lesion	C44.80	—	—	—	—	—
basal cell carcinoma	C44.81	—	—	—	—	—
specified type NEC	C44.89	—	—	—	—	—
squamous cell carcinoma	C44.82	—	—	—	—	—
palm — see also Neoplasm, skin, limb, upper	C44.60-☑	C79.2	D04.6-☑	D23.6-☑	D48.5	D49.2
palpebra	C44.10-☑	C79.2	D04.1-☑	D23.1-☑	D48.5	D49.2
skin — continued						
palpebra — continued						
basal cell carcinoma	C44.11-☑	—	—	—	—	—
specified type NEC	C44.19-☑	—	—	—	—	—
squamous cell carcinoma	C44.12-☑	—	—	—	—	—
penis NEC	C60.9	C79.82	D07.4	D29.0	D40.8	D49.59
perianal — see also Neoplasm, skin, anus	C44.500	C79.2	D04.5	D23.5	D48.5	D49.2
perineum — see also Neoplasm, skin, anus	C44.500	C79.2	D04.5	D23.5	D48.5	D49.2
pinna — see also Neoplasm, skin, ear	C44.20-☑	C79.2	D04.2-☑	D23.2-☑	D48.5	D49.2
plantar — see also Neoplasm, skin, limb, lower	C44.70-☑	C79.2	D04.7-☑	D23.7-☑	D48.5	D49.2
popliteal fossa or space — see also Neoplasm, skin, limb, lower	C44.70-☑	C79.2	D04.7-☑	D23.7-☑	D48.5	D49.2
prepuce	C60.0	C79.82	D07.4	D29.0	D40.8	D49.59
pubes — see also Neoplasm, skin, trunk	C44.509	C79.2	D04.5	D23.5	D48.5	D49.2
sacrococcygeal region — see also Neoplasm, skin, trunk	C44.509	C79.2	D04.5	D23.5	D48.5	D49.2
scalp	C44.40	C79.2	D04.4	D23.4	D48.5	D49.2
basal cell carcinoma	C44.41	—	—	—	—	—
specified type NEC	C44.49	—	—	—	—	—
squamous cell carcinoma	C44.42	—	—	—	—	—
scapular region — see also Neoplasm, skin, trunk	C44.509	C79.2	D04.5	D23.5	D48.5	D49.2
scrotum	C63.2	C79.82	D07.61	D29.4	D40.8	D49.59
shoulder — see also Neoplasm, skin, limb, upper	C44.60-☑	C79.2	D04.6-☑	D23.6-☑	D48.5	D49.2
sole (foot) — see also Neoplasm, skin, limb, lower	C44.70-☑	C79.2	D04.7-☑	D23.7-☑	D48.5	D49.2
specified sites NEC	C44.80	C79.2	D04.8	D23.9	D48.5	D49.2
basal cell carcinoma	C44.81	—	—	—	—	—
specified type NEC	C44.89	—	—	—	—	—
squamous cell carcinoma	C44.82	—	—	—	—	—
specified type NEC	C44.99	—	—	—	—	—
squamous cell carcinoma	C44.92	—	—	—	—	—
submammary fold — see also Neoplasm, skin, trunk	C44.509	C79.2	D04.5	D23.5	D48.5	D49.2
supraclavicular region — see also Neoplasm, skin, neck	C44.40	C79.2	D04.4	D23.4	D48.5	D49.2
temple — see also Neoplasm, skin, face	C44.309	C79.2	D04.39	D23.39	D48.5	D49.2
thigh — see also Neoplasm, skin, limb, lower	C44.70-☑	C79.2	D04.7-☑	D23.7-☑	D48.5	D49.2
thoracic wall — see also Neoplasm, skin, trunk	C44.509	C79.2	D04.5	D23.5	D48.5	D49.2
thumb — see also Neoplasm, skin, limb, upper	C44.60-☑	C79.2	D04.6-☑	D23.6-☑	D48.5	D49.2
toe — see also Neoplasm, skin, limb, lower	C44.70-☑	C79.2	D04.7-☑	D23.7-☑	D48.5	D49.2

Neoplasm Table

Neoplasm, skin NOS — Neoplasm, tongue

Neoplasm, neoplastic —	Malignant Primary	Malignant Secondary	Ca in situ	Benign	Uncertain	Unspecified Behavior
continued						
skin — *continued*						
tragus — *see also* Neoplasm, skin,						
ear	C44.20-☑	C79.2	D04.2-☑	D23.2-☑	D48.5	D49.2
trunk	C44.509	C79.2	D04.5	D23.5	D48.5	D49.2
basal cell carcinoma	C44.519	—	—	—	—	—
specified type NEC	C44.599	—	—	—	—	—
squamous cell carcinoma	C44.529	—	—	—	—	—
umbilicus — *see also* Neoplasm, skin, trunk	C44.509	C79.2	D04.5	D23.5	D48.5	D49.2
vulva	C51.9	C79.82	D07.1	D28.0	D39.8	D49.59
overlapping lesion	C51.8	—	—	—	—	—
wrist — *see also* Neoplasm, skin, limb, upper	C44.60-☑	C79.2	D04.6-☑	D23.6-☑	D48.5	D49.2
skull	C41.0	C79.51	—	D16.4	D48.0	D49.2
soft parts or tissues — *see* Neoplasm, connective tissue						
specified site NEC	C76.8	C79.89	D09.8	D36.7	D48.7	D49.89
spermatic cord	C63.1-☑	C79.82	D07.69	D29.8	D40.8	D49.59
sphenoid	C31.3	C78.39	D02.3	D14.0	D38.5	D49.1
bone	C41.0	C79.51	—	D16.4	D48.0	D49.2
sinus	C31.3	C78.39	D02.3	D14.0	D38.5	D49.1
sphincter						
anal	C21.1	C78.5	D01.3	D12.9	D37.8	D49.0
of Oddi	C24.0	C78.89	D01.5	D13.5	D37.6	D49.0
spine, spinal (column)	C41.2	C79.51	—	D16.6	D48.0	D49.2
bulb	C71.7	C79.31	—	D33.1	D43.1	D49.6
coccyx	C41.4	C79.51	—	D16.8	D48.0	D49.2
cord (cervical) (lumbar) (sacral) (thoracic)	C72.0	C79.49	—	D33.4	D43.4	D49.7
dura mater	C70.1	C79.49	—	D32.1	D42.1	D49.7
lumbosacral	C41.2	C79.51	—	D16.6	D48.0	D49.2
marrow NEC	C96.9	C79.52	—	—	D47.9	D49.89
membrane	C70.1	C79.49	—	D32.1	D42.1	D49.7
meninges	C70.1	C79.49	—	D32.1	D42.1	D49.7
nerve (root)	C47.9	C79.89	—	D36.10	D48.2	D49.2
pia mater	C70.1	C79.49	—	D32.1	D42.1	D49.7
root	C47.9	C79.89	—	D36.10	D48.2	D49.2
sacrum	C41.4	C79.51	—	D16.8	D48.0	D49.2
spleen, splenic NEC	C26.1	C78.89	D01.7	D13.9	D37.8	D49.0
flexure (colon)	C18.5	C78.5	D01.0	D12.3	D37.4	D49.0
stem, brain	C71.7	C79.31	—	D33.1	D43.1	D49.6
Stensen's duct	C07	C79.89	D00.00	D11.0	D37.030	D49.0
sternum	C41.3	C79.51	—	D16.7	D48.0	D49.2
stomach	C16.9	C78.89	D00.2	D13.1	D37.1	D49.0
antrum (pyloric)	C16.3	C78.89	D00.2	D13.1	D37.1	D49.0
body	C16.2	C78.89	D00.2	D13.1	D37.1	D49.0
cardia	C16.0	C78.89	D00.2	D13.1	D37.1	D49.0
cardiac orifice	C16.0	C78.89	D00.2	D13.1	D37.1	D49.0
corpus	C16.2	C78.89	D00.2	D13.1	D37.1	D49.0
fundus	C16.1	C78.89	D00.2	D13.1	D37.1	D49.0
greater curvature NEC	C16.6	C78.89	D00.2	D13.1	D37.1	D49.0
lesser curvature NEC	C16.5	C78.89	D00.2	D13.1	D37.1	D49.0
overlapping lesion	C16.8	—	—	—	—	—
prepylorus	C16.4	C78.89	D00.2	D13.1	D37.1	D49.0
pylorus	C16.4	C78.89	D00.2	D13.1	D37.1	D49.0
wall NEC	C16.9	C78.89	D00.2	D13.1	D37.1	D49.0
anterior NEC	C16.8	C78.89	D00.2	D13.1	D37.1	D49.0
posterior NEC	C16.8	C78.89	D00.2	D13.1	D37.1	D49.0
stroma, endometrial	C54.1	C79.82	D07.0	D26.1	D39.0	D49.59
stump, cervical	C53.8	C79.82	D06.7	D26.0	D39.0	D49.59
subcutaneous (nodule) (tissue) NEC — *see* Neoplasm, connective tissue						
subdural	C70.9	C79.32	—	D32.9	D42.9	D49.7
subglottis, subglottic	C32.2	C78.39	D02.0	D14.1	D38.0	D49.1
sublingual	C04.9	C79.89	D00.06	D10.2	D37.09	D49.0
gland or duct	C08.1	C79.89	D00.00	D11.7	D37.031	D49.0

Neoplasm, neoplastic —	Malignant Primary	Malignant Secondary	Ca in situ	Benign	Uncertain	Unspecified Behavior
continued						
submandibular gland	C08.0	C79.89	D00.00	D11.7	D37.032	D49.0
submaxillary gland or duct	C08.0	C79.89	D00.00	D11.7	D37.032	D49.0
submental	C76.0	C79.89	D09.8	D36.7	D48.7	D49.89
subpleural	C34.9-☑	C78.0-☑	D02.2-☑	D14.3-☑	D38.1	D49.1
substernal	C38.1	C78.1	—	D15.2	D38.3	D49.89
sudoriferous, sudoriparous gland, site unspecified	C44.90	C79.2	D04.9	D23.9	D48.5	D49.2
specified site — *see* Neoplasm, skin						
supraclavicular region	C76.0	C79.89	D09.8	D36.7	D48.7	D49.89
supraglottis	C32.1	C78.39	D02.0	D14.1	D38.0	D49.1
suprarenal	C74.9-☑	C79.7-☑	D09.3	D35.0-☑	D44.1-☑	D49.7
capsule	C74.9-☑	C79.7-☑	D09.3	D35.0-☑	D44.1-☑	D49.7
cortex	C74.0-☑	C79.7-☑	D09.3	D35.0-☑	D44.1-☑	D49.7
gland	C74.9-☑	C79.7-☑	D09.3	D35.0-☑	D44.1-☑	D49.7
medulla	C74.1-☑	C79.7-☑	D09.3	D35.0-☑	D44.1-☑	D49.7
suprasellar (region)	C71.9	C79.31	—	D33.2	D43.2	D49.6
supratentorial (brain) NEC	C71.0	C79.31	—	D33.0	D43.0	D49.6
sweat gland (apocrine) (eccrine), site unspecified	C44.90	C79.2	D04.9	D23.9	D48.5	D49.2
specified site — *see* Neoplasm, skin						
sympathetic nerve or nervous system NEC	C47.9	C79.89	—	D36.10	D48.2	D49.2
symphysis pubis	C41.4	C79.51	—	D16.8	D48.0	D49.2
synovial membrane — *see* Neoplasm, connective tissue						
tapetum, brain	C71.8	C79.31	—	D33.2	D43.2	D49.6
tarsus (any bone)	C40.3-☑	C79.51	—	D16.3-☑	—	—
temple (skin) — *see also* Neoplasm, skin, face	C44.309	C79.2	D04.39	D23.39	D48.5	D49.2
temporal						
bone	C41.0	C79.51	—	D16.4	D48.0	D49.2
lobe or pole	C71.2	C79.31	—	D33.0	D43.0	D49.6
region	C76.0	C79.89	D09.8	D36.7	D48.7	D49.89
skin — *see also* Neoplasm, skin, face	C44.309	C79.2	D04.39	D23.39	D48.5	D49.2
tendon (sheath) — *see* Neoplasm, connective tissue						
tentorium (cerebelli)	C70.0	C79.32	—	D32.0	D42.0	D49.7
testis, testes	C62.9-☑	C79.82	D07.69	D29.2-☑	D40.1-☑	D49.59
descended	C62.1-☑	C79.82	D07.69	D29.2-☑	D40.1-☑	D49.59
ectopic	C62.0-☑	C79.82	D07.69	D29.2-☑	D40.1-☑	D49.59
retained	C62.0-☑	C79.82	D07.69	D29.2-☑	D40.1-☑	D49.59
scrotal	C62.1-☑	C79.82	D07.69	D29.2-☑	D40.1-☑	D49.59
undescended	C62.0-☑	C79.82	D07.69	D29.2-☑	D40.1-☑	D49.59
unspecified whether descended or undescended	C62.9-☑	C79.82	D07.69	D29.2-☑	D40.1-☑	D49.59
thalamus	C71.0	C79.31	—	D33.0	D43.0	D49.6
thigh NEC	C76.5-☑	C79.89	D04.7-☑	D36.7	D48.7	D49.89
thorax, thoracic (cavity) (organs NEC)	C76.1	C79.89	D09.8	D36.7	D48.7	D49.89
duct	C49.3	C79.89	—	D21.3	D48.1	D49.2
wall NEC	C76.1	C79.89	D09.8	D36.7	D48.7	D49.89
throat	C14.0	C79.89	D00.08	D10.9	D37.05	D49.0
thumb NEC	C76.4-☑	C79.89	D04.6-☑	D36.7	D48.7	D49.89
thymus (gland)	C37	C79.89	D09.3	D15.0	D38.4	D49.89
thyroglossal duct	C73	C79.89	D09.3	D34	D44.0	D49.7
thyroid (gland)	C73	C79.89	D09.3	D34	D44.0	D49.7
cartilage	C32.3	C78.39	D02.0	D14.1	D38.0	D49.1
tibia (any part)	C40.2-☑	C79.51	—	D16.2-☑	—	—
toe NEC	C76.5-☑	C79.89	D04.7-☑	D36.7	D48.7	D49.89
tongue	C02.9	C79.89	D00.07	D10.1	D37.02	D49.0
anterior (two-thirds) NEC	C02.3	C79.89	D00.07	D10.1	D37.02	D49.0
dorsal surface	C02.0	C79.89	D00.07	D10.1	D37.02	D49.0
ventral surface	C02.2	C79.89	D00.07	D10.1	D37.02	D49.0

☑ Additional Character Required — Refer to the Tabular List for Character Selection   ▽ Subterms under main terms may continue to next column or page

	Malignant Primary	Malignant Secondary	Ca in situ	Benign	Uncertain	Unspecified Behavior
Neoplasm, neoplastic — *continued*						
tongue — *continued*						
base (dorsal surface)	C01	C79.89	D00.07	D10.1	D37.02	D49.0
border (lateral)	C02.1	C79.89	D00.07	D10.1	D37.02	D49.0
dorsal surface NEC	C02.0	C79.89	D00.07	D10.1	D37.02	D49.0
fixed part NEC	C01	C79.89	D00.07	D10.1	D37.02	D49.0
foreamen cecum	C02.0	C79.89	D00.07	D10.1	D37.02	D49.0
frenulum linguae	C02.2	C79.89	D00.07	D10.1	D37.02	D49.0
junctional zone	C02.8	C79.89	D00.07	D10.1	D37.02	D49.0
margin (lateral)	C02.1	C79.89	D00.07	D10.1	D37.02	D49.0
midline NEC	C02.0	C79.89	D00.07	D10.1	D37.02	D49.0
mobile part NEC	C02.3	C79.89	D00.07	D10.1	D37.02	D49.0
overlapping lesion	C02.8	—	—	—	—	—
posterior (third)	C01	C79.89	D00.07	D10.1	D37.02	D49.0
root	C01	C79.89	D00.07	D10.1	D37.02	D49.0
surface (dorsal)	C02.0	C79.89	D00.07	D10.1	D37.02	D49.0
base	C01	C79.89	D00.07	D10.1	D37.02	D49.0
ventral	C02.2	C79.89	D00.07	D10.1	D37.02	D49.0
tip	C02.1	C79.89	D00.07	D10.1	D37.02	D49.0
tonsil	C02.4	C79.89	D00.07	D10.1	D37.02	D49.0
tonsil	C09.9	C79.89	D00.08	D10.4	D37.05	D49.0
fauces, faucial	C09.9	C79.89	D00.08	D10.4	D37.05	D49.0
lingual	C02.4	C79.89	D00.07	D10.1	D37.02	D49.0
overlapping sites	C09.8	—	—	—	—	—
palatine	C09.9	C79.89	D00.08	D10.4	D37.05	D49.0
pharyngeal	C11.1	C79.89	D00.08	D10.6	D37.05	D49.0
pillar (anterior) (posterior)	C09.1	C79.89	D00.08	D10.5	D37.05	D49.0
tonsillar fossa	C09.0	C79.89	D00.08	D10.5	D37.05	D49.0
tooth socket NEC	C03.9	C79.89	D00.03	D10.39	D37.09	D49.0
trachea (cartilage) (mucosa)	C33	C78.39	D02.1	D14.2	D38.1	D49.1
overlapping lesion with bronchus or lung	C34.8-☑	—	—	—	—	—
tracheobronchial	C34.8-☑	C78.39	D02.1	D14.2	D38.1	D49.1
overlapping lesion with lung	C34.8-☑	—	—	—	—	—
tragus — *see also* Neoplasm, skin, ear	C44.20-☑	C79.2	D04.2-☑	D23.2-☑	D48.5	D49.2
trunk NEC	C76.8	C79.89	D04.5	D36.7	D48.7	D49.89
tubo-ovarian	C57.8	C79.82	D07.39	D28.7	D39.8	D49.59
tunica vaginalis	C63.7	C79.82	D07.69	D29.8	D40.8	D49.59
turbinate (bone)	C41.0	C79.51	—	D16.4	D48.0	D49.2
nasal	C30.0	C78.39	D02.3	D14.0	D38.5	D49.1
tympanic cavity	C30.1	C78.39	D02.3	D14.0	D38.5	D49.1
ulna (any part)	C40.0-☑	C79.51	—	D16.0-☑	—	—
umbilicus, umbilical — *see also* Neoplasm, skin, trunk	C44.509	C79.2	D04.5	D23.5	D48.5	D49.2
uncus, brain	C71.2	C79.31	—	D33.0	D43.0	D49.6
unknown site or unspecified	C80.1	C79.9	D09.9	D36.9	D48.9	D49.9
urachus	C67.7	C79.11	D09.0	D30.3	D41.4	D49.4
ureter-bladder (junction)	C67.6	C79.11	D09.0	D30.3	D41.4	D49.4
ureter, ureteral	C66.-☑	C79.19	D09.19	D30.2-☑	D41.2-☑	D49.59
orifice (bladder)	C67.6	C79.11	D09.0	D30.3	D41.4	D49.4
urethra, urethral (gland)	C68.0	C79.19	D09.19	D30.4	D41.3	D49.59
orifice, internal	C67.5	C79.11	D09.0	D30.3	D41.4	D49.4
urethrovaginal (septum)	C57.9	C79.82	D07.30	D28.9	D39.8	D49.59
urinary organ or system	C68.9	C79.10	D09.10	D30.9	D41.9	D49.59
bladder — *see* Neoplasm, bladder						
overlapping lesion	C68.8	—	—	—	—	—
specified sites NEC	C68.8	C79.19	D09.19	D30.8	D41.8	D49.59
utero-ovarian	C57.8	C79.82	D07.39	D28.7	D39.8	D49.59
ligament	C57.1-☑	C79.82	D07.39	D28.2	D39.8	D49.59
uterosacral ligament	C57.3	C79.82	—	D28.2	D39.8	D49.59
uterus, uteri, uterine	C55	C79.82	D07.0	D26.9	D39.0	D49.59
adnexa NEC	C57.4	C79.82	D07.39	D28.7	D39.8	D49.59
body	C54.9	C79.82	D07.0	D26.1	D39.0	D49.59
cervix	C53.9	C79.82	D06.9	D26.0	D39.0	D49.59
cornu	C54.9	C79.82	D07.0	D26.1	D39.0	D49.59
corpus	C54.9	C79.82	D07.0	D26.1	D39.0	D49.59
endocervix (canal) (gland)	C53.0	C79.82	D06.0	D26.0	D39.0	D49.59

	Malignant Primary	Malignant Secondary	Ca in situ	Benign	Uncertain	Unspecified Behavior
Neoplasm, neoplastic — *continued*						
uterus, uteri, uterine — *continued*						
endometrium	C54.1	C79.82	D07.0	D26.1	D39.0	D49.59
exocervix	C53.1	C79.82	D06.1	D26.0	D39.0	D49.59
external os	C53.1	C79.82	D06.1	D26.0	D39.0	D49.59
fundus	C54.3	C79.82	D07.0	D26.1	D39.0	D49.59
internal os	C53.0	C79.82	D06.0	D26.0	D39.0	D49.59
isthmus	C54.0	C79.82	D07.0	D26.1	D39.0	D49.59
ligament	C57.3	C79.82	—	D28.2	D39.8	D49.59
broad	C57.1-☑	C79.82	D07.39	D28.2	D39.8	D49.59
round	C57.2-☑	C79.82	—	D28.2	D39.8	D49.59
lower segment	C54.0	C79.82	D07.0	D26.1	D39.0	D49.59
myometrium	C54.2	C79.82	D07.0	D26.1	D39.0	D49.59
overlapping sites	C54.8	—	—	—	—	—
squamocolumnar junction	C53.8	C79.82	D06.7	D26.0	D39.0	D49.59
tube	C57.0-☑	C79.82	D07.39	D28.2	D39.8	D49.59
utricle, prostatic	C68.0	C79.19	D09.19	D30.4	D41.3	D49.59
uveal tract	C69.4-☑	C79.49	D09.2-☑	D31.4-☑	D48.7	D49.89
uvula	C05.2	C79.89	D00.04	D10.39	D37.09	D49.0
vagina, vaginal (fornix) (vault) (wall)	C52	C79.82	D07.2	D28.1	D39.8	D49.59
vaginovesical	C57.9	C79.82	D07.30	D28.9	D39.9	D49.59
septum	C57.9	C79.82	D07.30	D28.9	D39.9	D49.59
vallecula (epiglottis)	C10.0	C79.89	D00.08	D10.5	D37.05	D49.0
vascular — *see* Neoplasm, connective tissue						
vas deferens	C63.1-☑	C79.82	D07.69	D29.8	D40.8	D49.59
Vater's ampulla	C24.1	C78.89	D01.5	D13.5	D37.6	D49.0
vein, venous — *see* Neoplasm, connective tissue						
vena cava (abdominal) (inferior)	C49.4	C79.89	—	D21.4	D48.1	D49.2
superior	C49.3	C79.89	—	D21.3	D48.1	D49.2
ventricle (cerebral) (floor) (lateral) (third)	C71.5	C79.31	—	D33.0	D43.0	D49.6
cardiac (left) (right)	C38.0	C79.89	—	D15.1	D48.7	D49.89
fourth	C71.7	C79.31	—	D33.1	D43.1	D49.6
ventricular band of larynx	C32.1	C78.39	D02.0	D14.1	D38.0	D49.1
ventriculus — *see* Neoplasm, stomach						
vermillion border — *see* Neoplasm, lip						
vermis, cerebellum	C71.6	C79.31	—	D33.1	D43.1	D49.6
vertebra (column)	C41.2	C79.51	—	D16.6	D48.0	D49.2
coccyx	C41.4	C79.51	—	D16.8	D48.0	D49.2
marrow NEC	C96.9	C79.52	—	—	D47.9	D49.89
sacrum	C41.4	C79.51	—	D16.8	D48.0	D49.2
vesical — *see* Neoplasm, bladder						
vesicle, seminal	C63.7	C79.82	D07.69	D29.8	D40.8	D49.59
vesicocervical tissue	C57.9	C79.82	D07.30	D28.9	D39.9	D49.59
vesicorectal	C76.3	C79.82	D09.8	D36.7	D48.7	D49.89
vesicovaginal	C57.9	C79.82	D07.30	D28.9	D39.9	D49.59
septum	C57.9	C79.82	D07.30	D28.9	D39.8	D49.59
vessel (blood) — *see* Neoplasm, connective tissue						
vestibular gland, greater	C51.0	C79.82	D07.1	D28.0	D39.8	D49.59
vestibule						
mouth	C06.1	C79.89	D00.00	D10.39	D37.09	D49.0
nose	C30.0	C78.39	D02.3	D14.0	D38.5	D49.1
Virchow's gland	C77.0	C77.0	—	D36.0	D48.7	D49.89
viscera NEC	C76.8	C79.89	D09.8	D36.7	D48.7	D49.89
vocal cords (true)	C32.0	C78.39	D02.0	D14.1	D38.0	D49.1
false	C32.1	C78.39	D02.0	D14.1	D38.0	D49.1
vomer	C41.0	C79.51	—	D16.4	D48.0	D49.2
vulva	C51.9	C79.82	D07.1	D28.0	D39.8	D49.59
vulvovaginal gland	C51.0	C79.82	D07.1	D28.0	D39.8	D49.59
Waldeyer's ring	C14.2	C79.89	D00.08	D10.9	D37.05	D49.0
Wharton's duct	C08.0	C79.89	D00.00	D11.7	D37.032	D49.0
white matter (central) (cerebral)	C71.9	C79.31	—	D33.0	D43.0	D49.6
windpipe	C33	C78.39	D02.1	D14.2	D38.1	D49.1
Wirsung's duct	C25.3	C78.89	D01.7	D13.6	D37.8	D49.0
wolffian (body) (duct) female	C57.7	C79.82	D07.39	D28.7	D39.8	D49.59

☑ Subterms under main terms may continue to next column or page   ☑ Additional Character Required — Refer to the Tabular List for Character Selection

	Malignant Primary	Malignant Secondary	Ca in situ	Benign	Uncertain	Unspecified Behavior
Neoplasm, neoplastic — *continued*						
wolffian — *continued*						
male	C63.7	C79.82	D07.69	D29.8	D40.8	D49.59
womb — *see* Neoplasm, uterus						
wrist NEC	C76.4-☑	C79.89	D04.6-☑	D36.7	D48.7	D49.89
xiphoid process	C41.3	C79.51	—	D16.7	D48.0	D49.2
Zuckerkandl organ	C75.5	C79.89	—	D35.6	D44.7	D49.7

☑ Additional Character Required — Refer to the Tabular List for Character Selection   ▽ Subterms under main terms may continue to next column or page

Substance	Poisoning, Accidental (unintentional)	Poisoning, Intentional Self-harm	Poisoning, Assault	Poisoning, Undetermined	Adverse Effect	Under-dosing
14-Hydroxydihydromorphinone	T40.2X1	T40.2X2	T40.2X3	T40.2X4	T40.2X5	T40.2X6
1-Propanol	T51.3X1	T51.3X2	T51.3X3	T51.3X4	—	—
2,3,7,8-Tetrachlorodibenzo-p-dioxin	T53.7X1	T53.7X2	T53.7X3	T53.7X4	—	—
2,4,5-T (trichlorophenoxyacetic acid)	T60.1X1	T60.1X2	T60.1X3	T60.1X4	—	—
2,4,5-Trichlorophenoxyacetic acid	T60.3X1	T60.3X2	T60.3X3	T60.3X4	—	—
2,4-D (dichlorophenoxyacetic acid)	T60.3X1	T60.3X2	T60.3X3	T60.3X4	—	—
2,4-Toluene diisocyanate	T65.0X1	T65.0X2	T65.0X3	T65.0X4	—	—
2-Deoxy-5-fluorouridine	T45.1X1	T45.1X2	T45.1X3	T45.1X4	T45.1X5	T45.1X6
2-Ethoxyethanol	T52.3X1	T52.3X2	T52.3X3	T52.3X4	—	—
2-Methoxyethanol	T52.3X1	T52.3X2	T52.3X3	T52.3X4	—	—
2-Propanol	T51.2X1	T51.2X2	T51.2X3	T51.2X4	—	—
4-Aminobutyric acid	T43.8X1	T43.8X2	T43.8X3	T43.8X4	T43.8X5	T43.8X6
4-Aminophenol derivatives	T39.1X1	T39.1X2	T39.1X3	T39.1X4	T39.1X5	T39.1X6
5-Deoxy-5-fluorouridine	T45.1X1	T45.1X2	T45.1X3	T45.1X4	T45.1X5	T45.1X6
5-Methoxypsoralen (5-MOP)	T50.991	T50.992	T50.993	T50.994	T50.995	T50.996
8-Aminoquinoline drugs	T37.2X1	T37.2X2	T37.2X3	T37.2X4	T37.2X5	T37.2X6
8-Methoxypsoralen (8-MOP)	T50.991	T50.992	T50.993	T50.994	T50.995	T50.996
ABOB	T37.5X1	T37.5X2	T37.5X3	T37.5X4	T37.5X5	T37.5X6
Abrine	T62.2X1	T62.2X2	T62.2X3	T62.2X4	—	—
Abrus (seed)	T62.2X1	T62.2X2	T62.2X3	T62.2X4	—	—
Absinthe	T51.0X1	T51.0X2	T51.0X3	T51.0X4	—	—
beverage	T51.0X1	T51.0X2	T51.0X3	T51.0X4	—	—
Acaricide	T60.8X1	T60.8X2	T60.8X3	T60.8X4	—	—
Acebutolol	T44.7X1	T44.7X2	T44.7X3	T44.7X4	T44.7X5	T44.7X6
Acecarbromal	T42.6X1	T42.6X2	T42.6X3	T42.6X4	T42.6X5	T42.6X6
Aceclidine	T44.1X1	T44.1X2	T44.1X3	T44.1X4	T44.1X5	T44.1X6
Acedapsone	T37.0X1	T37.0X2	T37.0X3	T37.0X4	T37.0X5	T37.0X6
Acefylline piperazine	T48.6X1	T48.6X2	T48.6X3	T48.6X4	T48.6X5	T48.6X6
Acemorphan	T40.2X1	T40.2X2	T40.2X3	T40.2X4	T40.2X5	T40.2X6
Acenocoumarin	T45.511	T45.512	T45.513	T45.514	T45.515	T45.516
Acenocoumarol	T45.511	T45.512	T45.513	T45.514	T45.515	T45.516
Acepifylline	T48.6X1	T48.6X2	T48.6X3	T48.6X4	T48.6X5	T48.6X6
Acepromazine	T43.3X1	T43.3X2	T43.3X3	T43.3X4	T43.3X5	T43.3X6
Acesulfamethoxypyridazine	T37.0X1	T37.0X2	T37.0X3	T37.0X4	T37.0X5	T37.0X6
Acetal	T52.8X1	T52.8X2	T52.8X3	T52.8X4	—	—
Acetaldehyde (vapor)	T52.8X1	T52.8X2	T52.8X3	T52.8X4	—	—
liquid	T65.891	T65.892	T65.893	T65.894	—	—
Acetaminophen	T39.1X1	T39.1X2	T39.1X3	T39.1X4	T39.1X5	T39.1X6
Acetaminosalol	T39.1X1	T39.1X2	T39.1X3	T39.1X4	T39.1X5	T39.1X6
Acetanilide	T39.1X1	T39.1X2	T39.1X3	T39.1X4	T39.1X5	T39.1X6
Acetarsol	T37.3X1	T37.3X2	T37.3X3	T37.3X4	T37.3X5	T37.3X6
Acetazolamide	T50.2X1	T50.2X2	T50.2X3	T50.2X4	T50.2X5	T50.2X6
Acetiamine	T45.2X1	T45.2X2	T45.2X3	T45.2X4	T45.2X5	T45.2X6
Acetic						
acid	T54.2X1	T54.2X2	T54.2X3	T54.2X4	—	—
with sodium acetate (ointment)	T49.3X1	T49.3X2	T49.3X3	T49.3X4	T49.3X5	T49.3X6
ester (solvent)(vapor)	T52.8X1	T52.8X2	T52.8X3	T52.8X4	—	—
irrigating solution	T50.3X1	T50.3X2	T50.3X3	T50.3X4	T50.3X5	T50.3X6
medicinal (lotion)	T49.2X1	T49.2X2	T49.2X3	T49.2X4	T49.2X5	T49.2X6
anhydride	T65.891	T65.892	T65.893	T65.894	—	—
ether (vapor)	T52.8X1	T52.8X2	T52.8X3	T52.8X4	—	—
Acetohexamide	T38.3X1	T38.3X2	T38.3X3	T38.3X4	T38.3X5	T38.3X6
Acetohydroxamic acid	T50.991	T50.992	T50.993	T50.994	T50.995	T50.996
Acetomenaphthone	T45.7X1	T45.7X2	T45.7X3	T45.7X4	T45.7X5	T45.7X6
Acetomorphine	T40.1X1	T40.1X2	T40.1X3	T40.1X4	—	—
Acetone (oils)	T52.4X1	T52.4X2	T52.4X3	T52.4X4	—	—
chlorinated	T52.4X1	T52.4X2	T52.4X3	T52.4X4	—	—
vapor	T52.4X1	T52.4X2	T52.4X3	T52.4X4	—	—
Acetonitrile	T52.8X1	T52.8X2	T52.8X3	T52.8X4	—	—
Acetophenazine	T43.3X1	T43.3X2	T43.3X3	T43.3X4	T43.3X5	T43.3X6
Acetophenetedin	T39.1X1	T39.1X2	T39.1X3	T39.1X4	T39.1X5	T39.1X6
Acetophenone	T52.4X1	T52.4X2	T52.4X3	T52.4X4	—	—
Acetorphine	T40.2X1	T40.2X2	T40.2X3	T40.2X4	—	—
Acetosulfone (sodium)	T37.1X1	T37.1X2	T37.1X3	T37.1X4	T37.1X5	T37.1X6
Acetrizoate (sodium)	T50.8X1	T50.8X2	T50.8X3	T50.8X4	T50.8X5	T50.8X6
Acetrizoic acid	T50.8X1	T50.8X2	T50.8X3	T50.8X4	T50.8X5	T50.8X6
Acetyl						
bromide	T53.6X1	T53.6X2	T53.6X3	T53.6X4	—	—
chloride	T53.6X1	T53.6X2	T53.6X3	T53.6X4	—	—
Acetylcarbromal	T42.6X1	T42.6X2	T42.6X3	T42.6X4	T42.6X5	T42.6X6
Acetylcholine						
chloride	T44.1X1	T44.1X2	T44.1X3	T44.1X4	T44.1X5	T44.1X6
derivative	T44.1X1	T44.1X2	T44.1X3	T44.1X4	T44.1X5	T44.1X6
Acetylcysteine	T48.4X1	T48.4X2	T48.4X3	T48.4X4	T48.4X5	T48.4X6
Acetyldigitoxin	T46.0X1	T46.0X2	T46.0X3	T46.0X4	T46.0X5	T46.0X6
Acetyldigoxin	T46.0X1	T46.0X2	T46.0X3	T46.0X4	T46.0X5	T46.0X6

Substance	Poisoning, Accidental (unintentional)	Poisoning, Intentional Self-harm	Poisoning, Assault	Poisoning, Undetermined	Adverse Effect	Under-dosing
Acetyldihydrocodeine	T40.2X1	T40.2X2	T40.2X3	T40.2X4	—	—
Acetyldihydrocodeinone	T40.2X1	T40.2X2	T40.2X3	T40.2X4	—	—
Acetylene (gas)	T59.891	T59.892	T59.893	T59.894	—	—
dichloride	T53.6X1	T53.6X2	T53.6X3	T53.6X4	—	—
incomplete combustion of	T58.11	T58.12	T58.13	T58.14	—	—
industrial	T59.891	T59.892	T59.893	T59.894	—	—
tetrachloride	T53.6X1	T53.6X2	T53.6X3	T53.6X4	—	—
vapor	T53.6X1	T53.6X2	T53.6X3	T53.6X4	—	—
Acetylpheneturide	T42.6X1	T42.6X2	T42.6X3	T42.6X4	T42.6X5	T42.6X6
Acetylphenylhydrazine	T39.8X1	T39.8X2	T39.8X3	T39.8X4	T39.8X5	T39.8X6
Acetylsalicylic acid (salts)	T39.011	T39.012	T39.013	T39.014	T39.015	T39.016
enteric coated	T39.011	T39.012	T39.013	T39.014	T39.015	T39.016
Acetylsulfamethoxypyridazine	T37.0X1	T37.0X2	T37.0X3	T37.0X4	T37.0X5	T37.0X6
Achromycin	T36.4X1	T36.4X2	T36.4X3	T36.4X4	T36.4X5	T36.4X6
ophthalmic preparation	T49.5X1	T49.5X2	T49.5X3	T49.5X4	T49.5X5	T49.5X6
topical NEC	T49.0X1	T49.0X2	T49.0X3	T49.0X4	T49.0X5	T49.0X6
Aciclovir	T37.5X1	T37.5X2	T37.5X3	T37.5X4	T37.5X5	T37.5X6
Acidifying agent NEC	T50.901	T50.902	T50.903	T50.904	T50.905	T50.906
Acid (corrosive) NEC	T54.2X1	T54.2X2	T54.2X3	T54.2X4	—	—
Acipimox	T46.6X1	T46.6X2	T46.6X3	T46.6X4	T46.6X5	T46.6X6
Acitretin	T50.991	T50.992	T50.993	T50.994	T50.995	T50.996
Aclarubicin	T45.1X1	T45.1X2	T45.1X3	T45.1X4	T45.1X5	T45.1X6
Aclatonium napadisilate	T48.1X1	T48.1X2	T48.1X3	T48.1X4	T48.1X5	T48.1X6
Aconite (wild)	T46.991	T46.992	T46.993	T46.994	T46.995	T46.996
Aconitine	T46.991	T46.992	T46.993	T46.994	T46.995	T46.996
Aconitum ferox	T46.991	T46.992	T46.993	T46.994	T46.995	T46.996
Acridine	T65.6X1	T65.6X2	T65.6X3	T65.6X4	—	—
vapor	T59.891	T59.892	T59.893	T59.894	—	—
Acriflavine	T37.91	T37.92	T37.93	T37.94	T37.95	T37.96
Acriflavinium chloride	T49.0X1	T49.0X2	T49.0X3	T49.0X4	T49.0X5	T49.0X6
Acrinol	T49.0X1	T49.0X2	T49.0X3	T49.0X4	T49.0X5	T49.0X6
Acrisorcin	T49.0X1	T49.0X2	T49.0X3	T49.0X4	T49.0X5	T49.0X6
Acrivastine	T45.0X1	T45.0X2	T45.0X3	T45.0X4	T45.0X5	T45.0X6
Acrolein (gas)	T59.891	T59.892	T59.893	T59.894	—	—
liquid	T54.1X1	T54.1X2	T54.1X3	T54.1X4	—	—
Acrylamide	T65.891	T65.892	T65.893	T65.894	—	—
Acrylic resin	T49.3X1	T49.3X2	T49.3X3	T49.3X4	T49.3X5	T49.3X6
Acrylonitrile	T65.891	T65.892	T65.893	T65.894	—	—
Actaea spicata	T62.2X1	T62.2X2	T62.2X3	T62.2X4	—	—
berry	T62.1X1	T62.1X2	T62.1X3	T62.1X4	—	—
Acterol	T37.3X1	T37.3X2	T37.3X3	T37.3X4	T37.3X5	T37.3X6
ACTH	T38.811	T38.812	T38.813	T38.814	T38.815	T38.816
Actinomycin C	T45.1X1	T45.1X2	T45.1X3	T45.1X4	T45.1X5	T45.1X6
Actinomycin D	T45.1X1	T45.1X2	T45.1X3	T45.1X4	T45.1X5	T45.1X6
Activated charcoal — see also Charcoal, medicinal	T47.6X1	T47.6X2	T47.6X3	T47.6X4	T47.6X5	T47.6X6
Acyclovir	T37.5X1	T37.5X2	T37.5X3	T37.5X4	T37.5X5	T37.5X6
Adenine	T45.2X1	T45.2X2	T45.2X3	T45.2X4	T45.2X5	T45.2X6
arabinoside	T37.5X1	T37.5X2	T37.5X3	T37.5X4	T37.5X5	T37.5X6
Adenosine (phosphate)	T46.2X1	T46.2X2	T46.2X3	T46.2X4	T46.2X5	T46.2X6
ADH	T38.891	T38.892	T38.893	T38.894	T38.895	T38.896
Adhesive NEC	T65.891	T65.892	T65.893	T65.894	—	—
Adicillin	T36.0X1	T36.0X2	T36.0X3	T36.0X4	T36.0X5	T36.0X6
Adiphenine	T44.3X1	T44.3X2	T44.3X3	T44.3X4	T44.3X5	T44.3X6
Adipiodone	T50.8X1	T50.8X2	T50.8X3	T50.8X4	T50.8X5	T50.8X6
Adjunct, pharmaceutical	T50.901	T50.902	T50.903	T50.904	T50.905	T50.906
Adrenal (extract, cortex or medulla) (glucocorticoids) (hormones) (mineralocorticoids)	T38.0X1	T38.0X2	T38.0X3	T38.0X4	T38.0X5	T38.0X6
ENT agent	T49.6X1	T49.6X2	T49.6X3	T49.6X4	T49.6X5	T49.6X6
ophthalmic preparation	T49.5X1	T49.5X2	T49.5X3	T49.5X4	T49.5X5	T49.5X6
topical NEC	T49.0X1	T49.0X2	T49.0X3	T49.0X4	T49.0X5	T49.0X6
Adrenalin — see Adrenaline						
Adrenaline	T44.5X1	T44.5X2	T44.5X3	T44.5X4	T44.5X5	T44.5X6
Adrenergic NEC	T44.901	T44.902	T44.903	T44.904	T44.905	T44.906
blocking agent NEC	T44.8X1	T44.8X2	T44.8X3	T44.8X4	T44.8X5	T44.8X6
beta, heart†	T44.7X1	T44.7X2	T44.7X3	T44.7X4	T44.7X5	T44.7X6
specified NEC	T44.991	T44.992	T44.993	T44.994	T44.995	T44.996
Adrenochrome						
derivative	T46.991	T46.992	T46.993	T46.994	T46.995	T46.996
(mono) semicarbazone	T46.991	T46.992	T46.993	T46.994	T46.995	T46.996
Adrenocorticotrophic hormone	T38.811	T38.812	T38.813	T38.814	T38.815	T38.816
Adrenocorticotrophin	T38.811	T38.812	T38.813	T38.814	T38.815	T38.816
Adriamycin	T45.1X1	T45.1X2	T45.1X3	T45.1X4	T45.1X5	T45.1X6
Aerosol spray NEC	T65.91	T65.92	T65.93	T65.94	—	—
Aerosporin	T36.8X1	T36.8X2	T36.8X3	T36.8X4	T36.8X5	T36.8X6
ENT agent	T49.6X1	T49.6X2	T49.6X3	T49.6X4	T49.6X5	T49.6X6
ophthalmic preparation	T49.5X1	T49.5X2	T49.5X3	T49.5X4	T49.5X5	T49.5X6
topical NEC	T49.0X1	T49.0X2	T49.0X3	T49.0X4	T49.0X5	T49.0X6
Aethusa cynapium	T62.2X1	T62.2X2	T62.2X3	T62.2X4	—	—
Afghanistan black	T40.7X1	T40.7X2	T40.7X3	T40.7X4	T40.7X5	T40.7X6

Substance	Poisoning, Accidental (unintentional)	Poisoning, Intentional Self-harm	Poisoning, Assault	Poisoning, Undetermined	Adverse Effect	Under-dosing
Aflatoxin	T64.01	T64.02	T64.03	T64.04	—	—
Afloqualone	T42.8X1	T42.8X2	T42.8X3	T42.8X4	T42.8X5	T42.8X6
African boxwood	T62.2X1	T62.2X2	T62.2X3	T62.2X4		
Agar	T47.4X1	T47.4X2	T47.4X3	T47.4X4	T47.4X5	T47.4X6
Agonist						
predominantly						
alpha-adrenoreceptor	T44.4X1	T44.4X2	T44.4X3	T44.4X4	T44.4X5	T44.4X6
beta-adrenoreceptor	T44.5X1	T44.5X2	T44.5X3	T44.5X4	T44.5X5	T44.5X6
Agricultural agent NEC	T65.91	T65.92	T65.93	T65.94	—	—
Agrypnal	T42.3X1	T42.3X2	T42.3X3	T42.3X4	T42.3X5	T42.3X6
AHLG	T50.Z11	T50.Z12	T50.Z13	T50.Z14	T50.Z15	T50.Z16
Air contaminant(s), source/type NOS	T65.91	T65.92	T65.93	T65.94	—	—
Ajmaline	T46.2X1	T46.2X2	T46.2X3	T46.2X4	T46.2X5	T46.2X6
Akee	T62.1X1	T62.1X2	T62.1X3	T62.1X4		
Akrinol	T49.0X1	T49.0X2	T49.0X3	T49.0X4	T49.0X5	T49.0X6
Akritoin	T37.8X1	T37.8X2	T37.8X3	T37.8X4	T37.8X5	T37.8X6
Alacepril	T46.4X1	T46.4X2	T46.4X3	T46.4X4	T46.4X5	T46.4X6
Alantolactone	T37.4X1	T37.4X2	T37.4X3	T37.4X4	T37.4X5	T37.4X6
Albamycin	T36.8X1	T36.8X2	T36.8X3	T36.8X4	T36.8X5	T36.8X6
Albendazole	T37.4X1	T37.4X2	T37.4X3	T37.4X4	T37.4X5	T37.4X6
Albumin						
bovine	T45.8X1	T45.8X2	T45.8X3	T45.8X4	T45.8X5	T45.8X6
human serum	T45.8X1	T45.8X2	T45.8X3	T45.8X4	T45.8X5	T45.8X6
salt-poor	T45.8X1	T45.8X2	T45.8X3	T45.8X4	T45.8X5	T45.8X6
normal human serum	T45.8X1	T45.8X2	T45.8X3	T45.8X4	T45.8X5	T45.8X6
Albuterol	T48.6X1	T48.6X2	T48.6X3	T48.6X4	T48.6X5	T48.6X6
Albutoin	T42.0X1	T42.0X2	T42.0X3	T42.0X4	T42.0X5	T42.0X6
Aclometasone	T49.0X1	T49.0X2	T49.0X3	T49.0X4	T49.0X5	T49.0X6
Alcohol	T51.91	T51.92	T51.93	T51.94	—	—
absolute	T51.0X1	T51.0X2	T51.0X3	T51.0X4	—	—
beverage	T51.0X1	T51.0X2	T51.0X3	T51.0X4	—	—
allyl	T51.8X1	T51.8X2	T51.8X3	T51.8X4	—	—
amyl	T51.3X1	T51.3X2	T51.3X3	T51.3X4	—	—
antifreeze	T51.1X1	T51.1X2	T51.1X3	T51.1X4	—	—
beverage	T51.0X1	T51.0X2	T51.0X3	T51.0X4	—	—
butyl	T51.3X1	T51.3X2	T51.3X3	T51.3X4	—	—
dehydrated	T51.0X1	T51.0X2	T51.0X3	T51.0X4	—	—
beverage	T51.0X1	T51.0X2	T51.0X3	T51.0X4	—	—
denatured	T51.0X1	T51.0X2	T51.0X3	T51.0X4	—	—
deterrent NEC	T50.6X1	T50.6X2	T50.6X3	T50.6X4	T50.6X5	T50.6X6
diagnostic (gastric function)	T50.8X1	T50.8X2	T50.8X3	T50.8X4	T50.8X5	T50.8X6
ethyl	T51.0X1	T51.0X2	T51.0X3	T51.0X4	—	—
beverage	T51.0X1	T51.0X2	T51.0X3	T51.0X4	—	—
grain	T51.0X1	T51.0X2	T51.0X3	T51.0X4	—	—
beverage	T51.0X1	T51.0X2	T51.0X3	T51.0X4	—	—
industrial	T51.0X1	T51.0X2	T51.0X3	T51.0X4	—	—
isopropyl	T51.2X1	T51.2X2	T51.2X3	T51.2X4	—	—
methyl	T51.1X1	T51.1X2	T51.1X3	T51.1X4	—	—
preparation for consumption	T51.0X1	T51.0X2	T51.0X3	T51.0X4	—	—
propyl	T51.3X1	T51.3X2	T51.3X3	T51.3X4	—	—
secondary	T51.2X1	T51.2X2	T51.2X3	T51.2X4	—	—
radiator	T51.1X1	T51.1X2	T51.1X3	T51.1X4	—	—
rubbing	T51.2X1	T51.2X2	T51.2X3	T51.2X4	—	—
specified type NEC	T51.8X1	T51.8X2	T51.8X3	T51.8X4	—	—
surgical	T51.0X1	T51.0X2	T51.0X3	T51.0X4	—	—
vapor (from any type of Alcohol)	T59.891	T59.892	T59.893	T59.894	—	—
wood	T51.1X1	T51.1X2	T51.1X3	T51.1X4	—	—
Alcuronium (chloride)	T48.1X1	T48.1X2	T48.1X3	T48.1X4	T48.1X5	T48.1X6
Aldactone	T50.0X1	T50.0X2	T50.0X3	T50.0X4	T50.0X5	T50.0X6
Aldesulfone sodium	T37.1X1	T37.1X2	T37.1X3	T37.1X4	T37.1X5	T37.1X6
Aldicarb	T60.0X1	T60.0X2	T60.0X3	T60.0X4		
Aldomet	T46.5X1	T46.5X2	T46.5X3	T46.5X4	T46.5X5	T46.5X6
Aldosterone	T50.0X1	T50.0X2	T50.0X3	T50.0X4	T50.0X5	T50.0X6
Aldrin (dust)	T60.1X1	T60.1X2	T60.1X3	T60.1X4		
Aleve — *see* Naproxen						
Alexitol sodium	T47.1X1	T47.1X2	T47.1X3	T47.1X4	T47.1X5	T47.1X6
Alfacalcidol	T45.2X1	T45.2X2	T45.2X3	T45.2X4	T45.2X5	T45.2X6
Alfadolone	T41.1X1	T41.1X2	T41.1X3	T41.1X4	T41.1X5	T41.1X6
Alfaxalone	T41.1X1	T41.1X2	T41.1X3	T41.1X4	T41.1X5	T41.1X6
Alfentanil	T40.4X1	T40.4X2	T40.4X3	T40.4X4	T40.4X5	T40.4X6
Alfuzosin (hydrochloride)	T44.8X1	T44.8X2	T44.8X3	T44.8X4	T44.8X5	T44.8X6
Algae (harmful) (toxin)	T65.821	T65.822	T65.823	T65.824	—	—
Algeldrate	T47.1X1	T47.1X2	T47.1X3	T47.1X4	T47.1X5	T47.1X6
Algin	T47.8X1	T47.8X2	T47.8X3	T47.8X4	T47.8X5	T47.8X6
Alglucerase	T45.3X1	T45.3X2	T45.3X3	T45.3X4	T45.3X5	T45.3X6
Alidase	T45.3X1	T45.3X2	T45.3X3	T45.3X4	T45.3X5	T45.3X6
Alimemazine	T43.3X1	T43.3X2	T43.3X3	T43.3X4	T43.3X5	T43.3X6
Aliphatic thiocyanates	T65.0X1	T65.0X2	T65.0X3	T65.0X4	—	—
Alizapride	T45.0X1	T45.0X2	T45.0X3	T45.0X4	T45.0X5	T45.0X6
Alkali (caustic)	T54.3X1	T54.3X2	T54.3X3	T54.3X4		
Alkaline antiseptic solution (aromatic)	T49.6X1	T49.6X2	T49.6X3	T49.6X4	T49.6X5	T49.6X6
Alkalinizing agents (medicinal)	T50.901	T50.902	T50.903	T50.904	T50.905	T50.906
Alkalizing agent NEC	T50.901	T50.902	T50.903	T50.904	T50.905	T50.906
Alka-seltzer	T39.011	T39.012	T39.013	T39.014	T39.015	T39.016
Alkavervir	T46.5X1	T46.5X2	T46.5X3	T46.5X4	T46.5X5	T46.5X6
Alkonium (bromide)	T49.0X1	T49.0X2	T49.0X3	T49.0X4	T49.0X5	T49.0X6
Alkylating drug NEC	T45.1X1	T45.1X2	T45.1X3	T45.1X4	T45.1X5	T45.1X6
antimyeloproliferative	T45.1X1	T45.1X2	T45.1X3	T45.1X4	T45.1X5	T45.1X6
lymphatic	T45.1X1	T45.1X2	T45.1X3	T45.1X4	T45.1X5	T45.1X6
Alkylisocyanate	T65.0X1	T65.0X2	T65.0X3	T65.0X4	—	—
Allantoin	T49.4X1	T49.4X2	T49.4X3	T49.4X4	T49.4X5	T49.4X6
Allegron	T43.011	T43.012	T43.013	T43.014	T43.015	T43.016
Allethrin	T49.0X1	T49.0X2	T49.0X3	T49.0X4	T49.0X5	T49.0X6
Allobarbital	T42.3X1	T42.3X2	T42.3X3	T42.3X4	T42.3X5	T42.3X6
Allopurinol	T50.4X1	T50.4X2	T50.4X3	T50.4X4	T50.4X5	T50.4X6
Allyl						
alcohol	T51.8X1	T51.8X2	T51.8X3	T51.8X4	—	—
disulfide	T46.6X1	T46.6X2	T46.6X3	T46.6X4	T46.6X5	T46.6X6
Allylestrenol	T38.5X1	T38.5X2	T38.5X3	T38.5X4	T38.5X5	T38.5X6
Allylisopropylacetylurea	T42.6X1	T42.6X2	T42.6X3	T42.6X4	T42.6X5	T42.6X6
Allylisopropylmalonylurea	T42.3X1	T42.3X2	T42.3X3	T42.3X4	T42.3X5	T42.3X6
Allylthiourea	T49.3X1	T49.3X2	T49.3X3	T49.3X4	T49.3X5	T49.3X6
Allyltribromide	T42.6X1	T42.6X2	T42.6X3	T42.6X4	T42.6X5	T42.6X6
Allypropymal	T42.3X1	T42.3X2	T42.3X3	T42.3X4	T42.3X5	T42.3X6
Almagate	T47.1X1	T47.1X2	T47.1X3	T47.1X4	T47.1X5	T47.1X6
Almasilate	T47.1X1	T47.1X2	T47.1X3	T47.1X4	T47.1X5	T47.1X6
Almitrine	T50.7X1	T50.7X2	T50.7X3	T50.7X4	T50.7X5	T50.7X6
Aloes	T47.2X1	T47.2X2	T47.2X3	T47.2X4	T47.2X5	T47.2X6
Aloglutamol	T47.1X1	T47.1X2	T47.1X3	T47.1X4	T47.1X5	T47.1X6
Aloin	T47.2X1	T47.2X2	T47.2X3	T47.2X4	T47.2X5	T47.2X6
Aloxidone	T42.2X1	T42.2X2	T42.2X3	T42.2X4	T42.2X5	T42.2X6
Alpha						
acetyldigoxin	T46.0X1	T46.0X2	T46.0X3	T46.0X4	T46.0X5	T46.0X6
adrenergic blocking drug	T44.6X1	T44.6X2	T44.6X3	T44.6X4	T44.6X5	T44.6X6
amylase	T45.3X1	T45.3X2	T45.3X3	T45.3X4	T45.3X5	T45.3X6
tocoferol (acetate)	T45.2X1	T45.2X2	T45.2X3	T45.2X4	T45.2X5	T45.2X6
tocopherol	T45.2X1	T45.2X2	T45.2X3	T45.2X4	T45.2X5	T45.2X6
Alphadolone	T41.1X1	T41.1X2	T41.1X3	T41.1X4	T41.1X5	T41.1X6
Alphaprodine	T40.4X1	T40.4X2	T40.4X3	T40.4X4	T40.4X5	T40.4X6
Alphaxalone	T41.1X1	T41.1X2	T41.1X3	T41.1X4	T41.1X5	T41.1X6
Alprazolam	T42.4X1	T42.4X2	T42.4X3	T42.4X4	T42.4X5	T42.4X6
Alprenolol	T44.7X1	T44.7X2	T44.7X3	T44.7X4	T44.7X5	T44.7X6
Alprostadil	T46.7X1	T46.7X2	T46.7X3	T46.7X4	T46.7X5	T46.7X6
Alsactide	T38.811	T38.812	T38.813	T38.814	T38.815	T38.816
Alseroxylon	T46.5X1	T46.5X2	T46.5X3	T46.5X4	T46.5X5	T46.5X6
Alteplase	T45.611	T45.612	T45.613	T45.614	T45.615	T45.616
Altizide	T50.2X1	T50.2X2	T50.2X3	T50.2X4	T50.2X5	T50.2X6
Altretamine	T45.1X1	T45.1X2	T45.1X3	T45.1X4	T45.1X5	T45.1X6
Alum (medicinal)	T49.4X1	T49.4X2	T49.4X3	T49.4X4	T49.4X5	T49.4X6
nonmedicinal (ammonium) (potassium)	T56.891	T56.892	T56.893	T56.894	—	—
Aluminium, aluminum						
acetate	T49.2X1	T49.2X2	T49.2X3	T49.2X4	T49.2X5	T49.2X6
solution	T49.0X1	T49.0X2	T49.0X3	T49.0X4	T49.0X5	T49.0X6
aspirin	T39.011	T39.012	T39.013	T39.014	T39.015	T39.016
bis (acetylsalicylate)	T39.011	T39.012	T39.013	T39.014	T39.015	T39.016
carbonate (gel, basic)	T47.1X1	T47.1X2	T47.1X3	T47.1X4	T47.1X5	T47.1X6
chlorhydroxide-complex	T47.1X1	T47.1X2	T47.1X3	T47.1X4	T47.1X5	T47.1X6
chloride	T49.2X1	T49.2X2	T49.2X3	T49.2X4	T49.2X5	T49.2X6
clofibrate	T46.6X1	T46.6X2	T46.6X3	T46.6X4	T46.6X5	T46.6X6
diacetate	T49.2X1	T49.2X2	T49.2X3	T49.2X4	T49.2X5	T49.2X6
glycinate	T47.1X1	T47.1X2	T47.1X3	T47.1X4	T47.1X5	T47.1X6
hydroxide (gel)	T47.1X1	T47.1X2	T47.1X3	T47.1X4	T47.1X5	T47.1X6
hydroxide-magnesium carb. gel	T47.1X1	T47.1X2	T47.1X3	T47.1X4	T47.1X5	T47.1X6
magnesium silicate	T47.1X1	T47.1X2	T47.1X3	T47.1X4	T47.1X5	T47.1X6
nicotinate	T46.7X1	T46.7X2	T46.7X3	T46.7X4	T46.7X5	T46.7X6
ointment (surgical) (topical)	T49.3X1	T49.3X2	T49.3X3	T49.3X4	T49.3X5	T49.3X6
phosphate	T47.1X1	T47.1X2	T47.1X3	T47.1X4	T47.1X5	T47.1X6
salicylate	T39.091	T39.092	T39.093	T39.094	T39.095	T39.096
silicate	T47.1X1	T47.1X2	T47.1X3	T47.1X4	T47.1X5	T47.1X6
sodium silicate	T47.1X1	T47.1X2	T47.1X3	T47.1X4	T47.1X5	T47.1X6
subacetate	T49.2X1	T49.2X2	T49.2X3	T49.2X4	T49.2X5	T49.2X6
sulfate	T49.0X1	T49.0X2	T49.0X3	T49.0X4	T49.0X5	T49.0X6
tannate	T47.6X1	T47.6X2	T47.6X3	T47.6X4	T47.6X5	T47.6X6
topical NEC	T49.3X1	T49.3X2	T49.3X3	T49.3X4	T49.3X5	T49.3X6
Alurate	T42.3X1	T42.3X2	T42.3X3	T42.3X4	T42.3X5	T42.3X6
Alverine	T44.3X1	T44.3X2	T44.3X3	T44.3X4	T44.3X5	T44.3X6
Alvodine	T40.2X1	T40.2X2	T40.2X3	T40.2X4	T40.2X5	T40.2X6
Amanita phalloides	T62.0X1	T62.0X2	T62.0X3	T62.0X4	—	—

Additional Character May Be Required — Refer to the Tabular List for Character Selection   ▼ Subterms under main terms may continue to next column or page

Substance	Poisoning, Accidental (unintentional)	Poisoning, Intentional Self-harm	Poisoning, Assault	Poisoning, Undetermined	Adverse Effect	Under-dosing
Amanitine	T62.0X1	T62.0X2	T62.0X3	T62.0X4	—	—
Amantadine	T42.8X1	T42.8X2	T42.8X3	T42.8X4	T42.8X5	T42.8X6
Ambazone	T49.6X1	T49.6X2	T49.6X3	T49.6X4	T49.6X5	T49.6X6
Ambenonium (chloride)	T44.0X1	T44.0X2	T44.0X3	T44.0X4	T44.0X5	T44.0X6
Ambroxol	T48.4X1	T48.4X2	T48.4X3	T48.4X4	T48.4X5	T48.4X6
Ambuphylline	T48.6X1	T48.6X2	T48.6X3	T48.6X4	T48.6X5	T48.6X6
Ambutonium bromide	T44.3X1	T44.3X2	T44.3X3	T44.3X4	T44.3X5	T44.3X6
Amcinonide	T49.0X1	T49.0X2	T49.0X3	T49.0X4	T49.0X5	T49.0X6
Amdinocilline	T36.0X1	T36.0X2	T36.0X3	T36.0X4	T36.0X5	T36.0X6
Ametazole	T50.8X1	T50.8X2	T50.8X3	T50.8X4	T50.8X5	T50.8X6
Amethocaine	T41.3X1	T41.3X2	T41.3X3	T41.3X4	T41.3X5	T41.3X6
regional	T41.3X1	T41.3X2	T41.3X3	T41.3X4	T41.3X5	T41.3X6
spinal	T41.3X1	T41.3X2	T41.3X3	T41.3X4	T41.3X5	T41.3X6
Amethopterin	T45.1X1	T45.1X2	T45.1X3	T45.1X4	T45.1X5	T45.1X6
Amezinium metilsulfate	T44.991	T44.992	T44.993	T44.994	T44.995	T44.996
Amfebutamone	T43.291	T43.292	T43.293	T43.294	T43.295	T43.296
Amfepramone	T50.5X1	T50.5X2	T50.5X3	T50.5X4	T50.5X5	T50.5X6
Amfetamine	T43.621	T43.622	T43.623	T43.624	T43.625	T43.626
Amfetaminil	T43.621	T43.622	T43.623	T43.624	T43.625	T43.626
Amfomycin	T36.8X1	T36.8X2	T36.8X3	T36.8X4	T36.8X5	T36.8X6
Amidefrine mesilate	T48.5X1	T48.5X2	T48.5X3	T48.5X4	T48.5X5	T48.5X6
Amidone	T40.3X1	T40.3X2	T40.3X3	T40.3X4	T40.3X5	T40.3X6
Amidopyrine	T39.2X1	T39.2X2	T39.2X3	T39.2X4	T39.2X5	T39.2X6
Amidotrizoate	T50.8X1	T50.8X2	T50.8X3	T50.8X4	T50.8X5	T50.8X6
Amiflamine	T43.1X1	T43.1X2	T43.1X3	T43.1X4	T43.1X5	T43.1X6
Amikacin	T36.5X1	T36.5X2	T36.5X3	T36.5X4	T36.5X5	T36.5X6
Amikhelline	T46.3X1	T46.3X2	T46.3X3	T46.3X4	T46.3X5	T46.3X6
Amiloride	T50.2X1	T50.2X2	T50.2X3	T50.2X4	T50.2X5	T50.2X6
Aminacrine	T49.0X1	T49.0X2	T49.0X3	T49.0X4	T49.0X5	T49.0X6
Amineptine	T43.011	T43.012	T43.013	T43.014	T43.015	T43.016
Aminitrozole	T37.3X1	T37.3X2	T37.3X3	T37.3X4	T37.3X5	T37.3X6
Aminoacetic acid (derivatives)	T50.3X1	T50.3X2	T50.3X3	T50.3X4	T50.3X5	T50.3X6
Amino acids	T50.3X1	T50.3X2	T50.3X3	T50.3X4	T50.3X5	T50.3X6
Aminoacridine	T49.0X1	T49.0X2	T49.0X3	T49.0X4	T49.0X5	T49.0X6
Aminobenzoic acid (-p)	T49.3X1	T49.3X2	T49.3X3	T49.3X4	T49.3X5	T49.3X6
Aminocaproic acid	T45.621	T45.622	T45.623	T45.624	T45.625	T45.626
Aminoethylisothiourium	T45.8X1	T45.8X2	T45.8X3	T45.8X4	T45.8X5	T45.8X6
Aminofenazone	T39.2X1	T39.2X2	T39.2X3	T39.2X4	T39.2X5	T39.2X6
Aminoglutethimide	T45.1X1	T45.1X2	T45.1X3	T45.1X4	T45.1X5	T45.1X6
Aminohippuric acid	T50.8X1	T50.8X2	T50.8X3	T50.8X4	T50.8X5	T50.8X6
Aminomethylbenzoic acid	T45.691	T45.692	T45.693	T45.694	T45.695	T45.696
Aminometradine	T50.2X1	T50.2X2	T50.2X3	T50.2X4	T50.2X5	T50.2X6
Aminopentamide	T44.3X1	T44.3X2	T44.3X3	T44.3X4	T44.3X5	T44.3X6
Aminophenazone	T39.2X1	T39.2X2	T39.2X3	T39.2X4	T39.2X5	T39.2X6
Aminophenol	T54.0X1	T54.0X2	T54.0X3	T54.0X4	—	—
Aminophenylpyridone	T43.591	T43.592	T43.593	T43.594	T43.595	T43.596
Aminophylline	T48.6X1	T48.6X2	T48.6X3	T48.6X4	T48.6X5	T48.6X6
Aminopterin sodium	T45.1X1	T45.1X2	T45.1X3	T45.1X4	T45.1X5	T45.1X6
Aminopyrine	T39.2X1	T39.2X2	T39.2X3	T39.2X4	T39.2X5	T39.2X6
Aminorex	T50.5X1	T50.5X2	T50.5X3	T50.5X4	T50.5X5	T50.5X6
Aminosalicylic acid	T37.1X1	T37.1X2	T37.1X3	T37.1X4	T37.1X5	T37.1X6
Aminosalylum	T37.1X1	T37.1X2	T37.1X3	T37.1X4	T37.1X5	T37.1X6
Amiodarone	T46.2X1	T46.2X2	T46.2X3	T46.2X4	T46.2X5	T46.2X6
Amiphenazole	T50.7X1	T50.7X2	T50.7X3	T50.7X4	T50.7X5	T50.7X6
Amiquinsin	T46.5X1	T46.5X2	T46.5X3	T46.5X4	T46.5X5	T46.5X6
Amisometradine	T50.2X1	T50.2X2	T50.2X3	T50.2X4	T50.2X5	T50.2X6
Amisulpride	T43.591	T43.592	T43.593	T43.594	T43.595	T43.596
Amitriptyline	T43.011	T43.012	T43.013	T43.014	T43.015	T43.016
Amitriptylinoxide	T43.011	T43.012	T43.013	T43.014	T43.015	T43.016
Amlexanox	T48.6X1	T48.6X2	T48.6X3	T48.6X4	T48.6X5	T48.6X6
Ammonia (fumes) (gas) (vapor)	T59.891	T59.892	T59.893	T59.894	—	—
aromatic spirit	T48.991	T48.992	T48.993	T48.994	T48.995	T48.996
liquid (household)	T54.3X1	T54.3X2	T54.3X3	T54.3X4	—	—
Ammoniated mercury	T49.0X1	T49.0X2	T49.0X3	T49.0X4	T49.0X5	T49.0X6
Ammonium						
acid tartrate	T49.5X1	T49.5X2	T49.5X3	T49.5X4	T49.5X5	T49.5X6
bromide	T42.6X1	T42.6X2	T42.6X3	T42.6X4	T42.6X5	T42.6X6
carbonate	T54.3X1	T54.3X2	T54.3X3	T54.3X4	—	—
chloride	T50.991	T50.992	T50.993	T50.994	T50.995	T50.996
expectorant	T48.4X1	T48.4X2	T48.4X3	T48.4X4	T48.4X5	T48.4X6
compounds (household) NEC	T54.3X1	T54.3X2	T54.3X3	T54.3X4	—	—
fumes (any usage)	T59.891	T59.892	T59.893	T59.894	—	—
industrial	T54.3X1	T54.3X2	T54.3X3	T54.3X4	—	—
ichthyosulronate	T49.4X1	T49.4X2	T49.4X3	T49.4X4	T49.4X5	T49.4X6
mandelate	T37.91	T37.92	T37.93	T37.94	T37.95	T37.96
sulfamate	T60.3X1	T60.3X2	T60.3X3	T60.3X4	—	—
sulfonate resin	T47.8X1	T47.8X2	T47.8X3	T47.8X4	T47.8X5	T47.8X6
Amobarbital (sodium)	T42.3X1	T42.3X2	T42.3X3	T42.3X4	T42.3X5	T42.3X6
Amodiaquine	T37.2X1	T37.2X2	T37.2X3	T37.2X4	T37.2X5	T37.2X6
Amopyroquin (e)	T37.2X1	T37.2X2	T37.2X3	T37.2X4	T37.2X5	T37.2X6
Amoxapine	T43.011	T43.012	T43.013	T43.014	T43.015	T43.016
Amoxicillin	T36.0X1	T36.0X2	T36.0X3	T36.0X4	T36.0X5	T36.0X6
Amperozide	T43.591	T43.592	T43.593	T43.594	T43.595	T43.596
Amphenidone	T43.591	T43.592	T43.593	T43.594	T43.595	T43.596
Amphetamine NEC	T43.621	T43.622	T43.623	T43.624	T43.625	T43.626
Amphomycin	T36.8X1	T36.8X2	T36.8X3	T36.8X4	T36.8X5	T36.8X6
Amphotalide	T37.4X1	T37.4X2	T37.4X3	T37.4X4	T37.4X5	T37.4X6
Amphotericin B	T36.7X1	T36.7X2	T36.7X3	T36.7X4	T36.7X5	T36.7X6
topical	T49.0X1	T49.0X2	T49.0X3	T49.0X4	T49.0X5	T49.0X6
Ampicillin	T36.0X1	T36.0X2	T36.0X3	T36.0X4	T36.0X5	T36.0X6
Amprotropine	T44.3X1	T44.3X2	T44.3X3	T44.3X4	T44.3X5	T44.3X6
Amsacrine	T45.1X1	T45.1X2	T45.1X3	T45.1X4	T45.1X5	T45.1X6
Amygdaline	T62.2X1	T62.2X2	T62.2X3	T62.2X4	—	—
Amyl						
acetate	T52.8X1	T52.8X2	T52.8X3	T52.8X4	—	—
vapor	T59.891	T59.892	T59.893	T59.894	—	—
alcohol	T51.3X1	T51.3X2	T51.3X3	T51.3X4	—	—
chloride	T53.6X1	T53.6X2	T53.6X3	T53.6X4	—	—
formate	T52.8X1	T52.8X2	T52.8X3	T52.8X4	—	—
nitrite	T46.3X1	T46.3X2	T46.3X3	T46.3X4	T46.3X5	T46.3X6
propionate	T65.891	T65.892	T65.893	T65.894	—	—
Amylase	T47.5X1	T47.5X2	T47.5X3	T47.5X4	T47.5X5	T47.5X6
Amyleine, regional	T41.3X1	T41.3X2	T41.3X3	T41.3X4	T41.3X5	T41.3X6
Amylene						
dichloride	T53.6X1	T53.6X2	T53.6X3	T53.6X4	—	—
hydrate	T51.3X1	T51.3X2	T51.3X3	T51.3X4	—	—
Amylmetacresol	T49.6X1	T49.6X2	T49.6X3	T49.6X4	T49.6X5	T49.6X6
Amylobarbitone	T42.3X1	T42.3X2	T42.3X3	T42.3X4	T42.3X5	T42.3X6
Amylocaine, regional	T41.3X1	T41.3X2	T41.3X3	T41.3X4	T41.3X5	T41.3X6
infiltration (subcutaneous)	T41.3X1	T41.3X2	T41.3X3	T41.3X4	T41.3X5	T41.3X6
nerve block (peripheral) (plexus)	T41.3X1	T41.3X2	T41.3X3	T41.3X4	T41.3X5	T41.3X6
spinal	T41.3X1	T41.3X2	T41.3X3	T41.3X4	T41.3X5	T41.3X6
topical (surface)	T41.3X1	T41.3X2	T41.3X3	T41.3X4	T41.3X5	T41.3X6
Amylopectin	T47.6X1	T47.6X2	T47.6X3	T47.6X4	T47.6X5	T47.6X6
Amytal (sodium)	T42.3X1	T42.3X2	T42.3X3	T42.3X4	T42.3X5	T42.3X6
Anabolic steroid	T38.7X1	T38.7X2	T38.7X3	T38.7X4	T38.7X5	T38.7X6
Analeptic NEC	T50.7X1	T50.7X2	T50.7X3	T50.7X4	T50.7X5	T50.7X6
Analgesic	T39.91	T39.92	T39.93	T39.94	T39.95	T39.96
anti-inflammatory NEC	T39.91	T39.92	T39.93	T39.94	T39.95	T39.96
propionic acid derivative	T39.311	T39.312	T39.313	T39.314	T39.315	T39.316
antirheumatic NEC	T39.4X1	T39.4X2	T39.4X3	T39.4X4	T39.4X5	T39.4X6
aromatic NEC	T39.1X1	T39.1X2	T39.1X3	T39.1X4	T39.1X5	T39.1X6
narcotic NEC	T40.601	T40.602	T40.603	T40.604	T40.605	T40.606
combination	T40.601	T40.602	T40.603	T40.604	T40.605	T40.606
obstetric	T40.601	T40.602	T40.603	T40.604	T40.605	T40.606
non-narcotic NEC	T39.91	T39.92	T39.93	T39.94	T39.95	T39.96
combination	T39.91	T39.92	T39.93	T39.94	T39.95	T39.96
pyrazole	T39.2X1	T39.2X2	T39.2X3	T39.2X4	T39.2X5	T39.2X6
specified NEC	T39.8X1	T39.8X2	T39.8X3	T39.8X4	T39.8X5	T39.8X6
Analgin	T39.2X1	T39.2X2	T39.2X3	T39.2X4	T39.2X5	T39.2X6
Anamirta cocculus	T62.1X1	T62.1X2	T62.1X3	T62.1X4	—	—
Ancillin	T36.0X1	T36.0X2	T36.0X3	T36.0X4	T36.0X5	T36.0X6
Ancrod	T45.691	T45.692	T45.693	T45.694	T45.695	T45.696
Androgen	T38.7X1	T38.7X2	T38.7X3	T38.7X4	T38.7X5	T38.7X6
Androgen-estrogen mixture	T38.7X1	T38.7X2	T38.7X3	T38.7X4	T38.7X5	T38.7X6
Androstalone	T38.7X1	T38.7X2	T38.7X3	T38.7X4	T38.7X5	T38.7X6
Androstanolone	T38.7X1	T38.7X2	T38.7X3	T38.7X4	T38.7X5	T38.7X6
Androsterone	T38.7X1	T38.7X2	T38.7X3	T38.7X4	T38.7X5	T38.7X6
Anemone pulsatilla	T62.2X1	T62.2X2	T62.2X3	T62.2X4	—	—
Anesthesia						
caudal	T41.3X1	T41.3X2	T41.3X3	T41.3X4	T41.3X5	T41.3X6
endotracheal	T41.0X1	T41.0X2	T41.0X3	T41.0X4	T41.0X5	T41.0X6
epidural	T41.3X1	T41.3X2	T41.3X3	T41.3X4	T41.3X5	T41.3X6
inhalation	T41.0X1	T41.0X2	T41.0X3	T41.0X4	T41.0X5	T41.0X6
local	T41.3X1	T41.3X2	T41.3X3	T41.3X4	T41.3X5	T41.3X6
mucosal	T41.3X1	T41.3X2	T41.3X3	T41.3X4	T41.3X5	T41.3X6
muscle relaxation	T48.1X1	T48.1X2	T48.1X3	T48.1X4	T48.1X5	T48.1X6
nerve blocking	T41.3X1	T41.3X2	T41.3X3	T41.3X4	T41.3X5	T41.3X6
plexus blocking	T41.3X1	T41.3X2	T41.3X3	T41.3X4	T41.3X5	T41.3X6
potentiated	T41.201	T41.202	T41.203	T41.204	T41.205	T41.206
rectal	T41.201	T41.202	T41.203	T41.204	T41.205	T41.206
general	T41.201	T41.202	T41.203	T41.204	T41.205	T41.206
local	T41.3X1	T41.3X2	T41.3X3	T41.3X4	T41.3X5	T41.3X6
regional	T41.3X1	T41.3X2	T41.3X3	T41.3X4	T41.3X5	T41.3X6
surface	T41.3X1	T41.3X2	T41.3X3	T41.3X4	T41.3X5	T41.3X6
Anesthetic NEC — see also Anesthesia	T41.41	T41.42	T41.43	T41.44	T41.45	T41.46
with muscle relaxant	T41.201	T41.202	T41.203	T41.204	T41.205	T41.206
general	T41.201	T41.202	T41.203	T41.204	T41.205	T41.206
local	T41.3X1	T41.3X2	T41.3X3	T41.3X4	T41.3X5	T41.3X6
gaseous NEC	T41.0X1	T41.0X2	T41.0X3	T41.0X4	T41.0X5	T41.0X6

▽ **Subterms under main terms may continue to next column or page**   Additional Character May Be Required — Refer to the Tabular List for Character Selection   **351**

Amanitine — Anesthetic NEC

Table of Drugs and Chemicals

Anesthetic NEC — Antihemophilic

Substance	Poisoning, Accidental (unintentional)	Poisoning, Intentional Self-harm	Poisoning, Assault	Poisoning, Undetermined	Adverse Effect	Under-dosing
Anesthetic — *see also* Anesthesia — *continued*						
general NEC	T41.201	T41.202	T41.203	T41.204	T41.205	T41.206
halogenated hydrocarbon derivatives NEC	T41.0X1	T41.0X2	T41.0X3	T41.0X4	T41.0X5	T41.0X6
infiltration NEC	T41.3X1	T41.3X2	T41.3X3	T41.3X4	T41.3X5	T41.3X6
intravenous NEC	T41.1X1	T41.1X2	T41.1X3	T41.1X4	T41.1X5	T41.1X6
local NEC	T41.3X1	T41.3X2	T41.3X3	T41.3X4	T41.3X5	T41.3X6
rectal	T41.201	T41.202	T41.203	T41.204	T41.205	T41.206
general	T41.201	T41.202	T41.203	T41.204	T41.205	T41.206
local	T41.3X1	T41.3X2	T41.3X3	T41.3X4	T41.3X5	T41.3X6
regional NEC	T41.3X1	T41.3X2	T41.3X3	T41.3X4	T41.3X5	T41.3X6
spinal NEC	T41.3X1	T41.3X2	T41.3X3	T41.3X4	T41.3X5	T41.3X6
thiobarbiturate	T41.1X1	T41.1X2	T41.1X3	T41.1X4	T41.1X5	T41.1X6
topical	T41.3X1	T41.3X2	T41.3X3	T41.3X4	T41.3X5	T41.3X6
Aneurine	T45.2X1	T45.2X2	T45.2X3	T45.2X4	T45.2X5	T45.2X6
Angio-Conray	T50.8X1	T50.8X2	T50.8X3	T50.8X4	T50.8X5	T50.8X6
Angiotensin	T44.5X1	T44.5X2	T44.5X3	T44.5X4	T44.5X5	T44.5X6
Angiotensinamide	T44.991	T44.992	T44.993	T44.994	T44.995	T44.996
Anhydrohydroxy-progesterone	T38.5X1	T38.5X2	T38.5X3	T38.5X4	T38.5X5	T38.5X6
Anhydron	T50.2X1	T50.2X2	T50.2X3	T50.2X4	T50.2X5	T50.2X6
Anileridine	T40.4X1	T40.4X2	T40.4X3	T40.4X4	T40.4X5	T40.4X6
Aniline (dye) (liquid)	T65.3X1	T65.3X2	T65.3X3	T65.3X4	—	—
analgesic	T39.1X1	T39.1X2	T39.1X3	T39.1X4	T39.1X5	T39.1X6
derivatives, therapeutic NEC	T39.1X1	T39.1X2	T39.1X3	T39.1X4	T39.1X5	T39.1X6
vapor	T65.3X1	T65.3X2	T65.3X3	T65.3X4	—	—
Aniscoropine	T44.3X1	T44.3X2	T44.3X3	T44.3X4	T44.3X5	T44.3X6
Anise oil	T47.5X1	T47.5X2	T47.5X3	T47.5X4	T47.5X5	T47.5X6
Anisidine	T65.3X1	T65.3X2	T65.3X3	T65.3X4	—	—
Anisindione	T45.511	T45.512	T45.513	T45.514	T45.515	T45.516
Anisotropine methyl-bromide	T44.3X1	T44.3X2	T44.3X3	T44.3X4	T44.3X5	T44.3X6
Anistreplase	T45.611	T45.612	T45.613	T45.614	T45.615	T45.616
Anorexiant (central)	T50.5X1	T50.5X2	T50.5X3	T50.5X4	T50.5X5	T50.5X6
Anorexic agents	T50.5X1	T50.5X2	T50.5X3	T50.5X4	T50.5X5	T50.5X6
Ansamycin	T36.6X1	T36.6X2	T36.6X3	T36.6X4	T36.6X5	T36.6X6
Ant (bite) (sting)	T63.421	T63.422	T63.423	T63.424		
Antabuse	T50.6X1	T50.6X2	T50.6X3	T50.6X4	T50.6X5	T50.6X6
Antacid NEC	T47.1X1	T47.1X2	T47.1X3	T47.1X4	T47.1X5	T47.1X6
Antagonist						
Aldosterone	T50.0X1	T50.0X2	T50.0X3	T50.0X4	T50.0X5	T50.0X6
alpha-adrenoreceptor	T44.6X1	T44.6X2	T44.6X3	T44.6X4	T44.6X5	T44.6X6
anticoagulant	T45.7X1	T45.7X2	T45.7X3	T45.7X4	T45.7X5	T45.7X6
beta-adrenoreceptor	T44.7X1	T44.7X2	T44.7X3	T44.7X4	T44.7X5	T44.7X6
extrapyramidal NEC	T44.3X1	T44.3X2	T44.3X3	T44.3X4	T44.3X5	T44.3X6
folic acid	T45.1X1	T45.1X2	T45.1X3	T45.1X4	T45.1X5	T45.1X6
H2 receptor	T47.0X1	T47.0X2	T47.0X3	T47.0X4	T47.0X5	T47.0X6
heavy metal	T45.8X1	T45.8X2	T45.8X3	T45.8X4	T45.8X5	T45.8X6
narcotic analgesic	T50.7X1	T50.7X2	T50.7X3	T50.7X4	T50.7X5	T50.7X6
opiate	T50.7X1	T50.7X2	T50.7X3	T50.7X4	T50.7X5	T50.7X6
pyrimidine	T45.1X1	T45.1X2	T45.1X3	T45.1X4	T45.1X5	T45.1X6
serotonin	T46.5X1	T46.5X2	T46.5X3	T46.5X4	T46.5X5	T46.5X6
Antazolin (e)	T45.0X1	T45.0X2	T45.0X3	T45.0X4	T45.0X5	T45.0X6
Anterior pituitary hormone NEC	T38.811	T38.812	T38.813	T38.814	T38.815	T38.816
Anthelmintic NEC	T37.4X1	T37.4X2	T37.4X3	T37.4X4	T37.4X5	T37.4X6
Anthiolimine	T37.4X1	T37.4X2	T37.4X3	T37.4X4	T37.4X5	T37.4X6
Anthralin	T49.4X1	T49.4X2	T49.4X3	T49.4X4	T49.4X5	T49.4X6
Anthramycin	T45.1X1	T45.1X2	T45.1X3	T45.1X4	T45.1X5	T45.1X6
Antiadrenergic NEC	T44.8X1	T44.8X2	T44.8X3	T44.8X4	T44.8X5	T44.8X6
Antiallergic NEC	T45.0X1	T45.0X2	T45.0X3	T45.0X4	T45.0X5	T45.0X6
Antiandrogen NEC	T38.6X1	T38.6X2	T38.6X3	T38.6X4	T38.6X5	T38.6X6
Anti-anemic (drug) (preparation)	T45.8X1	T45.8X2	T45.8X3	T45.8X4	T45.8X5	T45.8X6
Antianxiety drug NEC	T43.501	T43.502	T43.503	T43.504	T43.505	T43.506
Antiaris toxicaria	T65.891	T65.892	T65.893	T65.894	—	—
Antiarteriosclerotic drug	T46.6X1	T46.6X2	T46.6X3	T46.6X4	T46.6X5	T46.6X6
Antiasthmatic drug NEC	T48.6X1	T48.6X2	T48.6X3	T48.6X4	T48.6X5	T48.6X6
Antibiotic NEC	T36.91	T36.92	T36.93	T36.94	T36.95	T36.96
aminoglycoside	T36.5X1	T36.5X2	T36.5X3	T36.5X4	T36.5X5	T36.5X6
anticancer	T45.1X1	T45.1X2	T45.1X3	T45.1X4	T45.1X5	T45.1X6
antifungal	T36.7X1	T36.7X2	T36.7X3	T36.7X4	T36.7X5	T36.7X6
antimycobacterial	T36.5X1	T36.5X2	T36.5X3	T36.5X4	T36.5X5	T36.5X6
antineoplastic	T45.1X1	T45.1X2	T45.1X3	T45.1X4	T45.1X5	T45.1X6
b-lactam NEC	T36.1X1	T36.1X2	T36.1X3	T36.1X4	T36.1X5	T36.1X6
cephalosporin (group)	T36.1X1	T36.1X2	T36.1X3	T36.1X4	T36.1X5	T36.1X6
chloramphenicol (group)	T36.2X1	T36.2X2	T36.2X3	T36.2X4	T36.2X5	T36.2X6
ENT	T49.6X1	T49.6X2	T49.6X3	T49.6X4	T49.6X5	T49.6X6
eye	T49.5X1	T49.5X2	T49.5X3	T49.5X4	T49.5X5	T49.5X6
fungicidal (local)	T49.0X1	T49.0X2	T49.0X3	T49.0X4	T49.0X5	T49.0X6
intestinal	T36.8X1	T36.8X2	T36.8X3	T36.8X4	T36.8X5	T36.8X6
local	T49.0X1	T49.0X2	T49.0X3	T49.0X4	T49.0X5	T49.0X6
Antibiotic — *continued*						
macrolides	T36.3X1	T36.3X2	T36.3X3	T36.3X4	T36.3X5	T36.3X6
polypeptide	T36.8X1	T36.8X2	T36.8X3	T36.8X4	T36.8X5	T36.8X6
specified NEC	T36.8X1	T36.8X2	T36.8X3	T36.8X4	T36.8X5	T36.8X6
tetracycline (group)	T36.4X1	T36.4X2	T36.4X3	T36.4X4	T36.4X5	T36.4X6
throat	T49.6X1	T49.6X2	T49.6X3	T49.6X4	T49.6X5	T49.6X6
Anticancer agents NEC	T45.1X1	T45.1X2	T45.1X3	T45.1X4	T45.1X5	T45.1X6
Anticholesterolemic drug NEC	T46.6X1	T46.6X2	T46.6X3	T46.6X4	T46.6X5	T46.6X6
Anticholinergic NEC	T44.3X1	T44.3X2	T44.3X3	T44.3X4	T44.3X5	T44.3X6
Anticholinesterase	T44.0X1	T44.0X2	T44.0X3	T44.0X4	T44.0X5	T44.0X6
organophosphorus						
insecticide	T60.0X1	T60.0X2	T60.0X3	T60.0X4	—	—
nerve gas	T59.891	T59.892	T59.893	T59.894	—	—
reversible	T44.0X1	T44.0X2	T44.0X3	T44.0X4	T44.0X5	T44.0X6
ophthalmological	T49.5X1	T49.5X2	T49.5X3	T49.5X4	T49.5X5	T49.5X6
Anticoagulant NEC	T45.511	T45.512	T45.513	T45.514	T45.515	T45.516
Antagonist	T45.7X1	T45.7X2	T45.7X3	T45.7X4	T45.7X5	T45.7X6
Anti-common-cold drug NEC	T48.5X1	T48.5X2	T48.5X3	T48.5X4	T48.5X5	T48.5X6
Anticonvulsant	T42.71	T42.72	T42.73	T42.74	T42.75	T42.76
barbiturate	T42.3X1	T42.3X2	T42.3X3	T42.3X4	T42.3X5	T42.3X6
combination (with barbiturate)	T42.3X1	T42.3X2	T42.3X3	T42.3X4	T42.3X5	T42.3X6
hydantoin	T42.0X1	T42.0X2	T42.0X3	T42.0X4	T42.0X5	T42.0X6
hypnotic NEC	T42.6X1	T42.6X2	T42.6X3	T42.6X4	T42.6X5	T42.6X6
oxazolidinedione	T42.2X1	T42.2X2	T42.2X3	T42.2X4	T42.2X5	T42.2X6
pyrimidinedione	T42.6X1	T42.6X2	T42.6X3	T42.6X4	T42.6X5	T42.6X6
specified NEC	T42.6X1	T42.6X2	T42.6X3	T42.6X4	T42.6X5	T42.6X6
succinimide	T42.2X1	T42.2X2	T42.2X3	T42.2X4	T42.2X5	T42.2X6
Antidepressant	T43.201	T43.202	T43.203	T43.204	T43.205	T43.206
monoamine oxidase inhibitor	T43.1X1	T43.1X2	T43.1X3	T43.1X4	T43.1X5	T43.1X6
selective serotonin norepinephrine reuptake inhibitor	T43.211	T43.212	T43.213	T43.214	T43.215	T43.216
selective serotonin reuptake inhibitor	T43.221	T43.222	T43.223	T43.224	T43.225	T43.226
specified NEC	T43.291	T43.292	T43.293	T43.294	T43.295	T43.296
tetracyclic	T43.021	T43.022	T43.023	T43.024	T43.025	T43.026
triazolopyridine	T43.211	T43.212	T43.213	T43.214	T43.215	T43.216
tricyclic	T43.011	T43.012	T43.013	T43.014	T43.015	T43.016
Antidiabetic NEC	T38.3X1	T38.3X2	T38.3X3	T38.3X4	T38.3X5	T38.3X6
biguanide	T38.3X1	T38.3X2	T38.3X3	T38.3X4	T38.3X5	T38.3X6
and sulfonyl combined	T38.3X1	T38.3X2	T38.3X3	T38.3X4	T38.3X5	T38.3X6
combined	T38.3X1	T38.3X2	T38.3X3	T38.3X4	T38.3X5	T38.3X6
sulfonylurea	T38.3X1	T38.3X2	T38.3X3	T38.3X4	T38.3X5	T38.3X6
Antidiarrheal drug NEC	T47.6X1	T47.6X2	T47.6X3	T47.6X4	T47.6X5	T47.6X6
absorbent	T47.6X1	T47.6X2	T47.6X3	T47.6X4	T47.6X5	T47.6X6
Anti-D immunoglobulin (human)	T50.Z11	T50.Z12	T50.Z13	T50.Z14	T50.Z15	T50.Z16
Antidiphtheria serum	T50.Z11	T50.Z12	T50.Z13	T50.Z14	T50.Z15	T50.Z16
Antidiuretic hormone	T38.891	T38.892	T38.893	T38.894	T38.895	T38.896
Antidote NEC	T50.6X1	T50.6X2	T50.6X3	T50.6X4	T50.6X5	T50.6X6
heavy metal	T45.8X1	T45.8X2	T45.8X3	T45.8X4	T45.8X5	T45.8X6
Antidysrhythmic NEC	T46.2X1	T46.2X2	T46.2X3	T46.2X4	T46.2X5	T46.2X6
Antiemetic drug	T45.0X1	T45.0X2	T45.0X3	T45.0X4	T45.0X5	T45.0X6
Antiepilepsy agent	T42.71	T42.72	T42.73	T42.74	T42.75	T42.76
combination	T42.5X1	T42.5X2	T42.5X3	T42.5X4	T42.5X5	T42.5X6
mixed	T42.5X1	T42.5X2	T42.5X3	T42.5X4	T42.5X5	T42.5X6
specified, NEC	T42.6X1	T42.6X2	T42.6X3	T42.6X4	T42.6X5	T42.6X6
Antiestrogen NEC	T38.6X1	T38.6X2	T38.6X3	T38.6X4	T38.6X5	T38.6X6
Antifertility pill	T38.4X1	T38.4X2	T38.4X3	T38.4X4	T38.4X5	T38.4X6
Antifibrinolytic drug	T45.621	T45.622	T45.623	T45.624	T45.625	T45.626
Antifilarial drug	T37.4X1	T37.4X2	T37.4X3	T37.4X4	T37.4X5	T37.4X6
Antiflatulent	T47.5X1	T47.5X2	T47.5X3	T47.5X4	T47.5X5	T47.5X6
Antifreeze	T65.91	T65.92		T65.94	—	—
alcohol	T51.1X1	T51.1X2	T51.1X3	T51.1X4	—	—
ethylene glycol	T51.8X1	T51.8X2	T51.8X3	T51.8X4	—	—
Antifungal						
antibiotic (systemic)	T36.7X1	T36.7X2	T36.7X3	T36.7X4	T36.7X5	T36.7X6
anti-infective NEC	T37.91	T37.92	T37.93	T37.94	T37.95	T37.96
disinfectant, local	T49.0X1	T49.0X2	T49.0X3	T49.0X4	T49.0X5	T49.0X6
nonmedicinal (spray)	T60.3X1	T60.3X2	T60.3X3	T60.3X4	—	—
topical	T49.0X1	T49.0X2	T49.0X3	T49.0X4	T49.0X5	T49.0X6
Anti-gastric-secretion drug NEC	T47.1X1	T47.1X2	T47.1X3	T47.1X4	T47.1X5	T47.1X6
Antigonadotrophin NEC	T38.6X1	T38.6X2	T38.6X3	T38.6X4	T38.6X5	T38.6X6
Antihallucinogen	T43.501	T43.502	T43.503	T43.504	T43.505	T43.506
Antihelmintics	T37.4X1	T37.4X2	T37.4X3	T37.4X4	T37.4X5	T37.4X6
Antihemophilic						
factor	T45.8X1	T45.8X2	T45.8X3	T45.8X4	T45.8X5	T45.8X6
fraction	T45.8X1	T45.8X2	T45.8X3	T45.8X4	T45.8X5	T45.8X6

Additional Character May Be Required — Refer to the Tabular List for Character Selection ▽ Subterms under main terms may continue to next column or page

Substance	Poisoning, Accidental (unintentional)	Poisoning, Intentional Self-harm	Poisoning, Assault	Poisoning, Undetermined	Adverse Effect	Under-dosing
Antihemophilic — continued						
globulin concentrate	T45.7X1	T45.7X2	T45.7X3	T45.7X4	T45.7X5	T45.7X6
human plasma	T45.8X1	T45.8X2	T45.8X3	T45.8X4	T45.8X5	T45.8X6
plasma, dried	T45.7X1	T45.7X2	T45.7X3	T45.7X4	T45.7X5	T45.7X6
Antihemorrhoidal preparation	T49.2X1	T49.2X2	T49.2X3	T49.2X4	T49.2X5	T49.2X6
Antiheparin drug	T45.7X1	T45.7X2	T45.7X3	T45.7X4	T45.7X5	T45.7X6
Antihistamine	T45.0X1	T45.0X2	T45.0X3	T45.0X4	T45.0X5	T45.0X6
Antihookworm drug	T37.4X1	T37.4X2	T37.4X3	T37.4X4	T37.4X5	T37.4X6
Anti-human lymphocytic globulin	T50.Z11	T50.Z12	T50.Z13	T50.Z14	T50.Z15	T50.Z16
Antihyperlipidemic drug	T46.6X1	T46.6X2	T46.6X3	T46.6X4	T46.6X5	T46.6X6
Antihypertensive drug NEC	T46.5X1	T46.5X2	T46.5X3	T46.5X4	T46.5X5	T46.5X6
Anti-infective NEC	T37.91	T37.92	T37.93	T37.94	T37.95	T37.96
anthelmintic	T37.4X1	T37.4X2	T37.4X3	T37.4X4	T37.4X5	T37.4X6
antibiotics	T36.91	T36.92	T36.93	T36.94	T36.95	T36.96
specified NEC	T36.8X1	T36.8X2	T36.8X3	T36.8X4	T36.8X5	T36.8X6
antimalarial	T37.2X1	T37.2X2	T37.2X3	T37.2X4	T37.2X5	T37.2X6
antimycobacterial NEC	T37.1X1	T37.1X2	T37.1X3	T37.1X4	T37.1X5	T37.1X6
antibiotics	T36.5X1	T36.5X2	T36.5X3	T36.5X4	T36.5X5	T36.5X6
antiprotozoal NEC	T37.3X1	T37.3X2	T37.3X3	T37.3X4	T37.3X5	T37.3X6
blood	T37.2X1	T37.2X2	T37.2X3	T37.2X4	T37.2X5	T37.2X6
antiviral	T37.5X1	T37.5X2	T37.5X3	T37.5X4	T37.5X5	T37.5X6
arsenical	T37.8X1	T37.8X2	T37.8X3	T37.8X4	T37.8X5	T37.8X6
bismuth, local	T49.0X1	T49.0X2	T49.0X3	T49.0X4	T49.0X5	T49.0X6
ENT	T49.6X1	T49.6X2	T49.6X3	T49.6X4	T49.6X5	T49.6X6
eye NEC	T49.5X1	T49.5X2	T49.5X3	T49.5X4	T49.5X5	T49.5X6
heavy metals NEC	T37.8X1	T37.8X2	T37.8X3	T37.8X4	T37.8X5	T37.8X6
local NEC	T49.0X1	T49.0X2	T49.0X3	T49.0X4	T49.0X5	T49.0X6
specified NEC	T49.0X1	T49.0X2	T49.0X3	T49.0X4	T49.0X5	T49.0X6
mixed	T37.91	T37.92	T37.93	T37.94	T37.95	T37.96
ophthalmic preparation	T49.5X1	T49.5X2	T49.5X3	T49.5X4	T49.5X5	T49.5X6
topical NEC	T49.0X1	T49.0X2	T49.0X3	T49.0X4	T49.0X5	T49.0X6
Anti-inflammatory drug NEC	T39.391	T39.392	T39.393	T39.394	T39.395	T39.396
local	T49.0X1	T49.0X2	T49.0X3	T49.0X4	T49.0X5	T49.0X6
nonsteroidal NEC	T39.391	T39.392	T39.393	T39.394	T39.395	T39.396
propionic acid derivative	T39.311	T39.312	T39.313	T39.314	T39.315	T39.316
specified NEC	T39.391	T39.392	T39.393	T39.394	T39.395	T39.396
Antikaluretic	T50.3X1	T50.3X2	T50.3X3	T50.3X4	T50.3X5	T50.3X6
Antiknock (tetraethyl lead)	T56.0X1	T56.0X2	T56.0X3	T56.0X4	—	—
Antilipemic drug NEC	T46.6X1	T46.6X2	T46.6X3	T46.6X4	T46.6X5	T46.6X6
Antimalarial	T37.2X1	T37.2X2	T37.2X3	T37.2X4	T37.2X5	T37.2X6
prophylactic NEC	T37.2X1	T37.2X2	T37.2X3	T37.2X4	T37.2X5	T37.2X6
pyrimidine derivative	T37.2X1	T37.2X2	T37.2X3	T37.2X4	T37.2X5	T37.2X6
Antimetabolite	T45.1X1	T45.1X2	T45.1X3	T45.1X4	T45.1X5	T45.1X6
Antimitotic agent	T45.1X1	T45.1X2	T45.1X3	T45.1X4	T45.1X5	T45.1X6
Antimony (compounds) (vapor) **NEC**	T56.891	T56.892	T56.893	T56.894	—	—
anti-infectives	T37.8X1	T37.8X2	T37.8X3	T37.8X4	T37.8X5	T37.8X6
dimercaptosuccinate	T37.3X1	T37.3X2	T37.3X3	T37.3X4	T37.3X5	T37.3X6
hydride	T56.891	T56.892	T56.893	T56.894	—	—
pesticide (vapor)	T60.8X1	T60.8X2	T60.8X3	T60.8X4	—	—
potassium (sodium) tartrate	T37.8X1	T37.8X2	T37.8X3	T37.8X4	T37.8X5	T37.8X6
sodium dimercaptosuccinate	T37.3X1	T37.3X2	T37.3X3	T37.3X4	T37.3X5	T37.3X6
tartrated	T37.8X1	T37.8X2	T37.8X3	T37.8X4	T37.8X5	T37.8X6
Antimuscarinic NEC	T44.3X1	T44.3X2	T44.3X3	T44.3X4	T44.3X5	T44.3X6
Antimycobacterial drug NEC	T37.1X1	T37.1X2	T37.1X3	T37.1X4	T37.1X5	T37.1X6
antibiotics	T36.5X1	T36.5X2	T36.5X3	T36.5X4	T36.5X5	T36.5X6
combination	T37.1X1	T37.1X2	T37.1X3	T37.1X4	T37.1X5	T37.1X6
Antinausea drug	T45.0X1	T45.0X2	T45.0X3	T45.0X4	T45.0X5	T45.0X6
Antinematode drug	T37.4X1	T37.4X2	T37.4X3	T37.4X4	T37.4X5	T37.4X6
Antineoplastic NEC	T45.1X1	T45.1X2	T45.1X3	T45.1X4	T45.1X5	T45.1X6
alkaloidal	T45.1X1	T45.1X2	T45.1X3	T45.1X4	T45.1X5	T45.1X6
antibiotics	T45.1X1	T45.1X2	T45.1X3	T45.1X4	T45.1X5	T45.1X6
combination	T45.1X1	T45.1X2	T45.1X3	T45.1X4	T45.1X5	T45.1X6
estrogen	T38.5X1	T38.5X2	T38.5X3	T38.5X4	T38.5X5	T38.5X6
steroid	T38.7X1	T38.7X2	T38.7X3	T38.7X4	T38.7X5	T38.7X6
Antiparasitic drug (systemic)	T37.91	T37.92	T37.93	T37.94	T37.95	T37.96
local	T49.0X1	T49.0X2	T49.0X3	T49.0X4	T49.0X5	T49.0X6
specified NEC	T37.8X1	T37.8X2	T37.8X3	T37.8X4	T37.8X5	T37.8X6
Antiparkinsonism drug NEC	T42.8X1	T42.8X2	T42.8X3	T42.8X4	T42.8X5	T42.8X6
Antiperspirant NEC	T49.2X1	T49.2X2	T49.2X3	T49.2X4	T49.2X5	T49.2X6
Antiphlogistic NEC	T39.4X1	T39.4X2	T39.4X3	T39.4X4	T39.4X5	T39.4X6
Antiplatyhelmintic drug	T37.4X1	T37.4X2	T37.4X3	T37.4X4	T37.4X5	T37.4X6
Antiprotozoal drug NEC	T37.3X1	T37.3X2	T37.3X3	T37.3X4	T37.3X5	T37.3X6
blood	T37.2X1	T37.2X2	T37.2X3	T37.2X4	T37.2X5	T37.2X6
local	T49.0X1	T49.0X2	T49.0X3	T49.0X4	T49.0X5	T49.0X6

Substance	Poisoning, Accidental (unintentional)	Poisoning, Intentional Self-harm	Poisoning, Assault	Poisoning, Undetermined	Adverse Effect	Under-dosing
Antipruritic drug NEC	T49.1X1	T49.1X2	T49.1X3	T49.1X4	T49.1X5	T49.1X6
Antipsychotic drug	T43.501	T43.502	T43.503	T43.504	T43.505	T43.506
specified NEC	T43.591	T43.592	T43.593	T43.594	T43.595	T43.596
Antipyretic	T39.91	T39.92	T39.93	T39.94	T39.95	T39.96
specified NEC	T39.8X1	T39.8X2	T39.8X3	T39.8X4	T39.8X5	T39.8X6
Antipyrine	T39.2X1	T39.2X2	T39.2X3	T39.2X4	T39.2X5	T39.2X6
Antirabies hyperimmune serum	T50.Z11	T50.Z12	T50.Z13	T50.Z14	T50.Z15	T50.Z16
Antirheumatic NEC	T39.4X1	T39.4X2	T39.4X3	T39.4X4	T39.4X5	T39.4X6
Antirigidity drug NEC	T42.8X1	T42.8X2	T42.8X3	T42.8X4	T42.8X5	T42.8X6
Antischistosomal drug	T37.4X1	T37.4X2	T37.4X3	T37.4X4	T37.4X5	T37.4X6
Antiscorpion sera	T50.Z11	T50.Z12	T50.Z13	T50.Z14	T50.Z15	T50.Z16
Antiseborrheics	T49.4X1	T49.4X2	T49.4X3	T49.4X4	T49.4X5	T49.4X6
Antiseptics (external) (medicinal)	T49.0X1	T49.0X2	T49.0X3	T49.0X4	T49.0X5	T49.0X6
Antistine	T45.0X1	T45.0X2	T45.0X3	T45.0X4	T45.0X5	T45.0X6
Antitapeworm drug	T37.4X1	T37.4X2	T37.4X3	T37.4X4	T37.4X5	T37.4X6
Antitetanus immunoglobulin	T50.Z11	T50.Z12	T50.Z13	T50.Z14	T50.Z15	T50.Z16
Antithrombotic	T45.521	T45.522	T45.523	T45.524	T45.525	T45.526
Antithyroid drug NEC	T38.2X1	T38.2X2	T38.2X3	T38.2X4	T38.2X5	T38.2X6
Antitoxin	T50.Z11	T50.Z12	T50.Z13	T50.Z14	T50.Z15	T50.Z16
diphtheria	T50.Z11	T50.Z12	T50.Z13	T50.Z14	T50.Z15	T50.Z16
gas gangrene	T50.Z11	T50.Z12	T50.Z13	T50.Z14	T50.Z15	T50.Z16
tetanus	T50.Z11	T50.Z12	T50.Z13	T50.Z14	T50.Z15	T50.Z16
Antitrichomonal drug	T37.3X1	T37.3X2	T37.3X3	T37.3X4	T37.3X5	T37.3X6
Antituberculars	T37.1X1	T37.1X2	T37.1X3	T37.1X4	T37.1X5	T37.1X6
antibiotics	T36.5X1	T36.5X2	T36.5X3	T36.5X4	T36.5X5	T36.5X6
Antitussive NEC	T48.3X1	T48.3X2	T48.3X3	T48.3X4	T48.3X5	T48.3X6
codeine mixture	T40.2X1	T40.2X2	T40.2X3	T40.2X4	T40.2X5	T40.2X6
opiate	T40.2X1	T40.2X2	T40.2X3	T40.2X4	T40.2X5	T40.2X6
Antivaricose drug	T46.8X1	T46.8X2	T46.8X3	T46.8X4	T46.8X5	T46.8X6
Antivenin, antivenom (sera)	T50.Z11	T50.Z12	T50.Z13	T50.Z14	T50.Z15	T50.Z16
crotaline	T50.Z11	T50.Z12	T50.Z13	T50.Z14	T50.Z15	T50.Z16
spider bite	T50.Z11	T50.Z12	T50.Z13	T50.Z14	T50.Z15	T50.Z16
Antivertigo drug	T45.0X1	T45.0X2	T45.0X3	T45.0X4	T45.0X5	T45.0X6
Antiviral drug NEC	T37.5X1	T37.5X2	T37.5X3	T37.5X4	T37.5X5	T37.5X6
eye	T49.5X1	T49.5X2	T49.5X3	T49.5X4	T49.5X5	T49.5X6
Antiwhipworm drug	T37.4X1	T37.4X2	T37.4X3	T37.4X4	T37.4X5	T37.4X6
Ant poison — see Insecticide						
Antrol — see also by specific chemical substance	T60.91	T60.92	T60.93	T60.94	—	—
fungicide	T60.91	T60.92	T60.93	T60.94	—	—
ANTU (alpha naphthylthiourea)	T60.4X1	T60.4X2	T60.4X3	T60.4X4	—	—
Apalcillin	T36.0X1	T36.0X2	T36.0X3	T36.0X4	T36.0X5	T36.0X6
APC	T48.5X1	T48.5X2	T48.5X3	T48.5X4	T48.5X5	T48.5X6
Aplonidine	T44.4X1	T44.4X2	T44.4X3	T44.4X4	T44.4X5	T44.4X6
Apomorphine	T47.7X1	T47.7X2	T47.7X3	T47.7X4	T47.7X5	T47.7X6
Appetite depressants, central	T50.5X1	T50.5X2	T50.5X3	T50.5X4	T50.5X5	T50.5X6
Apraclonidine (hydrochloride)	T44.4X1	T44.4X2	T44.4X3	T44.4X4	T44.4X5	T44.4X6
Apresoline	T46.5X1	T46.5X2	T46.5X3	T46.5X4	T46.5X5	T46.5X6
Aprindine	T46.2X1	T46.2X2	T46.2X3	T46.2X4	T46.2X5	T46.2X6
Aprobarbital	T42.3X1	T42.3X2	T42.3X3	T42.3X4	T42.3X5	T42.3X6
Aapronalide	T42.6X1	T42.6X2	T42.6X3	T42.6X4	T42.6X5	T42.6X6
Aprotinin	T45.621	T45.622	T45.623	T45.624	T45.625	T45.626
Aptocaine	T41.3X1	T41.3X2	T41.3X3	T41.3X4	T41.3X5	T41.3X6
Aqua fortis	T54.2X1	T54.2X2	T54.2X3	T54.2X4	—	—
Ara-A	T37.5X1	T37.5X2	T37.5X3	T37.5X4	T37.5X5	T37.5X6
Ara-C	T45.1X1	T45.1X2	T45.1X3	T45.1X4	T45.1X5	T45.1X6
Arachis oil	T49.3X1	T49.3X2	T49.3X3	T49.3X4	T49.3X5	T49.3X6
cathartic	T47.4X1	T47.4X2	T47.4X3	T47.4X4	T47.4X5	T47.4X6
Aralen	T37.2X1	T37.2X2	T37.2X3	T37.2X4	T37.2X5	T37.2X6
Arecoline	T44.1X1	T44.1X2	T44.1X3	T44.1X4	T44.1X5	T44.1X6
Arginine	T50.991	T50.992	T50.993	T50.994	T50.995	T50.996
glutamate	T50.991	T50.992	T50.993	T50.994	T50.995	T50.996
Argyrol	T49.0X1	T49.0X2	T49.0X3	T49.0X4	T49.0X5	T49.0X6
ENT agent	T49.6X1	T49.6X2	T49.6X3	T49.6X4	T49.6X5	T49.6X6
ophthalmic preparation	T49.5X1	T49.5X2	T49.5X3	T49.5X4	T49.5X5	T49.5X6
Aristocort	T38.0X1	T38.0X2	T38.0X3	T38.0X4	T38.0X5	T38.0X6
ENT agent	T49.6X1	T49.6X2	T49.6X3	T49.6X4	T49.6X5	T49.6X6
ophthalmic preparation	T49.5X1	T49.5X2	T49.5X3	T49.5X4	T49.5X5	T49.5X6
topical NEC	T49.0X1	T49.0X2	T49.0X3	T49.0X4	T49.0X5	T49.0X6
Aromatics, corrosive	T54.1X1	T54.1X2	T54.1X3	T54.1X4	—	—
disinfectants	T54.1X1	T54.1X2	T54.1X3	T54.1X4	—	—
Arsenate of lead	T57.0X1	T57.0X2	T57.0X3	T57.0X4	—	—
herbicide	T57.0X1	T57.0X2	T57.0X3	T57.0X4	—	—
Arsenic, arsenicals (compounds) (dust) (vapor) **NEC**	T57.0X1	T57.0X2	T57.0X3	T57.0X4	—	—
anti-infectives	T37.8X1	T37.8X2	T37.8X3	T37.8X4	T37.8X5	T37.8X6
pesticide (dust) (fumes)	T57.0X1	T57.0X2	T57.0X3	T57.0X4	—	—

Subterms under main terms may continue to next column or page — Additional Character May Be Required — Refer to the Tabular List for Character Selection — 353

Antihemophilic — Arsenic, arsenicals

Table of Drugs and Chemicals

Substance	Poisoning, Accidental (unintentional)	Poisoning, Intentional Self-harm	Poisoning, Assault	Poisoning, Undetermined	Adverse Effect	Under-dosing
Arsine (gas)	T57.0X1	T57.0X2	T57.0X3	T57.0X4	—	—
Arsphenamine (silver)	T37.8X1	T37.8X2	T37.8X3	T37.8X4	T37.8X5	T37.8X6
Arsthinol	T37.3X1	T37.3X2	T37.3X3	T37.3X4	T37.3X5	T37.3X6
Artane	T44.3X1	T44.3X2	T44.3X3	T44.3X4	T44.3X5	T44.3X6
Arthropod (venomous) NEC	T63.481	T63.482	T63.483	T63.484		
Articaine	T41.3X1	T41.3X2	T41.3X3	T41.3X4	T41.3X5	T41.3X6
Asbestos	T57.8X1	T57.8X2	T57.8X3	T57.8X4		
Ascaridole	T37.4X1	T37.4X2	T37.4X3	T37.4X4	T37.4X5	T37.4X6
Ascorbic acid	T45.2X1	T45.2X2	T45.2X3	T45.2X4	T45.2X5	T45.2X6
Asiaticoside	T49.0X1	T49.0X2	T49.0X3	T49.0X4	T49.0X5	T49.0X6
Asparaginase	T45.1X1	T45.1X2	T45.1X3	T45.1X4	T45.1X5	T45.1X6
Aspidium (oleoresin)	T37.4X1	T37.4X2	T37.4X3	T37.4X4	T37.4X5	T37.4X6
Aspirin (aluminum) (soluble)	T39.011	T39.012	T39.013	T39.014	T39.015	T39.016
Aspoxicillin	T36.0X1	T36.0X2	T36.0X3	T36.0X4	T36.0X5	T36.0X6
Astemizole	T45.0X1	T45.0X2	T45.0X3	T45.0X4	T45.0X5	T45.0X6
Astringent (local)	T49.2X1	T49.2X2	T49.2X3	T49.2X4	T49.2X5	T49.2X6
specified NEC	T49.2X1	T49.2X2	T49.2X3	T49.2X4	T49.2X5	T49.2X6
Astromicin	T36.5X1	T36.5X2	T36.5X3	T36.5X4	T36.5X5	T36.5X6
Ataractic drug NEC	T43.501	T43.502	T43.503	T43.504	T43.505	T43.506
Atenolol	T44.7X1	T44.7X2	T44.7X3	T44.7X4	T44.7X5	T44.7X6
Atonia drug, intestinal	T47.4X1	T47.4X2	T47.4X3	T47.4X4	T47.4X5	T47.4X6
Atophan	T50.4X1	T50.4X2	T50.4X3	T50.4X4	T50.4X5	T50.4X6
Atracurium besilate	T48.1X1	T48.1X2	T48.1X3	T48.1X4	T48.1X5	T48.1X6
Atropine	T44.3X1	T44.3X2	T44.3X3	T44.3X4	T44.3X5	T44.3X6
derivative	T44.3X1	T44.3X2	T44.3X3	T44.3X4	T44.3X5	T44.3X6
methonitrate	T44.3X1	T44.3X2	T44.3X3	T44.3X4	T44.3X5	T44.3X6
Attapulgite	T47.6X1	T47.6X2	T47.6X3	T47.6X4	T47.6X5	T47.6X6
Auramine	T65.891	T65.892	T65.893	T65.894	—	—
dye	T65.6X1	T65.6X2	T65.6X3	T65.6X4	—	—
fungicide	T60.3X1	T60.3X2	T60.3X3	T60.3X4	—	—
Auranofin	T39.4X1	T39.4X2	T39.4X3	T39.4X4	T39.4X5	T39.4X6
Aurantiin	T46.991	T46.992	T46.993	T46.994	T46.995	T46.996
Aureomycin	T36.4X1	T36.4X2	T36.4X3	T36.4X4	T36.4X5	T36.4X6
ophthalmic preparation	T49.5X1	T49.5X2	T49.5X3	T49.5X4	T49.5X5	T49.5X6
topical NEC	T49.0X1	T49.0X2	T49.0X3	T49.0X4	T49.0X5	T49.0X6
Aurothioglucose	T39.4X1	T39.4X2	T39.4X3	T39.4X4	T39.4X5	T39.4X6
Aurothioglycanide	T39.4X1	T39.4X2	T39.4X3	T39.4X4	T39.4X5	T39.4X6
Aurothiomalate sodium	T39.4X1	T39.4X2	T39.4X3	T39.4X4	T39.4X5	T39.4X6
Aurotioprol	T39.4X1	T39.4X2	T39.4X3	T39.4X4	T39.4X5	T39.4X6
Automobile fuel	T52.0X1	T52.0X2	T52.0X3	T52.0X4	—	—
Autonomic nervous system agent NEC	T44.901	T44.902	T44.903	T44.904	T44.905	T44.906
Avlosulfon	T37.1X1	T37.1X2	T37.1X3	T37.1X4	T37.1X5	T37.1X6
Avomine	T42.6X1	T42.6X2	T42.6X3	T42.6X4	T42.6X5	T42.6X6
Axerophthol	T45.2X1	T45.2X2	T45.2X3	T45.2X4	T45.2X5	T45.2X6
Azacitidine	T45.1X1	T45.1X2	T45.1X3	T45.1X4	T45.1X5	T45.1X6
Azacyclonol	T43.591	T43.592	T43.593	T43.594	T43.595	T43.596
Azadirachta	T60.2X1	T60.2X2	T60.2X3	T60.2X4	—	—
Azanidazole	T37.3X1	T37.3X2	T37.3X3	T37.3X4	T37.3X5	T37.3X6
Azapetine	T46.7X1	T46.7X2	T46.7X3	T46.7X4	T46.7X5	T46.7X6
Azapropazone	T39.2X1	T39.2X2	T39.2X3	T39.2X4	T39.2X5	T39.2X6
Azaribine	T45.1X1	T45.1X2	T45.1X3	T45.1X4	T45.1X5	T45.1X6
Azaserine	T45.1X1	T45.1X2	T45.1X3	T45.1X4	T45.1X5	T45.1X6
Azatadine	T45.0X1	T45.0X2	T45.0X3	T45.0X4	T45.0X5	T45.0X6
Azatepa	T45.1X1	T45.1X2	T45.1X3	T45.1X4	T45.1X5	T45.1X6
Azathioprine	T45.1X1	T45.1X2	T45.1X3	T45.1X4	T45.1X5	T45.1X6
Azelaic acid	T49.0X1	T49.0X2	T49.0X3	T49.0X4	T49.0X5	T49.0X6
Azelastine	T45.0X1	T45.0X2	T45.0X3	T45.0X4	T45.0X5	T45.0X6
Azidocillin	T36.0X1	T36.0X2	T36.0X3	T36.0X4	T36.0X5	T36.0X6
Azidothymidine	T37.5X1	T37.5X2	T37.5X3	T37.5X4	T37.5X5	T37.5X6
Azinphos (ethyl) (methyl)	T60.0X1	T60.0X2	T60.0X3	T60.0X4	—	—
Aziridine (chelating)	T54.1X1	T54.1X2	T54.1X3	T54.1X4	—	—
Azithromycin	T36.3X1	T36.3X2	T36.3X3	T36.3X4	T36.3X5	T36.3X6
Azlocillin	T36.0X1	T36.0X2	T36.0X3	T36.0X4	T36.0X5	T36.0X6
Azobenzene smoke	T65.3X1	T65.3X2	T65.3X3	T65.3X4	—	—
acaricide	T60.8X1	T60.8X2	T60.8X3	T60.8X4	—	—
Azosulfamide	T37.0X1	T37.0X2	T37.0X3	T37.0X4	T37.0X5	T37.0X6
AZT	T37.5X1	T37.5X2	T37.5X3	T37.5X4	T37.5X5	T37.5X6
Aztreonam	T36.1X1	T36.1X2	T36.1X3	T36.1X4	T36.1X5	T36.1X6
Azulfidine	T37.0X1	T37.0X2	T37.0X3	T37.0X4	T37.0X5	T37.0X6
Azuresin	T50.8X1	T50.8X2	T50.8X3	T50.8X4	T50.8X5	T50.8X6
b-acetyldigoxin	T46.0X1	T46.0X2	T46.0X3	T46.0X4	T46.0X5	T46.0X6
P-Acetamidophenol	T39.1X1	T39.1X2	T39.1X3	T39.1X4	T39.1X5	T39.1X6
Bacampicillin	T36.0X1	T36.0X2	T36.0X3	T36.0X4	T36.0X5	T36.0X6
Bacillus						
lactobacillus	T47.8X1	T47.8X2	T47.8X3	T47.8X4	T47.8X5	T47.8X6
subtilis	T47.6X1	T47.6X2	T47.6X3	T47.6X4	T47.6X5	T47.6X6
Bacimycin	T49.0X1	T49.0X2	T49.0X3	T49.0X4	T49.0X5	T49.0X6
ophthalmic preparation	T49.5X1	T49.5X2	T49.5X3	T49.5X4	T49.5X5	T49.5X6
Bacitracin zinc	T49.0X1	T49.0X2	T49.0X3	T49.0X4	T49.0X5	T49.0X6
with neomycin	T49.0X1	T49.0X2	T49.0X3	T49.0X4	T49.0X5	T49.0X6
ENT agent	T49.6X1	T49.6X2	T49.6X3	T49.6X4	T49.6X5	T49.6X6
ophthalmic preparation	T49.5X1	T49.5X2	T49.5X3	T49.5X4	T49.5X5	T49.5X6

Substance	Poisoning, Accidental (unintentional)	Poisoning, Intentional Self-harm	Poisoning, Assault	Poisoning, Undetermined	Adverse Effect	Under-dosing
Bacitracin zinc — *continued*						
topical NEC	T49.0X1	T49.0X2	T49.0X3	T49.0X4	T49.0X5	T49.0X6
Baclofen	T42.8X1	T42.8X2	T42.8X3	T42.8X4	T42.8X5	T42.8X6
Baking soda	T50.991	T50.992	T50.993	T50.994	T50.995	T50.996
BAL	T45.8X1	T45.8X2	T45.8X3	T45.8X4	T45.8X5	T45.8X6
Bambuterol	T48.6X1	T48.6X2	T48.6X3	T48.6X4	T48.6X5	T48.6X6
Bamethan (sulfate)	T46.7X1	T46.7X2	T46.7X3	T46.7X4	T46.7X5	T46.7X6
Bamifylline	T48.6X1	T48.6X2	T48.6X3	T48.6X4	T48.6X5	T48.6X6
Bamipine	T45.0X1	T45.0X2	T45.0X3	T45.0X4	T45.0X5	T45.0X6
Baneberry — *see* Actaea spicata						
Banewort — *see* Belladonna						
Barbenyl	T42.3X1	T42.3X2	T42.3X3	T42.3X4	T42.3X5	T42.3X6
Barbexaclone	T42.6X1	T42.6X2	T42.6X3	T42.6X4	T42.6X5	T42.6X6
Barbital	T42.3X1	T42.3X2	T42.3X3	T42.3X4	T42.3X5	T42.3X6
sodium	T42.3X1	T42.3X2	T42.3X3	T42.3X4	T42.3X5	T42.3X6
Barbitone	T42.3X1	T42.3X2	T42.3X3	T42.3X4	T42.3X5	T42.3X6
Barbiturate NEC	T42.3X1	T42.3X2	T42.3X3	T42.3X4	T42.3X5	T42.3X6
with tranquilizer	T42.3X1	T42.3X2	T42.3X3	T42.3X4	T42.3X5	T42.3X6
anesthetic (intravenous)	T41.1X1	T41.1X2	T41.1X3	T41.1X4	T41.1X5	T41.1X6
Barium (carbonate) (chloride) (sulfite)	T57.8X1	T57.8X2	T57.8X3	T57.8X4	—	—
diagnostic agent	T50.8X1	T50.8X2	T50.8X3	T50.8X4	T50.8X5	T50.8X6
pesticide	T60.4X1	T60.4X2	T60.4X3	T60.4X4	—	—
rodenticide	T60.4X1	T60.4X2	T60.4X3	T60.4X4	—	—
sulfate (medicinal)	T50.8X1	T50.8X2	T50.8X3	T50.8X4	T50.8X5	T50.8X6
Barrier cream	T49.3X1	T49.3X2	T49.3X3	T49.3X4	T49.3X5	T49.3X6
Basic fuchsin	T49.0X1	T49.0X2	T49.0X3	T49.0X4	T49.0X5	T49.0X6
Battery acid or fluid	T54.2X1	T54.2X2	T54.2X3	T54.2X4	—	—
Bay rum	T51.8X1	T51.8X2	T51.8X3	T51.8X4	—	—
b-benzalbutyramide	T46.6X1	T46.6X2	T46.6X3	T46.6X4	T46.6X5	T46.6X6
BCG (vaccine)	T50.A91	T50.A92	T50.A93	T50.A94	T50.A95	T50.A96
BCNU	T45.1X1	T45.1X2	T45.1X3	T45.1X4	T45.1X5	T45.1X6
Bearsfoot	T62.2X1	T62.2X2	T62.2X3	T62.2X4	—	—
Beclamide	T42.6X1	T42.6X2	T42.6X3	T42.6X4	T42.6X5	T42.6X6
Beclomethasone	T44.5X1	T44.5X2	T44.5X3	T44.5X4	T44.5X5	T44.5X6
Bee (sting) (venom)	T63.441	T63.442	T63.443	T63.444	—	—
Befunolol	T49.5X1	T49.5X2	T49.5X3	T49.5X4	T49.5X5	T49.5X6
Bekanamycin	T36.5X1	T36.5X2	T36.5X3	T36.5X4	T36.5X5	T36.5X6
Belladonna — *see also* Nightshade						
alkaloids	T44.3X1	T44.3X2	T44.3X3	T44.3X4	T44.3X5	T44.3X6
extract	T44.3X1	T44.3X2	T44.3X3	T44.3X4	T44.3X5	T44.3X6
herb	T44.3X1	T44.3X2	T44.3X3	T44.3X4	T44.3X5	T44.3X6
Bemegride	T50.7X1	T50.7X2	T50.7X3	T50.7X4	T50.7X5	T50.7X6
Benactyzine	T44.3X1	T44.3X2	T44.3X3	T44.3X4	T44.3X5	T44.3X6
Benadryl	T45.0X1	T45.0X2	T45.0X3	T45.0X4	T45.0X5	T45.0X6
Benaprizine	T44.3X1	T44.3X2	T44.3X3	T44.3X4	T44.3X5	T44.3X6
Benazepril	T46.4X1	T46.4X2	T46.4X3	T46.4X4	T46.4X5	T46.4X6
Bencyclane	T46.7X1	T46.7X2	T46.7X3	T46.7X4	T46.7X5	T46.7X6
Bendazol	T46.3X1	T46.3X2	T46.3X3	T46.3X4	T46.3X5	T46.3X6
Bendrofluazide	T50.2X1	T50.2X2	T50.2X3	T50.2X4	T50.2X5	T50.2X6
Bendroflumethiazide	T50.2X1	T50.2X2	T50.2X3	T50.2X4	T50.2X5	T50.2X6
Benemid	T50.4X1	T50.4X2	T50.4X3	T50.4X4	T50.4X5	T50.4X6
Benethamine penicillin	T36.0X1	T36.0X2	T36.0X3	T36.0X4	T36.0X5	T36.0X6
Benexate	T47.1X1	T47.1X2	T47.1X3	T47.1X4	T47.1X5	T47.1X6
Benfluorex	T46.6X1	T46.6X2	T46.6X3	T46.6X4	T46.6X5	T46.6X6
Benfotiamine	T45.2X1	T45.2X2	T45.2X3	T45.2X4	T45.2X5	T45.2X6
Benisone	T49.0X1	T49.0X2	T49.0X3	T49.0X4	T49.0X5	T49.0X6
Benomyl	T60.0X1	T60.0X2	T60.0X3	T60.0X4	—	—
Benoquin	T49.8X1	T49.8X2	T49.8X3	T49.8X4	T49.8X5	T49.8X6
Benoxinate	T41.3X1	T41.3X2	T41.3X3	T41.3X4	T41.3X5	T41.3X6
Benperidol	T43.4X1	T43.4X2	T43.4X3	T43.4X4	T43.4X5	T43.4X6
Benproperine	T48.3X1	T48.3X2	T48.3X3	T48.3X4	T48.3X5	T48.3X6
Benserazide	T42.8X1	T42.8X2	T42.8X3	T42.8X4	T42.8X5	T42.8X6
Bentazepam	T42.4X1	T42.4X2	T42.4X3	T42.4X4	T42.4X5	T42.4X6
Bentiromide	T50.8X1	T50.8X2	T50.8X3	T50.8X4	T50.8X5	T50.8X6
Bentonite	T49.3X1	T49.3X2	T49.3X3	T49.3X4	T49.3X5	T49.3X6
Benzalbutyramide	T46.6X1	T46.6X2	T46.6X3	T46.6X4	T46.6X5	T46.6X6
Benzalkonium (chloride)	T49.0X1	T49.0X2	T49.0X3	T49.0X4	T49.0X5	T49.0X6
ophthalmic preparation	T49.5X1	T49.5X2	T49.5X3	T49.5X4	T49.5X5	T49.5X6
Benzamidosalicylate (calcium)	T37.1X1	T37.1X2	T37.1X3	T37.1X4	T37.1X5	T37.1X6
Benzamine	T41.3X1	T41.3X2	T41.3X3	T41.3X4	T41.3X5	T41.3X6
lactate	T49.1X1	T49.1X2	T49.1X3	T49.1X4	T49.1X5	T49.1X6
Benzamphetamine	T50.5X1	T50.5X2	T50.5X3	T50.5X4	T50.5X5	T50.5X6
Benzapril hydrochloride	T46.5X1	T46.5X2	T46.5X3	T46.5X4	T46.5X5	T46.5X6
Benzathine benzylpenicillin	T36.0X1	T36.0X2	T36.0X3	T36.0X4	T36.0X5	T36.0X6
Benzathine penicillin	T36.0X1	T36.0X2	T36.0X3	T36.0X4	T36.0X5	T36.0X6
Benzatropine	T42.8X1	T42.8X2	T42.8X3	T42.8X4	T42.8X5	T42.8X6
Benzbromarone	T50.4X1	T50.4X2	T50.4X3	T50.4X4	T50.4X5	T50.4X6
Benzcarbimine	T45.1X1	T45.1X2	T45.1X3	T45.1X4	T45.1X5	T45.1X6
Benzedrex	T44.991	T44.992	T44.993	T44.994	T44.995	T44.996

Table of Drugs and Chemicals

Substance	Poisoning, Accidental (unintentional)	Poisoning, Intentional Self-harm	Poisoning, Assault	Poisoning, Undetermined	Adverse Effect	Under-dosing
Benzedrine (amphetamine)	T43.621	T43.622	T43.623	T43.624	T43.625	T43.626
Benzenamine	T65.3X1	T65.3X2	T65.3X3	T65.3X4	—	—
Benzene	T52.1X1	T52.1X2	T52.1X3	T52.1X4	—	—
homologues (acetyl) (dimethyl) (methyl) (solvent)	T52.2X1	T52.2X2	T52.2X3	T52.2X4	—	—
Benzethonium (chloride)	T49.0X1	T49.0X2	T49.0X3	T49.0X4	T49.0X5	T49.0X6
Benzfetamine	T50.5X1	T50.5X2	T50.5X3	T50.5X4	T50.5X5	T50.5X6
Benzhexol	T44.3X1	T44.3X2	T44.3X3	T44.3X4	T44.3X5	T44.3X6
Benzhydramine (chloride)	T45.0X1	T45.0X2	T45.0X3	T45.0X4	T45.0X5	T45.0X6
Benzidine	T65.891	T65.892	T65.893	T65.894	—	—
Benzilonium bromide	T44.3X1	T44.3X2	T44.3X3	T44.3X4	T44.3X5	T44.3X6
Benzimidazole	T60.3X1	T60.3X2	T60.3X3	T60.3X4	—	—
Benzin (e) — see Ligroin						
Benziodarone	T46.3X1	T46.3X2	T46.3X3	T46.3X4	T46.3X5	T46.3X6
Benznidazole	T37.3X1	T37.3X2	T37.3X3	T37.3X4	T37.3X5	T37.3X6
Benzocaine	T41.3X1	T41.3X2	T41.3X3	T41.3X4	T41.3X5	T41.3X6
Benzodiapin	T42.4X1	T42.4X2	T42.4X3	T42.4X4	T42.4X5	T42.4X6
Benzodiazepine NEC	T42.4X1	T42.4X2	T42.4X3	T42.4X4	T42.4X5	T42.4X6
Benzoic acid	T49.0X1	T49.0X2	T49.0X3	T49.0X4	T49.0X5	T49.0X6
with salicylic acid	T49.0X1	T49.0X2	T49.0X3	T49.0X4	T49.0X5	T49.0X6
Benzoin (tincture)	T48.5X1	T48.5X2	T48.5X3	T48.5X4	T48.5X5	T48.5X6
Benzol (benzene)	T52.1X1	T52.1X2	T52.1X3	T52.1X4	—	—
vapor	T52.0X1	T52.0X2	T52.0X3	T52.0X4	—	—
Benzomorphan	T40.2X1	T40.2X2	T40.2X3	T40.2X4	T40.2X5	T40.2X6
Benzonatate	T48.3X1	T48.3X2	T48.3X3	T48.3X4	T48.3X5	T48.3X6
Benzophenones	T49.3X1	T49.3X2	T49.3X3	T49.3X4	T49.3X5	T49.3X6
Benzopyrone	T46.991	T46.992	T46.993	T46.994	T46.995	T46.996
Benzothiadiazides	T50.2X1	T50.2X2	T50.2X3	T50.2X4	T50.2X5	T50.2X6
Benzoxonium chloride	T49.0X1	T49.0X2	T49.0X3	T49.0X4	T49.0X5	T49.0X6
Benzoylpas calcium	T37.1X1	T37.1X2	T37.1X3	T37.1X4	T37.1X5	T37.1X6
Benzoyl peroxide	T49.0X1	T49.0X2	T49.0X3	T49.0X4	T49.0X5	T49.0X6
Benzperidin	T43.591	T43.592	T43.593	T43.594	T43.595	T43.596
Benzperidol	T43.591	T43.592	T43.593	T43.594	T43.595	T43.596
Benzphetamine	T50.5X1	T50.5X2	T50.5X3	T50.5X4	T50.5X5	T50.5X6
Benzpyrinium bromide	T44.1X1	T44.1X2	T44.1X3	T44.1X4	T44.1X5	T44.1X6
Benzquinamide	T45.0X1	T45.0X2	T45.0X3	T45.0X4	T45.0X5	T45.0X6
Benzthiazide	T50.2X1	T50.2X2	T50.2X3	T50.2X4	T50.2X5	T50.2X6
Benztropine						
anticholinergic	T44.3X1	T44.3X2	T44.3X3	T44.3X4	T44.3X5	T44.3X6
antiparkinson	T42.8X1	T42.8X2	T42.8X3	T42.8X4	T42.8X5	T42.8X6
Benzydamine	T49.0X1	T49.0X2	T49.0X3	T49.0X4	T49.0X5	T49.0X6
Benzyl						
acetate	T52.8X1	T52.8X2	T52.8X3	T52.8X4	—	—
alcohol	T49.0X1	T49.0X2	T49.0X3	T49.0X4	T49.0X5	T49.0X6
benzoate	T49.0X1	T49.0X2	T49.0X3	T49.0X4	T49.0X5	T49.0X6
Benzoic acid	T49.0X1	T49.0X2	T49.0X3	T49.0X4	T49.0X5	T49.0X6
morphine	T40.2X1	T40.2X2	T40.2X3	T40.2X4	—	—
nicotinate	T46.6X1	T46.6X2	T46.6X3	T46.6X4	T46.6X5	T46.6X6
penicillin	T36.0X1	T36.0X2	T36.0X3	T36.0X4	T36.0X5	T36.0X6
Benzylhydrochlorthiazide	T50.2X1	T50.2X2	T50.2X3	T50.2X4	T50.2X5	T50.2X6
Benzylpenicillin	T36.0X1	T36.0X2	T36.0X3	T36.0X4	T36.0X5	T36.0X6
Benzylthiouracil	T38.2X1	T38.2X2	T38.2X3	T38.2X4	T38.2X5	T38.2X6
Bephenium hydroxynaphthoate	T37.4X1	T37.4X2	T37.4X3	T37.4X4	T37.4X5	T37.4X6
Bepridil	T46.1X1	T46.1X2	T46.1X3	T46.1X4	T46.1X5	T46.1X6
Bergamot oil	T65.891	T65.892	T65.893	T65.894	—	—
Bergapten	T50.991	T50.992	T50.993	T50.994	T50.995	T50.996
Berries, poisonous	T62.1X1	T62.1X2	T62.1X3	T62.1X4	—	—
Beryllium (compounds)	T56.7X1	T56.7X2	T56.7X3	T56.7X4	—	—
beta adrenergic blocking agent, heart	T44.7X1	T44.7X2	T44.7X3	T44.7X4	T44.7X5	T44.7X6
Betacarotene	T45.2X1	T45.2X2	T45.2X3	T45.2X4	T45.2X5	T45.2X6
Beta-Chlor	T42.6X1	T42.6X2	T42.6X3	T42.6X4	T42.6X5	T42.6X6
Betahistine	T46.7X1	T46.7X2	T46.7X3	T46.7X4	T46.7X5	T46.7X6
Betaine	T47.5X1	T47.5X2	T47.5X3	T47.5X4	T47.5X5	T47.5X6
Betamethasone	T49.0X1	T49.0X2	T49.0X3	T49.0X4	T49.0X5	T49.0X6
topical	T49.0X1	T49.0X2	T49.0X3	T49.0X4	T49.0X5	T49.0X6
Betamicin	T36.8X1	T36.8X2	T36.8X3	T36.8X4	T36.8X5	T36.8X6
Betanidine	T46.5X1	T46.5X2	T46.5X3	T46.5X4	T46.5X5	T46.5X6
Betaxolol	T44.7X1	T44.7X2	T44.7X3	T44.7X4	T44.7X5	T44.7X6
Betazole	T50.8X1	T50.8X2	T50.8X3	T50.8X4	T50.8X5	T50.8X6
Bethanechol	T44.1X1	T44.1X2	T44.1X3	T44.1X4	T44.1X5	T44.1X6
chloride	T44.1X1	T44.1X2	T44.1X3	T44.1X4	T44.1X5	T44.1X6
Bethanidine	T46.5X1	T46.5X2	T46.5X3	T46.5X4	T46.5X5	T46.5X6
Betoxycaine	T41.3X1	T41.3X2	T41.3X3	T41.3X4	T41.3X5	T41.3X6
Betula oil	T49.3X1	T49.3X2	T49.3X3	T49.3X4	T49.3X5	T49.3X6
Bevantolol	T44.7X1	T44.7X2	T44.7X3	T44.7X4	T44.7X5	T44.7X6
Bevonium metilsulfate	T44.3X1	T44.3X2	T44.3X3	T44.3X4	T44.3X5	T44.3X6
Bezafibrate	T46.6X1	T46.6X2	T46.6X3	T46.6X4	T46.6X5	T46.6X6
Bezitramide	T40.4X1	T40.4X2	T40.4X3	T40.4X4	T40.4X5	T40.4X6
BHA	T50.991	T50.992	T50.993	T50.994	T50.995	T50.996
Bhang	T40.7X1	T40.7X2	T40.7X3	T40.7X4	T40.7X5	T40.7X6
BHC (medicinal)	T49.0X1	T49.0X2	T49.0X3	T49.0X4	T49.0X5	T49.0X6

Substance	Poisoning, Accidental (unintentional)	Poisoning, Intentional Self-harm	Poisoning, Assault	Poisoning, Undetermined	Adverse Effect	Under-dosing
BHC — continued						
nonmedicinal (vapor)	T53.6X1	T53.6X2	T53.6X3	T53.6X4	—	—
Bialamicol	T37.3X1	T37.3X2	T37.3X3	T37.3X4	T37.3X5	T37.3X6
Bibenzonium bromide	T48.3X1	T48.3X2	T48.3X3	T48.3X4	T48.3X5	T48.3X6
Bibrocathol	T49.5X1	T49.5X2	T49.5X3	T49.5X4	T49.5X5	T49.5X6
Bichloride of mercury — see Mercury, chloride						
Bichromates (calcium) (potassium)(sodium) (crystals)	T57.8X1	T57.8X2	T57.8X3	T57.8X4		
fumes	T56.2X1	T56.2X2	T56.2X3	T56.2X4		
Biclotymol	T49.6X1	T49.6X2	T49.6X3	T49.6X4	T49.6X5	T49.6X6
Bicucculine	T50.7X1	T50.7X2	T50.7X3	T50.7X4	T50.7X5	T50.7X6
Bifemelane	T43.291	T43.292	T43.293	T43.294	T43.295	T43.296
Biguanide derivatives, oral	T38.3X1	T38.3X2	T38.3X3	T38.3X4	T38.3X5	T38.3X6
Bile salts	T47.5X1	T47.5X2	T47.5X3	T47.5X4	T47.5X5	T47.5X6
Biligrafin	T50.8X1	T50.8X2	T50.8X3	T50.8X4	T50.8X5	T50.8X6
Bilopaque	T50.8X1	T50.8X2	T50.8X3	T50.8X4	T50.8X5	T50.8X6
Binifibrate	T46.6X1	T46.6X2	T46.6X3	T46.6X4	T46.6X5	T46.6X6
Binitrobenzol	T65.3X1	T65.3X2	T65.3X3	T65.3X4	—	—
Bioflavonoid(s)	T46.991	T46.992	T46.993	T46.994	T46.995	T46.996
Biological substance NEC	T50.901	T50.902	T50.903	T50.904	T50.905	T50.906
Biotin	T45.2X1	T45.2X2	T45.2X3	T45.2X4	T45.2X5	T45.2X6
Biperiden	T44.3X1	T44.3X2	T44.3X3	T44.3X4	T44.3X5	T44.3X6
Bisacodyl	T47.2X1	T47.2X2	T47.2X3	T47.2X4	T47.2X5	T47.2X6
Bisbentiamine	T45.2X1	T45.2X2	T45.2X3	T45.2X4	T45.2X5	T45.2X6
Bisbutiamine	T45.2X1	T45.2X2	T45.2X3	T45.2X4	T45.2X5	T45.2X6
Bisdequalinium (salts) (diacetate)	T49.6X1	T49.6X2	T49.6X3	T49.6X4	T49.6X5	T49.6X6
Bishydroxycoumarin	T45.511	T45.512	T45.513	T45.514	T45.515	T45.516
Bismarsen	T37.8X1	T37.8X2	T37.8X3	T37.8X4	T37.8X5	T37.8X6
Bismuth salts	T47.6X1	T47.6X2	T47.6X3	T47.6X4	T47.6X5	T47.6X6
aluminate	T47.1X1	T47.1X2	T47.1X3	T47.1X4	T47.1X5	T47.1X6
anti-infectives	T37.8X1	T37.8X2	T37.8X3	T37.8X4	T37.8X5	T37.8X6
formic iodide	T49.0X1	T49.0X2	T49.0X3	T49.0X4	T49.0X5	T49.0X6
glycolylarsenate	T49.0X1	T49.0X2	T49.0X3	T49.0X4	T49.0X5	T49.0X6
nonmedicinal (compounds) NEC	T65.91	T65.92	T65.93	T65.94	—	—
subcarbonate	T47.6X1	T47.6X2	T47.6X3	T47.6X4	T47.6X5	T47.6X6
subsalicylate	T37.8X1	T37.8X2	T37.8X3	T37.8X4	T37.8X5	T37.8X6
sulfarsphenamine	T37.8X1	T37.8X2	T37.8X3	T37.8X4	T37.8X5	T37.8X6
Bisoprolol	T44.7X1	T44.7X2	T44.7X3	T44.7X4	T44.7X5	T44.7X6
Bisoxatin	T47.2X1	T47.2X2	T47.2X3	T47.2X4	T47.2X5	T47.2X6
Bisulepin (hydrochloride)	T45.0X1	T45.0X2	T45.0X3	T45.0X4	T45.0X5	T45.0X6
Bithionol	T37.8X1	T37.8X2	T37.8X3	T37.8X4	T37.8X5	T37.8X6
anthelminthic	T37.4X1	T37.4X2	T37.4X3	T37.4X4	T37.4X5	T37.4X6
Bitolterol	T48.6X1	T48.6X2	T48.6X3	T48.6X4	T48.6X5	T48.6X6
Bitoscanate	T37.4X1	T37.4X2	T37.4X3	T37.4X4	T37.4X5	T37.4X6
Bitter almond oil	T62.8X1	T62.8X2	T62.8X3	T62.8X4	—	—
Bittersweet	T62.2X1	T62.2X2	T62.2X3	T62.2X4	—	—
Black						
flag	T60.91	T60.92	T60.93	T60.94	—	—
henbane	T62.2X1	T62.2X2	T62.2X3	T62.2X4	—	—
leaf (40)	T60.91	T60.92	T60.93	T60.94	—	—
widow spider (bite)	T63.311	T63.312	T63.313	T63.314		
antivenin	T50.Z11	T50.Z12	T50.Z13	T50.Z14	T50.Z15	T50.Z16
Blast furnace gas (carbon monoxide from)	T58.8X1	T58.8X2	T58.8X3	T58.8X4		
Bleach	T54.91	T54.92	T54.93	T54.94		
Bleaching agent (medicinal)	T49.4X1	T49.4X2	T49.4X3	T49.4X4	T49.4X5	T49.4X6
Bleomycin	T45.1X1	T45.1X2	T45.1X3	T45.1X4	T45.1X5	T45.1X6
Blockain	T41.3X1	T41.3X2	T41.3X3	T41.3X4	T41.3X5	T41.3X6
infiltration (subcutaneous)	T41.3X1	T41.3X2	T41.3X3	T41.3X4	T41.3X5	T41.3X6
nerve block (peripheral) (plexus)	T41.3X1	T41.3X2	T41.3X3	T41.3X4	T41.3X5	T41.3X6
topical (surface)	T41.3X1	T41.3X2	T41.3X3	T41.3X4	T41.3X5	T41.3X6
Blockers, calcium channel	T46.1X1	T46.1X2	T46.1X3	T46.1X4	T46.1X5	T46.1X6
Blood (derivatives) (natural) (plasma) (whole)	T45.8X1	T45.8X2	T45.8X3	T45.8X4	T45.8X5	T45.8X6
dried	T45.8X1	T45.8X2	T45.8X3	T45.8X4	T45.8X5	T45.8X6
drug affecting NEC	T45.91	T45.92	T45.93	T45.94	T45.95	T45.96
expander NEC	T45.8X1	T45.8X2	T45.8X3	T45.8X4	T45.8X5	T45.8X6
fraction NEC	T45.8X1	T45.8X2	T45.8X3	T45.8X4	T45.8X5	T45.8X6
substitute (macromolecular)	T45.8X1	T45.8X2	T45.8X3	T45.8X4	T45.8X5	T45.8X6
Blue velvet	T40.2X1	T40.2X2	T40.2X3	T40.2X4	—	—
Bone meal	T62.8X1	T62.8X2	T62.8X3	T62.8X4	—	—
Bonine	T45.0X1	T45.0X2	T45.0X3	T45.0X4	T45.0X5	T45.0X6
Bopindolol	T44.7X1	T44.7X2	T44.7X3	T44.7X4	T44.7X5	T44.7X6
Boracic acid	T49.0X1	T49.0X2	T49.0X3	T49.0X4	T49.0X5	T49.0X6
ENT agent	T49.6X1	T49.6X2	T49.6X3	T49.6X4	T49.6X5	T49.6X6
ophthalmic preparation	T49.5X1	T49.5X2	T49.5X3	T49.5X4	T49.5X5	T49.5X6
Borane complex	T57.8X1	T57.8X2	T57.8X3	T57.8X4	—	—

Benzedrine — Borane complex

Table of Drugs and Chemicals

Substance	Poisoning, Accidental (unintentional)	Poisoning, Intentional Self-harm	Poisoning, Assault	Poisoning, Undetermined	Adverse Effect	Under-dosing
Borate(s)	T57.8X1	T57.8X2	T57.8X3	T57.8X4	—	—
buffer	T50.991	T50.992	T50.993	T50.994	T50.995	T50.996
cleanser	T54.91	T54.92	T54.93	T54.94	—	—
sodium	T57.8X1	T57.8X2	T57.8X3	T57.8X4	—	—
Borax (cleanser)	T54.91	T54.92	T54.93	T54.94	—	—
Bordeaux mixture	T60.3X1	T60.3X2	T60.3X3	T60.3X4	—	—
Boric acid	T49.0X1	T49.0X2	T49.0X3	T49.0X4	T49.0X5	T49.0X6
ENT agent	T49.6X1	T49.6X2	T49.6X3	T49.6X4	T49.6X5	T49.6X6
ophthalmic preparation	T49.5X1	T49.5X2	T49.5X3	T49.5X4	T49.5X5	T49.5X6
Bornaprine	T44.3X1	T44.3X2	T44.3X3	T44.3X4	T44.3X5	T44.3X6
Boron	T57.8X1	T57.8X2	T57.8X3	T57.8X4	—	—
hydride NEC	T57.8X1	T57.8X2	T57.8X3	T57.8X4	—	—
fumes or gas	T57.8X1	T57.8X2	T57.8X3	T57.8X4	—	—
trifluoride	T59.891	T59.892	T59.893	T59.894	—	—
Botox	T48.291	T48.292	T48.293	T48.294	T48.295	T48.296
Botulinus anti-toxin (type A, B)	T50.Z11	T50.Z12	T50.Z13	T50.Z14	T50.Z15	T50.Z16
Brake fluid vapor	T59.891	T59.892	T59.893	T59.894	—	—
Brallobarbital	T42.3X1	T42.3X2	T42.3X3	T42.3X4	T42.3X5	T42.3X6
Bran (wheat)	T47.4X1	T47.4X2	T47.4X3	T47.4X4	T47.4X5	T47.4X6
Brass (fumes)	T56.891	T56.892	T56.893	T56.894	—	—
Brasso	T52.0X1	T52.0X2	T52.0X3	T52.0X4	—	—
Bretylium tosilate	T46.2X1	T46.2X2	T46.2X3	T46.2X4	T46.2X5	T46.2X6
Brevital (sodium)	T41.1X1	T41.1X2	T41.1X3	T41.1X4	T41.1X5	T41.1X6
Brinase	T45.3X1	T45.3X2	T45.3X3	T45.3X4	T45.3X5	T45.3X6
British antilewisite	T45.8X1	T45.8X2	T45.8X3	T45.8X4	T45.8X5	T45.8X6
Brodifacoum	T60.4X1	T60.4X2	T60.4X3	T60.4X4	—	—
Bromal (hydrate)	T42.6X1	T42.6X2	T42.6X3	T42.6X4	T42.6X5	T42.6X6
Bromazepam	T42.4X1	T42.4X2	T42.4X3	T42.4X4	T42.4X5	T42.4X6
Bromazine	T45.0X1	T45.0X2	T45.0X3	T45.0X4	T45.0X5	T45.0X6
Brombenzylcyanide	T59.3X1	T59.3X2	T59.3X3	T59.3X4	—	—
Bromelains	T45.3X1	T45.3X2	T45.3X3	T45.3X4	T45.3X5	T45.3X6
Bromethalin	T60.4X1	T60.4X2	T60.4X3	T60.4X4	—	—
Bromhexine	T48.4X1	T48.4X2	T48.4X3	T48.4X4	T48.4X5	T48.4X6
Bromide salts	T42.6X1	T42.6X2	T42.6X3	T42.6X4	T42.6X5	T42.6X6
Bromindione	T45.511	T45.512	T45.513	T45.514	T45.515	T45.516
Bromine	T42.6X1	T42.6X2	T42.6X3	T42.6X4	T42.6X5	T42.6X6
compounds (medicinal)	T42.6X1	T42.6X2	T42.6X3	T42.6X4	T42.6X5	T42.6X6
sedative	T42.6X1	T42.6X2	T42.6X3	T42.6X4	T42.6X5	T42.6X6
vapor	T59.891	T59.892	T59.893	T59.894	—	—
Bromisoval	T42.6X1	T42.6X2	T42.6X3	T42.6X4	T42.6X5	T42.6X6
Bromisovalum	T42.6X1	T42.6X2	T42.6X3	T42.6X4	T42.6X5	T42.6X6
Bromobenzylcyanide	T59.3X1	T59.3X2	T59.3X3	T59.3X4	—	—
Bromochlorosalicylani-lide	T49.0X1	T49.0X2	T49.0X3	T49.0X4	T49.0X5	T49.0X6
Bromocriptine	T42.8X1	T42.8X2	T42.8X3	T42.8X4	T42.8X5	T42.8X6
Bromodiphenhydramine	T45.0X1	T45.0X2	T45.0X3	T45.0X4	T45.0X5	T45.0X6
Bromoform	T42.6X1	T42.6X2	T42.6X3	T42.6X4	T42.6X5	T42.6X6
Bromophenol blue reagent	T50.991	T50.992	T50.993	T50.994	T50.995	T50.996
Bromopride	T47.8X1	T47.8X2	T47.8X3	T47.8X4	T47.8X5	T47.8X6
Bromosalicylchloranitide	T49.0X1	T49.0X2	T49.0X3	T49.0X4	T49.0X5	T49.0X6
Bromosalicylhydroxamic acid	T37.1X1	T37.1X2	T37.1X3	T37.1X4	T37.1X5	T37.1X6
Bromo-seltzer	T39.1X1	T39.1X2	T39.1X3	T39.1X4	T39.1X5	T39.1X6
Bromoxynil	T60.3X1	T60.3X2	T60.3X3	T60.3X4	—	—
Bromperidol	T43.4X1	T43.4X2	T43.4X3	T43.4X4	T43.4X5	T43.4X6
Brompheniramine	T45.0X1	T45.0X2	T45.0X3	T45.0X4	T45.0X5	T45.0X6
Bromsulfophthalein	T50.8X1	T50.8X2	T50.8X3	T50.8X4	T50.8X5	T50.8X6
Bromural	T42.6X1	T42.6X2	T42.6X3	T42.6X4	T42.6X5	T42.6X6
Bromvaletone	T42.6X1	T42.6X2	T42.6X3	T42.6X4	T42.6X5	T42.6X6
Bronchodilator NEC	T48.6X1	T48.6X2	T48.6X3	T48.6X4	T48.6X5	T48.6X6
Brotizolam	T42.4X1	T42.4X2	T42.4X3	T42.4X4	T42.4X5	T42.4X6
Brovincamine	T46.7X1	T46.7X2	T46.7X3	T46.7X4	T46.7X5	T46.7X6
Brown recluse spider (bite) (venom)	T63.331	T63.332	T63.333	T63.334	—	—
Brown spider (bite) (venom)	T63.391	T63.392	T63.393	T63.394	—	—
Broxaterol	T48.6X1	T48.6X2	T48.6X3	T48.6X4	T48.6X5	T48.6X6
Broxuridine	T45.1X1	T45.1X2	T45.1X3	T45.1X4	T45.1X5	T45.1X6
Broxyquinoline	T37.8X1	T37.8X2	T37.8X3	T37.8X4	T37.8X5	T37.8X6
Bruceine	T48.291	T48.292	T48.293	T48.294	T48.295	T48.296
Brucia	T62.2X1	T62.2X2	T62.2X3	T62.2X4	—	—
Brucine	T65.1X1	T65.1X2	T65.1X3	T65.1X4	—	—
Brunswick green — see Copper						
Bruten — see Ibuprofen						
Bryonia	T47.2X1	T47.2X2	T47.2X3	T47.2X4	T47.2X5	T47.2X6
Buclizine	T45.0X1	T45.0X2	T45.0X3	T45.0X4	T45.0X5	T45.0X6
Buclosamide	T49.0X1	T49.0X2	T49.0X3	T49.0X4	T49.0X5	T49.0X6
Budesonide	T44.5X1	T44.5X2	T44.5X3	T44.5X4	T44.5X5	T44.5X6
Budralazine	T46.5X1	T46.5X2	T46.5X3	T46.5X4	T46.5X5	T46.5X6
Bufferin	T39.011	T39.012	T39.013	T39.014	T39.015	T39.016
Buflomedil	T46.7X1	T46.7X2	T46.7X3	T46.7X4	T46.7X5	T46.7X6
Buformin	T38.3X1	T38.3X2	T38.3X3	T38.3X4	T38.3X5	T38.3X6
Bufotenine	T40.991	T40.992	T40.993	T40.994	—	—
Bufrolin	T48.6X1	T48.6X2	T48.6X3	T48.6X4	T48.6X5	T48.6X6
Bufylline	T48.6X1	T48.6X2	T48.6X3	T48.6X4	T48.6X5	T48.6X6
Bulk filler	T50.5X1	T50.5X2	T50.5X3	T50.5X4	T50.5X5	T50.5X6
cathartic	T47.4X1	T47.4X2	T47.4X3	T47.4X4	T47.4X5	T47.4X6
Bumetanide	T50.1X1	T50.1X2	T50.1X3	T50.1X4	T50.1X5	T50.1X6
Bunaftine	T46.2X1	T46.2X2	T46.2X3	T46.2X4	T46.2X5	T46.2X6
Bunamiodyl	T50.8X1	T50.8X2	T50.8X3	T50.8X4	T50.8X5	T50.8X6
Bunazosin	T44.6X1	T44.6X2	T44.6X3	T44.6X4	T44.6X5	T44.6X6
Bunitrolol	T44.7X1	T44.7X2	T44.7X3	T44.7X4	T44.7X5	T44.7X6
Buphenine	T46.7X1	T46.7X2	T46.7X3	T46.7X4	T46.7X5	T46.7X6
Bupivacaine	T41.3X1	T41.3X2	T41.3X3	T41.3X4	T41.3X5	T41.3X6
infiltration (subcutaneous)	T41.3X1	T41.3X2	T41.3X3	T41.3X4	T41.3X5	T41.3X6
nerve block (peripheral) (plexus)	T41.3X1	T41.3X2	T41.3X3	T41.3X4	T41.3X5	T41.3X6
spinal	T41.3X1	T41.3X2	T41.3X3	T41.3X4	T41.3X5	T41.3X6
Bupranolol	T44.7X1	T44.7X2	T44.7X3	T44.7X4	T44.7X5	T44.7X6
Buprenorphine	T40.4X1	T40.4X2	T40.4X3	T40.4X4	T40.4X5	T40.4X6
Bupropion	T43.291	T43.292	T43.293	T43.294	T43.295	T43.296
Burimamide	T47.1X1	T47.1X2	T47.1X3	T47.1X4	T47.1X5	T47.1X6
Buserelin	T38.891	T38.892	T38.893	T38.894	T38.895	T38.896
Buspirone	T43.591	T43.592	T43.593	T43.594	T43.595	T43.596
Busulfan, busulphan	T45.1X1	T45.1X2	T45.1X3	T45.1X4	T45.1X5	T45.1X6
Butabarbital (sodium)	T42.3X1	T42.3X2	T42.3X3	T42.3X4	T42.3X5	T42.3X6
Butabarbitone	T42.3X1	T42.3X2	T42.3X3	T42.3X4	T42.3X5	T42.3X6
Butabarpal	T42.3X1	T42.3X2	T42.3X3	T42.3X4	T42.3X5	T42.3X6
Butacaine	T41.3X1	T41.3X2	T41.3X3	T41.3X4	T41.3X5	T41.3X6
Butalamine	T46.7X1	T46.7X2	T46.7X3	T46.7X4	T46.7X5	T46.7X6
Butalbital	T42.3X1	T42.3X2	T42.3X3	T42.3X4	T42.3X5	T42.3X6
Butallylonal	T42.3X1	T42.3X2	T42.3X3	T42.3X4	T42.3X5	T42.3X6
Butamben	T41.3X1	T41.3X2	T41.3X3	T41.3X4	T41.3X5	T41.3X6
Butamirate	T48.3X1	T48.3X2	T48.3X3	T48.3X4	T48.3X5	T48.3X6
Butane (distributed in mobile container)	T59.891	T59.892	T59.893	T59.894	—	—
distributed through pipes	T59.891	T59.892	T59.893	T59.894	—	—
incomplete combustion	T58.11	T58.12	T58.13	T58.14	—	—
Butanilicaine	T41.3X1	T41.3X2	T41.3X3	T41.3X4	T41.3X5	T41.3X6
Butanol	T51.3X1	T51.3X2	T51.3X3	T51.3X4	—	—
Butanone, 2-butanone	T52.4X1	T52.4X2	T52.4X3	T52.4X4	—	—
Butantrone	T49.4X1	T49.4X2	T49.4X3	T49.4X4	T49.4X5	T49.4X6
Butaperazine	T43.3X1	T43.3X2	T43.3X3	T43.3X4	T43.3X5	T43.3X6
Butazolidin	T39.2X1	T39.2X2	T39.2X3	T39.2X4	T39.2X5	T39.2X6
Butetamate	T48.6X1	T48.6X2	T48.6X3	T48.6X4	T48.6X5	T48.6X6
Butethal	T42.3X1	T42.3X2	T42.3X3	T42.3X4	T42.3X5	T42.3X6
Butethamate	T44.3X1	T44.3X2	T44.3X3	T44.3X4	T44.3X5	T44.3X6
Buthalitone (sodium)	T41.1X1	T41.1X2	T41.1X3	T41.1X4	T41.1X5	T41.1X6
Butisol (sodium)	T42.3X1	T42.3X2	T42.3X3	T42.3X4	T42.3X5	T42.3X6
Butizide	T50.2X1	T50.2X2	T50.2X3	T50.2X4	T50.2X5	T50.2X6
Butobarbital	T42.3X1	T42.3X2	T42.3X3	T42.3X4	T42.3X5	T42.3X6
sodium	T42.3X1	T42.3X2	T42.3X3	T42.3X4	T42.3X5	T42.3X6
Butobarbitone	T42.3X1	T42.3X2	T42.3X3	T42.3X4	T42.3X5	T42.3X6
Butoconazole (nitrate)	T49.0X1	T49.0X2	T49.0X3	T49.0X4	T49.0X5	T49.0X6
Butorphanol	T40.4X1	T40.4X2	T40.4X3	T40.4X4	T40.4X5	T40.4X6
Butriptyline	T43.011	T43.012	T43.013	T43.014	T43.015	T43.016
Butropium bromide	T44.3X1	T44.3X2	T44.3X3	T44.3X4	T44.3X5	T44.3X6
Buttercups	T62.2X1	T62.2X2	T62.2X3	T62.2X4	—	—
Butter of antimony — see Antimony						
Butyl						
acetate (secondary)	T52.8X1	T52.8X2	T52.8X3	T52.8X4	—	—
alcohol	T51.3X1	T51.3X2	T51.3X3	T51.3X4	—	—
aminobenzoate	T41.3X1	T41.3X2	T41.3X3	T41.3X4	T41.3X5	T41.3X6
butyrate	T52.8X1	T52.8X2	T52.8X3	T52.8X4	—	—
carbinol	T51.3X1	T51.3X2	T51.3X3	T51.3X4	—	—
carbitol	T52.3X1	T52.3X2	T52.3X3	T52.3X4	—	—
cellosolve	T52.3X1	T52.3X2	T52.3X3	T52.3X4	—	—
chloral (hydrate)	T42.6X1	T42.6X2	T42.6X3	T42.6X4	T42.6X5	T42.6X6
formate	T52.8X1	T52.8X2	T52.8X3	T52.8X4	—	—
lactate	T52.8X1	T52.8X2	T52.8X3	T52.8X4	—	—
propionate	T52.8X1	T52.8X2	T52.8X3	T52.8X4	—	—
scopolamine bromide	T44.3X1	T44.3X2	T44.3X3	T44.3X4	T44.3X5	T44.3X6
thiobarbital sodium	T41.1X1	T41.1X2	T41.1X3	T41.1X4	T41.1X5	T41.1X6
Butylated hydroxyanisole	T50.991	T50.992	T50.993	T50.994	T50.995	T50.996
Butylchloral hydrate	T42.6X1	T42.6X2	T42.6X3	T42.6X4	T42.6X5	T42.6X6
Butyltoluene	T52.2X1	T52.2X2	T52.2X3	T52.2X4	—	—
Butyn	T41.3X1	T41.3X2	T41.3X3	T41.3X4	T41.3X5	T41.3X6
Butyrophenone (-based tranquilizers)	T43.4X1	T43.4X2	T43.4X3	T43.4X4	T43.4X5	T43.4X6
Cabergoline	T42.8X1	T42.8X2	T42.8X3	T42.8X4	T42.8X5	T42.8X6
Cacodyl, cacodylic acid	T57.0X1	T57.0X2	T57.0X3	T57.0X4	—	—
Cactinomycin	T45.1X1	T45.1X2	T45.1X3	T45.1X4	T45.1X5	T45.1X6
Cade oil	T49.4X1	T49.4X2	T49.4X3	T49.4X4	T49.4X5	T49.4X6
Cadexomer iodine	T49.0X1	T49.0X2	T49.0X3	T49.0X4	T49.0X5	T49.0X6
Cadmium (chloride) (fumes) (oxide)	T56.3X1	T56.3X2	T56.3X3	T56.3X4	—	—

Table of Drugs and Chemicals

Borate — Cadmium

Additional Character May Be Required — Refer to the Tabular List for Character Selection   ▽ Subterms under main terms may continue to next column or page

Substance	Poisoning, Accidental (unintentional)	Poisoning, Intentional Self-harm	Poisoning, Assault	Poisoning, Undetermined	Adverse Effect	Under-dosing
Cadmium — *continued*						
sulfide (medicinal) NEC	T49.4X1	T49.4X2	T49.4X3	T49.4X4	T49.4X5	T49.4X6
Cadralazine	T46.5X1	T46.5X2	T46.5X3	T46.5X4	T46.5X5	T46.5X6
Caffeine	T43.611	T43.612	T43.613	T43.614	T43.615	T43.616
Calabar bean	T62.2X1	T62.2X2	T62.2X3	T62.2X4	—	—
Caladium seguinum	T62.2X1	T62.2X2	T62.2X3	T62.2X4	—	—
Calamine (lotion)	T49.3X1	T49.3X2	T49.3X3	T49.3X4	T49.3X5	T49.3X6
Calcifediol	T45.2X1	T45.2X2	T45.2X3	T45.2X4	T45.2X5	T45.2X6
Calciferol	T45.2X1	T45.2X2	T45.2X3	T45.2X4	T45.2X5	T45.2X6
Calcitonin	T50.991	T50.992	T50.993	T50.994	T50.995	T50.996
Calcitriol	T45.2X1	T45.2X2	T45.2X3	T45.2X4	T45.2X5	T45.2X6
Calcium	T50.3X1	T50.3X2	T50.3X3	T50.3X4	T50.3X5	T50.3X6
actylsalicylate	T39.011	T39.012	T39.013	T39.014	T39.015	T39.016
benzamidosalicylate	T37.1X1	T37.1X2	T37.1X3	T37.1X4	T37.1X5	T37.1X6
bromide	T42.6X1	T42.6X2	T42.6X3	T42.6X4	T42.6X5	T42.6X6
bromolactobionate	T42.6X1	T42.6X2	T42.6X3	T42.6X4	T42.6X5	T42.6X6
carbaspirin	T39.011	T39.012	T39.013	T39.014	T39.015	T39.016
carbimide	T50.6X1	T50.6X2	T50.6X3	T50.6X4	T50.6X5	T50.6X6
carbonate	T47.1X1	T47.1X2	T47.1X3	T47.1X4	T47.1X5	T47.1X6
chloride	T50.991	T50.992	T50.993	T50.994	T50.995	T50.996
anhydrous	T50.991	T50.992	T50.993	T50.994	T50.995	T50.996
cyanide	T57.8X1	T57.8X2	T57.8X3	T57.8X4	—	—
dioctyl sulfosuccinate	T47.4X1	T47.4X2	T47.4X3	T47.4X4	T47.4X5	T47.4X6
disodium edathamil	T45.8X1	T45.8X2	T45.8X3	T45.8X4	T45.8X5	T45.8X6
disodium edetate	T45.8X1	T45.8X2	T45.8X3	T45.8X4	T45.8X5	T45.8X6
dobesilate	T46.991	T46.992	T46.993	T46.994	T46.995	T46.996
EDTA	T45.8X1	T45.8X2	T45.8X3	T45.8X4	T45.8X5	T45.8X6
ferrous citrate	T45.4X1	T45.4X2	T45.4X3	T45.4X4	T45.4X5	T45.4X6
folinate	T45.8X1	T45.8X2	T45.8X3	T45.8X4	T45.8X5	T45.8X6
glubionate	T50.3X1	T50.3X2	T50.3X3	T50.3X4	T50.3X5	T50.3X6
gluconate	T50.3X1	T50.3X2	T50.3X3	T50.3X4	T50.3X5	T50.3X6
gluconogalactogluconate	T50.3X1	T50.3X2	T50.3X3	T50.3X4	T50.3X5	T50.3X6
hydrate, hydroxide	T54.3X1	T54.3X2	T54.3X3	T54.3X4	—	—
hypochlorite	T54.3X1	T54.3X2	T54.3X3	T54.3X4	—	—
iodide	T48.4X1	T48.4X2	T48.4X3	T48.4X4	T48.4X5	T48.4X6
ipodate	T50.8X1	T50.8X2	T50.8X3	T50.8X4	T50.8X5	T50.8X6
lactate	T50.3X1	T50.3X2	T50.3X3	T50.3X4	T50.3X5	T50.3X6
leucovorin	T45.8X1	T45.8X2	T45.8X3	T45.8X4	T45.8X5	T45.8X6
mandelate	T37.91	T37.92	T37.93	T37.94	T37.95	T37.96
oxide	T54.3X1	T54.3X2	T54.3X3	T54.3X4	—	—
pantothenate	T45.2X1	T45.2X2	T45.2X3	T45.2X4	T45.2X5	T45.2X6
phosphate	T50.3X1	T50.3X2	T50.3X3	T50.3X4	T50.3X5	T50.3X6
salicylate	T39.091	T39.092	T39.093	T39.094	T39.095	T39.096
salts	T50.3X1	T50.3X2	T50.3X3	T50.3X4	T50.3X5	T50.3X6
Calculus-dissolving drug	T50.991	T50.992	T50.993	T50.994	T50.995	T50.996
Calomel	T49.0X1	T49.0X2	T49.0X3	T49.0X4	T49.0X5	T49.0X6
Caloric agent	T50.3X1	T50.3X2	T50.3X3	T50.3X4	T50.3X5	T50.3X6
Calusterone	T38.7X1	T38.7X2	T38.7X3	T38.7X4	T38.7X5	T38.7X6
Camazepam	T42.4X1	T42.4X2	T42.4X3	T42.4X4	T42.4X5	T42.4X6
Camomile	T49.0X1	T49.0X2	T49.0X3	T49.0X4	T49.0X5	T49.0X6
Camoquin	T37.2X1	T37.2X2	T37.2X3	T37.2X4	T37.2X5	T37.2X6
Camphor						
insecticide	T60.2X1	T60.2X2	T60.2X3	T60.2X4	—	—
medicinal	T49.8X1	T49.8X2	T49.8X3	T49.8X4	T49.8X5	T49.8X6
Camylofin	T44.3X1	T44.3X2	T44.3X3	T44.3X4	T44.3X5	T44.3X6
Cancer chemotherapy drug regimen	T45.1X1	T45.1X2	T45.1X3	T45.1X4	T45.1X5	T45.1X6
Candeptin	T49.0X1	T49.0X2	T49.0X3	T49.0X4	T49.0X5	T49.0X6
Candicidin	T49.0X1	T49.0X2	T49.0X3	T49.0X4	T49.0X5	T49.0X6
Cannabinol	T40.7X1	T40.7X2	T40.7X3	T40.7X4	T40.7X5	T40.7X6
Cannabis (derivatives)	T40.7X1	T40.7X2	T40.7X3	T40.7X4	T40.7X5	T40.7X6
Canned heat	T51.1X1	T51.1X2	T51.1X3	T51.1X4	—	—
Canrenoic acid	T50.0X1	T50.0X2	T50.0X3	T50.0X4	T50.0X5	T50.0X6
Canrenone	T50.0X1	T50.0X2	T50.0X3	T50.0X4	T50.0X5	T50.0X6
Cantharides, cantharidin, cantharis	T49.8X1	T49.8X2	T49.8X3	T49.8X4	T49.8X5	T49.8X6
Canthaxanthin	T50.991	T50.992	T50.993	T50.994	T50.995	T50.996
Capillary-active drug NEC	T46.901	T46.902	T46.903	T46.904	T46.905	T46.906
Capreomycin	T36.8X1	T36.8X2	T36.8X3	T36.8X4	T36.8X5	T36.8X6
Capsicum	T49.4X1	T49.4X2	T49.4X3	T49.4X4	T49.4X5	T49.4X6
Captafol	T60.3X1	T60.3X2	T60.3X3	T60.3X4	—	—
Captan	T60.3X1	T60.3X2	T60.3X3	T60.3X4	—	—
Captodiame, captodiamine	T43.591	T43.592	T43.593	T43.594	T43.595	T43.596
Captopril	T46.4X1	T46.4X2	T46.4X3	T46.4X4	T46.4X5	T46.4X6
Caramiphen	T44.3X1	T44.3X2	T44.3X3	T44.3X4	T44.3X5	T44.3X6
Carazolol	T44.7X1	T44.7X2	T44.7X3	T44.7X4	T44.7X5	T44.7X6
Carbachol	T44.1X1	T44.1X2	T44.1X3	T44.1X4	T44.1X5	T44.1X6
Carbacrylamine (resin)	T50.3X1	T50.3X2	T50.3X3	T50.3X4	T50.3X5	T50.3X6
Carbamate (insecticide)	T60.0X1	T60.0X2	T60.0X3	T60.0X4	—	—
Carbamate (sedative)	T42.6X1	T42.6X2	T42.6X3	T42.6X4	T42.6X5	T42.6X6
herbicide	T60.0X1	T60.0X2	T60.0X3	T60.0X4	—	—
insecticide	T60.0X1	T60.0X2	T60.0X3	T60.0X4	—	—
Carbamazepine	T42.1X1	T42.1X2	T42.1X3	T42.1X4	T42.1X5	T42.1X6

Substance	Poisoning, Accidental (unintentional)	Poisoning, Intentional Self-harm	Poisoning, Assault	Poisoning, Undetermined	Adverse Effect	Under-dosing
Carbamide	T47.3X1	T47.3X2	T47.3X3	T47.3X4	T47.3X5	T47.3X6
peroxide	T49.0X1	T49.0X2	T49.0X3	T49.0X4	T49.0X5	T49.0X6
topical	T49.8X1	T49.8X2	T49.8X3	T49.8X4	T49.8X5	T49.8X6
Carbamylcholine chloride	T44.1X1	T44.1X2	T44.1X3	T44.1X4	T44.1X5	T44.1X6
Carbaril	T60.0X1	T60.0X2	T60.0X3	T60.0X4	—	—
Carbarsone	T37.3X1	T37.3X2	T37.3X3	T37.3X4	T37.3X5	T37.3X6
Carbaryl	T60.0X1	T60.0X2	T60.0X3	T60.0X4	—	—
Carbaspirin	T39.011	T39.012	T39.013	T39.014	T39.015	T39.016
Carbazochrome (salicylate) (sodium sulfonate)	T49.4X1	T49.4X2	T49.4X3	T49.4X4	T49.4X5	T49.4X6
Carbenicillin	T36.0X1	T36.0X2	T36.0X3	T36.0X4	T36.0X5	T36.0X6
Carbenoxolone	T47.1X1	T47.1X2	T47.1X3	T47.1X4	T47.1X5	T47.1X6
Carbetapentane	T48.3X1	T48.3X2	T48.3X3	T48.3X4	T48.3X5	T48.3X6
Carbethyl salicylate	T39.091	T39.092	T39.093	T39.094	T39.095	T39.096
Carbidopa (with levodopa)	T42.8X1	T42.8X2	T42.8X3	T42.8X4	T42.8X5	T42.8X6
Carbimazole	T38.2X1	T38.2X2	T38.2X3	T38.2X4	T38.2X5	T38.2X6
Carbinol	T51.1X1	T51.1X2	T51.1X3	T51.1X4	—	—
Carbinoxamine	T45.0X1	T45.0X2	T45.0X3	T45.0X4	T45.0X5	T45.0X6
Carbiphene	T39.8X1	T39.8X2	T39.8X3	T39.8X4	T39.8X5	T39.8X6
Carbitol	T52.3X1	T52.3X2	T52.3X3	T52.3X4	—	—
Carbocaine	T41.3X1	T41.3X2	T41.3X3	T41.3X4	T41.3X5	T41.3X6
infiltration (subcutaneous)	T41.3X1	T41.3X2	T41.3X3	T41.3X4	T41.3X5	T41.3X6
nerve block (peripheral) (plexus)	T41.3X1	T41.3X2	T41.3X3	T41.3X4	T41.3X5	T41.3X6
topical (surface)	T41.3X1	T41.3X2	T41.3X3	T41.3X4	T41.3X5	T41.3X6
Carbocisteine	T48.4X1	T48.4X2	T48.4X3	T48.4X4	T48.4X5	T48.4X6
Carbocromen	T46.3X1	T46.3X2	T46.3X3	T46.3X4	T46.3X5	T46.3X6
Carbol fuchsin	T49.0X1	T49.0X2	T49.0X3	T49.0X4	T49.0X5	T49.0X6
Carbolic acid — *see also* Phenol	T54.0X1	T54.0X2	T54.0X3	T54.0X4	—	—
Carbolonium (bromide)	T48.1X1	T48.1X2	T48.1X3	T48.1X4	T48.1X5	T48.1X6
Carbo medicinalis	T47.6X1	T47.6X2	T47.6X3	T47.6X4	T47.6X5	T47.6X6
Carbomycin	T36.8X1	T36.8X2	T36.8X3	T36.8X4	T36.8X5	T36.8X6
Carbon						
bisulfide (liquid)	T65.4X1	T65.4X2	T65.4X3	T65.4X4	—	—
vapor	T65.4X1	T65.4X2	T65.4X3	T65.4X4	—	—
dioxide (gas)	T59.7X1	T59.7X2	T59.7X3	T59.7X4	—	—
medicinal	T41.5X1	T41.5X2	T41.5X3	T41.5X4	T41.5X5	T41.5X6
nonmedicinal	T59.7X1	T59.7X2	T59.7X3	T59.7X4	—	—
snow	T49.4X1	T49.4X2	T49.4X3	T49.4X4	T49.4X5	T49.4X6
disulfide (liquid)	T65.4X1	T65.4X2	T65.4X3	T65.4X4	—	—
vapor	T65.4X1	T65.4X2	T65.4X3	T65.4X4	—	—
monoxide (from incomplete combustion)	T58.91	T58.92	T58.93	T58.94	—	—
blast furnace gas	T58.8X1	T58.8X2	T58.8X3	T58.8X4	—	—
butane (distributed in mobile container)	T58.11	T58.12	T58.13	T58.14	—	—
distributed through pipes	T58.11	T58.12	T58.13	T58.14	—	—
charcoal fumes	T58.2X1	T58.2X2	T58.2X3	T58.2X4	—	—
coal	T58.2X1	T58.2X2	T58.2X3	T58.2X4	—	—
coke (in domestic stoves, fireplaces)	T58.2X1	T58.2X2	T58.2X3	T58.2X4	—	—
exhaust gas (motor) not in transit	T58.01	T58.02	T58.03	T58.04	—	—
combustion engine, any not in watercraft	T58.01	T58.02	T58.03	T58.04	—	—
farm tractor, not in transit	T58.01	T58.02	T58.03	T58.04	—	—
gas engine	T58.01	T58.02	T58.03	T58.04	—	—
motor pump	T58.01	T58.02	T58.03	T58.04	—	—
motor vehicle, not in transit	T58.01	T58.02	T58.03	T58.04	—	—
fuel (in domestic use)	T58.2X1	T58.2X2	T58.2X3	T58.2X4	—	—
gas (piped)	T58.11	T58.12	T58.13	T58.14	—	—
in mobile container	T58.11	T58.12	T58.13	T58.14	—	—
piped (natural)	T58.11	T58.12	T58.13	T58.14	—	—
utility	T58.11	T58.12	T58.13	T58.14	—	—
in mobile container	T58.11	T58.12	T58.13	T58.14	—	—
gas (piped)	T58.11	T58.12	T58.13	T58.14	—	—
illuminating gas	T58.11	T58.12	T58.13	T58.14	—	—
industrial fuels or gases, any	T58.8X1	T58.8X2	T58.8X3	T58.8X4	—	—
kerosene (in domestic stoves, fireplaces)	T58.2X1	T58.2X2	T58.2X3	T58.2X4	—	—
kiln gas or vapor	T58.8X1	T58.8X2	T58.8X3	T58.8X4	—	—
motor exhaust gas, not in transit	T58.01	T58.02	T58.03	T58.04	—	—
piped gas (manufactured) (natural)	T58.11	T58.12	T58.13	T58.14	—	—
producer gas	T58.8X1	T58.8X2	T58.8X3	T58.8X4	—	—
propane (distributed in mobile container)	T58.11	T58.12	T58.13	T58.14	—	—

Substance	Poisoning, Accidental (unintentional)	Poisoning, Intentional Self-harm	Poisoning, Assault	Poisoning, Undetermined	Adverse Effect	Under-dosing
Carbon — *continued*						
monoxide — *continued*						
propane — *continued*						
distributed through pipes	T58.11	T58.12	T58.13	T58.14	—	—
solid (in domestic stoves, fireplaces)	T58.2X1	T58.2X2	T58.2X3	T58.2X4	—	—
specified source NEC	T58.8X1	T58.8X2	T58.8X3	T58.8X4	—	—
stove gas	T58.11	T58.12	T58.13	T58.14	—	—
piped	T58.11	T58.12	T58.13	T58.14	—	—
utility gas	T58.11	T58.12	T58.13	T58.14	—	—
piped	T58.11	T58.12	T58.13	T58.14	—	—
water gas	T58.11	T58.12	T58.13	T58.14	—	—
wood (in domestic stoves, fireplaces)	T58.2X1	T58.2X2	T58.2X3	T58.2X4	—	—
tetrachloride (vapor) NEC	T53.0X1	T53.0X2	T53.0X3	T53.0X4	—	—
liquid (cleansing agent) NEC	T53.0X1	T53.0X2	T53.0X3	T53.0X4	—	—
solvent	T53.0X1	T53.0X2	T53.0X3	T53.0X4	—	—
Carbonic acid gas	T59.7X1	T59.7X2	T59.7X3	T59.7X4	—	—
anhydrase inhibitor NEC	T50.2X1	T50.2X2	T50.2X3	T50.2X4	T50.2X5	T50.2X6
Carbophenothion	T60.0X1	T60.0X2	T60.0X3	T60.0X4	—	—
Carboplatin	T45.1X1	T45.1X2	T45.1X3	T45.1X4	T45.1X5	T45.1X6
Carboprost	T48.0X1	T48.0X2	T48.0X3	T48.0X4	T48.0X5	T48.0X6
Carboquone	T45.1X1	T45.1X2	T45.1X3	T45.1X4	T45.1X5	T45.1X6
Carbowax	T49.3X1	T49.3X2	T49.3X3	T49.3X4	T49.3X5	T49.3X6
Carboxymethylcellulose	T47.4X1	T47.4X2	T47.4X3	T47.4X4	T47.4X5	T47.4X6
Carbrital	T42.3X1	T42.3X2	T42.3X3	T42.3X4	T42.3X5	T42.3X6
Carbromal	T42.6X1	T42.6X2	T42.6X3	T42.6X4	T42.6X5	T42.6X6
Carbutamide	T38.3X1	T38.3X2	T38.3X3	T38.3X4	T38.3X5	T38.3X6
Carbuterol	T48.6X1	T48.6X2	T48.6X3	T48.6X4	T48.6X5	T48.6X6
Cardiac						
depressants	T46.2X1	T46.2X2	T46.2X3	T46.2X4	T46.2X5	T46.2X6
rhythm regulator	T46.2X1	T46.2X2	T46.2X3	T46.2X4	T46.2X5	T46.2X6
specified NEC	T46.2X1	T46.2X2	T46.2X3	T46.2X4	T46.2X5	T46.2X6
Cardiografin	T50.8X1	T50.8X2	T50.8X3	T50.8X4	T50.8X5	T50.8X6
Cardiogreen	T50.8X1	T50.8X2	T50.8X3	T50.8X4	T50.8X5	T50.8X6
Cardiotonic (glycoside) **NEC**	T46.0X1	T46.0X2	T46.0X3	T46.0X4	T46.0X5	T46.0X6
Cardiovascular drug NEC	T46.901	T46.902	T46.903	T46.904	T46.905	T46.906
Cardrase	T50.2X1	T50.2X2	T50.2X3	T50.2X4	T50.2X5	T50.2X6
Carfecillin	T36.0X1	T36.0X2	T36.0X3	T36.0X4	T36.0X5	T36.0X6
Carfenazine	T43.3X1	T43.3X2	T43.3X3	T43.3X4	T43.3X5	T43.3X6
Carfusin	T49.0X1	T49.0X2	T49.0X3	T49.0X4	T49.0X5	T49.0X6
Carindacillin	T36.0X1	T36.0X2	T36.0X3	T36.0X4	T36.0X5	T36.0X6
Carisoprodol	T42.8X1	T42.8X2	T42.8X3	T42.8X4	T42.8X5	T42.8X6
Carmellose	T47.4X1	T47.4X2	T47.4X3	T47.4X4	T47.4X5	T47.4X6
Carminative	T47.5X1	T47.5X2	T47.5X3	T47.5X4	T47.5X5	T47.5X6
Carmofur	T45.1X1	T45.1X2	T45.1X3	T45.1X4	T45.1X5	T45.1X6
Carmustine	T45.1X1	T45.1X2	T45.1X3	T45.1X4	T45.1X5	T45.1X6
Carotene	T45.2X1	T45.2X2	T45.2X3	T45.2X4	T45.2X5	T45.2X6
Carphenazine	T43.3X1	T43.3X2	T43.3X3	T43.3X4	T43.3X5	T43.3X6
Carpipramine	T42.4X1	T42.4X2	T42.4X3	T42.4X4	T42.4X5	T42.4X6
Carprofen	T39.311	T39.312	T39.313	T39.314	T39.315	T39.316
Carpronium chloride	T44.3X1	T44.3X2	T44.3X3	T44.3X4	T44.3X5	T44.3X6
Carrageenan	T47.8X1	T47.8X2	T47.8X3	T47.8X4	T47.8X5	T47.8X6
Carteolol	T44.7X1	T44.7X2	T44.7X3	T44.7X4	T44.7X5	T44.7X6
Carter's Little Pills	T47.2X1	T47.2X2	T47.2X3	T47.2X4	T47.2X5	T47.2X6
Cascara (sagrada)	T47.2X1	T47.2X2	T47.2X3	T47.2X4	T47.2X5	T47.2X6
Cassava	T62.2X1	T62.2X2	T62.2X3	T62.2X4	—	—
Castellani's paint	T49.0X1	T49.0X2	T49.0X3	T49.0X4	T49.0X5	T49.0X6
Castor						
bean	T62.2X1	T62.2X2	T62.2X3	T62.2X4	—	—
oil	T47.2X1	T47.2X2	T47.2X3	T47.2X4	T47.2X5	T47.2X6
Catalase	T45.3X1	T45.3X2	T45.3X3	T45.3X4	T45.3X5	T45.3X6
Caterpillar (sting)	T63.431	T63.432	T63.433	T63.434	—	—
Catha (edulis) (tea)	T43.691	T43.692	T43.693	T43.694	—	—
Cathartic NEC	T47.4X1	T47.4X2	T47.4X3	T47.4X4	T47.4X5	T47.4X6
anthacene derivative	T47.2X1	T47.2X2	T47.2X3	T47.2X4	T47.2X5	T47.2X6
bulk	T47.4X1	T47.4X2	T47.4X3	T47.4X4	T47.4X5	T47.4X6
contact	T47.2X1	T47.2X2	T47.2X3	T47.2X4	T47.2X5	T47.2X6
emollient NEC	T47.4X1	T47.4X2	T47.4X3	T47.4X4	T47.4X5	T47.4X6
irritant NEC	T47.2X1	T47.2X2	T47.2X3	T47.2X4	T47.2X5	T47.2X6
mucilage	T47.4X1	T47.4X2	T47.4X3	T47.4X4	T47.4X5	T47.4X6
saline	T47.3X1	T47.3X2	T47.3X3	T47.3X4	T47.3X5	T47.3X6
vegetable	T47.2X1	T47.2X2	T47.2X3	T47.2X4	T47.2X5	T47.2X6
Cathine	T50.5X1	T50.5X2	T50.5X3	T50.5X4	T50.5X5	T50.5X6
Cathomycin	T36.8X1	T36.8X2	T36.8X3	T36.8X4	T36.8X5	T36.8X6
Cation exchange resin	T50.3X1	T50.3X2	T50.3X3	T50.3X4	T50.3X5	T50.3X6
Caustic(s) NEC	T54.91	T54.92	T54.93	T54.94	—	—
alkali	T54.3X1	T54.3X2	T54.3X3	T54.3X4	—	—
hydroxide	T54.3X1	T54.3X2	T54.3X3	T54.3X4	—	—
potash	T54.3X1	T54.3X2	T54.3X3	T54.3X4	—	—
soda	T54.3X1	T54.3X2	T54.3X3	T54.3X4	—	—

Substance	Poisoning, Accidental (unintentional)	Poisoning, Intentional Self-harm	Poisoning, Assault	Poisoning, Undetermined	Adverse Effect	Under-dosing
Caustic(s) NEC — *continued*						
specified NEC	T54.91	T54.92	T54.93	T54.94	—	—
Ceepryn	T49.0X1	T49.0X2	T49.0X3	T49.0X4	T49.0X5	T49.0X6
ENT agent	T49.6X1	T49.6X2	T49.6X3	T49.6X4	T49.6X5	T49.6X6
lozenges	T49.6X1	T49.6X2	T49.6X3	T49.6X4	T49.6X5	T49.6X6
Cefacetrile	T36.1X1	T36.1X2	T36.1X3	T36.1X4	T36.1X5	T36.1X6
Cefaclor	T36.1X1	T36.1X2	T36.1X3	T36.1X4	T36.1X5	T36.1X6
Cefadroxil	T36.1X1	T36.1X2	T36.1X3	T36.1X4	T36.1X5	T36.1X6
Cefalexin	T36.1X1	T36.1X2	T36.1X3	T36.1X4	T36.1X5	T36.1X6
Cefaloglycin	T36.1X1	T36.1X2	T36.1X3	T36.1X4	T36.1X5	T36.1X6
Cefaloridine	T36.1X1	T36.1X2	T36.1X3	T36.1X4	T36.1X5	T36.1X6
Cefalosporins	T36.1X1	T36.1X2	T36.1X3	T36.1X4	T36.1X5	T36.1X6
Cefalotin	T36.1X1	T36.1X2	T36.1X3	T36.1X4	T36.1X5	T36.1X6
Cefamandole	T36.1X1	T36.1X2	T36.1X3	T36.1X4	T36.1X5	T36.1X6
Cefamycin antibiotic	T36.1X1	T36.1X2	T36.1X3	T36.1X4	T36.1X5	T36.1X6
Cefapirin	T36.1X1	T36.1X2	T36.1X3	T36.1X4	T36.1X5	T36.1X6
Cefatrizine	T36.1X1	T36.1X2	T36.1X3	T36.1X4	T36.1X5	T36.1X6
Cefazedone	T36.1X1	T36.1X2	T36.1X3	T36.1X4	T36.1X5	T36.1X6
Cefazolin	T36.1X1	T36.1X2	T36.1X3	T36.1X4	T36.1X5	T36.1X6
Cefbuperazone	T36.1X1	T36.1X2	T36.1X3	T36.1X4	T36.1X5	T36.1X6
Cefetamet	T36.1X1	T36.1X2	T36.1X3	T36.1X4	T36.1X5	T36.1X6
Cefixime	T36.1X1	T36.1X2	T36.1X3	T36.1X4	T36.1X5	T36.1X6
Cefmenoxime	T36.1X1	T36.1X2	T36.1X3	T36.1X4	T36.1X5	T36.1X6
Cefmetazole	T36.1X1	T36.1X2	T36.1X3	T36.1X4	T36.1X5	T36.1X6
Cefminox	T36.1X1	T36.1X2	T36.1X3	T36.1X4	T36.1X5	T36.1X6
Cefonicid	T36.1X1	T36.1X2	T36.1X3	T36.1X4	T36.1X5	T36.1X6
Cefoperazone	T36.1X1	T36.1X2	T36.1X3	T36.1X4	T36.1X5	T36.1X6
Ceforanide	T36.1X1	T36.1X2	T36.1X3	T36.1X4	T36.1X5	T36.1X6
Cefotaxime	T36.1X1	T36.1X2	T36.1X3	T36.1X4	T36.1X5	T36.1X6
Cefotetan	T36.1X1	T36.1X2	T36.1X3	T36.1X4	T36.1X5	T36.1X6
Cefotiam	T36.1X1	T36.1X2	T36.1X3	T36.1X4	T36.1X5	T36.1X6
Cefoxitin	T36.1X1	T36.1X2	T36.1X3	T36.1X4	T36.1X5	T36.1X6
Cefpimizole	T36.1X1	T36.1X2	T36.1X3	T36.1X4	T36.1X5	T36.1X6
Cefpiramide	T36.1X1	T36.1X2	T36.1X3	T36.1X4	T36.1X5	T36.1X6
Cefradine	T36.1X1	T36.1X2	T36.1X3	T36.1X4	T36.1X5	T36.1X6
Cefroxadine	T36.1X1	T36.1X2	T36.1X3	T36.1X4	T36.1X5	T36.1X6
Cefsulodin	T36.1X1	T36.1X2	T36.1X3	T36.1X4	T36.1X5	T36.1X6
Ceftazidime	T36.1X1	T36.1X2	T36.1X3	T36.1X4	T36.1X5	T36.1X6
Cefteram	T36.1X1	T36.1X2	T36.1X3	T36.1X4	T36.1X5	T36.1X6
Ceftezole	T36.1X1	T36.1X2	T36.1X3	T36.1X4	T36.1X5	T36.1X6
Ceftizoxime	T36.1X1	T36.1X2	T36.1X3	T36.1X4	T36.1X5	T36.1X6
Ceftriaxone	T36.1X1	T36.1X2	T36.1X3	T36.1X4	T36.1X5	T36.1X6
Cefuroxime	T36.1X1	T36.1X2	T36.1X3	T36.1X4	T36.1X5	T36.1X6
Cefuzonam	T36.1X1	T36.1X2	T36.1X3	T36.1X4	T36.1X5	T36.1X6
Celestone	T38.0X1	T38.0X2	T38.0X3	T38.0X4	T38.0X5	T38.0X6
topical	T49.0X1	T49.0X2	T49.0X3	T49.0X4	T49.0X5	T49.0X6
Celiprolol	T44.7X1	T44.7X2	T44.7X3	T44.7X4	T44.7X5	T44.7X6
Cellosolve	T52.91	T52.92	T52.93	T52.94	—	—
Cell stimulants and proliferants	T49.8X1	T49.8X2	T49.8X3	T49.8X4	T49.8X5	T49.8X6
Cellulose						
cathartic	T47.4X1	T47.4X2	T47.4X3	T47.4X4	T47.4X5	T47.4X6
hydroxyethyl	T47.4X1	T47.4X2	T47.4X3	T47.4X4	T47.4X5	T47.4X6
nitrates (topical)	T49.3X1	T49.3X2	T49.3X3	T49.3X4	T49.3X5	T49.3X6
oxidized	T49.4X1	T49.4X2	T49.4X3	T49.4X4	T49.4X5	T49.4X6
Centipede (bite)	T63.411	T63.412	T63.413	T63.414	—	—
Central nervous system						
depressants	T42.71	T42.72	T42.73	T42.74	T42.75	T42.76
anesthetic (general) NEC	T41.201	T41.202	T41.203	T41.204	T41.205	T41.206
gases NEC	T41.0X1	T41.0X2	T41.0X3	T41.0X4	T41.0X5	T41.0X6
intravenous	T41.1X1	T41.1X2	T41.1X3	T41.1X4	T41.1X5	T41.1X6
barbiturates	T42.3X1	T42.3X2	T42.3X3	T42.3X4	T42.3X5	T42.3X6
benzodiazepines	T42.4X1	T42.4X2	T42.4X3	T42.4X4	T42.4X5	T42.4X6
bromides	T42.6X1	T42.6X2	T42.6X3	T42.6X4	T42.6X5	T42.6X6
cannabis sativa	T40.7X1	T40.7X2	T40.7X3	T40.7X4	T40.7X5	T40.7X6
chloral hydrate	T42.6X1	T42.6X2	T42.6X3	T42.6X4	T42.6X5	T42.6X6
ethanol	T51.0X1	T51.0X2	T51.0X3	T51.0X4	—	—
hallucinogenics	T40.901	T40.902	T40.903	T40.904	T40.905	T40.906
hypnotics	T42.71	T42.72	T42.73	T42.74	T42.75	T42.76
specified NEC	T42.6X1	T42.6X2	T42.6X3	T42.6X4	T42.6X5	T42.6X6
muscle relaxants	T42.8X1	T42.8X2	T42.8X3	T42.8X4	T42.8X5	T42.8X6
paraldehyde	T42.6X1	T42.6X2	T42.6X3	T42.6X4	T42.6X5	T42.6X6
sedatives; sedative-hypnotics	T42.71	T42.72	T42.73	T42.74	T42.75	T42.76
mixed NEC	T42.6X1	T42.6X2	T42.6X3	T42.6X4	T42.6X5	T42.6X6
specified NEC	T42.6X1	T42.6X2	T42.6X3	T42.6X4	T42.6X5	T42.6X6
muscle-tone depressants	T42.8X1	T42.8X2	T42.8X3	T42.8X4	T42.8X5	T42.8X6
stimulants	T43.601	T43.602	T43.603	T43.604	T43.605	T43.606
amphetamines	T43.621	T43.622	T43.623	T43.624	T43.625	T43.626
analeptics	T50.7X1	T50.7X2	T50.7X3	T50.7X4	T50.7X5	T50.7X6
antidepressants	T43.201	T43.202	T43.203	T43.204	T43.205	T43.206
opiate antagonists	T50.7X1	T50.7X2	T50.7X3	T50.7X4	T50.7X5	T50.7X6
specified NEC	T43.691	T43.692	T43.693	T43.694	T43.695	T43.696

Substance	Poisoning, Accidental (unintentional)	Poisoning, Intentional Self-harm	Poisoning, Assault	Poisoning, Undetermined	Adverse Effect	Under-dosing
Cephalexin	T36.1X1	T36.1X2	T36.1X3	T36.1X4	T36.1X5	T36.1X6
Cephaloglycin	T36.1X1	T36.1X2	T36.1X3	T36.1X4	T36.1X5	T36.1X6
Cephaloridine	T36.1X1	T36.1X2	T36.1X3	T36.1X4	T36.1X5	T36.1X6
Cephalosporins	T36.1X1	T36.1X2	T36.1X3	T36.1X4	T36.1X5	T36.1X6
N (adicillin)	T36.0X1	T36.0X2	T36.0X3	T36.0X4	T36.0X5	T36.0X6
Cephalothin	T36.1X1	T36.1X2	T36.1X3	T36.1X4	T36.1X5	T36.1X6
Cephalotin	T36.1X1	T36.1X2	T36.1X3	T36.1X4	T36.1X5	T36.1X6
Cephradine	T36.1X1	T36.1X2	T36.1X3	T36.1X4	T36.1X5	T36.1X6
Cerbera (odallam)	T62.2X1	T62.2X2	T62.2X3	T62.2X4	—	—
Cerberin	T46.0X1	T46.0X2	T46.0X3	T46.0X4	T46.0X5	T46.0X6
Cerebral stimulants	T43.601	T43.602	T43.603	T43.604	T43.605	T43.606
psychotherapeutic	T43.601	T43.602	T43.603	T43.604	T43.605	T43.606
specified NEC	T43.691	T43.692	T43.693	T43.694	T43.695	T43.696
Cerium oxalate	T45.0X1	T45.0X2	T45.0X3	T45.0X4	T45.0X5	T45.0X6
Cerous oxalate	T45.0X1	T45.0X2	T45.0X3	T45.0X4	T45.0X5	T45.0X6
Ceruletide	T50.8X1	T50.8X2	T50.8X3	T50.8X4	T50.8X5	T50.8X6
Cetalkonium (chloride)	T49.0X1	T49.0X2	T49.0X3	T49.0X4	T49.0X5	T49.0X6
Cethexonium chloride	T49.0X1	T49.0X2	T49.0X3	T49.0X4	T49.0X5	T49.0X6
Cetiedil	T46.7X1	T46.7X2	T46.7X3	T46.7X4	T46.7X5	T46.7X6
Cetirizine	T45.0X1	T45.0X2	T45.0X3	T45.0X4	T45.0X5	T45.0X6
Cetomacrogol	T50.991	T50.992	T50.993	T50.994	T50.995	T50.996
Cetotiamine	T45.2X1	T45.2X2	T45.2X3	T45.2X4	T45.2X5	T45.2X6
Cetoxime	T45.0X1	T45.0X2	T45.0X3	T45.0X4	T45.0X5	T45.0X6
Cetraxate	T47.1X1	T47.1X2	T47.1X3	T47.1X4	T47.1X5	T47.1X6
Cetrimide	T49.0X1	T49.0X2	T49.0X3	T49.0X4	T49.0X5	T49.0X6
Cetrimonium (bromide)	T49.0X1	T49.0X2	T49.0X3	T49.0X4	T49.0X5	T49.0X6
Cetylpyridinium chloride	T49.0X1	T49.0X2	T49.0X3	T49.0X4	T49.0X5	T49.0X6
ENT agent	T49.6X1	T49.6X2	T49.6X3	T49.6X4	T49.6X5	T49.6X6
lozenges	T49.6X1	T49.6X2	T49.6X3	T49.6X4	T49.6X5	T49.6X6
Cevadilla — see Sabadilla						
Cevitamic acid	T45.2X1	T45.2X2	T45.2X3	T45.2X4	T45.2X5	T45.2X6
Chalk, precipitated	T47.1X1	T47.1X2	T47.1X3	T47.1X4	T47.1X5	T47.1X6
Chamomile	T49.0X1	T49.0X2	T49.0X3	T49.0X4		T49.0X6
Ch'an su	T46.0X1	T46.0X2	T46.0X3	T46.0X4	T46.0X5	T46.0X6
Charcoal	T47.6X1	T47.6X2	T47.6X3	T47.6X4	T47.6X5	T47.6X6
activated — see also Charcoal, medicinal	T47.6X1	T47.6X2	T47.6X3	T47.6X4	T47.6X5	T47.6X6
fumes (Carbon monoxide)	T58.2X1	T58.2X2	T58.2X3	T58.2X4	—	—
industrial	T58.8X1	T58.8X2	T58.8X3	T58.8X4	—	—
medicinal (activated)	T47.6X1	T47.6X2	T47.6X3	T47.6X4	T47.6X5	T47.6X6
antidiarrheal	T47.6X1	T47.6X2	T47.6X3	T47.6X4	T47.6X5	T47.6X6
poison control	T47.8X1	T47.8X2	T47.8X3	T47.8X4	T47.8X5	T47.8X6
specified use other than for diarrhea	T47.8X1	T47.8X2	T47.8X3	T47.8X4	T47.8X5	T47.8X6
topical	T49.8X1	T49.8X2	T49.8X3	T49.8X4	T49.8X5	T49.8X6
Chaulmosulfone	T37.1X1	T37.1X2	T37.1X3	T37.1X4	T37.1X5	T37.1X6
Chelating agent NEC	T50.6X1	T50.6X2	T50.6X3	T50.6X4	T50.6X5	T50.6X6
Chelidonium majus	T62.2X1	T62.2X2	T62.2X3	T62.2X4	—	—
Chemical substance NEC	T65.91	T65.92	T65.93	T65.94	—	—
Chenodeoxycholic acid	T47.5X1	T47.5X2	T47.5X3	T47.5X4	T47.5X5	T47.5X6
Chenodiol	T47.5X1	T47.5X2	T47.5X3	T47.5X4	T47.5X5	T47.5X6
Chenopodium	T37.4X1	T37.4X2	T37.4X3	T37.4X4	T37.4X5	T37.4X6
Cherry laurel	T62.2X1	T62.2X2	T62.2X3	T62.2X4	—	—
Chinidin (e)	T46.2X1	T46.2X2	T46.2X3	T46.2X4	T46.2X5	T46.2X6
Chiniofon	T37.8X1	T37.8X2	T37.8X3	T37.8X4	T37.8X5	T37.8X6
Chlophedianol	T48.3X1	T48.3X2	T48.3X3	T48.3X4	T48.3X5	T48.3X6
Chloral	T42.6X1	T42.6X2	T42.6X3	T42.6X4	T42.6X5	T42.6X6
derivative	T42.6X1	T42.6X2	T42.6X3	T42.6X4	T42.6X5	T42.6X6
hydrate	T42.6X1	T42.6X2	T42.6X3	T42.6X4	T42.6X5	T42.6X6
Chloralamide	T42.6X1	T42.6X2	T42.6X3	T42.6X4	T42.6X5	T42.6X6
Chloralodol	T42.6X1	T42.6X2	T42.6X3	T42.6X4	T42.6X5	T42.6X6
Chloralose	T60.4X1	T60.4X2	T60.4X3	T60.4X4	—	—
Chlorambucil	T45.1X1	T45.1X2	T45.1X3	T45.1X4	T45.1X5	T45.1X6
Chloramine	T57.8X1	T57.8X2	T57.8X3	T57.8X4	—	—
T	T49.0X1	T49.0X2	T49.0X3	T49.0X4	T49.0X5	T49.0X6
topical	T49.0X1	T49.0X2	T49.0X3	T49.0X4	T49.0X5	T49.0X6
Chloramphenicol	T36.2X1	T36.2X2	T36.2X3	T36.2X4	T36.2X5	T36.2X6
ENT agent	T49.6X1	T49.6X2	T49.6X3	T49.6X4	T49.6X5	T49.6X6
ophthalmic preparation	T49.5X1	T49.5X2	T49.5X3	T49.5X4	T49.5X5	T49.5X6
topical NEC	T49.0X1	T49.0X2	T49.0X3	T49.0X4	T49.0X5	T49.0X6
Chlorate (potassium) (sodium) NEC	T60.3X1	T60.3X2	T60.3X3	T60.3X4	—	—
herbicide	T60.3X1	T60.3X2	T60.3X3	T60.3X4	—	—
Chlorazanil	T50.2X1	T50.2X2	T50.2X3	T50.2X4	T50.2X5	T50.2X6
Chlorbenzene, chlorbenzol	T53.7X1	T53.7X2	T53.7X3	T53.7X4	—	—
Chlorbenzoxamine	T44.3X1	T44.3X2	T44.3X3	T44.3X4	T44.3X5	T44.3X6
Chlorbutol	T42.6X1	T42.6X2	T42.6X3	T42.6X4	T42.6X5	T42.6X6
Chlorcyclizine	T45.0X1	T45.0X2	T45.0X3	T45.0X4	T45.0X5	T45.0X6
Chlordan (e) (dust)	T60.1X1	T60.1X2	T60.1X3	T60.1X4	—	—
Chlordantoin	T49.0X1	T49.0X2	T49.0X3	T49.0X4	T49.0X5	T49.0X6
Chlordiazepoxide	T42.4X1	T42.4X2	T42.4X3	T42.4X4	T42.4X5	T42.4X6
Chlordiethyl benzamide	T49.3X1	T49.3X2	T49.3X3	T49.3X4	T49.3X5	T49.3X6
Chloresium	T49.8X1	T49.8X2	T49.8X3	T49.8X4	T49.8X5	T49.8X6
Chlorethiazol	T42.6X1	T42.6X2	T42.6X3	T42.6X4	T42.6X5	T42.6X6
Chlorethyl — see Ethyl chloride						
Chloretone	T42.6X1	T42.6X2	T42.6X3	T42.6X4	T42.6X5	T42.6X6
Chlorex	T53.6X1	T53.6X2	T53.6X3	T53.6X4	—	—
insecticide	T60.1X1	T60.1X2	T60.1X3	T60.1X4	—	—
Chlorfenvinphos	T60.0X1	T60.0X2	T60.0X3	T60.0X4	—	—
Chlorhexadol	T42.6X1	T42.6X2	T42.6X3	T42.6X4	T42.6X5	T42.6X6
Chlorhexamide	T45.1X1	T45.1X2	T45.1X3	T45.1X4	T45.1X5	T45.1X6
Chlorhexidine	T49.0X1	T49.0X2	T49.0X3	T49.0X4	T49.0X5	T49.0X6
Chlorhydroxyquinolin	T49.0X1	T49.0X2	T49.0X3	T49.0X4	T49.0X5	T49.0X6
Chloride of lime (bleach)	T54.3X1	T54.3X2	T54.3X3	T54.3X4	—	—
Chlorimipramine	T43.011	T43.012	T43.013	T43.014	T43.015	T43.016
Chlorinated						
camphene	T53.6X1	T53.6X2	T53.6X3	T53.6X4	—	—
diphenyl	T53.7X1	T53.7X2	T53.7X3	T53.7X4	—	—
hydrocarbons NEC	T53.91	T53.92	T53.93	T53.94	—	—
solvents	T53.91	T53.92	T53.93	T53.94	—	—
lime (bleach)	T54.3X1	T54.3X2	T54.3X3	T54.3X4	—	—
and boric acid solution	T49.0X1	T49.0X2	T49.0X3	T49.0X4	T49.0X5	T49.0X6
naphthalene (insecticide)	T60.1X1	T60.1X2	T60.1X3	T60.1X4	—	—
industrial (non-pesticide)	T53.7X1	T53.7X2	T53.7X3	T53.7X4	—	—
pesticide NEC	T60.8X1	T60.8X2	T60.8X3	T60.8X4	—	—
soda — see also sodium hypochlorite						
solution	T49.0X1	T49.0X2	T49.0X3	T49.0X4	T49.0X5	T49.0X6
Chlorine (fumes) (gas)	T59.4X1	T59.4X2	T59.4X3	T59.4X4	—	—
bleach	T54.3X1	T54.3X2	T54.3X3	T54.3X4	—	—
compound gas NEC	T59.4X1	T59.4X2	T59.4X3	T59.4X4	—	—
disinfectant	T59.4X1	T59.4X2	T59.4X3	T59.4X4	—	—
releasing agents NEC	T59.4X1	T59.4X2	T59.4X3	T59.4X4	—	—
Chlorisondamine chloride	T46.991	T46.992	T46.993	T46.994	T46.995	T46.996
Chlormadinone	T38.5X1	T38.5X2	T38.5X3	T38.5X4	T38.5X5	T38.5X6
Chlormephos	T60.0X1	T60.0X2	T60.0X3	T60.0X4	—	—
Chlormerodrin	T50.2X1	T50.2X2	T50.2X3	T50.2X4	T50.2X5	T50.2X6
Chlormethiazole	T42.6X1	T42.6X2	T42.6X3	T42.6X4	T42.6X5	T42.6X6
Chlormethine	T45.1X1	T45.1X2	T45.1X3	T45.1X4	T45.1X5	T45.1X6
Chlormethylenecycline	T36.4X1	T36.4X2	T36.4X3	T36.4X4	T36.4X5	T36.4X6
Chlormezanone	T42.6X1	T42.6X2	T42.6X3	T42.6X4	T42.6X5	T42.6X6
Chloroacetic acid	T60.3X1	T60.3X2	T60.3X3	T60.3X4	—	—
Chloroacetone	T59.3X1	T59.3X2	T59.3X3	T59.3X4	—	—
Chloroacetophenone	T59.3X1	T59.3X2	T59.3X3	T59.3X4	—	—
Chloroaniline	T53.7X1	T53.7X2	T53.7X3	T53.7X4	—	—
Chlorobenzene, chlorobenzol	T53.7X1	T53.7X2	T53.7X3	T53.7X4	—	—
Chlorobromomethane (fire extinguisher)	T53.6X1	T53.6X2	T53.6X3	T53.6X4	—	—
Chlorobutanol	T49.0X1	T49.0X2	T49.0X3	T49.0X4	T49.0X5	T49.0X6
Chlorocresol	T49.0X1	T49.0X2	T49.0X3	T49.0X4	T49.0X5	T49.0X6
Chlorodehydromethyltestosterone	T38.7X1	T38.7X2	T38.7X3	T38.7X4	T38.7X5	T38.7X6
Chlorodinitrobenzene	T53.7X1	T53.7X2	T53.7X3	T53.7X4	—	—
dust or vapor	T53.7X1	T53.7X2	T53.7X3	T53.7X4	—	—
Chlorodiphenyl	T53.7X1	T53.7X2	T53.7X3	T53.7X4	—	—
Chloroethane — see Ethyl chloride						
Chloroethylene	T53.6X1	T53.6X2	T53.6X3	T53.6X4	—	—
Chlorofluorocarbons	T53.5X1	T53.5X2	T53.5X3	T53.5X4	—	—
Chloroform (fumes) (vapor)	T53.1X1	T53.1X2	T53.1X3	T53.1X4	—	—
anesthetic	T41.0X1	T41.0X2	T41.0X3	T41.0X4	T41.0X5	T41.0X6
solvent	T53.1X1	T53.1X2	T53.1X3	T53.1X4	—	—
water, concentrated	T41.0X1	T41.0X2	T41.0X3	T41.0X4	T41.0X5	T41.0X6
Chloroguanide	T37.2X1	T37.2X2	T37.2X3	T37.2X4	T37.2X5	T37.2X6
Chloromycetin	T36.2X1	T36.2X2	T36.2X3	T36.2X4	T36.2X5	T36.2X6
ENT agent	T49.6X1	T49.6X2	T49.6X3	T49.6X4	T49.6X5	T49.6X6
ophthalmic preparation	T49.5X1	T49.5X2	T49.5X3	T49.5X4	T49.5X5	T49.5X6
otic solution	T49.6X1	T49.6X2	T49.6X3	T49.6X4	T49.6X5	T49.6X6
topical NEC	T49.0X1	T49.0X2	T49.0X3	T49.0X4	T49.0X5	T49.0X6
Chloronitrobenzene	T53.7X1	T53.7X2	T53.7X3	T53.7X4	—	—
dust or vapor	T53.7X1	T53.7X2	T53.7X3	T53.7X4	—	—
Chlorophacinone	T60.4X1	T60.4X2	T60.4X3	T60.4X4	—	—
Chlorophenol	T53.7X1	T53.7X2	T53.7X3	T53.7X4	—	—
Chlorophenothane	T60.1X1	T60.1X2	T60.1X3	T60.1X4	—	—
Chlorophyll	T50.991	T50.992	T50.993	T50.994	T50.995	T50.996
Chloropicrin (fumes)	T53.6X1	T53.6X2	T53.6X3	T53.6X4	—	—
fumigant	T60.8X1	T60.8X2	T60.8X3	T60.8X4	—	—
fungicide	T60.3X1	T60.3X2	T60.3X3	T60.3X4	—	—
pesticide	T60.8X1	T60.8X2	T60.8X3	T60.8X4	—	—
Chloroprocaine	T41.3X1	T41.3X2	T41.3X3	T41.3X4	T41.3X5	T41.3X6
infiltration (subcutaneous)	T41.3X1	T41.3X2	T41.3X3	T41.3X4	T41.3X5	T41.3X6
nerve block (peripheral) (plexus)	T41.3X1	T41.3X2	T41.3X3	T41.3X4	T41.3X5	T41.3X6
spinal	T41.3X1	T41.3X2	T41.3X3	T41.3X4	T41.3X5	T41.3X6
Chloroptic	T49.5X1	T49.5X2	T49.5X3	T49.5X4	T49.5X5	T49.5X6
Chloropurine	T45.1X1	T45.1X2	T45.1X3	T45.1X4	T45.1X5	T45.1X6

Table of Drugs and Chemicals

Substance	Poisoning, Accidental (unintentional)	Poisoning, Intentional Self-harm	Poisoning, Assault	Poisoning, Undetermined	Adverse Effect	Under-dosing
Chloropyramine	T45.0X1	T45.0X2	T45.0X3	T45.0X4	T45.0X5	T45.0X6
Chloropyrifos	T60.0X1	T60.0X2	T60.0X3	T60.0X4		
Chloropyrilene	T45.0X1	T45.0X2	T45.0X3	T45.0X4	T45.0X5	T45.0X6
Chloroquine	T37.2X1	T37.2X2	T37.2X3	T37.2X4	T37.2X5	T37.2X6
Chlorothalonil	T60.3X1	T60.3X2	T60.3X3	T60.3X4		
Chlorothen	T45.0X1	T45.0X2	T45.0X3	T45.0X4	T45.0X5	T45.0X6
Chlorothiazide	T50.2X1	T50.2X2	T50.2X3	T50.2X4	T50.2X5	T50.2X6
Chlorothymol	T49.4X1	T49.4X2	T49.4X3	T49.4X4	T49.4X5	T49.4X6
Chlorotrianisene	T38.5X1	T38.5X2	T38.5X3	T38.5X4	T38.5X5	T38.5X6
Chlorovinyldichloroarsine, not in war	T57.0X1	T57.0X2	T57.0X3	T57.0X4	—	—
Chloroxine	T49.4X1	T49.4X2	T49.4X3	T49.4X4	T49.4X5	T49.4X6
Chloroxylenol	T49.0X1	T49.0X2	T49.0X3	T49.0X4	T49.0X5	T49.0X6
Chlorphenamine	T45.0X1	T45.0X2	T45.0X3	T45.0X4	T45.0X5	T45.0X6
Chlorphenesin	T42.8X1	T42.8X2	T42.8X3	T42.8X4	T42.8X5	T42.8X6
topical (antifungal)	T49.0X1	T49.0X2	T49.0X3	T49.0X4	T49.0X5	T49.0X6
Chlorpheniramine	T45.0X1	T45.0X2	T45.0X3	T45.0X4	T45.0X5	T45.0X6
Chlorphenoxamine	T45.0X1	T45.0X2	T45.0X3	T45.0X4	T45.0X5	T45.0X6
Chlorphentermine	T50.5X1	T50.5X2	T50.5X3	T50.5X4	T50.5X5	T50.5X6
Chlorprocaine — see Chloroprocaine						
Chlorproguanil	T37.2X1	T37.2X2	T37.2X3	T37.2X4	T37.2X5	T37.2X6
Chlorpromazine	T43.3X1	T43.3X2	T43.3X3	T43.3X4	T43.3X5	T43.3X6
Chlorpropamide	T38.3X1	T38.3X2	T38.3X3	T38.3X4	T38.3X5	T38.3X6
Chlorprothixene	T43.4X1	T43.4X2	T43.4X3	T43.4X4	T43.4X5	T43.4X6
Chlorquinaldol	T49.0X1	T49.0X2	T49.0X3	T49.0X4	T49.0X5	T49.0X6
Chlorquinol	T49.0X1	T49.0X2	T49.0X3	T49.0X4	T49.0X5	T49.0X6
Chlortalidone	T50.2X1	T50.2X2	T50.2X3	T50.2X4	T50.2X5	T50.2X6
Chlortetracycline	T36.4X1	T36.4X2	T36.4X3	T36.4X4	T36.4X5	T36.4X6
Chlorthalidone	T50.2X1	T50.2X2	T50.2X3	T50.2X4	T50.2X5	T50.2X6
Chlorthion	T60.0X1	T60.0X2	T60.0X3	T60.0X4	—	—
Chlorthiophos	T60.0X1	T60.0X2	T60.0X3	T60.0X4	—	—
Chlortrianisene	T38.5X1	T38.5X2	T38.5X3	T38.5X4	T38.5X5	T38.5X6
Chlor-Trimeton	T45.0X1	T45.0X2	T45.0X3	T45.0X4	T45.0X5	T45.0X6
Chlorzoxazone	T42.8X1	T42.8X2	T42.8X3	T42.8X4	T42.8X5	T42.8X6
Choke damp	T59.7X1	T59.7X2	T59.7X3	T59.7X4	—	—
Cholagogues	T47.5X1	T47.5X2	T47.5X3	T47.5X4	T47.5X5	T47.5X6
Cholebrine	T50.8X1	T50.8X2	T50.8X3	T50.8X4	T50.8X5	T50.8X6
Cholecalciferol	T45.2X1	T45.2X2	T45.2X3	T45.2X4	T45.2X5	T45.2X6
Cholecystokinin	T50.8X1	T50.8X2	T50.8X3	T50.8X4	T50.8X5	T50.8X6
Cholera vaccine	T50.A91	T50.A92	T50.A93	T50.A94	T50.A95	T50.A96
Choleretic	T47.5X1	T47.5X2	T47.5X3	T47.5X4	T47.5X5	T47.5X6
Cholesterol-lowering agents	T46.6X1	T46.6X2	T46.6X3	T46.6X4	T46.6X5	T46.6X6
Cholestyramine (resin)	T46.6X1	T46.6X2	T46.6X3	T46.6X4	T46.6X5	T46.6X6
Cholic acid	T47.5X1	T47.5X2	T47.5X3	T47.5X4	T47.5X5	T47.5X6
Choline	T48.6X1	T48.6X2	T48.6X3	T48.6X4	T48.6X5	T48.6X6
chloride	T50.991	T50.992	T50.993	T50.994	T50.995	T50.996
dihydrogen citrate	T50.991	T50.992	T50.993	T50.994	T50.995	T50.996
salicylate	T39.091	T39.092	T39.093	T39.094	T39.095	T39.096
theophyllinate	T48.6X1	T48.6X2	T48.6X3	T48.6X4	T48.6X5	T48.6X6
Cholinergic (drug) **NEC**	T44.1X1	T44.1X2	T44.1X3	T44.1X4	T44.1X5	T44.1X6
muscle tone enhancer	T44.1X1	T44.1X2	T44.1X3	T44.1X4	T44.1X5	T44.1X6
organophosphorus	T44.0X1	T44.0X2	T44.0X3	T44.0X4	T44.0X5	T44.0X6
insecticide	T60.0X1	T60.0X2	T60.0X3	T60.0X4	—	—
nerve gas	T59.891	T59.892	T59.893	T59.894	—	—
trimethyl ammonium propanediol	T44.1X1	T44.1X2	T44.1X3	T44.1X4	T44.1X5	T44.1X6
Cholinesterase reactivator	T50.6X1	T50.6X2	T50.6X3	T50.6X4	T50.6X5	T50.6X6
Cholografin	T50.8X1	T50.8X2	T50.8X3	T50.8X4	T50.8X5	T50.8X6
Chorionic gonadotropin	T38.891	T38.892	T38.893	T38.894	T38.895	T38.896
Chromate	T56.2X1	T56.2X2	T56.2X3	T56.2X4	—	—
dust or mist	T56.2X1	T56.2X2	T56.2X3	T56.2X4	—	—
lead — see also lead	T56.0X1	T56.0X2	T56.0X3	T56.0X4	—	—
paint	T56.0X1	T56.0X2	T56.0X3	T56.0X4	—	—
Chromic						
acid	T56.2X1	T56.2X2	T56.2X3	T56.2X4	—	—
dust or mist	T56.2X1	T56.2X2	T56.2X3	T56.2X4	—	—
phosphate 32P	T45.1X1	T45.1X2	T45.1X3	T45.1X4	T45.1X5	T45.1X6
Chromium	T56.2X1	T56.2X2	T56.2X3	T56.2X4	—	—
compounds — see Chromate						
sesquioxide	T50.8X1	T50.8X2	T50.8X3	T50.8X4	T50.8X5	T50.8X6
Chromomycin A3	T45.1X1	T45.1X2	T45.1X3	T45.1X4	T45.1X5	T45.1X6
Chromonar	T46.3X1	T46.3X2	T46.3X3	T46.3X4	T46.3X5	T46.3X6
Chromyl chloride	T56.2X1	T56.2X2	T56.2X3	T56.2X4	—	—
Chrysarobin	T49.4X1	T49.4X2	T49.4X3	T49.4X4	T49.4X5	T49.4X6
Chrysazin	T47.2X1	T47.2X2	T47.2X3	T47.2X4	T47.2X5	T47.2X6
Chymar	T45.3X1	T45.3X2	T45.3X3	T45.3X4	T45.3X5	T45.3X6
ophthalmic preparation	T49.5X1	T49.5X2	T49.5X3	T49.5X4	T49.5X5	T49.5X6
Chymopapain	T45.3X1	T45.3X2	T45.3X3	T45.3X4	T45.3X5	T45.3X6
Chymotrypsin	T45.3X1	T45.3X2	T45.3X3	T45.3X4	T45.3X5	T45.3X6
ophthalmic preparation	T49.5X1	T49.5X2	T49.5X3	T49.5X4	T49.5X5	T49.5X6
Cianidanol	T50.991	T50.992	T50.993	T50.994	T50.995	T50.996
Cianopramine	T43.011	T43.012	T43.013	T43.014	T43.015	T43.016
Cibenzoline	T46.2X1	T46.2X2	T46.2X3	T46.2X4	T46.2X5	T46.2X6
Ciclacillin	T36.0X1	T36.0X2	T36.0X3	T36.0X4	T36.0X5	T36.0X6
Ciclobarbital — see Hexobarbital						
Ciclonicate	T46.7X1	T46.7X2	T46.7X3	T46.7X4	T46.7X5	T46.7X6
Ciclopirox (olamine)	T49.0X1	T49.0X2	T49.0X3	T49.0X4	T49.0X5	T49.0X6
Ciclosporin	T45.1X1	T45.1X2	T45.1X3	T45.1X4	T45.1X5	T45.1X6
Cicuta maculata or virosa	T62.2X1	T62.2X2	T62.2X3	T62.2X4		
Cicutoxin	T62.2X1	T62.2X2	T62.2X3	T62.2X4		
Cigarette lighter fluid	T52.0X1	T52.0X2	T52.0X3	T52.0X4		
Cigarettes (tobacco)	T65.221	T65.222	T65.223	T65.224		
Ciguatoxin	T61.01	T61.02	T61.03	T61.04		
Cilazapril	T46.4X1	T46.4X2	T46.4X3	T46.4X4	T46.4X5	T46.4X6
Cimetidine	T47.0X1	T47.0X2	T47.0X3	T47.0X4	T47.0X5	T47.0X6
Cimetropium bromide	T44.3X1	T44.3X2	T44.3X3	T44.3X4	T44.3X5	T44.3X6
Cinchocaine	T41.3X1	T41.3X2	T41.3X3	T41.3X4	T41.3X5	T41.3X6
topical (surface)	T41.3X1	T41.3X2	T41.3X3	T41.3X4	T41.3X5	T41.3X6
Cinchona	T37.2X1	T37.2X2	T37.2X3	T37.2X4	T37.2X5	T37.2X6
Cinchonine alkaloids	T37.2X1	T37.2X2	T37.2X3	T37.2X4	T37.2X5	T37.2X6
Cinchophen	T50.4X1	T50.4X2	T50.4X3	T50.4X4	T50.4X5	T50.4X6
Cinepazide	T46.7X1	T46.7X2	T46.7X3	T46.7X4	T46.7X5	T46.7X6
Cinnamedrine	T48.5X1	T48.5X2	T48.5X3	T48.5X4	T48.5X5	T48.5X6
Cinnarizine	T45.0X1	T45.0X2	T45.0X3	T45.0X4	T45.0X5	T45.0X6
Cinoxacin	T37.8X1	T37.8X2	T37.8X3	T37.8X4	T37.8X5	T37.8X6
Ciprofibrate	T46.6X1	T46.6X2	T46.6X3	T46.6X4	T46.6X5	T46.6X6
Ciprofloxacin	T36.8X1	T36.8X2	T36.8X3	T36.8X4	T36.8X5	T36.8X6
Cisapride	T47.8X1	T47.8X2	T47.8X3	T47.8X4	T47.8X5	T47.8X6
Cisplatin	T45.1X1	T45.1X2	T45.1X3	T45.1X4	T45.1X5	T45.1X6
Citalopram	T43.221	T43.222	T43.223	T43.224	T43.225	T43.226
Citanest	T41.3X1	T41.3X2	T41.3X3	T41.3X4	T41.3X5	T41.3X6
infiltration (subcutaneous)	T41.3X1	T41.3X2	T41.3X3	T41.3X4	T41.3X5	T41.3X6
nerve block (peripheral) (plexus)	T41.3X1	T41.3X2	T41.3X3	T41.3X4	T41.3X5	T41.3X6
Citric acid	T47.5X1	T47.5X2	T47.5X3	T47.5X4	T47.5X5	T47.5X6
Citrovorum (factor)	T45.8X1	T45.8X2	T45.8X3	T45.8X4	T45.8X5	T45.8X6
Claviceps purpurea	T62.2X1	T62.2X2	T62.2X3	T62.2X4	—	—
Clavulanic acid	T36.1X1	T36.1X2	T36.1X3	T36.1X4	T36.1X5	T36.1X6
Cleaner, cleansing agent, type not specified	T65.891	T65.892	T65.893	T65.894		
of paint or varnish	T52.91	T52.92	T52.93	T52.94		
specified type NEC	T65.891	T65.892	T65.893	T65.894		
Clebopride	T47.8X1	T47.8X2	T47.8X3	T47.8X4	T47.8X5	T47.8X6
Clefamide	T37.3X1	T37.3X2	T37.3X3	T37.3X4	T37.3X5	T37.3X6
Clemastine	T45.0X1	T45.0X2	T45.0X3	T45.0X4	T45.0X5	T45.0X6
Clematis vitalba	T62.2X1	T62.2X2	T62.2X3	T62.2X4	—	—
Clemizole	T45.0X1	T45.0X2	T45.0X3	T45.0X4	T45.0X5	T45.0X6
penicillin	T36.0X1	T36.0X2	T36.0X3	T36.0X4	T36.0X5	T36.0X6
Clenbuterol	T48.6X1	T48.6X2	T48.6X3	T48.6X4	T48.6X5	T48.6X6
Clidinium bromide	T44.3X1	T44.3X2	T44.3X3	T44.3X4	T44.3X5	T44.3X6
Clindamycin	T36.8X1	T36.8X2	T36.8X3	T36.8X4	T36.8X5	T36.8X6
Clinofibrate	T46.6X1	T46.6X2	T46.6X3	T46.6X4	T46.6X5	T46.6X6
Clioquinol	T37.8X1	T37.8X2	T37.8X3	T37.8X4	T37.8X5	T37.8X6
Cliradon	T40.2X1	T40.2X2	T40.2X3	T40.2X4	—	—
Clobazam	T42.4X1	T42.4X2	T42.4X3	T42.4X4	T42.4X5	T42.4X6
Clobenzorex	T50.5X1	T50.5X2	T50.5X3	T50.5X4	T50.5X5	T50.5X6
Clobetasol	T49.0X1	T49.0X2	T49.0X3	T49.0X4	T49.0X5	T49.0X6
Clobetasone	T49.0X1	T49.0X2	T49.0X3	T49.0X4	T49.0X5	T49.0X6
Clobutinol	T48.3X1	T48.3X2	T48.3X3	T48.3X4	T48.3X5	T48.3X6
Clocortolone	T38.0X1	T38.0X2	T38.0X3	T38.0X4	T38.0X5	T38.0X6
Clodantoin	T49.0X1	T49.0X2	T49.0X3	T49.0X4	T49.0X5	T49.0X6
Clodronic acid	T50.991	T50.992	T50.993	T50.994	T50.995	T50.996
Clofazimine	T37.1X1	T37.1X2	T37.1X3	T37.1X4	T37.1X5	T37.1X6
Clofedanol	T48.3X1	T48.3X2	T48.3X3	T48.3X4	T48.3X5	T48.3X6
Clofenamide	T50.2X1	T50.2X2	T50.2X3	T50.2X4	T50.2X5	T50.2X6
Clofenotane	T49.0X1	T49.0X2	T49.0X3	T49.0X4	T49.0X5	T49.0X6
Clofezone	T39.2X1	T39.2X2	T39.2X3	T39.2X4	T39.2X5	T39.2X6
Clofibrate	T46.6X1	T46.6X2	T46.6X3	T46.6X4	T46.6X5	T46.6X6
Clofibride	T46.6X1	T46.6X2	T46.6X3	T46.6X4	T46.6X5	T46.6X6
Cloforex	T50.5X1	T50.5X2	T50.5X3	T50.5X4	T50.5X5	T50.5X6
Clomethiazole	T42.6X1	T42.6X2	T42.6X3	T42.6X4	T42.6X5	T42.6X6
Clometocillin	T36.0X1	T36.0X2	T36.0X3	T36.0X4	T36.0X5	T36.0X6
Clomifene	T38.5X1	T38.5X2	T38.5X3	T38.5X4	T38.5X5	T38.5X6
Clomiphene	T38.5X1	T38.5X2	T38.5X3	T38.5X4	T38.5X5	T38.5X6
Clomipramine	T43.011	T43.012	T43.013	T43.014	T43.015	T43.016
Clomocycline	T36.4X1	T36.4X2	T36.4X3	T36.4X4	T36.4X5	T36.4X6
Clonazepam	T42.4X1	T42.4X2	T42.4X3	T42.4X4	T42.4X5	T42.4X6
Clonidine	T46.5X1	T46.5X2	T46.5X3	T46.5X4	T46.5X5	T46.5X6
Clonixin	T39.8X1	T39.8X2	T39.8X3	T39.8X4	T39.8X5	T39.8X6
Clopamide	T50.2X1	T50.2X2	T50.2X3	T50.2X4	T50.2X5	T50.2X6
Clopenthixol	T43.4X1	T43.4X2	T43.4X3	T43.4X4	T43.4X5	T43.4X6
Cloperastine	T48.3X1	T48.3X2	T48.3X3	T48.3X4	T48.3X5	T48.3X6
Clophedianol	T48.3X1	T48.3X2	T48.3X3	T48.3X4	T48.3X5	T48.3X6
Cloponone	T36.2X1	T36.2X2	T36.2X3	T36.2X4	T36.2X5	T36.2X6

Additional Character May Be Required — Refer to the Tabular List for Character Selection ▽ Subterms under main terms may continue to next column or page

Chloropyramine — Cloponone

Substance	Poisoning, Accidental (unintentional)	Poisoning, Intentional Self-harm	Poisoning, Assault	Poisoning, Undetermined	Adverse Effect	Under-dosing
Cloprednol	T38.0X1	T38.0X2	T38.0X3	T38.0X4	T38.0X5	T38.0X6
Cloral betaine	T42.6X1	T42.6X2	T42.6X3	T42.6X4	T42.6X5	T42.6X6
Cloramfenicol	T36.2X1	T36.2X2	T36.2X3	T36.2X4	T36.2X5	T36.2X6
Clorazepate (dipotassium)	T42.4X1	T42.4X2	T42.4X3	T42.4X4	T42.4X5	T42.4X6
Clorexolone	T50.2X1	T50.2X2	T50.2X3	T50.2X4	T50.2X5	T50.2X6
Clorfenamine	T45.0X1	T45.0X2	T45.0X3	T45.0X4	T45.0X5	T45.0X6
Clorgiline	T43.1X1	T43.1X2	T43.1X3	T43.1X4	T43.1X5	T43.1X6
Clorotepine	T44.3X1	T44.3X2	T44.3X3	T44.3X4	T44.3X5	T44.3X6
Clorox (bleach)	T54.91	T54.92	T54.93	T54.94	—	—
Clorprenaline	T48.6X1	T48.6X2	T48.6X3	T48.6X4	T48.6X5	T48.6X6
Clortermine	T50.5X1	T50.5X2	T50.5X3	T50.5X4	T50.5X5	T50.5X6
Clotiapine	T43.591	T43.592	T43.593	T43.594	T43.595	T43.596
Clotiazepam	T42.4X1	T42.4X2	T42.4X3	T42.4X4	T42.4X5	T42.4X6
Clotibric acid	T46.6X1	T46.6X2	T46.6X3	T46.6X4	T46.6X5	T46.6X6
Clotrimazole	T49.0X1	T49.0X2	T49.0X3	T49.0X4	T49.0X5	T49.0X6
Cloxacillin	T36.0X1	T36.0X2	T36.0X3	T36.0X4	T36.0X5	T36.0X6
Cloxazolam	T42.4X1	T42.4X2	T42.4X3	T42.4X4	T42.4X5	T42.4X6
Cloxiquine	T49.0X1	T49.0X2	T49.0X3	T49.0X4	T49.0X5	T49.0X6
Clozapine	T42.4X1	T42.4X2	T42.4X3	T42.4X4	T42.4X5	T42.4X6
Coagulant NEC	T45.7X1	T45.7X2	T45.7X3	T45.7X4	T45.7X5	T45.7X6
Coal (carbon monoxide from) — see also Carbon, monoxide, coal	T58.2X1	T58.2X2	T58.2X3	T58.2X4	—	—
oil — see Kerosene						
tar	T49.1X1	T49.1X2	T49.1X3	T49.1X4	T49.1X5	T49.1X6
fumes	T59.891	T59.892	T59.893	T59.894	—	—
medicinal (ointment)	T49.4X1	T49.4X2	T49.4X3	T49.4X4	T49.4X5	T49.4X6
analgesics NEC	T39.2X1	T39.2X2	T39.2X3	T39.2X4	T39.2X5	T39.2X6
naphtha (solvent)	T52.0X1	T52.0X2	T52.0X3	T52.0X4	—	—
Cobalamine	T45.2X1	T45.2X2	T45.2X3	T45.2X4	T45.2X5	T45.2X6
Cobalt (nonmedicinal) (fumes) (industrial)	T56.891	T56.892	T56.893	T56.894	—	—
medicinal (trace) (chloride)	T45.8X1	T45.8X2	T45.8X3	T45.8X4	T45.8X5	T45.8X6
Cobra (venom)	T63.041	T63.042	T63.043	T63.044	—	—
Coca (leaf)	T40.5X1	T40.5X2	T40.5X3	T40.5X4	T40.5X5	T40.5X6
Cocaine	T40.5X1	T40.5X2	T40.5X3	T40.5X4	T40.5X5	T40.5X6
topical anesthetic	T41.3X1	T41.3X2	T41.3X3	T41.3X4	T41.3X5	T41.3X6
Cocarboxylase	T45.3X1	T45.3X2	T45.3X3	T45.3X4	T45.3X5	T45.3X6
Coccidioidin	T50.8X1	T50.8X2	T50.8X3	T50.8X4	T50.8X5	T50.8X6
Cocculus indicus	T62.1X1	T62.1X2	T62.1X3	T62.1X4	—	—
Cochineal	T65.6X1	T65.6X2	T65.6X3	T65.6X4	—	—
medicinal products	T50.991	T50.992	T50.993	T50.994	T50.995	T50.996
Codeine	T40.2X1	T40.2X2	T40.2X3	T40.2X4	T40.2X5	T40.2X6
Cod-liver oil	T45.2X1	T45.2X2	T45.2X3	T45.2X4	T45.2X5	T45.2X6
Coenzyme A	T50.991	T50.992	T50.993	T50.994	T50.995	T50.996
Coffee	T62.8X1	T62.8X2	T62.8X3	T62.8X4	—	—
Cogalactoisomerase	T50.991	T50.992	T50.993	T50.994	T50.995	T50.996
Cogentin	T44.3X1	T44.3X2	T44.3X3	T44.3X4	T44.3X5	T44.3X6
Coke fumes or gas (carbon monoxide)	T58.2X1	T58.2X2	T58.2X3	T58.2X4	—	—
industrial use	T58.8X1	T58.8X2	T58.8X3	T58.8X4	—	—
Colace	T47.4X1	T47.4X2	T47.4X3	T47.4X4	T47.4X5	T47.4X6
Colaspase	T45.1X1	T45.1X2	T45.1X3	T45.1X4	T45.1X5	T45.1X6
Colchicine	T50.4X1	T50.4X2	T50.4X3	T50.4X4	T50.4X5	T50.4X6
Colchicum	T62.2X1	T62.2X2	T62.2X3	T62.2X4	—	—
Cold cream	T49.3X1	T49.3X2	T49.3X3	T49.3X4	T49.3X5	T49.3X6
Colecalciferol	T45.2X1	T45.2X2	T45.2X3	T45.2X4	T45.2X5	T45.2X6
Colestipol	T46.6X1	T46.6X2	T46.6X3	T46.6X4	T46.6X5	T46.6X6
Colestyramine	T46.6X1	T46.6X2	T46.6X3	T46.6X4	T46.6X5	T46.6X6
Colimycin	T36.8X1	T36.8X2	T36.8X3	T36.8X4	T36.8X5	T36.8X6
Colistimethate	T36.8X1	T36.8X2	T36.8X3	T36.8X4	T36.8X5	T36.8X6
Colistin	T36.8X1	T36.8X2	T36.8X3	T36.8X4	T36.8X5	T36.8X6
sulfate (eye preparation)	T49.5X1	T49.5X2	T49.5X3	T49.5X4	T49.5X5	T49.5X6
Collagen	T50.991	T50.992	T50.993	T50.994	T50.995	T50.996
Collagenase	T49.4X1	T49.4X2	T49.4X3	T49.4X4	T49.4X5	T49.4X6
Collodion	T49.3X1	T49.3X2	T49.3X3	T49.3X4	T49.3X5	T49.3X6
Colocynth	T47.2X1	T47.2X2	T47.2X3	T47.2X4	T47.2X5	T47.2X6
Colophony adhesive	T49.3X1	T49.3X2	T49.3X3	T49.3X4	T49.3X5	T49.3X6
Colorant — see also Dye	T50.991	T50.992	T50.993	T50.994	T50.995	T50.996
Coloring matter — see Dye(s)						
Combustion gas (after combustion) — see Carbon, monoxide						
prior to combustion	T59.891	T59.892	T59.893	T59.894	—	—
Compazine	T43.3X1	T43.3X2	T43.3X3	T43.3X4	T43.3X5	T43.3X6
Compound						
42 (warfarin)	T60.4X1	T60.4X2	T60.4X3	T60.4X4	—	—
269 (endrin)	T60.1X1	T60.1X2	T60.1X3	T60.1X4	—	—
497 (dieldrin)	T60.1X1	T60.1X2	T60.1X3	T60.1X4	—	—
1080 (sodium fluoroacetate)	T60.4X1	T60.4X2	T60.4X3	T60.4X4	—	—
3422 (parathion)	T60.0X1	T60.0X2	T60.0X3	T60.0X4	—	—
3911 (phorate)	T60.0X1	T60.0X2	T60.0X3	T60.0X4	—	—

Substance	Poisoning, Accidental (unintentional)	Poisoning, Intentional Self-harm	Poisoning, Assault	Poisoning, Undetermined	Adverse Effect	Under-dosing
Compound — continued						
3956 (toxaphene)	T60.1X1	T60.1X2	T60.1X3	T60.1X4	—	—
4049 (malathion)	T60.0X1	T60.0X2	T60.0X3	T60.0X4	—	—
4069 (malathion)	T60.0X1	T60.0X2	T60.0X3	T60.0X4	—	—
4124 (dicapthon)	T60.0X1	T60.0X2	T60.0X3	T60.0X4	—	—
E (cortisone)	T38.0X1	T38.0X2	T38.0X3	T38.0X4	T38.0X5	T38.0X6
F (hydrocortisone)	T38.0X1	T38.0X2	T38.0X3	T38.0X4	T38.0X5	T38.0X6
Congener, anabolic	T38.7X1	T38.7X2	T38.7X3	T38.7X4	T38.7X5	T38.7X6
Congo red	T50.8X1	T50.8X2	T50.8X3	T50.8X4	T50.8X5	T50.8X6
Coniine, conine	T62.2X1	T62.2X2	T62.2X3	T62.2X4	—	—
Conium (maculatum)	T62.2X1	T62.2X2	T62.2X3	T62.2X4	—	—
Conjugated estrogenic substances	T38.5X1	T38.5X2	T38.5X3	T38.5X4	T38.5X5	T38.5X6
Contac	T48.5X1	T48.5X2	T48.5X3	T48.5X4	T48.5X5	T48.5X6
Contact lens solution	T49.5X1	T49.5X2	T49.5X3	T49.5X4	T49.5X5	T49.5X6
Contraceptive (oral)	T38.4X1	T38.4X2	T38.4X3	T38.4X4	T38.4X5	T38.4X6
vaginal	T49.8X1	T49.8X2	T49.8X3	T49.8X4	T49.8X5	T49.8X6
Contrast medium, radiography	T50.8X1	T50.8X2	T50.8X3	T50.8X4	T50.8X5	T50.8X6
Convallaria glycosides	T46.0X1	T46.0X2	T46.0X3	T46.0X4	T46.0X5	T46.0X6
Convallaria majalis	T62.2X1	T62.2X2	T62.2X3	T62.2X4	—	—
berry	T62.1X1	T62.1X2	T62.1X3	T62.1X4	—	—
Copperhead snake (bite) (venom)	T63.061	T63.062	T63.063	T63.064	—	—
Copper (dust) (fumes) (nonmedicinal) NEC	T56.4X1	T56.4X2	T56.4X3	T56.4X4	—	—
arsenate, arsenite	T57.0X1	T57.0X2	T57.0X3	T57.0X4	—	—
insecticide	T60.2X1	T60.2X2	T60.2X3	T60.2X4	—	—
emetic	T47.7X1	T47.7X2	T47.7X3	T47.7X4	T47.7X5	T47.7X6
fungicide	T60.3X1	T60.3X2	T60.3X3	T60.3X4	—	—
gluconate	T49.0X1	T49.0X2	T49.0X3	T49.0X4	T49.0X5	T49.0X6
insecticide	T60.2X1	T60.2X2	T60.2X3	T60.2X4	—	—
medicinal (trace)	T45.8X1	T45.8X2	T45.8X3	T45.8X4	T45.8X5	T45.8X6
oleate	T49.0X1	T49.0X2	T49.0X3	T49.0X4	T49.0X5	T49.0X6
sulfate	T56.4X1	T56.4X2	T56.4X3	T56.4X4	—	—
cupric	T56.4X1	T56.4X2	T56.4X3	T56.4X4	—	—
fungicide	T60.3X1	T60.3X2	T60.3X3	T60.3X4	—	—
medicinal						
ear	T49.6X1	T49.6X2	T49.6X3	T49.6X4	T49.6X5	T49.6X6
emetic	T47.7X1	T47.7X2	T47.7X3	T47.7X4	T47.7X5	T47.7X6
eye	T49.5X1	T49.5X2	T49.5X3	T49.5X4	T49.5X5	T49.5X6
cuprous	T56.4X1	T56.4X2	T56.4X3	T56.4X4	—	—
fungicide	T60.3X1	T60.3X2	T60.3X3	T60.3X4	—	—
medicinal						
ear	T49.6X1	T49.6X2	T49.6X3	T49.6X4	T49.6X5	T49.6X6
emetic	T47.7X1	T47.7X2	T47.7X3	T47.7X4	T47.7X5	T47.7X6
eye	T49.5X1	T49.5X2	T49.5X3	T49.5X4	T49.5X5	T49.5X6
Coral (sting)	T63.691	T63.692	T63.693	T63.694	—	—
snake (bite) (venom)	T63.021	T63.022	T63.023	T63.024	—	—
Corbadrine	T49.6X1	T49.6X2	T49.6X3	T49.6X4	T49.6X5	T49.6X6
Cordite	T65.891	T65.892	T65.893	T65.894	—	—
vapor	T59.891	T59.892	T59.893	T59.894	—	—
Cordran	T49.0X1	T49.0X2	T49.0X3	T49.0X4	T49.0X5	T49.0X6
Corn cures	T49.4X1	T49.4X2	T49.4X3	T49.4X4	T49.4X5	T49.4X6
Cornhusker's lotion	T49.3X1	T49.3X2	T49.3X3	T49.3X4	T49.3X5	T49.3X6
Corn starch	T49.3X1	T49.3X2	T49.3X3	T49.3X4	T49.3X5	T49.3X6
Coronary vasodilator NEC	T46.3X1	T46.3X2	T46.3X3	T46.3X4	T46.3X5	T46.3X6
Corrosive NEC	T54.91	T54.92	T54.93	T54.94	—	—
acid NEC	T54.2X1	T54.2X2	T54.2X3	T54.2X4	—	—
aromatics	T54.1X1	T54.1X2	T54.1X3	T54.1X4	—	—
disinfectant	T54.1X1	T54.1X2	T54.1X3	T54.1X4	—	—
fumes NEC	T54.91	T54.92	T54.93	T54.94	—	—
specified NEC	T54.91	T54.92	T54.93	T54.94	—	—
sublimate	T56.1X1	T56.1X2	T56.1X3	T56.1X4	—	—
Cortate	T38.0X1	T38.0X2	T38.0X3	T38.0X4	T38.0X5	T38.0X6
Cort-Dome	T38.0X1	T38.0X2	T38.0X3	T38.0X4	T38.0X5	T38.0X6
ENT agent	T49.6X1	T49.6X2	T49.6X3	T49.6X4	T49.6X5	T49.6X6
ophthalmic preparation	T49.5X1	T49.5X2	T49.5X3	T49.5X4	T49.5X5	T49.5X6
topical NEC	T49.0X1	T49.0X2	T49.0X3	T49.0X4	T49.0X5	T49.0X6
Cortef	T38.0X1	T38.0X2	T38.0X3	T38.0X4	T38.0X5	T38.0X6
ENT agent	T49.6X1	T49.6X2	T49.6X3	T49.6X4	T49.6X5	T49.6X6
ophthalmic preparation	T49.5X1	T49.5X2	T49.5X3	T49.5X4	T49.5X5	T49.5X6
topical NEC	T49.0X1	T49.0X2	T49.0X3	T49.0X4	T49.0X5	T49.0X6
Corticosteroid	T38.0X1	T38.0X2	T38.0X3	T38.0X4	T38.0X5	T38.0X6
ENT agent	T49.6X1	T49.6X2	T49.6X3	T49.6X4	T49.6X5	T49.6X6
mineral	T50.0X1	T50.0X2	T50.0X3	T50.0X4	T50.0X5	T50.0X6
ophthalmic	T49.5X1	T49.5X2	T49.5X3	T49.5X4	T49.5X5	T49.5X6
topical NEC	T49.0X1	T49.0X2	T49.0X3	T49.0X4	T49.0X5	T49.0X6
Corticotropin	T38.811	T38.812	T38.813	T38.814	T38.815	T38.816
Cortisol	T49.0X1	T49.0X2	T49.0X3	T49.0X4	T49.0X5	T49.0X6
ENT agent	T49.6X1	T49.6X2	T49.6X3	T49.6X4	T49.6X5	T49.6X6
ophthalmic preparation	T49.5X1	T49.5X2	T49.5X3	T49.5X4	T49.5X5	T49.5X6
topical NEC	T49.0X1	T49.0X2	T49.0X3	T49.0X4	T49.0X5	T49.0X6

⬇ Subterms under main terms may continue to next column or page   Additional Character May Be Required — Refer to the Tabular List for Character Selection   361

Cloprednol — Cortisol

Table of Drugs and Chemicals

Cortisone—DDAVP

Substance	Poisoning, Accidental (unintentional)	Poisoning, Intentional Self-harm	Poisoning, Assault	Poisoning, Undetermined	Adverse Effect	Under-dosing
Cortisone (acetate)	T38.0X1	T38.0X2	T38.0X3	T38.0X4	T38.0X5	T38.0X6
ENT agent	T49.6X1	T49.6X2	T49.6X3	T49.6X4	T49.6X5	T49.6X6
ophthalmic preparation	T49.5X1	T49.5X2	T49.5X4	T49.5X4	T49.5X5	T49.5X6
topical NEC	T49.0X1	T49.0X2	T49.0X3	T49.0X4	T49.0X5	T49.0X6
Cortivazol	T38.0X1	T38.0X2	T38.0X3	T38.0X4	T38.0X5	T38.0X6
Cortogen	T38.0X1	T38.0X2	T38.0X3	T38.0X4	T38.0X5	T38.0X6
ENT agent	T49.6X1	T49.6X2	T49.6X3	T49.6X4	T49.6X5	T49.6X6
ophthalmic preparation	T49.5X1	T49.5X2	T49.5X3	T49.5X4	T49.5X5	T49.5X6
Cortone	T38.0X1	T38.0X2	T38.0X3	T38.0X4	T38.0X5	T38.0X6
ENT agent	T49.6X1	T49.6X2	T49.6X3	T49.6X4	T49.6X5	T49.6X6
ophthalmic preparation	T49.5X1	T49.5X2	T49.5X3	T49.5X4	T49.5X5	T49.5X6
Cortril	T38.0X1	T38.0X2	T38.0X3	T38.0X4	T38.0X5	T38.0X6
ENT agent	T49.6X1	T49.6X2	T49.6X3	T49.6X4	T49.6X5	T49.6X6
ophthalmic preparation	T49.5X1	T49.5X2	T49.5X3	T49.5X4	T49.5X5	T49.5X6
topical NEC	T49.0X1	T49.0X2	T49.0X3	T49.0X4	T49.0X5	T49.0X6
Corynebacterium parvum	T45.1X1	T45.1X2	T45.1X3	T45.1X4	T45.1X5	T45.1X6
Cosmetic preparation	T49.8X1	T49.8X2	T49.8X3	T49.8X4	T49.8X5	T49.8X6
Cosmetics	T49.8X1	T49.8X2	T49.8X3	T49.8X4	T49.8X5	T49.8X6
Cosyntropin	T38.811	T38.812	T38.813	T38.814	T38.815	T38.816
Cotarnine	T45.7X1	T45.7X2	T45.7X3	T45.7X4	T45.7X5	T45.7X6
Co-trimoxazole	T36.8X1	T36.8X2	T36.8X3	T36.8X4	T36.8X5	T36.8X6
Cottonseed oil	T49.3X1	T49.3X2	T49.3X3	T49.3X4	T49.3X5	T49.3X6
Cough mixture (syrup)	T48.4X1	T48.4X2	T48.4X3	T48.4X4	T48.4X5	T48.4X6
containing opiates	T40.2X1	T40.2X2	T40.2X3	T40.2X4	T40.2X5	T40.2X6
expectorants	T48.4X1	T48.4X2	T48.4X3	T48.4X4	T48.4X5	T48.4X6
Coumadin	T45.511	T45.512	T45.513	T45.514	T45.515	T45.516
rodenticide	T60.4X1	T60.4X2	T60.4X3	T60.4X4	—	—
Coumaphos	T60.0X1	T60.0X2	T60.0X3	T60.0X4	—	—
Coumarin	T45.511	T45.512	T45.513	T45.514	T45.515	T45.516
Coumetarol	T45.511	T45.512	T45.513	T45.514	T45.515	T45.516
Cowbane	T62.2X1	T62.2X2	T62.2X3	T62.2X4	—	—
Cozyme	T45.2X1	T45.2X2	T45.2X3	T45.2X4	T45.2X5	T45.2X6
Crack	T40.5X1	T40.5X2	T40.5X3	T40.5X4	—	—
Crataegus extract	T46.0X1	T46.0X2	T46.0X3	T46.0X4	T46.0X5	T46.0X6
Creolin	T54.1X1	T54.1X2	T54.1X3	T54.1X4	—	—
disinfectant	T54.1X1	T54.1X2	T54.1X3	T54.1X4	—	—
Creosol (compound)	T49.0X1	T49.0X2	T49.0X3	T49.0X4	T49.0X5	T49.0X6
Creosote (coal tar)	T49.0X1	T49.0X2	T49.0X3	T49.0X4	T49.0X5	T49.0X6
(beechwood)						
medicinal (expectorant)	T48.4X1	T48.4X2	T48.4X3	T48.4X4	T48.4X5	T48.4X6
syrup	T48.4X1	T48.4X2	T48.4X3	T48.4X4	T48.4X5	T48.4X6
Cresol(s)	T49.0X1	T49.0X2	T49.0X3	T49.0X4	T49.0X5	T49.0X6
and soap solution	T49.0X1	T49.0X2	T49.0X3	T49.0X4	T49.0X5	T49.0X6
Cresyl acetate	T49.0X1	T49.0X2	T49.0X3	T49.0X4	T49.0X5	T49.0X6
Cresylic acid	T49.0X1	T49.0X2	T49.0X3	T49.0X4	T49.0X5	T49.0X6
Crimidine	T60.4X1	T60.4X2	T60.4X3	T60.4X4	—	—
Croconazole	T37.8X1	T37.8X2	T37.8X3	T37.8X4	T37.8X5	T37.8X6
Cromoglicic acid	T48.6X1	T48.6X2	T48.6X3	T48.6X4	T48.6X5	T48.6X6
Cromolyn	T48.6X1	T48.6X2	T48.6X3	T48.6X4	T48.6X5	T48.6X6
Cromonar	T46.3X1	T46.3X2	T46.3X3	T46.3X4	T46.3X5	T46.3X6
Cropropamide	T39.8X1	T39.8X2	T39.8X3	T39.8X4	T39.8X5	T39.8X6
with crotethamide	T50.7X1	T50.7X2	T50.7X3	T50.7X4	T50.7X5	T50.7X6
Crotamiton	T49.0X1	T49.0X2	T49.0X3	T49.0X4	T49.0X5	T49.0X6
Crotethamide	T39.8X1	T39.8X2	T39.8X3	T39.8X4	T39.8X5	T39.8X6
with cropropamide	T50.7X1	T50.7X2	T50.7X3	T50.7X4	T50.7X5	T50.7X6
Croton (oil)	T47.2X1	T47.2X2	T47.2X3	T47.2X4	T47.2X5	T47.2X6
chloral	T42.6X1	T42.6X2	T42.6X3	T42.6X4	T42.6X5	T42.6X6
Crude oil	T52.0X1	T52.0X2	T52.0X3	T52.0X4	—	—
Cryogenine	T39.8X1	T39.8X2	T39.8X3	T39.8X4	T39.8X5	T39.8X6
Cryolite (vapor)	T60.1X1	T60.1X2	T60.1X3	T60.1X4	—	—
insecticide	T60.1X1	T60.1X2	T60.1X3	T60.1X4	—	—
Cryptenamine (tannates)	T46.5X1	T46.5X2	T46.5X3	T46.5X4	T46.5X5	T46.5X6
Crystal violet	T49.0X1	T49.0X2	T49.0X3	T49.0X4	T49.0X5	T49.0X6
Cuckoopint	T62.2X1	T62.2X2	T62.2X3	T62.2X4	—	—
Cumetharol	T45.511		T45.513	T45.514	T45.515	T45.516
Cupric						
acetate	T60.3X1	T60.3X2	T60.3X3	T60.3X4	—	—
acetoarsenite	T57.0X1	T57.0X2	T57.0X3	T57.0X4	—	—
arsenate	T57.0X1	T57.0X2	T57.0X3	T57.0X4	—	—
gluconate	T49.0X1	T49.0X2	T49.0X3	T49.0X4	T49.0X5	T49.0X6
oleate	T49.0X1	T49.0X2	T49.0X3	T49.0X4	T49.0X5	T49.0X6
sulfate	T56.4X1	T56.4X2	T56.4X3	T56.4X4	—	—
Cuprous sulfate — see also	T56.4X1	T56.4X2	T56.4X3	T56.4X4	—	—
Copper sulfate						
Curare, curarine	T48.1X1	T48.1X2	T48.1X3	T48.1X4	T48.1X5	T48.1X6
Cyamemazine	T43.3X1	T43.3X2	T43.3X3	T43.3X4	T43.3X5	T43.3X6
Cyamopsis tetragonoloba	T46.6X1	T46.6X2	T46.6X3	T46.6X4	T46.6X5	T46.6X6
Cyanacetyl hydrazide	T37.1X1	T37.1X2	T37.1X3	T37.1X4	T37.1X5	T37.1X6
Cyanic acid (gas)	T59.891	T59.892	T59.893	T59.894	—	—
Cyanide(s) (compounds)	T65.0X1	T65.0X2	T65.0X3	T65.0X4		
(potassium) (sodium)						
NEC	T65.0X1	T65.0X2	T65.0X3	T65.0X4		
dust or gas (inhalation) NEC	T57.3X1	T57.3X2	T57.3X3	T57.3X4	—	—

Substance	Poisoning, Accidental (unintentional)	Poisoning, Intentional Self-harm	Poisoning, Assault	Poisoning, Undetermined	Adverse Effect	Under-dosing
Cyanide(s) (compounds) (potassium) (sodium) **NEC** — *continued*						
fumigant	T65.0X1	T65.0X2	T65.0X3	T65.0X4		
hydrogen	T57.3X1	T57.3X2	T57.3X3	T57.3X4		
mercuric — *see* Mercury						
pesticide (dust) (fumes)	T65.0X1	T65.0X2	T65.0X3	T65.0X4		
Cyanoacrylate adhesive	T49.3X1	T49.3X2	T49.3X3	T49.3X4	T49.3X5	T49.3X6
Cyanocobalamin	T45.8X1	T45.8X2	T45.8X3	T45.8X4	T45.8X5	T45.8X6
Cyanogen (chloride) (gas)	T59.891	T59.892	T59.893	T59.894		
NEC						
Cyclacillin	T36.0X1	T36.0X2	T36.0X3	T36.0X4	T36.0X5	T36.0X6
Cyclaine	T41.3X1	T41.3X2	T41.3X3	T41.3X4	T41.3X5	T41.3X6
Cyclamate	T50.991	T50.992	T50.993	T50.994	T50.995	T50.996
Cyclamen europaeum	T62.2X1	T62.2X2	T62.2X3	T62.2X4	—	—
Cyclandelate	T46.7X1	T46.7X2	T46.7X3	T46.7X4	T46.7X5	T46.7X6
Cyclazocine	T50.7X1	T50.7X2	T50.7X3	T50.7X4	T50.7X5	T50.7X6
Cyclizine	T45.0X1	T45.0X2	T45.0X3	T45.0X4	T45.0X5	T45.0X6
Cyclobarbital	T42.3X1	T42.3X2	T42.3X3	T42.3X4	T42.3X5	T42.3X6
Cyclobarbitone	T42.3X1	T42.3X2	T42.3X3	T42.3X4	T42.3X5	T42.3X6
Cyclobenzaprine	T48.1X1	T48.1X2	T48.1X3	T48.1X4	T48.1X5	T48.1X6
Cyclodrine	T44.3X1	T44.3X2	T44.3X3	T44.3X4	T44.3X5	T44.3X6
Cycloguanil embonate	T37.2X1	T37.2X2	T37.2X3	T37.2X4	T37.2X5	T37.2X6
Cyclohexane	T52.8X1	T52.8X2	T52.8X3	T52.8X4	—	—
Cyclohexanol	T51.8X1	T51.8X2	T51.8X3	T51.8X4	—	—
Cyclohexanone	T52.4X1	T52.4X2	T52.4X3	T52.4X4	—	—
Cycloheximide	T60.3X1	T60.3X2	T60.3X3	T60.3X4	—	—
Cyclohexyl acetate	T52.8X1	T52.8X2	T52.8X3	T52.8X4	—	—
Cycloleucin	T45.1X1	T45.1X2	T45.1X3	T45.1X4	T45.1X5	T45.1X6
Cyclomethycaine	T41.3X1	T41.3X2	T41.3X3	T41.3X4	T41.3X5	T41.3X6
Cyclopentamine	T44.4X1	T44.4X2	T44.4X3	T44.4X4	T44.4X5	T44.4X6
Cyclopenthiazide	T50.2X1	T50.2X2	T50.2X3	T50.2X4	T50.2X5	T50.2X6
Cyclopentolate	T44.3X1	T44.3X2	T44.3X3	T44.3X4	T44.3X5	T44.3X6
Cyclophosphamide	T45.1X1	T45.1X2	T45.1X3	T45.1X4	T45.1X5	T45.1X6
Cycloplegic drug	T49.5X1	T49.5X2	T49.5X3	T49.5X4	T49.5X5	T49.5X6
Cyclopropane	T41.291	T41.292	T41.293	T41.294	T41.295	T41.296
Cyclopyrabital	T39.8X1	T39.8X2	T39.8X3	T39.8X4	T39.8X5	T39.8X6
Cycloserine	T37.1X1	T37.1X2	T37.1X3	T37.1X4	T37.1X5	T37.1X6
Cyclosporin	T45.1X1	T45.1X2	T45.1X3	T45.1X4	T45.1X5	T45.1X6
Cyclothiazide	T50.2X1	T50.2X2	T50.2X3	T50.2X4	T50.2X5	T50.2X6
Cycrimine	T44.3X1	T44.3X2	T44.3X3	T44.3X4	T44.3X5	T44.3X6
Cyhalothrin	T60.1X1	T60.1X2	T60.1X3	T60.1X4	—	—
Cymarin	T46.0X1	T46.0X2	T46.0X3	T46.0X4	T46.0X5	T46.0X6
Cypermethrin	T60.1X1	T60.1X2	T60.1X3	T60.1X4	—	—
Cyphenothrin	T60.2X1	T60.2X2	T60.2X3	T60.2X4	—	—
Cyproheptadine	T45.0X1	T45.0X2	T45.0X3	T45.0X4	T45.0X5	T45.0X6
Cyproterone	T38.6X1	T38.6X2	T38.6X3	T38.6X4	T38.6X5	T38.6X6
Cysteamine	T50.6X1	T50.6X2	T50.6X3	T50.6X4	T50.6X5	T50.6X6
Cytarabine	T45.1X1	T45.1X2	T45.1X3	T45.1X4	T45.1X5	T45.1X6
Cytisus						
laburnum	T62.2X1	T62.2X2	T62.2X3	T62.2X4	—	—
scoparius	T62.2X1	T62.2X2	T62.2X3	T62.2X4	—	—
Cytochrome C	T47.5X1	T47.5X2	T47.5X3	T47.5X4	T47.5X5	T47.5X6
Cytomel	T38.1X1	T38.1X2	T38.1X3	T38.1X4	T38.1X5	T38.1X6
Cytosine arabinoside	T45.1X1	T45.1X2	T45.1X3	T45.1X4	T45.1X5	T45.1X6
Cytoxan	T45.1X1	T45.1X2	T45.1X3	T45.1X4	T45.1X5	T45.1X6
Cytozyme	T45.7X1	T45.7X2	T45.7X3	T45.7X4	T45.7X5	T45.7X6
S-Carboxymethylcysteine	T48.4X1	T48.4X2	T48.4X3	T48.4X4	T48.4X5	T48.4X6
Dacarbazine	T45.1X1	T45.1X2	T45.1X3	T45.1X4	T45.1X5	T45.1X6
Dactinomycin	T45.1X1	T45.1X2	T45.1X3	T45.1X4	T45.1X5	T45.1X6
DADPS	T37.1X1	T37.1X2	T37.1X3	T37.1X4	T37.1X5	T37.1X6
Dakin's solution	T49.0X1	T49.0X2	T49.0X3	T49.0X4	T49.0X5	T49.0X6
Dalapon (sodium)	T60.3X1	T60.3X2	T60.3X3	T60.3X4	—	—
Dalmane	T42.4X1	T42.4X2	T42.4X3	T42.4X4	T42.4X5	T42.4X6
Danazol	T38.6X1	T38.6X2	T38.6X3	T38.6X4	T38.6X5	T38.6X6
Danilone	T45.511	T45.512	T45.513	T45.514	T45.515	T45.516
Danthron	T47.2X1	T47.2X2	T47.2X3	T47.2X4	T47.2X5	T47.2X6
Dantrolene	T42.8X1	T42.8X2	T42.8X3	T42.8X4	T42.8X5	T42.8X6
Dantron	T47.2X1	T47.2X2	T47.2X3	T47.2X4	T47.2X5	T47.2X6
Daphne (gnidium)	T62.2X1	T62.2X2	T62.2X3	T62.2X4	—	—
(mezereum)						
berry	T62.1X1	T62.1X2	T62.1X3	T62.1X4	—	—
Dapsone	T37.1X1	T37.1X2	T37.1X3	T37.1X4	T37.1X5	T37.1X6
Daraprim	T37.2X1	T37.2X2	T37.2X3	T37.2X4	T37.2X5	T37.2X6
Darnel	T62.2X1	T62.2X2	T62.2X3	T62.2X4	—	—
Darvon	T39.8X1	T39.8X2	T39.8X3	T39.8X4	T39.8X5	T39.8X6
Daunomycin	T45.1X1	T45.1X2	T45.1X3	T45.1X4	T45.1X5	T45.1X6
Daunorubicin	T45.1X1	T45.1X2	T45.1X3	T45.1X4	T45.1X5	T45.1X6
DBI	T38.3X1	T38.3X2	T38.3X3	T38.3X4	T38.3X5	T38.3X6
D-Con	T60.91	T60.92	T60.93	T60.94	—	—
insecticide	T60.2X1	T60.2X2	T60.2X3	T60.2X4	—	—
rodenticide	T60.4X1	T60.4X2	T60.4X3	T60.4X4	—	—
DDAVP	T38.891	T38.892	T38.893	T38.894	T38.895	T38.896

Substance	Poisoning, Accidental (unintentional)	Poisoning, Intentional Self-harm	Poisoning, Assault	Poisoning, Undetermined	Adverse Effect	Under-dosing
DDE (bis(chlorophenyl)-dichloroethylene)	T60.2X1	T60.2X2	T60.2X3	T60.2X4	—	—
DDS	T37.1X1	T37.1X2	T37.1X3	T37.1X4	T37.1X5	T37.1X6
DDT (dust)	T60.1X1	T60.1X2	T60.1X3	T60.1X4	—	—
Deadly nightshade — see also	T62.2X1	T62.2X2	T62.2X3	T62.2X4	—	—
Belladonna						
berry	T62.1X1	T62.1X2	T62.1X3	T62.1X4	—	—
Deamino-D-arginine vasopressin	T38.891	T38.892	T38.893	T38.894	T38.895	T38.896
Deanol (aceglumate)	T50.991	T50.992	T50.993	T50.994	T50.995	T50.996
Debrisoquine	T46.5X1	T46.5X2	T46.5X3	T46.5X4	T46.5X5	T46.5X6
Decaborane	T57.8X1	T57.8X2	T57.8X3	T57.8X4	—	—
fumes	T59.891	T59.892	T59.893	T59.894	—	—
Decadron	T38.0X1	T38.0X2	T38.0X3	T38.0X4	T38.0X5	T38.0X6
ENT agent	T49.6X1	T49.6X2	T49.6X3	T49.6X4	T49.6X5	T49.6X6
ophthalmic preparation	T49.5X1	T49.5X2	T49.5X3	T49.5X4	T49.5X5	T49.5X6
topical NEC	T49.0X1	T49.0X2	T49.0X3	T49.0X4	T49.0X5	T49.0X6
Decahydronaphthalene	T52.8X1	T52.8X2	T52.8X3	T52.8X4	—	—
Decalin	T52.8X1	T52.8X2	T52.8X3	T52.8X4	—	—
Decamethonium (bromide)	T48.1X1	T48.1X2	T48.1X3	T48.1X4	T48.1X5	T48.1X6
Decholin	T47.5X1	T47.5X2	T47.5X3	T47.5X4	T47.5X5	T47.5X6
Declomycin	T36.4X1	T36.4X2	T36.4X3	T36.4X4	T36.4X5	T36.4X6
Decongestant, nasal (mucosa)	T48.5X1	T48.5X2	T48.5X3	T48.5X4	T48.5X5	T48.5X6
combination	T48.5X1	T48.5X2	T48.5X3	T48.5X4	T48.5X5	T48.5X6
Deet	T60.8X1	T60.8X2	T60.8X3	T60.8X4	—	—
Deferoxamine	T45.8X1	T45.8X2	T45.8X3	T45.8X4	T45.8X5	T45.8X6
Deflazacort	T38.0X1	T38.0X2	T38.0X3	T38.0X4	T38.0X5	T38.0X6
Deglycyrrhizinized extract of licorice	T48.4X1	T48.4X2	T48.4X3	T48.4X4	T48.4X5	T48.4X6
Dehydrocholic acid	T47.5X1	T47.5X2	T47.5X3	T47.5X4	T47.5X5	T47.5X6
Dehydroemetine	T37.3X1	T37.3X2	T37.3X3	T37.3X4	T37.3X5	T37.3X6
Dekalin	T52.8X1	T52.8X2	T52.8X3	T52.8X4	—	—
Delalutin	T38.5X1	T38.5X2	T38.5X3	T38.5X4	T38.5X5	T38.5X6
Delorazepam	T42.4X1	T42.4X2	T42.4X3	T42.4X4	T42.4X5	T42.4X6
Delphinium	T62.2X1	T62.2X2	T62.2X3	T62.2X4	—	—
Deltamethrin	T60.1X1	T60.1X2	T60.1X3	T60.1X4	—	—
Deltasone	T38.0X1	T38.0X2	T38.0X3	T38.0X4	T38.0X5	T38.0X6
Deltra	T38.0X1	T38.0X2	T38.0X3	T38.0X4	T38.0X5	T38.0X6
Delvinal	T42.3X1	T42.3X2	T42.3X3	T42.3X4	T42.3X5	T42.3X6
Demecarium (bromide)	T49.5X1	T49.5X2	T49.5X3	T49.5X4	T49.5X5	T49.5X6
Demeclocycline	T36.4X1	T36.4X2	T36.4X3	T36.4X4	T36.4X5	T36.4X6
Demecolcine	T45.1X1	T45.1X2	T45.1X3	T45.1X4	T45.1X5	T45.1X6
Demegestone	T38.5X1	T38.5X2	T38.5X3	T38.5X4	T38.5X5	T38.5X6
Demelanizing agents	T49.8X1	T49.8X2	T49.8X3	T49.8X4	T49.8X5	T49.8X6
Demephion -O and -S	T60.0X1	T60.0X2	T60.0X3	T60.0X4	—	—
Demerol	T40.2X1	T40.2X2	T40.2X3	T40.2X4	T40.2X5	T40.2X6
Demethylchlortetracycline	T36.4X1	T36.4X2	T36.4X3	T36.4X4	T36.4X5	T36.4X6
Demethyltetracycline	T36.4X1	T36.4X2	T36.4X3	T36.4X4	T36.4X5	T36.4X6
Demeton -O and -S	T60.0X1	T60.0X2	T60.0X3	T60.0X4	—	—
Demulcent (external)	T49.3X1	T49.3X2	T49.3X3	T49.3X4	T49.3X5	T49.3X6
specified NEC	T49.3X1	T49.3X2	T49.3X3	T49.3X4	T49.3X5	T49.3X6
Demulen	T38.4X1	T38.4X2	T38.4X3	T38.4X4	T38.4X5	T38.4X6
Denatured alcohol	T51.0X1	T51.0X2	T51.0X3	T51.0X4	—	—
Dendrid	T49.5X1	T49.5X2	T49.5X3	T49.5X4	T49.5X5	T49.5X6
Dental drug, topical application NEC	T49.7X1	T49.7X2	T49.7X3	T49.7X4	T49.7X5	T49.7X6
Dentifrice	T49.7X1	T49.7X2	T49.7X3	T49.7X4	T49.7X5	T49.7X6
Deodorant spray (feminine hygiene)	T49.8X1	T49.8X2	T49.8X3	T49.8X4	T49.8X5	T49.8X6
Deoxycortone	T50.0X1	T50.0X2	T50.0X3	T50.0X4	T50.0X5	T50.0X6
Deoxyribonuclease (pancreatic)	T45.3X1	T45.3X2	T45.3X3	T45.3X4	T45.3X5	T45.3X6
Depilatory	T49.4X1	T49.4X2	T49.4X3	T49.4X4	T49.4X5	T49.4X6
Deprenalin	T42.8X1	T42.8X2	T42.8X3	T42.8X4	T42.8X5	T42.8X6
Deprenyl	T42.8X1	T42.8X2	T42.8X3	T42.8X4	T42.8X5	T42.8X6
Depressant						
appetite (central)	T50.5X1	T50.5X2	T50.5X3	T50.5X4	T50.5X5	T50.5X6
cardiac	T46.2X1	T46.2X2	T46.2X3	T46.2X4	T46.2X5	T46.2X6
central nervous system (anesthetic) — see also Central nervous system, depressants	T42.71	T42.72	T42.73	T42.74	T42.75	T42.76
general anesthetic	T41.201	T41.202	T41.203	T41.204	T41.205	T41.206
muscle tone	T42.8X1	T42.8X2	T42.8X3	T42.8X4	T42.8X5	T42.8X6
muscle tone, central	T42.8X1	T42.8X2	T42.8X3	T42.8X4	T42.8X5	T42.8X6
psychotherapeutic	T43.501	T43.502	T43.503	T43.504	T43.505	T43.506
Depressant, appetite	T50.5X1	T50.5X2	T50.5X3	T50.5X4	T50.5X5	T50.5X6
Deptropine	T45.0X1	T45.0X2	T45.0X3	T45.0X4	T45.0X5	T45.0X6
Dequalinium (chloride)	T49.0X1	T49.0X2	T49.0X3	T49.0X4	T49.0X5	T49.0X6
Derris root	T60.2X1	T60.2X2	T60.2X3	T60.2X4	—	—
Deserpidine	T46.5X1	T46.5X2	T46.5X3	T46.5X4	T46.5X5	T46.5X6
Desferrioxamine	T45.8X1	T45.8X2	T45.8X3	T45.8X4	T45.8X5	T45.8X6

Substance	Poisoning, Accidental (unintentional)	Poisoning, Intentional Self-harm	Poisoning, Assault	Poisoning, Undetermined	Adverse Effect	Under-dosing
Desipramine	T43.011	T43.012	T43.013	T43.014	T43.015	T43.016
Deslanoside	T46.0X1	T46.0X2	T46.0X3	T46.0X4	T46.0X5	T46.0X6
Desloughing agent	T49.4X1	T49.4X2	T49.4X3	T49.4X4	T49.4X5	T49.4X6
Desmethylimipramine	T43.011	T43.012	T43.013	T43.014	T43.015	T43.016
Desmopressin	T38.891	T38.892	T38.893	T38.894	T38.895	T38.896
Desocodeine	T40.2X1	T40.2X2	T40.2X3	T40.2X4	T40.2X5	T40.2X6
Desogestrel	T38.5X1	T38.5X2	T38.5X3	T38.5X4	T38.5X5	T38.5X6
Desomorphine	T40.2X1	T40.2X2	T40.2X3	T40.2X4	—	—
Desonide	T49.0X1	T49.0X2	T49.0X3	T49.0X4	T49.0X5	T49.0X6
Desoximetasone	T49.0X1	T49.0X2	T49.0X3	T49.0X4	T49.0X5	T49.0X6
Desoxycorticosteroid	T50.0X1	T50.0X2	T50.0X3	T50.0X4	T50.0X5	T50.0X6
Desoxycortone	T50.0X1	T50.0X2	T50.0X3	T50.0X4	T50.0X5	T50.0X6
Desoxyephedrine	T43.621	T43.622	T43.623	T43.624	T43.625	T43.626
Detaxtran	T46.6X1	T46.6X2	T46.6X3	T46.6X4	T46.6X5	T46.6X6
Detergent	T49.2X1	T49.2X2	T49.2X3	T49.2X4	T49.2X5	T49.2X6
external medication	T49.2X1	T49.2X2	T49.2X3	T49.2X4	T49.2X5	T49.2X6
local	T49.2X1	T49.2X2	T49.2X3	T49.2X4	T49.2X5	T49.2X6
medicinal	T49.2X1	T49.2X2	T49.2X3	T49.2X4	T49.2X5	T49.2X6
nonmedicinal	T55.1X1	T55.1X2	T55.1X3	T55.1X4	—	—
specified NEC	T55.1X1	T55.1X2	T55.1X3	T55.1X4	—	—
Deterrent, alcohol	T50.6X1	T50.6X2	T50.6X3	T50.6X4	T50.6X5	T50.6X6
Detoxifying agent	T50.6X1	T50.6X2	T50.6X3	T50.6X4	T50.6X5	T50.6X6
Detrothyronine	T38.1X1	T38.1X2	T38.1X3	T38.1X4	T38.1X5	T38.1X6
Dettol (external medication)	T49.0X1	T49.0X2	T49.0X3	T49.0X4	T49.0X5	T49.0X6
Dexamethasone	T38.0X1	T38.0X2	T38.0X3	T38.0X4	T38.0X5	T38.0X6
ENT agent	T49.6X1	T49.6X2	T49.6X3	T49.6X4	T49.6X5	T49.6X6
ophthalmic preparation	T49.5X1	T49.5X2	T49.5X3	T49.5X4	T49.5X5	T49.5X6
topical NEC	T49.0X1	T49.0X2	T49.0X3	T49.0X4	T49.0X5	T49.0X6
Dexamfetamine	T43.621	T43.622	T43.623	T43.624	T43.625	T43.626
Dexamphetamine	T43.621	T43.622	T43.623	T43.624	T43.625	T43.626
Dexbrompheniramine	T45.0X1	T45.0X2	T45.0X3	T45.0X4	T45.0X5	T45.0X6
Dexchlorpheniramine	T45.0X1	T45.0X2	T45.0X3	T45.0X4	T45.0X5	T45.0X6
Dexedrine	T43.621	T43.622	T43.623	T43.624	T43.625	T43.626
Dexetimide	T44.3X1	T44.3X2	T44.3X3	T44.3X4	T44.3X5	T44.3X6
Dexfenfluramine	T50.5X1	T50.5X2	T50.5X3	T50.5X4	T50.5X5	T50.5X6
Dexpanthenol	T45.2X1	T45.2X2	T45.2X3	T45.2X4	T45.2X5	T45.2X6
Dextran (40) (70) (150)	T45.8X1	T45.8X2	T45.8X3	T45.8X4	T45.8X5	T45.8X6
Dextriferron	T45.4X1	T45.4X2	T45.4X3	T45.4X4	T45.4X5	T45.4X6
Dextroamphetamine	T43.621	T43.622	T43.623	T43.624	T43.625	T43.626
Dextro calcium pantothenate	T45.2X1	T45.2X2	T45.2X3	T45.2X4	T45.2X5	T45.2X6
Dextromethorphan	T48.3X1	T48.3X2	T48.3X3	T48.3X4	T48.3X5	T48.3X6
Dextromoramide	T40.4X1	T40.4X2	T40.4X3	T40.4X4	—	—
topical	T49.8X1	T49.8X2	T49.8X3	T49.8X4	T49.8X5	T49.8X6
Dextro pantothenyl alcohol	T45.2X1	T45.2X2	T45.2X3	T45.2X4	T45.2X5	T45.2X6
Dextropropoxyphene	T40.4X1	T40.4X2	T40.4X3	T40.4X4	—	—
Dextrorphan	T40.2X1	T40.2X2	T40.2X3	T40.2X4	T40.2X5	T40.2X6
Dextrose	T50.3X1	T50.3X2	T50.3X3	T50.3X4	T50.3X5	T50.3X6
concentrated solution, intravenous	T46.8X1	T46.8X2	T46.8X3	T46.8X4	T46.8X5	T46.8X6
Dextrothyroxin	T38.1X1	T38.1X2	T38.1X3	T38.1X4	T38.1X5	T38.1X6
Dextrothyroxine sodium	T38.1X1	T38.1X2	T38.1X3	T38.1X4	T38.1X5	T38.1X6
DFP	T44.0X1	T44.0X2	T44.0X3	T44.0X4	T44.0X5	T44.0X6
DHE	T37.3X1	T37.3X2	T37.3X3	T37.3X4	T37.3X5	T37.3X6
45	T46.5X1	T46.5X2	T46.5X3	T46.5X4	T46.5X5	T46.5X6
Diabinese	T38.3X1	T38.3X2	T38.3X3	T38.3X4	T38.3X5	T38.3X6
Diacetone alcohol	T52.4X1	T52.4X2	T52.4X3	T52.4X4	—	—
Diacetyl monoxime	T50.991	T50.992	T50.993	T50.994	—	—
Diacetylmorphine	T40.1X1	T40.1X2	T40.1X3	T40.1X4	—	—
Diachylon plaster	T49.4X1	T49.4X2	T49.4X3	T49.4X4	T49.4X5	T49.4X6
Diaethylstilboestrolum	T38.5X1	T38.5X2	T38.5X3	T38.5X4	T38.5X5	T38.5X6
Diagnostic agent NEC	T50.8X1	T50.8X2	T50.8X3	T50.8X4	T50.8X5	T50.8X6
Dial (soap)	T49.2X1	T49.2X2	T49.2X3	T49.2X4	T49.2X5	T49.2X6
sedative	T42.3X1	T42.3X2	T42.3X3	T42.3X4	T42.3X5	T42.3X6
Dialkyl carbonate	T52.91	T52.92	T52.93	T52.94	—	—
Diallylbarbituric acid	T42.3X1	T42.3X2	T42.3X3	T42.3X4	T42.3X5	T42.3X6
Diallymal	T42.3X1	T42.3X2	T42.3X3	T42.3X4	T42.3X5	T42.3X6
Dialysis solution (intraperitoneal)	T50.3X1	T50.3X2	T50.3X3	T50.3X4	T50.3X5	T50.3X6
Diaminodiphenylsulfone	T37.1X1	T37.1X2	T37.1X3	T37.1X4	T37.1X5	T37.1X6
Diamorphine	T40.1X1	T40.1X2	T40.1X3	T40.1X4	—	—
Diamox	T50.2X1	T50.2X2	T50.2X3	T50.2X4	T50.2X5	T50.2X6
Diamthazole	T49.0X1	T49.0X2	T49.0X3	T49.0X4	T49.0X5	T49.0X6
Dianthone	T47.2X1	T47.2X2	T47.2X3	T47.2X4	T47.2X5	T47.2X6
Diaphenylsulfone	T37.0X1	T37.0X2	T37.0X3	T37.0X4	T37.0X5	T37.0X6
Diasone (sodium)	T37.1X1	T37.1X2	T37.1X3	T37.1X4	T37.1X5	T37.1X6
Diastase	T47.5X1	T47.5X2	T47.5X3	T47.5X4	T47.5X5	T47.5X6
Diatrizoate	T50.8X1	T50.8X2	T50.8X3	T50.8X4	T50.8X5	T50.8X6
Diazepam	T42.4X1	T42.4X2	T42.4X3	T42.4X4	T42.4X5	T42.4X6
Diazinon	T60.0X1	T60.0X2	T60.0X3	T60.0X4	—	—
Diazomethane (gas)	T59.891	T59.892	T59.893	T59.894	—	—
Diazoxide	T46.5X1	T46.5X2	T46.5X3	T46.5X4	T46.5X5	T46.5X6
Dibekacin	T36.5X1	T36.5X2	T36.5X3	T36.5X4	T36.5X5	T36.5X6

Substance	Poisoning, Accidental (unintentional)	Poisoning, Intentional Self-harm	Poisoning, Assault	Poisoning, Undetermined	Adverse Effect	Under-dosing
Dibenamine	T44.6X1	T44.6X2	T44.6X3	T44.6X4	T44.6X5	T44.6X6
Dibenzepin	T43.011	T43.012	T43.013	T43.014	T43.015	T43.016
Dibenzheptropine	T45.0X1	T45.0X2	T45.0X3	T45.0X4	T45.0X5	T45.0X6
Dibenzyline	T44.6X1	T44.6X2	T44.6X3	T44.6X4	T44.6X5	T44.6X6
Diborane (gas)	T59.891	T59.892	T59.893	T59.894	—	—
Dibromochloropropane	T60.8X1	T60.8X2	T60.8X3	T60.8X4	—	—
Dibromodulcitol	T45.1X1	T45.1X2	T45.1X3	T45.1X4	T45.1X5	T45.1X6
Dibromoethane	T53.6X1	T53.6X2	T53.6X3	T53.6X4	—	—
Dibromomannitol	T45.1X1	T45.1X2	T45.1X3	T45.1X4	T45.1X5	T45.1X6
Dibromopropamidine isethionate	T49.0X1	T49.0X2	T49.0X3	T49.0X4	T49.0X5	T49.0X6
Dibrompropamidine	T49.0X1	T49.0X2	T49.0X3	T49.0X4	T49.0X5	T49.0X6
Dibucaine	T41.3X1	T41.3X2	T41.3X3	T41.3X4	T41.3X5	T41.3X6
topical (surface)	T41.3X1	T41.3X2	T41.3X3	T41.3X4	T41.3X5	T41.3X6
Dibunate sodium	T48.3X1	T48.3X2	T48.3X3	T48.3X4	T48.3X5	T48.3X6
Dibutoline sulfate	T44.3X1	T44.3X2	T44.3X3	T44.3X4	T44.3X5	T44.3X6
Dicamba	T60.3X1	T60.3X2	T60.3X3	T60.3X4	—	—
Dicapthon	T60.0X1	T60.0X2	T60.0X3	T60.0X4	—	—
Dichlobenil	T60.3X1	T60.3X2	T60.3X3	T60.3X4	—	—
Dichlone	T60.3X1	T60.3X2	T60.3X3	T60.3X4	—	—
Dichloralphenozone	T42.6X1	T42.6X2	T42.6X3	T42.6X4	T42.6X5	T42.6X6
Dichlorbenzidine	T65.3X1	T65.3X2	T65.3X3	T65.3X4	—	—
Dichlorhydrin	T52.8X1	T52.8X2	T52.8X3	T52.8X4	—	—
Dichlorhydroxyquinoline	T37.8X1	T37.8X2	T37.8X3	T37.8X4	T37.8X5	T37.8X6
Dichlorobenzene	T53.7X1	T53.7X2	T53.7X3	T53.7X4	—	—
Dichlorobenzyl alcohol	T49.6X1	T49.6X2	T49.6X3	T49.6X4	T49.6X5	T49.6X6
Dichlorodifluoromethane	T53.5X1	T53.5X2	T53.5X3	T53.5X4	—	—
Dichloroethane	T52.8X1	T52.8X2	T52.8X3	T52.8X4	—	—
Dichloroethylene	T53.6X1	T53.6X2	T53.6X3	T53.6X4	—	—
Dichloroethyl sulfide, not in war	T59.891	T59.892	T59.893	T59.894	—	—
Dichloroformoxine, not in war	T59.891	T59.892	T59.893	T59.894	—	—
Dichlorohydrin, alpha-dichlorohydrin	T52.8X1	T52.8X2	T52.8X3	T52.8X4	—	—
Dichloromethane (solvent)	T53.4X1	T53.4X2	T53.4X3	T53.4X4	—	—
vapor	T53.4X1	T53.4X2	T53.4X3	T53.4X4	—	—
Dichloronaphthoquinone	T60.3X1	T60.3X2	T60.3X3	T60.3X4	—	—
Dichlorophen	T37.4X1	T37.4X2	T37.4X3	T37.4X4	T37.4X5	T37.4X6
Dichloropropene	T60.3X1	T60.3X2	T60.3X3	T60.3X4	—	—
Dichloropropionic acid	T60.3X1	T60.3X2	T60.3X3	T60.3X4	—	—
Dichlorphenamide	T50.2X1	T50.2X2	T50.2X3	T50.2X4	T50.2X5	T50.2X6
Dichlorvos	T60.0X1	T60.0X2	T60.0X3	T60.0X4	—	—
Diclofenac	T39.391	T39.392	T39.393	T39.394	T39.395	T39.396
Diclofenamide	T50.2X1	T50.2X2	T50.2X3	T50.2X4	T50.2X5	T50.2X6
Diclofensine	T43.291	T43.292	T43.293	T43.294	T43.295	T43.296
Diclonixine	T39.8X1	T39.8X2	T39.8X3	T39.8X4	T39.8X5	T39.8X6
Dicloxacillin	T36.0X1	T36.0X2	T36.0X3	T36.0X4	T36.0X5	T36.0X6
Dicophane	T49.0X1	T49.0X2	T49.0X3	T49.0X4	T49.0X5	T49.0X6
Dicoumarol, dicoumarin, dicumarol	T45.511	T45.512	T45.513	T45.514	T45.515	T45.516
Dicrotophos	T60.0X1	T60.0X2	T60.0X3	T60.0X4	—	—
Dicyanogen (gas)	T65.0X1	T65.0X2	T65.0X3	T65.0X4	—	—
Dicyclomine	T44.3X1	T44.3X2	T44.3X3	T44.3X4	T44.3X5	T44.3X6
Dicycloverine	T44.3X1	T44.3X2	T44.3X3	T44.3X4	T44.3X5	T44.3X6
Dideoxycytidine	T37.5X1	T37.5X2	T37.5X3	T37.5X4	T37.5X5	T37.5X6
Dideoxyinosine	T37.5X1	T37.5X2	T37.5X3	T37.5X4	T37.5X5	T37.5X6
Dieldrin (vapor)	T60.1X1	T60.1X2	T60.1X3	T60.1X4	—	—
Diemal	T42.3X1	T42.3X2	T42.3X3	T42.3X4	T42.3X5	T42.3X6
Dienestrol	T38.5X1	T38.5X2	T38.5X3	T38.5X4	T38.5X5	T38.5X6
Dienoestrol	T38.5X1	T38.5X2	T38.5X3	T38.5X4	T38.5X5	T38.5X6
Dietetic drug NEC	T50.901	T50.902	T50.903	T50.904	T50.905	T50.906
Diethazine	T42.8X1	T42.8X2	T42.8X3	T42.8X4	T42.8X5	T42.8X6
Diethyl						
barbituric acid	T42.3X1	T42.3X2	T42.3X3	T42.3X4	T42.3X5	T42.3X6
carbamazine	T37.4X1	T37.4X2	T37.4X3	T37.4X4	T37.4X5	T37.4X6
carbinol	T51.3X1	T51.3X2	T51.3X3	T51.3X4	—	—
carbonate	T52.8X1	T52.8X2	T52.8X3	T52.8X4	—	—
ether (vapor) — see also ether	T41.0X1	T41.0X2	T41.0X3	T41.0X4	T41.0X5	T41.0X6
oxide	T52.8X1	T52.8X2	T52.8X3	T52.8X4	—	—
propion	T50.5X1	T50.5X2	T50.5X3	T50.5X4	T50.5X5	T50.5X6
stilbestrol	T38.5X1	T38.5X2	T38.5X3	T38.5X4	T38.5X5	T38.5X6
toluamide (nonmedicinal)	T60.8X1	T60.8X2	T60.8X3	T60.8X4	—	—
medicinal	T49.3X1	T49.3X2	T49.3X3	T49.3X4	T49.3X5	T49.3X6
Diethylcarbamazine	T37.4X1	T37.4X2	T37.4X3	T37.4X4	T37.4X5	T37.4X6
Diethylene						
dioxide	T52.8X1	T52.8X2	T52.8X3	T52.8X4	—	—
glycol (monoacetate) (monobutyl ether) (monoethyl ether)	T52.3X1	T52.3X2	T52.3X3	T52.3X4	—	—
Diethylhexylphthalate	T65.891	T65.892	T65.893	T65.894	—	—
Diethylpropion	T50.5X1	T50.5X2	T50.5X3	T50.5X4	T50.5X5	T50.5X6

Substance	Poisoning, Accidental (unintentional)	Poisoning, Intentional Self-harm	Poisoning, Assault	Poisoning, Undetermined	Adverse Effect	Under-dosing
Diethylstilbestrol	T38.5X1	T38.5X2	T38.5X3	T38.5X4	T38.5X5	T38.5X6
Diethylstilboestrol	T38.5X1	T38.5X2	T38.5X3	T38.5X4	T38.5X5	T38.5X6
Diethylsulfone-diethylmethane	T42.6X1	T42.6X2	T42.6X3	T42.6X4	T42.6X5	T42.6X6
Diethyltoluamide	T49.0X1	T49.0X2	T49.0X3	T49.0X4	T49.0X5	T49.0X6
Diethyltryptamine (DET)	T40.991	T40.992	T40.993	T40.994	—	—
Difebarbamate	T42.3X1	T42.3X2	T42.3X3	T42.3X4	T42.3X5	T42.3X6
Difencloxazine	T40.2X1	T40.2X2	T40.2X3	T40.2X4	T40.2X5	T40.2X6
Difenidol	T45.0X1	T45.0X2	T45.0X3	T45.0X4	T45.0X5	T45.0X6
Difenoxin	T47.6X1	T47.6X2	T47.6X3	T47.6X4	T47.6X5	T47.6X6
Difetarsone	T37.3X1	T37.3X2	T37.3X3	T37.3X4	T37.3X5	T37.3X6
Diffusin	T45.3X1	T45.3X2	T45.3X3	T45.3X4	T45.3X5	T45.3X6
Diflorasone	T49.0X1	T49.0X2	T49.0X3	T49.0X4	T49.0X5	T49.0X6
Diflos	T44.0X1	T44.0X2	T44.0X3	T44.0X4	T44.0X5	T44.0X6
Diflubenzuron	T60.1X1	T60.1X2	T60.1X3	T60.1X4	—	—
Diflucortolone	T49.0X1	T49.0X2	T49.0X3	T49.0X4	T49.0X5	T49.0X6
Diflunisal	T39.091	T39.092	T39.093	T39.094	T39.095	T39.096
Difluoromethyldopa	T42.8X1	T42.8X2	T42.8X3	T42.8X4	T42.8X5	T42.8X6
Difluorophate	T44.0X1	T44.0X2	T44.0X3	T44.0X4	T44.0X5	T44.0X6
Digestant NEC	T47.5X1	T47.5X2	T47.5X3	T47.5X4	T47.5X5	T47.5X6
Digitalin (e)	T46.0X1	T46.0X2	T46.0X3	T46.0X4	T46.0X5	T46.0X6
Digitalis (leaf)(glycoside)	T46.0X1	T46.0X2	T46.0X3	T46.0X4	T46.0X5	T46.0X6
lanata	T46.0X1	T46.0X2	T46.0X3	T46.0X4	T46.0X5	T46.0X6
purpurea	T46.0X1	T46.0X2	T46.0X3	T46.0X4	T46.0X5	T46.0X6
Digitoxin	T46.0X1	T46.0X2	T46.0X3	T46.0X4	T46.0X5	T46.0X6
Digitoxose	T46.0X1	T46.0X2	T46.0X3	T46.0X4	T46.0X5	T46.0X6
Digoxin	T46.0X1	T46.0X2	T46.0X3	T46.0X4	T46.0X5	T46.0X6
Digoxine	T46.0X1	T46.0X2	T46.0X3	T46.0X4	T46.0X5	T46.0X6
Dihydralazine	T46.5X1	T46.5X2	T46.5X3	T46.5X4	T46.5X5	T46.5X6
Dihydrazine	T46.5X1	T46.5X2	T46.5X3	T46.5X4	T46.5X5	T46.5X6
Dihydrocodeine	T40.2X1	T40.2X2	T40.2X3	T40.2X4	T40.2X5	T40.2X6
Dihydrocodeinone	T40.2X1	T40.2X2	T40.2X3	T40.2X4	T40.2X5	T40.2X6
Dihydroergocornine	T46.7X1	T46.7X2	T46.7X3	T46.7X4	T46.7X5	T46.7X6
Dihydroergocristine (mesilate)	T46.7X1	T46.7X2	T46.7X3	T46.7X4	T46.7X5	T46.7X6
Dihydroergokryptine	T46.7X1	T46.7X2	T46.7X3	T46.7X4	T46.7X5	T46.7X6
Dihydroergotamine	T46.5X1	T46.5X2	T46.5X3	T46.5X4	T46.5X5	T46.5X6
Dihydroergotoxine mesilate	T46.7X1	T46.7X2	T46.7X3	T46.7X4	T46.7X5	T46.7X6
Dihydrohydroxycodeinone	T40.2X1	T40.2X2	T40.2X3	T40.2X4	T40.2X5	T40.2X6
Dihydrohydroxymorphinone	T40.2X1	T40.2X2	T40.2X3	T40.2X4	T40.2X5	T40.2X6
Dihydroisocodeine	T40.2X1	T40.2X2	T40.2X3	T40.2X4	T40.2X5	T40.2X6
Dihydromorphine	T40.2X1	T40.2X2	T40.2X3	T40.2X4	—	T40.2X6
Dihydromorphinone	T40.2X1	T40.2X2	T40.2X3	T40.2X4	T40.2X5	T40.2X6
Dihydrostreptomycin	T36.5X1	T36.5X2	T36.5X3	T36.5X4	T36.5X5	T36.5X6
Dihydrotachysterol	T45.2X1	T45.2X2	T45.2X3	T45.2X4	T45.2X5	T45.2X6
Dihydroxyaluminum aminoacetate	T47.1X1	T47.1X2	T47.1X3	T47.1X4	T47.1X5	T47.1X6
Dihydroxyaluminum sodium carbonate	T47.1X1	T47.1X2	T47.1X3	T47.1X4	T47.1X5	T47.1X6
Dihydroxyanthraquinone	T47.2X1	T47.2X2	T47.2X3	T47.2X4	T47.2X5	T47.2X6
Dihydroxycodeinone	T40.2X1	T40.2X2	T40.2X3	T40.2X4	T40.2X5	T40.2X6
Dihydroxypropyl theophylline	T50.2X1	T50.2X2	T50.2X3	T50.2X4	T50.2X5	T50.2X6
Diiodohydroxyquin	T37.8X1	T37.8X2	T37.8X3	T37.8X4	T37.8X5	T37.8X6
topical	T49.0X1	T49.0X2	T49.0X3	T49.0X4	T49.0X5	T49.0X6
Diiodohydroxyquinoline	T37.8X1	T37.8X2	T37.8X3	T37.8X4	T37.8X5	T37.8X6
Diiodotyrosine	T38.2X1	T38.2X2	T38.2X3	T38.2X4	T38.2X5	T38.2X6
Diisopromine	T44.3X1	T44.3X2	T44.3X3	T44.3X4	T44.3X5	T44.3X6
Diisopropylamine	T46.3X1	T46.3X2	T46.3X3	T46.3X4	T46.3X5	T46.3X6
Diisopropylfluorophosphonate	T44.0X1	T44.0X2	T44.0X3	T44.0X4	T44.0X5	T44.0X6
Dilantin	T42.0X1	T42.0X2	T42.0X3	T42.0X4	T42.0X5	T42.0X6
Dilaudid	T40.2X1	T40.2X2	T40.2X3	T40.2X4	T40.2X5	T40.2X6
Dilazep	T46.3X1	T46.3X2	T46.3X3	T46.3X4	T46.3X5	T46.3X6
Dill	T47.5X1	T47.5X2	T47.5X3	T47.5X4	T47.5X5	T47.5X6
Diloxanide	T37.3X1	T37.3X2	T37.3X3	T37.3X4	T37.3X5	T37.3X6
Diltiazem	T46.1X1	T46.1X2	T46.1X3	T46.1X4	T46.1X5	T46.1X6
Dimazole	T49.0X1	T49.0X2	T49.0X3	T49.0X4	T49.0X5	T49.0X6
Dimefline	T50.7X1	T50.7X2	T50.7X3	T50.7X4	T50.7X5	T50.7X6
Dimefox	T60.0X1	T60.0X2	T60.0X3	T60.0X4	—	—
Dimemorfan	T48.3X1	T48.3X2	T48.3X3	T48.3X4	T48.3X5	T48.3X6
Dimenhydrinate	T45.0X1	T45.0X2	T45.0X3	T45.0X4	T45.0X5	T45.0X6
Dimercaprol (British anti-lewisite)	T45.8X1	T45.8X2	T45.8X3	T45.8X4	T45.8X5	T45.8X6
Dimercaptopropanol	T45.8X1	T45.8X2	T45.8X3	T45.8X4	T45.8X5	T45.8X6
Dimestrol	T38.5X1	T38.5X2	T38.5X3	T38.5X4	T38.5X5	T38.5X6
Dimetane	T45.0X1	T45.0X2	T45.0X3	T45.0X4	T45.0X5	T45.0X6
Dimethicone	T47.1X1	T47.1X2	T47.1X3	T47.1X4	T47.1X5	T47.1X6
Dimethindene	T45.0X1	T45.0X2	T45.0X3	T45.0X4	T45.0X5	T45.0X6
Dimethisoquin	T49.1X1	T49.1X2	T49.1X3	T49.1X4	T49.1X5	T49.1X6
Dimethisterone	T38.5X1	T38.5X2	T38.5X3	T38.5X4	T38.5X5	T38.5X6
Dimethoate	T60.0X1	T60.0X2	T60.0X3	T60.0X4	—	—
Dimethocaine	T41.3X1	T41.3X2	T41.3X3	T41.3X4	T41.3X5	T41.3X6
Dimethoxanate	T48.3X1	T48.3X2	T48.3X3	T48.3X4	T48.3X5	T48.3X6

Additional Character May Be Required — Refer to the Tabular List for Character Selection ▽ Subterms under main terms may continue to next column or page

Substance	Poisoning, Accidental (unintentional)	Poisoning, Intentional Self-harm	Poisoning, Assault	Poisoning, Undetermined	Adverse Effect	Under-dosing
Dimethyl						
arsine, arsinic acid	T57.0X1	T57.0X2	T57.0X3	T57.0X4	—	—
carbinol	T51.2X1	T51.2X2	T51.2X3	T51.2X4	—	—
carbonate	T52.8X1	T52.8X2	T52.8X3	T52.8X4	—	—
diguanide	T38.3X1	T38.3X2	T38.3X3	T38.3X4	T38.3X5	T38.3X6
ketone	T52.4X1	T52.4X2	T52.4X3	T52.4X4	—	—
vapor	T52.4X1	T52.4X2	T52.4X3	T52.4X4	—	—
meperidine	T40.2X1	T40.2X2	T40.2X3	T40.2X4	T40.2X5	T40.2X6
parathion	T60.0X1	T60.0X2	T60.0X3	T60.0X4	—	—
phthlate	T49.3X1	T49.3X2	T49.3X3	T49.3X4	T49.3X5	T49.3X6
polysiloxane	T47.8X1	T47.8X2	T47.8X3	T47.8X4	T47.8X5	T47.8X6
sulfate (fumes)	T59.891	T59.892	T59.893	T59.894	—	—
liquid	T65.891	T65.892	T65.893	T65.894	—	—
sulfoxide (nonmedicinal)	T52.8X1	T52.8X2	T52.8X3	T52.8X4	—	—
medicinal	T49.4X1	T49.4X2	T49.4X3	T49.4X4	T49.4X5	T49.4X6
tryptamine	T40.991	T40.992	T40.993	T40.994	—	—
tubocurarine	T48.1X1	T48.1X2	T48.1X3	T48.1X4	T48.1X5	T48.1X6
Dimethylamine sulfate	T49.4X1	T49.4X2	T49.4X3	T49.4X4	T49.4X5	T49.4X6
Dimethylformamide	T52.8X1	T52.8X2	T52.8X3	T52.8X4	—	—
Dimethyltubocurarinium chloride	T48.1X1	T48.1X2	T48.1X3	T48.1X4	T48.1X5	T48.1X6
Dimeticone	T47.1X1	T47.1X2	T47.1X3	T47.1X4	T47.1X5	T47.1X6
Dimetilan	T60.0X1	T60.0X2	T60.0X3	T60.0X4	—	—
Dimetindene	T45.0X1	T45.0X2	T45.0X3	T45.0X4	T45.0X5	T45.0X6
Dimetotiazine	T43.3X1	T43.3X2	T43.3X3	T43.3X4	T43.3X5	T43.3X6
Dimorpholamine	T50.7X1	T50.7X2	T50.7X3	T50.7X4	T50.7X5	T50.7X6
Dimoxyline	T46.3X1	T46.3X2	T46.3X3	T46.3X4	T46.3X5	T46.3X6
Dinitrobenzene	T65.3X1	T65.3X2	T65.3X3	T65.3X4	—	—
vapor	T59.891	T59.892	T59.893	T59.894	—	—
Dinitrobenzol	T65.3X1	T65.3X2	T65.3X3	T65.3X4	—	—
vapor	T59.891	T59.892	T59.893	T59.894	—	—
Dinitrobutylphenol	T65.3X1	T65.3X2	T65.3X3	T65.3X4	—	—
Dinitro (-ortho-)cresol (pesticide)	T65.3X1	T65.3X2	T65.3X3	T65.3X4	—	—
(spray)						
Dinitrocyclohexylphenol	T65.3X1	T65.3X2	T65.3X3	T65.3X4	—	—
Dinitrophenol	T65.3X1	T65.3X2	T65.3X3	T65.3X4	—	—
Dinoprost	T48.0X1	T48.0X2	T48.0X3	T48.0X4	T48.0X5	T48.0X6
Dinoprostone	T48.0X1	T48.0X2	T48.0X3	T48.0X4	T48.0X5	T48.0X6
Dinoseb	T60.3X1	T60.3X2	T60.3X3	T60.3X4	—	—
Dioctyl sulfosuccinate (calcium)	T47.4X1	T47.4X2	T47.4X3	T47.4X4	T47.4X5	T47.4X6
(sodium)						
Diodone	T50.8X1	T50.8X2	T50.8X3	T50.8X4	T50.8X5	T50.8X6
Diodoquin	T37.8X1	T37.8X2	T37.8X3	T37.8X4	T37.8X5	T37.8X6
Dionin	T40.2X1	T40.2X2	T40.2X3	T40.2X4	T40.2X5	T40.2X6
Diosmin	T46.991	T46.992	T46.993	T46.994	T46.995	T46.996
Dioxane	T52.8X1	T52.8X2	T52.8X3	T52.8X4	—	—
Dioxathion	T60.0X1	T60.0X2	T60.0X3	T60.0X4	—	—
Dioxin	T53.7X1	T53.7X2	T53.7X3	T53.7X4	—	—
Dioxopromethazine	T43.3X1	T43.3X2	T43.3X3	T43.3X4	T43.3X5	T43.3X6
Dioxyline	T46.3X1	T46.3X2	T46.3X3	T46.3X4	T46.3X5	T46.3X6
Dipentene	T52.8X1	T52.8X2	T52.8X3	T52.8X4	—	—
Diperodon	T41.3X1	T41.3X2	T41.3X3	T41.3X4	T41.3X5	T41.3X6
Diphacinone	T60.4X1	T60.4X2	T60.4X3	T60.4X4	—	—
Diphemanil	T44.3X1	T44.3X2	T44.3X3	T44.3X4	T44.3X5	T44.3X6
metilsulfate	T44.3X1	T44.3X2	T44.3X3	T44.3X4	T44.3X5	T44.3X6
Diphenadione	T45.511	T45.512	T45.513	T45.514	T45.515	T45.516
rodenticide	T60.4X1	T60.4X2	T60.4X3	T60.4X4	—	—
Diphenhydramine	T45.0X1	T45.0X2	T45.0X3	T45.0X4	T45.0X5	T45.0X6
Diphenidol	T45.0X1	T45.0X2	T45.0X3	T45.0X4	T45.0X5	T45.0X6
Diphenoxylate	T47.6X1	T47.6X2	T47.6X3	T47.6X4	T47.6X5	T47.6X6
Diphenylamine	T65.3X1	T65.3X2	T65.3X3	T65.3X4	—	—
Diphenylbutazone	T39.2X1	T39.2X2	T39.2X3	T39.2X4	T39.2X5	T39.2X6
Diphenylchloroarsine, not in war	T57.0X1	T57.0X2	T57.0X3	T57.0X4	—	—
Diphenylhydantoin	T42.0X1	T42.0X2	T42.0X3	T42.0X4	T42.0X5	T42.0X6
Diphenylmethane dye	T52.1X1	T52.1X2	T52.1X3	T52.1X4	—	—
Diphenylpyraline	T45.0X1	T45.0X2	T45.0X3	T45.0X4	T45.0X5	T45.0X6
Diphtheria						
antitoxin	T50.Z11	T50.Z12	T50.Z13	T50.Z14	T50.Z15	T50.Z16
toxoid	T50.A91	T50.A92	T50.A93	T50.A94	T50.A95	T50.A96
with tetanus toxoid	T50.A21	T50.A22	T50.A23	T50.A24	T50.A25	T50.A26
with pertussis component	T50.A11	T50.A12	T50.A13	T50.A14	T50.A15	T50.A16
vaccine	T50.A91	T50.A92	T50.A93	T50.A94	T50.A95	T50.A96
combination						
without pertussis	T50.A21	T50.A22	T50.A23	T50.A24	T50.A25	T50.A26
including pertussis	T50.A11	T50.A12	T50.A13	T50.A14	T50.A15	T50.A16
Diphylline	T50.2X1	T50.2X2	T50.2X3	T50.2X4	T50.2X5	T50.2X6
Dipipanone	T40.4X1	T40.4X2	T40.4X3	T40.4X4	—	—
Dipivefrine	T49.5X1	T49.5X2	T49.5X3	T49.5X4	T49.5X5	T49.5X6
Diplovax	T50.B91	T50.B92	T50.B93	T50.B94	T50.B95	T50.B96
Diprophylline	T50.2X1	T50.2X2	T50.2X3	T50.2X4	T50.2X5	T50.2X6
Dipropyline	T48.291	T48.292	T48.293	T48.294	T48.295	T48.296

Substance	Poisoning, Accidental (unintentional)	Poisoning, Intentional Self-harm	Poisoning, Assault	Poisoning, Undetermined	Adverse Effect	Under-dosing
Dipyridamole	T46.3X1	T46.3X2	T46.3X3	T46.3X4	T46.3X5	T46.3X6
Dipyrone	T39.2X1	T39.2X2	T39.2X3	T39.2X4	T39.2X5	T39.2X6
Diquat (dibromide)	T60.3X1	T60.3X2	T60.3X3	T60.3X4	—	—
Disinfectant	T65.891	T65.892	T65.893	T65.894	—	—
alkaline	T54.3X1	T54.3X2	T54.3X3	T54.3X4	—	—
aromatic	T54.1X1	T54.1X2	T54.1X3	T54.1X4	—	—
intestinal	T37.8X1	T37.8X2	T37.8X3	T37.8X4	T37.8X5	T37.8X6
Disipal	T42.8X1	T42.8X2	T42.8X3	T42.8X4	T42.8X5	T42.8X6
Disodium edetate	T50.6X1	T50.6X2	T50.6X3	T50.6X4	T50.6X5	T50.6X6
Disoprofol	T41.291	T41.292	T41.293	T41.294	T41.295	T41.296
Disopyramide	T46.2X1	T46.2X2	T46.2X3	T46.2X4	T46.2X5	T46.2X6
Distigmine (bromide)	T44.0X1	T44.0X2	T44.0X3	T44.0X4	T44.0X5	T44.0X6
Disulfamide	T50.2X1	T50.2X2	T50.2X3	T50.2X4	T50.2X5	T50.2X6
Disulfanilamide	T37.0X1	T37.0X2	T37.0X3	T37.0X4	T37.0X5	T37.0X6
Disulfiram	T50.6X1	T50.6X2	T50.6X3	T50.6X4	T50.6X5	T50.6X6
Disulfoton	T60.0X1	T60.0X2	T60.0X3	T60.0X4	—	—
Dithiazanine iodide	T37.4X1	T37.4X2	T37.4X3	T37.4X4	T37.4X5	T37.4X6
Dithiocarbamate	T60.0X1	T60.0X2	T60.0X3	T60.0X4	—	—
Dithranol	T49.4X1	T49.4X2	T49.4X3	T49.4X4	T49.4X5	T49.4X6
Diucardin	T50.2X1	T50.2X2	T50.2X3	T50.2X4	T50.2X5	T50.2X6
Diupres	T50.2X1	T50.2X2	T50.2X3	T50.2X4	T50.2X5	T50.2X6
Diuretic NEC	T50.2X1	T50.2X2	T50.2X3	T50.2X4	T50.2X5	T50.2X6
benzothiadiazine	T50.2X1	T50.2X2	T50.2X3	T50.2X4	T50.2X5	T50.2X6
carbonic acid anhydrase inhibitors	T50.2X1	T50.2X2	T50.2X3	T50.2X4	T50.2X5	T50.2X6
furfuryl NEC	T50.2X1	T50.2X2	T50.2X3	T50.2X4	T50.2X5	T50.2X6
loop (high-ceiling)	T50.1X1	T50.1X2	T50.1X3	T50.1X4	T50.1X5	T50.1X6
mercurial NEC	T50.2X1	T50.2X2	T50.2X3	T50.2X4	T50.2X5	T50.2X6
osmotic	T50.2X1	T50.2X2	T50.2X3	T50.2X4	T50.2X5	T50.2X6
purine NEC	T50.2X1	T50.2X2	T50.2X3	T50.2X4	T50.2X5	T50.2X6
saluretic NEC	T50.2X1	T50.2X2	T50.2X3	T50.2X4	T50.2X5	T50.2X6
sulfonamide	T50.2X1	T50.2X2	T50.2X3	T50.2X4	T50.2X5	T50.2X6
thiazide NEC	T50.2X1	T50.2X2	T50.2X3	T50.2X4	T50.2X5	T50.2X6
xanthine	T50.2X1	T50.2X2	T50.2X3	T50.2X4	T50.2X5	T50.2X6
Diurgin	T50.2X1	T50.2X2	T50.2X3	T50.2X4	T50.2X5	T50.2X6
Diuril	T50.2X1	T50.2X2	T50.2X3	T50.2X4	T50.2X5	T50.2X6
Diuron	T60.3X1	T60.3X2	T60.3X3	T60.3X4	—	—
Divalproex	T42.6X1	T42.6X2	T42.6X3	T42.6X4	T42.6X5	T42.6X6
Divinyl ether	T41.0X1	T41.0X2	T41.0X3	T41.0X4	T41.0X5	T41.0X6
Dixanthogen	T49.0X1	T49.0X2	T49.0X3	T49.0X4	T49.0X5	T49.0X6
Dixyrazine	T43.3X1	T43.3X2	T43.3X3	T43.3X4	T43.3X5	T43.3X6
D-lysergic acid diethylamide	T40.8X1	T40.8X2	T40.8X3	T40.8X4	—	—
DMCT	T36.4X1	T36.4X2	T36.4X3	T36.4X4	T36.4X5	T36.4X6
DMSO — see Dimethyl sulfoxide						
DNBP	T60.3X1	T60.3X2	T60.3X3	T60.3X4	—	—
DNOC	T65.3X1	T65.3X2	T65.3X3	T65.3X4	—	—
Dobutamine	T44.5X1	T44.5X2	T44.5X3	T44.5X4	T44.5X5	T44.5X6
DOCA	T38.0X1	T38.0X2	T38.0X3	T38.0X4	T38.0X5	T38.0X6
Docusate sodium	T47.4X1	T47.4X2	T47.4X3	T47.4X4	T47.4X5	T47.4X6
Dodicin	T49.0X1	T49.0X2	T49.0X3	T49.0X4	T49.0X5	T49.0X6
Dofamium chloride	T49.0X1	T49.0X2	T49.0X3	T49.0X4	T49.0X5	T49.0X6
Dolophine	T40.3X1	T40.3X2	T40.3X3	T40.3X4	T40.3X5	T40.3X6
Doloxene	T39.8X1	T39.8X2	T39.8X3	T39.8X4	T39.8X5	T39.8X6
Domestic gas (after combustion) — see Gas, utility						
prior to combustion	T59.891	T59.892	T59.893	T59.894	—	—
Domiodol	T48.4X1	T48.4X2	T48.4X3	T48.4X4	T48.4X5	T48.4X6
Domiphen (bromide)	T49.0X1	T49.0X2	T49.0X3	T49.0X4	T49.0X5	T49.0X6
Domperidone	T45.0X1	T45.0X2	T45.0X3	T45.0X4	T45.0X5	T45.0X6
Dopa	T42.8X1	T42.8X2	T42.8X3	T42.8X4	T42.8X5	T42.8X6
Dopamine	T44.991	T44.992	T44.993	T44.994	T44.995	T44.996
Doriden	T42.6X1	T42.6X2	T42.6X3	T42.6X4	T42.6X5	T42.6X6
Dormiral	T42.3X1	T42.3X2	T42.3X3	T42.3X4	T42.3X5	T42.3X6
Dormison	T42.6X1	T42.6X2	T42.6X3	T42.6X4	T42.6X5	T42.6X6
Dornase	T48.4X1	T48.4X2	T48.4X3	T48.4X4	T48.4X5	T48.4X6
Dorsacaine	T41.3X1	T41.3X2	T41.3X3	T41.3X4	T41.3X5	T41.3X6
Dosulepin	T43.011	T43.012	T43.013	T43.014	T43.015	T43.016
Dothiepin	T43.011	T43.012	T43.013	T43.014	T43.015	T43.016
Doxantrazole	T48.6X1	T48.6X2	T48.6X3	T48.6X4	T48.6X5	T48.6X6
Doxapram	T50.7X1	T50.7X2	T50.7X3	T50.7X4	T50.7X5	T50.7X6
Doxazosin	T44.6X1	T44.6X2	T44.6X3	T44.6X4	T44.6X5	T44.6X6
Doxepin	T43.011	T43.012	T43.013	T43.014	T43.015	T43.016
Doxifluridine	T45.1X1	T45.1X2	T45.1X3	T45.1X4	T45.1X5	T45.1X6
Doxorubicin	T45.1X1	T45.1X2	T45.1X3	T45.1X4	T45.1X5	T45.1X6
Doxycycline	T36.4X1	T36.4X2	T36.4X3	T36.4X4	T36.4X5	T36.4X6
Doxylamine	T45.0X1	T45.0X2	T45.0X3	T45.0X4	T45.0X5	T45.0X6
Dramamine	T45.0X1	T45.0X2	T45.0X3	T45.0X4	T45.0X5	T45.0X6
Drano (drain cleaner)	T54.3X1	T54.3X2	T54.3X3	T54.3X4	—	—
Dressing, live pulp	T49.7X1	T49.7X2	T49.7X3	T49.7X4	T49.7X5	T49.7X6
Drocode	T40.2X1	T40.2X2	T40.2X3	T40.2X4	T40.2X5	T40.2X6
Dromoran	T40.2X1	T40.2X2	T40.2X3	T40.2X4	T40.2X5	T40.2X6
Dromostanolone	T38.7X1	T38.7X2	T38.7X3	T38.7X4	T38.7X5	T38.7X6

Substance	Poisoning, Accidental (unintentional)	Poisoning, Intentional Self-harm	Poisoning, Assault	Poisoning, Undetermined	Adverse Effect	Under-dosing
Dronabinol	T40.7X1	T40.7X2	T40.7X3	T40.7X4	T40.7X5	T40.7X6
Droperidol	T43.591	T43.592	T43.593	T43.594	T43.595	T43.596
Dropropizine	T48.3X1	T48.3X2	T48.3X3	T48.3X4	T48.3X5	T48.3X6
Drostanolone	T38.7X1	T38.7X2	T38.7X3	T38.7X4	T38.7X5	T38.7X6
Drotaverine	T44.3X1	T44.3X2	T44.3X3	T44.3X4	T44.3X5	T44.3X6
Drotrecogin alfa	T45.511	T45.512	T45.513	T45.514	T45.515	T45.516
Drug NEC	T50.901	T50.902	T50.903	T50.904	T50.905	T50.906
specified NEC	T50.991	T50.992	T50.993	T50.994	T50.995	T50.996
DTIC	T45.1X1	T45.1X2	T45.1X3	T45.1X4	T45.1X5	T45.1X6
Duboisine	T44.3X1	T44.3X2	T44.3X3	T44.3X4	T44.3X5	T44.3X6
Dulcolax	T47.2X1	T47.2X2	T47.2X3	T47.2X4	T47.2X5	T47.2X6
Duponol (C) (EP)	T49.2X1	T49.2X2	T49.2X3	T49.2X4	T49.2X5	T49.2X6
Durabolin	T38.7X1	T38.7X2	T38.7X3	T38.7X4	T38.7X5	T38.7X6
Dyclone	T41.3X1	T41.3X2	T41.3X3	T41.3X4	T41.3X5	T41.3X6
Dyclonine	T41.3X1	T41.3X2	T41.3X3	T41.3X4	T41.3X5	T41.3X6
Dydrogesterone	T38.5X1	T38.5X2	T38.5X3	T38.5X4	T38.5X5	T38.5X6
Dye NEC	T65.6X1	T65.6X2	T65.6X3	T65.6X4	—	—
antiseptic	T49.0X1	T49.0X2	T49.0X3	T49.0X4	T49.0X5	T49.0X6
diagnostic agents	T50.8X1	T50.8X2	T50.8X3	T50.8X4	T50.8X5	T50.8X6
pharmaceutical NEC	T50.901	T50.902	T50.903	T50.904	T50.905	T50.906
Dyflos	T44.0X1	T44.0X2	T44.0X3	T44.0X4	T44.0X5	T44.0X6
Dymelor	T38.3X1	T38.3X2	T38.3X3	T38.3X4	T38.3X5	T38.3X6
Dynamite	T65.3X1	T65.3X2	T65.3X3	T65.3X4	—	—
fumes	T59.891	T59.892	T59.893	T59.894	—	—
Dyphylline	T44.3X1	T44.3X2	T44.3X3	T44.3X4	T44.3X5	T44.3X6
b-eucaine	T49.1X1	T49.1X2	T49.1X3	T49.1X4	T49.1X5	T49.1X6
Ear drug NEC	T49.6X1	T49.6X2	T49.6X3	T49.6X4	T49.6X5	T49.6X6
Ear preparations	T49.6X1	T49.6X2	T49.6X3	T49.6X4	T49.6X5	T49.6X6
Echothiophate, echothiophate, ecothiophate	T49.5X1	T49.5X2	T49.5X3	T49.5X4	T49.5X5	T49.5X6
Econazole	T49.0X1	T49.0X2	T49.0X3	T49.0X4	T49.0X5	T49.0X6
Ecothiopate iodide	T49.5X1	T49.5X2	T49.5X3	T49.5X4	T49.5X5	T49.5X6
Ecstasy	T43.621	T43.622	T43.623	T43.624	T43.625	T43.626
Ectylurea	T42.6X1	T42.6X2	T42.6X3	T42.6X4	T42.6X5	T42.6X6
Edathamil disodium	T45.8X1	T45.8X2	T45.8X3	T45.8X4	T45.8X5	T45.8X6
Edecrin	T50.1X1	T50.1X2	T50.1X3	T50.1X4	T50.1X5	T50.1X6
Edetate, disodium (calcium)	T45.8X1	T45.8X2	T45.8X3	T45.8X4	T45.8X5	T45.8X6
Edoxudine	T49.5X1	T49.5X2	T49.5X3	T49.5X4	T49.5X5	T49.5X6
Edrophonium	T44.0X1	T44.0X2	T44.0X3	T44.0X4	T44.0X5	T44.0X6
chloride	T44.0X1	T44.0X2	T44.0X3	T44.0X4	T44.0X5	T44.0X6
EDTA	T50.6X1	T50.6X2	T50.6X3	T50.6X4	T50.6X5	T50.6X6
Eflornithine	T37.2X1	T37.2X2	T37.2X3	T37.2X4	T37.2X5	T37.2X6
Efloxate	T46.3X1	T46.3X2	T46.3X3	T46.3X4	T46.3X5	T46.3X6
Elase	T49.8X1	T49.8X2	T49.8X3	T49.8X4	T49.8X5	T49.8X6
Elastase	T47.5X1	T47.5X2	T47.5X3	T47.5X4	T47.5X5	T47.5X6
Elaterium	T47.2X1	T47.2X2	T47.2X3	T47.2X4	T47.2X5	T47.2X6
Elcatonin	T50.991	T50.992	T50.993	T50.994	T50.995	T50.996
Elder	T62.2X1	T62.2X2	T62.2X3	T62.2X4	—	—
berry, (unripe)	T62.1X1	T62.1X2	T62.1X3	T62.1X4	—	—
Electrolyte balance drug	T50.3X1	T50.3X2	T50.3X3	T50.3X4	T50.3X5	T50.3X6
Electrolytes NEC	T50.3X1	T50.3X2	T50.3X3	T50.3X4	T50.3X5	T50.3X6
Electrolytic agent NEC	T50.3X1	T50.3X2	T50.3X3	T50.3X4	T50.3X5	T50.3X6
Elemental diet	T50.901	T50.902	T50.903	T50.904	T50.905	T50.906
Elliptinium acetate	T45.1X1	T45.1X2	T45.1X3	T45.1X4	T45.1X5	T45.1X6
Embramine	T45.0X1	T45.0X2	T45.0X3	T45.0X4	T45.0X5	T45.0X6
Emepronium (salts)	T44.3X1	T44.3X2	T44.3X3	T44.3X4	T44.3X5	T44.3X6
bromide	T44.3X1	T44.3X2	T44.3X3	T44.3X4	T44.3X5	T44.3X6
Emetic NEC	T47.7X1	T47.7X2	T47.7X3	T47.7X4	T47.7X5	T47.7X6
Emetine	T37.3X1	T37.3X2	T37.3X3	T37.3X4	T37.3X5	T37.3X6
Emollient NEC	T49.3X1	T49.3X2	T49.3X3	T49.3X4	T49.3X5	T49.3X6
Emorfazone	T39.8X1	T39.8X2	T39.8X3	T39.8X4	T39.8X5	T39.8X6
Emylcamate	T43.591	T43.592	T43.593	T43.594	T43.595	T43.596
Enalapril	T46.4X1	T46.4X2	T46.4X3	T46.4X4	T46.4X5	T46.4X6
Enalaprilat	T46.4X1	T46.4X2	T46.4X3	T46.4X4	T46.4X5	T46.4X6
Encainide	T46.2X1	T46.2X2	T46.2X3	T46.2X4	T46.2X5	T46.2X6
Endocaine	T41.3X1	T41.3X2	T41.3X3	T41.3X4	T41.3X5	T41.3X6
Endosulfan	T60.2X1	T60.2X2	T60.2X3	T60.2X4	—	—
Endothall	T60.3X1	T60.3X2	T60.3X3	T60.3X4	—	—
Endralazine	T46.5X1	T46.5X2	T46.5X3	T46.5X4	T46.5X5	T46.5X6
Endrin	T60.1X1	T60.1X2	T60.1X3	T60.1X4	—	—
Enflurane	T41.0X1	T41.0X2	T41.0X3	T41.0X4	T41.0X5	T41.0X6
Enhexymal	T42.3X1	T42.3X2	T42.3X3	T42.3X4	T42.3X5	T42.3X6
Enocitabine	T45.1X1	T45.1X2	T45.1X3	T45.1X4	T45.1X5	T45.1X6
Enovid	T38.4X1	T38.4X2	T38.4X3	T38.4X4	T38.4X5	T38.4X6
Enoxacin	T36.8X1	T36.8X2	T36.8X3	T36.8X4	T36.8X5	T36.8X6
Enoxaparin (sodium)	T45.511	T45.512	T45.513	T45.514	T45.515	T45.516
Enpiprazole	T43.591	T43.592	T43.593	T43.594	T43.595	T43.596
Enprofylline	T48.6X1	T48.6X2	T48.6X3	T48.6X4	T48.6X5	T48.6X6
Enprostil	T47.1X1	T47.1X2	T47.1X3	T47.1X4	T47.1X5	T47.1X6
Enterogastrone	T38.891	T38.892	T38.893	T38.894	T38.895	T38.896
ENT preparations (anti-infectives)	T49.6X1	T49.6X2	T49.6X3	T49.6X4	T49.6X5	T49.6X6
Enviomycin	T36.8X1	T36.8X2	T36.8X3	T36.8X4	T36.8X5	T36.8X6
Enzodase	T45.3X1	T45.3X2	T45.3X3	T45.3X4	T45.3X5	T45.3X6
Enzyme NEC	T45.3X1	T45.3X2	T45.3X3	T45.3X4	T45.3X5	T45.3X6
depolymerizing	T49.8X1	T49.8X2	T49.8X3	T49.8X4	T49.8X5	T49.8X6
fibrolytic	T45.3X1	T45.3X2	T45.3X3	T45.3X4	T45.3X5	T45.3X6
gastric	T47.5X1	T47.5X2	T47.5X3	T47.5X4	T47.5X5	T47.5X6
intestinal	T47.5X1	T47.5X2	T47.5X3	T47.5X4	T47.5X5	T47.5X6
local action	T49.4X1	T49.4X2	T49.4X3	T49.4X4	T49.4X5	T49.4X6
proteolytic	T49.4X1	T49.4X2	T49.4X3	T49.4X4	T49.4X5	T49.4X6
thrombolytic	T45.3X1	T45.3X2	T45.3X3	T45.3X4	T45.3X5	T45.3X6
EPAB	T41.3X1	T41.3X2	T41.3X3	T41.3X4	T41.3X5	T41.3X6
Epanutin	T42.0X1	T42.0X2	T42.0X3	T42.0X4	T42.0X5	T42.0X6
Ephedra	T44.991	T44.992	T44.993	T44.994	T44.995	T44.996
Ephedrine	T44.991	T44.992	T44.993	T44.994	T44.995	T44.996
Epichlorhydrin, epichlorohydrin	T52.8X1	T52.8X2	T52.8X3	T52.8X4	—	—
Epicillin	T36.0X1	T36.0X2	T36.0X3	T36.0X4	T36.0X5	T36.0X6
Epiestriol	T38.5X1	T38.5X2	T38.5X3	T38.5X4	T38.5X5	T38.5X6
Epilim — *see* Sodium valproate						
Epimestrol	T38.5X1	T38.5X2	T38.5X3	T38.5X4	T38.5X5	T38.5X6
Epinephrine	T44.5X1	T44.5X2	T44.5X3	T44.5X4	T44.5X5	T44.5X6
Epirubicin	T45.1X1	T45.1X2	T45.1X3	T45.1X4	T45.1X5	T45.1X6
Epitiostanol	T38.7X1	T38.7X2	T38.7X3	T38.7X4	T38.7X5	T38.7X6
Epitizide	T50.2X1	T50.2X2	T50.2X3	T50.2X4	T50.2X5	T50.2X6
EPN	T60.0X1	T60.0X2	T60.0X3	T60.0X4	—	—
EPO	T45.8X1	T45.8X2	T45.8X3	T45.8X4	T45.8X5	T45.8X6
Epoetin alpha	T45.8X1	T45.8X2	T45.8X3	T45.8X4	T45.8X5	T45.8X6
Epomediol	T50.991	T50.992	T50.993	T50.994	T50.995	T50.996
Epoprostenol	T45.521	T45.522	T45.523	T45.524	T45.525	T45.526
Epoxy resin	T65.891	T65.892	T65.893	T65.894	—	—
Eprazinone	T48.4X1	T48.4X2	T48.4X3	T48.4X4	T48.4X5	T48.4X6
Epsilon aminocaproic acid	T45.621	T45.622	T45.623	T45.624	T45.625	T45.626
Epsom salt	T47.3X1	T47.3X2	T47.3X3	T47.3X4	T47.3X5	T47.3X6
Eptazocine	T40.4X1	T40.4X2	T40.4X3	T40.4X4	T40.4X5	T40.4X6
Equanil	T43.591	T43.592	T43.593	T43.594	T43.595	T43.596
Equisetum	T62.2X1	T62.2X2	T62.2X3	T62.2X4	—	—
diuretic	T50.2X1	T50.2X2	T50.2X3	T50.2X4	T50.2X5	T50.2X6
Ergobasine	T48.0X1	T48.0X2	T48.0X3	T48.0X4	T48.0X5	T48.0X6
Ergocalciferol	T45.2X1	T45.2X2	T45.2X3	T45.2X4	T45.2X5	T45.2X6
Ergoloid mesylates	T46.7X1	T46.7X2	T46.7X3	T46.7X4	T46.7X5	T46.7X6
Ergometrine	T48.0X1	T48.0X2	T48.0X3	T48.0X4	T48.0X5	T48.0X6
Ergonovine	T48.0X1	T48.0X2	T48.0X3	T48.0X4	T48.0X5	T48.0X6
Ergotamine	T46.5X1	T46.5X2	T46.5X3	T46.5X4	T46.5X5	T46.5X6
Ergotocine	T48.0X1	T48.0X2	T48.0X3	T48.0X4	T48.0X5	T48.0X6
Ergotrate	T48.0X1	T48.0X2	T48.0X3	T48.0X4	T48.0X5	T48.0X6
Ergot NEC	T64.81	T64.82	T64.83	T64.84	—	—
derivative	T48.0X1	T48.0X2	T48.0X3	T48.0X4	T48.0X5	T48.0X6
medicinal (alkaloids)	T48.0X1	T48.0X2	T48.0X3	T48.0X4	T48.0X5	T48.0X6
prepared	T48.0X1	T48.0X2	T48.0X3	T48.0X4	T48.0X5	T48.0X6
Erititryl tetranitrate	T46.3X1	T46.3X2	T46.3X3	T46.3X4	T46.3X5	T46.3X6
Erythrityl tetranitrate	T46.3X1	T46.3X2	T46.3X3	T46.3X4	T46.3X5	T46.3X6
Erythrol tetranitrate	T46.3X1	T46.3X2	T46.3X3	T46.3X4	T46.3X5	T46.3X6
Erythromycin (salts)	T36.3X1	T36.3X2	T36.3X3	T36.3X4	T36.3X5	T36.3X6
ophthalmic preparation	T49.5X1	T49.5X2	T49.5X3	T49.5X4	T49.5X5	T49.5X6
topical NEC	T49.0X1	T49.0X2	T49.0X3	T49.0X4	T49.0X5	T49.0X6
Erythropoietin	T45.8X1	T45.8X2	T45.8X3	T45.8X4	T45.8X5	T45.8X6
human	T45.8X1	T45.8X2	T45.8X3	T45.8X4	T45.8X5	T45.8X6
Escin	T46.991	T46.992	T46.993	T46.994	T46.995	T46.996
Esculin	T45.2X1	T45.2X2	T45.2X3	T45.2X4	T45.2X5	T45.2X6
Esculoside	T45.2X1	T45.2X2	T45.2X3	T45.2X4	T45.2X5	T45.2X6
ESDT (ether-soluble tar distillate)	T49.1X1	T49.1X2	T49.1X3	T49.1X4	T49.1X5	T49.1X6
Eserine	T49.5X1	T49.5X2	T49.5X3	T49.5X4	T49.5X5	T49.5X6
Esflurbiprofen	T39.311	T39.312	T39.313	T39.314	T39.315	T39.316
Eskabarb	T42.3X1	T42.3X2	T42.3X3	T42.3X4	T42.3X5	T42.3X6
Eskalith	T43.8X1	T43.8X2	T43.8X3	T43.8X4	T43.8X5	T43.8X6
Esmolol	T44.7X1	T44.7X2	T44.7X3	T44.7X4	T44.7X5	T44.7X6
Estanozolol	T38.7X1	T38.7X2	T38.7X3	T38.7X4	T38.7X5	T38.7X6
Estazolam	T42.4X1	T42.4X2	T42.4X3	T42.4X4	T42.4X5	T42.4X6
Estradiol	T38.5X1	T38.5X2	T38.5X3	T38.5X4	T38.5X5	T38.5X6
with testosterone	T38.7X1	T38.7X2	T38.7X3	T38.7X4	T38.7X5	T38.7X6
benzoate	T38.5X1	T38.5X2	T38.5X3	T38.5X4	T38.5X5	T38.5X6
Estramustine	T45.1X1	T45.1X2	T45.1X3	T45.1X4	T45.1X5	T45.1X6
Estriol	T38.5X1	T38.5X2	T38.5X3	T38.5X4	T38.5X5	T38.5X6
Estrogen	T38.5X1	T38.5X2	T38.5X3	T38.5X4	T38.5X5	T38.5X6
with progesterone	T38.5X1	T38.5X2	T38.5X3	T38.5X4	T38.5X5	T38.5X6
conjugated	T38.5X1	T38.5X2	T38.5X3	T38.5X4	T38.5X5	T38.5X6
Estrone	T38.5X1	T38.5X2	T38.5X3	T38.5X4	T38.5X5	T38.5X6
Estropipate	T38.5X1	T38.5X2	T38.5X3	T38.5X4	T38.5X5	T38.5X6
Etacrynate sodium	T50.1X1	T50.1X2	T50.1X3	T50.1X4	T50.1X5	T50.1X6
Etacrynic acid	T50.1X1	T50.1X2	T50.1X3	T50.1X4	T50.1X5	T50.1X6
Etafedrine	T48.6X1	T48.6X2	T48.6X3	T48.6X4	T48.6X5	T48.6X6
Etafenone	T46.3X1	T46.3X2	T46.3X3	T46.3X4	T46.3X5	T46.3X6
Etambutol	T37.1X1	T37.1X2	T37.1X3	T37.1X4	T37.1X5	T37.1X6

Additional Character May Be Required — Refer to the Tabular List for Character Selection

▽ Subterms under main terms may continue to next column or page

Substance	Poisoning, Accidental (unintentional)	Poisoning, Intentional Self-harm	Poisoning, Assault	Poisoning, Undetermined	Adverse Effect	Under-dosing
Etamiphyllin	T48.6X1	T48.6X2	T48.6X3	T48.6X4	T48.6X5	T48.6X6
Etamivan	T50.7X1	T50.7X2	T50.7X3	T50.7X4	T50.7X5	T50.7X6
Etamsylate	T45.7X1	T45.7X2	T45.7X3	T45.7X4	T45.7X5	T45.7X6
Etebenecid	T50.4X1	T50.4X2	T50.4X3	T50.4X4	T50.4X5	T50.4X6
Ethacridine	T49.0X1	T49.0X2	T49.0X3	T49.0X4	T49.0X5	T49.0X6
Ethacrynic acid	T50.1X1	T50.1X2	T50.1X3	T50.1X4	T50.1X5	T50.1X6
Ethadione	T42.2X1	T42.2X2	T42.2X3	T42.2X4	T42.2X5	T42.2X6
Ethambutol	T37.1X1	T37.1X2	T37.1X3	T37.1X4	T37.1X5	T37.1X6
Ethamide	T50.2X1	T50.2X2	T50.2X3	T50.2X4	T50.2X5	T50.2X6
Ethamivan	T50.7X1	T50.7X2	T50.7X3	T50.7X4	T50.7X5	T50.7X6
Ethamsylate	T45.7X1	T45.7X2	T45.7X3	T45.7X4	T45.7X5	T45.7X6
Ethanol	T51.0X1	T51.0X2	T51.0X3	T51.0X4	—	—
beverage	T51.0X1	T51.0X2	T51.0X3	T51.0X4		
Ethanolamine oleate	T46.8X1	T46.8X2	T46.8X3	T46.8X4	T46.8X5	T46.8X6
Ethaverine	T44.3X1	T44.3X2	T44.3X3	T44.3X4	T44.3X5	T44.3X6
Ethchlorvynol	T42.6X1	T42.6X2	T42.6X3	T42.6X4	T42.6X5	T42.6X6
Ethebenecid	T50.4X1	T50.4X2	T50.4X3	T50.4X4	T50.4X5	T50.4X6
Ether (vapor)	T41.0X1	T41.0X2	T41.0X3	T41.0X4	T41.0X5	T41.0X6
anesthetic	T41.0X1	T41.0X2	T41.0X3	T41.0X4	T41.0X5	T41.0X6
divinyl	T41.0X1	T41.0X2	T41.0X3	T41.0X4	T41.0X5	T41.0X6
ethyl (medicinal)	T41.0X1	T41.0X2	T41.0X3	T41.0X4	T41.0X5	T41.0X6
nonmedicinal	T52.8X1	T52.8X2	T52.8X3	T52.8X4		
petroleum — see Ligroin						
solvent	T52.8X1	T52.8X2	T52.8X3	T52.8X4	—	—
Ethiazide	T50.2X1	T50.2X2	T50.2X3	T50.2X4	T50.2X5	T50.2X6
Ethidium chloride (vapor)	T59.891	T59.892	T59.893	T59.894		
Ethinamate	T42.6X1	T42.6X2	T42.6X3	T42.6X4	T42.6X5	T42.6X6
Ethinylestradiol, ethinyloestradiol	T38.5X1	T38.5X2	T38.5X3	T38.5X4	T38.5X5	T38.5X6
with						
levonorgestrel	T38.4X1	T38.4X2	T38.4X3	T38.4X4	T38.4X5	T38.4X6
norethisterone	T38.4X1	T38.4X2	T38.4X3	T38.4X4	T38.4X5	T38.4X6
Ethiodized oil (131 I)	T50.8X1	T50.8X2	T50.8X3	T50.8X4	T50.8X5	T50.8X6
Ethion	T60.0X1	T60.0X2	T60.0X3	T60.0X4		
Ethionamide	T37.1X1	T37.1X2	T37.1X3	T37.1X4	T37.1X5	T37.1X6
Ethioniamide	T37.1X1	T37.1X2	T37.1X3	T37.1X4	T37.1X5	T37.1X6
Ethisterone	T38.5X1	T38.5X2	T38.5X3	T38.5X4	T38.5X5	T38.5X6
Ethobral	T42.3X1	T42.3X2	T42.3X3	T42.3X4	T42.3X5	T42.3X6
Ethocaine (infiltration) (topical)	T41.3X1	T41.3X2	T41.3X3	T41.3X4	T41.3X5	T41.3X6
nerve block (peripheral) (plexus)	T41.3X1	T41.3X2	T41.3X3	T41.3X4	T41.3X5	T41.3X6
spinal	T41.3X1	T41.3X2	T41.3X3	T41.3X4	T41.3X5	T41.3X6
Ethoheptazine	T40.4X1	T40.4X2	T40.4X3	T40.4X4	T40.4X5	T40.4X6
Ethopropazine	T44.3X1	T44.3X2	T44.3X3	T44.3X4	T44.3X5	T44.3X6
Ethosuximide	T42.2X1	T42.2X2	T42.2X3	T42.2X4	T42.2X5	T42.2X6
Ethotoin	T42.0X1	T42.0X2	T42.0X3	T42.0X4	T42.0X5	T42.0X6
Ethoxazene	T37.91	T37.92	T37.93	T37.94	T37.95	T37.96
Ethoxazorutoside	T46.991	T46.992	T46.993	T46.994	T46.995	T46.996
Ethoxzolamide	T50.2X1	T50.2X2	T50.2X3	T50.2X4	T50.2X5	T50.2X6
Ethyl						
acetate	T52.8X1	T52.8X2	T52.8X3	T52.8X4	—	—
alcohol	T51.0X1	T51.0X2	T51.0X3	T51.0X4	—	—
beverage	T51.0X1	T51.0X2	T51.0X3	T51.0X4	—	—
aldehyde (vapor)	T59.891	T59.892	T59.893	T59.894	—	—
liquid	T52.8X1	T52.8X2	T52.8X3	T52.8X4	—	—
aminobenzoate	T41.3X1	T41.3X2	T41.3X3	T41.3X4	T41.3X5	T41.3X6
aminophenothiazine	T43.3X1	T43.3X2	T43.3X3	T43.3X4	T43.3X5	T43.3X6
benzoate	T52.8X1	T52.8X2	T52.8X3	T52.8X4	—	—
biscoumacetate	T45.511	T45.512	T45.513	T45.514	T45.515	T45.516
bromide (anesthetic)	T41.0X1	T41.0X2	T41.0X3	T41.0X4	T41.0X5	T41.0X6
carbamate	T45.1X1	T45.1X2	T45.1X3	T45.1X4	T45.1X5	T45.1X6
carbinol	T51.3X1	T51.3X2	T51.3X3	T51.3X4	—	—
carbonate	T52.8X1	T52.8X2	T52.8X3	T52.8X4	—	—
chaulmoograte	T37.1X1	T37.1X2	T37.1X3	T37.1X4	T37.1X5	T37.1X6
chloride (anesthetic)	T41.0X1	T41.0X2	T41.0X3	T41.0X4	T41.0X5	T41.0X6
anesthetic (local)	T41.3X1	T41.3X2	T41.3X3	T41.3X4	T41.3X5	T41.3X6
inhaled	T41.0X1	T41.0X2	T41.0X3	T41.0X4	T41.0X5	T41.0X6
local	T49.4X1	T49.4X2	T49.4X3	T49.4X4	T49.4X5	T49.4X6
solvent	T53.6X1	T53.6X2	T53.6X3	T53.6X4	—	—
dibunate	T48.3X1	T48.3X2	T48.3X3	T48.3X4	T48.3X5	T48.3X6
dichloroarsine (vapor)	T57.0X1	T57.0X2	T57.0X3	T57.0X4	—	—
estranol	T38.7X1	T38.7X2	T38.7X3	T38.7X4	T38.7X5	T38.7X6
ether — see also ether	T52.8X1	T52.8X2	T52.8X3	T52.8X4	—	—
formate NEC (solvent)	T52.0X1	T52.0X2	T52.0X3	T52.0X4	—	—
fumarate	T49.4X1	T49.4X2	T49.4X3	T49.4X4	T49.4X5	T49.4X6
hydroxyisobutyrate NEC (solvent)	T52.8X1	T52.8X2	T52.8X3	T52.8X4	—	—
iodoacetate	T59.3X1	T59.3X2	T59.3X3	T59.3X4	—	—
lactate NEC (solvent)	T52.8X1	T52.8X2	T52.8X3	T52.8X4	—	—
loflazepate	T42.4X1	T42.4X2	T42.4X3	T42.4X4	T42.4X5	T42.4X6
mercuric chloride	T56.1X1	T56.1X2	T56.1X3	T56.1X4	—	—
methylcarbinol	T51.8X1	T51.8X2	T51.8X3	T51.8X4	—	—

Substance	Poisoning, Accidental (unintentional)	Poisoning, Intentional Self-harm	Poisoning, Assault	Poisoning, Undetermined	Adverse Effect	Under-dosing
Ethyl — continued						
morphine	T40.2X1	T40.2X2	T40.2X3	T40.2X4	T40.2X5	T40.2X6
noradrenaline	T48.6X1	T48.6X2	T48.6X3	T48.6X4	T48.6X5	T48.6X6
oxybutyrate NEC (solvent)	T52.8X1	T52.8X2	T52.8X3	T52.8X4		
Ethylene (gas)	T59.891	T59.892	T59.893	T59.894		
anesthetic (general)	T41.0X1	T41.0X2	T41.0X3	T41.0X4	T41.0X5	T41.0X6
chlorohydrin	T52.8X1	T52.8X2	T52.8X3	T52.8X4	—	—
vapor	T53.6X1	T53.6X2	T53.6X3	T53.6X4	—	—
dichloride	T52.8X1	T52.8X2	T52.8X3	T52.8X4	—	—
vapor	T53.6X1	T53.6X2	T53.6X3	T53.6X4	—	—
dinitrate	T52.3X1	T52.3X2	T52.3X3	T52.3X4	—	—
glycol(s)	T52.8X1	T52.8X2	T52.8X3	T52.8X4	—	—
dinitrate	T52.3X1	T52.3X2	T52.3X3	T52.3X4	—	—
monobutyl ether	T52.3X1	T52.3X2	T52.3X3	T52.3X4	—	—
imine	T54.1X1	T54.1X2	T54.1X3	T54.1X4	—	—
oxide (fumigant) (nonmedicinal)	T59.891	T59.892	T59.893	T59.894	—	—
medicinal	T49.0X1	T49.0X2	T49.0X3	T49.0X4	T49.0X5	T49.0X6
Ethylenediaminetetra-acetic acid	T50.6X1	T50.6X2	T50.6X3	T50.6X4	T50.6X5	T50.6X6
Ethylenediamine theophylline	T48.6X1	T48.6X2	T48.6X3	T48.6X4	T48.6X5	T48.6X6
Ethylenedinitrilotetra-acetate	T50.6X1	T50.6X2	T50.6X3	T50.6X4	T50.6X5	T50.6X6
Ethylestrenol	T38.7X1	T38.7X2	T38.7X3	T38.7X4	T38.7X5	T38.7X6
Ethylhydroxycellulose	T47.4X1	T47.4X2	T47.4X3	T47.4X4	T47.4X5	T47.4X6
Ethylidene						
chloride NEC	T53.6X1	T53.6X2	T53.6X3	T53.6X4	—	—
diacetate	T60.3X1	T60.3X2	T60.3X3	T60.3X4	—	—
dicoumarin	T45.511	T45.512	T45.513	T45.514	T45.515	T45.516
dicoumarol	T45.511	T45.512	T45.513	T45.514	T45.515	T45.516
diethyl ether	T52.0X1	T52.0X2	T52.0X3	T52.0X4	—	—
Ethylmorphine	T40.2X1	T40.2X2	T40.2X3	T40.2X4	T40.2X5	T40.2X6
Ethylnorepinephrine	T48.6X1	T48.6X2	T48.6X3	T48.6X4	T48.6X5	T48.6X6
Ethylparachlorophen-oxyisobutyrate	T46.6X1	T46.6X2	T46.6X3	T46.6X4	T46.6X5	T46.6X6
Ethynodiol	T38.4X1	T38.4X2	T38.4X3	T38.4X4	T38.4X5	T38.4X6
with mestranol diacetate	T38.4X1	T38.4X2	T38.4X3	T38.4X4	T38.4X5	T38.4X6
Etidocaine	T41.3X1	T41.3X2	T41.3X3	T41.3X4	T41.3X5	T41.3X6
infiltration (subcutaneous)	T41.3X1	T41.3X2	T41.3X3	T41.3X4	T41.3X5	T41.3X6
nerve (peripheral) (plexus)	T41.3X1	T41.3X2	T41.3X3	T41.3X4	T41.3X5	T41.3X6
Etidronate	T50.991	T50.992	T50.993	T50.994	T50.995	T50.996
Etidronic acid (disodium salt)	T50.991	T50.992	T50.993	T50.994	T50.995	T50.996
Etifoxine	T42.6X1	T42.6X2	T42.6X3	T42.6X4	T42.6X5	T42.6X6
Etilefrine	T44.4X1	T44.4X2	T44.4X3	T44.4X4	T44.4X5	T44.4X6
Etilfen	T42.3X1	T42.3X2	T42.3X3	T42.3X4	T42.3X5	T42.3X6
Etinodiol	T38.4X1	T38.4X2	T38.4X3	T38.4X4	T38.4X5	T38.4X6
Etiroxate	T46.6X1	T46.6X2	T46.6X3	T46.6X4	T46.6X5	T46.6X6
Etizolam	T42.4X1	T42.4X2	T42.4X3	T42.4X4	T42.4X5	T42.4X6
Etodolac	T39.391	T39.392	T39.393	T39.394	T39.395	T39.396
Etofamide	T37.3X1	T37.3X2	T37.3X3	T37.3X4	T37.3X5	T37.3X6
Etofibrate	T46.6X1	T46.6X2	T46.6X3	T46.6X4	T46.6X5	T46.6X6
Etofylline	T46.7X1	T46.7X2	T46.7X3	T46.7X4	T46.7X5	T46.7X6
clofibrate	T46.6X1	T46.6X2	T46.6X3	T46.6X4	T46.6X5	T46.6X6
Etoglucid	T45.1X1	T45.1X2	T45.1X3	T45.1X4	T45.1X5	T45.1X6
Etomidate	T41.1X1	T41.1X2	T41.1X3	T41.1X4	T41.1X5	T41.1X6
Etomide	T39.8X1	T39.8X2	T39.8X3	T39.8X4	T39.8X5	T39.8X6
Etomidoline	T44.3X1	T44.3X2	T44.3X3	T44.3X4	T44.3X5	T44.3X6
Etoposide	T45.1X1	T45.1X2	T45.1X3	T45.1X4	T45.1X5	T45.1X6
Etorphine	T40.2X1	T40.2X2	T40.2X3	T40.2X4	T40.2X5	T40.2X6
Etoval	T42.3X1	T42.3X2	T42.3X3	T42.3X4	T42.3X5	T42.3X6
Etozolin	T50.1X1	T50.1X2	T50.1X3	T50.1X4	T50.1X5	T50.1X6
Etretinate	T50.991	T50.992	T50.993	T50.994	T50.995	T50.996
Etryptamine	T43.691	T43.692	T43.693	T43.694	T43.695	T43.696
Etybenzatropine	T44.3X1	T44.3X2	T44.3X3	T44.3X4	T44.3X5	T44.3X6
Etynodiol	T38.4X1	T38.4X2	T38.4X3	T38.4X4	T38.4X5	T38.4X6
Eucaine	T41.3X1	T41.3X2	T41.3X3	T41.3X4	T41.3X5	T41.3X6
Eucalyptus oil	T49.7X1	T49.7X2	T49.7X3	T49.7X4	T49.7X5	T49.7X6
Eucatropine	T49.5X1	T49.5X2	T49.5X3	T49.5X4	T49.5X5	T49.5X6
Eucodal	T40.2X1	T40.2X2	T40.2X3	T40.2X4	T40.2X5	T40.2X6
Euneryl	T42.3X1	T42.3X2	T42.3X3	T42.3X4	T42.3X5	T42.3X6
Euphthalmine	T44.3X1	T44.3X2	T44.3X3	T44.3X4	T44.3X5	T44.3X6
Eurax	T49.0X1	T49.0X2	T49.0X3	T49.0X4	T49.0X5	T49.0X6
Euresol	T49.4X1	T49.4X2	T49.4X3	T49.4X4	T49.4X5	T49.4X6
Euthroid	T38.1X1	T38.1X2	T38.1X3	T38.1X4	T38.1X5	T38.1X6
Evans blue	T50.8X1	T50.8X2	T50.8X3	T50.8X4	T50.8X5	T50.8X6
Evipal	T42.3X1	T42.3X2	T42.3X3	T42.3X4	T42.3X5	T42.3X6
sodium	T41.1X1	T41.1X2	T41.1X3	T41.1X4	T41.1X5	T41.1X6
Evipan	T42.3X1	T42.3X2	T42.3X3	T42.3X4	T42.3X5	T42.3X6
sodium	T41.1X1	T41.1X2	T41.1X3	T41.1X4	T41.1X5	T41.1X6
Exalamide	T49.0X1	T49.0X2	T49.0X3	T49.0X4	T49.0X5	T49.0X6
Exalgin	T39.1X1	T39.1X2	T39.1X3	T39.1X4	T39.1X5	T39.1X6
Excipients, pharmaceutical	T50.901	T50.902	T50.903	T50.904	T50.905	T50.906

Table of Drugs and Chemicals

Exhaust gas — Fluorinated corticosteroids

Substance	Poisoning, Accidental (unintentional)	Poisoning, Intentional Self-harm	Poisoning, Assault	Poisoning, Undetermined	Adverse Effect	Under-dosing
Exhaust gas (engine) (motor vehicle)	T58.01	T58.02	T58.03	T58.04	—	—
Ex-Lax (phenolphthalein)	T47.2X1	T47.2X2	T47.2X3	T47.2X4	T47.2X5	T47.2X6
Expectorant NEC	T48.4X1	T48.4X2	T48.4X3	T48.4X4	T48.4X5	T48.4X6
Extended insulin zinc suspension	T38.3X1	T38.3X2	T38.3X3	T38.3X4	T38.3X5	T38.3X6
External medications (skin) (mucous membrane)	T49.91	T49.92	T49.93	T49.94	T49.95	T49.96
dental agent	T49.7X1	T49.7X2	T49.7X3	T49.7X4	T49.7X5	T49.7X6
ENT agent	T49.6X1	T49.6X2	T49.6X3	T49.6X4	T49.6X5	T49.6X6
ophthalmic preparation	T49.5X1	T49.5X2	T49.5X3	T49.5X4	T49.5X5	T49.5X6
specified NEC	T49.8X1	T49.8X2	T49.8X3	T49.8X4	T49.8X5	T49.8X6
Extrapyramidal antagonist NEC	T44.3X1	T44.3X2	T44.3X3	T44.3X4	T44.3X5	T44.3X6
Eye agents (anti-infective)	T49.5X1	T49.5X2	T49.5X3	T49.5X4	T49.5X5	T49.5X6
Eye drug NEC	T49.5X1	T49.5X2	T49.5X3	T49.5X4	T49.5X5	T49.5X6
FAC (fluorouracil + doxorubicin + cyclophosphamide)	T45.1X1	T45.1X2	T45.1X3	T45.1X4	T45.1X5	T45.1X6
Factor						
I (fibrinogen)	T45.8X1	T45.8X2	T45.8X3	T45.8X4	T45.8X5	T45.8X6
III (thromboplastin)	T45.8X1	T45.8X2	T45.8X3	T45.8X4	T45.8X5	T45.8X6
VIII (antihemophilic Factor) (concentrate)	T45.8X1	T45.8X2	T45.8X3	T45.8X4	T45.8X5	T45.8X6
IX complex	T45.7X1	T45.7X2	T45.7X3	T45.7X4	T45.7X5	T45.7X6
human	T45.8X1	T45.8X2	T45.8X3	T45.8X4	T45.8X5	T45.8X6
Famotidine	T47.0X1	T47.0X2	T47.0X3	T47.0X4	T47.0X5	T47.0X6
Fat suspension, intravenous	T50.991	T50.992	T50.993	T50.994	T50.995	T50.996
Fazadinium bromide	T48.1X1	T48.1X2	T48.1X3	T48.1X4	T48.1X5	T48.1X6
Febarbamate	T42.3X1	T42.3X2	T42.3X3	T42.3X4	T42.3X5	T42.3X6
Fecal softener	T47.4X1	T47.4X2	T47.4X3	T47.4X4	T47.4X5	T47.4X6
Fedrilate	T48.3X1	T48.3X2	T48.3X3	T48.3X4	T48.3X5	T48.3X6
Felodipine	T46.1X1	T46.1X2	T46.1X3	T46.1X4	T46.1X5	T46.1X6
Felypressin	T38.892	T38.892	T38.893	T38.894	T38.895	T38.896
Femoxetine	T43.221	T43.222	T43.223	T43.224	T43.225	T43.226
Fenalcomine	T46.3X1	T46.3X2	T46.3X3	T46.3X4	T46.3X5	T46.3X6
Fenamisal	T37.1X1	T37.1X2	T37.1X3	T37.1X4	T37.1X5	T37.1X6
Fenazone	T39.2X1	T39.2X2	T39.2X3	T39.2X4	T39.2X5	T39.2X6
Fenbendazole	T37.4X1	T37.4X2	T37.4X3	T37.4X4	T37.4X5	T37.4X6
Fenbutrazate	T50.5X1	T50.5X2	T50.5X3	T50.5X4	T50.5X5	T50.5X6
Fencamfamine	T43.691	T43.692	T43.693	T43.694	T43.695	T43.696
Fendiline	T46.1X1	T46.1X2	T46.1X3	T46.1X4	T46.1X5	T46.1X6
Fenetylline	T43.691	T43.692	T43.693	T43.694	T43.695	T43.696
Fenflumizole	T39.391	T39.392	T39.393	T39.394	T39.395	T39.396
Fenfluramine	T50.5X1	T50.5X2	T50.5X3	T50.5X4	T50.5X5	T50.5X6
Fenobarbital	T42.3X1	T42.3X2	T42.3X3	T42.3X4	T42.3X5	T42.3X6
Fenofibrate	T46.6X1	T46.6X2	T46.6X3	T46.6X4	T46.6X5	T46.6X6
Fenoprofen	T39.311	T39.312	T39.313	T39.314	T39.315	T39.316
Fenoterol	T48.6X1	T48.6X2	T48.6X3	T48.6X4	T48.6X5	T48.6X6
Fenoverine	T44.3X1	T44.3X2	T44.3X3	T44.3X4	T44.3X5	T44.3X6
Fenoxazoline	T48.5X1	T48.5X2	T48.5X3	T48.5X4	T48.5X5	T48.5X6
Fenproporex	T50.5X1	T50.5X2	T50.5X3	T50.5X4	T50.5X5	T50.5X6
Fenquizone	T50.2X1	T50.2X2	T50.2X3	T50.2X4	T50.2X5	T50.2X6
Fentanyl	T40.4X1	T40.4X2	T40.4X3	T40.4X4	T40.4X5	T40.4X6
Fentazin	T43.3X1	T43.3X2	T43.3X3	T43.3X4	T43.3X5	T43.3X6
Fenthion	T60.0X1	T60.0X2	T60.0X3	T60.0X4	—	—
Fenticlor	T49.0X1	T49.0X2	T49.0X3	T49.0X4	T49.0X5	T49.0X6
Fenylbutazone	T39.2X1	T39.2X2	T39.2X3	T39.2X4	T39.2X5	T39.2X6
Feprazone	T39.2X1	T39.2X2	T39.2X3	T39.2X4	T39.2X5	T39.2X6
Fer de lance (bite) (venom)	T63.061	T63.062	T63.063	T63.064	—	—
Ferric — *see also* Iron						
chloride	T45.4X1	T45.4X2	T45.4X3	T45.4X4	T45.4X5	T45.4X6
citrate	T45.4X1	T45.4X2	T45.4X3	T45.4X4	T45.4X5	T45.4X6
hydroxide						
colloidal	T45.4X1	T45.4X2	T45.4X3	T45.4X4	T45.4X5	T45.4X6
polymaltose	T45.4X1	T45.4X2	T45.4X3	T45.4X4	T45.4X5	T45.4X6
pyrophosphate	T45.4X1	T45.4X2	T45.4X3	T45.4X4	T45.4X5	T45.4X6
Ferritin	T45.4X1	T45.4X2	T45.4X3	T45.4X4	T45.4X5	T45.4X6
Ferrocholinate	T45.4X1	T45.4X2	T45.4X3	T45.4X4	T45.4X5	T45.4X6
Ferrodextrane	T45.4X1	T45.4X2	T45.4X3	T45.4X4	T45.4X5	T45.4X6
Ferropolimaler	T45.4X1	T45.4X2	T45.4X3	T45.4X4	T45.4X5	T45.4X6
Ferrous — *see also* Iron						
phosphate	T45.4X1	T45.4X2	T45.4X3	T45.4X4	T45.4X5	T45.4X6
salt	T45.4X1	T45.4X2	T45.4X3	T45.4X4	T45.4X5	T45.4X6
with folic acid	T45.4X1	T45.4X2	T45.4X3	T45.4X4	T45.4X5	T45.4X6
Ferrous fumerate, gluconate, lactate, salt NEC, sulfate (medicinal)	T45.4X1	T45.4X2	T45.4X3	T45.4X4	T45.4X5	T45.4X6
Ferrovanadium (fumes)	T59.891	T59.892	T59.893	T59.894	—	—
Ferrum — *see* Iron						
Fertilizers NEC	T65.891	T65.892	T65.893	T65.894	—	—
with herbicide mixture	T60.3X1	T60.3X2	T60.3X3	T60.3X4	—	—
Fetoxilate	T47.6X1	T47.6X2	T47.6X3	T47.6X4	T47.6X5	T47.6X6
Fiber, dietary	T47.4X1	T47.4X2	T47.4X3	T47.4X4	T47.4X5	T47.4X6
Fiberglass	T65.831	T65.832	T65.833	T65.834	—	—
Fibrinogen (human)	T45.8X1	T45.8X2	T45.8X3	T45.8X4	T45.8X5	T45.8X6
Fibrinolysin (human)	T45.691	T45.692	T45.693	T45.694	T45.695	T45.696
Fibrinolysis						
affecting drug	T45.601	T45.602	T45.603	T45.604	T45.605	T45.606
inhibitor NEC	T45.621	T45.622	T45.623	T45.624	T45.625	T45.626
Fibrinolytic drug	T45.611	T45.612	T45.613	T45.614	T45.615	T45.616
Filix mas	T37.4X1	T37.4X2	T37.4X3	T37.4X4	T37.4X5	T37.4X6
Filtering cream	T49.3X1	T49.3X2	T49.3X3	T49.3X4	T49.3X5	T49.3X6
Fiorinal	T39.011	T39.012	T39.013	T39.014	T39.015	T39.016
Firedamp	T59.891	T59.892	T59.893	T59.894	—	—
Fish, noxious, nonbacterial	T61.91	T61.92	T61.93	T61.94	—	—
ciguatera	T61.01	T61.02	T61.03	T61.04	—	—
scombroid	T61.11	T61.12	T61.13	T61.14	—	—
shell	T61.781	T61.782	T61.783	T61.784	—	—
specified NEC	T61.771	T61.772	T61.773	T61.774	—	—
Flagyl	T37.3X1	T37.3X2	T37.3X3	T37.3X4	T37.3X5	T37.3X6
Flavine adenine dinucleotide	T45.2X1	T45.2X2	T45.2X3	T45.2X4	T45.2X5	T45.2X6
Flavodic acid	T46.991	T46.992	T46.993	T46.994	T46.995	T46.996
Flavoxate	T44.3X1	T44.3X2	T44.3X3	T44.3X4	T44.3X5	T44.3X6
Flaxedil	T48.1X1	T48.1X2	T48.1X3	T48.1X4	T48.1X5	T48.1X6
Flaxseed (medicinal)	T49.3X1	T49.3X2	T49.3X3	T49.3X4	T49.3X5	T49.3X6
Flecainide	T46.2X1	T46.2X2	T46.2X3	T46.2X4	T46.2X5	T46.2X6
Fleroxacin	T36.8X1	T36.8X2	T36.8X3	T36.8X4	T36.8X5	T36.8X6
Floctafenine	T39.8X1	T39.8X2	T39.8X3	T39.8X4	T39.8X5	T39.8X6
Flomax	T44.6X1	T44.6X2	T44.6X3	T44.6X4	T44.6X5	T44.6X6
Flomoxef	T36.1X1	T36.1X2	T36.1X3	T36.1X4	T36.1X5	T36.1X6
Flopropione	T44.3X1	T44.3X2	T44.3X3	T44.3X4	T44.3X5	T44.3X6
Florantyrone	T47.5X1	T47.5X2	T47.5X3	T47.5X4	T47.5X5	T47.5X6
Floraquin	T37.8X1	T37.8X2	T37.8X3	T37.8X4	T37.8X5	T37.8X6
Florinef	T38.0X1	T38.0X2	T38.0X3	T38.0X4	T38.0X5	T38.0X6
ENT agent	T49.6X1	T49.6X2	T49.6X3	T49.6X4	T49.6X5	T49.6X6
ophthalmic preparation	T49.5X1	T49.5X2	T49.5X3	T49.5X4	T49.5X5	T49.5X6
topical NEC	T49.0X1	T49.0X2	T49.0X3	T49.0X4	T49.0X5	T49.0X6
Flowers of sulfur	T49.4X1	T49.4X2	T49.4X3	T49.4X4	T49.4X5	T49.4X6
Floxuridine	T45.1X1	T45.1X2	T45.1X3	T45.1X4	T45.1X5	T45.1X6
Fluanisone	T43.4X1	T43.4X2	T43.4X3	T43.4X4	T43.4X5	T43.4X6
Flubendazole	T37.4X1	T37.4X2	T37.4X3	T37.4X4	T37.4X5	T37.4X6
Fluclorolone acetonide	T49.0X1	T49.0X2	T49.0X3	T49.0X4	T49.0X5	T49.0X6
Flucloxacillin	T36.0X1	T36.0X2	T36.0X3	T36.0X4	T36.0X5	T36.0X6
Fluconazole	T37.8X1	T37.8X2	T37.8X3	T37.8X4	T37.8X5	T37.8X6
Flucytosine	T37.8X1	T37.8X2	T37.8X3	T37.8X4	T37.8X5	T37.8X6
Fludeoxyglucose (18F)	T50.8X1	T50.8X2	T50.8X3	T50.8X4	T50.8X5	T50.8X6
Fludiazepam	T42.4X1	T42.4X2	T42.4X3	T42.4X4	T42.4X5	T42.4X6
Fludrocortisone	T50.0X1	T50.0X2	T50.0X3	T50.0X4	T50.0X5	T50.0X6
ENT agent	T49.6X1	T49.6X2	T49.6X3	T49.6X4	T49.6X5	T49.6X6
ophthalmic preparation	T49.5X1	T49.5X2	T49.5X3	T49.5X4	T49.5X5	T49.5X6
topical NEC	T49.0X1	T49.0X2	T49.0X3	T49.0X4	T49.0X5	T49.0X6
Fludroxycortide	T49.0X1	T49.0X2	T49.0X3	T49.0X4	T49.0X5	T49.0X6
Flufenamic acid	T39.391	T39.392	T39.393	T39.394	T39.395	T39.396
Fluindione	T45.511	T45.512	T45.513	T45.514	T45.515	T45.516
Flumequine	T37.8X1	T37.8X2	T37.8X3	T37.8X4	T37.8X5	T37.8X6
Flumethasone	T49.0X1	T49.0X2	T49.0X3	T49.0X4	T49.0X5	T49.0X6
Flumethiazide	T50.2X1	T50.2X2	T50.2X3	T50.2X4	T50.2X5	T50.2X6
Flumidin	T37.5X1	T37.5X2	T37.5X3	T37.5X4	T37.5X5	T37.5X6
Flunarizine	T46.7X1	T46.7X2	T46.7X3	T46.7X4	T46.7X5	T46.7X6
Flunidazole	T37.8X1	T37.8X2	T37.8X3	T37.8X4	T37.8X5	T37.8X6
Flunisolide	T48.6X1	T48.6X2	T48.6X3	T48.6X4	T48.6X5	T48.6X6
Flunitrazepam	T42.4X1	T42.4X2	T42.4X3	T42.4X4	T42.4X5	T42.4X6
Fluocinolone (acetonide)	T49.0X1	T49.0X2	T49.0X3	T49.0X4	T49.0X5	T49.0X6
Fluocinonide	T49.0X1	T49.0X2	T49.0X3	T49.0X4	T49.0X5	T49.0X6
Fluocortin (butyl)	T49.0X1	T49.0X2	T49.0X3	T49.0X4	T49.0X5	T49.0X6
Fluocortolone	T49.0X1	T49.0X2	T49.0X3	T49.0X4	T49.0X5	T49.0X6
Fluohydrocortisone	T38.0X1	T38.0X2	T38.0X3	T38.0X4	T38.0X5	T38.0X6
ENT agent	T49.6X1	T49.6X2	T49.6X3	T49.6X4	T49.6X5	T49.6X6
ophthalmic preparation	T49.5X1	T49.5X2	T49.5X3	T49.5X4	T49.5X5	T49.5X6
topical NEC	T49.0X1	T49.0X2	T49.0X3	T49.0X4	T49.0X5	T49.0X6
Fluonid	T49.0X1	T49.0X2	T49.0X3	T49.0X4	T49.0X5	T49.0X6
Fluopromazine	T43.3X1	T43.3X2	T43.3X3	T43.3X4	T43.3X5	T43.3X6
Fluoracetate	T60.8X1	T60.8X2	T60.8X3	T60.8X4	—	—
Fluorescein	T50.8X1	T50.8X2	T50.8X3	T50.8X4	T50.8X5	T50.8X6
Fluorhydrocortisone	T50.0X1	T50.0X2	T50.0X3	T50.0X4	T50.0X5	T50.0X6
Fluoride (nonmedicinal) (pesticide) (sodium) **NEC**	T60.8X1	T60.8X2	T60.8X3	T60.8X4	—	—
hydrogen — *see* Hydrofluoric acid						
medicinal NEC	T50.991	T50.992	T50.993	T50.994	T50.995	T50.996
dental use	T49.7X1	T49.7X2	T49.7X3	T49.7X4	T49.7X5	T49.7X6
not pesticide NEC	T54.91	T54.92	T54.93	T54.94	—	—
stannous	T49.7X1	T49.7X2	T49.7X3	T49.7X4	T49.7X5	T49.7X6
Fluorinated corticosteroids	T38.0X1	T38.0X2	T38.0X3	T38.0X4	T38.0X5	T38.0X6

Substance	Poisoning, Accidental (unintentional)	Poisoning, Intentional Self-harm	Poisoning, Assault	Poisoning, Undetermined	Adverse Effect	Under-dosing
Fluorine (gas)	T59.5X1	T59.5X2	T59.5X3	T59.5X4	—	—
salt — *see* Fluoride(s)						
Fluoristan	T49.7X1	T49.7X2	T49.7X3	T49.7X4	T49.7X5	T49.7X6
Fluormetholone	T49.0X1	T49.0X2	T49.0X3	T49.0X4	T49.0X5	T49.0X6
Fluoroacetate	T60.8X1	T60.8X2	T60.8X3	T60.8X4	—	—
Fluorocarbon monomer	T53.6X1	T53.6X2	T53.6X3	T53.6X4	—	—
Fluorocytosine	T37.8X1	T37.8X2	T37.8X3	T37.8X4	T37.8X5	T37.8X6
Fluorodeoxyuridine	T45.1X1	T45.1X2	T45.1X3	T45.1X4	T45.1X5	T45.1X6
Fluoromentholone	T49.0X1	T49.0X2	T49.0X3	T49.0X4	T49.0X5	T49.0X6
ophthalmic preparation	T49.5X1	T49.5X2	T49.5X3	T49.5X4	T49.5X5	T49.5X6
Fluorophosphate	T60.0X1	T60.0X2	T60.0X3	T60.0X4	—	—
insecticide						
Fluorosol	T46.3X1	T46.3X2	T46.3X3	T46.3X4	T46.3X5	T46.3X6
Fluorouracil	T45.1X1	T45.1X2	T45.1X3	T45.1X4	T45.1X5	T45.1X6
Fluorphenylalanine	T49.5X1	T49.5X2	T49.5X3	T49.5X4	T49.5X5	T49.5X6
Fluothane	T41.0X1	T41.0X2	T41.0X3	T41.0X4	T41.0X5	T41.0X6
Fluoxetine	T43.221	T43.222	T43.223	T43.224	T43.225	T43.226
Fluoxymesterone	T38.7X1	T38.7X2	T38.7X3	T38.7X4	T38.7X5	T38.7X6
Flupenthixol	T43.4X1	T43.4X2	T43.4X3	T43.4X4	T43.4X5	T43.4X6
Flupentixol	T43.4X1	T43.4X2	T43.4X3	T43.4X4	T43.4X5	T43.4X6
Fluphenazine	T43.3X1	T43.3X2	T43.3X3	T43.3X4	T43.3X5	T43.3X6
Fluprednidene	T49.0X1	T49.0X2	T49.0X3	T49.0X4	T49.0X5	T49.0X6
Fluprednisolone	T38.0X1	T38.0X2	T38.0X3	T38.0X4	T38.0X5	T38.0X6
Fluradoline	T39.8X1	T39.8X2	T39.8X3	T39.8X4	T39.8X5	T39.8X6
Flurandrenolide	T49.0X1	T49.0X2	T49.0X3	T49.0X4	T49.0X5	T49.0X6
Flurandrenolone	T49.0X1	T49.0X2	T49.0X3	T49.0X4	T49.0X5	T49.0X6
Flurazepam	T42.4X1	T42.4X2	T42.4X3	T42.4X4	T42.4X5	T42.4X6
Flurbiprofen	T39.311	T39.312	T39.313	T39.314	T39.315	T39.316
Flurobate	T49.0X1	T49.0X2	T49.0X3	T49.0X4	T49.0X5	T49.0X6
Fluroxene	T41.0X1	T41.0X2	T41.0X3	T41.0X4	T41.0X5	T41.0X6
Fluspirilene	T43.591	T43.592	T43.593	T43.594	T43.595	T43.596
Flutamide	T38.6X1	T38.6X2	T38.6X3	T38.6X4	T38.6X5	T38.6X6
Flutazolam	T38.0X1	T38.0X2	T38.0X3	T38.0X4	T38.0X5	T38.0X6
Fluticasone propionate	T38.0X1	T38.0X2	T38.0X3	T38.0X4	T38.0X5	T38.0X6
Flutoprazepam	T42.4X1	T42.4X2	T42.4X3	T42.4X4	T42.4X5	T42.4X6
Flutropium bromide	T48.6X1	T48.6X2	T48.6X3	T48.6X4	T48.6X5	T48.6X6
Fluvoxamine	T43.221	T43.222	T43.223	T43.224	T43.225	T43.226
Folacin	T45.8X1	T45.8X2	T45.8X3	T45.8X4	T45.8X5	T45.8X6
Folic acid	T45.8X1	T45.8X2	T45.8X3	T45.8X4	T45.8X5	T45.8X6
with ferrous salt	T45.2X1	T45.2X2	T45.2X3	T45.2X4	T45.2X5	T45.2X6
antagonist	T45.1X1	T45.1X2	T45.1X3	T45.1X4	T45.1X5	T45.1X6
Folinic acid	T45.8X1	T45.8X2	T45.8X3	T45.8X4	T45.8X5	T45.8X6
Folium stramoniae	T48.6X1	T48.6X2	T48.6X3	T48.6X4	T48.6X5	T48.6X6
Follicle-stimulating hormone, human	T38.811	T38.812	T38.813	T38.814	T38.815	T38.816
Folpet	T60.3X1	T60.3X2	T60.3X3	T60.3X4	—	—
Fominoben	T48.3X1	T48.3X2	T48.3X3	T48.3X4	T48.3X5	T48.3X6
Food, foodstuffs, noxious, nonbacterial, NEC	T62.91	T62.92	T62.93	T62.94	—	—
berries	T62.1X1	T62.1X2	T62.1X3	T62.1X4	—	—
fish — *see also* Fish	T61.91	T61.92	T61.93	T61.94	—	—
mushrooms	T62.0X1	T62.0X2	T62.0X3	T62.0X4	—	—
plants	T62.2X1	T62.2X2	T62.2X3	T62.2X4	—	—
seafood	T61.91	T61.92	T61.93	T61.94	—	—
specified NEC	T61.8X1	T61.8X2	T61.8X3	T61.8X4	—	—
seeds	T62.2X1	T62.2X2	T62.2X3	T62.2X4	—	—
shellfish	T61.781	T61.782	T61.783	T61.784	—	—
specified NEC	T62.8X1	T62.8X2	T62.8X3	T62.8X4	—	—
Fool's parsley	T62.2X1	T62.2X2	T62.2X3	T62.2X4	—	—
Formaldehyde (solution), gas or	T59.2X1	T59.2X2	T59.2X3	T59.2X4	—	—
vapor						
fungicide	T60.3X1	T60.3X2	T60.3X3	T60.3X4	—	—
Formalin	T59.2X1	T59.2X2	T59.2X3	T59.2X4	—	—
fungicide	T60.3X1	T60.3X2	T60.3X3	T60.3X4	—	—
vapor	T59.2X1	T59.2X2	T59.2X3	T59.2X4	—	—
Formic acid	T54.2X1	T54.2X2	T54.2X3	T54.2X4	—	—
vapor	T59.891	T59.892	T59.893	T59.894	—	—
Foscarnet sodium	T37.5X1	T37.5X2	T37.5X3	T37.5X4	T37.5X5	T37.5X6
Fosfestrol	T38.5X1	T38.5X2	T38.5X3	T38.5X4	T38.5X5	T38.5X6
Fosfomycin	T36.8X1	T36.8X2	T36.8X3	T36.8X4	T36.8X5	T36.8X6
Fosfonet sodium	T37.5X1	T37.5X2	T37.5X3	T37.5X4	T37.5X5	T37.5X6
Fosinopril	T46.4X1	T46.4X2	T46.4X3	T46.4X4	T46.4X5	T46.4X6
sodium	T46.4X1	T46.4X2	T46.4X3	T46.4X4	T46.4X5	T46.4X6
Fowler's solution	T57.0X1	T57.0X2	T57.0X3	T57.0X4	—	—
Foxglove	T62.2X1	T62.2X2	T62.2X3	T62.2X4	—	—
Framycetin	T36.5X1	T36.5X2	T36.5X3	T36.5X4	T36.5X5	T36.5X6
Frangula	T47.2X1	T47.2X2	T47.2X3	T47.2X4	T47.2X5	T47.2X6
extract	T47.2X1	T47.2X2	T47.2X3	T47.2X4	T47.2X5	T47.2X6
Frei antigen	T50.8X1	T50.8X2	T50.8X3	T50.8X4	T50.8X5	T50.8X6
Freon	T53.5X1	T53.5X2	T53.5X3	T53.5X4	—	—
Fructose	T50.3X1	T50.3X2	T50.3X3	T50.3X4	T50.3X5	T50.3X6
Frusemide	T50.1X1	T50.1X2	T50.1X3	T50.1X4	T50.1X5	T50.1X6
FSH	T38.811	T38.812	T38.813	T38.814	T38.815	T38.816

Substance	Poisoning, Accidental (unintentional)	Poisoning, Intentional Self-harm	Poisoning, Assault	Poisoning, Undetermined	Adverse Effect	Under-dosing
Ftorafur	T45.1X1	T45.1X2	T45.1X3	T45.1X4	T45.1X5	T45.1X6
Fuel						
automobile	T52.0X1	T52.0X2	T52.0X3	T52.0X4	—	—
exhaust gas, not in transit	T58.01	T58.02	T58.03	T58.04	—	—
vapor NEC	T52.0X1	T52.0X2	T52.0X3	T52.0X4	—	—
gas (domestic use) — *see also* Carbon, monoxide, fuel, utility	T59.891	T59.892	T59.893	T59.894	—	—
utility	T59.891	T59.892	T59.893	T59.894	—	—
incomplete combustion of — *see* Carbon, monoxide, fuel, utility						
in mobile container	T59.891	T59.892	T59.893	T59.894	—	—
piped (natural)	T59.891	T59.892	T59.893	T59.894	—	—
industrial, incomplete combustion	T58.8X1	T58.8X2	T58.8X3	T58.8X4	—	—
Fugillin	T36.8X1	T36.8X2	T36.8X3	T36.8X4	T36.8X5	T36.8X6
Fulminate of mercury	T56.1X1	T56.1X2	T56.1X3	T56.1X4	—	—
Fulvicin	T36.7X1	T36.7X2	T36.7X3	T36.7X4	T36.7X5	T36.7X6
Fumadil	T36.8X1	T36.8X2	T36.8X3	T36.8X4	T36.8X5	T36.8X6
Fumagillin	T36.8X1	T36.8X2	T36.8X3	T36.8X4	T36.8X5	T36.8X6
Fumaric acid	T49.4X1	T49.4X2	T49.4X3	T49.4X4	T49.4X5	T49.4X6
Fumes (from)	T59.91	T59.92	T59.93	T59.94	—	—
carbon monoxide — *see* Carbon, monoxide						
charcoal (domestic use) — *see* Charcoal, fumes						
chloroform — *see* Chloroform						
coke (in domestic stoves, fireplaces) — *see* Coke fumes						
corrosive NEC	T54.91	T54.92	T54.93	T54.94	—	—
ether — *see* ether						
freons	T53.5X1	T53.5X2	T53.5X3	T53.5X4	—	—
hydrocarbons	T59.891	T59.892	T59.893	T59.894	—	—
petroleum (liquefied)	T59.891	T59.892	T59.893	T59.894	—	—
distributed through pipes (pure or mixed with air)	T59.891	T59.892	T59.893	T59.894	—	—
lead — *see* lead						
metal — *see* Metals, or the specified metal						
nitrogen dioxide	T59.0X1	T59.0X2	T59.0X3	T59.0X4	—	—
pesticides — *see* Pesticides						
petroleum (liquefied)	T59.891	T59.892	T59.893	T59.894	—	—
distributed through pipes (pure or mixed with air)	T59.891	T59.892	T59.893	T59.894	—	—
polyester	T59.891	T59.892	T59.893	T59.894	—	—
specified source NEC — *see also* substance specified	T59.891	T59.892	T59.893	T59.894	—	—
sulfur dioxide	T59.1X1	T59.1X2	T59.1X3	T59.1X4	—	—
Fumigant NEC	T60.91	T60.92	T60.93	T60.94	—	—
Fungicide NEC (nonmedicinal)	T60.3X1	T60.3X2	T60.3X3	T60.3X4	—	—
Fungi, noxious, used as food	T62.0X1	T62.0X2	T62.0X3	T62.0X4	—	—
Fungizone	T36.7X1	T36.7X2	T36.7X3	T36.7X4	T36.7X5	T36.7X6
topical	T49.0X1	T49.0X2	T49.0X3	T49.0X4	T49.0X5	T49.0X6
Furacin	T49.0X1	T49.0X2	T49.0X3	T49.0X4	T49.0X5	T49.0X6
Furadantin	T37.91	T37.92	T37.93	T37.94	T37.95	T37.96
Furazolidone	T37.8X1	T37.8X2	T37.8X3	T37.8X4	T37.8X5	T37.8X6
Furazolium chloride	T49.0X1	T49.0X2	T49.0X3	T49.0X4	T49.0X5	T49.0X6
Furfural	T52.8X1	T52.8X2	T52.8X3	T52.8X4	—	—
Furnace (coal burning) (domestic), gas from	T58.2X1	T58.2X2	T58.2X3	T58.2X4	—	—
industrial	T58.8X1	T58.8X2	T58.8X3	T58.8X4	—	—
Furniture polish	T65.891	T65.892	T65.893	T65.894	—	—
Furosemide	T50.1X1	T50.1X2	T50.1X3	T50.1X4	T50.1X5	T50.1X6
Furoxone	T37.91	T37.92	T37.93	T37.94	T37.95	T37.96
Fursultiamine	T45.2X1	T45.2X2	T45.2X3	T45.2X4	T45.2X5	T45.2X6
Fusafungine	T36.8X1	T36.8X2	T36.8X3	T36.8X4	T36.8X5	T36.8X6
Fusel oil (any) (amyl) (butyl) (propyl), vapor	T51.3X1	T51.3X2	T51.3X3	T51.3X4	—	—
Fusidate (ethanolamine) (sodium)	T36.8X1	T36.8X2	T36.8X3	T36.8X4	T36.8X5	T36.8X6
Fusidic acid	T36.8X1	T36.8X2	T36.8X3	T36.8X4	T36.8X5	T36.8X6
Fytic acid, nonasodium	T50.6X1	T50.6X2	T50.6X3	T50.6X4	T50.6X5	T50.6X6
b-Galactosidase	T47.5X1	T47.5X2	T47.5X3	T47.5X4	T47.5X5	T47.5X6
GABA	T43.8X1	T43.8X2	T43.8X3	T43.8X4	T43.8X5	T43.8X6
Gadopentetic acid	T50.8X1	T50.8X2	T50.8X3	T50.8X4	T50.8X5	T50.8X6
Galactose	T50.3X1	T50.3X2	T50.3X3	T50.3X4	T50.3X5	T50.3X6
Galantamine	T44.0X1	T44.0X2	T44.0X3	T44.0X4	T44.0X5	T44.0X6

Substance	Poisoning, Accidental (unintentional)	Poisoning, Intentional Self-harm	Poisoning, Assault	Poisoning, Undetermined	Adverse Effect	Under-dosing
Gallamine (triethiodide)	T48.1X1	T48.1X2	T48.1X3	T48.1X4	T48.1X5	T48.1X6
Gallium citrate	T50.991	T50.992	T50.993	T50.994	T50.995	T50.996
Gallopamil	T46.1X1	T46.1X2	T46.1X3	T46.1X4	T46.1X5	T46.1X6
Gamboge	T47.2X1	T47.2X2	T47.2X3	T47.2X4	T47.2X5	T47.2X6
Gamimune	T50.Z11	T50.Z12	T50.Z13	T50.Z14	T50.Z15	T50.Z16
Gamma-aminobutyric acid	T43.8X1	T43.8X2	T43.8X3	T43.8X4	T43.8X5	T43.8X6
Gamma-benzene hexachloride (medicinal)	T49.0X1	T49.0X2	T49.0X3	T49.0X4	T49.0X5	T49.0X6
nonmedicinal, vapor	T53.6X1	T53.6X2	T53.6X3	T53.6X4	—	—
Gamma-BHC (medicinal) — see also Gamma-benzene hexachloride	T49.0X1	T49.0X2	T49.0X3	T49.0X4	T49.0X5	T49.0X6
Gamma globulin	T50.Z11	T50.Z12	T50.Z13	T50.Z14	T50.Z15	T50.Z16
Gamulin	T50.Z11	T50.Z12	T50.Z13	T50.Z14	T50.Z15	T50.Z16
Ganciclovir (sodium)	T37.5X1	T37.5X2	T37.5X3	T37.5X4	T37.5X5	T37.5X6
Ganglionic blocking drug NEC	T44.2X1	T44.2X2	T44.2X3	T44.2X4	T44.2X5	T44.2X6
specified NEC	T44.2X1	T44.2X2	T44.2X3	T44.2X4	T44.2X5	T44.2X6
Ganja	T40.7X1	T40.7X2	T40.7X3	T40.7X4	T40.7X5	T40.7X6
Garamycin	T36.5X1	T36.5X2	T36.5X3	T36.5X4	T36.5X5	T36.5X6
ophthalmic preparation	T49.5X1	T49.5X2	T49.5X3	T49.5X4	T49.5X5	T49.5X6
topical NEC	T49.0X1	T49.0X2	T49.0X3	T49.0X4	T49.0X5	T49.0X6
Gardenal	T42.3X1	T42.3X2	T42.3X3	T42.3X4	T42.3X5	T42.3X6
Gardepanyl	T42.3X1	T42.3X2	T42.3X3	T42.3X4	T42.3X5	T42.3X6
Gaseous substance — see Gas						
Gasoline	T52.0X1	T52.0X2	T52.0X3	T52.0X4	—	—
vapor	T52.0X1	T52.0X2	T52.0X3	T52.0X4	—	—
Gastric enzymes	T47.5X1	T47.5X2	T47.5X3	T47.5X4	T47.5X5	T47.5X6
Gastrografin	T50.8X1	T50.8X2	T50.8X3	T50.8X4	T50.8X5	T50.8X6
Gastrointestinal drug	T47.91	T47.92	T47.93	T47.94	T47.95	T47.96
biological	T47.8X1	T47.8X2	T47.8X3	T47.8X4	T47.8X5	T47.8X6
specified NEC	T47.8X1	T47.8X2	T47.8X3	T47.8X4	T47.8X5	T47.8X6
Gas NEC	T59.91	T59.92	T59.93	T59.94	—	—
acetylene	T59.891	T59.892	T59.893	T59.894	—	—
incomplete combustion of	T58.11	T58.12	T58.13	T58.14	—	—
air contaminants, source or type not specified	T59.91	T59.92	T59.93	T59.94	—	—
anesthetic	T41.0X1	T41.0X2	T41.0X3	T41.0X4	T41.0X5	T41.0X6
blast furnace	T58.8X1	T58.8X2	T58.8X3	T58.8X4	—	—
butane — see butane						
carbon monoxide — see Carbon, monoxide						
chlorine	T59.4X1	T59.4X2	T59.4X3	T59.4X4	—	—
coal	T58.2X1	T58.2X2	T58.2X3	T58.2X4	—	—
cyanide	T57.3X1	T57.3X2	T57.3X3	T57.3X4	—	—
dicyanogen	T65.0X1	T65.0X2	T65.0X3	T65.0X4	—	—
domestic — see Domestic gas						
exhaust	T58.01	T58.02	T58.03	T58.04	—	—
from utility (for cooking, heating, or lighting) (after combustion) — see Carbon, monoxide, fuel, utility						
prior to combustion	T59.891	T59.892	T59.893	T59.894	—	—
from wood- or coal-burning stove or fireplace	T58.2X1	T58.2X2	T58.2X3	T58.2X4	—	—
fuel (domestic use) (after combustion) — see also Carbon, monoxide, fuel						
industrial use	T58.8X1	T58.8X2	T58.8X3	T58.8X4	—	—
prior to combustion	T59.891	T59.892	T59.893	T59.894	—	—
utility	T59.891	T59.892	T59.893	T59.894	—	—
incomplete combustion of — see Carbon, monoxide, fuel, utility						
in mobile container	T59.891	T59.892	T59.893	T59.894	—	—
piped (natural)	T59.891	T59.892	T59.893	T59.894	—	—
garage	T58.01	T58.02	T58.03	T58.04	—	—
hydrocarbon NEC	T59.891	T59.892	T59.893	T59.894	—	—
incomplete combustion of — see Carbon, monoxide, fuel, utility						
liquefied — see butane						
piped	T59.891	T59.892	T59.893	T59.894	—	—
hydrocyanic acid	T65.0X1	T65.0X2	T65.0X3	T65.0X4	—	—
illuminating (after combustion)	T58.11	T58.12	T58.13	T58.14	—	—
prior to combustion	T59.891	T59.892	T59.893	T59.894	—	—
incomplete combustion, any — see Carbon, monoxide						
kiln	T58.8X1	T58.8X2	T58.8X3	T58.8X4	—	—
lacrimogenic	T59.3X1	T59.3X2	T59.3X3	T59.3X4	—	—
Gas — continued						
liquefied petroleum — see butane						
marsh	T59.891	T59.892	T59.893	T59.894	—	—
motor exhaust, not in transit	T58.01	T58.02	T58.03	T58.04	—	—
mustard, not in war	T59.891	T59.892	T59.893	T59.894	—	—
natural	T59.891	T59.892	T59.893	T59.894	—	—
nerve, not in war	T59.91	T59.92	T59.93	T59.94	—	—
oil	T52.0X1	T52.0X2	T52.0X3	T52.0X4	—	—
petroleum (liquefied) (distributed in mobile containers)	T59.891	T59.892	T59.893	T59.894	—	—
piped (pure or mixed with air)	T59.891	T59.892	T59.893	T59.894	—	—
piped (manufactured) (natural) NEC	T59.891	T59.892	T59.893	T59.894	—	—
producer	T58.8X1	T58.8X2	T58.8X3	T58.8X4	—	—
propane — see propane						
refrigerant (chlorofluoro-carbon)	T53.5X1	T53.5X2	T53.5X3	T53.5X4	—	—
not chlorofluoro-carbon	T59.891	T59.892	T59.893	T59.894	—	—
sewer	T59.91	T59.92	T59.93	T59.94	—	—
specified source NEC	T59.91	T59.92	T59.93	T59.94	—	—
stove (after combustion)	T58.11	T58.12	T58.13	T58.14	—	—
prior to combustion	T59.891	T59.892	T59.893	T59.894	—	—
tear	T59.3X1	T59.3X2	T59.3X3	T59.3X4	—	—
therapeutic	T41.5X1	T41.5X2	T41.5X3	T41.5X4	T41.5X5	T41.5X6
utility (for cooking, heating, or lighting) (piped) NEC	T59.891	T59.892	T59.893	T59.894	—	—
incomplete combustion of — see Carbon, monoxide, fuel, utilty						
in mobile container	T59.891	T59.892	T59.893	T59.894	—	—
piped (natural)	T59.891	T59.892	T59.893	T59.894	—	—
water	T58.11	T58.12	T58.13	T58.14	—	—
incomplete combustion of — see Carbon, monoxide, fuel, utility						
Gaultheria procumbens	T62.2X1	T62.2X2	T62.2X3	T62.2X4	—	—
Gefarnate	T44.3X1	T44.3X2	T44.3X3	T44.3X4	T44.3X5	T44.3X6
Gelatin (intravenous)	T45.8X1	T45.8X2	T45.8X3	T45.8X4	T45.8X5	T45.8X6
absorbable (sponge)	T45.7X1	T45.7X2	T45.7X3	T45.7X4	T45.7X5	T45.7X6
Gelfilm	T49.8X1	T49.8X2	T49.8X3	T49.8X4	T49.8X5	T49.8X6
Gelfoam	T45.7X1	T45.7X2	T45.7X3	T45.7X4	T45.7X5	T45.7X6
Gelsemine	T50.991	T50.992	T50.993	T50.994	T50.995	T50.996
Gelsemium (sempervirens)	T62.2X1	T62.2X2	T62.2X3	T62.2X4	—	—
Gemeprost	T48.0X1	T48.0X2	T48.0X3	T48.0X4	T48.0X5	T48.0X6
Gemfibrozil	T46.6X1	T46.6X2	T46.6X3	T46.6X4	T46.6X5	T46.6X6
Gemonil	T42.3X1	T42.3X2	T42.3X3	T42.3X4	T42.3X5	T42.3X6
Gentamicin	T36.5X1	T36.5X2	T36.5X3	T36.5X4	T36.5X5	T36.5X6
ophthalmic preparation	T49.5X1	T49.5X2	T49.5X3	T49.5X4	T49.5X5	T49.5X6
topical NEC	T49.0X1	T49.0X2	T49.0X3	T49.0X4	T49.0X5	T49.0X6
Gentian	T47.5X1	T47.5X2	T47.5X3	T47.5X4	T47.5X5	T47.5X6
violet	T49.0X1	T49.0X2	T49.0X3	T49.0X4	T49.0X5	T49.0X6
Gepefrine	T44.4X1	T44.4X2	T44.4X3	T44.4X4	T44.4X5	T44.4X6
Gestonorone caproate	T38.5X1	T38.5X2	T38.5X3	T38.5X4	T38.5X5	T38.5X6
Gexane	T49.0X1	T49.0X2	T49.0X3	T49.0X4	T49.0X5	T49.0X6
Gila monster (venom)	T63.111	T63.112	T63.113	T63.114	—	—
Ginger	T47.5X1	T47.5X2	T47.5X3	T47.5X4	T47.5X5	T47.5X6
Jamaica — see Jamaica, ginger						
Gitalin	T46.0X1	T46.0X2	T46.0X3	T46.0X4	T46.0X5	T46.0X6
amorphous	T46.0X1	T46.0X2	T46.0X3	T46.0X4	T46.0X5	T46.0X6
Gitaloxin	T46.0X1	T46.0X2	T46.0X3	T46.0X4	T46.0X5	T46.0X6
Gitoxin	T46.0X1	T46.0X2	T46.0X3	T46.0X4	T46.0X5	T46.0X6
Glafenine	T39.8X1	T39.8X2	T39.8X3	T39.8X4	T39.8X5	T39.8X6
Glandular extract (medicinal) NEC	T50.Z91	T50.Z92	T50.Z93	T50.Z94	T50.Z95	T50.Z96
Glaucarubin	T37.3X1	T37.3X2	T37.3X3	T37.3X4	T37.3X5	T37.3X6
Glibenclamide	T38.3X1	T38.3X2	T38.3X3	T38.3X4	T38.3X5	T38.3X6
Glibornuride	T38.3X1	T38.3X2	T38.3X3	T38.3X4	T38.3X5	T38.3X6
Gliclazide	T38.3X1	T38.3X2	T38.3X3	T38.3X4	T38.3X5	T38.3X6
Glimidine	T38.3X1	T38.3X2	T38.3X3	T38.3X4	T38.3X5	T38.3X6
Glipizide	T38.3X1	T38.3X2	T38.3X3	T38.3X4	T38.3X5	T38.3X6
Gliquidone	T38.3X1	T38.3X2	T38.3X3	T38.3X4	T38.3X5	T38.3X6
Glisolamide	T38.3X1	T38.3X2	T38.3X3	T38.3X4	T38.3X5	T38.3X6
Glisoxepide	T38.3X1	T38.3X2	T38.3X3	T38.3X4	T38.3X5	T38.3X6
Globin zinc insulin	T38.3X1	T38.3X2	T38.3X3	T38.3X4	T38.3X5	T38.3X6
Globulin						
antilymphocytic	T50.Z11	T50.Z12	T50.Z13	T50.Z14	T50.Z15	T50.Z16
antirhesus	T50.Z11	T50.Z12	T50.Z13	T50.Z14	T50.Z15	T50.Z16
antivenin	T50.Z11	T50.Z12	T50.Z13	T50.Z14	T50.Z15	T50.Z16
antiviral	T50.Z11	T50.Z12	T50.Z13	T50.Z14	T50.Z15	T50.Z16

Substance	Poisoning, Accidental (unintentional)	Poisoning, Intentional Self-harm	Poisoning, Assault	Poisoning, Undetermined	Adverse Effect	Under-dosing
Glucagon	T38.3X1	T38.3X2	T38.3X3	T38.3X4	T38.3X5	T38.3X6
Glucocorticoids	T38.0X1	T38.0X2	T38.0X3	T38.0X4	T38.0X5	T38.0X6
Glucocorticosteroid	T38.0X1	T38.0X2	T38.0X3	T38.0X4	T38.0X5	T38.0X6
Gluconic acid	T50.991	T50.992	T50.993	T50.994	T50.995	T50.996
Glucosamine sulfate	T39.4X1	T39.4X2	T39.4X3	T39.4X4	T39.4X5	T39.4X6
Glucose	T50.3X1	T50.3X2	T50.3X3	T50.3X4	T50.3X5	T50.3X6
with sodium chloride	T50.3X1	T50.3X2	T50.3X3	T50.3X4	T50.3X5	T50.3X6
Glucosulfone sodium	T37.1X1	T37.1X2	T37.1X3	T37.1X4	T37.1X5	T37.1X6
Glucurolactone	T47.8X1	T47.8X2	T47.8X3	T47.8X4	T47.8X5	T47.8X6
Glue NEC	T52.8X1	T52.8X2	T52.8X3	T52.8X4	—	—
Glutamic acid	T47.5X1	T47.5X2	T47.5X3	T47.5X4	T47.5X5	T47.5X6
Glutaral (medicinal)	T49.0X1	T49.0X2	T49.0X3	T49.0X4	T49.0X5	T49.0X6
nonmedicinal	T65.891	T65.892	T65.893	T65.894	—	—
Glutaraldehyde (nonmedicinal)	T65.891	T65.892	T65.893	T65.894	—	—
medicinal	T49.0X1	T49.0X2	T49.0X3	T49.0X4	T49.0X5	T49.0X6
Glutathione	T50.6X1	T50.6X2	T50.6X3	T50.6X4	T50.6X5	T50.6X6
Glutethimide	T42.6X1	T42.6X2	T42.6X3	T42.6X4	T42.6X5	T42.6X6
Glyburide	T38.3X1	T38.3X2	T38.3X3	T38.3X4	T38.3X5	T38.3X6
Glycerin	T47.4X1	T47.4X2	T47.4X3	T47.4X4	T47.4X5	T47.4X6
Glycerol	T47.4X1	T47.4X2	T47.4X3	T47.4X4	T47.4X5	T47.4X6
borax	T49.6X1	T49.6X2	T49.6X3	T49.6X4	T49.6X5	T49.6X6
intravenous	T50.3X1	T50.3X2	T50.3X3	T50.3X4	T50.3X5	T50.3X6
iodinated	T48.4X1	T48.4X2	T48.4X3	T48.4X4	T48.4X5	T48.4X6
Glycerophosphate	T50.991	T50.992	T50.993	T50.994	T50.995	T50.996
Glyceryl						
gualacolate	T48.4X1	T48.4X2	T48.4X3	T48.4X4	T48.4X5	T48.4X6
nitrate	T46.3X1	T46.3X2	T46.3X3	T46.3X4	T46.3X5	T46.3X6
triacetate (topical)	T49.0X1	T49.0X2	T49.0X3	T49.0X4	T49.0X5	T49.0X6
trinitrate	T46.3X1	T46.3X2	T46.3X3	T46.3X4	T46.3X5	T46.3X6
Glycine	T50.3X1	T50.3X2	T50.3X3	T50.3X4	T50.3X5	T50.3X6
Glyclopyramide	T38.3X1	T38.3X2	T38.3X3	T38.3X4	T38.3X5	T38.3X6
Glycobiarsol	T37.3X1	T37.3X2	T37.3X3	T37.3X4	T37.3X5	T37.3X6
Glycols (ether)	T52.3X1	T52.3X2	T52.3X3	T52.3X4	—	—
Glyconiazide	T37.1X1	T37.1X2	T37.1X3	T37.1X4	T37.1X5	T37.1X6
Glycopyrrolate	T44.3X1	T44.3X2	T44.3X3	T44.3X4	T44.3X5	T44.3X6
Glycopyrronium	T44.3X1	T44.3X2	T44.3X3	T44.3X4	T44.3X5	T44.3X6
bromide	T44.3X1	T44.3X2	T44.3X3	T44.3X4	T44.3X5	T44.3X6
Glycoside, cardiac (stimulant)	T46.0X1	T46.0X2	T46.0X3	T46.0X4	T46.0X5	T46.0X6
Glycyclamide	T38.3X1	T38.3X2	T38.3X3	T38.3X4	T38.3X5	T38.3X6
Glycyrrhiza extract	T48.4X1	T48.4X2	T48.4X3	T48.4X4	T48.4X5	T48.4X6
Glycyrrhizic acid	T48.4X1	T48.4X2	T48.4X3	T48.4X4	T48.4X5	T48.4X6
Glycyrrhizinate potassium	T48.4X1	T48.4X2	T48.4X3	T48.4X4	T48.4X5	T48.4X6
Glymidine sodium	T38.3X1	T38.3X2	T38.3X3	T38.3X4	T38.3X5	T38.3X6
Glyphosate	T60.3X1	T60.3X2	T60.3X3	T60.3X4	—	—
Glyphylline	T48.6X1	T48.6X2	T48.6X3	T48.6X4	T48.6X5	T48.6X6
Gold						
colloidal (198Au)	T45.1X1	T45.1X2	T45.1X3	T45.1X4	T45.1X5	T45.1X6
salts	T39.4X1	T39.4X2	T39.4X3	T39.4X4	T39.4X5	T39.4X6
Golden sulfide of antimony	T56.891	T56.892	T56.893	T56.894	—	—
Goldylocks	T62.2X1	T62.2X2	T62.2X3	T62.2X4	—	—
Gonadal tissue extract	T38.901	T38.902	T38.903	T38.904	T38.905	T38.906
female	T38.5X1	T38.5X2	T38.5X3	T38.5X4	T38.5X5	T38.5X6
male	T38.7X1	T38.7X2	T38.7X3	T38.7X4	T38.7X5	T38.7X6
Gonadorelin	T38.891	T38.892	T38.893	T38.894	T38.895	T38.896
Gonadotropin	T38.891	T38.892	T38.893	T38.894	T38.895	T38.896
chorionic	T38.891	T38.892	T38.893	T38.894	T38.895	T38.896
pituitary	T38.811	T38.812	T38.813	T38.814	T38.815	T38.816
Goserelin	T45.1X1	T45.1X2	T45.1X3	T45.1X4	T45.1X5	T45.1X6
Grain alcohol	T51.0X1	T51.0X2	T51.0X3	T51.0X4	—	—
Gramicidin	T49.0X1	T49.0X2	T49.0X3	T49.0X4	T49.0X5	T49.0X6
Granisetron	T45.0X1	T45.0X2	T45.0X3	T45.0X4	T45.0X5	T45.0X6
Gratiola officinalis	T62.2X1	T62.2X2	T62.2X3	T62.2X4	—	—
Grease	T65.891	T65.892	T65.893	T65.894	—	—
Green hellebore	T62.2X1	T62.2X2	T62.2X3	T62.2X4	—	—
Green soap	T49.2X1	T49.2X2	T49.2X3	T49.2X4	T49.2X5	T49.2X6
Grifulvin	T36.7X1	T36.7X2	T36.7X3	T36.7X4	T36.7X5	T36.7X6
Griseofulvin	T36.7X1	T36.7X2	T36.7X3	T36.7X4	T36.7X5	T36.7X6
Growth hormone	T38.811	T38.812	T38.813	T38.814	T38.815	T38.816
Guaiacol derivatives	T48.4X1	T48.4X2	T48.4X3	T48.4X4	T48.4X5	T48.4X6
Guaiac reagent	T50.991	T50.992	T50.993	T50.994	T50.995	T50.996
Guaifenesin	T48.4X1	T48.4X2	T48.4X3	T48.4X4	T48.4X5	T48.4X6
Guaimesal	T48.4X1	T48.4X2	T48.4X3	T48.4X4	T48.4X5	T48.4X6
Guaiphenesin	T48.4X1	T48.4X2	T48.4X3	T48.4X4	T48.4X5	T48.4X6
Guamecycline	T36.4X1	T36.4X2	T36.4X3	T36.4X4	T36.4X5	T36.4X6
Guanabenz	T46.5X1	T46.5X2	T46.5X3	T46.5X4	T46.5X5	T46.5X6
Guanacline	T46.5X1	T46.5X2	T46.5X3	T46.5X4	T46.5X5	T46.5X6
Guanadrel	T46.5X1	T46.5X2	T46.5X3	T46.5X4	T46.5X5	T46.5X6
Guanatol	T37.2X1	T37.2X2	T37.2X3	T37.2X4	T37.2X5	T37.2X6
Guanethidine	T46.5X1	T46.5X2	T46.5X3	T46.5X4	T46.5X5	T46.5X6
Guanfacine	T46.5X1	T46.5X2	T46.5X3	T46.5X4	T46.5X5	T46.5X6
Guano	T65.891	T65.892	T65.893	T65.894	—	—
Guanochlor	T46.5X1	T46.5X2	T46.5X3	T46.5X4	T46.5X5	T46.5X6
Guanoclor	T46.5X1	T46.5X2	T46.5X3	T46.5X4	T46.5X5	T46.5X6
Guanoctine	T46.5X1	T46.5X2	T46.5X3	T46.5X4	T46.5X5	T46.5X6
Guanoxabenz	T46.5X1	T46.5X2	T46.5X3	T46.5X4	T46.5X5	T46.5X6
Guanoxan	T46.5X1	T46.5X2	T46.5X3	T46.5X4	T46.5X5	T46.5X6
Guar gum (medicinal)	T46.6X1	T46.6X2	T46.6X3	T46.6X4	T46.6X5	T46.6X6
Hachimycin	T36.7X1	T36.7X2	T36.7X3	T36.7X4	T36.7X5	T36.7X6
Hair						
dye	T49.4X1	T49.4X2	T49.4X3	T49.4X4	T49.4X5	T49.4X6
preparation NEC	T49.4X1	T49.4X2	T49.4X3	T49.4X4	T49.4X5	T49.4X6
Halazepam	T42.4X1	T42.4X2	T42.4X3	T42.4X4	T42.4X5	T42.4X6
Halcinolone	T49.0X1	T49.0X2	T49.0X3	T49.0X4	T49.0X5	T49.0X6
Halcinonide	T49.0X1	T49.0X2	T49.0X3	T49.0X4	T49.0X5	T49.0X6
Halethazole	T49.0X1	T49.0X2	T49.0X3	T49.0X4	T49.0X5	T49.0X6
Hallucinogen NEC	T40.901	T40.902	T40.903	T40.904	T40.905	T40.906
Halofantrine	T37.2X1	T37.2X2	T37.2X3	T37.2X4	T37.2X5	T37.2X6
Halofenate	T46.6X1	T46.6X2	T46.6X3	T46.6X4	T46.6X5	T46.6X6
Halometasone	T49.0X1	T49.0X2	T49.0X3	T49.0X4	T49.0X5	T49.0X6
Haloperidol	T43.4X1	T43.4X2	T43.4X3	T43.4X4	T43.4X5	T43.4X6
Haloprogin	T49.0X1	T49.0X2	T49.0X3	T49.0X4	T49.0X5	T49.0X6
Halotex	T49.0X1	T49.0X2	T49.0X3	T49.0X4	T49.0X5	T49.0X6
Halothane	T41.0X1	T41.0X2	T41.0X3	T41.0X4	T41.0X5	T41.0X6
Haloxazolam	T42.4X1	T42.4X2	T42.4X3	T42.4X4	T42.4X5	T42.4X6
Halquinols	T49.0X1	T49.0X2	T49.0X3	T49.0X4	T49.0X5	T49.0X6
Hamamelis	T49.2X1	T49.2X2	T49.2X3	T49.2X4	T49.2X5	T49.2X6
Haptendextran	T45.8X1	T45.8X2	T45.8X3	T45.8X4	T45.8X5	T45.8X6
Harmonyl	T46.5X1	T46.5X2	T46.5X3	T46.5X4	T46.5X5	T46.5X6
Hartmann's solution	T50.3X1	T50.3X2	T50.3X3	T50.3X4	T50.3X5	T50.3X6
Hashish	T40.7X1	T40.7X2	T40.7X3	T40.7X4	T40.7X5	T40.7X6
Hawaiian Woodrose seeds	T40.991	T40.992	T40.993	T40.994	—	—
HCB	T60.3X1	T60.3X2	T60.3X3	T60.3X4	—	—
HCH	T53.6X1	T53.6X2	T53.6X3	T53.6X4	—	—
medicinal	T49.0X1	T49.0X2	T49.0X3	T49.0X4	T49.0X5	T49.0X6
HCN	T57.3X1	T57.3X2	T57.3X3	T57.3X4	—	—
Headache cures, drugs, powders NEC	T50.901	T50.902	T50.903	T50.904	T50.905	T50.906
Heavenly Blue (morning glory)	T40.991	T40.992	T40.993	T40.994	—	—
Heavy metal antidote	T45.8X1	T45.8X2	T45.8X3	T45.8X4	T45.8X5	T45.8X6
Hedaquinium	T49.0X1	T49.0X2	T49.0X3	T49.0X4	T49.0X5	T49.0X6
Hedge hyssop	T62.2X1	T62.2X2	T62.2X3	T62.2X4	—	—
Heet	T49.8X1	T49.8X2	T49.8X3	T49.8X4	T49.8X5	T49.8X6
Helenin	T37.4X1	T37.4X2	T37.4X3	T37.4X4	T37.4X5	T37.4X6
Helium (nonmedicinal) NEC	T59.891	T59.892	T59.893	T59.894	—	—
medicinal	T48.991	T48.992	T48.993	T48.994	T48.995	T48.996
Hellebore (black) (green) (white)	T62.2X1	T62.2X2	T62.2X3	T62.2X4	—	—
Hematin	T45.8X1	T45.8X2	T45.8X3	T45.8X4	T45.8X5	T45.8X6
Hematinic preparation	T45.8X1	T45.8X2	T45.8X3	T45.8X4	T45.8X5	T45.8X6
Hematological agent	T45.91	T45.92	T45.93	T45.94	T45.95	T45.96
specified NEC	T45.8X1	T45.8X2	T45.8X3	T45.8X4	T45.8X5	T45.8X6
Hemlock	T62.2X1	T62.2X2	T62.2X3	T62.2X4	—	—
Hemostatic	T45.621	T45.622	T45.623	T45.624	T45.625	T45.626
drug, systemic	T45.621	T45.622	T45.623	T45.624	T45.625	T45.626
Hemostyptic	T49.4X1	T49.4X2	T49.4X3	T49.4X4	T49.4X5	T49.4X6
Henbane	T62.2X1	T62.2X2	T62.2X3	T62.2X4	—	—
Heparin (sodium)	T45.511	T45.512	T45.513	T45.514	T45.515	T45.516
action reverser	T45.7X1	T45.7X2	T45.7X3	T45.7X4	T45.7X5	T45.7X6
Heparin-fraction	T45.511	T45.512	T45.513	T45.514	T45.515	T45.516
Heparinoid (systemic)	T45.511	T45.512	T45.513	T45.514	T45.515	T45.516
Hepatic secretion stimulant	T47.8X1	T47.8X2	T47.8X3	T47.8X4	T47.8X5	T47.8X6
Hepatitis B						
immune globulin	T50.Z11	T50.Z12	T50.Z13	T50.Z14	T50.Z15	T50.Z16
vaccine	T50.B91	T50.B92	T50.B93	T50.B94	T50.B95	T50.B96
Hepronicate	T46.7X1	T46.7X2	T46.7X3	T46.7X4	T46.7X5	T46.7X6
Heptabarb	T42.3X1	T42.3X2	T42.3X3	T42.3X4	T42.3X5	T42.3X6
Heptabarbital	T42.3X1	T42.3X2	T42.3X3	T42.3X4	T42.3X5	T42.3X6
Heptabarbitone	T42.3X1	T42.3X2	T42.3X3	T42.3X4	T42.3X5	T42.3X6
Heptachlor	T60.1X1	T60.1X2	T60.1X3	T60.1X4	—	—
Heptalgin	T40.2X1	T40.2X2	T40.2X3	T40.2X4	T40.2X5	T40.2X6
Heptaminol	T46.3X1	T46.3X2	T46.3X3	T46.3X4	T46.3X5	T46.3X6
Herbicide NEC	T60.3X1	T60.3X2	T60.3X3	T60.3X4	—	—
Heroin	T40.1X1	T40.1X2	T40.1X3	T40.1X4	—	—
Herplex	T49.5X1	T49.5X2	T49.5X3	T49.5X4	T49.5X5	T49.5X6
HES	T45.8X1	T45.8X2	T45.8X3	T45.8X4	T45.8X5	T45.8X6
Hesperidin	T46.991	T46.992	T46.993	T46.994	T46.995	T46.996
Hetacillin	T36.0X1	T36.0X2	T36.0X3	T36.0X4	T36.0X5	T36.0X6
Hetastarch	T45.8X1	T45.8X2	T45.8X3	T45.8X4	T45.8X5	T45.8X6
HETP	T60.0X1	T60.0X2	T60.0X3	T60.0X4	—	—
Hexachlorobenzene (vapor)	T60.3X1	T60.3X2	T60.3X3	T60.3X4	—	—
Hexachlorocyclohexane	T53.6X1	T53.6X2	T53.6X3	T53.6X4	—	—
Hexachlorophene	T49.0X1	T49.0X2	T49.0X3	T49.0X4	T49.0X5	T49.0X6

Table of Drugs and Chemicals

Hexadiline — Hydroxyprogesterone

Substance	Poisoning, Accidental (unintentional)	Poisoning, Intentional Self-harm	Poisoning, Assault	Poisoning, Undetermined	Adverse Effect	Under-dosing
Hexadiline	T46.3X1	T46.3X2	T46.3X3	T46.3X4	T46.3X5	T46.3X6
Hexadimethrine (bromide)	T45.7X1	T45.7X2	T45.7X3	T45.7X4	T45.7X5	T45.7X6
Hexadylamine	T46.3X1	T46.3X2	T46.3X3	T46.3X4	T46.3X5	T46.3X6
Hexaethyl tetraphosphate	T60.0X1	T60.0X2	T60.0X3	T60.0X4	—	—
Hexafluorenium bromide	T48.1X1	T48.1X2	T48.1X3	T48.1X4	T48.1X5	T48.1X6
Hexafluronium (bromide)	T48.1X1	T48.1X2	T48.1X3	T48.1X4	T48.1X5	T48.1X6
Hexa-germ	T49.2X1	T49.2X2	T49.2X3	T49.2X4	T49.2X5	T49.2X6
Hexahydrobenzol	T52.8X1	T52.8X2	T52.8X3	T52.8X4	—	—
Hexahydrocresol(s)	T51.8X1	T51.8X2	T51.8X3	T51.8X4	—	—
arsenide	T57.0X1	T57.0X2	T57.0X3	T57.0X4	—	—
arseniurated	T57.0X1	T57.0X2	T57.0X3	T57.0X4	—	—
cyanide	T57.3X1	T57.3X2	T57.3X3	T57.3X4	—	—
gas	T59.891	T59.892	T59.893	T59.894	—	—
Fluoride (liquid)	T57.8X1	T57.8X2	T57.8X3	T57.8X4	—	—
vapor	T59.891	T59.892	T59.893	T59.894	—	—
phophorated	T60.0X1	T60.0X2	T60.0X3	T60.0X4	—	—
sulfate	T57.8X1	T57.8X2	T57.8X3	T57.8X4	—	—
sulfide (gas)	T59.6X1	T59.6X2	T59.6X3	T59.6X4	—	—
arseniurated	T57.0X1	T57.0X2	T57.0X3	T57.0X4	—	—
sulfurated	T57.8X1	T57.8X2	T57.8X3	T57.8X4	—	—
Hexahydrophenol	T51.8X1	T51.8X2	T51.8X3	T51.8X4	—	—
Hexalen	T51.8X1	T51.8X2	T51.8X3	T51.8X4	—	—
Hexamethonium bromide	T44.2X1	T44.2X2	T44.2X3	T44.2X4	T44.2X5	T44.2X6
Hexamethylene	T52.8X1	T52.8X2	T52.8X3	T52.8X4	—	—
Hexamethylmelamine	T45.1X1	T45.1X2	T45.1X3	T45.1X4	T45.1X5	T45.1X6
Hexamidine	T49.0X1	T49.0X2	T49.0X3	T49.0X4	T49.0X5	T49.0X6
Hexamine (mandelate)	T37.8X1	T37.8X2	T37.8X3	T37.8X4	T37.8X5	T37.8X6
Hexanone, 2-hexanone	T52.4X1	T52.4X2	T52.4X3	T52.4X4	—	—
Hexanuorenium	T48.1X1	T48.1X2	T48.1X3	T48.1X4	T48.1X5	T48.1X6
Hexapropymate	T42.6X1	T42.6X2	T42.6X3	T42.6X4	T42.6X5	T42.6X6
Hexasonium iodide	T44.3X1	T44.3X2	T44.3X3	T44.3X4	T44.3X5	T44.3X6
Hexcarbacholine bromide	T48.1X1	T48.1X2	T48.1X3	T48.1X4	T48.1X5	T48.1X6
Hexemal	T42.3X1	T42.3X2	T42.3X3	T42.3X4	T42.3X5	T42.3X6
Hexestrol	T38.5X1	T38.5X2	T38.5X3	T38.5X4	T38.5X5	T38.5X6
Hexethal (sodium)	T42.3X1	T42.3X2	T42.3X3	T42.3X4	T42.3X5	T42.3X6
Hexetidine	T37.8X1	T37.8X2	T37.8X3	T37.8X4	T37.8X5	T37.8X6
Hexobarbital	T42.3X1	T42.3X2	T42.3X3	T42.3X4	T42.3X5	T42.3X6
rectal	T41.291	T41.292	T41.293	T41.294	T41.295	T41.296
sodium	T41.1X1	T41.1X2	T41.1X3	T41.1X4	T41.1X5	T41.1X6
Hexobendine	T46.3X1	T46.3X2	T46.3X3	T46.3X4	T46.3X5	T46.3X6
Hexocyclium	T44.3X1	T44.3X2	T44.3X3	T44.3X4	T44.3X5	T44.3X6
metilsulfate	T44.3X1	T44.3X2	T44.3X3	T44.3X4	T44.3X5	T44.3X6
Hexoestrol	T38.5X1	T38.5X2	T38.5X3	T38.5X4	T38.5X5	T38.5X6
Hexone	T52.4X1	T52.4X2	T52.4X3	T52.4X4	—	—
Hexoprenaline	T48.6X1	T48.6X2	T48.6X3	T48.6X4	T48.6X5	T48.6X6
Hexylcaine	T41.3X1	T41.3X2	T41.3X3	T41.3X4	T41.3X5	T41.3X6
Hexylresorcinol	T52.2X1	T52.2X2	T52.2X3	T52.2X4	—	—
HGH (human growth hormone)	T38.811	T38.812	T38.813	T38.814	T38.815	T38.816
Hinkle's pills	T47.2X1	T47.2X2	T47.2X3	T47.2X4	T47.2X5	T47.2X6
Histalog	T50.8X1	T50.8X2	T50.8X3	T50.8X4	T50.8X5	T50.8X6
Histamine (phosphate)	T50.8X1	T50.8X2	T50.8X3	T50.8X4	T50.8X5	T50.8X6
Histoplasmin	T50.8X1	T50.8X2	T50.8X3	T50.8X4	T50.8X5	T50.8X6
Holly berries	T62.2X1	T62.2X2	T62.2X3	T62.2X4	—	—
Homatropine	T44.3X1	T44.3X2	T44.3X3	T44.3X4	T44.3X5	T44.3X6
methylbromide	T44.3X1	T44.3X2	T44.3X3	T44.3X4	T44.3X5	T44.3X6
Homochlorcyclizine	T45.0X1	T45.0X2	T45.0X3	T45.0X4	T45.0X5	T45.0X6
Homosalate	T49.3X1	T49.3X2	T49.3X3	T49.3X4	T49.3X5	T49.3X6
Homo-tet	T50.Z11	T50.Z12	T50.Z13	T50.Z14	T50.Z15	T50.Z16
Hormone	T38.801	T38.802	T38.803	T38.804	T38.805	T38.806
adrenal cortical steroids	T38.0X1	T38.0X2	T38.0X3	T38.0X4	T38.0X5	T38.0X6
androgenic	T38.7X1	T38.7X2	T38.7X3	T38.7X4	T38.7X5	T38.7X6
anterior pituitary NEC	T38.811	T38.813	T38.814	T38.815	T38.816	
antidiabetic agents	T38.3X1	T38.3X2	T38.3X3	T38.3X4	T38.3X5	T38.3X6
antidiuretic	T38.891	T38.892	T38.893	T38.894	T38.895	T38.896
cancer therapy	T45.1X1	T45.1X2	T45.1X3	T45.1X4	T45.1X5	T45.1X6
follicle stimulating	T38.811	T38.812	T38.813	T38.814	T38.815	T38.816
gonadotropic	T38.891	T38.892	T38.893	T38.894	T38.895	T38.896
pituitary	T38.811	T38.812	T38.813	T38.814	T38.815	T38.816
growth	T38.811	T38.812	T38.813	T38.814	T38.815	T38.816
luteinizing	T38.811	T38.812	T38.813	T38.814	T38.815	T38.816
ovarian	T38.5X1	T38.5X2	T38.5X3	T38.5X4	T38.5X5	T38.5X6
oxytocic	T48.0X1	T48.0X2	T48.0X3	T48.0X4	T48.0X5	T48.0X6
parathyroid (derivatives)	T50.991	T50.992	T50.993	T50.994	T50.995	T50.996
pituitary (posterior) NEC	T38.891	T38.892	T38.893	T38.894	T38.895	T38.896
anterior	T38.811	T38.812	T38.813	T38.814	T38.815	T38.816
specified, NEC	T38.891	T38.892	T38.893	T38.894	T38.895	T38.896
thyroid	T38.1X1	T38.1X2	T38.1X3	T38.1X4	T38.1X5	T38.1X6
Hornet (sting)	T63.451	T63.452	T63.453	T63.454	—	—
Horse anti-human lymphocytic serum	T50.Z11	T50.Z12	T50.Z13	T50.Z14	T50.Z15	T50.Z16
Horticulture agent NEC	T65.91	T65.92	T65.93	T65.94	—	—
with pesticide	T60.91	T60.92	T60.93	T60.94	—	—
Human						
albumin	T45.8X1	T45.8X2	T45.8X3	T45.8X4	T45.8X5	T45.8X6
growth hormone (HGH)	T38.811	T38.812	T38.813	T38.814	T38.815	T38.816
immune serum	T50.Z11	T50.Z12	T50.Z13	T50.Z14	T50.Z15	T50.Z16
Hyaluronidase	T45.3X1	T45.3X2	T45.3X3	T45.3X4	T45.3X5	T45.3X6
Hyazyme	T45.3X1	T45.3X2	T45.3X3	T45.3X4	T45.3X5	T45.3X6
Hycodan	T40.2X1	T40.2X2	T40.2X3	T40.2X4	T40.2X5	T40.2X6
Hydantoin derivative NEC	T42.0X1	T42.0X2	T42.0X3	T42.0X4	T42.0X5	T42.0X6
Hydeltra	T38.0X1	T38.0X2	T38.0X3	T38.0X4	T38.0X5	T38.0X6
Hydergine	T44.6X1	T44.6X2	T44.6X3	T44.6X4	T44.6X5	T44.6X6
Hydrabamine penicillin	T36.0X1	T36.0X2	T36.0X3	T36.0X4	T36.0X5	T36.0X6
Hydralazine	T46.5X1	T46.5X2	T46.5X3	T46.5X4	T46.5X5	T46.5X6
Hydrargaphen	T49.0X1	T49.0X2	T49.0X3	T49.0X4	T49.0X5	T49.0X6
Hydrargyri aminochloridum	T49.0X1	T49.0X2	T49.0X3	T49.0X4	T49.0X5	T49.0X6
Hydrastine	T48.291	T48.292	T48.293	T48.294	T48.295	T48.296
Hydrazine	T54.1X1	T54.1X2	T54.1X3	T54.1X4	—	—
monoamine oxidase inhibitors	T43.1X1	T43.1X2	T43.1X3	T43.1X4	T43.1X5	T43.1X6
Hydrazoic acid, azides	T54.2X1	T54.2X2	T54.2X3	T54.2X4	—	—
Hydriodic acid	T48.4X1	T48.4X2	T48.4X3	T48.4X4	T48.4X5	T48.4X6
Hydrocarbon gas	T59.891	T59.892	T59.893	T59.894	—	—
incomplete combustion of — see Carbon, monoxide, fuel, utility						
liquefied (mobile container)	T59.891	T59.892	T59.893	T59.894	—	—
piped (natural)	T59.891	T59.892	T59.893	T59.894	—	—
Hydrochloric acid (liquid)	T54.2X1	T54.2X2	T54.2X3	T54.2X4	—	—
medicinal (digestant)	T47.5X1	T47.5X2	T47.5X3	T47.5X4	T47.5X5	T47.5X6
vapor	T59.891	T59.892	T59.893	T59.894	—	—
Hydrochlorothiazide	T50.2X1	T50.2X2	T50.2X3	T50.2X4	T50.2X5	T50.2X6
Hydrocodone	T40.2X1	T40.2X2	T40.2X3	T40.2X4	T40.2X5	T40.2X6
Hydrocortisone (derivatives)	T38.0X1	T38.0X2	T38.0X3	T38.0X4	T38.0X5	T38.0X6
aceponate	T49.0X1	T49.0X2	T49.0X3	T49.0X4	T49.0X5	T49.0X6
ENT agent	T49.6X1	T49.6X2	T49.6X3	T49.6X4	T49.6X5	T49.6X6
ophthalmic preparation	T49.5X1	T49.5X2	T49.5X3	T49.5X4	T49.5X5	T49.5X6
topical NEC	T49.0X1	T49.0X2	T49.0X3	T49.0X4	T49.0X5	T49.0X6
Hydrocortone	T38.0X1	T38.0X2	T38.0X3	T38.0X4	T38.0X5	T38.0X6
ENT agent	T49.6X1	T49.6X2	T49.6X3	T49.6X4	T49.6X5	T49.6X6
ophthalmic preparation	T49.5X1	T49.5X2	T49.5X3	T49.5X4	T49.5X5	T49.5X6
topical NEC	T49.0X1	T49.0X2	T49.0X3	T49.0X4	T49.0X5	T49.0X6
Hydrocyanic acid (liquid)	T57.3X1	T57.3X2	T57.3X3	T57.3X4	—	—
gas	T65.0X1	T65.0X2	T65.0X3	T65.0X4	—	—
Hydroflumethiazide	T50.2X1	T50.2X2	T50.2X3	T50.2X4	T50.2X5	T50.2X6
Hydrofluoric acid (liquid)	T54.2X1	T54.2X2	T54.2X3	T54.2X4	—	—
vapor	T59.891	T59.892	T59.893	T59.894	—	—
Hydrogen	T59.891	T59.892	T59.893	T59.894	—	—
arsenide	T57.0X1	T57.0X2	T57.0X3	T57.0X4	—	—
arseniureted	T57.0X1	T57.0X2	T57.0X3	T57.0X4	—	—
chloride	T57.8X1	T57.8X2	T57.8X3	T57.8X4	—	—
cyanide (salts)	T57.3X1	T57.3X2	T57.3X3	T57.3X4	—	—
gas	T57.3X1	T57.3X2	T57.3X3	T57.3X4	—	—
Fluoride	T59.5X1	T59.5X2	T59.5X3	T59.5X4	—	—
vapor	T59.5X1	T59.5X2	T59.5X3	T59.5X4	—	—
peroxide	T49.0X1	T49.0X2	T49.0X3	T49.0X4	T49.0X5	T49.0X6
phosphureted	T57.1X1	T57.1X2	T57.1X3	T57.1X4	—	—
sulfide	T59.6X1	T59.6X2	T59.6X3	T59.6X4	—	—
arseniureted	T57.0X1	T57.0X2	T57.0X3	T57.0X4	—	—
sulfureted	T59.6X1	T59.6X2	T59.6X3	T59.6X4	—	—
Hydromethylpyridine	T46.7X1	T46.7X2	T46.7X3	T46.7X4	T46.7X5	T46.7X6
Hydromorphinol	T40.2X1	T40.2X2	T40.2X3	T40.2X4	—	—
Hydromorphinone	T40.2X1	T40.2X2	T40.2X3	T40.2X4	T40.2X5	T40.2X6
Hydromorphone	T40.2X1	T40.2X2	T40.2X3	T40.2X4	T40.2X5	T40.2X6
Hydromox	T50.2X1	T50.2X2	T50.2X3	T50.2X4	T50.2X5	T50.2X6
Hydrophilic lotion	T49.3X1	T49.3X2	T49.3X3	T49.3X4	T49.3X5	T49.3X6
Hydroquinidine	T46.2X1	T46.2X2	T46.2X3	T46.2X4	T46.2X5	T46.2X6
Hydroquinone	T52.2X1	T52.2X2	T52.2X3	T52.2X4	—	—
vapor	T59.891	T59.892	T59.893	T59.894	—	—
Hydrosulfuric acid (gas)	T59.6X1	T59.6X2	T59.6X3	T59.6X4	—	—
Hydrotalcite	T47.1X1	T47.1X2	T47.1X3	T47.1X4	T47.1X5	T47.1X6
Hydrous wool fat	T49.3X1	T49.3X2	T49.3X3	T49.3X4	T49.3X5	T49.3X6
Hydroxide, caustic	T54.3X1	T54.3X2	T54.3X3	T54.3X4	—	—
Hydroxocobalamin	T45.8X1	T45.8X2	T45.8X3	T45.8X4	T45.8X5	T45.8X6
Hydroxyamphetamine	T49.5X1	T49.5X2	T49.5X3	T49.5X4	T49.5X5	T49.5X6
Hydroxycarbamide	T45.1X1	T45.1X2	T45.1X3	T45.1X4	T45.1X5	T45.1X6
Hydroxychloroquine	T37.8X1	T37.8X2	T37.8X3	T37.8X4	T37.8X5	T37.8X6
Hydroxydihydrocodeinone	T40.2X1	T40.2X2	T40.2X3	T40.2X4	T40.2X5	T40.2X6
Hydroxyestrone	T38.5X1	T38.5X2	T38.5X3	T38.5X4	T38.5X5	T38.5X6
Hydroxyethyl starch	T45.8X1	T45.8X2	T45.8X3	T45.8X4	T45.8X5	T45.8X6
Hydroxymethylpentanone	T52.4X1	T52.4X2	T52.4X3	T52.4X4	—	—
Hydroxyphenamate	T43.591	T43.592	T43.593	T43.594	T43.595	T43.596
Hydroxyphenylbutazone	T39.2X1	T39.2X2	T39.2X3	T39.2X4	T39.2X5	T39.2X6
Hydroxyprogesterone	T38.5X1	T38.5X2	T38.5X3	T38.5X4	T38.5X5	T38.5X6

Additional Character May Be Required — Refer to the Tabular List for Character Selection ▽ Subterms under main terms may continue to next column or page

Substance	Poisoning, Accidental (unintentional)	Poisoning, Intentional Self-harm	Poisoning, Assault	Poisoning, Undetermined	Adverse Effect	Under-dosing
Hydroxyprogesterone — continued						
caproate	T38.5X1	T38.5X2	T38.5X3	T38.5X4	T38.5X5	T38.5X6
Hydroxyquinoline (derivatives) NEC	T37.8X1	T37.8X2	T37.8X3	T37.8X4	T37.8X5	T37.8X6
Hydroxystilbamidine	T37.3X1	T37.3X2	T37.3X3	T37.3X4	T37.3X5	T37.3X6
Hydroxytoluene (nonmedicinal)	T54.0X1	T54.0X2	T54.0X3	T54.0X4	—	—
medicinal	T49.0X1	T49.0X2	T49.0X3	T49.0X4	T49.0X5	T49.0X6
Hydroxyurea	T45.1X1	T45.1X2	T45.1X3	T45.1X4	T45.1X5	T45.1X6
Hydroxyzine	T43.591	T43.592	T43.593	T43.594	T43.595	T43.596
Hyoscine	T44.3X1	T44.3X2	T44.3X3	T44.3X4	T44.3X5	T44.3X6
Hyoscyamine	T44.3X1	T44.3X2	T44.3X3	T44.3X4	T44.3X5	T44.3X6
Hyoscyamus	T44.3X1	T44.3X2	T44.3X3	T44.3X4	T44.3X5	T44.3X6
dry extract	T44.3X1	T44.3X2	T44.3X3	T44.3X4	T44.3X5	T44.3X6
Hypaque	T50.8X1	T50.8X2	T50.8X3	T50.8X4	T50.8X5	T50.8X6
Hypertussis	T50.Z11	T50.Z12	T50.Z13	T50.Z14	T50.Z15	T50.Z16
Hypnotic	T42.71	T42.72	T42.73	T42.74	T42.75	T42.76
anticonvulsant	T42.71	T42.72	T42.73	T42.74	T42.75	T42.76
specified NEC	T42.6X1	T42.6X2	T42.6X3	T42.6X4	T42.6X5	T42.6X6
Hypochlorite	T49.0X1	T49.0X2	T49.0X3	T49.0X4	T49.0X5	T49.0X6
Hypophysis, posterior	T38.891	T38.892	T38.893	T38.894	T38.895	T38.896
Hypotensive NEC	T46.5X1	T46.5X2	T46.5X3	T46.5X4	T46.5X5	T46.5X6
Hypromellose	T49.5X1	T49.5X2	T49.5X3	T49.5X4	T49.5X5	T49.5X6
Ibacitabine	T37.5X1	T37.5X2	T37.5X3	T37.5X4	T37.5X5	T37.5X6
Ibopamine	T44.991	T44.992	T44.993	T44.994	T44.995	T44.996
Ibufenac	T39.311	T39.312	T39.313	T39.314	T39.315	T39.316
Ibuprofen	T39.311	T39.312	T39.313	T39.314	T39.315	T39.316
Ibuproxam	T39.311	T39.312	T39.313	T39.314	T39.315	T39.316
Ibuterol	T48.6X1	T48.6X2	T48.6X3	T48.6X4	T48.6X5	T48.6X6
Ichthammol	T49.0X1	T49.0X2	T49.0X3	T49.0X4	T49.0X5	T49.0X6
Ichthyol	T49.4X1	T49.4X2	T49.4X3	T49.4X4	T49.4X5	T49.4X6
Idarubicin	T45.1X1	T45.1X2	T45.1X3	T45.1X4	T45.1X5	T45.1X6
Idrocilamide	T42.8X1	T42.8X2	T42.8X3	T42.8X4	T42.8X5	T42.8X6
Ifenprodil	T46.7X1	T46.7X2	T46.7X3	T46.7X4	T46.7X5	T46.7X6
Ifosfamide	T45.1X1	T45.1X2	T45.1X3	T45.1X4	T45.1X5	T45.1X6
Iletin	T38.3X1	T38.3X2	T38.3X3	T38.3X4	T38.3X5	T38.3X6
Ilex	T62.2X1	T62.2X2	T62.2X3	T62.2X4	—	—
Illuminating gas (after combustion)	T58.11	T58.12	T58.13	T58.14	—	—
prior to combustion	T59.891	T59.892	T59.893	T59.894	—	—
Ilopan	T45.2X1	T45.2X2	T45.2X3	T45.2X4	T45.2X5	T45.2X6
Iloprost	T46.7X1	T46.7X2	T46.7X3	T46.7X4	T46.7X5	T46.7X6
Ilotycin	T36.3X1	T36.3X2	T36.3X3	T36.3X4	T36.3X5	T36.3X6
ophthalmic preparation	T49.5X1	T49.5X2	T49.5X3	T49.5X4	T49.5X5	T49.5X6
topical NEC	T49.0X1	T49.0X2	T49.0X3	T49.0X4	T49.0X5	T49.0X6
Imidazole-4-carboxamide	T45.1X1	T45.1X2	T45.1X3	T45.1X4	T45.1X5	T45.1X6
Iminostilbene	T42.1X1	T42.1X2	T42.1X3	T42.1X4	T42.1X5	T42.1X6
Imipenem	T36.0X1	T36.0X2	T36.0X3	T36.0X4	T36.0X5	T36.0X6
Imipramine	T43.011	T43.012	T43.013	T43.014	T43.015	T43.016
Immu-G	T50.Z11	T50.Z12	T50.Z13	T50.Z14	T50.Z15	T50.Z16
Immuglobin	T50.Z11	T50.Z12	T50.Z13	T50.Z14	T50.Z15	T50.Z16
Immune						
globulin	T50.Z11	T50.Z12	T50.Z13	T50.Z14	T50.Z15	T50.Z16
serum globulin	T50.Z11	T50.Z12	T50.Z13	T50.Z14	T50.Z15	T50.Z16
Immunoglobin human	T50.Z11	T50.Z12	T50.Z13	T50.Z14	T50.Z15	T50.Z16
(intravenous) (normal)						
unmodified	T50.Z11	T50.Z12	T50.Z13	T50.Z14	T50.Z15	T50.Z16
Immunosuppressive drug	T45.1X1	T45.1X2	T45.1X3	T45.1X4	T45.1X5	T45.1X6
Immu-tetanus	T50.Z11	T50.Z12	T50.Z13	T50.Z14	T50.Z15	T50.Z16
Indalpine	T43.221	T43.222	T43.223	T43.224	T43.225	T43.226
Indanazoline	T48.5X1	T48.5X2	T48.5X3	T48.5X4	T48.5X5	T48.5X6
Indandione (derivatives)	T45.511	T45.512	T45.513	T45.514	T45.515	T45.516
Indapamide	T46.5X1	T46.5X2	T46.5X3	T46.5X4	T46.5X5	T46.5X6
Indendione (derivatives)	T45.511	T45.512	T45.513	T45.514	T45.515	T45.516
Indenolol	T44.7X1	T44.7X2	T44.7X3	T44.7X4	T44.7X5	T44.7X6
Inderal	T44.7X1	T44.7X2	T44.7X3	T44.7X4	T44.7X5	T44.7X6
Indian						
hemp	T40.7X1	T40.7X2	T40.7X3	T40.7X4	T40.7X5	T40.7X6
tobacco	T62.2X1	T62.2X2	T62.2X3	T62.2X4	—	—
Indigo carmine	T50.8X1	T50.8X2	T50.8X3	T50.8X4	T50.8X5	T50.8X6
Indobufen	T45.521	T45.522	T45.523	T45.524	T45.525	T45.526
Indocin	T39.2X1	T39.2X2	T39.2X3	T39.2X4	T39.2X5	T39.2X6
Indocyanine green	T50.8X1	T50.8X2	T50.8X3	T50.8X4	T50.8X5	T50.8X6
Indometacin	T39.391	T39.392	T39.393	T39.394	T39.395	T39.396
Indomethacin	T39.391	T39.392	T39.393	T39.394	T39.395	T39.396
farnesil	T39.4X1	T39.4X2	T39.4X3	T39.4X4	T39.4X5	T39.4X6
Indoramin	T44.6X1	T44.6X2	T44.6X3	T44.6X4	T44.6X5	T44.6X6
Industrial						
alcohol	T51.0X1	T51.0X2	T51.0X3	T51.0X4	—	—
fumes	T59.891	T59.892	T59.893	T59.894	—	—
solvents (fumes) (vapors)	T52.91	T52.92	T52.93	T52.94	—	—
Influenza vaccine	T50.B91	T50.B92	T50.B93	T50.B94	T50.B95	T50.B96

Substance	Poisoning, Accidental (unintentional)	Poisoning, Intentional Self-harm	Poisoning, Assault	Poisoning, Undetermined	Adverse Effect	Under-dosing
Ingested substance NEC	T65.91	T65.92	T65.93	T65.94	—	—
INH	T37.1X1	T37.1X2	T37.1X3	T37.1X4	T37.1X5	T37.1X6
Inhalation, gas (noxious) — see Gas						
Inhibitor						
angiotensin-converting enzyme	T46.4X1	T46.4X2	T46.4X3	T46.4X4	T46.4X5	T46.4X6
carbonic anhydrase	T50.2X1	T50.2X2	T50.2X3	T50.2X4	T50.2X5	T50.2X6
fibrinolysis	T45.621	T45.622	T45.623	T45.624	T45.625	T45.626
monoamine oxidase NEC	T43.1X1	T43.1X2	T43.1X3	T43.1X4	T43.1X5	T43.1X6
hydrazine	T43.1X1	T43.1X2	T43.1X3	T43.1X4	T43.1X5	T43.1X6
postsynaptic	T43.8X1	T43.8X2	T43.8X3	T43.8X4	T43.8X5	T43.8X6
prothrombin synthesis	T45.511	T45.512	T45.513	T45.514	T45.515	T45.516
Ink	T65.891	T65.892	T65.893	T65.894	—	—
Inorganic substance NEC	T57.91	T57.92	T57.93	T57.94	—	—
Inosine pranobex	T37.5X1	T37.5X2	T37.5X3	T37.5X4	T37.5X5	T37.5X6
Inositol	T50.991	T50.992	T50.993	T50.994	T50.995	T50.996
nicotinate	T46.7X1	T46.7X2	T46.7X3	T46.7X4	T46.7X5	T46.7X6
Inproquone	T45.1X1	T45.1X2	T45.1X3	T45.1X4	T45.1X5	T45.1X6
Insecticide NEC	T60.91	T60.92	T60.93	T60.94	—	—
carbamate	T60.0X1	T60.0X2	T60.0X3	T60.0X4	—	—
chlorinated	T60.1X1	T60.1X2	T60.1X3	T60.1X4	—	—
mixed	T60.91	T60.92	T60.93	T60.94	—	—
organochlorine	T60.1X1	T60.1X2	T60.1X3	T60.1X4	—	—
organophosphorus	T60.0X1	T60.0X2	T60.0X3	T60.0X4	—	—
Insect (sting), venomous	T63.481	T63.482	T63.483	T63.484	—	—
ant	T63.421	T63.422	T63.423	T63.424	—	—
bee	T63.441	T63.442	T63.443	T63.444	—	—
caterpillar	T63.431	T63.432	T63.433	T63.434	—	—
hornet	T63.451	T63.452	T63.453	T63.454	—	—
wasp	T63.461	T63.462	T63.463	T63.464	—	—
Insular tissue extract	T38.3X1	T38.3X2	T38.3X3	T38.3X4	T38.3X5	T38.3X6
Insulin (amorphous) (globin) (isophane) (Lente) (NPH) (Semilente) (Ultralente)	T38.3X1	T38.3X2	T38.3X3	T38.3X4	T38.3X5	T38.3X6
defalan	T38.3X1	T38.3X2	T38.3X3	T38.3X4	T38.3X5	T38.3X6
human	T38.3X1	T38.3X2	T38.3X3	T38.3X4	T38.3X5	T38.3X6
injection, soluble	T38.3X1	T38.3X2	T38.3X3	T38.3X4	T38.3X5	T38.3X6
biphasic	T38.3X1	T38.3X2	T38.3X3	T38.3X4	T38.3X5	T38.3X6
intermediate acting	T38.3X1	T38.3X2	T38.3X3	T38.3X4	T38.3X5	T38.3X6
protamine zinc	T38.3X1	T38.3X2	T38.3X3	T38.3X4	T38.3X5	T38.3X6
slow acting	T38.3X1	T38.3X2	T38.3X3	T38.3X4	T38.3X5	T38.3X6
zinc						
protamine injection	T38.3X1	T38.3X2	T38.3X3	T38.3X4	T38.3X5	T38.3X6
suspension (amorphous) (crystalline)	T38.3X1	T38.3X2	T38.3X3	T38.3X4	T38.3X5	T38.3X6
Interferon (alpha) (beta) (gamma)	T37.5X1	T37.5X2	T37.5X3	T37.5X4	T37.5X5	T37.5X6
Intestinal motility control drug	T47.6X1	T47.6X2	T47.6X3	T47.6X4	T47.6X5	T47.6X6
biological	T47.8X1	T47.8X2	T47.8X3	T47.8X4	T47.8X5	T47.8X6
Intranarcon	T41.1X1	T41.1X2	T41.1X3	T41.1X4	T41.1X5	T41.1X6
Intravenous						
amino acids	T50.991	T50.992	T50.993	T50.994	T50.995	T50.996
fat suspension	T50.991	T50.992	T50.993	T50.994	T50.995	T50.996
Inulin	T50.8X1	T50.8X2	T50.8X3	T50.8X4	T50.8X5	T50.8X6
Invert sugar	T50.3X1	T50.3X2	T50.3X3	T50.3X4	T50.3X5	T50.3X6
Inza — see Naproxen						
Iobenzamic acid	T50.8X1	T50.8X2	T50.8X3	T50.8X4	T50.8X5	T50.8X6
Iocarmic acid	T50.8X1	T50.8X2	T50.8X3	T50.8X4	T50.8X5	T50.8X6
Iocetamic acid	T50.8X1	T50.8X2	T50.8X3	T50.8X4	T50.8X5	T50.8X6
Iodamide	T50.8X1	T50.8X2	T50.8X3	T50.8X4	T50.8X5	T50.8X6
Iodide NEC — see also Iodine	T49.0X1	T49.0X2	T49.0X3	T49.0X4	T49.0X5	T49.0X6
mercury (ointment)	T49.0X1	T49.0X2	T49.0X3	T49.0X4	T49.0X5	T49.0X6
methylate	T49.0X1	T49.0X2	T49.0X3	T49.0X4	T49.0X5	T49.0X6
potassium (expectorant) NEC	T48.4X1	T48.4X2	T48.4X3	T48.4X4	T48.4X5	T48.4X6
Iodinated						
contrast medium	T50.8X1	T50.8X2	T50.8X3	T50.8X4	T50.8X5	T50.8X6
glycerol	T48.4X1	T48.4X2	T48.4X3	T48.4X4	T48.4X5	T48.4X6
human serum albumin (131I)	T50.8X1	T50.8X2	T50.8X3	T50.8X4	T50.8X5	T50.8X6
Iodine (antiseptic, external) (tincture) NEC	T49.0X1	T49.0X2	T49.0X3	T49.0X4	T49.0X5	T49.0X6
125 — see also Radiation sickness, and Exposure to radioactive isotopes						
therapeutic	T50.8X1	T50.8X2	T50.8X3	T50.8X4	T50.8X5	T50.8X6
131 — see also Radiation sickness, and Exposure to radioactive isotopes	T50.991	T50.992	T50.993	T50.994	T50.995	T50.996
therapeutic	T38.2X1	T38.2X2	T38.2X3	T38.2X4	T38.2X5	T38.2X6
diagnostic	T50.8X1	T50.8X2	T50.8X3	T50.8X4	T50.8X5	T50.8X6

Substance	Poisoning, Accidental (unintentional)	Poisoning, Intentional Self-harm	Poisoning, Assault	Poisoning, Undetermined	Adverse Effect	Under-dosing
Iodine (antiseptic, external) (tincture) **NEC** — *continued*						
for thyroid conditions (antithyroid)	T38.2X1	T38.2X2	T38.2X3	T38.2X4	T38.2X5	T38.2X6
solution	T49.0X1	T49.0X2	T49.0X3	T49.0X4	T49.0X5	T49.0X6
vapor	T59.891	T59.892	T59.893	T59.894	—	—
Iodipamide	T50.8X1	T50.8X2	T50.8X3	T50.8X4	T50.8X5	T50.8X6
Iodized (poppy seed) oil	T50.8X1	T50.8X2	T50.8X3	T50.8X4	T50.8X5	T50.8X6
Iodobismitol	T37.8X1	T37.8X2	T37.8X3	T37.8X4	T37.8X5	T37.8X6
Iodochlorhydroxyquin	T37.8X1	T37.8X2	T37.8X3	T37.8X4	T37.8X5	T37.8X6
topical	T49.0X1	T49.0X2	T49.0X3	T49.0X4	T49.0X5	T49.0X6
Iodochlorhydroxyquinoline	T37.8X1	T37.8X2	T37.8X3	T37.8X4	T37.8X5	T37.8X6
Iodocholesterol (131I)	T50.8X1	T50.8X2	T50.8X3	T50.8X4	T50.8X5	T50.8X6
Iodoform	T49.0X1	T49.0X2	T49.0X3	T49.0X4	T49.0X5	T49.0X6
Iodohippuric acid	T50.8X1	T50.8X2	T50.8X3	T50.8X4	T50.8X5	T50.8X6
Iodopanoic acid	T50.8X1	T50.8X2	T50.8X3	T50.8X4	T50.8X5	T50.8X6
Iodophthalein (sodium)	T50.8X1	T50.8X2	T50.8X3	T50.8X4	T50.8X5	T50.8X6
Iodopyracet	T50.8X1	T50.8X2	T50.8X3	T50.8X4	T50.8X5	T50.8X6
Iodoquinol	T37.8X1	T37.8X2	T37.8X3	T37.8X4	T37.8X5	T37.8X6
Iodoxamic acid	T50.8X1	T50.8X2	T50.8X3	T50.8X4	T50.8X5	T50.8X6
Iofendylate	T50.8X1	T50.8X2	T50.8X3	T50.8X4	T50.8X5	T50.8X6
Ioglycamic acid	T50.8X1	T50.8X2	T50.8X3	T50.8X4	T50.8X5	T50.8X6
Iohexol	T50.8X1	T50.8X2	T50.8X3	T50.8X4	T50.8X5	T50.8X6
Ion exchange resin						
anion	T47.8X1	T47.8X2	T47.8X3	T47.8X4	T47.8X5	T47.8X6
cation	T50.3X1	T50.3X2	T50.3X3	T50.3X4	T50.3X5	T50.3X6
cholestyramine	T46.6X1	T46.6X2	T46.6X3	T46.6X4	T46.6X5	T46.6X6
intestinal	T47.8X1	T47.8X2	T47.8X3	T47.8X4	T47.8X5	T47.8X6
Iopamidol	T50.8X1	T50.8X2	T50.8X3	T50.8X4	T50.8X5	T50.8X6
Iopanoic acid	T50.8X1	T50.8X2	T50.8X3	T50.8X4	T50.8X5	T50.8X6
Iophenoic acid	T50.8X1	T50.8X2	T50.8X3	T50.8X4	T50.8X5	T50.8X6
Iopodate, sodium	T50.8X1	T50.8X2	T50.8X3	T50.8X4	T50.8X5	T50.8X6
Iopodic acid	T50.8X1	T50.8X2	T50.8X3	T50.8X4	T50.8X5	T50.8X6
Iopromide	T50.8X1	T50.8X2	T50.8X3	T50.8X4	T50.8X5	T50.8X6
Iopydol	T50.8X1	T50.8X2	T50.8X3	T50.8X4	T50.8X5	T50.8X6
Iotalamic acid	T50.8X1	T50.8X2	T50.8X3	T50.8X4	T50.8X5	T50.8X6
Iothalamate	T50.8X1	T50.8X2	T50.8X3	T50.8X4	T50.8X5	T50.8X6
Iothiouracil	T38.2X1	T38.2X2	T38.2X3	T38.2X4	T38.2X5	T38.2X6
Iotrol	T50.8X1	T50.8X2	T50.8X3	T50.8X4	T50.8X5	T50.8X6
Iotrolan	T50.8X1	T50.8X2	T50.8X3	T50.8X4	T50.8X5	T50.8X6
Iotroxate	T50.8X1	T50.8X2	T50.8X3	T50.8X4	T50.8X5	T50.8X6
Iotroxic acid	T50.8X1	T50.8X2	T50.8X3	T50.8X4	T50.8X5	T50.8X6
Ioversol	T50.8X1	T50.8X2	T50.8X3	T50.8X4	T50.8X5	T50.8X6
Ioxaglate	T50.8X1	T50.8X2	T50.8X3	T50.8X4	T50.8X5	T50.8X6
Ioxaglic acid	T50.8X1	T50.8X2	T50.8X3	T50.8X4	T50.8X5	T50.8X6
Ioxitalamic acid	T50.8X1	T50.8X2	T50.8X3	T50.8X4	T50.8X5	T50.8X6
Ipecac	T47.7X1	T47.7X2	T47.7X3	T47.7X4	T47.7X5	T47.7X6
Ipecacuanha	T48.4X1	T48.4X2	T48.4X3	T48.4X4	T48.4X5	T48.4X6
Ipodate, calcium	T50.8X1	T50.8X2	T50.8X3	T50.8X4	T50.8X5	T50.8X6
Ipral	T42.3X1	T42.3X2	T42.3X3	T42.3X4	T42.3X5	T42.3X6
Ipratropium (bromide)	T48.6X1	T48.6X2	T48.6X3	T48.6X4	T48.6X5	T48.6X6
Ipriflavone	T46.3X1	T46.3X2	T46.3X3	T46.3X4	T46.3X5	T46.3X6
Iprindole	T43.011	T43.012	T43.013	T43.014	T43.015	T43.016
Iproclozide	T43.1X1	T43.1X2	T43.1X3	T43.1X4	T43.1X5	T43.1X6
Iprofenin	T50.8X1	T50.8X2	T50.8X3	T50.8X4	T50.8X5	T50.8X6
Iproheptine	T49.2X1	T49.2X2	T49.2X3	T49.2X4	T49.2X5	T49.2X6
Iproniazid	T43.1X1	T43.1X2	T43.1X3	T43.1X4	T43.1X5	T43.1X6
Iproplatin	T45.1X1	T45.1X2	T45.1X3	T45.1X4	T45.1X5	T45.1X6
Iproveratril	T46.1X1	T46.1X2	T46.1X3	T46.1X4	T46.1X5	T46.1X6
Iron (compounds) (medicinal) **NEC**	T45.4X1	T45.4X2	T45.4X3	T45.4X4	T45.4X5	T45.4X6
ammonium	T45.4X1	T45.4X2	T45.4X3	T45.4X4	T45.4X5	T45.4X6
dextran injection	T45.4X1	T45.4X2	T45.4X3	T45.4X4	T45.4X5	T45.4X6
nonmedicinal	T56.891	T56.892	T56.893	T56.894	—	—
salts	T45.4X1	T45.4X2	T45.4X3	T45.4X4	T45.4X5	T45.4X6
sorbitex	T45.4X1	T45.4X2	T45.4X3	T45.4X4	T45.4X5	T45.4X6
sorbitol citric acid complex	T45.4X1	T45.4X2	T45.4X3	T45.4X4	T45.4X5	T45.4X6
Irrigating fluid (vaginal)	T49.8X1	T49.8X2	T49.8X3	T49.8X4	T49.8X5	T49.8X6
eye	T49.5X1	T49.5X2	T49.5X3	T49.5X4	T49.5X5	T49.5X6
Isepamicin	T36.5X1	T36.5X2	T36.5X3	T36.5X4	T36.5X5	T36.5X6
Isoamnile (citrate)	T48.3X1	T48.3X2	T48.3X3	T48.3X4	T48.3X5	T48.3X6
Isoamyl nitrite	T46.3X1	T46.3X2	T46.3X3	T46.3X4	T46.3X5	T46.3X6
Isobenzan	T60.1X1	T60.1X2	T60.1X3	T60.1X4		
Isobutyl acetate	T52.8X1	T52.8X2	T52.8X3	T52.8X4	—	—
Isocarboxazid	T43.1X1	T43.1X2	T43.1X3	T43.1X4	T43.1X5	T43.1X6
Isoconazole	T49.0X1	T49.0X2	T49.0X3	T49.0X4	T49.0X5	T49.0X6
Isocyanate	T65.0X1	T65.0X2	T65.0X3	T65.0X4	—	—
Isoephedrine	T44.991	T44.992	T44.993	T44.994	T44.995	T44.996
Isoetarine	T48.6X1	T48.6X2	T48.6X3	T48.6X4	T48.6X5	T48.6X6
Isoethadione	T42.2X1	T42.2X2	T42.2X3	T42.2X4	T42.2X5	T42.2X6
Isoetharine	T44.5X1	T44.5X2	T44.5X3	T44.5X4	T44.5X5	T44.5X6
Isoflurane	T41.0X1	T41.0X2	T41.0X3	T41.0X4	T41.0X5	T41.0X6
Isoflurophate	T44.0X1	T44.0X2	T44.0X3	T44.0X4	T44.0X5	T44.0X6

Substance	Poisoning, Accidental (unintentional)	Poisoning, Intentional Self-harm	Poisoning, Assault	Poisoning, Undetermined	Adverse Effect	Under-dosing
Isomaltose, ferric complex	T45.4X1	T45.4X2	T45.4X3	T45.4X4	T45.4X5	T45.4X6
Isometheptene	T44.3X1	T44.3X2	T44.3X3	T44.3X4	T44.3X5	T44.3X6
Isoniazid	T37.1X1	T37.1X2	T37.1X3	T37.1X4	T37.1X5	T37.1X6
with						
rifampicin	T36.6X1	T36.6X2	T36.6X3	T36.6X4	T36.6X5	T36.6X6
thioacetazone	T37.1X1	T37.1X2	T37.1X3	T37.1X4	T37.1X5	T37.1X6
Isonicotinic acid hydrazide	T37.1X1	T37.1X2	T37.1X3	T37.1X4	T37.1X5	T37.1X6
Isonipecaine	T40.4X1	T40.4X2	T40.4X3	T40.4X4	T40.4X5	T40.4X6
Isopentaquine	T37.2X1	T37.2X2	T37.2X3	T37.2X4	T37.2X5	T37.2X6
Isophane insulin	T38.3X1	T38.3X2	T38.3X3	T38.3X4	T38.3X5	T38.3X6
Isophorone	T65.891	T65.892	T65.893	T65.894	—	—
Isophosphamide	T45.1X1	T45.1X2	T45.1X3	T45.1X4	T45.1X5	T45.1X6
Isopregnenone	T38.5X1	T38.5X2	T38.5X3	T38.5X4	T38.5X5	T38.5X6
Isoprenaline	T48.6X1	T48.6X2	T48.6X3	T48.6X4	T48.6X5	T48.6X6
Isopromethazine	T43.3X1	T43.3X2	T43.3X3	T43.3X4	T43.3X5	T43.3X6
Isopropamide	T44.3X1	T44.3X2	T44.3X3	T44.3X4	T44.3X5	T44.3X6
iodide	T44.3X1	T44.3X2	T44.3X3	T44.3X4	T44.3X5	T44.3X6
Isopropanol	T51.2X1	T51.2X2	T51.2X3	T51.2X4	—	—
Isopropyl						
acetate	T52.8X1	T52.8X2	T52.8X3	T52.8X4	—	—
alcohol	T51.2X1	T51.2X2	T51.2X3	T51.2X4	—	—
medicinal	T49.4X1	T49.4X2	T49.4X3	T49.4X4	T49.4X5	T49.4X6
ether	T52.8X1	T52.8X2	T52.8X3	T52.8X4	—	—
Isopropylaminophenazone	T39.2X1	T39.2X2	T39.2X3	T39.2X4	T39.2X5	T39.2X6
Isoproterenol	T48.6X1	T48.6X2	T48.6X3	T48.6X4	T48.6X5	T48.6X6
Isosorbide dinitrate	T46.3X1	T46.3X2	T46.3X3	T46.3X4	T46.3X5	T46.3X6
Isothipendyl	T45.0X1	T45.0X2	T45.0X3	T45.0X4	T45.0X5	T45.0X6
Isotretinoin	T50.991	T50.992	T50.993	T50.994	T50.995	T50.996
Isoxazolyl penicillin	T36.0X1	T36.0X2	T36.0X3	T36.0X4	T36.0X5	T36.0X6
Isoxicam	T39.391	T39.392	T39.393	T39.394	T39.395	T39.396
Isoxsuprine	T46.7X1	T46.7X2	T46.7X3	T46.7X4	T46.7X5	T46.7X6
Ispagula	T47.4X1	T47.4X2	T47.4X3	T47.4X4	T47.4X5	T47.4X6
husk	T47.4X1	T47.4X2	T47.4X3	T47.4X4	T47.4X5	T47.4X6
Isradipine	T46.1X1	T46.1X2	T46.1X3	T46.1X4	T46.1X5	T46.1X6
l-thyroxine sodium	T38.1X1	T38.1X2	T38.1X3	T38.1X4	T38.1X5	T38.1X6
Itraconazole	T37.8X1	T37.8X2	T37.8X3	T37.8X4	T37.8X5	T37.8X6
Itramin tosilate	T46.3X1	T46.3X2	T46.3X3	T46.3X4	T46.3X5	T46.3X6
Ivermectin	T37.4X1	T37.4X2	T37.4X3	T37.4X4	T37.4X5	T37.4X6
Izoniazid	T37.1X1	T37.1X2	T37.1X3	T37.1X4	T37.1X5	T37.1X6
with thioacetazone	T37.1X1	T37.1X2	T37.1X3	T37.1X4	T37.1X5	T37.1X6
Jalap	T47.2X1	T47.2X2	T47.2X3	T47.2X4	T47.2X5	T47.2X6
Jamaica						
dogwood (bark)	T39.8X1	T39.8X2	T39.8X3	T39.8X4	T39.8X5	T39.8X6
ginger	T65.891	T65.892	T65.893	T65.894	—	—
root	T62.2X1	T62.2X2	T62.2X3	T62.2X4	—	—
Jatropha	T62.2X1	T62.2X2	T62.2X3	T62.2X4	—	—
curcas	T62.2X1	T62.2X2	T62.2X3	T62.2X4	—	—
Jectofer	T45.4X1	T45.4X2	T45.4X3	T45.4X4	T45.4X5	T45.4X6
Jellyfish (sting)	T63.621	T63.622	T63.623	T63.624	—	—
Jequirity (bean)	T62.2X1	T62.2X2	T62.2X3	T62.2X4	—	—
Jimson weed (stramonium)	T62.2X1	T62.2X2	T62.2X3	T62.2X4	—	—
seeds	T62.2X1	T62.2X2	T62.2X3	T62.2X4	—	—
Josamycin	T36.3X1	T36.3X2	T36.3X3	T36.3X4	T36.3X5	T36.3X6
Juniper tar	T49.1X1	T49.1X2	T49.1X3	T49.1X4	T49.1X5	T49.1X6
Kallidinogenase	T46.7X1	T46.7X2	T46.7X3	T46.7X4	T46.7X5	T46.7X6
Kallikrein	T46.7X1	T46.7X2	T46.7X3	T46.7X4	T46.7X5	T46.7X6
Kanamycin	T36.5X1	T36.5X2	T36.5X3	T36.5X4	T36.5X5	T36.5X6
Kantrex	T36.5X1	T36.5X2	T36.5X3	T36.5X4	T36.5X5	T36.5X6
Kaolin	T47.6X1	T47.6X2	T47.6X3	T47.6X4	T47.6X5	T47.6X6
light	T47.6X1	T47.6X2	T47.6X3	T47.6X4	T47.6X5	T47.6X6
Karaya (gum)	T47.4X1	T47.4X2	T47.4X3	T47.4X4	T47.4X5	T47.4X6
Kebuzone	T39.2X1	T39.2X2	T39.2X3	T39.2X4	T39.2X5	T39.2X6
Kelevan	T60.1X1	T60.1X2	T60.1X3	T60.1X4	—	—
Kemithal	T41.1X1	T41.1X2	T41.1X3	T41.1X4	T41.1X5	T41.1X6
Kenacort	T38.0X1	T38.0X2	T38.0X3	T38.0X4	T38.0X5	T38.0X6
Keratolytic drug NEC	T49.4X1	T49.4X2	T49.4X3	T49.4X4	T49.4X5	T49.4X6
anthracene	T49.4X1	T49.4X2	T49.4X3	T49.4X4	T49.4X5	T49.4X6
Keratoplastic NEC	T49.4X1	T49.4X2	T49.4X3	T49.4X4	T49.4X5	T49.4X6
Kerosene, kerosine (fuel) (solvent) **NEC**	T52.0X1	T52.0X2	T52.0X3	T52.0X4	—	—
insecticide	T52.0X1	T52.0X2	T52.0X3	T52.0X4	—	—
vapor	T52.0X1	T52.0X2	T52.0X3	T52.0X4	—	—
Ketamine	T41.291	T41.292	T41.293	T41.294	T41.295	T41.296
Ketazolam	T42.4X1	T42.4X2	T42.4X3	T42.4X4	T42.4X5	T42.4X6
Ketazon	T39.2X1	T39.2X2	T39.2X3	T39.2X4	T39.2X5	T39.2X6
Ketobemidone	T40.4X1	T40.4X2	T40.4X3	T40.4X4	—	—
Ketoconazole	T49.0X1	T49.0X2	T49.0X3	T49.0X4	T49.0X5	T49.0X6
Ketols	T52.4X1	T52.4X2	T52.4X3	T52.4X4	—	—
Ketone oils	T52.4X1	T52.4X2	T52.4X3	T52.4X4	—	—
Ketoprofen	T39.311	T39.312	T39.313	T39.314	T39.315	T39.316
Ketorolac	T39.8X1	T39.8X2	T39.8X3	T39.8X4	T39.8X5	T39.8X6
Ketotifen	T45.0X1	T45.0X2	T45.0X3	T45.0X4	T45.0X5	T45.0X6
Khat	T43.691	T43.692	T43.693	T43.694	—	—

Substance	Poisoning, Accidental (unintentional)	Poisoning, Intentional Self-harm	Poisoning, Assault	Poisoning, Undetermined	Adverse Effect	Under-dosing
Khellin	T46.3X1	T46.3X2	T46.3X3	T46.3X4	T46.3X5	T46.3X6
Khelloside	T46.3X1	T46.3X2	T46.3X3	T46.3X4	T46.3X5	T46.3X6
Kiln gas or vapor (carbon monoxide)	T58.8X1	T58.8X2	T58.8X3	T58.8X4	—	—
Kitasamycin	T36.3X1	T36.3X2	T36.3X3	T36.3X4	T36.3X5	T36.3X6
Konsyl	T47.4X1	T47.4X2	T47.4X3	T47.4X4	T47.4X5	T47.4X6
Kosam seed	T62.2X1	T62.2X2	T62.2X3	T62.2X4	—	—
Krait (venom)	T63.091	T63.092	T63.093	T63.094	—	—
Kwell (insecticide)	T60.1X1	T60.1X2	T60.1X3	T60.1X4	—	—
anti-infective (topical)	T49.0X1	T49.0X2	T49.0X3	T49.0X4	T49.0X5	T49.0X6
Labetalol	T44.8X1	T44.8X2	T44.8X3	T44.8X4	T44.8X5	T44.8X6
Laburnum (seeds)	T62.2X1	T62.2X2	T62.2X3	T62.2X4	—	—
leaves	T62.2X1	T62.2X2	T62.2X3	T62.2X4	—	—
Lachesine	T49.5X1	T49.5X2	T49.5X3	T49.5X4	T49.5X5	T49.5X6
Lacidipine	T46.5X1	T46.5X2	T46.5X3	T46.5X4	T46.5X5	T46.5X6
Lacquer	T65.6X1	T65.6X2	T65.6X3	T65.6X4	—	—
Lacrimogenic gas	T59.3X1	T59.3X2	T59.3X3	T59.3X4	—	—
Lactated potassic saline	T50.3X1	T50.3X2	T50.3X3	T50.3X4	T50.3X5	T50.3X6
Lactic acid	T49.8X1	T49.8X2	T49.8X3	T49.8X4	T49.8X5	T49.8X6
Lactobacillus						
acidophilus	T47.6X1	T47.6X2	T47.6X3	T47.6X4	T47.6X5	T47.6X6
compound	T47.6X1	T47.6X2	T47.6X3	T47.6X4	T47.6X5	T47.6X6
bifidus, lyophilized	T47.6X1	T47.6X2	T47.6X3	T47.6X4	T47.6X5	T47.6X6
bulgaricus	T47.6X1	T47.6X2	T47.6X3	T47.6X4	T47.6X5	T47.6X6
sporogenes	T47.6X1	T47.6X2	T47.6X3	T47.6X4	T47.6X5	T47.6X6
Lactoflavin	T45.2X1	T45.2X2	T45.2X3	T45.2X4	T45.2X5	T45.2X6
Lactose (as excipient)	T50.901	T50.902	T50.903	T50.904	T50.905	T50.906
Lactuca (virosa) (extract)	T42.6X1	T42.6X2	T42.6X3	T42.6X4	T42.6X5	T42.6X6
Lactucarium	T42.6X1	T42.6X2	T42.6X3	T42.6X4	T42.6X5	T42.6X6
Lactulose	T47.3X1	T47.3X2	T47.3X3	T47.3X4	T47.3X5	T47.3X6
Laevo — see Levo-						
Lanatosides	T46.0X1	T46.0X2	T46.0X3	T46.0X4	T46.0X5	T46.0X6
Lanolin	T49.3X1	T49.3X2	T49.3X3	T49.3X4	T49.3X5	T49.3X6
Largactil	T43.3X1	T43.3X2	T43.3X3	T43.3X4	T43.3X5	T43.3X6
Larkspur	T62.2X1	T62.2X2	T62.2X3	T62.2X4	—	—
Laroxyl	T43.011	T43.012	T43.013	T43.014	T43.015	T43.016
Lasix	T50.1X1	T50.1X2	T50.1X3	T50.1X4	T50.1X5	T50.1X6
Lassar's paste	T49.4X1	T49.4X2	T49.4X3	T49.4X4	T49.4X5	T49.4X6
Latamoxef	T36.1X1	T36.1X2	T36.1X3	T36.1X4	T36.1X5	T36.1X6
Latex	T65.811	T65.812	T65.813	T65.814	—	—
Lathyrus (seed)	T62.2X1	T62.2X2	T62.2X3	T62.2X4	—	—
Laudanum	T40.0X1	T40.0X2	T40.0X3	T40.0X4	T40.0X5	T40.0X6
Laudexium	T48.1X1	T48.1X2	T48.1X3	T48.1X4	T48.1X5	T48.1X6
Laughing gas	T41.0X1	T41.0X2	T41.0X3	T41.0X4	T41.0X5	T41.0X6
Laurel, black or cherry	T62.2X1	T62.2X2	T62.2X3	T62.2X4	—	—
Laurolinium	T49.0X1	T49.0X2	T49.0X3	T49.0X4	T49.0X5	T49.0X6
Lauryl sulfoacetate	T49.2X1	T49.2X2	T49.2X3	T49.2X4	T49.2X5	T49.2X6
Laxative NEC	T47.4X1	T47.4X2	T47.4X3	T47.4X4	T47.4X5	T47.4X6
osmotic	T47.3X1	T47.3X2	T47.3X3	T47.3X4	T47.3X5	T47.3X6
saline	T47.3X1	T47.3X2	T47.3X3	T47.3X4	T47.3X5	T47.3X6
stimulant	T47.2X1	T47.2X2	T47.2X3	T47.2X4	T47.2X5	T47.2X6
L-dopa	T42.8X1	T42.8X2	T42.8X3	T42.8X4	T42.8X5	T42.8X6
Lead (dust) (fumes) (vapor)	T56.0X1	T56.0X2	T56.0X3	T56.0X4	—	—
NEC						
acetate	T49.2X1	T49.2X2	T49.2X3	T49.2X4	T49.2X5	T49.2X6
alkyl (fuel additive)	T56.0X1	T56.0X2	T56.0X3	T56.0X4	—	—
anti-infectives	T37.8X1	T37.8X2	T37.8X3	T37.8X4	T37.8X5	T37.8X6
antiknock compound (tetraethyl)	T56.0X1	T56.0X2	T56.0X3	T56.0X4	—	—
arsenate, arsenite (dust)(herbicide)(insecticide) (vapor)	T57.0X1	T57.0X2	T57.0X3	T57.0X4		
carbonate	T56.0X1	T56.0X2	T56.0X3	T56.0X4	—	—
paint	T56.0X1	T56.0X2	T56.0X3	T56.0X4	—	—
chromate	T56.0X1	T56.0X2	T56.0X3	T56.0X4	—	—
paint	T56.0X1	T56.0X2	T56.0X3	T56.0X4	—	—
dioxide	T56.0X1	T56.0X2	T56.0X3	T56.0X4	—	—
inorganic	T56.0X1	T56.0X2	T56.0X3	T56.0X4	—	—
iodide	T56.0X1	T56.0X2	T56.0X3	T56.0X4	—	—
pigment (paint)	T56.0X1	T56.0X2	T56.0X3	T56.0X4	—	—
monoxide (dust)	T56.0X1	T56.0X2	T56.0X3	T56.0X4	—	—
paint	T56.0X1	T56.0X2	T56.0X3	T56.0X4	—	—
organic	T56.0X1	T56.0X2	T56.0X3	T56.0X4	—	—
oxide	T56.0X1	T56.0X2	T56.0X3	T56.0X4	—	—
paint	T56.0X1	T56.0X2	T56.0X3	T56.0X4	—	—
paint	T56.0X1	T56.0X2	T56.0X3	T56.0X4	—	—
salts	T56.0X1	T56.0X2	T56.0X3	T56.0X4	—	—
specified compound NEC	T56.0X1	T56.0X2	T56.0X3	T56.0X4	—	—
tetra-ethyl	T56.0X1	T56.0X2	T56.0X3	T56.0X4	—	—
Lebanese red	T40.7X1	T40.7X2	T40.7X3	T40.7X4	T40.7X5	T40.7X6
Lefetamine	T39.8X1	T39.8X2	T39.8X3	T39.8X4	T39.8X5	T39.8X6
Lenperone	T43.4X1	T43.4X2	T43.4X3	T43.4X4	T43.4X5	T43.4X6
Lente lietin (insulin)	T38.3X1	T38.3X2	T38.3X3	T38.3X4	T38.3X5	T38.3X6

Substance	Poisoning, Accidental (unintentional)	Poisoning, Intentional Self-harm	Poisoning, Assault	Poisoning, Undetermined	Adverse Effect	Under-dosing
Leptazol	T50.7X1	T50.7X2	T50.7X3	T50.7X4	T50.7X5	T50.7X6
Leptophos	T60.0X1	T60.0X2	T60.0X3	T60.0X4	—	—
Leritine	T40.2X1	T40.2X2	T40.2X3	T40.2X4	T40.2X5	T40.2X6
Letosteine	T48.4X1	T48.4X2	T48.4X3	T48.4X4	T48.4X5	T48.4X6
Letter	T38.1X1	T38.1X2	T38.1X3	T38.1X4	T38.1X5	T38.1X6
Lettuce opium	T42.6X1	T42.6X2	T42.6X3	T42.6X4	T42.6X5	T42.6X6
Leucinocaine	T41.3X1	T41.3X2	T41.3X3	T41.3X4	T41.3X5	T41.3X6
Leucocianidol	T46.991	T46.992	T46.993	T46.994	T46.995	T46.996
Leucovorin (factor)	T45.8X1	T45.8X2	T45.8X3	T45.8X4	T45.8X5	T45.8X6
Leukeran	T45.1X1	T45.1X2	T45.1X3	T45.1X4	T45.1X5	T45.1X6
Leuprolide	T38.891	T38.892	T38.893	T38.894	T38.895	T38.896
Levalbuterol	T48.6X1	T48.6X2	T48.6X3	T48.6X4	T48.6X5	T48.6X6
Levallorphan	T50.7X1	T50.7X2	T50.7X3	T50.7X4	T50.7X5	T50.7X6
Levamisole	T37.4X1	T37.4X2	T37.4X3	T37.4X4	T37.4X5	T37.4X6
Levanil	T42.6X1	T42.6X2	T42.6X3	T42.6X4	T42.6X5	T42.6X6
Levarterenol	T44.4X1	T44.4X2	T44.4X3	T44.4X4	T44.4X5	T44.4X6
Levdropropizine	T48.3X1	T48.3X2	T48.3X3	T48.3X4	T48.3X5	T48.3X6
Levobunolol	T49.5X1	T49.5X2	T49.5X3	T49.5X4	T49.5X5	T49.5X6
Levocabastine (hydrochloride)	T45.0X1	T45.0X2	T45.0X3	T45.0X4	T45.0X5	T45.0X6
Levocarnitine	T50.991	T50.992	T50.993	T50.994	T50.995	T50.996
Levodopa	T42.8X1	T42.8X2	T42.8X3	T42.8X4	T42.8X5	T42.8X6
with carbidopa	T42.8X1	T42.8X2	T42.8X3	T42.8X4	T42.8X5	T42.8X6
Levo-dromoran	T40.2X1	T40.2X2	T40.2X3	T40.2X4	T40.2X5	T40.2X6
Levoglutamide	T50.991	T50.992	T50.993	T50.994	T50.995	T50.996
Levoid	T38.1X1	T38.1X2	T38.1X3	T38.1X4	T38.1X5	T38.1X6
Levo-isomethadone	T40.3X1	T40.3X2	T40.3X3	T40.3X4	T40.3X5	T40.3X6
Levomepromazine	T43.3X1	T43.3X2	T43.3X3	T43.3X4	T43.3X5	T43.3X6
Levonordefrin	T49.6X1	T49.6X2	T49.6X3	T49.6X4	T49.6X5	T49.6X6
Levonorgestrel	T38.4X1	T38.4X2	T38.4X3	T38.4X4	T38.4X5	T38.4X6
with ethinylestradiol	T38.5X1	T38.5X2	T38.5X3	T38.5X4	T38.5X5	T38.5X6
Levopromazine	T43.3X1	T43.3X2	T43.3X3	T43.3X4	T43.3X5	T43.3X6
Levoprome	T42.6X1	T42.6X2	T42.6X3	T42.6X4	T42.6X5	T42.6X6
Levopropoxyphene	T40.4X1	T40.4X2	T40.4X3	T40.4X4	T40.4X5	T40.4X6
Levopropylhexedrine	T50.5X1	T50.5X2	T50.5X3	T50.5X4	T50.5X5	T50.5X6
Levoproxyphylline	T48.6X1	T48.6X2	T48.6X3	T48.6X4	T48.6X5	T48.6X6
Levorphanol	T40.4X1	T40.4X2	T40.4X3	T40.4X4	T40.4X5	T40.4X6
Levothyroxine	T38.1X1	T38.1X2	T38.1X3	T38.1X4	T38.1X5	T38.1X6
sodium	T38.1X1	T38.1X2	T38.1X3	T38.1X4	T38.1X5	T38.1X6
Levsin	T44.3X1	T44.3X2	T44.3X3	T44.3X4	T44.3X5	T44.3X6
Levulose	T50.3X1	T50.3X2	T50.3X3	T50.3X4	T50.3X5	T50.3X6
Lewisite (gas), not in war	T57.0X1	T57.0X2	T57.0X3	T57.0X4	—	—
Librium	T42.4X1	T42.4X2	T42.4X3	T42.4X4	T42.4X5	T42.4X6
Lidex	T49.0X1	T49.0X2	T49.0X3	T49.0X4	T49.0X5	T49.0X6
Lidocaine	T41.3X1	T41.3X2	T41.3X3	T41.3X4	T41.3X5	T41.3X6
regional	T41.3X1	T41.3X2	T41.3X3	T41.3X4	T41.3X5	T41.3X6
spinal	T41.3X1	T41.3X2	T41.3X3	T41.3X4	T41.3X5	T41.3X6
Lidofenin	T50.8X1	T50.8X2	T50.8X3	T50.8X4	T50.8X5	T50.8X6
Lidoflazine	T46.1X1	T46.1X2	T46.1X3	T46.1X4	T46.1X5	T46.1X6
Lighter fluid	T52.0X1	T52.0X2	T52.0X3	T52.0X4	—	—
Lignin hemicellulose	T47.6X1	T47.6X2	T47.6X3	T47.6X4	T47.6X5	T47.6X6
Lignocaine	T41.3X1	T41.3X2	T41.3X3	T41.3X4	T41.3X5	T41.3X6
regional	T41.3X1	T41.3X2	T41.3X3	T41.3X4	T41.3X5	T41.3X6
spinal	T41.3X1	T41.3X2	T41.3X3	T41.3X4	T41.3X5	T41.3X6
Ligroin(e) (solvent)	T52.0X1	T52.0X2	T52.0X3	T52.0X4	—	—
vapor	T59.891	T59.892	T59.893	T59.894	—	—
Ligustrum vulgare	T62.2X1	T62.2X2	T62.2X3	T62.2X4	—	—
Lily of the valley	T62.2X1	T62.2X2	T62.2X3	T62.2X4	—	—
Lime (chloride)	T54.3X1	T54.3X2	T54.3X3	T54.3X4	—	—
Limonene	T52.8X1	T52.8X2	T52.8X3	T52.8X4	—	—
Lincomycin	T36.8X1	T36.8X2	T36.8X3	T36.8X4	T36.8X5	T36.8X6
Lindane (insecticide) (nonmedicinal) (vapor)	T53.6X1	T53.6X2	T53.6X3	T53.6X4	—	—
medicinal	T49.0X1	T49.0X2	T49.0X3	T49.0X4	T49.0X5	T49.0X6
Liniments NEC	T49.91	T49.92	T49.93	T49.94	T49.95	T49.96
Linoleic acid	T46.6X1	T46.6X2	T46.6X3	T46.6X4	T46.6X5	T46.6X6
Linolenic acid	T46.6X1	T46.6X2	T46.6X3	T46.6X4	T46.6X5	T46.6X6
Linseed	T47.4X1	T47.4X2	T47.4X3	T47.4X4	T47.4X5	T47.4X6
Liothyronine	T38.1X1	T38.1X2	T38.1X3	T38.1X4	T38.1X5	T38.1X6
Liotrix	T38.1X1	T38.1X2	T38.1X3	T38.1X4	T38.1X5	T38.1X6
Lipancreatin	T47.5X1	T47.5X2	T47.5X3	T47.5X4	T47.5X5	T47.5X6
Lipo-alprostadil	T46.7X1	T46.7X2	T46.7X3	T46.7X4	T46.7X5	T46.7X6
Lipo-Lutin	T38.5X1	T38.5X2	T38.5X3	T38.5X4	T38.5X5	T38.5X6
Lipotropic drug NEC	T50.901	T50.902	T50.903	T50.904	T50.905	T50.906
Liquefied petroleum gases	T59.891	T59.892	T59.893	T59.894	—	—
piped (pure or mixed with air)	T59.891	T59.892	T59.893	T59.894	—	—
Liquid						
paraffin	T47.4X1	T47.4X2	T47.4X3	T47.4X4	T47.4X5	T47.4X6
petrolatum	T47.4X1	T47.4X2	T47.4X3	T47.4X4	T47.4X5	T47.4X6
topical	T49.3X1	T49.3X2	T49.3X3	T49.3X4	T49.3X5	T49.3X6
specified NEC	T65.891	T65.892	T65.893	T65.894	—	—
substance	T65.91	T65.92	T65.93	T65.94	—	—

Substance	Poisoning, Accidental (unintentional)	Poisoning, Intentional Self-harm	Poisoning, Assault	Poisoning, Undetermined	Adverse Effect	Under-dosing
Liquor creosolis compositus	T65.891	T65.892	T65.893	T65.894	—	—
Liquorice	T48.4X1	T48.4X2	T48.4X3	T48.4X4	T48.4X5	T48.4X6
extract	T47.8X1	T47.8X2	T47.8X3	T47.8X4	T47.8X5	T47.8X6
Lisinopril	T46.4X1	T46.4X2	T46.4X3	T46.4X4	T46.4X5	T46.4X6
Lisuride	T42.8X1	T42.8X2	T42.8X3	T42.8X4	T42.8X5	T42.8X6
Lithane	T43.8X1	T43.8X2	T43.8X3	T43.8X4	T43.8X5	T43.8X6
Lithium	T56.891	T56.892	T56.893	T56.894		
gluconate	T43.591	T43.592	T43.593	T43.594	T43.595	T43.596
salts (carbonate)	T43.591	T43.592	T43.593	T43.594	T43.595	T43.596
Lithonate	T43.8X1	T43.8X2	T43.8X3	T43.8X4	T43.8X5	T43.8X6
Liver						
extract	T45.8X1	T45.8X2	T45.8X3	T45.8X4	T45.8X5	T45.8X6
for parenteral use	T45.8X1	T45.8X2	T45.8X3	T45.8X4	T45.8X5	T45.8X6
fraction 1	T45.8X1	T45.8X2	T45.8X3	T45.8X4	T45.8X5	T45.8X6
hydrolysate	T45.8X1	T45.8X2	T45.8X3	T45.8X4	T45.8X5	T45.8X6
Lizard (bite) (venom)	T63.121	T63.122	T63.123	T63.124	—	—
LMD	T45.8X1	T45.8X2	T45.8X3	T45.8X4	T45.8X5	T45.8X6
Lobelia	T62.2X1	T62.2X2	T62.2X3	T62.2X4	—	—
Lobeline	T50.7X1	T50.7X2	T50.7X3	T50.7X4	T50.7X5	T50.7X6
Local action drug NEC	T49.8X1	T49.8X2	T49.8X3	T49.8X4	T49.8X5	T49.8X6
Locorten	T49.0X1	T49.0X2	T49.0X3	T49.0X4	T49.0X5	T49.0X6
Lofepramine	T43.011	T43.012	T43.013	T43.014	T43.015	T43.016
Lolium temulentum	T62.2X1	T62.2X2	T62.2X3	T62.2X4	—	—
Lomotil	T47.6X1	T47.6X2	T47.6X3	T47.6X4	T47.6X5	T47.6X6
Lomustine	T45.1X1	T45.1X2	T45.1X3	T45.1X4	T45.1X5	T45.1X6
Lonidamine	T45.1X1	T45.1X2	T45.1X3	T45.1X4	T45.1X5	T45.1X6
Loperamide	T47.6X1	T47.6X2	T47.6X3	T47.6X4	T47.6X5	T47.6X6
Loprazolam	T42.4X1	T42.4X2	T42.4X3	T42.4X4	T42.4X5	T42.4X6
Lorajmine	T46.2X1	T46.2X2	T46.2X3	T46.2X4	T46.2X5	T46.2X6
Loratidine	T45.0X1	T45.0X2	T45.0X3	T45.0X4	T45.0X5	T45.0X6
Lorazepam	T42.4X1	T42.4X2	T42.4X3	T42.4X4	T42.4X5	T42.4X6
Lorcainide	T46.2X1	T46.2X2	T46.2X3	T46.2X4	T46.2X5	T46.2X6
Lormetazepam	T42.4X1	T42.4X2	T42.4X3	T42.4X4	T42.4X5	T42.4X6
Lotions NEC	T49.91	T49.92	T49.93	T49.94	T49.95	T49.96
Lotusate	T42.3X1	T42.3X2	T42.3X3	T42.3X4	T42.3X5	T42.3X6
Lovastatin	T46.6X1	T46.6X2	T46.6X3	T46.6X4	T46.6X5	T46.6X6
Lowila	T49.2X1	T49.2X2	T49.2X3	T49.2X4	T49.2X5	T49.2X6
Loxapine	T43.591	T43.592	T43.593	T43.594	T43.595	T43.596
Lozenges (throat)	T49.6X1	T49.6X2	T49.6X3	T49.6X4	T49.6X5	T49.6X6
LSD	T40.8X1	T40.8X2	T40.8X3	T40.8X4	—	—
L-Tryptophan — see amino acid						
Lubricant, eye	T49.5X1	T49.5X2	T49.5X3	T49.5X4	T49.5X5	T49.5X6
Lubricating oil NEC	T52.0X1	T52.0X2	T52.0X3	T52.0X4	—	—
Lucanthone	T37.4X1	T37.4X2	T37.4X3	T37.4X4	T37.4X5	T37.4X6
Luminal	T42.3X1	T42.3X2	T42.3X3	T42.3X4	T42.3X5	T42.3X6
Lung irritant (gas) NEC	T59.91	T59.92	T59.93	T59.94		
Luteinizing hormone	T38.811	T38.812	T38.813	T38.814	T38.815	T38.816
Lutocylol	T38.5X1	T38.5X2	T38.5X3	T38.5X4	T38.5X5	T38.5X6
Lutromone	T38.5X1	T38.5X2	T38.5X3	T38.5X4	T38.5X5	T38.5X6
Lututrin	T48.291	T48.292	T48.293	T48.294	T48.295	T48.296
Lye (concentrated)	T54.3X1	T54.3X2	T54.3X3	T54.3X4	—	—
Lygranum (skin test)	T50.8X1	T50.8X2	T50.8X3	T50.8X4	T50.8X5	T50.8X6
Lymecycline	T36.4X1	T36.4X2	T36.4X3	T36.4X4	T36.4X5	T36.4X6
Lymphogranuloma venereum antigen	T50.8X1	T50.8X2	T50.8X3	T50.8X4	T50.8X5	T50.8X6
Lynestrenol	T38.4X1	T38.4X2	T38.4X3	T38.4X4	T38.4X5	T38.4X6
Lyovac Sodium Edecrin	T50.1X1	T50.1X2	T50.1X3	T50.1X4	T50.1X5	T50.1X6
Lypressin	T38.891	T38.892	T38.893	T38.894	T38.895	T38.896
Lysergic acid diethylamide	T40.8X1	T40.8X2	T40.8X3	T40.8X4	—	—
Lysergide	T40.8X1	T40.8X2	T40.8X3	T40.8X4	—	—
Lysine vasopressin	T38.891	T38.892	T38.893	T38.894	T38.895	T38.896
Lysol	T54.1X1	T54.1X2	T54.1X3	T54.1X4	—	—
Lysozyme	T49.0X1	T49.0X2	T49.0X3	T49.0X4	T49.0X5	T49.0X6
Lytta (vitatta)	T49.8X1	T49.8X2	T49.8X3	T49.8X4	T49.8X5	T49.8X6
Mace	T59.3X1	T59.3X2	T59.3X3	T59.3X4		
Macrogol	T50.991	T50.992	T50.993	T50.994	T50.995	T50.996
Macrolide						
anabolic drug	T38.7X1	T38.7X2	T38.7X3	T38.7X4	T38.7X5	T38.7X6
antibiotic	T36.3X1	T36.3X2	T36.3X3	T36.3X4	T36.3X5	T36.3X6
Mafenide	T49.0X1	T49.0X2	T49.0X3	T49.0X4	T49.0X5	T49.0X6
Magaldrate	T47.1X1	T47.1X2	T47.1X3	T47.1X4	T47.1X5	T47.1X6
Magic mushroom	T40.991	T40.992	T40.993	T40.994		
Magnamycin	T36.8X1	T36.8X2	T36.8X3	T36.8X4	T36.8X5	T36.8X6
Magnesia magma	T47.1X1	T47.1X2	T47.1X3	T47.1X4	T47.1X5	T47.1X6
Magnesium NEC	T56.891	T56.892	T56.893	T56.894		
carbonate	T47.1X1	T47.1X2	T47.1X3	T47.1X4	T47.1X5	T47.1X6
citrate	T47.4X1	T47.4X2	T47.4X3	T47.4X4	T47.4X5	T47.4X6
hydroxide	T47.1X1	T47.1X2	T47.1X3	T47.1X4	T47.1X5	T47.1X6
oxide	T47.1X1	T47.1X2	T47.1X3	T47.1X4	T47.1X5	T47.1X6
peroxide	T49.0X1	T49.0X2	T49.0X3	T49.0X4	T49.0X5	T49.0X6
salicylate	T39.091	T39.092	T39.093	T39.094	T39.095	T39.096
silicofluoride	T50.3X1	T50.3X2	T50.3X3	T50.3X4	T50.3X5	T50.3X6

Substance	Poisoning, Accidental (unintentional)	Poisoning, Intentional Self-harm	Poisoning, Assault	Poisoning, Undetermined	Adverse Effect	Under-dosing
Magnesium — continued						
sulfate	T47.4X1	T47.4X2	T47.4X3	T47.4X4	T47.4X5	T47.4X6
thiosulfate	T45.0X1	T45.0X2	T45.0X3	T45.0X4	T45.0X5	T45.0X6
trisilicate	T47.1X1	T47.1X2	T47.1X3	T47.1X4	T47.1X5	T47.1X6
Malathion (medicinal)	T49.0X1	T49.0X2	T49.0X3	T49.0X4	T49.0X5	T49.0X6
insecticide	T60.0X1	T60.0X2	T60.0X3	T60.0X4		
Male fern extract	T37.4X1	T37.4X2	T37.4X3	T37.4X4	T37.4X5	T37.4X6
M-AMSA	T45.1X1	T45.1X2	T45.1X3	T45.1X4	T45.1X5	T45.1X6
Mandelic acid	T37.8X1	T37.8X2	T37.8X3	T37.8X4	T37.8X5	T37.8X6
Manganese (dioxide) (salts)	T57.2X1	T57.2X2	T57.2X3	T57.2X4	—	—
medicinal	T50.991	T50.992	T50.993	T50.994	T50.995	T50.996
Mannitol	T47.3X1	T47.3X2	T47.3X3	T47.3X4	T47.3X5	T47.3X6
hexanitrate	T46.3X1	T46.3X2	T46.3X3	T46.3X4	T46.3X5	T46.3X6
Mannomustine	T45.1X1	T45.1X2	T45.1X3	T45.1X4	T45.1X5	T45.1X6
MAO inhibitors	T43.1X1	T43.1X2	T43.1X3	T43.1X4	T43.1X5	T43.1X6
Mapharsen	T37.8X1	T37.8X2	T37.8X3	T37.8X4	T37.8X5	T37.8X6
Maphenide	T49.0X1	T49.0X2	T49.0X3	T49.0X4	T49.0X5	T49.0X6
Maprotiline	T43.021	T43.022	T43.023	T43.024	T43.025	T43.026
Marcaine	T41.3X1	T41.3X2	T41.3X3	T41.3X4	T41.3X5	T41.3X6
infiltration (subcutaneous)	T41.3X1	T41.3X2	T41.3X3	T41.3X4	T41.3X5	T41.3X6
nerve block (peripheral) (plexus)	T41.3X1	T41.3X2	T41.3X3	T41.3X4	T41.3X5	T41.3X6
Marezine	T45.0X1	T45.0X2	T45.0X3	T45.0X4	T45.0X5	T45.0X6
Marihuana	T40.7X1	T40.7X2	T40.7X3	T40.7X4	T40.7X5	T40.7X6
Marijuana	T40.7X1	T40.7X2	T40.7X3	T40.7X4	T40.7X5	T40.7X6
Marine (sting)	T63.691	T63.692	T63.693	T63.694	—	—
animals (sting)	T63.691	T63.692	T63.693	T63.694	—	—
plants (sting)	T63.711	T63.712	T63.713	T63.714	—	—
Marplan	T43.1X1	T43.1X2	T43.1X3	T43.1X4	T43.1X5	T43.1X6
Marsh gas	T59.891	T59.892	T59.893	T59.894		
Marsilid	T43.1X1	T43.1X2	T43.1X3	T43.1X4	T43.1X5	T43.1X6
Matulane	T45.1X1	T45.1X2	T45.1X3	T45.1X4	T45.1X5	T45.1X6
Mazindol	T50.5X1	T50.5X2	T50.5X3	T50.5X4	T50.5X5	T50.5X6
MCPA	T60.3X1	T60.3X2	T60.3X3	T60.3X4		
MDMA	T43.621	T43.622	T43.623	T43.624	T43.625	T43.626
Meadow saffron	T62.2X1	T62.2X2	T62.2X3	T62.2X4	—	—
Measles virus vaccine (attenuated)	T50.B91	T50.B92	T50.B93	T50.B94	T50.B95	T50.B96
Meat, noxious	T62.8X1	T62.8X2	T62.8X3	T62.8X4		
Meballymal	T42.3X1	T42.3X2	T42.3X3	T42.3X4	T42.3X5	T42.3X6
Mebanazine	T43.1X1	T43.1X2	T43.1X3	T43.1X4	T43.1X5	T43.1X6
Mebaral	T42.3X1	T42.3X2	T42.3X3	T42.3X4	T42.3X5	T42.3X6
Mebendazole	T37.4X1	T37.4X2	T37.4X3	T37.4X4	T37.4X5	T37.4X6
Mebeverine	T44.3X1	T44.3X2	T44.3X3	T44.3X4	T44.3X5	T44.3X6
Mebhydrolin	T45.0X1	T45.0X2	T45.0X3	T45.0X4	T45.0X5	T45.0X6
Mebumal	T42.3X1	T42.3X2	T42.3X3	T42.3X4	T42.3X5	T42.3X6
Mebutamate	T43.591	T43.592	T43.593	T43.594	T43.595	T43.596
Mecamylamine	T44.2X1	T44.2X2	T44.2X3	T44.2X4	T44.2X5	T44.2X6
Mechlorethamine	T45.1X1	T45.1X2	T45.1X3	T45.1X4	T45.1X5	T45.1X6
Mecillinam	T36.0X1	T36.0X2	T36.0X3	T36.0X4	T36.0X5	T36.0X6
Meclizine (hydrochloride)	T45.0X1	T45.0X2	T45.0X3	T45.0X4	T45.0X5	T45.0X6
Meclocycline	T36.4X1	T36.4X2	T36.4X3	T36.4X4	T36.4X5	T36.4X6
Meclofenamate	T39.391	T39.392	T39.393	T39.394	T39.395	T39.396
Meclofenamic acid	T39.391	T39.392	T39.393	T39.394	T39.395	T39.396
Meclofenoxate	T43.691	T43.692	T43.693	T43.694	T43.695	T43.696
Meclozine	T45.0X1	T45.0X2	T45.0X3	T45.0X4	T45.0X5	T45.0X6
Mecobalamin	T45.8X1	T45.8X2	T45.8X3	T45.8X4	T45.8X5	T45.8X6
Mecoprop	T60.3X1	T60.3X2	T60.3X3	T60.3X4	—	—
Mecrilate	T49.3X1	T49.3X2	T49.3X3	T49.3X4	T49.3X5	T49.3X6
Mecysteine	T48.4X1	T48.4X2	T48.4X3	T48.4X4	T48.4X5	T48.4X6
Medazepam	T42.4X1	T42.4X2	T42.4X3	T42.4X4	T42.4X5	T42.4X6
Medicament NEC	T50.901	T50.902	T50.903	T50.904	T50.905	T50.906
Medinal	T42.3X1	T42.3X2	T42.3X3	T42.3X4	T42.3X5	T42.3X6
Medomin	T42.3X1	T42.3X2	T42.3X3	T42.3X4	T42.3X5	T42.3X6
Medrogestone	T38.5X1	T38.5X2	T38.5X3	T38.5X4	T38.5X5	T38.5X6
Medroxalol	T44.8X1	T44.8X2	T44.8X3	T44.8X4	T44.8X5	T44.8X6
Medroxyprogesterone acetate (depot)	T38.5X1	T38.5X2	T38.5X3	T38.5X4	T38.5X5	T38.5X6
Medrysone	T49.0X1	T49.0X2	T49.0X3	T49.0X4	T49.0X5	T49.0X6
Mefenamic acid	T39.391	T39.392	T39.393	T39.394	T39.395	T39.396
Mefenorex	T50.5X1	T50.5X2	T50.5X3	T50.5X4	T50.5X5	T50.5X6
Mefloquine	T37.2X1	T37.2X2	T37.2X3	T37.2X4	T37.2X5	T37.2X6
Mefruside	T50.2X1	T50.2X2	T50.2X3	T50.2X4	T50.2X5	T50.2X6
Megahallucinogen	T40.901	T40.902	T40.903	T40.904	T40.905	T40.906
Megestrol	T38.5X1	T38.5X2	T38.5X3	T38.5X4	T38.5X5	T38.5X6
Meglumine						
antimoniate	T37.8X1	T37.8X2	T37.8X3	T37.8X4	T37.8X5	T37.8X6
diatrizoate	T50.8X1	T50.8X2	T50.8X3	T50.8X4	T50.8X5	T50.8X6
iodipamide	T50.8X1	T50.8X2	T50.8X3	T50.8X4	T50.8X5	T50.8X6
iotroxate	T50.8X1	T50.8X2	T50.8X3	T50.8X4	T50.8X5	T50.8X6
MEK (methyl ethyl ketone)	T52.4X1	T52.4X2	T52.4X3	T52.4X4		
Meladinin	T49.3X1	T49.3X2	T49.3X3	T49.3X4	T49.3X5	T49.3X6
Meladrazine	T44.3X1	T44.3X2	T44.3X3	T44.3X4	T44.3X5	T44.3X6

376

Additional Character May Be Required — Refer to the Tabular List for Character Selection   ▼ Subterms under main terms may continue to next column or page

Substance	Poisoning, Accidental (unintentional)	Poisoning, Intentional Self-harm	Poisoning, Assault	Poisoning, Undetermined	Adverse Effect	Under-dosing
Melaleuca alternifolia oil	T49.0X1	T49.0X2	T49.0X3	T49.0X4	T49.0X5	T49.0X6
Melanizing agents	T49.3X1	T49.3X2	T49.3X3	T49.3X4	T49.3X5	T49.3X6
Melanocyte-stimulating hormone	T38.891	T38.892	T38.893	T38.894	T38.895	T38.896
Melarsonyl potassium	T37.3X1	T37.3X2	T37.3X3	T37.3X4	T37.3X5	T37.3X6
Melarsoprol	T37.3X1	T37.3X2	T37.3X3	T37.3X4	T37.3X5	T37.3X6
Melia azedarach	T62.2X1	T62.2X2	T62.2X3	T62.2X4	—	—
Melitracen	T43.011	T43.012	T43.013	T43.014	T43.015	T43.016
Mellaril	T43.3X1	T43.3X2	T43.3X3	T43.3X4	T43.3X5	T43.3X6
Meloxine	T49.3X1	T49.3X2	T49.3X3	T49.3X4	T49.3X5	T49.3X6
Melperone	T43.4X1	T43.4X2	T43.4X3	T43.4X4	T43.4X5	T43.4X6
Melphalan	T45.1X1	T45.1X2	T45.1X3	T45.1X4	T45.1X5	T45.1X6
Memantine	T43.8X1	T43.8X2	T43.8X3	T43.8X4	T43.8X5	T43.8X6
Menadiol	T45.7X1	T45.7X2	T45.7X3	T45.7X4	T45.7X5	T45.7X6
sodium sulfate	T45.7X1	T45.7X2	T45.7X3	T45.7X4	T45.7X5	T45.7X6
Menadione	T45.7X1	T45.7X2	T45.7X3	T45.7X4	T45.7X5	T45.7X6
sodium bisulfite	T45.7X1	T45.7X2	T45.7X3	T45.7X4	T45.7X5	T45.7X6
Menaphthone	T45.7X1	T45.7X2	T45.7X3	T45.7X4	T45.7X5	T45.7X6
Menaquinone	T45.7X1	T45.7X2	T45.7X3	T45.7X4	T45.7X5	T45.7X6
Menatetrenone	T45.7X1	T45.7X2	T45.7X3	T45.7X4	T45.7X5	T45.7X6
Meningococcal vaccine	T50.A91	T50.A92	T50.A93	T50.A94	T50.A95	T50.A96
Menningovax (-AC) (-C)	T50.A91	T50.A92	T50.A93	T50.A94	T50.A95	T50.A96
Menotropins	T38.811	T38.812	T38.813	T38.814	T38.815	T38.816
Menthol	T48.5X1	T48.5X2	T48.5X3	T48.5X4	T48.5X5	T48.5X6
Mepacrine	T37.2X1	T37.2X2	T37.2X3	T37.2X4	T37.2X5	T37.2X6
Meparfynol	T42.6X1	T42.6X2	T42.6X3	T42.6X4	T42.6X5	T42.6X6
Mepartricin	T36.7X1	T36.7X2	T36.7X3	T36.7X4	T36.7X5	T36.7X6
Mepazine	T43.3X1	T43.3X2	T43.3X3	T43.3X4	T43.3X5	T43.3X6
Mepenzolate	T44.3X1	T44.3X2	T44.3X3	T44.3X4	T44.3X5	T44.3X6
bromide	T44.3X1	T44.3X2	T44.3X3	T44.3X4	T44.3X5	T44.3X6
Meperidine	T40.4X1	T40.4X2	T40.4X3	T40.4X4	T40.4X5	T40.4X6
Mephebarbital	T42.3X1	T42.3X2	T42.3X3	T42.3X4	T42.3X5	T42.3X6
Mephenamin (e)	T42.8X1	T42.8X2	T42.8X3	T42.8X4	T42.8X5	T42.8X6
Mephenesin	T42.8X1	T42.8X2	T42.8X3	T42.8X4	T42.8X5	T42.8X6
Mephenhydramine	T45.0X1	T45.0X2	T45.0X3	T45.0X4	T45.0X5	T45.0X6
Mephenoxalone	T42.8X1	T42.8X2	T42.8X3	T42.8X4	T42.8X5	T42.8X6
Mephentermine	T44.991	T44.992	T44.993	T44.994	T44.995	T44.996
Mephenytoin	T42.0X1	T42.0X2	T42.0X3	T42.0X4	T42.0X5	T42.0X6
with phenobarbital	T42.3X1	T42.3X2	T42.3X3	T42.3X4	T42.3X5	T42.3X6
Mephobarbital	T42.3X1	T42.3X2	T42.3X3	T42.3X4	T42.3X5	T42.3X6
Mephosfolan	T60.0X1	T60.0X2	T60.0X3	T60.0X4	—	—
Mepindolol	T44.7X1	T44.7X2	T44.7X3	T44.7X4	T44.7X5	T44.7X6
Mepiperphenidol	T44.3X1	T44.3X2	T44.3X3	T44.3X4	T44.3X5	T44.3X6
Mepitiostane	T38.7X1	T38.7X2	T38.7X3	T38.7X4	T38.7X5	T38.7X6
Mepivacaine	T41.3X1	T41.3X2	T41.3X3	T41.3X4	T41.3X5	T41.3X6
epidural	T41.3X1	T41.3X2	T41.3X3	T41.3X4	T41.3X5	T41.3X6
Meprednisone	T38.0X1	T38.0X2	T38.0X3	T38.0X4	T38.0X5	T38.0X6
Meprobam	T43.591	T43.592	T43.593	T43.594	T43.595	T43.596
Meprobamate	T43.591	T43.592	T43.593	T43.594	T43.595	T43.596
Meproscillarin	T46.0X1	T46.0X2	T46.0X3	T46.0X4	T46.0X5	T46.0X6
Meprylcaine	T41.3X1	T41.3X2	T41.3X3	T41.3X4	T41.3X5	T41.3X6
Meptazinol	T39.8X1	T39.8X2	T39.8X3	T39.8X4	T39.8X5	T39.8X6
Mepyramine	T45.0X1	T45.0X2	T45.0X3	T45.0X4	T45.0X5	T45.0X6
Mequitazine	T43.3X1	T43.3X2	T43.3X3	T43.3X4	T43.3X5	T43.3X6
Meralluride	T50.2X1	T50.2X2	T50.2X3	T50.2X4	T50.2X5	T50.2X6
Merbaphen	T50.2X1	T50.2X2	T50.2X3	T50.2X4	T50.2X5	T50.2X6
Merbromin	T49.0X1	T49.0X2	T49.0X3	T49.0X4	T49.0X5	T49.0X6
Mercaptobenzothiazole salts	T49.0X1	T49.0X2	T49.0X3	T49.0X4	T49.0X5	T49.0X6
Mercaptomerin	T50.2X1	T50.2X2	T50.2X3	T50.2X4	T50.2X5	T50.2X6
Mercaptopurine	T45.1X1	T45.1X2	T45.1X3	T45.1X4	T45.1X5	T45.1X6
Mercumatilin	T50.2X1	T50.2X2	T50.2X3	T50.2X4	T50.2X5	T50.2X6
Mercuramide	T50.2X1	T50.2X2	T50.2X3	T50.2X4	T50.2X5	T50.2X6
Mercurochrome	T49.0X1	T49.0X2	T49.0X3	T49.0X4	T49.0X5	T49.0X6
Mercurophylline	T50.2X1	T50.2X2	T50.2X3	T50.2X4	T50.2X5	T50.2X6
Mercury, mercurial, mercuric, mercurous (compounds) (cyanide) (fumes) (nonmedicinal) (vapor) NEC	T56.1X1	T56.1X2	T56.1X3	T56.1X4	—	—
ammoniated	T49.0X1	T49.0X2	T49.0X3	T49.0X4	T49.0X5	T49.0X6
anti-infective						
local	T49.0X1	T49.0X2	T49.0X3	T49.0X4	T49.0X5	T49.0X6
systemic	T37.8X1	T37.8X2	T37.8X3	T37.8X4	T37.8X5	T37.8X6
topical	T49.0X1	T49.0X2	T49.0X3	T49.0X4	T49.0X5	T49.0X6
chloride (ammoniated)	T49.0X1	T49.0X2	T49.0X3	T49.0X4	T49.0X5	T49.0X6
fungicide	T56.1X1	T56.1X2	T56.1X3	T56.1X4	—	—
diuretic NEC	T50.2X1	T50.2X2	T50.2X3	T50.2X4	T50.2X5	T50.2X6
fungicide	T56.1X1	T56.1X2	T56.1X3	T56.1X4	—	—
organic (fungicide)	T56.1X1	T56.1X2	T56.1X3	T56.1X4	—	—
oxide, yellow	T49.0X1	T49.0X2	T49.0X3	T49.0X4	T49.0X5	T49.0X6
Mersalyl	T50.2X1	T50.2X2	T50.2X3	T50.2X4	T50.2X5	T50.2X6
Merthiolate	T49.0X1	T49.0X2	T49.0X3	T49.0X4	T49.0X5	T49.0X6

Substance	Poisoning, Accidental (unintentional)	Poisoning, Intentional Self-harm	Poisoning, Assault	Poisoning, Undetermined	Adverse Effect	Under-dosing
Merthiolate — continued						
ophthalmic preparation	T49.5X1	T49.5X2	T49.5X3	T49.5X4	T49.5X5	T49.5X6
Meruvax	T50.B91	T50.B92	T50.B93	T50.B94	T50.B95	T50.B96
Mesalazine	T47.8X1	T47.8X2	T47.8X3	T47.8X4	T47.8X5	T47.8X6
Mescal buttons	T40.991	T40.992	T40.993	T40.994	—	—
Mescaline	T40.991	T40.992	T40.993	T40.994	—	—
Mesna	T48.4X1	T48.4X2	T48.4X3	T48.4X4	T48.4X5	T48.4X6
Mesoglycan	T46.6X1	T46.6X2	T46.6X3	T46.6X4	T46.6X5	T46.6X6
Mesoridazine	T43.3X1	T43.3X2	T43.3X3	T43.3X4	T43.3X5	T43.3X6
Mestanolone	T38.7X1	T38.7X2	T38.7X3	T38.7X4	T38.7X5	T38.7X6
Mesterolone	T38.7X1	T38.7X2	T38.7X3	T38.7X4	T38.7X5	T38.7X6
Mestranol	T38.5X1	T38.5X2	T38.5X3	T38.5X4	T38.5X5	T38.5X6
Mesulergine	T42.8X1	T42.8X2	T42.8X3	T42.8X4	T42.8X5	T42.8X6
Mesulfen	T49.0X1	T49.0X2	T49.0X3	T49.0X4	T49.0X5	T49.0X6
Mesuximide	T42.2X1	T42.2X2	T42.2X3	T42.2X4	T42.2X5	T42.2X6
Metabutethamine	T41.3X1	T41.3X2	T41.3X3	T41.3X4	T41.3X5	T41.3X6
Metactesylacetate	T49.0X1	T49.0X2	T49.0X3	T49.0X4	T49.0X5	T49.0X6
Metacycline	T36.4X1	T36.4X2	T36.4X3	T36.4X4	T36.4X5	T36.4X6
Metaldehyde (snail killer) NEC	T60.8X1	T60.8X2	T60.8X3	T60.8X4	—	—
Metals (heavy) (nonmedicinal)	T56.91	T56.92	T56.93	T56.94	—	—
dust, fumes, or vapor NEC	T56.91	T56.92	T56.93	T56.94	—	—
light NEC	T56.91	T56.92	T56.93	T56.94	—	—
dust, fumes, or vapor NEC	T56.91	T56.92	T56.93	T56.94	—	—
specified NEC	T56.891	T56.892	T56.893	T56.894	—	—
thallium	T56.811	T56.812	T56.813	T56.814	—	—
Metamfetamine	T43.621	T43.622	T43.623	T43.624	T43.625	T43.626
Metamizole sodium	T39.2X1	T39.2X2	T39.2X3	T39.2X4	T39.2X5	T39.2X6
Metampicillin	T36.0X1	T36.0X2	T36.0X3	T36.0X4	T36.0X5	T36.0X6
Metamucil	T47.4X1	T47.4X2	T47.4X3	T47.4X4	T47.4X5	T47.4X6
Metandienone	T38.7X1	T38.7X2	T38.7X3	T38.7X4	T38.7X5	T38.7X6
Metandrostenolone	T38.7X1	T38.7X2	T38.7X3	T38.7X4	T38.7X5	T38.7X6
Metaphen	T49.0X1	T49.0X2	T49.0X3	T49.0X4	T49.0X5	T49.0X6
Metaphos	T60.0X1	T60.0X2	T60.0X3	T60.0X4	—	—
Metapramine	T43.011	T43.012	T43.013	T43.014	T43.015	T43.016
Metaproterenol	T48.291	T48.292	T48.293	T48.294	T48.295	T48.296
Metaraminol	T44.4X1	T44.4X2	T44.4X3	T44.4X4	T44.4X5	T44.4X6
Metaxalone	T42.8X1	T42.8X2	T42.8X3	T42.8X4	T42.8X5	T42.8X6
Metenolone	T38.7X1	T38.7X2	T38.7X3	T38.7X4	T38.7X5	T38.7X6
Metergoline	T42.8X1	T42.8X2	T42.8X3	T42.8X4	T42.8X5	T42.8X6
Metescufylline	T46.991	T46.992	T46.993	T46.994	T46.995	T46.996
Metetoin	T42.0X1	T42.0X2	T42.0X3	T42.0X4	T42.0X5	T42.0X6
Metformin	T38.3X1	T38.3X2	T38.3X3	T38.3X4	T38.3X5	T38.3X6
Methacholine	T44.1X1	T44.1X2	T44.1X3	T44.1X4	T44.1X5	T44.1X6
Methacycline	T36.4X1	T36.4X2	T36.4X3	T36.4X4	T36.4X5	T36.4X6
Methadone	T40.3X1	T40.3X2	T40.3X3	T40.3X4	T40.3X5	T40.3X6
Methallenestril	T38.5X1	T38.5X2	T38.5X3	T38.5X4	T38.5X5	T38.5X6
Methallenoestril	T38.5X1	T38.5X2	T38.5X3	T38.5X4	T38.5X5	T38.5X6
Methamphetamine	T43.621	T43.622	T43.623	T43.624	T43.625	T43.626
Methampyrone	T39.2X1	T39.2X2	T39.2X3	T39.2X4	T39.2X5	T39.2X6
Methandienone	T38.7X1	T38.7X2	T38.7X3	T38.7X4	T38.7X5	T38.7X6
Methandriol	T38.7X1	T38.7X2	T38.7X3	T38.7X4	T38.7X5	T38.7X6
Methandrostenolone	T38.7X1	T38.7X2	T38.7X3	T38.7X4	T38.7X5	T38.7X6
Methane	T59.891	T59.892	T59.893	T59.894	—	—
Methanethiol	T59.891	T59.892	T59.893	T59.894	—	—
Methaniazide	T37.1X1	T37.1X2	T37.1X3	T37.1X4	T37.1X5	T37.1X6
Methanol (vapor)	T51.1X1	T51.1X2	T51.1X3	T51.1X4	—	—
Methantheline	T44.3X1	T44.3X2	T44.3X3	T44.3X4	T44.3X5	T44.3X6
Methanthelinium bromide	T44.3X1	T44.3X2	T44.3X3	T44.3X4	T44.3X5	T44.3X6
Methaphenilene	T45.0X1	T45.0X2	T45.0X3	T45.0X4	T45.0X5	T45.0X6
Methapyrilene	T45.0X1	T45.0X2	T45.0X3	T45.0X4	T45.0X5	T45.0X6
Methaqualone (compound)	T42.6X1	T42.6X2	T42.6X3	T42.6X4	T42.6X5	T42.6X6
Metharbital	T42.3X1	T42.3X2	T42.3X3	T42.3X4	T42.3X5	T42.3X6
Methazolamide	T50.2X1	T50.2X2	T50.2X3	T50.2X4	T50.2X5	T50.2X6
Methdilazine	T43.3X1	T43.3X2	T43.3X3	T43.3X4	T43.3X5	T43.3X6
Methedrine	T43.621	T43.622	T43.623	T43.624	T43.625	T43.626
Methenamine (mandelate)	T37.8X1	T37.8X2	T37.8X3	T37.8X4	T37.8X5	T37.8X6
Methenolone	T38.7X1	T38.7X2	T38.7X3	T38.7X4	T38.7X5	T38.7X6
Methergine	T48.0X1	T48.0X2	T48.0X3	T48.0X4	T48.0X5	T48.0X6
Methetoin	T42.0X1	T42.0X2	T42.0X3	T42.0X4	T42.0X5	T42.0X6
Methiacil	T38.2X1	T38.2X2	T38.2X3	T38.2X4	T38.2X5	T38.2X6
Methicillin	T36.0X1	T36.0X2	T36.0X3	T36.0X4	T36.0X5	T36.0X6
Methimazole	T38.2X1	T38.2X2	T38.2X3	T38.2X4	T38.2X5	T38.2X6
Methiodal sodium	T50.8X1	T50.8X2	T50.8X3	T50.8X4	T50.8X5	T50.8X6
Methionine	T50.991	T50.992	T50.993	T50.994	T50.995	T50.996
Methisazone	T37.5X1	T37.5X2	T37.5X3	T37.5X4	T37.5X5	T37.5X6
Methisoprinol	T37.5X1	T37.5X2	T37.5X3	T37.5X4	T37.5X5	T37.5X6
Methitural	T42.3X1	T42.3X2	T42.3X3	T42.3X4	T42.3X5	T42.3X6
Methixene	T44.3X1	T44.3X2	T44.3X3	T44.3X4	T44.3X5	T44.3X6
Methobarbital, methobarbitone	T42.3X1	T42.3X2	T42.3X3	T42.3X4	T42.3X5	T42.3X6
Methocarbamol	T42.8X1	T42.8X2	T42.8X3	T42.8X4	T42.8X5	T42.8X6

Table of Drugs and Chemicals

Methocarbamol — Milk of magnesia

Substance	Poisoning, Accidental (unintentional)	Poisoning, Intentional Self-harm	Poisoning, Assault	Poisoning, Undetermined	Adverse Effect	Under-dosing
Methocarbamol — continued						
skeletal muscle relaxant	T48.1X1	T48.1X2	T48.1X3	T48.1X4	T48.1X5	T48.1X6
Methohexital	T41.1X1	T41.1X2	T41.1X3	T41.1X4	T41.1X5	T41.1X6
Methohexitone	T41.1X1	T41.1X2	T41.1X3	T41.1X4	T41.1X5	T41.1X6
Methoin	T42.0X1	T42.0X2	T42.0X3	T42.0X4	T42.0X5	T42.0X6
Methopholine	T39.8X1	T39.8X2	T39.8X3	T39.8X4	T39.8X5	T39.8X6
Methopromazine	T43.3X1	T43.3X2	T43.3X3	T43.3X4	T43.3X5	T43.3X6
Methorate	T48.3X1	T48.3X2	T48.3X3	T48.3X4	T48.3X5	T48.3X6
Methoserpidine	T46.5X1	T46.5X2	T46.5X3	T46.5X4	T46.5X5	T46.5X6
Methotrexate	T45.1X1	T45.1X2	T45.1X3	T45.1X4	T45.1X5	T45.1X6
Methotrimeprazine	T43.3X1	T43.3X2	T43.3X3	T43.3X4	T43.3X5	T43.3X6
Methoxa-Dome	T49.3X1	T49.3X2	T49.3X3	T49.3X4	T49.3X5	T49.3X6
Methoxamine	T44.4X1	T44.4X2	T44.4X3	T44.4X4	T44.4X5	T44.4X6
Methoxsalen	T50.991	T50.992	T50.993	T50.994	T50.995	T50.996
Methoxyaniline	T65.3X1	T65.3X2	T65.3X3	T65.3X4	—	—
Methoxybenzyl penicillin	T36.0X1	T36.0X2	T36.0X3	T36.0X4	T36.0X5	T36.0X6
Methoxychlor	T53.7X1	T53.7X2	T53.7X3	T53.7X4	—	—
Methoxy-DDT	T53.7X1	T53.7X2	T53.7X3	T53.7X4	—	—
Methoxyflurane	T41.0X1	T41.0X2	T41.0X3	T41.0X4	T41.0X5	T41.0X6
Methoxyphenamine	T48.6X1	T48.6X2	T48.6X3	T48.6X4	T48.6X5	T48.6X6
Methoxypromazine	T43.3X1	T43.3X2	T43.3X3	T43.3X4	T43.3X5	T43.3X6
Methscopolamine bromide	T44.3X1	T44.3X2	T44.3X3	T44.3X4	T44.3X5	T44.3X6
Methsuximide	T42.2X1	T42.2X2	T42.2X3	T42.2X4	T42.2X5	T42.2X6
Methyclothiazide	T50.2X1	T50.2X2	T50.2X3	T50.2X4	T50.2X5	T50.2X6
Methyl						
acetate	T52.4X1	T52.4X2	T52.4X3	T52.4X4	—	—
acetone	T52.4X1	T52.4X2	T52.4X3	T52.4X4	—	—
acrylate	T65.891	T65.892	T65.893	T65.894	—	—
alcohol	T51.1X1	T51.1X2	T51.1X3	T51.1X4	—	—
aminophenol	T65.3X1	T65.3X2	T65.3X3	T65.3X4	—	—
amphetamine	T43.621	T43.622	T43.623	T43.624	T43.625	T43.626
androstanolone	T38.7X1	T38.7X2	T38.7X3	T38.7X4	T38.7X5	T38.7X6
atropine	T44.3X1	T44.3X2	T44.3X3	T44.3X4	T44.3X5	T44.3X6
benzene	T52.2X1	T52.2X2	T52.2X3	T52.2X4	—	—
benzoate	T52.8X1	T52.8X2	T52.8X3	T52.8X4	—	—
benzol	T52.2X1	T52.2X2	T52.2X3	T52.2X4	—	—
bromide (gas)	T59.891	T59.892	T59.893	T59.894	—	—
fumigant	T60.8X1	T60.8X2	T60.8X3	T60.8X4	—	—
butanol	T51.3X1	T51.3X2	T51.3X3	T51.3X4	—	—
carbinol	T51.1X1	T51.1X2	T51.1X3	T51.1X4	—	—
carbonate	T52.8X1	T52.8X2	T52.8X3	T52.8X4	—	—
CCNU	T45.1X1	T45.1X2	T45.1X3	T45.1X4	T45.1X5	T45.1X6
cellosolve	T52.91	T52.92	T52.93	T52.94	—	—
cellulose	T47.4X1	T47.4X2	T47.4X3	T47.4X4	T47.4X5	T47.4X6
chloride (gas)	T59.891	T59.892	T59.893	T59.894	—	—
chloroformate	T59.3X1	T59.3X2	T59.3X3	T59.3X4	—	—
cyclohexane	T52.8X1	T52.8X2	T52.8X3	T52.8X4	—	—
cyclohexanol	T51.8X1	T51.8X2	T51.8X3	T51.8X4	—	—
cyclohexanone	T52.8X1	T52.8X2	T52.8X3	T52.8X4	—	—
cyclohexyl acetate	T52.8X1	T52.8X2	T52.8X3	T52.8X4	—	—
demeton	T60.0X1	T60.0X2	T60.0X3	T60.0X4	—	—
dihydromorphinone	T40.2X1	T40.2X2	T40.2X3	T40.2X4	T40.2X5	T40.2X6
ergometrine	T48.0X1	T48.0X2	T48.0X3	T48.0X4	T48.0X5	T48.0X6
ergonovine	T48.0X1	T48.0X2	T48.0X3	T48.0X4	T48.0X5	T48.0X6
ethyl ketone	T52.4X1	T52.4X2	T52.4X3	T52.4X4	—	—
glucamine antimonate	T37.8X1	T37.8X2	T37.8X3	T37.8X4	T37.8X5	T37.8X6
hydrazine	T65.891	T65.892	T65.893	T65.894	—	—
iodide	T65.891	T65.892	T65.893	T65.894	—	—
isobutyl ketone	T52.4X1	T52.4X2	T52.4X3	T52.4X4	—	—
isothiocyanate	T60.3X1	T60.3X2	T60.3X3	T60.3X4	—	—
mercaptan	T59.891	T59.892	T59.893	T59.894	—	—
morphine NEC	T40.2X1	T40.2X2	T40.2X3	T40.2X4	T40.2X5	T40.2X6
nicotinate	T49.4X1	T49.4X2	T49.4X3	T49.4X4	T49.4X5	T49.4X6
paraben	T49.0X1	T49.0X2	T49.0X3	T49.0X4	T49.0X5	T49.0X6
parafynol	T42.6X1	T42.6X2	T42.6X3	T42.6X4	T42.6X5	T42.6X6
parathion	T60.0X1	T60.0X2	T60.0X3	T60.0X4	—	—
peridol	T43.4X1	T43.4X2	T43.4X3	T43.4X4	T43.4X5	T43.4X6
phenidate	T43.631	T43.632	T43.633	T43.634	T43.635	T43.636
prednisolone	T38.0X1	T38.0X2	T38.0X3	T38.0X4	T38.0X5	T38.0X6
ENT agent	T49.6X1	T49.6X2	T49.6X3	T49.6X4	T49.6X5	T49.6X6
ophthalmic preparation	T49.5X1	T49.5X2	T49.5X3	T49.5X4	T49.5X5	T49.5X6
topical NEC	T49.0X1	T49.0X2	T49.0X3	T49.0X4	T49.0X5	T49.0X6
propylcarbinol	T51.3X1	T51.3X2	T51.3X3	T51.3X4	—	—
rosaniline NEC	T49.0X1	T49.0X2	T49.0X3	T49.0X4	T49.0X5	T49.0X6
salicylate	T49.2X1	T49.2X2	T49.2X3	T49.2X4	T49.2X5	T49.2X6
sulfate (fumes)	T59.891	T59.892	T59.893	T59.894	—	—
liquid	T52.8X1	T52.8X2	T52.8X3	T52.8X4	—	—
sulfonal	T42.6X1	T42.6X2	T42.6X3	T42.6X4	T42.6X5	T42.6X6
testosterone	T38.7X1	T38.7X2	T38.7X3	T38.7X4	T38.7X5	T38.7X6
thiouracil	T38.2X1	T38.2X2	T38.2X3	T38.2X4	T38.2X5	T38.2X6
Methylamphetamine	T43.621	T43.622	T43.623	T43.624	T43.625	T43.626
Methylated spirit	T51.1X1	T51.1X2	T51.1X3	T51.1X4	—	—
Methylatropine nitrate	T44.3X1	T44.3X2	T44.3X3	T44.3X4	T44.3X5	T44.3X6

Substance	Poisoning, Accidental (unintentional)	Poisoning, Intentional Self-harm	Poisoning, Assault	Poisoning, Undetermined	Adverse Effect	Under-dosing
Methylbenactyzium bromide	T44.3X1	T44.3X2	T44.3X3	T44.3X4	T44.3X5	T44.3X6
Methylbenzethonium chloride	T49.0X1	T49.0X2	T49.0X3	T49.0X4	T49.0X5	T49.0X6
Methylcellulose	T47.4X1	T47.4X2	T47.4X3	T47.4X4	T47.4X5	T47.4X6
laxative	T47.4X1	T47.4X2	T47.4X3	T47.4X4	T47.4X5	T47.4X6
Methylchlorophenoxyacetic acid	T60.3X1	T60.3X2	T60.3X3	T60.3X4	—	—
Methyldopa	T46.5X1	T46.5X2	T46.5X3	T46.5X4	T46.5X5	T46.5X6
Methyldopate	T46.5X1	T46.5X2	T46.5X3	T46.5X4	T46.5X5	T46.5X6
Methylene						
blue	T50.6X1	T50.6X2	T50.6X3	T50.6X4	T50.6X5	T50.6X6
chloride or dichloride (solvent) NEC	T53.4X1	T53.4X2	T53.4X3	T53.4X4	—	—
Methylenedioxyamphetamine	T43.621	T43.622	T43.623	T43.624	T43.625	T43.626
Methylenedioxymethamphetamine	T43.621	T43.622	T43.623	T43.624	T43.625	T43.626
Methylergometrine	T48.0X1	T48.0X2	T48.0X3	T48.0X4	T48.0X5	T48.0X6
Methylergonovine	T48.0X1	T48.0X2	T48.0X3	T48.0X4	T48.0X5	T48.0X6
Methylestrenolone	T38.5X1	T38.5X2	T38.5X3	T38.5X4	T38.5X5	T38.5X6
Methylethyl cellulose	T50.991	T50.992	T50.993	T50.994	T50.995	T50.996
Methylhexabital	T42.3X1	T42.3X2	T42.3X3	T42.3X4	T42.3X5	T42.3X6
Methylmorphine	T40.2X1	T40.2X2	T40.2X3	T40.2X4	T40.2X5	T40.2X6
Methylparaben (ophthalmic)	T49.5X1	T49.5X2	T49.5X3	T49.5X4	T49.5X5	T49.5X6
Methylparafynol	T42.6X1	T42.6X2	T42.6X3	T42.6X4	T42.6X5	T42.6X6
Methylpentynol, methylpenthynol	T42.6X1	T42.6X2	T42.6X3	T42.6X4	T42.6X5	T42.6X6
Methylphenidate	T43.631	T43.632	T43.633	T43.634	T43.635	T43.636
Methylphenobarbital	T42.3X1	T42.3X2	T42.3X3	T42.3X4	T42.3X5	T42.3X6
Methylpolysiloxane	T47.1X1	T47.1X2	T47.1X3	T47.1X4	T47.1X5	T47.1X6
Methylprednisolone — see Methyl, prednisolone						
Methylrosaniline	T49.0X1	T49.0X2	T49.0X3	T49.0X4	T49.0X5	T49.0X6
Methylrosanilinium chloride	T49.0X1	T49.0X2	T49.0X3	T49.0X4	T49.0X5	T49.0X6
Methyltestosterone	T38.7X1	T38.7X2	T38.7X3	T38.7X4	T38.7X5	T38.7X6
Methylthionine chloride	T50.6X1	T50.6X2	T50.6X3	T50.6X4	T50.6X5	T50.6X6
Methylthioninium chloride	T50.6X1	T50.6X2	T50.6X3	T50.6X4	T50.6X5	T50.6X6
Methylthiouracil	T38.2X1	T38.2X2	T38.2X3	T38.2X4	T38.2X5	T38.2X6
Methyprylon	T42.6X1	T42.6X2	T42.6X3	T42.6X4	T42.6X5	T42.6X6
Methysergide	T46.5X1	T46.5X2	T46.5X3	T46.5X4	T46.5X5	T46.5X6
Metiamide	T47.1X1	T47.1X2	T47.1X3	T47.1X4	T47.1X5	T47.1X6
Meticillin	T36.0X1	T36.0X2	T36.0X3	T36.0X4	T36.0X5	T36.0X6
Meticrane	T50.2X1	T50.2X2	T50.2X3	T50.2X4	T50.2X5	T50.2X6
Metildigoxin	T46.0X1	T46.0X2	T46.0X3	T46.0X4	T46.0X5	T46.0X6
Metipranolol	T49.5X1	T49.5X2	T49.5X3	T49.5X4	T49.5X5	T49.5X6
Metirosine	T46.5X1	T46.5X2	T46.5X3	T46.5X4	T46.5X5	T46.5X6
Metisazone	T37.5X1	T37.5X2	T37.5X3	T37.5X4	T37.5X5	T37.5X6
Metixene	T44.3X1	T44.3X2	T44.3X3	T44.3X4	T44.3X5	T44.3X6
Metizoline	T48.5X1	T48.5X2	T48.5X3	T48.5X4	T48.5X5	T48.5X6
Metoclopramide	T45.0X1	T45.0X2	T45.0X3	T45.0X4	T45.0X5	T45.0X6
Metofenazate	T43.3X1	T43.3X2	T43.3X3	T43.3X4	T43.3X5	T43.3X6
Metofoline	T39.8X1	T39.8X2	T39.8X3	T39.8X4	T39.8X5	T39.8X6
Metolazone	T50.2X1	T50.2X2	T50.2X3	T50.2X4	T50.2X5	T50.2X6
Metopon	T40.2X1	T40.2X2	T40.2X3	T40.2X4	T40.2X5	T40.2X6
Metoprine	T45.1X1	T45.1X2	T45.1X3	T45.1X4	T45.1X5	T45.1X6
Metoprolol	T44.7X1	T44.7X2	T44.7X3	T44.7X4	T44.7X5	T44.7X6
Metrifonate	T60.0X1	T60.0X2	T60.0X3	T60.0X4	—	—
Metrizamide	T50.8X1	T50.8X2	T50.8X3	T50.8X4	T50.8X5	T50.8X6
Metrizoic acid	T50.8X1	T50.8X2	T50.8X3	T50.8X4	T50.8X5	T50.8X6
Metronidazole	T37.8X1	T37.8X2	T37.8X3	T37.8X4	T37.8X5	T37.8X6
Metycaine	T41.3X1	T41.3X2	T41.3X3	T41.3X4	T41.3X5	T41.3X6
infiltration (subcutaneous)	T41.3X1	T41.3X2	T41.3X3	T41.3X4	T41.3X5	T41.3X6
nerve block (peripheral) (plexus)	T41.3X1	T41.3X2	T41.3X3	T41.3X4	T41.3X5	T41.3X6
topical (surface)	T41.3X1	T41.3X2	T41.3X3	T41.3X4	T41.3X5	T41.3X6
Metyrapone	T50.8X1	T50.8X2	T50.8X3	T50.8X4	T50.8X5	T50.8X6
Mevinphos	T60.0X1	T60.0X2	T60.0X3	T60.0X4	—	—
Mexazolam	T42.4X1	T42.4X2	T42.4X3	T42.4X4	T42.4X5	T42.4X6
Mexenone	T49.3X1	T49.3X2	T49.3X3	T49.3X4	T49.3X5	T49.3X6
Mexiletine	T46.2X1	T46.2X2	T46.2X3	T46.2X4	T46.2X5	T46.2X6
Mezereon	T62.2X1	T62.2X2	T62.2X3	T62.2X4	—	—
berries	T62.1X1	T62.1X2	T62.1X3	T62.1X4	—	—
Mezlocillin	T36.0X1	T36.0X2	T36.0X3	T36.0X4	T36.0X5	T36.0X6
Mianserin	T43.021	T43.022	T43.023	T43.024	T43.025	T43.026
Micatin	T49.0X1	T49.0X2	T49.0X3	T49.0X4	T49.0X5	T49.0X6
Miconazole	T49.0X1	T49.0X2	T49.0X3	T49.0X4	T49.0X5	T49.0X6
Micronomicin	T36.5X1	T36.5X2	T36.5X3	T36.5X4	T36.5X5	T36.5X6
Midazolam	T42.4X1	T42.4X2	T42.4X3	T42.4X4	T42.4X5	T42.4X6
Midecamycin	T36.3X1	T36.3X2	T36.3X3	T36.3X4	T36.3X5	T36.3X6
Mifepristone	T38.6X1	T38.6X2	T38.6X3	T38.6X4	T38.6X5	T38.6X6
Milk of magnesia	T47.1X1	T47.1X2	T47.1X3	T47.1X4	T47.1X5	T47.1X6

Additional Character May Be Required — Refer to the Tabular List for Character Selection ▽ Subterms under main terms may continue to next column or page

Substance	Poisoning, Accidental (unintentional)	Poisoning, Intentional Self-harm	Poisoning, Assault	Poisoning, Undetermined	Adverse Effect	Under-dosing
Millipede (tropical)	T63.411	T63.412	T63.413	T63.414	—	—
(venomous)						
Miltown	T43.591	T43.592	T43.593	T43.594	T43.595	T43.596
Milverine	T44.3X1	T44.3X2	T44.3X3	T44.3X4	T44.3X5	T44.3X6
Minaprine	T43.291	T43.292	T43.293	T43.294	T43.295	T43.296
Minaxolone	T41.291	T41.292	T41.293	T41.294	T41.295	T41.296
Mineral						
acids	T54.2X1	T54.2X2	T54.2X3	T54.2X4	—	—
oil (laxative)(medicinal)	T47.4X1	T47.4X2	T47.4X3	T47.4X4	T47.4X5	T47.4X6
emulsion	T47.2X1	T47.2X2	T47.2X3	T47.2X4	T47.2X5	T47.2X6
nonmedicinal	T52.0X1	T52.0X2	T52.0X3	T52.0X4	—	—
topical	T49.3X1	T49.3X2	T49.3X3	T49.3X4	T49.3X5	T49.3X6
salt NEC	T50.3X1	T50.3X2	T50.3X3	T50.3X4	T50.3X5	T50.3X6
spirits	T52.0X1	T52.0X2	T52.0X3	T52.0X4	—	—
Mineralocorticosteroid	T50.0X1	T50.0X2	T50.0X3	T50.0X4	T50.0X5	T50.0X6
Minocycline	T36.4X1	T36.4X2	T36.4X3	T36.4X4	T36.4X5	T36.4X6
Minoxidil	T46.7X1	T46.7X2	T46.7X3	T46.7X4	T46.7X5	T46.7X6
Miokamycin	T36.3X1	T36.3X2	T36.3X3	T36.3X4	T36.3X5	T36.3X6
Miotic drug	T49.5X1	T49.5X2	T49.5X3	T49.5X4	T49.5X5	T49.5X6
Mipafox	T60.0X1	T60.0X2	T60.0X3	T60.0X4	—	—
Mirex	T60.1X1	T60.1X2	T60.1X3	T60.1X4	—	—
Mirtazapine	T43.021	T43.022	T43.023	T43.024	T43.025	T43.026
Misonidazole	T37.3X1	T37.3X2	T37.3X3	T37.3X4	T37.3X5	T37.3X6
Misoprostol	T47.1X1	T47.1X2	T47.1X3	T47.1X4	T47.1X5	T47.1X6
Mithramycin	T45.1X1	T45.1X2	T45.1X3	T45.1X4	T45.1X5	T45.1X6
Mitobronitol	T45.1X1	T45.1X2	T45.1X3	T45.1X4	T45.1X5	T45.1X6
Mitoguazone	T45.1X1	T45.1X2	T45.1X3	T45.1X4	T45.1X5	T45.1X6
Mitolactol	T45.1X1	T45.1X2	T45.1X3	T45.1X4	T45.1X5	T45.1X6
Mitomycin	T45.1X1	T45.1X2	T45.1X3	T45.1X4	T45.1X5	T45.1X6
Mitopodozide	T45.1X1	T45.1X2	T45.1X3	T45.1X4	T45.1X5	T45.1X6
Mitotane	T45.1X1	T45.1X2	T45.1X3	T45.1X4	T45.1X5	T45.1X6
Mitoxantrone	T45.1X1	T45.1X2	T45.1X3	T45.1X4	T45.1X5	T45.1X6
Mivacurium chloride	T48.1X1	T48.1X2	T48.1X3	T48.1X4	T48.1X5	T48.1X6
Miyari bacteria	T47.6X1	T47.6X2	T47.6X3	T47.6X4	T47.6X5	T47.6X6
Moclobemide	T43.1X1	T43.1X2	T43.1X3	T43.1X4	T43.1X5	T43.1X6
Moderil	T46.5X1	T46.5X2	T46.5X3	T46.5X4	T46.5X5	T46.5X6
Mofebutazone	T39.2X1	T39.2X2	T39.2X3	T39.2X4	T39.2X5	T39.2X6
Mogadon — see Nitrazepam						
Molindone	T43.591	T43.592	T43.593	T43.594	T43.595	T43.596
Molsidomine	T46.3X1	T46.3X2	T46.3X3	T46.3X4	T46.3X5	T46.3X6
Mometasone	T49.0X1	T49.0X2	T49.0X3	T49.0X4	T49.0X5	T49.0X6
Monistat	T49.0X1	T49.0X2	T49.0X3	T49.0X4	T49.0X5	T49.0X6
Monkshood	T62.2X1	T62.2X2	T62.2X3	T62.2X4	—	—
Monoamine oxidase inhibitor NEC	T43.1X1	T43.1X2	T43.1X3	T43.1X4	T43.1X5	T43.1X6
hydrazine	T43.1X1	T43.1X2	T43.1X3	T43.1X4	T43.1X5	T43.1X6
Monobenzone	T49.4X1	T49.4X2	T49.4X3	T49.4X4	T49.4X5	T49.4X6
Monochloroacetic acid	T60.3X1	T60.3X2	T60.3X3	T60.3X4	—	—
Monochlorobenzene	T53.7X1	T53.7X2	T53.7X3	T53.7X4	—	—
Monoethanolamine	T46.8X1	T46.8X2	T46.8X3	T46.8X4	T46.8X5	T46.8X6
oleate	T46.8X1	T46.8X2	T46.8X3	T46.8X4	T46.8X5	T46.8X6
Monooctanoin	T50.991	T50.992	T50.993	T50.994	T50.995	T50.996
Monophenylbutazone	T39.2X1	T39.2X2	T39.2X3	T39.2X4	T39.2X5	T39.2X6
Monosodium glutamate	T65.891	T65.892	T65.893	T65.894	—	—
Monosulfiram	T49.0X1	T49.0X2	T49.0X3	T49.0X4	T49.0X5	T49.0X6
Monoxide, carbon — see Carbon, monoxide						
Monoxidine hydrochloride	T46.1X1	T46.1X2	T46.1X3	T46.1X4	T46.1X5	T46.1X6
Monuron	T60.3X1	T60.3X2	T60.3X3	T60.3X4	—	—
Moperone	T43.4X1	T43.4X2	T43.4X3	T43.4X4	T43.4X5	T43.4X6
Mopidamol	T45.1X1	T45.1X2	T45.1X3	T45.1X4	T45.1X5	T45.1X6
MOPP (mechloreth-amine + vincristine + prednisone + procarba-zine)	T45.1X1	T45.1X2	T45.1X3	T45.1X4	T45.1X5	T45.1X6
Morfin	T40.2X1	T40.2X2	T40.2X3	T40.2X4	T40.2X5	T40.2X6
Morinamide	T37.1X1	T37.1X2	T37.1X3	T37.1X4	T37.1X5	T37.1X6
Morning glory seeds	T40.991	T40.992	T40.993	T40.994	—	—
Moroxydine	T37.5X1	T37.5X2	T37.5X3	T37.5X4	T37.5X5	T37.5X6
Morphazinamide	T37.1X1	T37.1X2	T37.1X3	T37.1X4	T37.1X5	T37.1X6
Morphine	T40.2X1	T40.2X2	T40.2X3	T40.2X4	T40.2X5	T40.2X6
antagonist	T50.7X1	T50.7X2	T50.7X3	T50.7X4	T50.7X5	T50.7X6
Morpholinylethylmorphine	T40.2X1	T40.2X2	T40.2X3	T40.2X4	—	—
Morsuximide	T42.2X1	T42.2X2	T42.2X3	T42.2X4	T42.2X5	T42.2X6
Mosapramine	T43.591	T43.592	T43.593	T43.594	T43.595	T43.596
Moth balls — see also Pesticides	T60.2X1	T60.2X2	T60.2X3	T60.2X4	—	—
naphthalene	T60.2X1	T60.2X2	T60.2X3	T60.2X4	—	—
paradichlorobenzene	T60.1X1	T60.1X2	T60.1X3	T60.1X4	—	—
Motor exhaust gas	T58.01	T58.02	T58.03	T58.04	—	—
Mouthwash (antiseptic) (zinc chloride)	T49.6X1	T49.6X2	T49.6X3	T49.6X4	T49.6X5	T49.6X6
Moxastine	T45.0X1	T45.0X2	T45.0X3	T45.0X4	T45.0X5	T45.0X6
Moxaverine	T44.3X1	T44.3X2	T44.3X3	T44.3X4	T44.3X5	T44.3X6
Moxisylyte	T46.7X1	T46.7X2	T46.7X3	T46.7X4	T46.7X5	T46.7X6
Mucilage, plant	T47.4X1	T47.4X2	T47.4X3	T47.4X4	T47.4X5	T47.4X6
Mucolytic drug	T48.4X1	T48.4X2	T48.4X3	T48.4X4	T48.4X5	T48.4X6
Mucomyst	T48.4X1	T48.4X2	T48.4X3	T48.4X4	T48.4X5	T48.4X6
Mucous membrane agents (external)	T49.91	T49.92	T49.93	T49.94	T49.95	T49.96
specified NEC	T49.8X1	T49.8X2	T49.8X3	T49.8X4	T49.8X5	T49.8X6
Mumps						
immune globulin (human)	T50.Z11	T50.Z12	T50.Z13	T50.Z14	T50.Z15	T50.Z16
skin test antigen	T50.8X1	T50.8X2	T50.8X3	T50.8X4	T50.8X5	T50.8X6
vaccine	T50.B91	T50.B92	T50.B93	T50.B94	T50.B95	T50.B96
Mumpsvax	T50.B91	T50.B92	T50.B93	T50.B94	T50.B95	T50.B96
Mupirocin	T49.0X1	T49.0X2	T49.0X3	T49.0X4	T49.0X5	T49.0X6
Muriatic acid — see Hydrochloric acid						
Muromonab-CD3	T45.1X1	T45.1X2	T45.1X3	T45.1X4	T45.1X5	T45.1X6
Muscle-action drug NEC	T48.201	T48.202	T48.203	T48.204	T48.205	T48.206
Muscle affecting agents NEC	T48.201	T48.202	T48.203	T48.204	T48.205	T48.206
oxytocic	T48.0X1	T48.0X2	T48.0X3	T48.0X4	T48.0X5	T48.0X6
relaxants	T48.201	T48.202	T48.203	T48.204	T48.205	T48.206
central nervous system	T42.8X1	T42.8X2	T42.8X3	T42.8X4	T42.8X5	T42.8X6
skeletal	T48.1X1	T48.1X2	T48.1X3	T48.1X4	T48.1X5	T48.1X6
smooth	T44.3X1	T44.3X2	T44.3X3	T44.3X4	T44.3X5	T44.3X6
Muscle relaxant — see Relaxant, muscle						
Muscle-tone depressant, central NEC	T42.8X1	T42.8X2	T42.8X3	T42.8X4	T42.8X5	T42.8X6
specified NEC	T42.8X1	T42.8X2	T42.8X3	T42.8X4	T42.8X5	T42.8X6
Mushroom, noxious	T62.0X1	T62.0X2	T62.0X3	T62.0X4	—	—
Mussel, noxious	T61.781	T61.782	T61.783	T61.784	—	—
Mustard (emetic)	T47.7X1	T47.7X2	T47.7X3	T47.7X4	T47.7X5	T47.7X6
black	T47.7X1	T47.7X2	T47.7X3	T47.7X4	T47.7X5	T47.7X6
gas, not in war	T59.91	T59.92	T59.93	T59.94	—	—
nitrogen	T45.1X1	T45.1X2	T45.1X3	T45.1X4	T45.1X5	T45.1X6
Mustine	T45.1X1	T45.1X2	T45.1X3	T45.1X4	T45.1X5	T45.1X6
M-vac	T45.1X1	T45.1X2	T45.1X3	T45.1X4	T45.1X5	T45.1X6
Mycifradin	T36.5X1	T36.5X2	T36.5X3	T36.5X4	T36.5X5	T36.5X6
topical	T49.0X1	T49.0X2	T49.0X3	T49.0X4	T49.0X5	T49.0X6
Mycitracin	T36.8X1	T36.8X2	T36.8X3	T36.8X4	T36.8X5	T36.8X6
ophthalmic preparation	T49.5X1	T49.5X2	T49.5X3	T49.5X4	T49.5X5	T49.5X6
Mycostatin	T36.7X1	T36.7X2	T36.7X3	T36.7X4	T36.7X5	T36.7X6
topical	T49.0X1	T49.0X2	T49.0X3	T49.0X4	T49.0X5	T49.0X6
Mycotoxins	T64.81	T64.82	T64.83	T64.84	—	—
aflatoxin	T64.01	T64.02	T64.03	T64.04	—	—
specified NEC	T64.81	T64.82	T64.83	T64.84	—	—
Mydriacyl	T44.3X1	T44.3X2	T44.3X3	T44.3X4	T44.3X5	T44.3X6
Mydriatic drug	T49.5X1	T49.5X2	T49.5X3	T49.5X4	T49.5X5	T49.5X6
Myelobromal	T45.1X1	T45.1X2	T45.1X3	T45.1X4	T45.1X5	T45.1X6
Myleran	T45.1X1	T45.1X2	T45.1X3	T45.1X4	T45.1X5	T45.1X6
Myochrysin (e)	T39.2X1	T39.2X2	T39.2X3	T39.2X4	T39.2X5	T39.2X6
Myoneural blocking agents	T48.1X1	T48.1X2	T48.1X3	T48.1X4	T48.1X5	T48.1X6
Myralact	T49.0X1	T49.0X2	T49.0X3	T49.0X4	T49.0X5	T49.0X6
Myristica fragrans	T62.2X1	T62.2X2	T62.2X3	T62.2X4	—	—
Myristicin	T65.891	T65.892	T65.893	T65.894	—	—
Mysoline	T42.3X1	T42.3X2	T42.3X3	T42.3X4	T42.3X5	T42.3X6
Nabilone	T40.7X1	T40.7X2	T40.7X3	T40.7X4	T40.7X5	T40.7X6
Nabumetone	T39.391	T39.392	T39.393	T39.394	T39.395	T39.396
Nadolol	T44.7X1	T44.7X2	T44.7X3	T44.7X4	T44.7X5	T44.7X6
Nafcillin	T36.0X1	T36.0X2	T36.0X3	T36.0X4	T36.0X5	T36.0X6
Nafoxidine	T38.6X1	T38.6X2	T38.6X3	T38.6X4	T38.6X5	T38.6X6
Naftazone	T46.991	T46.992	T46.993	T46.994	T46.995	T46.996
Naftidrofuryl (oxalate)	T46.7X1	T46.7X2	T46.7X3	T46.7X4	T46.7X5	T46.7X6
Naftifine	T49.0X1	T49.0X2	T49.0X3	T49.0X4	T49.0X5	T49.0X6
Nail polish remover	T52.91	T52.92	T52.93	T52.94	—	—
Nalbuphine	T40.4X1	T40.4X2	T40.4X3	T40.4X4	T40.4X5	T40.4X6
Naled	T60.0X1	T60.0X2	T60.0X3	T60.0X4	—	—
Nalidixic acid	T37.8X1	T37.8X2	T37.8X3	T37.8X4	T37.8X5	T37.8X6
Nalorphine	T50.7X1	T50.7X2	T50.7X3	T50.7X4	T50.7X5	T50.7X6
Naloxone	T50.7X1	T50.7X2	T50.7X3	T50.7X4	T50.7X5	T50.7X6
Naltrexone	T50.7X1	T50.7X2	T50.7X3	T50.7X4	T50.7X5	T50.7X6
Namenda	T43.8X1	T43.8X2	T43.8X3	T43.8X4	T43.8X5	T43.8X6
Nandrolone	T38.7X1	T38.7X2	T38.7X3	T38.7X4	T38.7X5	T38.7X6
Naphazoline	T48.5X1	T48.5X2	T48.5X3	T48.5X4	T48.5X5	T48.5X6
Naphtha (painters') (petroleum)	T52.0X1	T52.0X2	T52.0X3	T52.0X4	—	—
solvent	T52.0X1	T52.0X2	T52.0X3	T52.0X4	—	—
vapor	T52.0X1	T52.0X2	T52.0X3	T52.0X4	—	—
Naphthalene (non-chlorinated)	T60.2X1	T60.2X2	T60.2X3	T60.2X4	—	—
chlorinated	T60.1X1	T60.1X2	T60.1X3	T60.1X4	—	—
vapor	T60.1X1	T60.1X2	T60.1X3	T60.1X4	—	—

▽ Subterms under main terms may continue to next column or page   Additional Character May Be Required — Refer to the Tabular List for Character Selection

Table of Drugs and Chemicals

Naphthalene — Nonoxinol

Substance	Poisoning, Accidental (unintentional)	Poisoning, Intentional Self-harm	Poisoning, Assault	Poisoning, Undetermined	Adverse Effect	Under-dosing
Naphthalene — *continued*						
insecticide or moth repellent	T60.2X1	T60.2X2	T60.2X3	T60.2X4	—	—
chlorinated	T60.1X1	T60.1X2	T60.1X3	T60.1X4	—	—
vapor	T60.2X1	T60.2X2	T60.2X3	T60.2X4	—	—
chlorinated	T60.1X1	T60.1X2	T60.1X3	T60.1X4	—	—
Naphthol	T65.891	T65.892	T65.893	T65.894	—	—
Naphthylamine	T65.891	T65.892	T65.893	T65.894	—	—
Naphthylthiourea (ANTU)	T60.4X1	T60.4X2	T60.4X3	T60.4X4	—	—
Naprosyn — *see* Naproxen						
Naproxen	T39.311	T39.312	T39.313	T39.314	T39.315	T39.316
Narcotic (drug)	T40.601	T40.602	T40.603	T40.604	T40.605	T40.606
analgesic NEC	T40.601	T40.602	T40.603	T40.604	T40.605	T40.606
antagonist	T50.7X1	T50.7X2	T50.7X3	T50.7X4	T50.7X5	T50.7X6
specified NEC	T40.691	T40.692	T40.693	T40.694	T40.695	T40.696
synthetic	T40.4X1	T40.4X2	T40.4X3	T40.4X4	T40.4X5	T40.4X6
Narcotine	T48.3X1	T48.3X2	T48.3X3	T48.3X4	T48.3X5	T48.3X6
Nardil	T43.1X1	T43.1X2	T43.1X3	T43.1X4	T43.1X5	T43.1X6
Nasal drug NEC	T49.6X1	T49.6X2	T49.6X3	T49.6X4	T49.6X5	T49.6X6
Natamycin	T49.0X1	T49.0X2	T49.0X3	T49.0X4	T49.0X5	T49.0X6
Natrium cyanide — *see* Cyanide(s)						
Natural						
blood (product)	T45.8X1	T45.8X2	T45.8X3	T45.8X4	T45.8X5	T45.8X6
gas (piped)	T59.891	T59.892	T59.893	T59.894	—	—
incomplete combustion	T58.11	T58.12	T58.13	T58.14	—	—
Nealbarbital	T42.3X1	T42.3X2	T42.3X3	T42.3X4	T42.3X5	T42.3X6
Nectadon	T48.3X1	T48.3X2	T48.3X3	T48.3X4	T48.3X5	T48.3X6
Nedocromil	T48.6X1	T48.6X2	T48.6X3	T48.6X4	T48.6X5	T48.6X6
Nefopam	T39.8X1	T39.8X2	T39.8X3	T39.8X4	T39.8X5	T39.8X6
Nematocyst (sting)	T63.691	T63.692	T63.693	T63.694	—	—
Nembutal	T42.3X1	T42.3X2	T42.3X3	T42.3X4	T42.3X5	T42.3X6
Nemonapride	T43.591	T43.592	T43.593	T43.594	T43.595	T43.596
Neoarsphenamine	T37.8X1	T37.8X2	T37.8X3	T37.8X4	T37.8X5	T37.8X6
Neocinchophen	T50.4X1	T50.4X2	T50.4X3	T50.4X4	T50.4X5	T50.4X6
Neomycin (derivatives)	T36.5X1	T36.5X2	T36.5X3	T36.5X4	T36.5X5	T36.5X6
with						
bacitracin	T49.0X1	T49.0X2	T49.0X3	T49.0X4	T49.0X5	T49.0X6
neostigmine	T44.0X1	T44.0X2	T44.0X3	T44.0X4	T44.0X5	T44.0X6
ENT agent	T49.6X1	T49.6X2	T49.6X3	T49.6X4	T49.6X5	T49.6X6
ophthalmic preparation	T49.5X1	T49.5X2	T49.5X3	T49.5X4	T49.5X5	T49.5X6
topical NEC	T49.0X1	T49.0X2	T49.0X3	T49.0X4	T49.0X5	T49.0X6
Neonal	T42.3X1	T42.3X2	T42.3X3	T42.3X4	T42.3X5	T42.3X6
Neoprontosil	T37.0X1	T37.0X2	T37.0X3	T37.0X4	T37.0X5	T37.0X6
Neosalvarsan	T37.8X1	T37.8X2	T37.8X3	T37.8X4	T37.8X5	T37.8X6
Neosilversalvarsan	T37.8X1	T37.8X2	T37.8X3	T37.8X4	T37.8X5	T37.8X6
Neosporin	T36.8X1	T36.8X2	T36.8X3	T36.8X4	T36.8X5	T36.8X6
ENT agent	T49.6X1	T49.6X2	T49.6X3	T49.6X4	T49.6X5	T49.6X6
opthalmic preparation	T49.5X1	T49.5X2	T49.5X3	T49.5X4	T49.5X5	T49.5X6
topical NEC	T49.0X1	T49.0X2	T49.0X3	T49.0X4	T49.0X5	T49.0X6
Neostigmine bromide	T44.0X1	T44.0X2	T44.0X3	T44.0X4	T44.0X5	T44.0X6
Neraval	T42.3X1	T42.3X2	T42.3X3	T42.3X4	T42.3X5	T42.3X6
Neravan	T42.3X1	T42.3X2	T42.3X3	T42.3X4	T42.3X5	T42.3X6
Nerium oleander	T62.2X1	T62.2X2	T62.2X3	T62.2X4	—	—
Nerve gas, not in war	T59.91	T59.92	T59.93	T59.94	—	—
Nesacaine	T41.3X1	T41.3X2	T41.3X3	T41.3X4	T41.3X5	T41.3X6
infiltration (subcutaneous)	T41.3X1	T41.3X2	T41.3X3	T41.3X4	T41.3X5	T41.3X6
nerve block (peripheral) (plexus)	T41.3X1	T41.3X2	T41.3X3	T41.3X4	T41.3X5	T41.3X6
Netilmicin	T36.5X1	T36.5X2	T36.5X3	T36.5X4	T36.5X5	T36.5X6
Neurobarb	T42.3X1	T42.3X2	T42.3X3	T42.3X4	T42.3X5	T42.3X6
Neuroleptic drug NEC	T43.501	T43.502	T43.503	T43.504	T43.505	T43.506
Neuromuscular blocking drug	T48.1X1	T48.1X2	T48.1X3	T48.1X4	T48.1X5	T48.1X6
Neutral insulin injection	T38.3X1	T38.3X2	T38.3X3	T38.3X4	T38.3X5	T38.3X6
Neutral spirits	T51.0X1	T51.0X2	T51.0X3	T51.0X4	—	—
beverage	T51.0X1	T51.0X2	T51.0X3	T51.0X4	—	—
Niacin	T46.7X1	T46.7X2	T46.7X3	T46.7X4	T46.7X5	T46.7X6
Niacinamide	T45.2X1	T45.2X2	T45.2X3	T45.2X4	T45.2X5	T45.2X6
Nialamide	T43.1X1	T43.1X2	T43.1X3	T43.1X4	T43.1X5	T43.1X6
Niaprazine	T42.6X1	T42.6X2	T42.6X3	T42.6X4	T42.6X5	T42.6X6
Nicametate	T46.7X1	T46.7X2	T46.7X3	T46.7X4	T46.7X5	T46.7X6
Nicardipine	T46.1X1	T46.1X2	T46.1X3	T46.1X4	T46.1X5	T46.1X6
Nicergoline	T46.7X1	T46.7X2	T46.7X3	T46.7X4	T46.7X5	T46.7X6
Nickel (carbonyl) (tetra-carbonyl) (fumes) (vapor)	T56.891	T56.892	T56.893	T56.894	—	—
Nickelocene	T56.891	T56.892	T56.893	T56.894	—	—
Niclosamide	T37.4X1	T37.4X2	T37.4X3	T37.4X4	T37.4X5	T37.4X6
Nicofuranose	T46.7X1	T46.7X2	T46.7X3	T46.7X4	T46.7X5	T46.7X6
Nicomorphine	T40.2X1	T40.2X2	T40.2X3	T40.2X4	—	—
Nicorandil	T46.3X1	T46.3X2	T46.3X3	T46.3X4	T46.3X5	T46.3X6
Nicotiana (plant)	T62.2X1	T62.2X2	T62.2X3	T62.2X4	—	—
Nicotinamide	T45.2X1	T45.2X2	T45.2X3	T45.2X4	T45.2X5	T45.2X6
Nicotine (insecticide) (spray) (sulfate) NEC	T60.2X1	T60.2X2	T60.2X3	T60.2X4	—	—
from tobacco	T65.291	T65.292	T65.293	T65.294	—	—
cigarettes	T65.221	T65.222	T65.223	T65.224	—	—
not insecticide	T65.291	T65.292	T65.293	T65.294	—	—
Nicotinic acid	T46.7X1	T46.7X2	T46.7X3	T46.7X4	T46.7X5	T46.7X6
Nicotinyl alcohol	T46.7X1	T46.7X2	T46.7X3	T46.7X4	T46.7X5	T46.7X6
Nicoumalone	T45.511	T45.512	T45.513	T45.514	T45.515	T45.516
Nifedipine	T46.1X1	T46.1X2	T46.1X3	T46.1X4	T46.1X5	T46.1X6
Nifenazone	T39.2X1	T39.2X2	T39.2X3	T39.2X4	T39.2X5	T39.2X6
Nifuraldezone	T37.91	T37.92	T37.93	T37.94	T37.95	T37.96
Nifuratel	T37.8X1	T37.8X2	T37.8X3	T37.8X4	T37.8X5	T37.8X6
Nifurtimox	T37.3X1	T37.3X2	T37.3X3	T37.3X4	T37.3X5	T37.3X6
Nifurtoinol	T37.8X1	T37.8X2	T37.8X3	T37.8X4	T37.8X5	T37.8X6
Nightshade, deadly (solanum) — *see also* Belladonna	T62.2X1	T62.2X2	T62.2X3	T62.2X4	—	—
berry	T62.1X1	T62.1X2	T62.1X3	T62.1X4	—	—
Nikethamide	T50.7X1	T50.7X2	T50.7X3	T50.7X4	T50.7X5	T50.7X6
Nilstat	T36.7X1	T36.7X2	T36.7X3	T36.7X4	T36.7X5	T36.7X6
topical	T49.0X1	T49.0X2	T49.0X3	T49.0X4	T49.0X5	T49.0X6
Nilutamide	T38.6X1	T38.6X2	T38.6X3	T38.6X4	T38.6X5	T38.6X6
Nimesulide	T39.391	T39.392	T39.393	T39.394	T39.395	T39.396
Nimetazepam	T42.4X1	T42.4X2	T42.4X3	T42.4X4	T42.4X5	T42.4X6
Nimodipine	T46.1X1	T46.1X2	T46.1X3	T46.1X4	T46.1X5	T46.1X6
Nimorazole	T37.3X1	T37.3X2	T37.3X3	T37.3X4	T37.3X5	T37.3X6
Nimustine	T45.1X1	T45.1X2	T45.1X3	T45.1X4	T45.1X5	T45.1X6
Niridazole	T37.4X1	T37.4X2	T37.4X3	T37.4X4	T37.4X5	T37.4X6
Nisentil	T40.2X1	T40.2X2	T40.2X3	T40.2X4	T40.2X5	T40.2X6
Nisoldipine	T46.1X1	T46.1X2	T46.1X3	T46.1X4	T46.1X5	T46.1X6
Nitramine	T65.3X1	T65.3X2	T65.3X3	T65.3X4	—	—
Nitrate, organic	T46.3X1	T46.3X2	T46.3X3	T46.3X4	T46.3X5	T46.3X6
Nitrazepam	T42.4X1	T42.4X2	T42.4X3	T42.4X4	T42.4X5	T42.4X6
Nitrefazole	T50.6X1	T50.6X2	T50.6X3	T50.6X4	T50.6X5	T50.6X6
Nitrendipine	T46.1X1	T46.1X2	T46.1X3	T46.1X4	T46.1X5	T46.1X6
Nitric						
acid (liquid)	T54.2X1	T54.2X2	T54.2X3	T54.2X4	—	—
vapor	T59.891	T59.892	T59.893	T59.894	—	—
oxide (gas)	T59.0X1	T59.0X2	T59.0X3	T59.0X4	—	—
Nitrimidazine	T37.3X1	T37.3X2	T37.3X3	T37.3X4	T37.3X5	T37.3X6
Nitrite, amyl (medicinal) (vapor)	T46.3X1	T46.3X2	T46.3X3	T46.3X4	T46.3X5	T46.3X6
Nitroaniline	T65.3X1	T65.3X2	T65.3X3	T65.3X4	—	—
vapor	T59.891	T59.892	T59.893	T59.894	—	—
Nitrobenzene, nitrobenzol	T65.3X1	T65.3X2	T65.3X3	T65.3X4	—	—
vapor	T65.3X1	T65.3X2	T65.3X3	T65.3X4	—	—
Nitrocellulose	T65.891	T65.892	T65.893	T65.894	—	—
lacquer	T65.891	T65.892	T65.893	T65.894	—	—
Nitrodiphenyl	T65.3X1	T65.3X2	T65.3X3	T65.3X4	—	—
Nitrofural	T49.0X1	T49.0X2	T49.0X3	T49.0X4	T49.0X5	T49.0X6
Nitrofurantoin	T37.8X1	T37.8X2	T37.8X3	T37.8X4	T37.8X5	T37.8X6
Nitrofurazone	T49.0X1	T49.0X2	T49.0X3	T49.0X4	T49.0X5	T49.0X6
Nitrogen	T59.0X1	T59.0X2	T59.0X3	T59.0X4	—	—
mustard	T45.1X1	T45.1X2	T45.1X3	T45.1X4	T45.1X5	T45.1X6
Nitroglycerin, nitroglycerol (medicinal)	T46.3X1	T46.3X2	T46.3X3	T46.3X4	T46.3X5	T46.3X6
nonmedicinal	T65.5X1	T65.5X2	T65.5X3	T65.5X4	—	—
fumes	T65.5X1	T65.5X2	T65.5X3	T65.5X4	—	—
Nitroglycol	T52.3X1	T52.3X2	T52.3X3	T52.3X4	—	—
Nitrohydrochloric acid	T54.2X1	T54.2X2	T54.2X3	T54.2X4	—	—
Nitromersol	T49.0X1	T49.0X2	T49.0X3	T49.0X4	T49.0X5	T49.0X6
Nitronaphthalene	T65.891	T65.892	T65.893	T65.894	—	—
Nitrophenol	T54.0X1	T54.0X2	T54.0X3	T54.0X4	—	—
Nitropropane	T52.8X1	T52.8X2	T52.8X3	T52.8X4	—	—
Nitroprusside	T46.5X1	T46.5X2	T46.5X3	T46.5X4	T46.5X5	T46.5X6
Nitrosodimethylamine	T65.3X1	T65.3X2	T65.3X3	T65.3X4	—	—
Nitrothiazol	T37.4X1	T37.4X2	T37.4X3	T37.4X4	T37.4X5	T37.4X6
Nitrotoluene, nitrotoluol	T65.3X1	T65.3X2	T65.3X3	T65.3X4	—	—
vapor	T65.3X1	T65.3X2	T65.3X3	T65.3X4	—	—
Nitrous						
acid (liquid)	T54.2X1	T54.2X2	T54.2X3	T54.2X4	—	—
fumes	T59.891	T59.892	T59.893	T59.894	—	—
ether spirit	T46.3X1	T46.3X2	T46.3X3	T46.3X4	T46.3X5	T46.3X6
oxide	T41.0X1	T41.0X2	T41.0X3	T41.0X4	T41.0X5	T41.0X6
Nitroxoline	T37.8X1	T37.8X2	T37.8X3	T37.8X4	T37.8X5	T37.8X6
Nitrozone	T49.0X1	T49.0X2	T49.0X3	T49.0X4	T49.0X5	T49.0X6
Nizatidine	T47.0X1	T47.0X2	T47.0X3	T47.0X4	T47.0X5	T47.0X6
Nizofenone	T43.8X1	T43.8X2	T43.8X3	T43.8X4	T43.8X5	T43.8X6
Noctec	T42.6X1	T42.6X2	T42.6X3	T42.6X4	T42.6X5	T42.6X6
Noludar	T42.6X1	T42.6X2	T42.6X3	T42.6X4	T42.6X5	T42.6X6
Nomegestrol	T38.5X1	T38.5X2	T38.5X3	T38.5X4	T38.5X5	T38.5X6
Nomifensine	T43.291	T43.292	T43.293	T43.294	T43.295	T43.296
Nonoxinol	T49.8X1	T49.8X2	T49.8X3	T49.8X4	T49.8X5	T49.8X6

Additional Character May Be Required — Refer to the Tabular List for Character Selection ▼ **Subterms under main terms may continue to next column or page**

Substance	Poisoning, Accidental (unintentional)	Poisoning, Intentional Self-harm	Poisoning, Assault	Poisoning, Undetermined	Adverse Effect	Underdosing
Nonylphenoxy	T49.8X1	T49.8X2	T49.8X3	T49.8X4	T49.8X5	T49.8X6
(polyethoxyethanol)						
Noptil	T42.3X1	T42.3X2	T42.3X3	T42.3X4	T42.3X5	T42.3X6
Noradrenaline	T44.4X1	T44.4X2	T44.4X3	T44.4X4	T44.4X5	T44.4X6
Noramidopyrine	T39.2X1	T39.2X2	T39.2X3	T39.2X4	T39.2X5	T39.2X6
methanesulfonate sodium	T39.2X1	T39.2X2	T39.2X3	T39.2X4	T39.2X5	T39.2X6
Norbormide	T60.4X1	T60.4X2	T60.4X3	T60.4X4	—	—
Nordazepam	T42.4X1	T42.4X2	T42.4X3	T42.4X4	T42.4X5	T42.4X6
Norepinephrine	T44.4X1	T44.4X2	T44.4X3	T44.4X4	T44.4X5	T44.4X6
Norethandrolone	T38.7X1	T38.7X2	T38.7X3	T38.7X4	T38.7X5	T38.7X6
Norethindrone	T38.4X1	T38.4X2	T38.4X3	T38.4X4	T38.4X5	T38.4X6
Norethisterone (acetate)	T38.4X1	T38.4X2	T38.4X3	T38.4X4	T38.4X5	T38.4X6
(enantate)						
with ethinylestradiol	T38.5X1	T38.5X2	T38.5X3	T38.5X4	T38.5X5	T38.5X6
Noretynodrel	T38.5X1	T38.5X2	T38.5X3	T38.5X4	T38.5X5	T38.5X6
Norfenefrine	T44.4X1	T44.4X2	T44.4X3	T44.4X4	T44.4X5	T44.4X6
Norfloxacin	T36.8X1	T36.8X2	T36.8X3	T36.8X4	T36.8X5	T36.8X6
Norgestrel	T38.4X1	T38.4X2	T38.4X3	T38.4X4	T38.4X5	T38.4X6
Norgestrienone	T38.4X1	T38.4X2	T38.4X3	T38.4X4	T38.4X5	T38.4X6
Norlestrin	T38.4X1	T38.4X2	T38.4X3	T38.4X4	T38.4X5	T38.4X6
Norlutin	T38.4X1	T38.4X2	T38.4X3	T38.4X4	T38.4X5	T38.4X6
Normal serum albumin (human),	T45.8X1	T45.8X2	T45.8X4		T45.8X5	T45.8X6
salt-poor						
Normethandrone	T38.5X1	T38.5X2	T38.5X3	T38.5X4	T38.5X5	T38.5X6
Normison — see						
Benzodiazepines						
Normorphine	T40.2X1	T40.2X2	T40.2X3	T40.2X4	—	—
Norpseudoephedrine	T50.5X1	T50.5X2	T50.5X3	T50.5X4	T50.5X5	T50.5X6
Nortestosterone	T38.7X1	T38.7X2	T38.7X3	T38.7X4	T38.7X5	T38.7X6
(furanpropionate)						
Nortriptyline	T43.011	T43.012	T43.013	T43.014	T43.015	T43.016
Noscapine	T48.3X1	T48.3X2	T48.3X3	T48.3X4	T48.3X5	T48.3X6
Nose preparations	T49.6X1	T49.6X2	T49.6X3	T49.6X4	T49.6X5	T49.6X6
Novobiocin	T36.5X1	T36.5X2	T36.5X3	T36.5X4	T36.5X5	T36.5X6
Novocain (infiltration)	T41.3X1	T41.3X2	T41.3X3	T41.3X4	T41.3X5	T41.3X6
(topical)						
nerve block (peripheral)	T41.3X1	T41.3X2	T41.3X3	T41.3X4	T41.3X5	T41.3X6
(plexus)						
spinal	T41.3X1	T41.3X2	T41.3X3	T41.3X4	T41.3X5	T41.3X6
Noxious foodstuff	T62.91	T62.92	T62.93	T62.94	—	—
specified NEC	T62.8X1	T62.8X2	T62.8X3	T62.8X4	—	—
Noxiptiline	T43.011	T43.012	T43.013	T43.014	T43.015	T43.016
Noxytiolin	T49.0X1	T49.0X2	T49.0X3	T49.0X4	T49.0X5	T49.0X6
NPH Iletin (insulin)	T38.3X1	T38.3X2	T38.3X3	T38.3X4	T38.3X5	T38.3X6
Numorphan	T40.2X1	T40.2X2	T40.2X3	T40.2X4	T40.2X5	T40.2X6
Nunol	T42.3X1	T42.3X2	T42.3X3	T42.3X4	T42.3X5	T42.3X6
Nupercaine (spinal	T41.3X1	T41.3X2	T41.3X3	T41.3X4	T41.3X5	T41.3X6
anesthetic)						
topical (surface)	T41.3X1	T41.3X2	T41.3X3	T41.3X4	T41.3X5	T41.3X6
Nutmeg oil (liniment)	T49.3X1	T49.3X2	T49.3X3	T49.3X4	T49.3X5	T49.3X6
Nutritional supplement	T50.901	T50.902	T50.903	T50.904	T50.905	T50.906
Nux vomica	T65.1X1	T65.1X2	T65.1X3	T65.1X4	—	—
Nydrazid	T37.1X1	T37.1X2	T37.1X3	T37.1X4	T37.1X5	T37.1X6
Nylidrin	T46.7X1	T46.7X2	T46.7X3	T46.7X4	T46.7X5	T46.7X6
Nystatin	T36.7X1	T36.7X2	T36.7X3	T36.7X4	T36.7X5	T36.7X6
topical	T49.0X1	T49.0X2	T49.0X3	T49.0X4	T49.0X5	T49.0X6
Nytol	T45.0X1	T45.0X2	T45.0X3	T45.0X4	T45.0X5	T45.0X6
Obidoxime chloride	T50.6X1	T50.6X2	T50.6X3	T50.6X4	T50.6X5	T50.6X6
Octafonium (chloride)	T49.3X1	T49.3X2	T49.3X3	T49.3X4	T49.3X5	T49.3X6
Octamethyl	T60.0X1	T60.0X2	T60.0X3	T60.0X4	—	—
pyrophosphoramide						
Octanoin	T50.991	T50.992	T50.993	T50.994	T50.995	T50.996
Octatropine	T44.3X1	T44.3X2	T44.3X3	T44.3X4	T44.3X5	T44.3X6
methylbromide						
Octotiamine	T45.2X1	T45.2X2	T45.2X3	T45.2X4	T45.2X5	T45.2X6
Octoxinol (9)	T49.8X1	T49.8X2	T49.8X3	T49.8X4	T49.8X5	T49.8X6
Octreotide	T38.991	T38.992	T38.993	T38.994	T38.995	T38.996
Octyl nitrite	T46.3X1	T46.3X2	T46.3X3	T46.3X4	T46.3X5	T46.3X6
Oestradiol	T38.5X1	T38.5X2	T38.5X3	T38.5X4	T38.5X5	T38.5X6
Oestriol	T38.5X1	T38.5X2	T38.5X3	T38.5X4	T38.5X5	T38.5X6
Oestrogen	T38.5X1	T38.5X2	T38.5X3	T38.5X4	T38.5X5	T38.5X6
Oestrone	T38.5X1	T38.5X2	T38.5X3	T38.5X4	T38.5X5	T38.5X6
Ofloxacin	T36.8X1	T36.8X2	T36.8X3	T36.8X4	T36.8X5	T36.8X6
Oil (of)	T65.891	T65.892	T65.893	T65.894	—	—
bitter almond	T62.8X1	T62.8X2	T62.8X3	T62.8X4	—	—
cloves	T49.7X1	T49.7X2	T49.7X3	T49.7X4	T49.7X5	T49.7X6
colors	T65.6X1	T65.6X2	T65.6X3	T65.6X4	—	—
fumes	T59.891	T59.892	T59.893	T59.894	—	—
lubricating	T52.0X1	T52.0X2	T52.0X3	T52.0X4	—	—
Niobe	T52.8X1	T52.8X2	T52.8X3	T52.8X4	—	—
vitriol (liquid)	T54.2X1	T54.2X2	T54.2X3	T54.2X4	—	—
fumes	T54.2X1	T54.2X2	T54.2X3	T54.2X4	—	—
wintergreen (bitter) NEC	T49.3X1	T49.3X2	T49.3X3	T49.3X4	T49.3X5	T49.3X6
Oily preparation (for skin)	T49.3X1	T49.3X2	T49.3X3	T49.3X4	T49.3X5	T49.3X6
Ointment NEC	T49.3X1	T49.3X2	T49.3X3	T49.3X4	T49.3X5	T49.3X6
Olanzapine	T43.591	T43.592	T43.593		T43.595	T43.596
Oleander	T62.2X1	T62.2X2	T62.2X3	T62.2X4	—	—
Oleandomycin	T36.3X1	T36.3X2	T36.3X3	T36.3X4	T36.3X5	T36.3X6
Oleandrin	T46.0X1	T46.0X2	T46.0X3	T46.0X4	T46.0X5	T46.0X6
Oleic acid	T46.6X1	T46.6X2	T46.6X3	T46.6X4	T46.6X5	T46.6X6
Oleovitamin A	T45.2X1	T45.2X2	T45.2X3	T45.2X4	T45.2X5	T45.2X6
Oleum ricini	T47.2X1	T47.2X2	T47.2X3	T47.2X4	T47.2X5	T47.2X6
Olive oil (medicinal) NEC	T47.4X1	T47.4X2	T47.4X3	T47.4X4	T47.4X5	T47.4X6
Olivomycin	T45.1X1	T45.1X2	T45.1X3	T45.1X4	T45.1X5	T45.1X6
Olsalazine	T47.8X1	T47.8X2	T47.8X3	T47.8X4	T47.8X5	T47.8X6
Omeprazole	T47.1X1	T47.1X2	T47.1X3	T47.1X4	T47.1X5	T47.1X6
OMPA	T60.0X1	T60.0X2	T60.0X3	T60.0X4	—	—
Oncovin	T45.1X1	T45.1X2	T45.1X3	T45.1X4	T45.1X5	T45.1X6
Ondansetron	T45.0X1	T45.0X2	T45.0X3	T45.0X4	T45.0X5	T45.0X6
Ophthaine	T41.3X1	T41.3X2	T41.3X3	T41.3X4	T41.3X5	T41.3X6
Ophthetic	T41.3X1	T41.3X2	T41.3X3	T41.3X4	T41.3X5	T41.3X6
Opiate NEC	T40.601	T40.602	T40.603	T40.604	T40.605	T40.606
antagonists	T50.7X1	T50.7X2	T50.7X3	T50.7X4	T50.7X5	T50.7X6
Opioid NEC	T40.2X1	T40.2X2	T40.2X3	T40.2X4	T40.2X5	T40.2X6
Opipramol	T43.011	T43.012	T43.013	T43.014	T43.015	T43.016
Opium alkaloids (total)	T40.0X1	T40.0X2	T40.0X3	T40.0X4	T40.0X5	T40.0X6
standardized powdered	T40.0X1	T40.0X2	T40.0X3	T40.0X4	T40.0X5	T40.0X6
tincture (camphorated)	T40.0X1	T40.0X2	T40.0X3	T40.0X4	T40.0X5	T40.0X6
Oracon	T38.4X1	T38.4X2	T38.4X3	T38.4X4	T38.4X5	T38.4X6
Oragrafin	T50.8X1	T50.8X2	T50.8X3	T50.8X4	T50.8X5	T50.8X6
Oral contraceptives	T38.4X1	T38.4X2	T38.4X3	T38.4X4	T38.4X5	T38.4X6
Oral rehydration salts	T50.3X1	T50.3X2	T50.3X3	T50.3X4	T50.3X5	T50.3X6
Orazamide	T50.991	T50.992	T50.993	T50.994	T50.995	T50.996
Orciprenaline	T48.291	T48.292	T48.293	T48.294	T48.295	T48.296
Organidin	T48.4X1	T48.4X2	T48.4X3	T48.4X4	T48.4X5	T48.4X6
Organonitrate NEC	T46.3X1	T46.3X2	T46.3X3	T46.3X4	T46.3X5	T46.3X6
Organophosphates	T60.0X1	T60.0X2	T60.0X3	T60.0X4	—	—
Orimune	T50.B91	T50.B92	T50.B93	T50.B94	T50.B95	T50.B96
Orinase	T38.3X1	T38.3X2	T38.3X3	T38.3X4	T38.3X5	T38.3X6
Ormeloxifene	T38.6X1	T38.6X2	T38.6X3	T38.6X4	T38.6X5	T38.6X6
Ornidazole	T37.3X1	T37.3X2	T37.3X3	T37.3X4	T37.3X5	T37.3X6
Ornithine aspartate	T50.991	T50.992	T50.993	T50.994	T50.995	T50.996
Ornoprostil	T47.1X1	T47.1X2	T47.1X3	T47.1X4	T47.1X5	T47.1X6
Orphenadrine	T42.8X1	T42.8X2	T42.8X3	T42.8X4	T42.8X5	T42.8X6
(hydrochloride)						
Ortal (sodium)	T42.3X1	T42.3X2	T42.3X3	T42.3X4	T42.3X5	T42.3X6
Orthoboric acid	T49.0X1	T49.0X2	T49.0X3	T49.0X4	T49.0X5	T49.0X6
ENT agent	T49.6X1	T49.6X2	T49.6X3	T49.6X4	T49.6X5	T49.6X6
ophthalmic preparation	T49.5X1	T49.5X2	T49.5X3	T49.5X4	T49.5X5	T49.5X6
Orthocaine	T41.3X1	T41.3X2	T41.3X3	T41.3X4	T41.3X5	T41.3X6
Orthodichlorobenzene	T53.7X1	T53.7X2	T53.7X3	T53.7X4	—	—
Ortho-Novum	T38.4X1	T38.4X2	T38.4X3	T38.4X4	T38.4X5	T38.4X6
Orthotolidine (reagent)	T54.2X1	T54.2X2	T54.2X3	T54.2X4	—	—
Osmic acid (liquid)	T54.2X1	T54.2X2	T54.2X3	T54.2X4	—	—
fumes	T54.2X1	T54.2X2	T54.2X3	T54.2X4	—	—
Osmotic diuretics	T50.2X1	T50.2X2	T50.2X3	T50.2X4	T50.2X5	T50.2X6
Otilonium bromide	T44.3X1	T44.3X2	T44.3X3	T44.3X4	T44.3X5	T44.3X6
Otorhinolaryngological drug	T49.6X1	T49.6X2	T49.6X3	T49.6X4	T49.6X5	T49.6X6
NEC						
Ouabain (e)	T46.0X1	T46.0X2	T46.0X3	T46.0X4	T46.0X5	T46.0X6
Ovarian						
hormone	T38.5X1	T38.5X2	T38.5X3	T38.5X4	T38.5X5	T38.5X6
stimulant	T38.5X1	T38.5X2	T38.5X3	T38.5X4	T38.5X5	T38.5X6
Ovral	T38.4X1	T38.4X2	T38.4X3	T38.4X4	T38.4X5	T38.4X6
Ovulen	T38.4X1	T38.4X2	T38.4X3	T38.4X4	T38.4X5	T38.4X6
Oxacillin	T36.0X1	T36.0X2	T36.0X3	T36.0X4	T36.0X5	T36.0X6
Oxalic acid	T54.2X1	T54.2X2	T54.2X3	T54.2X4	—	—
ammonium salt	T50.991	T50.992	T50.993	T50.994	T50.995	T50.996
Oxamniquine	T37.4X1	T37.4X2	T37.4X3	T37.4X4	T37.4X5	T37.4X6
Oxanamide	T43.591	T43.592	T43.593	T43.594	T43.595	T43.596
Oxandrolone	T38.7X1	T38.7X2	T38.7X3	T38.7X4	T38.7X5	T38.7X6
Oxantel	T37.4X1	T37.4X2	T37.4X3	T37.4X4	T37.4X5	T37.4X6
Oxapium iodide	T44.3X1	T44.3X2	T44.3X3	T44.3X4	T44.3X5	T44.3X6
Oxaprotiline	T43.021	T43.022	T43.023	T43.024	T43.025	T43.026
Oxaprozin	T39.311	T39.312	T39.313	T39.314	T39.315	T39.316
Oxatomide	T45.0X1	T45.0X2	T45.0X3	T45.0X4	T45.0X5	T45.0X6
Oxazepam	T42.4X1	T42.4X2	T42.4X3	T42.4X4	T42.4X5	T42.4X6
Oxazimedrine	T50.5X1	T50.5X2	T50.5X3	T50.5X4	T50.5X5	T50.5X6
Oxazolam	T42.4X1	T42.4X2	T42.4X3	T42.4X4	T42.4X5	T42.4X6
Oxazolidine derivatives	T42.2X1	T42.2X2	T42.2X3	T42.2X4	T42.2X5	T42.2X6
Oxazolidinedione	T42.2X1	T42.2X2	T42.2X3	T42.2X4	T42.2X5	T42.2X6
(derivative)						
Ox bile extract	T47.5X1	T47.5X2	T47.5X3	T47.5X4	T47.5X5	T47.5X6
Oxcarbazepine	T42.1X1	T42.1X2	T42.1X3	T42.1X4	T42.1X5	T42.1X6
Oxedrine	T44.4X1	T44.4X2	T44.4X3	T44.4X4	T44.4X5	T44.4X6
Oxeladin (citrate)	T48.3X1	T48.3X2	T48.3X3	T48.3X4	T48.3X5	T48.3X6

Substance	Poisoning, Accidental (unintentional)	Poisoning, Intentional Self-harm	Poisoning, Assault	Poisoning, Undetermined	Adverse Effect	Under-dosing
Oxendolone	T38.5X1	T38.5X2	T38.5X3	T38.5X4	T38.5X5	T38.5X6
Oxetacaine	T41.3X1	T41.3X2	T41.3X3	T41.3X4	T41.3X5	T41.3X6
Oxethazine	T41.3X1	T41.3X2	T41.3X3	T41.3X4	T41.3X5	T41.3X6
Oxetorone	T39.8X1	T39.8X2	T39.8X3	T39.8X4	T39.8X5	T39.8X6
Oxiconazole	T49.0X1	T49.0X2	T49.0X3	T49.0X4	T49.0X5	T49.0X6
Oxidizing agent NEC	T54.91	T54.92	T54.93	T54.94	—	—
Oxipurinol	T50.4X1	T50.4X2	T50.4X3	T50.4X4	T50.4X5	T50.4X6
Oxitriptan	T43.291	T43.292	T43.293	T43.294	T43.295	T43.296
Oxitropium bromide	T48.6X1	T48.6X2	T48.6X3	T48.6X4	T48.6X5	T48.6X6
Oxodipine	T46.1X1	T46.1X2	T46.1X3	T46.1X4	T46.1X5	T46.1X6
Oxolamine	T48.3X1	T48.3X2	T48.3X3	T48.3X4	T48.3X5	T48.3X6
Oxolinic acid	T37.8X1	T37.8X2	T37.8X3	T37.8X4	T37.8X5	T37.8X6
Oxomemazine	T43.3X1	T43.3X2	T43.3X3	T43.3X4	T43.3X5	T43.3X6
Oxophenarsine	T37.3X1	T37.3X2	T37.3X3	T37.3X4	T37.3X5	T37.3X6
Oxprenolol	T44.7X1	T44.7X2	T44.7X3	T44.7X4	T44.7X5	T44.7X6
Oxsoralen	T49.3X1	T49.3X2	T49.3X3	T49.3X4	T49.3X5	T49.3X6
Oxtriphylline	T48.6X1	T48.6X2	T48.6X3	T48.6X4	T48.6X5	T48.6X6
Oxybate sodium	T41.291	T41.292	T41.293	T41.294	T41.295	T41.296
Oxybuprocaine	T41.3X1	T41.3X2	T41.3X3	T41.3X4	T41.3X5	T41.3X6
Oxybutynin	T44.3X1	T44.3X2	T44.3X3	T44.3X4	T44.3X5	T44.3X6
Oxychlorosene	T49.0X1	T49.0X2	T49.0X3	T49.0X4	T49.0X5	T49.0X6
Oxycodone	T40.2X1	T40.2X2	T40.2X3	T40.2X4	T40.2X5	T40.2X6
Oxyfedrine	T46.3X1	T46.3X2	T46.3X3	T46.3X4	T46.3X5	T46.3X6
Oxygen	T41.5X1	T41.5X2	T41.5X3	T41.5X4	T41.5X5	T41.5X6
Oxylone	T49.0X1	T49.0X2	T49.0X3	T49.0X4	T49.0X5	T49.0X6
ophthalmic preparation	T49.5X1	T49.5X2	T49.5X3	T49.5X4	T49.5X5	T49.5X6
Oxymesterone	T38.7X1	T38.7X2	T38.7X3	T38.7X4	T38.7X5	T38.7X6
Oxymetazoline	T48.5X1	T48.5X2	T48.5X3	T48.5X4	T48.5X5	T48.5X6
Oxymetholone	T38.7X1	T38.7X2	T38.7X3	T38.7X4	T38.7X5	T38.7X6
Oxymorphone	T40.2X1	T40.2X2	T40.2X3	T40.2X4	T40.2X5	T40.2X6
Oxypertine	T43.591	T43.592	T43.593	T43.594	T43.595	T43.596
Oxyphenbutazone	T39.2X1	T39.2X2	T39.2X3	T39.2X4	T39.2X5	T39.2X6
Oxyphencyclimine	T44.3X1	T44.3X2	T44.3X3	T44.3X4	T44.3X5	T44.3X6
Oxyphenisatine	T47.2X1	T47.2X2	T47.2X3	T47.2X4	T47.2X5	T47.2X6
Oxyphenonium bromide	T44.3X1	T44.3X2	T44.3X3	T44.3X4	T44.3X5	T44.3X6
Oxypolygelatin	T45.8X1	T45.8X2	T45.8X3	T45.8X4	T45.8X5	T45.8X6
Oxyquinoline (derivatives)	T37.8X1	T37.8X2	T37.8X3	T37.8X4	T37.8X5	T37.8X6
Oxytetracycline	T36.4X1	T36.4X2	T36.4X3	T36.4X4	T36.4X5	T36.4X6
Oxytocic drug NEC	T48.0X1	T48.0X2	T48.0X3	T48.0X4	T48.0X5	T48.0X6
Oxytocin (synthetic)	T48.0X1	T48.0X2	T48.0X3	T48.0X4	T48.0X5	T48.0X6
Ozone	T59.891	T59.892	T59.893	T59.894	—	—
PABA	T49.3X1	T49.3X2	T49.3X3	T49.3X4	T49.3X5	T49.3X6
Packed red cells	T45.8X1	T45.8X2	T45.8X3	T45.8X4	T45.8X5	T45.8X6
Padimate	T49.3X1	T49.3X2	T49.3X3	T49.3X4	T49.3X5	T49.3X6
Paint NEC	T65.6X1	T65.6X2	T65.6X3	T65.6X4	—	—
cleaner	T52.91	T52.92	T52.93	T52.94	—	—
fumes NEC	T59.891	T59.892	T59.893	T59.894	—	—
lead (fumes)	T56.0X1	T56.0X2	T56.0X3	T56.0X4	—	—
solvent NEC	T52.8X1	T52.8X2	T52.8X3	T52.8X4	—	—
stripper	T52.8X1	T52.8X2	T52.8X3	T52.8X4	—	—
Palfium	T40.2X1	T40.2X2	T40.2X3	T40.2X4	—	—
Palm kernel oil	T50.991	T50.992	T50.993	T50.994	T50.995	T50.996
Paludrine	T37.2X1	T37.2X2	T37.2X3	T37.2X4	T37.2X5	T37.2X6
Pamaquine (naphthoute)	T37.2X1	T37.2X2	T37.2X3	T37.2X4	T37.2X5	T37.2X6
Panadol	T39.1X1	T39.1X2	T39.1X3	T39.1X4	T39.1X5	T39.1X6
Pancreatic						
digestive secretion stimulant	T47.8X1	T47.8X2	T47.8X3	T47.8X4	T47.8X5	T47.8X6
dornase	T45.3X1	T45.3X2	T45.3X3	T45.3X4	T45.3X5	T45.3X6
Pancreatin	T47.5X1	T47.5X2	T47.5X3	T47.5X4	T47.5X5	T47.5X6
Pancrelipase	T47.5X1	T47.5X2	T47.5X3	T47.5X4	T47.5X5	T47.5X6
Pancuronium (bromide)	T48.1X1	T48.1X2	T48.1X3	T48.1X4	T48.1X5	T48.1X6
Pangamic acid	T45.2X1	T45.2X2	T45.2X3	T45.2X4	T45.2X5	T45.2X6
Panthenol	T45.2X1	T45.2X2	T45.2X3	T45.2X4	T45.2X5	T45.2X6
topical	T49.8X1	T49.8X2	T49.8X3	T49.8X4	T49.8X5	T49.8X6
Pantopon	T40.0X1	T40.0X2	T40.0X3	T40.0X4	T40.0X5	T40.0X6
Pantothenic acid	T45.2X1	T45.2X2	T45.2X3	T45.2X4	T45.2X5	T45.2X6
Panwarfin	T45.511	T45.512	T45.513	T45.514	T45.515	T45.516
Papain	T47.5X1	T47.5X2	T47.5X3	T47.5X4	T47.5X5	T47.5X6
digestant	T47.5X1	T47.5X2	T47.5X3	T47.5X4	T47.5X5	T47.5X6
Papaveretum	T40.0X1	T40.0X2	T40.0X3	T40.0X4	T40.0X5	T40.0X6
Papaverine	T44.3X1	T44.3X2	T44.3X3	T44.3X4	T44.3X5	T44.3X6
Para-acetamidophenol	T39.1X1	T39.1X2	T39.1X3	T39.1X4	T39.1X5	T39.1X6
Para-aminobenzoic acid	T49.3X1	T49.3X2	T49.3X3	T49.3X4	T49.3X5	T49.3X6
Para-aminophenol	T39.1X1	T39.1X2	T39.1X3	T39.1X4	T39.1X5	T39.1X6
derivatives						
Para-aminosalicylic acid	T37.1X1	T37.1X2	T37.1X3	T37.1X4	T37.1X5	T37.1X6
Paracetaldehyde	T42.6X1	T42.6X2	T42.6X3	T42.6X4	T42.6X5	T42.6X6
Paracetamol	T39.1X1	T39.1X2	T39.1X3	T39.1X4	T39.1X5	T39.1X6
Parachlorophenol (camphorated)	T49.0X1	T49.0X2	T49.0X3	T49.0X4	T49.0X5	T49.0X6
Paracodin	T40.2X1	T40.2X2	T40.2X3	T40.2X4	T40.2X5	T40.2X6

Substance	Poisoning, Accidental (unintentional)	Poisoning, Intentional Self-harm	Poisoning, Assault	Poisoning, Undetermined	Adverse Effect	Under-dosing
Paradione	T42.2X1	T42.2X2	T42.2X3	T42.2X4	T42.2X5	T42.2X6
Paraffin(s) (wax)	T52.0X1	T52.0X2	T52.0X3	T52.0X4	—	—
liquid (medicinal)	T47.4X1	T47.4X2	T47.4X3	T47.4X4	T47.4X5	T47.4X6
nonmedicinal	T52.0X1	T52.0X2	T52.0X3	T52.0X4	—	—
Paraformaldehyde	T60.3X1	T60.3X2	T60.3X3	T60.3X4	—	—
Paraldehyde	T42.6X1	T42.6X2	T42.6X3	T42.6X4	T42.6X5	T42.6X6
Paramethadione	T42.2X1	T42.2X2	T42.2X3	T42.2X4	T42.2X5	T42.2X6
Paramethasone	T38.0X1	T38.0X2	T38.0X3	T38.0X4	T38.0X5	T38.0X6
acetate	T49.0X1	T49.0X2	T49.0X3	T49.0X4	T49.0X5	T49.0X6
Paraoxon	T60.0X1	T60.0X2	T60.0X3	T60.0X4	—	—
Paraquat	T60.3X1	T60.3X2	T60.3X3	T60.3X4	—	—
Parasympatholytic NEC	T44.3X1	T44.3X2	T44.3X3	T44.3X4	T44.3X5	T44.3X6
Parasympathomimetic drug NEC	T44.1X1	T44.1X2	T44.1X3	T44.1X4	T44.1X5	T44.1X6
Parathion	T60.0X1	T60.0X2	T60.0X3	T60.0X4	—	—
Parathormone	T50.991	T50.992	T50.993	T50.994	T50.995	T50.996
Parathyroid extract	T50.991	T50.992	T50.993	T50.994	T50.995	T50.996
Paratyphoid vaccine	T50.A91	T50.A92	T50.A93	T50.A94	T50.A95	T50.A96
Paredrine	T44.4X1	T44.4X2	T44.4X3	T44.4X4	T44.4X5	T44.4X6
Paregoric	T40.0X1	T40.0X2	T40.0X3	T40.0X4	T40.0X5	T40.0X6
Pargyline	T46.5X1	T46.5X2	T46.5X3	T46.5X4	T46.5X5	T46.5X6
Paris green	T57.0X1	T57.0X2	T57.0X3	T57.0X4	—	—
insecticide	T57.0X1	T57.0X2	T57.0X3	T57.0X4	—	—
Parnate	T43.1X1	T43.1X2	T43.1X3	T43.1X4	T43.1X5	T43.1X6
Paromomycin	T36.5X1	T36.5X2	T36.5X3	T36.5X4	T36.5X5	T36.5X6
Paroxypropione	T45.1X1	T45.1X2	T45.1X3	T45.1X4	T45.1X5	T45.1X6
Parzone	T40.2X1	T40.2X2	T40.2X3	T40.2X4	T40.2X5	T40.2X6
PAS	T37.1X1	T37.1X2	T37.1X3	T37.1X4	T37.1X5	T37.1X6
Pasiniazid	T37.1X1	T37.1X2	T37.1X3	T37.1X4	T37.1X5	T37.1X6
PBB (polybrominated biphenyls)	T65.891	T65.892	T65.893	T65.894		
PCB	T65.891	T65.892	T65.893	T65.894		
PCP						
meaning pentachlorophenol	T60.1X1	T60.1X2	T60.1X3	T60.1X4		
fungicide	T60.3X1	T60.3X2	T60.3X3	T60.3X4		
herbicide	T60.3X1	T60.3X2	T60.3X3	T60.3X4		
insecticide	T60.1X1	T60.1X2	T60.1X3	T60.1X4		
meaning phencyclidine	T40.991	T40.992	T40.993	T40.994		
Peach kernel oil (emulsion)	T47.4X1	T47.4X2	T47.4X3	T47.4X4	T47.4X5	T47.4X6
Peanut oil (emulsion) NEC	T47.4X1	T47.4X2	T47.4X3	T47.4X4	T47.4X5	T47.4X6
topical	T49.3X1	T49.3X2	T49.3X3	T49.3X4	T49.3X5	T49.3X6
Pearly Gates (morning glory seeds)	T40.991	T40.992	T40.993	T40.994		
Pecazine	T43.3X1	T43.3X2	T43.3X3	T43.3X4	T43.3X5	T43.3X6
Pectin	T47.6X1	T47.6X2	T47.6X3	T47.6X4	T47.6X5	T47.6X6
Pefloxacin	T37.8X1	T37.8X2	T37.8X3	T37.8X4	T37.8X5	T37.8X6
Pegademase, bovine	T50.Z91	T50.Z92	T50.Z93	T50.Z94	T50.Z95	T50.Z96
Pelletierine tannate	T37.4X1	T37.4X2	T37.4X3	T37.4X4	T37.4X5	T37.4X6
Pemirolast (potassium)	T48.6X1	T48.6X2	T48.6X3	T48.6X4	T48.6X5	T48.6X6
Pemoline	T50.7X1	T50.7X2	T50.7X3	T50.7X4	T50.7X5	T50.7X6
Pempidine	T44.2X1	T44.2X2	T44.2X3	T44.2X4	T44.2X5	T44.2X6
Penamecillin	T36.0X1	T36.0X2	T36.0X3	T36.0X4	T36.0X5	T36.0X6
Penbutolol	T44.7X1	T44.7X2	T44.7X3	T44.7X4	T44.7X5	T44.7X6
Penethamate	T36.0X1	T36.0X2	T36.0X3	T36.0X4	T36.0X5	T36.0X6
Penfluridol	T43.591	T43.592	T43.593	T43.594	T43.595	T43.596
Penflutizide	T50.2X1	T50.2X2	T50.2X3	T50.2X4	T50.2X5	T50.2X6
Pengitoxin	T46.0X1	T46.0X2	T46.0X3	T46.0X4	T46.0X5	T46.0X6
Penicillamine	T50.6X1	T50.6X2	T50.6X3	T50.6X4	T50.6X5	T50.6X6
Penicillin (any)	T36.0X1	T36.0X2	T36.0X3	T36.0X4	T36.0X5	T36.0X6
Penicillinase	T45.3X1	T45.3X2	T45.3X3	T45.3X4	T45.3X5	T45.3X6
Penicilloyl polylysine	T50.8X1	T50.8X2	T50.8X3	T50.8X4	T50.8X5	T50.8X6
Penimepicycline	T36.4X1	T36.4X2	T36.4X3	T36.4X4	T36.4X5	T36.4X6
Pentachloroethane	T53.6X1	T53.6X2	T53.6X3	T53.6X4	—	—
Pentachloronaphthalene	T53.7X1	T53.7X2	T53.7X3	T53.7X4	—	—
Pentachlorophenol (pesticide)	T60.1X1	T60.1X2	T60.1X3	T60.1X4	—	—
fungicide	T60.3X1	T60.3X2	T60.3X3	T60.3X4	—	—
herbicide	T60.3X1	T60.3X2	T60.3X3	T60.3X4	—	—
insecticide	T60.1X1	T60.1X2	T60.1X3	T60.1X4	—	—
Pentaerythritol	T46.3X1	T46.3X2	T46.3X3	T46.3X4	T46.3X5	T46.3X6
chloral	T42.6X1	T42.6X2	T42.6X3	T42.6X4	T42.6X5	T42.6X6
tetranitrate NEC	T46.3X1	T46.3X2	T46.3X3	T46.3X4	T46.3X5	T46.3X6
Pentaerythrityl tetranitrate	T46.3X1	T46.3X2	T46.3X3	T46.3X4	T46.3X5	T46.3X6
Pentagastrin	T50.8X1	T50.8X2	T50.8X3	T50.8X4	T50.8X5	T50.8X6
Pentalin	T53.6X1	T53.6X2	T53.6X3	T53.6X4	—	—
Pentamethonium bromide	T44.2X1	T44.2X2	T44.2X3	T44.2X4	T44.2X5	T44.2X6
Pentamidine	T37.3X1	T37.3X2	T37.3X3	T37.3X4	T37.3X5	T37.3X6
Pentanol	T51.3X1	T51.3X2	T51.3X3	T51.3X4	—	—
Pentapyrrolinium (bitartrate)	T44.2X1	T44.2X2	T44.2X3	T44.2X4	T44.2X5	T44.2X6
Pentaquine	T37.2X1	T37.2X2	T37.2X3	T37.2X4	T37.2X5	T37.2X6

Additional Character May Be Required — Refer to the Tabular List for Character Selection   ▽ Subterms under main terms may continue to next column or page

Substance	Poisoning, Accidental (unintentional)	Poisoning, Intentional Self-harm	Poisoning, Assault	Poisoning, Undetermined	Adverse Effect	Under-dosing
Pentazocine	T40.4X1	T40.4X2	T40.4X3	T40.4X4	T40.4X5	T40.4X6
Pentetrazole	T50.7X1	T50.7X2	T50.7X3	T50.7X4	T50.7X5	T50.7X6
Penthienate bromide	T44.3X1	T44.3X2	T44.3X3	T44.3X4	T44.3X5	T44.3X6
Pentifylline	T46.7X1	T46.7X2	T46.7X3	T46.7X4	T46.7X5	T46.7X6
Pentobarbital	T42.3X1	T42.3X2	T42.3X3	T42.3X4	T42.3X5	T42.3X6
sodium	T42.3X1	T42.3X2	T42.3X3	T42.3X4	T42.3X5	T42.3X6
Pentobarbitone	T42.3X1	T42.3X2	T42.3X3	T42.3X4	T42.3X5	T42.3X6
Pentolonium tartrate	T44.2X1	T44.2X2	T44.2X3	T44.2X4	T44.2X5	T44.2X6
Pentosan polysulfate	T39.8X1	T39.8X2	T39.8X3	T39.8X4	T39.8X5	T39.8X6
(sodium)						
Pentostatin	T45.1X1	T45.1X2	T45.1X3	T45.1X4	T45.1X5	T45.1X6
Pentothal	T41.1X1	T41.1X2	T41.1X3	T41.1X4	T41.1X5	T41.1X6
Pentoxifylline	T46.7X1	T46.7X2	T46.7X3	T46.7X4	T46.7X5	T46.7X6
Pentoxyverine	T48.3X1	T48.3X2	T48.3X3	T48.3X4	T48.3X5	T48.3X6
Pentrinat	T46.3X1	T46.3X2	T46.3X3	T46.3X4	T46.3X5	T46.3X6
Pentylenetetrazole	T50.7X1	T50.7X2	T50.7X3	T50.7X4	T50.7X5	T50.7X6
Pentylsalicylamide	T37.1X1	T37.1X2	T37.1X3	T37.1X4	T37.1X5	T37.1X6
Pentymal	T42.3X1	T42.3X2	T42.3X3	T42.3X4	T42.3X5	T42.3X6
Peplomycin	T45.1X1	T45.1X2	T45.1X3	T45.1X4	T45.1X5	T45.1X6
Peppermint (oil)	T47.5X1	T47.5X2	T47.5X3	T47.5X4	T47.5X5	T47.5X6
Pepsin	T47.5X1	T47.5X2	T47.5X3	T47.5X4	T47.5X5	T47.5X6
digestant	T47.5X1	T47.5X2	T47.5X3	T47.5X4	T47.5X5	T47.5X6
Pepstatin	T47.1X1	T47.1X2	T47.1X3	T47.1X4	T47.1X5	T47.1X6
Peptavlon	T50.8X1	T50.8X2	T50.8X3	T50.8X4	T50.8X5	T50.8X6
Perazine	T43.3X1	T43.3X2	T43.3X3	T43.3X4	T43.3X5	T43.3X6
Percaine (spinal)	T41.3X1	T41.3X2	T41.3X3	T41.3X4	T41.3X5	T41.3X6
topical (surface)	T41.3X1	T41.3X2	T41.3X3	T41.3X4	T41.3X5	T41.3X6
Perchloroethylene	T53.3X1	T53.3X2	T53.3X3	T53.3X4	—	—
medicinal	T37.4X1	T37.4X2	T37.4X3	T37.4X4	T37.4X5	T37.4X6
vapor	T53.3X1	T53.3X2	T53.3X3	T53.3X4	—	—
Percodan	T40.2X1	T40.2X2	T40.2X3	T40.2X4	T40.2X5	T40.2X6
Percogesic — see also acetaminophen	T45.0X1	T45.0X2	T45.0X3	T45.0X4	T45.0X5	T45.0X6
Percorten	T38.0X1	T38.0X2	T38.0X3	T38.0X4	T38.0X5	T38.0X6
Pergolide	T42.8X1	T42.8X2	T42.8X3	T42.8X4	T42.8X5	T42.8X6
Pergonal	T38.811	T38.812	T38.813	T38.814	T38.815	T38.816
Perhexilene	T46.3X1	T46.3X2	T46.3X3	T46.3X4	T46.3X5	T46.3X6
Perhexiline (maleate)	T46.3X1	T46.3X2	T46.3X3	T46.3X4	T46.3X5	T46.3X6
Periactin	T45.0X1	T45.0X2	T45.0X3	T45.0X4	T45.0X5	T45.0X6
Periciazine	T43.3X1	T43.3X2	T43.3X3	T43.3X4	T43.3X5	T43.3X6
Periclor	T42.6X1	T42.6X2	T42.6X3	T42.6X4	T42.6X5	T42.6X6
Periclor	T46.4X1	T46.4X2	T46.4X3	T46.4X4	T46.4X5	T46.4X6
Perindopril	T46.4X1	T46.4X2	T46.4X3	T46.4X4	T46.4X5	T46.4X6
Perisoxal	T39.8X1	T39.8X2	T39.8X3	T39.8X4	T39.8X5	T39.8X6
Peritoneal dialysis solution	T50.3X1	T50.3X2	T50.3X3	T50.3X4	T50.3X5	T50.3X6
Peritrate	T46.3X1	T46.3X2	T46.3X3	T46.3X4	T46.3X5	T46.3X6
Perlapine	T42.4X1	T42.4X2	T42.4X3	T42.4X4	T42.4X5	T42.4X6
Permanganate	T65.891	T65.892	T65.893	T65.894	—	—
Permethrin	T60.1X1	T60.1X2	T60.1X3	T60.1X4	—	—
Pernocton	T42.3X1	T42.3X2	T42.3X3	T42.3X4	T42.3X5	T42.3X6
Pernoston	T42.3X1	T42.3X2	T42.3X3	T42.3X4	T42.3X5	T42.3X6
Peronine	T40.2X1	T40.2X2	T40.2X3	T40.2X4	—	—
Perphenazine	T43.3X1	T43.3X2	T43.3X3	T43.3X4	T43.3X5	T43.3X6
Pertofrane	T43.011	T43.012	T43.013	T43.014	T43.015	T43.016
Pertussis						
immune serum (human)	T50.Z11	T50.Z12	T50.Z13	T50.Z14	T50.Z15	T50.Z16
vaccine (with diphtheria toxoid)	T50.A11	T50.A12	T50.A13	T50.A14	T50.A15	T50.A16
(with tetanus toxoid)						
Peruvian balsam	T49.0X1	T49.0X2	T49.0X3	T49.0X4	T49.0X5	T49.0X6
Peruvoside	T46.0X1	T46.0X2	T46.0X3	T46.0X4	T46.0X5	T46.0X6
Pesticide (dust) (fumes) (vapor)	T60.91	T60.92	T60.93	T60.94	—	—
NEC						
arsenic	T57.0X1	T57.0X2	T57.0X3	T57.0X4	—	—
chlorinated	T60.1X1	T60.1X2	T60.1X3	T60.1X4	—	—
cyanide	T65.0X1	T65.0X2	T65.0X3	T65.0X4	—	—
kerosene	T52.0X1	T52.0X2	T52.0X3	T52.0X4	—	—
mixture (of compounds)	T60.91	T60.92	T60.93	T60.94	—	—
naphthalene	T60.2X1	T60.2X2	T60.2X3	T60.2X4	—	—
organochlorine (compounds)	T60.1X1	T60.1X2	T60.1X3	T60.1X4	—	—
petroleum (distillate) (products) NEC	T60.8X1	T60.8X2	T60.8X3	T60.8X4	—	—
specified ingredient NEC	T60.8X1	T60.8X2	T60.8X3	T60.8X4	—	—
strychnine	T65.1X1	T65.1X2	T65.1X3	T65.1X4	—	—
thallium	T60.4X1	T60.4X2	T60.4X3	T60.4X4	—	—
Pethidine	T40.4X1	T40.4X2	T40.4X3	T40.4X4	T40.4X5	T40.4X6
Petrichloral	T42.6X1	T42.6X2	T42.6X3	T42.6X4	T42.6X5	T42.6X6
Petrol	T52.0X1	T52.0X2	T52.0X3	T52.0X4	—	—
vapor	T52.0X1	T52.0X2	T52.0X3	T52.0X4	—	—
Petrolatum	T49.3X1	T49.3X2	T49.3X3	T49.3X4	T49.3X5	T49.3X6
hydrophilic	T49.3X1	T49.3X2	T49.3X3	T49.3X4	T49.3X5	T49.3X6
liquid	T47.4X1	T47.4X2	T47.4X3	T47.4X4	T47.4X5	T47.4X6
topical	T49.3X1	T49.3X2	T49.3X3	T49.3X4	T49.3X5	T49.3X6
nonmedicinal	T52.0X1	T52.0X2	T52.0X3	T52.0X4	—	—

Substance	Poisoning, Accidental (unintentional)	Poisoning, Intentional Self-harm	Poisoning, Assault	Poisoning, Undetermined	Adverse Effect	Under-dosing
Petrolatum — continued						
red veterinary	T49.3X1	T49.3X2	T49.3X3	T49.3X4	T49.3X5	T49.3X6
white	T49.3X1	T49.3X2	T49.3X3	T49.3X4	T49.3X5	T49.3X6
Petroleum (products) NEC	T52.0X1	T52.0X2	T52.0X3	T52.0X4	—	—
benzine(s) — see Ligroin						
ether — see Ligroin						
jelly — see Petrolatum						
naphtha — see Ligroin						
pesticide	T60.8X1	T60.8X2	T60.8X3	T60.8X4	—	—
solids	T52.0X1	T52.0X2	T52.0X3	T52.0X4	—	—
solvents	T52.0X1	T52.0X2	T52.0X3	T52.0X4	—	—
vapor	T52.0X1	T52.0X2	T52.0X3	T52.0X4	—	—
Peyote	T40.991	T40.992	T40.993	T40.994	—	—
Phanodorm, phanodorn	T42.3X1	T42.3X2	T42.3X3	T42.3X4	T42.3X5	T42.3X6
Phanquinone	T37.3X1	T37.3X2	T37.3X3	T37.3X4	T37.3X5	T37.3X6
Phanquone	T37.3X1	T37.3X2	T37.3X3	T37.3X4	T37.3X5	T37.3X6
Pharmaceutical						
adjunct NEC	T50.901	T50.902	T50.903	T50.904	T50.905	T50.906
excipient NEC	T50.901	T50.902	T50.903	T50.904	T50.905	T50.906
sweetener	T50.901	T50.902	T50.903	T50.904	T50.905	T50.906
viscous agent	T50.901	T50.902	T50.903	T50.904	T50.905	T50.906
Phemitone	T42.3X1	T42.3X2	T42.3X3	T42.3X4	T42.3X5	T42.3X6
Phenacaine	T41.3X1	T41.3X2	T41.3X3	T41.3X4	T41.3X5	T41.3X6
Phenacemide	T42.6X1	T42.6X2	T42.6X3	T42.6X4	T42.6X5	T42.6X6
Phenacetin	T39.1X1	T39.1X2	T39.1X3	T39.1X4	T39.1X5	T39.1X6
Phenadoxone	T40.2X1	T40.2X2	T40.2X3	T40.2X4	—	—
Phenaglycodol	T43.591	T43.592	T43.593	T43.594	T43.595	T43.596
Phenantoin	T42.0X1	T42.0X2	T42.0X3	T42.0X4	T42.0X5	T42.0X6
Phenaphthazine reagent	T50.991	T50.992	T50.993	T50.994	T50.995	T50.996
Phenazocine	T40.4X1	T40.4X2	T40.4X3	T40.4X4	T40.4X5	T40.4X6
Phenazone	T39.2X1	T39.2X2	T39.2X3	T39.2X4	T39.2X5	T39.2X6
Phenazopyridine	T39.8X1	T39.8X2	T39.8X3	T39.8X4	T39.8X5	T39.8X6
Phenbenicillin	T36.0X1	T36.0X2	T36.0X3	T36.0X4	T36.0X5	T36.0X6
Phenbutrazate	T50.5X1	T50.5X2	T50.5X3	T50.5X4	T50.5X5	T50.5X6
Phencyclidine	T40.991	T40.992	T40.993	T40.994	T40.995	T40.996
Phendimetrazine	T50.5X1	T50.5X2	T50.5X3	T50.5X4	T50.5X5	T50.5X6
Phenelzine	T43.1X1	T43.1X2	T43.1X3	T43.1X4	T43.1X5	T43.1X6
Phenemal	T42.3X1	T42.3X2	T42.3X3	T42.3X4	T42.3X5	T42.3X6
Phenergan	T42.6X1	T42.6X2	T42.6X3	T42.6X4	T42.6X5	T42.6X6
Pheneticillin	T36.0X1	T36.0X2	T36.0X3	T36.0X4	T36.0X5	T36.0X6
Pheneturide	T42.6X1	T42.6X2	T42.6X3	T42.6X4	T42.6X5	T42.6X6
Phenformin	T38.3X1	T38.3X2	T38.3X3	T38.3X4	T38.3X5	T38.3X6
Phenglutarimide	T44.3X1	T44.3X2	T44.3X3	T44.3X4	T44.3X5	T44.3X6
Phenicarbazide	T39.8X1	T39.8X2	T39.8X3	T39.8X4	T39.8X5	T39.8X6
Phenindamine	T45.0X1	T45.0X2	T45.0X3	T45.0X4	T45.0X5	T45.0X6
Phenindione	T45.511	T45.512	T45.513	T45.514	T45.515	T45.516
Pheniprazine	T43.1X1	T43.1X2	T43.1X3	T43.1X4	T43.1X5	T43.1X6
Pheniramine	T45.0X1	T45.0X2	T45.0X3	T45.0X4	T45.0X5	T45.0X6
Phenisatin	T47.2X1	T47.2X2	T47.2X3	T47.2X4	T47.2X5	T47.2X6
Phenmetrazine	T50.5X1	T50.5X2	T50.5X3	T50.5X4	T50.5X5	T50.5X6
Phenobal	T42.3X1	T42.3X2	T42.3X3	T42.3X4	T42.3X5	T42.3X6
Phenobarbital	T42.3X1	T42.3X2	T42.3X3	T42.3X4	T42.3X5	T42.3X6
with						
mephenytoin	T42.3X1	T42.3X2	T42.3X3	T42.3X4	T42.3X5	T42.3X6
phenytoin	T42.3X1	T42.3X2	T42.3X3	T42.3X4	T42.3X5	T42.3X6
sodium	T42.3X1	T42.3X2	T42.3X3	T42.3X4	T42.3X5	T42.3X6
Phenobarbitone	T42.3X1	T42.3X2	T42.3X3	T42.3X4	T42.3X5	T42.3X6
Phenobutiodil	T50.8X1	T50.8X2	T50.8X3	T50.8X4	T50.8X5	T50.8X6
Phenoctide	T49.0X1	T49.0X2	T49.0X3	T49.0X4	T49.0X5	T49.0X6
Phenol	T49.0X1	T49.0X2	T49.0X3	T49.0X4	T49.0X5	T49.0X6
disinfectant	T54.0X1	T54.0X2	T54.0X3	T54.0X4	—	—
in oil injection	T46.8X1	T46.8X2	T46.8X3	T46.8X4	T46.8X5	T46.8X6
medicinal	T49.1X1	T49.1X2	T49.1X3	T49.1X4	T49.1X5	T49.1X6
nonmedicinal NEC	T54.0X1	T54.0X2	T54.0X3	T54.0X4	—	—
pesticide	T60.8X1	T60.8X2	T60.8X3	T60.8X4	—	—
red	T50.8X1	T50.8X2	T50.8X3	T50.8X4	T50.8X5	T50.8X6
Phenolic preparation	T49.1X1	T49.1X2	T49.1X3	T49.1X4	T49.1X5	T49.1X6
Phenolphthalein	T47.2X1	T47.2X2	T47.2X3	T47.2X4	T47.2X5	T47.2X6
Phenolsulfonphthalein	T50.8X1	T50.8X2	T50.8X3	T50.8X4	T50.8X5	T50.8X6
Phenomorphan	T40.2X1	T40.2X2	T40.2X3	T40.2X4	—	—
Phenonyl	T42.3X1	T42.3X2	T42.3X3	T42.3X4	T42.3X5	T42.3X6
Phenoperidine	T40.4X1	T40.4X2	T40.4X3	T40.4X4	—	—
Phenopyrazone	T46.991	T46.992	T46.993	T46.994	T46.995	T46.996
Phenoquin	T50.4X1	T50.4X2	T50.4X3	T50.4X4	T50.4X5	T50.4X6
Phenothiazine (psychotropic)	T43.3X1	T43.3X2	T43.3X3	T43.3X4	T43.3X5	T43.3X6
NEC						
insecticide	T60.2X1	T60.2X2	T60.2X3	T60.2X4	—	—
Phenothrin	T49.0X1	T49.0X2	T49.0X3	T49.0X4	T49.0X5	T49.0X6
Phenoxybenzamine	T46.7X1	T46.7X2	T46.7X3	T46.7X4	T46.7X5	T46.7X6
Phenoxyethanol	T49.0X1	T49.0X2	T49.0X3	T49.0X4	T49.0X5	T49.0X6
Phenoxymethyl penicillin	T36.0X1	T36.0X2	T36.0X3	T36.0X4	T36.0X5	T36.0X6
Phenprobamate	T42.8X1	T42.8X2	T42.8X3	T42.8X4	T42.8X5	T42.8X6
Phenprocoumon	T45.511	T45.512	T45.513	T45.514	T45.515	T45.516

Substance	Poisoning, Accidental (unintentional)	Poisoning, Intentional Self-harm	Poisoning, Assault	Poisoning, Undetermined	Adverse Effect	Under-dosing
Phensuximide	T42.2X1	T42.2X2	T42.2X3	T42.2X4	T42.2X5	T42.2X6
Phentermine	T50.5X1	T50.5X2	T50.5X3	T50.5X4	T50.5X5	T50.5X6
Phenthicillin	T36.0X1	T36.0X2	T36.0X3	T36.0X4	T36.0X5	T36.0X6
Phentolamine	T46.7X1	T46.7X2	T46.7X3	T46.7X4	T46.7X5	T46.7X6
Phenyl						
butazone	T39.2X1	T39.2X2	T39.2X3	T39.2X4	T39.2X5	T39.2X6
enediamine	T65.3X1	T65.3X2	T65.3X3	T65.3X4	—	—
hydrazine	T65.3X1	T65.3X2	T65.3X3	T65.3X4	—	—
antineoplastic	T45.1X1	T45.1X2	T45.1X3	T45.1X4	T45.1X5	T45.1X6
mercuric compounds — *see* Mercury						
salicylate	T49.3X1	T49.3X2	T49.3X3	T49.3X4	T49.3X5	T49.3X6
Phenylalanine mustard	T45.1X1	T45.1X2	T45.1X3	T45.1X4	T45.1X5	T45.1X6
Phenylbutazone	T39.2X1	T39.2X2	T39.2X3	T39.2X4	T39.2X5	T39.2X6
Phenylenediamine	T65.3X1	T65.3X2	T65.3X3	T65.3X4	—	—
Phenylephrine	T44.4X1	T44.4X2	T44.4X3	T44.4X4	T44.4X5	T44.4X6
Phenylethylbiguanide	T38.3X1	T38.3X2	T38.3X3	T38.3X4	T38.3X5	T38.3X6
Phenylmercuric						
acetate	T49.0X1	T49.0X2	T49.0X3	T49.0X4	T49.0X5	T49.0X6
borate	T49.0X1	T49.0X2	T49.0X3	T49.0X4	T49.0X5	T49.0X6
nitrate	T49.0X1	T49.0X2	T49.0X3	T49.0X4	T49.0X5	T49.0X6
Phenylmethylbarbitone	T42.3X1	T42.3X2	T42.3X3	T42.3X4	T42.3X5	T42.3X6
Phenylpropanol	T47.5X1	T47.5X2	T47.5X3	T47.5X4	T47.5X5	T47.5X6
Phenylpropanolamine	T44.991	T44.992	T44.993	T44.994	T44.995	T44.996
Phenylsulfthion	T60.0X1	T60.0X2	T60.0X3	T60.0X4	—	—
Phenyltoloxamine	T45.0X1	T45.0X2	T45.0X3	T45.0X4	T45.0X5	T45.0X6
Phenyramidol, phenyramidon	T39.8X1	T39.8X2	T39.8X3	T39.8X4	T39.8X5	T39.8X6
Phenytoin	T42.0X1	T42.0X2	T42.0X3	T42.0X4	T42.0X5	T42.0X6
with Phenobarbital	T42.3X1	T42.3X2	T42.3X3	T42.3X4	T42.3X5	T42.3X6
pHisoHex	T49.2X1	T49.2X2	T49.2X3	T49.2X4	T49.2X5	T49.2X6
Pholcodine	T48.3X1	T48.3X2	T48.3X3	T48.3X4	T48.3X5	T48.3X6
Pholedrine	T46.991	T46.992	T46.993	T46.994	T46.995	T46.996
Phorate	T60.0X1	T60.0X2	T60.0X3	T60.0X4	—	—
Phosdrin	T60.0X1	T60.0X2	T60.0X3	T60.0X4	—	—
Phosfolan	T60.0X1	T60.0X2	T60.0X3	T60.0X4	—	—
Phosgene (gas)	T59.891	T59.892	T59.893	T59.894	—	—
Phosphamidon	T60.0X1	T60.0X2	T60.0X3	T60.0X4	—	—
Phosphate	T65.891	T65.892	T65.893	T65.894	—	—
laxative	T47.4X1	T47.4X2	T47.4X3	T47.4X4	T47.4X5	T47.4X6
organic	T60.0X1	T60.0X2	T60.0X3	T60.0X4	—	—
solvent	T52.91	T52.92	T52.93	T52.94	—	—
tricresyl	T65.891	T65.892	T65.893	T65.894	—	—
Phosphine	T57.1X1	T57.1X2	T57.1X3	T57.1X4	—	—
fumigant	T57.1X1	T57.1X2	T57.1X3	T57.1X4	—	—
Phospholine	T49.5X1	T49.5X2	T49.5X3	T49.5X4	T49.5X5	T49.5X6
Phosphoric acid	T54.2X1	T54.2X2	T54.2X3	T54.2X4	—	—
Phosphorus (compound) NEC	T57.1X1	T57.1X2	T57.1X3	T57.1X4	—	—
pesticide	T60.0X1	T60.0X2	T60.0X3	T60.0X4	—	—
Phthalates	T65.891	T65.892	T65.893	T65.894	—	—
Phthalic anhydride	T65.891	T65.892	T65.893	T65.894	—	—
Phthalimidoglutarimide	T42.6X1	T42.6X2	T42.6X3	T42.6X4	T42.6X5	T42.6X6
Phthalylsulfathiazole	T37.0X1	T37.0X2	T37.0X3	T37.0X4	T37.0X5	T37.0X6
Phylloquinone	T45.7X1	T45.7X2	T45.7X3	T45.7X4	T45.7X5	T45.7X6
Physeptone	T40.3X1	T40.3X2	T40.3X3	T40.3X4	T40.3X5	T40.3X6
Physostigma venenosum	T62.2X1	T62.2X2	T62.2X3	T62.2X4	—	—
Physostigmine	T49.5X1	T49.5X2	T49.5X3	T49.5X4	T49.5X5	T49.5X6
Phytolacca decandra	T62.2X1	T62.2X2	T62.2X3	T62.2X4	—	—
berries	T62.1X1	T62.1X2	T62.1X3	T62.1X4	—	—
Phytomenadione	T45.7X1	T45.7X2	T45.7X3	T45.7X4	T45.7X5	T45.7X6
Phytonadione	T45.7X1	T45.7X2	T45.7X3	T45.7X4	T45.7X5	T45.7X6
Picoperine	T48.3X1	T48.3X2	T48.3X3	T48.3X4	T48.3X5	T48.3X6
Picosulfate (sodium)	T47.2X1	T47.2X2	T47.2X3	T47.2X4	T47.2X5	T47.2X6
Picric (acid)	T54.2X1	T54.2X2	T54.2X3	T54.2X4	—	—
Picrotoxin	T50.7X1	T50.7X2	T50.7X3	T50.7X4	T50.7X5	T50.7X6
Piketoprofen	T49.0X1	T49.0X2	T49.0X3	T49.0X4	T49.0X5	T49.0X6
Pilocarpine	T44.1X1	T44.1X2	T44.1X3	T44.1X4	T44.1X5	T44.1X6
Pilocarpus (jaborandi)	T44.1X1	T44.1X2	T44.1X3	T44.1X4	T44.1X5	T44.1X6
extract						
Pilsicainide (hydrochloride)	T46.2X1	T46.2X2	T46.2X3	T46.2X4	T46.2X5	T46.2X6
Pimaricin	T36.7X1	T36.7X2	T36.7X3	T36.7X4	T36.7X5	T36.7X6
Pimeclone	T50.7X1	T50.7X2	T50.7X3	T50.7X4	T50.7X5	T50.7X6
Pimelic ketone	T52.8X1	T52.8X2	T52.8X3	T52.8X4	—	—
Pimethixene	T45.0X1	T45.0X2	T45.0X3	T45.0X4	T45.0X5	T45.0X6
Piminodine	T40.2X1	T40.2X2	T40.2X3	T40.2X4	T40.2X5	T40.2X6
Pimozide	T43.591	T43.592	T43.593	T43.594	T43.595	T43.596
Pinacidil	T46.5X1	T46.5X2	T46.5X3	T46.5X4	T46.5X5	T46.5X6
Pinaverium bromide	T44.3X1	T44.3X2	T44.3X3	T44.3X4	T44.3X5	T44.3X6
Pinazepam	T42.4X1	T42.4X2	T42.4X3	T42.4X4	T42.4X5	T42.4X6
Pindolol	T44.7X1	T44.7X2	T44.7X3	T44.7X4	T44.7X5	T44.7X6
Pindone	T60.4X1	T60.4X2	T60.4X3	T60.4X4	—	—
Pine oil (disinfectant)	T65.891	T65.892	T65.893	T65.894	—	—

Substance	Poisoning, Accidental (unintentional)	Poisoning, Intentional Self-harm	Poisoning, Assault	Poisoning, Undetermined	Adverse Effect	Under-dosing
Pinkroot	T37.4X1	T37.4X2	T37.4X3	T37.4X4	T37.4X5	T37.4X6
Pipadone	T40.2X1	T40.2X2	T40.2X3	T40.2X4	—	—
Pipamazine	T45.0X1	T45.0X2	T45.0X3	T45.0X4	T45.0X5	T45.0X6
Pipamperone	T43.4X1	T43.4X2	T43.4X3	T43.4X4	T43.4X5	T43.4X6
Pipazetate	T48.3X1	T48.3X2	T48.3X3	T48.3X4	T48.3X5	T48.3X6
Pipemidic acid	T37.8X1	T37.8X2	T37.8X3	T37.8X4	T37.8X5	T37.8X6
Pipenzolate bromide	T44.3X1	T44.3X2	T44.3X3	T44.3X4	T44.3X5	T44.3X6
Piperacetazine	T43.3X1	T43.3X2	T43.3X3	T43.3X4	T43.3X5	T43.3X6
Piperacillin	T36.0X1	T36.0X2	T36.0X3	T36.0X4	T36.0X5	T36.0X6
Piperazine	T37.4X1	T37.4X2	T37.4X3	T37.4X4	T37.4X5	T37.4X6
estrone sulfate	T38.5X1	T38.5X2	T38.5X3	T38.5X4	T38.5X5	T38.5X6
Piper cubeba	T62.2X1	T62.2X2	T62.2X3	T62.2X4	—	—
Piperidione	T48.3X1	T48.3X2	T48.3X3	T48.3X4	T48.3X5	T48.3X6
Piperidolate	T44.3X1	T44.3X2	T44.3X3	T44.3X4	T44.3X5	T44.3X6
Piperocaine	T41.3X1	T41.3X2	T41.3X3	T41.3X4	T41.3X5	T41.3X6
infiltration (subcutaneous)	T41.3X1	T41.3X2	T41.3X3	T41.3X4	T41.3X5	T41.3X6
nerve block (peripheral) (plexus)	T41.3X1	T41.3X2	T41.3X3	T41.3X4	T41.3X5	T41.3X6
topical (surface)	T41.3X1	T41.3X2	T41.3X3	T41.3X4	T41.3X5	T41.3X6
Piperonyl butoxide	T60.8X1	T60.8X2	T60.8X3	T60.8X4	—	—
Pipethanate	T44.3X1	T44.3X2	T44.3X3	T44.3X4	T44.3X5	T44.3X6
Pipobroman	T45.1X1	T45.1X2	T45.1X3	T45.1X4	T45.1X5	T45.1X6
Pipotiazine	T43.3X1	T43.3X2	T43.3X3	T43.3X4	T43.3X5	T43.3X6
Pipoxizine	T45.0X1	T45.0X2	T45.0X3	T45.0X4	T45.0X5	T45.0X6
Pipradrol	T43.691	T43.692	T43.693	T43.694	T43.695	T43.696
Piprinhydrinate	T45.0X1	T45.0X2	T45.0X3	T45.0X4	T45.0X5	T45.0X6
Pirarubicin	T45.1X1	T45.1X2	T45.1X3	T45.1X4	T45.1X5	T45.1X6
Pirazinamide	T37.1X1	T37.1X2	T37.1X3	T37.1X4	T37.1X5	T37.1X6
Pirbuterol	T48.6X1	T48.6X2	T48.6X3	T48.6X4	T48.6X5	T48.6X6
Pirenzepine	T47.1X1	T47.1X2	T47.1X3	T47.1X4	T47.1X5	T47.1X6
Piretanide	T50.1X1	T50.1X2	T50.1X3	T50.1X4	T50.1X5	T50.1X6
Piribedil	T42.8X1	T42.8X2	T42.8X3	T42.8X4	T42.8X5	T42.8X6
Piridoxilate	T46.3X1	T46.3X2	T46.3X3	T46.3X4	T46.3X5	T46.3X6
Piritramide	T40.4X1	T40.4X2	T40.4X3	T40.4X4	—	—
Piromidic acid	T37.8X1	T37.8X2	T37.8X3	T37.8X4	T37.8X5	T37.8X6
Piroxicam	T39.391	T39.392	T39.393	T39.394	T39.395	T39.396
beta-cyclodextrin complex	T39.8X1	T39.8X2	T39.8X3	T39.8X4	T39.8X5	T39.8X6
Pirozadil	T46.6X1	T46.6X2	T46.6X3	T46.6X4	T46.6X5	T46.6X6
Piscidia (bark) (erythrina)	T39.8X1	T39.8X2	T39.8X3	T39.8X4	T39.8X5	T39.8X6
Pitch	T65.891	T65.892	T65.893	T65.894	—	—
Pitkin's solution	T41.3X1	T41.3X2	T41.3X3	T41.3X4	T41.3X5	T41.3X6
Pitocin	T48.0X1	T48.0X2	T48.0X3	T48.0X4	T48.0X5	T48.0X6
Pitressin (tannate)	T38.891	T38.892	T38.893	T38.894	T38.895	T38.896
Pituitary extracts (posterior)	T38.891	T38.892	T38.893	T38.894	T38.895	T38.896
anterior	T38.811	T38.812	T38.813	T38.814	T38.815	T38.816
Pituitrin	T38.891	T38.892	T38.893	T38.894	T38.895	T38.896
Pivampicillin	T36.0X1	T36.0X2	T36.0X3	T36.0X4	T36.0X5	T36.0X6
Pivmecillinam	T36.0X1	T36.0X2	T36.0X3	T36.0X4	T36.0X5	T36.0X6
Placental hormone	T38.891	T38.892	T38.893	T38.894	T38.895	T38.896
Placidyl	T42.6X1	T42.6X2	T42.6X3	T42.6X4	T42.6X5	T42.6X6
Plague vaccine	T50.A91	T50.A92	T50.A93	T50.A94	T50.A95	T50.A96
Plant						
food or fertilizer NEC	T65.891	T65.892	T65.893	T65.894	—	—
containing herbicide	T60.3X1	T60.3X2	T60.3X3	T60.3X4	—	—
noxious, used as food	T62.2X1	T62.2X2	T62.2X3	T62.2X4	—	—
berries	T62.1X1	T62.1X2	T62.1X3	T62.1X4	—	—
seeds	T62.2X1	T62.2X2	T62.2X3	T62.2X4	—	—
specified type NEC	T62.2X1	T62.2X2	T62.2X3	T62.2X4	—	—
Plasma	T45.8X1	T45.8X2	T45.8X3	T45.8X4	T45.8X5	T45.8X6
expander NEC	T45.8X1	T45.8X2	T45.8X3	T45.8X4	T45.8X5	T45.8X6
protein fraction (human)	T45.8X1	T45.8X2	T45.8X3	T45.8X4	T45.8X5	T45.8X6
Plasmanate	T45.8X1	T45.8X2	T45.8X3	T45.8X4	T45.8X5	T45.8X6
Plasminogen (tissue) activator	T45.611	T45.612	T45.613	T45.614	T45.615	T45.616
Plaster dressing	T49.3X1	T49.3X2	T49.3X3	T49.3X4	T49.3X5	T49.3X6
Plastic dressing	T49.3X1	T49.3X2	T49.3X3	T49.3X4	T49.3X5	T49.3X6
Plegicil	T43.3X1	T43.3X2	T43.3X3	T43.3X4	T43.3X5	T43.3X6
Plicamycin	T45.1X1	T45.1X2	T45.1X3	T45.1X4	T45.1X5	T45.1X6
Podophyllotoxin	T49.8X1	T49.8X2	T49.8X3	T49.8X4	T49.8X5	T49.8X6
Podophyllum (resin)	T49.4X1	T49.4X2	T49.4X3	T49.4X4	T49.4X5	T49.4X6
Poisonous berries	T62.1X1	T62.1X2	T62.1X3	T62.1X4	—	—
Poison NEC	T65.91	T65.92	T65.93	T65.94	—	—
Pokeweed (any part)	T62.2X1	T62.2X2	T62.2X3	T62.2X4	—	—
Poldine metilsulfate	T44.3X1	T44.3X2	T44.3X3	T44.3X4	T44.3X5	T44.3X6
Polidexide (sulfate)	T46.6X1	T46.6X2	T46.6X3	T46.6X4	T46.6X5	T46.6X6
Polidocanol	T46.8X1	T46.8X2	T46.8X3	T46.8X4	T46.8X5	T46.8X6
Poliomyelitis vaccine	T50.B91	T50.B92	T50.B93	T50.B94	T50.B95	T50.B96
Polish (car) (floor) (furniture) (metal) (porcelain) (silver)	T65.891	T65.892	T65.893	T65.894	—	—
abrasive	T65.891	T65.892	T65.893	T65.894	—	—
porcelain	T65.891	T65.892	T65.893	T65.894	—	—
Poloxalkol	T47.4X1	T47.4X2	T47.4X3	T47.4X4	T47.4X5	T47.4X6
Poloxamer	T47.4X1	T47.4X2	T47.4X3	T47.4X4	T47.4X5	T47.4X6

Additional Character May Be Required — Refer to the Tabular List for Character Selection ▽ Subterms under main terms may continue to next column or page

Substance	Poisoning, Accidental (unintentional)	Poisoning, Intentional Self-harm	Poisoning, Assault	Poisoning, Undetermined	Adverse Effect	Under-dosing
Polyaminostyrene resins	T50.3X1	T50.3X2	T50.3X3	T50.3X4	T50.3X5	T50.3X6
Polycarbophil	T47.4X1	T47.4X2	T47.4X3	T47.4X4	T47.4X5	T47.4X6
Polychlorinated biphenyl	T65.891	T65.892	T65.893	T65.894	—	—
Polycycline	T36.4X1	T36.4X2	T36.4X3	T36.4X4	T36.4X5	T36.4X6
Polyester fumes	T59.891	T59.892	T59.893	T59.894	—	—
Polyester resin hardener	T52.91	T52.92	T52.93	T52.94	—	—
fumes	T59.891	T59.892	T59.893	T59.894	—	—
Polyestradiol phosphate	T38.5X1	T38.5X2	T38.5X3	T38.5X4	T38.5X5	T38.5X6
Polyethanolamine alkyl sulfate	T49.2X1	T49.2X2	T49.2X3	T49.2X4	T49.2X5	T49.2X6
Polyethylene adhesive	T49.3X1	T49.3X2	T49.3X3	T49.3X4	T49.3X5	T49.3X6
Polyferose	T45.4X1	T45.4X2	T45.4X3	T45.4X4	T45.4X5	T45.4X6
Polygeline	T45.8X1	T45.8X2	T45.8X3	T45.8X4	T45.8X5	T45.8X6
Polymyxin	T36.8X1	T36.8X2	T36.8X3	T36.8X4	T36.8X5	T36.8X6
B	T36.8X1	T36.8X2	T36.8X3	T36.8X4	T36.8X5	T36.8X6
ENT agent	T49.6X1	T49.6X2	T49.6X3	T49.6X4	T49.6X5	T49.6X6
ophthalmic preparation	T49.5X1	T49.5X2	T49.5X3	T49.5X4	T49.5X5	T49.5X6
topical NEC	T49.0X1	T49.0X2	T49.0X3	T49.0X4	T49.0X5	T49.0X6
E sulfate (eye preparation)	T49.5X1	T49.5X2	T49.5X3	T49.5X4	T49.5X5	T49.5X6
Polynoxylin	T49.0X1	T49.0X2	T49.0X3	T49.0X4	T49.0X5	T49.0X6
Polyoestradiol phosphate	T38.5X1	T38.5X2	T38.5X3	T38.5X4	T38.5X5	T38.5X6
Polyoxymethyleneurea	T49.0X1	T49.0X2	T49.0X3	T49.0X4	T49.0X5	T49.0X6
Polysilane	T47.8X1	T47.8X2	T47.8X3	T47.8X4	T47.8X5	T47.8X6
Polytetrafluoroethylene (inhaled)	T59.891	T59.892	T59.893	T59.894	—	—
Polythiazide	T50.2X1	T50.2X2	T50.2X3	T50.2X4	T50.2X5	T50.2X6
Polyvidone	T45.8X1	T45.8X2	T45.8X3	T45.8X4	T45.8X5	T45.8X6
Polyvinylpyrrolidone	T45.8X1	T45.8X2	T45.8X3	T45.8X4	T45.8X5	T45.8X6
Pontocaine (hydrochloride) (infiltration) (topical)	T41.3X1	T41.3X2	T41.3X3	T41.3X4	T41.3X5	T41.3X6
nerve block (peripheral) (plexus)	T41.3X1	T41.3X2	T41.3X3	T41.3X4	T41.3X5	T41.3X6
spinal	T41.3X1	T41.3X2	T41.3X3	T41.3X4	T41.3X5	T41.3X6
Porfiromycin	T45.1X1	T45.1X2	T45.1X3	T45.1X4	T45.1X5	T45.1X6
Posterior pituitary hormone NEC	T38.891	T38.892	T38.893	T38.894	T38.895	T38.896
Pot	T40.7X1	T40.7X2	T40.7X3	T40.7X4	T40.7X5	T40.7X6
Potash (caustic)	T54.3X1	T54.3X2	T54.3X3	T54.3X4	—	—
Potassic saline injection (lactated)	T50.3X1	T50.3X2	T50.3X3	T50.3X4	T50.3X5	T50.3X6
Potassium-removing resin	T50.3X1	T50.3X2	T50.3X3	T50.3X4	T50.3X5	T50.3X6
Potassium-retaining drug	T50.3X1	T50.3X2	T50.3X3	T50.3X4	T50.3X5	T50.3X6
Potassium (salts) NEC	T50.3X1	T50.3X2	T50.3X3	T50.3X4	T50.3X5	T50.3X6
aminobenzoate	T45.8X1	T45.8X2	T45.8X3	T45.8X4	T45.8X5	T45.8X6
aminosalicylate	T37.1X1	T37.1X2	T37.1X3	T37.1X4	T37.1X5	T37.1X6
antimony ' tartrate'	T37.8X1	T37.8X2	T37.8X3	T37.8X4	T37.8X5	T37.8X6
arsenite (solution)	T57.0X1	T57.0X2	T57.0X3	T57.0X4	—	—
bichromate	T56.2X1	T56.2X2	T56.2X3	T56.2X4	—	—
bisulfate	T47.3X1	T47.3X2	T47.3X3	T47.3X4	T47.3X5	T47.3X6
bromide	T42.6X1	T42.6X2	T42.6X3	T42.6X4	T42.6X5	T42.6X6
canrenoate	T50.0X1	T50.0X2	T50.0X3	T50.0X4	T50.0X5	T50.0X6
carbonate	T54.3X1	T54.3X2	T54.3X3	T54.3X4	—	—
chlorate NEC	T65.891	T65.892	T65.893	T65.894	—	—
chloride	T50.3X1	T50.3X2	T50.3X3	T50.3X4	T50.3X5	T50.3X6
citrate	T50.991	T50.992	T50.993	T50.994	T50.995	T50.996
cyanide	T65.0X1	T65.0X2	T65.0X3	T65.0X4	—	—
ferric hexacyanoferrate (medicinal)	T50.6X1	T50.6X2	T50.6X3	T50.6X4	T50.6X5	T50.6X6
nonmedicinal	T65.891	T65.892	T65.893	T65.894	—	—
Fluoride	T57.8X1	T57.8X2	T57.8X3	T57.8X4	—	—
glucaldrate	T47.1X1	T47.1X2	T47.1X3	T47.1X4	T47.1X5	T47.1X6
hydroxide	T54.3X1	T54.3X2	T54.3X3	T54.3X4	—	—
iodate	T49.0X1	T49.0X2	T49.0X3	T49.0X4	T49.0X5	T49.0X6
iodide	T48.4X1	T48.4X2	T48.4X3	T48.4X4	T48.4X5	T48.4X6
nitrate	T57.8X1	T57.8X2	T57.8X3	T57.8X4	—	—
oxalate	T65.891	T65.892	T65.893	T65.894	—	—
perchlorate (nonmedicinal) NEC	T65.891	T65.892	T65.893	T65.894	—	—
antithyroid	T38.2X1	T38.2X2	T38.2X3	T38.2X4	T38.2X5	T38.2X6
medicinal	T38.2X1	T38.2X2	T38.2X3	T38.2X4	T38.2X5	T38.2X6
Permanganate (nonmedicinal)	T65.891	T65.892	T65.893	T65.894	—	—
medicinal	T49.0X1	T49.0X2	T49.0X3	T49.0X4	T49.0X5	T49.0X6
sulfate	T47.2X1	T47.2X2	T47.2X3	T47.2X4	T47.2X5	T47.2X6
Povidone	T45.8X1	T45.8X2	T45.8X3	T45.8X4	T45.8X5	T45.8X6
iodine	T49.0X1	T49.0X2	T49.0X3	T49.0X4	T49.0X5	T49.0X6
Practolol	T44.7X1	T44.7X2	T44.7X3	T44.7X4	T44.7X5	T44.7X6
Prajmalium bitartrate	T46.2X1	T46.2X2	T46.2X3	T46.2X4	T46.2X5	T46.2X6
Pralidoxime (iodide)	T50.6X1	T50.6X2	T50.6X3	T50.6X4	T50.6X5	T50.6X6
chloride	T50.6X1	T50.6X2	T50.6X3	T50.6X4	T50.6X5	T50.6X6
Pramiverine	T44.3X1	T44.3X2	T44.3X3	T44.3X4	T44.3X5	T44.3X6
Pramocaine	T49.1X1	T49.1X2	T49.1X3	T49.1X4	T49.1X5	T49.1X6
Pramoxine	T49.1X1	T49.1X2	T49.1X3	T49.1X4	T49.1X5	T49.1X6
Prasterone	T38.7X1	T38.7X2	T38.7X3	T38.7X4	T38.7X5	T38.7X6
Pravastatin	T46.6X1	T46.6X2	T46.6X3	T46.6X4	T46.6X5	T46.6X6
Prazepam	T42.4X1	T42.4X2	T42.4X3	T42.4X4	T42.4X5	T42.4X6
Praziquantel	T37.4X1	T37.4X2	T37.4X3	T37.4X4	T37.4X5	T37.4X6
Prazitone	T43.291	T43.292	T43.293	T43.294	T43.295	T43.296
Prazosin	T44.6X1	T44.6X2	T44.6X3	T44.6X4	T44.6X5	T44.6X6
Prednicarbate	T49.0X1	T49.0X2	T49.0X3	T49.0X4	T49.0X5	T49.0X6
Prednimustine	T45.1X1	T45.1X2	T45.1X3	T45.1X4	T45.1X5	T45.1X6
Prednisolone	T38.0X1	T38.0X2	T38.0X3	T38.0X4	T38.0X5	T38.0X6
ENT agent	T49.6X1	T49.6X2	T49.6X3	T49.6X4	T49.6X5	T49.6X6
ophthalmic preparation	T49.5X1	T49.5X2	T49.5X3	T49.5X4	T49.5X5	T49.5X6
steaglate	T38.0X1	T38.0X2	T38.0X3	T38.0X4	T38.0X5	T38.0X6
topical NEC	T49.0X1	T49.0X2	T49.0X3	T49.0X4	T49.0X5	T49.0X6
Prednisone	T38.0X1	T38.0X2	T38.0X3	T38.0X4	T38.0X5	T38.0X6
Prednylidene	T38.0X1	T38.0X2	T38.0X3	T38.0X4	T38.0X5	T38.0X6
Pregnandiol	T38.5X1	T38.5X2	T38.5X3	T38.5X4	T38.5X5	T38.5X6
Pregneninolone	T38.5X1	T38.5X2	T38.5X3	T38.5X4	T38.5X5	T38.5X6
Preludin	T43.691	T43.692	T43.693	T43.694	T43.695	T43.696
Premarin	T38.5X1	T38.5X2	T38.5X3	T38.5X4	T38.5X5	T38.5X6
Premedication anesthetic	T41.201	T41.202	T41.203	T41.204	T41.205	T41.206
Prenalterol	T44.5X1	T44.5X2	T44.5X3	T44.5X4	T44.5X5	T44.5X6
Prenoxdiazine	T48.3X1	T48.3X2	T48.3X3	T48.3X4	T48.3X5	T48.3X6
Prenylamine	T46.3X1	T46.3X2	T46.3X3	T46.3X4	T46.3X5	T46.3X6
Preparation H	T49.8X1	T49.8X2	T49.8X3	T49.8X4	T49.8X5	T49.8X6
Preparation, local	T49.4X1	T49.4X2	T49.4X3	T49.4X4	T49.4X5	T49.4X6
Preservative (nonmedicinal)	T65.891	T65.892	T65.893	T65.894	—	—
medicinal	T50.901	T50.902	T50.903	T50.904	T50.905	T50.906
wood	T60.91	T60.92	T60.93	T60.94	—	—
Prethcamide	T50.7X1	T50.7X2	T50.7X3	T50.7X4	T50.7X5	T50.7X6
Pride of China	T62.2X1	T62.2X2	T62.2X3	T62.2X4	—	—
Pridinol	T44.3X1	T44.3X2	T44.3X3	T44.3X4	T44.3X5	T44.3X6
Prifinium bromide	T44.3X1	T44.3X2	T44.3X3	T44.3X4	T44.3X5	T44.3X6
Prilocaine	T41.3X1	T41.3X2	T41.3X3	T41.3X4	T41.3X5	T41.3X6
infiltration (subcutaneous)	T41.3X1	T41.3X2	T41.3X3	T41.3X4	T41.3X5	T41.3X6
nerve block (peripheral) (plexus)	T41.3X1	T41.3X2	T41.3X3	T41.3X4	T41.3X5	T41.3X6
regional	T41.3X1	T41.3X2	T41.3X3	T41.3X4	T41.3X5	T41.3X6
Primaquine	T37.2X1	T37.2X2	T37.2X3	T37.2X4	T37.2X5	T37.2X6
Primidone	T42.6X1	T42.6X2	T42.6X3	T42.6X4	T42.6X5	T42.6X6
Primula (veris)	T62.2X1	T62.2X2	T62.2X3	T62.2X4	—	—
Prinadol	T40.2X1	T40.2X2	T40.2X3	T40.2X4	T40.2X5	T40.2X6
Priscol, Priscoline	T44.6X1	T44.6X2	T44.6X3	T44.6X4	T44.6X5	T44.6X6
Pristinamycin	T36.3X1	T36.3X2	T36.3X3	T36.3X4	T36.3X5	T36.3X6
Privet	T62.2X1	T62.2X2	T62.2X3	T62.2X4	—	—
berries	T62.1X1	T62.1X2	T62.1X3	T62.1X4	—	—
Privine	T44.4X1	T44.4X2	T44.4X3	T44.4X4	T44.4X5	T44.4X6
Pro-Banthine	T44.3X1	T44.3X2	T44.3X3	T44.3X4	T44.3X5	T44.3X6
Probarbital	T42.3X1	T42.3X2	T42.3X3	T42.3X4	T42.3X5	T42.3X6
Probenecid	T50.4X1	T50.4X2	T50.4X3	T50.4X4	T50.4X5	T50.4X6
Probucol	T46.6X1	T46.6X2	T46.6X3	T46.6X4	T46.6X5	T46.6X6
Procainamide	T46.2X1	T46.2X2	T46.2X3	T46.2X4	T46.2X5	T46.2X6
Procaine	T41.3X1	T41.3X2	T41.3X3	T41.3X4	T41.3X5	T41.3X6
benzylpenicillin	T36.0X1	T36.0X2	T36.0X3	T36.0X4	T36.0X5	T36.0X6
nerve block (periphreal) (plexus)	T41.3X1	T41.3X2	T41.3X3	T41.3X4	T41.3X5	T41.3X6
penicillin G	T36.0X1	T36.0X2	T36.0X3	T36.0X4	T36.0X5	T36.0X6
regional	T41.3X1	T41.3X2	T41.3X3	T41.3X4	T41.3X5	T41.3X6
spinal	T41.3X1	T41.3X2	T41.3X3	T41.3X4	T41.3X5	T41.3X6
Procalmidol	T43.591	T43.592	T43.593	T43.594	T43.595	T43.596
Procarbazine	T45.1X1	T45.1X2	T45.1X3	T45.1X4	T45.1X5	T45.1X6
Procaterol	T44.5X1	T44.5X2	T44.5X3	T44.5X4	T44.5X5	T44.5X6
Prochlorperazine	T43.3X1	T43.3X2	T43.3X3	T43.3X4	T43.3X5	T43.3X6
Procyclidine	T44.3X1	T44.3X2	T44.3X3	T44.3X4	T44.3X5	T44.3X6
Producer gas	T58.8X1	T58.8X2	T58.8X3	T58.8X4	—	—
Profadol	T40.4X1	T40.4X2	T40.4X3	T40.4X4	T40.4X5	T40.4X6
Profenamine	T44.3X1	T44.3X2	T44.3X3	T44.3X4	T44.3X5	T44.3X6
Profenil	T44.3X1	T44.3X2	T44.3X3	T44.3X4	T44.3X5	T44.3X6
Proflavine	T49.0X1	T49.0X2	T49.0X3	T49.0X4	T49.0X5	T49.0X6
Progabide	T42.6X1	T42.6X2	T42.6X3	T42.6X4	T42.6X5	T42.6X6
Progesterone	T38.5X1	T38.5X2	T38.5X3	T38.5X4	T38.5X5	T38.5X6
Progestin	T38.5X1	T38.5X2	T38.5X3	T38.5X4	T38.5X5	T38.5X6
oral contraceptive	T38.4X1	T38.4X2	T38.4X3	T38.4X4	T38.4X5	T38.4X6
Progestogen NEC	T38.5X1	T38.5X2	T38.5X3	T38.5X4	T38.5X5	T38.5X6
Progestone	T38.5X1	T38.5X2	T38.5X3	T38.5X4	T38.5X5	T38.5X6
Proglumide	T47.1X1	T47.1X2	T47.1X3	T47.1X4	T47.1X5	T47.1X6
Proguanil	T37.2X1	T37.2X2	T37.2X3	T37.2X4	T37.2X5	T37.2X6
Prolactin	T38.811	T38.812	T38.813	T38.814	T38.815	T38.816
Prolintane	T43.691	T43.692	T43.693	T43.694	T43.695	T43.696
Proloid	T38.1X1	T38.1X2	T38.1X3	T38.1X4	T38.1X5	T38.1X6
Proluton	T38.5X1	T38.5X2	T38.5X3	T38.5X4	T38.5X5	T38.5X6
Promacetin	T37.1X1	T37.1X2	T37.1X3	T37.1X4	T37.1X5	T37.1X6
Promazine	T43.3X1	T43.3X2	T43.3X3	T43.3X4	T43.3X5	T43.3X6
Promedol	T40.2X1	T40.2X2	T40.2X3	T40.2X4	—	—

Substance	Poisoning, Accidental (unintentional)	Poisoning, Intentional Self-harm	Poisoning, Assault	Poisoning, Undetermined	Adverse Effect	Underdosing
Promegestone	T38.5X1	T38.5X2	T38.5X3	T38.5X4	T38.5X5	T38.5X6
Promethazine (teoclate)	T43.3X1	T43.3X2	T43.3X3	T43.3X4	T43.3X5	T43.3X6
Promin	T37.1X1	T37.1X2	T37.1X3	T37.1X4	T37.1X5	T37.1X6
Pronase	T45.3X1	T45.3X2	T45.3X3	T45.3X4	T45.3X5	T45.3X6
Pronestyl (hydrochloride)	T46.2X1	T46.2X2	T46.2X3	T46.2X4	T46.2X5	T46.2X6
Pronetalol	T44.7X1	T44.7X2	T44.7X3	T44.7X4	T44.7X5	T44.7X6
Prontosil	T37.0X1	T37.0X2	T37.0X3	T37.0X4	T37.0X5	T37.0X6
Propachlor	T60.3X1	T60.3X2	T60.3X3	T60.3X4	—	—
Propafenone	T46.2X1	T46.2X2	T46.2X3	T46.2X4	—	T46.2X6
Propallylonal	T42.3X1	T42.3X2	T42.3X3	T42.3X4	T42.3X5	T42.3X6
Propamidine	T49.0X1	T49.0X2	T49.0X3	T49.0X4	T49.0X5	T49.0X6
Propane (distributed in mobile container)	T59.891	T59.892	T59.893	T59.894		
distributed through pipes	T59.891	T59.892	T59.893	T59.894	—	—
incomplete combustion	T58.11	T58.12	T58.13	T58.14	—	—
Propanidid	T41.291	T41.292	T41.293	T41.294	T41.295	T41.296
Propanil	T60.3X1	T60.3X2	T60.3X3	T60.3X4	—	—
Propantheline	T44.3X1	T44.3X2	T44.3X3	T44.3X4	T44.3X5	T44.3X6
bromide	T44.3X1	T44.3X2	T44.3X3	T44.3X4	T44.3X5	T44.3X6
Proparacaine	T41.3X1	T41.3X2	T41.3X3	T41.3X4	T41.3X5	T41.3X6
Propatylnitrate	T46.3X1	T46.3X2	T46.3X3	T46.3X4	T46.3X5	T46.3X6
Propicillin	T36.0X1	T36.0X2	T36.0X3	T36.0X4	T36.0X5	T36.0X6
Propiolactone	T49.0X1	T49.0X2	T49.0X3	T49.0X4	T49.0X5	T49.0X6
Propiomazine	T45.0X1	T45.0X2	T45.0X3	T45.0X4	T45.0X5	T45.0X6
Propionaldehyde (medicinal)	T42.6X1	T42.6X2	T42.6X3	T42.6X4	T42.6X5	T42.6X6
Propionate (calcium) (sodium)	T49.0X1	T49.0X2	T49.0X3	T49.0X4	T49.0X5	T49.0X6
Propion gel	T49.0X1	T49.0X2	T49.0X3	T49.0X4	T49.0X5	T49.0X6
Propitocaine	T41.3X1	T41.3X2	T41.3X3	T41.3X4	T41.3X5	T41.3X6
infiltration (subcutaneous)	T41.3X1	T41.3X2	T41.3X3	T41.3X4	T41.3X5	T41.3X6
nerve block (peripheral) (plexus)	T41.3X1	T41.3X2	T41.3X3	T41.3X4	T41.3X5	T41.3X6
Propofol	T41.291	T41.292	T41.293	T41.294	T41.295	T41.296
Propoxur	T60.0X1	T60.0X2	T60.0X3	T60.0X4	—	—
Propoxycaine	T41.3X1	T41.3X2	T41.3X3	T41.3X4	T41.3X5	T41.3X6
infiltration (subcutaneous)	T41.3X1	T41.3X2	T41.3X3	T41.3X4	T41.3X5	T41.3X6
nerve block (peripheral) (plexus)	T41.3X1	T41.3X2	T41.3X3	T41.3X4	T41.3X5	T41.3X6
topical (surface)	T41.3X1	T41.3X2	T41.3X3	T41.3X4	T41.3X5	T41.3X6
Propoxyphene	T40.4X1	T40.4X2	T40.4X3	T40.4X4	T40.4X5	T40.4X6
Propranolol	T44.7X1	T44.7X2	T44.7X3	T44.7X4	T44.7X5	T44.7X6
Propyl						
alcohol	T51.3X1	T51.3X2	T51.3X3	T51.3X4	—	—
carbinol	T51.3X1	T51.3X2	T51.3X3	T51.3X4	—	—
hexadrine	T44.4X1	T44.4X2	T44.4X3	T44.4X4	T44.4X5	T44.4X6
iodone	T50.8X1	T50.8X2	T50.8X3	T50.8X4	T50.8X5	T50.8X6
thiouracil	T38.2X1	T38.2X2	T38.2X3	T38.2X4	T38.2X5	T38.2X6
Propylaminophenothiazine	T43.3X1	T43.3X2	T43.3X3	T43.3X4	T43.3X5	T43.3X6
Propylene	T59.891	T59.892	T59.893	T59.894	—	—
Propylhexedrine	T48.5X1	T48.5X2	T48.5X3	T48.5X4	T48.5X5	T48.5X6
Propyliodone	T50.8X1	T50.8X2	T50.8X3	T50.8X4	T50.8X5	T50.8X6
Propylparaben (ophthalmic)	T49.5X1	T49.5X2	T49.5X3	T49.5X4	T49.5X5	T49.5X6
Propylthiouracil	T38.2X1	T38.2X2	T38.2X3	T38.2X4	T38.2X5	T38.2X6
Propyphenazone	T39.2X1	T39.2X2	T39.2X3	T39.2X4	T39.2X5	T39.2X6
Proquazone	T39.391	T39.392	T39.393	T39.394	T39.395	T39.396
Proscillaridin	T46.0X1	T46.0X2	T46.0X3	T46.0X4	T46.0X5	T46.0X6
Prostacyclin	T45.521	T45.522	T45.523	T45.524	T45.525	T45.526
Prostaglandin (I2)	T45.521	T45.522	T45.523	T45.524	T45.525	T45.526
E1	T46.7X1	T46.7X2	T46.7X3	T46.7X4	T46.7X5	T46.7X6
E2	T48.0X1	T48.0X2	T48.0X3	T48.0X4	T48.0X5	T48.0X6
F2 alpha	T48.0X1	T48.0X2	T48.0X3	T48.0X4	T48.0X5	T48.0X6
Prostigmin	T44.0X1	T44.0X2	T44.0X3	T44.0X4	T44.0X5	T44.0X6
Prosultiamine	T45.2X1	T45.2X2	T45.2X3	T45.2X4	T45.2X5	T45.2X6
Protamine sulfate	T45.7X1	T45.7X2	T45.7X3	T45.7X4	T45.7X5	T45.7X6
zinc insulin	T38.3X1	T38.3X2	T38.3X3	T38.3X4	T38.3X5	T38.3X6
Protease	T47.5X1	T47.5X2	T47.5X3	T47.5X4	T47.5X5	T47.5X6
Protectant, skin NEC	T49.3X1	T49.3X2	T49.3X3	T49.3X4	T49.3X5	T49.3X6
Protein hydrolysate	T50.991	T50.992	T50.993	T50.994	T50.995	T50.996
Prothiaden — see Dothiepin hydrochloride						
Prothionamide	T37.1X1	T37.1X2	T37.1X3	T37.1X4	T37.1X5	T37.1X6
Prothipendyl	T43.591	T43.592	T43.593	T43.594	T43.595	T43.596
Prothoate	T60.0X1	T60.0X2	T60.0X3	T60.0X4	—	—
Prothrombin						
activator	T45.7X1	T45.7X2	T45.7X3	T45.7X4	T45.7X5	T45.7X6
synthesis inhibitor	T45.511	T45.512	T45.513	T45.514	T45.515	T45.516
Protionamide	T37.1X1	T37.1X2	T37.1X3	T37.1X4	T37.1X5	T37.1X6
Protirelin	T38.891	T38.892	T38.893	T38.894	T38.895	T38.896
Protokylol	T48.6X1	T48.6X2	T48.6X3	T48.6X4	T48.6X5	T48.6X6
Protopam	T50.6X1	T50.6X2	T50.6X3	T50.6X4	T50.6X5	T50.6X6
Protoveratrine(s) (A) (B)	T46.5X1	T46.5X2	T46.5X3	T46.5X4	T46.5X5	T46.5X6
Protriptyline	T43.011	T43.012	T43.013	T43.014	T43.015	T43.016

Substance	Poisoning, Accidental (unintentional)	Poisoning, Intentional Self-harm	Poisoning, Assault	Poisoning, Undetermined	Adverse Effect	Underdosing
Provera	T38.5X1	T38.5X2	T38.5X3	T38.5X4	T38.5X5	T38.5X6
Provitamin A	T45.2X1	T45.2X2	T45.2X3	T45.2X4	T45.2X5	T45.2X6
Proxibarbal	T42.3X1	T42.3X2	T42.3X3	T42.3X4	T42.3X5	T42.3X6
Proxymetacaine	T41.3X1	T41.3X2	T41.3X3	T41.3X4	T41.3X5	T41.3X6
Proxyphylline	T48.6X1	T48.6X2	T48.6X3	T48.6X4	T48.6X5	T48.6X6
Prozac — see Fluoxetine hydrochloride						
Prunus						
laurocerasus	T62.2X1	T62.2X2	T62.2X3	T62.2X4	—	—
virginiana	T62.2X1	T62.2X2	T62.2X3	T62.2X4	—	—
Prussian blue						
commercial	T65.891	T65.892	T65.893	T65.894	—	—
therapeutic	T50.6X1	T50.6X2	T50.6X3	T50.6X4	T50.6X5	T50.6X6
Prussic acid	T65.0X1	T65.0X2	T65.0X3	T65.0X4	—	—
vapor	T57.3X1	T57.3X2	T57.3X3	T57.3X4	—	—
Pseudoephedrine	T44.991	T44.992	T44.993	T44.994	T44.995	T44.996
Psilocin	T40.991	T40.992	T40.993	T40.994	—	—
Psilocybin	T40.991	T40.992	T40.993	T40.994	—	—
Psilocybine	T40.991	T40.992	T40.993	T40.994	—	—
Psoralene (nonmedicinal)	T65.891	T65.892	T65.893	T65.894	—	—
Psoralens (medicinal)	T50.991	T50.992	T50.993	T50.994	T50.995	T50.996
PSP (phenolsulfonphthalein)	T50.8X1	T50.8X2	T50.8X3	T50.8X4	T50.8X5	T50.8X6
Psychodysleptic drug NEC	T40.901	T40.902	T40.903	T40.904	T40.905	T40.906
Psychostimulant	T43.601	T43.602	T43.603	T43.604	T43.605	T43.606
amphetamine	T43.621	T43.622	T43.623	T43.624	T43.625	T43.626
caffeine	T43.611	T43.612	T43.613	T43.614	T43.615	T43.616
methylphenidate	T43.631	T43.632	T43.633	T43.634	T43.635	T43.636
specified NEC	T43.691	T43.692	T43.693	T43.694	T43.695	T43.696
Psychotherapeutic drug NEC	T43.91	T43.92	T43.93	T43.94	T43.95	T43.96
antidepressants — see also Antidepressant	T43.201	T43.202	T43.203	T43.204	T43.205	T43.206
specified NEC	T43.8X1	T43.8X2	T43.8X3	T43.8X4	T43.8X5	T43.8X6
tranquilizers NEC	T43.501	T43.502	T43.503	T43.504	T43.505	T43.506
Psychotomimetic agents	T40.901	T40.902	T40.903	T40.904	T40.905	T40.906
Psychotropic drug NEC	T43.91	T43.92	T43.93	T43.94	T43.95	T43.96
specified NEC	T43.8X1	T43.8X2	T43.8X3	T43.8X4	T43.8X5	T43.8X6
Psyllium hydrophilic mucilloid	T47.4X1	T47.4X2	T47.4X3	T47.4X4	T47.4X5	T47.4X6
Pteroylglutamic acid	T45.8X1	T45.8X2	T45.8X3	T45.8X4	T45.8X5	T45.8X6
Pteroyltriglutamate	T45.1X1	T45.1X2	T45.1X3	T45.1X4	T45.1X5	T45.1X6
PTFE — see Polytetrafluoroethylene						
Pulp						
devitalizing paste	T49.7X1	T49.7X2	T49.7X3	T49.7X4	T49.7X5	T49.7X6
dressing	T49.7X1	T49.7X2	T49.7X3	T49.7X4	T49.7X5	T49.7X6
Pulsatilla	T62.2X1	T62.2X2	T62.2X3	T62.2X4	—	—
Pumpkin seed extract	T37.4X1	T37.4X2	T37.4X3	T37.4X4	T37.4X5	T37.4X6
Purex (bleach)	T54.91	T54.92	T54.93	T54.94	—	—
Purgative NEC — see also Cathartic	T47.4X1	T47.4X2	T47.4X3	T47.4X4	T47.4X5	T47.4X6
Purine analogue (antineoplastic)	T45.1X1	T45.1X2	T45.1X3	T45.1X4	T45.1X5	T45.1X6
Purine diuretics	T50.2X1	T50.2X2	T50.2X3	T50.2X4	T50.2X5	T50.2X6
Purinethol	T45.1X1	T45.1X2	T45.1X3	T45.1X4	T45.1X5	T45.1X6
PVP	T45.8X1	T45.8X2	T45.8X3	T45.8X4	T45.8X5	T45.8X6
Pyrabital	T39.8X1	T39.8X2	T39.8X3	T39.8X4	T39.8X5	T39.8X6
Pyramidon	T39.2X1	T39.2X2	T39.2X3	T39.2X4	T39.2X5	T39.2X6
Pyrantel	T37.4X1	T37.4X2	T37.4X3	T37.4X4	T37.4X5	T37.4X6
Pyrathiazine	T45.0X1	T45.0X2	T45.0X3	T45.0X4	T45.0X5	T45.0X6
Pyrazinamide	T37.1X1	T37.1X2	T37.1X3	T37.1X4	T37.1X5	T37.1X6
Pyrazinoic acid (amide)	T37.1X1	T37.1X2	T37.1X3	T37.1X4	T37.1X5	T37.1X6
Pyrazole (derivatives)	T39.2X1	T39.2X2	T39.2X3	T39.2X4	T39.2X5	T39.2X6
Pyrazolone analgesic NEC	T39.2X1	T39.2X2	T39.2X3	T39.2X4	T39.2X5	T39.2X6
Pyrethrin, pyrethrum (nonmedicinal)	T60.2X1	T60.2X2	T60.2X3	T60.2X4	—	—
Pyrethrum extract	T49.0X1	T49.0X2	T49.0X3	T49.0X4	T49.0X5	T49.0X6
Pyribenzamine	T45.0X1	T45.0X2	T45.0X3	T45.0X4	T45.0X5	T45.0X6
Pyridine	T52.8X1	T52.8X2	T52.8X3	T52.8X4	—	—
aldoxime methiodide	T50.6X1	T50.6X2	T50.6X3	T50.6X4	T50.6X5	T50.6X6
aldoxime methyl chloride	T50.6X1	T50.6X2	T50.6X3	T50.6X4	T50.6X5	T50.6X6
vapor	T59.891	T59.892	T59.893	T59.894	—	—
Pyridium	T39.8X1	T39.8X2	T39.8X3	T39.8X4	T39.8X5	T39.8X6
Pyridostigmine bromide	T44.0X1	T44.0X2	T44.0X3	T44.0X4	T44.0X5	T44.0X6
Pyridoxal phosphate	T45.2X1	T45.2X2	T45.2X3	T45.2X4	T45.2X5	T45.2X6
Pyridoxine	T45.2X1	T45.2X2	T45.2X3	T45.2X4	T45.2X5	T45.2X6
Pyrilamine	T45.0X1	T45.0X2	T45.0X3	T45.0X4	T45.0X5	T45.0X6
Pyrimethamine	T37.2X1	T37.2X2	T37.2X3	T37.2X4	T37.2X5	T37.2X6
with sulfadoxine	T37.2X1	T37.2X2	T37.2X3	T37.2X4	T37.2X5	T37.2X6
Pyrimidine antagonist	T45.1X1	T45.1X2	T45.1X3	T45.1X4	T45.1X5	T45.1X6
Pyriminil	T60.4X1	T60.4X2	T60.4X3	T60.4X4	—	—
Pyrithione zinc	T49.4X1	T49.4X2	T49.4X3	T49.4X4	T49.4X5	T49.4X6
Pyrithyldione	T42.6X1	T42.6X2	T42.6X3	T42.6X4	T42.6X5	T42.6X6

Substance	Poisoning, Accidental (unintentional)	Poisoning, Intentional Self-harm	Poisoning, Assault	Poisoning, Undetermined	Adverse Effect	Under-dosing
Pyrogallic acid	T49.0X1	T49.0X2	T49.0X3	T49.0X4	T49.0X5	T49.0X6
Pyrogallol	T49.0X1	T49.0X2	T49.0X3	T49.0X4	T49.0X5	T49.0X6
Pyroxylin	T49.3X1	T49.3X2	T49.3X3	T49.3X4	T49.3X5	T49.3X6
Pyrrobutamine	T45.0X1	T45.0X2	T45.0X3	T45.0X4	T45.0X5	T45.0X6
Pyrrolizidine alkaloids	T62.8X1	T62.8X2	T62.8X3	T62.8X4	—	—
Pyrvinium chloride	T37.4X1	T37.4X2	T37.4X3	T37.4X4	T37.4X5	T37.4X6
PZI	T38.3X1	T38.3X2	T38.3X3	T38.3X4	T38.3X5	T38.3X6
Quaalude	T42.6X1	T42.6X2	T42.6X3	T42.6X4	T42.6X5	T42.6X6
Quarternary ammonium						
anti-infective	T49.0X1	T49.0X2	T49.0X3	T49.0X4	T49.0X5	T49.0X6
ganglion blocking	T44.2X1	T44.2X2	T44.2X3	T44.2X4	T44.2X5	T44.2X6
parasympatholytic	T44.3X1	T44.3X2	T44.3X3	T44.3X4	T44.3X5	T44.3X6
Quazepam	T42.4X1	T42.4X2	T42.4X3	T42.4X4	T42.4X5	T42.4X6
Quicklime	T54.3X1	T54.3X2	T54.3X3	T54.3X4	—	—
Quillaja extract	T48.4X1	T48.4X2	T48.4X3	T48.4X4	T48.4X5	T48.4X6
Quinacrine	T37.2X1	T37.2X2	T37.2X3	T37.2X4	T37.2X5	T37.2X6
Quinaglute	T46.2X1	T46.2X2	T46.2X3	T46.2X4	T46.2X5	T46.2X6
Quinalbarbital	T42.3X1	T42.3X2	T42.3X3	T42.3X4	T42.3X5	T42.3X6
Quinalbarbitone sodium	T42.3X1	T42.3X2	T42.3X3	T42.3X4	T42.3X5	T42.3X6
Quinalphos	T60.0X1	T60.0X2	T60.0X3	T60.0X4	—	—
Quinapril	T46.4X1	T46.4X2	T46.4X3	T46.4X4	T46.4X5	T46.4X6
Quinestradiol	T38.5X1	T38.5X2	T38.5X3	T38.5X4	T38.5X5	T38.5X6
Quinestradol	T38.5X1	T38.5X2	T38.5X3	T38.5X4	T38.5X5	T38.5X6
Quinestrol	T38.5X1	T38.5X2	T38.5X3	T38.5X4	T38.5X5	T38.5X6
Quinethazone	T50.2X1	T50.2X2	T50.2X3	T50.2X4	T50.2X5	T50.2X6
Quingestanol	T38.4X1	T38.4X2	T38.4X3	T38.4X4	T38.4X5	T38.4X6
Quinidine	T46.2X1	T46.2X2	T46.2X3	T46.2X4	T46.2X5	T46.2X6
Quinine	T37.2X1	T37.2X2	T37.2X3	T37.2X4	T37.2X5	T37.2X6
Quiniobine	T37.8X1	T37.8X2	T37.8X3	T37.8X4	T37.8X5	T37.8X6
Quinisocaine	T49.1X1	T49.1X2	T49.1X3	T49.1X4	T49.1X5	T49.1X6
Quinocide	T37.2X1	T37.2X2	T37.2X3	T37.2X4	T37.2X5	T37.2X6
Quinoline (derivatives) NEC	T37.8X1	T37.8X2	T37.8X3	T37.8X4	T37.8X5	T37.8X6
Quinupramine	T43.011	T43.012	T43.013	T43.014	T43.015	T43.016
Quotane	T41.3X1	T41.3X2	T41.3X3	T41.3X4	T41.3X5	T41.3X6
Rabies						
immune globulin (human)	T50.Z11	T50.Z12	T50.Z13	T50.Z14	T50.Z15	T50.Z16
vaccine	T50.B91	T50.B92	T50.B93	T50.B94	T50.B95	T50.B96
Racemoramide	T40.2X1	T40.2X2	T40.2X3	T40.2X4	—	—
Racemorphan	T40.2X1	T40.2X2	T40.2X3	T40.2X4	T40.2X5	T40.2X6
Racepinefrin	T44.5X1	T44.5X2	T44.5X3	T44.5X4	T44.5X5	T44.5X6
Raclopride	T43.591	T43.592	T43.593	T43.594	T43.595	T43.596
Radiator alcohol	T51.1X1	T51.1X2	T51.1X3	T51.1X4	—	—
Radioactive drug NEC	T50.8X1	T50.8X2	T50.8X3	T50.8X4	T50.8X5	T50.8X6
Radio-opaque (drugs) (materials)	T50.8X1	T50.8X2	T50.8X3	T50.8X4	T50.8X5	T50.8X6
Ramifenazone	T39.2X1	T39.2X2	T39.2X3	T39.2X4	T39.2X5	T39.2X6
Ramipril	T46.4X1	T46.4X2	T46.4X3	T46.4X4	T46.4X5	T46.4X6
Ranitidine	T47.0X1	T47.0X2	T47.0X3	T47.0X4	T47.0X5	T47.0X6
Ranunculus	T62.2X1	T62.2X2	T62.2X3	T62.2X4	—	—
Rat poison NEC	T60.4X1	T60.4X2	T60.4X3	T60.4X4	—	—
Rattlesnake (venom)	T63.011	T63.012	T63.013	T63.014		
Raubasine	T46.7X1	T46.7X2	T46.7X3	T46.7X4	T46.7X5	T46.7X6
Raudixin	T46.5X1	T46.5X2	T46.5X3	T46.5X4	T46.5X5	T46.5X6
Rautensin	T46.5X1	T46.5X2	T46.5X3	T46.5X4	T46.5X5	T46.5X6
Rautina	T46.5X1	T46.5X2	T46.5X3	T46.5X4	T46.5X5	T46.5X6
Rautotal	T46.5X1	T46.5X2	T46.5X3	T46.5X4	T46.5X5	T46.5X6
Rauwiloid	T46.5X1	T46.5X2	T46.5X3	T46.5X4	T46.5X5	T46.5X6
Rauwoldin	T46.5X1	T46.5X2	T46.5X3	T46.5X4	T46.5X5	T46.5X6
Rauwolfia (alkaloids)	T46.5X1	T46.5X2	T46.5X3	T46.5X4	T46.5X5	T46.5X6
Razoxane	T45.1X1	T45.1X2	T45.1X3	T45.1X4	T45.1X5	T45.1X6
Realgar	T57.0X1	T57.0X2	T57.0X3	T57.0X4	—	—
Recombinant (R) — see specific protein						
Red blood cells, packed	T45.8X1	T45.8X2	T45.8X3	T45.8X4	T45.8X5	T45.8X6
Red squill (scilliroside)	T60.4X1	T60.4X2	T60.4X3	T60.4X4	—	—
Reducing agent, industrial NEC	T65.891	T65.892	T65.893	T65.894	—	—
Refrigerant gas (chlorofluorocarbon)	T53.5X1	T53.5X2	T53.5X3	T53.5X4	—	—
not chlorofluorocarbon	T59.891	T59.892	T59.893	T59.894	—	—
Regroton	T50.2X1	T50.2X2	T50.2X3	T50.2X4	T50.2X5	T50.2X6
Rehydration salts (oral)	T50.3X1	T50.3X2	T50.3X3	T50.3X4	T50.3X5	T50.3X6
Rela	T42.8X1	T42.8X2	T42.8X3	T42.8X4	T42.8X5	T42.8X6
Relaxant, muscle						
anesthetic	T48.1X1	T48.1X2	T48.1X3	T48.1X4	T48.1X5	T48.1X6
central nervous system	T42.8X1	T42.8X2	T42.8X3	T42.8X4	T42.8X5	T42.8X6
skeletal NEC	T48.1X1	T48.1X2	T48.1X3	T48.1X4	T48.1X5	T48.1X6
smooth NEC	T44.3X1	T44.3X2	T44.3X3	T44.3X4	T44.3X5	T44.3X6
Remoxipride	T43.591	T43.592	T43.593	T43.594	T43.595	T43.596
Renese	T50.2X1	T50.2X2	T50.2X3	T50.2X4	T50.2X5	T50.2X6
Renografin	T50.8X1	T50.8X2	T50.8X3	T50.8X4	T50.8X5	T50.8X6
Replacement solution	T50.3X1	T50.3X2	T50.3X3	T50.3X4	T50.3X5	T50.3X6
Reproterol	T48.6X1	T48.6X2	T48.6X3	T48.6X4	T48.6X5	T48.6X6
Rescinnamine	T46.5X1	T46.5X2	T46.5X3	T46.5X4	T46.5X5	T46.5X6
Reserpin (e)	T46.5X1	T46.5X2	T46.5X3	T46.5X4	T46.5X5	T46.5X6
Resorcin, resorcinol (nonmedicinal)	T65.891	T65.892	T65.893	T65.894	—	—
medicinal	T49.4X1	T49.4X2	T49.4X3	T49.4X4	T49.4X5	T49.4X6
Respaire	T48.4X1	T48.4X2	T48.4X3	T48.4X4	T48.4X5	T48.4X6
Respiratory drug NEC	T48.901	T48.902	T48.903	T48.904	T48.905	T48.906
antiasthmatic NEC	T48.6X1	T48.6X2	T48.6X3	T48.6X4	T48.6X5	T48.6X6
anti-common-cold NEC	T48.5X1	T48.5X2	T48.5X3	T48.5X4	T48.5X5	T48.5X6
expectorant NEC	T48.4X1	T48.4X2	T48.4X3	T48.4X4	T48.4X5	T48.4X6
stimulant	T48.901	T48.902	T48.903	T48.904	T48.905	T48.906
Retinoic acid	T49.0X1	T49.0X2	T49.0X3	T49.0X4	T49.0X5	T49.0X6
Retinol	T45.2X1	T45.2X2	T45.2X3	T45.2X4	T45.2X5	T45.2X6
Rh (D) immune globulin (human)	T50.Z11	T50.Z12	T50.Z13	T50.Z14	T50.Z15	T50.Z16
Rhodine	T39.011	T39.012	T39.013	T39.014	T39.015	T39.016
RhoGAM	T50.Z11	T50.Z12	T50.Z13	T50.Z14	T50.Z15	T50.Z16
Rhubarb						
dry extract	T47.2X1	T47.2X2	T47.2X3	T47.2X4	T47.2X5	T47.2X6
tincture, compound	T47.2X1	T47.2X2	T47.2X3	T47.2X4	T47.2X5	T47.2X6
Ribavirin	T37.5X1	T37.5X2	T37.5X3	T37.5X4	T37.5X5	T37.5X6
Riboflavin	T45.2X1	T45.2X2	T45.2X3	T45.2X4	T45.2X5	T45.2X6
Ribostamycin	T36.5X1	T36.5X2	T36.5X3	T36.5X4	T36.5X5	T36.5X6
Ricin	T62.2X1	T62.2X2	T62.2X3	T62.2X4	—	—
Ricinus communis	T62.2X1	T62.2X2	T62.2X3	T62.2X4	—	—
Rickettsial vaccine NEC	T50.A91	T50.A92	T50.A93	T50.A94	T50.A95	T50.A96
Rifabutin	T36.6X1	T36.6X2	T36.6X3	T36.6X4	T36.6X5	T36.6X6
Rifamide	T36.6X1	T36.6X2	T36.6X3	T36.6X4	T36.6X5	T36.6X6
Rifampicin	T36.6X1	T36.6X2	T36.6X3	T36.6X4	T36.6X5	T36.6X6
with isoniazid	T37.1X1	T37.1X2	T37.1X3	T37.1X4	T37.1X5	T37.1X6
Rifampin	T36.6X1	T36.6X2	T36.6X3	T36.6X4	T36.6X5	T36.6X6
Rifamycin	T36.6X1	T36.6X2	T36.6X3	T36.6X4	T36.6X5	T36.6X6
Rifaximin	T36.6X1	T36.6X2	T36.6X3	T36.6X4	T36.6X5	T36.6X6
Rimantadine	T37.5X1	T37.5X2	T37.5X3	T37.5X4	T37.5X5	T37.5X6
Rimazolium metilsulfate	T39.8X1	T39.8X2	T39.8X3	T39.8X4	T39.8X5	T39.8X6
Rimifon	T37.1X1	T37.1X2	T37.1X3	T37.1X4	T37.1X5	T37.1X6
Rimiterol	T48.6X1	T48.6X2	T48.6X3	T48.6X4	T48.6X5	T48.6X6
Ringer (lactate) solution	T50.3X1	T50.3X2	T50.3X3	T50.3X4	T50.3X5	T50.3X6
Ristocetin	T36.8X1	T36.8X2	T36.8X3	T36.8X4	T36.8X5	T36.8X6
Ritalin	T43.631	T43.632	T43.633	T43.634	T43.635	T43.636
Ritodrine	T44.5X1	T44.5X2	T44.5X3	T44.5X4	T44.5X5	T44.5X6
Roach killer — see Insecticide						
Rociverine	T44.3X1	T44.3X2	T44.3X3	T44.3X4	T44.3X5	T44.3X6
Rocky Mountain spotted fever vaccine	T50.A91	T50.A92	T50.A93	T50.A94	T50.A95	T50.A96
Rodenticide NEC	T60.4X1	T60.4X2	T60.4X3	T60.4X4	—	—
Rohypnol	T42.4X1	T42.4X2	T42.4X3	T42.4X4	T42.4X5	T42.4X6
Rokitamycin	T36.3X1	T36.3X2	T36.3X3	T36.3X4	T36.3X5	T36.3X6
Rolaids	T47.1X1	T47.1X2	T47.1X3	T47.1X4	T47.1X5	T47.1X6
Roletetracycline	T36.4X1	T36.4X2	T36.4X3	T36.4X4	T36.4X5	T36.4X6
Romilar	T48.3X1	T48.3X2	T48.3X3	T48.3X4	T48.3X5	T48.3X6
Ronifibrate	T46.6X1	T46.6X2	T46.6X3	T46.6X4	T46.6X5	T46.6X6
Rosaprostol	T47.1X1	T47.1X2	T47.1X3	T47.1X4	T47.1X5	T47.1X6
Rose bengal sodium (131I)	T50.8X1	T50.8X2	T50.8X3	T50.8X4	T50.8X5	T50.8X6
Rose water ointment	T49.3X1	T49.3X2	T49.3X3	T49.3X4	T49.3X5	T49.3X6
Rosoxacin	T37.8X1	T37.8X2	T37.8X3	T37.8X4	T37.8X5	T37.8X6
Rotenone	T60.2X1	T60.2X2	T60.2X3	T60.2X4	—	—
Rotoxamine	T45.0X1	T45.0X2	T45.0X3	T45.0X4	T45.0X5	T45.0X6
Rough-on-rats	T60.4X1	T60.4X2	T60.4X3	T60.4X4	—	—
Roxatidine	T47.0X1	T47.0X2	T47.0X3	T47.0X4	T47.0X5	T47.0X6
Roxithromycin	T36.3X1	T36.3X2	T36.3X3	T36.3X4	T36.3X5	T36.3X6
Rt-PA	T45.611	T45.612	T45.613	T45.614	T45.615	T45.616
Rubbing alcohol	T51.2X1	T51.2X2	T51.2X3	T51.2X4		
Rubefacient	T49.4X1	T49.4X2	T49.4X3	T49.4X4	T49.4X5	T49.4X6
Rubella vaccine	T50.B91	T50.B92	T50.B93	T50.B94	T50.B95	T50.B96
Rubeola vaccine	T50.B91	T50.B92	T50.B93	T50.B94	T50.B95	T50.B96
Rubidium chloride Rb82	T50.8X1	T50.8X2	T50.8X3	T50.8X4	T50.8X5	T50.8X6
Rubidomycin	T45.1X1	T45.1X2	T45.1X3	T45.1X4	T45.1X5	T45.1X6
Rue	T62.2X1	T62.2X2	T62.2X3	T62.2X4	—	—
Rufocromomycin	T45.1X1	T45.1X2	T45.1X3	T45.1X4	T45.1X5	T45.1X6
Russel's viper venin	T45.7X1	T45.7X2	T45.7X3	T45.7X4	T45.7X5	T45.7X6
Ruta (graveolens)	T62.2X1	T62.2X2	T62.2X3	T62.2X4	—	—
Rutinum	T46.991	T46.992	T46.993	T46.994	T46.995	T46.996
Rutoside	T46.991	T46.992	T46.993	T46.994	T46.995	T46.996
b-sitosterol(s)	T46.6X1	T46.6X2	T46.6X3	T46.6X4	T46.6X5	T46.6X6
Sabadilla (plant)	T62.2X1	T62.2X2	T62.2X3	T62.2X4	—	—
pesticide	T60.2X1	T60.2X2	T60.2X3	T60.2X4	—	—
Saccharated iron oxide	T45.8X1	T45.8X2	T45.8X3	T45.8X4	T45.8X5	T45.8X6
Saccharin	T50.901	T50.902	T50.903	T50.904	T50.905	T50.906
Saccharomyces boulardii	T47.6X1	T47.6X2	T47.6X3	T47.6X4	T47.6X5	T47.6X6
Safflower oil	T46.6X1	T46.6X2	T46.6X3	T46.6X4	T46.6X5	T46.6X6
Safrazine	T43.1X1	T43.1X2	T43.1X3	T43.1X4	T43.1X5	T43.1X6
Salazosulfapyridine	T37.0X1	T37.0X2	T37.0X3	T37.0X4	T37.0X5	T37.0X6

Table of Drugs and Chemicals

Pyrogallic acid — Salazosulfapyridine

Substance	Poisoning, Accidental (unintentional)	Poisoning, Intentional Self-harm	Poisoning, Assault	Poisoning, Undetermined	Adverse Effect	Under-dosing
Salbutamol	T48.6X1	T48.6X2	T48.6X3	T48.6X4	T48.6X5	T48.6X6
Salicylamide	T39.091	T39.092	T39.093	T39.094	T39.095	T39.096
Salicylate NEC	T39.091	T39.092	T39.093	T39.094	T39.095	T39.096
methyl	T49.3X1	T49.3X2	T49.3X3	T49.3X4	T49.3X5	T49.3X6
theobromine calcium	T50.2X1	T50.2X2	T50.2X3	T50.2X4	T50.2X5	T50.2X6
Salicylazosulfapyridine	T37.0X1	T37.0X2	T37.0X3	T37.0X4	T37.0X5	T37.0X6
Salicylhydroxamic acid	T49.0X1	T49.0X2	T49.0X3	T49.0X4	T49.0X5	T49.0X6
Salicylic acid	T49.4X1	T49.4X2	T49.4X3	T49.4X4	T49.4X5	T49.4X6
with benzoic acid	T49.4X1	T49.4X2	T49.4X3	T49.4X4	T49.4X5	T49.4X6
congeners	T39.091	T39.092	T39.093	T39.094	T39.095	T39.096
derivative	T39.091	T39.092	T39.093	T39.094	T39.095	T39.096
salts	T39.091	T39.092	T39.093	T39.094	T39.095	T39.096
Salinazid	T37.1X1	T37.1X2	T37.1X3	T37.1X4	T37.1X5	T37.1X6
Salmeterol	T48.6X1	T48.6X2	T48.6X3	T48.6X4	T48.6X5	T48.6X6
Salol	T49.3X1	T49.3X2	T49.3X3	T49.3X4	T49.3X5	T49.3X6
Salsalate	T39.091	T39.092	T39.093	T39.094	T39.095	T39.096
Salt-replacing drug	T50.901	T50.902	T50.903	T50.904	T50.905	T50.906
Salt-retaining mineralocorticoid	T50.0X1	T50.0X2	T50.0X3	T50.0X4	T50.0X5	T50.0X6
Salt substitute	T50.901	T50.902	T50.903	T50.904	T50.905	T50.906
Saluretic NEC	T50.2X1	T50.2X2	T50.2X3	T50.2X4	T50.2X5	T50.2X6
Saluron	T50.2X1	T50.2X2	T50.2X3	T50.2X4	T50.2X5	T50.2X6
Salvarsan 606 (neosilver) (silver)	T37.8X1	T37.8X2	T37.8X3	T37.8X4	T37.8X5	T37.8X6
Sambucus canadensis	T62.2X1	T62.2X2	T62.2X3	T62.2X4	—	—
berry	T62.1X1	T62.1X2	T62.1X3	T62.1X4	—	—
Sandril	T46.5X1	T46.5X2	T46.5X3	T46.5X4	T46.5X5	T46.5X6
Sanguinaria canadensis	T62.2X1	T62.2X2	T62.2X3	T62.2X4	—	—
Saniflush (cleaner)	T54.2X1	T54.2X2	T54.2X3	T54.2X4	—	—
Santonin	T37.4X1	T37.4X2	T37.4X3	T37.4X4	T37.4X5	T37.4X6
Santyl	T49.8X1	T49.8X2	T49.8X3	T49.8X4	T49.8X5	T49.8X6
Saralasin	T46.5X1	T46.5X2	T46.5X3	T46.5X4	T46.5X5	T46.5X6
Sarcolysin	T45.1X1	T45.1X2	T45.1X3	T45.1X4	T45.1X5	T45.1X6
Sarkomycin	T45.1X1	T45.1X2	T45.1X3	T45.1X4	T45.1X5	T45.1X6
Saroten	T43.011	T43.012	T43.013	T43.014	T43.015	T43.016
Saturnine — see Lead						
Savin (oil)	T49.4X1	T49.4X2	T49.4X3	T49.4X4	T49.4X5	T49.4X6
Scammony	T47.2X1	T47.2X2	T47.2X3	T47.2X4	T47.2X5	T47.2X6
Scarlet red	T49.8X1	T49.8X2	T49.8X3	T49.8X4	T49.8X5	T49.8X6
Scheele's green	T57.0X1	T57.0X2	T57.0X3	T57.0X4	—	—
insecticide	T57.0X1	T57.0X2	T57.0X3	T57.0X4	—	—
Schizontozide (blood) (tissue)	T37.2X1	T37.2X2	T37.2X3	T37.2X4	T37.2X5	T37.2X6
Schradan	T60.0X1	T60.0X2	T60.0X3	T60.0X4	—	—
Schweinfurth green	T57.0X1	T57.0X2	T57.0X3	T57.0X4	—	—
insecticide	T57.0X1	T57.0X2	T57.0X3	T57.0X4	—	—
Scilla, rat poison	T60.4X1	T60.4X2	T60.4X3	T60.4X4	—	—
Scillaren	T60.4X1	T60.4X2	T60.4X3	T60.4X4	—	—
Sclerosing agent	T46.8X1	T46.8X2	T46.8X3	T46.8X4	T46.8X5	T46.8X6
Scombrotoxin	T61.11	T61.12	T61.13	T61.14		
Scopolamine	T44.3X1	T44.3X2	T44.3X3	T44.3X4	T44.3X5	T44.3X6
Scopolia extract	T44.3X1	T44.3X2	T44.3X3	T44.3X4	T44.3X5	T44.3X6
Scouring powder	T65.891	T65.892	T65.893	T65.894	—	—
Sea						
anemone (sting)	T63.631	T63.632	T63.633	T63.634	—	—
cucumber (sting)	T63.691	T63.692	T63.693	T63.694	—	—
snake (bite) (venom)	T63.091	T63.092	T63.093	T63.094	—	—
urchin spine (puncture)	T63.691	T63.692	T63.693	T63.694	—	—
Seafood	T61.91	T61.92	T61.93	T61.94	—	—
specified NEC	T61.8X1	T61.8X2	T61.8X3	T61.8X4	—	—
Secbutabarbital	T42.3X1	T42.3X2	T42.3X3	T42.3X4	T42.3X5	T42.3X6
Secbutabarbitone	T42.3X1	T42.3X2	T42.3X3	T42.3X4	T42.3X5	T42.3X6
Secnidazole	T37.3X1	T37.3X2	T37.3X3	T37.3X4	T37.3X5	T37.3X6
Secobarbital	T42.3X1	T42.3X2	T42.3X3	T42.3X4	T42.3X5	T42.3X6
Seconal	T42.3X1	T42.3X2	T42.3X3	T42.3X4	T42.3X5	T42.3X6
Secretin	T50.8X1	T50.8X2	T50.8X3	T50.8X4	T50.8X5	T50.8X6
Sedative NEC	T42.71	T42.72	T42.73	T42.74	T42.75	T42.76
mixed NEC	T42.6X1	T42.6X2	T42.6X3	T42.6X4	T42.6X5	T42.6X6
Sedormid	T42.6X1	T42.6X2	T42.6X3	T42.6X4	T42.6X5	T42.6X6
Seed disinfectant or dressing	T60.8X1	T60.8X2	T60.8X3	T60.8X4	—	—
Seeds (poisonous)	T62.2X1	T62.2X2	T62.2X3	T62.2X4	—	—
Selegiline	T42.8X1	T42.8X2	T42.8X3	T42.8X4	T42.8X5	T42.8X6
Selenium NEC	T56.891	T56.892	T56.893	T56.894	—	—
disulfide or sulfide	T49.4X1	T49.4X2	T49.4X3	T49.4X4	T49.4X5	T49.4X6
fumes	T59.891	T59.892	T59.893	T59.894	—	—
sulfide	T49.4X1	T49.4X2	T49.4X3	T49.4X4	T49.4X5	T49.4X6
Selenomethionine (75Se)	T50.8X1	T50.8X2	T50.8X3	T50.8X4	T50.8X5	T50.8X6
Selsun	T49.4X1	T49.4X2	T49.4X3	T49.4X4	T49.4X5	T49.4X6
Semustine	T45.1X1	T45.1X2	T45.1X3	T45.1X4	T45.1X5	T45.1X6
Senega syrup	T48.4X1	T48.4X2	T48.4X3	T48.4X4	T48.4X5	T48.4X6
Senna	T47.2X1	T47.2X2	T47.2X3	T47.2X4	T47.2X5	T47.2X6
Sennoside A+B	T47.2X1	T47.2X2	T47.2X3	T47.2X4	T47.2X5	T47.2X6
Septisol	T49.2X1	T49.2X2	T49.2X3	T49.2X4	T49.2X5	T49.2X6
Seractide	T38.811	T38.812	T38.813	T38.814	T38.815	T38.816
Serax	T42.4X1	T42.4X2	T42.4X3	T42.4X4	T42.4X5	T42.4X6
Serenesil	T42.6X1	T42.6X2	T42.6X3	T42.6X4	T42.6X5	T42.6X6
Serenium (hydrochloride)	T37.91	T37.92	T37.93	T37.94	T37.95	T37.96
Serepax — see Oxazepam						
Sermorelin	T38.891	T38.892	T38.893	T38.894	T38.895	T38.896
Sernyl	T41.1X1	T41.1X2	T41.1X3	T41.1X4	T41.1X5	T41.1X6
Serotonin	T50.991	T50.992	T50.993	T50.994	T50.995	T50.996
Serpasil	T46.5X1	T46.5X2	T46.5X3	T46.5X4	T46.5X5	T46.5X6
Serrapeptase	T45.3X1	T45.3X2	T45.3X3	T45.3X4	T45.3X5	T45.3X6
Serum						
antibotulinus	T50.Z11	T50.Z12	T50.Z13	T50.Z14	T50.Z15	T50.Z16
anticytotoxic	T50.Z11	T50.Z12	T50.Z13	T50.Z14	T50.Z15	T50.Z16
antidiphtheria	T50.Z11	T50.Z12	T50.Z13	T50.Z14	T50.Z15	T50.Z16
antimeningococcus	T50.Z11	T50.Z12	T50.Z13	T50.Z14	T50.Z15	T50.Z16
anti-Rh	T50.Z11	T50.Z12	T50.Z13	T50.Z14	T50.Z15	T50.Z16
anti-snake-bite	T50.Z11	T50.Z12	T50.Z13	T50.Z14	T50.Z15	T50.Z16
antitetanic	T50.Z11	T50.Z12	T50.Z13	T50.Z14	T50.Z15	T50.Z16
antitoxic	T50.Z11	T50.Z12	T50.Z13	T50.Z14	T50.Z15	T50.Z16
complement (inhibitor)	T45.8X1	T45.8X2	T45.8X3	T45.8X4	T45.8X5	T45.8X6
convalescent	T50.Z11	T50.Z12	T50.Z13	T50.Z14	T50.Z15	T50.Z16
hemolytic complement	T45.8X1	T45.8X2	T45.8X3	T45.8X4	T45.8X5	T45.8X6
immune (human)	T50.Z11	T50.Z12	T50.Z13	T50.Z14	T50.Z15	T50.Z16
protective NEC	T50.Z11	T50.Z12	T50.Z13	T50.Z14	T50.Z15	T50.Z16
Setastine	T45.0X1	T45.0X2	T45.0X3	T45.0X4	T45.0X5	T45.0X6
Setoperone	T43.591	T43.592	T43.593	T43.594	T43.595	T43.596
Sewer gas	T59.91	T59.92	T59.93	T59.94	—	—
Shampoo	T55.0X1	T55.0X2	T55.0X3	T55.0X4	—	—
Shellfish, noxious, nonbacterial	T61.781	T61.782	T61.783	T61.784	—	—
Sildenafil	T46.7X1	T46.7X2	T46.7X3	T46.7X4	T46.7X5	T46.7X6
Silibinin	T50.991	T50.992	T50.993	T50.994	T50.995	T50.996
Silicone NEC	T65.891	T65.892	T65.893	T65.894	—	—
medicinal	T49.3X1	T49.3X2	T49.3X3	T49.3X4	T49.3X5	T49.3X6
Silvadene	T49.0X1	T49.0X2	T49.0X3	T49.0X4	T49.0X5	T49.0X6
Silver	T49.0X1	T49.0X2	T49.0X3	T49.0X4	T49.0X5	T49.0X6
anti-infectives	T49.0X1	T49.0X2	T49.0X3	T49.0X4	T49.0X5	T49.0X6
arsphenamine	T37.8X1	T37.8X2	T37.8X3	T37.8X4	T37.8X5	T37.8X6
colloidal	T49.0X1	T49.0X2	T49.0X3	T49.0X4	T49.0X5	T49.0X6
nitrate	T49.0X1	T49.0X2	T49.0X3	T49.0X4	T49.0X5	T49.0X6
ophthalmic preparation	T49.5X1	T49.5X2	T49.5X3	T49.5X4	T49.5X5	T49.5X6
toughened (keratolytic)	T49.4X1	T49.4X2	T49.4X3	T49.4X4	T49.4X5	T49.4X6
nonmedicinal (dust)	T56.891	T56.892	T56.893	T56.894	—	—
protein	T49.5X1	T49.5X2	T49.5X3	T49.5X4	T49.5X5	T49.5X6
salvarsan	T37.8X1	T37.8X2	T37.8X3	T37.8X4	T37.8X5	T37.8X6
sulfadiazine	T49.4X1	T49.4X2	T49.4X3	T49.4X4	T49.4X5	T49.4X6
Silymarin	T50.991	T50.992	T50.993	T50.994	T50.995	T50.996
Simaldrate	T47.1X1	T47.1X2	T47.1X3	T47.1X4	T47.1X5	T47.1X6
Simazine	T60.3X1	T60.3X2	T60.3X3	T60.3X4	—	—
Simethicone	T47.1X1	T47.1X2	T47.1X3	T47.1X4	T47.1X5	T47.1X6
Simfibrate	T46.6X1	T46.6X2	T46.6X3	T46.6X4	T46.6X5	T46.6X6
Simvastatin	T46.6X1	T46.6X2	T46.6X3	T46.6X4	T46.6X5	T46.6X6
Sincalide	T50.8X1	T50.8X2	T50.8X3	T50.8X4	T50.8X5	T50.8X6
Sinequan	T43.011	T43.012	T43.013	T43.014	T43.015	T43.016
Singoserp	T46.5X1	T46.5X2	T46.5X3	T46.5X4	T46.5X5	T46.5X6
Sintrom	T45.511	T45.512	T45.513	T45.514	T45.515	T45.516
Sisomicin	T36.5X1	T36.5X2	T36.5X3	T36.5X4	T36.5X5	T36.5X6
Sitosterols	T46.6X1	T46.6X2	T46.6X3	T46.6X4	T46.6X5	T46.6X6
Skeletal muscle relaxants	T48.1X1	T48.1X2	T48.1X3	T48.1X4	T48.1X5	T48.1X6
Skin						
agents (external)	T49.91	T49.92	T49.93	T49.94	T49.95	T49.96
specified NEC	T49.8X1	T49.8X2	T49.8X3	T49.8X4	T49.8X5	T49.8X6
test antigen	T50.8X1	T50.8X2	T50.8X3	T50.8X4	T50.8X5	T50.8X6
Sleep-eze	T45.0X1	T45.0X2	T45.0X3	T45.0X4	T45.0X5	T45.0X6
Sleeping draught, pill	T42.71	T42.72	T42.73	T42.74	T42.75	T42.76
Smallpox vaccine	T50.B11	T50.B12	T50.B13	T50.B14	T50.B15	T50.B16
Smelter fumes NEC	T56.91	T56.92	T56.93	T56.94	—	—
Smog	T59.1X1	T59.1X2	T59.1X3	T59.1X4	—	—
Smoke NEC	T59.811	T59.812	T59.813	T59.814	—	—
Smooth muscle relaxant	T44.3X1	T44.3X2	T44.3X3	T44.3X4	T44.3X5	T44.3X6
Snail killer NEC	T60.8X1	T60.8X2	T60.8X3	T60.8X4	—	—
Snake venom or bite	T63.001	T63.002	T63.003	T63.004	—	—
hemocoagulase	T45.7X1	T45.7X2	T45.7X3	T45.7X4	T45.7X5	T45.7X6
Snuff	T65.211	T65.212	T65.213	T65.214	—	—
Soap (powder) (product)	T55.0X1	T55.0X2	T55.0X3	T55.0X4	—	—
enema	T47.4X1	T47.4X2	T47.4X3	T47.4X4	T47.4X5	T47.4X6
medicinal, soft	T49.2X1	T49.2X2	T49.2X3	T49.2X4	T49.2X5	T49.2X6
superfatted	T49.2X1	T49.2X2	T49.2X3	T49.2X4	T49.2X5	T49.2X6
Sobrerol	T48.4X1	T48.4X2	T48.4X3	T48.4X4	T48.4X5	T48.4X6
Soda (caustic)	T54.3X1	T54.3X2	T54.3X3	T54.3X4	—	—
bicarb	T47.1X1	T47.1X2	T47.1X3	T47.1X4	T47.1X5	T47.1X6

388

Additional Character May Be Required — Refer to the Tabular List for Character Selection ▽ Subterms under main terms may continue to next column or page

Substance	Poisoning, Accidental (unintentional)	Poisoning, Intentional Self-harm	Poisoning, Assault	Poisoning, Undetermined	Adverse Effect	Under-dosing
Soda — *continued*						
chlorinated — *see* Sodium, hypochlorite						
Sodium						
acetosulfone	T37.1X1	T37.1X2	T37.1X3	T37.1X4	T37.1X5	T37.1X6
acetrizoate	T50.8X1	T50.8X2	T50.8X3	T50.8X4	T50.8X5	T50.8X6
acid phosphate	T50.3X1	T50.3X2	T50.3X3	T50.3X4	T50.3X5	T50.3X6
alginate	T47.8X1	T47.8X2	T47.8X3	T47.8X4	T47.8X5	T47.8X6
amidotrizoate	T50.8X1	T50.8X2	T50.8X3	T50.8X4	T50.8X5	T50.8X6
aminopterin	T45.1X1	T45.1X2	T45.1X3	T45.1X4	T45.1X5	T45.1X6
amylosulfate	T47.8X1	T47.8X2	T47.8X3	T47.8X4	T47.8X5	T47.8X6
amytal	T42.3X1	T42.3X2	T42.3X3	T42.3X4	T42.3X5	T42.3X6
antimony gluconate	T37.3X1	T37.3X2	T37.3X3	T37.3X4	T37.3X5	T37.3X6
arsenate	T57.0X1	T57.0X2	T57.0X3	T57.0X4	—	—
aurothiomalate	T39.4X1	T39.4X2	T39.4X3	T39.4X4	T39.4X5	T39.4X6
aurothiosulfate	T39.4X1	T39.4X2	T39.4X3	T39.4X4	T39.4X5	T39.4X6
barbiturate	T42.3X1	T42.3X2	T42.3X3	T42.3X4	T42.3X5	T42.3X6
basic phosphate	T47.4X1	T47.4X2	T47.4X3	T47.4X4	T47.4X5	T47.4X6
bicarbonate	T47.1X1	T47.1X2	T47.1X3	T47.1X4	T47.1X5	T47.1X6
bichromate	T57.8X1	T57.8X2	T57.8X3	T57.8X4	—	—
biphosphate	T50.3X1	T50.3X2	T50.3X3	T50.3X4	T50.3X5	T50.3X6
bisulfate	T65.891	T65.892	T65.893	T65.894	—	—
borate						
cleanser	T57.8X1	T57.8X2	T57.8X3	T57.8X4	—	—
eye	T49.5X1	T49.5X2	T49.5X3	T49.5X4	T49.5X5	T49.5X6
therapeutic	T49.8X1	T49.8X2	T49.8X3	T49.8X4	T49.8X5	T49.8X6
bromide	T42.6X1	T42.6X2	T42.6X3	T42.6X4	T42.6X5	T42.6X6
cacodylate (nonmedicinal) NEC	T50.8X1	T50.8X2	T50.8X3	T50.8X4	T50.8X5	T50.8X6
anti-infective	T37.8X1	T37.8X2	T37.8X3	T37.8X4	T37.8X5	T37.8X6
herbicide	T60.3X1	T60.3X2	T60.3X3	T60.3X4	—	—
calcium edetate	T45.8X1	T45.8X2	T45.8X3	T45.8X4	T45.8X5	T45.8X6
carbonate NEC	T54.3X1	T54.3X2	T54.3X3	T54.3X4	—	—
chlorate NEC	T65.891	T65.892	T65.893	T65.894	—	—
herbicide	T54.91	T54.92	T54.93	T54.94	—	—
chloride	T50.3X1	T50.3X2	T50.3X3	T50.3X4	T50.3X5	T50.3X6
with glucose	T50.3X1	T50.3X2	T50.3X3	T50.3X4	T50.3X5	T50.3X6
chromate	T65.891	T65.892	T65.893	T65.894	—	—
citrate	T50.991	T50.992	T50.993	T50.994	T50.995	T50.996
cromoglicate	T48.6X1	T48.6X2	T48.6X3	T48.6X4	T48.6X5	T48.6X6
cyanide	T65.0X1	T65.0X2	T65.0X3	T65.0X4	—	—
cyclamate	T50.3X1	T50.3X2	T50.3X3	T50.3X4	T50.3X5	T50.3X6
dehydrocholate	T45.8X1	T45.8X2	T45.8X3	T45.8X4	T45.8X5	T45.8X6
diatrizoate	T50.8X1	T50.8X2	T50.8X3	T50.8X4	T50.8X5	T50.8X6
dibunate	T48.4X1	T48.4X2	T48.4X3	T48.4X4	T48.4X5	T48.4X6
dioctyl sulfosuccinate	T47.4X1	T47.4X2	T47.4X3	T47.4X4	T47.4X5	T47.4X6
dipantoyl ferrate	T45.8X1	T45.8X2	T45.8X3	T45.8X4	T45.8X5	T45.8X6
edetate	T45.8X1	T45.8X2	T45.8X3	T45.8X4	T45.8X5	T45.8X6
ethacrynate	T50.1X1	T50.1X2	T50.1X3	T50.1X4	T50.1X5	T50.1X6
feredetate	T45.8X1	T45.8X2	T45.8X3	T45.8X4	T45.8X5	T45.8X6
Fluoride — *see* Fluoride						
fluoroacetate (dust) (pesticide)	T60.4X1	T60.4X2	T60.4X3	T60.4X4	—	—
free salt	T50.3X1	T50.3X2	T50.3X3	T50.3X4	T50.3X5	T50.3X6
fusidate	T36.8X1	T36.8X2	T36.8X3	T36.8X4	T36.8X5	T36.8X6
glucaldrate	T47.1X1	T47.1X2	T47.1X3	T47.1X4	T47.1X5	T47.1X6
glucosulfone	T37.1X1	T37.1X2	T37.1X3	T37.1X4	T37.1X5	T37.1X6
glutamate	T45.8X1	T45.8X2	T45.8X3	T45.8X4	T45.8X5	T45.8X6
hydrogen carbonate	T50.3X1	T50.3X2	T50.3X3	T50.3X4	T50.3X5	T50.3X6
hydroxide	T54.3X1	T54.3X2	T54.3X3	T54.3X4	—	—
hypochlorite (bleach) NEC	T54.3X1	T54.3X2	T54.3X3	T54.3X4	—	—
disinfectant	T54.3X1	T54.3X2	T54.3X3	T54.3X4	—	—
medicinal (anti-infective) (external)	T49.0X1	T49.0X2	T49.0X3	T49.0X4	T49.0X5	T49.0X6
vapor	T54.3X1	T54.3X2	T54.3X3	T54.3X4	—	—
hyposulfite	T49.0X1	T49.0X2	T49.0X3	T49.0X4	T49.0X5	T49.0X6
indigotin disulfonate	T50.8X1	T50.8X2	T50.8X3	T50.8X4	T50.8X5	T50.8X6
iodide	T50.991	T50.992	T50.993	T50.994	T50.995	T50.996
I-131	T50.8X1	T50.8X2	T50.8X3	T50.8X4	T50.8X5	T50.8X6
therapeutic	T38.2X1	T38.2X2	T38.2X3	T38.2X4	T38.2X5	T38.2X6
iodohippurate (131I)	T50.8X1	T50.8X2	T50.8X3	T50.8X4	T50.8X5	T50.8X6
iopodate	T50.8X1	T50.8X2	T50.8X3	T50.8X4	T50.8X5	T50.8X6
iothalamate	T50.8X1	T50.8X2	T50.8X3	T50.8X4	T50.8X5	T50.8X6
iron edetate	T45.4X1	T45.4X2	T45.4X3	T45.4X4	T45.4X5	T45.4X6
lactate (compound solution)	T45.8X1	T45.8X2	T45.8X3	T45.8X4	T45.8X5	T45.8X6
lauryl (sulfate)	T49.2X1	T49.2X2	T49.2X3	T49.2X4	T49.2X5	T49.2X6
L-triiodothyronine	T38.1X1	T38.1X2	T38.1X3	T38.1X4	T38.1X5	T38.1X6
magnesium citrate	T50.991	T50.992	T50.993	T50.994	T50.995	T50.996
mersalate	T50.2X1	T50.2X2	T50.2X3	T50.2X4	T50.2X5	T50.2X6
metasilicate	T65.891	T65.892	T65.893	T65.894	—	—
metrizoate	T50.8X1	T50.8X2	T50.8X3	T50.8X4	T50.8X5	T50.8X6
Sodium — *continued*						
monofluoroacetate (pesticide)	T60.1X1	T60.1X2	T60.1X3	T60.1X4	—	—
morrhuate	T46.8X1	T46.8X2	T46.8X3	T46.8X4	T46.8X5	T46.8X6
nafcillin	T36.0X1	T36.0X2	T36.0X3	T36.0X4	T36.0X5	T36.0X6
nitrate (oxidizing agent)	T65.891	T65.892	T65.893	T65.894	—	—
nitrite	T50.6X1	T50.6X2	T50.6X3	T50.6X4	T50.6X5	T50.6X6
nitroferricyanide	T46.5X1	T46.5X2	T46.5X3	T46.5X4	T46.5X5	T46.5X6
nitroprusside	T46.5X1	T46.5X2	T46.5X3	T46.5X4	T46.5X5	T46.5X6
oxalate	T65.891	T65.892	T65.893	T65.894	—	—
oxide/peroxide	T65.891	T65.892	T65.893	T65.894	—	—
oxybate	T41.291	T41.292	T41.293	T41.294	T41.295	T41.296
para-aminohippurate	T50.8X1	T50.8X2	T50.8X3	T50.8X4	T50.8X5	T50.8X6
perborate (nonmedicinal) NEC	T65.891	T65.892	T65.893	T65.894	—	—
medicinal	T49.0X1	T49.0X2	T49.0X3	T49.0X4	T49.0X5	T49.0X6
soap	T55.0X1	T55.0X2	T55.0X3	T55.0X4	—	—
percarbonate — *see* Sodium, perborate						
pertechnetate Tc99m	T50.8X1	T50.8X2	T50.8X3	T50.8X4	T50.8X5	T50.8X6
phosphate						
cellulose	T45.8X1	T45.8X2	T45.8X3	T45.8X4	T45.8X5	T45.8X6
dibasic	T47.2X1	T47.2X2	T47.2X3	T47.2X4	T47.2X5	T47.2X6
monobasic	T47.2X1	T47.2X2	T47.2X3	T47.2X4	T47.2X5	T47.2X6
phytate	T50.6X1	T50.6X2	T50.6X3	T50.6X4	T50.6X5	T50.6X6
picosulfate	T47.2X1	T47.2X2	T47.2X3	T47.2X4	T47.2X5	T47.2X6
polyhydroxyaluminium monocarbonate	T47.1X1	T47.1X2	T47.1X3	T47.1X4	T47.1X5	T47.1X6
polystyrene sulfonate	T50.3X1	T50.3X2	T50.3X3	T50.3X4	T50.3X5	T50.3X6
propionate	T49.0X1	T49.0X2	T49.0X3	T49.0X4	T49.0X5	T49.0X6
propyl hydroxybenzoate	T50.991	T50.992	T50.993	T50.994	T50.995	T50.996
psylliate	T46.8X1	T46.8X2	T46.8X3	T46.8X4	T46.8X5	T46.8X6
removing resins	T50.3X1	T50.3X2	T50.3X3	T50.3X4	T50.3X5	T50.3X6
salicylate	T39.091	T39.092	T39.093	T39.094	T39.095	T39.096
salt NEC	T50.3X1	T50.3X2	T50.3X3	T50.3X4	T50.3X5	T50.3X6
selenate	T60.2X1	T60.2X2	T60.2X3	T60.2X4	—	—
stibogluconate	T37.3X1	T37.3X2	T37.3X3	T37.3X4	T37.3X5	T37.3X6
sulfate	T47.4X1	T47.4X2	T47.4X3	T47.4X4	T47.4X5	T47.4X6
sulfoxone	T37.1X1	T37.1X2	T37.1X3	T37.1X4	T37.1X5	T37.1X6
tetradecyl sulfate	T46.8X1	T46.8X2	T46.8X3	T46.8X4	T46.8X5	T46.8X6
thiopental	T41.1X1	T41.1X2	T41.1X3	T41.1X4	T41.1X5	T41.1X6
thiosalicylate	T39.091	T39.092	T39.093	T39.094	T39.095	T39.096
thiosulfate	T50.6X1	T50.6X2	T50.6X3	T50.6X4	T50.6X5	T50.6X6
tolbutamide	T38.3X1	T38.3X2	T38.3X3	T38.3X4	T38.3X5	T38.3X6
(L)-triiodothyronine	T38.1X1	T38.1X2	T38.1X3	T38.1X4	T38.1X5	T38.1X6
tyropanoate	T50.8X1	T50.8X2	T50.8X3	T50.8X4	T50.8X5	T50.8X6
valproate	T42.6X1	T42.6X2	T42.6X3	T42.6X4	T42.6X5	T42.6X6
versenate	T50.6X1	T50.6X2	T50.6X3	T50.6X4	T50.6X5	T50.6X6
Sodium-free salt	T50.901	T50.902	T50.903	T50.904	T50.905	T50.906
Sodium-removing resin	T50.3X1	T50.3X2	T50.3X3	T50.3X4	T50.3X5	T50.3X6
Soft soap	T55.0X1	T55.0X2	T55.0X3	T55.0X4	—	—
Solanine	T62.2X1	T62.2X2	T62.2X3	T62.2X4	—	—
berries	T62.1X1	T62.1X2	T62.1X3	T62.1X4	—	—
Solanum dulcamara	T62.2X1	T62.2X2	T62.2X3	T62.2X4	—	—
berries	T62.1X1	T62.1X2	T62.1X3	T62.1X4	—	—
Solapsone	T37.1X1	T37.1X2	T37.1X3	T37.1X4	T37.1X5	T37.1X6
Solar lotion	T49.3X1	T49.3X2	T49.3X3	T49.3X4	T49.3X5	T49.3X6
Solasulfone	T37.1X1	T37.1X2	T37.1X3	T37.1X4	T37.1X5	T37.1X6
Soldering fluid	T65.891	T65.892	T65.893	T65.894	—	—
Solid substance	T65.91	T65.92	T65.93	T65.94	—	—
specified NEC	T65.891	T65.892	T65.893	T65.894	—	—
Solvent, industrial NEC	T52.91	T52.92	T52.93	T52.94	—	—
naphtha	T52.0X1	T52.0X2	T52.0X3	T52.0X4	—	—
petroleum	T52.0X1	T52.0X2	T52.0X3	T52.0X4	—	—
specified NEC	T52.8X1	T52.8X2	T52.8X3	T52.8X4	—	—
Soma	T42.8X1	T42.8X2	T42.8X3	T42.8X4	T42.8X5	T42.8X6
Somatorelin	T38.891	T38.892	T38.893	T38.894	T38.895	T38.896
Somatostatin	T38.991	T38.992	T38.993	T38.994	T38.995	T38.996
Somatotropin	T38.811	T38.812	T38.813	T38.814	T38.815	T38.816
Somatrem	T38.811	T38.812	T38.813	T38.814	T38.815	T38.816
Somatropin	T38.811	T38.812	T38.813	T38.814	T38.815	T38.816
Sominex	T45.0X1	T45.0X2	T45.0X3	T45.0X4	T45.0X5	T45.0X6
Somnos	T42.6X1	T42.6X2	T42.6X3	T42.6X4	T42.6X5	T42.6X6
Somonal	T42.3X1	T42.3X2	T42.3X3	T42.3X4	T42.3X5	T42.3X6
Soneryl	T42.3X1	T42.3X2	T42.3X3	T42.3X4	T42.3X5	T42.3X6
Soothing syrup	T50.901	T50.902	T50.903	T50.904	T50.905	T50.906
Sopor	T42.6X1	T42.6X2	T42.6X3	T42.6X4	T42.6X5	T42.6X6
Soporific	T42.71	T42.72	T42.73	T42.74	T42.75	T42.76
Soporific drug	T42.71	T42.72	T42.73	T42.74	T42.75	T42.76
specified type NEC	T42.6X1	T42.6X2	T42.6X3	T42.6X4	T42.6X5	T42.6X6
Sorbide nitrate	T46.3X1	T46.3X2	T46.3X3	T46.3X4	T46.3X5	T46.3X6
Sorbitol	T47.4X1	T47.4X2	T47.4X3	T47.4X4	T47.4X5	T47.4X6
Sotalol	T44.7X1	T44.7X2	T44.7X3	T44.7X4	T44.7X5	T44.7X6

☞ Subterms under main terms may continue to next column or page   Additional Character May Be Required — Refer to the Tabular List for Character Selection   389

Soda — Sotalol

Substance	Poisoning, Accidental (unintentional)	Poisoning, Intentional Self-harm	Poisoning, Assault	Poisoning, Undetermined	Adverse Effect	Under-dosing
Sotradecol	T46.8X1	T46.8X2	T46.8X3	T46.8X4	T46.8X5	T46.8X6
Soysterol	T46.6X1	T46.6X2	T46.6X3	T46.6X4	T46.6X5	T46.6X6
Spacoline	T44.3X1	T44.3X2	T44.3X3	T44.3X4	T44.3X5	T44.3X6
Spanish fly	T49.8X1	T49.8X2	T49.8X3	T49.8X4	T49.8X5	T49.8X6
Sparine	T43.3X1	T43.3X2	T43.3X3	T43.3X4	T43.3X5	T43.3X6
Sparteine	T48.0X1	T48.0X2	T48.0X3	T48.0X4	T48.0X5	T48.0X6
Spasmolytic						
anticholinergics	T44.3X1	T44.3X2	T44.3X3	T44.3X4	T44.3X5	T44.3X6
autonomic	T44.3X1	T44.3X2	T44.3X3	T44.3X4	T44.3X5	T44.3X6
bronchial NEC	T48.6X1	T48.6X2	T48.6X3	T48.6X4	T48.6X5	T48.6X6
quaternary ammonium	T44.3X1	T44.3X2	T44.3X3	T44.3X4	T44.3X5	T44.3X6
skeletal muscle NEC	T48.1X1	T48.1X2	T48.1X3	T48.1X4	T48.1X5	T48.1X6
Spectinomycin	T36.5X1	T36.5X2	T36.5X3	T36.5X4	T36.5X5	T36.5X6
Speed	T43.621	T43.622	T43.623	T43.624	T43.625	T43.626
Spermicide	T49.8X1	T49.8X2	T49.8X3	T49.8X4	T49.8X5	T49.8X6
Spider (bite) (venom)	T63.391	T63.392	T63.393	T63.394	—	—
antivenin	T50.Z11	T50.Z12	T50.Z13	T50.Z14	T50.Z15	T50.Z16
Spigelia (root)	T37.4X1	T37.4X2	T37.4X3	T37.4X4	T37.4X5	T37.4X6
Spindle inactivator	T50.4X1	T50.4X2	T50.4X3	T50.4X4	T50.4X5	T50.4X6
Spiperone	T43.4X1	T43.4X2	T43.4X3	T43.4X4	T43.4X5	T43.4X6
Spiramycin	T36.3X1	T36.3X2	T36.3X3	T36.3X4	T36.3X5	T36.3X6
Spirapril	T46.4X1	T46.4X2	T46.4X3	T46.4X4	T46.4X5	T46.4X6
Spirilene	T43.591	T43.592	T43.593	T43.594	T43.595	T43.596
Spirit(s) (neutral) **NEC**	T51.0X1	T51.0X2	T51.0X3	T51.0X4	—	—
beverage	T51.0X1	T51.0X2	T51.0X3	T51.0X4	—	—
industrial	T51.0X1	T51.0X2	T51.0X3	T51.0X4	—	—
mineral	T52.0X1	T52.0X2	T52.0X3	T52.0X4	—	—
of salt — see Hydrochloric acid						
surgical	T51.0X1	T51.0X2	T51.0X3	T51.0X4	—	—
Spironolactone	T50.0X1	T50.0X2	T50.0X3	T50.0X4	T50.0X5	T50.0X6
Spiroperidol	T43.4X1	T43.4X2	T43.4X3	T43.4X4	T43.4X5	T43.4X6
Sponge, absorbable (gelatin)	T45.7X1	T45.7X2	T45.7X3	T45.7X4	T45.7X5	T45.7X6
Sporostacin	T49.0X1	T49.0X2	T49.0X3	T49.0X4	T49.0X5	T49.0X6
Spray (aerosol)	T65.91	T65.92	T65.93	T65.94		
cosmetic	T65.891	T65.892	T65.893	T65.894	—	—
medicinal NEC	T50.901	T50.902	T50.903	T50.904	T50.905	T50.906
pesticides — see Pesticides						
specified content — see specific substance						
Spurge flax	T62.2X1	T62.2X2	T62.2X3	T62.2X4		
Spurges	T62.2X1	T62.2X2	T62.2X3	T62.2X4		
Sputum viscosity-lowering drug	T48.4X1	T48.4X2	T48.4X3	T48.4X4	T48.4X5	T48.4X6
Squill	T46.0X1	T46.0X2	T46.0X3	T46.0X4	T46.0X5	T46.0X6
rat poison	T60.4X1	T60.4X2	T60.4X3	T60.4X4	—	—
Squirting cucumber (cathartic)	T47.2X1	T47.2X2	T47.2X3	T47.2X4	T47.2X5	T47.2X6
Stains	T65.6X1	T65.6X2	T65.6X3	T65.6X4	—	—
Stannous fluoride	T49.7X1	T49.7X2	T49.7X3	T49.7X4	T49.7X5	T49.7X6
Stanolone	T38.7X1	T38.7X2	T38.7X3	T38.7X4	T38.7X5	T38.7X6
Stanozolol	T38.7X1	T38.7X2	T38.7X3	T38.7X4	T38.7X5	T38.7X6
Staphisagria or stavesacre (pediculicide)	T49.0X1	T49.0X2	T49.0X3	T49.0X4	T49.0X5	T49.0X6
Starch	T50.901	T50.902	T50.903	T50.904	T50.905	T50.906
Stelazine	T43.3X1	T43.3X2	T43.3X3	T43.3X4	T43.3X5	T43.3X6
Stemetil	T43.3X1	T43.3X2	T43.3X3	T43.3X4	T43.3X5	T43.3X6
Stepronin	T48.4X1	T48.4X2	T48.4X3	T48.4X4	T48.4X5	T48.4X6
Sterculia	T47.4X1	T47.4X2	T47.4X3	T47.4X4	T47.4X5	T47.4X6
Sternutator gas	T59.891	T59.892	T59.893	T59.894		
Steroid	T38.0X1	T38.0X2	T38.0X3	T38.0X4	T38.0X5	T38.0X6
anabolic	T38.7X1	T38.7X2	T38.7X3	T38.7X4	T38.7X5	T38.7X6
androgenic	T38.7X1	T38.7X2	T38.7X3	T38.7X4	T38.7X5	T38.7X6
antineoplastic, hormone	T38.7X1	T38.7X2	T38.7X3	T38.7X4	T38.7X5	T38.7X6
estrogen	T38.5X1	T38.5X2	T38.5X3	T38.5X4	T38.5X5	T38.5X6
ENT agent	T49.6X1	T49.6X2	T49.6X3	T49.6X4	T49.6X5	T49.6X6
ophthalmic preparation	T49.5X1	T49.5X2	T49.5X3	T49.5X4	T49.5X5	T49.5X6
topical NEC	T49.0X1	T49.0X2	T49.0X3	T49.0X4	T49.0X5	T49.0X6
Stibine	T56.891	T56.892	T56.893	T56.894	—	—
Stibogluconate	T37.3X1	T37.3X2	T37.3X3	T37.3X4	T37.3X5	T37.3X6
Stibophen	T37.4X1	T37.4X2	T37.4X3	T37.4X4	T37.4X5	T37.4X6
Stilbamidine (isetionate)	T37.3X1	T37.3X2	T37.3X3	T37.3X4	T37.3X5	T37.3X6
Stilbestrol	T38.5X1	T38.5X2	T38.5X3	T38.5X4	T38.5X5	T38.5X6
Stilboestrol	T38.5X1	T38.5X2	T38.5X3	T38.5X4	T38.5X5	T38.5X6
Stimulant						
central nervous system — see also Psychostimulant	T43.601	T43.602	T43.603	T43.604	T43.605	T43.606
analeptics	T50.7X1	T50.7X2	T50.7X3	T50.7X4	T50.7X5	T50.7X6
opiate antagonist	T50.7X1	T50.7X2	T50.7X3	T50.7X4	T50.7X5	T50.7X6
psychotherapeutic NEC — see also Psychotherapeutic drug	T43.601	T43.602	T43.603	T43.604	T43.605	T43.606
specified NEC	T43.691	T43.692	T43.693	T43.694	T43.695	T43.696
Stimulant — continued						
respiratory	T48.901	T48.902	T48.903	T48.904	T48.905	T48.906
Stone-dissolving drug	T50.901	T50.902	T50.903	T50.904	T50.905	T50.906
Storage battery (cells) (acid)	T54.2X1	T54.2X2	T54.2X3	T54.2X4		
Stovaine	T41.3X1	T41.3X2	T41.3X3	T41.3X4	T41.3X5	T41.3X6
infiltration (subcutaneous)	T41.3X1	T41.3X2	T41.3X3	T41.3X4	T41.3X5	T41.3X6
nerve block (peripheral) (plexus)	T41.3X1	T41.3X2	T41.3X3	T41.3X4	T41.3X5	T41.3X6
spinal	T41.3X1	T41.3X2	T41.3X3	T41.3X4	T41.3X5	T41.3X6
topical (surface)	T41.3X1	T41.3X2	T41.3X3	T41.3X4	T41.3X5	T41.3X6
Stovarsal	T37.8X1	T37.8X2	T37.8X3	T37.8X4	T37.8X5	T37.8X6
Stove gas — see Gas, stove						
Stoxil	T49.5X1	T49.5X2	T49.5X3	T49.5X4	T49.5X5	T49.5X6
Stramonium	T48.6X1	T48.6X2	T48.6X3	T48.6X4	T48.6X5	T48.6X6
natural state	T62.2X1	T62.2X2	T62.2X3	T62.2X4	—	—
Streptodornase	T45.3X1	T45.3X2	T45.3X3	T45.3X4	T45.3X5	T45.3X6
Streptoduocin	T36.5X1	T36.5X2	T36.5X3	T36.5X4	T36.5X5	T36.5X6
Streptokinase	T45.611	T45.612	T45.613	T45.614	T45.615	T45.616
Streptomycin (derivative)	T36.5X1	T36.5X2	T36.5X3	T36.5X4	T36.5X5	T36.5X6
Streptonivicin	T36.5X1	T36.5X2	T36.5X3	T36.5X4	T36.5X5	T36.5X6
Streptovarycin	T36.5X1	T36.5X2	T36.5X3	T36.5X4	T36.5X5	T36.5X6
Streptozocin	T45.1X1	T45.1X2	T45.1X3	T45.1X4	T45.1X5	T45.1X6
Streptozotocin	T45.1X1	T45.1X2	T45.1X3	T45.1X4	T45.1X5	T45.1X6
Stripper (paint) (solvent)	T52.8X1	T52.8X2	T52.8X3	T52.8X4	—	—
Strobane	T60.1X1	T60.1X2	T60.1X3	T60.1X4	—	—
Strofantina	T46.0X1	T46.0X2	T46.0X3	T46.0X4	T46.0X5	T46.0X6
Strophanthin (g) (k)	T46.0X1	T46.0X2	T46.0X3	T46.0X4	T46.0X5	T46.0X6
Strophanthus	T46.0X1	T46.0X2	T46.0X3	T46.0X4	T46.0X5	T46.0X6
Strophantin	T46.0X1	T46.0X2	T46.0X3	T46.0X4	T46.0X5	T46.0X6
Strophantin-g	T46.0X1	T46.0X2	T46.0X3	T46.0X4	T46.0X5	T46.0X6
Strychnine (nonmedicinal) (pesticide) (salts)	T65.1X1	T65.1X2	T65.1X3	T65.1X4	—	—
medicinal	T48.291	T48.292	T48.293	T48.294	T48.295	T48.296
Strychnos (ignatii) — see Strychnine						
Styramate	T42.8X1	T42.8X2	T42.8X3	T42.8X4	T42.8X5	T42.8X6
Styrene	T65.891	T65.892	T65.893	T65.894	—	—
Succinimide, antiepileptic or anticonvulsant	T42.2X1	T42.2X2	T42.2X3	T42.2X4	T42.2X5	T42.2X6
mercuric — see Mercury						
Succinylcholine	T48.1X1	T48.1X2	T48.1X3	T48.1X4	T48.1X5	T48.1X6
Succinylsulfathiazole	T37.0X1	T37.0X2	T37.0X3	T37.0X4	T37.0X5	T37.0X6
Sucralfate	T47.1X1	T47.1X2	T47.1X3	T47.1X4	T47.1X5	T47.1X6
Sucrose	T50.3X1	T50.3X2	T50.3X3	T50.3X4	T50.3X5	T50.3X6
Sufentanil	T40.4X1	T40.4X2	T40.4X3	T40.4X4	T40.4X5	T40.4X6
Sulbactam	T36.0X1	T36.0X2	T36.0X3	T36.0X4	T36.0X5	T36.0X6
Sulbenicillin	T36.0X1	T36.0X2	T36.0X3	T36.0X4	T36.0X5	T36.0X6
Sulbentine	T49.0X1	T49.0X2	T49.0X3	T49.0X4	T49.0X5	T49.0X6
Sulfacetamide	T49.0X1	T49.0X2	T49.0X3	T49.0X4	T49.0X5	T49.0X6
ophthalmic preparation	T49.5X1	T49.5X2	T49.5X3	T49.5X4	T49.5X5	T49.5X6
Sulfachlorpyridazine	T37.0X1	T37.0X2	T37.0X3	T37.0X4	T37.0X5	T37.0X6
Sulfacitine	T37.0X1	T37.0X2	T37.0X3	T37.0X4	T37.0X5	T37.0X6
Sulfadiasulfone sodium	T37.0X1	T37.0X2	T37.0X3	T37.0X4	T37.0X5	T37.0X6
Sulfadiazine	T37.0X1	T37.0X2	T37.0X3	T37.0X4	T37.0X5	T37.0X6
silver (topical)	T49.0X1	T49.0X2	T49.0X3	T49.0X4	T49.0X5	T49.0X6
Sulfadimethoxine	T37.0X1	T37.0X2	T37.0X3	T37.0X4	T37.0X5	T37.0X6
Sulfadimidine	T37.0X1	T37.0X2	T37.0X3	T37.0X4	T37.0X5	T37.0X6
Sulfadoxine	T37.0X1	T37.0X2	T37.0X3	T37.0X4	T37.0X5	T37.0X6
with pyrimethamine	T37.2X1	T37.2X2	T37.2X3	T37.2X4	T37.2X5	T37.2X6
Sulfaethidole	T37.0X1	T37.0X2	T37.0X3	T37.0X4	T37.0X5	T37.0X6
Sulfafurazole	T37.0X1	T37.0X2	T37.0X3	T37.0X4	T37.0X5	T37.0X6
Sulfaguanidine	T37.0X1	T37.0X2	T37.0X3	T37.0X4	T37.0X5	T37.0X6
Sulfalene	T37.0X1	T37.0X2	T37.0X3	T37.0X4	T37.0X5	T37.0X6
Sulfaloxate	T37.0X1	T37.0X2	T37.0X3	T37.0X4	T37.0X5	T37.0X6
Sulfaloxic acid	T37.0X1	T37.0X2	T37.0X3	T37.0X4	T37.0X5	T37.0X6
Sulfamazone	T39.2X1	T39.2X2	T39.2X3	T39.2X4	T39.2X5	T39.2X6
Sulfamerazine	T37.0X1	T37.0X2	T37.0X3	T37.0X4	T37.0X5	T37.0X6
Sulfameter	T37.0X1	T37.0X2	T37.0X3	T37.0X4	T37.0X5	T37.0X6
Sulfamethazine	T37.0X1	T37.0X2	T37.0X3	T37.0X4	T37.0X5	T37.0X6
Sulfamethizole	T37.0X1	T37.0X2	T37.0X3	T37.0X4	T37.0X5	T37.0X6
Sulfamethoxazole	T37.0X1	T37.0X2	T37.0X3	T37.0X4	T37.0X5	T37.0X6
with trimethoprim	T36.8X1	T36.8X2	T36.8X3	T36.8X4	T36.8X5	T36.8X6
Sulfamethoxydiazine	T37.0X1	T37.0X2	T37.0X3	T37.0X4	T37.0X5	T37.0X6
Sulfamethoxypyridazine	T37.0X1	T37.0X2	T37.0X3	T37.0X4	T37.0X5	T37.0X6
Sulfamethylthiazole	T37.0X1	T37.0X2	T37.0X3	T37.0X4	T37.0X5	T37.0X6
Sulfametoxydiazine	T37.0X1	T37.0X2	T37.0X3	T37.0X4	T37.0X5	T37.0X6
Sulfamidopyrine	T39.2X1	T39.2X2	T39.2X3	T39.2X4	T39.2X5	T39.2X6
Sulfamonomethoxine	T37.0X1	T37.0X2	T37.0X3	T37.0X4	T37.0X5	T37.0X6
Sulfamoxole	T37.0X1	T37.0X2	T37.0X3	T37.0X4	T37.0X5	T37.0X6
Sulfamylon	T49.0X1	T49.0X2	T49.0X3	T49.0X4	T49.0X5	T49.0X6
Sulfan blue (diagnostic dye)	T50.8X1	T50.8X2	T50.8X3	T50.8X4	T50.8X5	T50.8X6
Sulfanilamide	T37.0X1	T37.0X2	T37.0X3	T37.0X4	T37.0X5	T37.0X6
Sulfanilylguanidine	T37.0X1	T37.0X2	T37.0X3	T37.0X4	T37.0X5	T37.0X6

Substance	Poisoning, Accidental (unintentional)	Poisoning, Intentional Self-harm	Poisoning, Assault	Poisoning, Undetermined	Adverse Effect	Under-dosing
Sulfaperin	T37.0X1	T37.0X2	T37.0X3	T37.0X4	T37.0X5	T37.0X6
Sulfaphenazole	T37.0X1	T37.0X2	T37.0X3	T37.0X4	T37.0X5	T37.0X6
Sulfaphenylthiazole	T37.0X1	T37.0X2	T37.0X3	T37.0X4	T37.0X5	T37.0X6
Sulfaproxyline	T37.0X1	T37.0X2	T37.0X3	T37.0X4	T37.0X5	T37.0X6
Sulfapyridine	T37.0X1	T37.0X2	T37.0X3	T37.0X4	T37.0X5	T37.0X6
Sulfapyrimidine	T37.0X1	T37.0X2	T37.0X3	T37.0X4	T37.0X5	T37.0X6
Sulfarsphenamine	T37.8X1	T37.8X2	T37.8X3	T37.8X4	T37.8X5	T37.8X6
Sulfasalazine	T37.0X1	T37.0X2	T37.0X3	T37.0X4	T37.0X5	T37.0X6
Sulfasuxidine	T37.0X1	T37.0X2	T37.0X3	T37.0X4	T37.0X5	T37.0X6
Sulfasymazine	T37.0X1	T37.0X2	T37.0X3	T37.0X4	T37.0X5	T37.0X6
Sulfated amylopectin	T47.8X1	T47.8X2	T47.8X3	T47.8X4	T47.8X5	T47.8X6
Sulfathiazole	T37.0X1	T37.0X2	T37.0X3	T37.0X4	T37.0X5	T37.0X6
Sulfatostearate	T49.2X1	T49.2X2	T49.2X3	T49.2X4	T49.2X5	T49.2X6
Sulfinpyrazone	T50.4X1	T50.4X2	T50.4X3	T50.4X4	T50.4X5	T50.4X6
Sulfiram	T49.0X1	T49.0X2	T49.0X3	T49.0X4	T49.0X5	T49.0X6
Sulfisomidine	T37.0X1	T37.0X2	T37.0X3	T37.0X4	T37.0X5	T37.0X6
Sulfisoxazole	T37.0X1	T37.0X2	T37.0X3	T37.0X4	T37.0X5	T37.0X6
ophthalmic preparation	T49.5X1	T49.5X2	T49.5X3	T49.5X4	T49.5X5	T49.5X6
Sulfobromophthalein (sodium)	T50.8X1	T50.8X2	T50.8X3	T50.8X4	T50.8X5	T50.8X6
Sulfobromphthalein	T50.8X1	T50.8X2	T50.8X3	T50.8X4	T50.8X5	T50.8X6
Sulfogaiacol	T48.4X1	T48.4X2	T48.4X3	T48.4X4	T48.4X5	T48.4X6
Sulfomyxin	T36.8X1	T36.8X2	T36.8X3	T36.8X4	T36.8X5	T36.8X6
Sulfonal	T42.6X1	T42.6X2	T42.6X3	T42.6X4	T42.6X5	T42.6X6
Sulfonamide NEC	T37.0X1	T37.0X2	T37.0X3	T37.0X4	T37.0X5	T37.0X6
eye	T49.5X1	T49.5X2	T49.5X3	T49.5X4	T49.5X5	T49.5X6
Sulfonazide	T37.1X1	T37.1X2	T37.1X3	T37.1X4	T37.1X5	T37.1X6
Sulfones	T37.1X1	T37.1X2	T37.1X3	T37.1X4	T37.1X5	T37.1X6
Sulfonethylmethane	T42.6X1	T42.6X2	T42.6X3	T42.6X4	T42.6X5	T42.6X6
Sulfonmethane	T42.6X1	T42.6X2	T42.6X3	T42.6X4	T42.6X5	T42.6X6
Sulfonphthal, sulfonphthol	T50.8X1	T50.8X2	T50.8X3	T50.8X4	T50.8X5	T50.8X6
Sulfonylurea derivatives, oral	T38.3X1	T38.3X2	T38.3X3	T38.3X4	T38.3X5	T38.3X6
Sulforidazine	T43.3X1	T43.3X2	T43.3X3	T43.3X4	T43.3X5	T43.3X6
Sulfoxone	T37.1X1	T37.1X2	T37.1X3	T37.1X4	T37.1X5	T37.1X6
Sulfuric acid	T54.2X1	T54.2X2	T54.2X3	T54.2X4	—	—
Sulfur, sulfurated, sulfuric, sulfurous, sulfuryl (compounds NEC) (medicinal)	T49.4X1	T49.4X2	T49.4X3	T49.4X4	T49.4X5	T49.4X6
acid	T54.2X1	T54.2X2	T54.2X3	T54.2X4	—	—
dioxide (gas)	T59.1X1	T59.1X2	T59.1X3	T59.1X4	—	—
ether — see Ether(s)						
hydrogen	T59.6X1	T59.6X2	T59.6X3	T59.6X4	—	—
medicinal (keratolytic) (ointment) NEC	T49.4X1	T49.4X2	T49.4X3	T49.4X4	T49.4X5	T49.4X6
ointment	T49.0X1	T49.0X2	T49.0X3	T49.0X4	T49.0X5	T49.0X6
pesticide (vapor)	T60.91	T60.92	T60.93	T60.94	—	—
vapor NEC	T59.891	T59.892	T59.893	T59.894	—	—
Sulglicotide	T47.1X1	T47.1X2	T47.1X3	T47.1X4	T47.1X5	T47.1X6
Sulindac	T39.391	T39.392	T39.393	T39.394	T39.395	T39.396
Sulisatin	T47.2X1	T47.2X2	T47.2X3	T47.2X4	T47.2X5	T47.2X6
Sulisobenzone	T49.3X1	T49.3X2	T49.3X3	T49.3X4	T49.3X5	T49.3X6
Sulkowitch's reagent	T50.8X1	T50.8X2	T50.8X3	T50.8X4	T50.8X5	T50.8X6
Sulmetozine	T44.3X1	T44.3X2	T44.3X3	T44.3X4	T44.3X5	T44.3X6
Suloctidil	T46.7X1	T46.7X2	T46.7X3	T46.7X4	T46.7X5	T46.7X6
Sulph- — see also Sulf-						
Sulphadiazine	T37.0X1	T37.0X2	T37.0X3	T37.0X4	T37.0X5	T37.0X6
Sulphadimethoxine	T37.0X1	T37.0X2	T37.0X3	T37.0X4	T37.0X5	T37.0X6
Sulphadimidine	T37.0X1	T37.0X2	T37.0X3	T37.0X4	T37.0X5	T37.0X6
Sulphadione	T37.1X1	T37.1X2	T37.1X3	T37.1X4	T37.1X5	T37.1X6
Sulphafurazole	T37.0X1	T37.0X2	T37.0X3	T37.0X4	T37.0X5	T37.0X6
Sulphamethizole	T37.0X1	T37.0X2	T37.0X3	T37.0X4	T37.0X5	T37.0X6
Sulphamethoxazole	T37.0X1	T37.0X2	T37.0X3	T37.0X4	T37.0X5	T37.0X6
Sulphan blue	T50.8X1	T50.8X2	T50.8X3	T50.8X4	T50.8X5	T50.8X6
Sulphaphenazole	T37.0X1	T37.0X2	T37.0X3	T37.0X4	T37.0X5	T37.0X6
Sulphapyridine	T37.0X1	T37.0X2	T37.0X3	T37.0X4	T37.0X5	T37.0X6
Sulphasalazine	T37.0X1	T37.0X2	T37.0X3	T37.0X4	T37.0X5	T37.0X6
Sulphinpyrazone	T50.4X1	T50.4X2	T50.4X3	T50.4X4	T50.4X5	T50.4X6
Sulpiride	T43.591	T43.592	T43.593	T43.594	T43.595	T43.596
Sulprostone	T48.0X1	T48.0X2	T48.0X3	T48.0X4	T48.0X5	T48.0X6
Sulpyrine	T39.2X1	T39.2X2	T39.2X3	T39.2X4	T39.2X5	T39.2X6
Sultamicillin	T36.0X1	T36.0X2	T36.0X3	T36.0X4	T36.0X5	T36.0X6
Sulthiame	T42.6X1	T42.6X2	T42.6X3	T42.6X4	T42.6X5	T42.6X6
Sultiame	T42.6X1	T42.6X2	T42.6X3	T42.6X4	T42.6X5	T42.6X6
Sultopride	T43.591	T43.592	T43.593	T43.594	T43.595	T43.596
Sumatriptan	T39.8X1	T39.8X2	T39.8X3	T39.8X4	T39.8X5	T39.8X6
Sunflower seed oil	T46.6X1	T46.6X2	T46.6X3	T46.6X4	T46.6X5	T46.6X6
Superinone	T48.4X1	T48.4X2	T48.4X3	T48.4X4	T48.4X5	T48.4X6
Suprofen	T39.311	T39.312	T39.313	T39.314	T39.315	T39.316
Suramin (sodium)	T37.4X1	T37.4X2	T37.4X3	T37.4X4	T37.4X5	T37.4X6
Surfacaine	T41.3X1	T41.3X2	T41.3X3	T41.3X4	T41.3X5	T41.3X6
Surital	T41.1X1	T41.1X2	T41.1X3	T41.1X4	T41.1X5	T41.1X6
Sutilains	T45.3X1	T45.3X2	T45.3X3	T45.3X4	T45.3X5	T45.3X6
Suxamethonium (chloride)	T48.1X1	T48.1X2	T48.1X3	T48.1X4	T48.1X5	T48.1X6
Suxethonium (chloride)	T48.1X1	T48.1X2	T48.1X3	T48.1X4	T48.1X5	T48.1X6
Suxibuzone	T39.2X1	T39.2X2	T39.2X3	T39.2X4	T39.2X5	T39.2X6
Sweetener	T50.901	T50.902	T50.903	T50.904	T50.905	T50.906
Sweet niter spirit	T46.3X1	T46.3X2	T46.3X3	T46.3X4	T46.3X5	T46.3X6
Sweet oil (birch)	T49.3X1	T49.3X2	T49.3X3	T49.3X4	T49.3X5	T49.3X6
Sym-dichloroethyl ether	T53.6X1	T53.6X2	T53.6X3	T53.6X4	—	—
Sympatholytic NEC	T44.8X1	T44.8X2	T44.8X3	T44.8X4	T44.8X5	T44.8X6
haloalkylamine	T44.8X1	T44.8X2	T44.8X3	T44.8X4	T44.8X5	T44.8X6
Sympathomimetic NEC	T44.901	T44.902	T44.903	T44.904	T44.905	T44.906
anti-common-cold	T48.5X1	T48.5X2	T48.5X3	T48.5X4	T48.5X5	T48.5X6
bronchodilator	T48.6X1	T48.6X2	T48.6X3	T48.6X4	T48.6X5	T48.6X6
specified NEC	T44.991	T44.992	T44.993	T44.994	T44.995	T44.996
Synagis	T50.B91	T50.B92	T50.B93	T50.B94	T50.B95	T50.B96
Synalar	T49.0X1	T49.0X2	T49.0X3	T49.0X4	T49.0X5	T49.0X6
Synthroid	T38.1X1	T38.1X2	T38.1X3	T38.1X4	T38.1X5	T38.1X6
Syntocinon	T48.0X1	T48.0X2	T48.0X3	T48.0X4	T48.0X5	T48.0X6
Syrosingopine	T46.5X1	T46.5X2	T46.5X3	T46.5X4	T46.5X5	T46.5X6
Systemic drug	T45.91	T45.92	T45.93	T45.94	T45.95	T45.96
specified NEC	T45.8X1	T45.8X2	T45.8X3	T45.8X4	T45.8X5	T45.8X6
Tablets — see also specified substance	T50.901	T50.902	T50.903	T50.904	T50.905	T50.906
Tace	T38.5X1	T38.5X2	T38.5X3	T38.5X4	T38.5X5	T38.5X6
Tacrine	T44.0X1	T44.0X2	T44.0X3	T44.0X4	T44.0X5	T44.0X6
Tadalafil	T46.7X1	T46.7X2	T46.7X3	T46.7X4	T46.7X5	T46.7X6
Talampicillin	T36.0X1	T36.0X2	T36.0X3	T36.0X4	T36.0X5	T36.0X6
Talbutal	T42.3X1	T42.3X2	T42.3X3	T42.3X4	T42.3X5	T42.3X6
Talc powder	T49.3X1	T49.3X2	T49.3X3	T49.3X4	T49.3X5	T49.3X6
Talcum	T49.3X1	T49.3X2	T49.3X3	T49.3X4	T49.3X5	T49.3X6
Taleranol	T38.6X1	T38.6X2	T38.6X3	T38.6X4	T38.6X5	T38.6X6
Tamoxifen	T38.6X1	T38.6X2	T38.6X3	T38.6X4	T38.6X5	T38.6X6
Tamsulosin	T44.6X1	T44.6X2	T44.6X3	T44.6X4	T44.6X5	T44.6X6
Tandearil, tanderil	T39.2X1	T39.2X2	T39.2X3	T39.2X4	T39.2X5	T39.2X6
Tannic acid	T49.2X1	T49.2X2	T49.2X3	T49.2X4	T49.2X5	T49.2X6
medicinal (astringent)	T49.2X1	T49.2X2	T49.2X3	T49.2X4	T49.2X5	T49.2X6
Tannin — see Tannic acid						
Tansy	T62.2X1	T62.2X2	T62.2X3	T62.2X4	—	—
TAO	T36.3X1	T36.3X2	T36.3X3	T36.3X4	T36.3X5	T36.3X6
Tapazole	T38.2X1	T38.2X2	T38.2X3	T38.2X4	T38.2X5	T38.2X6
Taractan	T43.591	T43.592	T43.593	T43.594	T43.595	T43.596
Tarantula (venomous)	T63.321	T63.322	T63.323	T63.324		
Tartar emetic	T37.8X1	T37.8X2	T37.8X3	T37.8X4	T37.8X5	T37.8X6
Tartaric acid	T65.891	T65.892	T65.893	T65.894		
Tartrated antimony (anti-infective)	T37.8X1	T37.8X2	T37.8X3	T37.8X4	T37.8X5	T37.8X6
Tartrate, laxative	T47.4X1	T47.4X2	T47.4X3	T47.4X4	T47.4X5	T47.4X6
Tar NEC	T52.0X1	T52.0X2	T52.0X3	T52.0X4	—	—
camphor	T60.1X1	T60.1X2	T60.1X3	T60.1X4	—	—
distillate	T49.1X1	T49.1X2	T49.1X3	T49.1X4	T49.1X5	T49.1X6
fumes	T59.891	T59.892	T59.893	T59.894	—	—
medicinal	T49.1X1	T49.1X2	T49.1X3	T49.1X4	T49.1X5	T49.1X6
ointment	T49.1X1	T49.1X2	T49.1X3	T49.1X4	T49.1X5	T49.1X6
Tauromustine	T45.1X1	T45.1X2	T45.1X3	T45.1X4	T45.1X5	T45.1X6
TCA — see Trichloroacetic acid						
TCDD	T53.7X1	T53.7X2	T53.7X3	T53.7X4	—	—
TDI (vapor)	T65.0X1	T65.0X2	T65.0X3	T65.0X4	—	—
Tear						
gas	T59.3X1	T59.3X2	T59.3X3	T59.3X4	—	—
solution	T49.5X1	T49.5X2	T49.5X3	T49.5X4	T49.5X5	T49.5X6
Teclothiazide	T50.2X1	T50.2X2	T50.2X3	T50.2X4	T50.2X5	T50.2X6
Teclozan	T37.3X1	T37.3X2	T37.3X3	T37.3X4	T37.3X5	T37.3X6
Tegafur	T45.1X1	T45.1X2	T45.1X3	T45.1X4	T45.1X5	T45.1X6
Tegretol	T42.1X1	T42.1X2	T42.1X3	T42.1X4	T42.1X5	T42.1X6
Teicoplanin	T36.8X1	T36.8X2	T36.8X3	T36.8X4	T36.8X5	T36.8X6
Telepaque	T50.8X1	T50.8X2	T50.8X3	T50.8X4	T50.8X5	T50.8X6
Tellurium	T56.891	T56.892	T56.893	T56.894	—	—
fumes	T56.891	T56.892	T56.893	T56.894	—	—
TEM	T45.1X1	T45.1X2	T45.1X3	T45.1X4	T45.1X5	T45.1X6
Temazepam	T42.4X1	T42.4X2	T42.4X3	T42.4X4	T42.4X5	T42.4X6
Temocillin	T36.0X1	T36.0X2	T36.0X3	T36.0X4	T36.0X5	T36.0X6
Tenamfetamine	T43.621	T43.622	T43.623	T43.624	T43.625	T43.626
Teniposide	T45.1X1	T45.1X2	T45.1X3	T45.1X4	T45.1X5	T45.1X6
Tenitramine	T46.3X1	T46.3X2	T46.3X3	T46.3X4	T46.3X5	T46.3X6
Tenoglicin	T48.4X1	T48.4X2	T48.4X3	T48.4X4	T48.4X5	T48.4X6
Tenonitrozole	T37.3X1	T37.3X2	T37.3X3	T37.3X4	T37.3X5	T37.3X6
Tenoxicam	T39.391	T39.392	T39.393	T39.394	T39.395	T39.396
TEPA	T45.1X1	T45.1X2	T45.1X3	T45.1X4	T45.1X5	T45.1X6
TEPP	T60.0X1	T60.0X2	T60.0X3	T60.0X4	—	—
Teprotide	T46.5X1	T46.5X2	T46.5X3	T46.5X4	T46.5X5	T46.5X6
Terazosin	T44.6X1	T44.6X2	T44.6X3	T44.6X4	T44.6X5	T44.6X6
Terbufos	T60.0X1	T60.0X2	T60.0X3	T60.0X4	—	—
Terbutaline	T48.6X1	T48.6X2	T48.6X3	T48.6X4	T48.6X5	T48.6X6

Substance	Poisoning, Accidental (unintentional)	Poisoning, Intentional Self-harm	Poisoning, Assault	Poisoning, Undetermined	Adverse Effect	Under-dosing
Terconazole	T49.0X1	T49.0X2	T49.0X3	T49.0X4	T49.0X5	T49.0X6
Terfenadine	T45.0X1	T45.0X2	T45.0X3	T45.0X4	T45.0X5	T45.0X6
Teriparatide (acetate)	T50.991	T50.992	T50.993	T50.994	T50.995	T50.996
Terizidone	T37.1X1	T37.1X2	T37.1X3	T37.1X4	T37.1X5	T37.1X6
Terlipressin	T38.891	T38.892	T38.893	T38.894	T38.895	T38.896
Terodiline	T46.3X1	T46.3X2	T46.3X3	T46.3X4	T46.3X5	T46.3X6
Teroxalene	T37.4X1	T37.4X2	T37.4X3	T37.4X4	T37.4X5	T37.4X6
Terpin (cis) hydrate	T48.4X1	T48.4X2	T48.4X3	T48.4X4	T48.4X5	T48.4X6
Terramycin	T36.4X1	T36.4X2	T36.4X3	T36.4X4	T36.4X5	T36.4X6
Tertatolol	T44.7X1	T44.7X2	T44.7X3	T44.7X4	T44.7X5	T44.7X6
Tessalon	T48.3X1	T48.3X2	T48.3X3	T48.3X4	T48.3X5	T48.3X6
Testolactone	T38.7X1	T38.7X2	T38.7X3	T38.7X4	T38.7X5	T38.7X6
Testosterone	T38.7X1	T38.7X2	T38.7X3	T38.7X4	T38.7X5	T38.7X6
Tetanus toxoid or vaccine	T50.A91	T50.A92	T50.A93	T50.A94	T50.A95	T50.A96
antitoxin	T50.Z11	T50.Z12	T50.Z13	T50.Z14	T50.Z15	T50.Z16
immune globulin (human)	T50.Z11	T50.Z12	T50.Z13	T50.Z14	T50.Z15	T50.Z16
toxoid	T50.A91	T50.A92	T50.A93	T50.A94	T50.A95	T50.A96
with diphtheria toxoid	T50.A21	T50.A22	T50.A23	T50.A24	T50.A25	T50.A26
with pertussis	T50.A11	T50.A12	T50.A13	T50.A14	T50.A15	T50.A16
Tetrabenazine	T43.591	T43.592	T43.593	T43.594	T43.595	T43.596
Tetracaine	T41.3X1	T41.3X2	T41.3X3	T41.3X4	T41.3X5	T41.3X6
nerve block (peripheral) (plexus)	T41.3X1	T41.3X2	T41.3X3	T41.3X4	T41.3X5	T41.3X6
regional	T41.3X1	T41.3X2	T41.3X3	T41.3X4	T41.3X5	T41.3X6
spinal	T41.3X1	T41.3X2	T41.3X3	T41.3X4	T41.3X5	T41.3X6
Tetrachlorethylene — see Tetrachloroethylene						
Tetrachlormethiazide	T50.2X1	T50.2X2	T50.2X3	T50.2X4	T50.2X5	T50.2X6
Tetrachloroethane	T53.6X1	T53.6X2	T53.6X3	T53.6X4	—	—
vapor	T53.6X1	T53.6X2	T53.6X3	T53.6X4	—	—
paint or varnish	T53.6X1	T53.6X2	T53.6X3	T53.6X4	—	—
Tetrachloroethylene (liquid)	T53.3X1	T53.3X2	T53.3X3	T53.3X4	—	—
medicinal	T37.4X1	T37.4X2	T37.4X3	T37.4X4	T37.4X5	T37.4X6
vapor	T53.3X1	T53.3X2	T53.3X3	T53.3X4	—	—
Tetrachloromethane — see Carbon tetrachloride						
Tetracosactide	T38.811	T38.812	T38.813	T38.814	T38.815	T38.816
Tetracosactrin	T38.811	T38.812	T38.813	T38.814	T38.815	T38.816
Tetracycline	T36.4X1	T36.4X2	T36.4X3	T36.4X4	T36.4X5	T36.4X6
ophthalmic preparation	T49.5X1	T49.5X2	T49.5X3	T49.5X4	T49.5X5	T49.5X6
topical NEC	T49.0X1	T49.0X2	T49.0X3	T49.0X4	T49.0X5	T49.0X6
Tetradifon	T60.8X1	T60.8X2	T60.8X3	T60.8X4	—	—
Tetradotoxin	T61.771	T61.772	T61.773	T61.774	—	—
Tetraethyl						
lead	T56.0X1	T56.0X2	T56.0X3	T56.0X4	—	—
pyrophosphate	T60.0X1	T60.0X2	T60.0X3	T60.0X4	—	—
Tetraethylammonium chloride	T44.2X1	T44.2X2	T44.2X3	T44.2X4	T44.2X5	T44.2X6
Tetraethylthiuram disulfide	T50.6X1	T50.6X2	T50.6X3	T50.6X4	T50.6X5	T50.6X6
Tetrahydroaminoacridine	T44.0X1	T44.0X2	T44.0X3	T44.0X4	T44.0X5	T44.0X6
Tetrahydrocannabinol	T40.7X1	T40.7X2	T40.7X3	T40.7X4	T40.7X5	T40.7X6
Tetrahydrofuran	T52.8X1	T52.8X2	T52.8X3	T52.8X4	—	—
Tetrahydronaphthalene	T52.8X1	T52.8X2	T52.8X3	T52.8X4	—	—
Tetrahydrozoline	T49.5X1	T49.5X2	T49.5X3	T49.5X4	T49.5X5	T49.5X6
Tetralin	T52.8X1	T52.8X2	T52.8X3	T52.8X4	—	—
Tetramethrin	T60.2X1	T60.2X2	T60.2X3	T60.2X4	—	—
Tetramethylthiuram (disulfide) NEC	T60.3X1	T60.3X2	T60.3X3	T60.3X4	—	—
medicinal	T49.0X1	T49.0X2	T49.0X3	T49.0X4	T49.0X5	T49.0X6
Tetramisole	T37.4X1	T37.4X2	T37.4X3	T37.4X4	T37.4X5	T37.4X6
Tetranicotinoyl fructose	T46.7X1	T46.7X2	T46.7X3	T46.7X4	T46.7X5	T46.7X6
Tetrazepam	T42.4X1	T42.4X2	T42.4X3	T42.4X4	T42.4X5	T42.4X6
Tetronal	T42.6X1	T42.6X2	T42.6X3	T42.6X4	T42.6X5	T42.6X6
Tetryl	T65.3X1	T65.3X2	T65.3X3	T65.3X4	—	—
Tetrylammonium chloride	T44.2X1	T44.2X2	T44.2X3	T44.2X4	T44.2X5	T44.2X6
Tetryzoline	T49.5X1	T49.5X2	T49.5X3	T49.5X4	T49.5X5	T49.5X6
Thalidomide	T45.1X1	T45.1X2	T45.1X3	T45.1X4	T45.1X5	T45.1X6
Thallium (compounds) (dust)	T56.811	T56.812	T56.813	T56.814	—	—
NEC						
pesticide	T60.4X1	T60.4X2	T60.4X3	T60.4X4	—	—
THC	T40.7X1	T40.7X2	T40.7X3	T40.7X4	T40.7X5	T40.7X6
Thebacon	T48.3X1	T48.3X2	T48.3X3	T48.3X4	T48.3X5	T48.3X6
Thebaine	T40.2X1	T40.2X2	T40.2X3	T40.2X4	T40.2X5	T40.2X6
Thenoic acid	T49.6X1	T49.6X2	T49.6X3	T49.6X4	T49.6X5	T49.6X6
Thenyldiamine	T45.0X1	T45.0X2	T45.0X3	T45.0X4	T45.0X5	T45.0X6
Theobromine (calcium salicylate)	T48.6X1	T48.6X2	T48.6X3	T48.6X4	T48.6X5	T48.6X6
sodium salicylate	T48.6X1	T48.6X2	T48.6X3	T48.6X4	T48.6X5	T48.6X6
Theophyllamine	T48.6X1	T48.6X2	T48.6X3	T48.6X4	T48.6X5	T48.6X6
Theophylline	T48.6X1	T48.6X2	T48.6X3	T48.6X4	T48.6X5	T48.6X6
aminobenzoic acid	T48.6X1	T48.6X2	T48.6X3	T48.6X4	T48.6X5	T48.6X6

Substance	Poisoning, Accidental (unintentional)	Poisoning, Intentional Self-harm	Poisoning, Assault	Poisoning, Undetermined	Adverse Effect	Under-dosing
Theophylline — continued						
ethylenediamine	T48.6X1	T48.6X2	T48.6X3	T48.6X4	T48.6X5	T48.6X6
piperazine	T48.6X1	T48.6X2	T48.6X3	T48.6X4	T48.6X5	T48.6X6
p-amino-benzoate						
Thiabendazole	T37.4X1	T37.4X2	T37.4X3	T37.4X4	T37.4X5	T37.4X6
Thialbarbital	T41.1X1	T41.1X2	T41.1X3	T41.1X4	T41.1X5	T41.1X6
Thiamazole	T38.2X1	T38.2X2	T38.2X3	T38.2X4	T38.2X5	T38.2X6
Thiambutosine	T37.1X1	T37.1X2	T37.1X3	T37.1X4	T37.1X5	T37.1X6
Thiamine	T45.2X1	T45.2X2	T45.2X3	T45.2X4	T45.2X5	T45.2X6
Thiamphenicol	T36.2X1	T36.2X2	T36.2X3	T36.2X4	T36.2X5	T36.2X6
Thiamylal	T41.1X1	T41.1X2	T41.1X3	T41.1X4	T41.1X5	T41.1X6
sodium	T41.1X1	T41.1X2	T41.1X3	T41.1X4	T41.1X5	T41.1X6
Thiazesim	T43.291	T43.292	T43.293	T43.294	T43.295	T43.296
Thiazides (diuretics)	T50.2X1	T50.2X2	T50.2X3	T50.2X4	T50.2X5	T50.2X6
Thiazinamium metilsulfate	T43.3X1	T43.3X2	T43.3X3	T43.3X4	T43.3X5	T43.3X6
Thiethylperazine	T43.3X1	T43.3X2	T43.3X3	T43.3X4	T43.3X5	T43.3X6
Thimerosal	T49.0X1	T49.0X2	T49.0X3	T49.0X4	T49.0X5	T49.0X6
ophthalmic preparation	T49.5X1	T49.5X2	T49.5X3	T49.5X4	T49.5X5	T49.5X6
Thioacetazone	T37.1X1	T37.1X2	T37.1X3	T37.1X4	T37.1X5	T37.1X6
with isoniazid	T37.1X1	T37.1X2	T37.1X3	T37.1X4	T37.1X5	T37.1X6
Thiobarbital sodium	T41.1X1	T41.1X2	T41.1X3	T41.1X4	T41.1X5	T41.1X6
Thiobarbiturate anesthetic	T41.1X1	T41.1X2	T41.1X3	T41.1X4	T41.1X5	T41.1X6
Thiobismol	T37.8X1	T37.8X2	T37.8X3	T37.8X4	T37.8X5	T37.8X6
Thiobutabarbital sodium	T41.1X1	T41.1X2	T41.1X3	T41.1X4	T41.1X5	T41.1X6
Thiocarbamate (insecticide)	T60.0X1	T60.0X2	T60.0X3	T60.0X4	—	—
Thiocarbamide	T38.2X1	T38.2X2	T38.2X3	T38.2X4	T38.2X5	T38.2X6
Thiocarbarsone	T37.8X1	T37.8X2	T37.8X3	T37.8X4	T37.8X5	T37.8X6
Thiocarlide	T37.1X1	T37.1X2	T37.1X3	T37.1X4	T37.1X5	T37.1X6
Thioctamide	T50.991	T50.992	T50.993	T50.994	T50.995	T50.996
Thioctic acid	T50.991	T50.992	T50.993	T50.994	T50.995	T50.996
Thiofos	T60.0X1	T60.0X2	T60.0X3	T60.0X4	—	—
Thioglycolate	T49.4X1	T49.4X2	T49.4X3	T49.4X4	T49.4X5	T49.4X6
Thioglycolic acid	T65.891	T65.892	T65.893	T65.894	—	—
Thioguanine	T45.1X1	T45.1X2	T45.1X3	T45.1X4	T45.1X5	T45.1X6
Thiomercaptomerin	T50.2X1	T50.2X2	T50.2X3	T50.2X4	T50.2X5	T50.2X6
Thiomerin	T50.2X1	T50.2X2	T50.2X3	T50.2X4	T50.2X5	T50.2X6
Thiomersal	T49.0X1	T49.0X2	T49.0X3	T49.0X4	T49.0X5	T49.0X6
Thionazin	T60.0X1	T60.0X2	T60.0X3	T60.0X4	—	—
Thiopental (sodium)	T41.1X1	T41.1X2	T41.1X3	T41.1X4	T41.1X5	T41.1X6
Thiopentone (sodium)	T41.1X1	T41.1X2	T41.1X3	T41.1X4	T41.1X5	T41.1X6
Thiopropazate	T43.3X1	T43.3X2	T43.3X3	T43.3X4	T43.3X5	T43.3X6
Thioproperazine	T43.3X1	T43.3X2	T43.3X3	T43.3X4	T43.3X5	T43.3X6
Thioridazine	T43.3X1	T43.3X2	T43.3X3	T43.3X4	T43.3X5	T43.3X6
Thiosinamine	T49.3X1	T49.3X2	T49.3X3	T49.3X4	T49.3X5	T49.3X6
Thiotepa	T45.1X1	T45.1X2	T45.1X3	T45.1X4	T45.1X5	T45.1X6
Thiothixene	T43.4X1	T43.4X2	T43.4X3	T43.4X4	T43.4X5	T43.4X6
Thiouracil (benzyl) (methyl) (propyl)	T38.2X1	T38.2X2	T38.2X3	T38.2X4	T38.2X5	T38.2X6
Thiourea	T38.2X1	T38.2X2	T38.2X3	T38.2X4	T38.2X5	T38.2X6
Thiphenamil	T44.3X1	T44.3X2	T44.3X3	T44.3X4	T44.3X5	T44.3X6
Thiram	T60.3X1	T60.3X2	T60.3X3	T60.3X4	—	—
medicinal	T49.2X1	T49.2X2	T49.2X3	T49.2X4	T49.2X5	T49.2X6
Thonzylamine (systemic)	T45.0X1	T45.0X2	T45.0X3	T45.0X4	T45.0X5	T45.0X6
mucosal decongestant	T48.5X1	T48.5X2	T48.5X3	T48.5X4	T48.5X5	T48.5X6
Thorazine	T43.3X1	T43.3X2	T43.3X3	T43.3X4	T43.3X5	T43.3X6
Thorium dioxide suspension	T50.8X1	T50.8X2	T50.8X3	T50.8X4	T50.8X5	T50.8X6
Thornapple	T62.2X1	T62.2X2	T62.2X3	T62.2X4	—	—
Throat drug NEC	T49.6X1	T49.6X2	T49.6X3	T49.6X4	T49.6X5	T49.6X6
Thrombin	T45.7X1	T45.7X2	T45.7X3	T45.7X4	T45.7X5	T45.7X6
Thrombolysin	T45.611	T45.612	T45.613	T45.614	T45.615	T45.616
Thromboplastin	T45.7X1	T45.7X2	T45.7X3	T45.7X4	T45.7X5	T45.7X6
Thurfyl nicotinate	T46.7X1	T46.7X2	T46.7X3	T46.7X4	T46.7X5	T46.7X6
Thymol	T49.0X1	T49.0X2	T49.0X3	T49.0X4	T49.0X5	T49.0X6
Thymopentin	T37.5X1	T37.5X2	T37.5X3	T37.5X4	T37.5X5	T37.5X6
Thymoxamine	T46.7X1	T46.7X2	T46.7X3	T46.7X4	T46.7X5	T46.7X6
Thymus extract	T38.891	T38.892	T38.893	T38.894	T38.895	T38.896
Thyreotrophic hormone	T38.811	T38.812	T38.813	T38.814	T38.815	T38.816
Thyroglobulin	T38.1X1	T38.1X2	T38.1X3	T38.1X4	T38.1X5	T38.1X6
Thyroid (hormone)	T38.1X1	T38.1X2	T38.1X3	T38.1X4	T38.1X5	T38.1X6
Thyrolar	T38.1X1	T38.1X2	T38.1X3	T38.1X4	T38.1X5	T38.1X6
Thyrotrophin	T38.811	T38.812	T38.813	T38.814	T38.815	T38.816
Thyrotropic hormone	T38.811	T38.812	T38.813	T38.814	T38.815	T38.816
Thyroxine	T38.1X1	T38.1X2	T38.1X3	T38.1X4	T38.1X5	T38.1X6
Tiabendazole	T37.4X1	T37.4X2	T37.4X3	T37.4X4	T37.4X5	T37.4X6
Tiamizide	T50.2X1	T50.2X2	T50.2X3	T50.2X4	T50.2X5	T50.2X6
Tianeptine	T43.291	T43.292	T43.293	T43.294	T43.295	T43.296
Tiapamil	T46.1X1	T46.1X2	T46.1X3	T46.1X4	T46.1X5	T46.1X6
Tiapride	T43.591	T43.592	T43.593	T43.594	T43.595	T43.596
Tiaprofenic acid	T39.311	T39.312	T39.313	T39.314	T39.315	T39.316
Tiaramide	T39.8X1	T39.8X2	T39.8X3	T39.8X4	T39.8X5	T39.8X6
Ticarcillin	T36.0X1	T36.0X2	T36.0X3	T36.0X4	T36.0X5	T36.0X6
Ticlatone	T49.0X1	T49.0X2	T49.0X3	T49.0X4	T49.0X5	T49.0X6

Additional Character May Be Required — Refer to the Tabular List for Character Selection

▽ Subterms under main terms may continue to next column or page

Substance	Poisoning, Accidental (unintentional)	Poisoning, Intentional Self-harm	Poisoning, Assault	Poisoning, Undetermined	Adverse Effect	Underdosing
Ticlopidine	T45.521	T45.522	T45.523	T45.524	T45.525	T45.526
Ticrynafen	T50.1X1	T50.1X2	T50.1X3	T50.1X4	T50.1X5	T50.1X6
Tidiacic	T50.991	T50.992	T50.993	T50.994	T50.995	T50.996
Tiemonium	T44.3X1	T44.3X2	T44.3X3	T44.3X4	T44.3X5	T44.3X6
iodide	T44.3X1	T44.3X2	T44.3X3	T44.3X4	T44.3X5	T44.3X6
Tienilic acid	T50.1X1	T50.1X2	T50.1X3	T50.1X4	T50.1X5	T50.1X6
Tifenamil	T44.3X1	T44.3X2	T44.3X3	T44.3X4	T44.3X5	T44.3X6
Tigan	T45.0X1	T45.0X2	T45.0X3	T45.0X4	T45.0X5	T45.0X6
Tigloidine	T44.3X1	T44.3X2	T44.3X3	T44.3X4	T44.3X5	T44.3X6
Tilactase	T47.5X1	T47.5X2	T47.5X3	T47.5X4	T47.5X5	T47.5X6
Tiletamine	T41.291	T41.292	T41.293	T41.294	T41.295	T41.296
Tilidine	T40.4X1	T40.4X2	T40.4X3	T40.4X4	—	—
Timepidium bromide	T44.3X1	T44.3X2	T44.3X3	T44.3X4	T44.3X5	T44.3X6
Timiperone	T43.4X1	T43.4X2	T43.4X3	T43.4X4	T43.4X5	T43.4X6
Timolol	T44.7X1	T44.7X2	T44.7X3	T44.7X4	T44.7X5	T44.7X6
Tincture, iodine — see Iodine						
Tindal	T43.3X1	T43.3X2	T43.3X3	T43.3X4	T43.3X5	T43.3X6
Tinidazole	T37.3X1	T37.3X2	T37.3X3	T37.3X4	T37.3X5	T37.3X6
Tinoridine	T39.8X1	T39.8X2	T39.8X3	T39.8X4	T39.8X5	T39.8X6
Tin (chloride) (dust) (oxide)	T56.6X1	T56.6X2	T56.6X3	T56.6X4	—	—
NEC						
anti-infectives	T37.8X1	T37.8X2	T37.8X3	T37.8X4	T37.8X5	T37.8X6
Tiocarlide	T37.1X1	T37.1X2	T37.1X3	T37.1X4	T37.1X5	T37.1X6
Tioclomarol	T45.511	T45.512	T45.513	T45.514	T45.515	T45.516
Tioconazole	T49.0X1	T49.0X2	T49.0X3	T49.0X4	T49.0X5	T49.0X6
Tioguanine	T45.1X1	T45.1X2	T45.1X3	T45.1X4	T45.1X5	T45.1X6
Tiopronin	T50.991	T50.992	T50.993	T50.994	T50.995	T50.996
Tiotixene	T43.4X1	T43.4X2	T43.4X3	T43.4X4	T43.4X5	T43.4X6
Tioxolone	T49.4X1	T49.4X2	T49.4X3	T49.4X4	T49.4X5	T49.4X6
Tipepidine	T48.3X1	T48.3X2	T48.3X3	T48.3X4	T48.3X5	T48.3X6
Tiquizium bromide	T44.3X1	T44.3X2	T44.3X3	T44.3X4	T44.3X5	T44.3X6
Tiratricol	T38.1X1	T38.1X2	T38.1X3	T38.1X4	T38.1X5	T38.1X6
Tisopurine	T50.4X1	T50.4X2	T50.4X3	T50.4X4	T50.4X5	T50.4X6
Titanium (compounds)	T56.891	T56.892	T56.893	T56.894	—	—
(vapor)						
dioxide	T49.3X1	T49.3X2	T49.3X3	T49.3X4	T49.3X5	T49.3X6
ointment	T49.3X1	T49.3X2	T49.3X3	T49.3X4	T49.3X5	T49.3X6
oxide	T49.3X1	T49.3X2	T49.3X3	T49.3X4	T49.3X5	T49.3X6
tetrachloride	T56.891	T56.892	T56.893	T56.894	—	—
Titanocene	T56.891	T56.892	T56.893	T56.894	—	—
Titroid	T38.1X1	T38.1X2	T38.1X3	T38.1X4	T38.1X5	T38.1X6
Tizanidine	T42.8X1	T42.8X2	T42.8X3	T42.8X4	T42.8X5	T42.8X6
TMTD	T60.3X1	T60.3X2	T60.3X3	T60.3X4	—	—
TNT (fumes)	T65.3X1	T65.3X2	T65.3X3	T65.3X4	—	—
Toadstool	T62.0X1	T62.0X2	T62.0X3	T62.0X4	—	—
Tobacco NEC	T65.291	T65.292	T65.293	T65.294	—	—
cigarettes	T65.221	T65.222	T65.223	T65.224	—	—
Indian	T62.2X1	T62.2X2	T62.2X3	T62.2X4	—	—
smoke, second-hand	T65.221	T65.222	T65.223	T65.224	—	—
Tobramycin	T36.5X1	T36.5X2	T36.5X3	T36.5X4	T36.5X5	T36.5X6
Tocainide	T46.2X1	T46.2X2	T46.2X3	T46.2X4	T46.2X5	T46.2X6
Tocoferol	T45.2X1	T45.2X2	T45.2X3	T45.2X4	T45.2X5	T45.2X6
Tocopherol	T45.2X1	T45.2X2	T45.2X3	T45.2X4	T45.2X5	T45.2X6
acetate	T45.2X1	T45.2X2	T45.2X3	T45.2X4	T45.2X5	T45.2X6
Tocosamine	T48.0X1	T48.0X2	T48.0X3	T48.0X4	T48.0X5	T48.0X6
Todralazine	T46.5X1	T46.5X2	T46.5X3	T46.5X4	T46.5X5	T46.5X6
Tofisopam	T42.4X1	T42.4X2	T42.4X3	T42.4X4	T42.4X5	T42.4X6
Tofranil	T43.011	T43.012	T43.013	T43.014	T43.015	T43.016
Toilet deodorizer	T65.891	T65.892	T65.893	T65.894	—	—
Tolamolol	T44.7X1	T44.7X2	T44.7X3	T44.7X4	T44.7X5	T44.7X6
Tolazamide	T38.3X1	T38.3X2	T38.3X3	T38.3X4	T38.3X5	T38.3X6
Tolazoline	T46.7X1	T46.7X2	T46.7X3	T46.7X4	T46.7X5	T46.7X6
Tolbutamide (sodium)	T38.3X1	T38.3X2	T38.3X3	T38.3X4	T38.3X5	T38.3X6
Tolciclate	T49.0X1	T49.0X2	T49.0X3	T49.0X4	T49.0X5	T49.0X6
Tolmetin	T39.391	T39.392	T39.393	T39.394	T39.395	T39.396
Tolnaftate	T49.0X1	T49.0X2	T49.0X3	T49.0X4	T49.0X5	T49.0X6
Tolonidine	T46.5X1	T46.5X2	T46.5X3	T46.5X4	T46.5X5	T46.5X6
Toloxatone	T42.6X1	T42.6X2	T42.6X3	T42.6X4	T42.6X5	T42.6X6
Tolperisone	T44.3X1	T44.3X2	T44.3X3	T44.3X4	T44.3X5	T44.3X6
Tolserol	T42.8X1	T42.8X2	T42.8X3	T42.8X4	T42.8X5	T42.8X6
Toluene (liquid)	T52.2X1	T52.2X2	T52.2X3	T52.2X4	—	—
diisocyanate	T65.0X1	T65.0X2	T65.0X3	T65.0X4	—	—
Toluidine	T65.891	T65.892	T65.893	T65.894	—	—
vapor	T59.891	T59.892	T59.893	T59.894	—	—
Toluol (liquid)	T52.2X1	T52.2X2	T52.2X3	T52.2X4	—	—
vapor	T52.2X1	T52.2X2	T52.2X3	T52.2X4	—	—
Toluylenediamine	T65.3X1	T65.3X2	T65.3X3	T65.3X4	—	—
Tolylene-2,4-diisocyanate	T65.0X1	T65.0X2	T65.0X3	T65.0X4	—	—
Tonic NEC	T50.901	T50.902	T50.903	T50.904	T50.905	T50.906
Topical action drug NEC	T49.91	T49.92	T49.93	T49.94	T49.95	T49.96
ear, nose or throat	T49.6X1	T49.6X2	T49.6X3	T49.6X4	T49.6X5	T49.6X6
eye	T49.5X1	T49.5X2	T49.5X3	T49.5X4	T49.5X5	T49.5X6
skin	T49.91	T49.92	T49.93	T49.94	T49.95	T49.96

Substance	Poisoning, Accidental (unintentional)	Poisoning, Intentional Self-harm	Poisoning, Assault	Poisoning, Undetermined	Adverse Effect	Underdosing
Topical action drug — continued						
specified NEC	T49.8X1	T49.8X2	T49.8X3	T49.8X4	T49.8X5	T49.8X6
Toquizine	T44.3X1	T44.3X2	T44.3X3	T44.3X4	T44.3X5	T44.3X6
Toremifene	T38.6X1	T38.6X2	T38.6X3	T38.6X4	T38.6X5	T38.6X6
Tosylchloramide sodium	T49.8X1	T49.8X2	T49.8X3	T49.8X4	T49.8X5	T49.8X6
Toxaphene (dust) (spray)	T60.1X1	T60.1X2	T60.1X3	T60.1X4	—	—
Toxin, diphtheria (Schick Test)	T50.8X1	T50.8X2	T50.8X3	T50.8X4	T50.8X5	T50.8X6
Toxoid						
combined	T50.A21	T50.A22	T50.A23	T50.A24	T50.A25	T50.A26
diphtheria	T50.A91	T50.A92	T50.A93	T50.A94	T50.A95	T50.A96
tetanus	T50.A91	T50.A92	T50.A93	T50.A94	T50.A95	T50.A96
Trace element NEC	T45.8X1	T45.8X2	T45.8X3	T45.8X4	T45.8X5	T45.8X6
Tractor fuel NEC	T52.0X1	T52.0X2	T52.0X3	T52.0X4	—	—
Tragacanth	T50.991	T50.992	T50.993	T50.994	T50.995	T50.996
Tramadol	T40.4X1	T40.4X2	T40.4X3	T40.4X4	T40.4X5	T40.4X6
Tramazoline	T48.5X1	T48.5X2	T48.5X3	T48.5X4	T48.5X5	T48.5X6
Tranexamic acid	T45.621	T45.622	T45.623	T45.624	T45.625	T45.626
Tranilast	T45.0X1	T45.0X2	T45.0X3	T45.0X4	T45.0X5	T45.0X6
Tranquilizer NEC	T43.501	T43.502	T43.503	T43.504	T43.505	T43.506
with hypnotic or sedative	T42.6X1	T42.6X2	T42.6X3	T42.6X4	T42.6X5	T42.6X6
benzodiazepine NEC	T42.4X1	T42.4X2	T42.4X3	T42.4X4	T42.4X5	T42.4X6
butyrophenone NEC	T43.4X1	T43.4X2	T43.4X3	T43.4X4	T43.4X5	T43.4X6
carbamate	T43.591	T43.592	T43.593	T43.594	T43.595	T43.596
dimethylamine	T43.3X1	T43.3X2	T43.3X3	T43.3X4	T43.3X5	T43.3X6
ethylamine	T43.3X1	T43.3X2	T43.3X3	T43.3X4	T43.3X5	T43.3X6
hydroxyzine	T43.591	T43.592	T43.593	T43.594	T43.595	T43.596
major NEC	T43.501	T43.502	T43.503	T43.504	T43.505	T43.506
penothiazine NEC	T43.3X1	T43.3X2	T43.3X3	T43.3X4	T43.3X5	T43.3X6
phenothiazine-based	T43.3X1	T43.3X2	T43.3X3	T43.3X4	T43.3X5	T43.3X6
piperazine NEC	T43.3X1	T43.3X2	T43.3X3	T43.3X4	T43.3X5	T43.3X6
piperidine	T43.3X1	T43.3X2	T43.3X3	T43.3X4	T43.3X5	T43.3X6
propylamine	T43.3X1	T43.3X2	T43.3X3	T43.3X4	T43.3X5	T43.3X6
specified NEC	T43.591	T43.592	T43.593	T43.594	T43.595	T43.596
thioxanthene NEC	T43.591	T43.592	T43.593	T43.594	T43.595	T43.596
Tranxene	T42.4X1	T42.4X2	T42.4X3	T42.4X4	T42.4X5	T42.4X6
Tranylcypromine	T43.1X1	T43.1X2	T43.1X3	T43.1X4	T43.1X5	T43.1X6
Trapidil	T46.3X1	T46.3X2	T46.3X3	T46.3X4	T46.3X5	T46.3X6
Trasentine	T44.3X1	T44.3X2	T44.3X3	T44.3X4	T44.3X5	T44.3X6
Travert	T50.3X1	T50.3X2	T50.3X3	T50.3X4	T50.3X5	T50.3X6
Trazodone	T43.211	T43.212	T43.213	T43.214	T43.215	T43.216
Trecator	T37.1X1	T37.1X2	T37.1X3	T37.1X4	T37.1X5	T37.1X6
Treosulfan	T45.1X1	T45.1X2	T45.1X3	T45.1X4	T45.1X5	T45.1X6
Tretamine	T45.1X1	T45.1X2	T45.1X3	T45.1X4	T45.1X5	T45.1X6
Tretinoin	T49.0X1	T49.0X2	T49.0X3	T49.0X4	T49.0X5	T49.0X6
Tretoquinol	T48.6X1	T48.6X2	T48.6X3	T48.6X4	T48.6X5	T48.6X6
Triacetin	T49.0X1	T49.0X2	T49.0X3	T49.0X4	T49.0X5	T49.0X6
Triacetoxyanthracene	T49.4X1	T49.4X2	T49.4X3	T49.4X4	T49.4X5	T49.4X6
Triacetyloleandomycin	T36.3X1	T36.3X2	T36.3X3	T36.3X4	T36.3X5	T36.3X6
Triamcinolone	T38.0X1	T38.0X2	T38.0X3	T38.0X4	T38.0X5	T38.0X6
ENT agent	T49.6X1	T49.6X2	T49.6X3	T49.6X4	T49.6X5	T49.6X6
hexacetonide	T49.0X1	T49.0X2	T49.0X3	T49.0X4	T49.0X5	T49.0X6
ophthalmic preparation	T49.5X1	T49.5X2	T49.5X3	T49.5X4	T49.5X5	T49.5X6
topical NEC	T49.0X1	T49.0X2	T49.0X3	T49.0X4	T49.0X5	T49.0X6
Triampyzine	T44.3X1	T44.3X2	T44.3X3	T44.3X4	T44.3X5	T44.3X6
Triamterene	T50.2X1	T50.2X2	T50.2X3	T50.2X4	T50.2X5	T50.2X6
Triazine (herbicide)	T60.3X1	T60.3X2	T60.3X3	T60.3X4	—	—
Triaziquone	T45.1X1	T45.1X2	T45.1X3	T45.1X4	T45.1X5	T45.1X6
Triazolam	T42.4X1	T42.4X2	T42.4X3	T42.4X4	T42.4X5	T42.4X6
Triazole (herbicide)	T60.3X1	T60.3X2	T60.3X3	T60.3X4	—	—
Tribenoside	T46.991	T46.992	T46.993	T46.994	T46.995	T46.996
Tribromacetaldehyde	T42.6X1	T42.6X2	T42.6X3	T42.6X4	T42.6X5	T42.6X6
Tribromoethanol, rectal	T41.291	T41.292	T41.293	T41.294	T41.295	T41.296
Tribromomethane	T42.6X1	T42.6X2	T42.6X3	T42.6X4	T42.6X5	T42.6X6
Trichlorethane	T53.2X1	T53.2X2	T53.2X3	T53.2X4	—	—
Trichlorethylene	T53.2X1	T53.2X2	T53.2X3	T53.2X4	—	—
Trichlorfon	T60.0X1	T60.0X2	T60.0X3	T60.0X4	—	—
Trichlormethiazide	T50.2X1	T50.2X2	T50.2X3	T50.2X4	T50.2X5	T50.2X6
Trichlormethine	T45.1X1	T45.1X2	T45.1X3	T45.1X4	T45.1X5	T45.1X6
Trichloroacetic acid, Trichloracetic acid	T54.2X1	T54.2X2	T54.2X3	T54.2X4	—	—
medicinal	T49.4X1	T49.4X2	T49.4X3	T49.4X4	T49.4X5	T49.4X6
Trichloroethane	T53.2X1	T53.2X2	T53.2X3	T53.2X4	—	—
Trichloroethanol	T42.6X1	T42.6X2	T42.6X3	T42.6X4	T42.6X5	T42.6X6
Trichloroethylene (liquid) (vapor)	T53.2X1	T53.2X2	T53.2X3	T53.2X4	—	—
anesthetic (gas)	T41.0X1	T41.0X2	T41.0X3	T41.0X4	T41.0X5	T41.0X6
vapor NEC	T53.2X1	T53.2X2	T53.2X3	T53.2X4	—	—
Trichloroethyl phosphate	T42.6X1	T42.6X2	T42.6X3	T42.6X4	T42.6X5	T42.6X6
Trichlorofluoromethane NEC	T53.5X1	T53.5X2	T53.5X3	T53.5X4	—	—
Trichloronate	T60.0X1	T60.0X2	T60.0X3	T60.0X4	—	—
Trichloropropane	T53.6X1	T53.6X2	T53.6X3	T53.6X4	—	—

Table of Drugs and C...

Trichlorotriethylamine — Vaccine NEC

Substance	Poisoning, Accidental (unintentional)	Poisoning, Intentional Self-harm	Poisoning, Assault	Poisoning, Undetermined	Adverse Effect	Under-dosing
Trichlorotriethylamine	T45.1X1	T45.1X2	T45.1X3	T45.1X4	T45.1X5	T45.1X6
Trichomonacides NEC	T37.3X1	T37.3X2	T37.3X3	T37.3X4	T37.3X5	T37.3X6
Trichomycin	T36.7X1	T36.7X2	T36.7X3	T36.7X4	T36.7X5	T36.7X6
Triclobisonium chloride	T49.0X1	T49.0X2	T49.0X3	T49.0X4	T49.0X5	T49.0X6
Triclocarban	T49.0X1	T49.0X2	T49.0X3	T49.0X4	T49.0X5	T49.0X6
Triclofos	T42.6X1	T42.6X2	T42.6X3	T42.6X4	T42.6X5	T42.6X6
Triclosan	T49.0X1	T49.0X2	T49.0X3	T49.0X4	T49.0X5	T49.0X6
Tricresyl phosphate	T65.891	T65.892	T65.893	T65.894	—	—
solvent	T52.91	T52.92	T52.93	T52.94	—	—
Tricyclamol chloride	T44.3X1	T44.3X2	T44.3X3	T44.3X4	T44.3X5	T44.3X6
Tridesilon	T49.0X1	T49.0X2	T49.0X3	T49.0X4	T49.0X5	T49.0X6
Tridihexethyl iodide	T44.3X1	T44.3X2	T44.3X3	T44.3X4	T44.3X5	T44.3X6
Tridione	T42.2X1	T42.2X2	T42.2X3	T42.2X4	T42.2X5	T42.2X6
Trientine	T45.8X1	T45.8X2	T45.8X3	T45.8X4	T45.8X5	T45.8X6
Triethanolamine NEC	T54.3X1	T54.3X2	T54.3X3	T54.3X4	—	—
detergent	T54.3X1	T54.3X2	T54.3X3	T54.3X4	—	—
trinitrate (biphosphate)	T46.3X1	T46.3X2	T46.3X3	T46.3X4	T46.3X5	T46.3X6
Triethanomelamine	T45.1X1	T45.1X2	T45.1X3	T45.1X4	T45.1X5	T45.1X6
Triethylenemelamine	T45.1X1	T45.1X2	T45.1X3	T45.1X4	T45.1X5	T45.1X6
Triethylenephosphoramide	T45.1X1	T45.1X2	T45.1X3	T45.1X4	T45.1X5	T45.1X6
Triethylenethiophosphoramide	T45.1X1	T45.1X2	T45.1X3	T45.1X4	T45.1X5	T45.1X6
Trifluoperazine	T43.3X1	T43.3X2	T43.3X3	T43.3X4	T43.3X5	T43.3X6
Trifluoroethyl vinyl ether	T41.0X1	T41.0X2	T41.0X3	T41.0X4	T41.0X5	T41.0X6
Trifluperidol	T43.4X1	T43.4X2	T43.4X3	T43.4X4	T43.4X5	T43.4X6
Triflupromazine	T43.3X1	T43.3X2	T43.3X3	T43.3X4	T43.3X5	T43.3X6
Trifluridine	T37.5X1	T37.5X2	T37.5X3	T37.5X4	T37.5X5	T37.5X6
Triflusal	T45.521	T45.522	T45.523	T45.524	T45.525	T45.526
Trihexyphenidyl	T44.3X1	T44.3X2	T44.3X3	T44.3X4	T44.3X5	T44.3X6
Triiodothyronine	T38.1X1	T38.1X2	T38.1X3	T38.1X4	T38.1X5	T38.1X6
Trilene	T41.0X1	T41.0X2	T41.0X3	T41.0X4	T41.0X5	T41.0X6
Trilostane	T38.991	T38.992	T38.993	T38.994	T38.995	T38.996
Trimebutine	T44.3X1	T44.3X2	T44.3X3	T44.3X4	T44.3X5	T44.3X6
Trimecaine	T41.3X1	T41.3X2	T41.3X3	T41.3X4	T41.3X5	T41.3X6
Trimeprazine (tartrate)	T44.3X1	T44.3X2	T44.3X3	T44.3X4	T44.3X5	T44.3X6
Trimetaphan camsilate	T44.2X1	T44.2X2	T44.2X3	T44.2X4	T44.2X5	T44.2X6
Trimetazidine	T46.7X1	T46.7X2	T46.7X3	T46.7X4	T46.7X5	T46.7X6
Trimethadione	T42.2X1	T42.2X2	T42.2X3	T42.2X4	T42.2X5	T42.2X6
Trimethaphan	T44.2X1	T44.2X2	T44.2X3	T44.2X4	T44.2X5	T44.2X6
Trimethidinium	T44.2X1	T44.2X2	T44.2X3	T44.2X4	T44.2X5	T44.2X6
Trimethobenzamide	T45.0X1	T45.0X2	T45.0X3	T45.0X4	T45.0X5	T45.0X6
Trimethoprim	T37.8X1	T37.8X2	T37.8X3	T37.8X4	T37.8X5	T37.8X6
with sulfamethoxazole	T36.8X1	T36.8X2	T36.8X3	T36.8X4	T36.8X5	T36.8X6
Trimethylcarbinol	T51.3X1	T51.3X2	T51.3X3	T51.3X4	—	—
Trimethylpsoralen	T49.3X1	T49.3X2	T49.3X3	T49.3X4	T49.3X5	T49.3X6
Trimeton	T45.0X1	T45.0X2	T45.0X3	T45.0X4	T45.0X5	T45.0X6
Trimetrexate	T45.1X1	T45.1X2	T45.1X3	T45.1X4	T45.1X5	T45.1X6
Trimipramine	T43.011	T43.012	T43.013	T43.014	T43.015	T43.016
Trimustine	T45.1X1	T45.1X2	T45.1X3	T45.1X4	T45.1X5	T45.1X6
Trinitrine	T46.3X1	T46.3X2	T46.3X3	T46.3X4	T46.3X5	T46.3X6
Trinitrobenzol	T65.3X1	T65.3X2	T65.3X3	T65.3X4	—	—
Trinitrophenol	T65.3X1	T65.3X2	T65.3X3	T65.3X4	—	—
Trinitrotoluene (fumes)	T65.3X1	T65.3X2	T65.3X3	T65.3X4	—	—
Trional	T42.6X1	T42.6X2	T42.6X3	T42.6X4	T42.6X5	T42.6X6
Triorthocresyl phosphate	T65.891	T65.892	T65.893	T65.894	—	—
Trioxide of arsenic	T57.0X1	T57.0X2	T57.0X3	T57.0X4	—	—
Trioxysalen	T49.4X1	T49.4X2	T49.4X3	T49.4X4	T49.4X5	T49.4X6
Tripamide	T50.2X1	T50.2X2	T50.2X3	T50.2X4	T50.2X5	T50.2X6
Triparanol	T46.6X1	T46.6X2	T46.6X3	T46.6X4	T46.6X5	T46.6X6
Tripelennamine	T45.0X1	T45.0X2	T45.0X3	T45.0X4	T45.0X5	T45.0X6
Triperiden	T44.3X1	T44.3X2	T44.3X3	T44.3X4	T44.3X5	T44.3X6
Triperidol	T43.4X1	T43.4X2	T43.4X3	T43.4X4	T43.4X5	T43.4X6
Triphenylphosphate	T65.891	T65.892	T65.893	T65.894	—	—
Triple						
bromides	T42.6X1	T42.6X2	T42.6X3	T42.6X4	T42.6X5	T42.6X6
carbonate	T47.1X1	T47.1X2	T47.1X3	T47.1X4	T47.1X5	T47.1X6
vaccine						
DPT	T50.A11	T50.A12	T50.A13	T50.A14	T50.A15	T50.A16
including pertussis	T50.A11	T50.A12	T50.A13	T50.A14	T50.A15	T50.A16
MMR	T50.B91	T50.B92	T50.B93	T50.B94	T50.B95	T50.B96
Triprolidine	T45.0X1	T45.0X2	T45.0X3	T45.0X4	T45.0X5	T45.0X6
Trisodium hydrogen edetate	T50.6X1	T50.6X2	T50.6X3	T50.6X4	T50.6X5	T50.6X6
Trisoralen	T49.3X1	T49.3X2	T49.3X3	T49.3X4	T49.3X5	T49.3X6
Trisulfapyrimidines	T37.0X1	T37.0X2	T37.0X3	T37.0X4	T37.0X5	T37.0X6
Trithiozine	T44.3X1	T44.3X2	T44.3X3	T44.3X4	T44.3X5	T44.3X6
Tritiozine	T44.3X1	T44.3X2	T44.3X3	T44.3X4	T44.3X5	T44.3X6
Tritoqualine	T45.0X1	T45.0X2	T45.0X3	T45.0X4	T45.0X5	T45.0X6
Trofosfamide	T45.1X1	T45.1X2	T45.1X3	T45.1X4	T45.1X5	T45.1X6
Troleandomycin	T36.3X1	T36.3X2	T36.3X3	T36.3X4	T36.3X5	T36.3X6
Trolnitrate (phosphate)	T46.3X1	T46.3X2	T46.3X3	T46.3X4	T46.3X5	T46.3X6
Tromantadine	T37.5X1	T37.5X2	T37.5X3	T37.5X4	T37.5X5	T37.5X6
Trometamol	T50.2X1	T50.2X2	T50.2X3	T50.2X4	T50.2X5	T50.2X6
Tromethamine	T50.2X1	T50.2X2	T50.2X3	T50.2X4	T50.2X5	T50.2X6
Tronothane	T41.3X1	T41.3X2	T41.3X3	T41.3X4	T41.3X5	T41.3X6
Tropacine	T44.3X1	T44.3X2	T44.3X3	T44.3X4	T44.3X5	T44.3X6
Tropatepine	T44.3X1	T44.3X2	T44.3X3	T44.3X4	T44.3X5	T44.3X6
Tropicamide	T44.3X1	T44.3X2	T44.3X3	T44.3X4	T44.3X5	T44.3X6
Trospium chloride	T44.3X1	T44.3X2	T44.3X3	T44.3X4	T44.3X5	T44.3X6
Troxerutin	T46.991	T46.992	T46.993	T46.994	T46.995	T46.996
Troxidone	T42.2X1	T42.2X2	T42.2X3	T42.2X4	T42.2X5	T42.2X6
Tryparsamide	T37.3X1	T37.3X2	T37.3X3	T37.3X4	T37.3X5	T37.3X6
Trypsin	T45.3X1	T45.3X2	T45.3X3	T45.3X4	T45.3X5	T45.3X6
Tryptizol	T43.011	T43.012	T43.013	T43.014	T43.015	T43.016
TSH	T38.811	T38.812	T38.813	T38.814	T38.815	T38.816
Tuaminoheptane	T48.5X1	T48.5X2	T48.5X3	T48.5X4	T48.5X5	T48.5X6
Tuberculin, purified protein derivative (PPD)	T50.8X1	T50.8X2	T50.8X3	T50.8X4	T50.8X5	T50.8X6
Tubocurare	T48.1X1	T48.1X2	T48.1X3	T48.1X4	T48.1X5	T48.1X6
Tubocurarine (chloride)	T48.1X1	T48.1X2	T48.1X3	T48.1X4	T48.1X5	T48.1X6
Tulobuterol	T48.6X1	T48.6X2	T48.6X3	T48.6X4	T48.6X5	T48.6X6
Turpentine (spirits of)	T52.8X1	T52.8X2	T52.8X3	T52.8X4	—	—
vapor	T52.8X1	T52.8X2	T52.8X3	T52.8X4	—	—
Tybamate	T43.591	T43.592	T43.593	T43.594	T43.595	T43.596
Tyloxapol	T48.4X1	T48.4X2	T48.4X3	T48.4X4	T48.4X5	T48.4X6
Tymazoline	T48.5X1	T48.5X2	T48.5X3	T48.5X4	T48.5X5	T48.5X6
Typhoid-paratyphoid vaccine	T50.A91	T50.A92	T50.A93	T50.A94	T50.A95	T50.A96
Typhus vaccine	T50.A91	T50.A92	T50.A93	T50.A94	T50.A95	T50.A96
Tyropanoate	T50.8X1	T50.8X2	T50.8X3	T50.8X4	T50.8X5	T50.8X6
Tyrothricin	T49.6X1	T49.6X2	T49.6X3	T49.6X4	T49.6X5	T49.6X6
ENT agent	T49.6X1	T49.6X2	T49.6X3	T49.6X4	T49.6X5	T49.6X6
ophthalmic preparation	T49.5X1	T49.5X2	T49.5X3	T49.5X4	T49.5X5	T49.5X6
Ufenamate	T39.391	T39.392	T39.393	T39.394	T39.395	T39.396
Ultraviolet light protectant	T49.3X1	T49.3X2	T49.3X3	T49.3X4	T49.3X5	T49.3X6
Undecenoic acid	T49.0X1	T49.0X2	T49.0X3	T49.0X4	T49.0X5	T49.0X6
Undecoylium	T49.0X1	T49.0X2	T49.0X3	T49.0X4	T49.0X5	T49.0X6
Undecylenic acid (derivatives)	T49.0X1	T49.0X2	T49.0X3	T49.0X4	T49.0X5	T49.0X6
Unna's boot	T49.3X1	T49.3X2	T49.3X3	T49.3X4	T49.3X5	T49.3X6
Unsaturated fatty acid	T46.6X1	T46.6X2	T46.6X3	T46.6X4	T46.6X5	T46.6X6
Uracil mustard	T45.1X1	T45.1X2	T45.1X3	T45.1X4	T45.1X5	T45.1X6
Uramustine	T45.1X1	T45.1X2	T45.1X3	T45.1X4	T45.1X5	T45.1X6
Urapidil	T46.5X1	T46.5X2	T46.5X3	T46.5X4	T46.5X5	T46.5X6
Urari	T48.1X1	T48.1X2	T48.1X3	T48.1X4	T48.1X5	T48.1X6
Urate oxidase	T50.4X1	T50.4X2	T50.4X3	T50.4X4	T50.4X5	T50.4X6
Urea	T47.3X1	T47.3X2	T47.3X3	T47.3X4	T47.3X5	T47.3X6
peroxide	T49.0X1	T49.0X2	T49.0X3	T49.0X4	T49.0X5	T49.0X6
stibamine	T37.4X1	T37.4X2	T37.4X3	T37.4X4	T37.4X5	T37.4X6
topical	T49.8X1	T49.8X2	T49.8X3	T49.8X4	T49.8X5	T49.8X6
Urethane	T45.1X1	T45.1X2	T45.1X3	T45.1X4	T45.1X5	T45.1X6
Urginea (maritima) (scilla) — see Squill						
Uric acid metabolism drug NEC	T50.4X1	T50.4X2	T50.4X3	T50.4X4	T50.4X5	T50.4X6
Uricosuric agent	T50.4X1	T50.4X2	T50.4X3	T50.4X4	T50.4X5	T50.4X6
Urinary anti-infective	T37.8X1	T37.8X2	T37.8X3	T37.8X4	T37.8X5	T37.8X6
Urofollitropin	T38.811	T38.812	T38.813	T38.814	T38.815	T38.816
Urokinase	T45.611	T45.612	T45.613	T45.614	T45.615	T45.616
Urokon	T50.8X1	T50.8X2	T50.8X3	T50.8X4	T50.8X5	T50.8X6
Ursodeoxycholic acid	T50.991	T50.992	T50.993	T50.994	T50.995	T50.996
Ursodiol	T50.991	T50.992	T50.993	T50.994	T50.995	T50.996
Urtica	T62.2X1	T62.2X2	T62.2X3	T62.2X4	—	—
Utility gas — see Gas, utility						
Vaccine NEC	T50.Z91	T50.Z92	T50.Z93	T50.Z94	T50.Z95	T50.Z96
antineoplastic	T50.Z91	T50.Z92	T50.Z93	T50.Z94	T50.Z95	T50.Z96
bacterial NEC	T50.A91	T50.A92	T50.A93	T50.A94	T50.A95	T50.A96
with						
other bacterial component	T50.A21	T50.A22	T50.A23	T50.A24	T50.A25	T50.A26
pertussis component	T50.A11	T50.A12	T50.A13	T50.A14	T50.A15	T50.A16
viral-rickettsial component	T50.A21	T50.A22	T50.A23	T50.A24	T50.A25	T50.A26
mixed NEC	T50.A21	T50.A22	T50.A23	T50.A24	T50.A25	T50.A26
BCG	T50.A91	T50.A92	T50.A93	T50.A94	T50.A95	T50.A96
cholera	T50.A91	T50.A92	T50.A93	T50.A94	T50.A95	T50.A96
diphtheria	T50.A91	T50.A92	T50.A93	T50.A94	T50.A95	T50.A96
with tetanus	T50.A21	T50.A22	T50.A23	T50.A24	T50.A25	T50.A26
and pertussis	T50.A11	T50.A12	T50.A13	T50.A14	T50.A15	T50.A16
influenza	T50.B91	T50.B92	T50.B93	T50.B94	T50.B95	T50.B96
measles	T50.B91	T50.B92	T50.B93	T50.B94	T50.B95	T50.B96
with mumps and rubella	T50.B91	T50.B92	T50.B93	T50.B94	T50.B95	T50.B96
meningococcal	T50.A91	T50.A92	T50.A93	T50.A94	T50.A95	T50.A96
mumps	T50.B91	T50.B92	T50.B93	T50.B94	T50.B95	T50.B96
paratyphoid	T50.A91	T50.A92	T50.A93	T50.A94	T50.A95	T50.A96
pertussis	T50.A11	T50.A12	T50.A13	T50.A14	T50.A15	T50.A16
with diphtheria	T50.A11	T50.A12	T50.A13	T50.A14	T50.A15	T50.A16

Additional Character May Be Required — Refer to the Tabular List for Character Selection   ▽ Subterms under main terms may continue to next column or page

Substance	Poisoning, Accidental (unintentional)	Poisoning, Intentional Self-harm	Poisoning, Assault	Poisoning, Undetermined	Adverse Effect	Under-dosing
Vaccine — continued						
pertussis — continued						
with diphtheria — continued						
and tetanus	T50.A11	T50.A12	T50.A13	T50.A14	T50.A15	T50.A16
with other component	T50.A11	T50.A12	T50.A13	T50.A14	T50.A15	T50.A16
plague	T50.A91	T50.A92	T50.A93	T50.A94	T50.A95	T50.A96
poliomyelitis	T50.B91	T50.B92	T50.B93	T50.B94	T50.B95	T50.B96
poliovirus	T50.B91	T50.B92	T50.B93	T50.B94	T50.B95	T50.B96
rabies	T50.B91	T50.B92	T50.B93	T50.B94	T50.B95	T50.B96
respiratory syncytial virus	T50.B91	T50.B92	T50.B93	T50.B94	T50.B95	T50.B96
rickettsial NEC	T50.A91	T50.A92	T50.A93	T50.A94	T50.A95	T50.A96
with						
bacterial component	T50.A21	T50.A22	T50.A23	T50.A24	T50.A25	T50.A26
Rocky Mountain spotted fever	T50.A91	T50.A92	T50.A93	T50.A94	T50.A95	T50.A96
rubella	T50.B91	T50.B92	T50.B93	T50.B94	T50.B95	T50.B96
sabin oral	T50.B91	T50.B92	T50.B93	T50.B94	T50.B95	T50.B96
smallpox	T50.B11	T50.B12	T50.B13	T50.B14	T50.B15	T50.B16
TAB	T50.A91	T50.A92	T50.A93	T50.A94	T50.A95	T50.A96
tetanus	T50.A91	T50.A92	T50.A93	T50.A94	T50.A95	T50.A96
typhoid	T50.A91	T50.A92	T50.A93	T50.A94	T50.A95	T50.A96
typhus	T50.A91	T50.A92	T50.A93	T50.A94	T50.A95	T50.A96
viral NEC	T50.B91	T50.B92	T50.B93	T50.B94	T50.B95	T50.B96
yellow fever	T50.B91	T50.B92	T50.B93	T50.B94	T50.B95	T50.B96
Vaccinia immune globulin	T50.Z11	T50.Z12	T50.Z13	T50.Z14	T50.Z15	T50.Z16
Vaginal contraceptives	T49.8X1	T49.8X2	T49.8X3	T49.8X4	T49.8X5	T49.8X6
Valerian						
root	T42.6X1	T42.6X2	T42.6X3	T42.6X4	T42.6X5	T42.6X6
tincture	T42.6X1	T42.6X2	T42.6X3	T42.6X4	T42.6X5	T42.6X6
Valethamate bromide	T44.3X1	T44.3X2	T44.3X3	T44.3X4	T44.3X5	T44.3X6
Valisone	T49.0X1	T49.0X2	T49.0X3	T49.0X4	T49.0X5	T49.0X6
Valium	T42.4X1	T42.4X2	T42.4X3	T42.4X4	T42.4X5	T42.4X6
Valmid	T42.6X1	T42.6X2	T42.6X3	T42.6X4	T42.6X5	T42.6X6
Valnoctamide	T42.6X1	T42.6X2	T42.6X3	T42.6X4	T42.6X5	T42.6X6
Valproate (sodium)	T42.6X1	T42.6X2	T42.6X3	T42.6X4	T42.6X5	T42.6X6
Valproic acid	T42.6X1	T42.6X2	T42.6X3	T42.6X4	T42.6X5	T42.6X6
Valpromide	T42.6X1	T42.6X2	T42.6X3	T42.6X4	T42.6X5	T42.6X6
Vanadium	T56.891	T56.892	T56.893	T56.894	—	—
Vancomycin	T36.8X1	T36.8X2	T36.8X3	T36.8X4	T36.8X5	T36.8X6
Vapor — see also Gas	T59.91	T59.92	T59.93	T59.94	—	—
kiln (carbon monoxide)	T58.8X1	T58.8X2	T58.8X3	T58.8X4	—	—
lead — see lead						
specified source NEC	T59.891	T59.892	T59.893	T59.894	—	—
Vardenafil	T46.7X1	T46.7X2	T46.7X3	T46.7X4	T46.7X5	T46.7X6
Varicose reduction drug	T46.8X1	T46.8X2	T46.8X3	T46.8X4	T46.8X5	T46.8X6
Varnish	T65.4X1	T65.4X2	T65.4X3	T65.4X4	—	—
cleaner	T52.91	T52.92	T52.93	T52.94	—	—
Vaseline	T49.3X1	T49.3X2	T49.3X3	T49.3X4	T49.3X5	T49.3X6
Vasodilan	T46.7X1	T46.7X2	T46.7X3	T46.7X4	T46.7X5	T46.7X6
Vasodilator						
coronary NEC	T46.3X1	T46.3X2	T46.3X3	T46.3X4	T46.3X5	T46.3X6
peripheral NEC	T46.7X1	T46.7X2	T46.7X3	T46.7X4	T46.7X5	T46.7X6
Vasopressin	T38.891	T38.892	T38.893	T38.894	T38.895	T38.896
Vasopressor drugs	T38.891	T38.892	T38.893	T38.894	T38.895	T38.896
Vecuronium bromide	T48.1X1	T48.1X2	T48.1X3	T48.1X4	T48.1X5	T48.1X6
Vegetable extract, astringent	T49.2X1	T49.2X2	T49.2X3	T49.2X4	T49.2X5	T49.2X6
Venlafaxine	T43.211	T43.212	T43.213	T43.214	T43.215	T43.216
Venom, venomous (bite) (sting)	T63.91	T63.92	T63.93	T63.94	—	—
amphibian NEC	T63.831	T63.832	T63.833	T63.834	—	—
animal NEC	T63.891	T63.892	T63.893	T63.894	—	—
ant	T63.421	T63.422	T63.423	T63.424	—	—
arthropod NEC	T63.481	T63.482	T63.483	T63.484	—	—
bee	T63.441	T63.442	T63.443	T63.444	—	—
centipede	T63.411	T63.412	T63.413	T63.414	—	—
fish	T63.591	T63.592	T63.593	T63.594	—	—
frog	T63.811	T63.812	T63.813	T63.814	—	—
hornet	T63.451	T63.452	T63.453	T63.454	—	—
insect NEC	T63.481	T63.482	T63.483	T63.484	—	—
lizard	T63.121	T63.122	T63.123	T63.124	—	—
marine						
animals	T63.691	T63.692	T63.693	T63.694	—	—
bluebottle	T63.611	T63.612	T63.613	T63.614	—	—
jellyfish NEC	T63.621	T63.622	T63.623	T63.624	—	—
Portugese Man-o-war	T63.611	T63.612	T63.613	T63.614	—	—
sea anemone	T63.631	T63.632	T63.633	T63.634	—	—
specified NEC	T63.691	T63.692	T63.693	T63.694	—	—
fish	T63.591	T63.592	T63.593	T63.594	—	—
plants	T63.711	T63.712	T63.713	T63.714	—	—
sting ray	T63.511	T63.512	T63.513	T63.514	—	—
millipede (tropical)	T63.411	T63.412	T63.413	T63.414	—	—
plant NEC	T63.791	T63.792	T63.793	T63.794	—	—
Venom, venomous — continued						
plant — continued						
marine	T63.711	T63.712	T63.713	T63.714	—	—
reptile	T63.191	T63.192	T63.193	T63.194	—	—
gila monster	T63.111	T63.112	T63.113	T63.114	—	—
lizard NEC	T63.121	T63.122	T63.123	T63.124	—	—
scorpion	T63.2X1	T63.2X2	T63.2X3	T63.2X4	—	—
snake	T63.001	T63.002	T63.003	T63.004	—	—
African NEC	T63.081	T63.082	T63.083	T63.084	—	—
American (North) (South) NEC	T63.061	T63.062	T63.063	T63.064	—	—
Asian	T63.081	T63.082	T63.083	T63.084	—	—
Australian	T63.071	T63.072	T63.073	T63.074	—	—
cobra	T63.041	T63.042	T63.043	T63.044	—	—
coral snake	T63.021	T63.022	T63.023	T63.024	—	—
rattlesnake	T63.011	T63.012	T63.013	T63.014	—	—
specified NEC	T63.091	T63.092	T63.093	T63.094	—	—
taipan	T63.031	T63.032	T63.033	T63.034	—	—
specified NEC	T63.891	T63.892	T63.893	T63.894	—	—
spider	T63.301	T63.302	T63.303	T63.304	—	—
black widow	T63.311	T63.312	T63.313	T63.314	—	—
brown recluse	T63.331	T63.332	T63.333	T63.334	—	—
specified NEC	T63.391	T63.392	T63.393	T63.394	—	—
tarantula	T63.321	T63.322	T63.323	T63.324	—	—
sting ray	T63.511	T63.512	T63.513	T63.514	—	—
toad	T63.821	T63.822	T63.823	T63.824	—	—
wasp	T63.461	T63.462	T63.463	T63.464	—	—
Venous sclerosing drug NEC	T46.8X1	T46.8X2	T46.8X3	T46.8X4	T46.8X5	T46.8X6
Ventolin — see Albuterol						
Veramon	T42.3X1	T42.3X2	T42.3X3	T42.3X4	T42.3X5	T42.3X6
Verapamil	T46.1X1	T46.1X2	T46.1X3	T46.1X4	T46.1X5	T46.1X6
Veratrine	T46.5X1	T46.5X2	T46.5X3	T46.5X4	T46.5X5	T46.5X6
Veratrum						
album	T62.2X1	T62.2X2	T62.2X3	T62.2X4	—	—
alkaloids	T46.5X1	T46.5X2	T46.5X3	T46.5X4	T46.5X5	T46.5X6
viride	T62.2X1	T62.2X2	T62.2X3	T62.2X4	—	—
Verdigris	T60.3X1	T60.3X2	T60.3X3	T60.3X4	—	—
Veronal	T42.3X1	T42.3X2	T42.3X3	T42.3X4	T42.3X5	T42.3X6
Veroxil	T37.4X1	T37.4X2	T37.4X3	T37.4X4	T37.4X5	T37.4X6
Versenate	T50.6X1	T50.6X2	T50.6X3	T50.6X4	T50.6X5	T50.6X6
Versidyne	T39.8X1	T39.8X2	T39.8X3	T39.8X4	T39.8X5	T39.8X6
Vetrabutine	T48.0X1	T48.0X2	T48.0X3	T48.0X4	T48.0X5	T48.0X6
Vidarabine	T37.5X1	T37.5X2	T37.5X3	T37.5X4	T37.5X5	T37.5X6
Vienna						
green	T57.0X1	T57.0X2	T57.0X3	T57.0X4	—	—
insecticide	T60.2X1	T60.2X2	T60.2X3	T60.2X4	—	—
red	T57.0X1	T57.0X2	T57.0X3	T57.0X4	—	—
pharmaceutical dye	T50.991	T50.992	T50.993	T50.994	T50.995	T50.996
Vigabatrin	T42.6X1	T42.6X2	T42.6X3	T42.6X4	T42.6X5	T42.6X6
Viloxazine	T43.291	T43.292	T43.293	T43.294	T43.295	T43.296
Viminol	T39.8X1	T39.8X2	T39.8X3	T39.8X4	T39.8X5	T39.8X6
Vinbarbital, vinbarbitone	T42.3X1	T42.3X2	T42.3X3	T42.3X4	T42.3X5	T42.3X6
Vinblastine	T45.1X1	T45.1X2	T45.1X3	T45.1X4	T45.1X5	T45.1X6
Vinburnine	T46.7X1	T46.7X2	T46.7X3	T46.7X4	T46.7X5	T46.7X6
Vincamine	T45.1X1	T45.1X2	T45.1X3	T45.1X4	T45.1X5	T45.1X6
Vincristine	T45.1X1	T45.1X2	T45.1X3	T45.1X4	T45.1X5	T45.1X6
Vindesine	T45.1X1	T45.1X2	T45.1X3	T45.1X4	T45.1X5	T45.1X6
Vinesthene, vinethene	T41.0X1	T41.0X2	T41.0X3	T41.0X4	T41.0X5	T41.0X6
Vinorelbine tartrate	T45.1X1	T45.1X2	T45.1X3	T45.1X4	T45.1X5	T45.1X6
Vinpocetine	T46.7X1	T46.7X2	T46.7X3	T46.7X4	T46.7X5	T46.7X6
Vinyl						
acetate	T65.891	T65.892	T65.893	T65.894	—	—
bital	T42.3X1	T42.3X2	T42.3X3	T42.3X4	T42.3X5	T42.3X6
bromide	T65.891	T65.892	T65.893	T65.894	—	—
chloride	T59.891	T59.892	T59.893	T59.894	—	—
ether	T41.0X1	T41.0X2	T41.0X3	T41.0X4	T41.0X5	T41.0X6
Vinylbital	T42.3X1	T42.3X2	T42.3X3	T42.3X4	T42.3X5	T42.3X6
Vinylidene chloride	T65.891	T65.892	T65.893	T65.894	—	—
Vioform	T37.8X1	T37.8X2	T37.8X3	T37.8X4	T37.8X5	T37.8X6
topical	T49.0X1	T49.0X2	T49.0X3	T49.0X4	T49.0X5	T49.0X6
Viomycin	T36.8X1	T36.8X2	T36.8X3	T36.8X4	T36.8X5	T36.8X6
Viosterol	T45.2X1	T45.2X2	T45.2X3	T45.2X4	T45.2X5	T45.2X6
Viper (venom)	T63.091	T63.092	T63.093	T63.094	—	—
Viprynium	T37.4X1	T37.4X2	T37.4X3	T37.4X4	T37.4X5	T37.4X6
Viquidil	T46.7X1	T46.7X2	T46.7X3	T46.7X4	T46.7X5	T46.7X6
Viral vaccine NEC	T50.B91	T50.B92	T50.B93	T50.B94	T50.B95	T50.B96
Virginiamycin	T36.8X1	T36.8X2	T36.8X3	T36.8X4	T36.8X5	T36.8X6
Virugon	T37.5X1	T37.5X2	T37.5X3	T37.5X4	T37.5X5	T37.5X6
Viscous agent	T50.901	T50.902	T50.903	T50.904	T50.905	T50.906
Visine	T49.5X1	T49.5X2	T49.5X3	T49.5X4	T49.5X5	T49.5X6
Visnadine	T46.3X1	T46.3X2	T46.3X3	T46.3X4	T46.3X5	T46.3X6
Vitamin NEC	T45.2X1	T45.2X2	T45.2X3	T45.2X4	T45.2X5	T45.2X6

Substance	Poisoning, Accidental (unintentional)	Poisoning, Intentional Self-harm	Poisoning, Assault	Poisoning, Undetermined	Adverse Effect	Underdosing
Vitamin — *continued*						
A	T45.2X1	T45.2X2	T45.2X3	T45.2X4	T45.2X5	T45.2X6
B1	T45.2X1	T45.2X2	T45.2X3	T45.2X4	T45.2X5	T45.2X6
B2	T45.2X1	T45.2X2	T45.2X3	T45.2X4	T45.2X5	T45.2X6
B6	T45.2X1	T45.2X2	T45.2X3	T45.2X4	T45.2X5	T45.2X6
B12	T45.2X1	T45.2X2	T45.2X3	T45.2X4	T45.2X5	T45.2X6
B15	T45.2X1	T45.2X2	T45.2X3	T45.2X4	T45.2X5	T45.2X6
B NEC	T45.2X1	T45.2X2	T45.2X3	T45.2X4	T45.2X5	T45.2X6
nicotinic acid	T46.7X1	T46.7X2	T46.7X3	T46.7X4	T46.7X5	T46.7X6
C	T45.2X1	T45.2X2	T45.2X3	T45.2X4	T45.2X5	T45.2X6
D	T45.2X1	T45.2X2	T45.2X3	T45.2X4	T45.2X5	T45.2X6
D2	T45.2X1	T45.2X2	T45.2X3	T45.2X4	T45.2X5	T45.2X6
D3	T45.2X1	T45.2X2	T45.2X3	T45.2X4	T45.2X5	T45.2X6
E	T45.2X1	T45.2X2	T45.2X3	T45.2X4	T45.2X5	T45.2X6
E acetate	T45.2X1	T45.2X2	T45.2X3	T45.2X4	T45.2X5	T45.2X6
hematopoietic	T45.8X1	T45.8X2	T45.8X3	T45.8X4	T45.8X5	T45.8X6
K1	T45.7X1	T45.7X2	T45.7X3	T45.7X4	T45.7X5	T45.7X6
K2	T45.7X1	T45.7X2	T45.7X3	T45.7X4	T45.7X5	T45.7X6
K NEC	T45.7X1	T45.7X2	T45.7X3	T45.7X4	T45.7X5	T45.7X6
PP	T45.2X1	T45.2X2	T45.2X3	T45.2X4	T45.2X5	T45.2X6
ulceroprotectant	T47.1X1	T47.1X2	T47.1X3	T47.1X4	T47.1X5	T47.1X6
Vleminckx's solution	T49.4X1	T49.4X2	T49.4X3	T49.4X4	T49.4X5	T49.4X6
Voltaren — *see* Diclofenac						
sodium						
Warfarin	T45.511	T45.512	T45.513	T45.514	T45.515	T45.516
rodenticide	T45.511	T45.512	T45.513	T45.514	T45.515	T45.516
sodium	T45.511	T45.512	T45.513	T45.514	T45.515	T45.516
Wasp (sting)	T63.461	T63.462	T63.463	T63.464	—	—
Water						
balance drug	T50.3X1	T50.3X2	T50.3X3	T50.3X4	T50.3X5	T50.3X6
distilled	T50.3X1	T50.3X2	T50.3X3	T50.3X4	T50.3X5	T50.3X6
gas — *see* Gas, water						
incomplete combustion of — *see* Carbon, monoxide, fuel, utility						
hemlock	T62.2X1	T62.2X2	T62.2X3	T62.2X4	—	—
moccasin (venom)	T63.061	T63.062	T63.063	T63.064	—	—
purified	T50.3X1	T50.3X2	T50.3X3	T50.3X4	T50.3X5	T50.3X6
Wax (paraffin) (petroleum)	T52.0X1	T52.0X2	T52.0X3	T52.0X4	—	—
automobile	T65.891	T65.892	T65.893	T65.894	—	—
floor	T52.0X1	T52.0X2	T52.0X3	T52.0X4	—	—
Weed killers NEC	T60.3X1	T60.3X2	T60.3X3	T60.3X4	—	—
Welldorm	T42.6X1	T42.6X2	T42.6X3	T42.6X4	T42.6X5	T42.6X6
White						
arsenic	T57.0X1	T57.0X2	T57.0X3	T57.0X4	—	—
hellebore	T62.2X1	T62.2X2	T62.2X3	T62.2X4	—	—
lotion (keratolytic)	T49.4X1	T49.4X2	T49.4X3	T49.4X4	T49.4X5	T49.4X6
spirit	T52.0X1	T52.0X2	T52.0X3	T52.0X4	—	—
Whitewash	T65.891	T65.892	T65.893	T65.894	—	—
Whole blood (human)	T45.8X1	T45.8X2	T45.8X3	T45.8X4	T45.8X5	T45.8X6
Wild						
black cherry	T62.2X1	T62.2X2	T62.2X3	T62.2X4	—	—
poisonous plants NEC	T62.2X1	T62.2X2	T62.2X3	T62.2X4	—	—
Window cleaning fluid	T65.891	T65.892	T65.893	T65.894	—	—
Wintergreen (oil)	T49.3X1	T49.3X2	T49.3X3	T49.3X4	T49.3X5	T49.3X6
Wisterine	T62.2X1	T62.2X2	T62.2X3	T62.2X4	—	—
Witch hazel	T49.2X1	T49.2X2	T49.2X3	T49.2X4	T49.2X5	T49.2X6
Wood alcohol or spirit	T51.1X1	T51.1X2	T51.1X3	T51.1X4	—	—
Wool fat (hydrous)	T49.3X1	T49.3X2	T49.3X3	T49.3X4	T49.3X5	T49.3X6
Woorali	T48.1X1	T48.1X2	T48.1X3	T48.1X4	T48.1X5	T48.1X6
Wormseed, American	T37.4X1	T37.4X2	T37.4X3	T37.4X4	T37.4X5	T37.4X6
Xamoterol	T44.5X1	T44.5X2	T44.5X3	T44.5X4	T44.5X5	T44.5X6
Xanthine diuretics	T50.2X1	T50.2X2	T50.2X3	T50.2X4	T50.2X5	T50.2X6
Xanthinol nicotinate	T46.7X1	T46.7X2	T46.7X3	T46.7X4	T46.7X5	T46.7X6
Xanthotoxin	T49.3X1	T49.3X2	T49.3X3	T49.3X4	T49.3X5	T49.3X6
Xantinol nicotinate	T46.7X1	T46.7X2	T46.7X3	T46.7X4	T46.7X5	T46.7X6
Xantocillin	T36.0X1	T36.0X2	T36.0X3	T36.0X4	T36.0X5	T36.0X6
Xenon (127Xe) (133Xe)	T50.8X1	T50.8X2	T50.8X3	T50.8X4	T50.8X5	T50.8X6
Xenysalate	T49.4X1	T49.4X2	T49.4X3	T49.4X4	T49.4X5	T49.4X6
Xibornol	T37.8X1	T37.8X2	T37.8X3	T37.8X4	T37.8X5	T37.8X6
Xigris	T45.511	T45.512	T45.513	T45.514	T45.515	T45.516
Xipamide	T50.2X1	T50.2X2	T50.2X3	T50.2X4	T50.2X5	T50.2X6
Xylene (vapor)	T52.2X1	T52.2X2	T52.2X3	T52.2X4	—	—
Xylocaine (infiltration) (topical)	T41.3X1	T41.3X2	T41.3X3	T41.3X4	T41.3X5	T41.3X6
nerve block (peripheral) (plexus)	T41.3X1	T41.3X2	T41.3X3	T41.3X4	T41.3X5	T41.3X6
spinal	T41.3X1	T41.3X2	T41.3X3	T41.3X4	T41.3X5	T41.3X6
Xylol (vapor)	T52.2X1	T52.2X2	T52.2X3	T52.2X4	—	—
Xylometazoline	T48.5X1	T48.5X2	T48.5X3	T48.5X4	T48.5X5	T48.5X6
Yeast	T45.2X1	T45.2X2	T45.2X3	T45.2X4	T45.2X5	T45.2X6
dried	T45.2X1	T45.2X2	T45.2X3	T45.2X4	T45.2X5	T45.2X6
Yellow						
fever vaccine	T50.B91	T50.B92	T50.B93	T50.B94	T50.B95	T50.B96
jasmine	T62.2X1	T62.2X2	T62.2X3	T62.2X4	—	—
phenolphthalein	T47.2X1	T47.2X2	T47.2X3	T47.2X4	T47.2X5	T47.2X6
Yew	T62.2X1	T62.2X2	T62.2X3	T62.2X4	—	—
Yohimbic acid	T40.991	T40.992	T40.993	T40.994	T40.995	T40.996
Zactane	T39.8X1	T39.8X2	T39.8X3	T39.8X4	T39.8X5	T39.8X6
Zalcitabine	T37.5X1	T37.5X2	T37.5X3	T37.5X4	T37.5X5	T37.5X6
Zaroxolyn	T50.2X1	T50.2X2	T50.2X3	T50.2X4	T50.2X5	T50.2X6
Zephiran (topical)	T49.0X1	T49.0X2	T49.0X3	T49.0X4	T49.0X5	T49.0X6
ophthalmic preparation	T49.5X1	T49.5X2	T49.5X3	T49.5X4	T49.5X5	T49.5X6
Zeranol	T38.7X1	T38.7X2	T38.7X3	T38.7X4	T38.7X5	T38.7X6
Zerone	T51.1X1	T51.1X2	T51.1X3	T51.1X4	—	—
Zidovudine	T37.5X1	T37.5X2	T37.5X3	T37.5X4	T37.5X5	T37.5X6
Zimeldine	T43.221	T43.222	T43.223	T43.224	T43.225	T43.226
Zinc (compounds) (fumes) (vapor)	T56.5X1	T56.5X2	T56.5X3	T56.5X4	—	—
NEC						
anti-infectives	T49.0X1	T49.0X2	T49.0X3	T49.0X4	T49.0X5	T49.0X6
antivaricose	T46.8X1	T46.8X2	T46.8X3	T46.8X4	T46.8X5	T46.8X6
bacitracin	T49.0X1	T49.0X2	T49.0X3	T49.0X4	T49.0X5	T49.0X6
chloride (mouthwash)	T49.6X1	T49.6X2	T49.6X3	T49.6X4	T49.6X5	T49.6X6
chromate	T56.5X1	T56.5X2	T56.5X3	T56.5X4	—	—
gelatin	T49.3X1	T49.3X2	T49.3X3	T49.3X4	T49.3X5	T49.3X6
oxide	T49.3X1	T49.3X2	T49.3X3	T49.3X4	T49.3X5	T49.3X6
plaster	T49.3X1	T49.3X2	T49.3X3	T49.3X4	T49.3X5	T49.3X6
peroxide	T49.0X1	T49.0X2	T49.0X3	T49.0X4	T49.0X5	T49.0X6
pesticides	T56.5X1	T56.5X2	T56.5X3	T56.5X4	—	—
phosphide	T60.4X1	T60.4X2	T60.4X3	T60.4X4	—	—
pyrithionate	T49.4X1	T49.4X2	T49.4X3	T49.4X4	T49.4X5	T49.4X6
stearate	T49.3X1	T49.3X2	T49.3X3	T49.3X4	T49.3X5	T49.3X6
sulfate	T49.5X1	T49.5X2	T49.5X3	T49.5X4	T49.5X5	T49.5X6
ENT agent	T49.6X1	T49.6X2	T49.6X3	T49.6X4	T49.6X5	T49.6X6
ophthalmic solution	T49.5X1	T49.5X2	T49.5X3	T49.5X4	T49.5X5	T49.5X6
topical NEC	T49.0X1	T49.0X2	T49.0X3	T49.0X4	T49.0X5	T49.0X6
undecylenate	T49.0X1	T49.0X2	T49.0X3	T49.0X4	T49.0X5	T49.0X6
Zineb	T60.0X1	T60.0X2	T60.0X3	T60.0X4	—	—
Zinostatin	T45.1X1	T45.1X2	T45.1X3	T45.1X4	T45.1X5	T45.1X6
Zipeprol	T48.3X1	T48.3X2	T48.3X3	T48.3X4	T48.3X5	T48.3X6
Zofenopril	T46.4X1	T46.4X2	T46.4X3	T46.4X4	T46.4X5	T46.4X6
Zolpidem	T42.6X1	T42.6X2	T42.6X3	T42.6X4	T42.6X5	T42.6X6
Zomepirac	T39.391	T39.392	T39.393	T39.394	T39.395	T39.396
Zopiclone	T42.6X1	T42.6X2	T42.6X3	T42.6X4	T42.6X5	T42.6X6
Zorubicin	T45.1X1	T45.1X2	T45.1X3	T45.1X4	T45.1X5	T45.1X6
Zotepine	T43.591	T43.592	T43.593	T43.594	T43.595	T43.596
Zovant	T45.511	T45.512	T45.513	T45.514	T45.515	T45.516
Zoxazolamine	T42.8X1	T42.8X2	T42.8X3	T42.8X4	T42.8X5	T42.8X6
Zuclopenthixol	T43.4X1	T43.4X2	T43.4X3	T43.4X4	T43.4X5	T43.4X6
Zygadenus (venenosus)	T62.2X1	T62.2X2	T62.2X3	T62.2X4	—	—
Zyprexa	T43.591	T43.592	T43.593	T43.594	T43.595	T43.596

Additional Character May Be Required — Refer to the Tabular List for Character Selection   ▽ Subterms under main terms may continue to next column or page

A

Abandonment (causing exposure to weather conditions) (with intent to injure or kill) NEC X58 ☑

Abuse (adult) (child) (mental) (physical) (sexual) X58 ☑

Accident (to) X58 ☑
 aircraft (in transit) (powered) (*see also* Accident, transport, aircraft)
  due to, caused by cataclysm — *see* Forces of nature, by type
 animal-drawn vehicle — *see* Accident, transport, animal-drawn vehicle occupant
 animal-rider — *see* Accident, transport, animal-rider
 automobile — *see* Accident, transport, car occupant
 bare foot water skier V94.4 ☑
 boat, boating (*see also* Accident, watercraft)
  striking swimmer
   powered V94.11 ☑
   unpowered V94.12 ☑
 bus — *see* Accident, transport, bus occupant
 cable car, not on rails V98.0 ☑
  on rails — *see* Accident, transport, streetcar occupant
 car — *see* Accident, transport, car occupant
 caused by, due to
  animal NEC W64 ☑
  chain hoist W24.0 ☑
  cold (excessive) — *see* Exposure, cold
  corrosive liquid, substance — *see* Table of Drugs and Chemicals
  cutting or piercing instrument — *see* Contact, with, by type of instrument
  drive belt W24.0 ☑
  electric
   current — *see* Exposure, electric current
   motor (*see also* Contact, with, by type of machine) W31.3 ☑
   current (of) W86.8 ☑
  environmental factor NEC X58 ☑
  explosive material — *see* Explosion
  fire, flames — *see* Exposure, fire
  firearm missile — *see* Discharge, firearm by type
  heat (excessive) — *see* Heat
  hot — *see* Contact, with, hot
  ignition — *see* Ignition
  lifting device W24.0 ☑
  lightning — *see* subcategory T75.0 ☑
   causing fire — *see* Exposure, fire
  machine, machinery — *see* Contact, with, by type of machine
  natural factor NEC X58 ☑
  pulley (block) W24.0 ☑
  radiation — *see* Radiation
  steam X13.1 ☑
   inhalation X13.0 ☑
   pipe X16 ☑
  thunderbolt — *see* subcategory T75.0 ☑
   causing fire — *see* Exposure, fire
  transmission device W24.1 ☑
 coach — *see* Accident, transport, bus occupant
 coal car — *see* Accident, transport, industrial vehicle occupant
 diving (*see also* Fall, into, water)
  with
   drowning or submersion — *see* Drowning
 forklift — *see* Accident, transport, industrial vehicle occupant
 heavy transport vehicle NOS — *see* Accident, transport, truck occupant
 ice yacht V98.2 ☑
 in
  medical, surgical procedure
   as, or due to misadventure — *see* Misadventure
   causing an abnormal reaction or later complication without mention of misadventure (*see also* Complication of or following, by type of procedure) Y84.9
 land yacht V98.1 ☑
 late effect of — *see* W00-X58 with 7th character S
 logging car — *see* Accident, transport, industrial vehicle occupant
 machine, machinery (*see also* Contact, with, by type of machine)
  on board watercraft V93.69 ☑
   explosion — *see* Explosion, in, watercraft

Accident — *continued*
 machine, machinery (*see also* Contact, with, by type of machine) — *continued*
  on board watercraft — *continued*
   fire — *see* Burn, on board watercraft
   powered craft V93.63 ☑
    ferry boat V93.61 ☑
    fishing boat V93.62 ☑
    jetskis V93.63 ☑
    liner V93.61 ☑
    merchant ship V93.60 ☑
    passenger ship V93.61 ☑
    sailboat V93.64 ☑
 mine tram — *see* Accident, transport, industrial vehicle occupant
 mobility scooter (motorized) — *see* Accident, transport, pedestrian, conveyance, specified type NEC
 motor scooter — *see* Accident, transport, motorcyclist
 motor vehicle NOS (traffic) (*see also* Accident, transport) V89.2 ☑
  nontraffic V89.0 ☑
  three-wheeled NOS — *see* Accident, transport, three-wheeled motor vehicle occupant
 motorcycle NOS — *see* Accident, transport, motorcyclist
 nonmotor vehicle NOS (nontraffic) (*see also* Accident, transport) V89.1 ☑
  traffic NOS V89.3 ☑
 nontraffic (victim's mode of transport NOS) V88.9 ☑
  collision (between) V88.7 ☑
   bus and truck V88.5 ☑
   car and:
    bus V88.3 ☑
    pickup V88.2 ☑
    three-wheeled motor vehicle V88.0 ☑
    train V88.6 ☑
    truck V88.4 ☑
    two-wheeled motor vehicle V88.0 ☑
    van V88.2 ☑
   specified vehicle NEC and:
    three-wheeled motor vehicle V88.1 ☑
    two-wheeled motor vehicle V88.1 ☑
  known mode of transport — *see* Accident, transport, by type of vehicle
  noncollision V88.8 ☑
 on board watercraft V93.89 ☑
  powered craft V93.83 ☑
   ferry boat V93.81 ☑
   fishing boat V93.82 ☑
   jetskis V93.83 ☑
   liner V93.81 ☑
   merchant ship V93.80 ☑
   passenger ship V93.81 ☑
  unpowered craft V93.88 ☑
   canoe V93.85 ☑
   inflatable V93.86 ☑
    in tow
     recreational V94.31 ☑
     specified NEC V94.32 ☑
   kayak V93.85 ☑
   sailboat V93.84 ☑
   surf-board V93.88 ☑
   water skis V93.87 ☑
   windsurfer V93.88 ☑
 parachutist V97.29 ☑
  entangled in object V97.21 ☑
  injured on landing V97.22 ☑
 pedal cycle — *see* Accident, transport, pedal cyclist
 pedestrian (on foot)
  with
   another pedestrian W51 ☑
    with fall W03 ☑
     due to ice or snow W00.0 ☑
   on pedestrian conveyance NEC V00.09 ☑
   roller skater (in-line) V00.01 ☑
   skate boarder V00.02 ☑
   transport vehicle — *see* Accident, transport
  on pedestrian conveyance — *see* Accident, transport, pedestrian, conveyance
 pick-up truck or van — *see* Accident, transport, pickup truck occupant
 quarry truck — *see* Accident, transport, industrial vehicle occupant
 railway vehicle (any) (in motion) — *see* Accident, transport, railway vehicle occupant
  due to cataclysm — *see* Forces of nature, by type

Accident — *continued*
 scooter (non-motorized) — *see* Accident, transport, pedestrian, conveyance, scooter
 sequelae of — *see* categories W00-X58 with 7th character S
 skateboard — *see* Accident, transport, pedestrian, conveyance, skateboard
 ski(ing) — *see* Accident, transport, pedestrian, conveyance
  lift V98.3 ☑
 specified cause NEC X58 ☑
 streetcar — *see* Accident, transport, streetcar occupant
 traffic (victim's mode of transport NOS) V87.9 ☑
  collision (between) V87.7 ☑
   bus and truck V87.5 ☑
   car and:
    bus V87.3 ☑
    pickup V87.2 ☑
    three-wheeled motor vehicle V87.0 ☑
    train V87.6 ☑
    truck V87.4 ☑
    two-wheeled motor vehicle V87.0 ☑
    van V87.2 ☑
   specified vehicle NEC and:
    three-wheeled motor vehicle V87.1 ☑
    two-wheeled motor vehicle V87.1 ☑
  known mode of transport — *see* Accident, transport, by type of vehicle
  noncollision V87.8 ☑
 transport (involving injury to) V99 ☑
  18 wheeler — *see* Accident, transport, truck occupant
  agricultural vehicle occupant (nontraffic) V84.9 ☑
   driver V84.5 ☑
   hanger-on V84.7 ☑
   passenger V84.6 ☑
   traffic V84.3 ☑
    driver V84.0 ☑
    hanger-on V84.2 ☑
    passenger V84.1 ☑
   while boarding or alighting V84.4 ☑
  aircraft NEC V97.89 ☑
   military NEC V97.818 ☑
    with civilian aircraft V97.810 ☑
    civilian injured by V97.811 ☑
   occupant injured (in)
    nonpowered craft accident V96.9 ☑
     balloon V96.00 ☑
      collision V96.03 ☑
      crash V96.01 ☑
      explosion V96.05 ☑
      fire V96.04 ☑
      forced landing V96.02 ☑
      specified type NEC V96.09 ☑
     glider V96.20 ☑
      collision V96.23 ☑
      crash V96.21 ☑
      explosion V96.25 ☑
      fire V96.24 ☑
      forced landing V96.22 ☑
      specified type NEC V96.29 ☑
     hang glider V96.10 ☑
      collision V96.13 ☑
      crash V96.11 ☑
      explosion V96.15 ☑
      fire V96.14 ☑
      forced landing V96.12 ☑
      specified type NEC V96.19 ☑
     specified craft NEC V96.8 ☑
    powered craft accident V95.9 ☑
     fixed wing NEC
      commercial V95.30 ☑
       collision V95.33 ☑
       crash V95.31 ☑
       explosion V95.35 ☑
       fire V95.34 ☑
       forced landing V95.32 ☑
       specified type NEC V95.39 ☑
      private V95.20 ☑
       collision V95.23 ☑
       crash V95.21 ☑
       explosion V95.25 ☑
       fire V95.24 ☑
       forced landing V95.22 ☑
       specified type NEC V95.29 ☑
     glider V95.10 ☑

Accident — *continued*
 transport — *continued*
  aircraft — *continued*
   occupant injured — *continued*
    powered craft accident — *continued*
     glider — *continued*
      collision V95.13 ☑
      crash V95.11 ☑
      explosion V95.15 ☑
      fire V95.14 ☑
      forced landing V95.12 ☑
      specified type NEC V95.19 ☑
     helicopter V95.00 ☑
      collision V95.03 ☑
      crash V95.01 ☑
      explosion V95.05 ☑
      fire V95.04 ☑
      forced landing V95.02 ☑
      specified type NEC V95.09 ☑
     spacecraft V95.40 ☑
      collision V95.43 ☑
      crash V95.41 ☑
      explosion V95.45 ☑
      fire V95.44 ☑
      forced landing V95.42 ☑
      specified type NEC V95.49 ☑
     specified craft NEC V95.8 ☑
     ultralight V95.10 ☑
      collision V95.13 ☑
      crash V95.11 ☑
      explosion V95.15 ☑
      fire V95.14 ☑
      forced landing V95.12 ☑
      specified type NEC V95.19 ☑
    specified accident NEC V97.0 ☑
    while boarding or alighting V97.1 ☑
   person (injured by)
    falling from, in or on aircraft V97.0 ☑
    machinery on aircraft V97.89 ☑
    on ground with aircraft involvement V97.39 ☑
    rotating propeller V97.32 ☑
    struck by object falling from aircraft V97.31 ☑
    sucked into aircraft jet V97.33 ☑
    while boarding or alighting aircraft V97.1 ☑
  airport (battery-powered) passenger vehicle — *see* Accident, transport, industrial vehicle occupant
  all-terrain vehicle occupant (nontraffic) V86.95 ☑
   driver V86.55 ☑
   dune buggy — *see* Accident, transport, dune buggy occupant
   hanger-on V86.75 ☑
   passenger V86.65 ☑
   snowmobile — *see* Accident, transport, snowmobile occupant
   specified type NEC V86.99 ☑
   traffic V86.35 ☑
    driver V86.05 ☑
    hanger-on V86.25 ☑
    passenger V86.15 ☑
   while boarding or alighting V86.45 ☑
  ambulance occupant (traffic) V86.31 ☑
   driver V86.01 ☑
   hanger-on V86.21 ☑
   nontraffic V86.91 ☑
    driver V86.51 ☑
    hanger-on V86.71 ☑
    passenger V86.61 ☑
   passenger V86.11 ☑
   while boarding or alighting V86.41 ☑
  animal-drawn vehicle occupant (in) V80.929 ☑
   collision (with)
    animal V80.12 ☑
     being ridden V80.711 ☑
    animal-drawn vehicle V80.721 ☑
    bus V80.42 ☑
    car V80.42 ☑
    fixed or stationary object V80.82 ☑
    military vehicle V80.920 ☑
    nonmotor vehicle V80.791 ☑
    pedal cycle V80.22 ☑
    pedestrian V80.12 ☑
    pickup V80.42 ☑
    railway train or vehicle V80.62 ☑

Accident — *continued*
 transport — *continued*
  animal-drawn vehicle occupant — *continued*
   collision — *continued*
    specified motor vehicle NEC V80.52 ☑
    streetcar V80.731 ☑
    truck V80.42 ☑
    two- or three-wheeled motor vehicle V80.32 ☑
    van V80.42 ☑
   noncollision V80.02 ☑
   specified circumstance NEC V80.928 ☑
  animal-rider V80.919 ☑
   collision (with)
    animal V80.11 ☑
     being ridden V80.710 ☑
    animal-drawn vehicle V80.720 ☑
    bus V80.41 ☑
    car V80.41 ☑
    fixed or stationary object V80.81 ☑
    military vehicle V80.910 ☑
    nonmotor vehicle V80.790 ☑
    pedal cycle V80.21 ☑
    pedestrian V80.11 ☑
    pickup V80.41 ☑
    railway train or vehicle V80.61 ☑
    specified motor vehicle NEC V80.51 ☑
    streetcar V80.730 ☑
    truck V80.41 ☑
    two- or three-wheeled motor vehicle V80.31 ☑
    van V80.41 ☑
   noncollision V80.018 ☑
    specified as horse rider V80.010 ☑
   specified circumstance NEC V80.918 ☑
  armored car — *see* Accident, transport, truck occupant
  battery-powered truck (baggage) (mail) — *see* Accident, transport, industrial vehicle occupant
  bus occupant V79.9 ☑
   collision (with)
    animal (traffic) V70.9 ☑
     being ridden (traffic) V76.9 ☑
      nontraffic V76.3 ☑
      while boarding or alighting V76.4 ☑
     nontraffic V70.3 ☑
     while boarding or alighting V70.4 ☑
    animal-drawn vehicle (traffic) V76.9 ☑
     nontraffic V76.3 ☑
     while boarding or alighting V76.4 ☑
    bus (traffic) V74.9 ☑
     nontraffic V74.3 ☑
     while boarding or alighting V74.4 ☑
    car (traffic) V73.9 ☑
     nontraffic V73.3 ☑
     while boarding or alighting V73.4 ☑
    motor vehicle NOS (traffic) V79.60 ☑
     nontraffic V79.20 ☑
     specified type NEC (traffic) V79.69 ☑
      nontraffic V79.29 ☑
    pedal cycle (traffic) V71.9 ☑
     nontraffic V71.3 ☑
     while boarding or alighting V71.4 ☑
    pickup truck (traffic) V73.9 ☑
     nontraffic V73.3 ☑
     while boarding or alighting V73.4 ☑
    railway vehicle (traffic) V75.9 ☑
     nontraffic V75.3 ☑
     while boarding or alighting V75.4 ☑
    specified vehicle NEC (traffic) V76.9 ☑
     nontraffic V76.3 ☑
     while boarding or alighting V76.4 ☑
    stationary object (traffic) V77.9 ☑
     nontraffic V77.3 ☑
     while boarding or alighting V77.4 ☑
    streetcar (traffic) V76.9 ☑
     nontraffic V76.3 ☑
     while boarding or alighting V76.4 ☑
    three wheeled motor vehicle (traffic) V72.9 ☑
     nontraffic V72.3 ☑
     while boarding or alighting V72.4 ☑
    truck (traffic) V74.9 ☑
     nontraffic V74.3 ☑
     while boarding or alighting V74.4 ☑

Accident — *continued*
 transport — *continued*
  bus occupant — *continued*
   collision — *continued*
    two wheeled motor vehicle (traffic) V72.9 ☑
     nontraffic V72.3 ☑
     while boarding or alighting V72.4 ☑
    van (traffic) V73.9 ☑
     nontraffic V73.3 ☑
     while boarding or alighting V73.4 ☑
   driver
    collision (with)
     animal (traffic) V70.5 ☑
      being ridden (traffic) V76.5 ☑
       nontraffic V76.0 ☑
      nontraffic V70.0 ☑
     animal-drawn vehicle (traffic) V76.5 ☑
      nontraffic V76.0 ☑
     bus (traffic) V74.5 ☑
      nontraffic V74.0 ☑
     car (traffic) V73.5 ☑
      nontraffic V73.0 ☑
     motor vehicle NOS (traffic) V79.40 ☑
      nontraffic V79.00 ☑
      specified type NEC (traffic) V79.49 ☑
       nontraffic V79.09 ☑
     pedal cycle (traffic) V71.5 ☑
      nontraffic V71.0 ☑
     pickup truck (traffic) V73.5 ☑
      nontraffic V73.0 ☑
     railway vehicle (traffic) V75.5 ☑
      nontraffic V75.0 ☑
     specified vehicle NEC (traffic) V76.5 ☑
      nontraffic V76.0 ☑
     stationary object (traffic) V77.5 ☑
      nontraffic V77.0 ☑
     streetcar (traffic) V76.5 ☑
      nontraffic V76.0 ☑
     three wheeled motor vehicle (traffic) V72.5 ☑
      nontraffic V72.0 ☑
     truck (traffic) V74.5 ☑
      nontraffic V74.0 ☑
     two wheeled motor vehicle (traffic) V72.5 ☑
      nontraffic V72.0 ☑
     van (traffic) V73.5 ☑
      nontraffic V73.0 ☑
    noncollision accident (traffic) V78.5 ☑
     nontraffic V78.0 ☑
   hanger-on
    collision (with)
     animal (traffic) V70.7 ☑
      being ridden (traffic) V76.7 ☑
       nontraffic V76.2 ☑
      nontraffic V70.2 ☑
     animal-drawn vehicle (traffic) V76.7 ☑
      nontraffic V76.2 ☑
     bus (traffic) V74.7 ☑
      nontraffic V74.2 ☑
     car (traffic) V73.7 ☑
      nontraffic V73.2 ☑
     pedal cycle (traffic) V71.7 ☑
      nontraffic V71.2 ☑
     pickup truck (traffic) V73.7 ☑
      nontraffic V73.2 ☑
     railway vehicle (traffic) V75.7 ☑
      nontraffic V75.2 ☑
     specified vehicle NEC (traffic) V76.7 ☑
      nontraffic V76.2 ☑
     stationary object (traffic) V77.7 ☑
      nontraffic V77.2 ☑
     streetcar (traffic) V76.7 ☑
      nontraffic V76.2 ☑
     three wheeled motor vehicle (traffic) V72.7 ☑
      nontraffic V72.2 ☑
     truck (traffic) V74.7 ☑
      nontraffic V74.2 ☑
     two wheeled motor vehicle (traffic) V72.7 ☑
      nontraffic V72.2 ☑
     van (traffic) V73.7 ☑
      nontraffic V73.2 ☑
    noncollision accident (traffic) V78.7 ☑
     nontraffic V78.2 ☑

Accident — *continued*
  transport — *continued*
    bus occupant — *continued*
      noncollision accident (traffic) V78.9 ☑
        nontraffic V78.3 ☑
        while boarding or alighting V78.4 ☑
      nontraffic V79.3 ☑
      passenger
        collision (with)
          animal (traffic) V70.6 ☑
            being ridden (traffic) V76.6 ☑
              nontraffic V76.1 ☑
            nontraffic V70.1 ☑
          animal-drawn vehicle (traffic) V76.6 ☑
            nontraffic V76.1 ☑
          bus (traffic) V74.6 ☑
            nontraffic V74.1 ☑
          car (traffic) V73.6 ☑
            nontraffic V73.1 ☑
          motor vehicle NOS (traffic) V79.50 ☑
            nontraffic V79.10 ☑
            specified type NEC (traffic) V79.59 ☑
              nontraffic V79.19 ☑
          pedal cycle (traffic) V71.6 ☑
            nontraffic V71.1 ☑
          pickup truck (traffic) V73.6 ☑
            nontraffic V73.1 ☑
          railway vehicle (traffic) V75.6 ☑
            nontraffic V75.1 ☑
          specified vehicle NEC (traffic) V76.6 ☑
            nontraffic V76.1 ☑
          stationary object (traffic) V77.6 ☑
            nontraffic V77.1 ☑
          streetcar (traffic) V76.6 ☑
            nontraffic V76.1 ☑
          three wheeled motor vehicle (traffic)
            V72.6 ☑
            nontraffic V72.1 ☑
          truck (traffic) V74.6 ☑
            nontraffic V74.1 ☑
          two wheeled motor vehicle (traffic)
            V72.6 ☑
            nontraffic V72.1 ☑
          van (traffic) V73.6 ☑
            nontraffic V73.1 ☑
        noncollision accident (traffic) V78.6 ☑
          nontraffic V78.1 ☑
      specified type NEC V79.88 ☑
      military vehicle V79.81 ☑
    cable car, not on rails V98.0 ☑
      on rails — *see* Accident, transport, streetcar
        occupant
    car occupant V49.9 ☑
      ambulance occupant — *see* Accident, transport,
        ambulance occupant
      collision (with)
        animal (traffic) V40.9 ☑
          being ridden (traffic) V46.9 ☑
            nontraffic V46.3 ☑
            while boarding or alighting V46.4 ☑
          nontraffic V40.3 ☑
          while boarding or alighting V40.4 ☑
        animal-drawn vehicle (traffic) V46.9 ☑
          nontraffic V46.3 ☑
          while boarding or alighting V46.4 ☑
        bus (traffic) V44.9 ☑
          nontraffic V44.3 ☑
          while boarding or alighting V44.4 ☑
        car (traffic) V43.92 ☑
          nontraffic V43.32 ☑
          while boarding or alighting V43.42 ☑
        motor vehicle NOS (traffic) V49.60 ☑
          nontraffic V49.20 ☑
          specified type NEC (traffic) V49.69 ☑
            nontraffic V49.29 ☑
        pedal cycle (traffic) V41.9 ☑
          nontraffic V41.3 ☑
          while boarding or alighting V41.4 ☑
        pickup truck (traffic) V43.93 ☑
          nontraffic V43.33 ☑
          while boarding or alighting V43.43 ☑
        railway vehicle (traffic) V45.9 ☑
          nontraffic V45.3 ☑
          while boarding or alighting V45.4 ☑
        specified vehicle NEC (traffic) V46.9 ☑
          nontraffic V46.3 ☑

car occupant — *continued*
  collision — *continued*
    specified vehicle — *continued*
      while boarding or alighting V46.4 ☑
    sport utility vehicle (traffic) V43.91 ☑
      nontraffic V43.31 ☑
      while boarding or alighting V43.41 ☑
    stationary object (traffic) V47.9 ☑
      nontraffic V47.3 ☑
      while boarding or alighting V47.4 ☑
    streetcar (traffic) V46.9 ☑
      nontraffic V46.3 ☑
      while boarding or alighting V46.4 ☑
    three wheeled motor vehicle (traffic)
      V42.9 ☑
      nontraffic V42.3 ☑
      while boarding or alighting V42.4 ☑
    truck (traffic) V44.9 ☑
      nontraffic V44.3 ☑
      while boarding or alighting V44.4 ☑
    two wheeled motor vehicle (traffic) V42.9 ☑
      nontraffic V42.3 ☑
      while boarding or alighting V42.4 ☑
    van (traffic) V43.94 ☑
      nontraffic V43.34 ☑
      while boarding or alighting V43.44 ☑
  driver
    collision (with)
      animal (traffic) V40.5 ☑
        being ridden (traffic) V46.5 ☑
          nontraffic V46.0 ☑
        nontraffic V40.0 ☑
      animal-drawn vehicle (traffic) V46.5 ☑
        nontraffic V46.0 ☑
      bus (traffic) V44.5 ☑
        nontraffic V44.0 ☑
      car (traffic) V43.52 ☑
        nontraffic V43.02 ☑
      motor vehicle NOS (traffic) V49.40 ☑
        nontraffic V49.00 ☑
        specified type NEC (traffic) V49.49 ☑
          nontraffic V49.09 ☑
      pedal cycle (traffic) V41.5 ☑
        nontraffic V41.0 ☑
      pickup truck (traffic) V43.53 ☑
        nontraffic V43.03 ☑
      railway vehicle (traffic) V45.5 ☑
        nontraffic V45.0 ☑
      specified vehicle NEC (traffic) V46.5 ☑
        nontraffic V46.0 ☑
      sport utility vehicle (traffic) V43.51 ☑
        nontraffic V43.01 ☑
      stationary object (traffic) V47.5 ☑
        nontraffic V47.0 ☑
      streetcar (traffic) V46.5 ☑
        nontraffic V46.0 ☑
      three wheeled motor vehicle (traffic)
        V42.5 ☑
        nontraffic V42.0 ☑
      truck (traffic) V44.5 ☑
        nontraffic V44.0 ☑
      two wheeled motor vehicle (traffic)
        V42.5 ☑
        nontraffic V42.0 ☑
      van (traffic) V43.54 ☑
        nontraffic V43.04 ☑
    noncollision accident (traffic) V48.5 ☑
      nontraffic V48.0 ☑
  hanger-on
    collision (with)
      animal (traffic) V40.7 ☑
        being ridden (traffic) V46.7 ☑
          nontraffic V46.2 ☑
        nontraffic V40.2 ☑
      animal-drawn vehicle (traffic) V46.7 ☑
        nontraffic V46.2 ☑
      bus (traffic) V44.7 ☑
        nontraffic V44.2 ☑
      car (traffic) V43.72 ☑
        nontraffic V43.22 ☑
      pedal cycle (traffic) V41.7 ☑
        nontraffic V41.2 ☑
      pickup truck (traffic) V43.73 ☑
        nontraffic V43.23 ☑

car occupant — *continued*
  hanger-on — *continued*
    collision — *continued*
      railway vehicle (traffic) V45.7 ☑
        nontraffic V45.2 ☑
      specified vehicle NEC (traffic) V46.7 ☑
        nontraffic V46.2 ☑
      sport utility vehicle (traffic) V43.71 ☑
        nontraffic V43.21 ☑
      stationary object (traffic) V47.7 ☑
        nontraffic V47.2 ☑
      streetcar (traffic) V46.7 ☑
        nontraffic V46.2 ☑
      three wheeled motor vehicle (traffic)
        V42.7 ☑
        nontraffic V42.2 ☑
      truck (traffic) V44.7 ☑
        nontraffic V44.2 ☑
      two wheeled motor vehicle (traffic)
        V42.7 ☑
        nontraffic V42.2 ☑
      van (traffic) V43.74 ☑
        nontraffic V43.24 ☑
    noncollision accident (traffic) V48.7 ☑
      nontraffic V48.2 ☑
  noncollision accident (traffic) V48.9 ☑
    nontraffic V48.3 ☑
    while boarding or alighting V48.4 ☑
  nontraffic V49.3 ☑
  passenger
    collision (with)
      animal (traffic) V40.6 ☑
        being ridden (traffic) V46.6 ☑
          nontraffic V46.1 ☑
        nontraffic V40.1 ☑
      animal-drawn vehicle (traffic) V46.6 ☑
        nontraffic V46.1 ☑
      bus (traffic) V44.6 ☑
        nontraffic V44.1 ☑
      car (traffic) V43.62 ☑
        nontraffic V43.12 ☑
      motor vehicle NOS (traffic) V49.50 ☑
        nontraffic V49.10 ☑
        specified type NEC (traffic) V49.59 ☑
          nontraffic V49.19 ☑
      pedal cycle (traffic) V41.6 ☑
        nontraffic V41.1 ☑
      pickup truck (traffic) V43.63 ☑
        nontraffic V43.13 ☑
      railway vehicle (traffic) V45.6 ☑
        nontraffic V45.1 ☑
      specified vehicle NEC (traffic) V46.6 ☑
        nontraffic V46.1 ☑
      sport utility vehicle (traffic) V43.61 ☑
        nontraffic V43.11 ☑
      stationary object (traffic) V47.6 ☑
        nontraffic V47.1 ☑
      streetcar (traffic) V46.6 ☑
        nontraffic V46.1 ☑
      three wheeled motor vehicle (traffic)
        V42.6 ☑
        nontraffic V42.1 ☑
      truck (traffic) V44.6 ☑
        nontraffic V44.1 ☑
      two wheeled motor vehicle (traffic)
        V42.6 ☑
        nontraffic V42.1 ☑
      van (traffic) V43.64 ☑
        nontraffic V43.14 ☑
    noncollision accident (traffic) V48.6 ☑
      nontraffic V48.1 ☑
  specified type NEC V49.88 ☑
  military vehicle V49.81 ☑
coal car — *see* Accident, transport, industrial vehi-cle occupant
construction vehicle occupant (nontraffic) V85.9 ☑
  driver V85.5 ☑
  hanger-on V85.7 ☑
  passenger V85.6 ☑
  traffic V85.3 ☑
    driver V85.0 ☑
    hanger-on V85.2 ☑
    passenger V85.1 ☑
  while boarding or alighting V85.4 ☑

Accident — *continued*
  transport — *continued*
    dirt bike rider (nontraffic) V86.96 ☑
      driver V86.56 ☑
      hanger-on V86.76 ☑
      passenger V86.66 ☑
      traffic V86.36 ☑
        driver V86.06 ☑
        hanger-on V86.26 ☑
        passenger V86.16 ☑
      while boarding or alighting V86.46 ☑
    due to cataclysm — *see* Forces of nature, by type
    dune buggy occupant (nontraffic) V86.93 ☑
      driver V86.53 ☑
      hanger-on V86.73 ☑
      passenger V86.63 ☑
      traffic V86.33 ☑
        driver V86.03 ☑
        hanger-on V86.23 ☑
        passenger V86.13 ☑
      while boarding or alighting V86.43 ☑
    forklift — *see* Accident, transport, industrial vehicle occupant
    go cart — *see* Accident, transport, all-terrain vehicle occupant
    golf cart — *see* Accident, transport, all-terrain vehicle occupant
    heavy transport vehicle occupant — *see* Accident, transport, truck occupant
    ice yacht V98.2 ☑
    industrial vehicle occupant (nontraffic) V83.9 ☑
      driver V83.5 ☑
      hanger-on V83.7 ☑
      passenger V83.6 ☑
      traffic V83.3 ☑
        driver V83.0 ☑
        hanger-on V83.2 ☑
        passenger V83.1 ☑
      while boarding or alighting V83.4 ☑
    interurban electric car — *see* Accident, transport, streetcar
    land yacht V98.1 ☑
    logging car — *see* Accident, transport, industrial vehicle occupant
    military vehicle occupant (traffic) V86.34 ☑
      driver V86.04 ☑
      hanger-on V86.24 ☑
      nontraffic V86.94 ☑
        driver V86.54 ☑
        hanger-on V86.74 ☑
        passenger V86.64 ☑
      passenger V86.14 ☑
      while boarding or alighting V86.44 ☑
    mine tram — *see* Accident, transport, industrial vehicle occupant
    motor vehicle NEC occupant (traffic) V89.2 ☑
    motorcoach — *see* Accident, transport, bus occupant
    motor/cross bike rider (*see also* Accident, transport, dirt bike rider) V86.96 ☑
    motorcyclist V29.9 ☑
      collision (with)
        animal (traffic) V20.9 ☑
          being ridden (traffic) V26.9 ☑
            nontraffic V26.2 ☑
              while boarding or alighting V26.3 ☑
          nontraffic V20.2 ☑
          while boarding or alighting V20.3 ☑
        animal-drawn vehicle (traffic) V26.9 ☑
          nontraffic V26.2 ☑
          while boarding or alighting V26.3 ☑
        bus (traffic) V24.9 ☑
          nontraffic V24.2 ☑
          while boarding or alighting V24.3 ☑
        car (traffic) V23.9 ☑
          nontraffic V23.2 ☑
          while boarding or alighting V23.3 ☑
        motor vehicle NOS (traffic) V29.60 ☑
          nontraffic V29.20 ☑
          specified type NEC (traffic) V29.69 ☑
            nontraffic V29.29 ☑
        pedal cycle (traffic) V21.9 ☑
          nontraffic V21.2 ☑
          while boarding or alighting V21.3 ☑
        pickup truck (traffic) V23.9 ☑
          nontraffic V23.2 ☑

Accident — *continued*
  transport — *continued*
    motorcyclist — *continued*
      collision — *continued*
        pickup truck — *continued*
          while boarding or alighting V23.3 ☑
        railway vehicle (traffic) V25.9 ☑
          nontraffic V25.2 ☑
          while boarding or alighting V25.3 ☑
        specified vehicle NEC (traffic) V26.9 ☑
          nontraffic V26.2 ☑
          while boarding or alighting V26.3 ☑
        stationary object (traffic) V27.9 ☑
          nontraffic V27.2 ☑
          while boarding or alighting V27.3 ☑
        streetcar (traffic) V26.9 ☑
          nontraffic V26.2 ☑
          while boarding or alighting V26.3 ☑
        three wheeled motor vehicle (traffic) V22.9 ☑
          nontraffic V22.2 ☑
          while boarding or alighting V22.3 ☑
        truck (traffic) V24.9 ☑
          nontraffic V24.2 ☑
          while boarding or alighting V24.3 ☑
        two wheeled motor vehicle (traffic) V22.9 ☑
          nontraffic V22.2 ☑
          while boarding or alighting V22.3 ☑
        van (traffic) V23.9 ☑
          nontraffic V23.2 ☑
          while boarding or alighting V23.3 ☑
      driver
        collision (with)
          animal (traffic) V20.4 ☑
            being ridden (traffic) V26.4 ☑
              nontraffic V26.0 ☑
            nontraffic V20.0 ☑
          animal-drawn vehicle (traffic) V26.4 ☑
            nontraffic V26.0 ☑
          bus (traffic) V24.4 ☑
            nontraffic V24.0 ☑
          car (traffic) V23.4 ☑
            nontraffic V23.0 ☑
          motor vehicle NOS (traffic) V29.40 ☑
            nontraffic V29.00 ☑
            specified type NEC (traffic) V29.49 ☑
              nontraffic V29.09 ☑
          pedal cycle (traffic) V21.4 ☑
            nontraffic V21.0 ☑
          pickup truck (traffic) V23.4 ☑
            nontraffic V23.0 ☑
          railway vehicle (traffic) V25.4 ☑
            nontraffic V25.0 ☑
          specified vehicle NEC (traffic) V26.4 ☑
            nontraffic V26.0 ☑
          stationary object (traffic) V27.4 ☑
            nontraffic V27.0 ☑
          streetcar (traffic) V26.4 ☑
            nontraffic V26.0 ☑
          three wheeled motor vehicle (traffic) V22.4 ☑
            nontraffic V22.0 ☑
          truck (traffic) V24.4 ☑
            nontraffic V24.0 ☑
          two wheeled motor vehicle (traffic) V22.4 ☑
            nontraffic V22.0 ☑
          van (traffic) V23.4 ☑
            nontraffic V23.0 ☑
        noncollision accident (traffic) V28.4 ☑
          nontraffic V28.0 ☑
      noncollision accident (traffic) V28.9 ☑
        nontraffic V28.2 ☑
        while boarding or alighting V28.3 ☑
      nontraffic V29.3 ☑
      passenger
        collision (with)
          animal (traffic) V20.5 ☑
            being ridden (traffic) V26.5 ☑
              nontraffic V26.1 ☑
            nontraffic V20.1 ☑
          animal-drawn vehicle (traffic) V26.5 ☑
            nontraffic V26.1 ☑
          bus (traffic) V24.5 ☑
            nontraffic V24.1 ☑
          car (traffic) V23.5 ☑

Accident — *continued*
  transport — *continued*
    motorcyclist — *continued*
      passenger — *continued*
        collision — *continued*
          car — *continued*
            nontraffic V23.1 ☑
          motor vehicle NOS (traffic) V29.50 ☑
            nontraffic V29.10 ☑
            specified type NEC (traffic) V29.59 ☑
              nontraffic V29.19 ☑
          pedal cycle (traffic) V21.5 ☑
            nontraffic V21.1 ☑
          pickup truck (traffic) V23.5 ☑
            nontraffic V23.1 ☑
          railway vehicle (traffic) V25.5 ☑
            nontraffic V25.1 ☑
          specified vehicle NEC (traffic) V26.5 ☑
            nontraffic V26.1 ☑
          stationary object (traffic) V27.5 ☑
            nontraffic V27.1 ☑
          streetcar (traffic) V26.5 ☑
            nontraffic V26.1 ☑
          three wheeled motor vehicle (traffic) V22.5 ☑
            nontraffic V22.1 ☑
          truck (traffic) V24.5 ☑
            nontraffic V24.1 ☑
          two wheeled motor vehicle (traffic) V22.5 ☑
            nontraffic V22.1 ☑
          van (traffic) V23.5 ☑
            nontraffic V23.1 ☑
        noncollision accident (traffic) V28.5 ☑
          nontraffic V28.1 ☑
    specified type NEC V29.88 ☑
      military vehicle V29.81 ☑
    occupant (of)
      aircraft (powered) V95.9 ☑
        fixed wing
          commercial — *see* Accident, transport, aircraft, occupant, powered, fixed wing, commercial
          private — *see* Accident, transport, aircraft, occupant, powered, fixed wing, private
        nonpowered V96.9 ☑
        specified NEC V95.8 ☑
      airport battery-powered vehicle — *see* Accident, transport, industrial vehicle occupant
      all-terrain vehicle (ATV) — *see* Accident, transport, all-terrain vehicle occupant
      animal-drawn vehicle — *see* Accident, transport, animal-drawn vehicle occupant
      automobile — *see* Accident, transport, car occupant
      balloon V96.00 ☑
      battery-powered vehicle — *see* Accident, transport, industrial vehicle occupant
      bicycle — *see* Accident, transport, pedal cyclist
        motorized — *see* Accident, transport, motorcycle rider
      boat NEC — *see* Accident, watercraft
      bulldozer — *see* Accident, transport, construction vehicle occupant
      bus — *see* Accident, transport, bus occupant
      cable car (on rails) (*see also* Accident, transport, streetcar occupant)
        not on rails V98.0 ☑
      car (*see also* Accident, transport, car occupant)
        cable (on rails) (*see also* Accident, transport, streetcar occupant)
          not on rails V98.0 ☑
      coach — *see* Accident, transport, bus occupant
      coal-car — *see* Accident, transport, industrial vehicle occupant
      digger — *see* Accident, transport, construction vehicle occupant
      dump truck — *see* Accident, transport, construction vehicle occupant
      earth-leveler — *see* Accident, transport, construction vehicle occupant
      farm machinery (self-propelled) — *see* Accident, transport, agricultural vehicle occupant

☑ **Additional Character Required — Refer to the Tabular List for Character Selection**   🔻 **Subterms under main terms may continue to next column or page**

Accident — *continued*
  transport — *continued*
    occupant — *continued*
      forklift — *see* Accident, transport, industrial vehicle occupant
      glider (unpowered) V96.20 ☑
        hang V96.10 ☑
        powered (microlight) (ultralight) — *see* Accident, transport, aircraft, occupant, powered, glider
      glider (unpowered) NEC V96.20 ☑
      hang-glider V96.10 ☑
      harvester — *see* Accident, transport, agricultural vehicle occupant
      heavy (transport) vehicle — *see* Accident, transport, truck occupant
      helicopter — *see* Accident, transport, aircraft, occupant, helicopter
      ice-yacht V98.2 ☑
      kite (carrying person) V96.8 ☑
      land-yacht V98.1 ☑
      logging car — *see* Accident, transport, industrial vehicle occupant
      mechanical shovel — *see* Accident, transport, construction vehicle occupant
      microlight — *see* Accident, transport, aircraft, occupant, powered, glider
      minibus — *see* Accident, transport, pickup truck occupant
      minivan — *see* Accident, transport, pickup truck occupant
      moped — *see* Accident, transport, motorcycle
      motor scooter — *see* Accident, transport, motorcycle
      motorcycle (with sidecar) — *see* Accident, transport, motorcycle
      off-road motor-vehicle (*see also* Accident, transport, all-terrain vehicle occupant) V86.99 ☑
      pedal cycle (*see also* Accident, transport, pedal cyclist)
      pick-up (truck) — *see* Accident, transport, pickup truck occupant
      railway (train) (vehicle) (subterranean) (elevated) — *see* Accident, transport, railway vehicle occupant
      rickshaw — *see* Accident, transport, pedal cycle
        motorized — *see* Accident, transport, three-wheeled motor vehicle
        pedal driven — *see* Accident, transport, pedal cyclist
      road-roller — *see* Accident, transport, construction vehicle occupant
      ship NOS V94.9 ☑
      ski-lift (chair) (gondola) V98.3 ☑
      snowmobile — *see* Accident, transport, snowmobile occupant
      spacecraft, spaceship — *see* Accident, transport, aircraft, occupant, spacecraft
      sport utility vehicle — *see* Accident, transport, pickup truck occupant
      streetcar (interurban) (operating on public street or highway) — *see* Accident, transport, streetcar occupant
      SUV — *see* Accident, transport, pickup truck occupant
      téléférique V98.0 ☑
      three-wheeled vehicle (motorized) (*see also* Accident, transport, three-wheeled motor vehicle occupant)
        nonmotorized — *see* Accident, transport, pedal cycle
      tractor (farm) (and trailer) — *see* Accident, transport, agricultural vehicle occupant
      train — *see* Accident, transport, railway vehicle occupant
      tram — *see* Accident, transport, streetcar occupant
        in mine or quarry — *see* Accident, transport, industrial vehicle occupant
      tricycle — *see* Accident, transport, pedal cycle
        motorized — *see* Accident, transport, three-wheeled motor vehicle
      trolley — *see* Accident, transport, streetcar occupant
        in mine or quarry — *see* Accident, transport, industrial vehicle occupant

Accident — *continued*
  transport — *continued*
    occupant — *continued*
      tub, in mine or quarry — *see* Accident, transport, industrial vehicle occupant
      ultralight — *see* Accident, transport, aircraft, occupant, powered, glider
      van — *see* Accident, transport, van occupant
      vehicle NEC V89.9 ☑
        heavy transport — *see* Accident, transport, truck occupant
        motor (traffic) NEC V89.2 ☑
        nontraffic NEC V89.0 ☑
      watercraft NOS V94.9 ☑
        causing drowning — *see* Drowning, resulting from accident to boat
    off-road motor-vehicle (*see also* Accident, transport, all-terrain vehicle occupant) V86.99 ☑
    parachutist V97.29 ☑
      after accident to aircraft — *see* Accident, transport, aircraft
      entangled in object V97.21 ☑
      injured on landing V97.22 ☑
    pedal cyclist V19.9 ☑
      collision (with)
        animal (traffic) V10.9 ☑
          being ridden (traffic) V16.9 ☑
            nontraffic V16.2 ☑
            while boarding or alighting V16.3 ☑
          nontraffic V10.2 ☑
          while boarding or alighting V10.3 ☑
        animal-drawn vehicle (traffic) V16.9 ☑
          nontraffic V16.2 ☑
          while boarding or alighting V16.3 ☑
        bus (traffic) V14.9 ☑
          nontraffic V14.2 ☑
          while boarding or alighting V14.3 ☑
        car (traffic) V13.9 ☑
          nontraffic V13.2 ☑
          while boarding or alighting V13.3 ☑
        motor vehicle NOS (traffic) V19.60 ☑
          nontraffic V19.20 ☑
          specified type NEC (traffic) V19.69 ☑
            nontraffic V19.29 ☑
        pedal cycle (traffic) V11.9 ☑
          nontraffic V11.2 ☑
          while boarding or alighting V11.3 ☑
        pickup truck (traffic) V13.9 ☑
          nontraffic V13.2 ☑
          while boarding or alighting V13.3 ☑
        railway vehicle (traffic) V15.9 ☑
          nontraffic V15.2 ☑
          while boarding or alighting V15.3 ☑
        specified vehicle NEC (traffic) V16.9 ☑
          nontraffic V16.2 ☑
          while boarding or alighting V16.3 ☑
        stationary object (traffic) V17.9 ☑
          nontraffic V17.2 ☑
          while boarding or alighting V17.3 ☑
        streetcar (traffic) V16.9 ☑
          nontraffic V16.2 ☑
          while boarding or alighting V16.3 ☑
        three wheeled motor vehicle (traffic) V12.9 ☑
          nontraffic V12.2 ☑
          while boarding or alighting V12.3 ☑
        truck (traffic) V14.9 ☑
          nontraffic V14.2 ☑
          while boarding or alighting V14.3 ☑
        two wheeled motor vehicle (traffic) V12.9 ☑
          nontraffic V12.2 ☑
          while boarding or alighting V12.3 ☑
        van (traffic) V13.9 ☑
          nontraffic V13.2 ☑
          while boarding or alighting V13.3 ☑
      driver
        collision (with)
          animal (traffic) V10.4 ☑
            being ridden (traffic) V16.4 ☑
              nontraffic V16.0 ☑
            nontraffic V10.0 ☑
          animal-drawn vehicle (traffic) V16.4 ☑
            nontraffic V16.0 ☑
          bus (traffic) V14.4 ☑
            nontraffic V14.0 ☑
          car (traffic) V13.4 ☑

Accident — *continued*
  transport — *continued*
    pedal cyclist — *continued*
      driver — *continued*
        collision — *continued*
          car — *continued*
            nontraffic V13.0 ☑
          motor vehicle NOS (traffic) V19.40 ☑
            nontraffic V19.00 ☑
            specified type NEC (traffic) V19.49 ☑
              nontraffic V19.09 ☑
          pedal cycle (traffic) V11.4 ☑
            nontraffic V11.0 ☑
          pickup truck (traffic) V13.4 ☑
            nontraffic V13.0 ☑
          railway vehicle (traffic) V15.4 ☑
            nontraffic V15.0 ☑
          specified vehicle NEC (traffic) V16.4 ☑
            nontraffic V16.0 ☑
          stationary object (traffic) V17.4 ☑
            nontraffic V17.0 ☑
          streetcar (traffic) V16.4 ☑
            nontraffic V16.0 ☑
          three wheeled motor vehicle (traffic) V12.4 ☑
            nontraffic V12.0 ☑
          truck (traffic) V14.4 ☑
            nontraffic V14.0 ☑
          two wheeled motor vehicle (traffic) V12.4 ☑
            nontraffic V12.0 ☑
          van (traffic) V13.4 ☑
            nontraffic V13.0 ☑
        noncollision accident (traffic) V18.4 ☑
          nontraffic V18.0 ☑
      noncollision accident (traffic) V18.9 ☑
        nontraffic V18.2 ☑
        while boarding or alighting V18.3 ☑
      nontraffic V19.3 ☑
      passenger
        collision (with)
          animal (traffic) V10.5 ☑
            being ridden (traffic) V16.5 ☑
              nontraffic V16.1 ☑
            nontraffic V10.1 ☑
          animal-drawn vehicle (traffic) V16.5 ☑
            nontraffic V16.1 ☑
          bus (traffic) V14.5 ☑
            nontraffic V14.1 ☑
          car (traffic) V13.5 ☑
            nontraffic V13.1 ☑
          motor vehicle NOS (traffic) V19.50 ☑
            nontraffic V19.10 ☑
            specified type NEC (traffic) V19.59 ☑
              nontraffic V19.19 ☑
          pedal cycle (traffic) V11.5 ☑
            nontraffic V11.1 ☑
          pickup truck (traffic) V13.5 ☑
            nontraffic V13.1 ☑
          railway vehicle (traffic) V15.5 ☑
            nontraffic V15.1 ☑
          specified vehicle NEC (traffic) V16.5 ☑
            nontraffic V16.1 ☑
          stationary object (traffic) V17.5 ☑
            nontraffic V17.1 ☑
          streetcar (traffic) V16.5 ☑
            nontraffic V16.1 ☑
          three wheeled motor vehicle (traffic) V12.5 ☑
            nontraffic V12.1 ☑
          truck (traffic) V14.5 ☑
            nontraffic V14.1 ☑
          two wheeled motor vehicle (traffic) V12.5 ☑
            nontraffic V12.1 ☑
          van (traffic) V13.5 ☑
            nontraffic V13.1 ☑
        noncollision accident (traffic) V18.5 ☑
          nontraffic V18.1 ☑
      specified type NEC V19.88 ☑
        military vehicle V19.81 ☑
    pedestrian
      conveyance (occupant) V09.9 ☑
        babystroller V00.828 ☑
          collision (with) V09.9 ☑

Accident — *continued*
transport — *continued*
pedestrian — *continued*
conveyance — *continued*
babystroller — *continued*
collision — *continued*
animal being ridden or animal drawn vehicle V06.99 ☑
nontraffic V06.09 ☑
traffic V06.19 ☑
bus or heavy transport V04.99 ☑
nontraffic V04.09 ☑
traffic V04.19 ☑
car V03.99 ☑
nontraffic V03.09 ☑
traffic V03.19 ☑
pedal cycle V01.99 ☑
nontraffic V01.09 ☑
traffic V01.19 ☑
pick-up truck or van V03.99 ☑
nontraffic V03.09 ☑
traffic V03.19 ☑
railway (train) (vehicle) V05.99 ☑
nontraffic V05.09 ☑
traffic V05.19 ☑
stationary object V00.822 ☑
streetcar V06.99 ☑
nontraffic V06.09 ☑
traffic V06.19 ☑
two- or three-wheeled motor vehicle V02.99 ☑
nontraffic V02.09 ☑
traffic V02.19 ☑
vehicle V09.9 ☑
animal-drawn V06.99 ☑
nontraffic V06.09 ☑
traffic V06.19 ☑
motor
nontraffic V09.00 ☑
traffic V09.20 ☑
fall V00.821 ☑
nontraffic V09.1 ☑
involving motor vehicle NEC V09.00 ☑
traffic V09.3 ☑
involving motor vehicle NEC V09.20 ☑
flat-bottomed NEC V00.388 ☑
collision (with) V09.9 ☑
animal being ridden or animal drawn vehicle V06.99 ☑
nontraffic V06.09 ☑
traffic V06.19 ☑
bus or heavy transport V04.99 ☑
nontraffic V04.09 ☑
traffic V04.19 ☑
car V03.99 ☑
nontraffic V03.09 ☑
traffic V03.19 ☑
pedal cycle V01.99 ☑
nontraffic V01.09 ☑
traffic V01.19 ☑
pick-up truck or van V03.99 ☑
nontraffic V03.09 ☑
traffic V03.19 ☑
railway (train) (vehicle) V05.99 ☑
nontraffic V05.09 ☑
traffic V05.19 ☑
stationary object V00.382 ☑
streetcar V06.99 ☑
nontraffic V06.09 ☑
traffic V06.19 ☑
two- or three-wheeled motor vehicle V02.99 ☑
nontraffic V02.09 ☑
traffic V02.19 ☑
vehicle V09.9 ☑
animal-drawn V06.99 ☑
nontraffic V06.09 ☑
traffic V06.19 ☑
motor
nontraffic V09.00 ☑
traffic V09.20 ☑
fall V00.381 ☑
nontraffic V09.1 ☑

Accident — *continued*
transport — *continued*
pedestrian — *continued*
conveyance — *continued*
flat-bottomed — *continued*
nontraffic — *continued*
involving motor vehicle NEC V09.00 ☑
snow
board — *see* Accident, transport, pedestrian, conveyance, snow board
ski — *see* Accident, transport, pedestrian, conveyance, skis (snow)
traffic V09.3 ☑
involving motor vehicle NEC V09.20 ☑
gliding type NEC V00.288 ☑
collision (with) V09.9 ☑
animal being ridden or animal drawn vehicle V06.99 ☑
nontraffic V06.09 ☑
traffic V06.19 ☑
bus or heavy transport V04.99 ☑
nontraffic V04.09 ☑
traffic V04.19 ☑
car V03.99 ☑
nontraffic V03.09 ☑
traffic V03.19 ☑
pedal cycle V01.99 ☑
nontraffic V01.09 ☑
traffic V01.19 ☑
pick-up truck or van V03.99 ☑
nontraffic V03.09 ☑
traffic V03.19 ☑
railway (train) (vehicle) V05.99 ☑
nontraffic V05.09 ☑
traffic V05.19 ☑
stationary object V00.282 ☑
streetcar V06.99 ☑
nontraffic V06.09 ☑
traffic V02.19 ☑
two- or three-wheeled motor vehicle V02.99 ☑
nontraffic V02.09 ☑
traffic V02.19 ☑
vehicle V09.9 ☑
animal-drawn V06.99 ☑
nontraffic V06.09 ☑
traffic V06.19 ☑
motor
nontraffic V09.00 ☑
traffic V09.20 ☑
fall V00.281 ☑
heelies — *see* Accident, transport, pedestrian, conveyance, heelies
ice skate — *see* Accident, transport, pedestrian, conveyance, ice skate
nontraffic V09.1 ☑
involving motor vehicle NEC V09.00 ☑
sled — *see* Accident, transport, pedestrian, conveyance, sled
traffic V09.3 ☑
involving motor vehicle NEC V09.20 ☑
wheelies — *see* Accident, transport, pedestrian, conveyance, heelies
heelies V00.158 ☑
colliding with stationary object V00.152 ☑
fall V00.151 ☑
ice skates V00.218 ☑
collision (with) V09.9 ☑
animal being ridden or animal drawn vehicle V06.99 ☑
nontraffic V06.09 ☑
traffic V06.19 ☑
bus or heavy transport V04.99 ☑
nontraffic V04.09 ☑
traffic V04.19 ☑
car V03.99 ☑
nontraffic V03.09 ☑
traffic V03.19 ☑

Accident — *continued*
transport — *continued*
pedestrian — *continued*
conveyance — *continued*
ice skates — *continued*
collision — *continued*
pedal cycle V01.99 ☑
nontraffic V01.09 ☑
traffic V01.19 ☑
pick-up truck or van V03.99 ☑
nontraffic V03.09 ☑
traffic V03.19 ☑
railway (train) (vehicle) V05.99 ☑
nontraffic V05.09 ☑
traffic V05.19 ☑
stationary object V00.212 ☑
streetcar V06.99 ☑
nontraffic V06.09 ☑
traffic V06.19 ☑
two- or three-wheeled motor vehicle V02.99 ☑
nontraffic V02.09 ☑
traffic V02.19 ☑
vehicle V09.9 ☑
animal-drawn V06.99 ☑
nontraffic V06.09 ☑
traffic V06.19 ☑
motor
nontraffic V09.00 ☑
traffic V09.20 ☑
fall V00.211 ☑
nontraffic V09.1 ☑
involving motor vehicle NEC V09.00 ☑
traffic V09.3 ☑
involving motor vehicle NEC V09.20 ☑
motorized mobility scooter V00.838 ☑
collision with stationary object V00.832 ☑
fall from V00.831 ☑
nontraffic V09.1 ☑
involving motor vehicle V09.00 ☑
military V09.01 ☑
specified type NEC V09.09 ☑
roller skates (non in-line) V00.128 ☑
collision (with) V09.9 ☑
animal being ridden or animal drawn vehicle V06.91 ☑
nontraffic V06.01 ☑
traffic V06.11 ☑
bus or heavy transport V04.91 ☑
nontraffic V04.01 ☑
traffic V04.11 ☑
car V03.91 ☑
nontraffic V03.01 ☑
traffic V03.11 ☑
pedal cycle V01.91 ☑
nontraffic V01.01 ☑
traffic V01.11 ☑
pick-up truck or van V03.91 ☑
nontraffic V03.01 ☑
traffic V03.11 ☑
railway (train) (vehicle) V05.91 ☑
nontraffic V05.01 ☑
traffic V05.11 ☑
stationary object V00.122 ☑
streetcar V06.91 ☑
nontraffic V06.01 ☑
traffic V06.11 ☑
two- or three-wheeled motor vehicle V02.91 ☑
nontraffic V02.01 ☑
traffic V02.11 ☑
vehicle V09.9 ☑
animal-drawn V06.91 ☑
nontraffic V06.01 ☑
traffic V06.11 ☑
motor
nontraffic V09.00 ☑
traffic V09.20 ☑
fall V00.121 ☑
in-line V00.118 ☑

Accident — *continued*
  transport — *continued*
    pedestrian — *continued*
      conveyance — *continued*
        roller skates — *continued*
          in-line — *continued*
            collision — *see also* Accident, transport, pedestrian, conveyance occupant, roller skates, collision
              with stationary object V00.112 ☑
            fall V00.111 ☑
          nontraffic V09.1 ☑
            involving motor vehicle NEC V09.00 ☑
          traffic V09.3 ☑
            involving motor vehicle NEC V09.20 ☑
        rolling shoes V00.158 ☑
          colliding with stationary object V00.152 ☑
          fall V00.151 ☑
        rolling type NEC V00.188 ☑
          collision (with) V09.9 ☑
            animal being ridden or animal drawn vehicle V06.99 ☑
              nontraffic V06.09 ☑
              traffic V06.19 ☑
            bus or heavy transport V04.99 ☑
              nontraffic V04.09 ☑
              traffic V04.19 ☑
            car V03.99 ☑
              nontraffic V03.09 ☑
              traffic V03.19 ☑
            pedal cycle V01.99 ☑
              nontraffic V01.09 ☑
              traffic V01.19 ☑
            pick-up truck or van V03.99 ☑
              nontraffic V03.09 ☑
              traffic V03.19 ☑
            railway (train) (vehicle) V05.99 ☑
              nontraffic V05.09 ☑
              traffic V05.19 ☑
            stationary object V00.182 ☑
            streetcar V06.99 ☑
              nontraffic V06.09 ☑
              traffic V06.19 ☑
            two- or three-wheeled motor vehicle V02.99 ☑
              nontraffic V02.09 ☑
              traffic V02.19 ☑
            vehicle V09.9 ☑
              animal-drawn V06.99 ☑
                nontraffic V06.09 ☑
                traffic V06.19 ☑
              motor
                nontraffic V09.00 ☑
                traffic V09.20 ☑
          fall V00.181 ☑
        in-line roller skate — *see* Accident, transport, pedestrian, conveyance, roller skate, in-line
        nontraffic V09.1 ☑
          involving motor vehicle NEC V09.00 ☑
        roller skate — *see* Accident, transport, pedestrian, conveyance, roller skate
        scooter (non-motorized) — *see* Accident, transport, pedestrian, conveyance, scooter
        skateboard — *see* Accident, transport, pedestrian, conveyance, skateboard
        traffic V09.3 ☑
          involving motor vehicle NEC V09.20 ☑
        scooter (non-motorized) V00.148 ☑
          collision (with) V09.9 ☑
            animal being ridden or animal drawn vehicle V06.99 ☑
              nontraffic V06.09 ☑
              traffic V06.19 ☑
            bus or heavy transport V04.99 ☑
              nontraffic V04.09 ☑
              traffic V04.19 ☑

Accident — *continued*
  transport — *continued*
    pedestrian — *continued*
      conveyance — *continued*
        scooter — *continued*
          collision — *continued*
            car V03.99 ☑
              nontraffic V03.09 ☑
              traffic V03.19 ☑
            pedal cycle V01.99 ☑
              nontraffic V01.09 ☑
              traffic V01.19 ☑
            pick-up truck or van V03.99 ☑
              nontraffic V03.09 ☑
              traffic V03.19 ☑
            railway (train) (vehicle) V05.99 ☑
              nontraffic V05.09 ☑
              traffic V05.19 ☑
            stationary object V00.142 ☑
            streetcar V06.99 ☑
              nontraffic V06.09 ☑
              traffic V06.19 ☑
            two- or three-wheeled motor vehicle V02.99 ☑
              nontraffic V02.09 ☑
              traffic V02.19 ☑
            vehicle V09.9 ☑
              animal-drawn V06.99 ☑
                nontraffic V06.09 ☑
                traffic V06.19 ☑
              motor
                nontraffic V09.00 ☑
                traffic V09.20 ☑
          fall V00.141 ☑
          nontraffic V09.1 ☑
            involving motor vehicle NEC V09.00 ☑
          traffic V09.3 ☑
            involving motor vehicle NEC V09.20 ☑
        skate board V00.138 ☑
          collision (with) V09.9 ☑
            animal being ridden or animal drawn vehicle V06.92 ☑
              nontraffic V06.02 ☑
              traffic V06.12 ☑
            bus or heavy transport V04.92 ☑
              nontraffic V04.02 ☑
              traffic V04.12 ☑
            car V03.92 ☑
              nontraffic V03.02 ☑
              traffic V03.12 ☑
            pedal cycle V01.92 ☑
              nontraffic V01.02 ☑
              traffic V01.12 ☑
            pick-up truck or van V03.92 ☑
              nontraffic V03.02 ☑
              traffic V03.12 ☑
            railway (train) (vehicle) V05.92 ☑
              nontraffic V05.02 ☑
              traffic V05.12 ☑
            stationary object V00.132 ☑
            streetcar V06.92 ☑
              nontraffic V06.02 ☑
              traffic V06.12 ☑
            two- or three-wheeled motor vehicle V02.92 ☑
              nontraffic V02.02 ☑
              traffic V02.12 ☑
            vehicle V09.9 ☑
              animal-drawn V06.92 ☑
                nontraffic V06.02 ☑
                traffic V06.12 ☑
              motor
                nontraffic V09.00 ☑
                traffic V09.20 ☑
          fall V00.131 ☑
          nontraffic V09.1 ☑
            involving motor vehicle NEC V09.00 ☑
          traffic V09.3 ☑
            involving motor vehicle NEC V09.20 ☑
        skis (snow) V00.328 ☑
          collision (with) V09.9 ☑

Accident — *continued*
  transport — *continued*
    pedestrian — *continued*
      conveyance — *continued*
        skis — *continued*
          collision — *continued*
            animal being ridden or animal drawn vehicle V06.99 ☑
              nontraffic V06.09 ☑
              traffic V06.19 ☑
            bus or heavy transport V04.99 ☑
              nontraffic V04.09 ☑
              traffic V04.19 ☑
            car V03.99 ☑
              nontraffic V03.09 ☑
              traffic V03.19 ☑
            pedal cycle V01.99 ☑
              nontraffic V01.09 ☑
              traffic V01.19 ☑
            pick-up truck or van V03.99 ☑
              nontraffic V03.09 ☑
              traffic V03.19 ☑
            railway (train) (vehicle) V05.99 ☑
              nontraffic V05.09 ☑
              traffic V05.19 ☑
            stationary object V00.322 ☑
            streetcar V06.99 ☑
              nontraffic V06.09 ☑
              traffic V06.19 ☑
            two- or three-wheeled motor vehicle V02.99 ☑
              nontraffic V02.09 ☑
              traffic V02.19 ☑
            vehicle V09.9 ☑
              animal-drawn V06.99 ☑
                nontraffic V06.09 ☑
                traffic V06.19 ☑
              motor
                nontraffic V09.00 ☑
                traffic V09.20 ☑
          fall V00.321 ☑
          nontraffic V09.1 ☑
            involving motor vehicle NEC V09.00 ☑
          traffic V09.3 ☑
            involving motor vehicle NEC V09.20 ☑
        sled V00.228 ☑
          collision (with) V09.9 ☑
            animal being ridden or animal drawn vehicle V06.99 ☑
              nontraffic V06.09 ☑
              traffic V06.19 ☑
            bus or heavy transport V04.99 ☑
              nontraffic V04.09 ☑
              traffic V04.19 ☑
            car V03.99 ☑
              nontraffic V03.09 ☑
              traffic V03.19 ☑
            pedal cycle V01.99 ☑
              nontraffic V01.09 ☑
              traffic V01.19 ☑
            pick-up truck or van V03.99 ☑
              nontraffic V03.09 ☑
              traffic V03.19 ☑
            railway (train) (vehicle) V05.99 ☑
              nontraffic V05.09 ☑
              traffic V05.19 ☑
            stationary object V00.222 ☑
            streetcar V06.99 ☑
              nontraffic V06.09 ☑
              traffic V06.19 ☑
            two- or three-wheeled motor vehicle V02.99 ☑
              nontraffic V02.09 ☑
              traffic V02.19 ☑
            vehicle V09.9 ☑
              animal-drawn V06.99 ☑
                nontraffic V06.09 ☑
                traffic V06.19 ☑
              motor
                nontraffic V09.00 ☑
                traffic V09.20 ☑
          fall V00.221 ☑
          nontraffic V09.1 ☑

Accident — *continued*
  transport — *continued*
    pedestrian — *continued*
      conveyance — *continued*
        sled — *continued*
          nontraffic — *continued*
            involving motor vehicle NEC V09.00 ☑
          traffic V09.3 ☑
            involving motor vehicle NEC V09.20 ☑
        snow board V00.318 ☑
          collision (with) V09.9 ☑
            animal being ridden or animal drawn vehicle V06.99 ☑
              nontraffic V06.09 ☑
              traffic V06.19 ☑
            bus or heavy transport V04.99 ☑
              nontraffic V04.09 ☑
              traffic V04.19 ☑
            car V03.99 ☑
              nontraffic V03.09 ☑
              traffic V03.19 ☑
            pedal cycle V01.99 ☑
              nontraffic V01.09 ☑
              traffic V01.19 ☑
            pick-up truck or van V03.99 ☑
              nontraffic V03.09 ☑
              traffic V03.19 ☑
            railway (train) (vehicle) V05.99 ☑
              nontraffic V05.09 ☑
              traffic V05.19 ☑
            stationary object V00.312 ☑
            streetcar V06.99 ☑
              nontraffic V06.09 ☑
              traffic V06.19 ☑
            two- or three-wheeled motor vehicle V02.99 ☑
              nontraffic V02.09 ☑
              traffic V02.19 ☑
            vehicle V09.9 ☑
              animal-drawn V06.99 ☑
                nontraffic V06.09 ☑
                traffic V06.19 ☑
              motor
                nontraffic V09.00 ☑
                traffic V09.20 ☑
        fall V00.311 ☑
        nontraffic V09.1 ☑
          involving motor vehicle NEC V09.00 ☑
        traffic V09.3 ☑
          involving motor vehicle NEC V09.20 ☑
        specified type NEC V00.898 ☑
          collision (with) V09.9 ☑
            animal being ridden or animal drawn vehicle V06.99 ☑
              nontraffic V06.09 ☑
              traffic V06.19 ☑
            bus or heavy transport V04.99 ☑
              nontraffic V04.09 ☑
              traffic V04.19 ☑
            car V03.99 ☑
              nontraffic V03.09 ☑
              traffic V03.19 ☑
            pedal cycle V01.99 ☑
              nontraffic V01.09 ☑
              traffic V01.19 ☑
            pick-up truck or van V03.99 ☑
              nontraffic V03.09 ☑
              traffic V03.19 ☑
            railway (train) (vehicle) V05.99 ☑
              nontraffic V05.09 ☑
              traffic V05.19 ☑
            stationary object V00.892 ☑
            streetcar V06.99 ☑
              nontraffic V06.09 ☑
              traffic V06.19 ☑
            two- or three-wheeled motor vehicle V02.99 ☑
              nontraffic V02.09 ☑
              traffic V02.19 ☑
            vehicle V09.9 ☑
              animal-drawn V06.99 ☑
                nontraffic V06.09 ☑

Accident — *continued*
  transport — *continued*
    pedestrian — *continued*
      conveyance — *continued*
        specified type — *continued*
          collision — *continued*
            vehicle — *continued*
              animal-drawn — *continued*
                traffic V06.19 ☑
              motor
                nontraffic V09.00 ☑
                traffic V09.20 ☑
          fall V00.891 ☑
          nontraffic V09.1 ☑
            involving motor vehicle NEC V09.00 ☑
          traffic V09.3 ☑
            involving motor vehicle NEC V09.20 ☑
        traffic V09.3 ☑
          involving motor vehicle V09.20 ☑
            military V09.21 ☑
            specified type NEC V09.29 ☑
        wheelchair (powered) V00.818 ☑
          collision (with) V09.9 ☑
            animal being ridden or animal drawn vehicle V06.99 ☑
              nontraffic V06.09 ☑
              traffic V06.19 ☑
            bus or heavy transport V04.99 ☑
              nontraffic V04.09 ☑
              traffic V04.19 ☑
            car V03.99 ☑
              nontraffic V03.09 ☑
              traffic V03.19 ☑
            pedal cycle V01.99 ☑
              nontraffic V01.09 ☑
              traffic V01.19 ☑
            pick-up truck or van V03.99 ☑
              nontraffic V03.09 ☑
              traffic V03.19 ☑
            railway (train) (vehicle) V05.99 ☑
              nontraffic V05.09 ☑
            stationary object V00.812 ☑
            streetcar V06.99 ☑
              nontraffic V06.09 ☑
              traffic V06.19 ☑
            two- or three-wheeled motor vehicle V02.99 ☑
              nontraffic V02.09 ☑
              traffic V02.19 ☑
            vehicle V09.9 ☑
              animal-drawn V06.99 ☑
                nontraffic V06.09 ☑
                traffic V06.19 ☑
              motor
                nontraffic V09.00 ☑
                traffic V09.20 ☑
         fall V00.811 ☑
        nontraffic V09.1 ☑
          involving motor vehicle NEC V09.00 ☑
        traffic V09.3 ☑
          involving motor vehicle NEC V09.20 ☑
        wheeled shoe V00.158 ☑
          colliding with stationary object V00.152 ☑
          fall V00.151 ☑
      on foot (*see also* Accident, pedestrian)
        collision (with)
          animal being ridden or animal drawn vehicle V06.90 ☑
            nontraffic V06.00 ☑
            traffic V06.10 ☑
          bus or heavy transport V04.90 ☑
            nontraffic V04.00 ☑
            traffic V04.10 ☑
          car V03.90 ☑
            nontraffic V03.00 ☑
            traffic V03.10 ☑
          pedal cycle V01.90 ☑
            nontraffic V01.00 ☑
            traffic V01.10 ☑
          pick-up truck or van V03.90 ☑

Accident — *continued*
  transport — *continued*
    pedestrian — *continued*
      on foot (*see also* Accident, pedestrian) — *continued*
        collision — *continued*
          pick-up truck or van — *continued*
            nontraffic V03.00 ☑
            traffic V03.10 ☑
          railway (train) (vehicle) V05.90 ☑
            nontraffic V05.00 ☑
            traffic V05.10 ☑
          streetcar V06.90 ☑
            nontraffic V06.00 ☑
            traffic V06.10 ☑
          two- or three-wheeled motor vehicle V02.90 ☑
            nontraffic V02.00 ☑
            traffic V02.10 ☑
          vehicle V09.9 ☑
            animal-drawn V06.90 ☑
              nontraffic V06.00 ☑
              traffic V06.10 ☑
            motor
        nontraffic V09.1 ☑
          involving motor vehicle V09.00 ☑
            military V09.01 ☑
            specified type NEC V09.09 ☑
        traffic V09.3 ☑
          involving motor vehicle V09.20 ☑
            military V09.21 ☑
            specified type NEC V09.29 ☑
    person NEC (unknown way or transportation) V99 ☑
    collision (between)
      bus (with)
        heavy transport vehicle (traffic) V87.5 ☑
          nontraffic V88.5 ☑
      car (with)
        bus (traffic) V87.3 ☑
          nontraffic V88.3 ☑
        heavy transport vehicle (traffic) V87.4 ☑
          nontraffic V88.4 ☑
          nontraffic V88.5 ☑
        pick-up truck or van (traffic) V87.2 ☑
          nontraffic V88.2 ☑
        train or railway vehicle (traffic) V87.6 ☑
          nontraffic V88.6 ☑
        two-or three-wheeled motor vehicle (traffic) V87.0 ☑
          nontraffic V88.0 ☑
        motor vehicle (traffic) NEC V87.7 ☑
          nontraffic V88.7 ☑
      two-or three-wheeled vehicle (with) (traffic)
        motor vehicle NEC V87.1 ☑
          nontraffic V88.1 ☑
      nonmotor vehicle (collision) (noncollision) (traffic) V87.9 ☑
        nontraffic V88.9 ☑
    pickup truck occupant V59.9 ☑
      collision (with)
        animal (traffic) V50.9 ☑
          being ridden (traffic) V56.9 ☑
            nontraffic V56.3 ☑
            while boarding or alighting V56.4 ☑
          nontraffic V50.3 ☑
          while boarding or alighting V50.4 ☑
        animal-drawn vehicle (traffic) V56.9 ☑
          nontraffic V56.3 ☑
          while boarding or alighting V56.4 ☑
        bus (traffic) V54.9 ☑
          nontraffic V54.3 ☑
          while boarding or alighting V54.4 ☑
        car (traffic) V53.9 ☑
          nontraffic V53.3 ☑
          while boarding or alighting V53.4 ☑
        motor vehicle NOS (traffic) V59.60 ☑
          nontraffic V59.20 ☑
          specified type NEC (traffic) V59.69 ☑
            nontraffic V59.29 ☑
        pedal cycle (traffic) V51.9 ☑
          nontraffic V51.3 ☑
          while boarding or alighting V51.4 ☑
        pickup truck (traffic) V53.9 ☑
          nontraffic V53.3 ☑
          while boarding or alighting V53.4 ☑

☑ Additional Character Required — Refer to the Tabular List for Character Selection   ▽ Subterms under main terms may continue to next column or page

Accident — *continued*
  transport — *continued*
    pickup truck occupant — *continued*
      collision — *continued*
        railway vehicle (traffic) V55.9 ☑
          nontraffic V55.3 ☑
          while boarding or alighting V55.4 ☑
        specified vehicle NEC (traffic) V56.9 ☑
          nontraffic V56.3 ☑
          while boarding or alighting V56.4 ☑
        stationary object (traffic) V57.9 ☑
          nontraffic V57.3 ☑
          while boarding or alighting V57.4 ☑
        streetcar (traffic) V56.9 ☑
          nontraffic V56.3 ☑
          while boarding or alighting V56.4 ☑
        three wheeled motor vehicle (traffic)
          V52.9 ☑
          nontraffic V52.3 ☑
          while boarding or alighting V52.4 ☑
        truck (traffic) V54.9 ☑
          nontraffic V54.3 ☑
          while boarding or alighting V54.4 ☑
        two wheeled motor vehicle (traffic) V52.9 ☑
          nontraffic V52.3 ☑
          while boarding or alighting V52.4 ☑
        van (traffic) V53.9 ☑
          nontraffic V53.3 ☑
          while boarding or alighting V53.4 ☑
    driver
      collision (with)
        animal (traffic) V50.5 ☑
          being ridden (traffic) V56.5 ☑
            nontraffic V56.0 ☑
          nontraffic V50.0 ☑
        animal-drawn vehicle (traffic) V56.5 ☑
          nontraffic V56.0 ☑
        bus (traffic) V54.5 ☑
          nontraffic V54.0 ☑
        car (traffic) V53.5 ☑
          nontraffic V53.0 ☑
        motor vehicle NOS (traffic) V59.40 ☑
          nontraffic V59.00 ☑
          specified type NEC (traffic) V59.49 ☑
            nontraffic V59.09 ☑
        pedal cycle (traffic) V51.5 ☑
          nontraffic V51.0 ☑
        pickup truck (traffic) V53.5 ☑
          nontraffic V53.0 ☑
        railway vehicle (traffic) V55.5 ☑
          nontraffic V55.0 ☑
        specified vehicle NEC (traffic) V56.5 ☑
          nontraffic V56.0 ☑
        stationary object (traffic) V57.5 ☑
          nontraffic V57.0 ☑
        streetcar (traffic) V56.5 ☑
          nontraffic V56.0 ☑
        three wheeled motor vehicle (traffic)
          V52.5 ☑
          nontraffic V52.0 ☑
        truck (traffic) V54.5 ☑
          nontraffic V54.0 ☑
        two wheeled motor vehicle (traffic)
          V52.5 ☑
          nontraffic V52.0 ☑
        van (traffic) V53.5 ☑
          nontraffic V53.0 ☑
      noncollision accident (traffic) V58.5 ☑
        nontraffic V58.0 ☑
    hanger-on
      collision (with)
        animal (traffic) V50.7 ☑
          being ridden (traffic) V56.7 ☑
            nontraffic V56.2 ☑
          nontraffic V50.2 ☑
        animal-drawn vehicle (traffic) V56.7 ☑
          nontraffic V56.2 ☑
        bus (traffic) V54.7 ☑
          nontraffic V54.2 ☑
        car (traffic) V53.7 ☑
          nontraffic V53.2 ☑
        pedal cycle (traffic) V51.7 ☑
          nontraffic V51.2 ☑
        pickup truck (traffic) V53.7 ☑
          nontraffic V53.2 ☑
        railway vehicle (traffic) V55.7 ☑

Accident — *continued*
  transport — *continued*
    pickup truck occupant — *continued*
      hanger-on — *continued*
        collision — *continued*
          railway vehicle — *continued*
            nontraffic V55.2 ☑
          specified vehicle NEC (traffic) V56.7 ☑
            nontraffic V56.2 ☑
          stationary object (traffic) V57.7 ☑
            nontraffic V57.2 ☑
          streetcar (traffic) V56.7 ☑
            nontraffic V56.2 ☑
          three wheeled motor vehicle (traffic)
            V52.7 ☑
            nontraffic V52.2 ☑
          truck (traffic) V54.7 ☑
            nontraffic V54.2 ☑
          two wheeled motor vehicle (traffic)
            V52.7 ☑
            nontraffic V52.2 ☑
          van (traffic) V53.7 ☑
            nontraffic V53.2 ☑
        noncollision accident (traffic) V58.7 ☑
          nontraffic V58.2 ☑
      noncollision accident (traffic) V58.9 ☑
        nontraffic V58.3 ☑
        while boarding or alighting V58.4 ☑
      nontraffic V59.3 ☑
      passenger
        collision (with)
          animal (traffic) V50.6 ☑
            being ridden (traffic) V56.6 ☑
              nontraffic V56.1 ☑
            nontraffic V50.1 ☑
          animal-drawn vehicle (traffic) V56.6 ☑
            nontraffic V56.1 ☑
          bus (traffic) V54.6 ☑
            nontraffic V54.1 ☑
          car (traffic) V53.6 ☑
            nontraffic V53.1 ☑
          motor vehicle NOS (traffic) V59.50 ☑
            nontraffic V59.10 ☑
            specified type NEC (traffic) V59.59 ☑
              nontraffic V59.19 ☑
          pedal cycle (traffic) V51.6 ☑
            nontraffic V51.1 ☑
          pickup truck (traffic) V53.6 ☑
            nontraffic V53.1 ☑
          railway vehicle (traffic) V55.6 ☑
            nontraffic V55.1 ☑
          specified vehicle NEC (traffic) V56.6 ☑
            nontraffic V56.1 ☑
          stationary object (traffic) V57.6 ☑
            nontraffic V57.1 ☑
          streetcar (traffic) V56.6 ☑
            nontraffic V56.1 ☑
          three wheeled motor vehicle (traffic)
            V52.6 ☑
            nontraffic V52.1 ☑
          truck (traffic) V54.6 ☑
            nontraffic V54.1 ☑
          two wheeled motor vehicle (traffic)
            V52.6 ☑
            nontraffic V52.1 ☑
          van (traffic) V53.6 ☑
            nontraffic V53.1 ☑
        noncollision accident (traffic) V58.6 ☑
          nontraffic V58.1 ☑
    specified type NEC V59.88 ☑
      military vehicle V59.81 ☑
    quarry truck — *see* Accident, transport, industrial
      vehicle occupant
    race car — *see* Accident, transport, motor vehicle
      NEC occupant
    railway vehicle occupant V81.9 ☑
      collision (with) V81.3 ☑
        motor vehicle (non-military) (traffic)
          V81.1 ☑
          military V81.83 ☑
          nontraffic V81.0 ☑
        rolling stock V81.2 ☑
        specified object NEC V81.3 ☑
      during derailment V81.7 ☑

Accident — *continued*
  transport — *continued*
    railway vehicle occupant — *continued*
      during derailment — *continued*
        with antecedent collision — *see* Accident,
          transport, railway vehicle occupant,
          collision
      explosion V81.81 ☑
      fall (in railway vehicle) V81.5 ☑
        during derailment V81.7 ☑
          with antecedent collision — *see* Acci-
            dent, transport, railway vehicle
            occupant, collision
        from railway vehicle V81.6 ☑
          during derailment V81.7 ☑
            with antecedent collision — *see* Ac-
              cident, transport, railway vehi-
              cle occupant, collision
        while boarding or alighting V81.4 ☑
      fire V81.81 ☑
      object falling onto train V81.82 ☑
      specified type NEC V81.89 ☑
      while boarding or alighting V81.4 ☑
    ski lift V98.3 ☑
    snowmobile occupant (nontraffic) V86.92 ☑
      driver V86.52 ☑
      hanger-on V86.72 ☑
      passenger V86.62 ☑
      traffic V86.32 ☑
        driver V86.02 ☑
        hanger-on V86.22 ☑
        passenger V86.12 ☑
      while boarding or alighting V86.42 ☑
    specified NEC V98.8 ☑
    sport utility vehicle occupant (*see also* Accident,
      transport, pickup truck occupant)
    streetcar occupant V82.9 ☑
      collision (with) V82.3 ☑
        motor vehicle (traffic) V82.1 ☑
          nontraffic V82.0 ☑
        rolling stock V82.2 ☑
      during derailment V82.7 ☑
        with antecedent collision — *see* Accident,
          transport, streetcar occupant, collision
      fall (in streetcar) V82.5 ☑
        during derailment V82.7 ☑
          with antecedent collision — *see* Acci-
            dent, transport, streetcar occu-
            pant, collision
        from streetcar V82.6 ☑
          during derailment V82.7 ☑
            with antecedent collision — *see* Ac-
              cident, transport, streetcar oc-
              cupant, collision
          while boarding or alighting V82.4 ☑
        while boarding or alighting V82.4 ☑
      specified type NEC V82.8 ☑
      while boarding or alighting V82.4 ☑
    three-wheeled motor vehicle occupant V39.9 ☑
      collision (with)
        animal (traffic) V30.9 ☑
          being ridden (traffic) V36.9 ☑
            nontraffic V36.3 ☑
            while boarding or alighting V36.4 ☑
          nontraffic V30.3 ☑
          while boarding or alighting V30.4 ☑
        animal-drawn vehicle (traffic) V36.9 ☑
          nontraffic V36.3 ☑
          while boarding or alighting V36.4 ☑
        bus (traffic) V34.9 ☑
          nontraffic V34.3 ☑
          while boarding or alighting V34.4 ☑
        car (traffic) V33.9 ☑
          nontraffic V33.3 ☑
          while boarding or alighting V33.4 ☑
        motor vehicle NOS (traffic) V39.60 ☑
          nontraffic V39.20 ☑
          specified type NEC (traffic) V39.69 ☑
            nontraffic V39.29 ☑
        pedal cycle (traffic) V31.9 ☑
          nontraffic V31.3 ☑
          while boarding or alighting V31.4 ☑
        pickup truck (traffic) V33.9 ☑
          nontraffic V33.3 ☑
          while boarding or alighting V33.4 ☑
        railway vehicle (traffic) V35.9 ☑

Accident — *continued*
  transport — *continued*
    three-wheeled motor vehicle occupant — *continued*
      collision — *continued*
        railway vehicle — *continued*
          nontraffic V35.3 ☑
          while boarding or alighting V35.4 ☑
        specified vehicle NEC (traffic) V36.9 ☑
          nontraffic V36.3 ☑
          while boarding or alighting V36.4 ☑
        stationary object (traffic) V37.9 ☑
          nontraffic V37.3 ☑
          while boarding or alighting V37.4 ☑
        streetcar (traffic) V36.9 ☑
          nontraffic V36.3 ☑
          while boarding or alighting V36.4 ☑
        three wheeled motor vehicle (traffic) V32.9 ☑
          nontraffic V32.3 ☑
          while boarding or alighting V32.4 ☑
         truck (traffic) V34.9 ☑
          nontraffic V34.3 ☑
          while boarding or alighting V34.4 ☑
        two wheeled motor vehicle (traffic) V32.9 ☑
          nontraffic V32.3 ☑
          while boarding or alighting V32.4 ☑
        van (traffic) V33.9 ☑
          nontraffic V33.3 ☑
          while boarding or alighting V33.4 ☑
      driver
        collision (with)
          animal (traffic) V30.5 ☑
            being ridden (traffic) V36.5 ☑
              nontraffic V36.0 ☑
            nontraffic V30.0 ☑
          animal-drawn vehicle (traffic) V36.5 ☑
            nontraffic V36.0 ☑
          bus (traffic) V34.5 ☑
            nontraffic V34.0 ☑
          car (traffic) V33.5 ☑
            nontraffic V33.0 ☑
          motor vehicle NOS (traffic) V39.40 ☑
            nontraffic V39.00 ☑
            specified type NEC (traffic) V39.49 ☑
              nontraffic V39.09 ☑
          pedal cycle (traffic) V31.5 ☑
            nontraffic V31.0 ☑
          pickup truck (traffic) V33.5 ☑
            nontraffic V33.0 ☑
          railway vehicle (traffic) V35.5 ☑
            nontraffic V35.0 ☑
          specified vehicle NEC (traffic) V36.5 ☑
            nontraffic V36.0 ☑
          stationary object (traffic) V37.5 ☑
            nontraffic V37.0 ☑
          streetcar (traffic) V36.5 ☑
            nontraffic V36.0 ☑
          three wheeled motor vehicle (traffic) V32.5 ☑
            nontraffic V32.0 ☑
          truck (traffic) V34.5 ☑
            nontraffic V34.0 ☑
          two wheeled motor vehicle (traffic) V32.5 ☑
            nontraffic V32.0 ☑
          van (traffic) V33.5 ☑
            nontraffic V33.0 ☑
        noncollision accident (traffic) V38.5 ☑
          nontraffic V38.0 ☑
      hanger-on
        collision (with)
          animal (traffic) V30.7 ☑
            being ridden (traffic) V36.7 ☑
              nontraffic V36.2 ☑
            nontraffic V30.2 ☑
          animal-drawn vehicle (traffic) V36.7 ☑
            nontraffic V36.2 ☑
          bus (traffic) V34.7 ☑
            nontraffic V34.2 ☑
          car (traffic) V33.7 ☑
            nontraffic V33.2 ☑
          pedal cycle (traffic) V31.7 ☑
            nontraffic V31.2 ☑
          pickup truck (traffic) V33.7 ☑
            nontraffic V33.2 ☑

Accident — *continued*
  transport — *continued*
    three-wheeled motor vehicle occupant — *continued*
      hanger-on — *continued*
        collision — *continued*
          railway vehicle (traffic) V35.7 ☑
            nontraffic V35.2 ☑
          specified vehicle NEC (traffic) V36.7 ☑
            nontraffic V36.2 ☑
          stationary object (traffic) V37.7 ☑
            nontraffic V37.2 ☑
          streetcar (traffic) V36.7 ☑
            nontraffic V36.2 ☑
          three wheeled motor vehicle (traffic) V32.7 ☑
            nontraffic V32.2 ☑
          truck (traffic) V34.7 ☑
            nontraffic V34.2 ☑
          two wheeled motor vehicle (traffic) V32.7 ☑
            nontraffic V32.2 ☑
          van (traffic) V33.7 ☑
            nontraffic V33.2 ☑
        noncollision accident (traffic) V38.7 ☑
          nontraffic V38.2 ☑
      noncollision accident (traffic) V38.9 ☑
        nontraffic V38.3 ☑
        while boarding or alighting V38.4 ☑
      nontraffic V39.3 ☑
      passenger
        collision (with)
          animal (traffic) V30.6 ☑
            being ridden (traffic) V36.6 ☑
              nontraffic V36.1 ☑
            nontraffic V30.1 ☑
          animal-drawn vehicle (traffic) V36.6 ☑
            nontraffic V36.1 ☑
          bus (traffic) V34.6 ☑
            nontraffic V34.1 ☑
          car (traffic) V33.6 ☑
            nontraffic V33.1 ☑
          motor vehicle NOS (traffic) V39.50 ☑
            nontraffic V39.10 ☑
            specified type NEC (traffic) V39.59 ☑
              nontraffic V39.19 ☑
          pedal cycle (traffic) V31.6 ☑
            nontraffic V31.1 ☑
          pickup truck (traffic) V33.6 ☑
            nontraffic V33.1 ☑
          railway vehicle (traffic) V35.6 ☑
            nontraffic V35.1 ☑
          specified vehicle NEC (traffic) V36.6 ☑
            nontraffic V36.1 ☑
          stationary object (traffic) V37.6 ☑
            nontraffic V37.1 ☑
          streetcar (traffic) V36.6 ☑
            nontraffic V36.1 ☑
          three wheeled motor vehicle (traffic) V32.6 ☑
            nontraffic V32.1 ☑
          truck (traffic) V34.6 ☑
            nontraffic V34.1 ☑
          two wheeled motor vehicle (traffic) V32.6 ☑
            nontraffic V32.1 ☑
          van (traffic) V33.6 ☑
            nontraffic V33.1 ☑
        noncollision accident (traffic) V38.6 ☑
          nontraffic V38.1 ☑
      specified type NEC V39.89 ☑
      military vehicle V39.81 ☑
    tractor (farm) (and trailer) — *see* Accident, transport, agricultural vehicle occupant
    tram — *see* Accident, transport, streetcar
      in mine or quarry — *see* Accident, transport, industrial vehicle occupant
    trolley — *see* Accident, transport, streetcar
      in mine or quarry — *see* Accident, transport, industrial vehicle occupant
    truck (heavy) occupant V69.9 ☑
      collision (with)
        animal (traffic) V60.9 ☑
          being ridden (traffic) V66.9 ☑
            nontraffic V66.3 ☑
            while boarding or alighting V66.4 ☑

Accident — *continued*
  transport — *continued*
    truck occupant — *continued*
      collision — *continued*
        animal — *continued*
          nontraffic V60.3 ☑
          while boarding or alighting V60.4 ☑
        animal-drawn vehicle (traffic) V66.9 ☑
          nontraffic V66.3 ☑
          while boarding or alighting V66.4 ☑
        bus (traffic) V64.9 ☑
          nontraffic V64.3 ☑
          while boarding or alighting V64.4 ☑
        car (traffic) V63.9 ☑
          nontraffic V63.3 ☑
          while boarding or alighting V63.4 ☑
        motor vehicle NOS (traffic) V69.60 ☑
          nontraffic V69.20 ☑
          specified type NEC (traffic) V69.69 ☑
            nontraffic V69.29 ☑
        pedal cycle (traffic) V61.9 ☑
          nontraffic V61.3 ☑
          while boarding or alighting V61.4 ☑
        pickup truck (traffic) V63.9 ☑
          nontraffic V63.3 ☑
          while boarding or alighting V63.4 ☑
        railway vehicle (traffic) V65.9 ☑
          nontraffic V65.3 ☑
          while boarding or alighting V65.4 ☑
        specified vehicle NEC (traffic) V66.9 ☑
          nontraffic V66.3 ☑
          while boarding or alighting V66.4 ☑
        stationary object (traffic) V67.9 ☑
          nontraffic V67.3 ☑
          while boarding or alighting V67.4 ☑
        streetcar (traffic) V66.9 ☑
          nontraffic V66.3 ☑
          while boarding or alighting V66.4 ☑
        three wheeled motor vehicle (traffic) V62.9 ☑
          nontraffic V62.3 ☑
          while boarding or alighting V62.4 ☑
        truck (traffic) V64.9 ☑
          nontraffic V64.3 ☑
          while boarding or alighting V64.4 ☑
        two wheeled motor vehicle (traffic) V62.9 ☑
          nontraffic V62.3 ☑
          while boarding or alighting V62.4 ☑
        van (traffic) V63.9 ☑
          nontraffic V63.3 ☑
          while boarding or alighting V63.4 ☑
      driver
        collision (with)
          animal (traffic) V60.5 ☑
            being ridden (traffic) V66.5 ☑
              nontraffic V66.0 ☑
            nontraffic V60.0 ☑
          animal-drawn vehicle (traffic) V66.5 ☑
            nontraffic V66.0 ☑
          bus (traffic) V64.5 ☑
            nontraffic V64.0 ☑
          car (traffic) V63.5 ☑
            nontraffic V63.0 ☑
          motor vehicle NOS (traffic) V69.40 ☑
            nontraffic V69.00 ☑
            specified type NEC (traffic) V69.49 ☑
              nontraffic V69.09 ☑
          pedal cycle (traffic) V61.5 ☑
            nontraffic V61.0 ☑
          pickup truck (traffic) V63.5 ☑
            nontraffic V63.0 ☑
          railway vehicle (traffic) V65.5 ☑
            nontraffic V65.0 ☑
          specified vehicle NEC (traffic) V66.5 ☑
            nontraffic V66.0 ☑
          stationary object (traffic) V67.5 ☑
            nontraffic V67.0 ☑
          streetcar (traffic) V66.5 ☑
            nontraffic V66.0 ☑
          three wheeled motor vehicle (traffic) V62.5 ☑
            nontraffic V62.0 ☑
          truck (traffic) V64.5 ☑
            nontraffic V64.0 ☑
          two wheeled motor vehicle (traffic) V62.5 ☑

☑ Additional Character Required — Refer to the Tabular List for Character Selection   ▽ Subterms under main terms may continue to next column or page

Accident — *continued*
  transport — *continued*
    truck occupant — *continued*
      driver — *continued*
        collision — *continued*
          two wheeled motor vehicle — *continued*
            nontraffic V62.0 ☑
          van (traffic) V63.5 ☑
            nontraffic V63.0 ☑
        noncollision accident (traffic) V68.5 ☑
          nontraffic V68.0 ☑
      dump — *see* Accident, transport, construction
        vehicle occupant
      hanger-on
        collision (with)
          animal (traffic) V60.7 ☑
            being ridden (traffic) V66.7 ☑
              nontraffic V66.2 ☑
            nontraffic V60.2 ☑
          animal-drawn vehicle (traffic) V66.7 ☑
            nontraffic V66.2 ☑
          bus (traffic) V64.7 ☑
            nontraffic V64.2 ☑
          car (traffic) V63.7 ☑
            nontraffic V63.2 ☑
          pedal cycle (traffic) V61.7 ☑
            nontraffic V61.2 ☑
          pickup truck (traffic) V63.7 ☑
            nontraffic V63.2 ☑
          railway vehicle (traffic) V65.7 ☑
            nontraffic V65.2 ☑
          specified vehicle NEC (traffic) V66.7 ☑
            nontraffic V66.2 ☑
          stationary object (traffic) V67.7 ☑
            nontraffic V67.2 ☑
          streetcar (traffic) V66.7 ☑
            nontraffic V66.2 ☑
          three wheeled motor vehicle (traffic)
            V62.7 ☑
            nontraffic V62.2 ☑
          truck (traffic) V64.7 ☑
            nontraffic V64.2 ☑
          two wheeled motor vehicle (traffic)
            V62.7 ☑
            nontraffic V62.2 ☑
          van (traffic) V63.7 ☑
            nontraffic V63.2 ☑
        noncollision accident (traffic) V68.7 ☑
          nontraffic V68.2 ☑
      noncollision accident (traffic) V68.9 ☑
        nontraffic V68.3 ☑
        while boarding or alighting V68.4 ☑
      nontraffic V69.3 ☑
      passenger
        collision (with)
          animal (traffic) V60.6 ☑
            being ridden (traffic) V66.6 ☑
              nontraffic V66.1- ☑
            nontraffic V60.1 ☑
          animal-drawn vehicle (traffic) V66.6 ☑
            nontraffic V66.1 ☑
          bus (traffic) V64.6 ☑
            nontraffic V64.1 ☑
          car (traffic) V63.6 ☑
            nontraffic V63.1 ☑
          motor vehicle NOS (traffic) V69.50 ☑
            nontraffic V69.10 ☑
            specified type NEC (traffic) V69.59 ☑
              nontraffic V69.19 ☑
          pedal cycle (traffic) V61.6 ☑
            nontraffic V61.1 ☑
          pickup truck (traffic) V63.6 ☑
            nontraffic V63.1 ☑
          railway vehicle (traffic) V65.6 ☑
            nontraffic V65.1 ☑
          specified vehicle NEC (traffic) V66.6 ☑
            nontraffic V66.1 ☑
          stationary object (traffic) V67.6 ☑
            nontraffic V67.1 ☑
          streetcar (traffic) V66.6 ☑
            nontraffic V66.1 ☑
          three wheeled motor vehicle (traffic)
            V62.6 ☑
            nontraffic V62.1 ☑
          truck (traffic) V64.6 ☑

Accident — *continued*
  transport — *continued*
    truck occupant — *continued*
      passenger — *continued*
        collision — *continued*
          truck — *continued*
            nontraffic V64.1 ☑
          two wheeled motor vehicle (traffic)
            V62.6 ☑
            nontraffic V62.1 ☑
          van (traffic) V63.6 ☑
            nontraffic V63.1 ☑
        noncollision accident (traffic) V68.6 ☑
          nontraffic V68.1 ☑
      pickup — *see* Accident, transport, pickup truck
        occupant
      specified type NEC V69.88 ☑
      military vehicle V69.81 ☑
    van occupant V59.9 ☑
      collision (with)
        animal (traffic) V50.9 ☑
          being ridden (traffic) V56.9 ☑
            nontraffic V56.3 ☑
            while boarding or alighting V56.4 ☑
          nontraffic V50.3 ☑
          while boarding or alighting V50.4 ☑
        animal-drawn vehicle (traffic) V56.9 ☑
          nontraffic V56.3 ☑
          while boarding or alighting V56.4 ☑
        bus (traffic) V54.9 ☑
          nontraffic V54.3 ☑
          while boarding or alighting V54.4 ☑
        car (traffic) V53.9 ☑
          nontraffic V53.3 ☑
          while boarding or alighting V53.4 ☑
        motor vehicle NOS (traffic) V59.60 ☑
          nontraffic V59.20 ☑
          specified type NEC (traffic) V59.69 ☑
            nontraffic V59.29 ☑
        pedal cycle (traffic) V51.9 ☑
          nontraffic V51.3 ☑
          while boarding or alighting V51.4 ☑
        pickup truck (traffic) V53.9 ☑
          nontraffic V53.3 ☑
          while boarding or alighting V53.4 ☑
        railway vehicle (traffic) V55.9 ☑
          nontraffic V55.3 ☑
          while boarding or alighting V55.4 ☑
        specified vehicle NEC (traffic) V56.9 ☑
          nontraffic V56.3 ☑
          while boarding or alighting V56.4 ☑
        stationary object (traffic) V57.9 ☑
          nontraffic V57.3 ☑
          while boarding or alighting V57.4 ☑
        streetcar (traffic) V56.9 ☑
          nontraffic V56.3 ☑
          while boarding or alighting V56.4 ☑
        three wheeled motor vehicle (traffic)
          V52.9 ☑
          nontraffic V52.3 ☑
          while boarding or alighting V52.4 ☑
        truck (traffic) V54.9 ☑
          nontraffic V54.3 ☑
          while boarding or alighting V54.4 ☑
        two wheeled motor vehicle (traffic) V52.9 ☑
          nontraffic V52.3 ☑
          while boarding or alighting V52.4 ☑
        van (traffic) V53.9 ☑
          nontraffic V53.3 ☑
          while boarding or alighting V53.4 ☑
      driver
        collision (with)
          animal (traffic) V50.5 ☑
            being ridden (traffic) V56.5 ☑
              nontraffic V56.0 ☑
            nontraffic V50.0 ☑
          animal-drawn vehicle (traffic) V56.5 ☑
            nontraffic V56.0 ☑
          bus (traffic) V54.5 ☑
            nontraffic V54.0 ☑
          car (traffic) V53.5 ☑
            nontraffic V53.0 ☑
          motor vehicle NOS (traffic) V59.40 ☑
            nontraffic V59.00 ☑
            specified type NEC (traffic) V59.49 ☑
              nontraffic V59.09 ☑

Accident — *continued*
  transport — *continued*
    van occupant — *continued*
      driver — *continued*
        collision — *continued*
          pedal cycle (traffic) V51.5 ☑
            nontraffic V51.0 ☑
          pickup truck (traffic) V53.5 ☑
            nontraffic V53.0 ☑
          railway vehicle (traffic) V55.5 ☑
            nontraffic V55.0 ☑
          specified vehicle NEC (traffic) V56.5 ☑
            nontraffic V56.0 ☑
          stationary object (traffic) V57.5 ☑
            nontraffic V57.0 ☑
          streetcar (traffic) V56.5 ☑
            nontraffic V56.0 ☑
          three wheeled motor vehicle (traffic)
          V52.5 ☑
          nontraffic V52.0 ☑
          truck (traffic) V54.5 ☑
            nontraffic V54.0 ☑
          two wheeled motor vehicle (traffic)
          V52.5 ☑
          nontraffic V52.0 ☑
          van (traffic) V53.5 ☑
            nontraffic V53.0 ☑
        noncollision accident (traffic) V58.5 ☑
          nontraffic V58.0 ☑
      hanger-on
        collision (with)
          animal (traffic) V50.7 ☑
            being ridden (traffic) V56.7 ☑
              nontraffic V56.2 ☑
            nontraffic V50.2 ☑
          animal-drawn vehicle (traffic) V56.7 ☑
            nontraffic V56.2 ☑
          bus (traffic) V54.7 ☑
            nontraffic V54.2 ☑
          car (traffic) V53.7 ☑
            nontraffic V53.2 ☑
          pedal cycle (traffic) V51.7 ☑
            nontraffic V51.2 ☑
          pickup truck (traffic) V53.7 ☑
            nontraffic V53.2 ☑
          railway vehicle (traffic) V55.7 ☑
            nontraffic V55.2 ☑
          specified vehicle NEC (traffic) V56.7 ☑
            nontraffic V56.2 ☑
          stationary object (traffic) V57.7 ☑
            nontraffic V57.2 ☑
          streetcar (traffic) V56.7 ☑
            nontraffic V56.2 ☑
          three wheeled motor vehicle (traffic)
          V52.7 ☑
          nontraffic V52.2 ☑
          truck (traffic) V54.7 ☑
            nontraffic V54.2 ☑
          two wheeled motor vehicle (traffic)
          V52.7 ☑
          nontraffic V52.2 ☑
          van (traffic) V53.7 ☑
            nontraffic V53.2 ☑
        noncollision accident (traffic) V58.7 ☑
          nontraffic V58.2 ☑
      noncollision accident (traffic) V58.9 ☑
        nontraffic V58.3 ☑
        while boarding or alighting V58.4 ☑
      nontraffic V59.3 ☑
      passenger
        collision (with)
          animal (traffic) V50.6 ☑
            being ridden (traffic) V56.6 ☑
              nontraffic V56.1 ☑
            nontraffic V50.1 ☑
          animal-drawn vehicle (traffic) V56.6 ☑
            nontraffic V56.1 ☑
          bus (traffic) V54.6 ☑
            nontraffic V54.1 ☑
          car (traffic) V53.6 ☑
            nontraffic V53.1 ☑
          motor vehicle NOS (traffic) V59.50 ☑
            nontraffic V59.10 ☑
            specified type NEC (traffic) V59.59 ☑
              nontraffic V59.19 ☑
          pedal cycle (traffic) V51.6 ☑

▼ **Subterms under main terms may continue to next column or page**   ☑ **Additional Character Required — Refer to the Tabular List for Character Selection**   **407**

Accident — Accident

Activity — *continued*
- handball Y93.73
- handcrafts NEC Y93.D9 (*following* Y93.7)
- hang gliding Y93.35
- hiking (on level or elevated terrain) Y93.01
- hockey (ice) Y93.22
  - field Y93.65
- horseback riding Y93.52
- household (interior) maintenance NEC Y93.E9 (*following* Y93.7)
- ice NEC Y93.29
  - dancing Y93.21
  - hockey Y93.22
  - skating Y93.21
- inline roller skating Y93.51
- ironing Y93.E4 (*following* Y93.7)
- judo Y93.75
- jumping jacks Y93.A2 (*following* Y93.7)
- jumping rope Y93.56
- jumping (off) NEC Y93.39
  - BASE (Building, Antenna, Span, Earth) Y93.33
  - bungee Y93.34
  - jacks Y93.A2 (*following* Y93.7)
  - rope Y93.56
- karate Y93.75
- kayaking (in calm and turbulent water) Y93.16
- keyboarding (computer) Y93.C1 (*following* Y93.7)
- kickball Y93.6A
- knitting Y93.D1 (*following* Y93.7)
- lacrosse Y93.65
- land maintenance NEC Y93.H9 (*following* Y93.7)
- landscaping Y93.H2 (*following* Y93.7)
- laundry Y93.E2 (*following* Y93.7)
- machines (exercise)
  - primarily for cardiorespiratory conditioning Y93.A1 (*following* Y93.7)
  - primarily for muscle strengthening Y93.B1 (*following* Y93.7)
- maintenance
  - exterior building NEC Y93.H9 (*following* Y93.7)
  - household (interior) NEC Y93.E9 (*following* Y93.7)
  - land Y93.H9 (*following* Y93.7)
  - property Y93.H9 (*following* Y93.7)
- marching (on level or elevated terrain) Y93.01
- martial arts Y93.75
- microwave oven Y93.G3 (*following* Y93.7)
- milking an animal Y93.K2 (*following* Y93.7)
- mopping (floor) Y93.E5 (*following* Y93.7)
- mountain climbing Y93.31
- muscle strengthening
  - exercises (non-machine) NEC Y93.B9 (*following* Y93.7)
  - machines Y93.B1 (*following* Y93.7)
- musical keyboard (electronic) playing Y93.J1 (*following* Y93.7)
- nordic skiing Y93.24
- obstacle course Y93.A5 (*following* Y93.7)
- oven (microwave) Y93.G3 (*following* Y93.7)
- packing up and unpacking in moving to a new residence Y93.E6 (*following* Y93.7)
- parasailing Y93.19
- pass out game Y93.85
- percussion instrument playing NEC Y93.J2 (*following* Y93.7)
- personal
  - bathing and showering Y93.E1 (*following* Y93.7)
  - hygiene NEC Y93.E8 (*following* Y93.7)
  - showering Y93.E1 (*following* Y93.7)
- physical games generally associated with school recess, summer camp and children Y93.6A
- physical training NEC Y93.A9 (*following* Y93.7)
- piano playing Y93.J1 (*following* Y93.7)
- pilates Y93.B4 (*following* Y93.7)
- platform diving Y93.12
- playing musical instrument
  - brass instrument Y93.J4 (*following* Y93.7)
  - drum Y93.J2 (*following* Y93.7)
  - musical keyboard (electronic) Y93.J1 (*following* Y93.7)
  - percussion instrument NEC Y93.J2 (*following* Y93.7)
  - piano Y93.J1 (*following* Y93.7)
  - string instrument Y93.J3 (*following* Y93.7)
  - winds instrument Y93.J4 (*following* Y93.7)
- property maintenance
  - exterior NEC Y93.H9 (*following* Y93.7)
  - interior NEC Y93.E9 (*following* Y93.7)
- pruning (garden and lawn) Y93.H2 (*following* Y93.7)
- pull-ups Y93.B2 (*following* Y93.7)
- push-ups Y93.B2 (*following* Y93.7)

Activity — *continued*
- racquetball Y93.73
- rafting (in calm and turbulent water) Y93.16
- raking (leaves) Y93.H1 (*following* Y93.7)
- rappelling Y93.32
- refereeing a sports activity Y93.81
- residential relocation Y93.E6 (*following* Y93.7)
- rhythmic gymnastics Y93.43
- rhythmic movement NEC Y93.49
- riding
  - horseback Y93.52
  - rollercoaster Y93.I1 (*following* Y93.7)
- rock climbing Y93.31
- roller skating (inline) Y93.51
- rollercoaster riding Y93.I1 (*following* Y93.7)
- rough housing and horseplay Y93.83
- rowing (in calm and turbulent water) Y93.16
- rugby Y93.63
- running Y93.02
- SCUBA diving Y93.15
- sewing Y93.D2 (*following* Y93.7)
- shoveling Y93.H1 (*following* Y93.7)
  - dirt Y93.H1 (*following* Y93.7)
  - snow Y93.H1 (*following* Y93.7)
- showering (personal) Y93.E1 (*following* Y93.7)
- sit-ups Y93.B2 (*following* Y93.7)
- skateboarding Y93.51
- skating (ice) Y93.21
  - roller Y93.51
- skiing (alpine) (downhill) Y93.23
  - cross country Y93.24
  - nordic Y93.24
  - water Y93.17
- sledding (snow) Y93.23
- sleeping (sleep) Y93.84
- smoking and grilling food Y93.G2 (*following* Y93.7)
- snorkeling Y93.15
- snow NEC Y93.29
  - boarding Y93.23
  - shoveling Y93.H1 (*following* Y93.7)
  - sledding Y93.23
  - tubing Y93.23
- soccer Y93.66
- softball Y93.64
- specified NEC Y93.89
- spectator at an event Y93.82
- sports NEC Y93.79
  - sports played as a team or group NEC Y93.69
  - sports played individually NEC Y93.59
- springboard diving Y93.12
- squash Y93.73
- stationary bike Y93.A1 (*following* Y93.7)
- step (stepping) exercise (class) Y93.A3 (*following* Y93.7)
- stepper machine Y93.A1 (*following* Y93.7)
- stove Y93.G3 (*following* Y93.7)
- string instrument playing Y93.J3 (*following* Y93.7)
- surfing Y93.18
  - wind Y93.18
- swimming Y93.11
- tackle football Y93.61
- tap dancing Y93.41
- tennis Y93.73
- tobogganing Y93.23
- touch football Y93.62
- track and field events (non-running) Y93.57
  - running Y93.02
- trampoline Y93.44
- treadmill Y93.A1 (*following* Y93.7)
- trimming shrubs Y93.H2 (*following* Y93.7)
- tubing (in calm and turbulent water) Y93.16
  - snow Y93.23
- ultimate frisbee Y93.74
- underwater diving Y93.15
- unpacking in moving to a new residence Y93.E6 (*following* Y93.7)
- use of stove, oven and microwave oven Y93.G3 (*following* Y93.7)
- vacuuming Y93.E3 (*following* Y93.7)
- volleyball (beach) (court) Y93.68
- wake boarding Y93.17
- walking (on level or elevated terrain) Y93.01
  - an animal Y93.K1 (*following* Y93.7)
- walking an animal Y93.K1 (*following* Y93.7)
- wall climbing Y93.31
- warm up and cool down exercises Y93.A2 (*following* Y93.7)
- water NEC Y93.19
  - aerobics Y93.14
  - craft NEC Y93.19

Activity — *continued*
- water — *continued*
  - exercise Y93.14
  - polo Y93.13
  - skiing Y93.17
  - sliding Y93.18
  - survival training and testing Y93.19
- weeding (garden and lawn) Y93.H2 (*following* Y93.7)
- wind instrument playing Y93.J4 (*following* Y93.7)
- windsurfing Y93.18
- wrestling Y93.72
- yoga Y93.42

Adverse effect of drugs — *see* Table of Drugs and Chemicals
Aerosinusitis — *see* Air, pressure
After-effect, late — *see* Sequelae
Air
- blast in war operations — *see* War operations, air blast
- pressure
  - change, rapid
    - during
      - ascent W94.29 ☑
        - while (in) (surfacing from)
          - aircraft W94.23 ☑
          - deep water diving W94.21 ☑
          - underground W94.22 ☑
      - descent W94.39 ☑
        - in
          - aircraft W94.31 ☑
          - water W94.32 ☑
  - high, prolonged W94.0 ☑
  - low, prolonged W94.12 ☑
    - due to residence or long visit at high altitude W94.11 ☑
Alpine sickness W94.11 ☑
Altitude sickness W94.11 ☑
Anaphylactic shock, anaphylaxis — *see* Table of Drugs and Chemicals
Andes disease W94.11 ☑
Arachnidism, arachnoidism X58 ☑
Arson (with intent to injure or kill) X97 ☑
Asphyxia, asphyxiation
- by
  - food (bone) (seed) — *see* categories T17 and T18 ☑
  - gas (*see also* Table of Drugs and Chemicals)
    - legal
      - execution — *see* Legal, intervention, gas
      - intervention — *see* Legal, intervention, gas
- from
  - fire (*see also* Exposure, fire)
    - in war operations — *see* War operations, fire
  - ignition — *see* Ignition
  - vomitus T17.81 ☑
- in war operations — *see* War operations, restriction of airway
Aspiration
- food (any type) (into respiratory tract) (with asphyxia, obstruction respiratory tract, suffocation) — *see* categories T17 and T18 ☑
- foreign body — *see* Foreign body, aspiration
- vomitus (with asphyxia, obstruction respiratory tract, suffocation) T17.81 ☑
Assassination (attempt) — *see* Assault
Assault (homicidal) (by) (in) Y09
- arson X97 ☑
- bite (of human being) Y04.1 ☑
- bodily force Y04.8 ☑
  - bite Y04.1 ☑
  - bumping into Y04.2 ☑
  - sexual — *see* subcategories T74.0, T76.0 ☑
  - unarmed fight Y04.0 ☑
- bomb X96.9 ☑
  - antipersonnel X96.0 ☑
  - fertilizer X96.3 ☑
  - gasoline X96.1 ☑
  - letter X96.2 ☑
  - petrol X96.1 ☑
  - pipe X96.3 ☑
  - specified NEC X96.8 ☑
- brawl (hand) (fists) (foot) (unarmed) Y04.0 ☑
- burning, burns (by fire) NEC X97 ☑
  - acid Y08.89 ☑
  - caustic, corrosive substance Y08.89 ☑
  - chemical from swallowing caustic, corrosive substance — *see* Table of Drugs and Chemicals

Assault — *continued*
  burning, burns — *continued*
    cigarette(s) X97 ☑
    hot object X98.9 ☑
      fluid NEC X98.2 ☑
      household appliance X98.3 ☑
      specified NEC X98.8 ☑
      steam X98.0 ☑
      tap water X98.1 ☑
      vapors X98.0 ☑
    scalding — *see* Assault, burning
    steam X98.0 ☑
    vitriol Y08.89 ☑
  caustic, corrosive substance (gas) Y08.89 ☑
  crashing of
    aircraft Y08.81 ☑
    motor vehicle Y03.8 ☑
      pushed in front of Y02.0 ☑
      run over Y03.0 ☑
      specified NEC Y03.8 ☑
  cutting or piercing instrument X99.9 ☑
    dagger X99.2 ☑
    glass X99.0 ☑
    knife X99.1 ☑
    specified NEC X99.8 ☑
    sword X99.2 ☑
  dagger X99.2 ☑
  drowning (in) X92.9 ☑
    bathtub X92.0 ☑
    natural water X92.3 ☑
    specified NEC X92.8 ☑
    swimming pool X92.1 ☑
      following fall X92.2 ☑
  dynamite X96.8 ☑
  explosive(s) (material) X96.9 ☑
  fight (hand) (fists) (foot) (unarmed) Y04.0 ☑
    with weapon — *see* Assault, by type of weapon
  fire X97 ☑
  firearm X95.9 ☑
    airgun X95.01 ☑
    handgun X93 ☑
    hunting rifle X94.1 ☑
    larger X94.9 ☑
      specified NEC X94.8 ☑
    machine gun X94.2 ☑
    shotgun X94.0 ☑
    specified NEC X95.8 ☑
  from high place Y01 ☑
  gunshot (wound) NEC — *see* Assault, firearm, by type
  incendiary device X97 ☑
  injury Y09
    to child due to criminal abortion attempt NEC Y08.89 ☑
  knife X99.1 ☑
  late effect of — *see* categories X92-Y08 with 7th character S
  placing before moving object NEC Y02.8 ☑
    motor vehicle Y02.0 ☑
  poisoning — *see* categories T36-T65 with 7th character S
  puncture, any part of body — *see* Assault, cutting or piercing instrument
  pushing
    before moving object NEC Y02.8 ☑
      motor vehicle Y02.0 ☑
      subway train Y02.1 ☑
      train Y02.1 ☑
    from high place Y01 ☑
  rape T74.2- ☑
  scalding — *see* Assault, burning
  sequelae of — *see* categories X92-Y08 with 7th character S
  sexual (by bodily force) T74.2- ☑
  shooting — *see* Assault, firearm
  specified means NEC Y08.89 ☑
  stab, any part of body — *see* Assault, cutting or piercing instrument
  steam X98.0 ☑
  striking against
    other person Y04.2 ☑
    sports equipment Y08.09 ☑
      baseball bat Y08.02 ☑
      hockey stick Y08.01 ☑
  struck by
    sports equipment Y08.09 ☑
      baseball bat Y08.02 ☑

Assault — *continued*
  struck by — *continued*
    sports equipment — *continued*
      hockey stick Y08.01 ☑
  submersion — *see* Assault, drowning
  violence Y09
  weapon Y09
    blunt Y00 ☑
    cutting or piercing — *see* Assault, cutting or piercing instrument
    firearm — *see* Assault, firearm
  wound Y09
    cutting — *see* Assault, cutting or piercing instrument
    gunshot — *see* Assault, firearm
    knife X99.1 ☑
    piercing — *see* Assault, cutting or piercing instrument
    puncture — *see* Assault, cutting or piercing instrument
    stab — *see* Assault, cutting or piercing instrument

Attack by mammals NEC W55.89 ☑
Avalanche — *see* Landslide
Aviator's disease — *see* Air, pressure

B

Barotitis, barodontalgia, barosinusitis, barotrauma (otitic) (sinus) — *see* Air, pressure
Battered (baby) (child) (person) (syndrome) X58 ☑
Bayonet wound W26.1 ☑
  in
    legal intervention — *see* Legal, intervention, sharp object, bayonet
    war operations — *see* War operations, combat
  stated as undetermined whether accidental or intentional Y28.8 ☑
  suicide (attempt) X78.2 ☑
Bean in nose — *see* categories T17 and T18 ☑
Bed set on fire NEC — *see* Exposure, fire, uncontrolled, building, bed
Beheading (by guillotine)
  homicide X99.9 ☑
  legal execution — *see* Legal, intervention
Bending, injury in (prolonged) (static) X50.1 ☑
Bends — *see* Air, pressure, change
Bite, bitten by
  alligator W58.01 ☑
  arthropod (nonvenomous) NEC W57 ☑
  bull W55.21 ☑
  cat W55.01 ☑
  cow W55.21 ☑
  crocodile W58.11 ☑
  dog W54.0 ☑
  goat W55.31 ☑
  hoof stock NEC W55.31 ☑
  horse W55.11 ☑
  human being (accidentally) W50.3 ☑
    with intent to injure or kill Y04.1 ☑
    as, or caused by, a crowd or human stampede (with fall) W52 ☑
    assault Y04.1 ☑
    homicide (attempt) Y04.1 ☑
    in
      fight Y04.1 ☑
  insect (nonvenomous) W57 ☑
  lizard (nonvenomous) W59.01 ☑
  mammal NEC W55.81 ☑
    marine W56.31 ☑
  marine animal (nonvenomous) W56.81 ☑
  millipede W57 ☑
  moray eel W56.51 ☑
  mouse W53.01 ☑
  person(s) (accidentally) W50.3 ☑
    with intent to injure or kill Y04.1 ☑
    as, or caused by, a crowd or human stampede (with fall) W52 ☑
    assault Y04.1 ☑
    homicide (attempt) Y04.1 ☑
    in
      fight Y04.1 ☑
  pig W55.41 ☑
  raccoon W55.51 ☑
  rat W53.11 ☑
  reptile W59.81 ☑
    lizard W59.01 ☑

Bite, bitten by — *continued*
  reptile — *continued*
    snake W59.11 ☑
    turtle W59.21 ☑
      terrestrial W59.81 ☑
  rodent W53.81 ☑
    mouse W53.01 ☑
    rat W53.11 ☑
    specified NEC W53.81 ☑
    squirrel W53.21 ☑
  shark W56.41 ☑
  sheep W55.31 ☑
  snake (nonvenomous) W59.11 ☑
  spider (nonvenomous) W57 ☑
  squirrel W53.21 ☑
Blast (air) in war operations — *see* War operations, blast
Blizzard X37.2 ☑
Blood alcohol level Y90.9
  less than 20mg/100ml Y90.0
  20-39mg/100ml Y90.1
  40-59mg/100ml Y90.2
  60-79mg/100ml Y90.3
  80-99mg/100ml Y90.4
  100-119mg/100ml Y90.5
  120-199mg/100ml Y90.6
  200-239mg/100ml Y90.7
  presence in blood, level not specified Y90.9
Blow X58 ☑
  by law-enforcing agent, police (on duty) — *see* Legal, intervention, manhandling
    blunt object — *see* Legal, intervention, blunt object
Blowing up — *see* Explosion
Brawl (hand) (fists) (foot) Y04.0 ☑
Breakage (accidental) (part of)
  ladder (causing fall) W11
  scaffolding (causing fall) W12
Broken
  glass, contact with — *see* Contact, with, glass
  power line (causing electric shock) W85 ☑
Bumping against, into (accidentally)
  object NEC W22.8 ☑
    with fall — *see* Fall, due to, bumping against, object
    caused by crowd or human stampede (with fall) W52
    sports equipment W21.9 ☑
  person(s) W51 ☑
    with fall W03
      due to ice or snow W00.0 ☑
    assault Y04.2 ☑
    caused by, a crowd or human stampede (with fall) W52 ☑
    homicide (attempt) Y04.2 ☑
    sports equipment W21.9 ☑
Burn, burned, burning (accidental) (by) (from) (on)
  acid NEC — *see* Table of Drugs and Chemicals
  bed linen — *see* Exposure, fire, uncontrolled, in building, bed
  blowtorch X08.8 ☑
    with ignition of clothing NEC X06.2 ☑
      nightwear X05 ☑
  bonfire, campfire (controlled) (*see also* Exposure, fire, controlled, not in building)
    uncontrolled — *see* Exposure, fire, uncontrolled, not in building
  candle X08.8 ☑
    with ignition of clothing NEC X06.2 ☑
      nightwear X05 ☑
  caustic liquid, substance (external) (internal) NEC — *see* Table of Drugs and Chemicals
  chemical (external) (internal) (*see also* Table of Drugs and Chemicals)
    in war operations — *see* War operations. fire
  cigar(s) or cigarette(s) X08.8 ☑
    with ignition of clothing NEC X06.2 ☑
      nightwear X05 ☑
  clothes, clothing NEC (from controlled fire) X06.2 ☑
    with conflagration — *see* Exposure, fire, uncontrolled, building
    not in building or structure — *see* Exposure, fire, uncontrolled, not in building
  cooker (hot) X15.8 ☑
    stated as undetermined whether accidental or intentional Y27.3 ☑
    suicide (attempt) X77.3 ☑
  electric blanket X16 ☑

Burn, burned, burning — *continued*
  engine (hot) X17 ☑
  fire, flames — *see* Exposure, fire
  flare, Very pistol — *see* Discharge, firearm NEC
  heat
    from appliance (electrical) (household) X15.8 ☑
      cooker X15.8 ☑
      hotplate X15.2 ☑
      kettle X15.8 ☑
      light bulb X15.8 ☑
      saucepan X15.3 ☑
      skillet X15.3 ☑
      stated as undetermined whether accidental or
        intentional Y27.3 ☑
      stove X15.0 ☑
      suicide (attempt) X77.3 ☑
      toaster X15.1 ☑
    in local application or packing during medical or
      surgical procedure Y63.5
  heating
    appliance, radiator or pipe X16 ☑
  homicide (attempt) — *see* Assault, burning
  hot
    air X14.1 ☑
    cooker X15.8 ☑
    drink X10.0 ☑
    engine X17 ☑
    fat X10.2 ☑
    fluid NEC X12 ☑
    food X10.1 ☑
    gases X14.1 ☑
    heating appliance X16 ☑
    household appliance NEC X15.8 ☑
    kettle X15.8 ☑
    liquid NEC X12 ☑
    machinery X17 ☑
    metal (molten) (liquid) NEC X18 ☑
    object (not producing fire or flames) NEC X19 ☑
    oil (cooking) X10.2 ☑
    pipe(s) X16 ☑
    radiator X16 ☑
    saucepan (glass) (metal) X15.3 ☑
    stove (kitchen) X15.0 ☑
    substance NEC X19 ☑
      caustic or corrosive NEC — *see* Table of Drugs
        and Chemicals
    toaster X15.1 ☑
    tool X17 ☑
    vapor X13.1 ☑
    water (tap) — *see* Contact, with, hot, tap water
  hotplate X15.2 ☑
    suicide (attempt) X77.3 ☑
  ignition — *see* Ignition
  in war operations — *see* War operations, fire
  inflicted by other person X97
    by hot objects, hot vapor, and steam — *see* Assault,
      burning, hot object
  internal, from swallowed caustic, corrosive liquid,
    substance — *see* Table of Drugs and Chemicals
  iron (hot) X15.8 ☑
    stated as undetermined whether accidental or in-
      tentional Y27.3 ☑
    suicide (attempt) X77.3 ☑
  kettle (hot) X15.8 ☑
    stated as undetermined whether accidental or in-
      tentional Y27.3 ☑
    suicide (attempt) X77.3 ☑
  lamp (flame) X08.8 ☑
    with ignition of clothing NEC X06.2 ☑
      nightwear X05 ☑
  lighter (cigar) (cigarette) X08.8 ☑
    with ignition of clothing NEC X06.2 ☑
      nightwear X05 ☑
  lightning — *see* subcategory T75.0 ☑
    causing fire — *see* Exposure, fire
  liquid (boiling) (hot) NEC X12 ☑
    stated as undetermined whether accidental or in-
      tentional Y27.2 ☑
    suicide (attempt) X77.2 ☑
  local application of externally applied substance in
    medical or surgical care Y63.5
  machinery (hot) X17 ☑
  matches X08.8 ☑
    with ignition of clothing NEC X06.2 ☑
      nightwear X05 ☑

Burn, burned, burning — *continued*
  mattress — *see* Exposure, fire, uncontrolled, building,
    bed
  medicament, externally applied Y63.5
  metal (hot) (liquid) (molten) NEC X18 ☑
  nightwear (nightclothes, nightdress, gown, pajamas,
    robe) X05 ☑
  object (hot) NEC X19 ☑
  on board watercraft
    due to
      accident to watercraft V91.09 ☑
        powered craft V91.03 ☑
          ferry boat V91.01 ☑
          fishing boat V91.02 ☑
          jetskis V91.03 ☑
          liner V91.01 ☑
          merchant ship V91.00 ☑
          passenger ship V91.01 ☑
        unpowered craft V91.08 ☑
          canoe V91.05 ☑
          inflatable V91.06 ☑
          kayak V91.05 ☑
          sailboat V91.04 ☑
          surf-board V91.08 ☑
          water skis V91.07 ☑
          windsurfer V91.08 ☑
      fire on board V93.09 ☑
        ferry boat V93.01 ☑
        fishing boat V93.02 ☑
        jetskis V93.03 ☑
        liner V93.01 ☑
        merchant ship V93.00 ☑
        passenger ship V93.01 ☑
        powered craft NEC V93.03 ☑
        sailboat V93.04 ☑
      specified heat source NEC on board V93.19 ☑
        ferry boat V93.11 ☑
        fishing boat V93.12 ☑
        jetskis V93.13 ☑
        liner V93.11 ☑
        merchant ship V93.10 ☑
        passenger ship V93.11 ☑
        powered craft NEC V93.13 ☑
        sailboat V93.14 ☑
  pipe (hot) X16 ☑
    smoking X08.8 ☑
      with ignition of clothing NEC X06.2 ☑
        nightwear X05 ☑
  powder — *see* Powder burn
  radiator (hot) X16 ☑
  saucepan (hot) (glass) (metal) X15.3 ☑
    stated as undetermined whether accidental or in-
      tentional Y27.3 ☑
    suicide (attempt) X77.3 ☑
  self-inflicted X76
    stated as undetermined whether accidental or in-
      tentional Y26 ☑
  stated as undetermined whether accidental or inten-
    tional Y27.0 ☑
  steam X13.1 ☑
    pipe X16 ☑
      stated as undetermined whether accidental or
        intentional Y27.8 ☑
    stated as undetermined whether accidental or in-
      tentional Y27.0 ☑
    suicide (attempt) X77.0 ☑
  stove (hot) (kitchen) X15.0 ☑
    stated as undetermined whether accidental or in-
      tentional Y27.3 ☑
    suicide (attempt) X77.3 ☑
  substance (hot) NEC X19 ☑
    boiling X12 ☑
      stated as undetermined whether accidental or
        intentional Y27.2 ☑
      suicide (attempt) X77.2 ☑
    molten (metal) X18 ☑
  suicide (attempt) NEC X76 ☑
    hot
      household appliance X77.3 ☑
      object X77.9 ☑
  therapeutic misadventure
    heat in local application or packing during medical
      or surgical procedure Y63.5
    overdose of radiation Y63.2
  toaster (hot) X15.1 ☑

Burn, burned, burning — *continued*
  toaster — *continued*
    stated as undetermined whether accidental or in-
      tentional Y27.3 ☑
    suicide (attempt) X77.3 ☑
  tool (hot) X17 ☑
  torch, welding X08.8 ☑
    with ignition of clothing NEC X06.2 ☑
      nightwear X05 ☑
  trash fire (controlled) — *see* Exposure, fire, controlled,
    not in building
    uncontrolled — *see* Exposure, fire, uncontrolled,
      not in building
  vapor (hot) X13.1 ☑
    stated as undetermined whether accidental or in-
      tentional Y27.0 ☑
    suicide (attempt) X77.0 ☑
  Very pistol — *see* Discharge, firearm NEC
Butted by animal W55.82 ☑
  bull W55.22 ☑
  cow W55.22 ☑
  goat W55.32 ☑
  horse W55.12 ☑
  pig W55.42 ☑
  sheep W55.32 ☑

C

Caisson disease — *see* Air, pressure, change
Campfire (exposure to) (controlled) (*see also* Exposure,
  fire, controlled, not in building)
  uncontrolled — *see* Exposure, fire, uncontrolled, not
    in building
Capital punishment (any means) — *see* Legal, intervention
Car sickness T75.3 ☑
Casualty (not due to war) NEC X58 ☑
  war — *see* War operations
Cat
  bite W55.01 ☑
  scratch W55.03 ☑
Cataclysm, cataclysmic (any injury) NEC — *see* Forces
  of nature
Catching fire — *see* Exposure, fire
Caught
  between
    folding object W23.0 ☑
    objects (moving) (stationary and moving) W23.0 ☑
    and machinery — *see* Contact, with, by type of
      machine
    stationary W23.1 ☑
    sliding door and door frame W23.0 ☑
  by, in
    machinery (moving parts of) — *see* Contact, with,
      by type of machine
    washing-machine wringer W23.0 ☑
  under packing crate (due to losing grip) W23.1 ☑
**Cave-in caused by cataclysmic earth surface move-
  ment or eruption** — *see* Landslide
Change(s) in air pressure — *see* Air, pressure, change
Choked, choking (on) (any object except food or vomitus)
  food (bone) (seed) — *see* categories T17 and T18 ☑
  vomitus T17.81- ☑
Civil insurrection — *see* War operations
Cloudburst (any injury) X37.8 ☑
Cold, exposure to (accidental) (excessive) (extreme)
  (natural) (place) NEC — *see* Exposure, cold
Collapse
  building W20.1 ☑
    burning (uncontrolled fire) X00.2 ☑
  dam or man-made structure (causing earth movement)
    X36.0 ☑
  machinery — *see* Contact, with, by type of machine
  structure W20.1 ☑
    burning (uncontrolled fire) X00.2 ☑
Collision (accidental) NEC (*see also* Accident, transport)
  V89.9 ☑
  pedestrian W51 ☑
    with fall W03 ☑
      due to ice or snow W00.0 ☑
      involving pedestrian conveyance — *see* Acci-
        dent, transport, pedestrian, conveyance
    and
      crowd or human stampede (with fall) W52 ☑
      object W22.8 ☑

Collision — *continued*
  pedestrian — *continued*
    and — *continued*
      object — *continued*
        with fall — *see* Fall, due to, bumping against, object
  person(s) — *see* Collision, pedestrian
  transport vehicle NEC V89.9 ☑
    and
      avalanche, fallen or not moving — *see* Accident, transport
        falling or moving — *see* Landslide
      landslide, fallen or not moving — *see* Accident, transport
        falling or moving — *see* Landslide
    due to cataclysm — *see* Forces of nature, by type
    intentional, purposeful suicide (attempt) — *see* Suicide, collision
Combustion, spontaneous — *see* Ignition
Complication (delayed) **of or following** (medical or surgical procedure) Y84.9
  with misadventure — *see* Misadventure
  amputation of limb(s) Y83.5
  anastomosis (arteriovenous) (blood vessel) (gastroje-junal) (tendon) (natural or artificial material) Y83.2
  aspiration (of fluid) Y84.4
    tissue Y84.8
  biopsy Y84.8
  blood
    sampling Y84.7
    transfusion
      procedure Y84.8
  bypass Y83.2
  catheterization (urinary) Y84.6
    cardiac Y84.0
  colostomy Y83.3
  cystostomy Y83.3
  dialysis (kidney) Y84.1
  drug — *see* Table of Drugs and Chemicals
  due to misadventure — *see* Misadventure
  duodenostomy Y83.3
  electroshock therapy Y84.3
  external stoma, creation of Y83.3
  formation of external stoma Y83.3
  gastrostomy Y83.3
  graft Y83.2
  hypothermia (medically-induced) Y84.8
  implant, implantation (of)
    artificial
      internal device (cardiac pacemaker) (electrodes in brain) (heart valve prosthesis) (ortho-pedic) Y83.1
      material or tissue (for anastomosis or bypass) Y83.2
        with creation of external stoma Y83.3
      natural tissues (for anastomosis or bypass) Y83.2
        with creation of external stoma Y83.3
  infusion
    procedure Y84.8
  injection — *see* Table of Drugs and Chemicals
    procedure Y84.8
  insertion of gastric or duodenal sound Y84.5
  insulin-shock therapy Y84.3
  paracentesis (abdominal) (thoracic) (aspirative) Y84.4
  procedures other than surgical operation — *see* Complication of or following, by type of proce-dure
  radiological procedure or therapy Y84.2
  removal of organ (partial) (total) NEC Y83.6
  sampling
    blood Y84.7
    fluid NEC Y84.4
    tissue Y84.8
  shock therapy Y84.3
  surgical operation NEC (*see also* Complication of or following, by type of operation) Y83.9
    reconstructive NEC Y83.4
      with
        anastomosis, bypass or graft Y83.2
        formation of external stoma Y83.3
    specified NEC Y83.8
  transfusion (*see also* Table of Drugs and Chemicals)
    procedure Y84.8
  transplant, transplantation (heart) (kidney) (liver) (whole organ, any) Y83.0
    partial organ Y83.4
  ureterostomy Y83.3

Complication (delayed) **of or following** — *continued*
  vaccination (*see also* Table of Drugs and Chemicals)
    procedure Y84.8
Compression
  divers' squeeze — *see* Air, pressure, change
  trachea by
    food (lodged in esophagus) — *see* categories T17 and T18 ☑
    vomitus (lodged in esophagus) T17.81- ☑
Conflagration — *see* Exposure, fire, uncontrolled
Constriction (external)
  hair W49.01 ☑
  jewelry W49.04 ☑
  ring W49.04 ☑
  rubber band W49.03 ☑
  specified item NEC W49.09 ☑
  string W49.02 ☑
  thread W49.02 ☑
Contact (accidental)
  with
    abrasive wheel (metalworking) W31.1 ☑
    alligator W58.09 ☑
      bite W58.01 ☑
      crushing W58.03 ☑
      strike W58.02 ☑
    amphibian W62.9 ☑
      frog W62.0 ☑
      toad W62.1 ☑
    animal (nonvenomous) NEC W64 ☑
      marine W56.89 ☑
        bite W56.81 ☑
        dolphin — *see* Contact, with, dolphin
        fish NEC — *see* Contact, with, fish
        mammal — *see* Contact, with, mammal, marine
        orca — *see* Contact, with, orca
        sea lion — *see* Contact, with, sea lion
        shark — *see* Contact, with, shark
        strike W56.82 ☑
    animate mechanical force NEC W64 ☑
    arrow W21.89 ☑
      not thrown, projected or falling W45.8 ☑
    arthropods (nonvenomous) W57 ☑
    axe W27.0 ☑
    band-saw (industrial) W31.2 ☑
    bayonet — *see* Bayonet wound
    bee(s) X58 ☑
    bench-saw (industrial) W31.2 ☑
    bird W61.99 ☑
      bite W61.91 ☑
      chicken — *see* Contact, with, chicken
      duck — *see* Contact, with, duck
      goose — *see* Contact, with, goose
      macaw — *see* Contact, with, macaw
      parrot — *see* Contact, with, parrot
      psittacine — *see* Contact, with, psittacine
      strike W61.92 ☑
      turkey — *see* Contact, with, turkey
    blender W29.0 ☑
    boiling water X12 ☑
      stated as undetermined whether accidental or intentional Y27.2 ☑
      suicide (attempt) X77.2 ☑
    bore, earth-drilling or mining (land) (seabed) W31.0 ☑
    buffalo — *see* Contact, with, hoof stock NEC
    bull W55.29 ☑
      bite W55.21 ☑
      gored W55.22 ☑
      strike W55.22 ☑
    bumper cars W31.81 ☑
    camel — *see* Contact, with, hoof stock NEC
    can
      lid W26.8 ☑
      opener W27.4 ☑
        powered W29.0 ☑
    cat W55.09 ☑
      bite W55.01 ☑
      scratch W55.03 ☑
    caterpillar (venomous) X58 ☑
    centipede (venomous) X58 ☑
    chain
      hoist W24.0 ☑
        agricultural operations W30.89 ☑
      saw W29.3 ☑

Contact — *continued*
  with — *continued*
    chicken W61.39 ☑
      peck W61.33 ☑
      strike W61.32 ☑
    chisel W27.0 ☑
    circular saw W31.2 ☑
    cobra X58 ☑
    combine (harvester) W30.0 ☑
    conveyer belt W24.1 ☑
    cooker (hot) X15.8 ☑
      stated as undetermined whether accidental or intentional Y27.3 ☑
      suicide (attempt) X77.3 ☑
    coral X58 ☑
    cotton gin W31.82 ☑
    cow W55.29 ☑
      bite W55.21 ☑
      strike W55.22 ☑
    crane W24.0 ☑
      agricultural operations W30.89 ☑
    crocodile W58.19 ☑
      bite W58.11 ☑
      crushing W58.13 ☑
      strike W58.12 ☑
    dagger W26.1 ☑
      stated as undetermined whether accidental or intentional Y28.2 ☑
      suicide (attempt) X78.2 ☑
    dairy equipment W31.82 ☑
    dart W21.89 ☑
      not thrown, projected or falling W45.8 ☑
    deer — *see* Contact, with, hoof stock NEC
    derrick W24.0 ☑
      agricultural operations W30.89 ☑
      hay W30.2 ☑
    dog W54.8 ☑
      bite W54.0 ☑
      strike W54.1 ☑
    dolphin W56.09 ☑
      bite W56.01 ☑
      strike W56.02 ☑
    donkey — *see* Contact, with, hoof stock NEC
    drill (powered) W29.8 ☑
      earth (land) (seabed) W31.0 ☑
      nonpowered W27.8 ☑
    drive belt W24.0 ☑
      agricultural operations W30.89 ☑
    dry ice — *see* Exposure, cold, man-made
    dryer (clothes) (powered) (spin) W29.2 ☑
    duck W61.69 ☑
      bite W61.61 ☑
      strike W61.62 ☑
    earth (-)
      drilling machine (industrial) W31.0 ☑
      scraping machine in stationary use W31.83 ☑
    edge of stiff paper W26.2 ☑
    electric
      beater W29.0 ☑
      blanket X16 ☑
      fan W29.2 ☑
        commercial W31.82 ☑
      knife W29.1 ☑
      mixer W29.0 ☑
    elevator (building) W24.0 ☑
      agricultural operations W30.89 ☑
        grain W30.3 ☑
    engine(s), hot NEC X17 ☑
    excavating machine W31.0 ☑
    farm machine W30.9 ☑
    feces — *see* Contact, with, by type of animal
    fer de lance X58 ☑
    fish W56.59 ☑
      bite W56.51 ☑
      shark — *see* Contact, with, shark
      strike W56.52 ☑
    flying horses W31.81 ☑
    forging (metalworking) machine W31.1 ☑
    fork W27.4 ☑
    forklift (truck) W24.0 ☑
      agricultural operations W30.89 ☑
    frog W62.0 ☑
    garden
      cultivator (powered) W29.3 ☑
        riding W30.89 ☑
      fork W27.1 ☑

Contact — *continued*
　with — *continued*
　　gas turbine W31.3 ☑
　　Gila monster X58 ☑
　　giraffe — *see* Contact, with, hoof stock NEC
　　glass (sharp) (broken) W25 ☑
　　　with subsequent fall W18.02 ☑
　　　assault X99.0 ☑
　　　due to fall — *see* Fall, by type
　　　stated as undetermined whether accidental or intentional Y28.0 ☑
　　　suicide (attempt) X78.0 ☑
　　goat W55.39 ☑
　　　bite W55.31 ☑
　　　strike W55.32 ☑
　　goose W61.59 ☑
　　　bite W61.51 ☑
　　　strike W61.52 ☑
　　hand
　　　saw W27.0 ☑
　　　tool (not powered) NEC W27.8 ☑
　　　　powered W29.8 ☑
　　harvester W30.0 ☑
　　hay-derrick W30.2 ☑
　　heating
　　　appliance (hot) X16 ☑
　　　pad (electric) X16 ☑
　　heat NEC X19 ☑
　　　from appliance (electrical) (household) — *see* Contact, with, hot, household appliance heating appliance X16 ☑
　　hedge-trimmer (powered) W29.3 ☑
　　hoe W27.1 ☑
　　hoist (chain) (shaft) NEC W24.0 ☑
　　　agricultural W30.89 ☑
　　hoof stock NEC W55.39 ☑
　　　bite W55.31 ☑
　　　strike W55.32 ☑
　　hornet(s) X58 ☑
　　horse W55.19 ☑
　　　bite W55.11 ☑
　　　strike W55.12 ☑
　　hot
　　　air X14.1 ☑
　　　　inhalation X14.0 ☑
　　　cooker X15.8 ☑
　　　drinks X10.0 ☑
　　　engine X17 ☑
　　　fats X10.2 ☑
　　　fluids NEC X12 ☑
　　　　assault X98.2 ☑
　　　　suicide (attempt) X77.2 ☑
　　　　undetermined whether accidental or intentional Y27.2 ☑
　　　food X10.1 ☑
　　　gases X14.1 ☑
　　　　inhalation X14.0 ☑
　　　heating appliance X16 ☑
　　　household appliance X15.8 ☑
　　　　assault X98.3 ☑
　　　　cooker X15.8 ☑
　　　　hotplate X15.2 ☑
　　　　kettle X15.8 ☑
　　　　light bulb X15.8 ☑
　　　　object NEC X19 ☑
　　　　　assault X98.8 ☑
　　　　　stated as undetermined whether accidental or intentional Y27.9 ☑
　　　　　suicide (attempt) X77.8 ☑
　　　　saucepan X15.3 ☑
　　　　skillet X15.3 ☑
　　　　stated as undetermined whether accidental or intentional Y27.3 ☑
　　　　stove X15.0 ☑
　　　　suicide (attempt) X77.3 ☑
　　　　toaster X15.1 ☑
　　　kettle X15.8 ☑
　　　light bulb X15.8 ☑
　　　liquid NEC (*see also* Burn) X12 ☑
　　　　drinks X10.0 ☑
　　　　stated as undetermined whether accidental or intentional Y27.2 ☑
　　　　suicide (attempt) X77.2 ☑
　　　　tap water X11.8 ☑
　　　　　stated as undetermined whether accidental or intentional Y27.1 ☑

Contact — *continued*
　with — *continued*
　　hot — *continued*
　　　liquid (*see also* Burn) — *continued*
　　　　tap water — *continued*
　　　　　suicide (attempt) X77.1 ☑
　　　machinery X17 ☑
　　　metal (molten) (liquid) NEC X18 ☑
　　　object (not producing fire or flames) NEC X19 ☑
　　　oil (cooking) X10.2 ☑
　　　pipe X16 ☑
　　　plate X15.2 ☑
　　　radiator X16 ☑
　　　saucepan (glass) (metal) X15.3 ☑
　　　skillet X15.3 ☑
　　　stove (kitchen) X15.0 ☑
　　　substance NEC X19 ☑
　　　tap-water X11.8 ☑
　　　　assault X98.1 ☑
　　　　heated on stove X12 ☑
　　　　　stated as undetermined whether accidental or intentional Y27.2 ☑
　　　　　suicide (attempt) X77.2 ☑
　　　　in bathtub X11.0 ☑
　　　　running X11.1 ☑
　　　　stated as undetermined whether accidental or intentional Y27.1 ☑
　　　　suicide (attempt) X77.1 ☑
　　　toaster X15.1 ☑
　　　tool X17 ☑
　　　vapors X13.1 ☑
　　　　inhalation X13.0 ☑
　　　water (tap) X11.8 ☑
　　　　boiling X12 ☑
　　　　　stated as undetermined whether accidental or intentional Y27.2 ☑
　　　　　suicide (attempt) X77.2 ☑
　　　　heated on stove X12 ☑
　　　　　stated as undetermined whether accidental or intentional Y27.2 ☑
　　　　　suicide (attempt) X77.2 ☑
　　　　in bathtub X11.0 ☑
　　　　running X11.1 ☑
　　　　stated as undetermined whether accidental or intentional Y27.1 ☑
　　　　suicide (attempt) X77.1 ☑
　　hotplate X15.2 ☑
　　ice-pick W27.4 ☑
　　insect (nonvenomous) NEC W57 ☑
　　kettle (hot) X15.8 ☑
　　knife W26.0 ☑
　　　assault X99.1 ☑
　　　electric W29.1 ☑
　　　stated as undetermined whether accidental or intentional Y28.1 ☑
　　　suicide (attempt) X78.1 ☑
　　lathe (metalworking) W31.1 ☑
　　　turnings W45.8 ☑
　　　woodworking W31.2 ☑
　　lawnmower (powered) (ridden) W28 ☑
　　　causing electrocution W86.8 ☑
　　　　suicide (attempt) X83.1 ☑
　　　unpowered W27.1 ☑
　　lift, lifting (devices) W24.0 ☑
　　　agricultural operations W30.89 ☑
　　　shaft W24.0 ☑
　　liquefied gas — *see* Exposure, cold, man-made
　　liquid air, hydrogen, nitrogen — *see* Exposure, cold, man-made
　　lizard (nonvenomous) W59.09 ☑
　　　bite W59.01 ☑
　　　strike W59.02 ☑
　　llama — *see* Contact, with, hoof stock NEC
　　macaw W61.19 ☑
　　　bite W61.11 ☑
　　　strike W61.12 ☑
　　machine, machinery W31.9 ☑
　　　abrasive wheel W31.1 ☑
　　　agricultural including animal-powered W30.9 ☑
　　　　combine harvester W30.0 ☑
　　　　grain storage elevator W30.3 ☑
　　　　hay derrick W30.2 ☑
　　　　power take-off device W30.1 ☑
　　　　reaper W30.0 ☑
　　　　specified NEC W30.89 ☑

Contact — *continued*
　with — *continued*
　　machine, machinery — *continued*
　　　agricultural including animal-powered — *continued*
　　　　thresher W30.0 ☑
　　　　transport vehicle, stationary W30.81 ☑
　　　band saw W31.2 ☑
　　　bench saw W31.2 ☑
　　　circular saw W31.2 ☑
　　　commercial NEC W31.82 ☑
　　　drilling, metal (industrial) W31.1 ☑
　　　earth-drilling W31.0 ☑
　　　earthmoving or scraping W31.89 ☑
　　　excavating W31.89 ☑
　　　forging machine W31.1 ☑
　　　gas turbine W31.3 ☑
　　　hot X17 ☑
　　　internal combustion engine W31.3 ☑
　　　land drill W31.0 ☑
　　　lathe W31.1 ☑
　　　lifting (devices) W24.0 ☑
　　　metal drill W31.1 ☑
　　　metalworking (industrial) W31.1 ☑
　　　milling, metal W31.1 ☑
　　　mining W31.0 ☑
　　　molding W31.2 ☑
　　　overhead plane W31.2 ☑
　　　power press, metal W31.1 ☑
　　　prime mover W31.3 ☑
　　　printing W31.89 ☑
　　　radial saw W31.2 ☑
　　　recreational W31.81 ☑
　　　roller-coaster W31.81 ☑
　　　rolling mill, metal W31.1 ☑
　　　sander W31.2 ☑
　　　seabed drill W31.0 ☑
　　　shaft
　　　　hoist W31.0 ☑
　　　　lift W31.0 ☑
　　　specified NEC W31.89 ☑
　　　spinning W31.89 ☑
　　　steam engine W31.3 ☑
　　　transmission W24.1 ☑
　　　undercutter W31.0 ☑
　　　water driven turbine W31.3 ☑
　　　weaving W31.89 ☑
　　　woodworking or forming (industrial) W31.2 ☑
　　mammal (feces) (urine) W55.89 ☑
　　　bull — *see* Contact, with, bull
　　　cat — *see* Contact, with, cat
　　　cow — *see* Contact, with, cow
　　　goat — *see* Contact, with, goat
　　　hoof stock — *see* Contact, with, hoof stock
　　　horse — *see* Contact, with, horse
　　　marine W56.39 ☑
　　　　dolphin — *see* Contact, with, dolphin
　　　　orca — *see* Contact, with, orca
　　　　sea lion — *see* Contact, with, sea lion
　　　　specified NEC W56.39 ☑
　　　　　bite W56.31 ☑
　　　　　strike W56.32 ☑
　　　pig — *see* Contact, with, pig
　　　raccoon — *see* Contact, with, raccoon
　　　rodent — *see* Contact, with, rodent
　　　sheep — *see* Contact, with, sheep
　　　specified NEC W55.89 ☑
　　　　bite W55.81 ☑
　　　　strike W55.82 ☑
　　marine
　　　animal W56.89 ☑
　　　　bite W56.81 ☑
　　　　dolphin — *see* Contact, with, dolphin
　　　　fish NEC — *see* Contact, with, fish
　　　　mammal — *see* Contact, with, mammal, marine
　　　　orca — *see* Contact, with, orca
　　　　sea lion — *see* Contact, with, sea lion
　　　　shark — *see* Contact, with, shark
　　　　strike W56.82 ☑
　　meat
　　　grinder (domestic) W29.0 ☑
　　　　industrial W31.82 ☑
　　　　nonpowered W27.4 ☑
　　　slicer (domestic) W29.0 ☑
　　　　industrial W31.82 ☑

Contact — *continued*
  with — *continued*
    merry go round W31.81 ☑
    metal, hot (liquid) (molten) NEC X18 ☑
    millipede W57 ☑
    nail W45.0 ☑
      gun W29.4 ☑
    needle (sewing) W27.3 ☑
      hypodermic W46.0 ☑
        contaminated W46.1 ☑
    object (blunt) NEC
      hot NEC X19 ☑
      legal intervention — *see* Legal, intervention,
        blunt object
      sharp NEC W45.8 ☑
        inflicted by other person NEC W45.8 ☑
          stated as
            intentional homicide (attempt) —
              see Assault, cutting or piercing
              instrument
        legal intervention — *see* Legal, intervention,
          sharp object
        self-inflicted X78.9 ☑
    orca W56.29 ☑
      bite W56.21 ☑
      strike W56.22 ☑
    overhead plane W31.2 ☑
    paper (as sharp object) W26.2 ☑
    paper-cutter W27.5 ☑
    parrot W61.09 ☑
      bite W61.01 ☑
      strike W61.02 ☑
    pig W55.49 ☑
      bite W55.41 ☑
      strike W55.42 ☑
    pipe, hot X16 ☑
    pitchfork W27.1 ☑
    plane (metal) (wood) W27.0 ☑
      overhead W31.2 ☑
    plant thorns, spines, sharp leaves or other mecha-
      nisms W60 ☑
    powered
      garden cultivator W29.3 ☑
      household appliance, implement, or machine
        W29.8 ☑
      saw (industrial) W31.2 ☑
        hand W29.8 ☑
    printing machine W31.89 ☑
    psittacine bird W61.29 ☑
      bite W61.21 ☑
      macaw — *see* Contact, with, macaw
      parrot — *see* Contact, with, parrot
      strike W61.22 ☑
    pulley (block) (transmission) W24.0 ☑
      agricultural operations W30.89 ☑
    raccoon W55.59 ☑
      bite W55.51 ☑
      strike W55.52 ☑
    radial-saw (industrial) W31.2 ☑
    radiator (hot) X16 ☑
    rake W27.1 ☑
    rattlesnake X58 ☑
    reaper W30.0 ☑
    reptile W59.89 ☑
      lizard — *see* Contact, with, lizard
      snake — *see* Contact, with, snake
      specified NEC W59.89 ☑
        bite W59.81 ☑
        crushing W59.83 ☑
        strike W59.82 ☑
      turtle — *see* Contact, with, turtle
    rivet gun (powered) W29.4 ☑
    road scraper — *see* Accident, transport, construc-
      tion vehicle
    rodent (feces) (urine) W53.89 ☑
      bite W53.81 ☑
      mouse W53.09 ☑
        bite W53.01 ☑
      rat W53.19 ☑
        bite W53.11 ☑
      specified NEC W53.89 ☑
        bite W53.81 ☑
      squirrel W53.29 ☑
        bite W53.21 ☑
    roller coaster W31.81 ☑
    rope NEC W24.0 ☑

Contact — *continued*
  with — *continued*
    rope — *continued*
      agricultural operations W30.89 ☑
    saliva — *see* Contact, with, by type of animal
    sander W29.8 ☑
      industrial W31.2 ☑
    saucepan (hot) (glass) (metal) X15.3 ☑
    saw W27.0 ☑
      band (industrial) W31.2 ☑
      bench (industrial) W31.2 ☑
      chain W29.3 ☑
      hand W27.0 ☑
    sawing machine, metal W31.1 ☑
    scissors W27.2 ☑
    scorpion X58 ☑
    screwdriver W27.0 ☑
      powered W29.8 ☑
    sea
      anemone, cucumber or urchin (spine) X58 ☑
      lion W56.19 ☑
        bite W56.11 ☑
        strike W56.12 ☑
    serpent — *see* Contact, with, snake, by type
    sewing-machine (electric) (powered) W29.2 ☑
      not powered W27.8 ☑
    shaft (hoist) (lift) (transmission) NEC W24.0 ☑
      agricultural W30.89 ☑
    shark W56.49 ☑
      bite W56.41 ☑
      strike W56.42 ☑
    sharp object(s) W26.9 ☑
      specified NEC W26.8 ☑
    shears (hand) W27.2 ☑
      powered (industrial) W31.1 ☑
        domestic W29.2 ☑
    sheep W55.39 ☑
      bite W55.31 ☑
      strike W55.32 ☑
    shovel W27.8 ☑
      steam — *see* Accident, transport, construction
        vehicle
    snake (nonvenomous) W59.19 ☑
      bite W59.11 ☑
      crushing W59.13 ☑
      strike W59.12 ☑
    spade W27.1 ☑
    spider (venomous) X58 ☑
    spin-drier W29.2 ☑
    spinning machine W31.89 ☑
    splinter W45.8 ☑
    sports equipment W21.9 ☑
    staple gun (powered) W29.8 ☑
    steam X13.1 ☑
      engine W31.3 ☑
      inhalation X13.0 ☑
      pipe X16 ☑
      shovel W31.89 ☑
    stove (hot) (kitchen) X15.0 ☑
    substance, hot NEC X19 ☑
      molten (metal) X18 ☑
    sword W26.1 ☑
      assault X99.2 ☑
      stated as undetermined whether accidental or
        intentional Y28.2 ☑
      suicide (attempt) X78.2 ☑
    tarantula X58 ☑
    thresher W30.0 ☑
    tin can lid W26.8 ☑
    toad W62.1 ☑
    toaster (hot) X15.1 ☑
    tool W27.8 ☑
      hand (not powered) W27.8 ☑
        auger W27.0 ☑
        axe W27.0 ☑
        can opener W27.4 ☑
        chisel W27.0 ☑
        fork W27.4 ☑
        garden W27.1 ☑
        handsaw W27.0 ☑
        hoe W27.1 ☑
        ice-pick W27.4 ☑
        kitchen utensil W27.4 ☑
        manual
          lawn mower W27.1 ☑
          sewing machine W27.8 ☑

Contact — *continued*
  with — *continued*
    tool — *continued*
      hand — *continued*
        meat grinder W27.4 ☑
        needle (sewing) W27.3 ☑
          hypodermic W46.0 ☑
            contaminated W46.1 ☑
        paper cutter W27.5 ☑
        pitchfork W27.1 ☑
        rake W27.1 ☑
        scissors W27.2 ☑
        screwdriver W27.0 ☑
        specified NEC W27.8 ☑
        workbench W27.0 ☑
      hot X17 ☑
      powered W29.8 ☑
        blender W29.0 ☑
          commercial W31.82 ☑
        can opener W29.0 ☑
          commercial W31.82 ☑
        chainsaw W29.3 ☑
        clothes dryer W29.2 ☑
          commercial W31.82 ☑
        dishwasher W29.2 ☑
          commercial W31.82 ☑
        edger W29.3 ☑
        electric fan W29.2 ☑
          commercial W31.82 ☑
        electric knife W29.1 ☑
        food processor W29.0 ☑
          commercial W31.82 ☑
        garbage disposal W29.0 ☑
          commercial W31.82 ☑
        garden tool W29.3 ☑
        hedge trimmer W29.3 ☑
        ice maker W29.0 ☑
          commercial W31.82 ☑
        kitchen appliance W29.0 ☑
          commercial W31.82 ☑
        lawn mower W28 ☑
        meat grinder W29.0 ☑
          commercial W31.82 ☑
        mixer W29.0 ☑
          commercial W31.82 ☑
        rototiller W29.3 ☑
        sewing machine W29.2 ☑
          commercial W31.82 ☑
        washing machine W29.2 ☑
          commercial W31.82 ☑
    transmission device (belt, cable, chain, gear, pinion,
      shaft) W24.1 ☑
      agricultural operations W30.89 ☑
    turbine (gas) (water-driven) W31.3 ☑
    turkey W61.49 ☑
      peck W61.43 ☑
      strike W61.42 ☑
    turtle (nonvenomous) W59.29 ☑
      bite W59.21 ☑
      strike W59.22 ☑
      terrestrial W59.89 ☑
        bite W59.81 ☑
        crushing W59.83 ☑
        strike W59.82 ☑
    under-cutter W31.0 ☑
    urine — *see* Contact, with, by type of animal
    vehicle
      agricultural use (transport) — *see* Accident,
        transport, agricultural vehicle
        not on public highway W30.81 ☑
      industrial use (transport) — *see* Accident,
        transport, industrial vehicle
        not on public highway W31.83 ☑
      off-road use (transport) — *see* Accident, trans-
        port, all-terrain or off-road vehicle
        not on public highway W31.83 ☑
      special construction use (transport) — *see* Acci-
        dent, transport, construction vehicle
        not on public highway W31.83 ☑
    venomous
      animal X58 ☑
      arthropods X58 ☑
      lizard X58 ☑
      marine animal NEC X58 ☑
      marine plant NEC X58 ☑
      millipedes (tropical) X58 ☑

☑ Additional Character Required — Refer to the Tabular List for Character Selection   ▽ Subterms under main terms may continue to next column or page

Contact — *continued*
　with — *continued*
　　venomous — *continued*
　　　plant(s) X58 ☑
　　　snake X58 ☑
　　　spider X58 ☑
　　　viper X58 ☑
　　　washing-machine (powered) W29.2 ☑
　　　wasp X58 ☑
　　　weaving-machine W31.89 ☑
　　　winch W24.0 ☑
　　　　agricultural operations W30.89 ☑
　　　wire NEC W24.0 ☑
　　　　agricultural operations W30.89 ☑
　　　wood slivers W45.8 ☑
　　　yellow jacket X58 ☑
　　　zebra — *see* Contact, with, hoof stock NEC
　　pressure X50.9 ☑
　　stress X50.9 ☑
Coup de soleil X32 ☑
Crash
　aircraft (in transit) (powered) V95.9 ☑
　　balloon V96.01 ☑
　　fixed wing NEC (private) V95.21 ☑
　　　commercial V95.31 ☑
　　glider V96.21 ☑
　　　hang V96.11 ☑
　　　powered V95.11 ☑
　　helicopter V95.01 ☑
　　in war operations — *see* War operations, destruction of aircraft
　　microlight V95.11 ☑
　　nonpowered V96.9 ☑
　　　specified NEC V96.8 ☑
　　powered NEC V95.8 ☑
　　stated as
　　　homicide (attempt) Y08.81 ☑
　　　suicide (attempt) X83.0 ☑
　　ultralight V95.11 ☑
　　spacecraft V95.41 ☑
　transport vehicle NEC (*see also* Accident, transport) V89.9 ☑
　　homicide (attempt) Y03.8 ☑
　　motor NEC (traffic) V89.2 ☑
　　　homicide (attempt) Y03.8 ☑
　　　suicide (attempt) — *see* Suicide, collision
Cruelty (mental) (physical) (sexual) X58 ☑
Crushed (accidentally) X58 ☑
　between objects (moving) (stationary and moving) W23.0 ☑
　　stationary W23.1 ☑
　by
　　alligator W58.03 ☑
　　avalanche NEC — *see* Landslide
　　cave-in W20.0 ☑
　　　caused by cataclysmic earth surface movement — *see* Landslide
　　crocodile W58.13 ☑
　　crowd or human stampede W52 ☑
　　falling
　　　aircraft V97.39 ☑
　　　　in war operations — *see* War operations, destruction of aircraft
　　　earth, material W20.0 ☑
　　　　caused by cataclysmic earth surface movement — *see* Landslide
　　　object NEC W20.8 ☑
　　landslide NEC — *see* Landslide
　　lizard (nonvenomous) W59.09 ☑
　　machinery — *see* Contact, with, by type of machine
　　reptile NEC W59.89 ☑
　　snake (nonvenomous) W59.13 ☑
　in
　　machinery — *see* Contact, with, by type of machine
Cut, cutting (any part of body) (accidental) (*see also* Contact, with, by object or machine)
　during medical or surgical treatment as misadventure — *see* Index to Diseases and Injuries, Complications
　homicide (attempt) — *see* Assault, cutting or piercing instrument
　inflicted by other person — *see* Assault, cutting or piercing instrument
　legal
　　execution — *see* Legal, intervention

Cut, cutting — *continued*
　legal — *continued*
　　intervention — *see* Legal, intervention, sharp object
　machine NEC (*see also* Contact, with, by type of machine) W31.9 ☑
　self-inflicted — *see* Suicide, cutting or piercing instrument
　suicide (attempt) — *see* Suicide, cutting or piercing instrument
Cyclone (any injury) X37.1 ☑

D

Decapitation (accidental circumstances) NEC X58 ☑
　homicide X99.9 ☑
　legal execution — *see* Legal, intervention
Dehydration from lack of water X58 ☑
Deprivation X58 ☑
Derailment (accidental)
　railway (rolling stock) (train) (vehicle) (without antecedent collision) V81.7 ☑
　　with antecedent collision — *see* Accident, transport, railway vehicle occupant
　streetcar (without antecedent collision) V82.7 ☑
　　with antecedent collision — *see* Accident, transport, streetcar occupant
Descent
　parachute (voluntary) (without accident to aircraft) V97.29 ☑
　　due to accident to aircraft — *see* Accident, transport, aircraft
Desertion X58 ☑
Destitution X58 ☑
Disability, late effect or sequela of injury — *see* Sequelae
Discharge (accidental)
　airgun W34.010 ☑
　　assault X95.01 ☑
　　homicide (attempt) X95.01 ☑
　　stated as undetermined whether accidental or intentional Y24.0 ☑
　　suicide (attempt) X74.01 ☑
　BB gun — *see* Discharge, airgun
　firearm (accidental) W34.00 ☑
　　assault X95.9 ☑
　　handgun (pistol) (revolver) W32.0 ☑
　　　assault X93 ☑
　　　homicide (attempt) X93 ☑
　　　legal intervention — *see* Legal, intervention, firearm, handgun
　　　stated as undetermined whether accidental or intentional Y22 ☑
　　　suicide (attempt) X72 ☑
　　homicide (attempt) X95.9 ☑
　　hunting rifle W33.02 ☑
　　　assault X94.1 ☑
　　　homicide (attempt) X94.1 ☑
　　　legal intervention
　　　　injuring
　　　　　bystander Y35.032 ☑
　　　　　law enforcement personnel Y35.031 ☑
　　　　　suspect Y35.033 ☑
　　　stated as undetermined whether accidental or intentional Y23.1 ☑
　　　suicide (attempt) X73.1 ☑
　　larger W33.00 ☑
　　　assault X94.9 ☑
　　　homicide (attempt) X94.9 ☑
　　　hunting rifle — *see* Discharge, firearm, hunting rifle
　　　legal intervention — *see* Legal, intervention, firearm by type of firearm
　　　machine gun — *see* Discharge, firearm, machine gun
　　　shotgun — *see* Discharge, firearm, shotgun
　　　specified NEC W33.09 ☑
　　　　assault X94.8 ☑
　　　　homicide (attempt) X94.8 ☑
　　　　legal intervention
　　　　　injuring
　　　　　　bystander Y35.092 ☑
　　　　　　law enforcement personnel Y35.091 ☑
　　　　　　suspect Y35.093 ☑

Discharge — *continued*
　firearm — *continued*
　　larger — *continued*
　　　specified — *continued*
　　　　stated as undetermined whether accidental or intentional Y23.8 ☑
　　　　suicide (attempt) X73.8 ☑
　　　stated as undetermined whether accidental or intentional Y23.9 ☑
　　　suicide (attempt) X73.9 ☑
　　legal intervention
　　　injuring
　　　　bystander Y35.002 ☑
　　　　law enforcement personnel Y35.001 ☑
　　　　suspect Y35.03 ☑
　　　using rubber bullet
　　　　injuring
　　　　　bystander Y35.042 ☑
　　　　　law enforcement personnel Y35.041 ☑
　　　　　suspect Y35.043 ☑
　　machine gun W33.03 ☑
　　　assault X94.2 ☑
　　　homicide (attempt) X94.2 ☑
　　　legal intervention — *see* Legal, intervention, firearm, machine gun
　　　stated as undetermined whether accidental or intentional Y23.3 ☑
　　　suicide (attempt) X73.2 ☑
　　pellet gun — *see* Discharge, airgun
　　shotgun W33.01 ☑
　　　assault X94.0 ☑
　　　homicide (attempt) X94.0 ☑
　　　legal intervention — *see* Legal, intervention, firearm, specified NEC
　　　stated as undetermined whether accidental or intentional Y23.0 ☑
　　　suicide (attempt) X73.0 ☑
　　specified NEC W34.09 ☑
　　　assault X95.8 ☑
　　　homicide (attempt) X95.8 ☑
　　　legal intervention — *see* Legal, intervention, firearm, specified NEC
　　　stated as undetermined whether accidental or intentional Y24.8 ☑
　　　suicide (attempt) X74.8 ☑
　　stated as undetermined whether accidental or intentional Y24.9 ☑
　　suicide (attempt) X74.9 ☑
　　Very pistol W34.09 ☑
　　　assault X95.8 ☑
　　　homicide (attempt) X95.8 ☑
　　　stated as undetermined whether accidental or intentional Y24.8 ☑
　　　suicide (attempt) X74.8 ☑
　firework(s) W39 ☑
　　stated as undetermined whether accidental or intentional Y25 ☑
　gas-operated gun NEC W34.018 ☑
　　airgun — *see* Discharge, airgun
　　assault X95.09 ☑
　　homicide (attempt) X95.09 ☑
　　paintball gun — *see* Discharge, paintball gun
　　stated as undetermined whether accidental or intentional Y24.8 ☑
　　suicide (attempt) X74.09 ☑
　gun NEC (*see also* Discharge, firearm NEC)
　　air — *see* Discharge, airgun
　　BB — *see* Discharge, airgun
　　for single hand use — *see* Discharge, firearm, handgun
　　hand — *see* Discharge, firearm, handgun
　　machine — *see* Discharge, firearm, machine gun
　　other specified — *see* Discharge, firearm NEC
　　paintball — *see* Discharge, paintball gun
　　pellet — *see* Discharge, airgun
　handgun — *see* Discharge, firearm, handgun
　machine gun — *see* Discharge, firearm, machine gun
　paintball gun W34.011 ☑
　　assault X95.02 ☑
　　homicide (attempt) X95.02 ☑
　　stated as undetermined whether accidental or intentional Y24.8 ☑
　　suicide (attempt) X74.02 ☑
　pistol — *see* Discharge, firearm, handgun
　　flare — *see* Discharge, firearm, Very pistol
　　pellet — *see* Discharge, airgun

Discharge — *continued*
pistol — *see* Discharge, firearm, handgun — *continued*
    Very — *see* Discharge, firearm, Very pistol
revolver — *see* Discharge, firearm, handgun
rifle (hunting) — *see* Discharge, firearm, hunting rifle
shotgun — *see* Discharge, firearm, shotgun
spring-operated gun NEC W34.018 ☑
    assault X95.09 ☑
    homicide (attempt) X95.09 ☑
    stated as undetermined whether accidental or intentional Y24.8 ☑
    suicide (attempt) X74.09 ☑
Disease
Andes W94.11 ☑
aviator's — *see* Air, pressure
range W94.11 ☑
Diver's disease, palsy, paralysis, squeeze — *see* Air, pressure
Diving (into water) — *see* Accident, diving
Dog bite W54.0 ☑
Dragged by transport vehicle NEC (*see also* Accident, transport) V09.9 ☑
Drinking poison (accidental) — *see* Table of Drugs and Chemicals
Dropped (accidentally) **while being carried or supported by other person** W04 ☑
Drowning (accidental) W74 ☑
assault X92.9 ☑
due to
    accident (to)
        machinery — *see* Contact, with, by type of machine
        watercraft V90.89 ☑
            burning V90.29 ☑
                powered V90.23 ☑
                    fishing boat V90.22 ☑
                    jetskis V90.23 ☑
                    merchant ship V90.20 ☑
                    passenger ship V90.21 ☑
                unpowered V90.28 ☑
                    canoe V90.25 ☑
                    inflatable V90.26 ☑
                    kayak V90.25 ☑
                    sailboat V90.24 ☑
                    water skis V90.27 ☑
             crushed V90.39 ☑
                powered V90.33 ☑
                    fishing boat V90.32 ☑
                    jetskis V90.33 ☑
                    merchant ship V90.30 ☑
                    passenger ship V90.31 ☑
                unpowered V90.38 ☑
                    canoe V90.35 ☑
                    inflatable V90.36 ☑
                    kayak V90.35 ☑
                    sailboat V90.34 ☑
                    water skis V90.37 ☑
             overturning V90.09 ☑
                powered V90.03 ☑
                    fishing boat V90.02 ☑
                    jetskis V90.03 ☑
                    merchant ship V90.00 ☑
                    passenger ship V90.01 ☑
                unpowered V90.08 ☑
                    canoe V90.05 ☑
                    inflatable V90.06 ☑
                    kayak V90.05 ☑
                    sailboat V90.04 ☑
             sinking V90.19 ☑
                powered V90.13 ☑
                    fishing boat V90.12 ☑
                    jetskis V90.13 ☑
                    merchant ship V90.10 ☑
                    passenger ship V90.11 ☑
                unpowered V90.18 ☑
                    canoe V90.15 ☑
                    inflatable V90.16 ☑
                    kayak V90.15 ☑
                    sailboat V90.14 ☑
             specified type NEC V90.89 ☑
                powered V90.83 ☑
                    fishing boat V90.82 ☑
                    jetskis V90.83 ☑
                    merchant ship V90.80 ☑
                    passenger ship V90.81 ☑

Drowning — *continued*
due to — *continued*
    accident — *continued*
        watercraft — *continued*
            specified type — *continued*
                unpowered V90.88 ☑
                    canoe V90.85 ☑
                    inflatable V90.86 ☑
                    kayak V90.85 ☑
                    sailboat V90.84 ☑
                    water skis V90.87 ☑
    avalanche — *see* Landslide
    cataclysmic
        earth surface movement NEC — *see* Forces of nature, earth movement
        storm — *see* Forces of nature, cataclysmic storm
    cloudburst X37.8 ☑
    cyclone X37.1 ☑
    fall overboard (from) V92.09 ☑
        powered craft V92.03 ☑
            ferry boat V92.01 ☑
            fishing boat V92.02 ☑
            jetskis V92.03 ☑
            liner V92.01 ☑
            merchant ship V92.00 ☑
            passenger ship V92.01 ☑
    resulting from
        accident to watercraft — *see* Drowning, due to, accident to, watercraft
        being washed overboard (from) V92.29 ☑
            powered craft V92.23 ☑
                ferry boat V92.21 ☑
                fishing boat V92.22 ☑
                jetskis V92.23 ☑
                liner V92.21 ☑
                merchant ship V92.20 ☑
                passenger ship V92.21 ☑
            unpowered craft V92.28 ☑
                canoe V92.25 ☑
                inflatable V92.26 ☑
                kayak V92.25 ☑
                sailboat V92.24 ☑
                surf-board V92.28 ☑
                water skis V92.27 ☑
                windsurfer V92.28 ☑
        motion of watercraft V92.19 ☑
            powered craft V92.13 ☑
                ferry boat V92.11 ☑
                fishing boat V92.12 ☑
                jetskis V92.13 ☑
                liner V92.11 ☑
                merchant ship V92.10 ☑
                passenger ship V92.11 ☑
            unpowered craft
                canoe V92.15 ☑
                inflatable V92.16 ☑
                kayak V92.15 ☑
                sailboat V92.14 ☑
        unpowered craft V92.08 ☑
            canoe V92.05 ☑
            inflatable V92.06 ☑
            kayak V92.05 ☑
            sailboat V92.04 ☑
            surf-board V92.08 ☑
            water skis V92.07 ☑
            windsurfer V92.08 ☑
    hurricane X37.0 ☑
    jumping into water from watercraft (involved in accident) (*see also* Drowning, due to, accident to, watercraft)
        without accident to or on watercraft W16.711 ☑
    tidal wave NEC — *see* Forces of nature, tidal wave
    torrential rain X37.8 ☑
following
    fall
        into
            bathtub W16.211 ☑
            bucket W16.221 ☑
            fountain — *see* Drowning, following, fall, into, water, specified NEC
            quarry — *see* Drowning, following, fall, into, water, specified NEC
            reservoir — *see* Drowning, following, fall, into, water, specified NEC

Drowning — *continued*
following — *continued*
    fall — *continued*
        into — *continued*
            swimming-pool W16.011 ☑
                stated as undetermined whether accidental or intentional Y21.3 ☑
                striking
                    bottom W16.021 ☑
                    wall W16.031 ☑
                suicide (attempt) X71.2 ☑
            water NOS W16.41 ☑
                natural (lake) (open sea) (river) (stream) (pond) W16.111 ☑
                    striking
                      bottom W16.121 ☑
                      side W16.131 ☑
                specified NEC W16.311 ☑
                  striking
                    bottom W16.321 ☑
                    wall W16.331 ☑
        overboard NEC — *see* Drowning, due to, fall overboard
    jump or dive
        from boat W16.711 ☑
            striking bottom W16.721 ☑
        into
            fountain — *see* Drowning, following, jump or dive, into, water, specified NEC
            quarry — *see* Drowning, following, jump or dive, into, water, specified NEC
            reservoir — *see* Drowning, following, jump or dive, into, water, specified NEC
            swimming-pool W16.511 ☑
                striking
                    bottom W16.521 ☑
                    wall W16.531 ☑
                suicide (attempt) X71.2 ☑
            water NOS W16.91 ☑
                natural (lake) (open sea) (river) (stream) (pond) W16.611 ☑
                specified NEC W16.811 ☑
                  bottom W16.821 ☑
                  striking
                    bottom W16.821 ☑
                    wall W16.831 ☑
                striking
                  bottom W16.821 ☑
                  wall W16.831 ☑
                striking bottom W16.621 ☑
homicide (attempt) X92.9 ☑
in
    bathtub (accidental) W65 ☑
        assault X92.0 ☑
        following fall W16.211 ☑
            stated as undetermined whether accidental or intentional Y21.1 ☑
        stated as undetermined whether accidental or intentional Y21.0 ☑
        suicide (attempt) X71.0 ☑
    lake — *see* Drowning, in, natural water
    natural water (lake) (open sea) (river) (stream) (pond) W69 ☑
        assault X92.3 ☑
        following
            dive or jump W16.611 ☑
                striking bottom W16.621 ☑
            fall W16.111 ☑
                striking
                  bottom W16.121 ☑
                  side W16.131 ☑
        stated as undetermined whether accidental or intentional Y21.4 ☑
        suicide (attempt) X71.3 ☑
    quarry — *see* Drowning, in, specified place NEC
    quenching tank — *see* Drowning, in, specified place NEC
    reservoir — *see* Drowning, in, specified place NEC
    river — *see* Drowning, in, natural water
    sea — *see* Drowning, in, natural water
    specified place NEC W73 ☑
        assault X92.8 ☑
        following
            dive or jump W16.811 ☑
                striking
                  bottom W16.821 ☑
                  wall W16.831 ☑

☑ **Additional Character Required** — **Refer to the Tabular List for Character Selection**   ⬇ **Subterms under main terms may continue to next column or page**

Drowning — *continued*
in — *continued*
  specified place — *continued*
    following — *continued*
      fall W16.311 ☑
        striking
          bottom W16.321 ☑
          wall W16.331 ☑
    stated as undetermined whether accidental or
      intentional Y21.8 ☑
    suicide (attempt) X71.8 ☑
  stream — *see* Drowning, in, natural water
  swimming-pool W67 ☑
    assault X92.1 ☑
      following fall X92.2 ☑
    following
      dive or jump W16.511 ☑
        striking
          bottom W16.521 ☑
          wall W16.531 ☑
      fall W16.011 ☑
        striking
          bottom W16.021 ☑
          wall W16.031 ☑
    stated as undetermined whether accidental or
      intentional Y21.2 ☑
      following fall Y21.3 ☑
    suicide (attempt) X71.1 ☑
      following fall X71.2 ☑
  war operations — *see* War operations, restriction
    of airway
  resulting from accident to watercraft — *see* Drowning,
    due to, accident, watercraft
  self-inflicted X71.9 ☑
  stated as undetermined whether accidental or inten-
    tional Y21.9 ☑
  suicide (attempt) X71.9 ☑

E

Earth falling (on) W20.0 ☑
  caused by cataclysmic earth surface movement or
    eruption — *see* Landslide
Earth (surface) **movement NEC** — *see* Forces of nature,
  earth movement
Earthquake (any injury) X34 ☑
Effect(s) (adverse) **of**
  air pressure (any) — *see* Air, pressure
  cold, excessive (exposure to) — *see* Exposure, cold
  heat (excessive) — *see* Heat
  hot place (weather) — *see* Heat
  insolation X30 ☑
  late — *see* Sequelae
  motion — *see* Motion
  nuclear explosion or weapon in war operations — *see*
    War operations, nuclear weapon
  radiation — *see* Radiation
  travel — *see* Travel
Electric shock (accidental) (by) (in) — *see* Exposure,
  electric current
Electrocution (accidental) — *see* Exposure, electric current
Endotracheal tube wrongly placed during anesthetic
  procedure
Entanglement
  in
    bed linen, causing suffocation T71 ☑
    wheel of pedal cycle V19.88 ☑
Entry of foreign body or material — *see* Foreign body
Environmental pollution related condition — *see*
  category Z57 ☑
Execution, legal (any method) — *see* Legal, intervention
Exhaustion
  cold — *see* Exposure, cold
  due to excessive exertion (*see also* Overexertion)
    X50.9 ☑
  heat — *see* Heat
Explosion (accidental) (of) (with secondary fire) W40.9 ☑
  acetylene W40.1 ☑
  aerosol can W36.1 ☑
  air tank (compressed) (in machinery) W36.2 ☑
  aircraft (in transit) (powered) NEC V95.9 ☑
    balloon V96.05 ☑
    fixed wing NEC (private) V95.25 ☑
      commercial V95.35 ☑
    glider V96.25 ☑

Explosion — *continued*
  aircraft — *continued*
    glider — *continued*
      hang V96.15 ☑
      powered V95.15 ☑
    helicopter V95.05 ☑
    in war operations — *see* War operations, destruc-
      tion of aircraft
    microlight V95.15 ☑
    nonpowered V96.9 ☑
      specified NEC V96.8 ☑
    powered NEC V95.8 ☑
    stated as
      homicide (attempt) Y03.8 ☑
      suicide (attempt) X83.0 ☑
    ultralight V95.15 ☑
  anesthetic gas in operating room W40.1 ☑
  antipersonnel bomb W40.8 ☑
    assault X96.0 ☑
    homicide (attempt) X96.0 ☑
    suicide (attempt) X75 ☑
  assault X96.9 ☑
  bicycle tire W37.0 ☑
  blasting (cap) (materials) W40.0 ☑
  boiler (machinery), not on transport vehicle W35 ☑
    on watercraft — *see* Explosion, in, watercraft
  butane W40.1 ☑
  caused by other person X96.9 ☑
  coal gas W40.1 ☑
  detonator W40.0 ☑
  dump (munitions) W40.8 ☑
  dynamite W40.0 ☑
    in
      assault X96.8 ☑
      homicide (attempt) X96.8 ☑
      legal intervention
        injuring
          bystander Y35.112 ☑
          law enforcement personnel Y35.111 ☑
          suspect Y35.113 ☑
      suicide (attempt) X75 ☑
  explosive (material) W40.9 ☑
    gas W40.1 ☑
    in blasting operation W40.0 ☑
    specified NEC W40.8 ☑
      in
        assault X96.8 ☑
        homicide (attempt) X96.8 ☑
        legal intervention
          injuring
            bystander Y35.192 ☑
            law enforcement personnel
              Y35.191 ☑
            suspect Y35.193 ☑
        suicide (attempt) X75 ☑
  factory (munitions) W40.8 ☑
  fertilizer bomb W40.8 ☑
    assault X96.3 ☑
    homicide (attempt) X96.3 ☑
    suicide (attempt) X75 ☑
  firearm (parts) NEC W34.19 ☑
    airgun W34.110 ☑
    BB gun W34.110 ☑
    gas, air or spring-operated gun NEC W34.118 ☑
    hangun W32.1 ☑
    hunting rifle W33.12 ☑
    larger firearm W33.10 ☑
      specified NEC W33.19 ☑
    machine gun W33.13 ☑
    paintball gun W34.111 ☑
    pellet gun W34.110 ☑
    shotgun W33.11 ☑
    Very pistol [flare] W34.19 ☑
  fire-damp W40.1 ☑
  fireworks W39 ☑
  gas (coal) (explosive) W40.1 ☑
    cylinder W36.9 ☑
      aerosol can W36.1 ☑
      air tank W36.2 ☑
      pressurized W36.3 ☑
      specified NEC W36.8 ☑
  gasoline (fumes) (tank) not in moving motor vehicle
    W40.1 ☑
    bomb W40.8 ☑
      assault X96.1 ☑
      homicide (attempt) X96.1 ☑

Explosion — *continued*
  gasoline not in moving motor vehicle — *continued*
    bomb — *continued*
      suicide (attempt) X75 ☑
    in motor vehicle — *see* Accident, transport, by type
      of vehicle
  grain store W40.8 ☑
  grenade W40.8 ☑
    in
      assault X96.8 ☑
      homicide (attempt) X96.8 ☑
      legal intervention
        injuring
          bystander Y35.192 ☑
          law enforcement personnel Y35.191 ☑
          suspect Y35.193 ☑
      suicide (attempt) X75 ☑
  handgun (parts) — *see* Explosion, firearm, hangun
    (parts)
  homicide (attempt) X96.9 ☑
    antipersonnel bomb — *see* Explosion, antiperson-
      nel bomb
    fertilizer bomb — *see* Explosion, fertilizer bomb
    gasoline bomb — *see* Explosion, gasoline bomb
    letter bomb — *see* Explosion, letter bomb
    pipe bomb — *see* Explosion, pipe bomb
    specified NEC X96.8 ☑
  hose, pressurized W37.8 ☑
  hot water heater, tank (in machinery) W35 ☑
    on watercraft — *see* Explosion, in, watercraft
  in, on
    dump W40.8 ☑
    factory W40.8 ☑
    mine (of explosive gases) NEC W40.1 ☑
    watercraft V93.59 ☑
      powered craft V93.53 ☑
        ferry boat V93.51 ☑
        fishing boat V93.52 ☑
        jetskis V93.53 ☑
        liner V93.51 ☑
        merchant ship V93.50 ☑
        passenger ship V93.51 ☑
        sailboat V93.54 ☑
  letter bomb W40.8 ☑
    assault X96.2 ☑
    homicide (attempt) X96.2 ☑
    suicide (attempt) X75 ☑
  machinery (*see also* Contact, with, by type of machine)
    on board watercraft — *see* Explosion, in, watercraft
    pressure vessel — *see* Explosion, by type of vessel
  methane W40.1 ☑
  mine W40.1 ☑
  missile NEC W40.8 ☑
  mortar bomb W40.8 ☑
    in
      assault X96.8 ☑
      homicide (attempt) X96.8 ☑
      legal intervention
        injuring
          bystander Y35.192 ☑
          law enforcement personnel Y35.191 ☑
          suspect Y35.193 ☑
      suicide (attempt) X75 ☑
  munitions (dump) (factory) W40.8 ☑
  pipe, pressurized W37.8 ☑
    bomb W40.8 ☑
      assault X96.4 ☑
      homicide (attempt) X96.4 ☑
      suicide (attempt) X75 ☑
  pressure, pressurized
    cooker W38 ☑
    gas tank (in machinery) W36.3 ☑
    hose W37.8 ☑
    pipe W37.8 ☑
    specified device NEC W38 ☑
    tire W37.8 ☑
      bicycle W37.0 ☑
    vessel (in machinery) W38 ☑
  propane W40.1 ☑
  self-inflicted X75 ☑
  shell (artillery) NEC W40.8 ☑
    during war operations — *see* War operations, ex-
      plosion

Explosion — continued
shell — continued
in
legal intervention
injuring
bystander Y35.122 ☑
law enforcement personnel Y35.121 ☑
suspect Y35.123 ☑
war — see War operations, explosion
spacecraft V95.45 ☑
stated as undetermined whether accidental or intentional Y25 ☑
steam or water lines (in machinery) W37.8 ☑
stove W40.9 ☑
suicide (attempt) X75 ☑
tire, pressurized W37.8 ☑
bicycle W37.0 ☑
undetermined whether accidental or intentional Y25 ☑
vehicle tire NEC W37.8 ☑
bicycle W37.0 ☑
war operations — see War operations, explosion
Exposure (to) X58 ☑
air pressure change — see Air, pressure
cold (accidental) (excessive) (extreme) (natural) (place) X31 ☑
assault Y08.89 ☑
due to
man-made conditions W93.8 ☑
dry ice (contact) W93.01 ☑
inhalation W93.02 ☑
liquid air (contact) (hydrogen) (nitrogen) W93.11 ☑
inhalation W93.12 ☑
refrigeration unit (deep freeze) W93.2 ☑
suicide (attempt) X83.2 ☑
weather (conditions) X31 ☑
homicide (attempt) Y08.89 ☑
self-inflicted X83.2 ☑
due to abandonment or neglect X58 ☑
electric current W86.8 ☑
appliance (faulty) W86.8 ☑
domestic W86.0 ☑
caused by other person Y08.89 ☑
conductor (faulty) W86.1 ☑
control apparatus (faulty) W86.1 ☑
electric power generating plant, distribution station W86.1 ☑
electroshock gun — see Exposure, electric current, taser
high-voltage cable W85 ☑
homicide (attempt) Y08.89 ☑
legal execution — see Legal, intervention, specified means NEC
lightning — see subcategory T75.0 ☑
live rail W86.8 ☑
misadventure in medical or surgical procedure in electroshock therapy Y63.4
motor (electric) (faulty) W86.8 ☑
domestic W86.0 ☑
self-inflicted X83.1 ☑
specified NEC W86.8 ☑
domestic W86.0 ☑
stun gun — see Exposure, electric current, taser
suicide (attempt) X83.1 ☑
taser W86.8 ☑
assault Y08.89 ☑
legal intervention — see category Y35 ☑
self-harm (intentional) X83.8 ☑
undetermined intent Y33 ☑
third rail W86.8 ☑
transformer (faulty) W86.1 ☑
transmission lines W85 ☑
environmental tobacco smoke X58 ☑
excessive
cold — see Exposure, cold
heat (natural) NEC X30 ☑
man-made W92 ☑
factor(s) NOS X58 ☑
environmental NEC X58 ☑
man-made NEC W99 ☑
natural NEC — see Forces of nature
specified NEC X58 ☑
fire, flames (accidental) X08.8 ☑
assault X97 ☑

Exposure — continued
fire, flames — continued
campfire — see Exposure, fire, controlled, not in building
controlled (in)
with ignition (of) clothing (see also Ignition, clothes) X06.2 ☑
nightwear X05 ☑
bonfire — see Exposure, fire, controlled, not in building
brazier (in building or structure) (see also Exposure, fire, controlled, building)
not in building or structure — see Exposure, fire, controlled, not in building
building or structure X02.0 ☑
with
fall from building X02.3 ☑
from building X02.5 ☑
injury due to building collapse X02.2 ☑
smoke inhalation X02.1 ☑
hit by object from building X02.4 ☑
specified mode of injury NEC X02.8 ☑
fireplace, furnace or stove — see Exposure, fire, controlled, building
not in building or structure X03.0 ☑
with
fall X03.3 ☑
smoke inhalation X03.1 ☑
hit by object X03.4 ☑
specified mode of injury NEC X03.8 ☑
trash — see Exposure, fire, controlled, not in building
fireplace — see Exposure, fire, controlled, building
fittings or furniture (in building or structure) (uncontrolled) — see Exposure, fire, uncontrolled, building
forest (uncontrolled) — see Exposure, fire, uncontrolled, not in building
grass (uncontrolled) — see Exposure, fire, uncontrolled, not in building
hay (uncontrolled) — see Exposure, fire, uncontrolled, not in building
homicide (attempt) X97 ☑
ignition of highly flammable material X04 ☑
in, of, on, starting in
machinery — see Contact, with, by type of machine
motor vehicle (in motion) (see also Accident, transport, occupant by type of vehicle) V87.8 ☑
with collision — see Collision
railway rolling stock, train, vehicle V81.81 ☑
with collision — see Accident, transport, railway vehicle occupant
street car (in motion) V82.8 ☑
with collision — see Accident, transport, streetcar occupant
transport vehicle NEC (see also Accident, transport)
with collision — see Collision
war operations (see also War operations, fire)
from nuclear explosion — see War operations, nuclear weapons
watercraft (in transit) (not in transit) V91.09 ☑
localized — see Burn, on board watercraft, due to, fire on board
powered craft V91.03 ☑
ferry boat V91.01 ☑
fishing boat V91.02 ☑
jet skis V91.03 ☑
liner V91.01 ☑
merchant ship V91.00 ☑
passenger ship V91.01 ☑
unpowered craft V91.08 ☑
canoe V91.05 ☑
inflatable V91.06 ☑
kayak V91.05 ☑
sailboat V91.04 ☑
surf-board V91.08 ☑
waterskis V91.07 ☑
windsurfer V91.08 ☑
lumber (uncontrolled) — see Exposure, fire, uncontrolled, not in building
mine (uncontrolled) — see Exposure, fire, uncontrolled, not in building
prairie (uncontrolled) — see Exposure, fire, uncontrolled, not in building

Exposure — continued
fire, flames — continued
resulting from
explosion — see Explosion
lightning X08.8 ☑
self-inflicted X76 ☑
specified NEC X08.8 ☑
started by other person X97 ☑
stated as undetermined whether accidental or intentional Y26 ☑
stove — see Exposure, fire, controlled, building
suicide (attempt) X76 ☑
tunnel (uncontrolled) — see Exposure, fire, uncontrolled, not in building
uncontrolled
in building or structure X00.0 ☑
with
fall from building X00.3 ☑
injury due to building collapse X00.2 ☑
jump from building X00.5 ☑
smoke inhalation X00.1 ☑
bed X08.00 ☑
due to
cigarette X08.01 ☑
specified material NEC X08.09 ☑
furniture NEC X08.20 ☑
due to
cigarette X08.21 ☑
specified material NEC X08.29 ☑
hit by object from building X00.4 ☑
sofa X08.10 ☑
due to
cigarette X08.11 ☑
specified material NEC X08.19 ☑
specified mode of injury NEC X00.8 ☑
not in building or structure (any) X01.0 ☑
with
fall X01.3 ☑
smoke inhalation X01.1 ☑
hit by object X01.4 ☑
specified mode of injury NEC X01.8 ☑
undetermined whether accidental or intentional Y26 ☑
forces of nature NEC — see Forces of nature
G-forces (abnormal) W49.9 ☑
gravitational forces (abnormal) W49.9 ☑
heat (natural) NEC — see Heat
high-pressure jet (hydraulic) (pneumatic) W49.9 ☑
hydraulic jet W49.9 ☑
inanimate mechanical force W49.9 ☑
jet, high-pressure (hydraulic) (pneumatic) W49.9 ☑
lightning — see subcategory T75.0 ☑
causing fire — see Exposure, fire
mechanical forces NEC W49.9 ☑
animate NEC W64 ☑
inanimate NEC W49.9 ☑
noise W42.9 ☑
supersonic W42.0 ☑
noxious substance — see Table of Drugs and Chemicals
pneumatic jet W49.9 ☑
prolonged in deep-freeze unit or refrigerator W93.2 ☑
radiation — see Radiation
smoke (see also Exposure, fire)
tobacco, second hand Z77.22
specified factors NEC X58 ☑
sunlight X32 ☑
man-made (sun lamp) W89.8 ☑
tanning bed W89.1 ☑
supersonic waves W42.0 ☑
transmission line(s), electric W85 ☑
vibration W49.9 ☑
waves
infrasound W49.9 ☑
sound W42.9 ☑
supersonic W42.0 ☑
weather NEC — see Forces of nature
External cause status Y99.9
child assisting in compensated work for family Y99.8
civilian activity done for financial or other compensation Y99.0
civilian activity done for income or pay Y99.0
family member assisting in compensated work for other family member Y99.8
hobby not done for income Y99.8
leisure activity Y99.8

☑ Additional Character Required — Refer to the Tabular List for Character Selection   ▽ Subterms under main terms may continue to next column or page

External cause status — *continued*
  military activity Y99.1
  off-duty activity of military personnel Y99.8
  recreation or sport not for income or while a student
    Y99.8
  specified NEC Y99.8
  student activity Y99.8
  volunteer activity Y99.2

F

Factors, supplemental
  alcohol
    blood level
      less than 20mg/100ml Y90.0
      20-39mg/100ml Y90.1
      40-59mg/100ml Y90.2
      60-79mg/100ml Y90.3
      80-99mg/100ml Y90.4
      100-119mg/100ml Y90.5
      120-199mg/100ml Y90.6
      200-239mg/100ml Y90.7
      240mg/100ml or more Y90.8
      presence in blood, level not specified Y90.9
    presence in blood, but level not specified Y90.9
  environmental-pollution-related condition- see Z57 ☑
  nosocomial condition Y95
  work-related condition Y99.0
Failure
  in suture or ligature during surgical procedure Y65.2
  mechanical, of instrument or apparatus (any) (during
    any medical or surgical procedure) Y65.8
  sterile precautions (during medical and surgical care)
    — *see* Misadventure, failure, sterile precautions,
    by type of procedure
  to
    introduce tube or instrument Y65.4
      endotracheal tube during anesthesia Y65.3
    make curve (transport vehicle) NEC — *see* Accident,
      transport
    remove tube or instrument Y65.4
Fall, falling (accidental) W19 ☑
  building W20.1 ☑
    burning (uncontrolled fire) X00.3 ☑
  down
    embankment W17.81 ☑
    escalator W10.0 ☑
    hill W17.81 ☑
    ladder W11 ☑
    ramp W10.2 ☑
    stairs, steps W10.9 ☑
  due to
    bumping against
      object W18.00 ☑
        sharp glass W18.02 ☑
        specified NEC W18.09 ☑
        sports equipment W18.01 ☑
      person W03 ☑
        due to ice or snow W00.0 ☑
        on pedestrian conveyance — *see* Accident,
          transport, pedestrian, conveyance
    collision with another person W03 ☑
      due to ice or snow W00.0 ☑
      involving pedestrian conveyance — *see* Acci-
        dent, transport, pedestrian, conveyance
    grocery cart tipping over W17.82 ☑
    ice or snow W00.9 ☑
      from one level to another W00.2 ☑
      on stairs or steps W00.1 ☑
      involving pedestrian conveyance — *see* Acci-
        dent, transport, pedestrian, conveyance
      on same level W00.0 ☑
    slipping (on moving sidewalk) W01.0 ☑
      with subsequent striking against object
        W01.10 ☑
        furniture W01.190 ☑
        sharp object W01.119 ☑
          glass W01.110 ☑
          power tool or machine W01.111 ☑
          specified NEC W01.118 ☑
        specified NEC W01.198 ☑
    striking against
      object W18.00 ☑
        sharp glass W18.02 ☑
        specified NEC W18.09 ☑
        sports equipment W18.01 ☑
      person W03 ☑

Fall, falling — *continued*
  due to — *continued*
    striking against — *continued*
      person — *continued*
        due to ice or snow W00.0 ☑
        on pedestrian conveyance — *see* Accident,
          transport, pedestrian, conveyance
  earth (with asphyxia or suffocation (by pressure)) —
    see Earth, falling
  from, off, out of
    aircraft NEC (with accident to aircraft NEC) V97.0 ☑
      while boarding or alighting V97.1 ☑
    balcony W13.0 ☑
    bed W06 ☑
    boat, ship, watercraft NEC (with drowning or sub-
      mersion) — *see* Drowning, due to, fall over-
      board
      with hitting bottom or object V94.0 ☑
    bridge W13.1 ☑
    building W13.9 ☑
      burning (uncontrolled fire) X00.3 ☑
    cavity W17.2 ☑
    chair W07 ☑
    cherry picker W17.89 ☑
    cliff W15 ☑
    dock W17.4 ☑
    embankment W17.81 ☑
    escalator W10.0 ☑
    flagpole W13.8 ☑
    furniture NEC W08 ☑
    grocery cart W17.82 ☑
    haystack W17.89 ☑
    high place NEC W17.89 ☑
      stated as undetermined whether accidental or
        intentional Y30 ☑
    hole W17.2 ☑
    incline W10.2 ☑
    ladder W11 ☑
    lifting device W17.89 ☑
    machine, machinery (*see also* Contact, with, by
      type of machine)
      not in operation W17.89 ☑
    manhole W17.1 ☑
    mobile elevated work platform [MEWP] W17.89 ☑
    motorized mobility scooter W05.2 ☑
    one level to another NEC W17.89 ☑
      intentional, purposeful, suicide (attempt)
        X80 ☑
      stated as undetermined whether accidental or
        intentional Y30 ☑
    pit W17.2 ☑
    playground equipment W09.8 ☑
      jungle gym W09.2 ☑
      slide W09.0 ☑
      swing W09.1 ☑
    quarry W17.89 ☑
    railing W13.9 ☑
    ramp W10.2 ☑
    roof W13.2 ☑
    scaffolding W12 ☑
    scooter (nonmotorized) W05.1 ☑
      motorized mobility W05.2 ☑
    sky lift W17.89 ☑
    stairs, steps W10.9 ☑
      curb W10.1 ☑
      due to ice or snow W00.1 ☑
      escalator W10.0 ☑
      incline W10.2 ☑
      ramp W10.2 ☑
      sidewalk curb W10.1 ☑
      specified NEC W10.8 ☑
    stepladder W11 ☑
    storm drain W17.1 ☑
    streetcar NEC V82.6 ☑
      with antecedent collision — *see* Accident,
        transport, streetcar occupant
      while boarding or alighting V82.4 ☑
    structure NEC W13.8 ☑
      burning (uncontrolled fire) X00.3 ☑
    table W08 ☑
    toilet W18.11 ☑
      with subsequent striking against object
        W18.12 ☑
    train NEC V81.6 ☑
      during derailment (without antecedent colli-
        sion) V81.7 ☑

Fall, falling — *continued*
  from, off, out of — *continued*
    train — *continued*
      during derailment — *continued*
        with antecedent collision — *see* Accident,
          transport, railway vehicle occupant
      while boarding or alighting V81.4 ☑
      transport vehicle after collision — *see* Accident,
        transport, by type of vehicle, collision
    tree W14 ☑
    vehicle (in motion) NEC (*see also* Accident, trans-
      port) V89.9 ☑
      motor NEC (*see also* Accident, transport, occu-
        pant, by type of vehicle) V87.8 ☑
      stationary W17.89 ☑
        while boarding or alighting — *see* Accident,
          transport, by type of vehicle, while
          boarding or alighting
    viaduct W13.8 ☑
    wall W13.8 ☑
    watercraft (*see also* Drowning, due to, fall over-
      board)
      with hitting bottom or object V94.0 ☑
    well W17.0 ☑
    wheelchair, non-moving W05.0 ☑
      powered — *see* Accident, transport, pedestrian,
        conveyance occupant, specified type NEC
    window W13.4 ☑
  in, on
    aircraft NEC V97.0 ☑
      with accident to aircraft V97.0 ☑
      while boarding or alighting V97.1 ☑
    bathtub (empty) W18.2 ☑
      filled W16.212 ☑
        causing drowning W16.211 ☑
    escalator W10.0 ☑
    incline W10.2 ☑
    ladder W11 ☑
    machine, machinery — *see* Contact, with, by type
      of machine
    object, edged, pointed or sharp (with cut) — *see*
      Fall, by type
    playground equipment W09.8 ☑
      jungle gym W09.2 ☑
      slide W09.0 ☑
      swing W09.1 ☑
    ramp W10.2 ☑
    scaffolding W12 ☑
    shower W18.2 ☑
      causing drowning W16.211 ☑
    staircase, stairs, steps W10.9 ☑
      curb W10.1 ☑
      due to ice or snow W00.1 ☑
      escalator W10.0 ☑
      incline W10.2 ☑
      specified NEC W10.8 ☑
    streetcar (without antecedent collision) V82.5 ☑
      with antecedent collision — *see* Accident,
        transport, streetcar occupant
      while boarding or alighting V82.4 ☑
    train (without antecedent collision) V81.5 ☑
      with antecedent collision — *see* Accident,
        transport, railway vehicle occupant
      during derailment (without antecedent colli-
        sion) V81.7 ☑
        with antecedent collision — *see* Accident,
          transport, railway vehicle occupant
      while boarding or alighting V81.4 ☑
    transport vehicle after collision — *see* Accident,
      transport, by type of vehicle, collision
    watercraft V93.39 ☑
      due to
        accident to craft V91.29 ☑
          powered craft V91.23 ☑
            ferry boat V91.21 ☑
            fishing boat V91.22 ☑
            jetskis V91.23 ☑
            liner V91.21 ☑
            merchant ship V91.20 ☑
            passenger ship V91.21 ☑
          unpowered craft
            canoe V91.25 ☑
            inflatable V91.26 ☑
            kayak V91.25 ☑
            sailboat V91.24 ☑
        powered craft V93.33 ☑

Fall, falling — *continued*
  in, on — *continued*
    watercraft — *continued*
      powered craft — *continued*
        ferry boat V93.31 ☑
        fishing boat V93.32 ☑
        jetskis V93.33 ☑
        liner V93.31 ☑
        merchant ship V93.30 ☑
        passenger ship V93.31 ☑
      unpowered craft V93.38 ☑
        canoe V93.35 ☑
        inflatable V93.36 ☑
        kayak V93.35 ☑
        sailboat V93.34 ☑
        surf-board V93.38 ☑
        windsurfer V93.38 ☑
  into
    cavity W17.2 ☑
    dock W17.4 ☑
    fire — *see* Exposure, fire, by type
    haystack W17.89 ☑
    hole W17.2 ☑
    lake — *see* Fall, into, water
    manhole W17.1 ☑
    moving part of machinery — *see* Contact, with, by
      type of machine
    ocean — *see* Fall, into, water
    opening in surface NEC W17.89 ☑
    pit W17.2 ☑
    pond — *see* Fall, into, water
    quarry W17.89 ☑
    river — *see* Fall, into, water
    shaft W17.89 ☑
    storm drain W17.1 ☑
    stream — *see* Fall, into, water
    swimming pool (*see also* Fall, into, water, in,
      swimming pool)
      empty W17.3 ☑
    tank W17.89 ☑
    water W16.42 ☑
      causing drowning W16.41 ☑
      from watercraft — *see* Drowning, due to, fall
        overboard
      hitting diving board W21.4 ☑
      in
        bathtub W16.212 ☑
          causing drowning W16.211 ☑
        bucket W16.222 ☑
          causing drowning W16.221 ☑
        natural body of water W16.112 ☑
          causing drowning W16.111 ☑
          striking
            bottom W16.122 ☑
              causing drowning W16.121 ☑
            side W16.132 ☑
              causing drowning W16.131 ☑
        specified water NEC W16.312 ☑
          causing drowning W16.311 ☑
          striking
            bottom W16.322 ☑
              causing drowning W16.321 ☑
            wall W16.332 ☑
              causing drowning W16.331 ☑
        swimming pool W16.012 ☑
          causing drowning W16.011 ☑
          striking
            bottom W16.022 ☑
              causing drowning W16.031 ☑
            wall W16.032 ☑
              causing drowning W16.021 ☑
        utility bucket W16.222 ☑
          causing drowning W16.221 ☑
    well W17.0 ☑
  involving
    bed W06 ☑
    chair W07 ☑
    furniture NEC W08 ☑
    glass — *see* Fall, by type
    playground equipment W09.8 ☑
      jungle gym W09.2 ☑
      slide W09.0 ☑
      swing W09.1 ☑
    roller blades — *see* Accident, transport, pedestrian,
      conveyance

Fall, falling — *continued*
  involving — *continued*
    skateboard(s) — *see* Accident, transport, pedestri-
      an, conveyance
    skates (ice) (in line) (roller) — *see* Accident, trans-
      port, pedestrian, conveyance
    skis — *see* Accident, transport, pedestrian, con-
      veyance
    table W08 ☑
    wheelchair, non-moving W05.0 ☑
      powered — *see* Accident, transport, pedestrian,
        conveyance, specified type NEC
  object — *see* Struck by, object, falling
  off
    toilet W18.11 ☑
      with subsequent striking against object
        W18.12 ☑
  on same level W18.30 ☑
    due to
      specified NEC W18.39 ☑
      stepping on an object W18.31 ☑
  out of
    bed W06 ☑
    building NEC W13.8 ☑
    chair W07 ☑
    furniture NEC W08 ☑
    wheelchair, non-moving W05.0 ☑
      powered — *see* Accident, transport, pedestrian,
        conveyance, specified type NEC
    window W13.4 ☑
  over
    animal W01.0 ☑
    cliff W15 ☑
    embankment W17.81 ☑
    small object W01.0 ☑
  rock W20.8 ☑
  same level W18.30 ☑
    from
      being crushed, pushed, or stepped on by a
        crowd or human stampede W52 ☑
      collision, pushing, shoving, by or with other
        person W03 ☑
      slipping, stumbling, tripping W01.0 ☑
      involving ice or snow W00.0 ☑
        involving skates (ice) (roller), skateboard, skis
          — *see* Accident, transport, pedestrian,
          conveyance
  snowslide (avalanche) — *see* Landslide
  stone W20.8 ☑
  structure W20.1 ☑
    burning (uncontrolled fire) X00.3 ☑
  through
    bridge W13.1 ☑
    floor W13.3 ☑
    roof W13.2 ☑
    wall W13.8 ☑
    window W13.4 ☑
  timber W20.8 ☑
  tree (caused by lightning) W20.8 ☑
  while being carried or supported by other person(s)
    W04 ☑
Fallen on by
  animal (not being ridden) NEC W55.89 ☑
Felo-de-se — *see* Suicide
Fight (hand) (fists) (foot) — *see* Assault, fight
Fire (accidental) — *see* Exposure, fire
Firearm discharge — *see* Discharge, firearm
**Fireball effects from nuclear explosion in war oper-
  ations** — *see* War operations, nuclear weapons
Fireworks (explosion) W39 ☑
Flash burns from explosion — *see* Explosion
Flood (any injury) (caused by) X38 ☑
  collapse of man-made structure causing earth move-
    ment X36.0 ☑
  tidal wave — *see* Forces of nature, tidal wave
Food (any type) **in**
  air passages (with asphyxia, obstruction, or suffoca-
    tion) — *see* categories T17 and T18
  alimentary tract causing asphyxia (due to compression
    of trachea) — *see* categories T17 and T18
Forces of nature X39.8 ☑
  avalanche X36.1 ☑
    causing transport accident — *see* Accident, trans-
      port, by type of vehicle
  blizzard X37.2 ☑
  cataclysmic storm X37.9 ☑

Forces of nature — *continued*
  cataclysmic storm — *continued*
    with flood X38 ☑
    blizzard X37.2 ☑
    cloudburst X37.8 ☑
    cyclone X37.1 ☑
    dust storm X37.3 ☑
    hurricane X37.0 ☑
    specified storm NEC X37.8 ☑
    storm surge X37.0 ☑
    tornado X37.1 ☑
    twister X37.1 ☑
    typhoon X37.0 ☑
  cloudburst X37.8 ☑
  cold (natural) X31 ☑
  cyclone X37.1 ☑
  dam collapse causing earth movement X36.0 ☑
  dust storm X37.3 ☑
  earth movement X36.1 ☑
    caused by dam or structure collapse X36.0 ☑
    earthquake X34 ☑
  earthquake X34 ☑
  flood (caused by) X38 ☑
    dam collapse X36.0 ☑
    tidal wave — *see* Forces of nature, tidal wave
  heat (natural) X30 ☑
  hurricane X37.0 ☑
  landslide X36.1 ☑
    causing transport accident — *see* Accident, trans-
      port, by type of vehicle
  lightning — *see* subcategory T75.0 ☑
    causing fire — *see* Exposure, fire
  mudslide X36.1 ☑
    causing transport accident — *see* Accident, trans-
      port, by type of vehicle
  radiation (natural) X39.08 ☑
    radon X39.01 ☑
  radon X39.01 ☑
  specified force NEC X39.8 ☑
  storm surge X37.0 ☑
  structure collapse causing earth movement X36.0 ☑
  sunlight X32 ☑
  tidal wave X37.41 ☑
    due to
      earthquake X37.41 ☑
      landslide X37.43 ☑
      storm X37.42 ☑
      volcanic eruption X37.41 ☑
  tornado X37.1 ☑
  tsunami X37.41 ☑
  twister X37.1 ☑
  typhoon X37.0 ☑
  volcanic eruption X35 ☑
Foreign body
  aspiration — *see* Index to Diseases and Injuries, For-
    eign body, respiratory tract
  embedded in skin W45 ☑
  entering through skin W45.8 ☑
    can lid W26.8 ☑
    nail W45.0 ☑
    paper W26.2 ☑
    specified NEC W45.8 ☑
    splinter W45.8 ☑
Forest fire (exposure to) — *see* Exposure, fire, uncontrolled, not in building
Found injured X58 ☑
  from exposure (to) — *see* Exposure
  on
    highway, road(way), street V89.9 ☑
    railway right of way V81.9 ☑
Fracture (circumstances unknown or unspecified) X58 ☑
  due to specified cause NEC X58 ☑
Freezing — *see* Exposure, cold
Frostbite X31 ☑
  due to man-made conditions — *see* Exposure, cold,
    man-made
Frozen — *see* Exposure, cold

G

Gored by bull W55.22 ☑
Gunshot wound W34.00 ☑

H

Hailstones, injured by X39.8 ☑

Hanged herself or himself — *see* Hanging, self-inflicted
Hanging (accidental) (*see also* category) T71 ☑
  legal execution — *see* Legal, intervention, specified
      means NEC
Heat (effects of) (excessive) X30 ☑
  due to
    man-made conditions W92 ☑
      on board watercraft V93.29 ☑
        fishing boat V93.22 ☑
        merchant ship V93.20 ☑
        passenger ship V93.21 ☑
        sailboat V93.24 ☑
        specified powered craft NEC V93.23 ☑
    weather (conditions) X30 ☑
  from
    electric heating apparatus causing burning X16 ☑
    nuclear explosion in war operations — *see* War
      operations, nuclear weapons
  inappropriate in local application or packing in medical
    or surgical procedure Y63.5
Hemorrhage
  delayed following medical or surgical treatment
      without mention of misadventure — *see* Index
      to Diseases and Injuries, Complication(s)
  during medical or surgical treatment as misadventure
      — *see* Index to Diseases and Injuries, Complica-
      tion(s)
High
  altitude (effects) — *see* Air, pressure, low
  level of radioactivity, effects — *see* Radiation
  pressure (effects) — *see* Air, pressure, high
  temperature, effects — *see* Heat
Hit, hitting (accidental) by — *see* Struck by
Hitting against — *see* Striking against
Homicide (attempt) (justifiable) — *see* Assault
Hot
  place, effects (*see also* Heat)
  weather, effects X30 ☑
House fire (uncontrolled) — *see* Exposure, fire, uncon-
    trolled, building
Humidity, causing problem X39.8 ☑
Hunger X58 ☑
Hurricane (any injury) X37.0 ☑
Hypobarism, hypobaropathy — *see* Air, pressure, low

I

Ictus
  caloris (*see also* Heat)
  solaris X30 ☑
Ignition (accidental) (*see also* Exposure, fire) X08.8 ☑
  anesthetic gas in operating room W40.1 ☑
  apparel X06.2 ☑
    from highly flammable material X04 ☑
    nightwear X05 ☑
  bed linen (sheets) (spreads) (pillows) (mattress) — *see*
    Exposure, fire, uncontrolled, building, bed
  benzine X04 ☑
  clothes, clothing NEC (from controlled fire) X06.2 ☑
    from
      highly flammable material X04 ☑
  ether X04 ☑
    in operating room W40.1 ☑
  explosive material — *see* Explosion
  gasoline X04 ☑
  jewelry (plastic) (any) X06.0 ☑
  kerosene X04 ☑
  material
    explosive — *see* Explosion
    highly flammable with secondary explosion X04 ☑
  nightwear X05 ☑
  paraffin X04 ☑
  petrol X04 ☑
Immersion (accidental) (*see also* Drowning)
  hand or foot due to cold (excessive) X31 ☑
Implantation of quills of porcupine W55.89 ☑
Inanition (from) (hunger) X58 ☑
  thirst X58 ☑
Inappropriate operation performed
  correct operation on wrong side or body part (wrong
    side) (wrong site) Y65.53
  operation intended for another patient done on wrong
    patient Y65.52
  wrong operation performed on correct patient Y65.51
Inattention after, at birth (homicidal intent) (infantici-
    dal intent) X58 ☑

Incident, adverse
  device
    anesthesiology Y70.8
      accessory Y70.2
      diagnostic Y70.0
      miscellaneous Y70.8
      monitoring Y70.0
      prosthetic Y70.2
      rehabilitative Y70.1
      surgical Y70.3
      therapeutic Y70.1
    cardiovascular Y71.8
      accessory Y71.2
      diagnostic Y71.0
      miscellaneous Y71.8
      monitoring Y71.0
      prosthetic Y71.2
      rehabilitative Y71.1
      surgical Y71.3
      therapeutic Y71.1
    gastroenterology Y73.8
      accessory Y73.2
      diagnostic Y73.0
      miscellaneous Y73.8
      monitoring Y73.0
      prosthetic Y73.2
      rehabilitative Y73.1
      surgical Y73.3
      therapeutic Y73.1
    general
      hospital Y74.8
        accessory Y74.2
        diagnostic Y74.0
        miscellaneous Y74.8
        monitoring Y74.0
        prosthetic Y74.2
        rehabilitative Y74.1
        surgical Y74.3
        therapeutic Y74.1
      surgical Y81.8
        accessory Y81.2
        diagnostic Y81.0
        miscellaneous Y81.8
        monitoring Y81.0
        prosthetic Y81.2
        rehabilitative Y81.1
        surgical Y81.3
        therapeutic Y81.1
    gynecological Y76.8
      accessory Y76.2
      diagnostic Y76.0
      miscellaneous Y76.8
      monitoring Y76.0
      prosthetic Y76.2
      rehabilitative Y76.1
      surgical Y76.3
      therapeutic Y76.1
    medical Y82.9
      specified type NEC Y82.8
    neurological Y75.8
      accessory Y75.2
      diagnostic Y75.0
      miscellaneous Y75.8
      monitoring Y75.0
      prosthetic Y75.2
      rehabilitative Y75.1
      surgical Y75.3
      therapeutic Y75.1
    obstetrical Y76.8
      accessory Y76.2
      diagnostic Y76.0
      miscellaneous Y76.8
      monitoring Y76.0
      prosthetic Y76.2
      rehabilitative Y76.1
      surgical Y76.3
      therapeutic Y76.1
    ophthalmic Y77.8
      accessory Y77.2
      diagnostic Y77.0
      miscellaneous Y77.8
      monitoring Y77.0
      prosthetic Y77.2
      rehabilitative Y77.1
      surgical Y77.3
      therapeutic Y77.1
    orthopedic Y79.8
      accessory Y79.2
      diagnostic Y79.0

Incident, adverse — *continued*
  device — *continued*
    orthopedic — *continued*
      miscellaneous Y79.8
      monitoring Y79.0
      prosthetic Y79.2
      rehabilitative Y79.1
      surgical Y79.3
      therapeutic Y79.1
    otorhinolaryngological Y72.8
      accessory Y72.2
      diagnostic Y72.0
      miscellaneous Y72.8
      monitoring Y72.0
      prosthetic Y72.2
      rehabilitative Y72.1
      surgical Y72.3
      therapeutic Y72.1
    personal use Y74.8
      accessory Y74.2
      diagnostic Y74.0
      miscellaneous Y74.8
      monitoring Y74.0
      prosthetic Y74.2
      rehabilitative Y74.1
      surgical Y74.3
      therapeutic Y74.1
    physical medicine Y80.8
      accessory Y80.2
      diagnostic Y80.0
      miscellaneous Y80.8
      monitoring Y80.0
      prosthetic Y80.2
      rehabilitative Y80.1
      surgical Y80.3
      therapeutic Y80.1
    plastic surgical Y81.8
      accessory Y81.2
      diagnostic Y81.0
      miscellaneous Y81.8
      monitoring Y81.0
      prosthetic Y81.2
      rehabilitative Y81.1
      surgical Y81.3
      therapeutic Y81.1
    radiological Y78.8
      accessory Y78.2
      diagnostic Y78.0
      miscellaneous Y78.8
      monitoring Y78.0
      prosthetic Y78.2
      rehabilitative Y78.1
      surgical Y78.3
      therapeutic Y78.1
    urology Y73.8
      accessory Y73.2
      diagnostic Y73.0
      miscellaneous Y73.8
      monitoring Y73.0
      prosthetic Y73.2
      rehabilitative Y73.1
      surgical Y73.3
      therapeutic Y73.1
Incineration (accidental) — *see* Exposure, fire
Infanticide — *see* Assault
Infrasound waves (causing injury) W49.9 ☑
Ingestion
  foreign body (causing injury) (with obstruction) — *see*
    Foreign body, alimentary canal
  poisonous
    plant(s) X58 ☑
    substance NEC — *see* Table of Drugs and Chemicals
Inhalation
  excessively cold substance, man-made — *see* Expo-
    sure, cold, man-made
  food (any type) (into respiratory tract) (with asphyxia,
    obstruction respiratory tract, suffocation) — *see*
    categories T17 and T18 ☑
  foreign body — *see* Foreign body, aspiration
  gastric contents (with asphyxia, obstruction respiratory
    passage, suffocation) T17.81- ☑
  hot air or gases X14.0 ☑
  liquid air, hydrogen, nitrogen W93.12 ☑
    suicide (attempt) X83.2 ☑
  steam X13.0 ☑
    assault X98.0 ☑
    stated as undetermined whether accidental or in-
      tentional Y27.0 ☑

Inhalation — *continued*
  steam — *continued*
    suicide (attempt) X77.0 ☑
  toxic gas — *see* Table of Drugs and Chemicals
  vomitus (with asphyxia, obstruction respiratory passage, suffocation) T17.81-
Injury, injured (accidental(ly)) NOS X58 ☑
  by, caused by, from
    assault — *see* Assault
    law-enforcing agent, police, in course of legal intervention — *see* Legal intervention
    suicide (attempt) X83.8 ☑
  due to, in
    civil insurrection — *see* War operations
    fight (*see also* Assault, fight) Y04.0 ☑
    war operations — *see* War operations
  homicide (*see also* Assault) Y09
  inflicted (by)
    in course of arrest (attempted), suppression of disturbance, maintenance of order, by law-enforcing agents — *see* Legal intervention
    other person
      stated as
        accidental X58 ☑
        intentional, homicide (attempt) — *see* Assault
        undetermined whether accidental or intentional Y33 ☑
    purposely (inflicted) by other person(s) — *see* Assault
  self-inflicted X83.8 ☑
    stated as accidental X58 ☑
  specified cause NEC X58 ☑
  undetermined whether accidental or intentional Y33 ☑
Insolation, effects X30 ☑
Insufficient nourishment X58 ☑
Interruption of respiration (by)
  food (lodged in esophagus) — *see* categories T17 and T18 ☑
  vomitus (lodged in esophagus) T17.81- ☑
Intervention, legal — *see* Legal intervention
Intoxication
  drug — *see* Table of Drugs and Chemicals
  poison — *see* Table of Drugs and Chemicals

J

Jammed (accidentally)
  between objects (moving) (stationary and moving) W23.0 ☑
  stationary W23.1 ☑
Jumped, jumping
  before moving object NEC X81.8 ☑
    motor vehicle X81.0 ☑
    subway train X81.1 ☑
    train X81.1 ☑
    undetermined whether accidental or intentional Y31 ☑
  from
    boat (into water) voluntarily, without accident (to or on boat) W16.712 ☑
      with
        accident to or on boat — *see* Accident, watercraft
        drowning or submersion W16.711 ☑
          suicide (attempt) X71.3 ☑
      striking bottom W16.722 ☑
        causing drowning W16.721 ☑
    building (*see also* Jumped, from, high place) W13.9 ☑
      burning (uncontrolled fire) X00.5 ☑
    high place NEC W17.89 ☑
      suicide (attempt) X80 ☑
      undetermined whether accidental or intentional Y30 ☑
    structure (*see also* Jumped, from, high place) W13.9 ☑
      burning (uncontrolled fire) X00.5 ☑
  into water W16.92 ☑
    causing drowning W16.91 ☑
    from, off watercraft — *see* Jumped, from, boat
    in
      natural body W16.612 ☑
        causing drowning W16.611 ☑
        striking bottom W16.622 ☑
          causing drowning W16.621 ☑

Jumped, jumping — *continued*
  into water — *continued*
    in — *continued*
      specified place NEC W16.812 ☑
        causing drowning W16.811 ☑
        striking
          bottom W16.822 ☑
            causing drowning W16.821 ☑
          wall W16.832 ☑
            causing drowning W16.831 ☑
      swimming pool W16.512 ☑
        causing drowning W16.511 ☑
        striking
          bottom W16.522 ☑
            causing drowning W16.521 ☑
          wall W16.532 ☑
            causing drowning W16.531 ☑
    suicide (attempt) X71.3 ☑

K

Kicked by
  animal NEC W55.82 ☑
  person(s) (accidentally) W50.1 ☑
    with intent to injure or kill Y04.0 ☑
    as, or caused by, a crowd or human stampede (with fall) W52 ☑
    assault Y04.0 ☑
    homicide (attempt) Y04.0 ☑
    in
      fight Y04.0 ☑
      legal intervention
        injuring
          bystander Y35.812 ☑
          law enforcement personnel Y35.811 ☑
          suspect Y35.813 ☑
Kicking
  against
    object W22.8 ☑
      sports equipment W21.9 ☑
      stationary W22.09 ☑
        sports equipment W21.89 ☑
    person — *see* Striking against, person
    sports equipment W21.9 ☑
  carpet stretcher with knee X50.3 ☑
Killed, killing (accidentally) NOS (*see also* Injury) X58 ☑
  in
    action — *see* War operations
    brawl, fight (hand) (fists) (foot) Y04.0 ☑
      by weapon (*see also* Assault)
        cutting, piercing — *see* Assault, cutting or piercing instrument
        firearm — *see* Discharge, firearm, by type, homicide
  self
    stated as
      accident NOS X58 ☑
      suicide — *see* Suicide
      undetermined whether accidental or intentional Y33 ☑
Kneeling (prolonged (static)) X50.1 ☑
Knocked down (accidentally) (by) NOS X58 ☑
  animal (not being ridden) NEC (*see also* Struck by, by type of animal)
  crowd or human stampede W52 ☑
  person W51 ☑
    in brawl, fight Y04.0 ☑
  transport vehicle NEC (*see also* Accident, transport) V09.9 ☑

L

Laceration NEC — *see* Injury
Lack of
  care (helpless person) (infant) (newborn) X58 ☑
  food except as result of abandonment or neglect X58 ☑
    due to abandonment or neglect X58 ☑
  water except as result of transport accident X58 ☑
    due to transport accident — *see* Accident, transport, by type
  helpless person, infant, newborn X58 ☑
Landslide (falling on transport vehicle) X36.1 ☑
  caused by collapse of man-made structure X36.0 ☑
Late effect — *see* Sequelae

Legal
  execution (any method) — *see* Legal, intervention
  intervention (by)
    baton — *see* Legal, intervention, blunt object, baton
    bayonet — *see* Legal, intervention, sharp object, bayonet
    blow — *see* Legal, intervention, manhandling
    blunt object
      baton
        injuring
          bystander Y35.312 ☑
          law enforcement personnel Y35.311 ☑
          suspect Y35.313 ☑
        injuring
          bystander Y35.302 ☑
          law enforcement personnel Y35.301 ☑
          suspect Y35.303 ☑
      specified NEC
        injuring
          bystander Y35.392 ☑
          law enforcement personnel Y35.391 ☑
          suspect Y35.393 ☑
      stave
        injuring
          bystander Y35.392 ☑
          law enforcement personnel Y35.391 ☑
          suspect Y35.393 ☑
    bomb — *see* Legal, intervention, explosive
    cutting or piercing instrument — *see* Legal, intervention, sharp object
    dynamite — *see* Legal, intervention, explosive, dynamite
    explosive(s)
      dynamite
        injuring
          bystander Y35.112 ☑
          law enforcement personnel Y35.111 ☑
          suspect Y35.113 ☑
      grenade
        injuring
          bystander Y35.192 ☑
          law enforcement personnel Y35.191 ☑
          suspect Y35.193 ☑
      injuring
        bystander Y35.102 ☑
        law enforcement personnel Y35.101 ☑
        suspect Y35.103 ☑
      mortar bomb
        injuring
          bystander Y35.192 ☑
          law enforcement personnel Y35.191 ☑
          suspect Y35.193 ☑
      shell
        injuring
          bystander Y35.122 ☑
          law enforcement personnel Y35.121 ☑
          suspect Y35.123 ☑
      specified NEC
        injuring
          bystander Y35.192 ☑
          law enforcement personnel Y35.191 ☑
          suspect Y35.193 ☑
    firearm(s) (discharge)
      handgun
        injuring
          bystander Y35.022 ☑
          law enforcement personnel Y35.021 ☑
          suspect Y35.023 ☑
      injuring
        bystander Y35.002 ☑
        law enforcement personnel Y35.001 ☑
        suspect Y35.003 ☑
      machine gun
        injuring
          bystander Y35.012 ☑
          law enforcement personnel Y35.011 ☑
          suspect Y35.013 ☑
      rifle pellet
        injuring
          bystander Y35.032 ☑
          law enforcement personnel Y35.031 ☑
          suspect Y35.033 ☑
      rubber bullet
        injuring
          bystander Y35.042 ☑
          law enforcement personnel Y35.041 ☑

Legal — *continued*
　intervention — *continued*
　　firearm(s) — *continued*
　　　rubber bullet — *continued*
　　　　injuring — *continued*
　　　　　suspect Y35.043 ☑
　　　shotgun — *see* Legal, intervention, firearm,
　　　　　specified NEC
　　　specified NEC
　　　　injuring
　　　　　bystander Y35.092 ☑
　　　　　law enforcement personnel Y35.091 ☑
　　　　　suspect Y35.093 ☑
　　gas (asphyxiation) (poisoning)
　　　injuring
　　　　bystander Y35.202 ☑
　　　　law enforcement personnel Y35.201 ☑
　　　　suspect Y35.203 ☑
　　　specified NEC
　　　　injuring
　　　　　bystander Y35.292 ☑
　　　　　law enforcement personnel Y35.291 ☑
　　　　　suspect Y35.293 ☑
　　　tear gas
　　　　injuring
　　　　　bystander Y35.212 ☑
　　　　　law enforcement personnel Y35.211 ☑
　　　　　suspect Y35.213 ☑
　　grenade — *see* Legal, intervention, explosive,
　　　　grenade
　　injuring
　　　bystander Y35.92 ☑
　　　law enforcement personnel Y35.91 ☑
　　　suspect Y35.93 ☑
　　late effect (of) — *see with 7th character S* Y35 ☑
　　manhandling
　　　injuring
　　　　bystander Y35.812 ☑
　　　　law enforcement personnel Y35.811 ☑
　　　　suspect Y35.813 ☑
　　sequelae (of) — *see with 7th character S* Y35 ☑
　　sharp objects
　　　bayonet
　　　　injuring
　　　　　bystander Y35.412 ☑
　　　　　law enforcement personnel Y35.411 ☑
　　　　　suspect Y35.413 ☑
　　　injuring
　　　　bystander Y35.402 ☑
　　　　law enforcement personnel Y35.401 ☑
　　　　suspect Y35.403 ☑
　　　specified NEC
　　　　injuring
　　　　　bystander Y35.492 ☑
　　　　　law enforcement personnel Y35.491 ☑
　　　　　suspect Y35.493 ☑
　　specified means NEC
　　　injuring
　　　　bystander Y35.892 ☑
　　　　law enforcement personnel Y35.891 ☑
　　　　suspect Y35.893 ☑
　　stabbing — *see* Legal, intervention, sharp object
　　stave — *see* Legal, intervention, blunt object, stave
　　tear gas — *see* Legal, intervention, gas, tear gas
　　truncheon — *see* Legal, intervention, blunt object,
　　　　stave

Lifting — *see also* Overexertion
　heavy objects X50.0 ☑
　weights X50.0 ☑
Lightning (shock) (stroke) (struck by) — *see subcategory*
　　T75.0 ☑
　causing fire — *see* Exposure, fire
Loss of control (transport vehicle) NEC — *see* Accident,
　　transport
Lost at sea NOS — *see* Drowning, due to, fall overboard
Low
　pressure (effects) — *see* Air, pressure, low
　temperature (effects) — *see* Exposure, cold
Lying before train, vehicle or other moving object
　　X81.8 ☑
　subway train X81.1 ☑
　train X81.1 ☑
　undetermined whether accidental or intentional
　　Y31 ☑
Lynching — *see* Assault

M

Malfunction (mechanism or component) (of)
　firearm W34.10 ☑
　　airgun W34.110 ☑
　　BB gun W34.110 ☑
　　gas, air or spring-operated gun NEC W34.118 ☑
　　handgun W32.1 ☑
　　hunting rifle W33.12 ☑
　　larger firearm W33.10 ☑
　　　specified NEC W33.19 ☑
　　machine gun W33.13 ☑
　　paintball gun W34.111 ☑
　　pellet gun W34.110 ☑
　　shotgun W33.11 ☑
　　specified NEC W34.19 ☑
　　Very pistol [flare] W34.19 ☑
　　handgun — *see* Malfunction, firearm, handgun
Maltreatment — *see* Perpetrator
Mangled (accidentally) NOS X58 ☑
Manhandling (in brawl, fight) Y04.0 ☑
　legal intervention — *see* Legal, intervention, manhan-
　　dling
Manslaughter (nonaccidental) — *see* Assault
Mauled by animal NEC W55.89 ☑
Medical procedure, complication of (delayed or as an
　　abnormal reaction without mention of misadven-
　　ture) — *see* Complication of or following, by speci-
　　fied type of procedure
　due to or as a result of misadventure — *see* Misadven-
　　ture
Melting (due to fire) (*see also* Exposure, fire)
　apparel NEC X06.3 ☑
　clothes, clothing NEC X06.3 ☑
　　nightwear X05 ☑
　fittings or furniture (burning building) (uncontrolled
　　fire) X00.8 ☑
　nightwear X05 ☑
　plastic jewelry X06.1 ☑
Mental cruelty X58 ☑
Military operations (injuries to military and civilians
　　occuring during peacetime on military property
　　and during routine military exercises and opera-
　　tions) (by) (from) (involving) Y37.90- ☑
　air blast Y37.20- ☑
　aircraft
　　destruction — *see* Military operations, destruction
　　　of aircraft
　airway restriction — *see* Military operations, restriction
　　of airways
　asphyxiation — *see* Military operations, restriction of
　　airways
　biological weapons Y37.6X- ☑
　blast Y37.20- ☑
　blast fragments Y37.20- ☑
　blast wave Y37.20- ☑
　blast wind Y37.20- ☑
　bomb Y37.20- ☑
　　dirty Y37.50- ☑
　　gasoline Y37.31- ☑
　　incendiary Y37.31- ☑
　　petrol Y37.31- ☑
　bullet Y37.43- ☑
　　incendiary Y37.32- ☑
　　rubber Y37.41- ☑
　chemical weapons Y37.7X- ☑
　combat
　　hand to hand (unarmed) combat Y37.44- ☑
　　using blunt or piercing object Y37.45- ☑
　conflagration — *see* Military operations, fire
　conventional warfare NEC Y37.49- ☑
　depth-charge Y37.01- ☑
　destruction of aircraft Y37.10- ☑
　　due to
　　　air to air missile Y37.11- ☑
　　　collision with other aircraft Y37.12- ☑
　　　detonation (accidental) of onboard munitions
　　　　and explosives Y37.14- ☑
　　　enemy fire or explosives Y37.11- ☑
　　　explosive placed on aircraft Y37.11- ☑
　　　onboard fire Y37.13- ☑
　　　rocket propelled grenade [RPG] Y37.11- ☑
　　　small arms fire Y37.11- ☑
　　　surface to air missile Y37.11- ☑
　　specified NEC Y37.19- ☑

Military operations — *continued*
　detonation (accidental) of
　　onboard marine weapons Y37.05- ☑
　　own munitions or munitions launch device
　　　Y37.24- ☑
　dirty bomb Y37.50- ☑
　explosion (of) Y37.20- ☑
　　aerial bomb Y37.21- ☑
　　bomb NOS (*see also* Military operations, bomb(s))
　　　Y37.20- ☑
　　fragments Y37.20- ☑
　　grenade Y37.29- ☑
　　guided missile Y37.22- ☑
　　improvised explosive device [IED] (person-borne)
　　　(roadside) (vehicle-borne) Y37.23- ☑
　　land mine Y37.29- ☑
　　marine mine (at sea) (in harbor) Y37.02- ☑
　　marine weapon Y37.00- ☑
　　　specified NEC Y37.09- ☑
　　own munitions or munitions launch device (acci-
　　　dental) Y37.24- ☑
　　sea-based artillery shell Y37.03- ☑
　　specified NEC Y37.29- ☑
　　torpedo Y37.04- ☑
　fire Y37.30- ☑
　　specified NEC Y37.39- ☑
　firearms
　　discharge Y37.43- ☑
　　pellets Y37.42- ☑
　flamethrower Y37.33- ☑
　fragments (from) (of)
　　improvised explosive device [IED] (person-borne)
　　　(roadside) (vehicle-borne) Y37.26- ☑
　　munitions Y37.25- ☑
　　specified NEC Y37.29- ☑
　　weapons Y37.27- ☑
　friendly fire Y37.92- ☑
　hand to hand (unarmed) combat Y37.44- ☑
　hot substances — *see* Military operations, fire
　incendiary bullet Y37.32- ☑
　nuclear weapon (effects of) Y37.50- ☑
　　acute radiation exposure Y37.54- ☑
　　blast pressure Y37.51- ☑
　　direct blast Y37.51- ☑
　　direct heat Y37.53- ☑
　　fallout exposure Y37.54- ☑
　　fireball Y37.53- ☑
　　indirect blast (struck or crushed by blast debris)
　　　(being thrown by blast) Y37.52- ☑
　　ionizing radiation (immediate exposure) Y37.54- ☑
　　nuclear radiation Y37.54- ☑
　　radiation
　　　ionizing (immediate exposure) Y37.54- ☑
　　　nuclear Y37.54- ☑
　　　thermal Y37.53- ☑
　　secondary effects Y37.54- ☑
　　specified NEC Y37.59- ☑
　　thermal radiation Y37.53- ☑
　restriction of air (airway)
　　intentional Y37.46- ☑
　　unintentional Y37.47- ☑
　rubber bullets Y37.41- ☑
　shrapnel NOS Y37.29- ☑
　suffocation — *see* Military operations, restriction of
　　airways
　unconventional warfare NEC Y37.7X- ☑
　underwater blast NOS Y37.00- ☑
　warfare
　　conventional NEC Y37.49- ☑
　　unconventional NEC Y37.7X- ☑
　weapon of mass destruction [WMD] Y37.91- ☑
　weapons
　　biological weapons Y37.6X- ☑
　　chemical Y37.7X- ☑
　　nuclear (effects of) Y37.50- ☑
　　　acute radiation exposure Y37.54- ☑
　　　blast pressure Y37.51- ☑
　　　direct blast Y37.51- ☑
　　　direct heat Y37.53- ☑
　　　fallout exposure Y37.54- ☑
　　　fireball Y37.53- ☑
　　　radiation
　　　　ionizing (immediate exposure) Y37.54- ☑
　　　　nuclear Y37.54- ☑
　　　　thermal Y37.53- ☑
　　　secondary effects Y37.54- ☑

Military operations — *continued*
  weapons — *continued*
    nuclear — *continued*
      specified NEC Y37.59- ☑
    of mass destruction [WMD] Y37.91- ☑
Misadventure(s) to patient(s) during surgical or medical care Y69
  contaminated medical or biological substance (blood, drug, fluid) Y64.9
    administered (by) NEC Y64.9
      immunization Y64.1
      infusion Y64.0
      injection Y64.1
      specified means NEC Y64.8
      transfusion Y64.0
      vaccination Y64.1
  excessive amount of blood or other fluid during transfusion or infusion Y63.0
  failure
    in dosage Y63.9
      electroshock therapy Y63.4
      inappropriate temperature (too hot or too cold) in local application and packing Y63.5
      infusion
        excessive amount of fluid Y63.0
        incorrect dilution of fluid Y63.1
      insulin-shock therapy Y63.4
      nonadministration of necessary drug or biological substance Y63.6
      overdose — *see* Table of Drugs and Chemicals radiation, in therapy Y63.2
      radiation
        overdose Y63.2
      specified procedure NEC Y63.8
      transfusion
        excessive amount of blood Y63.0
    mechanical, of instrument or apparatus (any) (during any procedure) Y65.8
    sterile precautions (during procedure) Y62.9
      aspiration of fluid or tissue (by puncture or catheterization, except heart) Y62.6
      biopsy (except needle aspiration) Y62.8
        needle (aspirating) Y62.6
      blood sampling Y62.6
      catheterization Y62.6
        heart Y62.5
      dialysis (kidney) Y62.2
      endoscopic examination Y62.4
      enema Y62.8
      immunization Y62.3
      infusion Y62.1
      injection Y62.3
      needle biopsy Y62.6
      paracentesis (abdominal) (thoracic) Y62.6
      perfusion Y62.2
      puncture (lumbar) Y62.6
      removal of catheter or packing Y62.8
      specified procedure NEC Y62.8
      surgical operation Y62.0
      transfusion Y62.1
      vaccination Y62.3
    suture or ligature during surgical procedure Y65.2
    to introduce or to remove tube or instrument — *see* Failure, to
  hemorrhage — *see* Index to Diseases and Injuries, Complication(s)
  inadvertent exposure of patient to radiation Y63.3
  inappropriate
    operation performed — *see* Inappropriate operation performed
    temperature (too hot or too cold) in local application or packing Y63.5
  infusion (*see also* Misadventure, by type, infusion) Y69
    excessive amount of fluid Y63.0
    incorrect dilution of fluid Y63.1
    wrong fluid Y65.1
  mismatched blood in transfusion Y65.0
  nonadministration of necessary drug or biological substance Y63.6
  overdose — *see* Table of Drugs and Chemicals radiation (in therapy) Y63.2
  perforation — *see* Index to Diseases and Injuries, Complication(s)
  performance of inappropriate operation — *see* Inappropriate operation performed
  puncture — *see* Index to Diseases and Injuries, Complication(s)
  specified type NEC Y65.8

Misadventure(s) to patient(s) during surgical or medical care — *continued*
  specified type — *continued*
    failure
      suture or ligature during surgical operation Y65.2
      to introduce or to remove tube or instrument — *see* Failure, to
    infusion of wrong fluid Y65.1
    performance of inappropriate operation — *see* Inappropriate operation performed
    transfusion of mismatched blood Y65.0
    wrong
      fluid in infusion Y65.1
      placement of endotracheal tube during anesthetic procedure Y65.3
  transfusion — *see* Misadventure, by type, transfusion
    excessive amount of blood Y63.0
    mismatched blood Y65.0
  wrong
    drug given in error — *see* Table of Drugs and Chemicals
    fluid in infusion Y65.1
    placement of endotracheal tube during anesthetic procedure Y65.3
Mismatched blood in transfusion Y65.0
Motion sickness T75.3 ☑
Mountain sickness W94.11 ☑
Mudslide (of cataclysmic nature) — *see* Landslide
Murder (attempt) — *see* Assault

N

Nail
  contact with W45.0 ☑
    gun W29.4 ☑
  embedded in skin W45.0 ☑
Neglect (criminal) (homicidal intent) X58 ☑
Noise (causing injury) (pollution) W42.9 ☑
  supersonic W42.0 ☑
Nonadministration (of)
  drug or biological substance (necessary) Y63.6
  surgical and medical care Y66
Nosocomial condition Y95

O

Object
  falling
    from, in, on, hitting
      machinery — *see* Contact, with, by type of machine
    set in motion by
      accidental explosion or rupture of pressure vessel W38 ☑
      firearm — *see* Discharge, firearm, by type
      machine(ry) — *see* Contact, with, by type of machine
Overdose (drug) — *see* Table of Drugs and Chemicals radiation Y63.2
Overexertion X50.9 ☑
  from
    prolonged static or awkward postures X50.1 ☑
    repetitive movements X50.3 ☑
    specified strenuous movements or postures NEC X50.9 ☑
    strenuous movement or load X50.0 ☑
Overexposure (accidental) (to)
  cold (*see also* Exposure, cold) X31 ☑
    due to man-made conditions — *see* Exposure, cold, man-made
  heat (*see also* Heat) X30 ☑
  radiation — *see* Radiation
  radioactivity W88.0 ☑
  sun (sunburn) X32 ☑
  weather NEC — *see* Forces of nature
  wind NEC — *see* Forces of nature
Overheated — *see* Heat
Overturning (accidental)
  machinery — *see* Contact, with, by type of machine
  transport vehicle NEC (*see also* Accident, transport) V89.9 ☑
  watercraft (causing drowning, submersion) (*see also* Drowning, due to, accident to, watercraft, overturning)
    causing injury except drowning or submersion — *see* Accident, watercraft, causing, injury NEC

P

Parachute descent (voluntary) (without accident to aircraft) V97.29 ☑
  due to accident to aircraft — *see* Accident, transport, aircraft
Pecked by bird W61.99 ☑
Perforation during medical or surgical treatment as misadventure — *see* Index to Diseases and Injuries, Complication(s)
Perpetrator, perpetration, of assault, maltreatment and neglect (by) Y07.9
  boyfriend Y07.03
  brother Y07.410
    stepbrother Y07.435
  coach Y07.53
  cousin
    female Y07.491
    male Y07.490
  daycare provider Y07.519
    at-home
      adult care Y07.512
      childcare Y07.510
    care center
      adult care Y07.513
      childcare Y07.511
  family member NEC Y07.499
  father Y07.11
    adoptive Y07.13
    foster Y07.420
    stepfather Y07.430
  foster father Y07.420
  foster mother Y07.421
  girl friend Y07.04
  healthcare provider Y07.529
    mental health Y07.521
    specified NEC Y07.528
  husband Y07.01
  instructor Y07.53
  mother Y07.12
    adoptive Y07.14
    foster Y07.421
    stepmother Y07.433
  nonfamily member Y07.50
    specified NEC Y07.59
  nurse Y07.528
  occupational therapist Y07.528
  partner of parent
    female Y07.434
    male Y07.432
  physical therapist Y07.528
  sister Y07.411
  speech therapist Y07.528
  stepbrother Y07.435
  stepfather Y07.430
  stepmother Y07.433
  stepsister Y07.436
  teacher Y07.53
  wife Y07.02
Piercing — *see* Contact, with, by type of object or machine
Pinched
  between objects (moving) (stationary and moving) W23.0 ☑
  stationary W23.1 ☑
Pinned under machine(ry) — *see* Contact, with, by type of machine
Place of occurrence Y92.9
  abandoned house Y92.89
  airplane Y92.813
  airport Y92.520
  ambulatory health services establishment NEC Y92.538
  ambulatory surgery center Y92.530
  amusement park Y92.831
  apartment (co-op) — *see* Place of occurrence, residence, apartment
  assembly hall Y92.29
  bank Y92.510
  barn Y92.71
  baseball field Y92.320
  basketball court Y92.310
  beach Y92.832
  boarding house — *see* Place of occurrence, residence, boarding house
  boat Y92.814
  bowling alley Y92.39
  bridge Y92.89

External Causes Index

Place of occurrence — Prolonged

Place of occurrence — *continued*
residence — *continued*
  institutional — *continued*
    school dormitory — *continued*
      dining room Y92.161
      kitchen Y92.160
      specified NEC Y92.168
    specified NEC Y92.199
      bathroom Y92.192
      bedroom Y92.193
      dining room Y92.191
      driveway Y92.194
      garage Y92.195
      garden Y92.197
      kitchen Y92.190
      specified NEC Y92.198
      swimming pool Y92.196
      yard Y92.197
  kitchen Y92.000
  mobile home Y92.029
    bathroom Y92.022
    bedroom Y92.023
    dining room Y92.021
    driveway Y92.024
    garage Y92.025
    garden Y92.027
    kitchen Y92.020
    specified NEC Y92.028
    swimming pool Y92.026
    yard Y92.027
  specified place in residence NEC Y92.008
  specified residence type NEC Y92.099
    bathroom Y92.091
    bedroom Y92.092
    driveway Y92.093
    garage Y92.094
    garden Y92.096
    kitchen Y92.090
    specified NEC Y92.098
    swimming pool Y92.095
    yard Y92.096
restaurant Y92.511
riding school Y92.39
river Y92.828
road Y92.488
rodeo ring Y92.39
rugby field Y92.328
same day surgery center Y92.530
sand pit Y92.64
school (private) (public) (state) Y92.219
  college Y92.214
  daycare center Y92.210
  elementary school Y92.211
  high school Y92.213
  kindergarten Y92.211
  middle school Y92.212
  specified NEC Y92.218
  trace school Y92.215
  university Y92.214
  vocational school Y92.215
sea (shore) Y92.832
senior citizen center Y92.29
service area
  airport Y92.520
  bus station Y92.521
  gas station Y92.524
  highway rest stop Y92.523
  railway station Y92.522
shipyard Y92.62
shop (commercial) Y92.513
sidewalk Y92.480
silo Y92.79
skating rink (roller) Y92.331
  ice Y92.330
slaughter house Y92.86
soccer field Y92.322
specified place NEC Y92.89
sports area Y92.39
  athletic
    court Y92.318
      basketball Y92.310
      specified NEC Y92.318
      squash Y92.311
      tennis Y92.312
    field Y92.328
      baseball Y92.320
      cricket ground Y92.328
      football Y92.321
      hockey Y92.328

Place of occurrence — *continued*
sports area — *continued*
  athletic — *continued*
    field — *continued*
      soccer Y92.322
      specified NEC Y92.328
  golf course Y92.39
  gymnasium Y92.39
  riding school Y92.39
  skating rink (roller) Y92.331
    ice Y92.330
  stadium Y92.39
  swimming pool Y92.34
squash court Y92.311
stadium Y92.39
steeplechasing course Y92.39
store Y92.512
stream Y92.828
street and highway Y92.410
  bike path Y92.482
  freeway Y92.411
  highway ramp Y92.415
  interstate highway Y92.411
  local residential or business street Y92.414
  motorway Y92.411
  parking lot Y92.481
  parkway Y92.412
  sidewalk Y92.480
  specified NEC Y92.488
  state road Y92.413
subway car Y92.816
supermarket Y92.512
swamp Y92.828
swimming pool (public) Y92.34
  private (at) Y92.095
    boarding house Y92.045
    military base Y92.136
    mobile home Y92.026
    nursing home Y92.125
    orphanage Y92.115
    prison Y92.146
    reform school Y92.156
    single family residence Y92.016
synagogue Y92.22
television station Y92.59
tennis court Y92.312
theater Y92.254
trade area Y92.59
  bank Y92.510
  cafe Y92.511
  casino Y92.59
  garage Y92.59
  hotel Y92.59
  market Y92.512
  office building Y92.59
  radio station Y92.59
  restaurant Y92.511
  shop Y92.513
  shopping mall Y92.59
  store Y92.512
  supermarket Y92.512
  television station Y92.59
  warehouse Y92.59
trailer park, residential — *see* Place of occurrence, residence, mobile home
trailer site NOS Y92.89
train Y92.815
  station Y92.522
truck Y92.812
tunnel under construction Y92.69
university Y92.214
urgent (health) care center Y92.532
vehicle (transport) Y92.818
  airplane Y92.813
  boat Y92.814
  bus Y92.811
  car Y92.810
  specified NEC Y92.818
  subway car Y92.816
  train Y92.815
  truck Y92.812
warehouse Y92.59
water reservoir Y92.89
wilderness area Y92.828
  desert Y92.820
  forest Y92.821
  marsh Y92.828
  mountain Y92.828
  prairie Y92.828

Place of occurrence — *continued*
wilderness area — *continued*
  specified NEC Y92.828
  swamp Y92.828
workshop Y92.69
yard, private Y92.096
  boarding house Y92.046
  mobile home Y92.027
  single family house Y92.017
youth center Y92.29
zoo (zoological garden) Y92.834

Plumbism — *see* Table of Drugs and Chemicals, lead
Poisoning (accidental) (by) (*see also* Table of Drugs and Chemicals)
by plant, thorns, spines, sharp leaves or other mechanisms NEC X58 ☑
carbon monoxide
  generated by
    motor vehicle — *see* Accident, transport
    watercraft (in transit) (not in transit) V93.89 ☑
      ferry boat V93.81 ☑
      fishing boat V93.82 ☑
      jet skis V93.83 ☑
      liner V93.81 ☑
      merchant ship V93.80 ☑
      passenger ship V93.81 ☑
      powered craft NEC V93.83 ☑
caused by injection of poisons into skin by plant thorns, spines, sharp leaves X58 ☑
  marine or sea plants (venomous) X58 ☑
execution — *see* Legal, intervention, gas
intervention
  by gas — *see* Legal, intervention, gas
  other specified means — *see* Legal, intervention, specified means NEC
exhaust gas
  generated by
    motor vehicle — *see* Accident, transport
    watercraft (in transit) (not in transit) V93.89 ☑
      ferry boat V93.81 ☑
      fishing boat V93.82 ☑
      jet skis V93.83 ☑
      liner V93.81 ☑
      merchant ship V93.80 ☑
      passenger ship V93.81 ☑
      powered craft NEC V93.83 ☑
fumes or smoke due to
  explosion (*see also* Explosion) W40.9 ☑
  fire — *see* Exposure, fire
  ignition — *see* Ignition
gas
  in legal intervention — *see* Legal, intervention, gas
  legal execution — *see* Legal, intervention, gas
in war operations — *see* War operations
legal
Powder burn (by) (from)
airgun W34.110 ☑
BB gun W34.110 ☑
firearm NEC W34.19 ☑
gas, air or spring-operated gun NEC W34.118 ☑
handgun W32.1 ☑
hunting rifle W33.12 ☑
larger firearm W33.10 ☑
  specified NEC W33.19 ☑
machine gun W33.13 ☑
paintball gun W34.111 ☑
pellet gun W34.110 ☑
shotgun W33.11 ☑
Very pistol [flare] W34.19 ☑
Premature cessation (of) **surgical and medical care** Y66
Privation (food) (water) X58 ☑
Procedure (operation)
correct, on wrong side or body part (wrong side) (wrong site) Y65.53
intended for another patient done on wrong patient Y65.52
performed on patient not scheduled for surgery Y65.52
performed on wrong patient Y65.52
wrong, performed on correct patient Y65.51
Prolonged
sitting in transport vehicle — *see* Travel, by type of vehicle
stay in
  high altitude as cause of anoxia, barodontalgia, barotitis or hypoxia W94.11 ☑
  weightless environment X52 ☑

Pulling, excessive (see also Overexertion) X50.9- ☑
Puncture, puncturing (see also Contact, with, by type of object or machine)
  by
    plant thorns, spines, sharp leaves or other mechanisms NEC W60 ☑
    during medical or surgical treatment as misadventure — see Index to Diseases and Injuries, Complication(s)
Pushed, pushing (accidental) (injury in)
  by other person(s) (accidental) W51 ☑
    with fall W03 ☑
      due to ice or snow W00.0 ☑
    as, or caused by, a crowd or human stampede (with fall) W52 ☑
    before moving object NEC Y02.8 ☑
      motor vehicle Y02.0 ☑
      subway train Y02.1 ☑
      train Y02.1 ☑
    from
      high place NEC
        in accidental circumstances W17.89 ☑
        stated as
          intentional, homicide (attempt) Y01 ☑
          undetermined whether accidental or intentional Y30 ☑
      transport vehicle NEC (see also Accident, transport) V89.9 ☑
        stated as
          intentional, homicide (attempt) Y08.89 ☑
    overexertion X50.9 ☑

R

Radiation (exposure to)
  arc lamps W89.0 ☑
  atomic power plant (malfunction) NEC W88.1 ☑
  complication of or abnormal reaction to medical radiotherapy Y84.2
  electromagnetic, ionizing W88.0 ☑
  gamma rays W88.1 ☑
  in
    war operations (from or following nuclear explosion) — see War operations
  inadvertent exposure of patient (receiving test or therapy) Y63.3
  infrared (heaters and lamps) W90.1 ☑
    excessive heat from W92 ☑
  ionized, ionizing (particles, artificially accelerated)
    radioisotopes W88.1 ☑
    specified NEC W88.8 ☑
    x-rays W88.0 ☑
  isotopes, radioactive — see Radiation, radioactive isotopes
  laser(s) W90.2 ☑
    in war operations — see War operations
    misadventure in medical care Y63.2
  light sources (man-made visible and ultraviolet) W89.9 ☑
    natural X32 ☑
    specified NEC W89.8 ☑
    tanning bed W89.1 ☑
    welding light W89.0 ☑
  man-made visible light W89.9 ☑
    specified NEC W89.8 ☑
    tanning bed W89.1 ☑
    welding light W89.0 ☑
  microwave W90.8 ☑
  misadventure in medical or surgical procedure Y63.2
  natural NEC X39.08 ☑
  radon X39.01 ☑
  overdose (in medical or surgical procedure) Y63.2
  radar W90.0 ☑
  radioactive isotopes (any) W88.1 ☑
    atomic power plant malfunction W88.1 ☑
    misadventure in medical or surgical treatment Y63.2
  radiofrequency W90.0 ☑
  radium NEC W88.1 ☑
  sun X32 ☑
  ultraviolet (light) (man-made) W89.9 ☑
    natural X32 ☑
    specified NEC W89.8 ☑
    tanning bed W89.1 ☑
    welding light W89.0 ☑

Radiation — continued
  welding arc, torch, or light W89.0 ☑
    excessive heat from W92 ☑
  x-rays (hard) (soft) W88.0 ☑
Range disease W94.11 ☑
Rape (attempted) T74.2- ☑
Rat bite W53.11 ☑
Reaching (prolonged) (static) X50.1 ☑
Reaction, abnormal to medical procedure (see also Complication of or following, by type of procedure) Y84.9
  with misadventure — see Misadventure
  biologicals — see Table of Drugs and Chemicals
  drugs — see Table of Drugs and Chemicals
  vaccine — see Table of Drugs and Chemicals
Recoil
  airgun W34.110 ☑
  BB gun W34.110 ☑
  firearm NEC W34.19 ☑
  gas, air or spring-operated gun NEC W34.118 ☑
  handgun W32.1 ☑
  hunting rifle W33.12 ☑
  larger firearm W33.10 ☑
    specified NEC W33.19 ☑
  machine gun W33.13 ☑
  paintball gun W34.111 ☑
  pellet W34.110 ☑
  shotgun W33.11 ☑
  Very pistol [flare] W34.19 ☑
Reduction in
  atmospheric pressure — see Air, pressure, change
Rock falling on or hitting (accidentally) (person) W20.8 ☑
  in cave-in W20.0 ☑
Run over (accidentally) (by)
  animal (not being ridden) NEC W55.89 ☑
  machinery — see Contact, with, by specified type of machine
  transport vehicle NEC (see also Accident, transport) V09.9 ☑
    intentional homicide (attempt) Y03.0 ☑
    motor NEC V09.20 ☑
      intentional homicide (attempt) Y03.0 ☑
Running
  before moving object X81.8 ☑
    motor vehicle X81.0 ☑
Running off, away
  animal (being ridden) (see also Accident, transport) V80.918 ☑
    not being ridden W55.89 ☑
  animal-drawn vehicle NEC (see also Accident, transport) V80.928 ☑
  highway, road(way), street
    transport vehicle NEC (see also Accident, transport) V89.9 ☑
Rupture pressurized devices — see Explosion, by type of device

S

Saturnism — see Table of Drugs and Chemicals, lead
Scald, scalding (accidental) (by) (from) (in) X19 ☑
  air (hot) X14.1 ☑
  gases (hot) X14.1 ☑
  homicide (attempt) — see Assault, burning, hot object
  inflicted by other person
    stated as intentional, homicide (attempt) — see Assault, burning, hot object
  liquid (boiling) (hot) NEC X12 ☑
    stated as undetermined whether accidental or intentional Y27.2 ☑
    suicide (attempt) X77.2 ☑
  local application of externally applied substance in medical or surgical care Y63.5
  metal (molten) (liquid) (hot) NEC X18 ☑
  self-inflicted X77.9 ☑
  stated as undetermined whether accidental or intentional Y27.8 ☑
  steam X13.1 ☑
    assault X98.0 ☑
    stated as undetermined whether accidental or intentional Y27.0 ☑
    suicide (attempt) X77.0 ☑
  suicide (attempt) X77.9 ☑
  vapor (hot) X13.1 ☑
    assault X98.0 ☑

Scald, scalding — continued
  vapor — continued
    stated as undetermined whether accidental or intentional Y27.0 ☑
    suicide (attempt) X77.0 ☑
Scratched by
  cat W55.03 ☑
  person(s) (accidentally) W50.4 ☑
    with intent to injure or kill Y04.0 ☑
    as, or caused by, a crowd or human stampede (with fall) W52 ☑
    assault Y04.0 ☑
    homicide (attempt) Y04.0 ☑
    in
      fight Y04.0 ☑
      legal intervention
        injuring
          bystander Y35.892 ☑
          law enforcement personnel Y35.891 ☑
          suspect Y35.893 ☑
Seasickness T75.3
Self-harm NEC (see also External cause by type, undetermined whether accidental or intentional)
  intentional — see Suicide
  poisoning NEC — see Table of Drugs and Chemicals, poisoning, accidental
Self-inflicted (injury) **NEC** (see also External cause by type, undetermined whether accidental or intentional)
  intentional — see Suicide
  poisoning NEC — see Table of Drugs and Chemicals, poisoning, accidental
Sequelae (of)
  accident NEC — see W00-X58 with 7th character S
  assault (homicidal) (any means) — see X92-Y08 with 7th character S
  homicide, attempt (any means) — see X92-Y08 with 7th character S
  injury undetermined whether accidentally or purposely inflicted — see Y21-Y33 with 7th character S
  intentional self-harm (classifiable to X71-X83) — see X71-X83 with 7th character S
  legal intervention — see with 7th character S Y35 ☑
  motor vehicle accident — see V00-V99 with 7th character S
  suicide, attempt (any means) — see X71-X83 with 7th character S
  transport accident — see V00-V99 with 7th character S
  war operations — see War operations
Shock
  electric — see Exposure, electric current
  from electric appliance (any) (faulty) W86.8 ☑
    domestic W86.0 ☑
    suicide (attempt) X83.1 ☑
Shooting, shot (accidental(ly)) (see also Discharge, firearm, by type)
  herself or himself — see Discharge, firearm by type, self-inflicted
  homicide (attempt) — see Discharge, firearm by type, homicide
  in war operations — see War operations
  inflicted by other person — see Discharge, firearm by type, homicide
    accidental — see Discharge, firearm, by type of firearm
  legal
    execution — see Legal, intervention, firearm
    intervention — see Legal, intervention, firearm
  self-inflicted — see Discharge, firearm by type, suicide
    accidental — see Discharge, firearm, by type of firearm
  suicide (attempt) — see Discharge, firearm by type, suicide
Shoving (accidentally) **by other person** — see Pushed, by other person
Sickness
  alpine W94.11 ☑
  motion — see Motion
  mountain W94.11 ☑
Sinking (accidental)
  watercraft (causing drowning, submersion) (see also Drowning, due to, accident to, watercraft, sinking)
    causing injury except drowning or submersion — see Accident, watercraft, causing, injury NEC
Siriasis X32 ☑

▼ Subterms under main terms may continue to next column or page   ☑ Additional Character Required — Refer to the Tabular List for Character Selection   **427**

Pulling, excessive — Siriasis

External Causes Index

Sitting — Struck

Sitting (prolonged) (static) X50.1 ☑
Slashed wrists — *see* Cut, self-inflicted
Slipping (accidental) (on same level) (with fall) W01.0 ☑
  without fall W18.40 ☑
    due to
      specified NEC W18.49 ☑
      stepping from one level to another W18.43 ☑
      stepping into hole or opening W18.42 ☑
      stepping on object W18.41 ☑
  on
    ice W00.0 ☑
      with skates — *see* Accident, transport, pedestrian, conveyance
    mud W01.0 ☑
    oil W01.0 ☑
    snow W00.0 ☑
      with skis — *see* Accident, transport, pedestrian, conveyance
    surface (slippery) (wet) NEC W01.0 ☑
Sliver, wood, contact with W45.8 ☑
Smoldering (due to fire) — *see* Exposure, fire
Sodomy (attempted) **by force** T74.2 ☑
Sound waves (causing injury) W42.9 ☑
  supersonic W42.0 ☑
Splinter, contact with W45.8 ☑
Stab, stabbing — *see* Cut
Standing (prolonged) (static) X50.1 ☑
Starvation X58 ☑
Status of external cause Y99.9
  child assisting in compensated work for family Y99.8
  civilian activity done for financial or other compensation Y99.0
  civilian activity done for income or pay Y99.0
  family member assisting in compensated work for other family member Y99.8
  hobby not done for income Y99.8
  leisure activity Y99.8
  military activity Y99.1
  off-duty activity of military personnel Y99.8
  recreation or sport not for income or while a student Y99.8
  specified NEC Y99.8
  student activity Y99.8
  volunteer activity Y99.2
Stepped on
  by
    animal (not being ridden) NEC W55.89 ☑
    crowd or human stampede W52 ☑
    person W50.0 ☑
Stepping on
  object W22.8 ☑
    with fall W18.31 ☑
    sports equipment W21.9 ☑
    stationary W22.09 ☑
      sports equipment W21.89 ☑
  person W51 ☑
    by crowd or human stampede W52 ☑
    sports equipment W21.9 ☑
Sting
  arthropod, nonvenomous W57 ☑
  insect, nonvenomous W57 ☑
Storm (cataclysmic) — *see* Forces of nature, cataclysmic storm
Straining, excessive (*see also* Overexertion) X50.9 ☑
Strangling — *see* Strangulation
Strangulation (accidental) T71 ☑
Strenuous movements (*see also* Overexertion) X50.9 ☑
Striking against
  airbag (automobile) W22.10 ☑
    driver side W22.11 ☑
    front passenger side W22.12 ☑
    specified NEC W22.19 ☑
  bottom when
    diving or jumping into water (in) W16.822 ☑
      causing drowning W16.821 ☑
      from boat W16.722 ☑
        causing drowning W16.721 ☑
      natural body W16.622 ☑
        causing drowning W16.821 ☑
      swimming pool W16.522 ☑
        causing drowning W16.521 ☑
    falling into water (in) W16.322 ☑
      causing drowning W16.321 ☑
      fountain — *see* Striking against, bottom when, falling into water, specified NEC
      natural body W16.122 ☑

Striking against — *continued*
  bottom when — *continued*
    falling into water — *continued*
      natural body — *continued*
        causing drowning W16.121 ☑
      reservoir — *see* Striking against, bottom when, falling into water, specified NEC
      specified NEC W16.322 ☑
        causing drowning W16.321 ☑
      swimming pool W16.022 ☑
        causing drowning W16.021 ☑
  diving board (swimming-pool) W21.4 ☑
  object W22.8 ☑
    with
      drowning or submersion — *see* Drowning
      fall — *see* Fall, due to, bumping against, object
    caused by crowd or human stampede (with fall) W52 ☑
    furniture W22.03 ☑
    lamppost W22.02 ☑
    sports equipment W21.9 ☑
    stationary W22.09 ☑
      sports equipment W21.89 ☑
    wall W22.01 ☑
  person(s) W51 ☑
    with fall W03 ☑
      due to ice or snow W00.0 ☑
    as, or caused by, a crowd or human stampede (with fall) W52 ☑
    assault Y04.2 ☑
    homicide (attempt) Y04.2 ☑
  sports equipment W21.9 ☑
  wall (when) W22.01 ☑
    diving or jumping into water (in) W16.832 ☑
      causing drowning W16.831 ☑
      swimming pool W16.532 ☑
        causing drowning W16.531 ☑
    falling into water (in) W16.332 ☑
      causing drowning W16.331 ☑
      fountain — *see* Striking against, wall when, falling into water, specified NEC
      natural body W16.132 ☑
        causing drowning W16.131 ☑
      reservoir — *see* Striking against, wall when, falling into water, specified NEC
      specified NEC W16.332 ☑
        causing drowning W16.331 ☑
      swimming pool W16.032 ☑
        causing drowning W16.031 ☑
    swimming pool (when) W22.042 ☑
      causing drowning W22.041 ☑
      diving or jumping into water W16.532 ☑
        causing drowning W16.531 ☑
      falling into water W16.032 ☑
        causing drowning W16.031 ☑
Struck (accidentally) **by**
  airbag (automobile) W22.10 ☑
    driver side W22.11 ☑
    front passenger side W22.12 ☑
    specified NEC W22.19 ☑
  alligator W58.02 ☑
  animal (not being ridden) NEC W55.89 ☑
  avalanche — *see* Landslide
  ball (hit) (thrown) W21.00 ☑
    assault Y08.09 ☑
    baseball W21.03 ☑
    basketball W21.05 ☑
    football W21.01 ☑
    golf ball W21.04 ☑
    soccer W21.02 ☑
    softball W21.07 ☑
    specified NEC W21.09 ☑
    volleyball W21.06 ☑
  bat or racquet
    baseball bat W21.11 ☑
      assault Y08.02 ☑
    golf club W21.13 ☑
      assault Y08.09 ☑
    specified NEC W21.19 ☑
      assault Y08.09 ☑
    tennis racquet W21.12 ☑
      assault Y08.09 ☑
  bullet (*see also* Discharge, firearm by type)
    in war operations — *see* War operations
  crocodile W58.12 ☑
  dog W54.1 ☑

Struck (accidentally) **by** — *continued*
  flare, Very pistol — *see* Discharge, firearm NEC
  hailstones X39.8 ☑
  hockey (ice)
    field
      puck W21.221 ☑
      stick W21.211 ☑
    puck W21.220 ☑
    stick W21.210 ☑
      assault Y08.01 ☑
  landslide — *see* Landslide
  law-enforcement agent (on duty) — *see* Legal, intervention, manhandling
    with blunt object — *see* Legal, intervention, blunt object
  lightning T75.0 ☑
    causing fire — *see* Exposure, fire
  machine — *see* Contact, with, by type of machine
  mammal NEC W55.89 ☑
    marine W56.32 ☑
  marine animal W56.82 ☑
  missile
    firearm — *see* Discharge, firearm by type
    in war operations — *see* War operations, missile
  object W22.8 ☑
    blunt W22.8 ☑
      assault Y00 ☑
      suicide (attempt) X79 ☑
      undetermined whether accidental or intentional Y29 ☑
    falling W20.8 ☑
      from, in, on
        building W20.1 ☑
          burning (uncontrolled fire) X00.4 ☑
        cataclysmic
          earth surface movement NEC — *see* Landslide
          storm — *see* Forces of nature, cataclysmic storm
        cave-in W20.0 ☑
        earthquake X34 ☑
        machine (in operation) — *see* Contact, with, by type of machine
        structure W20.1 ☑
          burning X00.4 ☑
        transport vehicle (in motion) — *see* Accident, transport, by type of vehicle
        watercraft V93.49 ☑
          due to
            accident to craft V91.39 ☑
              powered craft V91.33 ☑
                ferry boat V91.31 ☑
                fishing boat V91.32 ☑
                jetskis V91.33 ☑
                liner V91.31 ☑
                merchant ship V91.30 ☑
                passenger ship V91.31 ☑
              unpowered craft V91.38 ☑
                canoe V91.35 ☑
                inflatable V91.36 ☑
                kayak V91.35 ☑
                sailboat V91.34 ☑
                surf-board V91.38 ☑
                windsurfer V91.38 ☑
            powered craft V93.43 ☑
              ferry boat V93.41 ☑
              fishing boat V93.42 ☑
              jetskis V93.43 ☑
              liner V93.41 ☑
              merchant ship V93.40 ☑
              passenger ship V93.41 ☑
            unpowered craft V93.48 ☑
              sailboat V93.44 ☑
              surf-board V93.48 ☑
              windsurfer V93.48 ☑
    moving NEC W20.8 ☑
    projected W20.8 ☑
      assault Y00 ☑
      in sports W21.9 ☑
        assault Y08.09 ☑
        ball W21.00 ☑
          baseball W21.03 ☑
          basketball W21.05 ☑
          football W21.01 ☑
          golf ball W21.04 ☑
          soccer W21.02 ☑

Struck (accidentally) **by** — *continued*
　object — *continued*
　　projected — *continued*
　　　in sports — *continued*
　　　　ball — *continued*
　　　　　softball W21.07 ☑
　　　　　specified NEC W21.09 ☑
　　　　　volleyball W21.06 ☑
　　　　bat or racquet
　　　　　baseball bat W21.11 ☑
　　　　　　assault Y08.02 ☑
　　　　　golf club W21.13 ☑
　　　　　　assault Y08.09 ☑
　　　　　specified NEC W21.19 ☑
　　　　　　assault Y08.09 ☑
　　　　　tennis racquet W21.12 ☑
　　　　　　assault Y08.09 ☑
　　　　hockey (ice)
　　　　　field
　　　　　　puck W21.221 ☑
　　　　　　stick W21.211 ☑
　　　　　puck W21.220 ☑
　　　　　stick W21.210 ☑
　　　　　　assault Y08.01 ☑
　　　　specified NEC W21.89 ☑
　　set in motion by explosion — *see* Explosion
　　thrown W20.8 ☑
　　　assault Y00 ☑
　　　in sports W21.9 ☑
　　　　assault Y08.09 ☑
　　　　ball W21.00 ☑
　　　　　baseball W21.03 ☑
　　　　　basketball W21.05 ☑
　　　　　football W21.01 ☑
　　　　　golf ball W21.04 ☑
　　　　　soccer W21.02 ☑
　　　　　soft ball W21.07 ☑
　　　　　specified NEC W21.09 ☑
　　　　　volleyball W21.06 ☑
　　　　bat or racquet
　　　　　baseball bat W21.11 ☑
　　　　　　assault Y08.02 ☑
　　　　　golf club W21.13 ☑
　　　　　　assault Y08.09 ☑
　　　　　specified NEC W21.19 ☑
　　　　　　assault Y08.09 ☑
　　　　　tennis racquet W21.12 ☑
　　　　　　assault Y08.09 ☑
　　　　hockey (ice)
　　　　　field
　　　　　　puck W21.221 ☑
　　　　　　stick W21.211 ☑
　　　　　puck W21.220 ☑
　　　　　stick W21.210 ☑
　　　　　　assault Y08.01 ☑
　　　　specified NEC W21.89 ☑
　other person(s) W50.0 ☑
　　with
　　　blunt object W22.8 ☑
　　　　intentional, homicide (attempt) Y00 ☑
　　　　sports equipment W21.9 ☑
　　　　undetermined whether accidental or intentional Y29 ☑
　　　fall W03 ☑
　　　　due to ice or snow W00.0 ☑
　　as, or caused by, a crowd or human stampede (with fall) W52 ☑
　　assault Y04.2 ☑
　　homicide (attempt) Y04.2 ☑
　　in legal intervention
　　　injuring
　　　　bystander Y35.812 ☑
　　　　law enforcement personnel Y35.811 ☑
　　　　suspect Y35.813 ☑
　　sports equipment W21.9 ☑
　police (on duty) — *see* Legal, intervention, manhandling
　　with blunt object — *see* Legal, intervention, blunt object
　sports equipment W21.9 ☑
　　assault Y08.09 ☑
　　ball W21.00 ☑
　　　baseball W21.03 ☑
　　　basketball W21.05 ☑
　　　football W21.01 ☑
　　　golf ball W21.04 ☑

Struck (accidentally) **by** — *continued*
　sports equipment — *continued*
　　ball — *continued*
　　　soccer W21.02 ☑
　　　soft ball W21.07 ☑
　　　specified NEC W21.09 ☑
　　　volleyball W21.06 ☑
　　bat or racquet
　　　baseball bat W21.11 ☑
　　　　assault Y08.02 ☑
　　　golf club W21.13 ☑
　　　　assault Y08.09 ☑
　　　specified NEC W21.19 ☑
　　　tennis racquet W21.12 ☑
　　cleats (shoe) W21.31 ☑
　　foot wear NEC W21.39 ☑
　　football helmet W21.81 ☑
　　hockey (ice)
　　　field
　　　　puck W21.221 ☑
　　　　stick W21.211 ☑
　　　puck W21.220 ☑
　　　stick W21.210 ☑
　　　　assault Y08.01 ☑
　　skate blades W21.32 ☑
　　specified NEC W21.89 ☑
　　　assault Y08.09 ☑
　thunderbolt — *see* subcategory T75.0 ☑
　　causing fire — *see* Exposure, fire
　transport vehicle NEC (*see also* Accident, transport) V09.9 ☑
　　intentional, homicide (attempt) Y03.0 ☑
　　motor NEC (*see also* Accident, transport) V09.20 ☑
　　　homicide Y03.0 ☑
　vehicle (transport) NEC — *see* Accident, transport, by type of vehicle
　　stationary (falling from jack, hydraulic lift, ramp) W20.8 ☑

Stumbling
　without fall W18.40 ☑
　　due to
　　　specified NEC W18.49 ☑
　　　stepping from one level to another W18.43 ☑
　　　stepping into hole or opening W18.42 ☑
　　　stepping on object W18.41 ☑
　　over
　　　animal NEC W01.0 ☑
　　　　with fall W18.09 ☑
　　　carpet, rug or (small) object W22.8 ☑
　　　　with fall W18.09 ☑
　　　person W51 ☑
　　　　with fall W03 ☑
　　　　　due to ice or snow W00.0 ☑
Submersion (accidental) — *see* Drowning
Suffocation (accidental) (by external means) (by pressure) (mechanical) (*see also* category) T71 ☑
　due to, by
　　avalanche — *see* Landslide
　　explosion — *see* Explosion
　　fire — *see* Exposure, fire
　　food, any type (aspiration) (ingestion) (inhalation) — *see* categories T17 and T18 ☑
　　ignition — *see* Ignition
　　landslide — *see* Landslide
　　machine(ry) — *see* Contact, with, by type of machine
　　vomitus (aspiration) (inhalation) T17.81- ☑
　in
　　burning building X00.8 ☑
Suicide, suicidal (attempted) (by) X83.8 ☑
　blunt object X79 ☑
　burning, burns X76 ☑
　　hot object X77.9 ☑
　　　fluid NEC X77.2 ☑
　　　household appliance X77.3 ☑
　　　specified NEC X77.8 ☑
　　　steam X77.0 ☑
　　　tap water X77.1 ☑
　　　vapors X77.0 ☑
　caustic substance — *see* Table of Drugs and Chemicals
　cold, extreme X83.2 ☑
　collision of motor vehicle with
　　motor vehicle X82.0 ☑
　　specified NEC X82.8 ☑
　　train X82.1 ☑

Suicide, suicidal — *continued*
　collision of motor vehicle with — *continued*
　　tree X82.2 ☑
　crashing of aircraft X83.0 ☑
　cut (any part of body) X78.9 ☑
　cutting or piercing instrument X78.9 ☑
　　dagger X78.2 ☑
　　glass X78.0 ☑
　　knife X78.1 ☑
　　specified NEC X78.8 ☑
　　sword X78.2 ☑
　drowning (in) X71.9 ☑
　　bathtub X71.0 ☑
　　natural water X71.3 ☑
　　specified NEC X71.8 ☑
　　swimming pool X71.1 ☑
　　　following fall X71.2 ☑
　electrocution X83.1 ☑
　explosive(s) (material) X75 ☑
　fire, flames X76 ☑
　firearm X74.9 ☑
　　airgun X74.01 ☑
　　handgun X72 ☑
　　hunting rifle X73.1 ☑
　　larger X73.9 ☑
　　　specified NEC X73.8 ☑
　　machine gun X73.2 ☑
　　shotgun X73.0 ☑
　　specified NEC X74.8 ☑
　hanging X83.8 ☑
　hot object — *see* Suicide, burning, hot object
　jumping
　　before moving object X81.8 ☑
　　　motor vehicle X81.0 ☑
　　　subway train X81.1 ☑
　　　train X81.1 ☑
　　from high place X80 ☑
　late effect of attempt — *see* X71-X83 with 7th character S
　lying before moving object, train, vehicle X81.8 ☑
　poisoning — *see* Table of Drugs and Chemicals
　puncture (any part of body) — *see* Suicide, cutting or piercing instrument
　scald — *see* Suicide, burning, hot object
　sequelae of attempt — *see* X71-X83 with 7th character S
　sharp object (any) — *see* Suicide, cutting or piercing instrument
　shooting — *see* Suicide, firearm
　specified means NEC X83.8 ☑
　stab (any part of body) — *see* Suicide, cutting or piercing instrument
　steam, hot vapors X77.0 ☑
　strangulation X83.8 ☑
　submersion — *see* Suicide, drowning
　suffocation X83.8 ☑
　wound NEC X83.8 ☑
Sunstroke X32 ☑
Supersonic waves (causing injury) W42.0 ☑
Surgical procedure, complication of (delayed or as an abnormal reaction without mention of misadventure) (*see also* Complication of or following, by type of procedure)
　due to or as a result of misadventure — *see* Misadventure
Swallowed, swallowing
　foreign body — *see* Foreign body, alimentary canal
　poison — *see* Table of Drugs and Chemicals
　substance
　　caustic or corrosive — *see* Table of Drugs and Chemicals
　　poisonous — *see* Table of Drugs and Chemicals

T

Tackle in sport W03 ☑
Terrorism (involving) Y38.80 ☑
　biological weapons Y38.6X- ☑
　chemical weapons Y38.7X- ☑
　conflagration Y38.3X- ☑
　drowning and submersion Y38.89- ☑
　explosion Y38.2X- ☑
　　destruction of aircraft Y38.1X- ☑
　　marine weapons Y38.0X- ☑
　fire Y38.3X- ☑
　firearms Y38.4X- ☑

Terrorism — *continued*
  hot substances Y38.3X- ☑
  lasers Y38.89- ☑
  nuclear weapons Y38.5X- ☑
  piercing or stabbing instruments Y38.89- ☑
  secondary effects Y38.9X- ☑
  specified method NEC Y38.89- ☑
  suicide bomber Y38.81- ☑
Thirst X58 ☑
Threat to breathing
  aspiration — *see* Aspiration
  due to cave-in, falling earth or substance NEC T71 ☑
Thrown (accidentally)
  against part (any) of or object in transport vehicle (in motion) NEC (*see also* Accident, transport)
  from
    high place, homicide (attempt) Y01 ☑
    machinery — *see* Contact, with, by type of machine
    transport vehicle NEC (*see also* Accident, transport) V89.9 ☑
  off — *see* Thrown, from
Thunderbolt — *see* subcategory T75.0 ☑
  causing fire — *see* Exposure, fire
Tidal wave (any injury) **NEC** — *see* Forces of nature, tidal wave
Took
  overdose (drug) — *see* Table of Drugs and Chemicals
  poison — *see* Table of Drugs and Chemicals
Tornado (any injury) X37.1 ☑
Torrential rain (any injury) X37.8 ☑
Torture X58 ☑
Trampled by animal NEC W55.89 ☑
Trapped (accidentally)
  between objects (moving) (stationary and moving) — *see* Caught
  by part (any) of
    motorcycle V29.88 ☑
    pedal cycle V19.88 ☑
    transport vehicle NEC (*see also* Accident, transport) V89.9 ☑
Travel (effects) (sickness) T75.3 ☑
Tree falling on or hitting (accidentally) (person) W20.8 ☑
Tripping
  without fall W18.40 ☑
    due to
      specified NEC W18.49 ☑
      stepping from one level to another W18.43 ☑
      stepping into hole or opening W18.42 ☑
      stepping on object W18.41 ☑
    over
      animal W01.0 ☑
        with fall W01.0 ☑
      carpet, rug or (small) object W22.8 ☑
        with fall W18.09 ☑
      person W51 ☑
        with fall W03 ☑
          due to ice or snow W00.0 ☑
Twisted by person(s) (accidentally) W50.2 ☑
  with intent to injure or kill Y04.0 ☑
  as, or caused by, a crowd or human stampede (with fall) W52 ☑
  assault Y04.0 ☑
  homicide (attempt) Y04.0 ☑
  in
    fight Y04.0 ☑
    legal intervention — *see* Legal, intervention, manhandling
Twisting (prolonged) (static) X50.1- ☑

U

Underdosing of necessary drugs, medicaments or biological substances Y63.6
Undetermined intent (contact) (exposure)
  automobile collision Y32 ☑
  blunt object Y29 ☑
  drowning (submersion) (in) Y21.9 ☑
    bathtub Y21.0 ☑
      after fall Y21.1 ☑
    natural water (lake) (ocean) (pond) (river) (stream) Y21.4 ☑
    specified place NEC Y21.8 ☑
    swimming pool Y21.2 ☑
      after fall Y21.3 ☑
  explosive material Y25 ☑

Undetermined intent — *continued*
  fall, jump or push from high place Y30 ☑
  falling, lying or running before moving object Y31 ☑
  fire Y26 ☑
  firearm discharge Y24.9 ☑
    airgun (BB) (pellet) Y24.0 ☑
    handgun (pistol) (revolver) Y22 ☑
    hunting rifle Y23.1 ☑
    larger Y23.9 ☑
      hunting rifle Y23.1 ☑
      machine gun Y23.3 ☑
      military Y23.2 ☑
      shotgun Y23.0 ☑
      specified type NEC Y23.8 ☑
    machine gun Y23.3 ☑
    military Y23.2 ☑
    shotgun Y23.0 ☑
    specified type NEC Y24.8 ☑
    Very pistol Y24.8 ☑
  hot object Y27.9 ☑
    fluid NEC Y27.2 ☑
    household appliance Y27.3 ☑
    specified object NEC Y27.8 ☑
    steam Y27.0 ☑
    tap water Y27.1 ☑
    vapor Y27.0 ☑
  jump, fall or push from high place Y30 ☑
  lying, falling or running before moving object Y31 ☑
  motor vehicle crash Y32 ☑
  push, fall or jump from high place Y30 ☑
  running, falling or lying before moving object Y31 ☑
  sharp object Y28.9 ☑
    dagger Y28.2 ☑
    glass Y28.0 ☑
    knife Y28.1 ☑
    specified object NEC Y28.8 ☑
    sword Y28.2 ☑
  smoke Y26 ☑
  specified event NEC Y33 ☑
Use of hand as hammer X50.3 ☑

V

Vibration (causing injury) W49.9 ☑
Victim (of)
  avalanche — *see* Landslide
  earth movements NEC — *see* Forces of nature, earth movement
  earthquake X34 ☑
  flood — *see* Flood
  landslide — *see* Landslide
  lightning — *see* subcategory T75.0 ☑
    causing fire — *see* Exposure, fire
  storm (cataclysmic) NEC — *see* Forces of nature, cataclysmic storm
  volcanic eruption X35 ☑
Volcanic eruption (any injury) X35 ☑
Vomitus, gastric contents in air passages (with asphyxia, obstruction or suffocation) T17.81- ☑

W

Walked into stationary object (any) W22.09 ☑
  furniture W22.03 ☑
  lamppost W22.02 ☑
  wall W22.01 ☑
War operations (injuries to military personnel and civilians during war, civil insurrection and peacekeeping missions) (by) (from) (involving) Y36.90 ☑
  after cessation of hostilities Y36.89- ☑
    explosion (of)
      bomb placed during war operations Y36.82- ☑
      mine placed during war operations Y36.81- ☑
      specified NEC Y36.88- ☑
  air blast Y36.20- ☑
  aircraft
    destruction — *see* War operations, destruction of aircraft
    airway restriction — *see* War operations, restriction of airways
    asphyxiation — *see* War operations, restriction of airways
  biological weapons Y36.6X- ☑
  blast Y36.20- ☑
  blast fragments Y36.20- ☑
  blast wave Y36.20- ☑

War operations — *continued*
  blast wind Y36.20- ☑
  bomb Y36.20- ☑
    dirty Y36.50- ☑
    gasoline Y36.31- ☑
    incendiary Y36.31- ☑
    petrol Y36.31- ☑
  bullet Y36.43- ☑
    incendiary Y36.32- ☑
    rubber Y36.41- ☑
  chemical weapons Y36.7X- ☑
  combat
    hand to hand (unarmed) combat Y36.44- ☑
    using blunt or piercing object Y36.45- ☑
  conflagration — *see* War operations, fire
  conventional warfare NEC Y36.49- ☑
  depth-charge Y36.01- ☑
  destruction of aircraft Y36.10- ☑
    due to
      air to air missile Y36.11- ☑
      collision with other aircraft Y36.12- ☑
      detonation (accidental) of onboard munitions and explosives Y36.14- ☑
      enemy fire or explosives Y36.11- ☑
      explosive placed on aircraft Y36.11- ☑
      onboard fire Y36.13- ☑
      rocket propelled grenade [RPG] Y36.11- ☑
      small arms fire Y36.11- ☑
      surface to air missile Y36.11- ☑
    specified NEC Y36.19- ☑
  detonation (accidental) of
    onboard marine weapons Y36.05- ☑
    own munitions or munitions launch device Y36.24- ☑
  dirty bomb Y36.50- ☑
  explosion (of) Y36.20- ☑
    aerial bomb Y36.21- ☑
    after cessation of hostilities
      bomb placed during war operations Y36.82- ☑
      mine placed during war operations Y36.81- ☑
    bomb NOS (*see also* War operations, bomb(s)) Y36.20- ☑
    fragments Y36.20- ☑
    grenade Y36.29- ☑
    guided missile Y36.22- ☑
    improvised explosive device [IED] (person-borne) (roadside) (vehicle-borne) Y36.23- ☑
    land mine Y36.29- ☑
    marine mine (at sea) (in harbor) Y36.02- ☑
    marine weapon Y36.00- ☑
      specified NEC Y36.09- ☑
    own munitions or munitions launch device (accidental) Y36.24- ☑
    sea-based artillery shell Y36.03- ☑
    specified NEC Y36.29- ☑
    torpedo Y36.04- ☑
  fire Y36.30- ☑
    specified NEC Y36.39- ☑
  firearms
    discharge Y36.43- ☑
    pellets Y36.42- ☑
  flamethrower Y36.33- ☑
  fragments (from) (of)
    improvised explosive device [IED] (person-borne) (roadside) (vehicle-borne) Y36.26- ☑
    munitions Y36.25- ☑
    specified NEC Y36.29- ☑
    weapons Y36.27- ☑
  friendly fire Y36.92 ☑
  hand to hand (unarmed) combat Y36.44- ☑
  hot substances — *see* War operations, fire
  incendiary bullet Y36.32- ☑
  nuclear weapon (effects of) Y36.50- ☑
    acute radiation exposure Y36.54- ☑
    blast pressure Y36.51- ☑
    direct blast Y36.51- ☑
    direct heat Y36.53- ☑
    fallout exposure Y36.54- ☑
    fireball Y36.53- ☑
    indirect blast (struck or crushed by blast debris) (being thrown by blast) Y36.52- ☑
    ionizing radiation (immediate exposure) Y36.54- ☑
    nuclear radiation Y36.54- ☑
    radiation
      ionizing (immediate exposure) Y36.54- ☑
      nuclear Y36.54- ☑

☑ Additional Character Required — Refer to the Tabular List for Character Selection   ⬚ Subterms under main terms may continue to next column or page

War operations — *continued*
  nuclear weapon — *continued*
    radiation — *continued*
      thermal Y36.53- ☑
    secondary effects Y36.54- ☑
    specified NEC Y36.59- ☑
    thermal radiation Y36.53- ☑
  restriction of air (airway)
    intentional Y36.46- ☑
    unintentional Y36.47- ☑
  rubber bullets Y36.41- ☑
  shrapnel NOS Y36.29- ☑
  suffocation — *see* War operations, restriction of airways
  unconventional warfare NEC Y36.7X- ☑
  underwater blast NOS Y36.00- ☑
  warfare
    conventional NEC Y36.49- ☑
    unconventional NEC Y36.7X- ☑

War operations — *continued*
  weapon of mass destruction [WMD] Y36.91 ☑
  weapons
    biological weapons Y36.6X- ☑
    chemical Y36.7X- ☑
    nuclear (effects of) Y36.50- ☑
      acute radiation exposure Y36.54- ☑
      blast pressure Y36.51- ☑
      direct blast Y36.51- ☑
      direct heat Y36.53- ☑
      fallout exposure Y36.54- ☑
      fireball Y36.53- ☑
      radiation
        ionizing (immediate exposure) Y36.54- ☑
        nuclear Y36.54- ☑
        thermal Y36.53- ☑
      secondary effects Y36.54- ☑
      specified NEC Y36.59- ☑
  of mass destruction [WMD] Y36.91 ☑

Washed
  away by flood — *see* Flood
  off road by storm (transport vehicle) — *see* Forces of nature, cataclysmic storm
Weather exposure NEC — *see* Forces of nature
Weightlessness (causing injury) (effects of) (in spacecraft, real or simulated) X52 ☑
Work related condition Y99.0
Wound (accidental) NEC (*see also* Injury) X58 ☑
  battle (*see also* War operations) Y36.90 ☑
  gunshot — *see* Discharge, firearm by type
Wreck transport vehicle NEC (*see also* Accident, transport) V89.9 ☑
Wrong
  device implanted into correct surgical site Y65.51
  fluid in infusion Y65.1
  patient, procedure performed on Y65.52
  procedure (operation) on correct patient Y65.51

Chapter 1. Certain Infectious and Parasitic Diseases (AØØ–B99)

Chapter Specific Guidelines with Coding Examples

The chapter specific guidelines from the ICD-10-CM Official Guidelines for Coding and Reporting have been provided below. Along with these guidelines are coding examples, contained in the shaded boxes, that have been developed to help illustrate the coding and/or sequencing guidance found in these guidelines.

a. Human immunodeficiency virus (HIV) infections

1) Code only confirmed cases

Code only confirmed cases of HIV infection/illness. This is an exception to the hospital inpatient guideline Section II, H.

In this context, "confirmation" does not require documentation of positive serology or culture for HIV; the provider's diagnostic statement that the patient is HIV positive, or has an HIV-related illness is sufficient.

> Patient admitted with anemia with possible HIV infection
>
> **D64.9   Anemia, unspecified**
>
> *Explanation:* Only the anemia is coded in this scenario because it has not been confirmed that an HIV infection is present. This is an exception to the guideline Section II, H for hospital inpatient coding.

2) Selection and sequencing of HIV codes

(a) Patient admitted for HIV-related condition

If a patient is admitted for an HIV-related condition, the principal diagnosis should be B2Ø, Human immunodeficiency virus [HIV] disease followed by additional diagnosis codes for all reported HIV-related conditions.

> HIV with PCP
>
> **B2Ø   Human immunodeficiency virus [HIV] disease**
>
> **B59   Pneumocystosis**
>
> *Explanation:* Pneumonia due to *Pneumocystis carinii* is an HIV related condition, so the HIV diagnosis code is reported first, followed by the code for the pneumonia.

(b) Patient with HIV disease admitted for unrelated condition

If a patient with HIV disease is admitted for an unrelated condition (such as a traumatic injury), the code for the unrelated condition (e.g., the nature of injury code) should be the principal diagnosis. Other diagnoses would be B2Ø followed by additional diagnosis codes for all reported HIV-related conditions.

> Unstable angina, native coronary artery atherosclerosis, HIV
>
> **I25.11Ø   Atherosclerotic heart disease of native coronary artery with unstable angina pectoris**
>
> **B2Ø   Human immunodeficiency virus [HIV] disease**
>
> *Explanation:* The arteriosclerotic coronary artery disease and the unstable angina are not related to HIV, so those conditions are reported first using a combination code, and HIV is reported secondarily.

(c) Whether the patient is newly diagnosed

Whether the patient is newly diagnosed or has had previous admissions/encounters for HIV conditions is irrelevant to the sequencing decision.

> Newly diagnosed multiple cutaneous Kaposi's sarcoma lesions in previously diagnosed HIV disease
>
> **B2Ø   Human immunodeficiency virus [HIV] disease**
>
> **C46.Ø   Kaposi's sarcoma of skin**
>
> *Explanation:* Even though the HIV was diagnosed on a previous encounter, it is still sequenced first when coded with an HIV related condition. Kaposi's sarcoma is an HIV-related condition.

(d) Asymptomatic human immunodeficiency virus

Z21, Asymptomatic human immunodeficiency virus [HIV] infection status, is to be applied when the patient without any documentation of symptoms is listed as being "HIV positive," "known HIV," "HIV test positive," or similar terminology. Do not use this code if the term "AIDS" is used or if the patient is treated for any HIV-related illness or is described as having any condition(s) resulting from his/her HIV positive status; use B2Ø in these cases.

> Patient admitted with acute appendicitis. Status positive HIV test on Atripla, with no prior symptoms
>
> **K35.8Ø   Unspecified acute appendicitis**
>
> **Z21   Asymptomatic human immunodeficiency virus [HIV] infection status**
>
> *Explanation:* Code Z21 is sequenced second since documentation indicates that the patient has had a positive HIV test but has been asymptomatic. Being on medication for HIV is not an indication that code B2Ø is used instead of Z21. Unless there has been documentation that the patient has had current or prior symptoms or HIV-related complications, code B2Ø is not used. The appendicitis is not an AIDS-related complication and is sequenced first.

(e) Patients with inconclusive HIV serology

Patients with inconclusive HIV serology, but no definitive diagnosis or manifestations of the illness, may be assigned code R75, Inconclusive laboratory evidence of human immunodeficiency virus [HIV].

(f) Previously diagnosed HIV-related illness

Patients with any known prior diagnosis of an HIV-related illness should be coded to B2Ø. Once a patient has developed an HIV-related illness, the patient should always be assigned code B2Ø on every subsequent admission/encounter. Patients previously diagnosed with any HIV illness (B2Ø) should never be assigned to R75 or Z21, Asymptomatic human immunodeficiency virus [HIV] infection status.

(g) HIV infection in pregnancy, childbirth and the puerperium

During pregnancy, childbirth or the puerperium, a patient admitted (or presenting for a health care encounter) because of an HIV-related illness should receive a principal diagnosis code of O98.7-, Human immunodeficiency [HIV] disease complicating pregnancy, childbirth and the puerperium, followed by B2Ø and the code(s) for the HIV-related illness(es). Codes from Chapter 15 always take sequencing priority.

Patients with asymptomatic HIV infection status admitted (or presenting for a health care encounter) during pregnancy, childbirth, or the puerperium should receive codes of O98.7- and Z21.

(h) Encounters for testing for HIV

If a patient is being seen to determine his/her HIV status, use code Z11.4, Encounter for screening for human immunodeficiency virus [HIV]. Use additional codes for any associated high risk behavior.

If a patient with signs or symptoms is being seen for HIV testing, code the signs and symptoms. An additional counseling code Z71.7, Human immunodeficiency virus [HIV] counseling, may be used if counseling is provided during the encounter for the test.

When a patient returns to be informed of his/her HIV test results and the test result is negative, use code Z71.7, Human immunodeficiency virus [HIV] counseling.

If the results are positive, see previous guidelines and assign codes as appropriate.

b. Infectious agents as the cause of diseases classified to other chapters

Certain infections are classified in chapters other than Chapter 1 and no organism is identified as part of the infection code. In these instances, it is necessary to use an additional code from Chapter 1 to identify the organism. A code from category B95, Streptococcus, Staphylococcus, and Enterococcus as the cause of diseases classified to other chapters, B96, Other bacterial agents as the cause of diseases classified to other chapters, or B97, Viral agents as the cause of diseases classified to other chapters, is to be used as an additional code to identify the organism. An instructional note will be found at the infection code advising that an additional organism code is required.

E. coli UTI

| N39.Ø | Urinary tract infection, site not specified |
| B96.2Ø | Unspecified Escherichia coli [E.coli] as the cause of diseases classified elsewhere |

Explanation: An instructional note under the code for the urinary tract infection indicates to code also the specific organism.

c. Infections resistant to antibiotics

Many bacterial infections are resistant to current antibiotics. It is necessary to identify all infections documented as antibiotic resistant. Assign a code from category Z16, Resistance to antimicrobial drugs, following the infection code only if the infection code does not identify drug resistance.

d. Sepsis, severe sepsis, and septic shock

1) Coding of sepsis and severe sepsis

(a) Sepsis

For a diagnosis of sepsis, assign the appropriate code for the underlying systemic infection. If the type of infection or causal organism is not further specified, assign code A41.9, Sepsis, unspecified organism.

A code from subcategory R65.2, Severe sepsis, should not be assigned unless severe sepsis or an associated acute organ dysfunction is documented.

Gram-negative sepsis

| A41.5Ø | Gram-negative sepsis, unspecified |

Staphylococcal sepsis

| A41.2 | Sepsis due to unspecified staphylococcus |

Explanation: In both examples above the organism causing the sepsis is identified, therefore A41.9 Sepsis, unspecified organism, would not be appropriate as this code would not capture the highest degree of specificity found in the documentation. Do not use an additional code for severe sepsis unless an acute organ dysfunction was also documented as "associated with" or "due to" the sepsis or the sepsis was documented as "severe."

(i) Negative or inconclusive blood cultures and sepsis

Negative or inconclusive blood cultures do not preclude a diagnosis of sepsis in patients with clinical evidence of the condition; however, the provider should be queried.

(ii) Urosepsis

The term urosepsis is a nonspecific term. It is not to be considered synonymous with sepsis. It has no default code in the Alphabetic Index. Should a provider use this term, he/she must be queried for clarification.

(iii) Sepsis with organ dysfunction

If a patient has sepsis and associated acute organ dysfunction or multiple organ dysfunction (MOD), follow the instructions for coding severe sepsis.

(iv) Acute organ dysfunction that is not clearly associated with the sepsis

If a patient has sepsis and an acute organ dysfunction, but the medical record documentation indicates that the acute organ dysfunction is related to a medical condition other than the sepsis, do not assign a code from subcategory R65.2, Severe sepsis. An acute organ dysfunction must be associated with the sepsis in order to assign the severe sepsis code. If the documentation is not clear as to whether an acute organ dysfunction is related to the sepsis or another medical condition, query the provider.

Sepsis and acute respiratory failure due to COPD exacerbation

A41.9	Sepsis, unspecified organism
J44.1	Chronic obstructive pulmonary disease with (acute) exacerbation
J96.ØØ	Acute respiratory failure, unspecified whether with hypoxia or hypercapnia

Explanation: Although acute organ dysfunction is present in the form of acute respiratory failure, severe sepsis (R65.2) is not coded in this example, as the acute respiratory failure is attributed to the COPD exacerbation rather than the sepsis. Sequencing of these codes would be determined by the circumstances of the admission.

(b) Severe sepsis

The coding of severe sepsis requires a minimum of 2 codes: first a code for the underlying systemic infection, followed by a code from subcategory R65.2, Severe sepsis. If the causal organism is not documented, assign code A41.9, Sepsis, unspecified organism, for the infection. Additional code(s) for the associated acute organ dysfunction are also required.

Due to the complex nature of severe sepsis, some cases may require querying the provider prior to assignment of the codes.

2) Septic shock

(a) Septic shock generally refers to circulatory failure associated with severe sepsis, and therefore, it represents a type of acute organ dysfunction.

For cases of septic shock, the code for the systemic infection should be sequenced first, followed by code R65.21, Severe sepsis with septic shock or code T81.12, Postprocedural septic shock. Any additional codes for the other acute organ dysfunctions should also be assigned. As noted in the sequencing instructions in the Tabular List, the code for septic shock cannot be assigned as a principal diagnosis.

Sepsis with septic shock

| A41.9 | Sepsis, unspecified organism |
| R65.21 | Severe sepsis with septic shock |

Explanation: Documentation of septic shock automatically implies severe sepsis as it is a form of acute organ dysfunction. Septic shock is not coded as the principal diagnosis; it is always preceded by the code for the systemic infection.

3) Sequencing of severe sepsis

If severe sepsis is present on admission, and meets the definition of principal diagnosis, the underlying systemic infection should be assigned as principal diagnosis followed by the appropriate code from subcategory R65.2 as required by the sequencing rules in the Tabular List. A code from subcategory R65.2 can never be assigned as a principal diagnosis.

When severe sepsis develops during an encounter (it was not present on admission), the underlying systemic infection and the appropriate code from subcategory R65.2 should be assigned as secondary diagnoses.

Severe sepsis may be present on admission, but the diagnosis may not be confirmed until sometime after admission. If the documentation is not clear whether severe sepsis was present on admission, the provider should be queried.

4) Sepsis and severe sepsis with a localized infection

If the reason for admission is both sepsis or severe sepsis and a localized infection, such as pneumonia or cellulitis, a code(s) for the underlying systemic infection should be assigned first and the code for the localized infection should be assigned as a secondary diagnosis. If the patient has severe sepsis, a code from subcategory R65.2 should also be assigned as a secondary diagnosis. If the patient is admitted with a localized infection, such as pneumonia, and sepsis/severe sepsis doesn't develop until after admission, the localized infection should be assigned first, followed by the appropriate sepsis/severe sepsis codes.

Patient presents with acute renal failure due to severe sepsis from *Pseudomonas pneumonia*

A41.9	Sepsis, unspecified organism
J15.1	Pneumonia due to Pseudomonas
R65.2Ø	Severe sepsis without septic shock
N17.9	Acute kidney failure, unspecified

Explanation: If all conditions are present on admission, the systemic infection (sepsis) is sequenced first followed by the codes for the localized infection (pneumonia), severe sepsis and any organ dysfunction. If only the pneumonia was present on admission with the sepsis and resulting renal failure developing later in the admission, then the pneumonia would be sequenced first.

5) Sepsis due to a postprocedural infection

(a) Documentation of causal relationship

As with all postprocedural complications, code assignment is based on the provider's documentation of the relationship between the infection and the procedure.

(b) Sepsis due to a postprocedural infection

For such cases, the postprocedural infection code, such as T80.2, Infections following infusion, transfusion, and therapeutic injection, T81.4, Infection following a procedure, T88.Ø, Infection following immunization, or O86.Ø, Infection of obstetric surgical wound, should be coded first, followed by the code for the specific infection. If the patient has severe sepsis, the appropriate code from subcategory R65.2 should also be assigned with the additional code(s) for any acute organ dysfunction.

(c) Postprocedural infection and postprocedural septic shock

In cases where a postprocedural infection has occurred and has resulted in severe sepsis the code for the precipitating complication such as code T81.4, Infection following a procedure, or O86.0, Infection of obstetrical surgical wound should be coded first followed by code R65.20, Severe sepsis without septic shock. A code for the systemic infection should also be assigned.

If a postprocedural infection has resulted in postprocedural septic shock, the code for the precipitating complication such as code T81.4, Infection following a procedure, or O86.0, Infection of obstetrical surgical wound should be coded first followed by code T81.12-, Postprocedural septic shock. A code for the systemic infection should also be assigned.

6) Sepsis and severe sepsis associated with a noninfectious process (condition)

In some cases a noninfectious process (condition), such as trauma, may lead to an infection which can result in sepsis or severe sepsis. If sepsis or severe sepsis is documented as associated with a noninfectious condition, such as a burn or serious injury, and this condition meets the definition for principal diagnosis, the code for the noninfectious condition should be sequenced first, followed by the code for the resulting infection. If severe sepsis is present, a code from subcategory R65.2 should also be assigned with any associated organ dysfunction(s) codes. It is not necessary to assign a code from subcategory R65.1, Systemic inflammatory response syndrome (SIRS) of non-infectious origin, for these cases.

If the infection meets the definition of principal diagnosis, it should be sequenced before the non-infectious condition. When both the associated non-infectious condition and the infection meet the definition of principal diagnosis, either may be assigned as principal diagnosis.

Only one code from category R65, Symptoms and signs specifically associated with systemic inflammation and infection, should be assigned. Therefore, when a non-infectious condition leads to an infection resulting in severe sepsis, assign the appropriate code from subcategory R65.2, Severe sepsis. Do not additionally assign a code from subcategory R65.1, Systemic inflammatory response syndrome (SIRS) of non-infectious origin.

See Section I.C.18. SIRS due to non-infectious process

> Patient admitted with multiple third-degree burns of right upper arm develops severe MSSA sepsis with septic shock, three days into admission
>
> **T22.391A**   **Burn of third degree of multiple sites of right shoulder and upper arm limb, except wrist and hand, initial encounter**
>
> **A41.01**   **Sepsis due to Methicillin susceptible Staphylococcus aureus**
>
> **R65.21**   **Severe sepsis with septic shock**
>
> *Explanation:* Severe sepsis is coded rather than SIRS from R65 because it is documented as a severe systemic infectious response with septic shock to a noninfectious condition. The code for the systemic infection is not used as the principal diagnosis because it was not present on admission. The patient was admitted for the burn injury.

7) Sepsis and septic shock complicating abortion, pregnancy, childbirth, and the puerperium

See Section I.C.15. Sepsis and septic shock complicating abortion, pregnancy, childbirth and the puerperium

8) Newborn sepsis

See Section I.C.16. f. Bacterial sepsis of Newborn

e. Methicillin resistant Staphylococcus aureus (MRSA) conditions

1) Selection and sequencing of MRSA codes

(a) Combination codes for MRSA infection

When a patient is diagnosed with an infection that is due to methicillin resistant *Staphylococcus aureus* (MRSA), and that infection has a combination code that includes the causal organism (e.g., sepsis, pneumonia) assign the appropriate combination code for the condition (e.g., code A41.02, Sepsis due to Methicillin resistant Staphylococcus aureus or code J15.212, Pneumonia due to Methicillin resistant Staphylococcus aureus). Do not assign code B95.62, Methicillin resistant Staphylococcus aureus infection as the cause of diseases classified elsewhere, as an additional code, because the

combination code includes the type of infection and the MRSA organism. Do not assign a code from subcategory Z16.11, Resistance to penicillins, as an additional diagnosis.

See Section C.1. for instructions on coding and sequencing of sepsis and severe sepsis.

(b) Other codes for MRSA infection

When there is documentation of a current infection (e.g., wound infection, stitch abscess, urinary tract infection) due to MRSA, and that infection does not have a combination code that includes the causal organism, assign the appropriate code to identify the condition along with code B95.62, Methicillin resistant Staphylococcus aureus infection as the cause of diseases classified elsewhere for the MRSA infection. Do not assign a code from subcategory Z16.11, Resistance to penicillins.

(c) Methicillin susceptible Staphylococcus aureus (MSSA) and MRSA colonization

The condition or state of being colonized or carrying MSSA or MRSA is called colonization or carriage, while an individual person is described as being colonized or being a carrier. Colonization means that MSSA or MSRA is present on or in the body without necessarily causing illness. A positive MRSA colonization test might be documented by the provider as "MRSA screen positive" or "MRSA nasal swab positive".

Assign code Z22.322, Carrier or suspected carrier of Methicillin resistant Staphylococcus aureus, for patients documented as having MRSA colonization. Assign code Z22.321, Carrier or suspected carrier of Methicillin susceptible Staphylococcus aureus, for patient documented as having MSSA colonization. Colonization is not necessarily indicative of a disease process or as the cause of a specific condition the patient may have unless documented as such by the provider.

(d) MRSA colonization and infection

If a patient is documented as having both MRSA colonization and infection during a hospital admission, code Z22.322, Carrier or suspected carrier of Methicillin resistant Staphylococcus aureus, and a code for the MRSA infection may both be assigned.

f. Zika virus infections

1) Code only confirmed cases

Code only a confirmed diagnosis of Zika virus (A92.5, Zika virus disease) as documented by the provider. This is an exception to the hospital inpatient guideline Section II, H. In this context, "confirmation" does not require documentation of the type of test performed; the physician's diagnostic statement that the condition is confirmed is sufficient. This code should be assigned regardless of the stated mode of transmission.

If the provider documents "suspected", "possible" or "probable" Zika, do not assign code A92.5. Assign a code(s) explaining the reason for encounter (such as fever, rash, or joint pain) or Z20.828, Contact with and (suspected) exposure to other viral communicable diseases.

> A 45-year-old female recently returned from a Caribbean vacation complaining of fever, headache, joint and muscle aches and is admitted for suspected influenza. Infectious Disease consult diagnoses Zika virus. Patient discharged with Zika virus disease and instructions for hydration, rest, acetaminophen, and follow-up with Infectious Disease.
>
> **A92.5**   **Zika virus disease**
>
> *Explanation:* Although only a confirmed diagnosis should be coded, when a provider documents a diagnosis of Zika virus, code A92.5 Zika virus disease, is reported whether or not there is any indication of the type of tests performed. If the patient is pregnant, code first a code from category O98.5- Other viral diseases complicating pregnancy, childbirth and the puerperium, followed by code (A92.5) for the confirmed Zika virus. See also guideline 1.C.15.a.1.

Chapter 1. Certain Infectious and Parasitic Diseases (A00-B99)

INCLUDES diseases generally recognized as communicable or transmissible
Use additional code to identify resistance to antimicrobial drugs (Z16.-)
EXCLUDES 1 certain localized infections—see body system-related chapters
EXCLUDES 2 carrier or suspected carrier of infectious disease (Z22.-)
infectious and parasitic diseases complicating pregnancy, childbirth and the puerperium (O98.-)
infectious and parasitic diseases specific to the perinatal period (P35-P39)
influenza and other acute respiratory infections (J00-J22)

This chapter contains the following blocks:

A00-A09   Intestinal infectious diseases
A15-A19   Tuberculosis
A20-A28   Certain zoonotic bacterial diseases
A30-A49   Other bacterial diseases
A50-A64   Infections with a predominantly sexual mode of transmission
A65-A69   Other spirochetal diseases
A70-A74   Other diseases caused by chlamydiae
A75-A79   Rickettsioses
A80-A89   Viral infections of the central nervous system
A90-A99   Arthropod-borne viral fevers and viral hemorrhagic fevers
B00-B09   Viral infections characterized by skin and mucous membrane lesions
B10   Other human herpesviruses
B15-B19   Viral hepatitis
B20   Human immunodeficiency virus [HIV] disease
B25-B34   Other viral diseases
B35-B49   Mycoses
B50-B64   Protozoal diseases
B65-B83   Helminthiases
B85-B89   Pediculosis, acariasis and other infestations
B90-B94   Sequelae of infectious and parasitic diseases
B95-B97   Bacterial and viral infectious agents
B99   Other infectious diseases

Intestinal Infectious Diseases (A00-A09)

✓4ᵗʰ A00   Cholera

> **CC Excl: For CC codes in category A00:** PDX collection 2

A00.0   Cholera due to Vibrio cholerae 01, biovar cholerae   `CC`
Classical cholera

A00.1   Cholera due to Vibrio cholerae 01, biovar eltor   `CC`
Cholera eltor

A00.9   Cholera, unspecified   `CC`

✓4ᵗʰ A01   Typhoid and paratyphoid fevers
DEF: Typhoid fever: An acute generalized illness caused by *Salmonella typhi;* clinical features are fever, headache, abdominal pain, cough, toxemia, leukopenia, abnormal pulse, rose spots on the skin, bacteremia, hyperplasia of intestinal lymph nodes, mesenteric lymphadenopathy, and Peyer's patches in the intestines.
DEF: Paratyphoid fever: A prolonged febrile illness, caused by *Salmonella* serotypes other than *S. typhi*, especially *S. enterica* serotypes paratyphi A, B, and C.

> **CC Excl: For CC codes in category A01:** PDX collection 3

✓5ᵗʰ A01.0   Typhoid fever
Infection due to Salmonella typhi

A01.00   Typhoid fever, unspecified   `CC`
A01.01   Typhoid meningitis   `CC`
A01.02   Typhoid fever with heart involvement   `CC`
Typhoid endocarditis   Typhoid myocarditis
A01.03   Typhoid pneumonia   `CC` `HCC`
A01.04   Typhoid arthritis   `CC` `HCC`
A01.05   Typhoid osteomyelitis   `CC` `HCC`
A01.09   Typhoid fever with other complications   `CC`
A01.1   Paratyphoid fever A   `CC`
A01.2   Paratyphoid fever B   `CC`
A01.3   Paratyphoid fever C   `CC`
A01.4   Paratyphoid fever, unspecified   `CC`
Infection due to Salmonella paratyphi NOS

✓4ᵗʰ A02   Other salmonella infections
INCLUDES infection or foodborne intoxication due to any Salmonella species other than S. typhi and S. paratyphi

A02.0   Salmonella enteritis   `CC`
Salmonellosis
CC Excl: PDX collection 4

A02.1   Salmonella sepsis   `HIV` `MCC` `HCC`
CC Excl: PDX collection 5

✓5ᵗʰ A02.2   Localized salmonella infections
A02.20   Localized salmonella infection, unspecified   `HIV`
A02.21   Salmonella meningitis   `HIV` `MCC`
CC Excl: PDX collection 6
A02.22   Salmonella pneumonia   `HIV` `MCC` `HCC`
CC Excl: PDX collection 7
A02.23   Salmonella arthritis   `HIV` `CC` `HCC`
CC Excl: PDX collection 8
A02.24   Salmonella osteomyelitis   `HIV` `CC` `HCC`
CC Excl: PDX collection 9
A02.25   Salmonella pyelonephritis   `HIV` `CC`
Salmonella tubulo-interstitial nephropathy
CC Excl: PDX collection 10
A02.29   Salmonella with other localized infection   `HIV` `CC`
CC Excl: PDX collection 10

A02.8   Other specified salmonella infections   `HIV` `CC`
CC Excl: PDX collection 11

A02.9   Salmonella infection, unspecified   `HIV` `CC`
CC Excl: PDX collection 12

✓4ᵗʰ A03   Shigellosis
DEF: Infection caused by the genus *Shigella*, of the family *Enterobacteriaceae*; known to cause an acute dysenteric infection of the bowel with fever, drowsiness, anorexia, nausea, vomiting, bloody diarrhea, abdominal cramps, and distention.

A03.0   Shigellosis due to Shigella dysenteriae   `CC`
Group A shigellosis [Shiga-Kruse dysentery]
CC Excl: PDX collection 13

A03.1   Shigellosis due to Shigella flexneri
Group B shigellosis

A03.2   Shigellosis due to Shigella boydii
Group C shigellosis

A03.3   Shigellosis due to Shigella sonnei
Group D shigellosis

A03.8   Other shigellosis

A03.9   Shigellosis, unspecified
Bacillary dysentery NOS

✓4ᵗʰ A04   Other bacterial intestinal infections
EXCLUDES 1 bacterial foodborne intoxications, NEC (A05.-)
tuberculous enteritis (A18.32)

> **CC Excl: For CC codes in category A04, unless otherwise noted:**
> **For codes A04.0-A04.4:** PDX collection 14
> **For codes A04.5-A04.8:** PDX collection 15

A04.0   Enteropathogenic Escherichia coli infection   `CC`
A04.1   Enterotoxigenic Escherichia coli infection   `CC`
A04.2   Enteroinvasive Escherichia coli infection   `CC`
A04.3   Enterohemorrhagic Escherichia coli infection   `CC`
DEF: *E. coli* infection penetrating the intestinal mucosa, producing microscopic ulceration and bleeding.
A04.4   Other intestinal Escherichia coli infections   `CC`
Escherichia coli enteritis NOS
A04.5   Campylobacter enteritis   `CC`
A04.6   Enteritis due to Yersinia enterocolitica   `CC`
EXCLUDES 1 extraintestinal yersiniosis (A28.2)

✓5ᵗʰ A04.7   Enterocolitis due to Clostridium difficile
Foodborne intoxication by Clostridium difficile
Pseudomembraneous colitis

● **A04.71   Enterocolitis due to Clostridium difficile, recurrent**   `CC`
● **A04.72   Enterocolitis due to Clostridium difficile, not specified as recurrent**   `CC`

A04.8   Other specified bacterial intestinal infections   `CC`
A04.9   Bacterial intestinal infection, unspecified   `CC`
Bacterial enteritis NOS
CC Excl: PDX collection 16

✓4ᵗʰ A05   Other bacterial foodborne intoxications, not elsewhere classified
EXCLUDES 1 Clostridium difficile foodborne intoxication and infection ►(A04.7-)◄
Escherichia coli infection (A04.0-A04.4)
listeriosis (A32.-)
salmonella foodborne intoxication and infection (A02.-)
toxic effect of noxious foodstuffs (T61-T62)

A05.0   Foodborne staphylococcal intoxication   `CC`
CC Excl: PDX collection 17

N Newborn: 0   **P** Pediatric: 0-17   **M** Maternity: 12-55   **A** Adult: 15-124   **MCC** Major CC Condition   **PDxMCC** PDx acts as own MCC   **CC** CC Condition   **PDxCC** PDx acts as own CC

A05.1 Botulism food poisoning `CC`
Botulism NOS
Classical foodborne intoxication due to Clostridium botulinum
EXCLUDES 1 *infant botulism (A48.51)*
wound botulism (A48.52)
CC Excl: PDX collection 18

A05.2 Foodborne Clostridium perfringens [Clostridium welchii] `CC`
intoxication
Enteritis necroticans
Pig-bel
CC Excl: PDX collection 19

A05.3 Foodborne Vibrio parahaemolyticus intoxication `CC`
CC Excl: PDX collection 17

A05.4 Foodborne Bacillus cereus intoxication `CC`
CC Excl: PDX collection 17

A05.5 Foodborne Vibrio vulnificus intoxication `CC`
CC Excl: PDX collection 17

A05.8 Other specified bacterial foodborne intoxications `CC`
CC Excl: PDX collection 17

A05.9 Bacterial foodborne intoxication, unspecified

✓4ᵗʰ **A06 Amebiasis**
INCLUDES infection due to Entamoeba histolytica
EXCLUDES 1 *other protozoal intestinal diseases (A07.-)*
EXCLUDES 2 *acanthamebiasis (B60.1-)*
Naegleriasis (B60.2)

A06.0 Acute amebic dysentery `CC`
Acute amebiasis
Intestinal amebiasis NOS
CC Excl: PDX collection 20

A06.1 Chronic intestinal amebiasis `CC`
CC Excl: PDX collection 20

A06.2 Amebic nondysenteric colitis `CC`
CC Excl: PDX collection 21

A06.3 Ameboma of intestine `CC`
Ameboma NOS
CC Excl: PDX collection 22

A06.4 Amebic liver abscess `MCC`
Hepatic amebiasis
CC Excl: PDX collection 23

A06.5 Amebic lung abscess `MCC` `HCC`
Amebic abscess of lung (and liver)
CC Excl: PDX collection 24

A06.6 Amebic brain abscess `MCC`
Amebic abscess of brain (and liver) (and lung)
CC Excl: PDX collection 25

A06.7 Cutaneous amebiasis

✓5ᵗʰ **A06.8 Amebic infection of other sites**

CC Excl: For CC codes in subcategory A06.8:
PDX collection 22

A06.81 Amebic cystitis `CC`

A06.82 Other amebic genitourinary infections `CC`
Amebic balanitis
Amebic vesiculitis
Amebic vulvovaginitis

A06.89 Other amebic infections `CC`
Amebic appendicitis
Amebic splenic abscess

A06.9 Amebiasis, unspecified

✓4ᵗʰ **A07 Other protozoal intestinal diseases**

CC Excl: For CC codes in category A07, unless otherwise noted:
PDX collection 26

A07.0 Balantidiasis
Balantidial dysentery

A07.1 Giardiasis [lambliasis] `CC`

A07.2 Cryptosporidiosis `CC` `HCC`

A07.3 Isosporiasis `HIV` `CC`
Infection due to Isospora belli and Isospora hominis
Intestinal coccidiosis
Isosporosis

A07.4 Cyclosporiasis `CC`
CC Excl: PDX collection 27

A07.8 Other specified protozoal intestinal diseases `CC`
Intestinal microsporidiosis   Sarcocystosis
Intestinal trichomoniasis   Sarcosporidiosis

A07.9 Protozoal intestinal disease, unspecified `CC`
Flagellate diarrhea   Protozoal diarrhea
Protozoal colitis   Protozoal dysentery

✓4ᵗʰ **A08 Viral and other specified intestinal infections**
EXCLUDES 1 *influenza with involvement of gastrointestinal tract (J09.X3, J10.2, J11.2)*

CC Excl: For CC codes in category A08: PDX collection 28

A08.0 Rotaviral enteritis `CC`

✓5ᵗʰ **A08.1 Acute gastroenteropathy due to Norwalk agent and other small round viruses**

A08.11 Acute gastroenteropathy due to Norwalk agent `CC`
Acute gastroenteropathy due to Norovirus
Acute gastroenteropathy due to Norwalk-like agent

A08.19 Acute gastroenteropathy due to other small round viruses `CC`
Acute gastroenteropathy due to small round virus [SRV] NOS

A08.2 Adenoviral enteritis `CC`

✓5ᵗʰ **A08.3 Other viral enteritis**

A08.31 Calicivirus enteritis `CC`

A08.32 Astrovirus enteritis `CC`

A08.39 Other viral enteritis `CC`
Coxsackie virus enteritis
Echovirus enteritis
Enterovirus enteritis NEC
Torovirus enteritis

A08.4 Viral intestinal infection, unspecified
Viral enteritis NOS   Viral gastroenteropathy NOS
Viral gastroenteritis NOS
AHA: 2016, 3Q, 12

A08.8 Other specified intestinal infections

A09 Infectious gastroenteritis and colitis, unspecified `CC`
Infectious colitis NOS
Infectious enteritis NOS
Infectious gastroenteritis NOS
EXCLUDES 1 *colitis NOS (K52.9)*
diarrhea NOS (R19.7)
enteritis NOS (K52.9)
gastroenteritis NOS (K52.9)
noninfective gastroenteritis and colitis, unspecified (K52.9)
DEF: Colitis: An inflammation of mucous membranes of the colon.
DEF: Enteritis: An inflammation of mucous membranes of the small intestine.
DEF: Gastroenteritis: An inflammation of mucous membranes of stomach and intestines.
CC Excl: PDX collection 17

Tuberculosis (A15-A19)

INCLUDES infections due to Mycobacterium tuberculosis and Mycobacterium bovis
EXCLUDES 1 *congenital tuberculosis (P37.0)*
nonspecific reaction to test for tuberculosis without active tuberculosis (R76.1-)
pneumoconiosis associated with tuberculosis, any type in A15 (J65)
positive PPD (R76.11)
positive tuberculin skin test without active tuberculosis (R76.11)
sequelae of tuberculosis (B90.-)
silicotuberculosis (J65)

✓4ᵗʰ **A15 Respiratory tuberculosis**

A15.0 Tuberculosis of lung `HIV` `CC`
Tuberculous bronchiectasis
Tuberculous fibrosis of lung
Tuberculous pneumonia
Tuberculous pneumothorax
CC Excl: PDX collection 29

A15.4 Tuberculosis of intrathoracic lymph nodes `HIV` `CC`
Tuberculosis of hilar lymph nodes
Tuberculosis of mediastinal lymph nodes
Tuberculosis of tracheobronchial lymph nodes
EXCLUDES 1 *tuberculosis specified as primary (A15.7)*
CC Excl: PDX collection 29

✓ Additional Character Req   ✓x7ᵗʰ Placeholder Alert   Unacceptable PDx   Manifestation   H1-H14 HAC   HCC CMS-HCC Condition   EXCLUDES 1 Not Coded Here   EXCLUDES 2 Not Included Here

Tuberculosis of Lung

Granulomas from Mycobacterium tuberculosis

A15.5 Tuberculosis of larynx, trachea and bronchus　`HIV` `CC`
Tuberculosis of bronchus
Tuberculosis of glottis
Tuberculosis of larynx
Tuberculosis of trachea
CC Excl: PDX collection 29

A15.6 Tuberculous pleurisy　`HIV` `CC`
Tuberculosis of pleura Tuberculous empyema
EXCLUDES 1　*primary respiratory tuberculosis (A15.7)*
CC Excl: PDX collection 29

A15.7 Primary respiratory tuberculosis　`HIV` `CC`
CC Excl: PDX collection 30

A15.8 Other respiratory tuberculosis　`HIV` `CC`
Mediastinal tuberculosis
Nasopharyngeal tuberculosis
Tuberculosis of nose
Tuberculosis of sinus [any nasal]
CC Excl: PDX collection 31

A15.9 Respiratory tuberculosis unspecified　`HIV` `CC`
CC Excl: PDX collection 31

`✓4th` **A17 Tuberculosis of** nervous system

A17.0 Tuberculous meningitis　`HIV` `MCC`
Tuberculosis of meninges (cerebral)(spinal)
Tuberculous leptomeningitis
EXCLUDES 1　*tuberculous meningoencephalitis (A17.82)*
CC Excl: PDX collection 32

A17.1 Meningeal tuberculoma　`HIV` `MCC`
Tuberculoma of meninges (cerebral) (spinal)
EXCLUDES 2　*tuberculoma of brain and spinal cord (A17.81)*
CC Excl: PDX collection 32

`✓5th` **A17.8 Other tuberculosis of nervous system**

A17.81 Tuberculoma of brain and spinal cord　`HIV` `MCC`
Tuberculous abscess of brain and spinal cord
CC Excl: PDX collection 33

A17.82 Tuberculous meningoencephalitis　`HIV` `MCC`
Tuberculous myelitis
CC Excl: PDX collection 33

A17.83 Tuberculous neuritis　`HIV` `MCC`
Tuberculous mononeuropathy
CC Excl: No Excl

A17.89 Other tuberculosis of nervous system　`HIV` `MCC`
Tuberculous polyneuropathy
CC Excl: PDX collection 34

A17.9 Tuberculosis of nervous system, unspecified　`HIV` `CC`
CC Excl: PDX collection 35

`✓4th` **A18 Tuberculosis of** other organs

`✓5th` **A18.0 Tuberculosis of** bones and joints

A18.01 Tuberculosis of spine　`HIV` `CC`
Pott's disease or curvature of spine
Tuberculous arthritis
Tuberculous osteomyelitis of spine
Tuberculous spondylitis
CC Excl: PDX collection 36

A18.02 Tuberculous arthritis of other joints　`HIV` `CC`
Tuberculosis of hip (joint)
Tuberculosis of knee (joint)
CC Excl: PDX collection 37

A18.03 Tuberculosis of other bones　`HIV` `CC`
Tuberculous mastoiditis
Tuberculous osteomyelitis
CC Excl: PDX collection 38

A18.09 Other musculoskeletal tuberculosis　`HIV` `CC`
Tuberculous myositis
Tuberculous synovitis
Tuberculous tenosynovitis
CC Excl: PDX collection 39

`✓5th` **A18.1 Tuberculosis of** genitourinary system

A18.10 Tuberculosis of genitourinary system, unspecified　`HIV` `CC`
CC Excl: PDX collection 40

A18.11 Tuberculosis of kidney and ureter　`HIV` `CC`
CC Excl: PDX collection 41

A18.12 Tuberculosis of bladder　`HIV` `CC`
CC Excl: PDX collection 41

A18.13 Tuberculosis of other urinary organs　`HIV` `CC`
Tuberculous urethritis
CC Excl: PDX collection 41

A18.14 Tuberculosis of prostate　`HIV` `CC` `A` ♂
CC Excl: PDX collection 42

A18.15 Tuberculosis of other male genital organs　`HIV` `CC` ♂
CC Excl: PDX collection 42

A18.16 Tuberculosis of cervix　`HIV` `CC` ♀
CC Excl: PDX collection 43

A18.17 Tuberculous female pelvic inflammatory disease　`HIV` `CC` ♀
Tuberculous endometritis
Tuberculous oophoritis and salpingitis
CC Excl: PDX collection 43

A18.18 Tuberculosis of other female genital organs　`HIV` `CC` ♀
Tuberculous ulceration of vulva
CC Excl: PDX collection 43

A18.2 Tuberculous peripheral lymphadenopathy　`HIV` `CC`
Tuberculous adenitis
EXCLUDES 2　*tuberculosis of bronchial and mediastinal lymph nodes (A15.4)*
tuberculosis of mesenteric and retroperitoneal lymph nodes (A18.39)
tuberculous tracheobronchial adenopathy (A15.4)
CC Excl: PDX collection 44

`✓5th` **A18.3 Tuberculosis of** intestines, peritoneum and mesenteric glands

CC Excl: For CC/MCC codes in subcategory A18.3, unless otherwise noted: PDX collection 45

A18.31 Tuberculous peritonitis　`HIV` `MCC`
Tuberculous ascites
DEF: Tuberculous inflammation of the membrane lining the abdomen.

A18.32 Tuberculous enteritis　`HIV` `CC`
Tuberculosis of anus and rectum
Tuberculosis of intestine (large) (small)

A18.39 Retroperitoneal tuberculosis　`HIV` `CC`
Tuberculosis of mesenteric glands
Tuberculosis of retroperitoneal (lymph glands)

A18.4 Tuberculosis of skin and subcutaneous tissue　`HIV` `CC`
Erythema induratum, tuberculous
Lupus excedens
Lupus vulgaris NOS
Lupus vulgaris of eyelid
Scrofuloderma
Tuberculosis of external ear
EXCLUDES 2　*lupus erythematosus (L93.-)*
lupus NOS (M32.9)
systemic (M32.-)
CC Excl: PDX collection 30

`✓5th` **A18.5 Tuberculosis of** eye
EXCLUDES 2　*lupus vulgaris of eyelid (A18.4)*

CC Excl: For CC codes in subcategory A18.5, unless otherwise noted: PDX collection 46

A18.50 Tuberculosis of eye, unspecified　`HIV` `CC`

A18.51 Tuberculous episcleritis　`HIV` `CC`

A18.52 Tuberculous keratitis　`HIV` `CC`
Tuberculous interstitial keratitis
Tuberculous keratoconjunctivitis (interstitial) (phlyctenular)

A18.53 Tuberculous chorioretinitis　`HIV` `CC`

A18.54 Tuberculous iridocyclitis　`HIV` `CC`

    A18.59   Other **tuberculosis of eye**   `HIV` `CC`
         Tuberculous conjunctivitis

  A18.6 **Tuberculosis of (inner) (middle) ear**   `HIV` `CC`
       Tuberculous otitis media
       EXCLUDES 2   tuberculosis of external ear (A18.4)
                 tuberculous mastoiditis (A18.03)
       CC Excl: PDX collection 47

  A18.7 **Tuberculosis of adrenal glands**   `HIV` `CC`
       Tuberculous Addison's disease
       CC Excl: PDX collection 48

 ✓5ᵗʰ **A18.8** **Tuberculosis of other specified organs**
    A18.81   **Tuberculosis of thyroid gland**   `HIV` `CC`
         CC Excl: PDX collection 49

    A18.82   **Tuberculosis of other endocrine glands**   `HIV` `CC`
         Tuberculosis of pituitary gland
         Tuberculosis of thymus gland
         CC Excl: PDX collection 35

    A18.83   **Tuberculosis of digestive tract organs, not elsewhere classified**   `HIV` `CC`
         EXCLUDES 1   tuberculosis of intestine (A18.32)
         CC Excl: PDX collection 45

    A18.84   **Tuberculosis of heart**   `HIV` `CC`
         Tuberculous cardiomyopathy
         Tuberculous endocarditis
         Tuberculous myocarditis
         Tuberculous pericarditis
         CC Excl: PDX collection 35

    A18.85   **Tuberculosis of spleen**   `HIV` `CC`
         CC Excl: PDX collection 50

    A18.89   **Tuberculosis of other sites**   `HIV` `CC`
         Tuberculosis of muscle
         Tuberculous cerebral arteritis
         CC Excl: PDX collection 35

✓4ᵗʰ **A19** **Miliary tuberculosis**
    INCLUDES   disseminated tuberculosis
                generalized tuberculosis
                tuberculous polyserositis

    CC Excl: For MCC codes in category A19: PDX collection 51

  A19.0 **Acute miliary tuberculosis of a single specified site**   `HIV` `MCC`
  A19.1 **Acute miliary tuberculosis of multiple sites**   `HIV` `MCC`
  A19.2 **Acute miliary tuberculosis, unspecified**   `HIV` `MCC`
  A19.8 **Other miliary tuberculosis**   `HIV` `MCC`
  A19.9 **Miliary tuberculosis, unspecified**   `HIV` `MCC`

Certain zoonotic bacterial diseases (A20-A28)

✓4ᵗʰ **A20** **Plague**
    INCLUDES   infection due to Yersinia pestis
  A20.0 **Bubonic plague**   `MCC`
       CC Excl: PDX collection 52

  A20.1 **Cellulocutaneous plague**   `MCC`
       CC Excl: PDX collection 52

  A20.2 **Pneumonic plague**   `MCC` `HCC`
       CC Excl: PDX collection 53

  A20.3 **Plague meningitis**   `MCC`
       CC Excl: PDX collection 54

  A20.7 **Septicemic plague**   `MCC` `HCC`
       CC Excl: PDX collection 55

  A20.8 **Other forms of plague**   `MCC`
       Abortive plague
       Asymptomatic plague
       Pestis minor
       CC Excl: PDX collection 54

  A20.9 **Plague, unspecified**   `MCC`
       CC Excl: PDX collection 56

✓4ᵗʰ **A21** **Tularemia**
    INCLUDES   deer-fly fever
                infection due to Francisella tularensis
                rabbit fever
    DEF: A febrile disease transmitted to humans by the bites of deer flies, fleas, and ticks; by inhaling aerosolized *F. tularensis*; or by ingesting contaminated food or water. Patients quickly develop fever, chills, weakness, headache, backache, and malaise.

  A21.0 **Ulceroglandular tularemia**   `CC`
       CC Excl: PDX collection 57

  A21.1 **Oculoglandular tularemia**   `CC`
       Ophthalmic tularemia
       CC Excl: PDX collection 58

  A21.2 **Pulmonary tularemia**   `CC` `HCC`
       CC Excl: PDX collection 59

  A21.3 **Gastrointestinal tularemia**   `CC`
       Abdominal tularemia
       CC Excl: PDX collection 60

  A21.7 **Generalized tularemia**   `CC`
       CC Excl: PDX collection 61

  A21.8 **Other forms of tularemia**   `CC`
       CC Excl: PDX collection 61

  A21.9 **Tulamirea, unspecified**   `CC`
       CC Excl: PDX collection 61

✓4ᵗʰ **A22** **Anthrax**
    INCLUDES   infection due to Bacillus anthracis
  A22.0 **Cutaneous anthrax**   `CC`
       Malignant carbuncle
       Malignant pustule
       CC Excl: PDX collection 62

  A22.1 **Pulmonary anthrax**   `MCC` `HCC`
       Inhalation anthrax
       Ragpicker's disease
       Woolsorter's disease
       CC Excl: PDX collection 63

  A22.2 **Gastrointestinal anthrax**   `CC`
       CC Excl: PDX collection 64

  A22.7 **Anthrax sepsis**   `PDxMCC` `MCC` `HCC`
       CC Excl: PDX collection 5

  A22.8 **Other forms of anthrax**   `CC`
       Anthrax meningitis
       CC Excl: PDX collection 65

  A22.9 **Anthrax, unspecified**   `CC`
       CC Excl: PDX collection 66

✓4ᵗʰ **A23** **Brucellosis**
    INCLUDES   Malta fever
                Mediterranean fever
                undulant fever
  A23.0 **Brucellosis due to Brucella melitensis**
  A23.1 **Brucellosis due to Brucella abortus**
  A23.2 **Brucellosis due to Brucella suis**
  A23.3 **Brucellosis due to Brucella canis**
  A23.8 **Other brucellosis**   `CC`
       CC Excl: PDX collection 67

  A23.9 **Brucellosis, unspecified**   `CC`
       CC Excl: PDX collection 67

✓4ᵗʰ **A24** **Glanders and melioidosis**

    CC Excl: For CC codes in category A24, unless otherwise noted: PDX collection 69

  A24.0 **Glanders**   `CC`
       Infection due to Pseudomonas mallei
       Malleus
       CC Excl: PDX collection 68

  A24.1 **Acute and fulminating melioidosis**   `CC`
       Melioidosis pneumonia
       Melioidosis sepsis

  A24.2 **Subacute and chronic melioidosis**   `CC`
  A24.3 **Other melioidosis**   `CC`
  A24.9 **Melioidosis, unspecified**   `CC`
       Infection due to Pseudomonas pseudomallei NOS
       Whitmore's disease

✓4ᵗʰ **A25** **Rat-bite fevers**

    CC Excl: For CC codes in category A25, unless otherwise noted: PDX collection 70

  A25.0 **Spirillosis**   `CC`
       Sodoku

  A25.1 **Streptobacillosis**   `CC`
       Epidemic arthritic erythema   Streptobacillary rat-bite fever
       Haverhill fever

  A25.9 **Rat-bite fever, unspecified**   `CC`

✓4ᵗʰ **A26** **Erysipeloid**
  A26.0 **Cutaneous erysipeloid**
       Erythema migrans

  A26.7 **Erysipelothrix sepsis**   `PDxMCC` `MCC` `HCC`
       CC Excl: PDX collection 71

  A26.8 **Other forms of erysipeloid**
  A26.9 **Erysipeloid, unspecified**

✓Additional Character Req   ✓×7ᵗʰ Placeholder Alert   Unacceptable PDx   Manifestation   `H1`–`H14` HAC   `HCC` CMS-HCC Condition   **EXCLUDES 1** Not Coded Here   **EXCLUDES 2** Not Included Here

ICD-10-CM 2018   **439**

Chapter 1. Certain Infectious and Parasitic Diseases

✓4ᵗʰ **A27** **Leptospirosis**

> **CC Excl:** For CC codes in category A27, unless otherwise noted:
> PDX collection 72

  A27.0 **Leptospirosis** icterohemorrhagica   `CC`
    Leptospiral or spirochetal jaundice (hemorrhagic)
    Weil's disease

  ✓5ᵗʰ **A27.8** **Other** forms of leptospirosis

    A27.81 **Aseptic meningitis** in leptospirosis   `MCC`
        CC Excl: PDX collection 73

    A27.89 **Other** forms of leptospirosis   `CC`

  A27.9 **Leptospirosis,** unspecified   `CC`

✓4ᵗʰ **A28** **Other zoonotic bacterial diseases, not elsewhere classified**

> **CC Excl:** For CC codes in category A28, unless otherwise noted:
> PDX collection 74

  A28.0 **Pasteurellosis**   `CC`

  A28.1 **Cat-scratch disease**   `CC`
    Cat-scratch fever
    CC Excl: PDX collection 75

  A28.2 **Extraintestinal yersiniosis**   `CC`
    EXCLUDES 1   *enteritis due to Yersinia enterocolitica (A04.6)*
                 plague (A20.-)

  A28.8 **Other specified zoonotic bacterial diseases, not**   `CC`
    elsewhere classified

  A28.9 **Zoonotic bacterial disease, unspecified**   `CC`

Other bacterial diseases (A30-A49)

AHA: 2016, 3Q, 8-14

✓4ᵗʰ **A30** **Leprosy [Hansen's disease]**
  INCLUDES   infection due to Mycobacterium leprae
  EXCLUDES 1   *sequelae of leprosy (B92)*

  A30.0 **Indeterminate leprosy**   `CC`
    I leprosy
    CC Excl: PDX collection 76

  A30.1 **Tuberculoid leprosy**   `CC`
    TT leprosy
    CC Excl: PDX collection 77

  A30.2 **Borderline tuberculoid leprosy**   `CC`
    BT leprosy
    CC Excl: PDX collection 78

  A30.3 **Borderline leprosy**   `CC`
    BB leprosy
    CC Excl: PDX collection 78

  A30.4 **Borderline lepromatous leprosy**   `CC`
    BL leprosy
    CC Excl: PDX collection 78

  A30.5 **Lepromatous leprosy**   `CC`
    LL leprosy
    CC Excl: PDX collection 79

  A30.8 **Other forms of leprosy**   `CC`
    CC Excl: PDX collection 80

  A30.9 **Leprosy, unspecified**   `CC`
    CC Excl: PDX collection 81

✓4ᵗʰ **A31** **Infection due to other mycobacteria**
  EXCLUDES 2   *leprosy (A30.-)*
            tuberculosis (A15-A19)

> **CC Excl:** For CC codes in category A31, unless otherwise noted:
> PDX collection 83

  A31.0 **Pulmonary mycobacterial infection**   `CC` `HCC`
    Infection due to Mycobacterium avium
    Infection due to Mycobacterium intracellulare [Battey bacillus]
    Infection due to Mycobacterium kansasii
    CC Excl: PDX collection 82

  A31.1 **Cutaneous mycobacterial infection**   `CC`
    Buruli ulcer
    Infection due to Mycobacterium marinum
    Infection due to Mycobacterium ulcerans

  A31.2 **Disseminated mycobacterium avium-intracellulare**   `HIV` `CC` `HCC`
    complex (DMAC)
    MAC sepsis

  A31.8 **Other mycobacterial infections**   `HIV` `CC`

  A31.9 **Mycobacterial infection, unspecified**   `HIV` `CC`
    Atypical mycobacterial infection NOS
    Mycobacteriosis NOS

✓4ᵗʰ **A32** **Listeriosis**
  INCLUDES   listerial foodborne infection
  EXCLUDES 1   *neonatal (disseminated) listeriosis (P37.2)*

> **CC Excl:** For CC codes in category A32, unless otherwise noted:
> PDX collection 74

  A32.0 **Cutaneous listeriosis**   `CC`

  ✓5ᵗʰ **A32.1** **Listerial meningitis and meningoencephalitis**
    A32.11 **Listerial meningitis**   `CC`
    A32.12 **Listerial meningoencephalitis**   `CC`

  A32.7 **Listerial sepsis**   `PDxMCC` `MCC` `HCC`
    CC Excl: PDX collection 71

  ✓5ᵗʰ **A32.8** **Other forms of listeriosis**
    A32.81 **Oculoglandular listeriosis**   `CC`
    A32.82 **Listerial endocarditis**   `CC`
    A32.89 **Other forms of listeriosis**   `CC`
        Listerial cerebral arteritis

  A32.9 **Listeriosis, unspecified**   `CC`

A33 **Tetanus neonatorum**   `MCC` `N`
  CC Excl: PDX collection 84

A34 **Obstetrical tetanus**   `CC` `M` `Q`
  CC Excl: PDX collection 85

A35 **Other tetanus**   `MCC`
  Tetanus NOS
  EXCLUDES 1   *obstetrical tetanus (A34)*
            tetanus neonatorum (A33)
  CC Excl: PDX collection 86

✓4ᵗʰ **A36** **Diphtheria**

> **CC Excl:** For CC codes in category A36, unless otherwise noted:
> PDX collection 87

  A36.0 **Pharyngeal diphtheria**   `CC`
    Diphtheritic membranous angina
    Tonsillar diphtheria

  A36.1 **Nasopharyngeal diphtheria**   `CC`

  A36.2 **Laryngeal diphtheria**
    Diphtheritic laryngotracheitis

  A36.3 **Cutaneous diphtheria**   `CC`
    EXCLUDES 2   *erythrasma (L08.1)*

  ✓5ᵗʰ **A36.8** **Other diphtheria**
    A36.81 **Diphtheritic cardiomyopathy**   `CC` `HCC`
        Diphtheritic myocarditis
        CC Excl: PDX collection 88

    A36.82 **Diphtheritic radiculomyelitis**   `CC`
    A36.83 **Diphtheritic polyneuritis**   `CC`
    A36.84 **Diphtheritic tubulo-interstitial nephropathy**   `CC`
    A36.85 **Diphtheritic cystitis**   `CC`
    A36.86 **Diphtheritic conjunctivitis**   `CC`
    A36.89 **Other diphtheritic complications**   `CC`
        Diphtheritic peritonitis

  A36.9 **Diphtheria, unspecified**

✓4ᵗʰ **A37** **Whooping cough**

> **CC Excl:** For CC codes in category A37, unless otherwise noted:
> PDX collection 89
> **For MCC codes in category A37, unless otherwise noted:**
> PDX collection 90

  ✓5ᵗʰ **A37.0** **Whooping cough due to Bordetella pertussis**
    A37.00 **Whooping cough due to Bordetella pertussis**   `CC`
        without pneumonia

    A37.01 **Whooping cough due to Bordetella**   `PDxMCC` `MCC`
        pertussis with pneumonia

  ✓5ᵗʰ **A37.1** **Whooping cough due to Bordetella parapertussis**
    A37.10 **Whooping cough due to Bordetella**   `CC`
        parapertussis without pneumonia

    A37.11 **Whooping cough due to Bordetella**   `PDxMCC` `MCC`
        parapertussis with pneumonia

  ✓5ᵗʰ **A37.8** **Whooping cough due to other Bordetella species**
    A37.80 **Whooping cough due to other Bordetella**   `CC`
        species without pneumonia

    A37.81 **Whooping cough due to other Bordetella**   `PDxMCC` `MCC`
        species with pneumonia

`N` Newborn: 0   `P` Pediatric: 0-17   `M` Maternity: 12-55   `A` Adult: 15-124   `MCC` Major CC Condition   `PDxMCC` PDx acts as own MCC   `CC` CC Condition   `PDxCC` PDx acts as own CC

440   ICD-10-CM 2018

✓5th **A37.9** **Whooping cough,** unspecified **species**

    A37.90 **Whooping cough, unspecified species** without **pneumonia** `CC`

    A37.91 **Whooping cough, unspecified species** with **pneumonia** `PDx MCC` `MCC`

✓4th **A38** **Scarlet fever**

    INCLUDES   scarlatina
    EXCLUDES 2   streptococcal sore throat (J02.0)

    CC Excl: For CC codes in category A38: PDX collection 91

    A38.0 **Scarlet fever with** otitis media `CC`
    A38.1 **Scarlet fever with** myocarditis `CC`
    A38.8 **Scarlet fever with** other complications `CC`
    A38.9 **Scarlet fever,** uncomplicated `CC`
      Scarlet fever, NOS

✓4th **A39** **Meningococcal infection**

    A39.0 **Meningococcal** meningitis `MCC`
      CC Excl: PDX collection 92

    A39.1 **Waterhouse-Friderichsen** syndrome `MCC` `HCC`
      Meningococcal hemorrhagic adrenalitis
      Meningococcic adrenal syndrome
      CC Excl: PDX collection 93

    A39.2 **Acute** meningococcemia `MCC` `HCC`
      CC Excl: PDX collection 94

    A39.3 **Chronic** meningococcemia `MCC` `HCC`
      CC Excl: PDX collection 94

    A39.4 **Meningococcemia,** unspecified `MCC` `HCC`
      CC Excl: PDX collection 94

✓5th   **A39.5** **Meningococcal** heart disease

      A39.50 **Meningococcal carditis,** unspecified `MCC`
         CC Excl: PDX collection 95

      A39.51 **Meningococcal** endocarditis `MCC`
         CC Excl: PDX collection 96

      A39.52 **Meningococcal** myocarditis `MCC`
         CC Excl: PDX collection 97

      A39.53 **Meningococcal** pericarditis `MCC`
         CC Excl: PDX collection 98

✓5th   **A39.8** **Other meningococcal infections**

      A39.81 **Meningococcal** encephalitis `MCC`
         CC Excl: PDX collection 99

      A39.82 **Meningococcal** retrobulbar neuritis `CC`
         CC Excl: PDX collection 100

      A39.83 **Meningococcal** arthritis `CC` `HCC`
         CC Excl: PDX collection 101

      A39.84 **Postmeningococcal** arthritis `CC` `HCC`
         CC Excl: PDX collection 101

      A39.89 **Other meningococcal** infections `CC`
         Meningococcal conjunctivitis
         CC Excl: PDX collection 102

    A39.9 **Meningococcal infection,** unspecified `CC`
      Meningococcal disease NOS
      CC Excl: PDX collection 102

✓4th **A40** **Streptococcal sepsis**

    Code first: postprocedural streptococcal sepsis (T81.4-)
      streptococcal sepsis during labor (O75.3)
      streptococcal sepsis following abortion or ectopic or molar pregnancy (O03-O07, O08.0)
      streptococcal sepsis following immunization (T88.0)
      streptococcal sepsis following infusion, transfusion or therapeutic injection (T80.2-)

    EXCLUDES 1   neonatal (P36.0-P36.1)
      puerperal sepsis (O85)
      sepsis due to Streptococcus, group D (A41.81)

    AHA: 2016, 1Q, 32

    CC Excl: For MCC codes in category A40: PDX collection 71

    A40.0 **Sepsis due to streptococcus,** group A `MCC` `HCC`
    A40.1 **Sepsis due to streptococcus,** group B `MCC` `HCC`
    A40.3 **Sepsis due to Streptococcus** pneumoniae `MCC` `HCC`
      Pneumococcal sepsis
      CC Excl: No Excl
    A40.8 **Other streptococcal sepsis** `MCC` `HCC`
    A40.9 **Streptococcal sepsis,** unspecified `HIV` `MCC` `HCC`

✓4th **A41** **Other sepsis**

    Code first: postprocedural sepsis (T81.4-)sepsis during labor (O75.3)
      sepsis following abortion, ectopic or molar pregnancy (O03-O07, O08.0)
      sepsis following immunization (T88.0)
      sepsis following infusion, transfusion or therapeutic injection (T80.2-)

    EXCLUDES 1   bacteremia NOS (R78.81)
      neonatal (P36.-)
      puerperal sepsis (O85)
      streptococcal sepsis (A40.-)

    EXCLUDES 2   sepsis (due to) (in) actinomycotic (A42.7)
      sepsis (due to) (in) anthrax (A22.7)
      sepsis (due to) (in) candidal (B37.7)
      sepsis (due to) (in) Erysipelothrix (A26.7)
      sepsis (due to) (in) extraintestinal yersiniosis (A28.2)
      sepsis (due to) (in) gonococcal (A54.86)
      sepsis (due to) (in) herpesviral (B00.7)
      sepsis (due to) (in) listerial (A32.7)
      sepsis (due to) (in) melioidosis (A24.1)
      sepsis (due to) (in) meningococcal (A39.2-A39.4)
      sepsis (due to) (in) plague (A20.7)
      sepsis (due to) (in) tularemia (A21.7)
      toxic shock syndrome (A48.3)

    AHA: 2016, 1Q, 32; 2014, 2Q, 13

    CC Excl: For MCC codes in category A41: PDX collection 71

✓5th   **A41.0** **Sepsis due to** Staphylococcus aureus

      A41.01 **Sepsis due to** Methicillin susceptible Staphylococcus aureus `HIV` `MCC` `HCC`
         MSSA sepsis
         Staphylococcus aureus sepsis NOS

      A41.02 **Sepsis due to** Methicillin resistant Staphylococcus aureus `HIV` `MCC` `HCC`

    A41.1 **Sepsis due to** other specified staphylococcus `HIV` `MCC` `HCC`
      Coagulase negative staphylococcus sepsis

    A41.2 **Sepsis due to** unspecified staphylococcus `HIV` `MCC` `HCC`
    A41.3 **Sepsis due to** Hemophilus influenzae `HIV` `MCC` `HCC`
    A41.4 **Sepsis due to** anaerobes `HIV` `MCC` `HCC`
      EXCLUDES 1   gas gangrene (A48.0)

✓5th   **A41.5** **Sepsis due to other** Gram-negative organisms

      A41.50 **Gram-negative sepsis,** unspecified `HIV` `MCC` `HCC`
         Gram-negative sepsis NOS

      A41.51 **Sepsis due to** Escherichia coli [E. coli] `HIV` `MCC` `HCC`
      A41.52 **Sepsis due to** Pseudomonas `HIV` `MCC` `HCC`
         Pseudomonas aeroginosa

      A41.53 **Sepsis due to** Serratia `HIV` `MCC` `HCC`
      A41.59 **Other** Gram-negative sepsis `HIV` `MCC` `HCC`

✓5th   **A41.8** **Other specified sepsis**

      A41.81 **Sepsis due to** Enterococcus `HIV` `MCC` `HCC`
      A41.89 **Other specified sepsis** `HIV` `MCC` `HCC`
         AHA: 2017, 1Q, 51; 2016, 3Q, 8-14

    A41.9 **Sepsis,** unspecified **organism** `HIV` `MCC` `HCC`
      Septicemia NOS

✓4th **A42** **Actinomycosis**

    EXCLUDES 1   actinomycetoma (B47.1)

    A42.0 **Pulmonary** actinomycosis `HIV` `CC` `HCC`
      CC Excl: PDX collection 103

    A42.1 **Abdominal** actinomycosis `HIV` `CC`
      CC Excl: PDX collection 104

    A42.2 **Cervicofacial** actinomycosis `HIV` `CC`
      CC Excl: PDX collection 105

    A42.7 **Actinomycotic** sepsis `HIV` `MCC` `HCC`
      CC Excl: PDX collection 71

✓5th   **A42.8** **Other forms of actinomycosis**

      CC Excl: For CC codes in subcategory A42.8: PDX collection 106

      A42.81 **Actinomycotic** meningitis `HIV` `CC`
      A42.82 **Actinomycotic** encephalitis `HIV` `CC`
      A42.89 **Other forms of actinomycosis** `HIV` `CC`

    A42.9 **Actinomycosis,** unspecified `HIV` `CC`
      CC Excl: PDX collection 106

✓ Additional Character Req   ✓x7th Placeholder Alert   Unacceptable PDx   Manifestation   H1-H14 HAC   HCC CMS-HCC Condition   EXCLUDES 1 Not Coded Here   EXCLUDES 2 Not Included Here

Chapter 1. Certain Infectious and Parasitic Diseases

☑️⁴ᵗʰ **A43 Nocardiosis**

A43.0 Pulmonary nocardiosis `HIV` `CC` `HCC`
CC Excl: PDX collection 103

A43.1 Cutaneous nocardiosis `HIV` `CC`
CC Excl: PDX collection 107

A43.8 Other forms of nocardiosis `HIV` `CC`
CC Excl: PDX collection 106

A43.9 Nocardiosis, unspecified `HIV` `CC`
CC Excl: PDX collection 106

☑️⁴ᵗʰ **A44 Bartonellosis**

CC Excl: For CC codes in category A44: PDX collection 108

A44.0 Systemic bartonellosis `CC`
Oroya fever

A44.1 Cutaneous and mucocutaneous bartonellosis `CC`
Verruga peruana

A44.8 Other forms of bartonellosis `CC`

A44.9 Bartonellosis, unspecified `CC`

A46 Erysipelas
EXCLUDES 1   postpartum or puerperal erysipelas (O86.89)
DEF: A skin infection affecting the upper dermis and superficial dermal lymphatics; lesion edges are well demarcated with distinct raised borders; it is often caused by group A *Streptococci*.

☑️⁴ᵗʰ **A48 Other bacterial diseases, not elsewhere classified**
EXCLUDES 1   actinomycetoma (B47.1)

A48.0 Gas gangrene `MCC` `HCC`
Clostridial cellulitis
Clostridial myonecrosis
CC Excl: PDX collection 109

A48.1 Legionnaires' disease `HIV` `MCC` `HCC`
DEF: Severe and often fatal infection by *Legionella pneumophila*; symptoms include high fever, gastrointestinal pain, headache, myalgia, dry cough, and pneumonia; usually transmitted through airborne water droplets via air conditioning systems or hot tubs.
CC Excl: PDX collection 110

A48.2 Nonpneumonic Legionnaires' disease [Pontiac fever]

A48.3 Toxic shock syndrome `MCC` `HCC`
Use additional code to identify the organism (B95, B96)
EXCLUDES 1   endotoxic shock NOS (R57.8)
          sepsis NOS (A41.9)
CC Excl: PDX collection 111

A48.4 Brazilian purpuric fever
Systemic Hemophilus aegyptius infection

☑️⁵ᵗʰ **A48.5 Other specified botulism**
Non-foodborne intoxication due to toxins of Clostridium botulinum [C. botulinum]
EXCLUDES 1   food poisoning due to toxins of Clostridium botulinum (A05.1)

CC Excl: For CC codes in subcategory A48.5: PDX collection 18

A48.51 Infant botulism `CC` `P`

A48.52 Wound botulism `CC`
Non-foodborne botulism NOS
Use additional code for associated wound

A48.8 Other specified bacterial diseases

☑️⁴ᵗʰ **A49 Bacterial infection of unspecified site**
EXCLUDES 1   bacterial agents as the cause of diseases classified elsewhere (B95-B96)
          chlamydial infection NOS (A74.9)
          meningococcal infection NOS (A39.9)
          rickettsial infection NOS (A79.9)
          spirochetal infection NOS (A69.9)

☑️⁵ᵗʰ **A49.0 Staphylococcal infection, unspecified site**

A49.01 Methicillin susceptible Staphylococcus aureus infection, unspecified site
Methicillin susceptible Staphylococcus aureus (MSSA) infection
Staphylococcus aureus infection NOS

A49.02 Methicillin resistant Staphylococcus aureus infection, unspecified site
Methicillin resistant Staphylococcus aureus (MRSA) infection

A49.1 Streptococcal infection, unspecified site

A49.2 Hemophilus influenzae infection, unspecified site

A49.3 Mycoplasma infection, unspecified site

A49.8 Other bacterial infections of unspecified site

A49.9 Bacterial infection, unspecified
EXCLUDES 1   bacteremia NOS (R78.81)

Infections with a predominantly sexual mode of transmission (A50-A64)

EXCLUDES 1   human immunodeficiency virus [HIV] disease (B20)
          nonspecific and nongonococcal urethritis (N34.1)
          Reiter's disease (M02.3-)

☑️⁴ᵗʰ **A50 Congenital syphilis**

☑️⁵ᵗʰ **A50.0 Early congenital syphilis, symptomatic**
Any congenital syphilitic condition specified as early or manifest less than two years after birth.

CC Excl: For CC codes in subcategory A50.0: PDX collection 112

A50.01 Early congenital syphilitic oculopathy `CC`

A50.02 Early congenital syphilitic osteochondropathy `CC`

A50.03 Early congenital syphilitic pharyngitis `CC`
Early congenital syphilitic laryngitis

A50.04 Early congenital syphilitic pneumonia `CC`

A50.05 Early congenital syphilitic rhinitis `CC`

A50.06 Early cutaneous congenital syphilis `CC`

A50.07 Early mucocutaneous congenital syphilis `CC`

A50.08 Early visceral congenital syphilis `CC`

A50.09 Other early congenital syphilis, symptomatic `CC`

A50.1 Early congenital syphilis, latent
Congenital syphilis without clinical manifestations, with positive serological reaction and negative spinal fluid test, less than two years after birth.

A50.2 Early congenital syphilis, unspecified `CC`
Congenital syphilis NOS less than two years after birth.
CC Excl: PDX collection 113

☑️⁵ᵗʰ **A50.3 Late congenital syphilitic oculopathy**
EXCLUDES 1   Hutchinson's triad (A50.53)

CC Excl: For CC/MCC codes in subcategory A50.3, unless otherwise noted: PDX collection 112

A50.30 Late congenital syphilitic oculopathy, unspecified `CC`

A50.31 Late congenital syphilitic interstitial keratitis `CC`

A50.32 Late congenital syphilitic chorioretinitis `CC`

A50.39 Other late congenital syphilitic oculopathy `CC`

☑️⁵ᵗʰ **A50.4 Late congenital neurosyphilis [juvenile neurosyphilis]**
Use additional code to identify any associated mental disorder
EXCLUDES 1   Hutchinson's triad (A50.53)

A50.40 Late congenital neurosyphilis, unspecified `CC`
Juvenile neurosyphilis NOS
CC Excl: PDX collection 114

A50.41 Late congenital syphilitic meningitis `MCC`
CC Excl: PDX collection 115

A50.42 Late congenital syphilitic encephalitis `MCC`
CC Excl: PDX collection 114

A50.43 Late congenital syphilitic polyneuropathy `CC`
CC Excl: PDX collection 114

A50.44 Late congenital syphilitic optic nerve atrophy `CC`
CC Excl: PDX collection 112

A50.45 Juvenile general paresis `CC`
Dementia paralytica juvenilis
Juvenile tabetoparetic neurosyphilis
CC Excl: PDX collection 114

A50.49 Other late congenital neurosyphilis `CC`
Juvenile tabes dorsalis
CC Excl: PDX collection 114

☑️⁵ᵗʰ **A50.5 Other late congenital syphilis, symptomatic**
Any congenital syphilitic condition specified as late or manifest two years or more after birth.

CC Excl: For CC codes in subcategory A50.5: PDX collection 112

A50.51 Clutton's joints `CC`

A50.52 Hutchinson's teeth `CC`

A50.53 Hutchinson's triad `CC`

A50.54 Late congenital cardiovascular syphilis `CC`

A50.55 Late congenital syphilitic arthropathy `CC` `HCC`

A50.56 Late congenital syphilitic osteochondropathy `CC`

`N` Newborn: 0   `P` Pediatric: 0-17   `M` Maternity: 12-55   `A` Adult: 15-124   `MCC` Major CC Condition   `PDxMCC` PDx acts as own MCC   `CC` CC Condition   `PDxCC` PDx acts as own CC

442   ICD-10-CM 2018

        A50.57 Syphilitic saddle nose `CC`

        A50.59 Other late congenital syphilis, symptomatic `CC`

    A50.6 Late congenital syphilis, latent
        Congenital syphilis without clinical manifestations, with positive serological reaction and negative spinal fluid test, two years or more after birth.

    A50.7 Late congenital syphilis, unspecified
        Congenital syphilis NOS two years or more after birth.

    A50.9 Congenital syphilis, unspecified

✓4ᵗʰ **A51 Early syphilis**

    A51.0 Primary genital syphilis
        Syphilitic chancre NOS

    A51.1 Primary anal syphilis

    A51.2 Primary syphilis of other sites

✓5ᵗʰ **A51.3 Secondary syphilis of skin and mucous membranes**
        DEF: Transitory or chronic cutaneous eruptions that present within two to 10 weeks following initial syphilis infection that may include nontender lymphadenopathy along with alopecia and condylomata lata.

        A51.31 Condyloma latum `CC`
            CC Excl: PDX collection 112

        A51.32 Syphilitic alopecia `CC`
            CC Excl: PDX collection 116

        A51.39 Other secondary syphilis of skin `CC`
            Syphilitic leukoderma
            Syphilitic mucous patch
            EXCLUDES 1   late syphilitic leukoderma (A52.79)
            CC Excl: PDX collection 112

    ✓5ᵗʰ **A51.4 Other secondary syphilis**

        A51.41 Secondary syphilitic meningitis `MCC`
            CC Excl: PDX collection 117

        A51.42 Secondary syphilitic female pelvic disease `CC` ♀
            CC Excl: PDX collection 113

        A51.43 Secondary syphilitic oculopathy `CC`
            Secondary syphilitic chorioretinitis
            Secondary syphilitic iridocyclitis, iritis
            Secondary syphilitic uveitis
            CC Excl: PDX collection 112

        A51.44 Secondary syphilitic nephritis `CC`
            CC Excl: PDX collection 113

        A51.45 Secondary syphilitic hepatitis `CC`
            CC Excl: PDX collection 118

        A51.46 Secondary syphilitic osteopathy `CC`
            CC Excl: PDX collection 119

        A51.49 Other secondary syphilitic conditions `CC`
            Secondary syphilitic lymphadenopathy
            Secondary syphilitic myositis
            CC Excl: No Excl

    A51.5 Early syphilis, latent
        Syphilis (acquired) without clinical manifestations, with positive serological reaction and negative spinal fluid test, less than two years after infection.

    A51.9 Early syphilis, unspecified

✓4ᵗʰ **A52 Late syphilis**

    ✓5ᵗʰ **A52.0 Cardiovascular and cerebrovascular syphilis**

        CC Excl: For CC codes in subcategory A52.0: PDX collection 114

        A52.00 Cardiovascular syphilis, unspecified `CC`

        A52.01 Syphilitic aneurysm of aorta `CC`

        A52.02 Syphilitic aortitis `CC`

        A52.03 Syphilitic endocarditis `CC`
            Syphilitic aortic valve incompetence or stenosis
            Syphilitic mitral valve stenosis
            Syphilitic pulmonary valve regurgitation

        A52.04 Syphilitic cerebral arteritis `CC`

        A52.05 Other cerebrovascular syphilis `CC`
            Syphilitic cerebral aneurysm (ruptured) (non-ruptured)
            Syphilitic cerebral thrombosis

        A52.06 Other syphilitic heart involvement `CC`
            Syphilitic coronary artery disease
            Syphilitic myocarditis
            Syphilitic pericarditis

        A52.09 Other cardiovascular syphilis `CC`

    ✓5ᵗʰ **A52.1 Symptomatic neurosyphilis**

        CC Excl: For CC/MCC codes in subcategory A52.1, unless otherwise noted: PDX collection 114

        A52.10 Symptomatic neurosyphilis, unspecified `CC`

        A52.11 Tabes dorsalis `CC`
            Locomotor ataxia (progressive)
            Tabetic neurosyphilis

        A52.12 Other cerebrospinal syphilis `CC`

        A52.13 Late syphilitic meningitis `MCC`
            CC Excl: PDX collection 115

        A52.14 Late syphilitic encephalitis `MCC`

        A52.15 Late syphilitic neuropathy `CC`
            Late syphilitic acoustic neuritis
            Late syphilitic optic (nerve) atrophy
            Late syphilitic polyneuropathy
            Late syphilitic retrobulbar neuritis

        A52.16 Charcôt's arthropathy (tabetic) `CC`

        A52.17 General paresis `CC`
            Dementia paralytica

        A52.19 Other symptomatic neurosyphilis `CC`
            Syphilitic parkinsonism

    A52.2 Asymptomatic neurosyphilis `CC`
        CC Excl: PDX collection 114

    A52.3 Neurosyphilis, unspecified `CC`
        Gumma (syphilitic)
        Syphilis (late)
        Syphiloma
        CC Excl: PDX collection 114

    ✓5ᵗʰ **A52.7 Other symptomatic late syphilis**

        CC Excl: For CC codes in subcategory A52.7, unless otherwise noted: PDX collection 116

        A52.71 Late syphilitic oculopathy `CC`
            Late syphilitic chorioretinitis
            Late syphilitic episcleritis
            CC Excl: PDX collection 120

        A52.72 Syphilis of lung and bronchus `CC`

        A52.73 Symptomatic late syphilis of other respiratory organs `CC`

        A52.74 Syphilis of liver and other viscera `CC`
            Late syphilitic peritonitis

        A52.75 Syphilis of kidney and ureter `CC`
            Syphilitic glomerular disease

        A52.76 Other genitourinary symptomatic late syphilis `CC`
            Late syphilitic female pelvic inflammatory disease

        A52.77 Syphilis of bone and joint `CC`

        A52.78 Syphilis of other musculoskeletal tissue `CC`
            Late syphilitic bursitis
            Syphilis [stage unspecified] of bursa
            Syphilis [stage unspecified] of muscle
            Syphilis [stage unspecified] of synovium
            Syphilis [stage unspecified] of tendon

        A52.79 Other symptomatic late syphilis `CC`
            Late syphilitic leukoderma
            Syphilis of adrenal gland
            Syphilis of pituitary gland
            Syphilis of thyroid gland
            Syphilitic splenomegaly
            EXCLUDES 1   syphilitic leukoderma (secondary) (A51.39)

    A52.8 Late syphilis, latent
        Syphilis (acquired) without clinical manifestations, with positive serological reaction and negative spinal fluid test, two years or more after infection

    A52.9 Late syphilis, unspecified

✓4ᵗʰ **A53 Other and unspecified syphilis**

    A53.0 Latent syphilis, unspecified as early or late
        Latent syphilis NOS   Positive serological reaction for syphilis

    A53.9 Syphilis, unspecified
        Infection due to Treponema pallidum NOS
        Syphilis (acquired) NOS
        EXCLUDES 1   syphilis NOS under two years of age (A50.2)

☑ Additional Character Req   ✗ₓ7ᵗʰ Placeholder Alert   Unacceptable PDx   Manifestation   H1 – H14 HAC   HCC CMS-HCC Condition   *EXCLUDES 1* Not Coded Here   *EXCLUDES 2* Not Included Here

A54   Gonococcal infection ✓4th

   ✓5th **A54.0   Gonococcal infection of** lower genitourinary tract without periurethral or accessory gland abscess

     EXCLUDES 1   gonococcal infection with genitourinary gland abscess (A54.1)
                 gonococcal infection with periurethral abscess (A54.1)

     CC Excl: For CC codes in subcategory A54.0: PDX collection 121

     A54.00   Gonococcal infection of lower genitourinary tract, unspecified   CC

     A54.01   Gonococcal cystitis and urethritis, unspecified   CC

     A54.02   Gonococcal vulvovaginitis, unspecified   CC ♀

     A54.03   Gonococcal cervicitis, unspecified   CC ♀

     A54.09   Other gonococcal infection of lower genitourinary tract   CC

   A54.1   Gonococcal infection of lower genitourinary tract with periurethral and accessory gland abscess   CC
     Gonococcal Bartholin's gland abscess
     CC Excl: PDX collection 121

   ✓5th **A54.2   Gonococcal** pelviperitonitis **and other** gonococcal genitourinary infection

     CC Excl: For CC codes in subcategory A54.2: PDX collection 121

     A54.21   Gonococcal infection of kidney and ureter   CC

     A54.22   Gonococcal prostatitis   CC ♂

     A54.23   Gonococcal infection of other male genital organs   CC ♂
       Gonococcal epididymitis   Gonococcal orchitis

     A54.24   Gonococcal female pelvic inflammatory disease   CC ♀
       Gonococcal pelviperitonitis
       EXCLUDES 1   gonococcal peritonitis (A54.85)

     A54.29   Other gonococcal genitourinary infections   CC

   ✓5th **A54.3   Gonococcal infection of** eye

     CC Excl: For CC codes in subcategory A54.3: PDX collection 116

     A54.30   Gonococcal infection of eye, unspecified   CC

     A54.31   Gonococcal conjunctivitis   CC
       Ophthalmia neonatorum due to gonococcus

     A54.32   Gonococcal iridocyclitis   CC

     A54.33   Gonococcal keratitis   CC

     A54.39   Other gonococcal eye infection   CC
       Gonococcal endophthalmia

   ✓5th **A54.4   Gonococcal infection of** musculoskeletal system

     CC Excl: For CC codes in subcategory A54.4: PDX collection 122

     A54.40   Gonococcal infection of musculoskeletal system, unspecified   CC HCC

     A54.41   Gonococcal spondylopathy   CC HCC

     A54.42   Gonococcal arthritis   CC HCC
       EXCLUDES 2   gonococcal infection of spine (A54.41)

     A54.43   Gonococcal osteomyelitis   CC HCC
       EXCLUDES 2   gonococcal infection of spine (A54.41)

     A54.49   Gonococcal infection of other musculoskeletal tissue   CC HCC
       Gonococcal bursitis
       Gonococcal myositis
       Gonococcal synovitis
       Gonococcal tenosynovitis

   A54.5   Gonococcal pharyngitis

   A54.6   Gonococcal infection of anus and rectum

   ✓5th **A54.8   Other gonococcal infections**

     A54.81   Gonococcal meningitis   MCC
       CC Excl: PDX collection 117

     A54.82   Gonococcal brain abscess   CC
       CC Excl: PDX collection 123

     A54.83   Gonococcal heart infection   CC
       Gonococcal endocarditis
       Gonococcal myocarditis
       Gonococcal pericarditis
       CC Excl: PDX collection 124

     A54.84   Gonococcal pneumonia   CC HCC
       CC Excl: PDX collection 123

     A54.85   Gonococcal peritonitis   CC HCC
       EXCLUDES 1   gonococcal pelviperitonitis (A54.24)
       CC Excl: PDX collection 125

     A54.86   Gonococcal sepsis   PDxMCC MCC HCC
       CC Excl: PDX collection 71

     A54.89   Other gonococcal infections   CC
       Gonococcal keratoderma
       Gonococcal lymphadenitis
       CC Excl: PDX collection 123

   A54.9   Gonococcal infection, unspecified   CC
     CC Excl: PDX collection 123

A55   Chlamydial lymphogranuloma (venereum)
   Climatic or tropical bubo
   Durand-Nicolas-Favre disease
   Esthiomene
   Lymphogranuloma inguinale

A56   Other sexually transmitted chlamydial diseases ✓4th
   INCLUDES   sexually transmitted diseases due to Chlamydia trachomatis
   EXCLUDES 1   neonatal chlamydial conjunctivitis (P39.1)
            neonatal chlamydial pneumonia (P23.1)
   EXCLUDES 2   chlamydial lymphogranuloma (A55)
            conditions classified to A74-

   ✓5th **A56.0   Chlamydial infection of** lower genitourinary tract

     A56.00   Chlamydial infection of lower genitourinary tract, unspecified

     A56.01   Chlamydial cystitis and urethritis

     A56.02   Chlamydial vulvovaginitis   ♀

     A56.09   Other chlamydial infection of lower genitourinary tract
       Chlamydial cervicitis

   ✓5th **A56.1   Chlamydial infection of** pelviperitoneum and other genitourinary organs

     A56.11   Chlamydial female pelvic inflammatory disease   ♀

     A56.19   Other chlamydial genitourinary infection
       Chlamydial epididymitis
       Chlamydial orchitis

   A56.2   Chlamydial infection of genitourinary tract, unspecified

   A56.3   Chlamydial infection of anus and rectum

   A56.4   Chlamydial infection of pharynx

   A56.8   Sexually transmitted chlamydial infection of other sites

A57   Chancroid
   Ulcus molle

A58   Granuloma inguinale
   Donovanosis

A59   Trichomoniasis ✓4th
   EXCLUDES 2   intestinal trichomoniasis (A07.8)

   ✓5th **A59.0   Urogenital** trichomoniasis

     A59.00   Urogenital trichomoniasis, unspecified
       Fluor (vaginalis) due to Trichomonas
       Leukorrhea (vaginalis) due to Trichomonas

     A59.01   Trichomonal vulvovaginitis   ♀

     A59.02   Trichomonal prostatitis   ♂

     A59.03   Trichomonal cystitis and urethritis

     A59.09   Other urogenital trichomoniasis
       Trichomonas cervicitis

   A59.8   Trichomoniasis of other sites

   A59.9   Trichomoniasis, unspecified

A60   Anogenital herpesviral [herpes simplex] infections ✓4th

   ✓5th **A60.0   Herpesviral infection of** genitalia and urogenital tract

     A60.00   Herpesviral infection of urogenital system, unspecified   HIV

     A60.01   Herpesviral infection of penis   HIV ♂

     A60.02   Herpesviral infection of other male genital organs   ♂

     A60.03   Herpesviral cervicitis   ♀

     A60.04   Herpesviral vulvovaginitis   HIV ♀
       Herpesviral [herpes simplex] ulceration
       Herpesviral [herpes simplex] vaginitis
       Herpesviral [herpes simplex] vulvitis

     A60.09   Herpesviral infection of other urogenital tract   HIV

   A60.1   Herpesviral infection of perianal skin and rectum   HIV

   A60.9   Anogenital herpesviral infection, unspecified   HIV

N Newborn: 0   P Pediatric: 0-17   M Maternity: 12-55   A Adult: 15-124   MCC Major CC Condition   PDxMCC PDx acts as own MCC   CC CC Condition   PDxCC PDx acts as own CC

444   ICD-10-CM 2018

✓4ᵗʰ A63 Other predominantly sexually transmitted diseases, not elsewhere classified
> EXCLUDES 2   molluscum contagiosum (B08.1)
>   papilloma of cervix (D26.0)

A63.0 Anogenital (venereal) warts
> Anogenital warts due to (human) papillomavirus [HPV]
> Condyloma acuminatum

A63.8 Other specified predominantly sexually transmitted diseases

A64 Unspecified sexually transmitted disease

Other spirochetal diseases (A65-A69)

> EXCLUDES 2   leptospirosis (A27.-)
>   syphilis (A50-A53)

A65 Nonvenereal syphilis
> Bejel
> Endemic syphilis
> Njovera

✓4ᵗʰ A66 Yaws
> INCLUDES   bouba
>   frambesia (tropica)
>   pian

A66.0 Initial lesions of yaws
> Chancre of yaws
> Frambesia, initial or primary
> Initial frambesial ulcer
> Mother yaw

A66.1 Multiple papillomata and wet crab yaws
> Frambesioma
> Pianoma
> Plantar or palmar papilloma of yaws

A66.2 Other early skin lesions of yaws
> Cutaneous yaws, less than five years after infection
> Early yaws (cutaneous) (macular) (maculopapular) (micropapular) (papular)
> Frambeside of early yaws

A66.3 Hyperkeratosis of yaws
> Ghoul hand
> Hyperkeratosis, palmar or plantar (early) (late) due to yaws
> Worm-eaten soles

A66.4 Gummata and ulcers of yaws
> Gummatous frambeside
> Nodular late yaws (ulcerated)

A66.5 Gangosa
> Rhinopharyngitis mutilans

A66.6 Bone and joint lesions of yaws   HCC
> Yaws ganglion
> Yaws goundou
> Yaws gumma, bone
> Yaws gummatous osteitis or periostitis
> Yaws hydrarthrosis
> Yaws osteitis
> Yaws periostitis (hypertrophic)

A66.7 Other manifestations of yaws
> Juxta-articular nodules of yaws
> Mucosal yaws

A66.8 Latent yaws
> Yaws without clinical manifestations, with positive serology

A66.9 Yaws, unspecified

✓4ᵗʰ A67 Pinta [carate]

A67.0 Primary lesions of pinta
> Chancre (primary) of pinta
> Papule (primary) of pinta

A67.1 Intermediate lesions of pinta
> Erythematous plaques of pinta
> Hyperchromic lesions of pinta
> Hyperkeratosis of pinta
> Pintids

A67.2 Late lesions of pinta
> Achromic skin lesions of pinta
> Cicatricial skin lesions of pinta
> Dyschromic skin lesions of pinta

A67.3 Mixed lesions of pinta
> Achromic with hyperchromic skin lesions of pinta [carate]

A67.9 Pinta, unspecified

✓4ᵗʰ A68 Relapsing fevers
> INCLUDES   recurrent fever
> EXCLUDES 2   Lyme disease (A69.2-)

> **CC Excl: For CC codes in category A68: PDX collection 108**

A68.0 Louse-borne relapsing fever   CC
> Relapsing fever due to Borrelia recurrentis

A68.1 Tick-borne relapsing fever   CC
> Relapsing fever due to any Borrelia species other than Borrelia recurrentis

A68.9 Relapsing fever, unspecified   CC

✓4ᵗʰ A69 Other spirochetal infections

A69.0 Necrotizing ulcerative stomatitis
> Cancrum oris   Noma
> Fusospirochetal gangrene   Stomatitis gangrenosa

A69.1 Other Vincent's infections   CC
> Fusospirochetal pharyngitis
> Necrotizing ulcerative (acute) gingivitis
> Necrotizing ulcerative (acute) gingivostomatitis
> Spirochetal stomatitis
> Trench mouth
> Vincent's angina
> Vincent's gingivitis
> **CC Excl: PDX collection 126**

✓5ᵗʰ A69.2 Lyme disease
> Erythema chronicum migrans due to Borrelia burgdorferi
> **DEF:** A recurrent multisystem disorder through tick bites; begins with lesions of erythema chronicum migrans; followed by arthritis of the large joints, myalgia, malaise, and neurological and cardiac manifestations.

> **CC Excl: For CC codes in subcategory A69.2:** PDX collection 108

> **A69.20 Lyme disease, unspecified**   CC
> **A69.21 Meningitis due to Lyme disease**   CC
> **A69.22 Other neurologic disorders in Lyme disease**   CC
> > Cranial neuritis
> > Meningoencephalitis
> > Polyneuropathy
> **A69.23 Arthritis due to Lyme disease**   CC HCC
> **A69.29 Other conditions associated with Lyme disease**   CC
> > Myopericarditis due to Lyme disease
> > **AHA:** 2016, 3Q, 12

A69.8 Other specified spirochetal infections

A69.9 Spirochetal infection, unspecified

Other diseases caused by chlamydiae (A70-A74)

> EXCLUDES 1   sexually transmitted chlamydial diseases (A55-A56)

A70 Chlamydia psittaci infections   CC
> Ornithosis
> Parrot fever
> Psittacosis
> **CC Excl: PDX collection 127**

✓4ᵗʰ A71 Trachoma
> EXCLUDES 1   sequelae of trachoma (B94.0)

A71.0 Initial stage of trachoma
> Trachoma dubium

A71.1 Active stage of trachoma
> Granular conjunctivitis (trachomatous)
> Trachomatous follicular conjunctivitis
> Trachomatous pannus

A71.9 Trachoma, unspecified

✓4ᵗʰ A74 Other diseases caused by chlamydiae
> EXCLUDES 1   neonatal chlamydial conjunctivitis (P39.1)
>   neonatal chlamydial pneumonia (P23.1)
>   Reiter's disease (M02.3-)
>   sexually transmitted chlamydial diseases (A55-A56)
> EXCLUDES 2   chlamydial pneumonia (J16.0)

A74.0 Chlamydial conjunctivitis
> Paratrachoma

✓5ᵗʰ A74.8 Other chlamydial diseases
> **A74.81 Chlamydial peritonitis**
> **A74.89 Other chlamydial diseases**

A74.9 Chlamydial infection, unspecified
> Chlamydiosis NOS

✓ Additional Character Req   ✓x7ᵗʰ Placeholder Alert   Unacceptable PDx   Manifestation   H1 - H14 HAC   HCC CMS-HCC Condition   EXCLUDES 1 Not Coded Here   EXCLUDES 2 Not Included Here

ICD-10-CM 2018   445

Rickettsioses (A75-A79)

✓4th **A75 Typhus fever**
> EXCLUDES 1 *rickettsiosis due to Ehrlichia sennetsu (A79.81)*

> **CC Excl: For CC codes in category A75, unless otherwise noted:** PDX collection 108

A75.0 Epidemic louse-borne typhus fever due to Rickettsia prowazekii   CC
> Classical typhus (fever)
> Epidemic (louse-borne) typhus

A75.1 Recrudescent typhus [Brill's disease]   CC
> Brill-Zinsser disease

A75.2 Typhus fever due to Rickettsia typhi   CC
> Murine (flea-borne) typhus

A75.3 Typhus fever due to Rickettsia tsutsugamushi   CC
> Scrub (mite-borne) typhus
> Tsutsugamushi fever

A75.9 Typhus fever, unspecified   CC
> Typhus (fever) NOS
> **CC Excl:** PDX collection 128

✓4th **A77 Spotted fever [tick-borne rickettsioses]**

> **CC Excl: For CC codes in category A77:** PDX collection 108

A77.0 Spotted fever due to Rickettsia rickettsii   CC
> Rocky Mountain spotted fever
> Sao Paulo fever

A77.1 Spotted fever due to Rickettsia conorii   CC
> African tick typhus
> Boutonneuse fever
> India tick typhus
> Kenya tick typhus
> Marseilles fever
> Mediterranean tick fever

A77.2 Spotted fever due to Rickettsia siberica   CC
> North Asian tick fever
> Siberian tick typhus

A77.3 Spotted fever due to Rickettsia australis   CC
> Queensland tick typhus

✓5th **A77.4 Ehrlichiosis**
> EXCLUDES 1 *Rickettsiosis due to Ehrlichia sennetsu (A79.81)*

A77.40 Ehrlichiosis, unspecified   CC

A77.41 Ehrlichiosis chafeensis [E. chafeensis]   CC

A77.49 Other ehrlichiosis   CC

A77.8 Other spotted fevers   CC

A77.9 Spotted fever, unspecified   CC
> Tick-borne typhus NOS

A78 Q fever   CC
> Infection due to Coxiella burnetii
> Nine Mile fever
> Quadrilateral fever
> **CC Excl:** PDX collection 108

✓4th **A79 Other rickettsioses**

> **CC Excl: For CC codes in category A79, unless otherwise noted:** PDX collection 129

A79.0 Trench fever   CC
> Quintan fever
> Wolhynian fever
> **CC Excl:** PDX collection 108

A79.1 Rickettsialpox due to Rickettsia akari   CC
> Kew Garden fever
> Vesicular rickettsiosis

✓5th **A79.8 Other specified rickettsioses**

A79.81 Rickettsiosis due to Ehrlichia sennetsu   CC

A79.89 Other specified rickettsioses   CC

A79.9 Rickettsiosis, unspecified   CC
> Rickettsial infection NOS

Viral and prion infections of the central nervous system (A80-A89)

> EXCLUDES 1 *postpolio syndrome (G14)*
> *sequelae of poliomyelitis (B91)*
> *sequelae of viral encephalitis (B94.1)*

✓4th **A80 Acute poliomyelitis**

> **CC Excl: For MCC codes in category A80:** PDX collection 130

A80.0 Acute paralytic poliomyelitis, vaccine-associated   MCC

A80.1 Acute paralytic poliomyelitis, wild virus, imported   MCC

A80.2 Acute paralytic poliomyelitis, wild virus, indigenous   MCC

✓5th **A80.3 Acute paralytic poliomyelitis, other and unspecified**

A80.30 Acute paralytic poliomyelitis, unspecified   MCC

A80.39 Other acute paralytic poliomyelitis   MCC

A80.4 Acute nonparalytic poliomyelitis

A80.9 Acute poliomyelitis, unspecified

✓4th **A81 Atypical virus infections of central nervous system**
> INCLUDES diseases of the central nervous system caused by prions
> Use additional code to identify:
> dementia with behavioral disturbance (F02.81)
> dementia without behavioral disturbance (F02.80)

✓5th **A81.0 Creutzfeldt-Jakob disease**

> **CC Excl: For codes in subcategory A81.0:** PDX collection 131

A81.00 Creutzfeldt-Jakob disease, unspecified   CC
> Jakob-Creutzfeldt disease, unspecified

A81.01 Variant Creutzfeldt-Jakob disease   CC
> vCJD

A81.09 Other Creutzfeldt-Jakob disease   CC
> CJD
> Familial Creutzfeldt-Jakob disease
> Iatrogenic Creutzfeldt-Jakob disease
> Sporadic Creutzfeldt-Jakob disease
> Subacute spongiform encephalopathy (with dementia)

A81.1 Subacute sclerosing panencephalitis   CC
> Dawson's inclusion body encephalitis
> Van Bogaert's sclerosing leukoencephalopathy
> **CC Excl:** PDX collection 132

A81.2 Progressive multifocal leukoencephalopathy   HIV CC
> Multifocal leukoencephalopathy NOS
> **CC Excl:** PDX collection 133

✓5th **A81.8 Other atypical virus infections of central nervous system**

A81.81 Kuru   CC
> **CC Excl:** PDX collection 134

A81.82 Gerstmann-Sträussler-Scheinker syndrome   HIV CC
> GSS syndrome
> **CC Excl:** PDX collection 135

A81.83 Fatal familial insomnia   HIV CC
> FFI
> **CC Excl:** PDX collection 135

A81.89 Other atypical virus infections of central nervous system   HIV CC
> **CC Excl:** PDX collection 135

A81.9 Atypical virus infection of central nervous system, unspecified   HIV CC
> Prion diseases of the central nervous system NOS
> **CC Excl:** PDX collection 134

✓4th **A82 Rabies**

> **CC Excl: For CC codes in category A82:** PDX collection 136

A82.0 Sylvatic rabies   CC

A82.1 Urban rabies   CC

A82.9 Rabies, unspecified   CC

✓4th **A83 Mosquito-borne viral encephalitis**
> INCLUDES mosquito-borne viral meningoencephalitis
> EXCLUDES 2 *Venezuelan equine encephalitis (A92.2)*
> *West Nile fever (A92.3-)*
> *West Nile virus (A92.3-)*

> **CC Excl: For MCC codes in category A83:** PDX collection 137

A83.0 Japanese encephalitis   MCC

A83.1 Western equine encephalitis   MCC

A83.2 Eastern equine encephalitis   MCC

A83.3 St Louis encephalitis   MCC

A83.4 Australian encephalitis   MCC
> Kunjin virus disease

A83.5 California encephalitis   MCC
> California meningoencephalitis
> La Crosse encephalitis

A83.6 Rocio virus disease   MCC

A83.8 Other mosquito-borne viral encephalitis   MCC

A83.9 Mosquito-borne viral encephalitis, unspecified   MCC

N Newborn: 0   P Pediatric: 0-17   M Maternity: 12-55   A Adult: 15-124   MCC Major CC Condition   PDxMCC PDx acts as own MCC   CC CC Condition   PDxCC PDx acts as own CC

446   ICD-10-CM 2018

✓4ᵗʰ **A84** **Tick-borne viral encephalitis**
> INCLUDES   tick-borne viral meningoencephalitis

> **CC Excl: For MCC codes in category A84:** PDX collection 137

    A84.0   **Far Eastern tick-borne encephalitis [Russian spring-summer encephalitis]**   `MCC`

    A84.1   **Central European tick-borne encephalitis**   `MCC`

    A84.8   **Other tick-borne viral encephalitis**   `MCC`
       Louping ill
       Powassan virus disease

    A84.9   **Tick-borne viral encephalitis, unspecified**   `MCC`

✓4ᵗʰ **A85** **Other viral encephalitis, not elsewhere classified**
> INCLUDES   specified viral encephalomyelitis NEC
>   specified viral meningoencephalitis NEC
> EXCLUDES 1   benign myalgic encephalomyelitis (G93.3)
>   encephalitis due to cytomegalovirus (B25.8)
>   encephalitis due to herpesvirus NEC (B10.0-)
>   encephalitis due to herpesvirus [herpes simplex] (B00.4)
>   encephalitis due to measles virus (B05.0)
>   encephalitis due to mumps virus (B26.2)
>   encephalitis due to poliomyelitis virus (A80.-)
>   encephalitis due to zoster (B02.0)
>   lymphocytic choriomeningitis (A87.2)

> **CC Excl: For CC codes in category A85, unless otherwise noted:** PDX collection 138

    A85.0   **Enteroviral encephalitis**   `HIV` `CC`
       Enteroviral encephalomyelitis

    A85.1   **Adenoviral encephalitis**   `HIV` `CC`
       Adenoviral meningoencephalitis

    A85.2   **Arthropod-borne viral encephalitis, unspecified**   `MCC`
> EXCLUDES 1   West nile virus with encephalitis (A92.31)
       CC Excl: PDX collection 137

    A85.8   **Other specified viral encephalitis**   `HIV` `CC`
       Encephalitis lethargica
       Von Economo-Cruchet disease

   A86 **Unspecified viral encephalitis**   `HIV` `CC`
       Viral encephalomyelitis NOS
       Viral meningoencephalitis NOS
       CC Excl: PDX collection 139

✓4ᵗʰ **A87** **Viral meningitis**
> EXCLUDES 1   meningitis due to herpesvirus [herpes simplex] (B00.3)
>   meningitis due to measles virus (B05.1)
>   meningitis due to mumps virus (B26.1)
>   meningitis due to poliomyelitis virus (A80.-)
>   meningitis due to zoster (B02.1)

> **CC Excl: For CC codes in category A87, unless otherwise noted:** PDX collection 140

    A87.0   **Enteroviral meningitis**   `CC`
       Coxsackievirus meningitis
       Echovirus meningitis

    A87.1   **Adenoviral meningitis**   `CC`

    A87.2   **Lymphocytic choriomeningitis**   `CC`
       Lymphocytic meningoencephalitis
       CC Excl: PDX collection 141

    A87.8   **Other viral meningitis**   `CC`

    A87.9   **Viral meningitis, unspecified**   `CC`

✓4ᵗʰ **A88** **Other viral infections of central nervous system, not elsewhere classified**
> EXCLUDES 1   viral encephalitis NOS (A86)
>   viral meningitis NOS (A87.9)

    A88.0   **Enteroviral exanthematous fever [Boston exanthem]**   `CC`
       CC Excl: PDX collection 137

    A88.1   **Epidemic vertigo**

    A88.8   **Other specified viral infections of central nervous system**   `HIV` `CC`
       CC Excl: PDX collection 138

   A89 **Unspecified viral infection of central nervous system**   `HIV` `CC`
       CC Excl: PDX collection 139

Arthropod-borne viral fevers and viral hemorrhagic fevers (A90-A99)

   A90 **Dengue fever [classical dengue]**   `CC`
> EXCLUDES 1   dengue hemorrhagic fever (A91)
       AHA: 2016, 3Q, 13
       CC Excl: PDX collection 142

   A91 **Dengue hemorrhagic fever**   `CC`
       CC Excl: PDX collection 143

✓4ᵗʰ **A92** **Other mosquito-borne viral fevers**
> EXCLUDES 1   Ross River disease (B33.1)

    A92.0   **Chikungunya virus disease**   `CC`
       Chikungunya (hemorrhagic) fever
       CC Excl: PDX collection 143

    A92.1   **O'nyong-nyong fever**   `CC`
       CC Excl: PDX collection 144

    A92.2   **Venezuelan equine fever**   `CC`
       Venezuelan equine encephalitis
       Venezuelan equine encephalomyelitis virus disease
       CC Excl: PDX collection 144

✓5ᵗʰ   **A92.3**   **West Nile virus infection**
       West Nile fever
       AHA: 2016, 3Q, 12

> **CC Excl: For MCC codes in subcategory A92.3:** PDX collection 145

      A92.30   **West Nile virus infection, unspecified**   `MCC`
         West Nile fever NOS
         West Nile fever without complications
         West Nile virus NOS

      A92.31   **West Nile virus infection with encephalitis**   `MCC`
         West Nile encephalitis
         West Nile encephalomyelitis

      A92.32   **West Nile virus infection with other neurologic manifestation**   `MCC`
         Use additional code to specify the neurologic manifestation

      A92.39   **West Nile virus infection with other complications**   `MCC`
         Use additional code to specify the other conditions

    A92.4   **Rift Valley fever**   `CC`
       CC Excl: PDX collection 144

    A92.5   **Zika virus disease**   `CC`
       Zika virus fever
       Zika virus infection
       Zika NOS
       CC Excl: PDX collection 144

    A92.8   **Other specified mosquito-borne viral fevers**   `CC`
       CC Excl: PDX collection 144

    A92.9   **Mosquito-borne viral fever, unspecified**   `CC`
       CC Excl: PDX collection 143

✓4ᵗʰ **A93** **Other arthropod-borne viral fevers, not elsewhere classified**

> **CC Excl: For CC codes in category A93, unless otherwise noted:** PDX collection 143

    A93.0   **Oropouche virus disease**   `CC`
       Oropouche fever
       CC Excl: PDX collection 144

    A93.1   **Sandfly fever**   `CC`
       Pappataci fever
       Phlebotomus fever

    A93.2   **Colorado tick fever**   `CC`

    A93.8   **Other specified arthropod-borne viral fevers**   `CC`
       Piry virus disease
       Vesicular stomatitis virus disease [Indiana fever]

   A94 **Unspecified arthropod-borne viral fever**   `CC`
       Arboviral fever NOS
       Arbovirus infection NOS
       CC Excl: PDX collection 143

✓4ᵗʰ **A95** **Yellow fever**

> **CC Excl: For CC codes in category A95:** PDX collection 146

    A95.0   **Sylvatic yellow fever**   `CC`
       Jungle yellow fever

    A95.1   **Urban yellow fever**   `CC`

    A95.9   **Yellow fever, unspecified**   `CC`

✓4ᵗʰ **A96** **Arenaviral hemorrhagic feverr**

> **CC Excl: For CC codes in category A96:** PDX collection 147

    A96.0   **Junin hemorrhagic fever**   `CC`
       Argentinian hemorrhagic fever

    A96.1   **Machupo hemorrhagic fever**   `CC`
       Bolivian hemorrhagic fever

    A96.2   **Lassa fever**

    A96.8   **Other arenaviral hemorrhagic fevers**   `CC`

    A96.9   **Arenaviral hemorrhagic fever, unspecified**   `CC`

✓ Additional Character Req   ✓x7ᵗʰ Placeholder Alert   Unacceptable PDx   Manifestation   H1-H14 HAC   HCC CMS-HCC Condition   EXCLUDES 1 Not Coded Here   EXCLUDES 2 Not Included Here

☑4ᵗʰ A98　Other viral hemorrhagic fevers, not elsewhere classified
　　EXCLUDES 1　chikungunya hemorrhagic fever (A92.0)
　　　　　　　　dengue hemorrhagic fever (A91)

　　　CC Excl: For CC codes in category A98, unless otherwise noted:
　　　PDX collection 143

A98.0　Crimean-Congo hemorrhagic fever　　`CC`
　　　Central Asian hemorrhagic fever

A98.1　Omsk hemorrhagic fever　　`CC`

A98.2　Kyasanur Forest disease　　`CC`

A98.3　Marburg virus disease

A98.4　Ebola virus disease

A98.5　Hemorrhagic fever with renal syndrome　　`CC`
　　　Epidemic hemorrhagic fever
　　　Korean hemorrhagic fever
　　　Russian hemorrhagic fever
　　　Hantaan virus disease
　　　Hantavirus disease with renal manifestations
　　　Nephropathia epidemica
　　　Songo fever
　　　EXCLUDES 1　hantavirus (cardio)-pulmonary syndrome (B33.4)
　　　CC Excl: PDX collection 148

A98.8　Other specified viral hemorrhagic fevers　　`CC`

A99　Unspecified viral hemorrhagic fever　　`CC`
　　　CC Excl: PDX collection 143

Viral infections characterized by skin and mucous membrane lesions (B00-B09)

☑4ᵗʰ B00　Herpesviral [herpes simplex] infections
　　EXCLUDES 1　congenital herpesviral infections (P35.2)
　　EXCLUDES 2　anogenital herpesviral infection (A60.-)
　　　　　　　　gammaherpesviral mononucleosis (B27.0-)
　　　　　　　　herpangina (B08.5)

B00.0　Eczema herpeticum　　`HIV`
　　　Kaposi's varicelliform eruption

B00.1　Herpesviral vesicular dermatitis　　`HIV`
　　　Herpes simplex facialis
　　　Herpes simplex labialis
　　　Herpes simplex otitis externa
　　　Vesicular dermatitis of ear
　　　Vesicular dermatitis of lip

B00.2　Herpesviral gingivostomatitis and pharyngotonsillitis　　`HIV` `CC`
　　　Herpesviral pharyngitis
　　　CC Excl: PDX collection 149

B00.3　Herpesviral meningitis　　`HIV` `MCC`
　　　CC Excl: PDX collection 150

B00.4　Herpesviral encephalitis　　`HIV` `MCC`
　　　Herpesviral meningoencephalitis
　　　Simian B disease
　　　EXCLUDES 1　herpesviral encephalitis due to herpesvirus 6 and 7
　　　　　　　　(B10.01, B10.09)
　　　　　　　　non-simplex herpesviral encephalitis (B10.0-)
　　　CC Excl: PDX collection 151

☑5ᵗʰ B00.5　Herpesviral ocular disease

　　　CC Excl: For CC codes in subcategory B00.5:
　　　PDX collection 152

B00.50　Herpesviral ocular disease, unspecified　　`HIV` `CC`

B00.51　Herpesviral iridocyclitis　　`HIV` `CC`
　　　Herpesviral iritis
　　　Herpesviral uveitis, anterior

B00.52　Herpesviral keratitis　　`HIV` `CC`
　　　Herpesviral keratoconjunctivitis

B00.53　Herpesviral conjunctivitis　　`HIV` `CC`

B00.59　Other herpesviral disease of eye　　`HIV` `CC`
　　　Herpesviral dermatitis of eyelid

B00.7　Disseminated herpesviral disease　　`HIV` `MCC` `HCC`
　　　Herpesviral sepsis
　　　CC Excl: PDX collection 153

☑5ᵗʰ B00.8　Other forms of herpesviral infections

B00.81　Herpesviral hepatitis　　`HIV` `CC`
　　　CC Excl: PDX collection 154

B00.82　Herpes simplex myelitis　　`MCC` `HCC`
　　　CC Excl: PDX collection 155

B00.89　Other herpesviral infection　　`HIV` `CC`
　　　Herpesviral whitlow
　　　CC Excl: PDX collection 156

B00.9　Herpesviral infection, unspecified　　`HIV`
　　　Herpes simplex infection NOS

☑4ᵗʰ B01　Varicella [chickenpox]

B01.0　Varicella meningitis　　`CC`
　　　CC Excl: PDX collection 157

☑5ᵗʰ B01.1　Varicella encephalitis, myelitis and encephalomyelitis
　　　Postchickenpox encephalitis, myelitis and encephalomyelitis

B01.11　Varicella encephalitis and encephalomyelitis　　`MCC`
　　　Postchickenpox encephalitis and encephalomyelitis
　　　CC Excl: PDX collection 158

B01.12　Varicella myelitis　　`MCC` `HCC`
　　　Postchickenpox myelitis
　　　CC Excl: PDX collection 159

B01.2　Varicella pneumonia　　`MCC`
　　　CC Excl: PDX collection 160

☑5ᵗʰ B01.8　Varicella with other complications

B01.81　Varicella keratitis　　`CC`
　　　CC Excl: PDX collection 157

B01.89　Other varicella complications　　`CC`
　　　CC Excl: PDX collection 157

B01.9　Varicella without complication　　`CC`
　　　Varicella NOS
　　　CC Excl: PDX collection 157

☑4ᵗʰ B02　Zoster [herpes zoster]
　　INCLUDES　shingles
　　　　　　　zona

B02.0　Zoster encephalitis　　`HIV` `CC`
　　　Zoster meningoencephalitis
　　　CC Excl: PDX collection 161

B02.1　Zoster meningitis　　`HIV` `MCC`
　　　CC Excl: PDX collection 162

☑5ᵗʰ B02.2　Zoster with other nervous system involvement

　　　CC Excl: For CC codes in subcategory B02.2, unless
　　　otherwise noted: PDX collection 161

B02.21　Postherpetic geniculate ganglionitis　　`HIV` `CC`

B02.22　Postherpetic trigeminal neuralgia　　`HIV` `CC`

B02.23　Postherpetic polyneuropathy　　`HIV` `CC`

B02.24　Postherpetic myelitis　　`MCC` `HCC`
　　　Herpes zoster myelitis
　　　CC Excl: PDX collection 163

B02.29　Other postherpetic nervous system involvement　　`HIV` `CC`
　　　Postherpetic radiculopathy

☑5ᵗʰ B02.3　Zoster ocular disease

　　　CC Excl: For CC codes in subcategory B02.3:
　　　PDX collection 164

B02.30　Zoster ocular disease, unspecified　　`HIV` `CC`

B02.31　Zoster conjunctivitis　　`HIV` `CC`

B02.32　Zoster iridocyclitis　　`HIV` `CC`

B02.33　Zoster keratitis　　`HIV` `CC`
　　　Herpes zoster keratoconjunctivitis

B02.34　Zoster scleritis　　`HIV` `CC`

B02.39　Other herpes zoster eye disease　　`HIV` `CC`
　　　Zoster blepharitis

B02.7　Disseminated zoster　　`HIV` `CC`
　　　CC Excl: PDX collection 165

B02.8　Zoster with other complications　　`HIV` `CC`
　　　Herpes zoster otitis externa
　　　CC Excl: PDX collection 165

B02.9　Zoster without complications　　`HIV`
　　　Zoster NOS

B03　Smallpox　　`CC`
　　　NOTE　In 1980 the 33rd World Health Assembly declared that
　　　　　　smallpox had been eradicated.
　　　　　　The classification is maintained for surveillance purposes.
　　　CC Excl: PDX collection 166

B04　Monkeypox　　`CC`
　　　CC Excl: PDX collection 167

☑4ᵗʰ B05　Measles
　　INCLUDES　morbilli
　　EXCLUDES 1　subacute sclerosing panencephalitis (A81.1)

B05.0　Measles complicated by encephalitis　　`MCC`
　　　Postmeasles encephalitis
　　　CC Excl: PDX collection 168

B05.1　Measles complicated by meningitis　　`CC`
　　　Postmeasles meningitis
　　　CC Excl: PDX collection 169

`N` Newborn: 0　`P` Pediatric: 0-17　`M` Maternity: 12-55　`A` Adult: 15-124　`MCC` Major CC Condition　`PDxMCC` PDx acts as own MCC　`CC` CC Condition　`PDxCC` PDx acts as own CC

448　　　　　　　　　　　　　　　　　　　　　　　　　　　　　　　　　　　　ICD-10-CM 2018

B05.2 Measles complicated by pneumonia `MCC`
Postmeasles pneumonia
CC Excl: PDX collection 170

B05.3 Measles complicated by otitis media
Postmeasles otitis media

B05.4 Measles with intestinal complications `CC`
CC Excl: PDX collection 169

✓5th **B05.8 Measles with other complications**

    B05.81 Measles keratitis and keratoconjunctivitis `CC`
    CC Excl: PDX collection 171

    B05.89 Other measles complications `CC`
    CC Excl: PDX collection 169

B05.9 Measles without complication
Measles NOS

✓4th **B06 Rubella [German measles]**
    EXCLUDES 1   congenital rubella (P35.0)

✓5th **B06.0 Rubella with neurological complications**

    CC Excl: For CC/MCC codes in subcategory B06.0:
    PDX collection 172

    B06.00 Rubella with neurological complication, unspecified `CC`

    B06.01 Rubella encephalitis `MCC`
    Rubella meningoencephalitis

    B06.02 Rubella meningitis `CC`

    B06.09 Other neurological complications of rubella `CC`

✓5th **B06.8 Rubella with other complications**

    B06.81 Rubella pneumonia `CC`
    CC Excl: PDX collection 172

    B06.82 Rubella arthritis `CC` `HCC`
    CC Excl: PDX collection 173

    B06.89 Other rubella complications `CC`
    CC Excl: PDX collection 172

B06.9 Rubella without complication
Rubella NOS

✓4th **B07 Viral warts**
    INCLUDES   verruca simplex
               verruca vulgaris
               viral warts due to human papillomavirus
    EXCLUDES 2   anogenital (venereal) warts (A63.0)
               papilloma of bladder (D41.4)
               papilloma of cervix (D26.0)
               papilloma larynx (D14.1)

B07.0 Plantar wart
Verruca plantaris

B07.8 Other viral warts
Common wart
Flat wart
Verruca plana

B07.9 Viral wart, unspecified

✓4th **B08 Other viral infections characterized by skin and mucous membrane lesions, not elsewhere classified**
    EXCLUDES 1   vesicular stomatitis virus disease (A93.8)

✓5th **B08.0 Other orthopoxvirus infections**
    EXCLUDES 2   monkeypox (B04)

    ✓6th **B08.01 Cowpox and vaccinia not from vaccine**
        B08.010 Cowpox
        DEF: A disease contracted by milking infected cows; vesicles usually appear on the fingers, hands and adjacent areas and usually disappear without scarring; other symptoms: local edema, lymphangitis, and regional lymphadenitis with or without fever.

        B08.011 Vaccinia not from vaccine
        EXCLUDES 1   vaccinia (from vaccination) (generalized) (T88.1)

    B08.02 Orf virus disease
    Contagious pustular dermatitis
    Ecthyma contagiosum

    B08.03 Pseudocowpox [milker's node]

    B08.04 Paravaccinia, unspecified

    B08.09 Other orthopoxvirus infections
    Orthopoxvirus infection NOS

B08.1 Molluscum contagiosum
DEF: Benign poxvirus infection causing small bumps on the skin or conjunctiva; transmitted by close contact.

✓5th **B08.2 Exanthema subitum [sixth disease]**
Roseola infantum

    B08.20 Exanthema subitum [sixth disease], unspecified `P`
    Roseola infantum, unspecified

    B08.21 Exanthema subitum [sixth disease] due to human herpesvirus 6 `P`
    Roseola infantum due to human herpesvirus 6

    B08.22 Exanthema subitum [sixth disease] due to human herpesvirus 7 `P`
    Roseola infantum due to human herpesvirus 7

B08.3 Erythema infectiosum [fifth disease] `CC`
CC Excl: PDX collection 174

B08.4 Enteroviral vesicular stomatitis with exanthem
Hand, foot and mouth disease

B08.5 Enteroviral vesicular pharyngitis
Herpangina
DEF: Acute infectious Coxsackie virus infection causing throat lesions, fever, and vomiting; generally affects children in summer.

✓5th **B08.6 Parapoxvirus infections**

    B08.60 Parapoxvirus infection, unspecified

    B08.61 Bovine stomatitis

    B08.62 Sealpox

    B08.69 Other parapoxvirus infections

✓5th **B08.7 Yatapoxvirus infections**

    B08.70 Yatapoxvirus infection, unspecified

    B08.71 Tanapox virus disease `CC`
    CC Excl: PDX collection 167

    B08.72 Yaba pox virus disease
    Yaba monkey tumor disease

    B08.79 Other yatapoxvirus infections

B08.8 Other specified viral infections characterized by skin and mucous membrane lesions
Enteroviral lymphonodular pharyngitis
Foot-and-mouth disease
Poxvirus NEC

B09 Unspecified viral infection characterized by skin and mucous membrane lesions
Viral enanthema NOS
Viral exanthema NOS

Other human herpesviruses (B10)

✓4th **B10 Other human herpesviruses**
    EXCLUDES 2   cytomegalovirus (B25.9)
               Epstein-Barr virus (B27.0-)
               herpes NOS (B00.9)
               herpes simplex (B00.-)
               herpes zoster (B02.-)
               human herpesvirus NOS (B00.-)
               human herpesvirus 1 and 2 (B00.-)
               human herpesvirus 3 (B01.-, B02.-)
               human herpesvirus 4 (B27.0-)
               human herpesvirus 5 (B25.-)
               varicella (B01.-)
               zoster (B02.-)

✓5th **B10.0 Other human herpesvirus encephalitis**
    EXCLUDES 2   herpes encephalitis NOS (B00.4)
               herpes simplex encephalitis (B00.4)
               human herpesvirus encephalitis (B00.4)
               simian B herpes virus encephalitis (B00.4)

    B10.01 Human herpesvirus 6 encephalitis `HIV` `MCC`
    CC Excl: PDX collection 151

    B10.09 Other human herpesvirus encephalitis `HIV` `MCC`
    Human herpesvirus 7 encephalitis
    CC Excl: PDX collection 151

✓5th **B10.8 Other human herpesvirus infection**

    B10.81 Human herpesvirus 6 infection

    B10.82 Human herpesvirus 7 infection

    B10.89 Other human herpesvirus infection
    Human herpesvirus 8 infection
    Kaposi's sarcoma-associated herpesvirus infection

✓Additional Character Req   ✓x7th Placeholder Alert   Unacceptable PDx   Manifestation   H1-H14 HAC   HCC CMS-HCC Condition   EXCLUDES 1 Not Coded Here   EXCLUDES 2 Not Included Here

ICD-10-CM 2018   449

Chapter 1. Certain Infectious and Parasitic Diseases

Viral hepatitis (B15-B19)

EXCLUDES 1   sequelae of viral hepatitis (B94.2)
EXCLUDES 2   cytomegaloviral hepatitis (B25.1)
     herpesviral [herpes simplex] hepatitis (B00.81)

DEF: Hepatitis A: HAV infection is self-limiting with flulike symptoms; transmission, fecal-oral.
DEF: Hepatitis B: HBV infection can be chronic and systemic; transmission, bodily fluids.
DEF: Hepatitis C: HCV infection can be chronic and systemic; transmission, blood transfusion and unidentified agents.
DEF: Hepatitis D (delta): HDV occurs only in the presence of hepatitis B virus; transmission, contaminated blood in contact with mucous membranes.
DEF: Hepatitis E: HEV is epidemic form; transmission, fecal-oral, most often from contaminated water.

✓4th **B15**   **Acute hepatitis A**

     B15.0   **Hepatitis A with hepatic coma**   MCC
         CC Excl: PDX collection 175

     B15.9   **Hepatitis A without hepatic coma**   CC
         Hepatitis A (acute)(viral) NOS
         CC Excl: PDX collection 175

✓4th **B16**   **Acute hepatitis B**
     AHA: 2016, 3Q, 13

     CC Excl: For CC/MCC codes in category B16: PDX collection 175

     B16.0   **Acute hepatitis B with delta-agent with hepatic coma**   MCC
     B16.1   **Acute hepatitis B with delta-agent without hepatic coma**   CC
     B16.2   **Acute hepatitis B without delta-agent with hepatic coma**   MCC
     B16.9   **Acute hepatitis B without delta-agent and without hepatic coma**   CC
         Hepatitis B (acute) (viral) NOS

✓4th **B17**   **Other acute viral hepatitis**

     CC Excl: For CC/MCC codes in category B17: PDX collection 175

     B17.0   **Acute delta-(super) infection of hepatitis B carrier**   CC
✓5th   **B17.1**   **Acute hepatitis C**   CC
         B17.10   **Acute hepatitis C without hepatic coma**   CC
             Acute hepatitis C NOS
         B17.11   **Acute hepatitis C with hepatic coma**   MCC
     B17.2   **Acute hepatitis E**   CC
     B17.8   **Other specified acute viral hepatitis**   CC
         Hepatitis non-A non-B (acute) (viral) NEC
     B17.9   **Acute viral hepatitis, unspecified**   CC
         Acute hepatitis NOS
         Acute infectious hepatitis NOSb

✓4th **B18**   **Chronic viral hepatitis**
     INCLUDES   carrier of viral hepatitis
     AHA: 2017, 1Q, 41

     CC Excl: For CC codes in category B18: PDX collection 175

     B18.0   **Chronic viral hepatitis B with delta-agent**   CC HCC
     B18.1   **Chronic viral hepatitis B without delta-agent**   CC HCC
         Carrier of viral hepatitis B
         Chronic (viral) hepatitis B
     B18.2   **Chronic viral hepatitis C**   HCC
         Carrier of viral hepatitis C
     B18.8   **Other chronic viral hepatitis**   CC HCC
         Carrier of other viral hepatitis
     B18.9   **Chronic viral hepatitis, unspecified**   CC HCC
         Carrier of unspecified viral hepatitis

✓4th **B19**   **Unspecified viral hepatitis**

     CC Excl: For CC/MCC codes in category B19: PDX collection 175

     B19.0   **Unspecified viral hepatitis with hepatic coma**   MCC
✓5th   **B19.1**   **Unspecified viral hepatitis B**
         B19.10   **Unspecified viral hepatitis B without hepatic coma**   CC
             Unspecified viral hepatitis B NOS
         B19.11   **Unspecified viral hepatitis B with hepatic coma**   MCC
✓5th   **B19.2**   **Unspecified viral hepatitis C**
         B19.20   **Unspecified viral hepatitis C without hepatic coma**
             Viral hepatitis C NOS
         B19.21   **Unspecified viral hepatitis C with hepatic coma**   MCC
     B19.9   **Unspecified viral hepatitis without hepatic coma**   CC
         Viral hepatitis NOS

Human immunodeficiency virus [HIV] disease (B20)

B20   **Human immunodeficiency virus [HIV] disease**   MCC HCC
     INCLUDES   acquired immune deficiency syndrome [AIDS]
         AIDS-related complex [ARC]
         HIV infection, symptomatic
     Code first human immunodeficiency virus [HIV] disease complicating pregnancy, childbirth and the puerperium, if applicable (O98.7-)
     Use additional code(s) to identify all manifestations of HIV infection
     EXCLUDES 1   asymptomatic human immunodeficiency virus [HIV] infection status (Z21)
         exposure to HIV virus (Z20.6)
         inconclusive serologic evidence of HIV (R75)
     CC Excl: PDX collection 176

Other viral diseases (B25-B34)

✓4th **B25**   **Cytomegaloviral disease**
     EXCLUDES 1   congenital cytomegalovirus infection (P35.1)
         cytomegaloviral mononucleosis (B27.1-)

     B25.0   **Cytomegaloviral pneumonitis**   PDxMCC MCC HCC
         CC Excl: PDX collection 110
     B25.1   **Cytomegaloviral hepatitis**   PDxCC CC HCC
         CC Excl: No Excl
     B25.2   **Cytomegaloviral pancreatitis**   PDxMCC MCC HCC
         CC Excl: PDX collection 177
     B25.8   **Other cytomegaloviral diseases**   HIV CC HCC
         Cytomegaloviral encephalitis
         CC Excl: PDX collection 178
     B25.9   **Cytomegaloviral disease, unspecified**   HIV CC HCC
         CC Excl: PDX collection 178

✓4th **B26**   **Mumps**
     INCLUDES   epidemic parotitis
         infectious parotitis

     B26.0   **Mumps orchitis**   CC ♂
         CC Excl: PDX collection 179
     B26.1   **Mumps meningitis**   MCC
         CC Excl: PDX collection 180
     B26.2   **Mumps encephalitis**   MCC
         CC Excl: PDX collection 181
     B26.3   **Mumps pancreatitis**   CC
         CC Excl: PDX collection 182
✓5th   **B26.8**   **Mumps with other complications**
         B26.81   **Mumps hepatitis**   CC
             CC Excl: PDX collection 183
         B26.82   **Mumps myocarditis**   CC
             CC Excl: PDX collection 184
         B26.83   **Mumps nephritis**   CC
             CC Excl: PDX collection 184
         B26.84   **Mumps polyneuropathy**   CC
             CC Excl: PDX collection 185
         B26.85   **Mumps arthritis**   CC HCC
             CC Excl: PDX collection 184
         B26.89   **Other mumps complications**   CC
             CC Excl: PDX collection 184
     B26.9   **Mumps without complication**
         Mumps NOS
         Mumps parotitis NOS

✓4th **B27**   **Infectious mononucleosis**
     INCLUDES   glandular fever
         monocytic angina
         Pfeiffer's disease

✓5th   **B27.0**   **Gammaherpesviral mononucleosis**
         Mononucleosis due to Epstein-Barr virus
         B27.00   **Gammaherpesviral mononucleosis without complication**
         B27.01   **Gammaherpesviral mononucleosis with polyneuropathy**
         B27.02   **Gammaherpesviral mononucleosis with meningitis**
         B27.09   **Gammaherpesviral mononucleosis with other complications**
             Hepatomegaly in gammaherpesviral mononucleosis

N Newborn: 0   P Pediatric: 0-17   M Maternity: 12-55   A Adult: 15-124   MCC Major CC Condition   PDxMCC PDx acts as own MCC   CC CC Condition   PDxCC PDx acts as own CC

450   ICD-10-CM 2018

☑5ᵗʰ **B27.1** **Cytomegaloviral mononucleosis**

    B27.10 **Cytomegaloviral mononucleosis** without complications

    B27.11 **Cytomegaloviral mononucleosis** with polyneuropathy

    B27.12 **Cytomegaloviral mononucleosis** with meningitis

    B27.19 **Cytomegaloviral mononucleosis** with other complication
        Hepatomegaly in cytomegaloviral mononucleosis

☑5ᵗʰ **B27.8** **Other infectious mononucleosis**

    B27.80 **Other infectious mononucleosis** without complication

    B27.81 **Other infectious mononucleosis** with polyneuropathy

    B27.82 **Other infectious mononucleosis** with meningitis

    B27.89 **Other infectious mononucleosis with** other complication
        Hepatomegaly in other infectious mononucleosis

☑5ᵗʰ **B27.9** **Infectious mononucleosis, unspecified**

    B27.90 **Infectious mononucleosis, unspecified** without complication

    B27.91 **Infectious mononucleosis, unspecified** with polyneuropathy

    B27.92 **Infectious mononucleosis, unspecified** with meningitis

    B27.99 **Infectious mononucleosis, unspecified** with other complication
        Hepatomegaly in unspecified infectious mononucleosis

☑4ᵗʰ **B30** **Viral conjunctivitis**

    EXCLUDES 1   *herpesviral [herpes simplex] ocular disease (B00.5)*
            ocular zoster (B02.3)

    B30.0 **Keratoconjunctivitis due to adenovirus**
        Epidemic keratoconjunctivitis
        Shipyard eye

    B30.1 **Conjunctivitis due to adenovirus**
        Acute adenoviral follicular conjunctivitis
        Swimming-pool conjunctivitis

    B30.2 **Viral pharyngoconjunctivitis**

    B30.3 **Acute epidemic hemorrhagic conjunctivitis (enteroviral)**
        Conjunctivitis due to coxsackievirus 24
        Conjunctivitis due to enterovirus 70
        Hemorrhagic conjunctivitis (acute)(epidemic)

    B30.8 **Other viral conjunctivitis**
        Newcastle conjunctivitis

    B30.9 **Viral conjunctivitis, unspecified**

☑4ᵗʰ **B33** **Other viral diseases, not elsewhere classified**

    B33.0 **Epidemic myalgia**
        Bornholm disease

    B33.1 **Ross River disease**   `CC`
        Epidemic polyarthritis and exanthema
        Ross River fever
        CC Excl: PDX collection 144

Viral Conjunctivitis

Normal conjunctiva

Inflamed conjunctiva

☑5ᵗʰ **B33.2** **Viral carditis**
    Coxsackie (virus) carditis

    B33.20 **Viral carditis, unspecified**   `CC`
        CC Excl: PDX collection 186

    B33.21 **Viral endocarditis**   `CC`
        CC Excl: PDX collection 187

    B33.22 **Viral myocarditis**   `CC`
        CC Excl: PDX collection 186

    B33.23 **Viral pericarditis**   `CC`
        CC Excl: PDX collection 188

    B33.24 **Viral cardiomyopathy**   `HCC`

    B33.3 **Retrovirus infections, not elsewhere classified**
        Retrovirus infection NOS

    B33.4 **Hantavirus (cardio)-pulmonary syndrome [HPS] [HCPS]**   `CC`
        Hantavirus disease with pulmonary manifestations
        Sin nombre virus disease
        Use additional code to identify any associated acute kidney failure (N17.9)
        EXCLUDES 1 *hantavirus disease with renal manifestations (A98.5)*
               hemorrhagic fever with renal manifestations (A98.5)
        CC Excl: PDX collection 189

    B33.8 **Other specified viral diseases**
        EXCLUDES 1 *anogenital human papillomavirus infection (A63.0)*
               viral warts due to human papillomavirus infection (B07)

☑4ᵗʰ **B34** **Viral infection of unspecified site**

    EXCLUDES 1 *anogenital human papillomavirus infection (A63.0)*
           cytomegaloviral disease NOS (B25.9)
           herpesvirus [herpes simplex] infection NOS (B00.9)
           retrovirus infection NOS (B33.3)
           viral agents as the cause of diseases classified elsewhere (B97.-)
           viral warts due to human papillomavirus infection (B07)

    B34.0 **Adenovirus infection, unspecified**

    B34.1 **Enterovirus infection, unspecified**
        Coxsackievirus infection NOS
        Echovirus infection NOS

    B34.2 **Coronavirus infection, unspecified**
        EXCLUDES 1 *pneumonia due to SARS-associated coronavirus (J12.81)*

    B34.3 **Parvovirus infection, unspecified**   `CC`
        CC Excl: PDX collection 174

    B34.4 **Papovavirus infection, unspecified**

    B34.8 **Other viral infections of unspecified site**

    B34.9 **Viral infection, unspecified**
        Viremia NOS
        AHA: 2016, 3Q, 10

Mycoses (B35-B49)

    EXCLUDES 2 *hypersensitivity pneumonitis due to organic dust (J67.-)*
           mycosis fungoides (C84.0-)

☑4ᵗʰ **B35** **Dermatophytosis**

    INCLUDES favus
           infections due to species of Epidermophyton, Micro-sporum and Trichophyton
           tinea, any type except those in B36-
    DEF: Contagious superficial fungal infection of the skin that invades and grows in dead keratin.

    B35.0 **Tinea barbae and tinea capitis**
        Beard ringworm
        Kerion
        Scalp ringworm
        Sycosis, mycotic

    B35.1 **Tinea unguium**
        Dermatophytic onychia
        Dermatophytosis of nail
        Onychomycosis
        Ringworm of nails

    B35.2 **Tinea manuum**
        Dermatophytosis of hand
        Hand ringworm

    B35.3 **Tinea pedis**
        Athlete's foot
        Dermatophytosis of foot
        Foot ringworm

    B35.4 **Tinea corporis**
        Ringworm of the body

    B35.5 **Tinea imbricata**
        Tokelau

☑ Additional Character Req   ☑7ᵗʰ Placeholder Alert   Unacceptable PDx   Manifestation   `H1`-`H14` HAC   `HCC` CMS-HCC Condition   *EXCLUDES 1* Not Coded Here   *EXCLUDES 2* Not Included Here

ICD-10-CM 2018   **451**

B27.1–B35.5

B35.6   Tinea cruris
    Dhobi itch
    Groin ringworm
    Jock itch

B35.8   Other dermatophytoses
    Disseminated dermatophytosis
    Granulomatous dermatophytosis

B35.9   Dermatophytosis, unspecified
    Ringworm NOS

✓4th B36   Other superficial mycoses

B36.0   Pityriasis versicolor
    Tinea flava
    Tinea versicolor

B36.1   Tinea nigra
    Keratomycosis nigricans palmaris
    Microsporosis nigra
    Pityriasis nigra

B36.2   White piedra
    Tinea blanca

B36.3   Black piedra

B36.8   Other specified superficial mycoses

B36.9   Superficial mycosis, unspecified

✓4th B37   Candidiasis
    INCLUDES   candidosis
              moniliasis
    EXCLUDES 1   neonatal candidiasis (P37.5)

B37.0   Candidal stomatitis   HIV CC
    Oral thrush
    CC Excl: PDX collection 190

B37.1   Pulmonary candidiasis   HIV MCC HCC
    Candidal bronchitis
    Candidal pneumonia
    CC Excl: PDX collection 190

B37.2   Candidiasis of skin and nail   HIV
    Candidal onychia
    Candidal paronychia
    EXCLUDES 2   diaper dermatitis (L22)

B37.3   Candidiasis of vulva and vagina   ♀
    Candidal vulvovaginitis
    Monilial vulvovaginitis
    Vaginal thrush

✓5th B37.4   Candidiasis of other urogenital sites

    B37.41   Candidal cystitis and urethritis   CC H6
        CC Excl: PDX collection 191

    B37.42   Candidal balanitis   ♂

    B37.49   Other urogenital candidiasis   CC H6
        Candidal pyelonephritis
        CC Excl: PDX collection 191

B37.5   Candidal meningitis   HIV MCC
    CC Excl: PDX collection 192

B37.6   Candidal endocarditis   HIV MCC
    CC Excl: PDX collection 190

B37.7   Candidal sepsis   PDxMCC MCC HCC
    Disseminated candidiasis
    Systemic candidiasis
    AHA: 2014, 4Q, 46
    CC Excl: PDX collection 193

✓5th B37.8   Candidiasis of other sites

    CC Excl: For CC codes in subcategory B37.8, unless otherwise noted: PDX collection 190

    B37.81   Candidal esophagitis   HIV CC HCC

    B37.82   Candidal enteritis   HIV CC
        Candidal proctitis

    B37.83   Candidal cheilitis   HIV CC

    B37.84   Candidal otitis externa   HIV CC

    B37.89   Other sites of candidiasis   HIV CC
        Candidal osteomyelitis
        CC Excl: PDX collection 194

B37.9   Candidiasis, unspecified   HIV
    Thrush NOS

✓4th B38   Coccidioidomycosis

B38.0   Acute pulmonary coccidioidomycosis   HIV CC HCC
    CC Excl: PDX collection 195

B38.1   Chronic pulmonary coccidioidomycosis   HIV CC HCC
    CC Excl: PDX collection 195

B38.2   Pulmonary coccidioidomycosis, unspecified   HIV CC HCC
    CC Excl: PDX collection 196

B38.3   Cutaneous coccidioidomycosis   HIV CC
    CC Excl: PDX collection 197

B38.4   Coccidioidomycosis meningitis   HIV MCC
    DEF: *Coccidioides immitis* infection of the lining of the brain and/or spinal cord.
    CC Excl: PDX collection 198

B38.7   Disseminated coccidioidomycosis   HIV CC
    Generalized coccidioidomycosis
    CC Excl: PDX collection 199

✓5th B38.8   Other forms of coccidioidomycosis

    B38.81   Prostatic coccidioidomycosis   HIV CC ♂
        CC Excl: PDX collection 197

    B38.89   Other forms of coccidioidomycosis   HIV CC
        CC Excl: PDX collection 199

B38.9   Coccidioidomycosis, unspecified   HIV CC
    CC Excl: PDX collection 199

✓4th B39   Histoplasmosis
    Code first associated AIDS (B20)
    Use additional code for any associated manifestations, such as:
       endocarditis (I39)
       meningitis (G02)
       pericarditis (I32)
       retinititis (H32)
    DEF: Type of lung infection caused by breathing in fungal spores often found in the droppings of bats and birds or soil contaminated by their droppings.

    CC Excl: For MCC codes in category B39, unless otherwise noted: PDX collection 200

B39.0   Acute pulmonary histoplasmosis capsulati   HIV MCC HCC

B39.1   Chronic pulmonary histoplasmosis capsulati   HIV MCC HCC

B39.2   Pulmonary histoplasmosis capsulati, unspecified   HIV MCC HCC

B39.3   Disseminated histoplasmosis capsulati   HIV CC
    Generalized histoplasmosis capsulati
    CC Excl: PDX collection 201

B39.4   Histoplasmosis capsulati, unspecified   HIV
    American histoplasmosis

B39.5   Histoplasmosis duboisii   HIV
    African histoplasmosis

B39.9   Histoplasmosis, unspecified   HIV

✓4th B40   Blastomycosis
    EXCLUDES 1   Brazilian blastomycosis (B41.-)
               keloidal blastomycosis (B48.0)

    CC Excl: For CC codes in category B40: PDX collection 202

B40.0   Acute pulmonary blastomycosis   CC HCC

B40.1   Chronic pulmonary blastomycosis   CC HCC

B40.2   Pulmonary blastomycosis, unspecified   CC HCC

B40.3   Cutaneous blastomycosis   CC

Histoplasmosis

Histoplasma capsulatum spores

Spores

N Newborn: 0   P Pediatric: 0–17   M Maternity: 12–55   A Adult: 15–124   MCC Major CC Condition   PDxMCC PDx acts as own MCC   CC CC Condition   PDxCC PDx acts as own CC

452   ICD-10-CM 2018

B40.7 Disseminated **blastomycosis**   `CC`
    Generalized blastomycosis

☑5ᵗʰ **B40.8** Other **forms of blastomycosis**

    B40.81 **Blastomycotic** meningoencephalitis   `CC`
        Meningomyelitis due to blastomycosis

    B40.89 Other **forms of blastomycosis**   `CC`

B40.9 **Blastomycosis,** unspecified   `CC`

☑4ᵗʰ **B41** **Paracoccidioidomycosis**
    `INCLUDES` Brazilian blastomycosis
           Lutz' disease

    CC Excl: For CC codes in category B41: PDX collection 203

B41.0 Pulmonary **paracoccidioidomycosis**   `CC` `HCC`

B41.7 Disseminated **paracoccidioidomycosis**   `CC`
    Generalized paracoccidioidomycosis

B41.8 Other **forms of paracoccidioidomycosis**   `CC`

B41.9 **Paracoccidioidomycosis,** unspecified   `CC`

☑4ᵗʰ **B42** **Sporotrichosis**

B42.0 Pulmonary **sporotrichosis**

B42.1 Lymphocutaneous **sporotrichosis**

B42.7 Disseminated **sporotrichosis**
    Generalized sporotrichosis

☑5ᵗʰ **B42.8** Other **forms of sporotrichosis**

    B42.81 Cerebral **sporotrichosis**
        Meningitis due to sporotrichosis

    B42.82 **Sporotrichosis** arthritis   `HCC`

    B42.89 Other **forms of sporotrichosis**

B42.9 **Sporotrichosis,** unspecified

☑4ᵗʰ **B43** **Chromomycosis and pheomycotic abscess**

B43.0 Cutaneous **chromomycosis**
    Dermatitis verrucosa

B43.1 **Pheomycotic** brain abscess
    Cerebral chromomycosis

B43.2 Subcutaneous **pheomycotic** abscess and cyst

B43.8 Other **forms of chromomycosis**

B43.9 **Chromomycosis,** unspecified

☑4ᵗʰ **B44** **Aspergillosis**
    `INCLUDES` aspergilloma

    CC Excl: For CC codes in category B44, unless otherwise noted: PDX collection 204

B44.0 Invasive pulmonary **aspergillosis**   `PDxMCC` `MCC` `HCC`
    CC Excl: PDX collection 110

B44.1 Other pulmonary **aspergillosis**   `CC` `HCC`

B44.2 Tonsillar **aspergillosis**   `CC` `HCC`

B44.7 Disseminated **aspergillosis**   `CC` `HCC`
    Generalized aspergillosis

☑5ᵗʰ **B44.8** Other **forms of aspergillosis**

    B44.81 Allergic bronchopulmonary **aspergillosis**   `CC` `HCC`
        CC Excl: PDX collection 205

    B44.89 Other **forms of aspergillosis**   `CC` `HCC`

B44.9 **Aspergillosis,** unspecified   `CC` `HCC`

☑4ᵗʰ **B45** **Cryptococcosis**

    CC Excl: For CC codes in category B45, unless otherwise noted: PDX collection 206

B45.0 Pulmonary **cryptococcosis**   `HIV` `CC` `HCC`

B45.1 Cerebral **cryptococcosis**   `PDxMCC` `MCC` `HCC`
    Cryptococcal meningitis
    Cryptococcosis meningocerebralis
    CC Excl: PDX collection 207

B45.2 Cutaneous **cryptococcosis**   `HIV` `CC` `HCC`

B45.3 Osseous **cryptococcosis**   `HIV` `CC` `HCC`

B45.7 Disseminated **cryptococcosis**   `HIV` `CC` `HCC`
    Generalized cryptococcosis

B45.8 Other **forms of cryptococcosis**   `HIV` `CC` `HCC`

B45.9 **Cryptococcosis,** unspecified   `HIV` `CC` `HCC`

☑4ᵗʰ **B46** **Zygomycosis**

    CC Excl: For MCC codes in category B46: PDX collection 208

B46.0 Pulmonary **mucormycosis**   `MCC` `HCC`

B46.1 Rhinocerebral **mucormycosis**   `MCC` `HCC`

B46.2 Gastrointestinal **mucormycosis**   `MCC` `HCC`

B46.3 Cutaneous **mucormycosis**   `MCC` `HCC`
    Subcutaneous mucormycosis

B46.4 Disseminated **mucormycosis**   `MCC` `HCC`
    Generalized mucormycosis

B46.5 **Mucormycosis,** unspecified   `MCC` `HCC`

B46.8 Other **zygomycoses**   `MCC` `HCC`
    Entomophthoromycosis

B46.9 **Zygomycosis,** unspecified   `MCC` `HCC`
    Phycomycosis NOS

☑4ᵗʰ **B47** **Mycetoma**

B47.0 **Eumycetoma**   `CC`
    Madura foot, mycotic
    Maduromycosis
    CC Excl: PDX collection 209

B47.1 **Actinomycetoma**   `HIV` `CC`
    CC Excl: PDX collection 106

B47.9 **Mycetoma,** unspecified   `HIV` `CC`
    Madura foot NOS
    CC Excl: PDX collection 210

☑4ᵗʰ **B48** **Other mycoses, not elsewhere classified**

B48.0 **Lobomycosis**
    Keloidal blastomycosis
    Lobo's disease

B48.1 **Rhinosporidiosis**

B48.2 **Allescheriasis**   `CC`
    Infection due to Pseudallescheria boydii
    `EXCLUDES 1` *eumycetoma (B47.0)*
    CC Excl: PDX collection 211

B48.3 **Geotrichosis**   `CC`
    Geotrichum stomatitis
    CC Excl: PDX collection 212

B48.4 **Penicillosis**   `CC` `HCC`
    CC Excl: PDX collection 204

B48.8 Other specified **mycoses**   `HIV` `CC` `HCC`
    Adiaspiromycosis
    Infection of tissue and organs by Alternaria
    Infection of tissue and organs by Drechslera
    Infection of tissue and organs by Fusarium
    Infection of tissue and organs by saprophytic fungi NEC
    AHA: 2014, 4Q, 46; 2014, 2Q, 13
    CC Excl: PDX collection 213

B49 **Unspecified mycosis**   `CC`
    Fungemia NOS
    CC Excl: PDX collection 212

Protozoal diseases (B50-B64)

`EXCLUDES 1` *amebiasis (A06.-)*
        other protozoal intestinal diseases (A07.-)

☑4ᵗʰ **B50** **Plasmodium** falciparum **malaria**
    `INCLUDES` mixed infections of Plasmodium falciparum with any other Plasmodium species

    CC Excl: For CC/MCC codes in category B50: PDX collection 214

B50.0 **Plasmodium falciparum malaria** with cerebral complications   `CC`
    Cerebral malaria NOS

B50.8 Other severe and complicated **Plasmodium falciparum malaria**   `CC`
    Severe or complicated Plasmodium falciparum malaria NOS

B50.9 **Plasmodium falciparum malaria,** unspecified   `MCC`

☑4ᵗʰ **B51** **Plasmodium** vivax **malaria**
    `INCLUDES` mixed infections of Plasmodium vivax with other Plasmodium species, except Plasmodium falciparum
    `EXCLUDES 1` *plasmodium vivax with Plasmodium falciparum (B50.-)*

    CC Excl: For CC codes in category B51, unless otherwise noted: PDX collection 214

B51.0 **Plasmodium vivax malaria with** rupture of spleen   `CC`

B51.8 **Plasmodium vivax malaria with** other complications   `CC`

B51.9 **Plasmodium vivax malaria without** complication
    Plasmodium vivax malaria NOS
    CC Excl: PDX collection 215

☑ Additional Character Req 🔲x7ᵗʰ Placeholder Alert Unacceptable PDx Manifestation `H1`-`H14` HAC `HCC` CMS-HCC Condition `EXCLUDES 1` Not Coded Here `EXCLUDES 2` Not Included Here

Chapter 1. Certain Infectious and Parasitic Diseases

B40.7–B51.9

✓4th **B52** **Plasmodium** malariae **malaria**
     INCLUDES   mixed infections of Plasmodium malariae with other Plasmodium species, except Plasmodium falciparum and Plasmodium vivax
     EXCLUDES 1   *Plasmodium falciparum (B50.-)*
               Plasmodium vivax (B51.-)

> **CC Excl:** For CC codes in category B52, unless otherwise noted: PDX collection 214

    B52.0 **Plasmodium** malariae malaria with **nephropathy** `PDx CC` `CC`
         CC Excl: PDX collection 216

    B52.8 **Plasmodium** malariae malaria with **other complications** `CC`

    B52.9 **Plasmodium** malariae malaria **without complication** `CC`
         Plasmodium malariae malaria NOS

✓4th **B53** Other **specified malaria**

> **CC Excl:** For CC codes in subcategory B53: PDX collection 214

    B53.0 **Plasmodium** ovale **malaria** `CC`
         EXCLUDES 1   *Plasmodium ovale with Plasmodium falciparum (B50.-)*
               Plasmodium ovale with Plasmodium malariae (B52.-)
               Plasmodium ovale with Plasmodium vivax (B51.-)

    B53.1 **Malaria due to simian plasmodia** `CC`
         EXCLUDES 1   *Malaria due to simian plasmodia with Plasmodium falciparum (B50.-)*
               Malaria due to simian plasmodia with Plasmodium malariae (B52.-)
               Malaria due to simian plasmodia with Plasmodium ovale (B53.0)
               Malaria due to simian plasmodia with Plasmodium vivax (B51.-)

    B53.8 Other **malaria, not elsewhere classified** `CC`

    B54 Unspecified **malaria** `CC`
         CC Excl: PDX collection 217

✓4th **B55** **Leishmaniasis**

> **CC Excl:** For CC codes in category B55: PDX collection 218

    B55.0 **Visceral leishmaniasis** `CC`
         Kala-azar
         Post-kala-azar dermal leishmaniasis

    B55.1 **Cutaneous leishmaniasis** `CC`

    B55.2 **Mucocutaneous leishmaniasis** `CC`

    B55.9 **Leishmaniasis, unspecified** `CC`

✓4th **B56** **African trypanosomiasis**

> **CC Excl:** For CC codes in category B56: PDX collection 218

    B56.0 **Gambiense trypanosomiasis** `CC`
         Infection due to Trypanosoma brucei gambiense
         West African sleeping sickness

    B56.1 **Rhodesiense trypanosomiasis** `CC`
         East African sleeping sickness
         Infection due to Trypanosoma brucei rhodesiense

    B56.9 **African trypanosomiasis, unspecified** `CC`
         Sleeping sickness NOS

✓4th **B57** **Chagas' disease**
     INCLUDES   American trypanosomiasis
               infection due to Trypanosoma cruzi

> **CC Excl:** For CC codes in category B57, unless otherwise noted: PDX collection 218

    B57.0 **Acute Chagas' disease with heart involvement** `CC`
         Acute Chagas' disease with myocarditis
         CC Excl: PDX collection 219

    B57.1 **Acute Chagas' disease without heart involvement** `CC`
         Acute Chagas' disease NOS

    B57.2 **Chagas' disease (chronic) with heart involvement** `CC`
         American trypanosomiasis NOS
         Chagas' disease (chronic) NOS
         Chagas' disease (chronic) with myocarditis
         Trypanosomiasis NOS
         CC Excl: PDX collection 219

    ✓5th **B57.3** **Chagas' disease (chronic) with digestive system involvement**
       B57.30 **Chagas' disease with digestive system involvement, unspecified** `CC`
       B57.31 **Megaesophagus in Chagas' disease** `CC`
       B57.32 **Megacolon in Chagas' disease** `CC`
       B57.39 **Other digestive system involvement in Chagas' disease** `CC`

    ✓5th **B57.4** **Chagas' disease (chronic) with nervous system involvement**
       B57.40 **Chagas' disease with nervous system involvement, unspecified** `CC`
       B57.41 **Meningitis in Chagas' disease** `CC`
       B57.42 **Meningoencephalitis in Chagas' disease** `CC`
       B57.49 **Other nervous system involvement in Chagas' disease** `CC`

    B57.5 **Chagas' disease (chronic) with other organ involvement** `CC`

✓4th **B58** **Toxoplasmosis**
     INCLUDES   infection due to Toxoplasma gondii
     EXCLUDES 1   *congenital toxoplasmosis (P37.1)*

    ✓5th **B58.0** **Toxoplasma oculopathy**
       B58.00 **Toxoplasma oculopathy, unspecified** `HIV` `CC`
           CC Excl: PDX collection 220
       B58.01 **Toxoplasma chorioretinitis** `HIV` `CC`
           CC Excl: PDX collection 221
       B58.09 Other **toxoplasma oculopathy** `HIV` `CC`
           Toxoplasma uveitis
           CC Excl: PDX collection 222

    B58.1 **Toxoplasma hepatitis** `HIV` `CC`
         CC Excl: PDX collection 223

    B58.2 **Toxoplasma meningoencephalitis** `HIV` `MCC` `HCC`
         CC Excl: PDX collection 224

    B58.3 **Pulmonary toxoplasmosis** `HIV` `MCC` `HCC`
         CC Excl: PDX collection 225

    ✓5th **B58.8** **Toxoplasmosis with other organ involvement**

> **CC Excl:** For CC codes in subcategory B58.8, unless otherwise noted: PDX collection 220

       B58.81 **Toxoplasma myocarditis** `HIV` `MCC`
           CC Excl: PDX collection 226
       B58.82 **Toxoplasma myositis** `HIV` `CC`
       B58.83 **Toxoplasma tubulo-interstitial nephropathy** `HIV` `CC`
           Toxoplasma pyelonephritis
       B58.89 **Toxoplasmosis with other organ involvement** `HIV` `CC`

    B58.9 **Toxoplasmosis, unspecified** `HIV` `CC`
         CC Excl: PDX collection 227

    B59 **Pneumocystosis** `HIV` `MCC` `HCC`
         Pneumonia due to Pneumocystis carinii
         Pneumonia due to Pneumocystis jiroveci
         CC Excl: PDX collection 228

✓4th **B60** Other **protozoal diseases, not elsewhere classified**
     EXCLUDES 1   *cryptosporidiosis (A07.2)*
               intestinal microsporidiosis (A07.8)
               isosporiasis (A07.3)

    B60.0 **Babesiosis** `CC`
         Piroplasmosis
         CC Excl: PDX collection 218

    ✓5th **B60.1** **Acanthamebiasis**
       B60.10 **Acanthamebiasis, unspecified** `CC`
           CC Excl: PDX collection 229
       B60.11 **Meningoencephalitis due to Acanthamoeba (culbertsoni)**
       B60.12 **Conjunctivitis due to Acanthamoeba**
       B60.13 **Keratoconjunctivitis due to Acanthamoeba**
       B60.19 Other **acanthamebic disease** `CC`
           CC Excl: PDX collection 229

    B60.2 **Naegleriasis** `CC`
         Primary amebic meningoencephalitis
         CC Excl: PDX collection 229

    B60.8 Other **specified protozoal diseases** `HIV`
         Microsporidiosis

    B64 Unspecified **protozoal disease**

Helminthiases (B65-B83)

✓4th **B65** **Schistosomiasis [bilharziasis]**
     INCLUDES   snail fever

> **CC Excl:** For CC codes in category B65: PDX collection 230

    B65.0 **Schistosomiasis due to Schistosoma haematobium [urinary schistosomiasis]** `CC`

    B65.1 **Schistosomiasis due to Schistosoma mansoni [intestinal schistosomiasis]** `CC`

    B65.2 **Schistosomiasis due to Schistosoma japonicum** `CC`
         Asiatic schistosomiasis

N Newborn: 0   P Pediatric: 0-17   M Maternity: 12-55   A Adult: 15-124   MCC Major CC Condition   PDxMCC PDx acts as own MCC   CC CC Condition   PDxCC PDx acts as own CC

454   ICD-10-CM 2018

B65.3 Cercarial dermatitis `CC`
Swimmer's itch

B65.8 Other schistosomiasis `CC`
Infection due to Schistosoma intercalatum
Infection due to Schistosoma mattheei
Infection due to Schistosoma mekongi

B65.9 Schistosomiasis, unspecified `CC`

✓4ᵗʰ **B66 Other fluke infections**

> **CC Excl: For CC codes in category B66:** PDX collection 231

B66.0 Opisthorchiasis `CC`
Infection due to cat liver fluke
Infection due to Opisthorchis (felineus)(viverrini)

B66.1 Clonorchiasis `CC`
Chinese liver fluke disease
Infection due to Clonorchis sinensis
Oriental liver fluke disease

B66.2 Dicroceliasis `CC`
Infection due to Dicrocoelium dendriticum
Lancet fluke infection

B66.3 Fascioliasis `CC`
Infection due to Fasciola gigantica
Infection due to Fasciola hepatica
Infection due to Fasciola indica
Sheep liver fluke disease

B66.4 Paragonimiasis `CC` `HCC`
Infection due to Paragonimus species
Lung fluke disease
Pulmonary distomiasis

B66.5 Fasciolopsiasis `CC`
Infection due to Fasciolopsis buski
Intestinal distomiasis

B66.8 Other specified fluke infections `H1`
Echinostomiasis   Nanophyetiasis
Heterophyiasis   Watsoniasis
Metagonimiasis

B66.9 Fluke infection, unspecified

✓4ᵗʰ **B67 Echinococcosis**
INCLUDES hydatidosis

B67.0 Echinococcus granulosus infection of liver `CC`
CC Excl: PDX collection 232

B67.1 Echinococcus granulosus infection of lung `CC` `HCC`
CC Excl: PDX collection 233

B67.2 Echinococcus granulosus infection of bone `CC`
CC Excl: PDX collection 234

✓5ᵗʰ **B67.3 Echinococcus granulosus infection, other and multiple sites**

B67.31 Echinococcus granulosus infection, thyroid gland `CC`
CC Excl: PDX collection 235

B67.32 Echinococcus granulosus infection, multiple sites `CC`
CC Excl: PDX collection 234

B67.39 Echinococcus granulosus infection, other sites `CC`
CC Excl: PDX collection 234

B67.4 Echinococcus granulosus infection, unspecified `CC`
Dog tapeworm (infection)
CC Excl: PDX collection 236

B67.5 Echinococcus multilocularis infection of liver `CC`
CC Excl: PDX collection 237

✓5ᵗʰ **B67.6 Echinococcus multilocularis infection, other and multiple sites**

B67.61 Echinococcus multilocularis infection, multiple sites `CC`
CC Excl: PDX collection 238

B67.69 Echinococcus multilocularis infection, other sites `CC`
CC Excl: PDX collection 238

B67.7 Echinococcus multilocularis infection, unspecified `CC`
CC Excl: PDX collection 239

B67.8 Echinococcosis, unspecified, of liver `CC`
CC Excl: PDX collection 240

✓5ᵗʰ **B67.9 Echinococcosis, other and unspecified**

B67.90 Echinococcosis, unspecified `CC`
Echinococcosis NOS
CC Excl: PDX collection 240

B67.99 Other echinococcosis `CC`
CC Excl: PDX collection 240

✓4ᵗʰ **B68 Taeniasis**
EXCLUDES 1 cysticercosis (B69.-)

B68.0 Taenia solium taeniasis `CC`
Pork tapeworm (infection)
CC Excl: PDX collection 241

B68.1 Taenia saginata taeniasis `CC`
Beef tapeworm (infection)
Infection due to adult tapeworm Taenia saginata
CC Excl: PDX collection 242

B68.9 Taeniasis, unspecified `CC`
CC Excl: PDX collection 242

✓4ᵗʰ **B69 Cysticercosis**
INCLUDES cysticerciasis infection due to larval form of Taenia solium

> **CC Excl: For CC codes in category B69:** PDX collection 242

B69.0 Cysticercosis of central nervous system `CC`

B69.1 Cysticercosis of eye `CC`

✓5ᵗʰ **B69.8 Cysticercosis of other sites**

B69.81 Myositis in cysticercosis `CC`

B69.89 Cysticercosis of other sites `CC`

B69.9 Cysticercosis, unspecified `CC`

✓4ᵗʰ **B70 Diphyllobothriasis and sparganosis**

> **CC Excl: For CC codes in category B70:** PDX collection 242

B70.0 Diphyllobothriasis `CC`
Diphyllobothrium (adult) (latum) (pacificum) infection
Fish tapeworm (infection)
EXCLUDES 2 larval diphyllobothriasis (B70.1)

B70.1 Sparganosis `CC`
Infection due to Sparganum (mansoni) (proliferum)
Infection due to Spirometra larva
Larval diphyllobothriasis
Spirometrosis

✓4ᵗʰ **B71 Other cestode infections**

> **CC Excl: For CC codes in category B71:** PDX collection 242

B71.0 Hymenolepiasis `CC`
Dwarf tapeworm infection
Rat tapeworm (infection)

B71.1 Dipylidiasis `CC`

B71.8 Other specified cestode infections `CC`
Coenurosis

B71.9 Cestode infection, unspecified
Tapeworm (infection) NOS

B72 Dracunculiasis `CC`
INCLUDES guinea worm infection
infection due to Dracunculus medinensis
CC Excl: PDX collection 243

✓4ᵗʰ **B73 Onchocerciasis**
INCLUDES onchocerca volvulus infection
onchocercosis
river blindness

> **CC Excl: For CC codes in category B73:** PDX collection 243

✓5ᵗʰ **B73.0 Onchocerciasis with eye disease**

B73.00 Onchocerciasis with eye involvement, unspecified `CC`

B73.01 Onchocerciasis with endophthalmitis `CC`

B73.02 Onchocerciasis with glaucoma `CC`

B73.09 Onchocerciasis with other eye involvement `CC`
Infestation of eyelid due to onchocerciasis

B73.1 Onchocerciasis without eye disease `CC`

✓4ᵗʰ **B74 Filariasis**
EXCLUDES 2 onchocerciasis (B73)
tropical (pulmonary) eosinophilia NOS (J82)

> **CC Excl: For CC codes in category B74:** PDX collection 243

B74.0 Filariasis due to Wuchereria bancrofti `CC`
Bancroftian elephantiasis
Bancroftian filariasis

B74.1 Filariasis due to Brugia malayi `CC`

B74.2 Filariasis due to Brugia timori `CC`

B74.3 Loiasis `CC`
Calabar swelling
Eyeworm disease of Africa
Loa loa infection

B74.4 Mansonelliasis `CC`
Infection due to Mansonella ozzardi
Infection due to Mansonella perstans
Infection due to Mansonella streptocerca

B74.8 Other filariases `CC`
Dirofilariasis

B74.9 Filariasis, unspecified `CC`

B75 Trichinellosis `CC`
INCLUDES infection due to Trichinella species
trichiniasis
CC Excl: PDX collection 244

✓4ᵗʰ **B76 Hookworm diseases**
INCLUDES uncinariasis

CC Excl: For CC codes in category B76: PDX collection 245

B76.0 Ancylostomiasis `CC`
Infection due to Ancylostoma species

B76.1 Necatoriasis `CC`
Infection due to Necator americanus

B76.8 Other hookworm diseases `CC`

B76.9 Hookworm disease, unspecified `CC`
Cutaneous larva migrans NOS

✓4ᵗʰ **B77 Ascariasis**
INCLUDES ascaridiasis
roundworm infection

CC Excl: For CC codes in category B77, unless otherwise noted:
PDX collection 246

B77.0 Ascariasis with intestinal complications `CC`

✓5ᵗʰ **B77.8** Ascariasis with other complications
B77.81 Ascariasis pneumonia `PDxMCC` `MCC`
CC Excl: PDX collection 247

B77.89 Ascariasis with other complications `CC`

B77.9 Ascariasis, unspecified `CC`

✓4ᵗʰ **B78 Strongyloidiasis**
EXCLUDES1 trichostrongyliasis (B81.2)

CC Excl: For CC codes in category B78: PDX collection 246

B78.0 Intestinal strongyloidiasis `HIV` `CC`

B78.1 Cutaneous strongyloidiasis

B78.7 Disseminated strongyloidiasis `HIV` `CC`

B78.9 Strongyloidiasis, unspecified `HIV` `CC`

B79 Trichuriasis `CC`
INCLUDES trichocephaliasis
whipworm (disease)(infection)
CC Excl: PDX collection 246

B80 Enterobiasis `CC`
INCLUDES oxyuriasis
pinworm infection
threadworm infection
CC Excl: PDX collection 246

✓4ᵗʰ **B81 Other intestinal helminthiases, not elsewhere classified**
EXCLUDES1 ▶angiostrongyliasis due to:
angiostrongylus cantonensis (B83.2)
parastrongylus cantonensis (B83.2) ◄

B81.0 Anisakiasis `CC`
Infection due to Anisakis larva
CC Excl: PDX collection 246

B81.1 Intestinal capillariasis `CC`
Capillariasis NOS
Infection due to Capillaria philippinensis
EXCLUDES2 hepatic capillariasis (B83.8)
CC Excl: PDX collection 246

B81.2 Trichostrongyliasis `CC`
CC Excl: PDX collection 246

B81.3 Intestinal angiostrongyliasis `CC`
▶Angiostrongyliasis due to:
angiostrongylus costaricensis
parastrongylus costaricensis◄
CC Excl: PDX collection 248

B81.4 Mixed intestinal helminthiases `CC`
Infection due to intestinal helminths classified to more than one
of the categories B65.0-B81.3 and B81.8
Mixed helminthiasis NOS
CC Excl: PDX collection 248

B81.8 Other specified intestinal helminthiases `CC`
Infection due to Oesophagostomum species
[esophagostomiasis]
Infection due to Ternidens diminutus [ternidensiasis]
CC Excl: PDX collection 248

✓4ᵗʰ **B82 Unspecified intestinal parasitism**
B82.0 Intestinal helminthiasis, unspecified `CC`
CC Excl: PDX collection 248

B82.9 Intestinal parasitism, unspecified

✓4ᵗʰ **B83 Other helminthiases**
EXCLUDES1 capillariasis NOS (B81.1)
EXCLUDES2 intestinal capillariasis (B81.1)

B83.0 Visceral larva migrans
Toxocariasis

B83.1 Gnathostomiasis
Wandering swelling

B83.2 Angiostrongyliasis due to Parastrongylus cantonensis
Eosinophilic meningoencephalitis due to Parastrongylus
cantonensis
EXCLUDES2 intestinal angiostrongyliasis (B81.3)

B83.3 Syngamiasis
Syngamosis

B83.4 Internal hirudiniasis
EXCLUDES2 external hirudiniasis (B88.3)

B83.8 Other specified helminthiases
Acanthocephaliasis   Metastrongyliasis
Gongylonemiasis   Thelaziasis
Hepatic capillariasis

B83.9 Helminthiasis, unspecified
Worms NOS
EXCLUDES1 intestinal helminthiasis NOS (B82.0)

Pediculosis, acariasis and other infestations (B85-B89)

✓4ᵗʰ **B85 Pediculosis and phthiriasis**
B85.0 Pediculosis due to Pediculus humanus capitis
Head-louse infestation

B85.1 Pediculosis due to Pediculus humanus corporis
Body-louse infestation

B85.2 Pediculosis, unspecified

B85.3 Phthiriasis
Infestation by crab-louse
Infestation by Phthirus pubis

B85.4 Mixed pediculosis and phthiriasis
Infestation classifiable to more than one of the categories
B85.0-B85.3

B86 Scabies
Sarcoptic itch

✓4ᵗʰ **B87 Myiasis**
INCLUDES infestation by larva of flies

B87.0 Cutaneous myiasis
Creeping myiasis

B87.1 Wound myiasis
Traumatic myiasis

B87.2 Ocular myiasis

B87.3 Nasopharyngeal myiasis
Laryngeal myiasis

B87.4 Aural myiasis

✓5ᵗʰ **B87.8** Myiasis of other sites
B87.81 Genitourinary myiasis
B87.82 Intestinal myiasis
B87.89 Myiasis of other sites

B87.9 Myiasis, unspecified

✓4ᵗʰ **B88 Other infestations**
B88.0 Other acariasis
Acarine dermatitis
Dermatitis due to Demodex species
Dermatitis due to Dermanyssus gallinae
Dermatitis due to Liponyssoides sanguineus
Trombiculosis
EXCLUDES2 scabies (B86)

B88.1 Tungiasis [sandflea infestation]

B88.2 Other arthropod infestations
Scarabiasis

`N` Newborn: 0   `P` Pediatric: 0-17   `M` Maternity: 12-55   `A` Adult: 15-124   `MCC` Major CC Condition   `PDxMCC` PDx acts as own MCC   `CC` CC Condition   `PDxCC` PDx acts as own CC

456   ICD-10-CM 2018

B88.3 External hirudiniasis
Leech infestation NOS
EXCLUDES 2 *internal hirudiniasis (B83.4)*

B88.8 Other specified infestations
Ichthyoparasitism due to Vandellia cirrhosa
Linguatulosis
Porocephaliasis

B88.9 Infestation, unspecified
Infestation (skin) NOS   Skin parasites NOS
Infestation by mites NOS

B89 Unspecified parasitic disease

Sequelae of infectious and parasitic diseases (B90-B94)

NOTE Categories B90-B94 are to be used to indicate conditions in categories A00-B89 as the cause of sequelae, which are themselves classified elsewhere. The "sequelae" include conditions specified as such; they also include residuals of diseases classifiable to the above categories if there is evidence that the disease itself is no longer present. Codes from these categories are not to be used for chronic infections. Code chronic current infections to active infectious disease as appropriate.

Code first condition resulting from (sequela) the infectious or parasitic disease

√4th B90 Sequelae of tuberculosis
B90.0 Sequelae of central nervous system tuberculosis
B90.1 Sequelae of genitourinary tuberculosis
B90.2 Sequelae of tuberculosis of bones and joints
B90.8 Sequelae of tuberculosis of other organs
EXCLUDES 2 *sequelae of respiratory tuberculosis (B90.9)*
B90.9 Sequelae of respiratory and unspecified tuberculosis
Sequelae of tuberculosis NOS

B91 Sequelae of poliomyelitis
EXCLUDES 1 *postpolio syndrome (G14)*

B92 Sequelae of leprosy

√4th B94 Sequelae of other and unspecified infectious and parasitic diseases
B94.0 Sequelae of trachoma
B94.1 Sequelae of viral encephalitis
B94.2 Sequelae of viral hepatitis
B94.8 Sequelae of other specified infectious and parasitic diseases
B94.9 Sequelae of unspecified infectious and parasitic disease

Bacterial and viral infectious agents (B95-B97)

NOTE These categories are provided for use as supplementary or additional codes to identify the infectious agent(s) in diseases classified elsewhere.

√4th B95 Streptococcus, Staphylococcus, and Enterococcus as the cause of diseases classified elsewhere
B95.0 Streptococcus, group A, as the cause of diseases classified elsewhere
B95.1 Streptococcus, group B, as the cause of diseases classified elsewhere
B95.2 Enterococcus as the cause of diseases classified elsewhere
B95.3 Streptococcus pneumoniae as the cause of diseases classified elsewhere
B95.4 Other streptococcus as the cause of diseases classified elsewhere
B95.5 Unspecified streptococcus as the cause of diseases classified elsewhere
√5th B95.6 Staphylococcus aureus as the cause of diseases classified elsewhere
    B95.61 Methicillin susceptible Staphylococcus aureus infection as the cause of diseases classified elsewhere
Methicillin susceptible Staphylococcus aureus (MSSA) infection as the cause of diseases classified elsewhere
Staphylococcus aureus infection NOS as the cause of diseases classified elsewhere
    B95.62 Methicillin resistant Staphylococcus aureus infection as the cause of diseases classified elsewhere
Methicillin resistant Staphylococcus aureus (MRSA) infection as the cause of diseases classified elsewhere
AHA: 2016, 1Q, 12

B95.7 Other staphylococcus as the cause of diseases classified elsewhere
B95.8 Unspecified staphylococcus as the cause of diseases classified elsewhere

√4th B96 Other bacterial agents as the cause of diseases classified elsewhere
B96.0 Mycoplasma pneumoniae [M. pneumoniae] as the cause of diseases classified elsewhere
Pleuro-pneumonia-like-organism [PPLO]
B96.1 Klebsiella pneumoniae [K. pneumoniae] as the cause of diseases classified elsewhere
√5th B96.2 Escherichia coli [E. coli] as the cause of diseases classified elsewhere
    B96.20 Unspecified Escherichia coli [E. coli] as the cause of diseases classified elsewhere
Escherichia coli [E. coli] NOS
    B96.21 Shiga toxin-producing Escherichia coli [E. coli] (STEC) O157 as the cause of diseases classified elsewhere
E. coli O157:H- (nonmotile) with confirmation of Shiga toxin
E. coli O157 with confirmation of Shiga toxin when H antigen is unknown, or is not H7
O157:H7 Escherichia coli [E.coli] with or without confirmation of Shiga toxin-production
Shiga toxin-producing Escherichia coli [E.coli] O157:H7 with or without confirmation of Shiga toxin-production
STEC O157:H7 with or without confirmation of Shiga toxin-production
    B96.22 Other specified Shiga toxin-producing Escherichia coli [E. coli] (STEC) as the cause of diseases classified elsewhere
Non-O157 Shiga toxin-producing Escherichia coli [E.coli]
Non-O157 Shiga toxin-producing Escherichia coli [E.coli] with known O group
    B96.23 Unspecified Shiga toxin-producing Escherichia coli [E. coli] (STEC) as the cause of diseases classified elsewhere
Shiga toxin-producing Escherichia coli [E. coli] with unspecified O group
STEC NOS
    B96.29 Other Escherichia coli [E. coli] as the cause of diseases classified elsewhere
Non-Shiga toxin-producing E. coli
B96.3 Hemophilus influenzae [H. influenzae] as the cause of diseases classified elsewhere
B96.4 Proteus (mirabilis) (morganii) as the cause of diseases classified elsewhere
B96.5 Pseudomonas (aeruginosa) (mallei) (pseudomallei) as the cause of diseases classified elsewhere
AHA: 2015, 1Q, 18
B96.6 Bacteroides fragilis [B. fragilis] as the cause of diseases classified elsewhere
B96.7 Clostridium perfringens [C. perfringens] as the cause of diseases classified elsewhere
√5th B96.8 Other specified bacterial agents as the cause of diseases classified elsewhere
    B96.81 Helicobacter pylori [H. pylori] as the cause of diseases classified elsewhere
    B96.82 Vibrio vulnificus as the cause of diseases classified elsewhere
    B96.89 Other specified bacterial agents as the cause of diseases classified elsewhere

√4th B97 Viral agents as the cause of diseases classified elsewhere
AHA: 2016, 3Q, 8-10, 14
B97.0 Adenovirus as the cause of diseases classified elsewhere
√5th B97.1 Enterovirus as the cause of diseases classified elsewhere
    B97.10 Unspecified enterovirus as the cause of diseases classified elsewhere
    B97.11 Coxsackievirus as the cause of diseases classified elsewhere
    B97.12 Echovirus as the cause of diseases classified elsewhere
    B97.19 Other enterovirus as the cause of diseases classified elsewhere

✓5ᵗʰ **B97.2** **Coronavirus as the cause of diseases classified elsewhere**

    B97.21 Coronavirus as the cause of diseases classified elsewhere as the cause of diseases classified elsewhere **CC**

        EXCLUDES 1 pneumonia due to SARS-associated coronavirus (J12.81)

        CC Excl: PDX collection 249

    B97.29 Other coronavirus as the cause of diseases classified elsewhere

✓5ᵗʰ **B97.3** **Retrovirus as the cause of diseases classified elsewhere**

        EXCLUDES 1 human immunodeficiency virus [HIV] disease (B20)

    B97.30 Unspecified retrovirus as the cause of diseases classified elsewhere

    B97.31 Lentivirus as the cause of diseases classified elsewhere

    B97.32 Oncovirus as the cause of diseases classified elsewhere

    B97.33 Human T-cell lymphotrophic virus, type I [HTLV-I] as the cause of diseases classified elsewhere **CC**

        CC Excl: PDX collection 250

    B97.34 Human T-cell lymphotrophic virus, type II [HTLV-II] as the cause of diseases classified elsewhere **CC**

        CC Excl: PDX collection 251

    B97.35 Human immunodeficiency virus, type 2 [HIV 2] as the cause of diseases classified elsewhere **CC** **HCC**

        CC Excl: PDX collection 252

    B97.39 Other retrovirus as the cause of diseases classified elsewhere

B97.4 Respiratory syncytial virus as the cause of diseases classified elsewhere

B97.5 Reovirus as the cause of diseases classified elsewhere

B97.6 Parvovirus as the cause of diseases classified elsewhere

B97.7 Papillomavirus as the cause of diseases classified elsewhere

✓5ᵗʰ **B97.8** Other viral agents as the cause of diseases classified elsewhere

    B97.81 Human metapneumovirus as the cause of diseases classified elsewhere

    B97.89 Other viral agents as the cause of diseases classified elsewhere

Other infectious diseases (B99)

✓4ᵗʰ **B99** **Other and unspecified infectious diseases**

    B99.8 Other infectious disease **HIV**

    B99.9 Unspecified infectious disease

N Newborn: 0   P Pediatric: 0-17   M Maternity: 12-55   A Adult: 15-124   **MCC** Major CC Condition   **PDx MCC** PDx acts as own MCC   **CC** CC Condition   **PDx CC** PDx acts as own CC

458   ICD-10-CM 2018

Chapter 2. Neoplasms (C00–D49)

Chapter Specific Guidelines with Coding Examples

The chapter specific guidelines from the ICD-10-CM Official Guidelines for Coding and Reporting have been provided below. Along with these guidelines are coding examples, contained in the shaded boxes, that have been developed to help illustrate the coding and/or sequencing guidance found in these guidelines.

General guidelines

Chapter 2 of the ICD-10-CM contains the codes for most benign and all malignant neoplasms. Certain benign neoplasms, such as prostatic adenomas, may be found in the specific body system chapters. To properly code a neoplasm it is necessary to determine from the record if the neoplasm is benign, in-situ, malignant, or of uncertain histologic behavior. If malignant, any secondary (metastatic) sites should also be determined.

Primary malignant neoplasms overlapping site boundaries

A primary malignant neoplasm that overlaps two or more contiguous (next to each other) sites should be classified to the subcategory/code .8 ('overlapping lesion'), unless the combination is specifically indexed elsewhere. For multiple neoplasms of the same site that are not contiguous such as tumors in different quadrants of the same breast, codes for each site should be assigned.

> A 73-year-old white female with a large rapidly growing malignant tumor in the left breast extending from the upper outer quadrant into the axillary tail
>
> **C50.812   Malignant neoplasm of overlapping sites of left female breast**
>
> *Explanation*: Because this is a single large tumor that overlaps two contiguous sites, a single code for overlapping sites is assigned.

> A 52-year old white female with two distinct lesions of the right breast, one (0.5 cm) in the upper outer quadrant and a second (1.5 cm) in the lower outer quadrant; path report indicates both lesions are malignant
>
> **C50.411   Malignant neoplasm of upper-outer quadrant of right female breast**
>
> **C50.511   Malignant neoplasm of lower-outer quadrant of right female breast**
>
> *Explanation*: This patient has two distinct malignant lesions of right breast in adjacent quadrants. Because the lesions are not contiguous, two codes are reported.

Malignant neoplasm of ectopic tissue

Malignant neoplasms of ectopic tissue are to be coded to the site of origin mentioned, e.g., ectopic pancreatic malignant neoplasms involving the stomach are coded to **malignant neoplasm of** pancreas, unspecified (C25.9).

The neoplasm table in the Alphabetic Index should be referenced first. However, if the histological term is documented, that term should be referenced first, rather than going immediately to the Neoplasm Table, in order to determine which column in the Neoplasm Table is appropriate. For example, if the documentation indicates "adenoma," refer to the term in the Alphabetic Index to review the entries under this term and the instructional note to "see also neoplasm, by site, benign." The table provides the proper code based on the type of neoplasm and the site. It is important to select the proper column in the table that corresponds to the type of neoplasm. The Tabular List should then be referenced to verify that the correct code has been selected from the table and that a more specific site code does not exist.

See Section I.C.21. Factors influencing health status and contact with health services, Status, for information regarding Z15.0, codes for genetic susceptibility to cancer.

a. Treatment directed at the malignancy

If the treatment is directed at the malignancy, designate the malignancy as the principal diagnosis.

The only exception to this guideline is if a patient admission/encounter is solely for the administration of chemotherapy, immunotherapy or **external beam** radiation therapy, assign the appropriate Z51.-- code as the first-listed or principal diagnosis, and the diagnosis or problem for which the service is being performed as a secondary diagnosis.

b. Treatment of secondary site

When a patient is admitted because of a primary neoplasm with metastasis and treatment is directed toward the secondary site only, the secondary neoplasm is designated as the principal diagnosis even though the primary malignancy is still present.

> Patient with primary prostate cancer with metastasis to lungs admitted for wedge resection of mass in right lung
>
> **C78.01   Secondary malignant neoplasm of right lung**
>
> **C61   Malignant neoplasm of prostate**
>
> *Explanation*: Since the admission is for treatment of the lung metastasis, the secondary lung metastasis is sequenced before the primary prostate cancer.

c. Coding and sequencing of complications

Coding and sequencing of complications associated with the malignancies or with the therapy thereof are subject to the following guidelines:

1) Anemia associated with malignancy

When admission/encounter is for management of an anemia associated with the malignancy, and the treatment is only for anemia, the appropriate code for the malignancy is sequenced as the principal or first-listed diagnosis followed by the appropriate code for the anemia (such as code D63.0, Anemia in neoplastic disease).

> Patient is admitted for treatment of anemia in advanced colon cancer
>
> **C18.9   Malignant neoplasm of colon, unspecified**
>
> **D63.0   Anemia in neoplastic disease**
>
> *Explanation*: Even though the admission was solely to treat the anemia, this guideline indicates that the code for the malignancy is sequenced first.

2) Anemia associated with chemotherapy, immunotherapy and radiation therapy

When the admission/encounter is for management of an anemia associated with an adverse effect of the administration of chemotherapy or immunotherapy and the only treatment is for the anemia, the anemia code is sequenced first followed by the appropriate codes for the neoplasm and the adverse effect (T45.1X5, Adverse effect of antineoplastic and immunosuppressive drugs).

> A 56-year-old Hispanic male with grade II follicular lymphoma involving multiple lymph node sites referred for blood transfusion to treat anemia due to chemotherapy
>
> **D64.81   Anemia due to antineoplastic chemotherapy**
>
> **C82.18   Follicular lymphoma grade II, lymph nodes of multiple sites**
>
> **T45.1X5A   Adverse effect of antineoplastic and immunosuppressive drugs, initial encounter**
>
> *Explanation*: The code for the anemia is sequenced first followed by the code for the malignant neoplasm and lastly the code for the adverse effect.

When the admission/encounter is for management of an anemia associated with an adverse effect of radiotherapy, the anemia code should be sequenced first, followed by the appropriate neoplasm code and code Y84.2, Radiological procedure and radiotherapy as the cause of abnormal reaction of the patient, or of later complication, without mention of misadventure at the time of the procedure.

A 55-year-old male with a large malignant rectal tumor has been receiving external radiation therapy to shrink the tumor prior to planned surgery. He is admitted today for a blood transfusion to treat anemia related to radiation therapy.

D64.89   **Other specified anemias**

C20   **Malignant neoplasm of rectum**

Y84.2   **Radiological procedure and radiotherapy as the cause of abnormal reaction of the patient, or of later complication, without mention of misadventure at the time of the procedure**

Explanation: The code for the anemia is sequenced first, followed by the code for the malignancy, and lastly the code for the abnormal reaction due to radiotherapy.

3) Management of dehydration due to the malignancy

When the admission/encounter is for management of dehydration due to the malignancy and only the dehydration is being treated (intravenous rehydration), the dehydration is sequenced first, followed by the code(s) for the malignancy.

4) Treatment of a complication resulting from a surgical procedure

When the admission/encounter is for treatment of a complication resulting from a surgical procedure, designate the complication as the principal or first-listed diagnosis if treatment is directed at resolving the complication.

d. Primary malignancy previously excised

When a primary malignancy has been previously excised or eradicated from its site and there is no further treatment directed to that site and there is no evidence of any existing primary malignancy, a code from category Z85, Personal history of malignant neoplasm, should be used to indicate the former site of the malignancy. Any mention of extension, invasion, or metastasis to another site is coded as a secondary malignant neoplasm to that site. The secondary site may be the principal or first-listed with the Z85 code used as a secondary code.

History of breast cancer, left radical mastectomy 18 months ago with no current treatment; bronchoscopy with lung biopsy shows metastatic disease in the right lung

C78.01   **Secondary malignant neoplasm of right lung**

Z85.3   **Personal history of malignant neoplasm of breast**

Explanation: The patient has undergone a diagnostic procedure that revealed metastatic breast cancer in the right lung. The code for the secondary (metastatic) site is sequenced first followed by a personal history code to identify the former site of the primary malignancy.

e. Admissions/encounters involving chemotherapy, immunotherapy and radiation therapy

1) Episode of care involves surgical removal of neoplasm

When an episode of care involves the surgical removal of a neoplasm, primary or secondary site, followed by adjunct chemotherapy or radiation treatment during the same episode of care, the code for the neoplasm should be assigned as principal or first-listed diagnosis.

2) Patient admission/encounter solely for administration of chemotherapy, immunotherapy and radiation therapy

If a patient admission/encounter is solely for the administration of chemotherapy, immunotherapy or **external beam** radiation therapy assign code Z51.0, Encounter for antineoplastic radiation therapy, or Z51.11, Encounter for antineoplastic chemotherapy, or Z51.12, Encounter for antineoplastic immunotherapy as the first-listed or principal diagnosis. If a patient receives more than one of these therapies during the same admission more than one of these codes may be assigned, in any sequence.

The malignancy for which the therapy is being administered should be assigned as a secondary diagnosis.

Patient is admitted for second round of rituximab and fludarabine for his chronic B cell lymphocytic leukemia

Z51.11   **Encounter for antineoplastic chemotherapy**

Z51.12   **Encounter for antineoplastic immunotherapy**

C91.10   **Chronic lymphocytic leukemia of B-cell type not having achieved remission**

Explanation: Rituximab is an antineoplastic immunotherapy while fludarabine is an antineoplastic chemotherapy. The two treatments are often used together. The admission was solely for the purpose of administering this treatment and either can be sequenced first, before the neoplastic condition.

If a patient admission/encounter is for the insertion or implantation of radioactive elements (e.g., brachytherapy) the appropriate code for the malignancy is sequenced as the principal or first-listed diagnosis. Code Z51.0 should not be assigned.

3) Patient admitted for radiation therapy, chemotherapy or immunotherapy and develops complications

When a patient is admitted for the purpose of **external beam** radiotherapy, immunotherapy or chemotherapy and develops complications such as uncontrolled nausea and vomiting or dehydration, the principal or first-listed diagnosis is Z51.0, Encounter for antineoplastic radiation therapy, or Z51.11, Encounter for antineoplastic chemotherapy, or Z51.12, Encounter for antineoplastic immunotherapy followed by any codes for the complications.

When a patient is admitted for the purpose of insertion or implantation of radioactive elements (e.g., brachytherapy) and develops complications such as uncontrolled nausea and vomiting or dehydration, the principal or first-listed diagnosis is the appropriate code for the malignancy followed by any codes for the complications.

f. Admission/encounter to determine extent of malignancy

When the reason for admission/encounter is to determine the extent of the malignancy, or for a procedure such as paracentesis or thoracentesis, the primary malignancy or appropriate metastatic site is designated as the principal or first-listed diagnosis, even though chemotherapy or radiotherapy is administered.

Patient with left lung cancer with malignant pleural effusion admitted for paracentesis and initiation/administration of chemotherapy

C34.92   **Malignant neoplasm of unspecified part of left bronchus or lung**

J91.0   **Malignant pleural effusion**

Z51.11   **Encounter for antineoplastic chemotherapy**

Explanation: The lung cancer is sequenced before the chemotherapy in this instance because the paracentesis for the malignant effusion is also being performed. An instructional note under the malignant effusion instructs that the lung cancer be sequenced first.

g. Symptoms, signs, and abnormal findings listed in Chapter 18 associated with neoplasms

Symptoms, signs, and ill-defined conditions listed in Chapter 18 characteristic of, or associated with, an existing primary or secondary site malignancy cannot be used to replace the malignancy as principal or first-listed diagnosis, regardless of the number of admissions or encounters for treatment and care of the neoplasm.

See Section I.C.21. Factors influencing health status and contact with health services, Encounter for prophylactic organ removal.

h. Admission/encounter for pain control/management

See Section I.C.6. for information on coding admission/encounter for pain control/management.

i. Malignancy in two or more noncontiguous sites

A patient may have more than one malignant tumor in the same organ. These tumors may represent different primaries or metastatic disease, depending on the site. Should the documentation be unclear, the provider should be queried as to the status of each tumor so that the correct codes can be assigned.

j. Disseminated malignant neoplasm, unspecified

Code C80.0, Disseminated malignant neoplasm, unspecified, is for use only in those cases where the patient has advanced metastatic disease and no known primary or secondary sites are specified. It should not be used in place of assigning codes for the primary site and all known secondary sites.

Patient who has had no medical care for many years is seen today and diagnosed with carcinomatosis

C80.0   Disseminated malignant neoplasm, unspecified

Explanation: Carcinomatosis NOS is an "includes" note under this code. Should seldom be used but is available for use in cases such as this.

k. Malignant neoplasm without specification of site

Code C80.1, Malignant (primary) neoplasm, unspecified, equates to Cancer, unspecified. This code should only be used when no determination can be made as to the primary site of a malignancy. This code should rarely be used in the inpatient setting.

Evaluation of painful hip leads to diagnosis of a metastatic bone lesion from an unknown primary neoplasm source

C79.51   Secondary malignant neoplasm of bone

C80.1   Malignant (primary) neoplasm, unspecified

Explanation: If only the secondary site is known, use code C80.1 for the unknown primary site.

l. Sequencing of neoplasm codes

1) Encounter for treatment of primary malignancy

If the reason for the encounter is for treatment of a primary malignancy, assign the malignancy as the principal/first-listed diagnosis. The primary site is to be sequenced first, followed by any metastatic sites.

2) Encounter for treatment of secondary malignancy

When an encounter is for a primary malignancy with metastasis and treatment is directed toward the metastatic (secondary) site(s) only, the metastatic site(s) is designated as the principal/first-listed diagnosis. The primary malignancy is coded as an additional code.

Patient has primary colon cancer with metastasis to rib and is evaluated for possible excision of portion of rib bone

C79.51   Secondary malignant neoplasm of bone

C18.9   Malignant neoplasm of colon, unspecified

Explanation: The treatment for this encounter is focused on the metastasis to the rib bone rather than the primary colon cancer, thus indicating that the bone metastasis is sequenced as the first-listed code.

3) Malignant neoplasm in a pregnant patient

When a pregnant woman has a malignant neoplasm, a code from subcategory O9A.1-, Malignant neoplasm complicating pregnancy, childbirth, and the puerperium, should be sequenced first, followed by the appropriate code from Chapter 2 to indicate the type of neoplasm.

A 30-year-old pregnant female in second trimester evaluated for thyroid malignancy

O9A.112   Malignant neoplasm complicating pregnancy, second trimester

C73   Malignant neoplasm of thyroid gland

Explanation: Codes from chapter 15 describing complications of pregnancy are sequenced as first-listed codes, further specified by codes from other chapters such as neoplastic, unless the pregnancy is documented as incidental to the condition. See also guideline 1.C.15.a.1.

4) Encounter for complication associated with a neoplasm

When an encounter is for management of a complication associated with a neoplasm, such as dehydration, and the treatment is only for the complication, the complication is coded first, followed by the appropriate code(s) for the neoplasm.

The exception to this guideline is anemia. When the admission/encounter is for management of an anemia associated with the malignancy, and the treatment is only for anemia, the appropriate code for the malignancy is sequenced as the principal or first-listed diagnosis followed by code D63.0, Anemia in neoplastic disease.

Patient with pancreatic cancer is seen for initiation of TPN for cancer-related moderate protein-calorie malnutrition

E44.0   Moderate protein-calorie malnutrition

C25.9   Malignant neoplasm of pancreas, unspecified

Explanation: The encounter is to initiate treatment for malnutrition, a common complication of many types of neoplasms, and is sequenced first.

5) Complication from surgical procedure for treatment of a neoplasm

When an encounter is for treatment of a complication resulting from a surgical procedure performed for the treatment of the neoplasm, designate the complication as the principal/first-listed diagnosis. See guideline regarding the coding of a current malignancy versus personal history to determine if the code for the neoplasm should also be assigned.

6) Pathologic fracture due to a neoplasm

When an encounter is for a pathological fracture due to a neoplasm, and the focus of treatment is the fracture, a code from subcategory M84.5, Pathological fracture in neoplastic disease, should be sequenced first, followed by the code for the neoplasm.

If the focus of treatment is the neoplasm with an associated pathological fracture, the neoplasm code should be sequenced first, followed by a code from M84.5 for the pathological fracture.

m. Current malignancy versus personal history of malignancy

When a primary malignancy has been excised but further treatment, such as an additional surgery for the malignancy, radiation therapy or chemotherapy is directed to that site, the primary malignancy code should be used until treatment is completed.

When a primary malignancy has been previously excised or eradicated from its site, there is no further treatment (of the malignancy) directed to that site, and there is no evidence of any existing primary malignancy, a code from category Z85, Personal history of malignant neoplasm, should be used to indicate the former site of the malignancy.

See Section I.C.21. Factors influencing health status and contact with health services, History (of)

Female patient with ongoing chemotherapy after right mastectomy for breast cancer

C50.911   Malignant neoplasm of unspecified site of right female breast

Z90.11   Acquired absence of right breast and nipple

Explanation: Even though the breast has been removed, the breast cancer is still being treated with chemotherapy and therefore is still coded as a current condition rather than personal history.

n. Leukemia, multiple myeloma, and malignant plasma cell neoplasms in remission versus personal history

The categories for leukemia, and category C90, Multiple myeloma and malignant plasma cell neoplasms, have codes indicating whether or not the leukemia has achieved remission. There are also codes Z85.6, Personal history of leukemia, and Z85.79, Personal history of other malignant neoplasms of lymphoid, hematopoietic and related tissues. If the documentation is unclear as to whether the leukemia has achieved remission, the provider should be queried.

See Section I.C.21. Factors influencing health status and contact with health services, History (of)

o. Aftercare following surgery for neoplasm

See Section I.C.21. Factors influencing health status and contact with health services, Aftercare

p. Follow-up care for completed treatment of a malignancy

See Section I.C.21. Factors influencing health status and contact with health services, Follow-up

q. Prophylactic organ removal for prevention of malignancy

See Section I.C. 21, Factors influencing health status and contact with health services, Prophylactic organ removal

r. Malignant neoplasm associated with transplanted organ

A malignant neoplasm of a transplanted organ should be coded as a transplant complication. Assign first the appropriate code from category T86.-, Complications of transplanted organs and tissue, followed by code C80.2, Malignant neoplasm associated with transplanted organ. Use an additional code for the specific malignancy.

Chapter 2. Neoplasms (C00-D49)

NOTE

Functional activity

All neoplasms are classified in this chapter, whether they are functionally active or not. An additional code from Chapter 4 may be used, to identify functional activity associated with any neoplasm.

Morphology [Histology]

Chapter 2 classifies neoplasms primarily by site (topography), with broad groupings for behavior, malignant, in situ, benign, etc. The Table of Neoplasms should be used to identify the correct topography code. In a few cases, such as for malignant melanoma and certain neuroendocrine tumors, the morphology (histologic type) is included in the category and codes.

Primary malignant neoplasms overlapping site boundaries

A primary malignant neoplasm that overlaps two or more contiguous (next to each other) sites should be classified to the subcategory/code 8 ("overlapping lesion"), unless the combination is specifically indexed elsewhere. For multiple neoplasms of the same site that are not contiguous, such as tumors in different quadrants of the same breast, codes for each site should be assigned.

Malignant neoplasm of ectopic tissue

Malignant neoplasms of ectopic tissue are to be coded to the site mentioned, e.g., ectopic pancreatic malignant neoplasms are coded to pancreas, unspecified (C25.9).

AHA: 2017, 1Q, 4, 5-6, 8

This chapter contains the following blocks:

C00-C14	Malignant neoplasms of lip, oral cavity and pharynx
C15-C26	Malignant neoplasms of digestive organs
C30-C39	Malignant neoplasms of respiratory and intrathoracic organs
C40-C41	Malignant neoplasms of bone and articular cartilage
C43-C44	Melanoma and other malignant neoplasms of skin
C45-C49	Malignant neoplasms of mesothelial and soft tissue
C50	Malignant neoplasms of breast
C51-C58	Malignant neoplasms of female genital organs
C60-C63	Malignant neoplasms of male genital organs
C64-C68	Malignant neoplasms of urinary tract
C69-C72	Malignant neoplasms of eye, brain and other parts of central nervous system
C73-C75	Malignant neoplasms of thyroid and other endocrine glands
C7A	Malignant neuroendocrine tumors
C7B	Secondary neuroendocrine tumors
C76-C80	Malignant neoplasms of ill-defined, other secondary and unspecified sites
C81-C96	Malignant neoplasms of lymphoid, hematopoietic and related tissue
D00-D09	In situ neoplasms
D10-D36	Benign neoplasms, except benign neuroendocrine tumors
D3A	Benign neuroendocrine tumors
D37-D48	Neoplasms of uncertain behavior, polycythemia vera and myelodysplastic syndromes
D49	Neoplasms of unspecified behavior

MALIGNANT NEOPLASMS (C00-C96)

Malignant neoplasms, stated or presumed to be primary (of specified sites), and certain specified histologies, except neuroendocrine, and of lymphoid, hematopoietic and related tissue (C00-C75)

Malignant neoplasms of lip, oral cavity and pharynx (C00-C14)

✔4ᵗʰ **C00** **Malignant neoplasm of lip**

Use additional code to identify:
alcohol abuse and dependence (F10.-)
history of tobacco dependence (Z87.891)
tobacco dependence (F17.-)
tobacco use (Z72.0)

EXCLUDES 1 *malignant melanoma of lip (C43.0)*
Merkel cell carcinoma of lip (C4A.0)
other and unspecified malignant neoplasm of skin of lip (C44.0-)

  C00.0 **Malignant neoplasm of external upper lip**
Malignant neoplasm of lipstick area of upper lip
Malignant neoplasm of upper lip NOS
Malignant neoplasm of vermilion border of upper lip

  C00.1 **Malignant neoplasm of external lower lip**
Malignant neoplasm of lower lip NOS
Malignant neoplasm of lipstick area of lower lip
Malignant neoplasm of vermilion border of lower lip

  C00.2 **Malignant neoplasm of external lip, unspecified**
Malignant neoplasm of vermilion border of lip NOS

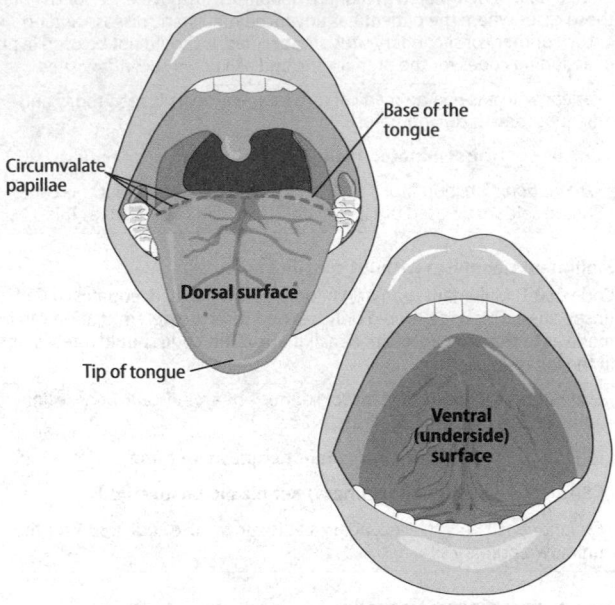

Malignant Neoplasm of Tongue

Base of the tongue
Circumvalate papillae
Dorsal surface
Tip of tongue
Ventral (underside) surface

  C00.3 **Malignant neoplasm of upper lip, inner aspect**
Malignant neoplasm of buccal aspect of upper lip
Malignant neoplasm of frenulum of upper lip
Malignant neoplasm of mucosa of upper lip
Malignant neoplasm of oral aspect of upper lip

  C00.4 **Malignant neoplasm of lower lip, inner aspect**
Malignant neoplasm of buccal aspect of lower lip
Malignant neoplasm of frenulum of lower lip
Malignant neoplasm of mucosa of lower lip
Malignant neoplasm of oral aspect of lower lip

  C00.5 **Malignant neoplasm of lip, unspecified, inner aspect**
Malignant neoplasm of buccal aspect of lip, unspecified
Malignant neoplasm of frenulum of lip, unspecified
Malignant neoplasm of mucosa of lip, unspecified
Malignant neoplasm of oral aspect of lip, unspecified

  C00.6 **Malignant neoplasm of commissure of lip, unspecified**

  C00.8 **Malignant neoplasm of overlapping sites of lip**

  C00.9 **Malignant neoplasm of lip, unspecified**

C01 **Malignant neoplasm of base of tongue**   HCC
Malignant neoplasm of dorsal surface of base of tongue
Malignant neoplasm of fixed part of tongue NOS
Malignant neoplasm of posterior third of tongue
Use additional code to identify:
alcohol abuse and dependence (F10.-)
history of tobacco dependence (Z87.891)
tobacco dependence (F17.-)
tobacco use (Z72.0)

✔4ᵗʰ **C02** **Malignant neoplasm of other and unspecified parts of tongue**
Use additional code to identify:
alcohol abuse and dependence (F10.-)
history of tobacco dependence (Z87.891)
tobacco dependence (F17.-)
tobacco use (Z72.0)

  C02.0 **Malignant neoplasm of dorsal surface of tongue**   HCC
Malignant neoplasm of anterior two-thirds of tongue, dorsal surface
EXCLUDES 2 *malignant neoplasm of dorsal surface of base of tongue (C01)*

  C02.1 **Malignant neoplasm of border of tongue**   HCC
Malignant neoplasm of tip of tongue

  C02.2 **Malignant neoplasm of ventral surface of tongue**   HCC
Malignant neoplasm of anterior two-thirds of tongue, ventral surface
Malignant neoplasm of frenulum linguae

  C02.3 **Malignant neoplasm of anterior two-thirds of tongue, part unspecified**   HCC
Malignant neoplasm of middle third of tongue NOS
Malignant neoplasm of mobile part of tongue NOS

  C02.4 **Malignant neoplasm of lingual tonsil**   HCC
EXCLUDES 2 *malignant neoplasm of tonsil NOS (C09.9)*

N Newborn: 0   P Pediatric: 0-17   M Maternity: 12-55   A Adult: 15-124   MCC Major CC Condition   PDxMCC PDx acts as own MCC   CC CC Condition   PDxCC PDx acts as own CC

462   ICD-10-CM 2018

C00-C02.4

C02.8 Malignant neoplasm of overlapping sites of tongue `HCC`
Malignant neoplasm of two or more contiguous sites of tongue

C02.9 Malignant neoplasm of tongue, unspecified `HCC`

✓4ᵗʰ **C03 Malignant neoplasm of gum**
`INCLUDES` malignant neoplasm of alveolar (ridge) mucosa
malignant neoplasm of gingiva
Use additional code to identify:
alcohol abuse and dependence (F10.-)
history of tobacco dependence (Z87.891)
tobacco dependence (F17.-)
tobacco use (Z72.0)
`EXCLUDES 2` malignant odontogenic neoplasms (C41.0-C41.1)

C03.0 Malignant neoplasm of upper gum `HCC`

C03.1 Malignant neoplasm of lower gum `HCC`

C03.9 Malignant neoplasm of gum, unspecified `HCC`

✓4ᵗʰ **C04 Malignant neoplasm of floor of mouth**
Use additional code to identify:
alcohol abuse and dependence (F10.-)
history of tobacco dependence (Z87.891)
tobacco dependence (F17.-)
tobacco use (Z72.0)

C04.0 Malignant neoplasm of anterior floor of mouth `HCC`
Malignant neoplasm of anterior to the premolar-canine junction

C04.1 Malignant neoplasm of lateral floor of mouth `HCC`

C04.8 Malignant neoplasm of overlapping sites of floor of mouth `HCC`

C04.9 Malignant neoplasm of floor of mouth, unspecified `HCC`

✓4ᵗʰ **C05 Malignant neoplasm of palate**
Use additional code to identify:
alcohol abuse and dependence (F10.-)
history of tobacco dependence (Z87.891)tobacco dependence (F17.-)
tobacco use (Z72.0)
`EXCLUDES 1` Kaposi's sarcoma of palate (C46.2)

C05.0 Malignant neoplasm of hard palate `HCC`

C05.1 Malignant neoplasm of soft palate `HCC`
`EXCLUDES 2` malignant neoplasm of nasopharyngeal surface of soft palate (C11.3)

C05.2 Malignant neoplasm of uvula `HCC`

C05.8 Malignant neoplasm of overlapping sites of palate `HCC`

C05.9 Malignant neoplasm of palate, unspecified `HCC`
Malignant neoplasm of roof of mouth

✓4ᵗʰ **C06 Malignant neoplasm of other and unspecified parts of mouth**
Use additional code to identify:
alcohol abuse and dependence (F10.-)
history of tobacco dependence (Z87.891)
tobacco dependence (F17.-)
tobacco use (Z72.0)

C06.0 Malignant neoplasm of cheek mucosa `HCC`
Malignant neoplasm of buccal mucosa NOS
Malignant neoplasm of internal cheek

C06.1 Malignant neoplasm of vestibule of mouth `HCC`
Malignant neoplasm of buccal sulcus (upper) (lower)
Malignant neoplasm of labial sulcus (upper) (lower)

C06.2 Malignant neoplasm of retromolar area `HCC`

✓5ᵗʰ **C06.8 Malignant neoplasm of overlapping sites of other and unspecified parts of mouth**

C06.80 Malignant neoplasm of overlapping sites of unspecified parts of mouth `HCC`

C06.89 Malignant neoplasm of overlapping sites of other parts of mouth `HCC`
"book leaf" neoplasm [ventral surface of tongue and floor of mouth]

C06.9 Malignant neoplasm of mouth, unspecified `HCC`
Malignant neoplasm of minor salivary gland, unspecified site
Malignant neoplasm of oral cavity NOS

C07 Malignant neoplasm of parotid gland `HCC`
Use additional code to identify:
alcohol abuse and dependence (F10.-)
exposure to environmental tobacco smoke (Z77.22)
exposure to tobacco smoke in the perinatal period (P96.81)
history of tobacco dependence (Z87.891)
occupational exposure to environmental tobacco smoke (Z57.31)
tobacco dependence (F17.-)
tobacco use (Z72.0)

✓4ᵗʰ **C08 Malignant neoplasm of other and unspecified major salivary glands**
`INCLUDES` malignant neoplasm of salivary ducts
Use additional code to identify:
alcohol abuse and dependence (F10.-)
exposure to environmental tobacco smoke (Z77.22)
exposure to tobacco smoke in the perinatal period (P96.81)
history of tobacco dependence (Z87.891)
occupational exposure to environmental tobacco smoke (Z57.31)
tobacco dependence (F17.-)
tobacco use (Z72.0)
`EXCLUDES 1` malignant neoplasms of specified minor salivary glands which are classified according to their anatomical location
`EXCLUDES 2` malignant neoplasms of minor salivary glands NOS (C06.9)
malignant neoplasm of parotid gland (C07)

C08.0 Malignant neoplasm of submandibular gland `HCC`
Malignant neoplasm of submaxillary gland

C08.1 Malignant neoplasm of sublingual gland `HCC`

C08.9 Malignant neoplasm of major salivary gland, unspecified `HCC`
Malignant neoplasm of salivary gland (major) NOS

✓4ᵗʰ **C09 Malignant neoplasm of tonsil**
Use additional code to identify:
alcohol abuse and dependence (F10.-)
exposure to environmental tobacco smoke (Z77.22)
exposure to tobacco smoke in the perinatal period (P96.81)
history of tobacco dependence (Z87.891)
occupational exposure to environmental tobacco smoke (Z57.31)
tobacco dependence (F17.-)
tobacco use (Z72.0)
`EXCLUDES 2` malignant neoplasm of lingual tonsil (C02.4)
malignant neoplasm of pharyngeal tonsil (C11.1)

C09.0 Malignant neoplasm of tonsillar fossa `HCC`

C09.1 Malignant neoplasm of tonsillar pillar (anterior) (posterior) `HCC`

C09.8 Malignant neoplasm of overlapping sites of tonsil `HCC`

C09.9 Malignant neoplasm of tonsil, unspecified `HCC`
Malignant neoplasm of tonsil NOS
Malignant neoplasm of faucial tonsils
Malignant neoplasm of palatine tonsils

✓4ᵗʰ **C10 Malignant neoplasm of oropharynx**
Use additional code to identify:
alcohol abuse and dependence (F10.-)
exposure to environmental tobacco smoke (Z77.22)
exposure to tobacco smoke in the perinatal period (P96.81)
history of tobacco dependence (Z87.891)
occupational exposure to environmental tobacco smoke (Z57.31)
tobacco dependence (F17.-)
tobacco use (Z72.0)
`EXCLUDES 2` malignant neoplasm of tonsil (C09.-)

C10.0 Malignant neoplasm of vallecula `HCC`

C10.1 Malignant neoplasm of anterior surface of epiglottis `HCC`
Malignant neoplasm of epiglottis, free border [margin]
Malignant neoplasm of glossoepiglottic fold(s)
`EXCLUDES 2` malignant neoplasm of epiglottis (suprahyoid portion) NOS (C32.1)

C10.2 Malignant neoplasm of lateral wall of oropharynx `HCC`

C10.3 Malignant neoplasm of posterior wall of oropharynx `HCC`

C10.4 Malignant neoplasm of branchial cleft `HCC`
Malignant neoplasm of branchial cyst [site of neoplasm]

C10.8 Malignant neoplasm of overlapping sites of oropharynx `HCC`
Malignant neoplasm of junctional region of oropharynx

C10.9 Malignant neoplasm of oropharynx, unspecified `HCC`

✓4ᵗʰ **C11 Malignant neoplasm of nasopharynx**
Use additional code to identify:
exposure to environmental tobacco smoke (Z77.22)
exposure to tobacco smoke in the perinatal period (P96.81)
history of tobacco dependence (Z87.891)
occupational exposure to environmental tobacco smoke (Z57.31)
tobacco dependence (F17.-)
tobacco use (Z72.0)

C11.0 Malignant neoplasm of superior wall of nasopharynx `HCC`
Malignant neoplasm of roof of nasopharynx

C11.1 Malignant neoplasm of posterior wall of nasopharynx `HCC`
Malignant neoplasm of adenoid
Malignant neoplasm of pharyngeal tonsil

C11.2 Malignant neoplasm of lateral wall of nasopharynx `HCC`
Malignant neoplasm of fossa of Rosenmüller
Malignant neoplasm of opening of auditory tube
Malignant neoplasm of pharyngeal recess

✓ Additional Character Req   ✓x7ᵗʰ Placeholder Alert   Unacceptable PDx   Manifestation   H1-H14 HAC   HCC CMS-HCC Condition   `EXCLUDES1` Not Coded Here   `EXCLUDES2` Not Included Here

C11.3   **Malignant neoplasm of** anterior wall **of nasopharynx** `HCC`
Malignant neoplasm of floor of nasopharynx
Malignant neoplasm of nasopharyngeal (anterior) (posterior) surface of soft palate
Malignant neoplasm of posterior margin of nasal choana
Malignant neoplasm of posterior margin of nasal septum

C11.8   **Malignant neoplasm of** overlapping sites **of nasopharynx** `HCC`

C11.9   **Malignant neoplasm of nasopharynx,** unspecified `HCC`
Malignant neoplasm of nasopharyngeal wall NOS

C12   **Malignant neoplasm of** pyriform sinus `HCC`
Malignant neoplasm of pyriform fossa
Use additional code to identify:
    exposure to environmental tobacco smoke (Z77.22)
    exposure to tobacco smoke in the perinatal period (P96.81)
    history of tobacco dependence (Z87.891)
    occupational exposure to environmental tobacco smoke (Z57.31)
    tobacco dependence (F17.-)
    tobacco use (Z72.0)

✓4ᵗʰ **C13**   **Malignant neoplasm of** hypopharynx
Use additional code to identify:
    exposure to environmental tobacco smoke (Z77.22)
    exposure to tobacco smoke in the perinatal period (P96.81)
    history of tobacco dependence (Z87.891)
    occupational exposure to environmental tobacco smoke (Z57.31)
    tobacco dependence (F17.-)
    tobacco use (Z72.0)
    EXCLUDES 2   *malignant neoplasm of pyriform sinus (C12)*

C13.0   **Malignant neoplasm of** postcricoid region `HCC`

C13.1   **Malignant neoplasm of** aryepiglottic fold, `HCC`
hypopharyngeal aspect
Malignant neoplasm of aryepiglottic fold, marginal zone
Malignant neoplasm of aryepiglottic fold NOS
Malignant neoplasm of interarytenoid fold, marginal zone
Malignant neoplasm of interarytenoid fold NOS
    EXCLUDES 2   *malignant neoplasm of aryepiglottic fold or interarytenoid fold, laryngeal aspect (C32.1)*

C13.2   **Malignant neoplasm of** posterior wall **of hypopharynx** `HCC`

C13.8   **Malignant neoplasm of** overlapping sites **of hypopharynx** `HCC`

C13.9   **Malignant neoplasm of hypopharynx,** unspecified `HCC`
Malignant neoplasm of hypopharyngeal wall NOS

✓4ᵗʰ **C14**   **Malignant neoplasm of** other and ill-defined sites in the lip, oral cavity and pharynx
Use additional code to identify:
    alcohol abuse and dependence (F10.-)
    exposure to environmental tobacco smoke (Z77.22)
    exposure to tobacco smoke in the perinatal period (P96.81)
    history of tobacco dependence (Z87.891)
    occupational exposure to environmental tobacco smoke (Z57.31)
    tobacco dependence (F17.-)
    tobacco use (Z72.0)
    EXCLUDES 1   *malignant neoplasm of oral cavity NOS (C06.9)*

C14.0   **Malignant neoplasm of pharynx,** unspecified `HCC`

C14.2   **Malignant neoplasm of** Waldeyer's ring `HCC`

C14.8   **Malignant neoplasm of** overlapping sites **of lip, oral cavity and pharynx** `HCC`
Primary malignant neoplasm of two or more contiguous sites of lip, oral cavity and pharynx
    EXCLUDES 1   *"book leaf" neoplasm [ventral surface of tongue and floor of mouth] (C06.89)*

Malignant neoplasms of digestive organs (C15-C26)

    EXCLUDES 1   *Kaposi's sarcoma of gastrointestinal sites (C46.4)*
    EXCLUDES 2   *gastrointestinal stromal tumors (C49.A-)*

✓4ᵗʰ **C15**   **Malignant neoplasm of** esophagus
Use additional code to identify:
    alcohol abuse and dependence (F10.-)

CC Excl: For CC codes in category C15: PDX collection 253

C15.3   **Malignant neoplasm of** upper third **of esophagus** `CC` `HCC`

C15.4   **Malignant neoplasm of** middle third **of esophagus** `CC` `HCC`

C15.5   **Malignant neoplasm of** lower third **of esophagus** `CC` `HCC`
    EXCLUDES 1   *malignant neoplasm of cardio-esophageal junction (C16.0)*

C15.8   **Malignant neoplasm of** overlapping sites **of esophagus** `CC` `HCC`

C15.9   **Malignant neoplasm of esophagus,** unspecified `CC` `HCC`

✓4ᵗʰ **C16**   **Malignant neoplasm of** stomach
Use additional code to identify:
    alcohol abuse and dependence (F10.-)
    EXCLUDES 2   *malignant carcinoid tumor of the stomach (C7A.092)*

CC Excl: For CC codes in category C16: PDX collection 254

C16.0   **Malignant neoplasm of** cardia `CC` `HCC`
Malignant neoplasm of cardiac orifice
Malignant neoplasm of cardio-esophageal junction
Malignant neoplasm of esophagus and stomach
Malignant neoplasm of gastro-esophageal junction

C16.1   **Malignant neoplasm of** fundus **of stomach** `CC` `HCC`

C16.2   **Malignant neoplasm of** body **of stomach** `CC` `HCC`

C16.3   **Malignant neoplasm of** pyloric antrum `CC` `HCC`
Malignant neoplasm of gastric antrum

C16.4   **Malignant neoplasm of** pylorus `CC` `HCC`
Malignant neoplasm of prepylorus
Malignant neoplasm of pyloric canal

C16.5   **Malignant neoplasm of** lesser curvature **of stomach, unspecified** `CC` `HCC`
Malignant neoplasm of lesser curvature of stomach, not classifiable to C16.1-C16.4

C16.6   **Malignant neoplasm of** greater curvature **of stomach, unspecified** `CC` `HCC`
Malignant neoplasm of greater curvature of stomach, not classifiable to C16.0-C16.4

C16.8   **Malignant neoplasm of** overlapping sites **of stomach** `CC` `HCC`

C16.9   **Malignant neoplasm of stomach,** unspecified `CC` `HCC`
Gastric cancer NOS

✓4ᵗʰ **C17**   **Malignant neoplasm of** small intestine
    EXCLUDES 1   *malignant carcinoid tumors of the small intestine (C7A.01)*
AHA: 2016, 1Q, 19

C17.0   **Malignant neoplasm of** duodenum `CC` `HCC`
    CC Excl: PDX collection 255

C17.1   **Malignant neoplasm of** jejunum `CC` `HCC`
    CC Excl: PDX collection 256

C17.2   **Malignant neoplasm of** ileum `CC` `HCC`
    EXCLUDES 1   *malignant neoplasm of ileocecal valve (C18.0)*
    CC Excl: PDX collection 257

C17.3   **Meckel's diverticulum, malignant** `CC` `HCC`
    EXCLUDES 1   *Meckel's diverticulum, congenital (Q43.0)*
    CC Excl: PDX collection 258

C17.8   **Malignant neoplasm of** overlapping sites **of small intestine** `CC` `HCC`
    CC Excl: PDX collection 259

C17.9   **Malignant neoplasm of small intestine,** unspecified `CC` `HCC`
    CC Excl: PDX collection 259

✓4ᵗʰ **C18**   **Malignant neoplasm of** colon
    EXCLUDES 1   *malignant carcinoid tumors of the colon (C7A.02-)*

C18.0   **Malignant neoplasm of** cecum `CC` `HCC`
Malignant neoplasm of ileocecal valve
    CC Excl: PDX collection 260

C18.1   **Malignant neoplasm of** appendix `CC` `HCC`
    CC Excl: PDX collection 261

C18.2   **Malignant neoplasm of** ascending colon `CC` `HCC`
    CC Excl: PDX collection 262

C18.3   **Malignant neoplasm of** hepatic flexure `CC` `HCC`
    CC Excl: PDX collection 263

C18.4   **Malignant neoplasm of** transverse colon `CC` `HCC`
    CC Excl: PDX collection 264

C18.5   **Malignant neoplasm of** splenic flexure `CC` `HCC`
    CC Excl: PDX collection 265

C18.6   **Malignant neoplasm of** descending colon `CC` `HCC`
    CC Excl: PDX collection 266

C18.7   **Malignant neoplasm of** sigmoid colon `CC` `HCC`
Malignant neoplasm of sigmoid (flexure)
    EXCLUDES 1   *malignant neoplasm of rectosigmoid junction (C19)*
    CC Excl: PDX collection 267

C18.8   **Malignant neoplasm of** overlapping sites **of colon** `CC` `HCC`
    CC Excl: PDX collection 268

C18.9   **Malignant neoplasm of colon,** unspecified `CC` `HCC`
Malignant neoplasm of large intestine NOS
    CC Excl: PDX collection 268

C19   **Malignant neoplasm of** rectosigmoid junction `CC` `HCC`
Malignant neoplasm of colon with rectum
Malignant neoplasm of rectosigmoid (colon)
    EXCLUDES 1   *malignant carcinoid tumors of the colon (C7A.02-)*
    CC Excl: PDX collection 269

N Newborn: 0   P Pediatric: 0-17   M Maternity: 12-55   A Adult: 15-124   MCC Major CC Condition   PDxMCC PDx acts as own MCC   CC CC Condition   PDxCC PDx acts as own CC

464   ICD-10-CM 2018

Colon

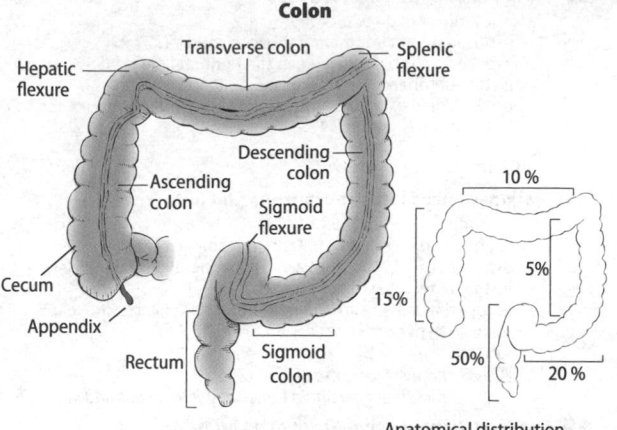

Anatomical distribution of large bowel cancers

C20 Malignant neoplasm of rectum `CC` `HCC`
Malignant neoplasm of rectal ampulla
EXCLUDES 1   *malignant carcinoid tumor of the rectum (C7A.026)*
CC Excl: PDX collection 270

✓4ᵗʰ C21 Malignant neoplasm of anus and anal canal
EXCLUDES 2   *malignant carcinoid tumors of the colon (C7A.02-)*
      malignant melanoma of anal margin (C43.51)
      malignant melanoma of anal skin (C43.51)
      malignant melanoma of perianal skin (C43.51)
      other and unspecified malignant neoplasm of anal margin
          (C44.500, C44.510, C44.520, C44.590)
      other and unspecified malignant neoplasm of anal skin
          (C44.500, C44.510, C44.520, C44.590)
      other and unspecified malignant neoplasm of perianal skin
          (C44.500, C44.510, C44.520, C44.590)

C21.0 Malignant neoplasm of anus, unspecified `CC` `HCC`
CC Excl: PDX collection 271

C21.1 Malignant neoplasm of anal canal `CC` `HCC`
Malignant neoplasm of anal sphincter
CC Excl: PDX collection 271

C21.2 Malignant neoplasm of cloacogenic zone `CC` `HCC`
CC Excl: PDX collection 272

C21.8 Malignant neoplasm of overlapping sites of rectum, `CC` `HCC`
anus and anal canal
Malignant neoplasm of anorectal junction
Malignant neoplasm of anorectum
Primary malignant neoplasm of two or more contiguous sites of
      rectum, anus and anal canal
CC Excl: PDX collection 272

✓4ᵗʰ C22 Malignant neoplasm of liver and intrahepatic bile ducts
Use additional code to identify:
    alcohol abuse and dependence (F10.-)
    hepatitis B (B16.-, B18.0-B18.1)
    hepatitis C (B17.1-, B18.2)
EXCLUDES 1   *malignant neoplasm of biliary tract NOS (C24.9)*
      secondary malignant neoplasm of liver and intrahepatic bile
          duct (C78.7)

CC Excl: For CC codes in category C22: PDX collection 273

C22.0 Liver cell carcinoma `CC` `HCC`
Hepatocellular carcinoma
Hepatoma
AHA: 2016, 1Q, 18

C22.1 Intrahepatic bile duct carcinoma `CC` `HCC`
Cholangiocarcinoma
EXCLUDES 1   *malignant neoplasm of hepatic duct (C24.0)*

C22.2 Hepatoblastoma `CC` `HCC`

C22.3 Angiosarcoma of liver `CC` `HCC`
Kupffer cell sarcoma

C22.4 Other sarcomas of liver `CC` `HCC`

C22.7 Other specified carcinomas of liver `CC` `HCC`

C22.8 Malignant neoplasm of liver, primary, unspecified `CC` `HCC`
as to type

C22.9 Malignant neoplasm of liver, not specified as primary `CC` `HCC`
or secondary

C23 Malignant neoplasm of gallbladder `CC` `HCC`
CC Excl: PDX collection 274

✓4ᵗʰ C24 Malignant neoplasm of other and unspecified parts of biliary
tract
EXCLUDES 1   *malignant neoplasm of intrahepatic bile duct (C22.1)*

C24.0 Malignant neoplasm of extrahepatic bile duct `CC` `HCC`
Malignant neoplasm of biliary duct or passage NOS
Malignant neoplasm of common bile duct
Malignant neoplasm of cystic duct
Malignant neoplasm of hepatic duct
CC Excl: PDX collection 275

C24.1 Malignant neoplasm of ampulla of Vater `CC` `HCC`
DEF: Malignant neoplasm in the area of dilation at the juncture of
the common bile and pancreatic ducts near the opening into the
lumen of the duodenum.
CC Excl: PDX collection 276

C24.8 Malignant neoplasm of overlapping sites of `CC` `HCC`
biliary tract
Malignant neoplasm involving both intrahepatic and
    extrahepatic bile ducts
Primary malignant neoplasm of two or more contiguous sites of
    biliary tract
CC Excl: PDX collection 277

C24.9 Malignant neoplasm of biliary tract, unspecified `CC` `HCC`
CC Excl: PDX collection 277

✓4ᵗʰ C25 Malignant neoplasm of pancreas
Code also exocrine pancreatic insufficiency (K86.81)
Use additional code to identify:
    alcohol abuse and dependence (F10.-)

CC Excl: For CC codes in category C25: PDX collection 278

C25.0 Malignant neoplasm of head of pancreas `CC` `HCC`

C25.1 Malignant neoplasm of body of pancreas `CC` `HCC`

C25.2 Malignant neoplasm of tail of pancreas `CC` `HCC`

C25.3 Malignant neoplasm of pancreatic duct `CC` `HCC`

C25.4 Malignant neoplasm of endocrine pancreas `CC` `HCC`
Malignant neoplasm of islets of Langerhans
Use additional code to identify any functional activity

C25.7 Malignant neoplasm of other parts of pancreas `CC` `HCC`
Malignant neoplasm of neck of pancreas

C25.8 Malignant neoplasm of overlapping sites of pancreas `CC` `HCC`

C25.9 Malignant neoplasm of pancreas, unspecified `CC` `HCC`

✓4ᵗʰ C26 Malignant neoplasm of other and ill-defined digestive organs
EXCLUDES 1   *malignant neoplasm of peritoneum and*
      retroperitoneum (C48.-)

C26.0 Malignant neoplasm of intestinal tract, part unspecified `HCC`
Malignant neoplasm of intestine NOS

C26.1 Malignant neoplasm of spleen `HCC`
EXCLUDES 1   *Hodgkin lymphoma (C81.-)*
      non-Hodgkin lymphoma (C82-C85)

C26.9 Malignant neoplasm of ill-defined sites within the `HCC`
digestive system
Malignant neoplasm of alimentary canal or tract NOS
Malignant neoplasm of gastrointestinal tract NOS
EXCLUDES 1   *malignant neoplasm of abdominal NOS (C76.2)*
      malignant neoplasm of intra-abdominal NOS (C76.2)

Pancreas

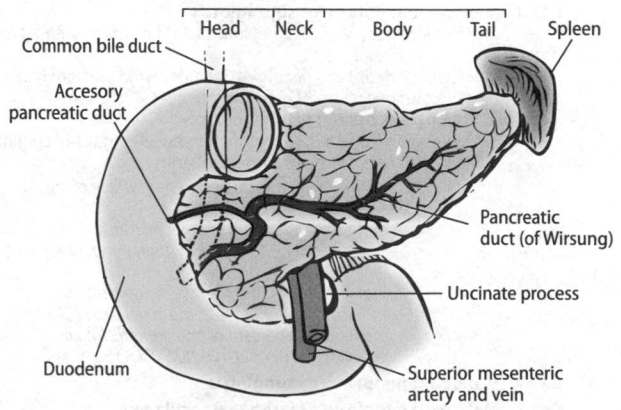

☑ Additional Character Req   ✓xⁿᵗʰ Placeholder Alert   Unacceptable PDx   Manifestation   **H1–H14** HAC   **HCC** CMS-HCC Condition   *EXCLUDES 1* Not Coded Here   *EXCLUDES 2* Not Included Here

Malignant neoplasms of respiratory and intrathoracic organs (C30-C39)

INCLUDES malignant neoplasm of middle ear
EXCLUDES1 mesothelioma (C45.-)

☑4ᵗʰ C30 Malignant neoplasm of nasal cavity and middle ear

C30.0 Malignant neoplasm of nasal cavity HCC
Malignant neoplasm of cartilage of nose
Malignant neoplasm of nasal concha
Malignant neoplasm of internal nose
Malignant neoplasm of septum of nose
Malignant neoplasm of vestibule of nose
EXCLUDES1 malignant melanoma of skin of nose (C43.31)
malignant neoplasm of nasal bone (C41.0)
malignant neoplasm of nose NOS (C76.0)
malignant neoplasm of olfactory bulb (C72.2-)
malignant neoplasm of posterior margin of nasal
septum and choana (C11.3)
malignant neoplasm of turbinates (C41.0)
other and unspecified malignant neoplasm of skin of
nose (C44.301, C44.311, C44.321, C44.391)

C30.1 Malignant neoplasm of middle ear HCC
Malignant neoplasm of antrum tympanicum
Malignant neoplasm of auditory tube
Malignant neoplasm of eustachian tube
Malignant neoplasm of inner ear
Malignant neoplasm of mastoid air cells
Malignant neoplasm of tympanic cavity
EXCLUDES1 malignant melanoma of skin of (external) ear (C43.2-)
malignant neoplasm of auricular canal (external)
(C43.2-,C44.2-)
malignant neoplasm of bone of ear (meatus) (C41.0)
malignant neoplasm of cartilage of ear (C49.0)
other and unspecified malignant neoplasm of skin of
(external) ear (C44.2-)

☑4ᵗʰ C31 Malignant neoplasm of accessory sinuses

C31.0 Malignant neoplasm of maxillary sinus HCC
Malignant neoplasm of antrum (Highmore) (maxillary)

C31.1 Malignant neoplasm of ethmoidal sinus HCC

C31.2 Malignant neoplasm of frontal sinus HCC

C31.3 Malignant neoplasm of sphenoid sinus HCC

C31.8 Malignant neoplasm of overlapping sites of accessory sinuses HCC

C31.9 Malignant neoplasm of accessory sinus, unspecified HCC

☑4ᵗʰ C32 Malignant neoplasm of larynx

Use additional code to identify:
alcohol abuse and dependence (F10.-)
exposure to environmental tobacco smoke (Z77.22)
exposure to tobacco smoke in the perinatal period (P96.81)
history of tobacco dependence (Z87.891)
occupational exposure to environmental tobacco smoke (Z57.31)
tobacco dependence (F17.-)
tobacco use (Z72.0)

C32.0 Malignant neoplasm of glottis HCC
Malignant neoplasm of intrinsic larynx
Malignant neoplasm of laryngeal commissure
(anterior)(posterior)
Malignant neoplasm of vocal cord (true) NOS

C32.1 Malignant neoplasm of supraglottis HCC
Malignant neoplasm of aryepiglottic fold or interarytenoid fold,
laryngeal aspect
Malignant neoplasm of epiglottis (suprahyoid portion) NOS
Malignant neoplasm of extrinsic larynx
Malignant neoplasm of false vocal cord
Malignant neoplasm of posterior (laryngeal) surface of epiglottis
Malignant neoplasm of ventricular bands
EXCLUDES2 malignant neoplasm of anterior surface of epiglottis
(C10.1)
malignant neoplasm of aryepiglottic fold or
interarytenoid fold, hypopharyngeal aspect
(C13.1)
malignant neoplasm of aryepiglottic fold or
interarytenoid fold, marginal zone (C13.1)
malignant neoplasm of aryepiglottic fold or
interarytenoid fold NOS (C13.1)

C32.2 Malignant neoplasm of subglottis HCC

C32.3 Malignant neoplasm of laryngeal cartilage HCC

C32.8 Malignant neoplasm of overlapping sites of larynx HCC

C32.9 Malignant neoplasm of larynx, unspecified HCC

C33 Malignant neoplasm of trachea CC HCC

Use additional code to identify:
exposure to environmental tobacco smoke (Z77.22)
exposure to tobacco smoke in the perinatal period (P96.81)
history of tobacco dependence (Z87.891)
occupational exposure to environmental tobacco smoke (Z57.31)
tobacco dependence (F17.-)
tobacco use (Z72.0)
CC Excl: PDX collection 279

☑4ᵗʰ C34 Malignant neoplasm of bronchus and lung

Use additional code to identify:
exposure to environmental tobacco smoke (Z77.22)
exposure to tobacco smoke in the perinatal period (P96.81)
history of tobacco dependence (Z87.891)
occupational exposure to environmental tobacco smoke (Z57.31)
tobacco dependence (F17.-)
tobacco use (Z72.0)
EXCLUDES1 Kaposi's sarcoma of lung (C46.5-)
malignant carcinoid tumor of the bronchus and lung (C7A.090)

☑5ᵗʰ C34.0 Malignant neoplasm of main bronchus
Malignant neoplasm of carina
Malignant neoplasm of hilus (of lung)

> **CC Excl: For CC codes in subcategory C34.0:**
> PDX collection 280

C34.00 Malignant neoplasm of unspecified main bronchus CC HCC

C34.01 Malignant neoplasm of right main bronchus CC HCC

C34.02 Malignant neoplasm of left main bronchus CC HCC

☑5ᵗʰ C34.1 Malignant neoplasm of upper lobe, bronchus or lung

> **CC Excl: For CC codes in subcategory C34.1:**
> PDX collection 281

C34.10 Malignant neoplasm of upper lobe, unspecified bronchus or lung CC HCC

C34.11 Malignant neoplasm of upper lobe, right bronchus or lung CC HCC

C34.12 Malignant neoplasm of upper lobe, left bronchus or lung CC HCC

C34.2 Malignant neoplasm of middle lobe, bronchus or lung CC HCC
CC Excl: PDX collection 282

☑5ᵗʰ C34.3 Malignant neoplasm of lower lobe, bronchus or lung

> **CC Excl: For CC codes in subcategory C34.3:**
> PDX collection 283

C34.30 Malignant neoplasm of lower lobe, unspecified bronchus or lung CC HCC

C34.31 Malignant neoplasm of lower lobe, right bronchus or lung CC HCC

C34.32 Malignant neoplasm of lower lobe, left bronchus or lung CC HCC

☑5ᵗʰ C34.8 Malignant neoplasm of overlapping sites of bronchus and lung

> **CC Excl: For CC codes in subcategory C34.8:**
> PDX collection 284

C34.80 Malignant neoplasm of overlapping sites of unspecified bronchus and lung CC HCC

C34.81 Malignant neoplasm of overlapping sites of right bronchus and lung CC HCC

C34.82 Malignant neoplasm of overlapping sites of left bronchus and lung CC HCC

☑5ᵗʰ C34.9 Malignant neoplasm of unspecified part of bronchus or lung

> **CC Excl: For CC codes in subcategory C34.9:**
> PDX collection 284

C34.90 Malignant neoplasm of unspecified part of unspecified bronchus or lung CC HCC
Lung cancer NOS

C34.91 Malignant neoplasm of unspecified part of right bronchus or lung CC HCC

C34.92 Malignant neoplasm of unspecified part of left bronchus or lung CC HCC

C37 Malignant neoplasm of thymus CC HCC
EXCLUDES1 malignant carcinoid tumor of the thymus (C7A.091)
CC Excl: PDX collection 285

N Newborn: 0 · P Pediatric: 0-17 · M Maternity: 12-55 · A Adult: 15-124 · MCC Major CC Condition · PDxMCC PDx acts as own MCC · CC CC Condition · PDxCC PDx acts as own CC

466 — ICD-10-CM 2018

☑4ᵗʰ **C38** **Malignant neoplasm of** heart, mediastinum and pleura
   EXCLUDES 1 *mesothelioma (C45.-)*

   CC Excl: For CC codes in category C38, unless otherwise noted:
   PDX collection 287

   C38.0 **Malignant neoplasm of** heart   CC HCC
      Malignant neoplasm of pericardium
      EXCLUDES 1 *malignant neoplasm of great vessels (C49.3)*
      CC Excl: PDX collection 286
   C38.1 **Malignant neoplasm of** anterior mediastinum   CC HCC
   C38.2 **Malignant neoplasm of** posterior mediastinum   CC HCC
   C38.3 **Malignant neoplasm of** mediastinum, part   CC HCC
      unspecified
   C38.4 **Malignant neoplasm of** pleura   CC HCC
   C38.8 **Malignant neoplasm of** overlapping sites of heart,   CC HCC
      mediastinum and pleura

☑4ᵗʰ **C39** **Malignant neoplasm of** other and ill-defined sites in the
   respiratory system and intrathoracic organs
      Use additional code to identify:
         exposure to environmental tobacco smoke (Z77.22)
         exposure to tobacco smoke in the perinatal period (P96.81)
         history of tobacco dependence (Z87.891)
         occupational exposure to environmental tobacco smoke (Z57.31)
         tobacco dependence (F17.-)
         tobacco use (Z72.0)
      EXCLUDES 1 *intrathoracic malignant neoplasm NOS (C76.1)*
            thoracic malignant neoplasm NOS (C76.1)
   C39.0 **Malignant neoplasm of** upper respiratory tract, part   HCC
      unspecified
   C39.9 **Malignant neoplasm of** lower respiratory tract, part   HCC
      unspecified
      Malignant neoplasm of respiratory tract NOS

Malignant neoplasms of bone and articular cartilage (C40-C41)
   INCLUDES malignant neoplasm of cartilage (articular) (joint)
         malignant neoplasm of periosteum
   EXCLUDES 1 *malignant neoplasm of bone marrow NOS (C96.9)*
         malignant neoplasm of synovia (C49.-)

☑4ᵗʰ **C40** **Malignant neoplasm of** bone and articular cartilage of limbs
      Use additional code to identify major osseous defect, if applicable
      (M89.7-)
   ☑5ᵗʰ **C40.0** **Malignant neoplasm of** scapula and long bones of upper limb

      CC Excl: For CC codes in subcategory C40.0:
      PDX collection 289

      C40.00 **Malignant neoplasm of** scapula and long   CC HCC
         bones of unspecified upper limb
      C40.01 **Malignant neoplasm of** scapula and long   CC HCC
         bones of right upper limb
      C40.02 **Malignant neoplasm of** scapula and long   CC HCC
         bones of left upper limb
   ☑5ᵗʰ **C40.1** **Malignant neoplasm of** short bones of upper limb

      CC Excl: For CC codes in subcategory C40.1:
      PDX collection 290

      C40.10 **Malignant neoplasm of** short bones of   CC HCC
         unspecified upper limb
      C40.11 **Malignant neoplasm of** short bones of right   CC HCC
         upper limb
      C40.12 **Malignant neoplasm of** short bones of left   CC HCC
         upper limb
   ☑5ᵗʰ **C40.2** **Malignant neoplasm of** long bones of lower limb

      CC Excl: For CC codes in subcategory C40.2:
      PDX collection 291

      C40.20 **Malignant neoplasm of** long bones of   CC HCC
         unspecified lower limb
      C40.21 **Malignant neoplasm of** long bones of right   CC HCC
         lower limb
      C40.22 **Malignant neoplasm of** long bones of left   CC HCC
         lower limb
   ☑5ᵗʰ **C40.3** **Malignant neoplasm of** short bones of lower limb

      CC Excl: For CC codes in subcategory C40.3:
      PDX collection 292

      C40.30 **Malignant neoplasm of** short bones of   CC HCC
         unspecified lower limb
      C40.31 **Malignant neoplasm of** short bones of right   CC HCC
         lower limb

      C40.32 **Malignant neoplasm of** short bones of left   CC HCC
         lower limb
   ☑5ᵗʰ **C40.8** **Malignant neoplasm of** overlapping sites of bone and
      articular cartilage of limb

      CC Excl: For CC codes in subcategory C40.8:
      PDX collection 293

      C40.80 **Malignant neoplasm of** overlapping sites of   CC HCC
         bone and articular cartilage of unspecified limb
      C40.81 **Malignant neoplasm of** overlapping sites of   CC HCC
         bone and articular cartilage of right limb
      C40.82 **Malignant neoplasm of** overlapping sites of   CC HCC
         bone and articular cartilage of left limb
   ☑5ᵗʰ **C40.9** **Malignant neoplasm of** unspecified bones and articular
      cartilage of limb

      CC Excl: For CC codes in subcategory C40.9:
      PDX collection 293

      C40.90 **Malignant neoplasm of** unspecified bones   CC HCC
         and articular cartilage of unspecified limb
      C40.91 **Malignant neoplasm of** unspecified bones   CC HCC
         and articular cartilage of right limb
      C40.92 **Malignant neoplasm of** unspecified bones   CC HCC
         and articular cartilage of left limb

☑4ᵗʰ **C41** **Malignant neoplasm of** bone and articular cartilage of other and
   unspecified sites
      EXCLUDES 1 *malignant neoplasm of bones of limbs (C40.-)*
            malignant neoplasm of cartilage of ear (C49.0)
            malignant neoplasm of cartilage of eyelid (C49.0)
            malignant neoplasm of cartilage of larynx (C32.3)
            malignant neoplasm of cartilage of limbs (C40.-)
            malignant neoplasm of cartilage of nose (C30.0)
   C41.0 **Malignant neoplasm of** bones of skull and face   CC HCC
      Malignant neoplasm of maxilla (superior)
      Malignant neoplasm of orbital bone
      EXCLUDES 2 *carcinoma, any type except intraosseous or*
            odontogenic of:
            maxillary sinus (C31.0)
            upper jaw (C03.0)
            malignant neoplasm of jaw bone (lower) (C41.1)
      CC Excl: PDX collection 294
   C41.1 **Malignant neoplasm of** mandible   CC HCC
      Malignant neoplasm of inferior maxilla
      Malignant neoplasm of lower jaw bone
      EXCLUDES 2 *carcinoma, any type except intraosseous or*
            odontogenic of:
            jaw NOS (C03.9)
            lower (C03.1)
            malignant neoplasm of upper jaw bone (C41.0)
      CC Excl: PDX collection 295
   C41.2 **Malignant neoplasm of** vertebral column   CC HCC
      EXCLUDES 1 *malignant neoplasm of sacrum and coccyx (C41.4)*
      CC Excl: PDX collection 296
   C41.3 **Malignant neoplasm of** ribs, sternum and clavicle   CC HCC
      CC Excl: PDX collection 297
   C41.4 **Malignant neoplasm of** pelvic bones, sacrum   CC HCC
      and coccyx
      CC Excl: PDX collection 298
   C41.9 **Malignant neoplasm of** bone and articular cartilage,   CC HCC
      unspecified
      CC Excl: PDX collection 293

Melanoma and other malignant neoplasms of skin (C43-C44)

☑4ᵗʰ **C43** **Malignant** melanoma of skin
      EXCLUDES 1 *melanoma in situ (D03.-)*
      EXCLUDES 2 *malignant melanoma of skin of genital organs (C51-C52, C60.-,*
            C63.-)
            Merkel cell carcinoma (C4A.-)
            sites other than skin—code to malignant neoplasm of the site
   C43.0 **Malignant melanoma of** lip   HCC
      EXCLUDES 1 *malignant neoplasm of vermilion border of lip (C00.0-*
            C00.2)
   ☑5ᵗʰ **C43.1** **Malignant melanoma of** eyelid, including canthus
      C43.10 **Malignant melanoma of** unspecified eyelid,   HCC
         including canthus
      C43.11 **Malignant melanoma of** right eyelid, including   HCC
         canthus
      C43.12 **Malignant melanoma of** left eyelid, including   HCC
         canthus

☑ Additional Character Req   ☑x 7ᵗʰ Placeholder Alert   Unacceptable PDx   Manifestation   H1-H14 HAC   HCC CMS-HCC Condition   EXCLUDES 1 Not Coded Here   EXCLUDES 2 Not Included Here

ICD-10-CM 2018   **467**

C38–C43.12

√5ᵗʰ **C43.2 Malignant melanoma of** ear and external auricular canal

    C43.20 Malignant melanoma of unspecified **ear and** HCC
    external auricular canal

    C43.21 Malignant melanoma of right **ear and external** HCC
    auricular canal

    C43.22 Malignant melanoma of left **ear and external** HCC
    auricular canal

√5ᵗʰ **C43.3 Malignant melanoma of other and unspecified** parts of face

    C43.30 Malignant melanoma of unspecified **part of face** HCC

    C43.31 Malignant melanoma of nose HCC

    C43.39 Malignant melanoma of other **parts of face** HCC

C43.4 Malignant melanoma of scalp and neck HCC

√5ᵗʰ **C43.5 Malignant melanoma of trunk**

    EXCLUDES 2   *malignant neoplasm of anus NOS (C21.0)*
             malignant neoplasm of scrotum (C63.2)

    C43.51 Malignant melanoma of anal skin HCC
        Malignant melanoma of anal margin
        Malignant melanoma of perianal skin

    C43.52 Malignant melanoma of skin of breast HCC

    C43.59 Malignant melanoma of other **part of trunk** HCC

√5ᵗʰ **C43.6 Malignant melanoma of** upper limb, including shoulder

    C43.60 Malignant melanoma of unspecified **upper limb,** HCC
    including shoulder

    C43.61 Malignant melanoma of right **upper limb,** HCC
    including shoulder

    C43.62 Malignant melanoma of left **upper limb,** HCC
    including shoulder

√5ᵗʰ **C43.7 Malignant melanoma of** lower limb, including hip

    C43.70 Malignant melanoma of unspecified **lower** HCC
    limb, including hip

    C43.71 Malignant melanoma of right **lower limb,** HCC
    including hip

    C43.72 Malignant melanoma of left **lower limb,** HCC
    including hip

C43.8 Malignant melanoma of overlapping sites **of skin** HCC

C43.9 Malignant melanoma of skin, unspecified HCC
     Malignant melanoma of unspecified site of skin
     Melanoma (malignant) NOS

√4ᵗʰ **C4A Merkel cell carcinoma**

   DEF: Malignant cutaneous cancer predominantly found in elderly patients with sun exposure that usually presents as a flesh-colored or bluish-red lump typically seen on the neck, head and face.

C4A.0 Merkel cell carcinoma of lip HCC

    EXCLUDES 1   *malignant neoplasm of vermilion border of lip (C00.0-*
             C00.2)

√5ᵗʰ **C4A.1 Merkel cell carcinoma of** eyelid, including canthus

    C4A.10 Merkel cell carcinoma of unspecified **eyelid,** HCC
    including canthus

    C4A.11 Merkel cell carcinoma of right **eyelid, including** HCC
    canthus

    C4A.12 Merkel cell carcinoma of left **eyelid, including** HCC
    canthus

√5ᵗʰ **C4A.2 Merkel cell carcinoma of** ear and external auricular canal

    C4A.20 Merkel cell carcinoma of unspecified **ear and** HCC
    external auricular canal

    C4A.21 Merkel cell carcinoma of right **ear and external** HCC
    auricular canal

    C4A.22 Merkel cell carcinoma of left **ear and external** HCC
    auricular canal

√5ᵗʰ **C4A.3 Merkel cell carcinoma of** other and unspecified **parts of face**

    C4A.30 Merkel cell carcinoma of unspecified **part of face** HCC

    C4A.31 Merkel cell carcinoma of nose HCC

    C4A.39 Merkel cell carcinoma of other **parts of face** HCC

C4A.4 Merkel cell carcinoma of scalp and neck HCC

√5ᵗʰ **C4A.5 Merkel cell carcinoma of trunk**

    EXCLUDES 2   *malignant neoplasm of anus NOS (C21.0)*
             malignant neoplasm of scrotum (C63.2)

    C4A.51 Merkel cell carcinoma of anal skin HCC
        Merkel cell carcinoma of anal margin
        Merkel cell carcinoma of perianal skin

    C4A.52 Merkel cell carcinoma of skin of breast HCC

    C4A.59 Merkel cell carcinoma of other **part of trunk** HCC

√5ᵗʰ **C4A.6 Merkel cell carcinoma of** upper limb, including shoulder

    C4A.60 Merkel cell carcinoma of unspecified **upper limb,** HCC
    including shoulder

    C4A.61 Merkel cell carcinoma of right **upper limb,** HCC
    including shoulder

    C4A.62 Merkel cell carcinoma of left **upper limb,** HCC
    including shoulder

√5ᵗʰ **C4A.7 Merkel cell carcinoma of** lower limb, including hip

    C4A.70 Merkel cell carcinoma of unspecified **lower** HCC
    limb, including hip

    C4A.71 Merkel cell carcinoma of right **lower limb,** HCC
    including hip

    C4A.72 Merkel cell carcinoma of left **lower limb,** HCC
    including hip

C4A.8 Merkel cell carcinoma of overlapping sites HCC

C4A.9 Merkel cell carcinoma, unspecified HCC
     Merkel cell carcinoma of unspecified site
     Merkel cell carcinoma (NOS)

√4ᵗʰ **C44 Other and unspecified malignant neoplasm of skin**

    INCLUDES   malignant neoplasm of sebaceous glands
             malignant neoplasm of sweat glands

    EXCLUDES 1   *Kaposi's sarcoma of skin (C46.0)*
             malignant melanoma of skin (C43.-)
             malignant neoplasm of skin of genital organs (C51-C52, C60-,
               C63.2)
             Merkel cell carcinoma (C4A.-)

   DEF: Basal cell carcinoma: An abnormal growth of skin cells that arises from the deepest layer of the epidermis and may present as an open sore, red patches, pink growth, or scar. One of the most common forms of skin cancer, typically caused by sun exposure.

   DEF: Squamous cell carcinoma: An uncontrolled growth of abnormal skin cells that arises from the skin's outer layers (epidermis) and may present as an open sore; firm, red nodule; elevated growth with a central depression; or flat sore with a scaly crust.

√5ᵗʰ **C44.0 Other and unspecified malignant neoplasm of skin of** lip

    EXCLUDES 1   *malignant neoplasm of lip (C00.-)*

    C44.00 Unspecified malignant neoplasm of skin of lip

    C44.01 Basal cell carcinoma of skin of lip

    C44.02 Squamous cell carcinoma of skin of lip

    C44.09 Other specified malignant neoplasm of skin of lip

√5ᵗʰ **C44.1 Other and unspecified malignant neoplasm of skin of** eyelid, including canthus

    EXCLUDES 1   *connective tissue of eyelid (C49.0)*

  √6ᵗʰ **C44.10 Unspecified malignant neoplasm of skin of eyelid, including canthus**

      C44.101 Unspecified malignant neoplasm of skin of unspecified **eyelid, including canthus**

      C44.102 Unspecified malignant neoplasm of skin of right **eyelid, including canthus**

      C44.109 Unspecified malignant neoplasm of skin of left **eyelid, including canthus**

  √6ᵗʰ **C44.11 Basal cell carcinoma of skin of eyelid, including canthus**

      C44.111 Basal cell carcinoma of skin of unspecified **eyelid, including canthus**

      C44.112 Basal cell carcinoma of skin of right **eyelid, including canthus**

      C44.119 Basal cell carcinoma of skin of left **eyelid, including canthus**

  √6ᵗʰ **C44.12 Squamous cell carcinoma of skin of eyelid, including canthus**

      C44.121 Squamous cell carcinoma of skin of unspecified **eyelid, including canthus**

      C44.122 Squamous cell carcinoma of skin of right **eyelid, including canthus**

      C44.129 Squamous cell carcinoma of skin of left **eyelid, including canthus**

  √6ᵗʰ **C44.19 Other specified malignant neoplasm of skin of eyelid, including canthus**

      C44.191 Other specified malignant neoplasm of skin of unspecified **eyelid, including canthus**

      C44.192 Other specified malignant neoplasm of skin of right **eyelid, including canthus**

      C44.199 Other specified malignant neoplasm of skin of left **eyelid, including canthus**

N Newborn: 0   P Pediatric: 0-17   M Maternity: 12-55   A Adult: 15-124   MCC Major CC Condition   PDxMCC PDx acts as own MCC   CC CC Condition   PDxCC PDx acts as own CC

468   ICD-10-CM 2018

✓5ᵗʰ **C44.2 Other and unspecified malignant neoplasm of** skin of ear and external auricular canal

     EXCLUDES 1   *connective tissue of ear (C49.Ø)*

✓6ᵗʰ   **C44.20**   Unspecified **malignant neoplasm of skin of ear and external auricular canal**

     C44.201   **Unspecified malignant neoplasm of skin of** unspecified **ear and external auricular canal**

     C44.202   **Unspecified malignant neoplasm of skin of** right **ear and external auricular canal**

     C44.209   **Unspecified malignant neoplasm of skin of** left **ear and external auricular canal**

✓6ᵗʰ   **C44.21**   Basal cell carcinoma **of skin of ear and external auricular canal**

     C44.211   **Basal cell carcinoma of skin of** unspecified **ear and external auricular canal**

     C44.212   **Basal cell carcinoma of skin of** right **ear and external auricular canal**

     C44.219   **Basal cell carcinoma of skin of** left **ear and external auricular canal**

✓6ᵗʰ   **C44.22**   Squamous cell carcinoma **of skin of ear and external auricular canal**

     C44.221   **Squamous cell carcinoma of skin of** unspecified **ear and external auricular canal**

     C44.222   **Squamous cell carcinoma of skin of** right **ear and external auricular canal**

     C44.229   **Squamous cell carcinoma of skin of** left **ear and external auricular canal**

✓6ᵗʰ   **C44.29**   Other **specified malignant neoplasm of skin of ear and external auricular canal**

     C44.291   **Other specified malignant neoplasm of skin of** unspecified **ear and external auricular canal**

     C44.292   **Other specified malignant neoplasm of skin of** right **ear and external auricular canal**

     C44.299   **Other specified malignant neoplasm of skin of** left **ear and external auricular canal**

✓5ᵗʰ **C44.3 Other and unspecified malignant neoplasm of skin of** other and unspecified parts of face

✓6ᵗʰ   **C44.30**   Unspecified **malignant neoplasm of skin of other and unspecified parts of face**

     C44.300   **Unspecified malignant neoplasm of skin of** unspecified **part of face**

     C44.301   **Unspecified malignant neoplasm of skin of** nose

     C44.309   **Unspecified malignant neoplasm of skin of** other **parts of face**

✓6ᵗʰ   **C44.31**   Basal cell carcinoma **of skin of other and unspecified parts of face**

     C44.310   **Basal cell carcinoma of skin of** unspecified **parts of face**

     C44.311   **Basal cell carcinoma of skin of** nose

     C44.319   **Basal cell carcinoma of skin of** other **parts of face**

✓6ᵗʰ   **C44.32**   Squamous cell carcinoma **of skin of other and unspecified parts of face**

     C44.320   **Squamous cell carcinoma of skin of** unspecified **parts of face**

     C44.321   **Squamous cell carcinoma of skin of** nose

     C44.329   **Squamous cell carcinoma of skin of** other **parts of face**

✓6ᵗʰ   **C44.39**   Other **specified malignant neoplasm of skin of other and unspecified parts of face**

     C44.390   **Other specified malignant neoplasm of skin of** unspecified **parts of face**

     C44.391   **Other specified malignant neoplasm of skin of** nose

     C44.399   **Other specified malignant neoplasm of skin of** other **parts of face**

✓5ᵗʰ **C44.4 Other and unspecified malignant neoplasm of skin of** scalp and neck

     C44.40   Unspecified **malignant neoplasm of skin of scalp and neck**

     C44.41   Basal cell carcinoma **of skin of scalp and neck**

     C44.42   Squamous cell carcinoma **of skin of scalp and neck**

     C44.49   **Other specified malignant neoplasm of skin of scalp and neck**

✓5ᵗʰ **C44.5 Other and unspecified malignant neoplasm of** skin of trunk

     EXCLUDES 1   *anus NOS (C21.Ø)*

                  scrotum (C63.2)

✓6ᵗʰ   **C44.50**   Unspecified **malignant neoplasm of skin of trunk**

     C44.500   **Unspecified malignant neoplasm of** anal **skin**

         Unspecified malignant neoplasm of anal margin

         Unspecified malignant neoplasm of perianal skin

     C44.501   **Unspecified malignant neoplasm of skin of breast**

     C44.509   **Unspecified malignant neoplasm of skin of** other **part of trunk**

✓6ᵗʰ   **C44.51**   Basal cell carcinoma **of skin of trunk**

     C44.510   **Basal cell carcinoma of** anal **skin**

         Basal cell carcinoma of anal margin

         Basal cell carcinoma of perianal skin

     C44.511   **Basal cell carcinoma of skin of breast**

     C44.519   **Basal cell carcinoma of skin of** other **part of trunk**

✓6ᵗʰ   **C44.52**   Squamous cell carcinoma **of skin of trunk**

     C44.520   **Squamous cell carcinoma of** anal **skin**

         Squamous cell carcinoma of anal margin

         Squamous cell carcinoma of perianal skin

     C44.521   **Squamous cell carcinoma of skin of breast**

     C44.529   **Squamous cell carcinoma of skin of** other **part of trunk**

✓6ᵗʰ   **C44.59**   Other **specified malignant neoplasm of skin of trunk**

     C44.590   **Other specified malignant neoplasm of** anal **skin**

         Other specified malignant neoplasm of anal margin

         Other specified malignant neoplasm of perianal skin

     C44.591   **Other specified malignant neoplasm of skin of breast**

     C44.599   **Other specified malignant neoplasm of skin of** other **part of trunk**

✓5ᵗʰ **C44.6 Other and unspecified malignant neoplasm of skin of** upper limb, including shoulder

✓6ᵗʰ   **C44.60**   Unspecified **malignant neoplasm of skin of upper limb, including shoulder**

     C44.601   **Unspecified malignant neoplasm of skin of** unspecified **upper limb, including shoulder**

     C44.602   **Unspecified malignant neoplasm of skin of** right **upper limb, including shoulder**

     C44.609   **Unspecified malignant neoplasm of skin of** left **upper limb, including shoulder**

✓6ᵗʰ   **C44.61**   Basal cell carcinoma **of skin of upper limb, including shoulder**

     C44.611   **Basal cell carcinoma of skin of** unspecified **upper limb, including shoulder**

     C44.612   **Basal cell carcinoma of skin of** right **upper limb, including shoulder**

     C44.619   **Basal cell carcinoma of skin of** left **upper limb, including shoulder**

✓6ᵗʰ   **C44.62**   Squamous cell carcinoma **of skin of upper limb, including shoulder**

     C44.621   **Squamous cell carcinoma of skin of** unspecified **upper limb, including shoulder**

     C44.622   **Squamous cell carcinoma of skin of** right **upper limb, including shoulder**

     C44.629   **Squamous cell carcinoma of skin of** left **upper limb, including shoulder**

✓6ᵗʰ   **C44.69**   Other **specified malignant neoplasm of skin of upper limb, including shoulder**

     C44.691   **Other specified malignant neoplasm of skin of** unspecified **upper limb, including shoulder**

     C44.692   **Other specified malignant neoplasm of skin of** right **upper limb, including shoulder**

     C44.699   **Other specified malignant neoplasm of skin of** left **upper limb, including shoulder**

✓5ᵗʰ **C44.7** **Other and unspecified malignant neoplasm of skin of** lower **limb, including hip**

    ✓6ᵗʰ **C44.70** Unspecified malignant neoplasm of skin of lower **limb, including hip**

        C44.701 **Unspecified malignant neoplasm of skin of** unspecified **lower limb, including hip**

        C44.702 **Unspecified malignant neoplasm of skin of** right **lower limb, including hip**

        C44.709 **Unspecified malignant neoplasm of skin of** left **lower limb, including hip**

    ✓6ᵗʰ **C44.71** Basal cell carcinoma of skin of lower limb, including **hip**

        C44.711 **Basal cell carcinoma of skin of** unspecified **lower limb, including hip**

        C44.712 **Basal cell carcinoma of skin of** right **lower limb, including hip**

        C44.719 **Basal cell carcinoma of skin of** left **lower limb, including hip**

    ✓6ᵗʰ **C44.72** Squamous cell carcinoma of skin of lower limb, **including hip**

        C44.721 **Squamous cell carcinoma of skin of** unspecified **lower limb, including hip**

        C44.722 **Squamous cell carcinoma of skin of** right **lower limb, including hip**

        C44.729 **Squamous cell carcinoma of skin of** left **lower limb, including hip**

    ✓6ᵗʰ **C44.79** Other specified malignant neoplasm of skin of lower **limb, including hip**

        C44.791 **Other specified malignant neoplasm of skin of** unspecified **lower limb, including hip**

        C44.792 **Other specified malignant neoplasm of skin of** right **lower limb, including hip**

        C44.799 **Other specified malignant neoplasm of skin of** left **lower limb, including hip**

✓5ᵗʰ **C44.8** **Other and unspecified malignant neoplasm of** overlapping **sites of skin**

    C44.80 **Unspecified malignant neoplasm of overlapping sites of skin**

    C44.81 **Basal cell carcinoma of overlapping sites of skin**

    C44.82 **Squamous cell carcinoma of overlapping sites of skin**

    C44.89 **Other specified malignant neoplasm of overlapping sites of skin**

✓5ᵗʰ **C44.9** **Other and unspecified malignant neoplasm of skin, unspecified**

    C44.90 **Unspecified malignant neoplasm of skin, unspecified**

        Malignant neoplasm of unspecified site of skin

    C44.91 **Basal cell carcinoma of skin, unspecified**

    C44.92 **Squamous cell carcinoma of skin, unspecified**

    C44.99 **Other specified malignant neoplasm of skin, unspecified**

Malignant neoplasms of mesothelial and soft tissue (C45-C49)

✓4ᵗʰ **C45** **Mesothelioma**

    DEF: Rare type of cancer that forms in the thin layer of protective tissue that covers the majority of internal organs (mesothelium).

    C45.0 **Mesothelioma of pleura**   CC HCC

        EXCLUDES 1   other malignant neoplasm of pleura (C38.4)

        AHA: 2017, 2Q, 11

        CC Excl: PDX collection 288

    C45.1 **Mesothelioma of peritoneum**   CC HCC

        Mesothelioma of cul-de-sac

        Mesothelioma of mesentery

        Mesothelioma of mesocolon

        Mesothelioma of omentum

        Mesothelioma of peritoneum (parietal) (pelvic)

        EXCLUDES 1   other malignant neoplasm of soft tissue of peritoneum (C48.-)

        CC Excl: PDX collection 299

    C45.2 **Mesothelioma of pericardium**   CC HCC

        EXCLUDES 1   other malignant neoplasm of pericardium (C38.0)

        CC Excl: PDX collection 286

    C45.7 **Mesothelioma of other sites**   HCC

    C45.9 **Mesothelioma, unspecified**   HCC

✓4ᵗʰ **C46** **Kaposi's sarcoma**

    Code first any human immunodeficiency virus [HIV] disease (B20)

    DEF: Malignant neoplasm that causes patches of abnormal tissue to grow under the skin, in the lining of the mouth, nose, and throat, in lymph nodes, or in other visceral organs. Kaposi's sarcoma is caused by human herpesvirus8 (HHV8).

    C46.0 **Kaposi's sarcoma of** skin   HIV CC HCC

        CC Excl: PDX collection 300

    C46.1 **Kaposi's sarcoma of** soft tissue   HIV CC HCC

        Kaposi's sarcoma of blood vessel

        Kaposi's sarcoma of connective tissue

        Kaposi's sarcoma of fascia

        Kaposi's sarcoma of ligament

        Kaposi's sarcoma of lymphatic(s) NEC

        Kaposi's sarcoma of muscle

        EXCLUDES 2   Kaposi's sarcoma of lymph glands and nodes (C46.3)

        CC Excl: PDX collection 301

    C46.2 **Kaposi's sarcoma of** palate   HIV CC HCC

        CC Excl: PDX collection 302

    C46.3 **Kaposi's sarcoma of** lymph nodes   HIV CC HCC

        CC Excl: PDX collection 303

    C46.4 **Kaposi's sarcoma of** gastrointestinal sites   HIV CC HCC

        CC Excl: PDX collection 304

    ✓5ᵗʰ **C46.5** **Kaposi's sarcoma of** lung

        CC Excl: For CC codes in subcategory C46.5: PDX collection 284

        C46.50 **Kaposi's sarcoma of** unspecified **lung**   HIV CC HCC

        C46.51 **Kaposi's sarcoma of** right **lung**   HIV CC HCC

        C46.52 **Kaposi's sarcoma of** left **lung**   HIV CC HCC

    C46.7 **Kaposi's sarcoma of** other sites   HIV CC HCC

        CC Excl: PDX collection 305

    C46.9 **Kaposi's sarcoma,** unspecified   HIV CC HCC

        Kaposi's sarcoma of unspecified site

        CC Excl: PDX collection 306

✓4ᵗʰ **C47** **Malignant neoplasm of peripheral nerves and autonomic nervous system**

    INCLUDES   malignant neoplasm of sympathetic and parasympathetic nerves and ganglia

    EXCLUDES 1   Kaposi's sarcoma of soft tissue (C46.1)

    CC Excl: For CC codes in category C47: PDX collection 307

    C47.0 **Malignant neoplasm of peripheral nerves of** head, **face and neck**   CC HCC

        EXCLUDES 1   malignant neoplasm of peripheral nerves of orbit (C69.6-)

    ✓5ᵗʰ **C47.1** **Malignant neoplasm of peripheral nerves of** upper limb, **including shoulder**

        C47.10 **Malignant neoplasm of peripheral nerves of** unspecified **upper limb, including shoulder**   CC HCC

        C47.11 **Malignant neoplasm of peripheral nerves of** right **upper limb, including shoulder**   CC HCC

        C47.12 **Malignant neoplasm of peripheral nerves of** left **upper limb, including shoulder**   CC HCC

    ✓5ᵗʰ **C47.2** **Malignant neoplasm of peripheral nerves of** lower limb, **including hip**

        C47.20 **Malignant neoplasm of peripheral nerves of** unspecified **lower limb, including hip**   CC HCC

        C47.21 **Malignant neoplasm of peripheral nerves of** right **lower limb, including hip**   CC HCC

        C47.22 **Malignant neoplasm of peripheral nerves of** left **lower limb, including hip**   CC HCC

    C47.3 **Malignant neoplasm of peripheral nerves of** thorax   CC HCC

    C47.4 **Malignant neoplasm of peripheral nerves of** abdomen   CC HCC

    C47.5 **Malignant neoplasm of peripheral nerves of** pelvis   CC HCC

    C47.6 **Malignant neoplasm of peripheral nerves of** trunk, **unspecified**   CC HCC

        Malignant neoplasm of peripheral nerves of unspecified part of trunk

    C47.8 **Malignant neoplasm of** overlapping sites of **peripheral nerves and autonomic nervous system**   CC HCC

    C47.9 **Malignant neoplasm of peripheral nerves and nervous autonomic system, unspecified**   CC HCC

        Malignant neoplasm of unspecified site of peripheral nerves and autonomic nervous system

---

☑4ᵗʰ C48 Malignant neoplasm of retroperitoneum and peritoneum
    EXCLUDES 1 *Kaposi's sarcoma of connective tissue (C46.1)*
        mesothelioma (C45.-)

    CC Excl: For CC codes in category C48, unless otherwise noted:
    PDX collection 299

    C48.0 Malignant neoplasm of retroperitoneum CC HCC
        CC Excl: PDX collection 308

    C48.1 Malignant neoplasm of specified parts of peritoneum CC HCC
        Malignant neoplasm of cul-de-sac
        Malignant neoplasm of mesentery
        Malignant neoplasm of mesocolon
        Malignant neoplasm of omentum
        Malignant neoplasm of parietal peritoneum
        Malignant neoplasm of pelvic peritoneum

    C48.2 Malignant neoplasm of peritoneum, unspecified CC HCC

    C48.8 Malignant neoplasm of overlapping sites of retroperitoneum and peritoneum CC HCC

☑4ᵗʰ C49 Malignant neoplasm of other connective and soft tissue
    INCLUDES malignant neoplasm of blood vessel
        malignant neoplasm of bursa
        malignant neoplasm of cartilage
        malignant neoplasm of fascia
        malignant neoplasm of fat
        malignant neoplasm of ligament, except uterine
        malignant neoplasm of lymphatic vessel
        malignant neoplasm of muscle
        malignant neoplasm of synovia
        malignant neoplasm of tendon (sheath)
    EXCLUDES 1 *malignant neoplasm of cartilage (of):*
        articular (C40-C41)   larynx (C32.3)   nose (C30.0)
        malignant neoplasm of connective tissue of breast (C50.-)
    EXCLUDES 2 *Kaposi's sarcoma of soft tissue (C46.1)*
        malignant neoplasm of heart (C38.0)
        malignant neoplasm of peripheral nerves and autonomic nervous system (C47.-)
        malignant neoplasm of peritoneum (C48.2)
        malignant neoplasm of retroperitoneum (C48.0)
        malignant neoplasm of uterine ligament (C57.3)
        mesothelioma (C45.-)

    CC Excl: For CC codes in category C49, unless otherwise noted:
    PDX collection 307

    C49.0 Malignant neoplasm of connective and soft tissue of head, face and neck CC HCC
        Malignant neoplasm of connective tissue of ear
        Malignant neoplasm of connective tissue of eyelid
        EXCLUDES 1 *connective tissue of orbit (C69.6-)*

    ☑5ᵗʰ C49.1 Malignant neoplasm of connective and soft tissue of upper limb, including shoulder
        C49.10 Malignant neoplasm of connective and soft tissue of unspecified upper limb, including shoulder CC HCC
        C49.11 Malignant neoplasm of connective and soft tissue of right upper limb, including shoulder CC HCC
        C49.12 Malignant neoplasm of connective and soft tissue of left upper limb, including shoulder CC HCC

    ☑5ᵗʰ C49.2 Malignant neoplasm of connective and soft tissue of lower limb, including hip
        C49.20 Malignant neoplasm of connective and soft tissue of unspecified lower limb, including hip CC HCC
        C49.21 Malignant neoplasm of connective and soft tissue of right lower limb, including hip CC HCC
        C49.22 Malignant neoplasm of connective and soft tissue of left lower limb, including hip CC HCC

    C49.3 Malignant neoplasm of connective and soft tissue of thorax CC HCC
        Malignant neoplasm of axilla
        Malignant neoplasm of diaphragm
        Malignant neoplasm of great vessels
        EXCLUDES 1 *malignant neoplasm of breast (C50.-)*
        malignant neoplasm of heart (C38.0)
        malignant neoplasm of mediastinum (C38.1-C38.3)
        malignant neoplasm of thymus (C37)
        AHA: 2015, 3Q, 19

    C49.4 Malignant neoplasm of connective and soft tissue of abdomen CC HCC
        Malignant neoplasm of abdominal wall
        Malignant neoplasm of hypochondrium

    C49.5 Malignant neoplasm of connective and soft tissue of pelvis CC HCC
        Malignant neoplasm of buttock
        Malignant neoplasm of groin
        Malignant neoplasm of perineum

    C49.6 Malignant neoplasm of connective and soft tissue of trunk, unspecified CC HCC
        Malignant neoplasm of back NOS

    C49.8 Malignant neoplasm of overlapping sites of connective and soft tissue CC HCC
        Primary malignant neoplasm of two or more contiguous sites of connective and soft tissue

    C49.9 Malignant neoplasm of connective and soft tissue, unspecified CC HCC

    ☑5ᵗʰ C49.A Gastrointestinal stromal tumor
        C49.A0 Gastrointestinal stromal tumor, unspecified site CC HCC
        C49.A1 Gastrointestinal stromal tumor of esophagus CC HCC
        C49.A2 Gastrointestinal stromal tumor of stomach CC HCC
            CC Excl: PDX collection 511
        C49.A3 Gastrointestinal stromal tumor of small intestine CC HCC
        C49.A4 Gastrointestinal stromal tumor of large intestine CC HCC
        C49.A5 Gastrointestinal stromal tumor of rectum CC HCC
        C49.A9 Gastrointestinal stromal tumor of other sites CC HCC

Malignant neoplasms of breast (C50)

☑4ᵗʰ C50 Malignant neoplasm of breast
    INCLUDES connective tissue of breast
        Paget's disease of breast
        Paget's disease of nipple
    Use additional code to identify estrogen receptor status (Z17.0, Z17.1)
    EXCLUDES 1 *skin of breast (C44.501, C44.511, C44.521, C44.591)*

    ☑5ᵗʰ C50.0 Malignant neoplasm of nipple and areola
        ☑6ᵗʰ C50.01 Malignant neoplasm of nipple and areola, female
            C50.011 Malignant neoplasm of nipple and areola, right female breast HCC ♀
            C50.012 Malignant neoplasm of nipple and areola, left female breast HCC ♀
            C50.019 Malignant neoplasm of nipple and areola, unspecified female breast HCC ♀
        ☑6ᵗʰ C50.02 Malignant neoplasm of nipple and areola, male
            C50.021 Malignant neoplasm of nipple and areola, right male breast HCC ♂
            C50.022 Malignant neoplasm of nipple and areola, left male breast HCC ♂
            C50.029 Malignant neoplasm of nipple and areola, unspecified male breast HCC ♂

    ☑5ᵗʰ C50.1 Malignant neoplasm of central portion of breast
        ☑6ᵗʰ C50.11 Malignant neoplasm of central portion of breast, female
            C50.111 Malignant neoplasm of central portion of right female breast HCC ♀
            C50.112 Malignant neoplasm of central portion of left female breast HCC ♀
            C50.119 Malignant neoplasm of central portion of unspecified female breast HCC ♀
        ☑6ᵗʰ C50.12 Malignant neoplasm of central portion of breast, male
            C50.121 Malignant neoplasm of central portion of right male breast HCC ♂
            C50.122 Malignant neoplasm of central portion of left male breast HCC ♂
            C50.129 Malignant neoplasm of central portion of unspecified male breast HCC ♂

    ☑5ᵗʰ C50.2 Malignant neoplasm of upper-inner quadrant of breast
        ☑6ᵗʰ C50.21 Malignant neoplasm of upper-inner quadrant of breast, female
            C50.211 Malignant neoplasm of upper-inner quadrant of right female breast HCC ♀
            C50.212 Malignant neoplasm of upper-inner quadrant of left female breast HCC ♀
            C50.219 Malignant neoplasm of upper-inner quadrant of unspecified female breast HCC ♀

☑ Additional Character Req   ☑7ᵗʰ Placeholder Alert   Unacceptable PDx   Manifestation   H1–H14 HAC   HCC CMS-HCC Condition   EXCLUDES 1 Not Coded Here   EXCLUDES 2 Not Included Here

ICD-10-CM 2018   471

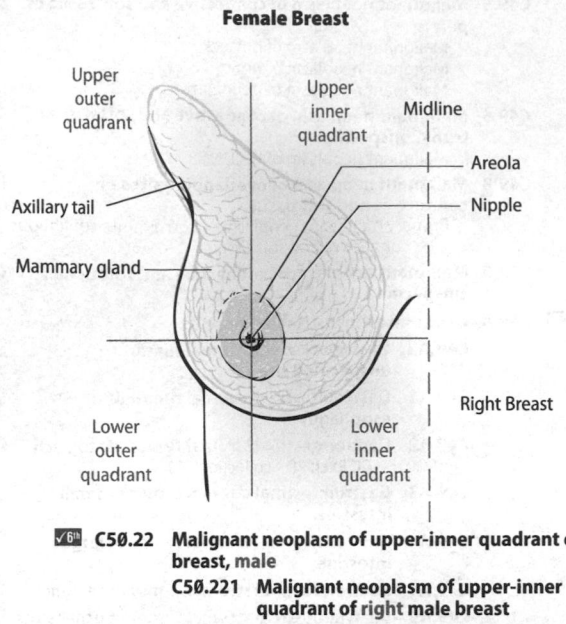

Female Breast

- Upper outer quadrant
- Upper inner quadrant
- Midline
- Areola
- Axillary tail
- Nipple
- Mammary gland
- Lower outer quadrant
- Lower inner quadrant
- Right Breast

√6ᵗʰ **C50.22** Malignant neoplasm of upper-inner quadrant of breast, male

    C50.221 Malignant neoplasm of upper-inner quadrant of right male breast HCC ♂

    C50.222 Malignant neoplasm of upper-inner quadrant of left male breast HCC ♂

    C50.229 Malignant neoplasm of upper-inner quadrant of unspecified male breast HCC ♂

√5ᵗʰ **C50.3** Malignant neoplasm of lower-inner quadrant of breast

  √6ᵗʰ **C50.31** Malignant neoplasm of lower-inner quadrant of breast, female

    C50.311 Malignant neoplasm of lower-inner quadrant of right female breast HCC ♀

    C50.312 Malignant neoplasm of lower-inner quadrant of left female breast HCC ♀

    C50.319 Malignant neoplasm of lower-inner quadrant of unspecified female breast HCC ♀

  √6ᵗʰ **C50.32** Malignant neoplasm of lower-inner quadrant of breast, male

    C50.321 Malignant neoplasm of lower-inner quadrant of right male breast HCC ♂

    C50.322 Malignant neoplasm of lower-inner quadrant of left male breast HCC ♂

    C50.329 Malignant neoplasm of lower-inner quadrant of unspecified male breast HCC ♂

√6ᵗʰ **C50.4** Malignant neoplasm of upper-outer quadrant of breast

  √6ᵗʰ **C50.41** Malignant neoplasm of upper-outer quadrant of breast, female

    C50.411 Malignant neoplasm of upper-outer quadrant of right female breast HCC ♀

    C50.412 Malignant neoplasm of upper-outer quadrant of left female breast HCC ♀

    C50.419 Malignant neoplasm of upper-outer quadrant of unspecified female breast HCC ♀

  √6ᵗʰ **C50.42** Malignant neoplasm of upper-outer quadrant of breast, male

    C50.421 Malignant neoplasm of upper-outer quadrant of right male breast HCC ♂

    C50.422 Malignant neoplasm of upper-outer quadrant of left male breast HCC ♂

    C50.429 Malignant neoplasm of upper-outer quadrant of unspecified male breast HCC ♂

√5ᵗʰ **C50.5** Malignant neoplasm of lower-outer quadrant of breast

  √6ᵗʰ **C50.51** Malignant neoplasm of lower-outer quadrant of breast, female

    C50.511 Malignant neoplasm of lower-outer quadrant of right female breast HCC ♀

    C50.512 Malignant neoplasm of lower-outer quadrant of left female breast HCC ♀

    C50.519 Malignant neoplasm of lower-outer quadrant of unspecified female breast HCC ♀

  √6ᵗʰ **C50.52** Malignant neoplasm of lower-outer quadrant of breast, male

    C50.521 Malignant neoplasm of lower-outer quadrant of right male breast HCC ♂

    C50.522 Malignant neoplasm of lower-outer quadrant of left male breast HCC ♂

    C50.529 Malignant neoplasm of lower-outer quadrant of unspecified male breast HCC ♂

√5ᵗʰ **C50.6** Malignant neoplasm of axillary tail of breast

  √6ᵗʰ **C50.61** Malignant neoplasm of axillary tail of breast, female

    C50.611 Malignant neoplasm of axillary tail of right female breast HCC ♀

    C50.612 Malignant neoplasm of axillary tail of left female breast HCC ♀

    C50.619 Malignant neoplasm of axillary tail of unspecified female breast HCC ♀

  √6ᵗʰ **C50.62** Malignant neoplasm of axillary tail of breast, male

    C50.621 Malignant neoplasm of axillary tail of right male breast HCC ♂

    C50.622 Malignant neoplasm of axillary tail of left male breast HCC ♂

    C50.629 Malignant neoplasm of axillary tail of unspecified male breast HCC ♂

√5ᵗʰ **C50.8** Malignant neoplasm of overlapping sites of breast

  √6ᵗʰ **C50.81** Malignant neoplasm of overlapping sites of breast, female

    C50.811 Malignant neoplasm of overlapping sites of right female breast HCC ♀

    C50.812 Malignant neoplasm of overlapping sites of left female breast HCC ♀

    C50.819 Malignant neoplasm of overlapping sites of unspecified female breast HCC ♀

  √6ᵗʰ **C50.82** Malignant neoplasm of overlapping sites of breast, male

    C50.821 Malignant neoplasm of overlapping sites of right male breast HCC ♂

    C50.822 Malignant neoplasm of overlapping sites of left male breast HCC ♂

    C50.829 Malignant neoplasm of overlapping sites of unspecified male breast HCC ♂

√5ᵗʰ **C50.9** Malignant neoplasm of breast of unspecified site

  √6ᵗʰ **C50.91** Malignant neoplasm of breast of unspecified site, female

    C50.911 Malignant neoplasm of unspecified site of right female breast HCC ♀

    C50.912 Malignant neoplasm of unspecified site of left female breast HCC ♀

    C50.919 Malignant neoplasm of unspecified site of unspecified female breast HCC ♀

  √6ᵗʰ **C50.92** Malignant neoplasm of breast of unspecified site, male

    C50.921 Malignant neoplasm of unspecified site of right male breast HCC ♂

    C50.922 Malignant neoplasm of unspecified site of left male breast HCC ♂

    C50.929 Malignant neoplasm of unspecified site of unspecified male breast HCC ♂

Malignant neoplasms of female genital organs (C51-C58)

INCLUDES   malignant neoplasm of skin of female genital organs

√4ᵗʰ **C51** Malignant neoplasm of vulva
    EXCLUDES 1   carcinoma in situ of vulva (D07.1)

  C51.0 Malignant neoplasm of labium majus HCC ♀
    Malignant neoplasm of Bartholin's [greater vestibular] gland

  C51.1 Malignant neoplasm of labium minus HCC ♀

  C51.2 Malignant neoplasm of clitoris HCC ♀

  C51.8 Malignant neoplasm of overlapping sites of vulva HCC ♀

  C51.9 Malignant neoplasm of vulva, unspecified HCC ♀
    Malignant neoplasm of external female genitalia NOS
    Malignant neoplasm of pudendum

C52 Malignant neoplasm of vagina HCC ♀
    EXCLUDES 1   carcinoma in situ of vagina (D07.2)

√4ᵗʰ **C53** Malignant neoplasm of cervix uteri
    EXCLUDES 1   carcinoma in situ of cervix uteri (D06.-)

  C53.0 Malignant neoplasm of endocervix HCC ♀

  C53.1 Malignant neoplasm of exocervix HCC ♀

  C53.8 Malignant neoplasm of overlapping sites of cervix uteri HCC ♀

  C53.9 Malignant neoplasm of cervix uteri, unspecified HCC ♀

N Newborn: 0   P Pediatric: 0-17   M Maternity: 12-55   A Adult: 15-124   MCC Major CC Condition   PDx MCC PDx acts as own MCC   CC CC Condition   PDx CC PDx acts as own CC

472   ICD-10-CM 2018

Chapter 2. Neoplasms

✓4ᵗʰ **C54** **Malignant neoplasm of** corpus uteri

     C54.0 **Malignant neoplasm of** isthmus uteri   HCC ♀
          Malignant neoplasm of lower uterine segment

     C54.1 **Malignant neoplasm of** endometrium   HCC ♀

     C54.2 **Malignant neoplasm of** myometrium   HCC ♀

     C54.3 **Malignant neoplasm of** fundus uteri   HCC ♀

     C54.8 **Malignant neoplasm of** overlapping sites **of corpus uteri**   HCC ♀

     C54.9 **Malignant neoplasm of corpus uteri,** unspecified   HCC ♀

C55 **Malignant neoplasm of uterus, part** unspecified   HCC ♀

✓4ᵗʰ **C56** **Malignant neoplasm of** ovary
     Use additional code to identify any functional activity

     CC Excl: For CC codes in category C56: PDX collection 309

     C56.1 **Malignant neoplasm of** right **ovary**   CC HCC ♀

     C56.2 **Malignant neoplasm of** left **ovary**   CC HCC ♀

     C56.9 **Malignant neoplasm of** unspecified **ovary**   CC HCC ♀

✓4ᵗʰ **C57** **Malignant neoplasm of** other and unspecified female genital organs

     ✓5ᵗʰ **C57.0** **Malignant neoplasm of** fallopian tube
          Malignant neoplasm of oviduct
          Malignant neoplasm of uterine tube

         C57.00 **Malignant neoplasm of** unspecified **fallopian tube**   HCC ♀

         C57.01 **Malignant neoplasm of** right **fallopian tube**   HCC ♀

         C57.02 **Malignant neoplasm of** left **fallopian tube**   HCC ♀

     ✓5ᵗʰ **C57.1** **Malignant neoplasm of** broad ligament

         C57.10 **Malignant neoplasm of** unspecified **broad ligament**   HCC ♀

         C57.11 **Malignant neoplasm of** right **broad ligament**   HCC ♀

         C57.12 **Malignant neoplasm of** left **broad ligament**   HCC ♀

     ✓5ᵗʰ **C57.2** **Malignant neoplasm of** round ligament

         C57.20 **Malignant neoplasm of** unspecified **round ligament**   HCC ♀

         C57.21 **Malignant neoplasm of** right **round ligament**   HCC ♀

         C57.22 **Malignant neoplasm of** left **round ligament**   HCC ♀

     C57.3 **Malignant neoplasm of** parametrium   HCC ♀
          Malignant neoplasm of uterine ligament NOS

     C57.4 **Malignant neoplasm of uterine adnexa,** unspecified   HCC ♀

     C57.7 **Malignant neoplasm of** other specified **female genital organs**   HCC ♀
          Malignant neoplasm of wolffian body or duct

     C57.8 **Malignant neoplasm of** overlapping sites **of female genital organs**   HCC ♀
          Primary malignant neoplasm of two or more contiguous sites of the female genital organs whose point of origin cannot be determined
          Primary tubo-ovarian malignant neoplasm whose point of origin cannot be determined
          Primary utero-ovarian malignant neoplasm whose point of origin cannot be determined

     C57.9 **Malignant neoplasm of female genital organ,** unspecified   HCC ♀
          Malignant neoplasm of female genitourinary tract NOS

C58 **Malignant neoplasm of** placenta   HCC M ♀
     INCLUDES   choriocarcinoma NOS
          chorionepithelioma NOS
     EXCLUDES 1   chorioadenoma (destruens) (D39.2)
          hydatidiform mole NOS (O01.9)
          invasive hydatidiform mole (D39.2)
          male choriocarcinoma NOS (C62.9-)
          malignant hydatidiform mole (D39.2)

Malignant neoplasms of male genital organs (C60-C63)

     INCLUDES   malignant neoplasm of skin of male genital organs

✓4ᵗʰ **C60** **Malignant neoplasm of** penis

     C60.0 **Malignant neoplasm of** prepuce   HCC ♂
          Malignant neoplasm of foreskin

     C60.1 **Malignant neoplasm of** glans **penis**   HCC ♂

     C60.2 **Malignant neoplasm of** body **of penis**   HCC ♂
          Malignant neoplasm of corpus cavernosum

     C60.8 **Malignant neoplasm of** overlapping sites **of penis**   HCC ♂

     C60.9 **Malignant neoplasm of penis,** unspecified   HCC ♂
          Malignant neoplasm of skin of penis NOS

C61 **Malignant neoplasm of** prostate   HCC ♂
     Use additional code to identify:
         hormone sensitivity status (Z19.1-Z19.2)
         rising PSA following treatment for malignant neoplasm of prostate (R97.21)
     EXCLUDES 1   malignant neoplasm of seminal vesicle (C63.7)
     AHA: 2017, 1Q, 17

✓4ᵗʰ **C62** **Malignant neoplasm of** testis
     Use additional code to identify any functional activity

     ✓5ᵗʰ **C62.0** **Malignant neoplasm of** undescended **testis**
          Malignant neoplasm of ectopic testis
          Malignant neoplasm of retained testis

         C62.00 **Malignant neoplasm of** unspecified **undescended testis**   HCC ♂

         C62.01 **Malignant neoplasm of undescended** right **testis**   HCC ♂

         C62.02 **Malignant neoplasm of undescended** left **testis**   HCC ♂

     ✓5ᵗʰ **C62.1** **Malignant neoplasm of** descended **testis**
          Malignant neoplasm of scrotal testis

         C62.10 **Malignant neoplasm of** unspecified **descended testis**   HCC ♂

         C62.11 **Malignant neoplasm of descended** right **testis**   HCC ♂

         C62.12 **Malignant neoplasm of descended** left **testis**   HCC ♂

     ✓5ᵗʰ **C62.9** **Malignant neoplasm of testis,** unspecified whether descended or undescended

         C62.90 **Malignant neoplasm of** unspecified **testis, unspecified whether descended or undescended**   HCC ♂
              Malignant neoplasm of testis NOS

         C62.91 **Malignant neoplasm of** right **testis, unspecified whether descended or undescended**   HCC ♂

         C62.92 **Malignant neoplasm of** left **testis, unspecified whether descended or undescended**   HCC ♂

✓4ᵗʰ **C63** **Malignant neoplasm of** other and unspecified male genital organs

     ✓5ᵗʰ **C63.0** **Malignant neoplasm of** epididymis

         C63.00 **Malignant neoplasm of** unspecified **epididymis**   HCC ♂

         C63.01 **Malignant neoplasm of** right **epididymis**   HCC ♂

         C63.02 **Malignant neoplasm of** left **epididymis**   HCC ♂

     ✓5ᵗʰ **C63.1** **Malignant neoplasm of** spermatic cord

         C63.10 **Malignant neoplasm of** unspecified **spermatic cord**   HCC ♂

         C63.11 **Malignant neoplasm of** right **spermatic cord**   HCC ♂

         C63.12 **Malignant neoplasm of** left **spermatic cord**   HCC ♂

     C63.2 **Malignant neoplasm of** scrotum   HCC ♂
          Malignant neoplasm of skin of scrotum

     C63.7 **Malignant neoplasm of** other specified **male genital organs**   HCC ♂
          Malignant neoplasm of seminal vesicle
          Malignant neoplasm of tunica vaginalis

     C63.8 **Malignant neoplasm of** overlapping sites **of male genital organs**   HCC ♂
          Primary malignant neoplasm of two or more contiguous sites of male genital organs whose point of origin cannot be determined

     C63.9 **Malignant neoplasm of male genital organ,** unspecified   HCC ♂
          Malignant neoplasm of male genitourinary tract NOS

Malignant neoplasms of urinary tract (C64-C68)

✓4ᵗʰ **C64** **Malignant neoplasm of** kidney, except renal pelvis
     EXCLUDES 1   malignant carcinoid tumor of the kidney (C7A.093)
         malignant neoplasm of renal calyces (C65.-)
         malignant neoplasm of renal pelvis (C65.-)

     CC Excl: For CC codes in category C64: PDX collection 310

     C64.1 **Malignant neoplasm of** right **kidney, except renal pelvis**   HCC CC

     C64.2 **Malignant neoplasm of** left **kidney, except renal pelvis**   HCC CC

     C64.9 **Malignant neoplasm of** unspecified **kidney, except renal pelvis**   HCC CC

✓ Additional Character Req   ✓x7ᵗʰ Placeholder Alert   Unacceptable PDx   Manifestation   H1 - H14 HAC   HCC CMS-HCC Condition   EXCLUDES 1 Not Coded Here   EXCLUDES 2 Not Included Here

ICD-10-CM 2018   473

Chapter 2. Neoplasms

C65–C71.9

✓4th **C65 Malignant neoplasm of renal pelvis**
  INCLUDES   malignant neoplasm of pelviureteric junction
       malignant neoplasm of renal calyces

  CC Excl: For CC codes in category C65: PDX collection 310

  C65.1 Malignant neoplasm of right renal pelvis CC HCC
  C65.2 Malignant neoplasm of left renal pelvis CC HCC
  C65.9 Malignant neoplasm of unspecified renal pelvis CC HCC

✓4th **C66 Malignant neoplasm of ureter**
  EXCLUDES 1   malignant neoplasm of ureteric orifice of bladder (C67.6)

  CC Excl: For CC codes in category C66: PDX collection 311

  C66.1 Malignant neoplasm of right ureter CC HCC
  C66.2 Malignant neoplasm of left ureter CC HCC
  C66.9 Malignant neoplasm of unspecified ureter CC HCC

✓4th **C67 Malignant neoplasm of bladder**
  C67.0 Malignant neoplasm of trigone of bladder HCC
  C67.1 Malignant neoplasm of dome of bladder HCC
  C67.2 Malignant neoplasm of lateral wall of bladder HCC
  C67.3 Malignant neoplasm of anterior wall of bladder HCC
  C67.4 Malignant neoplasm of posterior wall of bladder HCC
  C67.5 Malignant neoplasm of bladder neck HCC
       Malignant neoplasm of internal urethral orifice
  C67.6 Malignant neoplasm of ureteric orifice HCC
  C67.7 Malignant neoplasm of urachus HCC
  C67.8 Malignant neoplasm of overlapping sites of bladder HCC
  C67.9 Malignant neoplasm of bladder, unspecified HCC
       AHA: 2016, 1Q, 19

✓4th **C68 Malignant neoplasm of other and unspecified urinary organs**
  EXCLUDES 1   malignant neoplasm of female genitourinary tract NOS (C57.9)
       malignant neoplasm of male genitourinary tract NOS (C63.9)

  C68.0 Malignant neoplasm of urethra CC HCC
       EXCLUDES 1   malignant neoplasm of urethral orifice of bladder
         (C67.5)
       CC Excl: PDX collection 312
  C68.1 Malignant neoplasm of paraurethral glands CC HCC
       CC Excl: PDX collection 312
  C68.8 Malignant neoplasm of overlapping sites of urinary organs CC HCC
       Primary malignant neoplasm of two or more contiguous sites of
         urinary organs whose point of origin cannot be determined
       CC Excl: PDX collection 313
  C68.9 Malignant neoplasm of urinary organ, unspecified CC HCC
       Malignant neoplasm of urinary system NOS
       CC Excl: PDX collection 313

Malignant neoplasms of eye, brain and other parts of central nervous system (C69-C72)

✓4th **C69 Malignant neoplasm of eye and adnexa**
  EXCLUDES 1   malignant neoplasm of connective tissue of eyelid (C49.0)
       malignant neoplasm of eyelid (skin) (C43.1-, C44.1-)
       malignant neoplasm of optic nerve (C72.3-)

  ✓5th **C69.0 Malignant neoplasm of conjunctiva**
       C69.00 Malignant neoplasm of unspecified conjunctiva HCC
       C69.01 Malignant neoplasm of right conjunctiva HCC
       C69.02 Malignant neoplasm of left conjunctiva HCC

  ✓5th **C69.1 Malignant neoplasm of cornea**
       C69.10 Malignant neoplasm of unspecified cornea HCC
       C69.11 Malignant neoplasm of right cornea HCC
       C69.12 Malignant neoplasm of left cornea HCC

  ✓5th **C69.2 Malignant neoplasm of retina**
       EXCLUDES 1   dark area on retina (D49.81)
       neoplasm of unspecified behavior of retina and
         choroid (D49.81)
       retinal freckle (D49.81)
       C69.20 Malignant neoplasm of unspecified retina HCC
       C69.21 Malignant neoplasm of right retina HCC
       C69.22 Malignant neoplasm of left retina HCC

  ✓5th **C69.3 Malignant neoplasm of choroid**
       C69.30 Malignant neoplasm of unspecified choroid HCC
       C69.31 Malignant neoplasm of right choroid HCC
       C69.32 Malignant neoplasm of left choroid HCC

✓5th **C69.4 Malignant neoplasm of ciliary body**
       C69.40 Malignant neoplasm of unspecified ciliary body HCC
       C69.41 Malignant neoplasm of right ciliary body HCC
       C69.42 Malignant neoplasm of left ciliary body HCC

✓5th **C69.5 Malignant neoplasm of lacrimal gland and duct**
       Malignant neoplasm of lacrimal sac
       Malignant neoplasm of nasolacrimal duct
       C69.50 Malignant neoplasm of unspecified lacrimal gland and duct HCC
       C69.51 Malignant neoplasm of right lacrimal gland and duct HCC
       C69.52 Malignant neoplasm of left lacrimal gland and duct HCC

✓5th **C69.6 Malignant neoplasm of orbit**
       Malignant neoplasm of connective tissue of orbit
       Malignant neoplasm of extraocular muscle
       Malignant neoplasm of peripheral nerves of orbit
       Malignant neoplasm of retrobulbar tissue
       Malignant neoplasm of retro-ocular tissue
       EXCLUDES 1   malignant neoplasm of orbital bone (C41.0)
       C69.60 Malignant neoplasm of unspecified orbit HCC
       C69.61 Malignant neoplasm of right orbit HCC
       C69.62 Malignant neoplasm of left orbit HCC

✓5th **C69.8 Malignant neoplasm of overlapping sites of eye and adnexa**
       C69.80 Malignant neoplasm of overlapping sites of unspecified eye and adnexa HCC
       C69.81 Malignant neoplasm of overlapping sites of right eye and adnexa HCC
       C69.82 Malignant neoplasm of overlapping sites of left eye and adnexa HCC

✓5th **C69.9 Malignant neoplasm of unspecified site of eye**
       Malignant neoplasm of eyeball
       C69.90 Malignant neoplasm of unspecified site of unspecified eye HCC
       C69.91 Malignant neoplasm of unspecified site of right eye HCC
       C69.92 Malignant neoplasm of unspecified site of left eye HCC

✓4th **C70 Malignant neoplasm of meninges**
  C70.0 Malignant neoplasm of cerebral meninges CC HCC
       CC Excl: PDX collection 314
  C70.1 Malignant neoplasm of spinal meninges CC HCC
       CC Excl: PDX collection 315
  C70.9 Malignant neoplasm of meninges, unspecified CC HCC
       CC Excl: PDX collection 314

✓4th **C71 Malignant neoplasm of brain**
  EXCLUDES 1   malignant neoplasm of cranial nerves (C72.2-C72.5)
       retrobulbar malignant neoplasm (C69.6-)

  CC Excl: For CC codes in category C71: PDX collection 316

  C71.0 Malignant neoplasm of cerebrum, except lobes and ventricles CC HCC
       Malignant neoplasm of supratentorial NOS
  C71.1 Malignant neoplasm of frontal lobe CC HCC
  C71.2 Malignant neoplasm of temporal lobe CC HCC
  C71.3 Malignant neoplasm of parietal lobe CC HCC
  C71.4 Malignant neoplasm of occipital lobe CC HCC
  C71.5 Malignant neoplasm of cerebral ventricle CC HCC
       EXCLUDES 1   malignant neoplasm of fourth cerebral ventricle
         (C71.7)
  C71.6 Malignant neoplasm of cerebellum CC HCC
  C71.7 Malignant neoplasm of brain stem CC HCC
       Malignant neoplasm of fourth cerebral ventricle
       Infratentorial malignant neoplasm NOS
  C71.8 Malignant neoplasm of overlapping sites of brain CC HCC
  C71.9 Malignant neoplasm of brain, unspecified CC HCC
       AHA: 2014, 3Q, 3

N Newborn: 0   P Pediatric: 0-17   M Maternity: 12-55   A Adult: 15-124   MCC Major CC Condition   PDxMCC PDx acts as own MCC   CC CC Condition   PDxCC PDx acts as own CC

474   ICD-10-CM 2018

Lobes of the Brain

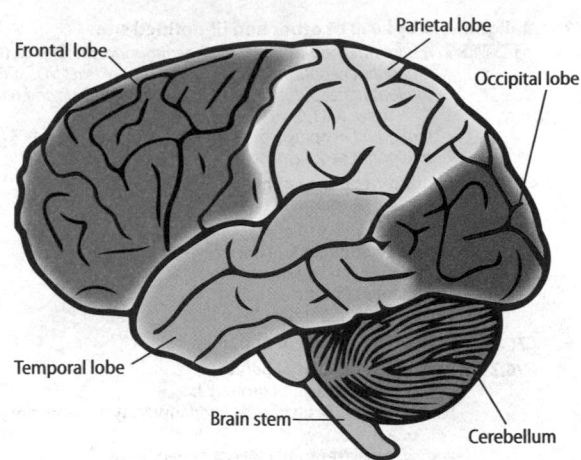

Frontal lobe
Parietal lobe
Occipital lobe
Temporal lobe
Brain stem
Cerebellum

✓4th C72 Malignant neoplasm of spinal cord, cranial nerves and other parts of central nervous system

> *EXCLUDES 1*   malignant neoplasm of meninges (C7Ø.-)
> malignant neoplasm of peripheral nerves and autonomic nervous system (C47.-)

CC Excl: For CC codes in category C72, unless otherwise noted: PDX collection 318

C72.Ø Malignant neoplasm of spinal cord   CC HCC
     CC Excl: PDX collection 317

C72.1 Malignant neoplasm of cauda equina   CC HCC
     CC Excl: PDX collection 317

✓5th C72.2 Malignant neoplasm of olfactory nerve
     Malignant neoplasm of olfactory bulb

     C72.2Ø Malignant neoplasm of unspecified olfactory nerve   CC HCC

     C72.21 Malignant neoplasm of right olfactory nerve   CC HCC
     C72.22 Malignant neoplasm of left olfactory nerve   CC HCC

✓5th C72.3 Malignant neoplasm of optic nerve

     C72.3Ø Malignant neoplasm of unspecified optic nerve   CC HCC

     C72.31 Malignant neoplasm of right optic nerve   CC HCC
     C72.32 Malignant neoplasm of left optic nerve   CC HCC

✓5th C72.4 Malignant neoplasm of acoustic nerve

     C72.4Ø Malignant neoplasm of unspecified acoustic nerve   CC HCC

     C72.41 Malignant neoplasm of right acoustic nerve   CC HCC
     C72.42 Malignant neoplasm of left acoustic nerve   CC HCC

✓5th C72.5 Malignant neoplasm of other and unspecified cranial nerves

     C72.5Ø Malignant neoplasm of unspecified cranial nerve   CC HCC
       Malignant neoplasm of cranial nerve NOS

     C72.59 Malignant neoplasm of other cranial nerves   CC HCC

C72.9 Malignant neoplasm of central nervous system, unspecified   CC HCC
     Malignant neoplasm of unspecified site of central nervous system
     Malignant neoplasm of nervous system NOS
     CC Excl: PDX collection 319

Malignant neoplasms of thyroid and other endocrine glands (C73-C75)

C73 Malignant neoplasm of thyroid gland   HCC
     Use additional code to identify any functional activity

✓4th C74 Malignant neoplasm of adrenal gland

CC Excl: For CC codes in category C74: PDX collection 32Ø

✓5th C74.Ø Malignant neoplasm of cortex of adrenal gland

     C74.ØØ Malignant neoplasm of cortex of unspecified adrenal gland   CC HCC

     C74.Ø1 Malignant neoplasm of cortex of right adrenal gland   CC HCC

     C74.Ø2 Malignant neoplasm of cortex of left adrenal gland   CC HCC

✓5th C74.1 Malignant neoplasm of medulla of adrenal gland

     C74.1Ø Malignant neoplasm of medulla of unspecified adrenal gland   CC HCC

     C74.11 Malignant neoplasm of medulla of right adrenal gland   CC HCC

     C74.12 Malignant neoplasm of medulla of left adrenal gland   CC HCC

✓5th C74.9 Malignant neoplasm of unspecified part of adrenal gland

     C74.9Ø Malignant neoplasm of unspecified part of unspecified adrenal gland   CC HCC

     C74.91 Malignant neoplasm of unspecified part of right adrenal gland   CC HCC

     C74.92 Malignant neoplasm of unspecified part of left adrenal gland   CC HCC

✓4th C75 Malignant neoplasm of other endocrine glands and related structures

> *EXCLUDES 1*   malignant carcinoid tumors (C7A.Ø-)
> malignant neoplasm of adrenal gland (C74.-)
> malignant neoplasm of endocrine pancreas (C25.4)
> malignant neoplasm of islets of Langerhans (C25.4)
> malignant neoplasm of ovary (C56.-)
> malignant neoplasm of testis (C62.-)
> malignant neoplasm of thymus (C37)
> malignant neoplasm of thyroid gland (C73)
> malignant neuroendocrine tumors (C7A.-)

C75.Ø Malignant neoplasm of parathyroid gland   CC HCC
     CC Excl: PDX collection 321

C75.1 Malignant neoplasm of pituitary gland   CC HCC
     CC Excl: PDX collection 322

C75.2 Malignant neoplasm of craniopharyngeal duct   CC HCC
     CC Excl: PDX collection 322

C75.3 Malignant neoplasm of pineal gland   CC HCC
     CC Excl: PDX collection 323

C75.4 Malignant neoplasm of carotid body   CC HCC
     CC Excl: PDX collection 324

C75.5 Malignant neoplasm of aortic body and other paraganglia   CC HCC
     CC Excl: PDX collection 325

C75.8 Malignant neoplasm with pluriglandular involvement, unspecified   CC HCC
     CC Excl: PDX collection 326

C75.9 Malignant neoplasm of endocrine gland, unspecified   CC HCC
     CC Excl: PDX collection 326

Malignant neuroendocrine tumors (C7A)

✓4th C7A Malignant neuroendocrine tumors

     Code also any associated multiple endocrine neoplasia [MEN] syndromes (E31.2-)
     Use additional code to identify any associated endocrine syndrome, such as:
       carcinoid syndrome (E34.Ø)

> *EXCLUDES 2*   malignant pancreatic islet cell tumors (C25.4)
> Merkel cell carcinoma (C4A.-)

✓5th C7A.Ø Malignant carcinoid tumors

     C7A.ØØ Malignant carcinoid tumor of unspecified site   CC HCC
       CC Excl: PDX collection 346

     ✓6th C7A.Ø1 Malignant carcinoid tumors of the small intestine

       C7A.Ø1Ø Malignant carcinoid tumor of the duodenum   CC HCC
         CC Excl: PDX collection 347

       C7A.Ø11 Malignant carcinoid tumor of the jejunum   CC HCC
         CC Excl: PDX collection 348

       C7A.Ø12 Malignant carcinoid tumor of the ileum   CC HCC
         CC Excl: PDX collection 349

       C7A.Ø19 Malignant carcinoid tumor of the small intestine, unspecified portion   CC HCC
         CC Excl: PDX collection 35Ø

     ✓6th C7A.Ø2 Malignant carcinoid tumors of the appendix, large intestine, and rectum

       C7A.Ø2Ø Malignant carcinoid tumor of the appendix   CC HCC
         CC Excl: PDX collection 351

       C7A.Ø21 Malignant carcinoid tumor of the cecum   CC HCC
         CC Excl: PDX collection 352

☑ Additional Character Req   ✓x7th Placeholder Alert   Unacceptable PDx   ■ Manifestation   H1 – H14 HAC   HCC CMS-HCC Condition   *EXCLUDES 1* Not Coded Here   *EXCLUDES 2* Not Included Here

ICD-10-CM 2018   **475**

C72–C7A.Ø21

C7A.Ø22 **Malignant carcinoid tumor of the ascending colon** `CC` `HCC`
CC Excl: PDX collection 353

C7A.Ø23 **Malignant carcinoid tumor of the transverse colon** `CC` `HCC`
CC Excl: PDX collection 354

C7A.Ø24 **Malignant carcinoid tumor of the descending colon** `CC` `HCC`
CC Excl: PDX collection 355

C7A.Ø25 **Malignant carcinoid tumor of the sigmoid colon** `CC` `HCC`
CC Excl: PDX collection 356

C7A.Ø26 **Malignant carcinoid tumor of the rectum** `CC` `HCC`
CC Excl: PDX collection 357

C7A.Ø29 **Malignant carcinoid tumor of the large, intestine, unspecified portion** `CC` `HCC`
Malignant carcinoid tumor of the colon NOS
CC Excl: PDX collection 358

√6th **C7A.Ø9** **Malignant carcinoid tumors of other sites**

C7A.Ø9Ø **Malignant carcinoid tumor of the bronchus and lung** `CC` `HCC`
CC Excl: PDX collection 359

C7A.Ø91 **Malignant carcinoid tumor of the thymus** `CC` `HCC`
CC Excl: PDX collection 36Ø

C7A.Ø92 **Malignant carcinoid tumor of the stomach** `CC` `HCC`
CC Excl: PDX collection 361

C7A.Ø93 **Malignant carcinoid tumor of the kidney** `CC` `HCC`
CC Excl: PDX collection 362

C7A.Ø94 **Malignant carcinoid tumor of the foregut, unspecified** `CC` `HCC`
CC Excl: PDX collection 361

C7A.Ø95 **Malignant carcinoid tumor of the midgut, unspecified** `CC` `HCC`
CC Excl: PDX collection 361

C7A.Ø96 **Malignant carcinoid tumor of the hindgut, unspecified** `CC` `HCC`
CC Excl: PDX collection 361

C7A.Ø98 **Malignant carcinoid tumors of other sites** `CC` `HCC`
CC Excl: PDX collection 346

C7A.1 **Malignant poorly differentiated neuroendocrine tumors** `CC` `HCC`
High grade neuroendocrine carcinoma, any site
Malignant poorly differentiated neuroendocrine tumor NOS
Malignant poorly differentiated neuroendocrine carcinoma, any site
CC Excl: PDX collection 346

C7A.8 **Other malignant neuroendocrine tumors** `CC` `HCC`
CC Excl: PDX collection 346

Secondary neuroendocrine tumors (C7B)

√4th **C7B** **Secondary neuroendocrine tumors**
Use additional code to identify any functional activity

√5th **C7B.Ø** **Secondary carcinoid tumors**

C7B.ØØ **Secondary carcinoid tumors, unspecified site** `HCC`

C7B.Ø1 **Secondary carcinoid tumors of distant lymph nodes** `CC` `HCC`
CC Excl: PDX collection 363

C7B.Ø2 **Secondary carcinoid tumors of liver** `CC` `HCC`
CC Excl: PDX collection 364

C7B.Ø3 **Secondary carcinoid tumors of bone** `CC` `HCC`
CC Excl: PDX collection 365

C7B.Ø4 **Secondary carcinoid tumors of peritoneum** `CC` `HCC`
Mesentery metastasis of carcinoid tumor
CC Excl: CPDX collection 366

C7B.Ø9 **Secondary carcinoid tumors of other sites** `CC` `HCC`
CC Excl: PDX collection 367

C7B.1 **Secondary Merkel cell carcinoma** `HCC`
Merkel cell carcinoma nodal presentation
Merkel cell carcinoma visceral metastatic presentation

C7B.8 **Other secondary neuroendocrine tumors** `CC` `HCC`
CC Excl: PDX collection 367

Malignant neoplasms of ill-defined, other secondary and unspecified sites (C76-C8Ø)

√4th **C76** **Malignant neoplasm of other and ill-defined sites**
EXCLUDES 1   malignant neoplasm of female genitourinary tract NOS (C57.9)
malignant neoplasm of male genitourinary tract NOS (C63.9)
malignant neoplasm of lymphoid, hematopoietic and related tissue (C81-C96)
malignant neoplasm of skin (C44.-)
malignant neoplasm of unspecified site NOS (C8Ø.1)

C76.Ø **Malignant neoplasm of head, face and neck** `HCC`
Malignant neoplasm of cheek NOS
Malignant neoplasm of nose NOS

C76.1 **Malignant neoplasm of thorax** `HCC`
Intrathoracic malignant neoplasm NOS
Malignant neoplasm of axilla NOS
Thoracic malignant neoplasm NOS

C76.2 **Malignant neoplasm of abdomen** `HCC`

C76.3 **Malignant neoplasm of pelvis** `HCC`
Malignant neoplasm of groin NOS
Malignant neoplasm of sites overlapping systems within the pelvis
Rectovaginal (septum) malignant neoplasm
Rectovesical (septum) malignant neoplasm

√5th **C76.4** **Malignant neoplasm of upper limb**

C76.4Ø **Malignant neoplasm of unspecified upper limb** `HCC`

C76.41 **Malignant neoplasm of right upper limb** `HCC`

C76.42 **Malignant neoplasm of left upper limb** `HCC`

√5th **C76.5** **Malignant neoplasm of lower limb**

C76.5Ø **Malignant neoplasm of unspecified lower limb** `HCC`

C76.51 **Malignant neoplasm of right lower limb** `HCC`

C76.52 **Malignant neoplasm of left lower limb** `HCC`

C76.8 **Malignant neoplasm of other specified ill-defined sites**
Malignant neoplasm of overlapping ill-defined sites

√4th **C77** **Secondary and unspecified malignant neoplasm of lymph nodes**
EXCLUDES 1   malignant neoplasm of lymph nodes, specified as primary (C81-C86, C88, C96.-)
mesentery metastasis of carcinoid tumor (C7B.Ø4)
secondary carcinoid tumors of distant lymph nodes (C7B.Ø1)

CC Excl: For CC codes in category C77: PDX collection 3Ø3

C77.Ø **Secondary and unspecified malignant neoplasm of lymph nodes of head, face and neck** `CC` `HCC`
Secondary and unspecified malignant neoplasm of supraclavicular lymph nodes

C77.1 **Secondary and unspecified malignant neoplasm of intrathoracic lymph nodes** `CC` `HCC`

C77.2 **Secondary and unspecified malignant neoplasm of intra-abdominal lymph nodes** `CC` `HCC`

C77.3 **Secondary and unspecified malignant neoplasm of axilla and upper limb lymph nodes** `CC` `HCC`
Secondary and unspecified malignant neoplasm of pectoral lymph nodes

C77.4 **Secondary and unspecified malignant neoplasm of inguinal and lower limb lymph nodes** `CC` `HCC`

C77.5 **Secondary and unspecified malignant neoplasm of intrapelvic lymph nodes** `CC` `HCC`

C77.8 **Secondary and unspecified malignant neoplasm of lymph nodes of multiple regions** `CC` `HCC`

C77.9 **Secondary and unspecified malignant neoplasm of lymph node, unspecified** `CC` `HCC`

√4th **C78** **Secondary malignant neoplasm of respiratory and digestive organs**
EXCLUDES 1   secondary carcinoid tumors of liver (C7B.Ø2)
secondary carcinoid tumors of peritoneum (C7B.Ø4)
EXCLUDES 2   lymph node metastases (C77.Ø)

√5th **C78.Ø** **Secondary malignant neoplasm of lung**

C78.ØØ **Secondary malignant neoplasm of unspecified lung** `CC` `HCC`
CC Excl: PDX collection 327

C78.Ø1 **Secondary malignant neoplasm of right lung** `CC` `HCC`
CC Excl: PDX collection 327

C78.Ø2 **Secondary malignant neoplasm of left lung** `CC` `HCC`
CC Excl: PDX collection 327

C78.1 **Secondary malignant neoplasm of mediastinum** `CC` `HCC`
CC Excl: PDX collection 328

C78.2 **Secondary malignant neoplasm of pleura** `CC` `HCC`
CC Excl: PDX collection 329

N Newborn: 0   P Pediatric: 0-17   M Maternity: 12-55   A Adult: 15-124   MCC Major CC Condition   PDxMCC PDx acts as own MCC   CC CC Condition   PDxCC PDx acts as own CC

476   ICD-10-CM 2018

✓5ᵗʰ **C78.3** **Secondary malignant neoplasm of** other and unspecified respiratory organs

     C78.30 **Secondary malignant neoplasm of** unspecified **respiratory organ** `CC` `HCC`
         CC Excl: PDX collection 330

     C78.39 **Secondary malignant neoplasm of** other respiratory organs `CC` `HCC`
         CC Excl: PDX collection 330

C78.4 **Secondary malignant neoplasm of** small intestine `CC` `HCC`
     CC Excl: PDX collection 331

C78.5 **Secondary malignant neoplasm of** large intestine and rectum `CC` `HCC`
     CC Excl: PDX collection 332

C78.6 **Secondary malignant neoplasm of** retroperitoneum and peritoneum `CC` `HCC`
     AHA: 2017, 2Q, 12
     CC Excl: PDX collection 333

C78.7 **Secondary malignant neoplasm of** liver and intrahepatic bile duct `CC` `HCC`
     CC Excl: PDX collection 334

✓5ᵗʰ **C78.8** **Secondary malignant neoplasm of** other and unspecified digestive organs

     C78.80 **Secondary malignant neoplasm of** digestive unspecified **organ** `CC` `HCC`
         CC Excl: PDX collection 335

     C78.89 **Secondary malignant neoplasm of** other digestive organs `CC` `HCC`
         Code also exocrine pancreatic insufficiency (K86.81)
         CC Excl: PDX collection 335

✓4ᵗʰ **C79** Secondary **malignant neoplasm of** other and unspecified sites
     EXCLUDES 1   secondary carcinoid tumors (C7B.-)
                 secondary neuroendocrine tumors (C7B.-)
     EXCLUDES 2   ~~lymph node metastases (C77.0)~~

✓5ᵗʰ **C79.0** **Secondary malignant neoplasm of** kidney and renal pelvis

     CC Excl: For CC codes in subcategory C79.0: PDX collection 336

     C79.00 **Secondary malignant neoplasm of** unspecified **kidney and renal pelvis** `CC` `HCC`

     C79.01 **Secondary malignant neoplasm of** right **kidney and renal pelvis** `CC` `HCC`

     C79.02 **Secondary malignant neoplasm of** left **kidney and renal pelvis** `CC` `HCC`

✓5ᵗʰ **C79.1** **Secondary malignant neoplasm of** bladder and other and unspecified urinary organs

     CC Excl: For CC codes in subcategory C79.1: PDX collection 336

     C79.10 **Secondary malignant neoplasm of** unspecified **urinary organs** `CC` `HCC`

     C79.11 **Secondary malignant neoplasm of** bladder `CC` `HCC`
         EXCLUDES 2 ▶lymph node metastases (C77.0)◄

     C79.19 **Secondary malignant neoplasm of** other urinary organs `CC` `HCC`

C79.2 **Secondary malignant neoplasm of** skin `CC` `HCC`
     EXCLUDES 1   secondary Merkel cell carcinoma (C7B.1)
     CC Excl: PDX collection 337

✓5ᵗʰ **C79.3** **Secondary malignant neoplasm of** brain and cerebral meninges

     C79.31 **Secondary malignant neoplasm of** brain `CC` `HCC`
         CC Excl: PDX collection 338

     C79.32 **Secondary malignant neoplasm of** cerebral meninges `CC` `HCC`
         CC Excl: PDX collection 339

✓5ᵗʰ **C79.4** **Secondary malignant neoplasm of** other and unspecified parts of nervous system

     C79.40 **Secondary malignant neoplasm of** unspecified **part of nervous system** `CC` `HCC`
         CC Excl: PDX collection 339

     C79.49 **Secondary malignant neoplasm of** other parts of nervous system `CC` `HCC`
         CC Excl: PDX collection 339

✓5ᵗʰ **C79.5** **Secondary malignant neoplasm of** bone and bone marrow
     EXCLUDES 1   secondary carcinoid tumors of bone (C7B.03)

     C79.51 **Secondary malignant neoplasm of** bone `CC` `HCC`
         CC Excl: PDX collection 340

     C79.52 **Secondary malignant neoplasm of** bone marrow `CC` `HCC`
         CC Excl: PDX collection 340

✓5ᵗʰ **C79.6** **Secondary malignant neoplasm of** ovary

     CC Excl: For CC codes in subcategory C79.6: PDX collection 341

     C79.60 **Secondary malignant neoplasm of** unspecified **ovary** `CC` `HCC` ♀

     C79.61 **Secondary malignant neoplasm of** right **ovary** `CC` `HCC` ♀

     C79.62 **Secondary malignant neoplasm of** left **ovary** `CC` `HCC` ♀

✓5ᵗʰ **C79.7** **Secondary malignant neoplasm of** adrenal gland

     CC Excl: For CC codes in subcategory C79.7: PDX collection 342

     C79.70 **Secondary malignant neoplasm of** unspecified **adrenal gland** `CC` `HCC`

     C79.71 **Secondary malignant neoplasm of** right **adrenal gland** `CC` `HCC`

     C79.72 **Secondary malignant neoplasm of** left **adrenal gland** `CC` `HCC`

✓5ᵗʰ **C79.8** **Secondary malignant neoplasm of** other specified sites

     C79.81 **Secondary malignant neoplasm of** breast `CC` `HCC`
         CC Excl: PDX collection 343

     C79.82 **Secondary malignant neoplasm of** genital organs `CC` `HCC`
         CC Excl: PDX collection 344

     C79.89 **Secondary malignant neoplasm of** other specified sites `CC` `HCC`
         AHA: 2017, 2Q, 11
         CC Excl: PDX collection 345

C79.9 **Secondary malignant neoplasm of** unspecified site `CC` `HCC`
     Metastatic cancer NOS
     Metastatic disease NOS
     EXCLUDES 1   carcinomatosis NOS (C80.0)
                 generalized cancer NOS (C80.0)
                 malignant (primary) neoplasm of unspecified site (C80.1)
     CC Excl: PDX collection 345

✓4ᵗʰ **C80** **Malignant neoplasm** without specification of site
     EXCLUDES 1   malignant carcinoid tumor of unspecified site (C7A.00)
                 malignant neoplasm of specified multiple sites—code to each site

C80.0 Disseminated **malignant neoplasm,** unspecified `CC` `HCC`
     Carcinomatosis NOS
     Generalized cancer, unspecified site (primary) (secondary)
     Generalized malignancy, unspecified site (primary) (secondary)
     CC Excl: PDX collection 345

C80.1 **Malignant** (primary) **neoplasm,** unspecified `HCC`
     Cancer NOS
     Cancer unspecified site (primary)
     Carcinoma unspecified site (primary)
     Malignancy unspecified site (primary)
     EXCLUDES 1   secondary malignant neoplasm of unspecified site (C79.9)

C80.2 **Malignant neoplasm associated with transplanted organ** `CC` `HCC`
     Code first complication of transplanted organ (T86.-)
     Use additional code to identify the specific malignancy
     CC Excl: PDX collection 345

Malignant neoplasms of lymphoid, hematopoietic and related tissue (C81-C96)

     EXCLUDES 2   Kaposi's sarcoma of lymph nodes (C46.3)
                 secondary and unspecified neoplasm of lymph nodes (C77.-)
                 secondary neoplasm of bone marrow (C79.52)
                 secondary neoplasm of spleen (C78.89)

✓4ᵗʰ **C81** **Hodgkin lymphoma**
     EXCLUDES 1   personal history of Hodgkin lymphoma (Z85.71)

✓5ᵗʰ **C81.0** Nodular lymphocyte predominant **Hodgkin lymphoma**

     C81.00 **Nodular lymphocyte predominant Hodgkin lymphoma,** unspecified **site** `CC` `HCC`
         CC Excl: PDX collection 368

     C81.01 **Nodular lymphocyte predominant Hodgkin lymphoma, lymph nodes of** head, face, and neck `CC` `HCC`
         CC Excl: PDX collection 369

     C81.02 **Nodular lymphocyte predominant Hodgkin lymphoma, intrathoracic lymph nodes** `CC` `HCC`
         CC Excl: PDX collection 370

C81.03 **Nodular lymphocyte predominant Hodgkin lymphoma, intra-abdominal lymph nodes** `CC` `HCC`
CC Excl: PDX collection 371

C81.04 **Nodular lymphocyte predominant Hodgkin lymphoma, lymph nodes of axilla and upper limb** `CC` `HCC`
CC Excl: PDX collection 372

C81.05 **Nodular lymphocyte predominant Hodgkin lymphoma, lymph nodes of inguinal region and lower limb** `CC` `HCC`
CC Excl: PDX collection 373

C81.06 **Nodular lymphocyte predominant Hodgkin lymphoma, intrapelvic lymph nodes** `CC` `HCC`
CC Excl: PDX collection 374

C81.07 **Nodular lymphocyte predominant Hodgkin lymphoma, spleen** `CC` `HCC`
CC Excl: PDX collection 375

C81.08 **Nodular lymphocyte predominant Hodgkin lymphoma, lymph nodes of multiple sites** `CC` `HCC`
CC Excl: PDX collection 368

C81.09 **Nodular lymphocyte predominant Hodgkin lymphoma, extranodal and solid organ sites** `CC` `HCC`
CC Excl: PDX collection 368

√5ᵗʰ **C81.1** **Nodular sclerosis Hodgkin lymphoma**
Nodular sclerosis classical Hodgkin lymphoma

C81.10 **Nodular sclerosis Hodgkin lymphoma, unspecified site** `CC` `HCC`
CC Excl: PDX collection 376

C81.11 **Nodular sclerosis Hodgkin lymphoma, lymph nodes of head, face, and neck** `CC` `HCC`
CC Excl: PDX collection 377

C81.12 **Nodular sclerosis Hodgkin lymphoma, intrathoracic lymph nodes** `CC` `HCC`
CC Excl: PDX collection 378

C81.13 **Nodular sclerosis Hodgkin lymphoma, intra-abdominal lymph nodes** `CC` `HCC`
CC Excl: PDX collection 379

C81.14 **Nodular sclerosis Hodgkin lymphoma, lymph nodes of axilla and upper limb** `CC` `HCC`
CC Excl: PDX collection 380

C81.15 **Nodular sclerosis Hodgkin lymphoma, lymph nodes of inguinal region and lower limb** `CC` `HCC`
CC Excl: PDX collection 381

C81.16 **Nodular sclerosis Hodgkin lymphoma, intrapelvic lymph nodes** `CC` `HCC`
CC Excl: PDX collection 382

C81.17 **Nodular sclerosis Hodgkin lymphoma, spleen** `CC` `HCC`
CC Excl: PDX collection 383

C81.18 **Nodular sclerosis Hodgkin lymphoma, lymph nodes of multiple sites** `CC` `HCC`
CC Excl: PDX collection 376

C81.19 **Nodular sclerosis Hodgkin lymphoma, extranodal and solid organ sites** `CC` `HCC`
CC Excl: PDX collection 376

√5ᵗʰ **C81.2** **Mixed cellularity Hodgkin lymphoma**
Mixed cellularity classical Hodgkin lymphoma

C81.20 **Mixed cellularity Hodgkin lymphoma, unspecified site** `CC` `HCC`
CC Excl: PDX collection 384

C81.21 **Mixed cellularity Hodgkin lymphoma, lymph nodes of head, face, and neck** `CC` `HCC`
CC Excl: PDX collection 385

C81.22 **Mixed cellularity Hodgkin lymphoma, intrathoracic lymph nodes** `CC` `HCC`
CC Excl: PDX collection 386

C81.23 **Mixed cellularity Hodgkin lymphoma, intra-abdominal lymph nodes** `CC` `HCC`
CC Excl: PDX collection 387

C81.24 **Mixed cellularity Hodgkin lymphoma, lymph nodes of axilla and upper limb** `CC` `HCC`
CC Excl: PDX collection 388

C81.25 **Mixed cellularity Hodgkin lymphoma, lymph nodes of inguinal region and lower limb** `CC` `HCC`
CC Excl: PDX collection 389

C81.26 **Mixed cellularity Hodgkin lymphoma, intrapelvic lymph nodes** `CC` `HCC`
CC Excl: CPDX collection 390

C81.27 **Mixed cellularity Hodgkin lymphoma, spleen** `CC` `HCC`
CC Excl: PDX collection 391

C81.28 **Mixed cellularity Hodgkin lymphoma, lymph nodes of multiple sites** `CC` `HCC`
CC Excl: PDX collection 384

C81.29 **Mixed cellularity Hodgkin lymphoma, extranodal and solid organ sites** `CC` `HCC`
CC Excl: PDX collection 384

√5ᵗʰ **C81.3** **Lymphocyte depleted Hodgkin lymphoma**
Lymphocyte depleted classical Hodgkin lymphoma

C81.30 **Lymphocyte depleted Hodgkin lymphoma, unspecified site** `CC` `HCC`
CC Excl: PDX collection 392

C81.31 **Lymphocyte depleted Hodgkin lymphoma, lymph nodes of head, face, and neck** `CC` `HCC`
CC Excl: PDX collection 393

C81.32 **Lymphocyte depleted Hodgkin lymphoma, intrathoracic lymph nodes** `CC` `HCC`
CC Excl: PDX collection 394

C81.33 **Lymphocyte depleted Hodgkin lymphoma, intra-abdominal lymph nodes** `CC` `HCC`
CC Excl: PDX collection 395

C81.34 **Lymphocyte depleted Hodgkin lymphoma, lymph nodes of axilla and upper limb** `CC` `HCC`
CC Excl: PDX collection 396

C81.35 **Lymphocyte depleted Hodgkin lymphoma, lymph nodes of inguinal region and lower limb** `CC` `HCC`
CC Excl: PDX collection 397

C81.36 **Lymphocyte depleted Hodgkin lymphoma, intrapelvic lymph nodes** `CC` `HCC`
CC Excl: PDX collection 398

C81.37 **Lymphocyte depleted Hodgkin lymphoma, spleen** `CC` `HCC`
CC Excl: PDX collection 399

C81.38 **Lymphocyte depleted Hodgkin lymphoma, lymph nodes of multiple sites** `CC` `HCC`
CC Excl: PDX collection 400

C81.39 **Lymphocyte depleted Hodgkin lymphoma, extranodal and solid organ sites** `CC` `HCC`
CC Excl: PDX collection 392

√5ᵗʰ **C81.4** **Lymphocyte-rich Hodgkin lymphoma**
Lymphocyte-rich classical Hodgkin lymphoma
EXCLUDES 1   *nodular lymphocyte predominant Hodgkin lymphoma (C81.0-)*

C81.40 **Lymphocyte-rich Hodgkin lymphoma, unspecified site** `CC` `HCC`
CC Excl: PDX collection 368

C81.41 **Lymphocyte-rich Hodgkin lymphoma, lymph nodes of head, face, and neck** `CC` `HCC`
CC Excl: PDX collection 369

C81.42 **Lymphocyte-rich Hodgkin lymphoma, intrathoracic lymph nodes** `CC` `HCC`
CC Excl: PDX collection 370

C81.43 **Lymphocyte-rich Hodgkin lymphoma, intra-abdominal lymph nodes** `CC` `HCC`
CC Excl: PDX collection 371

C81.44 **Lymphocyte-rich Hodgkin lymphoma, lymph nodes of axilla and upper limb** `CC` `HCC`
CC Excl: PDX collection 372

C81.45 **Lymphocyte-rich Hodgkin lymphoma, lymph nodes of inguinal region and lower limb** `CC` `HCC`
CC Excl: PDX collection 373

C81.46 **Lymphocyte-rich Hodgkin lymphoma, intrapelvic lymph nodes** `CC` `HCC`
CC Excl: PDX collection 374

C81.47 **Lymphocyte-rich Hodgkin lymphoma, spleen** `CC` `HCC`
CC Excl: CPDX collection 375

C81.48 **Lymphocyte-rich Hodgkin lymphoma, lymph nodes of multiple sites** `CC` `HCC`
CC Excl: PDX collection 368

C81.49 **Lymphocyte-rich Hodgkin lymphoma, extranodal and solid organ sites** `CC` `HCC`
CC Excl: PDX collection 368

√5ᵗʰ **C81.7** **Other Hodgkin lymphoma**
Classical Hodgkin lymphoma NOS
Other classical Hodgkin lymphoma

C81.70 **Other Hodgkin lymphoma, unspecified site** `CC` `HCC`
CC Excl: PDX collection 401

C81.71 **Other Hodgkin lymphoma, lymph nodes of head, face, and neck** `CC` `HCC`
CC Excl: PDX collection 402

C81.72 **Other Hodgkin lymphoma, intrathoracic lymph nodes** `CC` `HCC`
CC Excl: PDX collection 403

C81.73 **Other Hodgkin lymphoma,** intra-abdominal **lymph nodes** `CC` `HCC`
    CC Excl: PDX collection 404

C81.74 **Other Hodgkin lymphoma, lymph nodes of** axilla and upper limb `CC` `HCC`
    CC Excl: PDX collection 405

C81.75 **Other Hodgkin lymphoma, lymph nodes of** inguinal region and lower limb `CC` `HCC`
    CC Excl: PDX collection 406

C81.76 **Other Hodgkin lymphoma,** intrapelvic **lymph nodes** `CC` `HCC`
    CC Excl: PDX collection 407

C81.77 **Other Hodgkin lymphoma,** spleen `CC` `HCC`
    CC Excl: PDX collection 408

C81.78 **Other Hodgkin lymphoma, lymph nodes of** multiple sites `CC` `HCC`
    CC Excl: PDX collection 401

C81.79 **Other Hodgkin lymphoma,** extranodal and solid organ sites `CC` `HCC`
    CC Excl: PDX collection 401

✓6th **C81.9** **Hodgkin lymphoma,** unspecified

C81.90 **Hodgkin lymphoma, unspecified,** unspecified site `CC` `HCC`
    CC Excl: PDX collection 409

C81.91 **Hodgkin lymphoma, unspecified, lymph nodes of** head, face, and neck `CC` `HCC`
    CC Excl: PDX collection 410

C81.92 **Hodgkin lymphoma, unspecified,** intrathoracic **lymph nodes** `CC` `HCC`
    CC Excl: PDX collection 411

C81.93 **Hodgkin lymphoma, unspecified,** intra-abdominal **lymph nodes** `CC` `HCC`
    CC Excl: PDX collection 412

C81.94 **Hodgkin lymphoma, unspecified, lymph nodes of** axilla and upper limb `CC` `HCC`
    CC Excl: PDX collection 413

C81.95 **Hodgkin lymphoma, unspecified, lymph nodes of** inguinal region and lower limb `CC` `HCC`
    CC Excl: PDX collection 414

C81.96 **Hodgkin lymphoma, unspecified,** intrapelvic **lymph nodes** `CC` `HCC`
    CC Excl: PDX collection 415

C81.97 **Hodgkin lymphoma, unspecified,** spleen `CC` `HCC`
    CC Excl: PDX collection 416

C81.98 **Hodgkin lymphoma, unspecified, lymph nodes of** multiple sites `CC` `HCC`
    CC Excl: SPDX collection 409

C81.99 **Hodgkin lymphoma, unspecified,** extranodal and solid organ sites `CC` `HCC`
    CC Excl: No Excl

✓4th **C82** Follicular **lymphoma**
    INCLUDES   follicular lymphoma with or without diffuse areas
    EXCLUDES 1   *mature T/NK-cell lymphomas (C84.-)*
         personal history of non-Hodgkin lymphoma (Z85.72)

✓5th **C82.0** **Follicular lymphoma** grade I

C82.00 **Follicular lymphoma grade I,** unspecified site `CC` `HCC`
    CC Excl: PDX collection 417

C82.01 **Follicular lymphoma grade I, lymph nodes of** head, face, and neck `CC` `HCC`
    CC Excl: PDX collection 418

C82.02 **Follicular lymphoma grade I,** intrathoracic **lymph nodes** `CC` `HCC`
    CC Excl: PDX collection 419

C82.03 **Follicular lymphoma grade I,** intra-abdominal **lymph nodes** `CC` `HCC`
    CC Excl: PDX collection 420

C82.04 **Follicular lymphoma grade I, lymph nodes of** axilla and upper limb `CC` `HCC`
    CC Excl: PDX collection 421

C82.05 **Follicular lymphoma grade I, lymph nodes of** inguinal region and lower limb `CC` `HCC`
    CC Excl: PDX collection 422

C82.06 **Follicular lymphoma grade I,** intrapelvic **lymph nodes** `CC` `HCC`
    CC Excl: PDX collection 423

C82.07 **Follicular lymphoma grade I,** spleen `CC` `HCC`
    CC Excl: PDX collection 424

C82.08 **Follicular lymphoma grade I, lymph nodes of** multiple sites `CC` `HCC`
    CC Excl: PDX collection 425

C82.09 **Follicular lymphoma grade I,** extranodal and solid organ sites `CC` `HCC`
    CC Excl: PDX collection 417

✓5th **C82.1** **Follicular lymphoma** grade II

C82.10 **Follicular lymphoma grade II,** unspecified site `CC` `HCC`
    CC Excl: PDX collection 417

C82.11 **Follicular lymphoma grade II, lymph nodes of** head, face, and neck `CC` `HCC`
    CC Excl: PDX collection 418

C82.12 **Follicular lymphoma grade II,** intrathoracic **lymph nodes** `CC` `HCC`
    CC Excl: PDX collection 419

C82.13 **Follicular lymphoma grade II,** intra-abdominal **lymph nodes** `CC` `HCC`
    CC Excl: PDX collection 420

C82.14 **Follicular lymphoma grade II, lymph nodes of** axilla and upper limb `CC` `HCC`
    CC Excl: PDX collection 421

C82.15 **Follicular lymphoma grade II, lymph nodes of** inguinal region and lower limb `CC` `HCC`
    CC Excl: PDX collection 422

C82.16 **Follicular lymphoma grade II,** intrapelvic **lymph nodes** `CC` `HCC`
    CC Excl: PDX collection 423

C82.17 **Follicular lymphoma grade II,** spleen `CC` `HCC`
    CC Excl: PDX collection 424

C82.18 **Follicular lymphoma grade II, lymph nodes of** multiple sites `CC` `HCC`
    CC Excl: PDX collection 425

C82.19 **Follicular lymphoma grade II,** extranodal and solid organ sites `CC` `HCC`
    CC Excl: PDX collection 417

✓5th **C82.2** **Follicular lymphoma** grade III, unspecified

C82.20 **Follicular lymphoma, grade III, unspecified,** unspecified site `CC` `HCC`
    CC Excl: PDX collection 417

C82.21 **Follicular lymphoma grade III, unspecified, lymph nodes of** head, face, and neck `CC` `HCC`
    CC Excl: PDX collection 418

C82.22 **Follicular lymphoma grade III, unspecified,** intrathoracic **lymph nodes** `CC` `HCC`
    CC Excl: PDX collection 419

C82.23 **Follicular lymphoma grade III, unspecified,** intra-abdominal **lymph nodes** `CC` `HCC`
    CC Excl: PDX collection 420

C82.24 **Follicular lymphoma grade III, unspecified, lymph nodes of** axilla and upper limb `CC` `HCC`
    CC Excl: PDX collection 421

C82.25 **Follicular lymphoma grade III, unspecified, lymph nodes of** inguinal region and lower limb `CC` `HCC`
    CC Excl: PDX collection 422

C82.26 **Follicular lymphoma grade III, unspecified,** intrapelvic **lymph nodes** `CC` `HCC`
    CC Excl: PDX collection 423

C82.27 **Follicular lymphoma grade III, unspecified,** spleen `CC` `HCC`
    CC Excl: PDX collection 424

C82.28 **Follicular lymphoma grade III, unspecified, lymph nodes of** multiple sites `CC` `HCC`
    CC Excl: PDX collection 425

C82.29 **Follicular lymphoma grade III, unspecified,** extranodal and solid organ sites `CC` `HCC`
    CC Excl: PDX collection 417

✓5th **C82.3** **Follicular lymphoma** grade IIIa

C82.30 **Follicular lymphoma grade IIIa,** unspecified sitespleen `CC` `HCC`
    CC Excl: PDX collection 417

C82.31 **Follicular lymphoma grade IIIa, lymph nodes of** head, face, and neck `CC` `HCC`
    CC Excl: PDX collection 418

C82.32 **Follicular lymphoma grade IIIa,** intrathoracic **lymph nodes** `CC` `HCC`
    CC Excl: PDX collection 419

C82.33 **Follicular lymphoma grade IIIa,** intra-abdominal **lymph nodes** `CC` `HCC`
    CC Excl: PDX collection 420

C82.34 **Follicular lymphoma grade IIIa, lymph nodes of** axilla and upper limb `CC` `HCC`
    CC Excl: PDX collection 421

☑ Additional Character Req   ✓x7th Placeholder Alert   Unacceptable PDx   Manifestation   H1-H14 HAC   HCC CMS-HCC Condition   EXCLUDES 1 Not Coded Here   EXCLUDES 2 Not Included Here

ICD-10-CM 2018   479

C81.73–C82.34

Chapter 2. Neoplasms

C82.35 Follicular lymphoma grade IIIa, lymph nodes `CC` `HCC`
of inguinal region and lower limb
　CC Excl: PDX collection 422

C82.36 Follicular lymphoma grade IIIa, intrapelvic `CC` `HCC`
lymph nodes
　CC Excl: PDX collection 423

C82.37 Follicular lymphoma grade IIIa, spleen `CC` `HCC`
　CC Excl: PDX collection 424

C82.38 Follicular lymphoma grade IIIa, lymph nodes `CC` `HCC`
of multiple sites
　CC Excl: PDX collection 425

C82.39 Follicular lymphoma grade IIIa, extranodal `CC` `HCC`
and solid organ sites
　CC Excl: PDX collection 417

✓5th **C82.4** Follicular lymphoma grade IIIb

C82.40 Follicular lymphoma grade IIIb, `CC` `HCC`
unspecified site
　CC Excl: PDX collection 417

C82.41 Follicular lymphoma grade IIIb, lymph nodes `CC` `HCC`
of head, face, and neck
　CC Excl: PDX collection 418

C82.42 Follicular lymphoma grade IIIb, intrathoracic `CC` `HCC`
lymph nodes
　CC Excl: PDX collection 419

C82.43 Follicular lymphoma grade IIIb, `CC` `HCC`
intra-abdominal lymph nodes
　CC Excl: PDX collection 420

C82.44 Follicular lymphoma grade IIIb, lymph nodes `CC` `HCC`
of axilla and upper limb
　CC Excl: PDX collection 421

C82.45 Follicular lymphoma grade IIIb, lymph `CC` `HCC`
nodes of inguinal region and lower limb
　CC Excl: PDX collection 422

C82.46 Follicular lymphoma grade IIIb, intrapelvic `CC` `HCC`
lymph nodes
　CC Excl: PDX collection 423

C82.47 Follicular lymphoma grade IIIb, spleen `CC` `HCC`
　CC Excl: PDX collection 424

C82.48 Follicular lymphoma grade IIIb, lymph nodes `CC` `HCC`
of multiple sites
　CC Excl: PDX collection 425

C82.49 Follicular lymphoma grade IIIb, extranodal `CC` `HCC`
and solid organ sites
　CC Excl: PDX collection 417

✓5th **C82.5** Diffuse follicle center lymphoma

C82.50 Diffuse follicle center lymphoma, `HIV` `CC` `HCC`
unspecified site
　CC Excl: PDX collection 426

C82.51 Diffuse follicle center lymphoma, lymph `HIV` `CC` `HCC`
nodes of head, face, and neck
　CC Excl: PDX collection 427

C82.52 Diffuse follicle center lymphoma, `HIV` `CC` `HCC`
intrathoracic lymph nodes
　CC Excl: PDX collection 428

C82.53 Diffuse follicle center lymphoma, intra- `HIV` `CC` `HCC`
abdominal lymph nodes
　CC Excl: PDX collection 429

C82.54 Diffuse follicle center lymphoma, lymph `HIV` `CC` `HCC`
nodes of axilla and upper limb
　CC Excl: PDX collection 430

C82.55 Diffuse follicle center lymphoma, lymph `HIV` `CC` `HCC`
nodes of inguinal region and lower limb
　CC Excl: PDX collection 431

C82.56 Diffuse follicle center lymphoma, `HIV` `CC` `HCC`
intrapelvic lymph nodes
　CC Excl: PDX collection 432

C82.57 Diffuse follicle center lymphoma, spleen `HIV` `CC` `HCC`
　CC Excl: PDX collection 433

C82.58 Diffuse follicle center lymphoma, lymph `HIV` `CC` `HCC`
nodes of multiple sites
　CC Excl: PDX collection 434

C82.59 Diffuse follicle center lymphoma, `HIV` `CC` `HCC`
extranodal and solid organ sites
　CC Excl: PDX collection 426

✓5th **C82.6** Cutaneous follicle center lymphoma

C82.60 Cutaneous follicle center lymphoma, `CC` `HCC`
unspecified site
　CC Excl: PDX collection 417

C82.61 Cutaneous follicle center lymphoma, lymph `CC` `HCC`
nodes of head, face, and neck
　CC Excl: PDX collection 418

C82.62 Cutaneous follicle center lymphoma, `CC` `HCC`
intrathoracic lymph nodes
　CC Excl: PDX collection 419

C82.63 Cutaneous follicle center lymphoma, `CC` `HCC`
intra-abdominal lymph nodes
　CC Excl: PDX collection 420

C82.64 Cutaneous follicle center lymphoma, lymph `CC` `HCC`
nodes of axilla and upper limb
　CC Excl: PDX collection 421

C82.65 Cutaneous follicle center lymphoma, lymph `CC` `HCC`
nodes of inguinal region and lower limb
　CC Excl: PDX collection 422

C82.66 Cutaneous follicle center lymphoma, `CC` `HCC`
intrapelvic lymph nodes
　CC Excl: PDX collection 423

C82.67 Cutaneous follicle center lymphoma, spleen `CC` `HCC`
　CC Excl: PDX collection 424

C82.68 Cutaneous follicle center lymphoma, lymph `CC` `HCC`
nodes of multiple sites
　CC Excl: PDX collection 425

C82.69 Cutaneous follicle center lymphoma, `CC` `HCC`
extranodal and solid organ sites
　CC Excl: PDX collection 417

✓5th **C82.8** Other types of follicular lymphoma

C82.80 Other types of follicular lymphoma, `CC` `HCC`
unspecified site
　CC Excl: PDX collection 417

C82.81 Other types of follicular lymphoma, lymph `CC` `HCC`
nodes of head, face, and neck
　CC Excl: PDX collection 418

C82.82 Other types of follicular lymphoma, `CC` `HCC`
intrathoracic lymph nodes
　CC Excl: PDX collection 419

C82.83 Other types of follicular lymphoma, `CC` `HCC`
intra-abdominal lymph nodes
　CC Excl: PDX collection 420

C82.84 Other types of follicular lymphoma, lymph `CC` `HCC`
nodes of axilla and upper limb
　CC Excl: PDX collection 421

C82.85 Other types of follicular lymphoma, lymph `CC` `HCC`
nodes of inguinal region and lower limb
　CC Excl: PDX collection 422

C82.86 Other types of follicular lymphoma, `CC` `HCC`
intrapelvic lymph nodes
　CC Excl: PDX collection 423

C82.87 Other types of follicular lymphoma, spleen `CC` `HCC`
　CC Excl: PDX collection 424

C82.88 Other types of follicular lymphoma, lymph `CC` `HCC`
nodes of multiple sites
　CC Excl: PDX collection 425

C82.89 Other types of follicular lymphoma, `CC` `HCC`
extranodal and solid organ sites
　CC Excl: PDX collection 417

✓5th **C82.9** Follicular lymphoma, unspecified

C82.90 Follicular lymphoma, unspecified, `CC` `HCC`
unspecified site
　CC Excl: PDX collection 417

C82.91 Follicular lymphoma, unspecified, lymph `CC` `HCC`
nodes of head, face, and neck
　CC Excl: PDX collection 418

C82.92 Follicular lymphoma, unspecified, `CC` `HCC`
intrathoracic lymph nodes
　CC Excl: PDX collection 419

C82.93 Follicular lymphoma, unspecified, intra- `CC` `HCC`
abdominal lymph nodes
　CC Excl: PDX collection 420

C82.94 Follicular lymphoma, unspecified, lymph `CC` `HCC`
nodes of axilla and upper limb
　CC Excl: PDX collection 421

C82.95 Follicular lymphoma, unspecified, lymph `CC` `HCC`
nodes of inguinal region and lower limb
　CC Excl: PDX collection 422

C82.96 Follicular lymphoma, unspecified, `CC` `HCC`
intrapelvic lymph nodes
　CC Excl: PDX collection 423

C82.97 Follicular lymphoma, unspecified, spleen `CC` `HCC`
　CC Excl: PDX collection 424

C82.98 Follicular lymphoma, unspecified, lymph `CC` `HCC`
nodes of multiple sites
　CC Excl: PDX collection 425

`N` Newborn: 0　`P` Pediatric: 0-17　`M` Maternity: 12-55　`A` Adult: 15-124　`MCC` Major CC Condition　`PDxMCC` PDx acts as own MCC　`CC` CC Condition　`PDxCC` PDx acts as own CC

C82.99   **Follicular lymphoma, unspecified,** `CC` `HCC`
     extranodal and solid organ sites
      CC Excl: PDX collection 417

✓4ᵗʰ **C83**   **Non-follicular lymphoma**
    EXCLUDES 1   personal history of non-Hodgkin lymphoma (Z85.72)

✓5ᵗʰ **C83.0**   **Small cell B-cell lymphoma**
     Lymphoplasmacytic lymphoma
     Nodal marginal zone lymphoma
     Non-leukemic variant of B-CLL
     Splenic marginal zone lymphoma
     EXCLUDES 1   chronic lymphocytic leukemia (C91.1)
              mature T/NK-cell lymphomas (C84.-)
              Waldenström macroglobulinemia (C88.0)

C83.00   **Small cell B-cell lymphoma, unspecified** `HIV` `CC` `HCC`
     site
      CC Excl: PDX collection 435

C83.01   **Small cell B-cell lymphoma, lymph nodes** `HIV` `CC` `HCC`
     of head, face, and neck
      CC Excl: PDX collection 436

C83.02   **Small cell B-cell lymphoma, intrathoracic** `HIV` `CC` `HCC`
     lymph nodes
      CC Excl: PDX collection 437

C83.03   **Small cell B-cell lymphoma, intra-** `HIV` `CC` `HCC`
     abdominal lymph nodes
      CC Excl: PDX collection 438

C83.04   **Small cell B-cell lymphoma, lymph nodes** `HIV` `CC` `HCC`
     of axilla and upper limb
      CC Excl: PDX collection 439

C83.05   **Small cell B-cell lymphoma, lymph nodes** `HIV` `CC` `HCC`
     of inguinal region and lower limb
      CC Excl: CPDX collection 440

C83.06   **Small cell B-cell lymphoma, intrapelvic** `HIV` `CC` `HCC`
     lymph nodes
      CC Excl: PDX collection 441

C83.07   **Small cell B-cell lymphoma, spleen** `HIV` `CC` `HCC`
      CC Excl: PDX collection 442

C83.08   **Small cell B-cell lymphoma, lymph nodes** `HIV` `CC` `HCC`
     of multiple sites
      CC Excl: PDX collection 435

C83.09   **Small cell B-cell lymphoma, extranodal** `HIV` `CC` `HCC`
     and solid organ sites
      CC Excl: PDX collection 435

✓5ᵗʰ **C83.1**   **Mantle cell lymphoma**
     Centrocytic lymphoma
     Malignant lymphomatous polyposis
     DEF: Rare form of B-cell non-Hodgkin lymphoma named for the
     location of tumor cell production, the mantle zone of the lymph
     nodes.

C83.10   **Mantle cell lymphoma, unspecified site** `HIV` `CC` `HCC`
      CC Excl: PDX collection 426

C83.11   **Mantle cell lymphoma, lymph nodes of** `HIV` `CC` `HCC`
     head, face, and neck
      CC Excl: PDX collection 427

C83.12   **Mantle cell lymphoma, intrathoracic** `HIV` `CC` `HCC`
     lymph nodes
      CC Excl: PDX collection 428

C83.13   **Mantle cell lymphoma, intra-abdominal** `HIV` `CC` `HCC`
     lymph nodes
      CC Excl: PDX collection 429

C83.14   **Mantle cell lymphoma, lymph nodes of** `HIV` `CC` `HCC`
     axilla and upper limb
      CC Excl: PDX collection 430

C83.15   **Mantle cell lymphoma, lymph nodes of** `HIV` `CC` `HCC`
     inguinal region and lower limb
      CC Excl: PDX collection 431

C83.16   **Mantle cell lymphoma, intrapelvic lymph** `HIV` `CC` `HCC`
     nodes
      CC Excl: PDX collection 432

C83.17   **Mantle cell lymphoma, spleen** `HIV` `CC` `HCC`
      CC Excl: PDX collection 433

C83.18   **Mantle cell lymphoma, lymph nodes of** `HIV` `CC` `HCC`
     multiple sites
      CC Excl: PDX collection 434

C83.19   **Mantle cell lymphoma, extranodal and** `HIV` `CC` `HCC`
     solid organ sites
      CC Excl: PDX collection 426

✓5ᵗʰ **C83.3**   **Diffuse large B-cell lymphoma**
     Anaplastic diffuse large B-cell lymphoma
     CD30-positive diffuse large B-cell lymphoma
     Centroblastic diffuse large B-cell lymphoma
     Diffuse large B-cell lymphoma, subtype not specified
     Immunoblastic diffuse large B-cell lymphoma
     Plasmablastic diffuse large B-cell lymphoma
     T-cell rich diffuse large B-cell lymphoma
     EXCLUDES 1   mature T/NK-cell lymphomas (C84.-)
              mediastinal (thymic) large B-cell lymphoma (C85.2-)

C83.30   **Diffuse large B-cell lymphoma,** `HIV` `CC` `HCC`
     unspecified site
      CC Excl: PDX collection 443

C83.31   **Diffuse large B-cell lymphoma, lymph** `HIV` `CC` `HCC`
     nodes of head, face, and neck
      CC Excl: PDX collection 444

C83.32   **Diffuse large B-cell lymphoma,** `HIV` `CC` `HCC`
     intrathoracic lymph nodes
      CC Excl: PDX collection 445

C83.33   **Diffuse large B-cell lymphoma, intra-** `HIV` `CC` `HCC`
     abdominal lymph nodes
      CC Excl: PDX collection 446

C83.34   **Diffuse large B-cell lymphoma, lymph** `HIV` `CC` `HCC`
     nodes of axilla and upper limb
      CC Excl: PDX collection 447

C83.35   **Diffuse large B-cell lymphoma, lymph** `HIV` `CC` `HCC`
     nodes of inguinal region and lower limb
      CC Excl: PDX collection 448

C83.36   **Diffuse large B-cell lymphoma,** `HIV` `CC` `HCC`
     intrapelvic lymph nodes
      CC Excl: PDX collection 449

C83.37   **Diffuse large B-cell lymphoma, spleen** `HIV` `CC` `HCC`
      CC Excl: PDX collection 450

C83.38   **Diffuse large B-cell lymphoma, lymph** `HIV` `CC` `HCC`
     nodes of multiple sites
      CC Excl: PDX collection 443

C83.39   **Diffuse large B-cell lymphoma, extranodal** `HIV` `CC` `HCC`
     and solid organ sites
      CC Excl: PDX collection 443

✓5ᵗʰ **C83.5**   **Lymphoblastic (diffuse) lymphoma**
     B-precursor lymphoma
     Lymphoblastic B-cell lymphoma
     Lymphoblastic lymphoma NOS
     Lymphoblastic T-cell lymphoma
     T-precursor lymphoma

C83.50   **Lymphoblastic (diffuse) lymphoma,** `CC` `HCC`
     unspecified site
      CC Excl: PDX collection 451

C83.51   **Lymphoblastic (diffuse) lymphoma, lymph** `CC` `HCC`
     nodes of head, face, and neck
      CC Excl: PDX collection 452

C83.52   **Lymphoblastic (diffuse) lymphoma,** `CC` `HCC`
     intrathoracic lymph nodes
      CC Excl: PDX collection 453

C83.53   **Lymphoblastic (diffuse) lymphoma,** `CC` `HCC`
     intra-abdominal lymph nodes
      CC Excl: PDX collection 454

C83.54   **Lymphoblastic (diffuse) lymphoma, lymph** `CC` `HCC`
     nodes of axilla and upper limb
      CC Excl: PDX collection 455

C83.55   **Lymphoblastic (diffuse) lymphoma, lymph** `CC` `HCC`
     nodes of inguinal region and lower limb
      CC Excl: PDX collection 456

C83.56   **Lymphoblastic (diffuse) lymphoma,** `CC` `HCC`
     intrapelvic lymph nodes
      CC Excl: PDX collection 457

C83.57   **Lymphoblastic (diffuse) lymphoma, spleen** `CC` `HCC`
      CC Excl: PDX collection 458

C83.58   **Lymphoblastic (diffuse) lymphoma, lymph** `CC` `HCC`
     nodes of multiple sites
      CC Excl: PDX collection 451

C83.59   **Lymphoblastic (diffuse) lymphoma,** `CC` `HCC`
     extranodal and solid organ sites
      CC Excl: PDX collection 451

Chapter 2. Neoplasms

✓5th **C83.7 Burkitt lymphoma**
Atypical Burkitt lymphoma
Burkitt-like lymphoma
EXCLUDES 1   mature B-cell leukemia Burkitt type (C91.A-)
DEF: Malignancy of the lymphatic system, most often seen as a large bone-deteriorating lesion within the jaw or as an abdominal mass. It is a form of non-Hodgkin's lymphoma and is recognized as the fastest growing human tumor.

C83.70   **Burkitt lymphoma, unspecified site**   HIV CC HCC
    CC Excl: PDX collection 459

C83.71   **Burkitt lymphoma, lymph nodes of** head, face, and neck   HIV CC HCC
    CC Excl: PDX collection 460

C83.72   **Burkitt lymphoma, intrathoracic lymph nodes**   HIV CC HCC
    CC Excl: PDX collection 461

C83.73   **Burkitt lymphoma, intra-abdominal lymph nodes**   HIV CC HCC
    CC Excl: PDX collection 462

C83.74   **Burkitt lymphoma, lymph nodes of** axilla and upper limb   HIV CC HCC
    CC Excl: PDX collection 463

C83.75   **Burkitt lymphoma, lymph nodes of** inguinal region and lower limb   HIV CC HCC
    CC Excl: PDX collection 464

C83.76   **Burkitt lymphoma, intrapelvic lymph nodes**   HIV CC HCC
    CC Excl: PDX collection 465

C83.77   **Burkitt lymphoma, spleen**   HIV CC HCC
    CC Excl: PDX collection 466

C83.78   **Burkitt lymphoma, lymph nodes of** multiple sites   HIV CC HCC
    CC Excl: PDX collection 459

C83.79   **Burkitt lymphoma, extranodal and solid** organ sites   HIV CC HCC
    CC Excl: PDX collection 459

✓5th **C83.8 Other non-follicular lymphoma**
Intravascular large B-cell lymphoma
Lymphoid granulomatosis
Primary effusion B-cell lymphoma
EXCLUDES 1   mediastinal (thymic) large B-cell lymphoma (C85.2-)
        T-cell rich B-cell lymphoma (C83.3-)

C83.80   **Other non-follicular lymphoma, unspecified site**   HIV CC HCC
    CC Excl: PDX collection 435

C83.81   **Other non-follicular lymphoma, lymph nodes of** head, face, and neck   HIV CC HCC
    CC Excl: PDX collection 436

C83.82   **Other non-follicular lymphoma, intrathoracic lymph nodes**   HIV CC HCC
    CC Excl: PDX collection 437

C83.83   **Other non-follicular lymphoma, intra-abdominal lymph nodes**   HIV CC HCC
    CC Excl: PDX collection 438

C83.84   **Other non-follicular lymphoma, lymph nodes of** axilla and upper limb   HIV CC HCC
    CC Excl: PDX collection 439

C83.85   **Other non-follicular lymphoma, lymph nodes of** inguinal region and lower limb   HIV CC HCC
    CC Excl: PDX collection 440

C83.86   **Other non-follicular lymphoma, intrapelvic lymph nodes**   HIV CC HCC
    CC Excl: PDX collection 441

C83.87   **Other non-follicular lymphoma, spleen**   HIV CC HCC
    CC Excl: PDX collection 442

C83.88   **Other non-follicular lymphoma, lymph nodes of** multiple sites   HIV CC HCC
    CC Excl: PDX collection 435

C83.89   **Other non-follicular lymphoma, extranodal and solid organ sites**   HIV CC HCC
    CC Excl: SPDX collection 435

✓5th **C83.9 Non-follicular (diffuse) lymphoma, unspecified**

C83.90   **Non-follicular (diffuse) lymphoma, unspecified, unspecified site**   HIV CC HCC
    CC Excl: PDX collection 435

C83.91   **Non-follicular (diffuse) lymphoma, unspecified, lymph nodes of** head, face, and neck   HIV CC HCC
    CC Excl: PDX collection 436

C83.92   **Non-follicular (diffuse) lymphoma, unspecified, intrathoracic lymph nodes**   HIV CC HCC
    CC Excl: PDX collection 437

C83.93   **Non-follicular (diffuse) lymphoma, unspecified, intra-abdominal lymph nodes**   HIV CC HCC
    CC Excl: PDX collection 438

C83.94   **Non-follicular (diffuse) lymphoma, unspecified, lymph nodes of** axilla and upper limb   HIV CC HCC
    CC Excl: PDX collection 439

C83.95   **Non-follicular (diffuse) lymphoma, unspecified, lymph nodes of** inguinal region and lower limb   HIV CC HCC
    CC Excl: PDX collection 440

C83.96   **Non-follicular (diffuse) lymphoma, unspecified, intrapelvic lymph nodes**   HIV CC HCC
    CC Excl: PDX collection 441

C83.97   **Non-follicular (diffuse) lymphoma, unspecified, spleen**   HIV CC HCC
    CC Excl: PDX collection 442

C83.98   **Non-follicular (diffuse) lymphoma, unspecified, lymph nodes of** multiple sites   HIV CC HCC
    CC Excl: PDX collection 435

C83.99   **Non-follicular (diffuse) lymphoma, unspecified, extranodal and solid organ sites**   HIV CC HCC
    CC Excl: PDX collection 435

✓4th **C84 Mature T/NK-cell lymphomas**
EXCLUDES 1   personal history of non-Hodgkin lymphoma (Z85.72)

✓5th **C84.0 Mycosis fungoides**
EXCLUDES 1   peripheral T-cell lymphoma, not classified (C84.4-)
DEF: Most common form of cutaneous T-cell lymphoma, also known as Alibert-Bazin syndrome. A type of non-Hodgkin lymphoma in which white blood cells become cancerous and affect the skin and sometimes internal organs.

C84.00   **Mycosis fungoides, unspecified site**   CC HCC
    CC Excl: PDX collection 467

C84.01   **Mycosis fungoides, lymph nodes of** head, face, and neck   CC HCC
    CC Excl: PDX collection 468

C84.02   **Mycosis fungoides, intrathoracic lymph nodes**   CC HCC
    CC Excl: PDX collection 469

C84.03   **Mycosis fungoides, intra-abdominal lymph nodes**   CC HCC
    CC Excl: PDX collection 470

C84.04   **Mycosis fungoides, lymph nodes of** axilla and upper limb   CC HCC
    CC Excl: PDX collection 471

C84.05   **Mycosis fungoides, lymph nodes of** inguinal region and lower limb   CC HCC
    CC Excl: PDX collection 472

C84.06   **Mycosis fungoides, intrapelvic lymph nodes**   CC HCC
    CC Excl: PDX collection 473

C84.07   **Mycosis fungoides, spleen**   CC HCC
    CC Excl: PDX collection 474

C84.08   **Mycosis fungoides, lymph nodes of** multiple sites   CC HCC
    CC Excl: PDX collection 475

C84.09   **Mycosis fungoides, extranodal and solid organ sites**   CC HCC
    CC Excl: PDX collection 467

✓5th **C84.1 Sézary disease**

C84.10   **Sézary disease, unspecified site**   CC HCC
    CC Excl: PDX collection 476

C84.11   **Sézary disease, lymph nodes of** head, face, and neck   CC HCC
    CC Excl: PDX collection 477

C84.12   **Sézary disease, intrathoracic lymph nodes**   CC HCC
    CC Excl: PDX collection 478

C84.13   **Sézary disease, intra-abdominal lymph nodes**   CC HCC
    CC Excl: PDX collection 479

C84.14   **Sézary disease, lymph nodes of** axilla and upper limb   CC HCC
    CC Excl: PDX collection 480

C84.15   **Sézary disease, lymph nodes of** inguinal region and lower limb   CC HCC
    CC Excl: PDX collection 481

C84.16   **Sézary disease, intrapelvic lymph nodes**   CC HCC
    CC Excl: PDX collection 482

C84.17   **Sézary disease, spleen**   CC HCC
    CC Excl: PDX collection 483

C84.18   **Sézary disease, lymph nodes of** multiple sites   CC HCC
    CC Excl: PDX collection 484

N Newborn: 0   P Pediatric: 0-17   M Maternity: 12-55   A Adult: 15-124   MCC Major CC Condition   PDxMCC PDx acts as own MCC   CC CC Condition   PDxCC PDx acts as own CC

482   ICD-10-CM 2018

C84.19   **Sézary disease,** extranodal and solid organ sites   `CC` `HCC`
CC Excl: PDX collection 476

✓5ᵗʰ **C84.4**   **Peripheral T-cell lymphoma, not classified**
Lennert's lymphoma
Lymphoepithelioid lymphoma
Mature T-cell lymphoma, not elsewhere classified

C84.40   **Peripheral T-cell lymphoma, not classified,** unspecified site   `HIV` `CC` `HCC`
CC Excl: PDX collection 426

C84.41   **Peripheral T-cell lymphoma, not classified, lymph nodes of** head, face, and neck   `HIV` `CC` `HCC`
CC Excl: PDX collection 427

C84.42   **Peripheral T-cell lymphoma, not classified,** intrathoracic **lymph nodes**   `HIV` `CC` `HCC`
CC Excl: PDX collection 428

C84.43   **Peripheral T-cell lymphoma, not classified,** intra-abdominal **lymph nodes**   `HIV` `CC` `HCC`
CC Excl: PDX collection 429

C84.44   **Peripheral T-cell lymphoma, not classified, lymph nodes of** axilla and upper limb   `HIV` `CC` `HCC`
CC Excl: PDX collection 430

C84.45   **Peripheral T-cell lymphoma, not classified, lymph nodes of** inguinal region and lower limb   `HIV` `CC` `HCC`
CC Excl: PDX collection 431

C84.46   **Peripheral T-cell lymphoma, not classified,** intrapelvic **lymph nodes**   `HIV` `CC` `HCC`
CC Excl: PDX collection 432

C84.47   **Peripheral T-cell lymphoma, not classified,** spleen   `HIV` `CC` `HCC`
CC Excl: PDX collection 433

C84.48   **Peripheral T-cell lymphoma, not classified, lymph nodes of** multiple sites   `HIV` `CC` `HCC`
CC Excl: PDX collection 434

C84.49   **Peripheral T-cell lymphoma, not classified,** extranodal and solid organ sites   `HIV` `CC` `HCC`
CC Excl: PDX collection 426

✓5ᵗʰ **C84.6**   **Anaplastic large cell lymphoma,** ALK-positive
Anaplastic large cell lymphoma, CD30-positive

C84.60   **Anaplastic large cell lymphoma, ALK-positive,** unspecified site   `HIV` `CC` `HCC`
CC Excl: PDX collection 426

C84.61   **Anaplastic large cell lymphoma, ALK-positive, lymph nodes of** head, face, and neck   `HIV` `CC` `HCC`
CC Excl: PDX collection 427

C84.62   **Anaplastic large cell lymphoma, ALK-positive,** intrathoracic **lymph nodes**   `HIV` `CC` `HCC`
CC Excl: PDX collection 428

C84.63   **Anaplastic large cell lymphoma, ALK-positive,** intra-abdominal **lymph nodes**   `HIV` `CC` `HCC`
CC Excl: PDX collection 429

C84.64   **Anaplastic large cell lymphoma, ALK-positive, lymph nodes of** axilla and upper limb   `HIV` `CC` `HCC`
CC Excl: PDX collection 430

C84.65   **Anaplastic large cell lymphoma, ALK-positive, lymph nodes of** inguinal region and lower limb   `HIV` `CC` `HCC`
CC Excl: PDX collection 431

C84.66   **Anaplastic large cell lymphoma, ALK-positive,** intrapelvic **lymph nodes**   `HIV` `CC` `HCC`
CC Excl: PDX collection 432

C84.67   **Anaplastic large cell lymphoma, ALK-positive,** spleen   `HIV` `CC` `HCC`
CC Excl: PDX collection 433

C84.68   **Anaplastic large cell lymphoma, ALK-positive, lymph nodes of** multiple sites   `HIV` `CC` `HCC`
CC Excl: PDX collection 434

C84.69   **Anaplastic large cell lymphoma, ALK-positive,** extranodal and solid organ sites   `HIV` `CC` `HCC`
CC Excl: PDX collection 426

✓5ᵗʰ **C84.7**   **Anaplastic large cell lymphoma,** ALK-negative
EXCLUDES 1   *primary cutaneous CD30-positive T-cell proliferations (C86.6-)*

C84.70   **Anaplastic large cell lymphoma, ALK-negative,** unspecified site   `HIV` `CC` `HCC`
CC Excl: PDX collection 426

C84.71   **Anaplastic large cell lymphoma, ALK-negative, lymph nodes of** head, face, and neck   `HIV` `CC` `HCC`
CC Excl: PDX collection 427

C84.72   **Anaplastic large cell lymphoma, ALK-negative,** intrathoracic **lymph nodes**   `HIV` `CC` `HCC`
CC Excl: PDX collection 428

C84.73   **Anaplastic large cell lymphoma, ALK-negative,** intra-abdominal **lymph nodes**   `HIV` `CC` `HCC`
CC Excl: PDX collection 429

C84.74   **Anaplastic large cell lymphoma, ALK-negative, lymph nodes of** axilla and upper limb   `HIV` `CC` `HCC`
CC Excl: PDX collection 430

C84.75   **Anaplastic large cell lymphoma, ALK-negative, lymph nodes of** inguinal region and lower limb   `HIV` `CC` `HCC`
CC Excl: PDX collection 431

C84.76   **Anaplastic large cell lymphoma, ALK-negative,** intrapelvic **lymph nodes**   `HIV` `CC` `HCC`
CC Excl: PDX collection 432

C84.77   **Anaplastic large cell lymphoma, ALK-negative,** spleen   `HIV` `CC` `HCC`
CC Excl: PDX collection 433

C84.78   **Anaplastic large cell lymphoma, ALK-negative, lymph nodes of** multiple sites   `HIV` `CC` `HCC`
CC Excl: PDX collection 434

C84.79   **Anaplastic large cell lymphoma, ALK-negative,** extranodal and solid organ sites   `HIV` `CC` `HCC`
CC Excl: PDX collection 426

✓5ᵗʰ **C84.A**   **Cutaneous T-cell lymphoma, unspecified**

C84.A0   **Cutaneous T-cell lymphoma, unspecified,** unspecified site   `HIV` `CC` `HCC`
CC Excl: PDX collection 426

C84.A1   **Cutaneous T-cell lymphoma, unspecified, lymph nodes of** head, face, and neck   `HIV` `CC` `HCC`
CC Excl: PDX collection 427

C84.A2   **Cutaneous T-cell lymphoma, unspecified,** intrathoracic **lymph nodes**   `HIV` `CC` `HCC`
CC Excl: PDX collection 428

C84.A3   **Cutaneous T-cell lymphoma, unspecified,** intra-abdominal **lymph nodes**   `HIV` `CC` `HCC`
CC Excl: PDX collection 429

C84.A4   **Cutaneous T-cell lymphoma, unspecified, lymph nodes of** axilla and upper limb   `HIV` `CC` `HCC`
CC Excl: PDX collection 430

C84.A5   **Cutaneous T-cell lymphoma, unspecified, lymph nodes of** inguinal region and lower limb   `HIV` `CC` `HCC`
CC Excl: PDX collection 431

C84.A6   **Cutaneous T-cell lymphoma, unspecified,** intrapelvic **lymph nodes**   `HIV` `CC` `HCC`
CC Excl: PDX collection 432

C84.A7   **Cutaneous T-cell lymphoma, unspecified,** spleen   `HIV` `CC` `HCC`
CC Excl: PDX collection 433

C84.A8   **Cutaneous T-cell lymphoma, unspecified, lymph nodes of** multiple sites   `HIV` `CC` `HCC`
CC Excl: PDX collection 434

C84.A9   **Cutaneous T-cell lymphoma, unspecified,** extranodal and solid organ sites   `HIV` `CC` `HCC`
CC Excl: PDX collection 426

✓5ᵗʰ **C84.Z**   **Other** mature T/NK-cell lymphomas
NOTE   If T-cell lineage or involvement is mentioned in conjunction with a specific lymphoma, code to the more specific description.
EXCLUDES 1   *angioimmunoblastic T-cell lymphoma (C86.5)*
blastic NK-cell lymphoma (C86.4)
enteropathy-type T-cell lymphoma (C86.2)
extranodal NK-cell lymphoma, nasal type (C86.0)
hepatosplenic T-cell lymphoma (C86.1)
primary cutaneous CD30-positive T-cell proliferations (C86.6)
subcutaneous panniculitis-like T-cell lymphoma (C86.3)
T-cell leukemia (C91.1-)

C84.Z0   **Other mature T/NK-cell lymphomas,** unspecified site   `HIV` `CC` `HCC`
CC Excl: PDX collection 426

C84.Z1   **Other mature T/NK-cell lymphomas, lymph nodes of** head, face, and neck   `HIV` `CC` `HCC`
CC Excl: PDX collection 427

C84.Z2   **Other mature T/NK-cell lymphomas,** intrathoracic **lymph nodes**   `HIV` `CC` `HCC`
CC Excl: PDX collection 428

Chapter 2. Neoplasms

C84.Z3 **Other mature T/NK-cell lymphomas, intra-abdominal lymph nodes** `HIV` `CC` `HCC`
CC Excl: PDX collection 429

C84.Z4 **Other mature T/NK-cell lymphomas, lymph nodes of axilla and upper limb** `HIV` `CC` `HCC`
CC Excl: PDX collection 430

C84.Z5 **Other mature T/NK-cell lymphomas, lymph nodes of inguinal region and lower limb** `HIV` `CC` `HCC`
CC Excl: PDX collection 431

C84.Z6 **Other mature T/NK-cell lymphomas, intrapelvic lymph nodes** `HIV` `CC` `HCC`
CC Excl: PDX collection 432

C84.Z7 **Other mature T/NK-cell lymphomas, spleen** `HIV` `CC` `HCC`
CC Excl: PDX collection 433

C84.Z8 **Other mature T/NK-cell lymphomas, lymph ndoes of multiple sites** `HIV` `CC` `HCC`
CC Excl: PDX collection 434

C84.Z9 **Other mature T/NK-cell lymphomas, extranodal and solid organ sites** `HIV` `CC` `HCC`
CC Excl: PDX collection 426

✓5th **C84.9 Mature T/NK-cell lymphomas, unspecified**
NK/T cell lymphoma NOS
EXCLUDES 1   *mature T-cell lymphoma, not elsewhere classified (C84.4-)*

C84.90 **Mature T/NK-cell lymphomas, unspecified, unspecified site** `HIV` `CC` `HCC`
CC Excl: PDX collection 426

C84.91 **Mature T/NK-cell lymphomas, unspecified, lymph nodes of head, face, and neck** `HIV` `CC` `HCC`
CC Excl: PDX collection 427

C84.92 **Mature T/NK-cell lymphomas, unspecified, intrathoracic lymph nodes** `HIV` `CC` `HCC`
CC Excl: PDX collection 428

C84.93 **Mature T/NK-cell lymphomas, unspecified, intra-abdominal lymph nodes** `HIV` `CC` `HCC`
CC Excl: PDX collection 429

C84.94 **Mature T/NK-cell lymphomas, unspecified, lymph nodes of axilla and upper limb** `HIV` `CC` `HCC`
CC Excl: PDX collection 430

C84.95 **Mature T/NK-cell lymphomas, unspecified, lymph nodes of inguinal region and lower limb** `HIV` `CC` `HCC`
CC Excl: PDX collection 431

C84.96 **Mature T/NK-cell lymphomas, unspecified, intrapelvic lymph nodes** `HIV` `CC` `HCC`
CC Excl: PDX collection 432

C84.97 **Mature T/NK-cell lymphomas, unspecified, spleen** `HIV` `CC` `HCC`
CC Excl: PDX collection 433

C84.98 **Mature T/NK-cell lymphomas, unspecified, lymph nodes of multiple sites** `HIV` `CC` `HCC`
CC Excl: PDX collection 434

C84.99 **Mature T/NK-cell lymphomas, unspecified, extranodal and solid organ sites** `HIV` `CC` `HCC`
CC Excl: PDX collection 426

✓4th **C85 Other specified and unspecified types of non-Hodgkin lymphoma**
EXCLUDES 1   *other specified types of T/NK-cell lymphoma (C86.-)*
personal history of non-Hodgkin lymphoma (Z85.72)

✓5th **C85.1 Unspecified B-cell lymphoma**
NOTE   If B-cell lineage or involvement is mentioned in conjunction with a specific lymphoma, code to the more specific description.

C85.10 **Unspecified B-cell lymphoma, unspecified site** `HIV` `CC` `HCC`
CC Excl: PDX collection 426

C85.11 **Unspecified B-cell lymphoma, lymph nodes of head, face, and neck** `HIV` `CC` `HCC`
CC Excl: PDX collection 427

C85.12 **Unspecified B-cell lymphoma, intrathoracic lymph nodes** `HIV` `CC` `HCC`
CC Excl: PDX collection 428

C85.13 **Unspecified B-cell lymphoma, intra-abdominal lymph nodes** `HIV` `CC` `HCC`
CC Excl: PDX collection 429

C85.14 **Unspecified B-cell lymphoma, lymph nodes of axilla and upper limb** `HIV` `CC` `HCC`
CC Excl: PDX collection 430

C85.15 **Unspecified B-cell lymphoma, lymph nodes of inguinal region and lower limb** `HIV` `CC` `HCC`
CC Excl: PDX collection 431

C85.16 **Unspecified B-cell lymphoma, intrapelvic lymph nodes** `HIV` `CC` `HCC`
CC Excl: PDX collection 432

C85.17 **Unspecified B-cell lymphoma, spleen** `HIV` `CC` `HCC`
CC Excl: PDX collection 433

C85.18 **Unspecified B-cell lymphoma, lymph nodes of multiple sites** `HIV` `CC` `HCC`
CC Excl: PDX collection 434

C85.19 **Unspecified B-cell lymphoma, extranodal and solid organ sites** `HIV` `CC` `HCC`
CC Excl: PDX collection 426

✓5th **C85.2 Mediastinal (thymic) large B-cell lymphoma**

C85.20 **Mediastinal (thymic) large B-cell lymphoma, unspecified site** `HIV` `CC` `HCC`
CC Excl: PDX collection 426

C85.21 **Mediastinal (thymic) large B-cell lymphoma, lymph nodes of head, face, and neck** `HIV` `CC` `HCC`
CC Excl: PDX collection 427

C85.22 **Mediastinal (thymic) large B-cell lymphoma, intrathoracic lymph nodes** `HIV` `CC` `HCC`
CC Excl: PDX collection 428

C85.23 **Mediastinal (thymic) large B-cell lymphoma, intra-abdominal lymph nodes** `HIV` `CC` `HCC`
CC Excl: PDX collection 429

C85.24 **Mediastinal (thymic) large B-cell lymphoma, lymph nodes of axilla and upper limb** `HIV` `CC` `HCC`
CC Excl: PDX collection 430

C85.25 **Mediastinal (thymic) large B-cell lymphoma, lymph nodes of inguinal region and lower limb** `HIV` `CC` `HCC`
CC Excl: PDX collection 431

C85.26 **Mediastinal (thymic) large B-cell lymphoma, intrapelvic lymph nodes** `HIV` `CC` `HCC`
CC Excl: PDX collection 432

C85.27 **Mediastinal (thymic) large B-cell lymphoma, spleen** `HIV` `CC` `HCC`
CC Excl: PDX collection 433

C85.28 **Mediastinal (thymic) large B-cell lymphoma, lymph nodes of multiple sites** `HIV` `CC` `HCC`
CC Excl: PDX collection 434

C85.29 **Mediastinal (thymic) large B-cell lymphoma, extranodal and solid organ sites** `HIV` `CC` `HCC`
CC Excl: PDX collection 426

✓5th **C85.8 Other specified types of non-Hodgkin lymphoma**

C85.80 **Other specified types of non-Hodgkin lymphoma, unspecified site** `HIV` `CC` `HCC`
CC Excl: PDX collection 426

C85.81 **Other specified types of non-Hodgkin lymphoma, lymph nodes of head, face, and neck** `HIV` `CC` `HCC`
CC Excl: PDX collection 427

C85.82 **Other specified types of non-Hodgkin lymphoma, intrathoracic lymph nodes** `HIV` `CC` `HCC`
CC Excl: PDX collection 428

C85.83 **Other specified types of non-Hodgkin lymphoma, intra-abdominal lymph nodes** `HIV` `CC` `HCC`
CC Excl: PDX collection 429

C85.84 **Other specified types of non-Hodgkin lymphoma, lymph nodes of axilla and upper limb** `HIV` `CC` `HCC`
CC Excl: PDX collection 430

C85.85 **Other specified types of non-Hodgkin lymphoma, lymph nodes of inguinal region and lower limb** `HIV` `CC` `HCC`
CC Excl: PDX collection 431

C85.86 **Other specified types of non-Hodgkin lymphoma, intrapelvic lymph nodes** `HIV` `CC` `HCC`
CC Excl: PDX collection 432

C85.87 **Other specified types of non-Hodgkin lymphoma, spleen** `HIV` `CC` `HCC`
CC Excl: PDX collection 433

C85.88 **Other specified types of non-Hodgkin lymphoma, lymph nodes of multiple sites** `HIV` `CC` `HCC`
CC Excl: PDX collection 434

C85.89 **Other specified types of non-Hodgkin lymphoma, extranodal and solid organ sites** `HIV` `CC` `HCC`
CC Excl: PDX collection 426

N Newborn: 0   P Pediatric: 0-17   M Maternity: 12-55   A Adult: 15-124   MCC Major CC Condition   PDxMCC PDx acts as own MCC   CC CC Condition   PDxCC PDx acts as own CC

484   ICD-10-CM 2018

C84.Z3–C85.89

✓5th **C85.9 Non-Hodgkin lymphoma, unspecified**
Lymphoma NOS
Malignant lymphoma NOS
Non-Hodgkin lymphoma NOS

     C85.90 Non-Hodgkin lymphoma, unspecified, `HIV` `CC` `HCC`
unspecified site
CC Excl: PDX collection 426

     C85.91 Non-Hodgkin lymphoma, unspecified, `HIV` `CC` `HCC`
lymph nodes of head, face, and neck
CC Excl: PDX collection 427

     C85.92 Non-Hodgkin lymphoma, unspecified, `HIV` `CC` `HCC`
intrathoracic lymph nodes
CC Excl: PDX collection 428

     C85.93 Non-Hodgkin lymphoma, unspecified, `HIV` `CC` `HCC`
intra-abdominal lymph nodes
CC Excl: PDX collection 429

     C85.94 Non-Hodgkin lymphoma, unspecified, `HIV` `CC` `HCC`
lymph nodes of axilla and upper limb
CC Excl: PDX collection 430

     C85.95 Non-Hodgkin lymphoma, unspecified, `HIV` `CC` `HCC`
lymph nodes of inguinal region and lower limb
CC Excl: PDX collection 431

     C85.96 Non-Hodgkin lymphoma, unspecified, `HIV` `CC` `HCC`
intrapelvic lymph nodes
CC Excl: PDX collection 432

     C85.97 Non-Hodgkin lymphoma, unspecified, `HIV` `CC` `HCC`
spleen
CC Excl: PDX collection 433

     C85.98 Non-Hodgkin lymphoma, unspecified, `HIV` `CC` `HCC`
lymph nodes of multiple sites
CC Excl: PDX collection 434

     C85.99 Non-Hodgkin lymphoma, unspecified, `HIV` `CC` `HCC`
extranodal and solid organ sites
CC Excl: PDX collection 426

✓4th **C86 Other specified types of T/NK-cell lymphoma**
EXCLUDES1 anaplastic large cell lymphoma, ALK negative (C84.7-)
anaplastic large cell lymphoma, ALK positive (C84.6-)
mature T/NK-cell lymphomas (C84.-)
other specified types of non-Hodgkin lymphoma (C85.8-)

     C86.0 Extranodal NK/T-cell lymphoma, nasal type `HIV` `CC` `HCC`
CC Excl: PDX collection 427

     C86.1 Hepatosplenic T-cell lymphoma `HIV` `CC` `HCC`
Alpha-beta and gamma delta types
CC Excl: PDX collection 433

     C86.2 Enteropathy-type (intestinal) T-cell lymphoma `HIV` `CC` `HCC`
Enteropathy associated T-cell lymphoma
CC Excl: PDX collection 429

     C86.3 Subcutaneous panniculitis-like T-cell lymphoma `HIV` `CC` `HCC`
CC Excl: PDX collection 429

     C86.4 Blastic NK-cell lymphoma `HIV` `CC` `HCC`
▶Blastic plasmacytoid dendritic cell neoplasm (BPDCN)◀
CC Excl: PDX collection 426

     C86.5 Angioimmunoblastic T-cell lymphoma `HIV` `CC` `HCC`
Angioimmunoblastic lymphadenopathy with dysproteinemia [AILD]
CC Excl: PDX collection 435

     C86.6 Primary cutaneous CD30-positive T-cell `HIV` `CC` `HCC`
proliferations
Lymphomatoid papulosis
Primary cutaneous anaplastic large cell lymphoma
Primary cutaneous CD30-positive large T-cell lymphoma
CC Excl: PDX collection 435

✓4th **C88 Malignant immunoproliferative diseases and certain other B-cell lymphomas**
EXCLUDES1 B-cell lymphoma, unspecified (C85.1-)
personal history of other malignant neoplasms of lymphoid, hematopoietic and related tissues (Z85.79)

     C88.0 Waldenström macroglobulinemia `HCC`
Lymphoplasmacytic lymphoma with IgM-production
Macroglobulinemia (idiopathic) (primary)
EXCLUDES1 small cell B-cell lymphoma (C83.0)

     C88.2 Heavy chain disease `CC` `HCC`
Franklin disease
Gamma heavy chain disease
Mu heavy chain disease
CC Excl: PDX collection 485

     C88.3 Immunoproliferative small intestinal disease `CC` `HCC`
Alpha heavy chain disease
Mediterranean lymphoma
CC Excl: PDX collection 485

     C88.4 Extranodal marginal zone B-cell lymphoma of `HIV` `CC` `HCC`
mucosa-associated lymphoid tissue [MALT-lymphoma]
Lymphoma of skin-associated lymphoid tissue [SALT-lymphoma]
Lymphoma of bronchial-associated lymphoid tissue [BALT-lymphoma]
EXCLUDES1 high malignant (diffuse large B-cell) lymphoma (C83.3-)
CC Excl: PDX collection 426

     C88.8 Other malignant immunoproliferative diseases `CC` `HCC`
CC Excl: PDX collection 486

     C88.9 Malignant immunoproliferative disease, unspecified `CC` `HCC`
Immunoproliferative disease NOS
CC Excl: PDX collection 485

✓4th **C90 Multiple myeloma and malignant plasma cell neoplasms**
EXCLUDES1 personal history of other malignant neoplasms of lymphoid, hematopoietic and related tissues (Z85.79)

     CC Excl: For CC codes in category C90: PDX collection 485

✓5th **C90.0 Multiple myeloma**
Kahler's disease
Medullary plasmacytoma
Myelomatosis
Plasma cell myeloma
EXCLUDES1 solitary myeloma (C90.3-)
solitary plasmactyoma (C90.3-)

     C90.00 Multiple myeloma not having achieved `CC` `HCC`
remission
Multiple myeloma with failed remission
Multiple myeloma NOS

     C90.01 Multiple myeloma in remission `CC` `HCC`

     C90.02 Multiple myeloma in relapse `CC` `HCC`

✓5th **C90.1 Plasma cell leukemia**
Plasmacytic leukemia

     C90.10 Plasma cell leukemia not having achieved `CC` `HCC`
remission
Plasma cell leukemia with failed remission
Plasma cell leukemia NOS

     C90.11 Plasma cell leukemia in remission `CC` `HCC`

     C90.12 Plasma cell leukemia in relapse `CC` `HCC`

✓5th **C90.2 Extramedullary plasmacytoma**

     C90.20 Extramedullary plasmacytoma not having `CC` `HCC`
achieved remission
Extramedullary plasmacytoma with failed remission
Extramedullary plasmacytoma NOS

     C90.21 Extramedullary plasmacytoma in remission `CC` `HCC`

     C90.22 Extramedullary plasmacytoma in relapse `CC` `HCC`

✓5th **C90.3 Solitary plasmacytoma**
Localized malignant plasma cell tumor NOS
Plasmacytoma NOS
Solitary myeloma

     C90.30 Solitary plasmacytoma not having achieved `CC` `HCC`
remission
Solitary plasmacytoma with failed remission
Solitary plasmacytoma NOS

     C90.31 Solitary plasmacytoma in remission `CC` `HCC`

     C90.32 Solitary plasmacytoma in relapse `CC` `HCC`

✓4th **C91 Lymphoid leukemia**
EXCLUDES1 personal history of leukemia (Z85.6)

     CC Excl: For CC codes in category C91, unless otherwise noted: PDX collection 485

✓5th **C91.0 Acute lymphoblastic leukemia [ALL]**
NOTE Code C91.0 should only be used for T-cell and B-cell precursor leukemia

     C91.00 Acute lymphoblastic leukemia not having `CC` `HCC`
achieved remission
Acute lymphoblastic leukemia with failed remission
Acute lymphoblastic leukemia NOS

     C91.01 Acute lymphoblastic leukemia, in remission `CC` `HCC`

     C91.02 Acute lymphoblastic leukemia, in relapse `CC` `HCC`

√5th **C91.1** Chronic lymphocytic **leukemia of** B-cell type
Lymphoplasmacytic leukemia
Richter syndrome
EXCLUDES 1 *lymphoplasmacytic lymphoma (C83.0-)*

　C91.10 **Chronic lymphocytic leukemia of B-cell type** CC HCC
not having achieved remission
Chronic lymphocytic leukemia of B-cell type with
failed remission
Chronic lymphocytic leukemia of B-cell type NOS

　C91.11 **Chronic lymphocytic leukemia of B-cell type** CC HCC
in remission

　C91.12 **Chronic lymphocytic leukemia of B-cell type** CC HCC
in relapse

√5th **C91.3** Prolymphocytic **leukemia of** B-cell type

　C91.30 **Prolymphocytic leukemia of B-cell type** not CC HCC
having achieved remission
Prolymphocytic leukemia of B-cell type with failed
remission
Prolymphocytic leukemia of B-cell type NOS

　C91.31 **Prolymphocytic leukemia of B-cell type, in** CC HCC
remission

　C91.32 **Prolymphocytic leukemia of B-cell type, in** CC HCC
relapse

√5th **C91.4** Hairy cell **leukemia**
Leukemic reticuloendotheliosis

CC Excl: For CC codes in subcategory C91.4:
PDX collection 487

　C91.40 **Hairy cell leukemia not having achieved** CC HCC
remission
Hairy cell leukemia with failed remission
Hairy cell leukemia NOS

　C91.41 **Hairy cell leukemia, in remission** CC HCC

　C91.42 **Hairy cell leukemia, in relapse** CC HCC

√5th **C91.5** Adult T-cell **lymphoma/leukemia (HTLV-1-associated)**
Acute variant of adult T-cell lymphoma/leukemia (HTLV-1-
associated)
Chronic variant of adult T-cell lymphoma/leukemia (HTLV-1-
associated)
Lymphomatoid variant of adult T-cell lymphoma/leukemia
(HTLV-1-associated)
Smouldering variant of adult T-cell lymphoma/leukemia (HTLV-
1-associated)

　C91.50 **Adult T-cell lymphoma/leukemia (HTLV-1-** CC HCC A
associated) not having achieved remission
Adult T-cell lymphoma/leukemia (HTLV-1-associated)
with failed remission
Adult T-cell lymphoma/leukemia (HTLV-1-associated)
NOS

　C91.51 **Adult T-cell lymphoma/leukemia** CC HCC A
(HTLV-1-associated), in remission

　C91.52 **Adult T-cell lymphoma/leukemia** CC HCC A
(HTLV-1-associated), in relapse

√5th **C91.6** Prolymphocytic **leukemia of** T-cell type

　C91.60 **Prolymphocytic leukemia of T-cell type** not CC HCC
having achieved remission
Prolymphocytic leukemia of T-cell type with failed
remission
Prolymphocytic leukemia of T-cell type NOS

　C91.61 **Prolymphocytic leukemia of T-cell type, in** CC HCC
remission

　C91.62 **Prolymphocytic leukemia of T-cell type, in** CC HCC
relapse

√5th **C91.A** Mature B-cell **leukemia** Burkitt-type
EXCLUDES 1 *Burkitt lymphoma (C83.7-)*

　C91.A0 **Mature B-cell leukemia Burkitt-type** not CC HCC
having achieved remission
Mature B-cell leukemia Burkitt-type with failed
remission
Mature B-cell leukemia Burkitt-type NOS

　C91.A1 **Mature B-cell leukemia Burkitt-type, in** CC HCC
remission

　C91.A2 **Mature B-cell leukemia Burkitt-type,** CC HCC
in relapse

√5th **C91.Z** Other **lymphoid leukemia**
T-cell large granular lymphocytic leukemia (associated with
rheumatoid arthritis)

　C91.Z0 **Other lymphoid leukemia** not having CC HCC
achieved remission
Other lymphoid leukemia with failed remission
Other lymphoid leukemia NOS

　C91.Z1 **Other lymphoid leukemia, in remission** CC HCC

　C91.Z2 **Other lymphoid leukemia, in relapse** CC HCC

√5th **C91.9** Lymphoid leukemia, **unspecified**

　C91.90 **Lymphoid leukemia, unspecified not having** CC HCC
achieved remission
Lymphoid leukemia with failed remission
Lymphoid leukemia NOS

　C91.91 **Lymphoid leukemia, unspecified,** CC HCC
in remission

　C91.92 **Lymphoid leukemia, unspecified, in relapse** CC HCC

√4th **C92** **Myeloid leukemia**
INCLUDES　granulocytic leukemia
myelogenous leukemia
EXCLUDES 1 *personal history of leukemia (Z85.6)*

CC Excl: For CC codes in category C92: PDX collection 485

√5th **C92.0** Acute myeloblastic **leukemia**
Acute myeloblastic leukemia, minimal differentiation
Acute myeloblastic leukemia (with maturation)
Acute myeloblastic leukemia 1/ETO
Acute myeloblastic leukemia M0
Acute myeloblastic leukemia M1
Acute myeloblastic leukemia M2
Acute myeloblastic leukemia with t(8;21)
Acute myeloblastic leukemia (without a FAB classification) NOS
Refractory anemia with excess blasts in transformation [RAEB T]
EXCLUDES 1 *acute exacerbation of chronic myeloid leukemia*
(C92.10)
refractory anemia with excess of blasts not in
transformation (D46.2-)

　C92.00 **Acute myeloblastic leukemia, not having** CC HCC
achieved remission
Acute myeloblastic leukemia with failed remission
Acute myeloblastic leukemia NOS

　C92.01 **Acute myeloblastic leukemia, in remission** CC HCC

　C92.02 **Acute myeloblastic leukemia, in relapse** CC HCC

√5th **C92.1** Chronic myeloid leukemia, **BCR/ABL-positive**
Chronic myelogenous leukemia, Philadelphia chromosome
(Ph1) positive
Chronic myelogenous leukemia, t(9;22) (q34;q11)
Chronic myelogenous leukemia with crisis of blast cells
EXCLUDES 1 *atypical chronic myeloid leukemia BCR/ABL-negative*
(C92.2-)
chronic myelomonocytic leukemia (C93.1-)
chronic myeloproliferative disease (D47.1)

　C92.10 **Chronic myeloid leukemia, BCR/ABL-positive,** CC HCC
not having achieved remission
Chronic myeloid leukemia, BCR/ABL-positive with
failed remission
Chronic myeloid leukemia, BCR/ABL-positive NOS

　C92.11 **Chronic myeloid leukemia, BCR/ABL-positive,** CC HCC
in remission

　C92.12 **Chronic myeloid leukemia, BCR/ABL-positive,** CC HCC
in relapse

√5th **C92.2** Atypical chronic **myeloid leukemia, BCR/ABL-negative**

　C92.20 **Atypical chronic myeloid leukemia,** CC HCC
BCR/ABL-negative, not having achieved remission
Atypical chronic myeloid leukemia, BCR/ABL-
negative with failed remission
Atypical chronic myeloid leukemia, BCR/ABL-
negative NOS

　C92.21 **Atypical chronic myeloid leukemia,** CC HCC
BCR/ABL-negative, in remission

　C92.22 **Atypical chronic myeloid leukemia,** CC HCC
BCR/ABL-negative, in relapse

√5th **C92.3** Myeloid sarcoma
A malignant tumor of immature myeloid cells
Chloroma
Granulocytic sarcoma

　C92.30 **Myeloid sarcoma, not having achieved** CC HCC
remission
Myeloid sarcoma with failed remission
Myeloid sarcoma NOS

    C92.31   **Myeloid sarcoma,** in remission   `CC` `HCC`

    C92.32   **Myeloid sarcoma,** in relapse   `CC` `HCC`

✓5ᵗʰ **C92.4**   **Acute promyelocytic leukemia**
        AML M3
        AML Me with t(15;17) and variants

    C92.40   **Acute promyelocytic leukemia,** not having   `CC` `HCC`
        achieved remission
           Acute promyelocytic leukemia with failed remission
           Acute promyelocytic leukemia NOS

    C92.41   **Acute promyelocytic leukemia,** in remission   `CC` `HCC`

    C92.42   **Acute promyelocytic leukemia,** in relapse   `CC` `HCC`

✓5ᵗʰ **C92.5**   **Acute myelomonocytic leukemia**
        AML M4
        AML M4 Eo with inv(16) or t(16;16)

    C92.50   **Acute myelomonocytic leukemia,** not having   `CC` `HCC`
        achieved remission
           Acute myelomonocytic leukemia with failed remission
           Acute myelomonocytic leukemia NOS

    C92.51   **Acute myelomonocytic leukemia,** in   `CC` `HCC`
        remission

    C92.52   **Acute myelomonocytic leukemia,** in relapse   `CC` `HCC`

✓5ᵗʰ **C92.6**   **Acute myeloid leukemia with 11q23-abnormality**
        Acute myeloid leukemia with variation of MLL-gene

    C92.60   **Acute myeloid leukemia with**   `CC` `HCC`
        11q23-abnormality not having
        achieved remission
           Acute myeloid leukemia with 11q23-abnormality
           with failed remission
           Acute myeloid leukemia with 11q23-abnormality NOS

    C92.61   **Acute myeloid leukemia with**   `CC` `HCC`
        11q23-abnormality in remission

    C92.62   **Acute myeloid leukemia with**   `CC` `HCC`
        11q23-abnormality in relapse

✓5ᵗʰ **C92.A**   **Acute myeloid leukemia with multilineage dysplasia**
        Acute myeloid leukemia with dysplasia of remaining
        hematopoesis and/or myelodysplastic disease in its history

    C92.A0   **Acute myeloid leukemia with multilineage**   `CC` `HCC`
        dysplasia, not having achieved remission
           Acute myeloid leukemia with multilineage dysplasia
           with failed remission
           Acute myeloid leukemia with multilineage dysplasia
           NOS

    C92.A1   **Acute myeloid leukemia with multilineage**   `CC` `HCC`
        dysplasia, in remission

    C92.A2   **Acute myeloid leukemia with multilineage**   `CC` `HCC`
        dysplasia, in relapse

✓5ᵗʰ **C92.Z**   **Other myeloid leukemia**

    C92.Z0   **Other myeloid leukemia** not having achieved   `CC` `HCC`
        remission
           Myeloid leukemia NEC with failed remission
           Myeloid leukemia NEC

    C92.Z1   **Other myeloid leukemia,** in remission   `CC` `HCC`

    C92.Z2   **Other myeloid leukemia,** in relapse   `CC` `HCC`

✓5ᵗʰ **C92.9**   **Myeloid leukemia, unspecified**

    C92.90   **Myeloid leukemia, unspecified,** not having   `CC` `HCC`
        achieved remission
           Myeloid leukemia, unspecified with failed remission
           Myeloid leukemia, unspecified NOS

    C92.91   **Myeloid leukemia, unspecified** in remission   `CC` `HCC`

    C92.92   **Myeloid leukemia, unspecified** in relapse   `CC` `HCC`

✓4ᵗʰ **C93**   **Monocytic leukemia**
    `INCLUDES`   monocytoid leukemia
    `EXCLUDES 1`   *personal history of leukemia (Z85.6))*

    CC Excl: For CC codes in category C93: PDX collection 485

✓5ᵗʰ **C93.0**   **Acute monoblastic/monocytic leukemia**
        AML M5   AML M5b
        AML M5a

    C93.00   **Acute monoblastic/monocytic leukemia,** not   `CC` `HCC`
        having achieved remission
           Acute monoblastic/monocytic leukemia with failed
           remission
           Acute monoblastic/monocytic leukemia NOS

    C93.01   **Acute monoblastic/monocytic leukemia,** in   `CC` `HCC`
        remission

    C93.02   **Acute monoblastic/monocytic leukemia,** in   `CC` `HCC`
        relapse

✓5ᵗʰ **C93.1**   **Chronic myelomonocytic leukemia**
        Chronic monocytic leukemia
        CMML-1
        CMML-2
        CMML with eosinophilia

    C93.10   **Chronic myelomonocytic leukemia** not   `CC` `HCC`
        having achieved remission
           Chronic myelomonocytic leukemia with failed
           remission
           Chronic myelomonocytic leukemia NOS

    C93.11   **Chronic myelomonocytic leukemia,** in   `CC` `HCC`
        remission

    C93.12   **Chronic myelomonocytic leukemia,** in relapse `CC` `HCC`

✓5ᵗʰ **C93.3**   **Juvenile myelomonocytic leukemia**

    C93.30   **Juvenile myelomonocytic leukemia,** not   `CC` `HCC` `P`
        having achieved remission
           Juvenile myelomonocytic leukemia with failed
           remission
           Juvenile myelomonocytic leukemia NOS

    C93.31   **Juvenile myelomonocytic leukemia,** in   `CC` `HCC` `P`
        remission

    C93.32   **Juvenile myelomonocytic leukemia,** in   `CC` `HCC` `P`
        relapse

✓5ᵗʰ **C93.Z**   **Other monocytic leukemia**

    C93.Z0   **Other monocytic leukemia,** not having   `CC` `HCC`
        achieved remission
           Other monocytic leukemia NOS

    C93.Z1   **Other monocytic leukemia,** in remission   `CC` `HCC`

    C93.Z2   **Other monocytic leukemia,** in relapse   `CC` `HCC`

✓5ᵗʰ **C93.9**   **Monocytic leukemia, unspecified**

    C93.90   **Monocytic leukemia, unspecified,** not having   `CC` `HCC`
        achieved remission
           Monocytic leukemia, unspecified with failed remission
           Monocytic leukemia, unspecified NOS

    C93.91   **Monocytic leukemia, unspecified** in remission `CC` `HCC`

    C93.92   **Monocytic leukemia, unspecified** in relapse   `CC` `HCC`

✓4ᵗʰ **C94**   **Other leukemias of specified cell type**
    `EXCLUDES 1`   *leukemic reticuloendotheliosis (C91.4-)*
          myelodysplastic syndromes (D46.-)
          personal history of leukemia (Z85.6)
          plasma cell leukemia (C90.1-)

    CC Excl: For CC codes in category C94, unless otherwise noted:
     PDX collection 485

✓5ᵗʰ **C94.0**   **Acute erythroid leukemia**
        Acute myeloid leukemia M6(a)(b)
        Erythroleukemia
        DEF: Erythroleukemia: A malignant blood dyscrasia (a
        myeloproliferative disorder).

    C94.00   **Acute erythroid leukemia,** not having   `CC` `HCC`
        achieved remission
           Acute erythroid leukemia with failed remission
           Acute erythroid leukemia NOS

    C94.01   **Acute erythroid leukemia,** in remission   `CC` `HCC`

    C94.02   **Acute erythroid leukemia,** in relapse   `CC` `HCC`

✓5ᵗʰ **C94.2**   **Acute megakaryoblastic leukemia**
        Acute myeloid leukemia M7
        Acute megakaryocytic leukemia

    C94.20   **Acute megakaryoblastic leukemia** not having `CC` `HCC`
        achieved remission
           Acute megakaryoblastic leukemia with failed
           remission
           Acute megakaryoblastic leukemia NOS

    C94.21   **Acute megakaryoblastic leukemia,**   `CC` `HCC`
        in remission

    C94.22   **Acute megakaryoblastic leukemia,** in relapse `CC` `HCC`

✓5ᵗʰ **C94.3**   **Mast cell leukemia**

    C94.30   **Mast cell leukemia** not having achieved   `CC` `HCC`
        remission
           Mast cell leukemia with failed remission
           Mast cell leukemia NOS

    C94.31   **Mast cell leukemia,** in remission   `CC` `HCC`

    C94.32   **Mast cell leukemia,** in relapse   `CC` `HCC`

✔ Additional Character Req   ✓ˣ7ᵗʰ Placeholder Alert   Unacceptable PDx   Manifestation   `H1`-`H14` HAC   `HCC` CMS-HCC Condition   `EXCLUDES 1` Not Coded Here   `EXCLUDES 2` Not Included Here

ICD-10-CM 2018   **487**

✓5ᵗʰ **C94.4** **Acute panmyelosis with myelofibrosis**
Acute myelofibrosis
EXCLUDES 1   *myelofibrosis NOS (D75.81)*
secondary myelofibrosis NOS (D75.81)

C94.40 **Acute panmyelosis with myelofibrosis** not **having achieved remission**   `CC` `HCC`
Acute myelofibrosis NOS
Acute panmyelosis with myelofibrosis with failed remission
Acute panmyelosis NOS
CC Excl: PDX collection 488

C94.41 **Acute panmyelosis with myelofibrosis, in remission**   `CC` `HCC`
CC Excl: PDX collection 488

C94.42 **Acute panmyelosis with myelofibrosis, in relapse**   `CC` `HCC`
CC Excl: PDX collection 488

C94.6 **Myelodysplastic disease, not classified**   `CC` `HCC`
Myeloproliferative disease, not classified
CC Excl: PDX collection 488

✓5ᵗʰ **C94.8** **Other specified leukemias**
Aggressive NK-cell leukemia
Acute basophilic leukemia

C94.80 **Other specified leukemias** not having **achieved remission**   `CC` `HCC`
Other specified leukemia with failed remission
Other specified leukemias NOS

C94.81 **Other specified leukemias, in remission**   `CC` `HCC`

C94.82 **Other specified leukemias, in relapse**   `CC` `HCC`

✓4ᵗʰ **C95** **Leukemia of** unspecified cell type
EXCLUDES 1   *personal history of leukemia (Z85.6)*

CC Excl: For CC codes in category C95: PDX collection 485

✓5ᵗʰ **C95.0** **Acute** leukemia of unspecified cell type
Acute bilineal leukemia
Acute mixed lineage leukemia
Biphenotypic acute leukemia
Stem cell leukemia of unclear lineage
EXCLUDES 1   *acute exacerbation of unspecified chronic leukemia (C95.10)*

C95.00 **Acute leukemia of unspecified cell type** not **having achieved remission**   `CC` `HCC`
Acute leukemia of unspecified cell type with failed remission
Acute leukemia NOS

C95.01 **Acute leukemia of unspecified cell type, in remission**   `CC` `HCC`

C95.02 **Acute leukemia of unspecified cell type, in relapse**   `CC` `HCC`

✓5ᵗʰ **C95.1** **Chronic** leukemia of unspecified cell type

C95.10 **Chronic leukemia of unspecified cell type** not `CC` `HCC` **having achieved remission**
Chronic leukemia of unspecified cell type with failed remission
Chronic leukemia NOS

C95.11 **Chronic leukemia of unspecified cell type, in remission**   `CC` `HCC`

C95.12 **Chronic leukemia of unspecified cell type, in relapse**   `CC` `HCC`

✓5ᵗʰ **C95.9** **Leukemia,** unspecified

C95.90 **Leukemia, unspecified** not having achieved   `CC` `HCC` **remission**
Leukemia, unspecified with failed remission
Leukemia NOS

C95.91 **Leukemia, unspecified, in remission**   `CC` `HCC`

C95.92 **Leukemia, unspecified, in relapse**   `CC` `HCC`

✓4ᵗʰ **C96** **Other and unspecified malignant neoplasms of lymphoid, hematopoietic and related tissue**
EXCLUDES 1   *personal history of other malignant neoplasms of lymphoid, hematopoietic and related tissues (Z85.79)*

C96.0 **Multifocal and multisystemic (disseminated)**   `CC` `HCC` **Langerhans-cell histiocytosis**
Histiocytosis X, multisystemic
Letterer-Siwe disease
EXCLUDES 1   *adult pulmonary Langerhans cell histiocytosis (J84.82)*
multifocal and unisystemic Langerhans-cell histiocytosis (C96.5)
unifocal Langerhans-cell histiocytosis (C96.6)
CC Excl: PDX collection 489

▲ ✓5ᵗʰ **C96.2** **Malignant mast cell neoplasm**
~~Aggressive systemic mastocytosis~~
~~Mast cell sarcoma~~
EXCLUDES 1   *indolent mastocytosis ▶(D47.02)◀*
mast cell leukemia (C94.30)
mastocytosis (congenital) (cutaneous) (Q82.2)

CC Excl: For codes in subcategory C96.2:
PDX collection 490

• **C96.20** **Malignant mast cell neoplasm,** unspecified   `CC`

• **C96.21** **Aggressive systemic mastocytosis**   `CC`

• **C96.22** **Mast cell sarcoma**   `CC`

• **C96.29** **Other malignant mast cell neoplasm**   `CC`

C96.4 **Sarcoma of dendritic cells (accessory cells)**   `CC` `HCC`
Follicular dendritic cell sarcoma
Interdigitating dendritic cell sarcoma
Langerhans cell sarcoma
CC Excl: PDX collection 491

C96.5 **Multifocal and unisystemic Langerhans-cell**   `CC` `HCC` **histiocytosis**
Hand-Schüller-Christian disease
Histiocytosis X, multifocal
EXCLUDES 1   *multifocal and multisystemic (disseminated) Langerhans-cell histiocytosis (C96.0)*
unifocal Langerhans-cell histiocytosis (C96.6)
CC Excl: PDX collection 492

C96.6 **Unifocal Langerhans-cell histiocytosis**   `CC` `HCC`
Eosinophilic granuloma
Histiocytosis X, unifocal
Histiocytosis X NOS
Langerhans-cell histiocytosis NOS
EXCLUDES 1   *multifocal and multisysemic (disseminated) Langerhans-cell histiocytosis (C96.0)*
multifocal and unisystemic Langerhans-cell histiocytosis (C96.5)
CC Excl: PDX collection 492

C96.A **Histiocytic sarcoma**   `CC` `HCC`
Malignant histiocytosis
CC Excl: PDX collection 493

C96.Z **Other specified malignant neoplasms of lymphoid,**   `CC` `HCC` **hematopoietic and related tissue**
CC Excl: PDX collection 491

C96.9 **Malignant neoplasm of lymphoid, hematopoietic and**   `CC` `HCC` **related tissue, unspecified**
CC Excl: PDX collection 491

In situ neoplasms (D00-D09)

INCLUDES   Bowen's disease
erythroplasia
grade III intraepithelial neoplasia
Queyrat's erythroplasia

✓4ᵗʰ **D00** **Carcinoma in situ of** oral cavity, esophagus and stomach
EXCLUDES 1   *melanoma in situ (D03.-)*

✓5ᵗʰ **D00.0** **Carcinoma in situ of** lip, oral cavity and pharynx
Use additional code to identify:
exposure to environmental tobacco smoke (Z77.22)
exposure to tobacco smoke in the perinatal period (P96.81)
history of tobacco dependence (Z87.891)
occupational exposure to environmental tobacco smoke (Z57.31)
tobacco dependence (F17.-)
tobacco use (Z72.0)
EXCLUDES 1   *carcinoma in situ of aryepiglottic fold or interarytenoid fold, laryngeal aspect (D02.0)*
carcinoma in situ of epiglottis NOS (D02.0)
carcinoma in situ of epiglottis suprahyoid portion (D02.0)
carcinoma in situ of skin of lip (D03.0, D04.0)

D00.00 **Carcinoma in situ of oral cavity,** unspecified site

D00.01 **Carcinoma in situ of** labial mucosa and vermilion border

D00.02 **Carcinoma in situ of** buccal mucosa

D00.03 **Carcinoma in situ of** gingiva and edentulous alveolar ridge

D00.04 **Carcinoma in situ of** soft palate

D00.05 **Carcinoma in situ of** hard palate

D00.06 **Carcinoma in situ of** floor of mouth

D00.07 **Carcinoma in situ of** tongue

N Newborn: 0   P Pediatric: 0-17   M Maternity: 12-55   A Adult: 15-124   MCC Major CC Condition   PDxMCC PDx acts as own MCC   CC CC Condition   PDxCC PDx acts as own CC

488   ICD-10-CM 2018

D00.08 **Carcinoma in situ of** pharynx
    Carcinoma in situ of aryepiglottic fold NOS
    Carcinoma in situ of hypopharyngeal aspect of aryepiglottic fold
    Carcinoma in situ of marginal zone of aryepiglottic fold

D00.1 **Carcinoma in situ of** esophagus

D00.2 **Carcinoma in situ of** stomach

✓4ᵗʰ **D01** **Carcinoma in situ of** other and unspecified digestive organs
    EXCLUDES 1   melanoma in situ (D03.-)

D01.0 **Carcinoma in situ of** colon
    EXCLUDES 1   carcinoma in situ of rectosigmoid junction (D01.1)

D01.1 **Carcinoma in situ of** rectosigmoid junction

D01.2 **Carcinoma in situ of** rectum

D01.3 **Carcinoma in situ of** anus and anal canal
    Anal intraepithelial neoplasia III [AIN III]
    Severe dysplasia of anus
    EXCLUDES 1   anal intraepithelial neoplasia I and II [AIN I and AIN II] (K62.82)
       carcinoma in situ of anal margin (D04.5)
       carcinoma in situ of anal skin (D04.5)
       carcinoma in situ of perianal skin (D04.5)

✓5ᵗʰ **D01.4** **Carcinoma in situ of other and unspecified parts of** intestine
    EXCLUDES 1   carcinoma in situ of ampulla of Vater (D01.5)

D01.40 **Carcinoma in situ of** unspecified **part of intestine**

D01.49 **Carcinoma in situ of** other **parts of intestine**

D01.5 **Carcinoma in situ of** liver, gallbladder and bile ducts
    Carcinoma in situ of ampulla of Vater

D01.7 **Carcinoma in situ of** other **specified digestive organs**
    Carcinoma in situ of pancreas

D01.9 **Carcinoma in situ of digestive organ,** unspecified

✓4ᵗʰ **D02** **Carcinoma in situ of** middle ear and respiratory system
    Use additional code to identify:
    exposure to environmental tobacco smoke (Z77.22)
    exposure to tobacco smoke in the perinatal period (P96.81)
    history of tobacco dependence (Z87.891)
    occupational exposure to environmental tobacco smoke (Z57.31)
    tobacco dependence (F17.-)
    tobacco use (Z72.0)
    EXCLUDES 1   melanoma in situ (D03.-)

D02.0 **Carcinoma in situ of** larynx
    Carcinoma in situ of aryepiglottic fold or interarytenoid fold, laryngeal aspect
    Carcinoma in situ of epiglottis (suprahyoid portion)
    EXCLUDES 1   carcinoma in situ of aryepiglottic fold or interarytenoid fold NOS (D00.08)
       carcinoma in situ of hypopharyngeal aspect (D00.08)
       carcinoma in situ of marginal zone (D00.08)

D02.1 **Carcinoma in situ of** trachea

✓5ᵗʰ **D02.2** **Carcinoma in situ of** bronchus and lung

D02.20 **Carcinoma in situ of** unspecified **bronchus and lung**

D02.21 **Carcinoma in situ of** right **bronchus and lung**

D02.22 **Carcinoma in situ of** left **bronchus and lung**

D02.3 **Carcinoma in situ of** other **parts of respiratory system**
    Carcinoma in situ of accessory sinuses
    Carcinoma in situ of middle ear
    Carcinoma in situ of nasal cavities
    EXCLUDES 1   carcinoma in situ of ear (external) (skin) (D04.2-)
       carcinoma in situ of nose NOS (D09.8)
       carcinoma in situ of skin of nose (D04.3)

D02.4 **Carcinoma in situ of respiratory system,** unspecified

✓4ᵗʰ **D03** Melanoma **in situ**

D03.0 **Melanoma in situ of** lip   `HCC`

✓5ᵗʰ **D03.1** **Melanoma in situ of** eyelid, including canthus

D03.10 **Melanoma in situ of** unspecified **eyelid, including canthus**   `HCC`

D03.11 **Melanoma in situ of** right **eyelid, including canthus**   `HCC`

D03.12 **Melanoma in situ of** left **eyelid, including canthus**   `HCC`

✓5ᵗʰ **D03.2** **Melanoma in situ of** ear and external auricular canal

D03.20 **Melanoma in situ of** unspecified **ear and external auricular canal**   `HCC`

D03.21 **Melanoma in situ of** right **ear and external auricular canal**   `HCC`

D03.22 **Melanoma in situ of** left **ear and external auricular canal**   `HCC`

✓5ᵗʰ **D03.3** **Melanoma in situ of** other and unspecified parts of face

D03.30 **Melanoma in situ of** unspecified **part of face**   `HCC`

D03.39 **Melanoma in situ of** other **parts of face**   `HCC`

D03.4 **Melanoma in situ of** scalp and neck   `HCC`

✓5ᵗʰ **D03.5** **Melanoma in situ of** trunk

D03.51 **Melanoma in situ of** anal skin   `HCC`
    Melanoma in situ of anal margin
    Melanoma in situ of perianal skin

D03.52 **Melanoma in situ of** breast (skin) (soft tissue)   `HCC`

D03.59 **Melanoma in situ of** other **part of trunk**   `HCC`

✓5ᵗʰ **D03.6** **Melanoma in situ of** upper limb, including shoulder

D03.60 **Melanoma in situ of** unspecified **upper limb, including shoulder**   `HCC`

D03.61 **Melanoma in situ of** right **upper limb, including shoulder**   `HCC`

D03.62 **Melanoma in situ of** left **upper limb, including shoulder**   `HCC`

✓5ᵗʰ **D03.7** **Melanoma in situ of** lower limb, including hip

D03.70 **Melanoma in situ of** unspecified **lower limb, including hip**   `HCC`

D03.71 **Melanoma in situ of** right **lower limb, including hip**   `HCC`

D03.72 **Melanoma in situ of** left **lower limb, including hip**   `HCC`

D03.8 **Melanoma in situ of** other sites   `HCC`
    Melanoma in situ of scrotum
    EXCLUDES 1   carcinoma in situ of scrotum (D07.61)

D03.9 **Melanoma in situ,** unspecified   `HCC`

✓4ᵗʰ **D04** **Carcinoma in situ of** skin
    EXCLUDES 1   erythroplasia of Queyrat (penis) NOS (D07.4)
       melanoma in situ (D03.-)

D04.0 **Carcinoma in situ of skin of** lip
    EXCLUDES 1   carcinoma in situ of vermilion border of lip (D00.01)

✓5ᵗʰ **D04.1** **Carcinoma in situ of skin of** eyelid, including canthus

D04.10 **Carcinoma in situ of skin of** unspecified **eyelid, including canthus**

D04.11 **Carcinoma in situ of skin of** right **eyelid, including canthus**

D04.12 **Carcinoma in situ of skin of** left **eyelid, including canthus**

✓5ᵗʰ **D04.2** **Carcinoma in situ of skin of** ear and external auricular canal

D04.20 **Carcinoma in situ of skin of** unspecified **ear and external auricular canal**

D04.21 **Carcinoma in situ of skin of** right **ear and external auricular canal**

D04.22 **Carcinoma in situ of skin of** left **ear and external auricular canal**

✓5ᵗʰ **D04.3** **Carcinoma in situ of skin of** other and unspecified parts of face

D04.30 **Carcinoma in situ of skin of** unspecified **part of face**

D04.39 **Carcinoma in situ of skin of** other **parts of face**

D04.4 **Carcinoma in situ of skin of** scalp and neck

D04.5 **Carcinoma in situ of skin of** trunk
    Carcinoma in situ of anal margin
    Carcinoma in situ of anal skin
    Carcinoma in situ of perianal skin
    Carcinoma in situ of skin of breast
    EXCLUDES 1   carcinoma in situ of anus NOS (D01.3)
       carcinoma in situ of scrotum (D07.61)
       carcinoma in situ of skin of genital organs (D07.-)

✓5ᵗʰ **D04.6** **Carcinoma in situ of skin of** upper limb, including shoulder

D04.60 **Carcinoma in situ of skin of** unspecified **upper limb, including shoulder**

D04.61 **Carcinoma in situ of skin of** right **upper limb, including shoulder**

D04.62 **Carcinoma in situ of skin of** left **upper limb, including shoulder**

✓5ᵗʰ **D04.7** **Carcinoma in situ of skin of** lower limb, including hip

D04.70 **Carcinoma in situ of skin of** unspecified **lower limb, including hip**

D04.71 **Carcinoma in situ of skin of** right **lower limb, including hip**

✔ Additional Character Req   ✓x7ᵗʰ Placeholder Alert   Unacceptable PDx   Manifestation   H1 - H14 HAC   HCC CMS-HCC Condition   *EXCLUDES 1* Not Coded Here   *EXCLUDES 2* Not Included Here

ICD-10-CM 2018   489

Chapter 2. Neoplasms

D04.72 **Carcinoma in situ of skin of** left **lower limb, including** hip

D04.8 **Carcinoma in situ of skin of** other **sites**

D04.9 **Carcinoma in situ of skin,** unspecified

✓4ᵗʰ **D05 Carcinoma in situ of** breast

> EXCLUDES 1   *carcinoma in situ of skin of breast (D04.5)*
> *melanoma in situ of breast (skin) (D03.5)*
> *Paget's disease of breast or nipple (C50.-)*

✓5ᵗʰ **D05.0** Lobular **carcinoma in situ of breast**

D05.00 **Lobular carcinoma in situ of** unspecified **breast**

D05.01 **Lobular carcinoma in situ of** right **breast**

D05.02 **Lobular carcinoma in situ of** left **breast**

✓5ᵗʰ **D05.1** Intraductal **carcinoma in situ of breast**

D05.10 **Intraductal carcinoma in situ of** unspecified **breast**

D05.11 **Intraductal carcinoma in situ of** right **breast**

D05.12 **Intraductal carcinoma in situ of** left **breast**

✓5ᵗʰ **D05.8** Other **specified type of carcinoma in situ of breast**

D05.80 **Other specified type of carcinoma in situ of** unspecified **breast**

D05.81 **Other specified type of carcinoma in situ of** right **breast**

D05.82 **Other specified type of carcinoma in situ of** left **breast**

✓5ᵗʰ **D05.9** Unspecified **type of carcinoma in situ of breast**

D05.90 **Unspecified type of carcinoma in situ of** unspecified **breast**

D05.91 **Unspecified type of carcinoma in situ of** right **breast**

D05.92 **Unspecified type of carcinoma in situ of** left **breast**

✓4ᵗʰ **D06 Carcinoma in situ of** cervix uteri

> INCLUDES   cervical adenocarcinoma in situ
> cervical intraepithelial glandular neoplasia
> cervical intraepithelial neoplasia III [CIN III]
> severe dysplasia of cervix uteri

> EXCLUDES 1   *cervical intraepithelial neoplasia II [CIN II] (N87.1)*
> *cytologic evidence of malignancy of cervix without histologic confirmation (R87.614)*
> *high grade squamous intraepithelial lesion (HGSIL) of cervix (R87.613)*
> *melanoma in situ of cervix (D03.5)*
> *moderate cervical dysplasia (N87.1)*

D06.0 **Carcinoma in situ of** endocervix   ♀

D06.1 **Carcinoma in situ of** exocervix   ♀

D06.7 **Carcinoma in situ of** other parts **of cervix**   ♀

D06.9 **Carcinoma in situ of cervix,** unspecified   ♀

✓4ᵗʰ **D07 Carcinoma in situ of** other and unspecified genital organs

> EXCLUDES 1   *melanoma in situ of trunk (D03.5)*

D07.0 **Carcinoma in situ of** endometrium   ♀

D07.1 **Carcinoma in situ of** vulva   ♀
Severe dysplasia of vulva
Vulvar intraepithelial neoplasia III [VIN III]

> EXCLUDES 1   *moderate dysplasia of vulva (N90.1)*
> *vulvar intraepithelial neoplasia II [VIN II] (N90.1)*

D07.2 **Carcinoma in situ of** vagina   ♀
Severe dysplasia of vagina
Vaginal intraepithelial neoplasia III [VAIN III]

> EXCLUDES 1   *moderate dysplasia of vagina (N89.1)*
> *vaginal intraepithelial neoplasia II [VIN II] (N89.1)*

✓5ᵗʰ **D07.3 Carcinoma in situ of** other and unspecified female genital organs

D07.30 **Carcinoma in situ of** unspecified **female genital organs**   ♀

D07.39 **Carcinoma in situ of** other **female genital organs**   ♀

D07.4 **Carcinoma in situ of** penis   ♂
Erythroplasia of Queyrat NOS

D07.5 **Carcinoma in situ of** prostate   ♂
Prostatic intraepithelial neoplasia III (PIN III)
Severe dysplasia of prostate

> EXCLUDES 1   *dysplasia (mild) (moderate) of prostate (N42.3-)*
> *prostatic intraepithelial neoplasia II [PIN II] (N42.3-)*

✓5ᵗʰ **D07.6 Carcinoma in situ of** other and unspecified male genital organs

D07.60 **Carcinoma in situ of** unspecified **male genital organs**   ♂

D07.61 **Carcinoma in situ of** scrotum   ♂

D07.69 **Carcinoma in situ of** other **male genital organs**   ♂

✓4ᵗʰ **D09 Carcinoma in situ of** other and unspecified sites

> EXCLUDES 1   *melanoma in situ (D03.-)*

D09.0 **Carcinoma in situ of** bladder

✓5ᵗʰ **D09.1 Carcinoma in situ of** other and unspecified urinary organs

D09.10 **Carcinoma in situ of** unspecified **urinary organ**

D09.19 **Carcinoma in situ of** other **urinary organs**

✓5ᵗʰ **D09.2 Carcinoma in situ of** eye

> EXCLUDES 1   *carcinoma in situ of skin of eyelid (D04.1-)*

D09.20 **Carcinoma in situ of** unspecified **eye**

D09.21 **Carcinoma in situ of** right **eye**

D09.22 **Carcinoma in situ of** left **eye**

D09.3 **Carcinoma in situ of** thyroid and other endocrine glands

> EXCLUDES 1   *carcinoma in situ of endocrine pancreas (D01.7)*
> *carcinoma in situ of ovary (D07.39)*
> *carcinoma in situ of testis (D07.69)*

D09.8 **Carcinoma in situ of** other specified sites

D09.9 **Carcinoma in situ,** unspecified

Benign neoplasms, except benign neuroendocrine tumors (D10-D36)

✓4ᵗʰ **D10 Benign neoplasm of** mouth and pharynx

D10.0 **Benign neoplasm of** lip
Benign neoplasm of lip (frenulum) (inner aspect) (mucosa) (vermilion border)

> EXCLUDES 1   *benign neoplasm of skin of lip (D22.0, D23.0)*

D10.1 **Benign neoplasm of** tongue
Benign neoplasm of lingual tonsil

D10.2 **Benign neoplasm of** floor of mouth

✓5ᵗʰ **D10.3 Benign neoplasm of** other and unspecified parts of mouth

D10.30 **Benign neoplasm of** unspecified **part of mouth**

D10.39 **Benign neoplasm of** other parts of mouth
Benign neoplasm of minor salivary gland NOS

> EXCLUDES 1   *benign odontogenic neoplasms (D16.4-D16.5)*
> *benign neoplasm of mucosa of lip (D10.0)*
> *benign neoplasm of nasopharyngeal surface of soft palate (D10.6)*

D10.4 **Benign neoplasm of** tonsil
Benign neoplasm of tonsil (faucial) (palatine)

> EXCLUDES 1   *benign neoplasm of lingual tonsil (D10.1)*
> *benign neoplasm of pharyngeal tonsil (D10.6)*
> *benign neoplasm of tonsillar fossa (D10.5)*
> *benign neoplasm of tonsillar pillars (D10.5)*

D10.5 **Benign neoplasm of** other parts of oropharynx
Benign neoplasm of epiglottis, anterior aspect
Benign neoplasm of tonsillar fossa
Benign neoplasm of tonsillar pillars
Benign neoplasm of vallecula

> EXCLUDES 1   *benign neoplasm of epiglottis NOS (D14.1)*
> *benign neoplasm of epiglottis, suprahyoid portion (D14.1)*

D10.6 **Benign neoplasm of** nasopharynx
Benign neoplasm of pharyngeal tonsil
Benign neoplasm of posterior margin of septum and choanae

D10.7 **Benign neoplasm of** hypopharynx

D10.9 **Benign neoplasm of pharynx,** unspecified

✓4ᵗʰ **D11 Benign neoplasm of** major salivary glands

> EXCLUDES 1   *benign neoplasms of specified minor salivary glands which are classified according to their anatomical location*
> *benign neoplasms of minor salivary glands NOS (D10.39)*

D11.0 **Benign neoplasm of** parotid gland

D11.7 **Benign neoplasm of** other major salivary glands
Benign neoplasm of sublingual salivary gland
Benign neoplasm of submandibular salivary gland

D11.9 **Benign neoplasm of major salivary gland,** unspecified

✓4ᵗʰ **D12 Benign neoplasm of** colon, rectum, anus and anal canal

> EXCLUDES 1   *benign carcinoid tumors of the large intestine, and rectum (D3A.02-)*

AHA: 2017, 1Q, 15; 2015, 2Q, 14

D12.0 **Benign neoplasm of** cecum
Benign neoplasm of ileocecal valve

D12.1 **Benign neoplasm of** appendix

> EXCLUDES 1   *benign carcinoid tumor of the appendix (D3A.020)*

D12.2 **Benign neoplasm of** ascending colon

N Newborn: 0   P Pediatric: 0-17   M Maternity: 12-55   A Adult: 15-124   MCC Major CC Condition   PDxMCC PDx acts as own MCC   CC CC Condition   PDxCC PDx acts as own CC

490   ICD-10-CM 2018

D12.3 Benign neoplasm of transverse colon
Benign neoplasm of hepatic flexure
Benign neoplasm of splenic flexure
AHA: 2017, 1Q, 16

D12.4 Benign neoplasm of descending colon

D12.5 Benign neoplasm of sigmoid colon

D12.6 Benign neoplasm of colon, unspecified
Adenomatosis of colon
Benign neoplasm of large intestine NOS
Polyposis (hereditary) of colon
EXCLUDES 1   inflammatory polyp of colon (K51.4-)
          polyp of colon NOS (K63.5)

D12.7 Benign neoplasm of rectosigmoid junction

D12.8 Benign neoplasm of rectum
EXCLUDES 1   benign carcinoid tumor of the rectum (D3A.026)

D12.9 Benign neoplasm of anus and anal canal
Benign neoplasm of anus NOS
EXCLUDES 1   benign neoplasm of anal margin (D22.5, D23.5)
          benign neoplasm of anal skin (D22.5, D23.5)
          benign neoplasm of perianal skin (D22.5, D23.5)

✓4th D13 Benign neoplasm of other and ill-defined parts of digestive system
EXCLUDES 1   benign stromal tumors of digestive system (D21.4)

D13.0 Benign neoplasm of esophagus

D13.1 Benign neoplasm of stomach
EXCLUDES 1   benign carcinoid tumor of the stomach (D3A.092)

D13.2 Benign neoplasm of duodenum
EXCLUDES 1   benign carcinoid tumor of the duodenum (D3A.010)

✓5th D13.3 Benign neoplasm of other and unspecified parts of small intestine
EXCLUDES 1   benign carcinoid tumors of the small intestine (D3A.01)
          benign neoplasm of ileocecal valve (D12.0)

     D13.30 Benign neoplasm of unspecified part of small intestine

     D13.39 Benign neoplasm of other parts of small intestine

D13.4 Benign neoplasm of liver
Benign neoplasm of intrahepatic bile ducts

D13.5 Benign neoplasm of extrahepatic bile ducts

D13.6 Benign neoplasm of pancreas
EXCLUDES 1   benign neoplasm of endocrine pancreas (D13.7)

D13.7 Benign neoplasm of endocrine pancreas
Islet cell tumor
Benign neoplasm of islets of Langerhans
Use additional code to identify any functional activity

D13.9 Benign neoplasm of ill-defined sites within the digestive system
Benign neoplasm of digestive system NOS
Benign neoplasm of intestine NOS
Benign neoplasm of spleen

✓4th D14 Benign neoplasm of middle ear and respiratory system

D14.0 Benign neoplasm of middle ear, nasal cavity and accessory sinuses
Benign neoplasm of cartilage of nose
EXCLUDES 1   benign neoplasm of auricular canal (external) (D22.2-, D23.2-)
          benign neoplasm of bone of ear (D16.4)
          benign neoplasm of bone of nose (D16.4)
          benign neoplasm of cartilage of ear (D21.0)
          benign neoplasm of ear (external)(skin) (D22.2-, D23.2-)
          benign neoplasm of nose NOS (D36.7)
          benign neoplasm of skin of nose (D22.39, D23.39)
          benign neoplasm of olfactory bulb (D33.3)
          benign neoplasm of posterior margin of septum and choanae (D10.6)
          polyp of accessory sinus (J33.8)
          polyp of ear (middle) (H74.4)
          polyp of nasal (cavity) (J33.-)

D14.1 Benign neoplasm of larynx
Adenomatous polyp of larynx
Benign neoplasm of epiglottis (suprahyoid portion)
EXCLUDES 1   benign neoplasm of epiglottis, anterior aspect (D10.5)
          polyp (nonadenomatous) of vocal cord or larynx (J38.1)

D14.2 Benign neoplasm of trachea

✓5th D14.3 Benign neoplasm of bronchus and lung
EXCLUDES 1   benign carcinoid tumor of the bronchus and lung (D3A.090)

     D14.30 Benign neoplasm of unspecified bronchus and lung

     D14.31 Benign neoplasm of right bronchus and lung

     D14.32 Benign neoplasm of left bronchus and lung

D14.4 Benign neoplasm of respiratory system, unspecified

✓4th D15 Benign neoplasm of other and unspecified intrathoracic organs
EXCLUDES 1   benign neoplasm of mesothelial tissue (D19.-)

D15.0 Benign neoplasm of thymus
EXCLUDES 1   benign carcinoid tumor of the thymus (D3A.091)

D15.1 Benign neoplasm of heart
EXCLUDES 1   benign neoplasm of great vessels (D21.3)

D15.2 Benign neoplasm of mediastinum

D15.7 Benign neoplasm of other specified intrathoracic organs

D15.9 Benign neoplasm of intrathoracic organ, unspecified

✓4th D16 Benign neoplasm of bone and articular cartilage
EXCLUDES 1   benign neoplasm of connective tissue of ear (D21.0)
          benign neoplasm of connective tissue of eyelid (D21.0)
          benign neoplasm of connective tissue of larynx (D14.1)
          benign neoplasm of connective tissue of nose (D14.0)
          benign neoplasm of synovia (D21.-)

✓5th D16.0 Benign neoplasm of scapula and long bones of upper limb

     D16.00 Benign neoplasm of scapula and long bones of unspecified upper limb

     D16.01 Benign neoplasm of scapula and long bones of right upper limb

     D16.02 Benign neoplasm of scapula and long bones of left upper limb

✓5th D16.1 Benign neoplasm of short bones of upper limb

     D16.10 Benign neoplasm of short bones of unspecified upper limb

     D16.11 Benign neoplasm of short bones of right upper limb

     D16.12 Benign neoplasm of short bones of left upper limb

✓5th D16.2 Benign neoplasm of long bones of lower limb

     D16.20 Benign neoplasm of long bones of unspecified lower limb

     D16.21 Benign neoplasm of long bones of right lower limb

     D16.22 Benign neoplasm of long bones of left lower limb

✓5th D16.3 Benign neoplasm of short bones of lower limb

     D16.30 Benign neoplasm of short bones of unspecified lower limb

     D16.31 Benign neoplasm of short bones of right lower limb

     D16.32 Benign neoplasm of short bones of left lower limb

D16.4 Benign neoplasm of bones of skull and face
Benign neoplasm of maxilla (superior)
Benign neoplasm of orbital bone
Keratocyst of maxilla
Keratocystic odontogenic tumor of maxilla
EXCLUDES 2   benign neoplasm of lower jaw bone (D16.5)

D16.5 Benign neoplasm of lower jaw bone
Keratocyst of mandible
Keratocystic odontogenic tumor of mandible

D16.6 Benign neoplasm of vertebral column
EXCLUDES 1   benign neoplasm of sacrum and coccyx (D16.8)

D16.7 Benign neoplasm of ribs, sternum and clavicle

D16.8 Benign neoplasm of pelvic bones, sacrum and coccyx

D16.9 Benign neoplasm of bone and articular cartilage, unspecified

✓4th D17 Benign lipomatous neoplasm

D17.0 Benign lipomatous neoplasm of skin and subcutaneous tissue of head, face and neck

D17.1 Benign lipomatous neoplasm of skin and subcutaneous tissue of trunk

✓5th D17.2 Benign lipomatous neoplasm of skin and subcutaneous tissue of limb

     D17.20 Benign lipomatous neoplasm of skin and subcutaneous tissue of unspecified limb

     D17.21 Benign lipomatous neoplasm of skin and subcutaneous tissue of right arm

     D17.22 Benign lipomatous neoplasm of skin and subcutaneous tissue of left arm

     D17.23 Benign lipomatous neoplasm of skin and subcutaneous tissue of right leg

✓ Additional Character Req   ✓x7th Placeholder Alert   Unacceptable PDx   Manifestation   H1 - H14 HAC   HCC CMS-HCC Condition   *EXCLUDES 1* Not Coded Here   *EXCLUDES 2* Not Included Here

ICD-10-CM 2018   491

D17.24　**Benign lipomatous neoplasm of skin and subcutaneous tissue of** left leg

√5th D17.3　**Benign lipomatous neoplasm of** skin and subcutaneous tissue of other and unspecified sites

　　D17.30　**Benign lipomatous neoplasm of skin and subcutaneous tissue of** unspecified sites

　　D17.39　**Benign lipomatous neoplasm of skin and subcutaneous tissue of** other sites

D17.4　**Benign lipomatous neoplasm of** intrathoracic organs

D17.5　**Benign lipomatous neoplasm of** intra-abdominal organs
　　EXCLUDES 1　*benign lipomatous neoplasm of peritoneum and retroperitoneum (D17.79)*

D17.6　**Benign lipomatous neoplasm of** spermatic cord　　♂

√5th D17.7　**Benign lipomatous neoplasm of** other sites

　　D17.71　**Benign lipomatous neoplasm of** kidney

　　D17.72　**Benign lipomatous neoplasm of** other genitourinary organ

　　D17.79　**Benign lipomatous neoplasm of** other sites
　　　　Benign lipomatous neoplasm of peritoneum
　　　　Benign lipomatous neoplasm of retroperitoneum

D17.9　**Benign lipomatous neoplasm,** unspecified
　　Lipoma NOS

√4th **D18　Hemangioma and lymphangioma, any site**
　　EXCLUDES 1　*benign neoplasm of glomus jugulare (D35.6)*
　　　　blue or pigmented nevus (D22.-)
　　　　nevus NOS (D22.-)
　　　　vascular nevus (Q82.5)

√5th D18.0　**Hemangioma**
　　Angioma NOS
　　Cavernous nevus
　　DEF: A common benign tumor usually occurring in infancy; composed of newly formed blood vessels due to malformation of angioblastic tissue.

　　D18.00　**Hemangioma** unspecified site

　　D18.01　**Hemangioma of** skin and subcutaneous tissue

　　D18.02　**Hemangioma of** intracranial structures　　HCC

　　D18.03　**Hemangioma of** intra-abdominal structures

　　D18.09　**Hemangioma of** other sites

D18.1　**Lymphangioma, any site**

√4th **D19　Benign neoplasm of** mesothelial tissue

D19.0　**Benign neoplasm of mesothelial tissue of** pleura

D19.1　**Benign neoplasm of mesothelial tissue of** peritoneum

D19.7　**Benign neoplasm of mesothelial tissue of** other sites

D19.9　**Benign neoplasm of mesothelial tissue,** unspecified
　　Benign mesothelioma NOS

√4th **D20　Benign neoplasm of soft tissue of** retroperitoneum and peritoneum
　　EXCLUDES 1　*benign lipomatous neoplasm of peritoneum and retroperitoneum (D17.79)*
　　　　benign neoplasm of mesothelial tissue (D19.-)

D20.0　**Benign neoplasm of soft tissue of** retroperitoneum

D20.1　**Benign neoplasm of soft tissue of** peritoneum

√4th **D21　Other benign neoplasms of** connective and other soft tissue
　　INCLUDES　benign neoplasm of blood vessel
　　　　benign neoplasm of bursa
　　　　benign neoplasm of cartilage
　　　　benign neoplasm of fascia
　　　　benign neoplasm of fat
　　　　benign neoplasm of ligament, except uterine
　　　　benign neoplasm of lymphatic channel
　　　　benign neoplasm of muscle
　　　　benign neoplasm of synovia
　　　　benign neoplasm of tendon (sheath)
　　　　benign stromal tumors
　　EXCLUDES 1　*benign neoplasm of articular cartilage (D16.-)*
　　　　benign neoplasm of cartilage of larynx (D14.1)
　　　　benign neoplasm of cartilage of nose (D14.0)
　　　　benign neoplasm of connective tissue of breast (D24.-)
　　　　benign neoplasm of peripheral nerves and autonomic nervous system (D36.1-)
　　　　benign neoplasm of peritoneum (D20.1)
　　　　benign neoplasm of retroperitoneum (D20.0)
　　　　benign neoplasm of uterine ligament, any (D28.2)
　　　　benign neoplasm of vascular tissue (D18.-)
　　　　hemangioma (D18.0-)
　　　　lipomatous neoplasm (D17.-)
　　　　lymphangioma (D18.1)
　　　　uterine leiomyoma (D25.-)

D21.0　**Benign neoplasm of connective and other soft tissue of** head, face and neck
　　Benign neoplasm of connective tissue of ear
　　Benign neoplasm of connective tissue of eyelid
　　EXCLUDES 1　*benign neoplasm of connective tissue of orbit (D31.6-)*

√5th D21.1　**Benign neoplasm of connective and other soft tissue of** upper limb, including shoulder

　　D21.10　**Benign neoplasm of connective and other soft tissue of** unspecified upper limb, including shoulder

　　D21.11　**Benign neoplasm of connective and other soft tissue of** right upper limb, including shoulder

　　D21.12　**Benign neoplasm of connective and other soft tissue of** left upper limb, including shoulder

√5th D21.2　**Benign neoplasm of connective and other soft tissue of** lower limb, including hip

　　D21.20　**Benign neoplasm of connective and other soft tissue of** unspecified lower limb, including hip

　　D21.21　**Benign neoplasm of connective and other soft tissue of** right lower limb, including hip

　　D21.22　**Benign neoplasm of connective and other soft tissue of** left lower limb, including hip

D21.3　**Benign neoplasm of connective and other soft tissue of** thorax
　　Benign neoplasm of axilla
　　Benign neoplasm of diaphragm
　　Benign neoplasm of great vessels
　　EXCLUDES 1　*benign neoplasm of heart (D15.1)*
　　　　benign neoplasm of mediastinum (D15.2)
　　　　benign neoplasm of thymus (D15.0)

D21.4　**Benign neoplasm of connective and other soft tissue of** abdomen
　　Benign stromal tumors of abdomen

D21.5　**Benign neoplasm of connective and other soft tissue of** pelvis
　　EXCLUDES 1　*benign neoplasm of any uterine ligament (D28.2)*
　　　　uterine leiomyoma (D25.-)

D21.6　**Benign neoplasm of connective and other soft tissue of** trunk, unspecified
　　Benign neoplasm of back NOS

D21.9　**Benign neoplasm of connective and other soft tissue,** unspecified

√4th **D22　Melanocytic nevi**
　　INCLUDES　atypical nevus
　　　　blue hairy pigmented nevus
　　　　nevus NOS

D22.0　**Melanocytic nevi of** lip

√5th D22.1　**Melanocytic nevi of** eyelid, including canthus

　　D22.10　**Melanocytic nevi of** unspecified eyelid, including canthus

　　D22.11　**Melanocytic nevi of** right eyelid, including canthus

　　D22.12　**Melanocytic nevi of** left eyelid, including canthus

✓5th **D22.2** **Melanocytic nevi of** ear and external auricular canal

    D22.20 **Melanocytic nevi of** unspecified **ear and external auricular canal**

    D22.21 **Melanocytic nevi of** right **ear and external auricular canal**

    D22.22 **Melanocytic nevi of** left **ear and external auricular canal**

✓5th **D22.3** **Melanocytic nevi of** other and unspecified parts of face

    D22.30 **Melanocytic nevi of** unspecified **part of face**

    D22.39 **Melanocytic nevi of** other **parts of face**

D22.4 **Melanocytic nevi of** scalp and neck

D22.5 **Melanocytic nevi of** trunk

    Melanocytic nevi of anal margin
    Melanocytic nevi of anal skin
    Melanocytic nevi of perianal skin
    Melanocytic nevi of skin of breast

✓5th **D22.6** **Melanocytic nevi of** upper limb, including shoulder

    D22.60 **Melanocytic nevi of** unspecified **upper limb, including shoulder**

    D22.61 **Melanocytic nevi of** right **upper limb, including shoulder**

    D22.62 **Melanocytic nevi of** left **upper limb, including shoulder**

✓5th **D22.7** **Melanocytic nevi of** lower limb, including hip

    D22.70 **Melanocytic nevi of** unspecified **lower limb, including hip**

    D22.71 **Melanocytic nevi of** right **lower limb, including hip**

    D22.72 **Melanocytic nevi of** left **lower limb, including hip**

D22.9 **Melanocytic nevi,** unspecified

✓4th **D23** **Other benign neoplasms of** skin

    INCLUDES benign neoplasm of hair follicles
            benign neoplasm of sebaceous glands
            benign neoplasm of sweat glands

    EXCLUDES 1 *benign lipomatous neoplasms of skin (D17.0-D17.3)*
            melanocytic nevi (D22.-)

D23.0 **Other benign neoplasm of skin of** lip

    EXCLUDES 1 *benign neoplasm of vermilion border of lip (D10.0)*

✓5th **D23.1** **Other benign neoplasm of skin of** eyelid, including canthus

    D23.10 **Other benign neoplasm of skin of** unspecified **eyelid, including canthus**

    D23.11 **Other benign neoplasm of skin of** right **eyelid, including canthus**

    D23.12 **Other benign neoplasm of skin of** left **eyelid, including canthus**

✓5th **D23.2** **Other benign neoplasm of skin of** ear and external auricular canal

    D23.20 **Other benign neoplasm of skin of** unspecified **ear and external auricular canal**

    D23.21 **Other benign neoplasm of skin of** right **ear and external auricular canal**

    D23.22 **Other benign neoplasm of skin of** left **ear and external auricular canal**

✓5th **D23.3** **Other benign neoplasm of skin of** other and unspecified parts of face

    D23.30 **Other benign neoplasm of skin of** unspecified **part of face**

    D23.39 **Other benign neoplasm of skin of** other **parts of face**

D23.4 **Other benign neoplasm of skin of** scalp and neck

D23.5 **Other benign neoplasm of skin of** trunk

    Other benign neoplasm of anal margin
    Other benign neoplasm of anal skin
    Other benign neoplasm of perianal skin
    Other benign neoplasm of skin of breast

    EXCLUDES 1 *benign neoplasm of anus NOS (D12.9)*

✓5th **D23.6** **Other benign neoplasm of skin of** upper limb, including shoulder

    D23.60 **Other benign neoplasm of skin of** unspecified **upper limb, including shoulder**

    D23.61 **Other benign neoplasm of skin of** right **upper limb, including shoulder**

    D23.62 **Other benign neoplasm of skin of** left **upper limb, including shoulder**

✓5th **D23.7** **Other benign neoplasm of skin of** lower limb, including hip

    D23.70 **Other benign neoplasm of skin of** unspecified **lower limb, including hip**

    D23.71 **Other benign neoplasm of skin of** right **lower limb, including hip**

    D23.72 **Other benign neoplasm of skin of** left **lower limb, including hip**

D23.9 **Other benign neoplasm of skin,** unspecified

✓4th **D24** **Benign neoplasm of** breast

    INCLUDES benign neoplasm of connective tissue of breast
            benign neoplasm of soft parts of breast
            fibroadenoma of breast

    EXCLUDES 2 *adenofibrosis of breast (N60.2)*
            benign cyst of breast (N60.-)
            benign mammary dysplasia (N60.-)
            benign neoplasm of skin of breast (D22.5, D23.5)
            fibrocystic disease of breast (N60.-)

D24.1 **Benign neoplasm of** right **breast**

D24.2 **Benign neoplasm of** left **breast**

D24.9 **Benign neoplasm of** unspecified **breast**

✓4th **D25** **Leiomyoma of uterus**

    INCLUDES uterine fibroid
            uterine fibromyoma
            uterine myoma

D25.0 **Submucous leiomyoma of uterus** ♀

D25.1 **Intramural leiomyoma of uterus** ♀
    Interstitial leiomyoma of uterus

D25.2 **Subserosal leiomyoma of uterus** ♀
    Subperitoneal leiomyoma of uterus

D25.9 **Leiomyoma of uterus,** unspecified ♀

✓4th **D26** **Other benign neoplasms of** uterus

D26.0 **Other benign neoplasm of** cervix uteri ♀

D26.1 **Other benign neoplasm of** corpus uteri ♀

D26.7 **Other benign neoplasm of** other parts **of uterus** ♀

D26.9 **Other benign neoplasm of uterus,** unspecified ♀

✓4th **D27** **Benign neoplasm of** ovary

    Use additional code to identify any functional activity

    EXCLUDES 2 *corpus albicans cyst (N83.2-)*
            corpus luteum cyst (N83.1-)
            endometrial cyst (N80.1)
            follicular (atretic) cyst (N83.0-)
            graafian follicle cyst (N83.0-)
            ovarian cyst NEC (N83.2-)
            ovarian retention cyst (N83.2-)

D27.0 **Benign neoplasm of** right **ovary** ♀

D27.1 **Benign neoplasm of** left **ovary** ♀

D27.9 **Benign neoplasm of** unspecified **ovary** ♀

Uterine Leiomyomas (Fibroids)

Labels: Cornual, Pedunculated, Uterine cavity, Intramural, Subserosal, Submucosal, Cervical

✓ Additional Character Req ✓x7th Placeholder Alert Unacceptable PDx Manifestation H1 - H14 HAC HCC CMS-HCC Condition EXCLUDES 1 Not Coded Here EXCLUDES 2 Not Included Here

ICD-10-CM 2018   493

☑4ᵗʰ **D28** **Benign neoplasm of** other and unspecified female genital organs

INCLUDES   adenomatous polyp
benign neoplasm of skin of female genital organs
benign teratoma

EXCLUDES 1   *epoophoron cyst (Q50.5)*
fimbrial cyst (Q50.4)
Gartner's duct cyst (Q52.4)
parovarian cyst (Q50.5)

D28.0 **Benign neoplasm of** vulva   ♀

D28.1 **Benign neoplasm of** vagina   ♀

D28.2 **Benign neoplasm of** uterine tubes and ligaments   ♀
Benign neoplasm of fallopian tube
Benign neoplasm of uterine ligament (broad) (round)

D28.7 **Benign neoplasm of** other specified female genital organs   ♀

D28.9 **Benign neoplasm of** female genital organ, unspecified   ♀

☑4ᵗʰ **D29** **Benign neoplasm of** male genital organs

INCLUDES   benign neoplasm of skin of male genital organs

D29.0 **Benign neoplasm of** penis   ♂

D29.1 **Benign neoplasm of** prostate   ♂

EXCLUDES 1   *enlarged prostate (N40.-)*

☑5ᵗʰ **D29.2** **Benign neoplasm of** testis
Use additional code to identify any functional activity

D29.20 **Benign neoplasm of** unspecified testis   ♂

D29.21 **Benign neoplasm of** right testis   ♂

D29.22 **Benign neoplasm of** left testis   ♂

☑5ᵗʰ **D29.3** **Benign neoplasm of** epididymis

D29.30 **Benign neoplasm of** unspecified epididymis   ♂

D29.31 **Benign neoplasm of** right epididymis   ♂

D29.32 **Benign neoplasm of** left epididymis   ♂

D29.4 **Benign neoplasm of** scrotum   ♂
Benign neoplasm of skin of scrotum

D29.8 **Benign neoplasm of** other specified male genital organs   ♂
Benign neoplasm of seminal vesicle
Benign neoplasm of spermatic cord
Benign neoplasm of tunica vaginalis

D29.9 **Benign neoplasm of** male genital organ, unspecified   ♂

☑4ᵗʰ **D30** **Benign neoplasm of** urinary organs

☑5ᵗʰ **D30.0** **Benign neoplasm of** kidney

EXCLUDES 1   *benign carcinoid tumor of the kidney (D3A.093)*
benign neoplasm of renal calyces (D30.1-)
benign neoplasm of renal pelvis (D30.1-)

D30.00 **Benign neoplasm of** unspecified kidney

D30.01 **Benign neoplasm of** right kidney

D30.02 **Benign neoplasm of** left kidney

☑5ᵗʰ **D30.1** **Benign neoplasm of** renal pelvis

D30.10 **Benign neoplasm of** unspecified renal pelvis

D30.11 **Benign neoplasm of** right renal pelvis

D30.12 **Benign neoplasm of** left renal pelvis

☑5ᵗʰ **D30.2** **Benign neoplasm of** ureter

EXCLUDES 1   *benign neoplasm of ureteric orifice of bladder (D30.3)*

D30.20 **Benign neoplasm of** unspecified ureter

D30.21 **Benign neoplasm of** right ureter

D30.22 **Benign neoplasm of** left ureter

D30.3 **Benign neoplasm of** bladder
Benign neoplasm of ureteric orifice of bladder
Benign neoplasm of urethral orifice of bladder

D30.4 **Benign neoplasm of** urethra

EXCLUDES 1   *benign neoplasm of urethral orifice of bladder (D30.3)*

D30.8 **Benign neoplasm of** other specified urinary organs
Benign neoplasm of paraurethral glands

D30.9 **Benign neoplasm of** urinary organ, unspecified
Benign neoplasm of urinary system NOS

☑4ᵗʰ **D31** **Benign neoplasm of** eye and adnexa

EXCLUDES 1   *benign neoplasm of connective tissue of eyelid (D21.0)*
benign neoplasm of optic nerve (D33.3)
benign neoplasm of skin of eyelid (D22.1-, D23.1-)

☑5ᵗʰ **D31.0** **Benign neoplasm of** conjunctiva

D31.00 **Benign neoplasm of** unspecified conjunctiva

D31.01 **Benign neoplasm of** right conjunctiva

D31.02 **Benign neoplasm of** left conjunctiva

☑5ᵗʰ **D31.1** **Benign neoplasm of** cornea

D31.10 **Benign neoplasm of** unspecified cornea

D31.11 **Benign neoplasm of** right cornea

D31.12 **Benign neoplasm of** left cornea

☑5ᵗʰ **D31.2** **Benign neoplasm of** retina

EXCLUDES 1   *dark area on retina (D49.81)*
hemangioma of retina (D49.81)
neoplasm of unspecified behavior of retina and
choroid (D49.81)
retinal freckle (D49.81)

D31.20 **Benign neoplasm of** unspecified retina

D31.21 **Benign neoplasm of** right retina

D31.22 **Benign neoplasm of** left retina

☑5ᵗʰ **D31.3** **Benign neoplasm of** choroid

D31.30 **Benign neoplasm of** unspecified choroid

D31.31 **Benign neoplasm of** right choroid

D31.32 **Benign neoplasm of** left choroid

☑5ᵗʰ **D31.4** **Benign neoplasm of** ciliary body

D31.40 **Benign neoplasm of** unspecified ciliary body

D31.41 **Benign neoplasm of** right ciliary body

D31.42 **Benign neoplasm of** left ciliary body

☑5ᵗʰ **D31.5** **Benign neoplasm of** lacrimal gland and duct
Benign neoplasm of lacrimal sac
Benign neoplasm of nasolacrimal duct

D31.50 **Benign neoplasm of** unspecified lacrimal gland and
duct

D31.51 **Benign neoplasm of** right lacrimal gland and duct

D31.52 **Benign neoplasm of** left lacrimal gland and duct

☑5ᵗʰ **D31.6** **Benign neoplasm of** unspecified site of orbit
Benign neoplasm of connective tissue of orbit
Benign neoplasm of extraocular muscle
Benign neoplasm of peripheral nerves of orbit
Benign neoplasm of retrobulbar tissue
Benign neoplasm of retro-ocular tissue

EXCLUDES 1   *benign neoplasm of orbital bone (D16.4)*

D31.60 **Benign neoplasm of** unspecified site of unspecified
orbit

D31.61 **Benign neoplasm of** unspecified site of right orbit

D31.62 **Benign neoplasm of** unspecified site of left orbit

☑5ᵗʰ **D31.9** **Benign neoplasm of** unspecified part of eye
Benign neoplasm of eyeball

D31.90 **Benign neoplasm of** unspecified part of unspecified
eye

D31.91 **Benign neoplasm of** unspecified part of right eye

D31.92 **Benign neoplasm of** unspecified part of left eye

☑4ᵗʰ **D32** **Benign neoplasm of** meninges

D32.0 **Benign neoplasm of** cerebral meninges   HCC

D32.1 **Benign neoplasm of** spinal meninges   HCC

D32.9 **Benign neoplasm of** meninges, unspecified   HCC
Meningioma NOS

☑4ᵗʰ **D33** **Benign neoplasm of** brain and other parts of central nervous system

EXCLUDES 1   *angioma (D18.0-)*
benign neoplasm of meninges (D32.-)
benign neoplasm of peripheral nerves and autonomic nervous
system (D36.1-)
hemangioma (D18.0-)
neurofibromatosis (Q85.0-)
retro-ocular benign neoplasm (D31.6-)

D33.0 **Benign neoplasm of** brain, supratentorial   HCC
Benign neoplasm of cerebral ventricle
Benign neoplasm of cerebrum
Benign neoplasm of frontal lobe
Benign neoplasm of occipital lobe
Benign neoplasm of parietal lobe
Benign neoplasm of temporal lobe

EXCLUDES 1   *benign neoplasm of fourth ventricle (D33.1)*

D33.1 **Benign neoplasm of** brain, infratentorial   HCC
Benign neoplasm of brain stem
Benign neoplasm of cerebellum
Benign neoplasm of fourth ventricle

D33.2 **Benign neoplasm of** brain, unspecified   HCC

D33.3 **Benign neoplasm of** cranial nerves   HCC
Benign neoplasm of olfactory bulb

D33.4 **Benign neoplasm of** spinal cord   HCC

N Newborn: 0   **P** Pediatric: 0-17   **M** Maternity: 12-55   **A** Adult: 15-124   **MCC** Major CC Condition   **PDxMCC** PDx acts as own MCC   **CC** CC Condition   **PDxCC** PDx acts as own CC

494   ICD-10-CM 2018

D33.7 **Benign neoplasm of** other **specified parts of central nervous system** `HCC`

D33.9 **Benign neoplasm of central nervous system,** unspecified `HCC`
Benign neoplasm of nervous system (central) NOS

D34 **Benign neoplasm of** thyroid gland
Use additional code to identify any functional activity

✓4ᵗʰ **D35** **Benign neoplasm of** other and unspecified endocrine glands
Use additional code to identify any functional activity
`EXCLUDES 1` *benign neoplasm of endocrine pancreas (D13.7)*
benign neoplasm of ovary (D27.-)
benign neoplasm of testis (D29.2-)
benign neoplasm of thymus (D15.0)

✓5ᵗʰ **D35.0** **Benign neoplasm of** adrenal gland

D35.00 **Benign neoplasm of** unspecified **adrenal gland**

D35.01 **Benign neoplasm of** right **adrenal gland**

D35.02 **Benign neoplasm of** left **adrenal gland**

D35.1 **Benign neoplasm of** parathyroid gland

D35.2 **Benign neoplasm of** pituitary gland `HCC`
AHA: 2014, 3Q, 22

D35.3 **Benign neoplasm of** craniopharyngeal duct `HCC`

D35.4 **Benign neoplasm of** pineal gland `HCC`

D35.5 **Benign neoplasm of** carotid body

D35.6 **Benign neoplasm of** aortic body and other paraganglia
Benign tumor of glomus jugulare

D35.7 **Benign neoplasm of** other specified endocrine glands

D35.9 **Benign neoplasm of endocrine gland,** unspecified
Benign neoplasm of unspecified endocrine gland

✓4ᵗʰ **D36** **Benign neoplasm of** other and unspecified sites

D36.0 **Benign neoplasm of** lymph nodes
`EXCLUDES 1` *lymphangioma (D18.1)*

✓5ᵗʰ **D36.1** **Benign neoplasm of** peripheral nerves and autonomic nervous system
`EXCLUDES 1` *benign neoplasm of peripheral nerves of orbit (D31.6-)*
neurofibromatosis (Q85.0-)

D36.10 **Benign neoplasm of peripheral nerves and autonomic nervous system,** unspecified

D36.11 **Benign neoplasm of peripheral nerves and autonomic nervous system of** face, head, and neck

D36.12 **Benign neoplasm of peripheral nerves and autonomic nervous system,** upper limb, including shoulder

D36.13 **Benign neoplasm of peripheral nerves and autonomic nervous system of** lower limb, including hip

D36.14 **Benign neoplasm of peripheral nerves and autonomic nervous system of** thorax

D36.15 **Benign neoplasm of peripheral nerves and autonomic nervous system of** abdomen

D36.16 **Benign neoplasm of peripheral nerves and autonomic nervous system of** pelvis

D36.17 **Benign neoplasm of peripheral nerves and autonomic nervous system of** trunk, unspecified

D36.7 **Benign neoplasm of** other specified sites
Benign neoplasm of nose NOS

D36.9 **Benign neoplasm,** unspecified site

Benign neuroendocrine tumors (D3A)

✓4ᵗʰ **D3A** **Benign neuroendocrine tumors**
Code also any associated multiple endocrine neoplasia [MEN] syndromes (E31.2-)
Use additional code to identify any associated endocrine syndrome, such as:
carcinoid syndrome (E34.0)
`EXCLUDES 2` *benign pancreatic islet cell tumors (D13.7)*

✓5ᵗʰ **D3A.0** **Benign** carcinoid tumors

D3A.00 **Benign carcinoid tumor of** unspecified site
Carcinoid tumor NOS

✓6ᵗʰ **D3A.01** **Benign carcinoid tumors of the** small intestine

D3A.010 **Benign carcinoid tumor of the** duodenum

D3A.011 **Benign carcinoid tumor of the** jejunum

D3A.012 **Benign carcinoid tumor of the** ileum

D3A.019 **Benign carcinoid tumor of the small intestine,** unspecified portion

✓6ᵗʰ **D3A.02** **Benign carcinoid tumors of the** appendix, large intestine, and rectum

D3A.020 **Benign carcinoid tumor of the** appendix

D3A.021 **Benign carcinoid tumor of the** cecum

D3A.022 **Benign carcinoid tumor of the** ascending colon

D3A.023 **Benign carcinoid tumor of the** transverse colon

D3A.024 **Benign carcinoid tumor of the** descending colon

D3A.025 **Benign carcinoid tumor of the** sigmoid colon

D3A.026 **Benign carcinoid tumor of the** rectum

D3A.029 **Benign carcinoid tumor of the large intestine,** unspecified portion
Benign carcinoid tumor of the colon NOS

✓6ᵗʰ **D3A.09** **Benign carcinoid tumors of** other sites

D3A.090 **Benign carcinoid tumor of the** bronchus and lung

D3A.091 **Benign carcinoid tumor of the** thymus

D3A.092 **Benign carcinoid tumor of the** stomach

D3A.093 **Benign carcinoid tumor of the** kidney

D3A.094 **Benign carcinoid tumor of the** foregut, unspecified

D3A.095 **Benign carcinoid tumor of the** midgut, unspecified

D3A.096 **Benign carcinoid tumor of the** hindgut, unspecified

D3A.098 **Benign carcinoid tumors of** other sites

D3A.8 **Other benign neuroendocrine tumors**
Neuroendocrine tumor NOS

Neoplasms of uncertain behavior, polycythemia vera and myelodysplastic syndromes (D37-D48)

`NOTE` Categories D37-D44, and D48 classify by site neoplasms of uncertain behavior, i.e., histologic confirmation whether the neoplasm is malignant or benign cannot be made.
`EXCLUDES 1` *neoplasms of unspecified behavior (D49.-)*

✓4ᵗʰ **D37** **Neoplasm of uncertain behavior of** oral cavity and digestive organs
`EXCLUDES 1` *stromal tumors of uncertain behavior of digestive system (D48.1)*

✓5ᵗʰ **D37.0** **Neoplasm of uncertain behavior of** lip, oral cavity and pharynx
`EXCLUDES 1` *neoplasm of uncertain behavior of aryepiglottic fold or interarytenoid fold, laryngeal aspect (D38.0)*
neoplasm of uncertain behavior of epiglottis NOS (D38.0)
neoplasm of uncertain behavior of skin of lip (D48.5)
neoplasm of uncertain behavior of suprahyoid portion of epiglottis (D38.0)

D37.01 **Neoplasm of uncertain behavior of** lip
Neoplasm of uncertain behavior of vermilion border of lip

D37.02 **Neoplasm of uncertain behavior of** tongue

✓6ᵗʰ **D37.03** **Neoplasm of uncertain behavior of the** major salivary glands

D37.030 **Neoplasm of uncertain behavior of the** parotid **salivary glands**

D37.031 **Neoplasm of uncertain behavior of the** sublingual **salivary glands**

D37.032 **Neoplasm of uncertain behavior of the** submandibular **salivary glands**

D37.039 **Neoplasm of uncertain behavior of the** major salivary glands, **unspecified**

D37.04 **Neoplasm of uncertain behavior of the** minor salivary glands
Neoplasm of uncertain behavior of submucosal salivary glands of lip
Neoplasm of uncertain behavior of submucosal salivary glands of cheek
Neoplasm of uncertain behavior of submucosal salivary glands of hard palate
Neoplasm of uncertain behavior of submucosal salivary glands of soft palate

✓ Additional Character Req   ✓x7ᵗʰ Placeholder Alert   Unacceptable PDx   Manifestation   `H1`-`H14` HAC   `HCC` CMS-HCC Condition   `EXCLUDES 1` Not Coded Here   `EXCLUDES 2` Not Included Here

ICD-10-CM 2018   **495**

Chapter 2. Neoplasms (left margin)

D37.05 **Neoplasm of uncertain behavior of** pharynx
Neoplasm of uncertain behavior of aryepiglottic fold of pharynx NOS
Neoplasm of uncertain behavior of hypopharyngeal aspect of aryepiglottic fold of pharynx
Neoplasm of uncertain behavior of marginal zone of aryepiglottic fold of pharynx

D37.09 **Neoplasm of uncertain behavior of** other **specified sites of the oral cavity**

D37.1 **Neoplasm of uncertain behavior of** stomach

D37.2 **Neoplasm of uncertain behavior of** small intestine

D37.3 **Neoplasm of uncertain behavior of** appendix

D37.4 **Neoplasm of uncertain behavior of** colon

D37.5 **Neoplasm of uncertain behavior of** rectum
Neoplasm of uncertain behavior of rectosigmoid junction

D37.6 **Neoplasm of uncertain behavior of** liver, gallbladder and bile ducts
Neoplasm of uncertain behavior of ampulla of Vater

D37.8 **Neoplasm of uncertain behavior of** other **specified digestive organs**
Neoplasm of uncertain behavior of anal canal
Neoplasm of uncertain behavior of anal sphincter
Neoplasm of uncertain behavior of anus NOS
Neoplasm of uncertain behavior of esophagus
Neoplasm of uncertain behavior of intestine NOS
Neoplasm of uncertain behavior of pancreas
EXCLUDES 1 neoplasm of uncertain behavior of anal margin (D48.5)
neoplasm of uncertain behavior of anal skin (D48.5)
neoplasm of uncertain behavior of perianal skin (D48.5)

D37.9 **Neoplasm of uncertain behavior of digestive organ,** unspecified

✓4ᵗʰ **D38 Neoplasm of uncertain behavior of** middle ear and respiratory and intrathoracic organs
EXCLUDES 1 neoplasm of uncertain behavior of heart (D48.7)

D38.0 **Neoplasm of uncertain behavior of** larynx
Neoplasm of uncertain behavior of aryepiglottic fold or interarytenoid fold, laryngeal aspect
Neoplasm of uncertain behavior of epiglottis (suprahyoid portion)
EXCLUDES 1 neoplasm of uncertain behavior of aryepiglottic fold or interarytenoid fold NOS (D37.05)
neoplasm of uncertain behavior of hypopharyngeal aspect of aryepiglottic fold (D37.05)
neoplasm of uncertain behavior of marginal zone of aryepiglottic fold (D37.05)

D38.1 **Neoplasm of uncertain behavior of** trachea, bronchus and lung

D38.2 **Neoplasm of uncertain behavior of** pleura

D38.3 **Neoplasm of uncertain behavior of** mediastinum

D38.4 **Neoplasm of uncertain behavior of** thymus

D38.5 **Neoplasm of uncertain behavior of** other **respiratory organs**
Neoplasm of uncertain behavior of accessory sinuses
Neoplasm of uncertain behavior of cartilage of nose
Neoplasm of uncertain behavior of middle ear
Neoplasm of uncertain behavior of nasal cavities
EXCLUDES 1 neoplasm of uncertain behavior of ear (external) (skin) (D48.5)
neoplasm of uncertain behavior of nose NOS (D48.7)
neoplasm of uncertain behavior of skin of nose (D48.5)

D38.6 **Neoplasm of uncertain behavior of respiratory organ,** unspecified

✓4ᵗʰ **D39 Neoplasm of uncertain behavior of** female genital organs

D39.0 **Neoplasm of uncertain behavior of** uterus ♀

✓5ᵗʰ D39.1 **Neoplasm of uncertain behavior of** ovary ♀
Use additional code to identify any functional activity

D39.10 **Neoplasm of uncertain behavior of** unspecified ovary ♀

D39.11 **Neoplasm of uncertain behavior of** right ovary ♀

D39.12 **Neoplasm of uncertain behavior of** left ovary ♀

D39.2 **Neoplasm of uncertain behavior of** placenta Ⓜ♀
Chorioadenoma destruens
Invasive hydatidiform mole
Malignant hydatidiform mole
EXCLUDES 1 hydatidiform mole NOS (O01.9)

D39.8 **Neoplasm of uncertain behavior of** other specified female genital organs ♀
Neoplasm of uncertain behavior of skin of female genital organs

D39.9 **Neoplasm of uncertain behavior of female genital organ,** unspecified ♀

✓4ᵗʰ **D40 Neoplasm of uncertain behavior of** male genital organs

D40.0 **Neoplasm of uncertain behavior of** prostate ♂

✓5ᵗʰ D40.1 **Neoplasm of uncertain behavior of** testis ♂

D40.10 **Neoplasm of uncertain behavior of** unspecified testis ♂

D40.11 **Neoplasm of uncertain behavior of** right testis ♂

D40.12 **Neoplasm of uncertain behavior of** left testis ♂

D40.8 **Neoplasm of uncertain behavior of** other specified male genital organs ♂
Neoplasm of uncertain behavior of skin of male genital organs

D40.9 **Neoplasm of uncertain behavior of male genital organ,** unspecified ♂

✓4ᵗʰ **D41 Neoplasm of uncertain behavior of** urinary organs

✓5ᵗʰ D41.0 **Neoplasm of uncertain behavior of** kidney
EXCLUDES 1 neoplasm of uncertain behavior of renal pelvis (D41.1-)

D41.00 **Neoplasm of uncertain behavior of** unspecified kidney

D41.01 **Neoplasm of uncertain behavior of** right kidney

D41.02 **Neoplasm of uncertain behavior of** left kidney

✓5ᵗʰ D41.1 **Neoplasm of uncertain behavior of** renal pelvis

D41.10 **Neoplasm of uncertain behavior of** unspecified renal pelvis

D41.11 **Neoplasm of uncertain behavior of** right renal pelvis

D41.12 **Neoplasm of uncertain behavior of** left renal pelvis

✓5ᵗʰ D41.2 **Neoplasm of uncertain behavior of** ureter

D41.20 **Neoplasm of uncertain behavior of** unspecified ureter

D41.21 **Neoplasm of uncertain behavior of** right ureter

D41.22 **Neoplasm of uncertain behavior of** left ureter

D41.3 **Neoplasm of uncertain behavior of** urethra

D41.4 **Neoplasm of uncertain behavior of** bladder

D41.8 **Neoplasm of uncertain behavior of** other specified urinary organs

D41.9 **Neoplasm of uncertain behavior of** unspecified urinary organ

✓4ᵗʰ **D42 Neoplasm of uncertain behavior of** meninges

D42.0 **Neoplasm of uncertain behavior of** cerebral meninges HCC

D42.1 **Neoplasm of uncertain behavior of** spinal meninges HCC

D42.9 **Neoplasm of uncertain behavior of** meninges, unspecified HCC

✓4ᵗʰ **D43 Neoplasm of uncertain behavior of** brain and central nervous system
EXCLUDES 1 neoplasm of uncertain behavior of peripheral nerves and autonomic nervous system (D48.2)

D43.0 **Neoplasm of uncertain behavior of** brain, supratentorial HCC
Neoplasm of uncertain behavior of cerebral ventricle
Neoplasm of uncertain behavior of cerebrum
Neoplasm of uncertain behavior of frontal lobe
Neoplasm of uncertain behavior of occipital lobe
Neoplasm of uncertain behavior of parietal lobe
Neoplasm of uncertain behavior of temporal lobe
EXCLUDES 1 neoplasm of uncertain behavior of fourth ventricle (D43.1)

D43.1 **Neoplasm of uncertain behavior of** brain, infratentorial HCC
Neoplasm of uncertain behavior of brain stem
Neoplasm of uncertain behavior of cerebellum
Neoplasm of uncertain behavior of fourth ventricle

D43.2 **Neoplasm of uncertain behavior of** brain, unspecified HCC

D43.3 **Neoplasm of uncertain behavior of** cranial nerves HCC

D43.4 **Neoplasm of uncertain behavior of** spinal cord HCC

D43.8 **Neoplasm of uncertain behavior of** other specified parts of central nervous system HCC

D43.9 **Neoplasm of uncertain behavior of** central nervous system, unspecified HCC
Neoplasm of uncertain behavior of nervous system (central) NOS

Chapter 2. Neoplasms

✓4ᵗʰ **D44 Neoplasm of uncertain behavior of** endocrine glands

> EXCLUDES 1   *multiple endocrine adenomatosis (E31.2-)*
> *multiple endocrine neoplasia (E31.2-)*
> *neoplasm of uncertain behavior of endocrine pancreas (D37.8)*
> *neoplasm of uncertain behavior of ovary (D39.1-)*
> *neoplasm of uncertain behavior of testis (D40.1-)*
> *neoplasm of uncertain behavior of thymus (D38.4)*

   D44.0 Neoplasm of uncertain behavior of thyroid gland

✓5ᵗʰ **D44.1 Neoplasm of uncertain behavior of** adrenal gland
> Use additional code to identify any functional activity

     D44.10 Neoplasm of uncertain behavior of unspecified adrenal gland

     D44.11 Neoplasm of uncertain behavior of right adrenal gland

     D44.12 Neoplasm of uncertain behavior of left adrenal gland

   D44.2 Neoplasm of uncertain behavior of parathyroid gland

   D44.3 Neoplasm of uncertain behavior of pituitary gland   HCC
> Use additional code to identify any functional activity

   D44.4 Neoplasm of uncertain behavior of craniopharyngeal duct   HCC

   D44.5 Neoplasm of uncertain behavior of pineal gland   HCC

   D44.6 Neoplasm of uncertain behavior of carotid body   HCC

   D44.7 Neoplasm of uncertain behavior of aortic body and other paraganglia   HCC

   D44.9 Neoplasm of uncertain behavior of unspecified endocrine gland

D45 Polycythemia vera   HCC
> EXCLUDES 1   *familial polycythemia (D75.0)*
> *secondary polycythemia (D75.1)*
>
> **DEF:** Abnormal proliferation of all bone marrow elements, increased red cell mass, and total blood volume; unknown etiology, frequently associated with splenomegaly, leukocytosis, and thrombocythemia.

✓4ᵗʰ **D46 Myelodysplastic syndromes**
> Use additional code for adverse effect, if applicable, to identify drug (T36-T50 with fifth or sixth character 5)
> EXCLUDES 2   *drug-induced aplastic anemia (D61.1)*

   D46.0 Refractory anemia without ring sideroblasts, **so stated**   HCC
> Refractory anemia without sideroblasts, without excess of blasts

   D46.1 Refractory anemia with ring sideroblasts   HCC
> RARS

✓5ᵗʰ **D46.2 Refractory anemia** with excess of blasts [RAEB]

     D46.20 Refractory anemia with excess of blasts, unspecified   HCC
> RAEB NOS

     D46.21 Refractory anemia with excess of blasts 1   HCC
> RAEB 1

     D46.22 Refractory anemia with excess of blasts 2   CC HCC
> RAEB 2
> CC Excl: PDX collection 488

   D46.A Refractory cytopenia with multilineage dysplasia   HCC

   D46.B Refractory cytopenia with multilineage dysplasia and ring sideroblasts   HCC
> RCMD RS

   D46.C Myelodysplastic syndrome with isolated del(5q) chromosomal abnormality   CC HCC
> Myelodysplastic syndrome with 5q deletion
> 5q minus syndrome NOS
> CC Excl: PDX collection 488

   D46.4 Refractory anemia, unspecified   HCC

   D46.Z Other myelodysplastic syndromes   HCC
> EXCLUDES 1   *chronic myelomonocytic leukemia (C93.1-)*

   D46.9 Myelodysplastic syndrome, unspecified   HCC
> Myelodysplasia NOS

✓4ᵗʰ **D47 Other neoplasms of uncertain behavior of** lymphoid, hematopoietic and related tissue

> **CC Excl: For CC codes in category D47, unless otherwise noted:**
> PDX collection 488

▲   ✓5ᵗʰ **D47.0 Mast cell neoplasms of uncertain behavior**
> ~~Indolent systemic mastocytosis~~
> ~~Mast cell tumor NOS~~
> ~~Mastocytoma NOS~~
> EXCLUDES 1   ▶*congenital cutaneous mastocytosis (Q82.2-)*
> *histiocytic neoplasms of uncertain behavior (D47.Z9)*
> *malignant mast cell neoplasm (C96.2-)*◀
> ~~*mastocytosis (congenital) (cutaneous) (Q82.2)*~~

> **CC Excl: For codes in subcategory D47.0:**
> PDX collection 494

●   **D47.01 Cutaneous mastocytosis**   CC
> Diffuse cutaneous mastocytosis
> Maculopapular cutaneous mastocytosis
> Solitary mastocytoma
> Telangiectasia macularis eruptiva perstans
> Urticaria pigmentosa
> EXCLUDES 1   *congenital (diffuse) (maculopapular) cutaneous mastocytosis (Q82.2)*
> *congenital urticaria pigmentosa (Q82.2)*
> *extracutaneous mastocytoma (D47.09)*

●   **D47.02 Systemic mastocytosis**   CC
> Indolent systemic mastocytosis
> Isolated bone marrow mastocytosis
> Smoldering systemic mastocytosis
> Systemic mastocytosis, with an associated hematological non-mast cell lineage disease (SM-AHNMD)
> Code also, if applicable, any associated hematological non-mast cell lineage disease, such as:
> acute myeloid leukemia (C92.6-, C92.A-)
> chronic myelomonocytic leukemia (C93.1-)
> essential thrombocytosis (D47.3)
> hypereosinophilic syndrome (D72.1)
> myelodysplastic syndrome (D46.9)
> myeloproliferative syndrome (D47.1)
> non-Hodgkin lymphoma (C82-C85)
> plasma cell myeloma (C90.0-)
> polycythemia vera (D45)
> EXCLUDES 1   *aggressive systemic mastocytosis (C96.21)*
> *mast cell leukemia (C94.3-)*

●   **D47.09 Other mast cell neoplasms of uncertain behavior**   CC
> Extracutaneous mastocytoma
> Mast cell tumor NOS
> Mastocytoma NOS
> Mastocytosis NOS

   D47.1 Chronic myeloproliferative disease   CC HCC
> Chronic neutrophilic leukemia
> Myeloproliferative disease, unspecified
> EXCLUDES 1   *atypical chronic myeloid leukemia BCR/ABL-negative (C92.2-)*
> *chronic myeloid leukemia BCR/ABL-positive (C92.1-)*
> *myelofibrosis NOS (D75.81)*
> *myelophthisic anemia (D61.82)*
> *myelophthisis (D61.82)*
> *secondary myelofibrosis NOS (D75.81)*

   D47.2 Monoclonal gammopathy
> Monoclonal gammopathy of undetermined significance [MGUS]

   D47.3 Essential (hemorrhagic) thrombocythemia   HCC
> Essential thrombocytosis
> Idiopathic hemorrhagic thrombocythemia

   D47.4 Osteomyelofibrosis   HCC
> Chronic idiopathic myelofibrosis
> Myelofibrosis (idiopathic) (with myeloid metaplasia)
> Myelosclerosis (megakaryocytic) with myeloid metaplasia
> Secondary myelofibrosis in myeloproliferative disease
> EXCLUDES 1   *acute myelofibrosis (C94.4-)*

✓5ᵗʰ **D47.Z Other specified neoplasms of uncertain behavior of** lymphoid, hematopoietic and related tissue

     D47.Z1 Post-transplant lymphoproliferative disorder (PTLD)   CC HCC
> Code first complications of transplanted organs and tissue (T86.-)
> **DEF:** Excessive proliferation of B-cell lymphocytes following Epstein-Barr virus infection in organ transplant patients; may progress to non-Hodgkin lymphoma.
> CC Excl: PDX collection 495

☑ Additional Character Req   ✓x7ᵗʰ Placeholder Alert   Unacceptable PDx   Manifestation   H1 - H14 HAC   HCC CMS-HCC Condition   EXCLUDES 1 Not Coded Here   EXCLUDES 2 Not Included Here

ICD-10-CM 2018   **497**

    D47.Z2   **Castleman disease**   `CC` `HCC`
        Code also if applicable human herpesvirus 8 infection (B10.89)
        EXCLUDES 2   *Kaposi's sarcoma (C46-)*

    D47.Z9   **Other specified neoplasms of uncertain behavior of lymphoid, hematopoietic and related tissue**   `CC` `HCC`
        Histiocytic tumors of uncertain behavior

    D47.9   **Neoplasm of uncertain behavior of lymphoid, hematopoietic and related tissue, unspecified**   `CC` `HCC`
        Lymphoproliferative disease NOS

✓4th **D48**   **Neoplasm of uncertain behavior of other and unspecified sites**
    EXCLUDES 1   *neurofibromatosis (nonmalignant) (Q85.0-)*

    D48.0   **Neoplasm of uncertain behavior of bone and articular cartilage**
        EXCLUDES 1   *neoplasm of uncertain behavior of cartilage of ear (D48.1)*
                 neoplasm of uncertain behavior of cartilage of larynx (D38.0)
                 neoplasm of uncertain behavior of cartilage of nose (D38.5)
                 neoplasm of uncertain behavior of connective tissue of eyelid (D48.1)
                 neoplasm of uncertain behavior of synovia (D48.1)

    D48.1   **Neoplasm of uncertain behavior of connective and other soft tissue**
        Neoplasm of uncertain behavior of connective tissue of ear
        Neoplasm of uncertain behavior of connective tissue of eyelid
        Stromal tumors of uncertain behavior of digestive system
        EXCLUDES 1   *neoplasm of uncertain behavior of articular cartilage (D48.0)*
                 neoplasm of uncertain behavior of cartilage of larynx (D38.0)
                 neoplasm of uncertain behavior of cartilage of nose (D38.5)
                 neoplasm of uncertain behavior of connective tissue of breast (D48.6-)

    D48.2   **Neoplasm of uncertain behavior of peripheral nerves and autonomic nervous system**
        EXCLUDES 1   *neoplasm of uncertain behavior of peripheral nerves of orbit (D48.7)*

    D48.3   **Neoplasm of uncertain behavior of retroperitoneum**

    D48.4   **Neoplasm of uncertain behavior of peritoneum**

    D48.5   **Neoplasm of uncertain behavior of skin**
        Neoplasm of uncertain behavior of anal margin
        Neoplasm of uncertain behavior of anal skin
        Neoplasm of uncertain behavior of perianal skin
        Neoplasm of uncertain behavior of skin of breast
        EXCLUDES 1   *neoplasm of uncertain behavior of anus NOS (D37.8)*
                 neoplasm of uncertain behavior of skin of genital organs (D39.8, D40.8)
                 neoplasm of uncertain behavior of vermilion border of lip (D37.0)

✓5th **D48.6**   **Neoplasm of uncertain behavior of breast**
        Neoplasm of uncertain behavior of connective tissue of breast
        Cystosarcoma phyllodes
        EXCLUDES 1   *neoplasm of uncertain behavior of skin of breast (D48.5)*

        D48.60   **Neoplasm of uncertain behavior of unspecified breast**

        D48.61   **Neoplasm of uncertain behavior of right breast**

        D48.62   **Neoplasm of uncertain behavior of left breast**

    D48.7   **Neoplasm of uncertain behavior of other specified sites**
        Neoplasm of uncertain behavior of eye
        Neoplasm of uncertain behavior of heart
        Neoplasm of uncertain behavior of peripheral nerves of orbit
        EXCLUDES 1   *neoplasm of uncertain behavior of connective tissue (D48.1)*
                 neoplasm of uncertain behavior of skin of eyelid (D48.5)

    D48.9   **Neoplasm of uncertain behavior, unspecified**

Neoplasms of unspecified behavior (D49)

✓4th **D49**   **Neoplasms of unspecified behavior**
    `NOTE`   Category D49 classifies by site neoplasms of unspecified morphology and behavior. The term "mass", unless otherwise stated, is not to be regarded as a neoplastic growth.
    `INCLUDES`   "growth" NOS
                 neoplasm NOS
                 new growth NOS
                 tumor NOS
    EXCLUDES 1   *neoplasms of uncertain behavior (D37-D44, D48)*

    D49.0   **Neoplasm of unspecified behavior of digestive system**
        EXCLUDES 1   *neoplasm of unspecified behavior of margin of anus (D49.2)*
                 neoplasm of unspecified behavior of perianal skin (D49.2)
                 neoplasm of unspecified behavior of skin of anus (D49.2)

    D49.1   **Neoplasm of unspecified behavior of respiratory system**

    D49.2   **Neoplasm of unspecified behavior of bone, soft tissue, and skin**
        EXCLUDES 1   *neoplasm of unspecified behavior of anal canal (D49.0)*
                 neoplasm of unspecified behavior of anus NOS (D49.0)
                 neoplasm of unspecified behavior of bone marrow (D49.89)
                 neoplasm of unspecified behavior of cartilage of larynx (D49.1)
                 neoplasm of unspecified behavior of cartilage of nose (D49.1)
                 neoplasm of unspecified behavior of connective tissue of breast (D49.3)
                 neoplasm of unspecified behavior of skin of genital organs (D49.59)
                 neoplasm of unspecified behavior of vermilion border of lip (D49.0)

    D49.3   **Neoplasm of unspecified behavior of breast**
        EXCLUDES 1   *neoplasm of unspecified behavior of skin of breast (D49.2)*

    D49.4   **Neoplasm of unspecified behavior of bladder**

✓5th **D49.5**   **Neoplasm of unspecified behavior of other genitourinary organs**

    ✓6th **D49.51**   **Neoplasm of unspecified behavior of kidney**
        D49.511   **Neoplasm of unspecified behavior of right kidney**
        D49.512   **Neoplasm of unspecified behavior of left kidney**
        D49.519   **Neoplasm of unspecified behavior of unspecified kidney**

        D49.59   **Neoplasm of unspecified behavior of other genitourinary organ**

    D49.6   **Neoplasm of unspecified behavior of brain**   `HCC`
        EXCLUDES 1   *neoplasm of unspecified behavior of cerebral meninges (D49.7)*
                 neoplasm of unspecified behavior of cranial nerves (D49.7)

    D49.7   **Neoplasm of unspecified behavior of endocrine glands and other parts of nervous system**
        EXCLUDES 1   *neoplasm of unspecified behavior of peripheral, sympathetic, and parasympathetic nerves and ganglia (D49.2)*

✓5th **D49.8**   **Neoplasm of unspecified behavior of other specified sites**
        EXCLUDES 1   *neoplasm of unspecified behavior of eyelid (skin) (D49.2)*
                 neoplasm of unspecified behavior of eyelid cartilage (D49.2)
                 neoplasm of unspecified behavior of great vessels (D49.2)
                 neoplasm of unspecified behavior of optic nerve (D49.7)

        D49.81   **Neoplasm of unspecified behavior of retina and choroid**
                 Dark area on retina
                 Retinal freckle

        D49.89   **Neoplasm of unspecified behavior of other specified sites**

    D49.9   **Neoplasm of unspecified behavior of unspecified site**

Chapter 3. Diseases of the Blood and Blood-forming Organs and Certain Disorders Involving the Immune Mechanism (D5Ø–D89)

Chapter Specific Coding Guidelines and Examples
Reserved for future guideline expansion

Chapter 3. Diseases of the Blood and Blood-forming Organs and Certain Disorders Involving the Immune Mechanism (D50-D89)

> EXCLUDES 2   autoimmune disease (systemic) NOS (M35.9)
> certain conditions originating in the perinatal period (P00-P96)
> complications of pregnancy, childbirth and the puerperium (O00-O9A)
> congenital malformations, deformations and chromosomal abnormalities (Q00-Q99)
> endocrine, nutritional and metabolic diseases (E00-E88)
> human immunodeficiency virus [HIV] disease (B20)
> injury, poisoning and certain other consequences of external causes (S00-T88)
> neoplasms (C00-D49)
> symptoms, signs and abnormal clinical and laboratory findings, not elsewhere classified (R00-R94)

This chapter contains the following blocks:
D50-D53   Nutritional anemias
D55-D59   Hemolytic anemias
D60-D64   Aplastic and other anemias and other bone marrow failure syndromes
D65-D69   Coagulation defects, purpura and other hemorrhagic conditions
D70-D77   Other disorders of blood and blood-forming organs
D78   Intraoperative and postprocedural complications of the spleen
D80-D89   Certain disorders involving the immune mechanism

Nutritional anemias (D50-D53)

✓4ᵗʰ **D50   Iron deficiency anemia**
> INCLUDES   asiderotic anemia
> hypochromic anemia

D50.0   Iron deficiency anemia secondary to blood loss (chronic)
Posthemorrhagic anemia (chronic)
> EXCLUDES 1   acute posthemorrhagic anemia (D62)
> congenital anemia from fetal blood loss (P61.3)

D50.1   Sideropenic dysphagia
Kelly-Paterson syndrome   Plummer-Vinson syndrome

D50.8   Other iron deficiency anemias
Iron deficiency anemia due to inadequate dietary iron intake

D50.9   Iron deficiency anemia, unspecified

✓4ᵗʰ **D51   Vitamin B12 deficiency anemia**
> EXCLUDES 1   vitamin B12 deficiency (E53.8)

D51.0   Vitamin B12 deficiency anemia due to intrinsic factor deficiency
Addison anemia   Pernicious (congenital) anemia
Biermer anemia   Congenital intrinsic factor deficiency
DEF: Chronic progressive anemia due to vitamin B12 malabsorption; caused by lack of secretion of intrinsic factor, which is produced by the gastric mucosa of the stomach.

D51.1   Vitamin B12 deficiency anemia due to selective vitamin B12 malabsorption with proteinuria
Imerslund (Gräsbeck) syndrome
Megaloblastic hereditary anemia

D51.2   Transcobalamin II deficiency

D51.3   Other dietary vitamin B12 deficiency anemia
Vegan anemia

D51.8   Other vitamin B12 deficiency anemias

D51.9   Vitamin B12 deficiency anemia, unspecified

✓4ᵗʰ **D52   Folate deficiency anemia**
> EXCLUDES 1   folate deficiency without anemia (E53.8)

D52.0   Dietary folate deficiency anemia
Nutritional megaloblastic anemia
DEF: The result of a poor diet with inadequate intake of folate, which is needed to produce healthy red blood cells.

D52.1   Drug-induced folate deficiency anemia
Use additional code for adverse effect, if applicable, to identify drug (T36-T50 with fifth or sixth character 5)

D52.8   Other folate deficiency anemias

D52.9   Folate deficiency anemia, unspecified
Folic acid deficiency anemia NOS

✓4ᵗʰ **D53   Other nutritional anemias**
> INCLUDES   megaloblastic anemia unresponsive to vitamin B12 or folate therapy

D53.0   Protein deficiency anemia
Amino-acid deficiency anemia
Orotaciduric anemia
> EXCLUDES 1   Lesch-Nyhan syndrome (E79.1)

D53.1   Other megaloblastic anemias, not elsewhere classified
Megaloblastic anemia NOS
> EXCLUDES 1   Di Guglielmo's disease (C94.0)

D53.2   Scorbutic anemia
> EXCLUDES 1   scurvy (E54)

D53.8   Other specified nutritional anemias
Anemia associated with deficiency of copper
Anemia associated with deficiency of molybdenum
Anemia associated with deficiency of zinc
> EXCLUDES 1   nutritional deficiencies without anemia, such as:
> copper deficiency NOS (E61.0)
> molybdenum deficiency NOS (E61.5)
> zinc deficiency NOS (E60)

D53.9   Nutritional anemia, unspecified
Simple chronic anemia
> EXCLUDES 1   anemia NOS (D64.9)

Hemolytic anemias (D55-D59)

✓4ᵗʰ **D55   Anemia due to enzyme disorders**
> EXCLUDES 1   drug-induced enzyme deficiency anemia (D59.2)

D55.0   Anemia due to glucose-6-phosphate dehydrogenase [G6PD] deficiency   HCC
Favism
G6PD deficiency anemia

D55.1   Anemia due to other disorders of glutathione metabolism   HCC
Anemia (due to) enzyme deficiencies, except G6PD, related to the hexose monophosphate [HMP] shunt pathway
Anemia (due to) hemolytic nonspherocytic (hereditary), type I

D55.2   Anemia due to disorders of glycolytic enzymes   HCC
Hemolytic nonspherocytic (hereditary) anemia, type II
Hexokinase deficiency anemia
Pyruvate kinase [PK] deficiency anemia
Triose-phosphate isomerase deficiency anemia
> EXCLUDES 1   disorders of glycolysis not associated with anemia (E74.8)

D55.3   Anemia due to disorders of nucleotide metabolism   HCC

D55.8   Other anemias due to enzyme disorders   HCC

D55.9   Anemia due to enzyme disorder, unspecified   HCC

✓4ᵗʰ **D56   Thalassemia**
> EXCLUDES 1   sickle-cell thalassemia (D57.4-)

D56.0   Alpha thalassemia   HCC
Alpha thalassemia major
Hemoglobin H Constant Spring
Hemoglobin H disease
Hydrops fetalis due to alpha thalassemia
Severe alpha thalassemia
Triple gene defect alpha thalassemia
Use additional code, if applicable, for hydrops fetalis due to alpha thalassemia (P56.99)
> EXCLUDES 1   alpha thalassemia trait or minor (D56.3)
> asymptomatic alpha thalassemia (D56.3)
> hydrops fetalis due to isoimmunization (P56.0)
> hydrops fetalis not due to immune hemolysis (P83.2)
DEF: HBA1 and HBA2 genetic variant of chromosome 16 prevalent among those of African and Southeast Asian descent; associated with a wide spectrum of anemic presentation; includes hemoglobin H disease subtypes.

Thalassemia

Misshapen RBC

Misshapen RBC

Healthy RBC

N Newborn: 0   P Pediatric: 0-17   M Maternity: 12-55   A Adult: 15-124   MCC Major CC Condition   PDxMCC PDx acts as own MCC   CC CC Condition   PDxCC PDx acts as own CC

500   ICD-10-CM 2018

D56.1 Beta thalassemia `HCC`
  Beta thalassemia major   Severe beta thalassemia
  Cooley's anemia   Thalassemia intermedia
  Homozygous beta thalassemia   Thalassemia major
  EXCLUDES 1   beta thalassemia minor (D56.3)
           beta thalassemia trait (D56.3)
           delta-beta thalassemia (D56.2)
           hemoglobin E-beta thalassemia (D56.5)
           sickle-cell beta thalassemia (D57.4-)

D56.2 Delta-beta thalassemia `HCC`
  Homozygous delta-beta thalassemia
  EXCLUDES 1   delta-beta thalassemia minor (D56.3)
           delta-beta thalassemia trait (D56.3)

D56.3 Thalassemia minor
  Alpha thalassemia minor
  Alpha thalassemia silent carrier
  Alpha thalassemia trait
  Beta thalassemia minor
  Beta thalassemia trait
  Delta-beta thalassemia minor
  Delta-beta thalassemia trait
  Thalassemia trait NOS
  EXCLUDES 1   alpha thalassemia (D56.0)
           beta thalassemia (D56.1)
           delta-beta thalassemia (D56.2)
           hemoglobin E-beta thalassemia (D56.5)
           sickle-cell trait (D57.3)
  DEF: Solitary abnormal gene that identifies a carrier of the disease, yet with an absence of symptoms or a clinically mild anemic presentation.

D56.4 Hereditary persistence of fetal hemoglobin [HPFH] `HCC`

D56.5 Hemoglobin E-beta thalassemia `HCC`
  EXCLUDES 1   beta thalassemia (D56.1)
           beta thalassemia minor (D56.3)
           beta thalassemia trait (D56.3)
           delta-beta thalassemia (D56.2)
           delta-beta thalassemia trait (D56.3)
           hemoglobin E disease (D58.2)
           other hemoglobinopathies (D58.2)
           sickle-cell beta thalassemia (D57.4-)

D56.8 Other thalassemias `HCC`
  Dominant thalassemia
  Hemoglobin C thalassemia
  Mixed thalassemia
  Thalassemia with other hemoglobinopathy
  EXCLUDES 1   hemoglobin C disease (D58.2)
           hemoglobin E disease (D58.2)
           other hemoglobinopathies (D58.2)
           sickle-cell anemia (D57.-)
           sickle-cell thalassemia (D57.4)

D56.9 Thalassemia, unspecified
  Mediterranean anemia (with other hemoglobinopathy)

☑4th D57 Sickle-cell disorders
  Use additional code for any associated fever (R50.81)
  EXCLUDES 1   other hemoglobinopathies (D58.-)

  CC Excl: For MCC codes in category D57: PDX collection 496

  ☑5th D57.0 Hb-SS disease with crisis
  Sickle-cell disease NOS with crisis
  Hb-SS disease with vasoocclusive pain

  D57.00 Hb-SS disease with crisis, unspecified `MCC` `HCC`
  D57.01 Hb-SS disease with acute chest syndrome `MCC` `HCC`
  D57.02 Hb-SS disease with splenic sequestration `MCC` `HCC`

Sickle cell

Sickle cells

Normal RBCs

D57.1 Sickle-cell disease without crisis `HCC`
  Hb-SS disease without crisis
  Sickle-cell anemia NOS
  Sickle-cell disease NOS
  Sickle-cell disorder NOS

☑5th D57.2 Sickle-cell/Hb-C disease
  Hb-SC disease
  Hb-S/Hb-C disease

  D57.20 Sickle-cell/Hb-C disease without crisis `HCC`
  ☑6th D57.21 Sickle-cell/Hb-C disease with crisis
       D57.211 Sickle-cell/Hb-C disease with acute chest syndrome `PDxCC` `MCC` `HCC`
       D57.212 Sickle-cell/Hb-C disease with splenic sequestration `MCC` `HCC`
       D57.219 Sickle-cell/Hb-C disease with crisis, unspecified `MCC` `HCC`
           Sickle-cell/Hb-C disease with crisis NOS

D57.3 Sickle-cell trait `HCC`
  Hb-S trait
  Heterozygous hemoglobin S
  DEF: Heterozygous genetic makeup characterized by one gene for normal hemoglobin and one for sickle-cell hemoglobin; clinical disease rarely present.

☑5th D57.4 Sickle-cell thalassemia
  Sickle-cell beta thalassemia
  Thalassemia Hb-S disease

  D57.40 Sickle-cell thalassemia without crisis `HCC`
       Microdrepanocytosis
       Sickle-cell thalassemia NOS
  ☑6th D57.41 Sickle-cell thalassemia with crisis
       Sickle-cell thalassemia with vasoocclusive pain
       D57.411 Sickle-cell thalassemia with acute chest syndrome `PDxCC` `MCC` `HCC`
       D57.412 Sickle-cell thalassemia with splenic sequestration `MCC` `HCC`
       D57.419 Sickle-cell thalassemia with crisis, unspecified `MCC` `HCC`
           Sickle-cell thalassemia with crisis NOS

☑5th D57.8 Other sickle-cell disorders
  Hb-SD disease
  Hb-SE disease

  D57.80 Other sickle-cell disorders without crisis `HCC`
  ☑6th D57.81 Other sickle-cell disorders with crisis
       D57.811 Other sickle-cell disorders with acute chest syndrome `MCC` `HCC`
       D57.812 Other sickle-cell disorders with splenic sequestration `MCC` `HCC`
       D57.819 Other sickle-cell disorders with crisis, unspecified `MCC` `HCC`
           Other sickle-cell disorders with crisis NOS

☑4th D58 Other hereditary hemolytic anemias
  EXCLUDES 1   hemolytic anemia of the newborn (P55.-)

D58.0 Hereditary spherocytosis `HCC`
  Acholuric (familial) jaundice
  Congenital (spherocytic) hemolytic icterus
  Minkowski-Chauffard syndrome

D58.1 Hereditary elliptocytosis `HCC`
  Elliptocytosis (congenital)
  Ovalocytosis (congenital) (hereditary)

D58.2 Other hemoglobinopathies `HCC`
  Abnormal hemoglobin NOS
  Congenital Heinz body anemia
  Hb-C disease
  Hb-D disease
  Hb-E disease
  Hemoglobinopathy NOS
  Unstable hemoglobin hemolytic disease
  EXCLUDES 1   familial polycythemia (D75.0)
           Hb-M disease (D74.0)
           hemoglobin E-beta thalassemia (D56.5)
           hereditary persistence of fetal hemoglobin [HPFH] (D56.4)
           high-altitude polycythemia (D75.1)
           methemoglobinemia (D74.-)
           other hemoglobinopathies with thalassemia (D56.8)

D58.8 Other specified hereditary hemolytic anemias `CC` `HCC`
  Stomatocytosis
  CC Excl: PDX collection 497

D58.9 Hereditary hemolytic anemia, unspecified `CC` `HCC`
  CC Excl: PDX collection 497

☑ Additional Character Req   √x7th Placeholder Alert   Unacceptable PDx   Manifestation   `H1`-`H14` HAC   `HCC` CMS-HCC Condition   *EXCLUDES 1* Not Coded Here   *EXCLUDES 2* Not Included Here

✓4ᵗʰ **D59** **Acquired hemolytic anemia**

DEF: Non-hereditary anemia characterized by premature destruction of red blood cells; caused by infectious organisms, poisons, and physical agents.

> **CC Excl: For CC/MCC codes in category D59, unless otherwise noted:** PDX collection 496

D59.0 **Drug-induced autoimmune hemolytic anemia** `CC` `HCC`
> Use additional code for adverse effect, if applicable, to identify drug (T36-T50 with fifth or sixth character 5)

D59.1 **Other autoimmune hemolytic anemias** `CC` `HCC`
> Autoimmune hemolytic disease (cold type) (warm type)
> Chronic cold hemagglutinin disease
> Cold agglutinin disease
> Cold agglutinin hemoglobinuria
> Cold type (secondary) (symptomatic) hemolytic anemia
> Warm type (secondary) (symptomatic) hemolytic anemia
> *EXCLUDES 1*   Evans syndrome (D69.41)
>   hemolytic disease of newborn (P55.-)
>   paroxysmal cold hemoglobinuria (D59.6)

D59.2 **Drug-induced nonautoimmune hemolytic anemia** `CC` `HCC`
> Drug-induced enzyme deficiency anemia
> Use additional code for adverse effect, if applicable, to identify drug (T36-T50 with fifth or sixth character 5)

D59.3 **Hemolytic-uremic syndrome** `MCC` `HCC`
> Use additional code to identify associated:
>   E. coli infection (B96.2-)
>   Pneumococcal pneumonia (J13)
>   Shigella dysenteriae (A03.9)

D59.4 **Other nonautoimmune hemolytic anemias** `CC` `HCC`
> Mechanical hemolytic anemia
> Microangiopathic hemolytic anemia
> Toxic hemolytic anemia

D59.5 **Paroxysmal nocturnal hemoglobinuria** `HCC`
[Marchiafava-Micheli]
> *EXCLUDES 1*   hemoglobinuria NOS (R82.3)

D59.6 **Hemoglobinuria due to hemolysis from other external** `HCC`
causes
> Hemoglobinuria from exertion
> March hemoglobinuria
> Paroxysmal cold hemoglobinuria
> Use additional code (Chapter 20) to identify external cause
> *EXCLUDES 1*   hemoglobinuria NOS (R82.3)

D59.8 **Other acquired hemolytic anemias** `HCC`

D59.9 **Acquired hemolytic anemia, unspecified** `CC` `HCC`
> Idiopathic hemolytic anemia, chronic

Aplastic and other anemias and other bone marrow failure syndromes (D60-D64)

✓4ᵗʰ **D60** **Acquired pure red cell aplasia [erythroblastopenia]**
> *INCLUDES*   red cell aplasia (acquired) (adult) (with thymoma)
> *EXCLUDES 1*   congenital red cell aplasia (D61.01)

> **CC Excl: For MCC codes in category D60:** PDX collection 496

D60.0 **Chronic acquired pure red cell aplasia** `MCC` `HCC`

D60.1 **Transient acquired pure red cell aplasia** `MCC` `HCC`

D60.8 **Other acquired pure red cell aplasias** `MCC` `HCC`

D60.9 **Acquired pure red cell aplasia, unspecified** `MCC` `HCC`

✓4ᵗʰ **D61** **Other aplastic anemias and other bone marrow failure syndromes**
> *EXCLUDES 1*   neutropenia (D70.-)
> **AHA:** 2014, 4Q, 22

✓5ᵗʰ **D61.0** **Constitutional aplastic anemia**

    D61.01 **Constitutional (pure) red blood cell aplasia** `CC` `HCC`
> Blackfan-Diamond syndrome
> Congenital (pure) red cell aplasia
> Familial hypoplastic anemia
> Primary (pure) red cell aplasia
> Red cell (pure) aplasia of infants
> *EXCLUDES 1*   acquired red cell aplasia (D60.9)
> **CC Excl:** PDX collection 498

    D61.09 **Other constitutional aplastic anemia** `CC` `HCC`
> Fanconi's anemia
> Pancytopenia with malformations
> **CC Excl:** PDX collection 499

D61.1 **Drug-induced aplastic anemia** `MCC` `HCC`
> Use additional code for adverse effect, if applicable, to identify drug (T36-T50 with fifth or sixth character 5)
> **CC Excl:** PDX collection 496

D61.2 **Aplastic anemia due to other external agents** `MCC` `HCC`
> Code first, if applicable, toxic effects of substances chiefly nonmedicinal as to source (T51-T65)
> **CC Excl:** PDX collection 496

D61.3 **Idiopathic aplastic anemia** `MCC` `HCC`
> **CC Excl:** PDX collection 496

✓5ᵗʰ **D61.8** **Other specified aplastic anemias and other bone marrow failure syndromes**

> **CC Excl: For CC/MCC codes in subcategory D61.8:** PDX collection 500

    ✓6ᵗʰ **D61.81** **Pancytopenia**
> *EXCLUDES 1*   pancytopenia (due to) (with) aplastic anemia (D61.9)
>   pancytopenia (due to) (with) bone marrow infiltration (D61.82)
>   pancytopenia (due to) (with) congenital (pure) red cell aplasia (D61.01)
>   pancytopenia (due to) (with) hairy cell leukemia (C91.4-)
>   pancytopenia (due to) (with) human immunodeficiency virus disease (B20)
>   pancytopenia (due to) (with) leukoerythroblastic anemia (D61.82)
>   pancytopenia (due to) (with) myeloproliferative disease (D47.1)
> *EXCLUDES 2*   pancytopenia (due to) (with) myelodysplastic syndromes (D46.-)
> **DEF:** Occurs when a person has a shortage of all three blood cells: white, red, and platelets.

      D61.810 **Antineoplastic chemotherapy** `MCC` `HCC`
induced pancytopenia
> *EXCLUDES 2*   aplastic anemia due to antineoplastic chemotherapy (D61.1)

      D61.811 **Other drug-induced pancytopenia** `MCC` `HCC`
> *EXCLUDES 2*   aplastic anemia due to drugs (D61.1)

      D61.818 **Other pancytopenia** `CC` `HCC`

    D61.82 **Myelophthisis**
> Leukoerythroblastic anemia
> Myelophthisic anemia
> Panmyelophthisis
> Code also the underlying disorder, such as:
>   malignant neoplasm of breast (C50.-)
>   tuberculosis (A15.-)
> *EXCLUDES 1*   idiopathic myelofibrosis (D47.1)
>   myelofibrosis NOS (D75.81)
>   myelofibrosis with myeloid metaplasia (D47.4)
>   primary myelofibrosis (D47.1)
>   secondary myelofibrosis (D75.81)

    D61.89 **Other specified aplastic anemias and other** `MCC` `HCC`
bone marrow failure syndromes
> **CC Excl:** PDX collection 496

D61.9 **Aplastic anemia, unspecified** `CC` `HCC`
> Hypoplastic anemia NOS
> Medullary hypoplasia
> **CC Excl:** PDX collection 496

D62 **Acute posthemorrhagic anemia** `CC`
> *EXCLUDES 1*   anemia due to chronic blood loss (D50.0)
>   blood loss anemia NOS (D50.0)
>   congenital anemia from fetal blood loss (P61.3)
> **CC Excl:** PDX collection 501

✓4ᵗʰ **D63** **Anemia in chronic diseases classified elsewhere**

D63.0 *Anemia in neoplastic disease*
> Code first neoplasm (C00-D49)
> *EXCLUDES 1*   ~~anemia due to antineoplastic chemotherapy (D64.81)~~
>   aplastic anemia due to antineoplastic chemotherapy (D61.1)
> *EXCLUDES 2*   ▶anemia due to antineoplastic chemotherapy (D64.81)◀

D63.1 *Anemia in chronic kidney disease*
> Erythropoietin resistant anemia (EPO resistant anemia)
> Code first underlying chronic kidney disease (CKD) (N18.-)

N Newborn: 0   **P** Pediatric: 0-17   **M** Maternity: 12-55   **A** Adult: 15-124   **MCC** Major CC Condition   **PDxMCC** PDx acts as own MCC   **CC** CC Condition   **PDxCC** PDx acts as own CC

502   ICD-10-CM 2018

D63.8 **Anemia in** *other chronic diseases classified elsewhere*
Code first underlying disease, such as:
    diphyllobothriasis (B70.0)
    hookworm disease (B76.0-B76.9)
    hypothyroidism (E00.0-E03.9)
    malaria (B50.0-B54)
    symptomatic late syphilis (A52.79)
    tuberculosis (A18.89)

✅4ᵗʰ **D64 Other anemias**
> EXCLUDES 1   refractory anemia (D46.-)
>   refractory anemia with excess blasts in transformation
>   [RAEB T] (C92.0-)

D64.0 Hereditary sideroblastic anemia   HCC
    Sex-linked hypochromic sideroblastic anemia

D64.1 Secondary sideroblastic anemia due to disease   HCC
    Code first underlying disease

D64.2 Secondary sideroblastic anemia due to drugs and toxins   HCC
    Code first poisoning due to drug or toxin, if applicable (T36-T65
      with fifth or sixth character 1-4 or 6)
    Use additional code for adverse effect, if applicable, to identify
      drug (T36-T50 with fifth or sixth character 5)

D64.3 Other sideroblastic anemias   HCC
    Sideroblastic anemia NOS
    Pyridoxine-responsive sideroblastic anemia NEC

D64.4 Congenital dyserythropoietic anemia
    Dyshematopoietic anemia (congenital)
> EXCLUDES 1   Blackfan-Diamond syndrome (D61.01)
>   Di Guglielmo's disease (C94.0)

✅5ᵗʰ **D64.8 Other specified anemias**

    D64.81 Anemia due to antineoplastic chemotherapy
        Antineoplastic chemotherapy induced anemia
>   EXCLUDES 1   aplastic anemia due to antineoplastic
>   chemotherapy (D61.1)
>   EXCLUDES 2   anemia in neoplastic disease (D63.0)
        AHA: 2014, 4Q, 22
        DEF: Reversible adverse effect of chemotherapy,
        causing inhibition of bone marrow production; decrease
        in red blood cell production prevents adequate
        oxygenation of the tissues and organs causing fatigue,
        SOB, and exacerbation of other medical conditions.

    D64.89 Other specified anemias
        Infantile pseudoleukemia

D64.9 Anemia, unspecified
    AHA: 2017, 1Q, 7

Coagulation defects, purpura and other hemorrhagic conditions (D65-D69)

D65 Disseminated intravascular coagulation [defibrination   MCC HCC
syndrome]
    Afibrinogenemia, acquired
    Consumption coagulopathy
    Diffuse or disseminated intravascular coagulation [DIC]
    Fibrinolytic hemorrhage, acquired
    Fibrinolytic purpura
    Purpura fulminans
> EXCLUDES 1   disseminated intravascular coagulation (complicating):
>   abortion or ectopic or molar pregnancy (O00-O07, O08.1)
>   in newborn (P60)
>   pregnancy, childbirth and the puerperium (O45.0, O46.0,
>   O67.0, O72.3)
    CC Excl: PDX collection 502

D66 Hereditary factor VIII deficiency   MCC HCC
    Classical hemophilia
    Deficiency factor VIII (with functional defect)
    Hemophilia A
    Hemophilia NOS
> EXCLUDES 1   factor VIII deficiency with vascular defect (D68.0)
    DEF: Hereditary, sex-linked lack of antihemophilic globulin (AHG) (factor
    VIII); causes abnormal coagulation characterized by increased bleeding,
    large bruises of skin, bleeding in mouth, nose, gastrointestinal tract;
    hemorrhages into joints, resulting in swelling and impaired function.
    CC Excl: PDX collection 502

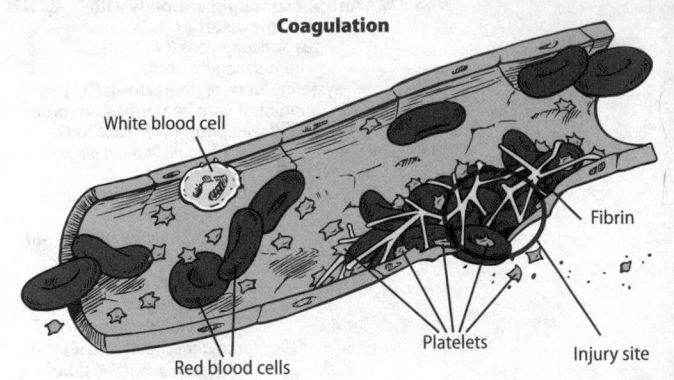

Coagulation

White blood cell

Fibrin

Platelets

Injury site

Red blood cells

D67 Hereditary factor IX deficiency   MCC HCC
    Christmas disease
    Factor IX deficiency (with functional defect)
    Hemophilia B
    Plasma thromboplastin component [PTC] deficiency
    CC Excl: PDX collection 502

✅4ᵗʰ **D68 Other coagulation defects**
> EXCLUDES 1   abnormal coagulation profile (R79.1)
>   coagulation defects complicating abortion or ectopic or molar
>   pregnancy (O00-O07, O08.1)
>   coagulation defects complicating pregnancy, childbirth and the
>   puerperium (O45.0, O46.0, O67.0, O72.3)
    AHA: 2016, 1Q, 14

> **CC Excl: For CC codes in category D68, unless otherwise noted:**
> PDX collection 502

D68.0 Von Willebrand's disease   CC HCC
    Angiohemophilia
    Factor VIII deficiency with vascular defect
    Vascular hemophilia
> EXCLUDES 1   capillary fragility (hereditary) (D69.8)
>   factor VIII deficiency NOS (D66)
>   factor VIII deficiency with functional defect (D66)
    DEF: Abnormal blood coagulation caused by deficient blood
    factor VII; congenital; symptoms include excess or prolonged
    bleeding.

D68.1 Hereditary factor XI deficiency   CC HCC
    Hemophilia C
    Plasma thromboplastin antecedent [PTA] deficiency
    Rosenthal's disease

D68.2 Hereditary deficiency of other clotting factors   CC HCC
    AC globulin deficiency
    Congenital afibrinogenemia
    Deficiency of factor I [fibrinogen]
    Deficiency of factor II [prothrombin]
    Deficiency of factor V [labile]
    Deficiency of factor VII [stable]
    Deficiency of factor X [Stuart-Prower]
    Deficiency of factor XII [Hageman]
    Deficiency of factor XIII [fibrin stabilizing]
    Dysfibrinogenemia (congenital)
    Hypoproconvertinemia
    Owren's disease
    Proaccelerin deficiency

✅5ᵗʰ **D68.3 Hemorrhagic disorder due to circulating anticoagulants**

    ✅6ᵗʰ **D68.31 Hemorrhagic disorder due to intrinsic circulating**
        anticoagulants, antibodies, or inhibitors

        D68.311 Acquired hemophilia   CC HCC
            Autoimmune hemophilia
            Autoimmune inhibitors to clotting factors
            Secondary hemophilia
            CC Excl: PDX collection 503

✅Additional Character Req   ✅x7ᵗʰ Placeholder Alert   Unacceptable PDx   Manifestation   H1 - H14 HAC   HCC CMS-HCC Condition   EXCLUDES 1 Not Coded Here   EXCLUDES 2 Not Included Here

D68.312 Antiphospholipid antibody with hemorrhagic disorder `CC` `HCC`
Lupus anticoagulant (LAC) with hemorrhagic disorder
Systemic lupus erythematosus [SLE] inhibitor with hemorrhagic disorder
EXCLUDES 1   *antiphospholipid antibody, finding without diagnosis (R76.0)*
antiphospholipid antibody syndrome (D68.61)
antiphospholipid antibody with hypercoagulable state (D68.61)
lupus anticoagulant (LAC) finding without diagnosis (R76.0)
lupus anticoagulant (LAC) with hypercoagulable state (D68.62)
systemic lupus erythematosus [SLE] inhibitor finding without diagnosis (R76.0)
systemic lupus erythematosus [SLE] inhibitor with hypercoagulable state (D68.62)
CC Excl: PDX collection 504

D68.318 Other hemorrhagic disorder due to `CC` `HCC` **intrinsic circulating anticoagulants, antibodies, or inhibitors**
Antithromboplastinemia
Antithromboplastinogenemia
Hemorrhagic disorder due to intrinsic increase in antithrombin
Hemorrhagic disorder due to intrinsic increase in anti-VIIIa
Hemorrhagic disorder due to intrinsic increase in anti-IXa
Hemorrhagic disorder due to intrinsic increase in anti-XIa
CC Excl: PDX collection 503

D68.32 Hemorrhagic disorder due to extrinsic `CC` `HCC` **circulating anticoagulants**
Drug-induced hemorrhagic disorder
Hemorrhagic disorder due to increase in anti-IIa
Hemorrhagic disorder due to increase in anti-Xa
Hyperheparinemia
Use additional code for adverse effect, if applicable, to identify drug (T45.515, T45.525)
AHA: 2016, 1Q, 14-15

D68.4 Acquired coagulation factor deficiency `CC` `HCC`
Deficiency of coagulation factor due to liver disease
Deficiency of coagulation factor due to vitamin K deficiency
EXCLUDES 1   *vitamin K deficiency of newborn (P53)*

✓5ᵗʰ **D68.5 Primary thrombophilia**
Primary hypercoagulable states
EXCLUDES 1   *antiphospholipid syndrome (D68.61)*
lupus anticoagulant (D68.62)
secondary activated protein C resistance (D68.69)
secondary antiphospholipid antibody syndrome (D68.69)
secondary lupus anticoagulant with hypercoagulable state (D68.69)
secondary systemic lupus erythematosus [SLE] inhibitor with hypercoagulable state (D68.69)
systemic lupus erythematosus [SLE] inhibitor finding without diagnosis (R76.0)
systemic lupus erythematosus [SLE] inhibitor with hemorrhagic disorder (D68.312)
thrombotic thrombocytopenic purpura (M31.1)

CC Excl: For CC codes in subcategory D68.5: PDX collection 505

D68.51 Activated protein C resistance `CC` `HCC`
Factor V Leiden mutation

D68.52 Prothrombin gene mutation `CC` `HCC`

D68.59 Other primary thrombophilia `CC` `HCC`
Antithrombin III deficiency
Hypercoagulable state NOS
Primary hypercoagulable state NEC
Primary thrombophilia NEC
Protein C deficiency
Protein S deficiency
Thrombophilia NOS

✓5ᵗʰ **D68.6 Other thrombophilia**
Other hypercoagulable states
EXCLUDES 1   *diffuse or disseminated intravascular coagulation [DIC] (D65)*
heparin induced thrombocytopenia (HIT) (D75.82)
hyperhomocysteinemia (E72.11)

CC Excl: For CC codes in subcategory D68.6: PDX collection 505

D68.61 Antiphospholipid syndrome `CC` `HCC`
Anticardiolipin syndrome
Antiphospholipid antibody syndrome
EXCLUDES 1   *antiphospholipid antibody, finding without diagnosis (R76.0)*
antiphospholipid antibody with hemorrhagic disorder (D68.312)
lupus anticoagulant syndrome (D68.62)

D68.62 Lupus anticoagulant syndrome `CC` `HCC`
Lupus anticoagulant
Presence of systemic lupus erythematosus [SLE] inhibitor
EXCLUDES 1   *anticardiolipin syndrome (D68.61)*
antiphospholipid syndrome (D68.61)
lupus anticoagulant (LAC) finding without diagnosis (R76.0)
lupus anticoagulant (LAC) with hemorrhagic disorder (D68.312)

D68.69 Other thrombophilia `CC` `HCC`
Hypercoagulable states NEC
Secondary hypercoagulable state NOS

D68.8 Other specified coagulation defects `CC` `HCC`
EXCLUDES 1   *hemorrhagic disease of newborn (P53)*

D68.9 Coagulation defect, unspecified `CC` `HCC`

✓4ᵗʰ **D69 Purpura and other hemorrhagic conditions**
EXCLUDES 1   *benign hypergammaglobulinemic purpura (D89.0)*
cryoglobulinemic purpura (D89.1)
essential (hemorrhagic) thrombocythemia (D47.3)
hemorrhagic thrombocythemia (D47.3)
purpura fulminans (D65)
thrombotic thrombocytopenic purpura (M31.1)
Waldenström hypergammaglobulinemic purpura (D89.0)

CC Excl: For CC codes in category D69: PDX collection 502

D69.0 Allergic purpura `CC` `HCC`
Allergic vasculitis
Nonthrombocytopenic hemorrhagic purpura
Nonthrombocytopenic idiopathic purpura
Purpura anaphylactoid
Purpura Henoch(-Schönlein)
Purpura rheumatica
Vascular purpura
EXCLUDES 1   *thrombocytopenic hemorrhagic purpura (D69.3)*
DEF: Any hemorrhagic condition, thrombocytic or nonthrombocytopenic in origin, caused by a presumed allergic reaction.

D69.1 Qualitative platelet defects `HCC`
Bernard-Soulier [giant platelet] syndrome
Glanzmann's disease
Grey platelet syndrome
Thromboasthenia (hemorrhagic) (hereditary)
Thrombocytopathy
EXCLUDES 1   *von Willebrand's disease (D68.0)*

D69.2 Other nonthrombocytopenic purpura `HCC`
Purpura NOS
Purpura simplex
Senile purpura

D69.3 Immune thrombocytopenic purpura `CC` `HCC`
Hemorrhagic (thrombocytopenic) purpura
Idiopathic thrombocytopenic purpura
Tidal platelet dysgenesis
DEF: Tidal platelet dysgenesis: Platelet counts fluctuate from normal to very low within periods of 20 to 40 days and may involve autoimmune platelet destruction.

✓5ᵗʰ **D69.4 Other primary thrombocytopenia**
EXCLUDES 1   *transient neonatal thrombocytopenia (P61.0)*
Wiskott-Aldrich syndrome (D82.0)

D69.41 Evans syndrome `CC` `HCC`

N Newborn: 0   P Pediatric: 0-17   M Maternity: 12-55   A Adult: 15-124   `MCC` Major CC Condition   `PDxMCC` PDx acts as own MCC   `CC` CC Condition   `PDxCC` PDx acts as own CC

D69.42 **Congenital and hereditary thrombocytopenia purpura** `CC` `HCC`
Congenital thrombocytopenia
Hereditary thrombocytopenia
Code first congenital or hereditary disorder, such as:
thrombocytopenia with absent radius (TAR syndrome) (Q87.2)

D69.49 **Other primary thrombocytopenia** `HCC`
Megakaryocytic hypoplasia
Primary thrombocytopenia NOS

✓5ᵗʰ **D69.5** **Secondary thrombocytopenia**
EXCLUDES 1   *heparin induced thrombocytopenia (HIT) (D75.82)*
transient thrombocytopenia of newborn (P61.0)

D69.51 **Posttransfusion purpura**
Posttransfusion purpura from whole blood (fresh) or blood products
PTP

D69.59 **Other secondary thrombocytopenia**
AHA: 2014, 4Q, 22

D69.6 **Thrombocytopenia, unspecified** `HCC`

D69.8 **Other specified hemorrhagic conditions** `HCC`
Capillary fragility (hereditary)
Vascular pseudohemophilia

D69.9 **Hemorrhagic condition, unspecified** `HCC`

Other disorders of blood and blood-forming organs (D70-D77)

✓4ᵗʰ **D70** **Neutropenia**
`INCLUDES`   agranulocytosis
decreased absolute neurophile count (ANC)
Use additional code for any associated:
fever (R50.81)
mucositis (J34.81, K12.3-, K92.81, N76.81)
EXCLUDES 1   *neutropenic splenomegaly (D73.81)*
transient neonatal neutropenia (P61.5)

D70.0 **Congenital agranulocytosis** `HCC`
Congenital neutropenia
Infantile genetic agranulocytosis
Kostmann's disease

D70.1 **Agranulocytosis secondary to cancer chemotherapy** `HCC`
Code also underlying neoplasm
Use additional code for adverse effect, if applicable, to identify drug (T45.1X5)
AHA: 2014, 4Q, 22

D70.2 **Other drug-induced agranulocytosis** `HCC`
Use additional code for adverse effect, if applicable, to identify drug (T36-T50 with fifth or sixth character 5)

D70.3 **Neutropenia due to infection** `HCC`

D70.4 **Cyclic neutropenia** `HCC`
Cyclic hematopoiesis
Periodic neutropenia

D70.8 **Other neutropenia** `HCC`

D70.9 **Neutropenia, unspecified** `HCC`

D71 **Functional disorders of polymorphonuclear neutrophils** `HCC`
Cell membrane receptor complex [CR3] defect
Chronic (childhood) granulomatous disease
Congenital dysphagocytosis
Progressive septic granulomatosis

✓4ᵗʰ **D72** **Other disorders of white blood cells**
EXCLUDES 1   *basophilia (D72.824)*
immunity disorders (D80-D89)
neutropenia (D70)
preleukemia (syndrome) (D46.9)

D72.0 **Genetic anomalies of leukocytes** `HCC`
Alder (granulation) (granulocyte) anomaly
Alder syndrome
Hereditary leukocytic hypersegmentation
Hereditary leukocytic hyposegmentation
Hereditary leukomelanopathy
May-Hegglin (granulation) (granulocyte) anomaly
May-Hegglin syndrome
Pelger-Huët (granulation) (granulocyte) anomaly
Pelger-Huët syndrome
EXCLUDES 1   *Chédiak (-Steinbrinck)-Higashi syndrome (E70.330)*

D72.1 **Eosinophilia**
Allergic eosinophilia
Hereditary eosinophilia
EXCLUDES 1   *Löffler's syndrome (J82)*
pulmonary eosinophilia (J82)

✓5ᵗʰ **D72.8** **Other specified disorders of white blood cells**
EXCLUDES 1   *leukemia (C91-C95)*

✓6ᵗʰ **D72.81** **Decreased white blood cell count**
EXCLUDES 1   *neutropenia (D70.-)*

D72.810 **Lymphocytopenia**
Decreased lymphocytes

D72.818 **Other decreased white blood cell count**
Basophilic leukopenia
Eosinophilic leukopenia
Monocytopenia
Other decreased leukocytes
Plasmacytopenia

D72.819 **Decreased white blood cell count, unspecified**
Decreased leukocytes, unspecified
Leukocytopenia, unspecified
Leukopenia
EXCLUDES 1   *malignant leukopenia (D70.9)*

✓6ᵗʰ **D72.82** **Elevated white blood cell count**
EXCLUDES 1   *eosinophilia (D72.1)*

D72.820 **Lymphocytosis (symptomatic)**
Elevated lymphocytes

D72.821 **Monocytosis (symptomatic)**
EXCLUDES 1   *infectious mononucleosis (B27.-)*

D72.822 **Plasmacytosis**

D72.823 **Leukemoid reaction**
Basophilic leukemoid reaction
Leukemoid reaction NOS
Lymphocytic leukemoid reaction
Monocytic leukemoid reaction
Myelocytic leukemoid reaction
Neutrophilic leukemoid reaction

D72.824 **Basophilia**

D72.825 **Bandemia**
Bandemia without diagnosis of specific infection
EXCLUDES 1   *confirmed infection—code to infection*
leukemia (C91.-, C92.-, C93.-, C94.-, C95.-)
DEF: Increase in early neutrophil cells, called band cells; may indicate infection.

D72.828 **Other elevated white blood cell count**

D72.829 **Elevated white blood cell count, unspecified**
Elevated leukocytes, unspecified
Leukocytosis, unspecified

D72.89 **Other specified disorders of white blood cells**
Abnormality of white blood cells NEC

D72.9 **Disorder of white blood cells, unspecified**
Abnormal leukocyte differential NOS

✓4ᵗʰ **D73** **Diseases of spleen**

D73.0 **Hyposplenism**
Atrophy of spleen
EXCLUDES 1   *asplenia (congenital) (Q89.01)*
postsurgical absence of spleen (Z90.81)

D73.1 **Hypersplenism**
EXCLUDES 1   *neutropenic splenomegaly (D73.81)*
primary splenic neutropenia (D73.81)
splenitis, splenomegaly in late syphilis (A52.79)
splenitis, splenomegaly in tuberculosis (A18.85)
splenomegaly NOS (R16.1)
splenomegaly congenital (Q89.0)

D73.2 **Chronic congestive splenomegaly**

D73.3 **Abscess of spleen**

D73.4 **Cyst of spleen**

D73.5 **Infarction of spleen**
Splenic rupture, nontraumatic
Torsion of spleen
EXCLUDES 1   *rupture of spleen due to Plasmodium vivax malaria (B51.0)*
traumatic rupture of spleen (S36.03-)

✓5ᵗʰ **D73.8** **Other diseases of spleen**

D73.81 **Neutropenic splenomegaly**
Werner-Schultz disease

D73.89 **Other diseases of spleen**
Fibrosis of spleen NOS
Perisplenitis
Splenitis NOS

✓ Additional Character Req   ✓x7ᵗʰ Placeholder Alert   Unacceptable PDx   Manifestation   `H1`-`H14` HAC   `HCC` CMS-HCC Condition   *EXCLUDES 1* Not Coded Here   *EXCLUDES 2* Not Included Here

ICD-10-CM 2018   **505**

Chapter 3. Diseases of the Blood and Blood-forming Organs

D73.9 Disease of spleen, unspecified

√4ᵗʰ **D74 Methemoglobinemia**

> **CC Excl: For CC codes in category D74:** PDX collection 506

D74.0 **Congenital methemoglobinemia**   CC
Congenital NADH-methemoglobin reductase deficiency
Hemoglobin-M [Hb-M] disease
Methemoglobinemia, hereditary

D74.8 Other **methemoglobinemias**   CC
Acquired methemoglobinemia (with sulfhemoglobinemia)
Toxic methemoglobinemia

D74.9 **Methemoglobinemia,** unspecified   CC

√4ᵗʰ **D75 Other and unspecified diseases of blood and blood-forming organs**

> EXCLUDES 2   acute lymphadenitis (L04.-)
> chronic lymphadenitis (I88.1)
> enlarged lymph nodes (R59.-)
> hypergammaglobulinemia NOS (D89.2)
> lymphadenitis NOS (I88.9)
> mesenteric lymphadenitis (acute) (chronic) (I88.0)

D75.0 **Familial erythrocytosis**
Benign polycythemia
Familial polycythemia
> EXCLUDES 1   hereditary ovalocytosis (D58.1)

D75.1 **Secondary polycythemia**
Acquired polycythemia
Emotional polycythemia
Erythrocytosis NOS
Hypoxemic polycythemia
Nephrogenous polycythemia
Polycythemia due to erythropoietin
Polycythemia due to fall in plasma volume
Polycythemia due to high altitude
Polycythemia due to stress
Polycythemia NOS
Relative polycythemia
> EXCLUDES 1   polycythemia neonatorum (P61.1)
> polycythemia vera (D45)

DEF: Elevated number of red blood cells in circulating blood as a result of reduced oxygen supply to the tissues.

√5ᵗʰ **D75.8** **Other specified diseases of blood and blood-forming organs**

D75.81 *Myelofibrosis*   CC HCC
Myelofibrosis NOS
Secondary myelofibrosis NOS
Code first the underlying disorder, such as:
    malignant neoplasm of breast (C50.-)
Use additional code, if applicable, for associated
    therapy-related myelodysplastic syndrome
    (D46.-)
Use additional code for adverse effect, if applicable, to
    identify drug (T45.1X5)
> EXCLUDES 1   acute myelofibrosis (C94.4-)
> idiopathic myelofibrosis (D47.1)
> leukoerythroblastic anemia (D61.82)
> myelofibrosis with myeloid metaplasia
>   (D47.4)
> myelophthisic anemia (D61.82)
> myelophthisis (D61.82)
> primary myelofibrosis (D47.1)

CC Excl: PDX collection 488

D75.82 **Heparin induced thrombocytopenia (HIT)**   HCC
DEF: Immune-mediated reaction to heparin therapy
causing an abrupt fall in platelet count and serious
complications such as pulmonary embolism, stroke,
AMI, or DVT.

D75.89 **Other specified diseases of blood and blood-forming organs**

D75.9 Disease of blood and blood-forming organs, unspecified

√4ᵗʰ **D76 Other specified diseases with participation of lymphoreticular and reticulohistiocytic tissue**

> EXCLUDES 1   (Abt-) Letterer-Siwe disease (C96.0)
> eosinophilic granuloma (C96.6)
> Hand-Schüller-Christian disease (C96.5)
> histiocytic medullary reticulosis (C96.9)
> histiocytic sarcoma (C96.A)
> histiocytosis X, multifocal (C96.5)
> histiocytosis X, unifocal (C96.6)
> Langerhans-cell histiocytosis, multifocal (C96.5)
> Langerhans-cell histiocytosis NOS (C96.6)
> Langerhans-cell histiocytosis, unifocal (C96.6)
> leukemic reticuloendotheliosis (C91.4-)
> lipomelanotic reticulosis (I89.8)
> malignant histiocytosis (C96.A)
> malignant reticulosis (C86.0)
> nonlipid reticuloendotheliosis (C96.0)

> **CC Excl: For CC codes in category D76, unless otherwise noted:** PDX collection 507

D76.1 **Hemophagocytic lymphohistiocytosis**   CC HCC
Familial hemophagocytic reticulosis
Histiocytoses of mononuclear phagocytes

D76.2 **Hemophagocytic syndrome, infection-associated**   CC HCC
Use additional code to identify infectious agent or disease

D76.3 **Other histiocytosis syndromes**   CC HCC
Reticulohistiocytoma (giant-cell)
Sinus histiocytosis with massive lymphadenopathy
Xanthogranuloma

D77 *Other disorders of blood and blood-forming organs in diseases classified elsewhere*
Code first underlying disease, such as:
    amyloidosis (E85.-)
    congenital early syphilis (A50.0)
    echinococcosis (B67.0-B67.9)
    malaria (B50.0-B54)
    schistosomiasis [bilharziasis] (B65.0-B65.9)
    vitamin C deficiency (E54)
> EXCLUDES 1   rupture of spleen due to Plasmodium vivax malaria (B51.0)
> splenitis, splenomegaly in late syphilis (A52.79)
> splenitis, splenomegaly in tuberculosis (A18.85)

Intraoperative and postprocedural complications of the spleen (D78)

√4ᵗʰ **D78 Intraoperative and postprocedural complications of the spleen**

> **CC Excl: For CC codes in category D78, unless otherwise noted:** PDX collection 508

√5ᵗʰ **D78.0** Intraoperative hemorrhage and hematoma **of the spleen complicating a procedure**
> EXCLUDES 1   intraoperative hemorrhage and hematoma of the
> spleen due to accidental puncture or laceration
> during a procedure (D78.1-)

D78.01 **Intraoperative hemorrhage and hematoma**   CC
of the spleen complicating a procedure on the
spleen

D78.02 **Intraoperative hemorrhage and hematoma**   CC
of the spleen complicating other procedure

√5ᵗʰ **D78.1** Accidental puncture and laceration **of the spleen during a procedure**

D78.11 **Accidental puncture and laceration of the**   CC
spleen during a procedure on the spleen
CC Excl: PDX collection 509

D78.12 **Accidental puncture and laceration of the**   CC
spleen during other procedure
CC Excl: PDX collection 509

√5ᵗʰ **D78.2** Postprocedural hemorrhage **of the spleen following a procedure**

D78.21 **Postprocedural hemorrhage of the spleen**   CC
following a procedure on the spleen

D78.22 **Postprocedural hemorrhage of the spleen**   CC
following other procedure

√5ᵗʰ **D78.3** Postprocedural hematoma and seroma **of the spleen following a procedure**

D78.31 **Postprocedural** hematoma **of the spleen**   CC
following a procedure on the spleen

D78.32 **Postprocedural** hematoma **of the spleen**   CC
following other procedure

D78.33 **Postprocedural** seroma **of the spleen following** CC
a procedure on the spleen

N Newborn: 0   P Pediatric: 0-17   M Maternity: 12-55   A Adult: 15-124   MCC Major CC Condition   PDxMCC PDx acts as own MCC   CC CC Condition   PDxCC PDx acts as own CC

506   ICD-10-CM 2018

D78.34 Postprocedural *seroma* of the spleen following other procedure   `CC`

✓5ᵗʰ **D78.8** Other **intraoperative and postprocedural complications of the spleen**
Use additional code, if applicable, to further specify disorder

     D78.81 Other **intraoperative** complications of the spleen   `CC`
        CC Excl: PDX collection 510

     D78.89 Other **postprocedural** complications of the spleen   `CC`
        CC Excl: PDX collection 510

Certain disorders involving the immune mechanism (D80-D89)

`INCLUDES`   defects in the complement system
immunodeficiency disorders, except human immunodeficiency virus [HIV] disease
sarcoidosis

`EXCLUDES 1`   *autoimmune disease (systemic) NOS (M35.9)*
functional disorders of polymorphonuclear neutrophils (D71)
human immunodeficiency virus [HIV] disease (B20)

✓4ᵗʰ **D80** **Immunodeficiency with predominantly antibody defects**

     CC Excl: For CC codes in category D80, unless otherwise noted: PDX collection 511

     D80.0 Hereditary **hypogammaglobulinemia**   `CC` `HCC`
        Autosomal recessive agammaglobulinemia (Swiss type)
        X-linked agammaglobulinemia [Bruton] (with growth hormone deficiency)

     D80.1 Nonfamilial **hypogammaglobulinemia**   `CC` `HCC`
        Agammaglobulinemia with immunoglobulin-bearing B-lymphocytes
        Common variable agammaglobulinemia [CVAgamma]
        Hypogammaglobulinemia NOS
        CC Excl: PDX collection 512

     D80.2 Selective deficiency of **immunoglobulin A [IgA]**   `CC` `HCC`
        CC Excl: PDX collection 512

     D80.3 Selective deficiency of **immunoglobulin G [IgG]** subclasses   `CC` `HCC`

     D80.4 Selective deficiency of **immunoglobulin M [IgM]**   `CC` `HCC`

     D80.5 Immunodeficiency with **increased immunoglobulin M [IgM]**   `CC` `HCC`

     D80.6 Antibody deficiency with **near-normal immunoglobulins or with hyperimmunoglobulinemia**   `CC` `HCC`

     D80.7 Transient **hypogammaglobulinemia of infancy**   `CC` `HCC`

     D80.8 Other **immunodeficiencies with predominantly antibody defects**   `CC` `HCC`
        Kappa light chain deficiency

     D80.9 Immunodeficiency with **predominantly antibody defects, unspecified**   `CC` `HCC`

✓4ᵗʰ **D81** **Combined immunodeficiencies**

     `EXCLUDES 1`   *autosomal recessive agammaglobulinemia (Swiss type) (D80.0)*

     CC Excl: For CC codes in category D81, unless otherwise noted: PDX collection 511

     D81.0 Severe **combined immunodeficiency [SCID] with reticular dysgenesis**   `CC` `HCC`

     D81.1 Severe **combined immunodeficiency [SCID] with low T- and B-cell numbers**   `CC` `HCC`

     D81.2 Severe **combined immunodeficiency [SCID] with low or normal B-cell numbers**   `CC` `HCC`

     D81.3 Adenosine deaminase **[ADA] deficiency**   `CC` `HCC`
        CC Excl: PDX collection 513

     D81.4 Nezelof's **syndrome**   `CC` `HCC`

     D81.5 Purine nucleoside phosphorylase **[PNP] deficiency**   `CC` `HCC`
        CC Excl: PDX collection 513

     D81.6 Major histocompatibility complex class I **deficiency**   `CC` `HCC`
        Bare lymphocyte syndrome

     D81.7 Major histocompatibility complex class II **deficiency**   `CC` `HCC`

     ✓5ᵗʰ **D81.8** Other **combined immunodeficiencies**

        ✓6ᵗʰ **D81.81** Biotin-dependent carboxylase **deficiency**
           Multiple carboxylase deficiency
           `EXCLUDES 1`   *biotin-dependent carboxylase deficiency due to dietary deficiency of biotin (E53.8)*

           D81.810 Biotinidase **deficiency**

           D81.818 Other **biotin-dependent carboxylase deficiency**
              Holocarboxylase synthetase deficiency
              Other multiple carboxylase deficiency

           D81.819 Biotin-dependent carboxylase deficiency, *unspecified*
              Multiple carboxylase deficiency, unspecified

     D81.89 Other **combined immunodeficiencies**   `CC` `HCC`

     D81.9 Combined immunodeficiency, *unspecified*   `CC` `HCC`
        Severe combined immunodeficiency disorder [SCID] NOS

✓4ᵗʰ **D82** **Immunodeficiency associated with other major defects**

     `EXCLUDES 1`   *ataxia telangiectasia [Louis-Bar] (G11.3)*

     D82.0 Wiskott-Aldrich syndrome   `CC` `HCC`
        Immunodeficiency with thrombocytopenia and eczema
        CC Excl: PDX collection 511

     D82.1 Di George's syndrome   `CC` `HCC`
        Pharyngeal pouch syndrome
        Thymic alymphoplasia
        Thymic aplasia or hypoplasia with immunodeficiency
        CC Excl: PDX collection 511

     D82.2 **Immunodeficiency with short-limbed stature**   `HCC`

     D82.3 **Immunodeficiency following hereditary defective response to Epstein-Barr virus**   `HCC`
        X-linked lymphoproliferative disease

     D82.4 **Hyperimmunoglobulin E [IgE] syndrome**   `HCC`

     D82.8 **Immunodeficiency associated with other specified major defects**   `HCC`

     D82.9 **Immunodeficiency associated with major defect, unspecified**   `HCC`

✓4ᵗʰ **D83** **Common variable immunodeficiency**

     CC Excl: For CC codes in category D83: PDX collection 511

     D83.0 **Common variable immunodeficiency with predominant abnormalities of B-cell numbers and function**   `CC` `HCC`

     D83.1 **Common variable immunodeficiency with predominant immunoregulatory T-cell disorders**   `CC` `HCC`

     D83.2 **Common variable immunodeficiency with autoantibodies to B- or T-cells**   `CC` `HCC`

     D83.8 Other **common variable immunodeficiencies**   `CC` `HCC`

     D83.9 **Common variable immunodeficiency, unspecified**   `CC` `HCC`

✓4ᵗʰ **D84** **Other immunodeficiencies**

     D84.0 Lymphocyte function antigen-1 **[LFA-1] defect**   `HCC`

     D84.1 Defects in the **complement system**   `HCC`
        C1 esterase inhibitor [C1-INH] deficiency

     D84.8 Other **specified immunodeficiencies**   `CC` `HCC`
        CC Excl: PDX collection 511

     D84.9 **Immunodeficiency, unspecified**   `CC` `HCC`
        CC Excl: PDX collection 511

✓4ᵗʰ **D86** **Sarcoidosis**

     D86.0 Sarcoidosis of **lung**   `HCC`

     D86.1 Sarcoidosis of **lymph nodes**

     D86.2 Sarcoidosis of **lung with sarcoidosis of lymph nodes**   `HCC`

     D86.3 Sarcoidosis of **skin**

     ✓5ᵗʰ **D86.8** Sarcoidosis of **other sites**

        D86.81 Sarcoid **meningitis**

        D86.82 Multiple cranial nerve palsies **in sarcoidosis**   `HCC`

        D86.83 Sarcoid **iridocyclitis**

        D86.84 Sarcoid **pyelonephritis**
           Tubulo-interstitial nephropathy in sarcoidosis

        D86.85 Sarcoid **myocarditis**

        D86.86 Sarcoid **arthropathy**
           Polyarthritis in sarcoidosis

        D86.87 Sarcoid **myositis**

        D86.89 Sarcoidosis of **other sites**
           Hepatic granuloma
           Uveoparotid fever [Heerfordt]

     D86.9 **Sarcoidosis, unspecified**

✓4ᵗʰ **D89** **Other disorders involving the immune mechanism, not elsewhere classified**

     `EXCLUDES 1`   *hyperglobulinemia NOS (R77.1)*
        monoclonal gammopathy (of undetermined significance) (D47.2)

     `EXCLUDES 2`   *transplant failure and rejection (T86.-)*

     D89.0 Polyclonal hypergammaglobulinemia
        Benign hypergammaglobulinemic purpura
        Polyclonal gammopathy NOS

✓ Additional Character Req   ✓x7ᵗʰ Placeholder Alert   Unacceptable PDx   Manifestation   `H1`-`H14` HAC   `HCC` CMS-HCC Condition   `EXCLUDES 1` Not Coded Here   `EXCLUDES 2` Not Included Here

D89.1   Cryoglobulinemia   `HCC`
     Cryoglobulinemic purpura
     Cryoglobulinemic vasculitis
     Essential cryoglobulinemia
     Idiopathic cryoglobulinemia
     Mixed cryoglobulinemia
     Primary cryoglobulinemia
     Secondary cryoglobulinemia

D89.2   Hypergammaglobulinemia, unspecified

D89.3   Immune reconstitution syndrome   `HCC`
     Immune reconstitution inflammatory syndrome [IRIS]
     Use additional code for adverse effect, if applicable, to identify drug (T36-T50 with fifth or sixth character 5)

☑5ᵗʰ **D89.4   Mast cell activation syndrome and related disorders**
     EXCLUDES 1   *aggressive systemic mastocytosis ▶(C96.21)◀*
               ▶congenital cutaneous mastocytosis◀ (Q82.2)
               ▶(non-congenital) cutaneous mastocytosis (D47.01)
               (indolent) systemic mastocytosis (D47.02)
               malignant mast cell neoplasm (C96.2-)◀
               malignant mastocytoma ▶(C96.29)◀
               mast cell leukemia (C94.3-)
               ▶mast cell sarcoma (C96.22)
               mastocytoma NOS (D47.09)
               other mast cell neoplasms of uncertain behavior (D47.09)◀
               systemic mastocytosis associated with a clonal hematologic non-mast cell lineage disease (SM-AHNMD)▶(D47.02)◀

     D89.40   Mast cell activation, unspecified   `HCC`
          Mast cell activation disorder, unspecified
          Mast cell activation syndrome, NOS

     D89.41   Monoclonal mast cell activation syndrome   `HCC`

     D89.42   Idiopathic mast cell activation syndrome   `HCC`

     D89.43   Secondary mast cell activation   `HCC`
          Secondary mast cell activation syndrome
          Code also underlying etiology, if known

     D89.49   Other mast cell activation disorder   `HCC`
          Other mast cell activation syndrome

☑5ᵗʰ **D89.8   Other specified disorders involving the immune mechanism, not elsewhere classified**

☑6ᵗʰ   **D89.81   Graft-versus-host disease**
          Code first underlying cause, such as:
             complications of transplanted organs and tissue (T86.-)
             complications of blood transfusion (T80.89)
          Use additional code to identify associated manifestations, such as:
             desquamative dermatitis (L30.8)
             diarrhea (R19.7)
             elevated bilirubin (R17)
             hair loss (L65.9)

         CC Excl: For CC codes in subcategory D89.81: PDX collection 514

         D89.810   Acute graft-versus-host disease   `CC` `HCC`
         D89.811   Chronic graft-versus-host disease   `CC` `HCC`
         D89.812   Acute on chronic graft-versus-host disease   `CC` `HCC`
         D89.813   Graft-versus-host disease, unspecified   `CC` `HCC`

     D89.82   Autoimmune lymphoproliferative syndrome [ALPS]   `HCC`
          DEF: Rare genetic alteration of the Fas protein; impairs normal cellular apoptosis (normal cell death), causing abnormal accumulation of lymphocytes in the lymph glands, liver, and spleen; symptoms include neutropenia, anemia, and thrombocytopenia.

     D89.89   Other specified disorders involving the immune mechanism, not elsewhere classified   `HCC`
          EXCLUDES 1   *human immunodeficiency virus disease (B20)*

D89.9   Disorder involving the immune mechanism, unspecified   `HCC`
     Immune disease NOS
     AHA: 2015, 3Q, 22

Ⓝ Newborn: 0   Ⓟ Pediatric: 0-17   Ⓜ Maternity: 12-55   Ⓐ Adult: 15-124   `MCC` Major CC Condition   `PDxMCC` PDx acts as own MCC   `CC` CC Condition   `PDxCC` PDx acts as own CC

508   ICD-10-CM 2018

Chapter 4. Endocrine, Nutritional and Metabolic Diseases (E00–E89)

Chapter Specific Guidelines with Coding Examples

The chapter specific guidelines from the ICD-10-CM Official Guidelines for Coding and Reporting have been provided below. Along with these guidelines are coding examples, contained in the shaded boxes, that have been developed to help illustrate the coding and/or sequencing guidance found in these guidelines.

a. Diabetes mellitus

The diabetes mellitus codes are combination codes that include the type of diabetes mellitus, the body system affected, and the complications affecting that body system. As many codes within a particular category as are necessary to describe all of the complications of the disease may be used. They should be sequenced based on the reason for a particular encounter. Assign as many codes from categories E08–E13 as needed to identify all of the associated conditions that the patient has.

> Patient is seen for poorly controlled diabetes, type 2, with diabetic polyneuropathy and diabetic retinopathy with macular edema
>
> **E11.65**   **Type 2 diabetes mellitus with hyperglycemia**
>
> **E11.311**   **Type 2 diabetes mellitus with unspecified diabetic retinopathy with macular edema**
>
> **E11.42**   **Type 2 diabetes mellitus with diabetic polyneuropathy**
>
> *Explanation*: Use as many codes to describe the diabetic complications as needed. Many are combination codes that describe more than one condition. Code first the reason for the encounter. "Poorly controlled" is described as "with hyperglycemia." Diabetes documented as "uncontrolled" is not assumed to be hyperglycemic but can be classified to either hyperglycemia or hypoglycemia. If documentation is not clear, the provider must be queried so that the appropriate code can be reported.

1) Type of diabetes

The age of a patient is not the sole determining factor, though most type 1 diabetics develop the condition before reaching puberty. For this reason type 1 diabetes mellitus is also referred to as juvenile diabetes.

> A 45-year-old patient is diagnosed with type 1 diabetes
>
> **E10.9**   **Type 1 diabetes mellitus without complications**
>
> *Explanation*: Although most type 1 diabetics are diagnosed in childhood or adolescence, it can also begin in adults.

2) Type of diabetes mellitus not documented

If the type of diabetes mellitus is not documented in the medical record the default is E11.-, Type 2 diabetes mellitus.

> H & P lists diabetes and hypertension on patient problem list
>
> **E11.9**   **Type 2 diabetes mellitus without complications**
>
> **I10**   **Essential (primary) hypertension**
>
> *Explanation*: Since the type of diabetes was not documented and no complications were noted, the default code is E11.9.

3) Diabetes mellitus and the use of insulin and oral hypoglycemics

If the documentation in a medical record does not indicate the type of diabetes but does indicate that the patient uses insulin, code E11-, Type 2 diabetes mellitus, should be assigned. **An additional code should be assigned from category Z79 to identify the long-term (current) use of insulin or oral hypoglycemic drugs. If the patient is treated with both oral medications and insulin, only the code for long-term (current) use of insulin should be assigned. Code Z79.4 should not be assigned if insulin is given temporarily to bring a type 2 patient's blood sugar under control during an encounter.**

> The H & P lists chronic diabetes and the use of daily metformin and nightly insulin.
>
> **E11.9**   **Type 2 diabetes mellitus without complications**
>
> **Z79.4**   **Long term (current) use of insulin**
>
> *Explanation*: Do not assume that a patient on insulin must have type 1 diabetes. The default for diabetes without further specification defaults to type 2. Patients with DM 2 often are prescribed both insulin and an oral hypoglycemic agent. Report only the code for the long-term use of insulin, when both are prescribed.

4) Diabetes mellitus in pregnancy and gestational diabetes

See Section I.C.15. Diabetes mellitus in pregnancy.
See Section I.C.15. Gestational (pregnancy induced) diabetes

5) Complications due to insulin pump malfunction

(a) Underdose of insulin due to insulin pump failure

An underdose of insulin due to an insulin pump failure should be assigned to a code from subcategory T85.6, Mechanical complication of other specified internal and external prosthetic devices, implants and grafts, that specifies the type of pump malfunction, as the principal or first-listed code, followed by code T38.3X6-, Underdosing of insulin and oral hypoglycemic [antidiabetic] drugs. Additional codes for the type of diabetes mellitus and any associated complications due to the underdosing should also be assigned.

> A 24-year-old type 1 diabetic male treated in ED for hyperglycemia; insulin pump found to be malfunctioning and underdosing
>
> **T85.614A**   **Breakdown (mechanical) of insulin pump, initial encounter**
>
> **T38.3X6A**   **Underdosing of insulin and oral hypoglycemic [antidiabetic] drugs, initial encounter**
>
> **E10.65**   **Type 1 diabetes mellitus with hyperglycemia**
>
> *Explanation*: The complication code for the mechanical breakdown of the pump is sequenced first, followed by the underdosing code and type of diabetes with complication. Code all other diabetic complication codes necessary to describe the patient's condition.

(b) Overdose of insulin due to insulin pump failure

The principal or first-listed code for an encounter due to an insulin pump malfunction resulting in an overdose of insulin, should also be T85.6-, Mechanical complication of other specified internal and external prosthetic devices, implants and grafts, followed by code T38.3X1-, Poisoning by insulin and oral hypoglycemic [antidiabetic] drugs, accidental (unintentional).

> A 24-year-old type 1 diabetic male found down with diabetic coma, brought into ED and treated for hypoglycemia; insulin pump found to be malfunctioning and overdosing
>
> **T85.614A**   **Breakdown (mechanical) of insulin pump, initial encounter**
>
> **T38.3X1A**   **Poisoning by insulin and oral hypoglycemic [antidiabetic] drugs, accidental (unintentional), initial encounter**
>
> **E10.641**   **Type 1 diabetes mellitus with hypoglycemia with coma**
>
> *Explanation*: The complication code for the mechanical breakdown of the pump is sequenced first, followed by the poisoning code and type of diabetes with complication. All the characters in the combination code must be used to form a valid code and to fully describe the type of diabetes, the hypoglycemia, and the coma.

6) Secondary diabetes mellitus

Codes under categories E08, Diabetes mellitus due to underlying condition, E09, Drug or chemical induced diabetes mellitus, and E13, Other specified diabetes mellitus, identify complications/manifestations associated with secondary diabetes mellitus. Secondary diabetes is always caused by another condition or event (e.g., cystic fibrosis, malignant neoplasm of pancreas, pancreatectomy, adverse effect of drug, or poisoning).

(a) Secondary diabetes mellitus and the use of insulin or *oral* hypoglycemic drugs

For patients with secondary diabetes mellitus who routinely use insulin or oral hypoglycemic drugs, an additional code from category Z79 should be assigned to identify the long-term (current) use of insulin or oral hypoglycemic drugs. If the patient is treated with both oral medications and insulin, only the code for long-term (current) use of insulin should be assigned. Code Z79.4 should not be assigned if insulin is given temporarily to bring a type 2 patient's blood sugar under control during an encounter.

Type 2 diabetic with no complications, normally only on oral metformin, is given insulin for three days to maintain glucose control while in the hospital recovering from surgery

E11.9   Type 2 diabetes mellitus without complications

Z79.84   Long term (current) use of oral hypoglycemic drugs

Explanation: Although the patient was given insulin for a short time during his hospital stay, the intent was only to maintain the patient's glucose levels while off his regular oral hypoglycemic medication, not for long term use. No code is needed for long term use of insulin, but a Z code for long term use of an oral hypoglycemic should be added to identify the chronic use of this drug.

Type 2 diabetic with diabetic polyneuropathy on insulin

E11.42   Type 2 diabetes mellitus with diabetic polyneuropathy

Z79.4   Long term (current) use of insulin

Explanation: Add the Z code for the long term use of insulin because the insulin is taken chronically.

(b) Assigning and sequencing secondary diabetes codes and its causes

The sequencing of the secondary diabetes codes in relationship to codes for the cause of the diabetes is based on the Tabular List instructions for categories E08, E09 and E13.

(i) Secondary diabetes mellitus due to pancreatectomy

For postpancreatectomy diabetes mellitus (lack of insulin due to the surgical removal of all or part of the pancreas), assign code E89.1, Postprocedural hypoinsulinemia. Assign a code from category E13 and a code from subcategory Z90.41, Acquired absence of pancreas, as additional codes.

Patient with newly diagnosed diabetes after surgical removal of part of pancreas is discharged with referral for consult to initiate insulin.

E89.1   Postprocedural hypoinsulinemia

E13.9   Other specified diabetes mellitus without complications

Z90.411   Acquired partial absence of pancreas

Explanation: Sequence the postprocedural complication of the hypoinsulinemia due to the partial removal of the pancreas as the first-listed code, followed by the other specified diabetes (NEC) with or without complications and the partial or total acquired absence of the pancreas. Code Z79.4 Long term (current) use of insulin, is not added because the insulin has not yet been started.

(ii) Secondary diabetes due to drugs

Secondary diabetes may be caused by an adverse effect of correctly administered medications, poisoning or sequela of poisoning.

See section I.C.19.e for coding of adverse effects and poisoning, and section I.C.20 for external cause code reporting.

Initial encounter for corticosteroid-induced diabetes mellitus

E09.9   Drug or chemical induced diabetes mellitus without complications

T38.0X5A   Adverse effect of glucocorticoids and synthetic analogues, initial encounter

Explanation: If the diabetes is caused by an adverse effect of a drug, the diabetic condition is coded first. If it occurs from a poisoning or overdose, the poisoning code causing the diabetes is sequenced first.

Chapter 4. Endocrine, Nutritional and Metabolic Diseases (E00-E89)

NOTE All neoplasms, whether functionally active or not, are classified in Chapter 2. Appropriate codes in this chapter (i.e. E05.8, E07.0, E16-E31, E34-) may be used as additional codes to indicate either functional activity by neoplasms and ectopic endocrine tissue or hyperfunction and hypofunction of endocrine glands associated with neoplasms and other conditions classified elsewhere.

EXCLUDES 1 *transitory endocrine and metabolic disorders specific to newborn (P70-P74)*

This chapter contains the following blocks:

E00-E07	Disorders of thyroid gland
E08-E13	Diabetes mellitus
E15-E16	Other disorders of glucose regulation and pancreatic internal secretion
E20-E35	Disorders of other endocrine glands
E36	Intraoperative complications of endocrine system
E40-E46	Malnutrition
E50-E64	Other nutritional deficiencies
E65-E68	Overweight, obesity and other hyperalimentation
E70-E88	Metabolic disorders
E89	Postprocedural endocrine and metabolic complications and disorders, not elsewhere classified

Disorders of thyroid gland (E00-E07)

✓4th E00 Congenital iodine-deficiency syndrome

Use additional code (F70-F79) to identify associated intellectual disabilities

EXCLUDES 1 *subclinical iodine-deficiency hypothyroidism (E02)*

E00.0 Congenital iodine-deficiency syndrome, neurological type
Endemic cretinism, neurological type

E00.1 Congenital iodine-deficiency syndrome, myxedematous type
Endemic hypothyroid cretinism
Endemic cretinism, myxedematous type

E00.2 Congenital iodine-deficiency syndrome, mixed type
Endemic cretinism, mixed type

E00.9 Congenital iodine-deficiency syndrome, unspecified
Congenital iodine-deficiency hypothyroidism NOS
Endemic cretinism NOS

✓4th E01 Iodine-deficiency related thyroid disorders and allied conditions

EXCLUDES 1 *congenital iodine-deficiency syndrome (E00.-)*
subclinical iodine-deficiency hypothyroidism (E02)

E01.0 Iodine-deficiency related diffuse (endemic) goiter

E01.1 Iodine-deficiency related multinodular (endemic) goiter
Iodine-deficiency related nodular goiter

E01.2 Iodine-deficiency related (endemic) goiter, unspecified
Endemic goiter NOS

E01.8 Other iodine-deficiency related thyroid disorders and allied conditions
Acquired iodine-deficiency hypothyroidism NOS

E02 Subclinical iodine-deficiency hypothyroidism

✓4th E03 Other hypothyroidism

EXCLUDES 1 *iodine-deficiency related hypothyroidism (E00-E02)*
postprocedural hypothyroidism (E89.0)

E03.0 Congenital hypothyroidism with diffuse goiter
Congenital parenchymatous goiter (nontoxic)
Congenital goiter (nontoxic) NOS

EXCLUDES 1 *transitory congenital goiter with normal function (P72.0)*

E03.1 Congenital hypothyroidism without goiter
Aplasia of thyroid (with myxedema)
Congenital atrophy of thyroid
Congenital hypothyroidism NOS

E03.2 Hypothyroidism due to medicaments and other exogenous substances
Code first poisoning due to drug or toxin, if applicable (T36-T65 with fifth or sixth character 1-4 or 6)
Use additional code for adverse effect, if applicable, to identify drug (T36-T50 with fifth or sixth character 5)

E03.3 Postinfectious hypothyroidism

E03.4 Atrophy of thyroid (acquired)

EXCLUDES 1 *congenital atrophy of thyroid (E03.1)*

E03.5 Myxedema coma **MCC HCC**
CC Excl: PDX collection 515

E03.8 Other specified hypothyroidism

E03.9 Hypothyroidism, unspecified
Myxedema NOS

✓4th E04 Other nontoxic goiter

EXCLUDES 1 *congenital goiter (NOS) (diffuse) (parenchymatous) (E03.0)*
iodine-deficiency related goiter (E00-E02)

E04.0 Nontoxic diffuse goiter
Diffuse (colloid) nontoxic goiter
Simple nontoxic goiter

E04.1 Nontoxic single thyroid nodule
Colloid nodule (cystic) (thyroid)   Thyroid (cystic) nodule NOS
Nontoxic uninodular goiter
DEF: Enlarged thyroid, commonly due to decreased thyroid production, with single nodule; no clinical hypothyroidism.

E04.2 Nontoxic multinodular goiter
Cystic goiter NOS
Multinodular (cystic) goiter NOS
DEF: Enlarged thyroid, commonly due to decreased thyroid production with multiple nodules; no clinical hypothyroidism.

E04.8 Other specified nontoxic goiter

E04.9 Nontoxic goiter, unspecified
Goiter NOS
Nodular goiter (nontoxic) NOS

✓4th E05 Thyrotoxicosis [hyperthyroidism]

EXCLUDES 1 *chronic thyroiditis with transient thyrotoxicosis (E06.2)*
neonatal thyrotoxicosis (P72.1)

CC Excl: For MCC codes in category E05: PDX collection 516

✓5th E05.0 Thyrotoxicosis with diffuse goiter
Exophthalmic or toxic goiter NOS
Graves' disease
Toxic diffuse goiter
DEF: Diffuse thyroid enlargement accompanied by hyperthyroidism, bulging eyes, and dermopathy.

E05.00 Thyrotoxicosis with diffuse goiter without thyrotoxic crisis or storm

E05.01 Thyrotoxicosis with diffuse goiter with thyrotoxic crisis or storm **MCC**

✓5th E05.1 Thyrotoxicosis with toxic single thyroid nodule
Thyrotoxicosis with toxic uninodular goiter
DEF: Symptomatic hyperthyroidism with a single nodule on the enlarged thyroid gland. Abrupt onset of symptoms include extreme nervousness, insomnia, weight loss, tremors, and psychosis or coma.

E05.10 Thyrotoxicosis with toxic single thyroid nodule without thyrotoxic crisis or storm

E05.11 Thyrotoxicosis with toxic single thyroid nodule with thyrotoxic crisis or storm **MCC**

✓5th E05.2 Thyrotoxicosis with toxic multinodular goiter
Toxic nodular goiter NOS

E05.20 Thyrotoxicosis with toxic multinodular goiter without thyrotoxic crisis or storm

E05.21 Thyrotoxicosis with toxic multinodular goiter with thyrotoxic crisis or storm **MCC**

✓5th E05.3 Thyrotoxicosis from ectopic thyroid tissue

E05.30 Thyrotoxicosis from ectopic thyroid tissue without thyrotoxic crisis or storm

E05.31 Thyrotoxicosis from ectopic thyroid tissue with thyrotoxic crisis or storm **MCC**

Goiter

Pyramidal lobe
Thyroid cartilage
Healthy thyroid
Goiter (hyperfunctioning thyroid)

✓ Additional Character Req ✓x7th Placeholder Alert Unacceptable PDx ■ Manifestation **H1 - H14** HAC **HCC** CMS-HCC Condition **EXCLUDES 1** Not Coded Here **EXCLUDES 2** Not Included Here

✓5ᵗʰ E05.4 Thyrotoxicosis factitia

  E05.40 Thyrotoxicosis factitia without thyrotoxic crisis or storm

  E05.41 Thyrotoxicosis factitia with thyrotoxic crisis or storm `MCC`

✓5ᵗʰ E05.8 Other thyrotoxicosis

  Overproduction of thyroid-stimulating hormone

  E05.80 Other thyrotoxicosis without thyrotoxic crisis or storm

  E05.81 Other thyrotoxicosis with thyrotoxic crisis or storm `MCC`

✓5ᵗʰ E05.9 Thyrotoxicosis, unspecified

  Hyperthyroidism NOS

  E05.90 Thyrotoxicosis, unspecified without thyrotoxic crisis or storm

  E05.91 Thyrotoxicosis, unspecified with thyrotoxic crisis or storm `MCC`

✓4ᵗʰ E06 Thyroiditis

  `EXCLUDES 1` *postpartum thyroiditis (O90.5)*

  E06.0 Acute thyroiditis `CC`

    Abscess of thyroid

    Pyogenic thyroiditis

    Suppurative thyroiditis

    Use additional code (B95-B97) to identify infectious agent

    CC Excl: PDX collection 517

  E06.1 Subacute thyroiditis

    de Quervain thyroiditis

    Giant-cell thyroiditis

    Granulomatous thyroiditis

    Nonsuppurative thyroiditis

    Viral thyroiditis

    `EXCLUDES 1` *autoimmune thyroiditis (E06.3)*

  E06.2 Chronic thyroiditis with transient thyrotoxicosis

    `EXCLUDES 1` *autoimmune thyroiditis (E06.3)*

  E06.3 Autoimmune thyroiditis

    Hashimoto's thyroiditis

    Hashitoxicosis (transient)

    Lymphadenoid goiter

    Lymphocytic thyroiditis

    Struma lymphomatosa

  E06.4 Drug-induced thyroiditis

    Use additional code for adverse effect, if applicable, to identify drug (T36-T50 with fifth or sixth character 5)

  E06.5 Other chronic thyroiditis

    Chronic fibrous thyroiditis

    Chronic thyroiditis NOS

    Ligneous thyroiditis

    Riedel thyroiditis

  E06.9 Thyroiditis, unspecified

✓4ᵗʰ E07 Other disorders of thyroid

  E07.0 Hypersecretion of calcitonin

    C-cell hyperplasia of thyroid

    Hypersecretion of thyrocalcitonin

  E07.1 Dyshormogenetic goiter

    Familial dyshormogenetic goiter

    Pendred's syndrome

    `EXCLUDES 1` *transitory congenital goiter with normal function (P72.0)*

✓5ᵗʰ E07.8 Other specified disorders of thyroid

  E07.81 Sick-euthyroid syndrome

    Euthyroid sick-syndrome

  E07.89 Other specified disorders of thyroid

    Abnormality of thyroid-binding globulin

    Hemorrhage of thyroid

    Infarction of thyroid

  E07.9 Disorder of thyroid, unspecified

Diabetes mellitus (E08-E13)

AHA: 2017, 1Q, 42; 2016, 2Q, 36; 2016, 1Q, 11-13

✓4ᵗʰ E08 Diabetes mellitus due to underlying condition

  Code first the underlying condition, such as:

    congenital rubella (P35.0)

    cushing's syndrome (E24.-)

    cystic fibrosis (E84.-)

    malignant neoplasm (C00-C96)

    malnutrition (E40-E46)

    pancreatitis and other diseases of the pancreas (K85.-, K86.-)

  Use additional code to identify control using:

    insulin (Z79.4)

    oral antidiabetic drugs (Z79.84)

    oral hypoglycemic drugs (Z79.84)

  `EXCLUDES 1` *drug or chemical induced diabetes mellitus (E09.-)*

    gestational diabetes (O24.4-)

    neonatal diabetes mellitus (P70.2)

    postpancreatectomy diabetes mellitus (E13.-)

    postprocedural diabetes mellitus (E13.-)

    secondary diabetes mellitus NEC (E13.-)

    type 1 diabetes mellitus (E10.-)

    type 2 diabetes mellitus (E11.-)

  AHA: 2013, 4Q, 114; 2013, 3Q, 20

> **CC Excl: For MCC codes in category E08, unless otherwise noted:** PDX collection 518

✓5ᵗʰ E08.0 Diabetes mellitus due to underlying condition with **hyperosmolarity**

  ***E08.00 Diabetes mellitus due to underlying condition with hyperosmolarity** without nonketotic hyperglycemic-hyperosmolar coma (NKHHC)* `MCC` `H9` `HCC`

  ***E08.01 Diabetes mellitus due to underlying condition with hyperosmolarity** with coma* `MCC` `H9` `HCC`

✓5ᵗʰ E08.1 Diabetes mellitus due to underlying condition with **ketoacidosis**

  ***E08.10 Diabetes mellitus due to underlying condition with ketoacidosis** without coma* `MCC` `H9` `HCC`

  ***E08.11 Diabetes mellitus due to underlying condition with ketoacidosis** with coma* `MCC` `HCC`

✓5ᵗʰ E08.2 Diabetes mellitus due to underlying condition with **kidney complications**

  ***E08.21 Diabetes mellitus due to underlying condition with diabetic** nephropathy* `HCC`

    Diabetes mellitus due to underlying condition with intercapillary glomerulosclerosis

    Diabetes mellitus due to underlying condition with intracapillary glomerulonephrosis

    Diabetes mellitus due to underlying condition with Kimmelstiel-Wilson disease

  ***E08.22 Diabetes mellitus due to underlying condition with diabetic** chronic kidney disease* `HCC`

    Use additional code to identify stage of chronic kidney disease (N18.1-N18.6)

  ***E08.29 Diabetes mellitus due to underlying condition with** other diabetic kidney complication* `HCC`

    Renal tubular degeneration in diabetes mellitus due to underlying condition

✓5ᵗʰ E08.3 Diabetes mellitus due to underlying condition with **ophthalmic complications**

> One of the following 7th characters is to be assigned to codes in subcategories E08.32, E08.33, E08.34, E08.35, and E08.37 to designate laterality of the disease:
>
> 1   right eye
>
> 2   left eye
>
> 3   bilateral
>
> 9   unspecified eye

✓6ᵗʰ E08.31 Diabetes mellitus due to underlying condition with **unspecified diabetic retinopathy**

  ***E08.311 Diabetes mellitus due to underlying condition with unspecified diabetic retinopathy** with macular edema* `HCC`

  ***E08.319 Diabetes mellitus due to underlying condition with unspecified diabetic retinopathy** without macular edema* `HCC`

N Newborn: 0   **P** Pediatric: 0-17   **M** Maternity: 12-55   **A** Adult: 15-124   `MCC` Major CC Condition   `PDxMCC` PDx acts as own MCC   `CC` CC Condition   `PDxCC` PDx acts as own CC

512   ICD-10-CM 2018

✓6th **E08.32 Diabetes mellitus due to underlying condition with** *mild nonproliferative diabetic retinopathy*
  Diabetes mellitus due to underlying condition with nonproliferative diabetic retinopathy NOS

 ✓7th *E08.321 Diabetes mellitus due to underlying condition with mild nonproliferative diabetic retinopathy with macular edema* HCC

 ✓7th *E08.329 Diabetes mellitus due to underlying condition with mild nonproliferative diabetic retinopathy without macular edema* HCC

✓6th **E08.33 Diabetes mellitus due to underlying condition with** *moderate nonproliferative diabetic retinopathy*

 ✓7th *E08.331 Diabetes mellitus due to underlying condition with moderate nonproliferative diabetic retinopathy with macular edema* HCC

 ✓7th *E08.339 Diabetes mellitus due to underlying condition with moderate nonproliferative diabetic retinopathy without macular edema* HCC

✓6th **E08.34 Diabetes mellitus due to underlying condition with** *severe nonproliferative diabetic retinopathy*

 ✓7th *E08.341 Diabetes mellitus due to underlying condition with severe nonproliferative diabetic retinopathy with macular edema* HCC

 ✓7th *E08.349 Diabetes mellitus due to underlying condition with severe nonproliferative diabetic retinopathy without macular edema* HCC

✓6th **E08.35 Diabetes mellitus due to underlying condition with** *proliferative diabetic retinopathy*

 ✓7th *E08.351 Diabetes mellitus due to underlying condition with proliferative diabetic retinopathy with macular edema* HCC

 ✓7th *E08.352 Diabetes mellitus due to underlying condition with proliferative diabetic retinopathy with traction retinal detachment involving the macula* HCC

 ✓7th *E08.353 Diabetes mellitus due to underlying condition with proliferative diabetic retinopathy with traction retinal detachment not involving the macula* HCC

 ✓7th *E08.354 Diabetes mellitus due to underlying condition with proliferative diabetic retinopathy with combined traction retinal detachment and rhegmatogenous retinal detachment* HCC

 ✓7th *E08.355 Diabetes mellitus due to underlying condition with stable proliferative diabetic retinopathy* HCC

 ✓7th *E08.359 Diabetes mellitus due to underlying condition with proliferative diabetic retinopathy without macular edema* HCC

E08.36 Diabetes mellitus due to underlying condition with diabetic cataract HCC
  AHA: 2016, 4Q, 142

✓x7th *E08.37 Diabetes mellitus due to underlying condition with diabetic macular edema, resolved following treatment* HCC

E08.39 Diabetes mellitus due to underlying condition with other diabetic ophthalmic complication HCC
  Use additional code to identify manifestation, such as: diabetic glaucoma (H40-H42)

✓5th **E08.4 Diabetes mellitus due to underlying condition with** *neurological complications*

 E08.40 Diabetes mellitus due to underlying condition with diabetic neuropathy, unspecified HCC

 E08.41 Diabetes mellitus due to underlying condition with diabetic mononeuropathy HCC

 E08.42 Diabetes mellitus due to underlying condition with diabetic polyneuropathy HCC
  Diabetes mellitus due to underlying condition with diabetic neuralgia

 E08.43 Diabetes mellitus due to underlying condition with diabetic autonomic (poly)neuropathy HCC
  Diabetes mellitus due to underlying condition with diabetic gastroparesis
  AHA: 2013, 4Q, 114

 E08.44 Diabetes mellitus due to underlying condition with diabetic amyotrophy HCC

E08.49 Diabetes mellitus due to underlying condition with other diabetic neurological complication HCC

✓5th **E08.5 Diabetes mellitus due to underlying condition with** *circulatory complications*

 E08.51 Diabetes mellitus due to underlying condition with diabetic peripheral angiopathy without gangrene HCC

 E08.52 Diabetes mellitus due to underlying condition with diabetic peripheral angiopathy with gangrene PDx CC CC HCC
  Diabetes mellitus due to underlying condition with diabetic gangrene
  CC Excl: PDX collection 519

 E08.59 Diabetes mellitus due to underlying condition with other circulatory complications HCC

✓5th **E08.6 Diabetes mellitus due to underlying condition with** *other specified complications*

 ✓6th **E08.61 Diabetes mellitus due to underlying condition with** *diabetic arthropathy*

  E08.610 Diabetes mellitus due to underlying condition with diabetic neuropathic arthropathy HCC
   Diabetes mellitus due to underlying condition with Charcôt's joints

  E08.618 Diabetes mellitus due to underlying condition with other diabetic arthropathy HCC

 ✓6th **E08.62 Diabetes mellitus due to underlying condition with** *skin complications*

  E08.620 Diabetes mellitus due to underlying condition with diabetic dermatitis HCC
   Diabetes mellitus due to underlying condition with diabetic necrobiosis lipoidica

  E08.621 Diabetes mellitus due to underlying condition with foot ulcer HCC
   Use additional code to identify site of ulcer (L97.4-, L97.5-)

  E08.622 Diabetes mellitus due to underlying condition with other skin ulcer HCC
   Use additional code to identify site of ulcer (L97.1-L97.9, L98.41-L98.49)

  E08.628 Diabetes mellitus due to underlying condition with other skin complications HCC

 ✓6th **E08.63 Diabetes mellitus due to underlying condition with** *oral complications*

  E08.630 Diabetes mellitus due to underlying condition with periodontal disease HCC

  E08.638 Diabetes mellitus due to underlying condition with other oral complications HCC

 ✓6th **E08.64 Diabetes mellitus due to underlying condition with** *hypoglycemia*

  E08.641 Diabetes mellitus due to underlying condition with hypoglycemia with coma MCC HCC

  E08.649 Diabetes mellitus due to underlying condition with hypoglycemia without coma HCC
   AHA: 2016, 3Q, 42; 2015, 3Q, 21

 E08.65 Diabetes mellitus due to underlying condition with hyperglycemia HCC

 E08.69 Diabetes mellitus due to underlying condition with other specified complication HCC
  Use additional code to identify complication
  AHA: 2016, 4Q, 141; 2016, 1Q, 13

E08.8 Diabetes mellitus due to underlying condition with unspecified complications HCC

E08.9 Diabetes mellitus due to underlying condition without complications HCC

✓ Additional Character Req ✓x7th Placeholder Alert Unacceptable PDx Manifestation H1 - H14 HAC HCC CMS-HCC Condition *EXCLUDES 1* Not Coded Here *EXCLUDES 2* Not Included Here

☑4ᵗʰ **E09** **Drug or chemical induced diabetes mellitus**

Code first poisoning due to drug or toxin, if applicable (T36-T65 with fifth or sixth character 1-4 or 6)

Use additional code for adverse effect, if applicable, to identify drug (T36-T50 with fifth or sixth character 5)

Use additional code to identify control using:
insulin (Z79.4)
oral antidiabetic drugs (Z79.84)
oral hypoglycemic drugs (Z79.84)

EXCLUDES 1   *diabetes mellitus due to underlying condition (E08.-)*
gestational diabetes (O24.4-)
neonatal diabetes mellitus (P70.2)
postpancreatectomy diabetes mellitus (E13.-)
postprocedural diabetes mellitus (E13.-)
secondary diabetes mellitus NEC (E13.-)
type 1 diabetes mellitus (E10.-)
type 2 diabetes mellitus (E11.-)

AHA: 2016, 1Q, 11-13; 2013, 4Q, 114; 2013, 3Q, 20

CC Excl: For MCC codes in category E09, unless otherwise noted: PDX collection 518

☑5ᵗʰ **E09.0** **Drug or chemical induced diabetes mellitus with hyperosmolarity**

    E09.00 **Drug or chemical induced diabetes mellituswith hyperosmolarity without nonketotic hyperglycemic-hyperosmolar coma (NKHHC)**   MCC H9 HCC

    E09.01 **Drug or chemical induced diabetes mellitus with hyperosmolarity with coma**   MCC H9 HCC

☑5ᵗʰ **E09.1** **Drug or chemical induced diabetes mellitus with ketoacidosis**

    E09.10 **Drug or chemical induced diabetes mellitus with ketoacidosis without coma**   MCC H9 HCC

    E09.11 **Drug or chemical induced diabetes mellitus with ketoacidosis with coma**   MCC HCC

☑5ᵗʰ **E09.2** **Drug or chemical induced diabetes mellitus with kidney complications**

    E09.21 **Drug or chemical induced diabetes mellitus with diabetic nephropathy**   HCC
Drug or chemical induced diabetes mellitus with intercapillary glomerulosclerosis
Drug or chemical induced diabetes mellitus with intracapillary glomerulonephrosis
Drug or chemical induced diabetes mellitus with Kimmelstiel-Wilson disease

    E09.22 **Drug or chemical induced diabetes mellitus with diabetic chronic kidney disease**   HCC
Use additional code to identify stage of chronic kidney disease (N18.1-N18.6)

    E09.29 **Drug or chemical induced diabetes mellitus with other diabetic kidney complication**   HCC
Drug or chemical induced diabetes mellitus with renal tubular degeneration

☑5ᵗʰ **E09.3** **Drug or chemical induced diabetes mellitus with ophthalmic complications**

One of the following 7th characters is to be assigned to codes in subcategories E09.32, E09.33, E09.34, E09.35, and E09.37 to designate laterality of the disease:
1   right eye
2   left eye
3   bilateral
9   unspecified eye

☑6ᵗʰ **E09.31** **Drug or chemical induced diabetes mellitus with unspecified diabetic retinopathy**

    E09.311 **Drug or chemical induced diabetes mellitus with unspecified diabetic retinopathy with macular edema**   HCC

    E09.319 **Drug or chemical induced diabetes mellitus with unspecified diabetic retinopathy without macular edema**   HCC

☑6ᵗʰ **E09.32** **Drug or chemical induced diabetes mellitus with mild nonproliferative diabetic retinopathy**
Drug or chemical induced diabetes mellitus with nonproliferative diabetic retinopathy NOS

    ☑7ᵗʰ **E09.321** **Drug or chemical induced diabetes mellitus with mild nonproliferative diabetic retinopathy with macular edema**   HCC

    ☑7ᵗʰ **E09.329** **Drug or chemical induced diabetes mellitus with mild nonproliferative diabetic retinopathy without macular edema**   HCC

☑6ᵗʰ **E09.33** **Drug or chemical induced diabetes mellitus with moderate nonproliferative diabetic retinopathy**

    ☑7ᵗʰ **E09.331** **Drug or chemical induced diabetes mellitus with moderate nonproliferative diabetic retinopathy with macular edema**   HCC

    ☑7ᵗʰ **E09.339** **Drug or chemical induced diabetes mellitus with moderate nonproliferative diabetic retinopathy without macular edema**   HCC

☑6ᵗʰ **E09.34** **Drug or chemical induced diabetes mellitus with severe nonproliferative diabetic retinopathy**

    ☑7ᵗʰ **E09.341** **Drug or chemical induced diabetes mellitus with severe nonproliferative diabetic retinopathy with macular edema**   HCC

    ☑7ᵗʰ **E09.349** **Drug or chemical induced diabetes mellitus with severe nonproliferative diabetic retinopathy without macular edema**   HCC

☑6ᵗʰ **E09.35** **Drug or chemical induced diabetes mellitus with proliferative diabetic retinopathy**

    ☑7ᵗʰ **E09.351** **Drug or chemical induced diabetes mellitus with proliferative diabetic retinopathy with macular edema**   HCC

    ☑7ᵗʰ **E09.352** **Drug or chemical induced diabetes mellitus with proliferative diabetic retinopathy with traction retinal detachment involving the macula**   HCC

    ☑7ᵗʰ **E09.353** **Drug or chemical induced diabetes mellitus with proliferative diabetic retinopathy with traction retinal detachment not involving the macula**   HCC

    ☑7ᵗʰ **E09.354** **Drug or chemical induced diabetes mellitus with proliferative diabetic retinopathy with combined traction retinal detachment and rhegmatogenous retinal detachment**   HCC

    ☑7ᵗʰ **E09.355** **Drug or chemical induced diabetes mellitus with stable proliferative diabetic retinopathy**   HCC

    ☑7ᵗʰ **E09.359** **Drug or chemical induced diabetes mellitus with proliferative diabetic retinopathy without macular edema**   HCC

    E09.36 **Drug or chemical induced diabetes mellitus with diabetic cataract**   HCC
AHA: 2016, 4Q, 142

☑x7ᵗʰ **E09.37** **Drug or chemical induced diabetes mellitus with diabetic macular edema, resolved following treatment**   HCC

    E09.39 **Drug or chemical induced diabetes mellitus with other diabetic ophthalmic complication**   HCC
Use additional code to identify manifestation, such as: diabetic glaucoma (H40-H42)

☑5ᵗʰ **E09.4** **Drug or chemical induced diabetes mellitus with neurological complications**

    E09.40 **Drug or chemical induced diabetes mellitus with neurological complications with diabetic neuropathy, unspecified**   HCC

    E09.41 **Drug or chemical induced diabetes mellitus with neurological complications with diabetic mononeuropathy**   HCC

    E09.42 **Drug or chemical induced diabetes mellitus with neurological complications with diabetic polyneuropathy**   HCC
Drug or chemical induced diabetes mellitus with diabetic neuralgia

    E09.43 **Drug or chemical induced diabetes mellitus with neurological complications with diabetic autonomic (poly)neuropathy**   HCC
Drug or chemical induced diabetes mellitus with diabetic gastroparesis
AHA: 2013, 4Q, 114

    E09.44 **Drug or chemical induced diabetes mellitus with neurological complications with diabetic amyotrophy**   HCC

    E09.49 **Drug or chemical induced diabetes mellitus with neurological complications with other diabetic neurological complication**   HCC

N Newborn: 0   P Pediatric: 0-17   M Maternity: 12-55   A Adult: 15-124   MCC Major CC Condition   PDxMCC PDx acts as own MCC   CC CC Condition   PDxCC PDx acts as own CC

514   ICD-10-CM 2018

✓5ᵗʰ E09.5 **Drug or chemical induced diabetes mellitus with circulatory complications**

    E09.51 **Drug or chemical induced diabetes mellitus with diabetic peripheral angiopathy without gangrene** `HCC`

    E09.52 **Drug or chemical induced diabetes mellitus with diabetic peripheral angiopathy with gangrene** `PDxCC` `CC` `HCC`

        Drug or chemical induced diabetes mellitus with diabetic gangrene

        CC Excl: PDX collection 519

    E09.59 **Drug or chemical induced diabetes mellitus with other circulatory complications** `HCC`

✓5ᵗʰ E09.6 **Drug or chemical induced diabetes mellitus with other specified complications**

    ✓6ᵗʰ E09.61 **Drug or chemical induced diabetes mellitus with diabetic arthropathy**

        E09.610 **Drug or chemical induced diabetes mellitus with diabetic neuropathic arthropathy** `HCC`

            Drug or chemical induced diabetes mellitus with Charcôt's joints

        E09.618 **Drug or chemical induced diabetes mellitus with other diabetic arthropathy** `HCC`

    ✓6ᵗʰ E09.62 **Drug or chemical induced diabetes mellitus with skin complications**

        E09.620 **Drug or chemical induced diabetes mellitus with diabetic dermatitis** `HCC`

            Drug or chemical induced diabetes mellitus with diabetic necrobiosis lipoidica

        E09.621 **Drug or chemical induced diabetes mellitus with foot ulcer** `HCC`

            Use additional code to identify site of ulcer (L97.4-, L97.5-)

        E09.622 **Drug or chemical induced diabetes mellitus with other skin ulcer** `HCC`

            Use additional code to identify site of ulcer (L97.1-L97.9, L98.41-L98.49)

        E09.628 **Drug or chemical induced diabetes mellitus with other skin complications** `HCC`

    ✓6ᵗʰ E09.63 **Drug or chemical induced diabetes mellitus with oral complications**

        E09.630 **Drug or chemical induced diabetes mellitus with periodontal disease** `HCC`

        E09.638 **Drug or chemical induced diabetes mellitus with other oral complications** `HCC`

    ✓6ᵗʰ E09.64 **Drug or chemical induced diabetes mellitus with hypoglycemia**

        E09.641 **Drug or chemical induced diabetes mellitus with hypoglycemia with coma** `MCC` `HCC`

        E09.649 **Drug or chemical induced diabetes mellitus with hypoglycemia without coma** `HCC`

            AHA: 2016, 3Q, 42; 2015, 3Q, 21

    E09.65 **Drug or chemical induced diabetes mellitus with hyperglycemia** `HCC`

    E09.69 **Drug or chemical induced diabetes mellitus with other specified complication** `HCC`

        Use additional code to identify complication

        AHA: 2016, 4Q, 141; 2016, 1Q, 13

E09.8 **Drug or chemical induced diabetes mellitus with unspecified complications** `HCC`

E09.9 **Drug or chemical induced diabetes mellitus without complications** `HCC`

✓4ᵗʰ E10 **Type 1 diabetes mellitus**

`INCLUDES` brittle diabetes (mellitus)
    diabetes (mellitus) due to autoimmune process
    diabetes (mellitus) due to immune mediated pancreatic islet beta-cell destruction
    idiopathic diabetes (mellitus)
    juvenile onset diabetes (mellitus)
    ketosis-prone diabetes (mellitus)

`EXCLUDES 1` *diabetes mellitus due to underlying condition (E08.-)*
    drug or chemical induced diabetes mellitus (E09.-)
    gestational diabetes (O24.4-)
    hyperglycemia NOS (R73.9)
    neonatal diabetes mellitus (P70.2)
    postpancreatectomy diabetes mellitus (E13.-)
    postprocedural diabetes mellitus (E13.-)
    secondary diabetes mellitus NEC (E13.-)
    type 2 diabetes mellitus (E11.-)

AHA: 2016, 1Q, 11-13; 2013, 4Q, 114; 2013, 3Q, 20

CC Excl: For MCC codes in category E10, unless otherwise noted: PDX collection 520

✓5ᵗʰ E10.1 **Type 1 diabetes mellitus with ketoacidosis**

    AHA: 2013, 3Q, 20

    E10.10 **Type 1 diabetes mellitus with ketoacidosis without coma** `MCC` `H9` `HCC`

    E10.11 **Type 1 diabetes mellitus with ketoacidosis with coma** `MCC` `HCC`

✓5ᵗʰ E10.2 **Type 1 diabetes mellitus with kidney complications**

    E10.21 **Type 1 diabetes mellitus with diabetic nephropathy** `HCC`

        Type 1 diabetes mellitus with intercapillary glomerulosclerosis

        Type 1 diabetes mellitus with intracapillary glomerulonephrosis

        Type 1 diabetes mellitus with Kimmelstiel-Wilson disease

    E10.22 **Type 1 diabetes mellitus with diabetic chronic kidney disease** `HCC`

        Use additional code to identify stage of chronic kidney disease (N18.1-N18.6)

    E10.29 **Type 1 diabetes mellitus with other diabetic kidney complication** `HCC`

        Type 1 diabetes mellitus with renal tubular degeneration

        AHA: 2016, 1Q, 13

✓5ᵗʰ E10.3 **Type 1 diabetes mellitus with ophthalmic complications**

One of the following 7th characters is to be assigned to codes in subcategories E10.32, E10.33, E10.34, E10.35, and E10.37 to designate laterality of the disease:
1   right eye
2   left eye
3   bilateral
9   unspecified eye

    ✓6ᵗʰ E10.31 **Type 1 diabetes mellitus with unspecified diabetic retinopathy**

        E10.311 **Type 1 diabetes mellitus with unspecified diabetic retinopathy with macular edema** `HCC`

        E10.319 **Type 1 diabetes mellitus with unspecified diabetic retinopathy without macular edema** `HCC`

    ✓6ᵗʰ E10.32 **Type 1 diabetes mellitus with mild nonproliferative diabetic retinopathy**

        Type 1 diabetes mellitus with nonproliferative diabetic retinopathy NOS

        ✓7ᵗʰ E10.321 **Type 1 diabetes mellitus with mild nonproliferative diabetic retinopathy with macular edema** `HCC`

        ✓7ᵗʰ E10.329 **Type 1 diabetes mellitus with mild nonproliferative diabetic retinopathy without macular edema** `HCC`

    ✓6ᵗʰ E10.33 **Type 1 diabetes mellitus with moderate nonproliferative diabetic retinopathy**

        ✓7ᵗʰ E10.331 **Type 1 diabetes mellitus with moderate nonproliferative diabetic retinopathy with macular edema** `HCC`

        ✓7ᵗʰ E10.339 **Type 1 diabetes mellitus with moderate nonproliferative diabetic retinopathy without macular edema** `HCC`

✓ Additional Character Req   ✓x7ᵗʰ Placeholder Alert   Unacceptable PDx   Manifestation   `H1`-`H14` HAC   `HCC` CMS-HCC Condition   `EXCLUDES 1` Not Coded Here   `EXCLUDES 2` Not Included Here

ICD-10-CM 2018   **515**

✓6ᵗʰ **E10.34** **Type 1 diabetes mellitus with** severe nonproliferative **diabetic** retinopathy

    ✓7ᵗʰ **E10.341** **Type 1 diabetes mellitus with severe** HCC **nonproliferative diabetic retinopathy with macular edema**

    ✓7ᵗʰ **E10.349** **Type 1 diabetes mellitus with severe** HCC **nonproliferative diabetic retinopathy without macular edema**

✓6ᵗʰ **E10.35** **Type 1 diabetes mellitus with** proliferative **diabetic** retinopathy

    ✓7ᵗʰ **E10.351** **Type 1 diabetes mellitus with** HCC **proliferative diabetic retinopathy with macular edema**

    ✓7ᵗʰ **E10.352** **Type 1 diabetes mellitus with** HCC **proliferative diabetic retinopathy with traction retinal detachment involving the macula**

    ✓7ᵗʰ **E10.353** **Type 1 diabetes mellitus with** HCC **proliferative diabetic retinopathy with traction retinal detachment not involving the macula**

    ✓7ᵗʰ **E10.354** **Type 1 diabetes mellitus with** HCC **proliferative diabetic retinopathy with combined traction retinal detachment and rhegmatogenous retinal detachment**

    ✓7ᵗʰ **E10.355** **Type 1 diabetes mellitus with stable** HCC **proliferative diabetic retinopathy**

    ✓7ᵗʰ **E10.359** **Type 1 diabetes mellitus with** HCC **proliferative diabetic retinopathy without macular edema**

E10.36 **Type 1 diabetes mellitus with diabetic** cataract HCC
    AHA: 2016, 4Q, 142

✓✗7ᵗʰ **E10.37** **Type 1 diabetes mellitus with diabetic** macular HCC **edema, resolved following treatment**

E10.39 **Type 1 diabetes mellitus with** other **diabetic** HCC **ophthalmic complication**
    Use additional code to identify manifestation, such as:
    diabetic glaucoma (H40-H42)

✓5ᵗʰ **E10.4** **Type 1 diabetes mellitus with** neurological complications

E10.40 **Type 1 diabetes mellitus with diabetic** HCC **neuropathy, unspecified**

E10.41 **Type 1 diabetes mellitus with diabetic** HCC **mononeuropathy**

E10.42 **Type 1 diabetes mellitus with diabetic** HCC **polyneuropathy**
    Type 1 diabetes mellitus with diabetic neuralgia

E10.43 **Type 1 diabetes mellitus with diabetic** HCC **autonomic (poly)neuropathy**
    Type 1 diabetes mellitus with diabetic gastroparesis
    AHA: 2013, 4Q, 114

E10.44 **Type 1 diabetes mellitus with diabetic** HCC **amyotrophy**

E10.49 **Type 1 diabetes mellitus with** other **diabetic** HCC **neurological complication**

✓5ᵗʰ **E10.5** **Type 1 diabetes mellitus with** circulatory complications

E10.51 **Type 1 diabetes mellitus with diabetic** HCC **peripheral angiopathy without gangrene**

E10.52 **Type 1 diabetes mellitus with diabetic** PDxCC CC HCC **peripheral angiopathy with gangrene**
    Type 1 diabetes mellitus with diabetic gangrene
    CC Excl: PDX collection 519

E10.59 **Type 1 diabetes mellitus with** other circulatory HCC **complications**

✓5ᵗʰ **E10.6** **Type 1 diabetes mellitus with** other specified complications

   ✓6ᵗʰ **E10.61** **Type 1 diabetes mellitus with diabetic** arthropathy

    E10.610 **Type 1 diabetes mellitus with diabetic** HCC **neuropathic arthropathy**
      Type 1 diabetes mellitus with Charcôt's joints

    E10.618 **Type 1 diabetes mellitus with** other HCC **diabetic arthropathy**

   ✓6ᵗʰ **E10.62** **Type 1 diabetes mellitus with** skin complications

    E10.620 **Type 1 diabetes mellitus with** HCC **diabetic dermatitis**
      Type 1 diabetes mellitus with diabetic necrobiosis lipoidica

E10.621 **Type 1 diabetes mellitus with** foot HCC **ulcer**
    Use additional code to identify site of ulcer (L97.4-, L97.5-)

E10.622 **Type 1 diabetes mellitus with** other HCC **skin ulcer**
    Use additional code to identify site of ulcer (L97.1-L97.9, L98.41-L98.49)

E10.628 **Type 1 diabetes mellitus with** other HCC **skin complications**

✓6ᵗʰ **E10.63** **Type 1 diabetes mellitus with** oral complications

E10.630 **Type 1 diabetes mellitus with** HCC **periodontal disease**

E10.638 **Type 1 diabetes mellitus with** other HCC **oral complications**

✓6ᵗʰ **E10.64** **Type 1 diabetes mellitus with** hypoglycemia

E10.641 **Type 1 diabetes mellitus with** MCC HCC **hypoglycemia with coma**

E10.649 **Type 1 diabetes mellitus with** HCC **hypoglycemia without coma**
    AHA: 2016, 3Q, 42; 2016, 1Q, 13; 2015, 3Q, 21

E10.65 **Type 1 diabetes mellitus with** hyperglycemia HCC
    AHA: 2013, 3Q, 20

E10.69 **Type 1 diabetes mellitus with** other specified HCC **complication**
    Use additional code to identify complication
    AHA: 2016, 4Q, 141; 2016, 1Q, 13

E10.8 **Type 1 diabetes mellitus with** unspecified complications HCC

E10.9 **Type 1 diabetes mellitus** without complications HCC

✓4ᵗʰ **E11** **Type 2 diabetes mellitus**
   INCLUDES   diabetes (mellitus) due to insulin secretory defect
     diabetes NOS
     insulin resistant diabetes (mellitus)
   Use additional code to identify control using:
     insulin (Z79.4)
     oral antidiabetic drugs (Z79.84)
     oral hypoglycemic drugs (Z79.84)
   EXCLUDES 1   *diabetes mellitus due to underlying condition (E08.-)*
     drug or chemical induced diabetes mellitus (E09.-)
     gestational diabetes (O24.4-)
     neonatal diabetes mellitus (P70.2)
     postpancreatectomy diabetes mellitus (E13.-)
     postprocedural diabetes mellitus (E13.-)
     secondary diabetes mellitus NEC (E13.-)
     type 1 diabetes mellitus (E10.-)
   AHA: 2016, 2Q, 10; 2016, 1Q, 11-13; 2013, 4Q, 114; 2013, 3Q, 20; 2013, 1Q, 26

CC Excl: For MCC codes in category E11, unless otherwise noted: PDX collection 518

✓5ᵗʰ **E11.0** **Type 2 diabetes mellitus with** hyperosmolarity

E11.00 **Type 2 diabetes mellitus with** MCC H9 HCC **hyperosmolarity without nonketotic hyperglycemic-hyperosmolar coma (NKHHC)**

E11.01 **Type 2 diabetes mellitus with** MCC H9 HCC **hyperosmolarity with coma**

● ✓5ᵗʰ **E11.1** **Type 2 diabetes mellitus with** ketoacidosis

●   **E11.10** **Type 2 diabetes mellitus with ketoacidosis** MCC **without coma**

●   **E11.11** **Type 2 diabetes mellitus with ketoacidosis** MCC **with coma**

✓5ᵗʰ **E11.2** **Type 2 diabetes mellitus with** kidney complications

E11.21 **Type 2 diabetes mellitus with diabetic** HCC **nephropathy**
    Type 2 diabetes mellitus with intercapillary glomerulosclerosis
    Type 2 diabetes mellitus with intracapillary glomerulonephrosis
    Type 2 diabetes mellitus with Kimmelstiel-Wilson disease

E11.22 **Type 2 diabetes mellitus with diabetic** chronic HCC **kidney disease**
    Use additional code to identify stage of chronic kidney disease (N18.1-N18.6)
    AHA: 2016, 1Q, 12

E11.29 **Type 2 diabetes mellitus with** other diabetic HCC **kidney complication**
    Type 2 diabetes mellitus with renal tubular degeneration

N Newborn: 0   P Pediatric: 0-17   M Maternity: 12-55   A Adult: 15-124   MCC Major CC Condition   PDxMCC PDx acts as own MCC   CC CC Condition   PDxCC PDx acts as own CC

516   ICD-10-CM 2018

☑5ᵗʰ **E11.3** **Type 2 diabetes mellitus with** ophthalmic complications

> One of the following 7th characters is to be assigned to codes in subcategories E11.32, E11.33, E11.34, E11.35, and E11.37 to designate laterality of the disease:
> 1   right eye
> 2   left eye
> 3   bilateral
> 9   unspecified eye

☑6ᵗʰ **E11.31** **Type 2 diabetes mellitus with** unspecified diabetic retinopathy

    E11.311 **Type 2 diabetes mellitus with** unspecified diabetic retinopathy **with macular edema** `HCC`

    E11.319 **Type 2 diabetes mellitus with** unspecified diabetic retinopathy **without macular edema** `HCC`

☑6ᵗʰ **E11.32** **Type 2 diabetes mellitus with** mild nonproliferative diabetic retinopathy

> Type 2 diabetes mellitus with nonproliferative diabetic retinopathy NOS

    ☑7ᵗʰ **E11.321** **Type 2 diabetes mellitus with mild** nonproliferative diabetic retinopathy **with macular edema** `HCC`

    ☑7ᵗʰ **E11.329** **Type 2 diabetes mellitus with mild** nonproliferative diabetic retinopathy **without macular edema** `HCC`

☑6ᵗʰ **E11.33** **Type 2 diabetes mellitus with** moderate nonproliferative **diabetic** retinopathy

    ☑7ᵗʰ **E11.331** **Type 2 diabetes mellitus with** moderate nonproliferative diabetic retinopathy **with macular edema** `HCC`

    ☑7ᵗʰ **E11.339** **Type 2 diabetes mellitus with** moderate nonproliferative diabetic retinopathy **without macular edema** `HCC`

☑6ᵗʰ **E11.34** **Type 2 diabetes mellitus with** severe nonproliferative **diabetic** retinopathy

    ☑7ᵗʰ **E11.341** **Type 2 diabetes mellitus with** severe nonproliferative diabetic retinopathy **with macular edema** `HCC`

    ☑7ᵗʰ **E11.349** **Type 2 diabetes mellitus with** severe nonproliferative diabetic retinopathy **without macular edema** `HCC`

☑6ᵗʰ **E11.35** **Type 2 diabetes mellitus with** proliferative diabetic retinopathy

    ☑7ᵗʰ **E11.351** **Type 2 diabetes mellitus with** proliferative diabetic retinopathy **with macular edema** `HCC`

    ☑7ᵗʰ **E11.352** **Type 2 diabetes mellitus with** proliferative diabetic retinopathy **with traction retinal detachment involving the macula** `HCC`

    ☑7ᵗʰ **E11.353** **Type 2 diabetes mellitus with** proliferative diabetic retinopathy **with traction retinal detachment not involving the macula** `HCC`

    ☑7ᵗʰ **E11.354** **Type 2 diabetes mellitus with** proliferative diabetic retinopathy **with combined traction retinal detachment and rhegmatogenous retinal detachment** `HCC`

    ☑7ᵗʰ **E11.355** **Type 2 diabetes mellitus with stable proliferative diabetic retinopathy** `HCC`

    ☑7ᵗʰ **E11.359** **Type 2 diabetes mellitus with** proliferative diabetic retinopathy **without macular edema** `HCC`

    E11.36 **Type 2 diabetes mellitus with diabetic** cataract `HCC`
> **AHA:** 2016, 4Q, 142

☑x7ᵗʰ **E11.37** **Type 2 diabetes mellitus with diabetic** macular edema, resolved following treatment `HCC`

    E11.39 **Type 2 diabetes mellitus with** other diabetic ophthalmic complication `HCC`
> Use additional code to identify manifestation, such as: diabetic glaucoma (H40-H42)

☑5ᵗʰ **E11.4** **Type 2 diabetes mellitus with** neurological complications

    E11.40 **Type 2 diabetes mellitus with diabetic neuropathy, unspecified** `HCC`
> **AHA:** 2013, 4Q, 129

    E11.41 **Type 2 diabetes mellitus with diabetic mononeuropathy** `HCC`

    E11.42 **Type 2 diabetes mellitus with diabetic polyneuropathy** `HCC`
> Type 2 diabetes mellitus with diabetic neuralgia
> **AHA:** 2016, 1Q, 12

    E11.43 **Type 2 diabetes mellitus with diabetic autonomic (poly)neuropathy** `HCC`
> Type 2 diabetes mellitus with diabetic gastroparesis
> **AHA:** 2013, 4Q, 114

    E11.44 **Type 2 diabetes mellitus with diabetic amyotrophy** `HCC`

    E11.49 **Type 2 diabetes mellitus with** other diabetic neurological complication `HCC`

☑5ᵗʰ **E11.5** **Type 2 diabetes mellitus with** circulatory complications

    E11.51 **Type 2 diabetes mellitus with diabetic peripheral angiopathy without gangrene** `HCC`

    E11.52 **Type 2 diabetes mellitus with diabetic peripheral angiopathy with gangrene** `PDxCC` `CC` `HCC`
> Type 2 diabetes mellitus with diabetic gangrene
> **CC Excl:** PDX collection 519

    E11.59 **Type 2 diabetes mellitus with** other circulatory complications `HCC`

☑5ᵗʰ **E11.6** **Type 2 diabetes mellitus with** other specified complications

    ☑6ᵗʰ **E11.61** **Type 2 diabetes mellitus with** diabetic arthropathy

        E11.610 **Type 2 diabetes mellitus with diabetic neuropathic arthropathy** `HCC`
> Type 2 diabetes mellitus with Charcôt's joints

        E11.618 **Type 2 diabetes mellitus with** other diabetic arthropathy `HCC`

    ☑6ᵗʰ **E11.62** **Type 2 diabetes mellitus with** skin complications

        E11.620 **Type 2 diabetes mellitus with diabetic dermatitis** `HCC`
> Type 2 diabetes mellitus with diabetic necrobiosis lipoidica

        E11.621 **Type 2 diabetes mellitus with foot ulcer** `HCC`
> Use additional code to identify site of ulcer (L97.4-, L97.5-)
> **AHA:** 2016, 1Q, 12

        E11.622 **Type 2 diabetes mellitus with** other skin ulcer `HCC`
> Use additional code to identify site of ulcer (L97.1-L97.9, L98.41-L98.49)

        E11.628 **Type 2 diabetes mellitus with** other skin complications `HCC`

    ☑6ᵗʰ **E11.63** **Type 2 diabetes mellitus with** oral complications

        E11.630 **Type 2 diabetes mellitus with periodontal disease** `HCC`

        E11.638 **Type 2 diabetes mellitus with** other oral complications `HCC`

    ☑6ᵗʰ **E11.64** **Type 2 diabetes mellitus with** hypoglycemia

        E11.641 **Type 2 diabetes mellitus with hypoglycemia with coma** `MCC` `HCC`

        E11.649 **Type 2 diabetes mellitus with hypoglycemia without coma** `HCC`
> **AHA:** 2016, 3Q, 42; 2015, 3Q, 21

    E11.65 **Type 2 diabetes mellitus with** hyperglycemia `HCC`
> **AHA:** 2013, 3Q, 20

    E11.69 **Type 2 diabetes mellitus with** other specified complication `HCC`
> Use additional code to identify complication
> **AHA:** 2016, 4Q, 141; 2016, 1Q, 13

E11.8 **Type 2 diabetes mellitus with** unspecified complications `HCC`

4 **E11.9** **Type 2 diabetes mellitus** without complications `HCC`

---

4   Questionable admission when used as PDx.

☑ Additional Character Req   ☑x7ᵗʰ Placeholder Alert   Unacceptable PDx   ■ Manifestation   `H1`-`H14` HAC   `HCC` CMS-HCC Condition   *EXCLUDES 1* Not Coded Here   *EXCLUDES 2* Not Included Here

Chapter 4. Endocrine, Nutritional and Metabolic Diseases

E13–E13.59

√4ᵗʰ **E13**   **Other specified diabetes mellitus**

    INCLUDES   diabetes mellitus due to genetic defects of beta-cell function
         diabetes mellitus due to genetic defects in insulin action
         postpancreatectomy diabetes mellitus
         postprocedural diabetes mellitus
         secondary diabetes mellitus NEC

    Use additional code to identify control using:
         insulin (Z79.4)
         oral antidiabetic drugs (Z79.84)
         oral hypoglycemic drugs (Z79.84)

    EXCLUDES 1   *diabetes (mellitus) due to autoimmune process (E10.-)*
         diabetes (mellitus) due to immune mediated pancreatic islet
           beta-cell destruction (E10.-)
         diabetes mellitus due to underlying condition (E08.-)
         drug or chemical induced diabetes mellitus (E09.-)
         gestational diabetes (O24.4-)
         neonatal diabetes mellitus (P70.2)
         type 1 diabetes mellitus (E10.-)
         ~~*type 2 diabetes mellitus (E11.-)*~~

    AHA: 2016, 1Q, 11-13; 2013, 4Q, 114; 2013, 3Q, 20

    CC Excl: For MCC codes in category E13, unless otherwise noted:
    PDX collection 518

√5ᵗʰ **E13.0**   **Other specified diabetes mellitus with** hyperosmolarity

     E13.00   **Other specified diabetes mellitus with**   MCC H9 HCC
          hyperosmolarity without nonketotic
          hyperglycemic-hyperosmolar coma (NKHHC)
            EXCLUDES 2 ▶*type 2 diabetes mellitus (E11.-)*◀

     E13.01   **Other specified diabetes mellitus with**   MCC H9 HCC
          hyperosmolarity with coma

√5ᵗʰ **E13.1**   **Other specified diabetes mellitus with** ketoacidosis
     AHA: 2016, 2Q, 10; 2013, 1Q, 26

     E13.10   **Other specified diabetes mellitus with**   MCC H9 HCC
          ketoacidosis without coma

     E13.11   **Other specified diabetes mellitus with**   MCC HCC
          ketoacidosis with coma

√5ᵗʰ **E13.2**   **Other specified diabetes mellitus with** kidney complications

     E13.21   **Other specified diabetes mellitus with diabetic**   HCC
          nephropathy
          Other specified diabetes mellitus with intercapillary
            glomerulosclerosis
          Other specified diabetes mellitus with intracapillary
            glomerulonephrosis
          Other specified diabetes mellitus with Kimmelstiel-
            Wilson disease

     E13.22   **Other specified diabetes mellitus with diabetic**   HCC
          chronic kidney disease
          Use additional code to identify stage of chronic kidney
            disease (N18.1-N18.6)

     E13.29   **Other specified diabetes mellitus with other**   HCC
          diabetic kidney complication
          Other specified diabetes mellitus with renal tubular
            degeneration

√5ᵗʰ **E13.3**   **Other specified diabetes mellitus with** ophthalmic
    complications

    One of the following 7th characters is to be assigned to codes
    in subcategories E13.32, E13.33, E13.34, E13.35, and E13.37 to
    designate laterality of the disease:
     1   right eye
     2   left eye
     3   bilateral
     9   unspecified eye

√6ᵗʰ   **E13.31**   **Other specified diabetes mellitus with** unspecified
          diabetic retinopathy

         E13.311   **Other specified diabetes mellitus with** HCC
            unspecified diabetic retinopathy with
            macular edema

         E13.319   **Other specified diabetes mellitus with** HCC
            unspecified diabetic retinopathy
            without macular edema

√6ᵗʰ   **E13.32**   **Other specified diabetes mellitus with** mild
          nonproliferative **diabetic** retinopathy
          Other specified diabetes mellitus with nonproliferative
            diabetic retinopathy NOS

         √7ᵗʰ **E13.321**   **Other specified diabetes mellitus with** HCC
            mild nonproliferative diabetic
            retinopathy with macular edema

         √7ᵗʰ **E13.329**   **Other specified diabetes mellitus with** HCC
            mild nonproliferative diabetic
            retinopathy without macular edema

√6ᵗʰ **E13.33**   **Other specified diabetes mellitus with** moderate
          nonproliferative **diabetic** retinopathy

         √7ᵗʰ **E13.331**   **Other specified diabetes mellitus with** HCC
            moderate nonproliferative diabetic
            retinopathy with macular edema

         √7ᵗʰ **E13.339**   **Other specified diabetes mellitus with** HCC
            moderate nonproliferative diabetic
            retinopathy without macular edema

√6ᵗʰ **E13.34**   **Other specified diabetes mellitus with** severe
          nonproliferative **diabetic** retinopathy

         √7ᵗʰ **E13.341**   **Other specified diabetes mellitus with** HCC
            severe nonproliferative diabetic
            retinopathy with macular edema

         √7ᵗʰ **E13.349**   **Other specified diabetes mellitus with** HCC
            severe nonproliferative diabetic
            retinopathy without macular edema

√6ᵗʰ **E13.35**   **Other specified diabetes mellitus with** proliferative
          diabetic retinopathy

         √7ᵗʰ **E13.351**   **Other specified diabetes mellitus with** HCC
            proliferative diabetic retinopathy with
            macular edema

         √7ᵗʰ **E13.352**   **Other specified diabetes mellitus with** HCC
            proliferative diabetic retinopathy with
            traction retinal detachment involving the
            macula

         √7ᵗʰ **E13.353**   **Other specified diabetes mellitus with** HCC
            proliferative diabetic retinopathy with
            traction retinal detachment not involving
            the macula

         √7ᵗʰ **E13.354**   **Other specified diabetes mellitus with** HCC
            proliferative diabetic retinopathy with
            combined traction retinal detachment and
            rhegmatogenous retinal detachment

         √7ᵗʰ **E13.355**   **Other specified diabetes mellitus with** HCC
            stable **proliferative diabetic retinopathy**

         √7ᵗʰ **E13.359**   **Other specified diabetes mellitus with** HCC
            proliferative diabetic retinopathy without
            macular edema

     E13.36   **Other specified diabetes mellitus with** diabetic   HCC
          cataract
          AHA: 2016, 4Q, 142

√x 7ᵗʰ **E13.37**   **Other specified diabetes mellitus with diabetic**   HCC
          macular edema, resolved following treatment

     E13.39   **Other specified diabetes mellitus with** other   HCC
          diabetic ophthalmic complication
          Use additional code to identify manifestation, such as:
            diabetic glaucoma (H40-H42)

√5ᵗʰ **E13.4**   **Other specified diabetes mellitus with** neurological
    complications

     E13.40   **Other specified diabetes mellitus with diabetic**   HCC
          neuropathy, unspecified

     E13.41   **Other specified diabetes mellitus with diabetic**   HCC
          mononeuropathy

     E13.42   **Other specified diabetes mellitus with diabetic**   HCC
          polyneuropathy
          Other specified diabetes mellitus with diabetic
            neuralgia

     E13.43   **Other specified diabetes mellitus with diabetic**   HCC
          autonomic (poly)neuropathy
          Other specified diabetes mellitus with diabetic
            gastroparesis
          AHA: 2013, 4Q, 114

     E13.44   **Other specified diabetes mellitus with diabetic**   HCC
          amyotrophy

     E13.49   **Other specified diabetes mellitus with** other   HCC
          diabetic neurological complication

√5ᵗʰ **E13.5**   **Other specified diabetes mellitus with** circulatory
    complications

     E13.51   **Other specified diabetes mellitus with diabetic**   HCC
          peripheral angiopathy without gangrene

     E13.52   **Other specified diabetes mellitus with**   PDxCC CC HCC
          diabetic peripheral angiopathy with gangrene
          Other specified diabetes mellitus with diabetic
            gangrene
          CC Excl: PDX collection 519

     E13.59   **Other specified diabetes mellitus with** other   HCC
          circulatory complications

N Newborn: 0   P Pediatric: 0-17   M Maternity: 12-55   A Adult: 15-124   MCC Major CC Condition   PDxMCC PDx acts as own MCC   CC CC Condition   PDxCC PDx acts as own CC

518   ICD-10-CM 2018

☑5ᵗʰ **E13.6 Other specified diabetes mellitus with** other specified complications

☑6ᵗʰ **E13.61 Other specified diabetes mellitus with diabetic** arthropathy

   E13.610 Other specified diabetes mellitus with HCC **diabetic** neuropathic **arthropathy**
      Other specified diabetes mellitus with Charcôt's joints

   E13.618 Other specified diabetes mellitus with HCC other **diabetic arthropathy**

☑6ᵗʰ **E13.62 Other specified diabetes mellitus with** skin complications

   E13.620 Other specified diabetes mellitus with HCC **diabetic** dermatitis
      Other specified diabetes mellitus with diabetic necrobiosis lipoidica

   E13.621 Other specified diabetes mellitus with HCC **foot ulcer**
      Use additional code to identify site of ulcer (L97.4-, L97.5-)

   E13.622 Other specified diabetes mellitus with HCC other **skin ulcer**
      Use additional code to identify site of ulcer (L97.1-L97.9, L98.41-L98.49)

   E13.628 Other specified diabetes mellitus with HCC other **skin complications**

☑6ᵗʰ **E13.63 Other specified diabetes mellitus with** oral complications

   E13.630 Other specified diabetes mellitus with HCC **periodontal disease**

   E13.638 Other specified diabetes mellitus with HCC other **oral complications**

☑6ᵗʰ **E13.64 Other specified diabetes mellitus with** hypoglycemia

   E13.641 Other specified diabetes mellitus MCC HCC **with hypoglycemia** with coma

   E13.649 Other specified diabetes mellitus with HCC **hypoglycemia** without coma
      AHA: 2016, 3Q, 42; 2015, 3Q, 21

   E13.65 Other specified diabetes mellitus with HCC **hyperglycemia**

   E13.69 Other specified diabetes mellitus with other HCC **specified complication**
      Use additional code to identify complication
      AHA: 2016, 4Q, 141; 2016, 1Q, 13

E13.8 Other specified diabetes mellitus with unspecified HCC **complications**

⁴ **E13.9 Other specified diabetes mellitus** without complications HCC

Other disorders of glucose regulation and pancreatic internal secretion (E15-E16)

E15 Nondiabetic hypoglycemic coma CC H9 HCC
INCLUDES drug-induced insulin coma in nondiabetic
hyperinsulinism with hypoglycemic coma
hypoglycemic coma NOS
CC Excl: PDX collection 520

☑4ᵗʰ **E16 Other disorders of pancreatic internal secretion**

E16.0 Drug-induced hypoglycemia without coma
    Use additional code for adverse effect, if applicable, to identify drug (T36-T50 with fifth or sixth character 5)
    EXCLUDES 1 diabetes with hypoglycemia without coma ▶(E09.649)◀

E16.1 Other hypoglycemia
    Functional hyperinsulinism
    Functional nonhyperinsulinemic hypoglycemia
    Hyperinsulinism NOS
    Hyperplasia of pancreatic islet beta cells NOS
    EXCLUDES 1 diabetes with hypoglycemia (E08.649, E10.649, E11.649, E13.649)
      hypoglycemia in infant of diabetic mother (P70.1)
      neonatal hypoglycemia (P70.4)

E16.2 Hypoglycemia, unspecified
    EXCLUDES 1 diabetes with hypoglycemia (E08.649, E10.649, E11.649, E13.649)
    AHA: 2016, 3Q, 42

E16.3 Increased secretion of glucagon
    Hyperplasia of pancreatic endocrine cells with glucagon excess

E16.4 Increased secretion of gastrin
    Hypergastrinemia
    Hyperplasia of pancreatic endocrine cells with gastrin excess
    Zollinger-Ellison syndrome

E16.8 Other specified disorders of pancreatic internal secretion
    Increased secretion from endocrine pancreas of growth hormone-releasing hormone
    Increased secretion from endocrine pancreas of pancreatic polypeptide
    Increased secretion from endocrine pancreas of somatostatin
    Increased secretion from endocrine pancreas of vasoactive-intestinal polypeptide

E16.9 Disorder of pancreatic internal secretion, unspecified
    Islet-cell hyperplasia NOS
    Pancreatic endocrine cell hyperplasia NOS

Disorders of other endocrine glands (E20-E35)

EXCLUDES 1 galactorrhea (N64.3)
    gynecomastia (N62)

☑4ᵗʰ **E20 Hypoparathyroidism**
    EXCLUDES 1 Di George's syndrome (D82.1)
      postprocedural hypoparathyroidism (E89.2)
      tetany NOS (R29.0)
      transitory neonatal hypoparathyroidism (P71.4)

E20.0 Idiopathic hypoparathyroidism HCC
    DEF: Abnormally low secretion of parathyroid hormones, with unknown cause, which causes decreased calcium and increased phosphorus in the blood, resulting in muscle cramps, tetany, tingling, or burning in lips, fingers, and toes, and cataracts.

E20.1 Pseudohypoparathyroidism

E20.8 Other hypoparathyroidism HCC

E20.9 Hypoparathyroidism, unspecified HCC
    Parathyroid tetany

☑4ᵗʰ **E21 Hyperparathyroidism and other disorders of parathyroid gland**
    EXCLUDES 1 adult osteomalacia (M83.-)
      ectopic hyperparathyroidism (E34.2)
      familial hypocalciuric hypercalcemia (E83.52)
      hungry bone syndrome (E83.81)
      infantile and juvenile osteomalacia (E55.0)

E21.0 Primary hyperparathyroidism HCC
    Hyperplasia of parathyroid
    Osteitis fibrosa cystica generalisata [von Recklinghausen's disease of bone]
    DEF: Parathyroid dysfunction commonly caused by hyperplasia of two or more glands; characteristic hypercalcemia and increased parathyroid hormone levels.

E21.1 Secondary hyperparathyroidism, not elsewhere classified HCC
    EXCLUDES 1 secondary hyperparathyroidism of renal origin (N25.81)

E21.2 Other hyperparathyroidism HCC
    Tertiary hyperparathyroidism
    EXCLUDES 1 familial hypocalciuric hypercalcemia (E83.52)

E21.3 Hyperparathyroidism, unspecified HCC

E21.4 Other specified disorders of parathyroid gland HCC

E21.5 Disorder of parathyroid gland, unspecified HCC

☑4ᵗʰ **E22 Hyperfunction of pituitary gland**
    EXCLUDES 1 Cushing's syndrome (E24.-)
      Nelson's syndrome (E24.1)
      overproduction of ACTH not associated with Cushing's disease (E27.0)
      overproduction of pituitary ACTH (E24.0)
      overproduction of thyroid-stimulating hormone (E05.8-)

CC Excl: For CC codes in category E22, unless otherwise noted: PDX collection 521

E22.0 Acromegaly and pituitary gigantism HCC
    Overproduction of growth hormone
    EXCLUDES 1 constitutional gigantism (E34.4)
      constitutional tall stature (E34.4)
      increased secretion from endocrine pancreas of growth hormone-releasing hormone (E16.8)

E22.1 Hyperprolactinemia CC HCC
    Use additional code for adverse effect, if applicable, to identify drug (T36-T50 with fifth or sixth character 5)

E22.2 Syndrome of inappropriate secretion of antidiuretic CC HCC **hormone**
    CC Excl: PDX collection 522

⁴ Questionable admission when used as PDx.

Chapter 4. Endocrine, Nutritional and Metabolic Diseases

E22.8   **Other hyperfunction of pituitary gland**   `CC` `HCC`
Central precocious puberty

E22.9   **Hyperfunction of pituitary gland, unspecified**   `CC` `HCC`

`✓4ᵗʰ` **E23**   **Hypofunction and other disorders of the pituitary gland**
`INCLUDES` the listed conditions whether the disorder is in the pituitary or the hypothalamus
`EXCLUDES 1` postprocedural hypopituitarism (E89.3)

E23.0   **Hypopituitarism**   `CC` `HCC`
Fertile eunuch syndrome
Hypogonadotropic hypogonadism
Idiopathic growth hormone deficiency
Isolated deficiency of gonadotropin
Isolated deficiency of growth hormone
Isolated deficiency of pituitary hormone
Kallmann's syndrome
Lorain-Levi short stature
Necrosis of pituitary gland (postpartum)
Panhypopituitarism
Pituitary cachexia
Pituitary insufficiency NOS
Pituitary short stature
Sheehan's syndrome
Simmonds' disease
CC Excl: PDX collection 523

E23.1   **Drug-induced hypopituitarism**   `HCC`
Use additional code for adverse effect, if applicable, to identify drug (T36-T50 with fifth or sixth character 5)

E23.2   **Diabetes insipidus**   `CC` `HCC`
`EXCLUDES 1` nephrogenic diabetes insipidus (N25.1)
CC Excl: PDX collection 524

E23.3   **Hypothalamic dysfunction, not elsewhere classified**   `HCC`
`EXCLUDES 1` Prader-Willi syndrome (Q87.1)
Russell-Silver syndrome (Q87.1)

E23.6   **Other disorders of pituitary gland**   `HCC`
Abscess of pituitary
Adiposogenital dystrophy

E23.7   **Disorder of pituitary gland, unspecified**   `HCC`

`✓4ᵗʰ` **E24**   **Cushing's syndrome**
`EXCLUDES 1` congenital adrenal hyperplasia (E25.0)

CC Excl: For CC codes in category E24: PDX collection 525

E24.0   **Pituitary-dependent Cushing's disease**   `CC` `HCC`
Overproduction of pituitary ACTH
Pituitary-dependent hypercorticalism

E24.1   **Nelson's syndrome**   `HCC`

E24.2   **Drug-induced Cushing's syndrome**   `CC` `HCC`
Use additional code for adverse effect, if applicable, to identify drug (T36-T50 with fifth or sixth character 5)

E24.3   **Ectopic ACTH syndrome**   `CC` `HCC`

E24.4   **Alcohol-induced pseudo-Cushing's syndrome**   `CC` `HCC`

E24.8   **Other Cushing's syndrome**   `CC` `HCC`

E24.9   **Cushing's syndrome, unspecified**   `CC` `HCC`

`✓4ᵗʰ` **E25**   **Adrenogenital disorders**
`INCLUDES` adrenogenital syndromes, virilizing or feminizing, whether acquired or due to adrenal hyperplasia consequent on inborn enzyme defects in hormone synthesis
female adrenal pseudohermaphroditism
female heterosexual precocious pseudopuberty
male isosexual precocious pseudopuberty
male macrogenitosomia praecox
male sexual precocity with adrenal hyperplasia
male virilization (female)
`EXCLUDES 1` indeterminate sex and pseudohermaphroditism (Q56)
chromosomal abnormalities (Q90-Q99)

E25.0   **Congenital adrenogenital disorders associated with enzyme deficiency**   `HCC`
Congenital adrenal hyperplasia
21-Hydroxylase deficiency
Salt-losing congenital adrenal hyperplasia

E25.8   **Other adrenogenital disorders**   `HCC`
Idiopathic adrenogenital disorder
Use additional code for adverse effect, if applicable, to identify drug (T36-T50 with fifth or sixth character 5)

E25.9   **Adrenogenital disorder, unspecified**   `HCC`
Adrenogenital syndrome NOS

`✓4ᵗʰ` **E26**   **Hyperaldosteronism**

`✓5ᵗʰ` **E26.0**   **Primary hyperaldosteronism**

E26.01   **Conn's syndrome**   `HCC`
Code also adrenal adenoma (D35.0-)

E26.02   **Glucocorticoid-remediable aldosteronism**   `HCC`
Familial aldosteronism type I
DEF: Rare autosomal dominant familial form of primary aldosteronism in which the secretion of aldosterone is under the influence of adrenocorticotrophic hormone (ACTH) rather than the renin-angiotensin mechanism; moderate hypersecretion of aldosterone and suppressed plasma renin activity that are rapidly reversed by administration of glucosteroids; symptoms include hypertension and mild hypokalemia.

E26.09   **Other primary hyperaldosteronism**   `HCC`
Primary aldosteronism due to adrenal hyperplasia (bilateral)

E26.1   **Secondary hyperaldosteronism**   `HCC`

`✓5ᵗʰ` **E26.8**   **Other hyperaldosteronism**

E26.81   **Bartter's syndrome**   `HCC`

E26.89   **Other hyperaldosteronism**   `HCC`

E26.9   **Hyperaldosteronism, unspecified**   `HCC`
Aldosteronism NOS
Hyperaldosteronism NOS

`✓4ᵗʰ` **E27**   **Other disorders of adrenal gland**

CC Excl: For CC codes in category E27: PDX collection 526

E27.0   **Other adrenocortical overactivity**   `CC` `HCC`
Overproduction of ACTH, not associated with Cushing's disease
Premature adrenarche
`EXCLUDES 1` Cushing's syndrome (E24.-)

E27.1   **Primary adrenocortical insufficiency**   `CC` `HCC`
Addison's disease
Autoimmune adrenalitis
`EXCLUDES 1` Addison only phenotype adrenoleukodystrophy (E71.528)
amyloidosis (E85.-)
tuberculous Addison's disease (A18.7)
Waterhouse-Friderichsen syndrome (A39.1)

E27.2   **Addisonian crisis**   `CC` `HCC`
Adrenal crisis
Adrenocortical crisis

E27.3   **Drug-induced adrenocortical insufficiency**   `CC` `HCC`
Use additional code for adverse effect, if applicable, to identify drug (T36-T50 with fifth or sixth character 5)

`✓5ᵗʰ` **E27.4**   **Other and unspecified adrenocortical insufficiency**
`EXCLUDES 1` adrenoleukodystrophy [Addison-Schilder] (E71.528)
Waterhouse-Friderichsen syndrome (A39.1)

E27.40   **Unspecified adrenocortical insufficiency**   `CC` `HCC`
Adrenocortical insufficiency NOS
Hypoaldosteronism

E27.49   **Other adrenocortical insufficiency**   `CC` `HCC`
Adrenal hemorrhage
Adrenal infarction

E27.5   **Adrenomedullary hyperfunction**   `CC` `HCC`
Adrenomedullary hyperplasia
Catecholamine hypersecretion

E27.8   **Other specified disorders of adrenal gland**   `HCC`
Abnormality of cortisol-binding globulin

E27.9   **Disorder of adrenal gland, unspecified**   `HCC`

`✓4ᵗʰ` **E28**   **Ovarian dysfunction**
`EXCLUDES 1` isolated gonadotropin deficiency (E23.0)
postprocedural ovarian failure (E89.4-)

E28.0   **Estrogen excess**   ♀
Use additional code for adverse effect, if applicable, to identify drug (T36-T50 with fifth or sixth character 5)

E28.1   **Androgen excess**   ♀
Hypersecretion of ovarian androgens
Use additional code for adverse effect, if applicable, to identify drug (T36-T50 with fifth or sixth character 5)

E28.2   **Polycystic ovarian syndrome**   ♀
Sclerocystic ovary syndrome
Stein-Leventhal syndrome

`N` Newborn: 0   `P` Pediatric: 0-17   `M` Maternity: 12-55   `A` Adult: 15-124   `MCC` Major CC Condition   `PDxMCC` PDx acts as own MCC   `CC` CC Condition   `PDxCC` PDx acts as own CC

√5th **E28.3 Primary ovarian failure**
EXCLUDES 1   *pure gonadal dysgenesis (Q99.1)*
            Turner's syndrome (Q96.-)

√6th   **E28.31 Premature menopause**

E28.310 Symptomatic premature menopause A♀
Symptoms such as flushing, sleeplessness, headache, lack of concentration, associated with premature menopause

E28.319 Asymptomatic premature menopause A♀
Premature menopause NOS

E28.39 Other primary ovarian failure ♀
Decreased estrogen
Resistant ovary syndrome

E28.8 Other ovarian dysfunction ♀
Ovarian hyperfunction NOS
EXCLUDES 1   *postprocedural ovarian failure (E89.4-)*

E28.9 Ovarian dysfunction, unspecified ♀

√4th **E29 Testicular dysfunction**
EXCLUDES 1   *androgen insensitivity syndrome (E34.5-)*
            azoospermia or oligospermia NOS (N46.0-N46.1)
            isolated gonadotropin deficiency (E23.0)
            Klinefelter's syndrome (Q98.0-Q98.1, Q98.4)

E29.0 Testicular hyperfunction ♂
Hypersecretion of testicular hormones

E29.1 Testicular hypofunction ♂
Defective biosynthesis of testicular androgen NOS
5-delta-Reductase deficiency (with male pseudohermaphroditism)
Testicular hypogonadism NOS
Use additional code for adverse effect, if applicable, to identify drug (T36-T50 with fifth or sixth character 5)
EXCLUDES 1   *postprocedural testicular hypofunction (E89.5)*

E29.8 Other testicular dysfunction ♂

E29.9 Testicular dysfunction, unspecified ♂

√4th **E30 Disorders of puberty, not elsewhere classified**

E30.0 Delayed puberty
Constitutional delay of puberty
Delayed sexual development

E30.1 Precocious puberty P
Precocious menstruation
EXCLUDES 1   *Albright (-McCune) (-Sternberg) syndrome (Q78.1)*
            central precocious puberty (E22.8)
            congenital adrenal hyperplasia (E25.0)
            female heterosexual precocious pseudopuberty (E25.-)
            male isosexual precocious pseudopuberty (E25.-)

E30.8 Other disorders of puberty P
Premature thelarche

E30.9 Disorder of puberty, unspecified

√4th **E31 Polyglandular dysfunction**
EXCLUDES 1   *ataxia telangiectasia [Louis-Bar] (G11.3)*
            dystrophia myotonica [Steinert] (G71.11)
            pseudohypoparathyroidism (E20.1)

E31.0 Autoimmune polyglandular failure HCC
Schmidt's syndrome

E31.1 Polyglandular hyperfunction HCC
EXCLUDES 1   *multiple endocrine adenomatosis (E31.2-)*
            multiple endocrine neoplasia (E31.2-)

√5th **E31.2 Multiple endocrine neoplasia [MEN] syndromes**
Multiple endocrine adenomatosis
Code also any associated malignancies and other conditions associated with the syndromes

E31.20 Multiple endocrine neoplasia [MEN] syndrome, unspecified HCC
Multiple endocrine adenomatosis NOS
Multiple endocrine neoplasia [MEN] syndrome NOS

E31.21 Multiple endocrine neoplasia [MEN] type I HCC
Wermer's syndrome

E31.22 Multiple endocrine neoplasia [MEN] type IIA HCC
Sipple's syndrome

E31.23 Multiple endocrine neoplasia [MEN] type IIB HCC

E31.8 Other polyglandular dysfunction HCC

E31.9 Polyglandular dysfunction, unspecified HCC

√4th **E32 Diseases of thymus**
EXCLUDES 1   *aplasia or hypoplasia of thymus with immunodeficiency (D82.1)*
            myasthenia gravis (G70.0)

E32.0 Persistent hyperplasia of thymus HCC
Hypertrophy of thymus

E32.1 Abscess of thymus CC HCC
CC Excl: PDX collection 527

E32.8 Other diseases of thymus HCC
EXCLUDES 1   *aplasia or hypoplasia with immunodeficiency (D82.1)*
            thymoma (D15.0)

E32.9 Disease of thymus, unspecified HCC

√4th **E34 Other endocrine disorders**
EXCLUDES 1   *pseudohypoparathyroidism (E20.1)*

E34.0 Carcinoid syndrome CC HCC
NOTE   May be used as an additional code to identify functional activity associated with a carcinoid tumor.
CC Excl: PDX collection 528

E34.1 Other hypersecretion of intestinal hormones

E34.2 Ectopic hormone secretion, not elsewhere classified
EXCLUDES 1   *ectopic ACTH syndrome (E24.3)*

E34.3 Short stature due to endocrine disorder
Constitutional short stature
Laron-type short stature
EXCLUDES 1   *achondroplastic short stature (Q77.4)*
            hypochondroplastic short stature (Q77.4)
            nutritional short stature (E45)
            pituitary short stature (E23.0)
            progeria (E34.8)
            renal short stature (N25.0)
            Russell-Silver syndrome (Q87.1)
            short-limbed stature with immunodeficiency (D82.2)
            short stature in specific dysmorphic syndromes— code to syndrome—see Alphabetical Index
            short stature NOS (R62.52)

E34.4 Constitutional tall stature HCC
Constitutional gigantism

√5th **E34.5 Androgen insensitivity syndrome**

E34.50 Androgen insensitivity syndrome, unspecified
Androgen insensitivity NOS

E34.51 Complete androgen insensitivity syndrome
Complete androgen insensitivity
de Quervain syndrome
Goldberg-Maxwell syndrome

E34.52 Partial androgen insensitivity syndrome
Partial androgen insensitivity
Reifenstein syndrome

E34.8 Other specified endocrine disorders
Pineal gland dysfunction   Progeria
EXCLUDES 2   *pseudohypoparathyroidism (E20.1)*

E34.9 Endocrine disorder, unspecified
Endocrine disturbance NOS
Hormone disturbance NOS

E35 *Disorders of endocrine glands in diseases classified elsewhere*
Code first underlying disease, such as:
late congenital syphilis of thymus gland [Dubois disease] (A50.5)
Use additional code, if applicable, to identify:
sequelae of tuberculosis of other organs (B90.8)
EXCLUDES 1   *Echinococcus granulosus infection of thyroid gland (B67.3)*
            meningococcal hemorrhagic adrenalitis (A39.1)
            syphilis of endocrine gland (A52.79)
            tuberculosis of adrenal gland, except calcification (A18.7)
            tuberculosis of endocrine gland NEC (A18.82)
            tuberculosis of thyroid gland (A18.81)
            Waterhouse-Friderichsen syndrome (A39.1)

Intraoperative Complications of Endocrine System (E36)

√4th **E36 Intraoperative complications of endocrine system**
EXCLUDES 2   *postprocedural endocrine and metabolic complications and disorders, not elsewhere classified (E89.-)*

√5th **E36.0 Intraoperative hemorrhage and hematoma of an endocrine system organ or structure complicating a procedure**
EXCLUDES 1   *intraoperative hemorrhage and hematoma of an endocrine system organ or structure due to accidental puncture or laceration during a procedure (E36.1-)*

E36.01 Intraoperative hemorrhage and hematoma of CC **an endocrine system organ or structure complicating an endocrine system procedure**
CC Excl: PDX collection 529

☑ Additional Character Req   √x7th Placeholder Alert   Unacceptable PDx   Manifestation   H1-H14 HAC   HCC CMS-HCC Condition   *EXCLUDES 1* Not Coded Here   *EXCLUDES 2* Not Included Here

ICD-10-CM 2018   521

Chapter 4. Endocrine, Nutritional and Metabolic Diseases

E36.02   Intraoperative hemorrhage and hematoma of an endocrine system organ or structure complicating other procedure   `CC`
CC Excl: PDX collection 529

✓5ᵗʰ **E36.1**   Accidental puncture and laceration of an endocrine system organ or structure during a procedure

E36.11   Accidental puncture and laceration of an endocrine system organ or structure during an endocrine system procedure   `CC`
CC Excl: PDX collection 509

E36.12   Accidental puncture and laceration of an endocrine system organ or structure during other procedure   `CC`
CC Excl: PDX collection 509

E36.8   Other intraoperative complications of endocrine system
Use additional code, if applicable, to further specify disorder

Malnutrition (E40-E46)

EXCLUDES 1   intestinal malabsorption (K90.-)
sequelae of protein-calorie malnutrition (E64.0)
EXCLUDES 2   nutritional anemias (D50-D53)
starvation (T73.0)

E40   Kwashiorkor   `MCC` `HCC`
Severe malnutrition with nutritional edema with dyspigmentation of skin and hair
EXCLUDES 1   marasmic kwashiorkor (E42)
CC Excl: PDX collection 530

E41   Nutritional marasmus   `MCC` `HCC`
Severe malnutrition with marasmus
EXCLUDES 1   marasmic kwashiorkor (E42)
DEF: Protein-calorie malabsorption or malnutrition in children; characterized by tissue wasting, dehydration, and subcutaneous fat depletion; may occur with infectious disease; also called infantile atrophy.
CC Excl: PDX collection 530

E42   Marasmic kwashiorkor   `MCC` `HCC`
Intermediate form severe protein-calorie malnutrition
Severe protein-calorie malnutrition with signs of both kwashiorkor and marasmus
CC Excl: PDX collection 530

E43   Unspecified severe protein-calorie malnutrition   `MCC` `HCC`
Starvation edema
CC Excl: PDX collection 530

✓4ᵗʰ **E44**   Protein-calorie malnutrition of moderate and mild degree

E44.0   Moderate protein-calorie malnutrition   `CC` `HCC`
CC Excl: PDX collection 530

E44.1   Mild protein-calorie malnutrition   `CC` `HCC`
CC Excl: PDX collection 530

E45   Retarded development following protein-calorie malnutrition   `CC` `HCC`
Nutritional short stature
Nutritional stunting
Physical retardation due to malnutrition
CC Excl: PDX collection 530

E46   Unspecified protein-calorie malnutrition   `CC` `HCC`
Malnutrition NOS
Protein-calorie imbalance NOS
EXCLUDES 1   nutritional deficiency NOS (E63.9)
CC Excl: PDX collection 530

Other nutritional deficiencies (E50-E64)

EXCLUDES 2   nutritional anemias (D50-D53)

✓4ᵗʰ **E50**   Vitamin A deficiency
EXCLUDES 1   sequelae of vitamin A deficiency (E64.1)

E50.0   Vitamin A deficiency with conjunctival xerosis

E50.1   Vitamin A deficiency with Bitot's spot and conjunctival xerosis
Bitot's spot in the young child
DEF: Vitamin A deficiency with conjunctival dryness, superficial spots of keratinized epithelium.

E50.2   Vitamin A deficiency with corneal xerosis

E50.3   Vitamin A deficiency with corneal ulceration and xerosis

E50.4   Vitamin A deficiency with keratomalacia
DEF: Vitamin A deficiency creating corneal dryness; progresses to corneal insensitivity, softness, and necrosis; usually bilateral.

E50.5   Vitamin A deficiency with night blindness

E50.6   Vitamin A deficiency with xerophthalmic scars of cornea

E50.7   Other ocular manifestations of vitamin A deficiency
Xerophthalmia NOS

E50.8   Other manifestations of vitamin A deficiency
Follicular keratosis
Xeroderma

E50.9   Vitamin A deficiency, unspecified
Hypovitaminosis A NOS

✓4ᵗʰ **E51**   Thiamine deficiency
EXCLUDES 1   sequelae of thiamine deficiency (E64.8)

CC Excl: For CC codes in category E51: PDX collection 531

✓5ᵗʰ **E51.1**   Beriberi

E51.11   Dry beriberi   `CC`
Beriberi NOS
Beriberi with polyneuropathy

E51.12   Wet beriberi   `CC`
Beriberi with cardiovascular manifestations
Cardiovascular beriberi
Shoshin disease

E51.2   Wernicke's encephalopathy   `CC`

E51.8   Other manifestations of thiamine deficiency   `CC`

E51.9   Thiamine deficiency, unspecified   `CC`

E52   Niacin deficiency [pellagra]
Niacin (-tryptophan) deficiency
Nicotinamide deficiency
Pellagra (alcoholic)
EXCLUDES 1   sequelae of niacin deficiency (E64.8)

✓4ᵗʰ **E53**   Deficiency of other B group vitamins
EXCLUDES 1   sequelae of vitamin B deficiency (E64.8)

E53.0   Riboflavin deficiency   `CC`
Ariboflavinosis
Vitamin B2 deficiency
CC Excl: PDX collection 531

E53.1   Pyridoxine deficiency
Vitamin B6 deficiency
EXCLUDES 1   pyridoxine-responsive sideroblastic anemia (D64.3)

E53.8   Deficiency of other specified B group vitamins
Biotin deficiency
Cyanocobalamin deficiency
Folate deficiency
Folic acid deficiency
Pantothenic acid deficiency
Vitamin B12 deficiency
EXCLUDES 1   folate deficiency anemia (D52.-)
vitamin B12 deficiency anemia (D51.-)

E53.9   Vitamin B deficiency, unspecified

E54   Ascorbic acid deficiency
Deficiency of vitamin C
Scurvy
EXCLUDES 1   scorbutic anemia (D53.2)
sequelae of vitamin C deficiency (E64.2)
DEF: Vitamin C deficiency causing swollen gums, myalgia, weight loss, and weakness.

✓4ᵗʰ **E55**   Vitamin D deficiency
EXCLUDES 1   adult osteomalacia (M83.-)
osteoporosis (M80.-)
sequelae of rickets (E64.3)

E55.0   Rickets, active   `CC`
Infantile osteomalacia
Juvenile osteomalacia
EXCLUDES 1   celiac rickets (K90.0)
Crohn's rickets (K50.-)
hereditary vitamin D-dependent rickets (E83.32)
inactive rickets (E64.3)
renal rickets (N25.0)
sequelae of rickets (E64.3)
vitamin D-resistant rickets (E83.31)
CC Excl: PDX collection 532

E55.9   Vitamin D deficiency, unspecified
Avitaminosis D

✓4ᵗʰ **E56**   Other vitamin deficiencies
EXCLUDES 1   sequelae of other vitamin deficiencies (E64.8)

E56.0   Deficiency of vitamin E

E56.1   Deficiency of vitamin K
EXCLUDES 1   deficiency of coagulation factor due to vitamin K deficiency (D68.4)
vitamin K deficiency of newborn (P53)

E56.8   Deficiency of other vitamins

E56.9   Vitamin deficiency, unspecified

`N` Newborn: 0   `P` Pediatric: 0-17   `M` Maternity: 12-55   `A` Adult: 15-124   `MCC` Major CC Condition   `PDxMCC` PDx acts as own MCC   `CC` CC Condition   `PDxCC` PDx acts as own CC

522   ICD-10-CM 2018

E58   **Dietary calcium deficiency**
> *EXCLUDES 1*   disorders of calcium metabolism (E83.5-)
> sequelae of calcium deficiency (E64.8)

E59   **Dietary selenium deficiency**
> Keshan disease
> *EXCLUDES 1*   sequelae of selenium deficiency (E64.8)

E60   **Dietary zinc deficiency**

✓4th **E61**   **Deficiency of other nutrient elements**
> Use additional code for adverse effect, if applicable, to identify drug (T36-T50 with fifth or sixth character 5)
> *EXCLUDES 1*   disorders of mineral metabolism (E83.-)
> iodine deficiency related thyroid disorders (E00-E02)
> sequelae of malnutrition and other nutritional deficiencies (E64.-)

   E61.0   **Copper deficiency**
   E61.1   **Iron deficiency**
> *EXCLUDES 1*   iron deficiency anemia (D50.-)

   E61.2   **Magnesium deficiency**
   E61.3   **Manganese deficiency**
   E61.4   **Chromium deficiency**
   E61.5   **Molybdenum deficiency**
   E61.6   **Vanadium deficiency**
   E61.7   **Deficiency of multiple nutrient elements**
   E61.8   **Deficiency of other specified nutrient elements**
   E61.9   **Deficiency of nutrient element, unspecified**

✓4th **E63**   **Other nutritional deficiencies**
> *EXCLUDES 1*   dehydration (E86.0)
> failure to thrive, adult (R62.7)
> failure to thrive, child (R62.51)
> feeding problems in newborn (P92.-)
> sequelae of malnutrition and other nutritional deficiencies (E64.-)

   E63.0   **Essential fatty acid [EFA] deficiency**
   E63.1   **Imbalance of constituents of food intake**
   E63.8   **Other specified nutritional deficiencies**
   E63.9   **Nutritional deficiency, unspecified**

✓4th **E64**   **Sequelae of malnutrition and other nutritional deficiencies**
> **NOTE**   This category is to be used to indicate conditions in categories E43, E44, E46, E50-E63 as the cause of sequelae, which are themselves classified elsewhere. The 'sequelae' include conditions specified as such; they also include the late effects of diseases classifiable to the above categories if the disease itself is no longer present
> Code first condition resulting from (sequela) of malnutrition and other nutritional deficiencies

   E64.0   **Sequelae of protein-calorie malnutrition**   CC HCC
> *EXCLUDES 2*   retarded development following protein-calorie malnutrition (E45)
> **CC Excl:** PDX collection 530

   E64.1   **Sequelae of vitamin A deficiency**
   E64.2   **Sequelae of vitamin C deficiency**
   E64.3   **Sequelae of rickets**
   E64.8   **Sequelae of other nutritional deficiencies**
   E64.9   **Sequelae of unspecified nutritional deficiency**

Overweight, obesity and other hyperalimentation (E65-E68)

E65   **Localized adiposity**
> Fat pad

✓4th **E66**   **Overweight and obesity**
> Code first obesity complicating pregnancy, childbirth and the puerperium, if applicable (O99.21-)
> Use additional code to identify body mass index (BMI), if known (Z68.-)
> *EXCLUDES 1*   adiposogenital dystrophy (E23.6)
> lipomatosis NOS (E88.2)
> lipomatosis dolorosa [Dercum] (E88.2)
> Prader-Willi syndrome (Q87.1)

   ✓5th **E66.0**   **Obesity due to excess calories**
     E66.01   **Morbid (severe) obesity due to excess calories**   H11 HCC
> *EXCLUDES 1*   morbid (severe) obesity with alveolar hypoventilation (E66.2)

     4 **E66.09**   **Other obesity due to excess calories**

4 **E66.1**   **Drug-induced obesity**
> Use additional code for adverse effect, if applicable, to identify drug (T36-T50 with fifth or sixth character 5)

   E66.2   **Morbid (severe) obesity with alveolar hypoventilation**   CC HCC
> Obesity hypoventilation syndrome (OHS)
> Pickwickian syndrome
> **CC Excl:** PDX collection 533

   E66.3   **Overweight**
4 **E66.8**   **Other obesity**
4 **E66.9**   **Obesity, unspecified**
> Obesity NOS

✓4th **E67**   **Other hyperalimentation**
> *EXCLUDES 1*   hyperalimentation NOS (R63.2)
> sequelae of hyperalimentation (E68)

   E67.0   **Hypervitaminosis A**
   E67.1   **Hypercarotinemia**
   E67.2   **Megavitamin-B6 syndrome**
   E67.3   **Hypervitaminosis D**
   E67.8   **Other specified hyperalimentation**

E68   **Sequelae of hyperalimentation**
> Code first condition resulting from (sequela) of hyperalimentation

Metabolic disorders (E70-E88)

> *EXCLUDES 1*   androgen insensitivity syndrome (E34.5-)
> congenital adrenal hyperplasia (E25.0)
> Ehlers-Danlos syndrome (Q79.6)
> hemolytic anemias attributable to enzyme disorders (D55.-)
> Marfan's syndrome (Q87.4)
> 5-alpha-reductase deficiency (E29.1)

✓4th **E70**   **Disorders of aromatic amino-acid metabolism**

> **CC Excl: For CC codes in category E70:** PDX collection 534

   E70.0   **Classical phenylketonuria**   CC HCC
   E70.1   **Other hyperphenylalaninemias**   CC HCC
   ✓5th **E70.2**   **Disorders of tyrosine metabolism**
> *EXCLUDES 1*   transitory tyrosinemia of newborn (P74.5)

     E70.20   **Disorder of tyrosine metabolism, unspecified**   CC HCC
     E70.21   **Tyrosinemia**   CC HCC
> Hypertyrosinemia

     E70.29   **Other disorders of tyrosine metabolism**   CC HCC
> Alkaptonuria
> Ochronosis

   ✓5th **E70.3**   **Albinism**
     E70.30   **Albinism, unspecified**   CC HCC
     ✓6th **E70.31**   **Ocular albinism**
       E70.310   **X-linked ocular albinism**   CC HCC
       E70.311   **Autosomal recessive ocular albinism**   CC HCC
       E70.318   **Other ocular albinism**   CC HCC
       E70.319   **Ocular albinism, unspecified**   CC HCC

     ✓6th **E70.32**   **Oculocutaneous albinism**
> *EXCLUDES 1*   Chediak-Higashi syndrome (E70.330)
> Hermansky-Pudlak syndrome (E70.331)

       E70.320   **Tyrosinase negative oculocutaneous albinism**   CC HCC
> Albinism I
> Oculocutaneous albinism ty-neg

       E70.321   **Tyrosinase positive oculocutaneous albinism**   CC HCC
> Albinism II
> Oculocutaneous albinism ty-pos

       E70.328   **Other oculocutaneous albinism**   CC HCC
> Cross syndrome

       E70.329   **Oculocutaneous albinism, unspecified**   CC HCC

     ✓6th **E70.33**   **Albinism with hematologic abnormality**
       E70.330   **Chediak-Higashi syndrome**   CC HCC
       E70.331   **Hermansky-Pudlak syndrome**   CC HCC
       E70.338   **Other albinism with hematologic abnormality**   CC HCC
       E70.339   **Albinism with hematologic abnormality, unspecified**   CC HCC

     E70.39   **Other specified albinism**   CC HCC
> Piebaldism

---

4   Questionable admission when used as PDx.

✓ Additional Character Req   ✓x7th Placeholder Alert   Unacceptable PDx   Manifestation   H1-H14 HAC   HCC CMS-HCC Condition   *EXCLUDES 1* Not Coded Here   *EXCLUDES 2* Not Included Here

Chapter 4. Endocrine, Nutritional and Metabolic Diseases

E70.4–E72.09

✓5th **E70.4** **Disorders of** histidine **metabolism**

     E70.40 **Disorders of histidine metabolism, unspecified** `CC` `HCC`

     E70.41 **Histidinemia** `CC` `HCC`

     E70.49 **Other** disorders of histidine metabolism `CC` `HCC`

E70.5 **Disorders of** tryptophan **metabolism** `CC` `HCC`

E70.8 **Other disorders of aromatic amino-acid metabolism** `CC` `HCC`

E70.9 **Disorder of aromatic amino-acid metabolism, unspecified** `CC` `HCC`

✓4th **E71** **Disorders of branched-chain amino-acid metabolism and fatty-acid metabolism**

     E71.0 **Maple-syrup-urine disease** `CC` `HCC`
         CC Excl: PDX collection 534

✓5th **E71.1** **Other disorders of** branched-chain amino-acid **metabolism**

     CC Excl: For CC codes in subcategory E71.1: PDX collection 534

     ✓6th **E71.11** **Branched-chain** organic acidurias

         E71.110 **Isovaleric acidemia** `CC` `HCC`

         E71.111 **3-methylglutaconic aciduria** `CC` `HCC`

         E71.118 **Other branched-chain organic acidurias** `CC` `HCC`

     ✓6th **E71.12** **Disorders of** propionate metabolism

         E71.120 **Methylmalonic acidemia** `CC` `HCC`

         E71.121 **Propionic acidemia** `CC` `HCC`

         E71.128 **Other disorders of propionate metabolism** `CC` `HCC`

     E71.19 **Other disorders of branched-chain amino-acid metabolism**
         Hyperleucine-isoleucinemia
         Hypervalinemia

E71.2 **Disorder of branched-chain amino-acid metabolism, unspecified** `CC` `HCC`
         CC Excl: PDX collection 534

✓5th **E71.3** **Disorders of fatty-acid metabolism**

     EXCLUDES 1   *peroxisomal disorders (E71.5)*
         Refsum's disease (G60.1)
         Schilder's disease (G37.0)

     EXCLUDES 2   *carnitine deficiency due to inborn error of metabolism (E71.42)*

     CC Excl: For CC codes in subcategory E71.3, unless otherwise noted: PDX collection 535

     E71.30 **Disorder of fatty-acid metabolism,** unspecified

     ✓6th **E71.31** **Disorders of fatty-acid** oxidation

         E71.310 **Long chain/very long chain acyl CoA dehydrogenase deficiency** `CC` `HCC`
             LCAD
             VLCAD

         E71.311 **Medium chain acyl CoA dehydrogenase deficiency** `CC` `HCC`
             MCAD

         E71.312 **Short chain acyl CoA dehydrogenase deficiency** `CC` `HCC`
             SCAD

         E71.313 **Glutaric aciduria type II** `CC` `HCC`
             Glutaric aciduria type II A
             Glutaric aciduria type II B
             Glutaric aciduria type II C
             EXCLUDES 1   *glutaric aciduria (type 1) NOS (E72.3)*

         E71.314 **Muscle carnitine palmitoyltransferase deficiency** `CC` `HCC`

         E71.318 **Other disorders of fatty-acid oxidation** `CC` `HCC`

     E71.32 **Disorders of** ketone metabolism `CC` `HCC`

     E71.39 **Other disorders of fatty-acid metabolism** `CC` `HCC`
         CC Excl: PDX collection 492

✓5th **E71.4** **Disorders of** carnitine **metabolism**

     EXCLUDES 1   *muscle carnitine palmitoyltransferase deficiency (E71.314)*

     E71.40 **Disorder of carnitine metabolism,** unspecified `HCC`

     E71.41 **Primary carnitine deficiency** `HCC`

     E71.42 **Carnitine deficiency due to inborn errors of metabolism** `HCC`
         Code also associated inborn error or metabolism

     E71.43 **Iatrogenic carnitine deficiency** `HCC`
         Carnitine deficiency due to hemodialysis
         Carnitine deficiency due to Valproic acid therapy

     ✓6th **E71.44** **Other secondary** carnitine deficiency

         E71.440 **Ruvalcaba-Myhre-Smith syndrome** `HCC`

         E71.448 **Other secondary carnitine deficiency** `HCC`

✓5th **E71.5** **Peroxisomal disorders**

     EXCLUDES 1   *Schilder's disease (G37.0)*

     CC Excl: For CC codes in subcategory E71.5: PDX collection 536

     E71.50 **Peroxisomal disorder,** unspecified `CC` `HCC`

     ✓6th **E71.51** **Disorders of peroxisome** biogenesis
         Group 1 peroxisomal disorders
         EXCLUDES 1   *Refsum's disease (G60.1)*

         E71.510 **Zellweger syndrome** `CC` `HCC`

         E71.511 **Neonatal adrenoleukodystrophy** `CC` `HCC`
             EXCLUDES 1   *X-linked adrenoleukodystrophy (E71.52-)*

         E71.518 **Other disorders of peroxisome biogenesis** `CC` `HCC`

     ✓6th **E71.52** **X-linked adrenoleukodystrophy**

         E71.520 **Childhood cerebral X-linked adrenoleukodystrophy** `CC` `HCC`

         E71.521 **Adolescent X-linked adrenoleukodystrophy** `CC` `HCC`

         E71.522 **Adrenomyeloneuropathy** `CC` `HCC`

         E71.528 **Other X-linked adrenoleukodystrophy** `CC` `HCC`
             Addison only phenotype adrenoleukodystrophy
             Addison-Schilder adrenoleukodystrophy

         E71.529 **X-linked adrenoleukodystrophy, unspecified type** `CC` `HCC`

     E71.53 **Other group 2 peroxisomal disorders** `CC` `HCC`

     ✓6th **E71.54** **Other peroxisomal disorders**

         E71.540 **Rhizomelic chondrodysplasia punctata** `CC` `HCC`
             EXCLUDES 1   *chondrodysplasia punctata NOS (Q77.3)*

         E71.541 **Zellweger-like syndrome** `CC` `HCC`

         E71.542 **Other group 3 peroxisomal disorders** `CC` `HCC`

         E71.548 **Other peroxisomal disorders** `CC` `HCC`

✓4th **E72** **Other disorders of amino-acid metabolism**

     EXCLUDES 1   *disorders of:*
         aromatic amino-acid metabolism (E70.-)
         branched-chain amino-acid metabolism (E71.0-E71.2)
         fatty-acid metabolism (E71.3)
         purine and pyrimidine metabolism (E79.-)
         gout (M1A.-, M10.-)

     CC Excl: For CC codes in category E72, unless otherwise noted: PDX collection 534

✓5th **E72.0** **Disorders of amino-acid** transport

     EXCLUDES 1   *disorders of tryptophan metabolism (E70.5)*

     E72.00 **Disorders of amino-acid transport, unspecified** `CC` `HCC`

     E72.01 **Cystinuria** `CC` `HCC`

     E72.02 **Hartnup's disease** `CC` `HCC`

     E72.03 **Lowe's syndrome** `CC` `HCC`
         Use additional code for associated glaucoma (H42)
         CC Excl: No Excl

     E72.04 **Cystinosis** `CC` `HCC`
         Fanconi (-de Toni) (-Debré) syndrome with cystinosis
         EXCLUDES 1   *Fanconi (-de Toni) (-Debré) syndrome without cystinosis (E72.09)*

     E72.09 **Other disorders of amino-acid transport** `CC` `HCC`
         Fanconi (-de Toni) (-Debré) syndrome, unspecified

N Newborn: 0   P Pediatric: 0-17   M Maternity: 12-55   A Adult: 15-124   `MCC` Major CC Condition   `PDxMCC` PDx acts as own MCC   `CC` CC Condition   `PDxCC` PDx acts as own CC

524   ICD-10-CM 2018

✓5ᵗʰ **E72.1   Disorders of sulfur-bearing amino-acid metabolism**

     EXCLUDES 1   *cystinosis (E72.04)*
                 cystinuria (E72.01)
                 transcobalamin II deficiency (D51.2)

     E72.10   Disorders of sulfur-bearing amino-acid metabolism, unspecified   CC HCC

     E72.11   Homocystinuria   CC HCC
                 Cystathionine synthase deficiency

     E72.12   Methylenetetrahydrofolate reductase deficiency   CC HCC

     E72.19   Other disorders of sulfur-bearing amino-acid metabolism   CC HCC
                 Cystathioninuria
                 Methioninemia
                 Sulfite oxidase deficiency

✓5ᵗʰ **E72.2   Disorders of urea cycle metabolism**

     EXCLUDES 1   *disorders of ornithine metabolism (E72.4)*

     E72.20   Disorder of urea cycle metabolism, unspecified   CC HCC
                 Hyperammonemia

         EXCLUDES 1   *hyperammonemia- hyperornithinemia-homocitrullinemia syndrome (E72.4)*
                       transient hyperammonemia of newborn (P74.6)

     E72.21   Argininemia   CC HCC

     E72.22   Arginosuccinic aciduria   CC HCC

     E72.23   Citrullinemia   CC HCC

     E72.29   Other disorders of urea cycle metabolism   CC HCC

E72.3   Disorders of lysine and hydroxylysine metabolism   CC HCC
     Glutaric aciduria NOS
     Glutaric aciduria (type I)
     Hydroxylysinemia
     Hyperlysinemia

     EXCLUDES 1   *glutaric aciduria type II (E71.313)*
                 Refsum's disease (G60.1)
                 Zellweger syndrome (E71.510)

E72.4   Disorders of ornithine metabolism   CC HCC
     Hyperammonemia-hyperornithinemia-homocitrullinemia syndrome
     Ornithinemia (types I, II)
     Ornithine transcarbamylase deficiency

     EXCLUDES 1   *hereditary choroidal dystrophy (H31.2-)*

✓5ᵗʰ **E72.5   Disorders of glycine metabolism**

     E72.50   Disorder of glycine metabolism, unspecified   CC HCC

     E72.51   Non-ketotic hyperglycinemia   CC HCC

     E72.52   Trimethylaminuria   CC HCC

     E72.53   Hyperoxaluria   CC HCC
                 Oxalosis
                 Oxaluria

     E72.59   Other disorders of glycine metabolism   CC HCC
                 D-glycericacidemia
                 Hyperhydroxyprolinemia
                 Hyperprolinemia (types I, II)
                 Sarcosinemia

E72.8   Other specified disorders of amino-acid metabolism   CC HCC
     Disorders of beta-amino-acid metabolism
     Disorders of gamma-glutamyl cycle

E72.9   Disorder of amino-acid metabolism, unspecified   CC HCC

✓4ᵗʰ **E73   Lactose intolerance**

E73.0   Congenital lactase deficiency

E73.1   Secondary lactase deficiency

E73.8   Other lactose intolerance

E73.9   Lactose intolerance, unspecified

✓4ᵗʰ **E74   Other disorders of carbohydrate metabolism**

     EXCLUDES 1   *diabetes mellitus (E08-E13)*
                 hypoglycemia NOS (E16.2)
                 increased secretion of glucagon (E16.3)
                 mucopolysaccharidosis (E76.0-E76.3)

     CC Excl: For CC codes in category E74: PDX collection 534

✓5ᵗʰ **E74.0   Glycogen storage disease**

     E74.00   Glycogen storage disease, unspecified   CC HCC

     E74.01   von Gierke disease   CC HCC
                 Type I glycogen storage disease

     E74.02   Pompe disease   CC HCC
                 Cardiac glycogenosis
                 Type II glycogen storage disease

     E74.03   Cori disease   CC HCC
                 Forbes disease
                 Type III glycogen storage disease

     E74.04   McArdle disease   CC HCC
                 Type V glycogen storage disease

     E74.09   Other glycogen storage disease   CC HCC
                 Andersen disease
                 Hers disease
                 Tauri disease
                 Glycogen storage disease, types 0, IV, VI-XI
                 Liver phosphorylase deficiency
                 Muscle phosphofructokinase deficiency

✓5ᵗʰ **E74.1   Disorders of fructose metabolism**

     EXCLUDES 1   *muscle phosphofructokinase deficiency (E74.09)*

     E74.10   Disorder of fructose metabolism, unspecified

     E74.11   Essential fructosuria
                 Fructokinase deficiency

     E74.12   Hereditary fructose intolerance
                 Fructosemia

     E74.19   Other disorders of fructose metabolism
                 Fructose-1, 6-diphosphatase deficiency

✓5ᵗʰ **E74.2   Disorders of galactose metabolism**

     E74.20   Disorders of galactose metabolism, unspecified   CC HCC

     E74.21   Galactosemia   CC HCC
           DEF: Any of three genetic disorders due to defective galactose metabolism; symptoms include failure to thrive in infancy, jaundice, liver and spleen damage, cataracts, and mental retardation.

     E74.29   Other disorders of galactose metabolism   CC HCC
                 Galactokinase deficiency

✓5ᵗʰ **E74.3   Other disorders of intestinal carbohydrate absorption**

     EXCLUDES 2   *lactose intolerance (E73.-)*

     E74.31   Sucrase-isomaltase deficiency

     E74.39   Other disorders of intestinal carbohydrate absorption
                 Disorder of intestinal carbohydrate absorption NOS
                 Glucose-galactose malabsorption
                 Sucrase deficiency

E74.4   Disorders of pyruvate metabolism and gluconeogenesis   CC HCC
     Deficiency of phosphoenolpyruvate carboxykinase
     Deficiency of pyruvate carboxylase
     Deficiency of pyruvate dehydrogenase

     EXCLUDES 1   *disorders of pyruvate metabolism and gluconeogenesis with anemia (D55.-)*
                       Leigh's syndrome (G31.82)

E74.8   Other specified disorders of carbohydrate metabolism   CC HCC
     Essential pentosuria
     Renal glycosuria

E74.9   Disorder of carbohydrate metabolism, unspecified   HCC

✔ Additional Character Req   ✔x7ᵗʰ Placeholder Alert   Unacceptable PDx   Manifestation   H1 - H14 HAC   HCC CMS-HCC Condition   EXCLUDES 1 Not Coded Here   EXCLUDES 2 Not Included Here

ICD-10-CM 2018   **525**

Tay-Sachs Disease

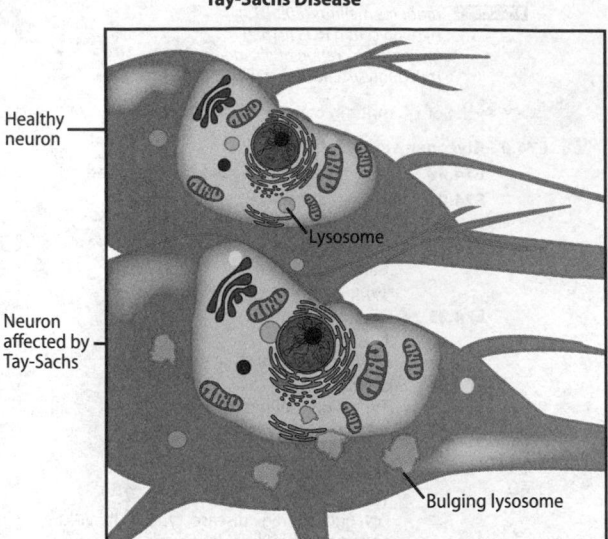

Healthy neuron

Lysosome

Neuron affected by Tay-Sachs

Bulging lysosome

√4th **E75** **Disorders of** sphingolipid **metabolism and** other lipid storage disorders
    EXCLUDES 1   *mucolipidosis, types I-III (E77.0-E77.1)*
                Refsum's disease (G60.1)

√5th **E75.0** **GM2 gangliosidosis**

    CC Excl: For CC codes in subcategory E75.0: PDX collection 537

    E75.00 **GM2 gangliosidosis,** unspecified   CC
    E75.01 **Sandhoff** disease   CC
    E75.02 **Tay-Sachs** disease   CC
         DEF: Genetic mutation of the HEXA gene that inhibits the breakdown of a toxic substance called ganglioside. The accumulation of ganglioside results in destruction of the neurons in the brain and spinal cord.
    E75.09 **Other GM2 gangliosidosis**   CC
         Adult GM2 gangliosidosis
         Juvenile GM2 gangliosidosis

√5th **E75.1** **Other and unspecified gangliosidosis**

    CC Excl: For CC codes in subcategory E75.1: PDX collection 537

    E75.10 **Unspecified gangliosidosis**   CC
         Gangliosidosis NOS
    E75.11 **Mucolipidosis IV**   CC
    E75.19 **Other gangliosidosis**   CC
         GM1 gangliosidosis
         GM3 gangliosidosis

√5th **E75.2** **Other sphingolipidosis**
    EXCLUDES 1   *adrenoleukodystrophy [Addison-Schilder] (E71.528)*

    CC Excl: For CC codes in subcategory E75.2: PDX collection 538

    E75.21 **Fabry (-Anderson) disease**   HCC
    E75.22 **Gaucher disease**   HCC
    E75.23 **Krabbe disease**   CC
   √6th **E75.24** **Niemann-Pick disease**
        E75.240 **Niemann-Pick disease** type A   HCC
        E75.241 **Niemann-Pick disease** type B   HCC
        E75.242 **Niemann-Pick disease** type C   HCC
        E75.243 **Niemann-Pick disease** type D   HCC
        E75.248 **Other Niemann-Pick disease**   HCC
        E75.249 **Niemann-Pick disease,** unspecified   HCC
    E75.25 **Metachromatic leukodystrophy**   CC
    E75.29 **Other sphingolipidosis**   CC
         Farber's syndrome
         Sulfatase deficiency
         Sulfatide lipidosis

   E75.3 **Sphingolipidosis, unspecified**   HCC

E75.4 **Neuronal ceroid lipofuscinosis**   CC
    Batten disease
    Bielschowsky-Jansky disease
    Kufs disease
    Spielmeyer-Vogt disease
    CC Excl: PDX collection 537

E75.5 **Other lipid storage disorders**
    Cerebrotendinous cholesterosis [van Bogaert-Scherer-Epstein]
    Wolman's disease

E75.6 **Lipid storage disorder, unspecified**

√4th **E76** **Disorders of** glycosaminoglycan **metabolism**

    CC Excl: For CC codes in category E76: PDX collection 539

√5th **E76.0** **Mucopolysaccharidosis,** type I
    E76.01 **Hurler's syndrome**   CC HCC
    E76.02 **Hurler-Scheie syndrome**   CC HCC
    E76.03 **Scheie's syndrome**   CC HCC

E76.1 **Mucopolysaccharidosis,** type II   CC HCC
    Hunter's syndrome

√5th **E76.2** **Other mucopolysaccharidoses**
   √6th **E76.21** **Morquio mucopolysaccharidoses**
        E76.210 **Morquio A mucopolysaccharidoses**   CC HCC
            Classic Morquio syndrome
            Morquio syndrome A
            Mucopolysaccharidosis, type IVA
        E76.211 **Morquio B mucopolysaccharidoses**   CC HCC
            Morquio-like mucopolysaccharidoses
            Morquio-like syndrome
            Morquio syndrome B
            Mucopolysaccharidosis, type IVB
        E76.219 **Morquio mucopolysaccharidoses,** unspecified   CC HCC
            Morquio syndrome
            Mucopolysaccharidosis, type IV
    E76.22 **Sanfilippo mucopolysaccharidoses**   CC HCC
         Mucopolysaccharidosis, type III (A) (B) (C) (D)
         Sanfilippo A syndrome
         Sanfilippo B syndrome
         Sanfilippo C syndrome
         Sanfilippo D syndrome
    E76.29 **Other mucopolysaccharidoses**   CC HCC
         beta-Glucuronidase deficiency
         Maroteaux-Lamy (mild) (severe) syndrome
         Mucopolysaccharidosis, types VI, VII

E76.3 **Mucopolysaccharidosis,** unspecified   CC HCC

E76.8 **Other disorders of glucosaminoglycan metabolism**   CC HCC

E76.9 **Glucosaminoglycan metabolism disorder,** unspecified   CC HCC

√4th **E77** **Disorders of** glycoprotein **metabolism**

E77.0 **Defects in post-translational modification of lysosomal enzymes**   HCC
    Mucolipidosis II [I-cell disease]
    Mucolipidosis III [pseudo-Hurler polydystrophy]

E77.1 **Defects in glycoprotein degradation**   HCC
    Aspartylglucosaminuria
    Fucosidosis
    Mannosidosis
    Sialidosis [mucolipidosis I]

E77.8 **Other disorders of glycoprotein metabolism**   HCC

E77.9 **Disorder of glycoprotein metabolism,** unspecified   HCC

√4th **E78** **Disorders of** lipoprotein metabolism and other lipidemias
    EXCLUDES 1   *sphingolipidosis (E75.0-E75.3)*

√5th **E78.0** **Pure hypercholesterolemia**
    E78.00 **Pure hypercholesterolemia, unspecified**
         Fredrickson's hyperlipoproteinemia, type IIa
         Hyperbetalipoproteinemia
         Low-density-lipoprotein-type [LDL] hyperlipoproteinemia
         ▶(Pure) hypercholesterolemia NOS◄
    E78.01 **Familial hypercholesterolemia**

E78.1 **Pure hyperglyceridemia**
    Elevated fasting triglycerides
    Endogenous hyperglyceridemia
    Fredrickson's hyperlipoproteinemia, type IV
    Hyperlipidemia, group B
    Hyperprebetalipoproteinemia
    Very-low-density-lipoprotein-type [VLDL] hyperlipoproteinemia

E78.2 **Mixed hyperlipidemia**
Broad- or floating-betalipoproteinemia
Combined hyperlipidemia NOS
Elevated cholesterol with elevated triglycerides NEC
Fredrickson's hyperlipoproteinemia, type IIb or III
Hyperbetalipoproteinemia with prebetalipoproteinemia
Hypercholesteremia with endogenous hyperglyceridemia
Hyperlipidemia, group C
Tubo-eruptive xanthoma
Xanthoma tuberosum
EXCLUDES 1   *cerebrotendinous cholesterosis [van Bogaert-Scherer-Epstein] (E75.5)*
familial combined hyperlipidemia (E78.4)

E78.3 **Hyperchylomicronemia**
Chylomicron retention disease
Fredrickson's hyperlipoproteinemia, type I or V
Hyperlipidemia, group D
Mixed hyperglyceridemia

E78.4 **Other hyperlipidemia**
Familial combined hyperlipidemia

E78.5 **Hyperlipidemia, unspecified**

E78.6 **Lipoprotein deficiency**
Abetalipoproteinemia
Depressed HDL cholesterol
High-density lipoprotein deficiency
Hypoalphalipoproteinemia
Hypobetalipoproteinemia (familial)
Lecithin cholesterol acyltransferase deficiency
Tangier disease

✓5ᵗʰ **E78.7** **Disorders of bile acid and cholesterol metabolism**
EXCLUDES 1   *Niemann-Pick disease type C (E75.242)*

E78.70 **Disorder of bile acid and cholesterol metabolism, unspecified**

E78.71 **Barth syndrome**   CC
CC Excl: PDX collection 540

E78.72 **Smith-Lemli-Opitz syndrome**   CC
CC Excl: PDX collection 540

E78.79 **Other disorders of bile acid and cholesterol metabolism**

✓5ᵗʰ **E78.8** **Other disorders of lipoprotein metabolism**

E78.81 **Lipoid dermatoarthritis**

E78.89 **Other lipoprotein metabolism disorders**

E78.9 **Disorder of lipoprotein metabolism, unspecified**

✓4ᵗʰ **E79** **Disorders of purine and pyrimidine metabolism**
EXCLUDES 1   *Ataxia-telangiectasia (Q87.1)*
Bloom's syndrome (Q82.8)
Cockayne's syndrome (Q87.1)
calculus of kidney (N20.0)
combined immunodeficiency disorders (D81.-)
Fanconi's anemia (D61.09)
gout (M1A.-, M10.-)
orotaciduric anemia (D53.0)
progeria (E34.8)
Werner's syndrome (E34.8)
xeroderma pigmentosum (Q82.1)

CC Excl: For CC codes in category E79: PDX collection 513

E79.0 **Hyperuricemia without signs of inflammatory arthritis and tophaceous disease**
Asymptomatic hyperuricemia

E79.1 **Lesch-Nyhan syndrome**   CC HCC
HGPRT deficiency

E79.2 **Myoadenylate deaminase deficiency**   CC HCC

E79.8 **Other disorders of purine and pyrimidine metabolism**   CC HCC
Hereditary xanthinuria

E79.9 **Disorder of purine and pyrimidine metabolism, unspecified**   CC HCC

✓4ᵗʰ **E80** **Disorders of porphyrin and bilirubin metabolism**
INCLUDES   defects of catalase and peroxidase

CC Excl: For CC codes in category E80, unless otherwise noted: PDX collection 513

E80.0 **Hereditary erythropoietic porphyria**   CC HCC
Congenital erythropoietic porphyria
Erythropoietic protoporphyria

E80.1 **Porphyria cutanea tarda**   CC HCC

✓5ᵗʰ **E80.2** **Other and unspecified porphyria**

E80.20 **Unspecified porphyria**   CC HCC
Porphyria NOS

E80.21 **Acute intermittent (hepatic) porphyria**   CC HCC

E80.29 **Other porphyria**   CC HCC
Hereditary coproporphyria

E80.3 **Defects of catalase and peroxidase**   CC HCC
Acatalasia [Takahara]
CC Excl: PDX collection 492

E80.4 **Gilbert syndrome**

E80.5 **Crigler-Najjar syndrome**

E80.6 **Other disorders of bilirubin metabolism**
Dubin-Johnson syndrome
Rotor's syndrome

E80.7 **Disorder of bilirubin metabolism, unspecified**

✓4ᵗʰ **E83** **Disorders of mineral metabolism**
EXCLUDES 1   *dietary mineral deficiency (E58-E61)*
parathyroid disorders (E20-E21)
vitamin D deficiency (E55.-)

✓5ᵗʰ **E83.0** **Disorders of copper metabolism**

E83.00 **Disorder of copper metabolism, unspecified**

E83.01 **Wilson's disease**
Code also associated Kayser Fleischer ring (H18.04-)

E83.09 **Other disorders of copper metabolism**
Menkes' (kinky hair) (steely hair) disease

✓5ᵗʰ **E83.1** **Disorders of iron metabolism**
EXCLUDES 1   *iron deficiency anemia (D50.-)*
sideroblastic anemia (D64.0-D64.3)

E83.10 **Disorder of iron metabolism, unspecified**

✓6ᵗʰ **E83.11** **Hemochromatosis**
EXCLUDES 1 ▶*GALD (P78.84)*
gestational alloimmune liver disease (P78.84)
neonatal hemochromatosis (P78.84)◀

E83.110 **Hereditary hemochromatosis**   HCC
Bronzed diabetes
Pigmentary cirrhosis (of liver)
Primary (hereditary) hemochromatosis

E83.111 **Hemochromatosis due to repeated red blood cell transfusions**
Iron overload due to repeated red blood cell transfusions
Transfusion (red blood cell) associated hemochromatosis

E83.118 **Other hemochromatosis**

E83.119 **Hemochromatosis, unspecified**

E83.19 **Other disorders of iron metabolism**
Use additional code, if applicable, for idiopathic pulmonary hemosiderosis (J84.03)

E83.2 **Disorders of zinc metabolism**
Acrodermatitis enteropathica

✓5ᵗʰ **E83.3** **Disorders of phosphorus metabolism and phosphatases**
EXCLUDES 1   *adult osteomalacia (M83.-)*
osteoporosis (M80.-)

E83.30 **Disorder of phosphorus metabolism, unspecified**

E83.31 **Familial hypophosphatemia**
Vitamin D-resistant osteomalacia
Vitamin D-resistant rickets
EXCLUDES 1   *vitamin D-deficiency rickets (E55.0)*

E83.32 **Hereditary vitamin D-dependent rickets (type 1) (type 2)**
25-hydroxyvitamin D 1-alpha-hydroxylase deficiency
Pseudovitamin D deficiency
Vitamin D receptor defect

E83.39 **Other disorders of phosphorus metabolism**
Acid phosphatase deficiency
Hypophosphatasia

✓5ᵗʰ **E83.4** **Disorders of magnesium metabolism**

E83.40 **Disorders of magnesium metabolism, unspecified**

E83.41 **Hypermagnesemia**

E83.42 **Hypomagnesemia**

E83.49 **Other disorders of magnesium metabolism**

✓5ᵗʰ **E83.5** **Disorders of calcium metabolism**
EXCLUDES 1   *chondrocalcinosis (M11.1-M11.2)*
hungry bone syndrome (E83.81)
hyperparathyroidism (E21.0-E21.3)

E83.50 **Unspecified disorder of calcium metabolism**

✓ Additional Character Req ✓x7ᵗʰ Placeholder Alert Unacceptable PDx Manifestation H1-H14 HAC HCC CMS-HCC Condition EXCLUDES 1 Not Coded Here EXCLUDES 2 Not Included Here

ICD-10-CM 2018 527

Chapter 4. Endocrine, Nutritional and Metabolic Diseases

E83.51–E88.2

E83.51   **Hypocalcemia**

E83.52   **Hypercalcemia**
Familial hypocalciuric hypercalcemia

E83.59   **Other disorders of calcium metabolism**
Idiopathic hypercalciuria

√5th **E83.8**   **Other disorders of mineral metabolism**

E83.81   **Hungry bone syndrome**

E83.89   **Other disorders of mineral metabolism**

E83.9   **Disorder of mineral metabolism, unspecified**

√4th **E84**   **Cystic fibrosis**
[INCLUDES] mucoviscidosis
Code also exocrine pancreatic insufficiency (K86.81)

CC Excl: For CC/MCC codes in category E84: PDX collection 541

E84.0   **Cystic fibrosis with pulmonary manifestations** [MCC] [HCC]
Use additional code to identify any infectious organism present, such as:
Pseudomonas (B96.5)

√5th **E84.1**   **Cystic fibrosis with intestinal manifestations**

E84.11   **Meconium ileus in cystic fibrosis** [MCC] [HCC] [N]
[EXCLUDES 1] meconium ileus not due to cystic fibrosis (P76.0)

E84.19   **Cystic fibrosis with other intestinal manifestations** [CC] [HCC]
Distal intestinal obstruction syndrome

E84.8   **Cystic fibrosis with other manifestations** [CC] [HCC]

E84.9   **Cystic fibrosis, unspecified** [CC] [HCC]

√4th **E85**   **Amyloidosis**
[EXCLUDES 1] Alzheimer's disease (G30.0)
[EXCLUDES 2] ▶Alzheimer's disease (G30.0-)◀
DEF: Conditions of diverse etiologies characterized by the accumulation of insoluble fibrillar proteins (amyloid) in various organs and tissues of the body, compromising vital functions.

CC Excl: For CC codes in category E85: PDX collection 542

E85.0   **Non-neuropathic heredofamilial amyloidosis** [CC] [HCC]
Hereditary amyloid nephropathy
▶Code also associated disorders, such as:
autoinflammatory syndromes (M04.-)◀
[EXCLUDES 2] ▶transthyretin-related (ATTR) familial amyloid cardiomyopathy (E85.4)◀

E85.1   **Neuropathic heredofamilial amyloidosis** [CC] [HCC]
Amyloid polyneuropathy (Portuguese)
▶Transthyretin-related (ATTR) familial amyloid polyneuropathy◀
AHA: 2012, 4Q, 99

E85.2   **Heredofamilial amyloidosis, unspecified** [CC] [HCC]

E85.3   **Secondary systemic amyloidosis** [CC] [HCC]
Hemodialysis-associated amyloidosis

E85.4   **Organ-limited amyloidosis** [CC] [HCC]
Localized amyloidosis
▶Transthyretin-related (ATTR) familial amyloid cardiomyopathy◀

√5th **E85.8**   **Other amyloidosis**

●   **E85.81**   **Light chain (AL) amyloidosis** [CC]

●   **E85.82**   **Wild-type transthyretin-related (ATTR) amyloidosis** [CC]
Senile systemic amyloidosis (SSA)

●   **E85.89**   **Other amyloidosis** [CC]

E85.9   **Amyloidosis, unspecified** [CC] [HCC]

√4th **E86**   **Volume depletion**
Use additional code(s) for any associated disorders of electrolyte and acid-base balance (E87.-)
[EXCLUDES 1] dehydration of newborn (P74.1)
hypovolemic shock NOS (R57.1)
postprocedural hypovolemic shock (T81.19)
traumatic hypovolemic shock (T79.4)

E86.0   **Dehydration**
AHA: 2014, 1Q, 7

E86.1   **Hypovolemia**
Depletion of volume of plasma

E86.9   **Volume depletion, unspecified**
DEF: Depletion of total body water (dehydration) and/or contraction of total intravascular plasma (hypovolemia).

√4th **E87**   **Other disorders of fluid, electrolyte and acid-base balance**
[EXCLUDES 1] diabetes insipidus (E23.2)
electrolyte imbalance associated with hyperemesis gravidarum (O21.1)
electrolyte imbalance following ectopic or molar pregnancy (O08.5)
familial periodic paralysis (G72.3)

CC Excl: For CC codes in category E87: PDX collection 543

E87.0   **Hyperosmolality and hypernatremia** [CC]
Sodium [Na] excess
Sodium [Na] overload
AHA: 2014, 1Q, 7

E87.1   **Hypo-osmolality and hyponatremia** [CC]
Sodium [Na] deficiency
[EXCLUDES 1] syndrome of inappropriate secretion of antidiuretic hormone (E22.2)
AHA: 2014, 1Q, 7

E87.2   **Acidosis** [CC]
Acidosis NOS
Lactic acidosis
Metabolic acidosis
Respiratory acidosis
[EXCLUDES 1] diabetic acidosis see categories E08-E10, E13 with ketoacidosis

E87.3   **Alkalosis** [CC]
Alkalosis NOS
Metabolic alkalosis
Respiratory alkalosis

E87.4   **Mixed disorder of acid-base balance** [CC]

E87.5   **Hyperkalemia**
Potassium [K] excess
Potassium [K] overload

E87.6   **Hypokalemia**
Potassium [K] deficiency

√5th **E87.7**   **Fluid overload**
[EXCLUDES 1] edema NOS (R60.9)
fluid retention (R60.9)

E87.70   **Fluid overload, unspecified**

E87.71   **Transfusion associated circulatory overload**
Fluid overload due to transfusion (blood) (blood components)
TACO

E87.79   **Other fluid overload**

E87.8   **Other disorders of electrolyte and fluid balance, not elsewhere classified**
Electrolyte imbalance NOS
Hyperchloremia
Hypochloremia

√4th **E88**   **Other and unspecified metabolic disorders**
Use additional codes for associated conditions
[EXCLUDES 1] histiocytosis X (chronic) (C96.6)

√5th **E88.0**   **Disorders of plasma-protein metabolism, not elsewhere classified**
[EXCLUDES 1] disorder of lipoprotein metabolism (E78.-)
monoclonal gammopathy (of undetermined significance) (D47.2)
polyclonal hypergammaglobulinemia (D89.0)
Waldenström's macroglobulinemia (C88.0)

E88.01   **Alpha-1-antitrypsin deficiency** [HCC]
AAT deficiency

E88.09   **Other disorders of plasma-protein metabolism, not elsewhere classified**
Bisalbuminemia

E88.1   **Lipodystrophy, not elsewhere classified**
Lipodystrophy NOS
[EXCLUDES 1] Whipple's disease (K90.81)

E88.2   **Lipomatosis, not elsewhere classified**
Lipomatosis NOS
Lipomatosis (Check) dolorosa [Dercum]

[N] Newborn: 0   [P] Pediatric: 0-17   [M] Maternity: 12-55   [A] Adult: 15-124   [MCC] Major CC Condition   [PDxMCC] PDx acts as own MCC   [CC] CC Condition   [PDxCC] PDx acts as own CC

528   ICD-10-CM 2018

E88.3 Tumor lysis syndrome `MCC`
Tumor lysis syndrome (spontaneous)
Tumor lysis syndrome following antineoplastic drug chemotherapy
Use additional code for adverse effect, if applicable, to identify drug (T45.1X5)
DEF: A potentially fatal metabolic complication of tumor necrosis caused by either spontaneous or treatment-related accumulation of byproducts from dying cancer cells; symptoms include hyperkalemia, hyperphosphatemia, hypocalcemia, hyperuricemia, and hyperuricosuria.
CC Excl: PDX collection 544

✓5ᵗʰ **E88.4 Mitochondrial metabolism disorders**
EXCLUDES 1   disorders of pyruvate metabolism (E74.4)
Kearns-Sayre syndrome (H49.81)
Leber's disease (H47.22)
Leigh's encephalopathy (G31.82)
Mitochondrial myopathy, NEC (G71.3)
Reye's syndrome (G93.7)

CC Excl: For CC codes in subcategory E88.4:
PDX collection 545

   E88.40 Mitochondrial metabolism disorder, unspecified `CC` `HCC`

   E88.41 MELAS syndrome `CC` `HCC`
Mitochondrial myopathy, encephalopathy, lactic acidosis and stroke-like episodes

   E88.42 MERRF syndrome `CC` `HCC`
Myoclonic epilepsy associated with ragged-red fibers
Code also progressive myoclonic epilepsy (G40.3-)

   E88.49 Other mitochondrial metabolism disorders `CC` `HCC`

✓5ᵗʰ **E88.8 Other specified metabolic disorders**
   E88.81 Metabolic syndrome
Dysmetabolic syndrome X
Use additional codes for associated manifestations, such as:
obesity (E66.-)

   E88.89 Other specified metabolic disorders `HCC`
Launois-Bensaude adenolipomatosis
EXCLUDES 1   adult pulmonary Langerhans cell histiocytosis (J84.82)

E88.9 Metabolic disorder, unspecified

Postprocedural endocrine and metabolic complications and disorders, not elsewhere classified (E89)

✓4ᵗʰ **E89 Postprocedural endocrine and metabolic complications and disorders, not elsewhere classified**
EXCLUDES 2   intraoperative complications of endocrine system organ or structure (E36.0-, E36.1-, E36.8)

E89.0 Postprocedural hypothyroidism
Postirradiation hypothyroidism
Postsurgical hypothyroidism

E89.1 Postprocedural hypoinsulinemia `CC`
Postpancreatectomy hyperglycemia
Postsurgical hypoinsulinemia
Use additional code, if applicable, to identify:
acquired absence of pancreas (Z90.41-)
diabetes mellitus (postpancreatectomy) (postprocedural) (E13.-)
insulin use (Z79.4)
EXCLUDES 1   transient postprocedural hyperglycemia (R73.9)
transient postprocedural hypoglycemia (E16.2)
CC Excl: PDX collection 520

E89.2 Postprocedural hypoparathyroidism `HCC`
Parathyroprival tetany

E89.3 Postprocedural hypopituitarism `HCC`
Postirradiation hypopituitarism

✓5ᵗʰ **E89.4 Postprocedural ovarian failure**
   E89.40 Asymptomatic postprocedural ovarian failure ♀
Postprocedural ovarian failure NOS

   E89.41 Symptomatic postprocedural ovarian failure ♀
Symptoms such as flushing, sleeplessness, headache, lack of concentration, associated with postprocedural menopause

E89.5 Postprocedural testicular hypofunction ♂

E89.6 Postprocedural adrenocortical (-medullary) hypofunction `CC` `HCC`
CC Excl: PDX collection 526

✓5ᵗʰ **E89.8 Other postprocedural endocrine and metabolic complications and disorders**

CC Excl: For CC codes in subcategory E89.8, unless otherwise noted: PDX collection 546

✓6ᵗʰ **E89.81 Postprocedural hemorrhage of an endocrine system organ or structure following a procedure**
   E89.810 Postprocedural hemorrhage of an endocrine system organ or structure following an endocrine system procedure `CC`
   E89.811 Postprocedural hemorrhage of an endocrine system organ or structure following other procedure `CC`

✓6ᵗʰ **E89.82 Postprocedural hematoma and seroma of an endocrine system organ or structure**
   E89.820 Postprocedural hematoma of an endocrine system organ or structure following an endocrine system procedure `CC`
   E89.821 Postprocedural hematoma of an endocrine system organ or structure following other procedure `CC`
   E89.822 Postprocedural seroma of an endocrine system organ or structure following an endocrine system procedure `CC`
   E89.823 Postprocedural seroma of an endocrine system organ or structure following other procedure `CC`

E89.89 Other postprocedural endocrine and metabolic complications and disorders `CC`
Use additional code, if applicable, to further specify disorder

Chapter 5. Mental, Behavioral and Neurodevelopmental Disorders (F01–F99)

Chapter Specific Guidelines with Coding Examples

The chapter specific guidelines from the ICD-10-CM Official Guidelines for Coding and Reporting have been provided below. Along with these guidelines are coding examples, contained in the shaded boxes, that have been developed to help illustrate the coding and/or sequencing guidance found in these guidelines.

a. Pain disorders related to psychological factors

Assign code F45.41, for pain that is exclusively related to psychological disorders. As indicated by the Excludes 1 note under category G89, a code from category G89 should not be assigned with code F45.41.

> Perceived abdominal pain determined to be persistent somatoform pain disorder
>
> **F45.41   Pain disorder exclusively related to psychological factors**
>
> *Explanation*: This pain was diagnosed as being exclusively psychological; therefore, no code from category G89 is added.

Code F45.42, Pain disorders with related psychological factors, should be used with a code from category G89, Pain, not elsewhere classified, if there is documentation of a psychological component for a patient with acute or chronic pain.

See Section I.C.6. Pain

b. Mental and behavioral disorders due to psychoactive substance use

1) In remission

Selection of codes for "in remission" for categories F10-F19, Mental and behavioral disorders due to psychoactive substance use (categories F10-F19 with **-11, -.21**) requires the provider's clinical judgment. The appropriate codes for "in remission" are assigned only on the basis of provider documentation (as defined in the Official Guidelines for Coding and Reporting)**, unless otherwise instructed by the classification.**

Mild substance use disorders in early or sustained remission are classified to the appropriate codes for substance abuse in remission, and moderate or severe substance use disorders in early or sustained remission are classified to the appropriate codes for substance dependence in remission.

2) Psychoactive substance use, abuse and dependence

When the provider documentation refers to use, abuse and dependence of the same substance (e.g. alcohol, opioid, cannabis, etc.), only one code should be assigned to identify the pattern of use based on the following hierarchy:

- If both use and abuse are documented, assign only the code for abuse
- If both abuse and dependence are documented, assign only the code for dependence
- If use, abuse and dependence are all documented, assign only the code for dependence
- If both use and dependence are documented, assign only the code for dependence.

> History and physical notes cannabis dependence; progress note says cannabis abuse
>
> **F12.20   Cannabis dependence, uncomplicated**
>
> *Explanation*: In the hierarchy, the dependence code is used if both abuse and dependence are documented.

> Discharge summary says cocaine abuse; progress notes list cocaine use
>
> **F14.10   Cocaine abuse, uncomplicated**
>
> *Explanation*: In the hierarchy, the abuse code is used if both abuse and use are documented.

3) Psychoactive substance use *disorders*

As with all other diagnoses, the codes for psychoactive substance use **disorders** (F10.9-, F11.9-, F12.9-, F13.9-, F14.9-, F15.9-, F16.9-) should only be assigned based on provider documentation and when they meet the definition of a reportable diagnosis (see Section III, Reporting Additional Diagnoses). The codes are to be used only when the psychoactive substance use is associated with a **physical,** mental or behavioral disorder, and such a relationship is documented by the provider.

> ED reports that a 27-year-old female tripped and broke her right ankle. Her friends reported that they were drinking and dancing at a nightclub.
>
> **S82.891A   Other fracture of right lower leg, initial encounter for closed fracture**
>
> **W01.0XXA   Fall on same level from slipping, tripping and stumbling, without subsequent striking against object, initial encounter**
>
> **Y92.252   Music hall as the place of occurrence of the external cause**
>
> **Y93.41   Activity, dancing**
>
> *Explanation*: Note that no code was added for alcohol use or abuse. Unless it is specifically associated with a diagnosis by provider documentation and meets the definition of a reportable diagnosis, it is not assigned. However, if the documentation from the provider stated: "The patient tripped, fell and fractured her right ankle while dancing due to her elevated blood alcohol, consistent with her ongoing alcohol abuse," the following code would be added:
>
> **F10.10   Alcohol abuse, uncomplicated**

Chapter 5. Mental, Behavioral and Neurodevelopmental Disorders

Chapter 5. Mental, Behavioral and Neurodevelopmental Disorders (F01-F99)

INCLUDES disorders of psychological development
EXCLUDES 2 *symptoms, signs and abnormal clinical laboratory findings, not elsewhere classified (R00-R99)*

This chapter contains the following blocks:

F01-F09	Mental disorders due to known physiological conditions
F10-F19	Mental and behavioral disorders due to psychoactive substance use
F20-F29	Schizophrenia, schizotypal, delusional, and other non-mood psychotic disorders
F30-F39	Mood [affective] disorders
F40-F48	Anxiety, dissociative, stress-related, somatoform and other nonpsychotic mental disorders
F50-F59	Behavioral syndromes associated with physiological disturbances and physical factors
F60-F69	Disorders of adult personality and behavior
F70-F79	Intellectual disabilities
F80-F89	Pervasive and specific developmental disorders
F90-F98	Behavioral and emotional disorders with onset usually occurring in childhood and adolescence
F99	Unspecified mental disorder

Mental disorders due to known physiological conditions (F01-F09)

NOTE This block comprises a range of mental disorders grouped together on the basis of their having in common a demonstrable etiology in cerebral disease, brain injury, or other insult leading to cerebral dysfunction. The dysfunction may be primary, as in diseases, injuries, and insults that affect the brain directly and selectively; or secondary, as in systemic diseases and disorders that attack the brain only as one of the multiple organs or systems of the body that are involved.

✓4ᵗʰ F01   Vascular dementia

Vascular dementia as a result of infarction of the brain due to vascular disease, including hypertensive cerebrovascular disease.
INCLUDES arteriosclerotic dementia
Code first the underlying physiological condition or sequelae of cerebrovascular disease.

✓5ᵗʰ F01.5   Vascular dementia

F01.50   Vascular dementia without behavioral disturbance   [A]
Major neurocognitive disorder without behavioral disturbance

F01.51   Vascular dementia with behavioral disturbance   [CC] [A]
Major neurocognitive disorder due to vascular disease, with behavioral disturbance
Major neurocognitive disorder with aggressive behavior
Major neurocognitive disorder with combative behavior
Major neurocognitive disorder with violent behavior
Vascular dementia with aggressive behavior
Vascular dementia with combative behavior
Vascular dementia with violent behavior
Use additional code, if applicable, to identify wandering in vascular dementia (Z91.83)
CC Excl: PDX collection 547

✓4ᵗʰ F02   Dementia in other diseases classified elsewhere

INCLUDES major neurocognitive disorder in other diseases classified elsewhere
Code first the underlying physiological condition, such as:
Alzheimer's (G30.-)
cerebral lipidosis (E75.4)
Creutzfeldt-Jakob disease (A81.0-)
dementia with Lewy bodies (G31.83)
dementia with Parkinsonism (G31.83)
epilepsy and recurrent seizures (G40.-)
frontotemporal dementia (G31.09)
hepatolenticular degeneration (E83.0)
human immunodeficiency virus [HIV] disease (B20)
Huntington's disease (G10)
hypercalcemia (E83.52)
hypothyroidism, acquired (E00-E03.-)
intoxications (T36-T65)
Jakob-Creutzfeldt disease (A81.0-)
multiple sclerosis (G35)
neurosyphilis (A52.17)
niacin deficiency [pellagra] (E52)
Parkinson's disease (G20)
Pick's disease (G31.01)
polyarteritis nodosa (M30.0)
prion disease (A81.9)
systemic lupus erythematosus (M32.-)
traumatic brain injury (S06.-)
trypanosomiasis (B56.-, B57.-)
vitamin B deficiency (E53.8)
EXCLUDES 2 *dementia in alcohol and psychoactive substance disorders (F10-F19, with .17, .27, .97)*
vascular dementia (F01.5-)

✓5ᵗʰ F02.8   Dementia in other diseases classified elsewhere
AHA: 2017, 2Q, 7; 2016, 4Q, 141; 2016, 2Q, 6

F02.80   Dementia in other diseases classified elsewhere without behavioral disturbance
Dementia in other diseases classified elsewhere NOS
Major neurocognitive disorder in other diseases classified elsewhere

F02.81   Dementia in other diseases classified elsewhere with behavioral disturbance   [CC]
Dementia in other diseases classified elsewhere with aggressive behavior
Dementia in other diseases classified elsewhere with combative behavior
Dementia in other diseases classified elsewhere with violent behavior
Major neurocognitive disorder in other diseases classified elsewhere with aggressive behavior
Major neurocognitive disorder in other diseases classified elsewhere with combative behavior
Major neurocognitive disorder in other diseases classified elsewhere with violent behavior
Use additional code, if applicable, to identify wandering in dementia in conditions classified elsewhere (Z91.83)
CC Excl: PDX collection 548

✓4ᵗʰ F03   Unspecified dementia

Presenile dementia NOS   Senile dementia NOS
Presenile psychosis NOS   Senile dementia depressed
Primary degenerative dementia NOS   or paranoid type
Senile dementia NOS   Senile psychosis NOS
EXCLUDES 1 *senility NOS (R41.81)*
EXCLUDES 2 *mild memory disturbance due to known physiological condition (F06.8)*
senile dementia with delirium or acute confusional state (F05)

✓5ᵗʰ F03.9   Unspecified dementia

F03.90   Unspecified dementia without behavioral disturbance   [HIV] [A]
Dementia NOS
AHA: 2012, 4Q, 92

F03.91   Unspecified dementia with behavioral disturbance   [CC] [A]
Unspecified dementia with aggressive behavior
Unspecified dementia with combative behavior
Unspecified dementia with violent behavior
Use additional code, if applicable, to identify wandering in unspecified dementia (Z91.83)
CC Excl: PDX collection 548

[N] Newborn: 0   [P] Pediatric: 0-17   [M] Maternity: 12-55   [A] Adult: 15-124   [MCC] Major CC Condition   [PDxMCC] PDx acts as own MCC   [CC] CC Condition   [PDxCC] PDx acts as own CC

532   ICD-10-CM 2018

F04   **Amnestic disorder due to known physiological condition**
    Korsakov's psychosis or syndrome, nonalcoholic
    Code first the underlying physiological condition
    EXCLUDES 1   amnesia NOS (R41.3)
              anterograde amnesia (R41.1)
              dissociative amnesia (F44.0)
              retrograde amnesia (R41.2)
    EXCLUDES 2   alcohol-induced or unspecified Korsakov's syndrome (F10.26, F10.96)
              Korsakov's syndrome induced by other psychoactive substances (F13.26, F13.96, F19.16, F19.26, F19.96)

F05   **Delirium due to known physiological condition**   **CC**
    Acute or subacute brain syndrome
    Acute or subacute confusional state (nonalcoholic)
    Acute or subacute infective psychosis
    Acute or subacute organic reaction
    Acute or subacute psycho-organic syndrome
    Delirium of mixed etiology
    Delirium superimposed on dementia
    Sundowning
    Code first the underlying physiological condition
    EXCLUDES 1   delirium NOS (R41.0)
    EXCLUDES 2   delirium tremens alcohol-induced or unspecified (F10.231, F10.921)
    CC Excl: PDX collection 549

☑4ᵗʰ **F06**   **Other mental disorders due to known physiological condition**
    INCLUDES   mental disorders due to endocrine disorder
              mental disorders due to exogenous hormone
              mental disorders due to exogenous toxic substance
              mental disorders due to primary cerebral disease
              mental disorders due to somatic illness
              mental disorders due to systemic disease affecting the brain
    Code first the underlying physiological condition
    EXCLUDES 1   unspecified dementia (F03)
    EXCLUDES 2   delirium due to known physiological condition (F05)
              dementia as classified in F01-F02
              other mental disorders associated with alcohol and other psychoactive substances (F10-F19)

    F06.0   **Psychotic disorder with hallucinations due to known physiological condition**   **CC**
        Organic hallucinatory state (nonalcoholic)
        EXCLUDES 2   hallucinations and perceptual disturbance induced by alcohol and other psychoactive substances (F10-F19 with .151, .251, .951)
                 schizophrenia (F20.-)
        CC Excl: PDX collection 550

    F06.1   **Catatonic disorder due to known physiological condition**
        Catatonia associated with another mental disorder
        Catatonia NOS
        EXCLUDES 1   catatonic stupor (R40.1)
                 stupor NOS (R40.1)
        EXCLUDES 2   catatonic schizophrenia (F20.2)
                 dissociative stupor (F44.2)

    F06.2   **Psychotic disorder with delusions due to known physiological condition**   **CC**
        Paranoid and paranoid-hallucinatory organic states
        Schizophrenia-like psychosis in epilepsy
        EXCLUDES 2   alcohol and drug-induced psychotic disorder (F10-F19 with .150, .250, .950)
                 brief psychotic disorder (F23)
                 delusional disorder (F22)
                 schizophrenia (F20.-)
        CC Excl: PDX collection 550

☑5ᵗʰ   **F06.3**   **Mood disorder due to known physiological condition**
        EXCLUDES 2   mood disorders due to alcohol and other psychoactive substances (F10-F19 with .14, .24, .94)
                 mood disorders, not due to known physiological condition or unspecified (F30-F39)

        F06.30   **Mood disorder due to known physiological condition, unspecified**

        F06.31   **Mood disorder due to known physiological condition with depressive features**
            ▶Depressive disorder due to known physiological condition, with depressive features◀

        F06.32   **Mood disorder due to known physiological condition with major depressive-like episode**
            ▶Depressive disorder due to known physiological condition, with major depressive–like episode◀

        F06.33   **Mood disorder due to known physiological condition with manic features**
            ▶Bipolar and related disorder due to a known physiological condition, with manic features
            Bipolar and related disorder due to known physiological condition, with manic- or hypomanic-like episodes◀

        F06.34   **Mood disorder due to known physiological condition with mixed features**
            ▶Bipolar and related disorder due to known physiological condition, with mixed features
            Depressive disorder due to known physiological condition, with mixed features◀

    F06.4   **Anxiety disorder due to known physiological condition**
        EXCLUDES 2   anxiety disorders due to alcohol and other psychoactive substances (F10-F19 with .180, .280, .980)
                 anxiety disorders, not due to known physiological condition or unspecified (F40.-, F41.-)

    F06.8   **Other specified mental disorders due to known physiological condition**   **HIV**
        Epileptic psychosis NOS
        ▶Obsessive-compulsive and related disorder due to a known physiological condition◀
        Organic dissociative disorder
        Organic emotionally labile [asthenic] disorder

☑4ᵗʰ **F07**   **Personality and behavioral disorders due to known physiological condition**
    Code first the underlying physiological condition

    F07.0   **Personality change due to known physiological condition**
        Frontal lobe syndrome
        Limbic epilepsy personality syndrome
        Lobotomy syndrome
        Organic personality disorder
        Organic pseudopsychopathic personality
        Organic pseudoretarded personality
        Postleucotomy syndrome
        Code first underlying physiological condition
        EXCLUDES 1   mild cognitive impairment (G31.84)
                 postconcussional syndrome (F07.81)
                 postencephalitic syndrome (F07.89)
                 signs and symptoms involving emotional state (R45.-)
        EXCLUDES 2   specific personality disorder (F60.-)

☑5ᵗʰ   **F07.8**   **Other personality and behavioral disorders due to known physiological condition**
        F07.81   **Postconcussional syndrome**
            Postcontusional syndrome (encephalopathy)
            Post-traumatic brain syndrome, nonpsychotic
            Use additional code to identify associated post-traumatic headache, if applicable (G44.3-)
            EXCLUDES 1   current concussion (brain) (S06.0-)
                    postencephalitic syndrome (F07.89)

        F07.89   **Other personality and behavioral disorders due to known physiological condition**
            Postencephalitic syndrome
            Right hemispheric organic affective disorder

    F07.9   **Unspecified personality and behavioral disorder due to known physiological condition**   **HIV**
        Organic psychosyndrome

F09   **Unspecified mental disorder due to known physiological condition**   **HIV**
    Mental disorder NOS due to known physiological condition
    Organic brain syndrome NOS
    Organic mental disorder NOS
    Organic psychosis NOS
    Symptomatic psychosis NOS
    Code first the underlying physiological condition
    EXCLUDES 1   psychosis NOS (F29)

☑ Additional Character Req   ✓x7ᵗʰ Placeholder Alert   Unacceptable PDx   Manifestation   **H1**-**H14** HAC   **HCC** CMS-HCC Condition   *EXCLUDES 1* Not Coded Here   *EXCLUDES 2* Not Included Here

Mental and behavioral disorders due to psychoactive substance use (F10-F19)

AHA: 2017, 2Q, 27

✓4th **F10   Alcohol related disorders**
Use additional code for blood alcohol level, if applicable (Y90.-)

CC Excl: For CC codes in category F10: PDX collection 550

✓5th **F10.1   Alcohol abuse**
  EXCLUDES 1   alcohol dependence (F10.2-)
  alcohol use, unspecified (F10.9-)
  AHA: 2015, 2Q, 15

  F10.10   Alcohol abuse, uncomplicated
  Alcohol use disorder, mild

  F10.11   Alcohol abuse, in remission
  Alcohol use disorder, mild, in early remission
  Alcohol use disorder, mild, in sustained remission

✓6th **F10.12   Alcohol abuse with intoxication**
  F10.120   Alcohol abuse with intoxication, uncomplicated HCC
  F10.121   Alcohol abuse with intoxication delirium CC HCC
  F10.129   Alcohol abuse with intoxication, unspecified HCC

  F10.14   Alcohol abuse with alcohol-induced mood disorder CC HCC
  Alcohol use disorder, mild, with alcohol-induced bipolar or related disorder
  Alcohol use disorder, mild, with alcohol-induced depressive disorder

✓6th **F10.15   Alcohol abuse with alcohol-induced psychotic disorder**
  F10.150   Alcohol abuse with alcohol-induced psychotic disorder with delusions HCC
  F10.151   Alcohol abuse with alcohol-induced psychotic disorder with hallucinations CC HCC HCC
  DEF: Psychosis lasting less than six months with slight or no clouding of consciousness in which auditory hallucinations predominate.
  F10.159   Alcohol abuse with alcohol-induced psychotic disorder, unspecified CC HCC

✓6th **F10.18   Alcohol abuse with other alcohol-induced disorders**
  F10.180   Alcohol abuse with alcohol-induced anxiety disorder CC HCC
  F10.181   Alcohol abuse with alcohol-induced sexual dysfunction CC HCC
  F10.182   Alcohol abuse with alcohol-induced sleep disorder CC HCC
  F10.188   Alcohol abuse with other alcohol-induced disorder CC HCC

  F10.19   Alcohol abuse with unspecified alcohol-induced disorder CC HCC

✓5th **F10.2   Alcohol dependence**
  EXCLUDES 1   alcohol abuse (F10.1-)
  alcohol use, unspecified (F10.9-)
  EXCLUDES 2   toxic effect of alcohol (T51.0-)

  F10.20   Alcohol dependence, uncomplicated HCC
  Alcohol use disorder, moderate
  Alcohol use disorder, severe

  F10.21   Alcohol dependence, in remission HCC
  ▶Alcohol use disorder, moderate, in early remission
  Alcohol use disorder, moderate, in sustained remission
  Alcohol use disorder, severe, in early remission
  Alcohol use disorder, severe, in sustained remission◄

✓6th **F10.22   Alcohol dependence with intoxication**
  Acute drunkenness (in alcoholism)
  EXCLUDES 2   alcohol dependence with withdrawal (F10.23-)
  F10.220   Alcohol dependence with intoxication, uncomplicated HCC
  F10.221   Alcohol dependence with intoxication delirium CC HCC
  F10.229   Alcohol dependence with intoxication, unspecified HCC

✓6th **F10.23   Alcohol dependence with withdrawal**
  EXCLUDES 2   alcohol dependence with intoxication (F10.22-)
  AHA: 2015, 2Q, 15
  F10.230   Alcohol dependence with withdrawal, uncomplicated CC HCC
  F10.231   Alcohol dependence with withdrawal delirium CC HCC
  F10.232   Alcohol dependence with withdrawal with perceptual disturbance CC HCC
  F10.239   Alcohol dependence with withdrawal, unspecified CC HCC

  F10.24   Alcohol dependence with alcohol-induced mood disorder CC HCC
  Alcohol use disorder, moderate, with alcohol-induced bipolar or related disorder
  Alcohol use disorder, moderate, with alcohol-induced depressive disorder
  Alcohol use disorder, severe, with alcohol-induced bipolar or related disorder
  Alcohol use disorder, severe, with alcohol-induced depressive disorder

✓6th **F10.25   Alcohol dependence with alcohol-induced psychotic disorder**
  F10.250   Alcohol dependence with alcohol-induced psychotic disorder with delusions HCC
  F10.251   Alcohol dependence with alcohol-induced psychotic disorder with hallucinations CC HCC
  F10.259   Alcohol dependence with alcohol-induced psychotic disorder, unspecified CC HCC

  F10.26   Alcohol dependence with alcohol-induced persisting amnestic disorder HCC
  Alcohol use disorder, moderate, with alcohol-induced major neurocognitive disorder, amnestic-confabulatory type
  Alcohol use disorder, severe, with alcohol-induced major neurocognitive disorder, amnestic-confabulatory type
  DEF: Prominent and lasting reduced memory span, disordered time appreciation and confabulation, occurs in alcoholics as sequel to acute alcoholic psychosis.

  F10.27   Alcohol dependence with alcohol-induced persisting dementia CC HCC
  Alcohol use disorder, moderate, with alcohol-induced major neurocognitive disorder, nonamnestic-confabulatory type
  Alcohol use disorder, severe, with alcohol-induced major neurocognitive disorder, nonamnestic-confabulatory type

✓6th **F10.28   Alcohol dependence with other alcohol-induced disorders**
  F10.280   Alcohol dependence with alcohol-induced anxiety disorder CC HCC
  F10.281   Alcohol dependence with alcohol-induced sexual dysfunction CC HCC
  F10.282   Alcohol dependence with alcohol-induced sleep disorder HCC
  F10.288   Alcohol dependence with other alcohol-induced disorder CC HCC
  Alcohol use disorder, moderate, with alcohol-induced mild neurocognitive disorder
  Alcohol use disorder, severe, with alcohol-induced mild neurocognitive disorder

  F10.29   Alcohol dependence with unspecified alcohol-induced disorder CC HCC

✓5th **F10.9   Alcohol use, unspecified**
  EXCLUDES 1   alcohol abuse (F10.1-)
  alcohol dependence (F10.2-)

✓6th **F10.92   Alcohol use, unspecified with intoxication**
  F10.920   Alcohol use, unspecified with intoxication, uncomplicated HCC
  F10.921   Alcohol use, unspecified with intoxication delirium CC HCC
  F10.929   Alcohol use, unspecified with intoxication, unspecified HCC

F10.94   **Alcohol use, unspecified with**   `CC` `HCC`
alcohol-induced mood disorder
     Alcohol induced bipolar or related disorder, without
     use disorder
     Alcohol induced depressive disorder, without use
     disorder

✓6ᵗʰ **F10.95**   **Alcohol use, unspecified with alcohol-induced
psychotic disorder**

    F10.950   **Alcohol use, unspecified with**   `HCC`
**alcohol-induced psychotic disorder
with delusions**

    F10.951   **Alcohol use, unspecified with**   `CC` `HCC`
**alcohol-induced psychotic disorder
with hallucinations**

    F10.959   **Alcohol use, unspecified with**   `CC` `HCC`
**alcohol-induced psychotic disorder,
unspecified**
       Alcohol-induced psychotic disorder
       without use disorder

F10.96   **Alcohol use, unspecified with alcohol-induced**   `HCC`
persisting amnestic disorder
     Alcohol-induced major neurocognitive disorder,
     amnestic-confabulatory type, without use
     disorder

F10.97   **Alcohol use, unspecified with alcohol-induced**   `HCC`
persisting dementia
     Alcohol-induced major neurocognitive disorder,
     nonamnestic-confabulatory type, without use
     disorder

✓6ᵗʰ **F10.98**   **Alcohol use, unspecified with other alcohol-induced
disorders**

    F10.980   **Alcohol use, unspecified with**   `CC` `HCC`
alcohol-induced anxiety disorder
       Alcohol induced anxiety disorder, without
       use disorder

    F10.981   **Alcohol use, unspecified with**   `CC` `HCC`
alcohol-induced sexual dysfunction
       Alcohol induced sexual dysfunction,
       without use disorder

    F10.982   **Alcohol use, unspecified with**   `HCC`
alcohol-induced sleep disorder
       Alcohol induced sleep disorder, without
       use disorder

    F10.988   **Alcohol use, unspecified with**   `CC` `HCC`
other alcohol-induced disorder
       Alcohol induced mild neurocognitive
       disorder, without use disorder

F10.99   **Alcohol use, unspecified with unspecified**   `CC` `HCC`
alcohol-induced disorder

✓4ᵗʰ **F11**   **Opioid related disorders**

> **CC Excl: For CC codes in category F11, unless otherwise noted:**
> PDX collection 550

✓5ᵗʰ **F11.1**   **Opioid abuse**
    EXCLUDES 1   *opioid dependence (F11.2-)*
             opioid use, unspecified (F11.9-)

    F11.10   **Opioid abuse, uncomplicated**
       Opioid use disorder, mild

●   **F11.11**   **Opioid abuse, in remission**
       Opioid use disorder, mild, in early remission
       Opioid use disorder, mild, in sustained remission

✓6ᵗʰ **F11.12**   **Opioid abuse with intoxication**

    F11.120   **Opioid abuse with intoxication,**   `HCC`
uncomplicated

    F11.121   **Opioid abuse with intoxication**   `CC` `HCC`
delirium

    F11.122   **Opioid abuse with intoxication with**   `HCC`
perceptual disturbance

    F11.129   **Opioid abuse with intoxication,**   `HCC`
unspecified

    F11.14   **Opioid abuse with opioid-induced mood**   `HCC`
disorder
       Opioid use disorder, mild, with opioid-induced
       depressive disorder

✓6ᵗʰ **F11.15**   **Opioid abuse with opioid-induced psychotic
disorder**

    F11.150   **Opioid abuse with opioid-induced**   `CC` `HCC`
psychotic disorder with delusions

    F11.151   **Opioid abuse with opioid-induced**   `CC` `HCC`
psychotic disorder with hallucinations

    F11.159   **Opioid abuse with opioid-induced**   `HCC`
psychotic disorder, unspecified

✓6ᵗʰ **F11.18**   **Opioid abuse with other opioid-induced disorder**

    F11.181   **Opioid abuse with opioid-induced**   `HCC`
sexual dysfunction

    F11.182   **Opioid abuse with opioid-induced**   `HCC`
sleep disorder

    F11.188   **Opioid abuse with other**   `HCC`
opioid-induced disorder

    F11.19   **Opioid abuse with unspecified opioid-induced**   `HCC`
disorder

✓5ᵗʰ **F11.2**   **Opioid dependence**
    EXCLUDES 1   *opioid abuse (F11.1-)*
             opioid use, unspecified (F11.9-)
    EXCLUDES 2   *opioid poisoning (T40.0-T40.2-)*

    F11.20   **Opioid dependence, uncomplicated**   `CC` `HCC`
       Opioid use disorder, moderate
       Opioid use disorder, severe
       CC Excl: No excl

    F11.21   **Opioid dependence, in remission**   `HCC`
       ▶Opioid use disorder, moderate, in early remission
       Opioid use disorder, moderate, in sustained remission
       Opioid use disorder, severe, in early remission
       Opioid use disorder, severe, in sustained remission◀

✓6ᵗʰ **F11.22**   **Opioid dependence with intoxication**
    EXCLUDES 1   *opioid dependence with withdrawal (F11.23)*

    F11.220   **Opioid dependence with intoxication,**   `HCC`
uncomplicated

    F11.221   **Opioid dependence with**   `CC` `HCC`
intoxication delirium

    F11.222   **Opioid dependence with**   `CC` `HCC`
**intoxication with perceptual
disturbance**
       CC Excl: No excl

    F11.229   **Opioid dependence with intoxication,**   `HCC`
unspecified

    F11.23   **Opioid dependence with withdrawal**   `CC` `HCC`
    EXCLUDES 1   *opioid dependence with intoxication
             (F11.22-)*

    F11.24   **Opioid dependence with opioid-induced**   `HCC`
mood disorder
       Opioid use disorder, moderate, with opioid induced
       depressive disorder

✓6ᵗʰ **F11.25**   **Opioid dependence with opioid-induced
psychotic disorder**

    F11.250   **Opioid dependence with**   `CC` `HCC`
**opioid-induced psychotic disorder
with delusions**

    F11.251   **Opioid dependence with opioid-**   `CC` `HCC`
**induced psychotic disorder
with hallucinations**

    F11.259   **Opioid dependence with opioid-**   `CC` `HCC`
induced psychotic disorder, unspecified
       CC Excl: No excl

✓6ᵗʰ **F11.28**   **Opioid dependence with other opioid-induced
disorder**

    F11.281   **Opioid dependence with opioid-**   `CC` `HCC`
induced sexual dysfunction
       CC Excl: No excl

    F11.282   **Opioid dependence with**   `CC` `HCC`
opioid-induced sleep disorder
       CC Excl: No excl

    F11.288   **Opioid dependence with other**   `CC` `HCC`
opioid-induced disorder
       CC Excl: No excl

    F11.29   **Opioid dependence with unspecified**   `HCC`
opioid-induced disorder

✓5ᵗʰ **F11.9**   **Opioid use, unspecified**
    EXCLUDES 1   *opioid abuse (F11.1-)*
             opioid dependence (F11.2-)

    F11.90   **Opioid use, unspecified, uncomplicated**

✓6ᵗʰ **F11.92**   **Opioid use, unspecified with intoxication**
    EXCLUDES 1   *opioid use, unspecified with withdrawal
             (F11.93)*

    F11.920   **Opioid use, unspecified with**   `HCC`
intoxication, uncomplicated

    F11.921   **Opioid use, unspecified with**   `CC` `HCC`
intoxication delirium
       Opioid-induced delirium

✓ Additional Character Req   ✓x7ᵗʰ Placeholder Alert   Unacceptable PDx   Manifestation   H1 - H14 HAC   `HCC` CMS-HCC Condition   *EXCLUDES 1* Not Coded Here   *EXCLUDES 2* Not Included Here

Chapter 5. Mental, Behavioral and Neurodevelopmental Disorders

F11.922 **Opioid use, unspecified with intoxication with** perceptual disturbance `HCC`

F11.929 **Opioid use, unspecified with intoxication,** unspecified `HCC`

F11.93 **Opioid use, unspecified with** withdrawal `CC` `HCC`
     EXCLUDES 1   *opioid use, unspecified with intoxication (F11.92-)*

F11.94 **Opioid use, unspecified with opioid-induced** mood disorder `HCC`
     Opioid induced depressive disorder, without use disorder

✓6th F11.95 **Opioid use, unspecified with opioid-induced** psychotic disorder

     F11.950 **Opioid use, unspecified with opioid-induced psychotic disorder with** delusions `CC` `HCC`

     F11.951 **Opioid use, unspecified with opioid-induced psychotic disorder with** hallucinations `CC` `HCC`

     F11.959 **Opioid use, unspecified with opioid-induced psychotic disorder,** unspecified `HCC`

✓6th F11.98 **Opioid use, unspecified with** other **specified opioid-induced disorder**

     F11.981 **Opioid use, unspecified with opioid-induced** sexual dysfunction `HCC`
         Opioid induced sexual dysfunction, without use disorder

     F11.982 **Opioid use, unspecified with opioid-induced** sleep disorder `HCC`
         Opioid induced sleep disorder, without use disorder

     F11.988 **Opioid use, unspecified with** other **opioid-induced disorder** `HCC`
         Opioid induced anxiety disorder, without use disorder

F11.99 **Opioid use, unspecified with** unspecified **opioid-induced disorder** `HCC`

✓4th **F12 Cannabis** related disorders
     INCLUDES   marijuana

     CC Excl: For CC codes in category F12: PDX collection 550

✓5th **F12.1 Cannabis** abuse
     EXCLUDES 1   *cannabis dependence (F12.2-)*
                  cannabis use, unspecified (F12.9-)

     F12.10 **Cannabis abuse,** uncomplicated
         Cannabis use disorder, mild

     F12.11 **Cannabis abuse,** in remission
         Cannabis use disorder, mild, in early remission
         Cannabis use disorder, mild, in sustained remission

  ✓6th F12.12 **Cannabis abuse with** intoxication

     F12.120 **Cannabis abuse with intoxication,** uncomplicated `HCC`

     F12.121 **Cannabis abuse with intoxication** delirium `CC` `HCC`

     F12.122 **Cannabis abuse with intoxication with** perceptual disturbance `HCC`

     F12.129 **Cannabis abuse with intoxication,** unspecified `HCC`

  ✓6th F12.15 **Cannabis abuse with** psychotic disorder

     F12.150 **Cannabis abuse with psychotic disorder with** delusions `CC` `HCC`

     F12.151 **Cannabis abuse with psychotic disorder with** hallucinations `CC` `HCC`

     F12.159 **Cannabis abuse with psychotic disorder,** unspecified `HCC`

  ✓6th F12.18 **Cannabis abuse with** other **cannabis-induced disorder**

     F12.180 **Cannabis abuse with cannabis-induced** anxiety disorder `HCC`

     F12.188 **Cannabis abuse with** other **cannabis-induced disorder** `HCC`
         Cannabis use disorder, mild, with cannabis-induced sleep disorder

     F12.19 **Cannabis abuse with** unspecified **cannabis-induced disorder** `HCC`

✓5th **F12.2 Cannabis** dependence
     EXCLUDES 1   *cannabis abuse (F12.1-)*
                  cannabis use, unspecified (F12.9-)
     EXCLUDES 2   *cannabis poisoning (T40.7-)*

     F12.20 **Cannabis dependence,** uncomplicated `HCC`
         Cannabis use disorder, moderate
         Cannabis use disorder, severe

     F12.21 **Cannabis dependence,** in remission `HCC`
         ▶Cannabis use disorder, moderate, in early remission
         Cannabis use disorder, moderate, in sustained remission
         Cannabis use disorder, severe, in early remission
         Cannabis use disorder, severe, in sustained remission◄

  ✓6th F12.22 **Cannabis dependence with** intoxication

     F12.220 **Cannabis dependence with intoxication,** uncomplicated `HCC`

     F12.221 **Cannabis dependence with intoxication** delirium `CC` `HCC`

     F12.222 **Cannabis dependence with intoxication with** perceptual disturbance `HCC`

     F12.229 **Cannabis dependence with intoxication,** unspecified `HCC`

  ✓6th F12.25 **Cannabis dependence with** psychotic disorder

     F12.250 **Cannabis dependence with psychotic disorder with** delusions `CC` `HCC`

     F12.251 **Cannabis dependence with psychotic disorder with** hallucinations `CC` `HCC`

     F12.259 **Cannabis dependence with psychotic disorder,** unspecified `HCC`

  ✓6th F12.28 **Cannabis dependence with** other **cannabis-induced disorder**

     F12.280 **Cannabis dependence with cannabis-induced** anxiety disorder `HCC`

     F12.288 **Cannabis dependence with** other **cannabis-induced disorder** `HCC`
         Cannabis use disorder, moderate, with cannabis-induced sleep disorder
         Cannabis use disorder, severe, with cannabis-induced sleep disorder
         Cannabis withdrawal

     F12.29 **Cannabis dependence with** unspecified **cannabis-induced disorder** `HCC`

✓5th **F12.9 Cannabis use,** unspecified
     EXCLUDES 1   *cannabis abuse (F12.1-)*
                  cannabis dependence (F12.2-)

     F12.90 **Cannabis use, unspecified,** uncomplicated

  ✓6th F12.92 **Cannabis use, unspecified with** intoxication

     F12.920 **Cannabis use, unspecified with intoxication,** uncomplicated `HCC`

     F12.921 **Cannabis use, unspecified with intoxication** delirium `CC` `HCC`

     F12.922 **Cannabis use, unspecified with intoxication with** perceptual disturbance `HCC`

     F12.929 **Cannabis use, unspecified with intoxication,** unspecified `HCC`

  ✓6th F12.95 **Cannabis use, unspecified with** psychotic disorder

     F12.950 **Cannabis use, unspecified with psychotic disorder with** delusions `CC` `HCC`

     F12.951 **Cannabis use, unspecified with psychotic disorder with** hallucinations `CC` `HCC`

     F12.959 **Cannabis use, unspecified with psychotic disorder,** unspecified `HCC`
         Cannabis induced psychotic disorder, without use disorder

  ✓6th F12.98 **Cannabis use, unspecified with** other **cannabis-induced disorder**

     F12.980 **Cannabis use, unspecified with** anxiety disorder `HCC`
         Cannabis induced anxiety disorder, without use disorder

     F12.988 **Cannabis use, unspecified with** other `HCC` **cannabis-induced disorder**
         Cannabis induced sleep disorder, without use disorder

     F12.99 **Cannabis use, unspecified with** unspecified **cannabis-induced disorder** `HCC`

N Newborn: 0   P Pediatric: 0-17   M Maternity: 12-55   A Adult: 15-124   MCC Major CC Condition   PDxMCC PDx acts as own MCC   CC CC Condition   PDxCC PDx acts as own CC

536   ICD-10-CM 2018

✓4th **F13** Sedative, hypnotic, or anxiolytic **related disorders**

> **CC Excl: For CC codes in category F13, unless otherwise noted:** PDX collection 550

✓5th **F13.1** **Sedative, hypnotic or anxiolytic-related** abuse

> EXCLUDES 1   *sedative, hypnotic or anxiolytic-related dependence (F13.2-)*
> *sedative, hypnotic, or anxiolytic use, unspecified (F13.9-)*

     F13.10 **Sedative, hypnotic or anxiolytic abuse, uncomplicated**
         Sedative, hypnotic, or anxiolytic use disorder, mild

•   **F13.11** **Sedative, hypnotic or anxiolytic abuse, in remission**
         Sedative, hypnotic, or anxiolytic use disorder, mild, in early remission
         Sedative, hypnotic, or anxiolytic use disorder, mild, in sustained remission

✓6th **F13.12** **Sedative, hypnotic or anxiolytic abuse with intoxication**
     F13.120 **Sedative, hypnotic or anxiolytic abuse** HCC **with intoxication, uncomplicated**
     F13.121 **Sedative, hypnotic or anxiolytic** CC HCC **abuse with intoxication** delirium
     F13.129 **Sedative, hypnotic or anxiolytic abuse** HCC **with intoxication, unspecified**

     F13.14 **Sedative, hypnotic or anxiolytic abuse with** HCC **sedative, hypnotic or anxiolytic-induced** mood disorder
       ▶Sedative, hypnotic, or anxiolytic use disorder, mild, with sedative, hypnotic, or anxiolytic-induced bipolar or related disorder
       Sedative, hypnotic, or anxiolytic use disorder, mild, with sedative, hypnotic, or anxiolytic-induced depressive disorder◀

✓6th **F13.15** **Sedative, hypnotic or anxiolytic abuse with sedative, hypnotic or anxiolytic-induced** psychotic disorder
     F13.150 **Sedative, hypnotic or anxiolytic** CC HCC **abuse with sedative, hypnotic or anxiolytic-induced psychotic disorder with** delusions
     F13.151 **Sedative, hypnotic or anxiolytic** CC HCC **abuse with sedative, hypnotic or anxiolytic-induced psychotic disorder with** hallucinations
     F13.159 **Sedative, hypnotic or anxiolytic abuse** HCC **with sedative, hypnotic or anxiolytic-induced psychotic disorder, unspecified**

✓6th **F13.18** **Sedative, hypnotic or anxiolytic abuse with** other **sedative, hypnotic or anxiolytic-induced disorders**
     F13.180 **Sedative, hypnotic or anxiolytic** HCC **abuse with sedative, hypnotic or anxiolytic-induced** anxiety disorder
     F13.181 **Sedative, hypnotic or anxiolytic** HCC **abuse with sedative, hypnotic or anxiolytic-induced** sexual dysfunction
     F13.182 **Sedative, hypnotic or anxiolytic** HCC **abuse with sedative, hypnotic or anxiolytic-induced** sleep disorder
     F13.188 **Sedative, hypnotic or anxiolytic** HCC **abuse with** other **sedative, hypnotic or anxiolytic-induced disorder**

     F13.19 **Sedative, hypnotic or anxiolytic abuse with** HCC **unspecified sedative, hypnotic or anxiolytic-induced disorder**

✓5th **F13.2** **Sedative, hypnotic or anxiolytic-related** dependence

> EXCLUDES 1   *sedative, hypnotic or anxiolytic-related abuse (F13.1-)*
> *sedative, hypnotic, or anxiolytic use, unspecified (F13.9-)*
> EXCLUDES 2   *sedative, hypnotic, or anxiolytic poisoning (T42.-)*

     F13.20 **Sedative, hypnotic or anxiolytic dependence,** CC HCC **uncomplicated**
         CC Excl: No excl

F13.21 **Sedative, hypnotic or anxiolytic dependence, in** HCC **remission**
     ▶Sedative, hypnotic or anxiolytic use disorder, moderate, in early remission
     Sedative, hypnotic or anxiolytic use disorder, moderate, in sustained remission
     Sedative, hypnotic or anxiolytic use disorder, severe, in early remission
     Sedative, hypnotic or anxiolytic use disorder, severe, in sustained remission◀

✓6th **F13.22** **Sedative, hypnotic or anxiolytic dependence with intoxication**
> EXCLUDES 1   *sedative, hypnotic or anxiolytic dependence with withdrawal (F13.23-)*

     F13.220 **Sedative, hypnotic or anxiolytic** HCC **dependence with intoxication, uncomplicated**
     F13.221 **Sedative, hypnotic or anxiolytic** CC HCC **dependence with intoxication** delirium
     F13.229 **Sedative, hypnotic or anxiolytic** HCC **dependence with intoxication, unspecified**

✓6th **F13.23** **Sedative, hypnotic or anxiolytic dependence with** withdrawal
     Sedative, hypnotic, or anxiolytic use disorder, moderate
     Sedative, hypnotic, or anxiolytic use disorder, severe
> EXCLUDES 1   *sedative, hypnotic or anxiolytic dependence with intoxication (F13.22-)*

     F13.230 **Sedative, hypnotic or anxiolytic** CC HCC **dependence with withdrawal, uncomplicated**
     F13.231 **Sedative, hypnotic or anxiolytic** CC HCC **dependence with withdrawal** delirium
     F13.232 **Sedative, hypnotic or anxiolytic** CC HCC **dependence with withdrawal with** perceptual disturbance
         Sedative, hypnotic, or anxiolytic withdrawal with perceptual disturbances
     F13.239 **Sedative, hypnotic or anxiolytic** CC HCC **dependence with withdrawal, unspecified**
         Sedative, hypnotic, or anxiolytic withdrawal without perceptual disturbances

     F13.24 **Sedative, hypnotic or anxiolytic dependence** HCC **with sedative, hypnotic or anxiolytic-induced** mood disorder
       ▶Sedative, hypnotic, or anxiolytic use disorder, moderate, with sedative, hypnotic, or anxiolytic-induced bipolar or related disorder
       Sedative, hypnotic, or anxiolytic use disorder, moderate, with sedative, hypnotic, or anxiolytic-induced depressive disorder◀
       Sedative, hypnotic, or anxiolytic use disorder, severe, with sedative, hypnotic, or anxiolytic-induced bipolar or related disorder
       ▶Sedative, hypnotic, or anxiolytic use disorder, severe, with sedative, hypnotic, or anxiolytic-induced depressive disorder◀

✓6th **F13.25** **Sedative, hypnotic or anxiolytic dependence with sedative, hypnotic or anxiolytic-induced** psychotic disorder
     F13.250 **Sedative, hypnotic or anxiolytic** CC HCC **dependence with sedative, hypnotic or anxiolytic-induced psychotic disorder with** delusions
     F13.251 **Sedative, hypnotic or anxiolytic** CC HCC **dependence with sedative, hypnotic or anxiolytic-induced psychotic disorder with** hallucinations
     F13.259 **Sedative, hypnotic or anxiolytic** CC HCC **dependence with sedative, hypnotic or anxiolytic-induced psychotic disorder, unspecified**
         CC Excl: No Excl

     F13.26 **Sedative, hypnotic or anxiolytic dependence** CC HCC **with sedative, hypnotic or anxiolytic-induced** persisting amnestic disorder
         CC Excl: No Excl

✓ Additional Character Req   ✓7th Placeholder Alert   Unacceptable PDx   Manifestation   H1 - H14 HAC   HCC CMS-HCC Condition   EXCLUDES 1 Not Coded Here   EXCLUDES 2 Not Included Here

ICD-10-CM 2018   **537**

F13.27 **Sedative, hypnotic or anxiolytic dependence** **CC HCC**
with sedative, hypnotic or anxiolytic-induced
persisting dementia
▶Sedative, hypnotic, or anxiolytic use disorder,
moderate, with sedative, hypnotic, or anxiolytic-
induced major neurocognitive disorder◀
Sedative, hypnotic, or anxiolytic use disorder, severe,
with sedative, hypnotic, or anxiolytic-induced
major neurocognitive disorder

✓6th **F13.28** **Sedative, hypnotic or anxiolytic dependence with**
other sedative, hypnotic or anxiolytic-induced
disorders
     F13.280 **Sedative, hypnotic or anxiolytic** **CC HCC**
dependence with sedative, hypnotic or
anxiolytic-induced anxiety disorder
       CC Excl: No Excl
     F13.281 **Sedative, hypnotic or anxiolytic** **CC HCC**
dependence with sedative, hypnotic or
anxiolytic-induced sexual dysfunction
       CC Excl: No Excl
     F13.282 **Sedative, hypnotic or anxiolytic** **CC HCC**
dependence with sedative, hypnotic or
anxiolytic-induced sleep disorder
       CC Excl: No Excl
     F13.288 **Sedative, hypnotic or anxiolytic** **CC HCC**
dependence with other sedative,
hypnotic or anxiolytic-induced disorder
▶Sedative, hypnotic, or anxiolytic use
disorder, moderate, with sedative,
hypnotic, or anxiolytic-induced mild
neurocognitive disorder
Sedative, hypnotic, or anxiolytic use
disorder, severe, with sedative,
hypnotic, or anxiolytic-induced mild
neurocognitive disorder◀
       CC Excl: No Excl

     F13.29 **Sedative, hypnotic or anxiolytic dependence** **HCC**
with unspecified sedative, hypnotic or anxiolytic-
induced disorder

✓5th **F13.9** **Sedative, hypnotic or anxiolytic-related use, unspecified**
     EXCLUDES 1 *sedative, hypnotic or anxiolytic-related abuse (F13.1-)*
sedative, hypnotic or anxiolytic-related dependence
(F13.2-)

     F13.90 **Sedative, hypnotic, or anxiolytic use, unspecified,**
uncomplicated

✓6th **F13.92** **Sedative, hypnotic or anxiolytic use, unspecified**
with intoxication
     EXCLUDES 1 *sedative, hypnotic or anxiolytic use,*
unspecified with withdrawal (F13.93-)
     F13.920 **Sedative, hypnotic or anxiolytic use,** **HCC**
unspecified with intoxication,
uncomplicated
     F13.921 **Sedative, hypnotic or anxiolytic** **CC HCC**
use, unspecified with intoxication
delirium
Sedative, hypnotic, or anxiolytic-induced
delirium
     F13.929 **Sedative, hypnotic or anxiolytic use,** **HCC**
unspecified with intoxication,
unspecified

✓6th **F13.93** **Sedative, hypnotic or anxiolytic use, unspecified**
with withdrawal
     EXCLUDES 1 *sedative, hypnotic or anxiolytic use,*
unspecified with intoxication (F13.92-)
     F13.930 **Sedative, hypnotic or anxiolytic** **CC HCC**
use, unspecified with withdrawal,
uncomplicated
     F13.931 **Sedative, hypnotic or anxiolytic** **CC HCC**
use, unspecified with withdrawal
delirium
     F13.932 **Sedative, hypnotic or anxiolytic** **CC HCC**
use, unspecified with withdrawal
with perceptual disturbances
     F13.939 **Sedative, hypnotic or anxiolytic** **CC HCC**
use, unspecified with withdrawal,
unspecified

F13.94 **Sedative, hypnotic or anxiolytic use,** **HCC**
unspecified with sedative, hypnotic or
anxiolytic-induced mood disorder
Sedative, hypnotic, or anxiolytic-induced bipolar or
related disorder, without use disorder
Sedative, hypnotic, or anxiolytic-induced depressive
disorder, without use disorder

✓6th **F13.95** **Sedative, hypnotic or anxiolytic use, unspecified**
with sedative, hypnotic or anxiolytic-induced
psychotic disorder
     F13.950 **Sedative, hypnotic or anxiolytic** **CC HCC**
use, unspecified with sedative, hypnotic
or anxiolytic-induced psychotic disorder
with delusions
     F13.951 **Sedative, hypnotic or anxiolytic** **CC HCC**
use, unspecified with sedative, hypnotic
or anxiolytic-induced psychotic disorder
with hallucinations
     F13.959 **Sedative, hypnotic or anxiolytic use,** **HCC**
unspecified with sedative, hypnotic or
anxiolytic-induced psychotic disorder,
unspecified
▶Sedative, hypnotic, or anxiolytic-induced
psychotic disorder, without use
disorder◀

F13.96 **Sedative, hypnotic or anxiolytic use, unspecified** **HCC**
with sedative, hypnotic or anxiolytic-induced
persisting amnestic disorder

F13.97 **Sedative, hypnotic or anxiolytic use,** **CC HCC**
unspecified with sedative, hypnotic or anxiolytic-
induced persisting dementia
▶Sedative, hypnotic, or anxiolytic-induced major
neurocognitive disorder, without use disorder◀

✓6th **F13.98** **Sedative, hypnotic or anxiolytic use, unspecified**
with other sedative, hypnotic or anxiolytic-induced
disorders
     F13.980 **Sedative, hypnotic or anxiolytic use,** **HCC**
unspecified with sedative, hypnotic or
anxiolytic-induced anxiety disorder
▶Sedative, hypnotic, or anxiolytic-induced
anxiety disorder, without use
disorder◀
     F13.981 **Sedative, hypnotic or anxiolytic use,** **HCC**
unspecified with sedative, hypnotic or
anxiolytic-induced sexual dysfunction
▶Sedative, hypnotic, or anxiolytic-induced
sexual dysfunction disorder, without
use disorder◀
     F13.982 **Sedative, hypnotic or anxiolytic use,** **HCC**
unspecified with sedative, hypnotic or
anxiolytic-induced sleep disorder
▶Sedative, hypnotic, or anxiolytic-induced
sleep disorder, without use disorder◀
     F13.988 **Sedative, hypnotic or anxiolytic use,** **HCC**
unspecified with other sedative,
hypnotic or anxiolytic-induced disorder
▶Sedative, hypnotic, or anxiolytic-induced
mild neurocognitive disorder◀

F13.99 **Sedative, hypnotic or anxiolytic use, unspecified** **HCC**
with unspecified sedative, hypnotic or anxiolytic-
induced disorder

✓4th **F14** **Cocaine related disorders**
     EXCLUDES 2 *other stimulant-related disorders (F15.-)*

     CC Excl: For CC codes in category F14, unless otherwise noted:
     PDX collection 550

✓5th **F14.1** **Cocaine abuse**
     EXCLUDES 1 *cocaine dependence (F14.2-)*
cocaine use, unspecified (F14.9-)
     F14.10 **Cocaine abuse, uncomplicated**
Cocaine use disorder, mild
●   **F14.11** **Cocaine abuse, in remission**
Cocaine use disorder, mild, in early remission
Cocaine use disorder, mild, in sustained remission
✓6th   **F14.12** **Cocaine abuse with intoxication**
     F14.120 **Cocaine abuse with intoxication,** **HCC**
uncomplicated
     F14.121 **Cocaine abuse with intoxication** **CC HCC**
with delirium
     F14.122 **Cocaine abuse with intoxication** **HCC**
with perceptual disturbance

N Newborn: 0   P Pediatric: 0-17   M Maternity: 12-55   A Adult: 15-124   **MCC** Major CC Condition   **PDxMCC** PDx acts as own MCC   **CC** CC Condition   **PDxCC** PDx acts as own CC

538   ICD-10-CM 2018

F14.129 Cocaine abuse with intoxication, HCC
unspecified

F14.14 Cocaine abuse with cocaine-induced mood HCC
disorder
Cocaine use disorder, mild, with cocaine-induced
bipolar or related disorder
Cocaine use disorder, mild, with cocaine-induced
depressive disorder

✓6ᵗʰ **F14.15 Cocaine abuse with cocaine-induced psychotic**
disorder

F14.150 Cocaine abuse with cocaine- CC HCC
induced psychotic disorder with delusions

F14.151 Cocaine abuse with cocaine- CC HCC
induced psychotic disorder with
hallucinations

F14.159 Cocaine abuse with cocaine-induced HCC
psychotic disorder, unspecified

✓6ᵗʰ **F14.18 Cocaine abuse with other cocaine-induced disorder**

F14.180 Cocaine abuse with cocaine-induced HCC
anxiety disorder

F14.181 Cocaine abuse with cocaine-induced HCC
sexual dysfunction

F14.182 Cocaine abuse with cocaine-induced HCC
sleep disorder

F14.188 Cocaine abuse with other cocaine- HCC
induced disorder
Cocaine use disorder, mild, with cocaine-
induced obsessive compulsive or
related disorder

F14.19 Cocaine abuse with unspecified cocaine- HCC
induced disorder

✓5ᵗʰ **F14.2 Cocaine dependence**
EXCLUDES 1 cocaine abuse (F14.1-)
cocaine use, unspecified (F14.9-)
EXCLUDES 2 cocaine poisoning (T40.5-)

F14.20 Cocaine dependence, uncomplicated CC HCC
Cocaine use disorder, moderate
Cocaine use disorder, severe
CC Excl: No Excl

F14.21 Cocaine dependence, in remission HCC
▶Cocaine use disorder, moderate, in early remission
Cocaine use disorder, moderate, in sustained
remission
Cocaine use disorder, severe, in early remission
Cocaine use disorder, severe, in sustained remission◀

✓6ᵗʰ **F14.22 Cocaine dependence with intoxication**
EXCLUDES 1 cocaine dependence with withdrawal
(F14.23)

F14.220 Cocaine dependence with HCC
intoxication, uncomplicated

F14.221 Cocaine dependence with CC HCC
intoxication delirium

F14.222 Cocaine dependence with CC HCC
intoxication with perceptual
disturbance
CC Excl: No Excl

F14.229 Cocaine dependence with CC HCC
intoxication, unspecified
CC Excl: No Excl

F14.23 Cocaine dependence with withdrawal CC HCC
EXCLUDES 1 cocaine dependence with intoxication
(F14.22-)

F14.24 Cocaine dependence with cocaine-induced HCC
mood disorder
Cocaine use disorder, moderate, with cocaine-induced
bipolar or related disorder
Cocaine use disorder, moderate, with cocaine-induced
depressive disorder
Cocaine use disorder, severe, with cocaine-induced
bipolar or related disorder
Cocaine use disorder, severe, with cocaine-induced
depressive disorder

✓6ᵗʰ **F14.25 Cocaine dependence with cocaine-induced**
psychotic disorder

F14.250 Cocaine dependence with CC HCC
cocaine-induced psychotic disorder
with delusions

F14.251 Cocaine dependence with CC HCC
cocaine-induced psychotic disorder
with hallucinations

F14.259 Cocaine dependence with CC HCC
cocaine-induced psychotic disorder,
unspecified
CC Excl: No Excl

✓6ᵗʰ **F14.28 Cocaine dependence with other cocaine-induced**
disorder

F14.280 Cocaine dependence with CC HCC
cocaine-induced anxiety disorder
CC Excl: No Excl

F14.281 Cocaine dependence with CC HCC
cocaine-induced sexual dysfunction
CC Excl: No Excl

F14.282 Cocaine dependence with CC HCC
cocaine-induced sleep disorder
CC Excl: No Excl

F14.288 Cocaine dependence with other CC HCC
cocaine-induced disorder
Cocaine use disorder, moderate, with
cocaine-induced obsessive
compulsive or related disorder
Cocaine use disorder, severe, with cocaine-
induced obsessive compulsive or
related disorder
CC Excl: No Excl

F14.29 Cocaine dependence with unspecified HCC
cocaine-induced disorder

✓5ᵗʰ **F14.9 Cocaine use, unspecified**
EXCLUDES 1 cocaine abuse (F14.1-)
cocaine dependence (F14.2-)

F14.90 Cocaine use, unspecified, uncomplicated

✓6ᵗʰ **F14.92 Cocaine use, unspecified with intoxication**

F14.920 Cocaine use, unspecified with HCC
intoxication, uncomplicated

F14.921 Cocaine use, unspecified with CC HCC
intoxication delirium

F14.922 Cocaine use, unspecified with HCC
intoxication with perceptual
disturbance

F14.929 Cocaine use, unspecified with HCC
intoxication, unspecified

F14.94 Cocaine use, unspecified with cocaine-induced HCC
mood disorder
Cocaine induced bipolar or related disorder, without
use disorder
Cocaine induced depressive disorder, without use
disorder

✓6ᵗʰ **F14.95 Cocaine use, unspecified with cocaine-induced**
psychotic disorder

F14.950 Cocaine use, unspecified with CC HCC
cocaine-induced psychotic disorder
with delusions

F14.951 Cocaine use, unspecified with CC HCC
cocaine-induced psychotic disorder
with hallucinations

F14.959 Cocaine use, unspecified with HCC
cocaine-induced psychotic disorder,
unspecified
Cocaine induced psychotic disorder,
without use disorder

✓6ᵗʰ **F14.98 Cocaine use, unspecified with other specified**
cocaine-induced disorder

F14.980 Cocaine use, unspecified with HCC
cocaine-induced anxiety disorder
Cocaine induced anxiety disorder, without
use disorder

F14.981 Cocaine use, unspecified with HCC
cocaine-induced sexual dysfunction
Cocaine induced sexual dysfunction,
without use disorder

F14.982 Cocaine use, unspecified with HCC
cocaine-induced sleep disorder
Cocaine induced sleep disorder, without
use disorder

F14.988 Cocaine use, unspecified with other HCC
cocaine-induced disorder
Cocaine induced obsessive compulsive or
related disorder

F14.99 Cocaine use, unspecified with unspecified HCC
cocaine-induced disorder

Chapter 5. Mental, Behavioral and Neurodevelopmental Disorders

✓4th F15 Other stimulant related disorders

> INCLUDES   amphetamine-related disorders
> caffeine
>
> EXCLUDES 2   cocaine-related disorders (F14.-)

> **CC Excl: For CC codes in category F15, unless otherwise noted:**
> PDX collection 55Ø

✓5th F15.1 Other stimulant abuse

> EXCLUDES 1   other stimulant dependence (F15.2-)
> other stimulant use, unspecified (F15.9-)

     F15.1Ø Other stimulant abuse, uncomplicated
Amphetamine type substance use disorder, mild
Other or unspecified stimulant use disorder, mild

     F15.11 Other stimulant abuse, in remission
Amphetamine type substance use disorder, mild, in early remission
Amphetamine type substance use disorder, mild, in sustained remission
Other or unspecified stimulant use disorder, mild, in early remission
Other or unspecified stimulant use disorder, mild, in sustained remission

     ✓6th F15.12 Other stimulant abuse with intoxication

         F15.12Ø Other stimulant abuse with intoxication, uncomplicated   HCC

         F15.121 Other stimulant abuse with intoxication delirium   CC HCC

         F15.122 Other stimulant abuse with intoxication with perceptual disturbance   HCC
Amphetamine or other stimulant use disorder, mild, with amphetamine or other stimulant intoxication, with perceptual disturbances

         F15.129 Other stimulant abuse with intoxication, unspecified   HCC
Amphetamine or other stimulant use disorder, mild, with amphetamine or other stimulant intoxication, without perceptual disturbances

     F15.14 Other stimulant abuse with stimulant-induced mood disorder   HCC
Amphetamine or other stimulant use disorder, mild, with amphetamine or other stimulant induced bipolar or related disorder
Amphetamine or other stimulant use disorder, mild, with amphetamine or other stimulant induced depressive disorder

     ✓6th F15.15 Other stimulant abuse with stimulant-induced psychotic disorder

         F15.15Ø Other stimulant abuse with stimulant-induced psychotic disorder with delusions   CC HCC

         F15.151 Other stimulant abuse with stimulant-induced psychotic disorder with hallucinations   CC HCC

         F15.159 Other stimulant abuse with stimulant-induced psychotic disorder, unspecified   HCC

     ✓6th F15.18 Other stimulant abuse with other stimulant-induced disorder

         F15.18Ø Other stimulant abuse with stimulant-induced anxiety disorder   HCC

         F15.181 Other stimulant abuse with stimulant-induced sexual dysfunction   HCC

         F15.182 Other stimulant abuse with stimulant-induced sleep disorder   HCC

         F15.188 Other stimulant abuse with other stimulant-induced disorder   HCC
Amphetamine or other stimulant use disorder, mild, with amphetamine or other stimulant induced obsessive-compulsive or related disorder

     F15.19 Other stimulant abuse with unspecified stimulant-induced disorder   HCC

✓5th F15.2 Other stimulant dependence

> EXCLUDES 1   other stimulant abuse (F15.1-)
> other stimulant use, unspecified (F15.9-)

     F15.2Ø Other stimulant dependence, uncomplicated   CC HCC
Amphetamine type substance use disorder, moderate
Amphetamine type substance use disorder, severe
Other or unspecified stimulant use disorder, moderate
Other or unspecified stimulant use disorder, severe
CC Excl: No Excl

     F15.21 Other stimulant dependence, in remission   HCC
▶Amphetamine type substance use disorder, moderate, in early remission
Amphetamine type substance use disorder, moderate, in sustained remission
Amphetamine type substance use disorder, severe, in early remission
Amphetamine type substance use disorder, severe, in sustained remission
Other or unspecified stimulant use disorder, moderate, in early remission
Other or unspecified stimulant use disorder, moderate, in sustained remission
Other or unspecified stimulant use disorder, severe, in early remission
Other or unspecified stimulant use disorder, severe, in sustained remission◀

     ✓6th F15.22 Other stimulant dependence with intoxication

> EXCLUDES 1   other stimulant dependence with withdrawal (F15.23)

         F15.22Ø Other stimulant dependence with intoxication, uncomplicated   HCC

         F15.221 Other stimulant dependence with intoxication delirium   CC HCC

         F15.222 Other stimulant dependence with intoxication with perceptual disturbance   CC HCC
Amphetamine or other stimulant use disorder, moderate, with amphetamine or other stimulant intoxication, with perceptual disturbances
Amphetamine or other stimulant use disorder, severe, with amphetamine or other stimulant intoxication, with perceptual disturbances
CC Excl: No Excl

         F15.229 Other stimulant dependence with intoxication, unspecified   HCC
Amphetamine or other stimulant use disorder, moderate, with amphetamine or other stimulant intoxication, without perceptual disturbances
Amphetamine or other stimulant use disorder, severe, with amphetamine or other stimulant intoxication, without perceptual disturbances

     F15.23 Other stimulant dependence with withdrawal   CC HCC
Amphetamine or other stimulant withdrawal
> EXCLUDES 1   other stimulant dependence with intoxication (F15.22-)

     F15.24 Other stimulant dependence with stimulant-induced mood disorder   HCC
Amphetamine or other stimulant use disorder, moderate, with amphetamine or other stimulant-induced bipolar or related disorder
Amphetamine or other stimulant use disorder, moderate, with amphetamine or other stimulant induced depressive disorder
Amphetamine or other stimulant use disorder, severe, with amphetamine or other stimulant-induced bipolar or related disorder
Amphetamine or other stimulant use disorder, severe, with amphetamine or other stimulant-induced depressive disorder

     ✓6th F15.25 Other stimulant dependence with stimulant-induced psychotic disorder

         F15.25Ø Other stimulant dependence with stimulant-induced psychotic disorder with delusions   CC HCC

         F15.251 Other stimulant dependence with stimulant-induced psychotic disorder with hallucinations   CC HCC

N Newborn: 0   P Pediatric: 0-17   M Maternity: 12-55   A Adult: 15-124   MCC Major CC Condition   PDxMCC PDx acts as own MCC   CC CC Condition   PDxCC PDx acts as own CC

540   ICD-10-CM 2018

F15.259 **Other stimulant dependence with stimulant-induced psychotic disorder, unspecified**
CC Excl: No Excl

✓6th F15.28 **Other stimulant dependence with other stimulant-induced disorder**

F15.280 **Other stimulant dependence with stimulant-induced anxiety disorder** `CC` `HCC`
CC Excl: No Excl

F15.281 **Other stimulant dependence with stimulant-induced sexual dysfunction** `CC` `HCC`
CC Excl: No Excl

F15.282 **Other stimulant dependence with stimulant-induced sleep disorder** `CC` `HCC`
CC Excl: No Excl

F15.288 **Other stimulant dependence with other stimulant-induced disorder** `CC` `HCC`
▶Amphetamine or other stimulant use disorder, moderate, with amphetamine or other stimulant induced obsessive compulsive or related disorder
Amphetamine or other stimulant use disorder, severe, with amphetamine or other stimulant induced obsessive compulsive or related disorder◀
CC Excl: No Excl

F15.29 **Other stimulant dependence with unspecified stimulant-induced disorder** `HCC`

✓5th F15.9 **Other stimulant use, unspecified**
EXCLUDES 1 other stimulant abuse (F15.1-)
other stimulant dependence (F15.2-)

F15.90 **Other stimulant use, unspecified, uncomplicated**

✓6th F15.92 **Other stimulant use, unspecified with intoxication**
EXCLUDES 1 other stimulant use, unspecified with withdrawal (F15.93)

F15.920 **Other stimulant use, unspecified with intoxication, uncomplicated** `HCC`

F15.921 **Other stimulant use, unspecified with intoxication delirium** `CC` `HCC`
Amphetamine or other stimulant-induced delirium

F15.922 **Other stimulant use, unspecified with intoxication with perceptual disturbance** `HCC`

F15.929 **Other stimulant use, unspecified with intoxication, unspecified** `HCC`
Caffeine intoxication

F15.93 **Other stimulant use, unspecified with withdrawal** `CC` `HCC`
Caffeine withdrawal
EXCLUDES 1 other stimulant use, unspecified with intoxication (F15.92-)

F15.94 **Other stimulant use, unspecified with stimulant-induced mood disorder** `HCC`
Amphetamine or other stimulant-induced bipolar or related disorder, without use disorder
Amphetamine or other stimulant-induced depressive disorder, without use disorder

✓6th F15.95 **Other stimulant use, unspecified with stimulant-induced psychotic disorder**

F15.950 **Other stimulant use, unspecified with stimulant-induced psychotic disorder with delusions** `CC` `HCC`

F15.951 **Other stimulant use, unspecified with stimulant-induced psychotic disorder with hallucinations** `CC` `HCC`

F15.959 **Other stimulant use, unspecified with stimulant-induced psychotic disorder, unspecified** `HCC`
▶Amphetamine or other stimulant-induced psychotic disorder, without use disorder◀

✓6th F15.98 **Other stimulant use, unspecified with other stimulant-induced disorder**

F15.980 **Other stimulant use, unspecified with stimulant-induced anxiety disorder** `HCC`
Amphetamine or other stimulant-induced anxiety disorder, without use disorder
Caffeine induced anxiety disorder, without use disorder

F15.981 **Other stimulant use, unspecified with stimulant-induced sexual dysfunction** `HCC`
Amphetamine or other stimulant-induced sexual dysfunction, without use disorder

F15.982 **Other stimulant use, unspecified with stimulant-induced sleep disorder** `HCC`
Amphetamine or other stimulant-induced sleep disorder, without use disorder
Caffeine induced sleep disorder, without use disorder

F15.988 **Other stimulant use, unspecified with other stimulant-induced disorder** `HCC`
Amphetamine or other stimulant-induced obsessive compulsive or related disorder, without use disorder

F15.99 **Other stimulant use, unspecified with unspecified stimulant-induced disorder** `HCC`

✓4th **F16** **Hallucinogen related disorders**
`INCLUDES` ecstasy
PCP
phencyclidine

CC Excl: For CC codes in category F16, unless otherwise noted:
PDX collection 550

✓5th F16.1 **Hallucinogen abuse**
EXCLUDES 1 hallucinogen dependence (F16.2-)
hallucinogen use, unspecified (F16.9-)

F16.10 **Hallucinogen abuse, uncomplicated**
Other hallucinogen use disorder, mild
Phencyclidine use disorder, mild

● F16.11 **Hallucinogen abuse, in remission**
Other hallucinogen use disorder, mild, in early remission
Other hallucinogen use disorder, mild, in sustained remission
Phencyclidine use disorder, mild, in early remission
Phencyclidine use disorder, mild, in sustained remission

✓6th F16.12 **Hallucinogen abuse with intoxication**

F16.120 **Hallucinogen abuse with intoxication, uncomplicated** `HCC`

F16.121 **Hallucinogen abuse with intoxication with delirium** `CC` `HCC`

F16.122 **Hallucinogen abuse with intoxication with perceptual disturbance** `HCC`

F16.129 **Hallucinogen abuse with intoxication, unspecified** `HCC`

F16.14 **Hallucinogen abuse with hallucinogen-induced mood disorder** `HCC`
Other hallucinogen use disorder, mild, with other hallucinogen induced bipolar or related disorder
Other hallucinogen use disorder, mild, with other hallucinogen induced depressive disorder
Phencyclidine use disorder, mild, with phencyclidine induced bipolar or related disorder
Phencyclidine use disorder, mild, with phencyclidine induced depressive disorder

✓6th F16.15 **Hallucinogen abuse with hallucinogen-induced psychotic disorder**

F16.150 **Hallucinogen abuse with hallucinogen-induced psychotic disorder with delusions** `CC` `HCC`

F16.151 **Hallucinogen abuse with hallucinogen-induced psychotic disorder with hallucinations** `CC` `HCC`

F16.159 **Hallucinogen abuse with hallucinogen-induced psychotic disorder, unspecified** `HCC`

✓6th F16.18 **Hallucinogen abuse with other hallucinogen-induced disorder**

F16.180 **Hallucinogen abuse with hallucinogen-induced anxiety disorder** `HCC`

F16.183 **Hallucinogen abuse with hallucinogen-induced persisting perception disorder (flashbacks)** `HCC`

F16.188 **Hallucinogen abuse with other hallucinogen-induced disorder** `HCC`

F16.19 **Hallucinogen abuse with unspecified hallucinogen-induced disorder** `HCC`

√5th F16.2 Hallucinogen dependence

> EXCLUDES 1   *hallucinogen abuse (F16.1-)*
> *hallucinoge n use, unspecified (F16.9-)*

F16.20 Hallucinogen dependence, uncomplicated   CC HCC
Other hallucinogen use disorder, moderate
Other hallucinogen use disorder, severe
Phencyclidine use disorder, moderate
Phencyclidine use disorder, severe
CC Excl: No Excl

F16.21 Hallucinogen dependence, in remission   HCC
▶Other hallucinogen use disorder, moderate, in early remission
Other hallucinogen use disorder, moderate, in sustained remission
Other hallucinogen use disorder, severe, in early remission
Other hallucinogen use disorder, severe, in sustained remission
Phencyclidine use disorder, moderate, in early remission
Phencyclidine use disorder, moderate, in sustained remission
Phencyclidine use disorder, severe, in early remission
Phencyclidine use disorder, severe, in sustained remission◀

√6th F16.22 Hallucinogen dependence with intoxication

F16.220 Hallucinogen dependence with intoxication, uncomplicated   HCC

F16.221 Hallucinogen dependence with intoxication with delirium   CC HCC

F16.229 Hallucinogen dependence with intoxication, unspecified   HCC

F16.24 Hallucinogen dependence with hallucinogen-induced mood disorder   HCC
Other hallucinogen use disorder, moderate, with other hallucinogen induced bipolar or related disorder
Other hallucinogen use disorder, moderate, with other hallucinogen induced depressive disorder
Other hallucinogen use disorder, severe, with other hallucinogen-induced bipolar or related disorder
Other hallucinogen use disorder, severe, with other hallucinogen-induced depressive disorder
Phencyclidine use disorder, moderate, with phencyclidine induced bipolar or related disorder
Phencyclidine use disorder, moderate, with phencyclidine induced depressive disorder
Phencyclidine use disorder, severe, with phencyclidine induced bipolar or related disorder
Phencyclidine use disorder, severe, with phencyclidine-induced depressive disorder

√6th F16.25 Hallucinogen dependence with hallucinogen-induced psychotic disorder

F16.250 Hallucinogen dependence with hallucinogen-induced psychotic disorder with delusions   CC HCC

F16.251 Hallucinogen dependence with hallucinogen-induced psychotic disorder with hallucinations   CC HCC

F16.259 Hallucinogen dependence with hallucinogen-induced psychotic disorder, unspecified   CC HCC
CC Excl: No Excl

√6th F16.28 Hallucinogen dependence with other hallucinogen-induced disorder

F16.280 Hallucinogen dependence with hallucinogen-induced anxiety disorder   CC HCC
CC Excl: No Excl

F16.283 Hallucinogen dependence with hallucinogen persisting perception disorder (flashbacks)   CC HCC
CC Excl: No Excl

F16.288 Hallucinogen dependence with other hallucinogen-induced disorder   CC HCC
CC Excl: No Excl

F16.29 Hallucinogen dependence with unspecified hallucinogen-induced disorder   HCC

√5th F16.9 Hallucinogen use, unspecified

> EXCLUDES 1   *hallucinogen abuse (F16.1-)*
> *hallucinogen dependence (F16.2-)*

F16.90 Hallucinogen use, unspecified, uncomplicated

√6th F16.92 Hallucinogen use, unspecified with intoxication

F16.920 Hallucinogen use, unspecified with intoxication, uncomplicated   HCC

F16.921 Hallucinogen use, unspecified with intoxication with delirium   CC HCC
Other hallucinogen intoxication delirium

F16.929 Hallucinogen use, unspecified with intoxication, unspecified   HCC

F16.94 Hallucinogen use, unspecified with hallucinogen-induced mood disorder   HCC
Other hallucinogen induced bipolar or related disorder, without use disorder
Other hallucinogen induced depressive disorder, without use disorder
Phencyclidine induced bipolar or related disorder, without use disorder
Phencyclidine induced depressive disorder, without use disorder

√6th F16.95 Hallucinogen use, unspecified with hallucinogen-induced psychotic disorder

F16.950 Hallucinogen use, unspecified with hallucinogen-induced psychotic disorder with delusions   CC HCC

F16.951 Hallucinogen use, unspecified with hallucinogen-induced psychotic disorder with hallucinations   CC HCC

F16.959 Hallucinogen use, unspecified with hallucinogen-induced psychotic disorder, unspecified   HCC
Other hallucinogen induced psychotic disorder, without use disorder
Phencyclidine induced psychotic disorder, without use disorder

√6th F16.98 Hallucinogen use, unspecified with other specified hallucinogen-induced disorder

F16.980 Hallucinogen use, unspecified with hallucinogen-induced anxiety disorder   HCC
Other hallucinogen-induced anxiety disorder, without use disorder
Phencyclidine induced anxiety disorder, without use disorder

F16.983 Hallucinogen use, unspecified with hallucinogen persisting perception disorder (flashbacks)   HCC

F16.988 Hallucinogen use, unspecified with other hallucinogen-induced disorder   HCC

F16.99 Hallucinogen use, unspecified with unspecified hallucinogen-induced disorder   HCC

√4th F17 Nicotine dependence

> EXCLUDES 1   *history of tobacco dependence (Z87.891)*
> *tobacco use NOS (Z72.0)*
> EXCLUDES 2   *tobacco use (smoking) during pregnancy, childbirth and the puerperium (O99.33-)*
> *toxic effect of nicotine (T65.2-)*
> **AHA:** 2013, 4Q, 108-109

> **CC Excl: For CC codes in category F17:** PDX collection 550

√5th F17.2 Nicotine dependence

√6th F17.20 Nicotine dependence, unspecified

F17.200 Nicotine dependence, unspecified, uncomplicated
Tobacco use disorder, mild
Tobacco use disorder, moderate
Tobacco use disorder, severe
AHA: 2016, 1Q, 36

F17.201 Nicotine dependence, unspecified, in remission
▶Tobacco use disorder, mild, in early remission
Tobacco use disorder, mild, in sustained remission
Tobacco use disorder, moderate, in early remission
Tobacco use disorder, moderate, in sustained remission
Tobacco use disorder, severe, in early remission
Tobacco use disorder, severe, in sustained remission◀

F17.203 Nicotine dependence unspecified, withdrawal   CC
Tobacco withdrawal

F17.208 Nicotine dependence, unspecified, with **other** nicotine-induced disorders

F17.209 Nicotine dependence, unspecified, with **unspecified** nicotine-induced disorders

✓6ᵗʰ **F17.21** Nicotine dependence, **cigarettes**

F17.210 **Nicotine dependence, cigarettes, uncomplicated**
AHA: 2017, 2Q, 28-29

F17.211 **Nicotine dependence, cigarettes, in remission**
▶Tobacco use disorder, cigarettes, mild, in early remission
Tobacco use disorder, cigarettes, mild, in sustained remission
Tobacco use disorder, cigarettes, moderate, in early remission
Tobacco use disorder, cigarettes, moderate, in sustained remission
Tobacco use disorder, cigarettes, severe, in early remission
Tobacco use disorder, cigarettes, severe, in sustained remission◀

F17.213 Nicotine dependence, cigarettes, with **withdrawal** `CC`

F17.218 Nicotine dependence, cigarettes, with **other** nicotine-induced disorders

F17.219 Nicotine dependence, cigarettes, with **unspecified** nicotine-induced disorders

✓6ᵗʰ **F17.22** Nicotine dependence, **chewing tobacco**

F17.220 **Nicotine dependence, chewing tobacco, uncomplicated**

F17.221 **Nicotine dependence, chewing tobacco, in remission**
▶Tobacco use disorder, chewing tobacco, mild, in early remission
Tobacco use disorder, chewing tobacco, mild, in sustained remission
Tobacco use disorder, chewing tobacco, moderate, in early remission
Tobacco use disorder, chewing tobacco, moderate, in sustained remission
Tobacco use disorder, chewing tobacco, severe, in early remission
Tobacco use disorder, chewing tobacco, severe, in sustained remission◀

F17.223 Nicotine dependence, chewing tobacco, with **withdrawal** `CC`

F17.228 Nicotine dependence, chewing tobacco, with **other** nicotine-induced disorders

F17.229 Nicotine dependence, chewing tobacco, with **unspecified** nicotine-induced disorders

✓6ᵗʰ **F17.29** Nicotine dependence, **other tobacco product**

F17.290 **Nicotine dependence, other tobacco product, uncomplicated**
AHA: 2017, 2Q, 28-29

F17.291 **Nicotine dependence, other tobacco product, in remission**
▶Tobacco use disorder, other tobacco product, mild, in early remission
Tobacco use disorder, other tobacco product, mild, in sustained remission
Tobacco use disorder, other tobacco product, moderate, in early remission
Tobacco use disorder, other tobacco product, moderate, in sustained remission
Tobacco use disorder, other tobacco product, severe, in early remission
Tobacco use disorder, other tobacco product, severe, in sustained remission◀

F17.293 Nicotine dependence, other tobacco product, with **withdrawal** `CC`

F17.298 Nicotine dependence, other tobacco product, with **other** nicotine-induced disorders

F17.299 Nicotine dependence, other tobacco product, with **unspecified** nicotine-induced disorders

✓4ᵗʰ **F18** **Inhalant related disorders**
`INCLUDES` volatile solvents

CC Excl: For CC codes in category F18, unless otherwise noted: PDX collection 550

✓5ᵗʰ **F18.1** Inhalant **abuse**
`EXCLUDES 1` inhalant dependence (F18.2-)
inhalant use, unspecified (F18.9-)

F18.10 **Inhalant abuse, uncomplicated**
Inhalant use disorder, mild

● **F18.11** **Inhalant abuse, in remission**
Inhalant use disorder, mild, in early remission
Inhalant use disorder, mild, in sustained remission

✓6ᵗʰ **F18.12** Inhalant abuse with **intoxication**

F18.120 **Inhalant abuse with intoxication, uncomplicated** `HCC`

F18.121 **Inhalant abuse with intoxication delirium** `CC` `HCC`

F18.129 **Inhalant abuse with intoxication, unspecified** `HCC`

F18.14 Inhalant abuse with inhalant-induced **mood** disorder `HCC`
Inhalant use disorder, mild, with inhalant induced depressive disorder

✓6ᵗʰ **F18.15** Inhalant abuse with inhalant-induced **psychotic** disorder

F18.150 **Inhalant abuse with inhalant-induced psychotic disorder with delusions** `CC` `HCC`

F18.151 **Inhalant abuse with inhalant-induced psychotic disorder with hallucinations** `CC` `HCC`

F18.159 **Inhalant abuse with inhalant-induced psychotic disorder, unspecified** `HCC`

F18.17 Inhalant abuse with inhalant-induced **dementia** `CC` `HCC`
Inhalant use disorder, mild, with inhalant induced major neurocognitive disorder

✓6ᵗʰ **F18.18** Inhalant abuse with **other** inhalant-induced disorders

F18.180 **Inhalant abuse with inhalant-induced anxiety disorder** `HCC`

F18.188 **Inhalant abuse with other inhalant-induced disorder** `HCC`
Inhalant use disorder, mild, with inhalant induced mild neurocognitive disorder

F18.19 Inhalant abuse with **unspecified** inhalant-induced disorder `HCC`

✓5ᵗʰ **F18.2** Inhalant **dependence**
`EXCLUDES 1` inhalant abuse (F18.1-)
inhalant use, unspecified (F18.9-)

F18.20 **Inhalant dependence, uncomplicated** `CC` `HCC`
Inhalant use disorder, moderate
Inhalant use disorder, severe
CC Excl: No Excl

F18.21 **Inhalant dependence, in remission** `HCC`
▶Inhalant use disorder, moderate, in early remission
Inhalant use disorder, moderate, in sustained remission
Inhalant use disorder, severe, in early remission
Inhalant use disorder, severe, in sustained remission◀

✓6ᵗʰ **F18.22** Inhalant dependence with **intoxication**

F18.220 **Inhalant dependence with intoxication, uncomplicated** `HCC`

F18.221 **Inhalant dependence with intoxication delirium** `CC` `HCC`

F18.229 **Inhalant dependence with intoxication, unspecified** `HCC`

F18.24 Inhalant dependence with inhalant-induced **mood disorder** `HCC`
Inhalant use disorder, moderate, with inhalant induced depressive disorder
Inhalant use disorder, severe, with inhalant induced depressive disorder

✓6ᵗʰ **F18.25** Inhalant dependence with inhalant-induced **psychotic disorder**

F18.250 **Inhalant dependence with inhalant-induced psychotic disorder with delusions** `CC` `HCC`

F18.251 Inhalant dependence with inhalant-induced psychotic disorder with **hallucinations** `CC` `HCC` ●

F18.259 Inhalant dependence with inhalant-induced psychotic disorder, **unspecified** `CC` `HCC`
CC Excl: No Excl

F18.27 Inhalant dependence with inhalant-induced `CC` `HCC` **dementia**
Inhalant use disorder, moderate, with inhalant induced major neurocognitive disorder
Inhalant use disorder, severe, with inhalant induced major neurocognitive disorder

✓6th **F18.28** Inhalant dependence with **other** inhalant-induced disorders

F18.280 Inhalant dependence with inhalant-induced **anxiety disorder** `CC` `HCC`
CC Excl: No Excl

F18.288 Inhalant dependence with **other** inhalant-induced disorder `CC` `HCC`
Inhalant use disorder, moderate, with inhalant-induced mild neurocognitive disorder
Inhalant use disorder, severe, with inhalant-induced mild neurocognitive disorder
CC Excl: No Excl

F18.29 Inhalant dependence with **unspecified** `HCC` inhalant-induced disorder

✓5th **F18.9** Inhalant use, **unspecified**
EXCLUDES 1 inhalant abuse (F18.1-)
inhalant dependence (F18.2-)

F18.90 Inhalant use, unspecified, **uncomplicated**

✓6th **F18.92** Inhalant use, unspecified with **intoxication**

F18.920 Inhalant use, unspecified with intoxication, **uncomplicated** `HCC`

F18.921 Inhalant use, unspecified with intoxication with **delirium** `CC` `HCC`

F18.929 Inhalant use, unspecified with intoxication, **unspecified** `HCC`

F18.94 Inhalant use, unspecified with inhalant-induced `HCC` **mood disorder**
Inhalant induced depressive disorder

✓6th **F18.95** Inhalant use, unspecified with inhalant-induced **psychotic disorder**

F18.950 Inhalant use, unspecified with inhalant-induced psychotic disorder with **delusions** `CC` `HCC`

F18.951 Inhalant use, unspecified with inhalant-induced psychotic disorder with **hallucinations** `CC` `HCC`

F18.959 Inhalant use, unspecified with inhalant-induced psychotic disorder, **unspecified** `HCC`

F18.97 Inhalant use, unspecified with inhalant-induced **persisting dementia** `CC` `HCC`
Inhalant-induced major neurocognitive disorder

✓6th **F18.98** Inhalant use, unspecified with **other** inhalant-induced disorders

F18.980 Inhalant use, unspecified with inhalant-induced **anxiety disorder** `HCC`

F18.988 Inhalant use, unspecified with **other** inhalant-induced disorder `HCC`
Inhalant-induced mild neurocognitive disorder

F18.99 Inhalant use, unspecified with **unspecified** inhalant-induced disorder `HCC`

✓4th **F19** Other psychoactive **substance related disorders**
INCLUDES polysubstance drug use (indiscriminate drug use)

CC Excl: For CC codes in category F19, unless otherwise noted: PDX collection 550

✓5th **F19.1** Other psychoactive substance **abuse**
EXCLUDES 1 other psychoactive substance dependence (F19.2-)
other psychoactive substance use, unspecified (F19.9-)

F19.10 Other psychoactive substance abuse, **uncomplicated**
Other (or unknown) substance use disorder, mild

F19.11 Other psychoactive substance abuse, **in remission**
Other (or unknown) substance use disorder, mild, in early remission
Other (or unknown) substance use disorder, mild, in sustained remission

✓6th **F19.12** Other psychoactive substance abuse with **intoxication**

F19.120 Other psychoactive substance abuse with intoxication, **uncomplicated**

F19.121 Other psychoactive substance abuse with intoxication **delirium** `CC` `HCC`

F19.122 Other psychoactive substance abuse with intoxication with **perceptual disturbances** `HCC`

F19.129 Other psychoactive substance abuse with intoxication, **unspecified** `HCC`

F19.14 Other psychoactive substance abuse with psychoactive substance-induced **mood disorder** `HCC`
Other (or unknown) substance use disorder, mild, with other (or unknown) substance-induced bipolar or related disorder
Other (or unknown) substance use disorder, mild, with other (or unknown) substance-induced depressive disorder

✓6th **F19.15** Other psychoactive substance abuse with psychoactive substance-induced **psychotic disorder**

F19.150 Other psychoactive substance abuse with psychoactive substance-induced psychotic disorder with **delusions** `CC` `HCC`

F19.151 Other psychoactive substance abuse with psychoactive substance-induced psychotic disorder with **hallucinations** `CC` `HCC`

F19.159 Other psychoactive substance abuse with psychoactive substance-induced psychotic disorder, **unspecified** `HCC`

F19.16 Other psychoactive substance abuse with psychoactive substance-induced **persisting amnestic disorder** `HCC`

F19.17 Other psychoactive substance abuse with psychoactive substance-induced **persisting dementia** `CC` `HCC`
Other (or unknown) substance use disorder, mild, with other (or unknown) substance-induced major neurocognitive disorder

✓6th **F19.18** Other psychoactive substance abuse with **other** psychoactive substance-induced disorders

F19.180 Other psychoactive substance abuse with psychoactive substance-induced **anxiety disorder** `HCC`

F19.181 Other psychoactive substance abuse with psychoactive substance-induced **sexual dysfunction** `HCC`

F19.182 Other psychoactive substance abuse with psychoactive substance-induced **sleep disorder** `HCC`

F19.188 Other psychoactive substance abuse with **other** psychoactive substance-induced disorder `HCC`
Other (or unknown) substance use disorder, mild, with other (or unknown) substance induced mild neurocognitive disorder
Other (or unknown) substance use disorder, mild, with other (or unknown) substance induced obsessive-compulsive or related disorder

F19.19 Other psychoactive substance abuse with **unspecified** psychoactive substance-induced disorder `HCC`

✓5th **F19.2** Other psychoactive substance **dependence**
EXCLUDES 1 other psychoactive substance abuse (F19.1-)
other psychoactive substance use, unspecified (F19.9-)

F19.20 Other psychoactive substance dependence, **uncomplicated** `CC` `HCC`
Other (or unknown) substance use disorder, moderate
Other (or unknown) substance use disorder, severe
CC Excl: No Excl

Ⓝ Newborn: 0 Ⓟ Pediatric: 0-17 Ⓜ Maternity: 12-55 Ⓐ Adult: 15-124 `MCC` Major CC Condition `PDxMCC` PDx acts as own MCC `CC` CC Condition `PDxCC` PDx acts as own CC

544 ICD-10-CM 2018

F19.21 **Other psychoactive substance dependence, in** `HCC`
remission
▶Other (or unknown) substance use disorder, moderate, in early remission
Other (or unknown) substance use disorder, moderate, in sustained remission
Other (or unknown) substance use disorder, severe, in early remission
Other (or unknown) substance use, severe, in sustained remission◀

✓6ᵗʰ **F19.22** **Other psychoactive substance dependence with intoxication**
> *EXCLUDES 1*   other psychoactive substance dependence with withdrawal (F19.23-)

    F19.220 **Other psychoactive substance** `HCC`
      dependence with intoxication, uncomplicated

    F19.221 **Other psychoactive substance** `CC` `HCC`
      dependence with intoxication delirium

    F19.222 **Other psychoactive substance** `CC` `HCC`
      dependence with intoxication with perceptual disturbance
      CC Excl: No Excl

    F19.229 **Other psychoactive substance** `HCC`
      dependence with intoxication, unspecified

✓6ᵗʰ **F19.23** **Other psychoactive substance dependence with withdrawal**
> *EXCLUDES 1*   other psychoactive substance dependence with intoxication (F19.22-)

    F19.230 **Other psychoactive substance** `CC` `HCC`
      dependence with withdrawal, uncomplicated

    F19.231 **Other psychoactive substance** `CC` `HCC`
      dependence with withdrawal delirium

    F19.232 **Other psychoactive substance** `CC` `HCC`
      dependence with withdrawal with perceptual disturbance

    F19.239 **Other psychoactive substance** `CC` `HCC`
      dependence with withdrawal, unspecified

F19.24 **Other psychoactive substance dependence** `HCC`
with psychoactive substance-induced mood disorder
Other (or unknown) substance use disorder, moderate, with other (or unknown) substance induced bipolar or related disorder
Other (or unknown) substance use disorder, moderate, with other (or unknown) substance induced depressive disorder
Other (or unknown) substance use disorder, severe, with other (or unknown) substance induced bipolar or related disorder
Other (or unknown) substance use disorder, severe, with other (or unknown) substance induced depressive disorder

✓6ᵗʰ **F19.25** **Other psychoactive substance dependence with psychoactive substance-induced psychotic disorder**

    F19.250 **Other psychoactive substance** `CC` `HCC`
      dependence with psychoactive substance-induced psychotic disorder with delusions

    F19.251 **Other psychoactive substance** `CC` `HCC`
      dependence with psychoactive substance-induced psychotic disorder with hallucinations

    F19.259 **Other psychoactive substance** `CC` `HCC`
      dependence with psychoactive substance-induced psychotic disorder, unspecified
      CC Excl: No Excl

F19.26 **Other psychoactive substance dependence** `CC` `HCC`
with psychoactive substance-induced persisting amnestic disorder
CC Excl: No Excl

F19.27 **Other psychoactive substance dependence** `CC` `HCC`
with psychoactive substance-induced persisting dementia
Other (or unknown) substance use disorder, moderate, with other (or unknown) substance induced major neurocognitive disorder
Other (or unknown) substance use disorder, severe, with other (or unknown) substance induced major neurocognitive disorder

✓6ᵗʰ **F19.28** **Other psychoactive substance dependence with other psychoactive substance-induced disorders**

    F19.280 **Other psychoactive substance** `CC` `HCC`
      dependence with psychoactive substance-induced anxiety disorder
      CC Excl: No Excl

    F19.281 **Other psychoactive substance** `CC` `HCC`
      dependence with psychoactive substance-induced sexual dysfunction
      CC Excl: No Excl

    F19.282 **Other psychoactive substance** `CC` `HCC`
      dependence with psychoactive substance-induced sleep disorder
      CC Excl: No Excl

    F19.288 **Other psychoactive substance** `CC` `HCC`
      dependence with other psychoactive substance-induced disorder
      Other (or unknown) substance use disorder, moderate, with other (or unknown) substance induced mild neurocognitive disorder
      Other (or unknown) substance use disorder, severe, with other (or unknown) substance induced mild neurocognitive disorder
      Other (or unknown) substance use disorder, moderate, with other (or unknown) substance induced obsessive compulsive or related disorder
      Other (or unknown) substance use disorder, severe, with other (or unknown) substance induced obsessive-compulsive or related disorder
      CC Excl: No Excl

F19.29 **Other psychoactive substance dependence** `HCC`
with unspecified psychoactive substance-induced disorder

✓5ᵗʰ **F19.9** **Other psychoactive substance use, unspecified**
> *EXCLUDES 1*   other psychoactive substance abuse (F19.1-)
>   other psychoactive substance dependence (F19.2-)

   F19.90 **Other psychoactive substance use, unspecified, uncomplicated**

✓6ᵗʰ **F19.92** **Other psychoactive substance use, unspecified with intoxication**
> *EXCLUDES 1*   other psychoactive substance use, unspecified with withdrawal (F19.93)

    F19.920 **Other psychoactive substance use,** `HCC`
      unspecified with intoxication, uncomplicated

    F19.921 **Other psychoactive substance use,** `CC` `HCC`
      unspecified with intoxication with delirium
      Other (or unknown) substance-induced delirium

    F19.922 **Other psychoactive substance use,** `HCC`
      unspecified with intoxication with perceptual disturbance

    F19.929 **Other psychoactive substance use,** `HCC`
      unspecified with intoxication, unspecified

✓6ᵗʰ **F19.93** **Other psychoactive substance use, unspecified with withdrawal**
> *EXCLUDES 1*   other psychoactive substance use, unspecified with intoxication (F19.92-)

    F19.930 **Other psychoactive substance use,** `CC` `HCC`
      unspecified with withdrawal, uncomplicated

    F19.931 **Other psychoactive substance use,** `CC` `HCC`
      unspecified with withdrawal delirium

    F19.932 **Other psychoactive substance use,** `CC` `HCC`
      unspecified with withdrawal with perceptual disturbance

    F19.939 **Other psychoactive substance use,** `CC` `HCC`
      unspecified with withdrawal, unspecified

F19.94 **Other psychoactive substance use, unspecified** `HCC`
with psychoactive substance-induced mood disorder
Other (or unknown) substance-induced bipolar or related disorder, without use disorder
Other (or unknown) substance-induced depressive disorder, without use disorder

---

✓ Additional Character Req   ✓x7ᵗʰ Placeholder Alert   Unacceptable PDx   Manifestation   **H1**-**H14** HAC   `HCC` CMS-HCC Condition   *EXCLUDES 1* Not Coded Here   *EXCLUDES 2* Not Included Here

√6th **F19.95** **Other psychoactive substance use, unspecified with psychoactive substance-induced psychotic disorder**

　　F19.950 **Other psychoactive substance use,** CC HCC **unspecified with psychoactive substance-induced psychotic disorder with delusions**

　　F19.951 **Other psychoactive substance use,** CC HCC **unspecified with psychoactive substance-induced psychotic disorder with hallucinations**

　　F19.959 **Other psychoactive substance use,** HCC **unspecified with psychoactive substance-induced psychotic disorder, unspecified**
　　　　Other or unknown substance-induced psychotic disorder, without use disorder

F19.96 **Other psychoactive substance use, unspecified** HCC **with psychoactive substance-induced persisting amnestic disorder**

F19.97 **Other psychoactive substance use,** CC HCC **unspecified with psychoactive substance-induced persisting dementia**
　　Other (or unknown) substance-induced major neurocognitive disorder, without use disorder

√6th **F19.98** **Other psychoactive substance use, unspecified with other psychoactive substance-induced disorders**

　　F19.980 **Other psychoactive substance use,** HCC **unspecified with psychoactive substance-induced anxiety disorder**
　　　　Other (or unknown) substance-induced anxiety disorder, without use disorder

　　F19.981 **Other psychoactive substance use,** HCC **unspecified with psychoactive substance-induced sexual dysfunction**
　　　　Other (or unknown) substance-induced sexual dysfunction, without use disorder

　　F19.982 **Other psychoactive substance use,** HCC **unspecified with psychoactive substance-induced sleep disorder**
　　　　Other (or unknown) substance-induced sleep disorder, without use disorder

　　F19.988 **Other psychoactive substance use,** HCC **unspecified with other psychoactive substance-induced disorder**
　　　　Other (or unknown) substance-induced mild neurocognitive disorder, without use disorder
　　　　Other (or unknown) substance-induced obsessive-compulsive or related disorder, without use disorder

F19.99 **Other psychoactive substance use, unspecified** HCC **with unspecified psychoactive substance-induced disorder**

Schizophrenia, schizotypal, delusional, and other non-mood psychotic disorders (F20-F29)

√4th **F20** **Schizophrenia**

EXCLUDES 1　brief psychotic disorder (F23)
　　　　cyclic schizophrenia (F25.0)
　　　　mood [affective] disorders with psychotic symptoms (F30.2, F31.2, F31.5, F31.64, F32.3, F33.3)
　　　　schizoaffective disorder (F25.-)
　　　　schizophrenic reaction NOS (F23)

EXCLUDES 2　schizophrenic reaction in:
　　　　alcoholism (F10.15-, F10.25-, F10.95-)
　　　　brain disease (F06.2)
　　　　epilepsy (F06.2)
　　　　psychoactive drug use (F11-F19 with .15..25, .95)
　　　　schizotypal disorder (F21)

DEF: Group of disorders with disturbances in thought (delusions, hallucinations), mood (blunted, flattened, inappropriate affect), sense of self; also bizarre, purposeless behavior, repetitive activity, or inactivity.

CC Excl: For CC codes in category F20: PDX collection 551

F20.0 **Paranoid schizophrenia** CC HCC
　　Paraphrenic schizophrenia
　　EXCLUDES 1　involutional paranoid state (F22)
　　　　paranoia (F22)
　　DEF: Preoccupied with delusional suspicions and auditory hallucinations related to single theme; usually hostile, grandiose, threatening, persecutory, occasionally hypochondriacal.

F20.1 **Disorganized schizophrenia** CC HCC
　　Hebephrenic schizophrenia
　　Hebephrenia

F20.2 **Catatonic schizophrenia** CC HCC
　　Schizophrenic catalepsy
　　Schizophrenic catatonia
　　Schizophrenic flexibilitas cerea
　　EXCLUDES 1　catatonic stupor (R40.1)
　　DEF: Extreme changes in motor activity; one extreme is decreased response or reaction to the environment and the other is spontaneous activity.

F20.3 **Undifferentiated schizophrenia** HCC
　　Atypical schizophrenia
　　EXCLUDES 1　acute schizophrenia-like psychotic disorder (F23)
　　EXCLUDES 2　post-schizophrenic depression (F32.89)

F20.5 **Residual schizophrenia** CC HCC
　　Restzustand (schizophrenic)
　　Schizophrenic residual state

√5th **F20.8** **Other schizophrenia**

　　F20.81 **Schizophreniform disorder** CC HCC
　　　　Schizophreniform psychosis NOS

　　F20.89 **Other schizophrenia** CC HCC
　　　　Cenesthopathic schizophrenia
　　　　Simple schizophrenia

F20.9 **Schizophrenia, unspecified** HCC

F21 **Schizotypal disorder**
　　Borderline schizophrenia
　　Latent schizophrenia
　　Latent schizophrenic reaction
　　Prepsychotic schizophrenia
　　Prodromal schizophrenia
　　Pseudoneurotic schizophrenia
　　Pseudopsychopathic schizophrenia
　　Schizotypal personality disorder
　　EXCLUDES 2　Asperger's syndrome (F84.5)
　　　　schizoid personality disorder (F60.1)

F22 **Delusional disorders** HCC
　　Delusional dysmorphophobia
　　Involutional paranoid state
　　Paranoia
　　Paranoia querulans
　　Paranoid psychosis
　　Paranoid state
　　Paraphrenia (late)
　　Sensitiver Beziehungswahn
　　EXCLUDES 1　mood [affective] disorders with psychotic symptoms (F30.2, F31.2, F31.5, F31.64, F32.3, F33.3)
　　　　paranoid schizophrenia (F20.0)
　　EXCLUDES 2　paranoid personality disorder (F60.0)
　　　　paranoid psychosis, psychogenic (F23)
　　　　paranoid reaction (F23)

F23 **Brief psychotic disorder** CC
　　Paranoid reaction
　　Psychogenic paranoid psychosis
　　EXCLUDES 2　mood [affective] disorders with psychotic symptoms (F30.2, F31.2, F31.5, F31.64, F32.3, F33.3)
　　CC Excl: No Excl

F24 **Shared psychotic disorder** HCC
　　Folie à deux
　　Induced paranoid disorder
　　Induced psychotic disorder

√4th **F25** **Schizoaffective disorders**
　　EXCLUDES 1　mood [affective] disorders with psychotic symptoms (F30.2, F31.2, F31.5, F31.64, F32.3, F33.3)
　　　　schizophrenia (F20.-)

F25.0 **Schizoaffective disorder, bipolar type** HCC
　　Cyclic schizophrenia
　　Schizoaffective disorder, manic type
　　Schizoaffective disorder, mixed type
　　Schizoaffective psychosis, bipolar type
　　~~Schizophreniform psychosis, manic type~~

F25.1 **Schizoaffective disorder, depressive type** HCC
　　Schizoaffective psychosis, depressive type
　　~~Schizophreniform psychosis, depressive type~~

F25.8 **Other schizoaffective disorders** HCC

F25.9 **Schizoaffective disorder, unspecified** HCC
　　Schizoaffective psychosis NOS

N Newborn: 0　P Pediatric: 0-17　M Maternity: 12-55　A Adult: 15-124　MCC Major CC Condition　PDxMCC PDx acts as own MCC　CC CC Condition　PDxCC PDx acts as own CC

546　　　　　　　　　　　　　　　　　　　　　　　　　　　　　　　　　ICD-10-CM 2018

F28   Other psychotic disorder not due to a substance or known `HIV`
physiological condition
    Chronic hallucinatory psychosis
    ▶Other specified schizophrenia spectrum and other psychotic disorder◀

F29   Unspecified psychosis not due to a substance or known `HIV`
physiological condition
    Chronic hallucinatory psychosis
    ▶Unspecified schizophrenia spectrum and other psychotic disorder◀
    `EXCLUDES 1`   *mental disorder NOS (F99)*
                unspecified mental disorder due to known physiological
                condition (F09)

Mood [affective] disorders (F30-F39)

`✓4ᵗʰ` **F30   Manic episode**
    `INCLUDES`   bipolar disorder, single manic episode
              mixed affective episode
    `EXCLUDES 1`   *bipolar disorder (F31.-)*
                major depressive disorder, recurrent (F33.-)
                major depressive disorder, single episode (F32.-)

    CC Excl: For CC codes in category F30, unless otherwise noted:
    PDX collection 551

`✓5ᵗʰ` **F30.1   Manic episode** without psychotic symptoms
        F30.10   Manic episode without psychotic symptoms, `CC` `HCC`
                unspecified
        F30.11   Manic episode without psychotic symptoms, `CC` `HCC`
                mild
        F30.12   Manic episode without psychotic symptoms, `CC` `HCC`
                moderate
        F30.13   Manic episode, severe, without psychotic `CC` `HCC`
                symptoms
                    CC Excl: PDX collection 552

    F30.2   Manic episode, severe with psychotic symptoms `CC` `HCC`
            Manic stupor
            Mania with mood-congruent psychotic symptoms
            Mania with mood-incongruent psychotic symptoms

    F30.3   Manic episode in partial remission   `HCC`

    F30.4   Manic episode in full remission   `HCC`

    F30.8   Other manic episodes   `HCC`
            Hypomania

    F30.9   Manic episode, unspecified   `CC` `HCC`
            Mania NOS

`✓4ᵗʰ` **F31   Bipolar disorder**
    `INCLUDES`   ▶bipolar I disorder
              bipolar type I disorder◀
              manic-depressive illness
              manic-depressive psychosis
              manic-depressive reaction
    `EXCLUDES 1`   *bipolar disorder, single manic episode (F30.-)*
                major depressive disorder, single episode (F32.-)
                major depressive disorder, recurrent (F33.-)
    `EXCLUDES 2`   *cyclothymia (F34.0)*

    CC Excl: For CC codes in category F31, unless otherwise noted:
    PDX collection 551

    F31.0   Bipolar disorder, current episode hypomanic   `CC` `HCC`

`✓5ᵗʰ` **F31.1   Bipolar disorder, current episode manic without psychotic**
        features
        F31.10   Bipolar disorder, current episode manic `CC` `HCC`
                without psychotic features, unspecified
        F31.11   Bipolar disorder, current episode manic `CC` `HCC`
                without psychotic features, mild
        F31.12   Bipolar disorder, current episode manic `CC` `HCC`
                without psychotic features, moderate
        F31.13   Bipolar disorder, current episode manic `CC` `HCC`
                without psychotic features, severe
                    CC Excl: PDX collection 553

    F31.2   Bipolar disorder, current episode manic severe with `CC` `HCC`
            psychotic features
            Bipolar disorder, current episode manic with mood-congruent
                psychotic symptoms
            Bipolar disorder, current episode manic with mood-incongruent
                psychotic symptoms
            ▶Bipolar I disorder, current or most recent episode manic with
                psychotic features◀

`✓5ᵗʰ` **F31.3   Bipolar disorder, current episode depressed, mild or**
        moderate severity
        F31.30   Bipolar disorder, current episode depressed, `CC` `HCC`
                mild or moderate severity, unspecified

        F31.31   Bipolar disorder, current episode depressed, `CC` `HCC`
                mild
        F31.32   Bipolar disorder, current episode depressed, `CC` `HCC`
                moderate

    F31.4   Bipolar disorder, current episode depressed, severe, `CC` `HCC`
            without psychotic features
                CC Excl: PDX collection 554

    F31.5   Bipolar disorder, current episode depressed, severe, `CC` `HCC`
            with psychotic features
            Bipolar disorder, current episode depressed with mood-
                incongruent psychotic symptoms
            Bipolar disorder, current episode depressed with mood-
                congruent psychotic symptoms
            ▶Bipolar I disorder, current or most recent episode depressed, with
                psychotic features◀

`✓5ᵗʰ` **F31.6   Bipolar disorder, current episode mixed**
        F31.60   Bipolar disorder, current episode mixed, `CC` `HCC`
                unspecified
        F31.61   Bipolar disorder, current episode mixed, `CC` `HCC`
                mild
        F31.62   Bipolar disorder, current episode mixed, `CC` `HCC`
                moderate
        F31.63   Bipolar disorder, current episode mixed, `CC` `HCC`
                severe, without psychotic features
                    CC Excl: PDX collection 554
        F31.64   Bipolar disorder, current episode mixed, `CC` `HCC`
                severe, with psychotic features
                Bipolar disorder, current episode mixed with mood-
                    congruent psychotic symptoms
                Bipolar disorder, current episode mixed with mood-
                    incongruent psychotic symptoms

`✓5ᵗʰ` **F31.7   Bipolar disorder, currently in remission**
        F31.70   Bipolar disorder, currently in remission, most `HCC`
                recent episode unspecified
        F31.71   Bipolar disorder, in partial remission, most `HCC`
                recent episode hypomanic
        F31.72   Bipolar disorder, in full remission, most `HCC`
                recent episode hypomanic
        F31.73   Bipolar disorder, in partial remission, most `HCC`
                recent episode manic
        F31.74   Bipolar disorder, in full remission, most `HCC`
                recent episode manic
        F31.75   Bipolar disorder, in partial remission, most `HCC`
                recent episode depressed
        F31.76   Bipolar disorder, in full remission, most `HCC`
                recent episode depressed
        F31.77   Bipolar disorder, in partial remission, most `HCC`
                recent episode mixed
        F31.78   Bipolar disorder, in full remission, most `HCC`
                recent episode mixed

`✓5ᵗʰ` **F31.8   Other bipolar disorders**
        F31.81   Bipolar II disorder `CC` `HCC`
                ▶Bipolar disorder, type 2◀
        F31.89   Other bipolar disorder `CC` `HCC`
                Recurrent manic episodes NOS

    F31.9   Bipolar disorder, unspecified `HCC`
            ▶Manic depression◀

`✓4ᵗʰ` **F32   Major depressive disorder, single episode**
    `INCLUDES`   single episode of agitated depression
              single episode of depressive reaction
              single episode of major depression
              single episode of psychogenic depression
              single episode of reactive depression
              single episode of vital depression
    `EXCLUDES 1`   *bipolar disorder (F31.-)*
                manic episode (F30.-)
                recurrent depressive disorder (F33.-)
    `EXCLUDES 2`   *adjustment disorder (F43.2)*
    DEF: Mood disorder that produces depression; may exhibit as sadness, low
    self-esteem, or guilt feelings; other manifestations may be withdrawal
    from friends and family and interrupted sleep.

    CC Excl: For CC codes in category F32: PDX collection 555

    F32.0   Major depressive disorder, single episode, mild `CC` `HCC`
    F32.1   Major depressive disorder, single episode, moderate `CC` `HCC`
    F32.2   Major depressive disorder, single episode, severe `CC` `HCC`
            without psychotic features

☑Additional Character Req   `✓x7ᵗʰ` Placeholder Alert   Unacceptable PDx   Manifestation   `H1`-`H14` HAC   `HCC` CMS-HCC Condition   `EXCLUDES 1` Not Coded Here   `EXCLUDES 2` Not Included Here

F32.3 **Major depressive disorder, single episode, severe** `CC` `HCC`
with psychotic features
Single episode of major depression with mood-congruent
psychotic symptoms
Single episode of major depression with mood-incongruent
psychotic symptoms
Single episode of major depression with psychotic symptoms
Single episode of psychogenic depressive psychosis
Single episode of psychotic depression
Single episode of reactive depressive psychosis

F32.4 **Major depressive disorder, single episode, in partial** `HCC`
remission

F32.5 **Major depressive disorder, single episode, in full** `HCC`
remission

√5th **F32.8** **Other depressive episodes**

F32.81 **Premenstrual dysphoric disorder** ♀
EXCLUDES 1   premenstrual tension syndrome (N94.3)

F32.89 **Other specified depressive episodes**
Atypical depression
Post-schizophrenic depression
Single episode of 'masked' depression NOS

F32.9 **Major depressive disorder, single episode, unspecified**
Depression NOS
Depressive disorder NOS
Major depression NOS
AHA: 2013, 4Q, 107

√4th **F33** **Major depressive disorder, recurrent**
`INCLUDES`   recurrent episodes of depressive reaction
recurrent episodes of endogenous depression
recurrent episodes of major depression
recurrent episodes of psychogenic depression
recurrent episodes of reactive depression
recurrent episodes of seasonal depressive disorder
recurrent episodes of vital depression
EXCLUDES 1   bipolar disorder (F31.-)
manic episode (F30.-)

CC Excl: For CC codes in category F33, unless otherwise noted:
PDX collection 555

F33.0 **Major depressive disorder, recurrent, mild** `CC` `HCC`

F33.1 **Major depressive disorder, recurrent, moderate** `CC` `HCC`

F33.2 **Major depressive disorder, recurrent, severe without** `CC` `HCC`
psychotic features

F33.3 **Major depressive disorder, recurrent, severe with** `CC` `HCC`
psychotic symptoms
Endogenous depression with psychotic symptoms
▶Major depressive disorder, recurrent, with psychotic features◀
Recurrent severe episodes of major depression with mood-
congruent psychotic symptoms
Recurrent severe episodes of major depression with mood-
incongruent psychotic symptoms
Recurrent severe episodes of major depression with psychotic
symptoms
Recurrent severe episodes of psychogenic depressive psychosis
Recurrent severe episodes of psychotic depression
Recurrent severe episodes of reactive depressive psychosis
CC Excl: PDX collection 551

√5th **F33.4** **Major depressive disorder, recurrent, in remission**

F33.40 **Major depressive disorder, recurrent, in** `CC` `HCC`
remission, unspecified

F33.41 **Major depressive disorder, recurrent, in partial** `HCC`
remission

F33.42 **Major depressive disorder, recurrent, in full** `HCC`
remission

F33.8 **Other recurrent depressive disorders** `HCC`
Recurrent brief depressive episodes
CC Excl: PDX collection 551

F33.9 **Major depressive disorder, recurrent, unspecified** `CC` `HCC`
Monopolar depression NOS

√4th **F34** **Persistent mood [affective] disorders**

F34.0 **Cyclothymic disorder**
Affective personality disorder
Cycloid personality
Cyclothymia
Cyclothymic personality

F34.1 **Dysthymic disorder**
Depressive neurosis
Depressive personality disorder
Dysthymia
Neurotic depression
Persistent anxiety depression
Persistent depressive disorder
EXCLUDES 2   anxiety depression (mild or not persistent) (F41.8)
DEF: Depression without psychosis; less severe but persistent
depression; is considered a mild to moderate chronic form of
depression.

√5th **F34.8** **Other persistent mood [affective] disorders**

F34.81 **Disruptive mood dysregulation disorder** `CC` `HCC`
CC Excl: PDX collection 551

F34.89 **Other specified persistent mood disorders** `CC` `HCC`
CC Excl: PDX collection 551

F34.9 **Persistent mood [affective] disorder, unspecified** `CC` `HCC`
CC Excl: PDX collection 551

F39 **Unspecified mood [affective] disorder** `HCC`
Affective psychosis NOS

Anxiety, dissociative, stress-related, somatoform and other nonpsychotic mental disorders (F40-F48)

√4th **F40** **Phobic anxiety disorders**

√5th **F40.0** **Agoraphobia**
DEF: Profound anxiety or fear of leaving familiar settings like
home, or being in unfamiliar locations or with strangers or crowds;
may or may not be preceded by recurrent panic attacks.

F40.00 **Agoraphobia, unspecified**

F40.01 **Agoraphobia with panic disorder**
Panic disorder with agoraphobia
EXCLUDES 1   panic disorder without agoraphobia (F41.0)

F40.02 **Agoraphobia without panic disorder**

√5th **F40.1** **Social phobias**
Anthropophobia
▶Social anxiety disorder◀
Social anxiety disorder of childhood
Social neurosis

F40.10 **Social phobia, unspecified**

F40.11 **Social phobia, generalized**

√5th **F40.2** **Specific (isolated) phobias**
EXCLUDES 2   dysmorphophobia (nondelusional) (F45.22)
nosophobia (F45.22)

√6th **F40.21** **Animal type phobia**

F40.210 **Arachnophobia**
Fear of spiders

F40.218 **Other animal type phobia**

√6th **F40.22** **Natural environment type phobia**

F40.220 **Fear of thunderstorms**

F40.228 **Other natural environment type phobia**

√6th **F40.23** **Blood, injection, injury type phobia**

F40.230 **Fear of blood**

F40.231 **Fear of injections and transfusions**

F40.232 **Fear of other medical care**

F40.233 **Fear of injury**

√6th **F40.24** **Situational type phobia**

F40.240 **Claustrophobia**

F40.241 **Acrophobia**

F40.242 **Fear of bridges**

F40.243 **Fear of flying**

F40.248 **Other situational type phobia**

√6th **F40.29** **Other specified phobia**

F40.290 **Androphobia**
Fear of men

F40.291 **Gynephobia**
Fear of women

F40.298 **Other specified phobia**

F40.8 **Other phobic anxiety disorders**
Phobic anxiety disorder of childhood

F40.9 **Phobic anxiety disorder, unspecified**
Phobia NOS
Phobic state NOS

N Newborn: 0   P Pediatric: 0-17   M Maternity: 12-55   A Adult: 15-124   `MCC` Major CC Condition   `PDxMCC` PDx acts as own MCC   `CC` CC Condition   `PDxCC` PDx acts as own CC

548   ICD-10-CM 2018

☑4ᵗʰ **F41 Other anxiety disorders**
> EXCLUDES 2 *anxiety in:*
>> *acute stress reaction (F43.0)*
>> *transient adjustment reaction (F43.2)*
>> *neurasthenia (F48.8)*
>> *psychophysiologic disorders (F45.-)*
>> *separation anxiety (F93.0)*

▲ **F41.0 Panic disorder [episodic paroxysmal anxiety]**
> Panic attack
> Panic state
> EXCLUDES 1 *panic disorder with agoraphobia (F40.01)*
> **DEF:** Neurotic disorder characterized by recurrent panic or anxiety, apprehension, fear, or terror; symptoms include shortness of breath, palpitations, dizziness, shakiness; fear of dying may persist.

F41.1 Generalized anxiety disorder
> Anxiety neurosis
> Anxiety reaction
> Anxiety state
> Overanxious disorder
> EXCLUDES 2 *neurasthenia (F48.8)*

F41.3 Other mixed anxiety disorders

F41.8 Other specified anxiety disorders
> Anxiety depression (mild or not persistent)
> Anxiety hysteria
> Mixed anxiety and depressive disorder

F41.9 Anxiety disorder, unspecified
> Anxiety NOS

☑4ᵗʰ **F42 Obsessive-compulsive disorder**
> EXCLUDES 2 *obsessive-compulsive personality (disorder) (F60.5)*
>> *obsessive-compulsive symptoms occurring in depression (F32-F33)*
>> *obsessive-compulsive symptoms occurring in schizophrenia (F20.-)*

F42.2 Mixed obsessional thoughts and acts

F42.3 Hoarding disorder

F42.4 Excoriation (skin-picking) disorder
> EXCLUDES 1 *factitial dermatitis (L98.1)*
>> *other specified behavioral and emotional disorders with onset usually occurring in early childhood and adolescence (F98.8)*

F42.8 Other obsessive-compulsive disorder
> Anancastic neurosis
> Obsessive-compulsive neurosis

F42.9 Obsessive-compulsive disorder, unspecified

☑4ᵗʰ **F43 Reaction to severe stress, and adjustment disorders**

F43.0 Acute stress reaction
> Acute crisis reaction
> Acute reaction to stress
> Combat and operational stress reaction
> Combat fatigue
> Crisis state
> Psychic shock

☑5ᵗʰ **F43.1 Post-traumatic stress disorder (PTSD)**
> Traumatic neurosis
> **DEF:** Preoccupation with traumatic events beyond normal experience; i.e., rape, personal assault, etc.; also recurring flashbacks of trauma; symptoms include difficulty remembering, sleeping, or concentrating, and guilt feelings for surviving.

F43.10 Post-traumatic stress disorder, unspecified

F43.11 Post-traumatic stress disorder, acute

F43.12 Post-traumatic stress disorder, chronic

☑5ᵗʰ **F43.2 Adjustment disorders**
> Culture shock
> Grief reaction
> Hospitalism in children
> EXCLUDES 2 *separation anxiety disorder of childhood (F93.0)*

F43.20 Adjustment disorder, unspecified

F43.21 Adjustment disorder with depressed mood
> **AHA:** 2014, 1Q, 25

F43.22 Adjustment disorder with anxiety

F43.23 Adjustment disorder with mixed anxiety and depressed mood

F43.24 Adjustment disorder with disturbance of conduct

F43.25 Adjustment disorder with mixed disturbance of emotions and conduct

F43.29 Adjustment disorder with other symptoms

F43.8 Other reactions to severe stress
> Other specified trauma and stressor-related disorder

F43.9 Reaction to severe stress, unspecified
> Trauma and stressor-related disorder, NOS

☑4ᵗʰ **F44 Dissociative and conversion disorders**
> INCLUDES conversion hysteria
>> conversion reaction
>> hysteria
>> hysterical psychosis
> EXCLUDES 2 *malingering [conscious simulation] (Z76.5)*

F44.0 Dissociative amnesia
> EXCLUDES 1 *amnesia NOS (R41.3)*
>> *anterograde amnesia (R41.1)*
>> *dissociative amnesia with dissociative fugue (F44.1)*
>> *retrograde amnesia (R41.2)*
> EXCLUDES 2 *alcohol-or other psychoactive substance-induced amnestic disorder (F10, F13, F19 with .26, .96)*
>> *amnestic disorder due to known physiological condition (F04)*
>> *postictal amnesia in epilepsy (G40.-)*

F44.1 Dissociative fugue
> Dissociative amnesia with dissociative fugue
> EXCLUDES 2 *postictal fugue in epilepsy (G40.-)*
> **DEF:** Dissociative hysteria; identified by loss of memory, flight from familiar surroundings to a completely separate environment, episodes may last hours or days; conscious activity is not associated with perception of surroundings and there is no later memory of episode.

F44.2 Dissociative stupor
> EXCLUDES 1 *catatonic stupor (R40.1)*
>> *stupor NOS (R40.1)*
> EXCLUDES 2 *catatonic disorder due to known physiological condition (F06.1)*
>> *depressive stupor (F32, F33)*
>> *manic stupor (F30, F31)*

F44.4 Conversion disorder with motor symptom or deficit
> ▶Conversion disorder with abnormal movement
> Conversion disorder with speech symptoms
> Conversion disorder with swallowing symptoms
> Conversion disorder with weakness/paralysis◀
> Dissociative motor disorders
> Psychogenic aphonia
> Psychogenic dysphonia

F44.5 Conversion disorder with seizures or convulsions
> ▶Conversion disorder with attacks or seizures◀
> Dissociative convulsions

F44.6 Conversion disorder with sensory symptom or deficit
> ▶Conversion disorder with anesthesia or sensory loss
> Conversion disorder with special sensory symptoms◀
> Dissociative anesthesia and sensory loss
> Psychogenic deafness

F44.7 Conversion disorder with mixed symptom presentation

☑5ᵗʰ **F44.8 Other dissociative and conversion disorders**

F44.81 Dissociative identity disorder
> Multiple personality disorder

F44.89 Other dissociative and conversion disorders
> Ganser's syndrome
> Psychogenic confusion
> Psychogenic twilight state
> Trance and possession disorders

F44.9 Dissociative and conversion disorder, unspecified
> Dissociative disorder NOS

☑4ᵗʰ **F45 Somatoform disorders**
> EXCLUDES 2 *dissociative and conversion disorders (F44.-)*
>> *factitious disorders (F68.1-)*
>> *hair-plucking (F63.3)*
>> *lalling (F80.0)*
>> *lisping (F80.0)*
>> *malingering [conscious simulation] (Z76.5)*
>> *nail-biting (F98.8)*
>> *psychological or behavioral factors associated with disorders or diseases classified elsewhere (F54)*
>> *sexual dysfunction, not due to a substance or known physiological condition (F52.-)*
>> *thumb-sucking (F98.8)*
>> *tic disorders (in childhood and adolescence) (F95.-)*
>> *Tourette's syndrome (F95.2)*
>> *trichotillomania (F63.3)*

F45.0 Somatization disorder
> Briquet's disorder
> Multiple psychosomatic disorder

☑ Additional Character Req √x7ᵗʰ Placeholder Alert Unacceptable PDx Manifestation H1 - H14 HAC HCC CMS-HCC Condition EXCLUDES 1 Not Coded Here EXCLUDES 2 Not Included Here

F45.1 Undifferentiated somatoform disorder
Somatic symptom disorder
Undifferentiated psychosomatic disorder

✓5th **F45.2 Hypochondriacal disorders**
EXCLUDES 2   *delusional dysmorphophobia (F22)*
fixed delusions about bodily functions or shape (F22)

F45.20 Hypochondriacal disorder, unspecified

F45.21 Hypochondriasis
Hypochondriacal neurosis
Illness anxiety disorder

F45.22 Body dysmorphic disorder
Dysmorphophobia (nondelusional)
Nosophobia

F45.29 Other hypochondriacal disorders

✓5th **F45.4 Pain disorders related to psychological factors**
EXCLUDES 1   *pain NOS (R52)*

F45.41 Pain disorder exclusively related to psychological factors
Somatoform pain disorder (persistent)

F45.42 Pain disorder with related psychological factors
Code also associated acute or chronic pain (G89.-)

F45.8 Other somatoform disorders
Psychogenic dysmenorrhea
Psychogenic dysphagia, including "globus hystericus"
Psychogenic pruritus
Psychogenic torticollis
Somatoform autonomic dysfunction
Teeth grinding
EXCLUDES 1   *sleep related teeth grinding (G47.63)*

F45.9 Somatoform disorder, unspecified
Psychosomatic disorder NOS

✓4th **F48 Other nonpsychotic mental disorders**
F48.1 Depersonalization-derealization syndrome
F48.2 Pseudobulbar affect
Involuntary emotional expression disorder
Code first underlying cause, if known, such as:
amyotrophic lateral sclerosis (G12.21)
multiple sclerosis (G35)
sequelae of cerebrovascular disease (I69.-)
sequelae of traumatic intracranial injury (S06.-)

F48.8 Other specified nonpsychotic mental disorders
Dhat syndrome
Neurasthenia
Occupational neurosis, including writer's cramp
Psychasthenia
Psychasthenic neurosis
Psychogenic syncope

F48.9 Nonpsychotic mental disorder, unspecified
Neurosis NOS

Behavioral syndromes associated with physiological disturbances and physical factors (F50-F59)

✓4th **F50 Eating disorders**
EXCLUDES 1   *anorexia NOS (R63.0)*
feeding difficulties (R63.3)
▶*feeding problems of newborn (P92.-)*◀
polyphagia (R63.2)
EXCLUDES 2   *feeding disorder in infancy or childhood (F98.2-)*

CC Excl: For CC codes in category F50, unless otherwise noted:
PDX collection 556

✓5th **F50.0 Anorexia nervosa**
EXCLUDES 1   *loss of appetite (R63.0)*
psychogenic loss of appetite (F50.89)

F50.00 Anorexia nervosa, unspecified   CC

F50.01 Anorexia nervosa, restricting type   CC

F50.02 Anorexia nervosa, binge eating/purging type   CC
EXCLUDES 1   *bulimia nervosa (F50.2)*

F50.2 Bulimia nervosa   CC
Bulimia NOS
Hyperorexia nervosa
EXCLUDES 1   *anorexia nervosa, binge eating/purging type (F50.02)*
CC Excl: PDX collection 557

✓5th **F50.8 Other eating disorders**
EXCLUDES 2   *pica of infancy and childhood (F98.3)*

F50.81 Binge eating disorder

● **F50.82 Avoidant/restrictive food intake disorder**

F50.89 Other specified eating disorder
Pica in adults
Psychogenic loss of appetite

F50.9 Eating disorder, unspecified
Atypical anorexia nervosa
Atypical bulimia nervosa
▶Feeding or eating disorder, unspecified
Other specified feeding disorder ◀

✓4th **F51 Sleep disorders not due to a substance or known physiological condition**
EXCLUDES 2   *organic sleep disorders (G47.-)*

✓5th **F51.0 Insomnia not due to a substance or known physiological condition**
EXCLUDES 2   *alcohol related insomnia (F10.182, F10.282, F10.982)*
drug-related insomnia (F11.182, F11.282, F11.982, F13.182, F13.282, F13.982, F14.182, F14.282, F14.982, F15.182, F15.282, F15.982, F19.182, F19.282, F19.982)
insomnia NOS (G47.0-)
insomnia due to known physiological condition (G47.0-)
organic insomnia (G47.0-)
sleep deprivation (Z72.820)

F51.01 Primary insomnia
Idiopathic insomnia

F51.02 Adjustment insomnia

F51.03 Paradoxical insomnia

F51.04 Psychophysiologic insomnia

F51.05 Insomnia due to other mental disorder
Code also associated mental disorder

F51.09 Other insomnia not due to a substance or known physiological condition

✓5th **F51.1 Hypersomnia not due to a substance or known physiological condition**
EXCLUDES 2   *alcohol related hypersomnia (F10.182, F10.282, F10.982)*
drug-related hypersomnia (F11.182, F11.282, F11.982, F13.182, F13.282, F13.982, F14.182, F14.282, F14.982, F15.182, F15.282, F15.982, F19.182, F19.282, F19.982)
hypersomnia NOS (G47.10)
hypersomnia due to known physiological condition (G47.10)
idiopathic hypersomnia (G47.11, G47.12)
narcolepsy (G47.4-)

F51.11 Primary hypersomnia

F51.12 Insufficient sleep syndrome
EXCLUDES 1   *sleep deprivation (Z72.820)*

F51.13 Hypersomnia due to other mental disorder
Code also associated mental disorder

F51.19 Other hypersomnia not due to a substance or known physiological condition

F51.3 Sleepwalking [somnambulism]
▶Non–rapid eye movement sleep arousal disorders, sleepwalking type◀

F51.4 Sleep terrors [night terrors]
▶Non–rapid eye movement sleep arousal disorders, sleep terror type◀

F51.5 Nightmare disorder
Dream anxiety disorder

F51.8 Other sleep disorders not due to a substance or known physiological condition

F51.9 Sleep disorder not due to a substance or known physiological condition, unspecified
Emotional sleep disorder NOS

✓4th **F52 Sexual dysfunction not due to a substance or known physiological condition**
EXCLUDES 2   *Dhat syndrome (F48.8)*

F52.0 Hypoactive sexual desire disorder
Lack or loss of sexual desire
▶Male hypoactive sexual desire disorder◀
Sexual anhedonia
EXCLUDES 1   *decreased libido (R68.82)*

F52.1 Sexual aversion disorder
Sexual aversion and lack of sexual enjoyment

✓5th **F52.2 Sexual arousal disorders**
Failure of genital response

F52.21   **Male erectile disorder**   ♂
▶Erectile disorder◀
Psychogenic impotence
EXCLUDES 1   *impotence of organic origin (N52.-)*
impotence NOS (N52.-)

F52.22   **Female sexual arousal disorder**   ♀
▶Female sexual interest/arousal disorder◀

✓5th   **F52.3 Orgasmic disorder**
Inhibited orgasm
Psychogenic anorgasmy

F52.31   **Female orgasmic disorder**   ♀

F52.32   **Male orgasmic disorder**   ♂
Delayed ejaculation

F52.4   **Premature ejaculation**   ♂

F52.5   **Vaginismus not due to a substance or known**   ♀
physiological condition
Psychogenic vaginismus
EXCLUDES 2   *vaginismus (due to a known physiological condition)*
(N94.2)
DEF: Psychogenic response resulting in painful contractions of vaginal canal muscles; can be severe enough to prevent sexual intercourse.

F52.6   **Dyspareunia not due to a substance or known physiological**
condition
Genito-pelvic pain penetration disorderPsychogenic
dyspareunia
EXCLUDES 2   *dyspareunia (due to a known physiological condition)*
(N94.1-)

F52.8   **Other sexual dysfunction not due to a substance or known**
physiological condition
Excessive sexual drive
Nymphomania
Satyriasis

F52.9   **Unspecified sexual dysfunction not due to a substance or**
known physiological condition
Sexual dysfunction NOS

F53   Puerperal psychosis   M♀
Postpartum depression
EXCLUDES 1   *mood disorders with psychotic features (F30.2, F31.2, F31.5,*
F31.64, F32.3, F33.3)
postpartum dysphoria (O90.6)
psychosis in schizophrenia, schizotypal, delusional, and other
psychotic disorders (F20-F29)

F54   *Psychological and behavioral factors associated with disorders or*
diseases classified elsewhere
Psychological factors affecting physical conditions
Code first the associated physical disorder, such as:
asthma (J45.-)
dermatitis (L23-L25)
gastric ulcer (K25.-)
mucous colitis (K58.-)
ulcerative colitis (K51.-)
urticaria (L50.-)
EXCLUDES 2   *tension-type headache (G44.2)*

✓4th   **F55   Abuse of non-psychoactive substances**
EXCLUDES 2   *abuse of psychoactive substances (F10-F19)*

F55.0   **Abuse of antacids**

F55.1   **Abuse of herbal or folk remedies**

F55.2   **Abuse of laxatives**

F55.3   **Abuse of steroids or hormones**

F55.4   **Abuse of vitamins**

F55.8   **Abuse of other non-psychoactive substances**

F59   Unspecified behavioral syndromes associated with physiological
disturbances and physical factors
Psychogenic physiological dysfunction NOS

Disorders of adult personality and behavior (F60-F69)

✓4th   **F60   Specific personality disorders**

F60.0   **Paranoid personality disorder**
Expansive paranoid personality (disorder)
Fanatic personality (disorder)
Paranoid personality (disorder)
Querulant personality (disorder)
Sensitive paranoid personality (disorder)
EXCLUDES 2   *paranoia (F22)*
paranoia querulans (F22)
paranoid psychosis (F22)
paranoid schizophrenia (F20.0)
paranoid state (F22)

F60.1   **Schizoid personality disorder**
EXCLUDES 2   *Asperger's syndrome (F84.5)*
delusional disorder (F22)
schizoid disorder of childhood (F84.5)
schizophrenia (F20.-)
schizotypal disorder (F21)

F60.2   **Antisocial personality disorder**
Amoral personality (disorder)
Asocial personality (disorder)
Dissocial personality disorder
Psychopathic personality (disorder)
Sociopathic personality (disorder)
EXCLUDES 1   *conduct disorders (F91.-)*
EXCLUDES 2   *borderline personality disorder (F60.3)*

F60.3   **Borderline personality disorder**
Aggressive personality (disorder)
Emotionally unstable personality disorder
Explosive personality (disorder)
EXCLUDES 2   *antisocial personality disorder (F60.2)*

F60.4   **Histrionic personality disorder**
Hysterical personality (disorder)
Psychoinfantile personality (disorder)

F60.5   **Obsessive-compulsive personality disorder**
Anankastic personality (disorder)
Compulsive personality (disorder)
Obsessional personality (disorder)
EXCLUDES 2   *obsessive-compulsive disorder (F42-)*

F60.6   **Avoidant personality disorder**
Anxious personality disorder

F60.7   **Dependent personality disorder**
Asthenic personality (disorder)
Inadequate personality (disorder)
Passive personality (disorder)

✓5th   **F60.8   Other specific personality disorders**

F60.81   **Narcissistic personality disorder**

F60.89   **Other specific personality disorders**
Eccentric personality disorder
"Haltlose" type personality disorder
Immature personality disorder
Passive-aggressive personality disorder
Psychoneurotic personality disorder
Self-defeating personality disorder

F60.9   **Personality disorder, unspecified**
Character disorder NOS
Character neurosis NOS
Pathological personality NOS

✓4th   **F63   Impulse disorders**
EXCLUDES 2   *habitual excessive use of alcohol or psychoactive substances*
(F10-F19)
impulse disorders involving sexual behavior (F65.-)

F63.0   **Pathological gambling**
Compulsive gambling
▶Gambling disorder◀
EXCLUDES 1   *gambling and betting NOS (Z72.6)*
EXCLUDES 2   *excessive gambling by manic patients (F30, F31)*
gambling in antisocial personality disorder (F60.2)

F63.1   **Pyromania**
Pathological fire-setting
EXCLUDES 2   *fire-setting (by) (in):*
adult with antisocial personality disorder (F60.2)
alcohol or psychoactive substance intoxication (F10-
F19)
conduct disorders (F91.-)
mental disorders due to known physiological
condition (F01-F09)
schizophrenia (F20.-)

☑Additional Character Req   ✓x 7th Placeholder Alert   Unacceptable PDx   Manifestation   H1-H14 HAC   HCC CMS-HCC Condition   EXCLUDES 1 Not Coded Here   EXCLUDES 2 Not Included Here

Chapter 5. Mental, Behavioral and Neurodevelopmental Disorders

F63.2 Kleptomania
Pathological stealing
EXCLUDES 1   *shoplifting as the reason for observation for suspected mental disorder (Z03.8)*
EXCLUDES 2   *depressive disorder with stealing (F31-F33)*
stealing due to underlying mental condition—code to mental condition
stealing in mental disorders due to known physiological condition (F01-F09)

F63.3 Trichotillomania
Hair plucking
EXCLUDES 2   *other stereotyped movement disorder (F98.4)*

☑5th **F63.8 Other impulse disorders**
   F63.81 Intermittent explosive disorder
   F63.89 Other impulse disorders

F63.9 Impulse disorder, unspecified
Impulse control disorder NOS

☑4th **F64 Gender identity disorders**
F64.0 Transsexualism
Gender identity disorder in adolescence and adulthood
Gender dysphoria in adolescents and adults

F64.1 Dual role transvestism
Use additional code to identify sex reassignment status (Z87.890)
EXCLUDES 1   *gender identity disorder in childhood (F64.2)*
EXCLUDES 2   *fetishistic transvestism (F65.1)*

F64.2 Gender identity disorder of childhood   P
Gender dysphoria in children
EXCLUDES 1   *gender identity disorder in adolescence and adulthood (F64.0)*
EXCLUDES 2   *sexual maturation disorder (F66)*

F64.8 Other gender identity disorders
▶Other specified gender dysphoria◀

F64.9 Gender identity disorder, unspecified
▶Gender dysphoria, unspecified◀
Gender-role disorder NOS

☑4th **F65 Paraphilias**
F65.0 Fetishism
▶Fetishistic disorder◀

F65.1 Transvestic fetishism
Fetishistic transvestism
▶Transvestic disorder◀

F65.2 Exhibitionism
▶Exhibitionistic disorder◀

F65.3 Voyeurism
▶Voyeuristic disorder◀

F65.4 Pedophilia
▶Pedophilic disorder◀

☑5th **F65.5 Sadomasochism**
   F65.50 Sadomasochism, unspecified
   F65.51 Sexual masochism
▶Sexual masochism disorder◀
   F65.52 Sexual sadism
▶Sexual sadism disorder◀

☑5th **F65.8 Other paraphilias**
   F65.81 Frotteurism
▶Frotteuristic disorder◀
   F65.89 Other paraphilias
Necrophilia
▶Other specified paraphilic disorder◀

F65.9 Paraphilia, unspecified
▶Paraphilic disorder, unspecified◀
Sexual deviation NOS

F66 Other sexual disorders
Sexual maturation disorder
Sexual relationship disorder

☑4th **F68 Other disorders of adult personality and behavior**
☑5th **F68.1 Factitious disorder**
Compensation neurosis
Elaboration of physical symptoms for psychological reasons
Hospital hopper syndrome
Münchhausen's syndrome
Peregrinating patient
EXCLUDES 2   *factitial dermatitis (L98.1)*
person feigning illness (with obvious motivation) (Z76.5)

   F68.10 Factitious disorder, unspecified   CC
CC Excl: PDX collection 551
   F68.11 Factitious disorder with predominantly psychological signs and symptoms
   F68.12 Factitious disorder with predominantly physical signs and symptoms   CC
CC Excl: PDX collection 551
   F68.13 Factitious disorder with combined psychological and physical signs and symptoms

F68.8 Other specified disorders of adult personality and behavior

F69 Unspecified disorder of adult personality and behavior   A

Intellectual Disabilities (F70-F79)

Code first any associated physical or developmental disorders
EXCLUDES 1   *borderline intellectual functioning, IQ above 70 to 84 (R41.83)*

F70 Mild intellectual disabilities
IQ level 50-55 to approximately 70
Mild mental subnormality

F71 Moderate intellectual disabilities
IQ level 35-40 to 50-55
Moderate mental subnormality

F72 Severe intellectual disabilities   CC
IQ 20-25 to 35-40
Severe mental subnormality
CC Excl: PDX collection 558

F73 Profound intellectual disabilities   CC
IQ level below 20-25
Profound mental subnormality
CC Excl: PDX collection 558

F78 Other intellectual disabilities

F79 Unspecified intellectual disabilities
Mental deficiency NOS
Mental subnormality NOS

Pervasive and specific developmental disorders (F80-F89)

☑4th **F80 Specific developmental disorders of speech and language**
F80.0 Phonological disorder
Dyslalia
Functional speech articulation disorder
Lalling
Lisping
Phonological developmental disorder
Speech articulation developmental disorder
Speech-sound disorder
EXCLUDES 1   *speech articulation impairment due to aphasia NOS (R47.01)*
speech articulation impairment due to apraxia (R48.2)
EXCLUDES 2   *speech articulation impairment due to hearing loss (F80.4)*
speech articulation impairment due to intellectual disabilities (F70-F79)
speech articulation impairment with expressive language developmental disorder (F80.1)
speech articulation impairment with mixed receptive expressive language developmental disorder (F80.2)

F80.1 Expressive language disorder
Developmental dysphasia or aphasia, expressive type
EXCLUDES 1   *dysphasia and aphasia NOS (R47.-)*
mixed receptive-expressive language disorder (F80.2)
EXCLUDES 2   *acquired aphasia with epilepsy [Landau-Kleffner] (G40.80-)*
intellectual disabilities (F70-F79)
pervasive developmental disorders (F84.-)
selective mutism (F94.0)

F80.2 Mixed receptive-expressive language disorder
Developmental dysphasia or aphasia, receptive type
Developmental Wernicke's aphasia
EXCLUDES 1   *central auditory processing disorder (H93.25)*
dysphasia or aphasia NOS (R47.-)
expressive language disorder (F80.1)
expressive type dysphasia or aphasia (F80.1)
word deafness (H93.25)
EXCLUDES 2   *acquired aphasia with epilepsy [Landau-Kleffner] (G40.80-)*
intellectual disabilities (F70-F79)
pervasive developmental disorders (F84.-)
selective mutism (F94.0)

N Newborn: 0   P Pediatric: 0-17   M Maternity: 12-55   A Adult: 15-124   MCC Major CC Condition   PDxMCC PDx acts as own MCC   CC CC Condition   PDxCC PDx acts as own CC

F80.4 **Speech and language development delay** due to hearing loss
Code also type of hearing loss (H90.-, H91.-)

√5ᵗʰ **F80.8** Other developmental disorders of speech and language
AHA: 2017, 1Q, 27

     F80.81 **Childhood onset fluency disorder**
Cluttering NOS
Stuttering NOS
EXCLUDES 1   *adult onset fluency disorder (F98.5)*
fluency disorder in conditions classified
elsewhere (R47.82)
fluency disorder (stuttering) following
cerebrovascular disease (I69. with final
characters-23)

     F80.82 **Social pragmatic communication disorder**
EXCLUDES 1   *Asperger's syndrome (F84.5)*
autistic disorder (F84.0)

     F80.89 **Other developmental disorders of speech and language**

     F80.9 **Developmental disorder of speech and language,** unspecified
Communication disorder NOS
Language disorder NOS

√4ᵗʰ **F81** **Specific developmental disorders of scholastic skills**

     F81.0 **Specific reading disorder**
"Backward reading"
Developmental dyslexia
▶Specific learning disorder, with impairment in reading◀
Specific reading retardation
EXCLUDES 1   *alexia NOS (R48.0)*
dyslexia NOS (R48.0)
DEF: Serious impairment of reading skills unexplained in relation
to general intelligence and teaching processes.

     F81.2 **Mathematics disorder**
Developmental acalculia
Developmental arithmetical disorder
Developmental Gerstmann's syndrome
▶Specific learning disorder, with impairment in mathmatics◀
EXCLUDES 1   *acalculia NOS (R48.8)*
EXCLUDES 2   *arithmetical difficulties associated with a reading*
disorder (F81.0)
arithmetical difficulties associated with a spelling
disorder (F81.81)
arithmetical difficulties due to inadequate teaching
(Z55.8)

√5ᵗʰ **F81.8** **Other developmental disorders of scholastic skills**

     F81.81 **Disorder of written expression**
▶Specific learning disorder, with impairment in written
expression◀
Specific spelling disorder

     F81.89 **Other developmental disorders of scholastic skills**

     F81.9 **Developmental disorder of scholastic skills, unspecified**
Knowledge acquisition disability NOS
Learning disability NOS
Learning disorder NOS

F82 **Specific developmental disorder of motor function**
Clumsy child syndrome
Developmental coordination disorder
Developmental dyspraxia
EXCLUDES 1   *abnormalities of gait and mobility (R26.-)*
lack of coordination (R27.-)
EXCLUDES 2   *lack of coordination secondary to intellectual disabilities*
(F70-F79)

√4ᵗʰ **F84** **Pervasive developmental disorders**
Use additional code to identify any associated medical condition and
intellectual disabilities

CC Excl: For CC codes in category F84, unless otherwise noted:
PDX collection 551

     F84.0 **Autistic disorder**   CC
Autism spectrum disorder
Infantile autism
Infantile psychosis
Kanner's syndrome
EXCLUDES 1   *Asperger's syndrome (F84.5)*
AHA: 2017, 1Q, 27

     F84.2 **Rett's syndrome**   CC
EXCLUDES 1   *Asperger's syndrome (F84.5)*
Autistic disorder (F84.0)
Other childhood disintegrative disorder (F84.3)
CC Excl: PDX collection 537

     F84.3 **Other childhood disintegrative disorder**   CC P
Dementia infantilis
Disintegrative psychosis
Heller's syndrome
Symbiotic psychosis
Use additional code to identify any associated neurological
condition
EXCLUDES 1   *Asperger's syndrome (F84.5)*
Autistic disorder (F84.0)
Rett's syndrome (F84.2)

     F84.5 **Asperger's syndrome**   CC
Asperger's disorder
Autistic psychopathy
Schizoid disorder of childhood

     F84.8 **Other pervasive developmental disorders**   CC
Overactive disorder associated with intellectual disabilities
and stereotyped movements

     F84.9 **Pervasive developmental disorder, unspecified**   CC
Atypical autism

F88 **Other disorders of psychological development**
Developmental agnosia
Global development delay
Other specified neurodevelopmental disorder

F89 **Unspecified disorder of psychological development**
Developmental disorder NOS
Neurodevelopmental disorder NOS

Behavioral and emotional disorders with onset usually occurring in childhood and adolescence (F90-F98)

NOTE   Codes within categories F90-F98 may be used regardless of the age
of a patient. These disorders generally have onset within the
childhood or adolescent years, but may continue throughout life or
not be diagnosed until adulthood

√4ᵗʰ **F90** **Attention-deficit hyperactivity disorders**
INCLUDES   attention deficit disorder with hyperactivity
attention deficit syndrome with hyperactivity
EXCLUDES 2   *anxiety disorders (F40.-, F41.-)*
mood [affective] disorders (F30-F39)
pervasive developmental disorders (F84.-)
schizophrenia (F20.-)

     F90.0 **Attention-deficit hyperactivity disorder,** predominantly
inattentive **type**
▶Attention-deficit/hyperactivity disorder, predominantly
inattentive presentation◀

     F90.1 **Attention-deficit hyperactivity disorder,** predominantly
hyperactive **type**
▶Attention-deficit/hyperactivity disorder, predominantly
hyperactive impulsive presentation◀

     F90.2 **Attention-deficit hyperactivity disorder,** combined **type**
▶Attention-deficit/hyperactivity disorder, combined presentation◀

     F90.8 **Attention-deficit hyperactivity disorder,** other **type**

     F90.9 **Attention-deficit hyperactivity disorder,** unspecified **type**
Attention-deficit hyperactivity disorder of childhood or
adolescence NOS
Attention-deficit hyperactivity disorder NOS

√4ᵗʰ **F91** **Conduct disorders**
EXCLUDES 1   *antisocial behavior (Z72.81-)*
antisocial personality disorder (F60.2)
EXCLUDES 2   *conduct problems associated with attention-deficit*
hyperactivity disorder (F90.-)
mood [affective] disorders (F30-F39)
pervasive developmental disorders (F84.-)
schizophrenia (F20.-)

     F91.0 **Conduct disorder** confined to family context

     F91.1 **Conduct disorder,** childhood-onset type
Unsocialized conduct disorder
Conduct disorder, solitary aggressive type
Unsocialized aggressive disorder

     F91.2 **Conduct disorder,** adolescent-onset type
Socialized conduct disorder
Conduct disorder, group type

     F91.3 **Oppositional defiant disorder**

     F91.8 **Other conduct disorders**
Other specified conduct disorder
Other specified disruptive disorder

✓ Additional Character Req   √x7ᵗʰ Placeholder Alert   Unacceptable PDx   Manifestation   H1-H14 HAC   HCC CMS-HCC Condition   *EXCLUDES 1* Not Coded Here   *EXCLUDES 2* Not Included Here

ICD-10-CM 2018   **553**

Chapter 5. Mental, Behavioral and Neurodevelopmental Disorders

F91.9   **Conduct disorder,** unspecified
Behavioral disorder NOS
Conduct disorder NOS
Disruptive behavior disorder NOS
Disruptive disorder NOS

√4ᵗʰ **F93**   **Emotional disorders with onset specific to childhood**

F93.0   **Separation anxiety disorder of childhood**
EXCLUDES 2   *mood [affective] disorders (F30-F39)*
nonpsychotic mental disorders (F40-F48)
phobic anxiety disorder of childhood (F40.8)
social phobia (F40.1)

F93.8   **Other childhood emotional disorders**
Identity disorder
EXCLUDES 2   *gender identity disorder of childhood (F64.2)*

F93.9   **Childhood emotional disorder, unspecified**

√4ᵗʰ **F94**   **Disorders of social functioning with onset specific to childhood and adolescence**

F94.0   **Selective mutism**
Elective mutism
EXCLUDES 2   *pervasive developmental disorders (F84.-)*
schizophrenia (F20.-)
specific developmental disorders of speech and language (F80.-)
transient mutism as part of separation anxiety in young children (F93.0)

F94.1   **Reactive attachment disorder of childhood**
Use additional code to identify any associated failure to thrive or growth retardation
EXCLUDES 1   *disinhibited attachment disorder of childhood (F94.1)*
normal variation in pattern of selective attachment
EXCLUDES 2   *Asperger's syndrome (F84.5)*
maltreatment syndromes (T74.-)
sexual or physical abuse in childhood, resulting in psychosocial problems (Z62.81-)

F94.2   **Disinhibited attachment disorder of childhood**
Affectionless psychopathy
Institutional syndrome
EXCLUDES 1   *reactive attachment disorder of childhood (F94.1)*
EXCLUDES 2   *Asperger's syndrome (F84.5)*
attention-deficit hyperactivity disorders (F90.-)
hospitalism in children (F43.2-)

F94.8   **Other childhood disorders of social functioning**

F94.9   **Childhood disorder of social functioning, unspecified**

√4ᵗʰ **F95**   **Tic disorder**

F95.0   **Transient tic disorder**
Provisional tic disorder

F95.1   **Chronic motor or vocal tic disorder**

F95.2   **Tourette's disorder**
Combined vocal and multiple motor tic disorder [de la Tourette]
Tourette's syndrome

F95.8   **Other tic disorders**

F95.9   **Tic disorder,** unspecified
Tic NOS

√4ᵗʰ **F98**   **Other behavioral and emotional disorders with onset usually occurring in childhood and adolescence**
EXCLUDES 2   *breath-holding spells (R06.89)*
gender identity disorder of childhood (F64.2)
Kleine-Levin syndrome (G47.13)
obsessive-compulsive disorder (F42-)
sleep disorders not due to a substance or known physiological condition (F51.-)

F98.0   **Enuresis not due to a substance or known physiological condition**
Enuresis (primary) (secondary) of nonorganic origin
Functional enuresis
Psychogenic enuresis
Urinary incontinence of nonorganic origin
EXCLUDES 1   *enuresis NOS (R32)*

F98.1   **Encopresis not due to a substance or known physiological condition**
Functional encopresis
Incontinence of feces of nonorganic origin
Psychogenic encopresis
Use additional code to identify the cause of any coexisting constipation
EXCLUDES 1   *encopresis NOS (R15.-)*

√5ᵗʰ **F98.2**   **Other feeding disorders of infancy and childhood**
EXCLUDES 1   *feeding difficulties (R63.3)*
EXCLUDES 2   *anorexia nervosa and other eating disorders (F50.-)*
feeding problems of newborn (P92.-)
pica of infancy or childhood (F98.3)

F98.21   **Rumination disorder of infancy**

F98.29   **Other feeding disorders of infancy and early childhood**

F98.3   **Pica of infancy and childhood**

F98.4   **Stereotyped movement disorders**
Stereotype/habit disorder
EXCLUDES 1   *abnormal involuntary movements (R25.-)*
EXCLUDES 2   *compulsions in obsessive-compulsive disorder (F42-)*
hair plucking (F63.3)
movement disorders of organic origin (G20-G25)
nail-biting (F98.8)
nose-picking (F98.8)
stereotypies that are part of a broader psychiatric condition (F01-F95)
thumb-sucking (F98.8)
tic disorders (F95.-)
trichotillomania (F63.3)

F98.5   **Adult onset fluency disorder**
EXCLUDES 1   *childhood onset fluency disorder (F80.81)*
dysphasia (R47.02)
fluency disorder in conditions classified elsewhere (R47.82)
fluency disorder (stuttering) following cerebrovascular disease (I69. with final characters -23)
tic disorders (F95.-)

F98.8   **Other specified behavioral and emotional disorders with onset usually occurring in childhood and adolescence**
Excessive masturbation
Nail-biting
Nose-picking
Thumb-sucking

F98.9   **Unspecified behavioral and emotional disorders with onset usually occurring in childhood and adolescence**

Unspecified mental disorder (F99)

F99   **Mental disorder, not otherwise specified**
Mental illness NOS
EXCLUDES 1   *unspecified mental disorder due to known physiological condition (F09)*

N Newborn: 0   P Pediatric: 0-17   M Maternity: 12-55   A Adult: 15-124   MCC Major CC Condition   PDx MCC PDx acts as own MCC   CC CC Condition   PDx CC PDx acts as own CC

554   ICD-10-CM 2018

Chapter 6. Diseases of the Nervous System (G00-G99)

Chapter Specific Guidelines with Coding Examples

The chapter specific guidelines from the ICD-10-CM Official Guidelines for Coding and Reporting have been provided below. Along with these guidelines are coding examples, contained in the shaded boxes, that have been developed to help illustrate the coding and/or sequencing guidance found in these guidelines.

a. Dominant/nondominant side

Codes from category G81, Hemiplegia and hemiparesis, and subcategories G83.1, Monoplegia of lower limb, G83.2, Monoplegia of upper limb, and G83.3, Monoplegia, unspecified, identify whether the dominant or nondominant side is affected. Should the affected side be documented, but not specified as dominant or nondominant, and the classification system does not indicate a default, code selection is as follows:

- For ambidextrous patients, the default should be dominant.
- If the left side is affected, the default is non-dominant.
- If the right side is affected, the default is dominant.

> Hemiplegia affecting left side of ambidextrous patient
>
> **G81.92　　Hemiplegia, unspecified affecting left dominant side**
>
> *Explanation*: Documentation states that the left side is affected and dominant is used for ambidextrous persons.

> Right spastic hemiplegia, unknown whether patient is right- or left-handed
>
> **G81.11　　Spastic hemiplegia affecting right dominant side**
>
> *Explanation*: Since it is unknown whether the patient is right- or left-handed, if the right side is affected, the default is dominant.

b. Pain—Category G89

1) General coding information

Codes in category G89, Pain, not elsewhere classified, may be used in conjunction with codes from other categories and chapters to provide more detail about acute or chronic pain and neoplasm-related pain, unless otherwise indicated below.

If the pain is not specified as acute or chronic, post-thoracotomy, postprocedural, or neoplasm-related, do not assign codes from category G89.

A code from category G89 should not be assigned if the underlying (definitive) diagnosis is known, unless the reason for the encounter is pain control/ management and not management of the underlying condition.

When an admission or encounter is for a procedure aimed at treating the underlying condition (e.g., spinal fusion, kyphoplasty), a code for the underlying condition (e.g., vertebral fracture, spinal stenosis) should be assigned as the principal diagnosis. No code from category G89 should be assigned.

> Elderly patient with back pain is admitted for kyphoplasty for age-related osteopathic compression fracture at vertebra T3
>
> **M80.08XA　　Age-related osteoporosis with current pathological fracture, vertebra(e), initial encounter for fracture**
>
> *Explanation*: No code is assigned for the pain as it is inherent in the underlying condition being treated.

(a) Category G89 codes as principal or first-listed diagnosis

Category G89 codes are acceptable as principal diagnosis or the first-listed code:

- When pain control or pain management is the reason for the admission/encounter (e.g., a patient with displaced intervertebral disc, nerve impingement and severe back pain presents for injection of steroid into the spinal canal). The underlying cause of the pain should be reported as an additional diagnosis, if known.

- When a patient is admitted for the insertion of a neurostimulator for pain control, assign the appropriate pain code as the principal or first-listed diagnosis. When an admission or encounter is for a procedure aimed at treating the underlying condition and a neurostimulator is inserted for pain control during the same admission/encounter, a code for the underlying condition should be assigned as the principal diagnosis and the appropriate pain code should be assigned as a secondary diagnosis.

> Patient with chronic pain from lumbar spondylosis with radiculopathy not relieved by surgery is admitted for insertion of neurostimulator.
>
> **G89.29　　Other chronic pain**
>
> **M47.26　　Other spondylosis with radiculopathy, lumbar region**
>
> *Explanation*: Since the patient is admitted specifically for a neurostimulator implantation for pain management and not to treat the underlying spondylosis, the chronic pain code is sequenced first, followed by the underlying condition. Neither code M54.16 nor M54.5 is necessary because M47.26 describes the radiculopathy and the site.

(b) Use of category G89 codes in conjunction with site specific pain codes

(i) Assigning category G89 and site-specific pain codes

Codes from category G89 may be used in conjunction with codes that identify the site of pain (including codes from chapter 18) if the category G89 code provides additional information. For example, if the code describes the site of the pain, but does not fully describe whether the pain is acute or chronic, then both codes should be assigned.

> During hospital stay, patient is seen by orthopaedics to evaluate chronic left shoulder pain.
>
> **M25.512　　Pain in left shoulder**
>
> **G89.29　　Other chronic pain**
>
> *Explanation*: No underlying condition has been determined yet so the pain would be the reason for the visit. The M25 pain code in this instance does not fully describe the condition as it does not represent that the pain is chronic. The G89 chronic pain code is assigned to provide specificity.

(ii) Sequencing of category G89 codes with site-specific pain codes

The sequencing of category G89 codes with site-specific pain codes (including chapter 18 codes), is dependent on the circumstances of the encounter/admission as follows:

- If the encounter is for pain control or pain management, assign the code from category G89 followed by the code identifying the specific site of pain (e.g., encounter for pain management for acute neck pain from trauma is assigned code G89.11, Acute pain due to trauma, followed by code M54.2, Cervicalgia, to identify the site of pain).

> Management of acute, traumatic right knee pain
>
> **G89.11　　Acute pain due to trauma**
>
> **M25.561　　Pain in right knee**
>
> *Explanation*: The reason for the encounter is to manage or control the pain, not to treat or evaluate an underlying condition. The G89 pain code is assigned as the principal diagnosis but in this instance does not fully describe the condition as it does not include the site and laterality. The M25 pain code is added to provide this information.

- If the encounter is for any other reason except pain control or pain management, and a related definitive diagnosis has not been established (confirmed) by the provider, assign the code for the specific site of pain first, followed by the appropriate code from category G89.

Tests are performed to investigate the source of the patient's chronic epigastric abdominal pain

R10.13	**Epigastric pain**
G89.29	**Other chronic pain**

Explanation: In this instance the patient's epigastric pain is not being treated; rather the source of the pain is being investigated. A code from chapter 18 for epigastric pain is sequenced before the additional specificity of the G89 code for the chronic pain.

2) Pain due to devices, implants and grafts
See Section I.C.19. Pain due to medical devices

3) Postoperative Pain
The provider's documentation should be used to guide the coding of postoperative pain, as well as *Section III. Reporting Additional Diagnoses* and *Section IV. Diagnostic Coding and Reporting in the Outpatient Setting.*

The default for post-thoracotomy and other postoperative pain not specified as acute or chronic is the code for the acute form.

Routine or expected postoperative pain immediately after surgery should not be coded.

Pain pump dose is increased for the patient's unexpected, extreme pain post-thoracotomy

G89.12	**Acute post-thoracotomy pain**

Explanation: When acute or chronic is not documented, default to acute. The use of "unexpected, extreme" and the increase of medication dosage indicate that the pain was more than routine or expected.

(a) Postoperative pain not associated with specific postoperative complication
Postoperative pain not associated with a specific postoperative complication is assigned to the appropriate postoperative pain code in category G89.

(b) Postoperative pain associated with specific postoperative complication
Postoperative pain associated with a specific postoperative complication (such as painful wire sutures) is assigned to the appropriate code(s) found in Chapter 19, Injury, poisoning, and certain other consequences of external causes. If appropriate, use additional code(s) from category G89 to identify acute or chronic pain (G89.18 or G89.28).

4) Chronic pain
Chronic pain is classified to subcategory G89.2. There is no time frame defining when pain becomes chronic pain. The provider's documentation should be used to guide use of these codes.

5) Neoplasm related pain
Code G89.3 is assigned to pain documented as being related, associated or due to cancer, primary or secondary malignancy, or tumor. This code is assigned regardless of whether the pain is acute or chronic.

This code may be assigned as the principal or first-listed code when the stated reason for the admission/encounter is documented as pain control/pain management. The underlying neoplasm should be reported as an additional diagnosis.

Pain medication adjustment for chronic pain from bone metastasis

G89.3	**Neoplasm related pain (acute)(chronic)**
C79.51	**Secondary malignant neoplasm of bone**

Explanation: Since the encounter was for pain medication management, the pain, rather than the neoplasm, was the reason for the encounter and is sequenced first. This "neoplasm-related pain" code includes both acute and chronic pain.

When the reason for the admission/encounter is management of the neoplasm and the pain associated with the neoplasm is also documented, code G89.3 may be assigned as an additional diagnosis. It is not necessary to assign an additional code for the site of the pain.

See Section I.C.2 for instructions on the sequencing of neoplasms for all other stated reasons for the admission/encounter (except for pain control/pain management).

Patient with lung cancer presents with acute hip pain and is evaluated and found to have iliac bone metastasis

C79.51	**Secondary malignant neoplasm of bone**
C34.90	**Malignant neoplasm of unspecified part of unspecified bronchus or lung**
G89.3	**Neoplasm related pain (acute)(chronic)**

Explanation: The reason for the encounter was the evaluation and diagnosis of the bone metastasis, whose code would be assigned as first-listed, followed by codes for the primary neoplasm and the pain due to the iliac bone metastasis.

6) Chronic pain syndrome
Central pain syndrome (G89.0) and chronic pain syndrome (G89.4) are different than the term "chronic pain," and therefore codes should only be used when the provider has specifically documented this condition.

See Section I.C.5. Pain disorders related to psychological factors

Chapter 6. Diseases of the Nervous System (G00-G99)

EXCLUDES 2 certain conditions originating in the perinatal period (P04-P96)
certain infectious and parasitic diseases (A00-B99)
complications of pregnancy, childbirth and the puerperium (O00-O9A)
congenital malformations, deformations, and chromosomal abnormalities (Q00-Q99)
endocrine, nutritional and metabolic diseases (E00-E88)
injury, poisoning and certain other consequences of external causes (S00-T88)
neoplasms (C00-D49)
symptoms, signs and abnormal clinical and laboratory findings, not elsewhere classified (R00-R94)

This chapter contains the following blocks:

G00-G09 Inflammatory diseases of the central nervous system
G10-G14 Systemic atrophies primarily affecting the central nervous system
G20-G26 Extrapyramidal and movement disorders
G30-G32 Other degenerative diseases of the nervous system
G35-G37 Demyelinating diseases of the central nervous system
G40-G47 Episodic and paroxysmal disorders
G50-G59 Nerve, nerve root and plexus disorders
G60-G65 Polyneuropathies and other disorders of the peripheral nervous system
G70-G73 Diseases of myoneural junction and muscle
G80-G83 Cerebral palsy and other paralytic syndromes
G89-G99 Other disorders of the nervous system

Inflammatory diseases of the central nervous system (G00-G09)

✓4th G00 Bacterial meningitis, not elsewhere classified

INCLUDES bacterial arachnoiditis
bacterial leptomeningitis
bacterial meningitis
bacterial pachymeningitis

EXCLUDES 1 ▶bacterial meningoencephalitis◄ (G04.2)
▶bacterial meningomyelitis◄ (G04.2)

CC Excl: For MCC codes in category G00: PDX collection 207

G00.0 Hemophilus meningitis MCC
Meningitis due to Hemophilus influenzae

G00.1 Pneumococcal meningitis MCC
Meningitis due to Streptococcal pneumoniae

G00.2 Streptococcal meningitis MCC
Use additional code to further identify organism (B95.0-B95.5)

G00.3 Staphylococcal meningitis MCC
Use additional code to further identify organism (B95.61-B95.8)

G00.8 Other bacterial meningitis MCC
Meningitis due to Escherichia coli
Meningitis due to Friedländer's bacillus
Meningitis due to Klebsiella
Use additional code to further identify organism (B96.-)

G00.9 Bacterial meningitis, unspecified MCC
Meningitis due to gram-negative bacteria, unspecified
Purulent meningitis NOS
Pyogenic meningitis NOS
Suppurative meningitis NOS

G01 Meningitis in bacterial diseases classified elsewhere MCC
Code first underlying disease
EXCLUDES 1 meningitis (in):
gonococcal (A54.81)
leptospirosis (A27.81)
listeriosis (A32.11)
Lyme disease (A69.21)
meningococcal (A39.0)
neurosyphilis (A52.13)
tuberculosis (A17.0)
meningoencephalitis and meningomyelitis in bacterial diseases classified elsewhere (G05)
CC Excl: PDX collection 207

G02 Meningitis in other infectious and parasitic diseases classified elsewhere MCC
Code first underlying disease, such as:
African trypanosomiasis (B56.-)
poliovirus infection (A80.-)
EXCLUDES 1 candidal meningitis (B37.5)
coccidioidomycosis meningitis (B38.4)
cryptococcal meningitis (B45.1)
herpesviral [herpes simplex] meningitis (B00.3)
infectious mononucleosis complicated by meningitis (B27.- with fourth character 2)
measles complicated by meningitis (B05.1)
meningoencephalitis and meningomyelitis in other infectious and parasitic diseases classified elsewhere (G05)
mumps meningitis (B26.1)
rubella meningitis (B06.02)
varicella [chickenpox] meningitis (B01.0)
zoster meningitis (B02.1)
CC Excl: PDX collection 559

✓4th G03 Meningitis due to other and unspecified causes
INCLUDES arachnoiditis NOS
leptomeningitis NOS
meningitis NOS
pachymeningitis NOS
EXCLUDES 1 meningoencephalitis (G04.-)
meningomyelitis (G04.-)

CC Excl: For CC/MCC codes in category G03, unless otherwise noted: PDX collection 207

G03.0 Nonpyogenic meningitis MCC
Aseptic meningitis
Nonbacterial meningitis

G03.1 Chronic meningitis CC

G03.2 Benign recurrent meningitis [Mollaret] CC
CC Excl: PDX collection 140

G03.8 Meningitis due to other specified causes MCC

G03.9 Meningitis, unspecified MCC
Arachnoiditis (spinal) NOS

✓4th G04 Encephalitis, myelitis and encephalomyelitis
INCLUDES acute ascending myelitis
meningoencephalitis
meningomyelitis
EXCLUDES 1 encephalopathy NOS (G93.40)
EXCLUDES 2 acute transverse myelitis (G37.3-)
alcoholic encephalopathy (G31.2)
benign myalgic encephalomyelitis (G93.3)
multiple sclerosis (G35)
subacute necrotizing myelitis (G37.4)
toxic encephalitis (G92)
toxic encephalopathy (G92)

✓5th G04.0 Acute disseminated encephalitis and encephalomyelitis (ADEM)
EXCLUDES 1 acute necrotizing hemorrhagic encephalopathy (G04.3-)
other noninfectious acute disseminated encephalomyelitis (noninfectious ADEM) (G04.81)

G04.00 Acute disseminated encephalitis and encephalomyelitis, unspecified MCC
CC Excl: PDX collection 560

G04.01 Postinfectious acute disseminated encephalitis and encephalomyelitis (postinfectious ADEM) MCC
EXCLUDES 1 post chickenpox encephalitis (B01.1)
post measles encephalitis (B05.0)
post measles myelitis (B05.1)
CC Excl: PDX collection 560

G04.02 Postimmunization acute disseminated encephalitis, myelitis and encephalomyelitis MCC
Encephalitis, postimmunization
Encephalomyelitis, postimmunization
Use additional code to identify the vaccine (T50.A-, T50.B-, T50Z-)
CC Excl: No Excl

G04.1 Tropical spastic paraplegia CC HCC
CC Excl: PDX collection 561

G04.2 Bacterial meningoencephalitis and meningomyelitis, not elsewhere classified MCC
CC Excl: PDX collection 207

Chapter 6. Diseases of the Nervous System

✓5ᵗʰ **G04.3 Acute necrotizing hemorrhagic encephalopathy**
EXCLUDES 1   acute disseminated encephalitis and encephalomyelitis (G04.0-)

G04.30 Acute necrotizing hemorrhagic encephalopathy, unspecified   MCC
CC Excl: No Excl

G04.31 Postinfectious acute necrotizing hemorrhagic encephalopathy   MCC
CC Excl: PDX collection 560

G04.32 Postimmunization acute necrotizing hemorrhagic encephalopathy   MCC
Use additional code to identify the vaccine (T50.A-, T50.B-, T50Z-)
CC Excl: No Excl

G04.39 Other acute necrotizing hemorrhagic encephalopathy   MCC
Code also underlying etiology, if applicable
CC Excl: No Excl

✓5ᵗʰ **G04.8 Other encephalitis, myelitis and encephalomyelitis**
Code also any associated seizure (G40.-, R56.9)

G04.81 Other encephalitis and encephalomyelitis   HIV MCC
Noninfectious acute disseminated encephalomyelitis (noninfectious ADEM)
CC Excl: PDX collection 560

G04.89 Other myelitis   HIV MCC HCC
CC Excl: PDX collection 560

✓5ᵗʰ **G04.9 Encephalitis, myelitis and encephalomyelitis, unspecified**

G04.90 Encephalitis and encephalomyelitis, unspecified   HIV MCC
Ventriculitis (cerebral) NOS
CC Excl: PDX collection 562

G04.91 Myelitis, unspecified   HIV MCC HCC
CC Excl: PDX collection 562

✓4ᵗʰ **G05 Encephalitis, myelitis and encephalomyelitis in diseases classified elsewhere**
Code first underlying disease, such as:
human immunodeficiency virus [HIV] disease (B20)
poliovirus (A80.-)
suppurative otitis media (H66.01-H66.4)
trichinellosis (B75)
EXCLUDES 1   adenoviral encephalitis, myelitis and encephalomyelitis (A85.1)
congenital toxoplasmosis encephalitis, myelitis and encephalomyelitis (P37.1)
cytomegaloviral encephalitis, myelitis and encephalomyelitis (B25.8)
encephalitis, myelitis and encephalomyelitis (in) measles (B05.0)
encephalitis, myelitis and encephalomyelitis (in) systemic lupus erythematosus (M32.19)
enteroviral encephalitis, myelitis and encephalomyelitis (A85.0)
eosinophilic meningoencephalitis (B83.2)
herpesviral [herpes simplex] encephalitis, myelitis and encephalomyelitis (B00.4)
listerial encephalitis, myelitis and encephalomyelitis (A32.12)
meningococcal encephalitis, myelitis and encephalomyelitis (A39.81)
mumps encephalitis, myelitis and encephalomyelitis (B26.2)
postchickenpox encephalitis, myelitis and encephalomyelitis (B01.1-)
rubella encephalitis, myelitis and encephalomyelitis (B06.01)
toxoplasmosis encephalitis, myelitis and encephalomyelitis (B58.2)
zoster encephalitis, myelitis and encephalomyelitis (B02.0)

G05.3 Encephalitis and encephalomyelitis in diseases classified elsewhere   MCC
Meningoencephalitis in diseases classified elsewhere
CC Excl: PDX collection 560

G05.4 Myelitis in diseases classified elsewhere   MCC HCC
Meningomyelitis in diseases classified elsewhere
CC Excl: PDX collection 560

✓4ᵗʰ **G06 Intracranial and intraspinal abscess and granuloma**
Use additional code (B95-B97) to identify infectious agent

G06.0 Intracranial abscess and granuloma   MCC
Brain [any part] abscess (embolic)
Cerebellar abscess (embolic)
Cerebral abscess (embolic)
Intracranial epidural abscess or granuloma
Intracranial extradural abscess or granuloma
Intracranial subdural abscess or granuloma
Otogenic abscess (embolic)
EXCLUDES 1   tuberculous intracranial abscess and granuloma (A17.81)
CC Excl: PDX collection 563

G06.1 Intraspinal abscess and granuloma   MCC
Abscess (embolic) of spinal cord [any part]
Intraspinal epidural abscess or granuloma
Intraspinal extradural abscess or granuloma
Intraspinal subdural abscess or granuloma
EXCLUDES 1   tuberculous intraspinal abscess and granuloma (A17.81)
CC Excl: PDX collection 564

G06.2 Extradural and subdural abscess, unspecified   MCC
CC Excl: PDX collection 565

G07 Intracranial and intraspinal abscess and granuloma in diseases classified elsewhere   MCC
Code first underlying disease, such as:
schistosomiasis granuloma of brain (B65.-)
EXCLUDES 1   abscess of brain:
amebic (A06.6)
chromomycotic (B43.1)
gonococcal (A54.82)
tuberculous (A17.81)
tuberculoma of meninges (A17.1)
CC Excl: PDX collection 565

G08 Intracranial and intraspinal phlebitis and thrombophlebitis   MCC
Septic embolism of intracranial or intraspinal venous sinuses and veins
Septic endophlebitis of intracranial or intraspinal venous sinuses and veins
Septic phlebitis of intracranial or intraspinal venous sinuses and veins
Septic thrombophlebitis of intracranial or intraspinal venous sinuses and veins
Septic thrombosis of intracranial or intraspinal venous sinuses and veins
EXCLUDES 1   intracranial phlebitis and thrombophlebitis complicating:
abortion, ectopic or molar pregnancy (O00-O07, O08.7)
pregnancy, childbirth and the puerperium (O22.5, O87.3)
nonpyogenic intracranial phlebitis and thrombophlebitis (I67.6)
EXCLUDES 2   intracranial phlebitis and thrombophlebitis complicating nonpyogenic intraspinal phlebitis and thrombophlebitis (G95.1)
DEF: Inflammation and formation of blood clot in a vein within the brain or spine, or their linings.
CC Excl: PDX collection 565

G09 Sequelae of inflammatory diseases of central nervous system
NOTE   Category G09 is to be used to indicate conditions whose primary classification is to G00-G08 as the cause of sequelae, themselves classifiable elsewhere. The "sequelae" include conditions specified as residuals.
Code first condition resulting from (sequela) of inflammatory diseases of central nervous system

Systemic atrophies primarily affecting the central nervous system (G10-G14)

G10 Huntington's disease   CC HCC
Huntington's chorea
Huntington's dementia
▶Code also dementia in other diseases classified elsewhere without behavioral disturbance (F02.80)◀
DEF: Genetic disease caused by degeneration of nerve cells in the brain, characterized by chronic progressive mental deterioration; dementia and death within 15 to 20 years of onset.
CC Excl: PDX collection 566

✓4ᵗʰ **G11 Hereditary ataxia**
EXCLUDES 2   cerebral palsy (G80.-)
hereditary and idiopathic neuropathy (G60.-)
metabolic disorders (E70-E88)

CC Excl: For CC codes in category G11, unless otherwise noted: PDX collection 567

G11.0 Congenital nonprogressive ataxia   CC HCC

N Newborn: 0   P Pediatric: 0-17   M Maternity: 12-55   A Adult: 15-124   MCC Major CC Condition   PDxMCC PDx acts as own MCC   CC CC Condition   PDxCC PDx acts as own CC

558   ICD-10-CM 2018

G11.1 Early-onset cerebellar ataxia `CC` `HCC`
Early-onset cerebellar ataxia with essential tremor
Early-onset cerebellar ataxia with myoclonus [Hunt's ataxia]
Early-onset cerebellar ataxia with retained tendon reflexes
Friedreich's ataxia (autosomal recessive)
X-linked recessive spinocerebellar ataxia

G11.2 Late-onset cerebellar ataxia `CC` `HCC` `A`

G11.3 Cerebellar ataxia with defective DNA repair `CC` `HCC`
Ataxia telangiectasia [Louis-Bar]
EXCLUDES 2   *Cockayne's syndrome (Q87.1)*
other disorders of purine and pyrimidine metabolism (E79.-)
xeroderma pigmentosum (Q82.1)

G11.4 Hereditary spastic paraplegia `CC` `HCC`
CC Excl: PDX collection 568

G11.8 Other hereditary ataxias `CC` `HCC`

G11.9 Hereditary ataxia, unspecified `CC` `HCC`
Hereditary cerebellar ataxia NOS
Hereditary cerebellar degeneration
Hereditary cerebellar disease
Hereditary cerebellar syndrome
CC Excl: PDX collection 569

✓4ᵗʰ G12 Spinal muscular atrophy and related syndromes

> **CC Excl: For CC codes in category G12:** PDX collection 570

G12.0 Infantile spinal muscular atrophy, type I [Werdnig-Hoffman] `CC` `HCC`

G12.1 Other inherited spinal muscular atrophy `CC` `HCC`
Adult form spinal muscular atrophy
Childhood form, type II spinal muscular atrophy
Distal spinal muscular atrophy
Juvenile form, type III spinal muscular atrophy [Kugelberg-Welander]
Progressive bulbar palsy of childhood [Fazio-Londe]
Scapuloperoneal form spinal muscular atrophy

✓5ᵗʰ G12.2 Motor neuron disease

    G12.20 Motor neuron disease, unspecified `CC` `HCC`

    G12.21 Amyotrophic lateral sclerosis `CC` `HCC` `A`
~~Progressive spinal muscle atrophy~~

    G12.22 Progressive bulbar palsy `CC` `HCC`

●   **G12.23 Primary lateral sclerosis** `CC`

●   **G12.24 Familial motor neuron disease** `CC`

●   **G12.25 Progressive spinal muscle atrophy** `CC`

    G12.29 Other motor neuron disease `CC` `HCC`
~~Familial motor neuron disease~~
~~Primary lateral sclerosis~~

G12.8 Other spinal muscular atrophies and related syndromes `CC` `HCC`

G12.9 Spinal muscular atrophy, unspecified `CC` `HCC`

✓4ᵗʰ G13 Systemic atrophies primarily affecting central nervous system in diseases classified elsewhere

G13.0 Paraneoplastic neuromyopathy and neuropathy `HCC`
Carcinomatous neuromyopathy
Sensorial paraneoplastic neuropathy [Denny Brown]
Code first underlying neoplasm (C00-D49)

G13.1 Other systemic atrophy primarily affecting central nervous system in neoplastic disease `HCC`
Paraneoplastic limbic encephalopathy
Code first underlying neoplasm (C00-D49)

G13.2 Systemic atrophy primarily affecting the central nervous system in myxedema
Code first underlying disease, such as:
hypothyroidism (E03.-)
myxedematous congenital iodine deficiency (E00.1)

G13.8 Systemic atrophy primarily affecting central nervous system in other diseases classified elsewhere
Code first underlying disease

G14 Postpolio syndrome
INCLUDES   postpolio myelitic syndrome
EXCLUDES 1   *sequelae of poliomyelitis (B91)*

Extrapyramidal and movement disorders (G20-G26)

G20 Parkinson's disease `HCC`
Hemiparkinsonism
Idiopathic Parkinsonism or Parkinson's disease
Paralysis agitans
Parkinsonism or Parkinson's disease NOS
Primary Parkinsonism or Parkinson's disease
EXCLUDES 1   *dementia with Parkinsonism (G31.83)*
AHA: 2017, 2Q, 7; 2016, 2Q, 6

✓4ᵗʰ G21 Secondary parkinsonism
EXCLUDES 1   *dementia with Parkinsonism (G31.83)*
Huntington's disease (G10)
Shy-Drager syndrome (G90.3)
syphilitic Parkinsonism (A52.19)

> **CC Excl: For CC codes in category G21, unless otherwise noted:** PDX collection 572

G21.0 Malignant neuroleptic syndrome `MCC`
Use additional code for adverse effect, if applicable, to identify drug (T43.3X5, T43.4X5, T43.505, T43.595)
EXCLUDES 1   *neuroleptic induced parkinsonism (G21.11)*
CC Excl: PDX collection 571

✓5ᵗʰ G21.1 Other drug-induced secondary parkinsonism

    G21.11 Neuroleptic induced parkinsonism `CC` `HCC`
Use additional code for adverse effect, if applicable, to identify drug (T43.3X5, T43.4X5, T43.505, T43.595)
EXCLUDES 1   *malignant neuroleptic syndrome (G21.0)*

    G21.19 Other drug induced secondary parkinsonism `CC` `HCC`
▶Other medication-induced parkinsonism◀
Use additional code for adverse effect, if applicable, to identify drug (T36-T50 with fifth or sixth character 5)

G21.2 Secondary parkinsonism due to other external agents `CC` `HCC`
Code first (T51-T65) to identify external agent

G21.3 Postencephalitic parkinsonism `CC` `HCC`

G21.4 Vascular parkinsonism `HCC`

G21.8 Other secondary parkinsonism `CC` `HCC`

G21.9 Secondary parkinsonism, unspecified `CC` `HCC`

✓4ᵗʰ G23 Other degenerative diseases of basal ganglia
EXCLUDES 2   *multi-system degeneration of the autonomic nervous system (G90.3)*

> **CC Excl: For CC codes in category G23:** PDX collection 573

G23.0 Hallervorden-Spatz disease `CC` `HCC`
Pigmentary pallidal degeneration

G23.1 Progressive supranuclear ophthalmoplegia [Steele-Richardson-Olszewski] `CC` `HCC`
Progressive supranuclear palsy

G23.2 Striatonigral degeneration `CC` `HCC`

G23.8 Other specified degenerative diseases of basal ganglia `CC` `HCC`
Calcification of basal ganglia

G23.9 Degenerative disease of basal ganglia, unspecified `CC` `HCC`

✓4ᵗʰ G24 Dystonia
INCLUDES   dyskinesia
EXCLUDES 2   *athetoid cerebral palsy (G80.3)*

> **CC Excl: For CC codes in category G24:** PDX collection 574

✓5ᵗʰ G24.0 Drug induced dystonia
Use additional code for adverse effect, if applicable, to identify drug (T36-T50 with fifth or sixth character5)

    G24.01 Drug induced subacute dyskinesia
Drug induced blepharospasm
Drug induced orofacial dyskinesia
Neuroleptic induced tardive dyskinesia
Tardive dyskinesia

    G24.02 Drug induced acute dystonia `CC`
Acute dystonic reaction to drugs
Neuroleptic induced acute dystonia

    G24.09 Other drug induced dystonia `CC`

G24.1 Genetic torsion dystonia
Dystonia deformans progressiva
Dystonia musculorum deformans
Familial torsion dystonia
Idiopathic familial dystonia
Idiopathic (torsion) dystonia NOS
(Schwalbe-) Ziehen-Oppenheim disease

✓ Additional Character Req   ✓x7ᵗʰ Placeholder Alert   Unacceptable PDx   Manifestation   `H1`-`H14` HAC   `HCC` CMS-HCC Condition   *EXCLUDES 1* Not Coded Here   *EXCLUDES 2* Not Included Here

ICD-10-CM 2018   559

Chapter 6. Diseases of the Nervous System

G24.2 **Idiopathic nonfamilial dystonia** `CC`

G24.3 **Spasmodic torticollis**
> EXCLUDES 1 congenital torticollis (Q68.0)
> hysterical torticollis (F44.4)
> ocular torticollis (R29.891)
> psychogenic torticollis (F45.8)
> torticollis NOS (M43.6)
> traumatic recurrent torticollis (S13.4)

G24.4 **Idiopathic orofacial dystonia**
> Orofacial dyskinesia
> EXCLUDES 1 drug induced orofacial dyskinesia (G24.01)

G24.5 **Blepharospasm**
> EXCLUDES 1 drug induced blepharospasm (G24.01)

G24.8 **Other dystonia** `CC`
> Acquired torsion dystonia NOS

G24.9 **Dystonia, unspecified**
> Dyskinesia NOS

✓4ᵗʰ G25 **Other extrapyramidal and movement disorders**
> EXCLUDES 2 sleep related movement disorders (G47.6-)

G25.0 **Essential tremor**
> Familial tremor
> EXCLUDES 1 tremor NOS (R25.1)

G25.1 **Drug-induced tremor**
> Use additional code for adverse effect, if applicable, to identify drug (T36-T50 with fifth or sixth character 5)

G25.2 **Other specified forms of tremor**
> Intention tremor

G25.3 **Myoclonus**
> Drug-induced myoclonus
> Palatal myoclonus
> Use additional code for adverse effect, if applicable, to identify drug (T36-T50 with fifth or sixth character 5)
> EXCLUDES 1 facial myokymia (G51.4)
> myoclonic epilepsy (G40.-)

G25.4 **Drug-induced chorea**
> Use additional code for adverse effect, if applicable, to identify drug (T36-T50 with fifth or sixth character 5)

G25.5 **Other chorea**
> Chorea NOS
> EXCLUDES 1 chorea NOS with heart involvement (I02.0)
> Huntington's chorea (G10)
> rheumatic chorea (I02.-)
> Sydenham's chorea (I02.-)

✓5ᵗʰ G25.6 **Drug induced tics and other tics of organic origin**

G25.61 **Drug induced tics**
> Use additional code for adverse effect, if applicable, to identify drug (T36-T50 with fifth or sixth character 5)

G25.69 **Other tics of organic origin**
> EXCLUDES 1 habit spasm (F95.9)
> tic NOS (F95.9)
> Tourette's syndrome (F95.2)

✓5ᵗʰ G25.7 **Other and unspecified drug induced movement disorders**
> Use additional code for adverse effect, if applicable, to identify drug (T36-T50 with fifth or sixth character 5)

G25.70 **Drug induced movement disorder, unspecified**

G25.71 **Drug induced akathisia**
> Drug induced acathisia
> Neuroleptic induced acute akathisia
> ►Tardive akathisia◄

G25.79 **Other drug induced movement disorders**

✓5ᵗʰ G25.8 **Other specified extrapyramidal and movement disorders**

G25.81 **Restless legs syndrome**
> DEF: Neurological disorder of unknown etiology creating an irresistible urge to move the legs, which may temporarily relieve the symptoms; is accompanied by motor restlessness and sensations of pain, burning, prickling, or tingling.

G25.82 **Stiff-man syndrome** `CC`
> CC Excl: PDX collection 575

G25.83 **Benign shuddering attacks**

G25.89 **Other specified extrapyramidal and movement disorders**

G25.9 **Extrapyramidal and movement disorder, unspecified** `CC`
> CC Excl: PDX collection 575

G26 *Extrapyramidal and movement disorders in diseases classified elsewhere*
> Code first underlying disease

Other degenerative diseases of the nervous system (G30-G32)

✓4ᵗʰ G30 **Alzheimer's disease**
> INCLUDES Alzheimer's dementia senile and presenile forms
> Use additional code to identify:
> delirium, if applicable (F05)
> dementia with behavioral disturbance (F02.81)
> dementia without behavioral disturbance (F02.80)
> EXCLUDES 1 senile degeneration of brain NEC (G31.1)
> senile dementia NOS (F03)
> senility NOS (R41.81)
> **AHA:** 2017, 1Q, 43

G30.0 **Alzheimer's disease with early onset**

G30.1 **Alzheimer's disease with late onset** `A`

G30.8 **Other Alzheimer's disease**

G30.9 **Alzheimer's disease, unspecified**
> **AHA:** 2016, 2Q, 6; 2012, 4Q, 95

✓4ᵗʰ G31 **Other degenerative diseases of nervous system, not elsewhere classified**
> Use additional code to identify:
> dementia with behavioral disturbance (F02.81)
> dementia without behavioral disturbance (F02.80)
> EXCLUDES 2 Reye's syndrome (G93.7)

✓5ᵗʰ G31.0 **Frontotemporal dementia**

G31.01 **Pick's disease**
> Primary progressive aphasia
> Progressive isolated aphasia
> DEF: A progressive frontotemporal dementia with asymmetrical atrophy of the frontal and temporal regions of the cerebral cortex, abnormal rounded brain cells called Pick cells with the presence of abnormal staining of protein (called tau); symptoms include prominent apathy, behavioral changes such as disinhibition and restlessness, echolalia, impairment of language, memory, and intellect, increased carelessness, poor personal hygiene, and decreased attention span.

G31.09 **Other frontotemporal dementia**
> Frontal dementia

G31.1 **Senile degeneration of brain, not elsewhere classified**
> EXCLUDES 1 Alzheimer's disease (G30.-)
> senility NOS (R41.81)

G31.2 **Degeneration of nervous system due to alcohol**
> Alcoholic cerebellar ataxia
> Alcoholic cerebellar degeneration
> Alcoholic cerebral degeneration
> Alcoholic encephalopathy
> Dysfunction of the autonomic nervous system due to alcohol
> Code also associated alcoholism (F10.-)

✓5ᵗʰ G31.8 **Other specified degenerative diseases of nervous system**

> **CC Excl: For CC codes in subcategory G31.8:** PDX collection 537

G31.81 **Alpers disease** `CC`
> Grey-matter degeneration

G31.82 **Leigh's disease** `CC`
> Subacute necrotizing encephalopathy

G31.83 **Dementia with Lewy bodies**
> Dementia with Parkinsonism
> Lewy body disease
> Lewy body dementia
> **AHA:** 2017, 2Q, 7; 2016, 4Q, 141
> DEF: A cerebral dementia with neurophysiologic changes, increased hippocampal volume, hypoperfusion in the occipital lobes, beta amyloid deposits with neurofibrillary tangles, and atrophy of cortex and brainstem. Hallmark neuropsychological characteristics include fluctuating cognition with pronounced variation in attention and alertness; recurrent hallucinations; and Parkinsonism.

N Newborn: 0   P Pediatric: 0-17   M Maternity: 12-55   A Adult: 15-124   MCC Major CC Condition   PDxMCC PDx acts as own MCC   CC CC Condition   PDxCC PDx acts as own CC

560   ICD-10-CM 2018

G31.84 Mild cognitive impairment, so stated
► Mild neurocognitive disorder◄
EXCLUDES 1 *age related cognitive decline (R41.81)*
altered mental status (R41.82)
cerebral degeneration (G31.9)
change in mental status (R41.82)
cognitive deficits following (sequelae of)
cerebral hemorrhage or infarction
(I69.01-, I69.11-, I69.21-, I69.31-, I69.81-,
I69.91-)
cognitive impairment due to intracranial or
head injury (S06.-)
dementia (F01.-, F02.-, F03)
mild memory disturbance (F06.8)
neurologic neglect syndrome (R41.4)
personality change, nonpsychotic (F68.8)

G31.85 Corticobasal degeneration

G31.89 Other specified degenerative diseases of nervous system

G31.9 Degenerative disease of nervous system, unspecified

✓4th **G32 Other degenerative disorders of nervous system in diseases classified elsewhere**

G32.0 Subacute combined degeneration of spinal cord in CC HCC
diseases classified elsewhere
Dana-Putnam syndrome
Sclerosis of spinal cord (combined) (dorsolateral) (posterolateral)
Code first underlying disease, such as:
anemia (D51.9)
dietary (D51.3)
pernicious (D51.0)
vitamin B12 deficiency (E53.8)
EXCLUDES 1 *syphilitic combined degeneration of spinal cord*
(A52.11)
CC Excl: PDX collection 576

✓5th **G32.8 Other specified degenerative disorders of nervous system in diseases classified elsewhere**
Code first underlying disease, such as:
amyloidosis cerebral degeneration (E85.-)
cerebral degeneration (due to) hypothyroidism (E00.0-E03.9)
cerebral degeneration (due to) neoplasm (C00-D49)
cerebral degeneration (due to) vitamin B deficiency, except thiamine (E52-E53.-)
EXCLUDES 1 *superior hemorrhagic polioencephalitis [Wernicke's*
encephalopathy] (E51.2)

G32.81 Cerebellar ataxia in diseases classified CC HCC
elsewhere
Code first underlying disease, such as:
celiac disease (with gluten ataxia) (K90.0)
cerebellar ataxia (in) neoplastic disease (para-neoplastic cerebellar degeneration) (C00-D49)
non-celiac gluten ataxia (M35.9)
EXCLUDES 1 *systemic atrophy primarily affecting the*
central nervous system in alcoholic
cerebellar ataxia (G31.2)
systemic atrophy primarily affecting the
central nervous system in myxedema
(G13.2)
CC Excl: PDX collection 567

G32.89 Other specified degenerative disorders of nervous system in diseases classified elsewhere
Degenerative encephalopathy in diseases classified elsewhere

Demyelinating diseases of the central nervous system (G35-G37)

G35 Multiple sclerosis HCC
Disseminated multiple sclerosis
Generalized multiple sclerosis
Multiple sclerosis NOS
Multiple sclerosis of brain stem
Multiple sclerosis of cord

✓4th **G36 Other acute disseminated demyelination**
EXCLUDES 1 *postinfectious encephalitis and encephalomyelitis NOS*
(G04.01)

CC Excl: For CC codes in category G36, unless otherwise noted:
PDX collection 578

G36.0 Neuromyelitis optica [Devic] CC HCC
Demyelination in optic neuritis
EXCLUDES 1 *optic neuritis NOS (H46)*
CC Excl: PDX collection 577

G36.1 Acute and subacute hemorrhagic leukoencephalitis CC HCC
[Hurst]

G36.8 Other specified acute disseminated demyelination CC HCC

G36.9 Acute disseminated demyelination, unspecified HIV CC HCC

✓4th **G37 Other demyelinating diseases of central nervous system**

G37.0 Diffuse sclerosis of central nervous system CC HCC
Periaxial encephalitis
Schilder's disease
EXCLUDES 1 *X linked adrenoleukodystrophy (E71.52-)*
CC Excl: PDX collection 579

G37.1 Central demyelination of corpus callosum CC HCC
CC Excl: PDX collection 578

G37.2 Central pontine myelinolysis CC HCC
CC Excl: PDX collection 578

G37.3 Acute transverse myelitis in demyelinating disease of CC HCC
central nervous system
Acute transverse myelitis NOS
Acute transverse myelopathy
EXCLUDES 1 *multiple sclerosis (G35)*
neuromyelitis optica [Devic] (G36.0)
CC Excl: PDX collection 580

G37.4 Subacute necrotizing myelitis of central nervous HIV MCC HCC
system
CC Excl: PDX collection 562

G37.5 Concentric sclerosis [Balo] of central nervous system CC HCC
CC Excl: PDX collection 579

G37.8 Other specified demyelinating diseases of central CC HCC
nervous system
CC Excl: PDX collection 578

G37.9 Demyelinating disease of central nervous system, HIV CC HCC
unspecified
CC Excl: PDX collection 578

Episodic and paroxysmal disorders (G40-G47)

✓4th **G40 Epilepsy and recurrent seizures**
NOTE The following terms are to be considered equivalent to intractable: pharmacoresistant (pharmacologically resistant), treatment resistant, refractory (medically) and poorly controlled
EXCLUDES 1 *conversion disorder with seizures (F44.5)*
convulsions NOS (R56.9)
post traumatic seizures (R56.1)
seizure (convulsive) NOS (R56.9)
seizure of newborn (P90)
EXCLUDES 2 *hippocampal sclerosis (G93.81)*
mesial temporal sclerosis (G93.81)
temporal sclerosis (G93.81)
Todd's paralysis (G83.84)

✓5th **G40.0 Localization-related (focal) (partial) idiopathic epilepsy and epileptic syndromes with seizures of localized onset**
Benign childhood epilepsy with centrotemporal EEG spikes
Childhood epilepsy with occipital EEG paroxysms
EXCLUDES 1 *adult onset localization-related epilepsy*
(G40.1-, G40.2-)

✓6th **G40.00 Localization-related (focal) (partial) idiopathic epilepsy and epileptic syndromes with seizures of localized onset, not intractable**
Localization-related (focal) (partial) idiopathic epilepsy and epileptic syndromes with seizures of localized onset without intractability

CC Excl: For CC codes in subcategory G40.00, unless otherwise noted: PDX collection 581

G40.001 Localization-related (focal) CC HCC
(partial) idiopathic epilepsy and epileptic syndromes with seizures of localized onset, not intractable, with status epilepticus

G40.009 Localization-related (focal) CC HCC
(partial) idiopathic epilepsy and epileptic syndromes with seizures of localized onset, not intractable, without status epilepticus
Localization-related (focal) (partial) idiopathic epilepsy and epileptic syndromes with seizures of localized onset NOS

✓ Additional Character Req ✓x7th Placeholder Alert Unacceptable PDx Manifestation **H1 -H14** HAC **HCC** CMS-HCC Condition *EXCLUDES 1* Not Coded Here *EXCLUDES 2* Not Included Here

ICD-10-CM 2018 **561**

✓6th **G40.01** **Localization-related (focal) (partial) idiopathic epilepsy and epileptic syndromes with seizures of localized onset**, intractable

> **CC Excl: For CC codes in subcategory G40.01:**
> PDX collection 582

    G40.011 **Localization-related (focal)** `CC` `HCC` **(partial) idiopathic epilepsy and epileptic syndromes with seizures of localized onset, intractable, with status epilepticus**

    G40.019 **Localization-related (focal)** `CC` `HCC` **(partial) idiopathic epilepsy and epileptic syndromes with seizures of localized onset, intractable, without status epilepticus**

✓5th **G40.1** **Localization-related (focal) (partial) symptomatic epilepsy and epileptic syndromes** with simple partial seizures
> Attacks without alteration of consciousness
> Epilepsia partialis continua [Kozhevnikof]
> Simple partial seizures developing into secondarily generalized seizures

✓6th **G40.10** **Localization-related (focal) (partial) symptomatic epilepsy and epileptic syndromes with simple partial seizures,** not intractable
> Localization-related (focal) (partial) symptomatic epilepsy and epileptic syndromes with simple partial seizures without intractability

> **CC Excl: For CC codes in subcategory G40.10:**
> PDX collection 581

    G40.101 **Localization-related (focal)** `CC` `HCC` **(partial) symptomatic epilepsy and epileptic syndromes with simple partial seizures, not intractable, with status epilepticus**

    G40.109 **Localization-related (focal)** `CC` `HCC` **(partial) symptomatic epilepsy and epileptic syndromes with simple partial seizures, not intractable, without status epilepticus**
> Localization-related (focal) (partial) symptomatic epilepsy and epileptic syndromes with simple partial seizures NOS

✓6th **G40.11** **Localization-related (focal) (partial) symptomatic epilepsy and epileptic syndromes with simple partial seizures,** intractable

> **CC Excl: For CC codes in subcategory G40.11:**
> PDX collection 582

    G40.111 **Localization-related (focal)** `CC` `HCC` **(partial) symptomatic epilepsy and epileptic syndromes with simple partial seizures, intractable, with status epilepticus**

    G40.119 **Localization-related (focal)** `CC` `HCC` **(partial) symptomatic epilepsy and epileptic syndromes with simple partial seizures, intractable, without status epilepticus**

✓5th **G40.2** **Localization-related (focal) (partial) symptomatic epilepsy and epileptic syndromes** with complex partial seizures
> Attacks with alteration of consciousness, often with automatisms
> Complex partial seizures developing into secondarily generalized seizures

✓6th **G40.20** **Localization-related (focal) (partial) symptomatic epilepsy and epileptic syndromes with complex partial seizures,** not intractable
> Localization-related (focal) (partial) symptomatic epilepsy and epileptic syndromes with complex partial seizures without intractability

> **CC Excl: For CC codes in subcategory G40.20:**
> PDX collection 581

    G40.201 **Localization-related (focal)** `CC` `HCC` **(partial) symptomatic epilepsy and epileptic syndromes with complex partial seizures, not intractable, with status epilepticus**

    G40.209 **Localization-related (focal)** `CC` `HCC` **(partial) symptomatic epilepsy and epileptic syndromes with complex partial seizures, not intractable,** without status epilepticus
> Localization-related (focal) (partial) symptomatic epilepsy and epileptic syndromes with complex partial seizures NOS

✓6th **G40.21** **Localization-related (focal) (partial) symptomatic epilepsy and epileptic syndromes with complex partial seizures,** intractable

> **CC Excl: For CC codes in subcategory G40.21:**
> PDX collection 582

    G40.211 **Localization-related (focal)** `CC` `HCC` **(partial) symptomatic epilepsy and epileptic syndromes with complex partial seizures, intractable, with status epilepticus**

    G40.219 **Localization-related (focal)** `CC` `HCC` **(partial) symptomatic epilepsy and epileptic syndromes with complex partial seizures, intractable, without status epilepticus**

✓5th **G40.3** Generalized **idiopathic epilepsy and epileptic syndromes**
> Code also MERRF syndrome, if applicable (E88.42)

> **CC Excl: For MCC codes in subcategory G40.3:**
> PDX collection 583

✓6th **G40.30** **Generalized idiopathic epilepsy and epileptic syndromes,** not intractable
> Generalized idiopathic epilepsy and epileptic syndromes without intractability

    G40.301 **Generalized idiopathic epilepsy** `MCC` `HCC` **and epileptic syndromes, not intractable,** with status epilepticus

    G40.309 **Generalized idiopathic epilepsy and** `HCC` **epileptic syndromes, not intractable,** without status epilepticus
> Generalized idiopathic epilepsy and epileptic syndromes NOS

✓6th **G40.31** **Generalized idiopathic epilepsy and epileptic syndromes,** intractable

    G40.311 **Generalized idiopathic epilepsy** `MCC` `HCC` **and epileptic syndromes, intractable,** with status epilepticus

    G40.319 **Generalized idiopathic epilepsy** `MCC` `HCC` **and epileptic syndromes, intractable,** without status epilepticus

✓5th **G40.A** **Absence epileptic syndrome**
> Childhood absence epilepsy [pyknolepsy]
> Juvenile absence epilepsy
> Absence epileptic syndrome, NOS

> **CC Excl: For CC codes in subcategory G40.A:**
> PDX collection 582

✓6th **G40.A0** **Absence epileptic syndrome,** not intractable

    G40.A01 **Absence epileptic syndrome, not** `HCC` **intractable,** with status epilepticus

    G40.A09 **Absence epileptic syndrome, not** `HCC` **intractable,** without status epilepticus

✓6th **G40.A1** **Absence epileptic syndrome,** intractable

    G40.A11 **Absence epileptic syndrome,** `CC` `HCC` **intractable,** with status epilepticus

    G40.A19 **Absence epileptic syndrome,** `CC` `HCC` **intractable,** without status epilepticus

✓5th **G40.B** Juvenile myoclonic epilepsy **[impulsive petit mal]**

> **CC Excl: For CC codes in subcategory G40.B:**
> PDX collection 582

✓6th **G40.B0** **Juvenile myoclonic epilepsy,** not intractable

    G40.B01 **Juvenile myoclonic epilepsy, not** `CC` `HCC` **intractable,** with status epilepticus

    G40.B09 **Juvenile myoclonic epilepsy, not** `CC` `HCC` **intractable,** without status epilepticus

✓6th **G40.B1** **Juvenile myoclonic epilepsy,** intractable

    G40.B11 **Juvenile myoclonic epilepsy,** `CC` `HCC` **intractable,** with status epilepticus

---

`N` Newborn: 0   `P` Pediatric: 0-17   `M` Maternity: 12-55   `A` Adult: 15-124   `MCC` Major CC Condition   `PDxMCC` PDx acts as own MCC   `CC` CC Condition   `PDxCC` PDx acts as own CC

562   ICD-10-CM 2018

G40.B19   **Juvenile myoclonic epilepsy,** `CC` `HCC`
intractable, without status epilepticus

√5th **G40.4**   **Other generalized epilepsy and epileptic syndromes**
Epilepsy with grand mal seizures on awakening
Epilepsy with myoclonic absences
Epilepsy with myoclonic-astatic seizures
Grand mal seizure NOS
Nonspecific atonic epileptic seizures
Nonspecific clonic epileptic seizures
Nonspecific myoclonic epileptic seizures
Nonspecific tonic epileptic seizures
Nonspecific tonic-clonic epileptic seizures
Symptomatic early myoclonic encephalopathy

√6th **G40.40**   **Other generalized epilepsy and epileptic syndromes, not intractable**
Other generalized epilepsy and epileptic syndromes without intractability
Other generalized epilepsy and epileptic syndromes NOS

     G40.401   **Other generalized epilepsy and** `HCC`
epileptic syndromes, not intractable, with status epilepticus

     G40.409   **Other generalized epilepsy and** `HCC`
epileptic syndromes, not intractable, without status epilepticus

√6th **G40.41**   **Other generalized epilepsy and epileptic syndromes, intractable**

> **CC Excl: For CC codes in subcategory G40.41:** PDX collection 582

     G40.411   **Other generalized epilepsy and** `CC` `HCC`
epileptic syndromes, intractable, with status epilepticus

     G40.419   **Other generalized epilepsy and** `CC` `HCC`
epileptic syndromes, intractable, without status epilepticus

√5th **G40.5**   **Epileptic seizures related to external causes**
Epileptic seizures related to alcohol
Epileptic seizures related to drugs
Epileptic seizures related to hormonal changes
Epileptic seizures related to sleep deprivation
Epileptic seizures related to stress
Use additional code for adverse effect, if applicable, to identify drug (T36-T50 with fifth or sixth character 5)
Code also, if applicable, associated epilepsy and recurrent seizures (G40.-)

> **CC Excl: For CC codes in subcategory G40.5:** PDX collection 582

√6th **G40.50**   **Epileptic seizures related to external causes, not intractable**

     G40.501   **Epileptic seizures related to** `CC` `HCC`
external causes, not intractable, with status epilepticus

     G40.509   **Epileptic seizures related to** `CC` `HCC`
external causes, not intractable, without status epilepticus
Epileptic seizures related to external causes, NOS

√5th **G40.8**   **Other epilepsy and recurrent seizures**
Epilepsies and epileptic syndromes undetermined as to whether they are focal or generalized
Landau-Kleffner syndrome

> **CC Excl: For CC codes in subcategory G40.8, unless otherwise noted:** PDX collection 582

√6th **G40.80**   **Other epilepsy**
     G40.801   **Other epilepsy, not intractable,** `CC` `HCC`
with status epilepticus
Other epilepsy without intractability with status epilepticus

     G40.802   **Other epilepsy, not intractable,** `CC` `HCC`
without status epilepticus
Other epilepsy without intractability without status epilepticus

     G40.803   **Other epilepsy, intractable,** `CC` `HCC`
with status epilepticus

     G40.804   **Other epilepsy, intractable,** `CC` `HCC`
without status epilepticus

√6th **G40.81**   **Lennox-Gastaut syndrome**
     G40.811   **Lennox-Gastaut syndrome, not** `CC` `HCC`
intractable, with status epilepticus

     G40.812   **Lennox-Gastaut syndrome, not** `CC` `HCC`
intractable, without status epilepticus

     G40.813   **Lennox-Gastaut syndrome,** `CC` `HCC`
intractable, with status epilepticus

     G40.814   **Lennox-Gastaut syndrome,** `CC` `HCC`
intractable, without status epilepticus

√6th **G40.82**   **Epileptic spasms**
Infantile spasms
Salaam attacks
West's syndrome

     G40.821   **Epileptic spasms, not intractable,** `CC` `HCC`
with status epilepticus
CC Excl: PDX collection 581

     G40.822   **Epileptic spasms, not intractable,** `CC` `HCC`
without status epilepticus
CC Excl: PDX collection 581

     G40.823   **Epileptic spasms, intractable,** `CC` `HCC`
with status epilepticus

     G40.824   **Epileptic spasms, intractable,** `CC` `HCC`
without status epilepticus

     G40.89   **Other seizures** `CC` `HCC`
> *EXCLUDES 1*   post traumatic seizures (R56.1)
> recurrent seizures NOS (G40.909)
> seizure NOS (R56.9)

√5th **G40.9**   **Epilepsy, unspecified**
√6th **G40.90**   **Epilepsy, unspecified, not intractable**
Epilepsy, unspecified, without intractability

     G40.901   **Epilepsy, unspecified, not intractable,** `HCC`
with status epilepticus

     G40.909   **Epilepsy, unspecified, not intractable,** `HCC`
without status epilepticus
Epilepsy NOS
Epileptic convulsions NOS
Epileptic fits NOS
Epileptic seizures NOS
Recurrent seizures NOS
Seizure disorder NOS

√6th **G40.91**   **Epilepsy, unspecified, intractable**
Intractable seizure disorder NOS

     G40.911   **Epilepsy, unspecified, intractable,** `CC` `HCC`
with status epilepticus
CC Excl: PDX collection 582

     G40.919   **Epilepsy, unspecified, intractable,** `CC` `HCC`
without status epilepticus
CC Excl: PDX collection 582

√4th **G43**   **Migraine**
NOTE   The following terms are to be considered equivalent to intractable: pharmacoresistant (pharmacologically resistant), treatment resistant, refractory (medically) and poorly controlled
Use additional code for adverse effect, if applicable, to identify drug (T36-T50 with fifth or sixth character 5)
> *EXCLUDES 1*   headache NOS (R51)
> lower half migraine (G44.00)
> *EXCLUDES 2*   headache syndromes (G44.-)

√5th **G43.0**   **Migraine without aura**
Common migraine
> *EXCLUDES 1*   chronic migraine without aura (G43.7-)

√6th **G43.00**   **Migraine without aura, not intractable**
Migraine without aura without mention of refractory migraine

     G43.001   **Migraine without aura, not intractable, with status migrainosus**

     G43.009   **Migraine without aura, not intractable, without status migrainosus**
Migraine without aura NOS

√6th **G43.01**   **Migraine without aura, intractable**
Migraine without aura with refractory migraine

     G43.011   **Migraine without aura, intractable, with status migrainosus**

     G43.019   **Migraine without aura, intractable, without status migrainosus**

Chapter 6. Diseases of the Nervous System

☑5ᵗʰ **G43.1** **Migraine** with aura
     Basilar migraine
     Classical migraine
     Migraine equivalents
     Migraine preceded or accompanied by transient focal
         neurological phenomena
     Migraine triggered seizures
     Migraine with acute-onset aura
     Migraine with aura without headache (migraine equivalents)
     Migraine with prolonged aura
     Migraine with typical aura
     Retinal migraine
     Code also any associated seizure (G40.-, R56.9)
     EXCLUDES 1   *persistent migraine aura (G43.5-, G43.6-)*

   ☑6ᵗʰ **G43.10** **Migraine with aura,** not intractable
       Migraine with aura without mention of refractory
       migraine

       G43.101 **Migraine with aura, not intractable,** with
               status migrainosus

       G43.109 **Migraine with aura, not intractable,**
               without status migrainosus
               Migraine with aura NOS

   ☑6ᵗʰ **G43.11** **Migraine with aura,** intractable
       Migraine with aura with refractory migraine

       G43.111 **Migraine with aura, intractable,** with
               status migrainosus

       G43.119 **Migraine with aura, intractable,** without
               status migrainosus

☑5ᵗʰ **G43.4** **Hemiplegic migraine**
     Familial migraine
     Sporadic migraine

   ☑6ᵗʰ **G43.40** **Hemiplegic migraine,** not intractable
       Hemiplegic migraine without refractory migraine

       G43.401 **Hemiplegic migraine, not intractable,** with
               status migrainosus

       G43.409 **Hemiplegic migraine, not intractable,**
               without status migrainosus
               Hemiplegic migraine NOS

   ☑6ᵗʰ **G43.41** **Hemiplegic migraine,** intractable
       Hemiplegic migraine with refractory migraine

       G43.411 **Hemiplegic migraine, intractable,** with
               status migrainosus

       G43.419 **Hemiplegic migraine, intractable,** without
               status migrainosus

☑5ᵗʰ **G43.5** **Persistent migraine** aura without cerebral infarction

   ☑6ᵗʰ **G43.50** **Persistent migraine aura without cerebral infarction,** not intractable
       Persistent migraine aura without cerebral infarction,
       without refractory migraine

       G43.501 **Persistent migraine aura without cerebral infarction, not intractable, with status migrainosus**

       G43.509 **Persistent migraine aura without cerebral infarction, not intractable, without status migrainosus**
               Persistent migraine aura NOS

   ☑6ᵗʰ **G43.51** **Persistent migraine aura without cerebral infarction,** intractable
       Persistent migraine aura without cerebral infarction,
       with refractory migraine

       G43.511 **Persistent migraine aura without cerebral infarction, intractable, with status migrainosus**

       G43.519 **Persistent migraine aura without cerebral infarction, intractable, without status migrainosus**

☑5ᵗʰ **G43.6** **Persistent migraine** aura with cerebral infarction
     Code also the type of cerebral infarction (I63.-)

     CC Excl: For CC codes in subcategory G43.6, unless otherwise noted: PDX collection 584

   ☑6ᵗʰ **G43.60** **Persistent migraine aura with cerebral infarction,** not intractable
       Persistent migraine aura with cerebral infarction,
       without refractory migraine

       G43.601 **Persistent migraine aura with cerebral** CC
               infarction, not intractable, with status migrainosus

       G43.609 **Persistent migraine aura with cerebral** CC
               infarction, not intractable, without status migrainosus
               CC Excl: PDX collection 585

   ☑6ᵗʰ **G43.61** **Persistent migraine aura with cerebral infarction,** intractable
       Persistent migraine aura with cerebral infarction, with
       refractory migraine

       G43.611 **Persistent migraine aura with cerebral** CC
               infarction, intractable, with status migrainosus

       G43.619 **Persistent migraine aura with cerebral** CC
               infarction, intractable, without status migrainosus

☑5ᵗʰ **G43.7** **Chronic migraine** without aura
     Transformed migraine
     EXCLUDES 1   *migraine without aura (G43.0-)*

   ☑6ᵗʰ **G43.70** **Chronic migraine without aura,** not intractable
       Chronic migraine without aura, without refractory
       migraine

       G43.701 **Chronic migraine without aura, not intractable, with status migrainosus**

       G43.709 **Chronic migraine without aura, not intractable, without status migrainosus**
               Chronic migraine without aura NOS

   ☑6ᵗʰ **G43.71** **Chronic migraine without aura,** intractable
       Chronic migraine without aura, with refractory
       migraine

       G43.711 **Chronic migraine without aura, intractable, with status migrainosus**

       G43.719 **Chronic migraine without aura, intractable, without status migrainosus**

☑5ᵗʰ **G43.A** **Cyclical vomiting**

     G43.A0 **Cyclical vomiting,** not intractable
       Cyclical vomiting, without refractory migraine

     G43.A1 **Cyclical vomiting,** intractable
       Cyclical vomiting, with refractory migraine

☑5ᵗʰ **G43.B** **Ophthalmoplegic migraine**

     G43.B0 **Ophthalmoplegic migraine,** not intractable
       Ophthalmoplegic migraine, without refractory
       migraine

     G43.B1 **Ophthalmoplegic migraine,** intractable
       Ophthalmoplegic migraine, with refractory migraine

☑5ᵗʰ **G43.C** **Periodic headache syndromes in child or adult**

     G43.C0 **Periodic headache syndromes in child or adult,** not intractable
       Periodic headache syndromes in child or adult,
       without refractory migraine

     G43.C1 **Periodic headache syndromes in child or adult,** intractable
       Periodic headache syndromes in child or adult, with
       refractory migraine

☑5ᵗʰ **G43.D** **Abdominal migraine**

     G43.D0 **Abdominal migraine,** not intractable
       Abdominal migraine, without refractory migraine

     G43.D1 **Abdominal migraine,** intractable
       Abdominal migraine, with refractory migraine

☑5ᵗʰ **G43.8** **Other migraine**

   ☑6ᵗʰ **G43.80** **Other migraine,** not intractable
       Other migraine, without refractory migraine

       G43.801 **Other migraine, not intractable,** with
               status migrainosus

       G43.809 **Other migraine, not intractable,** without
               status migrainosus

   ☑6ᵗʰ **G43.81** **Other migraine,** intractable
       Other migraine, with refractory migraine

       G43.811 **Other migraine, intractable,** with status
               migrainosus

       G43.819 **Other migraine, intractable,** without
               status migrainosus

N Newborn: 0   P Pediatric: 0-17   M Maternity: 12-55   A Adult: 15-124   MCC Major CC Condition   PDxMCC PDx acts as own MCC   CC CC Condition   PDxCC PDx acts as own CC

564   ICD-10-CM 2018

✓6ᵗʰ **G43.82 Menstrual migraine, not intractable**
     Menstrual headache, not intractable
     Menstrual migraine, without refractory migraine
     Menstrually related migraine, not intractable
     Pre-menstrual headache, not intractable
     Pre-menstrual migraine, not intractable
     Pure menstrual migraine, not intractable
     Code also associated premenstrual tension syndrome
       (N94.3)

     G43.821 Menstrual migraine, not intractable, ♀
           with status migrainosus

     G43.829 Menstrual migraine, not intractable, ♀
           without status migrainosus
           Menstrual migraine NOS

✓6ᵗʰ **G43.83 Menstrual migraine, intractable**
     Menstrual headache, intractable
     Menstrual migraine, with refractory migraine
     Menstrually related migraine, intractable
     Pre-menstrual headache, intractable
     Pre-menstrual migraine, intractable
     Pure menstrual migraine, intractable
     Code also associated premenstrual tension syndrome
       (N94.3)

     G43.831 Menstrual migraine, intractable, with ♀
           status migrainosus

     G43.839 Menstrual migraine, intractable, ♀
           without status migrainosus

✓5ᵗʰ **G43.9 Migraine, unspecified**

✓6ᵗʰ **G43.90 Migraine, unspecified, not intractable**
     Migraine, unspecified, without refractory migraine

     G43.901 Migraine, unspecified, not intractable,
           with status migrainosus
           Status migrainosus NOS

     G43.909 Migraine, unspecified, not intractable,
           without status migrainosus
           Migraine NOS

✓6ᵗʰ **G43.91 Migraine, unspecified, intractable**
     Migraine, unspecified, with refractory migraine

     G43.911 Migraine, unspecified, intractable, with
           status migrainosus

     G43.919 Migraine, unspecified, intractable,
           without status migrainosus

✓4ᵗʰ **G44 Other headache syndromes**
    EXCLUDES 1   *headache NOS (R51)*
    EXCLUDES 2   *atypical facial pain (G50.1)*
             headache due to lumbar puncture (G97.1)
             migraines (G43.-)
             trigeminal neuralgia (G50.0)

✓5ᵗʰ **G44.0 Cluster headaches and other trigeminal autonomic**
       cephalgias (TAC)

✓6ᵗʰ **G44.00 Cluster headache syndrome, unspecified**
     Ciliary neuralgia   Lower half migraine
     Cluster headache NOS   Migrainous neuralgia
     Histamine cephalgia

     G44.001 Cluster headache syndrome, unspecified,
           intractable

     G44.009 Cluster headache syndrome, unspecified,
           not intractable
           Cluster headache syndrome NOS

✓6ᵗʰ **G44.01 Episodic cluster headache**
     G44.011 Episodic cluster headache, intractable
     G44.019 Episodic cluster headache, not intractable
           Episodic cluster headache NOS

✓6ᵗʰ **G44.02 Chronic cluster headache**
     G44.021 Chronic cluster headache, intractable
     G44.029 Chronic cluster headache, not intractable
           Chronic cluster headache NOS

✓6ᵗʰ **G44.03 Episodic paroxysmal hemicrania**
     Paroxysmal hemicrania NOS

     G44.031 Episodic paroxysmal hemicrania,
           intractable

     G44.039 Episodic paroxysmal hemicrania, not
           intractable
           Episodic paroxysmal hemicrania NOS

✓6ᵗʰ **G44.04 Chronic paroxysmal hemicrania**
     G44.041 Chronic paroxysmal hemicrania,
           intractable

     G44.049 Chronic paroxysmal hemicrania, not
           intractable
           Chronic paroxysmal hemicrania NOS

✓6ᵗʰ **G44.05 Short lasting unilateral neuralgiform headache with**
       conjunctival injection and tearing (SUNCT)

     G44.051 Short lasting unilateral neuralgiform
           headache with conjunctival injection and
           tearing (SUNCT), intractable

     G44.059 Short lasting unilateral neuralgiform
           headache with conjunctival injection and
           tearing (SUNCT), not intractable
           Short lasting unilateral neuralgiform
             headache with conjunctival injection
             and tearing (SUNCT) NOS

✓6ᵗʰ **G44.09 Other trigeminal autonomic cephalgias (TAC)**
     G44.091 Other trigeminal autonomic cephalgias
           (TAC), intractable

     G44.099 Other trigeminal autonomic cephalgias
           syndrome (TAC), not intractable

G44.1 Vascular headache, not elsewhere classified
    EXCLUDES 2   *cluster headache (G44.0)*
             complicated headache syndromes (G44.5-)
             drug-induced headache (G44.4-)
             migraine (G43.-)
             other specified headache syndromes (G44.8-)
             post-traumatic headache (G44.3-)
             tension-type headache (G44.2-)

✓5ᵗʰ **G44.2 Tension-type headache**

✓6ᵗʰ **G44.20 Tension-type headache, unspecified**
     G44.201 Tension-type headache, unspecified,
           intractable

     G44.209 Tension-type headache, unspecified, not
           intractable
           Tension headache NOS

✓6ᵗʰ **G44.21 Episodic tension-type headache**
     G44.211 Episodic tension-type headache,
           intractable

     G44.219 Episodic tension-type headache, not
           intractable
           Episodic tension-type headache NOS

✓6ᵗʰ **G44.22 Chronic tension-type headache**
     G44.221 Chronic tension-type headache,
           intractable

     G44.229 Chronic tension-type headache, not
           intractable
           Chronic tension-type headache NOS

✓5ᵗʰ **G44.3 Post-traumatic headache**

✓6ᵗʰ **G44.30 Post-traumatic headache, unspecified**
     G44.301 Post-traumatic headache, unspecified,
           intractable

     G44.309 Post-traumatic headache, unspecified, not
           intractable
           Post-traumatic headache NOS

✓6ᵗʰ **G44.31 Acute post-traumatic headache**
     G44.311 Acute post-traumatic headache,
           intractable

     G44.319 Acute post-traumatic headache, not
           intractable
           Acute post-traumatic headache NOS

✓6ᵗʰ **G44.32 Chronic post-traumatic headache**
     G44.321 Chronic post-traumatic headache,
           intractable

     G44.329 Chronic post-traumatic headache, not
           intractable
           Chronic post-traumatic headache NOS

✓5ᵗʰ **G44.4 Drug-induced headache, not elsewhere classified**
     Medication overuse headache
     Use additional code for adverse effect, if applicable, to identify
       drug (T36-T50 with fifth or sixth character 5)

     G44.40 Drug-induced headache, not elsewhere classified,
         not intractable

     G44.41 Drug-induced headache, not elsewhere classified,
         intractable

✓5ᵗʰ **G44.5 Complicated headache syndromes**
     G44.51 Hemicrania continua
     G44.52 New daily persistent headache (NDPH)
     G44.53 Primary thunderclap headache

✓ Additional Character Req   ✓x7ᵗʰ Placeholder Alert   Unacceptable PDx   Manifestation   H1-H14 HAC   HCC CMS-HCC Condition   EXCLUDES 1 Not Coded Here   EXCLUDES 2 Not Included Here

ICD-10-CM 2018   **565**

Chapter 6. Diseases of the Nervous System

G44.59   Other complicated **headache syndrome**

☑5ᵗʰ **G44.8**   Other specified **headache syndromes**

     G44.81   Hypnic **headache**

     G44.82   Headache associated with **sexual activity**
          Orgasmic headache
          Preorgasmic headache

     G44.83   Primary **cough headache**

     G44.84   Primary **exertional headache**

     G44.85   Primary **stabbing headache**

     G44.89   Other **headache syndrome**

☑4ᵗʰ **G45**   **Transient cerebral ischemic attacks and related syndromes**
     EXCLUDES 1   neonatal cerebral ischemia (P91.0)
             transient retinal artery occlusion (H34.0-)

> **CC Excl: For CC codes in category G45, unless otherwise noted:**
> PDX collection 586

G45.0   **Vertebro-basilar artery syndrome**   CC

G45.1   **Carotid artery syndrome (hemispheric)**   CC

G45.2   **Multiple and bilateral precerebral artery syndromes**   CC

G45.3   **Amaurosis fugax**   CC
     CC Excl: PDX collection 587

G45.4   **Transient global amnesia**
     EXCLUDES 1   amnesia NOS (R41.3)

G45.8   **Other transient cerebral ischemic attacks and related syndromes**   CC

G45.9   **Transient cerebral ischemic attack, unspecified**   CC
     Spasm of cerebral artery
     TIA
     Transient cerebral ischemia NOS

☑4ᵗʰ **G46**   **Vascular syndromes of brain in cerebrovascular diseases**
     Code first underlying cerebrovascular disease (I60-I69)

> **CC Excl: For CC codes in category G46:** PDX collection 586

G46.0   **Middle cerebral artery syndrome**   CC

G46.1   **Anterior cerebral artery syndrome**   CC

G46.2   **Posterior cerebral artery syndrome**   CC

G46.3   **Brain stem stroke syndrome**
     Benedikt syndrome   Millard-Gubler syndrome
     Claude syndrome   Wallenberg syndrome
     Foville syndrome   Weber syndrome

G46.4   **Cerebellar stroke syndrome**

G46.5   **Pure motor lacunar syndrome**

G46.6   **Pure sensory lacunar syndrome**

G46.7   **Other lacunar syndromes**

G46.8   **Other vascular syndromes of brain in cerebrovascular diseases**

☑4ᵗʰ **G47**   **Sleep disorders**
     EXCLUDES 2   nightmares (F51.5)
             nonorganic sleep disorders (F51.-)
             sleep terrors (F51.4)
             sleepwalking (F51.3)

☑5ᵗʰ **G47.0**   **Insomnia**
     EXCLUDES 2   alcohol related insomnia (F10.182, F10.282, F10.982)
             drug-related insomnia (F11.182, F11.282, F11.982, F13.182, F13.282, F13.982, F14.182, F14.282, F14.982, F15.182, F15.282, F15.982, F19.182, F19.282, F19.982)
             idiopathic insomnia (F51.01)
             insomnia due to a mental disorder (F51.05)
             insomnia not due to a substance or known physiological condition (F51.0-)
             nonorganic insomnia (F51.0-)
             primary insomnia (F51.01)
             sleep apnea (G47.3-)

     G47.00   **Insomnia, unspecified**
          Insomnia NOS

     G47.01   **Insomnia due to medical condition**
          Code also associated medical condition

     G47.09   **Other insomnia**

☑5ᵗʰ **G47.1**   **Hypersomnia**
     EXCLUDES 2   alcohol-related hypersomnia (F10.182, F10.282, F10.982)
             drug-related hypersomnia (F11.182, F11.282, F11.982, F13.182, F13.282, F13.982, F14.182, F14.282, F14.982, F15.182, F15.282, F15.982, F19.182, F19.282, F19.982)
             hypersomnia due to a mental disorder (F51.13)
             hypersomnia not due to a substance or known physiological condition (F51.1-)
             primary hypersomnia (F51.11)
             sleep apnea (G47.3-)

     G47.10   **Hypersomnia, unspecified**
          Hypersomnia NOS

     G47.11   **Idiopathic hypersomnia with long sleep time**
          Idiopathic hypersomnia NOS

     G47.12   **Idiopathic hypersomnia without long sleep time**

     G47.13   **Recurrent hypersomnia**
          Kleine-Levin syndrome
          Menstrual related hypersomnia

     G47.14   **Hypersomnia due to medical condition**
          Code also associated medical condition

     G47.19   **Other hypersomnia**

☑5ᵗʰ **G47.2**   **Circadian rhythm sleep disorders**
     Disorders of the sleep wake schedule
     Inversion of nyctohemeral rhythm
     Inversion of sleep rhythm

     G47.20   **Circadian rhythm sleep disorder, unspecified type**
          Sleep wake schedule disorder NOS

     G47.21   **Circadian rhythm sleep disorder, delayed sleep phase type**
          Delayed sleep phase syndrome

     G47.22   **Circadian rhythm sleep disorder, advanced sleep phase type**

     G47.23   **Circadian rhythm sleep disorder, irregular sleep wake type**
          Irregular sleep-wake pattern

     G47.24   **Circadian rhythm sleep disorder, free running type**
          ▶Circadian rhythm sleep disorder, non-24-hour sleep-wake type◀

     G47.25   **Circadian rhythm sleep disorder, jet lag type**

     G47.26   **Circadian rhythm sleep disorder, shift work type**

     G47.27   *Circadian rhythm sleep disorder in conditions classified elsewhere*
          Code first underlying condition

     G47.29   **Other circadian rhythm sleep disorder**

☑5ᵗʰ **G47.3**   **Sleep apnea**
     Code also any associated underlying condition
     EXCLUDES 1   apnea NOS (R06.81)
             Cheyne-Stokes breathing (R06.3)
             pickwickian syndrome (E66.2)
             sleep apnea of newborn (P28.3)

     G47.30   **Sleep apnea, unspecified**
          Sleep apnea NOS

     G47.31   **Primary central sleep apnea**
          ▶Idiopathic central sleep apnea◀

     G47.32   **High altitude periodic breathing**

     G47.33   **Obstructive sleep apnea (adult) (pediatric)**
          ▶Obstructive sleep apnea hypopnea◀
          EXCLUDES 1   obstructive sleep apnea of newborn (P28.3)

     G47.34   **Idiopathic sleep related nonobstructive alveolar hypoventilation**
          Sleep related hypoxia

     G47.35   **Congenital central alveolar hypoventilation syndrome**

     G47.36   *Sleep related hypoventilation in conditions classified elsewhere*
          Sleep related hypoxemia in conditions classified elsewhere
          Code first underlying condition

     G47.37   *Central sleep apnea in conditions classified elsewhere*
          Code first underlying condition

     G47.39   **Other sleep apnea**

☑5ᵗʰ **G47.4**   **Narcolepsy and cataplexy**

     ☑6ᵗʰ **G47.41**   **Narcolepsy**

         G47.411   **Narcolepsy with cataplexy**

         G47.419   **Narcolepsy without cataplexy**
              Narcolepsy NOS

Ⓝ Newborn: 0   Ⓟ Pediatric: 0-17   Ⓜ Maternity: 12-55   Ⓐ Adult: 15-124   MCC Major CC Condition   PDxMCC PDx acts as own MCC   CC CC Condition   PDxCC PDx acts as own CC

566   ICD-10-CM 2018

✓6ᵗʰ **G47.42**   **Narcolepsy in conditions classified elsewhere**
Code first underlying condition

     G47.421   *Narcolepsy in conditions classified elsewhere with cataplexy*

     G47.429   *Narcolepsy in conditions classified elsewhere without cataplexy*

✓5ᵗʰ **G47.5**   **Parasomnia**
   EXCLUDES 1   *alcohol induced parasomnia (F10.182, F10.282, F10.982)*
      drug induced parasomnia (F11.182, F11.282, F11.982, F13.182, F13.282, F13.982, F14.182, F14.282, F14.982, F15.182, F15.282, F15.982, F19.182, F19.282, F19.982)
      parasomnia not due to a substance or known physiological condition (F51.8)

   G47.50   **Parasomnia, unspecified**
Parasomnia NOS

   G47.51   **Confusional arousals**

   G47.52   **REM sleep behavior disorder**

   G47.53   **Recurrent isolated sleep paralysis**

   G47.54   *Parasomnia in conditions classified elsewhere*
Code first underlying condition

   G47.59   **Other parasomnia**

✓5ᵗʰ **G47.6**   **Sleep related movement disorders**
   EXCLUDES 2   *restless legs syndrome (G25.81)*

   G47.61   **Periodic limb movement disorder**
~~Periodic limb movement disorder~~

   G47.62   **Sleep related leg cramps**

   G47.63   **Sleep related bruxism**
     EXCLUDES 1   *psychogenic bruxism (F45.8)*

   G47.69   **Other sleep related movement disorders**

G47.8   **Other sleep disorders**
▶Other specified sleep-wake disorder◀

G47.9   **Sleep disorder, unspecified**
Sleep disorder NOS
▶Unspecified sleep-wake disorder◀

Nerve, nerve root and plexus disorders (G50-G59)

EXCLUDES 1   *current traumatic nerve, nerve root and plexus disorders—see Injury, nerve by body region*
neuralgia NOS (M79.2)
neuritis NOS (M79.2)
peripheral neuritis in pregnancy (O26.82-)
radiculitis NOS (M54.1-)

✓4ᵗʰ **G50**   **Disorders of trigeminal nerve**
   INCLUDES   disorders of 5th cranial nerve

   G50.0   **Trigeminal neuralgia**
Syndrome of paroxysmal facial pain
Tic douloureux

   G50.1   **Atypical facial pain**

   G50.8   **Other disorders of trigeminal nerve**

   G50.9   **Disorder of trigeminal nerve, unspecified**

Trigeminal and Facial Nerve Branches

Supratrochlear nerve
Supraorbital nerve
V2 branch
Infraorbital nerve
V1 branch
Trigeminal nerve (CN V) branches in infratemporal fossa
V3 branch
Mental nerve
Mental foramen

✓4ᵗʰ **G51**   **Facial nerve disorders**
   INCLUDES   disorders of 7th cranial nerve

   G51.0   **Bell's palsy**
Facial palsy

   G51.1   **Geniculate ganglionitis**
     EXCLUDES 1   *postherpetic geniculate ganglionitis (B02.21)*

   G51.2   **Melkersson's syndrome**
Melkersson-Rosenthal syndrome

   G51.3   **Clonic hemifacial spasm**

   G51.4   **Facial myokymia**

   G51.8   **Other disorders of facial nerve**

   G51.9   **Disorder of facial nerve, unspecified**

✓4ᵗʰ **G52**   **Disorders of other cranial nerves**
   EXCLUDES 2   *disorders of acoustic [8th] nerve (H93.3)*
disorders of optic [2nd] nerve (H46, H47.0)
paralytic strabismus due to nerve palsy (H49.0-H49.2)

   G52.0   **Disorders of olfactory nerve**
Disorders of 1st cranial nerve

   G52.1   **Disorders of glossopharyngeal nerve**
Disorder of 9th cranial nerve
Glossopharyngeal neuralgia

   G52.2   **Disorders of vagus nerve**
Disorders of pneumogastric [10th] nerve

   G52.3   **Disorders of hypoglossal nerve**
Disorders of 12th cranial nerve

   G52.7   **Disorders of multiple cranial nerves**
Polyneuritis cranialis

   G52.8   **Disorders of other specified cranial nerves**

   G52.9   **Cranial nerve disorder, unspecified**

G53   *Cranial nerve disorders in diseases classified elsewhere*
Code first underlying disease, such as:
neoplasm (C00-D49)
   EXCLUDES 1   *multiple cranial nerve palsy in sarcoidosis (D86.82)*
multiple cranial nerve palsy in syphilis (A52.15)
postherpetic geniculate ganglionitis (B02.21)
postherpetic trigeminal neuralgia (B02.22)

✓4ᵗʰ **G54**   **Nerve root and plexus disorders**
   EXCLUDES 1   *current traumatic nerve root and plexus disorders—see nerve injury by body region*
intervertebral disc disorders (M50-M51)
neuritis or radiculitis brachial NOS (M54.13)
neuritis or radiculitis lumbar NOS (M54.16)
neuritis or radiculitis lumbosacral NOS (M54.17)
neuritis or radiculitis thoracic NOS (M54.14)
radiculitis NOS (M54.10)
radiculopathy NOS (M54.10)
spondylosis (M47.-)

   G54.0   **Brachial plexus disorders**
Thoracic outlet syndrome
DEF: Acquired disorder affecting the spinal nerves that send signals to the shoulder, arm, and hand; causes corresponding motor and sensory dysfunction; characterized by regional paresthesia, pain, and muscle weakness, and in severe cases paralysis.

   G54.1   **Lumbosacral plexus disorders**

   G54.2   **Cervical root disorders, not elsewhere classified**

   G54.3   **Thoracic root disorders, not elsewhere classified**

   G54.4   **Lumbosacral root disorders, not elsewhere classified**

   G54.5   **Neuralgic amyotrophy**
Parsonage-Aldren-Turner syndrome
Shoulder-girdle neuritis
     EXCLUDES 1   *neuralgic amyotrophy in diabetes mellitus (E08-E13 with .44)*

   G54.6   **Phantom limb syndrome with pain**   HCC

   G54.7   **Phantom limb syndrome without pain**   HCC
Phantom limb syndrome NOS

   G54.8   **Other nerve root and plexus disorders**

   G54.9   **Nerve root and plexus disorder, unspecified**

G55   *Nerve root and plexus compressions in diseases classified elsewhere*
Code first underlying disease, such as:
neoplasm (C00-D49)
   EXCLUDES 1   *nerve root compression (due to) (in) ankylosing spondylitis (M45.-)*
nerve root compression (due to) (in) dorsopathies (M53.-, M54.-)
nerve root compression (due to) (in) intervertebral disc disorders (M50.1-, M51.1-)
nerve root compression (due to) (in) spondylopathies (M46.-, M48.-)

☑Additional Character Req   ✓x7ᵗʰ Placeholder Alert   Unacceptable PDx   Manifestation   H1 - H14 HAC   HCC CMS-HCC Condition   EXCLUDES 1 Not Coded Here   EXCLUDES 2 Not Included Here

ICD-10-CM 2018   567

Chapter 6. Diseases of the Nervous System

Nerves of Upper Limb

- Radial
- Deep branch of radial
- Ulnar
- Superficial branch of radial
- Median

☑4ᵗʰ **G56 Mononeuropathies of upper limb**

> EXCLUDES 1   current traumatic nerve disorder—see nerve injury by body region

☑5ᵗʰ **G56.0 Carpal tunnel syndrome**

     G56.00   Carpal tunnel syndrome, unspecified upper limb

     G56.01   Carpal tunnel syndrome, right upper limb

     G56.02   Carpal tunnel syndrome, left upper limb

     G56.03   Carpal tunnel syndrome, bilateral upper limbs

☑5ᵗʰ **G56.1 Other lesions of median nerve**

     G56.10   Other lesions of median nerve, unspecified upper limb

     G56.11   Other lesions of median nerve, right upper limb

     G56.12   Other lesions of median nerve, left upper limb

     G56.13   Other lesions of median nerve, bilateral upper limbs

☑5ᵗʰ **G56.2 Lesion of ulnar nerve**

     Tardy ulnar nerve palsy

     G56.20   Lesion of ulnar nerve, unspecified upper limb

     G56.21   Lesion of ulnar nerve, right upper limb

     G56.22   Lesion of ulnar nerve, left upper limb

     G56.23   Lesion of ulnar nerve, bilateral upper limbs

☑5ᵗʰ **G56.3 Lesion of radial nerve**

     G56.30   Lesion of radial nerve, unspecified upper limb

     G56.31   Lesion of radial nerve, right upper limb

     G56.32   Lesion of radial nerve, left upper limb

     G56.33   Lesion of radial nerve, bilateral upper limbs

☑5ᵗʰ **G56.4 Causalgia of upper limb**

     Complex regional pain syndrome II of upper limb

> EXCLUDES 1   complex regional pain syndrome I of lower limb (G90.52-)
> complex regional pain syndrome I of upper limb (G90.51-)
> complex regional pain syndrome II of lower limb (G57.7-)
> reflex sympathetic dystrophy of lower limb (G90.52-)
> reflex sympathetic dystrophy of upper limb (G90.51-)

     G56.40   Causalgia of unspecified upper limb

     G56.41   Causalgia of right upper limb

     G56.42   Causalgia of left upper limb

     G56.43   Causalgia of bilateral upper limbs

☑5ᵗʰ **G56.8 Other specified mononeuropathies of upper limb**

     Interdigital neuroma of upper limb

     G56.80   Other specified mononeuropathies of unspecified upper limb

     G56.81   Other specified mononeuropathies of right upper limb

     G56.82   Other specified mononeuropathies of left upper limb

     G56.83   Other specified mononeuropathies of bilateral upper limbs

☑5ᵗʰ **G56.9 Unspecified mononeuropathy of upper limb**

     G56.90   Unspecified mononeuropathy of unspecified upper limb

     G56.91   Unspecified mononeuropathy of right upper limb

     G56.92   Unspecified mononeuropathy of left upper limb

     G56.93   Unspecified mononeuropathy of bilateral upper limbs

☑4ᵗʰ **G57 Mononeuropathies of lower limb**

> EXCLUDES 1   current traumatic nerve disorder—see nerve injury by body region

☑5ᵗʰ **G57.0 Lesion of sciatic nerve**

> EXCLUDES 1   sciatica NOS (M54.3-)
> EXCLUDES 2   sciatica attributed to intervertebral disc disorder (M51.1-)

     G57.00   Lesion of sciatic nerve, unspecified lower limb

     G57.01   Lesion of sciatic nerve, right lower limb

     G57.02   Lesion of sciatic nerve, left lower limb

     G57.03   Lesion of sciatic nerve, bilateral lower limbs

☑5ᵗʰ **G57.1 Meralgia paresthetica**

     Lateral cutaneous nerve of thigh syndrome

     G57.10   Meralgia paresthetica, unspecified lower limb

     G57.11   Meralgia paresthetica, right lower limb

     G57.12   Meralgia paresthetica, left lower limb

     G57.13   Meralgia paresthetica, bilateral lower limbs

☑5ᵗʰ **G57.2 Lesion of femoral nerve**

     G57.20   Lesion of femoral nerve, unspecified lower limb

     G57.21   Lesion of femoral nerve, right lower limb

     G57.22   Lesion of femoral nerve, left lower limb

     G57.23   Lesion of femoral nerve, bilateral lower limbs

☑5ᵗʰ **G57.3 Lesion of lateral popliteal nerve**

     Peroneal nerve palsy

     G57.30   Lesion of lateral popliteal nerve, unspecified lower limb

     G57.31   Lesion of lateral popliteal nerve, right lower limb

     G57.32   Lesion of lateral popliteal nerve, left lower limb

     G57.33   Lesion of lateral popliteal nerve, bilateral lower limbs

☑5ᵗʰ **G57.4 Lesion of medial popliteal nerve**

     G57.40   Lesion of medial popliteal nerve, unspecified lower limb

     G57.41   Lesion of medial popliteal nerve, right lower limb

Nerves of Lower Limb

- Obturator nerve
- Sciatic nerve
- Femoral nerve
- Saphenous nerve
- Common fibular (peroneal) nerve
- Deep fibular (peroneal) nerve
- Tibial nerve
- Superficial fibular (peroneal) nerve

Ⓝ Newborn: 0   Ⓟ Pediatric: 0-17   Ⓜ Maternity: 12-55   Ⓐ Adult: 15-124   **MCC** Major CC Condition   **PDxMCC** PDx acts as own MCC   **CC** CC Condition   **PDxCC** PDx acts as own CC

568   ICD-10-CM 2018

     G57.42   **Lesion of medial popliteal nerve, left lower limb**

     G57.43   **Lesion of medial popliteal nerve, bilateral lower limbs**

✓5th **G57.5**   **Tarsal tunnel syndrome**

     G57.50   **Tarsal tunnel syndrome, unspecified lower limb**

     G57.51   **Tarsal tunnel syndrome, right lower limb**

     G57.52   **Tarsal tunnel syndrome, left lower limb**

     G57.53   **Tarsal tunnel syndrome, bilateral lower limbs**

✓5th **G57.6**   **Lesion of plantar nerve**
     Morton's metatarsalgia

     G57.60   **Lesion of plantar nerve, unspecified lower limb**

     G57.61   **Lesion of plantar nerve, right lower limb**

     G57.62   **Lesion of plantar nerve, left lower limb**

     G57.63   **Lesion of plantar nerve, bilateral lower limbs**

✓5th **G57.7**   **Causalgia of lower limb**
     Complex regional pain syndrome II of lower limb

     EXCLUDES 1   *complex regional pain syndrome I of lower limb (G90.52-)*
         complex regional pain syndrome I of upper limb (G90.51-)
         complex regional pain syndrome II of upper limb (G56.4-)
         reflex sympathetic dystrophy of lower limb (G90.52-)
         reflex sympathetic dystrophy of upper limb (G90.51-)

     G57.70   **Causalgia of unspecified lower limb**

     G57.71   **Causalgia of right lower limb**

     G57.72   **Causalgia of left lower limb**

     G57.73   **Causalgia of bilateral lower limbs**

✓5th **G57.8**   **Other specified mononeuropathies of lower limb**
     Interdigital neuroma of lower limb

     G57.80   **Other specified mononeuropathies of unspecified lower limb**

     G57.81   **Other specified mononeuropathies of right lower limb**

     G57.82   **Other specified mononeuropathies of left lower limb**

     G57.83   **Other specified mononeuropathies of bilateral lower limbs**

✓5th **G57.9**   **Unspecified mononeuropathy of lower limb**

     G57.90   **Unspecified mononeuropathy of unspecified lower limb**

     G57.91   **Unspecified mononeuropathy of right lower limb**

     G57.92   **Unspecified mononeuropathy of left lower limb**

     G57.93   **Unspecified mononeuropathy of bilateral lower limbs**

✓4th **G58**   **Other mononeuropathies**

     G58.0   **Intercostal neuropathy**

     G58.7   **Mononeuritis multiplex**

     G58.8   **Other specified mononeuropathies**

     G58.9   **Mononeuropathy, unspecified**

G59   ***Mononeuropathy in diseases classified elsewhere***
     Code first underlying disease

     EXCLUDES 1   *diabetic mononeuropathy (E08-E13 with .41)*
         syphilitic nerve paralysis (A52.19)
         syphilitic neuritis (A52.15)
         tuberculous mononeuropathy (A17.83)

Polyneuropathies and other disorders of the peripheral nervous system (G60-G65)

     EXCLUDES 1   *neuralgia NOS (M79.2)*
         neuritis NOS (M79.2)
         peripheral neuritis in pregnancy (O26.82-)
         radiculitis NOS (M54.10)

✓4th **G60**   **Hereditary and idiopathic neuropathy**

     G60.0   **Hereditary motor and sensory neuropathy**
         Charcôt-Marie-Tooth disease
         Déjérine-Sottas disease
         Hereditary motor and sensory neuropathy, types I-IV
         Hypertrophic neuropathy of infancy
         Peroneal muscular atrophy (axonal type) (hypertrophic type)
         Roussy-Levy syndrome

     G60.1   **Refsum's disease**   CC
         Infantile Refsum disease
         AHA: 2014, 2Q, 4
         DEF: Genetic disorder of lipid metabolism; characterized by retinitis pigmentosa, degenerative nerve disease, ataxia, and dry, rough, scaly skin.
         CC Excl: PDX collection 588

     G60.2   **Neuropathy in association with hereditary ataxia**

     G60.3   **Idiopathic progressive neuropathy**

     G60.8   **Other hereditary and idiopathic neuropathies**
         Dominantly inherited sensory neuropathy
         Morvan's disease
         Nelaton's syndrome
         Recessively inherited sensory neuropathy

     G60.9   **Hereditary and idiopathic neuropathy, unspecified**

✓4th **G61**   **Inflammatory polyneuropathy**

     G61.0   **Guillain-Barre syndrome**   CC HCC
         Acute (post-)infective polyneuritis
         Miller Fisher syndrome
         AHA: 2014, 2Q, 4
         CC Excl: PDX collection 92

     G61.1   **Serum neuropathy**   HCC
         Use additional code for adverse effect, if applicable, to identify serum (T50.-)

✓5th **G61.8**   **Other inflammatory polyneuropathies**

     G61.81   **Chronic inflammatory demyelinating polyneuritis**   CC HCC
         CC Excl: PDX collection 589

     G61.82   **Multifocal motor neuropathy**   HCC
         MMN

     G61.89   **Other inflammatory polyneuropathies**   HCC

     G61.9   **Inflammatory polyneuropathy, unspecified**   HCC

✓4th **G62**   **Other and unspecified polyneuropathies**

     G62.0   **Drug-induced polyneuropathy**   HCC
         Use additional code for adverse effect, if applicable, to identify drug (T36-T50 with fifth or sixth character 5)

     G62.1   **Alcoholic polyneuropathy**   HCC

     G62.2   **Polyneuropathy due to other toxic agents**   HCC
         Code first (T51-T65) to identify toxic agent

✓5th **G62.8**   **Other specified polyneuropathies**

     G62.81   **Critical illness polyneuropathy**   CC HCC
         Acute motor neuropathy
         CC Excl: PDX collection 590

     G62.82   **Radiation-induced polyneuropathy**   HCC
         Use additional external cause code (W88-W90, X39.0-) to identify cause

     G62.89   **Other specified polyneuropathies**
         AHA: 2016, 2Q, 11

     G62.9   **Polyneuropathy, unspecified**
         Neuropathy NOS

G63   ***Polyneuropathy in diseases classified elsewhere***   HCC
     Code first underlying disease, such as:
         amyloidosis (E85.-)
         endocrine disease, except diabetes (E00-E07, E15-E16, E20-E34)
         metabolic diseases (E70-E88)
         neoplasm (C00-D49)
         nutritional deficiency (E40-E64)

     EXCLUDES 1   *polyneuropathy (in):*
         diabetes mellitus (E08-E13 with .42)
         diphtheria (A36.83)
         infectious mononucleosis (B27.0-B27.9 with 1)
         Lyme disease (A69.22)
         mumps (B26.84)
         postherpetic (B02.23)
         rheumatoid arthritis (M05.33)
         scleroderma (M34.83)
         systemic lupus erythematosus (M32.19)

     AHA: 2012, 4Q, 99

G64   **Other disorders of peripheral nervous system**
     Disorder of peripheral nervous system NOS

✓4th **G65**   **Sequelae of inflammatory and toxic polyneuropathies**
     Code first condition resulting from (sequela) of inflammatory and toxic polyneuropathies

     G65.0   **Sequelae of Guillain-Barré syndrome**   HCC

     G65.1   **Sequelae of other inflammatory polyneuropathy**   HCC

     G65.2   **Sequelae of toxic polyneuropathy**   HCC

✓ Additional Character Req   ✓x7th Placeholder Alert   Unacceptable PDx   Manifestation   H1-H14 HAC   HCC CMS-HCC Condition   EXCLUDES 1 Not Coded Here   EXCLUDES 2 Not Included Here

Chapter 6. Diseases of the Nervous System

Diseases of myoneural junction and muscle (G70-G73)

✓4ᵗʰ G70 Myasthenia gravis and other myoneural disorders
> EXCLUDES 1   botulism (A05.1, A48.51-A48.52)
> transient neonatal myasthenia gravis (P94.0)

CC Excl: For CC/MCC codes in category G70: PDX collection 591

✓5ᵗʰ G70.0 Myasthenia gravis
    G70.00 Myasthenia gravis without (acute) exacerbation `HCC`
        Myasthenia gravis NOS
    G70.01 Myasthenia gravis with (acute) exacerbation `MCC` `HCC`
        Myasthenia gravis in crisis

G70.1 Toxic myoneural disorders `HCC`
    Code first (T51-T65) to identify toxic agent

G70.2 Congenital and developmental myasthenia `HCC`

✓5ᵗʰ G70.8 Other specified myoneural disorders
    G70.80 Lambert-Eaton syndrome, unspecified `CC` `HCC`
        Lambert-Eaton syndrome NOS
    G70.81 Lambert-Eaton syndrome in disease classified elsewhere `CC` `HCC`
        Code first underlying disease
        > EXCLUDES 1   Lambert-Eaton syndrome in neoplastic disease (G73.1)
    G70.89 Other specified myoneural disorders `HCC`

G70.9 Myoneural disorder, unspecified `HCC`

✓4ᵗʰ G71 Primary disorders of muscles
> EXCLUDES 2   arthrogryposis multiplex congenita (Q74.3)
> metabolic disorders (E70-E88)
> myositis (M60.-)

G71.0 Muscular dystrophy `CC` `HCC`
    Autosomal recessive, childhood type, muscular dystrophy resembling Duchenne or Becker muscular dystrophy
    Benign [Becker] muscular dystrophy
    Benign scapuloperoneal muscular dystrophy with early contractures [Emery-Dreifuss]
    Congenital muscular dystrophy NOS
    Congenital muscular dystrophy with specific morphological abnormalities of the muscle fiber
    Distal muscular dystrophy
    Facioscapulohumeral muscular dystrophy
    Limb-girdle muscular dystrophy
    Ocular muscular dystrophy
    Oculopharyngeal muscular dystrophy
    Scapuloperoneal muscular dystrophy
    Severe [Duchenne] muscular dystrophy
    CC Excl: PDX collection 592

✓5ᵗʰ G71.1 Myotonic disorders
    G71.11 Myotonic muscular dystrophy `HCC`
        Dystrophia myotonica [Steinert]
        Myotonia atrophica
        Myotonic dystrophy
        Proximal myotonic myopathy (PROMM)
        Steinert disease
    G71.12 Myotonia congenita
        Acetazolamide responsive myotonia congenita
        Dominant myotonia congenita [Thomsen disease]
        Myotonia levior
        Recessive myotonia congenita [Becker disease]
    G71.13 Myotonic chondrodystrophy
        Chondrodystrophic myotonia
        Congenital myotonic chondrodystrophy
        Schwartz-Jampel disease
    G71.14 Drug induced myotonia
        Use additional code for adverse effect, if applicable, to identify drug (T36-T50 with fifth or sixth character 5)
    G71.19 Other specified myotonic disorders
        Myotonia fluctuans
        Myotonia permanens
        Neuromyotonia [Isaacs]
        Paramyotonia congenita (of von Eulenburg)
        Pseudomyotonia
        Symptomatic myotonia

G71.2 Congenital myopathies `CC` `HCC`
    Central core disease
    Fiber-type disproportion
    Minicore disease
    Multicore disease
    Myotubular (centronuclear) myopathy
    Nemaline myopathy
    > EXCLUDES 1   arthrogryposis multiplex congenita (Q74.3)
    CC Excl: PDX collection 592

G71.3 Mitochondrial myopathy, not elsewhere classified
    > EXCLUDES 1   Kearns-Sayre syndrome (H49.81)
        Leber's disease (H47.21)
        Leigh's encephalopathy (G31.82)
        mitochondrial metabolism disorders (E88.4-)
        Reye's syndrome (G93.7)

G71.8 Other primary disorders of muscles

G71.9 Primary disorder of muscle, unspecified
    Hereditary myopathy NOS

✓4ᵗʰ G72 Other and unspecified myopathies
> EXCLUDES 1   arthrogryposis multiplex congenita (Q74.3)
> dermatopolymyositis (M33.-)
> ischemic infarction of muscle (M62.2-)
> myositis (M60.-)
> polymyositis (M33.2-)

G72.0 Drug-induced myopathy `CC`
    Use additional code for adverse effect, if applicable, to identify drug (T36-T50 with fifth or sixth character 5)
    CC Excl: PDX collection 593

G72.1 Alcoholic myopathy `CC`
    Use additional code to identify alcoholism (F10.-)
    CC Excl: PDX collection 593

G72.2 Myopathy due to other toxic agents `CC`
    Code first (T51-T65) to identify toxic agent
    CC Excl: PDX collection 593

G72.3 Periodic paralysis
    Familial periodic paralysis
    Hyperkalemic periodic paralysis (familial)
    Hypokalemic periodic paralysis (familial)
    Myotonic periodic paralysis (familial)
    Normokalemic paralysis (familial)
    Potassium sensitive periodic paralysis
    > EXCLUDES 1   paramyotonia congenita (of von Eulenburg) (G71.19)

✓5ᵗʰ G72.4 Inflammatory and immune myopathies, not elsewhere classified
    G72.41 Inclusion body myositis [IBM]
    G72.49 Other inflammatory and immune myopathies, not elsewhere classified
        Inflammatory myopathy NOS

✓5ᵗʰ G72.8 Other specified myopathies
    G72.81 Critical illness myopathy `CC`
        Acute necrotizing myopathy
        Acute quadriplegic myopathy
        Intensive care (ICU) myopathy
        Myopathy of critical illness
        CC Excl: PDX collection 594
    G72.89 Other specified myopathies

G72.9 Myopathy, unspecified

✓4ᵗʰ G73 Disorders of myoneural junction and muscle in diseases classified elsewhere
    G73.1 Lambert-Eaton syndrome in neoplastic disease `CC` `HCC`
        Code first underlying neoplasm (C00-D49)
        > EXCLUDES 1   Lambert-Eaton syndrome not associated with neoplasm (G70.80-G70.81)
        CC Excl: PDX collection 591
    G73.3 Myasthenic syndromes in other diseases classified elsewhere `CC` `HCC`
        Code first underlying disease, such as:
        neoplasm (C00-D49)
        thyrotoxicosis (E05.-)
        CC Excl: PDX collection 591

N Newborn: 0   P Pediatric: 0-17   M Maternity: 12-55   A Adult: 15-124   MCC Major CC Condition   PDxMCC PDx acts as own MCC   CC CC Condition   PDxCC PDx acts as own CC

570   ICD-10-CM 2018

G73.7 *Myopathy in diseases classified elsewhere*
Code first underlying disease, such as:
    hyperparathyroidism (E21.0, E21.3)
    hypoparathyroidism (E20.-)
    glycogen storage disease (E74.0)
    lipid storage disorders (E75.-)
    EXCLUDES 1 *myopathy in:*
        rheumatoid arthritis (M05.4-)
        sarcoidosis (D86.87)
        scleroderma (M34.82)
        sicca syndrome [Sjögren] (M35.03)
        systemic lupus erythematosus (M32.19)

Cerebral palsy and other paralytic syndromes (G80-G83)

√4th G80 Cerebral palsy
    EXCLUDES 1 *hereditary spastic paraplegia (G11.4)*

G80.0 Spastic quadriplegic cerebral palsy   `MCC` `HCC`
    Congenital spastic paralysis (cerebral)
    CC Excl: PDX collection 595

G80.1 Spastic diplegic cerebral palsy   `CC` `HCC`
    Spastic cerebral palsy NOS
    CC Excl: PDX collection 596

G80.2 Spastic hemiplegic cerebral palsy   `CC` `HCC`
    CC Excl: PDX collection 597

G80.3 Athetoid cerebral palsy   `CC` `HCC`
    Double athetosis (syndrome)
    Dyskinetic cerebral palsy
    Dystonic cerebral palsy
    Vogt disease
    CC Excl: PDX collection 598

G80.4 Ataxic cerebral palsy   `HCC`

G80.8 Other cerebral palsy   `HCC`
    Mixed cerebral palsy syndromes

G80.9 Cerebral palsy, unspecified   `HCC`
    Cerebral palsy NOS

√4th G81 Hemiplegia and hemiparesis
    NOTE This category is to be used only when hemiplegia (complete)(incomplete) is reported without further specification, or is stated to be old or longstanding but of unspecified cause. The category is also for use in multiple coding to identify these types of hemiplegia resulting from any cause.
    EXCLUDES 1 *congenital cerebral palsy (G80.-)*
        hemiplegia and hemiparesis due to sequela of cerebrovascular disease (I69.05-, I69.15-, I69.25-, I69.35-, I69.85-, I69.95-)
    AHA: 2015, 1Q, 25

    CC Excl: For CC codes in category G81: PDX collection 561

√5th G81.0 Flaccid hemiplegia
  G81.00 Flaccid hemiplegia affecting unspecified side   `CC` `HCC`
  G81.01 Flaccid hemiplegia affecting right dominant side   `CC` `HCC`
  G81.02 Flaccid hemiplegia affecting left dominant side   `CC` `HCC`
  G81.03 Flaccid hemiplegia affecting right nondominant side   `CC` `HCC`
  G81.04 Flaccid hemiplegia affecting left nondominant side   `CC` `HCC`

√5th G81.1 Spastic hemiplegia
  G81.10 Spastic hemiplegia affecting unspecified side   `CC` `HCC`
  G81.11 Spastic hemiplegia affecting right dominant side   `CC` `HCC`
  G81.12 Spastic hemiplegia affecting left dominant side   `CC` `HCC`
  G81.13 Spastic hemiplegia affecting right nondominant side   `CC` `HCC`
  G81.14 Spastic hemiplegia affecting left nondominant side   `CC` `HCC`

√5th G81.9 Hemiplegia, unspecified
    AHA: 2014, 1Q, 23
  G81.90 Hemiplegia, unspecified affecting unspecified side   `CC` `HCC`
  G81.91 Hemiplegia, unspecified affecting right dominant side   `CC` `HCC`
  G81.92 Hemiplegia, unspecified affecting left dominant side   `CC` `HCC`

G81.93 Hemiplegia, unspecified affecting right nondominant side   `CC` `HCC`
G81.94 Hemiplegia, unspecified affecting left nondominant side   `CC` `HCC`

√4th G82 Paraplegia (paraparesis) and quadriplegia (quadriparesis)
    NOTE This category is to be used only when the listed conditions are reported without further specification, or are stated to be old or longstanding but of unspecified cause. The category is also for use in multiple coding to identify these conditions resulting from any cause
    EXCLUDES 1 *congenital cerebral palsy (G80.-)*
        functional quadriplegia (R53.2)
        hysterical paralysis (F44.4)

√5th G82.2 Paraplegia
    Paralysis of both lower limbs NOS
    Paraparesis (lower) NOS
    Paraplegia (lower) NOS

    CC Excl: For CC codes in subcategory G82.2: PDX collection 561

  G82.20 Paraplegia, unspecified   `CC` `HCC`
  G82.21 Paraplegia, complete   `CC` `HCC`
  G82.22 Paraplegia, incomplete   `CC` `HCC`

√5th G82.5 Quadriplegia

    CC Excl: For MCC codes in subcategory G82.5: PDX collection 595

  G82.50 Quadriplegia, unspecified   `MCC` `HCC`
  G82.51 Quadriplegia, C1-C4 complete   `MCC` `HCC`
  G82.52 Quadriplegia, C1-C4 incomplete   `MCC` `HCC`
  G82.53 Quadriplegia, C5-C7 complete   `MCC` `HCC`
  G82.54 Quadriplegia, C5-C7 incomplete   `MCC` `HCC`

√4th G83 Other paralytic syndromes
    NOTE This category is to be used only when the listed conditions are reported without further specification, or are stated to be old or longstanding but of unspecified cause. The category is also for use in multiple coding to identify these conditions resulting from any cause.
    INCLUDES paralysis (complete) (incomplete), except as in G80-G82

G83.0 Diplegia of upper limbs   `CC` `HCC`
    Diplegia (upper)
    Paralysis of both upper limbs
    CC Excl: PDX collection 599

√5th G83.1 Monoplegia of lower limb
    Paralysis of lower limb
    EXCLUDES 1 *monoplegia of lower limbs due to sequela of cerebrovascular disease (I69.04-, I69.14-, I69.24-, I69.34-, I69.84-, I69.94-)*
  G83.10 Monoplegia of lower limb affecting unspecified side   `HCC`
  G83.11 Monoplegia of lower limb affecting right dominant side   `HCC`
  G83.12 Monoplegia of lower limb affecting left dominant side   `HCC`
  G83.13 Monoplegia of lower limb affecting right nondominant side   `HCC`
  G83.14 Monoplegia of lower limb affecting left nondominant side   `HCC`

√5th G83.2 Monoplegia of upper limb
    Paralysis of upper limb
    EXCLUDES 1 *monoplegia of upper limbs due to sequela of cerebrovascular disease (I69.03-, I69.13-, I69.23-, I69.33-, I69.83-, I69.93-)*
  G83.20 Monoplegia of upper limb affecting unspecified side   `HCC`
  G83.21 Monoplegia of upper limb affecting right dominant side   `HCC`
  G83.22 Monoplegia of upper limb affecting left dominant side   `HCC`
  G83.23 Monoplegia of upper limb affecting right nondominant side   `HCC`
  G83.24 Monoplegia of upper limb affecting left nondominant side   `HCC`

√5th G83.3 Monoplegia, unspecified
  G83.30 Monoplegia, unspecified affecting unspecified side   `HCC`
  G83.31 Monoplegia, unspecified affecting right dominant side   `HCC`

☑Additional Character Req   √x7th Placeholder Alert   Unacceptable PDx   Manifestation   `H1`-`H14` HAC   `HCC` CMS-HCC Condition   *EXCLUDES 1* Not Coded Here   *EXCLUDES 2* Not Included Here

ICD-10-CM 2018   571

Chapter 6. Diseases of the Nervous System

G83.32   Monoplegia, unspecified affecting left dominant side   `HCC`

G83.33   Monoplegia, unspecified affecting right nondominant side   `HCC`

G83.34   Monoplegia, unspecified affecting left nondominant side   `HCC`

G83.4   Cauda equina syndrome   `CC` `HCC`
Neurogenic bladder due to cauda equina syndrome
> *EXCLUDES 1*   cord bladder NOS (G95.89)
> neurogenic bladder NOS (N31.9)

CC Excl: PDX collection 600

G83.5   Locked-in state   `MCC` `HCC`
CC Excl: PDX collection 601

✓5th **G83.8   Other specified paralytic syndromes**
> *EXCLUDES 1*   paralytic syndromes due to current spinal cord
> injury—code to spinal cord injury (S14, S24, S34)

G83.81   Brown-Séquard syndrome   `HCC`

G83.82   Anterior cord syndrome   `HCC`

G83.83   Posterior cord syndrome   `HCC`

G83.84   Todd's paralysis (postepileptic)   `HCC`

G83.89   Other specified paralytic syndromes   `HCC`

G83.9   Paralytic syndrome, unspecified   `HCC`

Other disorders of the nervous system (G89-G99)

✓4th **G89   Pain, not elsewhere classified**
Code also related psychological factors associated with pain (F45.42)
> *EXCLUDES 1*   generalized pain NOS (R52)
> pain disorders exclusively related to psychological factors
> (F45.41)
> pain NOS (R52)
> *EXCLUDES 2*   atypical face pain (G50.1)
> headache syndromes (G44.-)
> localized pain, unspecified type—code to pain by site, such as:
> abdomen pain (R10.-)
> back pain (M54.9)
> breast pain (N64.4)
> chest pain (R07.1-R07.9)
> ear pain (H92.0-)
> eye pain (H57.1)
> headache (R51)
> joint pain (M25.5-)
> limb pain (M79.6-)
> lumbar region pain (M54.5)
> painful urination (R30.9)
> pelvic and perineal pain (R10.2)
> renal colic (N23)
> shoulder pain (M25.51-)
> spine pain (M54.-)
> throat pain (R07.0)
> tongue pain (K14.6)
> tooth pain (K08.8)
> migraines (G43.-)
> myalgia (M79.1)
> pain from prosthetic devices, implants, and grafts (T82.84,
> T83.84, T84.84, T85.84-)
> phantom limb syndrome with pain (G54.6)
> vulvar vestibulitis (N94.810)
> vulvodynia (N94.81-)

G89.0   Central pain syndrome
Déjérine-Roussy syndrome
Myelopathic pain syndrome
Thalamic pain syndrome (hyperesthetic)

✓5th **G89.1   Acute pain, not elsewhere classified**

G89.11   Acute pain due to trauma

G89.12   Acute post-thoracotomy pain
Post-thoracotomy pain NOS

G89.18   Other acute postprocedural pain
Postoperative pain NOS
Postprocedural pain NOS

✓5th **G89.2   Chronic pain, not elsewhere classified**
> *EXCLUDES 1*   causalgia, lower limb (G57.7-)
> causalgia, upper limb (G56.4-)
> central pain syndrome (G89.0)
> chronic pain syndrome (G89.4)
> complex regional pain syndrome II, lower limb (G57.7-)
> complex regional pain syndrome II, upper limb (G56.4-)
> neoplasm related chronic pain (G89.3)
> reflex sympathetic dystrophy (G90.5-)

G89.21   Chronic pain due to trauma

G89.22   Chronic post-thoracotomy pain

G89.28   Other chronic postprocedural pain
Other chronic postoperative pain

G89.29   Other chronic pain

G89.3   Neoplasm related pain (acute) (chronic)
Cancer associated pain
Pain due to malignancy (primary) (secondary)
Tumor associated pain

G89.4   Chronic pain syndrome
Chronic pain associated with significant psychosocial dysfunction

✓4th **G90   Disorders of autonomic nervous system**
> *EXCLUDES 1*   dysfunction of the autonomic nervous system due to alcohol
> (G31.2)

✓5th **G90.0   Idiopathic peripheral autonomic neuropathy**

G90.01   Carotid sinus syncope
Carotid sinus syndrome
DEF: Vagal activation caused by pressure on the carotid sinus baroreceptors; sympathetic nerve impulses may cause sinus arrest or AV block.

G90.09   Other idiopathic peripheral autonomic neuropathy
Idiopathic peripheral autonomic neuropathy NOS

G90.1   Familial dysautonomia [Riley-Day]   `HCC`

G90.2   Horner's syndrome
Bernard(-Horner) syndrome
Cervical sympathetic dystrophy or paralysis

G90.3   Multi-system degeneration of the autonomic nervous   `CC` `HCC`
system
Neurogenic orthostatic hypotension [Shy-Drager]
> *EXCLUDES 1*   orthostatic hypotension NOS (I95.1)

CC Excl: PDX collection 573

G90.4   Autonomic dysreflexia
Use additional code to identify the cause, such as:
fecal impaction (K56.41)
pressure ulcer (pressure area) (L89.-)
urinary tract infection (N39.0)

✓5th **G90.5   Complex regional pain syndrome I (CRPS I)**
Reflex sympathetic dystrophy
> *EXCLUDES 1*   causalgia of lower limb (G57.7-)
> causalgia of upper limb (G56.4-)
> complex regional pain syndrome II of lower limb
> (G57.7-)
> complex regional pain syndrome II of upper limb
> (G56.4-)

> **CC Excl: For CC codes in subcategory G90.5, unless otherwise noted:** PDX collection 603

G90.50   Complex regional pain syndrome I, unspecified   `CC`
CC Excl: PDX collection 602

✓6th **G90.51   Complex regional pain syndrome I of upper limb**

G90.511   Complex regional pain syndrome I of right upper limb   `CC`

G90.512   Complex regional pain syndrome I of left upper limb   `CC`

G90.513   Complex regional pain syndrome I of upper limb, bilateral   `CC`

G90.519   Complex regional pain syndrome I of unspecified upper limb   `CC`

✓6th **G90.52   Complex regional pain syndrome I of lower limb**

G90.521   Complex regional pain syndrome I of right lower limb   `CC`

G90.522   Complex regional pain syndrome I of left lower limb   `CC`

G90.523   Complex regional pain syndrome I of lower limb, bilateral   `CC`

G90.529   Complex regional pain syndrome I of unspecified lower limb   `CC`

G90.59   Complex regional pain syndrome I of other specified site   `CC`

G90.8   Other disorders of autonomic nervous system

G90.9   Disorder of the autonomic nervous system, unspecified

N Newborn: 0   P Pediatric: 0-17   M Maternity: 12-55   A Adult: 15-124   `MCC` Major CC Condition   `PDxMCC` PDx acts as own MCC   `CC` CC Condition   `PDxCC` PDx acts as own CC

572   ICD-10-CM 2018

Hydrocephalus (Acquired)

Normal ventricles   Hydrocephalic ventricles

☑️4ᵗʰ **G91 Hydrocephalus**
    INCLUDES   acquired hydrocephalus
    EXCLUDES 1   *Arnold-Chiari syndrome with hydrocephalus (Q07.-)*
                congenital hydrocephalus (Q03.-)
                spina bifida with hydrocephalus (Q05.-)

> **CC Excl: For CC codes in category G91, unless otherwise noted:**
> PDX collection 605

G91.0 Communicating hydrocephalus   CC
     Secondary normal pressure hydrocephalus
     CC Excl: PDX collection 604

G91.1 Obstructive hydrocephalus   CC
     DEF: Obstruction of cerebrospinal fluid passage from brain into spinal canal; characterized by headaches, drowsiness, poor coordination, urinary incontinence, nausea, vomiting, and papilledema.

G91.2 (Idiopathic) normal pressure hydrocephalus   CC
     Normal pressure hydrocephalus NOS
     CC Excl: PDX collection 604

G91.3 Post-traumatic hydrocephalus, unspecified   CC

G91.4 Hydrocephalus in diseases classified elsewhere
     Code first underlying condition, such as:
         congenital syphilis (A50.4-)
         neoplasm (C00-D49)
         EXCLUDES 1   *hydrocephalus due to congenital toxoplasmosis (P37.1)*
     AHA: 2014, 3Q, 3

G91.8 Other hydrocephalus   CC

G91.9 Hydrocephalus, unspecified   CC

G92 Toxic encephalopathy   MCC
     Toxic encephalitis
     Toxic metabolic encephalopathy
     ▶Code first, if applicable, drug induced (T36-T50)◄
     Code first (T51-T65) to identify toxic agent
     AHA: 2017, 1Q, 39-40
     DEF: Brain tissue degeneration due to toxic substance.
     CC Excl: PDX collection 606

☑️4ᵗʰ **G93 Other disorders of brain**

G93.0 Cerebral cysts
     Arachnoid cyst
     Porencephalic cyst, acquired
     EXCLUDES 1   *acquired periventricular cysts of newborn (P91.1)*
                congenital cerebral cysts (Q04.6)

G93.1 Anoxic brain damage, not elsewhere classified   CC HCC
     EXCLUDES 1   *cerebral anoxia due to anesthesia during labor and delivery (O74.3)*
                cerebral anoxia due to anesthesia during the puerperium (O89.2)
                neonatal anoxia (P84)
     DEF: Brain injury not resulting from birth trauma that is due to lack of oxygen. Brain cells, when deprived of oxygen, begin to expire after 4 minutes.
     CC Excl: PDX collection 607

G93.2 Benign intracranial hypertension
     EXCLUDES 1   *hypertensive encephalopathy (I67.4)*

G93.3 Postviral fatigue syndrome
     Benign myalgic encephalomyelitis
     EXCLUDES 1   *chronic fatigue syndrome NOS (R53.82)*

☑️5ᵗʰ **G93.4 Other and unspecified encephalopathy**
     EXCLUDES 1   *alcoholic encephalopathy (G31.2)*
                encephalopathy in diseases classified elsewhere (G94)
                hypertensive encephalopathy (I67.4)
                toxic (metabolic) encephalopathy (G92)

     G93.40 Encephalopathy, unspecified   HIV MCC
         AHA: 2017, 2Q, 8
         CC Excl: PDX collection 608

     G93.41 Metabolic encephalopathy   HIV MCC
         Septic encephalopathy
         AHA: 2017, 2Q, 8; 2016, 3Q, 42; 2015, 3Q, 21
         CC Excl: GPDX collection 609

     G93.49 Other encephalopathy   HIV MCC
         Encephalopathy NEC
         AHA: 2017, 2Q, 9
         CC Excl: PDX collection 610

G93.5 Compression of brain   MCC HCC
     Arnold-Chiari type 1 compression of brain
     Compression of brain (stem)
     Herniation of brain (stem)
     EXCLUDES 1   *diffuse traumatic compression of brain (S06.2-)*
                focal traumatic compression of brain (S06.3-)
     CC Excl: PDX collection 611

G93.6 Cerebral edema   MCC HCC
     EXCLUDES 1   *cerebral edema due to birth injury (P11.0)*
                traumatic cerebral edema (S06.1-)
     CC Excl: PDX collection 612

G93.7 Reye's syndrome   MCC P
     ~~Code first (T39.0-), if salicylates-induced~~
     ▶Code first poisoning due to salicylates, if applicable (T39.0-, with sixth character 1-4)◄
     ▶Use additional code for adverse effect due to salicylates, if applicable (T39.0-, with sixth character 5)◄
     DEF: Rare childhood illness often developed after a viral upper respiratory infection; characterized by vomiting, elevated serum transaminase, brain swelling, disturbances of consciousness, seizures, and changes in liver and other viscera; can be fatal.
     CC Excl: PDX collection 613

☑️5ᵗʰ **G93.8 Other specified disorders of brain**

     G93.81 Temporal sclerosis
         Hippocampal sclerosis
         Mesial temporal sclerosis

     G93.82 Brain death   MCC
         CC Excl: PDX collection 515

     G93.89 Other specified disorders of brain
         Postradiation encephalopathy

G93.9 Disorder of brain, unspecified   HIV

G94 *Other disorders of brain in diseases classified elsewhere*
     Code first underlying disease
     EXCLUDES 1   *encephalopathy in congenital syphilis (A50.49)*
                encephalopathy in influenza (J09.X9, J10.81, J11.81)
                encephalopathy in syphilis (A52.19)
                hydrocephalus in diseases classified elsewhere (G91.4)

☑️4ᵗʰ **G95 Other and unspecified diseases of spinal cord**
     EXCLUDES 2   *myelitis (G04.-)*

G95.0 Syringomyelia and syringobulbia   CC HCC
     CC Excl: PDX collection 614

☑️5ᵗʰ **G95.1 Vascular myelopathies**
     EXCLUDES 2   *intraspinal phlebitis and thrombophlebitis, except non-pyogenic (G08)*

     G95.11 Acute infarction of spinal cord (embolic) (nonembolic)   MCC HCC
         Anoxia of spinal cord
         Arterial thrombosis of spinal cord
         CC Excl: PDX collection 603

     G95.19 Other vascular myelopathies   MCC HCC
         Edema of spinal cord
         Hematomyelia
         Nonpyogenic intraspinal phlebitis and thrombophlebitis
         Subacute necrotic myelopathy
         CC Excl: PDX collection 603

☑️Additional Character Req   ☑️x7ᵗʰ Placeholder Alert   Unacceptable PDx   Manifestation   **H1 - H14** HAC   **HCC** CMS-HCC Condition   **EXCLUDES 1** Not Coded Here   **EXCLUDES 2** Not Included Here

ICD-10-CM 2018   **573**

Chapter 6. Diseases of the Nervous System

☑5ᵗʰ **G95.2** **Other and unspecified cord compression**

     G95.20 **Unspecified cord compression**   HIV CC HCC
         CC Excl: PDX collection 615

     G95.29 **Other cord compression**   HIV CC HCC
         CC Excl: PDX collection 615

☑5ᵗʰ **G95.8** **Other specified diseases of spinal cord**
       EXCLUDES 1   *neurogenic bladder NOS (N31.9)*
                neurogenic bladder due to cauda equina syndrome
                    (G83.4)
                neuromuscular dysfunction of bladder without spinal
                    cord lesion (N31.-)

     G95.81 **Conus medullaris syndrome**   CC HCC
         CC Excl: PDX collection 603

     G95.89 **Other specified diseases of spinal cord**   CC HCC
         Cord bladder NOS
         Drug-induced myelopathy
         Radiation-induced myelopathy
         EXCLUDES 1   *myelopathy NOS (G95.9)*
         CC Excl: PDX collection 603

G95.9 **Disease of spinal cord, unspecified**   HIV CC HCC
     Myelopathy NOS
     CC Excl: PDX collection 615

☑4ᵗʰ **G96** **Other disorders of central nervous system**

     G96.0 **Cerebrospinal fluid leak**   CC
         EXCLUDES 1   *cerebrospinal fluid leak from spinal puncture (G97.0)*
         DEF: Cerebrospinal fluid discharging from the nose or the ear;
         caused by fracture of frontal bone with tearing of dura mater and
         arachnoid; characterized by watery drainage usually from only one
         side of the nose or one ear, headache, vision changes, and hearing
         loss.
         CC Excl: PDX collection 616

☑5ᵗʰ **G96.1** **Disorders of meninges, not elsewhere classified**

     G96.11 **Dural tear**   CC
         EXCLUDES 1   *accidental puncture or laceration of dura*
                    during a procedure (G97.41)
         AHA: 2014, 4Q, 24
         CC Excl: PDX collection 509

     G96.12 **Meningeal adhesions (cerebral) (spinal)**

     G96.19 **Other disorders of meninges, not elsewhere**
         classified

G96.8 **Other specified disorders of central nervous system**

G96.9 **Disorder of central nervous system, unspecified**   HIV

☑4ᵗʰ **G97** **Intraoperative and postprocedural complications and disorders of nervous system, not elsewhere classified**
     EXCLUDES 2   *intraoperative and postprocedural cerebrovascular infarction*
              (I97.81-, I97.82-)

     G97.0 **Cerebrospinal fluid leak from spinal puncture**   CC
         CC Excl: PDX collection 617

     G97.1 **Other reaction to spinal and lumbar puncture**
         Headache due to lumbar puncture

     G97.2 **Intracranial hypotension following ventricular shunting**   CC
         CC Excl: PDX collection 617

☑5ᵗʰ **G97.3** **Intraoperative hemorrhage and hematoma of a nervous system organ or structure complicating a procedure**
         EXCLUDES 1   *intraoperative hemorrhage and hematoma of a*
                  nervous system organ or structure due to
                  accidental puncture and laceration during a
                  procedure (G97.4-)

     G97.31 **Intraoperative hemorrhage and hematoma of a**   CC
         nervous system organ or structure complicating a
         nervous system procedure
         CC Excl: PDX collection 618

     G97.32 **Intraoperative hemorrhage and hematoma of a**   CC
         nervous system organ or structure complicating
         other procedure
         CC Excl: PDX collection 618

☑5ᵗʰ **G97.4** **Accidental puncture and laceration of a nervous system organ or structure during a procedure**

     CC Excl: For CC codes in subcategory G97.4:
     PDX collection 509

     G97.41 **Accidental puncture or laceration of dura**   CC
         during a procedure
         Incidental (inadvertent) durotomy
         AHA: 2014, 4Q, 24

     G97.48 **Accidental puncture and laceration of other**   CC
         nervous system organ or structure during a
         nervous system procedure

Spinal Puncture

- Spinal cord
- Epidural space
- Subarachnoid space
- Vertebra
- Spinal needle
- Lumbar area

     G97.49 **Accidental puncture and laceration of other**   CC
         nervous system organ or structure during
         other procedure

☑5ᵗʰ **G97.5** **Postprocedural hemorrhage of a nervous system organ or structure following a procedure**

     G97.51 **Postprocedural hemorrhage of a nervous**   CC
         system organ or structure following a nervous
         system procedure
         CC Excl: PDX collection 619

     G97.52 **Postprocedural hemorrhage of a nervous**   CC
         system organ or structure following other
         procedure
         CC Excl: PDX collection 619

☑5ᵗʰ **G97.6** **Postprocedural hematoma and seroma of a nervous system organ or structure following a procedure**

     CC Excl: For CC codes in subcategory G97.6, unless
     otherwise noted: PDX collection 619

     G97.61 **Postprocedural hematoma of a nervous system**   CC
         organ or structure following a nervous system
         procedure

     G97.62 **Postprocedural hematoma of a nervous system**   CC
         organ or structure following other procedure

     G97.63 **Postprocedural seroma of a nervous system**   CC
         organ or structure following a nervous system
         procedure

     G97.64 **Postprocedural seroma of a nervous system**   CC
         organ or structure following other procedure

☑5ᵗʰ **G97.8** **Other intraoperative and postprocedural complications and disorders of nervous system**
     Use additional code to further specify disorder

     G97.81 **Other intraoperative complications of nervous**   CC
         system
         CC Excl: PDX collection 617

     G97.82 **Other postprocedural complications and**   CC
         disorders of nervous system
         CC Excl: PDX collection 617

☑4ᵗʰ **G98** **Other disorders of nervous system not elsewhere classified**
     INCLUDES   nervous system disorder NOS

     G98.0 **Neurogenic arthritis, not elsewhere classified**
         Nonsyphilitic neurogenic arthropathy NEC
         Nonsyphilitic neurogenic spondylopathy NEC
         EXCLUDES 1   *spondylopathy (in):*
                  syringomyelia and syringobulbia (G95.0)
                  tabes dorsalis (A52.11)

     G98.8 **Other disorders of nervous system**   HIV
         Nervous system disorder NOS

☑4ᵗʰ **G99** **Other disorders of nervous system in diseases classified elsewhere**

     G99.0 *Autonomic neuropathy in diseases classified elsewhere*   CC
         Code first underlying disease, such as:
            amyloidosis (E85.-)
            gout (M1A.-, M10.-)
            hyperthyroidism (E05.-)
         EXCLUDES 1   *diabetic autonomic neuropathy (E08-E13 with .43)*
         CC Excl: PDX collection 620

N Newborn: 0   P Pediatric: 0-17   M Maternity: 12-55   A Adult: 15-124   MCC Major CC Condition   PDxMCC PDx acts as own MCC   CC CC Condition   PDxCC PDx acts as own CC

574   ICD-10-CM 2018

G99.2   *Myelopathy in diseases classified elsewhere*   `CC` `HCC`

     Code first underlying disease, such as:
        neoplasm (C00-D49)

     `EXCLUDES 1`   *myelopathy in:*
            intervertebral disease (M50.0-, M51.0-)
            spondylosis (M47.0-, M47.1-)

     CC Excl: PDX collection 603

G99.8   *Other specified disorders of nervous system in diseases classified elsewhere*

     Code first underlying disorder, such as:
        amyloidosis (E85.-)
        avitaminosis (E56.9)

     `EXCLUDES 1`   *nervous system involvement in:*
            cysticercosis (B69.0)
            rubella (B06.0-)
            syphilis (A52.1-)

☑ Additional Character Req   `√x7ᵗʰ` Placeholder Alert   Unacceptable PDx   Manifestation   `H1`-`H14` HAC   `HCC` CMS-HCC Condition   `EXCLUDES 1` Not Coded Here   `EXCLUDES 2` Not Included Here

ICD-10-CM 2018   **575**

Chapter 7. Diseases of the Eye and Adnexa (H00–H59)

Chapter Specific Guidelines with Coding Examples

The chapter specific guidelines from the ICD-10-CM Official Guidelines for Coding and Reporting have been provided below. Along with these guidelines are coding examples, contained in the shaded boxes, that have been developed to help illustrate the coding and/or sequencing guidance found in these guidelines.

a. Glaucoma

1) Assigning glaucoma codes

Assign as many codes from category H40, Glaucoma, as needed to identify the type of glaucoma, the affected eye, and the glaucoma stage.

2) Bilateral glaucoma with same type and stage

When a patient has bilateral glaucoma and both eyes are documented as being the same type and stage, and there is a code for bilateral glaucoma, report only the code for the type of glaucoma, bilateral, with the seventh character for the stage.

> Bilateral severe stage pigmentary glaucoma
>
> **H40.1333   Pigmentary glaucoma, bilateral, severe stage**
>
> *Explanation*: In this scenario, the patient has the same type and stage of glaucoma in both eyes. As this type of glaucoma has a code for bilateral, assign only the code for the bilateral glaucoma with the seventh character for the stage.

When a patient has bilateral glaucoma and both eyes are documented as being the same type and stage, and the classification does not provide a code for bilateral glaucoma (i.e. subcategories H40.10, H40.11 and H40.20) report only one code for the type of glaucoma with the appropriate seventh character for the stage.

> Bilateral open-angle glaucoma; not specified as to type and stage indeterminate in both eyes
>
> **H40.10X4   Unspecified open-angle glaucoma, indeterminate stage**
>
> *Explanation*: In this scenario, the patient has glaucoma of the same type and stage of both eyes, but there is no code specifically for bilateral glaucoma. Only one code is assigned with the appropriate seventh character for the stage.

3) Bilateral glaucoma stage with different types or stages

When a patient has bilateral glaucoma and each eye is documented as having a different type or stage, and the classification distinguishes laterality, assign the appropriate code for each eye rather than the code for bilateral glaucoma.

> Bilateral chronic angle-closure glaucoma; right eye is documented as mild stage and left eye as moderate stage
>
> **H40.2211   Chronic angle-closure glaucoma, right eye, mild stage**
>
> **H40.2222   Chronic angle-closure glaucoma, left eye, moderate stage**
>
> *Explanation*: In this scenario the patient has the same type of glaucoma in both eyes, but each eye is at a different stage. Because the subcategory for this condition identifies laterality, one code is assigned for the right eye and one code is assigned for the left eye, each with the appropriate seventh character for the stage appended.

When a patient has bilateral glaucoma and each eye is documented as having a different type, and the classification does not distinguish laterality (i.e. subcategories H40.10, H40.11 and H40.20), assign one code for each type of glaucoma with the appropriate seventh character for the stage.

> Documentation relates mild, unspecified primary angle-closure glaucoma of the left eye with mild unspecified open-angle glaucoma of the right eye
>
> **H40.20X1   Unspecified primary angle-closure glaucoma, mild stage**
>
> **H40.10X1   Unspecified open-angle glaucoma, mild stage**
>
> *Explanation*: In this scenario the patient has a different type of glaucoma in each eye and the classification does not distinguish laterality. A code for each type of glaucoma is assigned, each with the appropriate seventh character for the stage.

When a patient has bilateral glaucoma and each eye is documented as having the same type, but different stage, and the classification does not distinguish laterality (i.e. subcategories H40.10, H40.11 and H40.20), assign a code for the type of glaucoma for each eye with the seventh character for the specific glaucoma stage documented for each eye.

> Bilateral open-angle glaucoma, not specified as to type; the right eye is documented to be in mild stage and the left eye as being in moderate stage
>
> **H40.10X1   Unspecified open-angle glaucoma, mild stage**
>
> **H40.10X2   Unspecified open-angle glaucoma, moderate stage**
>
> *Explanation*: In this scenario the patient has the same type of glaucoma in each eye but each eye is at a different stage, and the classification does not distinguish laterality at this subcategory level. Two codes are assigned; both codes represent the same type of glaucoma but each has a different seventh character identifying the appropriate stage for each eye.

4) Patient admitted with glaucoma and stage evolves during the admission

If a patient is admitted with glaucoma and the stage progresses during the admission, assign the code for highest stage documented.

> Patient admitted with mild low-tension glaucoma of the right eye, which progresses to moderate stage during the patient's stay
>
> **H40.1212   Low-tension glaucoma, right eye, moderate stage**
>
> *Explanation*: When the glaucoma stage progresses during an admission, assign only the code for the highest stage documented.

5) Indeterminate stage glaucoma

Assignment of the seventh character "4" for "indeterminate stage" should be based on the clinical documentation. The seventh character "4" is used for glaucomas whose stage cannot be clinically determined. This seventh character should not be confused with the seventh character "0", unspecified, which should be assigned when there is no documentation regarding the stage of the glaucoma.

b. Blindness

If "blindness" or "low vision" of both eyes is documented but the visual impairment category is not documented, assign code H54.3, Unqualified visual loss, both eyes. If "blindness" or "low vision" in one eye is documented but the visual impairment category is not documented, assign a code from H54.6-, Unqualified visual loss, one eye. If "blindness" or "visual loss" is documented without any information about whether one or both eyes are affected, assign code H54.7, Unspecified visual loss.

Chapter 7. Diseases of the Eye and Adnexa (H00-H59)

NOTE   Use an external cause code following the code for the eye condition, if applicable, to identify the cause of the eye condition.

EXCLUDES 2   certain conditions originating in the perinatal period (P04-P96)
certain infectious and parasitic diseases (A00-B99)
complications of pregnancy, childbirth and the puerperium (O00-O9A)
congenital malformations, deformations, and chromosomal abnormalities (Q00-Q99)
diabetes mellitus related eye conditions (E09.3-, E10.3-, E11.3-, E13.3-)
endocrine, nutritional and metabolic diseases (E00-E88)
injury (trauma) of eye and orbit (S05.-)
injury, poisoning and certain other consequences of external causes (S00-T88)
neoplasms (C00-D49)
symptoms, signs and abnormal clinical and laboratory findings, not elsewhere classified (R00-R94)
syphilis related eye disorders (A50.01, A50.3-, A51.43, A52.71)

This chapter contains the following blocks:

H00-H05	Disorders of eyelid, lacrimal system and orbit
H10-H11	Disorders of conjunctiva
H15-H22	Disorders of sclera, cornea, iris and ciliary body
H25-H28	Disorders of lens
H30-H36	Disorders of choroid and retina
H40-H42	Glaucoma
H43-H44	Disorders of vitreous body and globe
H46-H47	Disorders of optic nerve and visual pathways
H49-H52	Disorders of ocular muscles, binocular movement, accommodation and refraction
H53-H54	Visual disturbances and blindness
H55-H57	Other disorders of eye and adnexa
H59	Intraoperative and postprocedural complications and disorders of eye and adnexa, not elsewhere classified

Disorders of eyelid, lacrimal system and orbit (H00-H05)

EXCLUDES 2   open wound of eyelid (S01.1-)
superficial injury of eyelid (S00.1-, S00.2-)

✓4ᵗʰ H00 Hordeolum and chalazion

   ✓5ᵗʰ H00.0 Hordeolum (externum) (internum) of eyelid

     ✓6ᵗʰ H00.01 Hordeolum externum
     Hordeolum NOS
     Stye

     H00.011 Hordeolum externum right upper eyelid
     H00.012 Hordeolum externum right lower eyelid
     H00.013 Hordeolum externum right eye, unspecified eyelid
     H00.014 Hordeolum externum left upper eyelid
     H00.015 Hordeolum externum left lower eyelid
     H00.016 Hordeolum externum left eye, unspecified eyelid
     H00.019 Hordeolum externum unspecified eye, unspecified eyelid

     ✓6ᵗʰ H00.02 Hordeolum internum
     Infection of meibomian gland

     H00.021 Hordeolum internum right upper eyelid
     H00.022 Hordeolum internum right lower eyelid
     H00.023 Hordeolum internum right eye, unspecified eyelid
     H00.024 Hordeolum internum left upper eyelid
     H00.025 Hordeolum internum left lower eyelid
     H00.026 Hordeolum internum left eye, unspecified eyelid
     H00.029 Hordeolum internum unspecified eye, unspecified eyelid

     ✓6ᵗʰ H00.03 Abscess of eyelid
     Furuncle of eyelid

     H00.031 Abscess of right upper eyelid
     H00.032 Abscess of right lower eyelid
     H00.033 Abscess of eyelid right eye, unspecified eyelid
     H00.034 Abscess of left upper eyelid
     H00.035 Abscess of left lower eyelid
     H00.036 Abscess of eyelid left eye, unspecified eyelid
     H00.039 Abscess of eyelid unspecified eye, unspecified eyelid

   ✓5ᵗʰ H00.1 Chalazion
   Meibomian (gland) cyst
   EXCLUDES 2 infected meibomian gland (H00.02-)

     H00.11 Chalazion right upper eyelid
     H00.12 Chalazion right lower eyelid
     H00.13 Chalazion right eye, unspecified eyelid
     H00.14 Chalazion left upper eyelid
     H00.15 Chalazion left lower eyelid
     H00.16 Chalazion left eye, unspecified eyelid
     H00.19 Chalazion unspecified eye, unspecified eyelid

✓4ᵗʰ H01 Other inflammation of eyelid

   ✓5ᵗʰ H01.0 Blepharitis
   EXCLUDES 1 blepharoconjunctivitis (H10.5-)

     ✓6ᵗʰ H01.00 Unspecified blepharitis
     H01.001 Unspecified blepharitis right upper eyelid
     H01.002 Unspecified blepharitis right lower eyelid
     H01.003 Unspecified blepharitis right eye, unspecified eyelid
     H01.004 Unspecified blepharitis left upper eyelid
     H01.005 Unspecified blepharitis left lower eyelid
     H01.006 Unspecified blepharitis left eye, unspecified eyelid
     H01.009 Unspecified blepharitis unspecified eye, unspecified eyelid

     ✓6ᵗʰ H01.01 Ulcerative blepharitis
     H01.011 Ulcerative blepharitis right upper eyelid
     H01.012 Ulcerative blepharitis right lower eyelid
     H01.013 Ulcerative blepharitis right eye, unspecified eyelid
     H01.014 Ulcerative blepharitis left upper eyelid
     H01.015 Ulcerative blepharitis left lower eyelid
     H01.016 Ulcerative blepharitis left eye, unspecified eyelid
     H01.019 Ulcerative blepharitis unspecified eye, unspecified eyelid

     ✓6ᵗʰ H01.02 Squamous blepharitis
     H01.021 Squamous blepharitis right upper eyelid
     H01.022 Squamous blepharitis right lower eyelid
     H01.023 Squamous blepharitis right eye, unspecified eyelid
     H01.024 Squamous blepharitis left upper eyelid
     H01.025 Squamous blepharitis left lower eyelid
     H01.026 Squamous blepharitis left eye, unspecified eyelid
     H01.029 Squamous blepharitis unspecified eye, unspecified eyelid

   ✓5ᵗʰ H01.1 Noninfectious dermatoses of eyelid

     ✓6ᵗʰ H01.11 Allergic dermatitis of eyelid
     Contact dermatitis of eyelid

     H01.111 Allergic dermatitis of right upper eyelid
     H01.112 Allergic dermatitis of right lower eyelid
     H01.113 Allergic dermatitis of right eye, unspecified eyelid
     H01.114 Allergic dermatitis of left upper eyelid
     H01.115 Allergic dermatitis of left lower eyelid
     H01.116 Allergic dermatitis of left eye, unspecified eyelid
     H01.119 Allergic dermatitis of unspecified eye, unspecified eyelid

     ✓6ᵗʰ H01.12 Discoid lupus erythematosus of eyelid
     H01.121 Discoid lupus erythematosus of right upper eyelid
     H01.122 Discoid lupus erythematosus of right lower eyelid
     H01.123 Discoid lupus erythematosus of right eye, unspecified eyelid
     H01.124 Discoid lupus erythematosus of left upper eyelid
     H01.125 Discoid lupus erythematosus of left lower eyelid
     H01.126 Discoid lupus erythematosus of left eye, unspecified eyelid
     H01.129 Discoid lupus erythematosus of unspecified eye, unspecified eyelid

   ✓6ᵗʰ **H01.13** **Eczematous dermatitis of eyelid**

       H01.131 **Eczematous dermatitis of right upper eyelid**

       H01.132 **Eczematous dermatitis of right lower eyelid**

       H01.133 **Eczematous dermatitis of right eye, unspecified eyelid**

       H01.134 **Eczematous dermatitis of left upper eyelid**

       H01.135 **Eczematous dermatitis of left lower eyelid**

       H01.136 **Eczematous dermatitis of left eye, unspecified eyelid**

       H01.139 **Eczematous dermatitis of unspecified eye, unspecified eyelid**

   ✓6ᵗʰ **H01.14** **Xeroderma of eyelid**

       H01.141 **Xeroderma of right upper eyelid**

       H01.142 **Xeroderma of right lower eyelid**

       H01.143 **Xeroderma of right eye, unspecified eyelid**

       H01.144 **Xeroderma of left upper eyelid**

       H01.145 **Xeroderma of left lower eyelid**

       H01.146 **Xeroderma of left eye, unspecified eyelid**

       H01.149 **Xeroderma of unspecified eye, unspecified eyelid**

   H01.8 **Other specified inflammations of eyelid**

   H01.9 **Unspecified inflammation of eyelid**
       Inflammation of eyelid NOS

✓4ᵗʰ **H02** **Other disorders of eyelid**

   EXCLUDES 1   congenital malformations of eyelid (Q10.0-Q10.3)

   ✓5ᵗʰ **H02.0** **Entropion and trichiasis of eyelid**

     ✓6ᵗʰ **H02.00** **Unspecified entropion of eyelid**

       H02.001 **Unspecified entropion of right upper eyelid**

       H02.002 **Unspecified entropion of right lower eyelid**

       H02.003 **Unspecified entropion of right eye, unspecified eyelid**

       H02.004 **Unspecified entropion of left upper eyelid**

       H02.005 **Unspecified entropion of left lower eyelid**

       H02.006 **Unspecified entropion of left eye, unspecified eyelid**

       H02.009 **Unspecified entropion of unspecified eye, unspecified eyelid**

     ✓6ᵗʰ **H02.01** **Cicatricial entropion of eyelid**

       H02.011 **Cicatricial entropion of right upper eyelid**

       H02.012 **Cicatricial entropion of right lower eyelid**

       H02.013 **Cicatricial entropion of right eye, unspecified eyelid**

       H02.014 **Cicatricial entropion of left upper eyelid**

       H02.015 **Cicatricial entropion of left lower eyelid**

       H02.016 **Cicatricial entropion of left eye, unspecified eyelid**

       H02.019 **Cicatricial entropion of unspecified eye, unspecified eyelid**

     ✓6ᵗʰ **H02.02** **Mechanical entropion of eyelid**

       H02.021 **Mechanical entropion of right upper eyelid**

       H02.022 **Mechanical entropion of right lower eyelid**

       H02.023 **Mechanical entropion of right eye, unspecified eyelid**

       H02.024 **Mechanical entropion of left upper eyelid**

       H02.025 **Mechanical entropion of left lower eyelid**

       H02.026 **Mechanical entropion of left eye, unspecified eyelid**

       H02.029 **Mechanical entropion of unspecified eye, unspecified eyelid**

     ✓6ᵗʰ **H02.03** **Senile entropion of eyelid**

       H02.031 **Senile entropion of right upper eyelid** Ⓐ

       H02.032 **Senile entropion of right lower eyelid** Ⓐ

       H02.033 **Senile entropion of right eye, unspecified eyelid** Ⓐ

       H02.034 **Senile entropion of left upper eyelid** Ⓐ

       H02.035 **Senile entropion of left lower eyelid** Ⓐ

       H02.036 **Senile entropion of left eye, unspecified eyelid** Ⓐ

       H02.039 **Senile entropion of unspecified eye, unspecified eyelid** Ⓐ

Entropion and Ectropion

Normal eyelid   Entropion   Ectropion

   ✓6ᵗʰ **H02.04** **Spastic entropion of eyelid**

       H02.041 **Spastic entropion of right upper eyelid**

       H02.042 **Spastic entropion of right lower eyelid**

       H02.043 **Spastic entropion of right eye, unspecified eyelid**

       H02.044 **Spastic entropion of left upper eyelid**

       H02.045 **Spastic entropion of left lower eyelid**

       H02.046 **Spastic entropion of left eye, unspecified eyelid**

       H02.049 **Spastic entropion of unspecified eye, unspecified eyelid**

 ▲ ✓6ᵗʰ **H02.05** **Trichiasis without entropion**

 ▲   **H02.051** **Trichiasis without entropion right upper eyelid**

 ▲   **H02.052** **Trichiasis without entropion right lower eyelid**

 ▲   **H02.053** **Trichiasis without entropion right eye, unspecified eyelid**

 ▲   **H02.054** **Trichiasis without entropion left upper eyelid**

 ▲   **H02.055** **Trichiasis without entropion left lower eyelid**

 ▲   **H02.056** **Trichiasis without entropion left eye, unspecified eyelid**

 ▲   **H02.059** **Trichiasis without entropion unspecified eye, unspecified eyelid**

   ✓5ᵗʰ **H02.1** **Ectropion of eyelid**

     ✓6ᵗʰ **H02.10** **Unspecified ectropion of eyelid**

       H02.101 **Unspecified ectropion of right upper eyelid**

       H02.102 **Unspecified ectropion of right lower eyelid**

       H02.103 **Unspecified ectropion of right eye, unspecified eyelid**

       H02.104 **Unspecified ectropion of left upper eyelid**

       H02.105 **Unspecified ectropion of left lower eyelid**

       H02.106 **Unspecified ectropion of left eye, unspecified eyelid**

       H02.109 **Unspecified ectropion of unspecified eye, unspecified eyelid**

     ✓6ᵗʰ **H02.11** **Cicatricial ectropion of eyelid**

       H02.111 **Cicatricial ectropion of right upper eyelid**

       H02.112 **Cicatricial ectropion of right lower eyelid**

       H02.113 **Cicatricial ectropion of right eye, unspecified eyelid**

       H02.114 **Cicatricial ectropion of left upper eyelid**

       H02.115 **Cicatricial ectropion of left lower eyelid**

       H02.116 **Cicatricial ectropion of left eye, unspecified eyelid**

       H02.119 **Cicatricial ectropion of unspecified eye, unspecified eyelid**

     ✓6ᵗʰ **H02.12** **Mechanical ectropion of eyelid**

       H02.121 **Mechanical ectropion of right upper eyelid**

       H02.122 **Mechanical ectropion of right lower eyelid**

       H02.123 **Mechanical ectropion of right eye, unspecified eyelid**

       H02.124 **Mechanical ectropion of left upper eyelid**

       H02.125 **Mechanical ectropion of left lower eyelid**

       H02.126 **Mechanical ectropion of left eye, unspecified eyelid**

       H02.129 **Mechanical ectropion of unspecified eye, unspecified eyelid**

✓ Additional Character Req   ✓×7ᵗʰ Placeholder Alert   Unacceptable PDx   Manifestation   **H1**-**H14** HAC   **HCC** CMS-HCC Condition   *EXCLUDES 1* Not Coded Here   *EXCLUDES 2* Not Included Here

ICD-10-CM 2018   **579**

Chapter 7. Diseases of the Eye and Adnexa

√6th **H02.13** Senile ectropion of eyelid
- H02.131 Senile ectropion of right upper eyelid   A
- H02.132 Senile ectropion of right lower eyelid   A
- H02.133 Senile ectropion of right eye, unspecified eyelid   A
- H02.134 Senile ectropion of left upper eyelid   A
- H02.135 Senile ectropion of left lower eyelid   A
- H02.136 Senile ectropion of left eye, unspecified eyelid   A
- H02.139 Senile ectropion of unspecified eye, unspecified eyelid   A

√6th **H02.14** Spastic ectropion of eyelid
- H02.141 Spastic ectropion of right upper eyelid
- H02.142 Spastic ectropion of right lower eyelid
- H02.143 Spastic ectropion of right eye, unspecified eyelid
- H02.144 Spastic ectropion of left upper eyelid
- H02.145 Spastic ectropion of left lower eyelid
- H02.146 Spastic ectropion of left eye, unspecified eyelid
- H02.149 Spastic ectropion of unspecified eye, unspecified eyelid

√5th **H02.2** Lagophthalmos

√6th **H02.20** Unspecified lagophthalmos
- H02.201 Unspecified lagophthalmos right upper eyelid
- H02.202 Unspecified lagophthalmos right lower eyelid
- H02.203 Unspecified lagophthalmos right eye, unspecified eyelid
- H02.204 Unspecified lagophthalmos left upper eyelid
- H02.205 Unspecified lagophthalmos left lower eyelid
- H02.206 Unspecified lagophthalmos left eye, unspecified eyelid
- H02.209 Unspecified lagophthalmos unspecified eye, unspecified eyelid

√6th **H02.21** Cicatricial lagophthalmos
- H02.211 Cicatricial lagophthalmos right upper eyelid
- H02.212 Cicatricial lagophthalmos right lower eyelid
- H02.213 Cicatricial lagophthalmos right eye, unspecified eyelid
- H02.214 Cicatricial lagophthalmos left upper eyelid
- H02.215 Cicatricial lagophthalmos left lower eyelid
- H02.216 Cicatricial lagophthalmos left eye, unspecified eyelid
- H02.219 Cicatricial lagophthalmos unspecified eye, unspecified eyelid

√6th **H02.22** Mechanical lagophthalmos
- H02.221 Mechanical lagophthalmos right upper eyelid
- H02.222 Mechanical lagophthalmos right lower eyelid
- H02.223 Mechanical lagophthalmos right eye, unspecified eyelid
- H02.224 Mechanical lagophthalmos left upper eyelid
- H02.225 Mechanical lagophthalmos left lower eyelid
- H02.226 Mechanical lagophthalmos left eye, unspecified eyelid
- H02.229 Mechanical lagophthalmos unspecified eye, unspecified eyelid

√6th **H02.23** Paralytic lagophthalmos
- H02.231 Paralytic lagophthalmos right upper eyelid
- H02.232 Paralytic lagophthalmos right lower eyelid
- H02.233 Paralytic lagophthalmos right eye, unspecified eyelid
- H02.234 Paralytic lagophthalmos left upper eyelid
- H02.235 Paralytic lagophthalmos left lower eyelid
- H02.236 Paralytic lagophthalmos left eye, unspecified eyelid
- H02.239 Paralytic lagophthalmos unspecified eye, unspecified eyelid

√5th **H02.3** Blepharochalasis
   Pseudoptosis
- H02.30 Blepharochalasis unspecified eye, unspecified eyelid
- H02.31 Blepharochalasis right upper eyelid
- H02.32 Blepharochalasis right lower eyelid
- H02.33 Blepharochalasis right eye, unspecified eyelid
- H02.34 Blepharochalasis left upper eyelid
- H02.35 Blepharochalasis left lower eyelid
- H02.36 Blepharochalasis left eye, unspecified eyelid

√5th **H02.4** Ptosis of eyelid

√6th **H02.40** Unspecified ptosis of eyelid
- H02.401 Unspecified ptosis of right eyelid
- H02.402 Unspecified ptosis of left eyelid
- H02.403 Unspecified ptosis of bilateral eyelids
- H02.409 Unspecified ptosis of unspecified eyelid

√6th **H02.41** Mechanical ptosis of eyelid
- H02.411 Mechanical ptosis of right eyelid
- H02.412 Mechanical ptosis of left eyelid
- H02.413 Mechanical ptosis of bilateral eyelids
- H02.419 Mechanical ptosis of unspecified eyelid

√6th **H02.42** Myogenic ptosis of eyelid
- H02.421 Myogenic ptosis of right eyelid
- H02.422 Myogenic ptosis of left eyelid
- H02.423 Myogenic ptosis of bilateral eyelids
- H02.429 Myogenic ptosis of unspecified eyelid

√6th **H02.43** Paralytic ptosis of eyelid
   Neurogenic ptosis of eyelid
- H02.431 Paralytic ptosis of right eyelid
- H02.432 Paralytic ptosis of left eyelid
- H02.433 Paralytic ptosis of bilateral eyelids
- H02.439 Paralytic ptosis unspecified eyelid

√5th **H02.5** Other disorders affecting eyelid function
   EXCLUDES 2   blepharospasm (G24.5)
           organic tic (G25.69)
           psychogenic tic (F95.-)

√6th **H02.51** Abnormal innervation syndrome
- H02.511 Abnormal innervation syndrome right upper eyelid
- H02.512 Abnormal innervation syndrome right lower eyelid
- H02.513 Abnormal innervation syndrome right eye, unspecified eyelid
- H02.514 Abnormal innervation syndrome left upper eyelid
- H02.515 Abnormal innervation syndrome left lower eyelid
- H02.516 Abnormal innervation syndrome left eye, unspecified eyelid
- H02.519 Abnormal innervation syndrome unspecified eye, unspecified eyelid

√6th **H02.52** Blepharophimosis
   Ankyloblepharon
- H02.521 Blepharophimosis right upper eyelid
- H02.522 Blepharophimosis right lower eyelid
- H02.523 Blepharophimosis right eye, unspecified eyelid
- H02.524 Blepharophimosis left upper eyelid
- H02.525 Blepharophimosis left lower eyelid
- H02.526 Blepharophimosis left eye, unspecified eyelid
- H02.529 Blepharophimosis unspecified eye, unspecified lid

√6th **H02.53** Eyelid retraction
   Eyelid lag
- H02.531 Eyelid retraction right upper eyelid
- H02.532 Eyelid retraction right lower eyelid
- H02.533 Eyelid retraction right eye, unspecified eyelid
- H02.534 Eyelid retraction left upper eyelid
- H02.535 Eyelid retraction left lower eyelid
- H02.536 Eyelid retraction left eye, unspecified eyelid

N Newborn: 0   P Pediatric: 0-17   M Maternity: 12-55   A Adult: 15-124   MCC Major CC Condition   PDxMCC PDx acts as own MCC   CC CC Condition   PDxCC PDx acts as own CC

580   ICD-10-CM 2018

H02.539   Eyelid retraction unspecified eye, unspecified lid

H02.59   Other disorders affecting eyelid function
Deficient blink reflex
Sensory disorders

✓5th **H02.6**   Xanthelasma of eyelid

H02.60   Xanthelasma of unspecified eye, unspecified eyelid

H02.61   Xanthelasma of right upper eyelid

H02.62   Xanthelasma of right lower eyelid

H02.63   Xanthelasma of right eye, unspecified eyelid

H02.64   Xanthelasma of left upper eyelid

H02.65   Xanthelasma of left lower eyelid

H02.66   Xanthelasma of left eye, unspecified eyelid

✓5th **H02.7**   Other and unspecified degenerative disorders of eyelid and periocular area

H02.70   Unspecified degenerative disorders of eyelid and periocular area

✓6th **H02.71**   Chloasma of eyelid and periocular area
Dyspigmentation of eyelid
Hyperpigmentation of eyelid

H02.711   Chloasma of right upper eyelid and periocular area

H02.712   Chloasma of right lower eyelid and periocular area

H02.713   Chloasma of right eye, unspecified eyelid and periocular area

H02.714   Chloasma of left upper eyelid and periocular area

H02.715   Chloasma of left lower eyelid and periocular area

H02.716   Chloasma of left eye, unspecified eyelid and periocular area

H02.719   Chloasma of unspecified eye, unspecified eyelid and periocular area

✓6th **H02.72**   Madarosis of eyelid and periocular area
Hypotrichosis of eyelid

H02.721   Madarosis of right upper eyelid and periocular area

H02.722   Madarosis of right lower eyelid and periocular area

H02.723   Madarosis of right eye, unspecified eyelid and periocular area

H02.724   Madarosis of left upper eyelid and periocular area

H02.725   Madarosis of left lower eyelid and periocular area

H02.726   Madarosis of left eye, unspecified eyelid and periocular area

H02.729   Madarosis of unspecified eye, unspecified eyelid and periocular area

✓6th **H02.73**   Vitiligo of eyelid and periocular area
Hypopigmentation of eyelid

H02.731   Vitiligo of right upper eyelid and periocular area

H02.732   Vitiligo of right lower eyelid and periocular area

H02.733   Vitiligo of right eye, unspecified eyelid and periocular area

H02.734   Vitiligo of left upper eyelid and periocular area

H02.735   Vitiligo of left lower eyelid and periocular area

H02.736   Vitiligo of left eye, unspecified eyelid and periocular area

H02.739   Vitiligo of unspecified eye, unspecified eyelid and periocular area

H02.79   Other degenerative disorders of eyelid and periocular area

✓5th **H02.8**   Other specified disorders of eyelid

✓6th **H02.81**   Retained foreign body in eyelid
Use additional code to identify the type of retained foreign body (Z18.-)

EXCLUDES 1   *laceration of eyelid with foreign body (S01.12-)*
retained intraocular foreign body (H44.6-, H44.7-)
superficial foreign body of eyelid and periocular area (S00.25-)

H02.811   Retained foreign body in right upper eyelid

H02.812   Retained foreign body in right lower eyelid

H02.813   Retained foreign body in right eye, unspecified eyelid

H02.814   Retained foreign body in left upper eyelid

H02.815   Retained foreign body in left lower eyelid

H02.816   Retained foreign body in left eye, unspecified eyelid

H02.819   Retained foreign body in unspecified eye, unspecified eyelid

✓6th **H02.82**   Cysts of eyelid
Sebaceous cyst of eyelid

H02.821   Cysts of right upper eyelid

H02.822   Cysts of right lower eyelid

H02.823   Cysts of right eye, unspecified eyelid

H02.824   Cysts of left upper eyelid

H02.825   Cysts of left lower eyelid

H02.826   Cysts of left eye, unspecified eyelid

H02.829   Cysts of unspecified eye, unspecified eyelid

✓6th **H02.83**   Dermatochalasis of eyelid
DEF: Acquired form of connective tissue disorder associated with decreased elastic tissue and abnormal elastin formation, resulting in loss of elasticity of the skin of the eyelid; generally associated with aging.

H02.831   Dermatochalasis of right upper eyelid

H02.832   Dermatochalasis of right lower eyelid

H02.833   Dermatochalasis of right eye, unspecified eyelid

H02.834   Dermatochalasis of left upper eyelid

H02.835   Dermatochalasis of left lower eyelid

H02.836   Dermatochalasis of left eye, unspecified eyelid

H02.839   Dermatochalasis of unspecified eye, unspecified eyelid

✓6th **H02.84**   Edema of eyelid
Hyperemia of eyelid

H02.841   Edema of right upper eyelid

H02.842   Edema of right lower eyelid

H02.843   Edema of right eye, unspecified eyelid

H02.844   Edema of left upper eyelid

H02.845   Edema of left lower eyelid

H02.846   Edema of left eye, unspecified eyelid

H02.849   Edema of unspecified eye, unspecified eyelid

✓6th **H02.85**   Elephantiasis of eyelid

H02.851   Elephantiasis of right upper eyelid

H02.852   Elephantiasis of right lower eyelid

H02.853   Elephantiasis of right eye, unspecified eyelid

H02.854   Elephantiasis of left upper eyelid

H02.855   Elephantiasis of left lower eyelid

H02.856   Elephantiasis of left eye, unspecified eyelid

H02.859   Elephantiasis of unspecified eye, unspecified eyelid

✓6th **H02.86**   Hypertrichosis of eyelid

H02.861   Hypertrichosis of right upper eyelid

H02.862   Hypertrichosis of right lower eyelid

H02.863   Hypertrichosis of right eye, unspecified eyelid

H02.864   Hypertrichosis of left upper eyelid

H02.865   Hypertrichosis of left lower eyelid

H02.866   Hypertrichosis of left eye, unspecified eyelid

✔ Additional Character Req   ✔x7th Placeholder Alert   Unacceptable PDx   Manifestation   H1 - H14 HAC   HCC CMS-HCC Condition   *EXCLUDES 1* Not Coded Here   *EXCLUDES 2* Not Included Here

ICD-10-CM 2018   581

       H02.869   **Hypertrichosis** of unspecified eye, unspecified eyelid

✓6ᵗʰ   **H02.87**   **Vascular anomalies of eyelid**
       H02.871   **Vascular anomalies of** right upper **eyelid**
       H02.872   **Vascular anomalies of** right lower **eyelid**
       H02.873   **Vascular anomalies of** right eye, unspecified **eyelid**
       H02.874   **Vascular anomalies of** left upper **eyelid**
       H02.875   **Vascular anomalies of** left lower **eyelid**
       H02.876   **Vascular anomalies of** left eye, unspecified **eyelid**
       H02.879   **Vascular anomalies of** unspecified eye, unspecified **eyelid**

   H02.89   **Other specified disorders of eyelid**
       Hemorrhage of eyelid

  H02.9   **Unspecified disorder of eyelid**
       Disorder of eyelid NOS

✓4ᵗʰ   **H04**   **Disorders of lacrimal system**
   EXCLUDES 1   *congenital malformations of lacrimal system (Q10.4-Q10.6)*

✓5ᵗʰ   **H04.0**   **Dacryoadenitis**

✓6ᵗʰ   **H04.00**   **Unspecified dacryoadenitis**
       H04.001   **Unspecified dacryoadenitis,** right lacrimal gland
       H04.002   **Unspecified dacryoadenitis,** left lacrimal gland
       H04.003   **Unspecified dacryoadenitis,** bilateral lacrimal glands
       H04.009   **Unspecified dacryoadenitis,** unspecified lacrimal gland

✓6ᵗʰ   **H04.01**   **Acute dacryoadenitis**
       H04.011   **Acute dacryoadenitis,** right lacrimal gland
       H04.012   **Acute dacryoadenitis,** left lacrimal gland
       H04.013   **Acute dacryoadenitis,** bilateral lacrimal glands
       H04.019   **Acute dacryoadenitis,** unspecified lacrimal gland

✓6ᵗʰ   **H04.02**   **Chronic dacryoadenitis**
       H04.021   **Chronic dacryoadenitis,** right lacrimal gland
       H04.022   **Chronic dacryoadenitis,** left lacrimal gland
       H04.023   **Chronic dacryoadenitis,** bilateral lacrimal glands
       H04.029   **Chronic dacryoadenitis,** unspecified lacrimal gland

✓6ᵗʰ   **H04.03**   **Chronic enlargement of lacrimal gland**
       H04.031   **Chronic enlargement of** right lacrimal gland
       H04.032   **Chronic enlargement of** left lacrimal gland
       H04.033   **Chronic enlargement of** bilateral lacrimal glands
       H04.039   **Chronic enlargement of** unspecified lacrimal gland

✓5ᵗʰ   **H04.1**   **Other disorders of lacrimal gland**

✓6ᵗʰ   **H04.11**   **Dacryops**
       H04.111   **Dacryops of** right lacrimal gland
       H04.112   **Dacryops of** left lacrimal gland
       H04.113   **Dacryops of** bilateral lacrimal glands
       H04.119   **Dacryops of** unspecified lacrimal gland

✓6ᵗʰ   **H04.12**   **Dry eye syndrome**
       Tear film insufficiency, NOS
       H04.121   **Dry eye syndrome of** right lacrimal gland
       H04.122   **Dry eye syndrome of** left lacrimal gland
       H04.123   **Dry eye syndrome of** bilateral lacrimal glands
       H04.129   **Dry eye syndrome of** unspecified lacrimal gland

✓6ᵗʰ   **H04.13**   **Lacrimal cyst**
       Lacrimal cystic degeneration
       H04.131   **Lacrimal cyst,** right lacrimal gland
       H04.132   **Lacrimal cyst,** left lacrimal gland
       H04.133   **Lacrimal cyst,** bilateral lacrimal glands
       H04.139   **Lacrimal cyst,** unspecified lacrimal gland

✓6ᵗʰ   **H04.14**   **Primary lacrimal gland atrophy**
       H04.141   **Primary lacrimal gland atrophy,** right lacrimal gland

       H04.142   **Primary lacrimal gland atrophy,** left lacrimal gland
       H04.143   **Primary lacrimal gland atrophy,** bilateral lacrimal glands
       H04.149   **Primary lacrimal gland atrophy,** unspecified lacrimal gland

✓6ᵗʰ   **H04.15**   **Secondary lacrimal gland atrophy**
       H04.151   **Secondary lacrimal gland atrophy,** right lacrimal gland
       H04.152   **Secondary lacrimal gland atrophy,** left lacrimal gland
       H04.153   **Secondary lacrimal gland atrophy,** bilateral lacrimal glands
       H04.159   **Secondary lacrimal gland atrophy,** unspecified lacrimal gland

✓6ᵗʰ   **H04.16**   **Lacrimal gland dislocation**
       H04.161   **Lacrimal gland dislocation,** right lacrimal gland
       H04.162   **Lacrimal gland dislocation,** left lacrimal gland
       H04.163   **Lacrimal gland dislocation,** bilateral lacrimal glands
       H04.169   **Lacrimal gland dislocation,** unspecified lacrimal gland

   H04.19   **Other specified disorders of lacrimal gland**

✓5ᵗʰ   **H04.2**   **Epiphora**

✓6ᵗʰ   **H04.20**   **Unspecified epiphora**
       H04.201   **Unspecified epiphora,** right lacrimal gland
       H04.202   **Unspecified epiphora,** left lacrimal gland
       H04.203   **Unspecified epiphora,** bilateral lacrimal glands
       H04.209   **Unspecified epiphora,** unspecified lacrimal gland

✓6ᵗʰ   **H04.21**   **Epiphora** due to excess lacrimation
       H04.211   **Epiphora due to excess lacrimation,** right lacrimal gland
       H04.212   **Epiphora due to excess lacrimation,** left lacrimal gland
       H04.213   **Epiphora due to excess lacrimation,** bilateral lacrimal glands
       H04.219   **Epiphora due to excess lacrimation,** unspecified lacrimal gland

✓6ᵗʰ   **H04.22**   **Epiphora** due to insufficient drainage
       H04.221   **Epiphora due to insufficient drainage,** right lacrimal gland
       H04.222   **Epiphora due to insufficient drainage,** left lacrimal gland
       H04.223   **Epiphora due to insufficient drainage,** bilateral lacrimal glands
       H04.229   **Epiphora due to insufficient drainage,** unspecified lacrimal gland

✓5ᵗʰ   **H04.3**   **Acute and unspecified inflammation of lacrimal passages**
   EXCLUDES 1   *neonatal dacryocystitis (P39.1)*

✓6ᵗʰ   **H04.30**   **Unspecified dacryocystitis**
       H04.301   **Unspecified dacryocystitis of** right lacrimal passage
       H04.302   **Unspecified dacryocystitis of** left lacrimal passage
       H04.303   **Unspecified dacryocystitis of** bilateral lacrimal passages
       H04.309   **Unspecified dacryocystitis of** unspecified lacrimal passage

✓6ᵗʰ   **H04.31**   **Phlegmonous dacryocystitis**
       H04.311   **Phlegmonous dacryocystitis of** right lacrimal passage
       H04.312   **Phlegmonous dacryocystitis of** left lacrimal passage
       H04.313   **Phlegmonous dacryocystitis of** bilateral lacrimal passages
       H04.319   **Phlegmonous dacryocystitis of** unspecified lacrimal passage

✓6ᵗʰ   **H04.32**   **Acute dacryocystitis**
       Acute dacryopericystitis
       H04.321   **Acute dacryocystitis of** right lacrimal passage
       H04.322   **Acute dacryocystitis of** left lacrimal passage

H04.323 Acute dacryocystitis of bilateral lacrimal passages

H04.329 Acute dacryocystitis of unspecified lacrimal passage

√6ᵗʰ **H04.33** Acute lacrimal canaliculitis

H04.331 Acute lacrimal canaliculitis of right lacrimal passage

H04.332 Acute lacrimal canaliculitis of left lacrimal passage

H04.333 Acute lacrimal canaliculitis of bilateral lacrimal passages

H04.339 Acute lacrimal canaliculitis of unspecified lacrimal passage

√5ᵗʰ **H04.4** Chronic inflammation of lacrimal passages

√6ᵗʰ **H04.41** Chronic dacryocystitis

H04.411 Chronic dacryocystitis of right lacrimal passage

H04.412 Chronic dacryocystitis of left lacrimal passage

H04.413 Chronic dacryocystitis of bilateral lacrimal passages

H04.419 Chronic dacryocystitis of unspecified lacrimal passage

√6ᵗʰ **H04.42** Chronic lacrimal canaliculitis

H04.421 Chronic lacrimal canaliculitis of right lacrimal passage

H04.422 Chronic lacrimal canaliculitis of left lacrimal passage

H04.423 Chronic lacrimal canaliculitis of bilateral lacrimal passages

H04.429 Chronic lacrimal canaliculitis of unspecified lacrimal passage

√6ᵗʰ **H04.43** Chronic lacrimal mucocele

H04.431 Chronic lacrimal mucocele of right lacrimal passage

H04.432 Chronic lacrimal mucocele of left lacrimal passage

H04.433 Chronic lacrimal mucocele of bilateral lacrimal passages

H04.439 Chronic lacrimal mucocele of unspecified lacrimal passage

√5ᵗʰ **H04.5** Stenosis and insufficiency of lacrimal passages

√6ᵗʰ **H04.51** Dacryolith

H04.511 Dacryolith of right lacrimal passage

H04.512 Dacryolith of left lacrimal passage

H04.513 Dacryolith of bilateral lacrimal passages

H04.519 Dacryolith of unspecified lacrimal passage

√6ᵗʰ **H04.52** Eversion of lacrimal punctum

H04.521 Eversion of right lacrimal punctum

H04.522 Eversion of left lacrimal punctum

H04.523 Eversion of bilateral lacrimal punctum

H04.529 Eversion of unspecified lacrimal punctum

√6ᵗʰ **H04.53** Neonatal obstruction of nasolacrimal duct

EXCLUDES 1   *congenital stenosis and stricture of lacrimal duct (Q10.5)*

H04.531 Neonatal obstruction of right nasolacrimal duct N

H04.532 Neonatal obstruction of left nasolacrimal duct N

H04.533 Neonatal obstruction of bilateral nasolacrimal duct N

H04.539 Neonatal obstruction of unspecified nasolacrimal duct N

√6ᵗʰ **H04.54** Stenosis of lacrimal canaliculi

H04.541 Stenosis of right lacrimal canaliculi

H04.542 Stenosis of left lacrimal canaliculi

H04.543 Stenosis of bilateral lacrimal canaliculi

H04.549 Stenosis of unspecified lacrimal canaliculi

√6ᵗʰ **H04.55** Acquired stenosis of nasolacrimal duct

H04.551 Acquired stenosis of right nasolacrimal duct

H04.552 Acquired stenosis of left nasolacrimal duct

H04.553 Acquired stenosis of bilateral nasolacrimal duct

H04.559 Acquired stenosis of unspecified nasolacrimal duct

√6ᵗʰ **H04.56** Stenosis of lacrimal punctum

H04.561 Stenosis of right lacrimal punctum

H04.562 Stenosis of left lacrimal punctum

H04.563 Stenosis of bilateral lacrimal punctum

H04.569 Stenosis of unspecified lacrimal punctum

√6ᵗʰ **H04.57** Stenosis of lacrimal sac

H04.571 Stenosis of right lacrimal sac

H04.572 Stenosis of left lacrimal sac

H04.573 Stenosis of bilateral lacrimal sac

H04.579 Stenosis of unspecified lacrimal sac

√5ᵗʰ **H04.6** Other changes of lacrimal passages

√6ᵗʰ **H04.61** Lacrimal fistula

H04.611 Lacrimal fistula right lacrimal passage

H04.612 Lacrimal fistula left lacrimal passage

H04.613 Lacrimal fistula bilateral lacrimal passages

H04.619 Lacrimal fistula unspecified lacrimal passage

H04.69 Other changes of lacrimal passages

√5ᵗʰ **H04.8** Other disorders of lacrimal system

√6ᵗʰ **H04.81** Granuloma of lacrimal passages

H04.811 Granuloma of right lacrimal passage

H04.812 Granuloma of left lacrimal passage

H04.813 Granuloma of bilateral lacrimal passages

H04.819 Granuloma of unspecified lacrimal passage

H04.89 Other disorders of lacrimal system

H04.9 Disorder of lacrimal system, unspecified

√4ᵗʰ **H05** Disorders of orbit

EXCLUDES 1   *congenital malformation of orbit (Q10.7)*

√5ᵗʰ **H05.0** Acute inflammation of orbit

H05.00 Unspecified acute inflammation of orbit

√6ᵗʰ **H05.01** Cellulitis of orbit

Abscess of orbit

> **CC Excl: For CC codes in subcategory H05.01:**
> PDX collection 621

H05.011 Cellulitis of right orbit CC

H05.012 Cellulitis of left orbit CC

H05.013 Cellulitis of bilateral orbits CC

H05.019 Cellulitis of unspecified orbit CC

√6ᵗʰ **H05.02** Osteomyelitis of orbit

> **CC Excl: For CC codes in subcategory H05.02:**
> PDX collection 622

H05.021 Osteomyelitis of right orbit CC

H05.022 Osteomyelitis of left orbit CC

H05.023 Osteomyelitis of bilateral orbits CC

H05.029 Osteomyelitis of unspecified orbit CC

√6ᵗʰ **H05.03** Periostitis of orbit

> **CC Excl: For CC codes in subcategory H05.03:**
> PDX collection 623

H05.031 Periostitis of right orbit CC

H05.032 Periostitis of left orbit CC

H05.033 Periostitis of bilateral orbits CC

H05.039 Periostitis of unspecified orbit CC

√6ᵗʰ **H05.04** Tenonitis of orbit

H05.041 Tenonitis of right orbit

H05.042 Tenonitis of left orbit

H05.043 Tenonitis of bilateral orbits

H05.049 Tenonitis of unspecified orbit

√5ᵗʰ **H05.1** Chronic inflammatory disorders of orbit

H05.10 Unspecified chronic inflammatory disorders of orbit

√6ᵗʰ **H05.11** Granuloma of orbit

Pseudotumor (inflammatory) of orbit

H05.111 Granuloma of right orbit

H05.112 Granuloma of left orbit

H05.113 Granuloma of bilateral orbits

H05.119 Granuloma of unspecified orbit

√6ᵗʰ **H05.12** Orbital myositis

H05.121 Orbital myositis, right orbit

H05.122 Orbital myositis, left orbit

H05.123 Orbital myositis, bilateral

✓ Additional Character Req   ✓x7ᵗʰ Placeholder Alert   Unacceptable PDx   Manifestation   H1 - H14 HAC   HCC CMS-HCC Condition   EXCLUDES 1 Not Coded Here   EXCLUDES 2 Not Included Here

ICD-10-CM 2018   583

H05.129   **Orbital myositis, unspecified orbit**

✓5th   **H05.2   Exophthalmic conditions**

H05.20   **Unspecified exophthalmos**

✓6th   **H05.21   Displacement (lateral) of globe**

H05.211   **Displacement (lateral) of globe, right eye**

H05.212   **Displacement (lateral) of globe, left eye**

H05.213   **Displacement (lateral) of globe, bilateral**

H05.219   **Displacement (lateral) of globe, unspecified eye**

✓6th   **H05.22   Edema of orbit**
Orbital congestion

H05.221   **Edema of right orbit**

H05.222   **Edema of left orbit**

H05.223   **Edema of bilateral orbit**

H05.229   **Edema of unspecified orbit**

✓6th   **H05.23   Hemorrhage of orbit**

H05.231   **Hemorrhage of right orbit**

H05.232   **Hemorrhage of left orbit**

H05.233   **Hemorrhage of bilateral orbit**

H05.239   **Hemorrhage of unspecified orbit**

✓6th   **H05.24   Constant exophthalmos**

H05.241   **Constant exophthalmos, right eye**

H05.242   **Constant exophthalmos, left eye**

H05.243   **Constant exophthalmos, bilateral**

H05.249   **Constant exophthalmos, unspecified eye**

✓6th   **H05.25   Intermittent exophthalmos**

H05.251   **Intermittent exophthalmos, right eye**

H05.252   **Intermittent exophthalmos, left eye**

H05.253   **Intermittent exophthalmos, bilateral**

H05.259   **Intermittent exophthalmos, unspecified eye**

✓6th   **H05.26   Pulsating exophthalmos**

H05.261   **Pulsating exophthalmos, right eye**

H05.262   **Pulsating exophthalmos, left eye**

H05.263   **Pulsating exophthalmos, bilateral**

H05.269   **Pulsating exophthalmos, unspecified eye**

✓5th   **H05.3   Deformity of orbit**

EXCLUDES 1   congenital deformity of orbit (Q10.7)
hypertelorism (Q75.2)

H05.30   **Unspecified deformity of orbit**

✓6th   **H05.31   Atrophy of orbit**

H05.311   **Atrophy of right orbit**

H05.312   **Atrophy of left orbit**

H05.313   **Atrophy of bilateral orbit**

H05.319   **Atrophy of unspecified orbit**

✓6th   **H05.32   Deformity of orbit due to bone disease**
Code also associated bone disease

H05.321   **Deformity of right orbit due to bone disease**

H05.322   **Deformity of left orbit due to bone disease**

H05.323   **Deformity of bilateral orbits due to bone disease**

H05.329   **Deformity of unspecified orbit due to bone disease**

✓6th   **H05.33   Deformity of orbit due to trauma or surgery**

H05.331   **Deformity of right orbit due to trauma or surgery**

H05.332   **Deformity of left orbit due to trauma or surgery**

H05.333   **Deformity of bilateral orbits due to trauma or surgery**

H05.339   **Deformity of unspecified orbit due to trauma or surgery**

✓6th   **H05.34   Enlargement of orbit**

H05.341   **Enlargement of right orbit**

H05.342   **Enlargement of left orbit**

H05.343   **Enlargement of bilateral orbits**

H05.349   **Enlargement of unspecified orbit**

✓6th   **H05.35   Exostosis of orbit**

H05.351   **Exostosis of right orbit**

H05.352   **Exostosis of left orbit**

H05.353   **Exostosis of bilateral orbits**

H05.359   **Exostosis of unspecified orbit**

✓5th   **H05.4   Enophthalmos**

✓6th   **H05.40   Unspecified enophthalmos**

H05.401   **Unspecified enophthalmos, right eye**

H05.402   **Unspecified enophthalmos, left eye**

H05.403   **Unspecified enophthalmos, bilateral**

H05.409   **Unspecified enophthalmos, unspecified eye**

✓6th   **H05.41   Enophthalmos due to atrophy of orbital tissue**

H05.411   **Enophthalmos due to atrophy of orbital tissue, right eye**

H05.412   **Enophthalmos due to atrophy of orbital tissue, left eye**

H05.413   **Enophthalmos due to atrophy of orbital tissue, bilateral**

H05.419   **Enophthalmos due to atrophy of orbital tissue, unspecified eye**

✓6th   **H05.42   Enophthalmos due to trauma or surgery**

H05.421   **Enophthalmos due to trauma or surgery, right eye**

H05.422   **Enophthalmos due to trauma or surgery, left eye**

H05.423   **Enophthalmos due to trauma or surgery, bilateral**

H05.429   **Enophthalmos due to trauma or surgery, unspecified eye**

✓5th   **H05.5   Retained (old) foreign body following penetrating wound of orbit**
Retrobulbar foreign body

Use additional code to identify the type of retained foreign body (Z18.-)

EXCLUDES 1   current penetrating wound of orbit (S05.4-)

EXCLUDES 2   retained foreign body of eyelid (H02.81-)
retained intraocular foreign body (H44.6-, H44.7-)

H05.50   **Retained (old) foreign body following penetrating wound of unspecified orbit**

H05.51   **Retained (old) foreign body following penetrating wound of right orbit**

H05.52   **Retained (old) foreign body following penetrating wound of left orbit**

H05.53   **Retained (old) foreign body following penetrating wound of bilateral orbits**

✓5th   **H05.8   Other disorders of orbit**

✓6th   **H05.81   Cyst of orbit**
Encephalocele of orbit

H05.811   **Cyst of right orbit**

H05.812   **Cyst of left orbit**

H05.813   **Cyst of bilateral orbits**

H05.819   **Cyst of unspecified orbit**

✓6th   **H05.82   Myopathy of extraocular muscles**

H05.821   **Myopathy of extraocular muscles, right orbit**

H05.822   **Myopathy of extraocular muscles, left orbit**

H05.823   **Myopathy of extraocular muscles, bilateral**

H05.829   **Myopathy of extraocular muscles, unspecified orbit**

H05.89   **Other disorders of orbit**

H05.9   **Unspecified disorder of orbit**

Disorders of conjunctiva (H10-H11)

✓4th   **H10   Conjunctivitis**

EXCLUDES 1   keratoconjunctivitis (H16.2-)

✓5th   **H10.0   Mucopurulent conjunctivitis**

✓6th   **H10.01   Acute follicular conjunctivitis**

H10.011   **Acute follicular conjunctivitis, right eye**

H10.012   **Acute follicular conjunctivitis, left eye**

H10.013   **Acute follicular conjunctivitis, bilateral**

H10.019   **Acute follicular conjunctivitis, unspecified eye**

✓6th   **H10.02   Other mucopurulent conjunctivitis**

H10.021   **Other mucopurulent conjunctivitis, right eye**

H10.022   **Other mucopurulent conjunctivitis, left eye**

        H10.023   **Other mucopurulent conjunctivitis, bilateral**

        H10.029   **Other mucopurulent conjunctivitis, unspecified eye**

✓5ᵗʰ **H10.1**   **Acute atopic conjunctivitis**
     Acute papillary conjunctivitis

     H10.10   **Acute atopic conjunctivitis,** unspecified eye
     H10.11   **Acute atopic conjunctivitis,** right eye
     H10.12   **Acute atopic conjunctivitis,** left eye
     H10.13   **Acute atopic conjunctivitis,** bilateral

✓5ᵗʰ **H10.2**   **Other acute conjunctivitis**

  ✓6ᵗʰ **H10.21**   **Acute toxic conjunctivitis**
     Acute chemical conjunctivitis
     Code first (T51-T65) to identify chemical and intent
     EXCLUDES 1   *burn and corrosion of eye and adnexa (T26.-)*

     H10.211   **Acute toxic conjunctivitis,** right eye
     H10.212   **Acute toxic conjunctivitis,** left eye
     H10.213   **Acute toxic conjunctivitis,** bilateral
     H10.219   **Acute toxic conjunctivitis,** unspecified eye

  ✓6ᵗʰ **H10.22**   **Pseudomembranous conjunctivitis**
     H10.221   **Pseudomembranous conjunctivitis,** right eye
     H10.222   **Pseudomembranous conjunctivitis,** left eye
     H10.223   **Pseudomembranous conjunctivitis, bilateral**
     H10.229   **Pseudomembranous conjunctivitis, unspecified eye**

  ✓6ᵗʰ **H10.23**   **Serous conjunctivitis, except viral**
     EXCLUDES 1   *viral conjunctivitis (B30.-)*
     H10.231   **Serous conjunctivitis, except viral,** right eye
     H10.232   **Serous conjunctivitis, except viral,** left eye
     H10.233   **Serous conjunctivitis, except viral, bilateral**
     H10.239   **Serous conjunctivitis, except viral, unspecified eye**

✓5ᵗʰ **H10.3**   **Unspecified acute conjunctivitis**
     EXCLUDES 1   *ophthalmia neonatorum NOS (P39.1)*

     H10.30   **Unspecified acute conjunctivitis,** unspecified eye
     H10.31   **Unspecified acute conjunctivitis,** right eye
     H10.32   **Unspecified acute conjunctivitis,** left eye
     H10.33   **Unspecified acute conjunctivitis,** bilateral

✓5ᵗʰ **H10.4**   **Chronic conjunctivitis**

  ✓6ᵗʰ **H10.40**   **Unspecified chronic conjunctivitis**
     H10.401   **Unspecified chronic conjunctivitis,** right eye
     H10.402   **Unspecified chronic conjunctivitis,** left eye
     H10.403   **Unspecified chronic conjunctivitis, bilateral**
     H10.409   **Unspecified chronic conjunctivitis, unspecified eye**

  ✓6ᵗʰ **H10.41**   **Chronic giant papillary conjunctivitis**
     H10.411   **Chronic giant papillary conjunctivitis, right eye**
     H10.412   **Chronic giant papillary conjunctivitis,** left eye
     H10.413   **Chronic giant papillary conjunctivitis, bilateral**
     H10.419   **Chronic giant papillary conjunctivitis, unspecified eye**

  ✓6ᵗʰ **H10.42**   **Simple chronic conjunctivitis**
     H10.421   **Simple chronic conjunctivitis,** right eye
     H10.422   **Simple chronic conjunctivitis,** left eye
     H10.423   **Simple chronic conjunctivitis,** bilateral
     H10.429   **Simple chronic conjunctivitis,** unspecified eye

  ✓6ᵗʰ **H10.43**   **Chronic follicular conjunctivitis**
     H10.431   **Chronic follicular conjunctivitis,** right eye
     H10.432   **Chronic follicular conjunctivitis,** left eye
     H10.433   **Chronic follicular conjunctivitis,** bilateral
     H10.439   **Chronic follicular conjunctivitis, unspecified eye**

     H10.44   **Vernal conjunctivitis**
     EXCLUDES 1   *vernal keratoconjunctivitis with limbar and corneal involvement (H16.26-)*

     H10.45   **Other chronic allergic conjunctivitis**

✓5ᵗʰ **H10.5**   **Blepharoconjunctivitis**

  ✓6ᵗʰ **H10.50**   **Unspecified blepharoconjunctivitis**
     H10.501   **Unspecified blepharoconjunctivitis,** right eye
     H10.502   **Unspecified blepharoconjunctivitis,** left eye
     H10.503   **Unspecified blepharoconjunctivitis, bilateral**
     H10.509   **Unspecified blepharoconjunctivitis, unspecified eye**

  ✓6ᵗʰ **H10.51**   **Ligneous conjunctivitis**
     H10.511   **Ligneous conjunctivitis,** right eye
     H10.512   **Ligneous conjunctivitis,** left eye
     H10.513   **Ligneous conjunctivitis,** bilateral
     H10.519   **Ligneous conjunctivitis,** unspecified eye

  ✓6ᵗʰ **H10.52**   **Angular blepharoconjunctivitis**
     H10.521   **Angular blepharoconjunctivitis,** right eye
     H10.522   **Angular blepharoconjunctivitis,** left eye
     H10.523   **Angular blepharoconjunctivitis,** bilateral
     H10.529   **Angular blepharoconjunctivitis, unspecified eye**

  ✓6ᵗʰ **H10.53**   **Contact blepharoconjunctivitis**
     H10.531   **Contact blepharoconjunctivitis,** right eye
     H10.532   **Contact blepharoconjunctivitis,** left eye
     H10.533   **Contact blepharoconjunctivitis,** bilateral
     H10.539   **Contact blepharoconjunctivitis, unspecified eye**

✓5ᵗʰ **H10.8**   **Other conjunctivitis**

  ✓6ᵗʰ **H10.81**   **Pingueculitis**
     EXCLUDES 1   *pinguecula (H11.15-)*
     H10.811   **Pingueculitis,** right eye
     H10.812   **Pingueculitis,** left eye
     H10.813   **Pingueculitis,** bilateral
     H10.819   **Pingueculitis,** unspecified eye

     H10.89   **Other conjunctivitis**

     H10.9   **Unspecified conjunctivitis**

✓4ᵗʰ **H11**   **Other disorders of conjunctiva**
     EXCLUDES 1   *keratoconjunctivitis (H16.2-)*

✓5ᵗʰ **H11.0**   **Pterygium of eye**
     EXCLUDES 1   *pseudopterygium (H11.81-)*

  ✓6ᵗʰ **H11.00**   **Unspecified pterygium of eye**
     H11.001   **Unspecified pterygium of** right eye
     H11.002   **Unspecified pterygium of** left eye
     H11.003   **Unspecified pterygium of eye,** bilateral
     H11.009   **Unspecified pterygium of** unspecified eye

  ✓6ᵗʰ **H11.01**   **Amyloid pterygium**
     H11.011   **Amyloid pterygium of** right eye
     H11.012   **Amyloid pterygium of** left eye
     H11.013   **Amyloid pterygium of eye,** bilateral
     H11.019   **Amyloid pterygium of** unspecified eye

  ✓6ᵗʰ **H11.02**   **Central pterygium of eye**
     H11.021   **Central pterygium of** right eye
     H11.022   **Central pterygium of** left eye
     H11.023   **Central pterygium of eye,** bilateral

Pterygium

Pterygium

✓ Additional Character Req   ✓×7ᵗʰ Placeholder Alert   Unacceptable PDx   Manifestation   **H1 - H14** HAC   **HCC** CMS-HCC Condition   *EXCLUDES 1* Not Coded Here   *EXCLUDES 2* Not Included Here

ICD-10-CM 2018   585

Chapter 7. Diseases of the Eye and Adnexa

H11.029   Central pterygium of unspecified eye

✓6th   **H11.03**   Double pterygium of eye
    H11.031   Double pterygium of right eye
    H11.032   Double pterygium of left eye
    H11.033   Double pterygium of eye, bilateral
    H11.039   Double pterygium of unspecified eye

✓6th   **H11.04**   Peripheral pterygium of eye, stationary
    H11.041   Peripheral pterygium, stationary, right eye
    H11.042   Peripheral pterygium, stationary, left eye
    H11.043   Peripheral pterygium, stationary, bilateral
    H11.049   Peripheral pterygium, stationary, unspecified eye

✓6th   **H11.05**   Peripheral pterygium of eye, progressive
    H11.051   Peripheral pterygium, progressive, right eye
    H11.052   Peripheral pterygium, progressive, left eye
    H11.053   Peripheral pterygium, progressive, bilateral
    H11.059   Peripheral pterygium, progressive, unspecified eye

✓6th   **H11.06**   Recurrent pterygium of eye
    H11.061   Recurrent pterygium of right eye
    H11.062   Recurrent pterygium of left eye
    H11.063   Recurrent pterygium of eye, bilateral
    H11.069   Recurrent pterygium of unspecified eye

✓5th   **H11.1**   Conjunctival degenerations and deposits
    EXCLUDES 2   *pseudopterygium (H11.81)*
    H11.10   Unspecified conjunctival degenerations

✓6th   **H11.11**   Conjunctival deposits
    H11.111   Conjunctival deposits, right eye
    H11.112   Conjunctival deposits, left eye
    H11.113   Conjunctival deposits, bilateral
    H11.119   Conjunctival deposits, unspecified eye

✓6th   **H11.12**   Conjunctival concretions
    H11.121   Conjunctival concretions, right eye
    H11.122   Conjunctival concretions, left eye
    H11.123   Conjunctival concretions, bilateral
    H11.129   Conjunctival concretions, unspecified eye

✓6th   **H11.13**   Conjunctival pigmentations
    Conjunctival argyrosis [argyria]
    H11.131   Conjunctival pigmentations, right eye
    H11.132   Conjunctival pigmentations, left eye
    H11.133   Conjunctival pigmentations, bilateral
    H11.139   Conjunctival pigmentations, unspecified eye

✓6th   **H11.14**   Conjunctival xerosis, unspecified
    EXCLUDES 1   *xerosis of conjunctiva due to vitamin A deficiency (E50.0, E50.1)*
    DEF: Abnormal dryness of conjunctiva due to lack of insufficient tears or conjunctival secretions.
    H11.141   Conjunctival xerosis, unspecified, right eye
    H11.142   Conjunctival xerosis , unspecified, left eye
    H11.143   Conjunctival xerosis, unspecified, bilateral
    H11.149   Conjunctival xerosis, unspecified, unspecified eyed

✓6th   **H11.15**   Pinguecula
    EXCLUDES 1   *pingueculitis (H10.81-)*
    H11.151   Pinguecula, right eye
    H11.152   Pinguecula, left eye
    H11.153   Pinguecula, bilateral
    H11.159   Pinguecula, unspecified eye

✓5th   **H11.2**   Conjunctival scars

✓6th   **H11.21**   Conjunctival adhesions and strands (localized)
    H11.211   Conjunctival adhesions and strands (localized), right eye
    H11.212   Conjunctival adhesions and strands (localized), left eye
    H11.213   Conjunctival adhesions and strands (localized), bilateral
    H11.219   Conjunctival adhesions and strands (localized), unspecified eye

Pinguecula

Pinguecula

✓6th   **H11.22**   Conjunctival granuloma
    H11.221   Conjunctival granuloma, right eye
    H11.222   Conjunctival granuloma, left eye
    H11.223   Conjunctival granuloma, bilateral
    H11.229   Conjunctival granuloma, unspecified

✓6th   **H11.23**   Symblepharon
    H11.231   Symblepharon, right eye
    H11.232   Symblepharon, left eye
    H11.233   Symblepharon, bilateral
    H11.239   Symblepharon, unspecified eye

✓6th   **H11.24**   Scarring of conjunctiva
    H11.241   Scarring of conjunctiva, right eye
    H11.242   Scarring of conjunctiva, left eye
    H11.243   Scarring of conjunctiva, bilateral
    H11.249   Scarring of conjunctiva, unspecified eye

✓5th   **H11.3**   Conjunctival hemorrhage
    Subconjunctival hemorrhage
    H11.30   Conjunctival hemorrhage, unspecified eye
    H11.31   Conjunctival hemorrhage, right eye
    H11.32   Conjunctival hemorrhage, left eye
    H11.33   Conjunctival hemorrhage, bilateral

✓5th   **H11.4**   Other conjunctival vascular disorders and cysts

✓6th   **H11.41**   Vascular abnormalities of conjunctiva
    Conjunctival aneurysm
    H11.411   Vascular abnormalities of conjunctiva, right eye
    H11.412   Vascular abnormalities of conjunctiva, left eye
    H11.413   Vascular abnormalities of conjunctiva, bilateral
    H11.419   Vascular abnormalities of conjunctiva, unspecified eye

✓6th   **H11.42**   Conjunctival edema
    H11.421   Conjunctival edema, right eye
    H11.422   Conjunctival edema, left eye
    H11.423   Conjunctival edema, bilateral
    H11.429   Conjunctival edema, unspecified eye

✓6th   **H11.43**   Conjunctival hyperemia
    H11.431   Conjunctival hyperemia, right eye
    H11.432   Conjunctival hyperemia, left eye
    H11.433   Conjunctival hyperemia, bilateral
    H11.439   Conjunctival hyperemia, unspecified eye

✓6th   **H11.44**   Conjunctival cysts
    H11.441   Conjunctival cysts, right eye
    H11.442   Conjunctival cysts, left eye
    H11.443   Conjunctival cysts, bilateral
    H11.449   Conjunctival cysts, unspecified eye

✓5th   **H11.8**   Other specified disorders of conjunctiva

✓6th   **H11.81**   Pseudopterygium of conjunctiva
    H11.811   Pseudopterygium of conjunctiva, right eye
    H11.812   Pseudopterygium of conjunctiva, left eye
    H11.813   Pseudopterygium of conjunctiva, bilateral
    H11.819   Pseudopterygium of conjunctiva, unspecified

✓6th   **H11.82**   Conjunctivochalasis
    H11.821   Conjunctivochalasis, right eye

N Newborn: 0   P Pediatric: 0-17   M Maternity: 12-55   A Adult: 15-124   MCC Major CC Condition   PDx MCC PDx acts as own MCC   CC CC Condition   PDx CC PDx acts as own CC

586   ICD-10-CM 2018

H11.822   **Conjunctivochalasis,** left eye
H11.823   **Conjunctivochalasis,** bilateral
H11.829   **Conjunctivochalasis,** unspecified eye
H11.89   **Other specified disorders of conjunctiva**
H11.9   **Unspecified disorder of conjunctiva**

Disorders of sclera, cornea, iris and ciliary body (H15-H22)

✓4th **H15   Disorders of sclera**
   ✓5th **H15.0   Scleritis**
     ✓6th **H15.00   Unspecified scleritis**
       H15.001   **Unspecified scleritis,** right eye
       H15.002   **Unspecified scleritis,** left eye
       H15.003   **Unspecified scleritis,** bilateral
       H15.009   **Unspecified scleritis,** unspecified eye
     ✓6th **H15.01   Anterior scleritis**
       H15.011   **Anterior scleritis,** right eye
       H15.012   **Anterior scleritis,** left eye
       H15.013   **Anterior scleritis,** bilateral
       H15.019   **Anterior scleritis,** unspecified eye
     ✓6th **H15.02   Brawny scleritis**
       H15.021   **Brawny scleritis,** right eye
       H15.022   **Brawny scleritis,** left eye
       H15.023   **Brawny scleritis,** bilateral
       H15.029   **Brawny scleritis,** unspecified eye
     ✓6th **H15.03   Posterior scleritis**
       Sclerotenonitis
       H15.031   **Posterior scleritis,** right eye
       H15.032   **Posterior scleritis,** left eye
       H15.033   **Posterior scleritis,** bilateral
       H15.039   **Posterior scleritis,** unspecified eye
     ✓6th **H15.04   Scleritis with corneal involvement**
       H15.041   **Scleritis with corneal involvement,** right eye
       H15.042   **Scleritis with corneal involvement,** left eye
       H15.043   **Scleritis with corneal involvement,** bilateral
       H15.049   **Scleritis with corneal involvement,** unspecified eye
     ✓6th **H15.05   Scleromalacia perforans**
       H15.051   **Scleromalacia perforans,** right eye
       H15.052   **Scleromalacia perforans,** left eye
       H15.053   **Scleromalacia perforans,** bilateral
       H15.059   **Scleromalacia perforans,** unspecified eye
     ✓6th **H15.09   Other scleritis**
       Scleral abscess
       H15.091   **Other scleritis,** right eye
       H15.092   **Other scleritis,** left eye
       H15.093   **Other scleritis,** bilateral
       H15.099   **Other scleritis,** unspecified eye
   ✓5th **H15.1   Episcleritis**
     ✓6th **H15.10   Unspecified episcleritis**
       H15.101   **Unspecified episcleritis,** right eye
       H15.102   **Unspecified episcleritis,** left eye
       H15.103   **Unspecified episcleritis,** bilateral
       H15.109   **Unspecified episcleritis,** unspecified eye
     ✓6th **H15.11   Episcleritis periodica fugax**
       H15.111   **Episcleritis periodica fugax,** right eye
       H15.112   **Episcleritis periodica fugax,** left eye
       H15.113   **Episcleritis periodica fugax,** bilateral
       H15.119   **Episcleritis periodica fugax,** unspecified eye
     ✓6th **H15.12   Nodular episcleritis**
       H15.121   **Nodular episcleritis,** right eye
       H15.122   **Nodular episcleritis,** left eye
       H15.123   **Nodular episcleritis,** bilateral
       H15.129   **Nodular episcleritis,** unspecified eye
   ✓5th **H15.8   Other disorders of sclera**
     EXCLUDES 2   blue sclera (Q13.5)
             degenerative myopia (H44.2-)
     ✓6th **H15.81   Equatorial staphyloma**
       H15.811   **Equatorial staphyloma,** right eye
       H15.812   **Equatorial staphyloma,** left eye

H15.813   **Equatorial staphyloma,** bilateral
H15.819   **Equatorial staphyloma,** unspecified eye
   ✓6th **H15.82   Localized anterior staphyloma**
     H15.821   **Localized anterior staphyloma,** right eye
     H15.822   **Localized anterior staphyloma,** left eye
     H15.823   **Localized anterior staphyloma,** bilateral
     H15.829   **Localized anterior staphyloma,** unspecified eye
   ✓6th **H15.83   Staphyloma posticum**
     H15.831   **Staphyloma posticum,** right eye
     H15.832   **Staphyloma posticum,** left eye
     H15.833   **Staphyloma posticum,** bilateral
     H15.839   **Staphyloma posticum,** unspecified eye
   ✓6th **H15.84   Scleral ectasia**
     H15.841   **Scleral ectasia,** right eye
     H15.842   **Scleral ectasia,** left eye
     H15.843   **Scleral ectasia,** bilateral
     H15.849   **Scleral ectasia,** unspecified eye
   ✓6th **H15.85   Ring staphyloma**
     H15.851   **Ring staphyloma,** right eye
     H15.852   **Ring staphyloma,** left eye
     H15.853   **Ring staphyloma,** bilateral
     H15.859   **Ring staphyloma,** unspecified eye
     H15.89   **Other disorders of sclera**
   H15.9   **Unspecified disorder of sclera**

✓4th **H16   Keratitis**
   ✓5th **H16.0   Corneal ulcer**
     ✓6th **H16.00   Unspecified corneal ulcer**
       H16.001   **Unspecified corneal ulcer,** right eye
       H16.002   **Unspecified corneal ulcer,** left eye
       H16.003   **Unspecified corneal ulcer,** bilateral
       H16.009   **Unspecified corneal ulcer,** unspecified eye
     ✓6th **H16.01   Central corneal ulcer**
       H16.011   **Central corneal ulcer,** right eye
       H16.012   **Central corneal ulcer,** left eye
       H16.013   **Central corneal ulcer,** bilateral
       H16.019   **Central corneal ulcer,** unspecified eye
     ✓6th **H16.02   Ring corneal ulcer**
       H16.021   **Ring corneal ulcer,** right eye
       H16.022   **Ring corneal ulcer,** left eye
       H16.023   **Ring corneal ulcer,** bilateral
       H16.029   **Ring corneal ulcer,** unspecified eye
     ✓6th **H16.03   Corneal ulcer with hypopyon**
       H16.031   **Corneal ulcer with hypopyon,** right eye
       H16.032   **Corneal ulcer with hypopyon,** left eye
       H16.033   **Corneal ulcer with hypopyon,** bilateral
       H16.039   **Corneal ulcer with hypopyon,** unspecified eye
     ✓6th **H16.04   Marginal corneal ulcer**
       H16.041   **Marginal corneal ulcer,** right eye
       H16.042   **Marginal corneal ulcer,** left eye
       H16.043   **Marginal corneal ulcer,** bilateral
       H16.049   **Marginal corneal ulcer,** unspecified eye
     ✓6th **H16.05   Mooren's corneal ulcer**
       H16.051   **Mooren's corneal ulcer,** right eye
       H16.052   **Mooren's corneal ulcer,** left eye
       H16.053   **Mooren's corneal ulcer,** bilateral
       H16.059   **Mooren's corneal ulcer,** unspecified eye
     ✓6th **H16.06   Mycotic corneal ulcer**
       H16.061   **Mycotic corneal ulcer,** right eye
       H16.062   **Mycotic corneal ulcer,** left eye
       H16.063   **Mycotic corneal ulcer,** bilateral
       H16.069   **Mycotic corneal ulcer,** unspecified eye
     ✓6th **H16.07   Perforated corneal ulcer**
       H16.071   **Perforated corneal ulcer,** right eye
       H16.072   **Perforated corneal ulcer,** left eye
       H16.073   **Perforated corneal ulcer,** bilateral
       H16.079   **Perforated corneal ulcer,** unspecified eye

✓5ᵗʰ **H16.1 Other and unspecified superficial keratitis without conjunctivitis**

  ✓6ᵗʰ **H16.10 Unspecified superficial keratitis**

    H16.101 Unspecified superficial keratitis, right eye

    H16.102 Unspecified superficial keratitis, left eye

    H16.103 Unspecified superficial keratitis, bilateral

    H16.109 Unspecified superficial keratitis, unspecified eye

  ✓6ᵗʰ **H16.11 Macular keratitis**

    Areolar keratitis

    Nummular keratitis

    Stellate keratitis

    Striate keratitis

    H16.111 Macular keratitis, right eye

    H16.112 Macular keratitis, left eye

    H16.113 Macular keratitis, bilateral

    H16.119 Macular keratitis, unspecified eye

  ✓6ᵗʰ **H16.12 Filamentary keratitis**

    H16.121 Filamentary keratitis, right eye

    H16.122 Filamentary keratitis, left eye

    H16.123 Filamentary keratitis, bilateral

    H16.129 Filamentary keratitis, unspecified eye

  ✓6ᵗʰ **H16.13 Photokeratitis**

    Snow blindness

    Welders keratitis

    H16.131 Photokeratitis, right eye

    H16.132 Photokeratitis, left eye

    H16.133 Photokeratitis, bilateral

    H16.139 Photokeratitis, unspecified eye

  ✓6ᵗʰ **H16.14 Punctate keratitis**

    H16.141 Punctate keratitis, right eye

    H16.142 Punctate keratitis, left eye

    H16.143 Punctate keratitis, bilateral

    H16.149 Punctate keratitis, unspecified eye

✓5ᵗʰ **H16.2 Keratoconjunctivitis**

  ✓6ᵗʰ **H16.20 Unspecified keratoconjunctivitis**

    Superficial keratitis with conjunctivitis NOS

    H16.201 Unspecified keratoconjunctivitis, right eye

    H16.202 Unspecified keratoconjunctivitis, left eye

    H16.203 Unspecified keratoconjunctivitis, bilateral

    H16.209 Unspecified keratoconjunctivitis, unspecified eye

  ✓6ᵗʰ **H16.21 Exposure keratoconjunctivitis**

    H16.211 Exposure keratoconjunctivitis, right eye

    H16.212 Exposure keratoconjunctivitis, left eye

    H16.213 Exposure keratoconjunctivitis, bilateral

    H16.219 Exposure keratoconjunctivitis, unspecified eye

  ✓6ᵗʰ **H16.22 Keratoconjunctivitis sicca, not specified as Sjögren's**

    EXCLUDES 1 *Sjögren's syndrome (M35.01)*

    H16.221 Keratoconjunctivitis sicca, not specified as Sjögren's, right eye

    H16.222 Keratoconjunctivitis sicca, not specified as Sjögren's, left eye

    H16.223 Keratoconjunctivitis sicca, not specified as Sjögren's, bilateral

    H16.229 Keratoconjunctivitis sicca, not specified as Sjögren's, unspecified eye

  ✓6ᵗʰ **H16.23 Neurotrophic keratoconjunctivitis**

    H16.231 Neurotrophic keratoconjunctivitis, right eye

    H16.232 Neurotrophic keratoconjunctivitis, left eye

    H16.233 Neurotrophic keratoconjunctivitis, bilateral

    H16.239 Neurotrophic keratoconjunctivitis, unspecified eye

  ✓6ᵗʰ **H16.24 Ophthalmia nodosa**

    H16.241 Ophthalmia nodosa, right eye

    H16.242 Ophthalmia nodosa, left eye

    H16.243 Ophthalmia nodosa, bilateral

    H16.249 Ophthalmia nodosa, unspecified eye

  ✓6ᵗʰ **H16.25 Phlyctenular keratoconjunctivitis**

    H16.251 Phlyctenular keratoconjunctivitis, right eye

    H16.252 Phlyctenular keratoconjunctivitis, left eye

    H16.253 Phlyctenular keratoconjunctivitis, bilateral

    H16.259 Phlyctenular keratoconjunctivitis, unspecified eye

  ✓6ᵗʰ **H16.26 Vernal keratoconjunctivitis, with limbar and corneal involvement**

    EXCLUDES 1 *vernal conjunctivitis without limbar and corneal involvement (H10.44)*

    H16.261 Vernal keratoconjunctivitis, with limbar and corneal involvement, right eye

    H16.262 Vernal keratoconjunctivitis, with limbar and corneal involvement, left eye

    H16.263 Vernal keratoconjunctivitis, with limbar and corneal involvement, bilateral

    H16.269 Vernal keratoconjunctivitis, with limbar and corneal involvement, unspecified eye

  ✓6ᵗʰ **H16.29 Other keratoconjunctivitis**

    H16.291 Other keratoconjunctivitis, right eye

    H16.292 Other keratoconjunctivitis, left eye

    H16.293 Other keratoconjunctivitis, bilateral

    H16.299 Other keratoconjunctivitis, unspecified eye

✓5ᵗʰ **H16.3 Interstitial and deep keratitis**

  ✓6ᵗʰ **H16.30 Unspecified interstitial keratitis**

    H16.301 Unspecified interstitial keratitis, right eye

    H16.302 Unspecified interstitial keratitis, left eye

    H16.303 Unspecified interstitial keratitis, bilateral

    H16.309 Unspecified interstitial keratitis, unspecified eye

  ✓6ᵗʰ **H16.31 Corneal abscess**

    H16.311 Corneal abscess, right eye

    H16.312 Corneal abscess, left eye

    H16.313 Corneal abscess, bilateral

    H16.319 Corneal abscess, unspecified eye

  ✓6ᵗʰ **H16.32 Diffuse interstitial keratitis**

    Cogan's syndrome

    H16.321 Diffuse interstitial keratitis, right eye

    H16.322 Diffuse interstitial keratitis, left eye

    H16.323 Diffuse interstitial keratitis, bilateral

    H16.329 Diffuse interstitial keratitis, unspecified eye

  ✓6ᵗʰ **H16.33 Sclerosing keratitis**

    H16.331 Sclerosing keratitis, right eye

    H16.332 Sclerosing keratitis, left eye

    H16.333 Sclerosing keratitis, bilateral

    H16.339 Sclerosing keratitis, unspecified eye

  ✓6ᵗʰ **H16.39 Other interstitial and deep keratitis**

    H16.391 Other interstitial and deep keratitis, right eye

    H16.392 Other interstitial and deep keratitis, left eye

    H16.393 Other interstitial and deep keratitis, bilateral

    H16.399 Other interstitial and deep keratitis, unspecified eye

✓5ᵗʰ **H16.4 Corneal neovascularization**

  ✓6ᵗʰ **H16.40 Unspecified corneal neovascularization**

    H16.401 Unspecified corneal neovascularization, right eye

    H16.402 Unspecified corneal neovascularization, left eye

    H16.403 Unspecified corneal neovascularization, bilateral

    H16.409 Unspecified corneal neovascularization, unspecified eye

  ✓6ᵗʰ **H16.41 Ghost vessels (corneal)**

    H16.411 Ghost vessels (corneal), right eye

    H16.412 Ghost vessels (corneal), left eye

    H16.413 Ghost vessels (corneal), bilateral

    H16.419 Ghost vessels (corneal), unspecified eye

✓6th **H16.42 Pannus (corneal)**
    H16.421 Pannus (corneal), right eye
    H16.422 Pannus (corneal), left eye
    H16.423 Pannus (corneal), bilateral
    H16.429 Pannus (corneal), unspecified eye

✓6th **H16.43 Localized vascularization of cornea**
    H16.431 Localized vascularization of cornea, right eye
    H16.432 Localized vascularization of cornea, left eye
    H16.433 Localized vascularization of cornea, bilateral
    H16.439 Localized vascularization of cornea, unspecified eye

✓6th **H16.44 Deep vascularization of cornea**
    H16.441 Deep vascularization of cornea, right eye
    H16.442 Deep vascularization of cornea, left eye
    H16.443 Deep vascularization of cornea, bilateral
    H16.449 Deep vascularization of cornea, unspecified eye

H16.8 Other keratitis
H16.9 Unspecified keratitis

✓4th **H17 Corneal scars and opacities**

✓5th **H17.0 Adherent leukoma**
    H17.00 Adherent leukoma, unspecified eye
    H17.01 Adherent leukoma, right eye
    H17.02 Adherent leukoma, left eye
    H17.03 Adherent leukoma, bilateral

✓5th **H17.1 Central corneal opacity**
    H17.10 Central corneal opacity, unspecified eye
    H17.11 Central corneal opacity, right eye
    H17.12 Central corneal opacity, left eye
    H17.13 Central corneal opacity, bilateral

✓5th **H17.8 Other corneal scars and opacities**
  ✓6th **H17.81 Minor opacity of cornea**
    Corneal nebula
    H17.811 Minor opacity of cornea, right eye
    H17.812 Minor opacity of cornea, left eye
    H17.813 Minor opacity of cornea, bilateral
    H17.819 Minor opacity of cornea, unspecified eye
  ✓6th **H17.82 Peripheral opacity of cornea**
    H17.821 Peripheral opacity of cornea, right eye
    H17.822 Peripheral opacity of cornea, left eye
    H17.823 Peripheral opacity of cornea, bilateral
    H17.829 Peripheral opacity of cornea, unspecified eye
  H17.89 Other corneal scars and opacities
H17.9 Unspecified corneal scar and opacity

✓4th **H18 Other disorders of cornea**

✓5th **H18.0 Corneal pigmentations and deposits**
  ✓6th **H18.00 Unspecified corneal deposit**
    H18.001 Unspecified corneal deposit, right eye
    H18.002 Unspecified corneal deposit, left eye
    H18.003 Unspecified corneal deposit, bilateral
    H18.009 Unspecified corneal deposit, unspecified eye
  ✓6th **H18.01 Anterior corneal pigmentations**
    Staehli's line
    H18.011 Anterior corneal pigmentations, right eye
    H18.012 Anterior corneal pigmentations, left eye
    H18.013 Anterior corneal pigmentations, bilateral
    H18.019 Anterior corneal pigmentations, unspecified eye
  ✓6th **H18.02 Argentous corneal deposits**
    H18.021 Argentous corneal deposits, right eye
    H18.022 Argentous corneal deposits, left eye
    H18.023 Argentous corneal deposits, bilateral
    H18.029 Argentous corneal deposits, unspecified eye

✓6th **H18.03 Corneal deposits in metabolic disorders**
    Code also associated metabolic disorder
    H18.031 Corneal deposits in metabolic disorders, right eye
    H18.032 Corneal deposits in metabolic disorders, left eye
    H18.033 Corneal deposits in metabolic disorders, bilateral
    H18.039 Corneal deposits in metabolic disorders, unspecified eye

✓6th **H18.04 Kayser-Fleischer ring**
    Code also associated Wilson's disease (E83.01)
    H18.041 Kayser-Fleischer ring, right eye
    H18.042 Kayser-Fleischer ring, left eye
    H18.043 Kayser-Fleischer ring, bilateral
    H18.049 Kayser-Fleischer ring, unspecified eye

✓6th **H18.05 Posterior corneal pigmentations**
    Krukenberg's spindle
    H18.051 Posterior corneal pigmentations, right eye
    H18.052 Posterior corneal pigmentations, left eye
    H18.053 Posterior corneal pigmentations, bilateral
    H18.059 Posterior corneal pigmentations, unspecified eye

✓6th **H18.06 Stromal corneal pigmentations**
    Hematocornea
    H18.061 Stromal corneal pigmentations, right eye
    H18.062 Stromal corneal pigmentations, left eye
    H18.063 Stromal corneal pigmentations, bilateral
    H18.069 Stromal corneal pigmentations, unspecified eye

✓5th **H18.1 Bullous keratopathy**
    DEF: Corneal swelling due to damaged corneal endothelium; characterized by recurring, rupturing epithelial "blisters"; occurs in glaucoma, iridocyclitis and Fuchs dystrophy.
    H18.10 Bullous keratopathy, unspecified eye
    H18.11 Bullous keratopathy, right eye
    H18.12 Bullous keratopathy, left eye
    H18.13 Bullous keratopathy, bilateral

✓5th **H18.2 Other and unspecified corneal edema**
    H18.20 Unspecified corneal edema
  ✓6th **H18.21 Corneal edema secondary to contact lens**
    EXCLUDES 2 other corneal disorders due to contact lens (H18.82-)
    H18.211 Corneal edema secondary to contact lens, right eye
    H18.212 Corneal edema secondary to contact lens, left eye
    H18.213 Corneal edema secondary to contact lens, bilateral
    H18.219 Corneal edema secondary to contact lens, unspecified eye
  ✓6th **H18.22 Idiopathic corneal edema**
    H18.221 Idiopathic corneal edema, right eye
    H18.222 Idiopathic corneal edema, left eye
    H18.223 Idiopathic corneal edema, bilateral
    H18.229 Idiopathic corneal edema, unspecified eye
  ✓6th **H18.23 Secondary corneal edema**
    H18.231 Secondary corneal edema, right eye
    H18.232 Secondary corneal edema, left eye
    H18.233 Secondary corneal edema, bilateral
    H18.239 Secondary corneal edema, unspecified eye

✓5th **H18.3 Changes of corneal membranes**
    H18.30 Unspecified corneal membrane change
  ✓6th **H18.31 Folds and rupture in Bowman's membrane**
    H18.311 Folds and rupture in Bowman's membrane, right eye
    H18.312 Folds and rupture in Bowman's membrane, left eye
    H18.313 Folds and rupture in Bowman's membrane, bilateral
    H18.319 Folds and rupture in Bowman's membrane, unspecified eye
  ✓6th **H18.32 Folds in Descemet's membrane**
    H18.321 Folds in Descemet's membrane, right eye
    H18.322 Folds in Descemet's membrane, left eye

H18.323 Folds in Descemet's membrane, bilateral

H18.329 Folds in Descemet's membrane, unspecified eye

✓6ᵗʰ **H18.33 Rupture in Descemet's membrane**

H18.331 Rupture in Descemet's membrane, right eye

H18.332 Rupture in Descemet's membrane, left eye

H18.333 Rupture in Descemet's membrane, bilateral

H18.339 Rupture in Descemet's membrane, unspecified eye

✓5ᵗʰ **H18.4 Corneal degeneration**

EXCLUDES 1   *Mooren's ulcer (H16.0-)*
           recurrent erosion of cornea (H18.83-)

H18.40 Unspecified corneal degeneration

✓6ᵗʰ **H18.41 Arcus senilis**
     Senile corneal changes

H18.411 Arcus senilis, right eye

H18.412 Arcus senilis, left eye

H18.413 Arcus senilis, bilateral

H18.419 Arcus senilis, unspecified eye

✓6ᵗʰ **H18.42 Band keratopathy**

H18.421 Band keratopathy, right eye

H18.422 Band keratopathy, left eye

H18.423 Band keratopathy, bilateral

H18.429 Band keratopathy, unspecified eye

H18.43 Other calcerous corneal degeneration

✓6ᵗʰ **H18.44 Keratomalacia**

EXCLUDES 1   *keratomalacia due to vitamin A deficiency (E50.4)*

H18.441 Keratomalacia, right eye

H18.442 Keratomalacia, left eye

H18.443 Keratomalacia, bilateral

H18.449 Keratomalacia, unspecified eye

✓6ᵗʰ **H18.45 Nodular corneal degeneration**

H18.451 Nodular corneal degeneration, right eye

H18.452 Nodular corneal degeneration, left eye

H18.453 Nodular corneal degeneration, bilateral

H18.459 Nodular corneal degeneration, unspecified eye

✓6ᵗʰ **H18.46 Peripheral corneal degeneration**

H18.461 Peripheral corneal degeneration, right eye

H18.462 Peripheral corneal degeneration, left eye

H18.463 Peripheral corneal degeneration, bilateral

H18.469 Peripheral corneal degeneration, unspecified eye

H18.49 Other corneal degeneration

✓5ᵗʰ **H18.5 Hereditary corneal dystrophies**

H18.50 Unspecified hereditary corneal dystrophies

H18.51 Endothelial corneal dystrophy
     Fuchs' dystrophy

H18.52 Epithelial (juvenile) corneal dystrophy

H18.53 Granular corneal dystrophy

H18.54 Lattice corneal dystrophy

H18.55 Macular corneal dystrophy

H18.59 Other hereditary corneal dystrophies

✓5ᵗʰ **H18.6 Keratoconus**

✓6ᵗʰ **H18.60 Keratoconus, unspecified**

H18.601 Keratoconus, unspecified, right eye

H18.602 Keratoconus, unspecified, left eye

H18.603 Keratoconus, unspecified, bilateral

H18.609 Keratoconus, unspecified, unspecified eye

✓6ᵗʰ **H18.61 Keratoconus, stable**

H18.611 Keratoconus, stable, right eye

H18.612 Keratoconus, stable, left eye

H18.613 Keratoconus, stable, bilateral

H18.619 Keratoconus, stable, unspecified eye

✓6ᵗʰ **H18.62 Keratoconus, unstable**
     Acute hydrops

H18.621 Keratoconus, unstable, right eye

H18.622 Keratoconus, unstable, left eye

H18.623 Keratoconus, unstable, bilateral

H18.629 Keratoconus, unstable, unspecified eye

✓5ᵗʰ **H18.7 Other and unspecified corneal deformities**

EXCLUDES 1   *congenital malformations of cornea (Q13.3-Q13.4)*

H18.70 Unspecified corneal deformity

✓6ᵗʰ **H18.71 Corneal ectasia**

H18.711 Corneal ectasia, right eye

H18.712 Corneal ectasia, left eye

H18.713 Corneal ectasia, bilateral

H18.719 Corneal ectasia, unspecified eye

✓6ᵗʰ **H18.72 Corneal staphyloma**

H18.721 Corneal staphyloma, right eye

H18.722 Corneal staphyloma, left eye

H18.723 Corneal staphyloma, bilateral

H18.729 Corneal staphyloma, unspecified eye

✓6ᵗʰ **H18.73 Descemetocele**

H18.731 Descemetocele, right eye

H18.732 Descemetocele, left eye

H18.733 Descemetocele, bilateral

H18.739 Descemetocele, unspecified eye

✓6ᵗʰ **H18.79 Other corneal deformities**

H18.791 Other corneal deformities, right eye

H18.792 Other corneal deformities, left eye

H18.793 Other corneal deformities, bilateral

H18.799 Other corneal deformities, unspecified eye

✓5ᵗʰ **H18.8 Other specified disorders of cornea**

✓6ᵗʰ **H18.81 Anesthesia and hypoesthesia of cornea**

H18.811 Anesthesia and hypoesthesia of cornea, right eye

H18.812 Anesthesia and hypoesthesia of cornea, left eye

H18.813 Anesthesia and hypoesthesia of cornea, bilateral

H18.819 Anesthesia and hypoesthesia of cornea, unspecified eye

✓6ᵗʰ **H18.82 Corneal disorder due to contact lens**

EXCLUDES 2   *corneal edema due to contact lens (H18.21-)*

H18.821 Corneal disorder due to contact lens, right eye

H18.822 Corneal disorder due to contact lens, left eye

H18.823 Corneal disorder due to contact lens, bilateral

H18.829 Corneal disorder due to contact lens, unspecified eye

✓6ᵗʰ **H18.83 Recurrent erosion of cornea**

H18.831 Recurrent erosion of cornea, right eye

H18.832 Recurrent erosion of cornea, left eye

H18.833 Recurrent erosion of cornea, bilateral

H18.839 Recurrent erosion of cornea, unspecified eye

✓6ᵗʰ **H18.89 Other specified disorders of cornea**

H18.891 Other specified disorders of cornea, right eye

H18.892 Other specified disorders of cornea, left eye

H18.893 Other specified disorders of cornea, bilateral

H18.899 Other specified disorders of cornea, unspecified eye

H18.9 Unspecified disorder of cornea

N Newborn: 0   P Pediatric: 0-17   M Maternity: 12-55   A Adult: 15-124   MCC Major CC Condition   PDxMCC PDx acts as own MCC   CC CC Condition   PDxCC PDx acts as own CC

590   ICD-10-CM 2018

✓4th **H20 Iridocyclitis**

> **CC Excl: For CC codes in category H20:** PDX collection 624

✓5th **H20.0 Acute and subacute iridocyclitis**
Acute anterior uveitis
Acute cyclitis
Acute iritis
Subacute anterior uveitis
Subacute cyclitis
Subacute iritis

> EXCLUDES 1 iridocyclitis, iritis, uveitis (due to) (in) diabetes mellitus (E08-E13 with .39)
> iridocyclitis, iritis, uveitis (due to) (in) diphtheria (A36.89)
> iridocyclitis, iritis, uveitis (due to) (in) gonococcal (A54.32)
> iridocyclitis, iritis, uveitis (due to) (in) herpes (simplex) (B00.51)
> iridocyclitis, iritis, uveitis (due to) (in) herpes zoster (B02.32)
> iridocyclitis, iritis, uveitis (due to) (in) late congenital syphilis (A50.39)
> iridocyclitis, iritis, uveitis (due to) (in) late syphilis (A52.71)
> iridocyclitis, iritis, uveitis (due to) (in) sarcoidosis (D86.83)
> iridocyclitis, iritis, uveitis (due to) (in) syphilis (A51.43)
> iridocyclitis, iritis, uveitis (due to) (in) toxoplasmosis (B58.09)
> iridocyclitis, iritis, uveitis (due to) (in) tuberculosis (A18.54)

    H20.00 Unspecified acute and subacute iridocyclitis `CC`

✓6th **H20.01 Primary iridocyclitis**
    H20.011 Primary iridocyclitis, right eye `CC`
    H20.012 Primary iridocyclitis, left eye `CC`
    H20.013 Primary iridocyclitis, bilateral `CC`
    H20.019 Primary iridocyclitis, unspecified eye `CC`

✓6th **H20.02 Recurrent acute iridocyclitis**
    H20.021 Recurrent acute iridocyclitis, right eye `CC`
    H20.022 Recurrent acute iridocyclitis, left eye `CC`
    H20.023 Recurrent acute iridocyclitis, bilateral `CC`
    H20.029 Recurrent acute iridocyclitis, unspecified eye `CC`

✓6th **H20.03 Secondary infectious iridocyclitis**
    H20.031 Secondary infectious iridocyclitis, right eye `CC`
    H20.032 Secondary infectious iridocyclitis, left eye `CC`
    H20.033 Secondary infectious iridocyclitis, bilateral `CC`
    H20.039 Secondary infectious iridocyclitis, unspecified eye `CC`

✓6th **H20.04 Secondary noninfectious iridocyclitis**
    H20.041 Secondary noninfectious iridocyclitis, right eye
    H20.042 Secondary noninfectious iridocyclitis, left eye
    H20.043 Secondary noninfectious iridocyclitis, bilateral
    H20.049 Secondary noninfectious iridocyclitis, unspecified eye

✓6th **H20.05 Hypopyon**
    H20.051 Hypopyon, right eye
    H20.052 Hypopyon, left eye
    H20.053 Hypopyon, bilateral
    H20.059 Hypopyon, unspecified eye

✓5th **H20.1 Chronic iridocyclitis**
Use additional code for any associated cataract (H26.21-)
> EXCLUDES 2 posterior cyclitis (H30.2-)

    H20.10 Chronic iridocyclitis, unspecified eye
    H20.11 Chronic iridocyclitis, right eye
    H20.12 Chronic iridocyclitis, left eye
    H20.13 Chronic iridocyclitis, bilateral

✓5th **H20.2 Lens-induced iridocyclitis**
    H20.20 Lens-induced iridocyclitis, unspecified eye
    H20.21 Lens-induced iridocyclitis, right eye
    H20.22 Lens-induced iridocyclitis, left eye
    H20.23 Lens-induced iridocyclitis, bilateral

Hyphema

Iris
Cornea
Hyphema

✓5th **H20.8 Other iridocyclitis**
> EXCLUDES 2 glaucomatocyclitis crises (H40.4-)
> posterior cyclitis (H30.2-)
> sympathetic uveitis (H44.13-)

✓6th **H20.81 Fuchs' heterochromic cyclitis**
    H20.811 Fuchs' heterochromic cyclitis, right eye
    H20.812 Fuchs' heterochromic cyclitis, left eye
    H20.813 Fuchs' heterochromic cyclitis, bilateral
    H20.819 Fuchs' heterochromic cyclitis, unspecified eye

✓6th **H20.82 Vogt-Koyanagi syndrome**
    H20.821 Vogt-Koyanagi syndrome, right eye
    H20.822 Vogt-Koyanagi syndrome, left eye
    H20.823 Vogt-Koyanagi syndrome, bilateral
    H20.829 Vogt-Koyanagi syndrome, unspecified eye

H20.9 Unspecified iridocyclitis `CC`
Uveitis NOS

✓4th **H21 Other disorders of iris and ciliary body**
> EXCLUDES 2 sympathetic uveitis (H44.1-)

✓5th **H21.0 Hyphema**
> EXCLUDES 1 traumatic hyphema (S05.1-)

    H21.00 Hyphema, unspecified eye
    H21.01 Hyphema, right eye
    H21.02 Hyphema, left eye
    H21.03 Hyphema, bilateral

✓5th **H21.1 Other vascular disorders of iris and ciliary body**
Neovascularization of iris or ciliary body
Rubeosis iridis
Rubeosis of iris

✓6th **H21.1X Other vascular disorders of iris and ciliary body**
    H21.1X1 Other vascular disorders of iris and ciliary body, right eye
    H21.1X2 Other vascular disorders of iris and ciliary body, left eye
    H21.1X3 Other vascular disorders of iris and ciliary body, bilateral
    H21.1X9 Other vascular disorders of iris and ciliary body, unspecified eye

✓5th **H21.2 Degeneration of iris and ciliary body**
✓6th **H21.21 Degeneration of chamber angle**
    H21.211 Degeneration of chamber angle, right eye
    H21.212 Degeneration of chamber angle, left eye
    H21.213 Degeneration of chamber angle, bilateral
    H21.219 Degeneration of chamber angle, unspecified eye

✓6th **H21.22 Degeneration of ciliary body**
    H21.221 Degeneration of ciliary body, right eye
    H21.222 Degeneration of ciliary body, left eye
    H21.223 Degeneration of ciliary body, bilateral
    H21.229 Degeneration of ciliary body, unspecified eye

✓6th **H21.23 Degeneration of iris (pigmentary)**
Translucency of iris
    H21.231 Degeneration of iris (pigmentary), right eye
    H21.232 Degeneration of iris (pigmentary), left eye
    H21.233 Degeneration of iris (pigmentary), bilateral

✓ Additional Character Req ✓7th Placeholder Alert Unacceptable PDx Manifestation H1-H14 HAC HCC CMS-HCC Condition EXCLUDES 1 Not Coded Here EXCLUDES 2 Not Included Here

ICD-10-CM 2018   591

H21.239   Degeneration of iris (pigmentary), unspecified eye

✓6th **H21.24   Degeneration of pupillary margin**

    H21.241   Degeneration of pupillary margin, right eye

    H21.242   Degeneration of pupillary margin, left eye

    H21.243   Degeneration of pupillary margin, bilateral

    H21.249   Degeneration of pupillary margin, unspecified eye

✓6th **H21.25   Iridoschisis**

    H21.251   Iridoschisis, right eye

    H21.252   Iridoschisis, left eye

    H21.253   Iridoschisis, bilateral

    H21.259   Iridoschisis, unspecified eye

✓6th **H21.26   Iris atrophy (essential) (progressive)**

    H21.261   Iris atrophy (essential) (progressive), right eye

    H21.262   Iris atrophy (essential) (progressive), left eye

    H21.263   Iris atrophy (essential) (progressive), bilateral

    H21.269   Iris atrophy (essential) (progressive), unspecified eye

✓6th **H21.27   Miotic pupillary cyst**

    H21.271   Miotic pupillary cyst, right eye

    H21.272   Miotic pupillary cyst, left eye

    H21.273   Miotic pupillary cyst, bilateral

    H21.279   Miotic pupillary cyst, unspecified eye

    H21.29   Other iris atrophy

✓5th **H21.3   Cyst of iris, ciliary body and anterior chamber**

    EXCLUDES 2   miotic pupillary cyst (H21.27-)

✓6th **H21.30   Idiopathic cysts of iris, ciliary body or anterior chamber**

    Cyst of iris, ciliary body or anterior chamber NOS

    H21.301   Idiopathic cysts of iris, ciliary body or anterior chamber, right eye

    H21.302   Idiopathic cysts of iris, ciliary body or anterior chamber, left eye

    H21.303   Idiopathic cysts of iris, ciliary body or anterior chamber, bilateral

    H21.309   Idiopathic cysts of iris, ciliary body or anterior chamber, unspecified eye

✓6th **H21.31   Exudative cysts of iris or anterior chamber**

    H21.311   Exudative cysts of iris or anterior chamber, right eye

    H21.312   Exudative cysts of iris or anterior chamber, left eye

    H21.313   Exudative cysts of iris or anterior chamber, bilateral

    H21.319   Exudative cysts of iris or anterior chamber, unspecified eye

✓6th **H21.32   Implantation cysts of iris, ciliary body or anterior chamber**

    H21.321   Implantation cysts of iris, ciliary body or anterior chamber, right eye

    H21.322   Implantation cysts of iris, ciliary body or anterior chamber, left eye

    H21.323   Implantation cysts of iris, ciliary body or anterior chamber, bilateral

    H21.329   Implantation cysts of iris, ciliary body or anterior chamber, unspecified eye

✓6th **H21.33   Parasitic cyst of iris, ciliary body or anterior chamber**

> **CC Excl: For CC codes in subcategory H21.33:**
> PDX collection 625

    H21.331   Parasitic cyst of iris, ciliary body or anterior chamber, right eye   `CC`

    H21.332   Parasitic cyst of iris, ciliary body or anterior chamber, left eye   `CC`

    H21.333   Parasitic cyst of iris, ciliary body or anterior chamber, bilateral   `CC`

    H21.339   Parasitic cyst of iris, ciliary body or anterior chamber, unspecified eye   `CC`

✓6th **H21.34   Primary cyst of pars plana**

    H21.341   Primary cyst of pars plana, right eye

    H21.342   Primary cyst of pars plana, left eye

    H21.343   Primary cyst of pars plana, bilateral

    H21.349   Primary cyst of pars plana, unspecified eye

✓6th **H21.35   Exudative cyst of pars plana**

    DEF: Protein, fatty-filled bullous elevation of nonpigmented outermost ciliary epithelium of pars plana; due to fluid leak from blood vessels.

    H21.351   Exudative cyst of pars plana, right eye

    H21.352   Exudative cyst of pars plana, left eye

    H21.353   Exudative cyst of pars plana, bilateral

    H21.359   Exudative cyst of pars plana, unspecified eye

✓5th **H21.4   Pupillary membranes**

    Iris bombé   Pupillary seclusion
    Pupillary occlusion

    EXCLUDES 1   congenital pupillary membranes (Q13.8)

    H21.40   Pupillary membranes, unspecified eye

    H21.41   Pupillary membranes, right eye

    H21.42   Pupillary membranes, left eye

    H21.43   Pupillary membranes, bilateral

✓5th **H21.5   Other and unspecified adhesions and disruptions of iris and ciliary body**

    EXCLUDES 1   corectopia (Q13.2)

✓6th **H21.50   Unspecified adhesions of iris**

    Synechia (iris) NOS

    H21.501   Unspecified adhesions of iris, right eye

    H21.502   Unspecified adhesions of iris, left eye

    H21.503   Unspecified adhesions of iris, bilateral

    H21.509   Unspecified adhesions of iris and ciliary body, unspecified eye

✓6th **H21.51   Anterior synechiae (iris)**

    H21.511   Anterior synechiae (iris), right eye

    H21.512   Anterior synechiae (iris), left eye

    H21.513   Anterior synechiae (iris), bilateral

    H21.519   Anterior synechiae (iris), unspecified eye

✓6th **H21.52   Goniosynechiae**

    H21.521   Goniosynechiae, right eye

    H21.522   Goniosynechiae, left eye

    H21.523   Goniosynechiae, bilateral

    H21.529   Goniosynechiae, unspecified eye

✓6th **H21.53   Iridodialysis**

    H21.531   Iridodialysis, right eye

    H21.532   Iridodialysis, left eye

    H21.533   Iridodialysis, bilateral

    H21.539   Iridodialysis, unspecified eye

✓6th **H21.54   Posterior synechiae (iris)**

    H21.541   Posterior synechiae (iris), right eye

    H21.542   Posterior synechiae (iris), left eye

    H21.543   Posterior synechiae (iris), bilateral

    H21.549   Posterior synechiae (iris), unspecified eye

✓6th **H21.55   Recession of chamber angle**

    H21.551   Recession of chamber angle, right eye

    H21.552   Recession of chamber angle, left eye

    H21.553   Recession of chamber angle, bilateral

    H21.559   Recession of chamber angle, unspecified eye

✓6th **H21.56   Pupillary abnormalities**

    Deformed pupil   Rupture of sphincter, pupil
    Ectopic pupil

    EXCLUDES 1   congenital deformity of pupil (Q13.2-)

    H21.561   Pupillary abnormality, right eye

    H21.562   Pupillary abnormality, left eye

    H21.563   Pupillary abnormality, bilateral

    H21.569   Pupillary abnormality, unspecified eye

✓5th **H21.8   Other specified disorders of iris and ciliary body**

    H21.81   Floppy iris syndrome

    Intraoperative floppy iris syndrome (IFIS)

    Use additional code for adverse effect, if applicable, to identify drug (T36-T50 with fifth or sixth character 5)

    H21.82   Plateau iris syndrome (post-iridectomy) (postprocedural)

N Newborn: 0   P Pediatric: 0-17   M Maternity: 12-55   A Adult: 15-124   MCC Major CC Condition   PDxMCC PDx acts as own MCC   CC CC Condition   PDxCC PDx acts as own CC

592

ICD-10-CM 2018

H21.89   Other specified disorders of iris and ciliary body

H21.9   Unspecified disorder of iris and ciliary body

H22   ***Disorders of iris and ciliary body in diseases classified elsewhere***
Code first underlying disease, such as:
gout (M1A.-, M10.-)
leprosy (A30.-)
parasitic disease (B89)

Disorders of lens (H25-H28)

✓4ᵗʰ **H25**   **Age-related cataract**
Senile cataract
EXCLUDES 2   *capsular glaucoma with pseudoexfoliation of lens (H40.1-)*

   ✓5ᵗʰ **H25.0**   **Age-related incipient cataract**

     ✓6ᵗʰ **H25.01**   **Cortical age-related cataract**

       H25.011   **Cortical age-related cataract, right eye** Ⓐ

       H25.012   **Cortical age-related cataract, left eye** Ⓐ

       H25.013   **Cortical age-related cataract, bilateral** Ⓐ

       H25.019   **Cortical age-related cataract, unspecified eye** Ⓐ

     ✓6ᵗʰ **H25.03**   **Anterior subcapsular polar age-related cataract**

       H25.031   **Anterior subcapsular polar age-related cataract, right eye** Ⓐ

       H25.032   **Anterior subcapsular polar age-related cataract, left eye** Ⓐ

       H25.033   **Anterior subcapsular polar age-related cataract, bilateral**

       H25.039   **Anterior subcapsular polar age-related cataract, unspecified eye** Ⓐ

     ✓6ᵗʰ **H25.04**   **Posterior subcapsular polar age-related cataract**

       H25.041   **Posterior subcapsular polar age-related cataract, right eye** Ⓐ

       H25.042   **Posterior subcapsular polar age-related cataract, left eye** Ⓐ

       H25.043   **Posterior subcapsular polar age-related cataract, bilateral** Ⓐ

       H25.049   **Posterior subcapsular polar age-related cataract, unspecified eye** Ⓐ

     ✓6ᵗʰ **H25.09**   **Other age-related incipient cataract**
Coronary age-related cataract
Punctate age-related cataract
Water clefts

       H25.091   **Other age-related incipient cataract, right eye** Ⓐ

       H25.092   **Other age-related incipient cataract, left eye** Ⓐ

       H25.093   **Other age-related incipient cataract, bilateral** Ⓐ

       H25.099   **Other age-related incipient cataract, unspecified eye** Ⓐ

   ✓5ᵗʰ **H25.1**   **Age-related nuclear cataract**
Cataracta brunescens
Nuclear sclerosis cataract
AHA: 2016, 1Q, 32

     H25.10   **Age-related nuclear cataract, unspecified eye** Ⓐ

     H25.11   **Age-related nuclear cataract, right eye** Ⓐ

Cataracts

Vitreous
Iris
Cornea
Retina
Pupil
Lens

Normal lens

Clouded lens

Lens affected by cataracts

H25.12   **Age-related nuclear cataract, left eye** Ⓐ

H25.13   **Age-related nuclear cataract, bilateral** Ⓐ

   ✓5ᵗʰ **H25.2**   **Age-related cataract, morgagnian type**
Age-related hypermature cataract

     H25.20   **Age-related cataract, morgagnian type, unspecified eye** Ⓐ

     H25.21   **Age-related cataract, morgagnian type, right eye** Ⓐ

     H25.22   **Age-related cataract, morgagnian type, left eye** Ⓐ

     H25.23   **Age-related cataract, morgagnian type, bilateral** Ⓐ

   ✓5ᵗʰ **H25.8**   **Other age-related cataract**

     ✓6ᵗʰ **H25.81**   **Combined forms of age-related cataract**

       H25.811   **Combined forms of age-related cataract, right eye** Ⓐ

       H25.812   **Combined forms of age-related cataract, left eye** Ⓐ

       H25.813   **Combined forms of age-related cataract, bilateral** Ⓐ

       H25.819   **Combined forms of age-related cataract, unspecified eye** Ⓐ

     H25.89   **Other age-related cataract** Ⓐ

   H25.9   **Unspecified age-related cataract** Ⓐ

✓4ᵗʰ **H26**   **Other cataract**
EXCLUDES 1   *congenital cataract (Q12.0)*

   ✓5ᵗʰ **H26.0**   **Infantile and juvenile cataract**

     ✓6ᵗʰ **H26.00**   **Unspecified infantile and juvenile cataract**

       H26.001   **Unspecified infantile and juvenile cataract, right eye** Ⓟ

       H26.002   **Unspecified infantile and juvenile cataract, left eye** Ⓟ

       H26.003   **Unspecified infantile and juvenile cataract, bilateral** Ⓟ

       H26.009   **Unspecified infantile and juvenile cataract, unspecified eye** Ⓟ

     ✓6ᵗʰ **H26.01**   **Infantile and juvenile cortical, lamellar, or zonular cataract**

       H26.011   **Infantile and juvenile cortical, lamellar, or zonular cataract, right eye** Ⓟ

       H26.012   **Infantile and juvenile cortical, lamellar, or zonular cataract, left eye** Ⓟ

       H26.013   **Infantile and juvenile cortical, lamellar, or zonular cataract, bilateral** Ⓟ

       H26.019   **Infantile and juvenile cortical, lamellar, or zonular cataract, unspecified eye** Ⓟ

     ✓6ᵗʰ **H26.03**   **Infantile and juvenile nuclear cataract**

       H26.031   **Infantile and juvenile nuclear cataract, right eye** Ⓟ

       H26.032   **Infantile and juvenile nuclear cataract, left eye** Ⓟ

       H26.033   **Infantile and juvenile nuclear cataract, bilateral** Ⓟ

       H26.039   **Infantile and juvenile nuclear cataract, unspecified eye** Ⓟ

     ✓6ᵗʰ **H26.04**   **Anterior subcapsular polar infantile and juvenile cataract**

       H26.041   **Anterior subcapsular polar infantile and juvenile cataract, right eye** Ⓟ

       H26.042   **Anterior subcapsular polar infantile and juvenile cataract, left eye** Ⓟ

       H26.043   **Anterior subcapsular polar infantile and juvenile cataract, bilateral** Ⓟ

       H26.049   **Anterior subcapsular polar infantile and juvenile cataract, unspecified eye** Ⓟ

     ✓6ᵗʰ **H26.05**   **Posterior subcapsular polar infantile and juvenile cataract**

       H26.051   **Posterior subcapsular polar infantile and juvenile cataract, right eye** Ⓟ

       H26.052   **Posterior subcapsular polar infantile and juvenile cataract, left eye** Ⓟ

       H26.053   **Posterior subcapsular polar infantile and juvenile cataract, bilateral** Ⓟ

       H26.059   **Posterior subcapsular polar infantile and juvenile cataract, unspecified eye** Ⓟ

     ✓6ᵗʰ **H26.06**   **Combined forms of infantile and juvenile cataract**

       H26.061   **Combined forms of infantile and juvenile cataract, right eye** Ⓟ

✓ Additional Character Req   ✓x7ᵗʰ Placeholder Alert   Unacceptable PDx   Manifestation   H1-H14 HAC   HCC CMS-HCC Condition   EXCLUDES 1 Not Coded Here   EXCLUDES 2 Not Included Here

       H26.Ø62   **Combined forms of infantile and juvenile cataract, left eye**   P

       H26.Ø63   **Combined forms of infantile and juvenile cataract, bilateral**   P

       H26.Ø69   **Combined forms of infantile and juvenile cataract, unspecified eye**   P

   H26.Ø9   Other **infantile and juvenile cataract**   P

✓5ᵗʰ **H26.1**   Traumatic **cataract**
Use additional code (Chapter 2Ø) to identify external cause

   ✓6ᵗʰ **H26.1Ø**   Unspecified **traumatic cataract**

       H26.1Ø1   **Unspecified traumatic cataract, right eye**

       H26.1Ø2   **Unspecified traumatic cataract, left eye**

       H26.1Ø3   **Unspecified traumatic cataract, bilateral**

       H26.1Ø9   **Unspecified traumatic cataract, unspecified eye**

   ✓6ᵗʰ **H26.11**   Localized **traumatic opacities**

       H26.111   **Localized traumatic opacities, right eye**

       H26.112   **Localized traumatic opacities, left eye**

       H26.113   **Localized traumatic opacities, bilateral**

       H26.119   **Localized traumatic opacities, unspecified eye**

   ✓6ᵗʰ **H26.12**   Partially resolved **traumatic cataract**

       H26.121   **Partially resolved traumatic cataract, right eye**

       H26.122   **Partially resolved traumatic cataract, left eye**

       H26.123   **Partially resolved traumatic cataract, bilateral**

       H26.129   **Partially resolved traumatic cataract, unspecified eye**

   ✓6ᵗʰ **H26.13**   Total **traumatic cataract**

       H26.131   **Total traumatic cataract, right eye**

       H26.132   **Total traumatic cataract, left eye**

       H26.133   **Total traumatic cataract, bilateral**

       H26.139   **Total traumatic cataract, unspecified eye**

✓5ᵗʰ **H26.2**   Complicated **cataract**

   H26.2Ø   Unspecified **complicated cataract**
Cataracta complicata NOS

   ✓6ᵗʰ **H26.21**   **Cataract** with neovascularization
Code also associated condition, such as:
chronic iridocyclitis (H2Ø.1-)

       H26.211   **Cataract with neovascularization, right eye**

       H26.212   **Cataract with neovascularization, left eye**

       H26.213   **Cataract with neovascularization, bilateral**

       H26.219   **Cataract with neovascularization, unspecified eye**

   ✓6ᵗʰ **H26.22**   **Cataract** secondary to ocular disorders (degenerative) (inflammatory)
Code also associated ocular disorder

       H26.221   **Cataract secondary to ocular disorders (degenerative) (inflammatory), right eye**

       H26.222   **Cataract secondary to ocular disorders (degenerative) (inflammatory), left eye**

       H26.223   **Cataract secondary to ocular disorders (degenerative) (inflammatory), bilateral**

       H26.229   **Cataract secondary to ocular disorders (degenerative) (inflammatory), unspecified eye**

   ✓6ᵗʰ **H26.23**   Glaucomatous flecks (subcapsular)
Code first underlying glaucoma (H4Ø-H42)

       H26.231   **Glaucomatous flecks (subcapsular), right eye**

       H26.232   **Glaucomatous flecks (subcapsular), left eye**

       H26.233   **Glaucomatous flecks (subcapsular), bilateral**

       H26.239   **Glaucomatous flecks (subcapsular), unspecified eye**

✓5ᵗʰ **H26.3**   Drug-induced **cataract**
Toxic cataract
Use additional code for adverse effect, if applicable, to identify drug (T36-T5Ø with fifth or sixth character 5)

   H26.3Ø   **Drug-induced cataract, unspecified eye**

   H26.31   **Drug-induced cataract, right eye**

   H26.32   **Drug-induced cataract, left eye**

   H26.33   **Drug-induced cataract, bilateral**

✓5ᵗʰ **H26.4**   Secondary **cataract**

   H26.4Ø   Unspecified **secondary cataract**

   ✓6ᵗʰ **H26.41**   **Soemmering's ring**

       H26.411   **Soemmering's ring, right eye**

       H26.412   **Soemmering's ring, left eye**

       H26.413   **Soemmering's ring, bilateral**

       H26.419   **Soemmering's ring, unspecified eye**

   ✓6ᵗʰ **H26.49**   Other **secondary cataract**

       H26.491   **Other secondary cataract, right eye**

       H26.492   **Other secondary cataract, left eye**

       H26.493   **Other secondary cataract, bilateral**

       H26.499   **Other secondary cataract, unspecified eye**

   H26.8   Other **specified cataract**

   H26.9   Unspecified **cataract**

✓4ᵗʰ **H27**   **Other disorders of lens**
   EXCLUDES 1   *congenital lens malformations (Q12.-)*
mechanical complications of intraocular lens implant (T85.2)
pseudophakia (Z96.1)

   ✓5ᵗʰ **H27.Ø**   **Aphakia**
Acquired absence of lens
Acquired aphakia
Aphakia due to trauma
   EXCLUDES 1   *cataract extraction status (Z98.4-)*
congenital absence of lens (Q12.3)
congenital aphakia (Q12.3)

       H27.ØØ   **Aphakia, unspecified eye**

       H27.Ø1   **Aphakia, right eye**

       H27.Ø2   **Aphakia, left eye**

       H27.Ø3   **Aphakia, bilateral**

   ✓5ᵗʰ **H27.1**   **Dislocation of lens**

       H27.1Ø   **Unspecified dislocation of lens**

   ✓6ᵗʰ **H27.11**   **Subluxation of lens**

       H27.111   **Subluxation of lens, right eye**

       H27.112   **Subluxation of lens, left eye**

       H27.113   **Subluxation of lens, bilateral**

       H27.119   **Subluxation of lens, unspecified eye**

   ✓6ᵗʰ **H27.12**   **Anterior dislocation of lens**

       H27.121   **Anterior dislocation of lens, right eye**

       H27.122   **Anterior dislocation of lens, left eye**

       H27.123   **Anterior dislocation of lens, bilateral**

       H27.129   **Anterior dislocation of lens, unspecified eye**

   ✓6ᵗʰ **H27.13**   **Posterior dislocation of lens**

       H27.131   **Posterior dislocation of lens, right eye**

       H27.132   **Posterior dislocation of lens, left eye**

       H27.133   **Posterior dislocation of lens, bilateral**

       H27.139   **Posterior dislocation of lens, unspecified eye**

   H27.8   Other **specified disorders of lens**

   H27.9   Unspecified **disorder of lens**

H28   *Cataract in diseases classified elsewhere*
Code first underlying disease, such as:
hypoparathyroidism (E2Ø.-)
myotonia (G71.1-)
myxedema (EØ3.-)
protein-calorie malnutrition (E4Ø-E46)
   EXCLUDES 1   *cataract in diabetes mellitus (EØ8.36, EØ9.36, E1Ø.36, E11.36, E13.36)*

N Newborn: 0   P Pediatric: 0-17   M Maternity: 12-55   A Adult: 15-124   MCC Major CC Condition   PDxMCC PDx acts as own MCC   CC CC Condition   PDxCC PDx acts as own CC

594   ICD-10-CM 2018

Disorders of choroid and retina (H30-H36)

✅4th **H30 Chorioretinal inflammation**

> **CC Excl: For CC codes in category H30:** PDX collection 626

✅5th **H30.0 Focal chorioretinal inflammation**
Focal chorioretinitis
Focal choroiditis
Focal retinitis
Focal retinochoroiditis

✅6th   **H30.00 Unspecified focal chorioretinal inflammation**
Focal chorioretinitis NOS
Focal choroiditis NOS
Focal retinitis NOS
Focal retinochoroiditis NOS

    H30.001 Unspecified focal chorioretinal inflammation, right eye

    H30.002 Unspecified focal chorioretinal inflammation, left eye

    H30.003 Unspecified focal chorioretinal inflammation, bilateral

    H30.009 Unspecified focal chorioretinal inflammation, unspecified eye

✅6th   **H30.01 Focal chorioretinal inflammation, juxtapapillary**

    H30.011 Focal chorioretinal inflammation, juxtapapillary, right eye

    H30.012 Focal chorioretinal inflammation, juxtapapillary, left eye

    H30.013 Focal chorioretinal inflammation, juxtapapillary, bilateral

    H30.019 Focal chorioretinal inflammation, juxtapapillary, unspecified eye

✅6th   **H30.02 Focal chorioretinal inflammation of posterior pole**

    H30.021 Focal chorioretinal inflammation of posterior pole, right eye

    H30.022 Focal chorioretinal inflammation of posterior pole, left eye

    H30.023 Focal chorioretinal inflammation of posterior pole, bilateral

    H30.029 Focal chorioretinal inflammation of posterior pole, unspecified eye

✅6th   **H30.03 Focal chorioretinal inflammation, peripheral**

    H30.031 Focal chorioretinal inflammation, peripheral, right eye

    H30.032 Focal chorioretinal inflammation, peripheral, left eye

    H30.033 Focal chorioretinal inflammation, peripheral, bilateral

    H30.039 Focal chorioretinal inflammation, peripheral, unspecified eye

✅6th   **H30.04 Focal chorioretinal inflammation, macular or paramacular**

    H30.041 Focal chorioretinal inflammation, macular or paramacular, right eye

    H30.042 Focal chorioretinal inflammation, macular or paramacular, left eye

    H30.043 Focal chorioretinal inflammation, macular or paramacular, bilateral

    H30.049 Focal chorioretinal inflammation, macular or paramacular, unspecified eye

✅5th **H30.1 Disseminated chorioretinal inflammation**
Disseminated chorioretinitis
Disseminated choroiditis
Disseminated retinitis
Disseminated retinochoroiditis
EXCLUDES 2   *exudative retinopathy (H35.02-)*

✅6th   **H30.10 Unspecified disseminated chorioretinal inflammation**
Disseminated chorioretinitis NOS
Disseminated choroiditis NOS
Disseminated retinitis NOS
Disseminated retinochoroiditis NOS

    H30.101 Unspecified disseminated chorioretinal inflammation, right eye `CC`

    H30.102 Unspecified disseminated chorioretinal inflammation, left eye `CC`

    H30.103 Unspecified disseminated chorioretinal inflammation, bilateral `CC`

    H30.109 Unspecified disseminated chorioretinal inflammation, unspecified eye `CC`

✅6th   **H30.11 Disseminated chorioretinal inflammation of posterior pole**

    H30.111 Disseminated chorioretinal inflammation of posterior pole, right eye `CC`

    H30.112 Disseminated chorioretinal inflammation of posterior pole, left eye `CC`

    H30.113 Disseminated chorioretinal inflammation of posterior pole, bilateral `CC`

    H30.119 Disseminated chorioretinal inflammation of posterior pole, unspecified eye `CC`

✅6th   **H30.12 Disseminated chorioretinal inflammation, peripheral**

    H30.121 Disseminated chorioretinal inflammation, peripheral right eye `CC`

    H30.122 Disseminated chorioretinal inflammation, peripheral, left eye `CC`

    H30.123 Disseminated chorioretinal inflammation, peripheral, bilateral `CC`

    H30.129 Disseminated chorioretinal inflammation, peripheral, unspecified eye `CC`

✅6th   **H30.13 Disseminated chorioretinal inflammation, generalized**

    H30.131 Disseminated chorioretinal inflammation, generalized, right eye `CC`

    H30.132 Disseminated chorioretinal inflammation, generalized, left eye `CC`

    H30.133 Disseminated chorioretinal inflammation, generalized, bilateral `CC`

    H30.139 Disseminated chorioretinal inflammation, generalized, unspecified eye `CC`

✅6th   **H30.14 Acute posterior multifocal placoid pigment epitheliopathy**

    H30.141 Acute posterior multifocal placoid pigment epitheliopathy, right eye `CC`

    H30.142 Acute posterior multifocal placoid pigment epitheliopathy, left eye `CC`

    H30.143 Acute posterior multifocal placoid pigment epitheliopathy, bilateral `CC`

    H30.149 Acute posterior multifocal placoid pigment epitheliopathy, unspecified eye `CC`

✅5th **H30.2 Posterior cyclitis**
Pars planitis

  H30.20 Posterior cyclitis, unspecified eye

  H30.21 Posterior cyclitis, right eye

  H30.22 Posterior cyclitis, left eye

  H30.23 Posterior cyclitis, bilateral

✅5th **H30.8 Other chorioretinal inflammations**

✅6th   **H30.81 Harada's disease**

    H30.811 Harada's disease, right eye

    H30.812 Harada's disease, left eye

    H30.813 Harada's disease, bilateral

    H30.819 Harada's disease, unspecified eye

✅6th   **H30.89 Other chorioretinal inflammations**

    H30.891 Other chorioretinal inflammations, right eye `CC`

    H30.892 Other chorioretinal inflammations, left eye `CC`

    H30.893 Other chorioretinal inflammations, bilateral `CC`

    H30.899 Other chorioretinal inflammations, unspecified eye `CC`

✅5th **H30.9 Unspecified chorioretinal inflammation**
Chorioretinitis NOS
Choroiditis NOS
Neuroretinitis NOS
Retinitis NOS
Retinochoroiditis NOS

  H30.90 Unspecified chorioretinal inflammation, unspecified eye `CC`

✅ Additional Character Req ✔x7th Placeholder Alert Unacceptable PDx Manifestation **H1**-**H14** HAC **HCC** CMS-HCC Condition *EXCLUDES 1* Not Coded Here *EXCLUDES 2* Not Included Here

Chapter 7. Diseases of the Eye and Adnexa

H30.91 Unspecified chorioretinal inflammation, right eye `CC`

H30.92 Unspecified chorioretinal inflammation, left eye `CC`

H30.93 Unspecified chorioretinal inflammation, bilateral `CC`

✓4th **H31 Other disorders of choroid**

> **CC Excl: For CC codes in category H31:** PDX collection 627

✓5th **H31.0 Chorioretinal scars**
> EXCLUDES 2   *postsurgical chorioretinal scars (H59.81-)*

  ✓6th **H31.00 Unspecified chorioretinal scars**
    H31.001 Unspecified chorioretinal scars, right eye
    H31.002 Unspecified chorioretinal scars, left eye
    H31.003 Unspecified chorioretinal scars, bilateral
    H31.009 Unspecified chorioretinal scars, unspecified eye

  ✓6th **H31.01 Macula scars of posterior pole (postinflammatory) (post-traumatic)**
> EXCLUDES 1   *postprocedural chorioretinal scar (H59.81-)*

    H31.011 Macula scars of posterior pole (postinflammatory) (post-traumatic), right eye
    H31.012 Macula scars of posterior pole (postinflammatory) (post-traumatic), left eye
    H31.013 Macula scars of posterior pole (postinflammatory) (post-traumatic), bilateral
    H31.019 Macula scars of posterior pole (postinflammatory) (post-traumatic), unspecified eye

  ✓6th **H31.02 Solar retinopathy**
    H31.021 Solar retinopathy, right eye
    H31.022 Solar retinopathy, left eye
    H31.023 Solar retinopathy, bilateral
    H31.029 Solar retinopathy, unspecified eye

  ✓6th **H31.09 Other chorioretinal scars**
    H31.091 Other chorioretinal scars, right eye
    H31.092 Other chorioretinal scars, left eye
    H31.093 Other chorioretinal scars, bilateral
    H31.099 Other chorioretinal scars, unspecified eye

✓5th **H31.1 Choroidal degeneration**
> EXCLUDES 2   *angioid streaks of macula (H35.33)*

  ✓6th **H31.10 Unspecified choroidal degeneration**
    Choroidal sclerosis NOS
    H31.101 Choroidal degeneration, unspecified, right eye
    H31.102 Choroidal degeneration, unspecified, left eye
    H31.103 Choroidal degeneration, unspecified, bilateral
    H31.109 Choroidal degeneration, unspecified, unspecified eye

  ✓6th **H31.11 Age-related choroidal atrophy**
    H31.111 Age-related choroidal atrophy, right eye `A`
    H31.112 Age-related choroidal atrophy, left eye `A`
    H31.113 Age-related choroidal atrophy, bilateral `A`
    H31.119 Age-related choroidal atrophy, unspecified eye `A`

  ✓6th **H31.12 Diffuse secondary atrophy of choroid**
    H31.121 Diffuse secondary atrophy of choroid, right eye
    H31.122 Diffuse secondary atrophy of choroid, left eye
    H31.123 Diffuse secondary atrophy of choroid, bilateral
    H31.129 Diffuse secondary atrophy of choroid, unspecified eye

✓5th **H31.2 Hereditary choroidal dystrophy**
> EXCLUDES 2   *hyperornithinemia (E72.4)*
>   *ornithinemia (E72.4)*

    H31.20 Hereditary choroidal dystrophy, unspecified

H31.21 Choroideremia

H31.22 Choroidal dystrophy (central areolar) (generalized) (peripapillary)

H31.23 Gyrate atrophy, choroid

H31.29 Other hereditary choroidal dystrophy

✓5th **H31.3 Choroidal hemorrhage and rupture**

  ✓6th **H31.30 Unspecified choroidal hemorrhage**
    H31.301 Unspecified choroidal hemorrhage, right eye
    H31.302 Unspecified choroidal hemorrhage, left eye
    H31.303 Unspecified choroidal hemorrhage, bilateral
    H31.309 Unspecified choroidal hemorrhage, unspecified eye

  ✓6th **H31.31 Expulsive choroidal hemorrhage**
    H31.311 Expulsive choroidal hemorrhage, right eye
    H31.312 Expulsive choroidal hemorrhage, left eye
    H31.313 Expulsive choroidal hemorrhage, bilateral
    H31.319 Expulsive choroidal hemorrhage, unspecified eye

  ✓6th **H31.32 Choroidal rupture**
    H31.321 Choroidal rupture, right eye `CC`
    H31.322 Choroidal rupture, left eye `CC`
    H31.323 Choroidal rupture, bilateral `CC`
    H31.329 Choroidal rupture, unspecified eye `CC`

✓5th **H31.4 Choroidal detachment**

  ✓6th **H31.40 Unspecified choroidal detachment**
    H31.401 Unspecified choroidal detachment, right eye `CC`
    H31.402 Unspecified choroidal detachment, left eye `CC`
    H31.403 Unspecified choroidal detachment, bilateral `CC`
    H31.409 Unspecified choroidal detachment, unspecified eye `CC`

  ✓6th **H31.41 Hemorrhagic choroidal detachment**
    H31.411 Hemorrhagic choroidal detachment, right eye `CC`
    H31.412 Hemorrhagic choroidal detachment, left eye `CC`
    H31.413 Hemorrhagic choroidal detachment, bilateral `CC`
    H31.419 Hemorrhagic choroidal detachment, unspecified eye `CC`

  ✓6th **H31.42 Serous choroidal detachment**
    H31.421 Serous choroidal detachment, right eye `CC`
    H31.422 Serous choroidal detachment, left eye `CC`
    H31.423 Serous choroidal detachment, bilateral `CC`
    H31.429 Serous choroidal detachment, unspecified eye `CC`

H31.8 Other specified disorders of choroid

H31.9 Unspecified disorder of choroid

H32 Chorioretinal disorders in diseases classified elsewhere
> Code first underlying disease, such as:
>   congenital toxoplasmosis (P37.1)
>   histoplasmosis (B39.-)
>   leprosy (A30.-)
> EXCLUDES 1   *chorioretinitis (in):*
>   *toxoplasmosis (acquired) (B58.01)*
>   *tuberculosis (A18.53)*

✓4th **H33 Retinal detachments and breaks**
> EXCLUDES 1   *detachment of retinal pigment epithelium (H35.72-, H35.73-)*

> **CC Excl: For CC codes in category H33, unless otherwise noted:** PDX collection 628

✓5th **H33.0 Retinal detachment with retinal break**
  Rhegmatogenous retinal detachment
> EXCLUDES 1   *serous retinal detachment (without retinal break) (H33.2-)*

  ✓6th **H33.00 Unspecified retinal detachment with retinal break**
    H33.001 Unspecified retinal detachment with retinal break, right eye

`N` Newborn: 0   `P` Pediatric: 0-17   `M` Maternity: 12-55   `A` Adult: 15-124   `MCC` Major CC Condition   `PDxMCC` PDx acts as own MCC   `CC` CC Condition   `PDxCC` PDx acts as own CC

596   ICD-10-CM 2018

Retinal Detachment

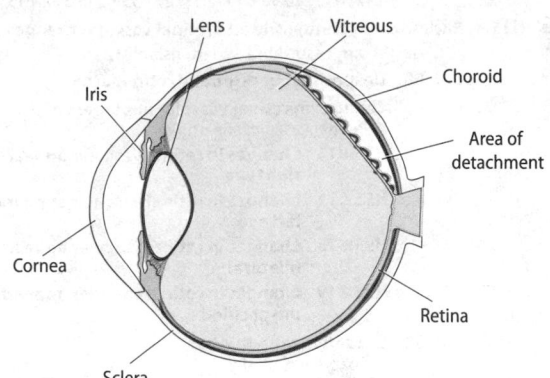

Labels: Lens, Vitreous, Choroid, Iris, Area of detachment, Cornea, Retina, Sclera

H33.002   Unspecified retinal detachment with retinal break, left eye

H33.003   Unspecified retinal detachment with retinal break, bilateral

H33.009   Unspecified retinal detachment with retinal break, unspecified eye

✓6ᵗʰ **H33.01**   Retinal detachment with single break

    H33.011   Retinal detachment with single break, right eye

    H33.012   Retinal detachment with single break, left eye

    H33.013   Retinal detachment with single break, bilateral

    H33.019   Retinal detachment with single break, unspecified eye

✓6ᵗʰ **H33.02**   Retinal detachment with multiple breaks

    H33.021   Retinal detachment with multiple breaks, right eye

    H33.022   Retinal detachment with multiple breaks, left eye

    H33.023   Retinal detachment with multiple breaks, bilateral

    H33.029   Retinal detachment with multiple breaks, unspecified eye

✓6ᵗʰ **H33.03**   Retinal detachment with giant retinal tear

    H33.031   Retinal detachment with giant retinal tear, right eye

    H33.032   Retinal detachment with giant retinal tear, left eye

    H33.033   Retinal detachment with giant retinal tear, bilateral

    H33.039   Retinal detachment with giant retinal tear, unspecified eye

✓6ᵗʰ **H33.04**   Retinal detachment with retinal dialysis

    H33.041   Retinal detachment with retinal dialysis, right eye

    H33.042   Retinal detachment with retinal dialysis, left eye

    H33.043   Retinal detachment with retinal dialysis, bilateral

    H33.049   Retinal detachment with retinal dialysis, unspecified eye

✓6ᵗʰ **H33.05**   Total retinal detachment

    H33.051   Total retinal detachment, right eye

    H33.052   Total retinal detachment, left eye

    H33.053   Total retinal detachment, bilateral

    H33.059   Total retinal detachment, unspecified eye

✓5ᵗʰ **H33.1**   Retinoschisis and retinal cysts

    EXCLUDES 1   congenital retinoschisis (Q14.1)
            microcystoid degeneration of retina (H35.42-)

✓6ᵗʰ **H33.10**   Unspecified retinoschisis

    H33.101   Unspecified retinoschisis, right eye

    H33.102   Unspecified retinoschisis, left eye

    H33.103   Unspecified retinoschisis, bilateral

    H33.109   Unspecified retinoschisis, unspecified eye

✓6ᵗʰ **H33.11**   Cyst of ora serrata

    H33.111   Cyst of ora serrata, right eye

    H33.112   Cyst of ora serrata, left eye

    H33.113   Cyst of ora serrata, bilateral

    H33.119   Cyst of ora serrata, unspecified eye

✓6ᵗʰ **H33.12**   Parasitic cyst of retina

    CC Excl: For CC codes in subcategory H33.12:
    PDX collection 625

    H33.121   Parasitic cyst of retina, right eye   `CC`

    H33.122   Parasitic cyst of retina, left eye   `CC`

    H33.123   Parasitic cyst of retina, bilateral   `CC`

    H33.129   Parasitic cyst of retina, unspecified eye   `CC`

✓6ᵗʰ **H33.19**   Other retinoschisis and retinal cysts
    Pseudocyst of retina

    H33.191   Other retinoschisis and retinal cysts, right eye

    H33.192   Other retinoschisis and retinal cysts, left eye

    H33.193   Other retinoschisis and retinal cysts, bilateral

    H33.199   Other retinoschisis and retinal cysts, unspecified eye

✓5ᵗʰ **H33.2**   Serous retinal detachment
    Retinal detachment NOS
    Retinal detachment without retinal break
    EXCLUDES 1   central serous chorioretinopathy (H35.71-)

    H33.20   Serous retinal detachment, unspecified eye   `CC`

    H33.21   Serous retinal detachment, right eye   `CC`

    H33.22   Serous retinal detachment, left eye   `CC`

    H33.23   Serous retinal detachment, bilateral   `CC`

✓5ᵗʰ **H33.3**   Retinal breaks without detachment
    EXCLUDES 1   chorioretinal scars after surgery for detachment (H59.81-)
            peripheral retinal degeneration without break (H35.4-)

✓6ᵗʰ **H33.30**   Unspecified retinal break

    H33.301   Unspecified retinal break, right eye

    H33.302   Unspecified retinal break, left eye

    H33.303   Unspecified retinal break, bilateral

    H33.309   Unspecified retinal break, unspecified eye

✓6ᵗʰ **H33.31**   Horseshoe tear of retina without detachment
    Operculum of retina without detachment

    H33.311   Horseshoe tear of retina without detachment, right eye

    H33.312   Horseshoe tear of retina without detachment, left eye

    H33.313   Horseshoe tear of retina without detachment, bilateral

    H33.319   Horseshoe tear of retina without detachment, unspecified eye

✓6ᵗʰ **H33.32**   Round hole of retina without detachment

    H33.321   Round hole, right eye

    H33.322   Round hole, left eye

    H33.323   Round hole, bilateral

    H33.329   Round hole, unspecified eye

✓6ᵗʰ **H33.33**   Multiple defects of retina without detachment

    H33.331   Multiple defects of retina without detachment, right eye

    H33.332   Multiple defects of retina without detachment, left eye

    H33.333   Multiple defects of retina without detachment, bilateral

    H33.339   Multiple defects of retina without detachment, unspecified eye

✓5ᵗʰ **H33.4**   Traction detachment of retina
    Proliferative vitreo-retinopathy with retinal detachment

    H33.40   Traction detachment of retina, unspecified eye   `CC`

    H33.41   Traction detachment of retina, right eye   `CC`

    H33.42   Traction detachment of retina, left eye   `CC`

    H33.43   Traction detachment of retina, bilateral   `CC`

H33.8   Other retinal detachments   `CC`

✓ Additional Character Req   ✓x7ᵗʰ Placeholder Alert   Unacceptable PDx   Manifestation   **H1**-**H14** HAC   **HCC** CMS-HCC Condition   *EXCLUDES 1* Not Coded Here   *EXCLUDES 2* Not Included Here

Chapter 7. Diseases of the Eye and Adnexa

H34–H35.1Ø9

✓4ᵗʰ **H34 Retinal vascular occlusions**

    EXCLUDES 1   *amaurosis fugax (G45.3)*

    CC Excl: For CC codes in category H34: PDX collection 587

✓5ᵗʰ **H34.Ø Transient retinal artery occlusion**

    H34.ØØ Transient retinal artery occlusion, unspecified eye CC

    H34.Ø1 Transient retinal artery occlusion, right eye CC

    H34.Ø2 Transient retinal artery occlusion, left eye CC

    H34.Ø3 Transient retinal artery occlusion, bilateral CC

✓5ᵗʰ **H34.1 Central retinal artery occlusion**

    H34.1Ø Central retinal artery occlusion, unspecified eye CC

    H34.11 Central retinal artery occlusion, right eye CC

    H34.12 Central retinal artery occlusion, left eye CC

    H34.13 Central retinal artery occlusion, bilateral CC

✓5ᵗʰ **H34.2 Other retinal artery occlusions**

    ✓6ᵗʰ **H34.21 Partial retinal artery occlusion**
        Hollenhorst's plaque
        Retinal microembolism

        H34.211 Partial retinal artery occlusion, right eye CC

        H34.212 Partial retinal artery occlusion, left eye CC

        H34.213 Partial retinal artery occlusion, bilateral CC

        H34.219 Partial retinal artery occlusion, unspecified eye CC

    ✓6ᵗʰ **H34.23 Retinal artery branch occlusion**

        H34.231 Retinal artery branch occlusion, right eye CC

        H34.232 Retinal artery branch occlusion, left eye CC

        H34.233 Retinal artery branch occlusion, bilateral CC

        H34.239 Retinal artery branch occlusion, unspecified eye CC

✓5ᵗʰ **H34.8 Other retinal vascular occlusions**

    ✓6ᵗʰ **H34.81 Central retinal vein occlusion**

        One of the following 7th characters is to be assigned to codes in subcategory H34.81 to designate the severity of the occlusion:
        Ø   with macular edema
        1   with retinal neovascularization
        2   stable
            old central retinal vein occlusion

        ✓7ᵗʰ **H34.811 Central retinal vein occlusion, right eye** CC

        ✓7ᵗʰ **H34.812 Central retinal vein occlusion, left eye** CC

        ✓7ᵗʰ **H34.813 Central retinal vein occlusion, bilateral** CC

        ✓7ᵗʰ **H34.819 Central retinal vein occlusion, unspecified eye** CC

    ✓6ᵗʰ **H34.82 Venous engorgement**
        Incipient retinal vein occlusion
        Partial retinal vein occlusion

        H34.821 Venous engorgement, right eye

        H34.822 Venous engorgement, left eye

        H34.823 Venous engorgement, bilateral

        H34.829 Venous engorgement, unspecified eye

    ✓6ᵗʰ **H34.83 Tributary (branch) retinal vein occlusion**

        One of the following 7th characters is to be assigned to codes in subcategory H34.83 to designate the severity of the occlusion:
        Ø   with macular edema
        1   with retinal neovascularization
        2   stable
            old tributary (branch) retinal vein occlusion

        ✓7ᵗʰ **H34.831 Tributary (branch) retinal vein occlusion, right eye**

        ✓7ᵗʰ **H34.832 Tributary (branch) retinal vein occlusion, left eye**

        ✓7ᵗʰ **H34.833 Tributary (branch) retinal vein occlusion, bilateral**

        ✓7ᵗʰ **H34.839 Tributary (branch) retinal vein occlusion, unspecified eye**

    H34.9 Unspecified retinal vascular occlusion CC

✓4ᵗʰ **H35 Other retinal disorders**

    EXCLUDES 2   *diabetic retinal disorders (E08.311- E08.359, E09.311- E09.359, E10.311- E10.359, E11.311- E11.359, E13.311- E13.359)*

✓5ᵗʰ **H35.Ø Background retinopathy and retinal vascular changes**
    Code also any associated hypertension (I1Ø.-)

    H35.ØØ Unspecified background retinopathy

    ✓6ᵗʰ **H35.Ø1 Changes in retinal vascular appearance**
        Retinal vascular sheathing

        H35.Ø11 Changes in retinal vascular appearance, right eye

        H35.Ø12 Changes in retinal vascular appearance, left eye

        H35.Ø13 Changes in retinal vascular appearance, bilateral

        H35.Ø19 Changes in retinal vascular appearance, unspecified eye

    ✓6ᵗʰ **H35.Ø2 Exudative retinopathy**
        Coats retinopathy

        H35.Ø21 Exudative retinopathy, right eye

        H35.Ø22 Exudative retinopathy, left eye

        H35.Ø23 Exudative retinopathy, bilateral

        H35.Ø29 Exudative retinopathy, unspecified eye

    ✓6ᵗʰ **H35.Ø3 Hypertensive retinopathy**

        H35.Ø31 Hypertensive retinopathy, right eye

        H35.Ø32 Hypertensive retinopathy, left eye

        H35.Ø33 Hypertensive retinopathy, bilateral

        H35.Ø39 Hypertensive retinopathy, unspecified eye

    ✓6ᵗʰ **H35.Ø4 Retinal micro-aneurysms, unspecified**

        H35.Ø41 Retinal micro-aneurysms, unspecified, right eye

        H35.Ø42 Retinal micro-aneurysms, unspecified, left eye

        H35.Ø43 Retinal micro-aneurysms, unspecified, bilateral

        H35.Ø49 Retinal micro-aneurysms, unspecified, unspecified eye

    ✓6ᵗʰ **H35.Ø5 Retinal neovascularization, unspecified**

        H35.Ø51 Retinal neovascularization, unspecified, right eye

        H35.Ø52 Retinal neovascularization, unspecified, left eye

        H35.Ø53 Retinal neovascularization, unspecified, bilateral

        H35.Ø59 Retinal neovascularization, unspecified, unspecified eye

    ✓6ᵗʰ **H35.Ø6 Retinal vasculitis**
        Eales disease
        Retinal perivasculitis
        DEF: Sight-threatening intraocular inflammation of the retinal blood vessels; causes minimal, partial, or even complete blindness.

        H35.Ø61 Retinal vasculitis, right eye

        H35.Ø62 Retinal vasculitis, left eye

        H35.Ø63 Retinal vasculitis, bilateral

        H35.Ø69 Retinal vasculitis, unspecified eye

    ✓6ᵗʰ **H35.Ø7 Retinal telangiectasis**

        H35.Ø71 Retinal telangiectasis, right eye

        H35.Ø72 Retinal telangiectasis, left eye

        H35.Ø73 Retinal telangiectasis, bilateral

        H35.Ø79 Retinal telangiectasis, unspecified eye

    H35.Ø9 Other intraretinal microvascular abnormalities
        Retinal varices

✓5ᵗʰ **H35.1 Retinopathy of prematurity**

    ✓6ᵗʰ **H35.1Ø Retinopathy of prematurity, unspecified**
        Retinopathy of prematurity NOS

        H35.1Ø1 Retinopathy of prematurity, unspecified, right eye

        H35.1Ø2 Retinopathy of prematurity, unspecified, left eye

        H35.1Ø3 Retinopathy of prematurity, unspecified, bilateral

        H35.1Ø9 Retinopathy of prematurity, unspecified, unspecified eye

---

N Newborn: 0   P Pediatric: 0-17   M Maternity: 12-55   A Adult: 15-124   MCC Major CC Condition   PDxMCC PDx acts as own MCC   CC CC Condition   PDxCC PDx acts as own CC

598   ICD-10-CM 2018

☑6ᵗʰ **H35.11** **Retinopathy of prematurity,** stage Ø

    H35.111 **Retinopathy of prematurity, stage Ø, right eye**

    H35.112 **Retinopathy of prematurity, stage Ø, left eye**

    H35.113 **Retinopathy of prematurity, stage Ø, bilateral**

    H35.119 **Retinopathy of prematurity, stage Ø, unspecified eye**

☑6ᵗʰ **H35.12** **Retinopathy of prematurity,** stage 1

    H35.121 **Retinopathy of prematurity, stage 1, right eye**

    H35.122 **Retinopathy of prematurity, stage 1, left eye**

    H35.123 **Retinopathy of prematurity, stage 1, bilateral**

    H35.129 **Retinopathy of prematurity, stage 1, unspecified eye**

☑6ᵗʰ **H35.13** **Retinopathy of prematurity,** stage 2

    H35.131 **Retinopathy of prematurity, stage 2, right eye**

    H35.132 **Retinopathy of prematurity, stage 2, left eye**

    H35.133 **Retinopathy of prematurity, stage 2, bilateral**

    H35.139 **Retinopathy of prematurity, stage 2, unspecified eye**

☑6ᵗʰ **H35.14** **Retinopathy of prematurity,** stage 3

    H35.141 **Retinopathy of prematurity, stage 3, right eye**

    H35.142 **Retinopathy of prematurity, stage 3, left eye**

    H35.143 **Retinopathy of prematurity, stage 3, bilateral**

    H35.149 **Retinopathy of prematurity, stage 3, unspecified eye**

☑6ᵗʰ **H35.15** **Retinopathy of prematurity,** stage 4

    H35.151 **Retinopathy of prematurity, stage 4, right eye**

    H35.152 **Retinopathy of prematurity, stage 4, left eye**

    H35.153 **Retinopathy of prematurity, stage 4, bilateral**

    H35.159 **Retinopathy of prematurity, stage 4, unspecified eye**

☑6ᵗʰ **H35.16** **Retinopathy of prematurity,** stage 5

    H35.161 **Retinopathy of prematurity, stage 5, right eye**

    H35.162 **Retinopathy of prematurity, stage 5, left eye**

    H35.163 **Retinopathy of prematurity, stage 5, bilateral**

    H35.169 **Retinopathy of prematurity, stage 5, unspecified eye**

☑6ᵗʰ **H35.17** **Retrolental fibroplasia**

    H35.171 **Retrolental fibroplasia,** right eye

    H35.172 **Retrolental fibroplasia,** left eye

    H35.173 **Retrolental fibroplasia,** bilateral

    H35.179 **Retrolental fibroplasia,** unspecified eye

☑5ᵗʰ **H35.2** **Other non-diabetic proliferative retinopathy**
    Proliferative vitreo-retinopathy
    EXCLUDES 1   proliferative vitreo-retinopathy with retinal detachment (H33.4-)

    H35.2Ø **Other non-diabetic proliferative retinopathy, unspecified eye**

    H35.21 **Other non-diabetic proliferative retinopathy,** right eye

    H35.22 **Other non-diabetic proliferative retinopathy,** left eye

    H35.23 **Other non-diabetic proliferative retinopathy, bilateral**

☑5ᵗʰ **H35.3** **Degeneration of macula and posterior pole**

    H35.3Ø **Unspecified macular degeneration**   Ⓐ
        Age-related macular degeneration

☑6ᵗʰ **H35.31** **Nonexudative age-related macular degeneration**
    Atrophic age-related macular degeneration
    Dry age-related macular degeneration
    AHA: 2016, 4Q, 21

> One of the following 7th characters is to be assigned to codes in subcategory H35.31 to designate the stage of the disease:
> Ø   stage unspecified
> 1   early dry stage
> 2   intermediate dry stage
> 3   advanced atrophic without subfoveal involvement
>   advanced dry stage
> 4   advanced atrophic with subfoveal involvement

    ☑7ᵗʰ **H35.311** **Nonexudative age-related macular degeneration,** right eye   Ⓐ

    ☑7ᵗʰ **H35.312** **Nonexudative age-related macular degeneration,** left eye   Ⓐ

    ☑7ᵗʰ **H35.313** **Nonexudative age-related macular degeneration,** bilateral   Ⓐ

    ☑7ᵗʰ **H35.319** **Nonexudative age-related macular degeneration,** unspecified eye   Ⓐ

☑6ᵗʰ **H35.32** **Exudative age-related macular degeneration**
    Wet age-related macular degeneration

> One of the following 7th characters is to be assigned to codes in subcategory H35.32 to designate the stage of the disease:
> Ø   stage unspecified
> 1   with active choroidal neovascularization
> 2   with inactive choroidal neovascularization
>   with involuted or regressed neovascularization
> 3   with inactive scar

    ☑7ᵗʰ **H35.321** **Exudative age-related macular degeneration,** right eye   HCC Ⓐ

    ☑7ᵗʰ **H35.322** **Exudative age-related macular degeneration,** left eye   HCC Ⓐ

    ☑7ᵗʰ **H35.323** **Exudative age-related macular degeneration,** bilateral   HCC Ⓐ

    ☑7ᵗʰ **H35.329** **Exudative age-related macular degeneration,** unspecified eye   HCC Ⓐ

    H35.33 **Angioid streaks of macula**
        DEF: Degeneration of choroid; characterized by broad, irregular, dark brown streaks radiating from optic disc; occurs with pseudoxanthoma elasticum or Paget's disease.

☑6ᵗʰ **H35.34** **Macular cyst, hole, or pseudohole**

    H35.341 **Macular cyst, hole, or pseudohole,** right eye

    H35.342 **Macular cyst, hole, or pseudohole,** left eye

    H35.343 **Macular cyst, hole, or pseudohole, bilateral**

    H35.349 **Macular cyst, hole, or pseudohole, unspecified eye**

☑6ᵗʰ **H35.35** **Cystoid macular degeneration**
    EXCLUDES 1   cystoid macular edema following cataract surgery (H59.Ø3-)

    H35.351 **Cystoid macular degeneration,** right eye

    H35.352 **Cystoid macular degeneration,** left eye

    H35.353 **Cystoid macular degeneration,** bilateral

    H35.359 **Cystoid macular degeneration, unspecified eye**

☑6ᵗʰ **H35.36** **Drusen (degenerative) of macula**
    AHA: 2017, 1Q, 51; 2016, 4Q, 21

    H35.361 **Drusen (degenerative) of macula,** right eye

    H35.362 **Drusen (degenerative) of macula,** left eye

    H35.363 **Drusen (degenerative) of macula,** bilateral

    H35.369 **Drusen (degenerative) of macula, unspecified eye**

☑6ᵗʰ **H35.37** **Puckering of macula**

    H35.371 **Puckering of macula,** right eye

    H35.372 **Puckering of macula,** left eye

    H35.373 **Puckering of macula,** bilateral

    H35.379 **Puckering of macula,** unspecified eye

☑6ᵗʰ **H35.38 Toxic maculopathy**
Code first poisoning due to drug or toxin, if applicable (T36-T65 with fifth or sixth character 1-4 or 6)
Use additional code for adverse effect, if applicable, to identify drug (T36-T50 with fifth or sixth character 5)

    H35.381 Toxic maculopathy, right eye
    H35.382 Toxic maculopathy, left eye
    H35.383 Toxic maculopathy, bilateral
    H35.389 Toxic maculopathy, unspecified eye

☑5ᵗʰ **H35.4 Peripheral retinal degeneration**
    EXCLUDES 1 hereditary retinal degeneration (dystrophy) (H35.5-)
    peripheral retinal degeneration with retinal break (H33.3-)

    H35.40 Unspecified peripheral retinal degeneration

☑6ᵗʰ **H35.41 Lattice degeneration of retina**
Palisade degeneration of retina
DEF: Degeneration of retina; often bilateral, usually benign; characterized by lines intersecting at irregular intervals in peripheral retina; retinal thinning and retinal holes may occur.

    H35.411 Lattice degeneration of retina, right eye
    H35.412 Lattice degeneration of retina, left eye
    H35.413 Lattice degeneration of retina, bilateral
    H35.419 Lattice degeneration of retina, unspecified eye

☑6ᵗʰ **H35.42 Microcystoid degeneration of retina**
    H35.421 Microcystoid degeneration of retina, right eye
    H35.422 Microcystoid degeneration of retina, left eye
    H35.423 Microcystoid degeneration of retina, bilateral
    H35.429 Microcystoid degeneration of retina, unspecified eye

☑6ᵗʰ **H35.43 Paving stone degeneration of retina**
    H35.431 Paving stone degeneration of retina, right eye
    H35.432 Paving stone degeneration of retina, left eye
    H35.433 Paving stone degeneration of retina, bilateral
    H35.439 Paving stone degeneration of retina, unspecified eye

☑6ᵗʰ **H35.44 Age-related reticular degeneration of retina**
    H35.441 Age-related reticular degeneration of retina, right eye A
    H35.442 Age-related reticular degeneration of retina, left eye A
    H35.443 Age-related reticular degeneration of retina, bilateral A
    H35.449 Age-related reticular degeneration of retina, unspecified eye A

☑6ᵗʰ **H35.45 Secondary pigmentary degeneration**
    H35.451 Secondary pigmentary degeneration, right eye
    H35.452 Secondary pigmentary degeneration, left eye
    H35.453 Secondary pigmentary degeneration, bilateral
    H35.459 Secondary pigmentary degeneration, unspecified eye

☑6ᵗʰ **H35.46 Secondary vitreoretinal degeneration**
    H35.461 Secondary vitreoretinal degeneration, right eye
    H35.462 Secondary vitreoretinal degeneration, left eye
    H35.463 Secondary vitreoretinal degeneration, bilateral
    H35.469 Secondary vitreoretinal degeneration, unspecified eye

☑5ᵗʰ **H35.5 Hereditary retinal dystrophy**
    EXCLUDES 1 dystrophies primarily involving Bruch's membrane (H31.1-)

    H35.50 Unspecified hereditary retinal dystrophy
    H35.51 Vitreoretinal dystrophy

    H35.52 Pigmentary retinal dystrophy
Albipunctate retinal dystrophy
Retinitis pigmentosa
Tapetoretinal dystrophy

    H35.53 Other dystrophies primarily involving the sensory retina
Stargardt's disease

    H35.54 Dystrophies primarily involving the retinal pigment epithelium
Vitelliform retinal dystrophy

☑5ᵗʰ **H35.6 Retinal hemorrhage**
    H35.60 Retinal hemorrhage, unspecified eye
    H35.61 Retinal hemorrhage, right eye
    H35.62 Retinal hemorrhage, left eye
    H35.63 Retinal hemorrhage, bilateral

☑5ᵗʰ **H35.7 Separation of retinal layers**
    EXCLUDES 1 retinal detachment (serous) (H33.2-)
    rhegmatogenous retinal detachment (H33.0-)

    CC Excl: For CC codes in subcategory H35.7:
PDX collection 628

    H35.70 Unspecified separation of retinal layers CC

☑6ᵗʰ **H35.71 Central serous chorioretinopathy**
    H35.711 Central serous chorioretinopathy, right eye
    H35.712 Central serous chorioretinopathy, left eye
    H35.713 Central serous chorioretinopathy, bilateral
    H35.719 Central serous chorioretinopathy, unspecified eye

☑6ᵗʰ **H35.72 Serous detachment of retinal pigment epithelium**
    H35.721 Serous detachment of retinal pigment epithelium, right eye CC
    H35.722 Serous detachment of retinal pigment epithelium, left eye CC
    H35.723 Serous detachment of retinal pigment epithelium, bilateral CC
    H35.729 Serous detachment of retinal pigment epithelium, unspecified eye CC

☑6ᵗʰ **H35.73 Hemorrhagic detachment of retinal pigment epithelium**
    H35.731 Hemorrhagic detachment of retinal pigment epithelium, right eye CC
    H35.732 Hemorrhagic detachment of retinal pigment epithelium, left eye CC
    H35.733 Hemorrhagic detachment of retinal pigment epithelium, bilateral CC
    H35.739 Hemorrhagic detachment of retinal pigment epithelium, unspecified eye CC

☑5ᵗʰ **H35.8 Other specified retinal disorders**
    EXCLUDES 2 retinal hemorrhage (H35.6-)

    H35.81 Retinal edema
Retinal cotton wool spots

    H35.82 Retinal ischemia CC
CC Excl: PDX collection 629

    H35.89 Other specified retinal disorders

    H35.9 Unspecified retinal disorder

H36 *Retinal disorders in diseases classified elsewhere*
Code first underlying disease, such as:
lipid storage disorders (E75.-)
sickle-cell disorders (D57.-)
    EXCLUDES 1 arteriosclerotic retinopathy (H35.0-)
    diabetic retinopathy (E08.3-, E09.3-, E10.3-, E11.3-, E13.3-)

Glaucoma (H40-H42)

☑4ᵗʰ **H40 Glaucoma**
    EXCLUDES 1 absolute glaucoma (H44.51-)
    congenital glaucoma (Q15.0)
    traumatic glaucoma due to birth injury (P15.3)

☑5ᵗʰ **H40.0 Glaucoma suspect**
☑6ᵗʰ   **H40.00 Preglaucoma, unspecified**
    H40.001 Preglaucoma, unspecified, right eye
    H40.002 Preglaucoma, unspecified, left eye
    H40.003 Preglaucoma, unspecified, bilateral
    H40.009 Preglaucoma, unspecified, unspecified eye

N Newborn: 0   P Pediatric: 0-17   M Maternity: 12-55   A Adult: 15-124   MCC Major CC Condition   PDxMCC PDx acts as own MCC   CC CC Condition   PDxCC PDx acts as own CC

600   ICD-10-CM 2018

✓6th **H40.01** Open angle **with borderline findings,** low risk
     Open angle, low risk

     H40.011 **Open angle with borderline findings, low risk,** right **eye**

     H40.012 **Open angle with borderline findings, low risk,** left **eye**

     H40.013 **Open angle with borderline findings, low risk,** bilateral

     H40.019 **Open angle with borderline findings, low risk,** unspecified **eye**

✓6th **H40.02** Open angle **with borderline findings,** high risk
     Open angle, high risk

     H40.021 **Open angle with borderline findings, high risk,** right **eye**

     H40.022 **Open angle with borderline findings, high risk,** left **eye**

     H40.023 **Open angle with borderline findings, high risk,** bilateral

     H40.029 **Open angle with borderline findings, high risk,** unspecified **eye**

✓6th **H40.03** Anatomical narrow **angle**
     Primary angle closure suspect

     H40.031 **Anatomical narrow angle,** right **eye**

     H40.032 **Anatomical narrow angle,** left **eye**

     H40.033 **Anatomical narrow angle,** bilateral

     H40.039 **Anatomical narrow angle,** unspecified **eye**

✓6th **H40.04** Steroid responder

     H40.041 **Steroid responder,** right **eye**

     H40.042 **Steroid responder,** left **eye**

     H40.043 **Steroid responder,** bilateral

     H40.049 **Steroid responder,** unspecified **eye**

✓6th **H40.05** Ocular hypertension

     H40.051 **Ocular hypertension,** right **eye**

     H40.052 **Ocular hypertension,** left **eye**

     H40.053 **Ocular hypertension,** bilateral

     H40.059 **Ocular hypertension,** unspecified **eye**

✓6th **H40.06** Primary angle **closure** without glaucoma damage

     H40.061 **Primary angle closure without glaucoma damage,** right **eye**

     H40.062 **Primary angle closure without glaucoma damage,** left **eye**

     H40.063 **Primary angle closure without glaucoma damage,** bilateral

     H40.069 **Primary angle closure without glaucoma damage,** unspecified **eye**

✓5th **H40.1** Open-angle glaucoma

     One of the following 7th characters is to be assigned to each code in subcategories H40.10, H40.11-, H40.12-, H40.13-, and H40.14- to designate the stage of glaucoma.
     0   stage unspecified
     1   mild stage
     2   moderate stage
     3   severe stage
     4   indeterminate stage

✓x7th **H40.10** Unspecified **open-angle glaucoma**

✓6th **H40.11** Primary **open-angle glaucoma**
     Chronic simple glaucoma

     ✓7th **H40.111** **Primary open-angle glaucoma,** right **eye**

     ✓7th **H40.112** **Primary open-angle glaucoma,** left **eye**

     ✓7th **H40.113** **Primary open-angle glaucoma,** bilateral

     ✓7th **H40.119** **Primary open-angle glaucoma, unspecified eye**

✓6th **H40.12** Low-tension **glaucoma**

     ✓7th **H40.121** **Low-tension glaucoma,** right **eye**

     ✓7th **H40.122** **Low-tension glaucoma,** left **eye**

     ✓7th **H40.123** **Low-tension glaucoma,** bilateral

     ✓7th **H40.129** **Low-tension glaucoma,** unspecified **eye**

✓6th **H40.13** Pigmentary **glaucoma**

     ✓7th **H40.131** **Pigmentary glaucoma,** right **eye**

     ✓7th **H40.132** **Pigmentary glaucoma,** left **eye**

     ✓7th **H40.133** **Pigmentary glaucoma,** bilateral

     ✓7th **H40.139** **Pigmentary glaucoma,** unspecified **eye**

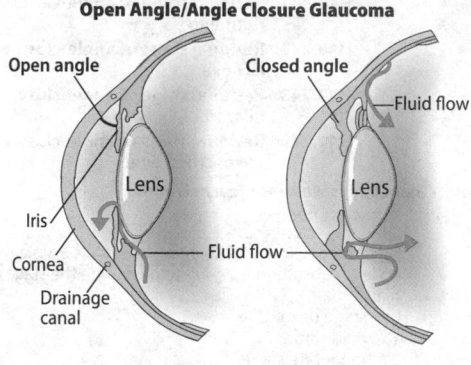

Open Angle/Angle Closure Glaucoma

Open angle — Closed angle — Fluid flow — Lens — Iris — Cornea — Fluid flow — Drainage canal

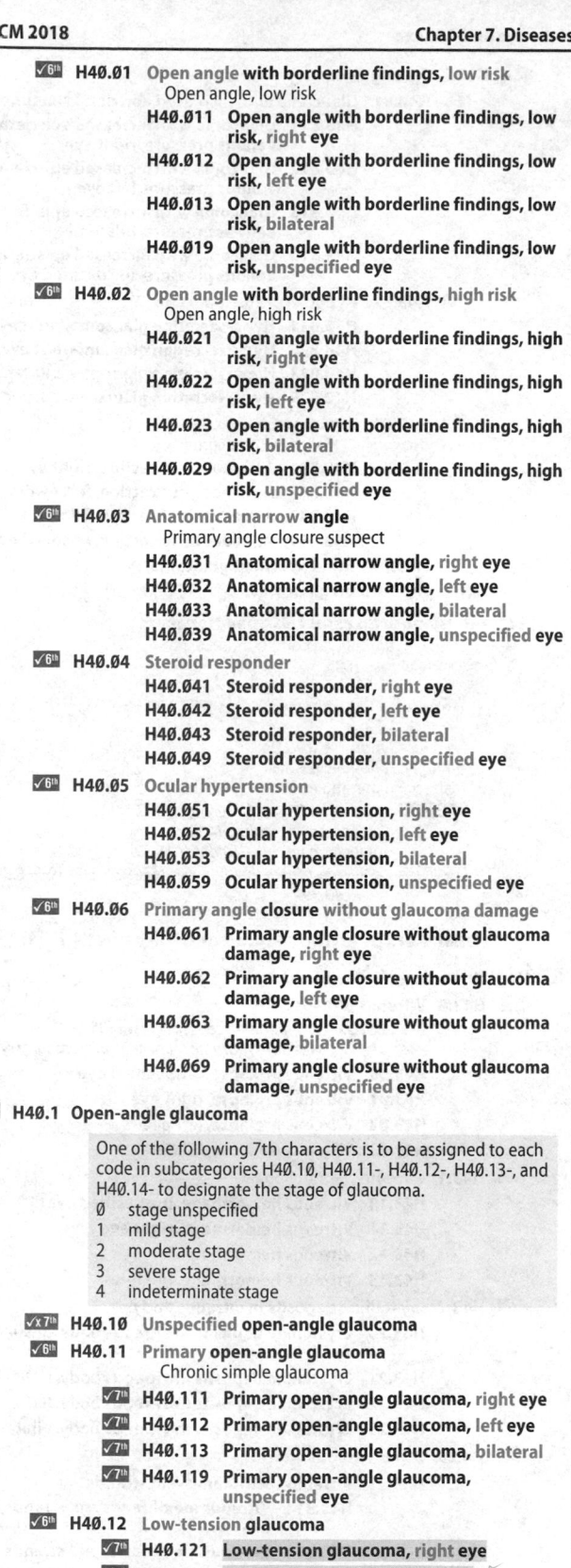

✓6th **H40.14** Capsular glaucoma with pseudoexfoliation **of lens**

     ✓7th **H40.141** **Capsular glaucoma with pseudoexfoliation of lens,** right **eye**

     ✓7th **H40.142** **Capsular glaucoma with pseudoexfoliation of lens,** left **eye**

     ✓7th **H40.143** **Capsular glaucoma with pseudoexfoliation of lens,** bilateral

     ✓7th **H40.149** **Capsular glaucoma with pseudoexfoliation of lens,** unspecified **eye**

✓6th **H40.15** Residual stage **of open-angle glaucoma**

     H40.151 **Residual stage of open-angle glaucoma, right eye**

     H40.152 **Residual stage of open-angle glaucoma, left eye**

     H40.153 **Residual stage of open-angle glaucoma, bilateral**

     H40.159 **Residual stage of open-angle glaucoma, unspecified eye**

✓5th **H40.2** Primary angle-closure glaucoma

     EXCLUDES 1   *aqueous misdirection (H40.83-)*
                     malignant glaucoma (H40.83-)

     One of the following 7th characters is to be assigned to each code in subcategories H40.20 and H40.22- to designate the stage of glaucoma.
     0   stage unspecified
     1   mild stage
     2   moderate stage
     3   severe stage
     4   indeterminate stage

✓x7th **H40.20** Unspecified **primary angle-closure glaucoma**

✓6th **H40.21** Acute **angle-closure glaucoma**
     Acute angle-closure glaucoma attack
     Acute angle-closure glaucoma crisis

     CC Excl: For CC codes in subcategory H40.21:
     PDX collection 630

     H40.211 **Acute angle-closure glaucoma,** right **eye**   `CC`

     H40.212 **Acute angle-closure glaucoma,** left **eye**   `CC`

     H40.213 **Acute angle-closure glaucoma,** bilateral   `CC`

     H40.219 **Acute angle-closure glaucoma,** unspecified **eye**   `CC`

✓6th **H40.22** Chronic **angle-closure glaucoma**
     Chronic primary angle-closure glaucoma

     ✓7th **H40.221** **Chronic angle-closure glaucoma,** right **eye**

     ✓7th **H40.222** **Chronic angle-closure glaucoma,** left **eye**

     ✓7th **H40.223** **Chronic angle-closure glaucoma,** bilateral

     ✓7th **H40.229** **Chronic angle-closure glaucoma, unspecified eye**

✓6th **H40.23** Intermittent **angle-closure glaucoma**

     H40.231 **Intermittent angle-closure glaucoma, right eye**

     H40.232 **Intermittent angle-closure glaucoma,** left **eye**

     H40.233 **Intermittent angle-closure glaucoma, bilateral**

     H40.239 **Intermittent angle-closure glaucoma, unspecified eye**

✓ Additional Character Req   ✓x7th Placeholder Alert   Unacceptable PDx   Manifestation   **H1–H14** HAC   HCC CMS-HCC Condition   *EXCLUDES 1* Not Coded Here   *EXCLUDES 2* Not Included Here

ICD-10-CM 2018   601

Chapter 7. Diseases of the Eye and Adnexa

H40.24–H43.399

✓6ᵗʰ **H40.24** Residual stage of angle-closure glaucoma

H40.241 Residual stage of angle-closure glaucoma, right eye

H40.242 Residual stage of angle-closure glaucoma, left eye

H40.243 Residual stage of angle-closure glaucoma, bilateral

H40.249 Residual stage of angle-closure glaucoma, unspecified eye

✓5ᵗʰ **H40.3** Glaucoma secondary to eye trauma

Code also underlying condition

One of the following 7th characters is to be assigned to each code in subcategory H40.3- to designate the stage of glaucoma.
- 0   stage unspecified
- 1   mild stage
- 2   moderate stage
- 3   severe stage
- 4   indeterminate stage

✓x7ᵗʰ **H40.30** Glaucoma secondary to eye trauma, unspecified eye

✓x7ᵗʰ **H40.31** Glaucoma secondary to eye trauma, right eye

✓x7ᵗʰ **H40.32** Glaucoma secondary to eye trauma, left eye

✓x7ᵗʰ **H40.33** Glaucoma secondary to eye trauma, bilateral

✓5ᵗʰ **H40.4** Glaucoma secondary to eye inflammation

Code also underlying condition

One of the following 7th characters is to be assigned to each code in subcategory H40.4- to designate the stage of glaucoma.
- 0   stage unspecified
- 1   mild stage
- 2   moderate stage
- 3   severe stage
- 4   indeterminate stage

✓x7ᵗʰ **H40.40** Glaucoma secondary to eye inflammation, unspecified eye

✓x7ᵗʰ **H40.41** Glaucoma secondary to eye inflammation, right eye

✓x7ᵗʰ **H40.42** Glaucoma secondary to eye inflammation, left eye

✓x7ᵗʰ **H40.43** Glaucoma secondary to eye inflammation, bilateral

✓5ᵗʰ **H40.5** Glaucoma secondary to other eye disorders

Code also underlying eye disorder

One of the following 7th characters is to be assigned to each code in subcategory H40.5- to designate the stage of glaucoma.
- 0   stage unspecified
- 1   mild stage
- 2   moderate stage
- 3   severe stage
- 4   indeterminate stage

✓x7ᵗʰ **H40.50** Glaucoma secondary to other eye disorders, unspecified eye

✓x7ᵗʰ **H40.51** Glaucoma secondary to other eye disorders, right eye

✓x7ᵗʰ **H40.52** Glaucoma secondary to other eye disorders, left eye

✓x7ᵗʰ **H40.53** Glaucoma secondary to other eye disorders, bilateral

✓5ᵗʰ **H40.6** Glaucoma secondary to drugs

Use additional code for adverse effect, if applicable, to identify drug (T36-T50 with fifth or sixth character 5)

One of the following 7th characters is to be assigned to each code in subcategory H40.6- to designate the stage of glaucoma.
- 0   stage unspecified
- 1   mild stage
- 2   moderate stage
- 3   severe stage
- 4   indeterminate stage

✓x7ᵗʰ **H40.60** Glaucoma secondary to drugs, unspecified eye

✓x7ᵗʰ **H40.61** Glaucoma secondary to drugs, right eye

✓x7ᵗʰ **H40.62** Glaucoma secondary to drugs, left eye

✓x7ᵗʰ **H40.63** Glaucoma secondary to drugs, bilateral

✓5ᵗʰ **H40.8** Other glaucoma

✓6ᵗʰ **H40.81** Glaucoma with increased episcleral venous pressure

H40.811 Glaucoma with increased episcleral venous pressure, right eye

H40.812 Glaucoma with increased episcleral venous pressure, left eye

H40.813 Glaucoma with increased episcleral venous pressure, bilateral

H40.819 Glaucoma with increased episcleral venous pressure, unspecified eye

✓6ᵗʰ **H40.82** Hypersecretion glaucoma

H40.821 Hypersecretion glaucoma, right eye

H40.822 Hypersecretion glaucoma, left eye

H40.823 Hypersecretion glaucoma, bilateral

H40.829 Hypersecretion glaucoma, unspecified eye

✓6ᵗʰ **H40.83** Aqueous misdirection

Malignant glaucoma

H40.831 Aqueous misdirection, right eye

H40.832 Aqueous misdirection, left eye

H40.833 Aqueous misdirection, bilateral

H40.839 Aqueous misdirection, unspecified eye

H40.89 Other specified glaucoma

H40.9 Unspecified glaucoma

H42 *Glaucoma in diseases classified elsewhere*

Code first underlying condition, such as:
- amyloidosis (E85.-)
- aniridia (Q13.1)
- ▶glaucoma (in) diabetes mellitus (E08.39, E09.39, E10.39, E11.39, E13.39)◀
- Lowe's syndrome (E72.03)
- Reiger's anomaly (Q13.81)
- specified metabolic disorder (E70-E88)

EXCLUDES 1   *glaucoma (in) onchocerciasis (B73.02)*
           glaucoma (in) syphilis (A52.71)
           glaucoma (in) tuberculous (A18.59)

EXCLUDES 2   ~~*glaucoma (in) diabetes mellitus (E08.39, E09.39, E10.39, E11.39, E13.39)*~~

Disorders of vitreous body and globe (H43-H44)

✓4ᵗʰ **H43** **Disorders of vitreous body**

✓5ᵗʰ **H43.0** Vitreous prolapse

EXCLUDES 1   *traumatic vitreous prolapse (S05.2-)*
           vitreous syndrome following cataract surgery (H59.0-)

H43.00 Vitreous prolapse, unspecified eye

H43.01 Vitreous prolapse, right eye

H43.02 Vitreous prolapse, left eye

H43.03 Vitreous prolapse, bilateral

✓5ᵗʰ **H43.1** Vitreous hemorrhage

H43.10 Vitreous hemorrhage, unspecified eye   HCC

H43.11 Vitreous hemorrhage, right eye   HCC

H43.12 Vitreous hemorrhage, left eye   HCC

H43.13 Vitreous hemorrhage, bilateral   HCC

✓5ᵗʰ **H43.2** Crystalline deposits in vitreous body

H43.20 Crystalline deposits in vitreous body, unspecified eye

H43.21 Crystalline deposits in vitreous body, right eye

H43.22 Crystalline deposits in vitreous body, left eye

H43.23 Crystalline deposits in vitreous body, bilateral

✓5ᵗʰ **H43.3** Other vitreous opacities

✓6ᵗʰ **H43.31** Vitreous membranes and strands

H43.311 Vitreous membranes and strands, right eye

H43.312 Vitreous membranes and strands, left eye

H43.313 Vitreous membranes and strands, bilateral

H43.319 Vitreous membranes and strands, unspecified eye

✓6ᵗʰ **H43.39** Other vitreous opacities

Vitreous floaters

H43.391 Other vitreous opacities, right eye

H43.392 Other vitreous opacities, left eye

H43.393 Other vitreous opacities, bilateral

H43.399 Other vitreous opacities, unspecified eye

N Newborn: 0   P Pediatric: 0-17   M Maternity: 12-55   A Adult: 15-124   MCC Major CC Condition   PDxMCC PDx acts as own MCC   CC CC Condition   PDxCC PDx acts as own CC

602   ICD-10-CM 2018

✓5ᵗʰ **H43.8** **Other** disorders of vitreous body

     EXCLUDES 1   proliferative vitreo-retinopathy with retinal detachment (H33.4-)

     EXCLUDES 2   vitreous abscess (H44.02-)

   ✓6ᵗʰ **H43.81** **Vitreous** degeneration
         Vitreous detachment

       H43.811 **Vitreous degeneration, right eye**
       H43.812 **Vitreous degeneration, left eye**
       H43.813 **Vitreous degeneration, bilateral**
       H43.819 **Vitreous degeneration, unspecified eye**

   ✓6ᵗʰ **H43.82** **Vitreomacular** adhesion
         Vitreomacular traction

       H43.821 **Vitreomacular adhesion, right eye**   A
       H43.822 **Vitreomacular adhesion, left eye**   A
       H43.823 **Vitreomacular adhesion, bilateral**   A
       H43.829 **Vitreomacular adhesion, unspecified eye**   A

       H43.89 **Other** disorders of vitreous body

     H43.9 **Unspecified** disorder of vitreous body

✓4ᵗʰ **H44** **Disorders of globe**

     INCLUDES   disorders affecting multiple structures of eye

✓5ᵗʰ **H44.0** **Purulent endophthalmitis**

       Use additional code to identify organism

     EXCLUDES 1   bleb associated endophthalmitis (H59.4-)

   ✓6ᵗʰ **H44.00** **Unspecified purulent endophthalmitis**

       CC Excl: For CC codes in subcategory H44.00: PDX collection 625

       H44.001 **Unspecified purulent endophthalmitis, right eye**   CC
       H44.002 **Unspecified purulent endophthalmitis, left eye**   CC
       H44.003 **Unspecified purulent endophthalmitis, bilateral**   CC
       H44.009 **Unspecified purulent endophthalmitis, unspecified eye**   CC

   ✓6ᵗʰ **H44.01** **Panophthalmitis (acute)**

       CC Excl: For CC codes in subcategory H44.01: PDX collection 625

       H44.011 **Panophthalmitis (acute), right eye**   CC
       H44.012 **Panophthalmitis (acute), left eye**   CC
       H44.013 **Panophthalmitis (acute), bilateral**   CC
       H44.019 **Panophthalmitis (acute), unspecified eye**   CC

   ✓6ᵗʰ **H44.02** **Vitreous abscess (chronic)**

       CC Excl: For CC codes in subcategory H44.02: PDX collection 631

       H44.021 **Vitreous abscess (chronic), right eye**   CC
       H44.022 **Vitreous abscess (chronic), left eye**   CC
       H44.023 **Vitreous abscess (chronic), bilateral**   CC
       H44.029 **Vitreous abscess (chronic), unspecified eye**   CC

✓5ᵗʰ **H44.1** **Other endophthalmitis**

     EXCLUDES 1   bleb associated endophthalmitis (H59.4-)

     EXCLUDES 2   ophthalmia nodosa (H16.2-)

   ✓6ᵗʰ **H44.11** **Panuveitis**
         DEF: Inflammation of all layers of uvea of eye, including choroid, iris, and ciliary body; also typically involves lens, retina, optic nerve, and vitreous; causes reduced vision or blindness.

       CC Excl: For CC codes in subcategory H44.11: PDX collection 632

       H44.111 **Panuveitis, right eye**   CC
       H44.112 **Panuveitis, left eye**   CC
       H44.113 **Panuveitis, bilateral**   CC
       H44.119 **Panuveitis, unspecified eye**   CC

   ✓6ᵗʰ **H44.12** **Parasitic endophthalmitis, unspecified**

       CC Excl: For CC codes in subcategory H44.12: PDX collection 625

       H44.121 **Parasitic endophthalmitis, unspecified, right eye**   CC
       H44.122 **Parasitic endophthalmitis, unspecified, left eye**   CC

       H44.123 **Parasitic endophthalmitis, unspecified, bilateral**   CC
       H44.129 **Parasitic endophthalmitis, unspecified, unspecified eye**   CC

   ✓6ᵗʰ **H44.13** **Sympathetic uveitis**

       CC Excl: For CC codes in subcategory H44.13: PDX collection 632

       H44.131 **Sympathetic uveitis, right eye**   CC
       H44.132 **Sympathetic uveitis, left eye**   CC
       H44.133 **Sympathetic uveitis, bilateral**   CC
       H44.139 **Sympathetic uveitis, unspecified eye**   CC

     H44.19 **Other endophthalmitis**   CC
       CC Excl: PDX collection 625

✓5ᵗʰ **H44.2** **Degenerative myopia**
       Malignant myopia

     H44.20 **Degenerative myopia, unspecified eye**
     H44.21 **Degenerative myopia, right eye**
     H44.22 **Degenerative myopia, left eye**
     H44.23 **Degenerative myopia, bilateral**

   ✓6ᵗʰ **H44.2A** **Degenerative myopia** with choroidal neovascularization
         Use additional code for any associated choroid disorders (H31.-)

       H44.2A1 **Degenerative myopia with choroidal neovascularization, right eye**
       H44.2A2 **Degenerative myopia with choroidal neovascularization, left eye**
       H44.2A3 **Degenerative myopia with choroidal neovascularization, bilateral eye**
       H44.2A9 **Degenerative myopia with choroidal neovascularization, unspecified eye**

   ✓6ᵗʰ **H44.2B** **Degenerative myopia** with macular hole
       H44.2B1 **Degenerative myopia with macular hole, right eye**
       H44.2B2 **Degenerative myopia with macular hole, left eye**
       H44.2B3 **Degenerative myopia with macular hole, bilateral eye**
       H44.2B9 **Degenerative myopia with macular hole, unspecified eye**

   ✓6ᵗʰ **H44.2C** **Degenerative myopia** with retinal detachment
         Use additional code to identify the retinal detachment (H33.-)
       H44.2C1 **Degenerative myopia with retinal detachment, right eye**
       H44.2C2 **Degenerative myopia with retinal detachment, left eye**
       H44.2C3 **Degenerative myopia with retinal detachment, bilateral eye**
       H44.2C9 **Degenerative myopia with retinal detachment, unspecified eye**

   ✓6ᵗʰ **H44.2D** **Degenerative myopia** with foveoschisis
       H44.2D1 **Degenerative myopia with foveoschisis, right eye**
       H44.2D2 **Degenerative myopia with foveoschisis, left eye**
       H44.2D3 **Degenerative myopia with foveoschisis, bilateral eye**
       H44.2D9 **Degenerative myopia with foveoschisis, unspecified eye**

   ✓6ᵗʰ **H44.2E** **Degenerative myopia** with other maculopathy
       H44.2E1 **Degenerative myopia with other maculopathy, right eye**
       H44.2E2 **Degenerative myopia with other maculopathy, left eye**
       H44.2E3 **Degenerative myopia with other maculopathy, bilateral eye**
       H44.2E9 **Degenerative myopia with other maculopathy, unspecified eye**

✓ Additional Character Req   ✓ˣ⁷ᵗʰ Placeholder Alert   Unacceptable PDx   ● Manifestation   H1 - H14 HAC   HCC CMS-HCC Condition   EXCLUDES 1 Not Coded Here   EXCLUDES 2 Not Included Here

ICD-10-CM 2018   **603**

✓5ᵗʰ H44.3 Other and unspecified degenerative disorders of globe

H44.30   Unspecified degenerative disorder of globe

✓6ᵗʰ H44.31 Chalcosis

H44.311   Chalcosis, right eye

H44.312   Chalcosis, left eye

H44.313   Chalcosis, bilateral

H44.319   Chalcosis, unspecified eye

✓6ᵗʰ H44.32 Siderosis of eye

DEF: Iron pigment deposits within tissue of eyeball; caused by high iron content of blood; characterized by cataract, rust-colored anterior subcapsular deposits, iris heterochromia, pupillary mydriasis, and depressed electroretinogram amplitudes.

H44.321   Siderosis of eye, right eye

H44.322   Siderosis of eye, left eye

H44.323   Siderosis of eye, bilateral

H44.329   Siderosis of eye, unspecified eye

✓6ᵗʰ H44.39 Other degenerative disorders of globe

H44.391   Other degenerative disorders of globe, right eye

H44.392   Other degenerative disorders of globe, left eye

H44.393   Other degenerative disorders of globe, bilateral

H44.399   Other degenerative disorders of globe, unspecified eye

✓5ᵗʰ H44.4 Hypotony of eye

H44.40   Unspecified hypotony of eye

✓6ᵗʰ H44.41 Flat anterior chamber hypotony of eye

H44.411   Flat anterior chamber hypotony of right eye

H44.412   Flat anterior chamber hypotony of left eye

H44.413   Flat anterior chamber hypotony of eye, bilateral

H44.419   Flat anterior chamber hypotony of unspecified eye

✓6ᵗʰ H44.42 Hypotony of eye due to ocular fistula

H44.421   Hypotony of right eye due to ocular fistula

H44.422   Hypotony of left eye due to ocular fistula

H44.423   Hypotony of eye due to ocular fistula, bilateral

H44.429   Hypotony of unspecified eye due to ocular fistula

✓6ᵗʰ H44.43 Hypotony of eye due to other ocular disorders

H44.431   Hypotony of eye due to other ocular disorders, right eye

H44.432   Hypotony of eye due to other ocular disorders, left eye

H44.433   Hypotony of eye due to other ocular disorders, bilateral

H44.439   Hypotony of eye due to other ocular disorders, unspecified eye

✓6ᵗʰ H44.44 Primary hypotony of eye

H44.441   Primary hypotony of right eye

H44.442   Primary hypotony of left eye

H44.443   Primary hypotony of eye, bilateral

H44.449   Primary hypotony of unspecified eye

✓5ᵗʰ H44.5 Degenerated conditions of globe

H44.50   Unspecified degenerated conditions of globe

✓6ᵗʰ H44.51 Absolute glaucoma

H44.511   Absolute glaucoma, right eye

H44.512   Absolute glaucoma, left eye

H44.513   Absolute glaucoma, bilateral

H44.519   Absolute glaucoma, unspecified eye

✓6ᵗʰ H44.52 Atrophy of globe

Phthisis bulbi

H44.521   Atrophy of globe, right eye

H44.522   Atrophy of globe, left eye

H44.523   Atrophy of globe, bilateral

H44.529   Atrophy of globe, unspecified eye

✓6ᵗʰ H44.53 Leucocoria

H44.531   Leucocoria, right eye

H44.532   Leucocoria, left eye

H44.533   Leucocoria, bilateral

H44.539   Leucocoria, unspecified eye

✓5ᵗʰ H44.6 Retained (old) intraocular foreign body, magnetic

Use additional code to identify magnetic foreign body (Z18.11)

EXCLUDES 1   current intraocular foreign body (S05.-)

EXCLUDES 2   retained foreign body in eyelid (H02.81-)

retained (old) foreign body following penetrating wound of orbit (H05.5-)

retained (old) intraocular foreign body, nonmagnetic (H44.7-)

✓6ᵗʰ H44.60 Unspecified retained (old) intraocular foreign body, magnetic

H44.601   Unspecified retained (old) intraocular foreign body, magnetic, right eye

H44.602   Unspecified retained (old) intraocular foreign body, magnetic, left eye

H44.603   Unspecified retained (old) intraocular foreign body, magnetic, bilateral

H44.609   Unspecified retained (old) intraocular foreign body, magnetic, unspecified eye

✓6ᵗʰ H44.61 Retained (old) magnetic foreign body in anterior chamber

H44.611   Retained (old) magnetic foreign body in anterior chamber, right eye

H44.612   Retained (old) magnetic foreign body in anterior chamber, left eye

H44.613   Retained (old) magnetic foreign body in anterior chamber, bilateral

H44.619   Retained (old) magnetic foreign body in anterior chamber, unspecified eye

✓6ᵗʰ H44.62 Retained (old) magnetic foreign body in iris or ciliary body

H44.621   Retained (old) magnetic foreign body in iris or ciliary body, right eye

H44.622   Retained (old) magnetic foreign body in iris or ciliary body, left eye

H44.623   Retained (old) magnetic foreign body in iris or ciliary body, bilateral

H44.629   Retained (old) magnetic foreign body in iris or ciliary body, unspecified eye

✓6ᵗʰ H44.63 Retained (old) magnetic foreign body in lens

H44.631   Retained (old) magnetic foreign body in lens, right eye

H44.632   Retained (old) magnetic foreign body in lens, left eye

H44.633   Retained (old) magnetic foreign body in lens, bilateral

H44.639   Retained (old) magnetic foreign body in lens, unspecified eye

✓6ᵗʰ H44.64 Retained (old) magnetic foreign body in posterior wall of globe

H44.641   Retained (old) magnetic foreign body in posterior wall of globe, right eye

H44.642   Retained (old) magnetic foreign body in posterior wall of globe, left eye

H44.643   Retained (old) magnetic foreign body in posterior wall of globe, bilateral

H44.649   Retained (old) magnetic foreign body in posterior wall of globe, unspecified eye

✓6ᵗʰ H44.65 Retained (old) magnetic foreign body in vitreous body

H44.651   Retained (old) magnetic foreign body in vitreous body, right eye

H44.652   Retained (old) magnetic foreign body in vitreous body, left eye

H44.653   Retained (old) magnetic foreign body in vitreous body, bilateral

H44.659   Retained (old) magnetic foreign body in vitreous body, unspecified eye

✓6ᵗʰ H44.69 Retained (old) intraocular foreign body, magnetic, in other or multiple sites

H44.691   Retained (old) intraocular foreign body, magnetic, in other or multiple sites, right eye

H44.692   Retained (old) intraocular foreign body, magnetic, in other or multiple sites, left eye

H44.693   Retained (old) intraocular foreign body, magnetic, in other or multiple sites, bilateral

---

N Newborn: 0   P Pediatric: 0-17   M Maternity: 12-55   A Adult: 15-124   MCC Major CC Condition   PDxMCC PDx acts as own MCC   CC CC Condition   PDxCC PDx acts as own CC

H44.699 Retained (old) intraocular foreign body, magnetic, in other or multiple sites, unspecified eye

✓5th **H44.7 Retained (old) intraocular foreign body, nonmagnetic**
Use additional code to identify nonmagnetic foreign body (Z18.01-Z18.10, Z18.12, Z18.2-Z18.9)
EXCLUDES 1 current intraocular foreign body (S05.-)
EXCLUDES 2 retained foreign body in eyelid (H02.81-)
retained (old) foreign body following penetrating wound of orbit (H05.5-)
retained (old) intraocular foreign body, magnetic (H44.6-)

✓6th **H44.70 Unspecified retained (old) intraocular foreign body, nonmagnetic**
H44.701 Unspecified retained (old) intraocular foreign body, nonmagnetic, right eye
H44.702 Unspecified retained (old) intraocular foreign body, nonmagnetic, left eye
H44.703 Unspecified retained (old) intraocular foreign body, nonmagnetic, bilateral
H44.709 Unspecified retained (old) intraocular foreign body, nonmagnetic, unspecified eye
Retained (old) intraocular foreign body NOS

✓6th **H44.71 Retained (nonmagnetic) (old) foreign body in anterior chamber**
H44.711 Retained (nonmagnetic) (old) foreign body in anterior chamber, right eye
H44.712 Retained (nonmagnetic) (old) foreign body in anterior chamber, left eye
H44.713 Retained (nonmagnetic) (old) foreign body in anterior chamber, bilateral
H44.719 Retained (nonmagnetic) (old) foreign body in anterior chamber, unspecified eye

✓6th **H44.72 Retained (nonmagnetic) (old) foreign body in iris or ciliary body**
H44.721 Retained (nonmagnetic) (old) foreign body in iris or ciliary body, right eye
H44.722 Retained (nonmagnetic) (old) foreign body in iris or ciliary body, left eye
H44.723 Retained (nonmagnetic) (old) foreign body in iris or ciliary body, bilateral
H44.729 Retained (nonmagnetic) (old) foreign body in iris or ciliary body, unspecified eye

✓6th **H44.73 Retained (nonmagnetic) (old) foreign body in lens**
H44.731 Retained (nonmagnetic) (old) foreign body in lens, right eye
H44.732 Retained (nonmagnetic) (old) foreign body in lens, left eye
H44.733 Retained (nonmagnetic) (old) foreign body in lens, bilateral
H44.739 Retained (nonmagnetic) (old) foreign body in lens, unspecified eye

✓6th **H44.74 Retained (nonmagnetic) (old) foreign body in posterior wall of globe**
H44.741 Retained (nonmagnetic) (old) foreign body in posterior wall of globe, right eye
H44.742 Retained (nonmagnetic) (old) foreign body in posterior wall of globe, left eye
H44.743 Retained (nonmagnetic) (old) foreign body in posterior wall of globe, bilateral
H44.749 Retained (nonmagnetic) (old) foreign body in posterior wall of globe, unspecified eye

✓6th **H44.75 Retained (nonmagnetic) (old) foreign body in vitreous body**
H44.751 Retained (nonmagnetic) (old) foreign body in vitreous body, right eye
H44.752 Retained (nonmagnetic) (old) foreign body in vitreous body, left eye
H44.753 Retained (nonmagnetic) (old) foreign body in vitreous body, bilateral
H44.759 Retained (nonmagnetic) (old) foreign body in vitreous body, unspecified eye

✓6th **H44.79 Retained (old) intraocular foreign body, nonmagnetic, in other or multiple sites**
H44.791 Retained (old) intraocular foreign body, nonmagnetic, in other or multiple sites, right eye
H44.792 Retained (old) intraocular foreign body, nonmagnetic, in other or multiple sites, left eye
H44.793 Retained (old) intraocular foreign body, nonmagnetic, in other or multiple sites, bilateral
H44.799 Retained (old) intraocular foreign body, nonmagnetic, in other or multiple sites, unspecified eye

✓5th **H44.8 Other disorders of globe**
✓6th **H44.81 Hemophthalmos**
DEF: Pool of blood within eyeball, not from current injury.
H44.811 Hemophthalmos, right eye
H44.812 Hemophthalmos, left eye
H44.813 Hemophthalmos, bilateral
H44.819 Hemophthalmos, unspecified eye

✓6th **H44.82 Luxation of globe**
H44.821 Luxation of globe, right eye
H44.822 Luxation of globe, left eye
H44.823 Luxation of globe, bilateral
H44.829 Luxation of globe, unspecified eye
H44.89 Other disorders of globe
H44.9 Unspecified disorder of globe

Disorders of optic nerve and visual pathways (H46-H47)

✓4th **H46 Optic neuritis**
EXCLUDES 2 ischemic optic neuropathy (H47.01-)
neuromyelitis optica [Devic] (G36.0)

CC Excl: For CC codes in category H46: PDX collection 633

✓5th **H46.0 Optic papillitis**
H46.00 Optic papillitis, unspecified eye `CC`
H46.01 Optic papillitis, right eye `CC`
H46.02 Optic papillitis, left eye `CC`
H46.03 Optic papillitis, bilateral `CC`

✓5th **H46.1 Retrobulbar neuritis**
Retrobulbar neuritis NOS
EXCLUDES 1 syphilitic retrobulbar neuritis (A52.15)
H46.10 Retrobulbar neuritis, unspecified eye `CC`
H46.11 Retrobulbar neuritis, right eye `CC`
H46.12 Retrobulbar neuritis, left eye `CC`
H46.13 Retrobulbar neuritis, bilateral `CC`

H46.2 Nutritional optic neuropathy
H46.3 Toxic optic neuropathy
Code first (T51-T65) to identify cause
H46.8 Other optic neuritis `CC`
H46.9 Unspecified optic neuritis `CC`

✓4th **H47 Other disorders of optic [2nd] nerve and visual pathways**
✓5th **H47.0 Disorders of optic nerve, not elsewhere classified**
✓6th **H47.01 Ischemic optic neuropathy**
H47.011 Ischemic optic neuropathy, right eye
H47.012 Ischemic optic neuropathy, left eye
H47.013 Ischemic optic neuropathy, bilateral
H47.019 Ischemic optic neuropathy, unspecified eye

✓6th **H47.02 Hemorrhage in optic nerve sheath**
H47.021 Hemorrhage in optic nerve sheath, right eye
H47.022 Hemorrhage in optic nerve sheath, left eye
H47.023 Hemorrhage in optic nerve sheath, bilateral
H47.029 Hemorrhage in optic nerve sheath, unspecified eye

✓6th **H47.03 Optic nerve hypoplasia**
H47.031 Optic nerve hypoplasia, right eye
H47.032 Optic nerve hypoplasia, left eye
H47.033 Optic nerve hypoplasia, bilateral
H47.039 Optic nerve hypoplasia, unspecified eye

✓6th **H47.09 Other** disorders of optic nerve, not elsewhere classified
Compression of optic nerve

H47.091 Other disorders of optic nerve, not elsewhere classified, **right eye**

H47.092 Other disorders of optic nerve, not elsewhere classified, **left eye**

H47.093 Other disorders of optic nerve, not elsewhere classified, **bilateral**

H47.099 Other disorders of optic nerve, not elsewhere classified, **unspecified eye**

✓5th **H47.1 Papilledema**

H47.10 Unspecified papilledema `CC`
CC Excl: PDX collection 634

H47.11 Papilledema associated with increased `CC`
intracranial pressure
CC Excl: PDX collection 634

H47.12 Papilledema associated with decreased ocular pressure

H47.13 Papilledema associated with retinal disorder

✓6th **H47.14 Foster-Kennedy syndrome**

H47.141 Foster-Kennedy syndrome, right eye

H47.142 Foster-Kennedy syndrome, left eye

H47.143 Foster-Kennedy syndrome, bilateral

H47.149 Foster-Kennedy syndrome, unspecified eye

✓5th **H47.2 Optic atrophy**

H47.20 Unspecified optic atrophy

✓6th **H47.21 Primary optic atrophy**

H47.211 Primary optic atrophy, right eye

H47.212 Primary optic atrophy, left eye

H47.213 Primary optic atrophy, bilateral

H47.219 Primary optic atrophy, unspecified eye

H47.22 Hereditary optic atrophy
Leber's optic atrophy

✓6th **H47.23 Glaucomatous optic atrophy**

H47.231 Glaucomatous optic atrophy, right eye

H47.232 Glaucomatous optic atrophy, left eye

H47.233 Glaucomatous optic atrophy, bilateral

H47.239 Glaucomatous optic atrophy, unspecified eye

✓6th **H47.29 Other optic atrophy**
Temporal pallor of optic disc

H47.291 Other optic atrophy, right eye

H47.292 Other optic atrophy, left eye

H47.293 Other optic atrophy, bilateral

H47.299 Other optic atrophy, unspecified eye

✓5th **H47.3 Other disorders of optic disc**

✓6th **H47.31 Coloboma of optic disc**

H47.311 Coloboma of optic disc, right eye

H47.312 Coloboma of optic disc, left eye

H47.313 Coloboma of optic disc, bilateral

H47.319 Coloboma of optic disc, unspecified eye

✓6th **H47.32 Drusen of optic disc**

H47.321 Drusen of optic disc, right eye

H47.322 Drusen of optic disc, left eye

H47.323 Drusen of optic disc, bilateral

H47.329 Drusen of optic disc, unspecified eye

✓6th **H47.33 Pseudopapilledema of optic disc**

H47.331 Pseudopapilledema of optic disc, right eye

H47.332 Pseudopapilledema of optic disc, left eye

H47.333 Pseudopapilledema of optic disc, bilateral

H47.339 Pseudopapilledema of optic disc, unspecified eye

✓6th **H47.39 Other disorders of optic disc**

H47.391 Other disorders of optic disc, right eye

H47.392 Other disorders of optic disc, left eye

H47.393 Other disorders of optic disc, bilateral

H47.399 Other disorders of optic disc, unspecified eye

✓5th **H47.4 Disorders of optic chiasm**
Code also underlying condition

CC Excl: For CC codes in subcategory H47.4:
PDX collection 635

H47.41 Disorders of optic chiasm in (due to) `CC`
inflammatory disorders

H47.42 Disorders of optic chiasm in (due to) neoplasm `CC`

H47.43 Disorders of optic chiasm in (due to) vascular `CC`
disorders

H47.49 Disorders of optic chiasm in (due to) other `CC`
disorders

✓5th **H47.5 Disorders of other visual pathways**
Disorders of optic tracts, geniculate nuclei and optic radiations
Code also underlying condition

CC Excl: For CC codes in subcategory H47.5:
PDX collection 635

✓6th **H47.51 Disorders of visual pathways in (due to)**
inflammatory disorders

H47.511 Disorders of visual pathways in `CC`
(due to) inflammatory disorders, right side

H47.512 Disorders of visual pathways in `CC`
(due to) inflammatory disorders, left side

H47.519 Disorders of visual pathways in `CC`
(due to) inflammatory disorders, unspecified side

✓6th **H47.52 Disorders of visual pathways in (due to) neoplasm**

H47.521 Disorders of visual pathways in `CC`
(due to) neoplasm, right side

H47.522 Disorders of visual pathways in `CC`
(due to) neoplasm, left side

H47.529 Disorders of visual pathways in `CC`
(due to) neoplasm, unspecified side

✓6th **H47.53 Disorders of visual pathways in (due to) vascular**
disorders

H47.531 Disorders of visual pathways in `CC`
(due to) vascular disorders, right side

H47.532 Disorders of visual pathways in `CC`
(due to) vascular disorders, left side

H47.539 Disorders of visual pathways in
(due to) vascular disorders, unspecified side

✓5th **H47.6 Disorders of visual cortex**
Code also underlying condition
EXCLUDES 1 injury to visual cortex S04.04

CC Excl: For CC codes in subcategory H47.6:
PDX collection 636

✓6th **H47.61 Cortical blindness**

H47.611 Cortical blindness, right side of brain

H47.612 Cortical blindness, left side of brain

H47.619 Cortical blindness, unspecified side of brain

✓6th **H47.62 Disorders of visual cortex in (due to) inflammatory**
disorders

H47.621 Disorders of visual cortex in (due to) `CC`
inflammatory disorders, right side of brain

H47.622 Disorders of visual cortex in (due to) `CC`
inflammatory disorders, left side of brain

H47.629 Disorders of visual cortex in (due to) `CC`
inflammatory disorders, unspecified side of brain

✓6th **H47.63 Disorders of visual cortex in (due to) neoplasm**

H47.631 Disorders of visual cortex in (due to) `CC`
neoplasm, right side of brain

H47.632 Disorders of visual cortex in (due to) `CC`
neoplasm, left side of brain

H47.639 Disorders of visual cortex in (due to) `CC`
neoplasm, unspecified side of brain

✓6th **H47.64 Disorders of visual cortex in (due to) vascular**
disorders

H47.641 Disorders of visual cortex in (due to) `CC`
vascular disorders, right side of brain

H47.642   **Disorders of visual cortex in (due to)** CC
vascular disorders, left **side of brain**

H47.649   **Disorders of visual cortex in (due to)** CC
vascular disorders, unspecified **side of**
brain

H47.9   Unspecified **disorder of visual pathways**

Disorders of ocular muscles, binocular movement, accommodation and refraction (H49-H52)

EXCLUDES 2   *nystagmus and other irregular eye movements (H55)*

✓4th **H49   Paralytic strabismus**

EXCLUDES 2   *internal ophthalmoplegia (H52.51-)*
internuclear ophthalmoplegia (H51.2-)
progressive supranuclear ophthalmoplegia (G23.1)

✓5th **H49.0   Third [oculomotor] nerve palsy**

H49.00   Third [oculomotor] nerve palsy, unspecified **eye**

H49.01   Third [oculomotor] nerve palsy, right **eye**

H49.02   Third [oculomotor] nerve palsy, left **eye**

H49.03   Third [oculomotor] nerve palsy, bilateral

✓5th **H49.1   Fourth [trochlear] nerve palsy**

H49.10   Fourth [trochlear] nerve palsy, unspecified **eye**

H49.11   Fourth [trochlear] nerve palsy, right **eye**

H49.12   Fourth [trochlear] nerve palsy, left **eye**

H49.13   Fourth [trochlear] nerve palsy, bilateral

✓5th **H49.2   Sixth [abducent] nerve palsy**

H49.20   Sixth [abducent] nerve palsy, unspecified **eye**

H49.21   Sixth [abducent] nerve palsy, right **eye**

H49.22   Sixth [abducent] nerve palsy, left **eye**

H49.23   Sixth [abducent] nerve palsy, bilateral

✓5th **H49.3   Total (external) ophthalmoplegia**

H49.30   Total (external) ophthalmoplegia, unspecified **eye**

H49.31   Total (external) ophthalmoplegia, right **eye**

H49.32   Total (external) ophthalmoplegia, left **eye**

H49.33   Total (external) ophthalmoplegia, bilateral

✓5th **H49.4   Progressive external ophthalmoplegia**

EXCLUDES 1   *Kearns-Sayre syndrome (H49.81-)*

H49.40   **Progressive external ophthalmoplegia, unspecified
eye**

H49.41   **Progressive external ophthalmoplegia, right eye**

H49.42   **Progressive external ophthalmoplegia, left eye**

H49.43   **Progressive external ophthalmoplegia, bilateral**

✓5th **H49.8   Other paralytic strabismus**

> **CC Excl: For CC codes in subcategory H49.8:**
> PDX collection 545

✓6th **H49.81   Kearns-Sayre syndrome**
Progressive external ophthalmoplegia with
pigmentary retinopathy
Use additional code for other manifestation, such as:
heart block (I45.9)

H49.811   Kearns-Sayre syndrome, right eye   CC HCC

H49.812   Kearns-Sayre syndrome, left eye   CC HCC

H49.813   Kearns-Sayre syndrome, bilateral   CC HCC

H49.819   Kearns-Sayre syndrome,   CC HCC
unspecified **eye**

✓6th **H49.88   Other paralytic strabismus**
External ophthalmoplegia NOS

H49.881   Other paralytic strabismus, right **eye**

H49.882   Other paralytic strabismus, left **eye**

H49.883   Other paralytic strabismus, bilateral

H49.889   Other paralytic strabismus, unspecified
eye

H49.9   Unspecified paralytic strabismus

✓4th **H50   Other strabismus**

✓5th **H50.0   Esotropia**
Convergent concomitant strabismus

EXCLUDES 1   *intermittent esotropia (H50.31-, H50.32)*

H50.00   Unspecified **esotropia**

✓6th **H50.01   Monocular esotropia**

H50.011   Monocular esotropia, right **eye**

H50.012   Monocular esotropia, left **eye**

Eye Muscle Diseases

R.   L.
Monocular (one eye only) esotropia (inward)

Monocular exotropia (outward)

Monocular hypertropia (upward)

✓6th **H50.02   Monocular esotropia with A pattern**

H50.021   **Monocular esotropia with A pattern,
right eye**

H50.022   **Monocular esotropia with A pattern,
left eye**

✓6th **H50.03   Monocular esotropia with V pattern**

H50.031   **Monocular esotropia with V pattern,
right eye**

H50.032   **Monocular esotropia with V pattern,
left eye**

✓6th **H50.04   Monocular esotropia with other noncomitancies**

H50.041   **Monocular esotropia with other
noncomitancies, right eye**

H50.042   **Monocular esotropia with other
noncomitancies, left eye**

H50.05   Alternating esotropia

H50.06   Alternating esotropia with A pattern

H50.07   Alternating esotropia with V pattern

H50.08   Alternating esotropia with other noncomitancies

✓5th **H50.1   Exotropia**
Divergent concomitant strabismus

EXCLUDES 1   *intermittent exotropia (H50.33-, H50.34)*

H50.10   Unspecified **exotropia**

✓6th **H50.11   Monocular exotropia**

H50.111   Monocular exotropia, right **eye**

H50.112   Monocular exotropia, left **eye**

✓6th **H50.12   Monocular exotropia with A pattern**

H50.121   **Monocular exotropia with A pattern,
right eye**

H50.122   **Monocular exotropia with A pattern,
left eye**

✓6th **H50.13   Monocular exotropia with V pattern**

H50.131   **Monocular exotropia with V pattern,
right eye**

H50.132   **Monocular exotropia with V pattern,
left eye**

✓6th **H50.14   Monocular exotropia with other noncomitancies**

H50.141   **Monocular exotropia with other
noncomitancies, right eye**

H50.142   **Monocular exotropia with other
noncomitancies, left eye**

H50.15   Alternating exotropia

H50.16   Alternating exotropia with A pattern

H50.17   Alternating exotropia with V pattern

H50.18   Alternating exotropia with other noncomitancies

✓5th **H50.2   Vertical strabismus**
Hypertropia

H50.21   Vertical strabismus, right **eye**

H50.22   Vertical strabismus, left **eye**

✓5th **H50.3   Intermittent heterotropia**

H50.30   Unspecified **intermittent heterotropia**

✓ Additional Character Req   ✓x7th Placeholder Alert   Unacceptable PDx   Manifestation   H1 - H14 HAC   HCC CMS-HCC Condition   EXCLUDES 1 Not Coded Here   EXCLUDES 2 Not Included Here

ICD-10-CM 2018   **607**

✓6th **H50.31** Intermittent monocular esotropia
    H50.311 Intermittent monocular esotropia, right eye
    H50.312 Intermittent monocular esotropia, left eye
    H50.32 Intermittent alternating esotropia
✓6th **H50.33** Intermittent monocular exotropia
    H50.331 Intermittent monocular exotropia, right eye
    H50.332 Intermittent monocular exotropia, left eye
    H50.34 Intermittent alternating exotropia
✓5th **H50.4** Other and unspecified heterotropia
    H50.40 Unspecified heterotropia
✓6th **H50.41** Cyclotropia
    H50.411 Cyclotropia, right eye
    H50.412 Cyclotropia, left eye
    H50.42 Monofixation syndrome
    H50.43 Accommodative component in esotropia
✓5th **H50.5** Heterophoria
    H50.50 Unspecified heterophoria
    H50.51 Esophoria
    H50.52 Exophoria
    H50.53 Vertical heterophoria
    H50.54 Cyclophoria
    H50.55 Alternating heterophoria
✓5th **H50.6** Mechanical strabismus
    H50.60 Mechanical strabismus, unspecified
✓6th **H50.61** Brown's sheath syndrome
    H50.611 Brown's sheath syndrome, right eye
    H50.612 Brown's sheath syndrome, left eye
    H50.69 Other mechanical strabismus
        Strabismus due to adhesions
        Traumatic limitation of duction of eye muscle
✓5th **H50.8** Other specified strabismus
✓6th **H50.81** Duane's syndrome
    H50.811 Duane's syndrome, right eye
    H50.812 Duane's syndrome, left eye
    H50.89 Other specified strabismus
    H50.9 Unspecified strabismus
✓4th **H51** Other disorders of binocular movement
    H51.0 Palsy (spasm) of conjugate gaze
✓5th **H51.1** Convergence insufficiency and excess
    H51.11 Convergence insufficiency
    H51.12 Convergence excess
✓5th **H51.2** Internuclear ophthalmoplegia
    H51.20 Internuclear ophthalmoplegia, unspecified eye
    H51.21 Internuclear ophthalmoplegia, right eye
    H51.22 Internuclear ophthalmoplegia, left eye
    H51.23 Internuclear ophthalmoplegia, bilateral
    H51.8 Other specified disorders of binocular movement
    H51.9 Unspecified disorder of binocular movement
✓4th **H52** Disorders of refraction and accommodation
✓5th **H52.0** Hypermetropia
    H52.00 Hypermetropia, unspecified eye
    H52.01 Hypermetropia, right eye
    H52.02 Hypermetropia, left eye
    H52.03 Hypermetropia, bilateral
✓5th **H52.1** Myopia
        EXCLUDES 1 *degenerative myopia (H44.2-)*
    H52.10 Myopia, unspecified eye
    H52.11 Myopia, right eye
    H52.12 Myopia, left eye
    H52.13 Myopia, bilateral
✓5th **H52.2** Astigmatism
✓6th **H52.20** Unspecified astigmatism
    H52.201 Unspecified astigmatism, right eye
    H52.202 Unspecified astigmatism, left eye
    H52.203 Unspecified astigmatism, bilateral
    H52.209 Unspecified astigmatism, unspecified eye

✓6th **H52.21** Irregular astigmatism
    H52.211 Irregular astigmatism, right eye
    H52.212 Irregular astigmatism, left eye
    H52.213 Irregular astigmatism, bilateral
    H52.219 Irregular astigmatism, unspecified eye
✓6th **H52.22** Regular astigmatism
    H52.221 Regular astigmatism, right eye
    H52.222 Regular astigmatism, left eye
    H52.223 Regular astigmatism, bilateral
    H52.229 Regular astigmatism, unspecified eye
✓5th **H52.3** Anisometropia and aniseikonia
    H52.31 Anisometropia
    H52.32 Aniseikonia
    H52.4 Presbyopia
✓5th **H52.5** Disorders of accommodation
✓6th **H52.51** Internal ophthalmoplegia (complete) (total)
    H52.511 Internal ophthalmoplegia (complete) (total), right eye
    H52.512 Internal ophthalmoplegia (complete) (total), left eye
    H52.513 Internal ophthalmoplegia (complete) (total), bilateral
    H52.519 Internal ophthalmoplegia (complete) (total), unspecified eye
✓6th **H52.52** Paresis of accommodation
    H52.521 Paresis of accommodation, right eye
    H52.522 Paresis of accommodation, left eye
    H52.523 Paresis of accommodation, bilateral
    H52.529 Paresis of accommodation, unspecified eye
✓6th **H52.53** Spasm of accommodation
    H52.531 Spasm of accommodation, right eye
    H52.532 Spasm of accommodation, left eye
    H52.533 Spasm of accommodation, bilateral
    H52.539 Spasm of accommodation, unspecified eye
    H52.6 Other disorders of refraction
    H52.7 Unspecified disorder of refraction

Visual disturbances and blindness (H53-H54)

✓4th **H53** Visual disturbances
✓5th **H53.0** Amblyopia ex anopsia
        EXCLUDES 1 *amblyopia due to vitamin A deficiency (E50.5)*
✓6th **H53.00** Unspecified amblyopia
    H53.001 Unspecified amblyopia, right eye
    H53.002 Unspecified amblyopia, left eye
    H53.003 Unspecified amblyopia, bilateral
    H53.009 Unspecified amblyopia, unspecified eye
✓6th **H53.01** Deprivation amblyopia
    H53.011 Deprivation amblyopia, right eye
    H53.012 Deprivation amblyopia, left eye
    H53.013 Deprivation amblyopia, bilateral
    H53.019 Deprivation amblyopia, unspecified eye
✓6th **H53.02** Refractive amblyopia
    H53.021 Refractive amblyopia, right eye
    H53.022 Refractive amblyopia, left eye
    H53.023 Refractive amblyopia, bilateral
    H53.029 Refractive amblyopia, unspecified eye
✓6th **H53.03** Strabismic amblyopia
        EXCLUDES 1 *strabismus (H50.-)*
    H53.031 Strabismic amblyopia, right eye
    H53.032 Strabismic amblyopia, left eye
    H53.033 Strabismic amblyopia, bilateral
    H53.039 Strabismic amblyopia, unspecified eye
✓6th **H53.04** Amblyopia suspect
    H53.041 Amblyopia suspect, right eye
    H53.042 Amblyopia suspect, left eye
    H53.043 Amblyopia suspect, bilateral
    H53.049 Amblyopia suspect, unspecified eye

N Newborn: 0   P Pediatric: 0-17   M Maternity: 12-55   A Adult: 15-124   MCC Major CC Condition   PDxMCC PDx acts as own MCC   CC CC Condition   PDxCC PDx acts as own CC

608   ICD-10-CM 2018

✓5ᵗʰ H53.1 Subjective visual disturbances

> **EXCLUDES 1** *subjective visual disturbances due to vitamin A deficiency (E50.5)*
> *visual hallucinations (R44.1)*

> **CC Excl: For CC codes in subcategory H53.1:**
> PDX collection 637

     H53.10 Unspecified subjective visual disturbances

     H53.11 Day blindness
         Hemeralopia

     ✓6ᵗʰ H53.12 Transient visual loss
         Scintillating scotoma

> **EXCLUDES 1** *amaurosis fugax (G45.3-)*
> *transient retinal artery occlusion (H34.0-)*

         H53.121 Transient visual loss, right eye `CC`
         H53.122 Transient visual loss, left eye `CC`
         H53.123 Transient visual loss, bilateral `CC`
         H53.129 Transient visual loss, unspecified eye `CC`

     ✓6ᵗʰ H53.13 Sudden visual loss
         H53.131 Sudden visual loss, right eye `CC`
         H53.132 Sudden visual loss, left eye `CC`
         H53.133 Sudden visual loss, bilateral `CC`
         H53.139 Sudden visual loss, unspecified eye `CC`

     ✓6ᵗʰ H53.14 Visual discomfort
         Asthenopia
         Photophobia
         H53.141 Visual discomfort, right eye
         H53.142 Visual discomfort, left eye
         H53.143 Visual discomfort, bilateral
         H53.149 Visual discomfort, unspecified

     H53.15 Visual distortions of shape and size
         Metamorphopsia

     H53.16 Psychophysical visual disturbances

     H53.19 Other subjective visual disturbances
         Visual halos

H53.2 Diplopia
     Double vision

✓5ᵗʰ H53.3 Other and unspecified disorders of binocular vision
     H53.30 Unspecified disorder of binocular vision
     H53.31 Abnormal retinal correspondence
     H53.32 Fusion with defective stereopsis
     H53.33 Simultaneous visual perception without fusion
     H53.34 Suppression of binocular vision

✓5ᵗʰ H53.4 Visual field defects
     H53.40 Unspecified visual field defects
     ✓6ᵗʰ H53.41 Scotoma involving central area
         Central scotoma
         H53.411 Scotoma involving central area, right eye
         H53.412 Scotoma involving central area, left eye
         H53.413 Scotoma involving central area, bilateral
         H53.419 Scotoma involving central area, unspecified eye

     ✓6ᵗʰ H53.42 Scotoma of blind spot area
         Enlarged blind spot
         H53.421 Scotoma of blind spot area, right eye
         H53.422 Scotoma of blind spot area, left eye
         H53.423 Scotoma of blind spot area, bilateral
         H53.429 Scotoma of blind spot area, unspecified eye

     ✓6ᵗʰ H53.43 Sector or arcuate defects
         Arcuate scotoma
         Bjerrum scotoma
         H53.431 Sector or arcuate defects, right eye
         H53.432 Sector or arcuate defects, left eye
         H53.433 Sector or arcuate defects, bilateral
         H53.439 Sector or arcuate defects, unspecified eye

     ✓6ᵗʰ H53.45 Other localized visual field defect
         Peripheral visual field defect
         Ring scotoma NOS
         Scotoma NOS
         H53.451 Other localized visual field defect, right eye
         H53.452 Other localized visual field defect, left eye
         H53.453 Other localized visual field defect, bilateral

         H53.459 Other localized visual field defect, unspecified eye

     ✓6ᵗʰ H53.46 Homonymous bilateral field defects
         Homonymous hemianopia
         Homonymous hemianopsia
         Quadrant anopia
         Quadrant anopsia
         H53.461 Homonymous bilateral field defects, right side
         H53.462 Homonymous bilateral field defects, left side
         H53.469 Homonymous bilateral field defects, unspecified side
           Homonymous bilateral field defects NOS

     H53.47 Heteronymous bilateral field defects
         Heteronymous hemianop(s)ia

     ✓6ᵗʰ H53.48 Generalized contraction of visual field
         H53.481 Generalized contraction of visual field, right eye
         H53.482 Generalized contraction of visual field, left eye
         H53.483 Generalized contraction of visual field, bilateral
         H53.489 Generalized contraction of visual field, unspecified eye

✓5ᵗʰ H53.5 Color vision deficiencies
     Color blindness

> **EXCLUDES 2** *day blindness (H53.11)*

     H53.50 Unspecified color vision deficiencies
         Color blindness NOS

     H53.51 Achromatopsia
         DEF: Nonprogressive genetic visual disorder; characterized by complete color blindness, decreased vision, and light sensitivity.

     H53.52 Acquired color vision deficiency

     H53.53 Deuteranomaly
         Deuteranopia
         DEF: Male-only genetic disorder; difficulty in distinguishing green and red, no shortened spectrum.

     H53.54 Protanomaly
         Protanopia

     H53.55 Tritanomaly
         Tritanopia

     H53.59 Other color vision deficiencies

✓5ᵗʰ H53.6 Night blindness

> **EXCLUDES 1** *night blindness due to vitamin A deficiency (E50.5)*

     H53.60 Unspecified night blindness
     H53.61 Abnormal dark adaptation curve
     H53.62 Acquired night blindness
     H53.63 Congenital night blindness
     H53.69 Other night blindness

✓5ᵗʰ H53.7 Vision sensitivity deficiencies
     H53.71 Glare sensitivity
     H53.72 Impaired contrast sensitivity

H53.8 Other visual disturbances

H53.9 Unspecified visual disturbance

✓4ᵗʰ H54 Blindness and low vision

> **NOTE** For definition of visual impairment categories see table below

> Code first any associated underlying cause of the blindness

> **EXCLUDES 1** *amaurosis fugax (G45.3)*

✓5ᵗʰ H54.0 Blindness, both eyes
     Visual impairment categories 3, 4, 5 in both eyes.

     ● **✓6ᵗʰ H54.0X Blindness, both eyes, different category levels**
     ●   **✓7ᵗʰ H54.0X3 Blindness right eye, category 3**
     ●   **H54.0X33 Blindness right eye category 3, blindness left eye category 3**
     ●   **H54.0X34 Blindness right eye category 3, blindness left eye category 4**
     ●   **H54.0X35 Blindness right eye category 3, blindness left eye category 5**
     ●   **✓7ᵗʰ H54.0X4 Blindness right eye, category 4**
     ●   **H54.0X43 Blindness right eye category 4, blindness left eye category 3**
     ●   **H54.0X44 Blindness right eye category 4, blindness left eye category 4**

✓ Additional Character Req   ✓7ᵗʰ Placeholder Alert   Unacceptable PDx   ■ Manifestation   **H1 -H14** HAC   **HCC** CMS-HCC Condition   **EXCLUDES 1** Not Coded Here   **EXCLUDES 2** Not Included Here

ICD-10-CM 2018   **609**

-      **H54.ØX45**   **Blindness right eye category 4, blindness left eye category 5**
- ✓7ᵗʰ **H54.ØX5**   **Blindness right eye, category 5**
-      **H54.ØX53**   **Blindness right eye category 5, blindness left eye category 3**
-      **H54.ØX54**   **Blindness right eye category 5, blindness left eye category 4**
-      **H54.ØX55**   **Blindness right eye category 5, blindness left eye category 5**

✓5ᵗʰ **H54.1**   **Blindness,** one eye, low vision other eye
     Visual impairment categories 3, 4, 5 in one eye, with categories 1 or 2 in the other eye.

     H54.1Ø   **Blindness, one eye, low vision other eye,** unspecified **eyes**

✓6ᵗʰ **H54.11**   Blindness, right eye, low vision left eye

- ✓7ᵗʰ **H54.113**   **Blindness right eye category 3, low vision left eye**
-      **H54.1131**   **Blindness right eye category 3, low vision left eye category 1**
-      **H54.1132**   **Blindness right eye category 3, low vision left eye category 2**
- ✓7ᵗʰ **H54.114**   **Blindness right eye category 4, low vision left eye**
-      **H54.1141**   **Blindness right eye category 4, low vision left eye category 1**
-      **H54.1142**   **Blindness right eye category 4, low vision left eye category 2**
- ✓7ᵗʰ **H54.115**   **Blindness right eye category 5, low vision left eye**
-      **H54.1151**   **Blindness right eye category 5, low vision left eye category 1**
-      **H54.1152**   **Blindness right eye category 5, low vision left eye category 2**

✓6ᵗʰ **H54.12**   Blindness, left eye, low vision right eye

- ✓7ᵗʰ **H54.121**   **Low vision right eye category 1, blindness left eye**
-      **H54.1213**   **Low vision right eye category 1, blindness left eye category 3**
-      **H54.1214**   **Low vision right eye category 1, blindness left eye category 4**
-      **H54.1215**   **Low vision right eye category 1, blindness left eye category 5**
- ✓7ᵗʰ **H54.122**   **Low vision right eye category 2, blindness left eye**
-      **H54.1223**   **Low vision right eye category 2, blindness left eye category 3**
-      **H54.1224**   **Low vision right eye category 2, blindness left eye category 4**
-      **H54.1225**   **Low vision right eye category 2, blindness left eye category 5**

✓5ᵗʰ **H54.2**   **Low vision, both eyes**
     Visual impairment categories 1 or 2 in both eyes.

- ✓6ᵗʰ **H54.2X**   Low vision, both eyes, different category levels
- ✓7ᵗʰ **H54.2X1**   **Low vision, right eye, category 1**
-      **H54.2X11**   **Low vision right eye category 1, low vision left eye category 1**
-      **H54.2X12**   **Low vision right eye category 1, low vision left eye category 2**

- ✓7ᵗʰ **H54.2X2**   **Low vision, right eye, category 2**
-      **H54.2X21**   **Low vision right eye category 2, low vision left eye category 1**
-      **H54.2X22**   **Low vision right eye category 2, low vision left eye category 2**

H54.3   Unqualified **visual loss, both eyes**
     Visual impairment category 9 in both eyes.

✓5ᵗʰ **H54.4**   Blindness**, one eye**
     Visual impairment categories 3, 4, 5 in one eye [normal vision in other eye].

     H54.4Ø   **Blindness, one eye,** unspecified **eye**

✓6ᵗʰ **H54.41**   Blindness, right eye, normal vision left eye

- ✓7ᵗʰ **H54.413**   **Blindness, right eye, category 3**
-      **H54.413A**   **Blindness right eye category 3, normal vision left eye**
- ✓7ᵗʰ **H54.414**   **Blindness, right eye, category 4**
-      **H54.414A**   **Blindness right eye category 4, normal vision left eye**
- ✓7ᵗʰ **H54.415**   **Blindness, right eye, category 5**
-      **H54.415A**   **Blindness right eye category 5, normal vision left eye**

✓6ᵗʰ **H54.42**   Blindness, left eye, normal vision right eye

- ✓7ᵗʰ **H54.42A**   **Blindness, left eye, category 3-5**
-      **H54.42A3**   **Blindness left eye category 3, normal vision right eye**
-      **H54.42A4**   **Blindness left eye category 4, normal vision right eye**
-      **H54.42A5**   **Blindness left eye category 5, normal vision right eye**

✓5ᵗʰ **H54.5**   **Low vision, one eye**
     Visual impairment categories 1 or 2 in one eye [normal vision in other eye].

     H54.5Ø   **Low vision, one eye,** unspecified **eye**

✓6ᵗʰ **H54.51**   Low vision, right eye, normal vision left eye

- ✓7ᵗʰ **H54.511**   **Low vision, right eye, category 1-2**
-      **H54.511A**   **Low vision right eye category 1, normal vision left eye**
-      **H54.512A**   **Low vision right eye category 2, normal vision left eye**

✓6ᵗʰ **H54.52**   Low vision, left eye, normal vision right eye

- ✓7ᵗʰ **H54.52A**   **Low vision, left eye, category 1-2**
-      **H54.52A1**   **Low vision left eye category 1, normal vision right eye**
-      **H54.52A2**   **Low vision left eye category 2, normal vision right eye**

✓5ᵗʰ **H54.6**   Unqualified visual loss**, one eye**
     Visual impairment category 9 in one eye [normal vision in other eye].

     H54.6Ø   **Unqualified visual loss, one eye,** unspecified

     H54.61   **Unqualified visual loss,** right **eye, normal vision** left **eye**

     H54.62   **Unqualified visual loss,** left **eye, normal vision** right **eye**

H54.7   Unspecified **visual loss**
     Visual impairment category 9 NOS

H54.8   Legal blindness**, as defined in USA**
     Blindness NOS according to USA definition
     EXCLUDES 1   *legal blindness with specification of impairment level (H54.Ø-H54.7)*

NOTE The table below gives a classification of severity of visual impairment recommended by a WHO Study Group on the Prevention of Blindness, Geneva, 6-10 November 1972.

The term "low vision" in category H54 comprises categories 1 and 2 of the table, the term "blindness" categories 3, 4 and 5, and the term "unqualified visual loss" category 9.

If the extent of the visual field is taken into account, patients with a field no greater than 10 but greater than 5 around central fixation should be placed in category 3 and patients with a field no greater than 5 around central fixation should be placed in category 4, even if the central acuity is not impaired.

Category of visual impairment	Visual acuity with best possible correction	
	Maximum less than:	**Minimum equal to or better than:**
1	6/18 3/10 (0.3) 20/70	6/60 1/10 (0.1) 20/200
2	6/60 1/10 (0.1) 20/200	3/60 1/20 (0.05) 20/400
3	3/60 1/20 (0.05) 20/400	1/60 (finger counting at one meter) 1/50 (0.02) 5/300 (20/1200)
4	1/60 (finger counting at one meter) 1/50 (0.02) 5/300	Light perception
5	No light perception	
9	Undetermined or unspecified	

Other disorders of eye and adnexa (H55-H57)

✓4ᵗʰ H55 **Nystagmus and other** irregular eye movements
    ✓5ᵗʰ H55.0 **Nystagmus**
        H55.00 **Unspecified nystagmus**
        H55.01 **Congenital nystagmus**
        H55.02 **Latent nystagmus**
        H55.03 **Visual deprivation nystagmus**
        H55.04 **Dissociated nystagmus**
        H55.09 **Other forms of nystagmus**
    ✓5ᵗʰ H55.8 **Other irregular eye movements**
        H55.81 **Saccadic eye movements**
        H55.89 **Other irregular eye movements**

✓4ᵗʰ H57 **Other disorders of eye and adnexa**
    ✓5ᵗʰ H57.0 **Anomalies of pupillary function**
        H57.00 **Unspecified anomaly of pupillary function**
        H57.01 **Argyll Robertson pupil, atypical**
            EXCLUDES 1 *syphilitic Argyll Robertson pupil (A52.19)*
        H57.02 **Anisocoria**
        H57.03 **Miosis**
        H57.04 **Mydriasis**
        ✓6ᵗʰ H57.05 **Tonic pupil**
            H57.051 **Tonic pupil, right eye**
            H57.052 **Tonic pupil, left eye**
            H57.053 **Tonic pupil, bilateral**
            H57.059 **Tonic pupil, unspecified eye**
        H57.09 **Other anomalies of pupillary function**
    ✓5ᵗʰ H57.1 **Ocular pain**
        H57.10 **Ocular pain, unspecified eye**
        H57.11 **Ocular pain, right eye**
        H57.12 **Ocular pain, left eye**
        H57.13 **Ocular pain, bilateral**
    H57.8 **Other specified disorders of eye and adnexa**
    H57.9 **Unspecified disorder of eye and adnexa**

Intraoperative and postprocedural complications and disorders of eye and adnexa, not elsewhere classified (H59)

✓4ᵗʰ H59 **Intraoperative and postprocedural complications and disorders of eye and adnexa, not elsewhere classified**
        EXCLUDES 1 *mechanical complication of intraocular lens (T85.2)*
                mechanical complication of other ocular prosthetic devices, implants and grafts (T85.3)
                pseudophakia (Z96.1)
                secondary cataracts (H26.4-)
    ✓5ᵗʰ H59.0 **Disorders of the eye** following cataract surgery

        CC Excl: For CC codes in subcategory H59.0: PDX collection 638

        ✓6ᵗʰ H59.01 **Keratopathy (bullous aphakic) following cataract surgery**
            Vitreal corneal syndrome
            Vitreous (touch) syndrome
            H59.011 **Keratopathy (bullous aphakic) following cataract surgery, right eye** `CC`
            H59.012 **Keratopathy (bullous aphakic) following cataract surgery, left eye** `CC`
            H59.013 **Keratopathy (bullous aphakic) following cataract surgery, bilateral**
            H59.019 **Keratopathy (bullous aphakic) following cataract surgery, unspecified eye** `CC`
        ✓6ᵗʰ H59.02 **Cataract (lens) fragments in eye following cataract surgery**
            H59.021 **Cataract (lens) fragments in eye following cataract surgery, right eye**
            H59.022 **Cataract (lens) fragments in eye following cataract surgery, left eye**
            H59.023 **Cataract (lens) fragments in eye following cataract surgery, bilateral**
            H59.029 **Cataract (lens) fragments in eye following cataract surgery, unspecified eye**
        ✓6ᵗʰ H59.03 **Cystoid macular edema following cataract surgery**
            H59.031 **Cystoid macular edema following cataract surgery, right eye** `CC`
            H59.032 **Cystoid macular edema following cataract surgery, left eye** `CC`
            H59.033 **Cystoid macular edema following cataract surgery, bilateral** `CC`
            H59.039 **Cystoid macular edema following cataract surgery, unspecified eye** `CC`
        ✓6ᵗʰ H59.09 **Other disorders of the eye following cataract surgery**
            H59.091 **Other disorders of the right eye following cataract surgery** `CC`
            H59.092 **Other disorders of the left eye following cataract surgery** `CC`
            H59.093 **Other disorders of the eye following cataract surgery, bilateral** `CC`
            H59.099 **Other disorders of unspecified eye following cataract surgery** `CC`
    ✓5ᵗʰ H59.1 **Intraoperative hemorrhage and hematoma of eye and adnexa complicating a procedure**
        EXCLUDES 1 *intraoperative hemorrhage and hematoma of eye and adnexa due to accidental puncture or laceration during a procedure (H59.2-)*

        CC Excl: For CC codes in subcategory H59.1: PDX collection 639

        ✓6ᵗʰ H59.11 **Intraoperative hemorrhage and hematoma of eye and adnexa complicating an** ophthalmic procedure
            H59.111 **Intraoperative hemorrhage and hematoma of right eye and adnexa complicating an ophthalmic procedure** `CC`
            H59.112 **Intraoperative hemorrhage and hematoma of left eye and adnexa complicating an ophthalmic procedure** `CC`
            H59.113 **Intraoperative hemorrhage and hematoma of eye and adnexa complicating an ophthalmic procedure, bilateral** `CC`
            H59.119 **Intraoperative hemorrhage and hematoma of unspecified eye and adnexa complicating an ophthalmic procedure** `CC`

✓ Additional Character Req   ✓x7ᵗʰ Placeholder Alert   Unacceptable PDx   Manifestation   **H1**-**H14** HAC   **HCC** CMS-HCC Condition   **EXCLUDES 1** Not Coded Here   **EXCLUDES 2** Not Included Here

ICD-10-CM 2018   **611**

☑6ᵗʰ H59.12 Intraoperative hemorrhage and hematoma of eye and adnexa complicating other procedure

H59.121 Intraoperative hemorrhage and hematoma of right eye and adnexa complicating other procedure `CC`

H59.122 Intraoperative hemorrhage and hematoma of left eye and adnexa complicating other procedure `CC`

H59.123 Intraoperative hemorrhage and hematoma of eye and adnexa complicating other procedure, bilateral `CC`

H59.129 Intraoperative hemorrhage and hematoma of unspecified eye and adnexa complicating other procedure `CC`

☑5ᵗʰ H59.2 Accidental puncture and laceration of eye and adnexa during a procedure

> **CC Excl:** For CC codes in subcategory H59.2:
> PDX collection 509

☑6ᵗʰ H59.21 Accidental puncture and laceration of eye and adnexa during an ophthalmic procedure

H59.211 Accidental puncture and laceration of right eye and adnexa during an ophthalmic procedure `CC`

H59.212 Accidental puncture and laceration of left eye and adnexa during an ophthalmic procedure `CC`

H59.213 Accidental puncture and laceration of eye and adnexa during an ophthalmic procedure, bilateral `CC`

H59.219 Accidental puncture and laceration of unspecified eye and adnexa during an ophthalmic procedure `CC`

☑6ᵗʰ H59.22 Accidental puncture and laceration of eye and adnexa during other procedure

H59.221 Accidental puncture and laceration of right eye and adnexa during other procedure `CC`

H59.222 Accidental puncture and laceration of left eye and adnexa during other procedure `CC`

H59.223 Accidental puncture and laceration of eye and adnexa during other procedure, bilateral `CC`

H59.229 Accidental puncture and laceration of unspecified eye and adnexa during other procedure `CC`

☑5ᵗʰ H59.3 Postprocedural hemorrhage, hematoma, and seroma of eye and adnexa following a procedure

> **CC Excl:** For CC codes in subcategory H59.3:
> PDX collection 639

☑6ᵗʰ H59.31 Postprocedural hemorrhage of eye and adnexa following an ophthalmic procedure

H59.311 Postprocedural hemorrhage of right eye and adnexa following an ophthalmic procedure `CC`

H59.312 Postprocedural hemorrhage of left eye and adnexa following an ophthalmic procedure `CC`

H59.313 Postprocedural hemorrhage of eye and adnexa following an ophthalmic procedure, bilateral `CC`

H59.319 Postprocedural hemorrhage of unspecified eye and adnexa following an ophthalmic procedure `CC`

☑6ᵗʰ H59.32 Postprocedural hemorrhage of eye and adnexa following other procedure

H59.321 Postprocedural hemorrhage of right eye and adnexa following other procedure `CC`

H59.322 Postprocedural hemorrhage of left eye and adnexa following other procedure `CC`

H59.323 Postprocedural hemorrhage of eye and adnexa following other procedure, bilateral `CC`

H59.329 Postprocedural hemorrhage of unspecified eye and adnexa following other procedure `CC`

☑6ᵗʰ H59.33 Postprocedural hematoma of eye and adnexa following an ophthalmic procedure

H59.331 Postprocedural hematoma of right eye and adnexa following an ophthalmic procedure `CC`

H59.332 Postprocedural hematoma of left eye and adnexa following an ophthalmic procedure `CC`

H59.333 Postprocedural hematoma of eye and adnexa following an ophthalmic procedure, bilateral `CC`

H59.339 Postprocedural hematoma of unspecified eye and adnexa following an ophthalmic procedure `CC`

☑6ᵗʰ H59.34 Postprocedural hematoma of eye and adnexa following other procedure

H59.341 Postprocedural hematoma of right eye and adnexa following other procedure `CC`

H59.342 Postprocedural hematoma of left eye and adnexa following other procedure `CC`

H59.343 Postprocedural hematoma of eye and adnexa following other procedure, bilateral `CC`

H59.349 Postprocedural hematoma of unspecified eye and adnexa following other procedure `CC`

☑6ᵗʰ H59.35 Postprocedural seroma of eye and adnexa following an ophthalmic procedure

H59.351 Postprocedural seroma of right eye and adnexa following an ophthalmic procedure `CC`

H59.352 Postprocedural seroma of left eye and adnexa following an ophthalmic procedure `CC`

H59.353 Postprocedural seroma of eye and adnexa following an ophthalmic procedure, bilateral `CC`

H59.359 Postprocedural seroma of unspecified eye and adnexa following an ophthalmic procedure `CC`

☑6ᵗʰ H59.36 Postprocedural seroma of eye and adnexa following other procedure

H59.361 Postprocedural seroma of right eye and adnexa following other procedure `CC`

H59.362 Postprocedural seroma of left eye and adnexa following other procedure `CC`

H59.363 Postprocedural seroma of eye and adnexa following other procedure, bilateral `CC`

H59.369 Postprocedural seroma of unspecified eye and adnexa following other procedurec `CC`

☑5ᵗʰ H59.4 Inflammation (infection) of postprocedural bleb
Postprocedural blebitis
> **EXCLUDES 1**   filtering (vitreous) bleb after glaucoma surgery status (Z98.83)

H59.40 Inflammation (infection) of postprocedural bleb, unspecified

H59.41 Inflammation (infection) of postprocedural bleb, stage 1

H59.42 Inflammation (infection) of postprocedural bleb, stage 2

H59.43 Inflammation (infection) of postprocedural bleb, stage 3
Bleb endophthalmitis

Ⓝ Newborn: 0   Ⓟ Pediatric: 0-17   Ⓜ Maternity: 12-55   Ⓐ Adult: 15-124   `MCC` Major CC Condition   `PDxMCC` PDx acts as own MCC   `CC` CC Condition   `PDxCC` PDx acts as own CC

612   ICD-10-CM 2018

☑5ᵗʰ H59.8 Other intraoperative and postprocedural complications and disorders of eye and adnexa, not elsewhere classified

> **CC Excl: For CC codes in subcategory H59.8:**
> PDX collection 638

☑6ᵗʰ H59.81 Chorioretinal scars after surgery for detachment

     H59.811 Chorioretinal scars after surgery for detachment, right eye   `CC`

     H59.812 Chorioretinal scars after surgery for detachment, left eye   `CC`

     H59.813 Chorioretinal scars after surgery for detachment, bilateral   `CC`

     H59.819 Chorioretinal scars after surgery for detachment, unspecified eye   `CC`

H59.88 Other intraoperative complications of eye and adnexa, not elsewhere classified   `CC`

H59.89 Other postprocedural complications and disorders of eye and adnexa, not elsewhere classified   `CC`

Chapter 8. Diseases of the Ear and Mastoid Process (H6Ø–H95)

Chapter Specific Coding Guidelines and Examples
Reserved for future guideline expansion.

Chapter 8. Diseases of the Ear and Mastoid Process (H60–H95)

NOTE   Use an external cause code following the code for the ear condition, if applicable, to identify the cause of the ear condition.

EXCLUDES 2   certain conditions originating in the perinatal period (P04–P96)
certain infectious and parasitic diseases (A00–B99)
complications of pregnancy, childbirth and the puerperium (O00–O9A)
congenital malformations, deformations and chromosomal abnormalities (Q00–Q99)
endocrine, nutritional and metabolic diseases (E00–E88)
injury, poisoning and certain other consequences of external causes (S00–T88)
neoplasms (C00–D49)
symptoms, signs and abnormal clinical and laboratory findings, not elsewhere classified (R00–R94)

This chapter contains the following blocks:

H60–H62	Diseases of external ear
H65–H75	Diseases of middle ear and mastoid
H80–H83	Diseases of inner ear
H90–H94	Other disorders of ear
H95	Intraoperative and postprocedural complications and disorders of ear and mastoid process, not elsewhere classified

Diseases of external ear (H60–H62)

H60 Otitis externa

H60.0 Abscess of external ear
Boil of external ear
Carbuncle of auricle or external auditory canal
Furuncle of external ear
- H60.00 Abscess of external ear, unspecified ear
- H60.01 Abscess of right external ear
- H60.02 Abscess of left external ear
- H60.03 Abscess of external ear, bilateral

H60.1 Cellulitis of external ear
Cellulitis of auricle
Cellulitis of external auditory canal
- H60.10 Cellulitis of external ear, unspecified ear
- H60.11 Cellulitis of right external ear
- H60.12 Cellulitis of left external ear
- H60.13 Cellulitis of external ear, bilateral

H60.2 Malignant otitis externa

CC Excl: For CC codes in subcategory H60.2:
PDX collection 640

- H60.20 Malignant otitis externa, unspecified ear **CC**
- H60.21 Malignant otitis externa, right ear **CC**
- H60.22 Malignant otitis externa, left ear **CC**
- H60.23 Malignant otitis externa, bilateral **CC**

H60.3 Other infective otitis externa

H60.31 Diffuse otitis externa
- H60.311 Diffuse otitis externa, right ear
- H60.312 Diffuse otitis externa, left ear
- H60.313 Diffuse otitis externa, bilateral
- H60.319 Diffuse otitis externa, unspecified ear

H60.32 Hemorrhagic otitis externa
- H60.321 Hemorrhagic otitis externa, right ear
- H60.322 Hemorrhagic otitis externa, left ear
- H60.323 Hemorrhagic otitis externa, bilateral
- H60.329 Hemorrhagic otitis externa, unspecified ear

H60.33 Swimmer's ear
DEF: Otitis externa; commonly occurs when water gets trapped in the ear after swimming.
- H60.331 Swimmer's ear, right ear
- H60.332 Swimmer's ear, left ear
- H60.333 Swimmer's ear, bilateral
- H60.339 Swimmer's ear, unspecified ear

H60.39 Other infective otitis externa
- H60.391 Other infective otitis externa, right ear
- H60.392 Other infective otitis externa, left ear
- H60.393 Other infective otitis externa, bilateral
- H60.399 Other infective otitis externa, unspecified ear

H60.4 Cholesteatoma of external ear
Keratosis obturans of external ear (canal)
EXCLUDES 2 cholesteatoma of middle ear (H71.-)
recurrent cholesteatoma of postmastoidectomy cavity (H95.0-)
- H60.40 Cholesteatoma of external ear, unspecified ear
- H60.41 Cholesteatoma of right external ear
- H60.42 Cholesteatoma of left external ear
- H60.43 Cholesteatoma of external ear, bilateral

H60.5 Acute noninfective otitis externa

H60.50 Unspecified acute noninfective otitis externa
Acute otitis externa NOS
- H60.501 Unspecified acute noninfective otitis externa, right ear
- H60.502 Unspecified acute noninfective otitis externa, left ear
- H60.503 Unspecified acute noninfective otitis externa, bilateral
- H60.509 Unspecified acute noninfective otitis externa, unspecified ear

H60.51 Acute actinic otitis externa
- H60.511 Acute actinic otitis externa, right ear
- H60.512 Acute actinic otitis externa, left ear
- H60.513 Acute actinic otitis externa, bilateral
- H60.519 Acute actinic otitis externa, unspecified ear

H60.52 Acute chemical otitis externa
- H60.521 Acute chemical otitis externa, right ear
- H60.522 Acute chemical otitis externa, left ear
- H60.523 Acute chemical otitis externa, bilateral
- H60.529 Acute chemical otitis externa, unspecified ear

H60.53 Acute contact otitis externa
- H60.531 Acute contact otitis externa, right ear
- H60.532 Acute contact otitis externa, left ear
- H60.533 Acute contact otitis externa, bilateral
- H60.539 Acute contact otitis externa, unspecified ear

H60.54 Acute eczematoid otitis externa
- H60.541 Acute eczematoid otitis externa, right ear
- H60.542 Acute eczematoid otitis externa, left ear
- H60.543 Acute eczematoid otitis externa, bilateral
- H60.549 Acute eczematoid otitis externa, unspecified ear

H60.55 Acute reactive otitis externa
- H60.551 Acute reactive otitis externa, right ear
- H60.552 Acute reactive otitis externa, left ear
- H60.553 Acute reactive otitis externa, bilateral
- H60.559 Acute reactive otitis externa, unspecified ear

H60.59 Other noninfective acute otitis externa
- H60.591 Other noninfective acute otitis externa, right ear
- H60.592 Other noninfective acute otitis externa, left ear
- H60.593 Other noninfective acute otitis externa, bilateral
- H60.599 Other noninfective acute otitis externa, unspecified ear

H60.6 Unspecified chronic otitis externa
- H60.60 Unspecified chronic otitis externa, unspecified ear
- H60.61 Unspecified chronic otitis externa, right ear
- H60.62 Unspecified chronic otitis externa, left ear
- H60.63 Unspecified chronic otitis externa, bilateral

H60.8 Other otitis externa

H60.8X Other otitis externa
- H60.8X1 Other otitis externa, right ear
- H60.8X2 Other otitis externa, left ear
- H60.8X3 Other otitis externa, bilateral
- H60.8X9 Other otitis externa, unspecified ear

N Newborn: 0   P Pediatric: 0-17   M Maternity: 12-55   A Adult: 15-124   MCC Major CC Condition   PDxMCC PDx acts as own MCC   CC CC Condition   PDxCC PDx acts as own CC

616   ICD-10-CM 2018

√5ᵗʰ **H60.9 Unspecified otitis externa**

    H60.90 Unspecified otitis externa, unspecified ear

    H60.91 Unspecified otitis externa, right ear

    H60.92 Unspecified otitis externa, left ear

    H60.93 Unspecified otitis externa, bilateral

√4ᵗʰ **H61 Other disorders of external ear**

  √5ᵗʰ **H61.0 Chondritis and perichondritis of external ear**

    Chondrodermatitis nodularis chronica helicis

    Perichondritis of auricle

    Perichondritis of pinna

    √6ᵗʰ **H61.00 Unspecified perichondritis of external ear**

      H61.001 Unspecified perichondritis of right external ear

      H61.002 Unspecified perichondritis of left external ear

      H61.003 Unspecified perichondritis of external ear, bilateral

      H61.009 Unspecified perichondritis of external ear, unspecified ear

    √6ᵗʰ **H61.01 Acute perichondritis of external ear**

      H61.011 Acute perichondritis of right external ear

      H61.012 Acute perichondritis of left external ear

      H61.013 Acute perichondritis of external ear, bilateral

      H61.019 Acute perichondritis of external ear, unspecified ear

    √6ᵗʰ **H61.02 Chronic perichondritis of external ear**

      H61.021 Chronic perichondritis of right external ear

      H61.022 Chronic perichondritis of left external ear

      H61.023 Chronic perichondritis of external ear, bilateral

      H61.029 Chronic perichondritis of external ear, unspecified ear

    √6ᵗʰ **H61.03 Chondritis of external ear**

      Chondritis of auricle   Chondritis of pinna

      AHA: 2015, 1Q, 18

      DEF: Infection that has progressed into the cartilage; presents as indurated and edematous skin over the pinna; vascular compromise occurs with tissue necrosis and deformity.

      H61.031 Chondritis of right external ear

      H61.032 Chondritis of left external ear

      H61.033 Chondritis of external ear, bilateral

      H61.039 Chondritis of external ear, unspecified ear

  √5ᵗʰ **H61.1 Noninfective disorders of pinna**

    EXCLUDES 2   *cauliflower ear (M95.1-)*

                gouty tophi of ear (M1A.-)

    √6ᵗʰ **H61.10 Unspecified noninfective disorders of pinna**

      Disorder of pinna NOS

      H61.101 Unspecified noninfective disorders of pinna, right ear

      H61.102 Unspecified noninfective disorders of pinna, left ear

      H61.103 Unspecified noninfective disorders of pinna, bilateral

      H61.109 Unspecified noninfective disorders of pinna, unspecified ear

    √6ᵗʰ **H61.11 Acquired deformity of pinna**

      Acquired deformity of auricle

      EXCLUDES 2   *cauliflower ear (M95.1-)*

      H61.111 Acquired deformity of pinna, right ear

      H61.112 Acquired deformity of pinna, left ear

      H61.113 Acquired deformity of pinna, bilateral

      H61.119 Acquired deformity of pinna, unspecified ear

    √6ᵗʰ **H61.12 Hematoma of pinna**

      Hematoma of auricle

      H61.121 Hematoma of pinna, right ear

      H61.122 Hematoma of pinna, left ear

      H61.123 Hematoma of pinna, bilateral

      H61.129 Hematoma of pinna, unspecified ear

    √6ᵗʰ **H61.19 Other noninfective disorders of pinna**

      H61.191 Noninfective disorders of pinna, right ear

      H61.192 Noninfective disorders of pinna, left ear

      H61.193 Noninfective disorders of pinna, bilateral

      H61.199 Noninfective disorders of pinna, unspecified ear

  √5ᵗʰ **H61.2 Impacted cerumen**

    Wax in ear

    ⁴ **H61.20 Impacted cerumen, unspecified ear**

    ⁴ **H61.21 Impacted cerumen, right ear**

    ⁴ **H61.22 Impacted cerumen, left ear**

    ⁴ **H61.23 Impacted cerumen, bilateral**

  √5ᵗʰ **H61.3 Acquired stenosis of external ear canal**

    Collapse of external ear canal

    EXCLUDES 1   *postprocedural stenosis of external ear canal (H95.81-)*

    √6ᵗʰ **H61.30 Acquired stenosis of external ear canal, unspecified**

      H61.301 Acquired stenosis of right external ear canal, unspecified

      H61.302 Acquired stenosis of left external ear canal, unspecified

      H61.303 Acquired stenosis of external ear canal, unspecified, bilateral

      H61.309 Acquired stenosis of external ear canal, unspecified, unspecified ear

    √6ᵗʰ **H61.31 Acquired stenosis of external ear canal secondary to trauma**

      H61.311 Acquired stenosis of right external ear canal secondary to trauma

      H61.312 Acquired stenosis of left external ear canal secondary to trauma

      H61.313 Acquired stenosis of external ear canal secondary to trauma, bilateral

      H61.319 Acquired stenosis of external ear canal secondary to trauma, unspecified ear

    √6ᵗʰ **H61.32 Acquired stenosis of external ear canal secondary to inflammation and infection**

      DEF: Narrowing of the external ear canal; due to chronic inflammation or infection.

      H61.321 Acquired stenosis of right external ear canal secondary to inflammation and infection

      H61.322 Acquired stenosis of left external ear canal secondary to inflammation and infection

      H61.323 Acquired stenosis of external ear canal secondary to inflammation and infection, bilateral

      H61.329 Acquired stenosis of external ear canal secondary to inflammation and infection, unspecified ear

    √6ᵗʰ **H61.39 Other acquired stenosis of external ear canal**

      H61.391 Other acquired stenosis of right external ear canal

      H61.392 Other acquired stenosis of left external ear canal

      H61.393 Other acquired stenosis of external ear canal, bilateral

      H61.399 Other acquired stenosis of external ear canal, unspecified ear

  √5ᵗʰ **H61.8 Other specified disorders of external ear**

    √6ᵗʰ **H61.81 Exostosis of external canal**

      H61.811 Exostosis of right external canal

      H61.812 Exostosis of left external canal

      H61.813 Exostosis of external canal, bilateral

      H61.819 Exostosis of external canal, unspecified ear

    √6ᵗʰ **H61.89 Other specified disorders of external ear**

      H61.891 Other specified disorders of right external ear

      H61.892 Other specified disorders of left external ear

      H61.893 Other specified disorders of external ear, bilateral

      H61.899 Other specified disorders of external ear, unspecified ear

---

⁴   Questionable admission when used as PDx.

✔Additional Character Req   ✔x7ᵗʰ Placeholder Alert   Unacceptable PDx   Manifestation   **H1 - H14** HAC   **HCC** CMS-HCC Condition   *EXCLUDES 1* Not Coded Here   *EXCLUDES 2* Not Included Here

✓5th H61.9 Disorder of external ear, unspecified
H61.90 Disorder of external ear, unspecified, unspecified ear
H61.91 Disorder of right external ear, unspecified
H61.92 Disorder of left external ear, unspecified
H61.93 Disorder of external ear, unspecified, bilateral

✓4th H62 Disorders of external ear in diseases classified elsewhere
✓5th H62.4 Otitis externa in other diseases classified elsewhere
Code first underlying disease, such as:
erysipelas (A46)
impetigo (L01.0)
EXCLUDES 1 otitis externa (in):
candidiasis (B37.84)
herpes viral [herpes simplex] (B00.1)
herpes zoster (B02.8)
H62.40 *Otitis externa in other diseases classified elsewhere, unspecified ear*
H62.41 *Otitis externa in other diseases classified elsewhere, right ear*
H62.42 *Otitis externa in other diseases classified elsewhere, left ear*
H62.43 *Otitis externa in other diseases classified elsewhere, bilateral*

✓5th H62.8 Other disorders of external ear in diseases classified elsewhere
Code first underlying disease, such as:
gout (M1A.-, M10.-)
✓6th H62.8X Other disorders of external ear in diseases classified elsewhere
H62.8X1 *Other disorders of right external ear in diseases classified elsewhere*
H62.8X2 *Other disorders of left external ear in diseases classified elsewhere*
H62.8X3 *Other disorders of external ear in diseases classified elsewhere, bilateral*
H62.8X9 *Other disorders of external ear in diseases classified elsewhere, unspecified ear*

Diseases of middle ear and mastoid (H65-H75)

✓4th H65 Nonsuppurative otitis media
INCLUDES nonsuppurative otitis media with myringitis
Use additional code for any associated perforated tympanic membrane (H72.-)
Use additional code to identify:
exposure to environmental tobacco smoke (Z77.22)
exposure to tobacco smoke in the perinatal period (P96.81)
history of tobacco dependence (Z87.891)
occupational exposure to environmental tobacco smoke (Z57.31)
tobacco dependence (F17.-)
tobacco use (Z72.0)

✓5th H65.0 Acute serous otitis media
Acute and subacute secretory otitis
H65.00 Acute serous otitis media, unspecified ear
H65.01 Acute serous otitis media, right ear
H65.02 Acute serous otitis media, left ear
H65.03 Acute serous otitis media, bilateral
H65.04 Acute serous otitis media, recurrent, right ear
H65.05 Acute serous otitis media, recurrent, left ear
H65.06 Acute serous otitis media, recurrent, bilateral
H65.07 Acute serous otitis media, recurrent, unspecified ear

✓5th H65.1 Other acute nonsuppurative otitis media
EXCLUDES 1 otitic barotrauma (T70.0)
otitis media (acute) NOS (H66.9)
✓6th H65.11 Acute and subacute allergic otitis media (mucoid) (sanguinous) (serous)
H65.111 Acute and subacute allergic otitis media (mucoid) (sanguinous) (serous), right ear
H65.112 Acute and subacute allergic otitis media (mucoid) (sanguinous) (serous), left ear
H65.113 Acute and subacute allergic otitis media (mucoid) (sanguinous) (serous), bilateral
H65.114 Acute and subacute allergic otitis media (mucoid) (sanguinous) (serous), recurrent, right ear

H65.115 Acute and subacute allergic otitis media (mucoid) (sanguinous) (serous), recurrent, left ear
H65.116 Acute and subacute allergic otitis media (mucoid) (sanguinous) (serous), recurrent, bilateral
H65.117 Acute and subacute allergic otitis media (mucoid) (sanguinous) (serous), recurrent, unspecified ear
H65.119 Acute and subacute allergic otitis media (mucoid) (sanguinous) (serous), unspecified ear

✓6th H65.19 Other acute nonsuppurative otitis media
Acute and subacute mucoid otitis media
Acute and subacute nonsuppurative otitis media NOS
Acute and subacute sanguinous otitis media
Acute and subacute seromucinous otitis media
H65.191 Other acute nonsuppurative otitis media, right ear
H65.192 Other acute nonsuppurative otitis media, left ear
H65.193 Other acute nonsuppurative otitis media, bilateral
H65.194 Other acute nonsuppurative otitis media, recurrent, right ear
H65.195 Other acute nonsuppurative otitis media, recurrent, left ear
H65.196 Other acute nonsuppurative otitis media, recurrent, bilateral
H65.197 Other acute nonsuppurative otitis media recurrent, unspecified ear
H65.199 Other acute nonsuppurative otitis media, unspecified ear

✓5th H65.2 Chronic serous otitis media
Chronic tubotympanal catarrh
H65.20 Chronic serous otitis media, unspecified ear
H65.21 Chronic serous otitis media, right ear
H65.22 Chronic serous otitis media, left ear
H65.23 Chronic serous otitis media, bilateral

✓5th H65.3 Chronic mucoid otitis media
Chronic mucinous otitis media
Chronic secretory otitis media
Chronic transudative otitis media
Glue ear
EXCLUDES 1 adhesive middle ear disease (H74.1)
H65.30 Chronic mucoid otitis media, unspecified ear
H65.31 Chronic mucoid otitis media, right ear
H65.32 Chronic mucoid otitis media, left ear
H65.33 Chronic mucoid otitis media, bilateral

✓5th H65.4 Other chronic nonsuppurative otitis media
✓6th H65.41 Chronic allergic otitis media
H65.411 Chronic allergic otitis media, right ear
H65.412 Chronic allergic otitis media, left ear
H65.413 Chronic allergic otitis media, bilateral
H65.419 Chronic allergic otitis media, unspecified ear
✓6th H65.49 Other chronic nonsuppurative otitis media
Chronic exudative otitis media
Chronic nonsuppurative otitis media NOS
Chronic otitis media with effusion (nonpurulent)
Chronic seromucinous otitis media
H65.491 Other chronic nonsuppurative otitis media, right ear
H65.492 Other chronic nonsuppurative otitis media, left ear
H65.493 Other chronic nonsuppurative otitis media, bilateral
H65.499 Other chronic nonsuppurative otitis media, unspecified ear

✓5th **H65.9** Unspecified **nonsuppurative otitis media**
     Allergic otitis media NOS
     Catarrhal otitis media NOS
     Exudative otitis media NOS
     Mucoid otitis media NOS
     Otitis media with effusion (nonpurulent) NOS
     Secretory otitis media NOS
     Seromucinous otitis media NOS
     Serous otitis media NOS
     Transudative otitis media NOS

    H65.90 Unspecified nonsuppurative otitis media, **unspecified ear**

    H65.91 Unspecified nonsuppurative otitis media, **right ear**

    H65.92 Unspecified nonsuppurative otitis media, **left ear**

    H65.93 Unspecified nonsuppurative otitis media, **bilateral**

✓4th **H66 Suppurative and unspecified otitis media**
   [INCLUDES] suppurative and unspecified otitis media with myringitis
   Use additional code to identify:
     exposure to environmental tobacco smoke (Z77.22)
     exposure to tobacco smoke in the perinatal period (P96.81)
     history of tobacco dependence (Z87.891)
     occupational exposure to environmental tobacco smoke (Z57.31)
     tobacco dependence (F17.-)
     tobacco use (Z72.0)
   AHA: 2016, 1Q, 34

✓5th **H66.0** Acute suppurative **otitis media**

   ✓6th **H66.00** Acute suppurative otitis media **without spontaneous rupture of ear drum**

     H66.001 Acute suppurative otitis media without spontaneous rupture of ear drum, **right ear**

     H66.002 Acute suppurative otitis media without spontaneous rupture of ear drum, **left ear**

     H66.003 Acute suppurative otitis media without spontaneous rupture of ear drum, **bilateral**

     H66.004 Acute suppurative otitis media without spontaneous rupture of ear drum, **recurrent, right ear**

     H66.005 Acute suppurative otitis media without spontaneous rupture of ear drum, **recurrent, left ear**

     H66.006 Acute suppurative otitis media without spontaneous rupture of ear drum, **recurrent, bilateral**

     H66.007 Acute suppurative otitis media without spontaneous rupture of ear drum, **recurrent, unspecified ear**

     H66.009 Acute suppurative otitis media without spontaneous rupture of ear drum, **unspecified ear**

   ✓6th **H66.01** Acute suppurative otitis media **with spontaneous rupture of ear drum**
     DEF: Sudden, severe inflammation of middle ear, with pressure causing the perforation of ear drum tissue.

     H66.011 Acute suppurative otitis media with spontaneous rupture of ear drum, **right ear**

     H66.012 Acute suppurative otitis media with spontaneous rupture of ear drum, **left ear**

     H66.013 Acute suppurative otitis media with spontaneous rupture of ear drum, **bilateral**

     H66.014 Acute suppurative otitis media with spontaneous rupture of ear drum, **recurrent, right ear**

     H66.015 Acute suppurative otitis media with spontaneous rupture of ear drum, **recurrent, left ear**

     H66.016 Acute suppurative otitis media with spontaneous rupture of ear drum, **recurrent, bilateral**

     H66.017 Acute suppurative otitis media with spontaneous rupture of ear drum, **recurrent, unspecified ear**

     H66.019 Acute suppurative otitis media with spontaneous rupture of ear drum, **unspecified ear**

✓5th **H66.1** Chronic tubotympanic **suppurative otitis media**
     Benign chronic suppurative otitis media
     Chronic tubotympanic disease
     Use additional code for any associated perforated tympanic membrane (H72.-)

    H66.10 Chronic tubotympanic suppurative otitis media, **unspecified**

    H66.11 Chronic tubotympanic suppurative otitis media, **right ear**

    H66.12 Chronic tubotympanic suppurative otitis media, **left ear**

    H66.13 Chronic tubotympanic suppurative otitis media, **bilateral**

✓5th **H66.2** Chronic atticoantral **suppurative otitis media**
     Chronic atticoantral disease
     Use additional code for any associated perforated tympanic membrane (H72.-)

    H66.20 Chronic atticoantral suppurative otitis media, **unspecified ear**

    H66.21 Chronic atticoantral suppurative otitis media, **right ear**

    H66.22 Chronic atticoantral suppurative otitis media, **left ear**

    H66.23 Chronic atticoantral suppurative otitis media, **bilateral**

✓5th **H66.3** Other **chronic suppurative otitis media**
     Chronic suppurative otitis media NOS
     Use additional code for any associated perforated tympanic membrane (H72.-)
     [EXCLUDES 1] *tuberculous otitis media (A18.6)*

   ✓6th **H66.3X** Other chronic suppurative otitis media

     H66.3X1 Other chronic suppurative otitis media, **right ear**

     H66.3X2 Other chronic suppurative otitis media, **left ear**

     H66.3X3 Other chronic suppurative otitis media, **bilateral**

     H66.3X9 Other chronic suppurative otitis media, **unspecified ear**

✓5th **H66.4 Suppurative otitis media, unspecified**
     Purulent otitis media NOS
     Use additional code for any associated perforated tympanic membrane (H72.-)

    H66.40 Suppurative otitis media, unspecified, **unspecified ear**

    H66.41 Suppurative otitis media, unspecified, **right ear**

    H66.42 Suppurative otitis media, unspecified, **left ear**

    H66.43 Suppurative otitis media, unspecified, **bilateral**

✓5th **H66.9 Otitis media, unspecified**
     Otitis media NOS
     Acute otitis media NOS
     Chronic otitis media NOS
     Use additional code for any associated perforated tympanic membrane (H72.-)

    H66.90 Otitis media, unspecified, **unspecified ear**

    H66.91 Otitis media, unspecified, **right ear**

    H66.92 Otitis media, unspecified, **left ear**

    H66.93 Otitis media, unspecified, **bilateral**

✓4th **H67 Otitis media in diseases classified elsewhere**
   Code first underlying disease, such as:
     viral disease NEC (B00-B34)
   Use additional code for any associated perforated tympanic membrane (H72.-)
   [EXCLUDES 1] *otitis media in:*
     influenza (J09.X9, J10.83, J11.83)
     measles (B05.3)
     scarlet fever (A38.0)
     tuberculosis (A18.6)

   H67.1 **Otitis media in diseases classified elsewhere, right ear**

   H67.2 **Otitis media in diseases classified elsewhere, left ear**

   H67.3 **Otitis media in diseases classified elsewhere, bilateral**

   H67.9 **Otitis media in diseases classified elsewhere, unspecified ear**

☑Additional Character Req   ✓x7th Placeholder Alert   Unacceptable PDx   Manifestation   H1–H14 HAC   HCC CMS-HCC Condition   EXCLUDES 1 Not Coded Here   EXCLUDES 2 Not Included Here

ICD-10-CM 2018   **619**

H65.9–H67.9

✓4ᵗʰ **H68 Eustachian salpingitis and obstruction**

✓5ᵗʰ **H68.0 Eustachian** salpingitis

✓6ᵗʰ **H68.00 Unspecified** Eustachian salpingitis

H68.001 Unspecified Eustachian salpingitis, **right ear**

H68.002 Unspecified Eustachian salpingitis, **left ear**

H68.003 Unspecified Eustachian salpingitis, **bilateral**

H68.009 Unspecified Eustachian salpingitis, **unspecified ear**

✓6ᵗʰ **H68.01 Acute** Eustachian salpingitis

H68.011 Acute Eustachian salpingitis, **right ear**

H68.012 Acute Eustachian salpingitis, **left ear**

H68.013 Acute Eustachian salpingitis, **bilateral**

H68.019 Acute Eustachian salpingitis, **unspecified ear**

✓6ᵗʰ **H68.02 Chronic** Eustachian salpingitis

H68.021 Chronic Eustachian salpingitis, **right ear**

H68.022 Chronic Eustachian salpingitis, **left ear**

H68.023 Chronic Eustachian salpingitis, **bilateral**

H68.029 Chronic Eustachian salpingitis, **unspecified ear**

✓5ᵗʰ **H68.1 Obstruction** of Eustachian tube
Stenosis of Eustachian tube
Stricture of Eustachian tube

✓6ᵗʰ **H68.10 Unspecified** obstruction of Eustachian tube

H68.101 Unspecified obstruction of Eustachian tube, **right ear**

H68.102 Unspecified obstruction of Eustachian tube, **left ear**

H68.103 Unspecified obstruction of Eustachian tube, **bilateral**

H68.109 Unspecified obstruction of Eustachian tube, **unspecified ear**

✓6ᵗʰ **H68.11 Osseous** obstruction of Eustachian tube

H68.111 Osseous obstruction of Eustachian tube, **right ear**

H68.112 Osseous obstruction of Eustachian tube, **left ear**

H68.113 Osseous obstruction of Eustachian tube, **bilateral**

H68.119 Osseous obstruction of Eustachian tube, **unspecified ear**

✓6ᵗʰ **H68.12 Intrinsic cartilagenous** obstruction of Eustachian tube

H68.121 Intrinsic cartilagenous obstruction of Eustachian tube, **right ear**

H68.122 Intrinsic cartilagenous obstruction of Eustachian tube, **left ear**

H68.123 Intrinsic cartilagenous obstruction of Eustachian tube, **bilateral**

H68.129 Intrinsic cartilagenous obstruction of Eustachian tube, **unspecified ear**

✓6ᵗʰ **H68.13 Extrinsic cartilagenous** obstruction of Eustachian tube
Compression of Eustachian tube

H68.131 Extrinsic cartilagenous obstruction of Eustachian tube, **right ear**

H68.132 Extrinsic cartilagenous obstruction of Eustachian tube, **left ear**

H68.133 Extrinsic cartilagenous obstruction of Eustachian tube, **bilateral**

H68.139 Extrinsic cartilagenous obstruction of Eustachian tube, **unspecified ear**

✓4ᵗʰ **H69 Other and unspecified disorders of Eustachian tube**

✓5ᵗʰ **H69.0 Patulous** Eustachian tube

H69.00 Patulous Eustachian tube, **unspecified ear**

H69.01 Patulous Eustachian tube, **right ear**

H69.02 Patulous Eustachian tube, **left ear**

H69.03 Patulous Eustachian tube, **bilateral**

✓5ᵗʰ **H69.8 Other specified** disorders of Eustachian tube

H69.80 Other specified disorders of Eustachian tube, **unspecified ear**

H69.81 Other specified disorders of Eustachian tube, **right ear**

H69.82 Other specified disorders of Eustachian tube, **left ear**

H69.83 Other specified disorders of Eustachian tube, **bilateral**

✓5ᵗʰ **H69.9 Unspecified** Eustachian tube disorder

H69.90 Unspecified Eustachian tube disorder, **unspecified ear**

H69.91 Unspecified Eustachian tube disorder, **right ear**

H69.92 Unspecified Eustachian tube disorder, **left ear**

H69.93 Unspecified Eustachian tube disorder, **bilateral**

✓4ᵗʰ **H70 Mastoiditis and related conditions**

✓5ᵗʰ **H70.0 Acute** mastoiditis
Abscess of mastoid
Empyema of mastoid

CC Excl: For CC codes in subcategory H70.0:
PDX collection 641

✓6ᵗʰ **H70.00 Acute mastoiditis** without complications

H70.001 Acute mastoiditis without complications, right ear `CC`

H70.002 Acute mastoiditis without complications, left ear `CC`

H70.003 Acute mastoiditis without complications, bilateral `CC`

H70.009 Acute mastoiditis without complications, unspecified ear `CC`

✓6ᵗʰ **H70.01 Subperiosteal abscess** of mastoid

H70.011 Subperiosteal abscess of mastoid, right ear `CC`

H70.012 Subperiosteal abscess of mastoid, left ear `CC`

H70.013 Subperiosteal abscess of mastoid, bilateral `CC`

H70.019 Subperiosteal abscess of mastoid, unspecified ear `CC`

✓6ᵗʰ **H70.09 Acute mastoiditis** with other complications

H70.091 Acute mastoiditis with other complications, right ear `CC`

H70.092 Acute mastoiditis with other complications, left ear `CC`

H70.093 Acute mastoiditis with other complications, bilateral `CC`

H70.099 Acute mastoiditis with other complications, unspecified ear `CC`

✓5ᵗʰ **H70.1 Chronic** mastoiditis
Caries of mastoid
Fistula of mastoid
EXCLUDES 1 *tuberculous mastoiditis (A18.03)*

H70.10 Chronic mastoiditis, unspecified ear

H70.11 Chronic mastoiditis, right ear

H70.12 Chronic mastoiditis, left ear

H70.13 Chronic mastoiditis, bilateral

✓5ᵗʰ **H70.2 Petrositis**
Inflammation of petrous bone

✓6ᵗʰ **H70.20 Unspecified** petrositis

H70.201 Unspecified petrositis, right ear

H70.202 Unspecified petrositis, left ear

H70.203 Unspecified petrositis, bilateral

H70.209 Unspecified petrositis, unspecified ear

✓6ᵗʰ **H70.21 Acute** petrositis
DEF: Sudden, severe inflammation of petrous temporal bone behind the ear; associated with middle ear infection.

H70.211 Acute petrositis, right ear

H70.212 Acute petrositis, left ear

H70.213 Acute petrositis, bilateral

H70.219 Acute petrositis, unspecified ear

✓6ᵗʰ **H70.22 Chronic** petrositis

H70.221 Chronic petrositis, right ear

H70.222 Chronic petrositis, left ear

H70.223 Chronic petrositis, bilateral

H70.229 Chronic petrositis, unspecified ear

✓5th **H70.8 Other mastoiditis and related conditions**
  EXCLUDES 1   *preauricular sinus and cyst (Q18.1)*
                     sinus, fistula, and cyst of branchial cleft (Q18.0)

  ✓6th **H70.81 Postauricular fistula**
      H70.811 Postauricular fistula, right ear
      H70.812 Postauricular fistula, left ear
      H70.813 Postauricular fistula, bilateral
      H70.819 Postauricular fistula, unspecified ear

  ✓6th **H70.89 Other mastoiditis and related conditions**
      H70.891 Other mastoiditis and related conditions, right ear
      H70.892 Other mastoiditis and related conditions, left ear
      H70.893 Other mastoiditis and related conditions, bilateral
      H70.899 Other mastoiditis and related conditions, unspecified ear

✓5th **H70.9 Unspecified mastoiditis**
    H70.90 Unspecified mastoiditis, unspecified ear
    H70.91 Unspecified mastoiditis, right ear
    H70.92 Unspecified mastoiditis, left ear
    H70.93 Unspecified mastoiditis, bilateral

✓4th **H71 Cholesteatoma of middle ear**
  EXCLUDES 2   *cholesteatoma of external ear (H60.4-)*
                     recurrent cholesteatoma of postmastoidectomy cavity (H95.0-)

✓5th **H71.0 Cholesteatoma of attic**
    H71.00 Cholesteatoma of attic, unspecified ear
    H71.01 Cholesteatoma of attic, right ear
    H71.02 Cholesteatoma of attic, left ear
    H71.03 Cholesteatoma of attic, bilateral

✓5th **H71.1 Cholesteatoma of tympanum**
    H71.10 Cholesteatoma of tympanum, unspecified ear
    H71.11 Cholesteatoma of tympanum, right ear
    H71.12 Cholesteatoma of tympanum, left ear
    H71.13 Cholesteatoma of tympanum, bilateral

✓5th **H71.2 Cholesteatoma of mastoid**
    H71.20 Cholesteatoma of mastoid, unspecified ear
    H71.21 Cholesteatoma of mastoid, right ear
    H71.22 Cholesteatoma of mastoid, left ear
    H71.23 Cholesteatoma of mastoid, bilateral

✓5th **H71.3 Diffuse cholesteatosis**
    H71.30 Diffuse cholesteatosis, unspecified ear
    H71.31 Diffuse cholesteatosis, right ear
    H71.32 Diffuse cholesteatosis, left ear
    H71.33 Diffuse cholesteatosis, bilateral

✓6th **H71.9 Unspecified cholesteatoma**
    H71.90 Unspecified cholesteatoma, unspecified ear
    H71.91 Unspecified cholesteatoma, right ear
    H71.92 Unspecified cholesteatoma, left ear
    H71.93 Unspecified cholesteatoma, bilateral

Cholesteatoma of Middle Ear

Middle ear chamber
Ear drum
Cholesteatoma sac

✓4th **H72 Perforation of tympanic membrane**
  INCLUDES   persistent post-traumatic perforation of ear drum
                postinflammatory perforation of ear drum
  Code first any associated otitis media (H65.-, H66.1-, H66.2-, H66.3-, H66.4-, H66.9-, H67.-)
  EXCLUDES 1   *acute suppurative otitis media with rupture of the tympanic membrane (H66.01-)*
                     traumatic rupture of ear drum (S09.2-)

✓5th **H72.0 Central perforation of tympanic membrane**
    H72.00 Central perforation of tympanic membrane, unspecified ear
    H72.01 Central perforation of tympanic membrane, right ear
    H72.02 Central perforation of tympanic membrane, left ear
    H72.03 Central perforation of tympanic membrane, bilateral

✓5th **H72.1 Attic perforation of tympanic membrane**
  Perforation of pars flaccida
    H72.10 Attic perforation of tympanic membrane, unspecified ear
    H72.11 Attic perforation of tympanic membrane, right ear
    H72.12 Attic perforation of tympanic membrane, left ear
    H72.13 Attic perforation of tympanic membrane, bilateral

✓5th **H72.2 Other marginal perforations of tympanic membrane**
  ✓6th **H72.2X Other marginal perforations of tympanic membrane**
      H72.2X1 Other marginal perforations of tympanic membrane, right ear
      H72.2X2 Other marginal perforations of tympanic membrane, left ear
      H72.2X3 Other marginal perforations of tympanic membrane, bilateral
      H72.2X9 Other marginal perforations of tympanic membrane, unspecified ear

✓5th **H72.8 Other perforations of tympanic membrane**
  ✓6th **H72.81 Multiple perforations of tympanic membrane**
      H72.811 Multiple perforations of tympanic membrane, right ear
      H72.812 Multiple perforations of tympanic membrane, left ear
      H72.813 Multiple perforations of tympanic membrane, bilateral
      H72.819 Multiple perforations of tympanic membrane, unspecified ear

  ✓6th **H72.82 Total perforations of tympanic membrane**
      H72.821 Total perforations of tympanic membrane, right ear
      H72.822 Total perforations of tympanic membrane, left ear
      H72.823 Total perforations of tympanic membrane, bilateral
      H72.829 Total perforations of tympanic membrane, unspecified ear

✓5th **H72.9 Unspecified perforation of tympanic membrane**
    H72.90 Unspecified perforation of tympanic membrane, unspecified ear
    H72.91 Unspecified perforation of tympanic membrane, right ear
    H72.92 Unspecified perforation of tympanic membrane, left ear
    H72.93 Unspecified perforation of tympanic membrane, bilateral

✓4th **H73 Other disorders of tympanic membrane**
  ✓5th **H73.0 Acute myringitis**
    EXCLUDES 1   *acute myringitis with otitis media (H65, H66)*

    ✓6th **H73.00 Unspecified acute myringitis**
      Acute tympanitis NOS
      H73.001 Acute myringitis, right ear
      H73.002 Acute myringitis, left ear
      H73.003 Acute myringitis, bilateral
      H73.009 Acute myringitis, unspecified ear

    ✓6th **H73.01 Bullous myringitis**
      DEF: Bacterial or viral otitis media; characterized by the appearance of serous or hemorrhagic blebs on the ear drum and sudden onset of severe pain in ear.
      H73.011 Bullous myringitis, right ear
      H73.012 Bullous myringitis, left ear

H73.013   Bullous myringitis, bilateral
H73.019   Bullous myringitis, unspecified ear
✓6th **H73.09   Other acute myringitis**
H73.091   Other acute myringitis, right ear
H73.092   Other acute myringitis, left ear
H73.093   Other acute myringitis, bilateral
H73.099   Other acute myringitis, unspecified ear

✓5th **H73.1   Chronic myringitis**
Chronic tympanitis
EXCLUDES 1   chronic myringitis with otitis media (H65, H66)
H73.10   Chronic myringitis, unspecified ear
H73.11   Chronic myringitis, right ear
H73.12   Chronic myringitis, left ear
H73.13   Chronic myringitis, bilateral

✓5th **H73.2   Unspecified myringitis**
H73.20   Unspecified myringitis, unspecified ear
H73.21   Unspecified myringitis, right ear
H73.22   Unspecified myringitis, left ear
H73.23   Unspecified myringitis, bilateral

✓5th **H73.8   Other specified disorders of tympanic membrane**
✓6th **H73.81   Atrophic flaccid tympanic membrane**
H73.811   Atrophic flaccid tympanic membrane, right ear
H73.812   Atrophic flaccid tympanic membrane, left ear
H73.813   Atrophic flaccid tympanic membrane, bilateral
H73.819   Atrophic flaccid tympanic membrane, unspecified ear
✓6th **H73.82   Atrophic nonflaccid tympanic membrane**
H73.821   Atrophic nonflaccid tympanic membrane, right ear
H73.822   Atrophic nonflaccid tympanic membrane, left ear
H73.823   Atrophic nonflaccid tympanic membrane, bilateral
H73.829   Atrophic nonflaccid tympanic membrane, unspecified ear
✓6th **H73.89   Other specified disorders of tympanic membrane**
H73.891   Other specified disorders of tympanic membrane, right ear
H73.892   Other specified disorders of tympanic membrane, left ear
H73.893   Other specified disorders of tympanic membrane, bilateral
H73.899   Other specified disorders of tympanic membrane, unspecified ear

✓5th **H73.9   Unspecified disorder of tympanic membrane**
H73.90   Unspecified disorder of tympanic membrane, unspecified ear
H73.91   Unspecified disorder of tympanic membrane, right ear
H73.92   Unspecified disorder of tympanic membrane, left ear
H73.93   Unspecified disorder of tympanic membrane, bilateral

✓4th **H74   Other disorders of middle ear mastoid**
EXCLUDES 2   mastoiditis (H70.-)

✓5th **H74.0   Tympanosclerosis**
DEF: Calcification of tissue in the ear drum, middle ear bones, and middle ear canal.
H74.01   Tympanosclerosis, right ear
H74.02   Tympanosclerosis, left ear
H74.03   Tympanosclerosis, bilateral
H74.09   Tympanosclerosis, unspecified ear

✓5th **H74.1   Adhesive middle ear disease**
Adhesive otitis
EXCLUDES 1   glue ear (H65.3-)
H74.11   Adhesive right middle ear disease
H74.12   Adhesive left middle ear disease
H74.13   Adhesive middle ear disease, bilateral
H74.19   Adhesive middle ear disease, unspecified ear

✓5th **H74.2   Discontinuity and dislocation of ear ossicles**
H74.20   Discontinuity and dislocation of ear ossicles, unspecified ear
H74.21   Discontinuity and dislocation of right ear ossicles
H74.22   Discontinuity and dislocation of left ear ossicles
H74.23   Discontinuity and dislocation of ear ossicles, bilateral

✓5th **H74.3   Other acquired abnormalities of ear ossicles**
✓6th **H74.31   Ankylosis of ear ossicles**
H74.311   Ankylosis of ear ossicles, right ear
H74.312   Ankylosis of ear ossicles, left ear
H74.313   Ankylosis of ear ossicles, bilateral
H74.319   Ankylosis of ear ossicles, unspecified ear
✓6th **H74.32   Partial loss of ear ossicles**
H74.321   Partial loss of ear ossicles, right ear
H74.322   Partial loss of ear ossicles, left ear
H74.323   Partial loss of ear ossicles, bilateral
H74.329   Partial loss of ear ossicles, unspecified ear
✓6th **H74.39   Other acquired abnormalities of ear ossicles**
H74.391   Other acquired abnormalities of right ear ossicles
H74.392   Other acquired abnormalities of left ear ossicles
H74.393   Other acquired abnormalities of ear ossicles, bilateral
H74.399   Other acquired abnormalities of ear ossicles, unspecified ear

✓5th **H74.4   Polyp of middle ear**
H74.40   Polyp of middle ear, unspecified ear
H74.41   Polyp of right middle ear
H74.42   Polyp of left middle ear
H74.43   Polyp of middle ear, bilateral

✓5th **H74.8   Other specified disorders of middle ear and mastoid**
✓6th **H74.8X   Other specified disorders of middle ear and mastoid**
H74.8X1   Other specified disorders of right middle ear and mastoid
H74.8X2   Other specified disorders of left middle ear and mastoid
H74.8X3   Other specified disorders of middle ear and mastoid, bilateral
H74.8X9   Other specified disorders of middle ear and mastoid, unspecified ear

✓5th **H74.9   Unspecified disorder of middle ear and mastoid**
H74.90   Unspecified disorder of middle ear and mastoid, unspecified ear
H74.91   Unspecified disorder of right middle ear and mastoid
H74.92   Unspecified disorder of left middle ear and mastoid
H74.93   Unspecified disorder of middle ear and mastoid, bilateral

✓4th **H75   Other disorders of middle ear and mastoid in diseases classified elsewhere**
Code first underlying disease

✓5th **H75.0   Mastoiditis in infectious and parasitic diseases classified elsewhere**
EXCLUDES 1   mastoiditis (in):
syphilis (A52.77)
tuberculosis (A18.03)
H75.00   *Mastoiditis in infectious and parasitic diseases classified elsewhere, unspecified ear*
H75.01   *Mastoiditis in infectious and parasitic diseases classified elsewhere, right ear*
H75.02   *Mastoiditis in infectious and parasitic diseases classified elsewhere, left ear*
H75.03   *Mastoiditis in infectious and parasitic diseases classified elsewhere, bilateral*

✓5th **H75.8   Other specified disorders of middle ear and mastoid in diseases classified elsewhere**
H75.80   *Other specified disorders of middle ear and mastoid in diseases classified elsewhere, unspecified ear*
H75.81   *Other specified disorders of right middle ear and mastoid in diseases classified elsewhere*
H75.82   *Other specified disorders of left middle ear and mastoid in diseases classified elsewhere*

N Newborn: 0   P Pediatric: 0-17   M Maternity: 12-55   A Adult: 15-124   MCC Major CC Condition   PDxMCC PDx acts as own MCC   CC CC Condition   PDxCC PDx acts as own CC

622   ICD-10-CM 2018

H75.83   *Other specified disorders of middle ear and mastoid in diseases classified elsewhere, bilateral*

Diseases of inner ear (H80-H83)

✓4ᵗʰ **H80**   **Otosclerosis**
     INCLUDES   otospongiosis

   ✓5ᵗʰ **H80.0**   **Otosclerosis involving oval window, nonobliterative**

       H80.00   **Otosclerosis involving oval window, nonobliterative, unspecified ear**

       H80.01   **Otosclerosis involving oval window, nonobliterative, right ear**

       H80.02   **Otosclerosis involving oval window, nonobliterative, left ear**

       H80.03   **Otosclerosis involving oval window, nonobliterative, bilateral**

   ✓5ᵗʰ **H80.1**   **Otosclerosis involving oval window, obliterative**

       H80.10   **Otosclerosis involving oval window, obliterative, unspecified ear**

       H80.11   **Otosclerosis involving oval window, obliterative, right ear**

       H80.12   **Otosclerosis involving oval window, obliterative, left ear**

       H80.13   **Otosclerosis involving oval window, obliterative, bilateral**

   ✓5ᵗʰ **H80.2**   **Cochlear otosclerosis**
       Otosclerosis involving otic capsule
       Otosclerosis involving round window

       H80.20   **Cochlear otosclerosis, unspecified ear**

       H80.21   **Cochlear otosclerosis, right ear**

       H80.22   **Cochlear otosclerosis, left ear**

       H80.23   **Cochlear otosclerosis, bilateral**

   ✓5ᵗʰ **H80.8**   **Other otosclerosis**

       H80.80   **Other otosclerosis, unspecified ear**

       H80.81   **Other otosclerosis, right ear**

       H80.82   **Other otosclerosis, left ear**

       H80.83   **Other otosclerosis, bilateral**

   ✓5ᵗʰ **H80.9**   **Unspecified otosclerosis**

       H80.90   **Unspecified otosclerosis, unspecified ear**

       H80.91   **Unspecified otosclerosis, right ear**

       H80.92   **Unspecified otosclerosis, left ear**

       H80.93   **Unspecified otosclerosis, bilateral**

✓4ᵗʰ **H81**   **Disorders of vestibular function**
     EXCLUDES 1   epidemic vertigo (A88.1)
                 vertigo NOS (R42)

   ✓5ᵗʰ **H81.0**   **Ménière's disease**
       Labyrinthine hydrops
       Ménière's syndrome or vertigo

       H81.01   **Ménière's disease, right ear**

       H81.02   **Ménière's disease, left ear**

       H81.03   **Ménière's disease, bilateral**

       H81.09   **Ménière's disease, unspecified ear**

   ✓5ᵗʰ **H81.1**   **Benign paroxysmal vertigo**

       H81.10   **Benign paroxysmal vertigo, unspecified ear**

       H81.11   **Benign paroxysmal vertigo, right ear**

       H81.12   **Benign paroxysmal vertigo, left ear**

       H81.13   **Benign paroxysmal vertigo, bilateral**

   ✓5ᵗʰ **H81.2**   **Vestibular neuronitis**
       DEF: Transient benign vertigo, caused by inflammation of the vestibular nerve; characterized by response to caloric stimulation on one side, nystagmus with rhythmic movement of eyes; normal auditory function present.

       H81.20   **Vestibular neuronitis, unspecified ear**

       H81.21   **Vestibular neuronitis, right ear**

       H81.22   **Vestibular neuronitis, left ear**

       H81.23   **Vestibular neuronitis, bilateral**

   ✓5ᵗʰ **H81.3**   **Other peripheral vertigo**

     ✓6ᵗʰ **H81.31**   **Aural vertigo**

         H81.311   **Aural vertigo, right ear**

         H81.312   **Aural vertigo, left ear**

         H81.313   **Aural vertigo, bilateral**

         H81.319   **Aural vertigo, unspecified ear**

     ✓6ᵗʰ **H81.39**   **Other peripheral vertigo**
         Lermoyez' syndrome
         Otogenic vertigo
         Peripheral vertigo NOS

         H81.391   **Other peripheral vertigo, right ear**

         H81.392   **Other peripheral vertigo, left ear**

         H81.393   **Other peripheral vertigo, bilateral**

         H81.399   **Other peripheral vertigo, unspecified ear**

   ✓5ᵗʰ **H81.4**   **Vertigo of central origin**
       Central positional nystagmus

       H81.41   **Vertigo of central origin, right ear**

       H81.42   **Vertigo of central origin, left ear**

       H81.43   **Vertigo of central origin, bilateral**

       H81.49   **Vertigo of central origin, unspecified ear**

   ✓5ᵗʰ **H81.8**   **Other disorders of vestibular function**

     ✓6ᵗʰ **H81.8X**   **Other disorders of vestibular function**

         H81.8X1   **Other disorders of vestibular function, right ear**

         H81.8X2   **Other disorders of vestibular function, left ear**

         H81.8X3   **Other disorders of vestibular function, bilateral**

         H81.8X9   **Other disorders of vestibular function, unspecified ear**

   ✓5ᵗʰ **H81.9**   **Unspecified disorder of vestibular function**
       Vertiginous syndrome NOS

       H81.90   **Unspecified disorder of vestibular function, unspecified ear**

       H81.91   **Unspecified disorder of vestibular function, right ear**

       H81.92   **Unspecified disorder of vestibular function, left ear**

       H81.93   **Unspecified disorder of vestibular function, bilateral**

✓4ᵗʰ **H82**   **Vertiginous syndromes in diseases classified elsewhere**
     Code first underlying disease
     EXCLUDES 1   epidemic vertigo (A88.1)

   H82.1   *Vertiginous syndromes in diseases classified elsewhere, right ear*

   H82.2   *Vertiginous syndromes in diseases classified elsewhere, left ear*

   H82.3   *Vertiginous syndromes in diseases classified elsewhere, bilateral*

   H82.9   *Vertiginous syndromes in diseases classified elsewhere, unspecified ear*

✓4ᵗʰ **H83**   **Other diseases of inner ear**

   ✓5ᵗʰ **H83.0**   **Labyrinthitis**
       DEF: Inflammation of the inner ear, or labyrinth; characterized by pus, vertigo, dizziness, nausea, and hearing loss.

       H83.01   **Labyrinthitis, right ear**

       H83.02   **Labyrinthitis, left ear**

       H83.03   **Labyrinthitis, bilateral**

       H83.09   **Labyrinthitis, unspecified ear**

   ✓5ᵗʰ **H83.1**   **Labyrinthine fistula**

       H83.11   **Labyrinthine fistula, right ear**

       H83.12   **Labyrinthine fistula, left ear**

       H83.13   **Labyrinthine fistula, bilateral**

       H83.19   **Labyrinthine fistula, unspecified ear**

   ✓5ᵗʰ **H83.2**   **Labyrinthine dysfunction**
       Labyrinthine hypersensitivity
       Labyrinthine hypofunction
       Labyrinthine loss of function
       DEF: Decreased function of the labyrinth sensors.

     ✓6ᵗʰ **H83.2X**   **Labyrinthine dysfunction**

         H83.2X1   **Labyrinthine dysfunction, right ear**

         H83.2X2   **Labyrinthine dysfunction, left ear**

         H83.2X3   **Labyrinthine dysfunction, bilateral**

         H83.2X9   **Labyrinthine dysfunction, unspecified ear**

   ✓5ᵗʰ **H83.3**   **Noise effects on inner ear**
       Acoustic trauma of inner ear
       Noise-induced hearing loss of inner ear

     ✓6ᵗʰ **H83.3X**   **Noise effects on inner ear**

         H83.3X1   **Noise effects on right inner ear**

         H83.3X2   **Noise effects on left inner ear**

         H83.3X3   **Noise effects on inner ear, bilateral**

         H83.3X9   **Noise effects on inner ear, unspecified ear**

✔ Additional Character Req   ✓x7ᵗʰ Placeholder Alert   Unacceptable PDx   Manifestation   **H1 - H14** HAC   **HCC** CMS-HCC Condition   **EXCLUDES 1** Not Coded Here   **EXCLUDES 2** Not Included Here

☑5ᵗʰ **H83.8** **Other specified diseases of inner ear**
 ☑6ᵗʰ **H83.8X** **Other specified diseases of inner ear**
  H83.8X1 **Other specified diseases of right inner ear**
  H83.8X2 **Other specified diseases of left inner ear**
  H83.8X3 **Other specified diseases of inner ear, bilateral**
  H83.8X9 **Other specified diseases of inner ear, unspecified ear**

☑5ᵗʰ **H83.9** **Unspecified disease of inner ear**
 H83.90 **Unspecified disease of inner ear, unspecified ear**
 H83.91 **Unspecified disease of right inner ear**
 H83.92 **Unspecified disease of left inner ear**
 H83.93 **Unspecified disease of inner ear, bilateral**

Other disorders of ear (H90-H94)

☑4ᵗʰ **H90** **Conductive and sensorineural hearing loss**
 EXCLUDES 1 *deaf nonspeaking NEC (H91.3)*
  deafness NOS (H91.9-)
  hearing loss NOS (H91.9-)
  noise-induced hearing loss (H83.3-)
  ototoxic hearing loss (H91.0-)
  sudden (idiopathic) hearing loss (H91.2-)
 AHA: 2015, 2Q, 7
 H90.0 **Conductive hearing loss, bilateral**

☑5ᵗʰ **H90.1** **Conductive hearing loss, unilateral with unrestricted hearing on the contralateral side**
 H90.11 **Conductive hearing loss, unilateral, right ear, with unrestricted hearing on the contralateral side**
 H90.12 **Conductive hearing loss, unilateral, left ear, with unrestricted hearing on the contralateral side**

 H90.2 **Conductive hearing loss, unspecified**
  Conductive deafness NOS

 H90.3 **Sensorineural hearing loss, bilateral**

☑5ᵗʰ **H90.4** **Sensorineural hearing loss, unilateral with unrestricted hearing on the contralateral side**
 H90.41 **Sensorineural hearing loss, unilateral, right ear, with unrestricted hearing on the contralateral side**
 H90.42 **Sensorineural hearing loss, unilateral, left ear, with unrestricted hearing on the contralateral side**

 H90.5 **Unspecified sensorineural hearing loss**
  Central hearing loss NOS Perceptive hearing loss NOS
  Congenital deafness NOS Sensorineural deafness NOS
  Neural hearing loss NOS Sensory hearing loss NOS
  EXCLUDES 1 *abnormal auditory perception (H93.2-)*
   psychogenic deafness (F44.6)

 H90.6 **Mixed conductive and sensorineural hearing loss, bilateral**
  AHA: 2015, 2Q, 7

☑5ᵗʰ **H90.7** **Mixed conductive and sensorineural hearing loss, unilateral with unrestricted hearing on the contralateral side**
 H90.71 **Mixed conductive and sensorineural hearing loss, unilateral, right ear, with unrestricted hearing on the contralateral side**
 H90.72 **Mixed conductive and sensorineural hearing loss, unilateral, left ear, with unrestricted hearing on the contralateral side**

 H90.8 **Mixed conductive and sensorineural hearing loss, unspecified**

☑5ᵗʰ **H90.A** **Conductive and sensorineural hearing loss with restricted hearing on the contralateral side**
 ☑6ᵗʰ **H90.A1** **Conductive hearing loss, unilateral, with restricted hearing on the contralateral side**
  H90.A11 **Conductive hearing loss, unilateral, right ear with restricted hearing on the contralateral side**
  H90.A12 **Conductive hearing loss, unilateral, left ear with restricted hearing on the contralateral side**
 ☑6ᵗʰ **H90.A2** **Sensorineural hearing loss, unilateral, with restricted hearing on the contralateral side**
  H90.A21 **Sensorineural hearing loss, unilateral, right ear, with restricted hearing on the contralateral side**
  H90.A22 **Sensorineural hearing loss, unilateral, left ear, with restricted hearing on the contralateral side**

☑6ᵗʰ **H90.A3** **Mixed conductive and sensorineural hearing loss, unilateral with restricted hearing on the contralateral side**
 H90.A31 **Mixed conductive and sensorineural hearing loss, unilateral, right ear with restricted hearing on the contralateral side**
 H90.A32 **Mixed conductive and sensorineural hearing loss, unilateral, left ear with restricted hearing on the contralateral side**

☑4ᵗʰ **H91** **Other and unspecified hearing loss**
 EXCLUDES 1 *abnormal auditory perception (H93.2-)*
  hearing loss as classified in H90-
  impacted cerumen (H61.2-)
  noise-induced hearing loss (H83.3-)
  psychogenic deafness (F44.6)
  transient ischemic deafness (H93.01-)

☑5ᵗʰ **H91.0** **Ototoxic hearing loss**
 Code first poisoning due to drug or toxin, if applicable (T36-T65 with fifth or sixth character 1-4 or 6)
 Use additional code for adverse effect, if applicable, to identify drug (T36-T50 with fifth or sixth character 5)
 H91.01 **Ototoxic hearing loss, right ear**
 H91.02 **Ototoxic hearing loss, left ear**
 H91.03 **Ototoxic hearing loss, bilateral**
 H91.09 **Ototoxic hearing loss, unspecified ear**

☑5ᵗʰ **H91.1** **Presbycusis**
 Presbyacusia
 H91.10 **Presbycusis, unspecified ear**
 H91.11 **Presbycusis, right ear**
 H91.12 **Presbycusis, left ear**
 H91.13 **Presbycusis, bilateral**

☑5ᵗʰ **H91.2** **Sudden idiopathic hearing loss**
 Sudden hearing loss NOS
 H91.20 **Sudden idiopathic hearing loss, unspecified ear**
 H91.21 **Sudden idiopathic hearing loss, right ear**
 H91.22 **Sudden idiopathic hearing loss, left ear**
 H91.23 **Sudden idiopathic hearing loss, bilateral**

 H91.3 **Deaf nonspeaking, not elsewhere classified**

☑5ᵗʰ **H91.8** **Other specified hearing loss**
 ☑6ᵗʰ **H91.8X** **Other specified hearing loss**
  H91.8X1 **Other specified hearing loss, right ear**
  H91.8X2 **Other specified hearing loss, left ear**
  H91.8X3 **Other specified hearing loss, bilateral**
  H91.8X9 **Other specified hearing loss, unspecified ear**

☑5ᵗʰ **H91.9** **Unspecified hearing loss**
 Deafness NOS
 High frequency deafness
 Low frequency deafness
 H91.90 **Unspecified hearing loss, unspecified ear**
 H91.91 **Unspecified hearing loss, right ear**
 H91.92 **Unspecified hearing loss, left ear**
 H91.93 **Unspecified hearing loss, bilateral**

☑4ᵗʰ **H92** **Otalgia and effusion of ear**
☑5ᵗʰ **H92.0** **Otalgia**
 H92.01 **Otalgia, right ear**
 H92.02 **Otalgia, left ear**
 H92.03 **Otalgia, bilateral**
 H92.09 **Otalgia, unspecified ear**

☑5ᵗʰ **H92.1** **Otorrhea**
 EXCLUDES 1 *leakage of cerebrospinal fluid through ear (G96.0)*
 H92.10 **Otorrhea, unspecified ear**
 H92.11 **Otorrhea, right ear**
 H92.12 **Otorrhea, left ear**
 H92.13 **Otorrhea, bilateral**

☑5ᵗʰ **H92.2** **Otorrhagia**
 EXCLUDES 1 *traumatic otorrhagia—code to injury*
 H92.20 **Otorrhagia, unspecified ear**
 H92.21 **Otorrhagia, right ear**
 H92.22 **Otorrhagia, left ear**
 H92.23 **Otorrhagia, bilateral**

☑4ᵗʰ **H93** **Other disorders of ear, not elsewhere classified**

☑5ᵗʰ **H93.0** **Degenerative and vascular disorders of ear**
     EXCLUDES 1   *presbycusis (H91.1)*

  ☑6ᵗʰ **H93.01** **Transient ischemic deafness**
       H93.011 **Transient ischemic deafness, right ear**
       H93.012 **Transient ischemic deafness, left ear**
       H93.013 **Transient ischemic deafness, bilateral**
       H93.019 **Transient ischemic deafness, unspecified ear**

  ☑6ᵗʰ **H93.09** **Unspecified degenerative and vascular disorders of ear**
       H93.091 **Unspecified degenerative and vascular disorders of right ear**
       H93.092 **Unspecified degenerative and vascular disorders of left ear**
       H93.093 **Unspecified degenerative and vascular disorders of ear, bilateral**
       H93.099 **Unspecified degenerative and vascular disorders of unspecified ear**

☑5ᵗʰ **H93.1** **Tinnitus**
       H93.11 **Tinnitus, right ear**
       H93.12 **Tinnitus, left ear**
       H93.13 **Tinnitus, bilateral**
       H93.19 **Tinnitus, unspecified ear**

☑5ᵗʰ **H93.A** **Pulsatile Tinnitus**
       H93.A1 **Pulsatile tinnitus, right ear**
       H93.A2 **Pulsatile tinnitus, left ear**
       H93.A3 **Pulsatile tinnitus, bilateral**
       H93.A9 **Pulsatile tinnitus, unspecified ear**

☑5ᵗʰ **H93.2** **Other abnormal auditory perceptions**
     EXCLUDES 2   *auditory hallucinations (R44.0)*

  ☑6ᵗʰ **H93.21** **Auditory recruitment**
       H93.211 **Auditory recruitment, right ear**
       H93.212 **Auditory recruitment, left ear**
       H93.213 **Auditory recruitment, bilateral**
       H93.219 **Auditory recruitment, unspecified ear**

  ☑6ᵗʰ **H93.22** **Diplacusis**
       H93.221 **Diplacusis, right ear**
       H93.222 **Diplacusis, left ear**
       H93.223 **Diplacusis, bilateral**
       H93.229 **Diplacusis, unspecified ear**

  ☑6ᵗʰ **H93.23** **Hyperacusis**
     DEF: Exceptionally acute sense of hearing caused by such conditions as Bell's palsy; this term may also refer to painful sensitivity to sounds.
       H93.231 **Hyperacusis, right ear**
       H93.232 **Hyperacusis, left ear**
       H93.233 **Hyperacusis, bilateral**
       H93.239 **Hyperacusis, unspecified ear**

  ☑6ᵗʰ **H93.24** **Temporary auditory threshold shift**
       H93.241 **Temporary auditory threshold shift, right ear**
       H93.242 **Temporary auditory threshold shift, left ear**
       H93.243 **Temporary auditory threshold shift, bilateral**
       H93.249 **Temporary auditory threshold shift, unspecified ear**

       H93.25 **Central auditory processing disorder**
         Congenital auditory imperception
         Word deafness
        EXCLUDES 1   *mixed receptive-expressive language disorder (F80.2)*

  ☑6ᵗʰ **H93.29** **Other abnormal auditory perceptions**
       H93.291 **Other abnormal auditory perceptions, right ear**
       H93.292 **Other abnormal auditory perceptions, left ear**
       H93.293 **Other abnormal auditory perceptions, bilateral**
       H93.299 **Other abnormal auditory perceptions, unspecified ear**

☑5ᵗʰ **H93.3** **Disorders of acoustic nerve**
     Disorder of 8th cranial nerve
     EXCLUDES 1   *acoustic neuroma (D33.3)*
           syphilitic acoustic neuritis (A52.15)

  ☑6ᵗʰ **H93.3X** **Disorders of acoustic nerve**
       H93.3X1 **Disorders of right acoustic nerve**
       H93.3X2 **Disorders of left acoustic nerve**
       H93.3X3 **Disorders of bilateral acoustic nerves**
       H93.3X9 **Disorders of unspecified acoustic nerve**

☑5ᵗʰ **H93.8** **Other specified disorders of ear**
  ☑6ᵗʰ **H93.8X** **Other specified disorders of ear**
       H93.8X1 **Other specified disorders of right ear**
       H93.8X2 **Other specified disorders of left ear**
       H93.8X3 **Other specified disorders of ear, bilateral**
       H93.8X9 **Other specified disorders of ear, unspecified ear**

☑5ᵗʰ **H93.9** **Unspecified disorder of ear**
       H93.90 **Unspecified disorder of ear, unspecified ear**
       H93.91 **Unspecified disorder of right ear**
       H93.92 **Unspecified disorder of left ear**
       H93.93 **Unspecified disorder of ear, bilateral**

☑4ᵗʰ **H94** **Other disorders of ear in diseases classified elsewhere**

☑5ᵗʰ **H94.0** **Acoustic neuritis in infectious and parasitic diseases classified elsewhere**
     Code first underlying disease, such as:
       parasitic disease (B65-B89)
     EXCLUDES 1   *acoustic neuritis (in):*
           herpes zoster (B02.29)
           syphilis (A52.15)

       H94.00   *Acoustic neuritis in infectious and parasitic diseases classified elsewhere, unspecified ear*
       H94.01   *Acoustic neuritis in infectious and parasitic diseases classified elsewhere, right ear*
       H94.02   *Acoustic neuritis in infectious and parasitic diseases classified elsewhere, left ear*
       H94.03   *Acoustic neuritis in infectious and parasitic diseases classified elsewhere, bilateral*

☑5ᵗʰ **H94.8** **Other specified disorders of ear in diseases classified elsewhere**
     Code first underlying disease, such as:
       congenital syphilis (A50.0)
     EXCLUDES 1   *aural myiasis (B87.4)*
           syphilitic labyrinthitis (A52.79)

       H94.80   *Other specified disorders of ear in diseases classified elsewhere, unspecified ear*
       H94.81   *Other specified disorders of right ear in diseases classified elsewhere*
       H94.82   *Other specified disorders of left ear in diseases classified elsewhere*
       H94.83   *Other specified disorders of ear in diseases classified elsewhere, bilateral*

Intraoperative and postprocedural complications and disorders of ear and mastoid process, not elsewhere classified (H95)

☑4ᵗʰ **H95** **Intraoperative and postprocedural complications and disorders of ear and mastoid process, not elsewhere classified**

☑5ᵗʰ **H95.0** **Recurrent cholesteatoma of postmastoidectomy cavity**
       H95.00 **Recurrent cholesteatoma of postmastoidectomy cavity, unspecified ear**
       H95.01 **Recurrent cholesteatoma of postmastoidectomy cavity, right ear**
       H95.02 **Recurrent cholesteatoma of postmastoidectomy cavity, left ear**
       H95.03 **Recurrent cholesteatoma of postmastoidectomy cavity, bilateral ears**

☑5ᵗʰ **H95.1** **Other disorders of ear and mastoid process following mastoidectomy**
  ☑6ᵗʰ **H95.11** **Chronic inflammation of postmastoidectomy cavity**
       H95.111 **Chronic inflammation of postmastoidectomy cavity, right ear**
       H95.112 **Chronic inflammation of postmastoidectomy cavity, left ear**
       H95.113 **Chronic inflammation of postmastoidectomy cavity, bilateral ears**

☑ Additional Character Req   ✓x7ᵗʰ Placeholder Alert   Unacceptable PDx   Manifestation   **H1**-**H14** HAC   **HCC** CMS-HCC Condition   **EXCLUDES 1** Not Coded Here   **EXCLUDES 2** Not Included Here

Chapter 8. Diseases of the Ear and Mastoid Process

      H95.119   **Chronic inflammation of postmastoidectomy cavity,** unspecified ear

✓6ᵗʰ   H95.12   **Granulation of postmastoidectomy cavity**

      H95.121   **Granulation of postmastoidectomy cavity,** right ear

      H95.122   **Granulation of postmastoidectomy cavity,** left ear

      H95.123   **Granulation of postmastoidectomy cavity,** bilateral ears

      H95.129   **Granulation of postmastoidectomy cavity,** unspecified ear

✓6ᵗʰ   H95.13   **Mucosal cyst of postmastoidectomy cavity**

      H95.131   **Mucosal cyst of postmastoidectomy cavity,** right ear

      H95.132   **Mucosal cyst of postmastoidectomy cavity,** left ear

      H95.133   **Mucosal cyst of postmastoidectomy cavity,** bilateral ears

      H95.139   **Mucosal cyst of postmastoidectomy cavity,** unspecified ear

✓6ᵗʰ   H95.19   **Other disorders following mastoidectomy**

      H95.191   **Other disorders following mastoidectomy,** right ear

      H95.192   **Other disorders following mastoidectomy,** left ear

      H95.193   **Other disorders following mastoidectomy,** bilateral ears

      H95.199   **Other disorders following mastoidectomy,** unspecified ear

✓5ᵗʰ   H95.2   **Intraoperative hemorrhage and hematoma** of ear and mastoid process complicating a procedure

      EXCLUDES 1   *intraoperative hemorrhage and hematoma of ear and mastoid process due to accidental puncture or laceration during a procedure (H95.3-)*

      H95.21   **Intraoperative hemorrhage and hematoma of ear and mastoid process complicating a procedure on the ear and mastoid process**   `CC`
           CC Excl: PDX collection 642

      H95.22   **Intraoperative hemorrhage and hematoma of of ear and mastoid process complicating** other procedure   `CC`
           CC Excl: PDX collection 642

✓5ᵗʰ   H95.3   **Accidental puncture and laceration** of ear and mastoid process during a procedure

      H95.31   **Accidental puncture and laceration of the ear and mastoid process** during a procedure on the ear and mastoid process   `CC`
           CC Excl: PDX collection 509

      H95.32   **Accidental puncture and laceration of the ear and mastoid process** during other procedure   `CC`
           CC Excl: PDX collection 509

✓5ᵗʰ   H95.4   **Postprocedural hemorrhage** of ear and mastoid process following a procedure

      H95.41   **Postprocedural hemorrhage of ear and mastoid process following a** procedure on the ear and mastoid process   `CC`
           CC Excl: PDX collection 642

      H95.42   **Postprocedural hemorrhage of ear and mastoid process following** other procedure   `CC`
           CC Excl: PDX collection 642

✓5ᵗʰ   H95.5   **Postprocedural hematoma and seroma** of ear and mastoid process following a procedure

      CC Excl: For CC codes in subcategory H95.5: PDX collection 642

      H95.51   **Postprocedural hematoma of ear and mastoid process following a** procedure on the ear and mastoid process   `CC`

      H95.52   **Postprocedural hematoma of ear and mastoid process following** other procedure   `CC`

      H95.53   **Postprocedural seroma of ear and mastoid process following a** procedure on the ear and mastoid process   `CC`

      H95.54   **Postprocedural seroma of ear and mastoid process following** other procedure   `CC`

✓5ᵗʰ   H95.8   **Other intraoperative and postprocedural complications and disorders of the ear and mastoid process, not elsewhere classified**

      EXCLUDES 2   *postprocedural complications and disorders following mastoidectomy (H95.0-, H95.1-)*

      CC Excl: For CC codes in subcategory H95.8: PDX collection 643

✓6ᵗʰ   H95.81   **Postprocedural stenosis** of external ear canal

      H95.811   **Postprocedural stenosis of** right **external ear canal**   `CC`

      H95.812   **Postprocedural stenosis of** left **external ear canal**   `CC`

      H95.813   **Postprocedural stenosis of external ear canal,** bilateral   `CC`

      H95.819   **Postprocedural stenosis of** unspecified **external ear canal**   `CC`

      H95.88   **Other intraoperative complications and disorders of the ear and mastoid process, not elsewhere classified**   `CC`
           Use additional code, if applicable, to further specify disorder

      H95.89   **Other postprocedural complications and disorders of the ear and mastoid process, not elsewhere classified**   `CC`
           Use additional code, if applicable, to further specify disorder

N Newborn: 0   P Pediatric: 0-17   M Maternity: 12-55   A Adult: 15-124   MCC Major CC Condition   PDxMCC PDx acts as own MCC   CC CC Condition   PDxCC PDx acts as own CC

626   ICD-10-CM 2018

Chapter 9. Diseases of the Circulatory System (I00–I99)

Chapter Specific Guidelines with Coding Examples

The chapter specific guidelines from the ICD-10-CM Official Guidelines for Coding and Reporting have been provided below. Along with these guidelines are coding examples, contained in the shaded boxes, that have been developed to help illustrate the coding and/or sequencing guidance found in these guidelines.

a. Hypertension

The classification presumes a causal relationship between hypertension and heart involvement and between hypertension and kidney involvement, as the two conditions are linked by the term "with" in the Alphabetic Index. These conditions should be coded as related even in the absence of provider documentation explicitly linking them, unless the documentation clearly states the conditions are unrelated.

For hypertension and conditions not specifically linked by relational terms such as "with," "associated with" or "due to" in the classification, provider documentation must link the conditions in order to code them as related.

1) Hypertension with heart disease

Hypertension with heart conditions classified to I50.- or I51.4-I51.9, are assigned to a code from category I11, Hypertensive heart disease. Use additional code(s) from category I50, Heart failure, to identify the type(s) of heart failure in those patients with heart failure.

The same heart conditions (I50.-, I51.4-I51.9) with hypertension are coded separately if the provider has specifically documented a different cause. Sequence according to the circumstances of the admission/encounter.

> Patient is admitted in left heart failure. Patient also has a history of hypertension managed by medication.
>
> **11.0**   **Hypertensive heart disease with heart failure**
>
> **I50.1**   **Left ventricular failure, unspecified**
>
> *Explanation*: Without a diagnostic statement to the contrary, hypertension and heart failure have an assumed causal relationship, and a combination code should be used. An additional code to identify the type of heart failure (I50.-) should also be provided.

2) Hypertensive chronic kidney disease

Assign codes from category I12, Hypertensive chronic kidney disease, when both hypertension and a condition classifiable to category N18, Chronic kidney disease (CKD), are present. CKD should not be coded as hypertensive if the physician has specifically documented a different cause.

The appropriate code from category N18 should be used as a secondary code with a code from category I12 to identify the stage of chronic kidney disease.

See Section I.C.14. Chronic kidney disease.

If a patient has hypertensive chronic kidney disease and acute renal failure, an additional code for the acute renal failure is required.

> Patient is admitted with stage IV chronic kidney disease (CKD). The patient also has documented hypertension secondary to primary hyperparathyroidism.
>
> **N18.4**   **Chronic kidney disease, stage 4 (severe)**
>
> **I10**   **Essential (primary) hypertension**
>
> **E21.0**   **Primary hyperparathyroidism**
>
> *Explanation*: A combination code describing a relationship between hypertension and CKD is not used due to the physician documentation identifying the primary hyperparathyroidism as the cause for the hypertension.

3) Hypertensive heart and chronic kidney disease

Assign codes from combination category I13, Hypertensive heart and chronic kidney disease, when there is hypertension with both heart and kidney involvement. If heart failure is present, assign an additional code from category I50 to identify the type of heart failure.

The appropriate code from category N18, Chronic kidney disease, should be used as a secondary code with a code from category I13 to identify the stage of chronic kidney disease.

See Section I.C.14. Chronic kidney disease.

The codes in category I13, Hypertensive heart and chronic kidney disease, are combination codes that include hypertension, heart disease and chronic kidney disease. The Includes note at I13 specifies that the conditions included at I11 and I12 are included together in I13. If a patient

has hypertension, heart disease and chronic kidney disease, then a code from I13 should be used, not individual codes for hypertension, heart disease and chronic kidney disease, or codes from I11 or I12.

For patients with both acute renal failure and chronic kidney disease, an additional code for acute renal failure is required.

> Hypertensive heart and kidney disease with congestive heart failure and stage 2 chronic kidney disease
>
> **I13.0**   **Hypertensive heart and chronic kidney disease with heart failure and stage 1 through stage 4 chronic kidney disease, or unspecified chronic kidney disease**
>
> **I50.9**   **Heart failure, unspecified**
>
> **N18.2**   **Chronic kidney disease, stage 2 (mild)**
>
> *Explanation*: Combination codes in category I13 are used to report conditions classifiable to *both* categories I11 and I12. Do not report conditions classifiable to I11 and I12 separately. Use additional codes to report type of heart failure and stage of CKD.

4) Hypertensive cerebrovascular disease

For hypertensive cerebrovascular disease, first assign the appropriate code from categories I60-I69, followed by the appropriate hypertension code.

> Rupture of cerebral aneurysm caused by malignant hypertension
>
> **I60.7**   **Nontraumatic subarachnoid hemorrhage from unspecified intracranial artery**
>
> **I10**   **Essential (primary) hypertension**
>
> *Explanation*: Hypertensive cerebrovascular disease requires two codes: the appropriate I60–I69 code followed by the appropriate hypertension code.

5) Hypertensive retinopathy

Subcategory H35.0, Background retinopathy and retinal vascular changes, should be used with a code from category I10 – I15, Hypertensive disease to include the systemic hypertension. The sequencing is based on the reason for the encounter.

> Hypertensive retinopathy of the right eye
>
> **H35.031**   **Hypertensive retinopathy, right eye**
>
> **I10**   **Essential (primary) hypertension**
>
> *Explanation*: Hypertensive retinopathy requires two codes: the appropriate subcategory H35.0 code and a code for the hypertension.

6) Hypertension, secondary

Secondary hypertension is due to an underlying condition. Two codes are required: one to identify the underlying etiology and one from category I15 to identify the hypertension. Sequencing of codes is determined by the reason for admission/encounter.

> Renovascular hypertension due to renal artery atherosclerosis
>
> **I15.0**   **Renovascular hypertension**
>
> **I70.1**   **Atherosclerosis of renal artery**
>
> *Explanation*: Secondary hypertension requires two codes: a code to identify the etiology and the appropriate I15 code.

7) Hypertension, transient

Assign code R03.0, Elevated blood pressure reading without diagnosis of hypertension, unless patient has an established diagnosis of hypertension. Assign code O13.-, Gestational [pregnancy-induced] hypertension without significant proteinuria, or O14.-, Pre-eclampsia, for transient hypertension of pregnancy.

8) Hypertension, controlled

This diagnostic statement usually refers to an existing state of hypertension under control by therapy. Assign the appropriate code from categories I10-I15, Hypertensive diseases.

9) Hypertension, uncontrolled

Uncontrolled hypertension may refer to untreated hypertension or hypertension not responding to current therapeutic regimen. In either case, assign the appropriate code from categories I10-I15, Hypertensive diseases.

10) Hypertensive crisis

Assign a code from category I16, Hypertensive crisis, for documented hypertensive urgency, hypertensive emergency or unspecified hypertensive crisis. Code also any identified hypertensive disease (I10-I15). The sequencing is based on the reason for the encounter.

10) Pulmonary hypertension

Pulmonary hypertension is classified to category I27, Other pulmonary heart diseases. For secondary pulmonary hypertension (I27.1, I27.2-), code also any associated conditions or adverse effects of drugs or toxins. The sequencing is based on the reason for the encounter.

b. Atherosclerotic coronary artery disease and angina

ICD-10-CM has combination codes for atherosclerotic heart disease with angina pectoris. The subcategories for these codes are I25.11, Atherosclerotic heart disease of native coronary artery with angina pectoris and I25.7, Atherosclerosis of coronary artery bypass graft(s) and coronary artery of transplanted heart with angina pectoris.

When using one of these combination codes it is not necessary to use an additional code for angina pectoris. A causal relationship can be assumed in a patient with both atherosclerosis and angina pectoris, unless the documentation indicates the angina is due to something other than the atherosclerosis.

If a patient with coronary artery disease is admitted due to an acute myocardial infarction (AMI), the AMI should be sequenced before the coronary artery disease.

See Section I.C.9. Acute myocardial infarction (AMI)

Patient is being seen for spastic angina pectoris. She also has a documented history of progressive coronary artery disease of the native vessels.

I25.111   **Atherosclerotic heart disease of native coronary artery with angina pectoris with documented spasm**

Explanation: Report the combination code for atherosclerotic heart disease (coronary artery disease) with angina pectoris. A causal relationship is assumed in a patient with both atherosclerosis and angina pectoris, unless the documentation indicates the angina is due to something other than the atherosclerosis. When using one of these combination codes, it is not necessary to use an additional code for angina pectoris.

c. Intraoperative and postprocedural cerebrovascular accident

Medical record documentation should clearly specify the cause- and- effect relationship between the medical intervention and the cerebrovascular accident in order to assign a code for intraoperative or postprocedural cerebrovascular accident.

Proper code assignment depends on whether it was an infarction or hemorrhage and whether it occurred intraoperatively or postoperatively. If it was a cerebral hemorrhage, code assignment depends on the type of procedure performed.

Embolic cerebral infarction of the right middle cerebral artery that occurred during hip replacement surgery. The surgeon documented as due to the surgery.

I97.811   **Intraoperative cerebrovascular infarction during other surgery**

I63.411   **Cerebral infarction due to embolism of right middle cerebral artery**

Explanation: Code assignment for intraoperative or postprocedural cerebrovascular accident is based on the provider's documentation of a cause-and-effect relationship between the condition and the procedure. Proper code assignment also depends on whether the cerebrovascular accident was an infarction or hemorrhage, occurred intraoperatively or postoperatively, and the type of procedure performed.

d. Sequelae of cerebrovascular disease

1) Category I69, Sequelae of cerebrovascular disease

Category I69 is used to indicate conditions classifiable to categories I60-I67 as the causes of sequela (neurologic deficits), themselves classified elsewhere. These "late effects" include neurologic deficits that persist after initial onset of conditions classifiable to categories I60-I67. The neurologic deficits caused by cerebrovascular disease may be present from the onset or may arise at any time after the onset of the condition classifiable to categories I60-I67.

Codes from category I69, Sequelae of cerebrovascular disease, that specify hemiplegia, hemiparesis and monoplegia identify whether the dominant or nondominant side is affected. Should the affected side be documented, but not specified as dominant or nondominant, and the classification system does not indicate a default, code selection is as follows:

- For ambidextrous patients, the default should be dominant.
- If the left side is affected, the default is non-dominant.
- If the right side is affected, the default is dominant.

2) Codes from category I69 with codes from I60–I67

Codes from category I69 may be assigned on a health care record with codes from I60-I67, if the patient has a current cerebrovascular disease and deficits from an old cerebrovascular disease.

3) Codes from category I69 and personal history of transient ischemic attack (TIA) and cerebral infarction (Z86.73)

Codes from category I69 should not be assigned if the patient does not have neurologic deficits.

See Section I.C.21. 4. History (of) for use of personal history codes

e. Acute myocardial infarction (AMI)

1) Type 1 ST elevation myocardial infarction (STEMI) and non ST elevation myocardial infarction (NSTEMI)

The ICD-10-CM codes for **type 1** acute myocardial infarction (AMI) identify the site, such as anterolateral wall or true posterior wall. Subcategories I21.0-I21.2 and code I21.3 are used for **type 1** ST elevation myocardial infarction (STEMI). Code I21.4, Non-ST elevation (NSTEMI) myocardial infarction, is used for **type 1** non ST elevation myocardial infarction (NSTEMI) and nontransmural MIs.

If **a type 1** NSTEMI evolves to STEMI, assign the STEMI code. If **a type 1** STEMI converts to NSTEMI due to thrombolytic therapy, it is still coded as STEMI.

For encounters occurring while the myocardial infarction is equal to, or less than, four weeks old, including transfers to another acute setting or a postacute setting, and the myocardial infarction meets the definition for "other diagnoses" (see Section III, Reporting Additional Diagnoses), codes from category I21 may continue to be reported. For encounters after the 4 week time frame and the patient is still receiving care related to the myocardial infarction, the appropriate aftercare code should be assigned, rather than a code from category I21. For old or healed myocardial infarctions not requiring further care, code I25.2, Old myocardial infarction, may be assigned.

2) Acute myocardial infarction, unspecified

Code **I21.9, Acute myocardial infarction, unspecified,** is the default for unspecified acute myocardial infarction **or unspecified type**. If only **type 1** STEMI or transmural MI without the site is documented, assign code I21.3, **ST elevation (STEMI) myocardial infarction of unspecified site**.

3) AMI documented as nontransmural or subendocardial but site provided

If an AMI is documented as nontransmural or subendocardial, but the site is provided, it is still coded as a subendocardial AMI.

See Section I.C.21.3 for information on coding status post administration of tPA in a different facility within the last 24 hours.

4) Subsequent acute myocardial infarction

A code from category I22, Subsequent ST elevation (STEMI) and non-ST elevation (NSTEMI) myocardial infarction, is to be used when a patient who has suffered **a type 1 or unspecified** AMI has a new AMI within the 4 week time frame of the initial AMI. A code from category I22 must be used in conjunction with a code from category I21. The sequencing of the I22 and I21 codes depends on the circumstances of the encounter.

Do not assign code I22 for subsequent myocardial infarctions other than type 1 or unspecified. For subsequent type 2 AMI assign only code I21.A1. For subsequent type 4 or type 5 AMI, assign only code I21.A9.

5) Other types of myocardial infarction

The ICD-10-CM provides codes for different types of myocardial infarction. Type 1 myocardial infarctions are assigned to codes I21.0-I21.4.

Type 2 myocardial infarction, and myocardial infarction due to demand ischemia or secondary to ischemic balance, is assigned to code I21.A1, Myocardial infarction type 2 with a code for the underlying cause. Do not assign code I24.8, Other forms of acute ischemic heart disease for the demand ischemia. Sequencing of type 2 AMI or the underlying cause is dependent on the circumstances of admission. When a type 2 AMI code is described as NSTEMI or STEMI, only assign code I21.A1. Codes I21.01-I21.4 should only be assigned for type 1 AMIs.

Acute myocardial infarctions type 3, 4a, 4b, 4c and 5 are assigned to code I21.A9, Other myocardial infarction type.

The "Code also" and "Code first" notes should be followed related to complications, and for coding of postprocedural myocardial infarctions during or following cardiac surgery.

Chapter 9. Diseases of the Circulatory System (I00-I99)

> **EXCLUDES 2**   certain conditions originating in the perinatal period (P04-P96)
> certain infectious and parasitic diseases (A00-B99)
> complications of pregnancy, childbirth and the puerperium (O00-O9A)
> congenital malformations, deformations, and chromosomal abnormalities (Q00-Q99)
> endocrine, nutritional and metabolic diseases (E00-E88)
> injury, poisoning and certain other consequences of external causes (S00-T88)
> neoplasms (C00-D49)
> symptoms, signs and abnormal clinical and laboratory findings, not elsewhere classified (R00-R94)
> systemic connective tissue disorders (M30-M36)
> transient cerebral ischemic attacks and related syndromes (G45.-)

This chapter contains the following blocks:

I00-I02	Acute rheumatic fever
I05-I09	Chronic rheumatic heart diseases
I10-I16	Hypertensive diseases
I20-I25	Ischemic heart diseases
I26-I28	Pulmonary heart disease and diseases of pulmonary circulation
I30-I52	Other forms of heart disease
I60-I69	Cerebrovascular diseases
I70-I79	Diseases of arteries, arterioles and capillaries
I80-I89	Diseases of veins, lymphatic vessels and lymph nodes, not elsewhere classified
I95-I99	Other and unspecified disorders of the circulatory system

Acute rheumatic fever (I00-I02)

I00   **Rheumatic fever without heart involvement**
> **INCLUDES**   arthritis, rheumatic, acute or subacute
> **EXCLUDES 1**   rheumatic fever with heart involvement (I01.0-I01.9)

✓4ᵗʰ I01   **Rheumatic fever with heart involvement**
> **EXCLUDES 1**   chronic diseases of rheumatic origin (I05-I09) unless rheumatic fever is also present or there is evidence of reactivation or activity of the rheumatic process.

   I01.0   **Acute rheumatic pericarditis**   **CC**
     Any condition in I00 with pericarditis
     Rheumatic pericarditis (acute)
>   **EXCLUDES 1**   acute pericarditis not specified as rheumatic (I30.-)
     CC Excl: PDX collection 188

   I01.1   **Acute rheumatic endocarditis**   **CC**
     Any condition in I00 with endocarditis or valvulitis
     Acute rheumatic valvulitis
     CC Excl: PDX collection 644

   I01.2   **Acute rheumatic myocarditis**   **CC**
     Any condition in I00 with myocarditis
     CC Excl: PDX collection 186

   I01.8   **Other acute rheumatic heart disease**   **CC**
     Any condition in I00 with other or multiple types of heart involvement
     Acute rheumatic pancarditis
     CC Excl: PDX collection 645

   I01.9   **Acute rheumatic heart disease, unspecified**   **CC**
     Any condition in I00 with unspecified type of heart involvement
     Rheumatic carditis, acute
     Rheumatic heart disease, active or acute
     CC Excl: PDX collection 646

✓4ᵗʰ I02   **Rheumatic chorea**
> **INCLUDES**   Sydenham's chorea
> **EXCLUDES 1**   chorea NOS (G25.5)
> Huntington's chorea (G10)

   I02.0   **Rheumatic chorea with heart involvement**   **CC**
     Chorea NOS with heart involvement
     Rheumatic chorea with heart involvement of any type classifiable under I01-
     CC Excl: PDX collection 645

   I02.9   **Rheumatic chorea without heart involvement**   **CC**
     Rheumatic chorea NOS
     CC Excl: PDX collection 646

Chronic rheumatic heart diseases (I05-I09)

✓4ᵗʰ I05   **Rheumatic mitral valve diseases**
> **INCLUDES**   conditions classifiable to both I05.0 and I05.2-I05.9, whether specified as rheumatic or not
> **EXCLUDES 1**   mitral valve disease specified as nonrheumatic (I34.-)
> mitral valve disease with aortic and/or tricuspid valve involvement (I08.-)

   I05.0   **Rheumatic mitral stenosis**
     Mitral (valve) obstruction (rheumatic)
     DEF: Narrowing of mitral valve between left atrium and left ventricle; due to rheumatic fever; characterized by shortness of breath during or after exercise, fatigue, palpitations, chest discomfort, and swelling of feet or legs.

   I05.1   **Rheumatic mitral insufficiency**
     Rheumatic mitral incompetence
     Rheumatic mitral regurgitation
>   **EXCLUDES 1**   mitral insufficiency not specified as rheumatic (I34.0)

   I05.2   **Rheumatic mitral stenosis with insufficiency**
     Rheumatic mitral stenosis with incompetence or regurgitation

   I05.8   **Other rheumatic mitral valve diseases**
     Rheumatic mitral (valve) failure

   I05.9   **Rheumatic mitral valve disease, unspecified**
     Rheumatic mitral (valve) disorder (chronic) NOS

✓4ᵗʰ I06   **Rheumatic aortic valve diseases**
> **EXCLUDES 1**   aortic valve disease not specified as rheumatic (I35.-)
> aortic valve disease with mitral and/or tricuspid valve involvement (I08.-)

   I06.0   **Rheumatic aortic stenosis**
     Rheumatic aortic (valve) obstruction

   I06.1   **Rheumatic aortic insufficiency**
     Rheumatic aortic incompetence
     Rheumatic aortic regurgitation

   I06.2   **Rheumatic aortic stenosis with insufficiency**
     Rheumatic aortic stenosis with incompetence or regurgitation

   I06.8   **Other rheumatic aortic valve diseases**

   I06.9   **Rheumatic aortic valve disease, unspecified**
     Rheumatic aortic (valve) disease NOS

✓4ᵗʰ I07   **Rheumatic tricuspid valve diseases**
> **INCLUDES**   rheumatic tricuspid valve diseases specified as rheumatic or unspecified
> **EXCLUDES 1**   tricuspid valve disease specified as nonrheumatic (I36.-)
> tricuspid valve disease with aortic and/or mitral valve involvement (I08.-)

   I07.0   **Rheumatic tricuspid stenosis**
     Tricuspid (valve) stenosis (rheumatic)

   I07.1   **Rheumatic tricuspid insufficiency**
     Tricuspid (valve) insufficiency (rheumatic)

   I07.2   **Rheumatic tricuspid stenosis and insufficiency**

   I07.8   **Other rheumatic tricuspid valve diseases**

   I07.9   **Rheumatic tricuspid valve disease, unspecified**
     Rheumatic tricuspid valve disorder NOS

✓4ᵗʰ I08   **Multiple valve diseases**
> **INCLUDES**   multiple valve diseases specified as rheumatic or unspecified
> **EXCLUDES 1**   endocarditis, valve unspecified (I38)
> multiple valve disease specified a nonrheumatic (I34.-, I35.-, I36.-, I37.-, I38.-, Q22.-, Q23.-, Q24.8-)
> rheumatic valve disease NOS (I09.1)

   I08.0   **Rheumatic disorders of both mitral and aortic valves**
     Involvement of both mitral and aortic valves specified as rheumatic or unspecified

   I08.1   **Rheumatic disorders of both mitral and tricuspid valves**

   I08.2   **Rheumatic disorders of both aortic and tricuspid valves**

   I08.3   **Combined rheumatic disorders of mitral, aortic and tricuspid valves**

   I08.8   **Other rheumatic multiple valve diseases**

   I08.9   **Rheumatic multiple valve disease, unspecified**

✓4ᵗʰ I09   **Other rheumatic heart diseases**

   I09.0   **Rheumatic myocarditis**   **CC**
>   **EXCLUDES 1**   myocarditis not specified as rheumatic (I51.4)
     CC Excl: PDX collection 647

   I09.1   **Rheumatic diseases of endocardium, valve unspecified**
     Rheumatic endocarditis (chronic)
     Rheumatic valvulitis (chronic)
>   **EXCLUDES 1**   endocarditis, valve unspecified (I38)

✅ Additional Character Req   ✓x7ᵗʰ Placeholder Alert   Unacceptable PDx   Manifestation   **H1**-**H14** HAC   **HCC** CMS-HCC Condition   **EXCLUDES 1** Not Coded Here   **EXCLUDES 2** Not Included Here

Chapter 9. Diseases of the Circulatory System

I09.2   **Chronic rheumatic pericarditis**   `CC`
     Adherent pericardium, rheumatic
     Chronic rheumatic mediastinopericarditis
     Chronic rheumatic myopericarditis
     EXCLUDES 1   *chronic pericarditis not specified as rheumatic (I31.-)*
     CC Excl: PDX collection 188

✓5ᵗʰ **I09.8**   **Other specified rheumatic heart diseases**

     I09.81   **Rheumatic heart failure**   `CC` `HCC`
         Use additional code to identify type of heart failure (I50.-)
         DEF: Decreased cardiac output, edema, and hypertension; due to rheumatic heart disease.
         CC Excl: PDX collection 648

     I09.89   **Other specified rheumatic heart diseases**
         Rheumatic disease of pulmonary valve

I09.9   **Rheumatic heart disease, unspecified**
     Rheumatic carditis
     EXCLUDES 1   *rheumatoid carditis (M05.31)*

Hypertensive diseases (I10-I16)

Use additional code to identify:
   exposure to environmental tobacco smoke (Z77.22)
   history of tobacco dependence (Z87.891)
   occupational exposure to environmental tobacco smoke (Z57.31)
   tobacco dependence (F17.-)
   tobacco use (Z72.0)
   EXCLUDES 1   *neonatal hypertension (P29.2)*
            primary pulmonary hypertension (I27.0)
   EXCLUDES 2   *hypertensive disease complicating pregnancy, childbirth and the puerperium (O10-O11, O13-O16)*

⁴ **I10**   **Essential (primary) hypertension**
     `INCLUDES`   high blood pressure
         hypertension (arterial) (benign) (essential) (malignant) (primary) (systemic)
     EXCLUDES 1   *hypertensive disease complicating pregnancy, childbirth and the puerperium (O10-O11, O13-O16)*
     EXCLUDES 2   *essential (primary) hypertension involving vessels of brain (I60-I69)*
              essential (primary) hypertension involving vessels of eye (H35.0-)
     AHA: 2016, 4Q, 27

✓4ᵗʰ **I11**   **Hypertensive heart disease**
     `INCLUDES`   ▶any condition in I50.-, I51.4-I51.9 due to hypertension◀

     I11.0   **Hypertensive heart disease with heart failure**   `HCC`
         Hypertensive heart failure
         Use additional code to identify type of heart failure (I50.-)
         AHA: 2017, 1Q, 47

     I11.9   **Hypertensive heart disease without heart failure**
         Hypertensive heart disease NOS

✓4ᵗʰ **I12**   **Hypertensive chronic kidney disease**
     `INCLUDES`   any condition in N18 and N26- due to hypertension
         arteriosclerosis of kidney
         arteriosclerotic nephritis (chronic) (interstitial)
         hypertensive nephropathy
         nephrosclerosis
     EXCLUDES 1   *hypertension due to kidney disease (I15.0, I15.1)*
              renovascular hypertension (I15.0)
              secondary hypertension (I15.-)
     EXCLUDES 2   *acute kidney failure (N17.-)*
     AHA: 2016, 3Q, 22

     I12.0   **Hypertensive chronic kidney disease with stage 5 chronic kidney disease or end stage renal disease**   `CC` `HCC`
         Use additional code to identify the stage of chronic kidney disease (N18.5, N18.6)
         CC Excl: PDX collection 649

     I12.9   **Hypertensive chronic kidney disease with stage 1 through stage 4 chronic kidney disease, or unspecified chronic kidney disease**
         Hypertensive chronic kidney disease NOS
         Hypertensive renal disease NOS
         Use additional code to identify the stage of chronic kidney disease (N18.1-N18.4, N18.9)

✓4ᵗʰ **I13**   **Hypertensive heart and chronic kidney disease**
     `INCLUDES`   any condition in I11.- with any condition in I12.-
         cardiorenal disease
         cardiovascular renal disease

     CC Excl: For CC codes in category I13: PDX collection 650

     I13.0   **Hypertensive heart and chronic kidney disease with heart failure and stage 1 through stage 4 chronic kidney disease, or unspecified chronic kidney disease**   `CC` `HCC`
         Use additional code to identify type of heart failure (I50.-)
         Use additional code to identify stage of chronic kidney disease (N18.1-N18.4, N18.9)

     ✓5ᵗʰ **I13.1**   **Hypertensive heart and chronic kidney disease without heart failure**

         I13.10   **Hypertensive heart and chronic kidney disease without heart failure, with stage 1 through stage 4 chronic kidney disease, or unspecified chronic kidney disease**
             Hypertensive heart disease and hypertensive chronic kidney disease NOS
             Use additional code to identify the stage of chronic kidney disease (N18.1-N18.4, N18.9)

         I13.11   **Hypertensive heart and chronic kidney disease without heart failure, with stage 5 chronic kidney disease, or end stage renal disease**   `CC` `HCC`
             Use additional code to identify the stage of chronic kidney disease (N18.5, N18.6)

     I13.2   **Hypertensive heart and chronic kidney disease with heart failure and with stage 5 chronic kidney disease, or end stage renal disease**   `CC` `HCC`
         Use additional code to identify type of heart failure (I50.-)
         Use additional code to identify the stage of chronic kidney disease (N18.5, N18.6)

✓4ᵗʰ **I15**   **Secondary hypertension**
     Code also underlying condition
     EXCLUDES 1   *postprocedural hypertension (I97.3)*
     EXCLUDES 2   *secondary hypertension involving vessels of brain (I60-I69)*
              secondary hypertension involving vessels of eye (H35.0-)

     I15.0   **Renovascular hypertension**

     I15.1   **Hypertension secondary to other renal disorders**
         AHA: 2016, 3Q, 22

     I15.2   **Hypertension secondary to endocrine disorders**

     I15.8   **Other secondary hypertension**

     I15.9   **Secondary hypertension, unspecified**

✓4ᵗʰ **I16**   **Hypertensive crisis**
     Code also any identified hypertensive disease (I10-I15)
     AHA: 2016, 4Q, 27

     I16.0   **Hypertensive urgency**

     I16.1   **Hypertensive emergency**   `CC`
         CC Excl: No Excl

     I16.9   **Hypertensive crisis, unspecified**   `CC`
         CC Excl: No Excl

Ischemic heart diseases (I20-I25)

Use additional code to identify presence of hypertension (I10-I16)

✓4ᵗʰ **I20**   **Angina pectoris**
     Use additional code to identify:
       exposure to environmental tobacco smoke (Z77.22)
       history of tobacco dependence (Z87.891)
       occupational exposure to environmental tobacco smoke (Z57.31)
       tobacco dependence (F17.-)
       tobacco use (Z72.0)
     EXCLUDES 1   *angina pectoris with atherosclerotic heart disease of native coronary arteries (I25.1-)*
              atherosclerosis of coronary artery bypass graft(s) and coronary artery of transplanted heart with angina pectoris (I25.7-)
              postinfarction angina (I23.7)

     I20.0   **Unstable angina**   `CC` `HCC`
         Accelerated angina
         Crescendo angina
         De novo effort angina
         Intermediate coronary syndrome
         Preinfarction syndrome
         Worsening effort angina
         DEF: A condition representing an intermediate stage between angina of effort and acute myocardial infarction.
         CC Excl: PDX collection 651

---

⁴   Questionable admission when used as PDx.

`N` Newborn: 0   `P` Pediatric: 0-17   `M` Maternity: 12-55   `A` Adult: 15-124   `MCC` Major CC Condition   `PDxMCC` PDx acts as own MCC   `CC` CC Condition   `PDxCC` PDx acts as own CC

630   ICD-10-CM 2018

I09.2–I20.0

I20.1   **Angina pectoris with documented spasm**   CC HCC
Angiospastic angina
Prinzmetal angina
Spasm-induced angina
Variant angina
CC Excl: PDX collection 652

I20.8   **Other forms of angina pectoris**   HCC
Angina equivalent
Angina of effort
Coronary slow flow syndrome
Stable angina
Stenocardia
Use additional code(s) for symptoms associated with angina equivalent

I20.9   **Angina pectoris, unspecified**   HCC
Angina NOS
Anginal syndrome
Cardiac angina
Ischemic chest pain

▲ ✓4th **I21 Acute myocardial infarction**

INCLUDES   cardiac infarction
coronary (artery) embolism
coronary (artery) occlusion
coronary (artery) rupture
coronary (artery) thrombosis
infarction of heart, myocardium, or ventricle
myocardial infarction specified as acute or with a stated duration of 4 weeks (28 days) or less from onset

Use additional code, if applicable, to identify:
exposure to environmental tobacco smoke (Z77.22)
history of tobacco dependence (Z87.891)
occupational exposure to environmental tobacco smoke (Z57.31)
status post administration of tPA (rtPA) in a different facility within the last 24 hours prior to admission to current facility (Z92.82)
tobacco dependence (F17.-)
tobacco use (Z72.0)

EXCLUDES 2   old myocardial infarction (I25.2)
postmyocardial infarction syndrome (I24.1)
▶subsequent type 1 myocardial infarction◀ (I22.-)

AHA: 2017, 1Q, 44-45; 2016, 4Q, 140; 2015, 2Q, 16; 2013, 1Q, 25; 2012, 4Q, 96, 102-103

CC Excl: For MCC codes in category I21: PDX collection 653

✓5th **I21.0**   **ST elevation (STEMI) myocardial infarction of anterior wall**
▶Type 1 ST elevation myocardial infarction of anterior wall◀

   I21.01   **ST elevation (STEMI) myocardial infarction involving left main coronary artery**   MCC HCC

   I21.02   **ST elevation (STEMI) myocardial infarction involving left anterior descending coronary artery**   MCC HCC
ST elevation (STEMI) myocardial infarction involving diagonal coronary artery
AHA: 2013, 1Q, 25

   I21.09   **ST elevation (STEMI) myocardial infarction involving other coronary artery of anterior wall**   MCC HCC
Acute transmural myocardial infarction of anterior wall
Anteroapical transmural (Q wave) infarction (acute)
Anterolateral transmural (Q wave) infarction (acute)
Anteroseptal transmural (Q wave) infarction (acute)
Transmural (Q wave) infarction (acute) (of) anterior (wall) NOS
AHA: 2012, 4Q, 102-103

✓5th **I21.1**   **ST elevation (STEMI) myocardial infarction of inferior wall**
▶Type 1 ST elevation myocardial infarction of inferior wall◀

   I21.11   **ST elevation (STEMI) myocardial infarction involving right coronary artery**   MCC HCC
Inferoposterior transmural (Q wave) infarction (acute)

   I21.19   **ST elevation (STEMI) myocardial infarction involving other coronary artery of inferior wall**   MCC HCC
Acute transmural myocardial infarction of inferior wall
Inferolateral transmural (Q wave) infarction (acute)
Transmural (Q wave) infarction (acute) (of) diaphragmatic wall
Transmural (Q wave) infarction (acute) (of) inferior (wall) NOS
EXCLUDES 2   ST elevation (STEMI) myocardial infarction involving left circumflex coronary artery (I21.21)
AHA: 2012, 4Q, 96

✓5th **I21.2**   **ST elevation (STEMI) myocardial infarction of other sites**
▶Type 1 ST elevation myocardial infarction of other sites◀

   I21.21   **ST elevation (STEMI) myocardial infarction involving left circumflex coronary artery**   MCC HCC
ST elevation (STEMI) myocardial infarction involving oblique marginal coronary artery

   I21.29   **ST elevation (STEMI) myocardial infarction involving other sites**   MCC HCC
Acute transmural myocardial infarction of other sites
Apical-lateral transmural (Q wave) infarction (acute)
Basal-lateral transmural (Q wave) infarction (acute)
High lateral transmural (Q wave) infarction (acute)
Lateral (wall) NOS transmural (Q wave) infarction (acute)
Posterior (true) transmural (Q wave) infarction (acute)
Posterobasal transmural (Q wave) infarction (acute)
Posterolateral transmural (Q wave) infarction (acute)
Posteroseptal transmural (Q wave) infarction (acute)
Septal transmural (Q wave) infarction (acute) NOS

I21.3   **ST elevation (STEMI) myocardial infarction of unspecified site**   MCC HCC
Acute transmural myocardial infarction of unspecified site
~~Myocardial infarction (acute) NOS~~
Transmural (Q wave) myocardial infarction NOS
▶Type 1 ST elevation myocardial infarction of unspecified site◀

I21.4   **Non-ST elevation (NSTEMI) myocardial infarction**   MCC HCC
Acute subendocardial myocardial infarction
Non-Q wave myocardial infarction NOS
Nontransmural myocardial infarction NOS
▶Type 1 non-ST elevation myocardial infarction◀
AHA: 2017, 1Q, 44-45

● **I21.9**   **Acute myocardial infarction, unspecified**
Myocardial infarction (acute) NOS

● ✓5th **I21.A**   **Other type of myocardial infarction**

●   **I21.A1**   **Myocardial infarction type 2**
Myocardial infarction due to demand ischemia
Myocardial infarction secondary to ischemic imbalance
Code also the underlying cause, if known and applicable, such as:
anemia (D50.0-D64.9)
chronic obstructive pulmonary disease (J44.-)
heart failure (I50.-)
paroxysmal tachycardia (I47.0-I47.9)
renal failure (N17.0-N19)
shock (R57.0-R57.9)

●   **I21.A9**   **Other myocardial infarction type**
Myocardial infarction associated with revascularization procedure
Myocardial infarction type 3
Myocardial infarction type 4a
Myocardial infarction type 4b
Myocardial infarction type 4c
Myocardial infarction type 5
Code first, if applicable, postprocedural myocardial infarction following cardiac surgery (I97.190), or postprocedural myocardial infarction during cardiac surgery (I97.790)
Code also complication, if known and applicable, such as:
(acute) stent occlusion (T82.897-)
(acute) stent stenosis (T82.857-)
(acute) stent thrombosis (T82.867-)
cardiac arrest due to underlying cardiac condition (I46.2)
complication of percutaneous coronary intervention (PCI) (I97.89)
occlusion of coronary artery bypass graft (T82.218-)

✓ Additional Character Req   ✓x7th Placeholder Alert   Unacceptable PDx   ■ Manifestation   H1 -H14 HAC   HCC CMS-HCC Condition   EXCLUDES 1 Not Coded Here   EXCLUDES 2 Not Included Here

Chapter 9. Diseases of the Circulatory System

☑4ᵗʰ **I22**   **Subsequent ST elevation (STEMI) and non-ST elevation (NSTEMI) myocardial infarction**

    INCLUDES   acute myocardial infarction occurring within four weeks (28 days) of a previous acute myocardial infarction, regardless of site
              cardiac infarction
              coronary (artery) embolism
              coronary (artery) occlusion
              coronary (artery) rupture
              coronary (artery) thrombosis
              infarction of heart, myocardium, or ventricle
              recurrent myocardial infarction
              reinfarction of myocardium
              rupture of heart, myocardium, or ventricle
              ▶subsequent type 1 myocardial infarction◀

Use additional code, if applicable, to identify:
    exposure to environmental tobacco smoke (Z77.22)
    history of tobacco dependence (Z87.891)
    occupational exposure to environmental tobacco smoke (Z57.31)
    status post administration of tPA (rtPA) in a different facility within the last 24 hours prior to admission to current facility (Z92.82)
    tobacco dependence (F17.-)
    tobacco use (Z72.0)

    EXCLUDES 1 ▶subsequent myocardial infarction, type 2 (I21.A1) subsequent myocardial infarction of other type (type 3) (type 4) (type 5) (I21.A9)◀

AHA: 2017, 2Q, 11; 2013, 1Q, 25; 2012, 4Q, 97, 102-103

    CC Excl: For MCC codes in category I22: PDX collection 653

I22.0   **Subsequent ST elevation (STEMI) myocardial infarction of anterior wall**   MCC HCC
    Subsequent acute transmural myocardial infarction of anterior wall
    Subsequent transmural (Q wave) infarction (acute)(of) anterior (wall) NOS
    Subsequent anteroapical transmural (Q wave) infarction (acute)
    Subsequent anterolateral transmural (Q wave) infarction (acute)
    Subsequent anteroseptal transmural (Q wave) infarction (acute)

I22.1   **Subsequent ST elevation (STEMI) myocardial infarction of inferior wall**   MCC HCC
    Subsequent acute transmural myocardial infarction of inferior wall
    Subsequent transmural (Q wave) infarction (acute)(of) diaphragmatic wall
    Subsequent transmural (Q wave) infarction (acute)(of) inferior (wall) NOS
    Subsequent inferolateral transmural (Q wave) infarction (acute)
    Subsequent inferoposterior transmural (Q wave) infarction (acute)
    AHA: 2012, 4Q, 102

I22.2   **Subsequent non-ST elevation (NSTEMI) myocardial infarction**   MCC HCC
    Subsequent acute subendocardial myocardial infarction
    Subsequent non-Q wave myocardial infarction NOS
    Subsequent nontransmural myocardial infarction NOS

I22.8   **Subsequent ST elevation (STEMI) myocardial infarction of other sites**   MCC HCC
    Subsequent acute transmural myocardial infarction of other sites
    Subsequent apical-lateral transmural (Q wave) myocardial infarction (acute)
    Subsequent basal-lateral transmural (Q wave) myocardial infarction (acute)
    Subsequent high lateral transmural (Q wave) myocardial infarction (acute)
    Subsequent transmural (Q wave) myocardial infarction (acute)(of) lateral (wall) NOS
    Subsequent posterior (true)transmural (Q wave) myocardial infarction (acute)
    Subsequent posterobasal transmural (Q wave) myocardial infarction (acute)
    Subsequent posterolateral transmural (Q wave) myocardial infarction (acute)
    Subsequent posteroseptal transmural (Q wave) myocardial infarction (acute)
    Subsequent septal NOS transmural (Q wave) myocardial infarction (acute)

I22.9   **Subsequent ST elevation (STEMI) myocardial infarction of unspecified site**   MCC HCC
    Subsequent acute myocardial infarction of unspecified site
    Subsequent myocardial infarction (acute) NOS

☑4ᵗʰ **I23**   **Certain current complications following ST elevation (STEMI) and non-ST elevation (NSTEMI) myocardial infarction (within the 28 day period)**
    AHA: 2017, 2Q, 11

    CC Excl: For CC codes in category I23, unless otherwise noted: PDX collection 654

I23.0   **Hemopericardium as current complication following acute myocardial infarction**   CC HCC A
    EXCLUDES 1 hemopericardium not specified as current complication following acute myocardial infarction (I31.2)

I23.1   **Atrial septal defect as current complication following acute myocardial infarction**   CC HCC A
    EXCLUDES 1 acquired atrial septal defect not specified as current complication following acute myocardial infarction (I51.0)

I23.2   **Ventricular septal defect as current complication following acute myocardial infarction**   CC HCC A
    EXCLUDES 1 acquired ventricular septal defect not specified as current complication following acute myocardial infarction (I51.0)

I23.3   **Rupture of cardiac wall without hemopericardium as current complication following acute myocardial infarction**   CC HCC A

I23.4   **Rupture of chordae tendineae as current complication following acute myocardial infarction**   MCC HCC
    EXCLUDES 1 rupture of chordae tendineae not specified as current complication following acute myocardial infarction (I51.1)
    CC Excl: PDX collection 655

I23.5   **Rupture of papillary muscle as current complication following acute myocardial infarction**   MCC HCC
    EXCLUDES 1 rupture of papillary muscle not specified as current complication following acute myocardial infarction (I51.2)
    CC Excl: PDX collection 656

I23.6   **Thrombosis of atrium, auricular appendage, and ventricle as current complications following acute myocardial infarction**   CC HCC A
    EXCLUDES 1 thrombosis of atrium, auricular appendage, and ventricle not specified as current complication following acute myocardial infarction (I51.3)

I23.7   **Postinfarction angina**   CC HCC A
    AHA: 2015, 2Q, 16

I23.8   **Other current complications following acute myocardial infarction**   CC HCC A

☑4ᵗʰ **I24**   **Other acute ischemic heart diseases**
    EXCLUDES 1 angina pectoris (I20.-)
                transient myocardial ischemia in newborn (P29.4)

    CC Excl: For CC codes in category I24, unless otherwise noted: PDX collection 657

I24.0   **Acute coronary thrombosis not resulting in myocardial infarction**   CC HCC
    Acute coronary (artery) (vein) embolism not resulting in myocardial infarction
    Acute coronary (artery) (vein) occlusion not resulting in myocardial infarction
    Acute coronary (artery) (vein) thromboembolism not resulting in myocardial infarction
    EXCLUDES 1 atherosclerotic heart disease (I25.1-)
    AHA: 2013, 1Q, 24

I24.1   **Dressler's syndrome**   CC HCC
    Postmyocardial infarction syndrome
    EXCLUDES 1 postinfarction angina (I23.7)
    CC Excl: PDX collection 658

I24.8   **Other forms of acute ischemic heart disease**   CC HCC
    EXCLUDES 1 ▶myocardial infarction due to demand ischemia (I21.A1)◀

I24.9   **Acute ischemic heart disease, unspecified**   CC HCC
    EXCLUDES 1 ischemic heart disease (chronic) NOS (I25.9)

N Newborn: 0   P Pediatric: 0-17   M Maternity: 12-55   A Adult: 15-124   MCC Major CC Condition   PDxMCC PDx acts as own MCC   CC CC Condition   PDxCC PDx acts as own CC

632   ICD-10-CM 2018

Atheromas

Atheromas (fatty tissue and/or plaque)   Lumen

✅4th **I25 Chronic ischemic heart disease**
Use additional code to identify:
chronic total occlusion of coronary artery (I25.82)
exposure to environmental tobacco smoke (Z77.22)
history of tobacco dependence (Z87.891)
occupational exposure to environmental tobacco smoke (Z57.31)
tobacco dependence (F17.-)
tobacco use (Z72.0)

✅5th **I25.1 Atherosclerotic heart disease of native coronary artery**
Atherosclerotic cardiovascular disease
Coronary (artery) atheroma
Coronary (artery) atherosclerosis
Coronary (artery) disease
Coronary (artery) sclerosis
Use additional code, if applicable, to identify:
coronary atherosclerosis due to calcified coronary lesion (I25.84)
coronary atherosclerosis due to lipid rich plaque (I25.83)
EXCLUDES 2   *atheroembolism (I75.-)*
atherosclerosis of coronary artery bypass graft(s) and transplanted heart (I25.7-)

I25.10 Atherosclerotic heart disease of native coronary   **A**
artery without angina pectoris
Atherosclerotic heart disease NOS
AHA: 2015, 2Q, 16; 2012, 4Q, 92

✅6th **I25.11 Atherosclerotic heart disease of native coronary**
artery with angina pectoris

I25.110 Atherosclerotic heart   PDxCC CC HCC A
disease of native coronary artery
with unstable angina pectoris
EXCLUDES 1   *unstable angina without atherosclerotic heart disease (I20.0)*
CC Excl: PDX collection 651

I25.111 Atherosclerotic heart disease of   HCC A
native coronary artery with angina
pectoris with documented spasm
EXCLUDES 1   *angina pectoris with documented spasm without atherosclerotic heart disease (I20.1)*

I25.118 Atherosclerotic heart disease of   HCC A
native coronary artery with other
forms of angina pectoris
EXCLUDES 1   *other forms of angina pectoris without atherosclerotic heart disease (I20.8)*
AHA: 2015, 2Q, 16

I25.119 Atherosclerotic heart disease of   HCC A
native coronary artery with
unspecified angina pectoris
Atherosclerotic heart disease with angina NOS
Atherosclerotic heart disease with ischemic chest pain
EXCLUDES 1   *unspecified angina pectoris without atherosclerotic heart disease (I20.9)*

I25.2 Old myocardial infarction
Healed myocardial infarction
Past myocardial infarction diagnosed by ECG or other investigation, but currently presenting no symptoms

I25.3 Aneurysm of heart   CC
Mural aneurysm
Ventricular aneurysm
CC Excl: PDX collection 659

✅5th **I25.4 Coronary artery aneurysm and dissection**
I25.41 Coronary artery aneurysm
Coronary arteriovenous fistula, acquired
EXCLUDES 1   *congenital coronary (artery) aneurysm (Q24.5)*

I25.42 Coronary artery dissection   MCC
DEF: A tear in the intimal arterial wall of a coronary artery resulting in the sudden intrusion of blood within the layers of the wall.
CC Excl: PDX collection 660

I25.5 Ischemic cardiomyopathy
EXCLUDES 2   *coronary atherosclerosis (I25.1-, I25.7-)*

I25.6 Silent myocardial ischemia

✅5th **I25.7 Atherosclerosis of coronary artery bypass graft(s) and coronary artery of transplanted heart with angina pectoris**
Use additional code, if applicable, to identify:
coronary atherosclerosis due to calcified coronary lesion (I25.84)
coronary atherosclerosis due to lipid rich plaque (I25.83)
EXCLUDES 1   *atherosclerosis of bypass graft(s) of transplanted heart without angina pectoris (I25.812)*
atherosclerosis of coronary artery bypass graft(s) without angina pectoris (I25.810)
atherosclerosis of native coronary artery of transplanted heart without angina pectoris (I25.811)
~~embolism or thrombus of coronary artery bypass graft(s) (T82.8-)~~

✅6th **I25.70 Atherosclerosis of coronary artery bypass graft(s), unspecified, with angina pectoris**
I25.700 Atherosclerosis of   PDxCC CC HCC A
coronary artery bypass graft(s), unspecified, with unstable angina pectoris
EXCLUDES 1   *unstable angina pectoris without atherosclerosis of coronary artery bypass graft (I20.0)*
CC Excl: PDX collection 651

I25.701 Atherosclerosis of coronary artery   HCC A
bypass graft(s), unspecified, with angina pectoris with documented spasm
EXCLUDES 1   *angina pectoris with documented spasm without atherosclerosis of coronary artery bypass graft (I20.1)*

I25.708 Atherosclerosis of coronary artery   HCC A
bypass graft(s), unspecified, with other forms of angina pectoris
EXCLUDES 1   *other forms of angina pectoris without atherosclerosis of coronary artery bypass graft (I20.8)*

I25.709 Atherosclerosis of coronary artery   HCC A
bypass graft(s), unspecified, with unspecified angina pectoris
EXCLUDES 1   *unspecified angina pectoris without atherosclerosis of coronary artery bypass graft (I20.9)*

✅6th **I25.71 Atherosclerosis of autologous vein coronary artery bypass graft(s) with angina pectoris**

CC Excl: For CC codes in subcategory I25.71, unless otherwise noted: PDX collection 662

I25.710 Atherosclerosis of   PDxCC CC HCC A
autologous vein coronary artery bypass graft(s) with unstable angina pectoris
EXCLUDES 1   *unstable angina without atherosclerosis of autologous vein coronary artery bypass graft(s) (I20.0)*
EXCLUDES 2   ▶*embolism or thrombus of coronary artery bypass graft(s) (T82.8-)*◀
CC Excl: PDX collection 661

I25.711 Atherosclerosis of autologous   CC HCC A
vein coronary artery bypass graft(s) with angina pectoris with documented spasm
EXCLUDES 1   *angina pectoris with documented spasm without atherosclerosis of autologous vein coronary artery bypass graft(s) (I20.1)*

I25.718   **Atherosclerosis of autologous** `CC` `HCC` `A` **vein coronary artery bypass graft(s) with other forms of angina pectoris**
> EXCLUDES 1   *other forms of angina pectoris without atherosclerosis of autologous vein coronary artery bypass graft(s) (I20.8)*

I25.719   **Atherosclerosis of autologous** `CC` `HCC` `A` **vein coronary artery bypass graft(s) with unspecified angina pectoris**
> EXCLUDES 1   *unspecified angina pectoris without atherosclerosis of autologous vein coronary artery bypass graft(s) (I20.9)*

✓6th **I25.72**   **Atherosclerosis of autologous artery coronary artery bypass graft(s) with angina pectoris**
Atherosclerosis of internal mammary artery graft with angina pectoris

> **CC Excl: For CC codes in subcategories I25.72, unless otherwise noted:** PDX collection 662

I25.720   **Atherosclerosis of** `PDxCC` `CC` `HCC` `A` **autologous artery coronary artery bypass graft(s) with unstable angina pectoris**
> EXCLUDES 1   *unstable angina without atherosclerosis of autologous artery coronary artery bypass graft(s) (I20.0)*
> **CC Excl:** PDX collection 661

I25.721   **Atherosclerosis of autologous** `CC` `HCC` `A` **artery coronary artery bypass graft(s) with angina pectoris with documented spasm**
> EXCLUDES 1   *angina pectoris with documented spasm without atherosclerosis of autologous artery coronary artery bypass graft(s) (I20.1)*

I25.728   **Atherosclerosis of autologous** `CC` `HCC` `A` **artery coronary artery bypass graft(s) with other forms of angina pectoris**
> EXCLUDES 1   *other forms of angina pectoris without atherosclerosis of autologous artery coronary artery bypass graft(s) (I20.8)*

I25.729   **Atherosclerosis of autologous** `CC` `HCC` `A` **artery coronary artery bypass graft(s) with unspecified angina pectoris**
> EXCLUDES 1   *unspecified angina pectoris without atherosclerosis of autologous artery coronary artery bypass graft(s) (I20.9)*

✓6th **I25.73**   **Atherosclerosis of nonautologous biological coronary artery bypass graft(s) with angina pectoris**

> **CC Excl: For CC codes in subcategories I25.73, unless otherwise noted:** PDX collection 662

I25.730   **Atherosclerosis of** `PDxCC` `CC` `HCC` `A` **nonautologous biological coronary artery bypass graft(s) with unstable angina pectoris**
> EXCLUDES 1   *unstable angina without atherosclerosis of nonautologous biological coronary artery bypass graft(s) (I20.0)*
> **CC Excl:** PDX collection 661

I25.731   **Atherosclerosis of** `CC` `HCC` `A` **nonautologous biological coronary artery bypass graft(s) with angina pectoris with documented spasm**
> EXCLUDES 1   *angina pectoris with documented spasm without atherosclerosis of nonautologous biological coronary artery bypass graft(s) (I20.1)*

I25.738   **Atherosclerosis of** `CC` `HCC` `A` **nonautologous biological coronary artery bypass graft(s) with other forms of angina pectoris**
> EXCLUDES 1   *other forms of angina pectoris without atherosclerosis of nonautologous biological coronary artery bypass graft(s) (I20.8)*

I25.739   **Atherosclerosis of** `CC` `HCC` `A` **nonautologous biological coronary artery bypass graft(s) with unspecified angina pectoris**
> EXCLUDES 1   *unspecified angina pectoris without atherosclerosis of nonautologous biological coronary artery bypass graft(s) (I20.9)*

✓6th **I25.75**   **Atherosclerosis of native coronary artery of transplanted heart with angina pectoris**
> EXCLUDES 1   *atherosclerosis of native coronary artery of transplanted heart without angina pectoris (I25.811)*

> **CC Excl: For CC codes in subcategory I25.75, unless otherwise noted:** PDX collection 664

I25.750   **Atherosclerosis of native** `PDxCC` `CC` `HCC` **coronary artery of transplanted heart with unstable angina**
> **CC Excl:** PDX collection 663

I25.751   **Atherosclerosis of native coronary** `CC` `HCC` **artery of transplanted heart with angina pectoris with documented spasm**

I25.758   **Atherosclerosis of native coronary** `CC` `HCC` **artery of transplanted heart with other forms of angina pectoris**

I25.759   **Atherosclerosis of native coronary** `CC` `HCC` **artery of transplanted heart with unspecified angina pectoris**

✓6th **I25.76**   **Atherosclerosis of bypass graft of coronary artery of transplanted heart with angina pectoris**
> EXCLUDES 1   *atherosclerosis of bypass graft of coronary artery of transplanted heart without angina pectoris (I25.812)*

> **CC Excl: For CC codes in subcategory I25.76, unless otherwise noted:** PDX collection 666

I25.760   **Atherosclerosis of bypass** `PDxCC` `CC` `HCC` `A` **graft of coronary artery of transplanted heart with unstable angina**
> **CC Excl:** PDX collection 665

I25.761   **Atherosclerosis of bypass graft** `CC` `HCC` `A` **of coronary artery of transplanted heart with angina pectoris with documented spasm**

I25.768   **Atherosclerosis of bypass graft** `CC` `HCC` `A` **of coronary artery of transplanted heart with other forms of angina pectoris**

I25.769   **Atherosclerosis of bypass graft** `CC` `HCC` `A` **of coronary artery of transplanted heart with unspecified angina pectoris**

✓6th **I25.79**   **Atherosclerosis of other coronary artery bypass graft(s) with angina pectoris**

I25.790   **Atherosclerosis of other** `PDxCC` `CC` `HCC` `A` **coronary artery bypass graft(s) with unstable angina pectoris**
> EXCLUDES 1   *unstable angina without atherosclerosis of other coronary artery bypass graft(s) (I20.0)*
> **CC Excl:** PDX collection 651

I25.791   **Atherosclerosis of other** `CC` `HCC` `A` **coronary artery bypass graft(s) with angina pectoris with documented spasm**
> EXCLUDES 1   *angina pectoris with documented spasm without atherosclerosis of other coronary artery bypass graft(s) (I20.1)*
> **CC Excl:** No Excl

I25.798   **Atherosclerosis of other** `CC` `HCC` `A` **coronary artery bypass graft(s) with other forms of angina pectoris**
> EXCLUDES 1   *other forms of angina pectoris without atherosclerosis of other coronary artery bypass graft(s) (I20.8)*
> **CC Excl:** No Excl

`N` Newborn: 0   `P` Pediatric: 0-17   `M` Maternity: 12-55   `A` Adult: 15-124   `MCC` Major CC Condition   `PDxMCC` PDx acts as own MCC   `CC` CC Condition   `PDxCC` PDx acts as own CC

634   ICD-10-CM 2018

I25.799   **Atherosclerosis of other**   `CC` `HCC` `A`
     coronary artery bypass graft(s) with
     unspecified angina pectoris
       EXCLUDES 1   unspecified angina pectoris
           without atherosclerosis of
           other coronary artery bypass
           graft(s) (I20.9)
       CC Excl: No Excl

✓5th **I25.8**   **Other forms of chronic ischemic heart disease**

   ✓6th **I25.81**   **Atherosclerosis of other coronary vessels without**
     angina pectoris
     Use additional code, if applicable, to identify:
       coronary atherosclerosis due to calcified coronary
         lesion (I25.84)
       coronary atherosclerosis due to lipid rich plaque
         (I25.83)
       EXCLUDES 1   atherosclerotic heart disease of native
           coronary artery without angina pectoris
           (I25.10)

     I25.810   **Atherosclerosis of coronary artery**   `CC` `A`
       bypass graft(s) without angina pectoris
       Atherosclerosis of coronary artery bypass
         graft NOS
       EXCLUDES 1   atherosclerosis of coronary
           bypass graft(s) with angina
           pectoris (I25.70--I25.73-,
           I25.79-)
       CC Excl: No Excl

     I25.811   **Atherosclerosis of native coronary**   `CC`
       artery of transplanted heart without
       angina pectoris
       Atherosclerosis of native coronary artery of
         transplanted heart NOS
       EXCLUDES 1   atherosclerosis of native coronary
           artery of transplanted heart
           with angina pectoris
           (I25.75-)
       CC Excl: PDX collection 664

     I25.812   **Atherosclerosis of bypass graft of**   `CC` `A`
       coronary artery of transplanted heart
       without angina pectoris
       Atherosclerosis of bypass graft of
         transplanted heart NOS
       EXCLUDES 1   atherosclerosis of bypass graft of
           transplanted heart with
           angina pectoris (I25.76)
       CC Excl: PDX collection 666

   I25.82   **Chronic total occlusion of coronary artery**
     Complete occlusion of coronary artery
     Total occlusion of coronary artery
     Code first coronary atherosclerosis (I25.1-, I25.7-,
       I25.81-)
     EXCLUDES 1 ▶acute coronary occlusion with myocardial
           infarction (I21.0-I21.9, I22.-)◀
           ▶acute coronary occlusion without
           myocardial infarction◀ (I24.0)
     DEF: Complete blockage of coronary artery due to
     plaque accumulation over an extended period of time;
     results in substantial reduction of blood flow;
     characterized by angina or chest pain.

   I25.83   **Coronary atherosclerosis due to lipid rich plaque**   `A`
     Code first coronary atherosclerosis (I25.1-, I25.7-,
       I25.81-)

   I25.84   **Coronary atherosclerosis due to calcified coronary**
     lesion
     Coronary atherosclerosis due to severely calcified
       coronary lesion
     Code first coronary atherosclerosis (I25.1-, I25.7-,
       I25.81-)

   I25.89   **Other forms of chronic ischemic heart disease**

I25.9   **Chronic ischemic heart disease, unspecified**
   Ischemic heart disease (chronic) NOS

Pulmonary heart disease and diseases of pulmonary circulation (I26-I28)

✓4th **I26**   **Pulmonary embolism**
   INCLUDES   pulmonary (acute) (artery)(vein) infarction
        pulmonary (acute) (artery)(vein) thromboembolism
        pulmonary (acute) (artery)(vein) thrombosis
   EXCLUDES 2   chronic pulmonary embolism (I27.82)
        personal history of pulmonary embolism (Z86.711)
        pulmonary embolism due to trauma (T79.0, T79.1)
        pulmonary embolism due to complications of surgical and
          medical care (T80.0, T81.7-, T82.8-)
        pulmonary embolism complicating abortion, ectopic or molar
          pregnancy (O00-O07, O08.2)
        pulmonary embolism complicating pregnancy, childbirth and
          the puerperium (O88.-)
        septic (non-pulmonary) arterial embolism (I76)

  ✓5th **I26.0**   **Pulmonary embolism with acute cor pulmonale**

     CC Excl: For MCC codes in subcategory I26.0, unless
     otherwise noted: PDX collection 667

   I26.01   **Septic pulmonary embolism with**   `PDxMCC` `MCC` `HCC`
     acute cor pulmonale
     Code first underlying infection

   I26.02   **Saddle embolus of pulmonary**   `PDxMCC` `MCC` `H10` `HCC`
     artery with acute cor pulmonale

   I26.09   **Other pulmonary embolism with**   `PDxMCC` `MCC` `H10` `HCC`
     acute cor pulmonale
     Acute cor pulmonale NOS
     AHA: 2014, 4Q, 21

  ✓5th **I26.9**   **Pulmonary embolism without acute cor pulmonale**

   I26.90   **Septic pulmonary embolism without acute**   `MCC` `HCC`
     cor pulmonale
     Code first underlying infection
     CC Excl: PDX collection 668

   I26.92   **Saddle embolus of pulmonary artery**   `MCC` `H10` `HCC`
     without acute cor pulmonale
     CC Excl: PDX collection 669

   I26.99   **Other pulmonary embolism without**   `MCC` `H10` `HCC`
     acute cor pulmonale
     Acute pulmonary embolism NOS
     Pulmonary embolism NOS
     CC Excl: PDX collection 670

✓4th **I27**   **Other pulmonary heart diseases**

  I27.0   **Primary pulmonary hypertension**   `CC` `HCC`
     ▶Heritable pulmonary arterial hypertension
     Idiopathic pulmonary arterial hypertension
     Primary group 1 pulmonary hypertension
     Primary pulmonary arterial hypertension◀
     EXCLUDES 1 ▶persistent pulmonary hypertension of newborn
           (P29.30)◀
           pulmonary hypertension NOS ▶(I27.20)◀
           ▶secondary pulmonary arterial hypertension (I27.21)◀
           secondary pulmonary hypertension ▶(I27.29)◀
     CC Excl: PDX collection 671

  I27.1   **Kyphoscoliotic heart disease**   `CC` `HCC`
     CC Excl: PDX collection 533

  ✓5th **I27.2**   **Other secondary pulmonary hypertension**
     ~~Pulmonary hypertension NOS~~
     Code also associated underlying condition
     EXCLUDES 1 ▶Eisenmenger's syndrome (I27.83)◀
     AHA: 2014, 4Q, 21

   ●   **I27.20**   **Pulmonary hypertension, unspecified**
     Pulmonary hypertension NOS

   ●   **I27.21**   **Secondary pulmonary arterial hypertension**
     (Associated) (drug-induced) (toxin-induced)
       pulmonary arterial hypertension NOS
     (Associated) (drug-induced) (toxin-induced)
       (secondary) group 1 pulmonary hypertension
     Code also associated conditions if applicable, or
       adverse effects of drugs or toxins, such as:
       adverse effect of appetite depressants (T50.5X5)
       congenital heart disease (Q20-Q28)
       human immunodeficiency virus [HIV] disease (B20)
       polymyositis (M33.2-)
       portal hypertension (K76.6)
       rheumatoid arthritis (M05.-)
       schistosomiasis (B65.-)
       Sjögren syndrome (M35.0-)
       systemic sclerosis (M34.-)

✓ Additional Character Req   ✓x7th Placeholder Alert   Unacceptable PDx   Manifestation   `H1`-`H14` HAC   `HCC` CMS-HCC Condition   *EXCLUDES 1* Not Coded Here   *EXCLUDES 2* Not Included Here

ICD-10-CM 2018   **635**

I27.22   **Pulmonary hypertension** due to left heart disease
Group 2 pulmonary hypertension
Code also associated left heart disease, if known, such as:
     multiple valve disease (I08.-)
     rheumatic mitral valve diseases (I05.-)
     rheumatic aortic valve diseases (I06.-)

I27.23   **Pulmonary hypertension** due to lung diseases and hypoxia
Group 3 pulmonary hypertension
Code also associated lung disease, if known, such as:
     bronchiectasis (J47.-)
     cystic fibrosis with pulmonary manifestations (E84.0)
     interstitial lung disease (J84.-)
     pleural effusion (J90)
     sleep apnea (G47.3-)

I27.24   **Chronic thromboembolic pulmonary hypertension**
Group 4 pulmonary hypertension
Code also associated pulmonary embolism, if applicable (I26.-, I27.82)

I27.29   **Other secondary pulmonary hypertension**
Group 5 pulmonary hypertension
Pulmonary hypertension with unclear multifactorial mechanisms
Pulmonary hypertension due to hematologic disorders
Pulmonary hypertension due to metabolic disorders
Pulmonary hypertension due to other systemic disorders
Code also other associated disorders, if known, such as:
     chronic myeloid leukemia (C92.10- C92.22)
     essential thrombocythemia (D47.3)
     Gaucher disease (E75.22)
     hypertensive chronic kidney disease with end stage renal disease (I12.0, I12.11, I13.2)
     hyperthyroidism (E05.-)
     hypothyroidism (E00-E03)
     polycythemia vera (D45)
     sarcoidosis (D86.-)
AHA: 2016, 2Q, 8

I27.8   **Other specified pulmonary heart diseases**

I27.81   **Cor pulmonale (chronic)**   `HCC`
Cor pulmonale NOS
EXCLUDES 1   *acute cor pulmonale (I26.0-)*
AHA: 2014, 4Q, 21

I27.82   **Chronic pulmonary embolism**   `CC` `HCC`
Use additional code, if applicable, for associated long-term (current) use of anticoagulants (Z79.01)
EXCLUDES 1   *personal history of pulmonary embolism (Z86.711)*
DEF: A long-standing condition commonly associated with pulmonary hypertension in which small blood clots travel to the lungs repeatedly over many weeks, months, or years, requiring continuation of established anticoagulant or thrombolytic therapy.
CC Excl: PDX collection 669

I27.83   **Eisenmenger's syndrome**
Eisenmenger's complex
(Irreversible) Eisenmenger's disease
Pulmonary hypertension with right to left shunt related to congenital heart disease
Code also underlying heart defect, if known, such as:
     atrial septal defect (Q21.1)
     Eisenmenger's defect (Q21.8)
     patent ductus arteriosus (Q25.0)
     ventricular septal defect (Q21.0)

I27.89   **Other specified pulmonary heart diseases**   `HCC`
~~Eisenmenger's complex~~
~~Eisenmenger's syndrome~~
EXCLUDES 1   ~~*Eisenmenger's defect (Q21.8)*~~

I27.9   **Pulmonary heart disease, unspecified**   `HCC`
Chronic cardiopulmonary disease

✓4th **I28**   **Other diseases of pulmonary vessels**

I28.0   **Arteriovenous fistula of pulmonary vessels**   `CC` `HCC`
EXCLUDES 1   *congenital arteriovenous fistula (Q25.72)*
CC Excl: PDX collection 672

I28.1   **Aneurysm of pulmonary artery**   `CC` `HCC`
EXCLUDES 1   *congenital aneurysm (Q25.79)*
           congenital arteriovenous aneurysm (Q25.72)
CC Excl: PDX collection 672

I28.8   **Other diseases of pulmonary vessels**   `HCC`
Pulmonary arteritis
Pulmonary endarteritis
Rupture of pulmonary vessels
Stenosis of pulmonary vessels
Stricture of pulmonary vessels

I28.9   **Disease of pulmonary vessels, unspecified**   `HCC`

Other forms of heart disease (I30-I52)

✓4th **I30**   **Acute pericarditis**
INCLUDES   acute mediastinopericarditis
          acute myopericarditis
          acute pericardial effusion
          acute pleuropericarditis
          acute pneumopericarditis
EXCLUDES 1   *Dressler's syndrome (I24.1)*
          rheumatic pericarditis (acute) (I01.0)
        ►*viral pericarditis due to Coxsakie virus (B33.23)*◄

CC Excl: For CC codes in category I30: PDX collection 673

I30.0   **Acute nonspecific idiopathic pericarditis**   `CC`

I30.1   **Infective pericarditis**   `CC`
Pneumococcal pericarditis
Pneumopyopericardium
Purulent pericarditis
Pyopericarditis
Pyopericardium
Pyopneumopericardium
Staphylococcal pericarditis
Streptococcal pericarditis
Suppurative pericarditis
Viral pericarditis
Use additional code (B95-B97) to identify infectious agent

I30.8   **Other forms of acute pericarditis**   `CC`

I30.9   **Acute pericarditis, unspecified**   `CC`

✓4th **I31**   **Other diseases of pericardium**
EXCLUDES 1   *diseases of pericardium specified as rheumatic (I09.2)*
          postcardiotomy syndrome (I97.0)
          traumatic injury to pericardium (S26.-)

I31.0   **Chronic adhesive pericarditis**   `CC`
Accretio cordis
Adherent pericardium
Adhesive mediastinopericarditis
CC Excl: PDX collection 674

I31.1   **Chronic constrictive pericarditis**   `CC`
Concretio cordis
Pericardial calcification
CC Excl: PDX collection 674

I31.2   **Hemopericardium, not elsewhere classified**   `CC`
EXCLUDES 1   *hemopericardium as current complication following acute myocardial infarction (I23.0)*
DEF: Presence of blood in the pericardial sac (pericardium). It can lead to potentially fatal cardiac tamponade if enough blood enters the pericardial cavity.
CC Excl: PDX collection 674

I31.3   **Pericardial effusion (noninflammatory)**   `CC`
Chylopericardium
EXCLUDES 1   *acute pericardial effusion (I30.9)*
CC Excl: PDX collection 188

I31.4   **Cardiac tamponade**   `CC`
Code first underlying cause
CC Excl: PDX collection 188

I31.8   **Other specified diseases of pericardium**   `CC`
Epicardial plaques   Focal pericardial adhesions
CC Excl: PDX collection 188

I31.9   **Disease of pericardium, unspecified**   `CC`
Pericarditis (chronic) NOS
CC Excl: PDX collection 188

`N` Newborn: 0   `P` Pediatric: 0-17   `M` Maternity: 12-55   `A` Adult: 15-124   `MCC` Major CC Condition   `PDxMCC` PDx acts as own MCC   `CC` CC Condition   `PDxCC` PDx acts as own CC

636   ICD-10-CM 2018

Cardiac Tamponade

Normal

Acute Pericardial Effusion with Cardiac Tamponade

Excessive fluid in pericardial space

Serous pericardium (visceral layer)

Fibrous pericardium

Pericardial space (potential)

Serous pericardium (parietal layer)

constricted areas

I32 Pericarditis in diseases classified elsewhere   CC

Code first underlying disease

EXCLUDES 1   pericarditis (in):
coxsackie (virus) (B33.23)
gonococcal (A54.83)
meningococcal (A39.53)
rheumatoid (arthritis) (M05.31)
syphilitic (A52.06)
systemic lupus erythematosus (M32.12)
tuberculosis (A18.84)

CC Excl: PDX collection 673

✓4th I33 Acute and subacute endocarditis

EXCLUDES 1   acute rheumatic endocarditis (I01.1)
endocarditis NOS (I38)

I33.0 Acute and subacute infective endocarditis   HIV MCC
Bacterial endocarditis (acute) (subacute)
Infective endocarditis (acute) (subacute) NOS
Endocarditis lenta (acute) (subacute)
Malignant endocarditis (acute) (subacute)
Purulent endocarditis (acute) (subacute)
Septic endocarditis (acute) (subacute)
Ulcerative endocarditis (acute) (subacute)
Vegetative endocarditis (acute) (subacute)
Use additional code (B95-B97) to identify infectious agent
CC Excl: PDX collection 675

I33.9 Acute and subacute endocarditis, unspecified   HIV MCC
Acute endocarditis NOS
Acute myoendocarditis NOS
Acute periendocarditis NOS
Subacute endocarditis NOS
Subacute myoendocarditis NOS
Subacute periendocarditis NOS
CC Excl: PDX collection 675

✓4th I34 Nonrheumatic mitral valve disorders

EXCLUDES 1   mitral valve disease (I05.9)
mitral valve failure (I05.8)
mitral valve stenosis (I05.0)
mitral valve disorder of unspecified cause with diseases of aortic and/or tricuspid valve(s) (I08.-)
mitral valve disorder of unspecified cause with mitral stenosis or obstruction (I05.0)
mitral valve disorder specified as congenital ▶(Q23.2, Q23.9)◀
mitral valve disorder specified as rheumatic (I05.-)

I34.0 Nonrheumatic mitral (valve) insufficiency
Nonrheumatic mitral (valve) incompetence NOS
Nonrheumatic mitral (valve) regurgitation NOS

I34.1 Nonrheumatic mitral (valve) prolapse
Floppy nonrheumatic mitral valve syndrome
EXCLUDES 1   Marfan's syndrome (Q87.4-)

I34.2 Nonrheumatic mitral (valve) stenosis

I34.8 Other nonrheumatic mitral valve disorders

I34.9 Nonrheumatic mitral valve disorder, unspecified

✓4th I35 Nonrheumatic aortic valve disorders

EXCLUDES 1   aortic valve disorder of unspecified cause but with diseases of mitral and/or tricuspid valve(s) (I08.-)
aortic valve disorder specified as congenital (Q23.0, Q23.1)
aortic valve disorder specified as rheumatic (I06.-)
hypertrophic subaortic stenosis (I42.1)

I35.0 Nonrheumatic aortic (valve) stenosis

I35.1 Nonrheumatic aortic (valve) insufficiency
Nonrheumatic aortic (valve) incompetence NOS
Nonrheumatic aortic (valve) regurgitation NOS

I35.2 Nonrheumatic aortic (valve) stenosis with insufficiency

I35.8 Other nonrheumatic aortic valve disorders

I35.9 Nonrheumatic aortic valve disorder, unspecified

✓4th I36 Nonrheumatic tricuspid valve disorders

EXCLUDES 1   tricuspid valve disorders of unspecified cause (I07.-)
tricuspid valve disorders specified as congenital (Q22.4, Q22.8, Q22.9)
tricuspid valve disorders specified as rheumatic (I07.-)
tricuspid valve disorders with aortic and/or mitral valve involvement (I08.-)

I36.0 Nonrheumatic tricuspid (valve) stenosis

I36.1 Nonrheumatic tricuspid (valve) insufficiency
Nonrheumatic tricuspid (valve) incompetence
Nonrheumatic tricuspid (valve) regurgitation

I36.2 Nonrheumatic tricuspid (valve) stenosis with insufficiency

I36.8 Other nonrheumatic tricuspid valve disorders

I36.9 Nonrheumatic tricuspid valve disorder, unspecified

✓4th I37 Nonrheumatic pulmonary valve disorders

EXCLUDES 1   pulmonary valve disorder specified as congenital (Q22.1, Q22.2, Q22.3)
pulmonary valve disorder specified as rheumatic (I09.89)

I37.0 Nonrheumatic pulmonary valve stenosis

I37.1 Nonrheumatic pulmonary valve insufficiency
Nonrheumatic pulmonary valve incompetence
Nonrheumatic pulmonary valve regurgitation

I37.2 Nonrheumatic pulmonary valve stenosis with insufficiency

I37.8 Other nonrheumatic pulmonary valve disorders

I37.9 Nonrheumatic pulmonary valve disorder, unspecified

I38 Endocarditis, valve unspecified   CC

INCLUDES   endocarditis (chronic) NOS
valvular incompetence NOS
valvular insufficiency NOS
valvular regurgitation NOS
valvular stenosis NOS
valvulitis (chronic) NOS

EXCLUDES 1   congenital insufficiency of cardiac valve NOS (Q24.8)
congenital stenosis of cardiac valve NOS (Q24.8)
endocardial fibroelastosis (I42.4)
endocarditis specified as rheumatic (I09.1)

CC Excl: PDX collection 676

I39 Endocarditis and heart valve disorders in diseases classified elsewhere   CC

Code first underlying disease, such as:
Q fever (A78)

EXCLUDES 1   endocardial involvement in:
candidiasis (B37.6)
gonococcal infection (A54.83)
Libman-Sacks disease (M32.11)
listerosis (A32.82)
meningococcal infection (A39.51)
rheumatoid arthritis (M05.31)
syphilis (A52.03)
tuberculosis (A18.84)
typhoid fever (A01.02)

CC Excl: PDX collection 676

✓4th I40 Acute myocarditis

INCLUDES   subacute myocarditis

EXCLUDES 1   acute rheumatic myocarditis (I01.2)

CC Excl: For MCC codes in category I40: PDX collection 677

I40.0 Infective myocarditis   HIV MCC
Septic myocarditis
Use additional code (B95-B97) to identify infectious agent

I40.1 Isolated myocarditis   HIV MCC
Fiedler's myocarditis
Giant cell myocarditis
Idiopathic myocarditis

I40.8 Other acute myocarditis   HIV MCC

I40.9 Acute myocarditis, unspecified   HIV MCC

I41　Myocarditis in diseases classified elsewhere　MCC

Code first underlying disease, such as:
typhus (A75.0-A75.9)

EXCLUDES 1　myocarditis (in):
Chagas' disease (chronic) (B57.2)
acute (B57.0)
coxsackie (virus) infection (B33.22)
diphtheritic (A36.81)
gonococcal (A54.83)
influenzal (J09.X9, J10.82, J11.82)
meningococcal (A39.52)
mumps (B26.82)
rheumatoid arthritis (M05.31)
sarcoid (D86.85)
syphilis (A52.06)
toxoplasmosis (B58.81)
tuberculous (A18.84)

CC Excl: PDX collection 677

✓4th I42　Cardiomyopathy

INCLUDES　myocardiopathy

Code first pre-existing cardiomyopathy complicating pregnancy and puerperium (O99.4)

EXCLUDES 2　ischemic cardiomyopathy (I25.5)
peripartum cardiomyopathy (O90.3)
ventricular hypertrophy (I51.7)

CC Excl: For CC codes in category I42: PDX collection 678

I42.0　**Dilated cardiomyopathy**　CC HCC
Congestive cardiomyopathy

I42.1　**Obstructive hypertrophic cardiomyopathy**　CC HCC
Hypertrophic subaortic stenosis (idiopathic)
DEF: Cardiomyopathy marked by left ventricle hypertrophy, enlarged septum; results in obstructed blood flow, arrhythmias, mitral regurgitation, and sudden cardiac death.

I42.2　**Other hypertrophic cardiomyopathy**　CC HCC
Nonobstructive hypertrophic cardiomyopathy

I42.3　**Endomyocardial (eosinophilic) disease**　CC HCC
Endomyocardial (tropical) fibrosis
Löffler's endocarditis

I42.4　**Endocardial fibroelastosis**　CC HCC
Congenital cardiomyopathy
Elastomyofibrosis

I42.5　**Other restrictive cardiomyopathy**　CC HCC
Constrictive cardiomyopathy NOS

I42.6　**Alcoholic cardiomyopathy**　CC HCC
Code also presence of alcoholism (F10.-)

I42.7　**Cardiomyopathy due to drug and external agent**　CC HCC
Code first poisoning due to drug or toxin, if applicable (T36-T65 with fifth or sixth character 1-4 or 6)
Use additional code for adverse effect, if applicable, to identify drug (T36-T50 with fifth or sixth character 5)

I42.8　**Other cardiomyopathies**　CC HCC

I42.9　**Cardiomyopathy, unspecified**　CC HCC
Cardiomyopathy (primary) (secondary) NOS

I43　Cardiomyopathy in diseases classified elsewhere　CC HCC

Code first underlying disease, such as:
amyloidosis (E85.-)
glycogen storage disease (E74.0)
gout (M10.0-)
thyrotoxicosis (E05.0-E05.9-)

EXCLUDES 1　cardiomyopathy (in):
coxsackie (virus) (B33.24)
diphtheria (A36.81)
sarcoidosis (D86.85)
tuberculosis (A18.84)

CC Excl: PDX collection 678

✓4th I44　Atrioventricular and left bundle-branch block

I44.0　**Atrioventricular block, first degree**

I44.1　**Atrioventricular block, second degree**
Atrioventricular block, type I and II
Möbitz block, type I and II
Second degree block, type I and II
Wenckebach's block

I44.2　**Atrioventricular block, complete**　CC HCC
Complete heart block NOS　　Third degree block
CC Excl: PDX collection 679

✓5th I44.3　**Other and unspecified atrioventricular block**
Atrioventricular block NOS

I44.30　**Unspecified atrioventricular block**

I44.39　Other **atrioventricular block**

4　I44.4　Left anterior fascicular **block**

4　I44.5　Left posterior fascicular **block**

✓5th I44.6　**Other and unspecified fascicular block**

4　I44.60　Unspecified fascicular block
Left bundle-branch hemiblock NOS

4　I44.69　Other **fascicular block**

4　I44.7　Left bundle-branch block, unspecified

✓4th I45　Other conduction disorders

CC Excl: For CC codes in category I45: PDX collection 679

4　I45.0　**Right fascicular block**

✓5th I45.1　**Other and unspecified right bundle-branch block**

4　I45.10　Unspecified right bundle-branch block
Right bundle-branch block NOS

4　I45.19　Other right bundle-branch block

I45.2　**Bifascicular block**　CC

I45.3　**Trifascicular block**　CC

I45.4　**Nonspecific intraventricular block**
Bundle-branch block NOS

I45.5　**Other specified heart block**
Sinoatrial block　　Sinoauricular block
EXCLUDES 1　heart block NOS (I45.9)

I45.6　**Pre-excitation syndrome**
Accelerated atrioventricular conduction
Accessory atrioventricular conduction
Anomalous atrioventricular excitation
Lown-Ganong-Levine syndrome
Pre-excitation atrioventricular conduction
Wolff-Parkinson-White syndrome

✓5th I45.8　**Other specified conduction disorders**

I45.81　**Long QT syndrome**
DEF: Condition characterized by recurrent syncope, malignant arrhythmias, and sudden death; characteristic prolonged Q-T interval on electrocardiogram.

I45.89　**Other specified conduction disorders**　CC
Atrioventricular [AV] dissociation
Interference dissociation
Isorhythmic dissociation
Nonparoxysmal AV nodal tachycardia
AHA: 2013, 2Q, 31

I45.9　**Conduction disorder, unspecified**
Heart block NOS
Stokes-Adams syndrome

Conduction Disorders

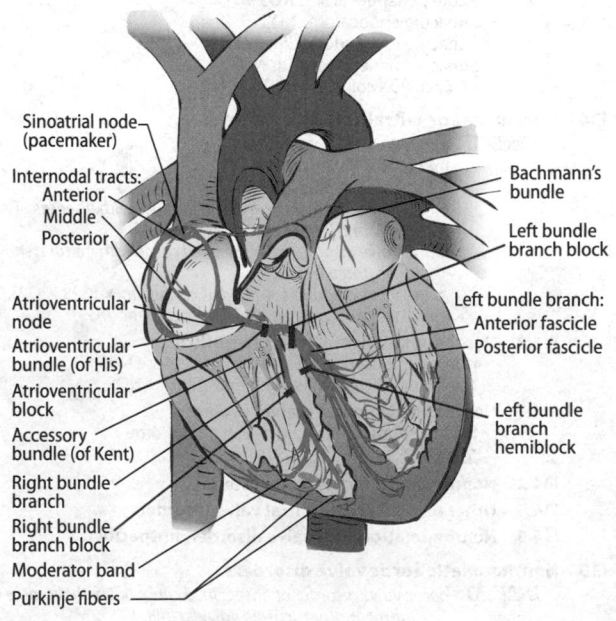

Sinoatrial node (pacemaker)
Internodal tracts:
Anterior
Middle
Posterior
Atrioventricular node
Atrioventricular bundle (of His)
Atrioventricular block
Accessory bundle (of Kent)
Right bundle branch
Right bundle branch block
Moderator band
Purkinje fibers
Bachmann's bundle
Left bundle branch block
Left bundle branch:
Anterior fascicle
Posterior fascicle
Left bundle branch hemiblock

4　Questionable admission when used as PDx.

N Newborn: 0　P Pediatric: 0-17　M Maternity: 12-55　A Adult: 15-124　MCC Major CC Condition　PDxMCC PDx acts as own MCC　CC CC Condition　PDxCC PDx acts as own CC

638　　ICD-10-CM 2018

✓4ᵗʰ **I46**   **Cardiac arrest**

> *EXCLUDES 1*   cardiogenic shock (R57.0)

> **CC Excl: For MCC codes in category I46:** PDX collection 680

¹ **I46.2**   **Cardiac arrest due to underlying cardiac condition**   `MCC` `HCC`
> Code first underlying cardiac condition

¹ **I46.8**   **Cardiac arrest due to other underlying condition**   `MCC` `HCC`
> Code first underlying condition

¹ **I46.9**   **Cardiac arrest, cause unspecified**   `MCC` `HCC`

✓4ᵗʰ **I47**   **Paroxysmal tachycardia**

> Code first tachycardia complicating:
> abortion or ectopic or molar pregnancy (O00-O07, O08.8)
> obstetric surgery and procedures (O75.4)

> *EXCLUDES 1*   tachycardia NOS (R00.0)
> sinoauricular tachycardia NOS (R00.0)
> sinus [sinusal] tachycardia NOS (R00.0)

> **CC Excl: For CC codes in category I47:** PDX collection 679

I47.0   **Re-entry ventricular arrhythmia**   `CC` `HCC`

I47.1   **Supraventricular tachycardia**   `CC` `HCC`
> Atrial (paroxysmal) tachycardia
> Atrioventricular [AV] (paroxysmal) tachycardia
> Atrioventricular re-entrant (nodal) tachycardia [AVNRT] [AVRT]
> Junctional (paroxysmal) tachycardia
> Nodal (paroxysmal) tachycardia

I47.2   **Ventricular tachycardia**   `CC` `HCC`
> **AHA:** 2013, 3Q, 23

I47.9   **Paroxysmal tachycardia, unspecified**   `HCC`
> Bouveret (-Hoffman) syndrome

✓4ᵗʰ **I48**   **Atrial fibrillation and flutter**

> **CC Excl: For CC codes in category I48:** PDX collection 679

I48.0   **Paroxysmal atrial fibrillation**   `HCC`

I48.1   **Persistent atrial fibrillation**   `CC` `HCC`

I48.2   **Chronic atrial fibrillation**   `HCC`
> Permanent atrial fibrillation

I48.3   **Typical atrial flutter**   `CC` `HCC`
> Type I atrial flutter

I48.4   **Atypical atrial flutter**   `CC` `HCC`
> Type II atrial flutter

✓5ᵗʰ **I48.9**   **Unspecified atrial fibrillation and atrial flutter**

> **I48.91**   **Unspecified atrial fibrillation**   `HCC`

> **I48.92**   **Unspecified atrial flutter**   `CC` `HCC`

✓4ᵗʰ **I49**   **Other cardiac arrhythmias**

> Code first cardiac arrhythmia complicating:
> abortion or ectopic or molar pregnancy (O00-O07, O08.8)
> obstetric surgery and procedures (O75.4)

> *EXCLUDES 1*   bradycardia NOS (R00.1)
> neonatal dysrhythmia (P29.1-)
> sinoatrial bradycardia (R00.1)
> sinus bradycardia (R00.1)
> vagal bradycardia (R00.1)

> *EXCLUDES 2* ▶bradycardia NOS (R00.1)◀

> **CC Excl: For CC/MCC codes in category I49:**
> PDX collection 679

✓5ᵗʰ **I49.0**   **Ventricular fibrillation and flutter**

> ¹ **I49.01**   **Ventricular fibrillation**   `MCC` `HCC`

> **I49.02**   **Ventricular flutter**   `MCC` `HCC`

I49.1   **Atrial premature depolarization**
> Atrial premature beats

I49.2   **Junctional premature depolarization**   `CC` `HCC`

I49.3   **Ventricular premature depolarization**

✓5ᵗʰ **I49.4**   **Other and unspecified premature depolarization**

> **I49.40**   **Unspecified premature depolarization**
> Premature beats NOS

> **I49.49**   **Other premature depolarization**
> Ectopic beats
> Extrasystoles
> Extrasystolic arrhythmias
> Premature contractions

I49.5   **Sick sinus syndrome**   `HCC`
> Tachycardia-bradycardia syndrome

I49.8   **Other specified cardiac arrhythmias**
> ▶Brugada syndrome◀
> Coronary sinus rhythm disorder
> Ectopic rhythm disorder
> Nodal rhythm disorder

I49.9   **Cardiac arrhythmia, unspecified**
> Arrhythmia (cardiac) NOS

✓4ᵗʰ **I50**   **Heart failure**

> Code first:
> heart failure complicating abortion or ectopic or molar pregnancy (O00-O07, O08.8)
> heart failure following surgery (I97.13-)
> heart failure due to hypertension (I11.0)
> heart failure due to hypertension with chronic kidney disease (I13.-)
> obstetric surgery and procedures (O75.4)
> rheumatic heart failure (I09.81)

> *EXCLUDES 1*   neonatal cardiac failure (P29.0)
> *EXCLUDES 2*   cardiac arrest (I46.-)
> **AHA:** 2017, 1Q, 47; 2014, 1Q, 25; 2013, 2Q, 33

> **CC Excl: For CC/MCC codes in category I50, unless otherwise noted:** PDX collection 682

▲ **I50.1**   **Left ventricular failure, unspecified**   `CC` `HCC`
> Cardiac asthma
> Edema of lung with heart disease NOS
> Edema of lung with heart failure
> Left heart failure
> Pulmonary edema with heart disease NOS
> Pulmonary edema with heart failure

> *EXCLUDES 1*   edema of lung without heart disease or heart failure (J81.-)
> pulmonary edema without heart disease or failure (J81.-)

> **CC Excl:** PDX collection 681

✓5ᵗʰ **I50.2**   **Systolic (congestive) heart failure**
> ▶Heart failure with reduced ejection fraction [HFrEF]
> Systolic left ventricular heart failure◀
> ▶Code also end stage heart failure, if applicable (I50.84)◀

> *EXCLUDES 1*   combined systolic (congestive) and diastolic (congestive) heart failure (I50.4-)
> **AHA:** 2017, 1Q, 46; 2016, 1Q, 10

> **I50.20**   **Unspecified systolic (congestive) heart failure**   `CC` `HCC`

> **I50.21**   **Acute systolic (congestive) heart failure**   `MCC` `HCC`

> **I50.22**   **Chronic systolic (congestive) heart failure**   `CC` `HCC`

> **I50.23**   **Acute on chronic systolic (congestive) heart failure**   `MCC` `HCC`

✓5ᵗʰ **I50.3**   **Diastolic (congestive) heart failure**
> ▶Diastolic left ventricular heart failure
> Heart failure with normal ejection fraction
> Heart failure with preserved ejection fraction [HFpEF]◀
> ▶Code also end stage heart failure, if applicable (I50.84)◀

> *EXCLUDES 1*   combined systolic (congestive) and diastolic (congestive) heart failure (I50.4-)
> **AHA:** 2017, 1Q, 46; 2016, 1Q, 10

> **I50.30**   **Unspecified diastolic (congestive) heart failure**   `CC` `HCC`

> **I50.31**   **Acute diastolic (congestive) heart failure**   `MCC` `HCC`

> **I50.32**   **Chronic diastolic (congestive) heart failure**   `CC` `HCC`

> **I50.33**   **Acute on chronic diastolic (congestive) heart failure**   `MCC` `HCC`

✓5ᵗʰ **I50.4**   **Combined systolic (congestive) and diastolic (congestive) heart failure**
> ▶Combined systolic and diastolic left ventricular heart failure
> Heart failure with reduced ejection fraction and diastolic dysfunction◀
> ▶Code also end stage heart failure, if applicable (I50.84)◀
> **AHA:** 2017, 1Q, 46; 2016, 1Q, 10

> **I50.40**   **Unspecified combined systolic (congestive) and diastolic (congestive) heart failure**   `CC` `HCC`

> **I50.41**   **Acute combined systolic (congestive) and diastolic (congestive) heart failure**   `MCC` `HCC`

> **I50.42**   **Chronic combined systolic (congestive) and diastolic (congestive) heart failure**   `CC` `HCC`

> **I50.43**   **Acute on chronic combined systolic (congestive) and diastolic (congestive) heart failure**   `MCC` `HCC`

---

¹ MCC only if patient is discharged alive.

☑ Additional Character Req   ✓x7ᵗʰ Placeholder Alert   Unacceptable PDx   Manifestation   `H1`-`H14` HAC   `HCC` CMS-HCC Condition   *EXCLUDES 1* Not Coded Here   *EXCLUDES 2* Not Included Here

Chapter 9. Diseases of the Circulatory System

- ✓5ᵗʰ **I50.8** **Other heart failure**
  - ✓6ᵗʰ **I50.81** **Right heart failure**
    Right ventricular failure
    - **I50.810** **Right heart failure, unspecified**
      Right heart failure without mention of left heart failure
      Right ventricular failure NOS
    - **I50.811** **Acute right heart failure**
      Acute isolated right heart failure
      Acute (isolated) right ventricular failure
    - **I50.812** **Chronic right heart failure**
      Chronic isolated right heart failure
      Chronic (isolated) right ventricular failure
    - **I50.813** **Acute on chronic right heart failure**
      Acute on chronic isolated right heart failure
      Acute on chronic (isolated) right ventricular failure
      Acute decompensation of chronic (isolated) right ventricular failure
      Acute exacerbation of chronic (isolated) right ventricular failure
    - **I50.814** **Right heart failure** due to left heart failure
      Right ventricular failure secondary to left ventricular failure
      Code also the type of left ventricular failure, if known (I50.2-I50.43)
      EXCLUDES 1 right heart failure with but not due to left heart failure (I50.82)
  - **I50.82** **Biventricular heart failure**
    Code also the type of left ventricular failure as systolic, diastolic, or combined, if known (I50.2-I50.43)
  - **I50.83** **High output heart failure**
  - **I50.84** **End stage heart failure**
    Stage D heart failure
    Code also the type of heart failure as systolic, diastolic, or combined, if known (I50.2-I50.43)
  - **I50.89** **Other heart failure**
- **I50.9** **Heart failure, unspecified** `HCC`
  Biventricular (heart) failure NOS
  Cardiac, heart or myocardial failure NOS
  Congestive heart disease
  Congestive heart failure NOS
  Right ventricular failure (secondary to left heart failure)
  EXCLUDES 2 fluid overload (E87.70)
  AHA: 2017, 1Q, 45-46; 2014, 4Q, 21; 2012, 4Q, 92
- ✓4ᵗʰ **I51** **Complications and ill-defined descriptions of heart disease**
  EXCLUDES 1 any condition in I51.4-I51.9 due to hypertension (I11.-)
  any condition in I51.4-I51.9 due to hypertension and chronic kidney disease (I13.-)
  heart disease specified as rheumatic (I00-I09)
  - **I51.0** **Cardiac septal defect, acquired** `CC` `A`
    Acquired septal atrial defect (old)
    Acquired septal auricular defect (old)
    Acquired septal ventricular defect (old)
    EXCLUDES 1 cardiac septal defect as current complication following acute myocardial infarction (I23.1, I23.2)
    DEF: Abnormal communication between opposite heart chambers due to defect of septum; not present at birth.
    CC Excl: PDX collection 654
  - **I51.1** **Rupture of chordae tendineae, not elsewhere classified** `MCC` `HCC`
    EXCLUDES 1 rupture of chordae tendineae as current complication following acute myocardial infarction (I23.4)
    CC Excl: PDX collection 655
  - **I51.2** **Rupture of papillary muscle, not elsewhere classified** `MCC` `HCC`
    EXCLUDES 1 rupture of papillary muscle as current complication following acute myocardial infarction (I23.5)
    CC Excl: PDX collection 656
  - **I51.3** **Intracardiac thrombosis, not elsewhere classified**
    Apical thrombosis (old)
    Atrial thrombosis (old)
    Auricular thrombosis (old)
    Mural thrombosis (old)
    Ventricular thrombosis (old)
    EXCLUDES 1 intracardiac thrombosis as current complication following acute myocardial infarction (I23.6)
    AHA: 2013, 1Q, 24

- **I51.4** **Myocarditis, unspecified** `HCC`
  Chronic (interstitial) myocarditis
  Myocardial fibrosis
  Myocarditis NOS
  EXCLUDES 1 acute or subacute myocarditis (I40.-)
- **I51.5** **Myocardial degeneration** `HCC`
  Fatty degeneration of heart or myocardium
  Myocardial disease
  Senile degeneration of heart or myocardium
- **I51.7** **Cardiomegaly**
  Cardiac dilatation
  Cardiac hypertrophy
  Ventricular dilatation
- ✓5ᵗʰ **I51.8** **Other ill-defined heart diseases**
  - **I51.81** **Takotsubo syndrome** `CC`
    Reversible left ventricular dysfunction following sudden emotional stress
    Stress induced cardiomyopathy
    Takotsubo cardiomyopathy
    Transient left ventricular apical ballooning syndrome
    CC Excl: PDX collection 683
  - **I51.89** **Other ill-defined heart diseases**
    Carditis (acute)(chronic)
    Pancarditis (acute)(chronic)
- **I51.9** **Heart disease, unspecified**
- **I52** ***Other heart disorders in diseases classified elsewhere***
  Code first underlying disease, such as:
  congenital syphilis (A50.5)
  mucopolysaccharidosis (E76.3)
  schistosomiasis (B65.0-B65.9)
  EXCLUDES 1 heart disease (in):
  gonococcal infection (A54.83)
  meningococcal infection (A39.50)
  rheumatoid arthritis (M05.31)
  syphilis (A52.06)

Cerebrovascular diseases (I60-I69)

Use additional code to identify presence of:
alcohol abuse and dependence (F10.-)
exposure to environmental tobacco smoke (Z77.22)
history of tobacco dependence (Z87.891)
hypertension (I10-I15)
occupational exposure to environmental tobacco smoke (Z57.31)
tobacco dependence (F17.-)
tobacco use (Z72.0)
EXCLUDES 1 transient cerebral ischemic attacks and related syndromes (G45.-)
traumatic intracranial hemorrhage (S06.-)
AHA: 2014, 3Q, 5; 2012, 4Q, 91-92

- ✓4ᵗʰ **I60** **Nontraumatic subarachnoid hemorrhage**
  INCLUDES ruptured cerebral aneurysm
  EXCLUDES 1 syphilitic ruptured cerebral aneurysm (A52.05)
  EXCLUDES 2 sequelae of subarachnoid hemorrhage (I69.0-)

  CC Excl: For MCC codes in category I60: PDX collection 684

  - ✓5ᵗʰ **I60.0** **Nontraumatic subarachnoid hemorrhage from** carotid siphon and bifurcation
    - **I60.00** **Nontraumatic subarachnoid hemorrhage from** unspecified **carotid siphon and bifurcation** `MCC` `HCC`
    - **I60.01** **Nontraumatic subarachnoid hemorrhage from** right **carotid siphon and bifurcation** `MCC` `HCC`
    - **I60.02** **Nontraumatic subarachnoid hemorrhage from** left **carotid siphon and bifurcation** `MCC` `HCC`
  - ✓5ᵗʰ **I60.1** **Nontraumatic subarachnoid hemorrhage from** middle cerebral artery
    - **I60.10** **Nontraumatic subarachnoid hemorrhage from** unspecified **middle cerebral artery** `MCC` `HCC`
    - **I60.11** **Nontraumatic subarachnoid hemorrhage from** right **middle cerebral artery** `MCC` `HCC`
    - **I60.12** **Nontraumatic subarachnoid hemorrhage from** left **middle cerebral artery** `MCC` `HCC`
  - **I60.2** **Nontraumatic subarachnoid hemorrhage from** anterior communicating artery `MCC` `HCC`
  - ✓5ᵗʰ **I60.3** **Nontraumatic subarachnoid hemorrhage from** posterior communicating artery
    - **I60.30** **Nontraumatic subarachnoid hemorrhage from** unspecified **posterior communicating artery** `MCC` `HCC`
    - **I60.31** **Nontraumatic subarachnoid hemorrhage from** right **posterior communicating artery** `MCC` `HCC`

N Newborn: 0　**P** Pediatric: 0-17　**M** Maternity: 12-55　**A** Adult: 15-124　**MCC** Major CC Condition　**PDxMCC** PDx acts as own MCC　**CC** CC Condition　**PDxCC** PDx acts as own CC

640　　　　　　　　　　　　　　　　　　　　　　　　　　　　ICD-10-CM 2018

I60.32   Nontraumatic subarachnoid hemorrhage from **left posterior communicating artery** `MCC` `HCC`

I60.4   Nontraumatic subarachnoid hemorrhage from **basilar artery** `MCC` `HCC`

✔5ᵗʰ **I60.5**   Nontraumatic subarachnoid hemorrhage from vertebral artery

     I60.50   Nontraumatic subarachnoid hemorrhage from unspecified vertebral artery `MCC` `HCC`

     I60.51   Nontraumatic subarachnoid hemorrhage from right vertebral artery `MCC` `HCC`

     I60.52   Nontraumatic subarachnoid hemorrhage from left vertebral artery `MCC` `HCC`

I60.6   Nontraumatic subarachnoid hemorrhage from other intracranial arteries `MCC` `HCC`

I60.7   Nontraumatic subarachnoid hemorrhage from unspecified intracranial artery `MCC` `HCC`
     Ruptured (congenital) berry aneurysm
     Ruptured (congenital) cerebral aneurysm
     Subarachnoid hemorrhage (nontraumatic) from cerebral artery NOS
     Subarachnoid hemorrhage (nontraumatic) from communicating artery NOS
     EXCLUDES 1   berry aneurysm, nonruptured (I67.1)

I60.8   Other nontraumatic subarachnoid hemorrhage `MCC` `HCC`
     Meningeal hemorrhage
     Rupture of cerebral arteriovenous malformation

I60.9   Nontraumatic subarachnoid hemorrhage, unspecified `MCC` `HCC`

✔4ᵗʰ **I61**   **Nontraumatic intracerebral hemorrhage**
     EXCLUDES 2   sequelae of intracerebral hemorrhage (I69.1-)
     AHA: 2017, 2Q, 9-10

     CC Excl: For MCC codes in category I61: PDX collection 684

     I61.0   Nontraumatic intracerebral hemorrhage in hemisphere, subcortical `MCC` `HCC`
        Deep intracerebral hemorrhage (nontraumatic)

     I61.1   Nontraumatic intracerebral hemorrhage in hemisphere, cortical `MCC` `HCC`
        Cerebral lobe hemorrhage (nontraumatic)
        Superficial intracerebral hemorrhage (nontraumatic)

     I61.2   Nontraumatic intracerebral hemorrhage in hemisphere, unspecified `MCC` `HCC`

     I61.3   Nontraumatic intracerebral hemorrhage in brain stem `MCC` `HCC`

     I61.4   Nontraumatic intracerebral hemorrhage in cerebellum `MCC` `HCC`

     I61.5   Nontraumatic intracerebral hemorrhage, intraventricular `MCC` `HCC`

     I61.6   Nontraumatic intracerebral hemorrhage, multiple localized `MCC` `HCC`

     I61.8   Other nontraumatic intracerebral hemorrhage `MCC` `HCC`

     I61.9   Nontraumatic intracerebral hemorrhage, unspecified `MCC` `HCC`

✔4ᵗʰ **I62**   **Other and unspecified nontraumatic intracranial hemorrhage**
     EXCLUDES 2   sequelae of intracranial hemorrhage (I69.2)

     CC Excl: For CC/MCC codes in category I62: PDX collection 684

     ✔5ᵗʰ **I62.0**   Nontraumatic subdural hemorrhage

        I62.00   Nontraumatic subdural hemorrhage, unspecified `MCC` `HCC`

        I62.01   Nontraumatic acute subdural hemorrhage `MCC` `HCC`

        I62.02   Nontraumatic subacute subdural hemorrhage `MCC` `HCC`

        I62.03   Nontraumatic chronic subdural hemorrhage `MCC` `HCC`

     I62.1   Nontraumatic extradural hemorrhage `MCC` `HCC`
        Nontraumatic epidural hemorrhage

     I62.9   Nontraumatic intracranial hemorrhage, unspecified `CC` `HCC`

✔4ᵗʰ **I63**   **Cerebral infarction**
     INCLUDES   occlusion and stenosis of cerebral and precerebral arteries, resulting in cerebral infarction
     Use additional code, if applicable, to identify status post administration of tPA (rtPA) in a different facility within the last 24 hours prior to admission to current facility (Z92.82)
     Use additional code, if known, to indicate National Institutes of Health Stroke Scale (NIHSS) score (R29.7-)
     EXCLUDES 2   sequelae of cerebral infarction (I69.3-)
     AHA: 2017, 2Q, 9-10; 2014, 1Q, 23

     ✔5ᵗʰ **I63.0**   Cerebral infarction due to thrombosis of precerebral arteries

        I63.00   Cerebral infarction due to thrombosis of unspecified precerebral artery `MCC` `HCC`
           CC Excl: PDX collection 685

        ✔6ᵗʰ **I63.01**   Cerebral infarction due to thrombosis of vertebral artery

           CC Excl: For MCC codes in subcategory I63.01: PDX collection 686

           I63.011   Cerebral infarction due to thrombosis of right vertebral artery `MCC` `HCC`

           I63.012   Cerebral infarction due to thrombosis of left vertebral artery `MCC` `HCC`

           I63.013   Cerebral infarction due to thrombosis of bilateral vertebral arteries `MCC` `HCC`

           I63.019   Cerebral infarction due to thrombosis of unspecified vertebral artery `MCC` `HCC`

        I63.02   Cerebral infarction due to thrombosis of basilar artery `MCC` `HCC`
           CC Excl: PDX collection 685

        ✔6ᵗʰ **I63.03**   Cerebral infarction due to thrombosis of carotid artery

           CC Excl: For MCC codes in subcategory I63.03: PDX collection 687

           I63.031   Cerebral infarction due to thrombosis of right carotid artery `MCC` `HCC`

           I63.032   Cerebral infarction due to thrombosis of left carotid artery `MCC` `HCC`

           I63.033   Cerebral infarction due to thrombosis of bilateral carotid arteries `MCC` `HCC`

           I63.039   Cerebral infarction due to thrombosis of unspecified carotid artery `MCC` `HCC`

        I63.09   Cerebral infarction due to thrombosis of other precerebral artery `MCC` `HCC`
           CC Excl: PDX collection 685

     ✔5ᵗʰ **I63.1**   Cerebral infarction due to embolism of precerebral arteries

        I63.10   Cerebral infarction due to embolism of unspecified precerebral artery `MCC` `HCC`
           CC Excl: PDX collection 685

        ✔6ᵗʰ **I63.11**   Cerebral infarction due to embolism of vertebral artery

           CC Excl: For MCC codes in subcategory I63.11: PDX collection 686

           I63.111   Cerebral infarction due to embolism of right vertebral artery `MCC` `HCC`

           I63.112   Cerebral infarction due to embolism of left vertebral artery `MCC` `HCC`

           I63.113   Cerebral infarction due to embolism of bilateral vertebral arteries `MCC` `HCC`

           I63.119   Cerebral infarction due to embolism of unspecified vertebral artery `MCC` `HCC`

        I63.12   Cerebral infarction due to embolism of basilar artery `MCC` `HCC`
           CC Excl: PDX collection 685

        ✔6ᵗʰ **I63.13**   Cerebral infarction due to embolism of carotid artery

           CC Excl: For MCC codes in subcategory I63.13: PDX collection 687

           I63.131   Cerebral infarction due to embolism of right carotid artery `MCC` `HCC`

           I63.132   Cerebral infarction due to embolism of left carotid artery `MCC` `HCC`

           I63.133   Cerebral infarction due to embolism of bilateral carotid arteries `MCC` `HCC`

           I63.139   Cerebral infarction due to embolism of unspecified carotid artery `MCC` `HCC`

✔ Additional Character Req   ✔x7ᵗʰ Placeholder Alert   Unacceptable PDx   Manifestation   **H1**-**H14** HAC   `HCC` CMS-HCC Condition   *EXCLUDES 1* Not Coded Here   *EXCLUDES 2* Not Included Here

ICD-10-CM 2018   641

I63.19 **Cerebral infarction due to embolism of other precerebral artery** `MCC` `HCC`
CC Excl: PDX collection 685

✓5ᵗʰ **I63.2** **Cerebral infarction due to unspecified occlusion or stenosis of precerebral arteries**

I63.20 **Cerebral infarction due to unspecified occlusion or stenosis of unspecified precerebral arteries** `MCC` `HCC`
CC Excl: PDX collection 685

✓6ᵗʰ **I63.21** **Cerebral infarction due to unspecified occlusion or stenosis of vertebral arteries**

CC Excl: For MCC codes in subcategory I63.21: PDX collection 686

▲ I63.211 **Cerebral infarction due to unspecified occlusion or stenosis of right vertebral artery** `MCC` `HCC`

▲ I63.212 **Cerebral infarction due to unspecified occlusion or stenosis of left vertebral artery** `MCC` `HCC`

I63.213 **Cerebral infarction due to unspecified occlusion or stenosis of bilateral vertebral arteries** `MCC` `HCC`

I63.219 **Cerebral infarction due to unspecified occlusion or stenosis of unspecified vertebral arteries** `MCC` `HCC`

▲ I63.22 **Cerebral infarction due to unspecified occlusion or stenosis of basilar artery** `MCC` `HCC`
CC Excl: PDX collection 685

✓6ᵗʰ **I63.23** **Cerebral infarction due to unspecified occlusion or stenosis of carotid arteries**

CC Excl: For MCC codes in subcategory I63.23: PDX collection 687

I63.231 **Cerebral infarction due to unspecified occlusion or stenosis of right carotid arteries** `MCC` `HCC`

I63.232 **Cerebral infarction due to unspecified occlusion or stenosis of left carotid arteries** `MCC` `HCC`

I63.233 **Cerebral infarction due to unspecified occlusion or stenosis of bilateral carotid arteries** `MCC` `HCC`

I63.239 **Cerebral infarction due to unspecified occlusion or stenosis of unspecified carotid arteries** `MCC` `HCC`

I63.29 **Cerebral infarction due to unspecified occlusion or stenosis of other precerebral arteries** `MCC` `HCC`
CC Excl: PDX collection 685

✓5ᵗʰ **I63.3** **Cerebral infarction due to thrombosis of cerebral arteries**

CC Excl: For MCC codes in subcategory I63.3: PDX collection 688

I63.30 **Cerebral infarction due to thrombosis of unspecified cerebral artery** `MCC` `HCC`

✓6ᵗʰ **I63.31** **Cerebral infarction due to thrombosis of middle cerebral artery**

I63.311 **Cerebral infarction due to thrombosis of right middle cerebral artery** `MCC` `HCC`

I63.312 **Cerebral infarction due to thrombosis of left middle cerebral artery** `MCC` `HCC`

I63.313 **Cerebral infarction due to thrombosis of bilateral middle cerebral arteries** `MCC` `HCC`

I63.319 **Cerebral infarction due to thrombosis of unspecified middle cerebral artery** `MCC` `HCC`

✓6ᵗʰ **I63.32** **Cerebral infarction due to thrombosis of anterior cerebral artery**

I63.321 **Cerebral infarction due to thrombosis of right anterior cerebral artery** `MCC` `HCC`

I63.322 **Cerebral infarction due to thrombosis of left anterior cerebral artery** `MCC` `HCC`

▲ I63.323 **Cerebral infarction due to thrombosis of bilateral anterior cerebral arteries** `MCC` `HCC`

I63.329 **Cerebral infarction due to thrombosis of unspecified anterior cerebral artery** `MCC` `HCC`

✓6ᵗʰ **I63.33** **Cerebral infarction due to thrombosis of posterior cerebral artery**

I63.331 **Cerebral infarction due to thrombosis of right posterior cerebral artery** `MCC` `HCC`

I63.332 **Cerebral infarction due to thrombosis of left posterior cerebral artery** `MCC` `HCC`

I63.333 **Cerebral infarction to thrombosis of bilateral posterior cerebral arteries** `MCC` `HCC`

I63.339 **Cerebral infarction due to thrombosis of unspecified posterior cerebral artery** `MCC` `HCC`

✓6ᵗʰ **I63.34** **Cerebral infarction due to thrombosis of cerebellar artery**

I63.341 **Cerebral infarction due to thrombosis of right cerebellar artery** `MCC` `HCC`

I63.342 **Cerebral infarction due to thrombosis of left cerebellar artery** `MCC` `HCC`

I63.343 **Cerebral infarction to thrombosis of bilateral cerebellar arteries** `MCC` `HCC`

I63.349 **Cerebral infarction due to thrombosis of unspecified cerebellar artery** `MCC` `HCC`

I63.39 **Cerebral infarction due to thrombosis of other cerebral artery** `MCC` `HCC`

✓5ᵗʰ **I63.4** **Cerebral infarction due to embolism of cerebral arteries**

CC Excl: For MCC codes in subcategory I63.4: PDX collection 688

I63.40 **Cerebral infarction due to embolism of unspecified cerebral artery** `MCC` `HCC`

✓6ᵗʰ **I63.41** **Cerebral infarction due to embolism of middle cerebral artery**

I63.411 **Cerebral infarction due to embolism of right middle cerebral artery** `MCC` `HCC`

I63.412 **Cerebral infarction due to embolism of left middle cerebral artery** `MCC` `HCC`

I63.413 **Cerebral infarction due to embolism of bilateral middle cerebral arteries** `MCC` `HCC`

I63.419 **Cerebral infarction due to embolism of unspecified middle cerebral artery** `MCC` `HCC`

✓6ᵗʰ **I63.42** **Cerebral infarction due to embolism of anterior cerebral artery**

I63.421 **Cerebral infarction due to embolism of right anterior cerebral artery** `MCC` `HCC`

I63.422 **Cerebral infarction due to embolism of left anterior cerebral artery** `MCC` `HCC`

I63.423 **Cerebral infarction due to embolism of bilateral anterior cerebral arteries** `MCC` `HCC`

I63.429 **Cerebral infarction due to embolism of unspecified anterior cerebral artery** `MCC` `HCC`

✓6ᵗʰ **I63.43** **Cerebral infarction due to embolism of posterior cerebral artery**

I63.431 **Cerebral infarction due to embolism of right posterior cerebral artery** `MCC` `HCC`

I63.432 **Cerebral infarction due to embolism of left posterior cerebral artery** `MCC` `HCC`

I63.433 **Cerebral infarction due to embolism of bilateral posterior cerebral arteries** `MCC` `HCC`

I63.439 **Cerebral infarction due to embolism of unspecified posterior cerebral artery** `MCC` `HCC`

N Newborn: 0   P Pediatric: 0-17   M Maternity: 12-55   A Adult: 15-124   `MCC` Major CC Condition   `PDxMCC` PDx acts as own MCC   `CC` CC Condition   `PDxCC` PDx acts as own CC

642   ICD-10-CM 2018

✓6th **I63.44** Cerebral infarction due to embolism of cerebellar artery

     I63.441 Cerebral infarction due to embolism of right cerebellar artery `MCC` `HCC`

     I63.442 Cerebral infarction due to embolism of left cerebellar artery `MCC` `HCC`

     I63.443 Cerebral infarction due to embolism of bilateral cerebellar arteries `MCC` `HCC`

     I63.449 Cerebral infarction due to embolism of unspecified cerebellar artery `MCC` `HCC`

   I63.49 Cerebral infarction due to embolism of other cerebral artery `MCC` `HCC`

✓5th **I63.5** Cerebral infarction due to unspecified occlusion or stenosis of cerebral arteries

> **CC Excl: For MCC codes in subcategory I63.5:**
> PDX collection 688

   I63.50 Cerebral infarction due to unspecified occlusion or stenosis of unspecified cerebral artery `MCC` `HCC`

✓6th **I63.51** Cerebral infarction due to unspecified occlusion or stenosis of middle cerebral artery

     I63.511 Cerebral infarction due to unspecified occlusion or stenosis of right middle cerebral artery `MCC` `HCC`

     I63.512 Cerebral infarction due to unspecified occlusion or stenosis of left middle cerebral artery `MCC` `HCC`

     ▲ **I63.513** Cerebral infarction due to unspecified occlusion or stenosis of bilateral middle cerebral arteries `MCC` `HCC`

     I63.519 Cerebral infarction due to unspecified occlusion or stenosis of unspecified middle cerebral artery `MCC` `HCC`

✓6th **I63.52** Cerebral infarction due to unspecified occlusion or stenosis of anterior cerebral artery

     I63.521 Cerebral infarction due to unspecified occlusion or stenosis of right anterior cerebral artery `MCC` `HCC`

     I63.522 Cerebral infarction due to unspecified occlusion or stenosis of left anterior cerebral artery `MCC` `HCC`

     ▲ **I63.523** Cerebral infarction due to unspecified occlusion or stenosis of bilateral anterior cerebral arteries `MCC` `HCC`

     I63.529 Cerebral infarction due to unspecified occlusion or stenosis of unspecified anterior cerebral artery `MCC` `HCC`

✓6th **I63.53** Cerebral infarction due to unspecified occlusion or stenosis of posterior cerebral artery

     I63.531 Cerebral infarction due to unspecified occlusion or stenosis of right posterior cerebral artery `MCC` `HCC`

     I63.532 Cerebral infarction due to unspecified occlusion or stenosis of left posterior cerebral artery `MCC` `HCC`

     ▲ **I63.533** Cerebral infarction due to unspecified occlusion or stenosis of bilateral posterior cerebral arteries `MCC` `HCC`

     I63.539 Cerebral infarction due to unspecified occlusion or stenosis of unspecified posterior cerebral artery `MCC` `HCC`

✓6th **I63.54** Cerebral infarction due to unspecified occlusion or stenosis of cerebellar artery

     I63.541 Cerebral infarction due to unspecified occlusion or stenosis of right cerebellar artery `MCC` `HCC`

     I63.542 Cerebral infarction due to unspecified occlusion or stenosis of left cerebellar artery `MCC` `HCC`

     I63.543 Cerebral infarction due to unspecified occlusion or stenosis of bilateral cerebellar arteries `MCC` `HCC`

     I63.549 Cerebral infarction due to unspecified occlusion or stenosis of unspecified cerebellar artery `MCC` `HCC`

   I63.59 Cerebral infarction due to unspecified occlusion or stenosis of other cerebral artery `MCC` `HCC`

I63.6 Cerebral infarction due to cerebral venous thrombosis, nonpyogenic `MCC` `HCC`
    CC Excl: PDX collection 688

I63.8 Other cerebral infarction `MCC` `HCC`
    CC Excl:.PDX collection 688

I63.9 Cerebral infarction, unspecified `MCC` `HCC`
    Stroke NOS
    EXCLUDES 2 ►transient cerebral ischemic attacks and related syndromes (G45.-)◄
    AHA: 2015, 1Q, 25
    CC Excl: PDX collection 688

✓4th **I65** Occlusion and stenosis of precerebral arteries, not resulting in cerebral infarction

    INCLUDES embolism of precerebral artery
            narrowing of precerebral artery
            obstruction (complete) (partial) of precerebral artery
            thrombosis of precerebral artery
    EXCLUDES 1 insufficiency, NOS, of precerebral artery (G45.-)
            insufficiency of precerebral arteries causing cerebral infarction (I63.0-I63.2)

✓5th **I65.0** Occlusion and stenosis of vertebral artery

   I65.01 Occlusion and stenosis of right vertebral artery

   I65.02 Occlusion and stenosis of left vertebral artery

   I65.03 Occlusion and stenosis of bilateral vertebral arteries

   I65.09 Occlusion and stenosis of unspecified vertebral artery

I65.1 Occlusion and stenosis of basilar artery

✓5th **I65.2** Occlusion and stenosis of carotid artery

   I65.21 Occlusion and stenosis of right carotid artery

   I65.22 Occlusion and stenosis of left carotid artery

   I65.23 Occlusion and stenosis of bilateral carotid arteries

   I65.29 Occlusion and stenosis of unspecified carotid artery

I65.8 Occlusion and stenosis of other precerebral arteries

I65.9 Occlusion and stenosis of unspecified precerebral artery
    Occlusion and stenosis of precerebral artery NOS

✓4th **I66** Occlusion and stenosis of cerebral arteries, not resulting in cerebral infarction

    INCLUDES embolism of cerebral artery
            narrowing of cerebral artery
            obstruction (complete) (partial) of cerebral artery
            thrombosis of cerebral artery
    EXCLUDES 1 occlusion and stenosis of cerebral artery causing cerebral infarction (I63.3-I63.5)

✓5th **I66.0** Occlusion and stenosis of middle cerebral artery

   I66.01 Occlusion and stenosis of right middle cerebral artery

   I66.02 Occlusion and stenosis of left middle cerebral artery

   I66.03 Occlusion and stenosis of bilateral middle cerebral arteries

   I66.09 Occlusion and stenosis of unspecified middle cerebral artery

✓5th **I66.1** Occlusion and stenosis of anterior cerebral artery

   I66.11 Occlusion and stenosis of right anterior cerebral artery

   I66.12 Occlusion and stenosis of left anterior cerebral artery

   I66.13 Occlusion and stenosis of bilateral anterior cerebral arteries

   I66.19 Occlusion and stenosis of unspecified anterior cerebral artery

✓5th **I66.2** Occlusion and stenosis of posterior cerebral artery

   I66.21 Occlusion and stenosis of right posterior cerebral artery

   I66.22 Occlusion and stenosis of left posterior cerebral artery

   I66.23 Occlusion and stenosis of bilateral posterior cerebral arteries

   I66.29 Occlusion and stenosis of unspecified posterior cerebral artery

I66.3 Occlusion and stenosis of cerebellar arteries

I66.8 Occlusion and stenosis of other cerebral arteries
    Occlusion and stenosis of perforating arteries

I66.9 Occlusion and stenosis of unspecified cerebral artery

✓ Additional Character Req   ✓x7th Placeholder Alert   Unacceptable PDx   Manifestation   H1 - H14 HAC   HCC CMS-HCC Condition   *EXCLUDES 1* Not Coded Here   *EXCLUDES 2* Not Included Here

ICD-10-CM 2018   643

I63.44–I66.9

Berry Aneurysm

Berry aneurysms form at the site of a weakness in an arterial wall, often at a junction

Berry aneurysm

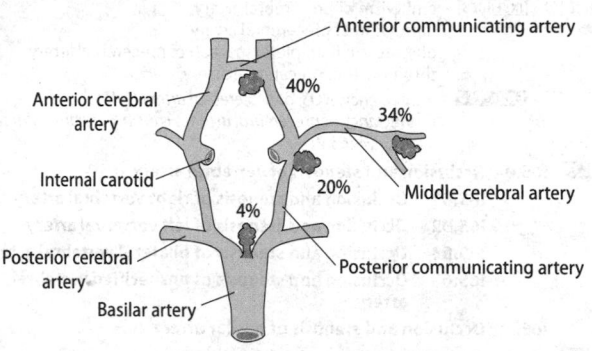

Anterior communicating artery

Anterior cerebral artery

Internal carotid

40%

34%

20%

4%

Middle cerebral artery

Posterior cerebral artery

Posterior communicating artery

Basilar artery

Common sites of berry aneurysms in the circle of Willis arteries

✓4ᵗʰ I67   Other cerebrovascular diseases
> *EXCLUDES 2*   *sequelae of the listed conditions (I69.8)*

I67.Ø   Dissection of cerebral arteries, nonruptured   `MCC` `HCC`
> *EXCLUDES 1*   *ruptured cerebral arteries (I6Ø.7)*
CC Excl: PDX collection 689

I67.1   Cerebral aneurysm, nonruptured
Cerebral aneurysm NOS
Cerebral arteriovenous fistula, acquired
Internal carotid artery aneurysm, intracranial portion
Internal carotid artery aneurysm, NOS
> *EXCLUDES 1*   *congenital cerebral aneurysm, nonruptured (Q28.-)*
> *ruptured cerebral aneurysm (I6Ø.7)*

I67.2   Cerebral atherosclerosis   `A`
Atheroma of cerebral and precerebral arteries

I67.3   Progressive vascular leukoencephalopathy   `HIV` `CC`
Binswanger's disease
CC Excl: PDX collection 133

I67.4   Hypertensive encephalopathy   `CC`
> *EXCLUDES 2* ▶*insufficiency, NOS, of precerebral arteries (G45.2)*◄
CC Excl: PDX collection 69Ø

I67.5   Moyamoya disease   `CC`
DEF: Cerebrovascular ischemia; vessels occlude and rupture, causing tiny hemorrhages at base of brain; affects predominantly Japanese people.
CC Excl: PDX collection 691

I67.6   Nonpyogenic thrombosis of intracranial venous system   `CC`
Nonpyogenic thrombosis of cerebral vein
Nonpyogenic thrombosis of intracranial venous sinus
> *EXCLUDES 1*   *nonpyogenic thrombosis of intracranial venous system causing infarction (I63.6)*
CC Excl: PDX collection 692

I67.7   Cerebral arteritis, not elsewhere classified   `CC`
Granulomatous angiitis of the nervous system
> *EXCLUDES 1*   *allergic granulomatous angiitis (M3Ø.1)*
CC Excl: PDX collection 693

✓5ᵗʰ I67.8   Other specified cerebrovascular diseases

I67.81   Acute cerebrovascular insufficiency   `CC`
Acute cerebrovascular insufficiency unspecified as to location or reversibility
CC Excl: PDX collection 694

I67.82   Cerebral ischemia   `CC`
Chronic cerebral ischemia
CC Excl: PDX collection 694

I67.83   Posterior reversible encephalopathy syndrome   `HIV` `MCC`
PRES
CC Excl: PDX collection 61Ø

✓6ᵗʰ I67.84   Cerebral vasospasm and vasoconstriction

I67.841   Reversible cerebrovascular vasoconstriction syndrome   `CC`
Call-Fleming syndrome
Code first underlying condition, if applicable, such as eclampsia (O15.ØØ-O15.9)
CC Excl: PDX collection 586

I67.848   Other cerebrovascular vasospasm and vasoconstriction   `CC`
CC Excl: PDX collection 586

I67.89   Other cerebrovascular disease   `CC`
CC Excl: PDX collection 694

I67.9   Cerebrovascular disease, unspecified

✓4ᵗʰ I68   Cerebrovascular disorders in diseases classified elsewhere

I68.Ø   *Cerebral amyloid angiopathy*
Code first underlying amyloidosis (E85.-)

I68.2   *Cerebral arteritis in other diseases classified elsewhere*   `CC`
Code first underlying disease
> *EXCLUDES 1*   *cerebral arteritis (in):*
> *listerosis (A32.89)*
> *systemic lupus erythematosus (M32.19)*
> *syphilis (A52.Ø4)*
> *tuberculosis (A18.89)*
CC Excl: PDX collection 693

I68.8   *Other cerebrovascular disorders in diseases classified elsewhere*
Code first underlying disease
> *EXCLUDES 1*   *syphilitic cerebral aneurysm (A52.Ø5)*

✓4ᵗʰ I69   Sequelae of cerebrovascular disease
> `NOTE`   Category I69 is to be used to indicate conditions in I6Ø-I67 as the cause of sequelae. The "sequelae" include conditions specified as such or as residuals which may occur at any time after the onset of the causal condition
> *EXCLUDES 1*   *personal history of cerebral infarction without residual deficit (Z86.73)*
> *personal history of prolonged reversible ischemic neurologic deficit (PRIND) (Z86.73)*
> *personal history of reversible ischemic neurologcial deficit (RIND) (Z86.73)*
> *sequelae of traumatic intracranial injury (SØ6.-)*
> ~~*transient ischemic attack (TIA) (G45.9)*~~
AHA: 2017, 1Q, 47; 2015, 1Q, 25; 2012, 4Q, 106

✓5ᵗʰ I69.Ø   Sequelae of nontraumatic subarachnoid hemorrhage

I69.ØØ   Unspecified sequelae of nontraumatic subarachnoid hemorrhage

✓6ᵗʰ I69.Ø1   Cognitive deficits following nontraumatic subarachnoid hemorrhage

I69.Ø1Ø   Attention and concentration deficit following nontraumatic subarachnoid hemorrhage

I69.Ø11   Memory deficit following nontraumatic subarachnoid hemorrhage

I69.Ø12   Visuospatial deficit and spatial neglect following nontraumatic subarachnoid hemorrhage

I69.Ø13   Psychomotor deficit following nontraumatic subarachnoid hemorrhage

I69.Ø14   Frontal lobe and executive function deficit following nontraumatic subarachnoid hemorrhage

I69.Ø15   Cognitive social or emotional deficit following nontraumatic subarachnoid hemorrhage

I69.Ø18   Other symptoms and signs involving cognitive functions following nontraumatic subarachnoid hemorrhage

I69.Ø19   Unspecified symptoms and signs involving cognitive functions following nontraumatic subarachnoid hemorrhage

✓6ᵗʰ I69.Ø2   Speech and language deficits following nontraumatic subarachnoid hemorrhage

I69.Ø2Ø   Aphasia following nontraumatic subarachnoid hemorrhage

I69.Ø21   Dysphasia following nontraumatic subarachnoid hemorrhage

I69.Ø22   Dysarthria following nontraumatic subarachnoid hemorrhage

`N` Newborn: 0   `P` Pediatric: 0-17   `M` Maternity: 12-55   `A` Adult: 15-124   `MCC` Major CC Condition   `PDxMCC` PDx acts as own MCC   `CC` CC Condition   `PDxCC` PDx acts as own CC

644   ICD-10-CM 2018

Chapter 9. Diseases of the Circulatory System

I69.023   **Fluency disorder** following nontraumatic subarachnoid hemorrhage
Stuttering following nontraumatic subarachnoid hemorrhage

I69.028   **Other speech and language deficits** following nontraumatic subarachnoid hemorrhage

✓6ᵗʰ **I69.03**   **Monoplegia** of upper limb following nontraumatic subarachnoid hemorrhage
AHA: 2017, 1Q, 47

I69.031   **Monoplegia of upper limb** following nontraumatic subarachnoid hemorrhage affecting **right dominant** side   HCC

I69.032   **Monoplegia of upper limb** following nontraumatic subarachnoid hemorrhage affecting **left dominant** side   HCC

I69.033   **Monoplegia of upper limb** following nontraumatic subarachnoid hemorrhage affecting **right non-dominant** side   HCC

I69.034   **Monoplegia of upper limb** following nontraumatic subarachnoid hemorrhage affecting **left non-dominant** side   HCC

I69.039   **Monoplegia of upper limb** following nontraumatic subarachnoid hemorrhage affecting **unspecified** side   HCC

✓6ᵗʰ **I69.04**   **Monoplegia** of lower limb following nontraumatic subarachnoid hemorrhage
AHA: 2017, 1Q, 47

I69.041   **Monoplegia of lower limb** following nontraumatic subarachnoid hemorrhage affecting **right dominant** side   HCC

I69.042   **Monoplegia of lower limb** following nontraumatic subarachnoid hemorrhage affecting **left dominant** side   HCC

I69.043   **Monoplegia of lower limb** following nontraumatic subarachnoid hemorrhage affecting **right non-dominant** side   HCC

I69.044   **Monoplegia of lower limb** following nontraumatic subarachnoid hemorrhage affecting **left non-dominant** side   HCC

I69.049   **Monoplegia of lower limb** following nontraumatic subarachnoid hemorrhage affecting **unspecified** side   HCC

✓6ᵗʰ **I69.05**   **Hemiplegia** and **hemiparesis** following nontraumatic subarachnoid hemorrhage
AHA: 2015, 1Q, 25

I69.051   **Hemiplegia and hemiparesis** following nontraumatic subarachnoid hemorrhage affecting **right dominant side**   CC HCC
CC Excl: PDX collection 695

I69.052   **Hemiplegia and hemiparesis** following nontraumatic subarachnoid hemorrhage affecting **left dominant side**   CC HCC
CC Excl: PDX collection 695

I69.053   **Hemiplegia and hemiparesis** following nontraumatic subarachnoid hemorrhage affecting **right non-dominant side**   CC HCC
CC Excl: PDX collection 696

I69.054   **Hemiplegia and hemiparesis** following nontraumatic subarachnoid hemorrhage affecting **left non-dominant side**   CC HCC
CC Excl: PDX collection 696

I69.059   **Hemiplegia and hemiparesis** following nontraumatic subarachnoid hemorrhage affecting **unspecified side**   CC HCC
CC Excl: PDX collection 697

✓6ᵗʰ **I69.06**   **Other paralytic syndrome** following nontraumatic subarachnoid hemorrhage
Use additional code to identify type of paralytic syndrome, such as:
locked-in state (G83.5)
quadriplegia (G82.5-)
EXCLUDES 1   *hemiplegia/hemiparesis following nontraumatic subarachnoid hemorrhage (I69.05-)*
monoplegia of lower limb following nontraumatic subarachnoid hemorrhage (I69.04-)
monoplegia of upper limb following nontraumatic subarachnoid hemorrhage (I69.03-)

I69.061   **Other paralytic syndrome** following nontraumatic subarachnoid hemorrhage affecting **right dominant side**   HCC

I69.062   **Other paralytic syndrome** following nontraumatic subarachnoid hemorrhage affecting **left dominant side**   HCC

I69.063   **Other paralytic syndrome** following nontraumatic subarachnoid hemorrhage affecting **right non-dominant side**   HCC

I69.064   **Other paralytic syndrome** following nontraumatic subarachnoid hemorrhage affecting **left non-dominant side**   HCC

I69.065   **Other paralytic syndrome** following nontraumatic subarachnoid hemorrhage, **bilateral**   HCC

I69.069   **Other paralytic syndrome** following nontraumatic subarachnoid hemorrhage affecting **unspecified** side   HCC

✓6ᵗʰ **I69.09**   **Other sequelae** of nontraumatic subarachnoid hemorrhage

I69.090   **Apraxia** following nontraumatic subarachnoid hemorrhage

I69.091   **Dysphagia** following nontraumatic subarachnoid hemorrhage
Use additional code to identify the type of dysphagia, if known (R13.1-)

I69.092   **Facial weakness** following nontraumatic subarachnoid hemorrhage
Facial droop following nontraumatic subarachnoid hemorrhage

I69.093   **Ataxia** following nontraumatic subarachnoid hemorrhage

I69.098   **Other sequelae** following nontraumatic subarachnoid hemorrhage
Alterations of sensation following nontraumatic subarachnoid hemorrhage
Disturbance of vision following nontraumatic subarachnoid hemorrhage
Use additional code to identify the sequelae

✓5ᵗʰ **I69.1**   **Sequelae** of nontraumatic **intracerebral** hemorrhage

I69.10   **Unspecified sequelae** of nontraumatic intracerebral hemorrhage

✓6ᵗʰ **I69.11**   **Cognitive deficits** following nontraumatic intracerebral hemorrhage

I69.110   **Attention and concentration deficit** following nontraumatic intracerebral hemorrhage

I69.111   **Memory deficit** following nontraumatic intracerebral hemorrhage

I69.112   **Visuospatial deficit and spatial neglect** following nontraumatic intracerebral hemorrhage

I69.113   **Psychomotor deficit** following nontraumatic intracerebral hemorrhage

I69.114   **Frontal lobe and executive function deficit** following nontraumatic intracerebral hemorrhage

I69.115   **Cognitive social or emotional deficit** following nontraumatic intracerebral hemorrhage

I69.118   **Other symptoms and signs involving cognitive functions** following nontraumatic intracerebral hemorrhage

I69.119   **Unspecified symptoms and signs involving cognitive functions** following nontraumatic intracerebral hemorrhage

✓6ᵗʰ **I69.12**   **Speech and language deficits** following nontraumatic intracerebral hemorrhage

I69.120   **Aphasia** following nontraumatic intracerebral hemorrhage

I69.121   **Dysphasia** following nontraumatic intracerebral hemorrhage

I69.122   **Dysarthria** following nontraumatic intracerebral hemorrhage

I69.123   **Fluency disorder** following nontraumatic intracerebral hemorrhage
Stuttering following nontraumatic intracerebral hemorrhage

Chapter 9. Diseases of the Circulatory System

I69.128–I69.223

I69.128   **Other speech and language deficits following nontraumatic intracerebral hemorrhage**

✓6ᵗʰ **I69.13**   **Monoplegia** of upper limb following nontraumatic intracerebral hemorrhage
AHA: 2017, 1Q, 47

   I69.131   **Monoplegia of upper limb following** `HCC` **nontraumatic intracerebral hemorrhage affecting** right dominant **side**

   I69.132   **Monoplegia of upper limb following** `HCC` **nontraumatic intracerebral hemorrhage affecting** left dominant **side**

   I69.133   **Monoplegia of upper limb following** `HCC` **nontraumatic intracerebral hemorrhage affecting** right non-dominant **side**

   I69.134   **Monoplegia of upper limb following** `HCC` **nontraumatic intracerebral hemorrhage affecting** left non-dominant **side**

   I69.139   **Monoplegia of upper limb following** `HCC` **nontraumatic intracerebral hemorrhage affecting** unspecified **side**

✓6ᵗʰ **I69.14**   **Monoplegia** of lower limb following nontraumatic intracerebral hemorrhage
AHA: 2017, 1Q, 47

   I69.141   **Monoplegia of lower limb following** `HCC` **nontraumatic intracerebral hemorrhage affecting** right dominant **side**

   I69.142   **Monoplegia of lower limb following** `HCC` **nontraumatic intracerebral hemorrhage affecting** left dominant **side**

   I69.143   **Monoplegia of lower limb following** `HCC` **nontraumatic intracerebral hemorrhage affecting** right non-dominant **side**

   I69.144   **Monoplegia of lower limb following** `HCC` **nontraumatic intracerebral hemorrhage affecting** left non-dominant **side**

   I69.149   **Monoplegia of lower limb following** `HCC` **nontraumatic intracerebral hemorrhage affecting** unspecified **side**

✓6ᵗʰ **I69.15**   **Hemiplegia** and hemiparesis following nontraumatic intracerebral hemorrhage
AHA: 2015, 1Q, 25

   I69.151   **Hemiplegia and hemiparesis** `CC` `HCC` **following nontraumatic intracerebral hemorrhage affecting** right dominant **side**
CC Excl: PDX collection 695

   I69.152   **Hemiplegia and hemiparesis** `CC` `HCC` **following nontraumatic intracerebral hemorrhage affecting** left dominant **side**
CC Excl: PDX collection 695

   I69.153   **Hemiplegia and hemiparesis** `CC` `HCC` **following nontraumatic intracerebral hemorrhage affecting** right non-dominant **side**
CC Excl: PDX collection 696

   I69.154   **Hemiplegia and hemiparesis** `CC` `HCC` **following nontraumatic intracerebral hemorrhage affecting** left non-dominant **side**
CC Excl: PDX collection 696

   I69.159   **Hemiplegia and hemiparesis** `CC` `HCC` **following nontraumatic intracerebral hemorrhage affecting** unspecified **side**
CC Excl: PDX collection 697

✓6ᵗʰ **I69.16**   **Other paralytic syndrome** following nontraumatic intracerebral hemorrhage
Use additional code to identify type of paralytic syndrome, such as:
    locked-in state (G83.5)
    quadriplegia (G82.5-)
   EXCLUDES 1   *hemiplegia/hemiparesis following nontraumatic intracerebral hemorrhage (I69.15-)*
         monoplegia of lower limb following nontraumatic intracerebral hemorrhage (I69.14-)
         monoplegia of upper limb following nontraumatic intracerebral hemorrhage (I69.13-)

   I69.161   **Other paralytic syndrome following** `HCC` **nontraumatic intracerebral hemorrhage affecting** right dominant **side**

   I69.162   **Other paralytic syndrome following** `HCC` **nontraumatic intracerebral hemorrhage affecting** left dominant **side**

   I69.163   **Other paralytic syndrome following** `HCC` **nontraumatic intracerebral hemorrhage affecting** right non-dominant **side**

   I69.164   **Other paralytic syndrome following** `HCC` **nontraumatic intracerebral hemorrhage affecting** left non-dominant **side**

   I69.165   **Other paralytic syndrome following** `HCC` **nontraumatic intracerebral hemorrhage, bilateral**

   I69.169   **Other paralytic syndrome following** `HCC` **nontraumatic intracerebral hemorrhage affecting** unspecified **side**

✓6ᵗʰ **I69.19**   **Other** sequelae of nontraumatic intracerebral hemorrhage

   I69.190   **Apraxia following nontraumatic intracerebral hemorrhage**

   I69.191   **Dysphagia following nontraumatic intracerebral hemorrhage**
Use additional code to identify the type of dysphagia, if known (R13.1-)

   I69.192   **Facial weakness following nontraumatic intracerebral hemorrhage**
Facial droop following nontraumatic intracerebral hemorrhage

   I69.193   **Ataxia following nontraumatic intracerebral hemorrhage**

   I69.198   **Other** sequelae of nontraumatic intracerebral hemorrhage
Alteration of sensations following nontraumatic intracerebral hemorrhage
Disturbance of vision following nontraumatic intracerebral hemorrhage
Use additional code to identify the sequelae

✓5ᵗʰ **I69.2**   **Sequelae of other nontraumatic** intracranial **hemorrhage**

   I69.20   **Unspecified** sequelae of other nontraumatic intracranial hemorrhage

✓6ᵗʰ **I69.21**   **Cognitive deficits** following other nontraumatic intracranial hemorrhage

   I69.210   **Attention and concentration** deficit following other nontraumatic intracranial hemorrhage

   I69.211   **Memory** deficit following other nontraumatic intracranial hemorrhage

   I69.212   **Visuospatial** deficit and spatial neglect following other nontraumatic intracranial hemorrhage

   I69.213   **Psychomotor** deficit following other nontraumatic intracranial hemorrhage

   I69.214   **Frontal lobe and executive function** deficit following other nontraumatic intracranial hemorrhage

   I69.215   **Cognitive social or emotional** deficit following other nontraumatic intracranial hemorrhage

   I69.218   **Other** symptoms and signs involving cognitive functions following other nontraumatic intracranial hemorrhage

   I69.219   **Unspecified** symptoms and signs involving cognitive functions following other nontraumatic intracranial hemorrhage

✓6ᵗʰ **I69.22**   **Speech and** language deficits following other nontraumatic intracranial hemorrhage

   I69.220   **Aphasia following other nontraumatic intracranial hemorrhage**

   I69.221   **Dysphasia following other nontraumatic intracranial hemorrhage**

   I69.222   **Dysarthria following other nontraumatic intracranial hemorrhage**

   I69.223   **Fluency disorder following other nontraumatic intracranial hemorrhage**
Stuttering following other nontraumatic intracranial hemorrhage

N Newborn: 0   P Pediatric: 0-17   M Maternity: 12-55   A Adult: 15-124   MCC Major CC Condition   PDxMCC PDx acts as own MCC   CC CC Condition   PDxCC PDx acts as own CC

646   ICD-10-CM 2018

I69.228   Other speech and language deficits following other nontraumatic intracranial hemorrhage

✓6ᵗʰ **I69.23**   Monoplegia of upper limb following other nontraumatic intracranial hemorrhage
    AHA: 2017, 1Q, 47

   I69.231   Monoplegia of upper limb following other nontraumatic intracranial hemorrhage affecting right dominant side   HCC

   I69.232   Monoplegia of upper limb following other nontraumatic intracranial hemorrhage affecting left dominant side   HCC

   I69.233   Monoplegia of upper limb following other nontraumatic intracranial hemorrhage affecting right non-dominant side   HCC

   I69.234   Monoplegia of upper limb following other nontraumatic intracranial hemorrhage affecting left non-dominant side   HCC

   I69.239   Monoplegia of upper limb following other nontraumatic intracranial hemorrhage affecting unspecified side   HCC

✓6ᵗʰ **I69.24**   Monoplegia of lower limb following other nontraumatic intracranial hemorrhage
    AHA: 2017, 1Q, 47

   I69.241   Monoplegia of lower limb following other nontraumatic intracranial hemorrhage affecting right dominant side   HCC

   I69.242   Monoplegia of lower limb following other nontraumatic intracranial hemorrhage affecting left dominant side   HCC

   I69.243   Monoplegia of lower limb following other nontraumatic intracranial hemorrhage affecting right non-dominant side   HCC

   I69.244   Monoplegia of lower limb following other nontraumatic intracranial hemorrhage affecting left non-dominant side   HCC

   I69.249   Monoplegia of lower limb following other nontraumatic intracranial hemorrhage affecting unspecified side   HCC

✓6ᵗʰ **I69.25**   Hemiplegia and hemiparesis following other nontraumatic intracranial hemorrhage
    AHA: 2015, 1Q, 25

   I69.251   Hemiplegia and hemiparesis following other nontraumatic intracranial hemorrhage affecting right dominant side   CC HCC
      CC Excl: PDX collection 695

   I69.252   Hemiplegia and hemiparesis following other nontraumatic intracranial hemorrhage affecting left dominant side   CC HCC
      CC Excl: PDX collection 695

   I69.253   Hemiplegia and hemiparesis following other nontraumatic intracranial hemorrhage affecting right non-dominant side   CC HCC
      CC Excl: PDX collection 696

   I69.254   Hemiplegia and hemiparesis following other nontraumatic intracranial hemorrhage affecting left non-dominant side   CC HCC
      CC Excl: PDX collection 696

   I69.259   Hemiplegia and hemiparesis following other nontraumatic intracranial hemorrhage affecting unspecified side   CC HCC
      CC Excl: PDX collection 697

✓6ᵗʰ **I69.26**   Other paralytic syndrome following other nontraumatic intracranial hemorrhage
    Use additional code to identify type of paralytic syndrome, such as:
     locked-in state (G83.5)
     quadriplegia (G82.5-)
    EXCLUDES 1   *hemiplegia/hemiparesis following other nontraumatic intracranial hemorrhage (I69.25-)*
      monoplegia of lower limb following other nontraumatic intracranial hemorrhage (I69.24-)
      monoplegia of upper limb following other nontraumatic intracranial hemorrhage (I69.23-)

   I69.261   Other paralytic syndrome following other nontraumatic intracranial hemorrhage affecting right dominant side   HCC

   I69.262   Other paralytic syndrome following other nontraumatic intracranial hemorrhage affecting left dominant side   HCC

   I69.263   Other paralytic syndrome following other nontraumatic intracranial hemorrhage affecting right non-dominant side   HCC

   I69.264   Other paralytic syndrome following other nontraumatic intracranial hemorrhage affecting left non-dominant side   HCC

   I69.265   Other paralytic syndrome following other nontraumatic intracranial hemorrhage, bilateral   HCC

   I69.269   Other paralytic syndrome following other nontraumatic intracranial hemorrhage affecting unspecified side   HCC

✓6ᵗʰ **I69.29**   Other sequelae of other nontraumatic intracranial hemorrhage

   I69.290   Apraxia following other nontraumatic intracranial hemorrhage

   I69.291   Dysphagia following other nontraumatic intracranial hemorrhage
      Use additional code to identify the type of dysphagia, if known (R13.1-)

   I69.292   Facial weakness following other nontraumatic intracranial hemorrhage
      Facial droop following other nontraumatic intracranial hemorrhage

   I69.293   Ataxia following other nontraumatic intracranial hemorrhage

   I69.298   Other sequelae of other nontraumatic intracranial hemorrhage
      Alteration of sensation following other nontraumatic intracranial hemorrhage
      Disturbance of vision following other nontraumatic intracranial hemorrhage
      Use additional code to identify the sequelae

✓5ᵗʰ **I69.3**   Sequelae of cerebral infarction
    Sequelae of stroke NOS
    AHA: 2013, 4Q, 127-128; 2012, 4Q, 92, 94

   I69.30   Unspecified sequelae of cerebral infarction

✓6ᵗʰ **I69.31**   Cognitive deficits following cerebral infarction

   I69.310   Attention and concentration deficit following cerebral infarction

   I69.311   Memory deficit following cerebral infarction

   I69.312   Visuospatial deficit and spatial neglect following cerebral infarction

   I69.313   Psychomotor deficit following cerebral infarction

   I69.314   Frontal lobe and executive function deficit following cerebral infarction

   I69.315   Cognitive social or emotional deficit following cerebral infarction

   I69.318   Other symptoms and signs involving cognitive functions following cerebral infarction

   I69.319   Unspecified symptoms and signs involving cognitive functions following cerebral infarction

✓ Additional Character Req   ✓ˣ7ᵗʰ Placeholder Alert   Unacceptable PDx   Manifestation   H1 - H14 HAC   HCC CMS-HCC Condition   *EXCLUDES 1* Not Coded Here   *EXCLUDES 2* Not Included Here

ICD-10-CM 2018   647

✓6ᵗʰ **I69.32** **Speech** and **language deficits** following cerebral infarction

I69.320 **Aphasia** following cerebral infarction

I69.321 **Dysphasia** following cerebral infarction
AHA: 2012, 4Q, 91

I69.322 **Dysarthria** following cerebral infarction
EXCLUDES 2 ▶*transient ischemic attack (TIA) (G45.9)*◀

I69.323 **Fluency disorder** following cerebral infarction
Stuttering following cerebral infarction

I69.328 **Other** speech and language deficits following cerebral infarction

✓6ᵗʰ **I69.33** **Monoplegia** of upper limb following cerebral infarction
AHA: 2017, 1Q, 47

I69.331 **Monoplegia of upper limb following cerebral infarction affecting right dominant side** HCC

I69.332 **Monoplegia of upper limb following cerebral infarction affecting left dominant side** HCC

I69.333 **Monoplegia of upper limb following cerebral infarction affecting right non-dominant side** HCC

I69.334 **Monoplegia of upper limb following cerebral infarction affecting left non-dominant side** HCC

I69.339 **Monoplegia of upper limb following cerebral infarction affecting unspecified side** HCC

✓6ᵗʰ **I69.34** **Monoplegia** of lower limb following cerebral infarction
AHA: 2017, 1Q, 47

I69.341 **Monoplegia of lower limb following cerebral infarction affecting right dominant side** HCC

I69.342 **Monoplegia of lower limb following cerebral infarction affecting left dominant side** HCC

I69.343 **Monoplegia of lower limb following cerebral infarction affecting right non-dominant side** HCC

I69.344 **Monoplegia of lower limb following cerebral infarction affecting left non-dominant side** HCC

I69.349 **Monoplegia of lower limb following cerebral infarction affecting unspecified side** HCC

✓6ᵗʰ **I69.35** **Hemiplegia** and **hemiparesis** following cerebral infarction
AHA: 2015, 1Q, 25

I69.351 **Hemiplegia and hemiparesis following cerebral infarction affecting right dominant side** CC HCC
EXCLUDES 2 ▶*transient ischemic attack (TIA) (G45.9)*◀
CC Excl: PDX collection 695

I69.352 **Hemiplegia and hemiparesis following cerebral infarction affecting left dominant side** CC HCC
CC Excl: PDX collection 695

I69.353 **Hemiplegia and hemiparesis following cerebral infarction affecting right non-dominant side** CC HCC
CC Excl: PDX collection 696

I69.354 **Hemiplegia and hemiparesis following cerebral infarction affecting left non-dominant side** CC HCC
AHA: 2012, 4Q, 91
CC Excl: PDX collection 696

I69.359 **Hemiplegia and hemiparesis following cerebral infarction affecting unspecified side** CC HCC
CC Excl: PDX collection 697

✓6ᵗʰ **I69.36** **Other paralytic syndrome** following cerebral infarction
Use additional code to identify type of paralytic syndrome, such as:
locked-in state (G83.5)
quadriplegia (G82.5-)
EXCLUDES 1 *hemiplegia/hemiparesis following cerebral infarction (I69.35-)*
monoplegia of lower limb following cerebral infarction (I69.34-)
monoplegia of upper limb following cerebral infarction (I69.33-)

I69.361 **Other paralytic syndrome following cerebral infarction affecting right dominant side** HCC

I69.362 **Other paralytic syndrome following cerebral infarction affecting left dominant side** HCC

I69.363 **Other paralytic syndrome following cerebral infarction affecting right non-dominant side** HCC

I69.364 **Other paralytic syndrome following cerebral infarction affecting left non-dominant side** HCC

I69.365 **Other paralytic syndrome following cerebral infarction, bilateral** HCC

I69.369 **Other paralytic syndrome following cerebral infarction affecting unspecified side** HCC

✓6ᵗʰ **I69.39** **Other sequelae of cerebral infarction**

I69.390 **Apraxia** following cerebral infarction

I69.391 **Dysphagia** following cerebral infarction
Use additional code to identify the type of dysphagia, if known (R13.1-)

I69.392 **Facial weakness** following cerebral infarction
Facial droop following cerebral infarction

I69.393 **Ataxia** following cerebral infarction

I69.398 **Other** sequelae of cerebral infarction
Alteration of sensation following cerebral infarction
Disturbance of vision following cerebral infarction
Use additional code to identify the sequelae

✓5ᵗʰ **I69.8** **Sequelae of** other cerebrovascular diseases
EXCLUDES 1 *sequelae of traumatic intracranial injury (S06.-)*

I69.80 **Unspecified** sequelae of other cerebrovascular disease

✓6ᵗʰ **I69.81** **Cognitive deficits** following other cerebrovascular disease

I69.810 **Attention and concentration deficit** following other cerebrovascular disease

I69.811 **Memory deficit** following other cerebrovascular disease

I69.812 **Visuospatial deficit and** spatial neglect following other cerebrovascular disease

I69.813 **Psychomotor deficit** following other cerebrovascular disease

I69.814 **Frontal lobe and executive function deficit** following other cerebrovascular disease

I69.815 **Cognitive social or emotional deficit** following other cerebrovascular disease

I69.818 **Other symptoms and signs involving cognitive functions** following other cerebrovascular disease

I69.819 **Unspecified symptoms and signs involving cognitive functions** following other cerebrovascular disease

✓6ᵗʰ **I69.82** **Speech** and **language deficits** following other cerebrovascular disease

I69.820 **Aphasia** following other cerebrovascular disease

I69.821 **Dysphasia** following other cerebrovascular disease

I69.822 **Dysarthria** following other cerebrovascular disease

I69.823   **Fluency disorder following other cerebrovascular disease**
     Stuttering following other cerebrovascular disease

I69.828   **Other speech and language deficits following other cerebrovascular disease**

✓6ᵗʰ **I69.83**   **Monoplegia of upper limb following other cerebrovascular disease**
     AHA: 2017, 1Q, 47

I69.831   **Monoplegia of upper limb following** HCC **other cerebrovascular disease affecting right dominant side**

I69.832   **Monoplegia of upper limb following** HCC **other cerebrovascular disease affecting left dominant side**

I69.833   **Monoplegia of upper limb following** HCC **other cerebrovascular disease affecting right non-dominant side**

I69.834   **Monoplegia of upper limb following** HCC **other cerebrovascular disease affecting left non-dominant side**

I69.839   **Monoplegia of upper limb following** HCC **other cerebrovascular disease affecting unspecified side**

✓6ᵗʰ **I69.84**   **Monoplegia of lower limb following other cerebrovascular disease**
     AHA: 2017, 1Q, 47

I69.841   **Monoplegia of lower limb following** HCC **other cerebrovascular disease affecting right dominant side**

I69.842   **Monoplegia of lower limb following** HCC **other cerebrovascular disease affecting left dominant side**

I69.843   **Monoplegia of lower limb following** HCC **other cerebrovascular disease affecting right non-dominant side**

I69.844   **Monoplegia of lower limb following** HCC **other cerebrovascular disease affecting left non-dominant side**

I69.849   **Monoplegia of lower limb following** HCC **other cerebrovascular disease affecting unspecified side**

✓6ᵗʰ **I69.85**   **Hemiplegia and hemiparesis following other cerebrovascular disease**
     AHA: 2015, 1Q, 25

I69.851   **Hemiplegia and hemiparesis** CC HCC **following other cerebrovascular disease affecting right dominant side**
     CC Excl: PDX collection 695

I69.852   **Hemiplegia and hemiparesis** CC HCC **following other cerebrovascular disease affecting left dominant side**
     CC Excl: PDX collection 695

I69.853   **Hemiplegia and hemiparesis** CC HCC **following other cerebrovascular disease affecting right non-dominant side**
     CC Excl: PDX collection 696

I69.854   **Hemiplegia and hemiparesis** CC HCC **following other cerebrovascular disease affecting left non-dominant side**
     CC Excl: PDX collection 696

I69.859   **Hemiplegia and hemiparesis** CC HCC **following other cerebrovascular disease affecting unspecified side**
     CC Excl: PDX collection 697

✓6ᵗʰ **I69.86**   **Other paralytic syndrome following other cerebrovascular disease**
     Use additional code to identify type of paralytic syndrome, such as:
       locked-in state (G83.5)
       quadriplegia (G82.5-)
     EXCLUDES 1   hemiplegia/hemiparesis following other cerebrovascular disease (I69.85-)
       monoplegia of lower limb following other cerebrovascular disease (I69.84-)
       monoplegia of upper limb following other cerebrovascular disease (I69.83-)

I69.861   **Other paralytic syndrome following** HCC **other cerebrovascular disease affecting right dominant side**

I69.862   **Other paralytic syndrome following** HCC **other cerebrovascular disease affecting left dominant side**

I69.863   **Other paralytic syndrome following** HCC **other cerebrovascular disease affecting right non-dominant side**

I69.864   **Other paralytic syndrome following** HCC **other cerebrovascular disease affecting left non-dominant side**

I69.865   **Other paralytic syndrome following** HCC **other cerebrovascular disease, bilateral**

I69.869   **Other paralytic syndrome following** HCC **other cerebrovascular disease affecting unspecified side**

✓6ᵗʰ **I69.89**   **Other sequelae of other cerebrovascular disease**

I69.890   **Apraxia following other cerebrovascular disease**

I69.891   **Dysphagia following other cerebrovascular disease**
     Use additional code to identify the type of dysphagia, if known (R13.1-)

I69.892   **Facial weakness following other cerebrovascular disease**
     Facial droop following other cerebrovascular disease

I69.893   **Ataxia following other cerebrovascular disease**

I69.898   **Other sequelae of other cerebrovascular disease**
     Alteration of sensation following other cerebrovascular disease
     Disturbance of vision following other cerebrovascular disease
     Use additional code to identify the sequelae

✓5ᵗʰ **I69.9**   **Sequelae of unspecified cerebrovascular diseases**
     EXCLUDES 1   sequelae of stroke (I69.3)
       sequelae of traumatic intracranial injury (S06.-)

I69.90   **Unspecified sequelae of unspecified cerebrovascular disease**

✓6ᵗʰ **I69.91**   **Cognitive deficits following unspecified cerebrovascular disease**

I69.910   **Attention and concentration deficit following unspecified cerebrovascular disease**

I69.911   **Memory deficit following unspecified cerebrovascular disease**

I69.912   **Visuospatial deficit and spatial neglect following unspecified cerebrovascular disease**

I69.913   **Psychomotor deficit following unspecified cerebrovascular disease**

I69.914   **Frontal lobe and executive function deficit following unspecified cerebrovascular disease**

I69.915   **Cognitive social or emotional deficit following unspecified cerebrovascular disease**

I69.918   **Other symptoms and signs involving cognitive functions following unspecified cerebrovascular disease**

I69.919   **Unspecified symptoms and signs involving cognitive functions following unspecified cerebrovascular disease**

✓6ᵗʰ **I69.92**   **Speech and language deficits following unspecified cerebrovascular disease**

I69.920   **Aphasia following unspecified cerebrovascular disease**

I69.921   **Dysphasia following unspecified cerebrovascular disease**

I69.922   **Dysarthria following unspecified cerebrovascular disease**

I69.923   **Fluency disorder following unspecified cerebrovascular disease**
     Stuttering following unspecified cerebrovascular disease

I69.928   **Other speech and language deficits following unspecified cerebrovascular disease**

✓ Additional Character Req   ✓x7ᵗʰ Placeholder Alert   Unacceptable PDx   Manifestation   H1-H14 HAC   HCC CMS-HCC Condition   *EXCLUDES 1* Not Coded Here   *EXCLUDES 2* Not Included Here

ICD-10-CM 2018   649

Chapter 9. Diseases of the Circulatory System

✓6ᵗʰ **I69.93 Monoplegia of upper limb following unspecified cerebrovascular disease**
AHA: 2017, 1Q, 47

I69.931 Monoplegia of upper limb following unspecified cerebrovascular disease affecting right dominant side   `HCC`

I69.932 Monoplegia of upper limb following unspecified cerebrovascular disease affecting left dominant side   `HCC`

I69.933 Monoplegia of upper limb following unspecified cerebrovascular disease affecting right non-dominant side   `HCC`

I69.934 Monoplegia of upper limb following unspecified cerebrovascular disease affecting left non-dominant side   `HCC`

I69.939 Monoplegia of upper limb following unspecified cerebrovascular disease affecting unspecified side   `HCC`

✓6ᵗʰ **I69.94 Monoplegia of lower limb following unspecified cerebrovascular disease**
AHA: 2017, 1Q, 47

I69.941 Monoplegia of lower limb following unspecified cerebrovascular disease affecting right dominant side   `HCC`

I69.942 Monoplegia of lower limb following unspecified cerebrovascular disease affecting left dominant side   `HCC`

I69.943 Monoplegia of lower limb following unspecified cerebrovascular disease affecting right non-dominant side   `HCC`

I69.944 Monoplegia of lower limb following unspecified cerebrovascular disease affecting left non-dominant side   `HCC`

I69.949 Monoplegia of lower limb following unspecified cerebrovascular disease affecting unspecified side   `HCC`

✓6ᵗʰ **I69.95 Hemiplegia and hemiparesis following unspecified cerebrovascular disease**
AHA: 2015, 1Q, 25

I69.951 Hemiplegia and hemiparesis following unspecified cerebrovascular disease affecting right dominant side   `CC` `HCC`
CC Excl: PDX collection 695

I69.952 Hemiplegia and hemiparesis following unspecified cerebrovascular disease affecting left dominant side   `CC` `HCC`
CC Excl: PDX collection 695

I69.953 Hemiplegia and hemiparesis following unspecified cerebrovascular disease affecting right non-dominant side   `CC` `HCC`
CC Excl: PDX collection 696

I69.954 Hemiplegia and hemiparesis following unspecified cerebrovascular disease affecting left non-dominant side   `CC` `HCC`
CC Excl: PDX collection 696

I69.959 Hemiplegia and hemiparesis following unspecified cerebrovascular disease affecting unspecified side   `CC` `HCC`
CC Excl: PDX collection 697

✓6ᵗʰ **I69.96 Other paralytic syndrome following unspecified cerebrovascular disease**
Use additional code to identify type of paralytic syndrome, such as:
  locked-in state (G83.5)
  quadriplegia (G82.5-)
EXCLUDES 1   hemiplegia/hemiparesis following unspecified cerebrovascular disease (I69.95-)
    monoplegia of lower limb following unspecified cerebrovascular disease (I69.94-)
    monoplegia of upper limb following unspecified cerebrovascular disease (I69.93-)

I69.961 Other paralytic syndrome following unspecified cerebrovascular disease affecting right dominant side   `HCC`

I69.962 Other paralytic syndrome following unspecified cerebrovascular disease affecting left dominant side   `HCC`

I69.963 Other paralytic syndrome following unspecified cerebrovascular disease affecting right non-dominant side   `HCC`

I69.964 Other paralytic syndrome following unspecified cerebrovascular disease affecting left non-dominant side   `HCC`

I69.965 Other paralytic syndrome following unspecified cerebrovascular disease, bilateral   `HCC`

I69.969 Other paralytic syndrome following unspecified cerebrovascular disease affecting unspecified side   `HCC`

✓6ᵗʰ **I69.99 Other sequelae of unspecified cerebrovascular disease**

I69.990 Apraxia following unspecified cerebrovascular disease

I69.991 Dysphagia following unspecified cerebrovascular disease
Use additional code to identify the type of dysphagia, if known (R13.1-)

I69.992 Facial weakness following unspecified cerebrovascular disease
Facial droop following unspecified cerebrovascular disease

I69.993 Ataxia following unspecified cerebrovascular disease

I69.998 Other sequelae following unspecified cerebrovascular disease
Alteration in sensation following unspecified cerebrovascular disease
Disturbance of vision following unspecified cerebrovascular disease
Use additional code to identify the sequelae

Diseases of arteries, arterioles and capillaries (I70-I79)

✓4ᵗʰ **I70 Atherosclerosis**
`INCLUDES`   arteriolosclerosis
    arterial degeneration
    arteriosclerosis
    arteriosclerotic vascular disease
    arteriovascular degeneration
    atheroma
    endarteritis deformans or obliterans
    senile arteritis
    senile endarteritis
    vascular degeneration
Use additional code to identify:
   exposure to environmental tobacco smoke (Z77.22)
   history of tobacco dependence (Z87.891)
   occupational exposure to environmental tobacco smoke (Z57.31)
   tobacco dependence (F17.-)
   tobacco use (Z72.0)
EXCLUDES 2   arteriosclerotic cardiovascular disease (I25.1-)
    arteriosclerotic heart disease (I25.1-)
    atheroembolism (I75.-)
    cerebral atherosclerosis (I67.2)
    coronary atherosclerosis (I25.1-)
    mesenteric atherosclerosis (K55.1)
    precerebral atherosclerosis (I67.2)
    primary pulmonary atherosclerosis (I27.0)

I70.0 Atherosclerosis of aorta   `HCC` `A`

I70.1 Atherosclerosis of renal artery   `HCC` `A`
Goldblatt's kidney
EXCLUDES 2   atherosclerosis of renal arterioles (I12.-)

✓5ᵗʰ **I70.2 Atherosclerosis of native arteries of the extremities**
Mönckeberg's (medial) sclerosis
Use additional code, if applicable, to identify chronic total occlusion of artery of extremity (I70.92)
EXCLUDES 2   atherosclerosis of bypass graft of extremities (I70.30-I70.79)

✓6ᵗʰ **I70.20 Unspecified atherosclerosis of native arteries of extremities**

I70.201 Unspecified atherosclerosis of native arteries of extremities, right leg   `HCC` `A`

I70.202 Unspecified atherosclerosis of native arteries of extremities, left leg   `HCC` `A`

I70.203 Unspecified atherosclerosis of native arteries of extremities, bilateral legs   `HCC` `A`

I70.208 Unspecified atherosclerosis of native arteries of extremities, other extremity   `HCC` `A`

N Newborn: 0   P Pediatric: 0-17   M Maternity: 12-55   A Adult: 15-124   MCC Major CC Condition   PDxMCC PDx acts as own MCC   CC CC Condition   PDxCC PDx acts as own CC

650   ICD-10-CM 2018

     I70.209 **Unspecified atherosclerosis of** HCC A **native arteries of extremities, unspecified extremity**

✓6ᵗʰ **I70.21** **Atherosclerosis of native arteries of extremities with intermittent claudication**

     I70.211 **Atherosclerosis of native arteries of** HCC A **extremities with intermittent claudication, right leg**

     I70.212 **Atherosclerosis of native arteries of** HCC A **extremities with intermittent claudication, left leg**

     I70.213 **Atherosclerosis of native arteries of** HCC A **extremities with intermittent claudication, bilateral legs**

     I70.218 **Atherosclerosis of native arteries of** HCC A **extremities with intermittent claudication, other extremity**

     I70.219 **Atherosclerosis of native arteries of** HCC A **extremities with intermittent claudication, unspecified extremity**

✓6ᵗʰ **I70.22** **Atherosclerosis of native arteries of extremities with rest pain**

     INCLUDES any condition classifiable to I70.21-

     I70.221 **Atherosclerosis of native arteries of** HCC A **extremities with rest pain, right leg**

     I70.222 **Atherosclerosis of native arteries of** HCC A **extremities with rest pain, left leg**

     I70.223 **Atherosclerosis of native arteries of** HCC A **extremities with rest pain, bilateral legs**

     I70.228 **Atherosclerosis of native arteries of** HCC A **extremities with rest pain, other extremity**

     I70.229 **Atherosclerosis of native arteries of** HCC A **extremities with rest pain, unspecified extremity**

✓6ᵗʰ **I70.23** **Atherosclerosis of native arteries of right leg with ulceration**

     INCLUDES any condition classifiable to I70.211 and I70.221

     Use additional code to identify severity of ulcer (L97.-)

     I70.231 **Atherosclerosis of native arteries of** HCC A **right leg with ulceration of thigh**

     I70.232 **Atherosclerosis of native arteries of** HCC A **right leg with ulceration of calf**

     I70.233 **Atherosclerosis of native arteries of** HCC A **right leg with ulceration of ankle**

     I70.234 **Atherosclerosis of native arteries of** HCC A **right leg with ulceration of heel and midfoot**

           Atherosclerosis of native arteries of right leg with ulceration of plantar surface of midfoot

     I70.235 **Atherosclerosis of native arteries of** HCC A **right leg with ulceration of other part of foot**

           Atherosclerosis of native arteries of right leg extremities with ulceration of toe

     I70.238 **Atherosclerosis of native arteries of** HCC A **right leg with ulceration of other part of lower right leg**

     I70.239 **Atherosclerosis of native arteries of** HCC A **right leg with ulceration of unspecified site**

✓6ᵗʰ **I70.24** **Atherosclerosis of native arteries of left leg with ulceration**

     INCLUDES any condition classifiable to I70.212 and I70.222

     Use additional code to identify severity of ulcer (L97.-)

     I70.241 **Atherosclerosis of native arteries of** HCC A **left leg with ulceration of thigh**

     I70.242 **Atherosclerosis of native arteries of** HCC A **left leg with ulceration of calf**

     I70.243 **Atherosclerosis of native arteries of** HCC A **left leg with ulceration of ankle**

     I70.244 **Atherosclerosis of native arteries of** HCC A **left leg with ulceration of heel and midfoot**

           Atherosclerosis of native arteries of left leg with ulceration of plantar surface of midfoot

     I70.245 **Atherosclerosis of native arteries** HCC A **of left leg with ulceration of other part of foot**

           Atherosclerosis of native arteries of left leg extremities with ulceration of toe

     I70.248 **Atherosclerosis of native arteries of** HCC A **left leg with ulceration of other part of lower left leg**

     I70.249 **Atherosclerosis of native arteries of** HCC A **left leg with ulceration of unspecified site**

     I70.25 **Atherosclerosis of native arteries of other** HCC A **extremities with ulceration**

     INCLUDES any condition classifiable to I70.218 and I70.228

     Use additional code to identify the severity of the ulcer (L98.49-)

✓6ᵗʰ **I70.26** **Atherosclerosis of native arteries of extremities with gangrene**

     INCLUDES any condition classifiable to I70.21-, I70.22-, I70.23-, I70.24-, and I70.25-

     Use additional code to identify the severity of any ulcer (L97.-, L98.49-), if applicable

     CC Excl: For CC codes in subcategory I70.26: PDX collection 519

     I70.261 **Atherosclerosis of native** CC HCC A **arteries of extremities with gangrene, right leg**

     I70.262 **Atherosclerosis of native** CC HCC A **arteries of extremities with gangrene, left leg**

     I70.263 **Atherosclerosis of native** CC HCC A **arteries of extremities with gangrene, bilateral legs**

     I70.268 **Atherosclerosis of native** CC HCC A **arteries of extremities with gangrene, other extremity**

     I70.269 **Atherosclerosis of native** CC HCC A **arteries of extremities with gangrene, unspecified extremity**

✓6ᵗʰ **I70.29** **Other atherosclerosis of native arteries of extremities**

     I70.291 **Other atherosclerosis of native** HCC A **arteries of extremities, right leg**

     I70.292 **Other atherosclerosis of native** HCC A **arteries of extremities, left leg**

     I70.293 **Other atherosclerosis of native** HCC A **arteries of extremities, bilateral legs**

     I70.298 **Other atherosclerosis of native** HCC A **arteries of extremities, other extremity**

     I70.299 **Other atherosclerosis of native** HCC A **arteries of extremities, unspecified extremity**

✓5ᵗʰ **I70.3** **Atherosclerosis of unspecified type of bypass graft(s) of the extremities**

     Use additional code, if applicable, to identify chronic total occlusion of artery of extremity (I70.92)

     EXCLUDES 1 *embolism or thrombus of bypass graft(s) of extremities (T82.8-)*

✓6ᵗʰ **I70.30** **Unspecified atherosclerosis of unspecified type of bypass graft(s) of the extremities**

     I70.301 **Unspecified atherosclerosis of** HCC A **unspecified type of bypass graft(s) of the extremities, right leg**

     I70.302 **Unspecified atherosclerosis of** HCC A **unspecified type of bypass graft(s) of the extremities, left leg**

     I70.303 **Unspecified atherosclerosis of** HCC A **unspecified type of bypass graft(s) of the extremities, bilateral legs**

     I70.308 **Unspecified atherosclerosis of** HCC A **unspecified type of bypass graft(s) of the extremities, other extremity**

     I70.309 **Unspecified atherosclerosis of** HCC A **unspecified type of bypass graft(s) of the extremities, unspecified extremity**

Chapter 9. Diseases of the Circulatory System

I70.31–I70.391

✓6ᵗʰ **I70.31 Atherosclerosis of unspecified type of bypass graft(s) of the extremities with intermittent claudication**

I70.311 Atherosclerosis of unspecified type ᴴᶜᶜ Ⓐ of bypass graft(s) of the extremities with intermittent claudication, right leg

I70.312 Atherosclerosis of unspecified type ᴴᶜᶜ Ⓐ of bypass graft(s) of the extremities with intermittent claudication, left leg

I70.313 Atherosclerosis of unspecified type ᴴᶜᶜ Ⓐ of bypass graft(s) of the extremities with intermittent claudication, bilateral legs

I70.318 Atherosclerosis of unspecified type ᴴᶜᶜ Ⓐ of bypass graft(s) of the extremities with intermittent claudication, other extremity

I70.319 Atherosclerosis of unspecified type ᴴᶜᶜ Ⓐ of bypass graft(s) of the extremities with intermittent claudication, unspecified extremity

✓6ᵗʰ **I70.32 Atherosclerosis of unspecified type of bypass graft(s) of the extremities with rest pain**
     INCLUDES any condition classifiable to I70.31-

I70.321 Atherosclerosis of unspecified type ᴴᶜᶜ Ⓐ of bypass graft(s) of the extremities with rest pain, right leg

I70.322 Atherosclerosis of unspecified type ᴴᶜᶜ Ⓐ of bypass graft(s) of the extremities with rest pain, left leg

I70.323 Atherosclerosis of unspecified type ᴴᶜᶜ Ⓐ of bypass graft(s) of the extremities with rest pain, bilateral legs

I70.328 Atherosclerosis of unspecified type ᴴᶜᶜ Ⓐ of bypass graft(s) of the extremities with rest pain, other extremity

I70.329 Atherosclerosis of unspecified type ᴴᶜᶜ Ⓐ of bypass graft(s) of the extremities with rest pain, unspecified extremity

✓6ᵗʰ **I70.33 Atherosclerosis of unspecified type of bypass graft(s) of the right leg with ulceration**
     INCLUDES any condition classifiable to I70.311 and I70.321
     Use additional code to identify severity of ulcer (L97.-)

CC Excl: For CC codes in subcategory I70.33: PDX collection 698

I70.331 Atherosclerosis of ᴾᴰˣᶜᶜ ᶜᶜ ᴴᶜᶜ Ⓐ unspecified type of bypass graft(s) of the right leg with ulceration of thigh

I70.332 Atherosclerosis of ᴾᴰˣᶜᶜ ᶜᶜ ᴴᶜᶜ Ⓐ unspecified type of bypass graft(s) of the right leg with ulceration of calf

I70.333 Atherosclerosis of ᴾᴰˣᶜᶜ ᶜᶜ ᴴᶜᶜ Ⓐ unspecified type of bypass graft(s) of the right leg with ulceration of ankle

I70.334 Atherosclerosis of ᴾᴰˣᶜᶜ ᶜᶜ ᴴᶜᶜ Ⓐ unspecified type of bypass graft(s) of the right leg with ulceration of heel and midfoot
     Atherosclerosis of unspecified type of bypass graft(s) of right leg with ulceration of plantar surface of midfoot

I70.335 Atherosclerosis of unspecified type ᴴᶜᶜ Ⓐ of bypass graft(s) of the right leg with ulceration of other part of foot
     Atherosclerosis of unspecified type of bypass graft(s) of the right leg with ulceration of toe

I70.338 Atherosclerosis of ᴾᴰˣᶜᶜ ᶜᶜ ᴴᶜᶜ Ⓐ unspecified type of bypass graft(s) of the right leg with ulceration of other part of lower leg

I70.339 Atherosclerosis of ᴾᴰˣᶜᶜ ᶜᶜ ᴴᶜᶜ Ⓐ unspecified type of bypass graft(s) of the right leg with ulceration of unspecified site

✓6ᵗʰ **I70.34 Atherosclerosis of unspecified type of bypass graft(s) of the left leg with ulceration**
     INCLUDES any condition classifiable to I70.312 and I70.322
     Use additional code to identify severity of ulcer (L97.-)

CC Excl: For CC codes in subcategory I70.34: PDX collection 698

I70.341 Atherosclerosis of ᴾᴰˣᶜᶜ ᶜᶜ ᴴᶜᶜ Ⓐ unspecified type of bypass graft(s) of the left leg with ulceration of thigh

I70.342 Atherosclerosis of ᴾᴰˣᶜᶜ ᶜᶜ ᴴᶜᶜ Ⓐ unspecified type of bypass graft(s) of the left leg with ulceration of calf

I70.343 Atherosclerosis of ᴾᴰˣᶜᶜ ᶜᶜ ᴴᶜᶜ Ⓐ unspecified type of bypass graft(s) of the left leg with ulceration of ankle

I70.344 Atherosclerosis of ᴾᴰˣᶜᶜ ᶜᶜ ᴴᶜᶜ Ⓐ unspecified type of bypass graft(s) of the left leg with ulceration of heel and midfoot
     Atherosclerosis of unspecified type of bypass graft(s) of left leg with ulceration of plantar surface of midfoot

I70.345 Atherosclerosis of unspecified ᴴᶜᶜ Ⓐ type of bypass graft(s) of the left leg with ulceration of other part of foot
     Atherosclerosis of unspecified type of bypass graft(s) of the left leg with ulceration of toe

I70.348 Atherosclerosis of ᴾᴰˣᶜᶜ ᶜᶜ ᴴᶜᶜ Ⓐ unspecified type of bypass graft(s) of the left leg with ulceration of other part of lower leg

I70.349 Atherosclerosis of ᴾᴰˣᶜᶜ ᶜᶜ ᴴᶜᶜ Ⓐ unspecified type of bypass graft(s) of the left leg with ulceration of unspecified site

I70.35 Atherosclerosis of unspecified type of bypass ᴴᶜᶜ Ⓐ graft(s) of other extremity with ulceration
     INCLUDES any condition classifiable to I70.318 and I70.328
     Use additional code to identify severity of ulcer (L98.49-)

✓6ᵗʰ **I70.36 Atherosclerosis of unspecified type of bypass graft(s) of the extremities with gangrene**
     INCLUDES any condition classifiable to I70.31-, I70.32-, I70.33-, I70.34-, I70.35
     Use additional code to identify the severity of any ulcer (L97.-, L98.49-), if applicable

CC Excl: For CC codes in subcategory I70.36, unless otherwise noted: PDX collection 519

I70.361 Atherosclerosis of ᴾᴰˣᶜᶜ ᶜᶜ ᴴᶜᶜ Ⓐ unspecified type of bypass graft(s) of the extremities with gangrene, right leg

I70.362 Atherosclerosis of ᴾᴰˣᶜᶜ ᶜᶜ ᴴᶜᶜ Ⓐ unspecified type of bypass graft(s) of the extremities with gangrene, left leg

I70.363 Atherosclerosis of ᴾᴰˣᶜᶜ ᶜᶜ ᴴᶜᶜ Ⓐ unspecified type of bypass graft(s) of the extremities with gangrene, bilateral legs

I70.368 Atherosclerosis of ᴾᴰˣᶜᶜ ᶜᶜ ᴴᶜᶜ Ⓐ unspecified type of bypass graft(s) of the extremities with gangrene, other extremity

I70.369 Atherosclerosis of ᴾᴰˣᶜᶜ ᶜᶜ ᴴᶜᶜ Ⓐ unspecified type of bypass graft(s) of the extremities with gangrene, unspecified extremity

✓6ᵗʰ **I70.39 Other atherosclerosis of unspecified type of bypass graft(s) of the extremities**

I70.391 Other atherosclerosis of ᴴᶜᶜ Ⓐ unspecified type of bypass graft(s) of the extremities, right leg

Ⓝ Newborn: 0   Ⓟ Pediatric: 0-17   Ⓜ Maternity: 12-55   Ⓐ Adult: 15-124   ᴹᶜᶜ Major CC Condition   ᴾᴰˣᴹᶜᶜ PDx acts as own MCC   ᶜᶜ CC Condition   ᴾᴰˣᶜᶜ PDx acts as own CC

652   ICD-10-CM 2018

I70.392 Other atherosclerosis of `HCC` `A`
unspecified type of bypass graft(s)
of the extremities, left leg

I70.393 Other atherosclerosis of `HCC` `A`
unspecified type of bypass graft(s)
of the extremities, bilateral legs

I70.398 Other atherosclerosis of `HCC` `A`
unspecified type of bypass graft(s)
of the extremities, other extremity

I70.399 Other atherosclerosis of `HCC` `A`
unspecified type of bypass graft(s)
of the extremities, unspecified extremity

✓5ᵗʰ **I70.4** Atherosclerosis of autologous vein bypass graft(s) of the
extremities
    Use additional code, if applicable, to identify chronic total
    occlusion of artery of extremity (I70.92)

  ✓6ᵗʰ **I70.40** Unspecified atherosclerosis of autologous vein
bypass graft(s) of the extremities

I70.401 Unspecified atherosclerosis of `HCC` `A`
autologous vein bypass graft(s) of the
extremities, right leg

I70.402 Unspecified atherosclerosis of `HCC` `A`
autologous vein bypass graft(s) of the
extremities, left leg

I70.403 Unspecified atherosclerosis of `HCC` `A`
autologous vein bypass graft(s) of the
extremities, bilateral legs

I70.408 Unspecified atherosclerosis of `HCC` `A`
autologous vein bypass graft(s) of the
extremities, other extremity

I70.409 Unspecified atherosclerosis of `HCC` `A`
autologous vein bypass graft(s) of the
extremities, unspecified extremity

  ✓6ᵗʰ **I70.41** Atherosclerosis of autologous vein bypass graft(s) of
the extremities with intermittent claudication

I70.411 Atherosclerosis of autologous vein `HCC` `A`
bypass graft(s) of the extremities with
intermittent claudication, right leg

I70.412 Atherosclerosis of autologous vein `HCC` `A`
bypass graft(s) of the extremities with
intermittent claudication, left leg

I70.413 Atherosclerosis of autologous vein `HCC` `A`
bypass graft(s) of the extremities with
intermittent claudication, bilateral legs

I70.418 Atherosclerosis of autologous vein `HCC` `A`
bypass graft(s) of the extremities with
intermittent claudication, other extremity

I70.419 Atherosclerosis of autologous vein `HCC` `A`
bypass graft(s) of the extremities with
intermittent claudication, unspecified
extremity

  ✓6ᵗʰ **I70.42** Atherosclerosis of autologous vein bypass graft(s) of
the extremities with rest pain
    `INCLUDES` any condition classifiable to I70.41-

I70.421 Atherosclerosis of autologous vein `HCC` `A`
bypass graft(s) of the extremities
with rest pain, right leg

I70.422 Atherosclerosis of autologous vein `HCC` `A`
bypass graft(s) of the extremities
with rest pain, left leg

I70.423 Atherosclerosis of autologous vein `HCC` `A`
bypass graft(s) of the extremities
with rest pain, bilateral legs

I70.428 Atherosclerosis of autologous vein `HCC` `A`
bypass graft(s) of the extremities
with rest pain, other extremity

I70.429 Atherosclerosis of autologous vein `HCC` `A`
bypass graft(s) of the extremities
with rest pain, unspecified extremity

  ✓6ᵗʰ **I70.43** Atherosclerosis of autologous vein bypass graft(s) of
the right leg with ulceration
    `INCLUDES` any condition classifiable to I70.411 and
        I70.421
    Use additional code to identify severity of ulcer (L97.-)

    CC Excl: For CC codes in subcategory I70.43:
    PDX collection 698

I70.431 Atherosclerosis of `PDxCC` `CC` `HCC` `A`
autologous vein bypass graft(s)
of the right leg with ulceration of thigh

I70.432 Atherosclerosis of `PDxCC` `CC` `HCC` `A`
autologous vein bypass graft(s)
of the right leg with ulceration of calf

I70.433 Atherosclerosis of `PDxCC` `CC` `HCC` `A`
autologous vein bypass graft(s)
of the right leg with ulceration of ankle

I70.434 Atherosclerosis of `PDxCC` `CC` `HCC` `A`
autologous vein bypass graft(s)
of the right leg with ulceration of
heel and midfoot
        Atherosclerosis of autologous vein bypass
        graft(s) of right leg with ulceration of
        plantar surface of midfoot

I70.435 Atherosclerosis of autologous vein `HCC` `A`
bypass graft(s) of the right leg with
ulceration of other part of foot
        Atherosclerosis of autologous vein bypass
        graft(s) of right leg with ulceration of
        toe

I70.438 Atherosclerosis of `PDxCC` `CC` `HCC` `A`
autologous vein bypass graft(s)
of the right leg with ulceration of
other part of lower leg

I70.439 Atherosclerosis of `PDxCC` `CC` `HCC` `A`
autologous vein bypass graft(s)
of the right leg with ulceration of
unspecified site

  ✓6ᵗʰ **I70.44** Atherosclerosis of autologous vein bypass graft(s) of
the left leg with ulceration
    `INCLUDES` any condition classifiable to I70.412 and
        I70.422
    Use additional code to identify severity of ulcer (L97.-)

    CC Excl: For CC codes in subcategory I70.44:
    PDX collection 698

I70.441 Atherosclerosis of `PDxCC` `CC` `HCC` `A`
autologous vein bypass graft(s)
of the left leg with ulceration of thigh

I70.442 Atherosclerosis of `PDxCC` `CC` `HCC` `A`
autologous vein bypass graft(s)
of the left leg with ulceration of calf

I70.443 Atherosclerosis of `PDxCC` `CC` `HCC` `A`
autologous vein bypass graft(s)
of the left leg with ulceration of ankle

I70.444 Atherosclerosis of `PDxCC` `CC` `HCC` `A`
autologous vein bypass graft(s)
of the left leg with ulceration of
heel and midfoot
        Atherosclerosis of autologous vein bypass
        graft(s) of left leg with ulceration of
        plantar surface of midfoot

I70.445 Atherosclerosis of autologous vein `HCC` `A`
bypass graft(s) of the left leg with
ulceration of other part of foot
        Atherosclerosis of autologous vein bypass
        graft(s) of left leg with ulceration of
        toe

I70.448 Atherosclerosis of `PDxCC` `CC` `HCC` `A`
autologous vein bypass graft(s)
of the left leg with ulceration of
other part of lower leg

I70.449 Atherosclerosis of `PDxCC` `CC` `HCC` `A`
autologous vein bypass graft(s)
of the left leg with ulceration of
unspecified site

  I70.45 Atherosclerosis of autologous vein bypass `HCC` `A`
graft(s) of other extremity with ulceration
    `INCLUDES` any condition classifiable to I70.418,
        I70.428, and I70.438
    Use additional code to identify severity of ulcer
    (L98.49)

  ✓6ᵗʰ **I70.46** Atherosclerosis of autologous vein bypass graft(s) of
the extremities with gangrene
    `INCLUDES` any condition classifiable to I70.41-, I70.42-,
        and I70.43-, I70.44-, I70.45
    Use additional code to identify the severity of any
    ulcer (L97.-, L98.49-), if applicable

    CC Excl: For CC codes in subcategory I70.46:
    PDX collection 519

I70.461 Atherosclerosis of `PDxCC` `CC` `HCC` `A`
autologous vein bypass graft(s)
of the extremities with gangrene,
right leg

✓Additional Character Req   ✓x7ᵗʰ Placeholder Alert   Unacceptable PDx   Manifestation   `H1`-`H14` HAC   `HCC` CMS-HCC Condition   `EXCLUDES1` Not Coded Here   `EXCLUDES2` Not Included Here

ICD-10-CM 2018   653

I70.462　Atherosclerosis of `PDxCC` `CC` `HCC` `A`
autologous vein bypass graft(s)
of the extremities with gangrene,
left leg

I70.463　Atherosclerosis of `PDxCC` `CC` `HCC` `A`
autologous vein bypass graft(s)
of the extremities with gangrene,
bilateral legs

I70.468　Atherosclerosis of `PDxCC` `CC` `HCC` `A`
autologous vein bypass graft(s)
of the extremities with gangrene,
other extremity

I70.469　Atherosclerosis of `PDxCC` `CC` `HCC` `A`
autologous vein bypass graft(s)
of the extremities with gangrene,
unspecified extremity

✓6ᵗʰ I70.49　Other atherosclerosis of autologous vein bypass
graft(s) of the extremities

I70.491　Other atherosclerosis of `HCC` `A`
autologous vein bypass graft(s)
of the extremities, right leg

I70.492　Other atherosclerosis of `HCC` `A`
autologous vein bypass graft(s)
of the extremities, left leg

I70.493　Other atherosclerosis of `HCC` `A`
autologous vein bypass graft(s)
of the extremities, bilateral legs

I70.498　Other atherosclerosis of `HCC` `A`
autologous vein bypass graft(s)
of the extremities, other extremity

I70.499　Other atherosclerosis of `HCC` `A`
autologous vein bypass graft(s) of the
extremities, unspecified extremity

✓5ᵗʰ I70.5　Atherosclerosis of nonautologous biological bypass graft(s)
of the extremities
　　Use additional code, if applicable, to identify chronic total
　　occlusion of artery of extremity (I70.92)

✓6ᵗʰ I70.50　Unspecified atherosclerosis of nonautologous
biological bypass graft(s) of the extremities

I70.501　Unspecified atherosclerosis of `HCC` `A`
nonautologous biological bypass
graft(s) of the extremities, right leg

I70.502　Unspecified atherosclerosis of `HCC` `A`
nonautologous biological bypass
graft(s) of the extremities, left leg

I70.503　Unspecified atherosclerosis of `HCC` `A`
nonautologous biological bypass
graft(s) of the extremities, bilateral legs

I70.508　Unspecified atherosclerosis of `HCC` `A`
nonautologous biological bypass
graft(s) of the extremities, other extremity

I70.509　Unspecified atherosclerosis of `HCC` `A`
nonautologous biological bypass
graft(s) of the extremities, unspecified
extremity

✓6ᵗʰ I70.51　Atherosclerosis of nonautologous biological bypass
graft(s) of the extremities with intermittent
claudication

I70.511　Atherosclerosis of nonautologous `HCC` `A`
biological bypass graft(s) of the
extremities with intermittent
claudication, right leg

I70.512　Atherosclerosis of nonautologous `HCC` `A`
biological bypass graft(s) of the
extremities with intermittent
claudication, left leg

I70.513　Atherosclerosis of nonautologous `HCC` `A`
biological bypass graft(s) of the
extremities with intermittent
claudication, bilateral legs

I70.518　Atherosclerosis of nonautologous `HCC` `A`
biological bypass graft(s) of the
extremities with intermittent
claudication, other extremity

I70.519　Atherosclerosis of nonautologous `HCC` `A`
biological bypass graft(s) of the
extremities with intermittent
claudication, unspecified extremity

✓6ᵗʰ I70.52　Atherosclerosis of nonautologous biological bypass
graft(s) of the extremities with rest pain
　　`INCLUDES`　any condition classifiable to I70.51-

I70.521　Atherosclerosis of nonautologous `HCC` `A`
biological bypass graft(s) of the
extremities with rest pain, right leg

I70.522　Atherosclerosis of nonautologous `HCC` `A`
biological bypass graft(s) of the
extremities with rest pain, left leg

I70.523　Atherosclerosis of nonautologous `HCC` `A`
biological bypass graft(s) of the
extremities with rest pain, bilateral legs

I70.528　Atherosclerosis of nonautologous `HCC` `A`
biological bypass graft(s) of the
extremities with rest pain, other extremity

I70.529　Atherosclerosis of nonautologous `HCC` `A`
biological bypass graft(s) of the
extremities with rest pain, unspecified
extremity

✓6ᵗʰ I70.53　Atherosclerosis of nonautologous biological bypass
graft(s) of the right leg with ulceration
　　`INCLUDES`　any condition classifiable to I70.511 and
　　　　　　　I70.521
　　Use additional code to identify severity of ulcer (L97.-)

CC Excl: For CC codes in subcategory I70.53:
PDX collection 698

I70.531　Atherosclerosis of `PDxCC` `CC` `HCC` `A`
biological nonautologous bypass graft(s)
of the right leg with ulceration of thigh

I70.532　Atherosclerosis of `PDxCC` `CC` `HCC` `A`
bilological nonautologous bypass graft(s)
of the right leg with ulceration of calf

I70.533　Atherosclerosis of `PDxCC` `CC` `HCC` `A`
nonautologous biological bypass graft(s)
of the right leg with ulceration of ankle

I70.534　Atherosclerosis of `PDxCC` `CC` `HCC` `A`
nonautologous biological bypass graft(s)
of the right leg with ulceration of heel and
midfoot
　　Atherosclerosis of nonautologous
　　　biological bypass graft(s) of right leg
　　　with ulceration of plantar surface of
　　　midfoot

I70.535　Atherosclerosis of nonautologous `HCC` `A`
biological bypass graft(s) of the right leg
with ulceration of other part of foot
　　Atherosclerosis of nonautologous
　　　biological bypass graft(s) of the right
　　　leg with ulceration of toe

I70.538　Atherosclerosis of `PDxCC` `CC` `HCC` `A`
nonautologous biological bypass graft(s)
of the right leg with ulceration of other
part of lower leg

I70.539　Atherosclerosis of `PDxCC` `CC` `HCC` `A`
nonautologous biological bypass graft(s)
of the right leg with ulceration of
unspecified site

✓6ᵗʰ I70.54　Atherosclerosis of nonautologous biological bypass
graft(s) of the left leg with ulceration
　　`INCLUDES`　any condition classifiable to I70.512 and
　　　　　　　I70.522
　　Use additional code to identify severity of ulcer (L97.-)

CC Excl: For CC codes in subcategory I70.54:
PDX collection 698

I70.541　Atherosclerosis of `PDxCC` `CC` `HCC` `A`
nonautologous biological bypass graft(s)
of the left leg with ulceration of thigh

I70.542　Atherosclerosis of `PDxCC` `CC` `HCC` `A`
nonautologous biological bypass graft(s)
of the left leg with ulceration of calf

I70.543　Atherosclerosis of `PDxCC` `CC` `HCC` `A`
nonautologous biological bypass graft(s)
of the left leg with ulceration of ankle

I70.544　Atherosclerosis of `PDxCC` `CC` `HCC` `A`
nonautologous biological bypass graft(s)
of the left leg with ulceration of heel and
midfoot
　　Atherosclerosis of nonautologous
　　　biological bypass graft(s) of left leg
　　　with ulceration of plantar surface of
　　　midfoot

`N` Newborn: 0　`P` Pediatric: 0-17　`M` Maternity: 12-55　`A` Adult: 15-124　`MCC` Major CC Condition　`PDxMCC` PDx acts as own MCC　`CC` CC Condition　`PDxCC` PDx acts as own CC

654　　　ICD-10-CM 2018

I70.545   **Atherosclerosis of nonautologous** `HCC` `A`
biological bypass graft(s) of the left leg
with ulceration of other part of foot
    Atherosclerosis of nonautologous
      biological bypass graft(s) of the left leg
      with ulceration of toe

I70.548   **Atherosclerosis of** `PDxCC` `CC` `HCC` `A`
nonautologous biological bypass
graft(s) of the left leg with ulceration
of other part of lower leg

I70.549   **Atherosclerosis of** `PDxCC` `CC` `HCC` `A`
nonautologous biological bypass
graft(s) of the left leg with ulceration
of unspecified site

I70.55   **Atherosclerosis of nonautologous biological** `HCC` `A`
bypass graft(s) of other **extremity with** ulceration
   `INCLUDES`   any condition classifiable to I70.518,
         I70.528, and I70.538
   Use additional code to identify severity of ulcer
     (L98.49)

`√6th` I70.56   **Atherosclerosis of nonautologous biological bypass**
graft(s) of the extremities with gangrene
   `INCLUDES`   any condition classifiable to I70.51-, I70.52-,
         and I70.53-, I70.54-, I70.55
   Use additional code to identify the severity of any
     ulcer (L97.-, L98.49-), if applicable

> **CC Excl: For CC codes in subcategory I70.56:**
> PDX collection 519

I70.561   **Atherosclerosis of** `PDxCC` `CC` `HCC` `A`
nonautologous biological bypass graft(s)
of the extremities with gangrene, right leg

I70.562   **Atherosclerosis of** `PDxCC` `CC` `HCC` `A`
nonautologous biological bypass graft(s)
of the extremities with gangrene, left leg

I70.563   **Atherosclerosis of** `PDxCC` `CC` `HCC` `A`
nonautologous biological bypass graft(s)
of the extremities with gangrene,
bilateral legs

I70.568   **Atherosclerosis of** `PDxCC` `CC` `HCC` `A`
nonautologous biological bypass graft(s)
of the extremities with gangrene, other
extremity

I70.569   **Atherosclerosis of** `PDxCC` `CC` `HCC` `A`
nonautologous biological bypass graft(s)
of the extremities with gangrene,
unspecified extremity

`√6th` I70.59   Other **atherosclerosis of nonautologous biological**
bypass graft(s) of the extremities

I70.591   **Other atherosclerosis of** `HCC` `A`
biological nonautologous bypass
graft(s) of the extremities, right leg

I70.592   **Other atherosclerosis of** `HCC` `A`
nonautologous biological bypass
graft(s) of the extremities, left leg

I70.593   **Other atherosclerosis of** `HCC` `A`
nonautologous biological bypass
graft(s) of the extremities,
bilateral legs

I70.598   **Other atherosclerosis of** `HCC` `A`
nonautologous biological bypass
graft(s) of the extremities,
other extremity

I70.599   **Other atherosclerosis of** `HCC` `A`
nonautologous biological bypass
graft(s) of the extremities,
unspecified extremity

`√5th` I70.6   **Atherosclerosis of** nonbiological bypass graft(s) **of the**
extremities
   Use additional code, if applicable, to identify chronic total
     occlusion of artery of extremity (I70.92)

`√6th` I70.60   Unspecified **atherosclerosis of nonbiological bypass**
graft(s) of the extremities

I70.601   **Unspecified atherosclerosis of** `HCC` `A`
nonbiological bypass graft(s) of the
extremities, right leg

I70.602   **Unspecified atherosclerosis of** `HCC` `A`
nonbiological bypass graft(s) of the
extremities, left leg

I70.603   **Unspecified atherosclerosis of** `HCC` `A`
nonbiological bypass graft(s) of the
extremities, bilateral legs

I70.608   **Unspecified atherosclerosis of** `HCC` `A`
nonbiological bypass graft(s) of the
extremities, other extremity

I70.609   **Unspecified atherosclerosis of** `HCC` `A`
nonbiological bypass graft(s) of the
extremities, unspecified extremity

`√6th` I70.61   **Atherosclerosis of nonbiological bypass graft(s) of**
the extremities with intermittent claudication

I70.611   **Atherosclerosis of nonbiological** `HCC` `A`
bypass graft(s) of the extremities with
intermittent claudication, right leg

I70.612   **Atherosclerosis of nonbiological** `HCC` `A`
bypass graft(s) of the extremities with
intermittent claudication, left leg

I70.613   **Atherosclerosis of nonbiological** `HCC` `A`
bypass graft(s) of the extremities with
intermittent claudication, bilateral legs

I70.618   **Atherosclerosis of nonbiological** `HCC` `A`
bypass graft(s) of the extremities with
intermittent claudication,
other extremity

I70.619   **Atherosclerosis of nonbiological** `HCC` `A`
bypass graft(s) of the extremities with
intermittent claudication, unspecified
extremity

`√6th` I70.62   **Atherosclerosis of nonbiological bypass graft(s) of**
the extremities with rest pain
   `INCLUDES`   any condition classifiable to I70.61-

I70.621   **Atherosclerosis of nonbiological** `HCC` `A`
bypass graft(s) of the extremities with
rest pain, right leg

I70.622   **Atherosclerosis of nonbiological** `HCC` `A`
bypass graft(s) of the extremities
with rest pain, left leg

I70.623   **Atherosclerosis of nonbiological** `HCC` `A`
bypass graft(s) of the extremities with rest
pain, bilateral legs

I70.628   **Atherosclerosis of nonbiological** `HCC` `A`
bypass graft(s) of the extremities
with rest pain, other extremity

I70.629   **Atherosclerosis of nonbiological** `HCC` `A`
bypass graft(s) of the extremities
with rest pain, unspecified extremity

`√6th` I70.63   **Atherosclerosis of nonbiological bypass graft(s) of**
the right leg with **ulceration**
   `INCLUDES`   any condition classifiable to I70.611 and
         I70.621
   Use additional code to identify severity of ulcer (L97.-)

> **CC Excl: For CC codes in subcategory I70.63:**
> PDX collection 698

I70.631   **Atherosclerosis of** `PDxCC` `CC` `HCC` `A`
nonbiological bypass graft(s) of the
right leg with ulceration of thigh

I70.632   **Atherosclerosis of** `PDxCC` `CC` `HCC` `A`
nonbiological bypass graft(s) of the
right leg with ulceration of calf

I70.633   **Atherosclerosis of** `PDxCC` `CC` `HCC` `A`
nonbiological bypass graft(s) of the
right leg with ulceration of ankle

I70.634   **Atherosclerosis of** `PDxCC` `CC` `HCC` `A`
nonbiological bypass graft(s) of the
right leg with ulceration of heel and
midfoot
    Atherosclerosis of nonbiological bypass
      graft(s) of right leg with ulceration of
      plantar surface of midfoot

I70.635   **Atherosclerosis of nonbiological** `HCC` `A`
bypass graft(s) of the right leg with
ulceration of other part of foot
    Atherosclerosis of nonbiological bypass
      graft(s) of the right leg with ulceration
      of toe

I70.638   **Atherosclerosis of** `PDxCC` `CC` `HCC` `A`
nonbiological bypass graft(s) of the
right leg with ulceration of other part
of lower leg

I70.639   **Atherosclerosis of** `PDxCC` `CC` `HCC` `A`
nonbiological bypass graft(s) of the
right leg with ulceration of unspecified
site

`√` Additional Character Req   `√x7th` Placeholder Alert   Unacceptable PDx   Manifestation   `H1`-`H14` HAC   `HCC` CMS-HCC Condition   `EXCLUDES1` Not Coded Here   `EXCLUDES2` Not Included Here

ICD-10-CM 2018   655

Chapter 9. Diseases of the Circulatory System (side margin)

I70.64–I70.733 (side margin)

✓6th **I70.64 Atherosclerosis of nonbiological bypass graft(s) of the left leg with ulceration**
INCLUDES any condition classifiable to I70.612 and I70.622
Use additional code to identify severity of ulcer (L97.-)

CC Excl: For CC codes in subcategory I70.64:
PDX collection 698

I70.641 **Atherosclerosis of nonbiological bypass graft(s) of the left leg with ulceration of thigh** PDxCC CC HCC A

I70.642 **Atherosclerosis of nonbiological bypass graft(s) of the left leg with ulceration of calf** PDxCC CC HCC A

I70.643 **Atherosclerosis of nonbiological bypass graft(s) of the left leg with ulceration of ankle** PDxCC CC HCC A

I70.644 **Atherosclerosis of nonbiological bypass graft(s) of the left leg with ulceration of heel and midfoot** PDxCC CC HCC A
Atherosclerosis of nonbiological bypass graft(s) of left leg with ulceration of plantar surface of midfoot

I70.645 **Atherosclerosis of nonbiological bypass graft(s) of the left leg with ulceration of other part of foot** HCC A
Atherosclerosis of nonbiological bypass graft(s) of the left leg with ulceration of toe

I70.648 **Atherosclerosis of nonbiological bypass graft(s) of the left leg with ulceration of other part of lower leg** PDxCC CC HCC A

I70.649 **Atherosclerosis of nonbiological bypass graft(s) of the left leg with ulceration of unspecified site** PDxCC CC HCC A

I70.65 **Atherosclerosis of nonbiological bypass graft(s) of other extremity with ulceration** HCC A
INCLUDES any condition classifiable to I70.618 and I70.628
Use additional code to identify severity of ulcer (L98.49)

✓6th **I70.66 Atherosclerosis of nonbiological bypass graft(s) of the extremities with gangrene**
INCLUDES any condition classifiable to I70.61-, I70.62-, I70.63-, I70.64-, I70.65
Use additional code to identify the severity of any ulcer (L97.-, L98.49-), if applicable

CC Excl: For CC codes in subcategory I70.66:
PDX collection 519

I70.661 **Atherosclerosis of nonbiological bypass graft(s) of the extremities with gangrene, right leg** PDxCC CC HCC A

I70.662 **Atherosclerosis of nonbiological bypass graft(s) of the extremities with gangrene, left leg** PDxCC CC HCC A

I70.663 **Atherosclerosis of nonbiological bypass graft(s) of the extremities with gangrene, bilateral legs** PDxCC CC HCC A

I70.668 **Atherosclerosis of nonbiological bypass graft(s) of the extremities with gangrene, other extremity** PDxCC CC HCC A

I70.669 **Atherosclerosis of nonbiological bypass graft(s) of the extremities with gangrene, unspecified extremity** PDxCC CC HCC A

✓6th **I70.69 Other atherosclerosis of nonbiological bypass graft(s) of the extremities**

I70.691 **Other atherosclerosis of nonbiological bypass graft(s) of the extremities, right leg** HCC A

I70.692 **Other atherosclerosis of nonbiological bypass graft(s) of the extremities, left leg** HCC A

I70.693 **Other atherosclerosis of nonbiological bypass graft(s) of the extremities, bilateral legs** HCC A

I70.698 **Other atherosclerosis of nonbiological bypass graft(s) of the extremities, other extremity** HCC A

I70.699 **Other atherosclerosis of nonbiological bypass graft(s) of the extremities, unspecified extremity** HCC A

✓5th **I70.7 Atherosclerosis of other type of bypass graft(s) of the extremities**
Use additional code, if applicable, to identify chronic total occlusion of artery of extremity (I70.92)

✓6th **I70.70 Unspecified atherosclerosis of other type of bypass graft(s) of the extremities**

I70.701 **Unspecified atherosclerosis of other type of bypass graft(s) of the extremities, right leg** HCC A

I70.702 **Unspecified atherosclerosis of other type of bypass graft(s) of the extremities, left leg** HCC A

I70.703 **Unspecified atherosclerosis of other type of bypass graft(s) of the extremities, bilateral legs** HCC A

I70.708 **Unspecified atherosclerosis of other type of bypass graft(s) of the extremities, other extremity** HCC A

I70.709 **Unspecified atherosclerosis of other type of bypass graft(s) of the extremities, unspecified extremity** HCC A

✓6th **I70.71 Atherosclerosis of other type of bypass graft(s) of the extremities with intermittent claudication**

I70.711 **Atherosclerosis of other type of bypass graft(s) of the extremities with intermittent claudication, right leg** HCC A

I70.712 **Atherosclerosis of other type of bypass graft(s) of the extremities with intermittent claudication, left leg** HCC A

I70.713 **Atherosclerosis of other type of bypass graft(s) of the extremities with intermittent claudication, bilateral legs** HCC A

I70.718 **Atherosclerosis of other type of bypass graft(s) of the extremities with intermittent claudication, other extremity** HCC A

I70.719 **Atherosclerosis of other type of bypass graft(s) of the extremities with intermittent claudication, unspecified extremity** HCC A

✓6th **I70.72 Atherosclerosis of other type of bypass graft(s) of the extremities with rest pain**
INCLUDES any condition classifiable to I70.71-

I70.721 **Atherosclerosis of other type of bypass graft(s) of the extremities with rest pain, right leg** HCC A

I70.722 **Atherosclerosis of other type of bypass graft(s) of the extremities with rest pain, left leg** HCC A

I70.723 **Atherosclerosis of other type of bypass graft(s) of the extremities with rest pain, bilateral legs** HCC A

I70.728 **Atherosclerosis of other type of bypass graft(s) of the extremities with rest pain, other extremity** HCC A

I70.729 **Atherosclerosis of other type of bypass graft(s) of the extremities with rest pain, unspecified extremity** HCC A

✓6th **I70.73 Atherosclerosis of other type of bypass graft(s) of the right leg with ulceration**
INCLUDES any condition classifiable to I70.711 and I70.721
Use additional code to identify severity of ulcer (L97.-)

CC Excl: For CC codes in subcategory I70.73:
PDX collection 698

I70.731 **Atherosclerosis of other type of bypass graft(s) of the right leg with ulceration of thigh** PDxCC CC HCC A

I70.732 **Atherosclerosis of other type of bypass graft(s) of the right leg with ulceration of calf** PDxCC CC HCC A

I70.733 **Atherosclerosis of other type of bypass graft(s) of the right leg with ulceration of ankle** PDxCC CC HCC A

I70.734   **Atherosclerosis of other** `PDxCC` `CC` `HCC` `A`
type of bypass graft(s) of the right leg with ulceration of heel and midfoot
Atherosclerosis of other type of bypass graft(s) of right leg with ulceration of plantar surface of midfoot

I70.735   **Atherosclerosis of other type of** `HCC` `A`
bypass graft(s) of the right leg with ulceration of other part of foot
Atherosclerosis of other type of bypass graft(s) of right leg with ulceration of toe

I70.738   **Atherosclerosis of other** `PDxCC` `CC` `HCC` `A`
type of bypass graft(s) of the right leg with ulceration of other part of lower leg

I70.739   **Atherosclerosis of other** `PDxCC` `CC` `HCC` `A`
type of bypass graft(s) of the right leg with ulceration of unspecified site

`✓6ᵗʰ` **I70.74**   **Atherosclerosis of other type of bypass graft(s) of the left leg with ulceration**
`INCLUDES`   any condition classifiable to I70.712 and I70.722
Use additional code to identify severity of ulcer (L97.-)

CC Excl: For CC codes in subcategory I70.74: PDX collection 698

I70.741   **Atherosclerosis of other** `PDxCC` `CC` `HCC` `A`
type of bypass graft(s) of the left leg with ulceration of thigh

I70.742   **Atherosclerosis of other** `PDxCC` `CC` `HCC` `A`
type of bypass graft(s) of the left leg with ulceration of calf

I70.743   **Atherosclerosis of other** `PDxCC` `CC` `HCC` `A`
type of bypass graft(s) of the left leg with ulceration of ankle

I70.744   **Atherosclerosis of other** `PDxCC` `CC` `HCC` `A`
type of bypass raft(s) of the left leg with ulceration of heel and midfoot
Atherosclerosis of other type of bypass graft(s) of left leg with ulceration of plantar surface of midfoot

I70.745   **Atherosclerosis of other type of** `HCC` `A`
bypass graft(s) of the left leg with ulceration of other part of foot
Atherosclerosis of other type of bypass graft(s) of left leg with ulceration of toe

I70.748   **Atherosclerosis of other** `PDxCC` `CC` `HCC` `A`
type of bypass graft(s) of the left leg with ulceration of other part of lower leg

I70.749   **Atherosclerosis of other** `PDxCC` `CC` `HCC` `A`
type of bypass graft(s) of the left leg with ulceration of unspecified site

I70.75   **Atherosclerosis of other type of bypass** `HCC` `A`
graft(s) of other extremity with ulceration
`INCLUDES`   any condition classifiable to I70.718 and I70.728
Use additional code to identify severity of ulcer (L98.49)

`✓6ᵗʰ` **I70.76**   **Atherosclerosis of other type of bypass graft(s) of the extremities with** gangrene
`INCLUDES`   any condition classifiable to I70.71-, I70.72-, I70.73-, I70.74-, I70.75
Use additional code to identify the severity of any ulcer (L97.-, L98.49-), if applicable

CC Excl: For CC codes in subcategory I70.76: PDX collection 519

I70.761   **Atherosclerosis of other** `PDxCC` `CC` `HCC` `A`
type of bypass graft(s) of the extremities with gangrene, right leg

I70.762   **Atherosclerosis of other** `PDxCC` `CC` `HCC` `A`
type of bypass graft(s) of the extremities with gangrene, left leg

I70.763   **Atherosclerosis of other** `PDxCC` `CC` `HCC` `A`
type of bypass graft(s) of the extremities with gangrene, bilateral legs

I70.768   **Atherosclerosis of other** `PDxCC` `CC` `HCC` `A`
type of bypass graft(s) of the extremities with gangrene, other extremity

I70.769   **Atherosclerosis of other** `PDxCC` `CC` `HCC` `A`
type of bypass graft(s) of the extremities with gangrene, unspecified extremity

`✓6ᵗʰ` **I70.79**   **Other atherosclerosis of other type of bypass graft(s) of the extremities**

I70.791   **Other atherosclerosis of other type** `HCC` `A`
of bypass graft(s) of the extremities, right leg

I70.792   **Other atherosclerosis of other type** `HCC` `A`
of bypass graft(s) of the extremities, left leg

I70.793   **Other atherosclerosis of other type** `HCC` `A`
of bypass graft(s) of the extremities, bilateral legs

I70.798   **Other atherosclerosis of other type** `HCC` `A`
of bypass graft(s) of the extremities, other extremity

I70.799   **Other atherosclerosis of other type** `HCC` `A`
of bypass graft(s) of the extremities, unspecified extremity

I70.8   **Atherosclerosis of** other arteries   `A`
TIP: Arteriosclerosis of the iliac arteries is coded here.

`✓5ᵗʰ` **I70.9**   **Other and unspecified atherosclerosis**

I70.90   **Unspecified** atherosclerosis   `A`

I70.91   **Generalized** atherosclerosis   `A`

I70.92   **Chronic total occlusion of artery of the** `CC` `HCC` `A`
extremities
Complete occlusion of artery of the extremities
Total occlusion of artery of the extremities
Code first atherosclerosis of arteries of the extremities (I70.2-, I70.3-, I70.4-, I70.5-, I70.6-, I70.7-)
CC Excl: PDX collection 699

`✓4ᵗʰ` **I71**   **Aortic aneurysm and dissection**
`EXCLUDES 1`   *aortic ectasia (I77.81-)*
syphilitic aortic aneurysm (A52.01)
traumatic aortic aneurysm (S25.09, S35.09)

CC Excl: For MCC codes in category I71: PDX collection 700

`✓5ᵗʰ` **I71.0**   **Dissection of** aorta

I71.00   **Dissection of** unspecified site of aorta   `MCC` `HCC`

I71.01   **Dissection of** thoracic aorta   `MCC` `HCC`

I71.02   **Dissection of** abdominal aorta   `MCC` `HCC`

I71.03   **Dissection of** thoracoabdominal aorta   `MCC` `HCC`

I71.1   **Thoracic** aortic aneurysm, ruptured   `MCC` `HCC`

I71.2   **Thoracic** aortic aneurysm, without rupture   `HCC`

I71.3   **Abdominal** aortic aneurysm, ruptured   `MCC` `HCC`

I71.4   **Abdominal** aortic aneurysm, without rupture   `HCC`

I71.5   **Thoracoabdominal** aortic aneurysm, ruptured   `MCC` `HCC`

I71.6   **Thoracoabdominal** aortic aneurysm, without rupture   `HCC`

I71.8   **Aortic aneurysm of** unspecified site, ruptured   `MCC` `HCC`
Rupture of aorta NOS

I71.9   **Aortic aneurysm of** unspecified site, without rupture   `HCC`
Aneurysm of aorta   Hyaline necrosis of aorta
Dilatation of aorta

`✓4ᵗʰ` **I72**   **Other aneurysm**
`INCLUDES`   aneurysm (cirsoid) (false) (ruptured)
`EXCLUDES 2`   *acquired aneurysm (I77.0)*
aneurysm (of) aorta (I71.-)
aneurysm (of) arteriovenous NOS (Q27.3-)
carotid artery dissection (I77.71)
cerebral (nonruptured) aneurysm (I67.1)
coronary aneurysm (I25.4)
coronary artery dissection (I25.42)
dissection of artery NEC (I77.79)
dissection of precerebral artery, congenital (nonruptured) (Q28.1)
heart aneurysm (I25.3)
iliac artery dissection (I77.72)
▶*precerebral artery, congenital (nonruptured) (Q28.1)*◀
pulmonary artery aneurysm (I28.1)
renal artery dissection (I77.73)
retinal aneurysm (H35.0)
ruptured cerebral aneurysm (I60.7)
varicose aneurysm (I77.0)
vertebral artery dissection (I77.74)

I72.0   **Aneurysm of** carotid artery   `HCC`
Aneurysm of common carotid artery
Aneurysm of external carotid artery
Aneurysm of internal carotid artery, extracranial portion
`EXCLUDES 1`   *aneurysm of internal carotid artery, intracranial portion (I67.1)*
aneurysm of internal carotid artery NOS (I67.1)

`✓` Additional Character Req   `✓x7ᵗʰ` Placeholder Alert   Unacceptable PDx   Manifestation   `H1`-`H14` HAC   `HCC` CMS-HCC Condition   `EXCLUDES1` Not Coded Here   `EXCLUDES2` Not Included Here

ICD-10-CM 2018   657

I70.734–I72.0

Aneurysm

Layers of muscular and elastic tissue

Outer layer

Inner layer

Aneurysm

I72.1	**Aneurysm of artery of upper extremity**	HCC
I72.2	**Aneurysm of renal artery**	HCC
I72.3	**Aneurysm of iliac artery**	HCC
I72.4	**Aneurysm of artery of lower extremity**	HCC
I72.5	**Aneurysm of other precerebral arteries**	HCC

Aneurysm of basilar artery (trunk)

EXCLUDES 2   aneurysm of carotid artery (I72.0)
           aneurysm of vertebral artery (I72.6)
           dissection of carotid artery (I77.71)
           dissection of other precerebral arteries (I77.75)
           dissection of vertebral artery (I77.74)

I72.6	**Aneurysm of vertebral artery**	HCC

EXCLUDES 2   dissection of vertebral artery (I77.74)

I72.8	**Aneurysm of other specified arteries**	HCC
I72.9	**Aneurysm of unspecified site**	HCC

✓4th   I73   Other peripheral vascular diseases

EXCLUDES 2   chilblains (T69.1)
           frostbite (T33- T34)
           immersion hand or foot (T69.0-)
           spasm of cerebral artery (G45.9)

✓5th   I73.0   Raynaud's syndrome

Raynaud's disease
Raynaud's phenomenon (secondary)

I73.00   Raynaud's syndrome without gangrene

I73.01   Raynaud's syndrome with gangrene   PDxCC CC HCC
     CC Excl: PDX collection 519

I73.1   Thromboangiitis obliterans [Buerger's disease]   HCC
     DEF: Inflammatory disease of extremity blood vessels, mainly the lower; associated with heavy tobacco use; arteries are more affected than veins; occurs primarily in young men and leads to tissue ischemia and gangrene.

✓5th   I73.8   Other specified peripheral vascular diseases

EXCLUDES 1   diabetic (peripheral) angiopathy (E08-E13 with .51-.52)

I73.81   Erythromelalgia   HCC

I73.89   Other specified peripheral vascular diseases   HCC
     Acrocyanosis
     Erythrocyanosis
     Simple acroparesthesia [Schultze's type]
     Vasomotor acroparesthesia [Nothnagel's type]

I73.9   Peripheral vascular disease, unspecified   HCC
     Intermittent claudication
     Peripheral angiopathy NOS
     Spasm of artery
     EXCLUDES 1   atherosclerosis of the extremities (I70.2--I70.7-)

✓4th   I74   Arterial embolism and thrombosis

INCLUDES   embolic infarction
          embolic occlusion
          thrombotic infarction
          thrombotic occlusion

Code first:
     embolism and thrombosis complicating abortion or ectopic or molar pregnancy (O00-O07, O08.2)
     embolism and thrombosis complicating pregnancy, childbirth and the puerperium (O88.-)

EXCLUDES 2   atheroembolism (I75.-)
           basilar embolism and thrombosis (I63.0-I63.2, I65.1)
           carotid embolism and thrombosis (I63.0-I63.2, I65.2)
           cerebral embolism and thrombosis (I63.3-I63.5, I66-)
           coronary embolism and thrombosis (I21-I25)
           mesenteric embolism and thrombosis (K55.0-)
           ophthalmic embolism and thrombosis (H34.-)
           precerebral embolism and thrombosis NOS (I63.0-I63.2, I65.9)
           pulmonary embolism and thrombosis (I26.-)
           renal embolism and thrombosis (N28.0)
           retinal embolism and thrombosis (H34.-)
           septic embolism and thrombosis (I76)
           vertebral embolism and thrombosis (I63.0-I63.2, I65.0)

✓5th   I74.0   Embolism and thrombosis of abdominal aorta

I74.01   Saddle embolus of abdominal aorta   MCC HCC
     CC Excl: PDX collection 669

I74.09   Other arterial embolism and thrombosis of abdominal aorta   CC HCC
     Aortic bifurcation syndrome   Leriche's syndrome
     Aortoiliac obstruction
     CC Excl: PDX collection 669

✓5th   I74.1   Embolism and thrombosis of other and unspecified parts of aorta

I74.10   Embolism and thrombosis of unspecified parts of aorta   CC HCC
     CC Excl: PDX collection 669

I74.11   Embolism and thrombosis of thoracic aorta   CC HCC
     CC Excl: PDX collection 701

I74.19   Embolism and thrombosis of other parts of aorta   CC HCC
     CC Excl: PDX collection 669

I74.2   Embolism and thrombosis of arteries of the upper extremities   CC HCC
     CC Excl: PDX collection 702

I74.3   Embolism and thrombosis of arteries of the lower extremities   CC HCC
     CC Excl: PDX collection 703

I74.4   Embolism and thrombosis of arteries of extremities, unspecified   CC HCC
     Peripheral arterial embolism NOS
     CC Excl: PDX collection 703

I74.5   Embolism and thrombosis of iliac artery   CC HCC
     CC Excl: PDX collection 704

I74.8   Embolism and thrombosis of other arteries   CC HCC
     CC Excl: PDX collection 705

I74.9   Embolism and thrombosis of unspecified artery   CC HCC
     CC Excl: PDX collection 705

✓4th   I75   Atheroembolism

INCLUDES   atherothrombotic microembolism
          cholesterol embolism

✓5th   I75.0   Atheroembolism of extremities

✓6th   I75.01   Atheroembolism of upper extremity

CC Excl: For CC codes in subcategory I75.01: PDX collection 706

I75.011   Atheroembolism of right upper extremity   CC HCC

I75.012   Atheroembolism of left upper extremity   CC HCC

I75.013   Atheroembolism of bilateral upper extremities   CC HCC

I75.019   Atheroembolism of unspecified upper extremity   CC HCC

✓6th   I75.02   Atheroembolism of lower extremity

CC Excl: For CC codes in subcategory I75.02: PDX collection 707

I75.021   Atheroembolism of right lower extremity   CC HCC

I75.022   Atheroembolism of left lower extremity   CC HCC

N Newborn: 0   P Pediatric: 0-17   M Maternity: 12-55   A Adult: 15-124   MCC Major CC Condition   PDxMCC PDx acts as own MCC   CC CC Condition   PDxCC PDx acts as own CC

658   ICD-10-CM 2018

    I75.Ø23 **Atheroembolism of** bilateral lower **CC HCC**
         extremities

    I75.Ø29 **Atheroembolism of** unspecified **CC HCC**
         lower extremity

✓5th **I75.8** **Atheroembolism of** other sites

    I75.81 **Atheroembolism of** kidney **CC HCC**
         Use additional code for any associated acute kidney
            failure and chronic kidney disease (N17.-, N18.-)
         CC Excl: PDX collection 7Ø8

    I75.89 **Atheroembolism of** other site **CC HCC**
         CC Excl: PDX collection 7Ø9

I76 **Septic arterial embolism** **CC HCC**
     Code first underlying infection, such as:
         infective endocarditis (I33.Ø)
         lung abscess (J85.-)
     Use additional code to identify the site of the embolism (I74.-)
     EXCLUDES 2   *septic pulmonary embolism (I26.Ø1, I26.9Ø)*
     CC Excl: PDX collection 7Ø5

✓4th **I77** **Other disorders of arteries and arterioles**
     EXCLUDES 2   *collagen (vascular) diseases (M3Ø-M36)*
         hypersensitivity angiitis (M31.Ø)
         pulmonary artery (I28.-)

    I77.Ø **Arteriovenous fistula, acquired** **HCC**
         Aneurysmal varix
         Arteriovenous aneurysm, acquired
         EXCLUDES 1   *arteriovenous aneurysm NOS (Q27.3-)*
             presence of arteriovenous shunt (fistula) for dialysis
                 (Z99.2)
             traumatic—see injury of blood vessel by body region
         EXCLUDES 2   *cerebral (I67.1)*
             coronary (I25.4)
         DEF: Communication between an artery and vein; caused by
         trauma or invasive procedures.

    I77.1 **Stricture of artery** **HCC**
         Narrowing of artery

    I77.2 **Rupture of artery** **CC HCC**
         Erosion of artery
         Fistula of artery
         Ulcer of artery
         EXCLUDES 1   *traumatic rupture of artery—see injury of blood vessel*
                 by body region
         CC Excl: PDX collection 71Ø

    I77.3 **Arterial fibromuscular dysplasia** **HCC**
         Fibromuscular hyperplasia (of) carotid artery
         Fibromuscular hyperplasia (of) renal artery

    I77.4 **Celiac artery compression syndrome** **CC HCC**
         CC Excl: PDX collection 711

    I77.5 **Necrosis of artery** **CC HCC**
         CC Excl: PDX collection 712

    I77.6 **Arteritis, unspecified** **HCC**
         Aortitis NOS
         Endarteritis NOS
         EXCLUDES 1   *arteritis or endarteritis:*
             aortic arch (M31.4)
             cerebral NEC (I67.7)
             coronary (I25.89)
             deformans (I7Ø.-)
             giant cell (M31.5., M31.6)
             obliterans (I7Ø.-)
             senile (I7Ø.-)

✓5th **I77.7** **Other arterial dissection**
         EXCLUDES 2   *dissection of aorta (I71.Ø-)*
             dissection of coronary artery (I25.42)

         CC Excl: For MCC codes in subcategory I77.7:
         PDX collection 689

    I77.7Ø **Dissection of** unspecified **artery** **MCC HCC**

    I77.71 **Dissection of** carotid **artery** **MCC HCC**

    I77.72 **Dissection of** iliac **artery** **MCC HCC**

    I77.73 **Dissection of** renal **artery** **MCC HCC**

    I77.74 **Dissection of** vertebral **artery** **MCC HCC**
         EXCLUDES 2   *aneurysm of vertebral artery (I72.6)*

    I77.75 **Dissection of** other precerebral **arteries** **MCC HCC**
         Dissection of basilar artery (trunk)
         EXCLUDES 2   *aneurysm of carotid artery (I72.Ø)*
             aneurysm of other precerebral arteries (I72.5)
             aneurysm of vertebral artery (I72.6)
             dissection of carotid artery (I77.71)
             dissection of vertebral artery (I77.74)

    I77.76 **Dissection of artery of** upper extremity **MCC HCC**

    I77.77 **Dissection of artery of** lower extremity **MCC HCC**

    I77.79 **Dissection of** other specified **artery** **MCC HCC**

✓5th **I77.8** **Other specified disorders of arteries and arterioles**

    ✓6th **I77.81** **Aortic ectasia**
         Ectasis aorta
         EXCLUDES 1   *aortic aneurysm and dissection (I71.Ø-)*

        I77.81Ø **Thoracic aortic ectasia** **HCC**

        I77.811 **Abdominal aortic ectasia** **HCC**

        I77.812 **Thoracoabdominal aortic ectasia** **HCC**

        I77.819 **Aortic ectasia, unspecified site** **HCC**

    I77.89 **Other specified disorders of arteries and** **HCC**
         arterioles

    I77.9 **Disorder of arteries and arterioles, unspecified** **HCC**

✓4th **I78** **Diseases of capillaries**

    I78.Ø **Hereditary hemorrhagic telangiectasia** **HCC**
         Rendu-Osler-Weber disease

    I78.1 **Nevus, non-neoplastic**
         Araneus nevus   Spider nevus
         Senile nevus   Stellar nevus
         EXCLUDES 1   *nevus NOS (D22.-)*
             vascular NOS (Q82.5)
         EXCLUDES 2   *blue nevus (D22.-)*
             flammeus nevus (Q82.5)
             hairy nevus (D22.-)
             melanocytic nevus (D22.-)
             pigmented nevus (D22.-)
             portwine nevus (Q82.5)
             sanguineous nevus (Q82.5)
             strawberry nevus (Q82.5)
             verrucous nevus (Q82.5)

    I78.8 **Other diseases of capillaries**

    I78.9 **Disease of capillaries, unspecified**

✓4th **I79** **Disorders of arteries, arterioles and capillaries in diseases classified elsewhere**

    I79.Ø *Aneurysm of aorta in diseases classified elsewhere* **HCC**
         Code first underlying disease
         EXCLUDES 1   *syphilitic aneurysm (A52.Ø1)*

    I79.1 *Aortitis in diseases classified elsewhere* **HCC**
         Code first underlying disease
         EXCLUDES 1   *syphilitic aortitis (A52.Ø2)*

    I79.8 *Other disorders of arteries, arterioles and capillaries* **HCC**
         in diseases classified elsewhere
         Code first underlying disease, such as:
            amyloidosis (E85.-)
         EXCLUDES 1   *diabetic (peripheral) angiopathy (EØ8-E13 with .51-*
                 .52)
             syphilitic endarteritis (A52.Ø9)
             tuberculous endarteritis (A18.89)

Diseases of veins, lymphatic vessels and lymph nodes, not elsewhere classified (I8Ø-I89)

✓4th **I8Ø** **Phlebitis and thrombophlebitis**
     INCLUDES   endophlebitis
               inflammation, vein
               periphlebitis
               suppurative phlebitis
     Code first:
         phlebitis and thrombophlebitis complicating abortion, ectopic or
            molar pregnancy (OØØ-OØ7, OØ8.7)
         phlebitis and thrombophlebitis complicating pregnancy, childbirth
            and the puerperium (O22.-, O87.-)
     EXCLUDES 1   *venous embolism and thrombosis of lower extremities (I82.4-,*
                 I82.5-, I82.81-)

     CC Excl: For CC codes in category I8Ø: PDX collection 713

✓5th **I8Ø.Ø** **Phlebitis and thrombophlebitis of** superficial vessels of lower extremities
         Phlebitis and thrombophlebitis of femoropopliteal vein

    I8Ø.ØØ **Phlebitis and thrombophlebitis of superficial vessels of** unspecified **lower extremity**

    I8Ø.Ø1 **Phlebitis and thrombophlebitis of superficial vessels of** right **lower extremity**

    I8Ø.Ø2 **Phlebitis and thrombophlebitis of superficial vessels of** left **lower extremity**

    I8Ø.Ø3 **Phlebitis and thrombophlebitis of superficial vessels of lower extremities,** bilateral

---

✓ Additional Character Req   ✓x7th Placeholder Alert   Unacceptable PDx   Manifestation   **H1**-**H14** HAC   **HCC** CMS-HCC Condition   *EXCLUDES 1* Not Coded Here   *EXCLUDES 2* Not Included Here

ICD-10-CM 2018   659

Chapter 9. Diseases of the Circulatory System *(side margin)*

I80.1 Phlebitis and thrombophlebitis of femoral vein
- **I80.10** Phlebitis and thrombophlebitis of unspecified femoral vein `CC` `HCC`
- **I80.11** Phlebitis and thrombophlebitis of right femoral vein `CC` `HCC`
- **I80.12** Phlebitis and thrombophlebitis of left femoral vein `CC` `HCC`
- **I80.13** Phlebitis and thrombophlebitis of femoral vein, bilateral `CC` `HCC`

I80.2 Phlebitis and thrombophlebitis of other and unspecified deep vessels of lower extremities
- **I80.20** Phlebitis and thrombophlebitis of unspecified deep vessels of lower extremities
  - **I80.201** Phlebitis and thrombophlebitis of unspecified deep vessels of right lower extremity `CC` `HCC`
  - **I80.202** Phlebitis and thrombophlebitis of unspecified deep vessels of left lower extremity `CC` `HCC`
  - **I80.203** Phlebitis and thrombophlebitis of unspecified deep vessels of lower extremities, bilateral `CC` `HCC`
  - **I80.209** Phlebitis and thrombophlebitis of unspecified deep vessels of unspecified lower extremity `CC` `HCC`
- **I80.21** Phlebitis and thrombophlebitis of iliac vein
  - **I80.211** Phlebitis and thrombophlebitis of right iliac vein `CC` `HCC`
  - **I80.212** Phlebitis and thrombophlebitis of left iliac vein `CC` `HCC`
  - **I80.213** Phlebitis and thrombophlebitis of iliac vein, bilateral `CC` `HCC`
  - **I80.219** Phlebitis and thrombophlebitis of unspecified iliac vein `CC` `HCC`
- **I80.22** Phlebitis and thrombophlebitis of popliteal vein
  - **I80.221** Phlebitis and thrombophlebitis of right popliteal vein `CC` `HCC`
  - **I80.222** Phlebitis and thrombophlebitis of left popliteal vein `CC` `HCC`
  - **I80.223** Phlebitis and thrombophlebitis of popliteal vein, bilateral `CC` `HCC`
  - **I80.229** Phlebitis and thrombophlebitis of unspecified popliteal vein `CC` `HCC`
- **I80.23** Phlebitis and thrombophlebitis of tibial vein
  - **I80.231** Phlebitis and thrombophlebitis of right tibial vein `CC` `HCC`
  - **I80.232** Phlebitis and thrombophlebitis of left tibial vein `CC` `HCC`
  - **I80.233** Phlebitis and thrombophlebitis of tibial vein, bilateral `CC` `HCC`
  - **I80.239** Phlebitis and thrombophlebitis of unspecified tibial vein `CC` `HCC`
- **I80.29** Phlebitis and thrombophlebitis of other deep vessels of lower extremities
  - **I80.291** Phlebitis and thrombophlebitis of other deep vessels of right lower extremity `CC` `HCC`
  - **I80.292** Phlebitis and thrombophlebitis of other deep vessels of left lower extremity `CC` `HCC`
  - **I80.293** Phlebitis and thrombophlebitis of other deep vessels of lower extremity, bilateral `CC` `HCC`
  - **I80.299** Phlebitis and thrombophlebitis of other deep vessels of unspecified lower extremity `CC` `HCC`

I80.3 Phlebitis and thrombophlebitis of lower extremities, unspecified

I80.8 Phlebitis and thrombophlebitis of other sites

I80.9 Phlebitis and thrombophlebitis of unspecified site

I81 Portal vein thrombosis `MCC`
Portal (vein) obstruction
> *EXCLUDES 2*   hepatic vein thrombosis (I82.0)
> phlebitis of portal vein (K75.1)

CC Excl: PDX collection 714

I82 Other venous embolism and thrombosis
Code first venous embolism and thrombosis complicating:
   abortion, ectopic or molar pregnancy (O00-O07, O08.7)
   pregnancy, childbirth and the puerperium (O22.-, O87.-)
> *EXCLUDES 2*   venous embolism and thrombosis (of):
>   cerebral (I63.6, I67.6)
>   coronary (I21-I25)
>   intracranial and intraspinal, septic or NOS (G08)
>   intracranial, nonpyogenic (I67.6)
>   intraspinal, nonpyogenic (G95.1)
>   mesenteric (K55.0-)
>   portal (I81)
>   pulmonary (I26.-)

- **I82.0 Budd-Chiari syndrome** `MCC` `HCC`
  Hepatic vein thrombosis
  DEF: Thrombosis or other obstruction of hepatic veins; symptoms include enlarged liver, extensive collateral vessels, intractable ascites, and severe portal hypertension.
  CC Excl: PDX collection 715

- **I82.1 Thrombophlebitis migrans** `CC`
  CC Excl: PDX collection 716

- **I82.2 Embolism and thrombosis of vena cava and other thoracic veins**
  > **CC Excl: For CC codes in subcategory I82.2, unless otherwise noted:** PDX collection 717
  - **I82.21 Embolism and thrombosis of superior vena cava**
    - **I82.210 Acute embolism and thrombosis of superior vena cava** `CC` `HCC`
      Embolism and thrombosis of superior vena cava NOS
    - **I82.211 Chronic embolism and thrombosis of superior vena cava** `CC` `HCC`
  - **I82.22 Embolism and thrombosis of inferior vena cava**
    - **I82.220 Acute embolism and thrombosis of inferior vena cava** `MCC` `HCC`
      Embolism and thrombosis of inferior vena cava NOS
      CC Excl: PDX collection 718
    - **I82.221 Chronic embolism and thromobosis of inferior vena cava** `MCC` `HCC`
      CC Excl: PDX collection 718
  - **I82.29 Embolism and thrombosis of other thoracic veins**
    Embolism and thrombosis of brachiocephalic (innominate) vein
    - **I82.290 Acute embolism and thrombosis of other thoracic veins** `CC` `HCC`
    - **I82.291 Chronic embolism and thrombosis of other thoracic veins** `CC` `HCC`

- **I82.3 Embolism and thrombosis of renal vein** `CC` `HCC`
  CC Excl: PDX collection 719

- **I82.4 Acute embolism and thrombosis of deep veins of lower extremity**
  > **CC Excl: For CC codes in subcategory I82.4:** PDX collection 717
  - **I82.40 Acute embolism and thrombosis of unspecified deep veins of lower extremity**
    Deep vein thrombosis NOS
    DVT NOS
    > *EXCLUDES 1*   acute embolism and thrombosis of unspecified deep veins of distal lower extremity (I82.4Z-)
    >   acute embolism and thrombosis of unspecified deep veins of proximal lower extremity (I82.4Y-)
    - **I82.401 Acute embolism and thrombosis of unspecified deep veins of right lower extremity** `CC` `H10` `HCC`
    - **I82.402 Acute embolism and thrombosis of unspecified deep veins of left lower extremity** `CC` `H10` `HCC`
    - **I82.403 Acute embolism and thrombosis of unspecified deep veins of lower extremity, bilateral** `CC` `H10` `HCC`
    - **I82.409 Acute embolism and thrombosis of unspecified deep veins of unspecified lower extremity** `CC` `H10` `HCC`
  - **I82.41 Acute embolism and thrombosis of femoral vein**
    - **I82.411 Acute embolism and thrombosis of right femoral vein** `CC` `H10` `HCC`
    - **I82.412 Acute embolism and thrombosis of left femoral vein** `CC` `H10` `HCC`

N Newborn: 0   **P** Pediatric: 0-17   **M** Maternity: 12-55   **A** Adult: 15-124   **MCC** Major CC Condition   **PDxMCC** PDx acts as own MCC   **CC** CC Condition   **PDxCC** PDx acts as own CC

660   ICD-10-CM 2018

I82.413   **Acute embolism and** `CC` `H10` `HCC`
thrombosis of femoral vein, bilateral

I82.419   **Acute embolism and** `CC` `H10` `HCC`
thrombosis of unspecified femoral vein

☑6ᵗʰ   **I82.42**   **Acute embolism and thrombosis of iliac vein**

I82.421   **Acute embolism and** `CC` `H10` `HCC`
thrombosis of right iliac vein

I82.422   **Acute embolism and** `CC` `H10` `HCC`
thrombosis of left iliac vein

I82.423   **Acute embolism and** `CC` `H10` `HCC`
thrombosis of iliac vein, bilateral

I82.429   **Acute embolism and** `CC` `H10` `HCC`
thrombosis of unspecified iliac vein

☑6ᵗʰ   **I82.43**   **Acute embolism and thrombosis of popliteal vein**

I82.431   **Acute embolism and** `CC` `H10` `HCC`
thrombosis of right popliteal vein

I82.432   **Acute embolism and** `CC` `H10` `HCC`
thrombosis of left popliteal vein

I82.433   **Acute embolism and** `CC` `H10` `HCC`
thrombosis of popliteal vein, bilateral

I82.439   **Acute embolism and** `CC` `H10` `HCC`
thrombosis of unspecified popliteal vein

☑6ᵗʰ   **I82.44**   **Acute embolism and thrombosis of tibial vein**

I82.441   **Acute embolism and** `CC` `H10` `HCC`
thrombosis of right tibial vein

I82.442   **Acute embolism and** `CC` `H10` `HCC`
thrombosis of left tibial vein

I82.443   **Acute embolism and** `CC` `H10` `HCC`
thrombosis of tibial vein, bilateral

I82.449   **Acute embolism and** `CC` `H10` `HCC`
unspecified tibial vein

☑6ᵗʰ   **I82.49**   **Acute embolism and thrombosis of other specified deep vein of lower extremity**

I82.491   **Acute embolism and** `CC` `H10` `HCC`
thrombosis of other specified deep vein of right lower extremity

I82.492   **Acute embolism and** `CC` `H10` `HCC`
thrombosis of other specified deep vein of left lower extremity

I82.493   **Acute embolism and** `CC` `H10` `HCC`
thrombosis of other specified deep vein of lower extremity, bilateral

I82.499   **Acute embolism and** `CC` `H10` `HCC`
thrombosis of other specified deep vein of unspecified lower extremity

☑6ᵗʰ   **I82.4Y**   **Acute embolism and thrombosis of unspecified deep veins of proximal lower extremity**
Acute embolism and thrombosis of deep vein of thigh NOS
Acute embolism and thrombosis of deep vein of upper leg NOS

I82.4Y1   **Acute embolism and** `CC` `H10` `HCC`
thrombosis of unspecified deep veins of right proximal lower extremity

I82.4Y2   **Acute embolism and** `CC` `H10` `HCC`
thrombosis of unspecified deep veins of left proximal lower extremity

I82.4Y3   **Acute embolism and** `CC` `H10` `HCC`
thrombosis of unspecified deep veins of proximal lower extremity, bilateral

I82.4Y9   **Acute embolism and** `CC` `H10` `HCC`
thrombosis of unspecified deep veins of unspecified proximal lower extremity

☑6ᵗʰ   **I82.4Z**   **Acute embolism and thrombosis of unspecified deep veins of distal lower extremity**
Acute embolism and thrombosis of deep vein of calf NOS
Acute embolism and thrombosis of deep vein of lower leg NOS

I82.4Z1   **Acute embolism and** `CC` `H10` `HCC`
thrombosis of unspecified deep veins of right distal lower extremity

I82.4Z2   **Acute embolism and** `CC` `H10` `HCC`
thrombosis of unspecified deep veins of left distal lower extremity

I82.4Z3   **Acute embolism and** `CC` `H10` `HCC`
thrombosis of unspecified deep veins of distal lower extremity, bilateral

I82.4Z9   **Acute embolism and** `CC` `H10` `HCC`
thrombosis of unspecified deep veins of unspecified distal lower extremity

☑5ᵗʰ   **I82.5**   **Chronic embolism and thrombosis of deep veins of lower extremity**
Use additional code, if applicable, for associated long-term (current) use of anticoagulants (Z79.01)

> *EXCLUDES 1*   personal history of venous embolism and thrombosis (Z86.718)

CC Excl: For CC codes in subcategory I82.5:
PDX collection 717

☑6ᵗʰ   **I82.50**   **Chronic embolism and thrombosis of unspecified deep veins of lower extremity**

> *EXCLUDES 1*   chronic embolism and thrombosis of unspecified deep veins of distal lower extremity (I82.5Z-)
> chronic embolism and thrombosis of unspecified deep veins of proximal lower extremity (I82.5Y-)

I82.501   **Chronic embolism and thrombosis** `CC` `HCC`
of unspecified deep veins of right lower extremity

I82.502   **Chronic embolism and thrombosis** `CC` `HCC`
of unspecified deep veins of left lower extremity

I82.503   **Chronic embolism and thrombosis** `CC` `HCC`
of unspecified deep veins of lower extremity, bilateral

I82.509   **Chronic embolism and thrombosis** `CC` `HCC`
of unspecified deep veins of unspecified lower extremity

☑6ᵗʰ   **I82.51**   **Chronic embolism and thrombosis of femoral vein**

I82.511   **Chronic embolism and thrombosis** `CC` `HCC`
of right femoral vein

I82.512   **Chronic embolism and thrombosis** `CC` `HCC`
left femoral vein

I82.513   **Chronic embolism and thrombosis** `CC` `HCC`
of femoral vein, bilateral

I82.519   **Chronic embolism and thrombosis** `CC` `HCC`
of unspecified femoral vein

☑6ᵗʰ   **I82.52**   **Chronic embolism and thrombosis of iliac vein**

I82.521   **Chronic embolism and thrombosis** `CC` `HCC`
of right iliac vein

I82.522   **Chronic embolism and thrombosis** `CC` `HCC`
of left iliac vein

I82.523   **Chronic embolism and thrombosis** `CC` `HCC`
of iliac vein, bilateral

I82.529   **Chronic embolism and thrombosis** `CC` `HCC`
of unspecified iliac vein

☑6ᵗʰ   **I82.53**   **Chronic embolism and thrombosis of popliteal vein**

I82.531   **Chronic embolism and thrombosis** `CC` `HCC`
of right popliteal vein

I82.532   **Chronic embolism and thrombosis** `CC` `HCC`
of left popliteal vein

I82.533   **Chronic embolism and thrombosis** `CC` `HCC`
of popliteal vein, bilateral

I82.539   **Chronic embolism and thrombosis** `CC` `HCC`
of unspecified popliteal vein

☑6ᵗʰ   **I82.54**   **Chronic embolism and thrombosis of tibial vein**

I82.541   **Chronic embolism and thrombosis** `CC` `HCC`
of right tibial vein

I82.542   **Chronic embolism and thrombosis** `CC` `HCC`
of left tibial vein

I82.543   **Chronic embolism and thrombosis** `CC` `HCC`
of tibial vein, bilateral

I82.549   **Chronic embolism and thrombosis** `CC` `HCC`
unspecified tibial vein

☑6ᵗʰ   **I82.59**   **Chronic embolism and thrombosis of other specified deep vein of lower extremity**

I82.591   **Chronic embolism and thrombosis** `CC` `HCC`
of other specified deep vein of right lower extremity

I82.592   **Chronic embolism and thrombosis** `CC` `HCC`
of other specified deep vein of left lower extremity

I82.593   **Chronic embolism and thrombosis** `CC` `HCC` **of other specified deep vein of lower extremity, bilateral**

I82.599   **Chronic embolism and thrombosis** `CC` `HCC` **of other specified deep vein of unspecified lower extremity**

✓6th   **I82.5Y**   **Chronic embolism and thrombosis of** unspecified **deep veins of** proximal lower extremity
Chronic embolism and thrombosis of deep veins of thigh NOS
Chronic embolism and thrombosis of deep veins of upper leg NOS

    I82.5Y1   **Chronic embolism and thrombosis** `CC` `HCC` **of unspecified deep veins of** right **proximal lower extremity**

    I82.5Y2   **Chronic embolism and thrombosis** `CC` `HCC` **of unspecified deep veins of** left **proximal lower extremity**

    I82.5Y3   **Chronic embolism and thrombosis** `CC` `HCC` **of unspecified deep veins of proximal lower extremity, bilateral**

    I82.5Y9   **Chronic embolism and thrombosis** `CC` `HCC` **of unspecified deep veins of** unspecified **proximal lower extremity**

✓6th   **I82.5Z**   **Chronic embolism and thrombosis of** unspecified **deep veins of** distal lower extremity
Chronic embolism and thrombosis of deep veins of calf NOS
Chronic embolism and thrombosis of deep veins of lower leg NOS

    I82.5Z1   **Chronic embolism and thrombosis** `CC` `HCC` **of unspecified deep veins of** right **distal lower extremity**

    I82.5Z2   **Chronic embolism and thrombosis** `CC` `HCC` **of unspecified deep veins of** left **distal lower extremity**

    I82.5Z3   **Chronic embolism and thrombosis** `CC` `HCC` **of unspecified deep veins of distal lower extremity, bilateral**

    I82.5Z9   **Chronic embolism and thrombosis** `CC` `HCC` **of unspecified deep veins of** unspecified **distal lower extremity**

✓5th   **I82.6**   **Acute embolism and thrombosis of veins of** upper extremity

CC Excl: For CC codes in subcategory I82.6:
PDX collection 717

✓6th   **I82.60**   **Acute embolism and thrombosis of** unspecified **veins of upper extremity**

    I82.601   **Acute embolism and thrombosis of** `CC` **unspecified veins of** right **upper extremity**

    I82.602   **Acute embolism and thrombosis of** `CC` **unspecified veins of** left **upper extremity**

    I82.603   **Acute embolism and thrombosis of** `CC` **unspecified veins of upper extremity, bilateral**

    I82.609   **Acute embolism and thrombosis of** `CC` **unspecified veins of** unspecified **upper extremity**

✓6th   **I82.61**   **Acute embolism and thrombosis of** superficial veins **of** upper extremity
Acute embolism and thrombosis of antecubital vein
Acute embolism and thrombosis of basilic vein
Acute embolism and thrombosis of cephalic vein

    I82.611   **Acute embolism and thrombosis of** `CC` **superficial veins of** right **upper extremity**

    I82.612   **Acute embolism and thrombosis of** `CC` **superficial veins of** left **upper extremity**

    I82.613   **Acute embolism and thrombosis of** `CC` **superficial veins of upper extremity, bilateral**

    I82.619   **Acute embolism and thrombosis of** `CC` **superficial veins of unspecified upper extremity**

✓6th   **I82.62**   **Acute embolism and thrombosis of** deep veins of upper extremity
Acute embolism and thrombosis of brachial vein
Acute embolism and thrombosis of radial vein
Acute embolism and thrombosis of ulnar vein

    I82.621   **Acute embolism and thrombosis of** `CC` `HCC` **deep veins of** right **upper extremity**

    I82.622   **Acute embolism and thrombosis of** `CC` `HCC` **deep veins of** left **upper extremity**

    I82.623   **Acute embolism and thrombosis of** `CC` `HCC` **deep veins of upper extremity, bilateral**

    I82.629   **Acute embolism and thrombosis of** `CC` `HCC` **deep veins of** unspecified **upper extremity**

✓5th   **I82.7**   **Chronic embolism and thrombosis of veins of** upper extremity
Use additional code, if applicable, for associated long-term (current) use of anticoagulants (Z79.01)

   `EXCLUDES 1`   *personal history of venous embolism and thrombosis (Z86.718)*

CC Excl: For CC codes in subcategory I82.7:
PDX collection 717

✓6th   **I82.70**   **Chronic embolism and thrombosis of** unspecified **veins of upper extremity**

    I82.701   **Chronic embolism and thrombosis of** `CC` **unspecified veins of** right **upper extremity**

    I82.702   **Chronic embolism and thrombosis of** `CC` **unspecified veins of** left **upper extremity**

    I82.703   **Chronic embolism and thrombosis of** `CC` **unspecified veins of upper extremity, bilateral**

    I82.709   **Chronic embolism and thrombosis of** `CC` **unspecified veins of** unspecified **upper extremity**

✓6th   **I82.71**   **Chronic embolism and thrombosis of** superficial **veins of upper extremity**
Chronic embolism and thrombosis of antecubital vein
Chronic embolism and thrombosis of basilic vein
Chronic embolism and thrombosis of cephalic vein

    I82.711   **Chronic embolism and thrombosis of** `CC` **superficial veins of** right **upper extremity**

    I82.712   **Chronic embolism and thrombosis of** `CC` **superficial veins of** left **upper extremity**

    I82.713   **Chronic embolism and thrombosis of** `CC` **superficial veins of upper extremity, bilateral**

    I82.719   **Chronic embolism and thrombosis of** `CC` **superficial veins of** unspecified **upper extremity**

✓6th   **I82.72**   **Chronic embolism and thrombosis of** deep veins of **upper extremity**
Chronic embolism and thrombosis of brachial vein
Chronic embolism and thrombosis of radial vein
Chronic embolism and thrombosis of ulnar vein

    I82.721   **Chronic embolism and thrombosis** `CC` `HCC` **of deep veins of** right **upper extremity**

    I82.722   **Chronic embolism and thrombosis** `CC` `HCC` **of deep veins of** left **upper extremity**

    I82.723   **Chronic embolism and thrombosis** `CC` `HCC` **of deep veins of** upper **extremity, bilateral**

    I82.729   **Chronic embolism and thrombosis** `CC` `HCC` **of deep veins of** unspecified **upper extremity**

✓5th   **I82.A**   **Embolism and thrombosis of** axillary vein

CC Excl: For CC codes in subcategory I82.A:
PDX collection 717

✓6th   **I82.A1**   **Acute embolism and thrombosis of axillary vein**

    I82.A11   **Acute embolism and thrombosis** `CC` `HCC` **of** right **axillary vein**

    I82.A12   **Acute embolism and thrombosis** `CC` `HCC` **of** left **axillary vein**

    I82.A13   **Acute embolism and thrombosis** `CC` `HCC` **of axillary vein, bilateral**

N Newborn: 0   P Pediatric: 0-17   M Maternity: 12-55   A Adult: 15-124   MCC Major CC Condition   PDxMCC PDx acts as own MCC   CC CC Condition   PDxCC PDx acts as own CC

662   ICD-10-CM 2018

         I82.A19   Acute embolism and thrombosis of unspecified axillary vein `CC` `HCC`

✓6ᵗʰ   I82.A2   Chronic embolism and thrombosis of axillary vein

         I82.A21   Chronic embolism and thrombosis of right axillary vein `CC` `HCC`

         I82.A22   Chronic embolism and thrombosis of left axillary vein `CC` `HCC`

         I82.A23   Chronic embolism and thrombosis of axillary vein, bilateral `CC` `HCC`

         I82.A29   Chronic embolism and thrombosis of unspecified axillary vein `CC` `HCC`

✓5ᵗʰ   **I82.B**   Embolism and thrombosis of subclavian vein

> **CC Excl: For CC codes in subcategory I82.B:**
> PDX collection 717

    ✓6ᵗʰ   **I82.B1**   Acute embolism and thrombosis of subclavian vein

         I82.B11   Acute embolism and thrombosis of right subclavian vein `CC` `HCC`

         I82.B12   Acute embolism and thrombosis of left subclavian vein `CC` `HCC`

         I82.B13   Acute embolism and thrombosis of subclavian vein, bilateral `CC` `HCC`

         I82.B19   Acute embolism and thrombosis of unspecified subclavian vein `CC` `HCC`

    ✓6ᵗʰ   **I82.B2**   Chronic embolism and thrombosis of subclavian vein

         I82.B21   Chronic embolism and thrombosis of right subclavian vein `CC` `HCC`

         I82.B22   Chronic embolism and thrombosis of left subclavian vein `CC` `HCC`

         I82.B23   Chronic embolism and thrombosis of subclavian vein, bilateral `CC` `HCC`

         I82.B29   Chronic embolism and thrombosis of unspecified subclavian vein `CC` `HCC`

✓5ᵗʰ   **I82.C**   Embolism and thrombosis of internal jugular vein

> **CC Excl: For CC codes in subcategory I82.C:**
> PDX collection 717

    ✓6ᵗʰ   **I82.C1**   Acute embolism and thrombosis of internal jugular vein

         I82.C11   Acute embolism and thrombosis of right internal jugular vein `CC` `HCC`

         I82.C12   Acute embolism and thrombosis of left internal jugular vein `CC` `HCC`

         I82.C13   Acute embolism and thrombosis of internal jugular vein, bilateral `CC` `HCC`

         I82.C19   Acute embolism and thrombosis of unspecified internal jugular vein `CC` `HCC`

    ✓6ᵗʰ   **I82.C2**   Chronic embolism and thrombosis of internal jugular vein

         I82.C21   Chronic embolism and thrombosis of right internal jugular vein `CC` `HCC`

         I82.C22   Chronic embolism and thrombosis of left internal jugular vein `CC` `HCC`

         I82.C23   Chronic embolism and thrombosis of internal jugular vein, bilateral `CC` `HCC`

         I82.C29   Chronic embolism and thrombosis of unspecified internal jugular vein `CC` `HCC`

✓5ᵗʰ   **I82.8**   Embolism and thrombosis of other specified veins

Use additional code, if applicable, for associated long-term (current) use of anticoagulants (Z79.01)

> **CC Excl: For CC codes in subcategory I82.8:**
> PDX collection 717

    ✓6ᵗʰ   **I82.81**   Embolism and thrombosis of superficial veins of lower extremities

Embolism and thrombosis of saphenous vein (greater) (lesser)

▲   I82.811   Embolism and thrombosis of superficial veins of right lower extremity `CC`

▲   I82.812   Embolism and thrombosis of superficial veins of left lower extremity `CC`

         I82.813   Embolism and thrombosis of superficial veins of lower extremities, bilateral `CC`

▲   I82.819   Embolism and thrombosis of superficial veins of unspecified lower extremity `CC`

    ✓6ᵗʰ   **I82.89**   Embolism and thrombosis of other specified veins

         I82.890   Acute embolism and thrombosis of other specified veins `CC`

         I82.891   Chronic embolism and thrombosis of other specified veins `CC`

✓5ᵗʰ   **I82.9**   Embolism and thrombosis of unspecified vein

> **CC Excl: For CC codes in subcategory I82.9:**
> PDX collection 717

         I82.90   Acute embolism and thrombosis of unspecified vein `CC`

Embolism of vein NOS
Thrombosis (vein) NOS

         I82.91   Chronic embolism and thrombosis of unspecified vein `CC`

✓4ᵗʰ   **I83**   **Varicose veins of lower extremities**

> *EXCLUDES 1*   varicose veins complicating pregnancy (O22.0-)
> varicose veins complicating the puerperium (O87.4)

✓5ᵗʰ   **I83.0**   Varicose veins of lower extremities with ulcer

Use additional code to identify severity of ulcer (L97.-)

    ✓6ᵗʰ   **I83.00**   Varicose veins of unspecified lower extremity with ulcer

         I83.001   Varicose veins of unspecified lower extremity with ulcer of thigh `HCC` `A`

         I83.002   Varicose veins of unspecified lower extremity with ulcer of calf `HCC` `A`

         I83.003   Varicose veins of unspecified lower extremity with ulcer of ankle `HCC` `A`

         I83.004   Varicose veins of unspecified lower extremity with ulcer of heel and midfoot `HCC` `A`

Varicose veins of unspecified lower extremity with ulcer of plantar surface of midfoot

         I83.005   Varicose veins of unspecified lower extremity with ulcer other part of foot `HCC` `A`

Varicose veins of unspecified lower extremity with ulcer of toe

         I83.008   Varicose veins of unspecified lower extremity with ulcer other part of lower leg `HCC` `A`

         I83.009   Varicose veins of unspecified lower extremity with ulcer of unspecified site `HCC` `A`

    ✓6ᵗʰ   **I83.01**   Varicose veins of right lower extremity with ulcer

         I83.011   Varicose veins of right lower extremity with ulcer of thigh `HCC` `A`

         I83.012   Varicose veins of right lower extremity with ulcer of calf `HCC` `A`

         I83.013   Varicose veins of right lower extremity with ulcer of ankle `HCC` `A`

         I83.014   Varicose veins of right lower extremity with ulcer of heel and midfoot `HCC` `A`

Varicose veins of right lower extremity with ulcer of plantar surface of midfoot

         I83.015   Varicose veins of right lower extremity with ulcer other part of foot `HCC` `A`

Varicose veins of right lower extremity with ulcer of toe

         I83.018   Varicose veins of right lower extremity with ulcer other part of lower leg `HCC` `A`

         I83.019   Varicose veins of right lower extremity with ulcer of unspecified site `HCC` `A`

    ✓6ᵗʰ   **I83.02**   Varicose veins of left lower extremity with ulcer

         I83.021   Varicose veins of left lower extremity with ulcer of thigh `HCC` `A`

         I83.022   Varicose veins of left lower extremity with ulcer of calf `HCC` `A`

         I83.023   Varicose veins of left lower extremity with ulcer of ankle `HCC` `A`

         I83.024   Varicose veins of left lower extremity with ulcer of heel and midfoot `HCC` `A`

Varicose veins of left lower extremity with ulcer of plantar surface of midfoot

I83.025 Varicose veins of left lower extremity with ulcer other part of foot `HCC` `A`
Varicose veins of left lower extremity with ulcer of toe

I83.028 Varicose veins of left lower extremity with ulcer other part of lower leg `HCC` `A`

I83.029 Varicose veins of left lower extremity with ulcer of unspecified site `HCC` `A`

✓5th **I83.1** Varicose veins of lower extremities with inflammation

I83.10 Varicose veins of unspecified lower extremity with inflammation `A`

I83.11 Varicose veins of right lower extremity with inflammation `A`

I83.12 Varicose veins of left lower extremity with inflammation `A`

✓5th **I83.2** Varicose veins of lower extremities with both ulcer and inflammation
Use additional code to identify severity of ulcer (L97.-)

CC Excl: For CC codes in subcategory I83.2:
PDX collection 720

✓6th **I83.20** Varicose veins of unspecified lower extremity with both ulcer and inflammation

I83.201 Varicose veins of unspecified lower extremity with both ulcer of thigh and inflammation `CC` `HCC` `A`

I83.202 Varicose veins of unspecified lower extremity with both ulcer of calf and inflammation `CC` `HCC` `A`

I83.203 Varicose veins of unspecified lower extremity with both ulcer of ankle and inflammation `CC` `HCC` `A`

I83.204 Varicose veins of unspecified lower extremity with both ulcer of heel and midfoot and inflammation `CC` `HCC` `A`
Varicose veins of unspecified lower extremity with both ulcer of plantar surface of midfoot and inflammation

I83.205 Varicose veins of unspecified lower extremity with both ulcer of other part of foot and inflammation `CC` `HCC` `A`
Varicose veins of unspecified lower extremity with both ulcer of toe and inflammation

I83.208 Varicose veins of unspecified lower extremity with both ulcer of other part of lower extremity and inflammation `CC` `HCC` `A`

I83.209 Varicose veins of unspecified lower extremity with both ulcer of unspecified site and inflammation `CC` `HCC` `A`

✓6th **I83.21** Varicose veins of right lower extremity with both ulcer and inflammation

I83.211 Varicose veins of right lower extremity with both ulcer of thigh and inflammation `CC` `HCC` `A`

I83.212 Varicose veins of right lower extremity with both ulcer of calf and inflammation `CC` `HCC` `A`

I83.213 Varicose veins of right lower extremity with both ulcer of ankle and inflammation `CC` `HCC` `A`

I83.214 Varicose veins of right lower extremity with both ulcer of heel and midfoot and inflammation `CC` `HCC` `A`
Varicose veins of right lower extremity with both ulcer of plantar surface of midfoot and inflammation

I83.215 Varicose veins of right lower extremity with both ulcer other part of foot and inflammation `CC` `HCC` `A`
Varicose veins of right lower extremity with both ulcer of toe and inflammation

I83.218 Varicose veins of right lower extremity with both ulcer of other part of lower extremity and inflammation `CC` `HCC` `A`

I83.219 Varicose veins of right lower extremity with both ulcer of unspecified site and inflammation `CC` `HCC` `A`

✓6th **I83.22** Varicose veins of left lower extremity with both ulcer and inflammation

I83.221 Varicose veins of left lower extremity with both ulcer of thigh and inflammation `CC` `HCC` `A`

I83.222 Varicose veins of left lower extremity with both ulcer of calf and inflammation `CC` `HCC` `A`

I83.223 Varicose veins of left lower extremity with both ulcer of ankle and inflammation `CC` `HCC` `A`

I83.224 Varicose veins of left lower extremity with both ulcer of heel and midfoot and inflammation `CC` `HCC` `A`
Varicose veins of left lower extremity with both ulcer of plantar surface of midfoot and inflammation

I83.225 Varicose veins of left lower extremity with both ulcer other part of foot and inflammation `CC` `HCC` `A`
Varicose veins of left lower extremity with both ulcer of toe and inflammation

I83.228 Varicose veins of left lower extremity with both ulcer of other part of lower extremity and inflammation `CC` `HCC` `A`

I83.229 Varicose veins of left lower extremity with both ulcer of unspecified site and inflammation `CC` `HCC` `A`

✓5th **I83.8** Varicose veins of lower extremities with other complications

✓6th **I83.81** Varicose veins of lower extremities with pain

▲ **I83.811** Varicose veins of right lower extremity with pain `A`

▲ **I83.812** Varicose veins of left lower extremity with pain `A`

I83.813 Varicose veins of bilateral lower extremities with pain `A`

▲ **I83.819** Varicose veins of unspecified lower extremity with pain `A`

✓6th **I83.89** Varicose veins of lower extremities with other complications
Varicose veins of lower extremities with edema
Varicose veins of lower extremities with swelling

▲ **I83.891** Varicose veins of right lower extremity with other complications `A`

▲ **I83.892** Varicose veins of left lower extremity with other complications `A`

I83.893 Varicose veins of bilateral lower extremities with other complications `A`

▲ **I83.899** Varicose veins of unspecified lower extremity with other complications `A`

✓5th **I83.9** Asymptomatic varicose veins of lower extremities
Phlebectasia of lower extremities
Varicose veins of lower extremities
Varix of lower extremities

I83.90 Asymptomatic varicose veins of unspecified lower extremity `A`
Varicose veins NOS

I83.91 Asymptomatic varicose veins of right lower extremity `A`

I83.92 Asymptomatic varicose veins of left lower extremity `A`

I83.93 Asymptomatic varicose veins of bilateral lower extremities `A`

✓4th **I85** Esophageal varices
Use additional code to identify:
alcohol abuse and dependence (F10.-)

✓5th **I85.0** Esophageal varices
Idiopathic esophageal varices
Primary esophageal varices

I85.00 Esophageal varices without bleeding `CC` `HCC`
Esophageal varices NOS
CC Excl: PDX collection 721

I85.01 Esophageal varices with bleeding `MCC` `HCC`
CC Excl: PDX collection 722

`N` Newborn: 0   `P` Pediatric: 0-17   `M` Maternity: 12-55   `A` Adult: 15-124   `MCC` Major CC Condition   `PDx MCC` PDx acts as own MCC   `CC` CC Condition   `PDx CC` PDx acts as own CC

664   ICD-10-CM 2018

✓5ᵗʰ **I85.1** **Secondary esophageal varices**
Esophageal varices secondary to alcoholic liver disease
Esophageal varices secondary to cirrhosis of liver
Esophageal varices secondary to schistosomiasis
Esophageal varices secondary to toxic liver disease
Code first underlying disease

I85.10 **Secondary esophageal varices without**   CC HCC
bleeding
CC Excl: PDX collection 723

I85.11 **Secondary esophageal varices with**   MCC HCC
bleeding
CC Excl: PDX collection 724

✓4ᵗʰ **I86** **Varicose veins of other sites**
EXCLUDES 1   varicose veins of unspecified site (I83.9-)
EXCLUDES 2   retinal varices (H35.0-)

I86.0 **Sublingual varices**
DEF: Distended, tortuous veins beneath tongue.

I86.1 **Scrotal varices**   ♂
Varicocele

I86.2 **Pelvic varices**

I86.3 **Vulval varices**   ♀
EXCLUDES 1   vulval varices complicating childbirth and the
puerperium (O87.8)
vulval varices complicating pregnancy (O22.1-)

I86.4 **Gastric varices**

I86.8 **Varicose veins of other specified sites**   A
Varicose ulcer of nasal septum

✓4ᵗʰ **I87** **Other disorders of veins**

✓5ᵗʰ **I87.0** **Postthrombotic syndrome**
Chronic venous hypertension due to deep vein thrombosis
Postphlebitic syndrome
EXCLUDES 1   chronic venous hypertension without deep vein
thrombosis (I87.3-)

CC Excl: For CC codes in subcategory I87.0:
PDX collection 725

✓6ᵗʰ **I87.00** **Postthrombotic syndrome without complications**
Asymptomatic postthrombotic syndrome

I87.001 **Postthrombotic syndrome without
complications of right lower extremity**

I87.002 **Postthrombotic syndrome without
complications of left lower extremity**

I87.003 **Postthrombotic syndrome without
complications of bilateral lower extremity**

I87.009 **Postthrombotic syndrome without
complications of unspecified extremity**
Postthrombotic syndrome NOS

✓6ᵗʰ **I87.01** **Postthrombotic syndrome with ulcer**
Use additional code to specify site and severity of ulcer
(L97.-)

I87.011 **Postthrombotic syndrome with**   CC HCC
ulcer of right lower extremity

I87.012 **Postthrombotic syndrome with**   CC HCC
ulcer of left lower extremity

I87.013 **Postthrombotic syndrome with**   CC HCC
ulcer of bilateral lower extremity

I87.019 **Postthrombotic syndrome with**   CC HCC
ulcer of unspecified lower extremity

✓6ᵗʰ **I87.02** **Postthrombotic syndrome with inflammation**

I87.021 **Postthrombotic syndrome with
inflammation of right lower extremity**

I87.022 **Postthrombotic syndrome with
inflammation of left lower extremity**

I87.023 **Postthrombotic syndrome with
inflammation of bilateral lower extremity**

I87.029 **Postthrombotic syndrome with
inflammation of unspecified lower
extremity**

✓6ᵗʰ **I87.03** **Postthrombotic syndrome with ulcer and
inflammation**
Use additional code to specify site and severity of ulcer
(L97.-)

I87.031 **Postthrombotic syndrome with**   CC HCC
**ulcer and inflammation of right lower
extremity**

I87.032 **Postthrombotic syndrome with**   CC HCC
**ulcer and inflammation of left lower
extremity**

I87.033 **Postthrombotic syndrome with**   CC HCC
**ulcer and inflammation of bilateral lower
extremity**

I87.039 **Postthrombotic syndrome with**   CC HCC
**ulcer and inflammation of unspecified
lower extremity**

✓6ᵗʰ **I87.09** **Postthrombotic syndrome with other complications**

I87.091 **Postthrombotic syndrome with other
complications of right lower extremity**

I87.092 **Postthrombotic syndrome with other
complications of left lower extremity**

I87.093 **Postthrombotic syndrome with other
complications of bilateral lower extremity**

I87.099 **Postthrombotic syndrome with other
complications of unspecified lower
extremity**

I87.1 **Compression of vein**   CC
Stricture of vein
Vena cava syndrome (inferior) (superior)
EXCLUDES 2   compression of pulmonary vein (I28.8)
CC Excl: PDX collection 726

I87.2 **Venous insufficiency (chronic) (peripheral)**
Stasis dermatitis
EXCLUDES 1   stasis dermatitis with varicose veins of lower
extremities (I83.1-, I83.2-)
DEF: Insufficient drainage of venous blood in any part of body;
results in edema or dermatosis.

✓5ᵗʰ **I87.3** **Chronic venous hypertension (idiopathic)**
Stasis edema
EXCLUDES 1   chronic venous hypertension due to deep vein
thrombosis (I87.0-)
varicose veins of lower extremities (I83.-)

CC Excl: For CC codes in subcategory I87.3:
PDX collection 727

✓6ᵗʰ **I87.30** **Chronic venous hypertension (idiopathic) without
complications**
Asymptomatic chronic venous hypertension
(idiopathic)

I87.301 **Chronic venous hypertension (idiopathic)
without complications of right lower
extremity**

I87.302 **Chronic venous hypertension (idiopathic)
without complications of left lower
extremity**

I87.303 **Chronic venous hypertension (idiopathic)
without complications of bilateral lower
extremity**

I87.309 **Chronic venous hypertension (idiopathic)
without complications of unspecified
lower extremity**
Chronic venous hypertension NOS

✓6ᵗʰ **I87.31** **Chronic venous hypertension (idiopathic) with ulcer**
Use additional code to specify site and severity of ulcer
(L97.-)

I87.311 **Chronic venous hypertension**   CC HCC
**(idiopathic) with ulcer of right lower
extremity**

I87.312 **Chronic venous hypertension**   CC HCC
**(idiopathic) with ulcer of left lower
extremity**

I87.313 **Chronic venous hypertension**   CC HCC
**(idiopathic) with ulcer of bilateral
lower extremity**

I87.319 **Chronic venous hypertension**   CC HCC
**(idiopathic) with ulcer of unspecified
lower extremity**

✓6ᵗʰ **I87.32** **Chronic venous hypertension (idiopathic) with
inflammation**

I87.321 **Chronic venous hypertension (idiopathic)
with inflammation of right lower
extremity**

I87.322 **Chronic venous hypertension (idiopathic)
with inflammation of left lower extremity**

I87.323 **Chronic venous hypertension (idiopathic)
with inflammation of bilateral lower
extremity**

I87.329 **Chronic venous hypertension (idiopathic)
with inflammation of unspecified lower
extremity**

Chapter 9. Diseases of the Circulatory System

☑6ᵗʰ **I87.33** **Chronic venous hypertension (idiopathic) with** ulcer and inflammation
Use additional code to specify site and severity of ulcer (L97.-)

I87.331 **Chronic venous hypertension (idiopathic) with ulcer and inflammation of** right lower **extremity** `CC` `HCC`

I87.332 **Chronic venous hypertension (idiopathic) with ulcer and inflammation of** left lower **extremity** `CC` `HCC`

I87.333 **Chronic venous hypertension (idiopathic) with ulcer and inflammation of** bilateral lower **extremity** `CC` `HCC`

I87.339 **Chronic venous hypertension (idiopathic) with ulcer and inflammation of** unspecified lower **extremity** `CC` `HCC`

☑6ᵗʰ **I87.39** **Chronic venous hypertension (idiopathic) with** other complications

I87.391 **Chronic venous hypertension (idiopathic) with other complications of** right lower **extremity**

I87.392 **Chronic venous hypertension (idiopathic) with other complications of** left lower **extremity**

I87.393 **Chronic venous hypertension (idiopathic) with other complications of** bilateral lower **extremity**

I87.399 **Chronic venous hypertension (idiopathic) with other complications of** unspecified lower **extremity**

I87.8 **Other specified disorders of veins**
Phlebosclerosis
Venofibrosis

I87.9 **Disorder of vein, unspecified**

☑4ᵗʰ **I88** **Nonspecific lymphadenitis**
EXCLUDES 1   *acute lymphadenitis, except mesenteric (L04.-)*
enlarged lymph nodes NOS (R59.-)
human immunodeficiency virus [HIV] disease resulting in generalized lymphadenopathy (B20)

I88.0 **Nonspecific mesenteric lymphadenitis**
Mesenteric lymphadenitis (acute)(chronic)

I88.1 **Chronic lymphadenitis, except mesenteric**
Adenitis
Lymphadenitis

I88.8 **Other nonspecific lymphadenitis**

I88.9 **Nonspecific lymphadenitis, unspecified**
Lymphadenitis NOS

☑4ᵗʰ **I89** **Other noninfective disorders of lymphatic vessels and lymph nodes**
EXCLUDES 1   *chylocele, tunica vaginalis (nonfilarial) NOS (N50.89)*
enlarged lymph nodes NOS (R59.-)
filarial chylocele (B74.-)
hereditary lymphedema (Q82.0)

I89.0 **Lymphedema, not elsewhere classified**
Elephantiasis (nonfilarial) NOS
Lymphangiectasis
Obliteration, lymphatic vessel
Praecox lymphedema
Secondary lymphedema
EXCLUDES 1   *postmastectomy lymphedema (I97.2)*

I89.1 **Lymphangitis**
Chronic lymphangitis
Lymphangitis NOS
Subacute lymphangitis
EXCLUDES 1   *acute lymphangitis (L03.-)*

I89.8 **Other specified noninfective disorders of lymphatic vessels and lymph nodes**
Chylocele (nonfilarial)
Chylous ascites
Chylous cyst
Lipomelanotic reticulosis
Lymph node or vessel fistula
Lymph node or vessel infarction
Lymph node or vessel rupture

I89.9 **Noninfective disorder of lymphatic vessels and lymph nodes, unspecified**
Disease of lymphatic vessels NOS

Other and unspecified disorders of the circulatory system (I95-I99)

☑4ᵗʰ **I95** **Hypotension**
EXCLUDES 1   *cardiovascular collapse (R57.9)*
maternal hypotension syndrome (O26.5-)
nonspecific low blood pressure reading NOS (R03.1)

I95.0 **Idiopathic** hypotension

I95.1 **Orthostatic** hypotension
Hypotension, postural
EXCLUDES 1   *neurogenic orthostatic hypotension [Shy-Drager] (G90.3)*
orthostatic hypotension due to drugs (I95.2)

I95.2 **Hypotension** due to drugs
Orthostatic hypotension due to drugs
Use additional code for adverse effect, if applicable, to identify drug (T36-T50 with fifth or sixth character 5)

I95.3 **Hypotension of** hemodialysis
Intra-dialytic hypotension

☑5ᵗʰ **I95.8** **Other hypotension**

I95.81 **Postprocedural** hypotension

I95.89 **Other** hypotension
Chronic hypotension

I95.9 **Hypotension,** unspecified

☑ **I96** **Gangrene, not elsewhere classified** `CC` `HCC`
Gangrenous cellulitis
EXCLUDES 1   *gangrene in atherosclerosis of native arteries of the extremities (I70.26)*
~~*gangrene in diabetes mellitus (E08-E13 with .52)*~~
gangrene in hernia (K40.1, K40.4, K41.1, K41.4, K42.1, K43.1-, K44.1, K45.1, K46.1)
gangrene in other peripheral vascular diseases (I73.-)
gangrene of certain specified sites—see Alphabetical Index
gas gangrene (A48.0)
pyoderma gangrenosum (L88)
EXCLUDES 2 ▶*gangrene in diabetes mellitus (E08-E13 with .52)*◀
AHA: 2013, 2Q, 34
CC Excl: PDX collection 519

☑4ᵗʰ **I97** **Intraoperative and postprocedural complications and disorders of circulatory system, not elsewhere classified**
EXCLUDES 2   *postprocedural shock (T81.1-)*

I97.0 **Postcardiotomy syndrome**

☑5ᵗʰ **I97.1** **Other** postprocedural cardiac **functional disturbances**
EXCLUDES 2   *acute pulmonary insufficiency following thoracic surgery (J95.1)*
intraoperative cardiac functional disturbances (I97.7-)

CC Excl: For CC codes in subcategory I97.1:
PDX collection 728

☑6ᵗʰ **I97.11** **Postprocedural** cardiac insufficiency

I97.110 **Postprocedural cardiac insufficiency following** cardiac surgery `CC`

I97.111 **Postprocedural cardiac insufficiency following** other surgery `CC`

☑6ᵗʰ **I97.12** **Postprocedural** cardiac arrest

I97.120 **Postprocedural cardiac arrest following** cardiac surgery `CC`

I97.121 **Postprocedural cardiac arrest following** other surgery `CC`

☑6ᵗʰ **I97.13** **Postprocedural** heart failure
Use additional code to identify the heart failure (I50.-)

I97.130 **Postprocedural heart failure following** cardiac surgery `CC`

I97.131 **Postprocedural heart failure following** other surgery `CC`

☑6ᵗʰ **I97.19** **Other** postprocedural cardiac functional disturbances
Use additional code, if applicable, to further specify disorder

I97.190 **Other postprocedural cardiac functional disturbances following** cardiac surgery `CC`
▶Use additional code, if applicable, for type 4 or type 5 myocardial infarction, to further specify disorder◀

I97.191 **Other postprocedural cardiac functional disturbances following** other surgery `CC`

Ⓝ Newborn: 0   Ⓟ Pediatric: 0-17   Ⓜ Maternity: 12-55   Ⓐ Adult: 15-124   `MCC` Major CC Condition   `PDxMCC` PDx acts as own MCC   `CC` CC Condition   `PDxCC` PDx acts as own CC

666   ICD-10-CM 2018

I97.2 Postmastectomy lymphedema syndrome   A
Elephantiasis due to mastectomy
Obliteration of lymphatic vessels

I97.3 Postprocedural hypertension

✓5ᵗʰ **I97.4 Intraoperative hemorrhage and hematoma of a circulatory system organ or structure complicating a procedure**
EXCLUDES 1   *intraoperative hemorrhage and hematoma of a circulatory system organ or structure due to accidental puncture and laceration during a procedure (I97.5-)*
EXCLUDES 2   *intraoperative cerebrovascular hemorrhage complicating a procedure (G97.3-)*

CC Excl: For CC codes in subcategory I97.4:
PDX collection 729

✓6ᵗʰ **I97.41 Intraoperative hemorrhage and hematoma of a circulatory system organ or structure complicating a circulatory system procedure**

    I97.410 Intraoperative hemorrhage and hematoma of a circulatory system organ or structure complicating a cardiac catheterization   CC

    I97.411 Intraoperative hemorrhage and hematoma of a circulatory system organ or structure complicating a cardiac bypass   CC

    I97.418 Intraoperative hemorrhage and hematoma of a circulatory system organ or structure complicating other circulatory system procedure   CC

I97.42 Intraoperative hemorrhage and hematoma of a circulatory system organ or structure complicating other procedure   CC

✓5ᵗʰ **I97.5 Accidental puncture and laceration of a circulatory system organ or structure during a procedure**
EXCLUDES 2   *accidental puncture and laceration of brain during a procedure (G97.4-)*

I97.51 Accidental puncture and laceration of a circulatory system organ or structure during a circulatory system procedure   CC
CC Excl: PDX collection 509

I97.52 Accidental puncture and laceration of a circulatory system organ or structure during other procedure   CC
CC Excl: PDX collection 509

✓5ᵗʰ **I97.6 Postprocedural hemorrhage, hematoma and seroma of a circulatory system organ or structure following a procedure**
EXCLUDES 2   *postprocedural cerebrovascular hemorrhage complicating a procedure (G97.5-)*

CC Excl: For CC codes in subcategory I97.6:
PDX collection 729

✓6ᵗʰ **I97.61 Postprocedural hemorrhage of a circulatory system organ or structure following a circulatory system procedure**

    I97.610 Postprocedural hemorrhage of a circulatory system organ or structure following a cardiac catheterization   CC

    I97.611 Postprocedural hemorrhage of a circulatory system organ or structure following cardiac bypass   CC

    I97.618 Postprocedural hemorrhage of a circulatory system organ or structure following other circulatory system procedure   CC

✓6ᵗʰ **I97.62 Postprocedural hemorrhage, hematoma and seroma of a circulatory system organ or structure following other procedure**

    I97.620 Postprocedural hemorrhage of a circulatory system organ or structure following other procedure   CC

    I97.621 Postprocedural hematoma of a circulatory system organ or structure following other procedure   CC

    I97.622 Postprocedural seroma of a circulatory system organ or structure following procedure   CC

✓6ᵗʰ **I97.63 Postprocedural hematoma of a circulatory system organ or structure following a circulatory system procedure**

    I97.630 Postprocedural hematoma of a circulatory system organ or structure following a cardiac catheterization   CC

    I97.631 Postprocedural hematoma of a circulatory system organ or structure following cardiac bypass   CC

    I97.638 Postprocedural hematoma of a circulatory system organ or structure following other circulatory system procedure   CC

✓6ᵗʰ **I97.64 Postprocedural seroma of a circulatory system organ or structure following a circulatory system procedure**

    I97.640 Postprocedural seroma of a circulatory system organ or structure following a cardiac catheterization   CC

    I97.641 Postprocedural seroma of a circulatory system organ or structure following cardiac bypass   CC

    I97.648 Postprocedural seroma of a circulatory system organ or structure following other circulatory system procedure   CC

✓5ᵗʰ **I97.7 Intraoperative cardiac functional disturbances**
EXCLUDES 2   *acute pulmonary insufficiency following thoracic surgery (J95.1)*
postprocedural cardiac functional disturbances (I97.1-)

CC Excl: For CC codes in subcategory I97.7:
PDX collection 728

✓6ᵗʰ **I97.71 Intraoperative cardiac arrest**

    I97.710 Intraoperative cardiac arrest during cardiac surgery   CC

    I97.711 Intraoperative cardiac arrest during other surgery   CC

✓6ᵗʰ **I97.79 Other intraoperative cardiac functional disturbances**
Use additional code, if applicable, to further specify disorder

    I97.790 Other intraoperative cardiac functional disturbances during cardiac surgery   CC

    I97.791 Other intraoperative cardiac functional disturbances during other surgery   CC

✓5ᵗʰ **I97.8 Other intraoperative and postprocedural complications and disorders of the circulatory system, not elsewhere classified**
Use additional code, if applicable, to further specify disorder

CC Excl: For CC codes in subcategory I97.8, unless otherwise noted: PDX collection 617

✓6ᵗʰ **I97.81 Intraoperative cerebrovascular infarction**

    I97.810 Intraoperative cerebrovascular infarction during cardiac surgery   CC HCC

    I97.811 Intraoperative cerebrovascular infarction during other surgery   CC HCC

✓6ᵗʰ **I97.82 Postprocedural cerebrovascular infarction**

    I97.820 Postprocedural cerebrovascular infarction following cardiac surgery   CC HCC

    I97.821 Postprocedural cerebrovascular infarction following other surgery   CC HCC

I97.88 Other intraoperative complications of the circulatory system, not elsewhere classified   CC
CC Excl: PDX collection 728

I97.89 Other postprocedural complications and disorders of the circulatory system, not elsewhere classified   CC
CC Excl: PDX collection 728

✓4ᵗʰ **I99 Other and unspecified disorders of circulatory system**

I99.8 Other disorder of circulatory system

I99.9 Unspecified disorder of circulatory system

✓ Additional Character Req   ✓x7ᵗʰ Placeholder Alert   Unacceptable PDx   Manifestation   H1 - H14 HAC   HCC CMS-HCC Condition   EXCLUDES 1 Not Coded Here   EXCLUDES 2 Not Included Here

Chapter 10. Diseases of the Respiratory System (J00–J99)

Chapter Specific Guidelines with Coding Examples

The chapter specific guidelines from the ICD-10-CM Official Guidelines for Coding and Reporting have been provided below. Along with these guidelines are coding examples, contained in the shaded boxes, that have been developed to help illustrate the coding and/or sequencing guidance found in these guidelines.

a. Chronic obstructive pulmonary disease [COPD] and asthma

1) Acute exacerbation of chronic obstructive bronchitis and asthma

The codes in categories J44 and J45 distinguish between uncomplicated cases and those in acute exacerbation. An acute exacerbation is a worsening or a decompensation of a chronic condition. An acute exacerbation is not equivalent to an infection superimposed on a chronic condition, though an exacerbation may be triggered by an infection.

Vancomycin IV was started to treat a patient with acute pneumonia due to *Streptococcus pneumoniae*. Patient also with acute exacerbation of COPD continued on home meds.

J13   **Pneumonia due to Streptococcus pneumoniae**

J44.0   **Chronic obstructive pulmonary disease with acute lower respiratory infection**

J44.1   **Chronic obstructive pulmonary disease with (acute) exacerbation**

Explanation: ICD-10-CM uses combination codes to create organism-specific classifications for acute pneumonia. Category J44 codes include combination codes with severity components, which differentiate between COPD with acute lower respiratory infection (acute pneumonia), COPD with acute exacerbation, and COPD without mention of a complication (unspecified).

An acute exacerbation is a worsening or a decompensation of a chronic condition. An acute exacerbation is not equivalent to an infection superimposed on a chronic condition, though an exacerbation may be triggered by an infection, as in this example. Treatment of the pneumonia necessitated the inpatient admission. Instructional notes at J44.0 say to "code also to identify the infection," which informs the coder that another code must be assigned if applicable. Sequencing of the pneumonia and COPD exacerbation are governed by the Section II, "Selection of Principal Diagnosis," guidelines. In this case it was the pneumonia that was "chiefly responsible for occasioning the admission" with the IV vancomycin treatment.

Exacerbation of moderate persistent asthma with status asthmaticus

J45.42   **Moderate persistent asthma with status asthmaticus**

Explanation: Category J45 Asthma includes severity-specific subcategories and fifth-character codes to distinguish between uncomplicated cases, those in acute exacerbation, and those with status asthmaticus.

---

b. Acute respiratory failure

1) Acute respiratory failure as principal diagnosis

A code from subcategory J96.0, Acute respiratory failure, or subcategory J96.2, Acute and chronic respiratory failure, may be assigned as a principal diagnosis when it is the condition established after study to be chiefly responsible for occasioning the admission to the hospital, and the selection is supported by the Alphabetic Index and Tabular List. However, chapter-specific coding guidelines (such as obstetrics, poisoning, HIV, newborn) that provide sequencing direction take precedence.

Acute hypoxic respiratory failure due to COPD exacerbation

J96.01   **Acute respiratory failure with hypoxia**

J44.1   **Chronic obstructive pulmonary disease with (acute) exacerbation**

Explanation: Category J96 classifies respiratory failure with combination codes that designate the severity and the presence of hypoxia and hypercapnia. Code J96.01 is sequenced as the first-listed diagnosis, as the reason for the admission. Respiratory failure may be assigned as a principal diagnosis when it is the condition established after study to be chiefly responsible for occasioning the admission to the hospital and the selection is supported by the Alphabetic Index and Tabular List.

---

2) Acute respiratory failure as secondary diagnosis

Respiratory failure may be listed as a secondary diagnosis if it occurs after admission, or if it is present on admission, but does not meet the definition of principal diagnosis.

Acute respiratory failure due to accidental oxycodone overdose

T40.2X1A   **Poisoning by other opioids, accidental (unintentional), initial encounter**

J96.00   **Acute respiratory failure, unspecified whether with hypoxia or hypercapnia**

Explanation: Respiratory failure may be assigned as a principal diagnosis when it is the condition established after study to be chiefly responsible for occasioning the admission to the hospital, and the selection is supported by the Alphabetic Index and Tabular List. However, chapter-specific coding guidelines, such as poisoning, that provide sequencing direction take precedence. When coding a poisoning or reaction to the improper use of a medication (e.g. overdose, wrong substance given or taken in error, wrong route of administration), first assign the appropriate code from categories T36–T50. Use additional code(s) for all manifestations of the poisoning. In this instance, the respiratory failure is a manifestation of the poisoning and is sequenced as a secondary diagnosis.

Acute pneumococcal pneumonia with subsequent development of acute respiratory failure

J13   **Pneumonia due to Streptococcus pneumoniae**

J96.00   **Acute respiratory failure, unspecified whether with hypoxia or hypercapnia**

Explanation: Acute respiratory failure may be listed as a secondary diagnosis if it occurs after admission, or if it is present on admission but does not meet the definition of principal diagnosis.

---

3) Sequencing of acute respiratory failure and another acute condition

When a patient is admitted with respiratory failure and another acute condition, (e.g., myocardial infarction, cerebrovascular accident, aspiration pneumonia), the principal diagnosis will not be the same in every situation. This applies whether the other acute condition is a respiratory or nonrespiratory condition. Selection of the principal diagnosis will be dependent on the circumstances of admission. If both the respiratory failure and the other acute condition are equally responsible for occasioning the admission to the hospital, and there are no chapter-specific sequencing rules, the guideline regarding two or more diagnoses that equally meet the definition for principal diagnosis (*Section II, C.*) may be applied in these situations.

If the documentation is not clear as to whether acute respiratory failure and another condition are equally responsible for occasioning the admission, query the provider for clarification.

Acute pneumococcal pneumonia and acute respiratory failure, both present on admission

J96.00   **Acute respiratory failure, unspecified whether with hypoxia or hypercapnia**

J13   **Pneumonia due to Streptococcus pneumoniae**

Explanation: When a patient is admitted with respiratory failure and another acute condition, such as a bacterial pneumonia, the principal diagnosis is not the same in every situation. This applies whether the other acute condition is a respiratory or nonrespiratory condition. The principal diagnosis depends on the circumstances of admission.

---

c. Influenza due to certain identified influenza viruses

Code only confirmed cases of influenza due to certain identified influenza viruses (category J09), and due to other identified influenza virus (category J10). This is an exception to the hospital inpatient guideline Section II, H. (Uncertain Diagnosis).

In this context, "confirmation" does not require documentation of positive laboratory testing specific for avian or other novel influenza A or other identified influenza virus. However, coding should be based on the provider's diagnostic statement that the patient has avian influenza, or other novel influenza A, for category J09, or has another particular identified strain of influenza, such as H1N1 or H3N2, but not identified as novel or variant, for category J10.

If the provider records "suspected" or "possible" or "probable" avian influenza, or novel influenza, or other identified influenza, then the appropriate influenza code from category J11, Influenza due to unidentified influenza virus, should be assigned. A code from category J09, Influenza due to certain identified influenza viruses, should not be assigned nor should a code from category J10, Influenza due to other identified influenza virus.

Influenza due to avian influenza virus with pneumonia

J09.X1   Influenza due to identified novel influenza A virus with pneumonia

Explanation: Codes in category J09 Influenza due to certain identified influenza viruses should be assigned only for confirmed cases. "Confirmation" does not require positive laboratory testing of a specific influenza virus but does need to be based on the provider's diagnostic statement, which should not include terms such as "possible," "probable," or "suspected."

---

d. Ventilator associated pneumonia

1) Documentation of ventilator associated pneumonia

As with all procedural or postprocedural complications, code assignment is based on the provider's documentation of the relationship between the condition and the procedure.

Code J95.851, Ventilator associated pneumonia, should be assigned only when the provider has documented ventilator associated pneumonia (VAP). An additional code to identify the organism (e.g., Pseudomonas aeruginosa, code B96.5) should also be assigned. Do not assign an additional code from categories J12-J18 to identify the type of pneumonia.

Code J95.851 should not be assigned for cases where the patient has pneumonia and is on a mechanical ventilator and the provider has not specifically stated that the pneumonia is ventilator-associated pneumonia. If the documentation is unclear as to whether the patient has a pneumonia that is a complication attributable to the mechanical ventilator, query the provider.

2) Ventilator associated pneumonia develops after admission

A patient may be admitted with one type of pneumonia (e.g., code J13, Pneumonia due to Streptococcus pneumonia) and subsequently develop VAP. In this instance, the principal diagnosis would be the appropriate code from categories J12-J18 for the pneumonia diagnosed at the time of admission. Code J95.851, Ventilator associated pneumonia, would be assigned as an additional diagnosis when the provider has also documented the presence of ventilator associated pneumonia.

Patient with pneumonia due to *Klebsiella pneumoniae* develops superimposed MRSA ventilator-associated pneumonia

J15.0   Pneumonia due to Klebsiella pneumoniae

J95.851   Ventilator associated pneumonia

B95.62   Methicillin resistant Staphylococcus aureus infection as the cause of diseases classified elsewhere

Explanation: Code assignment for ventilator-associated pneumonia is based on the provider's documentation of the relationship between the condition and the procedure and is reported only when the provider has documented ventilator-associated pneumonia (VAP).

A patient may be admitted with one type of pneumonia and subsequently develop VAP. In this example, the principal diagnosis code describes the pneumonia diagnosed at the time of admission, with code J95.851 Ventilator associated pneumonia, assigned as secondary.

Chapter 10. Diseases of the Respiratory System (J00-J99)

NOTE When a respiratory condition is described as occurring in more than one site and is not specifically indexed, it should be classified to the lower anatomic site (e.g. tracheobronchitis to bronchitis in J40).

Use additional code, where applicable, to identify:
exposure to environmental tobacco smoke (Z77.22)
exposure to tobacco smoke in the perinatal period (P96.81)
history of tobacco dependence (Z87.891)
occupational exposure to environmental tobacco smoke (Z57.31)
tobacco dependence (F17.-)
tobacco use (Z72.0)

EXCLUDES 2 *certain conditions originating in the perinatal period (P04-P96)*
certain infectious and parasitic diseases (A00-B99)
complications of pregnancy, childbirth and the puerperium (O00-O9A)
congenital malformations, deformations and chromosomal abnormalities (Q00-Q99)
endocrine, nutritional and metabolic diseases (E00-E88)
injury, poisoning and certain other consequences of external causes (S00-T88)
neoplasms (C00-D49)
smoke inhalation (T59.81-)
symptoms, signs and abnormal clinical and laboratory findings, not elsewhere classified (R00-R94)

This chapter contains the following blocks:
J00-J06   Acute upper respiratory infections
J09-J18   Influenza and pneumonia
J20-J22   Other acute lower respiratory infections
J30-J39   Other diseases of upper respiratory tract
J40-J47   Chronic lower respiratory diseases
J60-J70   Lung diseases due to external agents
J80-J84   Other respiratory diseases principally affecting the interstitium
J85-J86   Suppurative and necrotic conditions of the lower respiratory tract
J90-J94   Other diseases of the pleura
J95   Intraoperative and postprocedural complications and disorders of respiratory system, not elsewhere classified
J96-J99   Other diseases of the respiratory system

Acute upper respiratory infections (J00-J06)

EXCLUDES 1 *chronic obstructive pulmonary disease with acute lower respiratory infection (J44.0)*
influenza virus with other respiratory manifestations (J09.X2, J10.1, J11.1)

J00   Acute nasopharyngitis (common cold)
Acute rhinitis   Infective rhinitis
Coryza (acute)   Nasal catarrh, acute
Infective nasopharyngitis NOS   Nasopharyngitis NOS

EXCLUDES 1 *acute pharyngitis (J02.-)*
acute sore throat NOS (J02.9)
pharyngitis NOS (J02.9)
rhinitis NOS (J31.0)
sore throat NOS (J02.9)

EXCLUDES 2 *allergic rhinitis (J30.1-J30.9)*
chronic pharyngitis (J31.2)
chronic rhinitis (J31.0)
chronic sore throat (J31.2)
nasopharyngitis, chronic (J31.1)
vasomotor rhinitis (J30.0)

DEF: Acute inflammation of mucous membranes; extends from nares to pharynx; characterized by nasal obstruction, sneezing, runny nose, and sore throat.

✓4th J01   Acute sinusitis
INCLUDES acute abscess of sinus
acute empyema of sinus
acute infection of sinus
acute inflammation of sinus
acute suppuration of sinus
Use additional code (B95-B97) to identify infectious agent
EXCLUDES 1 *sinusitis NOS (J32.9)*
EXCLUDES 2 *chronic sinusitis (J32.0-J32.8)*

✓5th J01.0   Acute maxillary sinusitis
Acute antritis
J01.00   Acute maxillary sinusitis, unspecified
J01.01   Acute recurrent maxillary sinusitis

✓5th J01.1   Acute frontal sinusitis
J01.10   Acute frontal sinusitis, unspecified
J01.11   Acute recurrent frontal sinusitis

✓5th J01.2   Acute ethmoidal sinusitis
J01.20   Acute ethmoidal sinusitis, unspecified
J01.21   Acute recurrent ethmoidal sinusitis

✓5th J01.3   Acute sphenoidal sinusitis
J01.30   Acute sphenoidal sinusitis, unspecified
J01.31   Acute recurrent sphenoidal sinusitis

✓5th J01.4   Acute pansinusitis
J01.40   Acute pansinusitis, unspecified
J01.41   Acute recurrent pansinusitis

✓5th J01.8   Other acute sinusitis
J01.80   Other acute sinusitis
Acute sinusitis involving more than one sinus but not pansinusitis
J01.81   Other acute recurrent sinusitis
Acute recurrent sinusitis involving more than one sinus but not pansinusitis

✓5th J01.9   Acute sinusitis, unspecified
J01.90   Acute sinusitis, unspecified
J01.91   Acute recurrent sinusitis, unspecified

✓4th J02   Acute pharyngitis
INCLUDES acute sore throat
EXCLUDES 1 *acute laryngopharyngitis (J06.0)*
peritonsillar abscess (J36)
pharyngeal abscess (J39.1)
retropharyngeal abscess (J39.0)
EXCLUDES 2 *chronic pharyngitis (J31.2)*

J02.0   Streptococcal pharyngitis
Septic pharyngitis
Streptococcal sore throat
EXCLUDES 2 *scarlet fever (A38.-)*

J02.8   Acute pharyngitis due to other specified organisms
Use additional code (B95-B97) to identify infectious agent
EXCLUDES 1 *acute pharyngitis due to coxsackie virus (B08.5)*
acute pharyngitis due to gonococcus (A54.5)
acute pharyngitis due to herpes [simplex] virus (B00.2)
acute pharyngitis due to infectious mononucleosis (B27.-)
enteroviral vesicular pharyngitis (B08.5)

J02.9   Acute pharyngitis, unspecified
Gangrenous pharyngitis (acute)
Infective pharyngitis (acute) NOS
Pharyngitis (acute) NOS
Sore throat (acute) NOS
Suppurative pharyngitis (acute)
Ulcerative pharyngitis (acute)

✓4th J03   Acute tonsillitis
EXCLUDES 1 *acute sore throat (J02.-)*
hypertrophy of tonsils (J35.1)
peritonsillar abscess (J36)
sore throat NOS (J02.9)
streptococcal sore throat (J02.0)
EXCLUDES 2 *chronic tonsillitis (J35.0)*

✓5th J03.0   Streptococcal tonsillitis
J03.00   Acute streptococcal tonsillitis, unspecified
J03.01   Acute recurrent streptococcal tonsillitis

✓5th J03.8   Acute tonsillitis due to other specified organisms
Use additional code (B95-B97) to identify infectious agent
EXCLUDES 1 *diphtheritic tonsillitis (A36.0)*
herpesviral pharyngotonsillitis (B00.2)
streptococcal tonsillitis (J03.0)
tuberculous tonsillitis (A15.8)
Vincent's tonsillitis (A69.1)
J03.80   Acute tonsillitis due to other specified organisms
J03.81   Acute recurrent tonsillitis due to other specified organisms

✓5th J03.9   Acute tonsillitis, unspecified
Follicular tonsillitis (acute)
Gangrenous tonsillitis (acute)
Infective tonsillitis (acute)
Tonsillitis (acute) NOS
Ulcerative tonsillitis (acute)
J03.90   Acute tonsillitis, unspecified
J03.91   Acute recurrent tonsillitis, unspecified

Chapter 10. Diseases of the Respiratory System

✓4ᵗʰ **J04** **Acute laryngitis and tracheitis**
Use additional code (B95-B97) to identify infectious agent
> EXCLUDES 1 *acute obstructive laryngitis [croup] and epiglottitis (J05.-)*
> EXCLUDES 2 *laryngismus (stridulus) (J38.5)*

J04.0 **Acute laryngitis**
Edematous laryngitis (acute)
Laryngitis (acute) NOS
Subglottic laryngitis (acute)
Suppurative laryngitis (acute)
Ulcerative laryngitis (acute)
> EXCLUDES 1 *acute obstructive laryngitis (J05.0)*
> EXCLUDES 2 *chronic laryngitis (J37.0)*

✓5ᵗʰ **J04.1** **Acute tracheitis**
Acute viral tracheitis
Catarrhal tracheitis (acute)
Tracheitis (acute) NOS
> EXCLUDES 2 *chronic tracheitis (J42)*

J04.10 **Acute tracheitis without obstruction**

J04.11 **Acute tracheitis with obstruction** `MCC`
CC Excl: PDX collection 730

J04.2 **Acute laryngotracheitis**
Laryngotracheitis NOS
Tracheitis (acute) with laryngitis (acute)
> EXCLUDES 1 *acute obstructive laryngotracheitis (J05.0)*
> EXCLUDES 2 *chronic laryngotracheitis (J37.1)*

✓5ᵗʰ **J04.3** **Supraglottitis, unspecified**

J04.30 **Supraglottitis, unspecified, without obstruction**

J04.31 **Supraglottitis, unspecified, with obstruction** `MCC`
CC Excl: PDX collection 731

✓4ᵗʰ **J05** **Acute obstructive laryngitis [croup] and epiglottitis**
Use additional code (B95-B97) to identify infectious agent

J05.0 **Acute obstructive laryngitis [croup]**
Obstructive laryngitis (acute) NOS
Obstructive laryngotracheitis NOS
DEF: Acute laryngeal obstruction due to allergy, foreign body, or in the majority of cases a viral infection; symptoms include harsh, barking cough, hoarseness, and persistent high-pitched respiratory sound (stridor).

✓5ᵗʰ **J05.1** **Acute epiglottitis**
> EXCLUDES 2 *epiglottitis, chronic (J37.0)*

J05.10 **Acute epiglottitis without obstruction** `CC`
Epiglottitis NOS
CC Excl: PDX collection 732

J05.11 **Acute epiglottitis with obstruction** `MCC`
CC Excl: PDX collection 730

✓4ᵗʰ **J06** **Acute upper respiratory infections of multiple and unspecified sites**
> EXCLUDES 1 *acute respiratory infection NOS (J22)*
> *streptococcal pharyngitis (J02.0)*

J06.0 **Acute laryngopharyngitis**

J06.9 **Acute upper respiratory infection, unspecified**
Upper respiratory disease, acute
Upper respiratory infection NOS

Influenza and pneumonia (J09-J18)

> EXCLUDES 2 *allergic or eosinophilic pneumonia (J82)*
> *aspiration pneumonia NOS (J69.0)*
> *congenital pneumonia (P23.9)*
> *lipid pneumonia (J69.1)*
> *meconium pneumonia (P24.01)*
> *neonatal aspiration pneumonia (P24.-)*
> *pneumonia due to solids and liquids (J69.-)*
> *rheumatic pneumonia (I00)*
> *ventilator associated pneumonia (J95.851)*

✓4ᵗʰ **J09** **Influenza due to certain identified influenza viruses**
> EXCLUDES 1 ►*influenza A/H1N1 (J10.-)*◄
> *influenza due to other identified influenza virus (J10.-)*
> *influenza due to unidentified influenza virus (J11.-)*
> *seasonal influenza due to other identified influenza virus (J10.-)*
> *seasonal influenza due to unidentified influenza virus (J11.-)*

✓5ᵗʰ **J09.X** **Influenza due to identified novel influenza A virus**
Avian influenza
Bird influenza
Influenza A/H5N1
Influenza of other animal origin, not bird or swine
Swine influenza virus (viruses that normally cause infections in pigs)
AHA: 2016, 3Q, 10

J09.X1 **Influenza due to identified novel influenza A virus with pneumonia** `HIV` `MCC`
Code also, if applicable, associated:
lung abscess (J85.1)
other specified type of pneumonia
CC Excl: PDX collection 110

J09.X2 **Influenza due to identified novel influenza A virus with other respiratory manifestations**
Influenza due to identified novel influenza A virus NOS
Influenza due to identified novel influenza A virus with laryngitis
Influenza due to identified novel influenza A virus with pharyngitis
Influenza due to identified novel influenza A virus with upper respiratory symptoms
Use additional code, if applicable, for associated:
pleural effusion (J91.8)
sinusitis (J01.-)

J09.X3 **Influenza due to identified novel influenza A virus with gastrointestinal manifestations**
Influenza due to identified novel influenza A virus gastroenteritis
> EXCLUDES 1 *'intestinal flu' [viral gastroenteritis] (A08.-)*

J09.X9 **Influenza due to identified novel influenza A virus with other manifestations**
Influenza due to identified novel influenza A virus with encephalopathy
Influenza due to identified novel influenza A virus with myocarditis
Influenza due to identified novel influenza A virus with otitis media
Use additional code to identify manifestation

✓4ᵗʰ **J10** **Influenza due to other identified influenza virus**
> EXCLUDES 1 *influenza due to avian influenza virus (J09.X-)*
> *influenza due to swine flu (J09.X-)*
> *influenza due to unidentifed influenza virus (J11.-)*

✓5ᵗʰ **J10.0** **Influenza due to other identified influenza virus with pneumonia**
Code also associated lung abscess, if applicable (J85.1)

J10.00 **Influenza due to other identified influenza virus with unspecified type of pneumonia** `MCC`
CC Excl: PDX collection 110

J10.01 **Influenza due to other identified influenza virus with the same other identified influenza virus pneumonia** `MCC`
CC Excl: PDX collection 110

J10.08 **Influenza due to other identified influenza virus with other specified pneumonia** `HIV` `MCC`
Code also other specified type of pneumonia
CC Excl: PDX collection 733

Ⓝ Newborn: 0   Ⓟ Pediatric: 0-17   Ⓜ Maternity: 12-55   Ⓐ Adult: 15-124   `MCC` Major CC Condition   `PDx MCC` PDx acts as own MCC   `CC` CC Condition   `PDx CC` PDx acts as own CC

J10.1 **Influenza due to other identified influenza virus with** other **respiratory manifestations**
Influenza due to other identified influenza virus NOS
Influenza due to other identified influenza virus with laryngitis
Influenza due to other identified influenza virus with pharyngitis
Influenza due to other identified influenza virus with upper respiratory symptoms
Use additional code for associated pleural effusion, if applicable (J91.8)
Use additional code for associated sinusitis, if applicable (J01.-)
AHA: 2016, 3Q, 10-11

J10.2 **Influenza due to other identified influenza virus with** gastrointestinal manifestations
Influenza due to other identified influenza virus gastroenteritis
EXCLUDES 1   'intestinal flu' [viral gastroenteritis] (A08.-)

✓5ᵗʰ **J10.8** **Influenza due to other identified influenza virus with** other **manifestations**

  J10.81 **Influenza due to other identified influenza virus with** encephalopathy

  J10.82 **Influenza due to other identified influenza virus with** myocarditis

  J10.83 **Influenza due to other identified influenza virus with** otitis media
  Use additional code for any associated perforated tympanic membrane (H72.-)

  J10.89 **Influenza due to other identified influenza virus with** other **manifestations**
  Use additional codes to identify the manifestations

✓4ᵗʰ **J11** **Influenza due to** unidentified **influenza virus**

✓5ᵗʰ **J11.0** **Influenza due to unidentified influenza virus with** pneumonia
Code also associated lung abscess, if applicable (J85.1)
AHA: 2016, 3Q, 11

  J11.00 **Influenza due to unidentified influenza virus** `MCC` **with** unspecified type **of pneumonia**
  Influenza with pneumonia NOS
  CC Excl: PDX collection 110

  J11.08 **Influenza due to unidentified influenza virus** `MCC` **with** specified **pneumonia**
  Code also other specified type of pneumonia
  CC Excl: PDX collection 110

J11.1 **Influenza due to unidentified influenza virus with** other **respiratory manifestations**
Influenza NOS
Influenzal laryngitis NOS
Influenzal pharyngitis NOS
Influenza with upper respiratory symptoms NOS
Use additional code for associated pleural effusion, if applicable (J91.8)
Use additional code for associated sinusitis, if applicable (J01.-)

J11.2 **Influenza due to unidentified influenza virus with** gastrointestinal manifestations
Influenza gastroenteritis NOS
EXCLUDES 1   'intestinal flu' [viral gastroenteritis] (A08.-)

✓5ᵗʰ **J11.8** **Influenza due to unidentified influenza virus with** other **manifestations**

  J11.81 **Influenza due to unidentified influenza virus with** encephalopathy
  Influenzal encephalopathy NOS

  J11.82 **Influenza due to unidentified influenza virus with** myocarditis
  Influenzal myocarditis NOS

  J11.83 **Influenza due to unidentified influenza virus with** otitis media
  Influenzal otitis media NOS
  Use additional code for any associated perforated tympanic membrane (H72.-)

  J11.89 **Influenza due to unidentified influenza virus with** other **manifestations**
  Use additional codes to identify the manifestations

✓4ᵗʰ **J12** **Viral pneumonia, not elsewhere classified**
`INCLUDES`   bronchopneumonia due to viruses other than influenza viruses
Code first associated influenza, if applicable (J09.X1, J10.0-, J11.0-)
Code also associated abscess, if applicable (J85.1)
EXCLUDES 1   aspiration pneumonia due to anesthesia during labor and delivery (O74.0)
aspiration pneumonia due to anesthesia during pregnancy (O29)
aspiration pneumonia due to anesthesia during puerperium (O89.0)
aspiration pneumonia due to solids and liquids (J69.-)
aspiration pneumonia NOS (J69.0)
congenital pneumonia (P23.0)
congenital rubella pneumonitis (P35.0)
interstitial pneumonia NOS (J84.9)
lipid pneumonia (J69.1)
neonatal aspiration pneumonia (P24.-)
AHA: 2016, 3Q, 15; 2013, 4Q, 118

CC Excl: For MCC codes in category J12, unless otherwise noted: PDX collection 734

J12.0 **Adenoviral pneumonia** `MCC`
J12.1 **Respiratory syncytial virus pneumonia** `MCC`
J12.2 **Parainfluenza virus pneumonia** `MCC`
J12.3 **Human metapneumovirus pneumonia** `HIV` `MCC`

✓5ᵗʰ **J12.8** **Other viral pneumonia**

  J12.81 **Pneumonia due to SARS-associated** `HIV` `MCC` **coronavirus**
  Severe acute respiratory syndrome NOS
  DEF: A severe adult respiratory syndrome caused by the coronavirus, specified as inflammation of the lungs with consolidation.
  CC Excl: PDX collection 735

  J12.89 **Other viral pneumonia** `HIV` `MCC`

J12.9 **Viral pneumonia, unspecified** `HIV` `MCC`

J13 **Pneumonia due to** Streptococcus pneumoniae `HIV` `MCC` `HCC`
Bronchopneumonia due to S. pneumoniae
Code first associated influenza, if applicable (J09.X1, J10.0-, J11.0-)
Code also associated lung abscess, if applicable (J85.1)
EXCLUDES 1   congenital pneumonia due to S. pneumoniae (P23.6)
lobar pneumonia, unspecified organism (J18.1)
pneumonia due to other streptococci (J15.3-J15.4)
AHA: 2016, 3Q, 15; 2013, 4Q, 118
CC Excl: PDX collection 110

J14 **Pneumonia due to** Hemophilus influenzae `HIV` `MCC` `HCC`
Bronchopneumonia due to H. influenzae
Code first associated influenza, if applicable (J09.X1, J10.0-, J11.0-)
Code also associated lung abscess, if applicable (J85.1)
EXCLUDES 1   congenital pneumonia due to H. influenzae (P23.6)
AHA: 2016, 3Q, 15; 2013, 4Q, 118
CC Excl: PDX collection 110

✓4ᵗʰ **J15** **Bacterial pneumonia, not elsewhere classified**
`INCLUDES`   bronchopneumonia due to bacteria other than S. pneumoniae and H. influenzae
Code first associated influenza, if applicable (J09.X1, J10.0-, J11.0-)
Code also associated lung abscess, if applicable (J85.1)
EXCLUDES 1   chlamydial pneumonia (J16.0)
congenital pneumonia (P23.-)
Legionnaires' disease (A48.1)
spirochetal pneumonia (A69.8)
AHA: 2016, 3Q, 15; 2013, 4Q, 118

CC Excl: For MCC codes in category J15: PDX collection 110

J15.0 **Pneumonia due to** Klebsiella pneumoniae `HIV` `MCC` `HCC`
J15.1 **Pneumonia due to** Pseudomonas `HIV` `MCC` `HCC`

✓5ᵗʰ **J15.2** **Pneumonia due to** staphylococcus

  J15.20 **Pneumonia due to staphylococcus,** `HIV` `MCC` `HCC` **unspecified**

  ✓6ᵗʰ **J15.21** **Pneumonia due to Staphylococcus** aureus

    J15.211 **Pneumonia due to** Methicillin `HIV` `MCC` `HCC` **susceptible Staphylococcus aureus**
    MSSA pneumonia
    Pneumonia due to Staphylococcus aureus NOS

    J15.212 **Pneumonia due to** Methicillin `HIV` `MCC` `HCC` **resistant Staphylococcus aureus**

  J15.29 **Pneumonia due to** other **staphylococcus** `HIV` `MCC` `HCC`

J15.3 **Pneumonia due to streptococcus,** group B `HIV` `MCC` `HCC`

✔Additional Character Req   ✔x7ᵗʰ Placeholder Alert   Unacceptable PDx   Manifestation   `H1`-`H14` HAC   `HCC` CMS-HCC Condition   *EXCLUDES 1* Not Coded Here   *EXCLUDES 2* Not Included Here

Chapter 10. Diseases of the Respiratory System

J15.4   **Pneumonia due to** other **streptococci**   `HIV` `MCC` `HCC`
    EXCLUDES 1   *pneumonia due to streptococcus, group B (J15.3)*
         pneumonia due to Streptococcus pneumoniae (J13)

J15.5   **Pneumonia due to** **Escherichia coli**   `HIV` `MCC` `HCC`

▲   **J15.6**   **Pneumonia due to** other **Gram-negative bacteria**   `HIV` `MCC` `HCC`
    ►Pneumonia due to other aerobic Gram-negative bacteria◄
    Pneumonia due to Serratia marcescens

J15.7   **Pneumonia due to** **Mycoplasma pneumoniae**   `MCC`

J15.8   **Pneumonia due to** other **specified bacteria**   `HIV` `MCC` `HCC`

J15.9   **Unspecified** bacterial **pneumonia**   `HIV` `MCC`
    Pneumonia due to gram-positive bacteria

✓4ᵗʰ J16   **Pneumonia due to other infectious organisms, not elsewhere classified**
    Code first associated influenza, if applicable (J09.X1, J10.0-, J11.0-)
    Code also associated lung abscess, if applicable (J85.1)
    EXCLUDES 1   *congenital pneumonia (P23.-)*
         ornithosis (A70)
         pneumocystosis (B59)
         pneumonia NOS (J18.9)
    AHA: 2016, 3Q, 15; 2013, 4Q, 118

J16.0   **Chlamydial pneumonia**   `MCC`
    CC Excl: PDX collection 110

J16.8   **Pneumonia due to** other **specified infectious organisms**   `MCC`
    CC Excl: PDX collection 110

J17   *Pneumonia in diseases classified elsewhere*   `MCC`
    Code first underlying disease, such as:
    Q fever (A78)
    rheumatic fever (I00)
    schistosomiasis (B65.0-B65.9)
    EXCLUDES 1   *candidial pneumonia (B37.1)*
         chlamydial pneumonia (J16.0)
         gonorrheal pneumonia (A54.84)
         histoplasmosis pneumonia (B39.0-B39.2)
         measles pneumonia (B05.2)
         nocardiosis pneumonia (A43.0)
         pneumocystosis (B59)
         pneumonia due to Pneumocystis carinii (B59)
         pneumonia due to Pneumocystis jiroveci (B59)
         pneumonia in actinomycosis (A42.0)
         pneumonia in anthrax (A22.1)
         pneumonia in ascariasis (B77.81)
         pneumonia in aspergillosis (B44.0-B44.1)
         pneumonia in coccidioidomycosis (B38.0-B38.2)
         pneumonia in cytomegalovirus disease (B25.0)
         pneumonia in toxoplasmosis (B58.3)
         rubella pneumonia (B06.81)
         salmonella pneumonia (A02.22)
         spirochetal infection NEC with pneumonia (A69.8)
         tularemia pneumonia (A21.2)
         typhoid fever with pneumonia (A01.03)
         varicella pneumonia (B01.2)
         whooping cough with pneumonia (A37 with fifth-character 1)
    AHA: 2016, 3Q, 15; 2013, 4Q, 118
    CC Excl: PDX collection 110

✓4ᵗʰ J18   **Pneumonia, unspecified organism**
    Code first associated influenza, if applicable (J09.X1, J10.0-, J11.0-)
    EXCLUDES 1   *abscess of lung with pneumonia (J85.1)*
         aspiration pneumonia due to anesthesia during labor and delivery (O74.0)
         aspiration pneumonia due to anesthesia during pregnancy (O29)
         aspiration pneumonia due to anesthesia during puerperium (O89.0)
         aspiration pneumonia due to solids and liquids (J69.-)
         aspiration pneumonia NOS (J69.0)
         congenital pneumonia (P23.0)
         drug-induced interstitial lung disorder (J70.2-J70.4)
         interstitial pneumonia NOS (J84.9)
         lipid pneumonia (J69.1)
         neonatal aspiration pneumonia (P24.-)
         pneumonitis due to external agents (J67-J70)
         pneumonitis due to fumes and vapors (J68.0)
         usual interstitial pneumonia (J84.17)
    AHA: 2016, 3Q, 15; 2013, 4Q, 118

    CC Excl: For MCC codes in category J18, unless otherwise noted: PDX collection 110

J18.0   **Bronchopneumonia, unspecified organism**   `MCC`
    EXCLUDES 1   *hypostatic bronchopneumonia (J18.2)*
         lipid pneumonia (J69.1)
    EXCLUDES 2   *acute bronchiolitis (J21.-)*
         chronic bronchiolitis (J44.9)

J18.1   **Lobar** pneumonia, unspecified **organism**   `HIV` `MCC` `HCC`

J18.2   **Hypostatic** pneumonia, unspecified **organism**   `CC`
    Hypostatic bronchopneumonia
    Passive pneumonia
    CC Excl: PDX collection 736

J18.8   Other **pneumonia, unspecified organism**   `HIV` `MCC`

J18.9   **Pneumonia,** unspecified **organism**   `HIV` `MCC`
    AHA: 2014, 3Q, 4; 2013, 4Q, 119; 2012, 4Q, 94

Other acute lower respiratory infections (J20-J22)

    EXCLUDES 2   *chronic obstructive pulmonary disease with acute lower respiratory infection (J44.0)*

✓4ᵗʰ J20   **Acute bronchitis**
    `INCLUDES`   acute and subacute bronchitis (with) bronchospasm
         acute and subacute bronchitis (with) tracheitis
         acute and subacute bronchitis (with) tracheobronchitis, acute
         acute and subacute fibrinous bronchitis
         acute and subacute membranous bronchitis
         acute and subacute purulent bronchitis
         acute and subacute septic bronchitis
    EXCLUDES 1   *bronchitis NOS (J40)*
         tracheobronchitis NOS (J40)
    EXCLUDES 2   *acute bronchitis with bronchiectasis (J47.0)*
         acute bronchitis with chronic obstructive asthma (J44.0)
         acute bronchitis with chronic obstructive pulmonary disease (J44.0)
         allergic bronchitis NOS (J45.909)
         bronchitis due to chemicals, fumes and vapors (J68.0)
         chronic bronchitis NOS (J42)
         chronic mucopurulent bronchitis (J41.1)
         chronic obstructive bronchitis (J44.-)
         chronic obstructive tracheobronchitis (J44.-)
         chronic simple bronchitis (J41.0)
         chronic tracheobronchitis (J42)
    AHA: 2016, 3Q, 10, 16
    DEF: Acute inflammation of main branches of bronchial tree due to infectious or irritant agents; symptoms include cough with a varied production of sputum, fever, substernal soreness, and lung rales; usually last for three to 10 days.

J20.0   **Acute bronchitis due to** **Mycoplasma pneumoniae**

J20.1   **Acute bronchitis due to** **Hemophilus influenzae**

J20.2   **Acute bronchitis due to** **streptococcus**

J20.3   **Acute bronchitis due to** **coxsackievirus**

J20.4   **Acute bronchitis due to** **parainfluenza virus**

J20.5   **Acute bronchitis due to** **respiratory syncytial virus**

J20.6   **Acute bronchitis due to** **rhinovirus**

J20.7   **Acute bronchitis due to** **echovirus**

J20.8   **Acute bronchitis due to** other **specified organisms**

J20.9   **Acute bronchitis,** unspecified

✓4ᵗʰ J21   **Acute bronchiolitis**
    `INCLUDES`   acute bronchiolitis with bronchospasm
    EXCLUDES 2   *respiratory bronchiolitis interstitial lung disease (J84.115)*

    CC Excl: For CC codes in category J21, unless otherwise noted: PDX collection 738

J21.0   **Acute bronchiolitis due to** **respiratory syncytial virus**   `CC`
    CC Excl: PDX collection 737

J21.1   **Acute bronchiolitis due to** **human metapneumovirus**   `CC`

J21.8   **Acute bronchiolitis due to** other **specified organisms**   `CC`

J21.9   **Acute bronchiolitis,** unspecified   `CC`
    Bronchiolitis (acute)
    EXCLUDES 1   *chronic bronchiolitis (J44.-)*

J22   **Unspecified acute lower respiratory infection**
    Acute (lower) respiratory (tract) infection NOS
    EXCLUDES 1   *upper respiratory infection (acute) (J06.9)*

Other diseases of upper respiratory tract (J30-J39)

✓4ᵗʰ J30   **Vasomotor and allergic rhinitis**
    `INCLUDES`   spasmodic rhinorrhea
    EXCLUDES 1   *allergic rhinitis with asthma (bronchial) (J45.909)*
         rhinitis NOS (J31.0)

J30.0   **Vasomotor rhinitis**

J30.1   **Allergic rhinitis due to** pollen
    Allergy NOS due to pollen
    Hay fever
    Pollinosis

J30.2   **Other** seasonal allergic **rhinitis**

`N` Newborn: 0   `P` Pediatric: 0-17   `M` Maternity: 12-55   `A` Adult: 15-124   `MCC` Major CC Condition   `PDxMCC` PDx acts as own MCC   `CC` CC Condition   `PDxCC` PDx acts as own CC

674   ICD-10-CM 2018

Chapter 10. Diseases of the Respiratory System

J30.5   **Allergic rhinitis** due to food

✓5ᵗʰ **J30.8**   **Other allergic rhinitis**

     J30.81   **Allergic rhinitis due to animal** (cat) (dog) **hair and** dander

     J30.89   **Other allergic rhinitis**
         Perennial allergic rhinitis

J30.9   **Allergic rhinitis, unspecified**

✓4ᵗʰ **J31**   **Chronic rhinitis, nasopharyngitis and pharyngitis**

     Use additional code to identify:
     exposure to environmental tobacco smoke (Z77.22)
     exposure to tobacco smoke in the perinatal period (P96.81)
     history of tobacco dependence (Z87.891)
     occupational exposure to environmental tobacco smoke (Z57.31)
     tobacco dependence (F17.-)
     tobacco use (Z72.0)

     J31.0   **Chronic rhinitis**
         Atrophic rhinitis (chronic)
         Granulomatous rhinitis (chronic)
         Hypertrophic rhinitis (chronic)
         Obstructive rhinitis (chronic)
         Ozena
         Purulent rhinitis (chronic)
         Rhinitis (chronic) NOS
         Ulcerative rhinitis (chronic)
         EXCLUDES 1   allergic rhinitis (J30.1-J30.9)
                   vasomotor rhinitis (J30.0)
         DEF: Persistent inflammation of mucous membranes of nose; characterized by postnasal drip.

     J31.1   **Chronic nasopharyngitis**
         EXCLUDES 2   acute nasopharyngitis (J00)
         DEF: Persistent inflammation of mucous membranes extending from nares to pharynx; characterized by constant irritation in nasopharynx and postnasal drip.

     J31.2   **Chronic pharyngitis**
         Atrophic pharyngitis (chronic)
         Chronic sore throat
         Granular pharyngitis (chronic)
         Hypertrophic pharyngitis (chronic)
         EXCLUDES 2   acute pharyngitis (J02.9)

✓4ᵗʰ **J32**   **Chronic sinusitis**

     INCLUDES   sinus abscess
              sinus empyema
              sinus infection
              sinus suppuration

     Use additional code to identify:
     exposure to environmental tobacco smoke (Z77.22)
     exposure to tobacco smoke in the perinatal period (P96.81)
     history of tobacco dependence (Z87.891)
     infectious agent (B95-B97)
     occupational exposure to environmental tobacco smoke (Z57.31)
     tobacco dependence (F17.-)
     tobacco use (Z72.0)
     EXCLUDES 2   acute sinusitis (J01.-)

     J32.0   **Chronic maxillary sinusitis**
         Antritis (chronic)
         Maxillary sinusitis NOS

     J32.1   **Chronic frontal sinusitis**
         Frontal sinusitis NOS

     J32.2   **Chronic ethmoidal sinusitis**
         Ethmoidal sinusitis NOS
         EXCLUDES 1   Woakes' ethmoiditis (J33.1)

     J32.3   **Chronic sphenoidal sinusitis**
         Sphenoidal sinusitis NOS

     J32.4   **Chronic pansinusitis**
         Pansinusitis NOS

     J32.8   **Other chronic sinusitis**
         Sinusitis (chronic) involving more than one sinus but not pansinusitis

     J32.9   **Chronic sinusitis, unspecified**
         Sinusitis (chronic) NOS

✓4ᵗʰ **J33**   **Nasal polyp**

     Use additional code to identify:
     exposure to environmental tobacco smoke (Z77.22)
     exposure to tobacco smoke in the perinatal period (P96.81)
     history of tobacco dependence (Z87.891)
     occupational exposure to environmental tobacco smoke (Z57.31)
     tobacco dependence (F17.-)
     tobacco use (Z72.0)
     EXCLUDES 1   adenomatous polyps (D14.0)

     J33.0   **Polyp of nasal cavity**
         Choanal polyp
         Nasopharyngeal polyp

     J33.1   **Polypoid sinus degeneration**
         Woakes' syndrome or ethmoiditis

     J33.8   **Other polyp of sinus**
         Accessory polyp of sinus
         Ethmoidal polyp of sinus
         Maxillary polyp of sinus
         Sphenoidal polyp of sinus

     J33.9   **Nasal polyp, unspecified**

✓4ᵗʰ **J34**   **Other and unspecified disorders of nose and nasal sinuses**
     EXCLUDES 2   varicose ulcer of nasal septum (I86.8)

     J34.0   **Abscess, furuncle and carbuncle of nose**
         Cellulitis of nose   Ulceration of nose
         Necrosis of nose

     J34.1   **Cyst and mucocele of nose and nasal sinus**

     J34.2   **Deviated nasal septum**
         Deflection or deviation of septum (nasal) (acquired)
         EXCLUDES 1   congenital deviated nasal septum (Q67.4)

     J34.3   **Hypertrophy of nasal turbinates**

✓5ᵗʰ   **J34.8**   **Other specified disorders of nose and nasal sinuses**

         J34.81   **Nasal mucositis (ulcerative)**
              Code also type of associated therapy, such as:
                  antineoplastic and immunosuppressive drugs (T45.1X-)
                  radiological procedure and radiotherapy (Y84.2)
              EXCLUDES 2   gastrointestinal mucositis (ulcerative) (K92.81)
                         mucositis (ulcerative) of vagina and vulva (N76.81)
                         oral mucositis (ulcerative) (K12.3-)

         J34.89   **Other specified disorders of nose and nasal sinuses**
              Perforation of nasal septum NOS
              Rhinolith

     J34.9   **Unspecified disorder of nose and nasal sinuses**

✓4ᵗʰ **J35**   **Chronic diseases of tonsils and adenoids**

     Use additional code to identify:
     exposure to environmental tobacco smoke (Z77.22)
     exposure to tobacco smoke in the perinatal period (P96.81)
     history of tobacco dependence (Z87.891)
     occupational exposure to environmental tobacco smoke (Z57.31)
     tobacco dependence (F17.-)
     tobacco use (Z72.0)

✓5ᵗʰ   **J35.0**   **Chronic tonsillitis and adenoiditis**
         EXCLUDES 2   acute tonsillitis (J03.-)

         J35.01   **Chronic tonsillitis**

         J35.02   **Chronic adenoiditis**

         J35.03   **Chronic tonsillitis and adenoiditis**

     J35.1   **Hypertrophy of tonsils**
         Enlargement of tonsils
         EXCLUDES 1   hypertrophy of tonsils with tonsillitis (J35.0-)

     J35.2   **Hypertrophy of adenoids**
         Enlargement of adenoids
         EXCLUDES 1   hypertrophy of adenoids with adenoiditis (J35.0-)

     J35.3   **Hypertrophy of tonsils with hypertrophy of adenoids**
         EXCLUDES 1   hypertrophy of tonsils and adenoids with tonsillitis and adenoiditis (J35.03)

     J35.8   **Other chronic diseases of tonsils and adenoids**
         Adenoid vegetations   Tonsillar tag
         Amygdalolith   Ulcer of tonsil
         Calculus, tonsil
         Cicatrix of tonsil (and adenoid)

     J35.9   **Chronic disease of tonsils and adenoids, unspecified**
         Disease (chronic) of tonsils and adenoids NOS

✓ Additional Character Req   ✓x7ᵗʰ Placeholder Alert   Unacceptable PDx   Manifestation   H1 - H14 HAC   HCC CMS-HCC Condition   EXCLUDES 1 Not Coded Here   EXCLUDES 2 Not Included Here

ICD-10-CM 2018   **675**

J36 **Peritonsillar abscess**   CC
     INCLUDES   abscess of tonsil
               peritonsillar cellulitis
               quinsy
     Use additional code (B95-B97) to identify infectious agent
     EXCLUDES 1   *acute tonsillitis (J03.-)*
                chronic tonsillitis (J35.0)
                retropharyngeal abscess (J39.0)
                tonsillitis NOS (J03.9-)
     CC Excl: PDX collection 739

✓4th **J37** **Chronic laryngitis and laryngotracheitis**
     Use additional code to identify:
         exposure to environmental tobacco smoke (Z77.22)
         exposure to tobacco smoke in the perinatal period (P96.81)
         history of tobacco dependence (Z87.891)
         infectious agent (B95-B97)
         occupational exposure to environmental tobacco smoke (Z57.31)
         tobacco dependence (F17.-)
         tobacco use (Z72.0)

    J37.0 **Chronic laryngitis**
         Catarrhal laryngitis
         Hypertrophic laryngitis
         Sicca laryngitis
         EXCLUDES 2   *acute laryngitis (J04.0)*
                obstructive (acute) laryngitis (J05.0)

    J37.1 **Chronic laryngotracheitis**
         Laryngitis, chronic, with tracheitis (chronic)
         Tracheitis, chronic, with laryngitis
         EXCLUDES 1   *chronic tracheitis (J42)*
         EXCLUDES 2   *acute laryngotracheitis (J04.2)*
                acute tracheitis (J04.1)

✓4th **J38** **Diseases of vocal cords and larynx, not elsewhere classified**
     Use additional code to identify:
         exposure to environmental tobacco smoke (Z77.22)
         exposure to tobacco smoke in the perinatal period (P96.81)
         history of tobacco dependence (Z87.891)
         occupational exposure to environmental tobacco smoke (Z57.31)
         tobacco dependence (F17.-)
         tobacco use (Z72.0)
     EXCLUDES 1   *congenital laryngeal stridor (P28.89)*
                obstructive laryngitis (acute) (J05.0)
                postprocedural subglottic stenosis (J95.5)
                stridor (R06.1)
                ulcerative laryngitis (J04.0)

    ✓5th **J38.0** **Paralysis of vocal cords and larynx**
         Laryngoplegia
         Paralysis of glottis

       J38.00 **Paralysis of vocal cords and larynx, unspecified**
       J38.01 **Paralysis of vocal cords and larynx, unilateral**
       J38.02 **Paralysis of vocal cords and larynx, bilateral**

    J38.1 **Polyp of vocal cord and larynx**
         EXCLUDES 1   *adenomatous polyps (D14.1)*

    J38.2 **Nodules of vocal cords**
         Chorditis (fibrinous)(nodosa)(tuberosa)
         Singer's nodes
         Teacher's nodes

    J38.3 **Other diseases of vocal cords**
         Abscess of vocal cords
         Cellulitis of vocal cords
         Granuloma of vocal cords
         Leukokeratosis of vocal cords
         Leukoplakia of vocal cords

    J38.4 **Edema of larynx**
         Edema (of) glottis
         Subglottic edema
         Supraglottic edema
         EXCLUDES 1   *acute obstructive laryngitis [croup] (J05.0)*
                edematous laryngitis (J04.0)

    J38.5 **Laryngeal spasm**
         Laryngismus (stridulus)

    J38.6 **Stenosis of larynx**

    J38.7 **Other diseases of larynx**
         Abscess of larynx
         Cellulitis of larynx
         Disease of larynx NOS
         Necrosis of larynx
         Pachyderma of larynx
         Perichondritis of larynx
         Ulcer of larynx

✓4th **J39** **Other diseases of upper respiratory tract**
     EXCLUDES 1   *acute respiratory infection NOS (J22)*
                acute upper respiratory infection (J06.9)
                upper respiratory inflammation due to chemicals, gases, fumes
                  or vapors (J68.2)

    J39.0 **Retropharyngeal and parapharyngeal abscess**   CC
         Peripharyngeal abscess
         EXCLUDES 1   *peritonsillar abscess (J36)*
         DEF: Purulent infection behind pharynx and front of precerebral fascia; characterized by neck stiffness, cervical lymphadenopathy, sore throat, fever, and stridor.
         CC Excl: PDX collection 740

    J39.1 **Other abscess of pharynx**   CC
         Cellulitis of pharynx
         Nasopharyngeal abscess
         CC Excl: PDX collection 740

    J39.2 **Other diseases of pharynx**
         Cyst of pharynx
         Edema of pharynx
         EXCLUDES 2   *chronic pharyngitis (J31.2)*
                ulcerative pharyngitis (J02.9)

    J39.3 **Upper respiratory tract hypersensitivity reaction, site unspecified**
         EXCLUDES 1   *hypersensitivity reaction of upper respiratory tract,*
                  such as:
                     extrinsic allergic alveolitis (J67.9)
                     pneumoconiosis (J60-J67.9)

    J39.8 **Other specified diseases of upper respiratory tract**

    J39.9 **Disease of upper respiratory tract, unspecified**

Chronic lower respiratory diseases (J40-J47)

    EXCLUDES 1   *bronchitis due to chemicals, gases, fumes and vapors (J68.0)*
    EXCLUDES 2   *cystic fibrosis (E84.-)*

J40 **Bronchitis, not specified as acute or chronic**
     Bronchitis NOS
     Bronchitis with tracheitis NOS
     Catarrhal bronchitis
     Tracheobronchitis NOS
     Use additional code to identify:
         exposure to environmental tobacco smoke (Z77.22)
         exposure to tobacco smoke in the perinatal period (P96.81)
         history of tobacco dependence (Z87.891)
         occupational exposure to environmental tobacco smoke (Z57.31)
         tobacco dependence (F17.-)
         tobacco use (Z72.0)
     EXCLUDES 1   *acute bronchitis (J20.-)*
                allergic bronchitis NOS (J45.909)
                asthmatic bronchitis NOS (J45.9-)
                bronchitis due to chemicals, gases, fumes and vapors (J68.0)

✓4th **J41** **Simple and mucopurulent chronic bronchitis**
     Use additional code to identify:
         exposure to environmental tobacco smoke (Z77.22)
         exposure to tobacco smoke in the perinatal period (P96.81)
         history of tobacco dependence (Z87.891)
         occupational exposure to environmental tobacco smoke (Z57.31)
         tobacco dependence (F17.-)
         tobacco use (Z72.0)
     EXCLUDES 1   *chronic bronchitis NOS (J42)*
                chronic obstructive bronchitis (J44.-)

    J41.0 **Simple chronic bronchitis**   HCC
    J41.1 **Mucopurulent chronic bronchitis**   HCC
    J41.8 **Mixed simple and mucopurulent chronic bronchitis**   HCC

J42 **Unspecified chronic bronchitis**   HCC
     Chronic bronchitis NOS
     Chronic tracheitis
     Chronic tracheobronchitis
     Use additional code to identify:
         exposure to environmental tobacco smoke (Z77.22)
         exposure to tobacco smoke in the perinatal period (P96.81)
         history of tobacco dependence (Z87.891)
         occupational exposure to environmental tobacco smoke (Z57.31)
         tobacco dependence (F17.-)
         tobacco use (Z72.0)
     EXCLUDES 1   *chronic asthmatic bronchitis (J44.-)*
                chronic bronchitis with airways obstruction (J44.-)
                chronic emphysematous bronchitis (J44.-)
                chronic obstructive pulmonary disease NOS (J44.9)
                simple and mucopurulent chronic bronchitis (J41.-)

N Newborn: 0   P Pediatric: 0-17   M Maternity: 12-55   A Adult: 15-124   MCC Major CC Condition   PDxMCC PDx acts as own MCC   CC CC Condition   PDxCC PDx acts as own CC

676   ICD-10-CM 2018

J36–J42

Emphysema

Healthy alveoli   Alveoli w/ Emphysema

Patent bronchiole

Collapsed bronchiole

Well-vascularized

Dilated alveoli

Excess mucus

Alveolar membranes break down

Enlarged alveoli

Broken/ fewer capillaries

☑4ᵗʰ **J43** **Emphysema**

Use additional code to identify:
    exposure to environmental tobacco smoke (Z77.22)
    history of tobacco dependence (Z87.891)
    occupational exposure to environmental tobacco smoke (Z57.31)
    tobacco dependence (F17.-)
    tobacco use (Z72.0)

EXCLUDES 1 compensatory emphysema (J98.3)
    emphysema due to inhalation of chemicals, gases, fumes or
        vapors (J68.4)
    emphysema with chronic (obstructive) bronchitis (J44.-)
    emphysematous (obstructive) bronchitis (J44.-)
    interstitial emphysema (J98.2)
    mediastinal emphysema (J98.2)
    neonatal interstitial emphysema (P25.0)
    surgical (subcutaneous) emphysema (T81.82)
    traumatic subcutaneous emphysema (T79.7)

J43.0 **Unilateral pulmonary emphysema [MacLeod's syndrome]** ᴴᶜᶜ
    Swyer-James syndrome
    Unilateral emphysema
    Unilateral hyperlucent lung
    Unilateral pulmonary artery functional hypoplasia
    Unilateral transparency of lung

J43.1 **Panlobular emphysema**   ᴴᶜᶜ
    Panacinar emphysema

J43.2 **Centrilobular emphysema**   ᴴᶜᶜ

J43.8 **Other emphysema**   ᴴᶜᶜ

J43.9 **Emphysema, unspecified**   ᴴᶜᶜ
    Bullous emphysema (lung)(pulmonary)
    Emphysema (lung)(pulmonary) NOS
    Emphysematous bleb
    Vesicular emphysema (lung)(pulmonary)

☑4ᵗʰ **J44** **Other chronic obstructive pulmonary disease**
    INCLUDES asthma with chronic obstructive pulmonary disease
        chronic asthmatic (obstructive) bronchitis
        chronic bronchitis with airways obstruction
        chronic bronchitis with emphysema
        chronic emphysematous bronchitis
        chronic obstructive asthma
        chronic obstructive bronchitis
        chronic obstructive tracheobronchitis

Code also type of asthma, if applicable (J45.-)
Use additional code to identify:
    exposure to environmental tobacco smoke (Z77.22)
    history of tobacco dependence (Z87.891)
    occupational exposure to environmental tobacco smoke (Z57.31)
    tobacco dependence (F17.-)
    tobacco use (Z72.0)

EXCLUDES 1 bronchiectasis (J47.-)
    chronic bronchitis NOS (J42)
    chronic simple and mucopurulent bronchitis (J41.-)
    chronic tracheitis (J42)
    chronic tracheobronchitis (J42)
    emphysema without chronic bronchitis (J43.-)

EXCLUDES 2 ~~lung diseases due to external agents (J60–J70)~~
AHA: 2017, 1Q, 25-26; 2016, 3Q, 15-16; 2013, 4Q, 109

J44.0 **Chronic obstructive pulmonary disease with acute** ᶜᶜ ᴴᶜᶜ
    lower respiratory infection
    ►Code also to identify the infection◄
    ~~Use additional code to identify the infection~~
    AHA: 2017, 1Q, 24-25
    CC Excl: PDX collection 741

J44.1 **Chronic obstructive pulmonary disease with (acute)** ᶜᶜ ᴴᶜᶜ
    exacerbation
    Decompensated COPD
    Decompensated COPD with (acute) exacerbation
    EXCLUDES 2 chronic obstructive pulmonary disease [COPD] with
        acute bronchitis (J44.0)
        ►lung diseases due to external agents (J60-J70)◄
    AHA: 2017, 1Q, 26; 2016, 1Q, 36
    CC Excl: PDX collection 741

J44.9 **Chronic obstructive pulmonary disease, unspecified** ᴴᶜᶜ
    Chronic obstructive airway disease NOS
    Chronic obstructive lung disease NOS
    EXCLUDES 2 ►lung diseases due to external agents (J60-J70)◄
    AHA: 2016, 1Q, 36; 2014, 4Q, 21; 2013, 4Q, 109

☑4ᵗʰ **J45** **Asthma**
    INCLUDES   allergic (predominantly) asthma
        allergic bronchitis NOS
        allergic rhinitis with asthma
        atopic asthma
        extrinsic allergic asthma
        hay fever with asthma
        idiosyncratic asthma
        intrinsic nonallergic asthma
        nonallergic asthma

Use additional code to identify:
    exposure to environmental tobacco smoke (Z77.22)
    exposure to tobacco smoke in the perinatal period (P96.81)
    history of tobacco dependence (Z87.891)
    occupational exposure to environmental tobacco smoke (Z57.31)
    tobacco dependence (F17.-)
    tobacco use (Z72.0)

EXCLUDES 1 detergent asthma (J69.8)
    eosinophilic asthma (J82)
    ~~lung diseases due to external agents (J60-J70)~~
    miner's asthma (J60)
    wheezing NOS (R06.2)
    wood asthma (J67.8)

EXCLUDES 2 asthma with chronic obstructive pulmonary disease (J44.9)
    chronic asthmatic (obstructive) bronchitis (J44.9)
    chronic obstructive asthma (J44.9)

AHA: 2017, 1Q, 25-26; 2012, 4Q, 99
DEF: Status asthmaticus: Severe, intractable episode of asthma that is
unresponsive to normal therapeutic measures.

CC Excl: For CC codes in category J45: PDX collection 742

☑5ᵗʰ **J45.2** **Mild intermittent asthma**

J45.20 **Mild intermittent asthma, uncomplicated**
    Mild intermittent asthma NOS

J45.21 **Mild intermittent asthma with (acute)** ᶜᶜ
    exacerbation

J45.22 **Mild intermittent asthma with status** ᶜᶜ
    asthmaticus

☑5ᵗʰ **J45.3** **Mild persistent asthma**

J45.30 **Mild persistent asthma, uncomplicated**
    Mild persistent asthma NOS

J45.31 **Mild persistent asthma with (acute) exacerbation** ᶜᶜ
    AHA: 2016, 1Q, 35

J45.32 **Mild persistent asthma with status asthmaticus** ᶜᶜ

☑5ᵗʰ **J45.4** **Moderate persistent asthma**

J45.40 **Moderate persistent asthma, uncomplicated**
    Moderate persistent asthma NOS

J45.41 **Moderate persistent asthma with (acute)** ᶜᶜ
    exacerbation
    AHA: 2017, 1Q, 26

J45.42 **Moderate persistent asthma with status** ᶜᶜ
    asthmaticus

☑5ᵗʰ **J45.5** **Severe persistent asthma**

J45.50 **Severe persistent asthma, uncomplicated**
    Severe persistent asthma NOS

J45.51 **Severe persistent asthma with (acute)** ᶜᶜ
    exacerbation

J45.52 **Severe persistent asthma with status** ᶜᶜ
    asthmaticus

Asthma

Smooth muscle fibres

Contraction of smooth muscle fibres

Respiratory bronchiole

Mucus lining bronchial tubes

Alveoli

Extra mucus secretion in inflamed bronchial tubes

Air trapped within alveoli

Normal alveoli　　　　Asthmatic alveoli

☑5ᵗʰ **J45.9** **Other and unspecified asthma**

☑6ᵗʰ **J45.90** **Unspecified asthma**
Asthmatic bronchitis NOS
Childhood asthma NOS
Late onset asthma

J45.901 **Unspecified asthma with (acute) exacerbation** `CC`

J45.902 **Unspecified asthma with status asthmaticus** `CC`

J45.909 **Unspecified asthma, uncomplicated**
Asthma NOS
EXCLUDES 2 ▶*lung diseases due to external agents (J60-J70)*◀
AHA: 2017, 1Q, 25

☑6ᵗʰ **J45.99** **Other asthma**
J45.990 **Exercise induced bronchospasm**
J45.991 **Cough variant asthma**
J45.998 **Other asthma**

☑4ᵗʰ **J47** **Bronchiectasis**
INCLUDES bronchiolectasis
Use additional code to identify:
exposure to environmental tobacco smoke (Z77.22)
exposure to tobacco smoke in the perinatal period (P96.81)
history of tobacco dependence (Z87.891)
occupational exposure to environmental tobacco smoke (Z57.31)
tobacco dependence (F17.-)
tobacco use (Z72.0)
EXCLUDES 1 congenital bronchiectasis (Q33.4)
tuberculous bronchiectasis (current disease) (A15.0)

J47.0 **Bronchiectasis with acute lower respiratory infection** `CC` `HCC`
Bronchiectasis with acute bronchitis
Use additional code to identify the infection
CC Excl: PDX collection 743

J47.1 **Bronchiectasis with (acute) exacerbation** `CC` `HCC`
CC Excl: PDX collection 743

J47.9 **Bronchiectasis, uncomplicated** `HCC`
Bronchiectasis NOS

Lung diseases due to external agents (J60-J70)
EXCLUDES 2 asthma (J45.-)
malignant neoplasm of bronchus and lung (C34.-)

J60 **Coalworker's pneumoconiosis** `A` `HCC`
Anthracosilicosis
Anthracosis
Black lung disease
Coalworker's lung
EXCLUDES 1 coalworker pneumoconiosis with tuberculosis, any type in A15 (J65)

J61 **Pneumoconiosis due to asbestos and other mineral fibers** `A` `HCC`
Asbestosis
EXCLUDES 1 pleural plaque with asbestosis (J92.0)
pneumoconiosis with tuberculosis, any type in A15 (J65)

☑4ᵗʰ **J62** **Pneumoconiosis due to dust containing silica**
INCLUDES silicotic fibrosis (massive) of lung
EXCLUDES 1 pneumoconiosis with tuberculosis, any type in A15 (J65)

J62.0 **Pneumoconiosis due to talc dust** `HCC`
J62.8 **Pneumoconiosis due to other dust containing silica** `HCC`
Silicosis NOS

☑4ᵗʰ **J63** **Pneumoconiosis due to other inorganic dusts**
EXCLUDES 1 pneumoconiosis with tuberculosis, any type in A15 (J65)

J63.0 **Aluminosis (of lung)** `HCC`
J63.1 **Bauxite fibrosis (of lung)** `HCC`
J63.2 **Berylliosis** `HCC`
J63.3 **Graphite fibrosis (of lung)** `HCC`
J63.4 **Siderosis** `HCC`
J63.5 **Stannosis** `HCC`
J63.6 **Pneumoconiosis due to other specified inorganic dusts** `HCC`

J64 **Unspecified pneumoconiosis** `HCC`
EXCLUDES 1 pneumonoconiosis with tuberculosis, any type in A15 (J65)

J65 **Pneumoconiosis associated with tuberculosis** `HCC`
Any condition in J60-J64 with tuberculosis, any type in A15
Silicotuberculosis

☑4ᵗʰ **J66** **Airway disease due to specific organic dust**
EXCLUDES 2 allergic alveolitis (J67.-)
asbestosis (J61)
bagassosis (J67.1)
farmer's lung (J67.0)
hypersensitivity pneumonitis due to organic dust (J67.-)
reactive airways dysfunction syndrome (J68.3)

J66.0 **Byssinosis** `HCC`
Airway disease due to cotton dust
J66.1 **Flax-dressers' disease** `HCC`
J66.2 **Cannabinosis** `HCC`
J66.8 **Airway disease due to other specific organic dusts** `HCC`

☑4ᵗʰ **J67** **Hypersensitivity pneumonitis due to organic dust**
INCLUDES allergic alveolitis and pneumonitis due to inhaled organic dust and particles of fungal, actinomycetic or other origin
EXCLUDES 1 pneumonitis due to inhalation of chemicals, gases, fumes or vapors (J68.0)

CC Excl: For CC codes in category J67, unless otherwise noted:
PDX collection 110

J67.0 **Farmer's lung** `HCC`
Harvester's lung
Haymaker's lung
Moldy hay disease

J67.1 **Bagassosis** `HCC`
Bagasse disease
Bagasse pneumonitis

J67.2 **Bird fancier's lung** `HCC`
Budgerigar fancier's disease or lung
Pigeon fancier's disease or lung

J67.3 **Suberosis** `HCC`
Corkhandler's disease or lung
Corkworker's disease or lung

J67.4 **Maltworker's lung** `HCC`
Alveolitis due to Aspergillus clavatus

J67.5 **Mushroom-worker's lung** `HCC`

J67.6 **Maple-bark-stripper's lung** `HCC`
Alveolitis due to Cryptostroma corticale
Cryptostromosis

J67.7 **Air conditioner and humidifier lung** `CC` `HCC`
Allergic alveolitis due to fungal, thermophilic actinomycetes and other organisms growing in ventilation [air conditioning] systems

J67.8 **Hypersensitivity pneumonitis due to other organic dusts** `CC` `HCC`
Cheese-washer's lung
Coffee-worker's lung
Fish-meal worker's lung
Furrier's lung
Sequoiosis

J67.9 **Hypersensitivity pneumonitis due to unspecified organic dust** `CC` `HCC`
Allergic alveolitis (extrinsic) NOS
Hypersensitivity pneumonitis NOS

N Newborn: 0　　P Pediatric: 0-17　　M Maternity: 12-55　　A Adult: 15-124　　MCC Major CC Condition　　PDxMCC PDx acts as own MCC　　CC CC Condition　　PDxCC PDx acts as own CC

678　　　　　　　　　　　　　　　　　　　　　　　　　　　　　　ICD-10-CM 2018

✓4ᵗʰ **J68**   **Respiratory conditions due to inhalation of chemicals, gases, fumes and vapors**

Code first (T51-T65) to identify cause
Use additional code to identify associated respiratory conditions, such as:
   acute respiratory failure (J96.0-)

> **CC Excl: For CC/MCC codes in category J68:** PDX collection 110

J68.0   **Bronchitis and pneumonitis due to chemicals, gases, fumes and vapors**   `CC` `HCC`
   Chemical bronchitis (acute)

J68.1   **Pulmonary edema due to chemicals, gases, fumes and vapors**   `MCC` `HCC`
   Chemical pulmonary edema (acute) (chronic)
   EXCLUDES 1   *pulmonary edema (acute) (chronic) NOS (J81.-)*

J68.2   **Upper respiratory inflammation due to chemicals, gases, fumes and vapors, not elsewhere classified**   `HCC`

J68.3   **Other acute and subacute respiratory conditions due to chemicals, gases, fumes and vapors**   `HCC`
   Reactive airways dysfunction syndrome

J68.4   **Chronic respiratory conditions due to chemicals, gases, fumes and vapors**   `HCC`
   Emphysema (diffuse) (chronic) due to inhalation of chemicals, gases, fumes and vapors
   Obliterative bronchiolitis (chronic) (subacute) due to inhalation of chemicals, gases, fumes and vapors
   Pulmonary fibrosis (chronic) due to inhalation of chemicals, gases, fumes and vapors
   EXCLUDES 1   *chronic pulmonary edema due to chemicals, gases, fumes and vapors (J68.1)*

J68.8   **Other respiratory conditions due to chemicals, gases, fumes and vapors**   `HCC`

J68.9   **Unspecified respiratory condition due to chemicals, gases, fumes and vapors**   `HCC`

✓4ᵗʰ **J69**   **Pneumonitis due to solids and liquids**

   EXCLUDES 1   *neonatal aspiration syndromes (P24.-)*
           postprocedural pneumonitis (J95.4)
   AHA: 2017, 1Q, 24

> **CC Excl: For MCC codes in category J69:** PDX collection 110

J69.0   **Pneumonitis due to inhalation of food and vomit**   `MCC` `HCC`
   Aspiration pneumonia NOS
   Aspiration pneumonia (due to) food (regurgitated)
   Aspiration pneumonia (due to) gastric secretions
   Aspiration pneumonia (due to) milk
   Aspiration pneumonia (due to) vomit
   Code also any associated foreign body in respiratory tract (T17.-)
   EXCLUDES 1   *chemical pneumonitis due to anesthesia (J95.4)*
           obstetric aspiration pneumonia (O74.0)

J69.1   **Pneumonitis due to inhalation of oils and essences**   `MCC` `HCC`
   Exogenous lipoid pneumonia
   Lipid pneumonia NOS
   Code first (T51-T65) to identify substance
   EXCLUDES 1   *endogenous lipoid pneumonia (J84.89)*

J69.8   **Pneumonitis due to inhalation of other solids and liquids**   `MCC` `HCC`
   Pneumonitis due to aspiration of blood
   Pneumonitis due to aspiration of detergent
   Code first (T51-T65) to identify substance

✓4ᵗʰ **J70**   **Respiratory conditions due to other external agents**

> **CC Excl: For CC codes in category J70:** PDX collection 110

J70.0   **Acute pulmonary manifestations due to radiation**   `CC` `HCC`
   Radiation pneumonitis
   Use additional code (W88-W90, X39.0-) to identify the external cause

J70.1   **Chronic and other pulmonary manifestations due to radiation**   `CC` `HCC`
   Fibrosis of lung following radiation
   Use additional code (W88-W90, X39.0-) to identify the external cause

J70.2   **Acute drug-induced interstitial lung disorders**   `HCC`
   Use additional code for adverse effect, if applicable, to identify drug (T36-T50 with fifth or sixth character 5)
   EXCLUDES 1   *interstitial pneumonia NOS (J84.9)*
           lymphoid interstitial pneumonia (J84.2)

J70.3   **Chronic drug-induced interstitial lung disorders**   `HCC`
   Use additional code for adverse effect, if applicable, to identify drug (T36-T50 with fifth or sixth character 5)
   EXCLUDES 1   *interstitial pneumonia NOS (J84.9)*
           lymphoid interstitial pneumonia (J84.2)

J70.4   **Drug-induced interstitial lung disorders, unspecified**   `HCC`
   Use additional code for adverse effect, if applicable, to identify drug (T36-T50 with fifth or sixth character 5)
   EXCLUDES 1   *interstitial pneumonia NOS (J84.9)*
           lymphoid interstitial pneumonia (J84.2)

J70.5   **Respiratory conditions due to smoke inhalation**   `HCC`
   Smoke inhalation NOS
   EXCLUDES 1   *smoke inhalation due to chemicals, gases, fumes and vapors (J68.9)*
   AHA: 2013, 4Q, 121

J70.8   **Respiratory conditions due to other specified external agents**   `HCC`
   Code first (T51-T65) to identify the external agent

J70.9   **Respiratory conditions due to unspecified external agent**   `HCC`
   Code first (T51-T65) to identify the external agent

Other respiratory diseases principally affecting the interstitium (J80-J84)

J80   **Acute respiratory distress syndrome**   `CC` `HCC`
   Acute respiratory distress syndrome in adult or child
   Adult hyaline membrane disease
   EXCLUDES 1   *respiratory distress syndrome in newborn (perinatal) (P22.0)*
   AHA: 2017, 1Q, 26
   CC Excl: PDX collection 744

✓4ᵗʰ **J81**   **Pulmonary edema**
   Use additional code to identify:
      exposure to environmental tobacco smoke (Z77.22)
      history of tobacco dependence (Z87.891)
      occupational exposure to environmental tobacco smoke (Z57.31)
      tobacco dependence (F17.-)
      tobacco use (Z72.0)
   EXCLUDES 1   *chemical (acute) pulmonary edema (J68.1)*
           hypostatic pneumonia (J18.2)
           passive pneumonia (J18.2)
           pulmonary edema due to external agents (J60-J70)
           pulmonary edema with heart disease NOS (I50.1)
           pulmonary edema with heart failure (I50.1)

J81.0   **Acute pulmonary edema**   `MCC` `HCC`
   Acute edema of lung
   CC Excl: PDX collection 745

J81.1   **Chronic pulmonary edema**   `CC`
   Pulmonary congestion (chronic) (passive)
   Pulmonary edema NOS
   CC Excl: PDX collection 736

J82   **Pulmonary eosinophilia, not elsewhere classified**   `CC` `HCC`
   Allergic pneumonia
   Eosinophilic asthma
   Eosinophilic pneumonia
   Löffler's pneumonia
   Tropical (pulmonary) eosinophilia NOS
   EXCLUDES 1   *pulmonary eosinophilia due to aspergillosis (B44.-)*
           pulmonary eosinophilia due to drugs (J70.2-J70.4)
           pulmonary eosinophilia due to specified parasitic infection (B50-B83)
           pulmonary eosinophilia due to systemic connective tissue disorders (M30-M36)
           pulmonary infiltrate NOS (R91.8)
   CC Excl: PDX collection 746

✓4ᵗʰ **J84**   **Other interstitial pulmonary diseases**
   EXCLUDES 1   *drug-induced interstitial lung disorders (J70.2-J70.4)*
           interstitial emphysema (J98.2)
           ~~*lung diseases due to external agents (J60-J70)*~~
   EXCLUDES 2   ▶*lung diseases due to external agents (J60-J70)*◀

✓5ᵗʰ **J84.0**   **Alveolar and parieto-alveolar conditions**

> **CC Excl: For CC codes in subcategory J84.0:** PDX collection 747

J84.01   **Alveolar proteinosis**   `CC` `HCC`
   DEF: Reduced ventilation due to proteinaceous deposits on alveoli; symptoms include dyspnea, cough, chest pain, weakness, weight loss, and hemoptysis.

J84.02   **Pulmonary alveolar microlithiasis**   `CC` `HCC`

☑ Additional Character Req   ✓ₓ7ᵗʰ Placeholder Alert   Unacceptable PDx   Manifestation   `H1`-`H14` HAC   `HCC` CMS-HCC Condition   *EXCLUDES 1* Not Coded Here   *EXCLUDES 2* Not Included Here

Chapter 10. Diseases of the Respiratory System

J84.03   *Idiopathic pulmonary hemosiderosis*   `CC` `HCC`
Essential brown induration of lung
Code first underlying disease, such as:
  disorders of iron metabolism (E83.1-)
  EXCLUDES 1   *acute idiopathic pulmonary hemorrhage in infants [AIPHI] (R04.81)*
DEF: Fibrosis of alveolar walls; marked by abnormal accumulation of iron as hemosiderin in lungs; primarily affects children; symptoms include anemia, fluid in lungs, and blood in sputum; etiology unknown.

J84.09   **Other alveolar and parieto-alveolar conditions**   `CC` `HCC`

✓5ᵗʰ **J84.1**   **Other interstitial pulmonary diseases with fibrosis**
  EXCLUDES 1   *pulmonary fibrosis (chronic) due to inhalation of chemicals, gases, fumes or vapors (J68.4)*
    pulmonary fibrosis (chronic) following radiation (J70.1)

CC Excl: For CC codes in subcategory J84.1: PDX collection 747

J84.10   **Pulmonary fibrosis, unspecified**   `HCC`
Capillary fibrosis of lung
Cirrhosis of lung (chronic) NOS
Fibrosis of lung (atrophic) (chronic) (confluent) (massive) (perialveolar) (peribronchial) NOS
Induration of lung (chronic) NOS
Postinflammatory pulmonary fibrosis

✓6ᵗʰ **J84.11**   **Idiopathic interstitial pneumonia**
  EXCLUDES 1   *lymphoid interstitial pneumonia (J84.2)*
    pneumocystis pneumonia (B59)

  J84.111   **Idiopathic interstitial pneumonia, not otherwise specified**   `HCC`

  J84.112   **Idiopathic pulmonary fibrosis**   `HCC`
    Cryptogenic fibrosing alveolitis
    Idiopathic fibrosing alveolitis

  J84.113   **Idiopathic non-specific interstitial pneumonitis**   `HCC`
    EXCLUDES 1   *non-specific interstitial pneumonia NOS, or due to known underlying cause (J84.89)*

  J84.114   **Acute interstitial pneumonitis**   `CC` `HCC`
    Hamman-Rich syndrome
    EXCLUDES 1   *pneumocystis pneumonia (B59)*

  J84.115   **Respiratory bronchiolitis interstitial lung disease**   `HCC`

  J84.116   **Cryptogenic organizing pneumonia**   `CC` `HCC`
    EXCLUDES 1   *organizing pneumonia NOS, or due to known underlying cause (J84.89)*

  J84.117   **Desquamative interstitial pneumonia**   `CC` `HCC`

J84.17   *Other interstitial pulmonary diseases with fibrosis in diseases classified elsewhere*   `HCC`
Interstitial pneumonia (nonspecific) (usual) due to collagen vascular disease
Interstitial pneumonia (nonspecific) (usual) in diseases classified elsewhere
Organizing pneumonia due to collagen vascular disease
Organizing pneumonia in diseases classified elsewhere
Code first underlying disease, such as:
  progressive systemic sclerosis (M34.0)
  rheumatoid arthritis (M05.00-M06.9)
  systemic lupus erythematosis (M32.0-M32.9)

J84.2   **Lymphoid interstitial pneumonia**   `CC` `HCC`
Lymphoid interstitial pneumonitis
CC Excl: PDX collection 747

✓5ᵗʰ **J84.8**   **Other specified interstitial pulmonary diseases**
  EXCLUDES 1   *exogenous lipoid pneumonia (J69.1)*
    unspecified lipoid pneumonia (J69.1)

J84.81   **Lymphangioleiomyomatosis**   `MCC` `HCC`
Lymphangiomyomatosis
CC Excl: PDX collection 747

J84.82   **Adult pulmonary Langerhans cell histiocytosis**   `CC` `HCC` `A`
Adult PLCH
CC Excl: PDX collection 747

J84.83   **Surfactant mutations of the lung**   `MCC` `HCC`
DEF: Genetic disorder resulting in insufficient secretion of a complex mixture of phospholipids and proteins that reduce surface tension in the alveoli following the onset of breathing to facilitate lung expansion in the newborn; leading indication for pediatric lung transplantation.
CC Excl: PDX collection 748

✓6ᵗʰ **J84.84**   **Other interstitial lung diseases of childhood**

CC Excl: For MCC codes in subcategory J84.84, unless otherwise noted: PDX collection 748

  J84.841   **Neuroendocrine cell hyperplasia of infancy**   `MCC` `HCC`

  J84.842   **Pulmonary interstitial glycogenosis**   `MCC` `HCC`

  J84.843   **Alveolar capillary dysplasia with vein misalignment**   `MCC` `HCC`

  J84.848   **Other interstitial lung diseases of childhood**   `MCC` `HCC`

J84.89   **Other specified interstitial pulmonary diseases**   `HCC`
Endogenous lipoid pneumonia
Interstitial pneumonitis
Non-specific interstitial pneumonitis NOS
Organizing pneumonia NOS
Code first, if applicable:
  poisoning due to drug or toxin (T51-T65 with fifth or sixth character to indicate intent), for toxic pneumonopathy
  underlying cause of pneumonopathy, if known
Use additional code, for adverse effect, to identify drug (T36-T50 with fifth or sixth character 5), if drug-induced
  EXCLUDES 1   *cryptogenic organizing pneumonia (J84.116)*
    idiopathic non-specific interstitial pneumonitis (J84.113)
    lipoid pneumonia, exogenous or unspecified (J69.1)
    lymphoid interstitial pneumonia (J84.2)

J84.9   **Interstitial pulmonary disease, unspecified**   `CC` `HCC`
Interstitial pneumonia NOS
CC Excl: PDX collection 747

Suppurative and necrotic conditions of the lower respiratory tract (J85-J86)

✓4ᵗʰ **J85**   **Abscess of lung and mediastinum**
Use additional code (B95-B97) to identify infectious agent

CC Excl: For MCC codes in category J85, unless otherwise noted: PDX collection 749

J85.0   **Gangrene and necrosis of lung**   `MCC` `HCC`

J85.1   **Abscess of lung with pneumonia**   `MCC` `HCC`
Code also the type of pneumonia

J85.2   **Abscess of lung without pneumonia**   `MCC` `HCC`
Abscess of lung NOS

J85.3   **Abscess of mediastinum**   `MCC` `HCC`
CC Excl: PDX collection 750

✓4ᵗʰ **J86**   **Pyothorax**
Use additional code (B95-B97) to identify infectious agent
  EXCLUDES 1   *abscess of lung (J85.-)*
    pyothorax due to tuberculosis (A15.6)

J86.0   **Pyothorax with fistula**   `MCC` `HCC`
Bronchocutaneous fistula
Bronchopleural fistula
Hepatopleural fistula
Mediastinal fistula
Pleural fistula
Thoracic fistula
Any condition classifiable to J86.9 with fistula
DEF: Purulent infection of respiratory cavity, with communication from cavity to another structure.
CC Excl: PDX collection 751

J86.9   **Pyothorax without fistula**   `MCC` `HCC`
Abscess of pleura
Abscess of thorax
Empyema (chest) (lung) (pleura)
Fibrinopurulent pleurisy
Purulent pleurisy
Pyopneumothorax
Septic pleurisy
Seropurulent pleurisy
Suppurative pleurisy
CC Excl: PDX collection 751

`N` Newborn: 0   `P` Pediatric: 0-17   `M` Maternity: 12-55   `A` Adult: 15-124   `MCC` Major CC Condition   `PDxMCC` PDx acts as own MCC   `CC` CC Condition   `PDxCC` PDx acts as own CC

680   ICD-10-CM 2018

Pleural Effusion

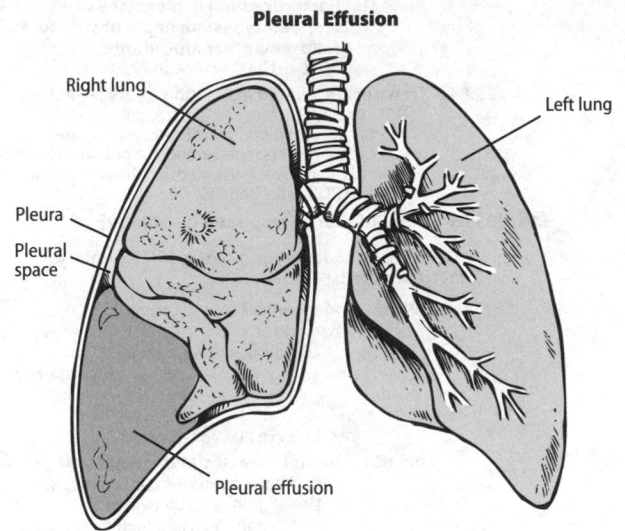

Right lung

Left lung

Pleura

Pleural space

Pleural effusion

Other diseases of the pleura (J90-J94)

J90   Pleural effusion, not elsewhere classified   `CC`
Encysted pleurisy
Pleural effusion NOS
Pleurisy with effusion (exudative) (serous)
> `EXCLUDES 1`   chylous (pleural) effusion (J94.0)
>   malignant pleural effusion (J91.0))
>   pleurisy NOS (R09.1)
>   tuberculous pleural effusion (A15.6)
CC Excl: PDX collection 752

✓4ᵗʰ J91   Pleural effusion in conditions classified elsewhere
> `EXCLUDES 2`   pleural effusion in heart failure (I50.-)
>   pleural effusion in systemic lupus erythematosus (M32.13)

   J91.0   *Malignant pleural effusion*   `CC`
     Code first underlying neoplasm
     CC Excl: PDX collection 753

   J91.8   *Pleural effusion in other conditions classified elsewhere*   `CC`
     Code first underlying disease, such as:
       filariasis (B74.0-B74.9)
       influenza (J09.X2, J10.1, J11.1)
     AHA: 2015, 2Q, 15
     CC Excl: PDX collection 752

✓4ᵗʰ J92   Pleural plaque
> `INCLUDES`   pleural thickening

   J92.0   Pleural plaque with presence of asbestos

   J92.9   Pleural plaque without asbestos
     Pleural plaque NOS

✓4ᵗʰ J93   Pneumothorax and air leak
> `EXCLUDES 1`   congenital or perinatal pneumothorax (P25.1)
>   postprocedural air leak (J95.812)
>   postprocedural pneumothorax (J95.811)
>   traumatic pneumothorax (S27.0)
>   tuberculous (current disease) pneumothorax (A15.-)
>   pyopneumothorax (J86.-)

   CC Excl: For CC/MCC codes in category J93: PDX collection 754

   J93.0   Spontaneous tension pneumothorax   `MCC`
     DEF: Leaking air from lung into lining, causing collapse.

   ✓5ᵗʰ J93.1   Other spontaneous pneumothorax

     J93.11   Primary spontaneous pneumothorax   `CC`

     J93.12   Secondary spontaneous pneumothorax   `CC`
       Code first underlying condition, such as:
         catamenial pneumothorax due to endometriosis
           (N80.8)
         cystic fibrosis (E84.-)
         eosinophilic pneumonia (J82)
         lymphangioleiomyomatosis (J84.81)
         malignant neoplasm of bronchus and lung (C34.-)
         Marfan's syndrome (Q87.4)
         pneumonia due to Pneumocystis carinii (B59)
         secondary malignant neoplasm of lung (C78.0-)
         spontaneous rupture of the esophagus (K22.3)

   ✓5ᵗʰ J93.8   Other pneumothorax and air leak

     J93.81   Chronic pneumothorax   `CC`

     J93.82   Other air leak   `CC`
       Persistent air leak

     J93.83   Other pneumothorax   `CC`
       Acute pneumothorax
       Spontaneous pneumothorax NOS

   J93.9   Pneumothorax, unspecified   `CC`
     Pneumothorax NOS

✓4ᵗʰ J94   Other pleural conditions
> `EXCLUDES 1`   pleurisy NOS (R09.1)
>   traumatic hemopneumothorax (S27.2)
>   traumatic hemothorax (S27.1)
>   tuberculous pleural conditions (current disease) (A15.-)

   J94.0   Chylous effusion   `CC`
     Chyliform effusion
     CC Excl: PDX collection 752

   J94.1   Fibrothorax

   J94.2   Hemothorax   `CC`
     Hemopneumothorax
     CC Excl: PDX collection 752

   J94.8   Other specified pleural conditions   `CC`
     Hydropneumothorax
     Hydrothorax
     CC Excl: No excl

   J94.9   Pleural condition, unspecified

Intraoperative and postprocedural complications and disorders of respiratory system, not elsewhere classified (J95)

✓4ᵗʰ J95   Intraoperative and postprocedural complications and disorders of respiratory system, not elsewhere classified
> `EXCLUDES 2`   aspiration pneumonia (J69.-)
>   emphysema (subcutaneous) resulting from a procedure
>   (T81.82)
>   hypostatic pneumonia (J18.2)
>   pulmonary manifestations due to radiation (J70.0- J70.1)

   ✓5ᵗʰ J95.0   Tracheostomy complications

     CC Excl: For CC codes in subcategory J95.0, unless otherwise noted: PDX collection 755

     J95.00   Unspecified tracheostomy complication   `CC` `HCC`

     J95.01   Hemorrhage from tracheostomy stoma   `CC` `HCC`

     J95.02   Infection of tracheostomy stoma   `CC` `HCC`
       Use additional code to identify type of infection, such as:
         cellulitis of neck ▶(L03.221)◀
         sepsis (A40, A41-)

     J95.03   Malfunction of tracheostomy stoma   `CC` `HCC`
       Mechanical complication of tracheostomy stoma
       Obstruction of tracheostomy airway
       Tracheal stenosis due to tracheostomy

Tracheostomy

Tracheostomy in place

Incision in trachea

Trachea

Tracheostomy tube

Chapter 10. Diseases of the Respiratory System

J95.04   **Tracheo-esophageal fistula following tracheostomy** `CC` `HCC`

J95.09   **Other tracheostomy complication** `CC` `HCC`

J95.1   **Acute pulmonary insufficiency following thoracic surgery** `MCC` `HCC`
- *EXCLUDES 2*   functional disturbances following cardiac surgery (I97.0, I97.1-)
- CC Excl: PDX collection 756

J95.2   **Acute pulmonary insufficiency following nonthoracic surgery** `MCC` `HCC`
- *EXCLUDES 2*   functional disturbances following cardiac surgery (I97.0, I97.1-)
- CC Excl: PDX collection 756

J95.3   **Chronic pulmonary insufficiency following surgery** `MCC` `HCC`
- *EXCLUDES 2*   functional disturbances following cardiac surgery (I97.0, I97.1-)
- CC Excl: PDX collection 756

J95.4   **Chemical pneumonitis due to anesthesia** `CC`
- Mendelson's syndrome
- Postprocedural aspiration pneumonia
- Use additional code for adverse effect, if applicable, to identify drug (T41.- with fifth or sixth character 5)
- *EXCLUDES 1*   aspiration pneumonitis due to anesthesia complicating labor and delivery (O74.0)
  - aspiration pneumonitis due to anesthesia complicating pregnancy (O29)
  - aspiration pneumonitis due to anesthesia complicating the puerperium (O89.01)
- CC Excl: PDX collection 757

J95.5   **Postprocedural subglottic stenosis** `CC`
- CC Excl: PDX collection 757

√5th J95.6   **Intraoperative hemorrhage and hematoma of a respiratory system organ or structure complicating a procedure**
- *EXCLUDES 1*   intraoperative hemorrhage and hematoma of a respiratory system organ or structure due to accidental puncture and laceration during procedure (J95.7-)

J95.61   **Intraoperative hemorrhage and hematoma of a respiratory system organ or structure complicating a respiratory system procedure** `CC`
- CC Excl: PDX collection 758

J95.62   **Intraoperative hemorrhage and hematoma of a respiratory system organ or structure complicating other procedure** `CC`
- CC Excl: PDX collection 758

√5th J95.7   **Accidental puncture and laceration of a respiratory system organ or structure during a procedure**
- *EXCLUDES 2*   postprocedural pneumothorax (J95.811)

J95.71   **Accidental puncture and laceration of a respiratory system organ or structure during a respiratory system procedure** `CC`
- CC Excl: PDX collection 509

J95.72   **Accidental puncture and laceration of a respiratory system organ or structure during other procedure** `CC`
- CC Excl: PDX collection 509

√5th J95.8   **Other intraoperative and postprocedural complications and disorders of respiratory system, not elsewhere classified**

√6th J95.81   **Postprocedural pneumothorax and air leak**

J95.811   **Postprocedural pneumothorax** `CC` `H14`
- CC Excl: PDX collection 754

J95.812   **Postprocedural air leak** `CC`
- CC Excl: PDX collection 754

√6th J95.82   **Postprocedural respiratory failure**
- *EXCLUDES 1*   respiratory failure in other conditions (J96.-)

J95.821   **Acute postprocedural respiratory failure** `MCC` `HCC`
- Postprocedural respiratory failure NOS
- CC Excl: PDX collection 756

J95.822   **Acute and chronic postprocedural respiratory failure** `MCC` `HCC`
- CC Excl: PDX collection 756

√6th J95.83   **Postprocedural hemorrhage of a respiratory system organ or structure following a procedure**

J95.830   **Postprocedural hemorrhage of a respiratory system organ or structure following a respiratory system procedure** `CC`
- CC Excl: PDX collection 758

J95.831   **Postprocedural hemorrhage of a respiratory system organ or structure following other procedure** `CC`
- CC Excl: PDX collection 758

J95.84   **Transfusion-related acute lung injury (TRALI)** `CC`
- DEF: A relatively rare, but serious, pulmonary complication of blood transfusion, with acute respiratory distress, noncardiogenic pulmonary edema, cyanosis, hypoxemia, hypotension, fever, and chills.
- CC Excl: PDX collection 757

√6th J95.85   **Complication of respirator [ventilator]**

CC Excl: For CC codes in subcategory J95.85, unless otherwise noted: PDX collection 757

J95.850   **Mechanical complication of respirator** `CC` `HCC`
- *EXCLUDES 1*   encounter for respirator [ventilator] dependence during power failure (Z99.12)
- CC Excl: PDX collection 759

J95.851   **Ventilator associated pneumonia** `HCC`
- Ventilator associated pneumonitis
- Use additional code to identify the organism, if known (B95.-, B96.-, B97.-)
- *EXCLUDES 1*   ventilator lung in newborn (P27.8)
- AHA: 2017, 1Q, 25

J95.859   **Other complication of respirator [ventilator]** `CC` `HCC`

√6th J95.86   **Postprocedural hematoma and seroma of a respiratory system organ or structure following a procedure**

CC Excl: For CC codes in subcategory J95.86: PDX collection 758

J95.860   **Postprocedural hematoma of a respiratory system organ or structure following a respiratory system procedure** `CC`

J95.861   **Postprocedural hematoma of a respiratory system organ or structure following other procedure** `CC`

J95.862   **Postprocedural seroma of a respiratory system organ or structure following a respiratory system procedure** `CC`

J95.863   **Postprocedural seroma of a respiratory system organ or structure following other procedure** `CC`

J95.88   **Other intraoperative complications of respiratory system, not elsewhere classified** `CC`
- CC Excl: PDX collection 757

J95.89   **Other postprocedural complications and disorders of respiratory system, not elsewhere classified** `CC`
- Use additional code to identify disorder, such as:
  - aspiration pneumonia (J69.-)
  - bacterial or viral pneumonia (J12-J18)
- *EXCLUDES 2*   acute pulmonary insufficiency following thoracic surgery (J95.1)
  - postprocedural subglottic stenosis (J95.5)
- CC Excl: PDX collection 757

Other diseases of the respiratory system (J96-J99)

√4th J96   **Respiratory failure, not elsewhere classified**
- *EXCLUDES 1*   acute respiratory distress syndrome (J80)
  - cardiorespiratory failure (R09.2)
  - newborn respiratory distress syndrome (P22.0)
  - postprocedural respiratory failure (J95.82-)
  - respiratory arrest (R09.2)
  - respiratory arrest of newborn (P28.81)
  - respiratory failure of newborn (P28.5)

CC Excl: For CC/MCC codes in category J96: PDX collection 744

√5th J96.0   **Acute respiratory failure**

J96.00   **Acute respiratory failure, unspecified whether with hypoxia or hypercapnia** `MCC` `HCC`
- AHA: 2016, 3Q, 14; 2013, 4Q, 121

J96.01   **Acute respiratory failure with hypoxia** `MCC` `HCC`

J96.02   **Acute respiratory failure with hypercapnia** `MCC` `HCC`

N Newborn: 0   P Pediatric: 0-17   M Maternity: 12-55   A Adult: 15-124   MCC Major CC Condition   PDxMCC PDx acts as own MCC   CC CC Condition   PDxCC PDx acts as own CC

682   ICD-10-CM 2018

✓5ᵗʰ J96.1 Chronic respiratory failure

    J96.10 Chronic respiratory failure, unspecified whether with hypoxia or hypercapnia `CC` `HCC`
        AHA: 2016, 1Q, 38; 2015, 1Q, 21

    J96.11 Chronic respiratory failure with hypoxia `CC` `HCC`
        AHA: 2013, 4Q, 129

    J96.12 Chronic respiratory failure with hypercapnia `CC` `HCC`

✓5ᵗʰ J96.2 Acute and chronic respiratory failure
    Acute on chronic respiratory failure

    J96.20 Acute and chronic respiratory failure, unspecified whether with hypoxia or hypercapnia `MCC` `HCC`

    J96.21 Acute and chronic respiratory failure with hypoxia `MCC` `HCC`

    J96.22 Acute and chronic respiratory failure with hypercapnia `MCC` `HCC`

✓5ᵗʰ J96.9 Respiratory failure, unspecified

    J96.90 Respiratory failure, unspecified, unspecified whether with hypoxia or hypercapnia `MCC` `HCC`

    J96.91 Respiratory failure, unspecified with hypoxia `MCC` `HCC`

    J96.92 Respiratory failure, unspecified with hypercapnia `MCC` `HCC`

✓4ᵗʰ J98 Other respiratory disorders
    Use additional code to identify:
      exposure to environmental tobacco smoke (Z77.22)
      exposure to tobacco smoke in the perinatal period (P96.81)
      history of tobacco dependence (Z87.891)
      occupational exposure to environmental tobacco smoke (Z57.31)
      tobacco dependence (F17.-)
      tobacco use (Z72.0)
    EXCLUDES 1   newborn apnea (P28.4)
             newborn sleep apnea (P28.3)
    EXCLUDES 2   apnea NOS (R06.81)
             sleep apnea (G47.3-)

✓5ᵗʰ J98.0 Diseases of bronchus, not elsewhere classified

    J98.01 Acute bronchospasm
      EXCLUDES 1   acute bronchiolitis with bronchospasm (J21.-)
               acute bronchitis with bronchospasm (J20.-)
               asthma (J45.-)
               exercise induced bronchospasm (J45.990)

    J98.09 Other diseases of bronchus, not elsewhere classified
      Broncholithiasis
      Calcification of bronchus
      Stenosis of bronchus
      Tracheobronchial collapse
      Tracheobronchial dyskinesia
      Ulcer of bronchus

✓5ᵗʰ J98.1 Pulmonary collapse
    EXCLUDES 1   therapeutic collapse of lung status (Z98.3)

    J98.11 Atelectasis `CC`
      EXCLUDES 1   newborn atelectasis
               tuberculous atelectasis (current disease) (A15)
      CC Excl: PDX collection 760

    J98.19 Other pulmonary collapse `CC`
      CC Excl: PDX collection 760

    J98.2 Interstitial emphysema `HCC`
      Mediastinal emphysema
      EXCLUDES 1   emphysema NOS (J43.9)
               emphysema in newborn (P25.0)
               surgical emphysema (subcutaneous) (T81.82)
               traumatic subcutaneous emphysema (T79.7)

    J98.3 Compensatory emphysema `HCC`
      DEF: Distention of all or part of the lung caused by disease processes or surgical intervention that decreased volume in another part of the lung; overcompensation reaction to the loss of capacity in another part of the lung; occurs in association with pneumonias, pleural effusions, atelectasis, empyema, and pneumothorax.

    J98.4 Other disorders of lung
      Calcification of lung
      Cystic lung disease (acquired)
      Lung disease NOS
      Pulmolithiasis
      EXCLUDES 1   acute interstitial pneumonitis (J84.114)
               pulmonary insufficiency following surgery (J95.1-J95.2)

✓5ᵗʰ J98.5 Diseases of mediastinum, not elsewhere classified
    EXCLUDES 2   abscess of mediastinum (J85.3)

    J98.51 Mediastinitis `MCC` `H8`
      Code first:
        underlying condition, if applicable, such as postoperative mediastinitis (T81.-)
      CC Excl: No Excl

    J98.59 Other diseases of mediastinum, not elsewhere classified `MCC` `H8`
      Fibrosis of mediastinum
      Hernia of mediastinum
      Retraction of mediastinum
      CC Excl: No Excl

    J98.6 Disorders of diaphragm
      Diaphragmatitis
      Paralysis of diaphragm
      Relaxation of diaphragm
      EXCLUDES 1   congenital malformation of diaphragm NEC (Q79.1)
               congenital diaphragmatic hernia (Q79.0)
      EXCLUDES 2   diaphragmatic hernia (K44.-)

    J98.8 Other specified respiratory disorders

    J98.9 Respiratory disorder, unspecified
      Respiratory disease (chronic) NOS

J99 Respiratory disorders in diseases classified elsewhere `HCC`
    Code first underlying disease, such as:
      amyloidosis (E85.-)
      ankylosing spondylitis (M45)
      congenital syphilis (A50.5)
      cryoglobulinemia (D89.1)
      early congenital syphilis (A50.0)
      schistosomiasis (B65.0-B65.9)
    EXCLUDES 1   respiratory disorders in:
        amebiasis (A06.5)
        blastomycosis (B40.0-B40.2)
        candidiasis (B37.1)
        coccidioidomycosis (B38.0-B38.2)
        cystic fibrosis with pulmonary manifestations (E84.0)
        dermatomyositis (M33.01, M33.11)
        histoplasmosis (B39.0-B39.2)
        late syphilis (A52.72, A52.73)
        polymyositis (M33.21)
        sicca syndrome (M35.02)
        systemic lupus erythematosus (M32.13)
        systemic sclerosis (M34.81)
        Wegener's granulomatosis (M31.30-M31.31)

☑Additional Character Req   ✓x7ᵗʰ Placeholder Alert   Unacceptable PDx   Manifestation   `H1`-`H14` HAC   `HCC` CMS-HCC Condition   *EXCLUDES 1* Not Coded Here   *EXCLUDES 2* Not Included Here

Chapter 11. Diseases of the Digestive System (KØØ–K95)

Chapter Specific Coding Guidelines and Examples
Reserved for future guideline expansion.

Chapter 11. Diseases of the Digestive System (K00-K95)

EXCLUDES 2   *certain conditions originating in the perinatal period (P04-P96)*
certain infectious and parasitic diseases (A00-B99)
complications of pregnancy, childbirth and the puerperium (O00-O9A)
congenital malformations, deformations and chromosomal abnormalities (Q00-Q99)
endocrine, nutritional and metabolic diseases (E00-E88)
injury, poisoning and certain other consequences of external causes (S00-T88)
neoplasms (C00-D49)
symptoms, signs and abnormal clinical and laboratory findings, not elsewhere classified (R00-R94)

This chapter contains the following blocks:

K00-K14	Diseases of oral cavity and salivary glands
K20-K31	Diseases of esophagus, stomach and duodenum
K35-K38	Diseases of appendix
K40-K46	Hernia
K50-K52	Noninfective enteritis and colitis
K55-K64	Other diseases of intestines
K65-K68	Diseases of peritoneum and retroperitoneum
K70-K77	Diseases of liver
K80-K87	Disorders of gallbladder, biliary tract and pancreas
K90-K95	Other diseases of the digestive system

Diseases of oral cavity and salivary glands (K00-K14)

✓4th **K00 Disorders of tooth development and eruption**
     EXCLUDES 2   *embedded and impacted teeth (K01.-)*

K00.0 Anodontia
     Hypodontia
     Oligodontia
     EXCLUDES 1   *acquired absence of teeth (K08.1-)*

K00.1 Supernumerary teeth
     Distomolar
     Fourth molar
     Mesiodens
     Paramolar
     Supplementary teeth
     EXCLUDES 2   *supernumerary roots (K00.2)*

K00.2 Abnormalities of size and form of teeth
     Concrescence of teeth
     Dens evaginatus
     Dens in dente
     Dens invaginatus
     Enamel pearls
     Fusion of teeth
     Gemination of teeth
     Macrodontia
     Microdontia
     Peg-shaped [conical] teeth
     Supernumerary roots
     Taurodontism
     Tuberculum paramolare
     EXCLUDES 1   *abnormalities of teeth due to congenital syphilis (A50.5)*
         tuberculum Carabelli, which is regarded as a normal variation and should not be coded

K00.3 Mottled teeth
     Dental fluorosis
     Mottling of enamel
     Nonfluoride enamel opacities
     EXCLUDES 2   *deposits [accretions] on teeth (K03.6)*

K00.4 Disturbances in tooth formation
     Aplasia and hypoplasia of cementum
     Dilaceration of tooth
     Enamel hypoplasia (neonatal) (postnatal) (prenatal)
     Regional odontodysplasia
     Turner's tooth
     EXCLUDES 1   *Hutchinson's teeth and mulberry molars in congenital syphilis (A50.5)*
     EXCLUDES 2   *mottled teeth (K00.3)*

K00.5 Hereditary disturbances in tooth structure, not elsewhere classified
     Amelogenesis imperfecta
     Dentinogenesis imperfecta
     Odontogenesis imperfecta
     Dentinal dysplasia
     Shell teeth

Tooth Anatomy

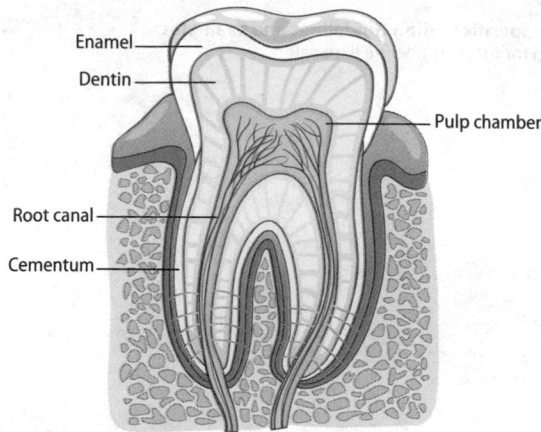

K00.6 Disturbances in tooth eruption
     Dentia praecox
     Natal tooth
     Neonatal tooth
     Premature eruption of tooth
     Premature shedding of primary [deciduous] tooth
     Prenatal teeth
     Retained [persistent] primary tooth
     EXCLUDES 2   *embedded and impacted teeth (K01.-)*

K00.7 Teething syndrome

K00.8 Other disorders of tooth development
     Color changes during tooth formation
     Intrinsic staining of teeth NOS
     EXCLUDES 2   *posteruptive color changes (K03.7)*

K00.9 Disorder of tooth development, unspecified
     Disorder of odontogenesis NOS

✓4th **K01 Embedded and impacted teeth**
     EXCLUDES 1   *abnormal position of fully erupted teeth (M26.3-)*

K01.0 Embedded teeth

K01.1 Impacted teeth

✓4th **K02 Dental caries**
     INCLUDES   caries of dentine
         dental cavities
         early childhood caries
         pre-eruptive caries
         recurrent caries (dentino enamel junction) (enamel) (to the pulp)
         tooth decay

K02.3 Arrested dental caries
     Arrested coronal and root caries

✓5th **K02.5 Dental caries on pit and fissure surface**
     Dental caries on chewing surface of tooth

     K02.51 Dental caries on pit and fissure surface limited to enamel
         White spot lesions [initial caries] on pit and fissure surface of tooth

     K02.52 Dental caries on pit and fissure surface penetrating into dentin
         Primary dental caries, cervical origin

     K02.53 Dental caries on pit and fissure surface penetrating into pulp

✓5th **K02.6 Dental caries on smooth surface**

     K02.61 Dental caries on smooth surface limited to enamel
         White spot lesions [initial caries] on smooth surface of tooth

     K02.62 Dental caries on smooth surface penetrating into dentin

     K02.63 Dental caries on smooth surface penetrating into pulp

K02.7 Dental root caries

K02.9 Dental caries, unspecified

N Newborn: 0   P Pediatric: 0-17   M Maternity: 12-55   A Adult: 15-124   MCC Major CC Condition   PDxMCC PDx acts as own MCC   CC CC Condition   PDxCC PDx acts as own CC

686   ICD-10-CM 2018

✓4th **K03** **Other diseases of hard tissues of teeth**
     EXCLUDES 2   *bruxism (F45.8)*
                dental caries (K02.-)
                teeth-grinding NOS (F45.8)

K03.0 **Excessive attrition of teeth**
     Approximal wear of teeth
     Occlusal wear of teeth

K03.1 **Abrasion of teeth**
     Dentifrice abrasion of teeth
     Habitual abrasion of teeth
     Occupational abrasion of teeth
     Ritual abrasion of teeth
     Traditional abrasion of teeth
     Wedge defect NOS

K03.2 **Erosion of teeth**
     Erosion of teeth due to diet
     Erosion of teeth due to drugs and medicaments
     Erosion of teeth due to persistent vomiting
     Erosion of teeth NOS
     Idiopathic erosion of teeth
     Occupational erosion of teeth

K03.3 **Pathological resorption of teeth**
     Internal granuloma of pulp
     Resorption of teeth (external)

K03.4 **Hypercementosis**
     Cementation hyperplasia

K03.5 **Ankylosis of teeth**

K03.6 **Deposits [accretions] on teeth**
     Betel deposits [accretions] on teeth
     Black deposits [accretions] on teeth
     Extrinsic staining of teeth NOS
     Green deposits [accretions] on teeth
     Materia alba deposits [accretions] on teeth
     Orange deposits [accretions] on teeth
     Staining of teeth NOS
     Subgingival dental calculus
     Supragingival dental calculus
     Tobacco deposits [accretions] on teeth

K03.7 **Posteruptive color changes of dental hard tissues**
     EXCLUDES 2   *deposits [accretions] on teeth (K03.6)*

✓5th **K03.8** **Other specified diseases of hard tissues of teeth**
     K03.81 **Cracked tooth**
         EXCLUDES 1   *asymptomatic craze lines in enamel—omit code*
                broken or fractured tooth due to trauma (S02.5)
     K03.89 **Other specified diseases of hard tissues of teeth**

K03.9 **Disease of hard tissues of teeth, unspecified**

✓4th **K04** **Diseases of pulp and periapical tissues**

     CC Excl: For CC codes in category K04: PDX collection 761

✓5th **K04.0** **Pulpitis**
     Acute pulpitis
     Chronic (hyperplastic) (ulcerative) pulpitis
     K04.01 **Reversible pulpitis**   CC
     K04.02 **Irreversible pulpitis**   CC

K04.1 **Necrosis of pulp**
     Pulpal gangrene

K04.2 **Pulp degeneration**
     Denticles
     Pulpal calcifications
     Pulpal stones

K04.3 **Abnormal hard tissue formation in pulp**
     Secondary or irregular dentine

K04.4 **Acute apical periodontitis of pulpal origin**   CC
     Acute apical periodontitis NOS
     EXCLUDES 1   *acute periodontitis (K05.2)*
     DEF: Severe inflammation of the area surrounding the tip of a tooth's root; often secondary to infection or trauma.
     CC Excl: PDX collection 761

K04.5 **Chronic apical periodontitis**
     Apical or periapical granuloma
     Apical periodontitis NOS
     EXCLUDES 1   *chronic periodontitis (K05.3-)*

K04.6 **Periapical abscess with sinus**
     Dental abscess with sinus
     Dentoalveolar abscess with sinus

K04.7 **Periapical abscess without sinus**
     Dental abscess without sinus
     Dentoalveolar abscess without sinus
     ~~Periapical abscess without sinus~~

K04.8 **Radicular cyst**
     Apical (periodontal) cyst
     Periapical cyst
     Residual radicular cyst
     EXCLUDES 2   *lateral periodontal cyst (K09.0)*
     DEF: Most common odontogenic cyst in tissue around tooth apex due to chronic inflammation of dental pulp.

✓5th **K04.9** **Other and unspecified diseases of pulp and periapical tissues**
     K04.90 **Unspecified diseases of pulp and periapical tissues**
     K04.99 **Other diseases of pulp and periapical tissues**

✓4th **K05** **Gingivitis and periodontal diseases**
     Use additional code to identify:
     alcohol abuse and dependence (F10.-)
     exposure to environmental tobacco smoke (Z77.22)
     exposure to tobacco smoke in the perinatal period (P96.81)
     history of tobacco dependence (Z87.891)
     occupational exposure to environmental tobacco smoke (Z57.31)
     tobacco dependence (F17.-)
     tobacco use (Z72.0)

✓5th **K05.0** **Acute gingivitis**
     EXCLUDES 1   *acute necrotizing ulcerative gingivitis (A69.1)*
                herpesviral [herpes simplex] gingivostomatitis (B00.2)
     K05.00 **Acute gingivitis, plaque induced**
         Acute gingivitis NOS
         Plaque induced gingival disease
     K05.01 **Acute gingivitis, non-plaque induced**

✓5th **K05.1** **Chronic gingivitis**
     Desquamative gingivitis (chronic)
     Gingivitis (chronic) NOS
     Hyperplastic gingivitis (chronic)
     Pregnancy associated gingivitis
     Simple marginal gingivitis (chronic)
     Ulcerative gingivitis (chronic)
     Code first, if applicable, diseases of the digestive system complicating pregnancy (O99.61-)
     K05.10 **Chronic gingivitis, plaque induced**
         Chronic gingivitis NOS
         Gingivitis NOS
     K05.11 **Chronic gingivitis, non-plaque induced**

✓5th **K05.2** **Aggressive periodontitis**
     Acute pericoronitis
     EXCLUDES 1   *acute apical periodontitis (K04.4)*
                periapical abscess (K04.7)
                periapical abscess with sinus (K04.6)
     K05.20 **Aggressive periodontitis, unspecified**
     ✓6th **K05.21** **Aggressive periodontitis, localized**
         Periodontal abscess
         K05.211 **Aggressive periodontitis, localized, slight**
         K05.212 **Aggressive periodontitis, localized, moderate**
         K05.213 **Aggressive periodontitis, localized, severe**
         K05.219 **Aggressive periodontitis, localized, unspecified severity**
     ✓6th **K05.22** **Aggressive periodontitis, generalized**
         K05.221 **Aggressive periodontitis, generalized, slight**
         K05.222 **Aggressive periodontitis, generalized, moderate**
         K05.223 **Aggressive periodontitis, generalized, severe**
         K05.229 **Aggressive periodontitis, generalized, unspecified severity**

✓5th **K05.3** **Chronic periodontitis**
     Chronic pericoronitis   Periodontitis NOS
     Complex periodontitis   Simplex periodontitis
     EXCLUDES 1   *chronic apical periodontitis (K04.5)*
     K05.30 **Chronic periodontitis, unspecified**
     ✓6th **K05.31** **Chronic periodontitis, localized**
         K05.311 **Chronic periodontitis, localized, slight**
         K05.312 **Chronic periodontitis, localized, moderate**

Chapter 11. Diseases of the Digestive System *(side margin)*

           K05.313   Chronic periodontitis, localized, severe

           K05.319   Chronic periodontitis, localized, unspecified severity

✓6ᵗʰ **K05.32**   Chronic periodontitis, generalized

           K05.321   Chronic periodontitis, generalized, slight

           K05.322   Chronic periodontitis, generalized, moderate

           K05.323   Chronic periodontitis, generalized, severe

           K05.329   Chronic periodontitis, generalized, unspecified severity

K05.4   Periodontosis
Juvenile periodontosis

K05.5   Other periodontal diseases
Combined periodontic-endodontic lesion
Narrow gingival width (of periodontal soft tissue)
EXCLUDES 2   *leukoplakia of gingiva (K13.21)*

K05.6   Periodontal disease, unspecified

✓4ᵗʰ **K06**   **Other disorders of gingiva and edentulous alveolar ridge**
EXCLUDES 2   *acute gingivitis (K05.0)*
atrophy of edentulous alveolar ridge (K08.2)
chronic gingivitis (K05.1)
gingivitis NOS (K05.1)

✓5ᵗʰ **K06.0**   Gingival recession
▶Gingival recession (postinfective) (postprocedural)◀

●   ✓6ᵗʰ **K06.01**   Gingival recession, localized

●   **K06.010**   Localized gingival recession, unspecified
Localized gingival recession, NOS

●   **K06.011**   Localized gingival recession, minimal

●   **K06.012**   Localized gingival recession, moderate

●   **K06.013**   Localized gingival recession, severe

●   ✓6ᵗʰ **K06.02**   Gingival recession, generalized

●   **K06.020**   Generalized gingival recession, unspecified
Generalized gingival recession, NOS

●   **K06.021**   Generalized gingival recession, minimal

●   **K06.022**   Generalized gingival recession, moderate

●   **K06.023**   Generalized gingival recession, severe

K06.1   Gingival enlargement
Gingival fibromatosis

K06.2   Gingival and edentulous alveolar ridge lesions associated with trauma
Irritative hyperplasia of edentulous ridge [denture hyperplasia]
Use additional code (Chapter 20) to identify external cause or denture status (Z97.2)

K06.3   Horizontal alveolar bone loss

K06.8   Other specified disorders of gingiva and edentulous alveolar ridge
Fibrous epulis
Flabby alveolar ridge
Giant cell epulis
Peripheral giant cell granuloma of gingiva
Pyogenic granuloma of gingiva
Vertical ridge deficiency
EXCLUDES 2   *gingival cyst (K09.0)*

K06.9   Disorder of gingiva and edentulous alveolar ridge, unspecified

✓4ᵗʰ **K08**   **Other disorders of teeth and supporting structures**
EXCLUDES 2   *dentofacial anomalies [including malocclusion] (M26.-)*
disorders of jaw (M27.-)

K08.0   Exfoliation of teeth due to systemic causes
Code also underlying systemic condition

✓5ᵗʰ **K08.1**   Complete loss of teeth
Acquired loss of teeth, complete
EXCLUDES 1   *congenital absence of teeth (K00.0)*
exfoliation of teeth due to systemic causes (K08.0)
partial loss of teeth (K08.4-)

✓6ᵗʰ **K08.10**   Complete loss of teeth, unspecified cause

       K08.101   Complete loss of teeth, unspecified cause, class I

       K08.102   Complete loss of teeth, unspecified cause, class II

       K08.103   Complete loss of teeth, unspecified cause, class III

       K08.104   Complete loss of teeth, unspecified cause, class IV

       K08.109   Complete loss of teeth, unspecified cause, unspecified class
Edentulism NOS

✓6ᵗʰ **K08.11**   Complete loss of teeth due to trauma

       K08.111   Complete loss of teeth due to trauma, class I

       K08.112   Complete loss of teeth due to trauma, class II

       K08.113   Complete loss of teeth due to trauma, class III

       K08.114   Complete loss of teeth due to trauma, class IV

       K08.119   Complete loss of teeth due to trauma, unspecified class

✓6ᵗʰ **K08.12**   Complete loss of teeth due to periodontal diseases

       K08.121   Complete loss of teeth due to periodontal diseases, class I

       K08.122   Complete loss of teeth due to periodontal diseases, class II

       K08.123   Complete loss of teeth due to periodontal diseases, class III

       K08.124   Complete loss of teeth due to periodontal diseases, class IV

       K08.129   Complete loss of teeth due to periodontal diseases, unspecified class

✓6ᵗʰ **K08.13**   Complete loss of teeth due to caries

       K08.131   Complete loss of teeth due to caries, class I

       K08.132   Complete loss of teeth due to caries, class II

       K08.133   Complete loss of teeth due to caries, class III

       K08.134   Complete loss of teeth due to caries, class IV

       K08.139   Complete loss of teeth due to caries, unspecified class

✓6ᵗʰ **K08.19**   Complete loss of teeth due to other specified cause

       K08.191   Complete loss of teeth due to other specified cause, class I

       K08.192   Complete loss of teeth due to other specified cause, class II

       K08.193   Complete loss of teeth due to other specified cause, class III

       K08.194   Complete loss of teeth due to other specified cause, class IV

       K08.199   Complete loss of teeth due to other specified cause, unspecified class

✓5ᵗʰ **K08.2**   Atrophy of edentulous alveolar ridge

       K08.20   Unspecified atrophy of edentulous alveolar ridge
Atrophy of the mandible NOS
Atrophy of the maxilla NOS

       K08.21   Minimal atrophy of the mandible
Minimal atrophy of the edentulous mandible

       K08.22   Moderate atrophy of the mandible
Moderate atrophy of the edentulous mandible

       K08.23   Severe atrophy of the mandible
Severe atrophy of the edentulous mandible

       K08.24   Minimal atrophy of the maxilla
Minimal atrophy of the edentulous maxilla

       K08.25   Moderate atrophy of the maxilla
Moderate atrophy of the edentulous maxilla

       K08.26   Severe atrophy of the maxilla
Severe atrophy of the edentulous maxilla

K08.3   Retained dental root

✓5ᵗʰ **K08.4**   Partial loss of teeth
Acquired loss of teeth, partial
EXCLUDES 1   *complete loss of teeth (K08.1-)*
congenital absence of teeth (K00.0)
EXCLUDES 2   *exfoliation of teeth due to systemic causes (K08.0)*

✓6ᵗʰ **K08.40**   Partial loss of teeth, unspecified cause

       K08.401   Partial loss of teeth, unspecified cause, class I

       K08.402   Partial loss of teeth, unspecified cause, class II

       K08.403   Partial loss of teeth, unspecified cause, class III

N Newborn: 0   P Pediatric: 0-17   M Maternity: 12-55   A Adult: 15-124   MCC Major CC Condition   PDxMCC PDx acts as own MCC   CC CC Condition   PDxCC PDx acts as own CC

688   ICD-10-CM 2018

K08.404   **Partial loss of teeth, unspecified cause, class IV**

K08.409   **Partial loss of teeth, unspecified cause, unspecified class**
Tooth extraction status NOS

✓6th   **K08.41**   **Partial loss of teeth due to** trauma

K08.411   **Partial loss of teeth due to trauma, class I**

K08.412   **Partial loss of teeth due to trauma, class II**

K08.413   **Partial loss of teeth due to trauma, class III**

K08.414   **Partial loss of teeth due to trauma, class IV**

K08.419   **Partial loss of teeth due to trauma, unspecified class**

✓6th   **K08.42**   **Partial loss of teeth due to** periodontal diseases

K08.421   **Partial loss of teeth due to periodontal diseases, class I**

K08.422   **Partial loss of teeth due to periodontal diseases, class II**

K08.423   **Partial loss of teeth due to periodontal diseases, class III**

K08.424   **Partial loss of teeth due to periodontal diseases, class IV**

K08.429   **Partial loss of teeth due to periodontal diseases, unspecified class**

✓6th   **K08.43**   **Partial loss of teeth due to** caries

K08.431   **Partial loss of teeth due to caries, class I**

K08.432   **Partial loss of teeth due to caries, class II**

K08.433   **Partial loss of teeth due to caries, class III**

K08.434   **Partial loss of teeth due to caries, class IV**

K08.439   **Partial loss of teeth due to caries, unspecified class**

✓6th   **K08.49**   **Partial loss of teeth due to** other specified cause

K08.491   **Partial loss of teeth due to other specified cause, class I**

K08.492   **Partial loss of teeth due to other specified cause, class II**

K08.493   **Partial loss of teeth due to other specified cause, class III**

K08.494   **Partial loss of teeth due to other specified cause, class IV**

K08.499   **Partial loss of teeth due to other specified cause, unspecified class**

✓5th   **K08.5**   **Unsatisfactory restoration of tooth**
Defective bridge, crown, filling
Defective dental restoration
EXCLUDES 1   *dental restoration status (Z98.811)*
EXCLUDES 2   *endosseous dental implant failure (M27.6-)*
unsatisfactory endodontic treatment (M27.5-)

K08.50   **Unsatisfactory restoration of tooth, unspecified**
Defective dental restoration NOS

K08.51   **Open restoration margins of tooth**
Dental restoration failure of marginal integrity
Open margin on tooth restoration
Poor gingival margin to tooth restoration

K08.52   **Unrepairable overhanging of dental restorative materials**
Overhanging of tooth restoration

✓6th   **K08.53**   **Fractured dental restorative material**
EXCLUDES 1   *cracked tooth (K03.81)*
traumatic fracture of tooth (S02.5)

K08.530   **Fractured dental restorative material without loss of material**

K08.531   **Fractured dental restorative material with loss of material**

K08.539   **Fractured dental restorative material, unspecified**

K08.54   **Contour of existing restoration of tooth biologically incompatible with oral health**
Dental restoration failure of periodontal anatomical integrity
Unacceptable contours of existing restoration of tooth
Unacceptable morphology of existing restoration of tooth

K08.55   **Allergy to existing dental restorative material**
Use additional code to identify the specific type of allergy

K08.56   **Poor aesthetic of existing restoration of tooth**
Dental restoration aesthetically inadequate or displeasing

K08.59   **Other unsatisfactory restoration of tooth**
Other defective dental restoration

✓5th   **K08.8**   **Other specified disorders of teeth and supporting structures**

K08.81   **Primary occlusal trauma**

K08.82   **Secondary occlusal trauma**

K08.89   **Other specified disorders of teeth and supporting structures**
Enlargement of alveolar ridge NOS
Insufficient anatomic crown height
Insufficient clinical crown length
Irregular alveolar process
Toothache NOS

K08.9   **Disorder of teeth and supporting structures, unspecified**

✓4th   **K09**   **Cysts of oral region, not elsewhere classified**
INCLUDES   lesions showing histological features both of aneurysmal cyst and of another fibro-osseous lesion
EXCLUDES 2   *cysts of jaw (M27.0-, M27.4-)*
radicular cyst (K04.8)

K09.0   **Developmental odontogenic cysts**
Dentigerous cyst
Eruption cyst
Follicular cyst
Gingival cyst
Lateral periodontal cyst
Primordial cyst
EXCLUDES 2   *keratocysts (D16.4, D16.5)*
odontogenic keratocystic tumors (D16.4, D16.5)

K09.1   **Developmental (nonodontogenic) cysts of oral region**
Cyst (of) incisive canal
Cyst (of) palatine of papilla
Globulomaxillary cyst
Median palatal cyst
Nasoalveolar cyst
Nasolabial cyst
Nasopalatine duct cyst

K09.8   **Other cysts of oral region, not elsewhere classified**
Dermoid cyst
Epidermoid cyst
Lymphoepithelial cyst
Epstein's pearl

K09.9   **Cyst of oral region, unspecified**

✓4th   **K11**   **Diseases of salivary glands**
Use additional code to identify:
alcohol abuse and dependence (F10.-)
exposure to environmental tobacco smoke (Z77.22)
exposure to tobacco smoke in the perinatal period (P96.81)
history of tobacco dependence (Z87.891)
occupational exposure to environmental tobacco smoke (Z57.31)
tobacco dependence (F17.-)
tobacco use (Z72.0)

K11.0   **Atrophy of salivary gland**

K11.1   **Hypertrophy of salivary gland**
DEF: Overgrowth of or enlarged salivary gland tissue; caused by infection, salivary duct blockage, autoimmune diseases, and benign and malignant tumors.

✓5th   **K11.2**   **Sialoadenitis**
Parotitis
EXCLUDES 1   *epidemic parotitis (B26.-)*
mumps (B26.-)
uveoparotid fever [Heerfordt] (D86.89)

K11.20   **Sialoadenitis, unspecified**

K11.21   **Acute sialoadenitis**
EXCLUDES 1   *acute recurrent sialoadenitis (K11.22)*

K11.22   **Acute recurrent sialoadenitis**

K11.23   **Chronic sialoadenitis**

K11.3   **Abscess of salivary gland**   CC
CC Excl: PDX collection 762

K11.4   **Fistula of salivary gland**   CC
EXCLUDES 1   *congenital fistula of salivary gland (Q38.4)*
CC Excl: PDX collection 762

K11.5   **Sialolithiasis**
Calculus of salivary gland or duct
Stone of salivary gland or duct

✔ Additional Character Req   ✓x7th Placeholder Alert   Unacceptable PDx   Manifestation   H1 - H14 HAC   HCC CMS-HCC Condition   EXCLUDES 1 Not Coded Here   EXCLUDES 2 Not Included Here

ICD-10-CM 2018   689

Chapter 11. Diseases of the Digestive System

K11.6   **Mucocele of salivary gland**
Mucous extravasation cyst of salivary gland
Mucous retention cyst of salivary gland
Ranula

K11.7   **Disturbances of salivary secretion**
Hypoptyalism
Ptyalism
Xerostomia
EXCLUDES 2   *dry mouth NOS (R68.2)*

K11.8   **Other diseases of salivary glands**
Benign lymphoepithelial lesion of salivary gland
Mikulicz' disease
Necrotizing sialometaplasia
Sialectasia
Stenosis of salivary duct
Stricture of salivary duct
EXCLUDES 1   *sicca syndrome [Sjögren] (M35.0-)*

K11.9   **Disease of salivary gland, unspecified**
Sialoadenopathy NOS

☑4ᵗʰ **K12**   **Stomatitis and related lesions**
Use additional code to identify:
alcohol abuse and dependence (F10.-)
exposure to environmental tobacco smoke (Z77.22)
exposure to tobacco smoke in the perinatal period (P96.81)
history of tobacco dependence (Z87.891)
occupational exposure to environmental tobacco smoke (Z57.31)
tobacco dependence (F17.-)
tobacco use (Z72.0)
EXCLUDES 1   *cancrum oris (A69.0)*
cheilitis (K13.0)
gangrenous stomatitis (A69.0)
herpesviral [herpes simplex] gingivostomatitis (B00.2)
noma (A69.0)

K12.0   **Recurrent oral aphthae**
Aphthous stomatitis (major) (minor)
Bednar's aphthae
Periadenitis mucosa necrotica recurrens
Recurrent aphthous ulcer
Stomatitis herpetiformis
DEF: Disorder of unknown etiology with small oval or round painful ulcers of the mouth marked by a grayish exudate and a red halo effect.

K12.1   **Other forms of stomatitis**
Stomatitis NOS
Denture stomatitis
Ulcerative stomatitis
Vesicular stomatitis
EXCLUDES 1   *acute necrotizing ulcerative stomatitis (A69.1)*
Vincent's stomatitis (A69.1)

K12.2   **Cellulitis and abscess of mouth**   CC
Cellulitis of mouth (floor)
Submandibular abscess
EXCLUDES 2   *abscess of salivary gland (K11.3)*
abscess of tongue (K14.0)
periapical abscess (K04.6-K04.7)
periodontal abscess (K05.21)
peritonsillar abscess (J36)
CC Excl: PDX collection 763

☑5ᵗʰ **K12.3**   **Oral mucositis (ulcerative)**
Mucositis (oral) (oropharyneal)
EXCLUDES 2   *gastrointestinal mucositis (ulcerative) (K92.81)*
mucositis (ulcerative) of vagina and vulva (N76.81)
nasal mucositis (ulcerative) (J34.81)

   K12.30   **Oral mucositis (ulcerative), unspecified**

   K12.31   **Oral mucositis (ulcerative) due to antineoplastic therapy**
Use additional code for adverse effect, if applicable, to identify antineoplastic and immunosuppressive drugs (T45.1X5)
Use additional code for other antineoplastic therapy, such as:
radiological procedure and radiotherapy (Y84.2)

   K12.32   **Oral mucositis (ulcerative) due to other drugs**
Use additional code for adverse effect, if applicable, to identify drug (T36-T50 with fifth or sixth character 5)

   K12.33   **Oral mucositis (ulcerative) due to radiation**
Use additional external cause code (W88-W90, X39.0-) to identify cause

   K12.39   **Other oral mucositis (ulcerative)**
Viral oral mucositis (ulcerative)

☑4ᵗʰ **K13**   **Other diseases of lip and oral mucosa**
INCLUDES   epithelial disturbances of tongue
Use additional code to identify:
alcohol abuse and dependence (F10.-)
exposure to environmental tobacco smoke (Z77.22)
exposure to tobacco smoke in the perinatal period (P96.81)
history of tobacco dependence (Z87.891)
occupational exposure to environmental tobacco smoke (Z57.31)
tobacco dependence (F17.-)
tobacco use (Z72.0)
EXCLUDES 2   *certain disorders of gingiva and edentulous alveolar ridge (K05-K06)*
cysts of oral region (K09.-)
diseases of tongue (K14.-)
stomatitis and related lesions (K12.-)

K13.0   **Diseases of lips**
Abscess of lips
Angular cheilitis
Cellulitis of lips
Cheilitis NOS
Cheilodynia
Cheilosis
Exfoliative cheilitis
Fistula of lips
Glandular cheilitis
Hypertrophy of lips
Perlèche NEC
EXCLUDES 1   *ariboflavinosis (E53.0)*
cheilitis due to radiation-related disorders (L55-L59)
congenital fistula of lips (Q38.0)
congenital hypertrophy of lips (Q18.6)
Perlèche due to candidiasis (B37.83)
Perlèche due to riboflavin deficiency (E53.0)

K13.1   **Cheek and lip biting**

☑5ᵗʰ **K13.2**   **Leukoplakia and other disturbances of oral epithelium, including tongue**
EXCLUDES 1   *carcinoma in situ of oral epithelium (D00.0-)*
hairy leukoplakia (K13.3)

   K13.21   **Leukoplakia of oral mucosa, including tongue**
Leukokeratosis of oral mucosa
Leukoplakia of gingiva, lips, tongue
EXCLUDES 1   *hairy leukoplakia (K13.3)*
leukokeratosis nicotina palati (K13.24)

   K13.22   **Minimal keratinized residual ridge mucosa**
Minimal keratinization of alveolar ridge mucosa

   K13.23   **Excessive keratinized residual ridge mucosa**
Excessive keratinization of alveolar ridge mucosa

   K13.24   **Leukokeratosis nicotina palati**
Smoker's palate

   K13.29   **Other disturbances of oral epithelium, including tongue**
Erythroplakia of mouth or tongue
Focal epithelial hyperplasia of mouth or tongue
Leukoedema of mouth or tongue
Other oral epithelium disturbances

K13.3   **Hairy leukoplakia**

K13.4   **Granuloma and granuloma-like lesions of oral mucosa**
Eosinophilic granuloma
Granuloma pyogenicum
Verrucous xanthoma

K13.5   **Oral submucous fibrosis**
Submucous fibrosis of tongue

K13.6   **Irritative hyperplasia of oral mucosa**
EXCLUDES 2   *irritative hyperplasia of edentulous ridge [denture hyperplasia] (K06.2)*

☑5ᵗʰ **K13.7**   **Other and unspecified lesions of oral mucosa**

   K13.70   **Unspecified lesions of oral mucosa**

   K13.79   **Other lesions of oral mucosa**
Focal oral mucinosis

Ⓝ Newborn: 0   Ⓟ Pediatric: 0-17   Ⓜ Maternity: 12-55   Ⓐ Adult: 15-124   MCC Major CC Condition   PDxMCC PDx acts as own MCC   CC CC Condition   PDxCC PDx acts as own CC

✓4th K14   Diseases of tongue

Use additional code to identify:
alcohol abuse and dependence (F10.-)
exposure to environmental tobacco smoke (Z77.22)
history of tobacco dependence (Z87.891)
occupational exposure to environmental tobacco smoke (Z57.31)
tobacco dependence (F17.-)
tobacco use (Z72.0)

EXCLUDES 2   *erythroplakia (K13.29)*
focal epithelial hyperplasia (K13.29)
leukedema of tongue (K13.29)
leukoplakia of tongue (K13.21)
hairy leukoplakia (K13.3)
macroglossia (congenital) (Q38.2)
submucous fibrosis of tongue (K13.5)

K14.0   Glossitis
Abscess of tongue
Ulceration (traumatic) of tongue
EXCLUDES 1   *atrophic glossitis (K14.4)*

K14.1   Geographic tongue
Benign migratory glossitis
Glossitis areata exfoliativa

K14.2   Median rhomboid glossitis

K14.3   Hypertrophy of tongue papillae
Black hairy tongue
Coated tongue
Hypertrophy of foliate papillae
Lingua villosa nigra

K14.4   Atrophy of tongue papillae
Atrophic glossitis

K14.5   Plicated tongue
Fissured tongue
Furrowed tongue
Scrotal tongue
EXCLUDES 1   *fissured tongue, congenital (Q38.3)*

K14.6   Glossodynia
Glossopyrosis
Painful tongue

K14.8   Other diseases of tongue
Atrophy of tongue
Crenated tongue
Enlargement of tongue
Glossocele
Glossoptosis
Hypertrophy of tongue

K14.9   Disease of tongue, unspecified
Glossopathy NOS

Diseases of esophagus, stomach and duodenum (K20-K31)

EXCLUDES 2   *hiatus hernia (K44.-)*

✓4th K20   Esophagitis

Use additional code to identify:
alcohol abuse and dependence (F10.-)
EXCLUDES 1   *erosion of esophagus (K22.1-)*
esophagitis with gastro-esophageal reflux disease (K21.0)
reflux esophagitis (K21.0)
ulcerative esophagitis (K22.1-)
EXCLUDES 2   *eosinophilic gastritis or gastroenteritis (K52.81)*

K20.0   Eosinophilic esophagitis

K20.8   Other esophagitis
Abscess of esophagus

K20.9   Esophagitis, unspecified
Esophagitis NOS

✓4th K21   Gastro-esophageal reflux disease

EXCLUDES 1   *newborn esophageal reflux (P78.83)*

K21.0   Gastro-esophageal reflux disease with esophagitis
Reflux esophagitis

K21.9   Gastro-esophageal reflux disease without esophagitis
Esophageal reflux NOS
AHA: 2016, 1Q, 18

✓4th K22   Other diseases of esophagus

EXCLUDES 2   *esophageal varices (I85.-)*

K22.0   Achalasia of cardia
Achalasia NOS
Cardiospasm
EXCLUDES 1   *congenital cardiospasm (Q39.5)*
DEF: Esophageal motility disorder; caused by absence of esophageal peristalsis and impaired relaxation of lower esophageal sphincter; characterized by dysphagia, regurgitation, and heartburn.

✓5th K22.1   Ulcer of esophagus
Barrett's ulcer
Erosion of esophagus
Fungal ulcer of esophagus
Peptic ulcer of esophagus
Ulcer of esophagus due to ingestion of chemicals
Ulcer of esophagus due to ingestion of drugs and medicaments
Ulcerative esophagitis
Code first poisoning due to drug or toxin, if applicable (T36-T65 with fifth or sixth character 1-4 or 6)
Use additional code for adverse effect, if applicable, to identify drug (T36-T50 with fifth or sixth character 5)
EXCLUDES 1   *Barrett's esophagus (K22.7-)*

     K22.10   Ulcer of esophagus without bleeding `CC`
Ulcer of esophagus NOS
CC Excl: PDX collection 764

     K22.11   Ulcer of esophagus with bleeding `MCC`
EXCLUDES 2   *bleeding esophageal varices (I85.01, I85.11)*
CC Excl: PDX collection 765

K22.2   Esophageal obstruction
Compression of esophagus
Constriction of esophagus
Stenosis of esophagus
Stricture of esophagus
EXCLUDES 1   *congenital stenosis or stricture of esophagus (Q39.3)*

K22.3   Perforation of esophagus `MCC`
Rupture of esophagus
EXCLUDES 1   *traumatic perforation of (thoracic) esophagus (S27.8-)*
CC Excl: PDX collection 766

K22.4   Dyskinesia of esophagus
Corkscrew esophagus
Diffuse esophageal spasm
Spasm of esophagus
EXCLUDES 1   *cardiospasm (K22.0)*

K22.5   Diverticulum of esophagus, acquired
Esophageal pouch, acquired
EXCLUDES 1   *diverticulum of esophagus (congenital) (Q39.6)*

K22.6   Gastro-esophageal laceration-hemorrhage syndrome `MCC`
Mallory-Weiss syndrome
CC Excl: PDX collection 767

✓5th K22.7   Barrett's esophagus
Barrett's disease
Barrett's syndrome
EXCLUDES 1   *Barrett's ulcer (K22.1)*
malignant neoplasm of esophagus (C15.)
DEF: A metaplastic disorder in which specialized columnar epithelial cells replace the normal squamous epithelial cells; secondary to chronic gastroesophageal reflux damage to the mucosa; increases risk of developing adenocarcinoma.

     K22.70   Barrett's esophagus without dysplasia
Barrett's esophagus NOS

     ✓6th **K22.71   Barrett's esophagus with dysplasia**
         K22.710   Barrett's esophagus with low grade dysplasia
         K22.711   Barrett's esophagus with high grade dysplasia
         K22.719   Barrett's esophagus with dysplasia, unspecified

K22.8   Other specified diseases of esophagus
Hemorrhage of esophagus NOS
EXCLUDES 2   *esophageal varices (I85.-)*
Paterson-Kelly syndrome (D50.1)

K22.9   Disease of esophagus, unspecified

Chapter 11. Diseases of the Digestive System

Gastrointestinal Ulcers

Esophagus
Esophageal ulcer
Stomach
Duodenal ulcer
Gastric ulcer
Small intestine

K23 Disorders of esophagus in diseases classified elsewhere

Code first underlying disease, such as:
  congenital syphilis (A50.5)

EXCLUDES 1   late syphilis (A52.79)
            megaesophagus due to Chagas' disease (B57.31)
            tuberculosis (A18.83)

✓4ᵗʰ K25 Gastric ulcer

INCLUDES   erosion (acute) of stomach
         pylorus ulcer (peptic)
         stomach ulcer (peptic)

Use additional code to identify:
  alcohol abuse and dependence (F10.-)

EXCLUDES 1   acute gastritis (K29.0-)
            peptic ulcer NOS (K27.-)

CC Excl: For CC/MCC codes in category K25: PDX collection 765

K25.0	Acute **gastric ulcer** with hemorrhage	MCC
K25.1	Acute **gastric ulcer** with perforation	MCC HCC
K25.2	Acute **gastric ulcer** with both hemorrhage and perforation	MCC HCC
K25.3	Acute **gastric ulcer** without hemorrhage or perforation	CC
K25.4	Chronic or unspecified **gastric ulcer** with hemorrhage	MCC
K25.5	Chronic or unspecified **gastric ulcer** with perforation	MCC HCC
K25.6	Chronic or unspecified **gastric ulcer** with both hemorrhage and perforation	MCC HCC
K25.7	Chronic **gastric ulcer** without hemorrhage or perforation	
K25.9	**Gastric ulcer, unspecified as acute or chronic,** without hemorrhage or perforation	

✓4ᵗʰ K26 Duodenal ulcer

INCLUDES   erosion (acute) of duodenum
         duodenum ulcer (peptic)
         postpyloric ulcer (peptic)

Use additional code to identify:
  alcohol abuse and dependence (F10.-)

EXCLUDES 1   peptic ulcer NOS (K27.-)

CC Excl: For MCC codes in category K26, unless otherwise noted: PDX collection 768

K26.0	Acute **duodenal ulcer** with hemorrhage	MCC
K26.1	Acute **duodenal ulcer** with perforation	MCC HCC
K26.2	Acute **duodenal ulcer** with both hemorrhage and perforation	MCC HCC
K26.3	Acute **duodenal ulcer** without hemorrhage or perforation	CC
	CC Excl: PDX collection 769	
K26.4	Chronic or unspecified **duodenal ulcer** with hemorrhage	MCC
	AHA: 2016, 1Q, 14	
K26.5	Chronic or unspecified **duodenal ulcer** with perforation	MCC HCC
K26.6	Chronic or unspecified **duodenal ulcer** with both hemorrhage and perforation	MCC HCC
K26.7	Chronic **duodenal ulcer** without hemorrhage or perforation	
K26.9	**Duodenal ulcer, unspecified as acute or chronic,** without hemorrhage or perforation	

✓4ᵗʰ K27 Peptic ulcer, site unspecified

INCLUDES   gastroduodenal ulcer NOS
         peptic ulcer NOS

Use additional code to identify:
  alcohol abuse and dependence (F10.-)

EXCLUDES 1   peptic ulcer of newborn (P78.82)

CC Excl: For CC/MCC codes in category K27: PDX collection 768

K27.0	Acute **peptic ulcer, site unspecified,** with hemorrhage	MCC
K27.1	Acute **peptic ulcer, site unspecified,** with perforation	MCC HCC
K27.2	Acute **peptic ulcer, site unspecified,** with both hemorrhage and perforation	MCC HCC
K27.3	Acute **peptic ulcer, site unspecified,** without hemorrhage or perforation	CC
K27.4	Chronic or unspecified **peptic ulcer, site unspecified,** with hemorrhage	MCC
K27.5	Chronic or unspecified **peptic ulcer, site unspecified,** with perforation	HCC
K27.6	Chronic or unspecified **peptic ulcer, site unspecified,** with both hemorrhage and perforation	MCC HCC
K27.7	Chronic **peptic ulcer, site unspecified,** without hemorrhage or perforation	
K27.9	**Peptic ulcer, site unspecified, unspecified as acute or chronic,** without hemorrhage or perforation	

✓4ᵗʰ K28 Gastrojejunal ulcer

INCLUDES   anastomotic ulcer (peptic) or erosion
         gastrocolic ulcer (peptic) or erosion
         gastrointestinal ulcer (peptic) or erosion
         gastrojejunal ulcer (peptic) or erosion
         jejunal ulcer (peptic) or erosion
         marginal ulcer (peptic) or erosion
         stomal ulcer (peptic) or erosion

Use additional code to identify:
  alcohol abuse and dependence (F10.-)

EXCLUDES 1   primary ulcer of small intestine (K63.3)

CC Excl: For CC/MCC codes in category K28: PDX collection 765

K28.0	Acute **gastrojejunal ulcer** with hemorrhage	MCC
K28.1	Acute **gastrojejunal ulcer** with perforation	MCC HCC
K28.2	Acute **gastrojejunal ulcer** with both hemorrhage and perforation	MCC HCC
K28.3	Acute **gastrojejunal ulcer** without hemorrhage or perforation	CC
K28.4	Chronic or unspecified **gastrojejunal ulcer** with hemorrhage	MCC
K28.5	Chronic or unspecified **gastrojejunal ulcer** with perforation	MCC HCC
K28.6	Chronic or unspecified **gastrojejunal ulcer** with both hemorrhage and perforation	MCC HCC
K28.7	Chronic **gastrojejunal ulcer** without hemorrhage or perforation	
K28.9	**Gastrojejunal ulcer, unspecified as acute or chronic,** without hemorrhage or perforation	

✓4ᵗʰ K29 Gastritis and duodenitis

EXCLUDES 1   eosinophilic gastritis or gastroenteritis (K52.81)
            Zollinger-Ellison syndrome (E16.4)

CC Excl: For MCC codes in category K29: PDX collection 770

✓5ᵗʰ **K29.0**	Acute **gastritis**	
	Use additional code to identify:	
	alcohol abuse and dependence (F10.-)	
	EXCLUDES 1 erosion (acute) of stomach (K25.-)	
K29.00	Acute **gastritis** without bleeding	
K29.01	Acute **gastritis** with bleeding	MCC
✓5ᵗʰ **K29.2**	Alcoholic **gastritis**	
	Use additional code to identify:	
	alcohol abuse and dependence (F10.-)	
K29.20	Alcoholic **gastritis** without bleeding	
K29.21	Alcoholic **gastritis** with bleeding	MCC
✓5ᵗʰ **K29.3**	Chronic superficial **gastritis**	
K29.30	Chronic superficial **gastritis** without bleeding	
K29.31	Chronic superficial **gastritis** with bleeding	MCC
✓5ᵗʰ **K29.4**	Chronic atrophic **gastritis**	
	Gastric atrophy	
K29.40	Chronic atrophic **gastritis** without bleeding	
K29.41	Chronic atrophic **gastritis** with bleeding	MCC

N Newborn: 0   P Pediatric: 0-17   M Maternity: 12-55   A Adult: 15-124   MCC Major CC Condition   PDxMCC PDx acts as own MCC   CC CC Condition   PDxCC PDx acts as own CC

692   ICD-10-CM 2018

✓5th **K29.5** **Unspecified chronic gastritis**
Chronic antral gastritis
Chronic fundal gastritis
　K29.50 **Unspecified chronic gastritis** without bleeding
　K29.51 **Unspecified chronic gastritis** with bleeding　MCC

✓5th **K29.6** **Other gastritis**
Giant hypertrophic gastritis
Granulomatous gastritis
Ménétrier's disease
　K29.60 **Other gastritis** without bleeding
　K29.61 **Other gastritis** with bleeding　MCC

✓5th **K29.7** **Gastritis, unspecified**
　K29.70 **Gastritis, unspecified, without bleeding**
　K29.71 **Gastritis, unspecified, with bleeding**　MCC

✓5th **K29.8** **Duodenitis**
　K29.80 **Duodenitis without bleeding**
　K29.81 **Duodenitis with bleeding**　MCC

✓5th **K29.9** **Gastroduodenitis, unspecified**
　K29.90 **Gastroduodenitis, unspecified, without bleeding**
　K29.91 **Gastroduodenitis, unspecified, with bleeding**　MCC

K30 **Functional dyspepsia**
Indigestion
　EXCLUDES 1　*dyspepsia NOS (R10.13)*
　　　heartburn (R12)
　　　nervous dyspepsia (F45.8)
　　　neurotic dyspepsia (F45.8)
　　　psychogenic dyspepsia (F45.8)

✓4th **K31** **Other diseases of stomach and duodenum**
　INCLUDES　functional disorders of stomach
　EXCLUDES 2　*diabetic gastroparesis (E08.43, E09.43, E10.43, E11.43, E13.43)*
　　　diverticulum of duodenum (K57.00-K57.13)

　K31.0 **Acute dilatation of stomach**　CC
　　Acute distention of stomach
　　CC Excl: PDX collection 771

　K31.1 **Adult hypertrophic pyloric stenosis**　CC A
　　Pyloric stenosis NOS
　　EXCLUDES 1　*congenital or infantile pyloric stenosis (Q40.0)*
　　CC Excl: PDX collection 772

　K31.2 **Hourglass stricture and stenosis of stomach**
　　EXCLUDES 1　*congenital hourglass stomach (Q40.2)*
　　　hourglass contraction of stomach (K31.89)

　K31.3 **Pylorospasm, not elsewhere classified**
　　EXCLUDES 1　*congenital or infantile pylorospasm (Q40.0)*
　　　neurotic pylorospasm (F45.8)
　　　psychogenic pylorospasm (F45.8)

　K31.4 **Gastric diverticulum**
　　EXCLUDES 1　*congenital diverticulum of stomach (Q40.2)*

　K31.5 **Obstruction of duodenum**　CC
　　Constriction of duodenum
　　Duodenal ileus (chronic)
　　Stenosis of duodenum
　　Stricture of duodenum
　　Volvulus of duodenum
　　EXCLUDES 1　*congenital stenosis of duodenum (Q41.0)*
　　CC Excl: PDX collection 773

　K31.6 **Fistula of stomach and duodenum**　CC
　　Gastrocolic fistula
　　Gastrojejunocolic fistula
　　CC Excl: PDX collection 774

　K31.7 **Polyp of stomach and duodenum**
　　EXCLUDES 1　*adenomatous polyp of stomach (D13.1)*

✓5th **K31.8** **Other specified diseases of stomach and duodenum**
　✓6th **K31.81** **Angiodysplasia of stomach and duodenum**
　　　K31.811 **Angiodysplasia of stomach and**　MCC
　　　　duodenum with bleeding
　　　　CC Excl: PDX collection 770
　　　K31.819 **Angiodysplasia of stomach and**
　　　　duodenum without bleeding
　　　　Angiodysplasia of stomach and duodenum NOS
　　K31.82 **Dieulafoy lesion (hemorrhagic) of stomach and**　MCC
　　　duodenum
　　　EXCLUDES 2　*Dieulafoy lesion of intestine (K63.81)*
　　　CC Excl: PDX collection 775

K31.83 **Achlorhydria**
　DEF: Absence of hydrochloric acid in gastric secretions due to gastric mucosa atrophy; unresponsive to histamines; also known as gastric anacidity.

K31.84 **Gastroparesis**
　Gastroparalysis
　Code first underlying disease, if known, such as:
　　anorexia nervosa (F50.0-)
　　diabetes mellitus (E08.43, E09.43, E10.43, E11.43, E13.43)
　　scleroderma (M34.-)
　AHA: 2013, 4Q, 114

K31.89 **Other diseases of stomach and duodenum**
　AHA: 2017, 1Q, 28

K31.9 **Disease of stomach and duodenum, unspecified**

Diseases of appendix (K35-K38)

✓4th **K35** **Acute appendicitis**

　CC Excl: For CC/MCC codes in category K35: PDX collection 776

　K35.2 **Acute appendicitis with generalized peritonitis**　MCC
　　Appendicitis (acute) with generalized (diffuse) peritonitis following rupture or perforation of appendix
　　Perforated appendix NOS
　　Ruptured appendix NOS

　K35.3 **Acute appendicitis with localized peritonitis**　MCC
　　Acute appendicitis with or without perforation or rupture with peritonitis NOS
　　Acute appendicitis with or without perforation or rupture with localized peritonitis
　　Acute appendicitis with peritoneal abscess

✓5th **K35.8** **Other and unspecified acute appendicitis**
　K35.80 **Unspecified acute appendicitis**　CC
　　Acute appendicitis NOS
　　Acute appendicitis without (localized) (generalized) peritonitis
　K35.89 **Other acute appendicitis**　CC

K36 **Other appendicitis**
　Chronic appendicitis
　Recurrent appendicitis

K37 **Unspecified appendicitis**
　EXCLUDES 1　*unspecified appendicitis with peritonitis (K35.2-K35.3)*

✓4th **K38** **Other diseases of appendix**
　K38.0 **Hyperplasia of appendix**
　K38.1 **Appendicular concretions**
　　Fecalith of appendix
　　Stercolith of appendix
　K38.2 **Diverticulum of appendix**
　K38.3 **Fistula of appendix**
　K38.8 **Other specified diseases of appendix**
　　Intussusception of appendix
　K38.9 **Disease of appendix, unspecified**

Hernia (K40-K46)

　NOTE　Hernia with both gangrene and obstruction is classified to hernia with gangrene.
　INCLUDES　acquired hernia
　　congenital [except diaphragmatic or hiatus] hernia
　　recurrent hernia

✓4th **K40** **Inguinal hernia**
　INCLUDES　bubonocele
　　direct inguinal hernia
　　double inguinal hernia
　　indirect inguinal hernia
　　inguinal hernia NOS
　　oblique inguinal hernia
　　scrotal hernia

　CC Excl: For CC/MCC codes in category K40: PDX collection 777

✓5th **K40.0** **Bilateral inguinal hernia, with obstruction, without gangrene**
　　Inguinal hernia (bilateral) causing obstruction without gangrene
　　Incarcerated inguinal hernia (bilateral) without gangrene
　　Irreducible inguinal hernia (bilateral) without gangrene
　　Strangulated inguinal hernia (bilateral) without gangrene
　K40.00 **Bilateral inguinal hernia, with obstruction, without gangrene, not specified as recurrent**
　　Bilateral inguinal hernia, with obstruction, without gangrene NOS

✓Additional Character Req　✓x7th Placeholder Alert　Unacceptable PDx　Manifestation　H1 -H14 HAC　HCC CMS-HCC Condition　EXCLUDES 1 Not Coded Here　EXCLUDES 2 Not Included Here

Chapter 11. Diseases of the Digestive System

Hernia Sites

K40.01 Bilateral inguinal hernia, with obstruction, without gangrene, recurrent `CC`

√5th **K40.1 Bilateral inguinal hernia, with gangrene**

K40.10 Bilateral inguinal hernia, with gangrene, not specified as recurrent `MCC`
Bilateral inguinal hernia, with gangrene NOS

K40.11 Bilateral inguinal hernia, with gangrene, recurrent `MCC`

√5th **K40.2 Bilateral inguinal hernia, without obstruction or gangrene**

K40.20 Bilateral inguinal hernia, without obstruction or gangrene, not specified as recurrent
Bilateral inguinal hernia NOS

K40.21 Bilateral inguinal hernia, without obstruction or gangrene, recurrent

√5th **K40.3 Unilateral inguinal hernia, with obstruction, without gangrene**
Inguinal hernia (unilateral) causing obstruction without gangrene
Incarcerated inguinal hernia (unilateral) without gangrene
Irreducible inguinal hernia (unilateral) without gangrene
Strangulated inguinal hernia (unilateral) without gangrene

K40.30 Unilateral inguinal hernia, with obstruction, without gangrene, not specified as recurrent `CC`
Inguinal hernia, with obstruction NOS
Unilateral inguinal hernia, with obstruction, without gangrene NOS

K40.31 Unilateral inguinal hernia, with obstruction, without gangrene, recurrent `CC`

√5th **K40.4 Unilateral inguinal hernia, with gangrene**

K40.40 Unilateral inguinal hernia, with gangrene, not specified as recurrent `MCC`
Inguinal hernia with gangrene NOS
Unilateral inguinal hernia with gangrene NOS

K40.41 Unilateral inguinal hernia, with gangrene, recurrent `MCC`

√5th **K40.9 Unilateral inguinal hernia, without obstruction or gangrene**

K40.90 Unilateral inguinal hernia, without obstruction or gangrene, not specified as recurrent
Inguinal hernia NOS
Unilateral inguinal hernia NOS

K40.91 Unilateral inguinal hernia, without obstruction or gangrene, recurrent

√4th **K41 Femoral hernia**

CC Excl: For CC/MCC codes in category K41, unless otherwise noted: PDX collection 778

√5th **K41.0 Bilateral femoral hernia, with obstruction, without gangrene**
Femoral hernia (bilateral) causing obstruction, without gangrene
Incarcerated femoral hernia (bilateral), without gangrene
Irreducible femoral hernia (bilateral), without gangrene
Strangulated femoral hernia (bilateral), without gangrene

K41.00 Bilateral femoral hernia, with obstruction, without gangrene, not specified as recurrent `CC`
Bilateral femoral hernia, with obstruction, without gangrene NOS

K41.01 Bilateral femoral hernia, with obstruction, without gangrene, recurrent `CC`

√5th **K41.1 Bilateral femoral hernia, with gangrene**

K41.10 Bilateral femoral hernia, with gangrene, not specified as recurrent `MCC`
Bilateral femoral hernia, with gangrene NOS
CC Excl: PDX collection 779

K41.11 Bilateral femoral hernia, with gangrene, recurrent `MCC`
CC Excl: PDX collection 779

√5th **K41.2 Bilateral femoral hernia, without obstruction or gangrene**

K41.20 Bilateral femoral hernia, without obstruction or gangrene, not specified as recurrent
Bilateral femoral hernia NOS

K41.21 Bilateral femoral hernia, without obstruction or gangrene, recurrent

√5th **K41.3 Unilateral femoral hernia, with obstruction, without gangrene**
Femoral hernia (unilateral) causing obstruction, without gangrene
Incarcerated femoral hernia (unilateral), without gangrene
Irreducible femoral hernia (unilateral), without gangrene
Strangulated femoral hernia (unilateral), without gangrene

K41.30 Unilateral femoral hernia, with obstruction, without gangrene, not specified as recurrent `CC`
Femoral hernia, with obstruction NOS
Unilateral femoral hernia, with obstruction NOS

K41.31 Unilateral femoral hernia, with obstruction, without gangrene, recurrent `CC`

√5th **K41.4 Unilateral femoral hernia, with gangrene**

K41.40 Unilateral femoral hernia, with gangrene, not specified as recurrent `MCC`
Femoral hernia, with gangrene NOS
Unilateral femoral hernia, with gangrene NOS
CC Excl: PDX collection 779

K41.41 Unilateral femoral hernia, with gangrene, recurrent `MCC`
CC Excl: PDX collection 779

√5th **K41.9 Unilateral femoral hernia, without obstruction or gangrene**

K41.90 Unilateral femoral hernia, without obstruction or gangrene, not specified as recurrent
Femoral hernia NOS
Unilateral femoral hernia NOS

K41.91 Unilateral femoral hernia, without obstruction or gangrene, recurrent

√4th **K42 Umbilical hernia**
`INCLUDES` paraumbilical hernia
`EXCLUDES 1` *omphalocele (Q79.2)*

K42.0 Umbilical hernia with obstruction, without gangrene `CC`
Umbilical hernia causing obstruction, without gangrene
Incarcerated umbilical hernia, without gangrene
Irreducible umbilical hernia, without gangrene
Strangulated umbilical hernia, without gangrene
CC Excl: PDX collection 780

K42.1 Umbilical hernia with gangrene `MCC`
Gangrenous umbilical hernia
CC Excl: PDX collection 781

K42.9 Umbilical hernia without obstruction or gangrene
Umbilical hernia NOS

√4th **K43 Ventral hernia**

K43.0 Incisional hernia with obstruction, without gangrene `CC`
Incisional hernia causing obstruction, without gangrene
Incarcerated incisional hernia, without gangrene
Irreducible incisional hernia, without gangrene
Strangulated incisional hernia, without gangrene
CC Excl: PDX collection 780

K43.1 Incisional hernia with gangrene `MCC`
Gangrenous incisional hernia
CC Excl: PDX collection 781

K43.2 Incisional hernia without obstruction or gangrene
Incisional hernia NOS

K43.3 Parastomal hernia with obstruction, without gangrene `CC`
Incarcerated parastomal hernia, without gangrene
Irreducible parastomal hernia, without gangrene
Parastomal hernia causing obstruction, without gangrene
Strangulated parastomal hernia, without gangrene
CC Excl: PDX collection 780

K43.4 Parastomal hernia with gangrene `MCC`
Gangrenous parastomal hernia
CC Excl: PDX collection 781

K43.5 Parastomal hernia without obstruction or gangrene
Parastomal hernia NOS

N Newborn: 0   P Pediatric: 0-17   M Maternity: 12-55   A Adult: 15-124   MCC Major CC Condition   PDxMCC PDx acts as own MCC   CC CC Condition   PDxCC PDx acts as own CC

694   ICD-10-CM 2018

K43.6 **Other and unspecified ventral hernia with obstruction, without gangrene** `CC`
     Epigastric hernia causing obstruction, without gangrene
     Hypogastric hernia causing obstruction, without gangrene
     Incarcerated epigastric hernia without gangrene
     Incarcerated hypogastric hernia without gangrene
     Incarcerated midline hernia without gangrene
     Incarcerated spigelian hernia without gangrene
     Incarcerated subxiphoid hernia without gangrene
     Irreducible epigastric hernia without gangrene
     Irreducible hypogastric hernia without gangrene
     Irreducible midline hernia without gangrene
     Irreducible spigelian hernia without gangrene
     Irreducible subxiphoid hernia without gangrene
     Midline hernia causing obstruction, without gangrene
     Spigelian hernia causing obstruction, without gangrene
     Strangulated epigastric hernia without gangrene
     Strangulated hypogastric hernia without gangrene
     Strangulated midline hernia without gangrene
     Strangulated spigelian hernia without gangrene
     Strangulated subxiphoid hernia without gangrene
     Subxiphoid hernia causing obstruction, without gangrene
     CC Excl: PDX collection 780

K43.7 **Other and unspecified ventral hernia with gangrene** `MCC`
     Any condition listed under K43.6 specified as gangrenous
     CC Excl: PDX collection 781

K43.9 **Ventral hernia without obstruction or gangrene**
     Epigastric hernia
     Ventral hernia NOS

✓4ᵗʰ **K44** **Diaphragmatic hernia**
     INCLUDES   hiatus hernia (esophageal) (sliding)
             paraesophageal hernia
     EXCLUDES 1   *congenital diaphragmatic hernia (Q79.0)*
             congenital hiatus hernia (Q40.1)

K44.0 **Diaphragmatic hernia with obstruction, without gangrene** `CC`
     Diaphragmatic hernia causing obstruction
     Incarcerated diaphragmatic hernia
     Irreducible diaphragmatic hernia
     Strangulated diaphragmatic hernia
     CC Excl: PDX collection 782

K44.1 **Diaphragmatic hernia with gangrene** `MCC`
     Gangrenous diaphragmatic hernia
     CC Excl: PDX collection 782

K44.9 **Diaphragmatic hernia without obstruction or gangrene**
     Diaphragmatic hernia NOS

Hiatal Hernia

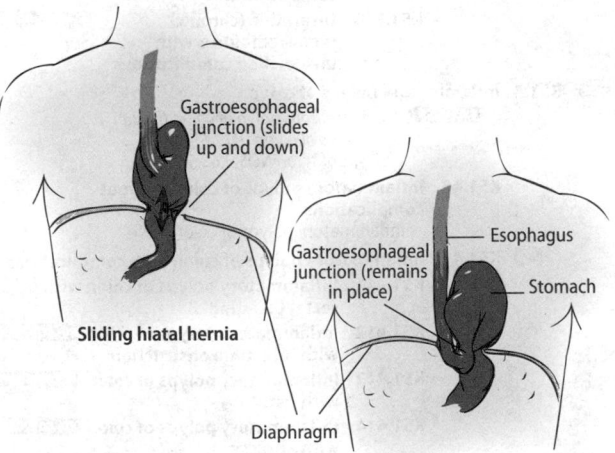

Gastroesophageal junction (slides up and down)

Sliding hiatal hernia

Esophagus

Gastroesophageal junction (remains in place)

Stomach

Diaphragm

Paraesophageal hiatal hernia

✓4ᵗʰ **K45** **Other abdominal hernia**
     INCLUDES   abdominal hernia, specified site NEC
             lumbar hernia
             obturator hernia
             pudendal hernia
             retroperitoneal hernia
             sciatic hernia

K45.0 **Other specified abdominal hernia with obstruction, without gangrene** `CC`
     Other specified abdominal hernia causing obstruction
     Other specified incarcerated abdominal hernia
     Other specified irreducible abdominal hernia
     Other specified strangulated abdominal hernia
     CC Excl: PDX collection 783

K45.1 **Other specified abdominal hernia with gangrene** `MCC`
     Any condition listed under K45 specified as gangrenous
     CC Excl: PDX collection 784

K45.8 **Other specified abdominal hernia without obstruction or gangrene**

✓4ᵗʰ **K46** **Unspecified abdominal hernia**
     INCLUDES   enterocele
             epiplocele
             hernia NOS
             interstitial hernia
             intestinal hernia
             intra-abdominal hernia
     EXCLUDES 1   *vaginal enterocele (N81.5)*

K46.0 **Unspecified abdominal hernia with obstruction, without gangrene** `CC`
     Unspecified abdominal hernia causing obstruction
     Unspecified incarcerated abdominal hernia
     Unspecified irreducible abdominal hernia
     Unspecified strangulated abdominal hernia
     CC Excl: PDX collection 783

K46.1 **Unspecified abdominal hernia with gangrene** `MCC`
     Any condition listed under K46 specified as gangrenous
     CC Excl: PDX collection 784

K46.9 **Unspecified abdominal hernia without obstruction or gangrene**
     Abdominal hernia NOS

Noninfective enteritis and colitis (K50-K52)

     INCLUDES   noninfective inflammatory bowel disease
     EXCLUDES 1   *irritable bowel syndrome (K58.-)*
             megacolon (K59.3-)

✓4ᵗʰ **K50** **Crohn's disease [regional enteritis]**
     INCLUDES   granulomatous enteritis
     Use additional code to identify manifestations, such as:
         pyoderma gangrenosum (L88)
     EXCLUDES 1   *ulcerative colitis (K51.-)*
     AHA: 2012, 4Q, 104

> **CC Excl: For CC codes in category K50, unless otherwise noted:** PDX collection 785

✓5ᵗʰ **K50.0** **Crohn's disease of small intestine**
     Crohn's disease [regional enteritis] of duodenum
     Crohn's disease [regional enteritis] of ileum
     Crohn's disease [regional enteritis] of jejunum
     Regional ileitis
     Terminal ileitis
     EXCLUDES 1   *Crohn's disease of both small and large intestine (K50.8-)*

     K50.00 **Crohn's disease of small intestine without complications** `CC` `HCC`

✓6ᵗʰ   **K50.01** **Crohn's disease of small intestine with complications**

         K50.011 **Crohn's disease of small intestine with rectal bleeding** `CC` `HCC`

         K50.012 **Crohn's disease of small intestine with intestinal obstruction** `PDxCC` `CC` `HCC`

         K50.013 **Crohn's disease of small intestine with fistula** `PDxCC` `CC` `HCC`

         K50.014 **Crohn's disease of small intestine with abscess** `PDxCC` `CC` `HCC`
             AHA: 2012, 4Q, 104

         K50.018 **Crohn's disease of small intestine with other complication** `CC` `HCC`

         K50.019 **Crohn's disease of small intestine with unspecified complications** `CC` `HCC`

✓ Additional Character Req   ✓x7ᵗʰ Placeholder Alert   Unacceptable PDx   Manifestation   H1 - H14 HAC   HCC CMS-HCC Condition   *EXCLUDES 1* Not Coded Here   *EXCLUDES 2* Not Included Here

✓5ᵗʰ K50.1 Crohn's disease of large intestine
Crohn's disease [regional enteritis] of colon
Crohn's disease [regional enteritis] of large bowel
Crohn's disease [regional enteritis] of rectum
Granulomatous colitis
Regional colitis

EXCLUDES 1 *Crohn's disease of both small and large intestine (K50.8)*

K50.10 Crohn's disease of large intestine without complications `CC` `HCC`

✓6ᵗʰ K50.11 Crohn's disease of large intestine with complications

K50.111 Crohn's disease of large intestine with rectal bleeding `CC` `HCC`

K50.112 Crohn's disease of large intestine with intestinal obstruction `PDxCC` `CC` `HCC`

K50.113 Crohn's disease of large intestine with fistula `PDxCC` `CC` `HCC`

K50.114 Crohn's disease of large intestinewith abscess `PDxCC` `CC` `HCC`

K50.118 Crohn's disease of large intestine with other complication `CC` `HCC`

K50.119 Crohn's disease of large intestine with unspecified complications `CC` `HCC`

✓5ᵗʰ K50.8 Crohn's disease of both small and large intestine

K50.80 Crohn's disease of both small and large intestine without complications `CC` `HCC`

✓6ᵗʰ K50.81 Crohn's disease of both small and large intestine with complications

K50.811 Crohn's disease of both small and large intestine with rectal bleeding `CC` `HCC`

K50.812 Crohn's disease of both small and large intestine with intestinal obstruction `PDxCC` `CC` `HCC`

K50.813 Crohn's disease of both small and large intestine with fistula `PDxCC` `CC` `HCC`

K50.814 Crohn's disease of both small and large intestine with abscess `PDxCC` `CC` `HCC`

K50.818 Crohn's disease of both small and large intestine with other complication `CC` `HCC`

K50.819 Crohn's disease of both small and large intestine with unspecified complications `CC` `HCC`

✓5ᵗʰ K50.9 Crohn's disease, unspecified

CC Excl: For CC codes in subcategory K50.9:
PDX collection 786

K50.90 Crohn's disease, unspecified, without complications `CC` `HCC`
Crohn's disease NOS
Regional enteritis NOS

✓6ᵗʰ K50.91 Crohn's disease, unspecified, with complications

K50.911 Crohn's disease, unspecified, with rectal bleeding `CC` `HCC`

K50.912 Crohn's disease, unspecified, with intestinal obstruction `PDxCC` `CC` `HCC`

K50.913 Crohn's disease, unspecified, with fistula `PDxCC` `CC` `HCC`

K50.914 Crohn's disease, unspecified, with abscess `PDxCC` `CC` `HCC`

K50.918 Crohn's disease, unspecified, with other complication `CC` `HCC`

K50.919 Crohn's disease, unspecified, with unspecified complications `CC` `HCC`

✓4ᵗʰ K51 Ulcerative colitis
Use additional code to identify manifestations, such as:
pyoderma gangrenosum (L88)

EXCLUDES 1 *Crohn's disease [regional enteritis] (K50.-)*

CC Excl: For CC codes in category K51, unless otherwise noted:
PDX collection 785

✓5ᵗʰ K51.0 Ulcerative (chronic) pancolitis
Backwash ileitis

K51.00 Ulcerative (chronic) pancolitis without complications `CC` `HCC`
Ulcerative (chronic) pancolitis NOS

✓6ᵗʰ K51.01 Ulcerative (chronic) pancolitis with complications

K51.011 Ulcerative (chronic) pancolitis with rectal bleeding `CC` `HCC`

K51.012 Ulcerative (chronic) pancolitis with intestinal obstruction `PDxCC` `CC` `HCC`

K51.013 Ulcerative (chronic) pancolitis with fistula `PDxCC` `CC` `HCC`

K51.014 Ulcerative (chronic) pancolitis with abscess `PDxCC` `CC` `HCC`

K51.018 Ulcerative (chronic) pancolitis with other complication `CC` `HCC`

K51.019 Ulcerative (chronic) pancolitis with unspecified complications `CC` `HCC`

✓5ᵗʰ K51.2 Ulcerative (chronic) proctitis

K51.20 Ulcerative (chronic) proctitis without complications `CC` `HCC`
Ulcerative (chronic) proctitis NOS

✓6ᵗʰ K51.21 Ulcerative (chronic) proctitis with complications

K51.211 Ulcerative (chronic) proctitis with rectal bleeding `CC` `HCC`

K51.212 Ulcerative (chronic) proctitis with intestinal obstruction `PDxCC` `CC` `HCC`

K51.213 Ulcerative (chronic) proctitis with fistula `PDxCC` `CC` `HCC`

K51.214 Ulcerative (chronic) proctitis with abscess `PDxCC` `CC` `HCC`

K51.218 Ulcerative (chronic) proctitis with other complication `CC` `HCC`

K51.219 Ulcerative (chronic) proctitis with unspecified complications `CC` `HCC`

✓5ᵗʰ K51.3 Ulcerative (chronic) rectosigmoiditis

K51.30 Ulcerative (chronic) rectosigmoiditis without complications `CC` `HCC`
Ulcerative (chronic) rectosigmoiditis NOS

✓6ᵗʰ K51.31 Ulcerative (chronic) rectosigmoiditis with complications

K51.311 Ulcerative (chronic) rectosigmoiditis with rectal bleeding `CC` `HCC`

K51.312 Ulcerative (chronic) rectosigmoiditis with intestinal obstruction `PDxCC` `CC` `HCC`

K51.313 Ulcerative (chronic) rectosigmoiditis with fistula `PDxCC` `CC` `HCC`

K51.314 Ulcerative (chronic) rectosigmoiditis with abscess `PDxCC` `CC` `HCC`

K51.318 Ulcerative (chronic) rectosigmoiditis with other complication `CC` `HCC`

K51.319 Ulcerative (chronic) rectosigmoiditis with unspecified complications `CC` `HCC`

✓5ᵗʰ K51.4 Inflammatory polyps of colon

EXCLUDES 1 *adenomatous polyp of colon (D12.6)*
polyposis of colon (D12.6)
polyps of colon NOS (K63.5)

K51.40 Inflammatory polyps of colon without complications `CC` `HCC`
Inflammatory polyps of colon NOS

✓6ᵗʰ K51.41 Inflammatory polyps of colon with complications

K51.411 Inflammatory polyps of colon with rectal bleeding `CC` `HCC`

K51.412 Inflammatory polyps of colon with intestinal obstruction `PDxCC` `CC` `HCC`

K51.413 Inflammatory polyps of colon with fistula `PDxCC` `CC` `HCC`

K51.414 Inflammatory polyps of colon with abscess `PDxCC` `CC` `HCC`

K51.418 Inflammatory polyps of colon with other complication `CC` `HCC`

K51.419 Inflammatory polyps of colon with unspecified complications `CC` `HCC`

✓5ᵗʰ K51.5 Left sided colitis
Left hemicolitis

K51.50 Left sided colitis without complications `CC` `HCC`
Left sided colitis NOS

✓6ᵗʰ K51.51 Left sided colitis with complications

K51.511 Left sided colitis with rectal bleeding `CC` `HCC`

K51.512 Left sided colitis with intestinal obstruction `PDxCC` `CC` `HCC`

Ⓝ Newborn: 0   Ⓟ Pediatric: 0-17   Ⓜ Maternity: 12-55   Ⓐ Adult: 15-124   `MCC` Major CC Condition   `PDxMCC` PDx acts as own MCC   `CC` CC Condition   `PDxCC` PDx acts as own CC

696

ICD-10-CM 2018

K51.513   **Left sided colitis with** fistula   `PDxCC` `CC` `HCC`
K51.514   **Left sided colitis with** abscess   `PDxCC` `CC` `HCC`
K51.518   **Left sided colitis with** other **complication**   `CC` `HCC`
K51.519   **Left sided colitis with** unspecified **complications**   `CC` `HCC`

✓5ᵗʰ **K51.8**   **Other ulcerative colitis**

K51.80   **Other ulcerative colitis** without complications `CC` `HCC`

✓6ᵗʰ **K51.81**   **Other ulcerative colitis with complications**

K51.811   **Other ulcerative colitis with** rectal **bleeding**   `CC` `HCC`
K51.812   **Other ulcerative colitis with intestinal obstruction**   `PDxCC` `CC` `HCC`
K51.813   **Other ulcerative colitis with** fistula   `PDxCC` `CC` `HCC`
K51.814   **Other ulcerative colitis with abscess**   `PDxCC` `CC` `HCC`
K51.818   **Other ulcerative colitis with** other **complication**   `CC` `HCC`
K51.819   **Other ulcerative colitis with unspecified complications**   `CC` `HCC`

✓5ᵗʰ **K51.9**   **Ulcerative colitis, unspecified**

CC Excl: For CC codes in subcategory K51.9:
PDX collection 787

K51.90   **Ulcerative colitis, unspecified,** without **complications**   `CC` `HCC`

✓6ᵗʰ **K51.91**   **Ulcerative colitis, unspecified, with complications**

K51.911   **Ulcerative colitis, unspecified with** `CC` `HCC` **rectal bleeding**
K51.912   **Ulcerative colitis, unspecified** `PDxCC` `CC` `HCC` **with intestinal obstruction**
K51.913   **Ulcerative colitis, unspecified** `PDxCC` `CC` `HCC` **with** fistula
K51.914   **Ulcerative colitis, unspecified** `PDxCC` `CC` `HCC` **with abscess**
K51.918   **Ulcerative colitis, unspecified with** `CC` `HCC` other **complication**
K51.919   **Ulcerative colitis, unspecified with** `CC` `HCC` **unspecified complications**

✓4ᵗʰ **K52**   **Other and unspecified noninfective gastroenteritis and colitis**

K52.0   **Gastroenteritis and colitis due to** radiation   `CC`
CC Excl: PDX collection 788

K52.1   **Toxic gastroenteritis and colitis**   `CC`
Drug-induced gastroenteritis and colitis
Code first (T51-T65) to identify toxic agent
Use additional code for adverse effect, if applicable, to identify drug (T36-T50 with fifth or sixth character 5)
CC Excl: PDX collection 789

✓5ᵗʰ **K52.2**   **Allergic and dietetic gastroenteritis and colitis**
Use additional code to identify type of food allergy (Z91.01-, Z91.02-)
EXCLUDES 2   allergic eosinophilic colitis (K52.82)
     allergic eosinophilic esophagitis (K20.0)
     allergic eosinophilic gastritis (K52.81)
     allergic eosinophilic gastroenteritis (K52.81)
     food protein-induced proctocolitis (K52.82)
DEF: True immunoglobulin E (IgE)-mediated allergic reaction of the lining of the stomach, intestines, or colon to food proteins; causes nausea, vomiting, diarrhea, and abdominal cramping.

K52.21   **Food protein-induced** enterocolitis syndrome
Use additional code for hypovolemic shock, if present (R57.1)

K52.22   **Food protein-induced** enteropathy

K52.29   **Other allergic and dietetic gastroenteritis and colitis**
Food hypersensitivity gastroenteritis or colitis
Immediate gastrointestinal hypersensitivity

K52.3   **Indeterminate colitis**
Colonic inflammatory bowel disease unclassified (IBDU)
EXCLUDES 1   unspecified colitis (K52.9)

✓5ᵗʰ **K52.8**   **Other specified noninfective gastroenteritis and colitis**

K52.81   **Eosinophilic gastritis or gastroenteritis**
Eosinophilic enteritis
EXCLUDES 2   eosinophilic esophagitis (K20.0)

K52.82   **Eosinophilic colitis**
Allergic proctocolitis
Food-induced eosinophilic proctocolitis
Food protein-induced proctocolitis
Milk protein-induced proctocolitis

✓6ᵗʰ **K52.83**   **Microscopic colitis**

K52.831   **Collagenous colitis**
K52.832   **Lymphocytic colitis**
K52.838   **Other microscopic colitis**
K52.839   **Microscopic colitis,** unspecified

K52.89   **Other specified noninfective gastroenteritis and colitis**

K52.9   **Noninfective gastroenteritis and colitis, unspecified**

Colitis NOS	Ileitis NOS
Enteritis NOS	Jejunitis NOS
Gastroenteritis NOS	Sigmoiditis NOS

EXCLUDES 1   diarrhea NOS (R19.7)
     functional diarrhea (K59.1)
     infectious gastroenteritis and colitis NOS (A09)
     neonatal diarrhea (noninfective) (P78.3)
     psychogenic diarrhea (F45.8)

Other diseases of intestines (K55-K64)

✓4ᵗʰ **K55**   **Vascular disorders of intestine**
EXCLUDES 1   necrotizing enterocolitis of newborn (P77.-)

CC Excl: For MCC codes in category K55, unless otherwise noted:
PDX collection 790

✓5ᵗʰ **K55.0**   **Acute vascular disorders of intestine**
Infarction of appendices epiploicae
Mesenteric (artery) (vein) embolism
Mesenteric (artery) (vein) infarction
Mesenteric (artery) (vein) thrombosis

✓6ᵗʰ **K55.01**   **Acute (reversible)** ischemia **of** small intestine

K55.011   **Focal (segmental) acute** `MCC` `HCC` **(reversible) ischemia of small intestine**
K55.012   **Diffuse acute (reversible)** `MCC` `HCC` **ischemia of small intestine**
K55.019   **Acute (reversible) ischemia of** `MCC` `HCC` **small intestine, extent unspecified**

✓6ᵗʰ **K55.02**   **Acute infarction of** small intestine
Gangrene of small intestine
Necrosis of small intestine

K55.021   **Focal (segmental) acute infarction** `MCC` `HCC` **of small intestine**
K55.022   **Diffuse acute infarction of small** `MCC` `HCC` **intestine**
K55.029   **Acute infarction of small intestine,** `MCC` `HCC` **extent unspecified**

✓6ᵗʰ **K55.03**   **Acute (reversible)** ischemia **of** large intestine
Acute fulminant ischemic colitis
Subacute ischemic colitis

K55.031   **Focal (segmental) acute** `MCC` `HCC` **(reversible) ischemia of large intestine**
K55.032   **Diffuse acute (reversible) ischemia** `MCC` `HCC` **of large intestine**
K55.039   **Acute (reversible) ischemia of** `MCC` `HCC` **large intestine, extent unspecified**

✓6ᵗʰ **K55.04**   **Acute** infarction **of** large intestine
Gangrene of large intestine
Necrosis of large intestine

K55.041   **Focal (segmental) acute infarction** `MCC` `HCC` **of large intestine**
K55.042   **Diffuse acute infarction of large** `MCC` `HCC` **intestine**
K55.049   **Acute infarction of large intestine,** `MCC` `HCC` **extent unspecified**

✓6ᵗʰ **K55.05**   **Acute (reversible)** ischemia **of intestine,** part unspecified

K55.051   **Focal (segmental) acute** `MCC` `HCC` **(reversible) ischemia of intestine, part unspecified**
K55.052   **Diffuse acute (reversible)** `MCC` `HCC` **ischemiaof intestine, part unspecified**
K55.059   **Acute (reversible) ischemia of** `MCC` `HCC` **intestine, part and extent unspecified**

√6th **K55.06**   **Acute infarction of intestine, part unspecified**
Acute intestinal infarction
Gangrene of intestine
Necrosis of intestine

     K55.061   **Focal (segmental) acute infarction** MCC HCC
of intestine, part unspecified

     K55.062   **Diffuse acute infarction of** MCC HCC
intestine, part unspecified

     K55.069   **Acute infarction of intestine, part** MCC HCC
and extent unspecified

K55.1   **Chronic vascular disorders of intestine** CC HCC
Chronic ischemic colitis
Chronic ischemic enteritis
Chronic ischemic enterocolitis
Ischemic stricture of intestine
Mesenteric atherosclerosis
Mesenteric vascular insufficiency
CC Excl: PDX collection 791

√5th **K55.2**   **Angiodysplasia of colon**

     K55.20   **Angiodysplasia of colon without hemorrhage**

     K55.21   **Angiodysplasia of colon with hemorrhage** MCC
DEF: Small vascular abnormalities due to fragile blood
vessels in the colon; results in blood loss from the
gastrointestinal (GI) tract.
CC Excl: PDX collection 770

√5th **K55.3**   **Necrotizing enterocolitis**
EXCLUDES 1   *necrotizing enterocolitis of newborn (P77.-)*
EXCLUDES 2   *necrotizing enterocolitis due to Clostridium difficile*
▶*(A04.7-)*◀

     K55.30   **Necrotizing enterocolitis, unspecified** MCC HCC
Necrotizing enterocolitis, NOS

     K55.31   **Stage 1 necrotizing enterocolitis** MCC HCC
Necrotizing enterocolitis without pneumatosis,
without perforation

     K55.32   **Stage 2 necrotizing enterocolitis** MCC HCC
Necrotizing enterocolitis with pneumatosis, without
perforation

     K55.33   **Stage 3 necrotizing enterocolitis** MCC HCC
Necrotizing enterocolitis with perforation
Necrotizing enterocolitis with pneumatosis and
perforation

K55.8   **Other vascular disorders of intestine** CC HCC
CC Excl: PDX collection 791

K55.9   **Vascular disorder of intestine, unspecified** CC HCC
Ischemic colitis
Ischemic enteritis
Ischemic enterocolitis
CC Excl: PDX collection 791

√4th **K56**   **Paralytic ileus and intestinal obstruction without hernia**
EXCLUDES 1   *congenital stricture or stenosis of intestine (Q41-Q42)*
cystic fibrosis with meconium ileus (E84.11)
intestinal obstruction with hernia (K40-K46)
ischemic stricture of intestine (K55.1)
meconium ileus NOS (P76.0)
neonatal intestinal obstructions classifiable to P76-
obstruction of duodenum (K31.5)
postprocedural intestinal obstruction ▶(K91.3-)◀
stenosis of anus or rectum (K62.4)

CC Excl: For CC/MCC codes in category K56: PDX collection 792

K56.0   **Paralytic ileus** CC HCC
Paralysis of bowel   Paralysis of intestine   Paralysis of colon
EXCLUDES 1   *gallstone ileus (K56.3)*
ileus NOS (K56.7)
obstructive ileus NOS ▶(K56.69-)◀

K56.1   **Intussusception** CC HCC
Intussusception or invagination of bowel
Intussusception or invagination of colon
Intussusception or invagination of intestine
Intussusception or invagination of rectum
EXCLUDES 2   *intussusception of appendix (K38.8)*
DEF: Intestinal obstruction due to prolapse of a bowel section into
adjacent section; occurs primarily in children; symptoms include
acute abdominal pain, vomiting, and passage of blood and mucus
from rectum.

K56.2   **Volvulus** MCC HCC
Strangulation of colon or intestine
Torsion of colon or intestine
Twist of colon or intestine
EXCLUDES 2   *volvulus of duodenum (K31.5)*

Volvulus

Knotted
intestine
(volvulus)

K56.3   **Gallstone ileus** CC HCC
Obstruction of intestine by gallstone

√5th **K56.4**   **Other impaction of intestine**

     K56.41   **Fecal impaction** HCC
EXCLUDES 1   *constipation (K59.0-)*
incomplete defecation (R15.0)

     K56.49   **Other impaction of intestine** CC HCC

▲ √5th **K56.5**   **Intestinal adhesions [bands] with obstruction**
(postinfection)
Abdominal hernia due to adhesions with obstruction
▶Peritoneal adhesions [bands] with intestinal obstruction
(postinfection)◀

●   **K56.50**   **Intestinal adhesions [bands], unspecified as** CC
to partial versus complete obstruction
Intestinal adhesions with obstruction NOS

●   **K56.51**   **Intestinal adhesions [bands], with partial** CC
obstruction
Intestinal adhesions with incomplete obstruction

●   **K56.52**   **Intestinal adhesions [bands] with complete** CC
obstruction

√5th **K56.6**   **Other and unspecified intestinal obstruction**
AHA: 2017, 2Q, 12

√6th   **K56.60**   **Unspecified intestinal obstruction**
~~Intestinal obstruction NOS~~
EXCLUDES 1   *intestinal obstruction due to specified*
condition—code to condition

●   **K56.600**   **Partial intestinal obstruction,** CC
unspecified as to cause
Incomplete intestinal obstruction, NOS

●   **K56.601**   **Complete intestinal obstruction,** CC
unspecified as to cause

●   **K56.609**   **Unspecified intestinal obstruction,** CC
unspecified as to partial versus
complete obstruction
Intestinal obstruction NOS

√6th   **K56.69**   **Other intestinal obstruction**
Enterostenosis NOS
Obstructive ileus NOS
Occlusion of colon or intestine NOS
Stenosis of colon or intestine NOS
Stricture of colon or intestine NOS
EXCLUDES 1   *intestinal obstruction due to specified*
condition—code to condition

●   **K56.690**   **Other partial intestinal obstruction** CC
Other incomplete intestinal obstruction

●   **K56.691**   **Other complete intestinal obstruction** CC

●   **K56.699**   **Other intestinal obstruction** CC
unspecified as to partial versus
complete obstruction
Other intestinal obstruction, NEC

K56.7   **Ileus, unspecified** CC HCC
EXCLUDES 1   *obstructive ileus ▶(K56.69-)◀*
EXCLUDES 2   ▶*intestinal obstruction with hernia (K40-K46)*◀
AHA: 2017, 1Q, 40

☑4ᵗʰ **K57 Diverticular disease of intestine**
> EXCLUDES 1   congenital diverticulum of intestine (Q43.8)
>   Meckel's diverticulum (Q43.0)
> EXCLUDES 2   diverticulum of appendix (K38.2)

CC Excl: For MCC codes in category K57, unless otherwise noted:
PDX collection 770

☑5ᵗʰ **K57.0 Diverticulitis of** small intestine with perforation and abscess
Diverticulitis of small intestine with peritonitis
> EXCLUDES 1   diverticulitis of both small and large intestine with
>   perforation and abscess (K57.4-)

     K57.00 Diverticulitis of small intestine with   `PDxCC` `CC`
           perforation and abscess without bleeding
           CC Excl: PDX collection 793

     K57.01 Diverticulitis of small intestine with   `PDxCC` `MCC`
           perforation and abscess with bleeding

☑5ᵗʰ **K57.1 Diverticular disease of** small intestine without perforation or abscess
> EXCLUDES 1   diverticular disease of both small and large intestine
>   without perforation or abscess (K57.5-)

     K57.10 Diverticulosis of small intestine without perforation
           or abscess without bleeding
           Diverticular disease of small intestine NOS

     K57.11 Diverticulosis of small intestine without   `MCC`
           perforation or abscess with bleeding

     K57.12 Diverticulitis of small intestine without   `CC`
           perforation or abscess without bleeding
           CC Excl: PDX collection 793

     K57.13 Diverticulitis of small intestine without   `MCC`
           perforation or abscess with bleeding

☑5ᵗʰ **K57.2 Diverticulitis of** large intestine with perforation and abscess
Diverticulitis of colon with peritonitis
> EXCLUDES 1   diverticulitis of both small and large intestine with
>   perforation and abscess (K57.4-)

     K57.20 Diverticulitis of large intestine with   `PDxCC` `CC`
           perforation and abscess without bleeding
           CC Excl: PDX collection 794

     K57.21 Diverticulitis of large intestine with   `PDxCC` `MCC`
           perforation and abscess with bleeding

☑5ᵗʰ **K57.3 Diverticular disease of** large intestine without perforation or abscess
> EXCLUDES 1   diverticular disease of both small and large intestine
>   without perforation or abscess (K57.5-)

     K57.30 Diverticulosis of large intestine without perforation
           or abscess without bleeding
           Diverticular disease of colon NOS

     K57.31 Diverticulosis of large intestine without   `MCC`
           perforation or abscess with bleeding

     K57.32 Diverticulitis of large intestine without   `CC`
           perforation or abscess without bleeding
           CC Excl: PDX collection 794

     K57.33 Diverticulitis of large intestine without   `MCC`
           perforation or abscess with bleeding

☑5ᵗʰ **K57.4 Diverticulitis of both** small and large intestine with perforation and abscess
Diverticulitis of both small and large intestine with peritonitis

     K57.40 Diverticulitis of both small and large   `PDxCC` `CC`
           intestine with perforation and abscess
           without bleeding
           CC Excl: PDX collection 794

     K57.41 Diverticulitis of both small and large   `PDxCC` `MCC`
           intestine with perforation and abscess
           with bleeding

☑5ᵗʰ **K57.5 Diverticular disease of** both small and large intestine without perforation or abscess

     K57.50 Diverticulosis of both small and large intestine
           without perforation or abscess without bleeding
           Diverticular disease of both small and large intestine
              NOS

     K57.51 Diverticulosis of both small and large intestine   `MCC`
           without perforation or abscess with bleeding

     K57.52 Diverticulitis of both small and large   `PDxCC` `CC`
           intestine without perforation or abscess
           without bleeding
           CC Excl: PDX collection 794

     K57.53 Diverticulitis of both small and large intestine   `MCC`
           without perforation or abscess with bleeding

☑5ᵗʰ **K57.8 Diverticulitis of intestine,** part unspecified, with perforation and abscess
Diverticulitis of intestine NOS with peritonitis

     K57.80 Diverticulitis of intestine, part unspecified,   `PDxCC` `CC`
           with perforation and abscess without bleeding
           CC Excl: PDX collection 794

     K57.81 Diverticulitis of intestine, part   `PDxCC` `MCC`
           unspecified, with perforation and abscess with
           bleeding

☑5ᵗʰ **K57.9 Diverticular disease of intestine,** part unspecified, without perforation or abscess

     K57.90 Diverticulosis of intestine, part unspecified, without
           perforation or abscess without bleeding
           Diverticular disease of intestine NOS

     K57.91 Diverticulosis of intestine, part unspecified,   `MCC`
           without perforation or abscess with bleeding

     K57.92 Diverticulitis of intestine, part unspecified,   `CC`
           without perforation or abscess without bleeding
           CC Excl: PDX collection 794

     K57.93 Diverticulitis of intestine, part unspecified,   `MCC`
           without perforation or abscess with bleeding

☑4ᵗʰ **K58 Irritable bowel syndrome**
> INCLUDES   irritable colon
>   spastic colon

     K58.0 Irritable bowel syndrome with diarrhea

     K58.1 Irritable bowel syndrome with constipation

     K58.2 Mixed irritable bowel syndrome

     K58.8 Other irritable bowel syndrome

     K58.9 Irritable bowel syndrome without diarrhea
         Irritable bowel syndrome NOS

☑4ᵗʰ **K59 Other functional intestinal disorders**
> EXCLUDES 1   change in bowel habit NOS (R19.4)
>   intestinal malabsorption (K90.-)
>   psychogenic intestinal disorders (F45.8)
> EXCLUDES 2   functional disorders of stomach (K31.-)

☑5ᵗʰ **K59.0 Constipation**
Use additional code for adverse effect, if applicable, to identify
drug (T36-T50 with fifth or sixth character 5)
> EXCLUDES 1   fecal impaction (K56.41)
>   incomplete defecation (R15.0)

     K59.00 Constipation, unspecified

     K59.01 Slow transit constipation
           DEF: Delay in the transit of fecal material through the
           colon secondary to smooth muscle dysfunction or
           decreased peristaltic contractions along the colon: also
           called colonic inertia or delayed transit.

     K59.02 Outlet dysfunction constipation

     K59.03 Drug induced constipation
           Use additional code for adverse effect, if applicable,
             to identify drug (T36-T50 with fifth or sixth
             character 5)

     K59.04 Chronic idiopathic constipation
           Functional constipation

     K59.09 Other constipation
           Chronic constipation

     K59.1 Functional diarrhea
> EXCLUDES 1   diarrhea NOS (R19.7)
>   irritable bowel syndrome with diarrhea (K58.0)

     K59.2 Neurogenic bowel, not elsewhere classified   `CC`
         DEF: Disorder of bowel due to spinal cord lesion due to injury or as
         a complication of conditions such as multiple sclerosis (MS) or
         spina bifida; loss of bowel control is the primary symptom,
         manifested as constipation or bowel incontinence.
         CC Excl: PDX collection 795

☑5ᵗʰ **K59.3 Megacolon, not elsewhere classified**
Dilatation of colon
Code first, if applicable (T51-T65) to identify toxic agent
> EXCLUDES 1   congenital megacolon (aganglionic) (Q43.1)
>   megacolon (due to) (in) Chagas' disease (B57.32)
>   megacolon (due to) (in) Clostridium difficile
>   ►(A04.7-)◄
>   megacolon (due to) (in) Hirschsprung's disease (Q43.1)

CC Excl: For CC codes in subcategory K59.3:
PDX collection 795

     K59.31 Toxic megacolon   `CC` `HCC`

     K59.39 Other megacolon   `CC`
         Megacolon NOS

☑ Additional Character Req   √x7ᵗʰ Placeholder Alert   Unacceptable PDx   Manifestation   H1 - H14 HAC   HCC CMS-HCC Condition   EXCLUDES 1 Not Coded Here   EXCLUDES 2 Not Included Here

ICD-10-CM 2018   699

K59.4   **Anal spasm**
Proctalgia fugax

K59.8   **Other specified functional intestinal disorders**
Atony of colon
Pseudo-obstruction (acute) (chronic) of intestine

K59.9   **Functional intestinal disorder, unspecified**

✓4ᵗʰ **K60**   **Fissure and fistula of anal and rectal regions**
> *EXCLUDES 1*   fissure and fistula of anal and rectal regions with abscess or cellulitis (K61.-)
> *EXCLUDES 2*   anal sphincter tear (healed) (nontraumatic) (old) (K62.81)

K60.0   **Acute anal fissure**

K60.1   **Chronic anal fissure**

K60.2   **Anal fissure, unspecified**

K60.3   **Anal fistula**

K60.4   **Rectal fistula**
Fistula of rectum to skin
> *EXCLUDES 1*   rectovaginal fistula (N82.3)
>   vesicorectal fistual (N32.1)

K60.5   **Anorectal fistula**

✓4ᵗʰ **K61**   **Abscess of anal and rectal regions**
> *INCLUDES*   abscess of anal and rectal regions
>   cellulitis of anal and rectal regions

CC Excl: For CC codes in category K61: PDX collection 796

K61.0   **Anal abscess**   `CC`
Perianal abscess
> *EXCLUDES 1*   intrasphincteric abscess (K61.4)

K61.1   **Rectal abscess**   `CC`
Perirectal abscess
> *EXCLUDES 1*   ischiorectal abscess (K61.3)
AHA: 2012, 4Q, 104

K61.2   **Anorectal abscess**   `CC`

K61.3   **Ischiorectal abscess**   `CC`
Abscess of ischiorectal fossa

K61.4   **Intrasphincteric abscess**   `CC`

✓4ᵗʰ **K62**   **Other diseases of anus and rectum**
> *INCLUDES*   anal canal
> *EXCLUDES 2*   colostomy and enterostomy malfunction (K94.0-, K94.1-)
>   fecal incontinence (R15.-)
>   hemorrhoids (K64.-)

K62.0   **Anal polyp**

K62.1   **Rectal polyp**
> *EXCLUDES 1*   adenomatous polyp (D12.8)

K62.2   **Anal prolapse**
Prolapse of anal canal

K62.3   **Rectal prolapse**
Prolapse of rectal mucosa

K62.4   **Stenosis of anus and rectum**
Stricture of anus (sphincter)

K62.5   **Hemorrhage of anus and rectum**   `CC`
> *EXCLUDES 1*   gastrointestinal bleeding NOS (K92.2)
>   melena (K92.1)
>   neonatal rectal hemorrhage (P54.2)
CC Excl: PDX collection 770

K62.6   **Ulcer of anus and rectum**   `CC`
Solitary ulcer of anus and rectum
Stercoral ulcer of anus and rectum
> *EXCLUDES 1*   fissure and fistula of anus and rectum (K60.-)
>   ulcerative colitis (K51.-)
CC Excl: PDX collection 797

K62.7   **Radiation proctitis**
Use additional code to identify the type of radiation (W90.-)

✓5ᵗʰ **K62.8**   **Other specified diseases of anus and rectum**
> *EXCLUDES 2*   ulcerative proctitis (K51.2)

     K62.81   **Anal sphincter tear (healed) (nontraumatic) (old)**
Tear of anus, nontraumatic
Use additional code for any associated fecal incontinence (R15.-)
> *EXCLUDES 2*   anal fissure (K60.-)
>   anal sphincter tear (healed) (old) complicating delivery (O34.7-)
>   traumatic tear of anal sphincter (S31.831)

     K62.82   **Dysplasia of anus**
Anal intraepithelial neoplasia I and II (AIN I and II) (histologically confirmed)
Dysplasia of anus NOS
Mild and moderate dysplasia of anus (histologically confirmed)
> *EXCLUDES 1*   abnormal results from anal cytologic examination without histologic confirmation (R85.61-)
>   anal intraepithelial neoplasia III (D01.3)
>   carcinoma in situ of anus (D01.3)
>   HGSIL of anus (R85.613)
>   severe dysplasia of anus (D01.3)

     K62.89   **Other specified diseases of anus and rectum**
Proctitis NOS
Use additional code for any associated fecal incontinence (R15.-)

K62.9   **Disease of anus and rectum, unspecified**

✓4ᵗʰ **K63**   **Other diseases of intestine**

K63.0   **Abscess of intestine**   `CC`
> *EXCLUDES 1*   abscess of intestine with Crohn's disease (K50.014, K50.114, K50.814, K50.914)
>   abscess of intestine with diverticular disease (K57.0, K57.2, K57.4, K57.8)
>   abscess of intestine with ulcerative colitis (K51.014, K51.214, K51.314, K51.414, K51.514, K51.814, K51.914)
> *EXCLUDES 2*   abscess of anal and rectal regions (K61.-)
>   abscess of appendix (K35.3)
CC Excl: PDX collection 798

K63.1   **Perforation of intestine (nontraumatic)**   `MCC` `HCC`
Perforation (nontraumatic) of rectum
> *EXCLUDES 1*   perforation (nontraumatic) of duodenum (K26.-)
>   perforation (nontraumatic) of intestine with diverticular disease (K57.0, K57.2, K57.4, K57.8)
> *EXCLUDES 2*   perforation (nontraumatic) of appendix (K35.2, K35.3)
CC Excl: PDX collection 799

K63.2   **Fistula of intestine**   `CC`
> *EXCLUDES 1*   fistula of duodenum (K31.6)
>   fistula of intestine with Crohn's disease (K50.013, K50.113, K50.813, K50.913)
>   fistula of intestine with ulcerative colitis (K51.013, K51.213, K51.313, K51.413, K51.513, K51.813, K51.913)
> *EXCLUDES 2*   fistula of anal and rectal regions (K60.-)
>   fistula of appendix (K38.3)
>   intestinal-genital fistula, female (N82.2-N82.4)
>   vesicointestinal fistula (N32.1)
CC Excl: PDX collection 800

K63.3   **Ulcer of intestine**   `CC`
Primary ulcer of small intestine
> *EXCLUDES 1*   duodenal ulcer (K26.-)
>   gastrointestinal ulcer (K28.-)
>   gastrojejunal ulcer (K28.-)
>   jejunal ulcer (K28.-)
>   peptic ulcer, site unspecified (K27.-)
>   ulcer of intestine with perforation (K63.1)
>   ulcer of anus or rectum (K62.6)
>   ulcerative colitis (K51.-)
CC Excl: PDX collection 801

K63.4   **Enteroptosis**

K63.5   **Polyp of colon**
> *EXCLUDES 1*   adenomatous polyp of colon (D12.6)
>   inflammatory polyp of colon (K51.4-)
>   polyposis of colon (D12.6)
AHA: 2017, 1Q, 15; 2015, 2Q, 14

✓5ᵗʰ **K63.8**   **Other specified diseases of intestine**

     K63.81   **Dieulafoy lesion of intestine**   `MCC`
> *EXCLUDES 2*   Dieulafoy lesion of stomach and duodenum (K31.82)
CC Excl: PDX collection 802

     K63.89   **Other specified diseases of intestine**
AHA: 2013, 2Q, 31

K63.9   **Disease of intestine, unspecified**

✓4ᵗʰ **K64**   **Hemorrhoids and perianal venous thrombosis**
> *INCLUDES*   piles
> *EXCLUDES 1*   hemorrhoids complicating childbirth and the puerperium (O87.2)
>   hemorrhoids complicating pregnancy (O22.4)

K64.0   **First degree hemorrhoids**
Grade/stage I hemorrhoids
Hemorrhoids (bleeding) without prolapse outside of anal canal

N Newborn: 0   P Pediatric: 0-17   M Maternity: 12-55   A Adult: 15-124   MCC Major CC Condition   PDxMCC PDx acts as own MCC   CC CC Condition   PDxCC PDx acts as own CC

700   ICD-10-CM 2018

Hemorrhoids

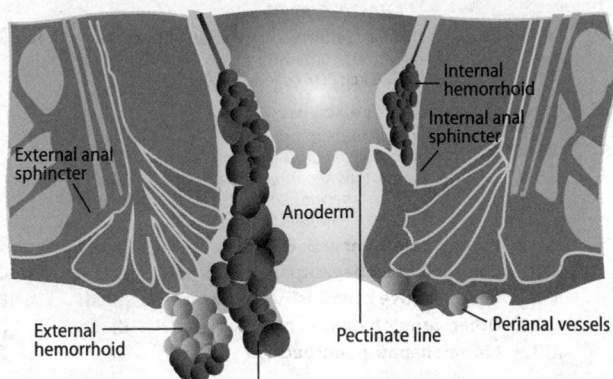

External anal sphincter

Internal hemorrhoid
Internal anal sphincter

Anoderm

External hemorrhoid

Pectinate line

Perianal vessels

Prolapsing internal hemorrhoid

K64.1 Second degree hemorrhoids
Grade/stage II hemorrhoids
Hemorrhoids (bleeding) that prolapse with straining, but retract spontaneously

K64.2 Third degree hemorrhoids
Grade/stage III hemorrhoids
Hemorrhoids (bleeding) that prolapse with straining and require manual replacement back inside anal canal

K64.3 Fourth degree hemorrhoids
Grade/stage IV hemorrhoids
Hemorrhoids (bleeding) with prolapsed tissue that cannot be manually replaced

K64.4 Residual hemorrhoidal skin tags
External hemorrhoids, NOS
Skin tags of anus

K64.5 Perianal venous thrombosis
External hemorrhoids with thrombosis
Perianal hematoma
Thrombosed hemorrhoids NOS

K64.8 Other hemorrhoids
Internal hemorrhoids, without mention of degree
Prolapsed hemorrhoids, degree not specified

K64.9 Unspecified hemorrhoids
Hemorrhoids (bleeding) NOS
Hemorrhoids (bleeding) without mention of degree

Diseases of peritoneum and retroperitoneum (K65-K68)

✓4th K65 Peritonitis
Use additional code (B95-B97), to identify infectious agent
EXCLUDES 1   acute appendicitis with generalized peritonitis (K35.2)
aseptic peritonitis (T81.6)
benign paroxysmal peritonitis (E85.0)
chemical peritonitis (T81.6)
diverticulitis of both small and large intestine with peritonitis (K57.4-)
diverticulitis of colon with peritonitis (K57.2-)
diverticulitis of intestine, NOS, with peritonitis (K57.8-)
diverticulitis of small intestine with peritonitis (K57.0-)
gonococcal peritonitis (A54.85)
neonatal peritonitis (P78.0-P78.1)
pelvic peritonitis, female (N73.3-N73.5)
periodic familial peritonitis (E85.0)
peritonitis due to talc or other foreign substance (T81.6)
peritonitis in chlamydia (A74.81)
peritonitis in diphtheria (A36.89)
peritonitis in syphilis (late) (A52.74)
peritonitis in tuberculosis (A18.31)
peritonitis with or following abortion or ectopic or molar pregnancy (O00-O07, O08.0)
peritonitis with or following appendicitis (K35.-)
peritonitis with or following diverticular disease of intestine (K57.-)
puerperal peritonitis (O85)
retroperitoneal infections (K68.-)

CC Excl: For CC/MCC codes in category K65: PDX collection 803

K65.0 Generalized (acute) peritonitis   `MCC` `HCC`
Pelvic peritonitis (acute), male
Subphrenic peritonitis (acute)
Suppurative peritonitis (acute)

K65.1 Peritoneal abscess   `MCC` `HCC`
Abdominopelvic abscess   Subdiaphragmatic abscess
Abscess (of) omentum   Subhepatic abscess
Abscess (of) peritoneum   Subphrenic abscess
Mesenteric abscess
Retrocecal abscess

K65.2 Spontaneous bacterial peritonitis   `MCC` `HCC`
EXCLUDES 1   bacterial peritonitis NOS (K65.9)

K65.3 Choleperitonitis   `MCC` `HCC`
Peritonitis due to bile
DEF: Inflammation of the peritoneum due to leakage of bile into the peritoneal cavity resulting from rupture of the bile passages or gallbladder.

K65.4 Sclerosing mesenteritis   `CC` `HCC`
Fat necrosis of peritoneum
(Idiopathic) sclerosing mesenteric fibrosis
Mesenteric lipodystrophy
Mesenteric panniculitis
Retractile mesenteritis

K65.8 Other peritonitis   `MCC` `HCC`
Chronic proliferative peritonitis   Peritonitis due to urine

K65.9 Peritonitis, unspecified   `MCC` `HCC`
Bacterial peritonitis NOS
AHA: 2013, 2Q, 31

✓4th K66 Other disorders of peritoneum
EXCLUDES 2   ascites (R18.-)
peritoneal effusion (chronic) (R18.8)

K66.0 Peritoneal adhesions (postprocedural) (postinfection)
Adhesions (of) abdominal (wall)   Adhesions (of) omentum
Adhesions (of) diaphragm   Adhesions (of) stomach
Adhesions (of) intestine   Adhesive bands
Adhesions (of) male pelvis   Mesenteric adhesions
EXCLUDES 1   female pelvic adhesions [bands] (N73.6)
peritoneal adhesions with intestinal obstruction ▶(K56.5-)◄

K66.1 Hemoperitoneum   `MCC`
EXCLUDES 1   traumatic hemoperitoneum (S36.8-)
CC Excl: PDX collection 804

K66.8 Other specified disorders of peritoneum

K66.9 Disorder of peritoneum, unspecified

K67 *Disorders of peritoneum in infectious diseases classified elsewhere*   `MCC` `HCC`
Code first underlying disease, such as:
congenital syphilis (A50.0)
helminthiasis (B65.0-B83.9)
EXCLUDES 1   peritonitis in chlamydia (A74.81)
peritonitis in diphtheria (A36.89)
peritonitis in gonococcal (A54.85)
peritonitis in syphilis (late) (A52.74)
peritonitis in tuberculosis (A18.31)
CC Excl: PDX collection 803

✓4th K68 Disorders of retroperitoneum
✓5th K68.1 Retroperitoneal abscess
K68.11 Postprocedural retroperitoneal abscess   `CC` `H11` `H12` `H13`
CC Excl: PDX collection 805
K68.12 Psoas muscle abscess   `MCC` `HCC`
CC Excl: PDX collection 806
K68.19 Other retroperitoneal abscess   `MCC` `HCC`
CC Excl: PDX collection 803
K68.9 Other disorders of retroperitoneum   `MCC`
CC Excl: PDX collection 803

Diseases of liver (K70-K77)

EXCLUDES 1   jaundice NOS (R17)
EXCLUDES 2   hemochromatosis (E83.11-)
Reye's syndrome (G93.7)
viral hepatitis (B15-B19)
Wilson's disease (E83.0)

✓4th K70 Alcoholic liver disease
Use additional code to identify:
alcohol abuse and dependence (F10.-)

K70.0 Alcoholic fatty liver   `A`

✓5th K70.1 Alcoholic hepatitis
K70.10 Alcoholic hepatitis without ascites   `A`
K70.11 Alcoholic hepatitis with ascites   `A`

K70.2 Alcoholic fibrosis and sclerosis of liver   `A`

✓ Additional Character Req   ✓x7th Placeholder Alert   Unacceptable PDx   Manifestation   H1 - H14 HAC   HCC CMS-HCC Condition   *EXCLUDES 1* Not Coded Here   *EXCLUDES 2* Not Included Here

ICD-10-CM 2018   701

K64.1–K70.2

Chapter 11. Diseases of the Digestive System

✓5ᵗʰ **K70.3 Alcoholic cirrhosis of liver**
Alcoholic cirrhosis NOS

     K70.30 Alcoholic cirrhosis of liver without ascites `HCC` `A`

     K70.31 Alcoholic cirrhosis of liver with ascites `HCC` `A`

✓5ᵗʰ **K70.4 Alcoholic hepatic failure**
Acute alcoholic hepatic failure
Alcoholic hepatic failure NOS
Chronic alcoholic hepatic failure
Subacute alcoholic hepatic failure

     K70.40 Alcoholic hepatic failure without coma `HCC` `A`

     K70.41 Alcoholic hepatic failure with coma `PDxMCC` `MCC` `HCC` `A`
         CC Excl: PDX collection 807

K70.9 Alcoholic liver disease, unspecified `HCC` `A`

✓4ᵗʰ **K71 Toxic liver disease**
     `INCLUDES` drug-induced idiosyncratic (unpredictable) liver disease
               drug-induced toxic (predictable) liver disease
     Code first poisoning due to drug or toxin, if applicable (T36-T65 with fifth or sixth character 1-4 or 6)
     Use additional code for adverse effect, if applicable, to identify drug (T36-T50 with fifth or sixth character 5)
     `EXCLUDES 2` *alcoholic liver disease (K70.-)*
               Budd-Chiari syndrome (I82.0)

K71.0 Toxic liver disease with cholestasis
Cholestasis with hepatocyte injury
"Pure" cholestasis

✓5ᵗʰ **K71.1 Toxic liver disease with hepatic necrosis**
Hepatic failure (acute) (chronic) due to drugs

     K71.10 Toxic liver disease with hepatic necrosis, without coma

     K71.11 Toxic liver disease with hepatic necrosis, with coma `PDxMCC` `MCC` `HCC`
         CC Excl: PDX collection 807

K71.2 Toxic liver disease with acute hepatitis

K71.3 Toxic liver disease with chronic persistent hepatitis

K71.4 Toxic liver disease with chronic lobular hepatitis

✓5ᵗʰ **K71.5 Toxic liver disease with chronic active hepatitis**
Toxic liver disease with lupoid hepatitis

     K71.50 Toxic liver disease with chronic active hepatitis without ascites

     K71.51 Toxic liver disease with chronic active hepatitis with ascites

K71.6 Toxic liver disease with hepatitis, not elsewhere classified

K71.7 Toxic liver disease with fibrosis and cirrhosis of liver

K71.8 Toxic liver disease with other disorders of liver
Toxic liver disease with focal nodular hyperplasia
Toxic liver disease with hepatic granulomas
Toxic liver disease with peliosis hepatis
Toxic liver disease with veno-occlusive disease of liver

K71.9 Toxic liver disease, unspecified

✓4ᵗʰ **K72 Hepatic failure, not elsewhere classified**
     `INCLUDES` fulminant hepatitis NEC, with hepatic failure
               hepatic encephalopathy NOS
               liver (cell) necrosis with hepatic failure
               malignant hepatitis NEC, with hepatic failure
               yellow liver atrophy or dystrophy
     `EXCLUDES 1` *alcoholic hepatic failure (K70.4)*
               hepatic failure with toxic liver disease (K71.1-)
               icterus of newborn (P55-P59)
               postprocedural hepatic failure (K91.82)
     `EXCLUDES 2` *hepatic failure complicating abortion or ectopic or molar pregnancy (O00-O07, O08.8)*
               hepatic failure complicating pregnancy, childbirth and the puerperium (O26.6-)
               viral hepatitis with hepatic coma (B15-B19)
     AHA: 2017, 1Q, 41

✓5ᵗʰ **K72.0 Acute and subacute hepatic failure**
Acute non-viral hepatitis NOS
AHA: 2015, 2Q, 17; 2014, 2Q, 13

     K72.00 Acute and subacute hepatic failure without coma `MCC`
         CC Excl: PDX collection 808

     K72.01 Acute and subacute hepatic failure with coma `PDxMCC` `MCC` `HCC`
         CC Excl: PDX collection 808

✓5ᵗʰ **K72.1 Chronic hepatic failure**

     K72.10 Chronic hepatic failure without coma `HCC`

     K72.11 Chronic hepatic failure with coma `PDxMCC` `MCC` `HCC`
         CC Excl: PDX collection 807

✓5ᵗʰ **K72.9 Hepatic failure, unspecified**

     K72.90 Hepatic failure, unspecified without coma `HCC`
         AHA: 2016, 2Q, 35

     K72.91 Hepatic failure, unspecified with coma `MCC` `HCC`
         Hepatic coma NOS
         CC Excl: PDX collection 807

✓4ᵗʰ **K73 Chronic hepatitis, not elsewhere classified**
     `EXCLUDES 1` *alcoholic hepatitis (chronic) (K70.1-)*
               drug-induced hepatitis (chronic) (K71.-)
               granulomatous hepatitis (chronic) NEC (K75.3)
               reactive, nonspecific hepatitis (chronic) (K75.2)
               viral hepatitis (chronic) (B15-B19)

K73.0 Chronic persistent hepatitis, not elsewhere classified `HCC`

K73.1 Chronic lobular hepatitis, not elsewhere classified `HCC`

K73.2 Chronic active hepatitis, not elsewhere classified `HCC`

K73.8 Other chronic hepatitis, not elsewhere classified `HCC`

K73.9 Chronic hepatitis, unspecified `HCC`

✓4ᵗʰ **K74 Fibrosis and cirrhosis of liver**
     Code also, if applicable, viral hepatitis (acute) (chronic) (B15-B19)
     `EXCLUDES 1` *alcoholic cirrhosis (of liver) (K70.3)*
               alcoholic fibrosis of liver (K70.2)
               cardiac sclerosis of liver (K76.1)
               cirrhosis (of liver) with toxic liver disease (K71.7)
               congenital cirrhosis (of liver) (P78.81)
               pigmentary cirrhosis (of liver) (E83.110)

K74.0 Hepatic fibrosis

K74.1 Hepatic sclerosis

K74.2 Hepatic fibrosis with hepatic sclerosis

K74.3 Primary biliary cirrhosis `HCC`
Chronic nonsuppurative destructive cholangitis

K74.4 Secondary biliary cirrhosis `HCC`

K74.5 Biliary cirrhosis, unspecified `HCC`

✓5ᵗʰ **K74.6 Other and unspecified cirrhosis of liver**

     K74.60 Unspecified cirrhosis of liver `HCC`
         Cirrhosis (of liver) NOS

     K74.69 Other cirrhosis of liver `HCC`
         Cryptogenic cirrhosis (of liver)
         Macronodular cirrhosis (of liver)
         Micronodular cirrhosis (of liver)
         Mixed type cirrhosis (of liver)
         Portal cirrhosis (of liver)
         Postnecrotic cirrhosis (of liver)

✓4ᵗʰ **K75 Other inflammatory liver diseases**
     `EXCLUDES 2` *toxic liver disease (K71.-)*

K75.0 Abscess of liver `MCC`
Cholangitic hepatic abscess
Hematogenic hepatic abscess
Hepatic abscess NOS
Lymphogenic hepatic abscess
Pylephlebitic hepatic abscess
     `EXCLUDES 2` *acute or subacute hepatitis NOS (B17.9)*
               acute or subacute non-viral hepatitis (K72.0)
               chronic hepatitis NEC (K73.8)
     CC Excl: PDX collection 809

K75.1 Phlebitis of portal vein `MCC`
Pylephlebitis
     `EXCLUDES 1` *pylephlebitic liver abscess (K75.0)*
     DEF: Inflammation of portal vein or branches; may be due to diverticulitis, perforated appendicitis, or peritonitis; symptoms include fever, chills, jaundice, sweating, and abscess in various body parts.
     CC Excl: PDX collection 809

K75.2 Nonspecific reactive hepatitis
     `EXCLUDES 1` *acute or subacute hepatitis (K72.0-)*
               chronic hepatitis NEC (K73.-)
               viral hepatitis (B15-B19)

K75.3 Granulomatous hepatitis, not elsewhere classified
     `EXCLUDES 1` *acute or subacute hepatitis (K72.0-)*
               chronic hepatitis NEC (K73.-)
               viral hepatitis (B15-B19)

K75.4 Autoimmune hepatitis `HCC`
Lupoid hepatitis NEC

✓5ᵗʰ **K75.8 Other specified inflammatory liver diseases**

     K75.81 Nonalcoholic steatohepatitis (NASH)

     K75.89 Other specified inflammatory liver diseases

`N` Newborn: 0   `P` Pediatric: 0-17   `M` Maternity: 12-55   `A` Adult: 15-124   `MCC` Major CC Condition   `PDxMCC` PDx acts as own MCC   `CC` CC Condition   `PDxCC` PDx acts as own CC

702   ICD-10-CM 2018

K75.9 Inflammatory liver disease, unspecified
Hepatitis NOS
> *EXCLUDES 1* *acute or subacute hepatitis (K72.0-)*
> *chronic hepatitis NEC (K73.-)*
> *viral hepatitis (B15-B19)*
AHA: 2015, 2Q, 17

✓4ᵗʰ **K76 Other diseases of liver**
> *EXCLUDES 2* *alcoholic liver disease (K70.-)*
> *amyloid degeneration of liver (E85.-)*
> *cystic disease of liver (congenital) (Q44.6)*
> *hepatic vein thrombosis (I82.0)*
> *hepatomegaly NOS (R16.0)*
> *pigmentary cirrhosis (of liver) (E83.110)*
> *portal vein thrombosis (I81)*
> *toxic liver disease (K71.-)*

K76.0 Fatty (change of) liver, not elsewhere classified
Nonalcoholic fatty liver disease (NAFLD)
> *EXCLUDES 1* *nonalcoholic steatohepatitis (NASH) (K75.81)*

K76.1 Chronic passive congestion of liver
Cardiac cirrhosis
Cardiac sclerosis

K76.2 Central hemorrhagic necrosis of liver   `MCC`
> *EXCLUDES 1* *liver necrosis with hepatic failure (K72.-)*
CC Excl: PDX collection 808

K76.3 Infarction of liver   `MCC`
CC Excl: PDX collection 808

K76.4 Peliosis hepatis
Hepatic angiomatosis

K76.5 Hepatic veno-occlusive disease
> *EXCLUDES 1* *Budd-Chiari syndrome (I82.0)*

K76.6 Portal hypertension   `CC` `HCC`
Use additional code for any associated complications, such as:
portal hypertensive gastropathy (K31.89)
CC Excl: PDX collection 810

K76.7 Hepatorenal syndrome   `MCC` `HCC`
> *EXCLUDES 1* *hepatorenal syndrome following labor and delivery*
> *(O90.4)*
> *postprocedural hepatorenal syndrome (K91.83)*
CC Excl: PDX collection 811

✓5ᵗʰ **K76.8 Other specified diseases of liver**

K76.81 Hepatopulmonary syndrome   `HCC`
Code first underlying liver disease, such as:
alcoholic cirrhosis of liver (K70.3-)
cirrhosis of liver without mention of alcohol (K74.6-)

K76.89 Other specified diseases of liver
Cyst (simple) of liver
Focal nodular hyperplasia of liver
Hepatoptosis

K76.9 Liver disease, unspecified

K77 Liver disorders in diseases classified elsewhere   `CC`
Code first underlying disease, such as:
amyloidosis (E85.-)
congenital syphilis (A50.0, A50.5)
congenital toxoplasmosis (P37.1)
schistosomiasis (B65.0-B65.9)
> *EXCLUDES 1* *alcoholic hepatitis (K70.1-)*
> *alcoholic liver disease (K70.-)*
> *cytomegaloviral hepatitis (B25.1)*
> *herpesviral [herpes simplex] hepatitis (B00.81)*
> *infectious mononucleosis with liver disease*
> *(B27.0-B27.9 with .9)*
> *mumps hepatitis (B26.81)*
> *sarcoidosis with liver disease (D86.89)*
> *secondary syphilis with liver disease (A51.45)*
> *syphilis (late) with liver disease (A52.74)*
> *toxoplasmosis (acquired) hepatitis (B58.1)*
> *tuberculosis with liver disease (A18.83)*
CC Excl: No Excl

Disorders of gallbladder, biliary tract and pancreas (K80-K87)

✓4ᵗʰ **K80 Cholelithiasis**
> *EXCLUDES 1* *retained cholelithiasis following cholecystectomy (K91.86)*

✓5ᵗʰ **K80.0 Calculus of gallbladder with acute cholecystitis**
Any condition listed in K80.2 with acute cholecystitis

K80.00 Calculus of gallbladder with acute cholecystitis   `CC`
without obstruction
CC Excl: PDX collection 812

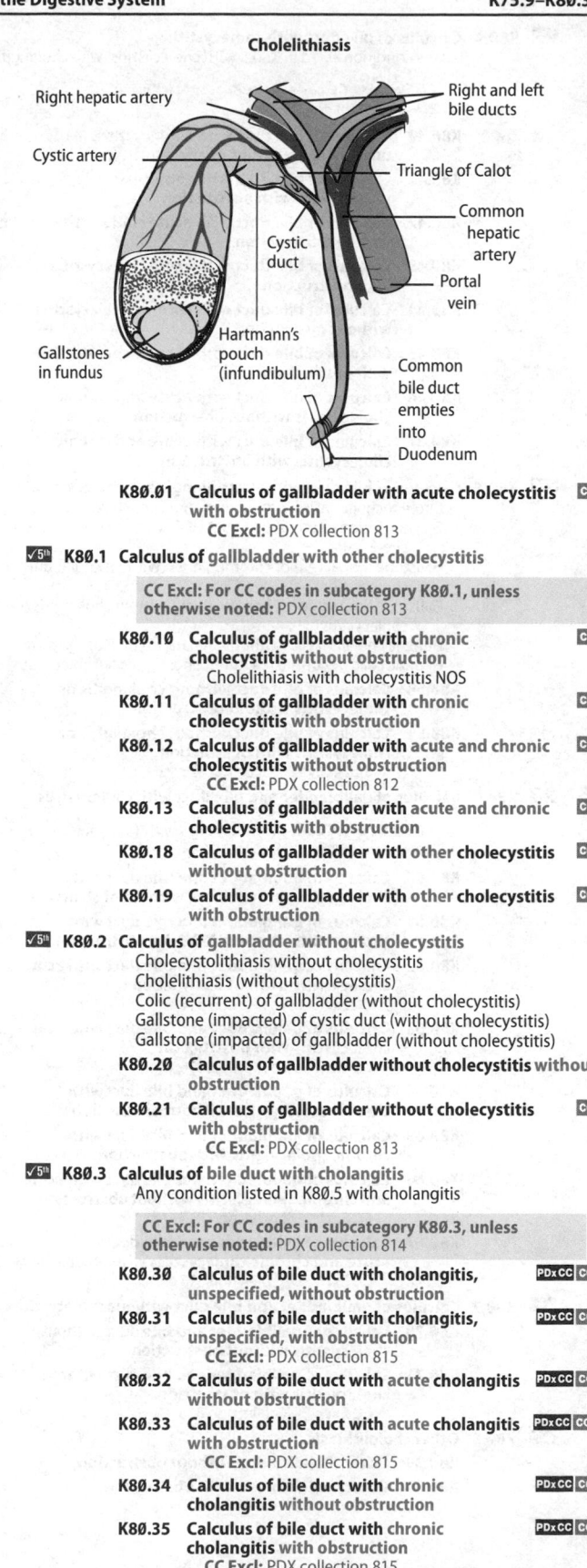

Cholelithiasis

Right hepatic artery
Cystic artery
Cystic duct
Gallstones in fundus
Hartmann's pouch (infundibulum)
Right and left bile ducts
Triangle of Calot
Common hepatic artery
Portal vein
Common bile duct empties into Duodenum

K80.01 Calculus of gallbladder with acute cholecystitis   `CC`
with obstruction
CC Excl: PDX collection 813

✓5ᵗʰ **K80.1 Calculus of gallbladder with other cholecystitis**

CC Excl: For CC codes in subcategory K80.1, unless otherwise noted: PDX collection 813

K80.10 Calculus of gallbladder with chronic   `CC`
cholecystitis without obstruction
Cholelithiasis with cholecystitis NOS

K80.11 Calculus of gallbladder with chronic   `CC`
cholecystitis with obstruction

K80.12 Calculus of gallbladder with acute and chronic   `CC`
cholecystitis without obstruction
CC Excl: PDX collection 812

K80.13 Calculus of gallbladder with acute and chronic   `CC`
cholecystitis with obstruction

K80.18 Calculus of gallbladder with other cholecystitis `CC`
without obstruction

K80.19 Calculus of gallbladder with other cholecystitis `CC`
with obstruction

✓5ᵗʰ **K80.2 Calculus of gallbladder without cholecystitis**
Cholecystolithiasis without cholecystitis
Cholelithiasis (without cholecystitis)
Colic (recurrent) of gallbladder (without cholecystitis)
Gallstone (impacted) of cystic duct (without cholecystitis)
Gallstone (impacted) of gallbladder (without cholecystitis)

K80.20 Calculus of gallbladder without cholecystitis without
obstruction

K80.21 Calculus of gallbladder without cholecystitis   `CC`
with obstruction
CC Excl: PDX collection 813

✓5ᵗʰ **K80.3 Calculus of bile duct with cholangitis**
Any condition listed in K80.5 with cholangitis

CC Excl: For CC codes in subcategory K80.3, unless otherwise noted: PDX collection 814

K80.30 Calculus of bile duct with cholangitis,   `PDx CC` `CC`
unspecified, without obstruction

K80.31 Calculus of bile duct with cholangitis,   `PDx CC` `CC`
unspecified, with obstruction
CC Excl: PDX collection 815

K80.32 Calculus of bile duct with acute cholangitis `PDx CC` `CC`
without obstruction

K80.33 Calculus of bile duct with acute cholangitis `PDx CC` `CC`
with obstruction
CC Excl: PDX collection 815

K80.34 Calculus of bile duct with chronic   `PDx CC` `CC`
cholangitis without obstruction

K80.35 Calculus of bile duct with chronic   `PDx CC` `CC`
cholangitis with obstruction
CC Excl: PDX collection 815

K80.36 Calculus of bile duct with acute and chronic `PDx CC` `CC`
cholangitis without obstruction

K80.37 Calculus of bile duct with acute and chronic `PDx CC` `CC`
cholangitis with obstruction
CC Excl: PDX collection 815

Chapter 11. Diseases of the Digestive System

✓5ᵗʰ **K80.4** **Calculus of** bile duct with cholecystitis
Any condition listed in K80.5 with cholecystitis (with cholangitis)

CC Excl: For CC codes in subcategory K80.4: PDX collection 815

K80.40 **Calculus of bile duct with cholecystitis, unspecified, without obstruction**   `CC`

K80.41 **Calculus of bile duct with cholecystitis, unspecified, with obstruction**   `CC`

K80.42 **Calculus of bile duct with** acute **cholecystitis** without obstruction   `CC`

K80.43 **Calculus of bile duct with** acute **cholecystitis** with obstruction   `CC`

K80.44 **Calculus of bile duct with** chronic **cholecystitis** without obstruction   `CC`

K80.45 **Calculus of bile duct with** chronic **cholecystitis** with obstruction   `CC`

K80.46 **Calculus of bile duct with** acute and chronic **cholecystitis** without obstruction   `CC`

K80.47 **Calculus of bile duct with** acute and chronic **cholecystitis** with obstruction   `CC`

✓5ᵗʰ **K80.5** **Calculus of** bile duct without cholangitis or cholecystitis
Choledocholithiasis (without cholangitis or cholecystitis)
Gallstone (impacted) of bile duct NOS (without cholangitis or cholecystitis)
Gallstone (impacted) of common duct (without cholangitis or cholecystitis)
Gallstone (impacted) of hepatic duct (without cholangitis or cholecystitis)
Hepatic cholelithiasis (without cholangitis or cholecystitis)
Hepatic colic (recurrent) (without cholangitis or cholecystitis)

K80.50 **Calculus of bile duct without cholangitis or cholecystitis** without obstruction

K80.51 **Calculus of bile duct without cholangitis or cholecystitis** with obstruction   `CC`
CC Excl: PDX collection 815

✓5ᵗʰ **K80.6** **Calculus of** gallbladder and bile duct with cholecystitis

CC Excl: For CC codes in subcategory K80.6, unless otherwise noted: PDX collection 815

K80.60 **Calculus of gallbladder and bile duct with cholecystitis, unspecified, without obstruction**   `CC`

K80.61 **Calculus of gallbladder and bile duct with cholecystitis, unspecified, with obstruction**   `CC`

K80.62 **Calculus of gallbladder and bile duct with** acute **cholecystitis** without obstruction   `CC`
CC Excl: PDX collection 816

K80.63 **Calculus of gallbladder and bile duct with** acute **cholecystitis** with obstruction   `CC`
CC Excl: PDX collection 816

K80.64 **Calculus of gallbladder and bile duct with** chronic **cholecystitis** without obstruction   `CC`

K80.65 **Calculus of gallbladder and bile duct with** chronic **cholecystitis** with obstruction   `CC`

K80.66 **Calculus of gallbladder and bile duct with** acute and chronic **cholecystitis** without obstruction   `CC`
CC Excl: PDX collection 817

K80.67 **Calculus of gallbladder and bile duct with** acute and chronic **cholecystitis** with obstruction   `MCC`
CC Excl: PDX collection 817

✓5ᵗʰ **K80.7** **Calculus of** gallbladder and bile duct without cholecystitis

K80.70 **Calculus of gallbladder and bile duct without cholecystitis** without obstruction

K80.71 **Calculus of gallbladder and bile duct without cholecystitis** with obstruction   `CC`
CC Excl: PDX collection 815

✓5ᵗʰ **K80.8** Other cholelithiasis

K80.80 **Other cholelithiasis** without obstruction

K80.81 **Other cholelithiasis** with obstruction   `CC`
CC Excl: PDX collection 815

✓4ᵗʰ **K81** **Cholecystitis**
EXCLUDES 1   cholecystitis with cholelithiasis (K80.-)

K81.0 **Acute cholecystitis**   `CC`
Abscess of gallbladder
Angiocholecystitis
Emphysematous (acute) cholecystitis
Empyema of gallbladder
Gangrene of gallbladder
Gangrenous cholecystitis
Suppurative cholecystitis
CC Excl: PDX collection 818

K81.1 **Chronic cholecystitis**

K81.2 **Acute cholecystitis with** chronic **cholecystitis**   `CC`
CC Excl: PDX collection 819

K81.9 **Cholecystitis, unspecified**

✓4ᵗʰ **K82** **Other diseases of gallbladder**
EXCLUDES 1   nonvisualization of gallbladder (R93.2)
postcholecystectomy syndrome (K91.5)

CC Excl: For CC/MCC codes in category K82: PDX collection 820

K82.0 **Obstruction of gallbladder**   `CC`
Occlusion of cystic duct or gallbladder without cholelithiasis
Stenosis of cystic duct or gallbladder without cholelithiasis
Stricture of cystic duct or gallbladder without cholelithiasis
EXCLUDES 1   obstruction of gallbladder with cholelithiasis (K80.-)

K82.1 **Hydrops of gallbladder**   `CC`
Mucocele of gallbladder

K82.2 **Perforation of gallbladder**   `MCC`
Rupture of cystic duct or gallbladder

K82.3 **Fistula of gallbladder**   `CC`
Cholecystocolic fistula
Cholecystoduodenal fistula

K82.4 **Cholesterolosis of gallbladder**
Strawberry gallbladder
EXCLUDES 1   cholesterolosis of gallbladder with cholecystitis (K81.-)
cholesterolosis of gallbladder with cholelithiasis (K80.-)

K82.8 **Other specified diseases of gallbladder**
Adhesions of cystic duct or gallbladder
Atrophy of cystic duct or gallbladder
Cyst of cystic duct or gallbladder
Dyskinesia of cystic duct or gallbladder
Hypertrophy of cystic duct or gallbladder
Nonfunctioning of cystic duct or gallbladder
Ulcer of cystic duct or gallbladder

K82.9 **Disease of gallbladder, unspecified**

✓4ᵗʰ **K83** **Other diseases of biliary tract**
EXCLUDES 1   postcholecystectomy syndrome (K91.5)
EXCLUDES 2   conditions involving the gallbladder (K81-K82)
conditions involving the cystic duct (K81-K82)

K83.0 **Cholangitis**   `CC`

Ascending cholangitis	Sclerosing cholangitis
Cholangitis NOS	Secondary cholangitis
Primary cholangitis	Stenosing cholangitis
Recurrent cholangitis	Suppurative cholangitis

EXCLUDES 1   cholangitic liver abscess (K75.0)
cholangitis with choledocholithiasis (K80.3-, K80.4-)
chronic nonsuppurative destructive cholangitis (K74.3)
CC Excl: PDX collection 814

K83.1 **Obstruction of bile duct**   `MCC`
Occlusion of bile duct without cholelithiasis
Stenosis of bile duct without cholelithiasis
Stricture of bile duct without cholelithiasis
EXCLUDES 1   congenital obstruction of bile duct (Q44.3)
obstruction of bile duct with cholelithiasis (K80.-)
AHA: 2016, 1Q, 18
CC Excl: PDX collection 821

K83.2 **Perforation of bile duct**   `MCC`
Rupture of bile duct
CC Excl: PDX collection 822

K83.3 **Fistula of bile duct**   `CC`
Choledochoduodenal fistula
CC Excl: PDX collection 822

K83.4 **Spasm of sphincter of Oddi**

K83.5 **Biliary cyst**

K83.8 **Other specified diseases of biliary tract**

Adhesions of biliary tract	Hypertrophy of biliary tract
Atrophy of biliary tract	Ulcer of biliary tract

K83.9 **Disease of biliary tract, unspecified**

Ⓝ Newborn: 0   Ⓟ Pediatric: 0-17   Ⓜ Maternity: 12-55   Ⓐ Adult: 15-124   `MCC` Major CC Condition   `PDxMCC` PDx acts as own MCC   `CC` CC Condition   `PDxCC` PDx acts as own CC

704   ICD-10-CM 2018

☑4ᵗʰ **K85** **Acute pancreatitis**
> INCLUDES   acute (recurrent) pancreatitis
>   subacute pancreatitis

> **CC Excl:** For MCC codes in category K85: PDX collection 177

☑5ᵗʰ **K85.0** Idiopathic **acute pancreatitis**
- **K85.00** **Idiopathic acute pancreatitis** without necrosis or infection   MCC
- **K85.01** **Idiopathic acute pancreatitis** with uninfected necrosis   MCC
- **K85.02** **Idiopathic acute pancreatitis** with infected necrosis   MCC

☑5ᵗʰ **K85.1** Biliary **acute pancreatitis**
> Gallstone pancreatitis
- **K85.10** **Biliary acute pancreatitis** without necrosis or infection   MCC
- **K85.11** **Biliary acute pancreatitis** with uninfected necrosis   MCC
- **K85.12** **Biliary acute pancreatitis** with infected necrosis   MCC

☑5ᵗʰ **K85.2** Alcohol induced **acute pancreatitis**
> EXCLUDES 2   alcohol induced chronic pancreatitis (K86.0)
- **K85.20** **Alcohol induced acute pancreatitis** without necrosis or infection   MCC
- **K85.21** **Alcohol induced acute pancreatitis** with uninfected necrosis   MCC
- **K85.22** **Alcohol induced acute pancreatitis** with infected necrosis   MCC

☑5ᵗʰ **K85.3** Drug induced **acute pancreatitis**
> Use additional code for adverse effect, if applicable, to identify drug (T36-T50 with fifth or sixth character 5)
> Use additional code to identify drug abuse and dependence (F11. – F17.-)
- **K85.30** **Drug induced acute pancreatitis** without necrosis or infection   MCC
- **K85.31** **Drug induced acute pancreatitis** with uninfected necrosis   MCC
- **K85.32** **Drug induced acute pancreatitis** with infected necrosis   MCC

☑5ᵗʰ **K85.8** Other **acute pancreatitis**
- **K85.80** **Other acute pancreatitis** without necrosis or infection   MCC
- **K85.81** **Other acute pancreatitis** with uninfected necrosis   MCC
- **K85.82** **Other acute pancreatitis** with infected necrosis   MCC

☑5ᵗʰ **K85.9** **Acute pancreatitis,** unspecified
> Pancreatitis NOS
- **K85.90** **Acute pancreatitis** without necrosis or infection, **unspecified**   MCC
- **K85.91** **Acute pancreatitis** with uninfected necrosis, **unspecified**   MCC
- **K85.92** **Acute pancreatitis** with infected necrosis, **unspecified**   MCC

☑4ᵗʰ **K86** **Other diseases of pancreas**
> EXCLUDES 2   fibrocystic disease of pancreas (E84.-)
>   islet cell tumor (of pancreas) (D13.7)
>   pancreatic steatorrhea (K90.3)

K86.0 **Alcohol-induced chronic pancreatitis**   CC HCC
> Code also exocrine pancreatic insufficiency (K86.81)
> Use additional code to identify:
>   alcohol abuse and dependence (F10.-)
> EXCLUDES 2   alcohol induced acute pancreatitis (K85.2-)
> **CC Excl:** PDX collection 823

K86.1 **Other chronic pancreatitis**   CC HCC
> Chronic pancreatitis NOS
> Infectious chronic pancreatitis
> Recurrent chronic pancreatitis
> Relapsing chronic pancreatitis
> Code also exocrine pancreatic insufficiency (K86.81)
> **CC Excl:** PDX collection 823

K86.2 **Cyst of pancreas**   CC
> **CC Excl:** PDX collection 824

K86.3 **Pseudocyst of pancreas**   CC
> **CC Excl:** PDX collection 824

☑5ᵗʰ **K86.8** **Other specified diseases of pancreas**
- **K86.81** **Exocrine pancreatic insufficiency**

K86.89 **Other specified diseases of pancreas**
> Aseptic pancreatic necrosis, unrelated to acute pancreatitis
> Atrophy of pancreas
> Calculus of pancreas
> Cirrhosis of pancreas
> Fibrosis of pancreas
> Pancreatic fat necrosis, unrelated to acute pancreatitis
> Pancreatic infantilism
> Pancreatic necrosis NOS, unrelated to acute pancreatitis

K86.9 **Disease of pancreas, unspecified**

K87 ***Disorders of gallbladder, biliary tract and pancreas in diseases classified elsewhere***
> Code first underlying disease
> EXCLUDES 1   cytomegaloviral pancreatitis (B25.2)
>   mumps pancreatitis (B26.3)
>   syphilitic gallbladder (A52.74)
>   syphilitic pancreas (A52.74)
>   tuberculosis of gallbladder (A18.83)
>   tuberculosis of pancreas (A18.83)

Other diseases of the digestive system (K90-K95)

☑4ᵗʰ **K90** **Intestinal malabsorption**
> EXCLUDES 1   intestinal malabsorption following gastrointestinal surgery (K91.2)

> **CC Excl:** For CC codes in category K90, unless otherwise noted: PDX collection 825

K90.0 **Celiac disease**
> Celiac disease with steatorrhea
> ►Celiac gluten-sensitive enteropathy◄
> Nontropical sprue
> Use additional code for associated disorders including:
>   dermatitis herpetiformis (L13.0)
>   gluten ataxia (G32.81)
> Code also exocrine pancreatic insufficiency (K86.81)
> **DEF:** Malabsorption syndrome due to gluten consumption; symptoms include fetid, bulky, frothy, oily stools, distended abdomen, gas, asthenia, electrolyte depletion, and vitamin B, D, and K deficiency.

K90.1 **Tropical sprue**   CC
> Sprue NOS
> Tropical steatorrhea

K90.2 **Blind loop syndrome, not elsewhere classified**   CC
> Blind loop syndrome NOS
> EXCLUDES 1   congenital blind loop syndrome (Q43.8)
>   postsurgical blind loop syndrome (K91.2)

K90.3 **Pancreatic steatorrhea**   CC

☑5ᵗʰ **K90.4** **Other malabsorption due to intolerance**
> EXCLUDES 2   ►celiac gluten-sensitive enteropathy◄ (K90.0)
>   lactose intolerance (E73.-)
- **K90.41** **Non-celiac gluten sensitivity**   CC
>   Gluten sensitivity NOS
>   Non-celiac gluten sensitive enteropathy
- **K90.49** **Malabsorption due to intolerance, not elsewhere classified**   CC
>   Malabsorption due to intolerance to carbohydrate
>   Malabsorption due to intolerance to fat
>   Malabsorption due to intolerance to protein
>   Malabsorption due to intolerance to starch

☑5ᵗʰ **K90.8** **Other intestinal malabsorption**
- **K90.81** **Whipple's disease**   CC
>   **CC Excl:** PDX collection 826
- **K90.89** **Other intestinal malabsorption**   CC

K90.9 **Intestinal malabsorption, unspecified**   CC

☑4ᵗʰ **K91** **Intraoperative and postprocedural complications and disorders of digestive system, not elsewhere classified**
> EXCLUDES 2   complications of artificial opening of digestive system (K94.-)
>   complications of bariatric procedures (K95.-)
>   gastrojejunal ulcer (K28.-)
>   postprocedural (radiation) retroperitoneal abscess (K68.11)
>   radiation colitis (K52.0)
>   radiation gastroenteritis (K52.0)
>   radiation proctitis (K62.7)

K91.0 **Vomiting following gastrointestinal surgery**

K91.1 **Postgastric surgery syndromes**
> Dumping syndrome
> Postgastrectomy syndrome
> Postvagotomy syndrome

☑ Additional Character Req   ✓ˣ7ᵗʰ Placeholder Alert   Unacceptable PDx   Manifestation   H1-H14 HAC   HCC CMS-HCC Condition   EXCLUDES 1 Not Coded Here   EXCLUDES 2 Not Included Here

K91.2　Postsurgical malabsorption, not elsewhere classified `CC`
　　Postsurgical blind loop syndrome
　　EXCLUDES 1　malabsorption osteomalacia in adults (M83.2)
　　　　　　malabsorption osteoporosis, postsurgical (M80.8-,
　　　　　　M81.8)
　　CC Excl: PDX collection 827

✓5th **K91.3　Postprocedural intestinal obstruction**
　　AHA: 2017, 1Q, 40

● 　**K91.30　Postprocedural intestinal obstruction,** `CC`
　　　　unspecified as to partial versus complete
　　　　Postprocedural intestinal obstruction NOS

● 　**K91.31　Postprocedural partial intestinal obstruction** `CC`
　　　　Postprocedural incomplete intestinal obstruction

● 　**K91.32　Postprocedural complete intestinal obstruction** `CC`

K91.5　Postcholecystectomy syndrome

✓5th **K91.6　Intraoperative hemorrhage and hematoma of a digestive**
　　system organ or structure complicating a procedure
　　　EXCLUDES 1　intraoperative hemorrhage and hematoma of a
　　　　　　digestive system organ or structure due to
　　　　　　accidental puncture and laceration during a
　　　　　　procedure (K91.7-)

　　K91.61　Intraoperative hemorrhage and hematoma of a `CC`
　　　　digestive system organ or structure complicating
　　　　a digestive system procedure
　　　　CC Excl: PDX collection 829

　　K91.62　Intraoperative hemorrhage and hematoma of a `CC`
　　　　digestive system organ or structure complicating
　　　　other procedure
　　　　CC Excl: PDX collection 829

✓5th **K91.7　Accidental puncture and laceration of a digestive system**
　　organ or structure during a procedure

　　K91.71　Accidental puncture and laceration of a digestive `CC`
　　　　system organ or structure during a digestive system
　　　　procedure
　　　　CC Excl: PDX collection 509

　　K91.72　Accidental puncture and laceration of a digestive `CC`
　　　　system organ or structure during other procedure
　　　　CC Excl: PDX collection 509

✓5th **K91.8　Other intraoperative and postprocedural complications and**
　　disorders of digestive system

　　　CC Excl: For CC codes in subcategory K91.8, unless
　　　otherwise noted: PDX collection 828

　　K91.81　Other intraoperative complications of digestive `CC`
　　　　system

　　K91.82　Postprocedural hepatic failure `CC`

　　K91.83　Postprocedural hepatorenal syndrome `CC`

✓6th **K91.84　Postprocedural hemorrhage of a digestive system**
　　　　organ or structure following a procedure

　　　　K91.840　Postprocedural hemorrhage of a `CC`
　　　　　　digestive system organ or structure
　　　　　　following a digestive system procedure
　　　　　　AHA: 2016, 1Q, 15
　　　　　　CC Excl: PDX collection 829

　　　　K91.841　Postprocedural hemorrhage of a `CC`
　　　　　　digestive system organ or structure
　　　　　　following other procedure
　　　　　　CC Excl: PDX collection 829

✓6th **K91.85　Complications of intestinal pouch**

　　　　K91.850　Pouchitis `CC` `HCC`
　　　　　　Inflammation of internal ileoanal pouch
　　　　　　DEF: Inflammatory complication of an
　　　　　　existing surgically created ileoanal pouch,
　　　　　　resulting in multiple GI complaints, including
　　　　　　diarrhea, abdominal pain, rectal bleeding,
　　　　　　fecal urgency, or incontinence.

　　　　K91.858　Other complications of intestinal `CC` `HCC`
　　　　　　pouch

　　K91.86　Retained cholelithiasis following `CC`
　　　　cholecystectomy

✓6th **K91.87　Postprocedural hematoma and seroma of a**
　　　　digestive system organ or structure following a
　　　　procedure

　　　　CC Excl: For CC codes in subcategory K91.87:
　　　　PDX collection 829

　　　　K91.870　Postprocedural hematoma of a `CC`
　　　　　　digestive system organ or structure
　　　　　　following a digestive system procedure

　　K91.871　Postprocedural hematoma of a `CC`
　　　　digestive system organ or structure
　　　　following other procedure

　　K91.872　Postprocedural seroma of a
　　　　digestive system organ or structure
　　　　following a digestive system procedure

　　K91.873　Postprocedural seroma of a
　　　　digestive system organ or structure
　　　　following other procedure

　　K91.89　Other postprocedural complications and `CC`
　　　　disorders of digestive system
　　　　Use additional code, if applicable, to further specify
　　　　　　disorder
　　　　EXCLUDES 2　postprocedural retroperitoneal abscess
　　　　　　(K68.11)
　　　　AHA: 2017, 1Q, 40
　　　　CC Excl: PDX collection 828

✓4th **K92　Other diseases of digestive system**
　　　EXCLUDES 1　neonatal gastrointestinal hemorrhage (P54.0-P54.3)

　　　CC Excl: For CC codes in category K92, unless otherwise noted:
　　　PDX collection 770

　　K92.0　Hematemesis `CC`

　　K92.1　Melena `CC`
　　　EXCLUDES 1　occult blood in feces (R19.5)

　　K92.2　Gastrointestinal hemorrhage, unspecified `CC`
　　　　Gastric hemorrhage NOS
　　　　Intestinal hemorrhage NOS
　　　EXCLUDES 1　acute hemorrhagic gastritis (K29.01)
　　　　　　hemorrhage of anus and rectum (K62.5)
　　　　　　angiodysplasia of stomach with hemorrhage (K31.811)
　　　　　　diverticular disease with hemorrhage (K57.-)
　　　　　　gastritis and duodenitis with hemorrhage (K29.-)
　　　　　　peptic ulcer with hemorrhage (K25-K28)

✓5th **K92.8　Other specified diseases of the digestive system**

　　K92.81　Gastrointestinal mucositis (ulcerative) `CC`
　　　　Code also type of associated therapy, such as:
　　　　　　antineoplastic and immunosuppressive drugs
　　　　　　(T45.1X-)
　　　　　　radiological procedure and radiotherapy (Y84.2)
　　　　EXCLUDES 2　mucositis (ulcerative) of vagina and vulva
　　　　　　(N76.81)
　　　　　　nasal mucositis (ulcerative) (J34.81)
　　　　　　oral mucositis (ulcerative) (K12.3-)
　　　　CC Excl: PDX collection 765

　　K92.89　Other specified diseases of the digestive system

　　K92.9　Disease of digestive system, unspecified

✓4th **K94　Complications of artificial openings of the digestive system**

✓5th **K94.0　Colostomy complications**

　　　CC Excl: For CC codes in subcategory K94.0, unless
　　　otherwise noted: PDX collection 830

　　K94.00　Colostomy complication, unspecified `HCC`

　　K94.01　Colostomy hemorrhage `CC` `HCC`

　　K94.02　Colostomy infection `CC` `HCC`
　　　　Use additional code to specify type of infection, such
　　　　　　as:
　　　　　　cellulitis of abdominal wall (L03.311)
　　　　　　sepsis (A40-, A41-)

　　K94.03　Colostomy malfunction `CC` `HCC`
　　　　Mechanical complication of colostomy
　　　　CC Excl: PDX collection 831

　　K94.09　Other complications of colostomy `CC` `HCC`

✓5th **K94.1　Enterostomy complicatiCC Excl: PDX collection 831ons**

　　　CC Excl: For CC codes in subcategory K94.1, unless
　　　otherwise noted: PDX collection 830

　　K94.10　Enterostomy complication, unspecified `HCC`

　　K94.11　Enterostomy hemorrhage `CC` `HCC`

　　K94.12　Enterostomy infection `CC` `HCC`
　　　　Use additional code to specify type of infection, such
　　　　　　as:
　　　　　　cellulitis of abdominal wall (L03.311)
　　　　　　sepsis (A40-, A41-)

　　K94.13　Enterostomy malfunction `CC` `HCC`
　　　　Mechanical complication of enterostomy
　　　　CC Excl: PDX collection 831

　　K94.19　Other complications of enterostomy `CC` `HCC`

N Newborn: 0　P Pediatric: 0-17　M Maternity: 12-55　A Adult: 15-124　MCC Major CC Condition　PDx MCC PDx acts as own MCC　CC CC Condition　PDx CC PDx acts as own CC

706　　　　　ICD-10-CM 2018

☑5ᵗʰ **K94.2** Gastrostomy complications

    K94.20 **Gastrostomy complication, unspecified** `HCC`

    K94.21 **Gastrostomy** hemorrhage `HCC`

    K94.22 **Gastrostomy** infection `CC` `HCC`
           Use additional code to specify type of infection, such as:
               cellulitis of abdominal wall (L03.311)
               sepsis (A40-, A41-)
           CC Excl: PDX collection 828

    K94.23 **Gastrostomy** malfunction `CC` `HCC`
           Mechanical complication of gastrostomy
           CC Excl: PDX collection 828

    K94.29 **Other complications of gastrostomy** `HCC`

☑5ᵗʰ **K94.3** Esophagostomy complications

> **CC Excl: For CC codes in subcategory K94.3:** PDX collection 828

    K94.30 **Esophagostomy complications, unspecified** `CC` `HCC`

    K94.31 **Esophagostomy** hemorrhage `CC` `HCC`

    K94.32 **Esophagostomy** infection `CC` `HCC`
           Use additional code to identify the infection

    K94.33 **Esophagostomy** malfunction `CC` `HCC`
           Mechanical complication of esophagostomy

    K94.39 **Other complications of esophagostomy** `CC` `HCC`

☑4ᵗʰ **K95** **Complications of bariatric procedures**

> **CC Excl: For CC codes in category K95:** PDX collection 828

☑5ᵗʰ **K95.0** **Complications of** gastric band procedure

    K95.01 **Infection due to gastric band procedure** `CC` `H11`
           Use additional code to specify type of infection or organism, such as:
               bacterial and viral infectious agents (B95.-, B96.-)
               cellulitis of abdominal wall (L03.311)
               sepsis (A40.-, A41.-)

    K95.09 **Other complications of gastric band procedure** `CC`
           Use additional code, if applicable, to further specify complication

☑5ᵗʰ **K95.8** **Complications of** other bariatric procedure
     EXCLUDES 1 complications of gastric band surgery (K95.0-)

    K95.81 **Infection due to other bariatric procedure** `CC` `H11`
           Use additional code to specify type of infection or organism, such as:
               bacterial and viral infectious agents (B95.-, B96.-)
               cellulitis of abdominal wall (L03.311)
               sepsis (A40.-, A41.-)

    K95.89 **Other complications of other bariatric procedure** `CC`
           Use additional code, if applicable, to further specify complication

---

☑ Additional Character Req   ☑x7ᵗʰ Placeholder Alert   Unacceptable PDx   Manifestation   `H1`-`H14` HAC   `HCC` CMS-HCC Condition   *EXCLUDES 1* Not Coded Here   *EXCLUDES 2* Not Included Here

Chapter 12. Diseases of the Skin and Subcutaneous Tissue (L00–L99)

Chapter Specific Guidelines with Coding Examples

The chapter specific guidelines from the ICD-10-CM Official Guidelines for Coding and Reporting have been provided below. Along with these guidelines are coding examples, contained in the shaded boxes, that have been developed to help illustrate the coding and/or sequencing guidance found in these guidelines.

a. Pressure ulcer stage codes

1) Pressure ulcer stages

Codes from category L89, Pressure ulcer, identify the site of the pressure ulcer as well as the stage of the ulcer.

The ICD-10-CM classifies pressure ulcer stages based on severity, which is designated by stages 1-4, unspecified stage and unstageable.

Assign as many codes from category L89 as needed to identify all the pressure ulcers the patient has, if applicable.

> Stage 4 pressure ulcer right heel, 9 x 10 cm that invades the muscle and fascia; stage 2 pressure ulcer of left elbow
>
> **L89.614**   **Pressure ulcer of right heel, stage 4**
>
> **L89.022**   **Pressure ulcer of left elbow, stage 2**
>
> *Explanation:* Patient has a right heel pressure ulcer documented as stage 4 and a left elbow pressure ulcer documented as stage 2. Combination codes from category L89 Pressure ulcer, identify the site of the pressure ulcer as well as the stage. Assign as many codes from category L89 as needed to identify all the pressure ulcers the patient has.

2) Unstageable pressure ulcers

Assignment of the code for unstageable pressure ulcer (L89.--0) should be based on the clinical documentation. These codes are used for pressure ulcers whose stage cannot be clinically determined (e.g., the ulcer is covered by eschar or has been treated with a skin or muscle graft) and pressure ulcers that are documented as deep tissue injury but not documented as due to trauma. This code should not be confused with the codes for unspecified stage (L89.--9). When there is no documentation regarding the stage of the pressure ulcer, assign the appropriate code for unspecified stage (L89.--9).

> Pressure ulcer of the right lower back documented as unstageable due to the presence of thick eschar covering the ulcer
>
> **L89.130**   **Pressure ulcer of right lower back, unstageable**
>
> *Explanation:* Codes for unstageable pressure ulcers are assigned when the stage cannot be clinically determined (e.g., the ulcer is covered by eschar or has been treated with a skin or muscle graft).

3) Documented pressure ulcer stage

Assignment of the pressure ulcer stage code should be guided by clinical documentation of the stage or documentation of the terms found in the Alphabetic Index. For clinical terms describing the stage that are not found in the Alphabetic Index, and there is no documentation of the stage, the provider should be queried.

> Left heel pressure ulcer with partial thickness skin loss involving the dermis
>
> **L89.622**   **Pressure ulcer of left heel, stage 2**
>
> *Explanation:* Code assignment for the pressure ulcer stage should be guided by either the clinical documentation of the stage or the documentation of terms found in the Alphabetic Index. The clinical documentation describing the left heel pressure ulcer "partial thickness skin loss involving the dermis" matches the ICD-10-CM index parenthetical description for stage 2 "(abrasion, blister, partial thickness skin loss involving epidermis and/or dermis)."

4) Patients admitted with pressure ulcers documented as healed

No code is assigned if the documentation states that the pressure ulcer is completely healed.

> Admission orders noted to watch closely for evolving pressure ulcers as patient history noted a healed pressure ulcer of the foot.
>
> **Z87.2**   **Personal history of diseases of the skin and subcutaneous tissue**
>
> *Explanation:* A code is assigned only for the personal history of the pressure ulcer. Personal history code Z87.2 includes conditions classifiable to L00–L99 such as pressure ulcer. No code is assigned for a pressure ulcer documented as completely healed.

5) Patients admitted with pressure ulcers documented as healing

Pressure ulcers described as healing should be assigned the appropriate pressure ulcer stage code based on the documentation in the medical record. If the documentation does not provide information about the stage of the healing pressure ulcer, assign the appropriate code for unspecified stage.

If the documentation is unclear as to whether the patient has a current (new) pressure ulcer or if the patient is being treated for a healing pressure ulcer, query the provider.

For ulcers that were present on admission but healed at the time of discharge, assign the code for the site and stage of the pressure ulcer at the time of admission.

> H & P noted healing stage 2 sacral pressure ulcer. Resolved at time of discharge summary.
>
> **L89.152**   **Pressure ulcer of sacral region, stage 2**
>
> *Explanation:* Although completely healed upon discharge, the pressure ulcer required observation and/or treatment and should be coded based on the site and stage upon admission.

6) Patient admitted with pressure ulcer evolving into another stage during the admission

If a patient is admitted **to an inpatient hospital** with a pressure ulcer at one stage and it progresses to a higher stage, two separate codes should be assigned: one code for the site and stage of the ulcer on admission and a second code for the same ulcer site and the highest stage reported during the stay.

> Stage 3 right hip pressure ulcer worsened during admission to a stage 4
>
> **L89.213**   **Pressure ulcer of right hip, stage 3**
>
> **L89.214**   **Pressure ulcer of right hip, stage 4**
>
> *Explanation:* A pressure ulcer that progresses from a lower stage to a higher stage is assigned two codes, one for the documented stage upon admission and one for the documented stage at discharge.

b. Non-pressure chronic ulcers

1) Patients admitted with non-pressure ulcers documented as healed

No code is assigned if the documentation states that the non-pressure ulcer is completely healed.

2) Patients admitted with non-pressure ulcers documented as healing

Non-pressure ulcers described as healing should be assigned the appropriate non-pressure ulcer code based on the documentation in the medical record. If the documentation does not provide information about the severity of the healing non-pressure ulcer, assign the appropriate code for unspecified severity.

If the documentation is unclear as to whether the patient has a current (new) non-pressure ulcer or if the patient is being treated for a healing non-pressure ulcer, query the provider.

For ulcers that were present on admission but healed at the time of discharge, assign the code for the site and severity of the non-pressure ulcer at the time of admission.

3) Patient admitted with non-pressure ulcer that progresses to another severity level during the admission

If a patient is admitted to an inpatient hospital with a non-pressure ulcer at one severity level and it progresses to a higher severity level, two separate codes should be assigned: one code for the site and severity level of the ulcer on admission and a second code for the same ulcer site and the highest severity level reported during the stay.

Chapter 12. Diseases of the Skin and Subcutaneous Tissue (L00-L99)

EXCLUDES 2 *certain conditions originating in the perinatal period (P04-P96)*
certain infectious and parasitic diseases (A00-B99)
complications of pregnancy, childbirth and the puerperium (O00-O9A)
congenital malformations, deformations, and chromosomal abnormalities (Q00-Q99)
endocrine, nutritional and metabolic diseases (E00-E88)
lipomelanotic reticulosis (I89.8)
neoplasms (C00-D49)
symptoms, signs and abnormal clinical and laboratory findings, not elsewhere classified (R00-R94)
systemic connective tissue disorders (M30-M36)
viral warts (B07.-)

This chapter contains the following blocks:

L00-L08   Infections of the skin and subcutaneous tissue
L10-L14   Bullous disorders
L20-L30   Dermatitis and eczema
L40-L45   Papulosquamous disorders
L49-L54   Urticaria and erythema
L55-L59   Radiation-related disorders of the skin and subcutaneous tissue
L60-L75   Disorders of skin appendages
L76   Intraoperative and postprocedural complications of skin and subcutaneous tissue
L80-L99   Other disorders of the skin and subcutaneous tissue

Infections of the skin and subcutaneous tissue (L00-L08)

Use additional code (B95-B97) to identify infectious agent

EXCLUDES 2 *hordeolum (H00.0)*
infective dermatitis (L30.3)
local infections of skin classified in Chapter 1
lupus panniculitis (L93.2)
panniculitis NOS (M79.3)
panniculitis of neck and back (M54.0-)
Perlèche NOS (K13.0)
Perlèche due to candidiasis (B37.0)
Perlèche due to riboflavin deficiency (E53.0)
pyogenic granuloma (L98.0)
relapsing panniculitis [Weber-Christian] (M35.6)
viral warts (B07.-)
zoster (B02.-)

L00   Staphylococcal scalded skin syndrome
Ritter's disease
Use additional code to identify percentage of skin exfoliation (L49.-)
EXCLUDES 1 *bullous impetigo (L01.03)*
pemphigus neonatorum (L01.03)
toxic epidermal necrolysis [Lyell] (L51.2)
DEF: Infectious skin disease of children younger than 5 years marked by eruptions ranging from a few localized blisters to widespread, easily ruptured, fine vesicles and bullae affecting almost the entire body; results in exfoliation of large planes of skin and leaves raw areas.

✓4ᵗʰ **L01   Impetigo**
EXCLUDES 1 *impetigo herpetiformis (L40.1)*

✓5ᵗʰ **L01.0   Impetigo**
Impetigo contagiosa
Impetigo vulgaris

L01.00   Impetigo, unspecified
Impetigo NOS

L01.01   Non-bullous impetigo

L01.02   Bockhart's impetigo
Impetigo follicularis
Perifolliculitis NOS
Superficial pustular perifolliculitis

L01.03   Bullous impetigo
Impetigo neonatorum
Pemphigus neonatorum

L01.09   Other impetigo
Ulcerative impetigo

L01.1   Impetiginization of other dermatoses

✓4ᵗʰ **L02   Cutaneous abscess, furuncle and carbuncle**
Use additional code to identify organism (B95-B96)
EXCLUDES 2 *abscess of anus and rectal regions (K61.-)*
abscess of female genital organs (external) (N76.4)
abscess of male genital organs (external) (N48.2, N49-)

✓5ᵗʰ **L02.0   Cutaneous abscess, furuncle and carbuncle of face**
EXCLUDES 2 *abscess of ear, external (H60.0)*
abscess of eyelid (H00.0)
abscess of head [any part, except face] (L02.8)
abscess of lacrimal gland (H04.0)
abscess of lacrimal passages (H04.3)
abscess of mouth (K12.2)
abscess of nose (J34.0)
abscess of orbit (H05.0)
submandibular abscess (K12.2)

L02.01   Cutaneous abscess of face   CC
CC Excl: No Excl

L02.02   Furuncle of face
Boil of face
Folliculitis of face

L02.03   Carbuncle of face

✓5ᵗʰ **L02.1   Cutaneous abscess, furuncle and carbuncle of neck**
L02.11   Cutaneous abscess of neck   CC
CC Excl: PDX collection 832

L02.12   Furuncle of neck
Boil of neck
Folliculitis of neck

L02.13   Carbuncle of neck

✓5ᵗʰ **L02.2   Cutaneous abscess, furuncle and carbuncle of trunk**
EXCLUDES 1 *non-newborn omphalitis (L08.82)*
omphalitis of newborn (P38.-)
EXCLUDES 2 *abscess of breast (N61.1)*
abscess of buttocks (L02.3)
abscess of female external genital organs (N76.4)
abscess of hip (L02.4)
abscess of male external genital organs (N48.2, N49-)

CC Excl: For CC codes in subcategory L02.2:
PDX collection 833

✓6ᵗʰ **L02.21   Cutaneous abscess of trunk**
L02.211   Cutaneous abscess of abdominal wall   CC
L02.212   Cutaneous abscess of back [any part, except buttock]   CC
L02.213   Cutaneous abscess of chest wall   CC
L02.214   Cutaneous abscess of groin   CC
L02.215   Cutaneous abscess of perineum   CC
L02.216   Cutaneous abscess of umbilicus   CC
L02.219   Cutaneous abscess of trunk, unspecified   CC

✓6ᵗʰ **L02.22   Furuncle of trunk**
Boil of trunk   Folliculitis of trunk
L02.221   Furuncle of abdominal wall
L02.222   Furuncle of back [any part, except buttock]
L02.223   Furuncle of chest wall
L02.224   Furuncle of groin
L02.225   Furuncle of perineum
L02.226   Furuncle of umbilicus
L02.229   Furuncle of trunk, unspecified

✓6ᵗʰ **L02.23   Carbuncle of trunk**
L02.231   Carbuncle of abdominal wall
L02.232   Carbuncle of back [any part, except buttock]
L02.233   Carbuncle of chest wall
L02.234   Carbuncle of groin
L02.235   Carbuncle of perineum
L02.236   Carbuncle of umbilicus
L02.239   Carbuncle of trunk, unspecified

✓5ᵗʰ **L02.3   Cutaneous abscess, furuncle and carbuncle of buttock**
EXCLUDES 1 *pilonidal cyst with abscess (L05.01)*

L02.31   Cutaneous abscess of buttock   CC
Cutaneous abscess of gluteal region
CC Excl: PDX collection 834

L02.32   Furuncle of buttock
Boil of buttock
Folliculitis of buttock
Furuncle of gluteal region

Ⓝ Newborn: 0   Ⓟ Pediatric: 0-17   Ⓜ Maternity: 12-55   Ⓐ Adult: 15-124   ᴹᶜᶜ Major CC Condition   ᴾᴰˣᴹᶜᶜ PDx acts as own MCC   ᶜᶜ CC Condition   ᴾᴰˣᶜᶜ PDx acts as own CC

710   ICD-10-CM 2018

L02.33   **Carbuncle of buttock**
Carbuncle of gluteal region

✓5ᵗʰ **L02.4**   **Cutaneous abscess, furuncle and carbuncle of limb**

> EXCLUDES 2   cutaneous abscess, furuncle and carbuncle of groin
> (L02.214, L02.224, L02.234)
> cutaneous abscess, furuncle and carbuncle of hand
> (L02.5-)
> cutaneous abscess, furuncle and carbuncle of foot
> (L02.6-)

> **CC Excl:** For CC codes in subcategory L02.4, unless
> otherwise noted: PDX collection 835

✓6ᵗʰ **L02.41**   **Cutaneous abscess of limb**
     L02.411   **Cutaneous abscess of right axilla**   CC
     L02.412   **Cutaneous abscess of left axilla**   CC
     L02.413   **Cutaneous abscess of right upper limb**   CC
     L02.414   **Cutaneous abscess of left upper limb**   CC
     L02.415   **Cutaneous abscess of right lower limb**   CC
         CC Excl: PDX collection 836
     L02.416   **Cutaneous abscess of left lower limb**   CC
         CC Excl: PDX collection 836
     L02.419   **Cutaneous abscess of limb,**   CC
         unspecified
         CC Excl: PDX collection 836

✓6ᵗʰ **L02.42**   **Furuncle of limb**
Boil of limb
Folliculitis of limb
     L02.421   **Furuncle of right axilla**
     L02.422   **Furuncle of left axilla**
     L02.423   **Furuncle of right upper limb**
     L02.424   **Furuncle of left upper limb**
     L02.425   **Furuncle of right lower limb**
     L02.426   **Furuncle of left lower limb**
     L02.429   **Furuncle of limb, unspecified**

✓6ᵗʰ **L02.43**   **Carbuncle of limb**
     L02.431   **Carbuncle of right axilla**
     L02.432   **Carbuncle of left axilla**
     L02.433   **Carbuncle of right upper limb**
     L02.434   **Carbuncle of left upper limb**
     L02.435   **Carbuncle of right lower limb**
     L02.436   **Carbuncle of left lower limb**
     L02.439   **Carbuncle of limb, unspecified**

✓5ᵗʰ **L02.5**   **Cutaneous abscess, furuncle and carbuncle of hand**

> **CC Excl:** For CC codes in subcategory L02.5:
> PDX collection 837

✓6ᵗʰ **L02.51**   **Cutaneous abscess of hand**
     L02.511   **Cutaneous abscess of right hand**   CC
     L02.512   **Cutaneous abscess of left hand**   CC
     L02.519   **Cutaneous abscess of unspecified**   CC
         hand

✓6ᵗʰ **L02.52**   **Furuncle hand**
Boil of hand
Folliculitis of hand
     L02.521   **Furuncle right hand**
     L02.522   **Furuncle left hand**
     L02.529   **Furuncle unspecified hand**

✓6ᵗʰ **L02.53**   **Carbuncle of hand**
     L02.531   **Carbuncle of right hand**
     L02.532   **Carbuncle of left hand**
     L02.539   **Carbuncle of unspecified hand**

✓5ᵗʰ **L02.6**   **Cutaneous abscess, furuncle and carbuncle of foot**

> **CC Excl:** For CC codes in subcategory L02.6:
> PDX collection 838

✓6ᵗʰ **L02.61**   **Cutaneous abscess of foot**
     L02.611   **Cutaneous abscess of right foot**   CC
     L02.612   **Cutaneous abscess of left foot**   CC
     L02.619   **Cutaneous abscess of unspecified**   CC
         foot

✓6ᵗʰ **L02.62**   **Furuncle of foot**
Boil of foot   Folliculitis of foot
     L02.621   **Furuncle of right foot**
     L02.622   **Furuncle of left foot**
     L02.629   **Furuncle of unspecified foot**

✓6ᵗʰ **L02.63**   **Carbuncle of foot**
     L02.631   **Carbuncle of right foot**
     L02.632   **Carbuncle of left foot**
     L02.639   **Carbuncle of unspecified foot**

✓5ᵗʰ **L02.8**   **Cutaneous abscess, furuncle and carbuncle of other sites**
✓6ᵗʰ **L02.81**   **Cutaneous abscess of other sites**
     L02.811   **Cutaneous abscess of head [any part,**   CC
         except face]
         CC Excl: PDX collection 839
     L02.818   **Cutaneous abscess of other sites**   CC
         CC Excl: PDX collection 839

✓6ᵗʰ **L02.82**   **Furuncle of other sites**
Boil of other sites   Folliculitis of other sites
     L02.821   **Furuncle of head [any part, except face]**
     L02.828   **Furuncle of other sites**

✓6ᵗʰ **L02.83**   **Carbuncle of other sites**
     L02.831   **Carbuncle of head [any part, except face]**
     L02.838   **Carbuncle of other sites**

✓5ᵗʰ **L02.9**   **Cutaneous abscess, furuncle and carbuncle, unspecified**
     L02.91   **Cutaneous abscess, unspecified**   CC
         CC Excl: PDX collection 839
     L02.92   **Furuncle, unspecified**
         Boil NOS   Furunculosis NOS
     L02.93   **Carbuncle, unspecified**

✓4ᵗʰ **L03**   **Cellulitis and acute lymphangitis**

> EXCLUDES 2   cellulitis of anal and rectal region (K61.-)
> cellulitis of external auditory canal (H60.1)
> cellulitis of eyelid (H00.03-)
> cellulitis of female external genital organs (N76.4)
> cellulitis of lacrimal apparatus (H04.3)
> cellulitis of male external genital organs (N48.2, N49-)
> cellulitis of mouth (K12.2)
> cellulitis of nose (J34.0)
> eosinophilic cellulitis [Wells] (L98.3)
> febrile neutrophilic dermatosis [Sweet] (L98.2)
> lymphangitis (chronic) (subacute) (I89.1)

✓5ᵗʰ **L03.0**   **Cellulitis and acute lymphangitis of finger and toe**
Infection of nail
Onychia
Paronychia
Perionychia
✓6ᵗʰ **L03.01**   **Cellulitis of finger**
Felon
Whitlow
> EXCLUDES 1   herpetic whitlow (B00.89)
DEF: Felon: Superficial bacterial skin infection at the tip
of the finger.
     L03.011   **Cellulitis of right finger**
     L03.012   **Cellulitis of left finger**
     L03.019   **Cellulitis of unspecified finger**

✓6ᵗʰ **L03.02**   **Acute lymphangitis of finger**
Hangnail with lymphangitis of finger
     L03.021   **Acute lymphangitis of right finger**
     L03.022   **Acute lymphangitis of left finger**
     L03.029   **Acute lymphangitis of unspecified finger**

✓6ᵗʰ **L03.03**   **Cellulitis of toe**
     L03.031   **Cellulitis of right toe**
     L03.032   **Cellulitis of left toe**
     L03.039   **Cellulitis of unspecified toe**

✓6ᵗʰ **L03.04**   **Acute lymphangitis of toe**
Hangnail with lymphangitis of toe
     L03.041   **Acute lymphangitis of right toe**
     L03.042   **Acute lymphangitis of left toe**
     L03.049   **Acute lymphangitis of unspecified toe**

✓5ᵗʰ **L03.1**   **Cellulitis and acute lymphangitis of other parts of limb**

> **CC Excl:** For CC codes in subcategory L03.1, unless
> otherwise noted: PDX collection 835

✓6ᵗʰ **L03.11**   **Cellulitis of other parts of limb**
> EXCLUDES 2   cellulitis of fingers (L03.01-)
> cellulitis of toes (L03.03-)
> groin (L03.314)
     L03.111   **Cellulitis of right axilla**   CC
     L03.112   **Cellulitis of left axilla**   CC
     L03.113   **Cellulitis of right upper limb**   CC
     L03.114   **Cellulitis of left upper limb**   CC

✓ Additional Character Req   ✓x7ᵗʰ Placeholder Alert   Unacceptable PDx   Manifestation   **H1**-**H14** HAC   **HCC** CMS-HCC Condition   EXCLUDES 1 Not Coded Here   EXCLUDES 2 Not Included Here

L03.115 Cellulitis of right lower limb `CC`
CC Excl: PDX collection 836

L03.116 Cellulitis of left lower limb `CC`
CC Excl: PDX collection 836

L03.119 Cellulitis of unspecified part of limb `CC`
CC Excl: PDX collection 836

✓6ᵗʰ **L03.12** Acute lymphangitis of other parts of limb
EXCLUDES 2 *acute lymphangitis of fingers (L03.02-)*
acute lymphangitis of groin (L03.324)
acute lymphangitis of toes (L03.04-)

L03.121 Acute lymphangitis of right axilla `CC`
L03.122 Acute lymphangitis of left axilla `CC`
L03.123 Acute lymphangitis of right upper limb `CC`
L03.124 Acute lymphangitis of left upper limb `CC`
L03.125 Acute lymphangitis of right lower limb `CC`
CC Excl: PDX collection 836

L03.126 Acute lymphangitis of left lower limb `CC`
CC Excl: PDX collection 836

L03.129 Acute lymphangitis of unspecified part of limb `CC`
CC Excl: PDX collection 836

✓5ᵗʰ **L03.2** Cellulitis and acute lymphangitis of face and neck

✓6ᵗʰ **L03.21** Cellulitis and acute lymphangitis of face

L03.211 Cellulitis of face `CC`
EXCLUDES 2 *abscess of orbit (H05.01-)*
cellulitis of ear (H60.1-)
cellulitis of eyelid (H00.03-)
cellulitis of head (L03.811)
cellulitis of lacrimal apparatus (H04.3)
cellulitis of lip (K13.0)
cellulitis of mouth (K12.2)
cellulitis of nose (internal) (J34.0)
cellulitis of orbit (H05.01-)
cellulitis of scalp (L03.811)
AHA: 2013, 4Q, 123
CC Excl: PDX collection 840

L03.212 Acute lymphangitis of face `CC`
CC Excl: No Excl

L03.213 Periorbital cellulitis `CC`
Preseptal cellulitis
CC Excl: PDX collection 840

✓6ᵗʰ **L03.22** Cellulitis and acute lymphangitis of neck

L03.221 Cellulitis of neck `CC`
CC Excl: PDX collection 832

L03.222 Acute lymphangitis of neck `CC`
CC Excl: PDX collection 832

✓5ᵗʰ **L03.3** Cellulitis and acute lymphangitis of trunk

CC Excl: For CC codes in subcategory L03.3, unless otherwise noted: PDX collection 833

✓6ᵗʰ **L03.31** Cellulitis of trunk
EXCLUDES 2 *cellulitis of anal and rectal regions (K61.-)*
cellulitis of breast NOS (N61.0)
cellulitis of female external genital organs (N76.4)
cellulitis of male external genital organs (N48.2, N49-)
omphalitis of newborn (P38.-)
puerperal cellulitis of breast (O91.2)

L03.311 Cellulitis of abdominal wall `CC`
EXCLUDES 2 *cellulitis of umbilicus (L03.316)*
cellulitis of groin (L03.314)

L03.312 Cellulitis of back [any part except buttock] `CC`

L03.313 Cellulitis of chest wall `CC`
L03.314 Cellulitis of groin `CC`
L03.315 Cellulitis of perineum `CC`
L03.316 Cellulitis of umbilicus `CC`
L03.317 Cellulitis of buttock `CC`
CC Excl: PDX collection 834

L03.319 Cellulitis of trunk, unspecified `CC`

✓6ᵗʰ **L03.32** Acute lymphangitis of trunk
L03.321 Acute lymphangitis of abdominal wall `CC`
L03.322 Acute lymphangitis of back [any part except buttock] `CC`
L03.323 Acute lymphangitis of chest wall `CC`
L03.324 Acute lymphangitis of groin `CC`
L03.325 Acute lymphangitis of perineum `CC`

L03.326 Acute lymphangitis of umbilicus `CC`
L03.327 Acute lymphangitis of buttock `CC`
CC Excl: PDX collection 834

L03.329 Acute lymphangitis of trunk, unspecified `CC`

✓5ᵗʰ **L03.8** Cellulitis and acute lymphangitis of other sites

CC Excl: For CC codes in subcategory L03.8:
PDX collection 839

✓6ᵗʰ **L03.81** Cellulitis of other sites

L03.811 Cellulitis of head [any part, except face] `CC`
Cellulitis of scalp
EXCLUDES 2 *cellulitis of face (L03.211)*

L03.818 Cellulitis of other sites `CC`

✓6ᵗʰ **L03.89** Acute lymphangitis of other sites
L03.891 Acute lymphangitis of head [any part, except face] `CC`
L03.898 Acute lymphangitis of other sites `CC`

✓5ᵗʰ **L03.9** Cellulitis and acute lymphangitis, unspecified

CC Excl: For CC codes in subcategory L03.9:
PDX collection 839

L03.90 Cellulitis, unspecified `CC`
L03.91 Acute lymphangitis, unspecified `CC`
EXCLUDES 1 *lymphangitis NOS (I89.1)*

✓4ᵗʰ **L04** Acute lymphadenitis
INCLUDES abscess (acute) of lymph nodes, except mesenteric
acute lymphadenitis, except mesenteric
EXCLUDES 1 *chronic or subacute lymphadenitis, except mesenteric (I88.1)*
enlarged lymph nodes (R59.-)
human immunodeficiency virus [HIV] disease resulting in generalized lymphadenopathy (B20)
lymphadenitis NOS (I88.9)
nonspecific mesenteric lymphadenitis (I88.0)

L04.0 Acute lymphadenitis of face, head and neck
L04.1 Acute lymphadenitis of trunk
L04.2 Acute lymphadenitis of upper limb
Acute lymphadenitis of axilla   Acute lymphadenitis of shoulder
L04.3 Acute lymphadenitis of lower limb
Acute lymphadenitis of hip
EXCLUDES 2 *acute lymphadenitis of groin (L04.1)*
L04.8 Acute lymphadenitis of other sites
L04.9 Acute lymphadenitis, unspecified

✓4ᵗʰ **L05** Pilonidal cyst and sinus

✓5ᵗʰ **L05.0** Pilonidal cyst and sinus with abscess

L05.01 Pilonidal cyst with abscess `CC`
Pilonidal abscess
Pilonidal dimple with abscess
Postanal dimple with abscess
EXCLUDES 2 *congenital sacral dimple (Q82.6)*
parasacral dimple (Q82.0)
CC Excl: PDX collection 841

L05.02 Pilonidal sinus with abscess `CC`
Coccygeal fistula with abscess
Coccygeal sinus with abscess
Pilonidal fistula with abscess
CC Excl: PDX collection 841

Pilonidal Cyst

Skin
Fistula
Pilonidal cyst
Fat
Bone

N Newborn: 0 P Pediatric: 0-17 M Maternity: 12-55 A Adult: 15-124 MCC Major CC Condition PDxMCC PDx acts as own MCC CC CC Condition PDxCC PDx acts as own CC

712   ICD-10-CM 2018

√5th **L05.9** **Pilonidal cyst and sinus** without abscess

L05.91 **Pilonidal cyst** without abscess
Pilonidal dimple
Postanal dimple
Pilonidal cyst NOS
EXCLUDES 2 *congenital sacral dimple (Q82.6)*
parasacral dimple (Q82.6)

L05.92 **Pilonidal sinus** without abscess
Coccygeal fistula
Coccygeal sinus without abscess
Pilonidal fistula

√4th **L08** **Other local infections of skin and subcutaneous tissue**

L08.0 **Pyoderma**
Dermatitis gangrenosa
Purulent dermatitis
Septic dermatitis
Suppurative dermatitis
EXCLUDES 1 *pyoderma gangrenosum (L88)*
pyoderma vegetans (L08.81)

L08.1 **Erythrasma** HIV CC
CC Excl: PDX collection 107

√5th **L08.8** **Other specified local infections of the skin and subcutaneous tissue**

L08.81 **Pyoderma vegetans**
EXCLUDES 1 *pyoderma gangrenosum (L88)*
pyoderma NOS (L08.0)

L08.82 **Omphalitis not of newborn**
EXCLUDES 1 *omphalitis of newborn (P38.-)*

L08.89 **Other specified local infections of the skin and subcutaneous tissue**

L08.9 **Local infection of the skin and subcutaneous tissue, unspecified**

Bullous disorders (L10-L14)

EXCLUDES 1 *benign familial pemphigus [Hailey-Hailey] (Q82.8)*
staphylococcal scalded skin syndrome (L00)
toxic epidermal necrolysis [Lyell] (L51.2)

√4th **L10** **Pemphigus**
EXCLUDES 1 *pemphigus neonatorum (L01.03)*

CC Excl: For CC codes in category L10: PDX collection 842

L10.0 **Pemphigus vulgaris** CC
L10.1 **Pemphigus vegetans** CC
L10.2 **Pemphigus foliaceous** CC
L10.3 **Brazilian pemphigus [fogo selvagem]** CC
L10.4 **Pemphigus erythematosus** CC
Senear-Usher syndrome
L10.5 **Drug-induced pemphigus** CC
Use additional code for adverse effect, if applicable, to identify drug (T36-T50 with fifth or sixth character 5)

√5th **L10.8** **Other pemphigus**
L10.81 **Paraneoplastic pemphigus** CC
L10.89 **Other pemphigus** CC
L10.9 **Pemphigus, unspecified** CC

√4th **L11** **Other acantholytic disorders**

L11.0 **Acquired keratosis follicularis**
EXCLUDES 1 *keratosis follicularis (congenital) [Darier-White] (Q82.8)*

L11.1 **Transient acantholytic dermatosis [Grover]**
L11.8 **Other specified acantholytic disorders**
L11.9 **Acantholytic disorder, unspecified**

√4th **L12** **Pemphigoid**
EXCLUDES 1 *herpes gestationis (O26.4-)*
impetigo herpetiformis (L40.1)

CC Excl: For CC codes in category L12, unless otherwise noted: PDX collection 842

L12.0 **Bullous pemphigoid** CC
L12.1 **Cicatricial pemphigoid**
Benign mucous membrane pemphigoid
DEF: Chronic autoimmune disease characterized by subepidermal blistering lesions of mucosa, including the conjunctiva; seen predominantly in the elderly; produces adhesions and scarring.
L12.2 **Chronic bullous disease of childhood** P
Juvenile dermatitis herpetiformis

√5th **L12.3** **Acquired epidermolysis bullosa**
EXCLUDES 1 *epidermolysis bullosa (congenital) (Q81.-)*

L12.30 **Acquired epidermolysis bullosa, unspecified** CC HCC
CC Excl: PDX collection 843

L12.31 **Epidermolysis bullosa due to drug** CC HCC
Use additional code for adverse effect, if applicable, to identify drug (T36-T50 with fifth or sixth character 5)
CC Excl: PDX collection 843

L12.35 **Other acquired epidermolysis bullosa** CC HCC
CC Excl: PDX collection 843

L12.8 **Other pemphigoid** CC
L12.9 **Pemphigoid, unspecified** CC

√4th **L13** **Other bullous disorders**

L13.0 **Dermatitis herpetiformis**
Duhring's disease
Hydroa herpetiformis
EXCLUDES 1 *juvenile dermatitis herpetiformis (L12.2)*
senile dermatitis herpetiformis (L12.0)
DEF: Skin disease to which people are genetically predisposed resulting from an immunological response to gluten; seen as an extremely pruritic eruption of various lesions that frequently heal, leaving hyperpigmentation or hypopigmentation and occasionally scarring; usually associated with an asymptomatic gluten-sensitive enteropathy.

L13.1 **Subcorneal pustular dermatitis**
Sneddon-Wilkinson disease

L13.8 **Other specified bullous disorders**
L13.9 **Bullous disorder, unspecified**

L14 *Bullous disorders in diseases classified elsewhere*
Code first underlying disease

Dermatitis and eczema (L20-L30)

NOTE In this block the terms dermatitis and eczema are used synonymously and interchangeably.

EXCLUDES 2 *chronic (childhood) granulomatous disease (D71)*
dermatitis gangrenosa (L08.0)
dermatitis herpetiformis (L13.0)
dry skin dermatitis (L85.3)
factitial dermatitis (L98.1)
perioral dermatitis (L71.0)
radiation-related disorders of the skin and subcutaneous tissue (L55-L59)
stasis dermatitis (I87.2)

√4th **L20** **Atopic dermatitis**
L20.0 **Besnier's prurigo**

√5th **L20.8** **Other atopic dermatitis**
EXCLUDES 2 *circumscribed neurodermatitis (L28.0)*

L20.81 **Atopic neurodermatitis**
Diffuse neurodermatitis
L20.82 **Flexural eczema**
L20.83 **Infantile (acute) (chronic) eczema** P
L20.84 **Intrinsic (allergic) eczema**
L20.89 **Other atopic dermatitis**
L20.9 **Atopic dermatitis, unspecified**

√4th **L21** **Seborrheic dermatitis**
EXCLUDES 2 *infective dermatitis (L30.3)*
seborrheic keratosis (L82.-)

L21.0 **Seborrhea capitis**
Cradle cap
L21.1 **Seborrheic infantile dermatitis** P
L21.8 **Other seborrheic dermatitis**
L21.9 **Seborrheic dermatitis, unspecified**
Seborrhea NOS

L22 **Diaper dermatitis**
Diaper erythema
Diaper rash
Psoriasiform diaper rash

Chapter 12. Diseases of the Skin and Subcutaneous Tissue

L23–L29.8

✓4ᵗʰ **L23 Allergic contact dermatitis**

EXCLUDES1   *allergy NOS (T78.40)*
contact dermatitis NOS (L25.9)
dermatitis NOS (L30.9)

EXCLUDES2   *dermatitis due to substances taken internally (L27.-)*
dermatitis of eyelid (H01.1-)
diaper dermatitis (L22)
eczema of external ear (H60.5-)
irritant contact dermatitis (L24.-)
perioral dermatitis (L71.0)
radiation-related disorders of the skin and subcutaneous tissue (L55-L59)

L23.0 Allergic contact dermatitis due to metals
Allergic contact dermatitis due to chromium
Allergic contact dermatitis due to nickel

L23.1 Allergic contact dermatitis due to adhesives

L23.2 Allergic contact dermatitis due to cosmetics

L23.3 Allergic contact dermatitis due to drugs in contact with skin
Use additional code for adverse effect, if applicable, to identify drug (T36-T50 with fifth or sixth character 5)
EXCLUDES2   *dermatitis due to ingested drugs and medicaments (L27.0-L27.1)*

L23.4 Allergic contact dermatitis due to dyes

L23.5 Allergic contact dermatitis due to other chemical products
Allergic contact dermatitis due to cement
Allergic contact dermatitis due to insecticide
Allergic contact dermatitis due to plastic
Allergic contact dermatitis due to rubber

L23.6 Allergic contact dermatitis due to food in contact with the skin
EXCLUDES2   *dermatitis due to ingested food (L27.2)*

L23.7 Allergic contact dermatitis due to plants, except food
EXCLUDES2   *allergy NOS due to pollen (J30.1)*

✓5ᵗʰ **L23.8 Allergic contact dermatitis due to other agents**

     L23.81 Allergic contact dermatitis due to animal (cat) (dog) dander
Allergic contact dermatitis due to animal (cat) (dog) hair

     L23.89 Allergic contact dermatitis due to other agents

L23.9 Allergic contact dermatitis, unspecified cause
Allergic contact eczema NOS

✓4ᵗʰ **L24 Irritant contact dermatitis**

EXCLUDES1   *allergy NOS (T78.40)*
contact dermatitis NOS (L25.9)
dermatitis NOS (L30.9)

EXCLUDES2   *allergic contact dermatitis (L23.-)*
dermatitis due to substances taken internally (L27.-)
dermatitis of eyelid (H01.1-)
diaper dermatitis (L22)
eczema of external ear (H60.5-)
perioral dermatitis (L71.0)
radiation-related disorders of the skin and subcutaneous tissue (L55-L59)

L24.0 Irritant contact dermatitis due to detergents

L24.1 Irritant contact dermatitis due to oils and greases

L24.2 Irritant contact dermatitis due to solvents
Irritant contact dermatitis due to chlorocompound
Irritant contact dermatitis due to cyclohexane
Irritant contact dermatitis due to ester
Irritant contact dermatitis due to glycol
Irritant contact dermatitis due to hydrocarbon
Irritant contact dermatitis due to ketone

L24.3 Irritant contact dermatitis due to cosmetics

L24.4 Irritant contact dermatitis due to drugs in contact with skin
Use additional code for adverse effect, if applicable, to identify drug (T36-T50 with fifth or sixth character 5)

L24.5 Irritant contact dermatitis due to other chemical products
Irritant contact dermatitis due to cement
Irritant contact dermatitis due to insecticide
Irritant contact dermatitis due to plastic
Irritant contact dermatitis due to rubber

L24.6 Irritant contact dermatitis due to food in contact with skin
EXCLUDES2   *dermatitis due to ingested food (L27.2)*

L24.7 Irritant contact dermatitis due to plants, except food
EXCLUDES2   *allergy NOS to pollen (J30.1)*

✓5ᵗʰ **L24.8 Irritant contact dermatitis due to other agents**

     L24.81 Irritant contact dermatitis due to metals
Irritant contact dermatitis due to chromium
Irritant contact dermatitis due to nickel

     L24.89 Irritant contact dermatitis due to other agents
Irritant contact dermatitis due to dyes

L24.9 Irritant contact dermatitis, unspecified cause
Irritant contact eczema NOS

✓4ᵗʰ **L25 Unspecified contact dermatitis**

EXCLUDES1   *allergic contact dermatitis (L23.-)*
allergy NOS (T78.40)
dermatitis NOS (L30.9)
irritant contact dermatitis (L24.-)

EXCLUDES2   *dermatitis due to ingested substances (L27.-)*
dermatitis of eyelid (H01.1-)
eczema of external ear (H60.5-)
perioral dermatitis (L71.0)
radiation-related disorders of the skin and subcutaneous tissue (L55-L59)

L25.0 Unspecified contact dermatitis due to cosmetics

L25.1 Unspecified contact dermatitis due to drugs in contact with skin
Use additional code for adverse effect, if applicable, to identify drug (T36-T50 with fifth or sixth character 5)
EXCLUDES2   *dermatitis due to ingested drugs and medicaments (L27.0-L27.1)*

L25.2 Unspecified contact dermatitis due to dyes

L25.3 Unspecified contact dermatitis due to other chemical products
Unspecified contact dermatitis due to cement
Unspecified contact dermatitis due to insecticide

L25.4 Unspecified contact dermatitis due to food in contact with skin
EXCLUDES2   *dermatitis due to ingested food (L27.2)*

L25.5 Unspecified contact dermatitis due to plants, except food
EXCLUDES1   *nettle rash (L50.9)*
EXCLUDES2   *allergy NOS due to pollen (J30.1)*

L25.8 Unspecified contact dermatitis due to other agents

L25.9 Unspecified contact dermatitis, unspecified cause
Contact dermatitis (occupational) NOS
Contact eczema (occupational) NOS

L26 Exfoliative dermatitis
Hebra's pityriasis
EXCLUDES1   *Ritter's disease (L00)*

✓4ᵗʰ **L27 Dermatitis due to substances taken internally**

EXCLUDES1   *allergy NOS (T78.40)*

EXCLUDES2   *adverse food reaction, except dermatitis (T78.0-T78.1)*
contact dermatitis (L23-L25)
drug photoallergic response (L56.1)
drug phototoxic response (L56.0)
urticaria (L50.-)

L27.0 Generalized skin eruption due to drugs and medicaments taken internally
Use additional code for adverse effect, if applicable, to identify drug (T36-T50 with fifth or sixth character 5)

L27.1 Localized skin eruption due to drugs and medicaments taken internally
Use additional code for adverse effect, if applicable, to identify drug (T36-T50 with fifth or sixth character 5)

L27.2 Dermatitis due to ingested food
EXCLUDES2   *dermatitis due to food in contact with skin (L23.6, L24.6, L25.4)*

L27.8 Dermatitis due to other substances taken internally

L27.9 Dermatitis due to unspecified substance taken internally

✓4ᵗʰ **L28 Lichen simplex chronicus and prurigo**

L28.0 Lichen simplex chronicus
Circumscribed neurodermatitis
Lichen NOS

L28.1 Prurigo nodularis

L28.2 Other prurigo
Prurigo NOS   Prurigo mitis
Prurigo Hebra   Urticaria papulosa

✓4ᵗʰ **L29 Pruritus**

EXCLUDES1   *neurotic excoriation (L98.1)*
psychogenic pruritus (F45.8)

L29.0 Pruritus ani

L29.1 Pruritus scroti   ♂

L29.2 Pruritus vulvae   ♀

L29.3 Anogenital pruritus, unspecified

L29.8 Other pruritus

N Newborn: 0   **P** Pediatric: 0-17   **M** Maternity: 12-55   **A** Adult: 15-124   **MCC** Major CC Condition   **PDxMCC** PDx acts as own MCC   **CC** CC Condition   **PDxCC** PDx acts as own CC

714   ICD-10-CM 2018

L29.9 **Pruritus, unspecified**
Itch NOS

☑4ᵗʰ **L30 Other and unspecified dermatitis**
EXCLUDES 2   *contact dermatitis (L23-L25)*
dry skin dermatitis (L85.3)
small plaque parapsoriasis (L41.3)
stasis dermatitis (I87.2)

L30.0 **Nummular dermatitis**

L30.1 **Dyshidrosis [pompholyx]**

L30.2 **Cutaneous autosensitization**
Candidid [levurid]
Dermatophytid
Eczematid

L30.3 **Infective dermatitis**
Infectious eczematoid dermatitis

L30.4 **Erythema intertrigo**

L30.5 **Pityriasis alba**

L30.8 **Other specified dermatitis**

L30.9 **Dermatitis, unspecified**
Eczema NOS

Papulosquamous disorders (L40-L45)

☑4ᵗʰ **L40 Psoriasis**

L40.0 **Psoriasis vulgaris**
Nummular psoriasis
Plaque psoriasis

L40.1 **Generalized pustular psoriasis**
Impetigo herpetiformis
Von Zumbusch's disease

L40.2 **Acrodermatitis continua**

L40.3 **Pustulosis palmaris et plantaris**

L40.4 **Guttate psoriasis**

☑5ᵗʰ **L40.5 Arthropathic psoriasis**

L40.50 **Arthropathic psoriasis, unspecified**   HCC

L40.51 **Distal interphalangeal psoriatic arthropathy**   HCC

L40.52 **Psoriatic arthritis mutilans**   HCC

L40.53 **Psoriatic spondylitis**   HCC

L40.54 **Psoriatic juvenile arthropathy**   HCC

L40.59 **Other psoriatic arthropathy**   HCC

L40.8 **Other psoriasis**
Flexural psoriasis

L40.9 **Psoriasis, unspecified**

☑4ᵗʰ **L41 Parapsoriasis**
EXCLUDES 1   *poikiloderma vasculare atrophicans (L94.5)*

L41.0 **Pityriasis lichenoides et varioliformis acuta**
Mucha-Habermann disease

L41.1 **Pityriasis lichenoides chronica**

L41.3 **Small plaque parapsoriasis**

L41.4 **Large plaque parapsoriasis**

L41.5 **Retiform parapsoriasis**

L41.8 **Other parapsoriasis**

L41.9 **Parapsoriasis, unspecified**

L42 **Pityriasis rosea**

☑4ᵗʰ **L43 Lichen planus**
EXCLUDES 1   *lichen planopilaris (L66.1)*

L43.0 **Hypertrophic lichen planus**

L43.1 **Bullous lichen planus**

L43.2 **Lichenoid drug reaction**
Use additional code for adverse effect, if applicable, to identify drug (T36-T50 with fifth or sixth character 5)

L43.3 **Subacute (active) lichen planus**
Lichen planus tropicus

L43.8 **Other lichen planus**

L43.9 **Lichen planus, unspecified**

☑4ᵗʰ **L44 Other papulosquamous disorders**

L44.0 **Pityriasis rubra pilaris**

L44.1 **Lichen nitidus**
DEF: Chronic, inflammatory, asymptomatic skin disorder, characterized by numerous glistening, flat-topped, discrete, skin-colored micropapules, most often on the penis, lower abdomen, inner thighs, wrists, forearms, breasts and buttocks.

L44.2 **Lichen striatus**

L44.3 **Lichen ruber moniliformis**

L44.4 **Infantile papular acrodermatitis [Gianotti-Crosti]**   P

L44.8 **Other specified papulosquamous disorders**

L44.9 **Papulosquamous disorder, unspecified**

L45 ***Papulosquamous disorders in diseases classified elsewhere***
Code first underlying disease

Urticaria and erythema (L49-L54)
EXCLUDES 1   *Lyme disease (A69.2-)*
rosacea (L71.-)

☑4ᵗʰ **L49 Exfoliation due to erythematous conditions according to extent of body surface involved**
Code first erythematous condition causing exfoliation, such as:
Ritter's disease (L00)
(Staphylococcal) scalded skin syndrom (L00)
Stevens-Johnson syndrome (L51.1)
Stevens-Johnson syndrome-toxic epidermal necrolysis overlap syndrome (L51.3)
toxic epidermal necrolysis (L51.2)

L49.0 **Exfoliation due to erythematous condition involving less than 10 percent of body surface**
Exfoliation due to erythematous condition NOS

L49.1 **Exfoliation due to erythematous condition involving 10-19 percent of body surface**

L49.2 **Exfoliation due to erythematous condition involving 20-29 percent of body surface**

L49.3 **Exfoliation due to erythematous condition involving 30-39 percent of body surface**   CC
CC Excl: PDX collection 844

L49.4 **Exfoliation due to erythematous condition involving 40-49 percent of body surface**   CC
CC Excl: PDX collection 845

L49.5 **Exfoliation due to erythematous condition involving 50-59 percent of body surface**   CC
CC Excl: PDX collection 846

L49.6 **Exfoliation due to erythematous condition involving 60-69 percent of body surface**   CC
CC Excl: PDX collection 847

L49.7 **Exfoliation due to erythematous condition involving 70-79 percent of body surface**   CC
CC Excl: PDX collection 848

L49.8 **Exfoliation due to erythematous condition involving 80-89 percent of body surface**   CC
CC Excl: PDX collection 849

L49.9 **Exfoliation due to erythematous condition involving 90 or more percent of body surface**   CC
CC Excl: PDX collection 850

☑4ᵗʰ **L50 Urticaria**
EXCLUDES 1   *allergic contact dermatitis (L23.-)*
angioneurotic edema (T78.3)
giant urticaria (T78.3)
hereditary angio-edema (D84.1)
Quincke's edema (T78.3)
serum urticaria (T80.6-)
solar urticaria (L56.3)
urticaria neonatorum (P83.8)
urticaria papulosa (L28.2)
urticaria pigmentosa (Q82.2)

L50.0 **Allergic urticaria**

L50.1 **Idiopathic urticaria**

L50.2 **Urticaria due to cold and heat**
EXCLUDES 2 *familial cold urticaria (M04.2)*

L50.3 **Dermatographic urticaria**

L50.4 **Vibratory urticaria**

L50.5 **Cholinergic urticaria**

L50.6 **Contact urticaria**

L50.8 **Other urticaria**
Chronic urticaria
Recurrent periodic urticaria

L50.9 **Urticaria, unspecified**

Chapter 12. Diseases of the Skin and Subcutaneous Tissue

L51–L60.0

✓4ᵗʰ **L51 Erythema multiforme**

Use additional code for adverse effect, if applicable, to identify drug (T36-T50 with fifth or sixth character 5)

Use additional code to identify associated manifestations, such as: arthropathy associated with dermatological disorders (M14.8-)
conjunctival edema (H11.42)
conjunctivitis (H10.22-)
corneal scars and opacities (H17.-)
corneal ulcer (H16.0-)
edema of eyelid (H02.84)
inflammation of eyelid (H01.8)
keratoconjunctivitis sicca (H16.22-)
mechanical lagophthalmos (H02.22-)
stomatitis (K12.-)
symblepharon (H11.23-)

Use additional code to identify percentage of skin exfoliation (L49.-)

EXCLUDES 1   *staphylococcal scalded skin syndrome (L00)*
Ritter's disease (L00)

L51.0 Nonbullous erythema multiforme

L51.1 Stevens-Johnson syndrome   CC HCC
CC Excl: PDX collection 843

L51.2 Toxic epidermal necrolysis [Lyell]   CC HCC
CC Excl: PDX collection 843

L51.3 Stevens-Johnson syndrome-toxic epidermal necrolysis overlap syndrome   CC HCC
SJS-TEN overlap syndrome
CC Excl: PDX collection 843

L51.8 Other erythema multiforme

L51.9 Erythema multiforme, unspecified
Erythema iris
Erythema multiforme major NOS
Erythema multiforme minor NOS
Herpes iris

L52 Erythema nodosum

EXCLUDES 1   *tuberculous erythema nodosum (A18.4)*
DEF: A form of panniculitis (inflammation of the fat layer beneath the skin) of particularly women, usually seen as a hypersensitivity reaction to infections, drugs, sarcoidosis, and specific enteropathies; the acute stage is associated with fever, malaise, and arthralgia; the lesions are pink to blue in color as tender nodules and are found on the front of the legs below the knees.

✓4ᵗʰ **L53 Other erythematous conditions**

EXCLUDES 1   *erythema ab igne (L59.0)*
erythema due to external agents in contact with skin (L23-L25)
erythema intertrigo (L30.4)

CC Excl: For CC codes in category L53: PDX collection 851

L53.0 Toxic erythema   CC
Code first poisoning due to drug or toxin, if applicable (T36-T65 with fifth or sixth character 1-4 or 6)
Use additional code for adverse effect, if applicable, to identify drug (T36-T50 with fifth or sixth character 5)
EXCLUDES 1   *neonatal erythema toxicum (P83.1)*

L53.1 Erythema annulare centrifugum   CC

L53.2 Erythema marginatum   CC

L53.3 Other chronic figurate erythema   CC

L53.8 Other specified erythematous conditions

L53.9 Erythematous condition, unspecified
Erythema NOS
Erythroderma NOS

L54 Erythema in diseases classified elsewhere
Code first underlying disease

Radiation-related disorders of the skin and subcutaneous tissue (L55-L59)

✓4ᵗʰ **L55 Sunburn**

L55.0 Sunburn of first degree

L55.1 Sunburn of second degree

L55.2 Sunburn of third degree

L55.9 Sunburn, unspecified

✓4ᵗʰ **L56 Other acute skin changes due to ultraviolet radiation**
Use additional code to identify the source of the ultraviolet radiation (W89, X32)

L56.0 Drug phototoxic response
Use additional code for adverse effect, if applicable, to identify drug (T36-T50 with fifth or sixth character 5)

L56.1 Drug photoallergic response
Use additional code for adverse effect, if applicable, to identify drug (T36-T50 with fifth or sixth character 5)

L56.2 Photocontact dermatitis [berloque dermatitis]

L56.3 Solar urticaria

L56.4 Polymorphous light eruption

L56.5 Disseminated superficial actinic porokeratosis (DSAP)
DEF: Autosomal dominant skin condition occurring in sun-exposed areas of the skin (particularly the arms and legs); characterized by superficial annular, keratotic, brownish-red spots or thickenings with depressed centers and sharp, ridged borders; may evolve into squamous cell carcinoma.

L56.8 Other specified acute skin changes due to ultraviolet radiation

L56.9 Acute skin change due to ultraviolet radiation, unspecified

✓4ᵗʰ **L57 Skin changes due to chronic exposure to nonionizing radiation**
Use additional code to identify the source of the ultraviolet radiation ▶(W89)◀

L57.0 Actinic keratosis
Keratosis NOS
Senile keratosis
Solar keratosis

L57.1 Actinic reticuloid

L57.2 Cutis rhomboidalis nuchae

L57.3 Poikiloderma of Civatte

L57.4 Cutis laxa senilis
Elastosis senilis

L57.5 Actinic granuloma

L57.8 Other skin changes due to chronic exposure to nonionizing radiation
Farmer's skin
Sailor's skin
Solar dermatitis

L57.9 Skin changes due to chronic exposure to nonionizing radiation, unspecified

✓4ᵗʰ **L58 Radiodermatitis**
Use additional code to identify the source of the radiation (W88, W90)

L58.0 Acute radiodermatitis

L58.1 Chronic radiodermatitis

L58.9 Radiodermatitis, unspecified

✓4ᵗʰ **L59 Other disorders of skin and subcutaneous tissue related to radiation**

L59.0 Erythema ab igne [dermatitis ab igne]

L59.8 Other specified disorders of the skin and subcutaneous tissue related to radiation
AHA: 2017, 1Q, 33

L59.9 Disorder of the skin and subcutaneous tissue related to radiation, unspecified

Disorders of skin appendages (L60-L75)

EXCLUDES 1   *congenital malformations of integument (Q84.-)*

✓4ᵗʰ **L60 Nail disorders**

EXCLUDES 2   *clubbing of nails (R68.3)*
onychia and paronychia (L03.0-)

L60.0 Ingrowing nail

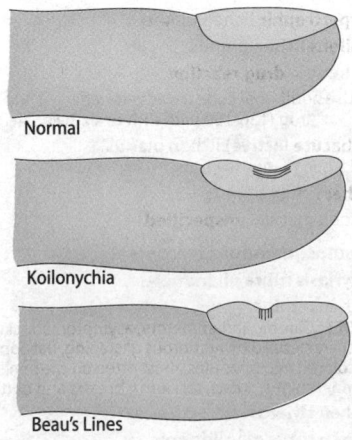

Nail Disorders

Normal

Koilonychia

Beau's Lines

N Newborn: 0   P Pediatric: 0-17   M Maternity: 12-55   A Adult: 15-124   MCC Major CC Condition   PDxMCC PDx acts as own MCC   CC CC Condition   PDxCC PDx acts as own CC

716   ICD-10-CM 2018

L60.1 **Onycholysis**

L60.2 **Onychogryphosis**

L60.3 **Nail dystrophy**

L60.4 **Beau's lines**

L60.5 **Yellow nail syndrome**

L60.8 **Other nail disorders**

L60.9 **Nail disorder, unspecified**

L62 *Nail disorders in diseases classified elsewhere*
Code first underlying disease, such as:
pachydermoperiostosis (M89.4-)

✓4ᵗʰ **L63 Alopecia areata**

L63.0 **Alopecia (capitis)** totalis

L63.1 **Alopecia** universalis

L63.2 **Ophiasis**

L63.8 **Other** alopecia areata

L63.9 **Alopecia areata,** unspecified

✓4ᵗʰ **L64 Androgenic alopecia**
INCLUDES male-pattern baldness

L64.0 **Drug-induced** androgenic alopecia
Use additional code for adverse effect, if applicable, to identify drug (T36-T50 with fifth or sixth character 5)

L64.8 **Other** androgenic alopecia

L64.9 **Androgenic alopecia,** unspecified

✓4ᵗʰ **L65 Other nonscarring hair loss**
Use additional code for adverse effect, if applicable, to identify drug (T36-T50 with fifth or sixth character 5)
EXCLUDES 1 trichotillomania (F63.3)

L65.0 **Telogen effluvium**
DEF: A form of nonscarring alopecia characterized by shedding of hair from premature telogen development in follicles due to stress, including shock, childbirth, surgery, drugs, or weight loss.

L65.1 **Anagen effluvium**

L65.2 **Alopecia mucinosa**

L65.8 **Other specified nonscarring hair loss**

L65.9 **Nonscarring hair loss, unspecified**
Alopecia NOS

✓4ᵗʰ **L66 Cicatricial alopecia [scarring hair loss]**

L66.0 **Pseudopelade**

L66.1 **Lichen planopilaris**
Follicular lichen planus

L66.2 **Folliculitis decalvans**

L66.3 **Perifolliculitis capitis abscedens**

L66.4 **Folliculitis ulerythematosa reticulata**

L66.8 **Other cicatricial alopecia**
AHA: 2015, 1Q, 19

L66.9 **Cicatricial alopecia, unspecified**

✓4ᵗʰ **L67 Hair color and hair shaft abnormalities**
EXCLUDES 1 monilethrix (Q84.1)
pili annulati (Q84.1)
telogen effluvium (L65.0)

L67.0 **Trichorrhexis nodosa**

L67.1 **Variations in hair color**
Canities
Greyness, hair (premature)
Heterochromia of hair
Poliosis circumscripta, acquired
Poliosis NOS

L67.8 **Other hair color and hair shaft abnormalities**
Fragilitas crinium

L67.9 **Hair color and hair shaft abnormality, unspecified**

✓4ᵗʰ **L68 Hypertrichosis**
INCLUDES excess hair
EXCLUDES 1 congenital hypertrichosis (Q84.2)
persistent lanugo (Q84.2)

L68.0 **Hirsutism**

L68.1 **Acquired hypertrichosis lanuginosa**

L68.2 **Localized hypertrichosis**

L68.3 **Polytrichia**

L68.8 **Other hypertrichosis**

L68.9 **Hypertrichosis, unspecified**

✓4ᵗʰ **L70 Acne**
EXCLUDES 2 acne keloid (L73.0)

L70.0 **Acne** vulgaris

L70.1 **Acne** conglobata

L70.2 **Acne** varioliformis
Acne necrotica miliaris
DEF: Rare form of acne characterized by development of persistent brown papulo-pustules followed by scar formation; usually on the brow and temporoparietal part of the scalp.

L70.3 **Acne** tropica

L70.4 **Infantile** acne   P

L70.5 **Acné excoriée**
Acné excoriée des jeunes filles
Picker's acne

L70.8 **Other** acne

L70.9 **Acne,** unspecified

✓4ᵗʰ **L71 Rosacea**
Use additional code for adverse effect, if applicable, to identify drug (T36-T50 with fifth or sixth character 5)

L71.0 **Perioral dermatitis**

L71.1 **Rhinophyma**

L71.8 **Other rosacea**

L71.9 **Rosacea, unspecified**

✓4ᵗʰ **L72 Follicular cysts of skin and subcutaneous tissue**

L72.0 **Epidermal cyst**

✓5ᵗʰ L72.1 **Pilar and trichodermal cyst**

L72.11 **Pilar cyst**

L72.12 **Trichodermal cyst**
Trichilemmal (proliferating) cyst

L72.2 **Steatocystoma multiplex**

L72.3 **Sebaceous cyst**
EXCLUDES 2 pilar cyst (L72.11)
trichilemmal (proliferating) cyst (L72.12)

L72.8 **Other follicular cysts of the skin and subcutaneous tissue**

L72.9 **Follicular cyst of the skin and subcutaneous tissue, unspecified**

✓4ᵗʰ **L73 Other follicular disorders**

L73.0 **Acne keloid**

L73.1 **Pseudofolliculitis barbae**

L73.2 **Hidradenitis suppurativa**

L73.8 **Other specified follicular disorders**
Sycosis barbae

L73.9 **Follicular disorder, unspecified**

✓4ᵗʰ **L74 Eccrine sweat disorders**
EXCLUDES 2 generalized hyperhidrosis (R61)

L74.0 **Miliaria** rubra

L74.1 **Miliaria** crystallina

L74.2 **Miliaria** profunda
Miliaria tropicalis

L74.3 **Miliaria,** unspecified

L74.4 **Anhidrosis**
Hypohidrosis

✓5ᵗʰ L74.5 **Focal hyperhidrosis**

✓6ᵗʰ L74.51 **Primary focal hyperhidrosis**

L74.510 **Primary focal hyperhidrosis,** axilla

L74.511 **Primary focal hyperhidrosis,** face

L74.512 **Primary focal hyperhidrosis,** palms

L74.513 **Primary focal hyperhidrosis,** soles

L74.519 **Primary focal hyperhidrosis,** unspecified

L74.52 **Secondary** focal hyperhidrosis
Frey's syndrome

L74.8 **Other eccrine sweat disorders**

L74.9 **Eccrine sweat disorder, unspecified**
Sweat gland disorder NOS

✓4ᵗʰ **L75 Apocrine sweat disorders**
EXCLUDES 1 dyshidrosis (L30.1)
hidradenitis suppurativa (L73.2)

L75.0 **Bromhidrosis**

L75.1 **Chromhidrosis**

Chapter 12. Diseases of the Skin and Subcutaneous Tissue

L75.2   Apocrine miliaria
Fox-Fordyce disease
DEF: Chronic, usually pruritic disease evidenced by small follicular papular eruptions, especially in the axillary and pubic areas; develops from the closure and rupture of the affected apocrine glands' intraepidermal portion of the ducts.

L75.8   Other apocrine sweat disorders

L75.9   Apocrine sweat disorder, unspecified

Intraoperative and postprocedural complications of skin and subcutaneous tissue (L76)

✓4ᵗʰ **L76   Intraoperative and postprocedural complications of skin and subcutaneous tissue**

> **CC Excl:** For CC codes in category L76, unless otherwise noted: PDX collection 852

✓5ᵗʰ **L76.0   Intraoperative hemorrhage and hematoma of skin and subcutaneous tissue complicating a procedure**
> *EXCLUDES 1*   *intraoperative hemorrhage and hematoma of skin and subcutaneous tissue due to accidental puncture and laceration during a procedure (L76.1-)*

    L76.01   Intraoperative hemorrhage and hematoma of skin and subcutaneous tissue complicating a dermatologic procedure   CC

    L76.02   Intraoperative hemorrhage and hematoma of skin and subcutaneous tissue complicating other procedure   CC

✓5ᵗʰ **L76.1   Accidental puncture and laceration of skin and subcutaneous tissue during a procedure**

    L76.11   Accidental puncture and laceration of skin and subcutaneous tissue during a dermatologic procedure   CC
        CC Excl: PDX collection 509

    L76.12   Accidental puncture and laceration of skin and subcutaneous tissue during other procedure   CC
        CC Excl: PDX collection 509

✓5ᵗʰ **L76.2   Postprocedural hemorrhage of skin and subcutaneous tissue following a procedure**

    L76.21   Postprocedural hemorrhage of skin and subcutaneous tissue following a dermatologic procedure   CC

    L76.22   Postprocedural hemorrhage of skin and subcutaneous tissue following other procedure   CC

✓5ᵗʰ **L76.3   Postprocedural hematoma and seroma of skin and subcutaneous tissue following a procedure**

    L76.31   Postprocedural hematoma of skin and subcutaneous tissue following a dermatologic procedure   CC

    L76.32   Postprocedural hematoma of skin and subcutaneous tissue following other procedure   CC

    L76.33   Postprocedural seroma of skin and subcutaneous tissue following a dermatologic procedure   CC

    L76.34   Postprocedural seroma of skin and subcutaneous tissue following other procedure   CC

✓5ᵗʰ **L76.8   Other intraoperative and postprocedural complications of skin and subcutaneous tissue**
Use additional code, if applicable, to further specify disorder

    L76.81   Other intraoperative complications of skin and subcutaneous tissue

    L76.82   Other postprocedural complications of skin and subcutaneous tissue

Other disorders of the skin and subcutaneous tissue (L80-L99)

L80   Vitiligo
> *EXCLUDES 2*   *vitiligo of eyelids (H02.73-)*
> *vitiligo of vulva (N90.89)*
DEF: Persistent, progressive development of nonpigmented white patches on otherwise normal skin.

✓4ᵗʰ **L81   Other disorders of pigmentation**
> *EXCLUDES 1*   *birthmark NOS (Q82.5)*
> *Peutz-Jeghers syndrome (Q85.8)*
> *EXCLUDES 2*   *nevus—see Alphabetical Index*

L81.0   Postinflammatory hyperpigmentation

L81.1   Chloasma

L81.2   Freckles

L81.3   Café au lait spots

L81.4   Other melanin hyperpigmentation
Lentigo

L81.5   Leukoderma, not elsewhere classified

L81.6   Other disorders of diminished melanin formation

L81.7   Pigmented purpuric dermatosis
Angioma serpiginosum

L81.8   Other specified disorders of pigmentation
Iron pigmentation
Tattoo pigmentation

L81.9   Disorder of pigmentation, unspecified

✓4ᵗʰ **L82   Seborrheic keratosis**
> *INCLUDES*   basal cell papilloma
> dermatosis papulosa nigra
> Leser-Trélat disease
> *EXCLUDES 2*   *seborrheic dermatitis (L21.-)*

L82.0   Inflamed seborrheic keratosis

L82.1   Other seborrheic keratosis
Seborrheic keratosis NOS

L83   Acanthosis nigricans
Confluent and reticulated papillomatosis
DEF: Diffuse, velvety hyperplasia of the spinous skin layer of the axilla and other body folds marked by gray, brown, or black pigmentation; in adult form often associated with malignant acanthosis nigricans in a benign, nevoid form relatively generalized.

L84   Corns and callosities
Callus   Clavus

✓4ᵗʰ **L85   Other epidermal thickening**
> *EXCLUDES 2*   *hypertrophic disorders of the skin (L91.-)*

L85.0   Acquired ichthyosis
> *EXCLUDES 1*   *congenital ichthyosis (Q80.-)*

L85.1   Acquired keratosis [keratoderma] palmaris et plantaris
> *EXCLUDES 1*   *inherited keratosis palmaris et plantaris (Q82.8)*

L85.2   Keratosis punctata (palmaris et plantaris)

L85.3   Xerosis cutis
Dry skin dermatitis

L85.8   Other specified epidermal thickening
Cutaneous horn

L85.9   Epidermal thickening, unspecified

L86   Keratoderma in diseases classified elsewhere
Code first underlying disease, such as:
    Reiter's disease (M02.3-)
> *EXCLUDES 1*   *gonococcal keratoderma (A54.89)*
> *gonococcal keratosis (A54.89)*
> *keratoderma due to vitamin A deficiency (E50.8)*
> *keratosis due to vitamin A deficiency (E50.8)*
> *xeroderma due to vitamin A deficiency (E50.8)*

✓4ᵗʰ **L87   Transepidermal elimination disorders**
> *EXCLUDES 1*   *granuloma annulare (perforating) (L92.0)*

L87.0   Keratosis follicularis et parafollicularis in cutem penetrans
Hyperkeratosis follicularis penetrans
Kyrle disease

L87.1   Reactive perforating collagenosis

L87.2   Elastosis perforans serpiginosa

L87.8   Other transepidermal elimination disorders

L87.9   Transepidermal elimination disorder, unspecified

L88   Pyoderma gangrenosum   CC
Phagedenic pyoderma
> *EXCLUDES 1*   *dermatitis gangrenosa (L08.0)*
DEF: Persistent debilitating skin disease characterized by irregular, boggy, blue-red ulcerations, with central healing and undermined edges.
CC Excl: PDX collection 853

N Newborn: 0   P Pediatric: 0-17   M Maternity: 12-55   A Adult: 15-124   MCC Major CC Condition   PDx MCC PDx acts as own MCC   CC CC Condition   PDx CC PDx acts as own CC

718   ICD-10-CM 2018

Four Stages of Pressure Ulcer

Stage 1
Persistent focal erythema

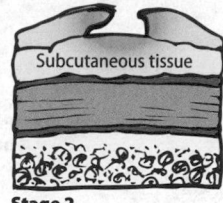

Subcutaneous tissue

Stage 2
Abrasion, blister, partial thickness skin loss involving epidermis and/or dermis

Epidermis
Dermis
Superficial fascia
Muscle

Stage 3
Full thickness skin loss involving damage or necrosis of subcutaneous tissue

Deep fascia
Bone

Stage 4
Necrosis of soft tissues through to underlying muscle, tendon, or bone

---

✓4ᵗʰ L89 Pressure ulcer

INCLUDES bed sore
decubitus ulcer
plaster ulcer
pressure area
pressure sore

Code first any associated gangrene (I96)

EXCLUDES 2 decubitus (trophic) ulcer of cervix (uteri) (N86)
diabetic ulcers (E08.621, E08.622, E09.621, E09.622, E10.621, E10.622, E11.621, E11.622, E13.621, E13.622)
non-pressure chronic ulcer of skin (L97.-)
skin infections (L00-L08)
varicose ulcer (I83.0, I83.2)

AHA: 2017, 1Q, 49; 2016, 4Q, 143

CC Excl: For MCC codes in category L89: PDX collection 854

✓5ᵗʰ L89.0 Pressure ulcer of elbow

✓6ᵗʰ L89.00 Pressure ulcer of unspecified elbow

L89.000 Pressure ulcer of unspecified elbow, unstageable HCC

L89.001 Pressure ulcer of unspecified elbow, stage 1
Healing pressure ulcer of unspecified elbow, stage 1
Pressure pre-ulcer skin changes limited to persistent focal edema, unspecified elbow

L89.002 Pressure ulcer of unspecified elbow, stage 2
Healing pressure ulcer of unspecified elbow, stage 2
Pressure ulcer with abrasion, blister, partial thickness skin loss involving epidermis and/or dermis, unspecified elbow

L89.003 Pressure ulcer of unspecified elbow, stage 3 PDxMCC MCC H4 HCC
Healing pressure ulcer of unspecified elbow, stage 3
Pressure ulcer with full thickness skin loss involving damage or necrosis of subcutaneous tissue, unspecified elbow

L89.004 Pressure ulcer of unspecified elbow, stage 4 PDxMCC MCC H4 HCC
Healing pressure ulcer of unspecified elbow, stage 4
Pressure ulcer with necrosis of soft tissues through to underlying muscle, tendon, or bone, unspecified elbow

L89.009 Pressure ulcer of unspecified elbow, unspecified stage
Healing pressure ulcer of elbow NOS
Healing pressure ulcer of unspecified elbow, unspecified stage

✓6ᵗʰ L89.01 Pressure ulcer of right elbow

L89.010 Pressure ulcer of right elbow, unstageable HCC

L89.011 Pressure ulcer of right elbow, stage 1
Healing pressure ulcer of right elbow, stage 1
Pressure pre-ulcer skin changes limited to persistent focal edema, right elbow

L89.012 Pressure ulcer of right elbow, stage 2
Healing pressure ulcer of right elbow, stage 2
Pressure ulcer with abrasion, blister, partial thickness skin loss involving epidermis and/or dermis, right elbow

L89.013 Pressure ulcer of right elbow, stage 3 PDxMCC MCC H4 HCC
Healing pressure ulcer of right elbow, stage 3
Pressure ulcer with full thickness skin loss involving damage or necrosis of subcutaneous tissue, right elbow

L89.014 Pressure ulcer of right elbow, stage 4 PDxMCC MCC H4 HCC
Healing pressure ulcer of right elbow, stage 4
Pressure ulcer with necrosis of soft tissues through to underlying muscle, tendon, or bone, right elbow

L89.019 Pressure ulcer of right elbow, unspecified stage
Healing pressure right of elbow NOS
▶Healing pressure ulcer of right elbow, unspecified stage◀

✓6ᵗʰ L89.02 Pressure ulcer of left elbow

L89.020 Pressure ulcer of left elbow, unstageable HCC

L89.021 Pressure ulcer of left elbow, stage 1
Healing pressure ulcer of left elbow, stage 1
Pressure pre-ulcer skin changes limited to persistent focal edema, left elbow

L89.022 Pressure ulcer of left elbow, stage 2
Healing pressure ulcer of left elbow, stage 2
Pressure ulcer with abrasion, blister, partial thickness skin loss involving epidermis and/or dermis, left elbow

L89.023 Pressure ulcer of left elbow, stage 3 PDxMCC MCC H4 HCC
Healing pressure ulcer of left elbow, stage 3
Pressure ulcer with full thickness skin loss involving damage or necrosis of subcutaneous tissue, left elbow

L89.024 Pressure ulcer of left elbow, stage 4 PDxMCC MCC H4 HCC
Healing pressure ulcer of left elbow, stage 4
Pressure ulcer with necrosis of soft tissues through to underlying muscle, tendon, or bone, left elbow

L89.029 Pressure ulcer of left elbow, unspecified stage
Healing pressure ulcer of left of elbow NOS
▶Healing pressure ulcer of left elbow, unspecified stage◀

✓5ᵗʰ L89.1 Pressure ulcer of back

✓6ᵗʰ L89.10 Pressure ulcer of unspecified part of back

L89.100 Pressure ulcer of unspecified part of back, unstageable HCC

L89.101 Pressure ulcer of unspecified part of back, stage 1
Healing pressure ulcer of unspecified part of back, stage 1
Pressure pre-ulcer skin changes limited to persistent focal edema, unspecified part of back

L89.102 Pressure ulcer of unspecified part of back, stage 2
Healing pressure ulcer of unspecified part of back, stage 2
Pressure ulcer with abrasion, blister, partial thickness skin loss involving epidermis and/or dermis, unspecified part of back

---

✔Additional Character Req   ✓x7ᵗʰ Placeholder Alert   Unacceptable PDx   Manifestation   H1 – H14 HAC   HCC CMS-HCC Condition   EXCLUDES 1 Not Coded Here   EXCLUDES 2 Not Included Here

L89.103 Pressure ulcer of unspecified part of back, stage 3 `PDxMCC` `MCC` `H4` `HCC`
Healing pressure ulcer of unspecified part of back, stage 3
Pressure ulcer with full thickness skin loss involving damage or necrosis of subcutaneous tissue, unspecified part of back

L89.104 Pressure ulcer of unspecified part of back, stage 4 `PDxMCC` `MCC` `H4` `HCC`
Healing pressure ulcer of unspecified part of back, stage 4
Pressure ulcer with necrosis of soft tissues through to underlying muscle, tendon, or bone, unspecified part of back

L89.109 Pressure ulcer of unspecified part of back, unspecified stage
Healing pressure ulcer of unspecified part of back NOS
Healing pressure ulcer of unspecified part of back, unspecified stage

✓6th **L89.11** Pressure ulcer of right upper back
Pressure ulcer of right shoulder blade

L89.110 Pressure ulcer of right upper back, unstageable `HCC`

L89.111 Pressure ulcer of right upper back, stage 1
Healing pressure ulcer of right upper back, stage 1
Pressure pre-ulcer skin changes limited to persistent focal edema, right upper back

L89.112 Pressure ulcer of right upper back, stage 2
Healing pressure ulcer of right upper back, stage 2
Pressure ulcer with abrasion, blister, partial thickness skin loss involving epidermis and/or dermis, right upper back

L89.113 Pressure ulcer of right upper back, stage 3 `PDxMCC` `MCC` `H4` `HCC`
Healing pressure ulcer of right upper back, stage 3
Pressure ulcer with full thickness skin loss involving damage or necrosis of subcutaneous tissue, right upper back

L89.114 Pressure ulcer of right upper back, stage 4 `PDxMCC` `MCC` `H4` `HCC`
Healing pressure ulcer of right upper back, stage 4
Pressure ulcer with necrosis of soft tissues through to underlying muscle, tendon, or bone, right upper back

L89.119 Pressure ulcer of right upper back, unspecified stage
Healing pressure ulcer of right upper back NOS
Healing pressure ulcer of right upper back, unspecified stage

✓6th **L89.12** Pressure ulcer of left upper back
Pressure ulcer of left shoulder blade

L89.120 Pressure ulcer of left upper back, unstageable `HCC`

L89.121 Pressure ulcer of left upper back, stage 1
Healing pressure ulcer of left upper back, stage 1
Pressure pre-ulcer skin changes limited to persistent focal edema, left upper back

L89.122 Pressure ulcer of left upper back, stage 2
Healing pressure ulcer of left upper back, stage 2
Pressure ulcer with abrasion, blister, partial thickness skin loss involving epidermis and/or dermis, left upper back

L89.123 Pressure ulcer of left upper back, stage 3 `PDxMCC` `MCC` `H4` `HCC`
Healing pressure ulcer of left upper back, stage 3
Pressure ulcer with full thickness skin loss involving damage or necrosis of subcutaneous tissue, left upper back

L89.124 Pressure ulcer of left upper back, stage 4 `PDxMCC` `MCC` `H4` `HCC`
Healing pressure ulcer of left upper back, stage 4
Pressure ulcer with necrosis of soft tissues through to underlying muscle, tendon, or bone, left upper back

L89.129 Pressure ulcer of left upper back, unspecified stage
Healing pressure ulcer of left upper back NOS
Healing pressure ulcer of left upper back, unspecified stage

✓6th **L89.13** Pressure ulcer of right lower back

L89.130 Pressure ulcer of right lower back, unstageable `HCC`

L89.131 Pressure ulcer of right lower back, stage 1
Healing pressure ulcer of right lower back, stage 1
Pressure pre-ulcer skin changes limited to persistent focal edema, right lower back

L89.132 Pressure ulcer of right lower back, stage 2
Healing pressure ulcer of right lower back, stage 2
Pressure ulcer with abrasion, blister, partial thickness skin loss involving epidermis and/or dermis, right lower back

L89.133 Pressure ulcer of right lower back, stage 3 `PDxMCC` `MCC` `H4` `HCC`
Healing pressure ulcer of right lower back, stage 3
Pressure ulcer with full thickness skin loss involving damage or necrosis of subcutaneous tissue, right lower back

L89.134 Pressure ulcer of right lower back, stage 4 `PDxMCC` `MCC` `H4` `HCC`
Healing pressure ulcer of right lower back, stage 4
Pressure ulcer with necrosis of soft tissues through to underlying muscle, tendon, or bone, right lower back

L89.139 Pressure ulcer of right lower back, unspecified stage
Healing pressure ulcer of right lower back NOS
Healing pressure ulcer of right lower back, unspecified stage

✓6th **L89.14** Pressure ulcer of left lower back

L89.140 Pressure ulcer of left lower back, unstageable `HCC`

L89.141 Pressure ulcer of left lower back, stage 1
Healing pressure ulcer of left lower back, stage 1
Pressure pre-ulcer skin changes limited to persistent focal edema, left lower back

L89.142 Pressure ulcer of left lower back, stage 2
Healing pressure ulcer of left lower back, stage 2
Pressure ulcer with abrasion, blister, partial thickness skin loss involving epidermis and/or dermis, left lower back

L89.143 Pressure ulcer of left lower back, stage 3 `PDxMCC` `MCC` `H4` `HCC`
Healing pressure ulcer of left lower back, stage 3
Pressure ulcer with full thickness skin loss involving damage or necrosis of subcutaneous tissue, left lower back

L89.144 Pressure ulcer of left lower back, stage 4 `PDxMCC` `MCC` `H4` `HCC`
Healing pressure ulcer of left lower back, stage 4
Pressure ulcer with necrosis of soft tissues through to underlying muscle, tendon, or bone, left lower back

L89.149 Pressure ulcer of left lower back, unspecified stage
Healing pressure ulcer of left lower back NOS
Healing pressure ulcer of left lower back, unspecified stage

N Newborn: 0   P Pediatric: 0-17   M Maternity: 12-55   A Adult: 15-124   `MCC` Major CC Condition   `PDxMCC` PDx acts as own MCC   `CC` CC Condition   `PDxCC` PDx acts as own CC

720   ICD-10-CM 2018

Chapter 12. Diseases of the Skin and Subcutaneous Tissue

√6th **L89.15** **Pressure ulcer of** sacral region
Pressure ulcer of coccyx
Pressure ulcer of tailbone

     L89.150 **Pressure ulcer of sacral region,** HCC
unstageable

     L89.151 **Pressure ulcer of sacral region,** stage 1
Healing pressure ulcer of sacral region, stage 1
Pressure pre-ulcer skin changes limited to persistent focal edema, sacral region

     L89.152 **Pressure ulcer of sacral region,** stage 2
Healing pressure ulcer of sacral region, stage 2
Pressure ulcer with abrasion, blister, partial thickness skin loss involving epidermis and/or dermis, sacral region

     L89.153 **Pressure ulcer of sacral** PDx MCC MCC H4 HCC
region, stage 3
Healing pressure ulcer of sacral region, stage 3
Pressure ulcer with full thickness skin loss involving damage or necrosis of subcutaneous tissue, sacral region

     L89.154 **Pressure ulcer of sacral** PDx MCC MCC H4 HCC
region, stage 4
Healing pressure ulcer of sacral region, stage 4
Pressure ulcer with necrosis of soft tissues through to underlying muscle, tendon, or bone, sacral region

     L89.159 **Pressure ulcer of sacral region,**
unspecified stage
Healing pressure ulcer of sacral region NOS
Healing pressure ulcer of sacral region, unspecified stage

√5th **L89.2** **Pressure ulcer of** hip

     √6th **L89.20** **Pressure ulcer of** unspecified hip

       L89.200 **Pressure ulcer of unspecified hip,** HCC
unstageable

       L89.201 **Pressure ulcer of unspecified hip,** stage 1
Healing pressure ulcer of unspecified hip back, stage 1
Pressure pre-ulcer skin changes limited to persistent focal edema, unspecified hip

       L89.202 **Pressure ulcer of unspecified hip,** stage 2
Healing pressure ulcer of unspecified hip, stage 2
Pressure ulcer with abrasion, blister, partial thickness skin loss involving epidermis and/or dermis, unspecified hip

       L89.203 **Pressure ulcer of** PDx MCC MCC H4 HCC
unspecified hip, stage 3
Healing pressure ulcer of unspecified hip, stage 3
Pressure ulcer with full thickness skin loss involving damage or necrosis of subcutaneous tissue, unspecified hip

       L89.204 **Pressure ulcer of** PDx MCC MCC H4 HCC
unspecified hip, stage 4
Healing pressure ulcer of unspecified hip, stage 4
Pressure ulcer with necrosis of soft tissues through to underlying muscle, tendon, or bone, unspecified hip

       L89.209 **Pressure ulcer of unspecified hip,**
unspecified stage
Healing pressure ulcer of unspecified hip NOS
Healing pressure ulcer of unspecified hip, unspecified stage

     √6th **L89.21** **Pressure ulcer of** right hip

       L89.210 **Pressure ulcer of right hip,** HCC
unstageable

       L89.211 **Pressure ulcer of right hip,** stage 1
Healing pressure ulcer of right hip back, stage 1
Pressure pre-ulcer skin changes limited to persistent focal edema, right hip

       L89.212 **Pressure ulcer of right hip,** stage 2
Healing pressure ulcer of right hip, stage 2
Pressure ulcer with abrasion, blister, partial thickness skin loss involving epidermis and/or dermis, right hip

     L89.213 **Pressure ulcer of right** PDx MCC MCC H4 HCC
hip, stage 3
Healing pressure ulcer of right hip, stage 3
Pressure ulcer with full thickness skin loss involving damage or necrosis of subcutaneous tissue, right hip

     L89.214 **Pressure ulcer of right** PDx MCC MCC H4 HCC
hip, stage 4
Healing pressure ulcer of right hip, stage 4
Pressure ulcer with necrosis of soft tissues through to underlying muscle, tendon, or bone, right hip

     L89.219 **Pressure ulcer of right hip,** unspecified
stage
Healing pressure ulcer of right hip NOS
Healing pressure ulcer of right hip, unspecified stage

√6th **L89.22** **Pressure ulcer of** left hip

     L89.220 **Pressure ulcer of left hip,** unstageable HCC

     L89.221 **Pressure ulcer of left hip,** stage 1
Healing pressure ulcer of left hip back, stage 1
Pressure pre-ulcer skin changes limited to persistent focal edema, left hip

     L89.222 **Pressure ulcer of left hip,** stage 2
Healing pressure ulcer of left hip, stage 2
Pressure ulcer with abrasion, blister, partial thickness skin loss involving epidermis and/or dermis, left hip

     L89.223 **Pressure ulcer of left** PDx MCC MCC H4 HCC
hip, stage 3
Healing pressure ulcer of left hip, stage 3
Pressure ulcer with full thickness skin loss involving damage or necrosis of subcutaneous tissue, left hip

     L89.224 **Pressure ulcer of left** PDx MCC MCC H4 HCC
hip, stage 4
Healing pressure ulcer of left hip, stage 4
Pressure ulcer with necrosis of soft tissues through to underlying muscle, tendon, or bone, left hip

     L89.229 **Pressure ulcer of left hip,** unspecified
stage
Healing pressure ulcer of left hip NOS
Healing pressure ulcer of left hip, unspecified stage

√5th **L89.3** **Pressure ulcer of** buttock

     √6th **L89.30** **Pressure ulcer of** unspecified buttock

       L89.300 **Pressure ulcer of unspecified buttock,** HCC
unstageable

       L89.301 **Pressure ulcer of unspecified buttock,**
stage 1
Healing pressure ulcer of unspecified buttock, stage 1
Pressure pre-ulcer skin changes limited to persistent focal edema, unspecified buttock

       L89.302 **Pressure ulcer of unspecified buttock,**
stage 2
Healing pressure ulcer of unspecified buttock, stage 2
Pressure ulcer with abrasion, blister, partial thickness skin loss involving epidermis and/or dermis, unspecified buttock

       L89.303 **Pressure ulcer of** PDx MCC MCC H4 HCC
unspecified buttock, stage 3
Healing pressure ulcer of unspecified buttock, stage 3
Pressure ulcer with full thickness skin loss involving damage or necrosis of subcutaneous tissue, unspecified buttock

       L89.304 **Pressure ulcer of** PDx MCC MCC H4 HCC
unspecified buttock, stage 4
Healing pressure ulcer of unspecified buttock, stage 4
Pressure ulcer with necrosis of soft tissues through to underlying muscle, tendon, or bone, unspecified buttock

---

√ Additional Character Req   √x7th Placeholder Alert   Unacceptable PDx   Manifestation   H1 - H14 HAC   HCC CMS-HCC Condition   *EXCLUDES 1* Not Coded Here   *EXCLUDES 2* Not Included Here

      L89.309 Pressure ulcer of unspecified buttock, unspecified stage
Healing pressure ulcer of unspecified buttock NOS
Healing pressure ulcer of unspecified buttock, unspecified stage

✓6th **L89.31 Pressure ulcer of right buttock**

      L89.310 Pressure ulcer of right buttock, unstageable `HCC`

      L89.311 Pressure ulcer of right buttock, stage 1
Healing pressure ulcer of right buttock, stage 1
Pressure pre-ulcer skin changes limited to persistent focal edema, right buttock

      L89.312 Pressure ulcer of right buttock, stage 2
Healing pressure ulcer of right buttock, stage 2
Pressure ulcer with abrasion, blister, partial thickness skin loss involving epidermis and/or dermis, right buttock

      L89.313 Pressure ulcer of right buttock, unspecified stage 3 `PDxMCC` `MCC` `H4` `HCC`
Healing pressure ulcer of right buttock, stage 3
Pressure ulcer with full thickness skin loss involving damage or necrosis of subcutaneous tissue, right buttock

      L89.314 Pressure ulcer of right buttock, unspecified stage 4 `PDxMCC` `MCC` `H4` `HCC`
Healing pressure ulcer of right buttock, stage 4
Pressure ulcer with necrosis of soft tissues through to underlying muscle, tendon, or bone, right buttock

      L89.319 Pressure ulcer of right buttock, unspecified stage
Healing pressure ulcer of right buttock NOS
Healing pressure ulcer of right buttock, unspecified stage

✓6th **L89.32 Pressure ulcer of left buttock**

      L89.320 Pressure ulcer of left buttock, unstageable `HCC`

      L89.321 Pressure ulcer of left buttock, stage 1
Healing pressure ulcer of left buttock, stage 1
Pressure pre-ulcer skin changes limited to persistent focal edema, left buttock

      L89.322 Pressure ulcer of left buttock, stage 2
Healing pressure ulcer of left buttock, stage 2
Pressure ulcer with abrasion, blister, partial thickness skin loss involving epidermis and/or dermis, left buttock

      L89.323 Pressure ulcer of left buttock, stage 3 `PDxMCC` `MCC` `H4` `HCC`
Healing pressure ulcer of left buttock, stage 3
Pressure ulcer with full thickness skin loss involving damage or necrosis of subcutaneous tissue, left buttock

      L89.324 Pressure ulcer of left buttock, stage 4 `PDxMCC` `MCC` `H4` `HCC`
Healing pressure ulcer of left buttock, stage 4
Pressure ulcer with necrosis of soft tissues through to underlying muscle, tendon, or bone, left buttock

      L89.329 Pressure ulcer of left buttock, unspecified stage
Healing pressure ulcer of left buttock NOS
Healing pressure ulcer of left buttock, unspecified stage

✓5th **L89.4 Pressure ulcer of contiguous site of back, buttock and hip**

      L89.40 Pressure ulcer of contiguous site of back, buttock and hip, unspecified stage
Healing pressure ulcer of contiguous site of back, buttock and hip NOS
Healing pressure ulcer of contiguous site of back, buttock and hip, unspecified stage

      L89.41 Pressure ulcer of contiguous site of back, buttock and hip, stage 1
Healing pressure ulcer of contiguous site of back, buttock and hip, stage 1
Pressure pre-ulcer skin changes limited to persistent focal edema, contiguous site of back, buttock and hip

      L89.42 Pressure ulcer of contiguous site of back, buttock and hip, stage 2
Healing pressure ulcer of contiguous site of back, buttock and hip, stage 2
Pressure ulcer with abrasion, blister, partial thickness skin loss involving epidermis and/or dermis, contiguous site of back, buttock and hip

      L89.43 Pressure ulcer of contiguous site of back, buttock and hip, stage 3 `PDxMCC` `MCC` `H4` `HCC`
Healing pressure ulcer of contiguous site of back, buttock and hip, stage 3
Pressure ulcer with full thickness skin loss involving damage or necrosis of subcutaneous tissue, contiguous site of back, buttock and hip

      L89.44 Pressure ulcer of contiguous site of back, buttock and hip, stage 4 `PDxMCC` `MCC` `H4` `HCC`
Healing pressure ulcer of contiguous site of back, buttock and hip, stage 4
Pressure ulcer with necrosis of soft tissues through to underlying muscle, tendon, or bone, contiguous site of back, buttock and hip

      L89.45 Pressure ulcer of contiguous site of back, buttock and hip, unstageable `HCC`

✓5th **L89.5 Pressure ulcer of ankle**

✓6th **L89.50 Pressure ulcer of unspecified ankle**

      L89.500 Pressure ulcer of unspecified ankle, unstageable `HCC`

      L89.501 Pressure ulcer of unspecified ankle, stage 1
Healing pressure ulcer of unspecified ankle, stage 1
Pressure pre-ulcer skin changes limited to persistent focal edema, unspecified ankle

      L89.502 Pressure ulcer of unspecified ankle, stage 2
Healing pressure ulcer of unspecified ankle, stage 2
Pressure ulcer with abrasion, blister, partial thickness skin loss involving epidermis and/or dermis, unspecified ankle

      L89.503 Pressure ulcer of unspecified ankle, stage 3 `PDxMCC` `MCC` `H4` `HCC`
Healing pressure ulcer of unspecified ankle, stage 3
Pressure ulcer with full thickness skin loss involving damage or necrosis of subcutaneous tissue, unspecified ankle

      L89.504 Pressure ulcer of unspecified ankle, stage 4 `PDxMCC` `MCC` `H4` `HCC`
Healing pressure ulcer of unspecified ankle, stage 4
Pressure ulcer with necrosis of soft tissues through to underlying muscle, tendon, or bone, unspecified ankle

      L89.509 Pressure ulcer of unspecified ankle, unspecified stage
Healing pressure ulcer of unspecified ankle NOS
Healing pressure ulcer of unspecified ankle, unspecified stage

✓6th **L89.51 Pressure ulcer of right ankle**

      L89.510 Pressure ulcer of right ankle, unstageable `HCC`

      L89.511 Pressure ulcer of right ankle, stage 1
Healing pressure ulcer of right ankle, stage 1
Pressure pre-ulcer skin changes limited to persistent focal edema, right ankle

      L89.512 Pressure ulcer of right ankle, stage 2
Healing pressure ulcer of right ankle, stage 2
Pressure pre-ulcer skin changes limited to persistent focal edema, right ankle

N Newborn: 0   P Pediatric: 0-17   M Maternity: 12-55   A Adult: 15-124   `MCC` Major CC Condition   `PDxMCC` PDx acts as own MCC   `CC` CC Condition   `PDxCC` PDx acts as own CC

722   ICD-10-CM 2018

L89.513   **Pressure ulcer of right ankle, stage 3**   `PDxMCC` `MCC` `H4` `HCC`
Healing pressure ulcer of right ankle, stage 3
Pressure ulcer with full thickness skin loss involving damage or necrosis of subcutaneous tissue, right ankle

L89.514   **Pressure ulcer of right ankle, stage 4**   `PDxMCC` `MCC` `H4` `HCC`
Healing pressure ulcer of right ankle, stage 4
Pressure ulcer with necrosis of soft tissues through to underlying muscle, tendon, or bone, right ankle

L89.519   **Pressure ulcer of right ankle, unspecified stage**
Healing pressure ulcer of right ankle NOS
Healing pressure ulcer of right ankle, unspecified stage

✓6th **L89.52**   **Pressure ulcer of left ankle**

L89.520   **Pressure ulcer of left ankle, unstageable**   `HCC`

L89.521   **Pressure ulcer of left ankle, stage 1**
Healing pressure ulcer of left ankle, stage 1
Pressure pre-ulcer skin changes limited to persistent focal edema, left ankle

L89.522   **Pressure ulcer of left ankle, stage 2**
Healing pressure ulcer of left ankle, stage 2
Pressure ulcer with abrasion, blister, partial thickness skin loss involving epidermis and/or dermis, left ankle

L89.523   **Pressure ulcer of left ankle, stage 3**   `PDxMCC` `MCC` `H4` `HCC`
Healing pressure ulcer of left ankle, stage 3
Pressure ulcer with full thickness skin loss involving damage or necrosis of subcutaneous tissue, left ankle

L89.524   **Pressure ulcer of left ankle, stage 4**   `PDxMCC` `MCC` `H4` `HCC`
Healing pressure ulcer of left ankle, stage 4
Pressure ulcer with necrosis of soft tissues through to underlying muscle, tendon, or bone, left ankle

L89.529   **Pressure ulcer of left ankle, unspecified stage**
Healing pressure ulcer of left ankle NOS
Healing pressure ulcer of left ankle, unspecified stage

✓5th **L89.6**   **Pressure ulcer of heel**

✓6th **L89.60**   **Pressure ulcer of unspecified heel**

L89.600   **Pressure ulcer of unspecified heel, unstageable**   `HCC`

L89.601   **Pressure ulcer of unspecified heel, stage 1**
Healing pressure ulcer of unspecified heel, stage 1
Pressure pre-ulcer skin changes limited to persistent focal edema, unspecified heel

L89.602   **Pressure ulcer of unspecified heel, stage 2**
Healing pressure ulcer of unspecified heel, stage 2
Pressure ulcer with abrasion, blister, partial thickness skin loss involving epidermis and/or dermis, unspecified heel

L89.603   **Pressure ulcer of unspecified heel, stage 3**   `PDxMCC` `MCC` `H4` `HCC`
Healing pressure ulcer of unspecified heel, stage 3
Pressure ulcer with full thickness skin loss involving damage or necrosis of subcutaneous tissue, unspecified heel

L89.604   **Pressure ulcer of unspecified heel, stage 4**   `PDxMCC` `MCC` `H4` `HCC`
Healing pressure ulcer of unspecified heel, stage 4
Pressure ulcer with necrosis of soft tissues through to underlying muscle, tendon, or bone, unspecified heel

L89.609   **Pressure ulcer of unspecified heel, unspecified stage**
Healing pressure ulcer of unspecified heel NOS
Healing pressure ulcer of unspecified heel, unspecified stage

✓6th **L89.61**   **Pressure ulcer of right heel**

L89.610   **Pressure ulcer of right heel, unstageable**   `HCC`

L89.611   **Pressure ulcer of right heel, stage 1**
Healing pressure ulcer of right heel, stage 1
Pressure pre-ulcer skin changes limited to persistent focal edema, right heel

L89.612   **Pressure ulcer of right heel, stage 2**
Healing pressure ulcer of right heel, stage 2
Pressure ulcer with abrasion, blister, partial thickness skin loss involving epidermis and/or dermis, right heel

L89.613   **Pressure ulcer of right heel, stage 3**   `PDxMCC` `MCC` `H4` `HCC`
Healing pressure ulcer of right heel, stage 3
Pressure ulcer with full thickness skin loss involving damage or necrosis of subcutaneous tissue, right heel

L89.614   **Pressure ulcer of right heel, stage 4**   `PDxMCC` `MCC` `H4` `HCC`
Healing pressure ulcer of right heel, stage 4
Pressure ulcer with necrosis of soft tissues through to underlying muscle, tendon, or bone, right heel

L89.619   **Pressure ulcer of right heel, unspecified stage**
Healing pressure ulcer of right heel NOS
▶Healing pressure ulcer of right heel, unspecified stage◀

✓6th **L89.62**   **Pressure ulcer of left heel**

L89.620   **Pressure ulcer of left heel, unstageable**   `HCC`

L89.621   **Pressure ulcer of left heel, stage 1**
Healing pressure ulcer of left heel, stage 1
Pressure pre-ulcer skin changes limited to persistent focal edema, left heel

L89.622   **Pressure ulcer of left heel, stage 2**
Healing pressure ulcer of left heel, stage 2
Pressure ulcer with abrasion, blister, partial thickness skin loss involving epidermis and/or dermis, left heel

L89.623   **Pressure ulcer of left heel, stage 3**   `PDxMCC` `MCC` `H4` `HCC`
Healing pressure ulcer of left heel, stage 3
Pressure ulcer with full thickness skin loss involving damage or necrosis of subcutaneous tissue, left heel

L89.624   **Pressure ulcer of left heel, stage 4**   `PDxMCC` `MCC` `H4` `HCC`
Healing pressure ulcer of left heel, stage 4
Pressure ulcer with necrosis of soft tissues through to underlying muscle, tendon, or bone, left heel

L89.629   **Pressure ulcer of left heel, unspecified stage**
Healing pressure ulcer of left heel NOS
Healing pressure ulcer of left heel, unspecified stage

✓5th **L89.8**   **Pressure ulcer of other site**

✓6th **L89.81**   **Pressure ulcer of head**
Pressure ulcer of face

L89.810   **Pressure ulcer of head, unstageable**   `HCC`

L89.811   **Pressure ulcer of head, stage 1**
Healing pressure ulcer of head, stage 1
Pressure pre-ulcer skin changes limited to persistent focal edema, head

L89.812   **Pressure ulcer of head, stage 2**
Healing pressure ulcer of head, stage 2
Pressure ulcer with abrasion, blister, partial thickness skin loss involving epidermis and/or dermis, head

---

✓ Additional Character Req   ✓x7th Placeholder Alert   Unacceptable PDx   Manifestation   `H1`-`H14` HAC   `HCC` CMS-HCC Condition   `EXCLUDES 1` Not Coded Here   `EXCLUDES 2` Not Included Here

Chapter 12. Diseases of the Skin and Subcutaneous Tissue

L89.813   Pressure ulcer of head, stage 3   `PDxMCC` `MCC` `H4` `HCC`
> Healing pressure ulcer of head, stage 3
> Pressure ulcer with full thickness skin loss involving damage or necrosis of subcutaneous tissue, head

L89.814   Pressure ulcer of head, stage 4   `PDxMCC` `MCC` `H4` `HCC`
> Healing pressure ulcer of head, stage 4
> Pressure ulcer with necrosis of soft tissues through to underlying muscle, tendon, or bone, head

L89.819   Pressure ulcer of head, unspecified stage
> Healing pressure ulcer of head NOS
> Healing pressure ulcer of head, unspecified stage

✓6ᵗʰ **L89.89   Pressure ulcer of other site**

L89.890   Pressure ulcer of other site, unstageable   `HCC`

L89.891   Pressure ulcer of other site, stage 1
> Healing pressure ulcer of other site, stage 1
> Pressure pre-ulcer skin changes limited to persistent focal edema, other site

L89.892   Pressure ulcer of other site, stage 2
> Healing pressure ulcer of other site, stage 2
> Pressure ulcer with abrasion, blister, partial thickness skin loss involving epidermis and/or dermis, other site

L89.893   Pressure ulcer of other site, stage 3   `PDxMCC` `MCC` `H4` `HCC`
> Healing pressure ulcer of other site, stage 3
> Pressure ulcer with full thickness skin loss involving damage or necrosis of subcutaneous tissue, other site

L89.894   Pressure ulcer of other site, stage 4   `PDxMCC` `MCC` `H4` `HCC`
> Healing pressure ulcer of other site, stage 4
> Pressure ulcer with necrosis of soft tissues through to underlying muscle, tendon, or bone, other site

L89.899   Pressure ulcer of other site, unspecified stage
> Healing pressure ulcer of other site NOS
> Healing pressure ulcer of other site, unspecified stage

✓5ᵗʰ **L89.9   Pressure ulcer of unspecified site**

L89.90   Pressure ulcer of unspecified site, unspecified stage
> Healing pressure ulcer of unspecified site NOS
> Healing pressure ulcer of unspecified site, unspecified stage

L89.91   Pressure ulcer of unspecified site, stage 1
> Healing pressure ulcer of unspecified site, stage 1
> Pressure pre-ulcer skin changes limited to persistent focal edema, unspecified site

L89.92   Pressure ulcer of unspecified site, stage 2
> Healing pressure ulcer of unspecified site, stage 2
> Pressure ulcer with abrasion, blister, partial thickness skin loss involving epidermis and/or dermis, unspecified site

L89.93   Pressure ulcer of unspecified site, stage 3   `PDxMCC` `MCC` `H4` `HCC`
> Healing pressure ulcer of unspecified site, stage 3
> Pressure ulcer with full thickness skin loss involving damage or necrosis of subcutaneous tissue, unspecified site

L89.94   Pressure ulcer of unspecified site, stage 4   `PDxMCC` `MCC` `H4` `HCC`
> Healing pressure ulcer of unspecified site, stage 4
> Pressure ulcer with necrosis of soft tissues through to underlying muscle, tendon, or bone, unspecified site

L89.95   Pressure ulcer of unspecified site, unstageable   `HCC`

✓4ᵗʰ **L90   Atrophic disorders of skin**

L90.0   Lichen sclerosus et atrophicus
> EXCLUDES 2   *lichen sclerosus of external female genital organs (N90.4)*
> *lichen sclerosus of external male genital organs (N48.0)*

L90.1   Anetoderma of Schweninger-Buzzi

L90.2   Anetoderma of Jadassohn-Pellizzari

L90.3   Atrophoderma of Pasini and Pierini

L90.4   Acrodermatitis chronica atrophicans

L90.5   Scar conditions and fibrosis of skin
> Adherent scar (skin)
> Cicatrix
> Disfigurement of skin due to scar
> Fibrosis of skin NOS
> Scar NOS
> EXCLUDES 2   *hypertrophic scar (L91.0)*
> *keloid scar (L91.0)*
> **AHA:** 2016, 2Q, 5; 2015, 1Q, 19

L90.6   Striae atrophicae

L90.8   Other atrophic disorders of skin

L90.9   Atrophic disorder of skin, unspecified

✓4ᵗʰ **L91   Hypertrophic disorders of skin**

L91.0   Hypertrophic scar
> Keloid
> Keloid scar
> EXCLUDES 2   *acne keloid (L73.0)*
> *scar NOS (L90.5)*
> **DEF:** Overgrowth of scar tissue due to excess amounts of collagen during connective tissue repair; occurs mainly on upper trunk, face.

L91.8   Other hypertrophic disorders of the skin

L91.9   Hypertrophic disorder of the skin, unspecified

✓4ᵗʰ **L92   Granulomatous disorders of skin and subcutaneous tissue**
> EXCLUDES 2   *actinic granuloma (L57.5)*

L92.0   Granuloma annulare
> Perforating granuloma annulare

L92.1   Necrobiosis lipoidica, not elsewhere classified
> EXCLUDES 1   *necrobiosis lipoidica associated with diabetes mellitus (E08-E13 with .620)*

L92.2   Granuloma faciale [eosinophilic granuloma of skin]

L92.3   Foreign body granuloma of the skin and subcutaneous tissue
> Use additional code to identify the type of retained foreign body (Z18.-)

L92.8   Other granulomatous disorders of the skin and subcutaneous tissue

L92.9   Granulomatous disorder of the skin and subcutaneous tissue, unspecified
> EXCLUDES 2   ▶*umbilical granuloma (P83.81)*◀

✓4ᵗʰ **L93   Lupus erythematosus**
> Use additional code for adverse effect, if applicable, to identify drug (T36-T50 with fifth or sixth character 5)
> EXCLUDES 1   *lupus exedens (A18.4)*
> *lupus vulgaris (A18.4)*
> *scleroderma (M34.-)*
> *systemic lupus erythematosus (M32.-)*

L93.0   Discoid lupus erythematosus
> Lupus erythematosus NOS

L93.1   Subacute cutaneous lupus erythematosus

L93.2   Other local lupus erythematosus
> Lupus erythematosus profundus
> Lupus panniculitis

✓4ᵗʰ **L94   Other localized connective tissue disorders**
> EXCLUDES 1   *systemic connective tissue disorders (M30-M36)*

L94.0   Localized scleroderma [morphea]
> Circumscribed scleroderma

L94.1   Linear scleroderma
> En coup de sabre lesion

L94.2   Calcinosis cutis

L94.3   Sclerodactyly

L94.4   Gottron's papules

L94.5   Poikiloderma vasculare atrophicans

L94.6   Ainhum

L94.8   Other specified localized connective tissue disorders

L94.9   Localized connective tissue disorder, unspecified

`N` Newborn: 0   `P` Pediatric: 0-17   `M` Maternity: 12-55   `A` Adult: 15-124   `MCC` Major CC Condition   `PDxMCC` PDx acts as own MCC   `CC` CC Condition   `PDxCC` PDx acts as own CC

724   ICD-10-CM 2018

☑️4ᵗʰ **L95** **Vasculitis limited to skin, not elsewhere classified**

    EXCLUDES 1   *angioma serpiginosum (L81.7)*
               Henoch(-Schönlein) purpura (D69.0)
               hypersensitivity angiitis (M31.0)
               lupus panniculitis (L93.2)
               panniculitis NOS (M79.3)
               panniculitis of neck and back (M54.0-)
               polyarteritis nodosa (M30.0)
               relapsing panniculitis (M35.6)
               rheumatoid vasculitis (M05.2)
               serum sickness (T80.6-)
               urticaria (L50.-)
               Wegener's granulomatosis (M31.3-)

    L95.0   **Livedoid vasculitis**
            Atrophie blanche (en plaque)

    L95.1   **Erythema elevatum diutinum**

    L95.8   **Other vasculitis limited to the skin**

    L95.9   **Vasculitis limited to the skin, unspecified**

☑️4ᵗʰ **L97** **Non-pressure chronic ulcer of lower limb, not elsewhere classified**

    INCLUDES   chronic ulcer of skin of lower limb NOS
               non-healing ulcer of skin
               non-infected sinus of skin
               trophic ulcer NOS
               tropical ulcer NOS
               ulcer of skin of lower limb NOS

    Code first any associated underlying condition, such as:
       any associated gangrene (I96)
       atherosclerosis of the lower extremities (I70.23-, I70.24-, I70.33-, I70.34-, I70.43-, I70.44-, I70.53-, I70.54-, I70.63-, I70.64-, I70.73-, I70.74-)
       chronic venous hypertension (I87.31-, I87.33-)
       diabetic ulcers (E08.621, E08.622, E09.621, E09.622, E10.621, E10.622, E11.621, E11.622, E13.621, E13.622)
       postphlebitic syndrome (I87.01-, I87.03-)
       postthrombotic syndrome (I87.01-, I87.03-)
       varicose ulcer (I83.0-, I83.2-)

    EXCLUDES 2   *pressure ulcer (pressure area) (L89.-)*
               skin infections (L00-L08)
               specific infections classified to A00-B99

    CC Excl: For CC codes in category L97: PDX collection 698

☑️5ᵗʰ **L97.1**   **Non-pressure chronic ulcer of** thigh

  ☑️6ᵗʰ **L97.10**   **Non-pressure chronic ulcer of** unspecified thigh

    L97.101   **Non-pressure chronic ulcer of** ᶜᶜ ᴴᶜᶜ **unspecified thigh** limited to breakdown of skin

    L97.102   **Non-pressure chronic ulcer of** ᶜᶜ ᴴᶜᶜ **unspecified thigh** with fat layer exposed

    L97.103   **Non-pressure chronic ulcer of** ᶜᶜ ᴴᶜᶜ **unspecified thigh** with necrosis of muscle

    L97.104   **Non-pressure chronic ulcer of** ᶜᶜ ᴴᶜᶜ **unspecified thigh** with necrosis of bone

●   **L97.105**   **Non-pressure chronic ulcer of** ᶜᶜ **unspecified thigh** with muscle involvement without evidence of necrosis

●   **L97.106**   **Non-pressure chronic ulcer of** ᶜᶜ **unspecified thigh** with bone involvement without evidence of necrosis

●   **L97.108**   **Non-pressure chronic ulcer of** ᶜᶜ **unspecified thigh** with other specified severity

    L97.109   **Non-pressure chronic ulcer of** ᶜᶜ ᴴᶜᶜ **unspecified thigh** with unspecified severity

  ☑️6ᵗʰ **L97.11**   **Non-pressure chronic ulcer of** right thigh

    L97.111   **Non-pressure chronic ulcer of right** ᶜᶜ ᴴᶜᶜ **thigh** limited to breakdown of skin

    L97.112   **Non-pressure chronic ulcer of right** ᶜᶜ ᴴᶜᶜ **thigh** with fat layer exposed

    L97.113   **Non-pressure chronic ulcer of right** ᶜᶜ ᴴᶜᶜ **thigh** with necrosis of muscle

    L97.114   **Non-pressure chronic ulcer of right** ᶜᶜ ᴴᶜᶜ **thigh** with necrosis of bone

●   **L97.115**   **Non-pressure chronic ulcer of right** ᶜᶜ **thigh** with muscle involvement without evidence of necrosis

●   **L97.116**   **Non-pressure chronic ulcer of right** ᶜᶜ **thigh** with bone involvement without evidence of necrosis

●   **L97.118**   **Non-pressure chronic ulcer of right** ᶜᶜ **thigh with other specified severity**

    L97.119   **Non-pressure chronic ulcer of right** ᶜᶜ ᴴᶜᶜ **thigh** with unspecified severity

  ☑️6ᵗʰ **L97.12**   **Non-pressure chronic ulcer of** left thigh

    L97.121   **Non-pressure chronic ulcer of left** ᶜᶜ ᴴᶜᶜ **thigh** limited to breakdown of skin

    L97.122   **Non-pressure chronic ulcer of left** ᶜᶜ ᴴᶜᶜ **thigh** with fat layer exposed

    L97.123   **Non-pressure chronic ulcer of left** ᶜᶜ ᴴᶜᶜ **thigh** with necrosis of muscle

    L97.124   **Non-pressure chronic ulcer of left** ᶜᶜ ᴴᶜᶜ **thigh** with necrosis of bone

●   **L97.125**   **Non-pressure chronic ulcer of left** ᶜᶜ **thigh** with muscle involvement without evidence of necrosis

●   **L97.126**   **Non-pressure chronic ulcer of left** ᶜᶜ **thigh** with bone involvement without evidence of necrosis

●   **L97.128**   **Non-pressure chronic ulcer of left** ᶜᶜ **thigh with other specified severity**

    L97.129   **Non-pressure chronic ulcer of left** ᶜᶜ ᴴᶜᶜ **thigh** with unspecified severity

☑️5ᵗʰ **L97.2**   **Non-pressure chronic ulcer of** calf

  ☑️6ᵗʰ **L97.20**   **Non-pressure chronic ulcer of** unspecified calf

    L97.201   **Non-pressure chronic ulcer of** ᶜᶜ ᴴᶜᶜ **unspecified calf** limited to breakdown of skin

    L97.202   **Non-pressure chronic ulcer of** ᶜᶜ ᴴᶜᶜ **unspecified calf** with fat layer exposed

    L97.203   **Non-pressure chronic ulcer of** ᶜᶜ ᴴᶜᶜ **unspecified calf** with necrosis of muscle

    L97.204   **Non-pressure chronic ulcer of** ᶜᶜ ᴴᶜᶜ **unspecified calf** with necrosis of bone

●   **L97.205**   **Non-pressure chronic ulcer of** ᶜᶜ **unspecified calf** with muscle involvement without evidence of necrosis

●   **L97.206**   **Non-pressure chronic ulcer of** ᶜᶜ **unspecified calf** with bone involvement without evidence of necrosis

●   **L97.208**   **Non-pressure chronic ulcer of** ᶜᶜ **unspecified calf with other specified severity**

    L97.209   **Non-pressure chronic ulcer of** ᶜᶜ ᴴᶜᶜ **unspecified calf** with unspecified severity

  ☑️6ᵗʰ **L97.21**   **Non-pressure chronic ulcer of** right calf

    L97.211   **Non-pressure chronic ulcer of right** ᶜᶜ ᴴᶜᶜ **calf** limited to breakdown of skin

    L97.212   **Non-pressure chronic ulcer of right** ᶜᶜ ᴴᶜᶜ **calf** with fat layer exposed

    L97.213   **Non-pressure chronic ulcer of right** ᶜᶜ ᴴᶜᶜ **calf** with necrosis of muscle

    L97.214   **Non-pressure chronic ulcer of right** ᶜᶜ ᴴᶜᶜ **calf** with necrosis of bone

●   **L97.215**   **Non-pressure chronic ulcer of right** ᶜᶜ **calf** with muscle involvement without evidence of necrosis

●   **L97.216**   **Non-pressure chronic ulcer of right** ᶜᶜ **calf** with bone involvement without evidence of necrosis

●   **L97.218**   **Non-pressure chronic ulcer of right** ᶜᶜ **calf with other specified severity**

    L97.219   **Non-pressure chronic ulcer of right** ᶜᶜ ᴴᶜᶜ **calf** with unspecified severity

  ☑️6ᵗʰ **L97.22**   **Non-pressure chronic ulcer of** left calf

    L97.221   **Non-pressure chronic ulcer of left** ᶜᶜ ᴴᶜᶜ **calf** limited to breakdown of skin

    L97.222   **Non-pressure chronic ulcer of left** ᶜᶜ ᴴᶜᶜ **calf** with fat layer exposed

    L97.223   **Non-pressure chronic ulcer of left** ᶜᶜ ᴴᶜᶜ **calf** with necrosis of muscle

    L97.224   **Non-pressure chronic ulcer of left** ᶜᶜ ᴴᶜᶜ **calf** with necrosis of bone

---

☑️Additional Character Req   ☑️x7ᵗʰ Placeholder Alert   Unacceptable PDx   Manifestation   **H1**-**H14** HAC   **HCC** CMS-HCC Condition   *EXCLUDES 1* Not Coded Here   *EXCLUDES 2* Not Included Here

Chapter 12. Diseases of the Skin and Subcutaneous Tissue

L97.225–L97.501

- L97.225   Non-pressure chronic ulcer of left calf with muscle involvement without evidence of necrosis   `CC`
- L97.226   Non-pressure chronic ulcer of left calf with bone involvement without evidence of necrosis   `CC`
- L97.228   Non-pressure chronic ulcer of left calf with other specified severity   `CC`
- L97.229   Non-pressure chronic ulcer of left calf with unspecified severity   `CC` `HCC`

√5th **L97.3 Non-pressure chronic ulcer of ankle**

√6th **L97.30 Non-pressure chronic ulcer of unspecified ankle**

- L97.301   Non-pressure chronic ulcer of unspecified ankle limited to breakdown of skin   `CC` `HCC`
- L97.302   Non-pressure chronic ulcer of unspecified ankle with fat layer exposed   `CC` `HCC`
- L97.303   Non-pressure chronic ulcer of unspecified ankle with necrosis of muscle   `CC` `HCC`
- L97.304   Non-pressure chronic ulcer of unspecified ankle with necrosis of bone   `CC` `HCC`
- L97.305   Non-pressure chronic ulcer of unspecified ankle with muscle involvement without evidence of necrosis   `CC`
- L97.306   Non-pressure chronic ulcer of unspecified ankle with bone involvement without evidence of necrosis   `CC`
- L97.308   Non-pressure chronic ulcer of unspecified ankle with other specified severity   `CC`
- L97.309   Non-pressure chronic ulcer of unspecified ankle with unspecified severity   `CC` `HCC`

√6th **L97.31 Non-pressure chronic ulcer of right ankle**

- L97.311   Non-pressure chronic ulcer of right ankle limited to breakdown of skin   `CC` `HCC`
- L97.312   Non-pressure chronic ulcer of right ankle with fat layer exposed   `CC` `HCC`
- L97.313   Non-pressure chronic ulcer of right ankle with necrosis of muscle   `CC` `HCC`
- L97.314   Non-pressure chronic ulcer of right ankle with necrosis of bone   `CC` `HCC`
- L97.315   Non-pressure chronic ulcer of right ankle with muscle involvement without evidence of necrosis   `CC`
- L97.316   Non-pressure chronic ulcer of right ankle with bone involvement without evidence of necrosis   `CC`
- L97.318   Non-pressure chronic ulcer of right ankle with other specified severity   `CC`
- L97.319   Non-pressure chronic ulcer of right ankle with unspecified severity   `CC` `HCC`

√6th **L97.32 Non-pressure chronic ulcer of left ankle**

- L97.321   Non-pressure chronic ulcer of left ankle limited to breakdown of skin   `CC` `HCC`
- L97.322   Non-pressure chronic ulcer of left ankle with fat layer exposed   `CC` `HCC`
- L97.323   Non-pressure chronic ulcer of left ankle with necrosis of muscle   `CC` `HCC`
- L97.324   Non-pressure chronic ulcer of left ankle with necrosis of bone   `CC` `HCC`
- L97.325   Non-pressure chronic ulcer of left ankle with muscle involvement without evidence of necrosis   `CC`
- L97.326   Non-pressure chronic ulcer of left ankle with bone involvement without evidence of necrosis   `CC`
- L97.328   Non-pressure chronic ulcer of left ankle with other specified severity   `CC`
- L97.329   Non-pressure chronic ulcer of left ankle with unspecified severity   `CC` `HCC`

√5th **L97.4 Non-pressure chronic ulcer of heel and midfoot**
Non-pressure chronic ulcer of plantar surface of midfoot

√6th **L97.40 Non-pressure chronic ulcer of unspecified heel and midfoot**

- L97.401   Non-pressure chronic ulcer of unspecified heel and midfoot limited to breakdown of skin   `CC` `HCC`
- L97.402   Non-pressure chronic ulcer of unspecified heel and midfoot with fat layer exposed   `CC` `HCC`
- L97.403   Non-pressure chronic ulcer of unspecified heel and midfoot with necrosis of muscle   `CC` `HCC`
- L97.404   Non-pressure chronic ulcer of unspecified heel and midfoot with necrosis of bone   `CC` `HCC`
- L97.405   Non-pressure chronic ulcer of unspecified heel and midfoot with muscle involvement without evidence of necrosis   `CC`
- L97.406   Non-pressure chronic ulcer of unspecified heel and midfoot with bone involvement without evidence of necrosis   `CC`
- L97.408   Non-pressure chronic ulcer of unspecified heel and midfoot with other specified severity   `CC`
- L97.409   Non-pressure chronic ulcer of unspecified heel and midfoot with unspecified severity   `CC` `HCC`

√6th **L97.41 Non-pressure chronic ulcer of right heel and midfoot**

- L97.411   Non-pressure chronic ulcer of right heel and midfoot limited to breakdown of skin   `CC` `HCC`
- L97.412   Non-pressure chronic ulcer of right heel and midfoot with fat layer exposed   `CC` `HCC`
- L97.413   Non-pressure chronic ulcer of right heel and midfoot with necrosis of muscle   `CC` `HCC`
- L97.414   Non-pressure chronic ulcer of right heel and midfoot with necrosis of bone   `CC` `HCC`
- L97.415   Non-pressure chronic ulcer of right heel and midfoot with muscle involvement without evidence of necrosis   `CC`
- L97.416   Non-pressure chronic ulcer of right heel and midfoot with bone involvement without evidence of necrosis   `CC`
- L97.418   Non-pressure chronic ulcer of right heel and midfoot with other specified severity   `CC`
- L97.419   Non-pressure chronic ulcer of right heel and midfoot with unspecified severity   `CC` `HCC`

√6th **L97.42 Non-pressure chronic ulcer of left heel and midfoot**

- L97.421   Non-pressure chronic ulcer of left heel and midfoot limited to breakdown of skin   `CC` `HCC`
  AHA: 2016, 1Q, 12
- L97.422   Non-pressure chronic ulcer of left heel and midfoot with fat layer exposed   `CC` `HCC`
- L97.423   Non-pressure chronic ulcer of left heel and midfoot with necrosis of muscle   `CC` `HCC`
- L97.424   Non-pressure chronic ulcer of left heel and midfoot with necrosis of bone   `CC` `HCC`
- L97.425   Non-pressure chronic ulcer of left heel and midfoot with muscle involvement without evidence of necrosis   `CC`
- L97.426   Non-pressure chronic ulcer of left heel and midfoot with bone involvement without evidence of necrosis   `CC`
- L97.428   Non-pressure chronic ulcer of left heel and midfoot with other specified severity   `CC`
- L97.429   Non-pressure chronic ulcer of left heel and midfoot with unspecified severity   `CC` `HCC`

√5th **L97.5 Non-pressure chronic ulcer of other part of foot**
Non-pressure chronic ulcer of toe

√6th **L97.50 Non-pressure chronic ulcer of other part of unspecified foot**

- L97.501   Non-pressure chronic ulcer of other part of unspecified foot limited to breakdown of skin   `HCC`

N Newborn: 0   P Pediatric: 0-17   M Maternity: 12-55   A Adult: 15-124   `MCC` Major CC Condition   `PDxMCC` PDx acts as own MCC   `CC` CC Condition   `PDxCC` PDx acts as own CC

726   ICD-10-CM 2018

L97.502 Non-pressure chronic ulcer of other part of unspecified foot with fat layer exposed `HCC`

L97.503 Non-pressure chronic ulcer of other part of unspecified foot with necrosis of muscle `HCC`

L97.504 Non-pressure chronic ulcer of other part of unspecified foot with necrosis of bone `HCC`

● **L97.505** Non-pressure chronic ulcer of other part of unspecified foot with muscle involvement without evidence of necrosis `CC`

● **L97.506** Non-pressure chronic ulcer of other part of unspecified foot with bone involvement without evidence of necrosis `CC`

● **L97.508** Non-pressure chronic ulcer of other part of unspecified foot with other specified severity `CC`

L97.509 Non-pressure chronic ulcer of other part of unspecified foot with unspecified severity `HCC`

√6ᵗʰ **L97.51** Non-pressure chronic ulcer of other part of right foot

L97.511 Non-pressure chronic ulcer of other part of right foot limited to breakdown of skin `HCC`

L97.512 Non-pressure chronic ulcer of other part of right foot with fat layer exposed `HCC`

L97.513 Non-pressure chronic ulcer of other part of right foot with necrosis of muscle `HCC`

L97.514 Non-pressure chronic ulcer of other part of right foot with necrosis of bone `HCC`

● **L97.515** Non-pressure chronic ulcer of other part of right foot with muscle involvement without evidence of necrosis `CC`

● **L97.516** Non-pressure chronic ulcer of other part of right foot with bone involvement without evidence of necrosis `CC`

● **L97.518** Non-pressure chronic ulcer of other part of right foot with other specified severity `CC`

L97.519 Non-pressure chronic ulcer of other part of right foot with unspecified severity `HCC`

√6ᵗʰ **L97.52** Non-pressure chronic ulcer of other part of left foot

L97.521 Non-pressure chronic ulcer of other part of left foot limited to breakdown of skin `HCC`

L97.522 Non-pressure chronic ulcer of other part of left foot with fat layer exposed `HCC`

L97.523 Non-pressure chronic ulcer of other part of left foot with necrosis of muscle `HCC`

L97.524 Non-pressure chronic ulcer of other part of left foot with necrosis of bone `HCC`

● **L97.525** Non-pressure chronic ulcer of other part of left foot with muscle involvement without evidence of necrosis `CC`

● **L97.526** Non-pressure chronic ulcer of other part of left foot with bone involvement without evidence of necrosis `CC`

● **L97.528** Non-pressure chronic ulcer of other part of left foot with other specified severity `CC`

L97.529 Non-pressure chronic ulcer of other part of left foot with unspecified severity `HCC`

√5ᵗʰ **L97.8** Non-pressure chronic ulcer of other part of lower leg

√6ᵗʰ **L97.80** Non-pressure chronic ulcer of other part of unspecified lower leg

L97.801 Non-pressure chronic ulcer of other part of unspecified lower leg limited to breakdown of skin `CC` `HCC`

L97.802 Non-pressure chronic ulcer of other part of unspecified lower leg with fat layer exposed `CC` `HCC`

L97.803 Non-pressure chronic ulcer of other part of unspecified lower leg with necrosis of muscle `CC` `HCC`

L97.804 Non-pressure chronic ulcer of other part of unspecified lower leg with necrosis of bone `CC` `HCC`

● **L97.805** Non-pressure chronic ulcer of other part of unspecified lower leg with muscle involvement without evidence of necrosis `CC`

● **L97.806** Non-pressure chronic ulcer of other part of unspecified lower leg with bone involvement without evidence of necrosis `CC`

● **L97.808** Non-pressure chronic ulcer of other part of unspecified lower leg with other specified severity `CC`

L97.809 Non-pressure chronic ulcer of other part of unspecified lower leg with unspecified severity `CC` `HCC`

√6ᵗʰ **L97.81** Non-pressure chronic ulcer of other part of right lower leg

L97.811 Non-pressure chronic ulcer of other part of right lower leg limited to breakdown of skin `CC` `HCC`

L97.812 Non-pressure chronic ulcer of other part of right lower leg with fat layer exposed `CC` `HCC`

L97.813 Non-pressure chronic ulcer of other part of right lower leg with necrosis of muscle `CC` `HCC`

L97.814 Non-pressure chronic ulcer of other part of right lower leg with necrosis of bone `CC` `HCC`

● **L97.815** Non-pressure chronic ulcer of other part of right lower leg with muscle involvement without evidence of necrosis `CC`

● **L97.816** Non-pressure chronic ulcer of other part of right lower leg with bone involvement without evidence of necrosis `CC`

● **L97.818** Non-pressure chronic ulcer of other part of right lower leg with other specified severity `CC`

L97.819 Non-pressure chronic ulcer of other part of right lower leg with unspecified severity `CC` `HCC`

√6ᵗʰ **L97.82** Non-pressure chronic ulcer of other part of left lower leg

L97.821 Non-pressure chronic ulcer of other part of left lower leg limited to breakdown of skin `CC` `HCC`

L97.822 Non-pressure chronic ulcer of other part of left lower leg with fat layer exposed `CC` `HCC`

L97.823 Non-pressure chronic ulcer of other part of left lower leg with necrosis of muscle `CC` `HCC`

L97.824 Non-pressure chronic ulcer of other part of left lower leg with necrosis of bone `CC` `HCC`

● **L97.825** Non-pressure chronic ulcer of other part of left lower leg with muscle involvement without evidence of necrosis `CC`

● **L97.826** Non-pressure chronic ulcer of other part of left lower leg with bone involvement without evidence of necrosis `CC`

● **L97.828** Non-pressure chronic ulcer of other part of left lower leg with other specified severity `CC`

L97.829 Non-pressure chronic ulcer of other part of left lower leg with unspecified severity `CC` `HCC`

√5ᵗʰ **L97.9** Non-pressure chronic ulcer of unspecified part of lower leg

√6ᵗʰ **L97.90** Non-pressure chronic ulcer of unspecified part of unspecified lower leg

L97.901 Non-pressure chronic ulcer of unspecified part of unspecified lower leg limited to breakdown of skin `CC` `HCC`

☑ Additional Character Req   √ˣ⁷ᵗʰ Placeholder Alert   Unacceptable PDx   Manifestation   H1 - H14 HAC   HCC CMS-HCC Condition   *EXCLUDES 1* Not Coded Here   *EXCLUDES 2* Not Included Here

ICD-10-CM 2018   727

Chapter 12. Diseases of the Skin and Subcutaneous Tissue

L97.502-L97.901

Chapter 12. Diseases of the Skin and Subcutaneous Tissue

L97.902   **Non-pressure chronic ulcer of unspecified part of unspecified lower leg with fat layer exposed** `CC` `HCC`

L97.903   **Non-pressure chronic ulcer of unspecified part of unspecified lower leg with necrosis of muscle** `CC` `HCC`

L97.904   **Non-pressure chronic ulcer of unspecified part of unspecified lower leg with necrosis of bone** `CC` `HCC`

● L97.905   **Non-pressure chronic ulcer of unspecified part of unspecified lower leg with muscle involvement without evidence of necrosis** `CC`

● L97.906   **Non-pressure chronic ulcer of unspecified part of unspecified lower leg with bone involvement without evidence of necrosis** `CC`

● L97.908   **Non-pressure chronic ulcer of unspecified part of unspecified lower leg with other specified severity** `CC`

L97.909   **Non-pressure chronic ulcer of unspecified part of unspecified lower leg with unspecified severity** `CC` `HCC`

√6ᵗʰ **L97.91**   **Non-pressure chronic ulcer of** unspecified part of right lower leg

L97.911   **Non-pressure chronic ulcer of unspecified part of right lower leg limited to breakdown of skin** `CC` `HCC`

L97.912   **Non-pressure chronic ulcer of unspecified part of right lower leg with fat layer exposed** `CC` `HCC`

L97.913   **Non-pressure chronic ulcer of unspecified part of right lower leg with necrosis of muscle** `CC` `HCC`

L97.914   **Non-pressure chronic ulcer of unspecified part of right lower leg with necrosis of bone** `CC` `HCC`

● L97.915   **Non-pressure chronic ulcer of unspecified part of right lower leg with muscle involvement without evidence of necrosis** `CC`

● L97.916   **Non-pressure chronic ulcer of unspecified part of right lower leg with bone involvement without evidence of necrosis** `CC`

● L97.918   **Non-pressure chronic ulcer of unspecified part of right lower leg with other specified severity** `CC`

L97.919   **Non-pressure chronic ulcer of unspecified part of right lower leg with unspecified severity** `CC` `HCC`

√6ᵗʰ **L97.92**   **Non-pressure chronic ulcer of** unspecified part of left lower leg

L97.921   **Non-pressure chronic ulcer of unspecified part of left lower leg limited to breakdown of skin** `CC` `HCC`

L97.922   **Non-pressure chronic ulcer of unspecified part of left lower leg with fat layer exposed** `CC` `HCC`

L97.923   **Non-pressure chronic ulcer of unspecified part of left lower leg with necrosis of muscle** `CC` `HCC`

L97.924   **Non-pressure chronic ulcer of unspecified part of left lower leg with necrosis of bone** `CC` `HCC`

● L97.925   **Non-pressure chronic ulcer of unspecified part of left lower leg with muscle involvement without evidence of necrosis** `CC`

● L97.926   **Non-pressure chronic ulcer of unspecified part of left lower leg with bone involvement without evidence of necrosis** `CC`

● L97.928   **Non-pressure chronic ulcer of unspecified part of left lower leg with other specified severity** `CC`

L97.929   **Non-pressure chronic ulcer of unspecified part of left lower leg with unspecified severity** `CC` `HCC`

√4ᵗʰ **L98**   **Other disorders of skin and subcutaneous tissue, not elsewhere classified**

L98.0   **Pyogenic granuloma**

> *EXCLUDES 2*   pyogenic granuloma of gingiva (K06.8)
> pyogenic granuloma of maxillary alveolar ridge (K04.5)
> pyogenic granuloma of oral mucosa (K13.4)

> **DEF:** Solitary polypoid capillary hemangioma often associated with local irritation, trauma, and superimposed inflammation; located on the skin and gingival or oral mucosa; they bleed easily and may ulcerate and form crusted sores.

L98.1   **Factitial dermatitis**

Neurotic excoriation

> *EXCLUDES 1*   excoriation (skin-picking) disorder (F42.4)

> **DEF:** Self-inflicted skin lesions to satisfy an unconscious psychological or emotional need; methods used to injure the skin include deep excoriations with a sharp instrument, scarification with a knife, or the application of caustic chemicals and burning, sometimes with a cigarette.

L98.2   **Febrile neutrophilic dermatosis [Sweet]**

L98.3   **Eosinophilic cellulitis [Wells]** `CC`

     CC Excl: PDX collection 839

√5ᵗʰ **L98.4**   **Non-pressure chronic ulcer of skin, not elsewhere classified**

Chronic ulcer of skin NOS

Tropical ulcer NOS

Ulcer of skin NOS

> *EXCLUDES 2*   pressure ulcer (pressure area) (L89.-)
> gangrene (I96)
> skin infections (L00-L08)
> specific infections classified to A00-B99
> ulcer of lower limb NEC (L97.-)
> varicose ulcer (I83.0-I82.2)

> **CC Excl: For CC codes in subcategory L98.4:**
> PDX collection 698

√6ᵗʰ **L98.41**   **Non-pressure chronic ulcer of** buttock

L98.411   **Non-pressure chronic ulcer of buttock limited to breakdown of skin** `HCC`

L98.412   **Non-pressure chronic ulcer of buttock with fat layer exposed** `HCC`

L98.413   **Non-pressure chronic ulcer of buttock with necrosis of muscle** `HCC`

L98.414   **Non-pressure chronic ulcer of buttock with necrosis of bone** `HCC`

● L98.415   **Non-pressure chronic ulcer of buttock with muscle involvement without evidence of necrosis** `CC`

● L98.416   **Non-pressure chronic ulcer of buttock with bone involvement without evidence of necrosis** `CC`

● L98.418   **Non-pressure chronic ulcer of buttock with other specified severity** `CC`

L98.419   **Non-pressure chronic ulcer of buttock with unspecified severity** `HCC`

√6ᵗʰ **L98.42**   **Non-pressure chronic ulcer of** back

L98.421   **Non-pressure chronic ulcer of back limited to breakdown of skin** `HCC`

L98.422   **Non-pressure chronic ulcer of back with fat layer exposed** `HCC`

L98.423   **Non-pressure chronic ulcer of back with necrosis of muscle** `HCC`

L98.424   **Non-pressure chronic ulcer of back with necrosis of bone** `HCC`

● L98.425   **Non-pressure chronic ulcer of back with muscle involvement without evidence of necrosis** `CC`

● L98.426   **Non-pressure chronic ulcer of back with bone involvement without evidence of necrosis** `CC`

● L98.428   **Non-pressure chronic ulcer of back with other specified severity** `CC`

L98.429   **Non-pressure chronic ulcer of back with unspecified severity** `HCC`

√6ᵗʰ **L98.49**   **Non-pressure chronic ulcer of** skin of other sites

Non-pressure chronic ulcer of skin NOS

L98.491   **Non-pressure chronic ulcer of skin of other sites limited to breakdown of skin** `HCC`

L98.492   **Non-pressure chronic ulcer of skin of other sites with fat layer exposed** `HCC`

Ⓝ Newborn: 0   Ⓟ Pediatric: 0-17   Ⓜ Maternity: 12-55   Ⓐ Adult: 15-124   `MCC` Major CC Condition   `PDxMCC` PDx acts as own MCC   `CC` CC Condition   `PDxCC` PDx acts as own CC

728   ICD-10-CM 2018

L98.493   **Non-pressure chronic ulcer of skin of other sites with necrosis of muscle** `HCC`

L98.494   **Non-pressure chronic ulcer of skin of other sites with necrosis of bone** `HCC`

-   L98.495   **Non-pressure chronic ulcer of other sites with muscle involvement without evidence of necrosis** `CC`

-   L98.496   **Non-pressure chronic ulcer of other sites with bone involvement without evidence of necrosis** `CC`

-   L98.498   **Non-pressure chronic ulcer of other sites with other specified severity** `CC`

L98.499   **Non-pressure chronic ulcer of skin of other sites with unspecified severity** `HCC`

L98.5   Mucinosis of the skin
     Focal mucinosis
     Lichen myxedematosus
     Reticular erythematous mucinosis
     EXCLUDES 1   focal oral mucinosis (K13.79)
                    myxedema (E03.9)

L98.6   Other infiltrative disorders of the skin and subcutaneous tissue
     EXCLUDES 1   hyalinosis cutis et mucosae (E78.89)

L98.7   Excessive and redundant skin and subcutaneous tissue
     Loose or sagging skin following bariatric surgery weight loss
     Loose or sagging skin following dietary weight loss
     Loose or sagging skin, NOS
     EXCLUDES 2   acquired excess or redundant skin of eyelid (H02.3-)
                    congenital excess or redundant skin of eyelid (Q10.3)
                    skin changes due to chronic exposure to nonionizing radiation (L57.-)

L98.8   Other specified disorders of the skin and subcutaneous tissue
     AHA: 2013, 2Q, 32

L98.9   Disorder of the skin and subcutaneous tissue, unspecified

L99   *Other disorders of skin and subcutaneous tissue in diseases classified elsewhere*
     Code first underlying disease, such as:
         amyloidosis (E85.-)
     EXCLUDES 1   skin disorders in diabetes (E08-E13 with .62)
                    skin disorders in gonorrhea (A54.89)
                    skin disorders in syphilis (A51.31, A52.79)

☑ Additional Character Req   `√x7ᵗʰ` Placeholder Alert   Unacceptable PDx   Manifestation   `H1`-`H14` HAC   `HCC` CMS-HCC Condition   *EXCLUDES 1* Not Coded Here   *EXCLUDES 2* Not Included Here

Chapter 13. Diseases of the Musculoskeletal System and Connective Tissue (MØØ–M99)

Chapter Specific Guidelines with Coding Examples

The chapter specific guidelines from the ICD-1Ø-CM Official Guidelines for Coding and Reporting have been provided below. Along with these guidelines are coding examples, contained in the shaded boxes, that have been developed to help illustrate the coding and/or sequencing guidance found in these guidelines.

a. Site and laterality

Most of the codes within Chapter 13 have site and laterality designations. The site represents the bone, joint or the muscle involved. For some conditions where more than one bone, joint or muscle is usually involved, such as osteoarthritis, there is a "multiple sites" code available. For categories where no multiple site code is provided and more than one bone, joint or muscle is involved, multiple codes should be used to indicate the different sites involved.

Rheumatoid arthritis of multiple sites without rheumatoid factor

MØ6.Ø9   **Rheumatoid arthritis without rheumatoid factor, multiple sites**

Explanation: For some conditions where more than one bone, joint or muscle is usually involved, such as osteoarthritis, there is a "multiple sites" code available.

Osteomyelitis of the fourth thoracic and second lumbar vertebrae

M46.24   **Osteomyelitis of vertebra, thoracic region**

M46.26   **Osteomyelitis of vertebra, lumbar region**

Explanation: For categories without a multiple site code and more than one bone, joint, or muscle is involved, multiple codes should be used to indicate the different sites involved.

1) Bone versus joint

For certain conditions, the bone may be affected at the upper or lower end, (e.g., avascular necrosis of bone, M87, Osteoporosis, M8Ø, M81). Though the portion of the bone affected may be at the joint, the site designation will be the bone, not the joint.

Idiopathic avascular necrosis of the femoral head of the left hip joint

M87.Ø52   **Idiopathic aseptic necrosis of left femur**

Explanation: For certain conditions such as avascular necrosis, the bone may be affected at the joint, but the site designation is the bone, not the joint.

b. Acute traumatic versus chronic or recurrent musculoskeletal conditions

Many musculoskeletal conditions are a result of previous injury or trauma to a site, or are recurrent conditions. Bone, joint or muscle conditions that are the result of a healed injury are usually found in chapter 13. Recurrent bone, joint or muscle conditions are also usually found in chapter 13. Any current, acute injury should be coded to the appropriate injury code from chapter 19. Chronic or recurrent conditions should generally be coded with a code from chapter 13. If it is difficult to determine from the documentation in the record which code is best to describe a condition, query the provider.

Acute traumatic bucket handle tear of right medial meniscus

S83.211A   **Bucket-handle tear of medial meniscus, current injury, right knee, initial encounter**

Explanation: Any current, acute injury is not coded in chapter 13. It should instead be coded to the appropriate injury code from chapter 19.

Old bucket handle tear of right medial meniscus

M23.2Ø3   **Derangement of unspecified medial meniscus due to old tear or injury, right knee**

Explanation: Chronic or recurrent conditions should generally be coded with a code from chapter 13.

c. Coding of pathologic fractures

7th character A is for use as long as the patient is receiving active treatment for the fracture. Examples of active treatment are: surgical treatment, emergency department encounter, evaluation and continuing treatment by the same or a different physician. While the patient may be seen by a new or different provider over the course of treatment for a pathological fracture, assignment of the 7th character is based on whether the patient is

undergoing active treatment and not whether the provider is seeing the patient for the first time.

Patient admitted for repair of pathologic fracture of left foot, unknown cause. The surgery will be performed by his orthopedic specialist who he has been seeing for this fracture for the past month.

M84.475A   **Pathological fracture, left foot, initial encounter for fracture**

Explanation: Seventh character A is for use as long as the patient is receiving active treatment for a pathologic fracture. Examples of active treatment are surgical treatment, emergency department encounter, evaluation, and continuing treatment by the same or a different physician.

The seventh character is based on whether the patient is undergoing active treatment such as surgery, and not whether the provider is seeing the patient for the first time.

7th character D is to be used for encounters after the patient has completed active treatment **for the fracture and is receiving routine care for the fracture during the healing or recovery phase.** The other 7th characters, listed under each subcategory in the Tabular List, are to be used for subsequent encounters for treatment of problems associated with the healing, such as malunions, nonunions, and sequelae.

Care for complications of surgical treatment for fracture repairs during the healing or recovery phase should be coded with the appropriate complication codes.

See Section I.C.19. Coding of traumatic fractures.

d. Osteoporosis

Osteoporosis is a systemic condition, meaning that all bones of the musculoskeletal system are affected. Therefore, site is not a component of the codes under category M81, Osteoporosis without current pathological fracture. The site codes under category M8Ø, Osteoporosis with current pathological fracture, identify the site of the fracture, not the osteoporosis.

1) Osteoporosis without pathological fracture

Category M81, Osteoporosis without current pathological fracture, is for use for patients with osteoporosis who do not currently have a pathologic fracture due to the osteoporosis, even if they have had a fracture in the past. For patients with a history of osteoporosis fractures, status code Z87.31Ø, Personal history of (healed) osteoporosis fracture, should follow the code from M81.

Age-related osteoporosis with healed osteoporotic fracture of the lumbar vertebra

M81.Ø   **Age-related osteoporosis without current pathological fracture**

Z87.31Ø   **Personal history of (healed) osteoporosis fracture**

Explanation: Category M81 is used for patients with osteoporosis who do not currently have a pathologic fracture due to the osteoporosis. To report a previous (healed) fracture, status code Z87.31Ø Personal history of (healed) osteoporosis fracture, should follow the code from M81.

2) Osteoporosis with current pathological fracture

Category M8Ø, Osteoporosis with current pathological fracture, is for patients who have a current pathologic fracture at the time of an encounter. The codes under M8Ø identify the site of the fracture. A code from category M8Ø, not a traumatic fracture code, should be used for any patient with known osteoporosis who suffers a fracture, even if the patient had a minor fall or trauma, if that fall or trauma would not usually break a normal, healthy bone.

Disuse osteoporosis with current fracture of right shoulder sustained lifting a grocery bag, initial encounter

M8Ø.811A   **Other osteoporosis with current pathological fracture, right shoulder, initial encounter for fracture**

Explanation: A code from category M8Ø, not a traumatic fracture code, should be used for any patient with known osteoporosis who suffers a fracture, even if the patient had a minor fall or trauma, if that fall or trauma would not usually break a normal, healthy bone.

Muscle/Tendon Table

ICD-10-CM categorizes certain muscles and tendons in the upper and lower extremities by their action (e.g., extension, flexion), their anatomical location (e.g., posterior, anterior), and/or whether they are intrinsic or extrinsic to a certain anatomical area. The Muscle/Tendon Table is provided at the beginning of chapters 13 and 19 as a resource to help users when code selection depends on one or more of these characteristics. Please note that this table is not all-inclusive, and proper code assignment should be based on the provider's documentation.

Body Region	Muscle	Extensor Tendon	Flexor Tendon	Other Tendon
Shoulder				
	Deltoid	Posterior deltoid	Anterior deltoid	
	Rotator cuff			
	Infraspinatus			Infraspinatus
	Subscapularis			Subscapularis
	Supraspinatus			Supraspinatus
	Teres minor			Teres minor
	Teres major	Teres major		
Upper arm				
	Anterior muscles			
	Biceps brachii — long head		Biceps brachii — long head	
	Biceps brachii — short head		Biceps brachii — short head	
	Brachialis		Brachialis	
	Coracobrachialis		Coracobrachialis	
	Posterior muscles			
	Triceps brachii	Triceps brachii		
Forearm				
	Anterior muscles			
	Flexors			
	Deep			
	Flexor digitorum profundus		Flexor digitorum profundus	
	Flexor pollicis longus		Flexor pollicis longus	
	Intermediate			
	Flexor digitorum superficialis		Flexor digitorum superficialis	
	Superficial			
	Flexor carpi radialis		Flexor carpi radialis	
	Flexor carpi ulnaris		Flexor carpi ulnaris	
	Palmaris longus		Palmaris longus	
	Pronators			
	Pronator quadratus			Pronator quadratus
	Pronator teres			Pronator teres
	Posterior muscles			
	Extensors			
	Deep			
	Abductor pollicis longus			Abductor pollicis longus
	Extensor indicis	Extensor indicis		
	Extensor pollicis brevis	Extensor pollicis brevis		
	Extensor pollicis longus	Extensor pollicis longus		
	Superficial			
	Brachioradialis			Brachioradialis
	Extensor carpi radialis brevis	Extensor carpi radialis brevis		
	Extensor carpi radialis longus	Extensor carpi radialis longus		
	Extensor carpi ulnaris	Extensor carpi ulnaris		
	Extensor digiti minimi	Extensor digiti minimi		
	Extensor digitorum	Extensor digitorum		
	Anconeus	Anconeus		
	Supinator			Supinator

Chapter 13. Diseases of the Musculoskeletal System and Connective Tissue

Body Region	Muscle	Extensor Tendon	Flexor Tendon	Other Tendon
Hand				
Extrinsic — attach to a site in the forearm as well as a site in the hand with action related to hand movement at the wrist				
	Extensor carpi radialis brevis	Extensor carpi radialis brevis		
	Extensor carpi radialis longus	Extensor carpie radialis longus		
	Extensor carpi ulnaris	Extensor carpi ulnaris		
	Flexor carpi radialis		Flexor carpi radialis	
	Flexor carpi ulnaris		Flexor carpi ulnaris	
	Flexor digitorum superficialis		Flexor digitorum superficialis	
	Palmaris longus		Palmaris longus	
Extrinsic — attach to a site in the forearm as well as a site in the hand with action in the hand related to finger movement				
	Adductor pollicis longus			Adductor pollicis longus
	Extensor digiti minimi	Extensor digiti minimi		
	Extensor digitorum	Extensor digitorum		
	Extensor indicis	Extensor indicis		
	Flexor digitorum profundus		Flexor digitorum profundus	
	Flexor digitorum superficialis		Flexor digitorum superficialis	
Extrinsic — attach to a site in the forearm as well as a site in the hand with action in the hand related to thumb movement				
	Extensor pollicis brevis	Extensor pollicis brevis		
	Extensor pollicis longus	Extensor pollicis longus		
	Flexor pollicis longus		Flexor pollicis longus	
Intrinsic — found within the hand only				
	Adductor pollicis			Adductor pollicis
	Dorsal interossei	Dorsal interossei	Dorsal interossei	
	Lumbricals	Lumbricals	Lumbricals	
	Palmaris brevis			Palmaris brevis
	Palmar interossei	Palmar interossei	Palmar interossei	
	Hypothenar muscles			
	Abductor digiti minimi			Abductor digiti minimi
	Flexor digiti minimi brevis		Flexor digiti minimi brevis	
	Oppenens digiti minimi		Oppenens digiti minimi	
	Thenar muscles			
	Abductor pollicis brevis			Abductor pollicis brevis
	Flexor pollicis brevis		Flexor pollicis brevis	
	Oppenens pollicis		Oppenens pollicis	
Thigh				
	Anterior muscles			
	Iliopsoas		Iliopsoas	
	Pectineus		Pectineus	
	Quadriceps	Quadriceps		
	Rectus femoris	Rectus femoris — Extends knee	Rectus femoris — Flexes hip	
	Vastus intermedius	Vastus intermedius		
	Vastus lateralis	Vastus lateralis		
	Vastus medialis	Vastus medialis		
	Sartorius		Sartorius	
	Medial muscles			
	Adductor brevis			Adductor brevis
	Adductor longus			Adductor longus
	Adductor magnus			Adductor magnus
	Gracilis			Gracilis
	Obturator externus			Obturator externus
	Posterior muscles			
	Hamstring	Hamstring — Extends hip	Hamstring — Flexes knee	
	Biceps femoris	Biceps femoris	Biceps femoris	
	Semimembranosus	Semimembranosus	Semimembranosus	
	Semitendinosus	Semitendinosus	Semitendinosus	

Chapter 13. Diseases of the Musculoskeletal System and Connective Tissue

Chapter 13. Diseases of the Musculoskeletal System and Connective Tissue

Body Region	Muscle	Extensor Tendon	Flexor Tendon	Other Tendon
Lower leg				
	Anterior muscles			
	Extensor digitorum longus	Extensor digitorum longus		
	Extensor hallucis longus	Extensor hallucis longus		
	Fibularis (peroneus) tertius	Fibularis (peroneus) tertius		
	Tibialis anterior	Tibialis anterior		Tibialis anterior
	Lateral muscles			
	Fibularis (peroneus) brevis		Fibularis (peroneus) brevis	
	Fibularis (peroneus) longus		Fibularis (peroneus) longus	
	Posterior muscles			
	Deep			
	Flexor digitorum longus		Flexor digitorum longus	
	Flexor hallucis longus		Flexor hallucis longus	
	Popliteus		Popliteus	
	Tibialis posterior		Tibialis posterior	
	Superficial			
	Gastrocnemius		Gastrocnemius	
	Plantaris		Plantaris	
	Soleus		Soleus	
				Calcaneal (Achilles)
Ankle/Foot				
Extrinsic — attach to a site in the lower leg as well as a site in the foot with action related to foot movement at the ankle				
	Plantaris		Plantaris	
	Soleus		Soleus	
	Tibialis anterior	Tibialis anterior		
	Tibialis posterior		Tibialis posterior	
Extrinsic — attach to a site in the lower leg as well as a site in the foot with action in the foot related to toe movement				
	Extensor digitorum longus	Extensor digitorum longus		
	Extensor hallicus longus	Extensor hallicus longus		
	Flexor digitorum longus		Flexor digitorum longus	
	Flexor hallucis longus		Flexor hallucis longus	
Intrinsic — found within the ankle/foot only				
	Dorsal muscles			
	Extensor digitorum brevis	Extensor digitorum brevis		
	Extensor hallucis brevis	Extensor hallucis brevis		
	Plantar muscles			
	Abductor digiti minimi		Abductor digiti minimi	
	Abductor hallucis		Abductor hallucis	
	Dorsal interossei	Dorsal interossei	Dorsal interossei	
	Flexor digiti minimi brevis		Flexor digiti minimi brevis	
	Flexor digitorum brevis		Flexor digitorum brevis	
	Flexor hallucis brevis		Flexor hallucis brevis	
	Lumbricals	Lumbricals	Lumbricals	
	Quadratus plantae		Quadratus plantae	
	Plantar interossei	Plantar interossei	Plantar interossei	

Chapter 13. Diseases of the Musculoskeletal System and Connective Tissue (M00-M99)

NOTE Use an external cause code following the code for the musculoskeletal condition, if applicable, to identify the cause of the musculoskeletal condition.

EXCLUDES 2 arthropathic psoriasis (L40.5-)
certain conditions originating in the perinatal period (P04-P96)
certain infectious and parasitic diseases (A00-B99)
compartment syndrome (traumatic) (T79.A-)
complications of pregnancy, childbirth and the puerperium (O00-O9A)
congenital malformations, deformations, and chromosomal abnormalities (Q00-Q99)
endocrine, nutritional and metabolic diseases (E00-E88)
injury, poisoning and certain other consequences of external causes (S00-T88)
neoplasms (C00-D49)
symptoms, signs and abnormal clinical and laboratory findings, not elsewhere classified (R00-R94)

This chapter contains the following blocks:

M00-M02	Infectious arthropathies
M04	~~Autoinflammatory syndromes~~
M05-M14	Inflammatory polyarthropathies
M15-M19	Osteoarthritis
M20-M25	Other joint disorders
M26-M27	Dentofacial anomalies [including malocclusion] and other disorders of jaw
M30-M36	Systemic connective tissue disorders
M40-M43	Deforming dorsopathies
M45-M49	Spondylopathies
M50-M54	Other dorsopathies
M60-M63	Disorders of muscles
M65-M67	Disorders of synovium and tendon
M70-M79	Other soft tissue disorders
M80-M85	Disorders of bone density and structure
M86-M90	Other osteopathies
M91-M94	Chondropathies
M95	Other disorders of the musculoskeletal system and connective tissue
M96	Intraoperative and postprocedural complications and disorders of musculoskeletal system, not elsewhere classified
M97	~~Periprosthetic fracture around internal prosthetic joint~~
M99	Biomechanical lesions, not elsewhere classified

ARTHROPATHIES (M00-M25)

INCLUDES disorders affecting predominantly peripheral (limb) joints

Infectious arthropathies (M00-M02)

NOTE This block comprises arthropathies due to microbiological agents. Distinction is made between the following types of etiological relationship:

a) direct infection of joint, where organisms invade synovial tissue and microbial antigen is present in the joint;

b) indirect infection, which may be of two types: a reactive arthropathy, where microbial infection of the body is established but neither organisms nor antigens can be identified in the joint, and a postinfective arthropathy, where microbial antigen is present but recovery of an organism is inconstant and evidence of local multiplication is lacking.

✓4th **M00 Pyogenic arthritis**

✓5th **M00.0 Staphylococcal arthritis and polyarthritis**
Use additional code (B95.61-B95.8) to identify bacterial agent
EXCLUDES 2 infection and inflammatory reaction due to internal joint prosthesis (T84.5-)

M00.00 Staphylococcal arthritis, unspecified joint CC HCC
CC Excl: PDX collection 855

✓6th **M00.01 Staphylococcal arthritis, shoulder**

CC Excl: For all CC codes in subcategory M00.01: PDX collection 856

M00.011 Staphylococcal arthritis, right shoulder CC HCC

M00.012 Staphylococcal arthritis, left shoulder CC HCC

M00.019 Staphylococcal arthritis, unspecified shoulder CC HCC

M00.02 Staphylococcal arthritis, elbow

CC Excl: For all CC codes in subcategory M00.02: PDX collection 857

M00.021 Staphylococcal arthritis, right elbow CC HCC

M00.022 Staphylococcal arthritis, left elbow CC HCC

M00.029 Staphylococcal arthritis, unspecified elbow CC HCC

✓6th **M00.03 Staphylococcal arthritis, wrist**
Staphylococcal arthritis of carpal bones

CC Excl: For all CC codes in subcategory M00.03: PDX collection 858

M00.031 Staphylococcal arthritis, right wrist CC HCC

M00.032 Staphylococcal arthritis, left wrist CC HCC

M00.039 Staphylococcal arthritis, unspecified wrist CC HCC

✓6th **M00.04 Staphylococcal arthritis, hand**
Staphylococcal arthritis of metacarpus and phalanges

CC Excl: For all CC codes in subcategory M00.04: PDX collection 859

M00.041 Staphylococcal arthritis, right hand CC HCC

M00.042 Staphylococcal arthritis, left hand CC HCC

M00.049 Staphylococcal arthritis, unspecified hand CC HCC

✓6th **M00.05 Staphylococcal arthritis, hip**

CC Excl: For all CC codes in subcategory M00.05: PDX collection 860

M00.051 Staphylococcal arthritis, right hip CC HCC
M00.052 Staphylococcal arthritis, left hip CC HCC
M00.059 Staphylococcal arthritis, unspecified hip CC HCC

✓6th **M00.06 Staphylococcal arthritis, knee**

CC Excl: For all CC codes in subcategory M00.06: PDX collection 861

M00.061 Staphylococcal arthritis, right knee CC HCC
M00.062 Staphylococcal arthritis, left knee CC HCC
M00.069 Staphylococcal arthritis, unspecified knee

✓6th **M00.07 Staphylococcal arthritis, ankle and foot**
Staphylococcal arthritis, tarsus, metatarsus and phalanges

CC Excl: For all CC codes in subcategory M00.07: PDX collection 862

M00.071 Staphylococcal arthritis, right ankle and foot CC HCC

M00.072 Staphylococcal arthritis, left ankle and foot CC HCC

M00.079 Staphylococcal arthritis, unspecified ankle and foot CC HCC

M00.08 Staphylococcal arthritis, vertebrae CC HCC
CC Excl: PDX collection 855

M00.09 Staphylococcal polyarthritis CC HCC
CC Excl: PDX collection 855

✓5th **M00.1 Pneumococcal arthritis and polyarthritis**

M00.10 Pneumococcal arthritis, unspecified joint CC HCC
CC Excl: PDX collection 855

✓6th **M00.11 Pneumococcal arthritis, shoulder**

CC Excl: For CC codes in subcategory M00.11: PDX collection 856

M00.111 Pneumococcal arthritis, right shoulder CC HCC

M00.112 Pneumococcal arthritis, left shoulder CC HCC

M00.119 Pneumococcal arthritis, unspecified shoulder CC HCC

√6ᵗʰ M00.12 Pneumococcal arthritis, elbow

> **CC Excl: For CC codes in subcategory M00.12:**
> PDX collection 857

    M00.121 Pneumococcal arthritis, right elbow `CC` `HCC`

    M00.122 Pneumococcal arthritis, left elbow `CC` `HCC`

    M00.129 Pneumococcal arthritis, unspecified elbow `CC` `HCC`

√6ᵗʰ M00.13 Pneumococcal arthritis, wrist
Pneumococcal arthritis of carpal bones

> **CC Excl: For CC codes in subcategory M00.13:**
> PDX collection 858

    M00.131 Pneumococcal arthritis, right wrist `CC` `HCC`

    M00.132 Pneumococcal arthritis, left wrist `CC` `HCC`

    M00.139 Pneumococcal arthritis, unspecified wrist `CC` `HCC`

√6ᵗʰ M00.14 Pneumococcal arthritis, hand
Pneumococcal arthritis of metacarpus and phalanges

> **CC Excl: For CC codes in subcategory M00.14:**
> PDX collection 859

    M00.141 Pneumococcal arthritis, right hand `CC` `HCC`

    M00.142 Pneumococcal arthritis, left hand `CC` `HCC`

    M00.149 Pneumococcal arthritis, unspecified hand `CC` `HCC`

√6ᵗʰ M00.15 Pneumococcal arthritis, hip

> **CC Excl: For CC codes in subcategory M00.15:**
> PDX collection 860

    M00.151 Pneumococcal arthritis, right hip `CC` `HCC`

    M00.152 Pneumococcal arthritis, left hip `CC` `HCC`

    M00.159 Pneumococcal arthritis, unspecified hip `CC` `HCC`

√6ᵗʰ M00.16 Pneumococcal arthritis, knee

> **CC Excl: For CC codes in subcategory M00.16:**
> PDX collection 861

    M00.161 Pneumococcal arthritis, right knee `CC` `HCC`

    M00.162 Pneumococcal arthritis, left knee `CC` `HCC`

    M00.169 Pneumococcal arthritis, unspecified knee `CC` `HCC`

√6ᵗʰ M00.17 Pneumococcal arthritis, ankle and foot
Pneumococcal arthritis, tarsus, metatarsus and phalanges

> **CC Excl: For CC codes in subcategory M00.17:**
> PDX collection 862

    M00.171 Pneumococcal arthritis, right ankle and foot `CC` `HCC`

    M00.172 Pneumococcal arthritis, left ankle and foot `CC` `HCC`

    M00.179 Pneumococcal arthritis, unspecified ankle and foot `CC` `HCC`

    M00.18 Pneumococcal arthritis, vertebrae `CC` `HCC`
           CC Excl: PDX collection 855

    M00.19 Pneumococcal polyarthritis `CC` `HCC`
           CC Excl: PDX collection 855

√5ᵗʰ M00.2 Other streptococcal arthritis and polyarthritis
Use additional code (B95.0-B95.2, B95.4-B95.5) to identify bacterial agent

    M00.20 Other streptococcal arthritis, unspecified joint `CC` `HCC`
           CC Excl: PDX collection 855

√6ᵗʰ M00.21 Other streptococcal arthritis, shoulder

> **CC Excl: For CC codes in subcategory M00.21:**
> PDX collection 856

    M00.211 Other streptococcal arthritis, right shoulder `CC` `HCC`

    M00.212 Other streptococcal arthritis, left shoulder `CC` `HCC`

    M00.219 Other streptococcal arthritis, unspecified shoulder `CC` `HCC`

√6ᵗʰ M00.22 Other streptococcal arthritis, elbow

> **CC Excl: For CC codes in subcategory M00.22:**
> PDX collection 857

    M00.221 Other streptococcal arthritis, right elbow `CC` `HCC`

    M00.222 Other streptococcal arthritis, left elbow `CC` `HCC`

    M00.229 Other streptococcal arthritis, unspecified elbow `CC` `HCC`

√6ᵗʰ M00.23 Other streptococcal arthritis, wrist
Other streptococcal arthritis of carpal bones

> **CC Excl: For CC codes in subcategory M00.23:**
> PDX collection 858

    M00.231 Other streptococcal arthritis, right wrist `CC` `HCC`

    M00.232 Other streptococcal arthritis, left wrist `CC` `HCC`

    M00.239 Other streptococcal arthritis, unspecified wrist `CC` `HCC`

√6ᵗʰ M00.24 Other streptococcal arthritis, hand
Other streptococcal arthritis metacarpus and phalanges

> **CC Excl: For CC codes in subcategory M00.24:**
> PDX collection 859

    M00.241 Other streptococcal arthritis, right hand `CC` `HCC`

    M00.242 Other streptococcal arthritis, left hand `CC` `HCC`

    M00.249 Other streptococcal arthritis, unspecified hand `CC` `HCC`

√6ᵗʰ M00.25 Other streptococcal arthritis, hip

> **CC Excl: For CC codes in subcategory M00.25:**
> PDX collection 860

    M00.251 Other streptococcal arthritis, right hip `CC` `HCC`

    M00.252 Other streptococcal arthritis, left hip `CC` `HCC`

    M00.259 Other streptococcal arthritis, unspecified hip `CC` `HCC`

√6ᵗʰ M00.26 Other streptococcal arthritis, knee

> **CC Excl: For CC codes in subcategory M00.26:**
> PDX collection 861

    M00.261 Other streptococcal arthritis, right knee `CC` `HCC`

    M00.262 Other streptococcal arthritis, left knee `CC` `HCC`

    M00.269 Other streptococcal arthritis, unspecified knee `CC` `HCC`

√6ᵗʰ M00.27 Other streptococcal arthritis, ankle and foot
Other streptococcal arthritis, tarsus, metatarsus and phalanges

> **CC Excl: For CC codes in subcategory M00.27:**
> PDX collection 862

    M00.271 Other streptococcal arthritis, right ankle and foot `CC` `HCC`

    M00.272 Other streptococcal arthritis, left ankle and foot `CC` `HCC`

    M00.279 Other streptococcal arthritis, unspecified ankle and foot `CC` `HCC`

    M00.28 Other streptococcal arthritis, vertebrae `CC` `HCC`
           CC Excl: PDX collection 855

    M00.29 Other streptococcal polyarthritis `CC` `HCC`
           CC Excl: PDX collection 855

√5ᵗʰ M00.8 Arthritis and polyarthritis due to other bacteria
Use additional code (B96) to identify bacteria

    M00.80 Arthritis due to other bacteria, unspecified joint `CC` `HCC`
           CC Excl: PDX collection 855

`N` Newborn: 0   `P` Pediatric: 0-17   `M` Maternity: 12-55   `A` Adult: 15-124   `MCC` Major CC Condition   `PDxMCC` PDx acts as own MCC   `CC` CC Condition   `PDxCC` PDx acts as own CC

✓6ᵗʰ **M00.81 Arthritis due to other bacteria, shoulder**

> **CC Excl: For CC codes in subcategory M00.81:** PDX collection 856

M00.811 Arthritis due to other bacteria, right shoulder `CC` `HCC`

M00.812 Arthritis due to other bacteria, left shoulder `CC` `HCC`

M00.819 Arthritis due to other bacteria, unspecified shoulder `CC` `HCC`

✓6ᵗʰ **M00.82 Arthritis due to other bacteria, elbow**

> **CC Excl: For CC codes in subcategory M00.82:** PDX collection 857

M00.821 Arthritis due to other bacteria, right elbow `CC` `HCC`

M00.822 Arthritis due to other bacteria, left elbow `CC` `HCC`

M00.829 Arthritis due to other bacteria, unspecified elbow `CC` `HCC`

✓6ᵗʰ **M00.83 Arthritis due to other bacteria, wrist**
Arthritis due to other bacteria, carpal bones

> **CC Excl: For CC codes in subcategory M00.83:** PDX collection 858

M00.831 Arthritis due to other bacteria, right wrist `CC` `HCC`

M00.832 Arthritis due to other bacteria, left wrist `CC` `HCC`

M00.839 Arthritis due to other bacteria, unspecified wrist `CC` `HCC`

✓6ᵗʰ **M00.84 Arthritis due to other bacteria, hand**
Arthritis due to other bacteria, metacarpus and phalanges

> **CC Excl: For CC codes in subcategory M00.84:** PDX collection 859

M00.841 Arthritis due to other bacteria, right hand `CC` `HCC`

M00.842 Arthritis due to other bacteria, left hand `CC` `HCC`

M00.849 Arthritis due to other bacteria, unspecified hand `CC` `HCC`

✓6ᵗʰ **M00.85 Arthritis due to other bacteria, hip**

> **CC Excl: For CC codes in subcategory M00.85:** PDX collection 860

M00.851 Arthritis due to other bacteria, right hip `CC` `HCC`

M00.852 Arthritis due to other bacteria, left hip `CC` `HCC`

M00.859 Arthritis due to other bacteria, unspecified hip `CC` `HCC`

✓6ᵗʰ **M00.86 Arthritis due to other bacteria, knee**

> **CC Excl: For CC codes in subcategory M00.86:** PDX collection 861

M00.861 Arthritis due to other bacteria, right knee `CC` `HCC`

M00.862 Arthritis due to other bacteria, left knee `CC` `HCC`

M00.869 Arthritis due to other bacteria, unspecified knee `CC` `HCC`

✓6ᵗʰ **M00.87 Arthritis due to other bacteria, ankle and foot**
Arthritis due to other bacteria, tarsus, metatarsus, and phalanges

> **CC Excl: For CC codes in subcategory M00.87:** PDX collection 862

M00.871 Arthritis due to other bacteria, right ankle and foot `CC` `HCC`

M00.872 Arthritis due to other bacteria, left ankle and foot `CC` `HCC`

M00.879 Arthritis due to other bacteria, unspecified ankle and foot `CC` `HCC`

M00.88 Arthritis due to other bacteria, vertebrae `CC` `HCC`
CC Excl: PDX collection 855

M00.89 Polyarthritis due to other bacteria `CC` `HCC`
CC Excl: PDX collection 855

M00.9 Pyogenic arthritis, unspecified `CC` `HCC`
Infective arthritis NOS
CC Excl: PDX collection 855

✓4ᵗʰ **M01 Direct infections of joint in infectious and parasitic diseases classified elsewhere**
Code first underlying disease, such as:
leprosy [Hansen's disease] (A30.-)
mycoses (B35-B49)
O'nyong-nyong fever (A92.1)
paratyphoid fever (A01.1-A01.4)

> *EXCLUDES 1*   arthropathy in Lyme disease (A69.23)
> gonococcal arthritis (A54.42)
> meningococcal arthritis (A39.83)
> mumps arthritis (B26.85)
> postinfective arthropathy (M02.-)
> postmeningococcal arthritis (A39.84)
> reactive arthritis (M02.3)
> rubella arthritis (B06.82)
> sarcoidosis arthritis (D86.86)
> typhoid fever arthritis (A01.04)
> tuberculosis arthritis (A18.01-A18.02)

> **CC Excl: For CC codes in category M01, unless otherwise noted:** PDX collection 863

✓5ᵗʰ **M01.X Direct infection of joint in infectious and parasitic diseases classified elsewhere**

M01.X0 Direct infection of unspecified joint in infectious and parasitic diseases classified elsewhere `CC` `HCC`

✓6ᵗʰ **M01.X1 Direct infection of shoulder joint in infectious and parasitic diseases classified elsewhere**

> **CC Excl: For CC codes in subcategory M01.X1, unless otherwise noted:** PDX collection 864

M01.X11 Direct infection of right shoulder in infectious and parasitic diseases classified elsewhere `CC` `HCC`

M01.X12 Direct infection of left shoulder in infectious and parasitic diseases classified elsewhere `CC` `HCC`

M01.X19 Direct infection of unspecified shoulder in infectious and parasitic diseases classified elsewhere `CC` `HCC`

✓6ᵗʰ **M01.X2 Direct infection of elbow in infectious and parasitic diseases classified elsewhere**

M01.X21 Direct infection of right elbow in infectious and parasitic diseases classified elsewhere `CC` `HCC`

M01.X22 Direct infection of left elbow in infectious and parasitic diseases classified elsewhere `CC` `HCC`

M01.X29 Direct infection of unspecified elbow in infectious and parasitic diseases classified elsewhere `CC` `HCC`

✓6ᵗʰ **M01.X3 Direct infection of wrist in infectious and parasitic diseases classified elsewhere**
Direct infection of carpal bones in infectious and parasitic diseases classified elsewhere

M01.X31 Direct infection of right wrist in infectious and parasitic diseases classified elsewhere `CC` `HCC`

M01.X32 Direct infection of left wrist in infectious and parasitic diseases classified elsewhere `CC` `HCC`

M01.X39 Direct infection of unspecified wrist in infectious and parasitic diseases classified elsewhere `CC` `HCC`

✓6ᵗʰ **M01.X4 Direct infection of hand in infectious and parasitic diseases classified elsewhere**
Direct infection of metacarpus and phalanges in infectious and parasitic diseases classified elsewhere

M01.X41 Direct infection of right hand in infectious and parasitic diseases classified elsewhere `CC` `HCC`

M01.X42 Direct infection of left hand in infectious and parasitic diseases classified elsewhere `CC` `HCC`

M01.X49 Direct infection of unspecified hand in infectious and parasitic diseases classified elsewhere `CC` `HCC`

✓ Additional Character Req   ✓x7ᵗʰ Placeholder Alert   Unacceptable PDx   Manifestation   H1 - H14 HAC   HCC CMS-HCC Condition   *EXCLUDES 1* Not Coded Here   *EXCLUDES 2* Not Included Here

Chapter 13. Diseases of the Musculoskeletal System and Connective Tissue

M01.X5–M02.152

✓6ᵗʰ **M01.X5** **Direct infection of hip in infectious and parasitic diseases classified elsewhere**

    M01.X51 *Direct infection of right hip in infectious and parasitic diseases classified elsewhere*   CC HCC

    M01.X52 *Direct infection of left hip in infectious and parasitic diseases classified elsewhere*   CC HCC

    M01.X59 *Direct infection of unspecified hip in infectious and parasitic diseases classified elsewhere*   CC HCC

✓6ᵗʰ **M01.X6** **Direct infection of knee in infectious and parasitic diseases classified elsewhere**

    M01.X61 *Direct infection of right knee in infectious and parasitic diseases classified elsewhere*   CC HCC

    M01.X62 *Direct infection of left knee in infectious and parasitic diseases classified elsewhere*   CC HCC

    M01.X69 *Direct infection of unspecified knee in infectious and parasitic diseases classified elsewhere*   CC HCC

✓6ᵗʰ **M01.X7** **Direct infection of ankle and foot in infectious and parasitic diseases classified elsewhere**

    Direct infection of tarsus, metatarsus and phalanges in infectious and parasitic diseases classified elsewhere

    M01.X71 *Direct infection of right ankle and foot in infectious and parasitic diseases classified elsewhere*   CC HCC

    M01.X72 *Direct infection of left ankle and foot in infectious and parasitic diseases classified elsewhere*   CC HCC

    M01.X79 *Direct infection of unspecified ankle and foot in infectious and parasitic diseases classified elsewhere*   CC HCC

    M01.X8 *Direct infection of vertebrae in infectious and parasitic diseases classified elsewhere*   CC HCC

    M01.X9 *Direct infection of multiple joints in infectious and parasitic diseases classified elsewhere*   CC HCC

✓4ᵗʰ **M02** **Postinfective and reactive arthropathies**

    Code first underlying disease, such as:
    congenital syphilis [Clutton's joints] (A50.5)
    enteritis due to Yersinia enterocolitica (A04.6)
    infective endocarditis (I33.0)
    viral hepatitis (B15-B19)

    EXCLUDES 1   *Behçet's disease (M35.2)*
      direct infections of joint in infectious and parasitic diseases classified elsewhere (M01.-)
      mumps arthritis (B26.85)
      postmeningococcal arthritis (A39.84)
      rheumatic fever (I00)
      rubella arthritis (B06.82)
      syphilis arthritis (late) (A52.77)
      tabetic arthropathy [Charcôt's] (A52.16)

✓5ᵗʰ **M02.0** **Arthropathy following intestinal bypass**

    M02.00 **Arthropathy following intestinal bypass, unspecified site**

✓6ᵗʰ   **M02.01** **Arthropathy following intestinal bypass, shoulder**

    M02.011 **Arthropathy following intestinal bypass, right shoulder**

    M02.012 **Arthropathy following intestinal bypass, left shoulder**

    M02.019 **Arthropathy following intestinal bypass, unspecified shoulder**

✓6ᵗʰ   **M02.02** **Arthropathy following intestinal bypass, elbow**

    M02.021 **Arthropathy following intestinal bypass, right elbow**

    M02.022 **Arthropathy following intestinal bypass, left elbow**

    M02.029 **Arthropathy following intestinal bypass, unspecified elbow**

✓6ᵗʰ   **M02.03** **Arthropathy following intestinal bypass, wrist**

    Arthropathy following intestinal bypass, carpal bones

    M02.031 **Arthropathy following intestinal bypass, right wrist**

    M02.032 **Arthropathy following intestinal bypass, left wrist**

    M02.039 **Arthropathy following intestinal bypass, unspecified wrist**

✓6ᵗʰ   **M02.04** **Arthropathy following intestinal bypass, hand**

    Arthropathy following intestinal bypass, metacarpals and phalanges

    M02.041 **Arthropathy following intestinal bypass, right hand**

    M02.042 **Arthropathy following intestinal bypass, left hand**

    M02.049 **Arthropathy following intestinal bypass, unspecified hand**

  M02.05 **Arthropathy following intestinal bypass, hip**

    M02.051 **Arthropathy following intestinal bypass, right hip**

    M02.052 **Arthropathy following intestinal bypass, left hip**

    M02.059 **Arthropathy following intestinal bypass, unspecified hip**

  M02.06 **Arthropathy following intestinal bypass, knee**

    M02.061 **Arthropathy following intestinal bypass, right knee**

    M02.062 **Arthropathy following intestinal bypass, left knee**

    M02.069 **Arthropathy following intestinal bypass, unspecified knee**

✓6ᵗʰ   **M02.07** **Arthropathy following intestinal bypass, ankle and foot**

    Arthropathy following intestinal bypass, tarsus, metatarsus and phalanges

    M02.071 **Arthropathy following intestinal bypass, right ankle and foot**

    M02.072 **Arthropathy following intestinal bypass, left ankle and foot**

    M02.079 **Arthropathy following intestinal bypass, unspecified ankle and foot**

  M02.08 **Arthropathy following intestinal bypass, vertebrae**

  M02.09 **Arthropathy following intestinal bypass, multiple sites**

✓5ᵗʰ **M02.1** **Postdysenteric arthropathy**

    CC Excl: For CC codes in subcategory M02.1, unless otherwise noted: PDX collection 863

    M02.10 **Postdysenteric arthropathy, unspecified site**   CC HCC

✓6ᵗʰ   **M02.11** **Postdysenteric arthropathy, shoulder**

    M02.111 **Postdysenteric arthropathy, right shoulder**   CC HCC

    M02.112 **Postdysenteric arthropathy, left shoulder**   CC HCC

    M02.119 **Postdysenteric arthropathy, unspecified shoulder**   CC HCC

✓6ᵗʰ   **M02.12** **Postdysenteric arthropathy, elbow**

    M02.121 **Postdysenteric arthropathy, right elbow**   CC HCC

    M02.122 **Postdysenteric arthropathy, left elbow**   CC HCC

    M02.129 **Postdysenteric arthropathy, unspecified elbow**   CC HCC

✓6ᵗʰ   **M02.13** **Postdysenteric arthropathy, wrist**

    Postdysenteric arthropathy, carpal bones

    M02.131 **Postdysenteric arthropathy, right wrist**   CC HCC

    M02.132 **Postdysenteric arthropathy, left wrist**   CC HCC

    M02.139 **Postdysenteric arthropathy, unspecified wrist**   CC HCC

✓6ᵗʰ   **M02.14** **Postdysenteric arthropathy, hand**

    Postdysenteric arthropathy, metacarpus and phalanges

    M02.141 **Postdysenteric arthropathy, right hand**   CC HCC

    M02.142 **Postdysenteric arthropathy, left hand**   CC HCC

    M02.149 **Postdysenteric arthropathy, unspecified hand**   CC HCC

✓6ᵗʰ   **M02.15** **Postdysenteric arthropathy, hip**

    M02.151 **Postdysenteric arthropathy, right hip**   CC HCC

    M02.152 **Postdysenteric arthropathy, left hip**   CC HCC

N Newborn: 0   P Pediatric: 0-17   M Maternity: 12-55   A Adult: 15-124   MCC Major CC Condition   PDx MCC PDx acts as own MCC   CC CC Condition   PDx CC PDx acts as own CC

738   ICD-10-CM 2018

M02.159   Postdysenteric arthropathy, unspecified **hip** `CC` `HCC`

☑6ᵗʰ **M02.16**   Postdysenteric arthropathy, **knee**

> **CC Excl: For CC codes in subcategory M02.16:** PDX collection 865

M02.161   Postdysenteric arthropathy, right **knee** `CC` `HCC`

M02.162   Postdysenteric arthropathy, left **knee** `CC` `HCC`

M02.169   Postdysenteric arthropathy, unspecified **knee** `CC` `HCC`

☑6ᵗʰ **M02.17**   Postdysenteric arthropathy, **ankle and foot**
Postdysenteric arthropathy, tarsus, metatarsus and phalanges

M02.171   Postdysenteric arthropathy, right **ankle and foot** `CC` `HCC`

M02.172   Postdysenteric arthropathy, left **ankle and foot** `CC` `HCC`

M02.179   Postdysenteric arthropathy, unspecified **ankle and foot** `CC` `HCC`

M02.18   Postdysenteric arthropathy, **vertebrae** `CC` `HCC`
CC Excl: PDX collection 866

M02.19   Postdysenteric arthropathy, **multiple sites** `CC` `HCC`

☑5ᵗʰ **M02.2**   **Postimmunization** arthropathy

M02.20   Postimmunization arthropathy, **unspecified site**

☑6ᵗʰ **M02.21**   Postimmunization arthropathy, **shoulder**

M02.211   Postimmunization arthropathy, right **shoulder**

M02.212   Postimmunization arthropathy, left **shoulder**

M02.219   Postimmunization arthropathy, unspecified **shoulder**

☑6ᵗʰ **M02.22**   Postimmunization arthropathy, **elbow**

M02.221   Postimmunization arthropathy, right **elbow**

M02.222   Postimmunization arthropathy, left **elbow**

M02.229   Postimmunization arthropathy, unspecified **elbow**

☑6ᵗʰ **M02.23**   Postimmunization arthropathy, **wrist**
Postimmunization arthropathy, carpal bones

M02.231   Postimmunization arthropathy, right **wrist**

M02.232   Postimmunization arthropathy, left **wrist**

M02.239   Postimmunization arthropathy, unspecified **wrist**

☑6ᵗʰ **M02.24**   Postimmunization arthropathy, **hand**
Postimmunization arthropathy, metacarpus and phalanges

M02.241   Postimmunization arthropathy, right **hand**

M02.242   Postimmunization arthropathy, left **hand**

M02.249   Postimmunization arthropathy, unspecified **hand**

☑6ᵗʰ **M02.25**   Postimmunization arthropathy, **hip**

M02.251   Postimmunization arthropathy, right **hip**

M02.252   Postimmunization arthropathy, left **hip**

M02.259   Postimmunization arthropathy, unspecified **hip**

☑6ᵗʰ **M02.26**   Postimmunization arthropathy, **knee**

M02.261   Postimmunization arthropathy, right **knee**

M02.262   Postimmunization arthropathy, left **knee**

M02.269   Postimmunization arthropathy, unspecified **knee**

☑6ᵗʰ **M02.27**   Postimmunization arthropathy, **ankle and foot**
Postimmunization arthropathy, tarsus, metatarsus and phalanges

M02.271   Postimmunization arthropathy, right **ankle and foot**

M02.272   Postimmunization arthropathy, left **ankle and foot**

M02.279   Postimmunization arthropathy, unspecified **ankle and foot**

M02.28   Postimmunization arthropathy, **vertebrae**

M02.29   Postimmunization arthropathy, **multiple sites**

☑5ᵗʰ **M02.3**   Reiter's disease
Reactive arthritis

> **CC Excl: For CC codes in subcategory M02.3:** PDX collection 863

M02.30   Reiter's disease, unspecified site `PDxCC` `CC` `HCC`

☑6ᵗʰ **M02.31**   Reiter's disease, **shoulder** `PDxCC` `CC` `HCC`

M02.311   Reiter's disease, right **shoulder** `PDxCC` `CC` `HCC`

M02.312   Reiter's disease, left **shoulder** `PDxCC` `CC` `HCC`

M02.319   Reiter's disease, unspecified **shoulder** `PDxCC` `CC` `HCC`

☑6ᵗʰ **M02.32**   Reiter's disease, **elbow**

M02.321   Reiter's disease, right **elbow** `PDxCC` `CC` `HCC`

M02.322   Reiter's disease, left **elbow** `PDxCC` `CC` `HCC`

M02.329   Reiter's disease, unspecified **elbow** `PDxCC` `CC` `HCC`

☑6ᵗʰ **M02.33**   Reiter's disease, **wrist**
Reiter's disease, carpal bones

M02.331   Reiter's disease, right **wrist** `PDxCC` `CC` `HCC`

M02.332   Reiter's disease, left **wrist** `PDxCC` `CC` `HCC`

M02.339   Reiter's disease, unspecified **wrist** `PDxCC` `CC` `HCC`

☑6ᵗʰ **M02.34**   Reiter's disease, **hand**
Reiter's disease, metacarpus and phalanges

M02.341   Reiter's disease, right **hand** `PDxCC` `CC` `HCC`

M02.342   Reiter's disease, left **hand** `PDxCC` `CC` `HCC`

M02.349   Reiter's disease, unspecified **hand** `PDxCC` `CC` `HCC`

☑6ᵗʰ **M02.35**   Reiter's disease, **hip**

M02.351   Reiter's disease, right **hip** `PDxCC` `CC` `HCC`

M02.352   Reiter's disease, left **hip** `PDxCC` `CC` `HCC`

M02.359   Reiter's disease, unspecified **hip** `PDxCC` `CC` `HCC`

☑6ᵗʰ **M02.36**   Reiter's disease, **knee**

M02.361   Reiter's disease, right **knee** `PDxCC` `CC` `HCC`

M02.362   Reiter's disease, left **knee** `PDxCC` `CC` `HCC`

M02.369   Reiter's disease, unspecified **knee** `PDxCC` `CC` `HCC`

☑6ᵗʰ **M02.37**   Reiter's disease, **ankle and foot**
Reiter's disease, tarsus, metatarsus and phalanges

M02.371   Reiter's disease, right **ankle and foot** `PDxCC` `CC` `HCC`

M02.372   Reiter's disease, left **ankle and foot** `PDxCC` `CC` `HCC`

M02.379   Reiter's disease, unspecified **ankle and foot** `PDxCC` `CC` `HCC`

M02.38   Reiter's disease, **vertebrae** `PDxCC` `CC` `HCC`

M02.39   Reiter's disease, **multiple sites** `PDxCC` `CC` `HCC`

☑5ᵗʰ **M02.8**   Other reactive **arthropathies**

> **CC Excl: For CC codes in subcategory M02.8, unless otherwise noted:** PDX collection 863

M02.80   *Other reactive arthropathies, unspecified site* `CC` `HCC`

☑6ᵗʰ **M02.81**   Other reactive arthropathies, **shoulder**

> **CC Excl: For CC codes in subcategory M02.81:** PDX collection 864

M02.811   *Other reactive arthropathies, right shoulder* `CC` `HCC`

M02.812   *Other reactive arthropathies, left shoulder* `CC` `HCC`

M02.819   *Other reactive arthropathies, unspecified shoulder* `CC` `HCC`

☑6ᵗʰ **M02.82**   Other reactive arthropathies, **elbow**

M02.821   *Other reactive arthropathies, right elbow* `CC` `HCC`

M02.822   *Other reactive arthropathies, left elbow* `CC` `HCC`

M02.829   *Other reactive arthropathies, unspecified elbow* `CC` `HCC`

✓6th **M02.83** **Other reactive arthropathies,** wrist
Other reactive arthropathies, carpal bones

     M02.831 *Other reactive arthropathies,*   CC HCC
right wrist

     M02.832 *Other reactive arthropathies,*   CC HCC
left wrist

     M02.839 *Other reactive arthropathies,*   CC HCC
unspecified wrist

✓6th **M02.84** **Other reactive arthropathies,** hand
Other reactive arthropathies, metacarpus and
phalanges

     M02.841 *Other reactive arthropathies,* right   CC HCC
hand

     M02.842 *Other reactive arthropathies,* left   CC HCC
hand

     M02.849 *Other reactive arthropathies,*   CC HCC
unspecified hand

✓6th **M02.85** **Other reactive arthropathies,** hip

     M02.851 *Other reactive arthropathies,*   CC HCC
right hip

     M02.852 *Other reactive arthropathies,*   CC HCC
left hip

     M02.859 *Other reactive arthropathies,*   CC HCC
unspecified hip

✓6th **M02.86** **Other reactive arthropathies,** knee

     M02.861 *Other reactive arthropathies,*   CC HCC
right knee

     M02.862 *Other reactive arthropathies,*   CC HCC
left knee

     M02.869 *Other reactive arthropathies,*   CC HCC
unspecified knee

✓6th **M02.87** **Other reactive arthropathies,** ankle and foot
Other reactive arthropathies, tarsus, metatarsus and
phalanges

     M02.871 *Other reactive arthropathies,* right   CC HCC
ankle and foot

     M02.872 *Other reactive arthropathies,* left   CC HCC
ankle and foot

     M02.879 *Other reactive arthropathies,*   CC HCC
unspecified ankle and foot

   M02.88 *Other reactive arthropathies,* vertebrae   CC HCC

   M02.89 *Other reactive arthropathies,* multiple sites   CC HCC

  M02.9 *Reactive arthropathy, unspecified*   HCC

Autoinflammatory syndromes (M04)

✓4th **M04** **Autoinflammatory syndromes**
    EXCLUDES 2   *Crohn's disease (K50.-)*

  M04.1 **Periodic fever syndromes**   HCC
    Familial Mediterranean fever
    Hyperimmunoglobin D syndrome
    Mevalonate kinase deficiency
    Tumor necrosis factor receptor associated periodic syndrome
    [TRAPS]

  M04.2 **Cryopyrin-associated periodic syndromes**   HCC
    Chronic infantile neurological, cutaneous and articular
     syndrome [CINCA]
    Familial cold autoinflammatory syndrome
    Familial cold urticaria
    Muckle-Wells syndrome
    Neonatal onset multisystemic inflammatory disorder [NOMID]

  M04.8 **Other autoinflammatory syndromes**   HCC
    Blau syndrome
    Deficiency of interleukin 1 receptor antagonist [DIRA]
    Majeed syndrome
    Periodic fever, aphthous stomatitis, pharyngitis, and
     adenopathy syndrome [PFAPA]
    Pyogenic arthritis, pyoderma gangrenosum, and acne syndrome
     [PAPA]

  M04.9 **Autoinflammatory syndrome, unspecified**   HCC

Inflammatory polyarthropathies (M05-M14)

✓4th **M05** **Rheumatoid arthritis with rheumatoid factor**
    EXCLUDES 1   *rheumatic fever (I00)*
        juvenile rheumatoid arthritis (M08.-)
        rheumatoid arthritis of spine (M45.-)
   DEF: Rheumatoid arthritis: Autoimmune systemic disease that causes
   chronic inflammation of joints and other areas of the body, manifested by
   inflammatory changes in articular structures and synovial membranes,
   atrophy, and loss in bone density.

✓5th **M05.0** **Felty's syndrome**
    Rheumatoid arthritis with splenoadenomegaly and leukopenia

    M05.00 **Felty's syndrome,** unspecified site   HCC

✓6th **M05.01** **Felty's syndrome,** shoulder
      M05.011 **Felty's syndrome,** right shoulder   HCC
      M05.012 **Felty's syndrome,** left shoulder   HCC
      M05.019 **Felty's syndrome,** unspecified   HCC
            shoulder

✓6th **M05.02** **Felty's syndrome,** elbow
      M05.021 **Felty's syndrome,** right elbow   HCC
      M05.022 **Felty's syndrome,** left elbow   HCC
      M05.029 **Felty's syndrome,** unspecified elbow   HCC

✓6th **M05.03** **Felty's syndrome,** wrist
      Felty's syndrome, carpal bones
      M05.031 **Felty's syndrome,** right wrist   HCC
      M05.032 **Felty's syndrome,** left wrist   HCC
      M05.039 **Felty's syndrome,** unspecified wrist   HCC

✓6th **M05.04** **Felty's syndrome,** hand
      Felty's syndrome, metacarpus and phalanges
      M05.041 **Felty's syndrome,** right hand   HCC
      M05.042 **Felty's syndrome,** left hand   HCC
      M05.049 **Felty's syndrome,** unspecified hand   HCC

✓6th **M05.05** **Felty's syndrome,** hip
      M05.051 **Felty's syndrome,** right hip   HCC
      M05.052 **Felty's syndrome,** left hip   HCC
      M05.059 **Felty's syndrome,** unspecified hip   HCC

✓6th **M05.06** **Felty's syndrome,** knee
      M05.061 **Felty's syndrome,** right knee   HCC
      M05.062 **Felty's syndrome,** left knee   HCC
      M05.069 **Felty's syndrome,** unspecified knee   HCC

✓6th **M05.07** **Felty's syndrome,** ankle and foot
      Felty's syndrome, tarsus, metatarsus and phalanges
      M05.071 **Felty's syndrome,** right ankle and   HCC
            foot
      M05.072 **Felty's syndrome,** left ankle and   HCC
            foot
      M05.079 **Felty's syndrome,** unspecified ankle   HCC
            and foot

    M05.09 **Felty's syndrome,** multiple sites   HCC

✓5th **M05.1** **Rheumatoid** lung disease with rheumatoid arthritis
    DEF: Lung disorders associated with rheumatoid arthritis.

    M05.10 **Rheumatoid lung disease with rheumatoid**   HCC
        arthritis of unspecified site

✓6th **M05.11** **Rheumatoid lung disease with rheumatoid arthritis**
of shoulder
      M05.111 **Rheumatoid lung disease with**   HCC
            rheumatoid arthritis of right shoulder
      M05.112 **Rheumatoid lung disease with**   HCC
            rheumatoid arthritis of left shoulder
      M05.119 **Rheumatoid lung disease with**   HCC
            rheumatoid arthritis of unspecified
            shoulder

✓6th **M05.12** **Rheumatoid lung disease with rheumatoid arthritis**
of elbow
      M05.121 **Rheumatoid lung disease with**   HCC
            rheumatoid arthritis of right elbow
      M05.122 **Rheumatoid lung disease with**   HCC
            rheumatoid arthritis of left elbow
      M05.129 **Rheumatoid lung disease with**   HCC
            rheumatoid arthritis of unspecified elbow

✓6th **M05.13** **Rheumatoid lung disease with rheumatoid arthritis of wrist**
Rheumatoid lung disease with rheumatoid arthritis, carpal bones

     M05.131 **Rheumatoid lung disease with rheumatoid arthritis of right wrist** `HCC`

     M05.132 **Rheumatoid lung disease with rheumatoid arthritis of left wrist** `HCC`

     M05.139 **Rheumatoid lung disease with rheumatoid arthritis of unspecified wrist** `HCC`

✓6th **M05.14** **Rheumatoid lung disease with rheumatoid arthritis of hand**
Rheumatoid lung disease with rheumatoid arthritis, metacarpus and phalanges

     M05.141 **Rheumatoid lung disease with rheumatoid arthritis of right hand** `HCC`

     M05.142 **Rheumatoid lung disease with rheumatoid arthritis of left hand** `HCC`

     M05.149 **Rheumatoid lung disease with rheumatoid arthritis of unspecified hand** `HCC`

✓6th **M05.15** **Rheumatoid lung disease with rheumatoid arthritis of hip**

     M05.151 **Rheumatoid lung disease with rheumatoid arthritis of right hip** `HCC`

     M05.152 **Rheumatoid lung disease with rheumatoid arthritis of left hip** `HCC`

     M05.159 **Rheumatoid lung disease with rheumatoid arthritis of unspecified hip** `HCC`

✓6th **M05.16** **Rheumatoid lung disease with rheumatoid arthritis of knee**

     M05.161 **Rheumatoid lung disease with rheumatoid arthritis of right knee** `HCC`

     M05.162 **Rheumatoid lung disease with rheumatoid arthritis of left knee** `HCC`

     M05.169 **Rheumatoid lung disease with rheumatoid arthritis of unspecified knee** `HCC`

✓6th **M05.17** **Rheumatoid lung disease with rheumatoid arthritis of ankle and foot**
Rheumatoid lung disease with rheumatoid arthritis, tarsus, metatarsus and phalanges

     M05.171 **Rheumatoid lung disease with rheumatoid arthritis of right ankle and foot** `HCC`

     M05.172 **Rheumatoid lung disease with rheumatoid arthritis of left ankle and foot** `HCC`

     M05.179 **Rheumatoid lung disease with rheumatoid arthritis of unspecified ankle and foot** `HCC`

   M05.19 **Rheumatoid lung disease with rheumatoid arthritis of multiple sites** `HCC`

✓5th **M05.2** **Rheumatoid vasculitis with rheumatoid arthritis**

   M05.20 **Rheumatoid vasculitis with rheumatoid arthritis of unspecified site** `HCC`

✓6th **M05.21** **Rheumatoid vasculitis with rheumatoid arthritis of shoulder**

     M05.211 **Rheumatoid vasculitis with rheumatoid arthritis of right shoulder** `HCC`

     M05.212 **Rheumatoid vasculitis with rheumatoid arthritis of left shoulder** `HCC`

     M05.219 **Rheumatoid vasculitis with rheumatoid arthritis of unspecified shoulder** `HCC`

✓6th **M05.22** **Rheumatoid vasculitis with rheumatoid arthritis of elbow**

     M05.221 **Rheumatoid vasculitis with rheumatoid arthritis of right elbow** `HCC`

     M05.222 **Rheumatoid vasculitis with rheumatoid arthritis of left elbow** `HCC`

     M05.229 **Rheumatoid vasculitis with rheumatoid arthritis of unspecified elbow** `HCC`

✓6th **M05.23** **Rheumatoid vasculitis with rheumatoid arthritis of wrist**
Rheumatoid vasculitis with rheumatoid arthritis, carpal bones

     M05.231 **Rheumatoid vasculitis with rheumatoid arthritis of right wrist** `HCC`

     M05.232 **Rheumatoid vasculitis with rheumatoid arthritis of left wrist** `HCC`

     M05.239 **Rheumatoid vasculitis with rheumatoid arthritis of unspecified wrist** `HCC`

✓6th **M05.24** **Rheumatoid vasculitis with rheumatoid arthritis of hand**
Rheumatoid vasculitis with rheumatoid arthritis, metacarpus and phalanges

     M05.241 **Rheumatoid vasculitis with rheumatoid arthritis of right hand** `HCC`

     M05.242 **Rheumatoid vasculitis with rheumatoid arthritis of left hand** `HCC`

     M05.249 **Rheumatoid vasculitis with rheumatoid arthritis of unspecified hand** `HCC`

✓6th **M05.25** **Rheumatoid vasculitis with rheumatoid arthritis of hip**

     M05.251 **Rheumatoid vasculitis with rheumatoid arthritis of right hip** `HCC`

     M05.252 **Rheumatoid vasculitis with rheumatoid arthritis of left hip** `HCC`

     M05.259 **Rheumatoid vasculitis with rheumatoid arthritis of unspecified hip** `HCC`

✓6th **M05.26** **Rheumatoid vasculitis with rheumatoid arthritis of knee**

     M05.261 **Rheumatoid vasculitis with rheumatoid arthritis of right knee** `HCC`

     M05.262 **Rheumatoid vasculitis with rheumatoid arthritis of left knee** `HCC`

     M05.269 **Rheumatoid vasculitis with rheumatoid arthritis of unspecified knee** `HCC`

✓6th **M05.27** **Rheumatoid vasculitis with rheumatoid arthritis of ankle and foot**
Rheumatoid vasculitis with rheumatoid arthritis, tarsus, metatarsus and phalanges

     M05.271 **Rheumatoid vasculitis with rheumatoid arthritis of right ankle and foot** `HCC`

     M05.272 **Rheumatoid vasculitis with rheumatoid arthritis of left ankle and foot** `HCC`

     M05.279 **Rheumatoid vasculitis with rheumatoid arthritis of unspecified ankle and foot** `HCC`

   M05.29 **Rheumatoid vasculitis with rheumatoid arthritis of multiple sites** `HCC`

✓5th **M05.3** **Rheumatoid heart disease with rheumatoid arthritis**
Rheumatoid carditis   Rheumatoid myocarditis
Rheumatoid endocarditis   Rheumatoid pericarditis

   M05.30 **Rheumatoid heart disease with rheumatoid arthritis of unspecified site** `HCC`

✓6th **M05.31** **Rheumatoid heart disease with rheumatoid arthritis of shoulder**

     M05.311 **Rheumatoid heart disease with rheumatoid arthritis of right shoulder** `HCC`

     M05.312 **Rheumatoid heart disease with rheumatoid arthritis of left shoulder** `HCC`

     M05.319 **Rheumatoid heart disease with rheumatoid arthritis of unspecified shoulder** `HCC`

✓6th **M05.32** **Rheumatoid heart disease with rheumatoid arthritis of elbow**

     M05.321 **Rheumatoid heart disease with rheumatoid arthritis of right elbow** `HCC`

     M05.322 **Rheumatoid heart disease with rheumatoid arthritis of left elbow** `HCC`

     M05.329 **Rheumatoid heart disease with rheumatoid arthritis of unspecified elbow** `HCC`

✓6th **M05.33** **Rheumatoid heart disease with rheumatoid arthritis of wrist**
Rheumatoid heart disease with rheumatoid arthritis, carpal bones

     M05.331 **Rheumatoid heart disease with rheumatoid arthritis of right wrist** `HCC`

     M05.332 **Rheumatoid heart disease with rheumatoid arthritis of left wrist** `HCC`

     M05.339 **Rheumatoid heart disease with rheumatoid arthritis of unspecified wrist** `HCC`

✓6th **M05.34 Rheumatoid heart disease with rheumatoid arthritis of hand**
　Rheumatoid heart disease with rheumatoid arthritis, metacarpus and phalanges

　M05.341 Rheumatoid heart disease with rheumatoid arthritis of **right** hand `HCC`

　M05.342 Rheumatoid heart disease with rheumatoid arthritis of **left** hand `HCC`

　M05.349 Rheumatoid heart disease with rheumatoid arthritis of **unspecified** hand `HCC`

✓6th **M05.35 Rheumatoid heart disease with rheumatoid arthritis of hip**

　M05.351 Rheumatoid heart disease with rheumatoid arthritis of **right** hip `HCC`

　M05.352 Rheumatoid heart disease with rheumatoid arthritis of **left** hip `HCC`

　M05.359 Rheumatoid heart disease with rheumatoid arthritis of **unspecified** hip `HCC`

✓6th **M05.36 Rheumatoid heart disease with rheumatoid arthritis of knee**

　M05.361 Rheumatoid heart disease with rheumatoid arthritis of **right** knee `HCC`

　M05.362 Rheumatoid heart disease with rheumatoid arthritis of **left** knee `HCC`

　M05.369 Rheumatoid heart disease with rheumatoid arthritis of **unspecified** knee `HCC`

✓6th **M05.37 Rheumatoid heart disease with rheumatoid arthritis of ankle and foot**
　Rheumatoid heart disease with rheumatoid arthritis, tarsus, metatarsus and phalanges

　M05.371 Rheumatoid heart disease with rheumatoid arthritis of **right** ankle and foot `HCC`

　M05.372 Rheumatoid heart disease with rheumatoid arthritis of **left** ankle and foot `HCC`

　M05.379 Rheumatoid heart disease with rheumatoid arthritis of **unspecified** ankle and foot `HCC`

M05.39 Rheumatoid heart disease with rheumatoid arthritis of multiple sites `HCC`

✓5th **M05.4 Rheumatoid myopathy with rheumatoid arthritis**

　CC Excl: For CC codes in subcategory M05.4:
　PDX collection 867

　M05.40 Rheumatoid myopathy with rheumatoid arthritis of unspecified site `PDxCC` `CC` `HCC`

✓6th **M05.41 Rheumatoid myopathy with rheumatoid arthritis of shoulder**

　M05.411 Rheumatoid myopathy with rheumatoid arthritis of **right** shoulder `PDxCC` `CC` `HCC`

　M05.412 Rheumatoid myopathy with rheumatoid arthritis of **left** shoulder `PDxCC` `CC` `HCC`

　M05.419 Rheumatoid myopathy with rheumatoid arthritis of **unspecified** shoulder `PDxCC` `CC` `HCC`

✓6th **M05.42 Rheumatoid myopathy with rheumatoid arthritis of elbow**

　M05.421 Rheumatoid myopathy with rheumatoid arthritis of **right** elbow `PDxCC` `CC` `HCC`

　M05.422 Rheumatoid myopathy with rheumatoid arthritis of **left** elbow `PDxCC` `CC` `HCC`

　M05.429 Rheumatoid myopathy with rheumatoid arthritis of **unspecified** elbow `PDxCC` `CC` `HCC`

✓6th **M05.43 Rheumatoid myopathy with rheumatoid arthritis of wrist**
　Rheumatoid myopathy with rheumatoid arthritis, carpal bones

　M05.431 Rheumatoid myopathy with rheumatoid arthritis of **right** wrist `PDxCC` `CC` `HCC`

　M05.432 Rheumatoid myopathy with rheumatoid arthritis of **left** wrist `PDxCC` `CC` `HCC`

　M05.439 Rheumatoid myopathy with rheumatoid arthritis of **unspecified** wrist `PDxCC` `CC` `HCC`

✓6th **M05.44 Rheumatoid myopathy with rheumatoid arthritis of hand**
　Rheumatoid myopathy with rheumatoid arthritis, metacarpus and phalanges

　M05.441 Rheumatoid myopathy with rheumatoid arthritis of **right** hand `PDxCC` `CC` `HCC`

　M05.442 Rheumatoid myopathy with rheumatoid arthritis of **left** hand `PDxCC` `CC` `HCC`

　M05.449 Rheumatoid myopathy with rheumatoid arthritis of **unspecified** hand `PDxCC` `CC` `HCC`

✓6th **M05.45 Rheumatoid myopathy with rheumatoid arthritis of hip**

　M05.451 Rheumatoid myopathy with rheumatoid arthritis of **right** hip `PDxCC` `CC` `HCC`

　M05.452 Rheumatoid myopathy with rheumatoid arthritis of **left** hip `PDxCC` `CC` `HCC`

　M05.459 Rheumatoid myopathy with rheumatoid arthritis of **unspecified** hip `PDxCC` `CC` `HCC`

✓6th **M05.46 Rheumatoid myopathy with rheumatoid arthritis of knee**

　M05.461 Rheumatoid myopathy with rheumatoid arthritis of **right** knee `PDxCC` `CC` `HCC`

　M05.462 Rheumatoid myopathy with rheumatoid arthritis of **left** knee `PDxCC` `CC` `HCC`

　M05.469 Rheumatoid myopathy with rheumatoid arthritis of **unspecified** knee `PDxCC` `CC` `HCC`

✓6th **M05.47 Rheumatoid myopathy with rheumatoid arthritis of ankle and foot**
　Rheumatoid myopathy with rheumatoid arthritis, tarsus, metatarsus and phalanges

　M05.471 Rheumatoid myopathy with rheumatoid arthritis of **right** ankle and foot `PDxCC` `CC` `HCC`

　M05.472 Rheumatoid myopathy with rheumatoid arthritis of **left** ankle and foot `PDxCC` `CC` `HCC`

　M05.479 Rheumatoid myopathy with rheumatoid arthritis of **unspecified** ankle and foot `PDxCC` `CC` `HCC`

　M05.49 Rheumatoid myopathy with rheumatoid arthritis of multiple sites `PDxCC` `CC` `HCC`

✓5th **M05.5 Rheumatoid polyneuropathy with rheumatoid arthritis**

　M05.50 Rheumatoid polyneuropathy with rheumatoid arthritis of unspecified site `HCC`

✓6th **M05.51 Rheumatoid polyneuropathy with rheumatoid arthritis of shoulder**

　M05.511 Rheumatoid polyneuropathy with rheumatoid arthritis of **right** shoulder `HCC`

　M05.512 Rheumatoid polyneuropathy with rheumatoid arthritis of **left** shoulder `HCC`

　M05.519 Rheumatoid polyneuropathy with rheumatoid arthritis of **unspecified** shoulder `HCC`

✓6th **M05.52 Rheumatoid polyneuropathy with rheumatoid arthritis of elbow**

　M05.521 Rheumatoid polyneuropathy with rheumatoid arthritis of **right** elbow `HCC`

　M05.522 Rheumatoid polyneuropathy with rheumatoid arthritis of **left** elbow `HCC`

　M05.529 Rheumatoid polyneuropathy with rheumatoid arthritis of **unspecified** elbow `HCC`

✓6th **M05.53 Rheumatoid polyneuropathy with rheumatoid arthritis of wrist**
　Rheumatoid polyneuropathy with rheumatoid arthritis, carpal bones

　M05.531 Rheumatoid polyneuropathy with rheumatoid arthritis of **right** wrist `HCC`

　M05.532 Rheumatoid polyneuropathy with rheumatoid arthritis of **left** wrist `HCC`

　M05.539 Rheumatoid polyneuropathy with rheumatoid arthritis of **unspecified** wrist `HCC`

Ⓝ Newborn: 0　Ⓟ Pediatric: 0-17　Ⓜ Maternity: 12-55　Ⓐ Adult: 15-124　`MCC` Major CC Condition　`PDxMCC` PDx acts as own MCC　`CC` CC Condition　`PDxCC` PDx acts as own CC

742

ICD-10-CM 2018

✓6ᵗʰ **M05.54** **Rheumatoid polyneuropathy with rheumatoid arthritis of hand**
Rheumatoid polyneuropathy with rheumatoid arthritis, metacarpus and phalanges

M05.541 Rheumatoid polyneuropathy with rheumatoid arthritis of right hand [HCC]

M05.542 Rheumatoid polyneuropathy with rheumatoid arthritis of left hand [HCC]

M05.549 Rheumatoid polyneuropathy with rheumatoid arthritis of unspecified hand [HCC]

✓6ᵗʰ **M05.55** **Rheumatoid polyneuropathy with rheumatoid arthritis of hip**

M05.551 Rheumatoid polyneuropathy with rheumatoid arthritis of right hip [HCC]

M05.552 Rheumatoid polyneuropathy with rheumatoid arthritis of left hip [HCC]

M05.559 Rheumatoid polyneuropathy with rheumatoid arthritis of unspecified hip [HCC]

✓6ᵗʰ **M05.56** **Rheumatoid polyneuropathy with rheumatoid arthritis of knee**

M05.561 Rheumatoid polyneuropathy with rheumatoid arthritis of right knee [HCC]

M05.562 Rheumatoid polyneuropathy with rheumatoid arthritis of left knee [HCC]

M05.569 Rheumatoid polyneuropathy with rheumatoid arthritis of unspecified knee [HCC]

✓6ᵗʰ **M05.57** **Rheumatoid polyneuropathy with rheumatoid arthritis of ankle and foot**
Rheumatoid polyneuropathy with rheumatoid arthritis, tarsus, metatarsus and phalanges

M05.571 Rheumatoid polyneuropathy with rheumatoid arthritis of right ankle and foot [HCC]

M05.572 Rheumatoid polyneuropathy with rheumatoid arthritis of left ankle and foot [HCC]

M05.579 Rheumatoid polyneuropathy with rheumatoid arthritis of unspecified ankle and foot [HCC]

M05.59 Rheumatoid polyneuropathy with rheumatoid arthritis of multiple sites [HCC]

✓5ᵗʰ **M05.6** **Rheumatoid arthritis with involvement of other organs and systems**

M05.60 Rheumatoid arthritis of unspecified site with involvement of other organs and systems [HCC]

✓6ᵗʰ **M05.61** **Rheumatoid arthritis of shoulder with involvement of other organs and systems**

M05.611 Rheumatoid arthritis of right shoulder with involvement of other organs and systems [HCC]

M05.612 Rheumatoid arthritis of left shoulder with involvement of other organs and systems [HCC]

M05.619 Rheumatoid arthritis of unspecified shoulder with involvement of other organs and systems [HCC]

✓6ᵗʰ **M05.62** **Rheumatoid arthritis of elbow with involvement of other organs and systems**

M05.621 Rheumatoid arthritis of right elbow with involvement of other organs and systems [HCC]

M05.622 Rheumatoid arthritis of left elbow with involvement of other organs and systems [HCC]

M05.629 Rheumatoid arthritis of unspecified elbow with involvement of other organs and systems [HCC]

✓6ᵗʰ **M05.63** **Rheumatoid arthritis of wrist with involvement of other organs and systems**
Rheumatoid arthritis of carpal bones with involvement of other organs and systems

M05.631 Rheumatoid arthritis of right wrist with involvement of other organs and systems [HCC]

M05.632 Rheumatoid arthritis of left wrist with involvement of other organs and systems [HCC]

M05.639 Rheumatoid arthritis of unspecified wrist with involvement of other organs and systems [HCC]

✓6ᵗʰ **M05.64** **Rheumatoid arthritis of hand with involvement of other organs and systems**
Rheumatoid arthritis of metacarpus and phalanges with involvement of other organs and systems

M05.641 Rheumatoid arthritis of right hand with involvement of other organs and systems [HCC]

M05.642 Rheumatoid arthritis of left hand with involvement of other organs and systems [HCC]

M05.649 Rheumatoid arthritis of unspecified hand with involvement of other organs and systems [HCC]

✓6ᵗʰ **M05.65** **Rheumatoid arthritis of hip with involvement of other organs and systems**

M05.651 Rheumatoid arthritis of right hip with involvement of other organs and systems [HCC]

M05.652 Rheumatoid arthritis of left hip with involvement of other organs and systems [HCC]

M05.659 Rheumatoid arthritis of unspecified hip with involvement of other organs and systems [HCC]

✓6ᵗʰ **M05.66** **Rheumatoid arthritis of knee with involvement of other organs and systems**

M05.661 Rheumatoid arthritis of right knee with involvement of other organs and systems [HCC]

M05.662 Rheumatoid arthritis of left knee with involvement of other organs and systems [HCC]

M05.669 Rheumatoid arthritis of unspecified knee with involvement of other organs and systems [HCC]

✓6ᵗʰ **M05.67** **Rheumatoid arthritis of ankle and foot with involvement of other organs and systems**
Rheumatoid arthritis of tarsus, metatarsus and phalanges with involvement of other organs and systems

M05.671 Rheumatoid arthritis of right ankle and foot with involvement of other organs and systems [HCC]

M05.672 Rheumatoid arthritis of left ankle and foot with involvement of other organs and systems [HCC]

M05.679 Rheumatoid arthritis of unspecified ankle and foot with involvement of other organs and systems [HCC]

M05.69 Rheumatoid arthritis of multiple sites with involvement of other organs and systems [HCC]

✓5ᵗʰ **M05.7** **Rheumatoid arthritis with rheumatoid factor without organ or systems involvement**

M05.70 Rheumatoid arthritis with rheumatoid factor of unspecified site without organ or systems involvement [HCC]

✓6ᵗʰ **M05.71** **Rheumatoid arthritis with rheumatoid factor of shoulder without organ or systems involvement**

M05.711 Rheumatoid arthritis with rheumatoid factor of right shoulder without organ or systems involvement [HCC]

M05.712 Rheumatoid arthritis with rheumatoid factor of left shoulder without organ or systems involvement [HCC]

M05.719 Rheumatoid arthritis with rheumatoid factor of unspecified shoulder without organ or systems involvement [HCC]

✓6ᵗʰ **M05.72** **Rheumatoid arthritis with rheumatoid factor of elbow without organ or systems involvement**

M05.721 Rheumatoid arthritis with rheumatoid factor of right elbow without organ or systems involvement [HCC]

M05.722 Rheumatoid arthritis with rheumatoid factor of left elbow without organ or systems involvement [HCC]

M05.729 Rheumatoid arthritis with rheumatoid factor of unspecified elbow without organ or systems involvement `HCC`

✓6ᵗʰ M05.73 **Rheumatoid arthritis with rheumatoid factor of wrist without organ or systems involvement**

M05.731 Rheumatoid arthritis with rheumatoid factor of right wrist without organ or systems involvement `HCC`

M05.732 Rheumatoid arthritis with rheumatoid factor of left wrist without organ or systems involvement `HCC`

M05.739 Rheumatoid arthritis with rheumatoid factor of unspecified wrist without organ or systems involvement `HCC`

✓6ᵗʰ M05.74 **Rheumatoid arthritis with rheumatoid factor of hand without organ or systems involvement**

M05.741 Rheumatoid arthritis with rheumatoid factor of right hand without organ or systems involvement `HCC`

M05.742 Rheumatoid arthritis with rheumatoid factor of left hand without organ or systems involvement `HCC`

M05.749 Rheumatoid arthritis with rheumatoid factor of unspecified hand without organ or systems involvement `HCC`

✓6ᵗʰ M05.75 **Rheumatoid arthritis with rheumatoid factor of hip without organ or systems involvement**

M05.751 Rheumatoid arthritis with rheumatoid factor of right hip without organ or systems involvement `HCC`

M05.752 Rheumatoid arthritis with rheumatoid factor of left hip without organ or systems involvement `HCC`

M05.759 Rheumatoid arthritis with rheumatoid factor of unspecified hip without organ or systems involvement `HCC`

✓6ᵗʰ M05.76 **Rheumatoid arthritis with rheumatoid factor of knee without organ or systems involvement**

M05.761 Rheumatoid arthritis with rheumatoid factor of right knee without organ or systems involvement `HCC`

M05.762 Rheumatoid arthritis with rheumatoid factor of left knee without organ or systems involvement `HCC`

M05.769 Rheumatoid arthritis with rheumatoid factor of unspecified knee without organ or systems involvement `HCC`

✓6ᵗʰ M05.77 **Rheumatoid arthritis with rheumatoid factor of ankle and foot without organ or systems involvement**

M05.771 Rheumatoid arthritis with rheumatoid factor of right ankle and foot without organ or systems involvement `HCC`

M05.772 Rheumatoid arthritis with rheumatoid factor of left ankle and foot without organ or systems involvement `HCC`

M05.779 Rheumatoid arthritis with heumatoid factor of unspecified ankle and foot without organ or systems involvement `HCC`

M05.79 Rheumatoid arthritis with rheumatoid factor of multiple sites without organ or systems involvement `HCC`

✓5ᵗʰ M05.8 **Other rheumatoid arthritis with rheumatoid factor**

M05.80 Other rheumatoid arthritis with rheumatoid actor of unspecified site `HCC`

✓6ᵗʰ M05.81 **Other rheumatoid arthritis with rheumatoid factor of shoulder**

M05.811 Other rheumatoid arthritis with rheumatoid factor of right shoulder `HCC`

M05.812 Other rheumatoid arthritis with rheumatoid factor of left shoulder `HCC`

M05.819 Other rheumatoid arthritis with rheumatoid factor of unspecified shoulder `HCC`

✓6ᵗʰ M05.82 **Other rheumatoid arthritis with rheumatoid factor of elbow**

M05.821 Other rheumatoid arthritis with rheumatoid factor of right elbow `HCC`

M05.822 Other rheumatoid arthritis with rheumatoid factor of left elbow `HCC`

M05.829 Other rheumatoid arthritis with rheumatoid factor of unspecified elbow `HCC`

✓6ᵗʰ M05.83 **Other rheumatoid arthritis with rheumatoid factor of wrist**

M05.831 Other rheumatoid arthritis with rheumatoid factor of right wrist `HCC`

M05.832 Other rheumatoid arthritis with rheumatoid factor of left wrist `HCC`

M05.839 Other rheumatoid arthritis with rheumatoid factor of unspecified wrist `HCC`

✓6ᵗʰ M05.84 **Other rheumatoid arthritis with rheumatoid factor of hand**

M05.841 Other rheumatoid arthritis with rheumatoid factor of right hand `HCC`

M05.842 Other rheumatoid arthritis with rheumatoid factor of left hand `HCC`

M05.849 Other rheumatoid arthritis with rheumatoid factor of unspecified hand `HCC`

✓6ᵗʰ M05.85 **Other rheumatoid arthritis with rheumatoid factor of hip**

M05.851 Other rheumatoid arthritis with rheumatoid factor of right hip `HCC`

M05.852 Other rheumatoid arthritis with rheumatoid factor of left hip `HCC`

M05.859 Other rheumatoid arthritis with rheumatoid factor of unspecified hip `HCC`

✓6ᵗʰ M05.86 **Other rheumatoid arthritis with rheumatoid factor of knee**

M05.861 Other rheumatoid arthritis with rheumatoid factor of right knee `HCC`

M05.862 Other rheumatoid arthritis with rheumatoid factor of left knee `HCC`

M05.869 Other rheumatoid arthritis with rheumatoid factor of unspecified knee `HCC`

✓6ᵗʰ M05.87 **Other rheumatoid arthritis with rheumatoid factor of ankle and foot**

M05.871 Other rheumatoid arthritis with rheumatoid factor of right ankle and foot `HCC`

M05.872 Other rheumatoid arthritis with rheumatoid factor of left ankle and foot `HCC`

M05.879 Other rheumatoid arthritis with rheumatoid factor of unspecified ankle and foot `HCC`

M05.89 Other rheumatoid arthritis with rheumatoid factor of multiple sites `HCC`

M05.9 **Rheumatoid arthritis with rheumatoid factor, unspecified** `HCC`

✓4ᵗʰ M06 **Other rheumatoid arthritis**

DEF: Rheumatoid arthritis: Autoimmune systemic disease that causes chronic inflammation of joints and other areas of the body, manifested by inflammatory changes in articular structures and synovial membranes, atrophy, and loss in bone density.

✓5ᵗʰ M06.0 **Rheumatoid arthritis without rheumatoid factor**

M06.00 Rheumatoid arthritis without rheumatoid factor, unspecified site `HCC`

✓6ᵗʰ M06.01 **Rheumatoid arthritis without rheumatoid factor, shoulder**

M06.011 Rheumatoid arthritis without rheumatoid factor, right shoulder `HCC`

M06.012 Rheumatoid arthritis without rheumatoid factor, left shoulder `HCC`

M06.019 Rheumatoid arthritis without rheumatoid factor, unspecified shoulder `HCC`

✓6ᵗʰ M06.02 **Rheumatoid arthritis without rheumatoid factor, elbow**

M06.021 Rheumatoid arthritis without rheumatoid factor, right elbow `HCC`

M06.022 Rheumatoid arthritis without rheumatoid factor, left elbow `HCC`

M06.029 Rheumatoid arthritis without rheumatoid factor, unspecified elbow `HCC`

Ⓝ Newborn: 0 Ⓟ Pediatric: 0-17 Ⓜ Maternity: 12-55 Ⓐ Adult: 15-124 **MCC** Major CC Condition **PDxMCC** PDx acts as own MCC **CC** CC Condition **PDxCC** PDx acts as own CC

744 ICD-10-CM 2018

✓6ᵗʰ **M06.03 Rheumatoid arthritis without rheumatoid factor, wrist**

    M06.031 Rheumatoid arthritis without rheumatoid factor, right wrist `HCC`

    M06.032 Rheumatoid arthritis without rheumatoid factor, left wrist `HCC`

    M06.039 Rheumatoid arthritis without rheumatoid factor, unspecified wrist `HCC`

✓6ᵗʰ **M06.04 Rheumatoid arthritis without rheumatoid factor, hand**

    M06.041 Rheumatoid arthritis without rheumatoid factor, right hand `HCC`

    M06.042 Rheumatoid arthritis without rheumatoid factor, left hand `HCC`

    M06.049 Rheumatoid arthritis without rheumatoid factor, unspecified hand `HCC`

✓6ᵗʰ **M06.05 Rheumatoid arthritis without rheumatoid factor, hip**

    M06.051 Rheumatoid arthritis without rheumatoid factor, right hip `HCC`

    M06.052 Rheumatoid arthritis without rheumatoid factor, left hip `HCC`

    M06.059 Rheumatoid arthritis without rheumatoid factor, unspecified hip `HCC`

✓6ᵗʰ **M06.06 Rheumatoid arthritis without rheumatoid factor, knee**

    M06.061 Rheumatoid arthritis without rheumatoid factor, right knee `HCC`

    M06.062 Rheumatoid arthritis without rheumatoid factor, left knee `HCC`

    M06.069 Rheumatoid arthritis without rheumatoid factor, unspecified knee `HCC`

✓6ᵗʰ **M06.07 Rheumatoid arthritis without rheumatoid factor, ankle and foot**

    M06.071 Rheumatoid arthritis without rheumatoid factor, right ankle and foot `HCC`

    M06.072 Rheumatoid arthritis without rheumatoid factor, left ankle and foot `HCC`

    M06.079 Rheumatoid arthritis without rheumatoid factor, unspecified ankle and foot `HCC`

M06.08 Rheumatoid arthritis without rheumatoid factor, vertebrae `HCC`

M06.09 Rheumatoid arthritis without rheumatoid factor, multiple sites `HCC`

M06.1 Adult-onset Still's disease `HCC` `A`

    EXCLUDES 1   *Still's disease NOS (M08.2-)*

✓5ᵗʰ **M06.2 Rheumatoid bursitis**

M06.20 Rheumatoid bursitis, unspecified site `HCC`

✓6ᵗʰ **M06.21 Rheumatoid bursitis, shoulder**

    M06.211 Rheumatoid bursitis, right shoulder `HCC`

    M06.212 Rheumatoid bursitis, left shoulder `HCC`

    M06.219 Rheumatoid bursitis, unspecified shoulder `HCC`

✓6ᵗʰ **M06.22 Rheumatoid bursitis, elbow**

    M06.221 Rheumatoid bursitis, right elbow `HCC`

    M06.222 Rheumatoid bursitis, left elbow `HCC`

    M06.229 Rheumatoid bursitis, unspecified elbow `HCC`

✓6ᵗʰ **M06.23 Rheumatoid bursitis, wrist**

    M06.231 Rheumatoid bursitis, right wrist `HCC`

    M06.232 Rheumatoid bursitis, left wrist `HCC`

    M06.239 Rheumatoid bursitis, unspecified wrist `HCC`

✓6ᵗʰ **M06.24 Rheumatoid bursitis, hand**

    M06.241 Rheumatoid bursitis, right hand `HCC`

    M06.242 Rheumatoid bursitis, left hand `HCC`

    M06.249 Rheumatoid bursitis, unspecified hand `HCC`

✓6ᵗʰ **M06.25 Rheumatoid bursitis, hip**

    M06.251 Rheumatoid bursitis, right hip `HCC`

    M06.252 Rheumatoid bursitis, left hip `HCC`

    M06.259 Rheumatoid bursitis, unspecified hip `HCC`

✓6ᵗʰ **M06.26 Rheumatoid bursitis, knee**

    M06.261 Rheumatoid bursitis, right knee `HCC`

    M06.262 Rheumatoid bursitis, left knee `HCC`

    M06.269 Rheumatoid bursitis, unspecified knee `HCC`

✓6ᵗʰ **M06.27 Rheumatoid bursitis, ankle and foot**

    M06.271 Rheumatoid bursitis, right ankle and foot `HCC`

    M06.272 Rheumatoid bursitis, left ankle and foot `HCC`

    M06.279 Rheumatoid bursitis, unspecified ankle and foot `HCC`

M06.28 Rheumatoid bursitis, vertebrae `HCC`

M06.29 Rheumatoid bursitis, multiple sites `HCC`

✓5ᵗʰ **M06.3 Rheumatoid nodule**

M06.30 Rheumatoid nodule, unspecified site `HCC`

✓6ᵗʰ **M06.31 Rheumatoid nodule, shoulder**

    M06.311 Rheumatoid nodule, right shoulder `HCC`

    M06.312 Rheumatoid nodule, left shoulder `HCC`

    M06.319 Rheumatoid nodule, unspecified shoulder `HCC`

✓6ᵗʰ **M06.32 Rheumatoid nodule, elbow**

    M06.321 Rheumatoid nodule, right elbow `HCC`

    M06.322 Rheumatoid nodule, left elbow `HCC`

    M06.329 Rheumatoid nodule, unspecified elbow `HCC`

✓6ᵗʰ **M06.33 Rheumatoid nodule, wrist**

    M06.331 Rheumatoid nodule, right wrist `HCC`

    M06.332 Rheumatoid nodule, left wrist `HCC`

    M06.339 Rheumatoid nodule, unspecified wrist `HCC`

✓6ᵗʰ **M06.34 Rheumatoid nodule, hand**

    M06.341 Rheumatoid nodule, right hand `HCC`

    M06.342 Rheumatoid nodule, left hand `HCC`

    M06.349 Rheumatoid nodule, unspecified hand `HCC`

✓6ᵗʰ **M06.35 Rheumatoid nodule, hip**

    M06.351 Rheumatoid nodule, right hip `HCC`

    M06.352 Rheumatoid nodule, left hip `HCC`

    M06.359 Rheumatoid nodule, unspecified hip `HCC`

✓6ᵗʰ **M06.36 Rheumatoid nodule, knee**

    M06.361 Rheumatoid nodule, right knee `HCC`

    M06.362 Rheumatoid nodule, left knee `HCC`

    M06.369 Rheumatoid nodule, unspecified knee `HCC`

✓6ᵗʰ **M06.37 Rheumatoid nodule, ankle and foot**

    M06.371 Rheumatoid nodule, right ankle and foot `HCC`

    M06.372 Rheumatoid nodule, left ankle and foot `HCC`

    M06.379 Rheumatoid nodule, unspecified ankle and foot `HCC`

M06.38 Rheumatoid nodule, vertebrae `HCC`

M06.39 Rheumatoid nodule, multiple sites `HCC`

M06.4 Inflammatory polyarthropathy

    EXCLUDES 1   *polyarthritis NOS (M13.0)*

✓5ᵗʰ **M06.8 Other specified rheumatoid arthritis**

M06.80 Other specified rheumatoid arthritis, unspecified site `HCC`

✓6ᵗʰ **M06.81 Other specified rheumatoid arthritis, shoulder**

    M06.811 Other specified rheumatoid arthritis, right shoulder `HCC`

    M06.812 Other specified rheumatoid arthritis, left shoulder `HCC`

    M06.819 Other specified rheumatoid arthritis, unspecified shoulder `HCC`

✓6ᵗʰ **M06.82 Other specified rheumatoid arthritis, elbow**

    M06.821 Other specified rheumatoid arthritis, right elbow `HCC`

    M06.822 Other specified rheumatoid arthritis, left elbow `HCC`

    M06.829 Other specified rheumatoid arthritis, unspecified elbow `HCC`

✓6ᵗʰ **M06.83 Other specified rheumatoid arthritis, wrist**

    M06.831 Other specified rheumatoid arthritis, right wrist `HCC`

M06.832   **Other specified rheumatoid arthritis, left wrist** `HCC`

M06.839   **Other specified rheumatoid arthritis, unspecified wrist** `HCC`

√6ᵗʰ **M06.84   Other specified rheumatoid arthritis, hand**

M06.841   **Other specified rheumatoid arthritis, right hand** `HCC`

M06.842   **Other specified rheumatoid arthritis, left hand** `HCC`

M06.849   **Other specified rheumatoid arthritis, unspecified hand** `HCC`

√6ᵗʰ **M06.85   Other specified rheumatoid arthritis, hip**

M06.851   **Other specified rheumatoid arthritis, right hip** `HCC`

M06.852   **Other specified rheumatoid arthritis, left hip** `HCC`

M06.859   **Other specified rheumatoid arthritis, unspecified hip** `HCC`

√6ᵗʰ **M06.86   Other specified rheumatoid arthritis, knee**

M06.861   **Other specified rheumatoid arthritis, right knee** `HCC`

M06.862   **Other specified rheumatoid arthritis, left knee** `HCC`

M06.869   **Other specified rheumatoid arthritis, unspecified knee** `HCC`

√6ᵗʰ **M06.87   Other specified rheumatoid arthritis, ankle and foot**

M06.871   **Other specified rheumatoid arthritis, right ankle and foot** `HCC`

M06.872   **Other specified rheumatoid arthritis, left ankle and foot** `HCC`

M06.879   **Other specified rheumatoid arthritis, unspecified ankle and foot** `HCC`

M06.88   **Other specified rheumatoid arthritis, vertebrae** `HCC`

M06.89   **Other specified rheumatoid arthritis, multiple sites** `HCC`

M06.9   **Rheumatoid arthritis, unspecified** `HCC`

√4ᵗʰ **M07   Enteropathic arthropathies**

Code also associated enteropathy, such as:
regional enteritis [Crohn's disease] (K50.-)
ulcerative colitis (K51.-)

EXCLUDES 1   *psoriatic arthropathies (L40.5-)*

√5ᵗʰ **M07.6   Enteropathic arthropathies**

M07.60   **Enteropathic arthropathies, unspecified site**

√6ᵗʰ **M07.61   Enteropathic arthropathies, shoulder**

M07.611   **Enteropathic arthropathies, right shoulder**

M07.612   **Enteropathic arthropathies, left shoulder**

M07.619   **Enteropathic arthropathies, unspecified shoulder**

√6ᵗʰ **M07.62   Enteropathic arthropathies, elbow**

M07.621   **Enteropathic arthropathies, right elbow**

M07.622   **Enteropathic arthropathies, left elbow**

M07.629   **Enteropathic arthropathies, unspecified elbow**

√6ᵗʰ **M07.63   Enteropathic arthropathies, wrist**

M07.631   **Enteropathic arthropathies, right wrist**

M07.632   **Enteropathic arthropathies, left wrist**

M07.639   **Enteropathic arthropathies, unspecified wrist**

√6ᵗʰ **M07.64   Enteropathic arthropathies, hand**

M07.641   **Enteropathic arthropathies, right hand**

M07.642   **Enteropathic arthropathies, left hand**

M07.649   **Enteropathic arthropathies, unspecified hand**

√6ᵗʰ **M07.65   Enteropathic arthropathies, hip**

M07.651   **Enteropathic arthropathies, right hip**

M07.652   **Enteropathic arthropathies, left hip**

M07.659   **Enteropathic arthropathies, unspecified hip**

√6ᵗʰ **M07.66   Enteropathic arthropathies, knee**

M07.661   **Enteropathic arthropathies, right knee**

M07.662   **Enteropathic arthropathies, left knee**

M07.669   **Enteropathic arthropathies, unspecified knee**

√6ᵗʰ **M07.67   Enteropathic arthropathies, ankle and foot**

M07.671   **Enteropathic arthropathies, right ankle and foot**

M07.672   **Enteropathic arthropathies, left ankle and foot**

M07.679   **Enteropathic arthropathies, unspecified ankle and foot**

M07.68   **Enteropathic arthropathies, vertebrae**

M07.69   **Enteropathic arthropathies, multiple sites**

√4ᵗʰ **M08   Juvenile arthritis**

Code also any associated underlying condition, such as:
regional enteritis [Crohn's disease] (K50.-)
ulcerative colitis (K51.-)

EXCLUDES 1   *arthropathy in Whipple's disease (M14.8)*
Felty's syndrome (M05.0)
juvenile dermatomyositis (M33.0-)
psoriatic juvenile arthropathy (L40.54)

√5ᵗʰ **M08.0   Unspecified juvenile rheumatoid arthritis**

Juvenile rheumatoid arthritis with or without rheumatoid factor

M08.00   **Unspecified juvenile rheumatoid arthritis of unspecified site** `HCC`

√6ᵗʰ **M08.01   Unspecified juvenile rheumatoid arthritis, shoulder**

M08.011   **Unspecified juvenile rheumatoid arthritis, right shoulder** `HCC`

M08.012   **Unspecified juvenile rheumatoid arthritis, left shoulder** `HCC`

M08.019   **Unspecified juvenile rheumatoid arthritis, unspecified shoulder** `HCC`

√6ᵗʰ **M08.02   Unspecified juvenile rheumatoid arthritis of elbow**

M08.021   **Unspecified juvenile rheumatoid arthritis, right elbow** `HCC`

M08.022   **Unspecified juvenile rheumatoid arthritis, left elbow** `HCC`

M08.029   **Unspecified juvenile rheumatoid arthritis, unspecified elbow** `HCC`

√6ᵗʰ **M08.03   Unspecified juvenile rheumatoid arthritis, wrist**

M08.031   **Unspecified juvenile rheumatoid arthritis, right wrist** `HCC`

M08.032   **Unspecified juvenile rheumatoid arthritis, left wrist** `HCC`

M08.039   **Unspecified juvenile rheumatoid arthritis, unspecified wrist** `HCC`

√6ᵗʰ **M08.04   Unspecified juvenile rheumatoid arthritis, hand**

M08.041   **Unspecified juvenile rheumatoid arthritis, right hand** `HCC`

M08.042   **Unspecified juvenile rheumatoid arthritis, left hand** `HCC`

M08.049   **Unspecified juvenile rheumatoid arthritis, unspecified hand** `HCC`

√6ᵗʰ **M08.05   Unspecified juvenile rheumatoid arthritis, hip**

M08.051   **Unspecified juvenile rheumatoid arthritis, right hip** `HCC`

M08.052   **Unspecified juvenile rheumatoid arthritis, left hip** `HCC`

M08.059   **Unspecified juvenile rheumatoid arthritis, unspecified hip** `HCC`

√6ᵗʰ **M08.06   Unspecified juvenile rheumatoid arthritis, knee**

M08.061   **Unspecified juvenile rheumatoid arthritis, right knee** `HCC`

M08.062   **Unspecified juvenile rheumatoid arthritis, left knee** `HCC`

M08.069   **Unspecified juvenile rheumatoid arthritis, unspecified knee** `HCC`

√6ᵗʰ **M08.07   Unspecified juvenile rheumatoid arthritis, ankle and foot**

M08.071   **Unspecified juvenile rheumatoid arthritis, right ankle and foot** `HCC`

M08.072   **Unspecified juvenile rheumatoid arthritis, left ankle and foot** `HCC`

M08.079   **Unspecified juvenile rheumatoid arthritis, unspecified ankle and foot** `HCC`

M08.08   **Unspecified juvenile rheumatoid arthritis, vertebrae** `HCC`

M08.09   **Unspecified juvenile rheumatoid arthritis, multiple sites** `HCC`

Ⓝ Newborn: 0   Ⓟ Pediatric: 0-17   Ⓜ Maternity: 12-55   Ⓐ Adult: 15-124   `MCC` Major CC Condition   `PDxMCC` PDx acts as own MCC   `CC` CC Condition   `PDxCC` PDx acts as own CC

746   ICD-10-CM 2018

M08.1 Juvenile ankylosing spondylitis `HCC`
   EXCLUDES 1   ankylosing spondylitis in adults (M45.0-)

✓5ᵗʰ **M08.2 Juvenile rheumatoid arthritis with systemic onset**
   Still's disease NOS
   EXCLUDES 1   adult-onset Still's disease (M06.1-)

   M08.20 Juvenile rheumatoid arthritis with systemic onset, unspecified site `HCC`

   ✓6ᵗʰ **M08.21** Juvenile rheumatoid arthritis with systemic onset, shoulder
      M08.211 Juvenile rheumatoid arthritis with systemic onset, right shoulder `HCC`
      M08.212 Juvenile rheumatoid arthritis with systemic onset, left shoulder `HCC`
      M08.219 Juvenile rheumatoid arthritis with systemic onset, unspecified shoulder `HCC`

   ✓6ᵗʰ **M08.22** Juvenile rheumatoid arthritis with systemic onset, elbow
      M08.221 Juvenile rheumatoid arthritis with systemic onset, right elbow `HCC`
      M08.222 Juvenile rheumatoid arthritis with systemic onset, left elbow `HCC`
      M08.229 Juvenile rheumatoid arthritis with systemic onset, unspecified elbow `HCC`

   ✓6ᵗʰ **M08.23** Juvenile rheumatoid arthritis with systemic onset, wrist
      M08.231 Juvenile rheumatoid arthritis with systemic onset, right wrist `HCC`
      M08.232 Juvenile rheumatoid arthritis with systemic onset, left wrist `HCC`
      M08.239 Juvenile rheumatoid arthritis with systemic onset, unspecified wrist `HCC`

   ✓6ᵗʰ **M08.24** Juvenile rheumatoid arthritis with systemic onset, hand
      M08.241 Juvenile rheumatoid arthritis with systemic onset, right hand `HCC`
      M08.242 Juvenile rheumatoid arthritis with systemic onset, left hand `HCC`
      M08.249 Juvenile rheumatoid arthritis with systemic onset, unspecified hand `HCC`

   ✓6ᵗʰ **M08.25** Juvenile rheumatoid arthritis with systemic onset, hip
      M08.251 Juvenile rheumatoid arthritis with systemic onset, right hip `HCC`
      M08.252 Juvenile rheumatoid arthritis with systemic onset, left hip `HCC`
      M08.259 Juvenile rheumatoid arthritis with systemic onset, unspecified hip `HCC`

   ✓6ᵗʰ **M08.26** Juvenile rheumatoid arthritis with systemic onset, knee
      M08.261 Juvenile rheumatoid arthritis with systemic onset, right knee `HCC`
      M08.262 Juvenile rheumatoid arthritis with systemic onset, left knee `HCC`
      M08.269 Juvenile rheumatoid arthritis with systemic onset, unspecified knee `HCC`

   ✓6ᵗʰ **M08.27** Juvenile rheumatoid arthritis with systemic onset, ankle and foot
      M08.271 Juvenile rheumatoid arthritis with systemic onset, right ankle and foot `HCC`
      M08.272 Juvenile rheumatoid arthritis with systemic onset, left ankle and foot `HCC`
      M08.279 Juvenile rheumatoid arthritis with systemic onset, unspecified ankle and foot `HCC`

   M08.28 Juvenile rheumatoid arthritis with systemic onset, vertebrae `HCC`

   M08.29 Juvenile rheumatoid arthritis with systemic onset, multiple sites `HCC`

M08.3 Juvenile rheumatoid polyarthritis (seronegative) `HCC`

✓5ᵗʰ **M08.4 Pauciarticular juvenile rheumatoid arthritis**

   M08.40 Pauciarticular juvenile rheumatoid arthritis, unspecified site `HCC`

   ✓6ᵗʰ **M08.41** Pauciarticular juvenile rheumatoid arthritis, shoulder
      M08.411 Pauciarticular juvenile rheumatoid arthritis, right shoulder `HCC`
      M08.412 Pauciarticular juvenile rheumatoid arthritis, left shoulder `HCC`
      M08.419 Pauciarticular juvenile rheumatoid arthritis, unspecified shoulder `HCC`

   ✓6ᵗʰ **M08.42** Pauciarticular juvenile rheumatoid arthritis, elbow
      M08.421 Pauciarticular juvenile rheumatoid arthritis, right elbow `HCC`
      M08.422 Pauciarticular juvenile rheumatoid arthritis, left elbow `HCC`
      M08.429 Pauciarticular juvenile rheumatoid arthritis, unspecified elbow `HCC`

   ✓6ᵗʰ **M08.43** Pauciarticular juvenile rheumatoid arthritis, wrist
      M08.431 Pauciarticular juvenile rheumatoid arthritis, right wrist `HCC`
      M08.432 Pauciarticular juvenile rheumatoid arthritis, left wrist `HCC`
      M08.439 Pauciarticular juvenile rheumatoid arthritis, unspecified wrist `HCC`

   ✓6ᵗʰ **M08.44** Pauciarticular juvenile rheumatoid arthritis, hand
      M08.441 Pauciarticular juvenile rheumatoid arthritis, right hand `HCC`
      M08.442 Pauciarticular juvenile rheumatoid arthritis, left hand `HCC`
      M08.449 Pauciarticular juvenile rheumatoid arthritis, unspecified hand `HCC`

   ✓6ᵗʰ **M08.45** Pauciarticular juvenile rheumatoid arthritis, hip
      M08.451 Pauciarticular juvenile rheumatoid arthritis, right hip `HCC`
      M08.452 Pauciarticular juvenile rheumatoid arthritis, left hip `HCC`
      M08.459 Pauciarticular juvenile rheumatoid arthritis, unspecified hip `HCC`

   ✓6ᵗʰ **M08.46** Pauciarticular juvenile rheumatoid arthritis, knee
      M08.461 Pauciarticular juvenile rheumatoid arthritis, right knee `HCC`
      M08.462 Pauciarticular juvenile rheumatoid arthritis, left knee `HCC`
      M08.469 Pauciarticular juvenile rheumatoid arthritis, unspecified knee `HCC`

   ✓6ᵗʰ **M08.47** Pauciarticular juvenile rheumatoid arthritis, ankle and foot
      M08.471 Pauciarticular juvenile rheumatoid arthritis, right ankle and foot `HCC`
      M08.472 Pauciarticular juvenile rheumatoid arthritis, left ankle and foot `HCC`
      M08.479 Pauciarticular juvenile rheumatoid arthritis, unspecified ankle and foot `HCC`

   M08.48 Pauciarticular juvenile rheumatoid arthritis, vertebrae `HCC`

✓5ᵗʰ **M08.8 Other juvenile arthritis**

   M08.80 Other juvenile arthritis, unspecified site `HCC`

   ✓6ᵗʰ **M08.81** Other juvenile arthritis, shoulder
      M08.811 Other juvenile arthritis, right shoulder `HCC`
      M08.812 Other juvenile arthritis, left shoulder `HCC`
      M08.819 Other juvenile arthritis, unspecified shoulder `HCC`

   ✓6ᵗʰ **M08.82** Other juvenile arthritis, elbow
      M08.821 Other juvenile arthritis, right elbow `HCC`
      M08.822 Other juvenile arthritis, left elbow `HCC`
      M08.829 Other juvenile arthritis, unspecified elbow `HCC`

   ✓6ᵗʰ **M08.83** Other juvenile arthritis, wrist
      M08.831 Other juvenile arthritis, right wrist `HCC`
      M08.832 Other juvenile arthritis, left wrist `HCC`
      M08.839 Other juvenile arthritis, unspecified wrist `HCC`

   ✓6ᵗʰ **M08.84** Other juvenile arthritis, hand
      M08.841 Other juvenile arthritis, right hand `HCC`
      M08.842 Other juvenile arthritis, left hand `HCC`
      M08.849 Other juvenile arthritis, unspecified hand `HCC`

   ✓6ᵗʰ **M08.85** Other juvenile arthritis, hip
      M08.851 Other juvenile arthritis, right hip `HCC`
      M08.852 Other juvenile arthritis, left hip `HCC`

✓ Additional Character Req   ✓x7ᵗʰ Placeholder Alert   Unacceptable PDx   Manifestation   H1 - H14 HAC   HCC CMS-HCC Condition   *EXCLUDES 1* Not Coded Here   *EXCLUDES 2* Not Included Here

M08.859   Other juvenile arthritis, unspecified hip   HCC

✓6ᵗʰ M08.86   Other juvenile arthritis, knee
   M08.861   Other juvenile arthritis, right knee   HCC
   M08.862   Other juvenile arthritis, left knee   HCC
   M08.869   Other juvenile arthritis, unspecified knee   HCC

✓6ᵗʰ M08.87   Other juvenile arthritis, ankle and foot
   M08.871   Other juvenile arthritis, right ankle and foot   HCC
   M08.872   Other juvenile arthritis, left ankle and foot   HCC
   M08.879   Other juvenile arthritis, unspecified ankle and foot   HCC

   M08.88   Other juvenile arthritis, other specified site   HCC
     Other juvenile arthritis, vertebrae

   M08.89   Other juvenile arthritis, multiple sites   HCC

✓5ᵗʰ M08.9   Juvenile arthritis, unspecified
   EXCLUDES 1   juvenile rheumatoid arthritis, unspecified (M08.0-)

   M08.90   Juvenile arthritis, unspecified, unspecified site   HCC

✓6ᵗʰ M08.91   Juvenile arthritis, unspecified, shoulder
   M08.911   Juvenile arthritis, unspecified, right shoulder   HCC
   M08.912   Juvenile arthritis, unspecified, left shoulder   HCC
   M08.919   Juvenile arthritis, unspecified, unspecified shoulder   HCC

✓6ᵗʰ M08.92   Juvenile arthritis, unspecified, elbow
   M08.921   Juvenile arthritis, unspecified, right elbow   HCC
   M08.922   Juvenile arthritis, unspecified, left elbow   HCC
   M08.929   Juvenile arthritis, unspecified, unspecified elbow   HCC

✓6ᵗʰ M08.93   Juvenile arthritis, unspecified, wrist
   M08.931   Juvenile arthritis, unspecified, right wrist   HCC
   M08.932   Juvenile arthritis, unspecified, left wrist   HCC
   M08.939   Juvenile arthritis, unspecified, unspecified wrist   HCC

✓6ᵗʰ M08.94   Juvenile arthritis, unspecified, hand
   M08.941   Juvenile arthritis, unspecified, right hand   HCC
   M08.942   Juvenile arthritis, unspecified, left hand   HCC
   M08.949   Juvenile arthritis, unspecified, unspecified hand   HCC

✓6ᵗʰ M08.95   Juvenile arthritis, unspecified, hip
   M08.951   Juvenile arthritis, unspecified, right hip   HCC
   M08.952   Juvenile arthritis, unspecified, left hip   HCC
   M08.959   Juvenile arthritis, unspecified, unspecified hip   HCC

✓6ᵗʰ M08.96   Juvenile arthritis, unspecified, knee
   M08.961   Juvenile arthritis, unspecified, right knee   HCC
   M08.962   Juvenile arthritis, unspecified, left knee   HCC
   M08.969   Juvenile arthritis, unspecified, unspecified knee   HCC

✓6ᵗʰ M08.97   Juvenile arthritis, unspecified, ankle and foot
   M08.971   Juvenile arthritis, unspecified, right ankle and foot   HCC
   M08.972   Juvenile arthritis, unspecified, left ankle and foot   HCC
   M08.979   Juvenile arthritis, unspecified, unspecified ankle and foot   HCC

   M08.98   Juvenile arthritis, unspecified, vertebrae   HCC

   M08.99   Juvenile arthritis, unspecified, multiple sites   HCC

✓4ᵗʰ M1A   Chronic gout
Use additional code to identify:
   autonomic neuropathy in diseases classified elsewhere (G99.0)
   calculus of urinary tract in diseases classified elsewhere (N22)
   cardiomyopathy in diseases classified elsewhere (I43)
   disorders of external ear in diseases classified elsewhere (H61.1-, H62.8-)
   disorders of iris and ciliary body in diseases classified elsewhere (H22)
   glomerular disorders in diseases classified elsewhere (N08)
   EXCLUDES 1   gout NOS (M10.-)
   EXCLUDES 2   acute gout (M10.-)

The appropriate 7th character is to be added to each code from category M1A.
   0   without tophus (tophi)
   1   with tophus (tophi)

✓5ᵗʰ M1A.0   Idiopathic chronic gout
   Chronic gouty bursitis
   Primary chronic gout

✓x 7ᵗʰ M1A.00   Idiopathic chronic gout, unspecified site

✓6ᵗʰ M1A.01   Idiopathic chronic gout, shoulder
   ✓7ᵗʰ M1A.011   Idiopathic chronic gout, right shoulder
   ✓7ᵗʰ M1A.012   Idiopathic chronic gout, left shoulder
   ✓7ᵗʰ M1A.019   Idiopathic chronic gout, unspecified shoulder

✓6ᵗʰ M1A.02   Idiopathic chronic gout, elbow
   ✓7ᵗʰ M1A.021   Idiopathic chronic gout, right elbow
   ✓7ᵗʰ M1A.022   Idiopathic chronic gout, left elbow
   ✓7ᵗʰ M1A.029   Idiopathic chronic gout, unspecified elbow

✓6ᵗʰ M1A.03   Idiopathic chronic gout, wrist
   ✓7ᵗʰ M1A.031   Idiopathic chronic gout, right wrist
   ✓7ᵗʰ M1A.032   Idiopathic chronic gout, left wrist
   ✓7ᵗʰ M1A.039   Idiopathic chronic gout, unspecified wrist

✓6ᵗʰ M1A.04   Idiopathic chronic gout, hand
   ✓7ᵗʰ M1A.041   Idiopathic chronic gout, right hand
   ✓7ᵗʰ M1A.042   Idiopathic chronic gout, left hand
   ✓7ᵗʰ M1A.049   Idiopathic chronic gout, unspecified hand

✓6ᵗʰ M1A.05   Idiopathic chronic gout, hip
   ✓7ᵗʰ M1A.051   Idiopathic chronic gout, right hip
   ✓7ᵗʰ M1A.052   Idiopathic chronic gout, left hip
   ✓7ᵗʰ M1A.059   Idiopathic chronic gout, unspecified hip

✓6ᵗʰ M1A.06   Idiopathic chronic gout, knee
   ✓7ᵗʰ M1A.061   Idiopathic chronic gout, right knee
   ✓7ᵗʰ M1A.062   Idiopathic chronic gout, left knee
   ✓7ᵗʰ M1A.069   Idiopathic chronic gout, unspecified knee

✓6ᵗʰ M1A.07   Idiopathic chronic gout, ankle and foot
   ✓7ᵗʰ M1A.071   Idiopathic chronic gout, right ankle and foot
   ✓7ᵗʰ M1A.072   Idiopathic chronic gout, left ankle and foot
   ✓7ᵗʰ M1A.079   Idiopathic chronic gout, unspecified ankle and foot

✓x 7ᵗʰ M1A.08   Idiopathic chronic gout, vertebrae

✓x 7ᵗʰ M1A.09   Idiopathic chronic gout, multiple sites

✓5ᵗʰ M1A.1   Lead-induced chronic gout
   Code first toxic effects of lead and its compounds (T56.0-)

✓x 7ᵗʰ M1A.10   Lead-induced chronic gout, unspecified site

✓6ᵗʰ M1A.11   Lead-induced chronic gout, shoulder
   ✓7ᵗʰ M1A.111   Lead-induced chronic gout, right shoulder
   ✓7ᵗʰ M1A.112   Lead-induced chronic gout, left shoulder
   ✓7ᵗʰ M1A.119   Lead-induced chronic gout, unspecified shoulder

✓6ᵗʰ M1A.12   Lead-induced chronic gout, elbow
   ✓7ᵗʰ M1A.121   Lead-induced chronic gout, right elbow
   ✓7ᵗʰ M1A.122   Lead-induced chronic gout, left elbow
   ✓7ᵗʰ M1A.129   Lead-induced chronic gout, unspecified elbow

✓6ᵗʰ M1A.13   Lead-induced chronic gout, wrist
   ✓7ᵗʰ M1A.131   Lead-induced chronic gout, right wrist
   ✓7ᵗʰ M1A.132   Lead-induced chronic gout, left wrist

N Newborn: 0   P Pediatric: 0-17   M Maternity: 12-55   A Adult: 15-124   MCC Major CC Condition   PDx MCC PDx acts as own MCC   CC CC Condition   PDx CC PDx acts as own CC

748   ICD-10-CM 2018

√7ᵗʰ **M1A.139** Lead-induced chronic gout, unspecified wrist

√6ᵗʰ **M1A.14** Lead-induced chronic gout, hand

    √7ᵗʰ **M1A.141** Lead-induced chronic gout, right hand

    √7ᵗʰ **M1A.142** Lead-induced chronic gout, left hand

    √7ᵗʰ **M1A.149** Lead-induced chronic gout, unspecified hand

√6ᵗʰ **M1A.15** Lead-induced chronic gout, hip

    √7ᵗʰ **M1A.151** Lead-induced chronic gout, right hip

    √7ᵗʰ **M1A.152** Lead-induced chronic gout, left hip

    √7ᵗʰ **M1A.159** Lead-induced chronic gout, unspecified hip

√6ᵗʰ **M1A.16** Lead-induced chronic gout, knee

    √7ᵗʰ **M1A.161** Lead-induced chronic gout, right knee

    √7ᵗʰ **M1A.162** Lead-induced chronic gout, left knee

    √7ᵗʰ **M1A.169** Lead-induced chronic gout, unspecified knee

√6ᵗʰ **M1A.17** Lead-induced chronic gout, ankle and foot

    √7ᵗʰ **M1A.171** Lead-induced chronic gout, right ankle and foot

    √7ᵗʰ **M1A.172** Lead-induced chronic gout, left ankle and foot

    √7ᵗʰ **M1A.179** Lead-induced chronic gout, unspecified ankle and foot

√x7ᵗʰ **M1A.18** Lead-induced chronic gout, vertebrae

√x7ᵗʰ **M1A.19** Lead-induced chronic gout, multiple sites

√5ᵗʰ **M1A.2** Drug-induced chronic gout

    Use additional code for adverse effect, if applicable, to identify drug (T36-T50 with fifth or sixth character 5)

√x7ᵗʰ **M1A.20** Drug-induced chronic gout, unspecified site

√6ᵗʰ **M1A.21** Drug-induced chronic gout, shoulder

    √7ᵗʰ **M1A.211** Drug-induced chronic gout, right shoulder

    √7ᵗʰ **M1A.212** Drug-induced chronic gout, left shoulder

    √7ᵗʰ **M1A.219** Drug-induced chronic gout, unspecified shoulder

√6ᵗʰ **M1A.22** Drug-induced chronic gout, elbow

    √7ᵗʰ **M1A.221** Drug-induced chronic gout, right elbow

    √7ᵗʰ **M1A.222** Drug-induced chronic gout, left elbow

    √7ᵗʰ **M1A.229** Drug-induced chronic gout, unspecified elbow

√6ᵗʰ **M1A.23** Drug-induced chronic gout, wrist

    √7ᵗʰ **M1A.231** Drug-induced chronic gout, right wrist

    √7ᵗʰ **M1A.232** Drug-induced chronic gout, left wrist

    √7ᵗʰ **M1A.239** Drug-induced chronic gout, unspecified wrist

√6ᵗʰ **M1A.24** Drug-induced chronic gout, hand

    √7ᵗʰ **M1A.241** Drug-induced chronic gout, right hand

    √7ᵗʰ **M1A.242** Drug-induced chronic gout, left hand

    √7ᵗʰ **M1A.249** Drug-induced chronic gout, unspecified hand

√6ᵗʰ **M1A.25** Drug-induced chronic gout, hip

    √7ᵗʰ **M1A.251** Drug-induced chronic gout, right hip

    √7ᵗʰ **M1A.252** Drug-induced chronic gout, left hip

    √7ᵗʰ **M1A.259** Drug-induced chronic gout, unspecified hip

√6ᵗʰ **M1A.26** Drug-induced chronic gout, knee

    √7ᵗʰ **M1A.261** Drug-induced chronic gout, right knee

    √7ᵗʰ **M1A.262** Drug-induced chronic gout, left knee

    √7ᵗʰ **M1A.269** Drug-induced chronic gout, unspecified knee

√6ᵗʰ **M1A.27** Drug-induced chronic gout, ankle and foot

    √7ᵗʰ **M1A.271** Drug-induced chronic gout, right ankle and foot

    √7ᵗʰ **M1A.272** Drug-induced chronic gout, left ankle and foot

    √7ᵗʰ **M1A.279** Drug-induced chronic gout, unspecified ankle and foot

√x7ᵗʰ **M1A.28** Drug-induced chronic gout, vertebrae

√x7ᵗʰ **M1A.29** Drug-induced chronic gout, multiple sites

√5ᵗʰ **M1A.3** Chronic gout due to renal impairment

    Code first associated renal disease

√x7ᵗʰ **M1A.30** Chronic gout due to renal impairment, unspecified site

√6ᵗʰ **M1A.31** Chronic gout due to renal impairment, shoulder

    √7ᵗʰ **M1A.311** Chronic gout due to renal impairment, right shoulder

    √7ᵗʰ **M1A.312** Chronic gout due to renal impairment, left shoulder

    √7ᵗʰ **M1A.319** Chronic gout due to renal impairment, unspecified shoulder

√6ᵗʰ **M1A.32** Chronic gout due to renal impairment, elbow

    √7ᵗʰ **M1A.321** Chronic gout due to renal impairment, right elbow

    √7ᵗʰ **M1A.322** Chronic gout due to renal impairment, left elbow

    √7ᵗʰ **M1A.329** Chronic gout due to renal impairment, unspecified elbow

√6ᵗʰ **M1A.33** Chronic gout due to renal impairment, wrist

    √7ᵗʰ **M1A.331** Chronic gout due to renal impairment, right wrist

    √7ᵗʰ **M1A.332** Chronic gout due to renal impairment, left wrist

    √7ᵗʰ **M1A.339** Chronic gout due to renal impairment, unspecified wrist

√6ᵗʰ **M1A.34** Chronic gout due to renal impairment, hand

    √7ᵗʰ **M1A.341** Chronic gout due to renal impairment, right hand

    √7ᵗʰ **M1A.342** Chronic gout due to renal impairment, left hand

    √7ᵗʰ **M1A.349** Chronic gout due to renal impairment, unspecified hand

√6ᵗʰ **M1A.35** Chronic gout due to renal impairment, hip

    √7ᵗʰ **M1A.351** Chronic gout due to renal impairment, right hip

    √7ᵗʰ **M1A.352** Chronic gout due to renal impairment, left hip

    √7ᵗʰ **M1A.359** Chronic gout due to renal impairment, unspecified hip

√6ᵗʰ **M1A.36** Chronic gout due to renal impairment, knee

    √7ᵗʰ **M1A.361** Chronic gout due to renal impairment, right knee

    √7ᵗʰ **M1A.362** Chronic gout due to renal impairment, left knee

    √7ᵗʰ **M1A.369** Chronic gout due to renal impairment, unspecified knee

√6ᵗʰ **M1A.37** Chronic gout due to renal impairment, ankle and foot

    √7ᵗʰ **M1A.371** Chronic gout due to renal impairment, right ankle and foot

    √7ᵗʰ **M1A.372** Chronic gout due to renal impairment, left ankle and foot

    √7ᵗʰ **M1A.379** Chronic gout due to renal impairment, unspecified ankle and foot

√x7ᵗʰ **M1A.38** Chronic gout due to renal impairment, vertebrae

√x7ᵗʰ **M1A.39** Chronic gout due to renal impairment, multiple sites

√5ᵗʰ **M1A.4** Other secondary chronic gout

    Code first associated condition

√x7ᵗʰ **M1A.40** Other secondary chronic gout, unspecified site

√6ᵗʰ **M1A.41** Other secondary chronic gout, shoulder

    √7ᵗʰ **M1A.411** Other secondary chronic gout, right shoulder

    √7ᵗʰ **M1A.412** Other secondary chronic gout, left shoulder

    √7ᵗʰ **M1A.419** Other secondary chronic gout, unspecified shoulder

√6ᵗʰ **M1A.42** Other secondary chronic gout, elbow

    √7ᵗʰ **M1A.421** Other secondary chronic gout, right elbow

    √7ᵗʰ **M1A.422** Other secondary chronic gout, left elbow

    √7ᵗʰ **M1A.429** Other secondary chronic gout, unspecified elbow

---

√ Additional Character Req   √x7ᵗʰ Placeholder Alert   Unacceptable PDx   Manifestation   **H1**-**H14** HAC   **HCC** CMS-HCC Condition   *EXCLUDES 1* Not Coded Here   *EXCLUDES 2* Not Included Here

✓6th **M1A.43 Other secondary chronic gout, wrist**
     ✓7th **M1A.431 Other secondary chronic gout, right wrist**
     ✓7th **M1A.432 Other secondary chronic gout, left wrist**
     ✓7th **M1A.439 Other secondary chronic gout, unspecified wrist**

✓6th **M1A.44 Other secondary chronic gout, hand**
     ✓7th **M1A.441 Other secondary chronic gout, right hand**
     ✓7th **M1A.442 Other secondary chronic gout, left hand**
     ✓7th **M1A.449 Other secondary chronic gout, unspecified hand**

✓6th **M1A.45 Other secondary chronic gout, hip**
     ✓7th **M1A.451 Other secondary chronic gout, right hip**
     ✓7th **M1A.452 Other secondary chronic gout, left hip**
     ✓7th **M1A.459 Other secondary chronic gout, unspecified hip**

✓6th **M1A.46 Other secondary chronic gout, knee**
     ✓7th **M1A.461 Other secondary chronic gout, right knee**
     ✓7th **M1A.462 Other secondary chronic gout, left knee**
     ✓7th **M1A.469 Other secondary chronic gout, unspecified knee**

✓6th **M1A.47 Other secondary chronic gout, ankle and foot**
     ✓7th **M1A.471 Other secondary chronic gout, right ankle and foot**
     ✓7th **M1A.472 Other secondary chronic gout, left ankle and foot**
     ✓7th **M1A.479 Other secondary chronic gout, unspecified ankle and foot**

✓x7th **M1A.48 Other secondary chronic gout, vertebrae**
✓x7th **M1A.49 Other secondary chronic gout, multiple sites**
✓x7th **M1A.9 Chronic gout, unspecified**

✓4th **M10 Gout**
Acute gout
Gout attack
Gout flare
Podagra
Use additional code to identify:
    autonomic neuropathy in diseases classified elsewhere (G99.0)
    calculus of urinary tract in diseases classified elsewhere (N22)
    cardiomyopathy in diseases classified elsewhere (I43)
    disorders of external ear in diseases classified elsewhere (H61.1-, H62.8-)
    disorders of iris and ciliary body in diseases classified elsewhere (H22)
    glomerular disorders in diseases classified elsewhere (N08)
EXCLUDES 2   *chronic gout (M1A.-)*
DEF: Purine and pyrimidine metabolic disorders; manifested by hyperuricemia and recurrent acute inflammatory arthritis; monosodium urate or monohydrate crystals may be deposited in and around the joints, leading to joint destruction and severe crippling.

✓5th **M10.0 Idiopathic gout**
Gouty bursitis
Primary gout
    M10.00 Idiopathic gout, unspecified site
    ✓6th **M10.01 Idiopathic gout, shoulder**
      M10.011 Idiopathic gout, right shoulder
      M10.012 Idiopathic gout, left shoulder
      M10.019 Idiopathic gout, unspecified shoulder
    ✓6th **M10.02 Idiopathic gout, elbow**
      M10.021 Idiopathic gout, right elbow
      M10.022 Idiopathic gout, left elbow
      M10.029 Idiopathic gout, unspecified elbow
    ✓6th **M10.03 Idiopathic gout, wrist**
      M10.031 Idiopathic gout, right wrist
      M10.032 Idiopathic gout, left wrist
      M10.039 Idiopathic gout, unspecified wrist
    ✓6th **M10.04 Idiopathic gout, hand**
      M10.041 Idiopathic gout, right hand
      M10.042 Idiopathic gout, left hand
      M10.049 Idiopathic gout, unspecified hand
    ✓6th **M10.05 Idiopathic gout, hip**
      M10.051 Idiopathic gout, right hip
      M10.052 Idiopathic gout, left hip
      M10.059 Idiopathic gout, unspecified hip

    ✓6th **M10.06 Idiopathic gout, knee**
      M10.061 Idiopathic gout, right knee
      M10.062 Idiopathic gout, left knee
      M10.069 Idiopathic gout, unspecified knee
    ✓6th **M10.07 Idiopathic gout, ankle and foot**
      M10.071 Idiopathic gout, right ankle and foot
      M10.072 Idiopathic gout, left ankle and foot
      M10.079 Idiopathic gout, unspecified ankle and foot
    M10.08 Idiopathic gout, vertebrae
    M10.09 Idiopathic gout, multiple sites

✓5th **M10.1 Lead-induced gout**
Code first toxic effects of lead and its compounds (T56.0-)
    M10.10 Lead-induced gout, unspecified site
    ✓6th **M10.11 Lead-induced gout, shoulder**
      M10.111 Lead-induced gout, right shoulder
      M10.112 Lead-induced gout, left shoulder
      M10.119 Lead-induced gout, unspecified shoulder
    ✓6th **M10.12 Lead-induced gout, elbow**
      M10.121 Lead-induced gout, right elbow
      M10.122 Lead-induced gout, left elbow
      M10.129 Lead-induced gout, unspecified elbow
    ✓6th **M10.13 Lead-induced gout, wrist**
      M10.131 Lead-induced gout, right wrist
      M10.132 Lead-induced gout, left wrist
      M10.139 Lead-induced gout, unspecified wrist
    ✓6th **M10.14 Lead-induced gout, hand**
      M10.141 Lead-induced gout, right hand
      M10.142 Lead-induced gout, left hand
      M10.149 Lead-induced gout, unspecified hand
    ✓6th **M10.15 Lead-induced gout, hip**
      M10.151 Lead-induced gout, right hip
      M10.152 Lead-induced gout, left hip
      M10.159 Lead-induced gout, unspecified hip
    ✓6th **M10.16 Lead-induced gout, knee**
      M10.161 Lead-induced gout, right knee
      M10.162 Lead-induced gout, left knee
      M10.169 Lead-induced gout, unspecified knee
    ✓6th **M10.17 Lead-induced gout, ankle and foot**
      M10.171 Lead-induced gout, right ankle and foot
      M10.172 Lead-induced gout, left ankle and foot
      M10.179 Lead-induced gout, unspecified ankle and foot
    M10.18 Lead-induced gout, vertebrae
    M10.19 Lead-induced gout, multiple sites

✓5th **M10.2 Drug-induced gout**
Use additional code for adverse effect, if applicable, to identify drug (T36-T50 with fifth or sixth character 5)
    M10.20 Drug-induced gout, unspecified site
    ✓6th **M10.21 Drug-induced gout, shoulder**
      M10.211 Drug-induced gout, right shoulder
      M10.212 Drug-induced gout, left shoulder
      M10.219 Drug-induced gout, unspecified shoulder
    ✓6th **M10.22 Drug-induced gout, elbow**
      M10.221 Drug-induced gout, right elbow
      M10.222 Drug-induced gout, left elbow
      M10.229 Drug-induced gout, unspecified elbow
    ✓6th **M10.23 Drug-induced gout, wrist**
      M10.231 Drug-induced gout, right wrist
      M10.232 Drug-induced gout, left wrist
      M10.239 Drug-induced gout, unspecified wrist
    ✓6th **M10.24 Drug-induced gout, hand**
      M10.241 Drug-induced gout, right hand
      M10.242 Drug-induced gout, left hand
      M10.249 Drug-induced gout, unspecified hand
    ✓6th **M10.25 Drug-induced gout, hip**
      M10.251 Drug-induced gout, right hip
      M10.252 Drug-induced gout, left hip
      M10.259 Drug-induced gout, unspecified hip

☑6ᵗʰ **M10.26 Drug-induced gout,** knee
     M10.261 **Drug-induced gout,** right **knee**
     M10.262 **Drug-induced gout,** left **knee**
     M10.269 **Drug-induced gout,** unspecified **knee**

☑6ᵗʰ **M10.27 Drug-induced gout,** ankle and foot
     M10.271 **Drug-induced gout,** right **ankle and foot**
     M10.272 **Drug-induced gout,** left **ankle and foot**
     M10.279 **Drug-induced gout,** unspecified **ankle and foot**

     M10.28 Drug-induced gout, vertebrae
     M10.29 Drug-induced gout, multiple sites

☑5ᵗʰ **M10.3 Gout due to** renal impairment
     Code first associated renal disease
     M10.30 Gout due to renal impairment, unspecified site

☑6ᵗʰ **M10.31 Gout due to renal impairment,** shoulder
     M10.311 **Gout due to renal impairment,** right **shoulder**
     M10.312 **Gout due to renal impairment,** left **shoulder**
     M10.319 **Gout due to renal impairment,** unspecified **shoulder**

☑6ᵗʰ **M10.32 Gout due to renal impairment,** elbow
     M10.321 **Gout due to renal impairment,** right **elbow**
     M10.322 **Gout due to renal impairment,** left **elbow**
     M10.329 **Gout due to renal impairment,** unspecified **elbow**

☑6ᵗʰ **M10.33 Gout due to renal impairment,** wrist
     M10.331 **Gout due to renal impairment,** right **wrist**
     M10.332 **Gout due to renal impairment,** left **wrist**
     M10.339 **Gout due to renal impairment,** unspecified **wrist**

☑6ᵗʰ **M10.34 Gout due to renal impairment,** hand
     M10.341 **Gout due to renal impairment,** right **hand**
     M10.342 **Gout due to renal impairment,** left **hand**
     M10.349 **Gout due to renal impairment,** unspecified **hand**

☑6ᵗʰ **M10.35 Gout due to renal impairment,** hip
     M10.351 **Gout due to renal impairment,** right **hip**
     M10.352 **Gout due to renal impairment,** left **hip**
     M10.359 **Gout due to renal impairment,** unspecified **hip**

☑6ᵗʰ **M10.36 Gout due to renal impairment,** knee
     M10.361 **Gout due to renal impairment,** right **knee**
     M10.362 **Gout due to renal impairment,** left **knee**
     M10.369 **Gout due to renal impairment,** unspecified **knee**

☑6ᵗʰ **M10.37 Gout due to renal impairment,** ankle and foot
     M10.371 **Gout due to renal impairment,** right **ankle and foot**
     M10.372 **Gout due to renal impairment,** left **ankle and foot**
     M10.379 **Gout due to renal impairment,** unspecified **ankle and foot**

     M10.38 Gout due to renal impairment, vertebrae
     M10.39 Gout due to renal impairment, multiple sites

☑5ᵗʰ **M10.4 Other secondary gout**
     Code first associated condition
     M10.40 Other secondary gout, unspecified site

☑6ᵗʰ **M10.41 Other secondary gout,** shoulder
     M10.411 **Other secondary gout,** right **shoulder**
     M10.412 **Other secondary gout,** left **shoulder**
     M10.419 **Other secondary gout,** unspecified **shoulder**

☑6ᵗʰ **M10.42 Other secondary gout,** elbow
     M10.421 **Other secondary gout,** right **elbow**
     M10.422 **Other secondary gout,** left **elbow**
     M10.429 **Other secondary gout,** unspecified **elbow**

☑6ᵗʰ **M10.43 Other secondary gout,** wrist
     M10.431 **Other secondary gout,** right **wrist**
     M10.432 **Other secondary gout,** left **wrist**
     M10.439 **Other secondary gout,** unspecified **wrist**

☑6ᵗʰ **M10.44 Other secondary gout,** hand
     M10.441 **Other secondary gout,** right **hand**
     M10.442 **Other secondary gout,** left **hand**
     M10.449 **Other secondary gout,** unspecified **hand**

☑6ᵗʰ **M10.45 Other secondary gout,** hip
     M10.451 **Other secondary gout,** right **hip**
     M10.452 **Other secondary gout,** left **hip**
     M10.459 **Other secondary gout,** unspecified **hip**

☑6ᵗʰ **M10.46 Other secondary gout,** knee
     M10.461 **Other secondary gout,** right **knee**
     M10.462 **Other secondary gout,** left **knee**
     M10.469 **Other secondary gout,** unspecified **knee**

☑6ᵗʰ **M10.47 Other secondary gout,** ankle and foot
     M10.471 **Other secondary gout,** right **ankle and foot**
     M10.472 **Other secondary gout,** left **ankle and foot**
     M10.479 **Other secondary gout,** unspecified **ankle and foot**

     M10.48 Other secondary gout, vertebrae
     M10.49 Other secondary gout, multiple sites

M10.9 Gout, unspecified
     Gout NOS

☑4ᵗʰ **M11 Other crystal arthropathies**

☑5ᵗʰ **M11.0 Hydroxyapatite deposition disease**
     M11.00 Hydroxyapatite deposition disease, unspecified site

☑6ᵗʰ **M11.01 Hydroxyapatite deposition disease,** shoulder
     M11.011 **Hydroxyapatite deposition disease,** right **shoulder**
     M11.012 **Hydroxyapatite deposition disease,** left **shoulder**
     M11.019 **Hydroxyapatite deposition disease,** unspecified **shoulder**

☑6ᵗʰ **M11.02 Hydroxyapatite deposition disease,** elbow
     M11.021 **Hydroxyapatite deposition disease,** right **elbow**
     M11.022 **Hydroxyapatite deposition disease,** left **elbow**
     M11.029 **Hydroxyapatite deposition disease,** unspecified **elbow**

☑6ᵗʰ **M11.03 Hydroxyapatite deposition disease,** wrist
     M11.031 **Hydroxyapatite deposition disease,** right **wrist**
     M11.032 **Hydroxyapatite deposition disease,** left **wrist**
     M11.039 **Hydroxyapatite deposition disease,** unspecified **wrist**

☑6ᵗʰ **M11.04 Hydroxyapatite deposition disease,** hand
     M11.041 **Hydroxyapatite deposition disease,** right **hand**
     M11.042 **Hydroxyapatite deposition disease,** left **hand**
     M11.049 **Hydroxyapatite deposition disease,** unspecified **hand**

☑6ᵗʰ **M11.05 Hydroxyapatite deposition disease,** hip
     M11.051 **Hydroxyapatite deposition disease,** right **hip**
     M11.052 **Hydroxyapatite deposition disease,** left **hip**
     M11.059 **Hydroxyapatite deposition disease,** unspecified **hip**

☑6ᵗʰ **M11.06 Hydroxyapatite deposition disease,** knee
     M11.061 **Hydroxyapatite deposition disease,** right **knee**
     M11.062 **Hydroxyapatite deposition disease,** left **knee**
     M11.069 **Hydroxyapatite deposition disease,** unspecified **knee**

☑6ᵗʰ **M11.07 Hydroxyapatite deposition disease,** ankle and foot
     M11.071 **Hydroxyapatite deposition disease,** right **ankle and foot**
     M11.072 **Hydroxyapatite deposition disease,** left **ankle and foot**
     M11.079 **Hydroxyapatite deposition disease,** unspecified **ankle and foot**

M11.08 Hydroxyapatite deposition disease, vertebrae

M11.09 Hydroxyapatite deposition disease, multiple sites

√5ᵗʰ **M11.1 Familial chondrocalcinosis**

    M11.10 Familial chondrocalcinosis, unspecified site

√6ᵗʰ **M11.11** Familial chondrocalcinosis, shoulder

    M11.111 Familial chondrocalcinosis, right shoulder

    M11.112 Familial chondrocalcinosis, left shoulder

    M11.119 Familial chondrocalcinosis, unspecified shoulder

√6ᵗʰ **M11.12** Familial chondrocalcinosis, elbow

    M11.121 Familial chondrocalcinosis, right elbow

    M11.122 Familial chondrocalcinosis, left elbow

    M11.129 Familial chondrocalcinosis, unspecified elbow

√6ᵗʰ **M11.13** Familial chondrocalcinosis, wrist

    M11.131 Familial chondrocalcinosis, right wrist

    M11.132 Familial chondrocalcinosis, left wrist

    M11.139 Familial chondrocalcinosis, unspecified wrist

√6ᵗʰ **M11.14** Familial chondrocalcinosis, hand

    M11.141 Familial chondrocalcinosis, right hand

    M11.142 Familial chondrocalcinosis, left hand

    M11.149 Familial chondrocalcinosis, unspecified hand

√6ᵗʰ **M11.15** Familial chondrocalcinosis, hip

    M11.151 Familial chondrocalcinosis, right hip

    M11.152 Familial chondrocalcinosis, left hip

    M11.159 Familial chondrocalcinosis, unspecified hip

√6ᵗʰ **M11.16** Familial chondrocalcinosis, knee

    M11.161 Familial chondrocalcinosis, right knee

    M11.162 Familial chondrocalcinosis, left knee

    M11.169 Familial chondrocalcinosis, unspecified knee

√6ᵗʰ **M11.17** Familial chondrocalcinosis, ankle and foot

    M11.171 Familial chondrocalcinosis, right ankle and foot

    M11.172 Familial chondrocalcinosis, left ankle and foot

    M11.179 Familial chondrocalcinosis, unspecified ankle and foot

    M11.18 Familial chondrocalcinosis, vertebrae

    M11.19 Familial chondrocalcinosis, multiple sites

√5ᵗʰ **M11.2 Other chondrocalcinosis**

    Chondrocalcinosis NOS

    M11.20 Other chondrocalcinosis, unspecified site

√6ᵗʰ **M11.21** Other chondrocalcinosis, shoulder

    M11.211 Other chondrocalcinosis, right shoulder

    M11.212 Other chondrocalcinosis, left shoulder

    M11.219 Other chondrocalcinosis, unspecified shoulder

√6ᵗʰ **M11.22** Other chondrocalcinosis, elbow

    M11.221 Other chondrocalcinosis, right elbow

    M11.222 Other chondrocalcinosis, left elbow

    M11.229 Other chondrocalcinosis, unspecified elbow

√6ᵗʰ **M11.23** Other chondrocalcinosis, wrist

    M11.231 Other chondrocalcinosis, right wrist

    M11.232 Other chondrocalcinosis, left wrist

    M11.239 Other chondrocalcinosis, unspecified wrist

√6ᵗʰ **M11.24** Other chondrocalcinosis, hand

    M11.241 Other chondrocalcinosis, right hand

    M11.242 Other chondrocalcinosis, left hand

    M11.249 Other chondrocalcinosis, unspecified hand

√6ᵗʰ **M11.25** Other chondrocalcinosis, hip

    M11.251 Other chondrocalcinosis, right hip

    M11.252 Other chondrocalcinosis, left hip

    M11.259 Other chondrocalcinosis, unspecified hip

√6ᵗʰ **M11.26** Other chondrocalcinosis, knee

    M11.261 Other chondrocalcinosis, right knee

    M11.262 Other chondrocalcinosis, left knee

    M11.269 Other chondrocalcinosis, unspecified knee

√6ᵗʰ **M11.27** Other chondrocalcinosis, ankle and foot

    M11.271 Other chondrocalcinosis, right ankle and foot

    M11.272 Other chondrocalcinosis, left ankle and foot

    M11.279 Other chondrocalcinosis, unspecified ankle and foot

    M11.28 Other chondrocalcinosis, vertebrae

    M11.29 Other chondrocalcinosis, multiple sites

√5ᵗʰ **M11.8 Other specified crystal arthropathies**

    M11.80 Other specified crystal arthropathies, unspecified site

√6ᵗʰ **M11.81** Other specified crystal arthropathies, shoulder

    M11.811 Other specified crystal arthropathies, right shoulder

    M11.812 Other specified crystal arthropathies, left shoulder

    M11.819 Other specified crystal arthropathies, unspecified shoulder

√6ᵗʰ **M11.82** Other specified crystal arthropathies, elbow

    M11.821 Other specified crystal arthropathies, right elbow

    M11.822 Other specified crystal arthropathies, left elbow

    M11.829 Other specified crystal arthropathies, unspecified elbow

√6ᵗʰ **M11.83** Other specified crystal arthropathies, wrist

    M11.831 Other specified crystal arthropathies, right wrist

    M11.832 Other specified crystal arthropathies, left wrist

    M11.839 Other specified crystal arthropathies, unspecified wrist

√6ᵗʰ **M11.84** Other specified crystal arthropathies, hand

    M11.841 Other specified crystal arthropathies, right hand

    M11.842 Other specified crystal arthropathies, left hand

    M11.849 Other specified crystal arthropathies, unspecified hand

√6ᵗʰ **M11.85** Other specified crystal arthropathies, hip

    M11.851 Other specified crystal arthropathies, right hip

    M11.852 Other specified crystal arthropathies, left hip

    M11.859 Other specified crystal arthropathies, unspecified hip

√6ᵗʰ **M11.86** Other specified crystal arthropathies, knee

    M11.861 Other specified crystal arthropathies, right knee

    M11.862 Other specified crystal arthropathies, left knee

    M11.869 Other specified crystal arthropathies, unspecified knee

√6ᵗʰ **M11.87** Other specified crystal arthropathies, ankle and foot

    M11.871 Other specified crystal arthropathies, right ankle and foot

    M11.872 Other specified crystal arthropathies, left ankle and foot

    M11.879 Other specified crystal arthropathies, unspecified ankle and foot

    M11.88 Other specified crystal arthropathies, vertebrae

    M11.89 Other specified crystal arthropathies, multiple sites

    M11.9 Crystal arthropathy, unspecified

√4ᵗʰ **M12 Other and unspecified arthropathy**

    EXCLUDES 1   arthrosis (M15-M19)
         cricoarytenoid arthropathy (J38.7)

√5ᵗʰ **M12.0 Chronic postrheumatic arthropathy [Jaccoud]**

    M12.00 Chronic postrheumatic arthropathy [Jaccoud], unspecified site   HCC

√6ᵗʰ **M12.01** Chronic postrheumatic arthropathy [Jaccoud], shoulder

    M12.011 Chronic postrheumatic arthropathy [Jaccoud], right shoulder   HCC

    M12.012 Chronic postrheumatic arthropathy [Jaccoud], left shoulder   HCC

N Newborn: 0   P Pediatric: 0-17   M Maternity: 12-55   A Adult: 15-124   MCC Major CC Condition   PDxMCC PDx acts as own MCC   CC CC Condition   PDxCC PDx acts as own CC

752   ICD-10-CM 2018

         M12.019   **Chronic postrheumatic arthropathy** `HCC`
                [Jaccoud], unspecified shoulder

   ✓6ᵗʰ   **M12.02**   **Chronic postrheumatic arthropathy [Jaccoud], elbow**
         M12.021   **Chronic postrheumatic arthropathy** `HCC`
                [Jaccoud], right elbow
         M12.022   **Chronic postrheumatic arthropathy** `HCC`
                [Jaccoud], left elbow
         M12.029   **Chronic postrheumatic arthropathy** `HCC`
                [Jaccoud], unspecified elbow

   ✓6ᵗʰ   **M12.03**   **Chronic postrheumatic arthropathy [Jaccoud], wrist**
         M12.031   **Chronic postrheumatic arthropathy** `HCC`
                [Jaccoud], right wrist
         M12.032   **Chronic postrheumatic arthropathy** `HCC`
                [Jaccoud], left wrist
         M12.039   **Chronic postrheumatic arthropathy** `HCC`
                [Jaccoud], unspecified wrist

   ✓6ᵗʰ   **M12.04**   **Chronic postrheumatic arthropathy [Jaccoud], hand**
         M12.041   **Chronic postrheumatic arthropathy** `HCC`
                [Jaccoud], right hand
         M12.042   **Chronic postrheumatic arthropathy** `HCC`
                [Jaccoud], left hand
         M12.049   **Chronic postrheumatic arthropathy** `HCC`
                [Jaccoud], unspecified hand

   ✓6ᵗʰ   **M12.05**   **Chronic postrheumatic arthropathy [Jaccoud], hip**
         M12.051   **Chronic postrheumatic arthropathy** `HCC`
                [Jaccoud], right hip
         M12.052   **Chronic postrheumatic arthropathy** `HCC`
                [Jaccoud], left hip
         M12.059   **Chronic postrheumatic arthropathy** `HCC`
                [Jaccoud], unspecified hip

   ✓6ᵗʰ   **M12.06**   **Chronic postrheumatic arthropathy [Jaccoud], knee**
         M12.061   **Chronic postrheumatic arthropathy** `HCC`
                [Jaccoud], right knee
         M12.062   **Chronic postrheumatic arthropathy** `HCC`
                [Jaccoud], left knee
         M12.069   **Chronic postrheumatic arthropathy** `HCC`
                [Jaccoud], unspecified knee

   ✓6ᵗʰ   **M12.07**   **Chronic postrheumatic arthropathy [Jaccoud], ankle and foot**
         M12.071   **Chronic postrheumatic arthropathy** `HCC`
                [Jaccoud], right ankle and foot
         M12.072   **Chronic postrheumatic arthropathy** `HCC`
                [Jaccoud], left ankle and foot
         M12.079   **Chronic postrheumatic arthropathy**
                [Jaccoud], unspecified ankle and foot `HCC`

       M12.08   **Chronic postrheumatic arthropathy [Jaccoud],** `HCC`
          other specified site
            Chronic postrheumatic arthropathy [Jaccoud], vertebrae

       M12.09   **Chronic postrheumatic arthropathy [Jaccoud],** `HCC`
          multiple sites

✓5ᵗʰ   **M12.1**   **Kaschin-Beck disease**
         Osteochondroarthrosis deformans endemica

       M12.10   **Kaschin-Beck disease, unspecified site**

   ✓6ᵗʰ   **M12.11**   **Kaschin-Beck disease, shoulder**
         M12.111   **Kaschin-Beck disease, right shoulder**
         M12.112   **Kaschin-Beck disease, left shoulder**
         M12.119   **Kaschin-Beck disease, unspecified shoulder**

   ✓6ᵗʰ   **M12.12**   **Kaschin-Beck disease, elbow**
         M12.121   **Kaschin-Beck disease, right elbow**
         M12.122   **Kaschin-Beck disease, left elbow**
         M12.129   **Kaschin-Beck disease, unspecified elbow**

   ✓6ᵗʰ   **M12.13**   **Kaschin-Beck disease, wrist**
         M12.131   **Kaschin-Beck disease, right wrist**
         M12.132   **Kaschin-Beck disease, left wrist**
         M12.139   **Kaschin-Beck disease, unspecified wrist**

   ✓6ᵗʰ   **M12.14**   **Kaschin-Beck disease, hand**
         M12.141   **Kaschin-Beck disease, right hand**
         M12.142   **Kaschin-Beck disease, left hand**
         M12.149   **Kaschin-Beck disease, unspecified hand**

   ✓6ᵗʰ   **M12.15**   **Kaschin-Beck disease, hip**
         M12.151   **Kaschin-Beck disease, right hip**
         M12.152   **Kaschin-Beck disease, left hip**
         M12.159   **Kaschin-Beck disease, unspecified hip**

   ✓6ᵗʰ   **M12.16**   **Kaschin-Beck disease, knee**
         M12.161   **Kaschin-Beck disease, right knee**
         M12.162   **Kaschin-Beck disease, left knee**
         M12.169   **Kaschin-Beck disease, unspecified knee**

   ✓6ᵗʰ   **M12.17**   **Kaschin-Beck disease, ankle and foot**
         M12.171   **Kaschin-Beck disease, right ankle and foot**
         M12.172   **Kaschin-Beck disease, left ankle and foot**
         M12.179   **Kaschin-Beck disease, unspecified ankle and foot**

       M12.18   **Kaschin-Beck disease, vertebrae**
       M12.19   **Kaschin-Beck disease, multiple sites**

✓5ᵗʰ   **M12.2**   **Villonodular synovitis (pigmented)**
       M12.20   **Villonodular synovitis (pigmented), unspecified site**

   ✓6ᵗʰ   **M12.21**   **Villonodular synovitis (pigmented), shoulder**
         M12.211   **Villonodular synovitis (pigmented), right shoulder**
         M12.212   **Villonodular synovitis (pigmented), left shoulder**
         M12.219   **Villonodular synovitis (pigmented), unspecified shoulder**

   ✓6ᵗʰ   **M12.22**   **Villonodular synovitis (pigmented), elbow**
         M12.221   **Villonodular synovitis (pigmented), right elbow**
         M12.222   **Villonodular synovitis (pigmented), left elbow**
         M12.229   **Villonodular synovitis (pigmented), unspecified elbow**

   ✓6ᵗʰ   **M12.23**   **Villonodular synovitis (pigmented), wrist**
         M12.231   **Villonodular synovitis (pigmented), right wrist**
         M12.232   **Villonodular synovitis (pigmented), left wrist**
         M12.239   **Villonodular synovitis (pigmented), unspecified wrist**

   ✓6ᵗʰ   **M12.24**   **Villonodular synovitis (pigmented), hand**
         M12.241   **Villonodular synovitis (pigmented), right hand**
         M12.242   **Villonodular synovitis (pigmented), left hand**
         M12.249   **Villonodular synovitis (pigmented), unspecified hand**

   ✓6ᵗʰ   **M12.25**   **Villonodular synovitis (pigmented), hip**
         M12.251   **Villonodular synovitis (pigmented), right hip**
         M12.252   **Villonodular synovitis (pigmented), left hip**
         M12.259   **Villonodular synovitis (pigmented), unspecified hip**

   ✓6ᵗʰ   **M12.26**   **Villonodular synovitis (pigmented), knee**
         M12.261   **Villonodular synovitis (pigmented), right knee**
         M12.262   **Villonodular synovitis (pigmented), left knee**
         M12.269   **Villonodular synovitis (pigmented), unspecified knee**

   ✓6ᵗʰ   **M12.27**   **Villonodular synovitis (pigmented), ankle and foot**
         M12.271   **Villonodular synovitis (pigmented), right ankle and foot**
         M12.272   **Villonodular synovitis (pigmented), left ankle and foot**
         M12.279   **Villonodular synovitis (pigmented), unspecified ankle and foot**

       M12.28   **Villonodular synovitis (pigmented), other specified site**
            Villonodular synovitis (pigmented), vertebrae

       M12.29   **Villonodular synovitis (pigmented), multiple sites**

✓5ᵗʰ   **M12.3**   **Palindromic rheumatism**
       M12.30   **Palindromic rheumatism, unspecified site**

   ✓6ᵗʰ   **M12.31**   **Palindromic rheumatism, shoulder**
         M12.311   **Palindromic rheumatism, right shoulder**
         M12.312   **Palindromic rheumatism, left shoulder**
         M12.319   **Palindromic rheumatism, unspecified shoulder**

✓6th **M12.32 Palindromic rheumatism,** elbow
    M12.321 Palindromic rheumatism, right **elbow**
    M12.322 Palindromic rheumatism, left **elbow**
    M12.329 Palindromic rheumatism, unspecified **elbow**

✓6th **M12.33 Palindromic rheumatism,** wrist
    M12.331 Palindromic rheumatism, right **wrist**
    M12.332 Palindromic rheumatism, left **wrist**
    M12.339 Palindromic rheumatism, unspecified **wrist**

✓6th **M12.34 Palindromic rheumatism,** hand
    M12.341 Palindromic rheumatism, right **hand**
    M12.342 Palindromic rheumatism, left **hand**
    M12.349 Palindromic rheumatism, unspecified **hand**

✓6th **M12.35 Palindromic rheumatism,** hip
    M12.351 Palindromic rheumatism, right **hip**
    M12.352 Palindromic rheumatism, left **hip**
    M12.359 Palindromic rheumatism, unspecified **hip**

✓6th **M12.36 Palindromic rheumatism,** knee
    M12.361 Palindromic rheumatism, right **knee**
    M12.362 Palindromic rheumatism, left **knee**
    M12.369 Palindromic rheumatism, unspecified **knee**

✓6th **M12.37 Palindromic rheumatism,** ankle and foot
    M12.371 Palindromic rheumatism, right **ankle and foot**
    M12.372 Palindromic rheumatism, left **ankle and foot**
    M12.379 Palindromic rheumatism, unspecified **ankle and foot**

M12.38 Palindromic rheumatism, other specified site
    Palindromic rheumatism, vertebrae

M12.39 Palindromic rheumatism, multiple sites

✓5th **M12.4 Intermittent hydrarthrosis**

M12.40 Intermittent hydrarthrosis, unspecified site

✓6th **M12.41 Intermittent hydrarthrosis,** shoulder
    M12.411 Intermittent hydrarthrosis, right **shoulder**
    M12.412 Intermittent hydrarthrosis, left **shoulder**
    M12.419 Intermittent hydrarthrosis, unspecified **shoulder**

✓6th **M12.42 Intermittent hydrarthrosis,** elbow
    M12.421 Intermittent hydrarthrosis, right **elbow**
    M12.422 Intermittent hydrarthrosis, left **elbow**
    M12.429 Intermittent hydrarthrosis, unspecified **elbow**

✓6th **M12.43 Intermittent hydrarthrosis,** wrist
    M12.431 Intermittent hydrarthrosis, right **wrist**
    M12.432 Intermittent hydrarthrosis, left **wrist**
    M12.439 Intermittent hydrarthrosis, unspecified **wrist**

✓6th **M12.44 Intermittent hydrarthrosis,** hand
    M12.441 Intermittent hydrarthrosis, right **hand**
    M12.442 Intermittent hydrarthrosis, left **hand**
    M12.449 Intermittent hydrarthrosis, unspecified **hand**

✓6th **M12.45 Intermittent hydrarthrosis,** hip
    M12.451 Intermittent hydrarthrosis, right **hip**
    M12.452 Intermittent hydrarthrosis, left **hip**
    M12.459 Intermittent hydrarthrosis, unspecified **hip**

✓6th **M12.46 Intermittent hydrarthrosis,** knee
    M12.461 Intermittent hydrarthrosis, right **knee**
    M12.462 Intermittent hydrarthrosis, left **knee**
    M12.469 Intermittent hydrarthrosis, unspecified **knee**

✓6th **M12.47 Intermittent hydrarthrosis,** ankle and foot
    M12.471 Intermittent hydrarthrosis, right **ankle and foot**
    M12.472 Intermittent hydrarthrosis, left **ankle and foot**
    M12.479 Intermittent hydrarthrosis, unspecified **ankle and foot**

M12.48 Intermittent hydrarthrosis, other site

M12.49 Intermittent hydrarthrosis, multiple sites

✓5th **M12.5 Traumatic arthropathy**
    EXCLUDES 1   current injury—see Alphabetic Index
       post-traumatic osteoarthritis NOS (M19.1-)
       post-traumatic osteoarthritis of first carpometacarpal joint (M18.2-M18.3)
       post-traumatic osteoarthritis of hip (M16.4-M16.5)
       post-traumatic osteoarthritis of knee (M17.2-M17.3)
       post-traumatic osteoarthritis of other single joints (M19.1-)
    AHA: 2015, 1Q, 17

M12.50 Traumatic arthropathy, unspecified site

✓6th **M12.51 Traumatic arthropathy,** shoulder
    M12.511 Traumatic arthropathy, right **shoulder**
    M12.512 Traumatic arthropathy, left **shoulder**
    M12.519 Traumatic arthropathy, unspecified **shoulder**

✓6th **M12.52 Traumatic arthropathy,** elbow
    M12.521 Traumatic arthropathy, right **elbow**
    M12.522 Traumatic arthropathy, left **elbow**
    M12.529 Traumatic arthropathy, unspecified **elbow**

✓6th **M12.53 Traumatic arthropathy,** wrist
    M12.531 Traumatic arthropathy, right **wrist**
    M12.532 Traumatic arthropathy, left **wrist**
    M12.539 Traumatic arthropathy, unspecified **wrist**

✓6th **M12.54 Traumatic arthropathy,** hand
    M12.541 Traumatic arthropathy, right **hand**
    M12.542 Traumatic arthropathy, left **hand**
    M12.549 Traumatic arthropathy, unspecified **hand**

✓6th **M12.55 Traumatic arthropathy,** hip
    M12.551 Traumatic arthropathy, right **hip**
    M12.552 Traumatic arthropathy, left **hip**
    M12.559 Traumatic arthropathy, unspecified **hip**

✓6th **M12.56 Traumatic arthropathy,** knee
    M12.561 Traumatic arthropathy, right **knee**
    M12.562 Traumatic arthropathy, left **knee**
    M12.569 Traumatic arthropathy, unspecified **knee**

✓6th **M12.57 Traumatic arthropathy,** ankle and foot
    M12.571 Traumatic arthropathy, right **ankle and foot**
    M12.572 Traumatic arthropathy, left **ankle and foot**
    M12.579 Traumatic arthropathy, unspecified **ankle and foot**

M12.58 Traumatic arthropathy, other specified site
    Traumatic arthropathy, vertebrae

M12.59 Traumatic arthropathy, multiple sites

✓5th **M12.8 Other specific arthropathies, not elsewhere classified**
    Transient arthropathy

M12.80 Other specific arthropathies, not elsewhere classified, unspecified site

✓6th **M12.81 Other specific arthropathies, not elsewhere classified,** shoulder
    M12.811 Other specific arthropathies, not elsewhere classified, right **shoulder**
    M12.812 Other specific arthropathies, not elsewhere classified, left **shoulder**
    M12.819 Other specific arthropathies, not elsewhere classified, unspecified **shoulder**

✓6th **M12.82 Other specific arthropathies, not elsewhere classified,** elbow
    M12.821 Other specific arthropathies, not elsewhere classified, right **elbow**
    M12.822 Other specific arthropathies, not elsewhere classified, left **elbow**
    M12.829 Other specific arthropathies, not elsewhere classified, unspecified **elbow**

✓6th **M12.83 Other specific arthropathies, not elsewhere classified,** wrist
    M12.831 Other specific arthropathies, not elsewhere classified, right **wrist**
    M12.832 Other specific arthropathies, not elsewhere classified, left **wrist**
    M12.839 Other specific arthropathies, not elsewhere classified, unspecified **wrist**

N Newborn: 0   P Pediatric: 0-17   M Maternity: 12-55   A Adult: 15-124   MCC Major CC Condition   PDxMCC PDx acts as own MCC   CC CC Condition   PDxCC PDx acts as own CC

754   ICD-10-CM 2018

☑6ᵗʰ **M12.84** **Other specific arthropathies, not elsewhere classified,** hand
     M12.841 Other specific arthropathies, not elsewhere classified, **right** hand
     M12.842 Other specific arthropathies, not elsewhere classified, **left** hand
     M12.849 Other specific arthropathies, not elsewhere classified, **unspecified** hand

☑6ᵗʰ **M12.85** **Other specific arthropathies, not elsewhere classified,** hip
     M12.851 Other specific arthropathies, not elsewhere classified, **right** hip
     M12.852 Other specific arthropathies, not elsewhere classified, **left** hip
     M12.859 Other specific arthropathies, not elsewhere classified, **unspecified** hip

☑6ᵗʰ **M12.86** **Other specific arthropathies, not elsewhere classified,** knee
     M12.861 Other specific arthropathies, not elsewhere classified, **right** knee
     M12.862 Other specific arthropathies, not elsewhere classified, **left** knee
     M12.869 Other specific arthropathies, not elsewhere classified, **unspecified** knee

☑6ᵗʰ **M12.87** **Other specific arthropathies, not elsewhere classified,** ankle and foot
     M12.871 Other specific arthropathies, not elsewhere classified, **right** ankle and foot
     M12.872 Other specific arthropathies, not elsewhere classified, **left** ankle and foot
     M12.879 Other specific arthropathies, not elsewhere classified, **unspecified** ankle and foot

M12.88 **Other specific arthropathies, not elsewhere classified,** other specified site
     Other specific arthropathies, not elsewhere classified, vertebrae

M12.89 **Other specific arthropathies, not elsewhere classified,** multiple sites

M12.9 **Arthropathy,** unspecified

☑4ᵗʰ **M13** **Other arthritis**
     EXCLUDES 1   arthrosis (M15-M19)
                 osteoarthritis (M15-M19)

M13.0 **Polyarthritis,** unspecified

☑5ᵗʰ **M13.1** **Monoarthritis, not elsewhere classified**
     M13.10 **Monoarthritis, not elsewhere classified,** unspecified site

     ☑6ᵗʰ **M13.11** **Monoarthritis, not elsewhere classified,** shoulder
         M13.111 Monoarthritis, not elsewhere classified, **right** shoulder
         M13.112 Monoarthritis, not elsewhere classified, **left** shoulder
         M13.119 Monoarthritis, not elsewhere classified, **unspecified shoulder**

     ☑6ᵗʰ **M13.12** **Monoarthritis, not elsewhere classified,** elbow
         M13.121 Monoarthritis, not elsewhere classified, **right** elbow
         M13.122 Monoarthritis, not elsewhere classified, **left** elbow
         M13.129 Monoarthritis, not elsewhere classified, **unspecified** elbow

     ☑6ᵗʰ **M13.13** **Monoarthritis, not elsewhere classified,** wrist
         M13.131 Monoarthritis, not elsewhere classified, **right** wrist
         M13.132 Monoarthritis, not elsewhere classified, **left** wrist
         M13.139 Monoarthritis, not elsewhere classified, **unspecified** wrist

     ☑6ᵗʰ **M13.14** **Monoarthritis, not elsewhere classified,** hand
         M13.141 Monoarthritis, not elsewhere classified, **right** hand
         M13.142 Monoarthritis, not elsewhere classified, **left** hand
         M13.149 Monoarthritis, not elsewhere classified, **unspecified** hand

☑6ᵗʰ **M13.15** **Monoarthritis, not elsewhere classified,** hip
     M13.151 Monoarthritis, not elsewhere classified, **right hip**
     M13.152 Monoarthritis, not elsewhere classified, **left hip**
     M13.159 Monoarthritis, not elsewhere classified, **unspecified hip**

☑6ᵗʰ **M13.16** **Monoarthritis, not elsewhere classified,** knee
     M13.161 Monoarthritis, not elsewhere classified, **right knee**
     M13.162 Monoarthritis, not elsewhere classified, **left knee**
     M13.169 Monoarthritis, not elsewhere classified, **unspecified knee**

☑6ᵗʰ **M13.17** **Monoarthritis, not elsewhere classified,** ankle and foot
     M13.171 Monoarthritis, not elsewhere classified, **right ankle and foot**
     M13.172 Monoarthritis, not elsewhere classified, **left ankle and foot**
     M13.179 Monoarthritis, not elsewhere classified, **unspecified ankle and foot**

☑5ᵗʰ **M13.8** **Other specified arthritis**
     Allergic arthritis
     EXCLUDES 1   osteoarthritis (M15-M19)

     M13.80 **Other specified arthritis,** unspecified site

     ☑6ᵗʰ **M13.81** **Other specified arthritis,** shoulder
         M13.811 Other specified arthritis, **right** shoulder
         M13.812 Other specified arthritis, **left** shoulder
         M13.819 Other specified arthritis, **unspecified shoulder**

     ☑6ᵗʰ **M13.82** **Other specified arthritis,** elbow
         M13.821 Other specified arthritis, **right** elbow
         M13.822 Other specified arthritis, **left** elbow
         M13.829 Other specified arthritis, **unspecified elbow**

     ☑6ᵗʰ **M13.83** **Other specified arthritis,** wrist
         M13.831 Other specified arthritis, **right** wrist
         M13.832 Other specified arthritis, **left** wrist
         M13.839 Other specified arthritis, **unspecified** wrist

     ☑6ᵗʰ **M13.84** **Other specified arthritis,** hand
         M13.841 Other specified arthritis, **right** hand
         M13.842 Other specified arthritis, **left** hand
         M13.849 Other specified arthritis, **unspecified** hand

     ☑6ᵗʰ **M13.85** **Other specified arthritis,** hip
         M13.851 Other specified arthritis, **right** hip
         M13.852 Other specified arthritis, **left** hip
         M13.859 Other specified arthritis, **unspecified** hip

     ☑6ᵗʰ **M13.86** **Other specified arthritis,** knee
         M13.861 Other specified arthritis, **right** knee
         M13.862 Other specified arthritis, **left** knee
         M13.869 Other specified arthritis, **unspecified** knee

     ☑6ᵗʰ **M13.87** **Other specified arthritis,** ankle and foot
         M13.871 Other specified arthritis, **right** ankle and foot
         M13.872 Other specified arthritis, **left** ankle and foot
         M13.879 Other specified arthritis, **unspecified** ankle and foot

     M13.88 **Other specified arthritis,** other site
     M13.89 **Other specified arthritis,** multiple sites

☑ Additional Character Req   ☑x7ᵗʰ Placeholder Alert   Unacceptable PDx   Manifestation   **H1**-**H14** HAC   **HCC** CMS-HCC Condition   *EXCLUDES 1* Not Coded Here   *EXCLUDES 2* Not Included Here

✓4ᵗʰ M14 Arthropathies in other diseases classified elsewhere

> *EXCLUDES 1*   arthropathy in:
> diabetes mellitus (E08-E13 with .61-)
> hematological disorders (M36.2-M36.3)
> hypersensitivity reactions (M36.4)
> neoplastic disease (M36.1)
> neurosyphillis (A52.16)
> sarcoidosis (D86.86)
> enteropathic arthropathies (M07.-)
> juvenile psoriatic arthropathy (L40.54)
> lipoid dermatoarthritis (E78.81)

✓5ᵗʰ M14.6 Charcôt's joint

> Neuropathic arthropathy
> *EXCLUDES 1*   Charcôt's joint in diabetes mellitus (E08-E13 with .610-)
> Charcôt's joint in tabes dorsalis (A52.16)

     M14.60 Charcôt's joint, unspecified site

     ✓6ᵗʰ M14.61 Charcôt's joint, shoulder

         M14.611 Charcôt's joint, right shoulder
         M14.612 Charcôt's joint, left shoulder
         M14.619 Charcôt's joint, unspecified shoulder

     ✓6ᵗʰ M14.62 Charcôt's joint, elbow

         M14.621 Charcôt's joint, right elbow
         M14.622 Charcôt's joint, left elbow
         M14.629 Charcôt's joint, unspecified elbow

     ✓6ᵗʰ M14.63 Charcôt's joint, wrist

         M14.631 Charcôt's joint, right wrist
         M14.632 Charcôt's joint, left wrist
         M14.639 Charcôt's joint, unspecified wrist

     ✓6ᵗʰ M14.64 Charcôt's joint, hand

         M14.641 Charcôt's joint, right hand
         M14.642 Charcôt's joint, left hand
         M14.649 Charcôt's joint, unspecified hand

     ✓6ᵗʰ M14.65 Charcôt's joint, hip

         M14.651 Charcôt's joint, right hip
         M14.652 Charcôt's joint, left hip
         M14.659 Charcôt's joint, unspecified hip

     ✓6ᵗʰ M14.66 Charcôt's joint, knee

         M14.661 Charcôt's joint, right knee
         M14.662 Charcôt's joint, left knee
         M14.669 Charcôt's joint, unspecified knee

     ✓6ᵗʰ M14.67 Charcôt's joint, ankle and foot

         M14.671 Charcôt's joint, right ankle and foot
         M14.672 Charcôt's joint, left ankle and foot
         M14.679 Charcôt's joint, unspecified ankle and foot

     M14.68 Charcôt's joint, vertebrae

     M14.69 Charcôt's joint, multiple sites

✓5ᵗʰ M14.8 Arthropathies in other specified diseases classified elsewhere

> Code first underlying disease, such as:
> amyloidosis (E85.-)
> erythema multiforme (L51.-)
> erythema nodosum (L52)
> hemochromatosis (E83.11-)
> hyperparathyroidism (E21.-)
> hypothyroidism (E00-E03)
> sickle-cell disorders (D57.-)
> thyrotoxicosis [hyperthyroidism] (E05.-)
> Whipple's disease (K90.81)

     M14.80 *Arthropathies in other specified diseases classified elsewhere, unspecified site*

     ✓6ᵗʰ M14.81 Arthropathies in other specified diseases classified elsewhere, shoulder

         M14.811 *Arthropathies in other specified diseases classified elsewhere, right shoulder*
         M14.812 *Arthropathies in other specified diseases classified elsewhere, left shoulder*
         M14.819 *Arthropathies in other specified diseases classified elsewhere, unspecified shoulder*

     ✓6ᵗʰ M14.82 Arthropathies in other specified diseases classified elsewhere, elbow

         M14.821 *Arthropathies in other specified diseases classified elsewhere, right elbow*
         M14.822 *Arthropathies in other specified diseases classified elsewhere, left elbow*
         M14.829 *Arthropathies in other specified diseases classified elsewhere, unspecified elbow*

     ✓6ᵗʰ M14.83 Arthropathies in other specified diseases classified elsewhere, wrist

         M14.831 *Arthropathies in other specified diseases classified elsewhere, right wrist*
         M14.832 *Arthropathies in other specified diseases classified elsewhere, left wrist*
         M14.839 *Arthropathies in other specified diseases classified elsewhere, unspecified wrist*

     ✓6ᵗʰ M14.84 Arthropathies in other specified diseases classified elsewhere, hand

         M14.841 *Arthropathies in other specified diseases classified elsewhere, right hand*
         M14.842 *Arthropathies in other specified diseases classified elsewhere, left hand*
         M14.849 *Arthropathies in other specified diseases classified elsewhere, unspecified hand*

     ✓6ᵗʰ M14.85 Arthropathies in other specified diseases classified elsewhere, hip

         M14.851 *Arthropathies in other specified diseases classified elsewhere, right hip*
         M14.852 *Arthropathies in other specified diseases classified elsewhere, left hip*
         M14.859 *Arthropathies in other specified diseases classified elsewhere, unspecified hip*

     ✓6ᵗʰ M14.86 Arthropathies in other specified diseases classified elsewhere, knee

         M14.861 *Arthropathies in other specified diseases classified elsewhere, right knee*
         M14.862 *Arthropathies in other specified diseases classified elsewhere, left knee*
         M14.869 *Arthropathies in other specified diseases classified elsewhere, unspecified knee*

     ✓6ᵗʰ M14.87 Arthropathies in other specified diseases classified elsewhere, ankle and foot

         M14.871 *Arthropathies in other specified diseases classified elsewhere, right ankle and foot*
         M14.872 *Arthropathies in other specified diseases classified elsewhere, left ankle and foot*
         M14.879 *Arthropathies in other specified diseases classified elsewhere, unspecified ankle and foot*

     M14.88 *Arthropathies in other specified diseases classified elsewhere, vertebrae*

     M14.89 *Arthropathies in other specified diseases classified elsewhere, multiple sites*

Osteoarthritis (M15-M19)

> *EXCLUDES 2*   osteoarthritis of spine (M47.-)

✓4ᵗʰ M15 Polyosteoarthritis

> *INCLUDES*   arthritis of multiple sites
> *EXCLUDES 1*   bilateral involvement of single joint (M16-M19)

     M15.0 Primary generalized (osteo)arthritis

     M15.1 Heberden's nodes (with arthropathy)
         Interphalangeal distal osteoarthritis

     M15.2 Bouchard's nodes (with arthropathy)
         Juxtaphalangeal distal osteoarthritis

     M15.3 Secondary multiple arthritis
         Post-traumatic polyosteoarthritis

     M15.4 Erosive (osteo)arthritis

     M15.8 Other polyosteoarthritis

     M15.9 Polyosteoarthritis, unspecified
         Generalized osteoarthritis NOS

✓4ᵗʰ M16 Osteoarthritis of hip

> **AHA:** 2016, 4Q, 146

     M16.0 Bilateral primary osteoarthritis of hip

     ✓5ᵗʰ M16.1 Unilateral primary osteoarthritis of hip
         Primary osteoarthritis of hip NOS

         M16.10 Unilateral primary osteoarthritis, unspecified hip
         M16.11 Unilateral primary osteoarthritis, right hip
         M16.12 Unilateral primary osteoarthritis, left hip

     M16.2 Bilateral osteoarthritis resulting from hip dysplasia

     ✓5ᵗʰ M16.3 Unilateral osteoarthritis resulting from hip dysplasia
         Dysplastic osteoarthritis of hip NOS

         M16.30 Unilateral osteoarthritis resulting from hip dysplasia, unspecified hip

N Newborn: 0   P Pediatric: 0-17   M Maternity: 12-55   A Adult: 15-124   MCC Major CC Condition   PDx MCC PDx acts as own MCC   CC CC Condition   PDx CC PDx acts as own CC

756   ICD-10-CM 2018

M16.31   **Unilateral osteoarthritis resulting from hip dysplasia, right hip**

M16.32   **Unilateral osteoarthritis resulting from hip dysplasia, left hip**

M16.4   **Bilateral post-traumatic osteoarthritis of hip**

√5ᵗʰ   M16.5   **Unilateral post-traumatic osteoarthritis of hip**
Post-traumatic osteoarthritis of hip NOS

     M16.50   **Unilateral post-traumatic osteoarthritis, unspecified hip**

     M16.51   **Unilateral post-traumatic osteoarthritis, right hip**

     M16.52   **Unilateral post-traumatic osteoarthritis, left hip**

M16.6   **Other bilateral secondary osteoarthritis of hip**

M16.7   **Other unilateral secondary osteoarthritis of hip**
Secondary osteoarthritis of hip NOS

M16.9   **Osteoarthritis of hip, unspecified**

√4ᵗʰ   **M17   Osteoarthritis of knee**
AHA: 2016, 4Q, 146-147

M17.0   **Bilateral primary osteoarthritis of knee**

√5ᵗʰ   M17.1   **Unilateral primary osteoarthritis of knee**
Primary osteoarthritis of knee NOS

     M17.10   **Unilateral primary osteoarthritis, unspecified knee**

     M17.11   **Unilateral primary osteoarthritis, right knee**

     M17.12   **Unilateral primary osteoarthritis, left knee**

M17.2   **Bilateral post-traumatic osteoarthritis of knee**

√5ᵗʰ   M17.3   **Unilateral post-traumatic osteoarthritis of knee**
Post-traumatic osteoarthritis of knee NOS

     M17.30   **Unilateral post-traumatic osteoarthritis, unspecified knee**

     M17.31   **Unilateral post-traumatic osteoarthritis, right knee**

     M17.32   **Unilateral post-traumatic osteoarthritis, left knee**

M17.4   **Other bilateral secondary osteoarthritis of knee**

M17.5   **Other unilateral secondary osteoarthritis of knee**
Secondary osteoarthritis of knee NOS

M17.9   **Osteoarthritis of knee, unspecified**

√4ᵗʰ   **M18   Osteoarthritis of first carpometacarpal joint**

M18.0   **Bilateral primary osteoarthritis of first carpometacarpal joints**

√5ᵗʰ   M18.1   **Unilateral primary osteoarthritis of first carpometacarpal joint**
Primary osteoarthritis of first carpometacarpal joint NOS

     M18.10   **Unilateral primary osteoarthritis of first carpometacarpal joint, unspecified hand**

     M18.11   **Unilateral primary osteoarthritis of first carpometacarpal joint, right hand**

     M18.12   **Unilateral primary osteoarthritis of first carpometacarpal joint, left hand**

M18.2   **Bilateral post-traumatic osteoarthritis of first carpometacarpal joints**

√5ᵗʰ   M18.3   **Unilateral post-traumatic osteoarthritis of first carpometacarpal joint**
Post-traumatic osteoarthritis of first carpometacarpal joint NOS

     M18.30   **Unilateral post-traumatic osteoarthritis of first carpometacarpal joint, unspecified hand**

     M18.31   **Unilateral post-traumatic osteoarthritis of first carpometacarpal joint, right hand**

     M18.32   **Unilateral post-traumatic osteoarthritis of first carpometacarpal joint, left hand**

M18.4   **Other bilateral secondary osteoarthritis of first carpometacarpal joints**

√5ᵗʰ   M18.5   **Other unilateral secondary osteoarthritis of first carpometacarpal joint**
Secondary osteoarthritis of first carpometacarpal joint NOS

     M18.50   **Other unilateral secondary osteoarthritis of first carpometacarpal joint, unspecified hand**

     M18.51   **Other unilateral secondary osteoarthritis of first carpometacarpal joint, right hand**

     M18.52   **Other unilateral secondary osteoarthritis of first carpometacarpal joint, left hand**

M18.9   **Osteoarthritis of first carpometacarpal joint, unspecified**

√4ᵗʰ   **M19   Other and unspecified osteoarthritis**
EXCLUDES 1   *polyarthritis (M15.-)*
EXCLUDES 2   *arthrosis of spine (M47.-)*
            hallux rigidus (M20.2)
            osteoarthritis of spine (M47.-)

√5ᵗʰ   M19.0   **Primary osteoarthritis of other joints**
AHA: 2016, 4Q, 145

   √6ᵗʰ   M19.01   **Primary osteoarthritis, shoulder**

     M19.011   **Primary osteoarthritis, right shoulder**

     M19.012   **Primary osteoarthritis, left shoulder**

     M19.019   **Primary osteoarthritis, unspecified shoulder**

   √6ᵗʰ   M19.02   **Primary osteoarthritis, elbow**

     M19.021   **Primary osteoarthritis, right elbow**

     M19.022   **Primary osteoarthritis, left elbow**

     M19.029   **Primary osteoarthritis, unspecified elbow**

   √6ᵗʰ   M19.03   **Primary osteoarthritis, wrist**

     M19.031   **Primary osteoarthritis, right wrist**

     M19.032   **Primary osteoarthritis, left wrist**

     M19.039   **Primary osteoarthritis, unspecified wrist**

   √6ᵗʰ   M19.04   **Primary osteoarthritis, hand**
EXCLUDES 2   *primary osteoarthritis of first carpometacarpal joint (M18.0-, M18.1-)*

     M19.041   **Primary osteoarthritis, right hand**

     M19.042   **Primary osteoarthritis, left hand**

     M19.049   **Primary osteoarthritis, unspecified hand**

   √6ᵗʰ   M19.07   **Primary osteoarthritis ankle and foot**

     M19.071   **Primary osteoarthritis, right ankle and foot**

     M19.072   **Primary osteoarthritis, left ankle and foot**

     M19.079   **Primary osteoarthritis, unspecified ankle and foot**

√5ᵗʰ   M19.1   **Post-traumatic osteoarthritis of other joints**

   √6ᵗʰ   M19.11   **Post-traumatic osteoarthritis, shoulder**

     M19.111   **Post-traumatic osteoarthritis, right shoulder**

     M19.112   **Post-traumatic osteoarthritis, left shoulder**

     M19.119   **Post-traumatic osteoarthritis, unspecified shoulder**

   √6ᵗʰ   M19.12   **Post-traumatic osteoarthritis, elbow**

     M19.121   **Post-traumatic osteoarthritis, right elbow**

     M19.122   **Post-traumatic osteoarthritis, left elbow**

     M19.129   **Post-traumatic osteoarthritis, unspecified elbow**

   √6ᵗʰ   M19.13   **Post-traumatic osteoarthritis, wrist**

     M19.131   **Post-traumatic osteoarthritis, right wrist**

     M19.132   **Post-traumatic osteoarthritis, left wrist**

     M19.139   **Post-traumatic osteoarthritis, unspecified wrist**

   √6ᵗʰ   M19.14   **Post-traumatic osteoarthritis, hand**
EXCLUDES 2   *post-traumatic osteoarthritis of first carpometacarpal joint (M18.2-, M18.3-)*

     M19.141   **Post-traumatic osteoarthritis, right hand**

     M19.142   **Post-traumatic osteoarthritis, left hand**

     M19.149   **Post-traumatic osteoarthritis, unspecified hand**

   √6ᵗʰ   M19.17   **Post-traumatic osteoarthritis, ankle and foot**

     M19.171   **Post-traumatic osteoarthritis, right ankle and foot**

     M19.172   **Post-traumatic osteoarthritis, left ankle and foot**

     M19.179   **Post-traumatic osteoarthritis, unspecified ankle and foot**

√5ᵗʰ   M19.2   **Secondary osteoarthritis of other joints**

   √6ᵗʰ   M19.21   **Secondary osteoarthritis, shoulder**

     M19.211   **Secondary osteoarthritis, right shoulder**

     M19.212   **Secondary osteoarthritis, left shoulder**

     M19.219   **Secondary osteoarthritis, unspecified shoulder**

   √6ᵗʰ   M19.22   **Secondary osteoarthritis, elbow**

     M19.221   **Secondary osteoarthritis, right elbow**

     M19.222   **Secondary osteoarthritis, left elbow**

M19.229 Secondary osteoarthritis, unspecified elbow

✓6th **M19.23** Secondary osteoarthritis, wrist
   M19.231 Secondary osteoarthritis, right wrist
   M19.232 Secondary osteoarthritis, left wrist
   M19.239 Secondary osteoarthritis, unspecified wrist

✓6th **M19.24** Secondary osteoarthritis, hand
   M19.241 Secondary osteoarthritis, right hand
   M19.242 Secondary osteoarthritis, left hand
   M19.249 Secondary osteoarthritis, unspecified hand

✓6th **M19.27** Secondary osteoarthritis, ankle and foot
   M19.271 Secondary osteoarthritis, right ankle and foot
   M19.272 Secondary osteoarthritis, left ankle and foot
   M19.279 Secondary osteoarthritis, unspecified ankle and foot

✓5th **M19.9** Osteoarthritis, unspecified site
   M19.90 Unspecified osteoarthritis, unspecified site
     Arthrosis NOS
     Arthritis NOS
     Osteoarthritis NOS
     AHA: 2016, 4Q, 147
   M19.91 Primary osteoarthritis, unspecified site
     Primary osteoarthritis NOS
   M19.92 Post-traumatic osteoarthritis, unspecified site
     Post-traumatic osteoarthritis NOS
   M19.93 Secondary osteoarthritis, unspecified site
     Secondary osteoarthritis NOS

Other joint disorders (M20-M25)
EXCLUDES 2 *joints of the spine (M40-M54)*

✓4th **M20 Acquired deformities of fingers and toes**
EXCLUDES 1 *acquired absence of fingers and toes (Z89.-)*
congenital absence of fingers and toes (Q71.3-, Q72.3-)
congenital deformities and malformations of fingers and toes (Q66-, Q68-Q70, Q74-)

✓5th **M20.0** Deformity of finger(s)
EXCLUDES 1 *clubbing of fingers (R68.3)*
palmar fascial fibromatosis [Dupuytren] (M72.0)
trigger finger (M65.3)

 ✓6th **M20.00** Unspecified deformity of finger(s)
   M20.001 Unspecified deformity of right finger(s)
   M20.002 Unspecified deformity of left finger(s)
   M20.009 Unspecified deformity of unspecified finger(s)

 ✓6th **M20.01** Mallet finger
   M20.011 Mallet finger of right finger(s)
   M20.012 Mallet finger of left finger(s)
   M20.019 Mallet finger of unspecified finger(s)d

 ✓6th **M20.02** Boutonnière deformity
   DEF: A deformity of the finger caused by flexion of the proximal interphalangeal joint and hyperextension of the distal joint; results from rheumatoid arthritis, osteoarthritis, or injury; also called buttonhole deformity.
   M20.021 Boutonnière deformity of right finger(s)
   M20.022 Boutonnière deformity of left finger(s)
   M20.029 Boutonnière deformity of unspecified finger(s)

 ✓6th **M20.03** Swan-neck deformity
   DEF: Flexed distal and hyperextended proximal interphalangeal joint; most commonly caused by rheumatoid arthritis.
   M20.031 Swan-neck deformity of right finger(s)
   M20.032 Swan-neck deformity of left finger(s)
   M20.039 Swan-neck deformity of unspecified finger(s)

 ✓6th **M20.09** Other deformity of finger(s)
   M20.091 Other deformity of right finger(s)
   M20.092 Other deformity of left finger(s)
   M20.099 Other deformity of finger(s), unspecified finger(s)

Hallux Valgus

Hallux valgus —

Medial eminence of metatarsal bone —

Right foot

✓5th **M20.1** Hallux valgus (acquired)
EXCLUDES 2 *bunion (M21.6-)*
   M20.10 Hallux valgus (acquired), unspecified foot
   M20.11 Hallux valgus (acquired), right foot
   M20.12 Hallux valgus (acquired), left foot

✓5th **M20.2** Hallux rigidus
   M20.20 Hallux rigidus, unspecified foot
   M20.21 Hallux rigidus, right foot
   M20.22 Hallux rigidus, left foot

✓5th **M20.3** Hallux varus (acquired)
   M20.30 Hallux varus (acquired), unspecified foot
   M20.31 Hallux varus (acquired), right foot
   M20.32 Hallux varus (acquired), left foot

✓5th **M20.4** Other hammer toe(s) (acquired)
   M20.40 Other hammer toe(s) (acquired), unspecified foot
   M20.41 Other hammer toe(s) (acquired), right foot
   M20.42 Other hammer toe(s) (acquired), left foot

✓5th **M20.5** Other deformities of toe(s) (acquired)
 ✓6th **M20.5X** Other deformities of toe(s) (acquired)
   M20.5X1 Other deformities of toe(s) (acquired), right foot
   M20.5X2 Other deformities of toe(s) (acquired), left foot
   M20.5X9 Other deformities of toe(s) (acquired), unspecified foot

✓5th **M20.6** Acquired deformities of toe(s), unspecified
   M20.60 Acquired deformities of toe(s), unspecified, unspecified foot
   M20.61 Acquired deformities of toe(s), unspecified, right foot
   M20.62 Acquired deformities of toe(s), unspecified, left foot

✓4th **M21 Other acquired deformities of limbs**
EXCLUDES 1 *acquired absence of limb (Z89.-)*
congenital absence of limbs (Q71-Q73)
congenital deformities and malformations of limbs (Q65-Q66, Q68-Q74)
EXCLUDES 2 *acquired deformities of fingers or toes (M20.-)*
coxa plana (M91.2)

✓5th **M21.0** Valgus deformity, not elsewhere classified
EXCLUDES 1 *metatarsus valgus (Q66.6)*
talipes calcaneovalgus (Q66.4)
   M21.00 Valgus deformity, not elsewhere classified, unspecified site
 ✓6th **M21.02** Valgus deformity, not elsewhere classified, elbow
   Cubitus valgus
   M21.021 Valgus deformity, not elsewhere classified, right elbow
   M21.022 Valgus deformity, not elsewhere classified, left elbow
   M21.029 Valgus deformity, not elsewhere classified, unspecified elbow

N Newborn: 0   P Pediatric: 0-17   M Maternity: 12-55   A Adult: 15-124   MCC Major CC Condition   PDxMCC PDx acts as own MCC   CC CC Condition   PDxCC PDx acts as own CC

758

ICD-10-CM 2018

Genu Valga (knock-knee)

Genu Varus (bowleg)

✓6th **M21.05** Valgus deformity, not elsewhere classified, hip
     M21.051 Valgus deformity, not elsewhere classified, right hip
     M21.052 Valgus deformity, not elsewhere classified, left hip
     M21.059 Valgus deformity, not elsewhere classified, unspecified hip

✓6th **M21.06** Valgus deformity, not elsewhere classified, knee
     Genu valgum
     Knock knee
     M21.061 Valgus deformity, not elsewhere classified, right knee
     M21.062 Valgus deformity, not elsewhere classified, left knee
     M21.069 Valgus deformity, not elsewhere classified, unspecified knee

✓6th **M21.07** Valgus deformity, not elsewhere classified, ankle
     M21.071 Valgus deformity, not elsewhere classified, right ankle
     M21.072 Valgus deformity, not elsewhere classified, left ankle
     M21.079 Valgus deformity, not elsewhere classified, unspecified ankle

✓5th **M21.1** Varus deformity, not elsewhere classified
     EXCLUDES 1   metatarsus varus (Q66.22)
             tibia vara (M92.5)
     M21.10 Varus deformity, not elsewhere classified, unspecified site

✓6th **M21.12** Varus deformity, not elsewhere classified, elbow
     Cubitus varus, elbow
     M21.121 Varus deformity, not elsewhere classified, right elbow
     M21.122 Varus deformity, not elsewhere classified, left elbow
     M21.129 Varus deformity, not elsewhere classified, unspecified elbow

✓6th **M21.15** Varus deformity, not elsewhere classified, hip
     M21.151 Varus deformity, not elsewhere classified, right hip
     M21.152 Varus deformity, not elsewhere classified, left hip
     M21.159 Varus deformity, not elsewhere classified, unspecified

✓6th **M21.16** Varus deformity, not elsewhere classified, knee
     Bow leg
     Genu varum
     M21.161 Varus deformity, not elsewhere classified, right knee
     M21.162 Varus deformity, not elsewhere classified, left knee
     M21.169 Varus deformity, not elsewhere classified, unspecified knee

✓6th **M21.17** Varus deformity, not elsewhere classified, ankle
     M21.171 Varus deformity, not elsewhere classified, right ankle
     M21.172 Varus deformity, not elsewhere classified, left ankle
     M21.179 Varus deformity, not elsewhere classified, unspecified ankle

✓5th **M21.2** Flexion deformity
     M21.20 Flexion deformity, unspecified site

✓6th **M21.21** Flexion deformity, shoulder
     M21.211 Flexion deformity, right shoulder
     M21.212 Flexion deformity, left shoulder
     M21.219 Flexion deformity, unspecified shoulder

✓6th **M21.22** Flexion deformity, elbow
     M21.221 Flexion deformity, right elbow
     M21.222 Flexion deformity, left elbow
     M21.229 Flexion deformity, unspecified elbow

✓6th **M21.23** Flexion deformity, wrist
     M21.231 Flexion deformity, right wrist
     M21.232 Flexion deformity, left wrist
     M21.239 Flexion deformity, unspecified wrist

✓6th **M21.24** Flexion deformity, finger joints
     M21.241 Flexion deformity, right finger joints
     M21.242 Flexion deformity, left finger joints
     M21.249 Flexion deformity, unspecified finger joints

✓6th **M21.25** Flexion deformity, hip
     M21.251 Flexion deformity, right hip
     M21.252 Flexion deformity, left hip
     M21.259 Flexion deformity, unspecified hip

✓6th **M21.26** Flexion deformity, knee
     M21.261 Flexion deformity, right knee
     M21.262 Flexion deformity, left knee
     M21.269 Flexion deformity, unspecified knee

✓6th **M21.27** Flexion deformity, ankle and toes
     M21.271 Flexion deformity, right ankle and toes
     M21.272 Flexion deformity, left ankle and toes
     M21.279 Flexion deformity, unspecified ankle and toes

✓5th **M21.3** Wrist or foot drop (acquired)

✓6th **M21.33** Wrist drop (acquired)
     M21.331 Wrist drop, right wrist
     M21.332 Wrist drop, left wrist
     M21.339 Wrist drop, unspecified wrist

✓6th **M21.37** Foot drop (acquired)
     M21.371 Foot drop, right foot
     M21.372 Foot drop, left foot
     M21.379 Foot drop, unspecified foot

✅ Additional Character Req   ✓x 7th Placeholder Alert   Unacceptable PDx   Manifestation   H1 - H14 HAC   HCC CMS-HCC Condition   *EXCLUDES 1* Not Coded Here   *EXCLUDES 2* Not Included Here

ICD-10-CM 2018   759

Chapter 13. Diseases of the Musculoskeletal System and Connective Tissue

✓5th **M21.4 Flat foot [pes planus] (acquired)**
     EXCLUDES 1   congenital pes planus (Q66.5-)
     M21.40 Flat foot [pes planus] (acquired), **unspecified** foot
     M21.41 Flat foot [pes planus] (acquired), **right** foot
     M21.42 Flat foot [pes planus] (acquired), **left** foot

✓5th **M21.5 Acquired clawhand, clubhand, clawfoot and clubfoot**
     EXCLUDES 1   clubfoot, not specified as acquired (Q66.89)
     ✓6th **M21.51 Acquired clawhand**
         M21.511 Acquired clawhand, **right** hand
         M21.512 Acquired clawhand, **left** hand
         M21.519 Acquired clawhand, **unspecified** hand
     ✓6th **M21.52 Acquired clubhand**
         M21.521 Acquired clubhand, **right** hand
         M21.522 Acquired clubhand, **left** hand
         M21.529 Acquired clubhand, **unspecified** hand
     ✓6th **M21.53 Acquired clawfoot**
         DEF: High foot arch with hyperextended toes at metatarsophalangeal joint and flexed toes at distal joints.
         M21.531 Acquired clawfoot, **right** foot
         M21.532 Acquired clawfoot, **left** foot
         M21.539 Acquired clawfoot, **unspecified** foot
     ✓6th **M21.54 Acquired clubfoot**
         M21.541 Acquired clubfoot, **right** foot
         M21.542 Acquired clubfoot, **left** foot
         M21.549 Acquired clubfoot, **unspecified** foot

✓5th **M21.6 Other acquired deformities of foot**
     EXCLUDES 2   deformities of toe (acquired) (M20.1-M20.6-)
     ✓6th **M21.61 Bunion**
         M21.611 Bunion of **right** foot
         M21.612 Bunion of **left** foot
         M21.619 Bunion of **unspecified** foot
     ✓6th **M21.62 Bunionette**
         M21.621 Bunionette of **right** foot
         M21.622 Bunionette of **left** foot
         M21.629 Bunionette of **unspecified** foot
     ✓6th **M21.6X Other acquired deformities of foot**
         M21.6X1 Other acquired deformities of **right** foot
         M21.6X2 Other acquired deformities of **left** foot
         M21.6X9 Other acquired deformities of **unspecified** foot

✓5th **M21.7 Unequal limb length (acquired)**
     NOTE   The site used should correspond to the shorter limb.
     M21.70 Unequal limb length (acquired), **unspecified** site
     ✓6th **M21.72 Unequal limb length (acquired), humerus**
         M21.721 Unequal limb length (acquired), **right** humerus
         M21.722 Unequal limb length (acquired), **left** humerus
         M21.729 Unequal limb length (acquired), **unspecified** humerus
     ✓6th **M21.73 Unequal limb length (acquired), ulna and radius**
         M21.731 Unequal limb length (acquired), **right ulna**
         M21.732 Unequal limb length (acquired), **left ulna**
         M21.733 Unequal limb length (acquired), **right radius**
         M21.734 Unequal limb length (acquired), **left radius**
         M21.739 Unequal limb length (acquired), **unspecified ulna and radius**
     ✓6th **M21.75 Unequal limb length (acquired), femur**
         M21.751 Unequal limb length (acquired), **right femur**
         M21.752 Unequal limb length (acquired), **left femur**
         M21.759 Unequal limb length (acquired), **unspecified femur**
     ✓6th **M21.76 Unequal limb length (acquired), tibia and fibula**
         M21.761 Unequal limb length (acquired), **right tibia**
         M21.762 Unequal limb length (acquired), **left tibia**
         M21.763 Unequal limb length (acquired), **right fibula**
         M21.764 Unequal limb length (acquired), **left fibula**
         M21.769 Unequal limb length (acquired), **unspecified tibia and fibula**

✓5th **M21.8 Other specified acquired deformities of limbs**
     EXCLUDES 2   coxa plana (M91.2)
     M21.80 Other specified acquired deformities of **unspecified limb**
     ✓6th **M21.82 Other specified acquired deformities of upper arm**
         M21.821 Other specified acquired deformities of **right upper arm**
         M21.822 Other specified acquired deformities of **left upper arm**
         M21.829 Other specified acquired deformities of **unspecified upper arm**
     ✓6th **M21.83 Other specified acquired deformities of forearm**
         M21.831 Other specified acquired deformities of **right forearm**
         M21.832 Other specified acquired deformities of **left forearm**
         M21.839 Other specified acquired deformities of **unspecified forearm**
     ✓6th **M21.85 Other specified acquired deformities of thigh**
         M21.851 Other specified acquired deformities of **right thigh**
         M21.852 Other specified acquired deformities of **left thigh**
         M21.859 Other specified acquired deformities of **unspecified thigh**
     ✓6th **M21.86 Other specified acquired deformities of lower leg**
         M21.861 Other specified acquired deformities of **right lower leg**
         M21.862 Other specified acquired deformities of **left lower leg**
         M21.869 Other specified acquired deformities of **unspecified lower leg**

✓5th **M21.9 Unspecified acquired deformity of limb and hand**
     M21.90 Unspecified acquired deformity of **unspecified limb**
     ✓6th **M21.92 Unspecified acquired deformity of upper arm**
         M21.921 Unspecified acquired deformity of **right upper arm**
         M21.922 Unspecified acquired deformity of **left upper arm**
         M21.929 Unspecified acquired deformity of **unspecified upper arm**
     ✓6th **M21.93 Unspecified acquired deformity of forearm**
         M21.931 Unspecified acquired deformity of **right forearm**
         M21.932 Unspecified acquired deformity of **left forearm**
         M21.939 Unspecified acquired deformity of **unspecified forearm**
     ✓6th **M21.94 Unspecified acquired deformity of hand**
         M21.941 Unspecified acquired deformity of hand, **right hand**
         M21.942 Unspecified acquired deformity of hand, **left hand**
         M21.949 Unspecified acquired deformity of hand, **unspecified hand**
     ✓6th **M21.95 Unspecified acquired deformity of thigh**
         M21.951 Unspecified acquired deformity of **right thigh**
         M21.952 Unspecified acquired deformity of **left thigh**
         M21.959 Unspecified acquired deformity of **unspecified thigh**
     ✓6th **M21.96 Unspecified acquired deformity of lower leg**
         M21.961 Unspecified acquired deformity of **right lower leg**
         M21.962 Unspecified acquired deformity of **left lower leg**
         M21.969 Unspecified acquired deformity of **unspecified lower leg**

N Newborn: 0   P Pediatric: 0-17   M Maternity: 12-55   A Adult: 15-124   MCC Major CC Condition   PDxMCC PDx acts as own MCC   CC CC Condition   PDxCC PDx acts as own CC

760   ICD-10-CM 2018

☑4ᵗʰ **M22 Disorder of patella**
> *EXCLUDES 1*   traumatic dislocation of patella (S83.0-)

☑5ᵗʰ **M22.0 Recurrent dislocation of patella**
- **M22.00** Recurrent dislocation of patella, unspecified knee
- **M22.01** Recurrent dislocation of patella, right knee
- **M22.02** Recurrent dislocation of patella, left knee

☑5ᵗʰ **M22.1 Recurrent subluxation of patella**
> Incomplete dislocation of patella
- **M22.10** Recurrent subluxation of patella, unspecified knee
- **M22.11** Recurrent subluxation of patella, right knee
- **M22.12** Recurrent subluxation of patella, left knee

☑5ᵗʰ **M22.2 Patellofemoral disorders**
- ☑6ᵗʰ **M22.2X** Patellofemoral disorders
  - **M22.2X1** Patellofemoral disorders, right knee
  - **M22.2X2** Patellofemoral disorders, left knee
  - **M22.2X9** Patellofemoral disorders, unspecified knee

☑5ᵗʰ **M22.3 Other derangements of patella**
- ☑6ᵗʰ **M22.3X** Other derangements of patella
  - **M22.3X1** Other derangements of patella, right knee
  - **M22.3X2** Other derangements of patella, left knee
  - **M22.3X9** Other derangements of patella, unspecified knee

☑5ᵗʰ **M22.4 Chondromalacia patellae**
- **M22.40** Chondromalacia patellae, unspecified knee
- **M22.41** Chondromalacia patellae, right knee
- **M22.42** Chondromalacia patellae, left knee

☑5ᵗʰ **M22.8 Other disorders of patella**
- ☑6ᵗʰ **M22.8X** Other disorders of patella
  - **M22.8X1** Other disorders of patella, right knee
  - **M22.8X2** Other disorders of patella, left knee
  - **M22.8X9** Other disorders of patella, unspecified knee

☑5ᵗʰ **M22.9 Unspecified disorder of patella**
- **M22.90** Unspecified disorder of patella, unspecified knee
- **M22.91** Unspecified disorder of patella, right knee
- **M22.92** Unspecified disorder of patella, left knee

☑4ᵗʰ **M23 Internal derangement of knee**
> *EXCLUDES 1*   ankylosis (M24.66)
> current injury—see injury of knee and lower leg (S80-S89)
> deformity of knee (M21.-)
> osteochondritis dissecans (M93.2)
> recurrent dislocation or subluxation of joints (M24.4)
> recurrent dislocation or subluxation of patella (M22.0-M22.1)

☑5ᵗʰ **M23.0 Cystic meniscus**
- ☑6ᵗʰ **M23.00** Cystic meniscus, unspecified meniscus
  > Cystic meniscus, unspecified lateral meniscus
  > Cystic meniscus, unspecified medial meniscus
  - **M23.000** Cystic meniscus, unspecified lateral meniscus, right knee
  - **M23.001** Cystic meniscus, unspecified lateral meniscus, left knee
  - **M23.002** Cystic meniscus, unspecified lateral meniscus, unspecified knee
  - **M23.003** Cystic meniscus, unspecified medial meniscus, right knee
  - **M23.004** Cystic meniscus, unspecified medial meniscus, left knee
  - **M23.005** Cystic meniscus, unspecified medial meniscus, unspecified knee
  - **M23.006** Cystic meniscus, unspecified meniscus, right knee
  - **M23.007** Cystic meniscus, unspecified meniscus, left knee
  - **M23.009** Cystic meniscus, unspecified meniscus, unspecified knee
- ☑6ᵗʰ **M23.01** Cystic meniscus, anterior horn of medial meniscus
  - **M23.011** Cystic meniscus, anterior horn of medial meniscus, right knee
  - **M23.012** Cystic meniscus, anterior horn of medial meniscus, left knee
  - **M23.019** Cystic meniscus, anterior horn of medial meniscus, unspecified knee

☑6ᵗʰ **M23.02 Cystic meniscus, posterior horn of medial meniscus**
- **M23.021** Cystic meniscus, posterior horn of medial meniscus, right knee
- **M23.022** Cystic meniscus, posterior horn of medial meniscus, left knee
- **M23.029** Cystic meniscus, posterior horn of medial meniscus, unspecified knee

☑6ᵗʰ **M23.03 Cystic meniscus, other medial meniscus**
- **M23.031** Cystic meniscus, other medial meniscus, right knee
- **M23.032** Cystic meniscus, other medial meniscus, left knee
- **M23.039** Cystic meniscus, other medial meniscus, unspecified knee

☑6ᵗʰ **M23.04 Cystic meniscus, anterior horn of lateral meniscus**
- **M23.041** Cystic meniscus, anterior horn of lateral meniscus, right knee
- **M23.042** Cystic meniscus, anterior horn of lateral meniscus, left knee
- **M23.049** Cystic meniscus, anterior horn of lateral meniscus, unspecified knee

☑6ᵗʰ **M23.05 Cystic meniscus, posterior horn of lateral meniscus**
- **M23.051** Cystic meniscus, posterior horn of lateral meniscus, right knee
- **M23.052** Cystic meniscus, posterior horn of lateral meniscus, left knee
- **M23.059** Cystic meniscus, posterior horn of lateral meniscus, unspecified knee

☑6ᵗʰ **M23.06 Cystic meniscus, other lateral meniscus**
- **M23.061** Cystic meniscus, other lateral meniscus, right knee
- **M23.062** Cystic meniscus, other lateral meniscus, left knee
- **M23.069** Cystic meniscus, other lateral meniscus, unspecified knee

☑5ᵗʰ **M23.2 Derangement of meniscus due to old tear or injury**
> Old bucket-handle tear
- ☑6ᵗʰ **M23.20** Derangement of unspecified meniscus due to old tear or injury
  > Derangement of unspecified lateral meniscus due to old tear or injury
  > Derangement of unspecified medial meniscus due to old tear or injury
  - **M23.200** Derangement of unspecified lateral meniscus due to old tear or injury, right knee
  - **M23.201** Derangement of unspecified lateral meniscus due to old tear or injury, left knee

Derangement of Meniscus

Overhead view of right knee

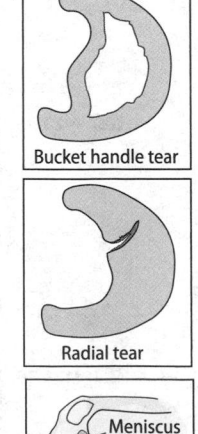

Bucket handle tear

Radial tear

Meniscus

☑ Additional Character Req   ☑x7ᵗʰ Placeholder Alert   Unacceptable PDx   Manifestation   H1 -H14 HAC   HCC CMS-HCC Condition   *EXCLUDES 1* Not Coded Here   *EXCLUDES 2* Not Included Here

ICD-10-CM 2018   **761**

M23.202   **Derangement of unspecified lateral meniscus due to old tear or injury, unspecified knee**

M23.203   **Derangement of unspecified medial meniscus due to old tear or injury, right knee**

M23.204   **Derangement of unspecified medial meniscus due to old tear or injury, left knee**

M23.205   **Derangement of unspecified medial meniscus due to old tear or injury, unspecified knee**

M23.206   **Derangement of unspecified meniscus due to old tear or injury, right knee**

M23.207   **Derangement of unspecified meniscus due to old tear or injury, left knee**

M23.209   **Derangement of unspecified meniscus due to old tear or injury, unspecified knee**

✓6th **M23.21**   **Derangement of anterior horn of medial meniscus due to old tear or injury**

M23.211   **Derangement of anterior horn of medial meniscus due to old tear or injury, right knee**

M23.212   **Derangement of anterior horn of medial meniscus due to old tear or injury, left knee**

M23.219   **Derangement of anterior horn of medial meniscus due to old tear or injury, unspecified knee**

✓6th **M23.22**   **Derangement of posterior horn of medial meniscus due to old tear or injury**

M23.221   **Derangement of posterior horn of medial meniscus due to old tear or injury, right knee**

M23.222   **Derangement of posterior horn of medial meniscus due to old tear or injury, left knee**

M23.229   **Derangement of posterior horn of medial meniscus due to old tear or injury, unspecified knee**

✓6th **M23.23**   **Derangement of other medial meniscus due to old tear or injury**

M23.231   **Derangement of other medial meniscus due to old tear or injury, right knee**

M23.232   **Derangement of other medial meniscus due to old tear or injury, left knee**

M23.239   **Derangement of other medial meniscus due to old tear or injury, unspecified knee**

✓6th **M23.24**   **Derangement of anterior horn of lateral meniscus due to old tear or injury**

M23.241   **Derangement of anterior horn of lateral meniscus due to old tear or injury, right knee**

M23.242   **Derangement of anterior horn of lateral meniscus due to old tear or injury, left knee**

M23.249   **Derangement of anterior horn of lateral meniscus due to old tear or injury, unspecified knee**

✓6th **M23.25**   **Derangement of posterior horn of lateral meniscus due to old tear or injury**

M23.251   **Derangement of posterior horn of lateral meniscus due to old tear or injury, right knee**

M23.252   **Derangement of posterior horn of lateral meniscus due to old tear or injury, left knee**

M23.259   **Derangement of posterior horn of lateral meniscus due to old tear or injury, unspecified knee**

✓6th **M23.26**   **Derangement of other lateral meniscus due to old tear or injury**

M23.261   **Derangement of other lateral meniscus due to old tear or injury, right knee**

M23.262   **Derangement of other lateral meniscus due to old tear or injury, left knee**

M23.269   **Derangement of other lateral meniscus due to old tear or injury, unspecified knee**

✓5th **M23.3**   **Other meniscus derangements**
Degenerate meniscus
Detached meniscus
Retained meniscus

✓6th **M23.30**   **Other meniscus derangements, unspecified meniscus**
Other meniscus derangements, unspecified lateral meniscus
Other meniscus derangements, unspecified medial meniscus

M23.300   **Other meniscus derangements, unspecified lateral meniscus, right knee**

M23.301   **Other meniscus derangements, unspecified lateral meniscus, left knee**

M23.302   **Other meniscus derangements, unspecified lateral meniscus, unspecified knee**

M23.303   **Other meniscus derangements, unspecified medial meniscus, right knee**

M23.304   **Other meniscus derangements, unspecified medial meniscus, left knee**

M23.305   **Other meniscus derangements, unspecified medial meniscus, unspecified knee**

M23.306   **Other meniscus derangements, unspecified meniscus, right knee**

M23.307   **Other meniscus derangements, unspecified meniscus, left knee**

M23.309   **Other meniscus derangements, unspecified meniscus, unspecified knee**

✓6th **M23.31**   **Other meniscus derangements, anterior horn of medial meniscus**

M23.311   **Other meniscus derangements, anterior horn of medial meniscus, right knee**

M23.312   **Other meniscus derangements, anterior horn of medial meniscus, left knee**

M23.319   **Other meniscus derangements, anterior horn of medial meniscus, unspecified knee**

✓6th **M23.32**   **Other meniscus derangements, posterior horn of medial meniscus**

M23.321   **Other meniscus derangements, posterior horn of medial meniscus, right knee**

M23.322   **Other meniscus derangements, posterior horn of medial meniscus, left knee**

M23.329   **Other meniscus derangements, posterior horn of medial meniscus, unspecified knee**

✓6th **M23.33**   **Other meniscus derangements, other medial meniscus**

M23.331   **Other meniscus derangements, other medial meniscus, right knee**

M23.332   **Other meniscus derangements, other medial meniscus, left knee**

M23.339   **Other meniscus derangements, other medial meniscus, unspecified knee**

✓6th **M23.34**   **Other meniscus derangements, anterior horn of lateral meniscus**

M23.341   **Other meniscus derangements, anterior horn of lateral meniscus, right knee**

M23.342   **Other meniscus derangements, anterior horn of lateral meniscus, left knee**

M23.349   **Other meniscus derangements, anterior horn of lateral meniscus, unspecified knee**

✓6th **M23.35**   **Other meniscus derangements, posterior horn of lateral meniscus**

M23.351   **Other meniscus derangements, posterior horn of lateral meniscus, right knee**

M23.352   **Other meniscus derangements, posterior horn of lateral meniscus, left knee**

M23.359   **Other meniscus derangements, posterior horn of lateral meniscus, unspecified knee**

✓6th **M23.36**   **Other meniscus derangements, other lateral meniscus**

M23.361   **Other meniscus derangements, other lateral meniscus, right knee**

M23.362   **Other meniscus derangements, other lateral meniscus, left knee**

M23.369   **Other meniscus derangements, other lateral meniscus, unspecified knee**

N Newborn: 0   P Pediatric: 0-17   M Maternity: 12-55   A Adult: 15-124   MCC Major CC Condition   PDx MCC PDx acts as own MCC   CC CC Condition   PDx CC PDx acts as own CC

762   ICD-10-CM 2018

√5ʰ **M23.4 Loose body in knee**
     M23.40 Loose body in knee, unspecified knee
     M23.41 Loose body in knee, right knee
     M23.42 Loose body in knee, left knee

√5ʰ **M23.5 Chronic instability of knee**
     M23.50 Chronic instability of knee, unspecified knee
     M23.51 Chronic instability of knee, right knee
     M23.52 Chronic instability of knee, left knee

√5ʰ **M23.6 Other spontaneous disruption of ligament(s) of knee**
   √6ʰ **M23.60 Other spontaneous disruption of unspecified ligament of knee**
     M23.601 Other spontaneous disruption of unspecified ligament of right knee
     M23.602 Other spontaneous disruption of unspecified ligament of left knee
     M23.609 Other spontaneous disruption of unspecified ligament of unspecified knee

   √6ʰ **M23.61 Other spontaneous disruption of anterior cruciate ligament of knee**
     M23.611 Other spontaneous disruption of anterior cruciate ligament of right knee
     M23.612 Other spontaneous disruption of anterior cruciate ligament of left knee
     M23.619 Other spontaneous disruption of anterior cruciate ligament of unspecified knee

   √6ʰ **M23.62 Other spontaneous disruption of posterior cruciate ligament of knee**
     M23.621 Other spontaneous disruption of posterior cruciate ligament of right knee
     M23.622 Other spontaneous disruption of posterior cruciate ligament of left knee
     M23.629 Other spontaneous disruption of posterior cruciate ligament of unspecified knee

   √6ʰ **M23.63 Other spontaneous disruption of medial collateral ligament of knee**
     M23.631 Other spontaneous disruption of medial collateral ligament of right knee
     M23.632 Other spontaneous disruption of medial collateral ligament of left knee
     M23.639 Other spontaneous disruption of medial collateral ligament of unspecified knee

   √6ʰ **M23.64 Other spontaneous disruption of lateral collateral ligament of knee**
     M23.641 Other spontaneous disruption of lateral collateral ligament of right knee
     M23.642 Other spontaneous disruption of lateral collateral ligament of left knee
     M23.649 Other spontaneous disruption of lateral collateral ligament of unspecified knee

   √6ʰ **M23.67 Other spontaneous disruption of capsular ligament of knee**
     M23.671 Other spontaneous disruption of capsular ligament of right knee
     M23.672 Other spontaneous disruption of capsular ligament of left knee
     M23.679 Other spontaneous disruption of capsular ligament of unspecified knee

√5ʰ **M23.8 Other internal derangements of knee**
     Laxity of ligament of knee
     Snapping knee
   √6ʰ **M23.8X Other internal derangements of knee**
     M23.8X1 Other internal derangements of right knee
     M23.8X2 Other internal derangements of left knee
     M23.8X9 Other internal derangements of unspecified knee

√5ʰ **M23.9 Unspecified internal derangement of knee**
     M23.90 Unspecified internal derangement of unspecified knee
     M23.91 Unspecified internal derangement of right knee
     M23.92 Unspecified internal derangement of left knee

√4ʰ **M24 Other specific joint derangements**
   EXCLUDES 1 current injury—see injury of joint by body region
   EXCLUDES 2 ganglion (M67.4)
     snapping knee (M23.8-)
     temporomandibular joint disorders (M26.6-)

√5ʰ **M24.0 Loose body in joint**
   EXCLUDES 2 loose body in knee (M23.4)
     M24.00 Loose body in unspecified joint
   √6ʰ **M24.01 Loose body in shoulder**
     M24.011 Loose body in right shoulder
     M24.012 Loose body in left shoulder
     M24.019 Loose body in unspecified shoulder
   √6ʰ **M24.02 Loose body in elbow**
     M24.021 Loose body in right elbow
     M24.022 Loose body in left elbow
     M24.029 Loose body in unspecified elbow
   √6ʰ **M24.03 Loose body in wrist**
     M24.031 Loose body in right wrist
     M24.032 Loose body in left wrist
     M24.039 Loose body in unspecified wrist
   √6ʰ **M24.04 Loose body in finger joints**
     M24.041 Loose body in right finger joint(s)
     M24.042 Loose body in left finger joint(s)
     M24.049 Loose body in unspecified finger joint(s)
   √6ʰ **M24.05 Loose body in hip**
     M24.051 Loose body in right hip
     M24.052 Loose body in left hip
     M24.059 Loose body in unspecified hip
   √6ʰ **M24.07 Loose body in ankle and toe joints**
     M24.071 Loose body in right ankle
     M24.072 Loose body in left ankle
     M24.073 Loose body in unspecified ankle
     M24.074 Loose body in right toe joint(s)
     M24.075 Loose body in left toe joint(s)
     M24.076 Loose body in unspecified toe joints
     M24.08 Loose body, other site

√5ʰ **M24.1 Other articular cartilage disorders**
   EXCLUDES 2 chondrocalcinosis (M11.1, M11.2-)
     internal derangement of knee (M23.-)
     metastatic calcification (E83.5)
     ochronosis (E70.2)
     M24.10 Other articular cartilage disorders, unspecified site
   √6ʰ **M24.11 Other articular cartilage disorders, shoulder**
     M24.111 Other articular cartilage disorders, right shoulder
     M24.112 Other articular cartilage disorders, left shoulder
     M24.119 Other articular cartilage disorders, unspecified shoulder
   √6ʰ **M24.12 Other articular cartilage disorders, elbow**
     M24.121 Other articular cartilage disorders, right elbow
     M24.122 Other articular cartilage disorders, left elbow
     M24.129 Other articular cartilage disorders, unspecified elbow
   √6ʰ **M24.13 Other articular cartilage disorders, wrist**
     M24.131 Other articular cartilage disorders, right wrist
     M24.132 Other articular cartilage disorders, left wrist
     M24.139 Other articular cartilage disorders, unspecified wrist
   √6ʰ **M24.14 Other articular cartilage disorders, hand**
     M24.141 Other articular cartilage disorders, right hand
     M24.142 Other articular cartilage disorders, left hand
     M24.149 Other articular cartilage disorders, unspecified hand

✓6ᵗʰ M24.15 Other articular cartilage disorders, hip
     M24.151 Other articular cartilage disorders, right hip
     M24.152 Other articular cartilage disorders, left hip
     M24.159 Other articular cartilage disorders, unspecified hip

✓6ᵗʰ M24.17 Other articular cartilage disorders, ankle and foot
     M24.171 Other articular cartilage disorders, right ankle
     M24.172 Other articular cartilage disorders, left ankle
     M24.173 Other articular cartilage disorders, unspecified ankle
     M24.174 Other articular cartilage disorders, right foot
     M24.175 Other articular cartilage disorders, left foot
     M24.176 Other articular cartilage disorders, unspecified foot

✓5ᵗʰ M24.2 Disorder of ligament
     Instability secondary to old ligament injury
     Ligamentous laxity NOS
     EXCLUDES 1   *familial ligamentous laxity (M35.7)*
     EXCLUDES 2   *internal derangement of knee (M23.5-M23.89)*

     M24.20 Disorder of ligament, unspecified site
✓6ᵗʰ M24.21 Disorder of ligament, shoulder
     M24.211 Disorder of ligament, right shoulder
     M24.212 Disorder of ligament, left shoulder
     M24.219 Disorder of ligament, unspecified shoulder
✓6ᵗʰ M24.22 Disorder of ligament, elbow
     M24.221 Disorder of ligament, right elbow
     M24.222 Disorder of ligament, left elbow
     M24.229 Disorder of ligament, unspecified elbow
✓6ᵗʰ M24.23 Disorder of ligament, wrist
     M24.231 Disorder of ligament, right wrist
     M24.232 Disorder of ligament, left wrist
     M24.239 Disorder of ligament, unspecified wrist
✓6ᵗʰ M24.24 Disorder of ligament, hand
     M24.241 Disorder of ligament, right hand
     M24.242 Disorder of ligament, left hand
     M24.249 Disorder of ligament, unspecified hand
✓6ᵗʰ M24.25 Disorder of ligament, hip
     M24.251 Disorder of ligament, right hip
     M24.252 Disorder of ligament, left hip
     M24.259 Disorder of ligament, unspecified hip
✓6ᵗʰ M24.27 Disorder of ligament, ankle and foot
     M24.271 Disorder of ligament, right ankle
     M24.272 Disorder of ligament, left ankle
     M24.273 Disorder of ligament, unspecified ankle
     M24.274 Disorder of ligament, right foot
     M24.275 Disorder of ligament, left foot
     M24.276 Disorder of ligament, unspecified foot
     M24.28 Disorder of ligament, vertebrae

✓5ᵗʰ M24.3 Pathological dislocation of joint, not elsewhere classified
     EXCLUDES 1   *congenital dislocation or displacement of joint—see congenital malformations and deformations of the musculoskeletal system (Q65-Q79)*
     current injury—see injury of joints and ligaments by body region
     recurrent dislocation of joint (M24.4-)

     M24.30 Pathological dislocation of unspecified joint, not elsewhere classified
✓6ᵗʰ M24.31 Pathological dislocation of shoulder, not elsewhere classified
     M24.311 Pathological dislocation of right shoulder, not elsewhere classified
     M24.312 Pathological dislocation of left shoulder, not elsewhere classified
     M24.319 Pathological dislocation of unspecified shoulder, not elsewhere classified
✓6ᵗʰ M24.32 Pathological dislocation of elbow, not elsewhere classified
     M24.321 Pathological dislocation of right elbow, not elsewhere classified

M24.322 Pathological dislocation of left elbow, not elsewhere classified
M24.329 Pathological dislocation of unspecified elbow, not elsewhere classified
✓6ᵗʰ M24.33 Pathological dislocation of wrist, not elsewhere classified
     M24.331 Pathological dislocation of right wrist, not elsewhere classified
     M24.332 Pathological dislocation of left wrist, not elsewhere classified
     M24.339 Pathological dislocation of unspecified wrist, not elsewhere classified
✓6ᵗʰ M24.34 Pathological dislocation of hand, not elsewhere classified
     M24.341 Pathological dislocation of right hand, not elsewhere classified
     M24.342 Pathological dislocation of left hand, not elsewhere classified
     M24.349 Pathological dislocation of unspecified hand, not elsewhere classified
✓6ᵗʰ M24.35 Pathological dislocation of hip, not elsewhere classified
     M24.351 Pathological dislocation of right hip, not elsewhere classified
     M24.352 Pathological dislocation of left hip, not elsewhere classified
     M24.359 Pathological dislocation of unspecified hip, not elsewhere classified
✓6ᵗʰ M24.36 Pathological dislocation of knee, not elsewhere classified
     M24.361 Pathological dislocation of right knee, not elsewhere classified
     M24.362 Pathological dislocation of left knee, not elsewhere classified
     M24.369 Pathological dislocation of unspecified knee, not elsewhere classified
✓6ᵗʰ M24.37 Pathological dislocation of ankle and foot, not elsewhere classified
     M24.371 Pathological dislocation of right ankle, not elsewhere classified
     M24.372 Pathological dislocation of left ankle, not elsewhere classified
     M24.373 Pathological dislocation of unspecified ankle, not elsewhere classified
     M24.374 Pathological dislocation of right foot, not elsewhere classified
     M24.375 Pathological dislocation of left foot, not elsewhere classified
     M24.376 Pathological dislocation of unspecified foot, not elsewhere classified

✓5ᵗʰ M24.4 Recurrent dislocation of joint
     Recurrent subluxation of joint
     EXCLUDES 2   *recurrent dislocation of patella (M22.0-M22.1)*
     recurrent vertebral dislocation (M43.3-, M43.4, M43.5-)

     M24.40 Recurrent dislocation, unspecified joint
✓6ᵗʰ M24.41 Recurrent dislocation, shoulder
     M24.411 Recurrent dislocation, right shoulder
     M24.412 Recurrent dislocation, left shoulder
     M24.419 Recurrent dislocation, unspecified shoulder
✓6ᵗʰ M24.42 Recurrent dislocation, elbow
     M24.421 Recurrent dislocation, right elbow
     M24.422 Recurrent dislocation, left elbow
     M24.429 Recurrent dislocation, unspecified elbow
✓6ᵗʰ M24.43 Recurrent dislocation, wrist
     M24.431 Recurrent dislocation, right wrist
     M24.432 Recurrent dislocation, left wrist
     M24.439 Recurrent dislocation, unspecified wrist
✓6ᵗʰ M24.44 Recurrent dislocation, hand and finger(s)
     M24.441 Recurrent dislocation, right hand
     M24.442 Recurrent dislocation, left hand
     M24.443 Recurrent dislocation, unspecified hand
     M24.444 Recurrent dislocation, right finger
     M24.445 Recurrent dislocation, left finger
     M24.446 Recurrent dislocation, unspecified finger

Ⓝ Newborn: 0   Ⓟ Pediatric: 0-17   Ⓜ Maternity: 12-55   Ⓐ Adult: 15-124   **MCC** Major CC Condition   **PDxMCC** PDx acts as own MCC   **CC** CC Condition   **PDxCC** PDx acts as own CC

✓6ᵗʰ **M24.45** Recurrent dislocation, hip
  M24.451 Recurrent dislocation, right hip
  M24.452 Recurrent dislocation, left hip
  M24.459 Recurrent dislocation, unspecified hip

✓6ᵗʰ **M24.46** Recurrent dislocation, knee
  M24.461 Recurrent dislocation, right knee
  M24.462 Recurrent dislocation, left knee
  M24.469 Recurrent dislocation, unspecified knee

✓6ᵗʰ **M24.47** Recurrent dislocation, ankle, foot and toes
  M24.471 Recurrent dislocation, right ankle
  M24.472 Recurrent dislocation, left ankle
  M24.473 Recurrent dislocation, unspecified ankle
  M24.474 Recurrent dislocation, right foot
  M24.475 Recurrent dislocation, left foot
  M24.476 Recurrent dislocation, unspecified foot
  M24.477 Recurrent dislocation, right toe(s)
  M24.478 Recurrent dislocation, left toe(s)
  M24.479 Recurrent dislocation, unspecified toe(s)

✓5ᵗʰ **M24.5** Contracture of joint
  EXCLUDES 1 contracture of muscle without contracture of joint (M62.4-)
  contracture of tendon (sheath) without contracture of joint (M62.4-)
  Dupuytren's contracture (M72.0)
  EXCLUDES 2 acquired deformities of limbs (M20-M21)
  AHA: 2016, 2Q, 6

  M24.50 Contracture, unspecified joint

✓6ᵗʰ **M24.51** Contracture, shoulder
  M24.511 Contracture, right shoulder
  M24.512 Contracture, left shoulder
  M24.519 Contracture, unspecified shoulder

✓6ᵗʰ **M24.52** Contracture, elbow
  M24.521 Contracture, right elbow
  M24.522 Contracture, left elbow
  M24.529 Contracture, unspecified elbow

✓6ᵗʰ **M24.53** Contracture, wrist
  M24.531 Contracture, right wrist
  M24.532 Contracture, left wrist
  M24.539 Contracture, unspecified wrist

✓6ᵗʰ **M24.54** Contracture, hand
  M24.541 Contracture, right hand
  M24.542 Contracture, left hand
  M24.549 Contracture, unspecified hand

✓6ᵗʰ **M24.55** Contracture, hip
  M24.551 Contracture, right hip
  M24.552 Contracture, left hip
  M24.559 Contracture, unspecified hip

✓6ᵗʰ **M24.56** Contracture, knee
  M24.561 Contracture, right knee
  M24.562 Contracture, left knee
  M24.569 Contracture, unspecified knee

✓6ᵗʰ **M24.57** Contracture, ankle and foot
  M24.571 Contracture, right ankle
  M24.572 Contracture, left ankle
  M24.573 Contracture, unspecified ankle
  M24.574 Contracture, right foot
  M24.575 Contracture, left foot
  M24.576 Contracture, unspecified foot

✓5ᵗʰ **M24.6** Ankylosis of joint
  EXCLUDES 1 stiffness of joint without ankylosis (M25.6-)
  EXCLUDES 2 spine (M43.2-)
  M24.60 Ankylosis, unspecified joint

✓6ᵗʰ **M24.61** Ankylosis, shoulder
  M24.611 Ankylosis, right shoulder
  M24.612 Ankylosis, left shoulder
  M24.619 Ankylosis, unspecified shoulder

✓6ᵗʰ **M24.62** Ankylosis, elbow
  M24.621 Ankylosis, right elbow
  M24.622 Ankylosis, left elbow
  M24.629 Ankylosis, unspecified elbow

✓6ᵗʰ **M24.63** Ankylosis, wrist
  M24.631 Ankylosis, right wrist

  M24.632 Ankylosis, left wrist
  M24.639 Ankylosis, unspecified wrist

✓6ᵗʰ **M24.64** Ankylosis, hand
  M24.641 Ankylosis, right hand
  M24.642 Ankylosis, left hand
  M24.649 Ankylosis, unspecified hand

✓6ᵗʰ **M24.65** Ankylosis, hip
  M24.651 Ankylosis, right hip
  M24.652 Ankylosis, left hip
  M24.659 Ankylosis, unspecified hip

✓6ᵗʰ **M24.66** Ankylosis, knee
  M24.661 Ankylosis, right knee
  M24.662 Ankylosis, left knee
  M24.669 Ankylosis, unspecified knee

✓6ᵗʰ **M24.67** Ankylosis, ankle and foot
  M24.671 Ankylosis, right ankle
  M24.672 Ankylosis, left ankle
  M24.673 Ankylosis, unspecified ankle
  M24.674 Ankylosis, right foot
  M24.675 Ankylosis, left foot
  M24.676 Ankylosis, unspecified foot

M24.7 Protrusio acetabuli

✓5ᵗʰ **M24.8** Other specific joint derangements, not elsewhere classified
  EXCLUDES 2 iliotibial band syndrome (M76.3)
  M24.80 Other specific joint derangements of unspecified joint, not elsewhere classified

✓6ᵗʰ **M24.81** Other specific joint derangements of shoulder, not elsewhere classified
  M24.811 Other specific joint derangements of right shoulder, not elsewhere classified
  M24.812 Other specific joint derangements of left shoulder, not elsewhere classified
  M24.819 Other specific joint derangements of unspecified shoulder, not elsewhere classified

✓6ᵗʰ **M24.82** Other specific joint derangements of elbow, not elsewhere classified
  M24.821 Other specific joint derangements of right elbow, not elsewhere classified
  M24.822 Other specific joint derangements of left elbow, not elsewhere classified
  M24.829 Other specific joint derangements of unspecified elbow, not elsewhere classified

✓6ᵗʰ **M24.83** Other specific joint derangements of wrist, not elsewhere classified
  M24.831 Other specific joint derangements of right wrist, not elsewhere classified
  M24.832 Other specific joint derangements of left wrist, not elsewhere classified
  M24.839 Other specific joint derangements of unspecified wrist, not elsewhere classified

✓6ᵗʰ **M24.84** Other specific joint derangements of hand, not elsewhere classified
  M24.841 Other specific joint derangements of right hand, not elsewhere classified
  M24.842 Other specific joint derangements of left hand, not elsewhere classified
  M24.849 Other specific joint derangements of unspecified hand, not elsewhere classified

✓6ᵗʰ **M24.85** Other specific joint derangements of hip, not elsewhere classified
  Irritable hip
  M24.851 Other specific joint derangements of right hip, not elsewhere classified
  M24.852 Other specific joint derangements of left hip, not elsewhere classified
  M24.859 Other specific joint derangements of unspecified hip, not elsewhere classified

✓6ᵗʰ **M24.87** Other specific joint derangements of ankle and foot, not elsewhere classified
  M24.871 Other specific joint derangements of right ankle, not elsewhere classified
  M24.872 Other specific joint derangements of left ankle, not elsewhere classified

---

✔ Additional Character Req ✓x7ᵗʰ Placeholder Alert Unacceptable PDx Manifestation H1–H14 HAC HCC CMS-HCC Condition EXCLUDES 1 Not Coded Here EXCLUDES 2 Not Included Here

M24.873   **Other specific joint derangements of unspecified ankle, not elsewhere classified**

M24.874   **Other specific joint derangements of right foot, not elsewhere classified**

M24.875   **Other specific joint derangements left foot, not elsewhere classified**

M24.876   **Other specific joint derangements of unspecified foot, not elsewhere classified**

M24.9   Joint derangement, unspecified

✓4ᵗʰ **M25   Other joint disorder, not elsewhere classified**

EXCLUDES 2   *abnormality of gait and mobility (R26.-)*
              acquired deformities of limb (M20-M21)
              calcification of bursa (M71.4-)
              calcification of shoulder (joint) (M75.3)
              calcification of tendon (M65.2-)
              difficulty in walking (R26.2)
              temporomandibular joint disorder (M26.6-)

✓5ᵗʰ **M25.0   Hemarthrosis**

EXCLUDES 1   *current injury—see injury of joint by body region*
              hemophilic arthropathy (M36.2)

M25.00   **Hemarthrosis, unspecified joint**   CC
     CC Excl: PDX collection 868

✓6ᵗʰ M25.01   **Hemarthrosis, shoulder**

     CC Excl: For CC codes in subcategory M25.01: PDX collection 869

M25.011   **Hemarthrosis, right shoulder**   CC
M25.012   **Hemarthrosis, left shoulder**   CC
M25.019   **Hemarthrosis, unspecified shoulder**   CC

✓6ᵗʰ M25.02   **Hemarthrosis, elbow**

     CC Excl: For CC codes in subcategory M25.02: PDX collection 870

M25.021   **Hemarthrosis, right elbow**   CC
M25.022   **Hemarthrosis, left elbow**   CC
M25.029   **Hemarthrosis, unspecified elbow**   CC

✓6ᵗʰ M25.03   **Hemarthrosis, wrist**

     CC Excl: For CC codes in subcategory M25.03: PDX collection 871

M25.031   **Hemarthrosis, right wrist**   CC
M25.032   **Hemarthrosis, left wrist**   CC
M25.039   **Hemarthrosis, unspecified wrist**   CC

✓6ᵗʰ M25.04   **Hemarthrosis, hand**

     CC Excl: For CC codes in subcategory M25.04: PDX collection 872

M25.041   **Hemarthrosis, right hand**   CC
M25.042   **Hemarthrosis, left hand**   CC
M25.049   **Hemarthrosis, unspecified hand**   CC

✓6ᵗʰ M25.05   **Hemarthrosis, hip**

     CC Excl: For CC codes in subcategory M25.05: PDX collection 868

M25.051   **Hemarthrosis, right hip**   CC
M25.052   **Hemarthrosis, left hip**   CC
M25.059   **Hemarthrosis, unspecified hip**   CC

✓6ᵗʰ M25.06   **Hemarthrosis, knee**

     CC Excl: For CC codes in subcategory M25.06: PDX collection 873

M25.061   **Hemarthrosis, right knee**   CC
M25.062   **Hemarthrosis, left knee**   CC
M25.069   **Hemarthrosis, unspecified knee**   CC

✓6ᵗʰ M25.07   **Hemarthrosis, ankle and foot**

     CC Excl: For CC codes in subcategory M25.07: PDX collection 873

M25.071   **Hemarthrosis, right ankle**   CC
M25.072   **Hemarthrosis, left ankle**   CC
M25.073   **Hemarthrosis, unspecified ankle**   CC
M25.074   **Hemarthrosis, right foot**   CC
M25.075   **Hemarthrosis, left foot**   CC
M25.076   **Hemarthrosis, unspecified foot**   CC

M25.08   **Hemarthrosis, other specified site**   CC
     Hemarthrosis, vertebrae
     CC Excl: PDX collection 868

✓5ᵗʰ **M25.1   Fistula of joint**

M25.10   **Fistula, unspecified joint**

✓6ᵗʰ M25.11   **Fistula, shoulder**

M25.111   **Fistula, right shoulder**
M25.112   **Fistula, left shoulder**
M25.119   **Fistula, unspecified shoulder**

✓6ᵗʰ M25.12   **Fistula, elbow**

M25.121   **Fistula, right elbow**
M25.122   **Fistula, left elbow**
M25.129   **Fistula, unspecified elbow**

✓6ᵗʰ M25.13   **Fistula, wrist**

M25.131   **Fistula, right wrist**
M25.132   **Fistula, left wrist**
M25.139   **Fistula, unspecified wrist**

✓6ᵗʰ M25.14   **Fistula, hand**

M25.141   **Fistula, right hand**
M25.142   **Fistula, left hand**
M25.149   **Fistula, unspecified hand**

✓6ᵗʰ M25.15   **Fistula, hip**

M25.151   **Fistula, right hip**
M25.152   **Fistula, left hip**
M25.159   **Fistula, unspecified hip**

✓6ᵗʰ M25.16   **Fistula, knee**

M25.161   **Fistula, right knee**
M25.162   **Fistula, left knee**
M25.169   **Fistula, unspecified knee**

✓6ᵗʰ M25.17   **Fistula, ankle and foot**

M25.171   **Fistula, right ankle**
M25.172   **Fistula, left ankle**
M25.173   **Fistula, unspecified ankle**
M25.174   **Fistula, right foot**
M25.175   **Fistula, left foot**
M25.176   **Fistula, unspecified foot**

M25.18   **Fistula, other specified site**
     Fistula, vertebrae

✓5ᵗʰ **M25.2   Flail joint**

M25.20   **Flail joint, unspecified joint**

✓6ᵗʰ M25.21   **Flail joint, shoulder**

M25.211   **Flail joint, right shoulder**
M25.212   **Flail joint, left shoulder**
M25.219   **Flail joint, unspecified shoulder**

✓6ᵗʰ M25.22   **Flail joint, elbow**

M25.221   **Flail joint, right elbow**
M25.222   **Flail joint, left elbow**
M25.229   **Flail joint, unspecified elbow**

✓6ᵗʰ M25.23   **Flail joint, wrist**

M25.231   **Flail joint, right wrist**
M25.232   **Flail joint, left wrist**
M25.239   **Flail joint, unspecified wrist**

✓6ᵗʰ M25.24   **Flail joint, hand**

M25.241   **Flail joint, right hand**
M25.242   **Flail joint, left hand**
M25.249   **Flail joint, unspecified hand**

✓6ᵗʰ M25.25   **Flail joint, hip**

M25.251   **Flail joint, right hip**
M25.252   **Flail joint, left hip**
M25.259   **Flail joint, unspecified hip**

✓6ᵗʰ M25.26   **Flail joint, knee**

M25.261   **Flail joint, right knee**
M25.262   **Flail joint, left knee**
M25.269   **Flail joint, unspecified knee**

✓6ᵗʰ M25.27   **Flail joint, ankle and foot**

M25.271   **Flail joint, right ankle and foot**
M25.272   **Flail joint, left ankle and foot**
M25.279   **Flail joint, unspecified ankle and foot**

M25.28   **Flail joint, other site**

✓5th **M25.3 Other instability of joint**
   EXCLUDES1   *instability of joint secondary to old ligament injury (M24.2-)*
   instability of joint secondary to removal of joint prosthesis (M96.8-)
   EXCLUDES2   *spinal instabilities (M53.2-)*
   M25.30 Other instability, unspecified joint
   ✓6th **M25.31 Other instability, shoulder**
      M25.311 Other instability, right shoulder
      M25.312 Other instability, left shoulder
      M25.319 Other instability, unspecified shoulder
   ✓6th **M25.32 Other instability, elbow**
      M25.321 Other instability, right elbow
      M25.322 Other instability, left elbow
      M25.329 Other instability, unspecified elbow
   ✓6th **M25.33 Other instability, wrist**
      M25.331 Other instability, right wrist
      M25.332 Other instability, left wrist
      M25.339 Other instability, unspecified wrist
   ✓6th **M25.34 Other instability, hand**
      M25.341 Other instability, right hand
      M25.342 Other instability, left hand
      M25.349 Other instability, unspecified hand
   ✓6th **M25.35 Other instability, hip**
      M25.351 Other instability, right hip
      M25.352 Other instability, left hip
      M25.359 Other instability, unspecified hip
   ✓6th **M25.36 Other instability, knee**
      M25.361 Other instability, right knee
      M25.362 Other instability, left knee
      M25.369 Other instability, unspecified knee
   ✓6th **M25.37 Other instability, ankle and foot**
      M25.371 Other instability, right ankle
      M25.372 Other instability, left ankle
      M25.373 Other instability, unspecified ankle
      M25.374 Other instability, right foot
      M25.375 Other instability, left foot
      M25.376 Other instability, unspecified foot

✓5th **M25.4 Effusion of joint**
   EXCLUDES1   *hydrarthrosis in yaws (A66.6)*
   intermittent hydrarthrosis (M12.4-)
   other infective (teno)synovitis (M65.1-)
   M25.40 Effusion, unspecified joint
   ✓6th **M25.41 Effusion, shoulder**
      M25.411 Effusion, right shoulder
      M25.412 Effusion, left shoulder
      M25.419 Effusion, unspecified shoulder
   ✓6th **M25.42 Effusion, elbow**
      M25.421 Effusion, right elbow
      M25.422 Effusion, left elbow
      M25.429 Effusion, unspecified elbow
   ✓6th **M25.43 Effusion, wrist**
      M25.431 Effusion, right wrist
      M25.432 Effusion, left wrist
      M25.439 Effusion, unspecified wrist
   ✓6th **M25.44 Effusion, hand**
      M25.441 Effusion, right hand
      M25.442 Effusion, left hand
      M25.449 Effusion, unspecified hand
   ✓6th **M25.45 Effusion, hip**
      M25.451 Effusion, right hip
      M25.452 Effusion, left hip
      M25.459 Effusion, unspecified hip
   ✓6th **M25.46 Effusion, knee**
      M25.461 Effusion, right knee
      M25.462 Effusion, left knee
      M25.469 Effusion, unspecified knee
   ✓6th **M25.47 Effusion, ankle and foot**
      M25.471 Effusion, right ankle
      M25.472 Effusion, left ankle
      M25.473 Effusion, unspecified ankle
      M25.474 Effusion, right foot

      M25.475 Effusion, left foot
      M25.476 Effusion, unspecified foot
   M25.48 Effusion, other site

✓5th **M25.5 Pain in joint**
   EXCLUDES2   *pain in hand (M79.64-)*
   pain in fingers (M79.64-)
   pain in foot (M79.67-)
   pain in limb (M79.6-)
   pain in toes (M79.67-)
   M25.50 Pain in unspecified joint
   ✓6th **M25.51 Pain in shoulder**
      M25.511 Pain in right shoulder
      M25.512 Pain in left shoulder
      M25.519 Pain in unspecified shoulder
   ✓6th **M25.52 Pain in elbow**
      M25.521 Pain in right elbow
      M25.522 Pain in left elbow
      M25.529 Pain in unspecified elbow
   ✓6th **M25.53 Pain in wrist**
      M25.531 Pain in right wrist
      M25.532 Pain in left wrist
      M25.539 Pain in unspecified wrist
   ✓6th **M25.54 Pain in joints of hand**
      M25.541 Pain in joints of right hand
      M25.542 Pain in joints of left hand
      M25.549 Pain in joints of unspecified hand
         Pain in joints of hand NOS
   ✓6th **M25.55 Pain in hip**
      M25.551 Pain in right hip
      M25.552 Pain in left hip
      M25.559 Pain in unspecified hip
   ✓6th **M25.56 Pain in knee**
      M25.561 Pain in right knee
      M25.562 Pain in left knee
      M25.569 Pain in unspecified knee
   ✓6th **M25.57 Pain in ankle and joints of foot**
      M25.571 Pain in right ankle and joints of right foot
      M25.572 Pain in left ankle and joints of left foot
      M25.579 Pain in unspecified ankle and joints of unspecified foot

✓5th **M25.6 Stiffness of joint, not elsewhere classified**
   EXCLUDES1   *ankylosis of joint (M24.6-)*
   contracture of joint (M24.5-)
   M25.60 Stiffness of unspecified joint, not elsewhere classified
   ✓6th **M25.61 Stiffness of shoulder, not elsewhere classified**
      M25.611 Stiffness of right shoulder, not elsewhere classified
      M25.612 Stiffness of left shoulder, not elsewhere classified
      M25.619 Stiffness of unspecified shoulder, not elsewhere classified
   ✓6th **M25.62 Stiffness of elbow, not elsewhere classified**
      M25.621 Stiffness of right elbow, not elsewhere classified
      M25.622 Stiffness of left elbow, not elsewhere classified
      M25.629 Stiffness of unspecified elbow, not elsewhere classified
   ✓6th **M25.63 Stiffness of wrist, not elsewhere classified**
      M25.631 Stiffness of right wrist, not elsewhere classified
      M25.632 Stiffness of left wrist, not elsewhere classified
      M25.639 Stiffness of unspecified wrist, not elsewhere classified
   ✓6th **M25.64 Stiffness of hand, not elsewhere classified**
      M25.641 Stiffness of right hand, not elsewhere classified
      M25.642 Stiffness of left hand, not elsewhere classified
      M25.649 Stiffness of unspecified hand, not elsewhere classified

☑6ᵗʰ **M25.65 Stiffness of hip, not elsewhere classified**
     M25.651 **Stiffness of right hip, not elsewhere classified**
     M25.652 **Stiffness of left hip, not elsewhere classified**
     M25.659 **Stiffness of unspecified hip, not elsewhere classified**

☑6ᵗʰ **M25.66 Stiffness of knee, not elsewhere classified**
     M25.661 **Stiffness of right knee, not elsewhere classified**
     M25.662 **Stiffness of left knee, not elsewhere classified**
     M25.669 **Stiffness of unspecified knee, not elsewhere classified**

☑6ᵗʰ **M25.67 Stiffness of ankle and foot, not elsewhere classified**
     M25.671 **Stiffness of right ankle, not elsewhere classified**
     M25.672 **Stiffness of left ankle, not elsewhere classified**
     M25.673 **Stiffness of unspecified ankle, not elsewhere classified**
     M25.674 **Stiffness of right foot, not elsewhere classified**
     M25.675 **Stiffness of left foot, not elsewhere classified**
     M25.676 **Stiffness of unspecified foot, not elsewhere classified**

☑5ᵗʰ **M25.7 Osteophyte**
     M25.70 **Osteophyte, unspecified joint**

☑6ᵗʰ **M25.71 Osteophyte, shoulder**
     M25.711 **Osteophyte, right shoulder**
     M25.712 **Osteophyte, left shoulder**
     M25.719 **Osteophyte, unspecified shoulder**

☑6ᵗʰ **M25.72 Osteophyte, elbow**
     M25.721 **Osteophyte, right elbow**
     M25.722 **Osteophyte, left elbow**
     M25.729 **Osteophyte, unspecified elbow**

☑6ᵗʰ **M25.73 Osteophyte, wrist**
     M25.731 **Osteophyte, right wrist**
     M25.732 **Osteophyte, left wrist**
     M25.739 **Osteophyte, unspecified wrist**

☑6ᵗʰ **M25.74 Osteophyte, hand**
     M25.741 **Osteophyte, right hand**
     M25.742 **Osteophyte, left hand**
     M25.749 **Osteophyte, unspecified hand**

☑6ᵗʰ **M25.75 Osteophyte, hip**
     M25.751 **Osteophyte, right hip**
     M25.752 **Osteophyte, left hip**
     M25.759 **Osteophyte, unspecified hip**

☑6ᵗʰ **M25.76 Osteophyte, knee**
     M25.761 **Osteophyte, right knee**
     M25.762 **Osteophyte, left knee**
     M25.769 **Osteophyte, unspecified knee**

☑6ᵗʰ **M25.77 Osteophyte, ankle and foot**
     M25.771 **Osteophyte, right ankle**
     M25.772 **Osteophyte, left ankle**
     M25.773 **Osteophyte, unspecified ankle**
     M25.774 **Osteophyte, right foot**
     M25.775 **Osteophyte, left foot**
     M25.776 **Osteophyte, unspecified foot**
     M25.78 **Osteophyte, vertebrae**

☑5ᵗʰ **M25.8 Other specified joint disorders**
     M25.80 **Other specified joint disorders, unspecified joint**

☑6ᵗʰ **M25.81 Other specified joint disorders, shoulder**
     M25.811 **Other specified joint disorders, right shoulder**
     M25.812 **Other specified joint disorders, left shoulder**
     M25.819 **Other specified joint disorders, unspecified shoulder**

☑6ᵗʰ **M25.82 Other specified joint disorders, elbow**
     M25.821 **Other specified joint disorders, right elbow**
     M25.822 **Other specified joint disorders, left elbow**

     M25.829 **Other specified joint disorders, unspecified elbow**

☑6ᵗʰ **M25.83 Other specified joint disorders, wrist**
     M25.831 **Other specified joint disorders, right wrist**
     M25.832 **Other specified joint disorders, left wrist**
     M25.839 **Other specified joint disorders, unspecified wrist**

☑6ᵗʰ **M25.84 Other specified joint disorders, hand**
     M25.841 **Other specified joint disorders, right hand**
     M25.842 **Other specified joint disorders, left hand**
     M25.849 **Other specified joint disorders, unspecified hand**

☑6ᵗʰ **M25.85 Other specified joint disorders, hip**
     AHA: 2014, 4Q, 25
     M25.851 **Other specified joint disorders, right hip**
     M25.852 **Other specified joint disorders, left hip**
     M25.859 **Other specified joint disorders, unspecified hip**

☑6ᵗʰ **M25.86 Other specified joint disorders, knee**
     M25.861 **Other specified joint disorders, right knee**
     M25.862 **Other specified joint disorders, left knee**
     M25.869 **Other specified joint disorders, unspecified knee**

☑6ᵗʰ **M25.87 Other specified joint disorders, ankle and foot**
     M25.871 **Other specified joint disorders, right ankle and foot**
     M25.872 **Other specified joint disorders, left ankle and foot**
     M25.879 **Other specified joint disorders, unspecified ankle and foot**

     M25.9 **Joint disorder, unspecified**

Dentofacial anomalies [including malocclusion] and other disorders of jaw (M26-M27)

EXCLUDES 1   *hemifacial atrophy or hypertrophy (Q67.4)*
     unilateral condylar hyperplasia or hypoplasia (M27.8)

☑4ᵗʰ **M26 Dentofacial anomalies [including malocclusion]**

☑5ᵗʰ **M26.0 Major anomalies of jaw size**
     EXCLUDES 1   *acromegaly (E22.0)*
         Robin's syndrome (Q87.0)
     M26.00 **Unspecified anomaly of jaw size**
     M26.01 **Maxillary hyperplasia**
     M26.02 **Maxillary hypoplasia**
         AHA: 2014, 3Q, 23
     M26.03 **Mandibular hyperplasia**
     M26.04 **Mandibular hypoplasia**
     M26.05 **Macrogenia**
     M26.06 **Microgenia**
     M26.07 **Excessive tuberosity of jaw**
         Entire maxillary tuberosity
     M26.09 **Other specified anomalies of jaw size**

☑5ᵗʰ **M26.1 Anomalies of jaw-cranial base relationship**
     M26.10 **Unspecified anomaly of jaw-cranial base relationship**
     M26.11 **Maxillary asymmetry**
     M26.12 **Other jaw asymmetry**
     M26.19 **Other specified anomalies of jaw-cranial base relationship**

☑5ᵗʰ **M26.2 Anomalies of dental arch relationship**
     M26.20 **Unspecified anomaly of dental arch relationship**

☑6ᵗʰ **M26.21 Malocclusion, Angle's class**
     M26.211 **Malocclusion, Angle's class I**
         Neutro-occlusion
     M26.212 **Malocclusion, Angle's class II**
         Disto-occlusion Division I
         Disto-occlusion Division II
     M26.213 **Malocclusion, Angle's class III**
         Mesio-occlusion
     M26.219 **Malocclusion, Angle's class, unspecified**

☑6ᵗʰ **M26.22 Open occlusal relationship**
     M26.220 **Open anterior occlusal relationship**
         Anterior openbite
     M26.221 **Open posterior occlusal relationship**
         Posterior openbite

Ⓝ Newborn: 0   Ⓟ Pediatric: 0-17   Ⓜ Maternity: 12-55   Ⓐ Adult: 15-124   MCC Major CC Condition   PDxMCC PDx acts as own MCC   CC CC Condition   PDxCC PDx acts as own CC

768   ICD-10-CM 2018

M26.23 **Excessive horizontal overlap**
Excessive horizontal overjet

M26.24 **Reverse articulation**
Crossbite (anterior) (posterior)

M26.25 **Anomalies of interarch distance**

M26.29 **Other anomalies of dental arch relationship**
Midline deviation of dental arch
Overbite (excessive) deep
Overbite (excessive) horizontal
Overbite (excessive) vertical
Posterior lingual occlusion of mandibular teeth

✓5ᵗʰ **M26.3 Anomalies of tooth position of fully erupted tooth or teeth**
EXCLUDES 2   embedded and impacted teeth (K01.-)

M26.30 **Unspecified anomaly of tooth position of fully erupted tooth or teeth**
Abnormal spacing of fully erupted tooth or teeth NOS
Displacement of fully erupted tooth or teeth NOS
Transposition of fully erupted tooth or teeth NOS

M26.31 **Crowding of fully erupted teeth**

M26.32 **Excessive spacing of fully erupted teeth**
Diastema of fully erupted tooth or teeth NOS

M26.33 **Horizontal displacement of fully erupted tooth or teeth**
Tipped tooth or teeth
Tipping of fully erupted tooth

M26.34 **Vertical displacement of fully erupted tooth or teeth**
Extruded tooth
Infraeruption of tooth or teeth
Supraeruption of tooth or teeth

M26.35 **Rotation of fully erupted tooth or teeth**

M26.36 **Insufficient interocclusal distance of fully erupted teeth (ridge)**
Lack of adequate intermaxillary vertical dimension of fully erupted teeth

M26.37 **Excessive interocclusal distance of fully erupted teeth**
Excessive intermaxillary vertical dimension of fully erupted teeth
Loss of occlusal vertical dimension of fully erupted teeth

M26.39 **Other anomalies of tooth position of fully erupted tooth or teeth**

M26.4 **Malocclusion, unspecified**

✓5ᵗʰ **M26.5 Dentofacial functional abnormalities**
EXCLUDES 1   bruxism (F45.8)
teeth-grinding NOS (F45.8)

M26.50 **Dentofacial functional abnormalities, unspecified**

M26.51 **Abnormal jaw closure**

M26.52 **Limited mandibular range of motion**

M26.53 **Deviation in opening and closing of the mandible**

M26.54 **Insufficient anterior guidance**
Insufficient anterior occlusal guidance

M26.55 **Centric occlusion maximum intercuspation discrepancy**
EXCLUDES 1   centric occlusion NOS (M26.59)

M26.56 **Non-working side interference**
Balancing side interference

M26.57 **Lack of posterior occlusal support**

M26.59 **Other dentofacial functional abnormalities**
Centric occlusion (of teeth) NOS
Malocclusion due to abnormal swallowing
Malocclusion due to mouth breathing
Malocclusion due to tongue, lip or finger habits

✓5ᵗʰ **M26.6 Temporomandibular joint disorders**
EXCLUDES 2   current temporomandibular joint dislocation (S03.0)
current temporomandibular joint sprain (S03.4)

✓6ᵗʰ M26.60 **Temporomandibular joint disorder, unspecified**

M26.601 **Right temporomandibular joint disorder, unspecified**

M26.602 **Left temporomandibular joint disorder, unspecified**

M26.603 **Bilateral temporomandibular joint disorder, unspecified**

M26.609 **Unspecified temporomandibular joint disorder, unspecified side**
Temporomandibular joint disorder NOS

Temporomandibular Joint

Cutaway detail
Upper joint space
Articular disc (meniscus)
Lower joint space
Condyle
Mandible   Cutaway view of temporomandibular joint (TMJ)

✓6ᵗʰ M26.61 **Adhesions and ankylosis of temporomandibular joint**

M26.611 **Adhesions and ankylosis of right temporomandibular joint**

M26.612 **Adhesions and ankylosis of left temporomandibular joint**

M26.613 **Adhesions and ankylosis of bilateral temporomandibular joint**

M26.619 **Adhesions and ankylosis of temporomandibular joint, unspecified side**

✓6ᵗʰ M26.62 **Arthralgia of temporomandibular joint**

M26.621 **Arthralgia of right temporomandibular joint**

M26.622 **Arthralgia of left temporomandibular joint**

M26.623 **Arthralgia of bilateral temporomandibular joint**

M26.629 **Arthralgia of temporomandibular joint, unspecified side**

✓6ᵗʰ M26.63 **Articular disc disorder of temporomandibular joint**

M26.631 **Articular disc disorder of right temporomandibular joint**

M26.632 **Articular disc disorder of left temporomandibular joint**

M26.633 **Articular disc disorder of bilateral temporomandibular joint**

M26.639 **Articular disc disorder of temporomandibular joint, unspecified side**

M26.69 **Other specified disorders of temporomandibular joint**

✓5ᵗʰ **M26.7 Dental alveolar anomalies**

M26.70 **Unspecified alveolar anomaly**

M26.71 **Alveolar maxillary hyperplasia**

M26.72 **Alveolar mandibular hyperplasia**

M26.73 **Alveolar maxillary hypoplasia**

M26.74 **Alveolar mandibular hypoplasia**

M26.79 **Other specified alveolar anomalies**

✓5ᵗʰ **M26.8 Other dentofacial anomalies**

M26.81 **Anterior soft tissue impingement**
Anterior soft tissue impingement on teeth

M26.82 **Posterior soft tissue impingement**
Posterior soft tissue impingement on teeth

M26.89 **Other dentofacial anomalies**

M26.9 **Dentofacial anomaly, unspecified**

✓4ᵗʰ **M27 Other diseases of jaws**

M27.0 **Developmental disorders of jaws**
Latent bone cyst of jaw
Stafne's cyst
Torus mandibularis
Torus palatinus

M27.1 **Giant cell granuloma, central**
Giant cell granuloma NOS
EXCLUDES 1   peripheral giant cell granuloma (K06.8)

✓ Additional Character Req   ✓x7ᵗʰ Placeholder Alert   Unacceptable PDx   Manifestation   **H1**-**H14** HAC   **HCC** CMS-HCC Condition   *EXCLUDES 1* Not Coded Here   *EXCLUDES 2* Not Included Here

ICD-10-CM 2018   769

Chapter 13. Diseases of the Musculoskeletal System and Connective Tissue

M27.2 Inflammatory conditions of jaws
Osteitis of jaw(s)
Osteomyelitis (neonatal) jaw(s)
Osteoradionecrosis jaw(s)
Periostitis jaw(s)
Sequestrum of jaw bone
Use additional code (W88-W90, X39.0) to identify radiation, if radiation-induced
EXCLUDES 2   osteonecrosis of jaw due to drug (M87.180)

M27.3 Alveolitis of jaws
Alveolar osteitis
Dry socket

✓5ᵗʰ **M27.4 Other and unspecified cysts of jaw**
EXCLUDES 1   cysts of oral region (K09.-)
latent bone cyst of jaw (M27.0)
Stafne's cyst (M27.0)

    M27.40 Unspecified cyst of jaw
       Cyst of jaw NOS

    M27.49 Other cysts of jaw
       Aneurysmal cyst of jaw
       Hemorrhagic cyst of jaw
       Traumatic cyst of jaw

✓5ᵗʰ **M27.5 Periradicular pathology associated with previous endodontic treatment**
    M27.51 Perforation of root canal space due to endodontic treatment
    M27.52 Endodontic overfill
    M27.53 Endodontic underfill
    M27.59 Other periradicular pathology associated with previous endodontic treatment

✓5ᵗʰ **M27.6 Endosseous dental implant failure**
    M27.61 Osseointegration failure of dental implant
       Hemorrhagic complications of dental implant placement
       Iatrogenic osseointegration failure of dental implant
       Osseointegration failure of dental implant due to complications of systemic disease
       Osseointegration failure of dental implant due to poor bone quality
       Pre-integration failure of dental implant NOS
       Pre-osseointegration failure of dental implant

    M27.62 Post-osseointegration biological failure of dental implant
       Failure of dental implant due to lack of attached gingiva
       Failure of dental implant due to occlusal trauma (caused by poor prosthetic design)
       Failure of dental implant due to parafunctional habits
       Failure of dental implant due to periodontal infection (peri-implantitis)
       Failure of dental implant due to poor oral hygiene
       Iatrogenic post-osseointegration failure of dental implant
       Post-osseointegration failure of dental implant due to complications of systemic disease

    M27.63 Post-osseointegration mechanical failure of dental implant
       Failure of dental prosthesis causing loss of dental implant
       Fracture of dental implant
       EXCLUDES 2   cracked tooth (K03.81)
                fractured dental restorative material with loss of material (K08.531)
                fractured dental restorative material without loss of material (K08.530)
                fractured tooth (S02.5)

    M27.69 Other endosseous dental implant failure
       Dental implant failure NOS

M27.8 Other specified diseases of jaws
Cherubism
Exostosis
Fibrous dysplasia
Unilateral condylar hyperplasia
Unilateral condylar hypoplasia
EXCLUDES 1   jaw pain (R68.84)

M27.9 Disease of jaws, unspecified

Systemic connective tissue disorders (M30-M36)

INCLUDES   autoimmune disease NOS
         collagen (vascular) disease NOS
         systemic autoimmune disease
         systemic collagen (vascular) disease
EXCLUDES 1   autoimmune disease, single organ or single cell-type—code to relevant condition category

✓4ᵗʰ **M30 Polyarteritis nodosa and related conditions**
EXCLUDES 1   microscopic polyarteritis (M31.7)

> **CC Excl: For CC codes in category M30, unless otherwise noted:** PDX collection 874

    M30.0 Polyarteritis nodosa `CC` `HCC`
    M30.1 Polyarteritis with lung involvement [Churg-Strauss] `CC` `HCC`
       Allergic granulomatous angiitis
    M30.2 Juvenile polyarteritis `CC` `HCC`
    M30.3 Mucocutaneous lymph node syndrome [Kawasaki] `CC` `HCC`
       CC Excl: PDX collection 875
    M30.8 Other conditions related to polyarteritis nodosa `CC` `HCC`
       Polyangiitis overlap syndrome

✓4ᵗʰ **M31 Other necrotizing vasculopathies**

> **CC Excl: For CC/MCC codes in category M31, unless otherwise noted:** PDX collection 874

    M31.0 Hypersensitivity angiitis `CC` `HCC`
       Goodpasture's syndrome
    M31.1 Thrombotic microangiopathy `MCC` `HCC`
       Thrombotic thrombocytopenic purpura
    M31.2 Lethal midline granuloma `CC` `HCC`
✓5ᵗʰ   **M31.3 Wegener's granulomatosis**
       Necrotizing respiratory granulomatosis
       M31.30 Wegener's granulomatosis without renal involvement `CC` `HCC`
          Wegener's granulomatosis NOS
       M31.31 Wegener's granulomatosis with renal involvement `CC` `HCC`
    M31.4 Aortic arch syndrome [Takayasu] `CC` `HCC`
    M31.5 Giant cell arteritis with polymyalgia rheumatica `HCC`
    M31.6 Other giant cell arteritis `HCC`
    M31.7 Microscopic polyangiitis `CC` `HCC`
       Microscopic polyarteritis
       EXCLUDES 1   polyarteritis nodosa (M30.0)
    M31.8 Other specified necrotizing vasculopathies `CC` `HCC`
       Hypocomplementemic vasculitis
       Septic vasculitis
       CC Excl: PDX collection 712
    M31.9 Necrotizing vasculopathy, unspecified `CC` `HCC`
       CC Excl: PDX collection 712

✓4ᵗʰ **M32 Systemic lupus erythematosus (SLE)**
EXCLUDES 1   lupus erythematosus (discoid) (NOS) (L93.0)

    M32.0 Drug-induced systemic lupus erythematosus `HCC`
       Use additional code for adverse effect, if applicable, to identify drug (T36-T50 with fifth or sixth character 5)

✓5ᵗʰ   **M32.1 Systemic lupus erythematosus with organ or system involvement**
       M32.10 Systemic lupus erythematosus, organ or system involvement unspecified `HCC`
       M32.11 Endocarditis in systemic lupus erythematosus `PDxCC` `CC` `HCC`
          Libman-Sacks disease
          CC Excl: PDX collection 676
       M32.12 Pericarditis in systemic lupus erythematosus `PDxCC` `CC` `HCC`
          Lupus pericarditis
          CC Excl: PDX collection 673
       M32.13 Lung involvement in systemic lupus erythematosus `HCC`
          Pleural effusion due to systemic lupus erythematosus
       M32.14 Glomerular disease in systemic lupus erythematosus `HCC`
          Lupus renal disease NOS
          AHA: 2013, 4Q, 125
       M32.15 Tubulo-interstitial nephropathy in systemic lupus erythematosus `HCC`
       M32.19 Other organ or system involvement in systemic lupus erythematosus `HCC`
    M32.8 Other forms of systemic lupus erythematosus `HCC`

N Newborn: 0   P Pediatric: 0-17   M Maternity: 12-55   A Adult: 15-124   **MCC** Major CC Condition   **PDxMCC** PDx acts as own MCC   **CC** CC Condition   **PDxCC** PDx acts as own CC

M32.9   **Systemic lupus erythematosus,** unspecified   `HCC`
     SLE NOS
     Systemic lupus erythematosus NOS
     Systemic lupus erythematosus without organ involvement

✓4th **M33**   **Dermatopolymyositis**

     CC Excl: For CC codes in category M33, unless otherwise noted:
     PDX collection 876

▲ ✓5th **M33.0**   **Juvenile** dermatomyositis

▲   **M33.00**   **Juvenile dermatomyositis, organ**   `CC` `HCC`
       involvement unspecified

▲   **M33.01**   **Juvenile dermatomyositis with** respiratory   `CC` `HCC`
       involvement

▲   **M33.02**   **Juvenile dermatomyositis with**   `PDxCC` `CC` `HCC`
       myopathy
       CC Excl: PDX collection 877

●   **M33.03**   **Juvenile dermatomyositis without myopathy**   `CC`

▲   **M33.09**   **Juvenile dermatomyositis with** other organ   `CC` `HCC`
       involvement

▲ ✓5th **M33.1**   **Other dermatomyositis**
     ►Adult dermatomyositis◄

▲   **M33.10**   **Other dermatomyositis, organ involvement**   `CC` `HCC`
       unspecified

▲   **M33.11**   **Other dermatomyositis with** respiratory   `CC` `HCC`
       involvement

▲   **M33.12**   **Other dermatomyositis with** myopathy   `PDxCC` `CC` `HCC`
       CC Excl: PDX collection 877

●   **M33.13**   **Other dermatomyositis without myopathy**   `CC`
       Dermatomyositis NOS

▲   **M33.19**   **Other dermatomyositis with** other organ   `CC` `HCC`
       involvement

✓5th **M33.2**   **Polymyositis**

     M33.20   **Polymyositis, organ involvement** unspecified `CC` `HCC`
       CC Excl: PDX collection 878

     M33.21   **Polymyositis with** respiratory **involvement** `CC` `HCC`
       CC Excl: PDX collection 878

     M33.22   **Polymyositis with** myopathy   `PDxCC` `CC` `HCC`
       CC Excl: PDX collection 879

     M33.29   **Polymyositis with** other organ **involvement** `CC` `HCC`
       CC Excl: PDX collection 878

✓5th **M33.9**   **Dermatopolymyositis,** unspecified

     M33.90   **Dermatopolymyositis, unspecified, organ**   `CC` `HCC`
       involvement unspecified

     M33.91   **Dermatopolymyositis, unspecified with**   `CC` `HCC`
       respiratory involvement

     M33.92   **Dermatopolymyositis, unspecified with**   `PDxCC` `CC` `HCC`
       myopathy
       CC Excl: PDX collection 877

●   **M33.93**   **Dermatopolymyositis, unspecified without**   `CC`
       myopathy

     M33.99   **Dermatopolymyositis, unspecified with**   `CC` `HCC`
       other organ involvement

✓4th **M34**   **Systemic sclerosis [scleroderma]**
     `EXCLUDES 1`   circumscribed scleroderma (L94.0)
       neonatal scleroderma (P83.8)

     M34.0   **Progressive** systemic sclerosis   `HCC`

     M34.1   **CR(E)ST syndrome**   `HCC`
       Combination of calcinosis, Raynaud's phenomenon, esophageal
       dysfunction, sclerodactyly, telangiectasia

     M34.2   **Systemic sclerosis** induced by drug and chemical   `HCC`
       Code first poisoning due to drug or toxin, if applicable (T36-T65
       with fifth or sixth character 1-4 or 6)
       Use additional code for adverse effect, if applicable, to identify
       drug (T36-T50 with fifth or sixth character 5)

✓5th **M34.8**   **Other forms** of systemic sclerosis

     M34.81   **Systemic sclerosis with** lung   `PDxCC` `CC` `HCC`
       involvement
       CC Excl: No excl

     M34.82   **Systemic sclerosis with** myopathy   `PDxCC` `CC` `HCC`
       CC Excl: PDX collection 867

     M34.83   **Systemic sclerosis with** polyneuropathy   `HCC`

     M34.89   **Other** systemic sclerosis   `HCC`

     M34.9   **Systemic sclerosis,** unspecified   `HCC`

✓4th **M35**   **Other systemic involvement of connective tissue**
     `EXCLUDES 1`   reactive perforating collagenosis (L87.1)

✓5th **M35.0**   **Sicca syndrome [Sjögren]**
     DEF: Autoimmune disease; associated with keratoconjunctivitis,
     laryngopharyngitis, rhinitis, dry mouth, enlarged parotid gland,
     and chronic polyarthritis.

     M35.00   **Sicca syndrome,** unspecified   `HCC`

     M35.01   **Sicca syndrome with** keratoconjunctivitis   `HCC`

     M35.02   **Sicca syndrome with** lung **involvement**   `HCC`

     M35.03   **Sicca syndrome with** myopathy   `PDxCC` `CC` `HCC`
       CC Excl: PDX collection 867

     M35.04   **Sicca syndrome with** tubulo-interstitial   `HCC`
       nephropathy
       Renal tubular acidosis in sicca syndrome

     M35.09   **Sicca syndrome with** other organ **involvement**   `HCC`

     M35.1   **Other overlap syndromes**   `CC` `HCC`
       Mixed connective tissue disease
       `EXCLUDES 1`   polyangiitis overlap syndrome (M30.8)
       CC Excl: PDX collection 880

     M35.2   **Behçet's disease**   `CC` `HCC`
       CC Excl: PDX collection 863

     M35.3   **Polymyalgia rheumatica**   `HCC`
       `EXCLUDES 1`   polymyalgia rheumatica with giant cell arteritis
         (M31.5)

     M35.4   **Diffuse (eosinophilic) fasciitis**

     M35.5   **Multifocal fibrosclerosis**   `CC` `HCC`
       CC Excl: PDX collection 880

     M35.6   **Relapsing panniculitis [Weber-Christian]**
       `EXCLUDES 1`   lupus panniculitis (L93.2)
         panniculitis NOS (M79.3-)

     M35.7   **Hypermobility syndrome**
       Familial ligamentous laxity
       `EXCLUDES 1`   Ehlers-Danlos syndrome (Q79.6)
         ligamentous laxity, NOS (M24.2-)

     M35.8   **Other specified systemic involvement of connective**   `CC` `HCC`
       tissue
       CC Excl: PDX collection 880

     M35.9   **Systemic involvement of connective tissue,** unspecified   `HCC`
       Autoimmune disease (systemic) NOS
       Collagen (vascular) disease NOS

✓4th **M36**   **Systemic disorders of connective tissue in diseases classified**
     elsewhere
     `EXCLUDES 2`   arthropathies in diseases classified elsewhere (M14.-)

     M36.0   *Dermato(poly)myositis in neoplastic disease*   `CC` `HCC`
       Code first underlying neoplasm (C00-D49)
       CC Excl: PDX collection 876

     M36.1   *Arthropathy in neoplastic disease*
       Code first underlying neoplasm, such as:
         leukemia (C91-C95)
         malignant histiocytosis (C96.A)
         multiple myeloma (C90.0)

     M36.2   *Hemophilic arthropathy*
       Hemarthrosis in hemophilic arthropathy
       Code first underlying disease, such as:
         factor VIII deficiency (D66)
           with vascular defect (D68.0)
         factor IX deficiency (D67)
         hemophilia (classical) (D66)
         hemophilia B (D67)
         hemophilia C (D68.1)

     M36.3   *Arthropathy in other blood disorders*

     M36.4   *Arthropathy in hypersensitivity reactions classified elsewhere*
       Code first underlying disease, such as:
         Henoch (-Schönlein) purpura (D69.0)
         serum sickness (T80.6-)

     M36.8   *Systemic disorders of connective tissue in other diseases*   `HCC`
       classified elsewhere
       Code first underlying disease, such as:
         alkaptonuria (E70.2)
         hypogammaglobulinemia (D80.-)
         ochronosis (E70.2)

✓ Additional Character Req   ✓x7th Placeholder Alert   Unacceptable PDx   Manifestation   H1 - H14 HAC   HCC CMS-HCC Condition   *EXCLUDES 1* Not Coded Here   *EXCLUDES 2* Not Included Here

ICD-10-CM 2018   **771**

Chapter 13. Diseases of the Musculoskeletal System and Connective Tissue

DORSOPATHIES (M40-M54)

Deforming dorsopathies (M40-M43)

✓4th M40 Kyphosis and lordosis
> EXCLUDES 1   congenital kyphosis and lordosis (Q76.4)
> kyphoscoliosis (M41.-)
> postprocedural kyphosis and lordosis (M96.-)

✓5th M40.0 Postural kyphosis
> EXCLUDES 1   osteochondrosis of spine (M42.-)

     M40.00   Postural kyphosis, site unspecified
     M40.03   Postural kyphosis, cervicothoracic region
     M40.04   Postural kyphosis, thoracic region
     M40.05   Postural kyphosis, thoracolumbar region

✓5th M40.1 Other secondary kyphosis
     M40.10   Other secondary kyphosis, site unspecified
     M40.12   Other secondary kyphosis, cervical region
     M40.13   Other secondary kyphosis, cervicothoracic region
     M40.14   Other secondary kyphosis, thoracic region
     M40.15   Other secondary kyphosis, thoracolumbar region

✓5th M40.2 Other and unspecified kyphosis
   ✓6th M40.20   Unspecified kyphosis
       M40.202   Unspecified kyphosis, cervical region
       M40.203   Unspecified kyphosis, cervicothoracic region
       M40.204   Unspecified kyphosis, thoracic region
       M40.205   Unspecified kyphosis, thoracolumbar region
       M40.209   Unspecified kyphosis, site unspecified
   ✓6th M40.29   Other kyphosis
       M40.292   Other kyphosis, cervical region
       M40.293   Other kyphosis, cervicothoracic region
       M40.294   Other kyphosis, thoracic region
       M40.295   Other kyphosis, thoracolumbar region
       M40.299   Other kyphosis, site unspecified

✓5th M40.3 Flatback syndrome
     M40.30   Flatback syndrome, site unspecified
     M40.35   Flatback syndrome, thoracolumbar region
     M40.36   Flatback syndrome, lumbar region
     M40.37   Flatback syndrome, lumbosacral region

✓5th M40.4 Postural lordosis
     Acquired lordosis
     M40.40   Postural lordosis, site unspecified
     M40.45   Postural lordosis, thoracolumbar region
     M40.46   Postural lordosis, lumbar region
     M40.47   Postural lordosis, lumbosacral region

✓5th M40.5 Lordosis, unspecified
     M40.50   Lordosis, unspecified, site unspecified
     M40.55   Lordosis, unspecified, thoracolumbar region
     M40.56   Lordosis, unspecified, lumbar region
     M40.57   Lordosis, unspecified, lumbosacral region

Kyphosis and Lordosis

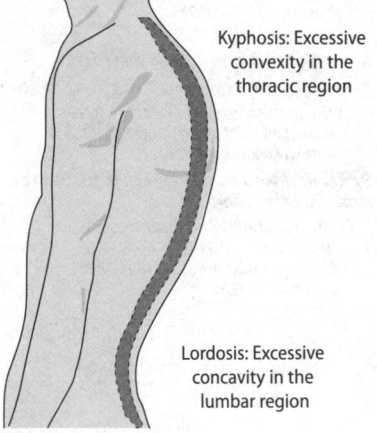

Kyphosis: Excessive convexity in the thoracic region

Lordosis: Excessive concavity in the lumbar region

✓4th M41 Scoliosis
> INCLUDES   kyphoscoliosis
> EXCLUDES 1   congenital scoliosis due to bony malformation (Q76.3)
> congenital scoliosis NOS (Q67.5)
> kyphoscoliotic heart disease (I27.1)
> postprocedural scoliosis (M96.-)
> postural congenital scoliosis (Q67.5)

✓5th M41.0 Infantile idiopathic scoliosis
     AHA: 2014, 4Q, 26
     M41.00   Infantile idiopathic scoliosis, site unspecified
     M41.02   Infantile idiopathic scoliosis, cervical region
     M41.03   Infantile idiopathic scoliosis, cervicothoracic region
     M41.04   Infantile idiopathic scoliosis, thoracic region
     M41.05   Infantile idiopathic scoliosis, thoracolumbar region
     M41.06   Infantile idiopathic scoliosis, lumbar region
     M41.07   Infantile idiopathic scoliosis, lumbosacral region
     M41.08   Infantile idiopathic scoliosis, sacral and sacrococcygeal region

✓5th M41.1 Juvenile and adolescent idiopathic scoliosis
   ✓6th M41.11   Juvenile idiopathic scoliosis
     AHA: 2014, 4Q, 28
       M41.112   Juvenile idiopathic scoliosis, cervical region
       M41.113   Juvenile idiopathic scoliosis, cervicothoracic region
       M41.114   Juvenile idiopathic scoliosis, thoracic region
       M41.115   Juvenile idiopathic scoliosis, thoracolumbar region
       M41.116   Juvenile idiopathic scoliosis, lumbar region
       M41.117   Juvenile idiopathic scoliosis, lumbosacral region
       M41.119   Juvenile idiopathic scoliosis, site unspecified
   ✓6th M41.12   Adolescent scoliosis
       M41.122   Adolescent idiopathic scoliosis, cervical region
       M41.123   Adolescent idiopathic scoliosis, cervicothoracic region
       M41.124   Adolescent idiopathic scoliosis, thoracic region
       M41.125   Adolescent idiopathic scoliosis, thoracolumbar region
       M41.126   Adolescent idiopathic scoliosis, lumbar region
       M41.127   Adolescent idiopathic scoliosis, lumbosacral region
       M41.129   Adolescent idiopathic scoliosis, site unspecified

✓5th M41.2 Other idiopathic scoliosis
     M41.20   Other idiopathic scoliosis, site unspecified
     M41.22   Other idiopathic scoliosis, cervical region

Scoliosis

Lateral curvature of spine

N Newborn: 0   P Pediatric: 0-17   M Maternity: 12-55   A Adult: 15-124   MCC Major CC Condition   PDxMCC PDx acts as own MCC   CC CC Condition   PDxCC PDx acts as own CC

M41.23 **Other idiopathic scoliosis, cervicothoracic region**
M41.24 **Other idiopathic scoliosis, thoracic region**
M41.25 **Other idiopathic scoliosis, thoracolumbar region**
M41.26 **Other idiopathic scoliosis, lumbar region**
M41.27 **Other idiopathic scoliosis, lumbosacral region**

✓5ᵗʰ **M41.3 Thoracogenic scoliosis**
M41.30 **Thoracogenic scoliosis, site unspecified**
M41.34 **Thoracogenic scoliosis, thoracic region**
M41.35 **Thoracogenic scoliosis, thoracolumbar region**

✓5ᵗʰ **M41.4 Neuromuscular scoliosis**
Scoliosis secondary to cerebral palsy, Friedreich's ataxia, poliomyelitis and other neuromuscular disorders
Code also underlying condition
AHA: 2014, 4Q, 27
M41.40 **Neuromuscular scoliosis, site unspecified**
M41.41 **Neuromuscular scoliosis, occipito-atlanto-axial region**
M41.42 **Neuromuscular scoliosis, cervical region**
M41.43 **Neuromuscular scoliosis, cervicothoracic region**
M41.44 **Neuromuscular scoliosis, thoracic region**
M41.45 **Neuromuscular scoliosis, thoracolumbar region**
M41.46 **Neuromuscular scoliosis, lumbar region**
M41.47 **Neuromuscular scoliosis, lumbosacral region**

✓5ᵗʰ **M41.5 Other secondary scoliosis**
M41.50 **Other secondary scoliosis, site unspecified**
M41.52 **Other secondary scoliosis, cervical region**
M41.53 **Other secondary scoliosis, cervicothoracic region**
M41.54 **Other secondary scoliosis, thoracic region**
M41.55 **Other secondary scoliosis, thoracolumbar region**
M41.56 **Other secondary scoliosis, lumbar region**
M41.57 **Other secondary scoliosis, lumbosacral region**

✓5ᵗʰ **M41.8 Other forms of scoliosis**
M41.80 **Other forms of scoliosis, site unspecified**
M41.82 **Other forms of scoliosis, cervical region**
M41.83 **Other forms of scoliosis, cervicothoracic region**
M41.84 **Other forms of scoliosis, thoracic region**
M41.85 **Other forms of scoliosis, thoracolumbar region**
M41.86 **Other forms of scoliosis, lumbar region**
M41.87 **Other forms of scoliosis, lumbosacral region**

M41.9 **Scoliosis, unspecified**

✓4ᵗʰ **M42 Spinal osteochondrosis**
✓5ᵗʰ **M42.0 Juvenile osteochondrosis of spine**
Calvé's disease
Scheuermann's disease
EXCLUDES 1 postural kyphosis (M40.0)
M42.00 **Juvenile osteochondrosis of spine, site unspecified**
M42.01 **Juvenile osteochondrosis of spine, occipito-atlanto-axial region**
M42.02 **Juvenile osteochondrosis of spine, cervical region**
M42.03 **Juvenile osteochondrosis of spine, cervicothoracic region**
M42.04 **Juvenile osteochondrosis of spine, thoracic region**
M42.05 **Juvenile osteochondrosis of spine, thoracolumbar region**
M42.06 **Juvenile osteochondrosis of spine, lumbar region**
M42.07 **Juvenile osteochondrosis of spine, lumbosacral region**
M42.08 **Juvenile osteochondrosis of spine, sacral and sacrococcygeal region**
M42.09 **Juvenile osteochondrosis of spine, multiple sites in spine**

✓5ᵗʰ **M42.1 Adult osteochondrosis of spine**
M42.10 **Adult osteochondrosis of spine, site unspecified** 🄰
M42.11 **Adult osteochondrosis of spine, occipito-atlanto-axial region** 🄰
M42.12 **Adult osteochondrosis of spine, cervical region** 🄰
M42.13 **Adult osteochondrosis of spine, cervicothoracic region** 🄰
M42.14 **Adult osteochondrosis of spine, thoracic region** 🄰
M42.15 **Adult osteochondrosis of spine, thoracolumbar region** 🄰
M42.16 **Adult osteochondrosis of spine, lumbar region** 🄰

M42.17 **Adult osteochondrosis of spine, lumbosacral region** 🄰
M42.18 **Adult osteochondrosis of spine, sacral and sacrococcygeal region** 🄰
M42.19 **Adult osteochondrosis of spine, multiple sites in spine** 🄰

M42.9 **Spinal osteochondrosis, unspecified**

✓4ᵗʰ **M43 Other deforming dorsopathies**
EXCLUDES 1 congenital spondylolysis and spondylolisthesis (Q76.2)
hemivertebra (Q76.3-Q76.4)
Klippel-Feil syndrome (Q76.1)
lumbarization and sacralization (Q76.4)
platyspondylisis (Q76.4)
spina bifida occulta (Q76.0)
spinal curvature in osteoporosis (M80.-)
spinal curvature in Paget's disease of bone [osteitis deformans] (M88.-)

✓5ᵗʰ **M43.0 Spondylolysis**
EXCLUDES 1 congenital spondylolysis (Q76.2)
spondylolisthesis (M43.1)
M43.00 **Spondylolysis, site unspecified**
M43.01 **Spondylolysis, occipito-atlanto-axial region**
M43.02 **Spondylolysis, cervical region**
M43.03 **Spondylolysis, cervicothoracic region**
M43.04 **Spondylolysis, thoracic region**
M43.05 **Spondylolysis, thoracolumbar region**
M43.06 **Spondylolysis, lumbar region**
M43.07 **Spondylolysis, lumbosacral region**
M43.08 **Spondylolysis, sacral and sacrococcygeal region**
M43.09 **Spondylolysis, multiple sites in spine**

✓5ᵗʰ **M43.1 Spondylolisthesis**
EXCLUDES 1 acute traumatic of lumbosacral region (S33.1)
acute traumatic of sites other than lumbosacral—code to Fracture, vertebra, by region
congenital spondylolisthesis (Q76.2)
M43.10 **Spondylolisthesis, site unspecified**
M43.11 **Spondylolisthesis, occipito-atlanto-axial region**
M43.12 **Spondylolisthesis, cervical region**
M43.13 **Spondylolisthesis, cervicothoracic region**
M43.14 **Spondylolisthesis, thoracic region**
M43.15 **Spondylolisthesis, thoracolumbar region**
M43.16 **Spondylolisthesis, lumbar region**
M43.17 **Spondylolisthesis, lumbosacral region**
M43.18 **Spondylolisthesis, sacral and sacrococcygeal region**
M43.19 **Spondylolisthesis, multiple sites in spine**

✓5ᵗʰ **M43.2 Fusion of spine**
Ankylosis of spinal joint
EXCLUDES 1 ankylosing spondylitis (M45.0-)
congenital fusion of spine (Q76.4)
EXCLUDES 2 arthrodesis status (Z98.1)
pseudoarthrosis after fusion or arthrodesis (M96.0)
M43.20 **Fusion of spine, site unspecified**
M43.21 **Fusion of spine, occipito-atlanto-axial region**
M43.22 **Fusion of spine, cervical region**
M43.23 **Fusion of spine, cervicothoracic region**
M43.24 **Fusion of spine, thoracic region**
M43.25 **Fusion of spine, thoracolumbar region**
M43.26 **Fusion of spine, lumbar region**
M43.27 **Fusion of spine, lumbosacral region**
M43.28 **Fusion of spine, sacral and sacrococcygeal region**

M43.3 **Recurrent atlantoaxial dislocation with myelopathy**
M43.4 **Other recurrent atlantoaxial dislocation**
✓5ᵗʰ **M43.5 Other recurrent vertebral dislocation**
EXCLUDES 1 biomechanical lesions NEC (M99.-)
✓6ᵗʰ **M43.5X Other recurrent vertebral dislocation**
M43.5X2 **Other recurrent vertebral dislocation, cervical region**
M43.5X3 **Other recurrent vertebral dislocation, cervicothoracic region**
M43.5X4 **Other recurrent vertebral dislocation, thoracic region**
M43.5X5 **Other recurrent vertebral dislocation, thoracolumbar region**

M43.5X6 **Other recurrent vertebral dislocation, lumbar region**

M43.5X7 **Other recurrent vertebral dislocation, lumbosacral region**

M43.5X8 **Other recurrent vertebral dislocation, sacral and sacrococcygeal region**

M43.5X9 **Other recurrent vertebral dislocation,** site unspecified

M43.6 Torticollis
> EXCLUDES 1 congenital (sternomastoid) torticollis (Q68.0)
> current injury—see Injury, of spine, by body region
> ocular torticollis (R29.891)
> psychogenic torticollis (F45.8)
> spasmodic torticollis (G24.3)
> torticollis due to birth injury (P15.2)

✓5th M43.8 Other specified deforming dorsopathies
> EXCLUDES 2 kyphosis and lordosis (M40.-)
> scoliosis (M41.-)

✓6th M43.8X Other specified deforming dorsopathies

M43.8X1 **Other specified deforming dorsopathies, occipito-atlanto-axial region**

M43.8X2 **Other specified deforming dorsopathies, cervical region**

M43.8X3 **Other specified deforming dorsopathies, cervicothoracic region**

M43.8X4 **Other specified deforming dorsopathies, thoracic region**

M43.8X5 **Other specified deforming dorsopathies, thoracolumbar region**

M43.8X6 **Other specified deforming dorsopathies, lumbar region**

M43.8X7 **Other specified deforming dorsopathies, lumbosacral region**

M43.8X8 **Other specified deforming dorsopathies, sacral and sacrococcygeal region**

M43.8X9 **Other specified deforming dorsopathies, site unspecified**

M43.9 Deforming dorsopathy, unspecified
Curvature of spine NOS

Spondylopathies (M45-M49)

✓4th M45 Ankylosing spondylitis
Rheumatoid arthritis of spine
> EXCLUDES 1 arthropathy in Reiter's disease (M02.3-)
> juvenile (ankylosing) spondylitis (M08.1)
> EXCLUDES 2 Behçet's disease (M35.2)

M45.0 **Ankylosing spondylitis of** multiple sites in spine `HCC`

M45.1 **Ankylosing spondylitis of** occipito-atlanto-axial region `HCC`

M45.2 **Ankylosing spondylitis of** cervical region `HCC`

M45.3 **Ankylosing spondylitis of** cervicothoracic region `HCC`

M45.4 **Ankylosing spondylitis of** thoracic region `HCC`

M45.5 **Ankylosing spondylitis of** thoracolumbar region `HCC`

M45.6 **Ankylosing spondylitis** lumbar region `HCC`

M45.7 **Ankylosing spondylitis of** lumbosacral region `HCC`

M45.8 **Ankylosing spondylitis** sacral and sacrococcygeal region `HCC`

M45.9 **Ankylosing spondylitis of** unspecified sites in spine `HCC`

✓4th M46 Other inflammatory spondylopathies

✓5th M46.0 Spinal enthesopathy
Disorder of ligamentous or muscular attachments of spine

M46.00 **Spinal enthesopathy,** site unspecified `HCC`

M46.01 **Spinal enthesopathy,** occipito-atlanto-axial region `HCC`

M46.02 **Spinal enthesopathy,** cervical region `HCC`

M46.03 **Spinal enthesopathy,** cervicothoracic region `HCC`

M46.04 **Spinal enthesopathy,** thoracic region `HCC`

M46.05 **Spinal enthesopathy,** thoracolumbar region `HCC`

M46.06 **Spinal enthesopathy,** lumbar region `HCC`

M46.07 **Spinal enthesopathy,** lumbosacral region `HCC`

M46.08 **Spinal enthesopathy,** sacral and sacrococcygeal region `HCC`

M46.09 **Spinal enthesopathy,** multiple sites in spine `HCC`

M46.1 Sacroiliitis, not elsewhere classified `HCC`
DEF: Inflammation of sacroiliac joint (situated at juncture of sacrum and hip); characterized by pain in buttocks or lower back that can extend down one or both legs.

✓5th M46.2 Osteomyelitis of vertebra

> **CC Excl: For CC codes in subcategory M46.2:**
> PDX collection 881

M46.20 **Osteomyelitis of vertebra,** site unspecified `CC` `HCC`

M46.21 **Osteomyelitis of vertebra,** occipito-atlanto-axial region `HCC`

M46.22 **Osteomyelitis of vertebra,** cervical region `CC` `HCC`

M46.23 **Osteomyelitis of vertebra,** cervicothoracic region `CC` `HCC`

M46.24 **Osteomyelitis of vertebra,** thoracic region `CC` `HCC`

M46.25 **Osteomyelitis of vertebra,** thoracolumbar region `CC` `HCC`

M46.26 **Osteomyelitis of vertebra,** lumbar region `CC` `HCC`

M46.27 **Osteomyelitis of vertebra,** lumbosacral region `CC` `HCC`

M46.28 **Osteomyelitis of vertebra,** sacral and sacrococcygeal region `CC` `HCC`

✓5th M46.3 Infection of intervertebral disc (pyogenic)
Use additional code (B95-B97) to identify infectious agent

> **CC Excl: For CC codes in subcategory M46.3:**
> PDX collection 882

M46.30 **Infection of intervertebral disc (pyogenic),** site unspecified `CC` `HCC`

M46.31 **Infection of intervertebral disc (pyogenic),** occipito-atlanto-axial region `HCC`

M46.32 **Infection of intervertebral disc (pyogenic),** cervical region `HCC`

M46.33 **Infection of intervertebral disc (pyogenic),** cervicothoracic region `CC` `HCC`

M46.34 **Infection of intervertebral disc (pyogenic),** thoracic region `CC` `HCC`

M46.35 **Infection of intervertebral disc (pyogenic),** thoracolumbar region `CC` `HCC`

M46.36 **Infection of intervertebral disc (pyogenic),** lumbar region `CC` `HCC`

M46.37 **Infection of intervertebral disc (pyogenic),** lumbosacral region `CC` `HCC`

M46.38 **Infection of intervertebral disc (pyogenic),** sacral and sacrococcygeal region `CC` `HCC`

M46.39 **Infection of intervertebral disc (pyogenic),** multiple sites in spine `CC` `HCC`

✓5th M46.4 Discitis, unspecified

M46.40 **Discitis, unspecified,** site unspecified

M46.41 **Discitis, unspecified,** occipito-atlanto-axial region

M46.42 **Discitis, unspecified,** cervical region

M46.43 **Discitis, unspecified,** cervicothoracic region

M46.44 **Discitis, unspecified,** thoracic region

M46.45 **Discitis, unspecified,** thoracolumbar region

M46.46 **Discitis, unspecified,** lumbar region

M46.47 **Discitis, unspecified,** lumbosacral region

M46.48 **Discitis, unspecified,** sacral and sacrococcygeal region

M46.49 **Discitis, unspecified,** multiple sites in spine

✓5th M46.5 Other infective spondylopathies

M46.50 **Other infective spondylopathies,** site unspecified `HCC`

M46.51 **Other infective spondylopathies,** occipito-atlanto-axial region `HCC`

M46.52 **Other infective spondylopathies,** cervical region `HCC`

M46.53 **Other infective spondylopathies,** cervicothoracic region `HCC`

M46.54 **Other infective spondylopathies,** thoracic region `HCC`

M46.55 **Other infective spondylopathies,** thoracolumbar region `HCC`

M46.56 **Other infective spondylopathies,** lumbar region `HCC`

M46.57 **Other infective spondylopathies,** lumbosacral region `HCC`

M46.58 **Other infective spondylopathies,** sacral and sacrococcygeal region `HCC`

M46.59 **Other infective spondylopathies,** multiple sites in spine `HCC`

N Newborn: 0   P Pediatric: 0-17   M Maternity: 12-55   A Adult: 15-124   MCC Major CC Condition   PDxMCC PDx acts as own MCC   CC CC Condition   PDxCC PDx acts as own CC

774   ICD-10-CM 2018

✓5ᵗʰ M46.8 Other specified inflammatory spondylopathies

M46.80 Other specified inflammatory spondylopathies, site unspecified `HCC`

M46.81 Other specified inflammatory spondylopathies, occipito-atlanto-axial region `HCC`

M46.82 Other specified inflammatory spondylopathies, cervical region `HCC`

M46.83 Other specified inflammatory spondylopathies, cervicothoracic region `HCC`

M46.84 Other specified inflammatory spondylopathies, thoracic region `HCC`

M46.85 Other specified inflammatory spondylopathies, thoracolumbar region `HCC`

M46.86 Other specified inflammatory spondylopathies, lumbar region `HCC`

M46.87 Other specified inflammatory spondylopathies, lumbosacral region `HCC`

M46.88 Other specified inflammatory spondylopathies, sacral and sacrococcygeal region `HCC`

M46.89 Other specified inflammatory spondylopathies, multiple sites in spine `HCC`

✓5ᵗʰ M46.9 Unspecified inflammatory spondylopathy

M46.90 Unspecified inflammatory spondylopathy, site unspecified `HCC`

M46.91 Unspecified inflammatory spondylopathy, occipito-atlanto-axial region `HCC`

M46.92 Unspecified inflammatory spondylopathy, cervical region `HCC`

M46.93 Unspecified inflammatory spondylopathy, cervicothoracic region `HCC`

M46.94 Unspecified inflammatory spondylopathy, thoracic region `HCC`

M46.95 Unspecified inflammatory spondylopathy, thoracolumbar region `HCC`

M46.96 Unspecified inflammatory spondylopathy, lumbar region `HCC`

M46.97 Unspecified inflammatory spondylopathy, lumbosacral region `HCC`

M46.98 Unspecified inflammatory spondylopathy, sacral and sacrococcygeal region `HCC`

M46.99 Unspecified inflammatory spondylopathy, multiple sites in spine `HCC`

✓4ᵗʰ M47 Spondylosis

   `INCLUDES` arthrosis or osteoarthritis of spine
         degeneration of facet joints

✓5ᵗʰ M47.0 Anterior spinal and vertebral artery compression syndromes

> **CC Excl: For CC codes in subcategory M47.0:**
> PDX collection 883

✓6ᵗʰ M47.01 Anterior spinal artery compression syndromes

M47.011 Anterior spinal artery compression syndromes, occipito-atlanto-axial region `CC`

M47.012 Anterior spinal artery compression syndromes, cervical region `CC`

M47.013 Anterior spinal artery compression syndromes, cervicothoracic region `CC`

M47.014 Anterior spinal artery compression syndromes, thoracic region `CC`

M47.015 Anterior spinal artery compression syndromes, thoracolumbar region `CC`

M47.016 Anterior spinal artery compression syndromes, lumbar region `CC`

M47.019 Anterior spinal artery compression syndromes, site unspecified `CC`

✓6ᵗʰ M47.02 Vertebral artery compression syndromes

M47.021 Vertebral artery compression syndromes, occipito-atlanto-axial region `CC`

M47.022 Vertebral artery compression syndromes, cervical region `CC`

M47.029 Vertebral artery compression syndromes, site unspecified `CC`

✓5ᵗʰ M47.1 Other spondylosis with myelopathy

    Spondylogenic compression of spinal cord
     EXCLUDES 1   vertebral subluxation (M43.3-M43.5X9)

M47.10 Other spondylosis with myelopathy, site unspecified `CC`
      CC Excl: PDX collection 884

M47.11 Other spondylosis with myelopathy, occipito-atlanto-axial region `CC`
      CC Excl: PDX collection 883

M47.12 Other spondylosis with myelopathy, cervical region `CC`
      CC Excl: PDX collection 883

M47.13 Other spondylosis with myelopathy, cervicothoracic region `CC`
      CC Excl: PDX collection 883

M47.14 Other spondylosis with myelopathy, thoracic region `CC`
      CC Excl: PDX collection 885

M47.15 Other spondylosis with myelopathy, thoracolumbar region `CC`
      CC Excl: PDX collection 885

M47.16 Other spondylosis with myelopathy, lumbar region `CC`
      CC Excl: PDX collection 886

✓5ᵗʰ M47.2 Other spondylosis with radiculopathy

M47.20 Other spondylosis with radiculopathy, site unspecified

M47.21 Other spondylosis with radiculopathy, occipito-atlanto-axial region

M47.22 Other spondylosis with radiculopathy, cervical region

M47.23 Other spondylosis with radiculopathy, cervicothoracic region

M47.24 Other spondylosis with radiculopathy, thoracic region

M47.25 Other spondylosis with radiculopathy, thoracolumbar region

M47.26 Other spondylosis with radiculopathy, lumbar region

M47.27 Other spondylosis with radiculopathy, lumbosacral region

M47.28 Other spondylosis with radiculopathy, sacral and sacrococcygeal region

✓5ᵗʰ M47.8 Other spondylosis

✓6ᵗʰ M47.81 Spondylosis without myelopathy or radiculopathy

M47.811 Spondylosis without myelopathy or radiculopathy, occipito-atlanto-axial region

M47.812 Spondylosis without myelopathy or radiculopathy, cervical region

M47.813 Spondylosis without myelopathy or radiculopathy, cervicothoracic region

M47.814 Spondylosis without myelopathy or radiculopathy, thoracic region

M47.815 Spondylosis without myelopathy or radiculopathy, thoracolumbar region

M47.816 Spondylosis without myelopathy or radiculopathy, lumbar region

M47.817 Spondylosis without myelopathy or radiculopathy, lumbosacral region

M47.818 Spondylosis without myelopathy or radiculopathy, sacral and sacrococcygeal region

M47.819 Spondylosis without myelopathy or radiculopathy, site unspecified

✓6ᵗʰ M47.89 Other spondylosis

M47.891 Other spondylosis, occipito-atlanto-axial region

M47.892 Other spondylosis, cervical region

M47.893 Other spondylosis, cervicothoracic region

M47.894 Other spondylosis, thoracic region

M47.895 Other spondylosis, thoracolumbar region

M47.896 Other spondylosis, lumbar region

M47.897 Other spondylosis, lumbosacral region

M47.898 Other spondylosis, sacral and sacrococcygeal region

M47.899 Other spondylosis, site unspecified

✓ Additional Character Req   ✓x7ᵗʰ Placeholder Alert   Unacceptable PDx   Manifestation   `H1`-`H14` HAC   `HCC` CMS-HCC Condition   *EXCLUDES 1* Not Coded Here   *EXCLUDES 2* Not Included Here

ICD-10-CM 2018   775

    M47.9   Spondylosis, unspecified

✓4ᵗʰ **M48   Other spondylopathies**

    ✓5ᵗʰ **M48.0   Spinal stenosis**
        Caudal stenosis

        M48.00   Spinal stenosis, site unspecified

        M48.01   Spinal stenosis, occipito-atlanto-axial region

        M48.02   Spinal stenosis, cervical region

        M48.03   Spinal stenosis, cervicothoracic region

        M48.04   Spinal stenosis, thoracic region

        M48.05   Spinal stenosis, thoracolumbar region

        ✓6ᵗʰ **M48.06   Spinal stenosis, lumbar region**
            DEF: Spinal canal narrowing in the lumbar area with nerve root compression, causing muscle pain, fatigue, and weakness during extension of the lumbar spine; pain is relieved by sitting or bending.

•   **M48.061   Spinal stenosis, lumbar region without neurogenic claudication**
            Spinal stenosis, lumbar region NOS

•   **M48.062   Spinal stenosis, lumbar region with neurogenic claudication**

        M48.07   Spinal stenosis, lumbosacral region

        M48.08   Spinal stenosis, sacral and sacrococcygeal region

    ✓5ᵗʰ **M48.1   Ankylosing hyperostosis [Forestier]**
        Diffuse idiopathic skeletal hyperostosis [DISH]

        M48.10   Ankylosing hyperostosis [Forestier], site unspecified

        M48.11   Ankylosing hyperostosis [Forestier], occipito-atlanto-axial region

        M48.12   Ankylosing hyperostosis [Forestier], cervical region

        M48.13   Ankylosing hyperostosis [Forestier], cervicothoracic region

        M48.14   Ankylosing hyperostosis [Forestier], thoracic region

        M48.15   Ankylosing hyperostosis [Forestier], thoracolumbar region

        M48.16   Ankylosing hyperostosis [Forestier], lumbar region

        M48.17   Ankylosing hyperostosis [Forestier], lumbosacral region

        M48.18   Ankylosing hyperostosis [Forestier], sacral and sacrococcygeal region

        M48.19   Ankylosing hyperostosis [Forestier], multiple sites in spine

    ✓5ᵗʰ **M48.2   Kissing spine**

        M48.20   Kissing spine, site unspecified

        M48.21   Kissing spine, occipito-atlanto-axial region

        M48.22   Kissing spine, cervical region

        M48.23   Kissing spine, cervicothoracic region

        M48.24   Kissing spine, thoracic region

        M48.25   Kissing spine, thoracolumbar region

        M48.26   Kissing spine, lumbar region

        M48.27   Kissing spine, lumbosacral region

    ✓5ᵗʰ **M48.3   Traumatic spondylopathy**

        CC Excl: For CC codes in subcategory M48.3:
        PDX collection 887

        M48.30   Traumatic spondylopathy, site unspecified   `CC`

        M48.31   Traumatic spondylopathy, occipito-atlanto-axial region   `CC`

        M48.32   Traumatic spondylopathy, cervical region   `CC`

        M48.33   Traumatic spondylopathy, cervicothoracic region   `CC`

        M48.34   Traumatic spondylopathy, thoracic region   `CC`

        M48.35   Traumatic spondylopathy, thoracolumbar region   `CC`

        M48.36   Traumatic spondylopathy, lumbar region   `CC`

        M48.37   Traumatic spondylopathy, lumbosacral region   `CC`

        M48.38   Traumatic spondylopathy, sacral and sacrococcygeal region   `CC`

    ✓5ᵗʰ **M48.4   Fatigue fracture of vertebra**
        Stress fracture of vertebra

        EXCLUDES 1   *pathological fracture NOS (M84.4-)*
            pathological fracture of vertebra due to neoplasm (M84.58)
            pathological fracture of vertebra due to other diagnosis (M84.68)
            pathological fracture of vertebra due to osteoporosis (M80.-)
            traumatic fracture of vertebrae (S12.0-S12.3-, S22.0-, S32.0-)

        The appropriate 7th character is to be added to each code from subcategory M48.4.
        A   initial encounter for fracture
        D   subsequent encounter for fracture with routine healing
        G   subsequent encounter for fracture with delayed healing
        S   sequela of fracture

        ✓x7ᵗʰ **M48.40   Fatigue fracture of vertebra, site unspecified**

        ✓x7ᵗʰ **M48.41   Fatigue fracture of vertebra, occipito-atlanto-axial region**

        ✓x7ᵗʰ **M48.42   Fatigue fracture of vertebra, cervical region**

        ✓x7ᵗʰ **M48.43   Fatigue fracture of vertebra, cervicothoracic region**

        ✓x7ᵗʰ **M48.44   Fatigue fracture of vertebra, thoracic region**

        ✓x7ᵗʰ **M48.45   Fatigue fracture of vertebra, thoracolumbar region**

        ✓x7ᵗʰ **M48.46   Fatigue fracture of vertebra, lumbar region**

        ✓x7ᵗʰ **M48.47   Fatigue fracture of vertebra, lumbosacral region**

        ✓x7ᵗʰ **M48.48   Fatigue fracture of vertebra, sacral and sacrococcygeal region**

    ✓5ᵗʰ **M48.5   Collapsed vertebra, not elsewhere classified**
        Collapsed vertebra NOS
        Compression fracture of vertebra NOS
        Wedging of vertebra NOS

        EXCLUDES 1   *current injury—see Injury of spine, by body region*
            fatigue fracture of vertebra (M48.4)
            pathological fracture of vertebra due to neoplasm (M84.58)
            pathological fracture of vertebra due to other diagnosis (M84.68)
            pathological fracture of vertebra due to osteoporosis (M80.-)
            pathological fracture NOS (M84.4-)
            stress fracture of vertebra (M48.4-)
            traumatic fracture of vertebra (S12-, S22-, S32-)

        The appropriate 7th character is to be added to each code from subcategory M48.5.
        A   initial encounter for fracture
        D   subsequent encounter for fracture with routine healing
        G   subsequent encounter for fracture with delayed healing
        S   sequela of fracture

        CC Excl: For CC codes in subcategory M48.5:
        PDX collection 888

    10 ✓x7ᵗʰ **M48.50   Collapsed vertebra, not elsewhere classified, site unspecified**   `CC` `HCC`

    10 ✓x7ᵗʰ **M48.51   Collapsed vertebra, not elsewhere classified, occipito-atlanto-axial region**   `CC` `HCC`

    10 ✓x7ᵗʰ **M48.52   Collapsed vertebra, not elsewhere classified, cervical region**   `CC` `HCC`

    10 ✓x7ᵗʰ **M48.53   Collapsed vertebra, not elsewhere classified, cervicothoracic region**   `CC` `HCC`

    10 ✓x7ᵗʰ **M48.54   Collapsed vertebra, not elsewhere classified, thoracic region**   `CC` `HCC`

    10 ✓x7ᵗʰ **M48.55   Collapsed vertebra, not elsewhere classified, thoracolumbar region**   `CC` `HCC`

    10 ✓x7ᵗʰ **M48.56   Collapsed vertebra, not elsewhere classified, lumbar region**   `CC` `HCC`

    10 ✓x7ᵗʰ **M48.57   Collapsed vertebra, not elsewhere classified, lumbosacral region**   `CC` `HCC`

    10 ✓x7ᵗʰ **M48.58   Collapsed vertebra, not elsewhere classified, sacral and sacrococcygeal region**   `CC` `HCC`

---

10 HCC with 7th character indicating initial encounter (A, B or C - specific to category).

N Newborn: 0   P Pediatric: 0-17   M Maternity: 12-55   A Adult: 15-124   `MCC` Major CC Condition   `PDxMCC` PDx acts as own MCC   `CC` CC Condition   `PDxCC` PDx acts as own CC

776   ICD-10-CM 2018

☑5th **M48.8 Other specified spondylopathies**
　　Ossification of posterior longitudinal ligament

　☑6th **M48.8X Other specified spondylopathies**

　　　M48.8X1 Other specified spondylopathies, `HCC`
　　　　　occipito-atlanto-axial region

　　　M48.8X2 Other specified spondylopathies, `HCC`
　　　　　cervical region

　　　M48.8X3 Other specified spondylopathies, `HCC`
　　　　　cervicothoracic region

　　　M48.8X4 Other specified spondylopathies, `HCC`
　　　　　thoracic region

　　　M48.8X5 Other specified spondylopathies, `HCC`
　　　　　thoracolumbar region

　　　M48.8X6 Other specified spondylopathies, `HCC`
　　　　　lumbar region

　　　M48.8X7 Other specified spondylopathies, `HCC`
　　　　　lumbosacral region

　　　M48.8X8 Other specified spondylopathies, `HCC`
　　　　　sacral and sacrococcygeal region

　　　M48.8X9 Other specified spondylopathies, `HCC`
　　　　　site unspecified

M48.9 Spondylopathy, unspecified

☑4th **M49 Spondylopathies in diseases classified elsewhere**
　　`INCLUDES` curvature of spine in diseases classified elsewhere
　　　　deformity of spine in diseases classified elsewhere
　　　　kyphosis in diseases classified elsewhere
　　　　scoliosis in diseases classified elsewhere
　　　　spondylopathy in diseases classified elsewhere
　　Code first underlying disease, such as:
　　　brucellosis (A23.-)
　　　Charcôt-Marie-Tooth disease (G60.0)
　　　enterobacterial infections (A01-A04)
　　　osteitis fibrosa cystica (E21.0)
　　`EXCLUDES 1` *curvature of spine in tuberculosis [Pott's] (A18.01)*
　　　　enteropathic arthropathies (M07.-)
　　　　gonococcal spondylitis (A54.41)
　　　　neuropathic [tabes dorsalis] spondylitis (A52.11)
　　　　neuropathic spondylopathy in syringomyelia (G95.0)
　　　　neuropathic spondylopathy in tabes dorsalis (A52.11)
　　　　nonsyphilitic neuropathic spondylopathy NEC (G98.0)
　　　　spondylitis in syphilis (acquired) (A52.77)
　　　　tuberculous spondylitis (A18.01)
　　　　typhoid fever spondylitis (A01.05)

☑5th **M49.8 Spondylopathy in diseases classified elsewhere**

　　　M49.80 *Spondylopathy in diseases classified elsewhere,* `HCC`
　　　　　site unspecified

　　　M49.81 *Spondylopathy in diseases classified elsewhere,* `HCC`
　　　　　occipito-atlanto-axial region

　　　M49.82 *Spondylopathy in diseases classified elsewhere,* `HCC`
　　　　　cervical region

　　　M49.83 *Spondylopathy in diseases classified elsewhere,* `HCC`
　　　　　cervicothoracic region

　　　M49.84 *Spondylopathy in diseases classified elsewhere,* `HCC`
　　　　　thoracic region

　　　M49.85 *Spondylopathy in diseases classified elsewhere,* `HCC`
　　　　　thoracolumbar region

　　　M49.86 *Spondylopathy in diseases classified elsewhere,* `HCC`
　　　　　lumbar region

　　　M49.87 *Spondylopathy in diseases classified elsewhere,* `HCC`
　　　　　lumbosacral region

　　　M49.88 *Spondylopathy in diseases classified elsewhere,* `HCC`
　　　　　sacral and sacrococcygeal region

　　　M49.89 *Spondylopathy in diseases classified elsewhere,* `HCC`
　　　　　multiple sites in spine

Other dorsopathies (M50-M54)

　`EXCLUDES 1` *current injury—see injury of spine by body region*
　　　discitis NOS (M46.4-)

☑4th **M50 Cervical disc disorders**
　　`NOTE` Code to the most superior level of disorder.
　　`INCLUDES` cervicothoracic disc disorders with cervicalgia
　　　　cervicothoracic disc disorders
　　AHA: 2016, 1Q, 17

☑5th **M50.0 Cervical disc disorder with myelopathy**

　　CC Excl: For CC codes in subcategory M50.0:
　　PDX collection 889

　　　M50.00 Cervical disc disorder with myelopathy, `CC`
　　　　　unspecified cervical region

M50.01 Cervical disc disorder with myelopathy, `CC`
　　high cervical region
　　　C2-C3 disc disorder with myelopathy
　　　C3-C4 disc disorder with myelopathy

☑6th **M50.02 Cervical disc disorder with myelopathy,**
　　mid-cervical region

　　　M50.020 Cervical disc disorder with `CC`
　　　　　myelopathy, mid-cervical region,
　　　　　unspecified level

　　　M50.021 Cervical disc disorder at C4-C5 level `CC`
　　　　　with myelopathy
　　　　　　C4-C5 disc disorder with myelopathy

　　　M50.022 Cervical disc disorder at C5-C6 level `CC`
　　　　　with myelopathy
　　　　　　C5-C6 disc disorder with myelopathy

　　　M50.023 Cervical disc disorder at C6-C7 level `CC`
　　　　　with myelopathy
　　　　　　C6-C7 disc disorder with myelopathy

　M50.03 Cervical disc disorder with myelopathy, `CC`
　　cervicothoracic region
　　　C7-T1 disc disorder with myelopathy

☑5th **M50.1 Cervical disc disorder with radiculopathy**
　　`EXCLUDES 2` *brachial radiculitis NOS (M54.13)*

　　M50.10 Cervical disc disorder with radiculopathy,
　　　unspecified cervical region

　　M50.11 Cervical disc disorder with radiculopathy, high
　　　cervical region
　　　　C2-C3 disc disorder with radiculopathy
　　　　C3 radiculopathy due to disc disorder
　　　　C3-C4 disc disorder with radiculopathy
　　　　C4 radiculopathy due to disc disorder

　☑6th **M50.12 Cervical disc disorder with radiculopathy, mid-**
　　　cervical region

　　　M50.120 Mid-cervical disc disorder, unspecified

　　　M50.121 Cervical disc disorder at C4-C5 level with
　　　　　radiculopathy
　　　　　　C4-C5 disc disorder with radiculopathy
　　　　　　C5 radiculopathy due to disc disorder

　　　M50.122 Cervical disc disorder at C5-C6 level with
　　　　　radiculopathy
　　　　　　C5-C6 disc disorder with radiculopathy
　　　　　　C6 radiculopathy due to disc disorder

　　　M50.123 Cervical disc disorder at C6-C7 level with
　　　　　radiculopathy
　　　　　　C6-C7 disc disorder with radiculopathy
　　　　　　C7 radiculopathy due to disc disorder

　　M50.13 Cervical disc disorder with radiculopathy,
　　　cervicothoracic region
　　　　C7-T1 disc disorder with radiculopathy
　　　　C8 radiculopathy due to disc disorder

☑5th **M50.2 Other cervical disc displacement**

　　M50.20 Other cervical disc displacement, unspecified
　　　cervical region

　　M50.21 Other cervical disc displacement, high cervical
　　　region
　　　　Other C2-C3 cervical disc displacement
　　　　Other C3-C4 cervical disc displacement

　☑6th **M50.22 Other cervical disc displacement, mid-cervical region**

　　　M50.220 Other cervical disc displacement,
　　　　　mid-cervical region, unspecified level

　　　M50.221 Other cervical disc displacement at C4-C5
　　　　　level
　　　　　　Other C4-C5 cervical disc displacement

　　　M50.222 Other cervical disc displacement at C5-C6
　　　　　level
　　　　　　Other C5-C6 cervical disc displacement

　　　M50.223 Other cervical disc displacement at C6-C7
　　　　　level
　　　　　　Other C6-C7 cervical disc displacement

　　M50.23 Other cervical disc displacement, cervicothoracic
　　　region
　　　　Other C7-T1 cervical disc displacement

☑5th **M50.3 Other cervical disc degeneration**

　　M50.30 Other cervical disc degeneration, unspecified
　　　cervical region

　　M50.31 Other cervical disc degeneration, high cervical
　　　region
　　　　Other C2-C3 cervical disc degeneration
　　　　Other C3-C4 cervical disc degeneration

☑ Additional Character Req   ☑x7th Placeholder Alert   Unacceptable PDx   Manifestation   `H1`-`H14` HAC   `HCC` CMS-HCC Condition   `EXCLUDES 1` Not Coded Here   `EXCLUDES 2` Not Included Here

√6th **M50.32** **Other cervical disc degeneration, mid-cervical region**

M50.320 **Other cervical disc degeneration, mid-cervical region, unspecified level**

M50.321 **Other cervical disc degeneration at C4-C5 level**
Other C4-C5 cervical disc degeneration

M50.322 **Other cervical disc degeneration at C5-C6 level**
Other C5-C6 cervical disc degeneration

M50.323 **Other cervical disc degeneration at C6-C7 level**
Other C6-C7 cervical disc degeneration

M50.33 **Other cervical disc degeneration, cervicothoracic region**
Other C7-T1 cervical disc degeneration

√5th **M50.8** **Other cervical disc disorders**

M50.80 **Other cervical disc disorders, unspecified cervical region**

M50.81 **Other cervical disc disorders, high cervical region**
Other C2-C3 cervical disc disorders
Other C3-C4 cervical disc disorders

√6th **M50.82** **Other cervical disc disorders, mid-cervical region**

M50.820 **Other cervical disc disorders, mid-cervical region, unspecified level**

M50.821 **Other cervical disc disorders at C4-C5 level**
Other C4-C5 cervical disc disorders

M50.822 **Other cervical disc disorders at C5-C6 level**
Other C5-C6 cervical disc disorders

M50.823 **Other cervical disc disorders at C6-C7 level**
Other C6-C7 cervical disc disorders

M50.83 **Other cervical disc disorders, cervicothoracic region**
Other C7-T1 cervical disc disorders

√5th **M50.9** **Cervical disc disorder, unspecified**

M50.90 **Cervical disc disorder, unspecified, unspecified cervical region**

M50.91 **Cervical disc disorder, unspecified, high cervical region**
C2-C3 cervical disc disorder, unspecified
C3-C4 cervical disc disorder, unspecified

√6th **M50.92** **Cervical disc disorder, unspecified, mid-cervical region**

M50.920 **Unspecified cervical disc disorder, mid-cervical region, unspecified level**

M50.921 **Unspecified cervical disc disorder at C4-C5 level**
Unspecified C4-C5 cervical disc disorder

M50.922 **Unspecified cervical disc disorder at C5-C6 level**
Unspecified C5-C6 cervical disc disorder

M50.923 **Unspecified cervical disc disorder at C6-C7 level**
Unspecified C6-C7 cervical disc disorder

M50.93 **Cervical disc disorder, unspecified, cervicothoracic region**
C7-T1 cervical disc disorder, unspecified

√4th **M51** **Thoracic, thoracolumbar, and lumbosacral intervertebral disc disorders**
EXCLUDES 2 *cervical and cervicothoracic disc disorders (M50.-)*
sacral and sacrococcygeal disorders (M53.3)

√5th **M51.0** **Thoracic, thoracolumbar and lumbosacral intervertebral disc disorders with myelopathy**

M51.04 **Intervertebral disc disorders with myelopathy, thoracic region** CC
CC Excl: PDX collection 890

M51.05 **Intervertebral disc disorders with myelopathy, thoracolumbar region** CC
CC Excl: PDX collection 890

M51.06 **Intervertebral disc disorders with myelopathy, lumbar region** CC
CC Excl: PDX collection 891

√5th **M51.1** **Thoracic, thoracolumbar and lumbosacral intervertebral disc disorders with radiculopathy**
Sciatica due to intervertebral disc disorder
EXCLUDES 1 *lumbar radiculitis NOS (M54.16)*
sciatica NOS (M54.3)

M51.14 **Intervertebral disc disorders with radiculopathy, thoracic region**

Displacement Intervertebral Disc

Normal Top View — Herniated Top View

Lamina
Ligamentum flavum
Nucleus pulposus
Spinal cord
Spinal nerve
Disc annulus
Nucleus pulposus
Herniates through annulus

M51.15 **Intervertebral disc disorders with radiculopathy, thoracolumbar region**

M51.16 **Intervertebral disc disorders with radiculopathy, lumbar region**

M51.17 **Intervertebral disc disorders with radiculopathy, lumbosacral region**

√5th **M51.2** **Other thoracic, thoracolumbar and lumbosacral intervertebral disc displacement**
Lumbago due to displacement of intervertebral disc

M51.24 **Other intervertebral disc displacement, thoracic region**

M51.25 **Other intervertebral disc displacement, thoracolumbar region**

M51.26 **Other intervertebral disc displacement, lumbar region**

M51.27 **Other intervertebral disc displacement, lumbosacral region**

√5th **M51.3** **Other thoracic, thoracolumbar and lumbosacral intervertebral disc degeneration**
AHA: 2013, 3Q, 22

M51.34 **Other intervertebral disc degeneration, thoracic region**

M51.35 **Other intervertebral disc degeneration, thoracolumbar region**

M51.36 **Other intervertebral disc degeneration, lumbar region**

M51.37 **Other intervertebral disc degeneration, lumbosacral region**

√5th **M51.4** **Schmorl's nodes**
DEF: Irregular bone defect in the margin of the vertebral body; causes herniation into end plate of vertebral body.

M51.44 **Schmorl's nodes, thoracic region**

M51.45 **Schmorl's nodes, thoracolumbar region**

M51.46 **Schmorl's nodes, lumbar region**

M51.47 **Schmorl's nodes, lumbosacral region**

√5th **M51.8** **Other thoracic, thoracolumbar and lumbosacral intervertebral disc disorders**

M51.84 **Other intervertebral disc disorders, thoracic region**

M51.85 **Other intervertebral disc disorders, thoracolumbar region**

M51.86 **Other intervertebral disc disorders, lumbar region**

M51.87 **Other intervertebral disc disorders, lumbosacral region**

M51.9 **Unspecified thoracic, thoracolumbar and lumbosacral intervertebral disc disorder**

√4th **M53** **Other and unspecified dorsopathies, not elsewhere classified**

M53.0 **Cervicocranial syndrome**
Posterior cervical sympathetic syndrome

M53.1 **Cervicobrachial syndrome**
EXCLUDES 2 *cervical disc disorder (M50.-)*
thoracic outlet syndrome (G54.0)

√5th **M53.2** **Spinal instabilities**

√6th **M53.2X** **Spinal instabilities**

M53.2X1 **Spinal instabilities, occipito-atlanto-axial region**

M53.2X2 **Spinal instabilities, cervical region**

M53.2X3 **Spinal instabilities, cervicothoracic region**

M53.2X4 **Spinal instabilities, thoracic region**

N Newborn: 0   P Pediatric: 0-17   M Maternity: 12-55   A Adult: 15-124   MCC Major CC Condition   PDxMCC PDx acts as own MCC   CC CC Condition   PDxCC PDx acts as own CC

778   ICD-10-CM 2018

M53.2X5   **Spinal instabilities, thoracolumbar region**
M53.2X6   **Spinal instabilities, lumbar region**
M53.2X7   **Spinal instabilities, lumbosacral region**
M53.2X8   **Spinal instabilities, sacral and sacrococcygeal region**
M53.2X9   **Spinal instabilities, site unspecified**

M53.3   **Sacrococcygeal disorders, not elsewhere classified**
Coccygodynia

✓5th   M53.8   **Other specified dorsopathies**
M53.80   **Other specified dorsopathies, site unspecified**
M53.81   **Other specified dorsopathies, occipito-atlanto-axial region**
M53.82   **Other specified dorsopathies, cervical region**
M53.83   **Other specified dorsopathies, cervicothoracic region**
M53.84   **Other specified dorsopathies, thoracic region**
M53.85   **Other specified dorsopathies, thoracolumbar region**
M53.86   **Other specified dorsopathies, lumbar region**
M53.87   **Other specified dorsopathies, lumbosacral region**
M53.88   **Other specified dorsopathies, sacral and sacrococcygeal region**

M53.9   **Dorsopathy, unspecified**

✓4th   **M54 Dorsalgia**
EXCLUDES 1   psychogenic dorsalgia (F45.41)

✓5th   M54.0   **Panniculitis affecting regions of neck and back**
EXCLUDES 1   lupus panniculitis (L93.2)
panniculitis NOS (M79.3)
relapsing [Weber-Christian] panniculitis (M35.6)

M54.00   **Panniculitis affecting regions of neck and back, site unspecified**
M54.01   **Panniculitis affecting regions of neck and back, occipito-atlanto-axial region**
M54.02   **Panniculitis affecting regions of neck and back, cervical region**
M54.03   **Panniculitis affecting regions of neck and back, cervicothoracic region**
M54.04   **Panniculitis affecting regions of neck and back, thoracic region**
M54.05   **Panniculitis affecting regions of neck and back, thoracolumbar region**
M54.06   **Panniculitis affecting regions of neck and back, lumbar region**
M54.07   **Panniculitis affecting regions of neck and back, lumbosacral region**
M54.08   **Panniculitis affecting regions of neck and back, sacral and sacrococcygeal region**
M54.09   **Panniculitis affecting regions, neck and back, multiple sites in spine**

✓5th   M54.1   **Radiculopathy**
Brachial neuritis or radiculitis NOS
Lumbar neuritis or radiculitis NOS
Lumbosacral neuritis or radiculitis NOS
Thoracic neuritis or radiculitis NOS
Radiculitis NOS
EXCLUDES 1   neuralgia and neuritis NOS (M79.2)
radiculopathy with cervical disc disorder (M50.1)
radiculopathy with lumbar and other intervertebral disc disorder (M51.1-)
radiculopathy with spondylosis (M47.2-)

M54.10   **Radiculopathy, site unspecified**
M54.11   **Radiculopathy, occipito-atlanto-axial region**
M54.12   **Radiculopathy, cervical region**
M54.13   **Radiculopathy, cervicothoracic region**
M54.14   **Radiculopathy, thoracic region**
M54.15   **Radiculopathy, thoracolumbar region**
M54.16   **Radiculopathy, lumbar region**
M54.17   **Radiculopathy, lumbosacral region**
M54.18   **Radiculopathy, sacral and sacrococcygeal region**

M54.2   **Cervicalgia**
EXCLUDES 1   cervicalgia due to intervertebral cervical disc disorder (M50.-)

✓5th   M54.3   **Sciatica**
EXCLUDES 1   lesion of sciatic nerve (G57.0)
sciatica due to intervertebral disc disorder (M51.1-)
sciatica with lumbago (M54.4-)

M54.30   **Sciatica, unspecified side**
M54.31   **Sciatica, right side**
M54.32   **Sciatica, left side**

✓5th   M54.4   **Lumbago with sciatica**
EXCLUDES 1   lumbago with sciatica due to intervertebral disc disorder (M51.1-)
AHA: 2016, 2Q, 7

M54.40   **Lumbago with sciatica, unspecified side**
M54.41   **Lumbago with sciatica, right side**
M54.42   **Lumbago with sciatica, left side**

M54.5   **Low back pain**
Loin pain
Lumbago NOS
EXCLUDES 1   low back strain (S39.012)
lumbago due to intervertebral disc displacement (M51.2-)
lumbago with sciatica (M54.4-)

M54.6   **Pain in thoracic spine**
EXCLUDES 1   pain in thoracic spine due to intervertebral disc disorder (M51.-)

✓5th   M54.8   **Other dorsalgia**
EXCLUDES 1   dorsalgia in thoracic region (M54.6)
low back pain (M54.5)

M54.81   **Occipital neuralgia**
M54.89   **Other dorsalgia**

M54.9   **Dorsalgia, unspecified**
Backache NOS
Back pain NOS

SOFT TISSUE DISORDERS (M60-M79)

Disorders of muscles (M60-M63)

EXCLUDES 1   dermatopolymyositis (M33.-)
muscular dystrophies and myopathies (G71-G72)
myopathy in amyloidosis (E85.-)
myopathy in polyarteritis nodosa (M30.0)
myopathy in rheumatoid arthritis (M05.32)
myopathy in scleroderma (M34.-)
myopathy in Sjögren's syndrome (M35.03)
myopathy in systemic lupus erythematosus (M32.-)

✓4th   **M60 Myositis**
EXCLUDES 2   inclusion body myositis [IBM] (G72.41)

✓5th   M60.0   **Infective myositis**
Tropical pyomyositis
Use additional code (B95-B97) to identify infectious agent

CC Excl: For CC codes in subcategory M60.0:
PDX collection 806

✓6th   M60.00   **Infective myositis, unspecified site**
M60.000   **Infective myositis, unspecified right arm**   CC
Infective myositis, right upper limb NOS
M60.001   **Infective myositis, unspecified left arm**   CC
Infective myositis, left upper limb NOS
M60.002   **Infective myositis, unspecified arm**   CC
Infective myositis, upper limb NOS
M60.003   **Infective myositis, unspecified right leg**   CC
Infective myositis, right lower limb NOS
M60.004   **Infective myositis, unspecified left leg**   CC
Infective myositis, left lower limb NOS
M60.005   **Infective myositis, unspecified leg**   CC
Infective myositis, lower limb NOS
M60.009   **Infective myositis, unspecified site**   CC

✓6th   M60.01   **Infective myositis, shoulder**
M60.011   **Infective myositis, right shoulder**   CC
M60.012   **Infective myositis, left shoulder**   CC
M60.019   **Infective myositis, unspecified shoulder**   CC

✓6th   M60.02   **Infective myositis, upper arm**
M60.021   **Infective myositis, right upper arm**   CC
M60.022   **Infective myositis, left upper arm**   CC

M60.029　Infective myositis, unspecified **upper arm** `CC`

✓6ᵗʰ M60.03　Infective myositis, **forearm**

M60.031　Infective myositis, right **forearm** `CC`

M60.032　Infective myositis, left **forearm** `CC`

M60.039　Infective myositis, unspecified **forearm** `CC`

✓6ᵗʰ M60.04　Infective myositis, **hand and fingers**

M60.041　Infective myositis, right **hand** `CC`

M60.042　Infective myositis, left **hand** `CC`

M60.043　Infective myositis, unspecified **hand** `CC`

M60.044　Infective myositis, right **finger(s)** `CC`

M60.045　Infective myositis, left **finger(s)** `CC`

M60.046　Infective myositis, unspecified **finger(s)** `CC`

✓6ᵗʰ M60.05　Infective myositis, **thigh**

M60.051　Infective myositis, right **thigh** `CC`

M60.052　Infective myositis, left **thigh** `CC`

M60.059　Infective myositis, unspecified **thigh** `CC`

✓6ᵗʰ M60.06　Infective myositis, **lower leg**

M60.061　Infective myositis, right **lower leg** `CC`

M60.062　Infective myositis, left **lower leg** `CC`

M60.069　Infective myositis, unspecified **lower leg** `CC`

✓6ᵗʰ M60.07　Infective myositis, **ankle, foot and toes**

M60.070　Infective myositis, right **ankle** `CC`

M60.071　Infective myositis, left **ankle** `CC`

M60.072　Infective myositis, unspecified **ankle** `CC`

M60.073　Infective myositis, right **foot** `CC`

M60.074　Infective myositis, left **foot** `CC`

M60.075　Infective myositis, unspecified **foot** `CC`

M60.076　Infective myositis, right **toe(s)** `CC`

M60.077　Infective myositis, left **toe(s)** `CC`

M60.078　Infective myositis, unspecified **toe(s)** `CC`

M60.08　Infective myositis, **other site** `CC`

M60.09　Infective myositis, **multiple sites** `CC`

M60.1 Interstitial myositis

M60.10　Interstitial myositis of **unspecified site**

✓6ᵗʰ M60.11　Interstitial myositis, **shoulder**

M60.111　Interstitial myositis, right **shoulder**

M60.112　Interstitial myositis, left **shoulder**

M60.119　Interstitial myositis, unspecified **shoulder**

✓6ᵗʰ M60.12　Interstitial myositis, **upper arm**

M60.121　Interstitial myositis, right **upper arm**

M60.122　Interstitial myositis, left **upper arm**

M60.129　Interstitial myositis, unspecified **upper arm**

✓6ᵗʰ M60.13　Interstitial myositis, **forearm**

M60.131　Interstitial myositis, right **forearm**

M60.132　Interstitial myositis, left **forearm**

M60.139　Interstitial myositis, unspecified **forearm**

✓6ᵗʰ M60.14　Interstitial myositis, **hand**

M60.141　Interstitial myositis, right **hand**

M60.142　Interstitial myositis, left **hand**

M60.149　Interstitial myositis, unspecified **hand**

✓6ᵗʰ M60.15　Interstitial myositis, **thigh**

M60.151　Interstitial myositis, right **thigh**

M60.152　Interstitial myositis, left **thigh**

M60.159　Interstitial myositis, unspecified **thigh**

✓6ᵗʰ M60.16　Interstitial myositis, **lower leg**

M60.161　Interstitial myositis, right **lower leg**

M60.162　Interstitial myositis, left **lower leg**

M60.169　Interstitial myositis, unspecified **lower leg**

✓6ᵗʰ M60.17　Interstitial myositis, **ankle and foot**

M60.171　Interstitial myositis, right **ankle and foot**

M60.172　Interstitial myositis, left **ankle and foot**

M60.179　Interstitial myositis, unspecified **ankle and foot**

M60.18　Interstitial myositis, **other site**

M60.19　Interstitial myositis, **multiple sites**

✓5ᵗʰ M60.2　Foreign body granuloma of soft tissue, not elsewhere classified

Use additional code to identify the type of retained foreign body (Z18.-)

EXCLUDES 1　*foreign body granuloma of skin and subcutaneous tissue (L92.3)*

M60.20　Foreign body granuloma of soft tissue, not elsewhere classified, **unspecified site**

✓6ᵗʰ M60.21　Foreign body granuloma of soft tissue, not elsewhere classified, **shoulder**

M60.211　Foreign body granuloma of soft tissue, not elsewhere classified, right **shoulder**

M60.212　Foreign body granuloma of soft tissue, not elsewhere classified, left **shoulder**

M60.219　Foreign body granuloma of soft tissue, not elsewhere classified, unspecified **shoulder**

✓6ᵗʰ M60.22　Foreign body granuloma of soft tissue, not elsewhere classified, **upper arm**

M60.221　Foreign body granuloma of soft tissue, not elsewhere classified, right **upper arm**

M60.222　Foreign body granuloma of soft tissue, not elsewhere classified, left **upper arm**

M60.229　Foreign body granuloma of soft tissue, not elsewhere classified, unspecified **upper arm**

✓6ᵗʰ M60.23　Foreign body granuloma of soft tissue, not elsewhere classified, **forearm**

M60.231　Foreign body granuloma of soft tissue, not elsewhere classified, right **forearm**

M60.232　Foreign body granuloma of soft tissue, not elsewhere classified, left **forearm**

M60.239　Foreign body granuloma of soft tissue, not elsewhere classified, unspecified **forearm**

✓6ᵗʰ M60.24　Foreign body granuloma of soft tissue, not elsewhere classified, **hand**

M60.241　Foreign body granuloma of soft tissue, not elsewhere classified, right **hand**

M60.242　Foreign body granuloma of soft tissue, not elsewhere classified, left **hand**

M60.249　Foreign body granuloma of soft tissue, not elsewhere classified, unspecified **hand**

✓6ᵗʰ M60.25　Foreign body granuloma of soft tissue, not elsewhere classified, **thigh**

M60.251　Foreign body granuloma of soft tissue, not elsewhere classified, right **thigh**

M60.252　Foreign body granuloma of soft tissue, not elsewhere classified, left **thigh**

M60.259　Foreign body granuloma of soft tissue, not elsewhere classified, unspecified **thigh**

✓6ᵗʰ M60.26　Foreign body granuloma of soft tissue, not elsewhere classified, **lower leg**

M60.261　Foreign body granuloma of soft tissue, not elsewhere classified, right **lower leg**

M60.262　Foreign body granuloma of soft tissue, not elsewhere classified, left **lower leg**

M60.269　Foreign body granuloma of soft tissue, not elsewhere classified, unspecified **lower leg**

✓6ᵗʰ M60.27　Foreign body granuloma of soft tissue, not elsewhere classified, **ankle and foot**

M60.271　Foreign body granuloma of soft tissue, not elsewhere classified, right **ankle and foot**

M60.272　Foreign body granuloma of soft tissue, not elsewhere classified, left **ankle and foot**

M60.279　Foreign body granuloma of soft tissue, not elsewhere classified, unspecified **ankle and foot**

M60.28　Foreign body granuloma of soft tissue, not elsewhere classified, **other site**

✓5ᵗʰ M60.8　**Other myositis**

M60.80　Other myositis, **unspecified site**

✓6ᵗʰ M60.81　Other myositis **shoulder**

M60.811　Other myositis, right **shoulder**

M60.812　Other myositis, left **shoulder**

M60.819　Other myositis, unspecified **shoulder**

✓6ᵗʰ M60.82　Other myositis, **upper arm**

M60.821　Other myositis, right **upper arm**

M60.822　Other myositis, left **upper arm**

N Newborn: 0　P Pediatric: 0-17　M Maternity: 12-55　A Adult: 15-124　MCC Major CC Condition　PDxMCC PDx acts as own MCC　CC CC Condition　PDxCC PDx acts as own CC

780　　ICD-10-CM 2018

M60.829   Other myositis, unspecified upper arm

✓6ᵗʰ   **M60.83**   **Other myositis, forearm**
     M60.831   Other myositis, right forearm
     M60.832   Other myositis, left forearm
     M60.839   Other myositis, unspecified forearm

✓6ᵗʰ   **M60.84**   **Other myositis, hand**
     M60.841   Other myositis, right hand
     M60.842   Other myositis, left hand
     M60.849   Other myositis, unspecified hand

✓6ᵗʰ   **M60.85**   **Other myositis, thigh**
     M60.851   Other myositis, right thigh
     M60.852   Other myositis, left thigh
     M60.859   Other myositis, unspecified thigh

✓6ᵗʰ   **M60.86**   **Other myositis, lower leg**
     M60.861   Other myositis, right lower leg
     M60.862   Other myositis, left lower leg
     M60.869   Other myositis, unspecified lower leg

✓6ᵗʰ   **M60.87**   **Other myositis, ankle and foot**
     M60.871   Other myositis, right ankle and foot
     M60.872   Other myositis, left ankle and foot
     M60.879   Other myositis, unspecified ankle and foot

     M60.88   Other myositis, other site
     M60.89   Other myositis, multiple sites

M60.9 Myositis, unspecified

✓4ᵗʰ **M61 Calcification and ossification of muscle**

✓5ᵗʰ   **M61.0 Myositis ossificans traumatica**
     M61.00   Myositis ossificans traumatica, unspecified site

✓6ᵗʰ   **M61.01**   **Myositis ossificans traumatica, shoulder**
     M61.011   Myositis ossificans traumatica, right shoulder
     M61.012   Myositis ossificans traumatica, left shoulder
     M61.019   Myositis ossificans traumatica, unspecified shoulder

✓6ᵗʰ   **M61.02**   **Myositis ossificans traumatica, upper arm**
     M61.021   Myositis ossificans traumatica, right upper arm
     M61.022   Myositis ossificans traumatica, left upper arm
     M61.029   Myositis ossificans traumatica, unspecified upper arm

✓6ᵗʰ   **M61.03**   **Myositis ossificans traumatica, forearm**
     M61.031   Myositis ossificans traumatica, right forearm
     M61.032   Myositis ossificans traumatica, left forearm
     M61.039   Myositis ossificans traumatica, unspecified forearm

✓6ᵗʰ   **M61.04**   **Myositis ossificans traumatica, hand**
     M61.041   Myositis ossificans traumatica, right hand
     M61.042   Myositis ossificans traumatica, left hand
     M61.049   Myositis ossificans traumatica, unspecified hand

✓6ᵗʰ   **M61.05**   **Myositis ossificans traumatica, thigh**
     M61.051   Myositis ossificans traumatica, right thigh
     M61.052   Myositis ossificans traumatica, left thigh
     M61.059   Myositis ossificans traumatica, unspecified thigh

✓6ᵗʰ   **M61.06**   **Myositis ossificans traumatica, lower leg**
     M61.061   Myositis ossificans traumatica, right lower leg
     M61.062   Myositis ossificans traumatica, left lower leg
     M61.069   Myositis ossificans traumatica, unspecified lower leg

✓6ᵗʰ   **M61.07**   **Myositis ossificans traumatica, ankle and foot**
     M61.071   Myositis ossificans traumatica, right ankle and foot
     M61.072   Myositis ossificans traumatica, left ankle and foot
     M61.079   Myositis ossificans traumatica, unspecified ankle and foot

     M61.08   Myositis ossificans traumatica, other site

     M61.09   Myositis ossificans traumatica, multiple sites

✓5ᵗʰ   **M61.1 Myositis ossificans progressiva**
     Fibrodysplasia ossificans progressiva
     M61.10   Myositis ossificans progressiva, unspecified site

✓6ᵗʰ   **M61.11**   **Myositis ossificans progressiva, shoulder**
     M61.111   Myositis ossificans progressiva, right shoulder
     M61.112   Myositis ossificans progressiva, left shoulder
     M61.119   Myositis ossificans progressiva, unspecified shoulder

✓6ᵗʰ   **M61.12**   **Myositis ossificans progressiva, upper arm**
     M61.121   Myositis ossificans progressiva, right upper arm
     M61.122   Myositis ossificans progressiva, left upper arm
     M61.129   Myositis ossificans progressiva, unspecified arm

✓6ᵗʰ   **M61.13**   **Myositis ossificans progressiva, forearm**
     M61.131   Myositis ossificans progressiva, right forearm
     M61.132   Myositis ossificans progressiva, left forearm
     M61.139   Myositis ossificans progressiva, unspecified forearm

✓6ᵗʰ   **M61.14**   **Myositis ossificans progressiva, hand and finger(s)**
     M61.141   Myositis ossificans progressiva, right hand
     M61.142   Myositis ossificans progressiva, left hand
     M61.143   Myositis ossificans progressiva, unspecified hand
     M61.144   Myositis ossificans progressiva, right finger(s)
     M61.145   Myositis ossificans progressiva, left finger(s)
     M61.146   Myositis ossificans progressiva, unspecified finger(s)

✓6ᵗʰ   **M61.15**   **Myositis ossificans progressiva, thigh**
     M61.151   Myositis ossificans progressiva, right thigh
     M61.152   Myositis ossificans progressiva, left thigh
     M61.159   Myositis ossificans progressiva, unspecified thigh

✓6ᵗʰ   **M61.16**   **Myositis ossificans progressiva, lower leg**
     M61.161   Myositis ossificans progressiva, right lower leg
     M61.162   Myositis ossificans progressiva, left lower leg
     M61.169   Myositis ossificans progressiva, unspecified lower leg

✓6ᵗʰ   **M61.17**   **Myositis ossificans progressiva, ankle, foot and toe(s)**
     M61.171   Myositis ossificans progressiva, right ankle
     M61.172   Myositis ossificans progressiva, left ankle
     M61.173   Myositis ossificans progressiva, unspecified ankle
     M61.174   Myositis ossificans progressiva, right foot
     M61.175   Myositis ossificans progressiva, left foot
     M61.176   Myositis ossificans progressiva, unspecified foot
     M61.177   Myositis ossificans progressiva, right toe(s)
     M61.178   Myositis ossificans progressiva, left toe(s)
     M61.179   Myositis ossificans progressiva, unspecified toe(s)

     M61.18   Myositis ossificans progressiva, other site
     M61.19   Myositis ossificans progressiva, multiple sites

✓5ᵗʰ   **M61.2 Paralytic calcification and ossification of muscle**
     Myositis ossificans associated with quadriplegia or paraplegia
     M61.20   Paralytic calcification and ossification of muscle, unspecified site

✓6ᵗʰ   **M61.21**   **Paralytic calcification and ossification of muscle, shoulder**
     M61.211   Paralytic calcification and ossification of muscle, right shoulder

✔Additional Character Req   ✓x7ᵗʰ Placeholder Alert   Unacceptable PDx   Manifestation   **H1**-**H14** HAC   **HCC** CMS-HCC Condition   *EXCLUDES 1* Not Coded Here   *EXCLUDES 2* Not Included Here

ICD-10-CM 2018   781

M61.212   Paralytic calcification and ossification of muscle, left shoulder

M61.219   Paralytic calcification and ossification of muscle, unspecified shoulder

✓6ᵗʰ   M61.22   Paralytic calcification and ossification of muscle, upper arm

M61.221   Paralytic calcification and ossification of muscle, right upper arm

M61.222   Paralytic calcification and ossification of muscle, left upper arm

M61.229   Paralytic calcification and ossification of muscle, unspecified upper arm

✓6ᵗʰ   M61.23   Paralytic calcification and ossification of muscle, forearm

M61.231   Paralytic calcification and ossification of muscle, right forearm

M61.232   Paralytic calcification and ossification of muscle, left forearm

M61.239   Paralytic calcification and ossification of muscle, unspecified forearm

✓6ᵗʰ   M61.24   Paralytic calcification and ossification of muscle, hand

M61.241   Paralytic calcification and ossification of muscle, right hand

M61.242   Paralytic calcification and ossification of muscle, left hand

M61.249   Paralytic calcification and ossification of muscle, unspecified hand

✓6ᵗʰ   M61.25   Paralytic calcification and ossification of muscle, thigh

M61.251   Paralytic calcification and ossification of muscle, right thigh

M61.252   Paralytic calcification and ossification of muscle, left thigh

M61.259   Paralytic calcification and ossification of muscle, unspecified thigh

✓6ᵗʰ   M61.26   Paralytic calcification and ossification of muscle, lower leg

M61.261   Paralytic calcification and ossification of muscle, right lower leg

M61.262   Paralytic calcification and ossification of muscle, left lower leg

M61.269   Paralytic calcification and ossification of muscle, unspecified lower leg

✓6ᵗʰ   M61.27   Paralytic calcification and ossification of muscle, ankle and foot

M61.271   Paralytic calcification and ossification of muscle, right ankle and foot

M61.272   Paralytic calcification and ossification of muscle, left ankle and foot

M61.279   Paralytic calcification and ossification of muscle, unspecified ankle and foot

M61.28   Paralytic calcification and ossification of muscle, other site

M61.29   Paralytic calcification and ossification of muscle, multiple sites

✓5ᵗʰ   M61.3   Calcification and ossification of muscles associated with burns

Myositis ossificans associated with burns

M61.30   Calcification and ossification of muscles associated with burns, unspecified site

✓6ᵗʰ   M61.31   Calcification and ossification of muscles associated with burns, shoulder

M61.311   Calcification and ossification of muscles associated with burns, right shoulder

M61.312   Calcification and ossification of muscles associated with burns, left shoulder

M61.319   Calcification and ossification of muscles associated with burns, unspecified shoulder

✓6ᵗʰ   M61.32   Calcification and ossification of muscles associated with burns, upper arm

M61.321   Calcification and ossification of muscles associated with burns, right upper arm

M61.322   Calcification and ossification of muscles associated with burns, left upper arm

M61.329   Calcification and ossification of muscles associated with burns, unspecified upper arm

✓6ᵗʰ   M61.33   Calcification and ossification of muscles associated with burns, forearm

M61.331   Calcification and ossification of muscles associated with burns, right forearm

M61.332   Calcification and ossification of muscles associated with burns, left forearm

M61.339   Calcification and ossification of muscles associated with burns, unspecified forearm

✓6ᵗʰ   M61.34   Calcification and ossification of muscles associated with burns, hand

M61.341   Calcification and ossification of muscles associated with burns, right hand

M61.342   Calcification and ossification of muscles associated with burns, left hand

M61.349   Calcification and ossification of muscles associated with burns, unspecified hand

✓6ᵗʰ   M61.35   Calcification and ossification of muscles associated with burns, thigh

M61.351   Calcification and ossification of muscles associated with burns, right thigh

M61.352   Calcification and ossification of muscles associated with burns, left thigh

M61.359   Calcification and ossification of muscles associated with burns, unspecified thigh

✓6ᵗʰ   M61.36   Calcification and ossification of muscles associated with burns, lower leg

M61.361   Calcification and ossification of muscles associated with burns, right lower leg

M61.362   Calcification and ossification of muscles associated with burns, left lower leg

M61.369   Calcification and ossification of muscles associated with burns, unspecified lower leg

✓6ᵗʰ   M61.37   Calcification and ossification of muscles associated with burns, ankle and foot

M61.371   Calcification and ossification of muscles associated with burns, right ankle and foot

M61.372   Calcification and ossification of muscles associated with burns, left ankle and foot

M61.379   Calcification and ossification of muscles associated with burns, unspecified ankle and foot

M61.38   Calcification and ossification of muscles associated with burns, other site

M61.39   Calcification and ossification of muscles associated with burns, multiple sites

✓5ᵗʰ   M61.4   Other calcification of muscle

> EXCLUDES 1   *calcific tendinitis NOS (M65.2-)*
> *calcific tendinitis of shoulder (M75.3)*

M61.40   Other calcification of muscle, unspecified site

✓6ᵗʰ   M61.41   Other calcification of muscle, shoulder

M61.411   Other calcification of muscle, right shoulder

M61.412   Other calcification of muscle, left shoulder

M61.419   Other calcification of muscle, unspecified shoulder

✓6ᵗʰ   M61.42   Other calcification of muscle, upper arm

M61.421   Other calcification of muscle, right upper arm

M61.422   Other calcification of muscle, left upper arm

M61.429   Other calcification of muscle, unspecified upper arm

✓6ᵗʰ   M61.43   Other calcification of muscle, forearm

M61.431   Other calcification of muscle, right forearm

M61.432   Other calcification of muscle, left forearm

M61.439   Other calcification of muscle, unspecified forearm

Ⓝ Newborn: 0   Ⓟ Pediatric: 0-17   Ⓜ Maternity: 12-55   Ⓐ Adult: 15-124   MCC Major CC Condition   PDx MCC PDx acts as own MCC   CC CC Condition   PDx CC PDx acts as own CC

782   ICD-10-CM 2018

✓6ᵗʰ M61.44 Other calcification of muscle, hand
  M61.441 Other calcification of muscle, right hand
  M61.442 Other calcification of muscle, left hand
  M61.449 Other calcification of muscle, unspecified hand

✓6ᵗʰ M61.45 Other calcification of muscle, thigh
  M61.451 Other calcification of muscle, right thigh
  M61.452 Other calcification of muscle, left thigh
  M61.459 Other calcification of muscle, unspecified thigh

✓6ᵗʰ M61.46 Other calcification of muscle, lower leg
  M61.461 Other calcification of muscle, right lower leg
  M61.462 Other calcification of muscle, left lower leg
  M61.469 Other calcification of muscle, unspecified lower leg

✓6ᵗʰ M61.47 Other calcification of muscle, ankle and foot
  M61.471 Other calcification of muscle, right ankle and foot
  M61.472 Other calcification of muscle, left ankle and foot
  M61.479 Other calcification of muscle, unspecified ankle and foot

M61.48 Other calcification of muscle, other site
M61.49 Other calcification of muscle, multiple sites

✓5ᵗʰ M61.5 Other ossification of muscle
  M61.50 Other ossification of muscle, unspecified site

✓6ᵗʰ M61.51 Other ossification of muscle, shoulder
  M61.511 Other ossification of muscle, right shoulder
  M61.512 Other ossification of muscle, left shoulder
  M61.519 Other ossification of muscle, unspecified shoulder

✓6ᵗʰ M61.52 Other ossification of muscle, upper arm
  M61.521 Other ossification of muscle, right upper arm
  M61.522 Other ossification of muscle, left upper arm
  M61.529 Other ossification of muscle, unspecified upper arm

✓6ᵗʰ M61.53 Other ossification of muscle, forearm
  M61.531 Other ossification of muscle, right forearm
  M61.532 Other ossification of muscle, left forearm
  M61.539 Other ossification of muscle, unspecified forearm

✓6ᵗʰ M61.54 Other ossification of muscle, hand
  M61.541 Other ossification of muscle, right hand
  M61.542 Other ossification of muscle, left hand
  M61.549 Other ossification of muscle, unspecified hand

✓6ᵗʰ M61.55 Other ossification of muscle, thigh
  M61.551 Other ossification of muscle, right thigh
  M61.552 Other ossification of muscle, left thigh
  M61.559 Other ossification of muscle, unspecified thigh

✓6ᵗʰ M61.56 Other ossification of muscle, lower leg
  M61.561 Other ossification of muscle, right lower leg
  M61.562 Other ossification of muscle, left lower leg
  M61.569 Other ossification of muscle, unspecified lower leg

✓6ᵗʰ M61.57 Other ossification of muscle, ankle and foot
  M61.571 Other ossification of muscle, right ankle and foot
  M61.572 Other ossification of muscle, left ankle and foot
  M61.579 Other ossification of muscle, unspecified ankle and foot

M61.58 Other ossification of muscle, other site
M61.59 Other ossification of muscle, multiple sites
M61.9 Calcification and ossification of muscle, unspecified

✓4ᵗʰ M62 Other disorders of muscle
  EXCLUDES 1   alcoholic myopathy (G72.1)
            cramp and spasm (R25.2)
            drug-induced myopathy (G72.0)
            myalgia (M79.1)
            stiff-man syndrome (G25.82)
  EXCLUDES 2   nontraumatic hematoma of muscle (M79.81)

✓5ᵗʰ M62.0 Separation of muscle (nontraumatic)
  Diastasis of muscle
  EXCLUDES 1   diastasis recti complicating pregnancy, labor and delivery (O71.8)
            traumatic separation of muscle—see strain of muscle by body region

  M62.00 Separation of muscle (nontraumatic), unspecified site

✓6ᵗʰ M62.01 Separation of muscle (nontraumatic), shoulder
  M62.011 Separation of muscle (nontraumatic), right shoulder
  M62.012 Separation of muscle (nontraumatic), left shoulder
  M62.019 Separation of muscle (nontraumatic), unspecified shoulder

✓6ᵗʰ M62.02 Separation of muscle (nontraumatic), upper arm
  M62.021 Separation of muscle (nontraumatic), right upper arm
  M62.022 Separation of muscle (nontraumatic), left upper arm
  M62.029 Separation of muscle (nontraumatic), unspecified upper arm

✓6ᵗʰ M62.03 Separation of muscle (nontraumatic), forearm
  M62.031 Separation of muscle (nontraumatic), right forearm
  M62.032 Separation of muscle (nontraumatic), left forearm
  M62.039 Separation of muscle (nontraumatic), unspecified forearm

✓6ᵗʰ M62.04 Separation of muscle (nontraumatic), hand
  M62.041 Separation of muscle (nontraumatic), right hand
  M62.042 Separation of muscle (nontraumatic), left hand
  M62.049 Separation of muscle (nontraumatic), unspecified hand

✓6ᵗʰ M62.05 Separation of muscle (nontraumatic), thigh
  M62.051 Separation of muscle (nontraumatic), right thigh
  M62.052 Separation of muscle (nontraumatic), left thigh
  M62.059 Separation of muscle (nontraumatic), unspecified thigh

✓6ᵗʰ M62.06 Separation of muscle (nontraumatic), lower leg
  M62.061 Separation of muscle (nontraumatic), right lower leg
  M62.062 Separation of muscle (nontraumatic), left lower leg
  M62.069 Separation of muscle (nontraumatic), unspecified lower leg

✓6ᵗʰ M62.07 Separation of muscle (nontraumatic), ankle and foot
  M62.071 Separation of muscle (nontraumatic), right ankle and foot
  M62.072 Separation of muscle (nontraumatic), left ankle and foot
  M62.079 Separation of muscle (nontraumatic), unspecified ankle and foot

  M62.08 Separation of muscle (nontraumatic), other site

✓5ᵗʰ M62.1 Other rupture of muscle (nontraumatic)
  EXCLUDES 1   traumatic rupture of muscle—see strain of muscle by body region
  EXCLUDES 2   rupture of tendon (M66.-)

  M62.10 Other rupture of muscle (nontraumatic), unspecified site

✓6ᵗʰ M62.11 Other rupture of muscle (nontraumatic), shoulder
  M62.111 Other rupture of muscle (nontraumatic), right shoulder
  M62.112 Other rupture of muscle (nontraumatic), left shoulder

---

        M62.119   **Other rupture of muscle (nontraumatic), unspecified shoulder**

✓6th   **M62.12**   **Other rupture of muscle (nontraumatic), upper arm**

        M62.121   **Other rupture of muscle (nontraumatic), right upper arm**

        M62.122   **Other rupture of muscle (nontraumatic), left upper arm**

        M62.129   **Other rupture of muscle (nontraumatic), unspecified upper arm**

✓6th   **M62.13**   **Other rupture of muscle (nontraumatic), forearm**

        M62.131   **Other rupture of muscle (nontraumatic), right forearm**

        M62.132   **Other rupture of muscle (nontraumatic), left forearm**

        M62.139   **Other rupture of muscle (nontraumatic), unspecified forearm**

✓6th   **M62.14**   **Other rupture of muscle (nontraumatic), hand**

        M62.141   **Other rupture of muscle (nontraumatic), right hand**

        M62.142   **Other rupture of muscle (nontraumatic), left hand**

        M62.149   **Other rupture of muscle (nontraumatic), unspecified hand**

✓6th   **M62.15**   **Other rupture of muscle (nontraumatic), thigh**

        M62.151   **Other rupture of muscle (nontraumatic), right thigh**

        M62.152   **Other rupture of muscle (nontraumatic), left thigh**

        M62.159   **Other rupture of muscle (nontraumatic), unspecified thigh**

✓6th   **M62.16**   **Other rupture of muscle (nontraumatic), lower leg**

        M62.161   **Other rupture of muscle (nontraumatic), right lower leg**

        M62.162   **Other rupture of muscle (nontraumatic), left lower leg**

        M62.169   **Other rupture of muscle (nontraumatic), unspecified lower leg**

✓6th   **M62.17**   **Other rupture of muscle (nontraumatic), ankle and foot**

        M62.171   **Other rupture of muscle (nontraumatic), right ankle and foot**

        M62.172   **Other rupture of muscle (nontraumatic), left ankle and foot**

        M62.179   **Other rupture of muscle (nontraumatic), unspecified ankle and foot**

    M62.18   **Other rupture of muscle (nontraumatic), other site**

✓5th   **M62.2**   **Nontraumatic ischemic infarction of muscle**

        EXCLUDES 1   *compartment syndrome (traumatic) (T79.A-)*
                  nontraumatic compartment syndrome (M79.A-)
                  rhabdomyolysis (M62.82)
                  traumatic ischemia of muscle (T79.6)
                  Volkmann's ischemic contracture (T79.6)

    M62.20   **Nontraumatic ischemic infarction of muscle, unspecified site**

✓6th   **M62.21**   **Nontraumatic ischemic infarction of muscle, shoulder**

        M62.211   **Nontraumatic ischemic infarction of muscle, right shoulder**

        M62.212   **Nontraumatic ischemic infarction of muscle, left shoulder**

        M62.219   **Nontraumatic ischemic infarction of muscle, unspecified shoulder**

✓6th   **M62.22**   **Nontraumatic ischemic infarction of muscle, upper arm**

        M62.221   **Nontraumatic ischemic infarction of muscle, right upper arm**

        M62.222   **Nontraumatic ischemic infarction of muscle, left upper arm**

        M62.229   **Nontraumatic ischemic infarction of muscle, unspecified upper arm**

✓6th   **M62.23**   **Nontraumatic ischemic infarction of muscle, forearm**

        M62.231   **Nontraumatic ischemic infarction of muscle, right forearm**

        M62.232   **Nontraumatic ischemic infarction of muscle, left forearm**

        M62.239   **Nontraumatic ischemic infarction of muscle, unspecified forearm**

✓6th   **M62.24**   **Nontraumatic ischemic infarction of muscle, hand**

        M62.241   **Nontraumatic ischemic infarction of muscle, right hand**

        M62.242   **Nontraumatic ischemic infarction of muscle, left hand**

        M62.249   **Nontraumatic ischemic infarction of muscle, unspecified hand**

✓6th   **M62.25**   **Nontraumatic ischemic infarction of muscle, thigh**

        M62.251   **Nontraumatic ischemic infarction of muscle, right thigh**

        M62.252   **Nontraumatic ischemic infarction of muscle, left thigh**

        M62.259   **Nontraumatic ischemic infarction of muscle, unspecified thigh**

✓6th   **M62.26**   **Nontraumatic ischemic infarction of muscle, lower leg**

        M62.261   **Nontraumatic ischemic infarction of muscle, right lower leg**

        M62.262   **Nontraumatic ischemic infarction of muscle, left lower leg**

        M62.269   **Nontraumatic ischemic infarction of muscle, unspecified lower leg**

✓6th   **M62.27**   **Nontraumatic ischemic infarction of muscle, ankle and foot**

        M62.271   **Nontraumatic ischemic infarction of muscle, right ankle and foot**

        M62.272   **Nontraumatic ischemic infarction of muscle, left ankle and foot**

        M62.279   **Nontraumatic ischemic infarction of muscle, unspecified ankle and foot**

    M62.28   **Nontraumatic ischemic infarction of muscle, other site**

    M62.3   **Immobility syndrome (paraplegic)**

✓5th   **M62.4**   **Contracture of muscle**

        Contracture of tendon (sheath)

        EXCLUDES 1   *contracture of joint (M24.5-)*

    M62.40   **Contracture of muscle, unspecified site**

✓6th   **M62.41**   **Contracture of muscle, shoulder**

        M62.411   **Contracture of muscle, right shoulder**

        M62.412   **Contracture of muscle, left shoulder**

        M62.419   **Contracture of muscle, unspecified shoulder**

✓6th   **M62.42**   **Contracture of muscle, upper arm**

        M62.421   **Contracture of muscle, right upper arm**

        M62.422   **Contracture of muscle, left upper arm**

        M62.429   **Contracture of muscle, unspecified upper arm**

✓6th   **M62.43**   **Contracture of muscle, forearm**

        M62.431   **Contracture of muscle, right forearm**

        M62.432   **Contracture of muscle, left forearm**

        M62.439   **Contracture of muscle, unspecified forearm**

✓6th   **M62.44**   **Contracture of muscle, hand**

        M62.441   **Contracture of muscle, right hand**

        M62.442   **Contracture of muscle, left hand**

        M62.449   **Contracture of muscle, unspecified hand**

✓6th   **M62.45**   **Contracture of muscle, thigh**

        M62.451   **Contracture of muscle, right thigh**

        M62.452   **Contracture of muscle, left thigh**

        M62.459   **Contracture of muscle, unspecified thigh**

✓6th   **M62.46**   **Contracture of muscle, lower leg**

        M62.461   **Contracture of muscle, right lower leg**

        M62.462   **Contracture of muscle, left lower leg**

        M62.469   **Contracture of muscle, unspecified lower leg**

✓6th   **M62.47**   **Contracture of muscle, ankle and foot**

        M62.471   **Contracture of muscle, right ankle and foot**

        M62.472   **Contracture of muscle, left ankle and foot**

        M62.479   **Contracture of muscle, unspecified ankle and foot**

    M62.48   **Contracture of muscle, other site**

    M62.49   **Contracture of muscle, multiple sites**

N Newborn: 0   P Pediatric: 0-17   M Maternity: 12-55   A Adult: 15-124   MCC Major CC Condition   PDx MCC PDx acts as own MCC   CC CC Condition   PDx CC PDx acts as own CC

784   ICD-10-CM 2018

✓5th **M62.5** **Muscle wasting and atrophy, not elsewhere classified**
Disuse atrophy NEC
EXCLUDES 1   neuralgic amyotrophy (G54.5)
           progressive muscular atrophy ▶(G12.21)◀
           sarcopenia (M62.84)
EXCLUDES 2   pelvic muscle wasting (N81.84)

     M62.50 **Muscle wasting and atrophy, not elsewhere classified, unspecified site**

✓6th **M62.51** **Muscle wasting and atrophy, not elsewhere classified, shoulder**

     M62.511 Muscle wasting and atrophy, not elsewhere classified, right shoulder

     M62.512 Muscle wasting and atrophy, not elsewhere classified, left shoulder

     M62.519 Muscle wasting and atrophy, not elsewhere classified, unspecified shoulder

✓6th **M62.52** **Muscle wasting and atrophy, not elsewhere classified, upper arm**

     M62.521 Muscle wasting and atrophy, not elsewhere classified, right upper arm

     M62.522 Muscle wasting and atrophy, not elsewhere classified, left upper arm

     M62.529 Muscle wasting and atrophy, not elsewhere classified, unspecified upper arm

✓6th **M62.53** **Muscle wasting and atrophy, not elsewhere classified, forearm**

     M62.531 Muscle wasting and atrophy, not elsewhere classified, right forearm

     M62.532 Muscle wasting and atrophy, not elsewhere classified, left forearm

     M62.539 Muscle wasting and atrophy, not elsewhere classified, unspecified forearm

✓6th **M62.54** **Muscle wasting and atrophy, not elsewhere classified, hand**

     M62.541 Muscle wasting and atrophy, not elsewhere classified, right hand

     M62.542 Muscle wasting and atrophy, not elsewhere classified, left hand

     M62.549 Muscle wasting and atrophy, not elsewhere classified, unspecified hand

✓6th **M62.55** **Muscle wasting and atrophy, not elsewhere classified, thigh**

     M62.551 Muscle wasting and atrophy, not elsewhere classified, right thigh

     M62.552 Muscle wasting and atrophy, not elsewhere classified, left thigh

     M62.559 Muscle wasting and atrophy, not elsewhere classified, unspecified thigh

✓6th **M62.56** **Muscle wasting and atrophy, not elsewhere classified, lower leg**

     M62.561 Muscle wasting and atrophy, not elsewhere classified, right lower leg

     M62.562 Muscle wasting and atrophy, not elsewhere classified, left lower leg

     M62.569 Muscle wasting and atrophy, not elsewhere classified, unspecified lower leg

✓6th **M62.57** **Muscle wasting and atrophy, not elsewhere classified, ankle and foot**

     M62.571 Muscle wasting and atrophy, not elsewhere classified, right ankle and foot

     M62.572 Muscle wasting and atrophy, not elsewhere classified, left ankle and foot

     M62.579 Muscle wasting and atrophy, not elsewhere classified, unspecified ankle and foot

     M62.58 **Muscle wasting and atrophy, not elsewhere classified, other site**

     M62.59 **Muscle wasting and atrophy, not elsewhere classified, multiple sites**

✓5th **M62.8** **Other specified disorders of muscle**
EXCLUDES 2   nontraumatic hematoma of muscle (M79.81)

     M62.81 **Muscle weakness (generalized)**
EXCLUDES 1   muscle weakness in sarcopenia (M62.84)

     M62.82 **Rhabdomyolysis**   CC
EXCLUDES 1   traumatic rhabdomyolysis (T79.6)
DEF: Rapid disintegration or destruction of skeletal muscle caused by direct or indirect injury; resulting in the excretion of muscle protein myoglobin into the urine.
CC Excl: PDX collection 892

✓6th **M62.83** **Muscle spasm**

     M62.830 **Muscle spasm of back**

     M62.831 **Muscle spasm of calf**
Charley-horse

     M62.838 **Other muscle spasm**

     M62.84 **Sarcopenia**
Age-related sarcopenia
Code first underlying disease, if applicable, such as:
   disorders of myoneural junction and muscle disease in diseases classified elsewhere (G73.-)
   other and unspecified myopathies (G72.-)
   primary disorders of muscles (G71.-)

     M62.89 **Other specified disorders of muscle**
Muscle (sheath) hernia

     M62.9 **Disorder of muscle, unspecified**

✓4th **M63** **Disorders of muscle in diseases classified elsewhere**
Code first underlying disease, such as:
   leprosy (A30.-)
   neoplasm (C49-, C79.89, D21-, D48.1)
   schistosomiasis (B65.-)
   trichinellosis (B75)
EXCLUDES 1   myopathy in cysticercosis (B69.81)
           myopathy in endocrine diseases (G73.7)
           myopathy in metabolic diseases (G73.7)
           myopathy in sarcoidosis (D86.87)
           myopathy in secondary syphilis (A51.49)
           myopathy in syphilis (late) (A52.78)
           myopathy in toxoplasmosis (B58.82)
           myopathy in tuberculosis (A18.09)

✓5th **M63.8** **Disorders of muscle in diseases classified elsewhere**

     M63.80 **Disorders of muscle in diseases classified elsewhere, unspecified site**

✓6th **M63.81** **Disorders of muscle in diseases classified elsewhere, shoulder**

     M63.811 *Disorders of muscle in diseases classified elsewhere, right shoulder*

     M63.812 *Disorders of muscle in diseases classified elsewhere, left shoulder*

     M63.819 *Disorders of muscle in diseases classified elsewhere, unspecified shoulder*

✓6th **M63.82** **Disorders of muscle in diseases classified elsewhere, upper arm**

     M63.821 *Disorders of muscle in diseases classified elsewhere, right upper arm*

     M63.822 *Disorders of muscle in diseases classified elsewhere, left upper arm*

     M63.829 *Disorders of muscle in diseases classified elsewhere, unspecified upper arm*

✓6th **M63.83** **Disorders of muscle in diseases classified elsewhere, forearm**

     M63.831 *Disorders of muscle in diseases classified elsewhere, right forearm*

     M63.832 *Disorders of muscle in diseases classified elsewhere, left forearm*

     M63.839 *Disorders of muscle in diseases classified elsewhere, unspecified forearm*

✓6th **M63.84** **Disorders of muscle in diseases classified elsewhere, hand**

     M63.841 *Disorders of muscle in diseases classified elsewhere, right hand*

     M63.842 *Disorders of muscle in diseases classified elsewhere, left hand*

     M63.849 *Disorders of muscle in diseases classified elsewhere, unspecified hand*

✓ Additional Character Req   ✓x7th Placeholder Alert   Unacceptable PDx   Manifestation   H1 - H14 HAC   HCC CMS-HCC Condition   EXCLUDES 1 Not Coded Here   EXCLUDES 2 Not Included Here

ICD-10-CM 2018   785

✓6ᵗʰ **M63.85** Disorders of muscle in diseases classified elsewhere, thigh

     M63.851   *Disorders of muscle in diseases classified elsewhere, right thigh*

     M63.852   *Disorders of muscle in diseases classified elsewhere, left thigh*

     M63.859   *Disorders of muscle in diseases classified elsewhere, unspecified thigh*

✓6ᵗʰ **M63.86** Disorders of muscle in diseases classified elsewhere, lower leg

     M63.861   *Disorders of muscle in diseases classified elsewhere, right lower leg*

     M63.862   *Disorders of muscle in diseases classified elsewhere, left lower leg*

     M63.869   *Disorders of muscle in diseases classified elsewhere, unspecified lower leg*

✓6ᵗʰ **M63.87** Disorders of muscle in diseases classified elsewhere, ankle and foot

     M63.871   *Disorders of muscle in diseases classified elsewhere, right ankle and foot*

     M63.872   *Disorders of muscle in diseases classified elsewhere, left ankle and foot*

     M63.879   *Disorders of muscle in diseases classified elsewhere, unspecified ankle and foot*

     M63.88   *Disorders of muscle in diseases classified elsewhere, other site*

     M63.89   *Disorders of muscle in diseases classified elsewhere, multiple sites*

Disorders of synovium and tendon (M65-M67)

✓4ᵗʰ **M65** **Synovitis and tenosynovitis**

     EXCLUDES 1   *chronic crepitant synovitis of hand and wrist (M70.0-)*
              current injury—see injury of ligament or tendon by body region
              soft tissue disorders related to use, overuse and pressure (M70.-)

✓5ᵗʰ **M65.0** Abscess of tendon sheath

     Use additional code (B95-B96) to identify bacterial agent.

     M65.00 Abscess of tendon sheath, unspecified site

✓6ᵗʰ   **M65.01** Abscess of tendon sheath, shoulder

     M65.011 Abscess of tendon sheath, right shoulder

     M65.012 Abscess of tendon sheath, left shoulder

     M65.019 Abscess of tendon sheath, unspecified shoulder

✓6ᵗʰ   **M65.02** Abscess of tendon sheath, upper arm

     M65.021 Abscess of tendon sheath, right upper arm

     M65.022 Abscess of tendon sheath, left upper arm

     M65.029 Abscess of tendon sheath, unspecified upper arm

✓6ᵗʰ   **M65.03** Abscess of tendon sheath, forearm

     M65.031 Abscess of tendon sheath, right forearm

     M65.032 Abscess of tendon sheath, left forearm

     M65.039 Abscess of tendon sheath, unspecified forearm

✓6ᵗʰ   **M65.04** Abscess of tendon sheath, hand

     M65.041 Abscess of tendon sheath, right hand

     M65.042 Abscess of tendon sheath, left hand

     M65.049 Abscess of tendon sheath, unspecified hand

✓6ᵗʰ   **M65.05** Abscess of tendon sheath, thigh

     M65.051 Abscess of tendon sheath, right thigh

     M65.052 Abscess of tendon sheath, left thigh

     M65.059 Abscess of tendon sheath, unspecified thigh

✓6ᵗʰ   **M65.06** Abscess of tendon sheath, lower leg

     M65.061 Abscess of tendon sheath, right lower leg

     M65.062 Abscess of tendon sheath, left lower leg

     M65.069 Abscess of tendon sheath, unspecified lower leg

✓6ᵗʰ   **M65.07** Abscess of tendon sheath, ankle and foot

     M65.071 Abscess of tendon sheath, right ankle and foot

     M65.072 Abscess of tendon sheath, left ankle and foot

     M65.079 Abscess of tendon sheath, unspecified ankle and foot

     M65.08 Abscess of tendon sheath, other site

✓5ᵗʰ **M65.1** Other infective (teno)synovitis

     M65.10 Other infective (teno)synovitis, unspecified site

✓6ᵗʰ   **M65.11** Other infective (teno)synovitis, shoulder

     M65.111 Other infective (teno)synovitis, right shoulder

     M65.112 Other infective (teno)synovitis, left shoulder

     M65.119 Other infective (teno)synovitis, unspecified shoulder

✓6ᵗʰ   **M65.12** Other infective (teno)synovitis, elbow

     M65.121 Other infective (teno)synovitis, right elbow

     M65.122 Other infective (teno)synovitis, left elbow

     M65.129 Other infective (teno)synovitis, unspecified elbow

✓6ᵗʰ   **M65.13** Other infective (teno)synovitis, wrist

     M65.131 Other infective (teno)synovitis, right wrist

     M65.132 Other infective (teno)synovitis, left wrist

     M65.139 Other infective (teno)synovitis, unspecified wrist

✓6ᵗʰ   **M65.14** Other infective (teno)synovitis, hand

     M65.141 Other infective (teno)synovitis, right hand

     M65.142 Other infective (teno)synovitis, left hand

     M65.149 Other infective (teno)synovitis, unspecified hand

✓6ᵗʰ   **M65.15** Other infective (teno)synovitis, hip

     M65.151 Other infective (teno)synovitis, right hip

     M65.152 Other infective (teno)synovitis, left hip

     M65.159 Other infective (teno)synovitis, unspecified hip

✓6ᵗʰ   **M65.16** Other infective (teno)synovitis, knee

     M65.161 Other infective (teno)synovitis, right knee

     M65.162 Other infective (teno)synovitis, left knee

     M65.169 Other infective (teno)synovitis, unspecified knee

✓6ᵗʰ   **M65.17** Other infective (teno)synovitis, ankle and foot

     M65.171 Other infective (teno)synovitis, right ankle and foot

     M65.172 Other infective (teno)synovitis, left ankle and foot

     M65.179 Other infective (teno)synovitis, unspecified ankle and foot

     M65.18 Other infective (teno)synovitis, other site

     M65.19 Other infective (teno)synovitis, multiple sites

✓5ᵗʰ **M65.2** Calcific tendinitis

     EXCLUDES 1   *tendinitis as classified in M75-M77*
              calcified tendinitis of shoulder (M75.3)

     M65.20 Calcific tendinitis, unspecified site

✓6ᵗʰ   **M65.22** Calcific tendinitis, upper arm

     M65.221 Calcific tendinitis, right upper arm

     M65.222 Calcific tendinitis, left upper arm

     M65.229 Calcific tendinitis, unspecified upper arm

✓6ᵗʰ   **M65.23** Calcific tendinitis, forearm

     M65.231 Calcific tendinitis, right forearm

     M65.232 Calcific tendinitis, left forearm

     M65.239 Calcific tendinitis, unspecified forearm

✓6ᵗʰ   **M65.24** Calcific tendinitis, hand

     M65.241 Calcific tendinitis, right hand

     M65.242 Calcific tendinitis, left hand

     M65.249 Calcific tendinitis, unspecified hand

✓6ᵗʰ   **M65.25** Calcific tendinitis, thigh

     M65.251 Calcific tendinitis, right thigh

     M65.252 Calcific tendinitis, left thigh

     M65.259 Calcific tendinitis, unspecified thigh

✓6ᵗʰ   **M65.26** Calcific tendinitis, lower leg

     M65.261 Calcific tendinitis, right lower leg

     M65.262 Calcific tendinitis, left lower leg

     M65.269 Calcific tendinitis, unspecified lower leg

✓6ᵗʰ   **M65.27** Calcific tendinitis, ankle and foot

     M65.271 Calcific tendinitis, right ankle and foot

     M65.272 Calcific tendinitis, left ankle and foot

     M65.279 Calcific tendinitis, unspecified ankle and foot

N Newborn: 0   P Pediatric: 0-17   M Maternity: 12-55   A Adult: 15-124   **MCC** Major CC Condition   **PDxMCC** PDx acts as own MCC   **CC** CC Condition   **PDxCC** PDx acts as own CC

786   ICD-10-CM 2018

M65.28   Calcific tendinitis, other site

M65.29   Calcific tendinitis, multiple sites

✓5ᵗʰ **M65.3   Trigger finger**
> Nodular tendinous disease

     M65.30   Trigger finger, unspecified finger

✓6ᵗʰ   **M65.31   Trigger thumb**

       M65.311   Trigger thumb, right thumb

       M65.312   Trigger thumb, left thumb

       M65.319   Trigger thumb, unspecified thumb

✓6ᵗʰ   **M65.32   Trigger finger, index finger**

       M65.321   Trigger finger, right index finger

       M65.322   Trigger finger, left index finger

       M65.329   Trigger finger, unspecified index finger

✓6ᵗʰ   **M65.33   Trigger finger, middle finger**

       M65.331   Trigger finger, right middle finger

       M65.332   Trigger finger, left middle finger

       M65.339   Trigger finger, unspecified middle finger

✓6ᵗʰ   **M65.34   Trigger finger, ring finger**

       M65.341   Trigger finger, right ring finger

       M65.342   Trigger finger, left ring finger

       M65.349   Trigger finger, unspecified ring finger

✓6ᵗʰ   **M65.35   Trigger finger, little finger**

       M65.351   Trigger finger, right little finger

       M65.352   Trigger finger, left little finger

       M65.359   Trigger finger, unspecified little finger

M65.4   Radial styloid tenosynovitis [de Quervain]

✓5ᵗʰ **M65.8   Other synovitis and tenosynovitis**

     M65.80   Other synovitis and tenosynovitis, unspecified site

✓6ᵗʰ   **M65.81   Other synovitis and tenosynovitis, shoulder**

       M65.811   Other synovitis and tenosynovitis, right shoulder

       M65.812   Other synovitis and tenosynovitis, left shoulder

       M65.819   Other synovitis and tenosynovitis, unspecified shoulder

✓6ᵗʰ   **M65.82   Other synovitis and tenosynovitis, upper arm**

       M65.821   Other synovitis and tenosynovitis, right upper arm

       M65.822   Other synovitis and tenosynovitis, left upper arm

       M65.829   Other synovitis and tenosynovitis, unspecified upper arm

✓6ᵗʰ   **M65.83   Other synovitis and tenosynovitis, forearm**

       M65.831   Other synovitis and tenosynovitis, right forearm

       M65.832   Other synovitis and tenosynovitis, left forearm

       M65.839   Other synovitis and tenosynovitis, unspecified forearm

✓6ᵗʰ   **M65.84   Other synovitis and tenosynovitis, hand**

       M65.841   Other synovitis and tenosynovitis, right hand

       M65.842   Other synovitis and tenosynovitis, left hand

       M65.849   Other synovitis and tenosynovitis, unspecified hand

✓6ᵗʰ   **M65.85   Other synovitis and tenosynovitis, thigh**

       M65.851   Other synovitis and tenosynovitis, right thigh

       M65.852   Other synovitis and tenosynovitis, left thigh

       M65.859   Other synovitis and tenosynovitis, unspecified thigh

✓6ᵗʰ   **M65.86   Other synovitis and tenosynovitis, lower leg**

       M65.861   Other synovitis and tenosynovitis, right lower leg

       M65.862   Other synovitis and tenosynovitis, left lower leg

       M65.869   Other synovitis and tenosynovitis, unspecified lower leg

✓6ᵗʰ   **M65.87   Other synovitis and tenosynovitis, ankle and foot**

       M65.871   Other synovitis and tenosynovitis, right ankle and foot

       M65.872   Other synovitis and tenosynovitis, left ankle and foot

       M65.879   Other synovitis and tenosynovitis, unspecified ankle and foot

     M65.88   Other synovitis and tenosynovitis, other site

     M65.89   Other synovitis and tenosynovitis, multiple sites

M65.9   Synovitis and tenosynovitis, unspecified

✓4ᵗʰ **M66   Spontaneous rupture of synovium and tendon**
> INCLUDES   rupture that occurs when a normal force is applied to tissues that are inferred to have less than normal strength
>
> EXCLUDES 2   rotator cuff syndrome (M75.1-)
> rupture where an abnormal force is applied to normal tissue—see injury of tendon by body region

M66.0   Rupture of popliteal cyst

✓5ᵗʰ **M66.1   Rupture of synovium**
> Rupture of synovial cyst
>
> EXCLUDES 2   rupture of popliteal cyst (M66.0)

     M66.10   Rupture of synovium, unspecified joint

✓6ᵗʰ   **M66.11   Rupture of synovium, shoulder**

       M66.111   Rupture of synovium, right shoulder

       M66.112   Rupture of synovium, left shoulder

       M66.119   Rupture of synovium, unspecified shoulder

✓6ᵗʰ   **M66.12   Rupture of synovium, elbow**

       M66.121   Rupture of synovium, right elbow

       M66.122   Rupture of synovium, left elbow

       M66.129   Rupture of synovium, unspecified elbow

✓6ᵗʰ   **M66.13   Rupture of synovium, wrist**

       M66.131   Rupture of synovium, right wrist

       M66.132   Rupture of synovium, left wrist

       M66.139   Rupture of synovium, unspecified wrist

✓6ᵗʰ   **M66.14   Rupture of synovium, hand and fingers**

       M66.141   Rupture of synovium, right hand

       M66.142   Rupture of synovium, left hand

       M66.143   Rupture of synovium, unspecified hand

       M66.144   Rupture of synovium, right finger(s)

       M66.145   Rupture of synovium, left finger(s)

       M66.146   Rupture of synovium, unspecified finger(s)

✓6ᵗʰ   **M66.15   Rupture of synovium, hip**

       M66.151   Rupture of synovium, right hip

       M66.152   Rupture of synovium, left hip

       M66.159   Rupture of synovium, unspecified hip

✓6ᵗʰ   **M66.17   Rupture of synovium, ankle, foot and toes**

       M66.171   Rupture of synovium, right ankle

       M66.172   Rupture of synovium, left ankle

       M66.173   Rupture of synovium, unspecified ankle

       M66.174   Rupture of synovium, right foot

       M66.175   Rupture of synovium, left foot

       M66.176   Rupture of synovium, unspecified foot

       M66.177   Rupture of synovium, right toe(s)

       M66.178   Rupture of synovium, left toe(s)

       M66.179   Rupture of synovium, unspecified toe(s)

     M66.18   Rupture of synovium, other site

✓5ᵗʰ **M66.2   Spontaneous rupture of extensor tendons**
> **TIP:** Refer to the Muscle/Tendon table at the beginning of this chapter.

     M66.20   Spontaneous rupture of extensor tendons, unspecified site

✓6ᵗʰ   **M66.21   Spontaneous rupture of extensor tendons, shoulder**

       M66.211   Spontaneous rupture of extensor tendons, right shoulder

       M66.212   Spontaneous rupture of extensor tendons, left shoulder

       M66.219   Spontaneous rupture of extensor tendons, unspecified shoulder

✓6ᵗʰ   **M66.22   Spontaneous rupture of extensor tendons, upper arm**

       M66.221   Spontaneous rupture of extensor tendons, right upper arm

       M66.222   Spontaneous rupture of extensor tendons, left upper arm

       M66.229   Spontaneous rupture of extensor tendons, unspecified upper arm

√6th **M66.23** Spontaneous rupture of extensor tendons, forearm

     M66.231 Spontaneous rupture of extensor tendons, right forearm

     M66.232 Spontaneous rupture of extensor tendons, left forearm

     M66.239 Spontaneous rupture of extensor tendons, unspecified forearm

√6th **M66.24** Spontaneous rupture of extensor tendons, hand

     M66.241 Spontaneous rupture of extensor tendons, right hand

     M66.242 Spontaneous rupture of extensor tendons, left hand

     M66.249 Spontaneous rupture of extensor tendons, unspecified hand

√6th **M66.25** Spontaneous rupture of extensor tendons, thigh

     M66.251 Spontaneous rupture of extensor tendons, right thigh

     M66.252 Spontaneous rupture of extensor tendons, left thigh

     M66.259 Spontaneous rupture of extensor tendons, unspecified thigh

√6th **M66.26** Spontaneous rupture of extensor tendons, lower leg

     M66.261 Spontaneous rupture of extensor tendons, right lower leg

     M66.262 Spontaneous rupture of extensor tendons, left lower leg

     M66.269 Spontaneous rupture of extensor tendons, unspecified lower leg

√6th **M66.27** Spontaneous rupture of extensor tendons, ankle and foot

     M66.271 Spontaneous rupture of extensor tendons, right ankle and foot

     M66.272 Spontaneous rupture of extensor tendons, left ankle and foot

     M66.279 Spontaneous rupture of extensor tendons, unspecified ankle and foot

M66.28 Spontaneous rupture of extensor tendons, other site

M66.29 Spontaneous rupture of extensor tendons, multiple sites

√5th **M66.3** Spontaneous rupture of flexor tendons

     TIP: Refer to the Muscle/Tendon table at the beginning of this chapter.

     M66.30 Spontaneous rupture of flexor tendons, unspecified site

√6th **M66.31** Spontaneous rupture of flexor tendons, shoulder

     M66.311 Spontaneous rupture of flexor tendons, right shoulder

     M66.312 Spontaneous rupture of flexor tendons, left shoulder

     M66.319 Spontaneous rupture of flexor tendons, unspecified shoulder

√6th **M66.32** Spontaneous rupture of flexor tendons, upper arm

     M66.321 Spontaneous rupture of flexor tendons, right upper arm

     M66.322 Spontaneous rupture of flexor tendons, left upper arm

     M66.329 Spontaneous rupture of flexor tendons, unspecified upper arm

√6th **M66.33** Spontaneous rupture of flexor tendons, forearm

     M66.331 Spontaneous rupture of flexor tendons, right forearm

     M66.332 Spontaneous rupture of flexor tendons, left forearm

     M66.339 Spontaneous rupture of flexor tendons, unspecified forearm

√6th **M66.34** Spontaneous rupture of flexor tendons, hand

     M66.341 Spontaneous rupture of flexor tendons, right hand

     M66.342 Spontaneous rupture of flexor tendons, left hand

     M66.349 Spontaneous rupture of flexor tendons, unspecified hand

√6th **M66.35** Spontaneous rupture of flexor tendons, thigh

     M66.351 Spontaneous rupture of flexor tendons, right thigh

     M66.352 Spontaneous rupture of flexor tendons, left thigh

     M66.359 Spontaneous rupture of flexor tendons, unspecified thigh

√6th **M66.36** Spontaneous rupture of flexor tendons, lower leg

     M66.361 Spontaneous rupture of flexor tendons, right lower leg

     M66.362 Spontaneous rupture of flexor tendons, left lower leg

     M66.369 Spontaneous rupture of flexor tendons, unspecified lower leg

√6th **M66.37** Spontaneous rupture of flexor tendons, ankle and foot

     M66.371 Spontaneous rupture of flexor tendons, right ankle and foot

     M66.372 Spontaneous rupture of flexor tendons, left ankle and foot

     M66.379 Spontaneous rupture of flexor tendons, unspecified ankle and foot

M66.38 Spontaneous rupture of flexor tendons, other site

M66.39 Spontaneous rupture of flexor tendons, multiple sites

√5th **M66.8** Spontaneous rupture of other tendons

     TIP: Refer to the Muscle/Tendon table at the beginning of this chapter.

     M66.80 Spontaneous rupture of other tendons, unspecified site

√6th **M66.81** Spontaneous rupture of other tendons, shoulder

     M66.811 Spontaneous rupture of other tendons, right shoulder

     M66.812 Spontaneous rupture of other tendons, left shoulder

     M66.819 Spontaneous rupture of other tendons, unspecified shoulder

√6th **M66.82** Spontaneous rupture of other tendons, upper arm

     M66.821 Spontaneous rupture of other tendons, right upper arm

     M66.822 Spontaneous rupture of other tendons, left upper arm

     M66.829 Spontaneous rupture of other tendons, unspecified upper arm

√6th **M66.83** Spontaneous rupture of other tendons, forearm

     M66.831 Spontaneous rupture of other tendons, right forearm

     M66.832 Spontaneous rupture of other tendons, left forearm

     M66.839 Spontaneous rupture of other tendons, unspecified forearm

√6th **M66.84** Spontaneous rupture of other tendons, hand

     M66.841 Spontaneous rupture of other tendons, right hand

     M66.842 Spontaneous rupture of other tendons, left hand

     M66.849 Spontaneous rupture of other tendons, unspecified hand

√6th **M66.85** Spontaneous rupture of other tendons, thigh

     M66.851 Spontaneous rupture of other tendons, right thigh

     M66.852 Spontaneous rupture of other tendons, left thigh

     M66.859 Spontaneous rupture of other tendons, unspecified thigh

√6th **M66.86** Spontaneous rupture of other tendons, lower leg

     M66.861 Spontaneous rupture of other tendons, right lower leg

     M66.862 Spontaneous rupture of other tendons, left lower leg

     M66.869 Spontaneous rupture of other tendons, unspecified lower leg

√6th **M66.87** Spontaneous rupture of other tendons, ankle and foot

     M66.871 Spontaneous rupture of other tendons, right ankle and foot

     M66.872 Spontaneous rupture of other tendons, left ankle and foot

     M66.879 Spontaneous rupture of other tendons, unspecified ankle and foot

M66.88 Spontaneous rupture of other tendons, other

N Newborn: 0   **P** Pediatric: 0-17   **M** Maternity: 12-55   **A** Adult: 15-124   **MCC** Major CC Condition   **PDxMCC** PDx acts as own MCC   **CC** CC Condition   **PDxCC** PDx acts as own CC

788   ICD-10-CM 2018

M66.89   **Spontaneous rupture of other tendons, multiple sites**

M66.9   **Spontaneous rupture of unspecified tendon**
Rupture at musculotendinous junction, nontraumatic

✔4ᵗʰ **M67**   **Other disorders of synovium and tendon**
EXCLUDES 1   palmar fascial fibromatosis [Dupuytren] (M72.0)
tendinitis NOS (M77.9-)
xanthomatosis localized to tendons (E78.2)

✔5ᵗʰ **M67.0**   **Short Achilles tendon (acquired)**

M67.00   **Short Achilles tendon (acquired), unspecified ankle**

M67.01   **Short Achilles tendon (acquired), right ankle**

M67.02   **Short Achilles tendon (acquired), left ankle**

✔5ᵗʰ **M67.2**   **Synovial hypertrophy, not elsewhere classified**
EXCLUDES 1   villonodular synovitis (pigmented) (M12.2-)

M67.20   **Synovial hypertrophy, not elsewhere classified, unspecified site**

✔6ᵗʰ M67.21   **Synovial hypertrophy, not elsewhere classified, shoulder**

M67.211   **Synovial hypertrophy, not elsewhere classified, right shoulder**

M67.212   **Synovial hypertrophy, not elsewhere classified, left shoulder**

M67.219   **Synovial hypertrophy, not elsewhere classified, unspecified shoulder**

✔6ᵗʰ M67.22   **Synovial hypertrophy, not elsewhere classified, upper arm**

M67.221   **Synovial hypertrophy, not elsewhere classified, right upper arm**

M67.222   **Synovial hypertrophy, not elsewhere classified, left upper arm**

M67.229   **Synovial hypertrophy, not elsewhere classified, unspecified upper arm**

✔6ᵗʰ M67.23   **Synovial hypertrophy, not elsewhere classified, forearm**

M67.231   **Synovial hypertrophy, not elsewhere classified, right forearm**

M67.232   **Synovial hypertrophy, not elsewhere classified, left forearm**

M67.239   **Synovial hypertrophy, not elsewhere classified, unspecified forearm**

✔6ᵗʰ M67.24   **Synovial hypertrophy, not elsewhere classified, hand**

M67.241   **Synovial hypertrophy, not elsewhere classified, right hand**

M67.242   **Synovial hypertrophy, not elsewhere classified, left hand**

M67.249   **Synovial hypertrophy, not elsewhere classified, unspecified hand**

✔6ᵗʰ M67.25   **Synovial hypertrophy, not elsewhere classified, thigh**

M67.251   **Synovial hypertrophy, not elsewhere classified, right thigh**

M67.252   **Synovial hypertrophy, not elsewhere classified, left thigh**

M67.259   **Synovial hypertrophy, not elsewhere classified, unspecified thigh**

✔6ᵗʰ M67.26   **Synovial hypertrophy, not elsewhere classified, lower leg**

M67.261   **Synovial hypertrophy, not elsewhere classified, right lower leg**

M67.262   **Synovial hypertrophy, not elsewhere classified, left lower leg**

M67.269   **Synovial hypertrophy, not elsewhere classified, unspecified lower leg**

✔6ᵗʰ M67.27   **Synovial hypertrophy, not elsewhere classified, ankle and foot**

M67.271   **Synovial hypertrophy, not elsewhere classified, right ankle and foot**

M67.272   **Synovial hypertrophy, not elsewhere classified, left ankle and foot**

M67.279   **Synovial hypertrophy, not elsewhere classified, unspecified ankle and foot**

M67.28   **Synovial hypertrophy, not elsewhere classified, other site**

M67.29   **Synovial hypertrophy, not elsewhere classified, multiple sites**

✔5ᵗʰ **M67.3**   **Transient synovitis**
Toxic synovitis
EXCLUDES 1   palindromic rheumatism (M12.3-)

M67.30   **Transient synovitis, unspecified site**

✔6ᵗʰ M67.31   **Transient synovitis, shoulder**

M67.311   **Transient synovitis, right shoulder**

M67.312   **Transient synovitis, left shoulder**

M67.319   **Transient synovitis, unspecified shoulder**

✔6ᵗʰ M67.32   **Transient synovitis, elbow**

M67.321   **Transient synovitis, right elbow**

M67.322   **Transient synovitis, left elbow**

M67.329   **Transient synovitis, unspecified elbow**

✔6ᵗʰ M67.33   **Transient synovitis, wrist**

M67.331   **Transient synovitis, right wrist**

M67.332   **Transient synovitis, left wrist**

M67.339   **Transient synovitis, unspecified wrist**

✔6ᵗʰ M67.34   **Transient synovitis, hand**

M67.341   **Transient synovitis, right hand**

M67.342   **Transient synovitis, left hand**

M67.349   **Transient synovitis, unspecified hand**

✔6ᵗʰ M67.35   **Transient synovitis, hip**

M67.351   **Transient synovitis, right hip**

M67.352   **Transient synovitis, left hip**

M67.359   **Transient synovitis, unspecified hip**

✔6ᵗʰ M67.36   **Transient synovitis, knee**

M67.361   **Transient synovitis, right knee**

M67.362   **Transient synovitis, left knee**

M67.369   **Transient synovitis, unspecified knee**

✔6ᵗʰ M67.37   **Transient synovitis, ankle and foot**

M67.371   **Transient synovitis, right ankle and foot**

M67.372   **Transient synovitis, left ankle and foot**

M67.379   **Transient synovitis, unspecified ankle and foot**

M67.38   **Transient synovitis, other site**

M67.39   **Transient synovitis, multiple sites**

✔5ᵗʰ **M67.4**   **Ganglion**
Ganglion of joint or tendon (sheath)
EXCLUDES 1   ganglion in yaws (A66.6)
EXCLUDES 2   cyst of bursa (M71.2-M71.3)
cyst of synovium (M71.2-M71.3)

M67.40   **Ganglion, unspecified site**

✔6ᵗʰ M67.41   **Ganglion, shoulder**

M67.411   **Ganglion, right shoulder**

M67.412   **Ganglion, left shoulder**

M67.419   **Ganglion, unspecified shoulder**

✔6ᵗʰ M67.42   **Ganglion, elbow**

M67.421   **Ganglion, right elbow**

M67.422   **Ganglion, left elbow**

M67.429   **Ganglion, unspecified elbow**

✔6ᵗʰ M67.43   **Ganglion, wrist**

M67.431   **Ganglion, right wrist**

Ganglion of Wrist

Extensor tendon sheaths

Ganglion of wrist (fluid-filled sac)

✔ Additional Character Req   ✔x7ᵗʰ Placeholder Alert   Unacceptable PDx   Manifestation   H1 - H14 HAC   HCC CMS-HCC Condition   *EXCLUDES 1* Not Coded Here   *EXCLUDES 2* Not Included Here

ICD-10-CM 2018   789

Chapter 13. Diseases of the Musculoskeletal System and Connective Tissue

M67.432 Ganglion, left wrist
M67.439 Ganglion, unspecified wrist

√6ᵗʰ **M67.44 Ganglion, hand**
M67.441 Ganglion, right hand
M67.442 Ganglion, left hand
M67.449 Ganglion, unspecified hand

√6ᵗʰ **M67.45 Ganglion, hip**
M67.451 Ganglion, right hip
M67.452 Ganglion, left hip
M67.459 Ganglion, unspecified hip

√6ᵗʰ **M67.46 Ganglion, knee**
M67.461 Ganglion, right knee
M67.462 Ganglion, left knee
M67.469 Ganglion, unspecified knee

√6ᵗʰ **M67.47 Ganglion, ankle and foot**
M67.471 Ganglion, right ankle and foot
M67.472 Ganglion, left ankle and foot
M67.479 Ganglion, unspecified ankle and foot

M67.48 Ganglion, other site
M67.49 Ganglion, multiple sites

√5ᵗʰ **M67.5 Plica syndrome**
Plica knee
M67.50 Plica syndrome, unspecified knee
M67.51 Plica syndrome, right knee
M67.52 Plica syndrome, left knee

√5ᵗʰ **M67.8 Other specified disorders of synovium and tendon**
M67.80 Other specified disorders of synovium and tendon, unspecified site

√6ᵗʰ **M67.81 Other specified disorders of synovium and tendon, shoulder**
M67.811 Other specified disorders of synovium, right shoulder
M67.812 Other specified disorders of synovium, left shoulder
M67.813 Other specified disorders of tendon, right shoulder
M67.814 Other specified disorders of tendon, left shoulder
M67.819 Other specified disorders of synovium and tendon, unspecified shoulder

√6ᵗʰ **M67.82 Other specified disorders of synovium and tendon, elbow**
M67.821 Other specified disorders of synovium, right elbow
M67.822 Other specified disorders of synovium, left elbow
M67.823 Other specified disorders of tendon, right elbow
M67.824 Other specified disorders of tendon, left elbow
M67.829 Other specified disorders of synovium and tendon, unspecified elbow

√6ᵗʰ **M67.83 Other specified disorders of synovium and tendon, wrist**
M67.831 Other specified disorders of synovium, right wrist
M67.832 Other specified disorders of synovium, left wrist
M67.833 Other specified disorders of tendon, right wrist
M67.834 Other specified disorders of tendon, left wrist
M67.839 Other specified disorders of synovium and tendon, unspecified forearm

√6ᵗʰ **M67.84 Other specified disorders of synovium and tendon, hand**
M67.841 Other specified disorders of synovium, right hand
M67.842 Other specified disorders of synovium, left hand
M67.843 Other specified disorders of tendon, right hand
M67.844 Other specified disorders of tendon, left hand
M67.849 Other specified disorders of synovium and tendon, unspecified hand

√6ᵗʰ **M67.85 Other specified disorders of synovium and tendon, hip**
M67.851 Other specified disorders of synovium, right hip
M67.852 Other specified disorders of synovium, left hip
M67.853 Other specified disorders of tendon, right hip
M67.854 Other specified disorders of tendon, left hip
M67.859 Other specified disorders of synovium and tendon, unspecified hip

√6ᵗʰ **M67.86 Other specified disorders of synovium and tendon, knee**
M67.861 Other specified disorders of synovium, right knee
M67.862 Other specified disorders of synovium, left knee
M67.863 Other specified disorders of tendon, right knee
M67.864 Other specified disorders of tendon, left knee
M67.869 Other specified disorders of synovium and tendon, unspecified knee

√6ᵗʰ **M67.87 Other specified disorders of synovium and tendon, ankle and foot**
M67.871 Other specified disorders of synovium, right ankle and foot
M67.872 Other specified disorders of synovium, left ankle and foot
M67.873 Other specified disorders of tendon, right ankle and foot
M67.874 Other specified disorders of tendon, left ankle and foot
M67.879 Other specified disorders of synovium and tendon, unspecified ankle and foot

M67.88 Other specified disorders of synovium and tendon, other site
M67.89 Other specified disorders of synovium and tendon, multiple sites

√5ᵗʰ **M67.9 Unspecified disorder of synovium and tendon**
M67.90 Unspecified disorder of synovium and tendon, unspecified site

√6ᵗʰ **M67.91 Unspecified disorder of synovium and tendon, shoulder**
M67.911 Unspecified disorder of synovium and tendon, right shoulder
M67.912 Unspecified disorder of synovium and tendon, left shoulder
M67.919 Unspecified disorder of synovium and tendon, unspecified shoulder

√6ᵗʰ **M67.92 Unspecified disorder of synovium and tendon, upper arm**
M67.921 Unspecified disorder of synovium and tendon, right upper arm
M67.922 Unspecified disorder of synovium and tendon, left upper arm
M67.929 Unspecified disorder of synovium and tendon, unspecified upper arm

√6ᵗʰ **M67.93 Unspecified disorder of synovium and tendon, forearm**
M67.931 Unspecified disorder of synovium and tendon, right forearm
M67.932 Unspecified disorder of synovium and tendon, left forearm
M67.939 Unspecified disorder of synovium and tendon, unspecified forearm

√6ᵗʰ **M67.94 Unspecified disorder of synovium and tendon, hand**
M67.941 Unspecified disorder of synovium and tendon, right hand
M67.942 Unspecified disorder of synovium and tendon, left hand
M67.949 Unspecified disorder of synovium and tendon, unspecified hand

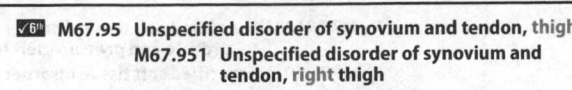

- ✓6ᵗʰ **M67.95** Unspecified disorder of synovium and tendon, thigh
    - **M67.951** Unspecified disorder of synovium and tendon, right thigh
    - **M67.952** Unspecified disorder of synovium and tendon, left thigh
    - **M67.959** Unspecified disorder of synovium and tendon, unspecified thigh
- ✓6ᵗʰ **M67.96** Unspecified disorder of synovium and tendon, lower leg
    - **M67.961** Unspecified disorder of synovium and tendon, right lower leg
    - **M67.962** Unspecified disorder of synovium and tendon, left lower leg
    - **M67.969** Unspecified disorder of synovium and tendon, unspecified lower leg
- ✓6ᵗʰ **M67.97** Unspecified disorder of synovium and tendon, ankle and foot
    - **M67.971** Unspecified disorder of synovium and tendon, right ankle and foot
    - **M67.972** Unspecified disorder of synovium and tendon, left ankle and foot
    - **M67.979** Unspecified disorder of synovium and tendon, unspecified ankle and foot
- **M67.98** Unspecified disorder of synovium and tendon, other site
- **M67.99** Unspecified disorder of synovium and tendon, multiple sites

Other soft tissue disorders (M70-M79)

- ✓4ᵗʰ **M70** Soft tissue disorders related to use, overuse and pressure
    - INCLUDES soft tissue disorders of occupational origin
    - Use additional external cause code to identify activity causing disorder (Y93.-)
    - EXCLUDES 1 bursitis NOS (M71.9-)
    - EXCLUDES 2 bursitis of shoulder (M75.5)
      enthesopathies (M76-M77)
      pressure ulcer (pressure area) (L89.-)
- ✓5ᵗʰ **M70.0** Crepitant synovitis (acute) (chronic) of hand and wrist
    - ✓6ᵗʰ **M70.03** Crepitant synovitis (acute) (chronic), wrist
        - **M70.031** Crepitant synovitis (acute) (chronic), right wrist
        - **M70.032** Crepitant synovitis (acute) (chronic), left wrist
        - **M70.039** Crepitant synovitis (acute) (chronic), unspecified wrist
    - ✓6ᵗʰ **M70.04** Crepitant synovitis (acute) (chronic), hand
        - **M70.041** Crepitant synovitis (acute) (chronic), right hand
        - **M70.042** Crepitant synovitis (acute) (chronic), left hand
        - **M70.049** Crepitant synovitis (acute) (chronic), unspecified hand
- ✓5ᵗʰ **M70.1** Bursitis of hand
    - **M70.10** Bursitis, unspecified hand
    - **M70.11** Bursitis, right hand
    - **M70.12** Bursitis, left hand
- ✓5ᵗʰ **M70.2** Olecranon bursitis
    - **M70.20** Olecranon bursitis, unspecified elbow
    - **M70.21** Olecranon bursitis, right elbow
    - **M70.22** Olecranon bursitis, left elbow
- ✓5ᵗʰ **M70.3** Other bursitis of elbow
    - **M70.30** Other bursitis of elbow, unspecified elbow
    - **M70.31** Other bursitis of elbow, right elbow
    - **M70.32** Other bursitis of elbow, left elbow
- ✓5ᵗʰ **M70.4** Prepatellar bursitis
    - **M70.40** Prepatellar bursitis, unspecified knee
    - **M70.41** Prepatellar bursitis, right knee
    - **M70.42** Prepatellar bursitis, left knee
- ✓5ᵗʰ **M70.5** Other bursitis of knee
    - **M70.50** Other bursitis of knee, unspecified knee
    - **M70.51** Other bursitis of knee, right knee
    - **M70.52** Other bursitis of knee, left knee

Knee Bursae

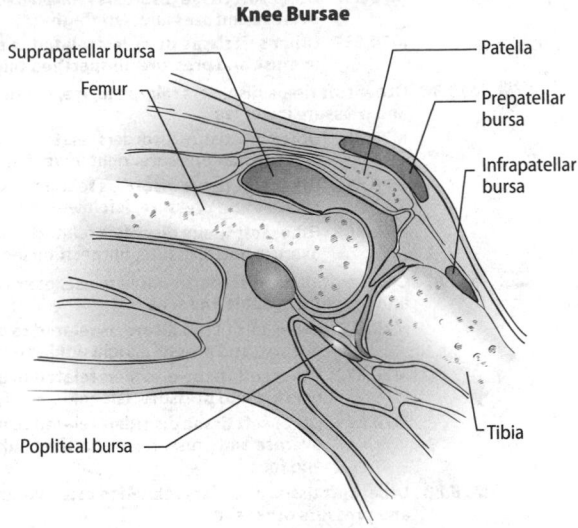

- ✓5ᵗʰ **M70.6** Trochanteric bursitis
    - Trochanteric tendinitis
    - **M70.60** Trochanteric bursitis, unspecified hip
    - **M70.61** Trochanteric bursitis, right hip
    - **M70.62** Trochanteric bursitis, left hip
- ✓5ᵗʰ **M70.7** Other bursitis of hip
    - Ischial bursitis
    - **M70.70** Other bursitis of hip, unspecified hip
    - **M70.71** Other bursitis of hip, right hip
    - **M70.72** Other bursitis of hip, left hip
- ✓5ᵗʰ **M70.8** Other soft tissue disorders related to use, overuse and pressure
    - **M70.80** Other soft tissue disorders related to use, overuse and pressure of unspecified site
    - ✓6ᵗʰ **M70.81** Other soft tissue disorders related to use, overuse and pressure of shoulder
        - **M70.811** Other soft tissue disorders related to use, overuse and pressure, right shoulder
        - **M70.812** Other soft tissue disorders related to use, overuse and pressure, left shoulder
        - **M70.819** Other soft tissue disorders related to use, overuse and pressure, unspecified shoulder
    - ✓6ᵗʰ **M70.82** Other soft tissue disorders related to use, overuse and pressure of upper arm
        - **M70.821** Other soft tissue disorders related to use, overuse and pressure, right upper arm
        - **M70.822** Other soft tissue disorders related to use, overuse and pressure, left upper arm
        - **M70.829** Other soft tissue disorders related to use, overuse and pressure, unspecified upper arms
    - ✓6ᵗʰ **M70.83** Other soft tissue disorders related to use, overuse and pressure of forearm
        - **M70.831** Other soft tissue disorders related to use, overuse and pressure, right forearm
        - **M70.832** Other soft tissue disorders related to use, overuse and pressure, left forearm
        - **M70.839** Other soft tissue disorders related to use, overuse and pressure, unspecified forearm
    - ✓6ᵗʰ **M70.84** Other soft tissue disorders related to use, overuse and pressure of hand
        - **M70.841** Other soft tissue disorders related to use, overuse and pressure, right hand
        - **M70.842** Other soft tissue disorders related to use, overuse and pressure, left hand
        - **M70.849** Other soft tissue disorders related to use, overuse and pressure, unspecified hand
    - ✓6ᵗʰ **M70.85** Other soft tissue disorders related to use, overuse and pressure of thigh
        - **M70.851** Other soft tissue disorders related to use, overuse and pressure, right thigh

---

✓ Additional Character Req   ✓x7ᵗʰ Placeholder Alert   Unacceptable PDx   Manifestation   H1 - H14 HAC   HCC CMS-HCC Condition   EXCLUDES 1 Not Coded Here   EXCLUDES 2 Not Included Here

M70.852 **Other soft tissue disorders related to use, overuse and pressure, left thigh**

M70.859 **Other soft tissue disorders related to use, overuse and pressure, unspecified thigh**

✓6ᵗʰ M70.86 **Other soft tissue disorders related to use, overuse and pressure lower leg**

   M70.861 **Other soft tissue disorders related to use, overuse and pressure, right lower leg**

   M70.862 **Other soft tissue disorders related to use, overuse and pressure, left lower leg**

   M70.869 **Other soft tissue disorders related to use, overuse and pressure, unspecified leg**

✓6ᵗʰ M70.87 **Other soft tissue disorders related to use, overuse and pressure of ankle and foot**

   M70.871 **Other soft tissue disorders related to use, overuse and pressure, right ankle and foot**

   M70.872 **Other soft tissue disorders related to use, overuse and pressure, left ankle and foot**

   M70.879 **Other soft tissue disorders related to use, overuse and pressure, unspecified ankle and foot**

M70.88 **Other soft tissue disorders related to use, overuse and pressure other site**

M70.89 **Other soft tissue disorders related to use, overuse and pressure multiple sites**

✓5ᵗʰ M70.9 **Unspecified soft tissue disorder related to use, overuse and pressure**

M70.90 **Unspecified soft tissue disorder related to use, overuse and pressure of unspecified site**

✓6ᵗʰ M70.91 **Unspecified soft tissue disorder related to use, overuse and pressure of shoulder**

   M70.911 **Unspecified soft tissue disorder related to use, overuse and pressure, right shoulder**

   M70.912 **Unspecified soft tissue disorder related to use, overuse and pressure, left shoulder**

   M70.919 **Unspecified soft tissue disorder related to use, overuse and pressure, unspecified shoulder**

✓6ᵗʰ M70.92 **Unspecified soft tissue disorder related to use, overuse and pressure of upper arm**

   M70.921 **Unspecified soft tissue disorder related to use, overuse and pressure, right upper arm**

   M70.922 **Unspecified soft tissue disorder related to use, overuse and pressure, left upper arm**

   M70.929 **Unspecified soft tissue disorder related to use, overuse and pressure, unspecified upper arm**

✓6ᵗʰ M70.93 **Unspecified soft tissue disorder related to use, overuse and pressure of forearm**

   M70.931 **Unspecified soft tissue disorder related to use, overuse and pressure, right forearm**

   M70.932 **Unspecified soft tissue disorder related to use, overuse and pressure, left forearm**

   M70.939 **Unspecified soft tissue disorder related to use, overuse and pressure, unspecified forearm**

✓6ᵗʰ M70.94 **Unspecified soft tissue disorder related to use, overuse and pressure of hand**

   M70.941 **Unspecified soft tissue disorder related to use, overuse and pressure, right hand**

   M70.942 **Unspecified soft tissue disorder related to use, overuse and pressure, left hand**

   M70.949 **Unspecified soft tissue disorder related to use, overuse and pressure, unspecified hand**

✓6ᵗʰ M70.95 **Unspecified soft tissue disorder related to use, overuse and pressure of thigh**

   M70.951 **Unspecified soft tissue disorder related to use, overuse and pressure, right thigh**

   M70.952 **Unspecified soft tissue disorder related to use, overuse and pressure, left thigh**

   M70.959 **Unspecified soft tissue disorder related to use, overuse and pressure, unspecified thigh**

✓6ᵗʰ M70.96 **Unspecified soft tissue disorder related to use, overuse and pressure lower leg**

   M70.961 **Unspecified soft tissue disorder related to use, overuse and pressure, right lower leg**

M70.962 **Unspecified soft tissue disorder related to use, overuse and pressure, left lower leg**

M70.969 **Unspecified soft tissue disorder related to use, overuse and pressure, unspecified lower leg**

✓6ᵗʰ M70.97 **Unspecified soft tissue disorder related to use, overuse and pressure of ankle and foot**

   M70.971 **Unspecified soft tissue disorder related to use, overuse and pressure, right ankle and foot**

   M70.972 **Unspecified soft tissue disorder related to use, overuse and pressure, left ankle and foot**

   M70.979 **Unspecified soft tissue disorder related to use, overuse and pressure, unspecified ankle and foot**

M70.98 **Unspecified soft tissue disorder related to use, overuse and pressure other**

M70.99 **Unspecified soft tissue disorder related to use, overuse and pressure multiple sites**

✓4ᵗʰ **M71 Other bursopathies**

  EXCLUDES 1 *bunion (M20.1)*
        bursitis related to use, overuse or pressure (M70.-)
        enthesopathies (M76-M77)

✓5ᵗʰ **M71.0 Abscess of bursa**

   Use additional code (B95.-, B96.-) to identify causative organism

M71.00 **Abscess of bursa, unspecified site**

✓6ᵗʰ M71.01 **Abscess of bursa, shoulder**

   M71.011 **Abscess of bursa, right shoulder**

   M71.012 **Abscess of bursa, left shoulder**

   M71.019 **Abscess of bursa, unspecified shoulder**

✓6ᵗʰ M71.02 **Abscess of bursa, elbow**

   M71.021 **Abscess of bursa, right elbow**

   M71.022 **Abscess of bursa, left elbow**

   M71.029 **Abscess of bursa, unspecified elbow**

✓6ᵗʰ M71.03 **Abscess of bursa, wrist**

   M71.031 **Abscess of bursa, right wrist**

   M71.032 **Abscess of bursa, left wrist**

   M71.039 **Abscess of bursa, unspecified wrist**

✓6ᵗʰ M71.04 **Abscess of bursa, hand**

   M71.041 **Abscess of bursa, right hand**

   M71.042 **Abscess of bursa, left hand**

   M71.049 **Abscess of bursa, unspecified hand**

✓6ᵗʰ M71.05 **Abscess of bursa, hip**

   M71.051 **Abscess of bursa, right hip**

   M71.052 **Abscess of bursa, left hip**

   M71.059 **Abscess of bursa, unspecified hip**

✓6ᵗʰ M71.06 **Abscess of bursa, knee**

   M71.061 **Abscess of bursa, right knee**

   M71.062 **Abscess of bursa, left knee**

   M71.069 **Abscess of bursa, unspecified knee**

✓6ᵗʰ M71.07 **Abscess of bursa, ankle and foot**

   M71.071 **Abscess of bursa, right ankle and foot**

   M71.072 **Abscess of bursa, left ankle and foot**

   M71.079 **Abscess of bursa, unspecified ankle and foot**

M71.08 **Abscess of bursa, other site**

M71.09 **Abscess of bursa, multiple sites**

✓5ᵗʰ **M71.1 Other infective bursitis**

   Use additional code (B95.-, B96.-) to identify causative organism

M71.10 **Other infective bursitis, unspecified site**

✓6ᵗʰ M71.11 **Other infective bursitis, shoulder**

   M71.111 **Other infective bursitis, right shoulder**

   M71.112 **Other infective bursitis, left shoulder**

   M71.119 **Other infective bursitis, unspecified shoulder**

✓6ᵗʰ M71.12 **Other infective bursitis, elbow**

   M71.121 **Other infective bursitis, right elbow**

   M71.122 **Other infective bursitis, left elbow**

   M71.129 **Other infective bursitis, unspecified elbow**

✓6ᵗʰ M71.13 **Other infective bursitis, wrist**

   M71.131 **Other infective bursitis, right wrist**

   M71.132 **Other infective bursitis, left wrist**

Ⓝ Newborn: 0   Ⓟ Pediatric: 0-17   Ⓜ Maternity: 12-55   Ⓐ Adult: 15-124   ᴹᶜᶜ Major CC Condition   ᴾᴰˣᴹᶜᶜ PDx acts as own MCC   ᶜᶜ CC Condition   ᴾᴰˣᶜᶜ PDx acts as own CC

792   ICD-10-CM 2018

     M71.139 Other infective bursitis, unspecified wrist

✓6th M71.14 Other infective bursitis, hand
     M71.141 Other infective bursitis, right hand
     M71.142 Other infective bursitis, left hand
     M71.149 Other infective bursitis, unspecified hand

✓6th M71.15 Other infective bursitis, hip
     M71.151 Other infective bursitis, right hip
     M71.152 Other infective bursitis, left hip
     M71.159 Other infective bursitis, unspecified hip

✓6th M71.16 Other infective bursitis, knee
     M71.161 Other infective bursitis, right knee
     M71.162 Other infective bursitis, left knee
     M71.169 Other infective bursitis, unspecified knee

✓6th M71.17 Other infective bursitis, ankle and foot
     M71.171 Other infective bursitis, right ankle and foot
     M71.172 Other infective bursitis, left ankle and foot
     M71.179 Other infective bursitis, unspecified ankle and foot

M71.18 Other infective bursitis, other site

M71.19 Other infective bursitis, multiple sites

✓5th M71.2 Synovial cyst of popliteal space [Baker]
     EXCLUDES 1   synovial cyst of popliteal space with rupture (M66.0)

M71.20 Synovial cyst of popliteal space [Baker], unspecified knee

M71.21 Synovial cyst of popliteal space [Baker], right knee

M71.22 Synovial cyst of popliteal space [Baker], left knee

✓5th M71.3 Other bursal cyst
     Synovial cyst NOS
     EXCLUDES 1   synovial cyst with rupture (M66.1-)

M71.30 Other bursal cyst, unspecified site

✓6th M71.31 Other bursal cyst, shoulder
     M71.311 Other bursal cyst, right shoulder
     M71.312 Other bursal cyst, left shoulder
     M71.319 Other bursal cyst, unspecified shoulder

✓6th M71.32 Other bursal cyst, elbow
     M71.321 Other bursal cyst, right elbow
     M71.322 Other bursal cyst, left elbow
     M71.329 Other bursal cyst, unspecified elbow

✓6th M71.33 Other bursal cyst, wrist
     M71.331 Other bursal cyst, right wrist
     M71.332 Other bursal cyst, left wrist
     M71.339 Other bursal cyst, unspecified wrist

✓6th M71.34 Other bursal cyst, hand
     M71.341 Other bursal cyst, right hand
     M71.342 Other bursal cyst, left hand
     M71.349 Other bursal cyst, unspecified hand

Baker's Cyst

Baker's cyst connected to knee joint synovial cavity

✓6th M71.35 Other bursal cyst, hip
     M71.351 Other bursal cyst, right hip
     M71.352 Other bursal cyst, left hip
     M71.359 Other bursal cyst, unspecified hip

✓6th M71.37 Other bursal cyst, ankle and foot
     M71.371 Other bursal cyst, right ankle and foot
     M71.372 Other bursal cyst, left ankle and foot
     M71.379 Other bursal cyst, unspecified ankle and foot

M71.38 Other bursal cyst, other site

M71.39 Other bursal cyst, multiple sites

✓5th M71.4 Calcium deposit in bursa
     EXCLUDES 2   calcium deposit in bursa of shoulder (M75.3)

M71.40 Calcium deposit in bursa, unspecified site

✓6th M71.42 Calcium deposit in bursa, elbow
     M71.421 Calcium deposit in bursa, right elbow
     M71.422 Calcium deposit in bursa, left elbow
     M71.429 Calcium deposit in bursa, unspecified elbow

✓6th M71.43 Calcium deposit in bursa, wrist
     M71.431 Calcium deposit in bursa, right wrist
     M71.432 Calcium deposit in bursa, left wrist
     M71.439 Calcium deposit in bursa, unspecified wrist

✓6th M71.44 Calcium deposit in bursa, hand
     M71.441 Calcium deposit in bursa, right hand
     M71.442 Calcium deposit in bursa, left hand
     M71.449 Calcium deposit in bursa, unspecified hand

✓6th M71.45 Calcium deposit in bursa, hip
     M71.451 Calcium deposit in bursa, right hip
     M71.452 Calcium deposit in bursa, left hip
     M71.459 Calcium deposit in bursa, unspecified hip

✓6th M71.46 Calcium deposit in bursa, knee
     M71.461 Calcium deposit in bursa, right knee
     M71.462 Calcium deposit in bursa, left knee
     M71.469 Calcium deposit in bursa, unspecified knee

✓6th M71.47 Calcium deposit in bursa, ankle and foot
     M71.471 Calcium deposit in bursa, right ankle and foot
     M71.472 Calcium deposit in bursa, left ankle and foot
     M71.479 Calcium deposit in bursa, unspecified ankle and foot

M71.48 Calcium deposit in bursa, other site

M71.49 Calcium deposit in bursa, multiple sites

✓5th M71.5 Other bursitis, not elsewhere classified
     EXCLUDES 1   bursitis NOS (M71.9-)
     EXCLUDES 2   bursitis of shoulder (M75.5)
          bursitis of tibial collateral [Pellegrini-Stieda] (M76.4-)

M71.50 Other bursitis, not elsewhere classified, unspecified site

✓6th M71.52 Other bursitis, not elsewhere classified, elbow
     M71.521 Other bursitis, not elsewhere classified, right elbow
     M71.522 Other bursitis, not elsewhere classified, left elbow
     M71.529 Other bursitis, not elsewhere classified, unspecified elbow

✓6th M71.53 Other bursitis, not elsewhere classified, wrist
     M71.531 Other bursitis, not elsewhere classified, right wrist
     M71.532 Other bursitis, not elsewhere classified, left wrist
     M71.539 Other bursitis, not elsewhere classified, unspecified wrist

✓6th M71.54 Other bursitis, not elsewhere classified, hand
     M71.541 Other bursitis, not elsewhere classified, right hand
     M71.542 Other bursitis, not elsewhere classified, left hand

✓ Additional Character Req   ✓x7th Placeholder Alert   Unacceptable PDx   Manifestation   H1 - H14 HAC   HCC CMS-HCC Condition   EXCLUDES 1 Not Coded Here   EXCLUDES 2 Not Included Here

ICD-10-CM 2018   793

      M71.549 Other bursitis, not elsewhere classified, unspecified hand

✓6ᵗʰ **M71.55 Other bursitis, not elsewhere classified, hip**
      M71.551 Other bursitis, not elsewhere classified, right hip
      M71.552 Other bursitis, not elsewhere classified, left hip
      M71.559 Other bursitis, not elsewhere classified, unspecified hip

✓6ᵗʰ **M71.56 Other bursitis, not elsewhere classified, knee**
      M71.561 Other bursitis, not elsewhere classified, right knee
      M71.562 Other bursitis, not elsewhere classified, left knee
      M71.569 Other bursitis, not elsewhere classified, unspecified knee

✓6ᵗʰ **M71.57 Other bursitis, not elsewhere classified, ankle and foot**
      M71.571 Other bursitis, not elsewhere classified, right ankle and foot
      M71.572 Other bursitis, not elsewhere classified, left ankle and foot
      M71.579 Other bursitis, not elsewhere classified, unspecified ankle and foot

  M71.58 Other bursitis, not elsewhere classified, other site

✓5ᵗʰ **M71.8 Other specified bursopathies**
  M71.80 Other specified bursopathies, unspecified site

✓6ᵗʰ **M71.81 Other specified bursopathies, shoulder**
      M71.811 Other specified bursopathies, right shoulder
      M71.812 Other specified bursopathies, left shoulder
      M71.819 Other specified bursopathies, unspecified shoulder

✓6ᵗʰ **M71.82 Other specified bursopathies, elbow**
      M71.821 Other specified bursopathies, right elbow
      M71.822 Other specified bursopathies, left elbow
      M71.829 Other specified bursopathies, unspecified elbow

✓6ᵗʰ **M71.83 Other specified bursopathies, wrist**
      M71.831 Other specified bursopathies, right wrist
      M71.832 Other specified bursopathies, left wrist
      M71.839 Other specified bursopathies, unspecified wrist

✓6ᵗʰ **M71.84 Other specified bursopathies, hand**
      M71.841 Other specified bursopathies, right hand
      M71.842 Other specified bursopathies, left hand
      M71.849 Other specified bursopathies, unspecified hand

✓6ᵗʰ **M71.85 Other specified bursopathies, hip**
      M71.851 Other specified bursopathies, right hip
      M71.852 Other specified bursopathies, left hip
      M71.859 Other specified bursopathies, unspecified hip

✓6ᵗʰ **M71.86 Other specified bursopathies, knee**
      M71.861 Other specified bursopathies, right knee
      M71.862 Other specified bursopathies, left knee
      M71.869 Other specified bursopathies, unspecified knee

✓6ᵗʰ **M71.87 Other specified bursopathies, ankle and foot**
      M71.871 Other specified bursopathies, right ankle and foot
      M71.872 Other specified bursopathies, left ankle and foot
      M71.879 Other specified bursopathies, unspecified ankle and foot

  M71.88 Other specified bursopathies, other site
  M71.89 Other specified bursopathies, multiple sites

M71.9 Bursopathy, unspecified
  Bursitis NOS

✓4ᵗʰ **M72 Fibroblastic disorders**
  EXCLUDES 2   retroperitoneal fibromatosis (D48.3)

M72.0 Palmar fascial fibromatosis [Dupuytren]   A
  DEF: Dupuytren's contracture: Flexion deformity of finger, due to shortened, thickened fibrosing of palmar fascia; cause unknown; associated with long-standing epilepsy.

M72.1 Knuckle pads

M72.2 Plantar fascial fibromatosis
  Plantar fasciitis
  DEF: Rapid-growing and multiplanar nodular swellings and pain in the foot; not associated with contractures.

M72.4 Pseudosarcomatous fibromatosis
  Nodular fasciitis

M72.6 Necrotizing fasciitis   MCC   HCC
  Use additional code (B95.-, B96.-) to identify causative organism
  CC Excl: PDX collection 806

M72.8 Other fibroblastic disorders
  Abscess of fascia
  Fasciitis NEC
  Other infective fasciitis
  Use additional code to (B95.-, B96.-) identify causative organism
  EXCLUDES 1   diffuse (eosinophilic) fasciitis (M35.4)
      necrotizing fasciitis (M72.6)
      nodular fasciitis (M72.4)
      perirenal fasciitis NOS (N13.5)
      perirenal fasciitis with infection (N13.6)
      plantar fasciitis (M72.2)

M72.9 Fibroblastic disorder, unspecified
  Fasciitis NOS
  Fibromatosis NOS

✓4ᵗʰ **M75 Shoulder lesions**
  EXCLUDES 2   shoulder-hand syndrome (M89.0-)

✓5ᵗʰ **M75.0 Adhesive capsulitis of shoulder**
  Frozen shoulder
  Periarthritis of shoulder
  AHA: 2015, 2Q, 23
  M75.00 Adhesive capsulitis of unspecified shoulder
  M75.01 Adhesive capsulitis of right shoulder
  M75.02 Adhesive capsulitis of left shoulder

✓5ᵗʰ **M75.1 Rotator cuff tear or rupture, not specified as traumatic**
  Rotator cuff syndrome
  Supraspinatus syndrome
  Supraspinatus tear or rupture, not specified as traumatic
  EXCLUDES 1   tear of rotator cuff, traumatic (S46.01-)

  ✓6ᵗʰ **M75.10 Unspecified rotator cuff tear or rupture, not specified as traumatic**
      M75.100 Unspecified rotator cuff tear or rupture of unspecified shoulder, not specified as traumatic
      M75.101 Unspecified rotator cuff tear or rupture of right shoulder, not specified as traumatic
      M75.102 Unspecified rotator cuff tear or rupture of left shoulder, not specified as traumatic

  ✓6ᵗʰ **M75.11 Incomplete rotator cuff tear or rupture not specified as traumatic**
      M75.110 Incomplete rotator cuff tear or rupture of unspecified shoulder, not specified as traumatic
      M75.111 Incomplete rotator cuff tear or rupture of right shoulder, not specified as traumatic
      M75.112 Incomplete rotator cuff tear or rupture of left shoulder, not specified as traumatic

  ✓6ᵗʰ **M75.12 Complete rotator cuff tear or rupture not specified as traumatic**
      M75.120 Complete rotator cuff tear or rupture of unspecified shoulder, not specified as traumatic
      M75.121 Complete rotator cuff tear or rupture of right shoulder, not specified as traumatic
      M75.122 Complete rotator cuff tear or rupture of left shoulder, not specified as traumatic

✓5ᵗʰ **M75.2 Bicipital tendinitis**
  M75.20 Bicipital tendinitis, unspecified shoulder
  M75.21 Bicipital tendinitis, right shoulder
  M75.22 Bicipital tendinitis, left shoulder

N Newborn: 0   P Pediatric: 0-17   M Maternity: 12-55   A Adult: 15-124   MCC Major CC Condition   PDxMCC PDx acts as own MCC   CC CC Condition   PDxCC PDx acts as own CC

794   ICD-10-CM 2018

✓5ᵗʰ **M75.3 Calcific tendinitis of shoulder**
    Calcified bursa of shoulder
    M75.30 Calcific tendinitis of unspecified shoulder
    M75.31 Calcific tendinitis of right shoulder
    M75.32 Calcific tendinitis of left shoulder

✓5ᵗʰ **M75.4 Impingement syndrome of shoulder**
    M75.40 Impingement syndrome of unspecified shoulder
    M75.41 Impingement syndrome of right shoulder
    M75.42 Impingement syndrome of left shoulder

✓5ᵗʰ **M75.5 Bursitis of shoulder**
    M75.50 Bursitis of unspecified shoulder
    M75.51 Bursitis of right shoulder
    M75.52 Bursitis of left shoulder

✓5ᵗʰ **M75.8 Other shoulder lesions**
    M75.80 Other shoulder lesions, unspecified shoulder
    M75.81 Other shoulder lesions, right shoulder
    M75.82 Other shoulder lesions, left shoulder

✓5ᵗʰ **M75.9 Shoulder lesion, unspecified**
    M75.90 Shoulder lesion, unspecified, unspecified shoulder
    M75.91 Shoulder lesion, unspecified, right shoulder
    M75.92 Shoulder lesion, unspecified, left shoulder

✓4ᵗʰ **M76 Enthesopathies, lower limb, excluding foot**
    EXCLUDES 2 bursitis due to use, overuse and pressure (M70.-)
    enthesopathies of ankle and foot (M77.5-)

✓5ᵗʰ **M76.0 Gluteal tendinitis**
    M76.00 Gluteal tendinitis, unspecified hip
    M76.01 Gluteal tendinitis, right hip
    M76.02 Gluteal tendinitis, left hip

✓5ᵗʰ **M76.1 Psoas tendinitis**
    M76.10 Psoas tendinitis, unspecified hip
    M76.11 Psoas tendinitis, right hip
    M76.12 Psoas tendinitis, left hip

✓5ᵗʰ **M76.2 Iliac crest spur**
    M76.20 Iliac crest spur, unspecified hip
    M76.21 Iliac crest spur, right hip
    M76.22 Iliac crest spur, left hip

✓5ᵗʰ **M76.3 Iliotibial band syndrome**
    M76.30 Iliotibial band syndrome, unspecified leg
    M76.31 Iliotibial band syndrome, right leg
    M76.32 Iliotibial band syndrome, left leg

✓5ᵗʰ **M76.4 Tibial collateral bursitis [Pellegrini-Stieda]**
    M76.40 Tibial collateral bursitis [Pellegrini-Stieda], unspecified leg
    M76.41 Tibial collateral bursitis [Pellegrini-Stieda], right leg
    M76.42 Tibial collateral bursitis [Pellegrini-Stieda], left leg

✓5ᵗʰ **M76.5 Patellar tendinitis**
    M76.50 Patellar tendinitis, unspecified knee
    M76.51 Patellar tendinitis, right knee
    M76.52 Patellar tendinitis, left knee

✓5ᵗʰ **M76.6 Achilles tendinitis**
    Achilles bursitis
    M76.60 Achilles tendinitis, unspecified leg
    M76.61 Achilles tendinitis, right leg
    M76.62 Achilles tendinitis, left leg

✓5ᵗʰ **M76.7 Peroneal tendinitis**
    M76.70 Peroneal tendinitis, unspecified leg
    M76.71 Peroneal tendinitis, right leg
    M76.72 Peroneal tendinitis, left leg

✓5ᵗʰ **M76.8 Other specified enthesopathies of lower limb, excluding foot**
    ✓6ᵗʰ **M76.81 Anterior tibial syndrome**
        M76.811 Anterior tibial syndrome, right leg
        M76.812 Anterior tibial syndrome, left leg
        M76.819 Anterior tibial syndrome, unspecified leg
    ✓6ᵗʰ **M76.82 Posterior tibial tendinitis**
        M76.821 Posterior tibial tendinitis, right leg
        M76.822 Posterior tibial tendinitis, left leg
        M76.829 Posterior tibial tendinitis, unspecified leg

✓6ᵗʰ **M76.89 Other specified enthesopathies of lower limb, excluding foot**
        M76.891 Other specified enthesopathies of right lower limb, excluding foot
        M76.892 Other specified enthesopathies of left lower limb, excluding foot
        M76.899 Other specified enthesopathies of unspecified lower limb, excluding foot
    M76.9 Unspecified enthesopathy, lower limb, excluding foot

✓4ᵗʰ **M77 Other enthesopathies**
    EXCLUDES 1 bursitis NOS (M71.9-)
    EXCLUDES 2 bursitis due to use, overuse and pressure (M70.-)
    osteophyte (M25.7)
    spinal enthesopathy (M46.0-)

✓5ᵗʰ **M77.0 Medial epicondylitis**
    M77.00 Medial epicondylitis, unspecified elbow
    M77.01 Medial epicondylitis, right elbow
    M77.02 Medial epicondylitis, left elbow

✓5ᵗʰ **M77.1 Lateral epicondylitis**
    Tennis elbow
    M77.10 Lateral epicondylitis, unspecified elbow
    M77.11 Lateral epicondylitis, right elbow
    M77.12 Lateral epicondylitis, left elbow

✓5ᵗʰ **M77.2 Periarthritis of wrist**
    M77.20 Periarthritis, unspecified wrist
    M77.21 Periarthritis, right wrist
    M77.22 Periarthritis, left wrist

✓5ᵗʰ **M77.3 Calcaneal spur**
    DEF: Overgrowth of calcaneus bone on underside of the heel; causes pain on walking; due to chronic avulsion injury of plantar fascia from calcaneus.
    M77.30 Calcaneal spur, unspecified foot
    M77.31 Calcaneal spur, right foot
    M77.32 Calcaneal spur, left foot

✓5ᵗʰ **M77.4 Metatarsalgia**
    EXCLUDES 1 Morton's metatarsalgia (G57.6)
    M77.40 Metatarsalgia, unspecified foot
    M77.41 Metatarsalgia, right foot
    M77.42 Metatarsalgia, left foot

✓5ᵗʰ **M77.5 Other enthesopathy of foot**
    M77.50 Other enthesopathy of unspecified foot
    M77.51 Other enthesopathy of right foot
    M77.52 Other enthesopathy of left foot
    M77.8 Other enthesopathies, not elsewhere classified
    M77.9 Enthesopathy, unspecified
    Bone spur NOS   Periarthritis NOS
    Capsulitis NOS   Tendinitis NOS

✓4ᵗʰ **M79 Other and unspecified soft tissue disorders, not elsewhere classified**
    EXCLUDES 1 psychogenic rheumatism (F45.8)
    soft tissue pain, psychogenic (F45.41)

    M79.0 Rheumatism, unspecified
    EXCLUDES 1 fibromyalgia (M79.7)
    palindromic rheumatism (M12.3-)

    M79.1 Myalgia
    Myofascial pain syndrome
    EXCLUDES 1 fibromyalgia (M79.7)
    myositis (M60.-)

    M79.2 Neuralgia and neuritis, unspecified
    EXCLUDES 1 brachial radiculitis NOS (M54.1)
    lumbosacral radiculitis NOS (M54.1)
    mononeuropathies (G56-G58)
    radiculitis NOS (M54.1)
    sciatica (M54.3-M54.4)

    M79.3 Panniculitis, unspecified
    EXCLUDES 1 lupus panniculitis (L93.2)
    neck and back panniculitis (M54.0-)
    relapsing [Weber-Christian] panniculitis (M35.6)

    M79.4 Hypertrophy of (infrapatellar) fat pad
    M79.5 Residual foreign body in soft tissue
    EXCLUDES 1 foreign body granuloma of skin and subcutaneous tissue (L92.3)
    foreign body granuloma of soft tissue (M60.2-)

✓5ᵗʰ **M79.6 Pain in limb, hand, foot, fingers and toes**
  EXCLUDES 2   pain in joint (M25.5-)

  ✓6ᵗʰ **M79.60 Pain in limb, unspecified**
     M79.601 Pain in right arm
              Pain in right upper limb NOS
     M79.602 Pain in left arm
              Pain in left upper limb NOS
     M79.603 Pain in arm, unspecified
              Pain in upper limb NOS
     M79.604 Pain in right leg
              Pain in right lower limb NOS
     M79.605 Pain in left leg
              Pain in left lower limb NOS
     M79.606 Pain in leg, unspecified
              Pain in lower limb NOS
     M79.609 Pain in unspecified limb
              Pain in limb NOS

  ✓6ᵗʰ **M79.62 Pain in upper arm**
              Pain in axillary region
     M79.621 Pain in right upper arm
     M79.622 Pain in left upper arm
     M79.629 Pain in unspecified upper arm

  ✓6ᵗʰ **M79.63 Pain in forearm**
     M79.631 Pain in right forearm
     M79.632 Pain in left forearm
     M79.639 Pain in unspecified forearm

  ✓6ᵗʰ **M79.64 Pain in hand and fingers**
     M79.641 Pain in right hand
     M79.642 Pain in left hand
     M79.643 Pain in unspecified hand
     M79.644 Pain in right finger(s)
     M79.645 Pain in left finger(s)
     M79.646 Pain in unspecified finger(s)

  ✓6ᵗʰ **M79.65 Pain in thigh**
     M79.651 Pain in right thigh
     M79.652 Pain in left thigh
     M79.659 Pain in unspecified thigh

  ✓6ᵗʰ **M79.66 Pain in lower leg**
     M79.661 Pain in right lower leg
     M79.662 Pain in left lower leg
     M79.669 Pain in unspecified lower leg

  ✓6ᵗʰ **M79.67 Pain in foot and toes**
     M79.671 Pain in right foot
     M79.672 Pain in left foot
     M79.673 Pain in unspecified foot
     M79.674 Pain in right toe(s)
     M79.675 Pain in left toe(s)
     M79.676 Pain in unspecified toe(s)

M79.7 Fibromyalgia
        Fibromyositis
        Fibrositis
        Myofibrositis

✓5ᵗʰ **M79.A Nontraumatic compartment syndrome**
        Code first, if applicable, associated postprocedural complication
        EXCLUDES 1   compartment syndrome NOS (T79.A-)
                 fibromyalgia (M79.7)
                 nontraumatic ischemic infarction of muscle (M62.2-)
                 traumatic compartment syndrome (T79.A-)

  ✓6ᵗʰ **M79.A1 Nontraumatic compartment syndrome of upper extremity**
              Nontraumatic compartment syndrome of shoulder, arm, forearm, wrist, hand, and fingers

        CC Excl: For CC codes in subcategory M79.A1:
        PDX collection 893

     M79.A11 Nontraumatic compartment syndrome CC
              of right upper extremity
     M79.A12 Nontraumatic compartment syndrome CC
              of left upper extremity
     M79.A19 Nontraumatic compartment syndrome CC
              of unspecified upper extremity

  ✓6ᵗʰ **M79.A2 Nontraumatic compartment syndrome of lower extremity**
              Nontraumatic compartment syndrome of hip, buttock, thigh, leg, foot, and toes

        CC Excl: For CC codes in subcategory M79.A2:
        PDX collection 894

     M79.A21 Nontraumatic compartment syndrome CC
              of right lower extremity
     M79.A22 Nontraumatic compartment syndrome CC
              of left lower extremity
     M79.A29 Nontraumatic compartment syndrome CC
              of unspecified lower extremity

     M79.A3 Nontraumatic compartment syndrome of CC
        abdomen
              CC Excl: PDX collection 895

     M79.A9 Nontraumatic compartment syndrome of other CC
        sites
              CC Excl: PDX collection 896

✓5ᵗʰ **M79.8 Other specified soft tissue disorders**
     M79.81 Nontraumatic hematoma of soft tissue
              Nontraumatic hematoma of muscle
              Nontraumatic seroma of muscle and soft tissue

     M79.89 Other specified soft tissue disorders
              Polyalgia

     M79.9 Soft tissue disorder, unspecified

OSTEOPATHIES AND CHONDROPATHIES (M80-M94)

Disorders of bone density and structure (M80-M85)

✓4ᵗʰ **M80 Osteoporosis with current pathological fracture**
        INCLUDES   osteoporosis with current fragility fracture
        Use additional code to identify major osseous defect, if applicable (M89.7-)
        EXCLUDES 1   collapsed vertebra NOS (M48.5)
                 pathological fracture NOS (M84.4)
                 wedging of vertebra NOS (M48.5)
        EXCLUDES 2   personal history of (healed) osteoporosis fracture (Z87.310)

        The appropriate 7th character is to be added to each code from category M80.
        A   initial encounter for fracture
        D   subsequent encounter for fracture with routine healing
        G   subsequent encounter for fracture with delayed healing
        K   subsequent encounter for fracture with nonunion
        P   subsequent encounter for fracture with malunion
        S   sequela

        CC Excl: For codes in category M80, unless otherwise noted:
        CC with 7th character A: PDX collection 888
        CC with 7th character K or P: PDX collection 897

✓5ᵗʰ **M80.0 Age-related osteoporosis with current pathological fracture**
              Involutional osteoporosis with current pathological fracture
              Osteoporosis NOS with current pathological fracture
              Postmenopausal osteoporosis with current pathological fracture
              Senile osteoporosis with current pathological fracture

  7 ✓x7ᵗʰ **M80.00 Age-related osteoporosis with current** CC A
              pathological fracture, unspecified site

  ✓6ᵗʰ **M80.01 Age-related osteoporosis with current**
              pathological fracture, shoulder
     7 ✓7ᵗʰ **M80.011 Age-related osteoporosis with** CC A
              current pathological fracture, right shoulder
     7 ✓7ᵗʰ **M80.012 Age-related osteoporosis with** CC A
              current pathological fracture, left shoulder
     7 ✓7ᵗʰ **M80.019 Age-related osteoporosis with** CC A
              current pathological fracture, unspecified shoulder

  ✓6ᵗʰ **M80.02 Age-related osteoporosis with current**
              pathological fracture, humerus
     7 ✓7ᵗʰ **M80.021 Age-related osteoporosis with** CC A
              current pathological fracture, right humerus
     7 ✓7ᵗʰ **M80.022 Age-related osteoporosis with** CC A
              current pathological fracture, left humerus

---

7   CC when reported as an initial encounter (7th character A, B, or C – specific to category) OR a subsequent encounter for nonunion or malunion (7th character K, M, N, P, Q, or R – specific to category).

7 ✓7ᵗʰ **M80.029 Age-related osteoporosis with current pathological fracture, unspecified humerus** CC A

✓6ᵗʰ **M80.03 Age-related osteoporosis with current pathological fracture, forearm**
Age-related osteoporosis with current pathological fracture of wrist

     7 ✓7ᵗʰ **M80.031 Age-related osteoporosis with current pathological fracture, right forearm** CC A

     7 ✓7ᵗʰ **M80.032 Age-related osteoporosis with current pathological fracture, left forearm** CC A

     7 ✓7ᵗʰ **M80.039 Age-related osteoporosis with current pathological fracture, unspecified forearm** CC A

✓6ᵗʰ **M80.04 Age-related osteoporosis with current pathological fracture, hand**

     7 ✓7ᵗʰ **M80.041 Age-related osteoporosis with current pathological fracture, right hand** CC A

     7 ✓7ᵗʰ **M80.042 Age-related osteoporosis with current pathological fracture, left hand** CC A

     7 ✓7ᵗʰ **M80.049 Age-related osteoporosis with current pathological fracture, unspecified hand** CC A

✓6ᵗʰ **M80.05 Age-related osteoporosis with current pathological fracture, femur**
Age-related osteoporosis with current pathological fracture of hip

     7, 10 ✓7ᵗʰ **M80.051 Age-related osteoporosis with current pathological fracture, right femur** CC HCC A

     7, 10 ✓7ᵗʰ **M80.052 Age-related osteoporosis with current pathological fracture, left femur** CC HCC A

     7, 10 ✓7ᵗʰ **M80.059 Age-related osteoporosis with current pathological fracture, unspecified femur** CC HCC A

✓6ᵗʰ **M80.06 Age-related osteoporosis with current pathological fracture, lower leg**

     7 ✓7ᵗʰ **M80.061 Age-related osteoporosis with current pathological fracture, right lower leg** CC A

     7 ✓7ᵗʰ **M80.062 Age-related osteoporosis with current pathological fracture, left lower leg** CC A

     7 ✓7ᵗʰ **M80.069 Age-related osteoporosis with current pathological fracture, unspecified lower leg** CC A

✓6ᵗʰ **M80.07 Age-related osteoporosis with current pathological fracture, ankle and foot**

     7 ✓7ᵗʰ **M80.071 Age-related osteoporosis with current pathological fracture, right ankle and foot** CC A

     7 ✓7ᵗʰ **M80.072 Age-related osteoporosis with current pathological fracture, left ankle and foot** CC A

     7 ✓7ᵗʰ **M80.079 Age-related osteoporosis with current pathological fracture, unspecified ankle and foot** CC A

7, 10 ✓x7ᵗʰ **M80.08 Age-related osteoporosis with current pathological fracture, vertebra(e)** CC HCC A

✓5ᵗʰ **M80.8 Other osteoporosis with current pathological fracture**
Drug-induced osteoporosis with current pathological fracture
Idiopathic osteoporosis with current pathological fracture
Osteoporosis of disuse with current pathological fracture
Postoophorectomy osteoporosis with current pathological fracture
Postsurgical malabsorption osteoporosis with current pathological fracture
Post-traumatic osteoporosis with current pathological fracture
Use additional code for adverse effect, if applicable, to identify drug (T36-T50 with fifth or sixth character 5)

     7 ✓x7ᵗʰ **M80.80 Other osteoporosis with current pathological fracture, unspecified site** CC

✓6ᵗʰ **M80.81 Other osteoporosis with current pathological fracture, shoulder**

     7 ✓7ᵗʰ **M80.811 Other osteoporosis with current pathological fracture, right shoulder** CC

     7 ✓7ᵗʰ **M80.812 Other osteoporosis with current pathological fracture, left shoulder** CC

     7 ✓7ᵗʰ **M80.819 Other osteoporosis with current pathological fracture, unspecified shoulder** CC

✓6ᵗʰ **M80.82 Other osteoporosis with current pathological fracture, humerus**

     7 ✓7ᵗʰ **M80.821 Other osteoporosis with current pathological fracture, right humerus** CC

     7 ✓7ᵗʰ **M80.822 Other osteoporosis with current pathological fracture, left humerus** CC

     7 ✓7ᵗʰ **M80.829 Other osteoporosis with current pathological fracture, unspecified humerus** CC

✓6ᵗʰ **M80.83 Other osteoporosis with current pathological fracture, forearm**
Other osteoporosis with current pathological fracture of wrist

     7 ✓7ᵗʰ **M80.831 Other osteoporosis with current pathological fracture, right forearm** CC

     7 ✓7ᵗʰ **M80.832 Other osteoporosis with current pathological fracture, left forearm** CC

     7 ✓7ᵗʰ **M80.839 Other osteoporosis with current pathological fracture, unspecified forearm** CC

✓6ᵗʰ **M80.84 Other osteoporosis with current pathological fracture, hand**

     7 ✓7ᵗʰ **M80.841 Other osteoporosis with current pathological fracture, right hand** CC

     7 ✓7ᵗʰ **M80.842 Other osteoporosis with current pathological fracture, left hand** CC

     7 ✓7ᵗʰ **M80.849 Other osteoporosis with current pathological fracture, unspecified hand** CC

✓6ᵗʰ **M80.85 Other osteoporosis with current pathological fracture, femur**
Other osteoporosis with current pathological fracture of hip

     7, 10 ✓7ᵗʰ **M80.851 Other osteoporosis with current pathological fracture, right femur** CC HCC

     7, 10 ✓7ᵗʰ **M80.852 Other osteoporosis with current pathological fracture, left femur** CC HCC

     7, 10 ✓7ᵗʰ **M80.859 Other osteoporosis with current pathological fracture, unspecified femur** CC HCC

✓6ᵗʰ **M80.86 Other osteoporosis with current pathological fracture, lower leg**

     7 ✓7ᵗʰ **M80.861 Other osteoporosis with current pathological fracture, right lower leg** CC

     7 ✓7ᵗʰ **M80.862 Other osteoporosis with current pathological fracture, left lower leg** CC

     7 ✓7ᵗʰ **M80.869 Other osteoporosis with current pathological fracture, unspecified lower leg** CC

✓6ᵗʰ **M80.87 Other osteoporosis with current pathological fracture, ankle and foot**

     7 ✓7ᵗʰ **M80.871 Other osteoporosis with current pathological fracture, right ankle and foot** CC

     7 ✓7ᵗʰ **M80.872 Other osteoporosis with current pathological fracture, left ankle and foot** CC

     7 ✓7ᵗʰ **M80.879 Other osteoporosis with current pathological fracture, unspecified ankle and foot** CC

7, 10 ✓x7ᵗʰ **M80.88 Other osteoporosis with current pathological fracture, vertebra(e)** CC HCC

---

7   CC when reported as an initial encounter (7th character A, B, or C – specific to category) OR a subsequent encounter for nonunion or malunion (7th character K, M, N, P, Q, or R – specific to category).

10   HCC with 7th character indicating initial encounter (A, B or C - specific to category).

✓ Additional Character Req   ✓x7ᵗʰ Placeholder Alert   Unacceptable PDx   Manifestation   H1 - H14 HAC   HCC CMS-HCC Condition   *EXCLUDES 1* Not Coded Here   *EXCLUDES 2* Not Included Here

✓4th **M81 Osteoporosis without current pathological fracture**
Use additional code to identify:
   major osseous defect, if applicable (M89.7-)
   personal history of (healed) osteoporosis fracture, if applicable (Z87.31Ø)
EXCLUDES 1   osteoporosis with current pathological fracture (M8Ø.-)
         Sudeck's atrophy (M89.Ø)

M81.Ø   Age-related osteoporosis without current pathological fracture   A
Involutional osteoporosis without current pathological fracture
Osteoporosis NOS
Postmenopausal osteoporosis without current pathological fracture
Senile osteoporosis without current pathological fracture

M81.6   Localized osteoporosis [Lequesne]
EXCLUDES 1   Sudeck's atrophy (M89.Ø)

M81.8   Other osteoporosis without current pathological fracture
Drug-induced osteoporosis without current pathological fracture
Idiopathic osteoporosis without current pathological fracture
Osteoporosis of disuse without current pathological fracture
Postoophorectomy osteoporosis without current pathological fracture
Postsurgical malabsorption osteoporosis without current pathological fracture
Post-traumatic osteoporosis without current pathological fracture
Use additional code for adverse effect, if applicable, to identify drug (T36-T5Ø with fifth or sixth character 5)

✓4th **M83 Adult osteomalacia**
EXCLUDES 1   infantile and juvenile osteomalacia (E55.Ø)
         renal osteodystrophy (N25.Ø)
         rickets (active) (E55.Ø)
         rickets (active) sequelae (E64.3)
         vitamin D-resistant osteomalacia (E83.3)
         vitamin D-resistant rickets (active) (E83.3)

M83.Ø   Puerperal osteomalacia   M♀

M83.1   Senile osteomalacia   A

M83.2   Adult osteomalacia due to malabsorption   A
Postsurgical malabsorption osteomalacia in adults

M83.3   Adult osteomalacia due to malnutrition   A

M83.4   Aluminum bone disease

M83.5   Other drug-induced osteomalacia in adults   A
Use additional code for adverse effect, if applicable, to identify drug (T36-T5Ø with fifth or sixth character 5)

M83.8   Other adult osteomalacia   A

M83.9   Adult osteomalacia, unspecified   A

✓4th **M84 Disorder of continuity of bone**
EXCLUDES 2   traumatic fracture of bone-see fracture, by site

✓5th **M84.3   Stress fracture**
Fatigue fracture   Stress fracture NOS
March fracture   Stress reaction
Use additional external cause code(s) to identify the cause of the stress fracture
EXCLUDES 1   pathological fracture NOS (M84.4-)
         pathological fracture due to osteoporosis (M8Ø.-)
         traumatic fracture (S12-, S22-, S32-, S42-, S52-, S62-, S72-, S82-, S92-)
EXCLUDES 2   personal history of (healed) stress (fatigue) fracture (Z87.312)
         stress fracture of vertebra (M48.4-)

> The appropriate 7th character is to be added to each code from subcategory M84.3.
> A   initial encounter for fracture
> D   subsequent encounter for fracture with routine healing
> G   subsequent encounter for fracture with delayed healing
> K   subsequent encounter for fracture with nonunion
> P   subsequent encounter for fracture with malunion
> S   sequela

CC Excl: For codes in subcategory M84.3:
CC with 7th character K or P: PDX collection 897

8   ✓x7th   **M84.3Ø   Stress fracture, unspecified site**   CC

✓6th **M84.31   Stress fracture, shoulder**
8   ✓7th   **M84.311   Stress fracture, right shoulder**   CC
8   ✓7th   **M84.312   Stress fracture, left shoulder**   CC
8   ✓7th   **M84.319   Stress fracture, unspecified shoulder**   CC

✓6th **M84.32   Stress fracture, humerus**
8   ✓7th   **M84.321   Stress fracture, right humerus**   CC
8   ✓7th   **M84.322   Stress fracture, left humerus**   CC
8   ✓7th   **M84.329   Stress fracture, unspecified humerus**   CC

✓6th **M84.33   Stress fracture, ulna and radius**
8   ✓7th   **M84.331   Stress fracture, right ulna**   CC
8   ✓7th   **M84.332   Stress fracture, left ulna**   CC
8   ✓7th   **M84.333   Stress fracture, right radius**   CC
8   ✓7th   **M84.334   Stress fracture, left radius**   CC
8   ✓7th   **M84.339   Stress fracture, unspecified ulna and radius**   CC

✓6th **M84.34   Stress fracture, hand and fingers**
8   ✓7th   **M84.341   Stress fracture, right hand**   CC
8   ✓7th   **M84.342   Stress fracture, left hand**   CC
8   ✓7th   **M84.343   Stress fracture, unspecified hand**   CC
8   ✓7th   **M84.344   Stress fracture, right finger(s)**   CC
8   ✓7th   **M84.345   Stress fracture, left finger(s)**   CC
8   ✓7th   **M84.346   Stress fracture, unspecified finger(s)**   CC

✓6th **M84.35   Stress fracture, pelvis and femur**
Stress fracture, hip
8   ✓7th   **M84.35Ø   Stress fracture, pelvis**   CC
8   ✓7th   **M84.351   Stress fracture, right femur**   CC
8   ✓7th   **M84.352   Stress fracture, left femur**   CC
8   ✓7th   **M84.353   Stress fracture, unspecified femur**   CC
8   ✓7th   **M84.359   Stress fracture, hip, unspecified**   CC

✓6th **M84.36   Stress fracture, tibia and fibula**
8   ✓7th   **M84.361   Stress fracture, right tibia**   CC
8   ✓7th   **M84.362   Stress fracture, left tibia**   CC
8   ✓7th   **M84.363   Stress fracture, right fibula**   CC
8   ✓7th   **M84.364   Stress fracture, left fibula**   CC
8   ✓7th   **M84.369   Stress fracture, unspecified tibia and fibula**   CC

✓6th **M84.37   Stress fracture, ankle, foot and toes**
8   ✓7th   **M84.371   Stress fracture, right ankle**   CC
8   ✓7th   **M84.372   Stress fracture, left ankle**   CC
8   ✓7th   **M84.373   Stress fracture, unspecified ankle**   CC
8   ✓7th   **M84.374   Stress fracture, right foot**   CC
8   ✓7th   **M84.375   Stress fracture, left foot**   CC
8   ✓7th   **M84.376   Stress fracture, unspecified foot**   CC
8   ✓7th   **M84.377   Stress fracture, right toe(s)**   CC
8   ✓7th   **M84.378   Stress fracture, left toe(s)**   CC
8   ✓7th   **M84.379   Stress fracture, unspecified toe(s)**   CC

8   ✓x7th   **M84.38   Stress fracture, other site**   CC
EXCLUDES 2   stress fracture of vertebra (M48.4-)

---

8   CC when reported as a subsequent encounter for nonunion or malunion (7th character K, M, N, P, Q, or R – specific to category).

N Newborn: 0   P Pediatric: 0-17   M Maternity: 12-55   A Adult: 15-124   MCC Major CC Condition   PDxMCC PDx acts as own MCC   CC CC Condition   PDxCC PDx acts as own CC

798   ICD-10-CM 2018

✓5th **M84.4 Pathological fracture,** not elsewhere classified
    Chronic fracture
    Pathological fracture NOS
    EXCLUDES 1   collapsed vertebra NEC (M48.5)
             pathological fracture in neoplastic disease (M84.5-)
             pathological fracture in osteoporosis (M80.-)
             pathological fracture in other disease (M84.6-)
             stress fracture (M84.3-)
             traumatic fracture (S12.-, S22.-, S32.-, S42.-, S52.-,
             S62.-, S72.-, S82.-, S92.-)
    EXCLUDES 2   personal history of (healed) pathological fracture
             (Z87.311)

The appropriate 7th character is to be added to each code from subcategory M84.4.
A   initial encounter for fracture
D   subsequent encounter for fracture with routine healing
G   subsequent encounter for fracture with delayed healing
K   subsequent encounter for fracture with nonunion
P   subsequent encounter for fracture with malunion
S   sequela

CC Excl: For codes in subcategory M84.4:
CC with 7th character A: PDX collection 888
CC with 7th character K or P: PDX collection 897

7   ✓x7th   **M84.40**   **Pathological fracture,** unspecified site   CC

✓6th   **M84.41**   **Pathological fracture,** shoulder
   7   ✓7th   **M84.411**   **Pathological fracture,** right shoulder   CC
   7   ✓7th   **M84.412**   **Pathological fracture,** left shoulder   CC
   7   ✓7th   **M84.419**   **Pathological fracture,** unspecified shoulder   CC

✓6th   **M84.42**   **Pathological fracture,** humerus
   7   ✓7th   **M84.421**   **Pathological fracture,** right humerus   CC
   7   ✓7th   **M84.422**   **Pathological fracture,** left humerus   CC
   7   ✓7th   **M84.429**   **Pathological fracture,** unspecified humerus   CC

✓6th   **M84.43**   **Pathological fracture,** ulna and radius
   7   ✓7th   **M84.431**   **Pathological fracture,** right ulna   CC
   7   ✓7th   **M84.432**   **Pathological fracture,** left ulna   CC
   7   ✓7th   **M84.433**   **Pathological fracture,** right radius   CC
   7   ✓7th   **M84.434**   **Pathological fracture,** left radius   CC
   7   ✓7th   **M84.439**   **Pathological fracture,** unspecified ulna and radius   CC

✓6th   **M84.44**   **Pathological fracture,** hand and fingers
   7   ✓7th   **M84.441**   **Pathological fracture,** right hand   CC
   7   ✓7th   **M84.442**   **Pathological fracture,** left hand   CC
   7   ✓7th   **M84.443**   **Pathological fracture,** unspecified hand   CC
   7   ✓7th   **M84.444**   **Pathological fracture,** right finger(s)   CC
   7   ✓7th   **M84.445**   **Pathological fracture,** left finger(s)   CC
   7   ✓7th   **M84.446**   **Pathological fracture,** unspecified finger(s)   CC

✓6th   **M84.45**   **Pathological fracture,** femur and pelvis
   7, 10   ✓7th   **M84.451**   **Pathological fracture,** right femur   CC HCC
   7, 10   ✓7th   **M84.452**   **Pathological fracture,** left femur   CC HCC
   7, 10   ✓7th   **M84.453**   **Pathological fracture,** unspecified femur   CC HCC
   7   ✓7th   **M84.454**   **Pathological fracture,** pelvis   CC
   7, 10   ✓7th   **M84.459**   **Pathological fracture,** hip, unspecified   CC HCC

✓6th   **M84.46**   **Pathological fracture,** tibia and fibula
   7   ✓7th   **M84.461**   **Pathological fracture,** right tibia   CC
   7   ✓7th   **M84.462**   **Pathological fracture,** left tibia   CC
   7   ✓7th   **M84.463**   **Pathological fracture,** right fibula   CC
   7   ✓7th   **M84.464**   **Pathological fracture,** left fibula   CC
   7   ✓7th   **M84.469**   **Pathological fracture,** unspecified tibia and fibula   CC

✓6th   **M84.47**   **Pathological fracture,** ankle, foot and toes
   7   ✓7th   **M84.471**   **Pathological fracture,** right ankle   CC
   7   ✓7th   **M84.472**   **Pathological fracture,** left ankle   CC
   7   ✓7th   **M84.473**   **Pathological fracture,** unspecified ankle   CC

---

   7   ✓7th   **M84.474**   **Pathological fracture,** right foot   CC
   7   ✓7th   **M84.475**   **Pathological fracture,** left foot   CC
   7   ✓7th   **M84.476**   **Pathological fracture,** unspecified foot   CC
   7   ✓7th   **M84.477**   **Pathological fracture,** right toe(s)   CC
   7   ✓7th   **M84.478**   **Pathological fracture,** left toe(s)   CC
   7   ✓7th   **M84.479**   **Pathological fracture,** unspecified toe(s)   CC

7   ✓x7th   **M84.48**   **Pathological fracture,** other site   CC

✓5th   **M84.5 Pathological fracture in** neoplastic disease
    Code also underlying neoplasm

The appropriate 7th character is to be added to each code from subcategory M84.5.
A   initial encounter for fracture
D   subsequent encounter for fracture with routine healing
G   subsequent encounter for fracture with delayed healing
K   subsequent encounter for fracture with nonunion
P   subsequent encounter for fracture with malunion
S   sequela

CC Excl: For codes in subcategory M84.5:
CC with 7th character A: PDX collection 888
CC with 7th character K or P: PDX collection 897

7   ✓x7th   **M84.50**   **Pathological fracture in neoplastic disease,** unspecified site   CC

✓6th   **M84.51**   **Pathological fracture in neoplastic disease,** shoulder
   7   ✓7th   **M84.511**   **Pathological fracture in neoplastic disease,** right shoulder   CC
   7   ✓7th   **M84.512**   **Pathological fracture in neoplastic disease,** left shoulder   CC
   7   ✓7th   **M84.519**   **Pathological fracture in neoplastic disease,** unspecified shoulder   CC

✓6th   **M84.52**   **Pathological fracture in neoplastic disease,** humerus
   7   ✓7th   **M84.521**   **Pathological fracture in neoplastic disease,** right humerus   CC
   7   ✓7th   **M84.522**   **Pathological fracture in neoplastic disease,** left humerus   CC
   7   ✓7th   **M84.529**   **Pathological fracture in neoplastic disease,** unspecified humerus   CC

✓6th   **M84.53**   **Pathological fracture in neoplastic disease,** ulna and radius
   7   ✓7th   **M84.531**   **Pathological fracture in neoplastic disease,** right ulna   CC
   7   ✓7th   **M84.532**   **Pathological fracture in neoplastic disease,** left ulna   CC
   7   ✓7th   **M84.533**   **Pathological fracture in neoplastic disease,** right radius   CC
   7   ✓7th   **M84.534**   **Pathological fracture in neoplastic disease,** left radius   CC
   7   ✓7th   **M84.539**   **Pathological fracture in neoplastic disease,** unspecified ulna and radius   CC

✓6th   **M84.54**   **Pathological fracture in neoplastic disease,** hand
   7   ✓7th   **M84.541**   **Pathological fracture in neoplastic disease,** right hand   CC
   7   ✓7th   **M84.542**   **Pathological fracture in neoplastic disease,** left hand   CC
   7   ✓7th   **M84.549**   **Pathological fracture in neoplastic disease,** unspecified hand   CC

✓6th   **M84.55**   **Pathological fracture in neoplastic disease,** pelvis and femur
   7   ✓7th   **M84.550**   **Pathological fracture in neoplastic disease,** pelvis   CC
   7, 10   ✓7th   **M84.551**   **Pathological fracture in neoplastic disease,** right femur   CC HCC
   7, 10   ✓7th   **M84.552**   **Pathological fracture in neoplastic disease,** left femur   CC HCC
   7, 10   ✓7th   **M84.553**   **Pathological fracture in neoplastic disease,** unspecified femur   CC HCC
   7, 10   ✓7th   **M84.559**   **Pathological fracture in neoplastic disease,** hip, unspecified   CC HCC

---

7   CC when reported as an initial encounter (7th character A, B, or C – specific to category) OR a subsequent encounter for nonunion or malunion (7th character K, M, N, P, Q, or R – specific to category).
10   HCC with 7th character indicating initial encounter (A, B or C - specific to category).

✓ Additional Character Req   ✓x7th Placeholder Alert   Unacceptable PDx   Manifestation   H1 - H14 HAC   HCC CMS-HCC Condition   *EXCLUDES 1* Not Coded Here   *EXCLUDES 2* Not Included Here

√6th **M84.56** **Pathological fracture in neoplastic disease, tibia and fibula**

  7 √7th **M84.561** **Pathological fracture in neoplastic disease, right tibia** `CC`

  7 √7th **M84.562** **Pathological fracture in neoplastic disease, left tibia** `CC`

  7 √7th **M84.563** **Pathological fracture in neoplastic disease, right fibula** `CC`

  7 √7th **M84.564** **Pathological fracture in neoplastic disease, left fibula** `CC`

  7 √7th **M84.569** **Pathological fracture in neoplastic disease, unspecified tibia and fibula** `CC`

√6th **M84.57** **Pathological fracture in neoplastic disease, ankle and foot**

  7 √7th **M84.571** **Pathological fracture in neoplastic disease, right ankle** `CC`

  7 √7th **M84.572** **Pathological fracture in neoplastic disease, left ankle** `CC`

  7 √7th **M84.573** **Pathological fracture in neoplastic disease, unspecified ankle** `CC`

  7 √7th **M84.574** **Pathological fracture in neoplastic disease, right foot** `CC`

  7 √7th **M84.575** **Pathological fracture in neoplastic disease, left foot** `CC`

  7 √7th **M84.576** **Pathological fracture in neoplastic disease, unspecified foot** `CC`

√x7th **M84.58** **Pathological fracture in neoplastic disease, other specified site** `CC`

    Pathological fracture in neoplastic disease, vertebrae

√5th **M84.6** **Pathological fracture in other disease**

  Code also underlying condition

  EXCLUDES 1 *pathological fracture in osteoporosis (M80.-)*

> The appropriate 7th character is to be added to each code from subcategory M84.6.
> A   initial encounter for fracture
> D   subsequent encounter for fracture with routine healing
> G   subsequent encounter for fracture with delayed healing
> K   subsequent encounter for fracture with nonunion
> P   subsequent encounter for fracture with malunion
> S   sequela

> **CC Excl: For codes in subcategory M84.6:**
> **CC with 7th character A:** PDX collection 888
> **CC with 7th character K or P:** PDX collection 897

  7 √x7th **M84.60** **Pathological fracture in other disease, unspecified site** `CC`

  √6th **M84.61** **Pathological fracture in other disease, shoulder**

    7 √7th **M84.611** **Pathological fracture in other disease, right shoulder** `CC`

    7 √7th **M84.612** **Pathological fracture in other disease, left shoulder** `CC`

    7 √7th **M84.619** **Pathological fracture in other disease, unspecified shoulder** `CC`

  √6th **M84.62** **Pathological fracture in other disease, humerus**

    7 √7th **M84.621** **Pathological fracture in other disease, right humerus** `CC`

    7 √7th **M84.622** **Pathological fracture in other disease, left humerus** `CC`

    7 √7th **M84.629** **Pathological fracture in other disease, unspecified humerus** `CC`

  √6th **M84.63** **Pathological fracture in other disease, ulna and radius**

    7 √7th **M84.631** **Pathological fracture in other disease, right ulna** `CC`

    7 √7th **M84.632** **Pathological fracture in other disease, left ulna** `CC`

    7 √7th **M84.633** **Pathological fracture in other disease, right radius** `CC`

    7 √7th **M84.634** **Pathological fracture in other disease, left radius** `CC`

    7 √7th **M84.639** **Pathological fracture in other disease, unspecified ulna and radius** `CC`

√6th **M84.64** **Pathological fracture in other disease, hand**

  7 √7th **M84.641** **Pathological fracture in other disease, right hand** `CC`

  7 √7th **M84.642** **Pathological fracture in other disease, left hand** `CC`

  7 √7th **M84.649** **Pathological fracture in other disease, unspecified hand** `CC`

√6th **M84.65** **Pathological fracture in other disease, pelvis and femur**

  7 √7th **M84.650** **Pathological fracture in other disease, pelvis** `CC`

  7, 10 √7th **M84.651** **Pathological fracture in other disease, right femur** `CC` `HCC`

  7, 10 √7th **M84.652** **Pathological fracture in other disease, left femur** `CC` `HCC`

  7, 10 √7th **M84.653** **Pathological fracture in other disease, unspecified femur** `CC` `HCC`

  7, 10 √7th **M84.659** **Pathological fracture in other disease, hip, unspecified** `CC` `HCC`

√6th **M84.66** **Pathological fracture in other disease, tibia and fibula**

  7 √7th **M84.661** **Pathological fracture in other disease, right tibia** `CC`

  7 √7th **M84.662** **Pathological fracture in other disease, left tibia** `CC`

  7 √7th **M84.663** **Pathological fracture in other disease, right fibula** `CC`

  7 √7th **M84.664** **Pathological fracture in other disease, left fibula** `CC`

  7 √7th **M84.669** **Pathological fracture in other disease, unspecified tibia and fibula** `CC`

√6th **M84.67** **Pathological fracture in other disease, ankle and foot**

  7 √7th **M84.671** **Pathological fracture in other disease, right ankle** `CC`

  7 √7th **M84.672** **Pathological fracture in other disease, left ankle** `CC`

  7 √7th **M84.673** **Pathological fracture in other disease, unspecified ankle** `CC`

  7 √7th **M84.674** **Pathological fracture in other disease, right foot** `CC`

  7 √7th **M84.675** **Pathological fracture in other disease, left foot** `CC`

  7 √7th **M84.676** **Pathological fracture in other disease, unspecified foot** `CC`

  7 √x7th **M84.68** **Pathological fracture in other disease, other site** `CC`

√5th **M84.7** **Nontraumatic fracture, not elsewhere classified**

  √6th **M84.75** **Atypical femoral fracture**

> The appropriate 7th character is to be added to each code from subcategory M84.75.
> A   initial encounter for fracture
> D   subsequent encounter for fracture with routine healing
> G   subsequent encounter for fracture with delayed healing
> K   subsequent encounter for fracture with nonunion
> P   subsequent encounter for fracture with malunion
> S   sequela

> **CC Excl: For CC codes in subcategory M84.75:**
> **CC with 7th character A:** PDX collection 888
> **CC with 7th character K or P:** PDX collection 897

    7 √7th **M84.750** **Atypical femoral fracture, unspecified** `CC`

    7 √7th **M84.751** **Incomplete atypical femoral fracture, right leg** `CC`

    7 √7th **M84.752** **Incomplete atypical femoral fracture, left leg** `CC`

    7 √7th **M84.753** **Incomplete atypical femoral fracture, unspecified leg** `CC`

---

7 CC when reported as an initial encounter (7th character A, B, or C – specific to category) OR a subsequent encounter for nonunion or malunion (7th character K, M, N, P, Q, or R – specific to category).

10 HCC with 7th character indicating initial encounter (A, B or C - specific to category).

`N` Newborn: 0   `P` Pediatric: 0-17   `M` Maternity: 12-55   `A` Adult: 15-124   `MCC` Major CC Condition   `PDxMCC` PDx acts as own MCC   `CC` CC Condition   `PDxCC` PDx acts as own CC

800   ICD-10-CM 2018

7, 10 ✔7ᵗʰ **M84.754** Complete transverse atypical femoral fracture, right leg   CC HCC

7, 10 ✔7ᵗʰ **M84.755** Complete transverse atypical femoral fracture, left leg   CC HCC

7, 10 ✔7ᵗʰ **M84.756** Complete transverse atypical femoral fracture, unspecified leg   CC HCC

7, 10 ✔7ᵗʰ **M84.757** Complete oblique atypical femoral fracture, right leg   CC HCC

7, 10 ✔7ᵗʰ **M84.758** Complete oblique atypical femoral fracture, left leg   CC HCC

7, 10 ✔7ᵗʰ **M84.759** Complete oblique atypical femoral fracture, unspecified leg   CC HCC

✔5ᵗʰ **M84.8** Other disorders of continuity of bone

   M84.80 Other disorders of continuity of bone, unspecified site

   ✔6ᵗʰ **M84.81** Other disorders of continuity of bone, shoulder

     M84.811 Other disorders of continuity of bone, right shoulder

     M84.812 Other disorders of continuity of bone, left shoulder

     M84.819 Other disorders of continuity of bone, unspecified shoulder

   ✔6ᵗʰ **M84.82** Other disorders of continuity of bone, humerus

     M84.821 Other disorders of continuity of bone, right humerus

     M84.822 Other disorders of continuity of bone, left humerus

     M84.829 Other disorders of continuity of bone, unspecified humerus

   ✔6ᵗʰ **M84.83** Other disorders of continuity of bone, ulna and radius

     M84.831 Other disorders of continuity of bone, right ulna

     M84.832 Other disorders of continuity of bone, left ulna

     M84.833 Other disorders of continuity of bone, right radius

     M84.834 Other disorders of continuity of bone, left radius

     M84.839 Other disorders of continuity of bone, unspecified ulna and radius

   ✔6ᵗʰ **M84.84** Other disorders of continuity of bone, hand

     M84.841 Other disorders of continuity of bone, right hand

     M84.842 Other disorders of continuity of bone, left hand

     M84.849 Other disorders of continuity of bone, unspecified hand

   ✔6ᵗʰ **M84.85** Other disorders of continuity of bone, pelvic region and thigh

     M84.851 Other disorders of continuity of bone, right pelvic region and thigh

     M84.852 Other disorders of continuity of bone, left pelvic region and thigh

     M84.859 Other disorders of continuity of bone, unspecified pelvic region and thigh

   ✔6ᵗʰ **M84.86** Other disorders of continuity of bone, tibia and fibula

     M84.861 Other disorders of continuity of bone, right tibia

     M84.862 Other disorders of continuity of bone, left tibia

     M84.863 Other disorders of continuity of bone, right fibula

     M84.864 Other disorders of continuity of bone, left fibula

     M84.869 Other disorders of continuity of bone, unspecified tibia and fibula

   ✔6ᵗʰ **M84.87** Other disorders of continuity of bone, ankle and foot

     M84.871 Other disorders of continuity of bone, right ankle and foot

     M84.872 Other disorders of continuity of bone, left ankle and foot

     M84.879 Other disorders of continuity of bone, unspecified ankle and foot

   M84.88 Other disorders of continuity of bone, other site

  M84.9 Disorder of continuity of bone, unspecified

✔4ᵗʰ **M85** Other disorders of bone density and structure

   EXCLUDES 1   osteogenesis imperfecta (Q78.0)
        osteopetrosis (Q78.2)
        osteopoikilosis (Q78.8)
        polyostotic fibrous dysplasia (Q78.1)

  ✔5ᵗʰ **M85.0** Fibrous dysplasia (monostotic)

     EXCLUDES 2   fibrous dysplasia of jaw (M27.8)

   M85.00 Fibrous dysplasia (monostotic), unspecified site

   ✔6ᵗʰ **M85.01** Fibrous dysplasia (monostotic), shoulder

     M85.011 Fibrous dysplasia (monostotic), right shoulder

     M85.012 Fibrous dysplasia (monostotic), left shoulder

     M85.019 Fibrous dysplasia (monostotic), unspecified shoulder

   ✔6ᵗʰ **M85.02** Fibrous dysplasia (monostotic), upper arm

     M85.021 Fibrous dysplasia (monostotic), right upper arm

     M85.022 Fibrous dysplasia (monostotic), left upper arm

     M85.029 Fibrous dysplasia (monostotic), unspecified upper arm

   ✔6ᵗʰ **M85.03** Fibrous dysplasia (monostotic), forearm

     M85.031 Fibrous dysplasia (monostotic), right forearm

     M85.032 Fibrous dysplasia (monostotic), left forearm

     M85.039 Fibrous dysplasia (monostotic), unspecified forearm

   ✔6ᵗʰ **M85.04** Fibrous dysplasia (monostotic), hand

     M85.041 Fibrous dysplasia (monostotic), right hand

     M85.042 Fibrous dysplasia (monostotic), left hand

     M85.049 Fibrous dysplasia (monostotic), unspecified hand

   ✔6ᵗʰ **M85.05** Fibrous dysplasia (monostotic), thigh

     M85.051 Fibrous dysplasia (monostotic), right thigh

     M85.052 Fibrous dysplasia (monostotic), left thigh

     M85.059 Fibrous dysplasia (monostotic), unspecified thigh

   ✔6ᵗʰ **M85.06** Fibrous dysplasia (monostotic), lower leg

     M85.061 Fibrous dysplasia (monostotic), right lower leg

     M85.062 Fibrous dysplasia (monostotic), left lower leg

     M85.069 Fibrous dysplasia (monostotic), unspecified lower leg

   ✔6ᵗʰ **M85.07** Fibrous dysplasia (monostotic), ankle and foot

     M85.071 Fibrous dysplasia (monostotic), right ankle and foot

     M85.072 Fibrous dysplasia (monostotic), left ankle and foot

     M85.079 Fibrous dysplasia (monostotic), unspecified ankle and foot

   M85.08 Fibrous dysplasia (monostotic), other site

   M85.09 Fibrous dysplasia (monostotic), multiple sites

  ✔5ᵗʰ **M85.1** Skeletal fluorosis

   M85.10 Skeletal fluorosis, unspecified site

   ✔6ᵗʰ **M85.11** Skeletal fluorosis, shoulder

     M85.111 Skeletal fluorosis, right shoulder

     M85.112 Skeletal fluorosis, left shoulder

     M85.119 Skeletal fluorosis, unspecified shoulder

   ✔6ᵗʰ **M85.12** Skeletal fluorosis, upper arm

     M85.121 Skeletal fluorosis, right upper arm

     M85.122 Skeletal fluorosis, left upper arm

     M85.129 Skeletal fluorosis, unspecified upper arm

   ✔6ᵗʰ **M85.13** Skeletal fluorosis, forearm

     M85.131 Skeletal fluorosis, right forearm

---

7   CC when reported as an initial encounter (7th character A, B, or C – specific to category) OR a subsequent encounter for nonunion or malunion (7th character K, M, N, P, Q, or R – specific to category).

10 HCC with 7th character indicating initial encounter (A, B or C - specific to category).

✔ Additional Character Req   ✔x7ᵗʰ Placeholder Alert   Unacceptable PDx   Manifestation   H1 - H14 HAC   HCC CMS-HCC Condition   EXCLUDES 1 Not Coded Here   EXCLUDES 2 Not Included Here

       M85.132   Skeletal fluorosis, left forearm
       M85.139   Skeletal fluorosis, unspecified forearm

✓6th   M85.14   Skeletal fluorosis, hand
       M85.141   Skeletal fluorosis, right hand
       M85.142   Skeletal fluorosis, left hand
       M85.149   Skeletal fluorosis, unspecified hand

✓6th   M85.15   Skeletal fluorosis, thigh
       M85.151   Skeletal fluorosis, right thigh
       M85.152   Skeletal fluorosis, left thigh
       M85.159   Skeletal fluorosis, unspecified thigh

✓6th   M85.16   Skeletal fluorosis, lower leg
       M85.161   Skeletal fluorosis, right lower leg
       M85.162   Skeletal fluorosis, left lower leg
       M85.169   Skeletal fluorosis, unspecified lower leg

✓6th   M85.17   Skeletal fluorosis, ankle and foot
       M85.171   Skeletal fluorosis, right ankle and foot
       M85.172   Skeletal fluorosis, left ankle and foot
       M85.179   Skeletal fluorosis, unspecified ankle and foot

    M85.18   Skeletal fluorosis, other site
    M85.19   Skeletal fluorosis, multiple sites

M85.2   Hyperostosis of skull
    DEF: Abnormal bone growth on inner aspect of cranial bones.

✓5th   M85.3   Osteitis condensans
    M85.30   Osteitis condensans, unspecified site

✓6th   M85.31   Osteitis condensans, shoulder
       M85.311   Osteitis condensans, right shoulder
       M85.312   Osteitis condensans, left shoulder
       M85.319   Osteitis condensans, unspecified shoulder

✓6th   M85.32   Osteitis condensans, upper arm
       M85.321   Osteitis condensans, right upper arm
       M85.322   Osteitis condensans, left upper arm
       M85.329   Osteitis condensans, unspecified upper arm

✓6th   M85.33   Osteitis condensans, forearm
       M85.331   Osteitis condensans, right forearm
       M85.332   Osteitis condensans, left forearm
       M85.339   Osteitis condensans, unspecified forearm

✓6th   M85.34   Osteitis condensans, hand
       M85.341   Osteitis condensans, right hand
       M85.342   Osteitis condensans, left hand
       M85.349   Osteitis condensans, unspecified hand

✓6th   M85.35   Osteitis condensans, thigh
       M85.351   Osteitis condensans, right thigh
       M85.352   Osteitis condensans, left thigh
       M85.359   Osteitis condensans, unspecified thigh

✓6th   M85.36   Osteitis condensans, lower leg
       M85.361   Osteitis condensans, right lower leg
       M85.362   Osteitis condensans, left lower leg
       M85.369   Osteitis condensans, unspecified lower leg

✓6th   M85.37   Osteitis condensans, ankle and foot
       M85.371   Osteitis condensans, right ankle and foot
       M85.372   Osteitis condensans, left ankle and foot
       M85.379   Osteitis condensans, unspecified ankle and foot

    M85.38   Osteitis condensans, other site
    M85.39   Osteitis condensans, multiple sites

✓5th   M85.4   Solitary bone cyst
    EXCLUDES 2   solitary cyst of jaw (M27.4)
    M85.40   Solitary bone cyst, unspecified site

✓6th   M85.41   Solitary bone cyst, shoulder
       M85.411   Solitary bone cyst, right shoulder
       M85.412   Solitary bone cyst, left shoulder
       M85.419   Solitary bone cyst, unspecified shoulder

✓6th   M85.42   Solitary bone cyst, humerus
       M85.421   Solitary bone cyst, right humerus
       M85.422   Solitary bone cyst, left humerus
       M85.429   Solitary bone cyst, unspecified humerus

✓6th   M85.43   Solitary bone cyst, ulna and radius
       M85.431   Solitary bone cyst, right ulna and radius
       M85.432   Solitary bone cyst, left ulna and radius

       M85.439   Solitary bone cyst, unspecified ulna and radius

✓6th   M85.44   Solitary bone cyst, hand
       M85.441   Solitary bone cyst, right hand
       M85.442   Solitary bone cyst, left hand
       M85.449   Solitary bone cyst, unspecified hand

✓6th   M85.45   Solitary bone cyst, pelvis
       M85.451   Solitary bone cyst, right pelvis
       M85.452   Solitary bone cyst, left pelvis
       M85.459   Solitary bone cyst, unspecified pelvis

✓6th   M85.46   Solitary bone cyst, tibia and fibula
       M85.461   Solitary bone cyst, right tibia and fibula
       M85.462   Solitary bone cyst, left tibia and fibula
       M85.469   Solitary bone cyst, unspecified tibia and fibula

✓6th   M85.47   Solitary bone cyst, ankle and foot
       M85.471   Solitary bone cyst, right ankle and foot
       M85.472   Solitary bone cyst, left ankle and foot
       M85.479   Solitary bone cyst, unspecified ankle and foot

    M85.48   Solitary bone cyst, other site

✓5th   M85.5   Aneurysmal bone cyst
    EXCLUDES 2   aneurysmal cyst of jaw (M27.4)
    DEF: Solitary bone lesion, bulges into periosteum; marked by calcified rim.
    M85.50   Aneurysmal bone cyst, unspecified site

✓6th   M85.51   Aneurysmal bone cyst, shoulder
       M85.511   Aneurysmal bone cyst, right shoulder
       M85.512   Aneurysmal bone cyst, left shoulder
       M85.519   Aneurysmal bone cyst, unspecified shoulder

✓6th   M85.52   Aneurysmal bone cyst, upper arm
       M85.521   Aneurysmal bone cyst, right upper arm
       M85.522   Aneurysmal bone cyst, left upper arm
       M85.529   Aneurysmal bone cyst, unspecified upper arm

✓6th   M85.53   Aneurysmal bone cyst, forearm
       M85.531   Aneurysmal bone cyst, right forearm
       M85.532   Aneurysmal bone cyst, left forearm
       M85.539   Aneurysmal bone cyst, unspecified forearm

✓6th   M85.54   Aneurysmal bone cyst, hand
       M85.541   Aneurysmal bone cyst, right hand
       M85.542   Aneurysmal bone cyst, left hand
       M85.549   Aneurysmal bone cyst, unspecified hand

✓6th   M85.55   Aneurysmal bone cyst, thigh
       M85.551   Aneurysmal bone cyst, right thigh
       M85.552   Aneurysmal bone cyst, left thigh
       M85.559   Aneurysmal bone cyst, unspecified thigh

✓6th   M85.56   Aneurysmal bone cyst, lower leg
       M85.561   Aneurysmal bone cyst, right lower leg
       M85.562   Aneurysmal bone cyst, left lower leg
       M85.569   Aneurysmal bone cyst, unspecified lower leg

✓6th   M85.57   Aneurysmal bone cyst, ankle and foot
       M85.571   Aneurysmal bone cyst, right ankle and foot
       M85.572   Aneurysmal bone cyst, left ankle and foot
       M85.579   Aneurysmal bone cyst, unspecified ankle and foot

    M85.58   Aneurysmal bone cyst, other site
    M85.59   Aneurysmal bone cyst, multiple sites

✓5th   M85.6   Other cyst of bone
    EXCLUDES 1   cyst of jaw NEC (M27.4)
              osteitis fibrosa cystica generalisata [von Recklinghausen's disease of bone] (E21.0)
    M85.60   Other cyst of bone, unspecified site

✓6th   M85.61   Other cyst of bone, shoulder
       M85.611   Other cyst of bone, right shoulder
       M85.612   Other cyst of bone, left shoulder
       M85.619   Other cyst of bone, unspecified shoulder

✓6th   M85.62   Other cyst of bone, upper arm
       M85.621   Other cyst of bone, right upper arm

N Newborn: 0   P Pediatric: 0-17   M Maternity: 12-55   A Adult: 15-124   MCC Major CC Condition   PDxMCC PDx acts as own MCC   CC CC Condition   PDxCC PDx acts as own CC

802   ICD-10-CM 2018

       M85.622   Other cyst of bone, left upper arm
       M85.629   Other cyst of bone, unspecified upper arm

✓6ᵗʰ   **M85.63**   **Other cyst of bone, forearm**
       M85.631   Other cyst of bone, right forearm
       M85.632   Other cyst of bone, left forearm
       M85.639   Other cyst of bone, unspecified forearm

✓6ᵗʰ   **M85.64**   **Other cyst of bone, hand**
       M85.641   Other cyst of bone, right hand
       M85.642   Other cyst of bone, left hand
       M85.649   Other cyst of bone, unspecified hand

✓6ᵗʰ   **M85.65**   **Other cyst of bone, thigh**
       M85.651   Other cyst of bone, right thigh
       M85.652   Other cyst of bone, left thigh
       M85.659   Other cyst of bone, unspecified thigh

✓6ᵗʰ   **M85.66**   **Other cyst of bone, lower leg**
       M85.661   Other cyst of bone, right lower leg
       M85.662   Other cyst of bone, left lower leg
       M85.669   Other cyst of bone, unspecified lower leg

✓6ᵗʰ   **M85.67**   **Other cyst of bone, ankle and foot**
       M85.671   Other cyst of bone, right ankle and foot
       M85.672   Other cyst of bone, left ankle and foot
       M85.679   Other cyst of bone, unspecified ankle and foot

     M85.68   **Other cyst of bone, other site**
     M85.69   **Other cyst of bone, multiple sites**

✓5ᵗʰ   **M85.8**   **Other specified disorders of bone density and structure**
       Hyperostosis of bones, except skull
       Osteosclerosis, acquired
       EXCLUDES 1   *diffuse idiopathic skeletal hyperostosis [DISH] (M48.1)*
                osteosclerosis congenita (Q77.4)
                osteosclerosis fragilitas (generalista) (Q78.2)
                osteosclerosis myelofibrosis (D75.81)

     M85.80   **Other specified disorders of bone density and structure, unspecified site**

✓6ᵗʰ   **M85.81**   **Other specified disorders of bone density and structure, shoulder**
       M85.811   Other specified disorders of bone density and structure, right shoulder
       M85.812   Other specified disorders of bone density and structure, left shoulder
       M85.819   Other specified disorders of bone density and structure, unspecified shoulder

✓6ᵗʰ   **M85.82**   **Other specified disorders of bone density and structure, upper arm**
       M85.821   Other specified disorders of bone density and structure, right upper arm
       M85.822   Other specified disorders of bone density and structure, left upper arm
       M85.829   Other specified disorders of bone density and structure, unspecified upper arm

✓6ᵗʰ   **M85.83**   **Other specified disorders of bone density and structure, forearm**
       M85.831   Other specified disorders of bone density and structure, right forearm
       M85.832   Other specified disorders of bone density and structure, left forearm
       M85.839   Other specified disorders of bone density and structure, unspecified forearm

✓6ᵗʰ   **M85.84**   **Other specified disorders of bone density and structure, hand**
       M85.841   Other specified disorders of bone density and structure, right hand
       M85.842   Other specified disorders of bone density and structure, left hand
       M85.849   Other specified disorders of bone density and structure, unspecified hand

✓6ᵗʰ   **M85.85**   **Other specified disorders of bone density and structure, thigh**
       M85.851   Other specified disorders of bone density and structure, right thigh
       M85.852   Other specified disorders of bone density and structure, left thigh
       M85.859   Other specified disorders of bone density and structure, unspecified thigh

✓6ᵗʰ   **M85.86**   **Other specified disorders of bone density and structure, lower leg**
       M85.861   Other specified disorders of bone density and structure, right lower leg
       M85.862   Other specified disorders of bone density and structure, left lower leg
       M85.869   Other specified disorders of bone density and structure, unspecified lower leg

✓6ᵗʰ   **M85.87**   **Other specified disorders of bone density and structure, ankle and foot**
       M85.871   Other specified disorders of bone density and structure, right ankle and foot
       M85.872   Other specified disorders of bone density and structure, left ankle and foot
       M85.879   Other specified disorders of bone density and structure, unspecified ankle and foot

     M85.88   **Other specified disorders of bone density and structure, other site**
     M85.89   **Other specified disorders of bone density and structure, multiple sites**

     M85.9   **Disorder of bone density and structure, unspecified**

Other osteopathies (M86-M90)

     EXCLUDES 1   *postprocedural osteopathies (M96.-)*

✓4ᵗʰ   **M86**   **Osteomyelitis**
       Use additional code (B95-B97) to identify infectious agent
       Use additional code to identify major osseous defect, if applicable (M89.7-)
       EXCLUDES 1   *osteomyelitis due to:*
                echinococcus (B67.2)
                gonococcus (A54.43)
                salmonella (A02.24)
       EXCLUDES 2   *ostemyelitis of:*
                orbit (H05.0-)
                petrous bone (H70.2-)
                vertebra (M46.2-)

✓5ᵗʰ   **M86.0**   **Acute hematogenous osteomyelitis**
     M86.00   **Acute hematogenous osteomyelitis, unspecified site**   CC   HCC
       CC Excl: PDX collection 898

✓6ᵗʰ   **M86.01**   **Acute hematogenous osteomyelitis, shoulder**
       CC Excl: For CC codes in subcategory M86.01: PDX collection 899
       M86.011   Acute hematogenous osteomyelitis, right shoulder   CC   HCC
       M86.012   Acute hematogenous osteomyelitis, left shoulder   CC   HCC
       M86.019   Acute hematogenous osteomyelitis, unspecified shoulder   CC   HCC

✓6ᵗʰ   **M86.02**   **Acute hematogenous osteomyelitis, humerus**
       CC Excl: For CC codes in subcategory M86.02: PDX collection 900
       M86.021   Acute hematogenous osteomyelitis, right humerus   CC   HCC
       M86.022   Acute hematogenous osteomyelitis, left humerus   CC   HCC
       M86.029   Acute hematogenous osteomyelitis, unspecified humerus   CC   HCC

✓6ᵗʰ   **M86.03**   **Acute hematogenous osteomyelitis, radius and ulna**
       CC Excl: For CC codes in subcategory M86.03: PDX collection 901
       M86.031   Acute hematogenous osteomyelitis, right radius and ulna   CC   HCC
       M86.032   Acute hematogenous osteomyelitis, left radius and ulna   CC   HCC
       M86.039   Acute hematogenous osteomyelitis, unspecified radius and ulna   CC   HCC

✓6ᵗʰ   **M86.04**   **Acute hematogenous osteomyelitis, hand**
       CC Excl: For CC codes in subcategory M86.04: PDX collection 902
       M86.041   Acute hematogenous osteomyelitis, right hand   CC   HCC
       M86.042   Acute hematogenous osteomyelitis, left hand   CC   HCC

M86.049   **Acute hematogenous osteomyelitis, unspecified hand** `CC` `HCC`

✓6ᵗʰ **M86.05 Acute hematogenous osteomyelitis, femur**

> **CC Excl: For CC codes in subcategory M86.05:**
> PDX collection 903

M86.051   **Acute hematogenous osteomyelitis, right femur** `CC` `HCC`

M86.052   **Acute hematogenous osteomyelitis, left femur** `CC` `HCC`

M86.059   **Acute hematogenous osteomyelitis, femur** `CC` `HCC`

✓6ᵗʰ **M86.06 Acute hematogenous osteomyelitis, tibia and fibula**

> **CC Excl: For CC codes in subcategory M86.06:**
> PDX collection 904

M86.061   **Acute hematogenous osteomyelitis, right tibia and fibula** `CC` `HCC`

M86.062   **Acute hematogenous osteomyelitis, left tibia and fibula** `CC` `HCC`

M86.069   **Acute hematogenous osteomyelitis, unspecified tibia and fibula** `CC` `HCC`

✓6ᵗʰ **M86.07 Acute hematogenous osteomyelitis, ankle and foot**

> **CC Excl: For CC codes in subcategory M86.07:**
> PDX collection 905

M86.071   **Acute hematogenous osteomyelitis, right ankle and foot** `CC` `HCC`

M86.072   **Acute hematogenous osteomyelitis, left ankle and foot** `CC` `HCC`

M86.079   **Acute hematogenous osteomyelitis, unspecified ankle and foot** `CC` `HCC`

M86.08   **Acute hematogenous osteomyelitis, other sites** `CC` `HCC`
> **CC Excl:** PDX collection 882

M86.09   **Acute hematogenous osteomyelitis, multiple sites** `CC` `HCC`
> **CC Excl:** PDX collection 898

✓5ᵗʰ **M86.1 Other acute osteomyelitis**

M86.10   **Other acute osteomyelitis, unspecified site** `CC` `HCC`
> **CC Excl:** PDX collection 898

✓6ᵗʰ **M86.11 Other acute osteomyelitis, shoulder**

> **CC Excl: For CC codes in subcategory M86.11:**
> PDX collection 899

M86.111   **Other acute osteomyelitis, right shoulder** `CC` `HCC`

M86.112   **Other acute osteomyelitis, left shoulder** `CC` `HCC`

M86.119   **Other acute osteomyelitis, unspecified shoulder** `CC` `HCC`

✓6ᵗʰ **M86.12 Other acute osteomyelitis, humerus**

> **CC Excl: For CC codes in subcategory M86.12:**
> PDX collection 900

M86.121   **Other acute osteomyelitis, right humerus** `CC` `HCC`

M86.122   **Other acute osteomyelitis, left humerus** `CC` `HCC`

M86.129   **Other acute osteomyelitis, unspecified humerus** `CC` `HCC`

✓6ᵗʰ **M86.13 Other acute osteomyelitis, radius and ulna**

> **CC Excl: For CC codes in subcategory M86.13:**
> PDX collection 901

M86.131   **Other acute osteomyelitis, right radius and ulna** `CC` `HCC`

M86.132   **Other acute osteomyelitis, left radius and ulna** `CC` `HCC`

M86.139   **Other acute osteomyelitis, unspecified radius and ulna** `CC` `HCC`

✓6ᵗʰ **M86.14 Other acute osteomyelitis, hand**

> **CC Excl: For CC codes in subcategory M86.14:**
> PDX collection 902

M86.141   **Other acute osteomyelitis, right hand** `CC` `HCC`

M86.142   **Other acute osteomyelitis, left hand** `CC` `HCC`

M86.149   **Other acute osteomyelitis, unspecified hand** `CC` `HCC`

✓6ᵗʰ **M86.15 Other acute osteomyelitis, femur**

> **CC Excl: For CC codes in subcategory M86.15:**
> PDX collection 903

M86.151   **Other acute osteomyelitis, right femur** `CC` `HCC`

M86.152   **Other acute osteomyelitis, left femur** `CC` `HCC`

M86.159   **Other acute osteomyelitis, unspecified femur** `CC` `HCC`

✓6ᵗʰ **M86.16 Other acute osteomyelitis, tibia and fibula**

> **CC Excl: For CC codes in subcategory M86.16:**
> PDX collection 904

M86.161   **Other acute osteomyelitis, right tibia and fibula** `CC` `HCC`

M86.162   **Other acute osteomyelitis, left tibia and fibula** `CC` `HCC`

M86.169   **Other acute osteomyelitis, unspecified tibia and fibula** `CC` `HCC`

✓6ᵗʰ **M86.17 Other acute osteomyelitis, ankle and foot**

> **CC Excl: For CC codes in subcategory M86.17:**
> PDX collection 905

M86.171   **Other acute osteomyelitis, right ankle and foot** `CC` `HCC`

M86.172   **Other acute osteomyelitis, left ankle and foot** `CC` `HCC`

M86.179   **Other acute osteomyelitis, unspecified ankle and foot** `CC` `HCC`

M86.18   **Other acute osteomyelitis, other site** `CC` `HCC`
> **CC Excl:** PDX collection 882

M86.19   **Other acute osteomyelitis, multiple sites** `CC` `HCC`
> **CC Excl:** PDX collection 898

✓5ᵗʰ **M86.2 Subacute osteomyelitis**

M86.20   **Subacute osteomyelitis, unspecified site** `CC` `HCC`
> **CC Excl:** PDX collection 898

✓6ᵗʰ **M86.21 Subacute osteomyelitis, shoulder**

> **CC Excl: For CC codes in subcategory M86.21:**
> PDX collection 899

M86.211   **Subacute osteomyelitis, right shoulder** `CC` `HCC`

M86.212   **Subacute osteomyelitis, left shoulder** `CC` `HCC`

M86.219   **Subacute osteomyelitis, unspecified shoulder** `CC` `HCC`

✓6ᵗʰ **M86.22 Subacute osteomyelitis, humerus**

> **CC Excl: For CC codes in subcategory M86.22:**
> PDX collection 900

M86.221   **Subacute osteomyelitis, right humerus** `CC` `HCC`

M86.222   **Subacute osteomyelitis, left humerus** `CC` `HCC`

M86.229   **Subacute osteomyelitis, unspecified humerus** `CC` `HCC`

✓6ᵗʰ **M86.23 Subacute osteomyelitis, radius and ulna**

> **CC Excl: For CC codes in subcategory M86.23:**
> PDX collection 901

M86.231   **Subacute osteomyelitis, right radius and ulna** `CC` `HCC`

M86.232   **Subacute osteomyelitis, left radius and ulna** `CC` `HCC`

M86.239   **Subacute osteomyelitis, unspecified radius and ulna** `CC` `HCC`

✓6ᵗʰ **M86.24 Subacute osteomyelitis, hand**

> **CC Excl: For CC codes in subcategory M86.24:**
> PDX collection 902

M86.241   **Subacute osteomyelitis, right hand** `CC` `HCC`

M86.242   **Subacute osteomyelitis, left hand** `CC` `HCC`

M86.249   **Subacute osteomyelitis, unspecified hand** `CC` `HCC`

Ⓝ Newborn: 0   Ⓟ Pediatric: 0-17   Ⓜ Maternity: 12-55   Ⓐ Adult: 15-124   `MCC` Major CC Condition   `PDxMCC` PDx acts as own MCC   `CC` CC Condition   `PDxCC` PDx acts as own CC

804   ICD-10-CM 2018

✓6ᵗʰ **M86.25** Subacute osteomyelitis, femur

> **CC Excl: For CC codes in subcategory M86.25:** PDX collection 903

　　M86.251 Subacute osteomyelitis, right femur　`CC` `HCC`

　　M86.252 Subacute osteomyelitis, left femur　`CC` `HCC`

　　M86.259 Subacute osteomyelitis, unspecified femur　`CC` `HCC`

✓6ᵗʰ **M86.26** Subacute osteomyelitis, tibia and fibula

> **CC Excl: For CC codes in subcategory M86.26:** PDX collection 904

　　M86.261 Subacute osteomyelitis, right tibia and fibula　`CC` `HCC`

　　M86.262 Subacute osteomyelitis, left tibia and fibula　`CC` `HCC`

　　M86.269 Subacute osteomyelitis, unspecified tibia and fibula　`CC` `HCC`

✓6ᵗʰ **M86.27** Subacute osteomyelitis, ankle and foot

> **CC Excl: For CC codes in subcategory M86.27:** PDX collection 905

　　M86.271 Subacute osteomyelitis, right ankle and foot　`CC` `HCC`

　　M86.272 Subacute osteomyelitis, left ankle and foot　`CC` `HCC`

　　M86.279 Subacute osteomyelitis, unspecified ankle and foot　`CC` `HCC`

　　M86.28 Subacute osteomyelitis, other site　`CC` `HCC`
　　　CC Excl: PDX collection 882

　　M86.29 Subacute osteomyelitis, multiple sites　`CC` `HCC`
　　　CC Excl: PDX collection 898

✓5ᵗʰ **M86.3** Chronic multifocal osteomyelitis

> **CC Excl: For CC codes in subcategory M86.3, unless otherwise noted:** PDX collection 881

　　M86.30 Chronic multifocal osteomyelitis, unspecified site　`CC` `HCC`
　　　CC Excl: PDX collection 906

✓6ᵗʰ **M86.31** Chronic multifocal osteomyelitis, shoulder

　　M86.311 Chronic multifocal osteomyelitis, right shoulder　`CC` `HCC`

　　M86.312 Chronic multifocal osteomyelitis, left shoulder　`CC` `HCC`

　　M86.319 Chronic multifocal osteomyelitis, unspecified shoulder　`CC` `HCC`

✓6ᵗʰ **M86.32** Chronic multifocal osteomyelitis, humerus

　　M86.321 Chronic multifocal osteomyelitis, right humerus　`CC` `HCC`

　　M86.322 Chronic multifocal osteomyelitis, left humerus　`CC` `HCC`

　　M86.329 Chronic multifocal osteomyelitis, unspecified humerus　`CC` `HCC`

✓6ᵗʰ **M86.33** Chronic multifocal osteomyelitis, radius and ulna

　　M86.331 Chronic multifocal osteomyelitis, right radius and ulna　`CC` `HCC`

　　M86.332 Chronic multifocal osteomyelitis, left radius and ulna　`CC` `HCC`

　　M86.339 Chronic multifocal osteomyelitis, unspecified radius and ulna　`CC` `HCC`

✓6ᵗʰ **M86.34** Chronic multifocal osteomyelitis, hand

　　M86.341 Chronic multifocal osteomyelitis, right hand　`CC` `HCC`

　　M86.342 Chronic multifocal osteomyelitis, left hand　`CC` `HCC`

　　M86.349 Chronic multifocal osteomyelitis, unspecified hand　`CC` `HCC`

✓6ᵗʰ **M86.35** Chronic multifocal osteomyelitis, femur

　　M86.351 Chronic multifocal osteomyelitis, right femur　`CC` `HCC`

　　M86.352 Chronic multifocal osteomyelitis, left femur　`CC` `HCC`

　　M86.359 Chronic multifocal osteomyelitis, unspecified femur　`CC` `HCC`

✓6ᵗʰ **M86.36** Chronic multifocal osteomyelitis, tibia and fibula

　　M86.361 Chronic multifocal osteomyelitis, right tibia and fibula　`CC` `HCC`

　　M86.362 Chronic multifocal osteomyelitis, left tibia and fibula　`CC` `HCC`

　　M86.369 Chronic multifocal osteomyelitis, unspecified tibia and fibula　`CC` `HCC`

✓6ᵗʰ **M86.37** Chronic multifocal osteomyelitis, ankle and foot

　　M86.371 Chronic multifocal osteomyelitis, right ankle and foot　`CC` `HCC`

　　M86.372 Chronic multifocal osteomyelitis, left ankle and foot　`CC` `HCC`

　　M86.379 Chronic multifocal osteomyelitis, unspecified ankle and foot　`CC` `HCC`

　　M86.38 Chronic multifocal osteomyelitis, other site　`CC` `HCC`

　　M86.39 Chronic multifocal osteomyelitis, multiple sites　`CC` `HCC`

✓5ᵗʰ **M86.4** Chronic osteomyelitis with draining sinus

> **CC Excl: For CC codes in subcategory M86.4, unless otherwise noted:** PDX collection 881

　　M86.40 Chronic osteomyelitis with draining sinus, unspecified site　`CC` `HCC`
　　　CC Excl: PDX collection 906

✓6ᵗʰ **M86.41** Chronic osteomyelitis with draining sinus, shoulder

　　M86.411 Chronic osteomyelitis with draining sinus, right shoulder　`CC` `HCC`

　　M86.412 Chronic osteomyelitis with draining sinus, left shoulder　`CC` `HCC`

　　M86.419 Chronic osteomyelitis with draining sinus, unspecified shoulder　`CC` `HCC`

✓6ᵗʰ **M86.42** Chronic osteomyelitis with draining sinus, humerus

　　M86.421 Chronic osteomyelitis with draining sinus, right humerus　`CC` `HCC`

　　M86.422 Chronic osteomyelitis with draining sinus, left humerus　`CC` `HCC`

　　M86.429 Chronic osteomyelitis with draining sinus, unspecified humerus　`CC` `HCC`

✓6ᵗʰ **M86.43** Chronic osteomyelitis with draining sinus, radius and ulna

　　M86.431 Chronic osteomyelitis with draining sinus, right radius and ulna　`CC` `HCC`

　　M86.432 Chronic osteomyelitis with draining sinus, left radius and ulna　`CC` `HCC`

　　M86.439 Chronic osteomyelitis with draining sinus, unspecified radius and ulna　`CC` `HCC`

✓6ᵗʰ **M86.44** Chronic osteomyelitis with draining sinus, hand

　　M86.441 Chronic osteomyelitis with draining sinus, right hand　`CC` `HCC`

　　M86.442 Chronic osteomyelitis with draining sinus, left hand　`CC` `HCC`

　　M86.449 Chronic osteomyelitis with draining sinus, unspecified hand　`CC` `HCC`

✓6ᵗʰ **M86.45** Chronic osteomyelitis with draining sinus, femur

　　M86.451 Chronic osteomyelitis with draining sinus, right femur　`CC` `HCC`

　　M86.452 Chronic osteomyelitis with draining sinus, left femur　`CC` `HCC`

　　M86.459 Chronic osteomyelitis with draining sinus, unspecified femur　`CC` `HCC`

✓6ᵗʰ **M86.46** Chronic osteomyelitis with draining sinus, tibia and fibula

　　M86.461 Chronic osteomyelitis with draining sinus, right tibia and fibula　`CC` `HCC`

　　M86.462 Chronic osteomyelitis with draining sinus, left tibia and fibula　`CC` `HCC`

　　M86.469 Chronic osteomyelitis with draining sinus, unspecified tibia and fibula　`CC` `HCC`

✓6ᵗʰ **M86.47** Chronic osteomyelitis with draining sinus, ankle and foot

　　M86.471 Chronic osteomyelitis with draining sinus, right ankle and foot　`CC` `HCC`

　　M86.472 Chronic osteomyelitis with draining sinus, left ankle and foot　`CC` `HCC`

✔ Additional Character Req　✓x7ᵗʰ Placeholder Alert　Unacceptable PDx　Manifestation　H1-H14 HAC　HCC CMS-HCC Condition　*EXCLUDES 1* Not Coded Here　*EXCLUDES 2* Not Included Here

ICD-10-CM 2018　　　　　　　　　　　　　　　　　　　　　　　　　　　　　　　　　　　　　　**805**

M86.479   **Chronic osteomyelitis with draining sinus, unspecified ankle and foot** `CC` `HCC`

M86.48   **Chronic osteomyelitis with draining sinus, other site** `CC` `HCC`

M86.49   **Chronic osteomyelitis with draining sinus, multiple sites** `CC` `HCC`

✓5ᵗʰ **M86.5**   Other chronic hematogenous **osteomyelitis**

> **CC Excl: For CC codes in subcategory M86.5, unless otherwise noted:** PDX collection 881

M86.50   **Other chronic hematogenous osteomyelitis, unspecified site** `CC` `HCC`
> **CC Excl:** PDX collection 906

✓6ᵗʰ **M86.51**   **Other chronic hematogenous osteomyelitis, shoulder**

M86.511   Other chronic hematogenous osteomyelitis, **right shoulder** `CC` `HCC`

M86.512   Other chronic hematogenous osteomyelitis, **left shoulder** `CC` `HCC`

M86.519   Other chronic hematogenous osteomyelitis, unspecified **shoulder** `CC` `HCC`

✓6ᵗʰ **M86.52**   **Other chronic hematogenous osteomyelitis, humerus**

M86.521   Other chronic hematogenous osteomyelitis, **right humerus** `CC` `HCC`

M86.522   Other chronic hematogenous osteomyelitis, **left humerus** `CC` `HCC`

M86.529   Other chronic hematogenous osteomyelitis, unspecified **humerus** `CC` `HCC`

✓6ᵗʰ **M86.53**   **Other chronic hematogenous osteomyelitis, radius and ulna**

M86.531   Other chronic hematogenous osteomyelitis, **right radius and ulna** `CC` `HCC`

M86.532   Other chronic hematogenous osteomyelitis, **left radius and ulna** `CC` `HCC`

M86.539   Other chronic hematogenous osteomyelitis, unspecified **radius and ulna** `CC` `HCC`

✓6ᵗʰ **M86.54**   Other chronic hematogenous osteomyelitis, **hand**

M86.541   Other chronic hematogenous osteomyelitis, **right hand** `CC` `HCC`

M86.542   Other chronic hematogenous osteomyelitis, **left hand** `CC` `HCC`

M86.549   Other chronic hematogenous osteomyelitis, unspecified **hand** `CC` `HCC`

✓6ᵗʰ **M86.55**   Other chronic hematogenous osteomyelitis, **femur**

M86.551   Other chronic hematogenous osteomyelitis, **right femur** `CC` `HCC`

M86.552   Other chronic hematogenous osteomyelitis, **left femur** `CC` `HCC`

M86.559   Other chronic hematogenous osteomyelitis, unspecified **femur** `CC` `HCC`

✓6ᵗʰ **M86.56**   Other chronic hematogenous osteomyelitis, **tibia and fibula**

M86.561   Other chronic hematogenous osteomyelitis, **right tibia and fibula** `CC` `HCC`

M86.562   Other chronic hematogenous osteomyelitis, **left tibia and fibula** `CC` `HCC`

M86.569   Other chronic hematogenous osteomyelitis, unspecified **tibia and fibula** `CC` `HCC`

✓6ᵗʰ **M86.57**   Other chronic hematogenous osteomyelitis, **ankle and foot**

M86.571   Other chronic hematogenous osteomyelitis, **right ankle and foot** `CC` `HCC`

M86.572   Other chronic hematogenous osteomyelitis, **left ankle and foot** `CC` `HCC`

M86.579   Other chronic hematogenous osteomyelitis, unspecified **ankle and foot** `CC` `HCC`

M86.58   **Other chronic hematogenous osteomyelitis, other site** `CC` `HCC`

M86.59   **Other chronic hematogenous osteomyelitis, multiple sites** `CC` `HCC`

✓5ᵗʰ **M86.6**   Other chronic **osteomyelitis**

> **CC Excl: For CC codes in subcategory M86.6, unless otherwise noted:** PDX collection 881

M86.60   **Other chronic osteomyelitis, unspecified site** `CC` `HCC`
> **CC Excl:** PDX collection 906

✓6ᵗʰ **M86.61**   Other chronic osteomyelitis, **shoulder**

M86.611   Other chronic osteomyelitis, **right shoulder** `CC` `HCC`

M86.612   Other chronic osteomyelitis, **left shoulder** `CC` `HCC`

M86.619   Other chronic osteomyelitis, unspecified **shoulder** `CC` `HCC`

✓6ᵗʰ **M86.62**   Other chronic osteomyelitis, **humerus**

M86.621   Other chronic osteomyelitis, **right humerus** `CC` `HCC`

M86.622   Other chronic osteomyelitis, **left humerus** `CC` `HCC`

M86.629   Other chronic osteomyelitis, unspecified **humerus** `CC` `HCC`

✓6ᵗʰ **M86.63**   Other chronic osteomyelitis, **radius and ulna**

M86.631   Other chronic osteomyelitis, **right radius and ulna** `CC` `HCC`

M86.632   Other chronic osteomyelitis, **left radius and ulna** `CC` `HCC`

M86.639   Other chronic osteomyelitis, unspecified **radius and ulna** `CC` `HCC`

✓6ᵗʰ **M86.64**   Other chronic osteomyelitis, **hand**

M86.641   Other chronic osteomyelitis, **right hand** `CC` `HCC`

M86.642   Other chronic osteomyelitis, **left hand** `CC` `HCC`

M86.649   Other chronic osteomyelitis, unspecified **hand** `CC` `HCC`

✓6ᵗʰ **M86.65**   Other chronic osteomyelitis, **thigh**

M86.651   Other chronic osteomyelitis, **right thigh** `CC` `HCC`

M86.652   Other chronic osteomyelitis, **left thigh** `CC` `HCC`

M86.659   Other chronic osteomyelitis, unspecified **thigh** `CC` `HCC`

✓6ᵗʰ **M86.66**   Other chronic osteomyelitis, **tibia and fibula**

M86.661   Other chronic osteomyelitis, **right tibia and fibula** `CC` `HCC`

M86.662   Other chronic osteomyelitis, **left tibia and fibula** `CC` `HCC`

M86.669   Other chronic osteomyelitis, unspecified **tibia and fibula** `CC` `HCC`

✓6ᵗʰ **M86.67**   Other chronic osteomyelitis, **ankle and foot**

M86.671   Other chronic osteomyelitis, **right ankle and foot** `CC` `HCC`
> **AHA:** 2016, 1Q, 13

M86.672   Other chronic osteomyelitis, **left ankle and foot** `CC` `HCC`

M86.679   Other chronic osteomyelitis, unspecified **ankle and foot** `CC` `HCC`

M86.68   **Other chronic osteomyelitis, other site** `CC` `HCC`

M86.69   **Other chronic osteomyelitis, multiple sites** `CC` `HCC`

✓5ᵗʰ **M86.8**   Other **osteomyelitis**
Brodie's abscess

> **CC Excl: For CC codes in subcategory M86.8, unless otherwise noted:** PDX collection 881

✓6ᵗʰ **M86.8X**   **Other osteomyelitis**

M86.8X0   Other osteomyelitis, **multiple sites** `CC` `HCC`

M86.8X1   Other osteomyelitis, **shoulder** `CC` `HCC`

M86.8X2   Other osteomyelitis, **upper arm** `CC` `HCC`

M86.8X3   Other osteomyelitis, **forearm** `CC` `HCC`

M86.8X4   Other osteomyelitis, **hand** `CC` `HCC`

M86.8X5   Other osteomyelitis, **thigh** `CC` `HCC`

M86.8X6   Other osteomyelitis, **lower leg** `CC` `HCC`

M86.8X7   Other osteomyelitis, **ankle and foot** `CC` `HCC`

M86.8X8   Other osteomyelitis, **other site** `CC` `HCC`

M86.8X9   Other osteomyelitis, unspecified **sites** `CC` `HCC`
> **CC Excl:** PDX collection 906

N Newborn: 0   P Pediatric: 0-17   M Maternity: 12-55   A Adult: 15-124   MCC Major CC Condition   PDxMCC PDx acts as own MCC   CC CC Condition   PDxCC PDx acts as own CC

806   ICD-10-CM 2018

M86.9 Osteomyelitis, unspecified   `CC` `HCC`
     Infection of bone NOS
     Periostitis without osteomyelitis
     CC Excl: PDX collection 906

`✓4ᵗʰ` **M87 Osteonecrosis**
     `INCLUDES` avascular necrosis of bone
     Use additional code to identify major osseous defect, if applicable
     (M89.7-)
     `EXCLUDES 1` *juvenile osteonecrosis (M91-M92)*
              osteochondropathies (M90-M93)

> **CC Excl: For CC codes in category M87, unless otherwise noted:** PDX collection 907

`✓5ᵗʰ` **M87.0 Idiopathic aseptic** necrosis of bone
     M87.00 Idiopathic aseptic necrosis of unspecified bone   `CC` `HCC`

     `✓6ᵗʰ` **M87.01 Idiopathic aseptic necrosis of** shoulder
         Idiopathic aseptic necrosis of clavicle and scapula

> **CC Excl: For CC codes in subcategory M87.01:** PDX collection 908

         M87.011 Idiopathic aseptic necrosis of right shoulder   `CC` `HCC`
         M87.012 Idiopathic aseptic necrosis of left shoulder   `CC` `HCC`
         M87.019 Idiopathic aseptic necrosis of unspecified shoulder   `CC` `HCC`

     `✓6ᵗʰ` **M87.02 Idiopathic aseptic necrosis of** humerus

> **CC Excl: For CC codes in subcategory M87.02:** PDX collection 908·

         M87.021 Idiopathic aseptic necrosis of right humerus   `CC` `HCC`
         M87.022 Idiopathic aseptic necrosis of left humerus   `CC` `HCC`
         M87.029 Idiopathic aseptic necrosis of unspecified humerus   `CC` `HCC`

     `✓6ᵗʰ` **M87.03 Idiopathic aseptic necrosis of** radius, ulna and carpus
         M87.031 Idiopathic aseptic necrosis of right radius   `CC` `HCC`
         M87.032 Idiopathic aseptic necrosis of left radius   `CC` `HCC`
         M87.033 Idiopathic aseptic necrosis of unspecified radius
         M87.034 Idiopathic aseptic necrosis of right ulna   `CC` `HCC`
         M87.035 Idiopathic aseptic necrosis of left ulna
         M87.036 Idiopathic aseptic necrosis of unspecified ulna
         M87.037 Idiopathic aseptic necrosis of right carpus   `CC` `HCC`
         M87.038 Idiopathic aseptic necrosis of left carpus   `CC` `HCC`
         M87.039 Idiopathic aseptic necrosis of unspecified carpus   `CC` `HCC`

     `✓6ᵗʰ` **M87.04 Idiopathic aseptic necrosis of** hand and fingers
         Idiopathic aseptic necrosis of metacarpals and phalanges of hands
         M87.041 Idiopathic aseptic necrosis of right hand   `CC` `HCC`
         M87.042 Idiopathic aseptic necrosis of left hand   `CC` `HCC`
         M87.043 Idiopathic aseptic necrosis of unspecified hand   `CC` `HCC`
         M87.044 Idiopathic aseptic necrosis of right finger(s)   `CC` `HCC`
         M87.045 Idiopathic aseptic necrosis of left finger(s)   `CC` `HCC`
         M87.046 Idiopathic aseptic necrosis of unspecified finger(s)   `CC` `HCC`

     `✓6ᵗʰ` **M87.05 Idiopathic aseptic necrosis of** pelvis and femur
         M87.050 Idiopathic aseptic necrosis of pelvis   `CC` `HCC`
         M87.051 Idiopathic aseptic necrosis of right femur   `CC` `HCC`
             CC Excl: PDX collection 909

M87.052 Idiopathic aseptic necrosis of left femur   `CC` `HCC`
     CC Excl: PDX collection 909
M87.059 Idiopathic aseptic necrosis of unspecified femur   `CC` `HCC`
     Idiopathic aseptic necrosis of hip NOS
     CC Excl: PDX collection 909

`✓6ᵗʰ` **M87.06 Idiopathic aseptic necrosis of** tibia and fibula
     M87.061 Idiopathic aseptic necrosis of right tibia   `CC` `HCC`
     M87.062 Idiopathic aseptic necrosis of left tibia   `CC` `HCC`
     M87.063 Idiopathic aseptic necrosis of unspecified tibia   `CC` `HCC`
     M87.064 Idiopathic aseptic necrosis of right fibula   `CC` `HCC`
     M87.065 Idiopathic aseptic necrosis of left fibula   `CC` `HCC`
     M87.066 Idiopathic aseptic necrosis of unspecified fibula   `CC` `HCC`

`✓6ᵗʰ` **M87.07 Idiopathic aseptic necrosis of** ankle, foot and toes
     Idiopathic aseptic necrosis of metatarsus, tarsus, and phalanges of toes
     M87.071 Idiopathic aseptic necrosis of right ankle   `CC` `HCC`
     M87.072 Idiopathic aseptic necrosis of left ankle   `CC` `HCC`
     M87.073 Idiopathic aseptic necrosis of unspecified ankle   `CC` `HCC`
     M87.074 Idiopathic aseptic necrosis of right foot   `CC` `HCC`
         CC Excl: PDX collection 910
     M87.075 Idiopathic aseptic necrosis of left foot   `CC` `HCC`
         CC Excl: PDX collection 910
     M87.076 Idiopathic aseptic necrosis of unspecified foot   `CC` `HCC`
         CC Excl: PDX collection 910
     M87.077 Idiopathic aseptic necrosis of right toe(s)   `CC` `HCC`
     M87.078 Idiopathic aseptic necrosis of left toe(s)   `CC` `HCC`
     M87.079 Idiopathic aseptic necrosis of unspecified toe(s)   `CC` `HCC`

M87.08 Idiopathic aseptic necrosis of bone, other site   `CC` `HCC`
M87.09 Idiopathic aseptic necrosis of bone, multiple sites   `CC` `HCC`

`✓5ᵗʰ` **M87.1 Osteonecrosis due to drugs**
     Use additional code for adverse effect, if applicable, to identify drug (T36-T50 with fifth or sixth character 5)
     M87.10 Osteonecrosis due to drugs, unspecified bone   `CC` `HCC`

     `✓6ᵗʰ` **M87.11 Osteonecrosis due to drugs, shoulder**
         M87.111 Osteonecrosis due to drugs, right shoulder   `CC` `HCC`
         M87.112 Osteonecrosis due to drugs, left shoulder   `CC` `HCC`
         M87.119 Osteonecrosis due to drugs, unspecified shoulder   `CC` `HCC`

     `✓6ᵗʰ` **M87.12 Osteonecrosis due to drugs, humerus**

> **CC Excl: For CC codes in subcategory M87.12:** PDX collection 908

         M87.121 Osteonecrosis due to drugs, right humerus   `CC` `HCC`
         M87.122 Osteonecrosis due to drugs, left humerus   `CC` `HCC`
         M87.129 Osteonecrosis due to drugs, unspecified humerus   `CC` `HCC`

     `✓6ᵗʰ` **M87.13 Osteonecrosis due to drugs of** radius, ulna and carpus
         M87.131 Osteonecrosis due to drugs of right radius   `CC` `HCC`
         M87.132 Osteonecrosis due to drugs of left radius   `CC` `HCC`
         M87.133 Osteonecrosis due to drugs of unspecified radius   `CC` `HCC`

`✓`Additional Character Req   `✓x7ᵗʰ` Placeholder Alert   Unacceptable PDx   Manifestation   `H1`-`H14` HAC   `HCC` CMS-HCC Condition   `EXCLUDES 1` Not Coded Here   `EXCLUDES 2` Not Included Here

ICD-10-CM 2018   **807**

M87.134 Osteonecrosis due to drugs of right ulna `CC` `HCC`

M87.135 Osteonecrosis due to drugs of left ulna `CC` `HCC`

M87.136 Osteonecrosis due to drugs of unspecified ulna `CC` `HCC`

M87.137 Osteonecrosis due to drugs of right carpus `CC` `HCC`

M87.138 Osteonecrosis due to drugs of left carpus `CC` `HCC`

M87.139 Osteonecrosis due to drugs of unspecified carpus `CC` `HCC`

✓6ᵗʰ M87.14 Osteonecrosis due to drugs, hand and fingers

M87.141 Osteonecrosis due to drugs, right hand `CC` `HCC`

M87.142 Osteonecrosis due to drugs, left hand `CC` `HCC`

M87.143 Osteonecrosis due to drugs, unspecified hand `CC` `HCC`

M87.144 Osteonecrosis due to drugs, right finger(s) `CC` `HCC`

M87.145 Osteonecrosis due to drugs, left finger(s) `CC` `HCC`

M87.146 Osteonecrosis due to drugs, unspecified finger(s) `CC` `HCC`

✓6ᵗʰ M87.15 Osteonecrosis due to drugs, pelvis and femur

> **CC Excl:** For CC codes in subcategory M87.15: PDX collection 909

M87.150 Osteonecrosis due to drugs, pelvis `CC` `HCC`

M87.151 Osteonecrosis due to drugs, right femur `CC` `HCC`

M87.152 Osteonecrosis due to drugs, left femur `CC` `HCC`

M87.159 Osteonecrosis due to drugs, unspecified femur `CC` `HCC`

✓6ᵗʰ M87.16 Osteonecrosis due to drugs, tibia and fibula

M87.161 Osteonecrosis due to drugs, right tibia `CC` `HCC`

M87.162 Osteonecrosis due to drugs, left tibia `CC` `HCC`

M87.163 Osteonecrosis due to drugs, unspecified tibia `CC` `HCC`

M87.164 Osteonecrosis due to drugs, right fibula `CC` `HCC`

M87.165 Osteonecrosis due to drugs, left fibula `CC` `HCC`

M87.166 Osteonecrosis due to drugs, unspecified fibula `CC` `HCC`

✓6ᵗʰ M87.17 Osteonecrosis due to drugs, ankle, foot and toes

M87.171 Osteonecrosis due to drugs, right ankle `CC` `HCC`

M87.172 Osteonecrosis due to drugs, left ankle `CC` `HCC`

M87.173 Osteonecrosis due to drugs, unspecified ankle `CC` `HCC`

M87.174 Osteonecrosis due to drugs, right foot `CC` `HCC`

> **CC Excl:** PDX collection 910

M87.175 Osteonecrosis due to drugs, left foot `CC` `HCC`

> **CC Excl:** PDX collection 910

M87.176 Osteonecrosis due to drugs, unspecified foot `CC` `HCC`

> **CC Excl:** PDX collection 910

M87.177 Osteonecrosis due to drugs, right toe(s) `CC` `HCC`

M87.178 Osteonecrosis due to drugs, left toe(s) `CC` `HCC`

M87.179 Osteonecrosis due to drugs, unspecified toe(s) `CC` `HCC`

✓6ᵗʰ M87.18 Osteonecrosis due to drugs, other site

M87.180 Osteonecrosis due to drugs, jaw `CC` `HCC`

M87.188 Osteonecrosis due to drugs, other site `CC` `HCC`

M87.19 Osteonecrosis due to drugs, multiple sites `CC` `HCC`

✓5ᵗʰ M87.2 Osteonecrosis due to previous trauma

M87.20 Osteonecrosis due to previous trauma, unspecified bone `CC` `HCC`

✓6ᵗʰ M87.21 Osteonecrosis due to previous trauma, shoulder

M87.211 Osteonecrosis due to previous trauma, right shoulder `CC` `HCC`

M87.212 Osteonecrosis due to previous trauma, left shoulder `CC` `HCC`

M87.219 Osteonecrosis due to previous trauma, unspecified shoulder `CC` `HCC`

✓6ᵗʰ M87.22 Osteonecrosis due to previous trauma, humerus

> **CC Excl:** For CC codes in subcategory M87.22: PDX collection 908

M87.221 Osteonecrosis due to previous trauma, right humerus `CC` `HCC`

M87.222 Osteonecrosis due to previous trauma, left humerus `CC` `HCC`

M87.229 Osteonecrosis due to previous trauma, unspecified humerus `CC` `HCC`

✓6ᵗʰ M87.23 Osteonecrosis due to previous trauma of radius, ulna and carpus

M87.231 Osteonecrosis due to previous trauma of right radius `CC` `HCC`

M87.232 Osteonecrosis due to previous trauma of left radius `CC` `HCC`

M87.233 Osteonecrosis due to previous trauma of unspecified radius `CC` `HCC`

M87.234 Osteonecrosis due to previous trauma of right ulna `CC` `HCC`

M87.235 Osteonecrosis due to previous trauma of left ulna `CC` `HCC`

M87.236 Osteonecrosis due to previous trauma of unspecified ulna `CC` `HCC`

M87.237 Osteonecrosis due to previous trauma of right carpus `CC` `HCC`

M87.238 Osteonecrosis due to previous trauma of left carpus `CC` `HCC`

M87.239 Osteonecrosis due to previous trauma of unspecified carpus `CC` `HCC`

✓6ᵗʰ M87.24 Osteonecrosis due to previous trauma, hand and fingers

M87.241 Osteonecrosis due to previous trauma, right hand `CC` `HCC`

M87.242 Osteonecrosis due to previous trauma, left hand `CC` `HCC`

M87.243 Osteonecrosis due to previous trauma, unspecified hand `CC` `HCC`

M87.244 Osteonecrosis due to previous trauma, right finger(s) `CC` `HCC`

M87.245 Osteonecrosis due to previous trauma, left finger(s) `CC` `HCC`

M87.246 Osteonecrosis due to previous trauma, unspecified finger(s) `CC` `HCC`

✓6ᵗʰ M87.25 Osteonecrosis due to previous trauma, pelvis and femur

M87.250 Osteonecrosis due to previous trauma, pelvis `CC` `HCC`

M87.251 Osteonecrosis due to previous trauma, right femur `CC` `HCC`

> **CC Excl:** PDX collection 909

M87.252 Osteonecrosis due to previous trauma, left femur `CC` `HCC`

> **CC Excl:** PDX collection 909

M87.256 Osteonecrosis due to previous trauma, unspecified femur `CC` `HCC`

> **CC Excl:** PDX collection 909

✓6ᵗʰ M87.26 Osteonecrosis due to previous trauma, tibia and fibula

M87.261 Osteonecrosis due to previous trauma, right tibia `CC` `HCC`

M87.262 Osteonecrosis due to previous trauma, left tibia `CC` `HCC`

M87.263 Osteonecrosis due to previous trauma, unspecified tibia `CC` `HCC`

M87.264 Osteonecrosis due to previous trauma, right fibula `CC` `HCC`

M87.265 Osteonecrosis due to previous trauma, left fibula `CC` `HCC`

N Newborn: 0   P Pediatric: 0-17   M Maternity: 12-55   A Adult: 15-124   MCC Major CC Condition   PDx MCC PDx acts as own MCC   CC CC Condition   PDx CC PDx acts as own CC

808   ICD-10-CM 2018

M87.266 Osteonecrosis due to previous trauma, unspecified fibula   `CC` `HCC`

✓6th **M87.27** Osteonecrosis due to previous trauma, ankle, foot and toes

     M87.271 Osteonecrosis due to previous trauma, right ankle   `CC` `HCC`

     M87.272 Osteonecrosis due to previous trauma, left ankle   `CC` `HCC`

     M87.273 Osteonecrosis due to previous trauma, unspecified ankle   `CC` `HCC`

     M87.274 Osteonecrosis due to previous trauma, right foot   `CC` `HCC`
       CC Excl: PDX collection 910

     M87.275 Osteonecrosis due to previous trauma, left foot   `CC` `HCC`
       CC Excl: PDX collection 910

     M87.276 Osteonecrosis due to previous trauma, unspecified foot   `CC` `HCC`
       CC Excl: PDX collection 910

     M87.277 Osteonecrosis due to previous trauma, right toe(s)   `CC` `HCC`

     M87.278 Osteonecrosis due to previous trauma, left toe(s)   `CC` `HCC`

     M87.279 Osteonecrosis due to previous trauma, unspecified toe(s)   `CC` `HCC`

M87.28 Osteonecrosis due to previous trauma, other site   `CC` `HCC`

M87.29 Osteonecrosis due to previous trauma, multiple sites   `CC` `HCC`

✓5th **M87.3** Other secondary osteonecrosis

     M87.30 Other secondary osteonecrosis, unspecified bone   `CC` `HCC`

✓6th **M87.31** Other secondary osteonecrosis, shoulder

     M87.311 Other secondary osteonecrosis, right shoulder   `CC` `HCC`

     M87.312 Other secondary osteonecrosis, left shoulder   `CC` `HCC`

     M87.319 Other secondary osteonecrosis, unspecified shoulder   `CC` `HCC`

✓6th **M87.32** Other secondary osteonecrosis, humerus

     CC Excl: For CC codes in subcategory M87.32: PDX collection 908

     M87.321 Other secondary osteonecrosis, right humerus   `CC` `HCC`

     M87.322 Other secondary osteonecrosis, left humerus   `CC` `HCC`

     M87.329 Other secondary osteonecrosis, unspecified humerus   `CC` `HCC`

✓6th **M87.33** Other secondary osteonecrosis of radius, ulna and carpus

     M87.331 Other secondary osteonecrosis of right radius   `CC` `HCC`

     M87.332 Other secondary osteonecrosis of left radius   `CC` `HCC`

     M87.333 Other secondary osteonecrosis of unspecified radius   `CC` `HCC`

     M87.334 Other secondary osteonecrosis of right ulna   `CC` `HCC`

     M87.335 Other secondary osteonecrosis of left ulna   `CC` `HCC`

     M87.336 Other secondary osteonecrosis of unspecified ulna   `CC` `HCC`

     M87.337 Other secondary osteonecrosis of right carpus   `CC` `HCC`

     M87.338 Other secondary osteonecrosis of left carpus   `CC` `HCC`

     M87.339 Other secondary osteonecrosis of unspecified carpus   `CC` `HCC`

✓6th **M87.34** Other secondary osteonecrosis, hand and fingers

     M87.341 Other secondary osteonecrosis, right hand   `CC` `HCC`

     M87.342 Other secondary osteonecrosis, left hand   `CC` `HCC`

     M87.343 Other secondary osteonecrosis, unspecified hand   `CC` `HCC`

     M87.344 Other secondary osteonecrosis, right finger(s)   `CC` `HCC`

     M87.345 Other secondary osteonecrosis, left finger(s)   `CC` `HCC`

     M87.346 Other secondary osteonecrosis, unspecified finger(s)   `CC` `HCC`

✓6th **M87.35** Other secondary osteonecrosis, pelvis and femur

     CC Excl: For CC codes in subcategory M87.35: PDX collection 909

     M87.350 Other secondary osteonecrosis, pelvis   `CC` `HCC`

     M87.351 Other secondary osteonecrosis, right femur   `CC` `HCC`

     M87.352 Other secondary osteonecrosis, left femur   `CC` `HCC`

     M87.353 Other secondary osteonecrosis, unspecified femur   `CC` `HCC`

✓6th **M87.36** Other secondary osteonecrosis, tibia and fibula

     M87.361 Other secondary osteonecrosis, right tibia   `CC` `HCC`

     M87.362 Other secondary osteonecrosis, left tibia   `CC` `HCC`

     M87.363 Other secondary osteonecrosis, unspecified tibia   `CC` `HCC`

     M87.364 Other secondary osteonecrosis, right fibula   `CC` `HCC`

     M87.365 Other secondary osteonecrosis, left fibula   `CC` `HCC`

     M87.366 Other secondary osteonecrosis, unspecified fibula   `CC` `HCC`

✓6th **M87.37** Other secondary osteonecrosis, ankle and foot

     M87.371 Other secondary osteonecrosis, right ankle   `CC` `HCC`

     M87.372 Other secondary osteonecrosis, left ankle   `CC` `HCC`

     M87.373 Other secondary osteonecrosis, unspecified ankle   `CC` `HCC`

     M87.374 Other secondary osteonecrosis, right foot   `CC` `HCC`
       CC Excl: PDX collection 910

     M87.375 Other secondary osteonecrosis, left foot   `CC` `HCC`
       CC Excl: PDX collection 910

     M87.376 Other secondary osteonecrosis, unspecified foot   `CC` `HCC`
       CC Excl: PDX collection 910

     M87.377 Other secondary osteonecrosis, right toe(s)   `CC` `HCC`

     M87.378 Other secondary osteonecrosis, left toe(s)   `CC` `HCC`

     M87.379 Other secondary osteonecrosis, unspecified toe(s)   `CC` `HCC`

M87.38 Other secondary osteonecrosis, other site   `CC` `HCC`

M87.39 Other secondary osteonecrosis, multiple sites   `CC` `HCC`

✓5th **M87.8** Other osteonecrosis

     M87.80 Other osteonecrosis, unspecified bone   `CC` `HCC`

✓6th **M87.81** Other osteonecrosis, shoulder

     M87.811 Other osteonecrosis, right shoulder   `CC` `HCC`

     M87.812 Other osteonecrosis, left shoulder   `CC` `HCC`

     M87.819 Other osteonecrosis, unspecified shoulder   `CC` `HCC`

✓6th **M87.82** Other osteonecrosis, humerus

     CC Excl: For CC codes in subcategory M87.82: PDX collection 908

     M87.821 Other osteonecrosis, right humerus   `CC` `HCC`

     M87.822 Other osteonecrosis, left humerus   `CC` `HCC`

     M87.829 Other osteonecrosis, unspecified humerus   `CC` `HCC`

✓6th **M87.83** Other osteonecrosis of radius, ulna and carpus

     M87.831 Other osteonecrosis of right radius   `CC` `HCC`

     M87.832 Other osteonecrosis of left radius   `CC` `HCC`

     M87.833 Other osteonecrosis of unspecified radius   `CC` `HCC`

✓ Additional Character Req   ✓x7th Placeholder Alert   Unacceptable PDx   Manifestation   H1-H14 HAC   HCC CMS-HCC Condition   *EXCLUDES 1* Not Coded Here   *EXCLUDES 2* Not Included Here

ICD-10-CM 2018   809

M87.834 Other osteonecrosis of right ulna `CC` `HCC`
M87.835 Other osteonecrosis of left ulna `CC` `HCC`
M87.836 Other osteonecrosis of unspecified ulna `CC` `HCC`
M87.837 Other osteonecrosis of right carpus `CC` `HCC`
M87.838 Other osteonecrosis of left carpus `CC` `HCC`
M87.839 Other osteonecrosis of unspecified carpus `CC` `HCC`

✓6th **M87.84 Other osteonecrosis, hand and fingers**
M87.841 Other osteonecrosis, right hand `CC` `HCC`
M87.842 Other osteonecrosis, left hand `CC` `HCC`
M87.843 Other osteonecrosis, unspecified hand `CC` `HCC`
M87.844 Other osteonecrosis, right finger(s) `CC` `HCC`
M87.845 Other osteonecrosis, left finger(s) `CC` `HCC`
M87.849 Other osteonecrosis, unspecified finger(s) `CC` `HCC`

✓6th **M87.85 Other osteonecrosis, pelvis and femur**

CC Excl: For CC codes in subcategory M87.85: PDX collection 909

M87.850 Other osteonecrosis, pelvis `CC` `HCC`
M87.851 Other osteonecrosis, right femur `CC` `HCC`
M87.852 Other osteonecrosis, left femur `CC` `HCC`
M87.859 Other osteonecrosis, unspecified femur `CC` `HCC`

✓6th **M87.86 Other osteonecrosis, tibia and fibula**
M87.861 Other osteonecrosis, right tibia `CC` `HCC`
M87.862 Other osteonecrosis, left tibia `CC` `HCC`
M87.863 Other osteonecrosis, unspecified tibia `CC` `HCC`
M87.864 Other osteonecrosis, right fibula `CC` `HCC`
M87.865 Other osteonecrosis, left fibula `CC` `HCC`
M87.869 Other osteonecrosis, unspecified fibula `CC` `HCC`

✓6th **M87.87 Other osteonecrosis, ankle, foot and toes**
M87.871 Other osteonecrosis, right ankle `CC` `HCC`
M87.872 Other osteonecrosis, left ankle `CC` `HCC`
M87.873 Other osteonecrosis, unspecified ankle `CC` `HCC`
M87.874 Other osteonecrosis, right foot `CC` `HCC`
CC Excl: PDX collection 910
M87.875 Other osteonecrosis, left foot `CC` `HCC`
CC Excl: PDX collection 910
M87.876 Other osteonecrosis, unspecified foot `CC` `HCC`
CC Excl: PDX collection 910
M87.877 Other osteonecrosis, right toe(s) `CC` `HCC`
M87.878 Other osteonecrosis, left toe(s) `CC` `HCC`
M87.879 Other osteonecrosis, unspecified toe(s) `CC` `HCC`

M87.88 Other osteonecrosis, other site `CC` `HCC`
M87.89 Other osteonecrosis, multiple sites `CC` `HCC`
M87.9 Osteonecrosis, unspecified `CC` `HCC`
Necrosis of bone NOS

✓4th **M88 Osteitis deformans [Paget's disease of bone]**
EXCLUDES 1 osteitis deformans in neoplastic disease (M90.6)

M88.0 Osteitis deformans of skull
M88.1 Osteitis deformans of vertebrae
✓5th **M88.8 Osteitis deformans of other bones**
✓6th **M88.81 Osteitis deformans of shoulder**
M88.811 Osteitis deformans of right shoulder
M88.812 Osteitis deformans of left shoulder
M88.819 Osteitis deformans of unspecified shoulder
✓6th **M88.82 Osteitis deformans of upper arm**
M88.821 Osteitis deformans of right upper arm
M88.822 Osteitis deformans of left upper arm
M88.829 Osteitis deformans of unspecified upper arm
✓6th **M88.83 Osteitis deformans of forearm**
M88.831 Osteitis deformans of right forearm
M88.832 Osteitis deformans of left forearm
M88.839 Osteitis deformans of unspecified forearm

✓6th **M88.84 Osteitis deformans of hand**
M88.841 Osteitis deformans of right hand
M88.842 Osteitis deformans of left hand
M88.849 Osteitis deformans of unspecified hand
✓6th **M88.85 Osteitis deformans of thigh**
M88.851 Osteitis deformans of right thigh
M88.852 Osteitis deformans of left thigh
M88.859 Osteitis deformans of unspecified thigh
✓6th **M88.86 Osteitis deformans of lower leg**
M88.861 Osteitis deformans of right lower leg
M88.862 Osteitis deformans of left lower leg
M88.869 Osteitis deformans of unspecified lower leg
✓6th **M88.87 Osteitis deformans of ankle and foot**
M88.871 Osteitis deformans of right ankle and foot
M88.872 Osteitis deformans of left ankle and foot
M88.879 Osteitis deformans of unspecified ankle and foot
M88.88 Osteitis deformans of other bones
EXCLUDES 2 osteitis deformans of skull (M88.0)
osteitis deformans of vertebrae (M88.1)
M88.89 Osteitis deformans of multiple sites
M88.9 Osteitis deformans of unspecified bone

✓4th **M89 Other disorders of bone**
✓5th **M89.0 Algoneurodystrophy**
Shoulder-hand syndrome
Sudeck's atrophy
EXCLUDES 1 causalgia, lower limb (G57.7-)
causalgia, upper limb (G56.4-)
complex regional pain syndrome II, lower limb (G57.7-)
complex regional pain syndrome II, upper limb (G56.4-)
reflex sympathetic dystrophy (G90.5-)

M89.00 Algoneurodystrophy, unspecified site
✓6th **M89.01 Algoneurodystrophy, shoulder**
M89.011 Algoneurodystrophy, right shoulder
M89.012 Algoneurodystrophy, left shoulder
M89.019 Algoneurodystrophy, unspecified shoulder
✓6th **M89.02 Algoneurodystrophy, upper arm**
M89.021 Algoneurodystrophy, right upper arm
M89.022 Algoneurodystrophy, left upper arm
M89.029 Algoneurodystrophy, unspecified upper arm
✓6th **M89.03 Algoneurodystrophy, forearm**
M89.031 Algoneurodystrophy, right forearm
M89.032 Algoneurodystrophy, left forearm
M89.039 Algoneurodystrophy, unspecified forearm
✓6th **M89.04 Algoneurodystrophy, hand**
M89.041 Algoneurodystrophy, right hand
M89.042 Algoneurodystrophy, left hand
M89.049 Algoneurodystrophy, unspecified hand
✓6th **M89.05 Algoneurodystrophy, thigh**
M89.051 Algoneurodystrophy, right thigh
M89.052 Algoneurodystrophy, left thigh
M89.059 Algoneurodystrophy, unspecified thigh
✓6th **M89.06 Algoneurodystrophy, lower leg**
M89.061 Algoneurodystrophy, right lower leg
M89.062 Algoneurodystrophy, left lower leg
M89.069 Algoneurodystrophy, unspecified lower leg
✓6th **M89.07 Algoneurodystrophy, ankle and foot**
M89.071 Algoneurodystrophy, right ankle and foot
M89.072 Algoneurodystrophy, left ankle and foot
M89.079 Algoneurodystrophy, unspecified ankle and foot
M89.08 Algoneurodystrophy, other site
M89.09 Algoneurodystrophy, multiple sites

☑5ᵗʰ **M89.1 Physeal arrest**
　　Arrest of growth plate
　　Epiphyseal arrest
　　Growth plate arrest

☑6ᵗʰ **M89.12 Physeal arrest, humerus**
　　M89.121 **Complete physeal arrest, right proximal humerus**
　　M89.122 **Complete physeal arrest, left proximal humerus**
　　M89.123 **Partial physeal arrest, right proximal humerus**
　　M89.124 **Partial physeal arrest, left proximal humerus**
　　M89.125 **Complete physeal arrest, right distal humerus**
　　M89.126 **Complete physeal arrest, left distal humerus**
　　M89.127 **Partial physeal arrest, right distal humerus**
　　M89.128 **Partial physeal arrest, left distal humerus**
　　M89.129 **Physeal arrest, humerus, unspecified**

☑6ᵗʰ **M89.13 Physeal arrest, forearm**
　　M89.131 **Complete physeal arrest, right distal radius**
　　M89.132 **Complete physeal arrest, left distal radius**
　　M89.133 **Partial physeal arrest, right distal radius**
　　M89.134 **Partial physeal arrest, left distal radius**
　　M89.138 **Other physeal arrest of forearm**
　　M89.139 **Physeal arrest, forearm, unspecified**

☑6ᵗʰ **M89.15 Physeal arrest, femur**
　　M89.151 **Complete physeal arrest, right proximal femur**
　　M89.152 **Complete physeal arrest, left proximal femur**
　　M89.153 **Partial physeal arrest, right proximal femur**
　　M89.154 **Partial physeal arrest, left proximal femur**
　　M89.155 **Complete physeal arrest, right distal femur**
　　M89.156 **Complete physeal arrest, left distal femur**
　　M89.157 **Partial physeal arrest, right distal femur**
　　M89.158 **Partial physeal arrest, left distal femur**
　　M89.159 **Physeal arrest, femur, unspecified**

☑6ᵗʰ **M89.16 Physeal arrest, lower leg**
　　M89.160 **Complete physeal arrest, right proximal tibia**
　　M89.161 **Complete physeal arrest, left proximal tibia**
　　M89.162 **Partial physeal arrest, right proximal tibia**
　　M89.163 **Partial physeal arrest, left proximal tibia**
　　M89.164 **Complete physeal arrest, right distal tibia**
　　M89.165 **Complete physeal arrest, left distal tibia**
　　M89.166 **Partial physeal arrest, right distal tibia**
　　M89.167 **Partial physeal arrest, left distal tibia**
　　M89.168 **Other physeal arrest of lower leg**
　　M89.169 **Physeal arrest, lower leg, unspecified**

　M89.18 **Physeal arrest, other site**

☑5ᵗʰ **M89.2 Other disorders of bone development and growth**
　M89.20 **Other disorders of bone development and growth, unspecified site**

☑6ᵗʰ **M89.21 Other disorders of bone development and growth, shoulder**
　　M89.211 **Other disorders of bone development and growth, right shoulder**
　　M89.212 **Other disorders of bone development and growth, left shoulder**
　　M89.219 **Other disorders of bone development and growth, unspecified shoulder**

☑6ᵗʰ **M89.22 Other disorders of bone development and growth, humerus**
　　M89.221 **Other disorders of bone development and growth, right humerus**
　　M89.222 **Other disorders of bone development and growth, left humerus**
　　M89.229 **Other disorders of bone development and growth, unspecified humerus**

☑6ᵗʰ **M89.23 Other disorders of bone development and growth, ulna and radius**
　　M89.231 **Other disorders of bone development and growth, right ulna**
　　M89.232 **Other disorders of bone development and growth, left ulna**
　　M89.233 **Other disorders of bone development and growth, right radius**
　　M89.234 **Other disorders of bone development and growth, left radius**
　　M89.239 **Other disorders of bone development and growth, unspecified ulna and radius**

☑6ᵗʰ **M89.24 Other disorders of bone development and growth, hand**
　　M89.241 **Other disorders of bone development and growth, right hand**
　　M89.242 **Other disorders of bone development and growth, left hand**
　　M89.249 **Other disorders of bone development and growth, unspecified hand**

☑6ᵗʰ **M89.25 Other disorders of bone development and growth, femur**
　　M89.251 **Other disorders of bone development and growth, right femur**
　　M89.252 **Other disorders of bone development and growth, left femur**
　　M89.259 **Other disorders of bone development and growth, unspecified femur**

☑6ᵗʰ **M89.26 Other disorders of bone development and growth, tibia and fibula**
　　M89.261 **Other disorders of bone development and growth, right tibia**
　　M89.262 **Other disorders of bone development and growth, left tibia**
　　M89.263 **Other disorders of bone development and growth, right fibula**
　　M89.264 **Other disorders of bone development and growth, left fibula**
　　M89.269 **Other disorders of bone development and growth, unspecified lower leg**

☑6ᵗʰ **M89.27 Other disorders of bone development and growth, ankle and foot**
　　M89.271 **Other disorders of bone development and growth, right ankle and foot**
　　M89.272 **Other disorders of bone development and growth, left ankle and foot**
　　M89.279 **Other disorders of bone development and growth, unspecified ankle and foot**

　M89.28 **Other disorders of bone development and growth, other site**
　M89.29 **Other disorders of bone development and growth, multiple sites**

☑5ᵗʰ **M89.3 Hypertrophy of bone**
　M89.30 **Hypertrophy of bone, unspecified site**

☑6ᵗʰ **M89.31 Hypertrophy of bone, shoulder**
　　M89.311 **Hypertrophy of bone, right shoulder**
　　M89.312 **Hypertrophy of bone, left shoulder**
　　M89.319 **Hypertrophy of bone, unspecified shoulder**

☑6ᵗʰ **M89.32 Hypertrophy of bone, humerus**
　　M89.321 **Hypertrophy of bone, right humerus**
　　M89.322 **Hypertrophy of bone, left humerus**
　　M89.329 **Hypertrophy of bone, unspecified humerus**

☑6ᵗʰ **M89.33 Hypertrophy of bone, ulna and radius**
　　M89.331 **Hypertrophy of bone, right ulna**
　　M89.332 **Hypertrophy of bone, left ulna**
　　M89.333 **Hypertrophy of bone, right radius**
　　M89.334 **Hypertrophy of bone, left radius**
　　M89.339 **Hypertrophy of bone, unspecified ulna and radius**

☑6ᵗʰ **M89.34 Hypertrophy of bone, hand**
　　M89.341 **Hypertrophy of bone, right hand**
　　M89.342 **Hypertrophy of bone, left hand**
　　M89.349 **Hypertrophy of bone, unspecified hand**

M89.35 Hypertrophy of bone, femur
M89.351 Hypertrophy of bone, right femur
M89.352 Hypertrophy of bone, left femur
M89.359 Hypertrophy of bone, unspecified femur

M89.36 Hypertrophy of bone, tibia and fibula
M89.361 Hypertrophy of bone, right tibia
M89.362 Hypertrophy of bone, left tibia
M89.363 Hypertrophy of bone, right fibula
M89.364 Hypertrophy of bone, left fibula
M89.369 Hypertrophy of bone, unspecified tibia and fibula

M89.37 Hypertrophy of bone, ankle and foot
M89.371 Hypertrophy of bone, right ankle and foot
M89.372 Hypertrophy of bone, left ankle and foot
M89.379 Hypertrophy of bone, unspecified ankle and foot

M89.38 Hypertrophy of bone, other site
M89.39 Hypertrophy of bone, multiple sites

M89.4 Other hypertrophic osteoarthropathy
Marie-Bamberger disease
Pachydermoperiostosis

M89.40 Other hypertrophic osteoarthropathy, unspecified site

M89.41 Other hypertrophic osteoarthropathy, shoulder
M89.411 Other hypertrophic osteoarthropathy, right shoulder
M89.412 Other hypertrophic osteoarthropathy, left shoulder
M89.419 Other hypertrophic osteoarthropathy, unspecified shoulder

M89.42 Other hypertrophic osteoarthropathy, upper arm
M89.421 Other hypertrophic osteoarthropathy, right upper arm
M89.422 Other hypertrophic osteoarthropathy, left upper arm
M89.429 Other hypertrophic osteoarthropathy, unspecified upper arm

M89.43 Other hypertrophic osteoarthropathy, forearm
M89.431 Other hypertrophic osteoarthropathy, right forearm
M89.432 Other hypertrophic osteoarthropathy, left forearm
M89.439 Other hypertrophic osteoarthropathy, unspecified forearm

M89.44 Other hypertrophic osteoarthropathy, hand
M89.441 Other hypertrophic osteoarthropathy, right hand
M89.442 Other hypertrophic osteoarthropathy, left hand
M89.449 Other hypertrophic osteoarthropathy, unspecified hand

M89.45 Other hypertrophic osteoarthropathy, thigh
M89.451 Other hypertrophic osteoarthropathy, right thigh
M89.452 Other hypertrophic osteoarthropathy, left thigh
M89.459 Other hypertrophic osteoarthropathy, unspecified thigh

M89.46 Other hypertrophic osteoarthropathy, lower leg
M89.461 Other hypertrophic osteoarthropathy, right lower leg
M89.462 Other hypertrophic osteoarthropathy, left lower leg
M89.469 Other hypertrophic osteoarthropathy, unspecified lower leg

M89.47 Other hypertrophic osteoarthropathy, ankle and foot
M89.471 Other hypertrophic osteoarthropathy, right ankle and foot
M89.472 Other hypertrophic osteoarthropathy, left ankle and foot
M89.479 Other hypertrophic osteoarthropathy, unspecified ankle and foot

M89.48 Other hypertrophic osteoarthropathy, other site
M89.49 Other hypertrophic osteoarthropathy, multiple sites

M89.5 Osteolysis
Use additional code to identify major osseous defect, if applicable (M89.7-)
EXCLUDES 2 periprosthetic osteolysis of internal prosthetic joint (T84.05-)

M89.50 Osteolysis, unspecified site
M89.51 Osteolysis, shoulder
M89.511 Osteolysis, right shoulder
M89.512 Osteolysis, left shoulder
M89.519 Osteolysis, unspecified shoulder

M89.52 Osteolysis, upper arm
M89.521 Osteolysis, right upper arm
M89.522 Osteolysis, left upper arm
M89.529 Osteolysis, unspecified upper arm

M89.53 Osteolysis, forearm
M89.531 Osteolysis, right forearm
M89.532 Osteolysis, left forearm
M89.539 Osteolysis, unspecified forearm

M89.54 Osteolysis, hand
M89.541 Osteolysis, right hand
M89.542 Osteolysis, left hand
M89.549 Osteolysis, unspecified hand

M89.55 Osteolysis, thigh
M89.551 Osteolysis, right thigh
M89.552 Osteolysis, left thigh
M89.559 Osteolysis, unspecified thigh

M89.56 Osteolysis, lower leg
M89.561 Osteolysis, right lower leg
M89.562 Osteolysis, left lower leg
M89.569 Osteolysis, unspecified lower leg

M89.57 Osteolysis, ankle and foot
M89.571 Osteolysis, right ankle and foot
M89.572 Osteolysis, left ankle and foot
M89.579 Osteolysis, unspecified ankle and foot

M89.58 Osteolysis, other site
M89.59 Osteolysis, multiple sites

M89.6 Osteopathy after poliomyelitis
Use additional code (B91) to identify previous poliomyelitis
EXCLUDES 1 postpolio syndrome (G14)

M89.60 Osteopathy after poliomyelitis, unspecified site HCC
M89.61 Osteopathy after poliomyelitis, shoulder
M89.611 Osteopathy after poliomyelitis, right shoulder HCC
M89.612 Osteopathy after poliomyelitis, left shoulder HCC
M89.619 Osteopathy after poliomyelitis, unspecified shoulder HCC

M89.62 Osteopathy after poliomyelitis, upper arm
M89.621 Osteopathy after poliomyelitis, right upper arm HCC
M89.622 Osteopathy after poliomyelitis, left upper arm HCC
M89.629 Osteopathy after poliomyelitis, unspecified upper arm HCC

M89.63 Osteopathy after poliomyelitis, forearm
M89.631 Osteopathy after poliomyelitis, right forearm HCC
M89.632 Osteopathy after poliomyelitis, left forearm HCC
M89.639 Osteopathy after poliomyelitis, unspecified forearm HCC

M89.64 Osteopathy after poliomyelitis, hand
M89.641 Osteopathy after poliomyelitis, right hand HCC
M89.642 Osteopathy after poliomyelitis, left hand HCC
M89.649 Osteopathy after poliomyelitis, unspecified hand HCC

M89.65 Osteopathy after poliomyelitis, thigh
M89.651 Osteopathy after poliomyelitis, right thigh HCC
M89.652 Osteopathy after poliomyelitis, left thigh HCC

N Newborn: 0 P Pediatric: 0-17 M Maternity: 12-55 A Adult: 15-124 MCC Major CC Condition PDxMCC PDx acts as own MCC CC CC Condition PDxCC PDx acts as own CC

812   ICD-10-CM 2018

M89.659   **Osteopathy after poliomyelitis, unspecified thigh**   `HCC`

✓6ᵗʰ   M89.66   **Osteopathy after poliomyelitis, lower leg**

M89.661   **Osteopathy after poliomyelitis, right lower leg**   `HCC`

M89.662   **Osteopathy after poliomyelitis, left lower leg**   `HCC`

M89.669   **Osteopathy after poliomyelitis, unspecified lower leg**   `HCC`

✓6ᵗʰ   M89.67   **Osteopathy after poliomyelitis, ankle and foot**

M89.671   **Osteopathy after poliomyelitis, right ankle and foot**   `HCC`

M89.672   **Osteopathy after poliomyelitis, left ankle and foot**   `HCC`

M89.679   **Osteopathy after poliomyelitis, unspecified ankle and foot**   `HCC`

M89.68   **Osteopathy after poliomyelitis, other site**   `HCC`

M89.69   **Osteopathy after poliomyelitis, multiple sites**   `HCC`

✓5ᵗʰ   **M89.7   Major osseous defect**

Code first underlying disease, if known, such as:
aseptic necrosis of bone (M87.-)
malignant neoplasm of bone (C40.-)
osteolysis (M89.5)
osteomyelitis (M86.-)
osteonecrosis (M87.-)
osteoporosis (M80.-, M81.-)
periprosthetic osteolysis (T84.05-)

M89.70   **Major osseous defect, unspecified site**

✓6ᵗʰ   M89.71   **Major osseous defect, shoulder region**
Major osseous defect clavicle or scapula

M89.711   **Major osseous defect, right shoulder region**

M89.712   **Major osseous defect, left shoulder region**

M89.719   **Major osseous defect, unspecified shoulder region**

✓6ᵗʰ   M89.72   **Major osseous defect, humerus**

M89.721   **Major osseous defect, right humerus**

M89.722   **Major osseous defect, left humerus**

M89.729   **Major osseous defect, unspecified humerus**

✓6ᵗʰ   M89.73   **Major osseous defect, forearm**
Major osseous defect of radius and ulna

M89.731   **Major osseous defect, right forearm**

M89.732   **Major osseous defect, left forearm**

M89.739   **Major osseous defect, unspecified forearm**

✓6ᵗʰ   M89.74   **Major osseous defect, hand**
Major osseous defect of carpus, fingers, metacarpus

M89.741   **Major osseous defect, right hand**

M89.742   **Major osseous defect, left hand**

M89.749   **Major osseous defect, unspecified hand**

✓6ᵗʰ   M89.75   **Major osseous defect, pelvic region and thigh**
Major osseous defect of femur and pelvis

M89.751   **Major osseous defect, right pelvic region and thigh**

M89.752   **Major osseous defect, left pelvic region and thigh**

M89.759   **Major osseous defect, unspecified pelvic region and thigh**

✓6ᵗʰ   M89.76   **Major osseous defect, lower leg**
Major osseous defect of fibula and tibia

M89.761   **Major osseous defect, right lower leg**

M89.762   **Major osseous defect, left lower leg**

M89.769   **Major osseous defect, unspecified lower leg**

✓6ᵗʰ   M89.77   **Major osseous defect, ankle and foot**
Major osseous defect of metatarsus, tarsus, toes

M89.771   **Major osseous defect, right ankle and foot**

M89.772   **Major osseous defect, left ankle and foot**

M89.779   **Major osseous defect, unspecified ankle and foot**

M89.78   **Major osseous defect, other site**

M89.79   **Major osseous defect, multiple sites**

✓5ᵗʰ   **M89.8   Other specified disorders of bone**
Infantile cortical hyperostoses
Post-traumatic subperiosteal ossification

✓6ᵗʰ   M89.8X   **Other specified disorders of bone**

M89.8X0   **Other specified disorders of bone, multiple sites**

M89.8X1   **Other specified disorders of bone, shoulder**

M89.8X2   **Other specified disorders of bone, upper arm**

M89.8X3   **Other specified disorders of bone, forearm**

M89.8X4   **Other specified disorders of bone, hand**

M89.8X5   **Other specified disorders of bone, thigh**

M89.8X6   **Other specified disorders of bone, lower leg**

M89.8X7   **Other specified disorders of bone, ankle and foot**

M89.8X8   **Other specified disorders of bone, other site**

M89.8X9   **Other specified disorders of bone, unspecified site**

M89.9   Disorder of bone, unspecified

✓4ᵗʰ   **M90   Osteopathies in diseases classified elsewhere**

EXCLUDES 1   osteochondritis, osteomyelitis, and osteopathy (in):
cryptococcosis (B45.3)
diabetes mellitus (E08-E13 with .69-)
gonococcal (A54.43)
neurogenic syphilis (A52.11)
renal osteodystrophy (N25.0)
salmonellosis (A02.24)
secondary syphilis (A51.46)
syphilis (late) (A52.77)

✓5ᵗʰ   **M90.5   Osteonecrosis in diseases classified elsewhere**
Code first underlying disease, such as:
caisson disease (T70.3)
hemoglobinopathy (D50-D64)

CC Excl: For CC codes in subcategory M90.5, unless otherwise noted: PDX collection 907

M90.50   *Osteonecrosis in diseases classified elsewhere, unspecified site*   `PDxCC` `CC` `HCC`

✓6ᵗʰ   M90.51   **Osteonecrosis in diseases classified elsewhere, shoulder**

CC Excl: For CC codes in subcategory M90.51: PDX collection 908

M90.511   *Osteonecrosis in diseases classified elsewhere, right shoulder*   `PDxCC` `CC` `HCC`

M90.512   *Osteonecrosis in diseases classified elsewhere, left shoulder*   `PDxCC` `CC` `HCC`

M90.519   *Osteonecrosis in diseases classified elsewhere, unspecified shoulder*   `PDxCC` `CC` `HCC`

✓6ᵗʰ   M90.52   **Osteonecrosis in diseases classified elsewhere, upper arm**

M90.521   *Osteonecrosis in diseases classified elsewhere, right upper arm*   `PDxCC` `CC` `HCC`

M90.522   *Osteonecrosis in diseases classified elsewhere, left upper arm*   `PDxCC` `CC` `HCC`

M90.529   *Osteonecrosis in diseases classified elsewhere, unspecified upper arm*   `PDxCC` `CC` `HCC`

✓6ᵗʰ   M90.53   **Osteonecrosis in diseases classified elsewhere, forearm**

M90.531   *Osteonecrosis in diseases classified elsewhere, right forearm*   `PDxCC` `CC` `HCC`

M90.532   *Osteonecrosis in diseases classified elsewhere, left forearm*   `PDxCC` `CC` `HCC`

M90.539   *Osteonecrosis in diseases classified elsewhere, unspecified forearm*   `PDxCC` `CC` `HCC`

✓6ᵗʰ   M90.54   **Osteonecrosis in diseases classified elsewhere, hand**

M90.541   *Osteonecrosis in diseases classified elsewhere, right hand*   `PDxCC` `CC` `HCC`

M90.542   *Osteonecrosis in diseases classified elsewhere, left hand*   `PDxCC` `CC` `HCC`

M90.549   *Osteonecrosis in diseases classified elsewhere, unspecified hand*   `PDxCC` `CC` `HCC`

✔ Additional Character Req   ✔x7ᵗʰ Placeholder Alert   Unacceptable PDx   Manifestation   H1-H14 HAC   HCC CMS-HCC Condition   *EXCLUDES 1* Not Coded Here   *EXCLUDES 2* Not Included Here

ICD-10-CM 2018   813

Chapter 13. Diseases of the Musculoskeletal System and Connective Tissue

✓6ᵗʰ **M90.55** Osteonecrosis in diseases classified elsewhere, thigh

> **CC Excl:** For CC codes in subcategory M90.55:
> PDX collection 909

> *M90.551* **Osteonecrosis in diseases** `PDxCC` `CC` `HCC`
> classified elsewhere, *right* thigh
>
> *M90.552* **Osteonecrosis in diseases** `PDxCC` `CC` `HCC`
> classified elsewhere, *left* thigh
>
> *M90.559* **Osteonecrosis in diseases** `PDxCC` `CC` `HCC`
> classified elsewhere, *unspecified*
> thigh

✓6ᵗʰ **M90.56** Osteonecrosis in diseases classified elsewhere, lower
leg

> *M90.561* **Osteonecrosis in diseases** `PDxCC` `CC` `HCC`
> classified elsewhere, *right* lower leg
>
> *M90.562* **Osteonecrosis in diseases** `PDxCC` `CC` `HCC`
> classified elsewhere, *left* lower leg
>
> *M90.569* **Osteonecrosis in diseases** `PDxCC` `CC` `HCC`
> classified elsewhere, *unspecified*
> lower leg

✓6ᵗʰ **M90.57** Osteonecrosis in diseases classified elsewhere, ankle
and foot

> *M90.571* **Osteonecrosis in diseases** `PDxCC` `CC` `HCC`
> classified elsewhere, *right* ankle
> and foot
>
> *M90.572* **Osteonecrosis in diseases** `PDxCC` `CC` `HCC`
> classified elsewhere, *left* ankle
> and foot
>
> *M90.579* **Osteonecrosis in diseases** `PDxCC` `CC` `HCC`
> classified elsewhere, *unspecified*
> ankle and foot

> *M90.58* **Osteonecrosis in diseases classified** `PDxCC` `CC` `HCC`
> elsewhere, *other site*
>
> *M90.59* **Osteonecrosis in diseases classified** `PDxCC` `CC` `HCC`
> elsewhere, *multiple sites*

✓5ᵗʰ **M90.6** Osteitis deformans in neoplastic diseases

> Osteitis deformans in malignant neoplasm of bone
> Code first the neoplasm (C40-, C41-)
>
> *EXCLUDES 1* osteitis deformans [Paget's disease of bone] (M88.-)

> *M90.60* **Osteitis deformans in neoplastic diseases, *unspecified***
> ***site***

✓6ᵗʰ **M90.61** Osteitis deformans in neoplastic diseases, shoulder

> *M90.611* **Osteitis deformans in neoplastic diseases,**
> ***right* shoulder**
>
> *M90.612* **Osteitis deformans in neoplastic diseases,**
> ***left* shoulder**
>
> *M90.619* **Osteitis deformans in neoplastic diseases,**
> ***unspecified* shoulder**

✓6ᵗʰ **M90.62** Osteitis deformans in neoplastic diseases, upper arm

> *M90.621* **Osteitis deformans in neoplastic diseases,**
> ***right* upper arm**
>
> *M90.622* **Osteitis deformans in neoplastic diseases,**
> ***left* upper arm**
>
> *M90.629* **Osteitis deformans in neoplastic diseases,**
> ***unspecified* upper arm**

✓6ᵗʰ **M90.63** Osteitis deformans in neoplastic diseases, forearm

> *M90.631* **Osteitis deformans in neoplastic diseases,**
> ***right* forearm**
>
> *M90.632* **Osteitis deformans in neoplastic diseases,**
> ***left* forearm**
>
> *M90.639* **Osteitis deformans in neoplastic diseases,**
> ***unspecified* forearm**

✓6ᵗʰ **M90.64** Osteitis deformans in neoplastic diseases, hand

> *M90.641* **Osteitis deformans in neoplastic diseases,**
> ***right* hand**
>
> *M90.642* **Osteitis deformans in neoplastic diseases,**
> ***left* hand**
>
> *M90.649* **Osteitis deformans in neoplastic diseases,**
> ***unspecified* hand**

✓6ᵗʰ **M90.65** Osteitis deformans in neoplastic diseases, thigh

> *M90.651* **Osteitis deformans in neoplastic diseases,**
> ***right* thigh**
>
> *M90.652* **Osteitis deformans in neoplastic diseases,**
> ***left* thigh**
>
> *M90.659* **Osteitis deformans in neoplastic diseases,**
> ***unspecified* thigh**

✓6ᵗʰ **M90.66** Osteitis deformans in neoplastic diseases, lower leg

> *M90.661* **Osteitis deformans in neoplastic diseases,**
> ***right* lower leg**
>
> *M90.662* **Osteitis deformans in neoplastic diseases,**
> ***left* lower leg**
>
> *M90.669* **Osteitis deformans in neoplastic diseases,**
> ***unspecified* lower leg**

✓6ᵗʰ **M90.67** Osteitis deformans in neoplastic diseases, ankle and
foot

> *M90.671* **Osteitis deformans in neoplastic diseases,**
> ***right* ankle and foot**
>
> *M90.672* **Osteitis deformans in neoplastic diseases,**
> ***left* ankle and foot**
>
> *M90.679* **Osteitis deformans in neoplastic diseases,**
> ***unspecified* ankle and foot**

> *M90.68* **Osteitis deformans in neoplastic diseases, *other site***
>
> *M90.69* **Osteitis deformans in neoplastic diseases, *multiple***
> ***sites***

✓5ᵗʰ **M90.8** Osteopathy in diseases classified elsewhere

> Code first underlying disease, such as:
> rickets (E55.0)
> vitamin-D-resistant rickets (E83.3)

> *M90.80* **Osteopathy in diseases classified elsewhere,**
> ***unspecified site***

✓6ᵗʰ **M90.81** Osteopathy in diseases classified elsewhere,
shoulder

> *M90.811* **Osteopathy in diseases classified elsewhere,**
> ***right* shoulder**
>
> *M90.812* **Osteopathy in diseases classified elsewhere,**
> ***left* shoulder**
>
> *M90.819* **Osteopathy in diseases classified elsewhere,**
> ***unspecified* shoulder**

✓6ᵗʰ **M90.82** Osteopathy in diseases classified elsewhere, upper
arm

> *M90.821* **Osteopathy in diseases classified elsewhere,**
> ***right* upper arm**
>
> *M90.822* **Osteopathy in diseases classified elsewhere,**
> ***left* upper arm**
>
> *M90.829* **Osteopathy in diseases classified elsewhere,**
> ***unspecified* upper arm**

✓6ᵗʰ **M90.83** Osteopathy in diseases classified elsewhere,
forearm

> *M90.831* **Osteopathy in diseases classified elsewhere,**
> ***right* forearm**
>
> *M90.832* **Osteopathy in diseases classified elsewhere,**
> ***left* forearm**
>
> *M90.839* **Osteopathy in diseases classified elsewhere,**
> ***unspecified* forearm**

✓6ᵗʰ **M90.84** Osteopathy in diseases classified elsewhere, hand

> *M90.841* **Osteopathy in diseases classified elsewhere,**
> ***right* hand**
>
> *M90.842* **Osteopathy in diseases classified elsewhere,**
> ***left* hand**
>
> *M90.849* **Osteopathy in diseases classified elsewhere,**
> ***unspecified* hand**

✓6ᵗʰ **M90.85** Osteopathy in diseases classified elsewhere, thigh

> *M90.851* **Osteopathy in diseases classified elsewhere,**
> ***right* thigh**
>
> *M90.852* **Osteopathy in diseases classified elsewhere,**
> ***left* thigh**
>
> *M90.859* **Osteopathy in diseases classified elsewhere,**
> ***unspecified* thigh**

✓6ᵗʰ **M90.86** Osteopathy in diseases classified elsewhere, lower
leg

> *M90.861* **Osteopathy in diseases classified elsewhere,**
> ***right* lower leg**
>
> *M90.862* **Osteopathy in diseases classified elsewhere,**
> ***left* lower leg**
>
> *M90.869* **Osteopathy in diseases classified elsewhere,**
> ***unspecified* lower leg**

✓6ᵗʰ **M90.87** Osteopathy in diseases classified elsewhere, ankle
and foot

> *M90.871* **Osteopathy in diseases classified elsewhere,**
> ***right* ankle and foot**
>
> *M90.872* **Osteopathy in diseases classified elsewhere,**
> ***left* ankle and foot**
>
> *M90.879* **Osteopathy in diseases classified elsewhere,**
> ***unspecified* ankle and foot**

Ⓝ Newborn: 0 Ⓟ Pediatric: 0-17 Ⓜ Maternity: 12-55 Ⓐ Adult: 15-124 `MCC` Major CC Condition `PDxMCC` PDx acts as own MCC `CC` CC Condition `PDxCC` PDx acts as own CC

814   ICD-10-CM 2018

M90.88   *Osteopathy in diseases classified elsewhere, other site*
M90.89   *Osteopathy in diseases classified elsewhere, multiple sites*

Chondropathies (M91-M94)

EXCLUDES 1   *postprocedural chondropathies (M96.-)*

☑4ᵗʰ **M91 Juvenile osteochondrosis of** hip and pelvis

EXCLUDES 1   *slipped upper femoral epiphysis (nontraumatic) (M93.0)*

M91.0 Juvenile osteochondrosis of pelvis
Osteochondrosis (juvenile) of acetabulum
Osteochondrosis (juvenile) of iliac crest [Buchanan]
Osteochondrosis (juvenile) of ischiopubic synchondrosis [van Neck]
Osteochondrosis (juvenile) of symphysis pubis [Pierson]

☑5ᵗʰ **M91.1 Juvenile osteochondrosis of** head of femur [Legg-Calvé-Perthes]
M91.10   **Juvenile osteochondrosis of head of femur [Legg-Calvé-Perthes],** unspecified **leg**
M91.11   **Juvenile osteochondrosis of head of femur [Legg-Calvé-Perthes],** right **leg**
M91.12   **Juvenile osteochondrosis of head of femur [Legg-Calvé-Perthes],** left **leg**

☑5ᵗʰ **M91.2** Coxa plana
Hip deformity due to previous juvenile osteochondrosis
M91.20   Coxa plana, unspecified **hip**
M91.21   Coxa plana, right **hip**
M91.22   Coxa plana, left **hip**

☑5ᵗʰ **M91.3** Pseudocoxalgia
M91.30   Pseudocoxalgia, unspecified **hip**
M91.31   Pseudocoxalgia, right **hip**
M91.32   Pseudocoxalgia, left **hip**

☑5ᵗʰ **M91.4** Coxa magna
M91.40   Coxa magna, unspecified **hip**
M91.41   Coxa magna, right **hip**
M91.42   Coxa magna, left **hip**

☑5ᵗʰ **M91.8** Other **juvenile osteochondrosis of hip and pelvis**
Juvenile osteochondrosis after reduction of congenital dislocation of hip
M91.80   **Other juvenile osteochondrosis of hip and pelvis,** unspecified **leg**
M91.81   **Other juvenile osteochondrosis of hip and pelvis,** right **leg**
M91.82   **Other juvenile osteochondrosis of hip and pelvis,** left **leg**

☑5ᵗʰ **M91.9 Juvenile osteochondrosis of hip and pelvis,** unspecified
M91.90   **Juvenile osteochondrosis of hip and pelvis, unspecified,** unspecified **leg**
M91.91   **Juvenile osteochondrosis of hip and pelvis, unspecified,** right **leg**
M91.92   **Juvenile osteochondrosis of hip and pelvis, unspecified,** left **leg**

☑4ᵗʰ **M92 Other juvenile osteochondrosis**

☑5ᵗʰ **M92.0 Juvenile osteochondrosis of** humerus
Osteochondrosis (juvenile) of capitulum of humerus [Panner]
Osteochondrosis (juvenile) of head of humerus [Haas]
M92.00   **Juvenile osteochondrosis of humerus,** unspecified **arm**
M92.01   **Juvenile osteochondrosis of humerus,** right **arm**
M92.02   **Juvenile osteochondrosis of humerus,** left **arm**

☑5ᵗʰ **M92.1 Juvenile osteochondrosis of** radius and ulna
Osteochondrosis (juvenile) of lower ulna [Burns]
Osteochondrosis (juvenile) of radial head [Brailsford]
M92.10   **Juvenile osteochondrosis of radius and ulna,** unspecified **arm**
M92.11   **Juvenile osteochondrosis of radius and ulna,** right **arm**
M92.12   **Juvenile osteochondrosis of radius and ulna,** left **arm**

☑5ᵗʰ **M92.2 Juvenile osteochondrosis,** hand
☑6ᵗʰ **M92.20**   Unspecified **juvenile osteochondrosis,** hand
M92.201   **Unspecified juvenile osteochondrosis,** right **hand**
M92.202   **Unspecified juvenile osteochondrosis,** left **hand**

M92.209   **Unspecified juvenile osteochondrosis,** unspecified **hand**

☑6ᵗʰ **M92.21**   **Osteochondrosis (juvenile) of** carpal lunate [Kienböck]
M92.211   **Osteochondrosis (juvenile) of carpal lunate [Kienböck],** right **hand**
M92.212   **Osteochondrosis (juvenile) of carpal lunate [Kienböck],** left **hand**
M92.219   **Osteochondrosis (juvenile) of carpal lunate [Kienböck],** unspecified **hand**

☑6ᵗʰ **M92.22**   **Osteochondrosis (juvenile) of** metacarpal heads [Mauclaire]
M92.221   **Osteochondrosis (juvenile) of metacarpal heads [Mauclaire],** right **hand**
M92.222   **Osteochondrosis (juvenile) of metacarpal heads [Mauclaire],** left **hand**
M92.229   **Osteochondrosis (juvenile) of metacarpal heads [Mauclaire],** unspecified **hand**

☑6ᵗʰ **M92.29**   Other **juvenile osteochondrosis,** hand
M92.291   **Other juvenile osteochondrosis,** right **hand**
M92.292   **Other juvenile osteochondrosis,** left **hand**
M92.299   **Other juvenile osteochondrosis,** unspecified **hand**

☑5ᵗʰ **M92.3 Other juvenile osteochondrosis,** upper limb
M92.30   **Other juvenile osteochondrosis,** unspecified **upper limb**
M92.31   **Other juvenile osteochondrosis,** right **upper limb**
M92.32   **Other juvenile osteochondrosis,** left **upper limb**

☑5ᵗʰ **M92.4 Juvenile osteochondrosis of** patella
Osteochondrosis (juvenile) of primary patellar center [Köhler]
Osteochondrosis (juvenile) of secondary patellar centre [Sinding Larsen]
M92.40   **Juvenile osteochondrosis of patella,** unspecified **knee**
M92.41   **Juvenile osteochondrosis of patella,** right **knee**
M92.42   **Juvenile osteochondrosis of patella,** left **knee**

☑5ᵗʰ **M92.5 Juvenile osteochondrosis of** tibia and fibula
Osteochondrosis (juvenile) of proximal tibia [Blount]
Osteochondrosis (juvenile) of tibial tubercle [Osgood-Schlatter]
Tibia vara
M92.50   **Juvenile osteochondrosis of tibia and fibula,** unspecified **leg**
M92.51   **Juvenile osteochondrosis of tibia and fibula,** right **leg**
M92.52   **Juvenile osteochondrosis of tibia and fibula,** left **leg**

☑5ᵗʰ **M92.6 Juvenile osteochondrosis of** tarsus
Osteochondrosis (juvenile) of calcaneum [Sever]
Osteochondrosis (juvenile) of os tibiale externum [Haglund]
Osteochondrosis (juvenile) of talus [Diaz]
Osteochondrosis (juvenile) of tarsal navicular [Köhler]
M92.60   **Juvenile osteochondrosis of tarsus,** unspecified **ankle**
M92.61   **Juvenile osteochondrosis of tarsus,** right **ankle**
M92.62   **Juvenile osteochondrosis of tarsus,** left **ankle**

☑5ᵗʰ **M92.7 Juvenile osteochondrosis of** metatarsus
Osteochondrosis (juvenile) of fifth metatarsus [Iselin]
Osteochondrosis (juvenile) of second metatarsus [Freiberg]
M92.70   **Juvenile osteochondrosis of metatarsus,** unspecified **foot**
M92.71   **Juvenile osteochondrosis of metatarsus,** right **foot**
M92.72   **Juvenile osteochondrosis of metatarsus,** left **foot**

M92.8 Other specified juvenile osteochondrosis
Calcaneal apophysitis

M92.9 Juvenile osteochondrosis, unspecified
Juvenile apophysitis NOS
Juvenile epiphysitis NOS
Juvenile osteochondritis NOS
Juvenile osteochondrosis NOS

☑ Additional Character Req   ☑x7ᵗʰ Placeholder Alert   Unacceptable PDx   Manifestation   **H1**-**H14** HAC   **HCC** CMS-HCC Condition   EXCLUDES 1 Not Coded Here   EXCLUDES 2 Not Included Here

ICD-10-CM 2018   815

✓4th **M93 Other osteochondropathies**
     EXCLUDES 2   *osteochondrosis of spine (M42.-)*

✓5th **M93.0 Slipped upper femoral epiphysis (nontraumatic)**
     Use additional code for associated chondrolysis (M94.3)

✓6th **M93.00 Unspecified slipped upper femoral epiphysis (nontraumatic)**
- **M93.001** Unspecified slipped upper femoral epiphysis (nontraumatic), right hip
- **M93.002** Unspecified slipped upper femoral epiphysis (nontraumatic), left hip
- **M93.003** Unspecified slipped upper femoral epiphysis (nontraumatic), unspecified hip

✓6th **M93.01 Acute slipped upper femoral epiphysis (nontraumatic)**
- **M93.011** Acute slipped upper femoral epiphysis (nontraumatic), right hip
- **M93.012** Acute slipped upper femoral epiphysis (nontraumatic), left hip
- **M93.013** Acute slipped upper femoral epiphysis (nontraumatic), unspecified hip

✓6th **M93.02 Chronic slipped upper femoral epiphysis (nontraumatic)**
- **M93.021** Chronic slipped upper femoral epiphysis (nontraumatic), right hip
- **M93.022** Chronic slipped upper femoral epiphysis (nontraumatic), left hip
- **M93.023** Chronic slipped upper femoral epiphysis (nontraumatic), unspecified hip

✓6th **M93.03 Acute on chronic slipped upper femoral epiphysis (nontraumatic)**
- **M93.031** Acute on chronic slipped upper femoral epiphysis (nontraumatic), right hip
- **M93.032** Acute on chronic slipped upper femoral epiphysis (nontraumatic), left hip
- **M93.033** Acute on chronic slipped upper femoral epiphysis (nontraumatic), unspecified hip

M93.1 Kienböck's disease of adults   A
     Adult osteochondrosis of carpal lunates

✓5th **M93.2 Osteochondritis dissecans**
- **M93.20** Osteochondritis dissecans of unspecified site

✓6th **M93.21 Osteochondritis dissecans of shoulder**
- **M93.211** Osteochondritis dissecans, right shoulder
- **M93.212** Osteochondritis dissecans, left shoulder
- **M93.219** Osteochondritis dissecans, unspecified shoulder

✓6th **M93.22 Osteochondritis dissecans of elbow**
- **M93.221** Osteochondritis dissecans, right elbow
- **M93.222** Osteochondritis dissecans, left elbow
- **M93.229** Osteochondritis dissecans, unspecified elbow

✓6th **M93.23 Osteochondritis dissecans of wrist**
- **M93.231** Osteochondritis dissecans, right wrist
- **M93.232** Osteochondritis dissecans, left wrist
- **M93.239** Osteochondritis dissecans, unspecified wrist

✓6th **M93.24 Osteochondritis dissecans of joints of hand**
- **M93.241** Osteochondritis dissecans, joints of right hand
- **M93.242** Osteochondritis dissecans, joints of left hand
- **M93.249** Osteochondritis dissecans, joints of unspecified hand

✓6th **M93.25 Osteochondritis dissecans of hip**
- **M93.251** Osteochondritis dissecans, right hip
- **M93.252** Osteochondritis dissecans, left hip
- **M93.259** Osteochondritis dissecans, unspecified hip

✓6th **M93.26 Osteochondritis dissecans knee**
- **M93.261** Osteochondritis dissecans, right knee
- **M93.262** Osteochondritis dissecans, left knee
- **M93.269** Osteochondritis dissecans, unspecified knee

✓6th **M93.27 Osteochondritis dissecans of ankle and joints of foot**
- **M93.271** Osteochondritis dissecans, right ankle and joints of right foot
- **M93.272** Osteochondritis dissecans, left ankle and joints of left foot
- **M93.279** Osteochondritis dissecans, unspecified ankle and joints of foot

- **M93.28** Osteochondritis dissecans other site
- **M93.29** Osteochondritis dissecans multiple sites

✓5th **M93.8 Other specified osteochondropathies**
- **M93.80** Other specified osteochondropathies of unspecified site

✓6th **M93.81 Other specified osteochondropathies of shoulder**
- **M93.811** Other specified osteochondropathies, right shoulder
- **M93.812** Other specified osteochondropathies, left shoulder
- **M93.819** Other specified osteochondropathies, unspecified shoulder

✓6th **M93.82 Other specified osteochondropathies of upper arm**
- **M93.821** Other specified osteochondropathies, right upper arm
- **M93.822** Other specified osteochondropathies, left upper arm
- **M93.829** Other specified osteochondropathies, unspecified upper arm

✓6th **M93.83 Other specified osteochondropathies of forearm**
- **M93.831** Other specified osteochondropathies, right forearm
- **M93.832** Other specified osteochondropathies, left forearm
- **M93.839** Other specified osteochondropathies, unspecified forearm

✓6th **M93.84 Other specified osteochondropathies of hand**
- **M93.841** Other specified osteochondropathies, right hand
- **M93.842** Other specified osteochondropathies, left hand
- **M93.849** Other specified osteochondropathies, unspecified hand

✓6th **M93.85 Other specified osteochondropathies of thigh**
- **M93.851** Other specified osteochondropathies, right thigh
- **M93.852** Other specified osteochondropathies, left thigh
- **M93.859** Other specified osteochondropathies, unspecified thigh

✓6th **M93.86 Other specified osteochondropathies lower leg**
- **M93.861** Other specified osteochondropathies, right lower leg
- **M93.862** Other specified osteochondropathies, left lower leg
- **M93.869** Other specified osteochondropathies, unspecified lower leg

✓6th **M93.87 Other specified osteochondropathies of ankle and foot**
- **M93.871** Other specified osteochondropathies, right ankle and foot
- **M93.872** Other specified osteochondropathies, left ankle and foot
- **M93.879** Other specified osteochondropathies, unspecified ankle and foot

- **M93.88** Other specified osteochondropathies other site
- **M93.89** Other specified osteochondropathies multiple sites

✓5th **M93.9 Osteochondropathy, unspecified**
     Apophysitis NOS   Osteochondritis NOS
     Epiphysitis NOS   Osteochondrosis NOS

- **M93.90** Osteochondropathy, unspecified of unspecified site

✓6th **M93.91 Osteochondropathy, unspecified of shoulder**
- **M93.911** Osteochondropathy, unspecified, right shoulder
- **M93.912** Osteochondropathy, unspecified, left shoulder
- **M93.919** Osteochondropathy, unspecified, unspecified shoulder

✓6th **M93.92 Osteochondropathy, unspecified of upper arm**
- **M93.921** Osteochondropathy, unspecified, right upper arm

N Newborn: 0   P Pediatric: 0-17   M Maternity: 12-55   A Adult: 15-124   MCC Major CC Condition   PDxMCC PDx acts as own MCC   CC CC Condition   PDxCC PDx acts as own CC

816   ICD-10-CM 2018

        M93.922 Osteochondropathy, unspecified, left upper arm

        M93.929 Osteochondropathy, unspecified, unspecified upper arm

✓6ᵗʰ M93.93 Osteochondropathy, unspecified of forearm

        M93.931 Osteochondropathy, unspecified, right forearm

        M93.932 Osteochondropathy, unspecified, left forearm

        M93.939 Osteochondropathy, unspecified, unspecified forearm

✓6ᵗʰ M93.94 Osteochondropathy, unspecified of hand

        M93.941 Osteochondropathy, unspecified, right hand

        M93.942 Osteochondropathy, unspecified, left hand

        M93.949 Osteochondropathy, unspecified, unspecified hand

✓6ᵗʰ M93.95 Osteochondropathy, unspecified of thigh

        M93.951 Osteochondropathy, unspecified, right thigh

        M93.952 Osteochondropathy, unspecified, left thigh

        M93.959 Osteochondropathy, unspecified, unspecified thigh

✓6ᵗʰ M93.96 Osteochondropathy, unspecified lower leg

        M93.961 Osteochondropathy, unspecified, right lower leg

        M93.962 Osteochondropathy, unspecified, left lower leg

        M93.969 Osteochondropathy, unspecified, unspecified lower leg

✓6ᵗʰ M93.97 Osteochondropathy, unspecified of ankle and foot

        M93.971 Osteochondropathy, unspecified, right ankle and foot

        M93.972 Osteochondropathy, unspecified, left ankle and foot

        M93.979 Osteochondropathy, unspecified, unspecified ankle and foot

    M93.98 Osteochondropathy, unspecified other site

    M93.99 Osteochondropathy, unspecified multiple sites

✓4ᵗʰ **M94** **Other disorders of cartilage**

    M94.0 **Chondrocostal junction syndrome [Tietze]**
        Costochondritis

    M94.1 **Relapsing polychondritis**

✓5ᵗʰ **M94.2** **Chondromalacia**
        EXCLUDES 1 chondromalacia patellae (M22.4)

    M94.20 **Chondromalacia, unspecified site**

✓6ᵗʰ **M94.21** **Chondromalacia, shoulder**

        M94.211 Chondromalacia, right shoulder

        M94.212 Chondromalacia, left shoulder

        M94.219 Chondromalacia, unspecified shoulder

✓6ᵗʰ **M94.22** **Chondromalacia, elbow**

        M94.221 Chondromalacia, right elbow

        M94.222 Chondromalacia, left elbow

        M94.229 Chondromalacia, unspecified elbow

✓6ᵗʰ **M94.23** **Chondromalacia, wrist**

        M94.231 Chondromalacia, right wrist

        M94.232 Chondromalacia, left wrist

        M94.239 Chondromalacia, unspecified wrist

✓6ᵗʰ **M94.24** **Chondromalacia, joints of hand**

        M94.241 Chondromalacia, joints of right hand

        M94.242 Chondromalacia, joints of left hand

        M94.249 Chondromalacia, joints of unspecified hand

✓6ᵗʰ **M94.25** **Chondromalacia, hip**

        M94.251 Chondromalacia, right hip

        M94.252 Chondromalacia, left hip

        M94.259 Chondromalacia, unspecified hip

✓6ᵗʰ **M94.26** **Chondromalacia, knee**

        M94.261 Chondromalacia, right knee

        M94.262 Chondromalacia, left knee

        M94.269 Chondromalacia, unspecified knee

✓6ᵗʰ **M94.27** **Chondromalacia, ankle and joints of foot**

        M94.271 Chondromalacia, right ankle and joints of right foot

        M94.272 Chondromalacia, left ankle and joints of left foot

        M94.279 Chondromalacia, unspecified ankle and joints of foot

    M94.28 **Chondromalacia, other site**

    M94.29 **Chondromalacia, multiple sites**

✓5ᵗʰ **M94.3** **Chondrolysis**
        Code first any associated slipped upper femoral epiphysis (nontraumatic) (M93.0-)

✓6ᵗʰ **M94.35** **Chondrolysis, hip**

        M94.351 Chondrolysis, right hip

        M94.352 Chondrolysis, left hip

        M94.359 Chondrolysis, unspecified hip

✓5ᵗʰ **M94.8** **Other specified disorders of cartilage**

✓6ᵗʰ **M94.8X** **Other specified disorders of cartilage**

        M94.8X0 Other specified disorders of cartilage, multiple sites

        M94.8X1 Other specified disorders of cartilage, shoulder

        M94.8X2 Other specified disorders of cartilage, upper arm

        M94.8X3 Other specified disorders of cartilage, forearm

        M94.8X4 Other specified disorders of cartilage, hand

        M94.8X5 Other specified disorders of cartilage, thigh

        M94.8X6 Other specified disorders of cartilage, lower leg

        M94.8X7 Other specified disorders of cartilage, ankle and foot

        M94.8X8 Other specified disorders of cartilage, other site

        M94.8X9 Other specified disorders of cartilage, unspecified sites

    M94.9 **Disorder of cartilage, unspecified**

Other disorders of the musculoskeletal system and connective tissue (M95)

✓4ᵗʰ **M95** **Other acquired deformities of musculoskeletal system and connective tissue**
        EXCLUDES 2 acquired absence of limbs and organs (Z89-Z90)
                    acquired deformities of limbs (M20-M21)
                    congenital malformations and deformations of the musculoskeletal system (Q65-Q79)
                    deforming dorsopathies (M40-M43)
                    dentofacial anomalies [including malocclusion] (M26.-)
                    postprocedural musculoskeletal disorders (M96.-)

    M95.0 **Acquired deformity of nose**
        EXCLUDES 2 deviated nasal septum (J34.2)

✓5ᵗʰ **M95.1** **Cauliflower ear**
        EXCLUDES 2 other acquired deformities of ear (H61.1)
        DEF: Acquired deformity of the external ear; due to injury, subsequent perichondritis.

    M95.10 **Cauliflower ear, unspecified ear**

    M95.11 **Cauliflower ear, right ear**

    M95.12 **Cauliflower ear, left ear**

    M95.2 **Other acquired deformity of head**

    M95.3 **Acquired deformity of neck**

    M95.4 **Acquired deformity of chest and rib**
        AHA: 2014, 4Q, 26-27

    M95.5 **Acquired deformity of pelvis**
        EXCLUDES 1 maternal care for known or suspected disproportion (O33.-)

    M95.8 **Other specified acquired deformities of musculoskeletal system**

    M95.9 **Acquired deformity of musculoskeletal system, unspecified**

✔ Additional Character Req   ✓x7ᵗʰ Placeholder Alert   Unacceptable PDx   Manifestation   H1-H14 HAC   HCC CMS-HCC Condition   *EXCLUDES 1* Not Coded Here   *EXCLUDES 2* Not Included Here

ICD-10-CM 2018   817

Intraoperative and postprocedural complications and disorders of musculoskeletal system, not elsewhere classified (M96)

√4th **M96** Intraoperative and postprocedural complications and disorders of musculoskeletal system, not elsewhere classified

> EXCLUDES 2 *arthropathy following intestinal bypass (M02.0-)*
> *complications of internal orthopedic prosthetic devices, implants and grafts (T84.-)*
> *disorders associated with osteoporosis (M80)*
> *periprosthetic fracture around internal prosthetic joint (M97.-)*
> *presence of functional implants and other devices (Z96-Z97)*

M96.0 Pseudarthrosis after fusion or arthrodesis　　CC
　　　　CC Excl: No Excl

M96.1 Postlaminectomy syndrome, not elsewhere classified

M96.2 Postradiation kyphosis

M96.3 Postlaminectomy kyphosis

M96.4 Postsurgical lordosis

M96.5 Postradiation scoliosis

√5th **M96.6** Fracture of bone following insertion of orthopedic implant, joint prosthesis, or bone plate
　　　　Intraoperative fracture of bone during insertion of orthopedic implant, joint prosthesis, or bone plate

> EXCLUDES 2 *complication of internal orthopedic devices, implants or grafts (T84.-)*

> **CC Excl: For CC codes in subcategory M96.6:** PDX collection 911

√6th **M96.62** Fracture of humerus following insertion of orthopedic implant, joint prosthesis, or bone plate

M96.621 Fracture of humerus following insertion of orthopedic implant, joint prosthesis, or bone plate, right arm　　CC HCC

M96.622 Fracture of humerus following insertion of orthopedic implant, joint prosthesis, or bone plate, left arm　　CC HCC

M96.629 Fracture of humerus following insertion of orthopedic implant, joint prosthesis, or bone plate, unspecified arm

√6th **M96.63** Fracture of radius or ulna following insertion of orthopedic implant, joint prosthesis, or bone plate

M96.631 Fracture of radius or ulna following nsertion of orthopedic implant, joint prosthesis, or bone plate, right arm　　CC HCC

M96.632 Fracture of radius or ulna following insertion of orthopedic implant, joint prosthesis, or bone plate, left arm　　CC HCC

M96.639 Fracture of radius or ulna following insertion of orthopedic implant, joint prosthesis, or bone plate, unspecified arm　　CC HCC

M96.65 Fracture of pelvis following insertion of orthopedic implant, joint prosthesis, or bone plate　　CC HCC

√6th **M96.66** Fracture of femur following insertion of orthopedic implant, joint prosthesis, or bone plate

M96.661 Fracture of femur following insertion of orthopedic implant, joint prosthesis, or bone plate, right leg　　CC HCC

M96.662 Fracture of femur following insertion of orthopedic implant, joint prosthesis, or bone plate, left leg　　CC HCC

M96.669 Fracture of femur following insertion of orthopedic implant, joint prosthesis, or bone plate, unspecified leg　　CC HCC

√6th **M96.67** Fracture of tibia or fibula following insertion of orthopedic implant, joint prosthesis, or bone plate

M96.671 Fracture of tibia or fibula following insertion of orthopedic implant, joint prosthesis, or bone plate, right leg　　CC HCC

M96.672 Fracture of tibia or fibula following insertion of orthopedic implant, joint prosthesis, or bone plate, left leg　　CC HCC

M96.679 Fracture of tibia or fibula following insertion of orthopedic implant, joint prosthesis, or bone plate, unspecified leg　　CC HCC

M96.69 Fracture of other bone following insertion of orthopedic implant, joint prosthesis, or bone plate　　CC HCC

√5th **M96.8** Other intraoperative and postprocedural complications and disorders of musculoskeletal system, not elsewhere classified

> **CC Excl: For CC codes in subcategory M96.8, unless otherwise noted:** PDX collection 912

√6th **M96.81** Intraoperative hemorrhage and hematoma of a musculoskeletal structure complicating a procedure

> EXCLUDES 1 *intraoperative hemorrhage and hematoma of a musculoskeletal structure due to accidental puncture and laceration during a procedure (M96.82-)*

M96.810 Intraoperative hemorrhage and hematoma of a musculoskeletal structure complicating a musculoskeletal system procedure　　CC

M96.811 Intraoperative hemorrhage and hematoma of a musculoskeletal structure complicating other procedure　　CC

√6th **M96.82** Accidental puncture and laceration of a musculoskeletal structure during a procedure

M96.820 Accidental puncture and laceration of a musculoskeletal structure during a musculoskeletal system procedure　　CC
　　　　CC Excl: PDX collection 509

M96.821 Accidental puncture and laceration of a musculoskeletal structure during other procedure　　CC
　　　　CC Excl: PDX collection 509

√6th **M96.83** Postprocedural hemorrhage of a musculoskeletal structure following a procedure

M96.830 Postprocedural hemorrhage of a musculoskeletal structure following a musculoskeletal system procedure　　CC

M96.831 Postprocedural hemorrhage of a musculoskeletal structure following other procedure　　CC

√6th **M96.84** Postprocedural hematoma and seroma of a musculoskeletal structure following a procedure

M96.840 Postprocedural hematoma of a musculoskeletal structure following a musculoskeletal system procedure　　CC

M96.841 Postprocedural hematoma of a musculoskeletal structure following other procedure　　CC

M96.842 Postprocedural seroma of a musculoskeletal structure following a musculoskeletal system procedure　　CC

M96.843 Postprocedural seroma of a musculoskeletal structure following other procedure　　CC

M96.89 Other intraoperative and postprocedural complications and disorders of the musculoskeletal system　　CC
　　　　Instability of joint secondary to removal of joint prosthesis
　　　　Use additional code, if applicable, to further specify disorder
　　　　CC Excl: PDX collection 643

Periprosthetic fracture around internal prosthetic joint (M97)

√4th **M97** Periprosthetic fracture around internal prosthetic joint

> EXCLUDES 2 *breakage (fracture) of prosthetic joint (T84.01-)*
> *fracture of bone following insertion of orthopedic implant, joint prosthesis or bone plate (M96.6-)*

> The appropriate 7th character is to be added to each code from category M97.
> A　initial encounter
> D　subsequent encounter
> S　sequela

> **CC Excl: For CC codes in category M97:** PDX collection 911

√5th **M97.0** Periprosthetic fracture around internal prosthetic hip joint

7, 10 √x7th **M97.01** Periprosthetic fracture around internal prosthetic right hip joint　　CC HCC

7, 10 √x7th **M97.02** Periprosthetic fracture around internal prosthetic left hip joint　　CC HCC

7　CC when reported as an initial encounter (7th character A, B, or C – specific to category) OR a subsequent encounter for nonunion or malunion (7th character K, M, N, P, Q, or R – specific to category).

10　HCC with 7th character indicating initial encounter (A, B or C - specific to category).

√5ᵗʰ **M97.1 Periprosthetic fracture around internal prosthetic** knee **joint**

    √x7ᵗʰ **M97.11 Periprosthetic fracture around internal prosthetic** right **knee joint** `CC`

    √x7ᵗʰ **M97.12 Periprosthetic fracture around internal prosthetic** left **knee joint** `CC`

√5ᵗʰ **M97.2 Periprosthetic fracture around internal prosthetic** ankle **joint**

    √x7ᵗʰ **M97.21 Periprosthetic fracture around internal prosthetic** right **ankle joint** `CC`

    √x7ᵗʰ **M97.22 Periprosthetic fracture around internal prosthetic** left **ankle joint** `CC`

√5ᵗʰ **M97.3 Periprosthetic fracture around internal prosthetic** shoulder **joint**

    √x7ᵗʰ **M97.31 Periprosthetic fracture around internal prosthetic** right **shoulder joint** `CC`

    √x7ᵗʰ **M97.32 Periprosthetic fracture around internal prosthetic** left **shoulder joint** `CC`

√5ᵗʰ **M97.4 Periprosthetic fracture around internal prosthetic** elbow **joint**

    √x7ᵗʰ **M97.41 Periprosthetic fracture around internal prosthetic** right **elbow joint** `CC`

    √x7ᵗʰ **M97.42 Periprosthetic fracture around internal prosthetic** left **elbow joint** `CC`

√x7ᵗʰ **M97.8 Periprosthetic fracture around** other **internal prosthetic joint** `CC`

    Periprosthetic fracture around internal prosthetic finger joint
    Periprosthetic fracture around internal prosthetic spinal joint
    Periprosthetic fracture around internal prosthetic toe joint
    Periprosthetic fracture around internal prosthetic wrist joint
    Use additional code to identify the joint (Z96.6-)

√x7ᵗʰ **M97.9 Periprosthetic fracture around** unspecified **internal prosthetic joint** `CC`

Biomechanical lesions, not elsewhere classified (M99)

√4ᵗʰ **M99 Biomechanical lesions, not elsewhere classified**

    NOTE   This category should not be used if the condition can be classified elsewhere.

√5ᵗʰ **M99.0 Segmental and somatic dysfunction**

    M99.00 Segmental and somatic dysfunction of head **region**

    M99.01 Segmental and somatic dysfunction of cervical **region**

    M99.02 Segmental and somatic dysfunction of thoracic **region**

    M99.03 Segmental and somatic dysfunction of lumbar **region**

    M99.04 Segmental and somatic dysfunction of sacral **region**

    M99.05 Segmental and somatic dysfunction of pelvic **region**

    M99.06 Segmental and somatic dysfunction of lower **extremity**

    M99.07 Segmental and somatic dysfunction of upper **extremity**

    M99.08 Segmental and somatic dysfunction of rib cage

    M99.09 Segmental and somatic dysfunction of abdomen and other **regions**

√5ᵗʰ **M99.1 Subluxation complex (vertebral)**

    CC Excl: For CC codes in subcategory M99.1, unless otherwise noted: PDX collection 913

    M99.10 Subluxation complex (vertebral) of head **region** `CC` `H5`

    M99.11 Subluxation complex (vertebral) of cervical **region** `CC` `H5`

    M99.12 Subluxation complex (vertebral) of thoracic **region**

    M99.13 Subluxation complex (vertebral) of lumbar **region**

    M99.14 Subluxation complex (vertebral) of sacral **region**

    M99.15 Subluxation complex (vertebral) of pelvic **region**

    M99.16 Subluxation complex (vertebral) of lower extremity

    M99.17 Subluxation complex (vertebral) of upper extremity

    M99.18 Subluxation complex (vertebral) of rib cage `CC` `H5`
        CC Excl: PDX collection 914

    M99.19 Subluxation complex (vertebral) of abdomen and other **regions**

√5ᵗʰ **M99.2 Subluxation stenosis of neural canal**

    M99.20 Subluxation stenosis of neural canal of head **region**

    M99.21 Subluxation stenosis of neural canal of cervical **region**

    M99.22 Subluxation stenosis of neural canal of thoracic **region**

    M99.23 Subluxation stenosis of neural canal of lumbar **region**

    M99.24 Subluxation stenosis of neural canal of sacral **region**

    M99.25 Subluxation stenosis of neural canal of pelvic **region**

    M99.26 Subluxation stenosis of neural canal of lower **extremity**

    M99.27 Subluxation stenosis of neural canal of upper **extremity**

    M99.28 Subluxation stenosis of neural canal of rib cage

    M99.29 Subluxation stenosis of neural canal of abdomen and other **regions**

√5ᵗʰ **M99.3 Osseous stenosis of neural canal**

    M99.30 Osseous stenosis of neural canal of head **region**

    M99.31 Osseous stenosis of neural canal of cervical **region**

    M99.32 Osseous stenosis of neural canal of thoracic **region**

    M99.33 Osseous stenosis of neural canal of lumbar **region**

    M99.34 Osseous stenosis of neural canal of sacral **region**

    M99.35 Osseous stenosis of neural canal of pelvic **region**

    M99.36 Osseous stenosis of neural canal of lower extremity

    M99.37 Osseous stenosis of neural canal of upper extremity

    M99.38 Osseous stenosis of neural canal of rib cage

    M99.39 Osseous stenosis of neural canal of abdomen and other **regions**

√5ᵗʰ **M99.4 Connective tissue stenosis of neural canal**

    M99.40 Connective tissue stenosis of neural canal of head **region**

    M99.41 Connective tissue stenosis of neural canal of cervical **region**

    M99.42 Connective tissue stenosis of neural canal of thoracic **region**

    M99.43 Connective tissue stenosis of neural canal of lumbar **region**

    M99.44 Connective tissue stenosis of neural canal of sacral **region**

    M99.45 Connective tissue stenosis of neural canal of pelvic **region**

    M99.46 Connective tissue stenosis of neural canal of lower **extremity**

    M99.47 Connective tissue stenosis of neural canal of upper **extremity**

    M99.48 Connective tissue stenosis of neural canal of rib cage

    M99.49 Connective tissue stenosis of neural canal of abdomen and other **regions**

√5ᵗʰ **M99.5 Intervertebral disc stenosis of neural canal**

    M99.50 Intervertebral disc stenosis of neural canal of head **region**

    M99.51 Intervertebral disc stenosis of neural canal of cervical **region**

    M99.52 Intervertebral disc stenosis of neural canal of thoracic **region**

    M99.53 Intervertebral disc stenosis of neural canal of lumbar **region**

    M99.54 Intervertebral disc stenosis of neural canal of sacral **region**

    M99.55 Intervertebral disc stenosis of neural canal of pelvic **region**

    M99.56 Intervertebral disc stenosis of neural canal of lower **extremity**

    M99.57 Intervertebral disc stenosis of neural canal of upper **extremity**

    M99.58 Intervertebral disc stenosis of neural canal of rib cage

    M99.59 Intervertebral disc stenosis of neural canal of abdomen and other **regions**

√5ᵗʰ **M99.6 Osseous and subluxation stenosis of intervertebral foramina**

    M99.60 Osseous and subluxation stenosis of intervertebral foramina of head **region**

    M99.61 Osseous and subluxation stenosis of intervertebral foramina of cervical **region**

    M99.62 Osseous and subluxation stenosis of intervertebral foramina of thoracic **region**

    M99.63 Osseous and subluxation stenosis of intervertebral foramina of lumbar **region**

✓ Additional Character Req   √x7ᵗʰ Placeholder Alert   Unacceptable PDx   Manifestation   H1-H14 HAC   HCC CMS-HCC Condition   *EXCLUDES 1* Not Coded Here   *EXCLUDES 2* Not Included Here

ICD-10-CM 2018   819

M99.64   **Osseous and subluxation stenosis of intervertebral foramina of sacral region**

M99.65   **Osseous and subluxation stenosis of intervertebral foramina of pelvic region**

M99.66   **Osseous and subluxation stenosis of intervertebral foramina of lower extremity**

M99.67   **Osseous and subluxation stenosis of intervertebral foramina of upper extremity**

M99.68   **Osseous and subluxation stenosis of intervertebral foramina of rib cage**

M99.69   **Osseous and subluxation stenosis of intervertebral foramina of abdomen and other regions**

✓5ᵗʰ   **M99.7   Connective tissue and disc stenosis of intervertebral foramina**

M99.70   **Connective tissue and disc stenosis of intervertebral foramina of head region**

M99.71   **Connective tissue and disc stenosis of intervertebral foramina of cervical region**

M99.72   **Connective tissue and disc stenosis of intervertebral foramina of thoracic region**

M99.73   **Connective tissue and disc stenosis of intervertebral foramina of lumbar region**

M99.74   **Connective tissue and disc stenosis of intervertebral foramina of sacral region**

M99.75   **Connective tissue and disc stenosis of intervertebral foramina of pelvic region**

M99.76   **Connective tissue and disc stenosis of intervertebral foramina of lower extremity**

M99.77   **Connective tissue and disc stenosis of intervertebral foramina of upper extremity**

M99.78   **Connective tissue and disc stenosis of intervertebral foramina of rib cage**

M99.79   **Connective tissue and disc stenosis of intervertebral foramina of abdomen and other regions**

✓5ᵗʰ   **M99.8   Other biomechanical lesions**

M99.80   **Other biomechanical lesions of head region**

M99.81   **Other biomechanical lesions of cervical region**

M99.82   **Other biomechanical lesions of thoracic region**

M99.83   **Other biomechanical lesions of lumbar region**

M99.84   **Other biomechanical lesions of sacral region**

M99.85   **Other biomechanical lesions of pelvic region**

M99.86   **Other biomechanical lesions of lower extremity**

M99.87   **Other biomechanical lesions of upper extremity**

M99.88   **Other biomechanical lesions of rib cage**

M99.89   **Other biomechanical lesions of abdomen and other regions**

M99.9   Biomechanical lesion, unspecified

Ⓝ Newborn: 0   Ⓟ Pediatric: 0-17   Ⓜ Maternity: 12-55   Ⓐ Adult: 15-124   **MCC** Major CC Condition   **PDxMCC** PDx acts as own MCC   **CC** CC Condition   **PDxCC** PDx acts as own CC

820   ICD-10-CM 2018

Chapter 14. Diseases of Genitourinary System (NØØ–N99)

Chapter Specific Guidelines with Coding Examples

The chapter specific guidelines from the ICD-10-CM Official Guidelines for Coding and Reporting have been provided below. Along with these guidelines are coding examples, contained in the shaded boxes, that have been developed to help illustrate the coding and/or sequencing guidance found in these guidelines.

a. Chronic kidney disease

1) Stages of chronic kidney disease (CKD)

The ICD-10-CM classifies CKD based on severity. The severity of CKD is designated by stages 1-5. Stage 2, code N18.2, equates to mild CKD; stage 3, code N18.3, equates to moderate CKD; and stage 4, code N18.4, equates to severe CKD. Code N18.6, End stage renal disease (ESRD), is assigned when the provider has documented end-stage-renal disease (ESRD).

If both a stage of CKD and ESRD are documented, assign code N18.6 only.

> Stage 5 chronic kidney disease with ESRD requiring chronic dialysis
>
> **N18.6**   **End stage renal disease**
>
> **Z99.2**   **Dependence on renal dialysis**
>
> *Explanation:* The diagnostic statement indicates the patient has chronic kidney disease, documented both as stage 5 and as ESRD requiring chronic dialysis. Code N18.6 End stage renal disease (ESRD), is assigned when the provider has documented end-stage-renal disease (ESRD). If both a stage of CKD and ESRD are documented, assign code N18.6 only.

2) Chronic kidney disease and kidney transplant status

Patients who have undergone kidney transplant may still have some form of chronic kidney disease (CKD) because the kidney transplant may not fully restore kidney function. Therefore, the presence of CKD alone does not constitute a transplant complication. Assign the appropriate N18 code for the patient's stage of CKD and code Z94.0, Kidney transplant status. If a transplant complication such as failure or rejection or other transplant complication is documented, see section I.C.19.g for information on coding complications of a kidney transplant. If the documentation is unclear as to whether the patient has a complication of the transplant, query the provider.

> Patient with residual chronic kidney disease stage 1 after kidney transplant
>
> **N18.1**   **Chronic kidney disease, stage 1**
>
> **Z94.Ø**   **Kidney transplant status**
>
> *Explanation:* Patients who have undergone kidney transplant may still have some form of chronic kidney disease (CKD) because the kidney transplant may not fully restore kidney function. The presence of CKD alone does not constitute a transplant complication. Assign the appropriate N18 code for the patient's stage of CKD and code Z94.0 Kidney transplant status.

3) Chronic kidney disease with other conditions

Patients with CKD may also suffer from other serious conditions, most commonly diabetes mellitus and hypertension. The sequencing of the CKD code in relationship to codes for other contributing conditions is based on the conventions in the Tabular List.

See I.C.9. Hypertensive chronic kidney disease.

See I.C.19. Chronic kidney disease and kidney transplant complications.

> Type 1 diabetic chronic kidney disease, stage 2
>
> **E1Ø.22**   **Type 1 diabetes mellitus with diabetic chronic kidney disease**
>
> **N18.2**   **Chronic kidney disease, stage 2 (mild)**
>
> *Explanation:* Patients with CKD may also suffer from other serious conditions such as diabetes mellitus. The sequencing of the CKD code in relationship to codes for other contributing conditions is based on the conventions in the Tabular List. Diabetic CKD code E10.22 includes an instructional note to "Use additional code to identify stage of chronic kidney disease (N18.1–N18.6)," thus providing sequencing direction.

Chapter 14. Diseases of the Genitourinary System (N00-N99)

EXCLUDES 2   certain conditions originating in the perinatal period (P04-P96)
certain infectious and parasitic diseases (A00-B99)
complications of pregnancy, childbirth and the puerperium (O00-O9A)
congenital malformations, deformations and chromosomal abnormalities (Q00-Q99)
endocrine, nutritional and metabolic diseases (E00-E88)
injury, poisoning and certain other consequences of external causes (S00-T88)
neoplasms (C00-D49)
symptoms, signs and abnormal clinical and laboratory findings, not elsewhere classified (R00-R94)

This chapter contains the following blocks:

N00-N08	Glomerular diseases
N10-N16	Renal tubulo-interstitial diseases
N17-N19	Acute kidney failure and chronic kidney disease
N20-N23	Urolithiasis
N25-N29	Other disorders of kidney and ureter
N30-N39	Other diseases of the urinary system
N40-N53	Diseases of male genital organs
N60-N65	Disorders of breast
N70-N77	Inflammatory diseases of female pelvic organs
N80-N98	Noninflammatory disorders of female genital tract
N99	Intraoperative and postprocedural complications and disorders of genitourinary system, not elsewhere classified

Glomerular diseases (N00-N08)

Code also any associated kidney failure (N17-N19).

EXCLUDES 1   hypertensive chronic kidney disease (I12.-)

✓4ᵗʰ N00   Acute nephritic syndrome

INCLUDES   acute glomerular disease
acute glomerulonephritis
acute nephritis

EXCLUDES 1   acute tubulo-interstitial nephritis (N10)
nephritic syndrome NOS (N05.-)

CC Excl: For MCC codes in category N00, unless otherwise noted: PDX collection 915

N00.0 Acute nephritic syndrome with minor glomerular abnormality   MCC
Acute nephritic syndrome with minimal change lesion

N00.1 Acute nephritic syndrome with focal and segmental glomerular lesions   MCC
Acute nephritic syndrome with focal and segmental hyalinosis
Acute nephritic syndrome with focal and segmental sclerosis
Acute nephritic syndrome with focal glomerulonephritis

N00.2 Acute nephritic syndrome with diffuse membranous glomerulonephritis   MCC

N00.3 Acute nephritic syndrome with diffuse mesangial proliferative glomerulonephritis   MCC

N00.4 Acute nephritic syndrome with diffuse endocapillary proliferative glomerulonephritis   MCC

N00.5 Acute nephritic syndrome with diffuse mesangiocapillary glomerulonephritis   MCC
Acute nephritic syndrome with membranoproliferative glomerulonephritis, types 1 and 3, or NOS

N00.6 Acute nephritic syndrome with dense deposit disease   MCC
Acute nephritic syndrome with membranoproliferative glomerulonephritis, type 2

N00.7 Acute nephritic syndrome with diffuse crescentic glomerulonephritis   MCC
Acute nephritic syndrome with extracapillary glomerulonephritis

N00.8 Acute nephritic syndrome with other morphologic changes   MCC
Acute nephritic syndrome with proliferative glomerulonephritis NOS
CC Excl: PDX collection 916

N00.9 Acute nephritic syndrome with unspecified morphologic changes   MCC

✓4ᵗʰ N01   Rapidly progressive nephritic syndrome

INCLUDES   rapidly progressive glomerular disease
rapidly progressive glomerulonephritis
rapidly progressive nephritis

EXCLUDES 1   nephritic syndrome NOS (N05.-)

CC Excl: For MCC codes in category N01: PDX collection 915

N01.0 Rapidly progressive nephritic syndrome with minor glomerular abnormality   MCC
Rapidly progressive nephritic syndrome with minimal change lesion

N01.1 Rapidly progressive nephritic syndrome with focal and segmental glomerular lesions   MCC
Rapidly progressive nephritic syndrome with focal and segmental hyalinosis
Rapidly progressive nephritic syndrome with focal and segmental sclerosis
Rapidly progressive nephritic syndrome with focal glomerulonephritis

N01.2 Rapidly progressive nephritic syndrome with diffuse membranous glomerulonephritis   MCC

N01.3 Rapidly progressive nephritic syndrome with diffuse mesangial proliferative glomerulonephritis   MCC

N01.4 Rapidly progressive nephritic syndrome with diffuse endocapillary proliferative glomerulonephritis   MCC

N01.5 Rapidly progressive nephritic syndrome with diffuse mesangiocapillary glomerulonephritis   MCC
Rapidly progressive nephritic syndrome with membranoproliferative glomerulonephritis, types 1 and 3, or NOS

N01.6 Rapidly progressive nephritic syndrome with dense deposit disease   MCC
Rapidly progressive nephritic syndrome with membranoproliferative glomerulonephritis, type 2

N01.7 Rapidly progressive nephritic syndrome with diffuse crescentic glomerulonephritis   MCC
Rapidly progressive nephritic syndrome with extracapillary glomerulonephritis

N01.8 Rapidly progressive nephritic syndrome with other morphologic changes   MCC
Rapidly progressive nephritic syndrome with proliferative glomerulonephritis NOS

N01.9 Rapidly progressive nephritic syndrome with unspecified morphologic changes   MCC

✓4ᵗʰ N02   Recurrent and persistent hematuria

EXCLUDES 1   acute cystitis with hematuria (N30.01)
hematuria NOS (R31.9)
hematuria not associated with specified morphologic lesions (R31.-)

CC Excl: For CC codes in category N02, unless otherwise noted: PDX collection 917

N02.0 Recurrent and persistent hematuria with minor glomerular abnormality   CC
Recurrent and persistent hematuria with minimal change lesion

N02.1 Recurrent and persistent hematuria with focal and segmental glomerular lesions   CC
Recurrent and persistent hematuria with focal and segmental hyalinosis
Recurrent and persistent hematuria with focal and segmental sclerosis
Recurrent and persistent hematuria with focal glomerulonephritis

N02.2 Recurrent and persistent hematuria with diffuse membranous glomerulonephritis   CC

N02.3 Recurrent and persistent hematuria with diffuse mesangial proliferative glomerulonephritis   CC

N02.4 Recurrent and persistent hematuria with diffuse endocapillary proliferative glomerulonephritis   CC

N02.5 Recurrent and persistent hematuria with diffuse mesangiocapillary glomerulonephritis   CC
Recurrent and persistent hematuria with membranoproliferative glomerulonephritis, types 1 and 3, or NOS

N02.6 Recurrent and persistent hematuria with dense deposit disease   CC
Recurrent and persistent hematuria with membranoproliferative glomerulonephritis, type 2

N02.7 **Recurrent and persistent hematuria with** diffuse crescentic glomerulonephritis `CC`
     Recurrent and persistent hematuria with extracapillary glomerulonephritis

N02.8 **Recurrent and persistent hematuria with** other morphologic changes `CC`
     Recurrent and persistent hematuria with proliferative glomerulonephritis NOS
     CC Excl: PDX collection 915

N02.9 **Recurrent and persistent hematuria with** unspecified morphologic changes `CC`
     AHA: 2017, 2Q, 5
     CC Excl: PDX collection 915

✓4ᵗʰ **N03** **Chronic** nephritic syndrome
     INCLUDES   chronic glomerular disease
                 chronic glomerulonephritis
                 chronic nephritis
     EXCLUDES 1   *chronic tubulo-interstitial nephritis (N11.-)*
                  diffuse sclerosing glomerulonephritis (N05.8-)
                  nephritic syndrome NOS (N05.-)
     DEF: Slow, progressive type of nephritis characterized by inflammation of the capillary loops in the glomeruli of the kidney, which leads to renal failure.

     CC Excl: For CC codes in catagory N03: PDX collection 918

N03.0 **Chronic nephritic syndrome with** minor glomerular abnormality `CC`
     Chronic nephritic syndrome with minimal change lesion

N03.1 **Chronic nephritic syndrome with** focal and segmental glomerular lesions `CC`
     Chronic nephritic syndrome with focal and segmental hyalinosis
     Chronic nephritic syndrome with focal and segmental sclerosis
     Chronic nephritic syndrome with focal glomerulonephritis

N03.2 **Chronic nephritic syndrome with** diffuse membranous glomerulonephritis `CC`

N03.3 **Chronic nephritic syndrome with** diffuse mesangial proliferative glomerulonephritis `CC`

N03.4 **Chronic nephritic syndrome with** diffuse endocapillary proliferative glomerulonephritis `CC`

N03.5 **Chronic nephritic syndrome with** diffuse mesangiocapillary glomerulonephritis `CC`
     Chronic nephritic syndrome with membranoproliferative glomerulonephritis, types 1 and 3, or NOS

N03.6 **Chronic nephritic syndrome with** dense deposit disease `CC`
     Chronic nephritic syndrome with membranoproliferative glomerulonephritis, type 2

N03.7 **Chronic nephritic syndrome with** diffuse crescentic glomerulonephritis `CC`
     Chronic nephritic syndrome with extracapillary glomerulonephritis

N03.8 **Chronic nephritic syndrome with** other morphologic changes `CC`
     Chronic nephritic syndrome with proliferative glomerulonephritis NOS

N03.9 **Chronic nephritic syndrome with** unspecified morphologic changes `CC`

✓4ᵗʰ **N04** **Nephrotic syndrome**
     INCLUDES   congenital nephrotic syndrome
                 lipoid nephrosis

     CC Excl: For CC codes in category N04, unless otherwise noted: PDX collection 917

N04.0 **Nephrotic syndrome with** minor glomerular abnormality `CC`
     Nephrotic syndrome with minimal change lesion

N04.1 **Nephrotic syndrome with** focal and segmental glomerular lesions `CC`
     Nephrotic syndrome with focal and segmental hyalinosis
     Nephrotic syndrome with focal and segmental sclerosis
     Nephrotic syndrome with focal glomerulonephritis

N04.2 **Nephrotic syndrome with** diffuse membranous glomerulonephritis `CC`

N04.3 **Nephrotic syndrome with** diffuse mesangial proliferative glomerulonephritis `CC`

N04.4 **Nephrotic syndrome with** diffuse endocapillary proliferative glomerulonephritis `CC`

N04.5 **Nephrotic syndrome with** diffuse mesangiocapillary glomerulonephritis `CC`
     Nephrotic syndrome with membranoproliferative glomerulonephritis, types 1 and 3, or NOS

N04.6 **Nephrotic syndrome with** dense deposit disease `CC`
     Nephrotic syndrome with membranoproliferative glomerulonephritis, type 2

N04.7 **Nephrotic syndrome with** diffuse crescentic glomerulonephritis `CC`
     Nephrotic syndrome with extracapillary glomerulonephritis
     CC Excl: PDX collection 915

N04.8 **Nephrotic syndrome with** other morphologic changes `CC`
     Nephrotic syndrome with proliferative glomerulonephritis NOS
     CC Excl: PDX collection 915

N04.9 **Nephrotic syndrome with** unspecified morphologic changes `CC`
     CC Excl: PDX collection 915

✓4ᵗʰ **N05** **Unspecified** nephritic syndrome
     INCLUDES   glomerular disease NOS
                 glomerulonephritis NOS
                 nephritis NOS
                 nephropathy NOS and renal disease NOS with morphological lesion specified in .0-.8
     EXCLUDES 1   *nephropathy NOS with no stated morphological lesion (N28.9)*
                  renal disease NOS with no stated morphological lesion (N28.9)
                  tubulo-interstitial nephritis NOS (N12)

     CC Excl: For CC codes in category N05: PDX collection 918

N05.0 **Unspecified nephritic syndrome with** minor glomerular abnormality
     Unspecified nephritic syndrome with minimal change lesion

N05.1 **Unspecified nephritic syndrome with** focal and segmental glomerular lesions
     Unspecified nephritic syndrome with focal and segmental hyalinosis
     Unspecified nephritic syndrome with focal and segmental sclerosis
     Unspecified nephritic syndrome with focal glomerulonephritis

N05.2 **Unspecified nephritic syndrome with** diffuse membranous glomerulonephritis `CC`

N05.3 **Unspecified nephritic syndrome with** diffuse mesangial proliferative glomerulonephritis `CC`

N05.4 **Unspecified nephritic syndrome with** diffuse endocapillary proliferative glomerulonephritis `CC`

N05.5 **Unspecified nephritic syndrome with** diffuse mesangiocapillary glomerulonephritis `CC`
     Unspecified nephritic syndrome with membranoproliferative glomerulonephritis, types 1 and 3, or NOS

N05.6 **Unspecified nephritic syndrome with** dense deposit disease
     Unspecified nephritic syndrome with membranoproliferative glomerulonephritis, type 2

N05.7 **Unspecified nephritic syndrome with** diffuse crescentic glomerulonephritis
     Unspecified nephritic syndrome with extracapillary glomerulonephritis

N05.8 **Unspecified nephritic syndrome with** other morphologic changes
     Unspecified nephritic syndrome with proliferative glomerulonephritis NOS

N05.9 **Unspecified nephritic syndrome with** unspecified morphologic changes

✓4ᵗʰ **N06** **Isolated proteinuria with specified morphological lesion**
     EXCLUDES 1   *proteinuria not associated with specific morphologic lesions (R80.0)*

     CC Excl: For CC codes in category N06: PDX collection 918

N06.0 **Isolated proteinuria with** minor glomerular abnormality
     Isolated proteinuria with minimal change lesion

N06.1 **Isolated proteinuria with** focal and segmental glomerular lesions
     Isolated proteinuria with focal and segmental hyalinosis
     Isolated proteinuria with focal and segmental sclerosis
     Isolated proteinuria with focal glomerulonephritis

N06.2 **Isolated proteinuria with** diffuse membranous glomerulonephritis `CC`

N06.3 **Isolated proteinuria with** diffuse mesangial proliferative glomerulonephritis `CC`

N06.4 **Isolated proteinuria with** diffuse endocapillary proliferative glomerulonephritis `CC`

N06.5 **Isolated proteinuria with** diffuse mesangiocapillary glomerulonephritis `CC`
     Isolated proteinuria with membranoproliferative glomerulonephritis, types 1 and 3, or NOS

Chapter 14. Diseases of Genitourinary System

N06.6 Isolated proteinuria with dense deposit disease
Isolated proteinuria with membranoproliferative glomerulonephritis, type 2

N06.7 Isolated proteinuria with diffuse crescentic glomerulonephritis
Isolated proteinuria with extracapillary glomerulonephritis

N06.8 Isolated proteinuria with other morphologic lesion
Isolated proteinuria with proliferative glomerulonephritis NOS

N06.9 Isolated proteinuria with unspecified morphologic lesion

☑4ᵗʰ N07 Hereditary nephropathy, not elsewhere classified
EXCLUDES 2 Alport's syndrome (Q87.81-)
hereditary amyloid nephropathy (E85.-)
nail patella syndrome (Q87.2)
non-neuropathic heredofamilial amyloidosis (E85.-)

CC Excl: For CC codes in category N07: PDX collection 918

N07.0 Hereditary nephropathy, not elsewhere classified with minor glomerular abnormality
Hereditary nephropathy, not elsewhere classified with minimal change lesion

N07.1 Hereditary nephropathy, not elsewhere classified with focal and segmental glomerular lesions
Hereditary nephropathy, not elsewhere classified with focal and segmental hyalinosis
Hereditary nephropathy, not elsewhere classified with focal and segmental sclerosis
Hereditary nephropathy, not elsewhere classified with focal glomerulonephritis

N07.2 Hereditary nephropathy, not elsewhere classified with diffuse membranous glomerulonephritis CC

N07.3 Hereditary nephropathy, not elsewhere classified with diffuse mesangial proliferative glomerulonephritis CC

N07.4 Hereditary nephropathy, not elsewhere classified with diffuse endocapillary proliferative glomerulonephritis CC

N07.5 Hereditary nephropathy, not elsewhere classified with diffuse mesangiocapillary glomerulonephritis CC
Hereditary nephropathy, not elsewhere classified with membranoproliferative glomerulonephritis, types 1 and 3, or NOS

N07.6 Hereditary nephropathy, not elsewhere classified with dense deposit disease
Hereditary nephropathy, not elsewhere classified with membranoproliferative glomerulonephritis, type 2

N07.7 Hereditary nephropathy, not elsewhere classified with diffuse crescentic glomerulonephritis
Hereditary nephropathy, not elsewhere classified with extracapillary glomerulonephritis

N07.8 Hereditary nephropathy, not elsewhere classified with other morphologic lesions
Hereditary nephropathy, not elsewhere classified with proliferative glomerulonephritis NOS

N07.9 Hereditary nephropathy, not elsewhere classified with unspecified morphologic lesions

N08 Glomerular disorders in diseases classified elsewhere
Glomerulonephritis
Nephritis
Nephropathy
Code first underlying disease, such as:
amyloidosis (E85.-)
congenital syphilis (A50.5)
cryoglobulinemia (D89.1)
disseminated intravascular coagulation (D65)
gout (M1A.-, M10.-)
microscopic polyangiitis (M31.7)
multiple myeloma (C90.0-)
sepsis (A40.0-A41.9)
sickle-cell disease (D57.0-D57.8)
EXCLUDES 1 glomerulonephritis, nephritis and nephropathy (in):
antiglomerular basement membrane disease (M31.0)
diabetes (E08-E13 with .21)
gonococcal (A54.21)
Goodpasture's syndrome (M31.0)
hemolytic-uremic syndrome (D59.3)
lupus (M32.14)
mumps (B26.83)
syphilis (A52.75)
systemic lupus erythematosus (M32.14)
Wegener's granulomatosis (M31.31)
pyelonephritis in diseases classified elsewhere (N16)
renal tubulo-interstitial disorders classified elsewhere (N16)

Renal tubulo-interstitial diseases (N10-N16)

INCLUDES pyelonephritis
EXCLUDES 1 pyeloureteritis cystica (N28.85)

N10 Acute pyelonephritis CC H6
Acute infectious interstitial nephritis
Acute pyelitis
Acute tubulo-interstitial nephritis
Hemoglobin nephrosis
Myoglobin nephrosis
Use additional code (B95-B97), to identify infectious agent
CC Excl: PDX collection 919

☑4ᵗʰ N11 Chronic tubulo-interstitial nephritis
INCLUDES chronic infectious interstitial nephritis
chronic pyelitis
chronic pyelonephritis
Use additional code (B95-B97), to identify infectious agent

N11.0 Nonobstructive reflux-associated chronic pyelonephritis
Pyelonephritis (chronic) associated with (vesicoureteral) reflux
EXCLUDES 1 vesicoureteral reflux NOS (N13.70)

N11.1 Chronic obstructive pyelonephritis PDx CC CC
Pyelonephritis (chronic) associated with anomaly of pelviureteric junction
Pyelonephritis (chronic) associated with anomaly of pyeloureteric junction
Pyelonephritis (chronic) associated with crossing of vessel
Pyelonephritis (chronic) associated with kinking of ureter
Pyelonephritis (chronic) associated with obstruction of ureter
Pyelonephritis (chronic) associated with stricture of pelviureteric junction
Pyelonephritis (chronic) associated with stricture of ureter
EXCLUDES 1 calculous pyelonephritis (N20.9)
obstructive uropathy (N13.-)
CC Excl: PDX collection 920

N11.8 Other chronic tubulo-interstitial nephritis CC
Nonobstructive chronic pyelonephritis NOS
CC Excl: PDX collection 921

N11.9 Chronic tubulo-interstitial nephritis, unspecified CC H6
Chronic interstitial nephritis NOS
Chronic pyelitis NOS
Chronic pyelonephritis NOS
CC Excl: PDX collection 922

N12 Tubulo-interstitial nephritis, not specified as acute or chronic CC H6
Interstitial nephritis NOS
Pyelitis NOS
Pyelonephritis NOS
EXCLUDES 1 calculous pyelonephritis (N20.9)
CC Excl: PDX collection 922

☑4ᵗʰ N13 Obstructive and reflux uropathy
EXCLUDES 2 calculus of kidney and ureter without hydronephrosis (N20.-)
congenital obstructive defects of renal pelvis and ureter (Q62.0-Q62.3)
hydronephrosis with ureteropelvic junction obstruction ▶(Q62.11)◄
obstructive pyelonephritis (N11.1)

CC Excl: For CC codes in category N13, unless otherwise noted: PDX collection 922

N13.0 Hydronephrosis with ureteropelvic junction obstruction PDx CC CC
Hydronephrosis due to acquired occlusion of ureteropelvic junction
EXCLUDES 2 hydronephrosis with ureteropelvic junction obstruction due to calculus (N13.2)

N13.1 Hydronephrosis with ureteral stricture, not elsewhere classified PDx CC CC
EXCLUDES 1 hydronephrosis with ureteral stricture with infection (N13.6)

N13.2 Hydronephrosis with renal and ureteral calculous obstruction PDx CC CC
EXCLUDES 1 hydronephrosis with renal and ureteral calculous obstruction with infection (N13.6)

☑5ᵗʰ N13.3 Other and unspecified hydronephrosis
EXCLUDES 1 hydronephrosis with infection (N13.6)

N13.30 Unspecified hydronephrosis CC

N13.39 Other hydronephrosis CC

N Newborn: 0 P Pediatric: 0-17 M Maternity: 12-55 A Adult: 15-124 MCC Major CC Condition PDxMCC PDx acts as own MCC CC CC Condition PDxCC PDx acts as own CC

N06.6–N13.39

824 ICD-10-CM 2018

Hydronephrosis/UPJ Obstruction

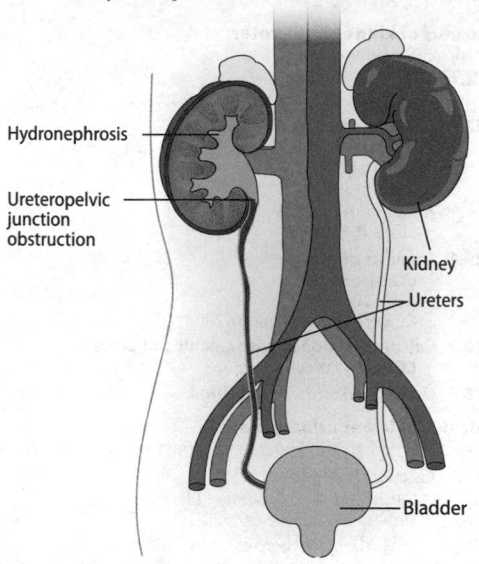

Hydronephrosis

Ureteropelvic junction obstruction

Kidney

Ureters

Bladder

N13.4 Hydroureter   `CC`
> EXCLUDES 1   *congenital hydroureter (Q62.3-)*
> *hydroureter with infection (N13.6)*
> *vesicoureteral-reflux with hydroureter (N13.73-)*
> **CC Excl:** PDX collection 923

N13.5 Crossing vessel and stricture of ureter without hydronephrosis
> Kinking and stricture of ureter without hydronephrosis
> EXCLUDES 1   *crossing vessel and stricture of ureter without hydronephrosis with infection (N13.6)*

N13.6 Pyonephrosis   `CC` `H6`
> Conditions in N13.0-N13.5 with infection
> Obstructive uropathy with infection
> Use additional code (B95-B97), to identify infectious agent

☑5ᵗʰ **N13.7 Vesicoureteral-reflux**
> EXCLUDES 1   *reflux-associated pyelonephritis (N11.0)*

     N13.70 Vesicoureteral-reflux, unspecified
> Vesicoureteral-reflux NOS

     N13.71 Vesicoureteral-reflux without reflux nephropathy

☑6ᵗʰ   **N13.72 Vesicoureteral-reflux** with reflux nephropathy without hydroureter

         N13.721 Vesicoureteral-reflux with reflux nephropathy without hydroureter, unilateral

         N13.722 Vesicoureteral-reflux with reflux nephropathy without hydroureter, bilateral

         N13.729 Vesicoureteral-reflux with reflux nephropathy without hydroureter, unspecified

Vesicoureteral Reflux

Kidneys

Ureters

Bladder

Normal flow of urine   Urine flowing the wrong way (VUR)

☑6ᵗʰ   **N13.73 Vesicoureteral-reflux** with reflux nephropathy with hydroureter

         N13.731 Vesicoureteral-reflux with reflux nephropathy with hydroureter, unilateral

         N13.732 Vesicoureteral-reflux with reflux nephropathy with hydroureter, bilateral

         N13.739 Vesicoureteral-reflux with reflux nephropathy with hydroureter, unspecified

N13.8 Other obstructive and reflux uropathy   `CC`
> Urinary tract obstruction due to specified cause
> Code first, if applicable, any causal condition, such as:
>   enlarged prostate (N40.1)
> **CC Excl:** PDX collection 920

N13.9 Obstructive and reflux uropathy, unspecified
> Urinary tract obstruction NOS

☑4ᵗʰ **N14 Drug- and heavy-metal-induced tubulo-interstitial and tubular conditions**
> Code first poisoning due to drug or toxin, if applicable (T36-T65 with fifth or sixth character 1-4 or 6)
> Use additional code for adverse effect, if applicable, to identify drug (T36-T50 with fifth or sixth character 5)

     N14.0 Analgesic nephropathy

     N14.1 Nephropathy induced by other drugs, medicaments and biological substances

     N14.2 Nephropathy induced by unspecified drug, medicament or biological substance

     N14.3 Nephropathy induced by heavy metals

     N14.4 Toxic nephropathy, not elsewhere classified

☑4ᵗʰ **N15 Other renal tubulo-interstitial diseases**

     N15.0 Balkan nephropathy
> Balkan endemic nephropathy

     N15.1 Renal and perinephric abscess   `MCC` `H6`
> **CC Excl:** PDX collection 919

     N15.8 Other specified renal tubulo-interstitial diseases

     N15.9 Renal tubulo-interstitial disease, unspecified
> Infection of kidney NOS
> EXCLUDES 1   *urinary tract infection NOS (N39.0)*

N16 *Renal tubulo-interstitial disorders in diseases classified elsewhere*
> Pyelonephritis
> Tubulo-interstitial nephritis
> Code first underlying disease, such as:
>   brucellosis (A23.0-A23.9)
>   cryoglobulinemia (D89.1)
>   glycogen storage disease (E74.0)
>   leukemia (C91-C95)
>   lymphoma (C81.0-C85.9, C96.0-C96.9)
>   multiple myeloma (C90.0-)
>   sepsis (A40.0-A41.9)
>   Wilson's disease (E83.0)
> EXCLUDES 1   *diphtheritic pyelonephritis and tubulo-interstitial nephritis (A36.84)*
> *pyelonephritis and tubulo-interstitial nephritis in candidiasis (B37.49)*
> *pyelonephritis and tubulo-interstitial nephritis in cystinosis (E72.04)*
> *pyelonephritis and tubulo-interstitial nephritis in salmonella infection (A02.25)*
> *pyelonephritis and tubulo-interstitial nephritis in sarcoidosis (D86.84)*
> *pyelonephritis and tubulo-interstitial nephritis in sicca syndrome [Sjogren's] (M35.04)*
> *pyelonephritis and tubulo-interstitial nephritis in systemic lupus erythematosus (M32.15)*
> *pyelonephritis and tubulo-interstitial nephritis in toxoplasmosis (B58.83)*
> *renal tubular degeneration in diabetes (E08-E13 with .29)*
> *syphilitic pyelonephritis and tubulo-interstitial nephritis (A52.75)*

☑ Additional Character Req   ☑x7ᵗʰ Placeholder Alert   Unacceptable PDx   Manifestation   `H1`-`H14` HAC   `HCC` CMS-HCC Condition   EXCLUDES 1 Not Coded Here   EXCLUDES 2 Not Included Here

ICD-10-CM 2018   825

Chapter 14. Diseases of Genitourinary System

Acute kidney failure and chronic kidney disease (N17-N19)

EXCLUDES 2   congenital renal failure (P96.0)
drug- and heavy-metal-induced tubulo-interstitial and tubular
    conditions (N14.-)
extrarenal uremia (R39.2)
hemolytic-uremic syndrome (D59.3)
hepatorenal syndrome (K76.7)
postpartum hepatorenal syndrome (O90.4)
posttraumatic renal failure (T79.5)
prerenal uremia (R39.2)
renal failure complicating abortion or ectopic or molar pregnancy (O00-
    O07, O08.4)
renal failure following labor and delivery (O90.4)
renal failure postprocedural (N99.0)

✓4ᵗʰ N17   Acute kidney failure

Code also associated underlying condition
EXCLUDES 1   posttraumatic renal failure (T79.5)
AHA: 2013, 4Q, 124

CC Excl: For CC/MCC codes in category N17: PDX collection 924

N17.0   Acute kidney failure with tubular necrosis   MCC HCC
Acute tubular necrosis
Renal tubular necrosis
Tubular necrosis NOS

N17.1   Acute kidney failure with acute cortical necrosis   MCC HCC
Acute cortical necrosis
Cortical necrosis NOS
Renal cortical necrosis

N17.2   Acute kidney failure with medullary necrosis   MCC HCC
Medullary [papillary] necrosis NOS
Acute medullary [papillary] necrosis
Renal medullary [papillary] necrosis

N17.8   Other acute kidney failure   CC HCC
CC Excl: PDX collection 925

N17.9   Acute kidney failure, unspecified   CC HCC
Acute kidney injury (nontraumatic)
EXCLUDES 2   traumatic kidney injury (S37.0-)

✓4ᵗʰ N18   Chronic kidney disease (CKD)

Code first any associated:
diabetic chronic kidney disease (E08.22, E09.22, E10.22, E11.22,
    E13.22)
hypertensive chronic kidney disease (I12-, I13-)
Use additional code to identify kidney transplant status, if applicable,
    (Z94.0)
AHA: 2013, 1Q, 24

N18.1   Chronic kidney disease, stage 1

N18.2   Chronic kidney disease, stage 2 (mild)

N18.3   Chronic kidney disease, stage 3 (moderate)

N18.4   Chronic kidney disease, stage 4 (severe)   CC HCC
CC Excl: PDX collection 926

N18.5   Chronic kidney disease, stage 5   CC HCC
EXCLUDES 1   chronic kidney disease, stage 5 requiring chronic
    dialysis (N18.6)
DEF: End-stage renal disease (ESRD) with GFR value of 15 ml/min
or less not yet requiring chronic dialysis.
CC Excl: PDX collection 926

N18.6   End stage renal disease   MCC HCC
Chronic kidney disease requiring chronic dialysis
Use additional code to identify dialysis status (Z99.2)
AHA: 2016, 3Q, 22; 2016, 1Q, 12; 2013, 4Q, 124-125
CC Excl: PDX collection 927

N18.9   Chronic kidney disease, unspecified
Chronic renal disease
Chronic renal failure NOS
Chronic renal insufficiency
▶Chronic uremia NOS
Diffuse sclerosing glomerulonephritis NOS◀

N19   Unspecified kidney failure

Uremia NOS
EXCLUDES 1   acute kidney failure (N17.-)
chronic kidney disease (N18.-)
chronic uremia (N18.9)
extrarenal uremia (R39.2)
prerenal uremia (R39.2)
renal insufficiency (acute) (N28.9)
uremia of newborn (P96.0)

Urolithiasis (N20-N23)

AHA: 2017, 1Q, 5; 2015, 2Q, 8

✓4ᵗʰ N20   Calculus of kidney and ureter

Calculous pyelonephritis
EXCLUDES 1   nephrocalcinosis (E83.5)
that with hydronephrosis (N13.2)

N20.0   Calculus of kidney
Nephrolithiasis NOS
Renal calculus
Renal stone
Staghorn calculus
Stone in kidney

N20.1   Calculus of ureter   CC
Ureteric stone
AHA: 2016, 3Q, 22
CC Excl: PDX collection 928

N20.2   Calculus of kidney with calculus of ureter   CC
CC Excl: PDX collection 928

N20.9   Urinary calculus, unspecified

✓4ᵗʰ N21   Calculus of lower urinary tract

INCLUDES   calculus of lower urinary tract with cystitis and urethritis

N21.0   Calculus in bladder
Calculus in diverticulum of bladder
Urinary bladder stone
EXCLUDES 2   staghorn calculus (N20.0)

N21.1   Calculus in urethra
EXCLUDES 2   calculus of prostate (N42.0)

N21.8   Other lower urinary tract calculus

N21.9   Calculus of lower urinary tract, unspecified
EXCLUDES 1   calculus of urinary tract NOS (N20.9)

N22   *Calculus of urinary tract in diseases classified elsewhere*

Code first underlying disease, such as:
gout (M1A.-, M10.-)
schistosomiasis (B65.0-B65.9)

N23   Unspecified renal colic

Other disorders of kidney and ureter (N25-N29)

EXCLUDES 2   disorders of kidney and ureter with urolithiasis (N20-N23)

✓4ᵗʰ N25   Disorders resulting from impaired renal tubular function

EXCLUDES 1   *metabolic disorders classifiable to E70-E88*

N25.0   Renal osteodystrophy
Azotemic osteodystrophy
Phosphate-losing tubular disorders
Renal rickets
Renal short stature
EXCLUDES 2   ▶metabolic disorders classifiable to E70-E88◀

N25.1   Nephrogenic diabetes insipidus   CC HCC
EXCLUDES 1   diabetes insipidus NOS (E23.2)
DEF: Type of diabetes due to inability of renal tubules to reabsorb
water back into the body; not responsive to vasopressin
(antidiuretic hormone); characterized by excessive thirst and
excessive urine production; may develop into chronic renal
insufficiency.
CC Excl: PDX collection 929

✓5ᵗʰ N25.8   Other disorders resulting from impaired renal tubular function

N25.81   Secondary hyperparathyroidism of renal origin   CC HCC
EXCLUDES 1   secondary hyperparathyroidism, non-renal
    (E21.1)
EXCLUDES 2   ▶metabolic disorders classifiable to
    E70-E88◀
DEF: Parathyroid dysfunction caused by chronic renal
failure; phosphate clearance is impaired, phosphate is
released from bone, vitamin D is not produced,
intestinal calcium absorption is low, and blood levels of
calcium are lowered, causing excessive production of
parathyroid hormone.
CC Excl: PDX collection 930

N25.89   Other disorders resulting from impaired renal tubular function
Hypokalemic nephropathy
Lightwood-Albright syndrome
Renal tubular acidosis NOS

N25.9   Disorder resulting from impaired renal tubular function, unspecified

N Newborn: 0   P Pediatric: 0-17   M Maternity: 12-55   A Adult: 15-124   MCC Major CC Condition   PDxMCC PDx acts as own MCC   CC CC Condition   PDxCC PDx acts as own CC

826   ICD-10-CM 2018

✓4ᵗʰ **N26 Unspecified contracted kidney**
- *EXCLUDES 1*   contracted kidney due to hypertension (I12.-)
  - diffuse sclerosing glomerulonephritis (N05.8-)
  - hypertensive nephrosclerosis (arteriolar) (arteriosclerotic) (I12.-)
  - small kidney of unknown cause (N27.-)

N26.1 Atrophy of kidney (terminal)

N26.2 Page kidney

N26.9 Renal sclerosis, unspecified

✓4ᵗʰ **N27 Small kidney of unknown cause**
- *INCLUDES*   oligonephronia

N27.0 Small kidney, unilateral

N27.1 Small kidney, bilateral

N27.9 Small kidney, unspecified

✓4ᵗʰ **N28 Other disorders of kidney and ureter, not elsewhere classified**

N28.0 Ischemia and infarction of kidney   CC HCC
- Renal artery embolism
- Renal artery obstruction
- Renal artery occlusion
- Renal artery thrombosis
- Renal infarct
- *EXCLUDES 1*   atherosclerosis of renal artery (extrarenal part) (I70.1)
  - congenital stenosis of renal artery (Q27.1)
  - Goldblatt's kidney (I70.1)
- **CC Excl:** PDX collection 931

N28.1 Cyst of kidney, acquired
- ▶Cyst (multiple) (solitary) of kidney (acquired)◄
- *EXCLUDES 1*   cystic kidney disease (congenital) (Q61.-)

✓5ᵗʰ **N28.8 Other specified disorders of kidney and ureter**
- *EXCLUDES 1*   hydroureter (N13.4)
  - ureteric stricture with hydronephrosis (N13.1)
  - ureteric stricture without hydronephrosis (N13.5)

   CC Excl: For CC codes in subcategory N28.8:
PDX collection 922

N28.81 Hypertrophy of kidney

N28.82 Megaloureter

N28.83 Nephroptosis

N28.84 Pyelitis cystica   CC H6

N28.85 Pyeloureteritis cystica   CC H6

N28.86 Ureteritis cystica   CC H6

N28.89 Other specified disorders of kidney and ureter

N28.9 Disorder of kidney and ureter, unspecified
- Nephropathy NOS
- Renal disease (acute) NOS
- Renal insufficiency (acute)
- *EXCLUDES 1*   chronic renal insufficiency (N18.9)
  - unspecified nephritic syndrome (N05.-)
- **AHA:** 2016, 1Q, 13

N29 Other disorders of kidney and ureter in diseases classified elsewhere
- Code first underlying disease, such as:
  - amyloidosis (E85.-)
  - nephrocalcinosis (E83.5)
  - schistosomiasis (B65.0-B65.9)
- *EXCLUDES 1*   disorders of kidney and ureter in:
  - cystinosis (E72.0)
  - gonorrhea (A54.21)
  - syphilis (A52.75)
  - tuberculosis (A18.11)

Other diseases of the urinary system (N30-N39)

- *EXCLUDES 1*   urinary infection (complicating):
  - abortion or ectopic or molar pregnancy (O00-O07, O08.8)
  - pregnancy, childbirth and the puerperium (O23-, O75.3, O86.2-)

✓4ᵗʰ **N30 Cystitis**
- Use additional code to identify infectious agent (B95-B97)
- *EXCLUDES 1*   prostatocystitis (N41.3)
- **AHA:** 2017, 1Q, 6

   CC Excl: For CC codes in category N30: PDX collection 932

✓5ᵗʰ **N30.0 Acute cystitis**
- *EXCLUDES 1*   irradiation cystitis (N30.4-)
  - trigonitis (N30.3-)

N30.00 Acute cystitis without hematuria   CC H6

N30.01 Acute cystitis with hematuria   CC H6

✓5ᵗʰ **N30.1 Interstitial cystitis (chronic)**

N30.10 Interstitial cystitis (chronic) without hematuria

N30.11 Interstitial cystitis (chronic) with hematuria

✓5ᵗʰ **N30.2 Other chronic cystitis**

N30.20 Other chronic cystitis without hematuria

N30.21 Other chronic cystitis with hematuria

✓5ᵗʰ **N30.3 Trigonitis**
- Urethrotrigonitis

N30.30 Trigonitis without hematuria

N30.31 Trigonitis with hematuria

✓5ᵗʰ **N30.4 Irradiation cystitis**

N30.40 Irradiation cystitis without hematuria   CC

N30.41 Irradiation cystitis with hematuria   CC

✓5ᵗʰ **N30.8 Other cystitis**
- Abscess of bladder

N30.80 Other cystitis without hematuria

N30.81 Other cystitis with hematuria

✓5ᵗʰ **N30.9 Cystitis, unspecified**

N30.90 Cystitis, unspecified without hematuria

N30.91 Cystitis, unspecified with hematuria

✓4ᵗʰ **N31 Neuromuscular dysfunction of bladder, not elsewhere classified**
- Use additional code to identify any associated urinary incontinence (N39.3-N39.4-)
- *EXCLUDES 1*   cord bladder NOS (G95.89)
  - neurogenic bladder due to cauda equina syndrome (G83.4)
  - neuromuscular dysfunction due to spinal cord lesion (G95.89)

N31.0 Uninhibited neuropathic bladder, not elsewhere classified

N31.1 Reflex neuropathic bladder, not elsewhere classified

N31.2 Flaccid neuropathic bladder, not elsewhere classified
- Atonic (motor) (sensory) neuropathic bladder
- Autonomous neuropathic bladder
- Nonreflex neuropathic bladder

N31.8 Other neuromuscular dysfunction of bladder

N31.9 Neuromuscular dysfunction of bladder, unspecified
- Neurogenic bladder dysfunction NOS

✓4ᵗʰ **N32 Other disorders of bladder**
- *EXCLUDES 2*   calculus of bladder (N21.0)
  - cystocele (N81.0)
  - hernia or prolapse of bladder, female (N81.1-)

N32.0 Bladder-neck obstruction
- Bladder-neck stenosis (acquired)
- *EXCLUDES 1*   congenital bladder-neck obstruction (Q64.3-)
- **DEF:** Bladder outlet and vesicourethral obstruction; occurs as a consequence of benign prostatic hypertrophy or prostatic cancer; may also occur in either sex due to strictures, radiation, cystoscopy, catheterization, injury, infection, blood clots, bladder cancer, impaction, or other disease that compresses the bladder neck.

N32.1 Vesicointestinal fistula   CC
- Vesicorectal fistula
- **CC Excl:** PDX collection 933

N32.2 Vesical fistula, not elsewhere classified   CC
- *EXCLUDES 1*   fistula between bladder and female genital tract (N82.0-N82.1)
- **CC Excl:** PDX collection 933

N32.3 Diverticulum of bladder
- *EXCLUDES 1*   congenital diverticulum of bladder (Q64.6)
  - diverticulitis of bladder (N30.8-)

✓5ᵗʰ **N32.8 Other specified disorders of bladder**

N32.81 Overactive bladder
- Detrusor muscle hyperactivity
- *EXCLUDES 1*   frequent urination due to specified bladder condition—code to condition
- **DEF:** Sudden involuntary contractions of the muscular wall of bladder; results in sudden, strong urge to urinate.

N32.89 Other specified disorders of bladder
- Bladder hemorrhage
- Bladder hypertrophy
- Calcified bladder
- Contracted bladder

N32.9 Bladder disorder, unspecified

N33   Bladder disorders in diseases classified elsewhere
Code first underlying disease, such as:
schistosomiasis (B65.0-B65.9)
> EXCLUDES 1   bladder disorder in syphilis (A52.76)
> bladder disorder in tuberculosis (A18.12)
> candidal cystitis (B37.41)
> chlamydial cystitis (A56.01)
> cystitis in gonorrhea (A54.01)
> cystitis in neurogenic bladder (N31.-)
> diphtheritic cystitis (A36.85)
> neurogenic bladder (N31.-)
> syphilitic cystitis (A52.76)
> trichomonal cystitis (A59.03)

✓4ᵗʰ N34   Urethritis and urethral syndrome
Use additional code (B95-B97), to identify infectious agent
> EXCLUDES 2   Reiter's disease (M02.3-)
> urethritis in diseases with a predominantly sexual mode of
> transmission (A50-A64)
> urethrotrigonitis (N30.3-)
AHA: 2017, 1Q, 6

N34.0   Urethral abscess   CC H6
Abscess (of) Cowper's gland
Abscess (of) Littrés gland
Abscess (of) urethral (gland)
Periurethral abscess
> EXCLUDES 1   urethral caruncle (N36.2)
CC Excl: PDX collection 934

N34.1   Nonspecific urethritis
Nongonococcal urethritis
Nonvenereal urethritis

N34.2   Other urethritis
Meatitis, urethral
Postmenopausal urethritis
Ulcer of urethra (meatus)
Urethritis NOS

N34.3   Urethral syndrome, unspecified

✓4ᵗʰ N35   Urethral stricture
> EXCLUDES 1   congenital urethral stricture (Q64.3-)
> postprocedural urethral stricture (N99.1-)

✓5ᵗʰ N35.0   Post-traumatic urethral stricture
Urethral stricture due to injury
> EXCLUDES 1   postprocedural urethral stricture (N99.1-)

✓6ᵗʰ N35.01   Post-traumatic urethral stricture, male
N35.010   Post-traumatic urethral stricture, ♂
male, meatal
N35.011   Post-traumatic bulbous urethral ♂
stricture
N35.012   Post-traumatic membranous urethral ♂
stricture
N35.013   Post-traumatic anterior urethral ♂
stricture
N35.014   Post-traumatic urethral stricture, ♂
male, unspecified

✓6ᵗʰ N35.02   Post-traumatic urethral stricture, female
N35.021   Urethral stricture due to childbirth ♀
N35.028   Other post-traumatic urethral stricture, ♀
female

✓5ᵗʰ N35.1   Postinfective urethral stricture, not elsewhere classified
> EXCLUDES 1   urethral stricture associated with schistosomiasis
> (B65-, N29)
> gonococcal urethral stricture (A54.01)
> syphilitic urethral stricture (A52.76)

✓6ᵗʰ N35.11   Postinfective urethral stricture, not elsewhere classified, male
N35.111   Postinfective urethral stricture, not ♂
elsewhere classified, male, meatal
▲   N35.112   Postinfective bulbous urethral ♂
stricture, not elsewhere classified, male
▲   N35.113   Postinfective membranous urethral ♂
stricture, not elsewhere classified, male
▲   N35.114   Postinfective anterior urethral ♂
stricture, not elsewhere classified, male
N35.119   Postinfective urethral stricture, not ♂
elsewhere classified, male, unspecified

N35.12   Postinfective urethral stricture, not elsewhere ♀
classified, female

N35.8   Other urethral stricture
> EXCLUDES 1   postprocedural urethral stricture (N99.1-)

N35.9   Urethral stricture, unspecified

✓4ᵗʰ N36   Other disorders of urethra
N36.0   Urethral fistula   CC
Urethroperineal fistula
Urethrorectal fistula
Urinary fistula NOS
> EXCLUDES 1   urethroscrotal fistula (N50.89)
> urethrovaginal fistula (N82.1)
> urethrovesicovaginal fistula (N82.1)
CC Excl: PDX collection 935

N36.1   Urethral diverticulum

N36.2   Urethral caruncle

✓5ᵗʰ N36.4   Urethral functional and muscular disorders
Use additional code to identify associated urinary stress
incontinence (N39.3)
N36.41   Hypermobility of urethra
N36.42   Intrinsic sphincter deficiency (ISD)
N36.43   Combined hypermobility of urethra and intrinsic
sphincter deficiency
N36.44   Muscular disorders of urethra
Bladder sphincter dyssynergy

N36.5   Urethral false passage

N36.8   Other specified disorders of urethra
> EXCLUDES 1   congenital urethrocele (Q64.7)
> female urethrocele (N81.0)

N36.9   Urethral disorder, unspecified

N37   Urethral disorders in diseases classified elsewhere
Code first underlying disease
> EXCLUDES 1   urethritis (in):
> candidal infection (B37.41)
> chlamydial (A56.01)
> gonorrhea (A54.01)
> syphilis (A52.76)
> trichomonal infection (A59.03)
> tuberculosis (A18.13)

✓4ᵗʰ N39   Other disorders of urinary system
> EXCLUDES 2   hematuria NOS (R31.-)
> recurrent or persistent hematuria (N02.-)
> recurrent or persistent hematuria with specified morphological
> lesion (N02.-)
> proteinuria NOS (R80.-)

N39.0   Urinary tract infection, site not specified   CC H6
Use additional code (B95-B97), to identify infectious agent
> EXCLUDES 1   candidiasis of urinary tract (B37.4-)
> neonatal urinary tract infection (P39.3)
> urinary tract infection of specified site, such as:
> cystitis (N30.-)
> urethritis (N34.-)
AHA: 2017, 1Q, 6; 2012, 4Q, 94
CC Excl: PDX collection 936

N39.3   Stress incontinence (female) (male)
Code also any associated overactive bladder (N32.81)
> EXCLUDES 1   mixed incontinence (N39.46)

✓5ᵗʰ N39.4   Other specified urinary incontinence
Code also any associated overactive bladder (N32.81)
> EXCLUDES 1   enuresis NOS (R32)
> functional urinary incontinence (R39.81)
> urinary incontinence associated with cognitive
> impairment (R39.81)
> urinary incontinence NOS (R32)
> urinary incontinence of nonorganic origin (F98.0)
N39.41   Urge incontinence
> EXCLUDES 1   mixed incontinence (N39.46)
N39.42   Incontinence without sensory awareness
Insensible (urinary) incontinence
N39.43   Post-void dribbling
N39.44   Nocturnal enuresis
N39.45   Continuous leakage
N39.46   Mixed incontinence
Urge and stress incontinence
✓6ᵗʰ N39.49   Other specified urinary incontinence
N39.490   Overflow incontinence
N39.491   Coital incontinence
N39.492   Postural (urinary) incontinence

N Newborn: 0   P Pediatric: 0-17   M Maternity: 12-55   A Adult: 15-124   MCC Major CC Condition   PDxMCC PDx acts as own MCC   CC CC Condition   PDxCC PDx acts as own CC

N39.498 Other specified urinary incontinence
Reflex incontinence
Total incontinence

N39.8 Other specified disorders of urinary system

N39.9 Disorder of urinary system, unspecified

Diseases of male genital organs (N40-N53)

☑4ᵗʰ N40 Benign prostatic hyperplasia
INCLUDES   adenofibromatous hypertrophy of prostate
benign hypertrophy of the prostate
benign prostatic hypertrophy
BPH
enlarged prostate
nodular prostate
polyp of prostate
EXCLUDES 1   benign neoplasms of prostate (adenoma, benign)
(fibroadenoma) (fibroma) (myoma) (D29.1)
EXCLUDES 2   malignant neoplasm of prostate (C61)

N40.0 Benign prostatic hyperplasia without lower   Ⓐ♂
urinary tract symptoms
Enlarged prostate NOS
Enlarged prostate without LUTS

N40.1 Benign prostatic hyperplasia with lower urinary tract   Ⓐ♂
symptoms
Enlarged prostate with LUTS
Use additional code for associated symptoms, when specified:
incomplete bladder emptying (R39.14)
nocturia (R35.1)
straining on urination (R39.16)
urinary frequency (R35.0)
urinary hesitancy (R39.11)
urinary incontinence (N39.4-)
urinary obstruction (N13.8)
urinary retention (R33.8)
urinary urgency (R39.15)
weak urinary stream (R39.12)

N40.2 Nodular prostate without lower urinary tract symptoms   Ⓐ♂
Nodular prostate without LUTS

N40.3 Nodular prostate with lower urinary tract symptoms   Ⓐ♂
Use additional code for associated symptoms, when specified:
incomplete bladder emptying (R39.14)
nocturia (R35.1)
straining on urination (R39.16)
urinary frequency (R35.0)
urinary hesitancy (R39.11)
urinary incontinence (N39.4-)
urinary obstruction (N13.8)
urinary retention (R33.8)
urinary urgency (R39.15)
weak urinary stream (R39.12)

☑4ᵗʰ N41 Inflammatory diseases of prostate
Use additional code (B95-B97), to identify infectious agent

N41.0 Acute prostatitis   CC Ⓐ♂
CC Excl: PDX collection 937

N41.1 Chronic prostatitis   Ⓐ♂

N41.2 Abscess of prostate   CC Ⓐ♂
CC Excl: PDX collection 937

N41.3 Prostatocystitis   Ⓐ♂

N41.4 Granulomatous prostatitis   Ⓐ♂

N41.8 Other inflammatory diseases of prostate   Ⓐ♂

N41.9 Inflammatory disease of prostate, unspecified   Ⓐ♂
Prostatitis NOS

☑4ᵗʰ N42 Other and unspecified disorders of prostate

N42.0 Calculus of prostate   Ⓐ♂
Prostatic stone
DEF: Formation of small, solid stone often composed of calcium
carbonate or calcium phosphate in the prostate gland.

N42.1 Congestion and hemorrhage of prostate   Ⓐ♂
EXCLUDES 1   enlarged prostate (N40.-)
hematuria (R31.-)
hyperplasia of prostate (N40.-)
inflammatory diseases of prostate (N41.-)

☑5ᵗʰ N42.3 Dysplasia of prostate
N42.30 Unspecified dysplasia of prostate   ♂

N42.31 Prostatic intraepithelial neoplasia   ♂
PIN
Prostatic intraepithelial neoplasia I (PIN I)
Prostatic intraepithelial neoplasia II (PIN II)
EXCLUDES 1   prostatic intraepithelial neoplasia III (PIN III)
(D07.5)
DEF: Abnormality of shape and size of the intraepithelial
tissues of the prostate; premalignant condition
characterized by stalks and absence of a basilar cell
layer; synonyms are intraductal dysplasia, large acinar
atypical hyperplasia, atypical primary hyperplasia,
hyperplasia with malignant changes, marked atypia, or
duct-acinar dysplasia.

N42.32 Atypical small acinar proliferation of prostate   ♂

N42.39 Other dysplasia of prostate   ♂

☑5ᵗʰ N42.8 Other specified disorders of prostate

N42.81 Prostatodynia syndrome   Ⓐ♂
Painful prostate syndrome

N42.82 Prostatosis syndrome   Ⓐ♂

N42.83 Cyst of prostate   Ⓐ♂

N42.89 Other specified disorders of prostate   Ⓐ♂

N42.9 Disorder of prostate, unspecified   Ⓐ♂

☑4ᵗʰ N43 Hydrocele and spermatocele
INCLUDES   hydrocele of spermatic cord, testis or tunica vaginalis
EXCLUDES 1   congenital hydrocele (P83.5)

N43.0 Encysted hydrocele   ♂

N43.1 Infected hydrocele   CC ♂
Use additional code (B95-B97), to identify infectious agent
CC Excl: PDX collection 938

N43.2 Other hydrocele   ♂

N43.3 Hydrocele, unspecified   ♂

☑5ᵗʰ N43.4 Spermatocele of epididymis
Spermatic cyst

N43.40 Spermatocele of epididymis, unspecified   ♂

N43.41 Spermatocele of epididymis, single   ♂

N43.42 Spermatocele of epididymis, multiple   ♂

☑4ᵗʰ N44 Noninflammatory disorders of testis

CC Excl: For CC codes in category N44: PDX collection 939

☑5ᵗʰ N44.0 Torsion of testis

N44.00 Torsion of testis, unspecified   CC ♂

N44.01 Extravaginal torsion of spermatic cord   CC ♂
DEF: Torsion of the spermatic cord just below the tunica
vaginalis attachments.

N44.02 Intravaginal torsion of spermatic cord   CC ♂
Torsion of spermatic cord NOS

N44.03 Torsion of appendix testis   CC ♂

N44.04 Torsion of appendix epididymis   CC ♂

N44.1 Cyst of tunica albuginea testis   ♂

N44.2 Benign cyst of testis   ♂

N44.8 Other noninflammatory disorders of the testis   ♂

☑4ᵗʰ N45 Orchitis and epididymitis
Use additional code (B95-B97), to identify infectious agent

N45.1 Epididymitis   ♂

N45.2 Orchitis   ♂

N45.3 Epididymo-orchitis   ♂

N45.4 Abscess of epididymis or testis   CC ♂
CC Excl: PDX collection 940

Hydrocele

Normal   Noncommunicating hydrocele   Communicating hydrocele   Hydrocele of the cord

Testicle
Scrotum

☑ Additional Character Req   ✓x7ᵗʰ Placeholder Alert   Unacceptable PDx   Manifestation   H1-H14 HAC   HCC CMS-HCC Condition   EXCLUDES 1 Not Coded Here   EXCLUDES 2 Not Included Here

ICD-10-CM 2018   829

Chapter 14. Diseases of Genitourinary System *(left margin)*

N46–N50.9 *(left margin bottom)*

✓4ᵗʰ **N46 Male infertility**
     EXCLUDES 1   vasectomy status (Z98.52)

   ✓5ᵗʰ **N46.0 Azoospermia**
      Absolute male infertility
      Male infertility due to germinal (cell) aplasia
      Male infertility due to spermatogenic arrest (complete)

      N46.01 Organic azoospermia   A♂
        Azoospermia NOS

     ✓6ᵗʰ **N46.02 Azoospermia due to extratesticular causes**
        Code also associated cause

        N46.021 Azoospermia due to drug therapy A♂
        N46.022 Azoospermia due to infection A♂
        N46.023 Azoospermia due to obstruction of efferent ducts A♂
        N46.024 Azoospermia due to radiation A♂
        N46.025 Azoospermia due to systemic disease A♂
        N46.029 Azoospermia due to other extratesticular causes A♂

   ✓5ᵗʰ **N46.1 Oligospermia**
      Male infertility due to germinal cell desquamation
      Male infertility due to hypospermatogenesis
      Male infertility due to incomplete spermatogenic arrest

      N46.11 Organic oligospermia   A♂
        Oligospermia NOS

     ✓6ᵗʰ **N46.12 Oligospermia due to extratesticular causes**
        Code also associated cause

        N46.121 Oligospermia due to drug therapy A♂
        N46.122 Oligospermia due to infection A♂
        N46.123 Oligospermia due to obstruction of efferent ducts A♂
        N46.124 Oligospermia due to radiation A♂
        N46.125 Oligospermia due to systemic disease A♂
        N46.129 Oligospermia due to other extratesticular causes A♂

   N46.8 Other male infertility A♂
   N46.9 Male infertility, unspecified A♂

✓4ᵗʰ **N47 Disorders of prepuce**
   N47.0 Adherent prepuce, newborn N♂
   N47.1 Phimosis ♂
   N47.2 Paraphimosis ♂
   N47.3 Deficient foreskin ♂
   N47.4 Benign cyst of prepuce ♂
   N47.5 Adhesions of prepuce and glans penis ♂
   N47.6 Balanoposthitis ♂
     Use additional code (B95-B97), to identify infectious agent
      EXCLUDES 1   balanitis (N48.1)
   N47.7 Other inflammatory diseases of prepuce ♂
     Use additional code (B95-B97), to identify infectious agent
   N47.8 Other disorders of prepuce ♂

✓4ᵗʰ **N48 Other disorders of penis**
   N48.0 Leukoplakia of penis ♂
     Balanitis xerotica obliterans
     Kraurosis of penis
     Lichen sclerosus of external male genital organs
      EXCLUDES 1   carcinoma in situ of penis (D07.4)
   N48.1 Balanitis ♂
     Use additional code (B95-B97), to identify infectious agent
      EXCLUDES 1   amebic balanitis (A06.8)
          balanitis xerotica obliterans (N48.0)
          candidal balanitis (B37.42)
          gonococcal balanitis (A54.23)
          herpesviral [herpes simplex] balanitis (A60.01)
   ✓5ᵗʰ **N48.2 Other inflammatory disorders of penis**
     Use additional code (B95-B97), to identify infectious agent
      EXCLUDES 1   balanitis (N48.1)
          balanitis xerotica obliterans (N48.0)
          balanoposthitis (N47.6)
      N48.21 Abscess of corpus cavernosum and penis ♂
      N48.22 Cellulitis of corpus cavernosum and penis ♂
      N48.29 Other inflammatory disorders of penis ♂

✓5ᵗʰ **N48.3 Priapism**
     Painful erection
     Code first underlying cause

     CC Excl: For CC codes in subcategory N48.3:
     PDX collection 941

     N48.30 Priapism, unspecified CC♂
     N48.31 Priapism due to trauma CC♂
     N48.32 Priapism due to disease classified elsewhere CC♂
     N48.33 Priapism, drug-induced CC♂
     N48.39 Other priapism CC♂
   N48.5 Ulcer of penis ♂
   N48.6 Induration penis plastica ♂
     Peyronie's disease
     Plastic induration of penis
   ✓5ᵗʰ **N48.8 Other specified disorders of penis**
     N48.81 Thrombosis of superficial vein of penis ♂
     N48.82 Acquired torsion of penis ♂
      Acquired torsion of penis NOS
      EXCLUDES 1   congenital torsion of penis (Q55.63)
     N48.83 Acquired buried penis ♂
      EXCLUDES 1   congenital hidden penis (Q55.64)
     N48.89 Other specified disorders of penis ♂
   N48.9 Disorder of penis, unspecified ♂

✓4ᵗʰ **N49 Inflammatory disorders of male genital organs, not elsewhere classified**
   Use additional code (B95-B97), to identify infectious agent
     EXCLUDES 1   inflammation of penis (N48.1, N48.2-)
          orchitis and epididymitis (N45.-)

   N49.0 Inflammatory disorders of seminal vesicle ♂
     Vesiculitis NOS
   N49.1 Inflammatory disorders of spermatic cord, tunica vaginalis and vas deferens ♂
     Vasitis
   N49.2 Inflammatory disorders of scrotum ♂
   N49.3 Fournier gangrene ♂
   N49.8 Inflammatory disorders of other specified male genital organs ♂
     Inflammation of multiple sites in male genital organs
   N49.9 Inflammatory disorder of unspecified male genital organ ♂
     Abscess of unspecified male genital organ
     Boil of unspecified male genital organ
     Carbuncle of unspecified male genital organ
     Cellulitis of unspecified male genital organ

✓4ᵗʰ **N50 Other and unspecified disorders of male genital organs**
     EXCLUDES 2   torsion of testis (N44.0-)
   N50.0 Atrophy of testis ♂
   N50.1 Vascular disorders of male genital organs ♂
     Hematocele, NOS, of male genital organs
     Hemorrhage of male genital organs
     Thrombosis of male genital organs
   N50.3 Cyst of epididymis ♂
   ✓5ᵗʰ **N50.8 Other specified disorders of male genital organs**
     ✓6ᵗʰ **N50.81 Testicular pain**
       N50.811 Right testicular pain ♂
       N50.812 Left testicular pain ♂
       N50.819 Testicular pain, unspecified ♂
     N50.82 Scrotal pain ♂
     N50.89 Other specified disorders of the male genital organs ♂
      Atrophy of scrotum, seminal vesicle, spermatic cord, tunica vaginalis and vas deferens
      Chylocele, tunica vaginalis (nonfilarial) NOS
      Edema of scrotum, seminal vesicle, spermatic cord, tunica vaginalis and vas deferens
      Hypertrophy of scrotum, seminal vesicle, spermatic cord, tunica vaginalis and vas deferens
      Stricture of spermatic cord, tunica vaginalis, and vas deferens
      Ulcer of scrotum, seminal vesicle, spermatic cord, testis, tunica vaginalis and vas deferens
      Urethroscrotal fistula
   N50.9 Disorder of male genital organs, unspecified ♂

N Newborn: 0   P Pediatric: 0-17   M Maternity: 12-55   A Adult: 15-124   MCC Major CC Condition   PDx MCC PDx acts as own MCC   CC CC Condition   PDx CC PDx acts as own CC

830   ICD-10-CM 2018

N51 *Disorders of male genital organs in diseases classified elsewhere* ♂

Code first underlying disease, such as:
    filariasis (B74.0-B74.9)
    EXCLUDES 1   amebic balanitis (A06.8)
            candidal balanitis (B37.42)
            gonococcal balanitis (A54.23)
            gonococcal prostatitis (A54.22)
            herpesviral [herpes simplex] balanitis (A60.01)
            trichomonal prostatitis (A59.02)
            tuberculous prostatitis (A18.14)

√4th **N52** **Male erectile dysfunction**
    EXCLUDES 1   psychogenic impotence (F52.21)

√5th   **N52.0** **Vasculogenic erectile dysfunction**
      N52.01 **Erectile dysfunction due to arterial insufficiency** ☒♂
      N52.02 **Corporo-venous occlusive erectile dysfunction** ☒♂
      N52.03 **Combined arterial insufficiency and corporo-venous occlusive erectile dysfunction** ☒♂

  N52.1 *Erectile dysfunction due to diseases classified elsewhere* ☒♂
      Code first underlying disease

  N52.2 **Drug-induced erectile dysfunction** ☒♂

√5th   **N52.3** **Postprocedural erectile dysfunction**
      N52.31 **Erectile dysfunction following radical prostatectomy** ☒♂
      N52.32 **Erectile dysfunction following radical cystectomy** ☒♂
      N52.33 **Erectile dysfunction following urethral surgery** ☒♂
      N52.34 **Erectile dysfunction following simple prostatectomy** ☒♂
      N52.35 **Erectile dysfunction following radiation therapy** ☒♂
      N52.36 **Erectile dysfunction following interstitial seed therapy** ☒♂
      N52.37 **Erectile dysfunction following prostate ablative therapy** ☒♂
          Erectile dysfunction following cryotherapy
          Erectile dysfunction following other prostate ablative therapies
          Erectile dysfunction following ultrasound ablative therapies
      N52.39 **Other and unspecified postprocedural erectile dysfunction** ☒♂

  N52.8 **Other male erectile dysfunction** ☒♂

  N52.9 **Male erectile dysfunction, unspecified** ☒♂
      Impotence NOS

√4th **N53** **Other male sexual dysfunction**
    EXCLUDES 1   psychogenic sexual dysfunction (F52.-)

√5th   **N53.1** **Ejaculatory dysfunction**
    EXCLUDES 1   premature ejaculation (F52.4)
      N53.11 **Retarded ejaculation** ♂
      N53.12 **Painful ejaculation** ♂
      N53.13 **Anejaculatory orgasm** ♂
      N53.14 **Retrograde ejaculation** ♂
          DEF: A form of male sexual dysfunction in which the semen enters the bladder instead of going out through the urethra during ejaculation.
      N53.19 **Other ejaculatory dysfunction** ♂
          Ejaculatory dysfunction NOS

  N53.8 **Other male sexual dysfunction** ♂

  N53.9 **Unspecified male sexual dysfunction** ♂

Disorders of breast (N60-N65)

EXCLUDES 1   disorders of breast associated with childbirth (O91-O92)

√4th **N60** **Benign mammary dysplasia**
    INCLUDES   fibrocystic mastopathy

√5th   **N60.0** **Solitary cyst of breast**
      Cyst of breast
      N60.01 **Solitary cyst of right breast**
      N60.02 **Solitary cyst of left breast**
      N60.09 **Solitary cyst of unspecified breast**

√5th   **N60.1** **Diffuse cystic mastopathy**
      Cystic breast
      Fibrocystic disease of breast
      EXCLUDES 1   diffuse cystic mastopathy with epithelial proliferation (N60.3-)
      N60.11 **Diffuse cystic mastopathy of right breast** ☒
      N60.12 **Diffuse cystic mastopathy of left breast** ☒
      N60.19 **Diffuse cystic mastopathy of unspecified breast** ☒

√5th   **N60.2** **Fibroadenosis of breast**
      Adenofibrosis of breast
      EXCLUDES 2   fibroadenoma of breast (D24.-)
      N60.21 **Fibroadenosis of right breast**
      N60.22 **Fibroadenosis of left breast**
      N60.29 **Fibroadenosis of unspecified breast**

√5th   **N60.3** **Fibrosclerosis of breast**
      Cystic mastopathy with epithelial proliferation
      N60.31 **Fibrosclerosis of right breast**
      N60.32 **Fibrosclerosis of left breast**
      N60.39 **Fibrosclerosis of unspecified breast**

√5th   **N60.4** **Mammary duct ectasia**
      N60.41 **Mammary duct ectasia of right breast**
      N60.42 **Mammary duct ectasia of left breast**
      N60.49 **Mammary duct ectasia of unspecified breast**

√5th   **N60.8** **Other benign mammary dysplasias**
      N60.81 **Other benign mammary dysplasias of right breast**
      N60.82 **Other benign mammary dysplasias of left breast**
      N60.89 **Other benign mammary dysplasias of unspecified breast**

√5th   **N60.9** **Unspecified benign mammary dysplasia**
      N60.91 **Unspecified benign mammary dysplasia of right breast**
      N60.92 **Unspecified benign mammary dysplasia of left breast**
      N60.99 **Unspecified benign mammary dysplasia of unspecified breast**

√4th **N61** **Inflammatory disorders of breast**
    EXCLUDES 1   inflammatory carcinoma of breast (C50.9)
            inflammatory disorder of breast associated with childbirth (O91.-)
            neonatal infective mastitis (P39.0)
            thrombophlebitis of breast [Mondor's disease] (I80.8)

  N61.0 **Mastitis without abscess**
      Infective mastitis (acute) (nonpuerperal) (subacute)
      Mastitis (acute) (nonpuerperal) (subacute) NOS
      Cellulitis (acute) (nonpuerperal) (subacute) of breast NOS
      Cellulitis (acute) (nonpuerperal) (subacute) of nipple NOS

  N61.1 **Abscess of the breast and nipple**
      Abscess (acute) (chronic) (nonpuerperal) of areola
      Abscess (acute) (chronic) (nonpuerperal) of breast
      Carbuncle of breast
      Mastitis with abscess

N62 **Hypertrophy of breast**
    Gynecomastia
    Hypertrophy of breast NOS
    Massive pubertal hypertrophy of breast
    EXCLUDES 1   breast engorgement of newborn (P83.4)
            disproportion of reconstructed breast (N65.1)

√4th **N63** **Unspecified lump in breast**
    Nodule(s) NOS in breast

●   **N63.0** **Unspecified lump in unspecified breast**

● √5th   **N63.1** **Unspecified lump in the right breast**
●   **N63.10** **Unspecified lump in the right breast, unspecified quadrant**
●   **N63.11** **Unspecified lump in the right breast, upper outer quadrant**
●   **N63.12** **Unspecified lump in the right breast, upper inner quadrant**
●   **N63.13** **Unspecified lump in the right breast, lower outer quadrant**
●   **N63.14** **Unspecified lump in the right breast, lower inner quadrant**

● √5th   **N63.2** **Unspecified lump in the left breast**
●   **N63.20** **Unspecified lump in the left breast, unspecified quadrant**
●   **N63.21** **Unspecified lump in the left breast, upper outer quadrant**

- **N63.22   Unspecified lump in the left breast, upper inner quadrant**
- **N63.23   Unspecified lump in the left breast, lower outer quadrant**
- **N63.24   Unspecified lump in the left breast, lower inner quadrant**
- ✓5th **N63.3 Unspecified lump in axillary tail**
- **N63.31   Unspecified lump in axillary tail of the right breast**
- **N63.32   Unspecified lump in axillary tail of the left breast**
- ✓5th **N63.4 Unspecified lump in breast, subareolar**
- **N63.41   Unspecified lump in right breast, subareolar**
- **N63.42   Unspecified lump in left breast, subareolar**

✓4th **N64   Other disorders of breast**
> EXCLUDES 2   *mechanical complication of breast prosthesis and implant (T85.4-)*

N64.0   Fissure and fistula of nipple

N64.1   Fat necrosis of breast
> Fat necrosis (segmental) of breast
> Code first breast necrosis due to breast graft (T85.898)

N64.2   Atrophy of breast

N64.3   Galactorrhea not associated with childbirth

N64.4   Mastodynia

✓5th **N64.5   Other signs and symptoms in breast**
> EXCLUDES 2   *abnormal findings on diagnostic imaging of breast (R92.-)*

N64.51   Induration of breast

N64.52   Nipple discharge
> EXCLUDES 1   *abnormal findings in nipple discharge (R89.-)*

N64.53   Retraction of nipple

N64.59   Other signs and symptoms in breast

✓5th **N64.8   Other specified disorders of breast**

N64.81   Ptosis of breast   A
> EXCLUDES 1   *ptosis of native breast in relation to reconstructed breast (N65.1)*

N64.82   Hypoplasia of breast   A
> Micromastia
> EXCLUDES 1   *congenital absence of breast (Q83.0)*
> *hypoplasia of native breast in relation to reconstructed breast (N65.1)*

N64.89   Other specified disorders of breast
> Galactocele
> Subinvolution of breast (postlactational)

N64.9   Disorder of breast, unspecified

✓4th **N65   Deformity and disproportion of reconstructed breast**

N65.0   Deformity of reconstructed breast   A
> Contour irregularity in reconstructed breast
> Excess tissue in reconstructed breast
> Misshapen reconstructed breast

N65.1   Disproportion of reconstructed breast   A
> Breast asymmetry between native breast and reconstructed breast
> Disproportion between native breast and reconstructed breast

Inflammatory diseases of female pelvic organs (N70-N77)

> EXCLUDES 1   *inflammatory diseases of female pelvic organs complicating:*
> *abortion or ectopic or molar pregnancy (O00-O07, O08.0)*
> *pregnancy, childbirth and the puerperium (O23-, O75.3, O85, O86-)*

✓4th **N70   Salpingitis and oophoritis**
> INCLUDES   abscess (of) fallopian tube
> abscess (of) ovary
> pyosalpinx
> salpingo-oophoritis
> tubo-ovarian abscess
> tubo-ovarian inflammatory disease
> Use additional code (B95-B97), to identify infectious agent
> EXCLUDES 1   *gonococcal infection (A54.24)*
> *tuberculous infection (A18.17)*

> **CC Excl: For CC codes in category N70:** PDX collection 942

✓5th **N70.0   Acute salpingitis and oophoritis**
> **N70.01   Acute salpingitis**   CC ♀
> **N70.02   Acute oophoritis**   CC ♀
> **N70.03   Acute salpingitis and oophoritis**   CC ♀

✓5th **N70.1   Chronic salpingitis and oophoritis**
> Hydrosalpinx
> **N70.11   Chronic salpingitis**   ♀
> **N70.12   Chronic oophoritis**   ♀
> **N70.13   Chronic salpingitis and oophoritis**   ♀

✓5th **N70.9   Salpingitis and oophoritis, unspecified**
> **N70.91   Salpingitis, unspecified**   ♀
> **N70.92   Oophoritis, unspecified**   ♀
> **N70.93   Salpingitis and oophoritis, unspecified**   ♀

✓4th **N71   Inflammatory disease of uterus, except cervix**
> INCLUDES   endo (myo) metritis
> metritis
> myometritis
> pyometra
> uterine abscess
> Use additional code (B95-B97), to identify infectious agent
> EXCLUDES 1   *hyperplastic endometritis (N85.0-)*
> *infection of uterus following delivery (O85, O86.-)*

N71.0   Acute inflammatory disease of uterus   CC ♀
> CC Excl: PDX collection 943

N71.1   Chronic inflammatory disease of uterus   ♀

N71.9   Inflammatory disease of uterus, unspecified   ♀

N72   Inflammatory disease of cervix uteri   ♀
> INCLUDES   cervicitis (with or without erosion or ectropion)
> endocervicitis (with or without erosion or ectropion)
> exocervicitis (with or without erosion or ectropion)
> Use additional code (B95-B97), to identify infectious agent
> EXCLUDES 1   *erosion and ectropion of cervix without cervicitis (N86)*

✓4th **N73   Other female pelvic inflammatory diseases**
> Use additional code (B95-B97), to identify infectious agent

> **CC Excl: For CC/MCC codes in category N73:** PDX collection 942

N73.0   Acute parametritis and pelvic cellulitis   CC ♀
> Abscess of broad ligament
> Abscess of parametrium
> Pelvic cellulitis, female
> **DEF:** Parametritis: Inflammation of the parametrium; pelvic cellulitis is a synonym for parametritis.

N73.1   Chronic parametritis and pelvic cellulitis   ♀
> Any condition in N73.0 specified as chronic
> EXCLUDES 1   *tuberculous parametritis and pelvic cellulitis (A18.17)*

N73.2   Unspecified parametritis and pelvic cellulitis   ♀
> Any condition in N73.0 unspecified whether acute or chronic

N73.3   Female acute pelvic peritonitis   MCC ♀

N73.4   Female chronic pelvic peritonitis   CC ♀
> EXCLUDES 1   *tuberculous pelvic (female) peritonitis (A18.17)*

N73.5   Female pelvic peritonitis, unspecified   ♀

N73.6   Female pelvic peritoneal adhesions (postinfective)   ♀
> EXCLUDES 2   *postprocedural pelvic peritoneal adhesions (N99.4)*
> **AHA:** 2014, 1Q, 6

N73.8   Other specified female pelvic inflammatory diseases   ♀

N73.9   Female pelvic inflammatory disease, unspecified   ♀
> Female pelvic infection or inflammation NOS

N74   Female pelvic inflammatory disorders in diseases classified elsewhere   ♀
> Code first underlying disease
> EXCLUDES 1   *chlamydial cervicitis (A56.02)*
> *chlamydial pelvic inflammatory disease (A56.11)*
> *gonococcal cervicitis (A54.03)*
> *gonococcal pelvic inflammatory disease (A54.24)*
> *herpesviral [herpes simplex] cervicitis (A60.03)*
> *herpesviral [herpes simplex] pelvic inflammatory disease (A60.09)*
> *syphilitic cervicitis (A52.76)*
> *syphilitic pelvic inflammatory disease (A52.76)*
> *trichomonal cervicitis (A59.09)*
> *tuberculous cervicitis (A18.16)*
> *tuberculous pelvic inflammatory disease (A18.17)*

✓4th **N75   Diseases of Bartholin's gland**

N75.0   Cyst of Bartholin's gland   ♀

N75.1   Abscess of Bartholin's gland   CC ♀
> CC Excl: PDX collection 944

N75.8   Other diseases of Bartholin's gland   ♀
> Bartholinitis

N75.9   Disease of Bartholin's gland, unspecified   ♀

✓4ᵗʰ **N76** **Other inflammation of vagina and vulva**
Use additional code (B95-B97), to identify infectious agent
EXCLUDES 2 *senile (atrophic) vaginitis (N95.2)*
vulvar vestibulitis (N94.810)

    N76.0 **Acute vaginitis** ♀
        Acute vulvovaginitis   Vulvovaginitis NOS
        Vaginitis NOS

    N76.1 **Subacute and chronic vaginitis** ♀
        Chronic vulvovaginitis
        Subacute vulvovaginitis

    N76.2 **Acute vulvitis** ♀
        Vulvitis NOS

    N76.3 **Subacute and chronic vulvitis** ♀

    N76.4 **Abscess of vulva** CC ♀
        Furuncle of vulva
        CC Excl: PDX collection 944

    N76.5 **Ulceration of vagina** ♀

    N76.6 **Ulceration of vulva** ♀

✓5ᵗʰ   **N76.8** **Other specified inflammation of vagina and vulva**
        N76.81 **Mucositis (ulcerative) of vagina and vulva** CC ♀
            Code also type of associated therapy, such as:
                antineoplastic and immunosuppressive drugs
                (T45.1X-)
                radiological procedure and radiotherapy (Y84.2)
            EXCLUDES 2 *gastrointestinal mucositis (ulcerative)*
                  (K92.81)
                nasal mucositis (ulcerative) (J34.81)
                oral mucositis (ulcerative) (K12.3-)
            CC Excl: PDX collection 945
        N76.89 **Other specified inflammation of vagina and vulva** ♀

✓4ᵗʰ **N77** **Vulvovaginal ulceration and inflammation in diseases classified elsewhere**

    N77.0 ***Ulceration of vulva in diseases classified elsewhere*** ♀
        Code first underlying disease, such as:
            Behçet's disease (M35.2)
        EXCLUDES 1 *ulceration of vulva in gonococcal infection (A54.02)*
            ulceration of vulva in herpesviral [herpes simplex]
               infection (A60.04)
            ulceration of vulva in syphilis (A51.0)
            ulceration of vulva in tuberculosis (A18.18)

    N77.1 ***Vaginitis, vulvitis and vulvovaginitis in diseases classified elsewhere*** ♀
        Code first underlying disease, such as:
            pinworm (B80)
        EXCLUDES 1 *candidal vulvovaginitis (B37.3)*
            chlamydial vulvovaginitis (A56.02)
            gonococcal vulvovaginitis (A54.02)
            herpesviral [herpes simplex] vulvovaginitis (A60.04)
            trichomonal vulvovaginitis (A59.01)
            tuberculous vulvovaginitis (A18.18)
            vulvovaginitis in early syphilis (A51.0)
            vulvovaginitis in late syphilis (A52.76)

Noninflammatory disorders of female genital tract (N80-N98)

✓4ᵗʰ **N80** **Endometriosis**

    N80.0 **Endometriosis of uterus** ♀
        Adenomyosis
        EXCLUDES 1 *stromal endometriosis (D39.0)*

    N80.1 **Endometriosis of ovary** ♀

    N80.2 **Endometriosis of fallopian tube** ♀

    N80.3 **Endometriosis of pelvic peritoneum** ♀

    N80.4 **Endometriosis of rectovaginal septum and vagina** ♀

    N80.5 **Endometriosis of intestine** ♀

    N80.6 **Endometriosis in cutaneous scar** ♀

    N80.8 **Other endometriosis** ♀
        ▶Endometriosis of thorax◀

    N80.9 **Endometriosis, unspecified** ♀

✓4ᵗʰ **N81** **Female genital prolapse**
    EXCLUDES 1 *genital prolapse complicating pregnancy, labor or delivery (O34.5-)*
        prolapse and hernia of ovary and fallopian tube (N83.4-)
        prolapse of vaginal vault after hysterectomy (N99.3)

    N81.0 **Urethrocele** ♀
        EXCLUDES 1 *urethrocele with cystocele (N81.1-)*
            urethrocele with prolapse of uterus (N81.2-N81.4)

Types of Pelvic Organ Prolapse

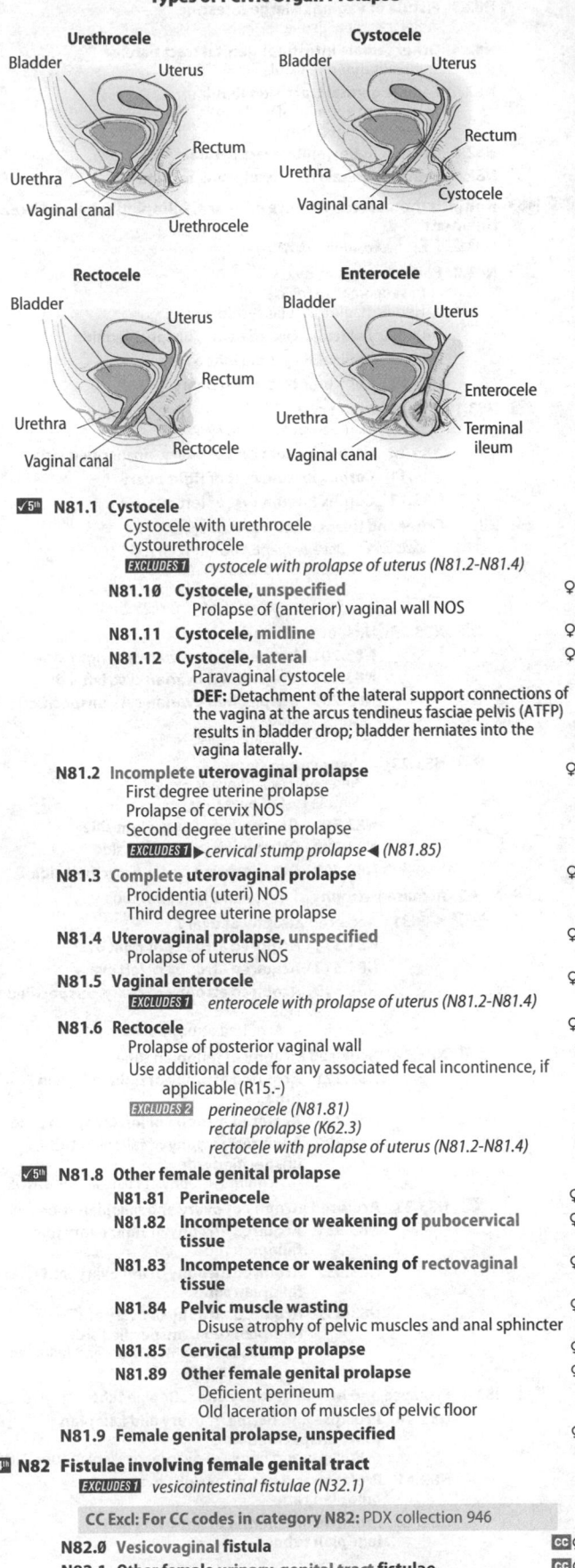

✓5ᵗʰ **N81.1** **Cystocele**
        Cystocele with urethrocele
        Cystourethrocele
        EXCLUDES 1 *cystocele with prolapse of uterus (N81.2-N81.4)*

        N81.10 **Cystocele, unspecified** ♀
            Prolapse of (anterior) vaginal wall NOS

        N81.11 **Cystocele, midline** ♀

        N81.12 **Cystocele, lateral** ♀
            Paravaginal cystocele
            DEF: Detachment of the lateral support connections of the vagina at the arcus tendineus fasciae pelvis (ATFP) results in bladder drop; bladder herniates into the vagina laterally.

    N81.2 **Incomplete uterovaginal prolapse** ♀
        First degree uterine prolapse
        Prolapse of cervix NOS
        Second degree uterine prolapse
        EXCLUDES 1 ▶*cervical stump prolapse*◀ *(N81.85)*

    N81.3 **Complete uterovaginal prolapse** ♀
        Procidentia (uteri) NOS
        Third degree uterine prolapse

    N81.4 **Uterovaginal prolapse, unspecified** ♀
        Prolapse of uterus NOS

    N81.5 **Vaginal enterocele** ♀
        EXCLUDES 1 *enterocele with prolapse of uterus (N81.2-N81.4)*

    N81.6 **Rectocele** ♀
        Prolapse of posterior vaginal wall
        Use additional code for any associated fecal incontinence, if applicable (R15.-)
        EXCLUDES 2 *perineocele (N81.81)*
            rectal prolapse (K62.3)
            rectocele with prolapse of uterus (N81.2-N81.4)

✓5ᵗʰ **N81.8** **Other female genital prolapse**
        N81.81 **Perineocele** ♀

        N81.82 **Incompetence or weakening of pubocervical tissue** ♀

        N81.83 **Incompetence or weakening of rectovaginal tissue** ♀

        N81.84 **Pelvic muscle wasting** ♀
            Disuse atrophy of pelvic muscles and anal sphincter

        N81.85 **Cervical stump prolapse** ♀

        N81.89 **Other female genital prolapse** ♀
            Deficient perineum
            Old laceration of muscles of pelvic floor

    N81.9 **Female genital prolapse, unspecified** ♀

✓4ᵗʰ **N82** **Fistulae involving female genital tract**
    EXCLUDES 1 *vesicointestinal fistulae (N32.1)*

    CC Excl: For CC codes in category N82: PDX collection 946

    N82.0 **Vesicovaginal fistula** CC ♀

    N82.1 **Other female urinary-genital tract fistulae** CC ♀
        Cervicovesical fistula   Uteroureteric fistula
        Ureterovaginal fistula   Uterovesical fistula
        Urethrovaginal fistula

✓ Additional Character Req   ✓x7ᵗʰ Placeholder Alert   Unacceptable PDx   Manifestation   H1-H14 HAC   HCC CMS-HCC Condition   EXCLUDES 1 Not Coded Here   EXCLUDES 2 Not Included Here

ICD-10-CM 2018   833

N76–N82.1

N82.2   **Fistula of vagina to small intestine**   CC ♀

N82.3   **Fistula of vagina to large intestine**   CC ♀
     Rectovaginal fistula

N82.4   **Other female intestinal-genital tract fistulae**   CC ♀
     Intestinouterine fistula

N82.5   **Female genital tract-skin fistulae**   CC ♀
     Uterus to abdominal wall fistula
     Vaginoperineal fistula

N82.8   **Other female genital tract fistulae**   CC ♀

N82.9   **Female genital tract fistula, unspecified**   CC ♀

√4ᵗʰ **N83**   **Noninflammatory disorders of ovary, fallopian tube and broad ligament**
     EXCLUDES 2   *hydrosalpinx (N70.1-)*

√5ᵗʰ **N83.0**   **Follicular cyst of ovary**
     Cyst of graafian follicle
     Hemorrhagic follicular cyst (of ovary)

     N83.00   **Follicular cyst of ovary, unspecified side**   ♀

     N83.01   **Follicular cyst of right ovary**   ♀

     N83.02   **Follicular cyst of left ovary**   ♀

√5ᵗʰ **N83.1**   **Corpus luteum cyst**
     Hemorrhagic corpus luteum cyst

     N83.10   **Corpus luteum cyst of ovary, unspecified side**   ♀

     N83.11   **Corpus luteum cyst of right ovary**   ♀

     N83.12   **Corpus luteum cyst of left ovary**   ♀

√5ᵗʰ **N83.2**   **Other and unspecified ovarian cysts**
     EXCLUDES 1   *developmental ovarian cyst (Q50.1)*
          neoplastic ovarian cyst (D27.-)
          polycystic ovarian syndrome (E28.2)
          Stein-Leventhal syndrome (E28.2)

     √6ᵗʰ **N83.20**   **Unspecified ovarian cysts**

         N83.201   **Unspecified ovarian cyst, right side**   ♀

         N83.202   **Unspecified ovarian cyst, left side**   ♀

         N83.209   **Unspecified ovarian cyst, unspecified side**   ♀
            Ovarian cyst, NOS

     √6ᵗʰ **N83.29**   **Other ovarian cysts**
         Retention cyst of ovary
         Simple cyst of ovary

         N83.291   **Other ovarian cyst, right side**   ♀

         N83.292   **Other ovarian cyst, left side**   ♀

         N83.299   **Other ovarian cyst, unspecified side**   ♀

√5ᵗʰ **N83.3**   **Acquired atrophy of ovary and fallopian tube**

     √6ᵗʰ **N83.31**   **Acquired atrophy of ovary**

         N83.311   **Acquired atrophy of right ovary**   ♀

         N83.312   **Acquired atrophy of left ovary**   ♀

         N83.319   **Acquired atrophy of ovary, unspecified side**   ♀
            Acquired atrophy of ovary, NOS

     √6ᵗʰ **N83.32**   **Acquired atrophy of fallopian tube**

         N83.321   **Acquired atrophy of right fallopian tube**   ♀

         N83.322   **Acquired atrophy of left fallopian tube**   ♀

         N83.329   **Acquired atrophy of fallopian tube, unspecified side**   ♀
            Acquired atrophy of fallopian tube, NOS

     √6ᵗʰ **N83.33**   **Acquired atrophy of ovary and fallopian tube**

         N83.331   **Acquired atrophy of right ovary and fallopian tube**   ♀

         N83.332   **Acquired atrophy of left ovary and fallopian tube**   ♀

         N83.339   **Acquired atrophy of ovary and fallopian tube, unspecified side**   ♀
            Acquired atrophy of ovary and fallopian tube, NOS

√5ᵗʰ **N83.4**   **Prolapse and hernia of ovary and fallopian tube**

     N83.40   **Prolapse and hernia of ovary and fallopian tube, unspecified side**   ♀
         Prolapse and hernia of ovary and fallopian tube, NOS

     N83.41   **Prolapse and hernia of right ovary and fallopian tube**   ♀

     N83.42   **Prolapse and hernia of left ovary and fallopian tube**   ♀

√5ᵗʰ **N83.5**   **Torsion of ovary, ovarian pedicle and fallopian tube**
     Torsion of accessory tube

     CC Excl: For CC codes in subcategory N83.5:
     PDX collection 947

     √6ᵗʰ **N83.51**   **Torsion of ovary and ovarian pedicle**

         N83.511   **Torsion of right ovary and ovarian pedicle**   CC ♀

         N83.512   **Torsion of left ovary and ovarian pedicle**   CC ♀

         N83.519   **Torsion of ovary and ovarian pedicle, unspecified side**   CC ♀
            Torsion of ovary and ovarian pedicle, NOS

     √6ᵗʰ **N83.52**   **Torsion of fallopian tube**
         Torsion of hydatid of Morgagni

         N83.521   **Torsion of right fallopian tube**   CC ♀

         N83.522   **Torsion of left fallopian tube**   CC ♀

         N83.529   **Torsion of fallopian tube, unspecified side**   CC ♀
            Torsion of fallopian tube, NOS

     N83.53   **Torsion of ovary, ovarian pedicle and fallopian tube**   CC ♀

N83.6   **Hematosalpinx**   ♀
     EXCLUDES 1   *hematosalpinx (with) (in):*
          hematocolpos (N89.7)
          hematometra (N85.7)
          tubal pregnancy (O00.1-)

N83.7   **Hematoma of broad ligament**   ♀

N83.8   **Other noninflammatory disorders of ovary, fallopian tube and broad ligament**   ♀
     Broad ligament laceration syndrome [Allen-Masters]

N83.9   **Noninflammatory disorder of ovary, fallopian tube and broad ligament, unspecified**

√4ᵗʰ **N84**   **Polyp of female genital tract**
     EXCLUDES 1   *adenomatous polyp (D28.-)*
          placental polyp (O90.89)

N84.0   **Polyp of corpus uteri**   ♀
     Polyp of endometrium   Polyp of uterus NOS
     EXCLUDES 1   *polypoid endometrial hyperplasia (N85.0-)*

N84.1   **Polyp of cervix uteri**   ♀
     Mucous polyp of cervix

N84.2   **Polyp of vagina**   ♀

N84.3   **Polyp of vulva**   ♀
     Polyp of labia

N84.8   **Polyp of other parts of female genital tract**   ♀

N84.9   **Polyp of female genital tract, unspecified**   ♀

√4ᵗʰ **N85**   **Other noninflammatory disorders of uterus, except cervix**
     EXCLUDES 1   *endometriosis (N80.-)*
          inflammatory diseases of uterus (N71.-)
          noninflammatory disorders of cervix, except malposition
            (N86-N88)
          polyp of corpus uteri (N84.0)
          uterine prolapse (N81.-)

     √5ᵗʰ **N85.0**   **Endometrial hyperplasia**

         N85.00   **Endometrial hyperplasia, unspecified**   ♀
            Hyperplasia (adenomatous) (cystic) (glandular) of endometrium
            Hyperplastic endometritis

         N85.01   **Benign endometrial hyperplasia**   ♀
            Endometrial hyperplasia (complex) (simple) without atypia

         N85.02   **Endometrial intraepithelial neoplasia [EIN]**   ♀
            Endometrial hyperplasia with atypia
            EXCLUDES 1   *malignant neoplasm of endometrium (with endometrial intraepithelial neoplasia [EIN]) (C54.1)*

     N85.2   **Hypertrophy of uterus**   ♀
         Bulky or enlarged uterus
         EXCLUDES 1   *puerperal hypertrophy of uterus (O90.89)*

     N85.3   **Subinvolution of uterus**   ♀
         EXCLUDES 1   *puerperal subinvolution of uterus (O90.89)*

     N85.4   **Malposition of uterus**   ♀
         Anteversion of uterus
         Retroflexion of uterus
         Retroversion of uterus
         EXCLUDES 1   *malposition of uterus complicating pregnancy, labor or delivery (O34.5-, O65.5)*

N Newborn: 0   P Pediatric: 0-17   M Maternity: 12-55   A Adult: 15-124   MCC Major CC Condition   PDxMCC PDx acts as own MCC   CC CC Condition   PDxCC PDx acts as own CC

Inversion of Uterus

Uterus

N85.5 Inversion of uterus ♀
- EXCLUDES 1 *current obstetric trauma (O71.2)*
  postpartum inversion of uterus (O71.2)

N85.6 Intrauterine synechiae ♀

N85.7 Hematometra ♀
- Hematosalpinx with hematometra
- EXCLUDES 1 *hematometra with hematocolpos (N89.7)*
- **DEF:** Accumulation of blood within the uterus.

N85.8 Other specified noninflammatory disorders of uterus ♀
- Atrophy of uterus, acquired
- Fibrosis of uterus NOS

N85.9 Noninflammatory disorder of uterus, unspecified ♀
- Disorder of uterus NOS

N86 Erosion and ectropion of cervix uteri ♀
- Decubitus (trophic) ulcer of cervix
- Eversion of cervix
- EXCLUDES 1 *erosion and ectropion of cervix with cervicitis (N72)*

✓4th N87 Dysplasia of cervix uteri
- EXCLUDES 1 *abnormal results from cervical cytologic examination without*
  histologic confirmation (R87.61-)
  carcinoma in situ of cervix uteri (D06.-)
  cervical intraepithelial neoplasia III [CIN III] (D06.-)
  HGSIL of cervix (R87.613)
  severe dysplasia of cervix uteri (D06.-)

N87.0 Mild cervical dysplasia ♀
- Cervical intraepithelial neoplasia I [CIN I]

N87.1 Moderate cervical dysplasia ♀
- Cervical intraepithelial neoplasia II [CIN II]

N87.9 Dysplasia of cervix uteri, unspecified ♀
- Anaplasia of cervix
- Cervical atypism
- Cervical dysplasia NOS

✓4th N88 Other noninflammatory disorders of cervix uteri
- EXCLUDES 2 *inflammatory disease of cervix (N72)*
  polyp of cervix (N84.1)

N88.0 Leukoplakia of cervix uteri ♀

N88.1 Old laceration of cervix uteri ♀
- Adhesions of cervix
- EXCLUDES 1 *current obstetric trauma (O71.3)*

N88.2 Stricture and stenosis of cervix uteri ♀
- EXCLUDES 1 *stricture and stenosis of cervix uteri complicating labor*
  (O65.5)

N88.3 Incompetence of cervix uteri ♀
- Investigation and management of (suspected) cervical
  incompetence in a nonpregnant woman
- EXCLUDES 1 *cervical incompetence complicating pregnancy*
  (O34.3-)

N88.4 Hypertrophic elongation of cervix uteri ♀

N88.8 Other specified noninflammatory disorders of cervix uteri ♀
- EXCLUDES 1 *current obstetric trauma (O71.3)*

N88.9 Noninflammatory disorder of cervix uteri, unspecified ♀

✓4th N89 Other noninflammatory disorders of vagina
- EXCLUDES 1 *abnormal results from vaginal cytologic examination without*
  histologic confirmation (R87.62-)
  carcinoma in situ of vagina (D07.2)
  HGSIL of vagina (R87.623)
  inflammation of vagina (N76.-)
  senile (atrophic) vaginitis (N95.2)
  severe dysplasia of vagina (D07.2)
  trichomonal leukorrhea (A59.00)
  vaginal intraepithelial neoplasia [VAIN], grade III (D07.2)

N89.0 Mild vaginal dysplasia ♀
- Vaginal intraepithelial neoplasia [VAIN], grade I

N89.1 Moderate vaginal dysplasia ♀
- Vaginal intraepithelial neoplasia [VAIN], grade II

N89.3 Dysplasia of vagina, unspecified ♀

N89.4 Leukoplakia of vagina ♀

N89.5 Stricture and atresia of vagina ♀
- Vaginal adhesions   Vaginal stenosis
- EXCLUDES 1 *congenital atresia or stricture (Q52.4)*
  postprocedural adhesions of vagina (N99.2)

N89.6 Tight hymenal ring ♀
- Rigid hymen
- Tight introitus
- EXCLUDES 1 *imperforate hymen (Q52.3)*

N89.7 Hematocolpos ♀
- Hematocolpos with hematometra or hematosalpinx

N89.8 Other specified noninflammatory disorders of vagina ♀
- Leukorrhea NOS
- Old vaginal laceration
- Pessary ulcer of vagina
- EXCLUDES 1 *current obstetric trauma (O70-, O71.4, O71.7-O71.8)*
  old laceration involving muscles of pelvic floor (N81.8)

N89.9 Noninflammatory disorder of vagina, unspecified ♀

✓4th N90 Other noninflammatory disorders of vulva and perineum
- EXCLUDES 1 *anogenital (venereal) warts (A63.0)*
  carcinoma in situ of vulva (D07.1)
  condyloma acuminatum (A63.0)
  current obstetric trauma (O70-, O71.7-O71.8)
  inflammation of vulva (N76.-)
  severe dysplasia of vulva (D07.1)
  vulvar intraepithelial neoplasm III [VIN III] (D07.1)

N90.0 Mild vulvar dysplasia ♀
- Vulvar intraepithelial neoplasia [VIN], grade I

N90.1 Moderate vulvar dysplasia ♀
- Vulvar intraepithelial neoplasia [VIN], grade II

N90.3 Dysplasia of vulva, unspecified ♀

N90.4 Leukoplakia of vulva ♀
- Dystrophy of vulva
- Kraurosis of vulva
- Lichen sclerosus of external female genital organs

N90.5 Atrophy of vulva ♀
- Stenosis of vulva

✓5th N90.6 Hypertrophy of vulva

    N90.60 Unspecified hypertrophy of vulva ♀
- Unspecified hypertrophy of labia

    N90.61 Childhood asymmetric labium majus enlargement ♀
- CALME

    N90.69 Other specified hypertrophy of vulva ♀
- Other specified hypertrophy of labia

N90.7 Vulvar cyst ♀

✓5th N90.8 Other specified noninflammatory disorders of vulva and perineum

    ✓6th N90.81 Female genital mutilation status
- Female genital cutting status

        N90.810 Female genital mutilation status, unspecified ♀
- Female genital cutting status, unspecified
- Female genital mutilation status NOS

        N90.811 Female genital mutilation Type I status ♀
- Clitorectomy status
- Female genital cutting Type I status

        N90.812 Female genital mutilation Type II status ♀
- Clitorectomy with excision of labia minora status
- Female genital cutting Type II status

        N90.813 Female genital mutilation Type III status ♀
- Female genital cutting Type III status
- Infibulation status

✓ Additional Character Req   Vx7th Placeholder Alert   Unacceptable PDx   Manifestation   H1 - H14 HAC   HCC CMS-HCC Condition   EXCLUDES 1 Not Coded Here   EXCLUDES 2 Not Included Here

ICD-10-CM 2018   835

Chapter 14. Diseases of Genitourinary System

N90.818 **Other female genital mutilation status** ♀
Female genital cutting Type IV status
Female genital mutilation Type IV status
Other female genital cutting status

N90.89 **Other specified noninflammatory disorders of vulva and perineum** ♀
Adhesions of vulva
Hypertrophy of clitoris

N90.9 **Noninflammatory disorder of vulva and perineum, unspecified** ♀

✓4ᵗʰ **N91** **Absent, scanty and rare menstruation**
EXCLUDES 1   *ovarian dysfunction (E28.-)*

N91.0 **Primary amenorrhea** ♀
N91.1 **Secondary amenorrhea** ♀
N91.2 **Amenorrhea, unspecified** ♀
N91.3 **Primary oligomenorrhea** ♀
N91.4 **Secondary oligomenorrhea** ♀
N91.5 **Oligomenorrhea, unspecified** ♀
Hypomenorrhea NOS

✓4ᵗʰ **N92** **Excessive, frequent and irregular menstruation**
EXCLUDES 1   *postmenopausal bleeding (N95.0)*
precocious puberty (menstruation) (E30.1)

N92.0 **Excessive and frequent menstruation with regular cycle** ♀
Heavy periods NOS
Menorrhagia NOS
Polymenorrhea

N92.1 **Excessive and frequent menstruation with irregular cycle** ♀
Irregular intermenstrual bleeding
Irregular, shortened intervals between menstrual bleeding
Menometrorrhagia
Metrorrhagia

N92.2 **Excessive menstruation at puberty** P♀
Excessive bleeding associated with onset of menstrual periods
Pubertal menorrhagia
Puberty bleeding

N92.3 **Ovulation bleeding** ♀
Regular intermenstrual bleeding

N92.4 **Excessive bleeding in the premenopausal period** ♀
Climacteric menorrhagia or metrorrhagia
Menopausal menorrhagia or metrorrhagia
Preclimacteric menorrhagia or metrorrhagia
Premenopausal menorrhagia or metrorrhagia

N92.5 **Other specified irregular menstruation** ♀
N92.6 **Irregular menstruation, unspecified** ♀
Irregular bleeding NOS
Irregular periods NOS
EXCLUDES 1   *irregular menstruation with:*
lengthened intervals or scanty bleeding (N91.3-N91.5)
shortened intervals or excessive bleeding (N92.1)

✓4ᵗʰ **N93** **Other abnormal uterine and vaginal bleeding**
EXCLUDES 1   *neonatal vaginal hemorrhage (P54.6)*
precocious puberty (menstruation) (E30.1)
pseudomenses (P54.6)

N93.0 **Postcoital and contact bleeding** ♀
N93.1 **Pre-pubertal vaginal bleeding** ♀
N93.8 **Other specified abnormal uterine and vaginal bleeding** ♀
Dysfunctional or functional uterine or vaginal bleeding NOS

N93.9 **Abnormal uterine and vaginal bleeding, unspecified** ♀

✓4ᵗʰ **N94** **Pain and other conditions associated with female genital organs and menstrual cycle**

N94.0 **Mittelschmerz** ♀
DEF: One-sided, lower abdominal pain occurring between menstrual periods; associated with ovulation.

✓5ᵗʰ **N94.1** **Dyspareunia**
EXCLUDES 1   *psychogenic dyspareunia (F52.6)*

N94.10 **Unspecified dyspareunia** ♀
N94.11 **Superficial (introital) dyspareunia** ♀
N94.12 **Deep dyspareunia** ♀
N94.19 **Other specified dyspareunia** ♀

N94.2 **Vaginismus** ♀
EXCLUDES 1   *psychogenic vaginismus (F52.5)*

N94.3 **Premenstrual tension syndrome** ♀
~~Premenstrual dysphoric disorder~~
Code also associated menstrual migraine (G43.82-, G43.83-)
EXCLUDES 1   *premenstrual dysphoric disorder (F32.81)*

N94.4 **Primary dysmenorrhea** ♀
N94.5 **Secondary dysmenorrhea** ♀
N94.6 **Dysmenorrhea, unspecified** ♀
EXCLUDES 1   *psychogenic dysmenorrhea (F45.8)*

✓5ᵗʰ **N94.8** **Other specified conditions associated with female genital organs and menstrual cycle**

✓6ᵗʰ **N94.81** **Vulvodynia**
N94.810 **Vulvar vestibulitis** ♀
N94.818 **Other vulvodynia** ♀
N94.819 **Vulvodynia, unspecified** ♀
Vulvodynia NOS

N94.89 **Other specified conditions associated with female genital organs and menstrual cycle** ♀

N94.9 **Unspecified condition associated with female genital organs and menstrual cycle** ♀

✓4ᵗʰ **N95** **Menopausal and other perimenopausal disorders**
Menopausal and other perimenopausal disorders due to naturally occurring (age-related) menopause and perimenopause
EXCLUDES 1   *excessive bleeding in the premenopausal period (N92.4)*
menopausal and perimenopausal disorders due to artificial or premature menopause (E89.4-, E28.31-)
premature menopause (E28.31-)
EXCLUDES 2   *postmenopausal osteoporosis (M81.0-)*
postmenopausal osteoporosis with current pathological fracture (M80.0-)
postmenopausal urethritis (N34.2)

N95.0 **Postmenopausal bleeding** ♀
N95.1 **Menopausal and female climacteric states** ♀
Symptoms such as flushing, sleeplessness, headache, lack of concentration, associated with natural (age-related) menopause
Use additional code for associated symptoms
EXCLUDES 1   *asymptomatic menopausal state (Z78.0)*
symptoms associated with artificial menopause (E89.41)
symptoms associated with premature menopause (E28.310)

N95.2 **Postmenopausal atrophic vaginitis** ♀
Senile (atrophic) vaginitis

N95.8 **Other specified menopausal and perimenopausal disorders** ♀

N95.9 **Unspecified menopausal and perimenopausal disorder** ♀

N96 **Recurrent pregnancy loss** ♀
Investigation or care in a nonpregnant woman with history of recurrent pregnancy loss
EXCLUDES 1   *recurrent pregnancy loss with current pregnancy (O26.2-)*

✓4ᵗʰ **N97** **Female infertility**
INCLUDES   inability to achieve a pregnancy
sterility, female NOS
EXCLUDES 1   *female infertility associated with:*
hypopituitarism (E23.0)
Stein-Leventhal syndrome (E28.2)
EXCLUDES 2   *incompetence of cervix uteri (N88.3)*
DEF: Infertility: Inability to conceive for at least one year with regular intercourse.
DEF: Primary infertility: Infertility occurring in patients who have never conceived.
DEF: Secondary infertility: Infertility occurring in patients who have previously conceived.

N97.0 **Female infertility associated with anovulation** ♀
N97.1 **Female infertility of tubal origin** ♀
Female infertility associated with congenital anomaly of tube
Female infertility due to tubal block
Female infertility due to tubal occlusion
Female infertility due to tubal stenosis

N97.2 **Female infertility of uterine origin** ♀
Female infertility associated with congenital anomaly of uterus
Female infertility due to nonimplantation of ovum

N97.8 **Female infertility of other origin** ♀
N97.9 **Female infertility, unspecified** ♀

✓4ᵗʰ **N98** **Complications associated with artificial fertilization**

CC Excl: For CC codes in category N98, unless otherwise noted:
PDX collection 643

N98.0 **Infection associated with artificial insemination** CC ♀
CC Excl: PDX collection 948

N98.1 **Hyperstimulation of ovaries** CC ♀
Hyperstimulation of ovaries NOS
Hyperstimulation of ovaries associated with induced ovulation

---

Ⓝ Newborn: 0   Ⓟ Pediatric: 0-17   Ⓜ Maternity: 12-55   Ⓐ Adult: 15-124   **MCC** Major CC Condition   **PDxMCC** PDx acts as own MCC   **CC** CC Condition   **PDxCC** PDx acts as own CC

N98.2   **Complications of attempted introduction of fertilized ovum following in vitro fertilization**   `CC` ♀

N98.3   **Complications of attempted introduction of embryo in embryo transfer**   `CC` ♀

N98.8   **Other complications associated with artificial fertilization**   `CC` ♀

N98.9   **Complication associated with artificial fertilization, unspecified**   `CC` ♀

Intraoperative and postprocedural complications and disorders of genitourinary system, not elsewhere classified (N99)

☑4ᵗʰ **N99**   **Intraoperative and postprocedural complications and disorders of genitourinary system, not elsewhere classified**

> *EXCLUDES 2*   irradiation cystitis (N30.4-)
> postoophorectomy osteoporosis with current pathological fracture (M80.8-)
> postoophorectomy osteoporosis without current pathological fracture (M81.8)

N99.0   **Postprocedural (acute) (chronic) kidney failure**
     Use additional code for type of kidney disease

☑5ᵗʰ **N99.1**   **Postprocedural urethral stricture**
     Postcatheterization urethral stricture

    ☑6ᵗʰ **N99.11**   **Postprocedural urethral stricture, male**

       N99.110   **Postprocedural urethral stricture, male, meatal**   ♂

▲   **N99.111**   **Postprocedural bulbous urethral stricture, male**   ♂

▲   **N99.112**   **Postprocedural membranous urethral stricture, male**   ♂

▲   **N99.113**   **Postprocedural anterior bulbous urethral stricture, male**   ♂

       N99.114   **Postprocedural urethral stricture, male, unspecified**   ♂

       N99.115   **Postprocedural fossa navicularis urethral stricture**   ♂

    N99.12   **Postprocedural urethral stricture, female**   ♀

N99.2   **Postprocedural adhesions of vagina**   ♀

N99.3   **Prolapse of vaginal vault after hysterectomy**   ♀

N99.4   **Postprocedural pelvic peritoneal adhesions**
> *EXCLUDES 2*   pelvic peritoneal adhesions NOS (N73.6)
> postinfective pelvic peritoneal adhesions (N73.6)

☑5ᵗʰ **N99.5**   **Complications of stoma of urinary tract**
> *EXCLUDES 2*   mechanical complication of urinary catheter (T83.0-)

    ☑6ᵗʰ **N99.51**   **Complication of cystostomy**

       N99.510   **Cystostomy hemorrhage**   `CC` `HCC`
          CC Excl: PDX collection 949

       N99.511   **Cystostomy infection**   `CC` `HCC`
          CC Excl: PDX collection 950

       N99.512   **Cystostomy malfunction**   `CC` `HCC`
          CC Excl: PDX collection 951

       N99.518   **Other cystostomy complication**   `CC` `HCC`
          CC Excl: PDX collection 949

    ☑6ᵗʰ **N99.52**   **Complication of incontinent external stoma of urinary tract**

       N99.520   **Hemorrhage of incontinent external stoma of urinary tract**   `HCC`

       N99.521   **Infection of incontinent external stoma of urinary tract**   `HCC`

       N99.522   **Malfunction of incontinent external stoma of urinary tract**   `HCC`

       N99.523   **Herniation of incontinent stoma of urinary tract**   `HCC`

       N99.524   **Stenosis of incontinent stoma of urinary tract**   `HCC`

       N99.528   **Other complication of incontinent external stoma of urinary tract**   `HCC`

    ☑6ᵗʰ **N99.53**   **Complication of continent stoma of urinary tract**

       N99.530   **Hemorrhage of continent stoma of urinary tract**   `HCC`

       N99.531   **Infection of continent stoma of urinary tract**   `HCC`

       N99.532   **Malfunction of continent stoma of urinary tract**   `HCC`

       N99.533   **Herniation of continent stoma of urinary tract**   `HCC`

       N99.534   **Stenosis of continent stoma of urinary tract**   `HCC`

       N99.538   **Other complication of continent stoma of urinary tract**   `HCC`

☑5ᵗʰ **N99.6**   **Intraoperative hemorrhage and hematoma of a genitourinary system organ or structure complicating a procedure**
> *EXCLUDES 1*   intraoperative hemorrhage and hematoma of a genitourinary system organ or structure due to accidental puncture or laceration during a procedure (N99.7-)

    N99.61   **Intraoperative hemorrhage and hematoma of a genitourinary system organ or structure complicating a genitourinary system procedure**   `CC`
       CC Excl: PDX collection 952

    N99.62   **Intraoperative hemorrhage and hematoma of a genitourinary system organ or structure complicating other procedure**   `CC`
       CC Excl: PDX collection 952

☑5ᵗʰ **N99.7**   **Accidental puncture and laceration of a genitourinary system organ or structure during a procedure**

    N99.71   **Accidental puncture and laceration of a genitourinary system organ or structure during a genitourinary system procedure**   `CC`
       CC Excl: PDX collection 509

    N99.72   **Accidental puncture and laceration of a genitourinary system organ or structure during other procedure**   `CC`
       CC Excl: PDX collection 509

☑5ᵗʰ **N99.8**   **Other intraoperative and postprocedural complications and disorders of genitourinary system**

> **CC Excl: For CC codes in subcategory N99.8, unless otherwise noted: PDX collection 952**

    N99.81   **Other intraoperative complications of genitourinary system**

    ☑6ᵗʰ **N99.82**   **Postprocedural hemorrhage of a genitourinary system organ or structure following a procedure**

       N99.820   **Postprocedural hemorrhage of a genitourinary system organ or structure following a genitourinary system procedure**   `CC`

       N99.821   **Postprocedural hemorrhage of a genitourinary system organ or structure following other procedure**   `CC`

    N99.83   **Residual ovary syndrome**   ♀

    ☑6ᵗʰ **N99.84**   **Postprocedural hematoma and seroma of a genitourinary system organ or structure following a procedure**

       N99.840   **Postprocedural hematoma of a genitourinary system organ or structure following a genitourinary system procedure**   `CC`

       N99.841   **Postprocedural hematoma of a genitourinary system organ or structure following other procedure**   `CC`

       N99.842   **Postprocedural seroma of a genitourinary system organ or structure following a genitourinary system procedure**   `CC`

       N99.843   **Postprocedural seroma of a genitourinary system organ or structure following other procedure**   `CC`

    N99.89   **Other postprocedural complications and disorders of genitourinary system**

Chapter 15. Pregnancy, Childbirth and the Puerperium (O00–O9A)

Chapter Specific Guidelines with Coding Examples

The chapter specific guidelines from the ICD-10-CM Official Guidelines for Coding and Reporting have been provided below. Along with these guidelines are coding examples, contained in the shaded boxes, that have been developed to help illustrate the coding and/or sequencing guidance found in these guidelines.

a. General rules for obstetric cases

1) Codes from Chapter 15 and sequencing priority

Obstetric cases require codes from chapter 15, codes in the range O00-O9A, Pregnancy, Childbirth, and the Puerperium. Chapter 15 codes have sequencing priority over codes from other chapters. Additional codes from other chapters may be used in conjunction with chapter 15 codes to further specify conditions. Should the provider document that the pregnancy is incidental to the encounter, then code Z33.1, Pregnant state, incidental, should be used in place of any chapter 15 codes. It is the provider's responsibility to state that the condition being treated is not affecting the pregnancy.

> Pregnant patient at 25 weeks' gestation admitted for bladder abscess.
>
> **O23.12**   **Infections of bladder in pregnancy, second trimester**
>
> **N30.80**   **Other cystitis without hematuria**
>
> **Z3A.25**   **25 weeks gestation of pregnancy**
>
> *Explanation:* The documentation does not indicate that the pregnancy is incidental or in any way unaffected by the bladder abscess; therefore, an obstetrics code should be sequenced first. An additional code was provided to identify the specific bladder condition as this information is not called out specifically in the obstetrics code.

2) Chapter 15 codes used only on the maternal record

Chapter 15 codes are to be used only on the maternal record, never on the record of the newborn.

3) Final character for trimester

The majority of codes in Chapter 15 have a final character indicating the trimester of pregnancy. The timeframes for the trimesters are indicated at the beginning of the chapter. If trimester is not a component of a code, it is because the condition always occurs in a specific trimester, or the concept of trimester of pregnancy is not applicable. Certain codes have characters for only certain trimesters because the condition does not occur in all trimesters, but it may occur in more than just one.

Assignment of the final character for trimester should be based on the provider's documentation of the trimester (or number of weeks) for the current admission/encounter. This applies to the assignment of trimester for pre-existing conditions as well as those that develop during or are due to the pregnancy. The provider's documentation of the number of weeks may be used to assign the appropriate code identifying the trimester.

Whenever delivery occurs during the current admission, and there is an "in childbirth" option for the obstetric complication being coded, the "in childbirth" code should be assigned.

> Pregnant patient at 21 weeks' gestation admitted with excessive vomiting
>
> **O21.2**   **Late vomiting of pregnancy**
>
> **Z3A.21**   **21 weeks gestation of pregnancy**
>
> *Explanation:* Category O21 classifies vomiting in pregnancy. Although code selection is based on whether the vomiting is before or after 20 completed weeks, these codes are not further classified by trimester. If vomiting only in the second trimester was documented, the provider should be queried for the specific week of gestation, as this will affect code selection.

4) Selection of trimester for inpatient admissions that encompass more than one trimester

In instances when a patient is admitted to a hospital for complications of pregnancy during one trimester and remains in the hospital into a subsequent trimester, the trimester character for the antepartum complication code should be assigned on the basis of the trimester when the complication developed, not the trimester of the discharge. If the condition developed prior to the current admission/encounter or represents a pre-existing condition, the trimester character for the trimester at the time of the admission/encounter should be assigned.

> Patient admitted at 27 6/7 weeks' gestation for hemorrhaging from partial placenta previa; three days after admission at 28 1/7 weeks' gestation, she developed gestational hypertension
>
> **O44.32**   **Partial placenta previa with hemorrhage, second trimester**
>
> **O13.3**   **Gestational [pregnancy-induced] hypertension without significant proteinuria, third trimester**
>
> **Z3A.27**   **27 weeks gestation of pregnancy**
>
> *Explanation:* The patient presented with hemorrhaging from partial placenta previa while still in her 27th week, which falls within the second trimester. The gestational hypertension did not occur until three days after admission, putting the patient in her 28th week of pregnancy or what is considered to be the third trimester. The weeks of gestation captured by a code from category Z3A should represent only the gestational weeks upon admission.

5) Unspecified trimester

Each category that includes codes for trimester has a code for "unspecified trimester." The "unspecified trimester" code should rarely be used, such as when the documentation in the record is insufficient to determine the trimester and it is not possible to obtain clarification.

6) 7th character for fetus identification

Where applicable, a 7th character is to be assigned for certain categories (O31, O32, O33.3 - O33.6, O35, O36, O40, O41, O60.1, O60.2, O64, and O69) to identify the fetus for which the complication code applies.

Assign 7th character "0":

- For single gestations
- When the documentation in the record is insufficient to determine the fetus affected and it is not possible to obtain clarification.
- When it is not possible to clinically determine which fetus is affected.

> Maternal patient with twin gestations is seen after ultrasound identifies fetus B to be in breech presentation
>
> **O32.1XX2**   **Maternal care for breech presentation, fetus 2**
>
> *Explanation:* The documentation indicates that although there are two fetuses, only one fetus is determined to be in breech presentation. Whether fetus 2 or fetus B is used, the coder can assign the seventh character of 2 to identify the second fetus as the one in breech.

b. Selection of OB principal or first-listed diagnosis

1) Routine outpatient prenatal visits

For routine outpatient prenatal visits when no complications are present, a code from category Z34, Encounter for supervision of normal pregnancy, should be used as the first-listed diagnosis. These codes should not be used in conjunction with chapter 15 codes.

2) Supervision of high-risk pregnancy

Codes from category O09, Supervision of high-risk pregnancy, are intended for use only during the prenatal period. For complications during the labor or delivery episode as a result of a high-risk pregnancy, assign the applicable complication codes from Chapter 15. If there are no complications during the labor or delivery episode, assign code O80, Encounter for full-term uncomplicated delivery.

For routine prenatal outpatient visits for patients with high-risk pregnancies, a code from category O09, Supervision of high-risk pregnancy, should be used as the first-listed diagnosis. Secondary chapter 15 codes may be used in conjunction with these codes if appropriate.

> 36-year-old admitted in labor with second child at 39 weeks' gestation, delivered a healthy baby, delivery complicated by tear of fourchette that was repaired
>
> **O70.0**   **First degree perineal laceration during delivery**
>
> **Z3A.39**   **39 weeks gestation of pregnancy**
>
> **Z37.0**   **Single live birth**
>
> Explanation: Although this patient is over 35 and having her second child (elderly multigravida), do not append a code from subcategory O09.52-. A code describing the tear of the fourchette, which complicated the delivery, should be used in addition to the applicable Z codes.

Chapter 15. Pregnancy, Childbirth and the Puerperium

3) Episodes when no delivery occurs

In episodes when no delivery occurs, the principal diagnosis should correspond to the principal complication of the pregnancy which necessitated the encounter. Should more than one complication exist, all of which are treated or monitored, any of the complications codes may be sequenced first.

4) When a delivery occurs

When an obstetric patient is admitted and delivers during that admission, the condition that prompted the admission should be sequenced as the principal diagnosis. If multiple conditions prompted the admission, sequence the one most related to the delivery as the principal diagnosis. A code for any complication of the delivery should be assigned as an additional diagnosis. In cases of cesarean delivery, if the patient was admitted with a condition that resulted in the performance of a cesarean procedure, that condition should be selected as the principal diagnosis. If the reason for the admission was unrelated to the condition resulting in the cesarean delivery, the condition related to the reason for the admission should be selected as the principal diagnosis.

Maternal patient with diet-controlled gestational diabetes was admitted at 38 weeks' gestation in obstructed labor due to footling presentation; cesarean performed for the malpresentation

O64.8XX0	Obstructed labor due to other malposition and malpresentation, not applicable or unspecified
O24.420	Gestational diabetes mellitus in childbirth, diet controlled
Z3A.38	38 weeks gestation of pregnancy
Z37.0	Single live birth

Explanation: The obstructed labor necessitated the cesarean procedure.

At 39 weeks' gestation, a maternal patient presents with hemorrhage with coagulation defect; the next day the patient goes into labor and eventually delivers via cesarean section due to arrested active phase of labor

O46.003	Antepartum hemorrhage with coagulation defect, unspecified, third trimester
O62.1	Secondary uterine inertia
Z3A.39	39 weeks gestation of pregnancy
Z37.0	Single live birth

Explanation: The patient was admitted because of the antepartum hemorrhage with coagulation defect. The arrested active phase, although the reason for the cesarean delivery, did not develop until later into the stay.

5) Outcome of delivery

A code from category Z37, Outcome of delivery, should be included on every maternal record when a delivery has occurred. These codes are not to be used on subsequent records or on the newborn record.

c. Pre-existing conditions versus conditions due to the pregnancy

Certain categories in Chapter 15 distinguish between conditions of the mother that existed prior to pregnancy (pre-existing) and those that are a direct result of pregnancy. When assigning codes from Chapter 15, it is important to assess if a condition was pre-existing prior to pregnancy or developed during or due to the pregnancy in order to assign the correct code.

Categories that do not distinguish between pre-existing and pregnancy-related conditions may be used for either. It is acceptable to use codes specifically for the puerperium with codes complicating pregnancy and childbirth if a condition arises postpartum during the delivery encounter.

d. Pre-existing hypertension in pregnancy

Category O10, Pre-existing hypertension complicating pregnancy, childbirth and the puerperium, includes codes for hypertensive heart and hypertensive chronic kidney disease. When assigning one of the O10 codes that includes hypertensive heart disease or hypertensive chronic kidney disease, it is necessary to add a secondary code from the appropriate hypertension category to specify the type of heart failure or chronic kidney disease.

See Section I.C.9. Hypertension.

e. Fetal conditions affecting the management of the mother

1) Codes from categories O35 and O36

Codes from categories O35, Maternal care for known or suspected fetal abnormality and damage, and O36, Maternal care for other fetal problems, are assigned only when the fetal condition is actually responsible for modifying the management of the mother, i.e., by requiring diagnostic studies, additional observation, special care, or termination of pregnancy. The fact that the fetal condition exists does not justify assigning a code from this series to the mother's record.

A patient is seen in ED for spotting 15 weeks into her pregnancy; the doctors also suspect fetal hydrocephalus.

O26.852	Spotting complicating pregnancy, second trimester
Z3A.15	15 weeks gestation of pregnancy

Explanation: Whether the fetal hydrocephalus was suspected or confirmed, an additional code is not warranted for this condition as the documentation does not indicate that this fetal condition is in any way altering the management of the mother or complicating her pregnancy.

2) In utero surgery

In cases when surgery is performed on the fetus, a diagnosis code from category O35, Maternal care for known or suspected fetal abnormality and damage, should be assigned identifying the fetal condition. Assign the appropriate procedure code for the procedure performed.

No code from Chapter 16, the perinatal codes, should be used on the mother's record to identify fetal conditions. Surgery performed in utero on a fetus is still to be coded as an obstetric encounter.

f. HIV infection in pregnancy, childbirth and the puerperium

During pregnancy, childbirth or the puerperium, a patient admitted because of an HIV-related illness should receive a principal diagnosis from subcategory O98.7-, Human immunodeficiency [HIV] disease complicating pregnancy, childbirth and the puerperium, followed by the code(s) for the HIV-related illness(es).

Patients with asymptomatic HIV infection status admitted during pregnancy, childbirth, or the puerperium should receive codes of O98.7- and Z21, Asymptomatic human immunodeficiency virus [HIV] infection status.

A previously asymptomatic HIV patient who is 13 weeks pregnant is admitted with oral thrush.

O98.711	Human immunodeficiency virus [HIV] disease complicating pregnancy, first trimester
B20	Human immunodeficiency virus [HIV] disease
B37.0	Candidal stomatitis
Z3A.13	13 weeks gestation of pregnancy

Explanation: Because oral thrush is an HIV-related condition, this patient is now considered to have HIV disease. An obstetrics code indicating that HIV is complicating the pregnancy is coded first, followed by B20 for HIV disease as well as a code for the oral thrush.

g. Diabetes mellitus in pregnancy

Diabetes mellitus is a significant complicating factor in pregnancy. Pregnant women who are diabetic should be assigned a code from category O24, Diabetes mellitus in pregnancy, childbirth, and the puerperium, first, followed by the appropriate diabetes code(s) (E08-E13) from Chapter 4.

h. Long term use of insulin and oral hypoglycemics

See section I.C.4.a.3 for information on the long term use of insulin and oral hypoglycemic.

i. Gestational (pregnancy induced) diabetes

Gestational (pregnancy induced) diabetes can occur during the second and third trimester of pregnancy in women who were not diabetic prior to pregnancy. Gestational diabetes can cause complications in the pregnancy similar to those of pre-existing diabetes mellitus. It also puts the woman at greater risk of developing diabetes after the pregnancy. Codes for gestational diabetes are in subcategory O24.4, Gestational diabetes mellitus. No other code from category O24, Diabetes mellitus in pregnancy, childbirth, and the puerperium, should be used with a code from O24.4.

The codes under subcategory O24.4 include diet controlled, insulin controlled, and controlled by oral hypoglycemic drugs. If a patient with gestational diabetes is treated with both diet and insulin, only the code for insulin-controlled is required. If a patient with gestational diabetes is treated with both diet and oral hypoglycemic medications, only the code for "controlled by oral hypoglycemic drugs" is required. Code Z79.4, Long-term (current) use of insulin or code Z79.84, Long-term (current) use of oral hypoglycemic drugs, should not be assigned with codes from subcategory O24.4.

An abnormal glucose tolerance in pregnancy is assigned a code from subcategory O99.81, Abnormal glucose complicating pregnancy, childbirth, and the puerperium.

> Patient at 39 weeks term pregnancy with gestational diabetes was admitted in labor and delivered a healthy newborn. Patient is on diabetes diet with daily metformin.
>
> **O24.425**   **Gestational diabetes mellitus in childbirth, controlled by oral hypoglycemic drugs**
>
> **Z3A.39**   **39 weeks gestation of pregnancy**
>
> **Z37.0**   **Single live birth**
>
> *Explanation:* When the patient is admitted for delivery and the patient's gestational diabetes is controlled by both diet and oral hypoglycemic medications, only the combination code in subcategory O24.4- Gestational diabetes mellitus, is reported. No code is added for diet controlled diabetes, and no Z code for long-term use of oral hypoglycemics is reported with the O24.4 combination codes.

j. Sepsis and septic shock complicating abortion, pregnancy, childbirth and the puerperium

When assigning a chapter 15 code for sepsis complicating abortion, pregnancy, childbirth, and the puerperium, a code for the specific type of infection should be assigned as an additional diagnosis. If severe sepsis is present, a code from subcategory R65.2, Severe sepsis, and code(s) for associated organ dysfunction(s) should also be assigned as additional diagnoses.

> Patient is seen several days after a miscarriage with sepsis; cultures return MSSA
>
> **O03.87**   **Sepsis following complete or unspecified spontaneous abortion**
>
> **B95.61**   **Methicillin susceptible Staphylococcus aureus infection as the cause of diseases classified elsewhere**
>
> *Explanation:* The type of infection that caused this patient to become septic was methicillin susceptible *Staphylococcus aureus* (MSSA), which as a secondary code helps capture all aspects related to this patient's septic condition.

k. Puerperal sepsis

Code O85, Puerperal sepsis, should be assigned with a secondary code to identify the causal organism (e.g., for a bacterial infection, assign a code from category B95-B96, Bacterial infections in conditions classified elsewhere). A code from category A40, Streptococcal sepsis, or A41, Other sepsis, should not be used for puerperal sepsis. If applicable, use additional codes to identify severe sepsis (R65.2-) and any associated acute organ dysfunction.

l. Alcohol and tobacco use during pregnancy, childbirth and the puerperium

1) Alcohol use during pregnancy, childbirth and the puerperium

Codes under subcategory O99.31, Alcohol use complicating pregnancy, childbirth, and the puerperium, should be assigned for any pregnancy case when a mother uses alcohol during the pregnancy or postpartum. A secondary code from category F10, Alcohol related disorders, should also be assigned to identify manifestations of the alcohol use.

2) Tobacco use during pregnancy, childbirth and the puerperium

Codes under subcategory O99.33, Smoking (tobacco) complicating pregnancy, childbirth, and the puerperium, should be assigned for any pregnancy case when a mother uses any type of tobacco product during the pregnancy or postpartum. A secondary code from category F17, Nicotine dependence, should also be assigned to identify the type of nicotine dependence.

m. Poisoning, toxic effects, adverse effects and underdosing in a pregnant patient

A code from subcategory O9A.2, Injury, poisoning and certain other consequences of external causes complicating pregnancy, childbirth, and the puerperium, should be sequenced first, followed by the appropriate injury, poisoning, toxic effect, adverse effect or underdosing code, and then the additional code(s) that specifies the condition caused by the poisoning, toxic effect, adverse effect or underdosing.

See Section I.C.19. Adverse effects, poisoning, underdosing and toxic effects.

> Patient admitted with accidental carbon monoxide poisoning from a gas heating implement; the patient is 18 weeks' pregnant
>
> **O9A.212**   **Injury, poisoning and certain other consequences of external causes complicating pregnancy, second trimester**
>
> **T58.11XA**   **Toxic effect of carbon monoxide from utility gas, accidental (unintentional), initial encounter**
>
> **Z3A.18**   **18 weeks gestation of pregnancy**
>
> *Explanation:* Although the carbon monoxide poisoning is the reason the patient was admitted, a code from the obstetrics chapter must be sequenced first. Chapter 15 codes have sequencing priority over codes from other chapters.

n. Normal delivery, code O80

1) Encounter for full term uncomplicated delivery

Code O80 should be assigned when a woman is admitted for a full-term normal delivery and delivers a single, healthy infant without any complications antepartum, during the delivery, or postpartum during the delivery episode. Code O80 is always a principal diagnosis. It is not to be used if any other code from chapter 15 is needed to describe a current complication of the antenatal, delivery, or perinatal period. Additional codes from other chapters may be used with code O80 if they are not related to or are in any way complicating the pregnancy.

2) Uncomplicated delivery with resolved antepartum complication

Code O80 may be used if the patient had a complication at some point during the pregnancy, but the complication is not present at the time of the admission for delivery.

> Patient presents in labor at 39 weeks' gestation and delivers a healthy newborn; patient had abnormal glucose levels in her first trimester, which have since resolved
>
> **O80**   **Encounter for full-term uncomplicated delivery**
>
> **Z37.0**   **Single live birth**
>
> *Explanation:* The abnormal glucose levels during the first trimester cannot be coded if they are not affecting the patient's current trimester. Without additional complications associated with the pregnancy, fetus, or mother, code O80 is appropriate.

3) Outcome of delivery for O80

Z37.0, Single live birth, is the only outcome of delivery code appropriate for use with O80.

o. The peripartum and postpartum periods

1) Peripartum and postpartum periods

The postpartum period begins immediately after delivery and continues for six weeks following delivery. The peripartum period is defined as the last month of pregnancy to five months postpartum.

2) Peripartum and postpartum complication

A postpartum complication is any complication occurring within the six-week period.

3) Pregnancy-related complications after 6 week period

Chapter 15 codes may also be used to describe pregnancy-related complications after the peripartum or postpartum period if the provider documents that a condition is pregnancy related.

> Patient admitted for varicose veins. She had a baby boy three months ago; the varicose veins started to appear one month ago. The doctor attributes the patient's pregnancy as the cause of the varicose veins, which continue to be painful and bother the patient. She is seeking surgical relief.
>
> **O87.4**   **Varicose veins of the lower extremity in the puerperium**
>
> *Explanation:* Although the varicose veins occurred several months after the delivery of the newborn, the doctor attributed the varicose veins to pregnancy and therefore a code from chapter 15 is appropriate.

4) Admission for routine postpartum care following delivery outside hospital

When the mother delivers outside the hospital prior to admission and is admitted for routine postpartum care and no complications are noted, code Z39.0, Encounter for care and examination of mother immediately after delivery, should be assigned as the principal diagnosis.

Chapter 15. Pregnancy, Childbirth and the Puerperium

5) Pregnancy associated cardiomyopathy

Pregnancy associated cardiomyopathy, code O90.3, is unique in that it may be diagnosed in the third trimester of pregnancy but may continue to progress months after delivery. For this reason, it is referred to as peripartum cardiomyopathy. Code O90.3 is only for use when the cardiomyopathy develops as a result of pregnancy in a woman who did not have pre-existing heart disease.

p. Code O94, Sequelae of complication of pregnancy, childbirth, and the puerperium

1) Code O94

Code O94, Sequelae of complication of pregnancy, childbirth, and the puerperium, is for use in those cases when an initial complication of a pregnancy develops a sequelae requiring care or treatment at a future date.

2) After the initial postpartum period

This code may be used at any time after the initial postpartum period.

3) Sequencing of code O94

This code, like all sequela codes, is to be sequenced following the code describing the sequelae of the complication.

q. Termination of pregnancy and spontaneous abortions

1) Abortion with liveborn fetus

When an attempted termination of pregnancy results in a liveborn fetus, assign code Z33.2, Encounter for elective termination of pregnancy and a code from category Z37, Outcome of Delivery.

2) Retained products of conception following an abortion

Subsequent encounters for retained products of conception following a spontaneous abortion or elective termination of pregnancy, **without complications** are assigned O03.**4, Incomplete spontaneous,** abortion **without complication**, or codes O07.4, Failed attempted termination of pregnancy without complication. This advice is appropriate even when the patient was discharged previously with a discharge diagnosis of complete abortion. **If the patient has a specific complication associated with the spontaneous abortion or elective termination of pregnancy in addition to retained products of conception, assign the appropriate complication in category O03 or O07 instead of code O03.4 or O07.4**

> Patient was seen two days ago for complete spontaneous abortion but returns today for urinary tract infection (UTI) with ultrasound showing retained products of conception
>
> **O03.38   Urinary tract infection following incomplete spontaneous abortion**
>
> *Explanation:* Although the diagnosis from the patient's previous stay indicated that the patient had a complete abortion, it is now determined that there were actually retained products of conception (POC). An abortion with retained POC is considered incomplete and in this case resulted in the patient developing a UTI.

3) Complications leading to abortion

Codes from Chapter 15 may be used as additional codes to identify any documented complications of the pregnancy in conjunction with codes in categories in **O04,** O07 and O08.

r. Abuse in a pregnant patient

For suspected or confirmed cases of abuse of a pregnant patient, a code(s) from subcategories O9A.3, Physical abuse complicating pregnancy, childbirth, and the puerperium, O9A.4, Sexual abuse complicating pregnancy, childbirth, and the puerperium, and O9A.5, Psychological abuse complicating pregnancy, childbirth, and the puerperium, should be sequenced first, followed by the appropriate codes (if applicable) to identify any associated current injury due to physical abuse, sexual abuse, and the perpetrator of abuse.

See Section I.C.19. Adult and child abuse, neglect and other maltreatment.

Chapter 15. Pregnancy, Childbirth and the Puerperium (O00-O9A)

NOTE   CODES FROM THIS CHAPTER ARE FOR USE ONLY ON MATERNAL RECORDS, NEVER ON NEWBORN RECORDS.

Codes from this chapter are for use for conditions related to or aggravated by the pregnancy, childbirth, or by the puerperium (maternal causes or obstetric causes).

NOTE   Trimesters are counted from the first day of the last menstrual period. They are defined as follows:

     1st trimester- less than 14 weeks 0 days
     2nd trimester- 14 weeks 0 days to less than 28 weeks 0 days
     3rd trimester- 28 weeks 0 days until delivery

Use additional code from category Z3A, Weeks of gestation, to identify the specific week of the pregnancy, if known

EXCLUDES 1   *supervision of normal pregnancy (Z34.-)*
EXCLUDES 2   *mental and behavioral disorders associated with the puerperium (F53)*
     dobstetrical tetanus (A34)
     postpartum necrosis of pituitary gland (E23.0)
     puerperal osteomalacia (M83.0)

AHA: 2016, 1Q, 3-5; 2014, 3Q, 17

This chapter contains the following blocks:

O00-O08   Pregnancy with abortive outcome
O09   Supervision of high risk pregnancy
O10-O16   Edema, proteinuria and hypertensive disorders in pregnancy, childbirth and the puerperium
O20-O29   Other maternal disorders predominantly related to pregnancy
O30-O48   Maternal care related to the fetus and amniotic cavity and possible delivery problems
O60-O77   Complications of labor and delivery
O80, O82   Encounter for delivery
O85-O92   Complications predominantly related to the puerperium
O94-O9A   Other obstetric conditions, not elsewhere classified

Pregnancy with abortive outcome (O00-O08)

EXCLUDES 1   *continuing pregnancy in multiple gestation after abortion of one fetus or more (O31.1-, O31.3-)*

✓4ᵗʰ O00   Ectopic pregnancy

INCLUDES   ruptured ectopic pregnancy

Use additional code from category O08 to identify any associated complication

AHA: 2014, 3Q, 17
DEF: Implantation of fertilized egg outside the uterus, usually in fallopian tube or abdomen; requires emergency treatment.

CC Excl: For CC codes in category O00: PDX collection 953

✓5ᵗʰ **O00.0   Abdominal pregnancy**
     EXCLUDES 1   *maternal care for viable fetus in abdominal pregnancy (O36.7-)*

     O00.00   Abdominal pregnancy without intrauterine pregnancy   CC M♀
         Abdominal pregnancy NOS

     O00.01   Abdominal pregnancy with intrauterine pregnancy   CC M♀

✓5ᵗʰ **O00.1   Tubal pregnancy**
     Fallopian pregnancy
     Rupture of (fallopian) tube due to pregnancy
     Tubal abortion

     ✓6ᵗʰ **O00.10   Tubal pregnancy without intrauterine pregnancy**
         Tubal pregnancy NOS

         O00.101   Right tubal pregnancy without intrauterine pregnancy   CC M

         O00.102   Left tubal pregnancy without intrauterine pregnancy   CC M

         O00.109   Unspecified tubal pregnancy without intrauterine pregnancy   CC M

     ✓6ᵗʰ **O00.11   Tubal pregnancy with intrauterine pregnancy**

         O00.111   Right tubal pregnancy with intrauterine pregnancy   CC M

         O00.112   Left tubal pregnancy with intrauterine pregnancy   CC M

         O00.119   Unspecified tubal pregnancy with intrauterine pregnancy   CC M

✓5ᵗʰ **O00.2   Ovarian pregnancy**

     ✓6ᵗʰ **O00.20   Ovarian pregnancy without intrauterine pregnancy**
         Ovarian pregnancy NOS

         O00.201   Right ovarian pregnancy without intrauterine pregnancy   CC M

         O00.202   Left ovarian pregnancy without intrauterine pregnancy   CC M

         O00.209   Unspecified ovarian pregnancy without intrauterine pregnancy   CC M

     ✓6ᵗʰ **O00.21   Ovarian pregnancy with intrauterine pregnancy**

         O00.211   Right ovarian pregnancy with intrauterine pregnancy   CC M

         O00.212   Left ovarian pregnancy with intrauterine pregnancy   CC M

         O00.219   Unspecified ovarian pregnancy with intrauterine pregnancy   CC M

✓5ᵗʰ **O00.8   Other ectopic pregnancy**
     Cervical pregnancy
     Cornual pregnancy
     Intraligamentous pregnancy
     Mural pregnancy

     O00.80   Other ectopic pregnancy without intrauterine pregnancy   CC M♀
         Other ectopic pregnancy NOS

     O00.81   Other ectopic pregnancy with intrauterine pregnancy   CC M♀

✓5ᵗʰ **O00.9   Ectopic pregnancy, unspecified**

     O00.90   Unspecified ectopic pregnancy without intrauterine pregnancy   CC M♀
         Ectopic pregnancy NOS

     O00.91   Unspecified ectopic pregnancy with intrauterine pregnancy   CC M♀

✓4ᵗʰ O01   Hydatidiform mole

Use additional code from category O08 to identify any associated complication

EXCLUDES 1   *chorioadenoma (destruens) (D39.2)*
     malignant hydatidiform mole (D39.2)

AHA: 2014, 3Q, 17
DEF: Abnormal product of pregnancy; marked by mass of cysts resembling bunch of grapes due to chorionic villi proliferation and dissolution; must be surgically removed.

     O01.0   Classical hydatidiform mole   M♀
         Complete hydatidiform mole

     O01.1   Incomplete and partial hydatidiform mole   M♀

     O01.9   Hydatidiform mole, unspecified   M♀
         Trophoblastic disease NOS
         Vesicular mole NOS

✓4ᵗʰ O02   Other abnormal products of conception

Use additional code from category O08 to identify any associated complication

EXCLUDES 1   *papyraceous fetus (O31.0-)*

AHA: 2014, 3Q, 17

     O02.0   Blighted ovum and nonhydatidiform mole   M♀
         Carneous mole
         Fleshy mole
         Intrauterine mole NOS
         Molar pregnancy NEC
         Pathological ovum

Ectopic Pregnancy

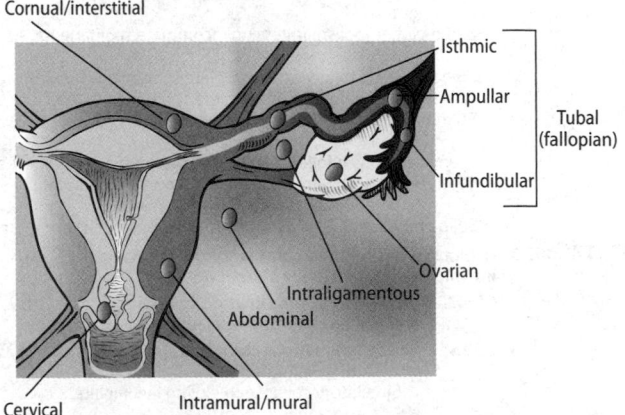

✓ Additional Character Req   ✓x7ᵗʰ Placeholder Alert   Unacceptable PDx   Manifestation   H1-H14 HAC   HCC CMS-HCC Condition   EXCLUDES 1 Not Coded Here   EXCLUDES 2 Not Included Here

ICD-10-CM 2018   843

Chapter 15. Pregnancy, Childbirth and the Puerperium

O02.1 Missed abortion M♀
Early fetal death, before completion of 20 weeks of gestation, with retention of dead fetus
EXCLUDES 1 *failed induced abortion (O07.-)*
fetal death (intrauterine) (late) (O36.4)
missed abortion with blighted ovum (O02.0)
missed abortion with hydatidiform mole (O01.-)
missed abortion with nonhydatidiform (O02.0)
missed abortion with other abnormal products of conception (O02.8-)
missed delivery (O36.4)
stillbirth (P95)

✓5th **O02.8 Other specified abnormal products of conception**
EXCLUDES 1 *abnormal products of conception with blighted ovum (O02.0)*
abnormal products of conception with hydatidiform mole (O01.-)
abnormal products of conception with nonhydatidiform mole (O02.0)

O02.81 Inappropriate change in quantitative human chorionic gonadotropin (hCG) in early pregnancy M♀
Biochemical pregnancy
Chemical pregnancy
Inappropriate level of quantitative human chorionic gonadotropin (hCG) for gestational age in early pregnancy

O02.89 Other abnormal products of conception M♀
O02.9 Abnormal product of conception, unspecified M♀

✓4th **O03 Spontaneous abortion**
NOTE Incomplete abortion includes retained products of conception following spontaneous abortion
INCLUDES miscarriage

CC Excl: For CC/MCC codes in category O03: PDX collection 954

O03.0 Genital tract and pelvic infection following incomplete spontaneous abortion CC M♀
Endometritis following incomplete spontaneous abortion
Oophoritis following incomplete spontaneous abortion
Parametritis following incomplete spontaneous abortion
Pelvic peritonitis following incomplete spontaneous abortion
Salpingitis following incomplete spontaneous abortion
Salpingo-oophoritis following incomplete spontaneous abortion
EXCLUDES 1 *sepsis following incomplete spontaneous abortion (O03.37)*
urinary tract infection following incomplete spontaneous abortion (O03.38)

O03.1 Delayed or excessive hemorrhage following incomplete spontaneous abortion M♀
Afibrinogenemia following incomplete spontaneous abortion
Defibrination syndrome following incomplete spontaneous abortion
Hemolysis following incomplete spontaneous abortion
Intravascular coagulation following incomplete spontaneous abortion

O03.2 Embolism following incomplete spontaneous abortion MCC M♀
Air embolism following incomplete spontaneous abortion
Amniotic fluid embolism following incomplete spontaneous abortion
Blood-clot embolism following incomplete spontaneous abortion
Embolism NOS following incomplete spontaneous abortion
Fat embolism following incomplete spontaneous abortion
Pulmonary embolism following incomplete spontaneous abortion
Pyemic embolism following incomplete spontaneous abortion
Septic or septicopyemic embolism following incomplete spontaneous abortion
Soap embolism following incomplete spontaneous abortion

✓5th **O03.3 Other and unspecified complications following incomplete spontaneous abortion**

O03.30 Unspecified complication following incomplete spontaneous abortion CC M♀

O03.31 Shock following incomplete spontaneous abortion MCC M♀
Circulatory collapse following incomplete spontaneous abortion
Shock (postprocedural) following incomplete spontaneous abortion
EXCLUDES 1 *shock due to infection following incomplete spontaneous abortion (O03.37)*

O03.32 Renal failure following incomplete spontaneous abortion MCC M♀
Kidney failure (acute) following incomplete spontaneous abortion
Oliguria following incomplete spontaneous abortion
Renal shutdown following incomplete spontaneous abortion
Renal tubular necrosis following incomplete spontaneous abortion
Uremia following incomplete spontaneous abortion

O03.33 Metabolic disorder following incomplete spontaneous abortion CC M♀

O03.34 Damage to pelvic organs following incomplete spontaneous abortion CC M♀
Laceration, perforation, tear or chemical damage of bladder following incomplete spontaneous abortion
Laceration, perforation, tear or chemical damage of bowel following incomplete spontaneous abortion
Laceration, perforation, tear or chemical damage of broad ligament following incomplete spontaneous abortion
Laceration, perforation, tear or chemical damage of cervix following incomplete spontaneous abortion
Laceration, perforation, tear or chemical damage of periurethral tissue following incomplete spontaneous abortion
Laceration, perforation, tear or chemical damage of uterus following incomplete spontaneous abortion
Laceration, perforation, tear or chemical damage of vagina following incomplete spontaneous abortion

O03.35 Other venous complications following incomplete spontaneous abortion CC M♀

O03.36 Cardiac arrest following incomplete spontaneous abortion CC M♀

O03.37 Sepsis following incomplete spontaneous abortion CC M♀
Use additional code to identify infectious agent (B95-B97)
Use additional code to identify severe sepsis, if applicable (R65.2-)
EXCLUDES 1 *septic or septicopyemic embolism following incomplete spontaneous abortion (O03.2)*

O03.38 Urinary tract infection following incomplete spontaneous abortion CC M♀
Cystitis following incomplete spontaneous abortion

O03.39 Incomplete spontaneous abortion with other complications CC M♀

O03.4 Incomplete spontaneous abortion without complication M♀

O03.5 Genital tract and pelvic infection following complete or unspecified spontaneous abortion CC M♀
Endometritis following complete or unspecified spontaneous abortion
Oophoritis following complete or unspecified spontaneous abortion
Parametritis following complete or unspecified spontaneous abortion
Pelvic peritonitis following complete or unspecified spontaneous abortion
Salpingitis following complete or unspecified spontaneous abortion
Salpingo-oophoritis following complete or unspecified spontaneous abortion
EXCLUDES 1 *sepsis following complete or unspecified spontaneous abortion (O03.87)*
urinary tract infection following complete or unspecified spontaneous abortion (O03.88)

O03.6 Delayed or excessive hemorrhage following complete or unspecified spontaneous abortion M♀
Afibrinogenemia following complete or unspecified spontaneous abortion
Defibrination syndrome following complete or unspecified spontaneous abortion
Hemolysis following complete or unspecified spontaneous abortion
Intravascular coagulation following complete or unspecified spontaneous abortion

O03.7 Embolism **following** complete or unspecified [cc][M][♀]
spontaneous abortion
    Air embolism following complete or unspecified spontaneous
      abortion
    Amniotic fluid embolism following complete or unspecified
      spontaneous abortion
    Blood-clot embolism following complete or unspecified
      spontaneous abortion
    Embolism NOS following complete or unspecified spontaneous
      abortion
    Fat embolism following complete or unspecified spontaneous
      abortion
    Pulmonary embolism following complete or unspecified
      spontaneous abortion
    Pyemic embolism following complete or unspecified
      spontaneous abortion
    Septic or septicopyemic embolism following complete or
      unspecified spontaneous abortion
    Soap embolism following complete or unspecified spontaneous
      abortion

[✓5th] **O03.8** Other **and unspecified** complications **following** complete or
unspecified **spontaneous abortion**

  O03.80 Unspecified **complication following complete** [cc][M]
    or unspecified spontaneous abortion

  O03.81 Shock **following complete or unspecified** [MCC][M]♀
    spontaneous abortion
      Circulatory collapse following complete or unspecified
        spontaneous abortion
      Shock (postprocedural) following complete or
        unspecified spontaneous abortion
      EXCLUDES 1   *shock due to infection following complete or*
          unspecified spontaneous abortion
          (O03.87)

  O03.82 Renal failure **following complete or** [MCC][M]♀
    unspecified spontaneous abortion
      Kidney failure (acute) following complete or
        unspecified spontaneous abortion
      Oliguria following complete or unspecified
        spontaneous abortion
      Renal shutdown following complete or unspecified
        spontaneous abortion
      Renal tubular necrosis following complete or
        unspecified spontaneous abortion
      Uremia following complete or unspecified
        spontaneous abortion

  O03.83 Metabolic **disorder following complete or** [cc][M]♀
    unspecified spontaneous abortion

  O03.84 Damage to pelvic organs **following complete** [cc][M]♀
    or unspecified spontaneous abortion
      Laceration, perforation, tear or chemical damage of
        bladder following complete or unspecified
        spontaneous abortion
      Laceration, perforation, tear or chemical damage of
        bowel following complete or unspecified
        spontaneous abortion
      Laceration, perforation, tear or chemical damage of
        broad ligament following complete or
        unspecified spontaneous abortion
      Laceration, perforation, tear or chemical damage of
        cervix following complete or unspecified
        spontaneous abortion
      Laceration, perforation, tear or chemical damage of
        periurethral tissue following complete or
        unspecified spontaneous abortion
      Laceration, perforation, tear or chemical damage of
        uterus following complete or unspecified
        spontaneous abortion
      Laceration, perforation, tear or chemical damage of
        vagina following complete or unspecified
        spontaneous abortion

  O03.85 Other venous **complications following** [cc][M]♀
    complete or unspecified spontaneous abortion

  O03.86 Cardiac arrest **following complete or** [cc][M]♀
    unspecified spontaneous abortion

  O03.87 Sepsis **following complete or unspecified** [cc][M]♀
    spontaneous abortion
      Use additional code to identify infectious agent
        (B95-B97)
      Use additional code to identify severe sepsis, if
        applicable (R65.2-)
      EXCLUDES 1   *septic or septicopyemic embolism following*
          complete or unspecified spontaneous
          abortion (O03.7)

O03.88 Urinary tract infection **following complete or** [cc][M]♀
unspecified spontaneous abortion
    Cystitis following complete or unspecified
      spontaneous abortion

O03.89 Complete or unspecified spontaneous [cc][M]♀
abortion with other **complications**

O03.9 Complete or unspecified spontaneous abortion without [M]♀
complication
    Miscarriage NOS
    Spontaneous abortion NOS

[✓4th] **O04** Complications **following (induced)** termination of pregnancy
    [INCLUDES] complications following (induced) termination of pregnancy
    EXCLUDES 1   *encounter for elective termination of pregnancy, uncomplicated*
        (Z33.2)
        failed attempted termination of pregnancy (O07.-)

> **CC Excl: For CC/MCC codes in category O04, unless otherwise noted:** PDX collection 954

O04.5 Genital tract and pelvic infection **following (induced)** [cc][M]♀
termination of pregnancy
    Endometritis following (induced) termination of pregnancy
    Oophoritis following (induced) termination of pregnancy
    Parametritis following (induced) termination of pregnancy
    Pelvic peritonitis following (induced) termination of pregnancy
    Salpingitis following (induced) termination of pregnancy
    Salpingo-oophoritis following (induced) termination of
      pregnancy
    EXCLUDES 1   *sepsis following (induced) termination of pregnancy*
        (O04.87)
        urinary tract infection following (induced) termination
        of pregnancy (O04.88)

O04.6 Delayed or excessive hemorrhage **following (induced)** [M]♀
termination of pregnancy
    Afibrinogenemia following (induced) termination of pregnancy
    Defibrination syndrome following (induced) termination of
      pregnancy
    Hemolysis following (induced) termination of pregnancy
    Intravascular coagulation following (induced) termination of
      pregnancy

O04.7 Embolism **following (induced) termination of** [MCC][M]♀
pregnancy
    Air embolism following (induced) termination of pregnancy
    Amniotic fluid embolism following (induced) termination of
      pregnancy
    Blood-clot embolism following (induced) termination of
      pregnancy
    Embolism NOS following (induced) termination of pregnancy
    Fat embolism following (induced) termination of pregnancy
    Pulmonary embolism following (induced) termination of
      pregnancy
    Pyemic embolism following (induced) termination of pregnancy
    Septic or septicopyemic embolism following (induced)
      termination of pregnancy
    Soap embolism following (induced) termination of pregnancy

[✓5th] **O04.8** (Induced) termination of pregnancy with other **and**
unspecified **complications**

  O04.80 (Induced) termination of pregnancy with [cc][M]♀
    unspecified **complications**

  O04.81 Shock **following (induced) termination of** [MCC][M]♀
    pregnancy
      Circulatory collapse following (induced) termination of
        pregnancy
      Shock (postprocedural) following (induced)
        termination of pregnancy
      EXCLUDES 1   *shock due to infection following (induced)*
          termination of pregnancy (O04.87)

  O04.82 Renal failure **following (induced)** [MCC][M]♀
    termination of pregnancy
      Kidney failure (acute) following (induced) termination
        of pregnancy
      Oliguria following (induced) termination of pregnancy
      Renal shutdown following (induced) termination of
        pregnancy
      Renal tubular necrosis following (induced) termination
        of pregnancy
      Uremia following (induced) termination of pregnancy

  O04.83 Metabolic disorder **following (induced)** [cc][M]♀
    termination of pregnancy

☑ Additional Character Req   [✓x7th] Placeholder Alert   Unacceptable PDx   Manifestation   [H1]-[H14] HAC   [HCC] CMS-HCC Condition   *EXCLUDES 1* Not Coded Here   *EXCLUDES 2* Not Included Here

ICD-10-CM 2018   **845**

O04.84   **Damage to pelvic organs following (induced)** `CC` `M`♀ **termination of pregnancy**
     Laceration, perforation, tear or chemical damage of bladder following (induced) termination of pregnancy
     Laceration, perforation, tear or chemical damage of bowel following (induced) termination of pregnancy
     Laceration, perforation, tear or chemical damage of broad ligament following (induced) termination of pregnancy
     Laceration, perforation, tear or chemical damage of cervix following (induced) termination of pregnancy
     Laceration, perforation, tear or chemical damage of periurethral tissue following (induced) termination of pregnancy
     Laceration, perforation, tear or chemical damage of uterus following (induced) termination of pregnancy
     Laceration, perforation, tear or chemical damage of vagina following (induced) termination of pregnancy

O04.85   **Other venous complications following** `CC` `M`♀ **(induced) termination of pregnancy**

O04.86   **Cardiac arrest following (induced)** `CC` `M`♀ **termination of pregnancy**

O04.87   **Sepsis following (induced) termination of** `CC` `M`♀ **pregnancy**
     Use additional code to identify infectious agent (B95-B97)
     Use additional code to identify severe sepsis, if applicable (R65.2-)
     EXCLUDES 1   *septic or septicopyemic embolism following (induced) termination of pregnancy (O04.7)*
     CC Excl: PDX collection 955

O04.88   **Urinary tract infection following (induced)** `CC` `M`♀ **termination of pregnancy**
     Cystitis following (induced) termination of pregnancy

O04.89   **(Induced) termination of pregnancy with** `CC` `M`♀ **other complications**

`√4th` **O07**   **Failed attempted termination of pregnancy**
     `INCLUDES`   failure of attempted induction of termination of pregnancy incomplete elective abortion
     EXCLUDES 1   *incomplete spontaneous abortion (O03.0-)*

O07.0   **Genital tract and pelvic infection following failed** `CC` `M`♀ **attempted termination of pregnancy**
     Endometritis following failed attempted termination of pregnancy
     Oophoritis following failed attempted termination of pregnancy
     Parametritis following failed attempted termination of pregnancy
     Pelvic peritonitis following failed attempted termination of pregnancy
     Salpingitis following failed attempted termination of pregnancy
     Salpingo-oophoritis following failed attempted termination of pregnancy
     EXCLUDES 1   *sepsis following failed attempted termination of pregnancy (O07.37)*
         urinary tract infection following failed attempted termination of pregnancy (O07.38)
     CC Excl: PDX collection 956

O07.1   **Delayed or excessive hemorrhage following failed** `CC` `M`♀ **attempted termination of pregnancy**
     Afibrinogenemia following failed attempted termination of pregnancy
     Defibrination syndrome following failed attempted termination of pregnancy
     Hemolysis following failed attempted termination of pregnancy
     Intravascular coagulation following failed attempted termination of pregnancy
     CC Excl: PDX collection 957

O07.2   **Embolism following failed attempted termination of** `MCC` `M`♀ **pregnancy**
     Air embolism following failed attempted termination of pregnancy
     Amniotic fluid embolism following failed attempted termination of pregnancy
     Blood-clot embolism following failed attempted termination of pregnancy
     Embolism NOS following failed attempted termination of pregnancy
     Fat embolism following failed attempted termination of pregnancy
     Pulmonary embolism following failed attempted termination of pregnancy
     Pyemic embolism following failed attempted termination of pregnancy
     Septic or septicopyemic embolism following failed attempted termination of pregnancy
     Soap embolism following failed attempted termination of pregnancy
     CC Excl: PDX collection 958

`√5th` **O07.3**   **Failed attempted termination of pregnancy with other and unspecified complications**

O07.30   **Failed attempted termination of pregnancy** `CC` `M`♀ **with unspecified complications**
     CC Excl: PDX collection 954

O07.31   **Shock following failed attempted** `MCC` `M`♀ **termination of pregnancy**
     Circulatory collapse following failed attempted termination of pregnancy
     Shock (postprocedural) following failed attempted termination of pregnancy
     EXCLUDES 1   *shock due to infection following failed attempted termination of pregnancy (O07.37)*
     CC Excl: PDX collection 959

O07.32   **Renal failure following failed attempted** `MCC` `M`♀ **termination of pregnancy**
     Kidney failure (acute) following failed attempted termination of pregnancy
     Oliguria following failed attempted termination of pregnancy
     Renal shutdown following failed attempted termination of pregnancy
     Renal tubular necrosis following failed attempted termination of pregnancy
     Uremia following failed attempted termination of pregnancy
     CC Excl: PDX collection 960

O07.33   **Metabolic disorder following failed** `CC` `M`♀ **attempted termination of pregnancy**
     CC Excl: PDX collection 954

O07.34   **Damage to pelvic organs following failed** `CC` `M`♀ **attempted termination of pregnancy**
     Laceration, perforation, tear or chemical damage of bladder following failed attempted termination of pregnancy
     Laceration, perforation, tear or chemical damage of bowel following failed attempted termination of pregnancy
     Laceration, perforation, tear or chemical damage of broad ligament following failed attempted termination of pregnancy
     Laceration, perforation, tear or chemical damage of cervix following failed attempted termination of pregnancy
     Laceration, perforation, tear or chemical damage of periurethral tissue following failed attempted termination of pregnancy
     Laceration, perforation, tear or chemical damage of uterus following failed attempted termination of pregnancy
     Laceration, perforation, tear or chemical damage of vagina following failed attempted termination of pregnancy
     CC Excl: PDX collection 961

O07.35   **Other venous complications following failed** `CC` `M`♀ **attempted termination of pregnancy**
     CC Excl: PDX collection 954

O07.36   **Cardiac arrest following failed attempted** `CC` `M`♀ **termination of pregnancy**
     CC Excl: PDX collection 954

Chapter 15. Pregnancy, Childbirth and the Puerperium

O07.37   **Sepsis following failed attempted**   CC M ♀
       termination of pregnancy
         Use additional code to identify infectious agent (B95-
          B97)
         Use additional code to identify severe sepsis, if
          applicable (R65.2-)
         EXCLUDES 1   *septic or septicopyemic embolism following*
            failed attempted termination of
            pregnancy (O07.2)
         CC Excl: PDX collection 956

O07.38   **Urinary tract infection following failed**   CC M ♀
       attempted termination of pregnancy
         Cystitis following failed attempted termination of
          pregnancy
         CC Excl: PDX collection 954

O07.39   **Failed attempted termination of pregnancy**   CC M ♀
       with other complications
         CC Excl: PDX collection 954

O07.4   **Failed attempted termination of pregnancy without**   M ♀
     complication

☑4ᵗʰ **O08**   **Complications following ectopic and molar pregnancy**
       This category is for use with categories O00–O02 to identify any
       associated complications

      CC Excl: For CC/MCC codes in category O08, unless otherwise
      noted: PDX collection 963

O08.0   **Genital tract and pelvic infection following ectopic**   CC M ♀
     and molar pregnancy
       Endometritis following ectopic and molar pregnancy
       Oophoritis following ectopic and molar pregnancy
       Parametritis following ectopic and molar pregnancy
       Pelvic peritonitis following ectopic and molar pregnancy
       Salpingitis following ectopic and molar pregnancy
       Salpingo-oophoritis following ectopic and molar pregnancy
       EXCLUDES 1   *sepsis following ectopic and molar pregnancy (O08.82)*
            urinary tract infection (O08.83)
      CC Excl: PDX collection 85

O08.1   **Delayed or excessive hemorrhage following ectopic**   CC M ♀
     and molar pregnancy
       Afibrinogenemia following ectopic and molar pregnancy
       Defibrination syndrome following ectopic and molar pregnancy
       Hemolysis following ectopic and molar pregnancy
       Intravascular coagulation following ectopic and molar
         pregnancy
       EXCLUDES 1   *delayed or excessive hemorrhage due to incomplete*
            abortion (O03.1)
      CC Excl: PDX collection 962

O08.2   **Embolism following ectopic and molar pregnancy**   MCC M ♀
       Air embolism following ectopic and molar pregnancy
       Amniotic fluid embolism following ectopic and molar pregnancy
       Blood-clot embolism following ectopic and molar pregnancy
       Embolism NOS following ectopic and molar pregnancy
       Fat embolism following ectopic and molar pregnancy
       Pulmonary embolism following ectopic and molar pregnancy
       Pyemic embolism following ectopic and molar pregnancy
       Septic or septicopyemic embolism following ectopic and molar
         pregnancy
       Soap embolism following ectopic and molar pregnancy

O08.3   **Shock following ectopic and molar pregnancy**   MCC M ♀
       Circulatory collapse following ectopic and molar pregnancy
       Shock (postprocedural) following ectopic and molar pregnancy
       EXCLUDES 1   *shock due to infection following ectopic and molar*
            pregnancy (O08.82)

O08.4   **Renal failure following ectopic and molar pregnancy**   MCC M ♀
       Kidney failure (acute) following ectopic and molar pregnancy
       Oliguria following ectopic and molar pregnancy
       Renal shutdown following ectopic and molar pregnancy
       Renal tubular necrosis following ectopic and molar pregnancy
       Uremia following ectopic and molar pregnancy

O08.5   **Metabolic disorders following an ectopic and molar**   CC M ♀
     pregnancy

O08.6   **Damage to pelvic organs and tissues following an**   CC M ♀
     ectopic and molar pregnancy
       Laceration, perforation, tear or chemical damage of bladder
         following an ectopic and molar pregnancy
       Laceration, perforation, tear or chemical damage of bowel
         following an ectopic and molar pregnancy
       Laceration, perforation, tear or chemical damage of broad
         ligament following an ectopic and molar pregnancy
       Laceration, perforation, tear or chemical damage of cervix
         following an ectopic and molar pregnancy
       Laceration, perforation, tear or chemical damage of periurethral
         tissue following an ectopic and molar pregnancy
       Laceration, perforation, tear or chemical damage of uterus
         following an ectopic and molar pregnancy
       Laceration, perforation, tear or chemical damage of vagina
         following an ectopic and molar pregnancy

O08.7   **Other venous complications following an ectopic**   CC M ♀
     and molar pregnancy

☑5ᵗʰ **O08.8**   **Other complications following an ectopic and molar**
     pregnancy

O08.81   **Cardiac arrest following an ectopic and molar**   CC M ♀
       pregnancy

O08.82   **Sepsis following ectopic and molar pregnancy**   CC M ♀
         Use additional code to identify infectious agent
          (B95-B97)
         Use additional code to identify severe sepsis, if
          applicable (R65.2-)
         EXCLUDES 1   *septic or septicopyemic embolism following*
            ectopic and molar pregnancy (O08.2)
         CC Excl: PDX collection 85

O08.83   **Urinary tract infection following an ectopic**   CC M ♀
       and molar pregnancy
         Cystitis following an ectopic and molar pregnancy

O08.89   **Other complications following an ectopic**   CC M ♀
       and molar pregnancy

O08.9   **Unspecified complication following an ectopic and**   CC M ♀
     molar pregnancy

Supervision of high risk pregnancy (O09)

☑4ᵗʰ **O09**   **Supervision of high risk pregnancy**
       AHA: 2016, 4Q, 150

☑5ᵗʰ **O09.0**   **Supervision of pregnancy with history of infertility**

O09.00   **Supervision of pregnancy with history of**   M ♀
       infertility, unspecified trimester

O09.01   **Supervision of pregnancy with history of**   M ♀
       infertility, first trimester

O09.02   **Supervision of pregnancy with history of**   M ♀
       infertility, second trimester

O09.03   **Supervision of pregnancy with history of**   M ♀
       infertility, third trimester

☑5ᵗʰ **O09.1**   **Supervision of pregnancy with history of ectopic**
     pregnancy

O09.10   **Supervision of pregnancy with history of**   M ♀
       ectopic pregnancy, unspecified trimester

O09.11   **Supervision of pregnancy with history of**   M ♀
       ectopic pregnancy, first trimester

O09.12   **Supervision of pregnancy with history of**   M ♀
       ectopic pregnancy, second trimester

O09.13   **Supervision of pregnancy with history of**   M ♀
       ectopic pregnancy, third trimester

☑5ᵗʰ **O09.A**   **Supervision of pregnancy with history of molar pregnancy**

O09.A0   **Supervision of pregnancy with history of molar**   M ♀
       pregnancy, unspecified trimester

O09.A1   **Supervision of pregnancy with history of molar**   M ♀
       pregnancy, first trimester

O09.A2   **Supervision of pregnancy with history of molar**   M ♀
       pregnancy, second trimester

O09.A3   **Supervision of pregnancy with history of molar**   M ♀
       pregnancy, third trimester

☑5ᵗʰ **O09.2**   **Supervision of pregnancy with other poor reproductive or**
     obstetric history
       EXCLUDES 2   *pregnancy care for patient with history of recurrent*
            pregnancy loss (O26.2-)

☑6ᵗʰ **O09.21**   **Supervision of pregnancy with history of pre-term**
       labor

O09.211   **Supervision of pregnancy with history**   M ♀
       of pre-term labor, first trimester

O09.212   **Supervision of pregnancy with history**   M ♀
       of pre-term labor, second trimester

O09.213 Supervision of pregnancy with history Ⓜ♀
of pre-term labor, **third trimester**

O09.219 Supervision of pregnancy with history Ⓜ♀
of pre-term labor, **unspecified trimester**

✓6ᵗʰ **O09.29** Supervision of pregnancy with **other** poor
reproductive or obstetric history
Supervision of pregnancy with history of neonatal
death
Supervision of pregnancy with history of stillbirth

O09.291 Supervision of pregnancy with other Ⓜ♀
poor reproductive or obstetric
history, **first trimester**

O09.292 Supervision of pregnancy with other Ⓜ♀
poor reproductive or obstetric
history, **second trimester**

O09.293 Supervision of pregnancy with other Ⓜ♀
poor reproductive or obstetric
history, **third trimester**

O09.299 Supervision of pregnancy with other Ⓜ♀
poor reproductive or obstetric
history, **unspecified trimester**

✓5ᵗʰ **O09.3** Supervision of pregnancy with **insufficient antenatal care**
Supervision of concealed pregnancy
Supervision of hidden pregnancy

O09.30 Supervision of pregnancy with insufficient Ⓜ♀
antenatal care, **unspecified trimester**

O09.31 Supervision of pregnancy with insufficient Ⓜ♀
antenatal care, **first trimester**

O09.32 Supervision of pregnancy with insufficient Ⓜ♀
antenatal care, **second trimester**

O09.33 Supervision of pregnancy with insufficient Ⓜ♀
antenatal care, **third trimester**

✓5ᵗʰ **O09.4** Supervision of pregnancy with **grand multiparity**

O09.40 Supervision of pregnancy with grand Ⓜ♀
multiparity, **unspecified trimester**

O09.41 Supervision of pregnancy with grand Ⓜ♀
multiparity, **first trimester**

O09.42 Supervision of pregnancy with grand Ⓜ♀
multiparity, **second trimester**

O09.43 Supervision of pregnancy with grand Ⓜ♀
multiparity, **third trimester**

✓5ᵗʰ **O09.5** Supervision of **elderly primigravida and multigravida**
Pregnancy for a female 35 years and older at expected date of
delivery

✓6ᵗʰ **O09.51** Supervision of **elderly primigravida**

O09.511 Supervision of elderly primigravida, Ⓜ♀
first trimester

O09.512 Supervision of elderly primigravida, Ⓜ♀
second trimester

O09.513 Supervision of elderly primigravida, Ⓜ♀
third trimester

O09.519 Supervision of elderly primigravida, Ⓜ♀
unspecified trimester

✓6ᵗʰ **O09.52** Supervision of **elderly multigravida**

O09.521 Supervision of elderly multigravida, Ⓜ♀
first trimester

O09.522 Supervision of elderly multigravida, Ⓜ♀
second trimester

O09.523 Supervision of elderly multigravida, Ⓜ♀
third trimester

O09.529 Supervision of elderly multigravida, Ⓜ♀
unspecified trimester

✓5ᵗʰ **O09.6** Supervision of **young primigravida and multigravida**
Supervision of pregnancy for a female less than 16 years old at
expected date of delivery

✓6ᵗʰ **O09.61** Supervision of **young primigravida**

O09.611 Supervision of young primigravida, Ⓜ♀
first trimester

O09.612 Supervision of young primigravida, Ⓜ♀
second trimester

O09.613 Supervision of young primigravida, Ⓜ♀
third trimester

O09.619 Supervision of young primigravida, Ⓜ♀
unspecified trimester

✓6ᵗʰ **O09.62** Supervision of young **multigravida**

O09.621 Supervision of young multigravida, Ⓜ♀
first trimester

O09.622 Supervision of young multigravida, Ⓜ♀
second trimester

O09.623 Supervision of young multigravida, Ⓜ♀
third trimester

O09.629 Supervision of young multigravida, Ⓜ♀
unspecified trimester

✓5ᵗʰ **O09.7** Supervision of high risk pregnancy due to **social problems**

O09.70 Supervision of high risk pregnancy due to Ⓜ♀
social problems, **unspecified trimester**

O09.71 Supervision of high risk pregnancy due to Ⓜ♀
social problems, **first trimester**

O09.72 Supervision of high risk pregnancy due to Ⓜ♀
social problems, **second trimester**

O09.73 Supervision of high risk pregnancy due to Ⓜ♀
social problems, **third trimester**

✓5ᵗʰ **O09.8** Supervision of **other** high risk pregnancies

✓6ᵗʰ **O09.81** Supervision of pregnancy **resulting from assisted reproductive technology**
Supervision of pregnancy resulting from in-vitro
fertilization
EXCLUDES 2 *gestational carrier status (Z33.3)*

O09.811 Supervision of pregnancy resulting Ⓜ♀
from assisted reproductive
technology, **first trimester**

O09.812 Supervision of pregnancy resulting Ⓜ♀
from assisted reproductive
technology, **second trimester**

O09.813 Supervision of pregnancy resulting Ⓜ♀
from assisted reproductive
technology, **third trimester**

O09.819 Supervision of pregnancy resulting Ⓜ♀
from assisted reproductive
technology, **unspecified trimester**

✓6ᵗʰ **O09.82** Supervision of pregnancy with **history of in utero procedure during previous pregnancy**

O09.821 Supervision of pregnancy with history Ⓜ♀
of in utero procedure during previous
pregnancy, **first trimester**

O09.822 Supervision of pregnancy with history Ⓜ♀
of in utero procedure during previous
pregnancy, **second trimester**

O09.823 Supervision of pregnancy with history Ⓜ♀
of in utero procedure during previous
pregnancy, **third trimester**

O09.829 Supervision of pregnancy with history Ⓜ♀
of in utero procedure during previous
pregnancy, **unspecified trimester**
EXCLUDES 1 *supervision of pregnancy affected
by in utero procedure during
current pregnancy (O35.7)*

✓6ᵗʰ **O09.89** Supervision of **other** high risk pregnancies

O09.891 Supervision of other high risk Ⓜ♀
pregnancies, **first trimester**

O09.892 Supervision of other high risk Ⓜ♀
pregnancies, **second trimester**

O09.893 Supervision of other high risk Ⓜ♀
pregnancies, **third trimester**

O09.899 Supervision of other high risk Ⓜ♀
pregnancies, **unspecified trimester**

✓5ᵗʰ **O09.9** Supervision of high risk pregnancy, **unspecified**

O09.90 Supervision of high risk pregnancy, Ⓜ♀
unspecified, **unspecified trimester**

O09.91 Supervision of high risk pregnancy, Ⓜ♀
unspecified, **first trimester**

O09.92 Supervision of high risk pregnancy, Ⓜ♀
unspecified, **second trimester**

O09.93 Supervision of high risk pregnancy, Ⓜ♀
unspecified, **third trimester**

Edema, proteinuria and hypertensive disorders in pregnancy, childbirth and the puerperium (O10-O16)

✓4ᵗʰ **O10** **Pre-existing hypertension complicating pregnancy, childbirth and the puerperium**

> INCLUDES   pre-existing hypertension with pre-existing proteinuria complicating pregnancy, childbirth and the puerperium
>
> EXCLUDES 2   *pre-existing hypertension with superimposed pre-eclampsia complicating pregnancy, childbirth and the puerperium (O11.-)*

> CC Excl: For CC/MCC codes in category O10: PDX collection 964

✓5ᵗʰ **O10.0** **Pre-existing essential hypertension complicating pregnancy, childbirth and the puerperium**
> Any condition in I10 specified as a reason for obstetric care during pregnancy, childbirth or the puerperium

     ✓6ᵗʰ **O10.01** **Pre-existing essential hypertension complicating pregnancy**

         O10.011 **Pre-existing essential hypertension complicating pregnancy, first trimester** CC M♀

         O10.012 **Pre-existing essential hypertension complicating pregnancy, second trimester** CC M♀

         O10.013 **Pre-existing essential hypertension complicating pregnancy, third trimester** CC M♀

         O10.019 **Pre-existing essential hypertension complicating pregnancy, unspecified trimester** M♀

     O10.02 **Pre-existing essential hypertension complicating childbirth** CC M♀

     O10.03 **Pre-existing essential hypertension complicating the puerperium** M♀

✓5ᵗʰ **O10.1** **Pre-existing hypertensive heart disease complicating pregnancy, childbirth and the puerperium**
> Any condition in I11 specified as a reason for obstetric care during pregnancy, childbirth or the puerperium
> Use additional code from I11 to identify the type of hypertensive heart disease

     ✓6ᵗʰ **O10.11** **Pre-existing hypertensive heart disease complicating pregnancy**

         O10.111 **Pre-existing hypertensive heart disease complicating pregnancy, first trimester** M♀

         O10.112 **Pre-existing hypertensive heart disease complicating pregnancy, second trimester** M♀

         O10.113 **Pre-existing hypertensive heart disease complicating pregnancy, third trimester** M♀

         O10.119 **Pre-existing hypertensive heart disease complicating pregnancy, unspecified trimester** M♀

     O10.12 **Pre-existing hypertensive heart disease complicating childbirth** M♀

     O10.13 **Pre-existing hypertensive heart disease complicating the puerperium** M♀

✓5ᵗʰ **O10.2** **Pre-existing hypertensive chronic kidney disease complicating pregnancy, childbirth and the puerperium**
> Any condition in I12 specified as a reason for obstetric care during pregnancy, childbirth or the puerperium
> Use additional code from I12 to identify the type of hypertensive chronic kidney disease

     ✓6ᵗʰ **O10.21** **Pre-existing hypertensive chronic kidney disease complicating pregnancy**

         O10.211 **Pre-existing hypertensive chronic kidney disease complicating pregnancy, first trimester** M♀

         O10.212 **Pre-existing hypertensive chronic kidney disease complicating pregnancy, second trimester** M♀

         O10.213 **Pre-existing hypertensive chronic kidney disease complicating pregnancy, third trimester** M♀

         O10.219 **Pre-existing hypertensive chronic kidney disease complicating pregnancy, unspecified trimester** M♀

     O10.22 **Pre-existing hypertensive chronic kidney disease complicating childbirth** M♀

     O10.23 **Pre-existing hypertensive chronic kidney disease complicating the puerperium** M♀

✓5ᵗʰ **O10.3** **Pre-existing hypertensive heart and chronic kidney disease complicating pregnancy, childbirth and the puerperium**
> Any condition in I13 specified as a reason for obstetric care during pregnancy, childbirth or the puerperium
> Use additional code from I13 to identify the type of hypertensive heart and chronic kidney disease

     ✓6ᵗʰ **O10.31** **Pre-existing hypertensive heart and chronic kidney disease complicating pregnancy**

         O10.311 **Pre-existing hypertensive heart and chronic kidney disease complicating pregnancy, first trimester** M♀

         O10.312 **Pre-existing hypertensive heart and chronic kidney disease complicating pregnancy, second trimester** M♀

         O10.313 **Pre-existing hypertensive heart and chronic kidney disease complicating pregnancy, third trimester** M♀

         O10.319 **Pre-existing hypertensive heart and chronic kidney disease complicating pregnancy, unspecified trimester** M♀

     O10.32 **Pre-existing hypertensive heart and chronic kidney disease complicating childbirth** M♀

     O10.33 **Pre-existing hypertensive heart and chronic kidney disease complicating the puerperium** M♀

✓5ᵗʰ **O10.4** **Pre-existing secondary hypertension complicating pregnancy, childbirth and the puerperium**
> Any condition in I15 specified as a reason for obstetric care during pregnancy, childbirth or the puerperium
> Use additional code from I15 to identify the type of secondary hypertension

     ✓6ᵗʰ **O10.41** **Pre-existing secondary hypertension complicating pregnancy**

         O10.411 **Pre-existing secondary hypertension complicating pregnancy, first trimester** CC M♀

         O10.412 **Pre-existing secondary hypertension complicating pregnancy, second trimester** CC M♀

         O10.413 **Pre-existing secondary hypertension complicating pregnancy, third trimester** CC M♀

         O10.419 **Pre-existing secondary hypertension complicating pregnancy, unspecified trimester** M♀

     O10.42 **Pre-existing secondary hypertension complicating childbirth** MCC M♀

     O10.43 **Pre-existing secondary hypertension complicating the puerperium** CC M♀

✓5ᵗʰ **O10.9** **Unspecified pre-existing hypertension complicating pregnancy, childbirth and the puerperium**

     ✓6ᵗʰ **O10.91** **Unspecified pre-existing hypertension complicating pregnancy**

         O10.911 **Unspecified pre-existing hypertension complicating pregnancy, first trimester** CC M♀

         O10.912 **Unspecified pre-existing hypertension complicating pregnancy, second trimester** CC M♀

         O10.913 **Unspecified pre-existing hypertension complicating pregnancy, third trimester** CC M♀

         O10.919 **Unspecified pre-existing hypertension complicating pregnancy, unspecified trimester** M♀

     O10.92 **Unspecified pre-existing hypertension complicating childbirth** CC M♀

     O10.93 **Unspecified pre-existing hypertension complicating the puerperium** M♀

✓4ᵗʰ **O11** **Pre-existing hypertension with pre-eclampsia**
> INCLUDES   conditions in O10 complicated by pre-eclampsia
>   pre-eclampsia superimposed pre-existing hypertension
> Use additional code from O10 to identify the type of hypertension

> CC Excl: For MCC codes in category O11: PDX collection 964

     O11.1 **Pre-existing hypertension with pre-eclampsia, first trimester** MCC M♀

Chapter 15. Pregnancy, Childbirth and the Puerperium

O11.2 **Pre-existing hypertension with pre-eclampsia, second trimester** `MCC` `M♀`

O11.3 **Pre-existing hypertension with pre-eclampsia, third trimester** `MCC` `M♀`

O11.4 **Pre-existing hypertension with pre-eclampsia, complicating childbirth** `M♀`

O11.5 **Pre-existing hypertension with pre-eclampsia, complicating the puerperium** `M♀`

O11.9 **Pre-existing hypertension with pre-eclampsia, unspecified trimester** `M♀`

√4ᵗʰ **O12 Gestational [pregnancy-induced] edema and proteinuria without hypertension**

CC Excl: For CC codes in category O12: PDX collection 965

√5ᵗʰ **O12.0 Gestational edema**

O12.00 **Gestational edema, unspecified trimester** `M♀`

O12.01 **Gestational edema, first trimester** `M♀`

O12.02 **Gestational edema, second trimester** `M♀`

O12.03 **Gestational edema, third trimester** `M♀`

O12.04 **Gestational edema, complicating childbirth** `M♀`

O12.05 **Gestational edema, complicating the puerperium** `M♀`

√5ᵗʰ **O12.1 Gestational proteinuria**

O12.10 **Gestational proteinuria, unspecified trimester** `M♀`

O12.11 **Gestational proteinuria, first trimester** `CC` `M♀`

O12.12 **Gestational proteinuria, second trimester** `CC` `M♀`

O12.13 **Gestational proteinuria, third trimester** `CC` `M♀`

O12.14 **Gestational proteinuria, complicating childbirth** `M♀`

O12.15 **Gestational proteinuria, complicating the puerperium** `M♀`

√5ᵗʰ **O12.2 Gestational edema with proteinuria**

O12.20 **Gestational edema with proteinuria, unspecified trimester** `M♀`

O12.21 **Gestational edema with proteinuria, first trimester** `PDxCC` `CC` `M♀`

O12.22 **Gestational edema with proteinuria, second trimester** `PDxCC` `CC` `M♀`

O12.23 **Gestational edema with proteinuria, third trimester** `PDxCC` `CC` `M♀`

O12.24 **Gestational edema with proteinuria, complicating childbirth** `M♀`

O12.25 **Gestational edema with proteinuria, complicating the puerperium** `M♀`

√4ᵗʰ **O13 Gestational [pregnancy-induced] hypertension without significant proteinuria**
INCLUDES   gestational hypertension NOS
     transient hypertension of pregnancy
AHA: 2016, 1Q, 5

O13.1 **Gestational [pregnancy-induced] hypertension without significant proteinuria, first trimester** `M♀`

O13.2 **Gestational [pregnancy-induced] hypertension without significant proteinuria, second trimester** `M♀`

O13.3 **Gestational [pregnancy-induced] hypertension without significant proteinuria, third trimester** `M♀`

O13.4 **Gestational [pregnancy-induced] hypertension without significant proteinuria, complicating childbirth** `M♀`

O13.5 **Gestational [pregnancy-induced] hypertension without significant proteinuria, complicating the puerperium** `M♀`

O13.9 **Gestational [pregnancy-induced] hypertension without significant proteinuria, unspecified trimester** `M♀`

√4ᵗʰ **O14 Pre-eclampsia**
EXCLUDES 1   pre-existing hypertension with pre-eclampsia (O11)

CC Excl: For CC /MCC codes in category O14: PDX collection 964

√5ᵗʰ **O14.0 Mild to moderate pre-eclampsia**

O14.00 **Mild to moderate pre-eclampsia, unspecified trimester** `M♀`

O14.02 **Mild to moderate pre-eclampsia, second trimester** `CC` `M♀`

O14.03 **Mild to moderate pre-eclampsia, third trimester** `CC` `M♀`

O14.04 **Mild to moderate pre-eclampsia, complicating childbirth** `M♀`

O14.05 **Mild to moderate pre-eclampsia, complicating the puerperium** `M♀`

√5ᵗʰ **O14.1 Severe pre-eclampsia**
EXCLUDES 1   HELLP syndrome (O14.2-)

O14.10 **Severe pre-eclampsia, unspecified trimester** `M♀`

O14.12 **Severe pre-eclampsia, second trimester** `MCC` `M♀`

O14.13 **Severe pre-eclampsia, third trimester** `MCC` `M♀`

O14.14 **Severe pre-eclampsia complicating childbirth** `M♀`

O14.15 **Severe pre-eclampsia, complicating the puerperium** `M♀`

√5ᵗʰ **O14.2 HELLP syndrome**
Severe pre-eclampsia with hemolysis, elevated liver enzymes and low platelet count (HELLP)

O14.20 **HELLP syndrome (HELLP), unspecified trimester** `M♀`

O14.22 **HELLP syndrome (HELLP), second trimester** `MCC` `M♀`

O14.23 **HELLP syndrome (HELLP), third trimester** `MCC` `M♀`

O14.24 **HELLP syndrome, complicating childbirth** `M♀`

O14.25 **HELLP syndrome, complicating the puerperium** `M♀`

√5ᵗʰ **O14.9 Unspecified pre-eclampsia**

O14.90 **Unspecified pre-eclampsia, unspecified trimester** `M♀`

O14.92 **Unspecified pre-eclampsia, second trimester** `CC` `M♀`

O14.93 **Unspecified pre-eclampsia, third trimester** `CC` `M♀`

O14.94 **Unspecified pre-eclampsia, complicating childbirth** `M♀`

O14.95 **Unspecified pre-eclampsia, complicating the puerperium** `M♀`

√4ᵗʰ **O15 Eclampsia**
INCLUDES   convulsions following conditions in O10-O14 and O16

CC Excl: For MCC codes in category O15: PDX collection 964

√5ᵗʰ **O15.0 Eclampsia complicating pregnancy**

O15.00 **Eclampsia complicating pregnancy, unspecified trimester** `M♀`

O15.02 **Eclampsia complicating pregnancy, second trimester** `MCC` `M♀`

O15.03 **Eclampsia complicating pregnancy, third trimester** `MCC` `M♀`

O15.1 **Eclampsia complicating labor** `MCC` `M♀`

O15.2 **Eclampsia complicating the puerperium** `MCC` `M♀`

O15.9 **Eclampsia, unspecified as to time period** `M♀`
Eclampsia NOS

√4ᵗʰ **O16 Unspecified maternal hypertension**

CC Excl: For CC codes in category O16: PDX collection 964

O16.1 **Unspecified maternal hypertension, first trimester** `CC` `M♀`

O16.2 **Unspecified maternal hypertension, second trimester** `CC` `M♀`

O16.3 **Unspecified maternal hypertension, third trimester** `CC` `M♀`

O16.4 **Unspecified maternal hypertension, complicating childbirth** `M♀`

O16.5 **Unspecified maternal hypertension, complicating the puerperium** `M♀`

O16.9 **Unspecified maternal hypertension, unspecified trimester** `M♀`

Other maternal disorders predominantly related to pregnancy (O20-O29)

EXCLUDES 2   maternal care related to the fetus and amniotic cavity and possible delivery problems (O30-O48)
maternal diseases classifiable elsewhere but complicating pregnancy, labor and delivery, and the puerperium (O98-O99)

√4ᵗʰ **O20 Hemorrhage in early pregnancy**
Hemorrhage before completion of 20 weeks gestation
EXCLUDES 1   pregnancy with abortive outcome (O00-O08)

O20.0 **Threatened abortion** `CC` `M♀`
Hemorrhage specified as due to threatened abortion
DEF: Bloody discharge during pregnancy; cervix may be dilated and pregnancy threatened, but the pregnancy is not terminated.
CC Excl: PDX collection 966

O20.8 **Other hemorrhage in early pregnancy** `M♀`

O20.9 **Hemorrhage in early pregnancy, unspecified** `CC` `M♀`
CC Excl: PDX collection 966

`N` Newborn: 0   `P` Pediatric: 0-17   `M` Maternity: 12-55   `A` Adult: 15-124   `MCC` Major CC Condition   `PDxMCC` PDx acts as own MCC   `CC` CC Condition   `PDxCC` PDx acts as own CC

850   ICD-10-CM 2018

✅4th **O21 Excessive vomiting in pregnancy**

  O21.0 Mild hyperemesis gravidarum   M♀
    Hyperemesis gravidarum, mild or unspecified, starting before the end of the 20th week of gestation

  O21.1 Hyperemesis gravidarum with metabolic disturbance   M♀
    Hyperemesis gravidarum, starting before the end of the 20th week of gestation, with metabolic disturbance such as carbohydrate depletion
    Hyperemesis gravidarum, starting before the end of the 20th week of gestation, with metabolic disturbance such as dehydration
    Hyperemesis gravidarum, starting before the end of the 20th week of gestation, with metabolic disturbance such as electrolyte imbalance

  O21.2 Late vomiting of pregnancy   M♀
    Excessive vomiting starting after 20 completed weeks of gestation

  O21.8 Other vomiting complicating pregnancy   M♀
    Vomiting due to diseases classified elsewhere, complicating pregnancy
    Use additional code to identify cause

  O21.9 Vomiting of pregnancy, unspecified   M♀

✅4th **O22 Venous complications and hemorrhoids in pregnancy**

  EXCLUDES 1   venous complications of:
    abortion NOS (O03.9)
    ectopic or molar pregnancy (O08.7)
    failed attempted abortion (O07.35)
    induced abortion (O04.85)
    spontaneous abortion (O03.89)
  EXCLUDES 2   obstetric pulmonary embolism (O88.-)
    venous complications and hemorrhoids of childbirth and the puerperium (O87.-)

  CC Excl: For CC/MCC codes in category O22: PDX collection 967

✅5th **O22.0 Varicose veins of lower extremity in pregnancy**
    Varicose veins NOS in pregnancy
    DEF: Distended, tortuous veins of lower extremities associated with pregnancy.

    O22.00 Varicose veins of lower extremity in pregnancy, M♀ **unspecified trimester**

    O22.01 Varicose veins of lower extremity in pregnancy, M♀ **first trimester**

    O22.02 Varicose veins of lower extremity in pregnancy, M♀ **second trimester**

    O22.03 Varicose veins of lower extremity in pregnancy, M♀ **third trimester**

✅5th **O22.1 Genital varices in pregnancy**
    Perineal varices in pregnancy
    Vaginal varices in pregnancy
    Vulval varices in pregnancy

    O22.10 Genital varices in pregnancy, unspecified M♀ **trimester**

    O22.11 Genital varices in pregnancy, first trimester M♀

    O22.12 Genital varices in pregnancy, second trimester M♀

    O22.13 Genital varices in pregnancy, third trimester M♀

✅5th **O22.2 Superficial thrombophlebitis in pregnancy**
    Phlebitis in pregnancy NOS
    Thrombophlebitis of legs in pregnancy
    Thrombosis in pregnancy NOS
    Use additional code to identify the superficial thrombophlebitis (I80.0-)

    O22.20 Superficial thrombophlebitis in pregnancy, CC M♀ **unspecified trimester**

    O22.21 Superficial thrombophlebitis in pregnancy, CC M♀ **first trimester**

    O22.22 Superficial thrombophlebitis in pregnancy, CC M♀ **second trimester**

    O22.23 Superficial thrombophlebitis in pregnancy, CC M♀ **third trimester**

✅5th **O22.3 Deep phlebothrombosis in pregnancy**
    Deep vein thrombosis, antepartum
    Use additional code to identify the deep vein thrombosis (I82.4-, I82.5-, I82.62-, I82.72-)
    Use additional code, if applicable, for associated long-term (current) use of anticoagulants (Z79.01)

    O22.30 Deep phlebothrombosis in pregnancy, CC M♀ **unspecified trimester**

    O22.31 Deep phlebothrombosis in pregnancy, MCC M♀ **first trimester**

    O22.32 Deep phlebothrombosis in pregnancy, MCC M♀ **second trimester**

    O22.33 Deep phlebothrombosis in pregnancy, MCC M♀ **third trimester**

✅5th **O22.4 Hemorrhoids in pregnancy**

    O22.40 Hemorrhoids in pregnancy, unspecified CC M♀ **trimester**

    O22.41 Hemorrhoids in pregnancy, first trimester CC M♀

    O22.42 Hemorrhoids in pregnancy, second trimester CC M♀

    O22.43 Hemorrhoids in pregnancy, third trimester CC M♀

✅5th **O22.5 Cerebral venous thrombosis in pregnancy**
    Cerebrovenous sinus thrombosis in pregnancy

    O22.50 Cerebral venous thrombosis in pregnancy, CC M♀ **unspecified trimester**

    O22.51 Cerebral venous thrombosis in pregnancy, CC M♀ **first trimester**

    O22.52 Cerebral venous thrombosis in pregnancy, CC M♀ **second trimester**

    O22.53 Cerebral venous thrombosis in pregnancy, CC M♀ **third trimester**

✅5th **O22.8 Other venous complications in pregnancy**

  ✅6th **O22.8X Other venous complications in pregnancy**

    O22.8X1 Other venous complications in CC M♀ **pregnancy, first trimester**

    O22.8X2 Other venous complications in CC M♀ **pregnancy, second trimester**

    O22.8X3 Other venous complications in CC M♀ **pregnancy, third trimester**

    O22.8X9 Other venous complications in CC M♀ **pregnancy, unspecified trimester**

✅5th **O22.9 Venous complication in pregnancy, unspecified**
    Gestational phlebitis NOS
    Gestational phlebopathy NOS
    Gestational thrombosis NOS

    O22.90 Venous complication in pregnancy, CC M♀ **unspecified, unspecified trimester**

    O22.91 Venous complication in pregnancy, M♀ **unspecified, first trimester**

    O22.92 Venous complication in pregnancy, M♀ **unspecified, second trimester**

    O22.93 Venous complication in pregnancy, M♀ **unspecified, third trimester**

✅4th **O23 Infections of genitourinary tract in pregnancy**
    Use additional code to identify organism (B95.-, B96.-)
  EXCLUDES 2   gonococcal infections complicating pregnancy, childbirth and the puerperium (O98.2)
    infections with a predominantly sexual mode of transmission NOS complicating pregnancy, childbirth and the puerperium (O98.3)
    syphilis complicating pregnancy, childbirth and the puerperium (O98.1)
    tuberculosis of genitourinary system complicating pregnancy, childbirth and the puerperium (O98.0)
    venereal disease NOS complicating pregnancy, childbirth and the puerperium (O98.3)

  CC Excl: For CC codes in category O23: PDX collection 968

✅5th **O23.0 Infections of kidney in pregnancy**
    Pyelonephritis in pregnancy

    O23.00 Infections of kidney in pregnancy, unspecified M♀ **trimester**

    O23.01 Infections of kidney in pregnancy, first CC M♀ **trimester**

    O23.02 Infections of kidney in pregnancy, second CC M♀ **trimester**

    O23.03 Infections of kidney in pregnancy, third CC M♀ **trimester**

✅5th **O23.1 Infections of bladder in pregnancy**

    O23.10 Infections of bladder in pregnancy, M♀ **unspecified trimester**

    O23.11 Infections of bladder in pregnancy, CC M♀ **first trimester**

    O23.12 Infections of bladder in pregnancy, CC M♀ **second trimester**

    O23.13 Infections of bladder in pregnancy, CC M♀ **third trimester**

Chapter 15. Pregnancy, Childbirth and the Puerperium *(side margin)*

☑5ᵗʰ **O23.2 Infections of urethra in pregnancy**

O23.20 Infections of urethra in pregnancy, unspecified trimester   Ⓜ♀

O23.21 Infections of urethra in pregnancy, first trimester   CC Ⓜ♀

O23.22 Infections of urethra in pregnancy, second trimester   CC Ⓜ♀

O23.23 Infections of urethra in pregnancy, third trimester   CC Ⓜ♀

☑5ᵗʰ **O23.3 Infections of other parts of urinary tract in pregnancy**

O23.30 Infections of other parts of urinary tract in pregnancy, unspecified trimester   Ⓜ♀

O23.31 Infections of other parts of urinary tract in pregnancy, first trimester   CC Ⓜ♀

O23.32 Infections of other parts of urinary tract in pregnancy, second trimester   CC Ⓜ♀

O23.33 Infections of other parts of urinary tract in pregnancy, third trimester   CC Ⓜ♀

☑5ᵗʰ **O23.4 Unspecified infection of urinary tract in pregnancy**

O23.40 Unspecified infection of urinary tract in pregnancy, unspecified trimester   Ⓜ♀

O23.41 Unspecified infection of urinary tract in pregnancy, first trimester   CC Ⓜ♀

O23.42 Unspecified infection of urinary tract in pregnancy, second trimester   CC Ⓜ♀

O23.43 Unspecified infection of urinary tract in pregnancy, third trimester   CC Ⓜ♀

☑5ᵗʰ **O23.5 Infections of the genital tract in pregnancy**

☑6ᵗʰ **O23.51 Infection of cervix in pregnancy**

O23.511 Infections of cervix in pregnancy, first trimester   CC Ⓜ♀

O23.512 Infections of cervix in pregnancy, second trimester   CC Ⓜ♀

O23.513 Infections of cervix in pregnancy, third trimester   CC Ⓜ♀

O23.519 Infections of cervix in pregnancy, unspecified trimester   Ⓜ♀

☑6ᵗʰ **O23.52 Salpingo-oophoritis in pregnancy**
Oophoritis in pregnancy
Salpingitis in pregnancy

O23.521 Salpingo-oophoritis in pregnancy, first trimester   CC Ⓜ♀

O23.522 Salpingo-oophoritis in pregnancy, second trimester   CC Ⓜ♀

O23.523 Salpingo-oophoritis in pregnancy, third trimester   CC Ⓜ♀

O23.529 Salpingo-oophoritis in pregnancy, unspecified trimester   Ⓜ♀

☑6ᵗʰ **O23.59 Infection of other part of genital tract in pregnancy**

O23.591 Infection of other part of genital tract in pregnancy, first trimester   CC Ⓜ♀

O23.592 Infection of other part of genital tract in pregnancy, second trimester   CC Ⓜ♀

O23.593 Infection of other part of genital tract in pregnancy, third trimester   CC Ⓜ♀

O23.599 Infection of other part of genital tract in pregnancy, unspecified trimester   Ⓜ♀

☑5ᵗʰ **O23.9 Unspecified genitourinary tract infection in pregnancy**
Genitourinary tract infection in pregnancy NOS

O23.90 Unspecified genitourinary tract infection in pregnancy, unspecified trimester   Ⓜ♀

O23.91 Unspecified genitourinary tract infection in pregnancy, first trimester   CC Ⓜ♀

O23.92 Unspecified genitourinary tract infection in pregnancy, second trimester   CC Ⓜ♀

O23.93 Unspecified genitourinary tract infection in pregnancy, third trimester   CC Ⓜ♀

☑4ᵗʰ **O24 Diabetes mellitus in pregnancy, childbirth, and the puerperium**

CC Excl: For CC/MCC codes in category O24: PDX collection 969

☑5ᵗʰ **O24.0 Pre-existing type 1 diabetes mellitus, in pregnancy, childbirth and the puerperium**
Juvenile onset diabetes mellitus, in pregnancy, childbirth and the puerperium
Ketosis-prone diabetes mellitus in pregnancy, childbirth and the puerperium
Use additional code from category E10 to further identify any manifestations

☑6ᵗʰ **O24.01 Pre-existing type 1 diabetes mellitus, in pregnancy**

O24.011 Pre-existing type 1 diabetes mellitus, in pregnancy, first trimester   CC Ⓜ♀

O24.012 Pre-existing type 1 diabetes mellitus, in pregnancy, second trimester   CC Ⓜ♀

O24.013 Pre-existing type 1 diabetes mellitus, in pregnancy, third trimester   CC Ⓜ♀

O24.019 Pre-existing type 1 diabetes mellitus, in pregnancy, unspecified trimester   CC Ⓜ♀

O24.02 Pre-existing type 1 diabetes mellitus, in childbirth   MCC Ⓜ♀

O24.03 Pre-existing type 1 diabetes mellitus, in the puerperium   CC Ⓜ♀

☑5ᵗʰ **O24.1 Pre-existing type 2 diabetes mellitus, in pregnancy, childbirth and the puerperium**
Insulin-resistant diabetes mellitus in pregnancy, childbirth and the puerperium
Use additional code (for):
    from category E11 to further identify any manifestations
    long-term (current) use of insulin (Z79.4)

☑6ᵗʰ **O24.11 Pre-existing type 2 diabetes mellitus, in pregnancy**

O24.111 Pre-existing type 2 diabetes mellitus, in pregnancy, first trimester   CC Ⓜ♀

O24.112 Pre-existing type 2 diabetes mellitus, in pregnancy, second trimester   CC Ⓜ♀

O24.113 Pre-existing type 2 diabetes mellitus, in pregnancy, third trimester   CC Ⓜ♀

O24.119 Pre-existing type 2 diabetes mellitus, in pregnancy, unspecified trimester   CC Ⓜ♀

O24.12 Pre-existing type 2 diabetes mellitus, in childbirth   MCC Ⓜ♀

O24.13 Pre-existing type 2 diabetes mellitus, in the puerperium   CC Ⓜ♀

☑5ᵗʰ **O24.3 Unspecified pre-existing diabetes mellitus in pregnancy, childbirth and the puerperium**
Use additional code (for):
    from category E11 to further identify any manifestation
    long-term (current) use of insulin (Z79.4)

☑6ᵗʰ **O24.31 Unspecified pre-existing diabetes mellitus in pregnancy**

O24.311 Unspecified pre-existing diabetes mellitus in pregnancy, first trimester   CC Ⓜ♀

O24.312 Unspecified pre-existing diabetes mellitus in pregnancy, second trimester   CC Ⓜ♀

O24.313 Unspecified pre-existing diabetes mellitus in pregnancy, third trimester   CC Ⓜ♀

O24.319 Unspecified pre-existing diabetes mellitus in pregnancy, unspecified trimester   CC Ⓜ♀

O24.32 Unspecified pre-existing diabetes mellitus in childbirth   MCC Ⓜ♀

O24.33 Unspecified pre-existing diabetes mellitus in the puerperium   CC Ⓜ♀

☑5ᵗʰ **O24.4 Gestational diabetes mellitus**
Diabetes mellitus arising in pregnancy
Gestational diabetes mellitus NOS

☑6ᵗʰ **O24.41 Gestational diabetes mellitus in pregnancy**

O24.41Ø Gestational diabetes mellitus in pregnancy, diet controlled   Ⓜ♀

Ⓝ Newborn: 0   Ⓟ Pediatric: 0-17   Ⓜ Maternity: 12-55   Ⓐ Adult: 15-124   MCC Major CC Condition   PDxMCC PDx acts as own MCC   CC CC Condition   PDxCC PDx acts as own CC

852   ICD-10-CM 2018

O24.414 Gestational diabetes mellitus in pregnancy, **insulin controlled** Ⓜ♀

O24.415 Gestational diabetes mellitus in pregnancy, **controlled by oral hypoglycemic drugs** Ⓜ♀
> Gestational diabetes mellitus in pregnancy, controlled by oral antidiabetic drugs

O24.419 Gestational diabetes mellitus in pregnancy, **unspecified control** Ⓜ♀
> AHA: 2015, 4Q, 34

✓6th **O24.42** Gestational diabetes mellitus in childbirth
> AHA: 2016, 1Q, 5

O24.420 Gestational diabetes mellitus in childbirth, **diet controlled** Ⓜ♀

O24.424 Gestational diabetes mellitus in childbirth, **insulin controlled** Ⓜ♀

O24.425 Gestational diabetes mellitus in childbirth, **controlled by oral hypoglycemic drugs** Ⓜ♀
> Gestational diabetes mellitus in childbirth, controlled by oral antidiabetic drugs

O24.429 Gestational diabetes mellitus in childbirth, **unspecified control** Ⓜ♀
> AHA: 2015, 4Q, 34

✓6th **O24.43** Gestational diabetes mellitus in the **puerperium**

O24.430 Gestational diabetes mellitus in the **puerperium, diet controlled** Ⓜ♀

O24.434 Gestational diabetes mellitus in the **puerperium, insulin controlled** Ⓜ♀

O24.435 Gestational diabetes mellitus in **puerperium, controlled by oral hypoglycemic drugs** Ⓜ♀
> Gestational diabetes mellitus in puerperium, controlled by oral antidiabetic drugs

O24.439 Gestational diabetes mellitus in the **puerperium, unspecified control** Ⓜ♀
> AHA: 2015, 4Q, 34

✓5th **O24.8** Other pre-existing **diabetes mellitus in pregnancy, childbirth, and the puerperium**
> Use additional code (for):
> from categories E08, E09 and E13 to further identify any manifestation
> long-term (current) use of insulin (Z79.4)

✓6th **O24.81** Other pre-existing diabetes mellitus in **pregnancy**

O24.811 Other pre-existing diabetes mellitus in pregnancy, **first trimester** CC Ⓜ♀

O24.812 Other pre-existing diabetes mellitus in pregnancy, **second trimester** CC Ⓜ♀

O24.813 Other pre-existing diabetes mellitus in pregnancy, **third trimester** CC Ⓜ♀

O24.819 Other pre-existing diabetes mellitus in pregnancy, **unspecified trimester** CC Ⓜ♀

O24.82 Other pre-existing diabetes mellitus in **childbirth** MCC Ⓜ♀

O24.83 Other pre-existing diabetes mellitus in the **puerperium** CC Ⓜ♀

✓5th **O24.9** Unspecified **diabetes mellitus in pregnancy, childbirth and the puerperium**
> Use additional code for long-term (current) use of insulin (Z79.4)

✓6th **O24.91** Unspecified diabetes mellitus in **pregnancy**

O24.911 Unspecified diabetes mellitus in pregnancy, **first trimester** CC Ⓜ♀

O24.912 Unspecified diabetes mellitus in pregnancy, **second trimester** CC Ⓜ♀

O24.913 Unspecified diabetes mellitus in pregnancy, **third trimester** CC Ⓜ♀

O24.919 Unspecified diabetes mellitus in pregnancy, **unspecified trimester** CC Ⓜ♀

O24.92 Unspecified diabetes mellitus in **childbirth** Ⓜ♀

O24.93 Unspecified diabetes mellitus in the **puerperium** CC Ⓜ♀

✓4th **O25** Malnutrition in pregnancy, childbirth and the puerperium

✓5th **O25.1** Malnutrition in **pregnancy**

O25.10 Malnutrition in pregnancy, **unspecified trimester** Ⓜ♀

O25.11 Malnutrition in pregnancy, **first trimester** Ⓜ♀

O25.12 Malnutrition in pregnancy, **second trimester** Ⓜ♀

O25.13 Malnutrition in pregnancy, **third trimester** Ⓜ♀

O25.2 Malnutrition in **childbirth** Ⓜ♀

O25.3 Malnutrition in the **puerperium** Ⓜ♀

✓4th **O26** Maternal care for other conditions predominantly related to pregnancy

✓5th **O26.0** Excessive weight gain in pregnancy
> EXCLUDES 2   gestational edema (O12.0, O12.2)

O26.00 Excessive weight gain in pregnancy, **unspecified trimester** Ⓜ♀

O26.01 Excessive weight gain in pregnancy, **first trimester** Ⓜ♀

O26.02 Excessive weight gain in pregnancy, **second trimester** Ⓜ♀

O26.03 Excessive weight gain in pregnancy, **third trimester** Ⓜ♀

✓5th **O26.1** Low weight gain in pregnancy

O26.10 Low weight gain in pregnancy, **unspecified trimester** Ⓜ♀

O26.11 Low weight gain in pregnancy, **first trimester** Ⓜ♀

O26.12 Low weight gain in pregnancy, **second trimester** Ⓜ♀

O26.13 Low weight gain in pregnancy, **third trimester** Ⓜ♀

✓5th **O26.2** Pregnancy care for patient with recurrent pregnancy loss

O26.20 Pregnancy care for patient with recurrent pregnancy loss, **unspecified trimester** Ⓜ♀

O26.21 Pregnancy care for patient with recurrent pregnancy loss, **first trimester** Ⓜ♀

O26.22 Pregnancy care for patient with recurrent pregnancy loss, **second trimester** Ⓜ♀

O26.23 Pregnancy care for patient with recurrent pregnancy loss, **third trimester** Ⓜ♀

✓5th **O26.3** Retained intrauterine contraceptive device in pregnancy

O26.30 Retained intrauterine contraceptive device in pregnancy, **unspecified trimester** Ⓜ♀

O26.31 Retained intrauterine contraceptive device in pregnancy, **first trimester** Ⓜ♀

O26.32 Retained intrauterine contraceptive device in pregnancy, **second trimester** Ⓜ♀

O26.33 Retained intrauterine contraceptive device in pregnancy, **third trimester** Ⓜ♀

✓5th **O26.4** Herpes gestationis

O26.40 Herpes gestationis, **unspecified trimester** Ⓜ♀

O26.41 Herpes gestationis, **first trimester** Ⓜ♀

O26.42 Herpes gestationis, **second trimester** Ⓜ♀

O26.43 Herpes gestationis, **third trimester** Ⓜ♀

✓5th **O26.5** Maternal hypotension syndrome
> Supine hypotensive syndrome

O26.50 Maternal hypotension syndrome, **unspecified trimester** Ⓜ♀

O26.51 Maternal hypotension syndrome, **first trimester** Ⓜ♀

O26.52 Maternal hypotension syndrome, **second trimester** Ⓜ♀

O26.53 Maternal hypotension syndrome, **third trimester** Ⓜ♀

✓5th **O26.6** Liver and biliary tract disorders in pregnancy, childbirth and the puerperium
> Use additional code to identify the specific disorder
> EXCLUDES 2   hepatorenal syndrome following labor and delivery (O90.4)

> **CC Excl: For CC codes in subcategory O26.6:**
> PDX collection 972

✓6th **O26.61** Liver and biliary tract disorders in **pregnancy**

O26.611 Liver and biliary tract disorders in pregnancy, **first trimester** CC Ⓜ♀

O26.612 Liver and biliary tract disorders in pregnancy, **second trimester** CC Ⓜ♀

O26.613 Liver and biliary tract disorders in pregnancy, **third trimester** CC Ⓜ♀

O26.619 Liver and biliary tract disorders in pregnancy, **unspecified trimester** Ⓜ♀

O26.62 Liver and biliary tract disorders in **childbirth** CC Ⓜ♀

O26.63 Liver and biliary tract disorders in the **puerperium** Ⓜ♀

✓ Additional Character Req   ✓x7th Placeholder Alert   Unacceptable PDx   Manifestation   H1–H14 HAC   HCC CMS-HCC Condition   EXCLUDES 1 Not Coded Here   EXCLUDES 2 Not Included Here

ICD-10-CM 2018   853

Chapter 15. Pregnancy, Childbirth and the Puerperium

O26.7–O29.Ø19

√5ᵗʰ **O26.7 Subluxation of symphysis (pubis) in pregnancy, childbirth and the puerperium**
> EXCLUDES 1   *traumatic separation of symphysis (pubis) during childbirth (O71.6)*

  √6ᵗʰ **O26.71 Subluxation of symphysis (pubis) in pregnancy**

    O26.711 Subluxation of symphysis (pubis) in pregnancy, first trimester Ⓜ♀

    O26.712 Subluxation of symphysis (pubis) in pregnancy, second trimester Ⓜ♀

    O26.713 Subluxation of symphysis (pubis) in pregnancy, third trimester Ⓜ♀

    O26.719 Subluxation of symphysis (pubis) in pregnancy, unspecified trimester Ⓜ♀

  O26.72 Subluxation of symphysis (pubis) in childbirth Ⓜ♀

  O26.73 Subluxation of symphysis (pubis) in the puerperium Ⓜ♀

√5ᵗʰ **O26.8 Other specified pregnancy related conditions**

  √6ᵗʰ **O26.81 Pregnancy related exhaustion and fatigue**

    O26.811 Pregnancy related exhaustion and fatigue, first trimester Ⓜ♀

    O26.812 Pregnancy related exhaustion and fatigue, second trimester Ⓜ♀

    O26.813 Pregnancy related exhaustion and fatigue, third trimester Ⓜ♀

    O26.819 Pregnancy related exhaustion and fatigue, unspecified trimester Ⓜ♀

  √6ᵗʰ **O26.82 Pregnancy related peripheral neuritis**

    O26.821 Pregnancy related peripheral neuritis, first trimester Ⓜ♀

    O26.822 Pregnancy related peripheral neuritis, second trimester Ⓜ♀

    O26.823 Pregnancy related peripheral neuritis, third trimester Ⓜ♀

    O26.829 Pregnancy related peripheral neuritis, unspecified trimester Ⓜ♀

  √6ᵗʰ **O26.83 Pregnancy related renal disease**
> Use additional code to identify the specific disorder

> **CC Excl: For CC codes in subcategory O26.83:** PDX collection 965

    O26.831 Pregnancy related renal disease, first trimester CC Ⓜ♀

    O26.832 Pregnancy related renal disease, second trimester CC Ⓜ♀

    O26.833 Pregnancy related renal disease, third trimester CC Ⓜ♀

    O26.839 Pregnancy related renal disease, unspecified trimester Ⓜ♀

  √6ᵗʰ **O26.84 Uterine size-date discrepancy complicating pregnancy**
> EXCLUDES 1   *encounter for suspected problem with fetal growth ruled out (ZØ3.74)*

    O26.841 Uterine size-date discrepancy, first trimester Ⓜ♀

    O26.842 Uterine size-date discrepancy, second trimester Ⓜ♀

    O26.843 Uterine size-date discrepancy, third trimester Ⓜ♀

    O26.849 Uterine size-date discrepancy, unspecified trimester Ⓜ♀

  √6ᵗʰ **O26.85 Spotting complicating pregnancy**

    O26.851 Spotting complicating pregnancy, first trimester Ⓜ♀

    O26.852 Spotting complicating pregnancy, second trimester Ⓜ♀

    O26.853 Spotting complicating pregnancy, third trimester Ⓜ♀

    O26.859 Spotting complicating pregnancy, unspecified trimester Ⓜ♀

  O26.86 Pruritic urticarial papules and plaques of pregnancy (PUPPP) Ⓜ♀
> Polymorphic eruption of pregnancy

√6ᵗʰ **O26.87 Cervical shortening**
> EXCLUDES 1   *encounter for suspected cervical shortening ruled out (ZØ3.75)*
> **DEF:** A cervix that has shortened to < 25 mm before the 24th week of pregnancy; warning sign for impending premature delivery; treated by cervical cerclage placement or progesterone.

> **CC Excl: For CC codes in subcategory O26.87:** PDX collection 973

    O26.872 Cervical shortening, second trimester CC Ⓜ♀

    O26.873 Cervical shortening, third trimester CC Ⓜ♀

    O26.879 Cervical shortening, unspecified trimester CC Ⓜ♀

√6ᵗʰ **O26.89 Other specified pregnancy related conditions**
> **AHA:** 2015, 3Q, 40

    O26.891 Other specified pregnancy related conditions, first trimester Ⓜ♀

    O26.892 Other specified pregnancy related conditions, second trimester Ⓜ♀

    O26.893 Other specified pregnancy related conditions, third trimester Ⓜ♀

    O26.899 Other specified pregnancy related conditions, unspecified trimester Ⓜ♀

√5ᵗʰ **O26.9 Pregnancy related conditions, unspecified**

  O26.90 Pregnancy related conditions, unspecified, unspecified trimester Ⓜ♀

  O26.91 Pregnancy related conditions, unspecified, first trimester Ⓜ♀

  O26.92 Pregnancy related conditions, unspecified, second trimester Ⓜ♀

  O26.93 Pregnancy related conditions, unspecified, third trimester Ⓜ♀

√4ᵗʰ **O28 Abnormal findings on antenatal screening of mother**
> EXCLUDES 1   *diagnostic findings classified elsewhere—see Alphabetical Index*

  O28.Ø Abnormal hematological finding on antenatal screening of mother Ⓜ♀

  O28.1 Abnormal biochemical finding on antenatal screening of mother Ⓜ♀

  O28.2 Abnormal cytological finding on antenatal screening of mother Ⓜ♀

  O28.3 Abnormal ultrasonic finding on antenatal screening of mother Ⓜ♀

  O28.4 Abnormal radiological finding on antenatal screening of mother Ⓜ♀

  O28.5 Abnormal chromosomal and genetic finding on antenatal screening of mother Ⓜ♀

  O28.8 Other abnormal findings on antenatal screening of mother Ⓜ♀

  O28.9 Unspecified abnormal findings on antenatal screening of mother Ⓜ♀

√4ᵗʰ **O29 Complications of anesthesia during pregnancy**
> INCLUDES   maternal complications arising from the administration of a general, regional or local anesthetic, analgesic or other sedation during pregnancy
> Use additional code, if necessary, to identify the complication
> EXCLUDES 2   *complications of anesthesia during labor and delivery (O74.-)*
> *complications of anesthesia during the puerperium (O89.-)*

√5ᵗʰ **O29.Ø Pulmonary complications of anesthesia during pregnancy**

  √6ᵗʰ **O29.Ø1 Aspiration pneumonitis due to anesthesia during pregnancy**
> Inhalation of stomach contents or secretions NOS due to anesthesia during pregnancy
> Mendelson's syndrome due to anesthesia during pregnancy

    O29.Ø11 Aspiration pneumonitis due to anesthesia during pregnancy, first trimester Ⓜ♀

    O29.Ø12 Aspiration pneumonitis due to anesthesia during pregnancy, second trimester Ⓜ♀

    O29.Ø13 Aspiration pneumonitis due to anesthesia during pregnancy, third trimester Ⓜ♀

    O29.Ø19 Aspiration pneumonitis due to anesthesia during pregnancy, unspecified trimester Ⓜ♀

Ⓝ Newborn: 0   Ⓟ Pediatric: 0-17   Ⓜ Maternity: 12-55   Ⓐ Adult: 15-124   ᴹᶜᶜ Major CC Condition   ᴾᴰˣᴹᶜᶜ PDx acts as own MCC   ᶜᶜ CC Condition   ᴾᴰˣᶜᶜ PDx acts as own CC

854   **ICD-10-CM 2018**

√6ᵗʰ **O29.Ø2 Pressure collapse of lung due to anesthesia during pregnancy**

O29.Ø21 Pressure collapse of lung due to anesthesia during pregnancy, first trimester Ⓜ♀

O29.Ø22 Pressure collapse of lung due to anesthesia during pregnancy, second trimester Ⓜ♀

O29.Ø23 Pressure collapse of lung due to anesthesia during pregnancy, third trimester Ⓜ♀

O29.Ø29 Pressure collapse of lung due to anesthesia during pregnancy, unspecified trimester Ⓜ♀

√6ᵗʰ **O29.Ø9 Other pulmonary complications of anesthesia during pregnancy**

O29.Ø91 Other pulmonary complications of anesthesia during pregnancy, first trimester Ⓜ♀

O29.Ø92 Other pulmonary complications of anesthesia during pregnancy, second trimester Ⓜ♀

O29.Ø93 Other pulmonary complications of anesthesia during pregnancy, third trimester Ⓜ♀

O29.Ø99 Other pulmonary complications of anesthesia during pregnancy, unspecified trimester Ⓜ♀

√5ᵗʰ **O29.1 Cardiac complications of anesthesia during pregnancy**

√6ᵗʰ **O29.11 Cardiac arrest due to anesthesia during pregnancy**

O29.111 Cardiac arrest due to anesthesia during pregnancy, first trimester Ⓜ♀

O29.112 Cardiac arrest due to anesthesia during pregnancy, second trimester Ⓜ♀

O29.113 Cardiac arrest due to anesthesia during pregnancy, third trimester Ⓜ♀

O29.119 Cardiac arrest due to anesthesia during pregnancy, unspecified trimester Ⓜ♀

√6ᵗʰ **O29.12 Cardiac failure due to anesthesia during pregnancy**

O29.121 Cardiac failure due to anesthesia during pregnancy, first trimester Ⓜ♀

O29.122 Cardiac failure due to anesthesia during pregnancy, second trimester Ⓜ♀

O29.123 Cardiac failure due to anesthesia during pregnancy, third trimester Ⓜ♀

O29.129 Cardiac failure due to anesthesia during pregnancy, unspecified trimester Ⓜ♀

√6ᵗʰ **O29.19 Other cardiac complications of anesthesia during pregnancy**

O29.191 Other cardiac complications of anesthesia during pregnancy, first trimester Ⓜ♀

O29.192 Other cardiac complications of anesthesia during pregnancy, second trimester Ⓜ♀

O29.193 Other cardiac complications of anesthesia during pregnancy, third trimester Ⓜ♀

O29.199 Other cardiac complications of anesthesia during pregnancy, unspecified trimester Ⓜ♀

√5ᵗʰ **O29.2 Central nervous system complications of anesthesia during pregnancy**

√6ᵗʰ **O29.21 Cerebral anoxia due to anesthesia during pregnancy**

O29.211 Cerebral anoxia due to anesthesia during pregnancy, first trimester Ⓜ♀

O29.212 Cerebral anoxia due to anesthesia during pregnancy, second trimester Ⓜ♀

O29.213 Cerebral anoxia due to anesthesia during pregnancy, third trimester Ⓜ♀

O29.219 Cerebral anoxia due to anesthesia during pregnancy, unspecified trimester Ⓜ♀

√6ᵗʰ **O29.29 Other central nervous system complications of anesthesia during pregnancy**

O29.291 Other central nervous system complications of anesthesia during pregnancy, first trimester Ⓜ♀

O29.292 Other central nervous system complications of anesthesia during pregnancy, second trimester Ⓜ♀

O29.293 Other central nervous system complications of anesthesia during pregnancy, third trimester Ⓜ♀

O29.299 Other central nervous system complications of anesthesia during pregnancy, unspecified trimester Ⓜ♀

√5ᵗʰ **O29.3 Toxic reaction to local anesthesia during pregnancy**

√6ᵗʰ **O29.3X Toxic reaction to local anesthesia during pregnancy**

O29.3X1 Toxic reaction to local anesthesia during pregnancy, first trimester Ⓜ♀

O29.3X2 Toxic reaction to local anesthesia during pregnancy, second trimester Ⓜ♀

O29.3X3 Toxic reaction to local anesthesia during pregnancy, third trimester Ⓜ♀

O29.3X9 Toxic reaction to local anesthesia during pregnancy, unspecified trimester Ⓜ♀

√5ᵗʰ **O29.4 Spinal and epidural anesthesia induced headache during pregnancy**

O29.4Ø Spinal and epidural anesthesia induced headache during pregnancy, unspecified trimester Ⓜ♀

O29.41 Spinal and epidural anesthesia induced headache during pregnancy, first trimester Ⓜ♀

O29.42 Spinal and epidural anesthesia induced headache during pregnancy, second trimester Ⓜ♀

O29.43 Spinal and epidural anesthesia induced headache during pregnancy, third trimester Ⓜ♀

√5ᵗʰ **O29.5 Other complications of spinal and epidural anesthesia during pregnancy**

√6ᵗʰ **O29.5X Other complications of spinal and epidural anesthesia during pregnancy**

O29.5X1 Other complications of spinal and epidural anesthesia during pregnancy, first trimester Ⓜ♀

O29.5X2 Other complications of spinal and epidural anesthesia during pregnancy, second trimester Ⓜ♀

O29.5X3 Other complications of spinal and epidural anesthesia during pregnancy, third trimester Ⓜ♀

O29.5X9 Other complications of spinal and epidural anesthesia during pregnancy, unspecified trimester Ⓜ♀

√5ᵗʰ **O29.6 Failed or difficult intubation for anesthesia during pregnancy**

O29.6Ø Failed or difficult intubation for anesthesia during pregnancy, unspecified trimester Ⓜ♀

O29.61 Failed or difficult intubation for anesthesia during pregnancy, first trimester Ⓜ♀

O29.62 Failed or difficult intubation for anesthesia during pregnancy, second trimester Ⓜ♀

O29.63 Failed or difficult intubation for anesthesia during pregnancy, third trimester Ⓜ♀

√5ᵗʰ **O29.8 Other complications of anesthesia during pregnancy**

√6ᵗʰ **O29.8X Other complications of anesthesia during pregnancy**

O29.8X1 Other complications of anesthesia during pregnancy, first trimester Ⓜ♀

O29.8X2 Other complications of anesthesia during pregnancy, second trimester Ⓜ♀

O29.8X3 Other complications of anesthesia during pregnancy, third trimester Ⓜ♀

O29.8X9 Other complications of anesthesia during pregnancy, unspecified trimester Ⓜ♀

√5ᵗʰ **O29.9 Unspecified complication of anesthesia during pregnancy**

O29.9Ø Unspecified complication of anesthesia during pregnancy, unspecified trimester Ⓜ♀

O29.91 Unspecified complication of anesthesia during pregnancy, first trimester Ⓜ♀

O29.92 Unspecified complication of anesthesia during pregnancy, second trimester Ⓜ♀

O29.93 Unspecified complication of anesthesia during pregnancy, third trimester Ⓜ♀

✔ Additional Character Req   √ₓ7ᵗʰ Placeholder Alert   Unacceptable PDx   Manifestation   H1-H14 HAC   HCC CMS-HCC Condition   *EXCLUDES 1* Not Coded Here   *EXCLUDES 2* Not Included Here

ICD-10-CM 2018   855

Chapter 15. Pregnancy, Childbirth and the Puerperium

O30–O30.111

Twin Gestation – Monochorionic/Monoamniotic

- 1 Chorionic sac
- 1 Amniotic sac
- 2 Fetuses
- 2 Umbilical cords
- 1 Placenta

Maternal care related to the fetus and amniotic cavity and possible delivery problems (O30-O48)

√4th **O30 Multiple gestation**

Code also any complications specific to multiple gestation

CC Excl: For CC codes in category O30: PDX collection 976

√5th **O30.0 Twin pregnancy**

√6th **O30.00 Twin pregnancy, unspecified number of placenta and unspecified number of amniotic sacs**

     O30.001 Twin pregnancy, unspecified number of placenta and unspecified number of amniotic sacs, **first trimester** M♀

     O30.002 Twin pregnancy, unspecified number of placenta and unspecified number of amniotic sacs, **second trimester** M♀

     O30.003 Twin pregnancy, unspecified number of placenta and unspecified number of amniotic sacs, **third trimester** M♀

     O30.009 Twin pregnancy, unspecified number of placenta and unspecified number of amniotic sacs, **unspecified trimester** M♀

√6th **O30.01 Twin pregnancy, monochorionic/monoamniotic**

Twin pregnancy, one placenta, one amniotic sac

EXCLUDES 1   conjoined twins (O30.02-)

     O30.011 Twin pregnancy, monochorionic/monoamniotic, **first trimester** M♀

     O30.012 Twin pregnancy, monochorionic/monoamniotic, **second trimester** M♀

     O30.013 Twin pregnancy, monochorionic/monoamniotic, **third trimester** M♀

     O30.019 Twin pregnancy, monochorionic/monoamniotic, **unspecified trimester** M♀

√6th **O30.02 Conjoined twin pregnancy**

     O30.021 Conjoined twin pregnancy, **first trimester** M♀

     O30.022 Conjoined twin pregnancy, **second trimester** M♀

     O30.023 Conjoined twin pregnancy, **third trimester** M♀

     O30.029 Conjoined twin pregnancy, **unspecified trimester** M♀

Twin Gestation – Dichorionic/Diamniotic

- 2 Chorionic sacs
- 2 Amniotic sacs
- 2 Fetuses
- 2 Umbilical cords
- 2 Placentas

Twin Gestation – Monochorionic/Diamniotic

- 1 Chorionic sac
- 2 Amniotic sacs
- 2 Fetuses
- 2 Umbilical cords
- 1 Placenta

√6th **O30.03 Twin pregnancy, monochorionic/diamniotic**

Twin pregnancy, one placenta, two amniotic sacs

     O30.031 Twin pregnancy, monochorionic/diamniotic, **first trimester** M♀

     O30.032 Twin pregnancy, monochorionic/diamniotic, **second trimester** M♀

     O30.033 Twin pregnancy, monochorionic/diamniotic, **third trimester** M♀

     O30.039 Twin pregnancy, monochorionic/diamniotic, **unspecified trimester** M♀

√6th **O30.04 Twin pregnancy, dichorionic/diamniotic**

Twin pregnancy, two placentae, two amniotic sacs

     O30.041 Twin pregnancy, dichorionic/diamniotic, **first trimester** M♀

     O30.042 Twin pregnancy, dichorionic/diamniotic, **second trimester** M♀

     O30.043 Twin pregnancy, dichorionic/diamniotic, **third trimester** M♀

     O30.049 Twin pregnancy, dichorionic/diamniotic, **unspecified trimester** M♀

√6th **O30.09 Twin pregnancy, unable to determine number of placenta and number of amniotic sacs**

     O30.091 Twin pregnancy, unable to determine number of placenta and number of amniotic sacs, **first trimester** M♀

     O30.092 Twin pregnancy, unable to determine number of placenta and number of amniotic sacs, **second trimester** M♀

     O30.093 Twin pregnancy, unable to determine number of placenta and number of amniotic sacs, **third trimester** M♀

     O30.099 Twin pregnancy, unable to determine number of placenta and number of amniotic sacs, **unspecified trimester** M♀

√5th **O30.1 Triplet pregnancy**

√6th **O30.10 Triplet pregnancy, unspecified number of placenta and unspecified number of amniotic sacs**

AHA: 2016, 2Q, 8

     O30.101 Triplet pregnancy, unspecified number of placenta and unspecified number of amniotic sacs, **first trimester** CC M♀

     O30.102 Triplet pregnancy, unspecified number of placenta and unspecified number of amniotic sacs, **second trimester** CC M♀

     O30.103 Triplet pregnancy, unspecified number of placenta and unspecified number of amniotic sacs, **third trimester** CC M♀

     O30.109 Triplet pregnancy, unspecified number of placenta and unspecified number of amniotic sacs, **unspecified trimester** M♀

√6th **O30.11 Triplet pregnancy with two or more monochorionic fetuses**

     O30.111 Triplet pregnancy with two or more monochorionic fetuses, **first trimester** CC M♀

N Newborn: 0   P Pediatric: 0-17   M Maternity: 12-55   A Adult: 15-124   MCC Major CC Condition   PDxMCC PDx acts as own MCC   CC CC Condition   PDxCC PDx acts as own CC

856   ICD-10-CM 2018

O30.112   **Triplet pregnancy with two or more** CC M ♀ **monochorionic fetuses, second trimester**

O30.113   **Triplet pregnancy with two or more** CC M ♀ **monochorionic fetuses, third trimester**

O30.119   **Triplet pregnancy with two or more** M ♀ **monochorionic fetuses, unspecified trimester**

✓6ᵗʰ   **O30.12**   **Triplet pregnancy with** two or more monoamniotic fetuses

O30.121   **Triplet pregnancy with two or more** CC M ♀ **monoamniotic fetuses, first trimester**

O30.122   **Triplet pregnancy with two or more** CC M ♀ **monoamniotic fetuses, second trimester**

O30.123   **Triplet pregnancy with two or more** CC M ♀ **monoamniotic fetuses, third trimester**

O30.129   **Triplet pregnancy with two or more** M ♀ **monoamniotic fetuses, unspecified trimester**

✓6ᵗʰ   **O30.19**   **Triplet pregnancy,** unable to determine number of placenta and number of amniotic sacs

O30.191   **Triplet pregnancy, unable to** CC M ♀ **determine number of placenta and number of amniotic sacs, first trimester**

O30.192   **Triplet pregnancy, unable to** CC M ♀ **determine number of placenta and number of amniotic sacs, second trimester**

O30.193   **Triplet pregnancy, unable to** CC M ♀ **determine number of placenta and number of amniotic sacs, third trimester**

O30.199   **Triplet pregnancy, unable to** M ♀ **determine number of placenta and number of amniotic sacs, unspecified trimester**

✓5ᵗʰ   **O30.2**   Quadruplet **pregnancy**

✓6ᵗʰ   **O30.20**   **Quadruplet pregnancy,** unspecified number of placenta and unspecified number of amniotic sacs

O30.201   **Quadruplet pregnancy, unspecified** CC M ♀ **number of placenta and unspecified number of amniotic sacs, first trimester**

O30.202   **Quadruplet pregnancy, unspecified** CC M ♀ **number of placenta and unspecified number of amniotic sacs, second trimester**

O30.203   **Quadruplet pregnancy, unspecified** CC ♀ **number of placenta and unspecified number of amniotic sacs, third trimester**

O30.209   **Quadruplet pregnancy, unspecified** M ♀ **number of placenta and unspecified number of amniotic sacs, unspecified trimester**

✓6ᵗʰ   **O30.21**   **Quadruplet pregnancy with** two or more monochorionic fetuses

O30.211   **Quadruplet pregnancy with two or** CC M ♀ **more monochorionic fetuses, first trimester**

O30.212   **Quadruplet pregnancy with two or** CC M ♀ **more monochorionic fetuses, second trimester**

O30.213   **Quadruplet pregnancy with two or** CC M ♀ **more monochorionic fetuses, third trimester**

O30.219   **Quadruplet pregnancy with two or** M ♀ **more monochorionic fetuses, unspecified trimester**

✓6ᵗʰ   **O30.22**   **Quadruplet pregnancy with** two or more monoamniotic fetuses

O30.221   **Quadruplet pregnancy with two or** CC M ♀ **more monoamniotic fetuses, first trimester**

O30.222   **Quadruplet pregnancy with two or** CC M ♀ **more monoamniotic fetuses, second trimester**

O30.223   **Quadruplet pregnancy with two or** CC M ♀ **more monoamniotic fetuses, third trimester**

O30.229   **Quadruplet pregnancy with two or** M ♀ **more monoamniotic fetuses, unspecified trimester**

✓6ᵗʰ   **O30.29**   **Quadruplet pregnancy,** unable to determine number of placenta and number of amniotic sacs

O30.291   **Quadruplet pregnancy, unable to** CC M ♀ **determine number of placenta and number of amniotic sacs, first trimester**

O30.292   **Quadruplet pregnancy, unable to** CC M ♀ **determine number of placenta and number of amniotic sacs, second trimester**

O30.293   **Quadruplet pregnancy, unable to** CC M ♀ **determine number of placenta and number of amniotic sacs, third trimester**

O30.299   **Quadruplet pregnancy, unable to** M ♀ **determine number of placenta and number of amniotic sacs, unspecified trimester**

✓5ᵗʰ   **O30.8**   Other **specified multiple gestation**
Multiple gestation pregnancy greater than quadruplets

✓6ᵗʰ   **O30.80**   **Other specified multiple gestation,** unspecified number of placenta and unspecified number of amniotic sacs

O30.801   **Other specified multiple gestation,** CC M ♀ **unspecified number of placenta and unspecified number of amniotic sacs, first trimester**

O30.802   **Other specified multiple gestation,** CC M ♀ **unspecified number of placenta and unspecified number of amniotic sacs, second trimester**

O30.803   **Other specified multiple gestation,** CC M ♀ **unspecified number of placenta and unspecified number of amniotic sacs, third trimester**

O30.809   **Other specified multiple gestation,** M ♀ **unspecified number of placenta and unspecified number of amniotic sacs, unspecified trimester**

✓6ᵗʰ   **O30.81**   **Other specified multiple gestation with** two or more monochorionic fetuses

O30.811   **Other specified multiple gestation** CC M ♀ **with two or more monochorionic fetuses, first trimester**

O30.812   **Other specified multiple gestation** CC M ♀ **with two or more monochorionic fetuses, second trimester**

O30.813   **Other specified multiple gestation** CC M ♀ **with two or more monochorionic fetuses, third trimester**

O30.819   **Other specified multiple gestation** M ♀ **with two or more monochorionic fetuses, unspecified trimester**

✓6ᵗʰ   **O30.82**   **Other specified multiple gestation with** two or more monoamniotic fetuses

O30.821   **Other specified multiple gestation** CC M ♀ **with two or more monoamniotic fetuses, first trimester**

O30.822   **Other specified multiple gestation** CC M ♀ **with two or more monoamniotic fetuses, second trimester**

O30.823   **Other specified multiple gestation** CC M ♀ **with two or more monoamniotic fetuses, third trimester**

O30.829   **Other specified multiple gestation** M ♀ **with two or more monoamniotic fetuses, unspecified trimester**

✔ Additional Character Req   ✔x7ᵗʰ Placeholder Alert   Unacceptable PDx   Manifestation   H1 - H14 HAC   HCC CMS-HCC Condition   EXCLUDES 1 Not Coded Here   EXCLUDES 2 Not Included Here

✔6ᵗʰ **O30.89** **Other specified multiple gestation,** unable to determine number of placenta and number of amniotic sacs

O30.891 **Other specified multiple gestation,** CC MQ unable to determine number of placenta and number of amniotic sacs, first trimester

O30.892 **Other specified multiple gestation,** CC MQ unable to determine number of placenta and number of amniotic sacs, second trimester

O30.893 **Other specified multiple gestation,** CC MQ unable to determine number of placenta and number of amniotic sacs, third trimester

O30.899 **Other specified multiple gestation,** MQ unable to determine number of placenta and number of amniotic sacs, unspecified trimester

✔5ᵗʰ **O30.9** **Multiple gestation, unspecified**
Multiple pregnancy NOS

O30.90 **Multiple gestation, unspecified,** unspecified MQ trimester

O30.91 **Multiple gestation, unspecified,** first trimester MQ

O30.92 **Multiple gestation, unspecified,** second MQ trimester

O30.93 **Multiple gestation, unspecified,** third trimester MQ

✔4ᵗʰ **O31** **Complications specific to multiple gestation**
EXCLUDES 2 *delayed delivery of second twin, triplet, etc. (O63.2)*
malpresentation of one fetus or more (O32.9)
placental transfusion syndromes (O43.0-)
AHA: 2012, 4Q, 107

> One of the following 7th characters is to be assigned to each code under category O31. 7th character 0 is for single gestations and multiple gestations where the fetus is unspecified. 7th characters 1 through 9 are for cases of multiple gestations to identify the fetus for which the code applies. The appropriate code from category O30, Multiple gestation, must also be assigned when assigning a code from category O31 that has a 7th character of 1 through 9.
>
> 0   not applicable or   3   fetus 3
>   unspecified   4   fetus 4
> 1   fetus 1   5   fetus 5
> 2   fetus 2   9   other fetus

✔5ᵗʰ **O31.0** **Papyraceous fetus**
Fetus compressus

✔7ᵗʰ **O31.00** **Papyraceous fetus,** unspecified trimester MQ

✔7ᵗʰ **O31.01** **Papyraceous fetus,** first trimester MQ

✔7ᵗʰ **O31.02** **Papyraceous fetus,** second trimester MQ

✔7ᵗʰ **O31.03** **Papyraceous fetus,** third trimester MQ

✔5ᵗʰ **O31.1** **Continuing pregnancy** after spontaneous abortion **of one fetus or more**

✔7ᵗʰ **O31.10** **Continuing pregnancy after spontaneous** MQ **abortion of one fetus or more,** unspecified trimester

✔7ᵗʰ **O31.11** **Continuing pregnancy after spontaneous** MQ **abortion of one fetus or more,** first trimester

✔7ᵗʰ **O31.12** **Continuing pregnancy after spontaneous** MQ **abortion of one fetus or more,** second trimester

✔7ᵗʰ **O31.13** **Continuing pregnancy after spontaneous** MQ **abortion of one fetus or more,** third trimester

✔5ᵗʰ **O31.2** **Continuing pregnancy** after intrauterine death **of one fetus or more**

✔7ᵗʰ **O31.20** **Continuing pregnancy after intrauterine death** MQ **of one fetus or more,** unspecified trimester

✔7ᵗʰ **O31.21** **Continuing pregnancy after intrauterine death** MQ **of one fetus or more,** first trimester

✔7ᵗʰ **O31.22** **Continuing pregnancy after intrauterine death** MQ **of one fetus or more,** second trimester

✔7ᵗʰ **O31.23** **Continuing pregnancy after intrauterine death** MQ **of one fetus or more,** third trimester

✔5ᵗʰ **O31.3** **Continuing pregnancy after** elective fetal reduction **of one fetus or more**
Continuing pregnancy after selective termination of one fetus or more

✔7ᵗʰ **O31.30** **Continuing pregnancy after elective fetal** MQ **reduction of one fetus or more,** unspecified trimester

✔7ᵗʰ **O31.31** **Continuing pregnancy after elective fetal** MQ **reduction of one fetus or more,** first trimester

✔7ᵗʰ **O31.32** **Continuing pregnancy after elective fetal** MQ **reduction of one fetus or more,** second trimester

✔7ᵗʰ **O31.33** **Continuing pregnancy after elective fetal** MQ **reduction of one fetus or more,** third trimester

✔5ᵗʰ **O31.8** **Other complications specific to multiple gestation**

✔6ᵗʰ **O31.8X** **Other complications specific to multiple gestation**

> **CC Excl: For CC codes in subcategory O31.8X:**
> PDX collection 976

✔7ᵗʰ **O31.8X1** **Other complications specific to** CC MQ **multiple gestation,** first trimester

✔7ᵗʰ **O31.8X2** **Other complications specific to** CC MQ **multiple gestation,** second trimester

✔7ᵗʰ **O31.8X3** **Other complications specific to** CC MQ **multiple gestation,** third trimester

✔7ᵗʰ **O31.8X9** **Other complications specific to** MQ **multiple gestation,** unspecified trimester

✔4ᵗʰ **O32** **Maternal care for malpresentation of fetus**
INCLUDES the listed conditions as a reason for observation, hospitalization or other obstetric care of the mother, or for cesarean delivery before onset of labor
EXCLUDES 1 *malpresentation of fetus with obstructed labor (O64.-)*
AHA: 2012, 4Q, 107

> One of the following 7th characters is to be assigned to each code under category O32. 7th character 0 is for single gestations and multiple gestations where the fetus is unspecified. 7th characters 1 through 9 are for cases of multiple gestations to identify the fetus for which the code applies. The appropriate code from category O30, Multiple gestation, must also be assigned when assigning a code from category O32 that has a 7th character of 1 through 9.
>
> 0   not applicable or   3   fetus 3
>   unspecified   4   fetus 4
> 1   fetus 1   5   fetus 5
> 2   fetus 2   9   other fetus

✔x7ᵗʰ **O32.0** **Maternal care for** unstable lie MQ

✔x7ᵗʰ **O32.1** **Maternal care for** breech presentation MQ
Maternal care for buttocks presentation
Maternal care for complete breech
Maternal care for frank breech
EXCLUDES 1 *footling presentation (O32.8)*
incomplete breech (O32.8)
DEF: Fetus presentation in a longitudinal lie with the buttocks or feet closest to birth canal; may require external cephalic version or cesarean delivery.

✔x7ᵗʰ **O32.2** **Maternal care for** transverse and oblique lie MQ
Maternal care for oblique presentation
Maternal care for transverse presentation

✔x7ᵗʰ **O32.3** **Maternal care for** face, brow and chin presentation MQ

✔x7ᵗʰ **O32.4** **Maternal care for** high head at term MQ
Maternal care for failure of head to enter pelvic brim

✔x7ᵗʰ **O32.6** **Maternal care for** compound presentation MQ

✔x7ᵗʰ **O32.8** **Maternal care for** other malpresentation of fetus MQ
Maternal care for footling presentation
Maternal care for incomplete breech

✔x7ᵗʰ **O32.9** **Maternal care for** malpresentation of fetus, unspecified MQ

Fetal Malpresentation

Breech

Mother's pelvis

Face (mentum)

Shoulder (arm prolapse)

Compound (extremity together with head)

Oblique

N Newborn: 0   P Pediatric: 0-17   M Maternity: 12-55   A Adult: 15-124   MCC Major CC Condition   PDxMCC PDx acts as own MCC   CC CC Condition   PDxCC PDx acts as own CC

858   ICD-10-CM 2018

✓4th **O33 Maternal care for disproportion**

INCLUDES the listed conditions as a reason for observation, hospitalization or other obstetric care of the mother, or for cesarean delivery before onset of labor

EXCLUDES 1 *disproportion with obstructed labor (O65-O66)*

O33.0 Maternal care for disproportion due to deformity of maternal pelvic bones CC M♀

Maternal care for disproportion due to pelvic deformity causing disproportion NOS

CC Excl: PDX collection 977

O33.1 Maternal care for disproportion due to generally contracted pelvis M♀

Maternal care for disproportion due to contracted pelvis NOS causing disproportion

O33.2 Maternal care for disproportion due to inlet contraction of pelvis M♀

Maternal care for disproportion due to inlet contraction (pelvis) causing disproportion

✓x7th **O33.3 Maternal care for disproportion due to outlet contraction of pelvis** M♀

Maternal care for disproportion due to mid-cavity contraction (pelvis)

Maternal care for disproportion due to outlet contraction (pelvis)

One of the following 7th characters is to be assigned to code O33.3. 7th character Ø is for single gestations and multiple gestations where the fetus is unspecified. 7th characters 1 through 9 are for cases of multiple gestations to identify the fetus for which the code applies. The appropriate code from category O30, Multiple gestation, must also be assigned when assigning code O33.3 with a 7th character of 1 through 9.

Ø	not applicable or unspecified	3	fetus 3
		4	fetus 4
1	fetus 1	5	fetus 5
2	fetus 2	9	other fetus

✓x7th **O33.4 Maternal care for disproportion of mixed maternal and fetal origin** M♀

One of the following 7th characters is to be assigned to code O33.4. 7th character Ø is for single gestations and multiple gestations where the fetus is unspecified. 7th characters 1 through 9 are for cases of multiple gestations to identify the fetus for which the code applies. The appropriate code from category O30, Multiple gestation, must also be assigned when assigning code O33.4 with a 7th character of 1 through 9.

Ø	not applicable or unspecified	3	fetus 3
		4	fetus 4
1	fetus 1	5	fetus 5
2	fetus 2	9	other fetus

✓x7th **O33.5 Maternal care for disproportion due to unusually large fetus** M♀

Maternal care for disproportion due to disproportion of fetal origin with normally formed fetus

Maternal care for disproportion due to fetal disproportion NOS

One of the following 7th characters is to be assigned to code O33.5. 7th character Ø is for single gestations and multiple gestations where the fetus is unspecified. 7th characters 1 through 9 are for cases of multiple gestations to identify the fetus for which the code applies. The appropriate code from category O30, Multiple gestation, must also be assigned when assigning code O33.5 with a 7th character of 1 through 9.

Ø	not applicable or unspecified	3	fetus 3
		4	fetus 4
1	fetus 1	5	fetus 5
2	fetus 2	9	other fetus

✓x7th **O33.6 Maternal care for disproportion due to hydrocephalic fetus** M♀

One of the following 7th characters is to be assigned to code O33.6. 7th character Ø is for single gestations and multiple gestations where the fetus is unspecified. 7th characters 1 through 9 are for cases of multiple gestations to identify the fetus for which the code applies. The appropriate code from category O30, Multiple gestation, must also be assigned when assigning code O33.6 with a 7th character of 1 through 9.

Ø	not applicable or unspecified	3	fetus 3
		4	fetus 4
1	fetus 1	5	fetus 5
2	fetus 2	9	other fetus

✓x7th **O33.7 Maternal care for disproportion due to other fetal deformities** M♀

Maternal care for disproportion due to fetal ascites

Maternal care for disproportion due to fetal hydrops

Maternal care for disproportion due to fetal meningomyelocele

Maternal care for disproportion due to fetal sacral teratoma

Maternal care for disproportion due to fetal tumor

EXCLUDES 1 *obstructed labor due to other fetal deformities (O66.3)*

One of the following 7th characters is to be assigned to code O33.7. 7th character Ø is for single gestations and multiple gestations where the fetus is unspecified. 7th characters 1 through 9 are for cases of multiple gestations to identify the fetus for which the code applies. The appropriate code from category O30, Multiple gestation, must also be assigned when assigning code O33.7 with a 7th character of 1 through 9.

Ø	not applicable or unspecified	3	fetus 3
		4	fetus 4
1	fetus 1	5	fetus 5
2	fetus 2	9	other fetus

O33.8 Maternal care for disproportion of other origin M♀

O33.9 Maternal care for disproportion, unspecified M♀

Maternal care for disproportion due to cephalopelvic disproportion NOS

Maternal care for disproportion due to fetopelvic disproportion NOS

✓4th **O34 Maternal care for abnormality of pelvic organs**

INCLUDES the listed conditions as a reason for hospitalization or other obstetric care of the mother, or for cesarean delivery before onset of labor

Code first any associated obstructed labor (O65.5)

Use additional code for specific condition

✓5th **O34.0 Maternal care for congenital malformation of uterus**

Maternal care for double uterus

Maternal care for uterus bicornis

O34.00 Maternal care for unspecified congenital malformation of uterus, unspecified trimester M♀

O34.01 Maternal care for unspecified congenital malformation of uterus, first trimester M♀

O34.02 Maternal care for unspecified congenital malformation of uterus, second trimester M♀

O34.03 Maternal care for unspecified congenital malformation of uterus, third trimester M♀

✓5th **O34.1 Maternal care for benign tumor of corpus uteri**

EXCLUDES 2 *maternal care for benign tumor of cervix (O34.4-)*

maternal care for malignant neoplasm of uterus (O9A.1-)

O34.10 Maternal care for benign tumor of corpus uteri, unspecified trimester M♀

O34.11 Maternal care for benign tumor of corpus uteri, first trimester M♀

O34.12 Maternal care for benign tumor of corpus uteri, second trimester M♀

O34.13 Maternal care for benign tumor of corpus uteri, third trimester M♀

✓5th **O34.2 Maternal care due to uterine scar from previous surgery**

✓6th **O34.21 Maternal care for scar from previous cesarean delivery**

O34.211 Maternal care for low transverse scar from previous cesarean delivery M♀

O34.212 Maternal care for vertical scar from previous cesarean delivery M♀

Maternal care for classical scar from previous cesarean delivery

O34.219 Maternal care for unspecified type scar from previous cesarean delivery M♀

O34.29 Maternal care due to uterine scar from other previous surgery M♀

Maternal care due to uterine scar from other transmural uterine incision

Chapter 15. Pregnancy, Childbirth and the Puerperium (left margin)

O34.3–O35.7 (left margin)

√5th **O34.3 Maternal care for** cervical incompetence

Maternal care for cerclage with or without cervical incompetence

Maternal care for Shirodkar suture with or without cervical incompetence

DEF: Inadequate functioning of cervix marked by abnormal widening during pregnancy that may cause premature birth or miscarriage.

CC Excl: For MCC codes in subcategory O34.3:
PDX collection 973

    O34.30 **Maternal care for cervical incompetence,** unspecified trimester   M♀

    O34.31 **Maternal care for cervical incompetence,** first trimester   MCC M♀

    O34.32 **Maternal care for cervical incompetence,** second trimester   MCC M♀

    O34.33 **Maternal care for cervical incompetence,** third trimester   MCC M♀

√5th **O34.4 Maternal care for** other abnormalities of cervix

    O34.40 **Maternal care for other abnormalities of cervix,** unspecified trimester   M♀

    O34.41 **Maternal care for other abnormalities of cervix,** first trimester   M♀

    O34.42 **Maternal care for other abnormalities of cervix,** second trimester   M♀

    O34.43 **Maternal care for other abnormalities of cervix,** third trimester   M♀

√5th **O34.5 Maternal care for** other abnormalities of gravid uterus

  √6th **O34.51** **Maternal care for** incarceration of gravid uterus

    O34.511 **Maternal care for incarceration of gravid uterus, first trimester**   M♀

    O34.512 **Maternal care for incarceration of gravid uterus, second trimester**   M♀

    O34.513 **Maternal care for incarceration of gravid uterus, third trimester**   M♀

    O34.519 **Maternal care for incarceration of gravid uterus, unspecified trimester**   M♀

  √6th **O34.52** **Maternal care for** prolapse of gravid uterus

    O34.521 **Maternal care for prolapse of gravid uterus, first trimester**   M♀

    O34.522 **Maternal care for prolapse of gravid uterus, second trimester**   M♀

    O34.523 **Maternal care for prolapse of gravid uterus, third trimester**   M♀

    O34.529 **Maternal care for prolapse of gravid uterus, unspecified trimester**   M♀

  √6th **O34.53** **Maternal care for** retroversion of gravid uterus

    O34.531 **Maternal care for retroversion of gravid uterus, first trimester**   M♀

    O34.532 **Maternal care for retroversion of gravid uterus, second trimester**   M♀

    O34.533 **Maternal care for retroversion of gravid uterus, third trimester**   M♀

    O34.539 **Maternal care for retroversion of gravid uterus, unspecified trimester**   M♀

  √6th **O34.59** **Maternal care for** other abnormalities of gravid uterus

    O34.591 **Maternal care for other abnormalities of gravid uterus, first trimester**   M♀

    O34.592 **Maternal care for other abnormalities of gravid uterus, second trimester**   M♀

    O34.593 **Maternal care for other abnormalities of gravid uterus, third trimester**   M♀

    O34.599 **Maternal care for other abnormalities of gravid uterus, unspecified trimester**   M♀

√5th **O34.6 Maternal care for** abnormality of vagina

    EXCLUDES 2   maternal care for vaginal varices in pregnancy (O22.1-)

    O34.60 **Maternal care for abnormality of vagina,** unspecified trimester   M♀

    O34.61 **Maternal care for abnormality of vagina,** first trimester   M♀

    O34.62 **Maternal care for abnormality of vagina,** second trimester   M♀

    O34.63 **Maternal care for abnormality of vagina,** third trimester   M♀

√5th **O34.7 Maternal care for** abnormality of vulva and perineum

    EXCLUDES 2   maternal care for perineal and vulval varices in pregnancy (O22.1-)

    O34.70 **Maternal care for abnormality of vulva and perineum,** unspecified trimester   M♀

    O34.71 **Maternal care for abnormality of vulva and perineum,** first trimester   M♀

    O34.72 **Maternal care for abnormality of vulva and perineum,** second trimester   M♀

    O34.73 **Maternal care for abnormality of vulva and perineum,** third trimester   M♀

√5th **O34.8 Maternal care for** other abnormalities of pelvic organs

    O34.80 **Maternal care for other abnormalities of pelvic organs,** unspecified trimester   M♀

    O34.81 **Maternal care for other abnormalities of pelvic organs,** first trimester   M♀

    O34.82 **Maternal care for other abnormalities of pelvic organs,** second trimester   M♀

    O34.83 **Maternal care for other abnormalities of pelvic organs,** third trimester   M♀

√5th **O34.9 Maternal care for** abnormality of pelvic organ, unspecified

    O34.90 **Maternal care for abnormality of pelvic organ, unspecified,** unspecified trimester   M♀

    O34.91 **Maternal care for abnormality of pelvic organ, unspecified,** first trimester   M♀

    O34.92 **Maternal care for abnormality of pelvic organ, unspecified,** second trimester   M♀

    O34.93 **Maternal care for abnormality of pelvic organ, unspecified,** third trimester   M♀

√4th **O35 Maternal care for known or suspected fetal abnormality and damage**

  INCLUDES   the listed conditions in the fetus as a reason for hospitalization or other obstetric care to the mother, or for termination of pregnancy

Code also any associated maternal condition

  EXCLUDES 1   encounter for suspected maternal and fetal conditions ruled out (Z03.7-)

One of the following 7th characters is to be assigned to each code under category O35. 7th character Ø is for single gestations and multiple gestations where the fetus is unspecified. 7th characters 1 through 9 are for cases of multiple gestations to identify the fetus for which the code applies. The appropriate code from category O30, Multiple gestation, must also be assigned when assigning a code from category O35 that has a 7th character of 1 through 9.

Ø	not applicable or unspecified	3	fetus 3
		4	fetus 4
1	fetus 1	5	fetus 5
2	fetus 2	9	other fetus

√x7th **O35.0 Maternal care for (suspected)** central nervous system malformation in fetus   M♀

Maternal care for fetal anencephaly

Maternal care for fetal hydrocephalus

Maternal care for fetal spina bifida

  EXCLUDES 2   chromosomal abnormality in fetus (O35.1)

√x7th **O35.1 Maternal care for (suspected)** chromosomal abnormality in fetus   M♀

√x7th **O35.2 Maternal care for (suspected)** hereditary disease in fetus   M♀

  EXCLUDES 2   chromosomal abnormality in fetus (O35.1)

√x7th **O35.3 Maternal care for (suspected)** damage to fetus from viral disease in mother   M♀

Maternal care for damage to fetus from maternal cytomegalovirus infection

Maternal care for damage to fetus from maternal rubella

√x7th **O35.4 Maternal care for (suspected)** damage to fetus from alcohol   M♀

√x7th **O35.5 Maternal care for (suspected)** damage to fetus by drugs   M♀

Maternal care for damage to fetus from drug addiction

√x7th **O35.6 Maternal care for (suspected)** damage to fetus by radiation   M♀

√x7th **O35.7 Maternal care for (suspected)** damage to fetus by other medical procedures   M♀

Maternal care for damage to fetus by amniocentesis

Maternal care for damage to fetus by biopsy procedures

Maternal care for damage to fetus by hematological investigation

Maternal care for damage to fetus by intrauterine contraceptive device

Maternal care for damage to fetus by intrauterine surgery

N Newborn: 0   P Pediatric: 0-17   M Maternity: 12-55   A Adult: 15-124   MCC Major CC Condition   PDxMCC PDx acts as own MCC   CC CC Condition   PDxCC PDx acts as own CC

860   ICD-10-CM 2018

√x7ᵗʰ **O35.8** **Maternal care for other (suspected)** fetal abnormality **and damage** Ⓜ♀
     Maternal care for damage to fetus from maternal listeriosis
     Maternal care for damage to fetus from maternal toxoplasmosis

√x7ᵗʰ **O35.9** **Maternal care for (suspected)** fetal abnormality and **damage, unspecified** Ⓜ♀

√4ᵗʰ **O36** **Maternal care for other fetal problems**
     INCLUDES   the listed conditions in the fetus as a reason for hospitalization or other obstetric care of the mother, or for termination of pregnancy
     EXCLUDES 1   encounter for suspected maternal and fetal conditions ruled out (Z03.7-)
         placental transfusion syndromes (O43.0-)
     EXCLUDES 2   labor and delivery complicated by fetal stress (O77.-)
     AHA: 2015, 3Q, 40

> One of the following 7th characters is to be assigned to each code under category O36. 7th character Ø is for single gestations and multiple gestations where the fetus is unspecified. 7th characters 1 through 9 are for cases of multiple gestations to identify the fetus for which the code applies. The appropriate code from category O30, Multiple gestation, must also be assigned when assigning a code from category O36 that has a 7th character of 1 through 9.
>
> Ø   not applicable or   3   fetus 3
>   unspecified   4   fetus 4
> 1   fetus 1   5   fetus 5
> 2   fetus 2   9   other fetus

√5ᵗʰ **O36.Ø** **Maternal care for rhesus isoimmunization**
     Maternal care for Rh incompatibility (with hydrops fetalis)

> **CC Excl:** For CC codes in subcategory O36.Ø:
> PDX collection 978

√6ᵗʰ **O36.Ø1** **Maternal care for** anti-D [Rh] antibodies
         AHA: 2014, 4Q, 17

     √7ᵗʰ **O36.Ø11** **Maternal care for anti-D [Rh] antibodies,** first trimester   cc Ⓜ♀

     √7ᵗʰ **O36.Ø12** **Maternal care for anti-D [Rh] antibodies,** second trimester   cc Ⓜ♀

     √7ᵗʰ **O36.Ø13** **Maternal care for anti-D [Rh] antibodies,** third trimester   cc Ⓜ♀

     √7ᵗʰ **O36.Ø19** **Maternal care for anti-D [Rh] antibodies, unspecified** trimester   Ⓜ♀

√6ᵗʰ **O36.Ø9** **Maternal care for** other rhesus isoimmunization

     √7ᵗʰ **O36.Ø91** **Maternal care for other rhesus isoimmunization,** first trimester   cc Ⓜ♀

     √7ᵗʰ **O36.Ø92** **Maternal care for other rhesus isoimmunization,** second trimester   cc Ⓜ♀

     √7ᵗʰ **O36.Ø93** **Maternal care for other rhesus isoimmunization,** third trimester   cc Ⓜ♀

     √7ᵗʰ **O36.Ø99** **Maternal care for other rhesus isoimmunization, unspecified trimester**   Ⓜ♀

√5ᵗʰ **O36.1** **Maternal care for other isoimmunization**
     Maternal care for ABO isoimmunization

√6ᵗʰ **O36.11** **Maternal care for** Anti-A sensitization
         Maternal care for isoimmunization NOS (with hydrops fetalis)

     √7ᵗʰ **O36.111** **Maternal care for Anti-A sensitization,** first trimester   Ⓜ♀

     √7ᵗʰ **O36.112** **Maternal care for Anti-A sensitization,** second trimester   Ⓜ♀

     √7ᵗʰ **O36.113** **Maternal care for Anti-A sensitization,** third trimester   Ⓜ♀

     √7ᵗʰ **O36.119** **Maternal care for Anti-A sensitization, unspecified trimester**   Ⓜ♀

√6ᵗʰ **O36.19** **Maternal care for** other isoimmunization
         Maternal care for Anti-B sensitization

     √7ᵗʰ **O36.191** **Maternal care for other isoimmunization,** first trimester   Ⓜ♀

     √7ᵗʰ **O36.192** **Maternal care for other isoimmunization,** second trimester   Ⓜ♀

     √7ᵗʰ **O36.193** **Maternal care for other isoimmunization,** third trimester   Ⓜ♀

     √7ᵗʰ **O36.199** **Maternal care for other isoimmunization,** unspecified trimester   Ⓜ♀

√5ᵗʰ **O36.2** **Maternal care for hydrops fetalis**
     Maternal care for hydrops fetalis NOS
     Maternal care for hydrops fetalis not associated with isoimmunization
     EXCLUDES 1   hydrops fetalis associated with ABO isoimmunization (O36.1-)
         hydrops fetalis associated with rhesus isoimmunization (O36.Ø-)

     √x7ᵗʰ **O36.2Ø** **Maternal care for hydrops fetalis, unspecified** trimester   Ⓜ♀

     √x7ᵗʰ **O36.21** **Maternal care for hydrops fetalis, first** trimester   Ⓜ♀

     √x7ᵗʰ **O36.22** **Maternal care for hydrops fetalis, second** trimester   Ⓜ♀

     √x7ᵗʰ **O36.23** **Maternal care for hydrops fetalis, third** trimester   Ⓜ♀

√x7ᵗʰ **O36.4** **Maternal care for intrauterine death**   cc Ⓜ♀
     Maternal care for intrauterine fetal death NOS
     Maternal care for intrauterine fetal death after completion of 20 weeks of gestation
     Maternal care for late fetal death
     Maternal care for missed delivery
     EXCLUDES 1   missed abortion (O02.1)
         stillbirth (P95)
     CC Excl: PDX collection 979

√5ᵗʰ **O36.5** **Maternal care for known or suspected poor fetal growth**

     √6ᵗʰ **O36.51** **Maternal care for known or suspected placental insufficiency**

         √7ᵗʰ **O36.511** **Maternal care for known or suspected placental insufficiency, first trimester**   Ⓜ♀

         √7ᵗʰ **O36.512** **Maternal care for known or suspected placental insufficiency, second trimester**   Ⓜ♀

         √7ᵗʰ **O36.513** **Maternal care for known or suspected placental insufficiency, third trimester**   Ⓜ♀

         √7ᵗʰ **O36.519** **Maternal care for known or suspected placental insufficiency, unspecified trimester**   Ⓜ♀

     √6ᵗʰ **O36.59** **Maternal care for other known or suspected poor fetal growth**
         Maternal care for known or suspected light-for-dates NOS
         Maternal care for known or suspected small-for-dates NOS

         √7ᵗʰ **O36.591** **Maternal care for other known or suspected poor fetal growth, first trimester**   Ⓜ♀

         √7ᵗʰ **O36.592** **Maternal care for other known or suspected poor fetal growth, second trimester**   Ⓜ♀

         √7ᵗʰ **O36.593** **Maternal care for other known or suspected poor fetal growth, third trimester**   Ⓜ♀

         √7ᵗʰ **O36.599** **Maternal care for other known or suspected poor fetal growth, unspecified trimester**   Ⓜ♀

√5ᵗʰ **O36.6** **Maternal care for excessive fetal growth**
     Maternal care for known or suspected large-for-dates

     √x7ᵗʰ **O36.6Ø** **Maternal care for excessive fetal growth, unspecified trimester**   Ⓜ♀

     √x7ᵗʰ **O36.61** **Maternal care for excessive fetal growth, first trimester**   Ⓜ♀

     √x7ᵗʰ **O36.62** **Maternal care for excessive fetal growth, second trimester**   Ⓜ♀

     √x7ᵗʰ **O36.63** **Maternal care for excessive fetal growth, third trimester**   Ⓜ♀

√5ᵗʰ **O36.7** **Maternal care for viable fetus in abdominal pregnancy**

     √x7ᵗʰ **O36.7Ø** **Maternal care for viable fetus in abdominal pregnancy, unspecified trimester**   Ⓜ♀

     √x7ᵗʰ **O36.71** **Maternal care for viable fetus in abdominal pregnancy, first trimester**   Ⓜ♀

     √x7ᵗʰ **O36.72** **Maternal care for viable fetus in abdominal pregnancy, second trimester**   Ⓜ♀

     √x7ᵗʰ **O36.73** **Maternal care for viable fetus in abdominal pregnancy, third trimester**   Ⓜ♀

✓ Additional Character Req   √x7ᵗʰ Placeholder Alert   Unacceptable PDx   Manifestation   H1 - H14 HAC   HCC CMS-HCC Condition   EXCLUDES 1 Not Coded Here   EXCLUDES 2 Not Included Here

ICD-10-CM 2018   861

Chapter 15. Pregnancy, Childbirth and the Puerperium

O36.8–O41.92

√5th **O36.8 Maternal care for other specified fetal problems**

√7th **O36.80 Pregnancy with inconclusive fetal viability** Ⓜ♀
Encounter to determine fetal viability of pregnancy

√6th **O36.81 Decreased fetal movements**

√7th **O36.812 Decreased fetal movements, second trimester** Ⓜ♀

√7th **O36.813 Decreased fetal movements, third trimester** Ⓜ♀

√7th **O36.819 Decreased fetal movements, unspecified trimester** Ⓜ♀

√6th **O36.82 Fetal anemia and thrombocytopenia**

√7th **O36.821 Fetal anemia and thrombocytopenia, first trimester** Ⓜ♀

√7th **O36.822 Fetal anemia and thrombocytopenia, second trimester** Ⓜ♀

√7th **O36.823 Fetal anemia and thrombocytopenia, third trimester** Ⓜ♀

√7th **O36.829 Fetal anemia and thrombocytopenia, unspecified trimester** Ⓜ♀

● √6th **O36.83 Maternal care for abnormalities of the fetal heart rate or rhythm**

● √7th **O36.831 Maternal care for abnormalities of the fetal heart rate or rhythm, first trimester** Ⓜ

● √7th **O36.832 Maternal care for abnormalities of the fetal heart rate or rhythm, second trimester** Ⓜ

● √7th **O36.833 Maternal care for abnormalities of the fetal heart rate or rhythm, third trimester** Ⓜ

● √7th **O36.839 Maternal care for abnormalities of the fetal heart rate or rhythm, unspecified trimester** Ⓜ

√6th **O36.89 Maternal care for other specified fetal problems**

√7th **O36.891 Maternal care for other specified fetal problems, first trimester** Ⓜ♀

√7th **O36.892 Maternal care for other specified fetal problems, second trimester** Ⓜ♀

√7th **O36.893 Maternal care for other specified fetal problems, third trimester** Ⓜ♀

√7th **O36.899 Maternal care for other specified fetal problems, unspecified trimester** Ⓜ♀

√5th **O36.9 Maternal care for fetal problem, unspecified**

√x7th **O36.90 Maternal care for fetal problem, unspecified, unspecified trimester** Ⓜ♀

√x7th **O36.91 Maternal care for fetal problem, unspecified, first trimester** Ⓜ♀

√x7th **O36.92 Maternal care for fetal problem, unspecified, second trimester** Ⓜ♀

√x7th **O36.93 Maternal care for fetal problem, unspecified, third trimester** Ⓜ♀

√4th **O40 Polyhydramnios**

INCLUDES hydramnios

EXCLUDES 1 encounter for suspected maternal and fetal conditions ruled out (Z03.7-)

AHA: 2016, 1Q, 4

One of the following 7th characters is to be assigned to each code under category O40. 7th character Ø is for single gestations and multiple gestations where the fetus is unspecified. 7th characters 1 through 9 are for cases of multiple gestations to identify the fetus for which the code applies. The appropriate code from category O30, Multiple gestation, must also be assigned when assigning a code from category O40 that has a 7th character of 1 through 9.

Ø	not applicable or unspecified	3	fetus 3
		4	fetus 4
1	fetus 1	5	fetus 5
2	fetus 2	9	other fetus

√x7th **O40.1 Polyhydramnios, first trimester** Ⓜ♀

√x7th **O40.2 Polyhydramnios, second trimester** Ⓜ♀

√x7th **O40.3 Polyhydramnios, third trimester** Ⓜ♀

√x7th **O40.9 Polyhydramnios, unspecified trimester** Ⓜ♀

√4th **O41 Other disorders of amniotic fluid and membranes**

EXCLUDES 1 encounter for suspected maternal and fetal conditions ruled out (Z03.7-)

One of the following 7th characters is to be assigned to each code under category O41. 7th character Ø is for single gestations and multiple gestations where the fetus is unspecified. 7th characters 1 through 9 are for cases of multiple gestations to identify the fetus for which the code applies. The appropriate code from category O30, Multiple gestation, must also be assigned when assigning a code from category O41 that has a 7th character of 1 through 9.

Ø	not applicable or unspecified	3	fetus 3
		4	fetus 4
1	fetus 1	5	fetus 5
2	fetus 2	9	other fetus

√5th **O41.0 Oligohydramnios**
Oligohydramnios without rupture of membranes

CC Excl: For CC codes in subcategory O41.0:
PDX collection 982

√x7th **O41.00 Oligohydramnios, unspecified trimester** Ⓜ♀

√x7th **O41.01 Oligohydramnios, first trimester** CC Ⓜ♀

√x7th **O41.02 Oligohydramnios, second trimester** CC Ⓜ♀

√x7th **O41.03 Oligohydramnios, third trimester** CC Ⓜ♀

√5th **O41.1 Infection of amniotic sac and membranes**

CC Excl: For MCC codes in subcategory O41.1:
PDX collection 983

√6th **O41.10 Infection of amniotic sac and membranes, unspecified**

√7th **O41.101 Infection of amniotic sac and membranes, unspecified, first trimester** MCC Ⓜ♀

√7th **O41.102 Infection of amniotic sac and membranes, unspecified, second trimester** MCC Ⓜ♀

√7th **O41.103 Infection of amniotic sac and membranes, unspecified, third trimester** MCC Ⓜ♀

√7th **O41.109 Infection of amniotic sac and membranes, unspecified, unspecified trimester** Ⓜ♀

√6th **O41.12 Chorioamnionitis**

√7th **O41.121 Chorioamnionitis, first trimester** MCC Ⓜ♀

√7th **O41.122 Chorioamnionitis, second trimester** MCC Ⓜ♀

√7th **O41.123 Chorioamnionitis, third trimester** MCC Ⓜ♀

√7th **O41.129 Chorioamnionitis, unspecified trimester** Ⓜ♀

√6th **O41.14 Placentitis**

√7th **O41.141 Placentitis, first trimester** MCC Ⓜ♀

√7th **O41.142 Placentitis, second trimester** MCC Ⓜ♀

√7th **O41.143 Placentitis, third trimester** MCC Ⓜ♀

√7th **O41.149 Placentitis, unspecified trimester** Ⓜ♀

√5th **O41.8 Other specified disorders of amniotic fluid and membranes**

√6th **O41.8X Other specified disorders of amniotic fluid and membranes**

√7th **O41.8X1 Other specified disorders of amniotic fluid and membranes, first trimester** Ⓜ♀

√7th **O41.8X2 Other specified disorders of amniotic fluid and membranes, second trimester** Ⓜ♀

√7th **O41.8X3 Other specified disorders of amniotic fluid and membranes, third trimester** Ⓜ♀

√7th **O41.8X9 Other specified disorders of amniotic fluid and membranes, unspecified trimester** Ⓜ♀

√5th **O41.9 Disorder of amniotic fluid and membranes, unspecified**

√x7th **O41.90 Disorder of amniotic fluid and membranes, unspecified, unspecified trimester** Ⓜ♀

√x7th **O41.91 Disorder of amniotic fluid and membranes, unspecified, first trimester** Ⓜ♀

√x7th **O41.92 Disorder of amniotic fluid and membranes, unspecified, second trimester** Ⓜ♀

Ⓝ Newborn: 0 Ⓟ Pediatric: 0-17 Ⓜ Maternity: 12-55 Ⓐ Adult: 15-124 MCC Major CC Condition PDxMCC PDx acts as own MCC CC CC Condition PDxCC PDx acts as own CC

862 ICD-10-CM 2018

✓x7ᵗʰ **O41.93** **Disorder of amniotic fluid and membranes, unspecified,** third trimester Ⓜ♀

✓4ᵗʰ **O42** **Premature rupture of membranes**
AHA: 2016, 1Q, 3

✓5ᵗʰ **O42.0** **Premature rupture of membranes,** onset of labor within 24 hours of rupture

   O42.00 **Premature rupture of membranes, onset of labor within 24 hours of rupture,** unspecified weeks of gestation Ⓜ♀

✓6ᵗʰ **O42.01** **Preterm premature rupture of membranes, onset of labor within 24 hours of rupture**
Premature rupture of membranes before 37 completed weeks of gestation

    O42.011 **Preterm premature rupture of membranes, onset of labor within 24 hours of rupture,** first trimester Ⓜ♀

    O42.012 **Preterm premature rupture of membranes, onset of labor within 24 hours of rupture,** second trimester Ⓜ♀

    O42.013 **Preterm premature rupture of membranes, onset of labor within 24 hours of rupture,** third trimester Ⓜ♀

    O42.019 **Preterm premature rupture of membranes, onset of labor within 24 hours of rupture,** unspecified trimester Ⓜ♀

   O42.02 **Full-term premature rupture of membranes, onset of labor within 24 hours of rupture** Ⓜ♀
Premature rupture of membranes at or after 37 completed weeks of gestation, onset of labor within 24 hours of rupture

✓5ᵗʰ **O42.1** **Premature rupture of membranes,** onset of labor more than 24 hours following rupture
AHA: 2016, 1Q, 5

   O42.10 **Premature rupture of membranes, onset of labor more than 24 hours following rupture,** unspecified weeks of gestation Ⓜ♀

✓6ᵗʰ **O42.11** **Preterm premature rupture of membranes, onset of labor more than 24 hours following rupture**
Premature rupture of membranes before 37 completed weeks of gestation

    O42.111 **Preterm premature rupture of membranes, onset of labor more than 24 hours following rupture,** first trimester Ⓜ♀

    O42.112 **Preterm premature rupture of membranes, onset of labor more than 24 hours following rupture,** second trimester Ⓜ♀

    O42.113 **Preterm premature rupture of membranes, onset of labor more than 24 hours following rupture,** third trimester Ⓜ♀

    O42.119 **Preterm premature rupture of membranes, onset of labor more than 24 hours following rupture,** unspecified trimester Ⓜ♀

   O42.12 **Full-term premature rupture of membranes, onset of labor more than 24 hours following rupture** Ⓜ♀
Premature rupture of membranes at or after 37 completed weeks of gestation, onset of labor more than 24 hours following rupture

✓5ᵗʰ **O42.9** **Premature rupture of membranes,** unspecified as to length of time between rupture and onset of labor

   O42.90 **Premature rupture of membranes, unspecified as to length of time between rupture and onset of labor,** unspecified weeks of gestation Ⓜ♀

✓6ᵗʰ **O42.91** **Preterm premature rupture of membranes, unspecified as to length of time between rupture and onset of labor**
Premature rupture of membranes before 37 completed weeks of gestation

    O42.911 **Preterm premature rupture of membranes, unspecified as to length of time between rupture and onset of labor,** first trimester Ⓜ♀

    O42.912 **Preterm premature rupture of membranes, unspecified as to length of time between rupture and onset of labor,** second trimester Ⓜ♀

    O42.913 **Preterm premature rupture of membranes, unspecified as to length of time between rupture and onset of labor,** third trimester Ⓜ♀

    O42.919 **Preterm premature rupture of membranes, unspecified as to length of time between rupture and onset of labor,** unspecified trimester Ⓜ♀

   O42.92 **Full-term premature rupture of membranes, unspecified as to length of time between rupture and onset of labor** Ⓜ♀
Premature rupture of membranes at or after 37 completed weeks of gestation, unspecified as to length of time between rupture and onset of labor

✓4ᵗʰ **O43** **Placental disorders**
EXCLUDES 2   maternal care for poor fetal growth due to placental insufficiency (O36.5-)
placenta previa (O44.-)
placental polyp (O90.89)
placentitis (O41.14-)
premature separation of placenta [abruptio placentae] (O45.-)

✓5ᵗʰ **O43.0** **Placental transfusion syndromes**

✓6ᵗʰ **O43.01** **Fetomaternal placental transfusion syndrome**
Maternofetal placental transfusion syndrome

    O43.011 **Fetomaternal placental transfusion syndrome,** first trimester Ⓜ♀

    O43.012 **Fetomaternal placental transfusion syndrome,** second trimester Ⓜ♀

    O43.013 **Fetomaternal placental transfusion syndrome,** third trimester Ⓜ♀

    O43.019 **Fetomaternal placental transfusion syndrome,** unspecified trimester Ⓜ♀

✓6ᵗʰ **O43.02** **Fetus-to-fetus placental transfusion syndrome**

    O43.021 **Fetus-to-fetus placental transfusion syndrome,** first trimester Ⓜ♀

    O43.022 **Fetus-to-fetus placental transfusion syndrome,** second trimester Ⓜ♀

    O43.023 **Fetus-to-fetus placental transfusion syndrome,** third trimester Ⓜ♀

    O43.029 **Fetus-to-fetus placental transfusion syndrome,** unspecified trimester Ⓜ♀

✓5ᵗʰ **O43.1** **Malformation of placenta**

✓6ᵗʰ **O43.10** **Malformation of placenta,** unspecified
Abnormal placenta NOS

    O43.101 **Malformation of placenta, unspecified,** first trimester Ⓜ♀

    O43.102 **Malformation of placenta, unspecified,** second trimester Ⓜ♀

    O43.103 **Malformation of placenta, unspecified,** third trimester Ⓜ♀

    O43.109 **Malformation of placenta, unspecified,** unspecified trimester Ⓜ♀

✓6ᵗʰ **O43.11** **Circumvallate placenta**

    O43.111 **Circumvallate placenta,** first trimester Ⓜ♀

    O43.112 **Circumvallate placenta,** second trimester Ⓜ♀

    O43.113 **Circumvallate placenta,** third trimester Ⓜ♀

Twin to Twin Transfusion Syndrome (TTTS)

Healthy twins   Twins with TTTS

　　　O43.119 **Circumvallate placenta,** unspecified Ⓜ♀
　　　　　　　trimester

✓6ᵗʰ **O43.12** Velamentous insertion of umbilical cord
　　　O43.121 **Velamentous insertion of umbilical** Ⓜ♀
　　　　　　　cord, first trimester
　　　O43.122 **Velamentous insertion of umbilical** Ⓜ♀
　　　　　　　cord, second trimester
　　　O43.123 **Velamentous insertion of umbilical** Ⓜ♀
　　　　　　　cord, third trimester
　　　O43.129 **Velamentous insertion of umbilical** Ⓜ♀
　　　　　　　cord, unspecified trimester

✓6ᵗʰ **O43.19** Other malformation of placenta
　　　O43.191 **Other malformation of placenta,** Ⓜ♀
　　　　　　　first trimester
　　　O43.192 **Other malformation of placenta,** Ⓜ♀
　　　　　　　second trimester
　　　O43.193 **Other malformation of placenta,** Ⓜ♀
　　　　　　　third trimester
　　　O43.199 **Other malformation of placenta,** Ⓜ♀
　　　　　　　unspecified trimester

✓5ᵗʰ **O43.2** **Morbidly adherent placenta**
　　　Code also associated third stage postpartum hemorrhage, if
　　　applicable (O72.0)
　　　EXCLUDES 1　retained placenta (O73.-)

✓6ᵗʰ **O43.21** Placenta accreta
　　　O43.211 **Placenta accreta,** first trimester Ⓜ♀
　　　O43.212 **Placenta accreta,** second trimester Ⓜ♀
　　　O43.213 **Placenta accreta,** third trimester Ⓜ♀
　　　O43.219 **Placenta accreta,** unspecified Ⓜ♀
　　　　　　　trimester

✓6ᵗʰ **O43.22** Placenta increta
　　　O43.221 **Placenta increta,** first trimester Ⓜ♀
　　　O43.222 **Placenta increta,** second trimester Ⓜ♀
　　　O43.223 **Placenta increta,** third trimester Ⓜ♀
　　　O43.229 **Placenta increta,** unspecified Ⓜ♀
　　　　　　　trimester

✓6ᵗʰ **O43.23** Placenta percreta
　　　O43.231 **Placenta percreta,** first trimester Ⓜ♀
　　　O43.232 **Placenta percreta,** second trimester Ⓜ♀
　　　O43.233 **Placenta percreta,** third trimester Ⓜ♀
　　　O43.239 **Placenta percreta,** unspecified Ⓜ♀
　　　　　　　trimester

✓5ᵗʰ **O43.8** **Other placental disorders**
✓6ᵗʰ **O43.81** Placental infarction
　　　O43.811 **Placental infarction,** first trimester Ⓜ♀
　　　O43.812 **Placental infarction,** second trimester Ⓜ♀
　　　O43.813 **Placental infarction,** third trimester Ⓜ♀
　　　O43.819 **Placental infarction,** unspecified Ⓜ♀
　　　　　　　trimester

✓6ᵗʰ **O43.89** Other placental disorders
　　　Placental dysfunction
　　　O43.891 **Other placental disorders,** first Ⓜ♀
　　　　　　　trimester
　　　O43.892 **Other placental disorders,** second Ⓜ♀
　　　　　　　trimester
　　　O43.893 **Other placental disorders,** third Ⓜ♀
　　　　　　　trimester
　　　O43.899 **Other placental disorders,** Ⓜ♀
　　　　　　　unspecified trimester

✓5ᵗʰ **O43.9** **Unspecified placental disorder**
　　　O43.90 **Unspecified placental disorder,** unspecified Ⓜ♀
　　　　　　trimester
　　　O43.91 **Unspecified placental disorder,** first trimester Ⓜ♀
　　　O43.92 **Unspecified placental disorder,** second Ⓜ♀
　　　　　　trimester
　　　O43.93 **Unspecified placental disorder,** third trimester Ⓜ♀

✓4ᵗʰ **O44** **Placenta previa**
　　　DEF: Placenta implanted in lower segment of uterus; commonly causes
　　　hemorrhage in the last trimester of pregnancy.

　　　CC Excl: For CC/MCC codes in category O44: PDX collection 966

✓5ᵗʰ **O44.0** **Complete placenta previa NOS or** without hemorrhage
　　　Placenta previa NOS
　　　O44.00 **Complete placenta previa NOS or without** Ⓜ♀
　　　　　　hemorrhage, unspecified trimester

　　　O44.01 **Complete placenta previa NOS or without** CC Ⓜ♀
　　　　　　hemorrhage, first trimester
　　　O44.02 **Complete placenta previa NOS or without** CC Ⓜ♀
　　　　　　hemorrhage, second trimester
　　　O44.03 **Complete placenta previa NOS or without** CC Ⓜ♀
　　　　　　hemorrhage, third trimester

✓5ᵗʰ **O44.1** **Complete** placenta previa with hemorrhage
　　　EXCLUDES 1　labor and delivery complicated by hemorrhage from
　　　　　　　　　vasa previa (O69.4)
　　　O44.10 **Complete placenta previa with hemorrhage,** Ⓜ♀
　　　　　　unspecified trimester
　　　O44.11 **Complete placenta previa with hemorrhage,** MCC Ⓜ♀
　　　　　　first trimester
　　　O44.12 **Complete placenta previa with hemorrhage,** MCC Ⓜ♀
　　　　　　second trimester
　　　O44.13 **Complete placenta previa with hemorrhage,** MCC Ⓜ♀
　　　　　　third trimester

✓5ᵗʰ **O44.2** **Partial** placenta previa without hemorrhage
　　　Marginal placenta previa, NOS or without hemorrhage
　　　O44.20 **Partial placenta previa NOS or without** Ⓜ♀
　　　　　　hemorrhage, unspecified trimester
　　　O44.21 **Partial placenta previa NOS or without** CC Ⓜ♀
　　　　　　hemorrhage, first trimester
　　　O44.22 **Partial placenta previa NOS or without** CC Ⓜ♀
　　　　　　hemorrhage, second trimester
　　　O44.23 **Partial placenta previa NOS or without** CC Ⓜ♀
　　　　　　hemorrhage, third trimester

✓5ᵗʰ **O44.3** **Partial** placenta previa with hemorrhage
　　　Marginal placenta previa with hemorrhage
　　　O44.30 **Partial placenta previa with hemorrhage,** Ⓜ♀
　　　　　　unspecified trimester
　　　O44.31 **Partial placenta previa with hemorrhage,** MCC Ⓜ♀
　　　　　　first trimester
　　　O44.32 **Partial placenta previa with hemorrhage,** MCC Ⓜ♀
　　　　　　second trimester
　　　O44.33 **Partial placenta previa with hemorrhage,** MCC Ⓜ♀
　　　　　　third trimester

✓5ᵗʰ **O44.4** **Low lying** placenta NOS or without hemorrhage
　　　Low implantation of placenta NOS or without hemorrhage
　　　O44.40 **Low lying placenta NOS or without** Ⓜ♀
　　　　　　hemorrhage, unspecified trimester
　　　O44.41 **Low lying placenta NOS or without** CC Ⓜ♀
　　　　　　hemorrhage, first trimester
　　　O44.42 **Low lying placenta NOS or without** CC Ⓜ♀
　　　　　　hemorrhage, second trimester
　　　O44.43 **Low lying placenta NOS or without** CC Ⓜ♀
　　　　　　hemorrhage, third trimester

✓5ᵗʰ **O44.5** **Low lying** placenta with hemorrhage
　　　Low implantation of placenta with hemorrhage
　　　O44.50 **Low lying placenta with hemorrhage,** Ⓜ♀
　　　　　　unspecified trimester
　　　O44.51 **Low lying placenta with hemorrhage,** first MCC Ⓜ♀
　　　　　　trimester
　　　O44.52 **Low lying placenta with hemorrhage,** MCC Ⓜ♀
　　　　　　second trimester
　　　O44.53 **Low lying placenta with hemorrhage,** third MCC Ⓜ♀
　　　　　　trimester

✓4ᵗʰ **O45** **Premature separation of placenta [abruptio placentae]**
✓5ᵗʰ **O45.0** **Premature separation of placenta with** coagulation defect

　　　CC Excl: For MCC codes in subcategory O45.0:
　　　PDX collection 985

✓6ᵗʰ **O45.00** **Premature separation of placenta with coagulation**
　　　defect, unspecified
　　　O45.001 **Premature separation of placenta** MCC Ⓜ♀
　　　　　　　with coagulation defect,
　　　　　　　unspecified, first trimester
　　　O45.002 **Premature separation of placenta** MCC Ⓜ♀
　　　　　　　with coagulation defect,
　　　　　　　unspecified, second trimester
　　　O45.003 **Premature separation of placenta** MCC Ⓜ♀
　　　　　　　with coagulation defect,
　　　　　　　unspecified, third trimester
　　　O45.009 **Premature separation of placenta** Ⓜ♀
　　　　　　　with coagulation defect, unspecified,
　　　　　　　unspecified trimester

✓6ᵗʰ **O45.01 Premature separation of placenta** with afibrinogenemia
     Premature separation of placenta with hypofibrinogenemia

     O45.011 Premature separation of placenta with afibrinogenemia, first trimester MCC M♀

     O45.012 Premature separation of placenta with afibrinogenemia, second trimester MCC M♀

     O45.013 Premature separation of placenta with afibrinogenemia, third trimester MCC M♀

     O45.019 Premature separation of placenta with afibrinogenemia, unspecified trimester M♀

✓6ᵗʰ **O45.02 Premature separation of placenta with** disseminated intravascular coagulation

     O45.021 Premature separation of placenta with disseminated intravascular coagulation, first trimester MCC M♀

     O45.022 Premature separation of placenta with disseminated intravascular coagulation, second trimester MCC M♀

     O45.023 Premature separation of placenta with disseminated intravascular coagulation, third trimester MCC M♀

     O45.029 Premature separation of placenta with disseminated intravascular coagulation, unspecified trimester M♀

✓6ᵗʰ **O45.09 Premature separation of placenta with** other coagulation defect

     O45.091 Premature separation of placenta with other coagulation defect, first trimester MCC M♀

     O45.092 Premature separation of placenta with other coagulation defect, second trimester MCC M♀

     O45.093 Premature separation of placenta with other coagulation defect, third trimester MCC M♀

     O45.099 Premature separation of placenta with other coagulation defect, unspecified trimester M♀

✓5ᵗʰ **O45.8 Other premature separation** of placenta

     CC Excl: For MCC codes in subcategory O45.8: PDX collection 986

✓6ᵗʰ **O45.8X Other premature separation of placenta**

     O45.8X1 Other premature separation of placenta, first trimester MCC M♀

     O45.8X2 Other premature separation of placenta, second trimester MCC M♀

     O45.8X3 Other premature separation of placenta, third trimester MCC M♀

     O45.8X9 Other premature separation of placenta, unspecified trimester M♀

✓5ᵗʰ **O45.9 Premature separation of placenta,** unspecified
     Abruptio placentae NOS

     CC Excl: For MCC codes in subcategory O45.9: PDX collection 986

     O45.90 Premature separation of placenta, unspecified, unspecified trimester M♀

     O45.91 Premature separation of placenta, unspecified, first trimester MCC M♀

     O45.92 Premature separation of placenta, unspecified, second trimester MCC M♀

     O45.93 Premature separation of placenta, unspecified, third trimester MCC M♀

✓4ᵗʰ **O46 Antepartum hemorrhage, not elsewhere classified**
     EXCLUDES 1   *hemorrhage in early pregnancy (O20.-)*
           intrapartum hemorrhage NEC (O67.-)
           placenta previa (O44.-)
           premature separation of placenta [abruptio placentae] (O45.-)
     DEF: Uterine hemorrhage prior to delivery; not related to placenta previa or abruptio placentae.

✓5ᵗʰ **O46.0 Antepartum hemorrhage with** coagulation defect

     CC Excl: For MCC codes in subcategory O46.0: PDX collection 985

✓6ᵗʰ **O46.00 Antepartum hemorrhage with coagulation defect, unspecified**

     O46.001 Antepartum hemorrhage with coagulation defect, unspecified, first trimester MCC M♀

     O46.002 Antepartum hemorrhage with coagulation defect, unspecified, second trimester MCC M♀

     O46.003 Antepartum hemorrhage with coagulation defect, unspecified, third trimester MCC M♀

     O46.009 Antepartum hemorrhage with coagulation defect, unspecified, unspecified trimester M♀

✓6ᵗʰ **O46.01 Antepartum hemorrhage with** afibrinogenemia
     Antepartum hemorrhage with hypofibrinogenemia

     O46.011 Antepartum hemorrhage with afibrinogenemia, first trimester MCC M♀

     O46.012 Antepartum hemorrhage with afibrinogenemia, second trimester MCC M♀

     O46.013 Antepartum hemorrhage with afibrinogenemia, third trimester MCC M♀

     O46.019 Antepartum hemorrhage with afibrinogenemia, unspecified trimester M♀

✓6ᵗʰ **O46.02 Antepartum hemorrhage with** disseminated intravascular coagulation

     O46.021 Antepartum hemorrhage with disseminated intravascular coagulation, first trimester MCC M♀

     O46.022 Antepartum hemorrhage with disseminated intravascular coagulation, second trimester MCC M♀

     O46.023 Antepartum hemorrhage with disseminated intravascular coagulation, third trimester MCC M♀

     O46.029 Antepartum hemorrhage with disseminated intravascular coagulation, unspecified trimester M♀

✓6ᵗʰ **O46.09 Antepartum hemorrhage with** other coagulation defect

     O46.091 Antepartum hemorrhage with other coagulation defect, first trimester MCC M♀

     O46.092 Antepartum hemorrhage with other coagulation defect, second trimester MCC M♀

     O46.093 Antepartum hemorrhage with other coagulation defect, third trimester MCC M♀

     O46.099 Antepartum hemorrhage with other coagulation defect, unspecified trimester M♀

✓5ᵗʰ **O46.8 Other** antepartum hemorrhage

✓6ᵗʰ **O46.8X Other** antepartum hemorrhage

     O46.8X1 Other antepartum hemorrhage, first trimester M♀

     O46.8X2 Other antepartum hemorrhage, second trimester M♀

     O46.8X3 Other antepartum hemorrhage, third trimester M♀

     O46.8X9 Other antepartum hemorrhage, unspecified trimester M♀

✓5ᵗʰ **O46.9 Antepartum hemorrhage,** unspecified

     O46.90 Antepartum hemorrhage, unspecified, unspecified trimester M♀

     O46.91 Antepartum hemorrhage, unspecified, first trimester M♀

✓ Additional Character Req   ✓x7ᵗʰ Placeholder Alert   Unacceptable PDx   Manifestation   H1-H14 HAC   HCC CMS-HCC Condition   *EXCLUDES 1* Not Coded Here   *EXCLUDES 2* Not Included Here

O46.92   **Antepartum hemorrhage, unspecified, second trimester**   M♀

O46.93   **Antepartum hemorrhage, unspecified, third trimester**   M♀

✓4ᵗʰ O47   False labor
> INCLUDES   Braxton Hicks contractions
> threatened labor
> EXCLUDES 1   *preterm labor (O60.-)*

> CC Excl: For CC codes in catagory O47: PDX collection 987

✓5ᵗʰ O47.0   False labor before 37 completed weeks of gestation

O47.00   **False labor before 37 completed weeks of gestation, unspecified trimester**   M♀

O47.02   **False labor before 37 completed weeks of gestation, second trimester**   CC M♀

O47.03   **False labor before 37 completed weeks of gestation, third trimester**   CC M♀

O47.1   **False labor at or after 37 completed weeks of gestation**   CC M♀

O47.9   **False labor, unspecified**   M♀

✓4ᵗʰ O48   Late pregnancy

O48.0   **Post-term pregnancy**   M♀
> Pregnancy over 40 completed weeks to 42 completed weeks gestation

O48.1   **Prolonged pregnancy**   M♀
> Pregnancy which has advanced beyond 42 completed weeks gestation
> AHA: 2016, 1Q, 5

Complications of labor and delivery (O60-O77)

✓4ᵗʰ O60   Preterm labor
> INCLUDES   onset (spontaneous) of labor before 37 completed weeks of gestation
> EXCLUDES 1   *false labor (O47.0-)*
> *threatened labor NOS (O47.0-)*

> CC Excl: For CC/MCC codes in category O60: PDX collection 987

✓5ᵗʰ O60.0   Preterm labor without delivery

O60.00   **Preterm labor without delivery, unspecified trimester**   M♀

O60.02   **Preterm labor without delivery, second trimester**   MCC M♀

O60.03   **Preterm labor without delivery, third trimester**   MCC M♀

✓5ᵗʰ O60.1   Preterm labor with preterm delivery
> AHA: 2016, 2Q, 10

> One of the following 7th characters is to be assigned to each code under subcategory O60.1. 7th character 0 is for single gestations and multiple gestations where the fetus is unspecified. 7th characters 1 through 9 are for cases of multiple gestations to identify the fetus for which the code applies. The appropriate code from category O30, Multiple gestation, must also be assigned when assigning a code from subcategory O60.1 that has a 7th character of 1 through 9.
> | | | | |
> |---|---|---|---|
> | 0 | not applicable or unspecified | 3 | fetus 3 |
> | 1 | fetus 1 | 4 | fetus 4 |
> | 2 | fetus 2 | 5 | fetus 5 |
> | | | 9 | other fetus |

✓x7ᵗʰ O60.10   **Preterm labor with preterm delivery, unspecified trimester**   CC M♀
> Preterm labor with delivery NOS

✓x7ᵗʰ O60.12   **Preterm labor second trimester with preterm delivery second trimester**   MCC M♀

✓x7ᵗʰ O60.13   **Preterm labor second trimester with preterm delivery third trimester**   MCC M♀

✓x7ᵗʰ O60.14   **Preterm labor third trimester with preterm delivery third trimester**   MCC M♀

✓5ᵗʰ O60.2   Term delivery with preterm labor

> One of the following 7th characters is to be assigned to each code under subcategory O60.2. 7th character 0 is for single gestations and multiple gestations where the fetus is unspecified. 7th characters 1 through 9 are for cases of multiple gestations to identify the fetus for which the code applies. The appropriate code from category O30, Multiple gestation, must also be assigned when assigning a code from subcategory O60.2 that has a 7th character of 1 through 9.
> | | | | |
> |---|---|---|---|
> | 0 | not applicable or unspecified | 3 | fetus 3 |
> | | | 4 | fetus 4 |
> | 1 | fetus 1 | 5 | fetus 5 |
> | 2 | fetus 2 | 9 | other fetus |

✓x7ᵗʰ O60.20   **Term delivery with preterm labor, unspecified trimester**   CC M♀

✓x7ᵗʰ O60.22   **Term delivery with preterm labor, second trimester**   MCC M♀

✓x7ᵗʰ O60.23   **Term delivery with preterm labor, third trimester**   MCC M♀

✓4ᵗʰ O61   Failed induction of labor

O61.0   **Failed medical induction of labor**   M♀
> Failed induction (of labor) by oxytocin
> Failed induction (of labor) by prostaglandins

O61.1   **Failed instrumental induction of labor**   M♀
> Failed mechanical induction (of labor)
> Failed surgical induction (of labor)

O61.8   **Other failed induction of labor**   M♀

O61.9   **Failed induction of labor, unspecified**   M♀

✓4ᵗʰ O62   Abnormalities of forces of labor

O62.0   **Primary inadequate contractions**   M♀
> Failure of cervical dilatation
> Primary hypotonic uterine dysfunction
> Uterine inertia during latent phase of labor

O62.1   **Secondary uterine inertia**   M♀
> Arrested active phase of labor
> Secondary hypotonic uterine dysfunction

O62.2   **Other uterine inertia**   M♀
> Atony of uterus without hemorrhage
> Atony of uterus NOS
> Desultory labor
> Hypotonic uterine dysfunction NOS
> Irregular labor
> Poor contractions
> Slow slope active phase of labor
> Uterine inertia NOS
> EXCLUDES 1   *atony of uterus with hemorrhage (postpartum) (O72.1)*
> *postpartum atony of uterus without hemorrhage (O75.89)*

O62.3   **Precipitate labor**   M♀

O62.4   **Hypertonic, incoordinate, and prolonged uterine contractions**   M♀
> Cervical spasm
> Contraction ring dystocia
> Dyscoordinate labor
> Hour-glass contraction of uterus
> Hypertonic uterine dysfunction
> Incoordinate uterine action
> Tetanic contractions
> Uterine dystocia NOS
> Uterine spasm
> EXCLUDES 1   *dystocia (fetal) (maternal) NOS (O66.9)*

O62.8   **Other abnormalities of forces of labor**   M♀

O62.9   **Abnormality of forces of labor, unspecified**   M♀

✓4ᵗʰ O63   Long labor

O63.0   **Prolonged first stage (of labor)**   M♀

O63.1   **Prolonged second stage (of labor)**   M♀

O63.2   **Delayed delivery of second twin, triplet, etc.**   M♀

O63.9   **Long labor, unspecified**   CC M♀
> Prolonged labor NOS
> CC Excl: PDX collection 988

N Newborn: 0   P Pediatric: 0-17   M Maternity: 12-55   A Adult: 15-124   MCC Major CC Condition   PDxMCC PDx acts as own MCC   CC CC Condition   PDxCC PDx acts as own CC

866   ICD-10-CM 2018

Fetal Malposition

Breech

Shoulder
(arm prolapse)

Mother's
pelvis

Compound
(extremity
together
with head)

Face
(mentum)

Oblique

☑4ᵗʰ **O64 Obstructed labor due to malposition and malpresentation of fetus**

One of the following 7th characters is to be assigned to each code under category O64. 7th character Ø is for single gestations and multiple gestations where the fetus is unspecified. 7th characters 1 through 9 are for cases of multiple gestations to identify the fetus for which the code applies. The appropriate code from category O30, Multiple gestation, must also be assigned when assigning a code from category O64 that has a 7th character of 1 through 9.

Ø	not applicable or unspecified	3	fetus 3
		4	fetus 4
1	fetus 1	5	fetus 5
2	fetus 2	9	other fetus

√x7ᵗʰ **O64.Ø Obstructed labor due to incomplete rotation of fetal head**   Ⓜ♀
   Deep transverse arrest
   Obstructed labor due to persistent occipitoiliac (position)
   Obstructed labor due to persistent occipitoposterior (position)
   Obstructed labor due to persistent occipitosacral (position)
   Obstructed labor due to persistent occipitotransverse (position)

√x7ᵗʰ **O64.1 Obstructed labor due to breech presentation**   Ⓜ♀
   Obstructed labor due to buttocks presentation
   Obstructed labor due to complete breech presentation
   Obstructed labor due to frank breech presentation

√x7ᵗʰ **O64.2 Obstructed labor due to face presentation**   Ⓜ♀
   Obstructed labor due to chin presentation

√x7ᵗʰ **O64.3 Obstructed labor due to brow presentation**   Ⓜ♀

√x7ᵗʰ **O64.4 Obstructed labor due to shoulder presentation**   Ⓜ♀
   Prolapsed arm
   EXCLUDES 1 impacted shoulders (O66.Ø)
            shoulder dystocia (O66.Ø)

√x7ᵗʰ **O64.5 Obstructed labor due to compound presentation**   Ⓜ♀

√x7ᵗʰ **O64.8 Obstructed labor due to other malposition and malpresentation**   Ⓜ♀
   Obstructed labor due to footling presentation
   Obstructed labor due to incomplete breech presentation

√x7ᵗʰ **O64.9 Obstructed labor due to malposition and malpresentation, unspecified**   Ⓜ♀

☑4ᵗʰ **O65 Obstructed labor due to maternal pelvic abnormality**

O65.Ø Obstructed labor due to deformed pelvis   Ⓜ♀

O65.1 Obstructed labor due to generally contracted pelvis   Ⓜ♀

O65.2 Obstructed labor due to pelvic inlet contraction   Ⓜ♀

O65.3 Obstructed labor due to pelvic outlet and mid-cavity contraction   Ⓜ♀

O65.4 Obstructed labor due to fetopelvic disproportion, unspecified   Ⓜ♀
   EXCLUDES 1 dystocia due to abnormality of fetus (O66.2-O66.3)

O65.5 Obstructed labor due to abnormality of maternal pelvic organs   Ⓜ♀
   Obstructed labor due to conditions listed in O34-
   Use additional code to identify abnormality of pelvic organs (O34.-)

O65.8 Obstructed labor due to other maternal pelvic abnormalities   Ⓜ♀

O65.9 Obstructed labor due to maternal pelvic abnormality, unspecified   Ⓜ♀

☑4ᵗʰ **O66 Other obstructed labor**

O66.Ø Obstructed labor due to shoulder dystocia   Ⓜ♀
   Impacted shoulders
   DEF: Obstructed labor due to impacted fetal shoulders; emergency condition that may require cesarean section, forceps delivery, vacuum extraction, or simphysiotomy.

O66.1 Obstructed labor due to locked twins   Ⓜ♀

O66.2 Obstructed labor due to unusually large fetus   Ⓜ♀

O66.3 Obstructed labor due to other abnormalities of fetus   Ⓜ♀
   Dystocia due to fetal ascites
   Dystocia due to fetal hydrops
   Dystocia due to fetal meningomyelocele
   Dystocia due to fetal sacral teratoma
   Dystocia due to fetal tumor
   Dystocia due to hydrocephalic fetus
   Use additional code to identify cause of obstruction

☑5ᵗʰ **O66.4 Failed trial of labor**

O66.40 Failed trial of labor, unspecified   Ⓜ♀

O66.41 Failed attempted vaginal birth after previous cesarean delivery   Ⓜ♀
   Code first rupture of uterus, if applicable (O71.Ø-, O71.1)

O66.5 Attempted application of vacuum extractor and forceps   Ⓜ♀
   Attempted application of vacuum or forceps, with subsequent delivery by forceps or cesarean delivery

O66.6 Obstructed labor due to other multiple fetuses   Ⓜ♀

O66.8 Other specified obstructed labor   Ⓜ♀
   Use additional code to identify cause of obstruction

O66.9 Obstructed labor, unspecified   Ⓜ♀
   Dystocia NOS
   Fetal dystocia NOS
   Maternal dystocia NOS

☑4ᵗʰ **O67 Labor and delivery complicated by intrapartum hemorrhage, not elsewhere classified**
   EXCLUDES 1 antepartum hemorrhage NEC (O46.-)
            placenta previa (O44.-)
            premature separation of placenta [abruptio placentae] (O45.-)
   EXCLUDES 2 postpartum hemorrhage (O72.-)

O67.Ø Intrapartum hemorrhage with coagulation defect   ᴹᶜᶜ Ⓜ♀
   Intrapartum hemorrhage (excessive) associated with afibrinogenemia
   Intrapartum hemorrhage (excessive) associated with disseminated intravascular coagulation
   Intrapartum hemorrhage (excessive) associated with hyperfibrinolysis
   Intrapartum hemorrhage (excessive) associated with hypofibrinogenemia
   CC Excl: PDX collection 985

O67.8 Other intrapartum hemorrhage   Ⓜ♀
   Excessive intrapartum hemorrhage

O67.9 Intrapartum hemorrhage, unspecified   Ⓜ♀

O68 Labor and delivery complicated by abnormality of fetal acid-base balance   ᶜᶜ Ⓜ♀
   Fetal acidemia complicating labor and delivery
   Fetal acidosis complicating labor and delivery
   Fetal alkalosis complicating labor and delivery
   Fetal metabolic acidemia complicating labor and delivery
   EXCLUDES 1 fetal stress NOS (O77.9)
            labor and delivery complicated by electrocardiographic evidence of fetal stress (O77.8)
            labor and delivery complicated by ultrasonic evidence of fetal stress (O77.8)
   EXCLUDES 2 abnormality in fetal heart rate or rhythm (O76)
            labor and delivery complicated by meconium in amniotic fluid (O77.Ø)
   CC Excl: PDX collection 989

☑ Additional Character Req   √x7ᵗʰ Placeholder Alert   Unacceptable PDx   Manifestation   ᴴ¹-ᴴ¹⁴ HAC   ᴴᶜᶜ CMS-HCC Condition   *EXCLUDES 1* Not Coded Here   *EXCLUDES 2* Not Included Here

✓4th O69 Labor and delivery complicated by umbilical cord complications
AHA: 2016, 1Q, 5

> One of the following 7th characters is to be assigned to each code under category O69. 7th character Ø is for single gestations and multiple gestations where the fetus is unspecified. 7th characters 1 through 9 are for cases of multiple gestations to identify the fetus for which the code applies. The appropriate code from category O3Ø, Multiple gestation, must also be assigned when assigning a code from category O69 that has a 7th character of 1 through 9.
>
> | | | | |
> |---|---|---|---|
> | Ø | not applicable or unspecified | 3 | fetus 3 |
> | | | 4 | fetus 4 |
> | 1 | fetus 1 | 5 | fetus 5 |
> | 2 | fetus 2 | 9 | other fetus |

✓x7th O69.Ø Labor and delivery complicated by prolapse of cord M♀
    DEF: Abnormal presentation of fetus; marked by protruding umbilical cord during labor; can cause fetal death.

✓x7th O69.1 Labor and delivery complicated by cord around neck, with compression M♀
    EXCLUDES 1   labor and delivery complicated by cord around neck, without compression (O69.81)

✓x7th O69.2 Labor and delivery complicated by other cord entanglement, with compression M♀
    Labor and delivery complicated by compression of cord NOS
    Labor and delivery complicated by entanglement of cords of twins in monoamniotic sac
    Labor and delivery complicated by knot in cord
    EXCLUDES 1   labor and delivery complicated by other cord entanglement, without compression (O69.82)

✓x7th O69.3 Labor and delivery complicated by short cord M♀

✓x7th O69.4 Labor and delivery complicated by vasa previa M♀
    Labor and delivery complicated by hemorrhage from vasa previa

✓x7th O69.5 Labor and delivery complicated by vascular lesion of cord M♀
    Labor and delivery complicated by cord bruising
    Labor and delivery complicated by cord hematoma
    Labor and delivery complicated by thrombosis of umbilical vessels

✓5th O69.8 Labor and delivery complicated by other cord complications

✓x7th O69.81 Labor and delivery complicated by cord around neck, without compression M♀
    AHA: 2016, 1Q, 5

✓x7th O69.82 Labor and delivery complicated by other cord entanglement, without compression M♀

✓x7th O69.89 Labor and delivery complicated by other cord complications M♀

✓x7th O69.9 Labor and delivery complicated by cord complication, unspecified M♀

✓4th O7Ø Perineal laceration during delivery
    INCLUDES   episiotomy extended by laceration
    EXCLUDES 1   obstetric high vaginal laceration alone (O71.4)
    AHA: 2016, 2Q, 34; 2016, 1Q, 3-4, 5

O7Ø.Ø First degree perineal laceration during delivery M♀
    Perineal laceration, rupture or tear involving fourchette during delivery
    Perineal laceration, rupture or tear involving labia during delivery
    Perineal laceration, rupture or tear involving skin during delivery
    Perineal laceration, rupture or tear involving vagina during delivery
    Perineal laceration, rupture or tear involving vulva during delivery
    Slight perineal laceration, rupture or tear during delivery

O7Ø.1 Second degree perineal laceration during delivery M♀
    Perineal laceration, rupture or tear during delivery as in O7Ø.Ø, also involving pelvic floor
    Perineal laceration, rupture or tear during delivery as in O7Ø.Ø, also involving perineal muscles
    Perineal laceration, rupture or tear during delivery as in O7Ø.Ø, also involving vaginal muscles
    EXCLUDES 1   perineal laceration involving anal sphincter (O7Ø.2)

✓5th O7Ø.2 Third degree perineal laceration during delivery
    Perineal laceration, rupture or tear during delivery as in O7Ø.1, also involving anal sphincter
    Perineal laceration, rupture or tear during delivery as in O7Ø.1, also involving rectovaginal septum
    Perineal laceration, rupture or tear during delivery as in O7Ø.1, also involving sphincter NOS
    EXCLUDES 1   anal sphincter tear during delivery without third degree perineal laceration (O7Ø.4)
               perineal laceration involving anal or rectal mucosa (O7Ø.3)

    CC Excl: For CC codes in subcategory O7Ø.2: PDX collection 99Ø

O7Ø.2Ø Third degree perineal laceration during delivery, unspecified CC M♀

O7Ø.21 Third degree perineal laceration during delivery, IIIa CC M♀
    Third degree perineal laceration during delivery with less than 50% of external anal sphincter (EAS) thickness torn

O7Ø.22 Third degree perineal laceration during delivery, IIIb CC M♀
    Third degree perineal laceration during delivery with more than 50% external anal sphincter (EAS) thickness torn

O7Ø.23 Third degree perineal laceration during delivery, IIIc CC M♀
    Third degree perineal laceration during delivery with both external anal sphincter (EAS) and internal anal sphincter (IAS) torn

O7Ø.3 Fourth degree perineal laceration during delivery CC M♀
    Perineal laceration, rupture or tear during delivery as in O7Ø.2, also involving anal mucosa
    Perineal laceration, rupture or tear during delivery as in O7Ø.2, also involving rectal mucosa
    CC Excl: PDX collection 991

O7Ø.4 Anal sphincter tear complicating delivery, not associated with third degree laceration CC M♀
    EXCLUDES 1   anal sphincter tear with third degree perineal laceration (O7Ø.2)
    CC Excl: PDX collection 992

O7Ø.9 Perineal laceration during delivery, unspecified M♀

✓4th O71 Other obstetric trauma
    Obstetric damage from instruments

✓5th O71.Ø Rupture of uterus (spontaneous) before onset of labor
    EXCLUDES 1   disruption of (current) cesarean delivery wound (O9Ø.Ø)
               laceration of uterus, NEC (O71.81)

O71.ØØ Rupture of uterus before onset of labor, unspecified trimester M♀

O71.Ø2 Rupture of uterus before onset of labor, second trimester MCC M♀
    CC Excl: PDX collection 993

O71.Ø3 Rupture of uterus before onset of labor, third trimester MCC M♀
    CC Excl: PDX collection 993

O71.1 Rupture of uterus during labor MCC M♀
    Rupture of uterus not stated as occurring before onset of labor
    EXCLUDES 1   disruption of cesarean delivery wound (O9Ø.Ø)
               laceration of uterus, NEC (O71.81)
    CC Excl: PDX collection 993

O71.2 Postpartum inversion of uterus CC M♀
    CC Excl: PDX collection 994

O71.3 Obstetric laceration of cervix CC M♀
    Annular detachment of cervix
    CC Excl: PDX collection 995

O71.4 Obstetric high vaginal laceration alone CC M♀
    Laceration of vaginal wall without perineal laceration
    EXCLUDES 1   obstetric high vaginal laceration with perineal laceration (O7Ø.-)
    AHA: 2016, 1Q, 5
    CC Excl: PDX collection 996

O71.5 Other obstetric injury to pelvic organs CC M♀
    Obstetric injury to bladder
    Obstetric injury to urethra
    EXCLUDES 2   obstetric periurethral trauma (O71.82)
    AHA: 2014, 4Q, 18
    CC Excl: PDX collection 993

N Newborn: 0   P Pediatric: 0-17   M Maternity: 12-55   A Adult: 15-124   MCC Major CC Condition   PDxMCC PDx acts as own MCC   CC CC Condition   PDxCC PDx acts as own CC

868   ICD-10-CM 2018

O71.6 Obstetric damage to pelvic joints and ligaments `CC` `M♀`
Obstetric avulsion of inner symphyseal cartilage
Obstetric damage to coccyx
Obstetric traumatic separation of symphysis (pubis)
CC Excl: PDX collection 997

O71.7 Obstetric hematoma of pelvis `CC` `M♀`
Obstetric hematoma of perineum
Obstetric hematoma of vagina
Obstetric hematoma of vulva
CC Excl: PDX collection 998

✓5ᵗʰ **O71.8 Other specified obstetric trauma**

     O71.81 Laceration of uterus, not elsewhere classified `M♀`

     O71.82 Other specified trauma to perineum and vulva `M♀`
         Obstetric periurethral trauma
         AHA: 2016, 1Q, 4; 2014, 4Q, 18

     O71.89 Other specified obstetric trauma `M♀`

O71.9 Obstetric trauma, unspecified `M♀`

✓4ᵗʰ **O72 Postpartum hemorrhage**
     `INCLUDES` hemorrhage after delivery of fetus or infant

O72.0 Third-stage hemorrhage `CC` `M♀`
Hemorrhage associated with retained, trapped or adherent
     placenta
Retained placenta NOS
Code also type of adherent placenta (O43.2-)
CC Excl: PDX collection 999

O72.1 Other immediate postpartum hemorrhage `CC` `M♀`
Hemorrhage following delivery of placenta
Postpartum hemorrhage (atonic) NOS
Uterine atony with hemorrhage
     `EXCLUDES 1` uterine atony NOS (O62.2)
         uterine atony without hemorrhage (O62.2)
         postpartum atony of uterus without hemorrhage
         (O75.89)
AHA: 2016, 1Q, 4
CC Excl: PDX collection 1000

O72.2 Delayed and secondary postpartum hemorrhage `CC` `M♀`
Hemorrhage associated with retained portions of placenta or
     membranes after the first 24 hours following delivery of
     placenta
Retained products of conception NOS, following delivery
CC Excl: PDX collection 1001

O72.3 Postpartum coagulation defects `M♀`
Postpartum afibrinogenemia
Postpartum fibrinolysis

✓4ᵗʰ **O73 Retained placenta and membranes, without hemorrhage**
     `EXCLUDES 1` placenta accreta (O43.21-)
         placenta increta (O43.22-)
         placenta percreta (O43.23-)
DEF: Postpartum condition resulting from failure to expel placental
membrane tissues due to failed contractions of uterine wall.

O73.0 Retained placenta without hemorrhage `M♀`
Adherent placenta, without hemorrhage
Trapped placenta without hemorrhage

O73.1 Retained portions of placenta and membranes, without `M♀`
hemorrhage
Retained products of conception following delivery, without
     hemorrhage

✓4ᵗʰ **O74 Complications of anesthesia during labor and delivery**
     `INCLUDES` maternal complications arising from the administration of a
         general, regional or local anesthetic, analgesic or other
         sedation during labor and delivery
Use additional code, if applicable, to identify specific complication

O74.0 Aspiration pneumonitis due to anesthesia during labor `M♀`
and delivery
Inhalation of stomach contents or secretions NOS due to
     anesthesia during labor and delivery
Mendelson's syndrome due to anesthesia during labor and
     delivery

O74.1 Other pulmonary complications of anesthesia during `M♀`
labor and delivery

O74.2 Cardiac complications of anesthesia during labor and `M♀`
delivery

O74.3 Central nervous system complications of anesthesia `M♀`
during labor and delivery

O74.4 Toxic reaction to local anesthesia during labor and `M♀`
delivery

O74.5 Spinal and epidural anesthesia-induced headache `M♀`
during labor and delivery

O74.6 Other complications of spinal and epidural anesthesia `M♀`
during labor and delivery

O74.7 Failed or difficult intubation for anesthesia during `M♀`
labor and delivery

O74.8 Other complications of anesthesia during labor and `M♀`
delivery

O74.9 Complication of anesthesia during labor and delivery, `M♀`
unspecified

✓4ᵗʰ **O75 Other complications of labor and delivery, not elsewhere**
classified
     `EXCLUDES 2` puerperal (postpartum) infection (O86.-)
         puerperal (postpartum) sepsis (O85)

O75.0 Maternal distress during labor and delivery `M♀`

O75.1 Shock during or following labor and delivery `MCC` `M♀`
Obstetric shock following labor and delivery
CC Excl: PDX collection 1002

O75.2 Pyrexia during labor, not elsewhere classified `CC` `M♀`
CC Excl: PDX collection 1003

O75.3 Other infection during labor `MCC` `M♀`
Sepsis during labor
Use additional code (B95-B97), to identify infectious agent
CC Excl: PDX collection 1004

O75.4 Other complications of obstetric surgery and procedures `M♀`
Cardiac arrest following obstetric surgery or procedures
Cardiac failure following obstetric surgery or procedures
Cerebral anoxia following obstetric surgery or procedures
Pulmonary edema following obstetric surgery or procedures
Use additional code to identify specific complication
     `EXCLUDES 2` complications of anesthesia during labor and delivery
         (O74.-)
         disruption of obstetrical (surgical) wound (O90.0-
         O90.1)
         hematoma of obstetrical (surgical) wound (O90.2)
         infection of obstetrical (surgical) wound (O86.0)

O75.5 Delayed delivery after artificial rupture of membranes `M♀`

✓5ᵗʰ **O75.8 Other specified complications of labor and delivery**

     O75.81 Maternal exhaustion complicating labor `M♀`
         and delivery

     O75.82 Onset (spontaneous) of labor after 37 `M♀`
         completedweeks of gestation but before 39
         completed weeks gestation, with delivery by
         (planned) cesarean section
         Delivery by (planned) cesarean section occurring after
             37 completed weeks of gestation but before 39
             completed weeks gestation due to (spontaneous)
             onset of labor
         Code first to specify reason for planned cesarean
             section such as:
             cephalopelvic disproportion (normally formed
                fetus) (O33.9)
             previous cesarean delivery (O34.21)

     O75.89 Other specified complications of labor `M♀`
         and delivery

O75.9 Complication of labor and delivery, unspecified `M♀`

O76 Abnormality in fetal heart rate and rhythm complicating `M♀`
labor and delivery
Depressed fetal heart rate tones complicating labor and delivery
Fetal bradycardia complicating labor and delivery
Fetal heart rate abnormal variability complicating labor and delivery
Fetal heart rate decelerations complicating labor and delivery
Fetal heart rate irregularity complicating labor and delivery
Fetal tachycardia complicating labor and delivery
Non-reassuring fetal heart rate or rhythm complicating labor and
     delivery
     `EXCLUDES 1` fetal stress NOS (O77.9)
         labor and delivery complicated by electrocardiographic
         evidence of fetal stress (O77.8)
         labor and delivery complicated by ultrasonic evidence of fetal
         stress (O77.8)
     `EXCLUDES 2` fetal metabolic acidemia (O68)
         other fetal stress (O77.0-O77.1)
AHA: 2013, 4Q, 118

✓4ᵗʰ **O77 Other fetal stress complicating labor and delivery**

O77.0 Labor and delivery complicated by meconium `M♀`
in amniotic fluid
AHA: 2013, 4Q, 117-118

O77.1 Fetal stress in labor or delivery due to drug `M♀`
administration

✓ Additional Character Req   ✓x7ᵗʰ Placeholder Alert   Unacceptable PDx   Manifestation   `H1`-`H14` HAC   `HCC` CMS-HCC Condition   `EXCLUDES 1` Not Coded Here   `EXCLUDES 2` Not Included Here

ICD-10-CM 2018   869

O77.8 **Labor and delivery complicated by other evidence of fetal stress** M♀
Labor and delivery complicated by electrocardiographic evidence of fetal stress
Labor and delivery complicated by ultrasonic evidence of fetal stress
> EXCLUDES 1   *abnormality in fetal heart rate or rhythm (O76)*
> *abnormality in fetal acid-base balance (O68)*
> *fetal metabolic acidemia (O68)*

O77.9 **Labor and delivery complicated by fetal stress, unspecified** M♀
> EXCLUDES 1   *abnormality in fetal heart rate or rhythm (O76)*
> *abnormality in fetal acid-base balance (O68)*
> *fetal metabolic acidemia (O68)*

Encounter for delivery (O80-O82)

O80 **Encounter for full-term uncomplicated delivery** M♀
> NOTE   Delivery requiring minimal or no assistance, with or without episiotomy, without fetal manipulation [e.g., rotation version] or instrumentation [forceps] of a spontaneous, cephalic, vaginal, full-term, single, live-born infant. This code is for use as a single diagnosis code and is not to be used with any other code from chapter 15.
> Use additional code to indicate outcome of delivery (Z37.0)
> **AHA:** 2016, 4Q, 150; 2014, 2Q, 9

O82 **Encounter for cesarean delivery without indication** M♀
Use additional code to indicate outcome of delivery (Z37.0)

Complications predominantly related to the puerperium (O85-O92)

> EXCLUDES 2   *mental and behavioral disorders associated with the puerperium (F53)*
> *obstetrical tetanus (A34)*
> *puerperal osteomalacia (M83.0)*

O85 **Puerperal sepsis** MCC M♀
Postpartum sepsis
Puerperal peritonitis
Puerperal pyemia
Use additional code (B95-B97), to identify infectious agent
Use additional code (R65.2-) to identify severe sepsis, if applicable
> EXCLUDES 1   *fever of unknown origin following delivery (O86.4)*
> *genital tract infection following delivery (O86.1-)*
> *obstetric pyemic and septic embolism (O88.3-)*
> *puerperal septic thrombophlebitis (O86.81)*
> *urinary tract infection following delivery (O86.2-)*
> EXCLUDES 2   *sepsis during labor (O75.3)*
> **CC Excl:** PDX collection 1005

✓4ᵗʰ **O86** **Other puerperal infections**
Use additional code (B95-B97), to identify infectious agent
> EXCLUDES 2   *infection during labor (O75.3)*
> *obstetrical tetanus (A34)*

> **CC Excl: For CC codes in category O86, unless otherwise noted:** PDX collection 968

O86.0 **Infection of obstetric surgical wound** M♀
Infected cesarean delivery wound following delivery
Infected perineal repair following delivery

✓5ᵗʰ **O86.1** **Other infection of genital tract following delivery**
    O86.11 **Cervicitis following delivery** CC M♀
    O86.12 **Endometritis following delivery** CC M♀
       CC Excl: PDX collection 1005
    O86.13 **Vaginitis following delivery** CC M♀
    O86.19 **Other infection of genital tract following delivery** CC M♀

✓5ᵗʰ **O86.2** **Urinary tract infection following delivery**
    O86.20 **Urinary tract infection following delivery, unspecified** CC M♀
       Puerperal urinary tract infection NOS
    O86.21 **Infection of kidney following delivery** CC M♀
    O86.22 **Infection of bladder following delivery** CC M♀
       Infection of urethra following delivery
    O86.29 **Other urinary tract infection following delivery** CC M♀

O86.4 **Pyrexia of unknown origin following delivery** CC M♀
Puerperal infection NOS following delivery
Puerperal pyrexia NOS following delivery
> EXCLUDES 2   *pyrexia during labor (O75.2)*
> **DEF:** Fever of unknown origin experienced by the mother after childbirth.
> **CC Excl:** PDX collection 1006

✓5ᵗʰ **O86.8** **Other specified puerperal infections**
    O86.81 **Puerperal septic thrombophlebitis** MCC M♀
       CC Excl: PDX collection 1005
    O86.89 **Other specified puerperal infections** MCC M♀
       CC Excl: PDX collection 1005

✓4ᵗʰ **O87** **Venous complications and hemorrhoids in the puerperium**
> INCLUDES   venous complications in labor, delivery and the puerperium
> EXCLUDES 2   *obstetric embolism (O88.-)*
> *puerperal septic thrombophlebitis (O86.81)*
> *venous complications in pregnancy (O22.-)*

> **CC Excl: For CC/MCC codes in category O87:** PDX collection 967

O87.0 **Superficial thrombophlebitis in the puerperium** CC M♀
Puerperal phlebitis NOS
Puerperal thrombosis NOS

O87.1 **Deep phlebothrombosis in the puerperium** MCC M♀
Deep vein thrombosis, postpartum
Pelvic thrombophlebitis, postpartum
Use additional code to identify the deep vein thrombosis (I82.4-, I82.5-, I82.62-. I82.72-)
Use additional code, if applicable, for associated long-term (current) use of anticoagulants (Z79.01)

O87.2 **Hemorrhoids in the puerperium** CC M♀

O87.3 **Cerebral venous thrombosis in the puerperium** CC M♀
Cerebrovenous sinus thrombosis in the puerperium

O87.4 **Varicose veins of lower extremity in the puerperium** M♀

O87.8 **Other venous complications in the puerperium** CC M♀
Genital varices in the puerperium

O87.9 **Venous complication in the puerperium, unspecified** M♀
Puerperal phlebopathy NOS

✓4ᵗʰ **O88** **Obstetric embolism**
> EXCLUDES 1   *embolism complicating abortion NOS (O03.2)*
> *embolism complicating ectopic or molar pregnancy (O08.2)*
> *embolism complicating failed attempted abortion (O07.2)*
> *embolism complicating induced abortion (O04.7)*
> *embolism complicating spontaneous abortion (O03.2, O03.7)*

> **CC Excl: For CC/MCC codes in category O88:** PDX collection 1007

✓5ᵗʰ **O88.0** **Obstetric air embolism**
> **DEF:** Sudden blocking of pulmonary artery or right ventricle with air or nitrogen bubbles.

    ✓6ᵗʰ **O88.01** **Obstetric air embolism in pregnancy**
       O88.011 **Air embolism in pregnancy, first trimester** MCC M♀
       O88.012 **Air embolism in pregnancy, second trimester** MCC M♀
       O88.013 **Air embolism in pregnancy, third trimester** MCC M♀
       O88.019 **Air embolism in pregnancy, unspecified trimester** M♀
    O88.02 **Air embolism in childbirth** MCC M♀
    O88.03 **Air embolism in the puerperium** MCC M♀

✓5ᵗʰ **O88.1** **Amniotic fluid embolism**
Anaphylactoid syndrome in pregnancy

    ✓6ᵗʰ **O88.11** **Amniotic fluid embolism in pregnancy**
       O88.111 **Amniotic fluid embolism in pregnancy, first trimester** MCC M♀
       O88.112 **Amniotic fluid embolism in pregnancy, second trimester** MCC M♀
       O88.113 **Amniotic fluid embolism in pregnancy, third trimester** MCC M♀
       O88.119 **Amniotic fluid embolism in pregnancy, unspecified trimester** M♀
    O88.12 **Amniotic fluid embolism in childbirth** MCC M♀
    O88.13 **Amniotic fluid embolism in the puerperium** MCC M♀

✓5ᵗʰ **O88.2** **Obstetric thromboembolism**

    ✓6ᵗʰ **O88.21** **Thromboembolism in pregnancy**
       Obstetric (pulmonary) embolism NOS
       O88.211 **Thromboembolism in pregnancy, first trimester** MCC M♀
       O88.212 **Thromboembolism in pregnancy, second trimester** MCC M♀
       O88.213 **Thromboembolism in pregnancy, third trimester** MCC M♀
       O88.219 **Thromboembolism in pregnancy, unspecified trimester** M♀
    O88.22 **Thromboembolism in childbirth** MCC M♀

O88.23 Thromboembolism in the puerperium   MCC M♀
Puerperal (pulmonary) embolism NOS

✓5th **O88.3 Obstetric** pyemic and septic embolism

✓6th **O88.31 Pyemic and septic embolism in** pregnancy

O88.311 Pyemic and septic embolism in pregnancy, first trimester   MCC M♀

O88.312 Pyemic and septic embolism in pregnancy, second trimester   MCC M♀

O88.313 Pyemic and septic embolism in pregnancy, third trimester   MCC M♀

O88.319 Pyemic and septic embolism in pregnancy, unspecified trimester   CC M♀

O88.32 Pyemic and septic embolism in childbirth   MCC M♀

O88.33 Pyemic and septic embolism in the puerperium   MCC M♀

✓5th **O88.8 Other** obstetric embolism
Obstetric fat embolism

✓6th **O88.81 Other embolism in** pregnancy

O88.811 Other embolism in pregnancy, first trimester   MCC M♀

O88.812 Other embolism in pregnancy, second trimester   MCC M♀

O88.813 Other embolism in pregnancy, third trimester   MCC M♀

O88.819 Other embolism in pregnancy, unspecified trimester   M♀

O88.82 Other embolism in childbirth   MCC M♀

O88.83 Other embolism in the puerperium   MCC M♀

✓4th **O89 Complications of anesthesia during the puerperium**
INCLUDES maternal complications arising from the administration of a general, regional or local anesthetic, analgesic or other sedation during the puerperium
Use additional code, if applicable, to identify specific complication

✓5th **O89.0 Pulmonary complications of anesthesia during the puerperium**

O89.01 Aspiration pneumonitis due to anesthesia during the puerperium   M♀
Inhalation of stomach contents or secretions NOS due to anesthesia during the puerperium
Mendelson's syndrome due to anesthesia during the puerperium

O89.09 Other pulmonary complications of anesthesia during the puerperium   M♀

O89.1 Cardiac complications of anesthesia during the puerperium   M♀

O89.2 Central nervous system complications of anesthesia during the puerperium   M♀

O89.3 Toxic reaction to local anesthesia during the puerperium   M♀

O89.4 Spinal and epidural anesthesia-induced headache during the puerperium   M♀

O89.5 Other complications of spinal and epidural anesthesia during the puerperium   M♀

O89.6 Failed or difficult intubation for anesthesia during the puerperium   M♀

O89.8 Other complications of anesthesia during the puerperium   M♀

O89.9 Complication of anesthesia during the puerperium, unspecified   M♀

✓4th **O90 Complications of the puerperium, not elsewhere classified**

O90.0 Disruption of cesarean delivery wound   M♀
Dehiscence of cesarean delivery wound
EXCLUDES 1   rupture of uterus (spontaneous) before onset of labor (O71.0-)
rupture of uterus during labor (O71.1)

O90.1 Disruption of perineal obstetric wound   M♀
Disruption of wound of episiotomy
Disruption of wound of perineal laceration
Secondary perineal tear

O90.2 Hematoma of obstetric wound   M♀

O90.3 Peripartum cardiomyopathy   MCC M♀
Conditions in I42- arising during pregnancy and the puerperium
EXCLUDES 1   pre-existing heart disease complicating pregnancy and the puerperium (O99.4-)
DEF: Any structural or functional abnormality of the ventricular myocardium, noninflammatory disease of obscure or unknown etiology with onset during the postpartum period.
CC Excl: PDX collection 1008

O90.4 Postpartum acute kidney failure   MCC M♀
Hepatorenal syndrome following labor and delivery
CC Excl: PDX collection 1009

O90.5 Postpartum thyroiditis   M♀

O90.6 Postpartum mood disturbance   M♀
Postpartum blues
Postpartum dysphoria
Postpartum sadness
EXCLUDES 1   postpartum depression (F53)
puerperal psychosis (F53)

✓5th **O90.8 Other complications of the puerperium, not elsewhere classified**

O90.81 Anemia of the puerperium
Postpartum anemia NOS
EXCLUDES 1   pre-existing anemia complicating the puerperium (O99.03)

O90.89 Other complications of the puerperium, not elsewhere classified   M♀
Placental polyp

O90.9 Complication of the puerperium, unspecified   M♀

✓4th **O91 Infections of breast associated with pregnancy, the puerperium and lactation**
Use additional code to identify infection

✓5th **O91.0 Infection of nipple associated with pregnancy, the puerperium and lactation**

✓6th **O91.01 Infection of nipple associated with** pregnancy
Gestational abscess of nipple

O91.011 Infection of nipple associated with pregnancy, first trimester   M♀

O91.012 Infection of nipple associated with pregnancy, second trimester   M♀

O91.013 Infection of nipple associated with pregnancy, third trimester   M♀

O91.019 Infection of nipple associated with pregnancy, unspecified trimester   M♀

O91.02 Infection of nipple associated with the puerperium   M♀
Puerperal abscess of nipple

O91.03 Infection of nipple associated with lactation   M♀
Abscess of nipple associated with lactation

✓5th **O91.1 Abscess of breast associated with pregnancy, the puerperium and lactation**

✓6th **O91.11 Abscess of breast associated with** pregnancy
Gestational mammary abscess
Gestational purulent mastitis
Gestational subareolar abscess

O91.111 Abscess of breast associated with pregnancy, first trimester   M♀

O91.112 Abscess of breast associated with pregnancy, second trimester   M♀

O91.113 Abscess of breast associated with pregnancy, third trimester   M♀

O91.119 Abscess of breast associated with pregnancy, unspecified trimester   M♀

O91.12 Abscess of breast associated with the puerperium   M♀
Puerperal mammary abscess
Puerperal purulent mastitis
Puerperal subareolar abscess

O91.13 Abscess of breast associated with lactation   M♀
Mammary abscess associated with lactation
Purulent mastitis associated with lactation
Subareolar abscess associated with lactation

✓5th **O91.2 Nonpurulent mastitis associated with pregnancy, the puerperium and lactation**

✓6th **O91.21 Nonpurulent mastitis associated with** pregnancy
Gestational interstitial mastitis
Gestational lymphangitis of breast
Gestational mastitis NOS
Gestational parenchymatous mastitis

O91.211 Nonpurulent mastitis associated with pregnancy, first trimester   M♀

O91.212 Nonpurulent mastitis associated with pregnancy, second trimester   M♀

O91.213 Nonpurulent mastitis associated with pregnancy, third trimester   M♀

O91.219 Nonpurulent mastitis associated with pregnancy, unspecified trimester   M♀

✓ Additional Character Req   ✓x7th Placeholder Alert   Unacceptable PDx   Manifestation   H1-H14 HAC   HCC CMS-HCC Condition   EXCLUDES1 Not Coded Here   EXCLUDES2 Not Included Here

O91.22   **Nonpurulent mastitis associated with the puerperium**   M♀
- Puerperal interstitial mastitis
- Puerperal lymphangitis of breast
- Puerperal mastitis NOS
- Puerperal parenchymatous mastitis

O91.23   **Nonpurulent mastitis associated with lactation**   M♀
- Interstitial mastitis associated with lactation
- Lymphangitis of breast associated with lactation
- Mastitis NOS associated with lactation
- Parenchymatous mastitis associated with lactation

√4th **O92 Other disorders of breast and disorders of lactation associated with pregnancy and the puerperium**

√5th **O92.0 Retracted nipple associated with pregnancy, the puerperium, and lactation**

√6th **O92.01 Retracted nipple associated with pregnancy**

O92.011 **Retracted nipple associated with pregnancy, first trimester**   M♀

O92.012 **Retracted nipple associated with pregnancy, second trimester**   M♀

O92.013 **Retracted nipple associated with pregnancy, third trimester**   M♀

O92.019 **Retracted nipple associated with pregnancy, unspecified trimester**   M♀

O92.02 **Retracted nipple associated with the puerperium**   M♀

O92.03 **Retracted nipple associated with lactation**   M♀

√5th **O92.1 Cracked nipple associated with pregnancy, the puerperium, and lactation**
- Fissure of nipple, gestational or puerperal

√6th **O92.11 Cracked nipple associated with pregnancy**

O92.111 **Cracked nipple associated with pregnancy, first trimester**   M♀

O92.112 **Cracked nipple associated with pregnancy, second trimester**   M♀

O92.113 **Cracked nipple associated with pregnancy, third trimester**   M♀

O92.119 **Cracked nipple associated with pregnancy, unspecified trimester**   M♀

O92.12 **Cracked nipple associated with the puerperium**   M♀

O92.13 **Cracked nipple associated with lactation**   M♀

√5th **O92.2 Other and unspecified disorders of breast associated with pregnancy and the puerperium**

O92.20 **Unspecified disorder of breast associated with pregnancy and the puerperium**   M♀

O92.29 **Other disorders of breast associated with pregnancy and the puerperium**   M♀

O92.3 **Agalactia**   M♀
- Primary agalactia
  - EXCLUDES 1   *elective agalactia (O92.5)*
    secondary agalactia (O92.5)
    therapeutic agalactia (O92.5)
- **DEF:** Absence of milk secretion in a female after delivery.

O92.4 **Hypogalactia**   M♀

O92.5 **Suppressed lactation**   M♀
- Elective agalactia
- Secondary agalactia
- Therapeutic agalactia
  - EXCLUDES 1   *primary agalactia (O92.3)*

O92.6 **Galactorrhea**   M♀
- **DEF:** Excessive or persistent milk secretion by breast; may occur in absence of nursing.

√5th **O92.7 Other and unspecified disorders of lactation**

O92.70 **Unspecified disorders of lactation**   M♀

O92.79 **Other disorders of lactation**   M♀
- Puerperal galactocele

Other obstetric conditions, not elsewhere classified (O94-O9A)

O94 Sequelae of complication of pregnancy, childbirth, and the puerperium   M♀
- NOTE   This category is to be used to indicate conditions in O00-O77.-, O85-O94 and O98-O9A.- as the cause of late effects. The sequelae include conditions specified as such, or as late effects, which may occur at any time after the puerperium.
- Code first condition resulting from (sequela) of complication of pregnancy, childbirth, and the puerperium

√4th **O98 Maternal infectious and parasitic diseases classifiable elsewhere but complicating pregnancy, childbirth and the puerperium**
- INCLUDES   the listed conditions when complicating the pregnant state, when aggravated by the pregnancy, or as a reason for obstetric care
- Use additional code (Chapter 1), to identify specific infectious or parasitic disease
- EXCLUDES 2   *herpes gestationis (O26.4-)*
  infectious carrier state (O99.82-, O99.83-)
  obstetrical tetanus (A34)
  puerperal infection (O86.-)
  puerperal sepsis (O85)
  when the reason for maternal care is that the disease is known or suspected to have affected the fetus (O35-O36)

√5th **O98.0 Tuberculosis complicating pregnancy, childbirth and the puerperium**
- Conditions in A15-A19

> **CC Excl: For CC codes in subcategory O98.0:**
> PDX collection 1011

√6th **O98.01 Tuberculosis complicating pregnancy**

O98.011 **Tuberculosis complicating pregnancy, first trimester**   CC M♀

O98.012 **Tuberculosis complicating pregnancy, second trimester**   CC M♀

O98.013 **Tuberculosis complicating pregnancy, third trimester**   CC M♀

O98.019 **Tuberculosis complicating pregnancy, unspecified trimester**   M♀

O98.02 **Tuberculosis complicating childbirth**   CC M♀

O98.03 **Tuberculosis complicating the puerperium**   CC M♀

√5th **O98.1 Syphilis complicating pregnancy, childbirth and the puerperium**
- Conditions in A50-A53

> **CC Excl: For CC codes in subcategory O98.1:**
> PDX collection 1012

√6th **O98.11 Syphilis complicating pregnancy**

O98.111 **Syphilis complicating pregnancy, first trimester**   CC M♀

O98.112 **Syphilis complicating pregnancy, second trimester**   CC M♀

O98.113 **Syphilis complicating pregnancy, third trimester**   CC M♀

O98.119 **Syphilis complicating pregnancy, unspecified trimester**   M♀

O98.12 **Syphilis complicating childbirth**   CC M♀

O98.13 **Syphilis complicating the puerperium**   CC M♀

√5th **O98.2 Gonorrhea complicating pregnancy, childbirth and the puerperium**
- Conditions in A54-

> **CC Excl: For CC codes in subcategory O98.2:**
> PDX collection 1012

√6th **O98.21 Gonorrhea complicating pregnancy**

O98.211 **Gonorrhea complicating pregnancy, first trimester**   CC M♀

O98.212 **Gonorrhea complicating pregnancy, second trimester**   CC M♀

O98.213 **Gonorrhea complicating pregnancy, third trimester**   CC M♀

O98.219 **Gonorrhea complicating pregnancy, unspecified trimester**   M♀

O98.22 **Gonorrhea complicating childbirth**   CC M♀

O98.23 **Gonorrhea complicating the puerperium**   CC M♀

√5th **O98.3 Other infections with a predominantly sexual mode of transmission complicating pregnancy, childbirth and the puerperium**
- Conditions in A55-A64

> **CC Excl: For CC codes in subcategory O98.3:**
> PDX collection 1012

√6th **O98.31 Other infections with a predominantly sexual mode of transmission complicating pregnancy**

O98.311 **Other infections with a predominantly sexual mode of transmission complicating pregnancy, first trimester**   CC M♀

N Newborn: 0   P Pediatric: 0-17   M Maternity: 12-55   A Adult: 15-124   MCC Major CC Condition   PDxMCC PDx acts as own MCC   CC CC Condition   PDxCC PDx acts as own CC

872   ICD-10-CM 2018

O98.312 Other infections with a predominantly sexual mode of transmission complicating pregnancy, second trimester ᴄᴄ Ⓜ♀

O98.313 Other infections with a predominantly sexual mode of transmission complicating pregnancy, third trimester ᴄᴄ Ⓜ♀

O98.319 Other infections with a predominantly sexual mode of transmission complicating pregnancy, unspecified trimester Ⓜ♀

O98.32 Other infections with a predominantly sexual mode of transmission complicating childbirth ᴄᴄ Ⓜ♀

O98.33 Other infections with a predominantly sexual mode of transmission complicating the puerperium ᴄᴄ Ⓜ♀

✓5ᵗʰ **O98.4** Viral hepatitis complicating pregnancy, childbirth and the puerperium
Conditions in B15-B19

CC Excl: For CC codes in subcategory O98.4: PDX collection 1013

✓6ᵗʰ **O98.41** Viral hepatitis complicating pregnancy

O98.411 Viral hepatitis complicating pregnancy, first trimester ᴄᴄ Ⓜ♀

O98.412 Viral hepatitis complicating pregnancy, second trimester ᴄᴄ Ⓜ♀

O98.413 Viral hepatitis complicating pregnancy, third trimester ᴄᴄ Ⓜ♀

O98.419 Viral hepatitis complicating pregnancy, unspecified trimester Ⓜ♀

O98.42 Viral hepatitis complicating childbirth ᴄᴄ Ⓜ♀

O98.43 Viral hepatitis complicating the puerperium ᴄᴄ Ⓜ♀

✓5ᵗʰ **O98.5** Other viral diseases complicating pregnancy, childbirth and the puerperium
Conditions in A80-B09, B25-B34, R87.81-, R87.82-
ᴇxᴄʟᴜᴅᴇs 1 human immunodeficiency virus [HIV] disease complicating pregnancy, childbirth and the puerperium (O98.7-)

CC Excl: For CC codes in subcategory O98.5: PDX collection 1013

✓6ᵗʰ **O98.51** Other viral diseases complicating pregnancy

O98.511 Other viral diseases complicating pregnancy, first trimester ᴄᴄ Ⓜ♀

O98.512 Other viral diseases complicating pregnancy, second trimester ᴄᴄ Ⓜ♀

O98.513 Other viral diseases complicating pregnancy, third trimester ᴄᴄ Ⓜ♀

O98.519 Other viral diseases complicating pregnancy, unspecified trimester Ⓜ♀

O98.52 Other viral diseases complicating childbirth ᴄᴄ Ⓜ♀

O98.53 Other viral diseases complicating the puerperium ᴄᴄ Ⓜ♀

✓5ᵗʰ **O98.6** Protozoal diseases complicating pregnancy, childbirth and the puerperium
Conditions in B50-B64

CC Excl: For CC codes in subcategory O98.6, unless otherwise noted: PDX collection 1014

✓6ᵗʰ **O98.61** Protozoal diseases complicating pregnancy

O98.611 Protozoal diseases complicating pregnancy, first trimester ᴄᴄ Ⓜ♀

O98.612 Protozoal diseases complicating pregnancy, second trimester ᴄᴄ Ⓜ♀

O98.613 Protozoal diseases complicating pregnancy, third trimester ᴄᴄ Ⓜ♀

O98.619 Protozoal diseases complicating pregnancy, unspecified trimester Ⓜ♀

O98.62 Protozoal diseases complicating childbirth ᴄᴄ Ⓜ♀
CC Excl: PDX collection 1015

O98.63 Protozoal diseases complicating the puerperium ᴄᴄ Ⓜ♀
CC Excl: PDX collection 1015

✓5ᵗʰ **O98.7** Human immunodeficiency virus [HIV] disease complicating pregnancy, childbirth and the puerperium
Use additional code to identify the type of HIV disease:
acquired immune deficiency syndrome (AIDS) (B20)
asymptomatic HIV status (Z21)
HIV positive NOS (Z21)
symptomatic HIV disease (B20)

CC Excl: For CC codes in subcategory O98.7: PDX collection 1013

✓6ᵗʰ **O98.71** Human immunodeficiency virus [HIV] disease complicating pregnancy

O98.711 Human immunodeficiency virus [HIV] disease complicating pregnancy, first trimester ᴄᴄ Ⓜ♀

O98.712 Human immunodeficiency virus [HIV] disease complicating pregnancy, second trimester ᴄᴄ Ⓜ♀

O98.713 Human immunodeficiency virus [HIV] disease complicating pregnancy, third trimester ᴄᴄ Ⓜ♀

O98.719 Human immunodeficiency virus [HIV] disease complicating pregnancy, unspecified trimester Ⓜ♀

O98.72 Human immunodeficiency virus [HIV] disease complicating childbirth ᴄᴄ Ⓜ♀

O98.73 Human immunodeficiency virus [HIV] disease complicating the puerperium ᴄᴄ Ⓜ♀

✓5ᵗʰ **O98.8** Other maternal infectious and parasitic diseases complicating pregnancy, childbirth and the puerperium

CC Excl: For CC codes in subcategory O98.8: PDX collection 1013

✓6ᵗʰ **O98.81** Other maternal infectious and parasitic diseases complicating pregnancy

O98.811 Other maternal infectious and parasitic diseases complicating pregnancy, first trimester ᴄᴄ Ⓜ♀

O98.812 Other maternal infectious and parasitic diseases complicating pregnancy, second trimester ᴄᴄ Ⓜ♀

O98.813 Other maternal infectious and parasitic diseases complicating pregnancy, third trimester ᴄᴄ Ⓜ♀

O98.819 Other maternal infectious and parasitic diseases complicating pregnancy, unspecified trimester Ⓜ♀

O98.82 Other maternal infectious and parasitic diseases complicating childbirth ᴄᴄ Ⓜ♀

O98.83 Other maternal infectious and parasitic diseases complicating the puerperium ᴄᴄ Ⓜ♀

✓5ᵗʰ **O98.9** Unspecified maternal infectious and parasitic disease complicating pregnancy, childbirth and the puerperium

CC Excl: For CC codes in subcategory O98.9: PDX collection 1013

✓6ᵗʰ **O98.91** Unspecified maternal infectious and parasitic disease complicating pregnancy

O98.911 Unspecified maternal infectious and parasitic disease complicating pregnancy, first trimester ᴄᴄ Ⓜ♀

O98.912 Unspecified maternal infectious and parasitic disease complicating pregnancy, second trimester ᴄᴄ Ⓜ♀

O98.913 Unspecified maternal infectious and parasitic disease complicating pregnancy, third trimester ᴄᴄ Ⓜ♀

O98.919 Unspecified maternal infectious and parasitic disease complicating pregnancy, unspecified trimester Ⓜ♀

O98.92 Unspecified maternal infectious and parasitic disease complicating childbirth ᴄᴄ Ⓜ♀

O98.93 Unspecified maternal infectious and parasitic disease complicating the puerperium ᴄᴄ Ⓜ♀

☑4ᵗʰ **O99 Other maternal diseases classifiable elsewhere but complicating pregnancy, childbirth and the puerperium**
> INCLUDES conditions which complicate the pregnant state, are aggravated by the pregnancy or are a main reason for obstetric care
>
> Use additional code to identify specific condition
> EXCLUDES 2 *when the reason for maternal care is that the condition is known or suspected to have affected the fetus (O35-O36)*

☑5ᵗʰ **O99.0 Anemia complicating pregnancy, childbirth and the puerperium**
> Conditions in D50-D64
> EXCLUDES 1 *anemia arising in the puerperium (O90.81)*
> *postpartum anemia NOS (O90.81)*

☑6ᵗʰ **O99.01 Anemia complicating pregnancy**
> AHA: 2016, 1Q, 4

     O99.011 Anemia complicating pregnancy, first trimester Ⓜ♀

     O99.012 Anemia complicating pregnancy, second trimester Ⓜ♀

     O99.013 Anemia complicating pregnancy, third trimester Ⓜ♀

     O99.019 Anemia complicating pregnancy, unspecified trimester Ⓜ♀

   O99.02 Anemia complicating childbirth Ⓜ♀

   O99.03 Anemia complicating the puerperium Ⓜ♀
> EXCLUDES 1 *postpartum anemia not pre-existing prior to delivery (O90.81)*

☑5ᵗʰ **O99.1 Other diseases of the blood and blood-forming organs and certain disorders involving the immune mechanism complicating pregnancy, childbirth and the puerperium**
> Conditions in D65-D89
> EXCLUDES 1 ▶*hemorrhage with coagulation defects (O45.-, O46.0-, O67.0, O72.3)*◀
> EXCLUDES 2 *hemorrhage with coagulation defects (O45.-, O46.0-, O67.0, O72.3)*

> **CC Excl: For CC codes in subcategory O99.1, unless otherwise noted:** PDX collection 1016

☑6ᵗʰ **O99.11 Other diseases of the blood and blood-forming organs and certain disorders involving the immune mechanism complicating pregnancy**

     O99.111 Other diseases of the blood and blood-forming organs and certain disorders involving the immune mechanism complicating pregnancy, first trimester CC Ⓜ♀

     O99.112 Other diseases of the blood and blood-forming organs and certain disorders involving the immune mechanism complicating pregnancy, second trimester CC Ⓜ♀

     O99.113 Other diseases of the blood and blood-forming organs and certain disorders involving the immune mechanism complicating pregnancy, third trimester CC Ⓜ♀

     O99.119 Other diseases of the blood and blood-forming organs and certain disorders involving the immune mechanism complicating pregnancy, unspecified trimester CC Ⓜ♀
> **CC Excl:** PDX collection 1017

   O99.12 Other diseases of the blood and blood-forming organs and certain disorders involving the immune mechanism complicating childbirth CC Ⓜ♀

   O99.13 Other diseases of the blood and blood-forming organs and certain disorders involving the immune mechanism complicating the puerperium CC Ⓜ♀

☑5ᵗʰ **O99.2 Endocrine, nutritional and metabolic diseases complicating pregnancy, childbirth and the puerperium**
> Conditions in E00-E88
> EXCLUDES 2 *diabetes mellitus (O24.-)*
> *malnutrition (O25.-)*
> *postpartum thyroiditis (O90.5)*

☑6ᵗʰ **O99.21 Obesity complicating pregnancy, childbirth, and the puerperium**
> Use additional code to identify the type of obesity (E66.-)

     O99.210 Obesity complicating pregnancy, unspecified trimester Ⓜ♀

     O99.211 Obesity complicating pregnancy, first trimester Ⓜ♀

     O99.212 Obesity complicating pregnancy, second trimester Ⓜ♀

     O99.213 Obesity complicating pregnancy, third trimester Ⓜ♀

     O99.214 Obesity complicating childbirth Ⓜ♀

     O99.215 Obesity complicating the puerperium Ⓜ♀

☑6ᵗʰ **O99.28 Other endocrine, nutritional and metabolic diseases complicating pregnancy, childbirth and the puerperium**

     O99.280 Endocrine, nutritional and metabolic diseases complicating pregnancy, unspecified trimester Ⓜ♀

     O99.281 Endocrine, nutritional and metabolic diseases complicating pregnancy, first trimester Ⓜ♀

     O99.282 Endocrine, nutritional and metabolic diseases complicating pregnancy, second trimester Ⓜ♀

     O99.283 Endocrine, nutritional and metabolic diseases complicating pregnancy, third trimester Ⓜ♀

     O99.284 Endocrine, nutritional and metabolic diseases complicating childbirth Ⓜ♀

     O99.285 Endocrine, nutritional and metabolic diseases complicating the puerperium Ⓜ♀

☑5ᵗʰ **O99.3 Mental disorders and diseases of the nervous system complicating pregnancy, childbirth and the puerperium**

> **CC Excl: For CC codes in subcategory O99.3, unless otherwise noted:** PDX collection 1018

☑6ᵗʰ **O99.31 Alcohol use complicating pregnancy, childbirth, and the puerperium**
> Use additional code(s) from F10 to identify manifestations of the alcohol use

     O99.310 Alcohol use complicating pregnancy, unspecified trimester Ⓜ♀

     O99.311 Alcohol use complicating pregnancy, first trimester Ⓜ♀

     O99.312 Alcohol use complicating pregnancy, second trimester Ⓜ♀

     O99.313 Alcohol use complicating pregnancy, third trimester Ⓜ♀

     O99.314 Alcohol use complicating childbirth Ⓜ♀

     O99.315 Alcohol use complicating the puerperium Ⓜ♀

☑6ᵗʰ **O99.32 Drug use complicating pregnancy, childbirth, and the puerperium**
> Use additional code(s) from F11-F16 and F18-F19 to identify manifestations of the drug use

     O99.320 Drug use complicating pregnancy, unspecified trimester Ⓜ♀

     O99.321 Drug use complicating pregnancy, first trimester CC Ⓜ♀

     O99.322 Drug use complicating pregnancy, second trimester CC Ⓜ♀

     O99.323 Drug use complicating pregnancy, third trimester CC Ⓜ♀

     O99.324 Drug use complicating childbirth CC Ⓜ♀

     O99.325 Drug use complicating the puerperium CC Ⓜ♀

Ⓝ Newborn: 0   Ⓟ Pediatric: 0-17   Ⓜ Maternity: 12-55   Ⓐ Adult: 15-124   MCC Major CC Condition   PDxMCC PDx acts as own MCC   CC CC Condition   PDxCC PDx acts as own CC

874   ICD-10-CM 2018

✓6ᵗʰ O99.33 Tobacco use disorder complicating pregnancy, childbirth, and the puerperium

Smoking complicating pregnancy, childbirth, and the puerperium

Use additional code from category F17 to identify type of tobacco nicotine dependence

O99.330 Smoking (tobacco) complicating pregnancy, unspecified trimester Ⓜ♀

O99.331 Smoking (tobacco) complicating pregnancy, first trimester Ⓜ♀

O99.332 Smoking (tobacco) complicating pregnancy, second trimester Ⓜ♀

O99.333 Smoking (tobacco) complicating pregnancy, third trimester Ⓜ♀

O99.334 Smoking (tobacco) complicating childbirth Ⓜ♀

O99.335 Smoking (tobacco) complicating the puerperium Ⓜ♀

✓6ᵗʰ O99.34 Other mental disorders complicating pregnancy, childbirth, and the puerperium

Conditions in F01-F09 and F20-F99

> EXCLUDES 2 *postpartum mood disturbance (O90.6)*
> *postnatal psychosis (F53)*
> *puerperal psychosis (F53)*

O99.340 Other mental disorders complicating pregnancy, unspecified trimester Ⓜ♀

O99.341 Other mental disorders complicating pregnancy, first trimester Ⓜ♀

O99.342 Other mental disorders complicating pregnancy, second trimester Ⓜ♀

O99.343 Other mental disorders complicating pregnancy, third trimester Ⓜ♀

O99.344 Other mental disorders complicating childbirth Ⓜ♀

O99.345 Other mental disorders complicating the puerperium Ⓜ♀

✓6ᵗʰ O99.35 Diseases of the nervous system complicating pregnancy, childbirth, and the puerperium

Conditions in G00-G99

> EXCLUDES 2 *pregnancy related peripheral neuritis (O26.8-)*

O99.350 Diseases of the nervous system complicating pregnancy, unspecified trimester Ⓜ♀

O99.351 Diseases of the nervous system complicating pregnancy, first trimester Ⓜ♀

O99.352 Diseases of the nervous system complicating pregnancy, second trimester Ⓜ♀

O99.353 Diseases of the nervous system complicating pregnancy, third trimester Ⓜ♀

O99.354 Diseases of the nervous system complicating childbirth CC Ⓜ♀
CC Excl: PDX collection 1016

O99.355 Diseases of the nervous system complicating the puerperium CC Ⓜ♀
CC Excl: PDX collection 1016

✓5ᵗʰ O99.4 Diseases of the circulatory system complicating pregnancy, childbirth and the puerperium

Conditions in I00-I99

> EXCLUDES 1 *peripartum cardiomyopathy (O90.3)*
> EXCLUDES 2 *hypertensive disorders (O10-O16)*
> *obstetric embolism (O88.-)*
> *venous complications and cerebrovenous sinus thrombosis in labor, childbirth and the puerperium (O87.-)*
> *venous complications and cerebrovenous sinus thrombosis in pregnancy (O22.-)*

AHA: 2016, 2Q, 8

> CC Excl: For CC codes in subcategory O99.4, unless otherwise noted: PDX collection 1019

✓6ᵗʰ O99.41 Diseases of the circulatory system complicating pregnancy

O99.411 Diseases of the circulatory system complicating pregnancy, first trimester CC Ⓜ♀

O99.412 Diseases of the circulatory system complicating pregnancy, second trimester CC Ⓜ♀

O99.413 Diseases of the circulatory system complicating pregnancy, third trimester CC Ⓜ♀

O99.419 Diseases of the circulatory system complicating pregnancy, unspecified trimester Ⓜ♀

O99.42 Diseases of the circulatory system complicating childbirth MCC Ⓜ♀
CC Excl: PDX collection 1008

O99.43 Diseases of the circulatory system complicating the puerperium CC Ⓜ♀

✓5ᵗʰ O99.5 Diseases of the respiratory system complicating pregnancy, childbirth and the puerperium

Conditions in J00-J99

✓6ᵗʰ O99.51 Diseases of the respiratory system complicating pregnancy

O99.511 Diseases of the respiratory system complicating pregnancy, first trimester Ⓜ♀

O99.512 Diseases of the respiratory system complicating pregnancy, second trimester Ⓜ♀

O99.513 Diseases of the respiratory system complicating pregnancy, third trimester Ⓜ♀

O99.519 Diseases of the respiratory system complicating pregnancy, unspecified trimester Ⓜ♀

O99.52 Diseases of the respiratory system complicating childbirth Ⓜ♀

O99.53 Diseases of the respiratory system complicating the puerperium Ⓜ♀

✓5ᵗʰ O99.6 Diseases of the digestive system complicating pregnancy, childbirth and the puerperium

Conditions in K00-K93

> EXCLUDES 2 *hemorrhoids in pregnancy (O22.4-)*
> *liver and biliary tract disorders in pregnancy, childbirth and the puerperium (O26.6-)*

✓6ᵗʰ O99.61 Diseases of the digestive system complicating pregnancy
AHA: 2016, 1Q, 4

O99.611 Diseases of the digestive system complicating pregnancy, first trimester Ⓜ♀

O99.612 Diseases of the digestive system complicating pregnancy, second trimester Ⓜ♀

O99.613 Diseases of the digestive system complicating pregnancy, third trimester Ⓜ♀

O99.619 Diseases of the digestive system complicating pregnancy, unspecified trimester Ⓜ♀

O99.62 Diseases of the digestive system complicating childbirth Ⓜ♀

O99.63 Diseases of the digestive system complicating the puerperium Ⓜ♀

✓5ᵗʰ O99.7 Diseases of the skin and subcutaneous tissue complicating pregnancy, childbirth and the puerperium

Conditions in L00-L99

> EXCLUDES 2 *herpes gestationis (O26.4)*
> *pruritic urticarial papules and plaques of pregnancy (PUPPP) (O26.86)*

✓6ᵗʰ O99.71 Diseases of the skin and subcutaneous tissue complicating pregnancy

O99.711 Diseases of the skin and subcutaneous tissue complicating pregnancy, first trimester Ⓜ♀

O99.712 Diseases of the skin and subcutaneous tissue complicating pregnancy, second trimester Ⓜ♀

O99.713 Diseases of the skin and subcutaneous tissue complicating pregnancy, third trimester Ⓜ♀

O99.719 Diseases of the skin and subcutaneous tissue complicating pregnancy, unspecified trimester Ⓜ♀

O99.72 Diseases of the skin and subcutaneous tissue complicating childbirth Ⓜ♀

O99.73 Diseases of the skin and subcutaneous tissue complicating the puerperium Ⓜ♀

✓ Additional Character Req   ✓x7ᵗʰ Placeholder Alert   Unacceptable PDx   Manifestation   H1-H14 HAC   HCC CMS-HCC Condition   EXCLUDES 1 Not Coded Here   EXCLUDES 2 Not Included Here

Chapter 15. Pregnancy, Childbirth and the Puerperium

O99.8–O9A.43

✓5ᵗʰ **O99.8** **Other** specified diseases and conditions complicating pregnancy, childbirth and the puerperium
Conditions in D00-D48, H00-H95, M00-N99, and Q00-Q99
Use additional code to identify condition
EXCLUDES 2   *genitourinary infections in pregnancy (O23.-)*
infection of genitourinary tract following delivery (O86.1-O86.3)
malignant neoplasm complicating pregnancy, childbirth and the puerperium (O9A.1-)
maternal care for known or suspected abnormality of maternal pelvic organs (O34.-)
postpartum acute kidney failure (O90.4)
traumatic injuries in pregnancy (O9A.2)

CC Excl: For CC codes in subcategory O99.8:
PDX collection 1013

✓6ᵗʰ **O99.81** Abnormal glucose complicating pregnancy, childbirth and the puerperium
EXCLUDES 1   *gestational diabetes (O24.4-)*

     O99.810 Abnormal glucose complicating pregnancy   Ⓜ♀

     O99.814 Abnormal glucose complicating childbirth   Ⓜ♀

     O99.815 Abnormal glucose complicating the puerperium   Ⓜ♀

✓6ᵗʰ **O99.82** Streptococcus B carrier state complicating pregnancy, childbirth and the puerperium
EXCLUDES 1   *carrier of streptococcus group B (GBS) in a nonpregnant woman (Z22.330)*

     O99.820 Streptococcus B carrier state complicating pregnancy   Ⓜ♀

     O99.824 Streptococcus B carrier state complicating childbirth   Ⓜ♀

     O99.825 Streptococcus B carrier state complicating the puerperium   Ⓜ♀

✓6ᵗʰ **O99.83** Other infection carrier state complicating pregnancy, childbirth and the puerperium
Use additional code to identify the carrier state (Z22.-)

     O99.830 Other infection carrier state complicating pregnancy   CC Ⓜ♀

     O99.834 Other infection carrier state complicating childbirth   CC Ⓜ♀

     O99.835 Other infection carrier state complicating the puerperium   CC Ⓜ♀

✓6ᵗʰ **O99.84** Bariatric surgery status complicating pregnancy, childbirth and the puerperium
Gastric banding status complicating pregnancy, childbirth and the puerperium
Gastric bypass status for obesity complicating pregnancy, childbirth and the puerperium
Obesity surgery status complicating pregnancy, childbirth and the puerperium

     O99.840 Bariatric surgery status complicating pregnancy, unspecified trimester   Ⓜ♀

     O99.841 Bariatric surgery status complicating pregnancy, first trimester   Ⓜ♀

     O99.842 Bariatric surgery status complicating pregnancy, second trimester   Ⓜ♀

     O99.843 Bariatric surgery status complicating pregnancy, third trimester   Ⓜ♀

     O99.844 Bariatric surgery status complicating childbirth   Ⓜ♀

     O99.845 Bariatric surgery status complicating the puerperium   Ⓜ♀

   O99.89 Other specified diseases and conditions complicating pregnancy, childbirth and the puerperium   Ⓜ♀

✓4ᵗʰ **O9A** Maternal malignant neoplasms, traumatic injuries and abuse classifiable elsewhere but complicating pregnancy, childbirth and the puerperium

✓5ᵗʰ **O9A.1** Malignant neoplasm complicating pregnancy, childbirth and the puerperium
Conditions in C00-C96
Use additional code to identify neoplasm
EXCLUDES 2   *maternal care for benign tumor of corpus uteri (O34.1-)*
maternal care for benign tumor of cervix (O34.4-)
AHA: 2015, 3Q, 19

✓6ᵗʰ **O9A.11** Malignant neoplasm complicating pregnancy

     O9A.111 Malignant neoplasm complicating pregnancy, first trimester   Ⓜ♀

     O9A.112 Malignant neoplasm complicating pregnancy, second trimester   Ⓜ♀

     O9A.113 Malignant neoplasm complicating pregnancy, third trimester   Ⓜ♀

     O9A.119 Malignant neoplasm complicating pregnancy, unspecified trimester   Ⓜ♀

   O9A.12 Malignant neoplasm complicating childbirth   Ⓜ♀

   O9A.13 Malignant neoplasm complicating the puerperium   Ⓜ♀

✓5ᵗʰ **O9A.2** Injury, poisoning and certain other consequences of external causes complicating pregnancy, childbirth and the puerperium
Conditions in S00-T88, except T74 and T76
Use additional code(s) to identify the injury or poisoning
EXCLUDES 2   *physical, sexual and psychological abuse complicating pregnancy, childbirth and the puerperium (O9A.3-, O9A.4-, O9A.5-)*

✓6ᵗʰ **O9A.21** Injury, poisoning and certain other consequences of external causes complicating pregnancy

     O9A.211 Injury, poisoning and certain other consequences of external causes complicating pregnancy, first trimester   Ⓜ♀

     O9A.212 Injury, poisoning and certain other consequences of external causes complicating pregnancy, second trimester   Ⓜ♀

     O9A.213 Injury, poisoning and certain other consequences of external causes complicating pregnancy, third trimester   Ⓜ♀

     O9A.219 Injury, poisoning and certain other consequences of external causes complicating pregnancy, unspecified trimester   Ⓜ♀

   O9A.22 Injury, poisoning and certain other consequences of external causes complicating childbirth   Ⓜ♀

   O9A.23 Injury, poisoning and certain other consequences of external causes complicating the puerperium   Ⓜ♀

✓5ᵗʰ **O9A.3** Physical abuse complicating pregnancy, childbirth and the puerperium
Conditions in T74.11 or T76.11
Use additional code (if applicable):
   to identify any associated current injury due to physical abuse
   to identify the perpetrator of abuse (Y07.-)
EXCLUDES 2   *sexual abuse complicating pregnancy, childbirth and the puerperium (O9A.4)*

✓6ᵗʰ **O9A.31** Physical abuse complicating pregnancy

     O9A.311 Physical abuse complicating pregnancy, first trimester   Ⓜ♀

     O9A.312 Physical abuse complicating pregnancy, second trimester   Ⓜ♀

     O9A.313 Physical abuse complicating pregnancy, third trimester   Ⓜ♀

     O9A.319 Physical abuse complicating pregnancy, unspecified trimester   Ⓜ♀

   O9A.32 Physical abuse complicating childbirth   Ⓜ♀

   O9A.33 Physical abuse complicating the puerperium   Ⓜ♀

✓5ᵗʰ **O9A.4** Sexual abuse complicating pregnancy, childbirth and the puerperium
Conditions in T74.21 or T76.21
Use additional code (if applicable):
   to identify any associated current injury due to sexual abuse
   to identify the perpetrator of abuse (Y07.-)

✓6ᵗʰ **O9A.41** Sexual abuse complicating pregnancy

     O9A.411 Sexual abuse complicating pregnancy, first trimester   Ⓜ♀

     O9A.412 Sexual abuse complicating pregnancy, second trimester   Ⓜ♀

     O9A.413 Sexual abuse complicating pregnancy, third trimester   Ⓜ♀

     O9A.419 Sexual abuse complicating pregnancy, unspecified trimester   Ⓜ♀

   O9A.42 Sexual abuse complicating childbirth   Ⓜ♀

   O9A.43 Sexual abuse complicating the puerperium   Ⓜ♀

Ⓝ Newborn: 0   Ⓟ Pediatric: 0-17   Ⓜ Maternity: 12-55   Ⓐ Adult: 15-124   MCC Major CC Condition   PDxMCC PDx acts as own MCC   CC CC Condition   PDxCC PDx acts as own CC

876   ICD-10-CM 2018

√5ᵗʰ **O9A.5** Psychological abuse **complicating pregnancy, childbirth and the puerperium**
    Conditions in T74.31 or T76.31
    Use additional code to identify the perpetrator of abuse (Y07.-)

  √6ᵗʰ **O9A.51** **Psychological abuse complicating** pregnancy

      O9A.511 **Psychological abuse complicating pregnancy,** first trimester   M♀

      O9A.512 **Psychological abuse complicating pregnancy,** second trimester   M♀

      O9A.513 **Psychological abuse complicating pregnancy,** third trimester   M♀

      O9A.519 **Psychological abuse complicating pregnancy,** unspecified trimester   M♀

  O9A.52 **Psychological abuse complicating** childbirth   M♀

  O9A.53 **Psychological abuse complicating the** puerperium   M♀

☑ Additional Character Req   √x7ᵗʰ Placeholder Alert   Unacceptable PDx   Manifestation   **H1** - **H14** HAC   **HCC** CMS-HCC Condition   *EXCLUDES 1* Not Coded Here   *EXCLUDES 2* Not Included Here

ICD-10-CM 2018   **877**

Chapter 16. Certain Conditions Originating in the Perinatal Period (P00–P96)

Chapter Specific Guidelines with Coding Examples

The chapter specific guidelines from the ICD-10-CM Official Guidelines for Coding and Reporting have been provided below. Along with these guidelines are coding examples, contained in the shaded boxes, that have been developed to help illustrate the coding and/or sequencing guidance found in these guidelines.

For coding and reporting purposes the perinatal period is defined as before birth through the 28th day following birth. The following guidelines are provided for reporting purposes

a. General perinatal rules

1) Use of Chapter 16 codes

Codes in this chapter are <u>never</u> for use on the maternal record. Codes from Chapter 15, the obstetric chapter, are never permitted on the newborn record. Chapter 16 codes may be used throughout the life of the patient if the condition is still present.

2) Principal diagnosis for birth record

When coding the birth episode in a newborn record, assign a code from category Z38, Liveborn infants according to place of birth and type of delivery, as the principal diagnosis. A code from category Z38 is assigned only once, to a newborn at the time of birth. If a newborn is transferred to another institution, a code from category Z38 should not be used at the receiving hospital.

A code from category Z38 is used only on the newborn record, not on the mother's record.

> Newborn delivered via vaginal delivery in Rural Hospital A, experienced meconium aspiration resulting in pneumonia. Rural Hospital A is not equipped to handle the extensive respiratory therapy this baby needs and transfers the patient to Metropolis Hospital B, where the pneumonia resolves and the newborn is eventually discharged.
>
> *Rural Hospital A*
>
> **Z38.00**   **Single liveborn infant, delivered vaginally**
>
> **P24.01**   **Meconium aspiration with respiratory symptoms**
>
> *Metropolis Hospital B*
>
> **P24.01**   **Meconium aspiration with respiratory symptoms**
>
> *Explanation:* A code from category Z38 is a one-time use only code. The hospital that actually delivered the newborn, in this case Rural Hospital A, can append a code from category Z38 but for the delivery admission only. Once the patient is transferred or discharged, the Z38 category no longer applies for that patient.
>
> The reason for the transfer to Metropolis Hospital B was for the respiratory symptoms (pneumonia) the newborn was exhibiting secondary to aspirating meconium.

3) Use of codes from other chapters with codes from Chapter 16

Codes from other chapters may be used with codes from chapter 16 if the codes from the other chapters provide more specific detail. Codes for signs and symptoms may be assigned when a definitive diagnosis has not been established. If the reason for the encounter is a perinatal condition, the code from chapter 16 should be sequenced first.

4) Use of Chapter 16 codes after the perinatal period

Should a condition originate in the perinatal period, and continue throughout the life of the patient, the perinatal code should continue to be used regardless of the patient's age.

> A 7-year-old patient with history of birth injury that resulted in Erb's palsy is seen for subscapularis release
>
> **P14.0**   **Erb's paralysis due to birth injury**
>
> *Explanation:* Although in this instance Erb's palsy is specifically related to a birth injury, it has not resolved and continues to be a health concern. A perinatal code is appropriate even though this patient is beyond the perinatal period.

5) Birth process or community acquired conditions

If a newborn has a condition that may be either due to the birth process or community acquired and the documentation does not indicate which it is, the default is due to the birth process and the code from Chapter 16 should be used. If the condition is community-acquired, a code from Chapter 16 should not be assigned.

6) Code all clinically significant conditions

All clinically significant conditions noted on routine newborn examination should be coded. A condition is clinically significant if it requires:

clinical evaluation; or

therapeutic treatment; or

diagnostic procedures; or

extended length of hospital stay; or

increased nursing care and/or monitoring; or

has implications for future health care needs

Note: The perinatal guidelines listed above are the same as the general coding guidelines for "additional diagnoses", except for the final point regarding implications for future health care needs. Codes should be assigned for conditions that have been specified by the provider as having implications for future health care needs.

b. Observation and evaluation of newborns for suspected conditions not found

1) *Use of Z05 codes*

Assign a code from category Z05, Observation and evaluation of newborns and infants for suspected conditions ruled out, to identify those instances when a healthy newborn is evaluated for a suspected condition that is determined after study not to be present. Do not use a code from category Z05 when the patient has identified signs or symptoms of a suspected problem; in such cases code the sign or symptom.

2) *Z05 on Other than the birth record*

A code from category Z05 may also be assigned as a principal or first-listed code for readmissions or encounters when the code from category Z38 code no longer applies. Codes from category Z05 are for use only for healthy newborns and infants for which no condition after study is found to be present.

3) Z05 on a birth record

A code from category Z05 is to be used as a secondary code after the code from category Z38, Liveborn infants according to place of birth and type of delivery.

> Newborn delivered via vaginal delivery; previous ultrasounds showed what appeared to be an abnormality of the right kidney. Kidney function tests were performed and ultrasounds taken and any genitourinary conditions ruled out.
>
> **Z38.00**   **Single liveborn infant, delivered vaginally**
>
> **Z05.6**   **Observation and evaluation of newborn for suspected genitourinary condition ruled out**
>
> Explanation: The newborn had no signs or symptoms of kidney or other genitourinary condition but was evaluated after delivery due to the abnormal prenatal ultrasound findings. A Z code describing the type and place of birth should be coded first, followed by a Z05 category code for the work performed to rule out a suspected genitourinary condition.

c. Coding additional perinatal diagnoses

1) Assigning codes for conditions that require treatment

Assign codes for conditions that require treatment or further investigation, prolong the length of stay, or require resource utilization.

2) **Codes for conditions specified as having implications for future health care needs**

Assign codes for conditions that have been specified by the provider as having implications for future health care needs.

Note: This guideline should not be used for adult patients.

> An abnormal noise was heard in the left hip of a post-term newborn during a physical examination. The pediatrician would like to follow the patient after discharge as a hip click can be an early sign of hip dysplasia. The newborn was delivered via cesarean at 41 weeks.
>
> **Z38.01**   **Single liveborn infant, delivered by cesarean**
>
> **P08.21**   **Post-term newborn**
>
> **R29.4**   **Clicking hip**
>
> *Explanation:* The abnormal hip noise or click is appended as a secondary diagnosis not only because it is an abnormal finding upon examination, but also due to its potential to be part of a bigger health issue. The hip dysplasia has not yet been diagnosed and does not warrant a code at this time.

d. Prematurity and fetal growth retardation

Providers utilize different criteria in determining prematurity. A code for prematurity should not be assigned unless it is documented. Assignment of codes in categories P05, Disorders of newborn related to slow fetal growth and fetal malnutrition, and P07, Disorders of newborn related to short gestation and low birth weight, not elsewhere classified, should be based on the recorded birth weight and estimated gestational age.

When both birth weight and gestational age are available, two codes from category P07 should be assigned, with the code for birth weight sequenced before the code for gestational age.

e. Low birth weight and immaturity status

Codes from category P07, Disorders of newborn related to short gestation and low birth weight, not elsewhere classified, are for use for a child or adult who was premature or had a low birth weight as a newborn and this is affecting the patient's current health status.

See Section I.C.21. Factors influencing health status and contact with health services, Status.

> A 35-year-old patient, who weighed 659 grams at birth, is seen for heart disease documented as being a consequence of the low birth weight
>
> **I51.9**   **Heart disease, unspecified**
>
> **P07.02**   **Extremely low birth weight newborn, 500–749 grams**
>
> *Explanation:* A code from subcategories P07.0- and P07.1- is appropriate, regardless of the age of the patient, as long as the documentation provides a clear link between the patient's current illness and the low birth weight.

f. Bacterial sepsis of newborn

Category P36, Bacterial sepsis of newborn, includes congenital sepsis. If a perinate is documented as having sepsis without documentation of congenital or community acquired, the default is congenital and a code from category P36 should be assigned. If the P36 code includes the causal organism, an additional code from category B95, Streptococcus, Staphylococcus, and Enterococcus as the cause of diseases classified elsewhere, or B96, Other bacterial agents as the cause of diseases classified elsewhere, should not be assigned. If the P36 code does not include the causal organism, assign an additional code from category B96. If applicable, use additional codes to identify severe sepsis (R65.2-) and any associated acute organ dysfunction.

> A full-term infant develops severe sepsis 24 hours after discharge from the hospital and is readmitted; cultures identified *E. coli* as the infective agent
>
> **P36.4**   **Sepsis of newborn due to Escherichia coli**
>
> **R65.20**   **Severe sepsis without septic shock**
>
> *Explanation:* Even though this newborn was discharged and could have acquired *E. coli* from his/her external environment, due to the lack of documentation specifying specifically how this pathogen was acquired, the default is to code the *E. coli* sepsis as congenital. A code from chapter 1, "Certain Infectious and Parasitic Diseases," is not required because the perinatal sepsis code identifies both the sepsis and the bacteria causing the sepsis.

g. Stillbirth

Code P95, Stillbirth, is only for use in institutions that maintain separate records for stillbirths. No other code should be used with P95. Code P95 should not be used on the mother's record.

Chapter 16. Certain Conditions Originating in the Perinatal Period (P00-P96)

NOTE   Codes from this chapter are for use on newborn records only, never on maternal records.

INCLUDES   conditions that have their origin in the fetal or perinatal period (before birth through the first 28 days after birth) even if morbidity occurs later

EXCLUDES 2   *congenital malformations, deformations and chromosomal abnormalities (Q00-Q99)*
endocrine, nutritional and metabolic diseases (E00-E88)
injury, poisoning and certain other consequences of external causes (S00-T88)
neoplasms (C00-D49)
tetanus neonatorum (A33)

This chapter contains the following blocks:

P00-P04	Newborn affected by maternal factors and by complications of pregnancy, labor, and delivery
P05-P08	Disorders of newborn related to length of gestation and fetal growth
P09	Abnormal findings on neonatal screening
P10-P15	Birth trauma
P19-P29	Respiratory and cardiovascular disorders specific to the perinatal period
P35-P39	Infections specific to the perinatal period
P50-P61	Hemorrhagic and hematological disorders of newborn
P70-P74	Transitory endocrine and metabolic disorders specific to newborn
P76-P78	Digestive system disorders of newborn
P80-P83	Conditions involving the integument and temperature regulation of newborn
P84	Other problems with newborn
P90-P96	Other disorders originating in the perinatal period

Newborn affected by maternal factors and by complications of pregnancy, labor, and delivery (P00-P04)

NOTE   These codes are for use when the listed maternal conditions are specified as the cause of confirmed morbidity or potential morbidity which have their origin in the perinatal period (before birth through the first 28 days after birth).

✓4th P00   Newborn affected by maternal conditions that may be unrelated to present pregnancy
Code first any current condition in newborn
EXCLUDES 2   *encounter for observation of newborn for suspected diseases and conditions ruled out (Z05.-)*
newborn affected by maternal complications of pregnancy (P01.-)
newborn affected by maternal endocrine and metabolic disorders (P70-P74)
newborn affected by noxious substances transmitted via placenta or breast milk (P04.-)

P00.0   Newborn affected by maternal hypertensive disorders
Newborn affected by maternal conditions classifiable to O10-O11, O13-O16

P00.1   Newborn affected by maternal renal and urinary tract diseases
Newborn affected by maternal conditions classifiable to N00-N39

P00.2   Newborn affected by maternal infectious and parasitic diseases
Newborn affected by maternal infectious disease classifiable to A00-B99, J09 and J10
EXCLUDES 1   *infections specific to the perinatal period (P35-P39)*
maternal genital tract or other localized infections (P00.8)
EXCLUDES 2   ▶*infections specific to the perinatal period (P35-P39)*◀
AHA: 2015, 3Q, 20

P00.3   Newborn affected by other maternal circulatory and respiratory diseases
Newborn affected by maternal conditions classifiable to I00-I99, J00-J99, Q20-Q34 and not included in P00.0, P00.2

P00.4   Newborn affected by maternal nutritional disorders
Newborn affected by maternal disorders classifiable to E40-E64
Maternal malnutrition NOS

P00.5   Newborn affected by maternal injury
Newborn affected by maternal conditions classifiable to O9A.2-

P00.6   Newborn affected by surgical procedure on mother
Newborn affected by amniocentesis
EXCLUDES 1   *Cesarean delivery for present delivery (P03.4)*
damage to placenta from amniocentesis, Cesarean delivery or surgical induction (P02.1)
previous surgery to uterus or pelvic organs (P03.89)
EXCLUDES 2   *newborn affected by complication of (fetal) intrauterine procedure (P96.5)*

P00.7   Newborn affected by other medical procedures on mother, not elsewhere classified
Newborn affected by radiation to mother
EXCLUDES 1   *damage to placenta from amniocentesis, cesarean delivery or surgical induction (P02.1)*
newborn affected by other complications of labor and delivery (P03.-)

✓5th P00.8   Newborn affected by other maternal conditions
P00.81   Newborn affected by periodontal disease in mother
P00.89   Newborn affected by other maternal conditions
Newborn affected by conditions classifiable to T80-T88
Newborn affected by maternal genital tract or other localized infections
Newborn affected by maternal systemic lupus erythematosus

P00.9   Newborn affected by unspecified maternal condition

✓4th P01   Newborn affected by maternal complications of pregnancy
Code first any current condition in newborn
EXCLUDES 2   *encounter for observation of newborn for suspected diseases and conditions ruled out (Z05.-)*

P01.0   Newborn affected by incompetent cervix

P01.1   Newborn affected by premature rupture of membranes

P01.2   Newborn affected by oligohydramnios
EXCLUDES 1   *oligohydramnios due to premature rupture of membranes (P01.1)*
DEF: Low amniotic fluid level, resulting in underdeveloped organs in the fetus.

P01.3   Newborn affected by polyhydramnios
Newborn affected by hydramnios

P01.4   Newborn affected by ectopic pregnancy
Newborn affected by abdominal pregnancy

P01.5   Newborn affected by multiple pregnancy
Newborn affected by triplet (pregnancy)
Newborn affected by twin (pregnancy)

P01.6   Newborn affected by maternal death

P01.7   Newborn affected by malpresentation before labor
Newborn affected by breech presentation before labor
Newborn affected by external version before labor
Newborn affected by face presentation before labor
Newborn affected by transverse lie before labor
Newborn affected by unstable lie before labor

P01.8   Newborn affected by other maternal complications of pregnancy

P01.9   Newborn affected by maternal complication of pregnancy, unspecified

✓4th P02   Newborn affected by complications of placenta, cord and membranes
Code first any current condition in newborn
EXCLUDES 2   *encounter for observation of newborn for suspected diseases and conditions ruled out (Z05.-)*

P02.0   Newborn affected by placenta previa
DEF: Placenta developed in lower segment of uterus; can cause hemorrhaging leading to preterm delivery.

P02.1   Newborn affected by other forms of placental separation and hemorrhage
Newborn affected by abruptio placenta
Newborn affected by accidental hemorrhage
Newborn affected by antepartum hemorrhage
Newborn affected by damage to placenta from amniocentesis, cesarean delivery or surgical induction
Newborn affected by maternal blood loss
Newborn affected by premature separation of placenta

✓5th P02.2   Newborn affected by other and unspecified morphological and functional abnormalities of placenta
P02.20   Newborn affected by unspecified morphological and functional abnormalities of placenta

---

✓ Additional Character Req   ✓x7th Placeholder Alert   Unacceptable PDx   Manifestation   H1 - H14 HAC   HCC CMS-HCC Condition   EXCLUDES 1 Not Coded Here   EXCLUDES 2 Not Included Here

ICD-10-CM 2018   881

P02.29   **Newborn affected by other** morphological **and functional** abnormalities **of placenta**
Newborn affected by placental dysfunction
Newborn affected by placental infarction
Newborn affected by placental insufficiency

P02.3   **Newborn affected by** placental transfusion syndromes
Newborn affected by placental and cord abnormalities resulting in twin-to-twin or other transplacental transfusion

P02.4   **Newborn affected by** prolapsed cord

P02.5   **Newborn affected by** other compression **of umbilical cord**
Newborn affected by umbilical cord (tightly) around neck
Newborn affected by entanglement of umbilical cord
Newborn affected by knot in umbilical cord

✓5th **P02.6**   **Newborn affected by other and unspecified** conditions of **umbilical cord**

P02.60   **Newborn affected by** unspecified **conditions of umbilical cord**

P02.69   **Newborn affected by** other **conditions of umbilical cord**
Newborn affected by short umbilical cord
Newborn affected by vasa previa
EXCLUDES 1   *newborn affected by single umbilical artery (Q27.0)*

P02.7   **Newborn affected by** chorioamnionitis
Newborn affected by amnionitis
Newborn affected by membranitis
Newborn affected by placentitis
DEF: Inflammation of the fetal membranes due to maternal infection; characterized by fetal tachycardia, respiratory distress, apnea, weak cries, and poor sucking.

P02.8   **Newborn affected by** other abnormalities of membranes

P02.9   **Newborn affected by** abnormality of membranes, **unspecified**

✓4th **P03**   **Newborn affected by other complications of** labor and delivery
Code first any current condition in newborn
EXCLUDES 2   *encounter for observation of newborn for suspected diseases and conditions ruled out (Z05.-)*

P03.0   **Newborn affected by** breech delivery and extraction

P03.1   **Newborn affected by other** malpresentation, malposition **and disproportion during labor and delivery**
Newborn affected by contracted pelvis
Newborn affected by conditions classifiable to O64-O66
Newborn affected by persistent occipitoposterior
Newborn affected by transverse lie

P03.2   **Newborn affected by** forceps delivery

Forceps Assisted Birth

Forceps extractor

Vacuum Assisted Birth

Vacuum extractor

P03.3   **Newborn affected by delivery by** vacuum extractor [ventouse]

P03.4   **Newborn affected by** Cesarean delivery

P03.5   **Newborn affected by** precipitate delivery
Newborn affected by rapid second stage

P03.6   **Newborn affected by** abnormal uterine contractions
Newborn affected by conditions classifiable to O62.-, except O62.3
Newborn affected by hypertonic labor
Newborn affected by uterine inertia

✓5th **P03.8**   **Newborn affected by** other **specified complications of labor and delivery**

✓6th **P03.81**   **Newborn affected by** abnormality in fetal (intrauterine) heart rate or rhythm
EXCLUDES 1   *neonatal cardiac dysrhythmia (P29.1-)*

P03.810   **Newborn affected by abnormality in fetal (intrauterine) heart rate or rhythm** before the onset of labor

P03.811   **Newborn affected by abnormality in fetal (intrauterine) heart rate or rhythm** during labor

P03.819   **Newborn affected by abnormality in fetal (intrauterine) heart rate or rhythm,** unspecified as to time of onset

P03.82   Meconium passage **during delivery**
EXCLUDES 1   *meconium aspiration (P24.00, P24.01)*
meconium staining (P96.83)
DEF: Fetal intestinal activity that increases in response to a fetomaternal distressed state during delivery; the anal sphincter relaxes, and meconium is passed into the amniotic fluid.

P03.89   **Newborn affected by** other specified complications of labor and delivery
Newborn affected by abnormality of maternal soft tissues
Newborn affected by conditions classifiable to O60-O75 and by procedures used in labor and delivery not included in P02.- and P03.0-P03.6
Newborn affected by induction of labor

P03.9   **Newborn affected by** complication of labor and delivery, **unspecified**

✓4th **P04**   **Newborn affected by** noxious substances transmitted via placenta or breast milk
INCLUDES   nonteratogenic effects of substances transmitted via placenta
EXCLUDES 2   *congenital malformations (Q00-Q99)*
encounter for observation of newborn for suspected diseases and conditions ruled out (Z05.-)
neonatal jaundice from excessive hemolysis due to drugs or toxins transmitted from mother (P58.4)
newborn in contact with and (suspected) exposures hazardous to health not transmitted via placenta or breast milk (Z77.-)

P04.0   **Newborn affected by maternal** anesthesia and analgesia **in pregnancy, labor and delivery**
Newborn affected by reactions and intoxications from maternal opiates and tranquilizers administered during labor and delivery

P04.1   **Newborn affected by** other maternal medication
Newborn affected by cancer chemotherapy
Newborn affected by cytotoxic drugs
EXCLUDES 1   *dysmorphism due to warfarin (Q86.2)*
fetal hydantoin syndrome (Q86.1)
maternal use of drugs of addiction (P04.4-)

P04.2   **Newborn affected by maternal** use of tobacco
Newborn affected by exposure in utero to tobacco smoke
EXCLUDES 2   *newborn exposure to environmental tobacco smoke (P96.81)*

P04.3   **Newborn affected by maternal** use of alcohol
EXCLUDES 1   *fetal alcohol syndrome (Q86.0)*

✓5th **P04.4**   **Newborn affected by maternal use of** drugs of addiction

P04.41   **Newborn affected by maternal** use of cocaine
"Crack baby"

P04.49   **Newborn affected by maternal** use of other drugs of addiction
EXCLUDES 2   *newborn affected by maternal anesthesia and analgesia (P04.0)*
withdrawal symptoms from maternal use of drugs of addiction (P96.1)

P04.5   **Newborn affected by maternal use of** nutritional chemical substances

P04.6   Newborn affected by maternal exposure to environmental chemical substances

P04.8   Newborn affected by other maternal noxious substances

P04.9   Newborn affected by maternal noxious substance, unspecified

Disorders of newborn related to length of gestation and fetal growth (P05-P08)

✓4ᵗʰ **P05   Disorders of newborn related to slow fetal growth and fetal malnutrition**

✓5ᵗʰ   **P05.0   Newborn light for gestational age**
Newborn light-for-dates
Weight below but length above 10th percentile for gestational age

   P05.00   Newborn light for gestational age, unspecified weight

   P05.01   Newborn light for gestational age, less than 500 grams

   P05.02   Newborn light for gestational age, 500-749 grams

   P05.03   Newborn light for gestational age, 750-999 grams

   P05.04   Newborn light for gestational age, 1000-1249 grams

   P05.05   Newborn light for gestational age, 1250-1499 grams

   P05.06   Newborn light for gestational age, 1500-1749 grams

   P05.07   Newborn light for gestational age, 1750-1999 grams

   P05.08   Newborn light for gestational age, 2000-2499 grams

   P05.09   Newborn light for gestational age, 2500 grams and over
Newborn light for gestational age, other

✓5ᵗʰ   **P05.1   Newborn small for gestational age**
Newborn small-and-light-for-dates
Newborn small-for-dates
Weight and length below 10th percentile for gestational age

   P05.10   Newborn small for gestational age, unspecified weight

   P05.11   Newborn small for gestational age, less than 500 grams

   P05.12   Newborn small for gestational age, 500-749 grams

   P05.13   Newborn small for gestational age, 750-999 grams

   P05.14   Newborn small for gestational age, 1000-1249 grams

   P05.15   Newborn small for gestational age, 1250-1499 grams

   P05.16   Newborn small for gestational age, 1500-1749 grams

   P05.17   Newborn small for gestational age, 1750-1999 grams

   P05.18   Newborn small for gestational age, 2000-2499 grams

   P05.19   Newborn small for gestational age, other
Newborn small for gestational age, 2500 grams and over

   P05.2   Newborn affected by fetal (intrauterine) malnutrition not light or small for gestational age
Infant, not light or small for gestational age, showing signs of fetal malnutrition, such as dry, peeling skin and loss of subcutaneous tissue
   EXCLUDES 1   newborn affected by fetal malnutrition with light for gestational age (P05.0-)
   newborn affected by fetal malnutrition with small for gestational age (P05.1-)

   P05.9   Newborn affected by slow intrauterine growth, unspecified
Newborn affected by fetal growth retardation NOS

✓4ᵗʰ **P07   Disorders of newborn related to short gestation and low birth weight, not elsewhere classified**
   NOTE   When both birth weight and gestational age of the newborn are available, both should be coded with birth weight sequenced before gestational age
   INCLUDES   the listed conditions, without further specification, as the cause of morbidity or additional care, in newborn

✓5ᵗʰ   **P07.0   Extremely low birth weight newborn**
Newborn birth weight 999 g. or less
   EXCLUDES 1   low birth weight due to slow fetal growth and fetal malnutrition (P05.-)

   P07.00   Extremely low birth weight newborn, unspecified weight

   P07.01   Extremely low birth weight newborn, less than 500 grams

   P07.02   Extremely low birth weight newborn, 500-749 grams

   P07.03   Extremely low birth weight newborn, 750-999 grams

✓5ᵗʰ   **P07.1   Other low birth weight newborn**
Newborn birth weight 1000-2499 g.
   EXCLUDES 1   low birth weight due to slow fetal growth and fetal malnutrition (P05.-)

   P07.10   Other low birth weight newborn, unspecified weight

   P07.14   Other low birth weight newborn, 1000-1249 grams

   P07.15   Other low birth weight newborn, 1250-1499 grams

   P07.16   Other low birth weight newborn, 1500-1749 grams

   P07.17   Other low birth weight newborn, 1750-1999 grams

   P07.18   Other low birth weight newborn, 2000-2499 grams

✓5ᵗʰ   **P07.2   Extreme immaturity of newborn**
Less than 28 completed weeks (less than 196 completed days) of gestation.

   P07.20   Extreme immaturity of newborn, unspecified weeks of gestation
Gestational age less than 28 completed weeks NOS

   P07.21   Extreme immaturity of newborn, gestational age less than 23 completed weeks
Extreme immaturity of newborn, gestational age less than 23 weeks, 0 days

   P07.22   Extreme immaturity of newborn, gestational age 23 completed weeks
Extreme immaturity of newborn, gestational age 23 weeks, 0 days through 23 weeks, 6 days

   P07.23   Extreme immaturity of newborn, gestational age 24 completed weeks
Extreme immaturity of newborn, gestational age 24 weeks, 0 days through 24 weeks, 6 days

   P07.24   Extreme immaturity of newborn, gestational age 25 completed weeks
Extreme immaturity of newborn, gestational age 25 weeks, 0 days through 25 weeks, 6 days

   P07.25   Extreme immaturity of newborn, gestational age 26 completed weeks
Extreme immaturity of newborn, gestational age 26 weeks, 0 days through 26 weeks, 6 days

   P07.26   Extreme immaturity of newborn, gestational age 27 completed weeks
Extreme immaturity of newborn, gestational age 27 weeks, 0 days through 27 weeks, 6 days

✓5ᵗʰ   **P07.3   Preterm [premature] newborn [other]**
28 completed weeks or more but less than 37 completed weeks (196 completed days but less than 259 completed days) of gestation
Prematurity NOS

   P07.30   Preterm newborn, unspecified weeks of gestation

   P07.31   Preterm newborn, gestational age 28 completed weeks
Preterm newborn, gestational age 28 weeks, 0 days through 28 weeks, 6 days

   P07.32   Preterm newborn, gestational age 29 completed weeks
Preterm newborn, gestational age 29 weeks, 0 days through 29 weeks, 6 days

   P07.33   Preterm newborn, gestational age 30 completed weeks
Preterm newborn, gestational age 30 weeks, 0 days through 30 weeks, 6 days

   P07.34   Preterm newborn, gestational age 31 completed weeks
Preterm newborn, gestational age 31 weeks, 0 days through 31 weeks, 6 days

   P07.35   Preterm newborn, gestational age 32 completed weeks
Preterm newborn, gestational age 32 weeks, 0 days through 32 weeks, 6 days

   P07.36   Preterm newborn, gestational age 33 completed weeks
Preterm newborn, gestational age 33 weeks, 0 days through 33 weeks, 6 days

   P07.37   Preterm newborn, gestational age 34 completed weeks
Preterm newborn, gestational age 34 weeks, 0 days through 34 weeks, 6 days

---

✓ Additional Character Req   ✓x7ᵗʰ Placeholder Alert   Unacceptable PDx   Manifestation   **H1**-**H14** HAC   **HCC** CMS-HCC Condition   *EXCLUDES 1* Not Coded Here   *EXCLUDES 2* Not Included Here

Chapter 16. Certain Conditions Originating in the Perinatal Period

P07.38   **Preterm newborn, gestational age 35 completed weeks**
Preterm newborn, gestational age 35 weeks, 0 days through 35 weeks, 6 days

P07.39   **Preterm newborn, gestational age 36 completed weeks**
Preterm newborn, gestational age 36 weeks, 0 days through 36 weeks, 6 days

✓4ᵗʰ P08 **Disorders of newborn related to long gestation and high birth weight**
NOTE   When both birth weight and gestational age of the newborn are available, priority of assignment should be given to birth weight
INCLUDES   the listed conditions, without further specification, as causes of morbidity or additional care, in newborn

P08.0   **Exceptionally large newborn baby**
Usually implies a birth weight of 4500 g. or more
EXCLUDES 1   syndrome of infant of diabetic mother (P70.1)
syndrome of infant of mother with gestational diabetes (P70.0)

P08.1   **Other heavy for gestational age newborn**
Other newborn heavy- or large-for-dates regardless of period of gestation
Usually implies a birth weight of 4000 g. to 4499 g.
EXCLUDES 1   newborn with a birth weight of 4500 or more (P08.0)
syndrome of infant of diabetic mother (P70.1)
syndrome of infant of mother with gestational diabetes (P70.0).

✓5ᵗʰ P08.2   **Late newborn, not heavy for gestational age**
AHA: 2014, 1Q, 14

P08.21   **Post-term newborn**
Newborn with gestation period over 40 completed weeks to 42 completed weeks

P08.22   **Prolonged gestation of newborn**
Newborn with gestation period over 42 completed weeks (294 days or more), not heavy- or large-for-dates.
Postmaturity NOS

Abnormal findings on neonatal screening (P09)

P09   **Abnormal findings on neonatal screening**
Use additional code to identify signs, symptoms and conditions associated with the screening
EXCLUDES 2   nonspecific serologic evidence of human immunodeficiency virus [HIV] (R75)

Birth trauma (P10-P15)

✓4ᵗʰ P10 **Intracranial laceration and hemorrhage due to birth injury**
EXCLUDES 1   intracranial hemorrhage of newborn NOS (P52.9)
intracranial hemorrhage of newborn due to anoxia or hypoxia (P52.-)
nontraumatic intracranial hemorrhage of newborn (P52.-)

CC Excl: For MCC codes in category P10, unless otherwise noted: PDX collection 1020

P10.0   **Subdural hemorrhage due to birth injury**   MCC
Subdural hematoma (localized) due to birth injury
EXCLUDES 1   subdural hemorrhage accompanying tentorial tear (P10.4)

P10.1   **Cerebral hemorrhage due to birth injury**   MCC
P10.2   **Intraventricular hemorrhage due to birth injury**   CC
CC Excl: PDX collection 1021
P10.3   **Subarachnoid hemorrhage due to birth injury**   MCC
CC Excl: PDX collection 1022
P10.4   **Tentorial tear due to birth injury**   MCC
P10.8   **Other intracranial lacerations and hemorrhages due to birth injury**   MCC
P10.9   **Unspecified intracranial laceration and hemorrhage due to birth injury**   MCC

✓4ᵗʰ P11 **Other birth injuries to central nervous system**

CC Excl: For MCC codes in category P11, unless otherwise noted: PDX collection 1020

P11.0   **Cerebral edema due to birth injury**   MCC
P11.1   **Other specified brain damage due to birth injury**
P11.2   **Unspecified brain damage due to birth injury**   MCC
P11.3   **Birth injury to facial nerve**
Facial palsy due to birth injury

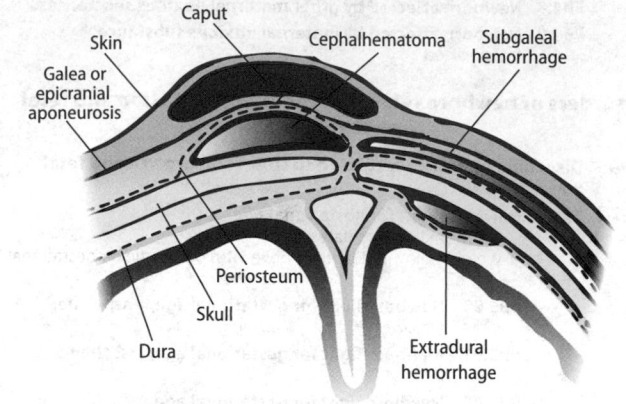
Birth Injuries to Scalp
Caput / Cephalhematoma / Subgaleal hemorrhage / Skin / Galea or epicranial aponeurosis / Periosteum / Skull / Dura / Extradural hemorrhage

P11.4   **Birth injury to other cranial nerves**
P11.5   **Birth injury to spine and spinal cord**
Fracture of spine due to birth injury
P11.9   **Birth injury to central nervous system, unspecified**   MCC

✓4ᵗʰ P12 **Birth injury to scalp**
P12.0   **Cephalhematoma due to birth injury**
P12.1   **Chignon (from vacuum extraction) due to birth injury**
P12.2   **Epicranial subaponeurotic hemorrhage due to birth injury**   CC
Subgaleal hemorrhage
CC Excl: PDX collection 1023
P12.3   **Bruising of scalp due to birth injury**
P12.4   **Injury of scalp of newborn due to monitoring equipment**
Sampling incision of scalp of newborn
Scalp clip (electrode) injury of newborn
✓5ᵗʰ P12.8   **Other birth injuries to scalp**
P12.81   **Caput succedaneum**
P12.89   **Other birth injuries to scalp**
P12.9   **Birth injury to scalp, unspecified**

✓4ᵗʰ P13 **Birth injury to skeleton**
EXCLUDES 2   birth injury to spine (P11.5)
P13.0   **Fracture of skull due to birth injury**
P13.1   **Other birth injuries to skull**
EXCLUDES 1   cephalhematoma (P12.0)
P13.2   **Birth injury to femur**
P13.3   **Birth injury to other long bones**
P13.4   **Fracture of clavicle due to birth injury**
P13.8   **Birth injuries to other parts of skeleton**
P13.9   **Birth injury to skeleton, unspecified**

✓4ᵗʰ P14 **Birth injury to peripheral nervous system**
P14.0   **Erb's paralysis due to birth injury**
P14.1   **Klumpke's paralysis due to birth injury**
P14.2   **Phrenic nerve paralysis due to birth injury**
P14.3   **Other brachial plexus birth injuries**
P14.8   **Birth injuries to other parts of peripheral nervous system**
P14.9   **Birth injury to peripheral nervous system, unspecified**

✓4ᵗʰ P15 **Other birth injuries**
P15.0   **Birth injury to liver**
Rupture of liver due to birth injury
P15.1   **Birth injury to spleen**
Rupture of spleen due to birth injury
P15.2   **Sternomastoid injury due to birth injury**
P15.3   **Birth injury to eye**
Subconjunctival hemorrhage due to birth injury
Traumatic glaucoma due to birth injury
P15.4   **Birth injury to face**
Facial congestion due to birth injury
P15.5   **Birth injury to external genitalia**
P15.6   **Subcutaneous fat necrosis due to birth injury**
P15.8   **Other specified birth injuries**
TIP: Use for any injury of newborn from scalpel.
P15.9   **Birth injury, unspecified**

N Newborn: 0   P Pediatric: 0-17   M Maternity: 12-55   A Adult: 15-124   MCC Major CC Condition   PDxMCC PDx acts as own MCC   CC CC Condition   PDxCC PDx acts as own CC

Respiratory and cardiovascular disorders specific to the perinatal period (P19-P29)

✓4ᵗʰ P19   Metabolic acidemia in newborn
   INCLUDES   metabolic acidemia in newborn

   P19.Ø   Metabolic acidemia in newborn first noted before onset of labor

   P19.1   Metabolic acidemia in newborn first noted during labor

   P19.2   Metabolic acidemia noted at birth

   P19.9   Metabolic acidemia, unspecified

✓4ᵗʰ P22   Respiratory distress of newborn
   EXCLUDES 1   *respiratory arrest of newborn (P28.81)*
        respiratory failure of newborn NOS (P28.5)

   P22.Ø   Respiratory distress syndrome of newborn   MCC
     Cardiorespiratory distress syndrome of newborn
     Hyaline membrane disease
     Idiopathic respiratory distress syndrome [IRDS or RDS] of newborn
     Pulmonary hypoperfusion syndrome
     Respiratory distress syndrome, type I
     DEF: Severe chest contractions upon air intake and expiratory grunting; infant appears blue due to oxygen deficiency and has rapid respiratory rate; formerly called hyaline membrane disease.
     CC Excl: PDX collection 748

   P22.1   Transient tachypnea of newborn
     Idiopathic tachypnea of newborn
     Respiratory distress syndrome, type II
     Wet lung syndrome
     DEF: Rapid, labored breathing of newborn; short-term problem that begins after birth and lasts about three days.

   P22.8   Other respiratory distress of newborn

   P22.9   Respiratory distress of newborn, unspecified

✓4ᵗʰ P23   Congenital pneumonia
   INCLUDES   infective pneumonia acquired in utero or during birth
   EXCLUDES 1   *neonatal pneumonia resulting from aspiration (P24.-)*

   CC Excl: For MCC codes in subcategory P23: PDX collection 748

   P23.Ø   Congenital pneumonia due to viral agent   MCC
     Use additional code (B97) to identify organism
     EXCLUDES 1   *congenital rubella pneumonitis (P35.Ø)*

   P23.1   Congenital pneumonia due to Chlamydia   MCC

   P23.2   Congenital pneumonia due to staphylococcus   MCC

   P23.3   Congenital pneumonia due to streptococcus, group B   MCC

   P23.4   Congenital pneumonia due to Escherichia coli   MCC

   P23.5   Congenital pneumonia due to Pseudomonas   MCC

   P23.6   Congenital pneumonia due to other bacterial agents   MCC
     Congenital pneumonia due to Hemophilus influenzae
     Congenital pneumonia due to Klebsiella pneumoniae
     Congenital pneumonia due to Mycoplasma
     Congenital pneumonia due to Streptococcus, except group B
     Use additional code (B95-B96) to identify organism

   P23.8   Congenital pneumonia due to other organisms   MCC

   P23.9   Congenital pneumonia, unspecified   MCC

✓4ᵗʰ P24   Neonatal aspiration
   INCLUDES   aspiration in utero and during delivery

   CC Excl: For MCC codes in category P24: PDX collection 748

   ✓5ᵗʰ P24.Ø   Meconium aspiration
     EXCLUDES 1   *meconium passage (without aspiration) during delivery (PØ3.82)*
        meconium staining (P96.83)

     P24.ØØ   Meconium aspiration without respiratory symptoms
       Meconium aspiration NOS

     P24.Ø1   Meconium aspiration with respiratory symptoms   MCC
       Meconium aspiration pneumonia
       Meconium aspiration pneumonitis
       Meconium aspiration syndrome NOS
       Use additional code to identify any secondary pulmonary hypertension, if applicable ▶(I27.2-)◀
       DEF: Aspiration of fetal intestinal material during or prior to delivery; usually a complication of placental insufficiency, causing pneumonitis and bronchial obstruction (inflammatory reaction of lungs).
       CC Excl: PDX collection 748

   ✓5ᵗʰ P24.1   Neonatal aspiration of (clear) amniotic fluid and mucus
     Neonatal aspiration of liquor (amnii)

     P24.1Ø   Neonatal aspiration of (clear) amniotic fluid and mucus without respiratory symptoms
       Neonatal aspiration of amniotic fluid and mucus NOS

     P24.11   Neonatal aspiration of (clear) amniotic fluid and mucus with respiratory symptoms   MCC
       Neonatal aspiration of amniotic fluid and mucus with pneumonia
       Neonatal aspiration of amniotic fluid and mucus with pneumonitis
       Use additional code to identify any secondary pulmonary hypertension, if applicable ▶(I27.2-)◀
       CC Excl: PDX collection 748

   ✓5ᵗʰ P24.2   Neonatal aspiration of blood

     P24.2Ø   Neonatal aspiration of blood without respiratory symptoms
       Neonatal aspiration of blood NOS

     P24.21   Neonatal aspiration of blood with respiratory symptoms   MCC
       Neonatal aspiration of blood with pneumonia
       Neonatal aspiration of blood with pneumonitis
       Use additional code to identify any secondary pulmonary hypertension, if applicable ▶(I27.2-)◀
       CC Excl: PDX collection 748

   ✓5ᵗʰ P24.3   Neonatal aspiration of milk and regurgitated food
     Neonatal aspiration of stomach contents

     P24.3Ø   Neonatal aspiration of milk and regurgitated food without respiratory symptoms
       Neonatal aspiration of milk and regurgitated food NOS

     P24.31   Neonatal aspiration of milk and regurgitated food with respiratory symptoms   MCC
       Neonatal aspiration of milk and regurgitated food with pneumonia
       Neonatal aspiration of milk and regurgitated food with pneumonitis
       Use additional code to identify any secondary pulmonary hypertension, if applicable ▶(I27.2-)◀
       CC Excl: PDX collection 748

   ✓5ᵗʰ P24.8   Other neonatal aspiration

     P24.8Ø   Other neonatal aspiration without respiratory symptoms
       Neonatal aspiration NEC

     P24.81   Other neonatal aspiration with respiratory symptoms   MCC
       Neonatal aspiration pneumonia NEC
       Neonatal aspiration with pneumonitis NEC
       Neonatal aspiration with pneumonia NOS
       Neonatal aspiration with pneumonitis NOS
       Use additional code to identify any secondary pulmonary hypertension, if applicable ▶(I27.2-)◀
       CC Excl: PDX collection 748

   P24.9   Neonatal aspiration, unspecified

✓4ᵗʰ P25   Interstitial emphysema and related conditions originating in the perinatal period

   CC Excl: For MCC codes in subcategory P25: PDX collection 748

   P25.Ø   Interstitial emphysema originating in the perinatal period   MCC

   P25.1   Pneumothorax originating in the perinatal period   MCC

   P25.2   Pneumomediastinum originating in the perinatal period   MCC

   P25.3   Pneumopericardium originating in the perinatal period   MCC

   P25.8   Other conditions related to interstitial emphysema originating in the perinatal period   MCC

✓4ᵗʰ P26   Pulmonary hemorrhage originating in the perinatal period
   EXCLUDES 1   *acute idiopathic hemorrhage in infants over 28 days old (RØ4.81)*

   CC Excl: For MCC codes in subcategory P26: PDX collection 748

   P26.Ø   Tracheobronchial hemorrhage originating in the perinatal period   MCC

   P26.1   Massive pulmonary hemorrhage originating in the perinatal period   MCC

   P26.8   Other pulmonary hemorrhages originating in the perinatal period   MCC

   P26.9   Unspecified pulmonary hemorrhage originating in the perinatal period   MCC

☑4ᵗʰ P27 Chronic respiratory disease originating in the perinatal period
- EXCLUDES 1 *respiratory distress of newborn (P22.0-P22.9)*
- EXCLUDES 2 ▶*respiratory distress of newborn (P22.0-P22.9)*◀

P27.0 Wilson-Mikity syndrome `MCC`
Pulmonary dysmaturity

P27.1 Bronchopulmonary dysplasia originating in the perinatal period `MCC`

P27.8 Other chronic respiratory diseases originating in the perinatal period `MCC`
Congenital pulmonary fibrosis   Ventilator lung in newborn

P27.9 Unspecified chronic respiratory disease originating in the perinatal period `MCC`

☑4ᵗʰ P28 Other respiratory conditions originating in the perinatal period
- EXCLUDES 1 *congenital malformations of the respiratory system (Q30-Q34)*

CC Excl: For CC/MCC codes in subcategory P28, unless otherwise noted: PDX collection 748

P28.0 Primary atelectasis of newborn `CC`
Primary failure to expand terminal respiratory units
Pulmonary hypoplasia associated with short gestation
Pulmonary immaturity NOS

☑5ᵗʰ P28.1 Other and unspecified atelectasis of newborn

P28.10 Unspecified atelectasis of newborn `CC`
Atelectasis of newborn NOS

P28.11 Resorption atelectasis without respiratory distress syndrome `CC`
- EXCLUDES 1 *resorption atelectasis with respiratory distress syndrome (P22.0)*

P28.19 Other atelectasis of newborn `CC`
Partial atelectasis of newborn
Secondary atelectasis of newborn

P28.2 Cyanotic attacks of newborn `CC`
- EXCLUDES 1 *apnea of newborn (P28.3-P28.4)*
CC Excl: PDX collection 1024

P28.3 Primary sleep apnea of newborn `CC`
Central sleep apnea of newborn
Obstructive sleep apnea of newborn
Sleep apnea of newborn NOS
DEF: Unexplained cessation of breathing when a neonate makes no respiratory effort for 20 seconds or longer, or when neonate's breathing cessation is accompanied by cyanosis, bradycardia, or hypotonia.
CC Excl: PDX collection 1025

P28.4 Other apnea of newborn `CC`
Apnea of prematurity
Obstructive apnea of newborn
- EXCLUDES 1 *obstructive sleep apnea of newborn (P28.3)*
CC Excl: PDX collection 1026

P28.5 Respiratory failure of newborn `MCC`
- EXCLUDES 1 *respiratory arrest of newborn (P28.81)*
respiratory distress of newborn (P22.0-)

☑5ᵗʰ P28.8 Other specified respiratory conditions of newborn

P28.81 Respiratory arrest of newborn `MCC`
CC Excl: PDX collection 1027

P28.89 Other specified respiratory conditions of newborn
Congenital laryngeal stridor
Sniffles in newborn
Snuffles in newborn
- EXCLUDES 1 *early congenital syphilitic rhinitis (A50.05)*

P28.9 Respiratory condition of newborn, unspecified
Respiratory depression in newborn

☑4ᵗʰ P29 Cardiovascular disorders originating in the perinatal period
- EXCLUDES 1 *congenital malformations of the circulatory system (Q20-Q28)*

P29.0 Neonatal cardiac failure

☑5ᵗʰ P29.1 Neonatal cardiac dysrhythmia

P29.11 Neonatal tachycardia

P29.12 Neonatal bradycardia

P29.2 Neonatal hypertension

☑5ᵗʰ P29.3 Persistent fetal circulation
~~Delayed closure of ductus arteriosus~~
~~(Persistent) pulmonary hypertension of newborn~~

CC Excl: For codes in subcategory P29.3: PDX collection 1028

● **P29.30 Pulmonary hypertension of newborn** `MCC`
Persistent pulmonary hypertension of newborn

● **P29.38 Other persistent fetal circulation** `MCC`
Delayed closure of ductus arteriosus

P29.4 Transient myocardial ischemia in newborn

☑5ᵗʰ P29.8 Other cardiovascular disorders originating in the perinatal period

P29.81 Cardiac arrest of newborn `MCC`
CC Excl: PDX collection 1029

P29.89 Other cardiovascular disorders originating in the perinatal period
AHA: 2014, 4Q, 23

P29.9 Cardiovascular disorder originating in the perinatal period, unspecified

Infections specific to the perinatal period (P35-P39)
Infections acquired in utero, during birth via the umbilicus, or during the first 28 days after birth
- EXCLUDES 2 *asymptomatic human immunodeficiency virus [HIV] infection status (Z21)*
congenital gonococcal infection (A54.-)
congenital pneumonia (P23.-)
congenital syphilis (A50.-)
human immunodeficiency virus [HIV] disease (B20)
infant botulism (A48.51)
infectious diseases not specific to the perinatal period (A00-B99, J09, J10-)
intestinal infectious disease (A00-A09)
laboratory evidence of human immunodeficiency virus [HIV] (R75)
tetanus neonatorum (A33)

☑4ᵗʰ P35 Congenital viral diseases
- INCLUDES infections acquired in utero or during birth

CC Excl: For MCC codes in category P35, unless otherwise noted: PDX collection 562

P35.0 Congenital rubella syndrome `CC`
Congenital rubella pneumonitis
CC Excl: PDX collection 1030

P35.1 Congenital cytomegalovirus infection `MCC`
CC Excl: PDX collection 1030

P35.2 Congenital herpesviral [herpes simplex] infection `MCC`

P35.3 Congenital viral hepatitis `MCC`

P35.8 Other congenital viral diseases `MCC`
Congenital varicella [chickenpox]

P35.9 Congenital viral disease, unspecified `MCC`

☑4ᵗʰ P36 Bacterial sepsis of newborn
- INCLUDES congenital sepsis
Use additional code(s), if applicable, to identify severe sepsis (R65.2-) and associated acute organ dysfunction(s)

CC Excl: For MCC codes in subcategory P36: PDX collection 1031

P36.0 Sepsis of newborn due to streptococcus, group B `MCC` `HCC`

☑5ᵗʰ P36.1 Sepsis of newborn due to other and unspecified streptococci

P36.10 Sepsis of newborn due to unspecified streptococci `MCC` `HCC`

P36.19 Sepsis of newborn due to other streptococci `MCC` `HCC`

P36.2 Sepsis of newborn due to Staphylococcus aureus `MCC` `HCC`

☑5ᵗʰ P36.3 Sepsis of newborn due to other and unspecified staphylococci

P36.30 Sepsis of newborn due to unspecified staphylococci `MCC` `HCC`

P36.39 Sepsis of newborn due to other staphylococci `MCC` `HCC`

P36.4 Sepsis of newborn due to Escherichia coli `MCC` `HCC`

P36.5 Sepsis of newborn due to anaerobes `MCC` `HCC`

P36.8 Other bacterial sepsis of newborn `MCC` `HCC`
Use additional code from category B96 to identify organism

P36.9 Bacterial sepsis of newborn, unspecified `MCC` `HCC`

☑4ᵗʰ P37 Other congenital infectious and parasitic diseases
- EXCLUDES 2 *congenital syphilis (A50.-)*
infectious neonatal diarrhea (A00-A09)
necrotizing enterocolitis in newborn (P77.-)
noninfectious neonatal diarrhea (P78.3)
ophthalmia neonatorum due to gonococcus (A54.31)
tetanus neonatorum (A33)

CC Excl: For MCC codes in subcategory P37: PDX collection 562

P37.0 Congenital tuberculosis `MCC`

P37.1 Congenital toxoplasmosis `MCC`
Hydrocephalus due to congenital toxoplasmosis

N Newborn: 0   P Pediatric: 0-17   M Maternity: 12-55   A Adult: 15-124   MCC Major CC Condition   PDxMCC PDx acts as own MCC   CC CC Condition   PDxCC PDx acts as own CC

886   ICD-10-CM 2018

P37.2	**Neonatal (disseminated) listeriosis**	MCC
P37.3	**Congenital** falciparum malaria	MCC
P37.4	**Other congenital** malaria	MCC
P37.5	**Neonatal** candidiasis	
P37.8	Other **specified congenital infectious and parasitic diseases**	MCC
P37.9	**Congenital infectious or parasitic disease,** unspecified	MCC

✓4ᵗʰ **P38 Omphalitis of newborn**
  EXCLUDES 1 omphalitis not of newborn (L08.82)
    tetanus omphalitis (A33)
    umbilical hemorrhage of newborn (P51.-)

P38.1	**Omphalitis with mild hemorrhage**	CC
	CC Excl: PDX collection 1032	
P38.9	**Omphalitis without hemorrhage**	CC
	Omphalitis of newborn NOS	
	CC Excl: PDX collection 1032	

✓4ᵗʰ **P39 Other infections specific to the perinatal period**
  Use additional code to identify organism or specific infection

  CC Excl: For CC codes in category P39, unless otherwise noted: PDX collection 1033

P39.0	**Neonatal infective** mastitis	CC
	EXCLUDES 1 breast engorgement of newborn (P83.4)	
	noninfective mastitis of newborn (P83.4)	
	CC Excl: PDX collection 1032	
P39.1	**Neonatal** conjunctivitis and dacryocystitis	
	Neonatal chlamydial conjunctivitis	
	Ophthalmia neonatorum NOS	
	EXCLUDES 1 gonococcal conjunctivitis (A54.31)	
P39.2	Intra-amniotic **infection affecting newborn, not elsewhere classified**	CC
P39.3	**Neonatal** urinary tract **infection**	CC
	CC Excl: PDX collection 1034	
P39.4	**Neonatal** skin **infection**	CC
	Neonatal pyoderma	
	EXCLUDES 1 pemphigus neonatorum (L00)	
	staphylococcal scalded skin syndrome (L00)	
P39.8	Other **specified infections specific to the perinatal period**	CC
P39.9	**Infection specific to the perinatal period,** unspecified	CC

Hemorrhagic and hematological disorders of newborn (P50-P61)

  EXCLUDES 1 congenital stenosis and stricture of bile ducts (Q44.3)
    Crigler-Najjar syndrome (E80.5)
    Dubin-Johnson syndrome (E80.6)
    Gilbert syndrome (E80.4)
    hereditary hemolytic anemias (D55-D58)

✓4ᵗʰ **P50 Newborn affected by intrauterine (fetal)** blood loss
  EXCLUDES 1 congenital anemia from intrauterine (fetal) blood loss (P61.3)

  P50.0 **Newborn affected by intrauterine (fetal) blood loss from** vasa previa
  P50.1 **Newborn affected by intrauterine (fetal) blood loss from** ruptured cord
  P50.2 **Newborn affected by intrauterine (fetal) blood loss from** placenta
  P50.3 **Newborn affected by hemorrhage into** co-twin
  P50.4 **Newborn affected by hemorrhage into** maternal circulation
  P50.5 **Newborn affected by intrauterine (fetal) blood loss from** cut end of co-twin's cord
  P50.8 **Newborn affected by** other **intrauterine (fetal) blood loss**
  P50.9 **Newborn affected by intrauterine (fetal) blood loss,** unspecified
    Newborn affected by fetal hemorrhage NOS

✓4ᵗʰ **P51 Umbilical hemorrhage of newborn**
  EXCLUDES 1 omphalitis with mild hemorrhage (P38.1)
    umbilical hemorrhage from cut end of co-twins cord (P50.5)

  P51.0 **Massive umbilical hemorrhage of newborn**
  P51.8 Other **umbilical hemorrhages of newborn**
    Slipped umbilical ligature NOS
  P51.9 **Umbilical hemorrhage of newborn,** unspecified

✓4ᵗʰ **P52 Intracranial nontraumatic hemorrhage of newborn** MCC
  INCLUDES intracranial hemorrhage due to anoxia or hypoxia
  EXCLUDES 1 intracranial hemorrhage due to birth injury (P10.-)
    intracranial hemorrhage due to other injury (S06.-)

P52.0	**Intraventricular (nontraumatic) hemorrhage, grade 1, of newborn**	CC
	Subependymal hemorrhage (without intraventricular extension)	
	Bleeding into germinal matrix	
	CC Excl: PDX collection 1021	
P52.1	**Intraventricular (nontraumatic) hemorrhage, grade 2, of newborn**	CC
	Subependymal hemorrhage with intraventricular extension	
	Bleeding into ventricle	
	CC Excl: PDX collection 1021	

✓5ᵗʰ P52.2 **Intraventricular (nontraumatic) hemorrhage, grade 3 and grade 4, of newborn**

P52.21	**Intraventricular (nontraumatic) hemorrhage, grade 3, of newborn**	MCC
	Subependymal hemorrhage with intraventricular extension with enlargement of ventricle	
	CC Excl: PDX collection 1021	
P52.22	**Intraventricular (nontraumatic) hemorrhage, grade 4, of newborn**	MCC
	Bleeding into cerebral cortex	
	Subependymal hemorrhage with intracerebral extension	
	CC Excl: PDX collection 1021	

P52.3	**Unspecified intraventricular (nontraumatic) hemorrhage of newborn**	CC
	CC Excl: PDX collection 1021	
P52.4	**Intracerebral (nontraumatic) hemorrhage of newborn**	MCC
	CC Excl: PDX collection 1020	
P52.5	**Subarachnoid (nontraumatic) hemorrhage of newborn**	MCC
	CC Excl: PDX collection 1022	
P52.6	**Cerebellar (nontraumatic) and posterior fossa hemorrhage of newborn**	MCC
	CC Excl: PDX collection 1020	
P52.8	**Other intracranial (nontraumatic) hemorrhages of newborn**	MCC
	CC Excl: PDX collection 1020	
P52.9	**Intracranial (nontraumatic) hemorrhage of newborn, unspecified**	MCC
	CC Excl: PDX collection 1020	

P53	**Hemorrhagic disease of newborn**	CC
	Vitamin K deficiency of newborn	
	CC Excl: PDX collection 1035	

✓4ᵗʰ **P54 Other neonatal hemorrhages**
  EXCLUDES 1 newborn affected by (intrauterine) blood loss (P50.-)
    pulmonary hemorrhage originating in the perinatal period (P26.-)

  CC Excl: For CC/MCC codes in category P54: PDX collection 1036

P54.0	**Neonatal hematemesis**	
	EXCLUDES 1 neonatal hematemesis due to swallowed maternal blood (P78.2)	
P54.1	**Neonatal melena**	MCC
	EXCLUDES 1 neonatal melena due to swallowed maternal blood (P78.2)	
P54.2	**Neonatal rectal hemorrhage**	MCC
P54.3	**Other neonatal gastrointestinal hemorrhage**	MCC
P54.4	**Neonatal adrenal hemorrhage**	CC
P54.5	**Neonatal cutaneous hemorrhage**	
	Neonatal bruising	
	Neonatal ecchymoses	
	Neonatal petechiae	
	Neonatal superficial hematomata	
	EXCLUDES 2 bruising of scalp due to birth injury (P12.3)	
	cephalhematoma due to birth injury (P12.0)	
P54.6	**Neonatal vaginal hemorrhage**	♀
	Neonatal pseudomenses	
P54.8	**Other specified neonatal hemorrhages**	
P54.9	**Neonatal hemorrhage, unspecified**	

✓ Additional Character Req ✓x7ᵗʰ Placeholder Alert Unacceptable PDx Manifestation H1 - H14 HAC HCC CMS-HCC Condition *EXCLUDES 1* Not Coded Here *EXCLUDES 2* Not Included Here

ICD-10-CM 2018   887

Chapter 16. Certain Conditions Originating in the Perinatal Period

P55–P71.8

✓4th **P55 Hemolytic disease of newborn**

    P55.0 Rh isoimmunization of newborn
        DEF: Incompatible Rh fetal-maternal blood grouping; prematurely destroys red blood cells; characterized by jaundice, asphyxia, pulmonary hypertension, edema, respiratory distress, kernicterus, and coagulopathies; detected by Coombs test.

    P55.1 ABO isoimmunization of newborn
        AHA: 2015, 3Q, 20

    P55.8 Other hemolytic diseases of newborn

    P55.9 Hemolytic disease of newborn, unspecified

✓4th **P56 Hydrops fetalis due to hemolytic disease**
    EXCLUDES 1 *hydrops fetalis NOS (P83.2)*

    CC Excl: For MCC codes in subcategory P56: PDX collection 1037

    P56.0 Hydrops fetalis due to isoimmunization   MCC

    ✓5th **P56.9 Hydrops fetalis due to other and unspecified hemolytic disease**

        P56.90 Hydrops fetalis due to unspecified hemolytic disease   MCC

        P56.99 Hydrops fetalis due to other hemolytic disease   MCC

✓4th **P57 Kernicterus**

    P57.0 Kernicterus due to isoimmunization   MCC
        DEF: Complication of erythroblastosis fetalis associated with severe neural symptoms, high blood bilirubin levels and nerve cell destruction; results in bilirubin-pigmented gray matter of central nervous system.
        CC Excl: PDX collection 1037

    P57.8 Other specified kernicterus   MCC
        EXCLUDES 1 *Crigler-Najjar syndrome (E80.5)*
        CC Excl: PDX collection 1038

    P57.9 Kernicterus, unspecified   MCC
        CC Excl: PDX collection 1038

✓4th **P58 Neonatal jaundice due to other excessive hemolysis**
    EXCLUDES 1 *jaundice due to isoimmunization (P55-P57)*

    P58.0 Neonatal jaundice due to bruising

    P58.1 Neonatal jaundice due to bleeding

    P58.2 Neonatal jaundice due to infection

    P58.3 Neonatal jaundice due to polycythemia

    ✓5th **P58.4 Neonatal jaundice due to drugs or toxins transmitted from mother or given to newborn**
        Code first poisoning due to drug or toxin, if applicable (T36-T65 with fifth or sixth character 1-4 or 6)
        Use additional code for adverse effect, if applicable, to identify drug (T36-T50 with fifth or sixth character 5)

        P58.41 Neonatal jaundice due to drugs or toxins transmitted from mother

        P58.42 Neonatal jaundice due to drugs or toxins given to newborn

    P58.5 Neonatal jaundice due to swallowed maternal blood

    P58.8 Neonatal jaundice due to other specified excessive hemolysis

    P58.9 Neonatal jaundice due to excessive hemolysis, unspecified

✓4th **P59 Neonatal jaundice from other and unspecified causes**
    EXCLUDES 1 *jaundice due to inborn errors of metabolism (E70-E88)*
        kernicterus (P57.-)

    CC Excl: For MCC codes in category P59: PDX collection 1038

    P59.0 Neonatal jaundice associated with preterm delivery
        Hyperbilirubinemia of prematurity
        Jaundice due to delayed conjugation associated with preterm delivery

    P59.1 Inspissated bile syndrome   MCC

    ✓5th **P59.2 Neonatal jaundice from other and unspecified hepatocellular damage**
        EXCLUDES 1 *congenital viral hepatitis (P35.3)*

        P59.20 Neonatal jaundice from unspecified hepatocellular damage   MCC

        P59.29 Neonatal jaundice from other hepatocellular damage   MCC
            Neonatal giant cell hepatitis
            Neonatal (idiopathic) hepatitis

    P59.3 Neonatal jaundice from breast milk inhibitor

    P59.8 Neonatal jaundice from other specified causes

    P59.9 Neonatal jaundice, unspecified
        Neonatal physiological jaundice (intense)(prolonged) NOS
        AHA: 2015, 3Q, 20

P60 Disseminated intravascular coagulation of newborn   MCC
    Defibrination syndrome of newborn
    CC Excl: PDX collection 1035

✓4th **P61 Other perinatal hematological disorders**
    EXCLUDES 1 *transient hypogammaglobulinemia of infancy (D80.7)*

    P61.0 Transient neonatal thrombocytopenia   MCC
        Neonatal thrombocytopenia due to exchange transfusion
        Neonatal thrombocytopenia due to idiopathic maternal thrombocytopenia
        Neonatal thrombocytopenia due to isoimmunization
        DEF: Temporary decrease in blood platelets of newborn; secondary to placental insufficiency.
        CC Excl: PDX collection 1035

    P61.1 Polycythemia neonatorum
        DEF: Abnormal increase of total red blood cells of newborn; results in hyperviscosity, which slows the flow of blood through small blood vessels.

    P61.2 Anemia of prematurity   CC
        CC Excl: PDX collection 1039

    P61.3 Congenital anemia from fetal blood loss   CC
        CC Excl: PDX collection 1039

    P61.4 Other congenital anemias, not elsewhere classified   CC
        Congenital anemia NOS
        CC Excl: PDX collection 1039

    P61.5 Transient neonatal neutropenia   MCC
        EXCLUDES 1 *congenital neutropenia (nontransient) (D70.0)*
        DEF: Low blood neutrophil counts of newborn; occurs due to maternal hypertension, sepsis, twin-twin transfusion, alloimmunization, and hemolytic disease.
        CC Excl: PDX collection 1040

    P61.6 Other transient neonatal disorders of coagulation   CC
        CC Excl: PDX collection 1035

    P61.8 Other specified perinatal hematological disorders

    P61.9 Perinatal hematological disorder, unspecified

Transitory endocrine and metabolic disorders specific to newborn (P70-P74)

    INCLUDES transitory endocrine and metabolic disturbances caused by the infant's response to maternal endocrine and metabolic factors, or its adjustment to extrauterine environment

✓4th **P70 Transitory disorders of carbohydrate metabolism specific to newborn**

    P70.0 Syndrome of infant of mother with gestational diabetes
        Newborn (with hypoglycemia) affected by maternal gestational diabetes
        EXCLUDES 1 *newborn (with hypoglycemia) affected by maternal (pre-existing) diabetes mellitus (P70.1)*
        syndrome of infant of a diabetic mother (P70.1)

    P70.1 Syndrome of infant of a diabetic mother
        Newborn (with hypoglycemia) affected by maternal (pre-existing) diabetes mellitus
        EXCLUDES 1 *newborn (with hypoglycemia) affected by maternal gestational diabetes (P70.0)*
        syndrome of infant of mother with gestational diabetes (P70.0)

    P70.2 Neonatal diabetes mellitus   CC
        CC Excl: PDX collection 1041

    P70.3 Iatrogenic neonatal hypoglycemia

    P70.4 Other neonatal hypoglycemia
        Transient neonatal hypoglycemia

    P70.8 Other transitory disorders of carbohydrate metabolism of newborn   CC
        CC Excl: PDX collection 1042

    P70.9 Transitory disorder of carbohydrate metabolism of newborn, unspecified

✓4th **P71 Transitory neonatal disorders of calcium and magnesium metabolism**

    CC Excl: For CC codes in category P71: PDX collection 1041

    P71.0 Cow's milk hypocalcemia in newborn   CC

    P71.1 Other neonatal hypocalcemia   CC
        EXCLUDES 1 *neonatal hypoparathyroidism (P71.4)*

    P71.2 Neonatal hypomagnesemia   CC

    P71.3 Neonatal tetany without calcium or magnesium deficiency   CC
        Neonatal tetany NOS

    P71.4 Transitory neonatal hypoparathyroidism   CC

    P71.8 Other transitory neonatal disorders of calcium and magnesium metabolism   CC

N Newborn: 0   P Pediatric: 0-17   M Maternity: 12-55   A Adult: 15-124   MCC Major CC Condition   PDxMCC PDx acts as own MCC   CC CC Condition   PDxCC PDx acts as own CC

888   ICD-10-CM 2018

P71.9   **Transitory neonatal disorder of calcium and magnesium metabolism,** unspecified   `CC`

✓4ᵗʰ **P72**   **Other transitory neonatal** endocrine disorders
- *EXCLUDES 1*   congenital hypothyroidism with or without goiter (E03.0-E03.1)
  - dyshormogenetic goiter (E07.1)
  - Pendred's syndrome (E07.1)

CC Excl: For CC codes in category P72: PDX collection 1042

P72.0   **Neonatal goiter, not elsewhere classified**   `CC`
- Transitory congenital goiter with normal functioning

P72.1   **Transitory** neonatal hyperthyroidism   `CC`
- Neonatal thyrotoxicosis
- **CC Excl:** PDX collection 1041

P72.2   **Other** transitory neonatal disorders of thyroid function, `CC`
not elsewhere classified
- Transitory neonatal hypothyroidism

P72.8   **Other** specified transitory neonatal endocrine disorders   `CC`

P72.9   **Transitory neonatal endocrine disorder,** unspecified

✓4ᵗʰ **P74**   **Other transitory neonatal** electrolyte and metabolic **disturbances**

CC Excl: For CC codes in category P74: PDX collection 1042

P74.0   **Late metabolic acidosis** of newborn   `MCC`
- *EXCLUDES 1*   (fetal) metabolic acidosis of newborn (P19)
- **CC Excl:** PDX collection 1041

P74.1   **Dehydration** of newborn

P74.2   **Disturbances of** sodium balance **of newborn**

P74.3   **Disturbances of** potassium balance **of newborn**

P74.4   **Other** transitory electrolyte disturbances of newborn

P74.5   **Transitory** tyrosinemia **of newborn**   `CC`

P74.6   **Transitory** hyperammonemia **of newborn**   `CC`

P74.8   **Other** transitory metabolic disturbances **of newborn**   `CC`
- Amino-acid metabolic disorders described as transitory

P74.9   **Transitory metabolic disturbance of newborn,** unspecified

Digestive system disorders of newborn (P76-P78)

✓4ᵗʰ **P76**   **Other intestinal obstruction of newborn**

P76.0   **Meconium plug syndrome**
- Meconium ileus NOS
- *EXCLUDES 1*   meconium ileus in cystic fibrosis (E84.11)

P76.1   **Transitory ileus of newborn**   `CC`
- *EXCLUDES 1*   Hirschsprung's disease (Q43.1)
- **CC Excl:** PDX collection 1043

P76.2   **Intestinal obstruction due to inspissated milk**

P76.8   **Other specified intestinal obstruction of newborn**
- *EXCLUDES 1*   intestinal obstruction classifiable to K56-.

P76.9   **Intestinal obstruction of newborn, unspecified**

✓4ᵗʰ **P77**   **Necrotizing enterocolitis of newborn**
- **DEF:** Serious intestinal infection and inflammation in preterm infants; severity is measured by stages and may progress to life-threatening perforation or peritonitis; resection surgical treatment may be necessary.

CC Excl: For MCC codes in category P77: PDX collection 1044

P77.1   **Stage 1 necrotizing enterocolitis in newborn**   `MCC`
- Necrotizing enterocolitis without pneumatosis, without perforation
- **DEF:** Broad-spectrum symptoms with nonspecific signs, including feeding intolerance, abdominal distention, bradycardia, and metabolic abnormalities.

P77.2   **Stage 2 necrotizing enterocolitis in newborn**   `MCC`
- Necrotizing enterocolitis with pneumatosis, without perforation
- **DEF:** Radiographic confirmation of necrotizing enterocolitis showing intestinal dilatation, fixed loops of bowels, pneumatosis intestinalis, metabolic acidosis, and thrombocytopenia.

P77.3   **Stage 3 necrotizing enterocolitis in newborn**   `MCC`
- Necrotizing enterocolitis with perforation
- Necrotizing enterocolitis with pneumatosis and perforation
- **DEF:** Advanced stage in which infant demonstrates signs of bowel perforation, septic shock, metabolic acidosis, ascites, disseminated intravascular coagulopathy, neutropenia.

P77.9   **Necrotizing enterocolitis in newborn,** unspecified   `MCC`
- Necrotizing enterocolitis in newborn, NOS

✓4ᵗʰ **P78**   **Other perinatal digestive system disorders**
- *EXCLUDES 1*   cystic fibrosis (E84.0-E84.9)
  - neonatal gastrointestinal hemorrhages (P54.0-P54.3)

P78.0   **Perinatal intestinal perforation**   `MCC`
- Meconium peritonitis
- **CC Excl:** PDX collection 1044

P78.1   **Other neonatal peritonitis**
- Neonatal peritonitis NOS

P78.2   **Neonatal hematemesis and melena due to swallowed maternal blood**

P78.3   **Noninfective neonatal diarrhea**
- Neonatal diarrhea NOS

✓5ᵗʰ **P78.8**   **Other specified perinatal digestive system disorders**

P78.81   **Congenital cirrhosis (of liver)**

P78.82   **Peptic ulcer of newborn**

P78.83   **Newborn esophageal reflux**
- Neonatal esophageal reflux

P78.84   **Gestational alloimmune liver disease**
- GALD
- Neonatal hemochromatosis
- *EXCLUDES 1*   hemochromatosis (E83.11-)

P78.89   **Other specified perinatal digestive system disorders**

P78.9   **Perinatal digestive system disorder, unspecified**

Conditions involving the integument and temperature regulation of newborn (P80-P83)

✓4ᵗʰ **P80**   **Hypothermia of newborn**

P80.0   **Cold injury syndrome**
- Severe and usually chronic hypothermia associated with a pink flushed appearance, edema and neurological and biochemical abnormalities.
- *EXCLUDES 1*   mild hypothermia of newborn (P80.8)

P80.8   **Other hypothermia of newborn**
- Mild hypothermia of newborn

P80.9   **Hypothermia of newborn, unspecified**

✓4ᵗʰ **P81**   **Other disturbances of temperature regulation of newborn**

P81.0   **Environmental hyperthermia of newborn**

P81.8   **Other specified disturbances of temperature regulation of newborn**

P81.9   **Disturbance of temperature regulation of newborn, unspecified**
- Fever of newborn NOS

✓4ᵗʰ **P83**   **Other conditions of integument specific to newborn**
- *EXCLUDES 1*   congenital malformations of skin and integument (Q80-Q84)
  - hydrops fetalis due to hemolytic disease (P56.-)
  - neonatal skin infection (P39.4)
  - staphylococcal scalded skin syndrome (L00)
- *EXCLUDES 2*   cradle cap (L21.0)
  - diaper [napkin] dermatitis (L22)

P83.0   **Sclerema neonatorum**   `CC`
- **DEF:** Diffuse, rapidly progressing white, waxy, nonpitting hardening of tissue, usually of legs and feet that is life-threatening; found in preterm or debilitated infants; unknown etiology.
- **CC Excl:** PDX collection 1045

P83.1   **Neonatal erythema toxicum**

P83.2   **Hydrops fetalis not due to hemolytic disease**   `MCC`
- Hydrops fetalis NOS
- **DEF:** Severe, life-threatening problem of newborn characterized by severe edema of entire body; unrelated to immune response.
- **CC Excl:** PDX collection 1046

✓5ᵗʰ **P83.3**   **Other and unspecified edema specific to newborn**

P83.30   **Unspecified edema specific to newborn**   `CC`
- **CC Excl:** PDX collection 1047

P83.39   **Other edema specific to newborn**   `CC`
- **CC Excl:** PDX collection 1047

P83.4   **Breast engorgement of newborn**
- Noninfective mastitis of newborn

P83.5   **Congenital hydrocele**   ♂

P83.6   **Umbilical polyp of newborn**

☑5ᵗʰ **P83.8** **Other specified conditions of integument specific to newborn**
~~Bronze baby syndrome~~
~~Neonatal scleroderma~~
~~Urticaria neonatorum~~

●   **P83.81** **Umbilical granuloma**
EXCLUDES 2 *granulomatous disorder of the skin and subcutaneous tissue, unspecified (L92.9)*

●   **P83.88** **Other specified conditions of integument specific to newborn**
Bronze baby syndrome
Neonatal scleroderma
Urticaria neonatorum

P83.9 **Condition of the integument specific to newborn, unspecified**

Other problems with newborn (P84)

P84 **Other problems with newborn**
Acidemia of newborn
Acidosis of newborn
Anoxia of newborn NOS
Asphyxia of newborn NOS
Hypercapnia of newborn
Hypoxemia of newborn
Hypoxia of newborn NOS
Mixed metabolic and respiratory acidosis of newborn
EXCLUDES 1 *intracranial hemorrhage due to anoxia or hypoxia (P52.-)*
hypoxic ischemic encephalopathy [HIE] (P91.6-)
late metabolic acidosis of newborn (P74.0)

Other disorders originating in the perinatal period (P90-P96)

P90 **Convulsions of newborn**   MCC
EXCLUDES 1 *benign myoclonic epilepsy in infancy (G40.3-)*
benign neonatal convulsions (familial) (G40.3-)
CC Excl: PDX collection 1048

☑4ᵗʰ **P91** **Other disturbances of cerebral status of newborn**

CC Excl: For CC/MCC codes in category P91, unless otherwise noted: PDX collection 1049

P91.0 **Neonatal cerebral ischemia**   MCC
P91.1 **Acquired periventricular cysts of newborn**   MCC
P91.2 **Neonatal cerebral leukomalacia**   MCC
Periventricular leukomalacia
CC Excl: PDX collection 1022
P91.3 **Neonatal cerebral irritability**   MCC
P91.4 **Neonatal cerebral depression**   MCC
P91.5 **Neonatal coma**   MCC

☑5ᵗʰ **P91.6** **Hypoxic ischemic encephalopathy [HIE]**
EXCLUDES 1 ►*neonatal cerebral depression (P91.4)*
neonatal cerebral irritability (P91.3)
neonatal coma (P91.5)◄

CC Excl: For CC/MCC codes in subcategory P91.6: PDX collection 1050

P91.60 **Hypoxic ischemic encephalopathy [HIE], unspecified**   CC
P91.61 **Mild hypoxic ischemic encephalopathy [HIE]**   CC
P91.62 **Moderate hypoxic ischemic encephalopathy [HIE]**   CC
P91.63 **Severe hypoxic ischemic encephalopathy [HIE]**   MCC

☑5ᵗʰ **P91.8** **Other specified disturbances of cerebral status of newborn**
●   ☑6ᵗʰ **P91.81** **Neonatal encephalopathy**
P91.811 **Neonatal encephalopathy in diseases classified elsewhere**
Code first underlying condition, if known, such as:
congenital cirrhosis (of liver) (P78.71)
intracranial nontraumatic hemorrhage of newborn (P52.-)
kernicterus (P57.-)
●   **P91.819** **Neonatal encephalopathy, unspecified**
●   **P91.88** **Other specified disturbances of cerebral status of newborn**
P91.9 **Disturbance of cerebral status of newborn, unspecified**

☑4ᵗʰ **P92** **Feeding problems of newborn**
EXCLUDES 1 ►*eating disorders (F50.-)*◄
feeding problems in child over 28 days old (R63.3)
AHA: 2016, 3Q, 19

☑5ᵗʰ **P92.0** **Vomiting of newborn**
EXCLUDES 1 *vomiting of child over 28 days old (R11.-)*
P92.01 **Bilious vomiting of newborn**   MCC
EXCLUDES 1 *bilious vomiting in child over 28 days old (R11.14)*
CC Excl: PDX collection 1051
P92.09 **Other vomiting of newborn**
EXCLUDES 1 *regurgitation of food in newborn (P92.1)*

P92.1 **Regurgitation and rumination of newborn**
P92.2 **Slow feeding of newborn**
P92.3 **Underfeeding of newborn**
P92.4 **Overfeeding of newborn**
P92.5 **Neonatal difficulty in feeding at breast**
AHA: 2017, 1Q, 28
P92.6 **Failure to thrive in newborn**
EXCLUDES 1 *failure to thrive in child over 28 days old (R62.51)*
P92.8 **Other feeding problems of newborn**
P92.9 **Feeding problem of newborn, unspecified**

☑4ᵗʰ **P93** **Reactions and intoxications due to drugs administered to newborn**
INCLUDES reactions and intoxications due to drugs administered to fetus affecting newborn
EXCLUDES 1 *jaundice due to drugs or toxins transmitted from mother or given to newborn (P58.4-)*
reactions and intoxications from maternal opiates, tranquilizers and other medication (P04.0-P04.1, P04.4)
withdrawal symptoms from maternal use of drugs of addiction (P96.1)
withdrawal symptoms from therapeutic use of drugs in newborn (P96.2)

P93.0 **Grey baby syndrome**   CC
Grey syndrome from chloramphenicol administration in newborn
CC Excl: PDX collection 1052
P93.8 **Other reactions and intoxications due to drugs administered to newborn**   CC
Use additional code for adverse effect, if applicable, to identify drug (T36-T50 with fifth or sixth character 5)
CC Excl: PDX collection 1052

☑4ᵗʰ **P94** **Disorders of muscle tone of newborn**
P94.0 **Transient neonatal myasthenia gravis**   CC
EXCLUDES 1 *myasthenia gravis (G70.0)*
CC Excl: PDX collection 1041
P94.1 **Congenital hypertonia**
P94.2 **Congenital hypotonia**
Floppy baby syndrome, unspecified
P94.8 **Other disorders of muscle tone of newborn**
P94.9 **Disorder of muscle tone of newborn, unspecified**

P95 **Stillbirth**
Deadborn fetus NOS
Fetal death of unspecified cause
Stillbirth NOS
EXCLUDES 1 *maternal care for intrauterine death (O36.4)*
missed abortion (O02.1)
outcome of delivery, stillbirth (Z37.1, Z37.3, Z37.4, Z37.7)

☑4ᵗʰ **P96** **Other conditions originating in the perinatal period**
P96.0 **Congenital renal failure**
Uremia of newborn
P96.1 **Neonatal withdrawal symptoms from maternal use of drugs of addiction**   CC
Drug withdrawal syndrome in infant of dependent mother
Neonatal abstinence syndrome
EXCLUDES 1 *reactions and intoxications from maternal opiates and tranquilizers administered during labor and delivery (P04.0)*
CC Excl: PDX collection 1052
P96.2 **Withdrawal symptoms from therapeutic use of drugs in newborn**   CC
CC Excl: PDX collection 1052
P96.3 **Wide cranial sutures of newborn**
Neonatal craniotabes

P96.5 **Complication to newborn due to (fetal) intrauterine procedure**
　　EXCLUDES 2　*newborn affected by amniocentesis (P00.6)*

✓6ᵗʰ **P96.8** **Other specified conditions originating in the perinatal period**

　　P96.81 **Exposure to (parental) (environmental) tobacco smoke in the perinatal period**
　　　EXCLUDES 2　*newborn affected by in utero exposure to tobacco (P04.2)*
　　　　　exposure to environmental tobacco smoke after the perinatal period (Z77.22)

　　P96.82 **Delayed separation of umbilical cord**

　　P96.83 **Meconium staining**
　　　EXCLUDES 1　*meconium aspiration (P24.00, P24.01)*
　　　　　meconium passage during delivery (P03.82)

　　P96.89 **Other specified conditions originating in the perinatal period**
　　　Use additional code to specify condition

P96.9 **Condition originating in the perinatal period, unspecified**
　　Congenital debility NOS

✓Additional Character Req　✓x7ᵗʰ Placeholder Alert　Unacceptable PDx　Manifestation　H1 - H14 HAC　HCC CMS-HCC Condition　*EXCLUDES 1* Not Coded Here　*EXCLUDES 2* Not Included Here

ICD-10-CM 2018　　　　　　　　891

Chapter 17. Congenital Malformations, Deformations and Chromosomal Abnormalities (Q00–Q99)

Chapter Specific Guidelines with Coding Examples

The chapter specific guidelines from the ICD-10-CM Official Guidelines for Coding and Reporting have been provided below. Along with these guidelines are coding examples, contained in the shaded boxes, that have been developed to help illustrate the coding and/or sequencing guidance found in these guidelines.

Assign an appropriate code(s) from categories Q00-Q99, Congenital malformations, deformations, and chromosomal abnormalities when a malformation/deformation or chromosomal abnormality is documented. A malformation/deformation/or chromosomal abnormality may be the principal/first-listed diagnosis on a record or a secondary diagnosis.

When a malformation/deformation/or chromosomal abnormality does not have a unique code assignment, assign additional code(s) for any manifestations that may be present.

When the code assignment specifically identifies the malformation/deformation/or chromosomal abnormality, manifestations that are an inherent component of the anomaly should not be coded separately. Additional codes should be assigned for manifestations that are not an inherent component.

8-day-old infant with tetralogy of Fallot and pulmonary stenosis

Q21.3   **Tetralogy of Fallot**

Explanation: Pulmonary stenosis is inherent in the disease process of tetralogy of Fallot. When the code assignment specifically identifies the malformation/deformation/or chromosomal abnormality, manifestations that are inherent components of the anomaly should not be coded separately.

7-month-old infant with Down syndrome and common atrioventricular canal

Q90.9   **Down syndrome, unspecified**

Q21.2   **Atrioventricular septal defect**

Explanation: While a common atrioventricular canal is often associated with patients with Down syndrome, this manifestation is not an inherent component and may be reported separately. When the code assignment specifically identifies the anomaly, manifestations that are inherent components of the condition should not be coded separately. Additional codes should be assigned for manifestations that are not inherent components.

Codes from Chapter 17 may be used throughout the life of the patient. If a congenital malformation or deformity has been corrected, a personal history code should be used to identify the history of the malformation or deformity. Although present at birth, malformation/deformation/or chromosomal abnormality may not be identified until later in life. Whenever the condition is diagnosed by the physician, it is appropriate to assign a code from codes Q00-Q99. For the birth admission, the appropriate code from category Z38, Liveborn infants, according to place of birth and type of delivery, should be sequenced as the principal diagnosis, followed by any congenital anomaly codes, Q00- Q99.

Three-year-old with history of corrected ventricular septal defect

Z87.74   **Personal history of (corrected) congenital malformations of heart and circulatory system**

Explanation: If a congenital malformation or deformity has been corrected, a personal history code should be used to identify the history of the malformation or deformity.

Forty-year-old man with headaches diagnosed with congenital arteriovenous malformation by brain scan

Q28.2   **Arteriovenous malformation of cerebral vessels**

Explanation: Although present at birth, malformations may not be identified until later in life. Whenever the condition is diagnosed by the physician, it is appropriate to assign a code from the range Q00–Q99.

Newborn with anencephaly delivered vaginally in hospital

Z38.00   **Single liveborn infant, delivered vaginally**

Q00.0   **Anencephaly**

Explanation: For the birth admission, the appropriate code from category Z38 Liveborn infants, according to place of birth and type of delivery, should be sequenced as the principal diagnosis, followed by any congenital anomaly codes, Q00–Q99.

Chapter 17. Congenital Malformations, Deformations and Chromosomal Abnormalities(Q00-Q99)

NOTE   Codes from this chapter are not for use on maternal or fetal records.

EXCLUDES 2   *inborn errors of metabolism (E70-E88)*

This chapter contains the following blocks:

Q00-Q07   Congenital malformations of the nervous system
Q10-Q18   Congenital malformations of eye, ear, face and neck
Q20-Q28   Congenital malformations of the circulatory system
Q30-Q34   Congenital malformations of the respiratory system
Q35-Q37   Cleft lip and cleft palate
Q38-Q45   Other congenital malformations of the digestive system
Q50-Q56   Congenital malformations of genital organs
Q60-Q64   Congenital malformations of the urinary system
Q65-Q79   Congenital malformations and deformations of the musculoskeletal system
Q80-Q89   Other congenital malformations
Q90-Q99   Chromosomal abnormalities, not elsewhere classified

Congenital malformations of the nervous system (Q00-Q07)

✓4ᵗʰ Q00 Anencephaly and similar malformations

CC Excl: For MCC codes in category Q00: PDX collection 1053

Q00.0 Anencephaly   `MCC` `HCC`
Acephaly
Acrania
Amyelencephaly
Hemianencephaly
Hemicephaly

Q00.1 Craniorachischisis   `MCC` `HCC`

Q00.2 Iniencephaly   `MCC` `HCC`

✓4ᵗʰ Q01 Encephalocele
INCLUDES   Arnold-Chiari syndrome, type III
encephalocystocele
encephalomyelocele
hydroencephalocele
hydromeningocele, cranial
meningocele, cerebral
meningoencephalocele
EXCLUDES 1   *Meckel-Gruber syndrome (Q61.9)*

CC Excl: For CC codes in category Q01: PDX collection 1054

Q01.0 Frontal encephalocele   `CC` `HCC`
Q01.1 Nasofrontal encephalocele   `CC` `HCC`
Q01.2 Occipital encephalocele   `CC` `HCC`
Q01.8 Encephalocele of other sites   `CC` `HCC`
Q01.9 Encephalocele, unspecified   `CC` `HCC`

Q02 Microcephaly   `HCC`
INCLUDES   hydromicrocephaly
micrencephalon
EXCLUDES 1   *Meckel-Gruber syndrome (Q61.9)*

✓4ᵗʰ Q03 Congenital hydrocephalus
INCLUDES   hydrocephalus in newborn
EXCLUDES 1   *Arnold-Chiari syndrome, type II (Q07.0-)*
acquired hydrocephalus (G91.-)
hydrocephalus due to congenital toxoplasmosis (P37.1)
hydrocephalus with spina bifida (Q05.0-Q05.4)

Q03.0 Malformations of aqueduct of Sylvius   `HCC`
Anomaly of aqueduct of Sylvius
Obstruction of aqueduct of Sylvius, congenital
Stenosis of aqueduct of Sylvius

Q03.1 Atresia of foramina of Magendie and Luschka   `HCC`
Dandy-Walker syndrome

Q03.8 Other congenital hydrocephalus   `HCC`
Q03.9 Congenital hydrocephalus, unspecified   `HCC`

✓4ᵗʰ Q04 Other congenital malformations of brain
EXCLUDES 1   *cyclopia (Q87.0)*
macrocephaly (Q75.3)

CC Excl: For MCC codes in category Q04, unless otherwise noted: PDX collection 1054

Q04.0 Congenital malformations of corpus callosum   `MCC` `HCC`
Agenesis of corpus callosum

Q04.1 Arhinencephaly   `MCC` `HCC`
Q04.2 Holoprosencephaly   `MCC` `HCC`

Congenital Hydrocephalus

Pressure

Normal ventricles   Hydrocephalic ventricles

Q04.3 Other reduction deformities of brain   `MCC` `HCC`
Absence of part of brain
Agenesis of part of brain
Agyria
Aplasia of part of brain
Hydranencephaly
Hypoplasia of part of brain
Lissencephaly
Microgyria
Pachygyria
EXCLUDES 1   *congenital malformations of corpus callosum (Q04.0)*

Q04.4 Septo-optic dysplasia of brain   `CC` `HCC`
CC Excl: PDX collection 1055

Q04.5 Megalencephaly   `CC` `HCC`
CC Excl: PDX collection 1055

Q04.6 Congenital cerebral cysts   `CC` `HCC`
Porencephaly
Schizencephaly
EXCLUDES 1   *acquired porencephalic cyst (G93.0)*
CC Excl: PDX collection 1055

Q04.8 Other specified congenital malformations of brain   `CC` `HCC`
Arnold-Chiari syndrome, type IV
Macrogyria
CC Excl: PDX collection 1055

Q04.9 Congenital malformation of brain, unspecified   `HCC`
Congenital anomaly NOS of brain
Congenital deformity NOS of brain
Congenital disease or lesion NOS of brain
Multiple anomalies NOS of brain, congenital

✓4ᵗʰ Q05 Spina bifida
Hydromeningocele (spinal)
Meningocele (spinal)
Meningomyelocele
Myelocele
Myelomeningocele
Rachischisis
Spina bifida (aperta)(cystica)
Syringomyelocele
Use additional code for any associated paraplegia (paraparesis) (G82.2-)
EXCLUDES 1   *Arnold-Chiari syndrome, type II (Q07.0-)*
spina bifida occulta (Q76.0)

CC Excl: For CC codes in category Q05: PDX collection 1056

Q05.0 Cervical spina bifida with hydrocephalus   `CC` `HCC`
Q05.1 Thoracic spina bifida with hydrocephalus   `CC` `HCC`
Dorsal spina bifida with hydrocephalus
Thoracolumbar spina bifida with hydrocephalus

Q05.2 Lumbar spina bifida with hydrocephalus   `CC` `HCC`
Lumbosacral spina bifida with hydrocephalus

Q05.3 Sacral spina bifida with hydrocephalus   `CC` `HCC`
Q05.4 Unspecified spina bifida with hydrocephalus   `CC` `HCC`
Q05.5 Cervical spina bifida without hydrocephalus   `HCC`
Q05.6 Thoracic spina bifida without hydrocephalus   `HCC`
Dorsal spina bifida NOS
Thoracolumbar spina bifida NOS

Q05.7 Lumbar spina bifida without hydrocephalus   `HCC`
Lumbosacral spina bifida NOS

Q05.8 Sacral spina bifida without hydrocephalus   `HCC`
Q05.9 Spina bifida, unspecified   `HCC`

N Newborn: 0   P Pediatric: 0-17   M Maternity: 12-55   A Adult: 15-124   `MCC` Major CC Condition   `PDxMCC` PDx acts as own MCC   `CC` CC Condition   `PDxCC` PDx acts as own CC

Spina Bifida

Spina bifida occulta   Meningocele   Myelomeningocele

☑4ᵗʰ **Q06 Other congenital malformations of spinal cord**

Q06.0 Amyelia `HCC`

Q06.1 Hypoplasia and dysplasia of spinal cord `HCC`
Atelomyelia
Myelatelia
Myelodysplasia of spinal cord

Q06.2 Diastematomyelia `HCC`
DEF: Rare congenital anomaly often associated with spina bifida; the spinal cord is separated into longitudinal halves by a bony, cartilaginous or fibrous septum, each half surrounded by a dural sac.

Q06.3 Other congenital cauda equina malformations `HCC`

Q06.4 Hydromyelia `HCC`
Hydrorachis

Q06.8 Other specified congenital malformations of spinal cord `HCC`

Q06.9 Congenital malformation of spinal cord, unspecified `HCC`
Congenital anomaly NOS of spinal cord
Congenital deformity NOS of spinal cord
Congenital disease or lesion NOS of spinal cord

☑4ᵗʰ **Q07 Other congenital malformations of nervous system**
EXCLUDES 2   congenital central alveolar hypoventilation syndrome (G47.35)
familial dysautonomia [Riley-Day] (G90.1)
neurofibromatosis (nonmalignant) (Q85.0-)

CC Excl: For CC codes in category Q07: PDX collection 1056

☑5ᵗʰ **Q07.0 Arnold-Chiari syndrome**
Arnold-Chiari syndrome, type II
EXCLUDES 1   Arnold-Chiari syndrome, type III (Q01.-)
Arnold-Chiari syndrome, type IV (Q04.8)

Q07.00 Arnold-Chiari syndrome without spina bifida or hydrocephalus `HCC`

Q07.01 Arnold-Chiari syndrome with spina bifida `HCC`

Q07.02 Arnold-Chiari syndrome with hydrocephalus `CC` `HCC`

Q07.03 Arnold-Chiari syndrome with spina bifida and hydrocephalus `CC` `HCC`

Q07.8 Other specified congenital malformations of nervous system `HCC`
Agenesis of nerve
Displacement of brachial plexus
Jaw-winking syndrome
Marcus Gunn's syndrome

Q07.9 Congenital malformation of nervous system, unspecified `HCC`
Congenital anomaly NOS of nervous system
Congenital deformity NOS of nervous system
Congenital disease or lesion NOS of nervous system

Congenital malformations of eye, ear, face and neck (Q10-Q18)

EXCLUDES 2   cleft lip and cleft palate (Q35-Q37)
congenital malformation of cervical spine (Q05.0, Q05.5, Q67.5, Q76.0-Q76.4)
congenital malformation of larynx (Q31.-)
congenital malformation of lip NEC (Q38.0)
congenital malformation of nose (Q30.-)
congenital malformation of parathyroid gland (Q89.2)
congenital malformation of thyroid gland (Q89.2)

☑4ᵗʰ **Q10 Congenital malformations of eyelid, lacrimal apparatus and orbit**
EXCLUDES 1   cryptophthalmos NOS (Q11.2)
cryptophthalmos syndrome (Q87.0)

Q10.0 Congenital ptosis
DEF: Congenital drooping of eyelid; mostly idiopathic, but may occur genetically.

Q10.1 Congenital ectropion

Q10.2 Congenital entropion

Q10.3 Other congenital malformations of eyelid
Ablepharon
Blepharophimosis, congenital
Coloboma of eyelid
Congenital absence or agenesis of cilia
Congenital absence or agenesis of eyelid
Congenital accessory eyelid
Congenital accessory eye muscle
Congenital malformation of eyelid NOS

Q10.4 Absence and agenesis of lacrimal apparatus
Congenital absence of punctum lacrimale

Q10.5 Congenital stenosis and stricture of lacrimal duct

Q10.6 Other congenital malformations of lacrimal apparatus
Congenital malformation of lacrimal apparatus NOS

Q10.7 Congenital malformation of orbit

☑4ᵗʰ **Q11 Anophthalmos, microphthalmos and macrophthalmos**

Q11.0 Cystic eyeball

Q11.1 Other anophthalmos
Anophthalmos NOS
Agenesis of eye
Aplasia of eye

Q11.2 Microphthalmos
Cryptophthalmos NOS
Dysplasia of eye
Hypoplasia of eye
Rudimentary eye
EXCLUDES 1   cryptophthalmos syndrome (Q87.0)

Q11.3 Macrophthalmos
EXCLUDES 1   macrophthalmos in congenital glaucoma (Q15.0)

☑4ᵗʰ **Q12 Congenital lens malformations**

Q12.0 Congenital cataract

Q12.1 Congenital displaced lens

Q12.2 Coloboma of lens

Q12.3 Congenital aphakia

Q12.4 Spherophakia

Q12.8 Other congenital lens malformations
Microphakia

Q12.9 Congenital lens malformation, unspecified

☑4ᵗʰ **Q13 Congenital malformations of anterior segment of eye**

Q13.0 Coloboma of iris
Coloboma NOS

Q13.1 Absence of iris
Aniridia
Use additional code for associated glaucoma (H42)
DEF: Incompletely formed or absent iris; affects both eyes; dominant trait.

Q13.2 Other congenital malformations of iris
Anisocoria, congenital
Atresia of pupil
Congenital malformation of iris NOS
Corectopia

Q13.3 Congenital corneal opacity

Q13.4 Other congenital corneal malformations
Congenital malformation of cornea NOS
Microcornea
Peter's anomaly

Q13.5 Blue sclera

Coloboma of Lens

Coloboma

☑ Additional Character Req   ✓ₓ7ᵗʰ Placeholder Alert   Unacceptable PDx   Manifestation   `H1`-`H14` HAC   `HCC` CMS-HCC Condition   *EXCLUDES 1* Not Coded Here   *EXCLUDES 2* Not Included Here

Chapter 17. Congenital Malformations, Deformations and Chromosomal Abnormalities

☑5ᵗʰ **Q13.8** **Other congenital malformations of anterior segment of eye**

     Q13.81 **Rieger's anomaly**
Use additional code for associated glaucoma (H42)

     Q13.89 **Other congenital malformations of anterior segment of eye**

Q13.9 **Congenital malformation of anterior segment of eye, unspecified**

☑4ᵗʰ **Q14** **Congenital malformations of posterior segment of eye**

     EXCLUDES 2   optic nerve hypoplasia (H47.03-)

Q14.0 **Congenital malformation of vitreous humor**
Congenital vitreous opacity

Q14.1 **Congenital malformation of retina**
Congenital retinal aneurysm

Q14.2 **Congenital malformation of optic disc**
Coloboma of optic disc

Q14.3 **Congenital malformation of choroid**

Q14.8 **Other congenital malformations of posterior segment of eye**
Coloboma of the fundus

Q14.9 **Congenital malformation of posterior segment of eye, unspecified**

☑4ᵗʰ **Q15** **Other congenital malformations of eye**

     EXCLUDES 1   congenital nystagmus (H55.01)
ocular albinism (E70.31-)
optic nerve hypoplasia (H47.03-)
retinitis pigmentosa (H35.52)

Q15.0 **Congenital glaucoma**
Axenfeld's anomaly
Buphthalmos
Glaucoma of childhood
Glaucoma of newborn
Hydrophthalmos
Keratoglobus, congenital, with glaucoma
Macrocornea with glaucoma
Macrophthalmos in congenital glaucoma
Megalocornea with glaucoma

Q15.8 **Other specified congenital malformations of eye**

Q15.9 **Congenital malformation of eye, unspecified**
Congenital anomaly of eye
Congenital deformity of eye

☑4ᵗʰ **Q16** **Congenital malformations of ear causing impairment of hearing**

     EXCLUDES 1   congenital deafness (H90.-)

Q16.0 **Congenital absence of (ear) auricle**

Q16.1 **Congenital absence, atresia and stricture of auditory canal (external)**
Congenital atresia or stricture of osseous meatus

Q16.2 **Absence of eustachian tube**

Q16.3 **Congenital malformation of ear ossicles**
Congenital fusion of ear ossicles

Q16.4 **Other congenital malformations of middle ear**
Congenital malformation of middle ear NOS

Q16.5 **Congenital malformation of inner ear**
Congenital anomaly of membranous labyrinth
Congenital anomaly of organ of Corti

Q16.9 **Congenital malformation of ear causing impairment of hearing, unspecified**
Congenital absence of ear NOS

☑4ᵗʰ **Q17** **Other congenital malformations of ear**

     EXCLUDES 1   congenital malformations of ear with impairment of hearing (Q16.0- Q16.9)
preauricular sinus (Q18.1)

Q17.0 **Accessory auricle**
Accessory tragus
Polyotia
Preauricular appendage or tag
Supernumerary ear
Supernumerary lobule

Q17.1 **Macrotia**
DEF: Birth defect characterized by abnormal enlargement of the pinna of the ear.

Q17.2 **Microtia**

Q17.3 **Other misshapen ear**
Pointed ear

Q17.4 **Misplaced ear**
Low-set ears
     EXCLUDES 1   cervical auricle (Q18.2)

Q17.5 **Prominent ear**
Bat ear

Q17.8 **Other specified congenital malformations of ear**
Congenital absence of lobe of ear

Q17.9 **Congenital malformation of ear, unspecified**
Congenital anomaly of ear NOS

☑4ᵗʰ **Q18** **Other congenital malformations of face and neck**

     EXCLUDES 1   cleft lip and cleft palate (Q35-Q37)
conditions classified to Q67.0-Q67.4
congenital malformations of skull and face bones (Q75.-)
cyclopia (Q87.0)
dentofacial anomalies [including malocclusion] (M26.-)
malformation syndromes affecting facial appearance (Q87.0)
persistent thyroglossal duct (Q89.2)

Q18.0 **Sinus, fistula and cyst of branchial cleft**
Branchial vestige

Q18.1 **Preauricular sinus and cyst**
Fistula of auricle, congenital
Cervicoaural fistula

Q18.2 **Other branchial cleft malformations**
Branchial cleft malformation NOS
Cervical auricle
Otocephaly

Q18.3 **Webbing of neck**
Pterygium colli
DEF: Congenital malformation characterized by thick, triangular skinfold that stretches from the lateral side of the neck across the shoulder; associated with genetic conditions Turner's and Noonan's syndromes.

Q18.4 **Macrostomia**
DEF: Rare congenital craniofacial bilateral or unilateral anomaly of mouth due to malformed maxillary and mandibular processes; results in abnormally large mouth extending towards ear.

Q18.5 **Microstomia**

Q18.6 **Macrocheilia**
Hypertrophy of lip, congenital

Q18.7 **Microcheilia**

Q18.8 **Other specified congenital malformations of face and neck**
Medial cyst of face and neck
Medial fistula of face and neck
Medial sinus of face and neck

Q18.9 **Congenital malformation of face and neck, unspecified**
Congenital anomaly NOS of face and neck

Congenital malformations of the circulatory system (Q20-Q28)

☑4ᵗʰ **Q20** **Congenital malformations of cardiac chambers and connections**

     EXCLUDES 1   dextrocardia with situs inversus (Q89.3)
mirror-image atrial arrangement with situs inversus (Q89.3)

CC Excl: For CC/MCC codes in category Q20: PDX collection 1057

Q20.0 **Common arterial trunk**   MCC
Persistent truncus arteriosus
     EXCLUDES 1   aortic septal defect (Q21.4)

Q20.1 **Double outlet right ventricle**   MCC
Taussig-Bing syndrome

Q20.2 **Double outlet left ventricle**   MCC

Q20.3 **Discordant ventriculoarterial connection**   MCC
Dextrotransposition of aorta
Transposition of great vessels (complete)

Q20.4 **Double inlet ventricle**   MCC
Common ventricle
Cor triloculare biatriatum
Single ventricle

Q20.5 **Discordant atrioventricular connection**   CC
Corrected transposition
Levotransposition
Ventricular inversion

Q20.6 **Isomerism of atrial appendages**
Isomerism of atrial appendages with asplenia or polysplenia

Q20.8 **Other congenital malformations of cardiac chambers and connections**
Cor binoculare

Q20.9 **Congenital malformation of cardiac chambers and connections, unspecified**

Ⓝ Newborn: 0   Ⓟ Pediatric: 0-17   Ⓜ Maternity: 12-55   Ⓐ Adult: 15-124   MCC Major CC Condition   PDx MCC PDx acts as own MCC   CC CC Condition   PDx CC PDx acts as own CC

896   ICD-10-CM 2018

Ventricular Septal Defect

Chapter 17. Congenital Malformations, Deformations and Chromosomal Abnormalities

Atrioventricular Septal Defect

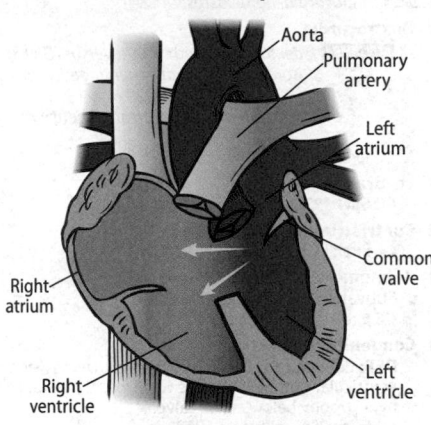

Labels: Aorta; Pulmonary artery; Left atrium; Common valve; Right atrium; Right ventricle; Left ventricle

✓4ᵗʰ Q21   Congenital malformations of cardiac septa
> **EXCLUDES 1**   *acquired cardiac septal defect (I51.0)*

CC Excl: For CC/MCC codes in category Q21, unless otherwise noted: PDX collection 1057

Q21.0   Ventricular septal defect   `CC`
Roger's disease

Q21.1   Atrial septal defect   `CC`
Coronary sinus defect
Patent or persistent foramen ovale
Patent or persistent ostium secundum defect (type II)
Patent or persistent sinus venosus defect
CC Excl: PDX collection 1058

Q21.2   Atrioventricular septal defect   `CC`
Common atrioventricular canal
Endocardial cushion defect
Ostium primum atrial septal defect (type I)

Q21.3   Tetralogy of Fallot   `MCC`
Ventricular septal defect with pulmonary stenosis or atresia, dextroposition of aorta and hypertrophy of right ventricle.
AHA: 2014, 3Q, 16

Q21.4   Aortopulmonary septal defect
Aortic septal defect
Aortopulmonary window

Q21.8   Other congenital malformations of cardiac septa
Eisenmenger's defect
Pentalogy of Fallot
▶Code also if applicable:
Eisenmenger's complex (I27.83)
Eisenmenger's syndrome (I27.83)◀
> **EXCLUDES 1**   *Eisenmenger's complex (I27.8)*
> *Eisenmenger's syndrome (I27.8)*

Q21.9   Congenital malformation of cardiac septum, unspecified
Septal (heart) defect NOS

Atrial Septal Defect

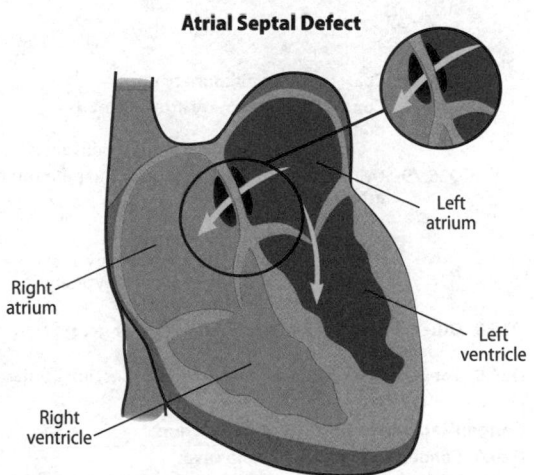

Labels: Left atrium; Left ventricle; Right atrium; Right ventricle

✓4ᵗʰ Q22   Congenital malformations of pulmonary and tricuspid valves

CC Excl: For MCC codes in category Q22, unless otherwise noted: PDX collection 1061

Q22.0   Pulmonary valve atresia   `MCC`
CC Excl: PDX collection 1059

Q22.1   Congenital pulmonary valve stenosis   `CC`
DEF: Stenosis of opening between pulmonary artery and right ventricle; causes obstructed blood outflow from right ventricle.
CC Excl: PDX collection 1059

Q22.2   Congenital pulmonary valve insufficiency   `CC`
Congenital pulmonary valve regurgitation
CC Excl: PDX collection 1060

Q22.3   Other congenital malformations of pulmonary valve   `CC`
Congenital malformation of pulmonary valve NOS
Supernumerary cusps of pulmonary valve
CC Excl: PDX collection 1060

Q22.4   Congenital tricuspid stenosis   `MCC`
Congenital tricuspid atresia

Q22.5   Ebstein's anomaly   `MCC`
DEF: Malformation of the tricuspid valve characterized by septal and posterior leaflets attaching to the wall of the right ventricle; causes the right ventricle to fuse with the atrium into a large right atrium and a small ventricle; leads to heart failure and abnormal cardiac rhythm.

Q22.6   Hypoplastic right heart syndrome   `MCC`

Q22.8   Other congenital malformations of tricuspid valve   `MCC`

Q22.9   Congenital malformation of tricuspid valve, unspecified   `MCC`

✓4ᵗʰ Q23   Congenital malformations of aortic and mitral valves

CC Excl: For CC/MCC codes in category Q23: PDX collection 1061

Q23.0   Congenital stenosis of aortic valve   `CC`
Congenital aortic atresia
Congenital aortic stenosis NOS
> **EXCLUDES 1**   *congenital stenosis of aortic valve in hypoplastic left heart syndrome (Q23.4)*
> *congenital subaortic stenosis (Q24.4)*
> *supravalvular aortic stenosis (congenital) (Q25.3)*

Q23.1   Congenital insufficiency of aortic valve   `CC`
Bicuspid aortic valve
Congenital aortic insufficiency

Q23.2   Congenital mitral stenosis   `CC`
Congenital mitral atresia
DEF: Congenital stenosis of mitral valve orifice between left atrium and ventricle; at the supravalvular, valvular, or subvalvular levels; causes obstruction to left ventricular filling.

Q23.3   Congenital mitral insufficiency   `CC`

Q23.4   Hypoplastic left heart syndrome   `MCC`

Q23.8   Other congenital malformations of aortic and mitral valves

Q23.9   Congenital malformation of aortic and mitral valves, unspecified

✔ Additional Character Req   ✔x7ᵗʰ Placeholder Alert   Unacceptable PDx   Manifestation   H1–H14 HAC   HCC CMS-HCC Condition   EXCLUDES 1 Not Coded Here   EXCLUDES 2 Not Included Here

ICD-10-CM 2018   897

Q21–Q23.9

☑4th Q24 Other congenital malformations of heart
     EXCLUDES 1 *endocardial fibroelastosis (I42.4)*

     Q24.Ø Dextrocardia   `CC`
         EXCLUDES 1 *dextrocardia with situs inversus (Q89.3)*
             isomerism of atrial appendages (with asplenia or
             polysplenia) (Q20.6)
             mirror-image atrial arrangement with situs inversus
             (Q89.3)
         CC Excl: PDX collection 1Ø62

     Q24.1 Levocardia   `CC`
         CC Excl: PDX collection 1Ø62

     Q24.2 Cor triatriatum   `MCC`
         CC Excl: PDX collection 1Ø63

     Q24.3 Pulmonary infundibular stenosis   `CC`
         Subvalvular pulmonic stenosis
         CC Excl: PDX collection 1Ø63

     Q24.4 Congenital subaortic stenosis   `MCC`
         DEF: Congenital heart defect characterized by stenosis of left
         ventricular outflow tract due to fibrous tissue ring or septal
         hypertrophy below aortic valve.
         CC Excl: PDX collection 1Ø63

     Q24.5 Malformation of coronary vessels   `CC`
         Congenital coronary (artery) aneurysm
         CC Excl: PDX collection 1Ø64

     Q24.6 Congenital heart block   `MCC`
         CC Excl: PDX collection 1Ø65

     Q24.8 Other specified congenital malformations of heart
         Congenital diverticulum of left ventricle
         Congenital malformation of myocardium
         Congenital malformation of pericardium
         Malposition of heart
         Uhl's disease

     Q24.9 Congenital malformation of heart, unspecified
         Congenital anomaly of heart
         Congenital disease of heart

☑4th Q25 Congenital malformations of great arteries

     Q25.Ø Patent ductus arteriosus   `CC`
         Patent ductus Botallo
         Persistent ductus arteriosus
         CC Excl: PDX collection 1Ø66

     Q25.1 Coarctation of aorta   `CC`
         Coarctation of aorta (preductal) (postductal)
         Stenosis of aorta
         CC Excl: PDX collection 1Ø67

     ☑5th Q25.2 Atresia of aorta

         Q25.21 Interruption of aortic arch   `CC`
             Atresia of aortic arch
             CC Excl: PDX collection 1Ø68

         Q25.29 Other atresia of aorta   `CC`
             Atresia of aorta
             CC Excl: PDX collection 1Ø68

     Q25.3 Supravalvular aortic stenosis   `CC`
         EXCLUDES 1 *congenital aortic stenosis NOS (Q23.Ø)*
             congenital stenosis of aortic valve (Q23.Ø)
         CC Excl: PDX collection 1Ø68

Patent Ductus Arteriosus

Patent ductus arteriosus
Aorta
Pulmonary artery
Superior vena cava
Atria
Septum
Patent foramen ovale
Right atrium
Left atrium
Schematic showing foramen ovale

Aortic Arch Anomalies

Aortic arch
Esophagus
Trachea
Normal aortic arch
Double aortic arch
Right aortic arch

☑5th Q25.4 Other congenital malformations of aorta
     EXCLUDES 1 *hypoplasia of aorta in hypoplastic left heart syndrome*
             (Q23.4)

     CC Excl: For CC codes in subcategory Q25.4:
     PDX collection 1Ø69

     Q25.40 Congenital malformation of aorta unspecified   `CC`
     Q25.41 Absence and aplasia of aorta   `CC`
     Q25.42 Hypoplasia of aorta   `CC`
     Q25.43 Congenital aneurysm of aorta   `CC`
         Congenital aneurysm of aortic root
         Congenital aneurysm of aortic sinus
     Q25.44 Congenital dilation of aorta   `CC`
     Q25.45 Double aortic arch   `CC`
         Vascular ring of aorta
     Q25.46 Tortuous aortic arch   `CC`
         Persistent convolutions of aortic arch
     Q25.47 Right aortic arch   `CC`
         Persistent right aortic arch
     Q25.48 Anomalous origin of subclavian artery   `CC`
     Q25.49 Other congenital malformations of aorta   `CC`
         ▶Aortic arch
         Bovine arch◀

     Q25.5 Atresia of pulmonary artery   `MCC`
         CC Excl: PDX collection 1Ø70

     Q25.6 Stenosis of pulmonary artery   `MCC`
         Supravalvular pulmonary stenosis
         CC Excl: PDX collection 1Ø70

     ☑5th Q25.7 Other congenital malformations of pulmonary artery

     CC Excl: For MCC codes in subcategory Q25.7:
     PDX collection 1Ø70

         Q25.71 Coarctation of pulmonary artery   `MCC`
         Q25.72 Congenital pulmonary arteriovenous malformation   `MCC`
             Congenital pulmonary arteriovenous aneurysm
         Q25.79 Other congenital malformations of pulmonary artery   `MCC`
             Aberrant pulmonary artery
             Agenesis of pulmonary artery
             Congenital aneurysm of pulmonary artery
             Congenital anomaly of pulmonary artery
             Hypoplasia of pulmonary artery

     Q25.8 Other congenital malformations of other great arteries   `CC`
         CC Excl: PDX collection 1Ø69

     Q25.9 Congenital malformation of great arteries, unspecified   `CC`
         CC Excl: PDX collection 1Ø69

☑4th Q26 Congenital malformations of great veins

     Q26.Ø Congenital stenosis of vena cava   `CC`
         Congenital stenosis of vena cava (inferior)(superior)
         CC Excl: PDX collection 1Ø71

N Newborn: 0   **P** Pediatric: 0-17   **M** Maternity: 12-55   **A** Adult: 15-124   **MCC** Major CC Condition   **PDx MCC** PDx acts as own MCC   **CC** CC Condition   **PDx CC** PDx acts as own CC

898   ICD-10-CM 2018

Q26.1 Persistent left superior vena cava   `CC`
　　CC Excl: PDX collection 1071

Q26.2 Total anomalous pulmonary venous connection   `CC`
　　Total anomalous pulmonary venous return [TAPVR],
　　　subdiaphragmatic
　　Total anomalous pulmonary venous return [TAPVR],
　　　supradiaphragmatic
　　CC Excl: PDX collection 1072

Q26.3 Partial anomalous pulmonary venous connection   `CC`
　　Partial anomalous pulmonary venous return
　　CC Excl: PDX collection 1073

Q26.4 Anomalous pulmonary venous connection, unspecified   `CC`
　　CC Excl: PDX collection 1073

Q26.5 Anomalous portal venous connection

Q26.6 Portal vein-hepatic artery fistula

Q26.8 Other congenital malformations of great veins   `CC`
　　Absence of vena cava (inferior) (superior)
　　Azygos continuation of inferior vena cava
　　Persistent left posterior cardinal vein
　　Scimitar syndrome
　　CC Excl: PDX collection 1071

Q26.9 Congenital malformation of great vein, unspecified   `CC`
　　Congenital anomaly of vena cava (inferior) (superior) NOS
　　CC Excl: PDX collection 1074

✓4ᵗʰ **Q27** Other congenital malformations of peripheral vascular system
　　EXCLUDES 2　anomalies of cerebral and precerebral vessels (Q28.0-Q28.3)
　　　　anomalies of coronary vessels (Q24.5)
　　　　anomalies of pulmonary artery (Q25.5-Q25.7)
　　　　congenital retinal aneurysm (Q14.1)
　　　　hemangioma and lymphangioma (D18.-)

Q27.0 Congenital absence and hypoplasia of umbilical artery
　　Single umbilical artery

Q27.1 Congenital renal artery stenosis

Q27.2 Other congenital malformations of renal artery
　　Congenital malformation of renal artery NOS
　　Multiple renal arteries

✓5ᵗʰ **Q27.3** Arteriovenous malformation (peripheral)
　　Arteriovenous aneurysm
　　EXCLUDES 1　acquired arteriovenous aneurysm (I77.0)
　　EXCLUDES 2　arteriovenous malformation of cerebral vessels (Q28.2)
　　　　arteriovenous malformation of precerebral vessels
　　　　　(Q28.0)

　　Q27.30 Arteriovenous malformation, site unspecified   `CC`
　　　　CC Excl: PDX collection 1075

　　Q27.31 Arteriovenous malformation of vessel of upper limb

　　Q27.32 Arteriovenous malformation of vessel of lower limb

　　Q27.33 Arteriovenous malformation of digestive system
　　　　vessel

　　Q27.34 Arteriovenous malformation of renal vessel

　　Q27.39 Arteriovenous malformation, other site

Q27.4 Congenital phlebectasia   `CC`
　　CC Excl: PDX collection 1075

Q27.8 Other specified congenital malformations of peripheral
　　vascular system
　　Absence of peripheral vascular system
　　Atresia of peripheral vascular system
　　Congenital aneurysm (peripheral)
　　Congenital stricture, artery
　　Congenital varix
　　EXCLUDES 1　arteriovenous malformation (Q27.3-)

Q27.9 Congenital malformation of peripheral vascular system,
　　unspecified
　　Anomaly of artery or vein NOS

✓4ᵗʰ **Q28** Other congenital malformations of circulatory system
　　EXCLUDES 1　congenital aneurysm NOS (Q27.8)
　　　　congenital coronary aneurysm (Q24.5)
　　　　ruptured cerebral arteriovenous malformation (I60.8)
　　　　ruptured malformation of precerebral vessels (I72.0)
　　EXCLUDES 2　congenital peripheral aneurysm (Q27.8)
　　　　congenital pulmonary aneurysm (Q25.79)
　　　　congenital retinal aneurysm (Q14.1)

　　CC Excl: For CC codes in category Q28, unless otherwise noted:
　　PDX collection 1075

Q28.0 Arteriovenous malformation of precerebral vessels   `CC`
　　Congenital arteriovenous precerebral aneurysm (nonruptured)

Q28.1 Other malformations of precerebral vessels   `CC`
　　Congenital malformation of precerebral vessels NOS
　　Congenital precerebral aneurysm (nonruptured)

Q28.2 Arteriovenous malformation of cerebral vessels   `MCC`
　　Arteriovenous malformation of brain NOS
　　Congenital arteriovenous cerebral aneurysm (nonruptured)
　　CC Excl: PDX collection 1076

Q28.3 Other malformations of cerebral vessels   `MCC`
　　Congenital cerebral aneurysm (nonruptured)
　　Congenital malformation of cerebral vessels NOS
　　Developmental venous anomaly
　　CC Excl: PDX collection 1076

Q28.8 Other specified congenital malformations of circulatory   `CC`
　　system
　　Congenital aneurysm, specified site NEC
　　Spinal vessel anomaly

Q28.9 Congenital malformation of circulatory system,   `CC`
　　unspecified
　　CC Excl: PDX collection 1077

Congenital malformations of the respiratory system (Q30-Q34)

✓4ᵗʰ **Q30** Congenital malformations of nose
　　EXCLUDES 1　congenital deviation of nasal septum (Q67.4)

Q30.0 Choanal atresia
　　Atresia of nares (anterior) (posterior)
　　Congenital stenosis of nares (anterior) (posterior)

Q30.1 Agenesis and underdevelopment of nose
　　Congenital absent of nose

Q30.2 Fissured, notched and cleft nose

Q30.3 Congenital perforated nasal septum

Q30.8 Other congenital malformations of nose
　　Accessory nose
　　Congenital anomaly of nasal sinus wall

Q30.9 Congenital malformation of nose, unspecified

✓4ᵗʰ **Q31** Congenital malformations of larynx
　　EXCLUDES 1　congenital laryngeal stridor NOS (P28.89)

　　CC Excl: For CC codes in category Q31: PDX collection 1078

Q31.0 Web of larynx
　　Glottic web of larynx
　　Subglottic web of larynx
　　Web of larynx NOS
　　DEF: Congenital malformation of larynx; marked by thin,
　　translucent, or thick, fibrotic membrane-like structure between
　　vocal folds; characterized by shortness of breath, and stridor.

Q31.1 Congenital subglottic stenosis   `CC`

Q31.2 Laryngeal hypoplasia   `CC`

Q31.3 Laryngocele   `CC`

Q31.5 Congenital laryngomalacia   `CC`

Q31.8 Other congenital malformations of larynx   `CC`
　　Absence of larynx
　　Agenesis of larynx
　　Atresia of larynx
　　Congenital cleft thyroid cartilage
　　Congenital fissure of epiglottis
　　Congenital stenosis of larynx NEC
　　Posterior cleft of cricoid cartilage

Q31.9 Congenital malformation of larynx, unspecified   `CC`

✓4ᵗʰ **Q32** Congenital malformations of trachea and bronchus
　　EXCLUDES 1　congenital bronchiectasis (Q33.4)

　　CC Excl: For CC codes in category Q32: PDX collection 1078

Q32.0 Congenital tracheomalacia   `CC`

Q32.1 Other congenital malformations of trachea   `CC`
　　Atresia of trachea
　　Congenital anomaly of tracheal cartilage
　　Congenital dilatation of trachea
　　Congenital malformation of trachea
　　Congenital stenosis of trachea
　　Congenital tracheocele

Q32.2 Congenital bronchomalacia   `CC`

Q32.3 Congenital stenosis of bronchus   `CC`

Q32.4 Other congenital malformations of bronchus   `CC`
　　Absence of bronchus
　　Agenesis of bronchus
　　Atresia of bronchus
　　Congenital diverticulum of bronchus
　　Congenital malformation of bronchus NOS

✓ Additional Character Req   ✓x7ᵗʰ Placeholder Alert   Unacceptable PDx   Manifestation   H1 - H14 HAC   HCC CMS-HCC Condition   *EXCLUDES 1* Not Coded Here   *EXCLUDES 2* Not Included Here

ICD-10-CM 2018   899

☑4ᵗʰ **Q33** **Congenital malformations of lung**

> **CC Excl: For CC/MCC codes in category Q33, unless otherwise noted:** PDX collection 1079

Q33.0 **Congenital cystic lung**   `CC`
Congenital cystic lung disease
Congenital honeycomb lung
Congenital polycystic lung disease
   `EXCLUDES 1`   cystic fibrosis (E84.0)
              cystic lung disease, acquired or unspecified (J98.4)

Q33.1 **Accessory lobe of lung**
Azygos lobe (fissured), lung

Q33.2 **Sequestration of lung**   `MCC`

Q33.3 **Agenesis of lung**   `MCC`
Congenital absence of lung (lobe)

Q33.4 **Congenital bronchiectasis**   `CC`
CC Excl: PDX collection 1080

Q33.5 **Ectopic tissue in lung**

Q33.6 **Congenital hypoplasia and dysplasia of lung**   `MCC`
   `EXCLUDES 1`   pulmonary hypoplasia associated with short gestation (P28.0)

Q33.8 **Other congenital malformations of lung**

Q33.9 **Congenital malformation of lung, unspecified**

☑4ᵗʰ **Q34** **Other congenital malformations of respiratory system**
   `EXCLUDES 2`   congenital central alveolar hypoventilation syndrome (G47.35)

Q34.0 **Anomaly of pleura**

Q34.1 **Congenital cyst of mediastinum**

Q34.8 **Other specified congenital malformations of respiratory system**
Atresia of nasopharynx

Q34.9 **Congenital malformation of respiratory system, unspecified**
Congenital absence of respiratory system
Congenital anomaly of respiratory system NOS

Cleft lip and cleft palate (Q35-Q37)

Use additional code to identify associated malformation of the nose (Q30.2)
   `EXCLUDES 1`   Robin's syndrome (Q87.0)

☑4ᵗʰ **Q35** **Cleft palate**
   `INCLUDES`   fissure of palate
             palatoschisis
   `EXCLUDES 1`   cleft palate with cleft lip (Q37.-)

Q35.1 **Cleft hard palate**

Q35.3 **Cleft soft palate**

Q35.5 **Cleft hard palate with cleft soft palate**

Q35.7 **Cleft uvula**

Q35.9 **Cleft palate, unspecified**
Cleft palate NOS

☑4ᵗʰ **Q36** **Cleft lip**
   `INCLUDES`   cheiloschisis
             congenital fissure of lip
             harelip
             labium leporinum
   `EXCLUDES 1`   cleft lip with cleft palate (Q37.-)

Q36.0 **Cleft lip, bilateral**

Q36.1 **Cleft lip, median**

Q36.9 **Cleft lip, unilateral**
Cleft lip NOS

Cleft Palate

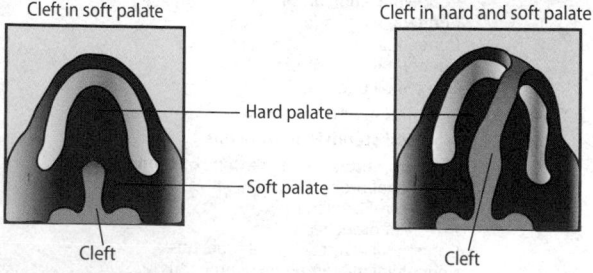

Cleft in soft palate   Cleft in hard and soft palate

Hard palate —
Soft palate —
Cleft   Cleft

Cleft Lip

Unilateral incomplete   Unilateral complete   Bilateral complete

☑4ᵗʰ **Q37** **Cleft palate with cleft lip**
   `INCLUDES`   cheilopalatoschisis

Q37.0 **Cleft hard palate with bilateral cleft lip**

Q37.1 **Cleft hard palate with unilateral cleft lip**
Cleft hard palate with cleft lip NOS

Q37.2 **Cleft soft palate with bilateral cleft lip**

Q37.3 **Cleft soft palate with unilateral cleft lip**
Cleft soft palate with cleft lip NOS

Q37.4 **Cleft hard and soft palate with bilateral cleft lip**

Q37.5 **Cleft hard and soft palate with unilateral cleft lip**
Cleft hard and soft palate with cleft lip NOS

Q37.8 **Unspecified cleft palate with bilateral cleft lip**

Q37.9 **Unspecified cleft palate with unilateral cleft lip**
Cleft palate with cleft lip NOS

Other congenital malformations of the digestive system (Q38-Q45)

☑4ᵗʰ **Q38** **Other congenital malformations of tongue, mouth and pharynx**
   `EXCLUDES 1`   dentofacial anomalies (M26.-)
             macrostomia (Q18.4)
             microstomia (Q18.5)

Q38.0 **Congenital malformations of lips, not elsewhere classified**
Congenital fistula of lip
Congenital malformation of lip NOS
Van der Woude's syndrome
   `EXCLUDES 1`   cleft lip (Q36.-)
             cleft lip with cleft palate (Q37.-)
             macrocheilia (Q18.6)
             microcheilia (Q18.7)

Q38.1 **Ankyloglossia**
Tongue tie

Q38.2 **Macroglossia**
Congenital hypertrophy of tongue

Q38.3 **Other congenital malformations of tongue**
Aglossia
Bifid tongue
Congenital adhesion of tongue
Congenital fissure of tongue
Congenital malformation of tongue NOS
Double tongue
Hypoglossia
Hypoplasia of tongue
Microglossia

Q38.4 **Congenital malformations of salivary glands and ducts**
Atresia of salivary glands and ducts
Congenital absence of salivary glands and ducts
Congenital accessory salivary glands and ducts
Congenital fistula of salivary gland

Q38.5 **Congenital malformations of palate, not elsewhere classified**
Congenital absence of uvula
Congenital malformation of palate NOS
Congenital high arched palate
   `EXCLUDES 1`   cleft palate (Q35.-)
             cleft palate with cleft lip (Q37.-)

Q38.6 **Other congenital malformations of mouth**
Congenital malformation of mouth NOS

Q38.7 **Congenital pharyngeal pouch**
Congenital diverticulum of pharynx
   `EXCLUDES 1`   pharyngeal pouch syndrome (D82.1)

Q38.8 **Other congenital malformations of pharynx**
Congenital malformation of pharynx NOS
Imperforate pharynx

N Newborn: 0   P Pediatric: 0-17   M Maternity: 12-55   A Adult: 15-124   `MCC` Major CC Condition   `PDxMCC` PDx acts as own MCC   `CC` CC Condition   `PDxCC` PDx acts as own CC

900   **ICD-10-CM 2018**

✓4ᵗʰ **Q39 Congenital malformations of esophagus**

CC Excl: For MCC codes in category Q39: PDX collection 1081
For CC codes in category Q39: PDX collection 1082

Q39.0 Atresia of esophagus without fistula `MCC`
Atresia of esophagus NOS

Q39.1 Atresia of esophagus with tracheo-esophageal fistula `MCC`
Atresia of esophagus with broncho-esophageal fistula

Q39.2 Congenital tracheo-esophageal fistula without atresia `MCC`
Congenital tracheo-esophageal fistula NOS

Q39.3 Congenital stenosis and stricture of esophagus `MCC`

Q39.4 Esophageal web `MCC`

Q39.5 Congenital dilatation of esophagus `CC`
Congenital cardiospasm

Q39.6 Congenital diverticulum of esophagus `CC`
Congenital esophageal pouch

Q39.8 Other congenital malformations of esophagus `CC`
Congenital absence of esophagus
Congenital displacement of esophagus
Congenital duplication of esophagus

Q39.9 Congenital malformation of esophagus, unspecified `CC`

✓4ᵗʰ **Q40 Other congenital malformations of upper alimentary tract**

Q40.0 Congenital hypertrophic pyloric stenosis
Congenital or infantile constriction
Congenital or infantile hypertrophy
Congenital or infantile spasm
Congenital or infantile stenosis
Congenital or infantile stricture

Q40.1 Congenital hiatus hernia
Congenital displacement of cardia through esophageal hiatus
EXCLUDES 1   congenital diaphragmatic hernia (Q79.0)

Q40.2 Other specified congenital malformations of stomach
Congenital displacement of stomach
Congenital diverticulum of stomach
Congenital hourglass stomach
Congenital duplication of stomach
Megalogastria
Microgastria

Q40.3 Congenital malformation of stomach, unspecified

Q40.8 Other specified congenital malformations of upper alimentary tract

Q40.9 Congenital malformation of upper alimentary tract, unspecified
Congenital anomaly of upper alimentary tract
Congenital deformity of upper alimentary tract

✓4ᵗʰ **Q41 Congenital absence, atresia and stenosis of small intestine**
INCLUDES   congenital obstruction, occlusion or stricture of small intestine or intestine NOS
EXCLUDES 1   cystic fibrosis with intestinal manifestation (E84.11)
meconium ileus NOS (without cystic fibrosis) (P76.0)

CC Excl: For CC codes in category Q41: PDX collection 1083

Q41.0 Congenital absence, atresia and stenosis of duodenum `CC`

Q41.1 Congenital absence, atresia and stenosis of jejunum `CC`
Apple peel syndrome
Imperforate jejunum

Q41.2 Congenital absence, atresia and stenosis of ileum `CC`

Q41.8 Congenital absence, atresia and stenosis of other specified parts of small intestine `CC`

Q41.9 Congenital absence, atresia and stenosis of small intestine, part unspecified `CC`
Congenital absence, atresia and stenosis of intestine NOS

✓4ᵗʰ **Q42 Congenital absence, atresia and stenosis of large intestine**
INCLUDES   congenital obstruction, occlusion and stricture of large intestine

CC Excl: For CC codes in category Q42: PDX collection 1084

Q42.0 Congenital absence, atresia and stenosis of rectum with fistula `CC`

Q42.1 Congenital absence, atresia and stenosis of rectum without fistula `CC`
Imperforate rectum

Q42.2 Congenital absence, atresia and stenosis of anus with fistula `CC`

Q42.3 Congenital absence, atresia and stenosis of anus without fistula `CC`
Imperforate anus

Q42.8 Congenital absence, atresia and stenosis of other parts of large intestine `CC`

Q42.9 Congenital absence, atresia and stenosis of large intestine, part unspecified `CC`

✓4ᵗʰ **Q43 Other congenital malformations of intestine**

CC Excl: For CC codes in category Q43, unless otherwise noted: PDX collection 1087

Q43.0 Meckel's diverticulum (displaced) (hypertrophic)
Persistent omphalomesenteric duct
Persistent vitelline duct

Q43.1 Hirschsprung's disease `CC`
Aganglionosis
Congenital (aganglionic) megacolon
CC Excl: PDX collection 1085

Q43.2 Other congenital functional disorders of colon `CC`
Congenital dilatation of colon
CC Excl: PDX collection 1085

Q43.3 Congenital malformations of intestinal fixation `CC`
Congenital omental, anomalous adhesions [bands]
Congenital peritoneal adhesions [bands]
Incomplete rotation of cecum and colon
Insufficient rotation of cecum and colon
Jackson's membrane
Malrotation of colon
Rotation failure of cecum and colon
Universal mesentery
CC Excl: DX collection 1086

Q43.4 Duplication of intestine `CC`

Q43.5 Ectopic anus `CC`

Q43.6 Congenital fistula of rectum and anus `CC`
EXCLUDES 1   congenital fistula of anus with absence, atresia and stenosis (Q42.2)
congenital fistula of rectum with absence, atresia and stenosis (Q42.0)
congenital rectovaginal fistula (Q52.2)
congenital urethrorectal fistula (Q64.73)
pilonidal fistula or sinus (L05.-)

Q43.7 Persistent cloaca `CC`
Cloaca NOS

Q43.8 Other specified congenital malformations of intestine `CC`
Congenital blind loop syndrome
Congenital diverticulitis, colon
Congenital diverticulum, intestine
Dolichocolon
Megaloappendix
Megaloduodenum
Microcolon
Transposition of appendix
Transposition of colon
Transposition of intestine
AHA: 2013, 2Q, 31

Q43.9 Congenital malformation of intestine, unspecified `CC`

✓4ᵗʰ **Q44 Congenital malformations of gallbladder, bile ducts and liver**

CC Excl: For CC codes in category Q44, unless otherwise noted: PDX collection 1088

Q44.0 Agenesis, aplasia and hypoplasia of gallbladder `CC`
Congenital absence of gallbladder

Q44.1 Other congenital malformations of gallbladder `CC`
Congenital malformation of gallbladder NOS
Intrahepatic gallbladder

Q44.2 Atresia of bile ducts `MCC`
CC Excl: PDX collection 1089

Q44.3 Congenital stenosis and stricture of bile ducts `MCC`
CC Excl: PDX collection 1089

Q44.4 Choledochal cyst `CC`

Q44.5 Other congenital malformations of bile ducts `CC`
Accessory hepatic duct
Biliary duct duplication
Congenital malformation of bile duct NOS
Cystic duct duplication

Q44.6 Cystic disease of liver `CC`
Fibrocystic disease of liver
CC Excl: PDX collection 1090

Q44.7 Other congenital malformations of liver `CC`
Accessory liver
Alagille's syndrome
Congenital absence of liver
Congenital hepatomegaly
Congenital malformation of liver NOS

✓4ᵗʰ Q45 Other congenital malformations of digestive system
EXCLUDES 2 congenital diaphragmatic hernia (Q79.0)
congenital hiatus hernia (Q40.1)

CC Excl: For CC codes in category Q45: PDX collection 1091

Q45.0 Agenesis, aplasia and hypoplasia of pancreas CC
Congenital absence of pancreas
Q45.1 Annular pancreas CC
Q45.2 Congenital pancreatic cyst CC
Q45.3 Other congenital malformations of pancreas and pancreatic duct CC
Accessory pancreas
Congenital malformation of pancreas or pancreatic duct NOS
EXCLUDES 1 congenital diabetes mellitus (E10.-)
cystic fibrosis (E84.0-E84.9)
fibrocystic disease of pancreas (E84.-)
neonatal diabetes mellitus (P70.2)
Q45.8 Other specified congenital malformations of digestive system
Absence (complete) (partial) of alimentary tract NOS
Duplication of digestive system
Malposition, congenital of digestive system
Q45.9 Congenital malformation of digestive system, unspecified
Congenital anomaly of digestive system
Congenital deformity of digestive system

Congenital malformations of genital organs (Q50-Q56)
EXCLUDES 1 androgen insensitivity syndrome (E34.5-)
syndromes associated with anomalies in the number and form of chromosomes (Q90-Q99)

✓4ᵗʰ Q50 Congenital malformations of ovaries, fallopian tubes and broad ligaments
✓5ᵗʰ Q50.0 Congenital absence of ovary
EXCLUDES 1 Turner's syndrome (Q96.-)
Q50.01 Congenital absence of ovary, unilateral ♀
Q50.02 Congenital absence of ovary, bilateral ♀
Q50.1 Developmental ovarian cyst ♀
Q50.2 Congenital torsion of ovary ♀
✓5ᵗʰ Q50.3 Other congenital malformations of ovary
Q50.31 Accessory ovary
Q50.32 Ovarian streak
46, XX with streak gonads
Q50.39 Other congenital malformation of ovary ♀
Congenital malformation of ovary NOS
Q50.4 Embryonic cyst of fallopian tube ♀
Fimbrial cyst
Q50.5 Embryonic cyst of broad ligament ♀
Epoophoron cyst
Parovarian cyst
Q50.6 Other congenital malformations of fallopian tube and broad ligament ♀
Absence of fallopian tube and broad ligament
Accessory fallopian tube and broad ligament
Atresia of fallopian tube and broad ligament
Congenital malformation of fallopian tube or broad ligament NOS

✓4ᵗʰ Q51 Congenital malformations of uterus and cervix
Q51.0 Agenesis and aplasia of uterus ♀
Congenital absence of uterus
✓5ᵗʰ Q51.1 Doubling of uterus with doubling of cervix and vagina
Q51.10 Doubling of uterus with doubling of cervix and vagina without obstruction ♀
Doubling of uterus with doubling of cervix and vagina NOS
Q51.11 Doubling of uterus with doubling of cervix and vagina with obstruction ♀
Q51.2 Other doubling of uterus ♀
Doubling of uterus NOS
Septate uterus, complete or partial
Q51.3 Bicornate uterus ♀
Bicornate uterus, complete or partial
Q51.4 Unicornate uterus ♀
Unicornate uterus with or without a separate uterine horn
Uterus with only one functioning horn
Q51.5 Agenesis and aplasia of cervix ♀
Congenital absence of cervix
Q51.6 Embryonic cyst of cervix ♀

Q51.7 Congenital fistulae between uterus and digestive and urinary tracts ♀
✓5ᵗʰ Q51.8 Other congenital malformations of uterus and cervix
✓6ᵗʰ Q51.81 Other congenital malformations of uterus
Q51.810 Arcuate uterus ♀
Arcuatus uterus
Q51.811 Hypoplasia of uterus ♀
Q51.818 Other congenital malformations of uterus ♀
Müllerian anomaly of uterus NEC
✓6ᵗʰ Q51.82 Other congenital malformations of cervix
Q51.820 Cervical duplication ♀
Q51.821 Hypoplasia of cervix ♀
Q51.828 Other congenital malformations of cervix ♀
Q51.9 Congenital malformation of uterus and cervix, unspecified ♀

✓4ᵗʰ Q52 Other congenital malformations of female genitalia
Q52.0 Congenital absence of vagina ♀
Vaginal agenesis, total or partial
✓5ᵗʰ Q52.1 Doubling of vagina
EXCLUDES 1 doubling of vagina with doubling of uterus and cervix (Q51.1-)
Q52.10 Doubling of vagina, unspecified ♀
Septate vagina NOS
Q52.11 Transverse vaginal septum ♀
✓6ᵗʰ Q52.12 Longitudinal vaginal septum
Q52.120 Longitudinal vaginal septum, nonobstructing ♀
Q52.121 Longitudinal vaginal septum, obstructing, right side ♀
Q52.122 Longitudinal vaginal septum, obstructing, left side ♀
Q52.123 Longitudinal vaginal septum, microperforate, right side ♀
Q52.124 Longitudinal vaginal septum, microperforate, left side ♀
Q52.129 Other and unspecified longitudinal vaginal septum ♀
Q52.2 Congenital rectovaginal fistula ♀
EXCLUDES 1 cloaca (Q43.7)
Q52.3 Imperforate hymen ♀
DEF: Obstructive anomaly of vagina, characterized by complete closure of membranous fold around external opening of vagina, obstructing the vaginal introitus.
Q52.4 Other congenital malformations of vagina ♀
Canal of Nuck cyst, congenital
Congenital malformation of vagina NOS
Embryonic vaginal cyst
Gartner's duct cyst
Q52.5 Fusion of labia ♀
Q52.6 Congenital malformation of clitoris ♀
✓5ᵗʰ Q52.7 Other and unspecified congenital malformations of vulva
Q52.70 Unspecified congenital malformations of vulva ♀
Congenital malformation of vulva NOS
Q52.71 Congenital absence of vulva ♀
Q52.79 Other congenital malformations of vulva ♀
Congenital cyst of vulva
Q52.8 Other specified congenital malformations of female genitalia ♀
Q52.9 Congenital malformation of female genitalia, unspecified ♀

✓4ᵗʰ Q53 Undescended and ectopic testicle
✓5ᵗʰ Q53.0 Ectopic testis
Q53.00 Ectopic testis, unspecified ♂
Q53.01 Ectopic testis, unilateral ♂
Q53.02 Ectopic testes, bilateral ♂
✓5ᵗʰ Q53.1 Undescended testicle, unilateral
Q53.10 Unspecified undescended testicle, unilateral ♂
✓6ᵗʰ Q53.11 Abdominal testis, unilateral
● **Q53.111 Unilateral intraabdominal testis** ♂
● **Q53.112 Unilateral inguinal testis** ♂
Q53.12 Ectopic perineal testis, unilateral ♂
● **Q53.13 Unilateral high scrotal testis** ♂

N Newborn: 0 **P** Pediatric: 0-17 **M** Maternity: 12-55 **A** Adult: 15-124 **MCC** Major CC Condition **PDxMCC** PDx acts as own MCC **CC** CC Condition **PDxCC** PDx acts as own CC

902 ICD-10-CM 2018

Hypospadias and Epispadias

Balanic (glanular, coronal) hypospadias
Subcoronal hypospadias
Penile hypospadias
Penile raphe
Scrotal hypospadias
Penoscrotal hypospadius
Scrotum
Scrotal raphe
Perineal hypospadias

Hypospadias (ventral view)

Normal external urethral orifice
Glans penis
Foreskin (retracted)
Epispadias

Epispadias (dorsal view)

√5th **Q53.2** Undescended **testicle,** bilateral
  Q53.20 Undescended testicle, unspecified, bilateral ♂
  √6th **Q53.21** Abdominal **testis, bilateral**
    • **Q53.211** Bilateral intraabdominal **testes** ♂
    • **Q53.212** Bilateral inguinal **testes** ♂
    • **Q53.22** Ectopic perineal **testis, bilateral** ♂
    • **Q53.23** Bilateral **high scrotal testes** ♂
  Q53.9 Undescended **testicle,** unspecified
    Cryptorchism NOS

√4th **Q54** Hypospadias
  EXCLUDES 1 *epispadias (Q64.0)*
  DEF: Abnormal opening of urethra on the ventral (underside) surface of the penis.
  Q54.0 Hypospadias, balanic ♂
    Hypospadias, coronal
    Hypospadias, glandular
  Q54.1 Hypospadias, penile ♂
  Q54.2 Hypospadias, penoscrotal ♂
  Q54.3 Hypospadias, perineal ♂
  Q54.4 Congenital chordee ♂
    Chordee without hypospadias
  Q54.8 Other hypospadias ♂
    Hypospadias with intersex state
  Q54.9 Hypospadias, unspecified ♂

√4th **Q55** Other congenital malformations of male genital organs
  EXCLUDES 1 *congenital hydrocele (P83.5)*
    hypospadias (Q54.-)
  Q55.0 Absence and aplasia of testis ♂
    Monorchism
  Q55.1 Hypoplasia of testis and scrotum ♂
    Fusion of testes
  √5th **Q55.2** Other and unspecified congenital malformations of testis and scrotum
    Q55.20 Unspecified congenital malformations of testis and scrotum ♂
      Congenital malformation of testis or scrotum NOS
    Q55.21 Polyorchism ♂
    Q55.22 Retractile **testis** ♂
    Q55.23 Scrotal transposition ♂
    Q55.29 Other congenital malformations of testis and scrotum ♂
  Q55.3 Atresia of **vas deferens** ♂
    Code first any associated cystic fibrosis (E84.-)
  Q55.4 Other congenital malformations of vas deferens, epididymis, seminal vesicles and prostate ♂
    Absence or aplasia of prostate
    Absence or aplasia of spermatic cord
    Congenital malformation of vas deferens, epididymis, seminal vesicles or prostate NOS
  Q55.5 Congenital absence and aplasia of penis ♂
  √5th **Q55.6** Other congenital malformations of penis
    Q55.61 Curvature of penis (lateral) ♂
    Q55.62 Hypoplasia of penis ♂
      Micropenis
    Q55.63 Congenital torsion of penis ♂
      EXCLUDES 1 *acquired torsion of penis (N48.82)*

    Q55.64 Hidden **penis** ♂
      Buried penis
      Concealed penis
      EXCLUDES 1 *acquired buried penis (N48.83)*
    Q55.69 Other congenital malformation of penis ♂
      Congenital malformation of penis NOS
  Q55.7 Congenital vasocutaneous fistula ♂
  Q55.8 Other specified congenital malformations of male ♂
    genital organs
  Q55.9 Congenital malformation of male genital organ, ♂
    unspecified
    Congenital anomaly of male genital organ
    Congenital deformity of male genital organ

√4th **Q56** Indeterminate sex and pseudohermaphroditism
  EXCLUDES 1 *46, XX true hermaphrodite (Q99.1)*
    androgen insensitivity syndrome (E34.5-)
    chimera 46, XX/46, XY true hermaphrodite (Q99.0)
    female pseudohermaphroditism with adrenocortical disorder (E25.-)
    pseudohermaphroditism with specified chromosomal anomaly (Q96-Q99)
    pure gonadal dysgenesis (Q99.1)
  Q56.0 Hermaphroditism, **not elsewhere classified**
    Ovotestis
  Q56.1 Male pseudohermaphroditism, not elsewhere classified ♂
    46, XY with streak gonads
    Male pseudohermaphroditism NOS
  Q56.2 Female **pseudohermaphroditism, not elsewhere** ♀
    classified
    Female pseudohermaphroditism NOS
  Q56.3 Pseudohermaphroditism, unspecified
  Q56.4 Indeterminate sex, unspecified
    Ambiguous genitalia

Congenital malformations of the urinary system (Q60-Q64)

√4th **Q60** Renal agenesis and other reduction defects of kidney
  INCLUDES congenital absence of kidney
    congenital atrophy of kidney
    infantile atrophy of kidney

  CC Excl: For CC codes in category Q60: PDX collection 1092

  Q60.0 Renal agenesis, unilateral CC
  Q60.1 Renal agenesis, bilateral CC
  Q60.2 Renal agenesis, unspecified CC
  Q60.3 Renal hypoplasia, unilateral CC
  Q60.4 Renal hypoplasia, bilateral CC
  Q60.5 Renal hypoplasia, unspecified CC
  Q60.6 Potter's syndrome CC

√4th **Q61** Cystic kidney disease
  EXCLUDES 1 *acquired cyst of kidney (N28.1)*
    Potter's syndrome (Q60.6)
  √5th **Q61.0** Congenital renal cyst
    Q61.00 Congenital renal cyst, unspecified CC
      Cyst of kidney NOS (congenital)
      CC Excl: PDX collection 1093
    Q61.01 Congenital single renal cyst CC
      CC Excl: PDX collection 1094
    Q61.02 Congenital multiple renal cysts CC
      CC Excl: PDX collection 1095
  √5th **Q61.1** Polycystic kidney, infantile type
    Polycystic kidney, autosomal recessive
    Q61.11 Cystic dilatation of collecting ducts CC
      CC Excl: PDX collection 1096
    Q61.19 Other polycystic kidney, infantile type CC
      CC Excl: PDX collection 1096
  Q61.2 Polycystic kidney, adult type CC
    Polycystic kidney, autosomal dominant
    CC Excl: PDX collection 1096
  Q61.3 Polycystic kidney, unspecified CC
    AHA: 2016, 3Q, 22
    CC Excl: PDX collection 1096
  Q61.4 Renal dysplasia CC
    Multicystic dysplastic kidney
    Multicystic kidney (development)
    Multicystic kidney disease
    Multicystic renal dysplasia
    EXCLUDES 1 *polycystic kidney disease (Q61.11-Q61.3)*
    CC Excl: PDX collection 1097

☑Additional Character Req √x7th Placeholder Alert Unacceptable PDx Manifestation H1-H14 HAC HCC CMS-HCC Condition EXCLUDES 1 Not Coded Here EXCLUDES 2 Not Included Here

ICD-10-CM 2018   **903**

Q61.5 **Medullary cystic kidney** `CC`
Nephronopthisis
Sponge kidney NOS
DEF: Sponge kidney: Dilated collecting tubules; usually asymptomatic but calcinosis in tubules may cause renal insufficiency.
CC Excl: PDX collection 1095

Q61.8 **Other cystic kidney diseases** `CC`
Fibrocystic kidney
Fibrocystic renal degeneration or disease
CC Excl: PDX collection 1095

Q61.9 **Cystic kidney disease, unspecified** `CC`
Meckel-Gruber syndrome
CC Excl: PDX collection 1093

✓4ᵗʰ **Q62** **Congenital obstructive defects of renal pelvis and congenital malformations of ureter**

> **CC Excl:** For CC codes in category Q62: PDX collection 1098

Q62.0 **Congenital hydronephrosis** `CC`

✓5ᵗʰ **Q62.1** **Congenital occlusion of ureter**
Atresia and stenosis of ureter

     Q62.10 **Congenital occlusion of ureter, unspecified** `CC`
     Q62.11 **Congenital occlusion of ureteropelvic junction** `CC`
     Q62.12 **Congenital occlusion of ureterovesical orifice** `CC`

Q62.2 **Congenital megaureter** `CC`
Congenital dilatation of ureter

✓5ᵗʰ **Q62.3** **Other obstructive defects of renal pelvis and ureter**

     Q62.31 **Congenital ureterocele, orthotopic** `CC`
     Q62.32 **Cecoureterocele** `CC`
     Ectopic ureterocele
     Q62.39 **Other obstructive defects of renal pelvis and ureter** `CC`
     Ureteropelvic junction obstruction NOS

Q62.4 **Agenesis of ureter**
Congenital absence ureter

Q62.5 **Duplication of ureter**
Accessory ureter
Double ureter

✓5ᵗʰ **Q62.6** **Malposition of ureter**

     Q62.60 **Malposition of ureter, unspecified**
     Q62.61 **Deviation of ureter**
     Q62.62 **Displacement of ureter**
     Q62.63 **Anomalous implantation of ureter**
     Ectopia of ureter
     Ectopic ureter
     Q62.69 **Other malposition of ureter**

Q62.7 **Congenital vesico-uretero-renal reflux**

Q62.8 **Other congenital malformations of ureter**
Anomaly of ureter NOS

✓4ᵗʰ **Q63** **Other congenital malformations of kidney**
> *EXCLUDES 1*   *congenital nephrotic syndrome (N04.-)*

Q63.0 **Accessory kidney**

Q63.1 **Lobulated, fused and horseshoe kidney**

Q63.2 **Ectopic kidney**
Congenital displaced kidney
Malrotation of kidney

Q63.3 **Hyperplastic and giant kidney**
Compensatory hypertrophy of kidney

Q63.8 **Other specified congenital malformations of kidney**
Congenital renal calculi

Q63.9 **Congenital malformation of kidney, unspecified**

✓4ᵗʰ **Q64** **Other congenital malformations of urinary system**

Q64.0 **Epispadias**
> *EXCLUDES 1*   *hypospadias (Q54.-)*

✓5ᵗʰ **Q64.1** **Exstrophy of urinary bladder**

> **CC Excl:** For CC codes in subcategory Q64.1:
> PDX collection 1099

     Q64.10 **Exstrophy of urinary bladder, unspecified** `CC`
     Ectopia vesicae
     Q64.11 **Supravesical fissure of urinary bladder** `CC`
     Q64.12 **Cloacal exstrophy of urinary bladder** `CC`
     Q64.19 **Other exstrophy of urinary bladder** `CC`
     Extroversion of bladder

Q64.2 **Congenital posterior urethral valves** `CC`
     CC Excl: PDX collection 1100

✓5ᵗʰ **Q64.3** **Other atresia and stenosis of urethra and bladder neck**

> **CC Excl:** For CC codes in subcategory Q64.3:
> PDX collection 1100

     Q64.31 **Congenital bladder neck obstruction** `CC`
     Congenital obstruction of vesicourethral orifice
     Q64.32 **Congenital stricture of urethra** `CC`
     Q64.33 **Congenital stricture of urinary meatus** `CC`
     Q64.39 **Other atresia and stenosis of urethra and bladder neck** `CC`
     Atresia and stenosis of urethra and bladder neck NOS

Q64.4 **Malformation of urachus**
Cyst of urachus
Patent urachus
Prolapse of urachus

Q64.5 **Congenital absence of bladder and urethra**

Q64.6 **Congenital diverticulum of bladder**

✓5ᵗʰ **Q64.7** **Other and unspecified congenital malformations of bladder and urethra**
> *EXCLUDES 1*   *congenital prolapse of bladder (mucosa) (Q79.4)*

     Q64.70 **Unspecified congenital malformation of bladder and urethra**
     Malformation of bladder or urethra NOS
     Q64.71 **Congenital prolapse of urethra**
     Q64.72 **Congenital prolapse of urinary meatus**
     Q64.73 **Congenital urethrorectal fistula**
     Q64.74 **Double urethra**
     Q64.75 **Double urinary meatus**
     Q64.79 **Other congenital malformations of bladder and urethra**

Q64.8 **Other specified congenital malformations of urinary system**

Q64.9 **Congenital malformation of urinary system, unspecified**
Congenital anomaly NOS of urinary system
Congenital deformity NOS of urinary system

Congenital malformations and deformations of the musculoskeletal system (Q65-Q79)

✓4ᵗʰ **Q65** **Congenital deformities of hip**
> *EXCLUDES 1*   *clicking hip (R29.4)*

✓5ᵗʰ **Q65.0** **Congenital dislocation of hip, unilateral**
     Q65.00 **Congenital dislocation of unspecified hip, unilateral**
     Q65.01 **Congenital dislocation of right hip, unilateral**
     Q65.02 **Congenital dislocation of left hip, unilateral**

Q65.1 **Congenital dislocation of hip, bilateral**

Q65.2 **Congenital dislocation of hip, unspecified**

✓5ᵗʰ **Q65.3** **Congenital partial dislocation of hip, unilateral**
     Q65.30 **Congenital partial dislocation of unspecified hip, unilateral**
     Q65.31 **Congenital partial dislocation of right hip, unilateral**
     Q65.32 **Congenital partial dislocation of left hip, unilateral**

Q65.4 **Congenital partial dislocation of hip, bilateral**

Q65.5 **Congenital partial dislocation of hip, unspecified**

Q65.6 **Congenital unstable hip**
Congenital dislocatable hip

✓5ᵗʰ **Q65.8** **Other congenital deformities of hip**
     Q65.81 **Congenital coxa valga**
     Q65.82 **Congenital coxa vara**
     Q65.89 **Other specified congenital deformities of hip**
     Anteversion of femoral neck
     Congenital acetabular dysplasia

Q65.9 **Congenital deformity of hip, unspecified**

✓4ᵗʰ **Q66** **Congenital deformities of feet**
> *EXCLUDES 1*   *reduction defects of feet (Q72.-)*
> *valgus deformities (acquired) (M21.0-)*
> *varus deformities (acquired) (M21.1-)*

Q66.0 **Congenital talipes equinovarus**

Q66.1 **Congenital talipes calcaneovarus**

✓5ᵗʰ **Q66.2** **Congenital metatarsus (primus) varus**
     Q66.21 **Congenital metatarsus primus varus**
     Q66.22 **Congenital metatarsus adductus**
     Congenital metatarsus varus

Q66.3 **Other congenital varus deformities of feet**
Hallux varus, congenital

N Newborn: 0   P Pediatric: 0-17   M Maternity: 12-55   A Adult: 15-124   MCC Major CC Condition   PDxMCC PDx acts as own MCC   CC CC Condition   PDxCC PDx acts as own CC

904   ICD-10-CM 2018

Q66.4 Congenital talipes calcaneovalgus

✓5th **Q66.5 Congenital** pes planus
    Congenital flat foot
    Congenital rigid flat foot
    Congenital spastic (everted) flat foot
    EXCLUDES 1   pes planus, acquired (M21.4)

    Q66.50 Congenital pes planus, unspecified **foot**

    Q66.51 Congenital pes planus, right **foot**

    Q66.52 Congenital pes planus, left **foot**

Q66.6 Other congenital valgus deformities of feet
    Congenital metatarsus valgus

Q66.7 Congenital pes cavus

✓5th **Q66.8 Other congenital deformities of feet**

    Q66.80 Congenital vertical talus deformity, unspecified **foot**

    Q66.81 Congenital vertical talus deformity, right **foot**

    Q66.82 Congenital vertical talus deformity, left **foot**

    Q66.89 Other specified congenital deformities of feet
        Congenital asymmetric talipes
        Congenital clubfoot NOS
        Congenital talipes NOS
        Congenital tarsal coalition
        Hammer toe, congenital

Q66.9 Congenital deformity of feet, unspecified

✓4th **Q67 Congenital musculoskeletal deformities of** head, face, spine and chest
    EXCLUDES 1   congenital malformation syndromes classified to Q87-
             Potter's syndrome (Q60.6)

Q67.0 Congenital facial asymmetry

Q67.1 Congenital compression facies

Q67.2 Dolichocephaly

Q67.3 Plagiocephaly

Q67.4 Other congenital deformities of skull, face and jaw
    Congenital depressions in skull
    Congenital hemifacial atrophy or hypertrophy
    Deviation of nasal septum, congenital
    Squashed or bent nose, congenital
    EXCLUDES 1   dentofacial anomalies [including malocclusion]
             (M26.-)
             syphilitic saddle nose (A50.5)

Q67.5 Congenital deformity of spine   CC
    Congenital postural scoliosis
    Congenital scoliosis NOS
    EXCLUDES 1   infantile idiopathic scoliosis (M41.0)
             scoliosis due to congenital bony malformation (Q76.3)
    AHA: 2014, 4Q, 26
    CC Excl: PDX collection 1101

Q67.6 Pectus excavatum
    Congenital funnel chest

Q67.7 Pectus carinatum
    Congenital pigeon chest

Q67.8 Other congenital deformities of chest   CC
    Congenital deformity of chest wall NOS
    CC Excl: PDX collection 1102

✓4th **Q68 Other congenital musculoskeletal deformities**
    EXCLUDES 1   reduction defects of limb(s) (Q71-Q73)
    EXCLUDES 2   congenital myotonic chondrodystrophy (G71.13)

Q68.0 Congenital deformity of sternocleidomastoid muscle
    Congenital contracture of sternocleidomastoid (muscle)
    Congenital (sternomastoid) torticollis
    Sternomastoid tumor (congenital)

Q68.1 Congenital deformity of finger(s) and hand   CC
    Congenital clubfinger
    Spade-like hand (congenital)
    CC Excl: PDX collection 1102

Q68.2 Congenital deformity of knee
    Congenital dislocation of knee
    Congenital genu recurvatum

Q68.3 Congenital bowing of femur
    EXCLUDES 1   anteversion of femur (neck) (Q65.89)

Q68.4 Congenital bowing of tibia and fibula

Q68.5 Congenital bowing of long bones of leg, unspecified

Q68.6 Discoid meniscus

Q68.8 Other specified congenital musculoskeletal deformities
    Congenital deformity of clavicle
    Congenital deformity of elbow
    Congenital deformity of forearm
    Congenital deformity of scapula
    Congenital deformity of wrist
    Congenital dislocation of elbow
    Congenital dislocation of shoulder
    Congenital dislocation of wrist

✓4th **Q69 Polydactyly**

    Q69.0 Accessory finger(s)

    Q69.1 Accessory thumb(s)

    Q69.2 Accessory toe(s)
        Accessory hallux

    Q69.9 Polydactyly, unspecified
        Supernumerary digit(s) NOS

✓4th **Q70 Syndactyly**

✓5th **Q70.0 Fused fingers**
    Complex syndactyly of fingers with synostosis

    Q70.00 Fused fingers, unspecified **hand**

    Q70.01 Fused fingers, right **hand**

    Q70.02 Fused fingers, left **hand**

    Q70.03 Fused fingers, bilateral

✓5th **Q70.1 Webbed fingers**
    Simple syndactyly of fingers without synostosis

    Q70.10 Webbed fingers, unspecified **hand**

    Q70.11 Webbed fingers, right **hand**

    Q70.12 Webbed fingers, left **hand**

    Q70.13 Webbed fingers, bilateral

✓5th **Q70.2 Fused toes**
    Complex syndactyly of toes with synostosis

    Q70.20 Fused toes, unspecified **foot**

    Q70.21 Fused toes, right **foot**

    Q70.22 Fused toes, left **foot**

    Q70.23 Fused toes, bilateral

✓5th **Q70.3 Webbed toes**
    Simple syndactyly of toes without synostosis

    Q70.30 Webbed toes, unspecified **foot**

    Q70.31 Webbed toes, right **foot**

    Q70.32 Webbed toes, left **foot**

    Q70.33 Webbed toes, bilateral

    Q70.4 Polysyndactyly, unspecified
        EXCLUDES 1   specified syndactyly of hand and feet—code to
                 specified conditions (Q70.0-Q70.3-)

    Q70.9 Syndactyly, unspecified
        Symphalangy NOS

✓4th **Q71 Reduction defects of** upper limb

✓5th **Q71.0 Congenital** complete absence **of upper limb**

    Q71.00 Congenital complete absence of unspecified **upper limb**

    Q71.01 Congenital complete absence of right **upper limb**

    Q71.02 Congenital complete absence of left **upper limb**

    Q71.03 Congenital complete absence of upper limb, bilateral

✓5th **Q71.1 Congenital** absence of upper arm and forearm with hand present

    Q71.10 Congenital absence of unspecified **upper arm and forearm with hand present**

    Q71.11 Congenital absence of right **upper arm and forearm with hand present**

    Q71.12 Congenital absence of left **upper arm and forearm with hand present**

    Q71.13 Congenital absence of upper arm and forearm with hand present, bilateral

✓5th **Q71.2 Congenital** absence of both forearm and hand

    Q71.20 Congenital absence of both forearm and hand, unspecified **upper limb**

    Q71.21 Congenital absence of both forearm and hand, right **upper limb**

    Q71.22 Congenital absence of both forearm and hand, left **upper limb**

    Q71.23 Congenital absence of both forearm and hand, bilateral

✓ Additional Character Req   ✓x7th Placeholder Alert   Unacceptable PDx   Manifestation   H1 - H14 HAC   HCC CMS-HCC Condition   EXCLUDES 1 Not Coded Here   EXCLUDES 2 Not Included Here

ICD-10-CM 2018   905

Chapter 17. Congenital Malformations, Deformations and Chromosomal Abnormalities

Q71.3–Q74.0

✓5ᵗʰ **Q71.3 Congenital absence of hand and finger**
     Q71.30 Congenital absence of unspecified hand and finger
     Q71.31 Congenital absence of right hand and finger
     Q71.32 Congenital absence of left hand and finger
     Q71.33 Congenital absence of hand and finger, bilateral

✓5ᵗʰ **Q71.4 Longitudinal reduction defect of radius**
     Clubhand (congenital)
     Radial clubhand
     Q71.40 Longitudinal reduction defect of unspecified radius
     Q71.41 Longitudinal reduction defect of right radius
     Q71.42 Longitudinal reduction defect of left radius
     Q71.43 Longitudinal reduction defect of radius, bilateral

✓5ᵗʰ **Q71.5 Longitudinal reduction defect of ulna**
     Q71.50 Longitudinal reduction defect of unspecified ulna
     Q71.51 Longitudinal reduction defect of right ulna
     Q71.52 Longitudinal reduction defect of left ulna
     Q71.53 Longitudinal reduction defect of ulna, bilateral

✓5ᵗʰ **Q71.6 Lobster-claw hand**
     Q71.60 Lobster-claw hand, unspecified hand
     Q71.61 Lobster-claw right hand
     Q71.62 Lobster-claw left hand
     Q71.63 Lobster-claw hand, bilateral

✓5ᵗʰ **Q71.8 Other reduction defects of upper limb**
     ✓6ᵗʰ **Q71.81** Congenital shortening of upper limb
         Q71.811 Congenital shortening of right upper limb
         Q71.812 Congenital shortening of left upper limb
         Q71.813 Congenital shortening of upper limb, bilateral
         Q71.819 Congenital shortening of unspecified upper limb
     ✓6ᵗʰ **Q71.89** Other reduction defects of upper limb
         Q71.891 Other reduction defects of right upper limb
         Q71.892 Other reduction defects of left upper limb
         Q71.893 Other reduction defects of upper limb, bilateral
         Q71.899 Other reduction defects of unspecified upper limb

✓5ᵗʰ **Q71.9 Unspecified reduction defect of upper limb**
     Q71.90 Unspecified reduction defect of unspecified upper limb
     Q71.91 Unspecified reduction defect of right upper limb
     Q71.92 Unspecified reduction defect of left upper limb
     Q71.93 Unspecified reduction defect of upper limb, bilateral

✓4ᵗʰ **Q72 Reduction defects of lower limb**

✓5ᵗʰ **Q72.0 Congenital complete absence of lower limb**
     Q72.00 Congenital complete absence of unspecified lower limb
     Q72.01 Congenital complete absence of right lower limb
     Q72.02 Congenital complete absence of left lower limb
     Q72.03 Congenital complete absence of lower limb, bilateral

✓5ᵗʰ **Q72.1 Congenital absence of thigh and lower leg with foot present**
     Q72.10 Congenital absence of unspecified thigh and lower leg with foot present
     Q72.11 Congenital absence of right thigh and lower leg with foot present
     Q72.12 Congenital absence of left thigh and lower leg with foot present
     Q72.13 Congenital absence of thigh and lower leg with foot present, bilateral

✓5ᵗʰ **Q72.2 Congenital absence of both lower leg and foot**
     Q72.20 Congenital absence of both lower leg and foot, unspecified lower limb
     Q72.21 Congenital absence of both lower leg and foot, right lower limb
     Q72.22 Congenital absence of both lower leg and foot, left lower limb
     Q72.23 Congenital absence of both lower leg and foot, bilateral

✓5ᵗʰ **Q72.3 Congenital absence of foot and toe(s)**
     Q72.30 Congenital absence of unspecified foot and toe(s)
     Q72.31 Congenital absence of right foot and toe(s)

     Q72.32 Congenital absence of left foot and toe(s)
     Q72.33 Congenital absence of foot and toe(s), bilateral

✓5ᵗʰ **Q72.4 Longitudinal reduction defect of femur**
     Proximal femoral focal deficiency
     Q72.40 Longitudinal reduction defect of unspecified femur
     Q72.41 Longitudinal reduction defect of right femur
     Q72.42 Longitudinal reduction defect of left femur
     Q72.43 Longitudinal reduction defect of femur, bilateral

✓5ᵗʰ **Q72.5 Longitudinal reduction defect of tibia**
     Q72.50 Longitudinal reduction defect of unspecified tibia
     Q72.51 Longitudinal reduction defect of right tibia
     Q72.52 Longitudinal reduction defect of left tibia
     Q72.53 Longitudinal reduction defect of tibia, bilateral

✓5ᵗʰ **Q72.6 Longitudinal reduction defect of fibula**
     Q72.60 Longitudinal reduction defect of unspecified fibula
     Q72.61 Longitudinal reduction defect of right fibula
     Q72.62 Longitudinal reduction defect of left fibula
     Q72.63 Longitudinal reduction defect of fibula, bilateral

✓5ᵗʰ **Q72.7 Split foot**
     Q72.70 Split foot, unspecified lower limb
     Q72.71 Split foot, right lower limb
     Q72.72 Split foot, left lower limb
     Q72.73 Split foot, bilateral

✓5ᵗʰ **Q72.8 Other reduction defects of lower limb**
     ✓6ᵗʰ **Q72.81** Congenital shortening of lower limb
         Q72.811 Congenital shortening of right lower limb
         Q72.812 Congenital shortening of left lower limb
         Q72.813 Congenital shortening of lower limb, bilateral
         Q72.819 Congenital shortening of unspecified lower limb
     ✓6ᵗʰ **Q72.89** Other reduction defects of lower limb
         Q72.891 Other reduction defects of right lower limb
         Q72.892 Other reduction defects of left lower limb
         Q72.893 Other reduction defects of lower limb, bilateral
         Q72.899 Other reduction defects of unspecified lower limb

✓5ᵗʰ **Q72.9 Unspecified reduction defect of lower limb**
     Q72.90 Unspecified reduction defect of unspecified lower limb
     Q72.91 Unspecified reduction defect of right lower limb
     Q72.92 Unspecified reduction defect of left lower limb
     Q72.93 Unspecified reduction defect of lower limb, bilateral

✓4ᵗʰ **Q73 Reduction defects of unspecified limb**

Q73.0 Congenital absence of unspecified limb(s)
     Amelia NOS

Q73.1 Phocomelia, unspecified limb(s)
     Phocomelia NOS

Q73.8 Other reduction defects of unspecified limb(s)
     Longitudinal reduction deformity of unspecified limb(s)
     Ectromelia of limb NOS
     Hemimelia of limb NOS
     Reduction defect of limb NOS

✓4ᵗʰ **Q74 Other congenital malformations of limb(s)**
     EXCLUDES 1   polydactyly (Q69.-)
         reduction defect of limb (Q71-Q73)
         syndactyly (Q70.-)

Q74.0 Other congenital malformations of upper limb(s), including shoulder girdle
     Accessory carpal bones
     Cleidocranial dysostosis
     Congenital pseudarthrosis of clavicle
     Macrodactylia (fingers)
     Madelung's deformity
     Radioulnar synostosis
     Sprengel's deformity
     Triphalangeal thumb

Ⓝ Newborn: 0   Ⓟ Pediatric: 0-17   Ⓜ Maternity: 12-55   Ⓐ Adult: 15-124   **MCC** Major CC Condition   **PDxMCC** PDx acts as own MCC   **CC** CC Condition   **PDxCC** PDx acts as own CC

906   ICD-10-CM 2018

Q74.1 Congenital malformation of knee
Congenital absence of patella
Congenital dislocation of patella
Congenital genu valgum
Congenital genu varum
Rudimentary patella
EXCLUDES 1   *congenital dislocation of knee (Q68.2)*
congenital genu recurvatum (Q68.2)
nail patella syndrome (Q87.2)

Q74.2 Other congenital malformations of lower limb(s), including pelvic girdle
Congenital fusion of sacroiliac joint
Congenital malformation of ankle joint
Congenital malformation of sacroiliac joint
EXCLUDES 1   *anteversion of femur (neck) (Q65.89)*

Q74.3 Arthrogryposis multiplex congenita   CC
CC Excl: PDX collection 1102

Q74.8 Other specified congenital malformations of limb(s)

Q74.9 Unspecified congenital malformation of limb(s)
Congenital anomaly of limb(s) NOS

✓4th **Q75 Other congenital malformations of skull and face bones**
EXCLUDES 1   *congenital malformation of face NOS (Q18.-)*
congenital malformation syndromes classified to Q87.-
dentofacial anomalies [including malocclusion] (M26.-)
musculoskeletal deformities of head and face (Q67.0-Q67.4)
skull defects associated with congenital anomalies of brain such as:
anencephaly (Q00.0)
encephalocele (Q01.-)
hydrocephalus (Q03.-)
microcephaly (Q02)

Q75.0 Craniosynostosis
Acrocephaly
Imperfect fusion of skull
Oxycephaly
Trigonocephaly

Q75.1 Craniofacial dysostosis
Crouzon's disease

Q75.2 Hypertelorism

Q75.3 Macrocephaly

Q75.4 Mandibulofacial dysostosis
Franceschetti syndrome
Treacher Collins syndrome

Q75.5 Oculomandibular dysostosis

Q75.8 Other specified congenital malformations of skull and face bones
Absence of skull bone, congenital
Congenital deformity of forehead
Platybasia

Q75.9 Congenital malformation of skull and face bones, unspecified
Congenital anomaly of face bones NOS
Congenital anomaly of skull NOS

✓4th **Q76 Congenital malformations of spine and bony thorax**
EXCLUDES 1   *congenital musculoskeletal deformities of spine and chest (Q67.5-Q67.8)*

Q76.0 Spina bifida occulta
EXCLUDES 1   *meningocele (spinal) (Q05.-)*
spina bifida (aperta) (cystica) (Q05.-)

Q76.1 Klippel-Feil syndrome
Cervical fusion syndrome

Q76.2 Congenital spondylolisthesis
Congenital spondylolysis
EXCLUDES 1   *spondylolisthesis (acquired) (M43.1-)*
spondylolysis (acquired) (M43.0-)

Q76.3 Congenital scoliosis due to congenital bony malformation   CC
Hemivertebra fusion or failure of segmentation with scoliosis
CC Excl: PDX collection 1101

✓5th **Q76.4 Other congenital malformations of spine, not associated with scoliosis**

CC Excl: For CC codes in subcategory Q76.4:
PDX collection 1101

✓6th **Q76.41 Congenital kyphosis**
Q76.411 Congenital kyphosis, occipito-atlanto-axial region
Q76.412 Congenital kyphosis, cervical region
Q76.413 Congenital kyphosis, cervicothoracic region
Q76.414 Congenital kyphosis, thoracic region

Q76.415 Congenital kyphosis, thoracolumbar region
Q76.419 Congenital kyphosis, unspecified region

✓6th **Q76.42 Congenital lordosis**
Q76.425 Congenital lordosis, thoracolumbar region   CC
Q76.426 Congenital lordosis, lumbar region   CC
Q76.427 Congenital lordosis, lumbosacral region   CC
Q76.428 Congenital lordosis, sacral and sacrococcygeal region   CC
Q76.429 Congenital lordosis, unspecified region   CC

Q76.49 Other congenital malformations of spine, not associated with scoliosis
Congenital absence of vertebra NOS
Congenital fusion of spine NOS
Congenital malformation of lumbosacral (joint) (region) NOS
Congenital malformation of spine NOS
Hemivertebra NOS
Malformation of spine NOS
Platyspondylisis NOS
Supernumerary vertebra NOS

Q76.5 Cervical rib
Supernumerary rib in cervical region

Q76.6 Other congenital malformations of ribs   CC
Accessory rib
Congenital absence of rib
Congenital fusion of ribs
Congenital malformation of ribs NOS
EXCLUDES 1   *short rib syndrome (Q77.2)*
CC Excl: PDX collection 1103

Q76.7 Congenital malformation of sternum   CC
Congenital absence of sternum
Sternum bifidum
CC Excl: PDX collection 1103

Q76.8 Other congenital malformations of bony thorax   CC
CC Excl: PDX collection 1103

Q76.9 Congenital malformation of bony thorax, unspecified   CC
CC Excl: PDX collection 1103

✓4th **Q77 Osteochondrodysplasia with defects of growth of tubular bones and spine**
EXCLUDES 1   *mucopolysaccharidosis (E76.0-E76.3)*
EXCLUDES 2   *congenital myotonic chondrodystrophy (G71.13)*

Q77.0 Achondrogenesis
Hypochondrogenesis

Q77.1 Thanatophoric short stature

Q77.2 Short rib syndrome   CC
Asphyxiating thoracic dysplasia [Jeune]
CC Excl: PDX collection 1103

Q77.3 Chondrodysplasia punctata
EXCLUDES 1   *Rhizomelic chondrodysplasia punctata (E71.43)*

Q77.4 Achondroplasia
Hypochondroplasia
Osteosclerosis congenita

Q77.5 Diastrophic dysplasia

Q77.6 Chondroectodermal dysplasia
Ellis-van Creveld syndrome

Q77.7 Spondyloepiphyseal dysplasia

Q77.8 Other osteochondrodysplasia with defects of growth of tubular bones and spine

Q77.9 Osteochondrodysplasia with defects of growth of tubular bones and spine, unspecified

✓4th **Q78 Other osteochondrodysplasias**
EXCLUDES 2   *congenital myotonic chondrodystrophy (G71.13)*

Q78.0 Osteogenesis imperfecta   CC
Fragilitas ossium
Osteopsathyrosis
CC Excl: PDX collection 1104

Q78.1 Polyostotic fibrous dysplasia
Albright(-McCune)(-Sternberg) syndrome

Q78.2 Osteopetrosis   CC
Albers-Schönberg syndrome
Osteosclerosis NOS
CC Excl: PDX collection 1104

Q78.3 Progressive diaphyseal dysplasia
Camurati-Engelmann syndrome

✓Additional Character Req   ✓x7th Placeholder Alert   Unacceptable PDx   Manifestation   H1-H14 HAC   HCC CMS-HCC Condition   *EXCLUDES 1* Not Coded Here   *EXCLUDES 2* Not Included Here

Chapter 17. Congenital Malformations, Deformations and Chromosomal Abnormalities

Q78.4–Q83

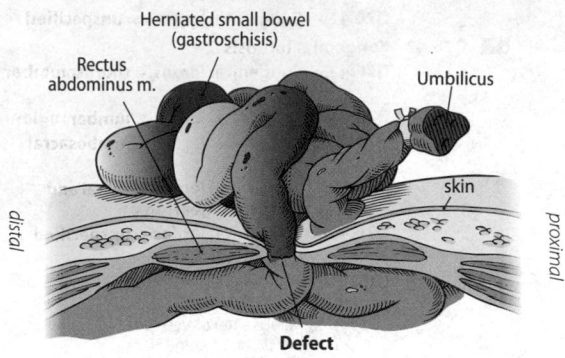

Gastroschisis

Herniated small bowel (gastroschisis)

Rectus abdominus m.

Umbilicus

skin

distal

proximal

Defect

Q78.4 Enchondromatosis
Maffucci's syndrome
Ollier's disease

Q78.5 Metaphyseal dysplasia
Pyle's syndrome

Q78.6 Multiple congenital exostoses
Diaphyseal aclasis

Q78.8 Other specified osteochondrodysplasias
Osteopoikilosis

Q78.9 Osteochondrodysplasia, unspecified
Chondrodystrophy NOS
Osteodystrophy NOS

☑4ᵗʰ **Q79 Congenital malformations of musculoskeletal system, not elsewhere classified**
EXCLUDES 2   *congenital (sternomastoid) torticollis (Q68.0)*

CC Excl: For MCC codes in category Q79, unless otherwise noted: PDX collection 1106

Q79.0 Congenital diaphragmatic hernia   MCC
EXCLUDES 1   *congenital hiatus hernia (Q40.1)*
CC Excl: PDX collection 1105

Q79.1 Other congenital malformations of diaphragm   MCC
Absence of diaphragm
Congenital malformation of diaphragm NOS
Eventration of diaphragm
CC Excl: PDX collection 1105

Q79.2 Exomphalos   MCC
Omphalocele
EXCLUDES 1   *umbilical hernia (K42.-)*

Q79.3 Gastroschisis   MCC

Q79.4 Prune belly syndrome   MCC
Congenital prolapse of bladder mucosa
Eagle-Barrett syndrome

☑5ᵗʰ **Q79.5 Other congenital malformations of abdominal wall**
EXCLUDES 1   *umbilical hernia (K42.-)*

   Q79.51 Congenital hernia of bladder   MCC

   Q79.59 Other congenital malformations of abdominal wall   MCC

Q79.6 Ehlers-Danlos syndrome   CC
DEF: Connective tissue disorder that causes hyperextended skin and joints; results in fragile blood vessels with bleeding, poor wound healing, and subcutaneous pseudotumors.
CC Excl: PDX collection 1107

Q79.8 Other congenital malformations of musculoskeletal system
Absence of muscle
Absence of tendon
Accessory muscle
Amyotrophia congenita
Congenital constricting bands
Congenital shortening of tendon
Poland syndrome

Q79.9 Congenital malformation of musculoskeletal system, unspecified
Congenital anomaly of musculoskeletal system NOS
Congenital deformity of musculoskeletal system NOS

Other congenital malformations (Q80-Q89)

☑4ᵗʰ **Q80 Congenital ichthyosis**
EXCLUDES 1   *Refsum's disease (G60.1)*

Q80.0 Ichthyosis vulgaris

Q80.1 X-linked ichthyosis

Q80.2 Lamellar ichthyosis
Collodion baby

Q80.3 Congenital bullous ichthyosiform erythroderma

Q80.4 Harlequin fetus

Q80.8 Other congenital ichthyosis

Q80.9 Congenital ichthyosis, unspecified

☑4ᵗʰ **Q81 Epidermolysis bullosa**

Q81.0 Epidermolysis bullosa simplex
EXCLUDES 1   *Cockayne's syndrome (Q87.1)*

Q81.1 Epidermolysis bullosa letalis
Herlitz' syndrome

Q81.2 Epidermolysis bullosa dystrophica

Q81.8 Other epidermolysis bullosa

Q81.9 Epidermolysis bullosa, unspecified

☑4ᵗʰ **Q82 Other congenital malformations of skin**
EXCLUDES 1   *acrodermatitis enteropathica (E83.2)*
congenital erythropoietic porphyria (E80.0)
pilonidal cyst or sinus (L05.-)
Sturge-Weber (-Dimitri) syndrome (Q85.8)

Q82.0 Hereditary lymphedema

Q82.1 Xeroderma pigmentosum

▲   **Q82.2 Congenital cutaneous mastocytosis**
▶Congenital diffuse cutaneous mastocytosis
Congenital maculopapular cutaneous mastocytosis
Congenital urticaria pigmentosa◀
Urticaria pigmentosa
EXCLUDES 1   ▶*cutaneous mastocytosis NOS (D47.01)*
diffuse cutaneous mastocytosis (with onset after newborn period) (D47.01)◀
malignant mastocytosis ▶(C96.2-)◀
▶*systemic mastocytosis (D47.02)*
urticaria pigmentosa (non-congenital) (with onset after newborn period) (D47.01)◀

Q82.3 Incontinentia pigmenti

Q82.4 Ectodermal dysplasia (anhidrotic)
EXCLUDES 1   *Ellis-van Creveld syndrome (Q77.6)*

Q82.5 Congenital non-neoplastic nevus
Birthmark NOS
Flammeus Nevus
Portwine Nevus
Sanguineous Nevus
Strawberry Nevus
Vascular Nevus NOS
Verrucous Nevus
EXCLUDES 2   *araneus nevus (I78.1)*
café au lait spots (L81.3)
lentigo (L81.4)
melanocytic nevus (D22.-)
nevus NOS (D22.-)
pigmented nevus (D22.-)
spider nevus (I78.1)
stellar nevus (I78.1)

Q82.6 Congenital sacral dimple
Parasacral dimple
EXCLUDES 2   *pilonidal cyst with abscess (L05.01)*
pilonidal cyst without abscess (L05.91)

Q82.8 Other specified congenital malformations of skin
Abnormal palmar creases
Accessory skin tags
Benign familial pemphigus [Hailey-Hailey]
Congenital poikiloderma
Cutis laxa (hyperelastica)
Dermatoglyphic anomalies
Inherited keratosis palmaris et plantaris
Keratosis follicularis [Darier-White]
EXCLUDES 1   *Ehlers-Danlos syndrome (Q79.6)*
AHA: 2016, 1Q, 17

Q82.9 Congenital malformation of skin, unspecified

☑4ᵗʰ **Q83 Congenital malformations of breast**
EXCLUDES 2   *absence of pectoral muscle (Q79.8)*
hypoplasia of breast (N64.82)
micromastia (N64.82)

N Newborn: 0   P Pediatric: 0-17   M Maternity: 12-55   A Adult: 15-124   MCC Major CC Condition   PDx MCC PDx acts as own MCC   CC CC Condition   PDx CC PDx acts as own CC

908   ICD-10-CM 2018

Q83.0 Congenital absence of breast with absent nipple

Q83.1 Accessory breast
Supernumerary breast

Q83.2 Absent nipple

Q83.3 Accessory nipple
Supernumerary nipple

Q83.8 Other congenital malformations of breast

Q83.9 Congenital malformation of breast, unspecified

☑4ᵗʰ **Q84** Other congenital malformations of integument

Q84.0 Congenital alopecia
Congenital atrichosis

Q84.1 Congenital morphological disturbances of hair, not elsewhere classified
Beaded hair
Monilethrix
Pili annulati
EXCLUDES 1   Menkes' kinky hair syndrome (E83.0)

Q84.2 Other congenital malformations of hair
Congenital hypertrichosis
Congenital malformation of hair NOS
Persistent lanugo

Q84.3 Anonychia
EXCLUDES 1   nail patella syndrome (Q87.2)

Q84.4 Congenital leukonychia

Q84.5 Enlarged and hypertrophic nails
Congenital onychauxis
Pachyonychia

Q84.6 Other congenital malformations of nails
Congenital clubnail
Congenital koilonychia
Congenital malformation of nail NOS

Q84.8 Other specified congenital malformations of integument
Aplasia cutis congenita

Q84.9 Congenital malformation of integument, unspecified
Congenital anomaly of integument NOS
Congenital deformity of integument NOS

☑4ᵗʰ **Q85** Phakomatoses, not elsewhere classified
EXCLUDES 1   ataxia telangiectasia [Louis-Bar] (G11.3)
familial dysautonomia [Riley-Day] (G90.1)

☑5ᵗʰ **Q85.0** Neurofibromatosis (nonmalignant)

Q85.00 Neurofibromatosis, unspecified   HCC

Q85.01 Neurofibromatosis, type 1   HCC
Von Recklinghausen disease

Q85.02 Neurofibromatosis, type 2   HCC
Acoustic neurofibromatosis
DEF: Inherited condition with cutaneous lesions, benign tumors of peripheral nerves, and bilateral 8th nerve masses.

Q85.03 Schwannomatosis   HCC
DEF: A genetic mutation (SMARCB1/INI1) causing multiple benign tumors along nerve pathways; characterized by the exception of 8th cranial nerve involvement.

Q85.09 Other neurofibromatosis   HCC

Q85.1 Tuberous sclerosis   CC HCC
Bourneville's disease
Epiloia
CC Excl: PDX collection 1108

Q85.8 Other phakomatoses, not elsewhere classified   CC HCC
Peutz-Jeghers Syndrome
Sturge-Weber(-Dimitri) syndrome
von Hippel-Lindau syndrome
EXCLUDES 1   Meckel-Gruber syndrome (Q61.9)
CC Excl: PDX collection 1109

Q85.9 Phakomatosis, unspecified   CC HCC
Hamartosis NOS
CC Excl: PDX collection 1109

☑4ᵗʰ **Q86** Congenital malformation syndromes due to known exogenous causes, not elsewhere classified
EXCLUDES 2   iodine-deficiency-related hypothyroidism (E00-E02)
nonteratogenic effects of substances transmitted via placenta or breast milk (P04.-)

Q86.0 Fetal alcohol syndrome (dysmorphic)

Q86.1 Fetal hydantoin syndrome
Meadow's syndrome

Q86.2 Dysmorphism due to warfarin

Q86.8 Other congenital malformation syndromes due to known exogenous causes

☑4ᵗʰ **Q87** Other specified congenital malformation syndromes affecting multiple systems
Use additional code(s) to identify all associated manifestations

CC Excl: For CC codes in category Q87, unless otherwise noted:
PDX collection 540

Q87.0 Congenital malformation syndromes predominantly affecting facial appearance
Acrocephalopolysyndactyly
Acrocephalosyndactyly [Apert]
Cryptophthalmos syndrome
Cyclopia
Goldenhar syndrome
Moebius syndrome
Oro-facial-digital syndrome
Robin syndrome
Whistling face

Q87.1 Congenital malformation syndromes predominantly associated with short stature   CC
Aarskog syndrome
Cockayne syndrome
De Lange syndrome
Dubowitz syndrome
Noonan syndrome
Prader-Willi syndrome
Robinow-Silverman-Smith syndrome
Russell-Silver syndrome
Seckel syndrome
EXCLUDES 1   Ellis-van Creveld syndrome (Q77.6)
Smith-Lemli-Opitz syndrome (E78.72)
CC Excl: PDX collection 1110

Q87.2 Congenital malformation syndromes predominantly involving limbs   CC
Holt-Oram syndrome
Klippel-Trenaunay-Weber syndrome
Nail patella syndrome
Rubinstein-Taybi syndrome
Sirenomelia syndrome
Thrombocytopenia with absent radius [TAR] syndrome
VATER syndrome

Q87.3 Congenital malformation syndromes involving early overgrowth   CC
Beckwith-Wiedemann syndrome
Sotos syndrome
Weaver syndrome

☑5ᵗʰ **Q87.4** Marfan's syndrome

CC Excl: For CC codes in subcategory Q87.4:
PDX collection 1110

Q87.40 Marfan's syndrome, unspecified   CC

☑6ᵗʰ **Q87.41** Marfan's syndrome with cardiovascular manifestations

Q87.410 Marfan's syndrome with aortic dilation   CC

Q87.418 Marfan's syndrome with other cardiovascular manifestations   CC

Q87.42 Marfan's syndrome with ocular manifestations   CC

Q87.43 Marfan's syndrome with skeletal manifestation   CC

Q87.5 Other congenital malformation syndromes with other skeletal changes   CC

☑5ᵗʰ **Q87.8** Other specified congenital malformation syndromes, not elsewhere classified
EXCLUDES 1   Zellweger syndrome (E71.510)

Q87.81 Alport syndrome   CC
Use additional code to identify stage of chronic kidney disease (N18.1-N18.6)

Q87.82 Arterial tortuosity syndrome   CC

Q87.89 Other specified congenital malformation syndromes, not elsewhere classified   CC
Laurence-Moon (-Bardet)-Biedl syndrome

☑4ᵗʰ **Q89** Other congenital malformations, not elsewhere classified

☑5ᵗʰ **Q89.0** Congenital absence and malformations of spleen
EXCLUDES 1   isomerism of atrial appendages (with asplenia or polysplenia) (Q20.6)

Q89.01 Asplenia (congenital)   CC
CC Excl: PDX collection 1111

Q89.09 Congenital malformations of spleen   CC
Congenital splenomegaly
CC Excl: PDX collection 1111

☑ Additional Character Req   ☑7ᵗʰ Placeholder Alert   Unacceptable PDx   Manifestation   H1-H14 HAC   HCC CMS-HCC Condition   EXCLUDES 1 Not Coded Here   EXCLUDES 2 Not Included Here

ICD-10-CM 2018   **909**

Q89.1 Congenital malformations of adrenal gland
> *EXCLUDES 1* adrenogenital disorders (E25.-)
> congenital adrenal hyperplasia (E2Ø.Ø)

Q89.2 Congenital malformations of other endocrine glands
Congenital malformation of parathyroid or thyroid gland
Persistent thyroglossal duct
Thyroglossal cyst
> *EXCLUDES 1* congenital goiter (EØ3.Ø)
> congenital hypothyroidism (EØ3.1)

Q89.3 Situs inversus   `CC`
Dextrocardia with situs inversus
Mirror-image atrial arrangement with situs inversus
Situs inversus or transversus abdominalis
Situs inversus or transversus thoracis
Transposition of abdominal viscera
Transposition of thoracic viscera
> *EXCLUDES 1* dextrocardia NOS (Q24.Ø)

CC Excl: PDX collection 1112

Q89.4 Conjoined twins   `MCC`
Craniopagus
Dicephaly
Pygopagus
Thoracopagus
CC Excl: PDX collection 1113

Q89.7 Multiple congenital malformations, not elsewhere classified   `CC`
Multiple congenital anomalies NOS
Multiple congenital deformities NOS
> *EXCLUDES 1* congenital malformation syndromes affecting multiple
> systems (Q87.-)

CC Excl: PDX collection 1112

Q89.8 Other specified congenital malformations   `CC`
Use additional code(s) to identify all associated manifestations
CC Excl: PDX collection 54Ø

Q89.9 Congenital malformation, unspecified
Congenital anomaly NOS
Congenital deformity NOS

Chromosomal abnormalities, not elsewhere classified (Q90-Q99)

> *EXCLUDES 2* mitochondrial metabolic disorders (E88.4-)

✓4ᵗʰ Q90 Down syndrome
Use additional code(s) to identify any associated physical conditions and degree of intellectual disabilities (F7Ø-F79)

Q90.0 Trisomy 21, nonmosaicism (meiotic nondisjunction)

Q90.1 Trisomy 21, mosaicism (mitotic nondisjunction)

Q90.2 Trisomy 21, translocation

Q90.9 Down syndrome, unspecified
Trisomy 21 NOS

✓4ᵗʰ Q91 Trisomy 18 and Trisomy 13

> CC Excl: For CC codes in category Q91: PDX collection 1114

Q91.0 Trisomy 18, nonmosaicism (meiotic nondisjunction) `CC`

Q91.1 Trisomy 18, mosaicism (mitotic nondisjunction)   `CC`

Q91.2 Trisomy 18, translocation   `CC`

Q91.3 Trisomy 18, unspecified   `CC`

Q91.4 Trisomy 13, nonmosaicism (meiotic nondisjunction) `CC`

Q91.5 Trisomy 13, mosaicism (mitotic nondisjunction)   `CC`

Q91.6 Trisomy 13, translocation   `CC`

Q91.7 Trisomy 13, unspecified   `CC`

✓4ᵗʰ Q92 Other trisomies and partial trisomies of the autosomes, not elsewhere classified
> *INCLUDES* unbalanced translocations and insertions
> *EXCLUDES 1* trisomies of chromosomes 13, 18, 21 (Q9Ø-Q91)

Q92.0 Whole chromosome trisomy, nonmosaicism (meiotic nondisjunction)

Q92.1 Whole chromosome trisomy, mosaicism (mitotic nondisjunction)

Q92.2 Partial trisomy
Less than whole arm duplicated
Whole arm or more duplicated
> *EXCLUDES 1* partial trisomy due to unbalanced translocation
> (Q92.5)

Q92.5 Duplications with other complex rearrangements
Partial trisomy due to unbalanced translocations
Code also any associated deletions due to unbalanced translocations, inversions and insertions (Q93.7)

✓5ᵗʰ Q92.6 Marker chromosomes
Trisomies due to dicentrics
Trisomies due to extra rings
Trisomies due to isochromosomes
Individual with marker heterochromatin

Q92.61 Marker chromosomes in normal individual

Q92.62 Marker chromosomes in abnormal individual

Q92.7 Triploidy and polyploidy

Q92.8 Other specified trisomies and partial trisomies of autosomes
Duplications identified by fluorescence in situ hybridization (FISH)
Duplications identified by in situ hybridization (ISH)
Duplications seen only at prometaphase

Q92.9 Trisomy and partial trisomy of autosomes, unspecified

✓4ᵗʰ Q93 Monosomies and deletions from the autosomes, not elsewhere classified

> CC Excl: For CC codes in category Q93, unless otherwise noted:
> PDX collection 1115

Q93.0 Whole chromosome monosomy, nonmosaicism (meiotic nondisjunction)

Q93.1 Whole chromosome monosomy, mosaicism (mitotic nondisjunction)

Q93.2 Chromosome replaced with ring, dicentric or isochromosome

Q93.3 Deletion of short arm of chromosome 4   `CC`
Wolff-Hirschorn syndrome

Q93.4 Deletion of short arm of chromosome 5   `CC`
Cri-du-chat syndrome
CC Excl: PDX collection 1116

Q93.5 Other deletions of part of a chromosome   `CC`
Angelman syndrome

Q93.7 Deletions with other complex rearrangements   `CC`
Deletions due to unbalanced translocations, inversions and insertions
Code also any associated duplications due to unbalanced translocations, inversions and insertions (Q92.5)

✓5ᵗʰ Q93.8 Other deletions from the autosomes

Q93.81 Velo-cardio-facial syndrome   `MCC`
Deletion 22q11.2
DEF: Microdeletion syndrome affecting multiple organs; characteristic cleft palate, heart defects, elongated face with almond-shaped eyes, wide nose, small ears, weak immune system, weak musculature, hypothyroidism, short stature, and scoliosis; deletion at q11.2 on the long arm of the chromosome 22.
CC Excl: PDX collection 1117

Q93.88 Other microdeletions   `CC`
Miller-Dieker syndrome
Smith-Magenis syndrome
CC Excl: PDX collection 1118

Q93.89 Other deletions from the autosomes   `CC`
Deletions identified by fluorescence in situ hybridization (FISH)
Deletions identified by in situ hybridization (ISH)
Deletions seen only at prometaphase

Q93.9 Deletion from autosomes, unspecified   `CC`

✓4ᵗʰ Q95 Balanced rearrangements and structural markers, not elsewhere classified
> *INCLUDES* Robertsonian and balanced reciprocal translocations and insertions

Q95.0 Balanced translocation and insertion in normal individual

Q95.1 Chromosome inversion in normal individual

Q95.2 Balanced autosomal rearrangement in abnormal individual

Q95.3 Balanced sex/autosomal rearrangement in abnormal individual

Q95.5 Individual with autosomal fragile site

Q95.8 Other balanced rearrangements and structural markers

Q95.9 Balanced rearrangement and structural marker, unspecified

✓4ᵗʰ Q96 Turner's syndrome
> *EXCLUDES 1* Noonan syndrome (Q87.1)

Q96.0 Karyotype 45, X   ♀

Q96.1 Karyotype 46, X iso (Xq)   ♀
Karyotype 46, isochromosome Xq

Q96.2 Karyotype 46, X with abnormal sex chromosome, except iso (Xq)   ♀
Karyotype 46, X with abnormal sex chromosome, except isochromosome Xq

Q96.3 Mosaicism, 45, X/46, XX or XY   ♀

N Newborn: 0   P Pediatric: 0-17   M Maternity: 12-55   A Adult: 15-124   `MCC` Major CC Condition   `PDx MCC` PDx acts as own MCC   `CC` CC Condition   `PDx CC` PDx acts as own CC

Q96.4 **Mosaicism, 45, X/other cell line(s) with abnormal sex chromosome** ♀

Q96.8 **Other variants of Turner's syndrome** ♀

Q96.9 **Turner's syndrome, unspecified** ♀

✓4ᵗʰ **Q97 Other sex chromosome abnormalities, female phenotype, not elsewhere classified**

　　EXCLUDES 1 Turner's syndrome (Q96.-)

Q97.0 **Karyotype 47, XXX** ♀

Q97.1 **Female with more than three X chromosomes** ♀

Q97.2 **Mosaicism, lines with various numbers of X chromosomes** ♀

Q97.3 **Female with 46, XY karyotype** ♀

Q97.8 **Other specified sex chromosome abnormalities, female phenotype** ♀

Q97.9 **Sex chromosome abnormality, female phenotype, unspecified** ♀

✓4ᵗʰ **Q98 Other sex chromosome abnormalities, male phenotype, not elsewhere classified**

Q98.0 **Klinefelter syndrome karyotype 47, XXY** ♂

Q98.1 **Klinefelter syndrome, male with more than two X chromosomes** ♂

Q98.3 **Other male with 46, XX karyotype** ♂

Q98.4 **Klinefelter syndrome, unspecified** ♂

Q98.5 **Karyotype 47, XYY**

Q98.6 **Male with structurally abnormal sex chromosome** ♂

Q98.7 **Male with sex chromosome mosaicism** ♂

Q98.8 **Other specified sex chromosome abnormalities, male phenotype** ♂

Q98.9 **Sex chromosome abnormality, male phenotype, unspecified** ♂

✓4ᵗʰ **Q99 Other chromosome abnormalities, not elsewhere classified**

Q99.0 **Chimera 46, XX/46, XY**
　　Chimera 46, XX/46, XY true hermaphrodite

Q99.1 **46, XX true hermaphrodite**
　　46, XX with streak gonads
　　46, XY with streak gonads
　　Pure gonadal dysgenesis

Q99.2 **Fragile X chromosome**
　　Fragile X syndrome

Q99.8 **Other specified chromosome abnormalities**

Q99.9 **Chromosomal abnormality, unspecified**

✓Additional Character Req ✓x7ᵗʰ Placeholder Alert Unacceptable PDx Manifestation **H1**-**H14** HAC **HCC** CMS-HCC Condition *EXCLUDES 1* Not Coded Here *EXCLUDES 2* Not Included Here

ICD-10-CM 2018   **911**

Chapter 18. Symptoms, Signs and Abnormal Clinical and Laboratory Findings, Not Elsewhere Classified (R00–R99)

Chapter Specific Guidelines with Coding Examples

The chapter specific guidelines from the ICD-10-CM Official Guidelines for Coding and Reporting have been provided below. Along with these guidelines are coding examples, contained in the shaded boxes, that have been developed to help illustrate the coding and/or sequencing guidance found in these guidelines.

Chapter 18 includes symptoms, signs, abnormal results of clinical or other investigative procedures, and ill-defined conditions regarding which no diagnosis classifiable elsewhere is recorded. Signs and symptoms that point to a specific diagnosis have been assigned to a category in other chapters of the classification.

a. Use of symptom codes

Codes that describe symptoms and signs are acceptable for reporting purposes when a related definitive diagnosis has not been established (confirmed) by the provider.

Chest pain of unknown origin

R07.9   Chest pain, unspecified

Explanation: Codes that describe symptoms such as chest pain are acceptable for reporting purposes when the provider has not established (confirmed) a related definitive diagnosis.

b. Use of a symptom code with a definitive diagnosis code

Codes for signs and symptoms may be reported in addition to a related definitive diagnosis when the sign or symptom is not routinely associated with that diagnosis, such as the various signs and symptoms associated with complex syndromes. The definitive diagnosis code should be sequenced before the symptom code.

Signs or symptoms that are associated routinely with a disease process should not be assigned as additional codes, unless otherwise instructed by the classification.

Pneumonia with hemoptysis

J18.9   Pneumonia, unspecified organism

R04.2   Hemoptysis

Explanation: Codes for signs and symptoms may be reported in addition to a related definitive diagnosis when the sign or symptom is not routinely associated with that diagnosis.

Abdominal pain due to acute appendicitis

K35.80   Unspecified acute appendicitis

Explanation: Codes for signs or symptoms routinely associated with a disease process should not be assigned unless the classification instructs otherwise.

c. Combination codes that include symptoms

ICD-10-CM contains a number of combination codes that identify both the definitive diagnosis and common symptoms of that diagnosis. When using one of these combination codes, an additional code should not be assigned for the symptom.

Acute gastritis with hemorrhage

K29.01   Acute gastritis with bleeding

Explanation: When a combination code identifies both the definitive diagnosis and the symptom, an additional code should not be assigned for the symptom.

d. Repeated falls

Code R29.6, Repeated falls, is for use for encounters when a patient has recently fallen and the reason for the fall is being investigated.

Code Z91.81, History of falling, is for use when a patient has fallen in the past and is at risk for future falls. When appropriate, both codes R29.6 and Z91.81 may be assigned together.

e. Coma scale

The coma scale codes (R40.2-) can be used in conjunction with traumatic brain injury codes, acute cerebrovascular disease or sequelae of cerebrovascular disease codes. These codes are primarily for use by trauma registries, but they may be used in any setting where this information is collected. The coma scale may also be used to assess the status of the central nervous system for other non-trauma conditions, such as monitoring patients in the intensive care unit regardless of medical condition. The coma scale codes should be sequenced after the diagnosis code(s).

These codes, one from each subcategory, are needed to complete the scale. The 7th character indicates when the scale was recorded. The 7th character should match for all three codes.

At a minimum, report the initial score documented on presentation at your facility. This may be a score from the emergency medicine technician (EMT) or in the emergency department. If desired, a facility may choose to capture multiple coma scale scores.

Assign code R40.24, Glasgow coma scale, total score, when only the total score is documented in the medical record and not the individual score(s).

23-year-old man found down after unknown injury with skull fracture and with concussion and loss of consciousness of unknown duration. EMS evaluated the patient in the field and reported the individual Glasgow coma scores:

Eye opening response—3: eyes open to speech

Verbal response—4: confused but coherent speech

Motor response—6: obeys commands fully

S02.0XXA   Fracture of vault of skull, initial encounter for closed fracture

S06.0X9A   Concussion with loss of consciousness of unspecified duration, initial encounter

R40.2131   Coma scale, eyes open, to sound, in the field [EMT or ambulance]

R40.2241   Coma scale, best verbal response, confused conversation, in the field [EMT or ambulance]

R40.2361   Coma scale, best motor response, obeys commands, in the field [EMT or ambulance]

Explanation: When individual scores for the Glasgow coma scale are documented, one code from each category is needed to complete the scale. The seventh character indicates when the scale was recorded and should match for all three codes. Assign a code from subcategory R40.24- Glasgow coma scale, total score, when only the total and not the individual score(s) is documented.

Patient with intractable epilepsy with status epilepticus arrives to ED with alteration of consciousness. Coma scale performed en route by EMT documented total coma score as 11. Another coma score was performed upon hospital admission that was documented as 14.

G40.911   Epilepsy, unspecified, intractable, with status epilepticus

R40.2421   lasgow coma scale score 9-12, in the field [EMT or ambulance]

R40.2413   Glasgow coma scale score 13-15, at hospital admission

Explanation: Coma scores may be used to assess mental status in non-trauma conditions. Use only code R40.24- Glasgow coma scale, total scores when individual scores are unavailable. Multiple scores may be reported with the seventh character representing where or when the assessment was made.

f. Functional quadriplegia
GUIDELINE HAS BEEN DELETED EFFECTIVE OCTOBER 1, 2017

g. SIRS due to non-infectious process

The systemic inflammatory response syndrome (SIRS) can develop as a result of certain non-infectious disease processes, such as trauma, malignant neoplasm, or pancreatitis. When SIRS is documented with a noninfectious condition, and no subsequent infection is documented, the code for the underlying condition, such as an injury, should be assigned, followed by code

R65.1Ø, Systemic inflammatory response syndrome (SIRS) of non-infectious origin without acute organ dysfunction, or code R65.11, Systemic inflammatory response syndrome (SIRS) of non-infectious origin with acute organ dysfunction. If an associated acute organ dysfunction is documented, the appropriate code(s) for the specific type of organ dysfunction(s) should be assigned in addition to code R65.11. If acute organ dysfunction is documented, but it cannot be determined if the acute organ dysfunction is associated with SIRS or due to another condition (e.g., directly due to the trauma), the provider should be queried.

Systemic inflammatory response syndrome (SIRS) due to acute gallstone pancreatitis

K85.1Ø   **Biliary acute pancreatitis without necrosis or infection**

R65.1Ø   **Systemic inflammatory response syndrome (SIRS) of noninfectious origin without acute organ dysfunction**

Explanation: When SIRS is documented with a noninfectious condition without subsequent infection documented, the code for the underlying condition such as pancreatitis should be assigned followed by the appropriate code for SIRS of noninfectious origin, either with or without associated organ dysfunction.

h. Death NOS

Code R99, Ill-defined and unknown cause of mortality, is only for use in the very limited circumstance when a patient who has already died is brought into an emergency department or other healthcare facility and is pronounced dead upon arrival. It does not represent the discharge disposition of death.

i. NIHSS stroke scale

The NIH stroke scale (NIHSS) codes (R29.7- -) can be used in conjunction with acute stroke codes (I63) to identify the patient's neurological status and the severity of the stroke. The stroke scale codes should be sequenced after the acute stroke diagnosis code(s).

At a minimum, report the initial score documented. If desired, a facility may choose to capture multiple stroke scale scores.

See Section I.B.14. for information concerning the medical record documentation that may be used for assignment of the NIHSS codes.

Patient admitted with CVA seen by neurology consult who documents moderate to severe stroke, 17 on NIHSS stroke scale.

I63.9   **Cerebral infarction, unspecified**

R29.717   **NIHSS score 17**

Explanation: Unspecified cerebral vascular accident (CVA) is sequenced before the NIHSS stroke scale score code. The stroke scale is an assessment tool to help measure stroke-related neurological deficits. Fifteen items are evaluated by trained observers and include such conditions as levels of consciousness, language, dysarthria, ataxia, and sensory loss. A facility may report multiple stroke scale scores if it wants to.

Chapter 18. Symptoms, Signs and Abnormal Clinical and Laboratory Findings, Not Elsewhere Classified (R00-R99)

NOTE   This chapter includes symptoms, signs, abnormal results of clinical or other investigative procedures, and ill-defined conditions regarding which no diagnosis classifiable elsewhere is recorded.

Signs and symptoms that point rather definitely to a given diagnosis have been assigned to a category in other chapters of the classification. In general, categories in this chapter include the less well-defined conditions and symptoms that, without the necessary study of the case to establish a final diagnosis, point perhaps equally to two or more diseases or to two or more systems of the body. Practically all categories in the chapter could be designated "not otherwise specified", "unknown etiology" or "transient". The Alphabetical Index should be consulted to determine which symptoms and signs are to be allocated here and which to other chapters. The residual subcategories, numbered .8, are generally provided for other relevant symptoms that cannot be allocated elsewhere in the classification.

The conditions and signs or symptoms included in categories R00-R94 consist of:

(a)   cases for which no more specific diagnosis can be made even after all the facts bearing on the case have been investigated;

(b)   signs or symptoms existing at the time of initial encounter that proved to be transient and whose causes could not be determined;

(c)   provisional diagnosis in a patient who failed to return for further investigation or care;

(d)   cases referred elsewhere for investigation or treatment before the diagnosis was made;

(e)   cases in which a more precise diagnosis was not available for any other reason;

(f)   certain symptoms, for which supplementary information is provided, that represent important problems in medical care in their own right.

EXCLUDES 2   *abnormal findings on antenatal screening of mother (O28.-)*
certain conditions originating in the perinatal period (P04-P96)
signs and symptoms classified in the body system chapters
signs and symptoms of breast (N63, N64.5)

AHA: 2017, 1Q, 6, 7

This chapter contains the following blocks:

R00-R09   Symptoms and signs involving the circulatory and respiratory systems
R10-R19   Symptoms and signs involving the digestive system and abdomen
R20-R23   Symptoms and signs involving the skin and subcutaneous tissue
R25-R29   Symptoms and signs involving the nervous and musculoskeletal systems
R30-R39   Symptoms and signs involving the genitourinary system
R40-R46   Symptoms and signs involving cognition, perception, emotional state and behavior
R47-R49   Symptoms and signs involving speech and voice
R50-R69   General symptoms and signs
R70-R79   Abnormal findings on examination of blood, without diagnosis
R80-R82   Abnormal findings on examination of urine, without diagnosis
R83-R89   Abnormal findings on examination of other body fluids, substances and tissues, without diagnosis
R90-R94   Abnormal findings on diagnostic imaging and in function studies, without diagnosis
R97   Abnormal tumor markers
R99   Ill-defined and unknown cause of mortality

Symptoms and signs involving the circulatory and respiratory systems (R00-R09)

☑4ᵗʰ R00   Abnormalities of heart beat
    EXCLUDES 1   *abnormalities originating in the perinatal period (P29.1-)*
    EXCLUDES 2   *specified arrhythmias (I47-I49)*

    R00.0   Tachycardia, unspecified
      Rapid heart beat
      Sinoauricular tachycardia NOS
      Sinus [sinusal] tachycardia NOS
      EXCLUDES 1   *neonatal tachycardia (P29.11)*
               paroxysmal tachycardia (I47.-)
      DEF: Excessively rapid heart rate of more than 100 beats per minute.

    R00.1   Bradycardia, unspecified
      Sinoatrial bradycardia
      Sinus bradycardia
      Slow heart beat
      Vagal bradycardia
      Use additional code for adverse effect, if applicable, to identify drug (T36-T50 with fifth or sixth character 5)
      EXCLUDES 1   *neonatal bradycardia (P29.12)*

    R00.2   Palpitations
      Awareness of heart beat

    R00.8   Other abnormalities of heart beat

    R00.9   Unspecified abnormalities of heart beat

☑4ᵗʰ R01   Cardiac murmurs and other cardiac sounds
    EXCLUDES 1   *cardiac murmurs and sounds originating in the perinatal period (P29.8)*

    R01.0   Benign and innocent cardiac murmurs
      Functional cardiac murmur

    R01.1   Cardiac murmur, unspecified
      Cardiac bruit NOS
      Heart murmur NOS
      Systolic murmur NOS

    R01.2   Other cardiac sounds
      Cardiac dullness, increased or decreased
      Precordial friction

☑4ᵗʰ R03   Abnormal blood-pressure reading, without diagnosis

   4   R03.0   Elevated blood-pressure reading, without diagnosis of hypertension
      NOTE   This category is to be used to record an episode of elevated blood pressure in a patient in whom no formal diagnosis of hypertension has been made, or as an isolated incidental finding.

    R03.1   Nonspecific low blood-pressure reading
      EXCLUDES 1   *hypotension (I95.-)*
               maternal hypotension syndrome (O26.5-)
               neurogenic orthostatic hypotension (G90.3)

☑4ᵗʰ R04   Hemorrhage from respiratory passages

    CC Excl: For CC codes in category R04: PDX collection 1119

    R04.0   Epistaxis
      Hemorrhage from nose
      Nosebleed

    R04.1   Hemorrhage from throat
      EXCLUDES 2   *hemoptysis (R04.2)*

    R04.2   Hemoptysis   **CC**
      Blood-stained sputum
      Cough with hemorrhage
      AHA: 2013, 4Q, 118

☑5ᵗʰ R04.8   Hemorrhage from other sites in respiratory passages

      R04.81   Acute idiopathic pulmonary hemorrhage in infants   **CC** **P**
         AIPHI
         Acute idiopathic hemorrhage in infants over 28 days old
         EXCLUDES 1   *perinatal pulmonary hemorrhage (P26.-)*
                  von Willebrand's disease (D68.0)

      R04.89   Hemorrhage from other sites in respiratory passages   **CC**
         Pulmonary hemorrhage NOS

    R04.9   Hemorrhage from respiratory passages, unspecified   **CC**

R05   Cough
    EXCLUDES 1   *cough with hemorrhage (R04.2)*
               smoker's cough (J41.0)
    AHA: 2016, 2Q, 33

☑4ᵗʰ R06   Abnormalities of breathing
    EXCLUDES 1   *acute respiratory distress syndrome (J80)*
               respiratory arrest (R09.2)
               respiratory arrest of newborn (P28.81)
               respiratory distress syndrome of newborn (P22.-)
               respiratory failure (J96.-)
               respiratory failure of newborn (P28.5)

☑5ᵗʰ R06.0   Dyspnea
    EXCLUDES 1   *tachypnea NOS (R06.82)*
               transient tachypnea of newborn (P22.1)

      R06.00   Dyspnea, unspecified
         AHA: 2017, 1Q, 26

      R06.01   Orthopnea

---

4   Questionable admission when used as PDx.

☑ Additional Character Req   ✓x7ᵗʰ Placeholder Alert   Unacceptable PDx   Manifestation   **H1**-**H14** HAC   **HCC** CMS-HCC Condition   *EXCLUDES 1* Not Coded Here   *EXCLUDES 2* Not Included Here

ICD-10-CM 2018   915

●
R06.02   **Shortness of breath**

R06.03   **Acute respiratory distress**

R06.09   **Other forms of dyspnea**

R06.1   **Stridor**
> EXCLUDES 1   *congenital laryngeal stridor (P28.89)*
> *laryngismus (stridulus) (J38.5)*

R06.2   **Wheezing**
> EXCLUDES 1   *asthma (J45.-)*

AHA: 2016, 2Q, 33
DEF: High-pitched whistling sound during breathing due to stenosis of respiratory passageway; associated with asthma, sleep apnea, bronchiectasis, bronchiolitis, COPD, and pleural effusion.

R06.3   **Periodic breathing**   CC
> Cheyne-Stokes breathing
> **CC Excl:** PDX collection 1120

R06.4   **Hyperventilation**
> EXCLUDES 1   *psychogenic hyperventilation (F45.8)*

R06.5   **Mouth breathing**
> EXCLUDES 2   *dry mouth NOS (R68.2)*

R06.6   **Hiccough**
> EXCLUDES 1   *psychogenic hiccough (F45.8)*

R06.7   **Sneezing**

√5th   R06.8   **Other abnormalities of breathing**

R06.81   **Apnea, not elsewhere classified**
> Apnea NOS
> EXCLUDES 1   *apnea (of) newborn (P28.4)*
> *sleep apnea (G47.3-)*
> *sleep apnea of newborn (primary) (P28.3)*

R06.82   **Tachypnea, not elsewhere classified**
> Tachypnea NOS
> EXCLUDES 1   *transitory tachypnea of newborn (P22.1)*

R06.83   **Snoring**

R06.89   **Other abnormalities of breathing**
> Breath-holding (spells)
> Sighing

R06.9   **Unspecified abnormalities of breathing**

√4th   **R07**   **Pain in throat and chest**
> EXCLUDES 1   *epidemic myalgia (B33.0)*
> EXCLUDES 2   *jaw pain (R68.84)*
> *pain in breast (N64.4)*

R07.0   **Pain in throat**
> EXCLUDES 1   *chronic sore throat (J31.2)*
> *sore throat (acute) NOS (J02.9)*
> EXCLUDES 2   *dysphagia (R13.1-)*
> *pain in neck (M54.2)*

R07.1   **Chest pain on breathing**
> Painful respiration

R07.2   **Precordial pain**

√5th   R07.8   **Other chest pain**

R07.81   **Pleurodynia**
> Pleurodynia NOS
> EXCLUDES 1   *epidemic pleurodynia (B33.0)*

R07.82   **Intercostal pain**

R07.89   **Other chest pain**
> Anterior chest-wall pain NOS

R07.9   **Chest pain, unspecified**

√4th   **R09**   **Other symptoms and signs involving the circulatory and respiratory system**
> EXCLUDES 1   *acute respiratory distress syndrome (J80)*
> *respiratory arrest of newborn (P28.81)*
> *respiratory distress syndrome of newborn (P22.0)*
> *respiratory failure (J96.-)*
> *respiratory failure of newborn (P28.5)*

√5th   R09.0   **Asphyxia and hypoxemia**
> EXCLUDES 1   *asphyxia due to carbon monoxide (T58.-)*
> *asphyxia due to foreign body in respiratory tract (T17.-)*
> *birth (intrauterine) asphyxia (P84)*
> *hypercapnia (R06.4)*
> *hyperventilation (R06.4)*
> *traumatic asphyxia (T71.-)*
> EXCLUDES 2 ▶ *hypercapnia (R06.89)* ◄

R09.01   **Asphyxia**   CC
> **CC Excl:** PDX collection 1121

R09.02   **Hypoxemia**

R09.1   **Pleurisy**
> EXCLUDES 1   *pleurisy with effusion (J90)*

1   R09.2   **Respiratory arrest**   MCC HCC
> Cardiorespiratory failure
> EXCLUDES 1   *cardiac arrest (I46.-)*
> *respiratory arrest of newborn (P28.81)*
> *respiratory distress of newborn (P22.0)*
> *respiratory failure (J96.-)*
> *respiratory failure of newborn (P28.5)*
> *respiratory insufficiency (R06.89)*
> *respiratory insufficiency of newborn (P28.5)*

CC Excl: PDX collection 1121

R09.3   **Abnormal sputum**
> Abnormal amount of sputum
> Abnormal color of sputum
> Abnormal odor of sputum
> Excessive sputum
> EXCLUDES 1   *blood-stained sputum (R04.2)*

√5th   R09.8   **Other specified symptoms and signs involving the circulatory and respiratory systems**

R09.81   **Nasal congestion**

R09.82   **Postnasal drip**

R09.89   **Other specified symptoms and signs involving the circulatory and respiratory systems**
> Abnormal chest percussion
> Bruit (arterial)
> Chest tympany
> Choking sensation
> Feeling of foreign body in throat
> Friction sounds in chest
> Rales
> Weak pulse
> EXCLUDES 2   *foreign body in throat (T17.2-)*
> *wheezing (R06.2)*

Symptoms and signs involving the digestive system and abdomen (R10-R19)

> EXCLUDES 2   *congenital or infantile pylorospasm (Q40.0)*
> *gastrointestinal hemorrhage (K92.0-K92.2)*
> *intestinal obstruction (K56.-)*
> *newborn gastrointestinal hemorrhage (P54.0-P54.3)*
> *newborn intestinal obstruction (P76.-)*
> *pylorospasm (K31.3)*
> *signs and symptoms involving the urinary system (R30-R39)*
> *symptoms referable to female genital organs (N94.-)*
> *symptoms referable to male genital organs (N48-N50)*

√4th   **R10**   **Abdominal and pelvic pain**
> EXCLUDES 1   *renal colic (N23)*
> EXCLUDES 2   *dorsalgia (M54.-)*
> *flatulence and related conditions (R14.-)*

R10.0   **Acute abdomen**
> Severe abdominal pain (generalized) (with abdominal rigidity)
> EXCLUDES 1   *abdominal rigidity NOS (R19.3)*
> *generalized abdominal pain NOS (R10.84)*
> *localized abdominal pain (R10.1-R10.3-)*

Abdominal Pain

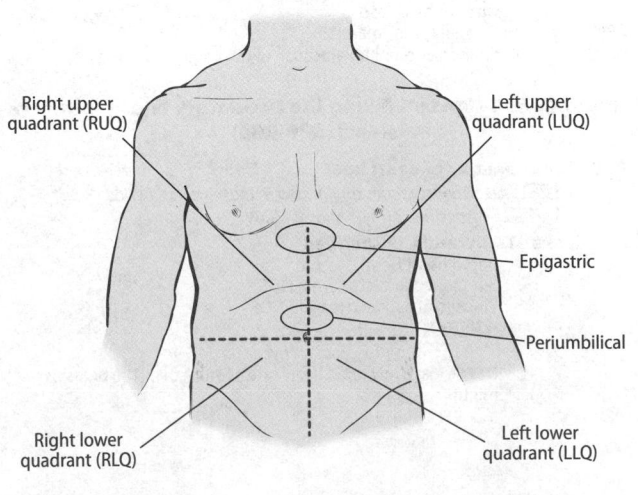

Right upper quadrant (RUQ)

Left upper quadrant (LUQ)

Epigastric

Periumbilical

Right lower quadrant (RLQ)

Left lower quadrant (LLQ)

---

1   MCC only if patient is discharged alive.

N Newborn: 0   P Pediatric: 0-17   M Maternity: 12-55   A Adult: 15-124   MCC Major CC Condition   PDxMCC PDx acts as own MCC   CC CC Condition   PDxCC PDx acts as own CC

✓5ᵗʰ **R10.1 Pain localized to upper abdomen**
     R10.10 Upper abdominal pain, unspecified
     R10.11 Right upper quadrant pain
     R10.12 Left upper quadrant pain
     R10.13 Epigastric pain
        Dyspepsia
        EXCLUDES 1   functional dyspepsia (K30)

R10.2 Pelvic and perineal pain
     EXCLUDES 1   vulvodynia (N94.81)

✓5ᵗʰ **R10.3 Pain localized to other parts of lower abdomen**
     R10.30 Lower abdominal pain, unspecified
     R10.31 Right lower quadrant pain
     R10.32 Left lower quadrant pain
     R10.33 Periumbilical pain

✓5ᵗʰ **R10.8 Other abdominal pain**
     ✓6ᵗʰ **R10.81 Abdominal tenderness**
        Abdominal tenderness NOS
        R10.811 Right upper quadrant abdominal tenderness
        R10.812 Left upper quadrant abdominal tenderness
        R10.813 Right lower quadrant abdominal tenderness
        R10.814 Left lower quadrant abdominal tenderness
        R10.815 Periumbilic abdominal tenderness
        R10.816 Epigastric abdominal tenderness
        R10.817 Generalized abdominal tenderness
        R10.819 Abdominal tenderness, unspecified site
     ✓6ᵗʰ **R10.82 Rebound abdominal tenderness**
        R10.821 Right upper quadrant rebound abdominal tenderness
        R10.822 Left upper quadrant rebound abdominal tenderness
        R10.823 Right lower quadrant rebound abdominal tenderness
        R10.824 Left lower quadrant rebound abdominal tenderness
        R10.825 Periumbilic rebound abdominal tenderness
        R10.826 Epigastric rebound abdominal tenderness
        R10.827 Generalized rebound abdominal tenderness
        R10.829 Rebound abdominal tenderness, unspecified site
     R10.83 Colic   P
        Colic NOS
        Infantile colic
        EXCLUDES 1   colic in adult and child over 12 months old (R10.84)
        DEF: Inconsolable crying in an otherwise well-fed and healthy infant for more than three hours a day, three days a week, for more than three weeks.
     R10.84 Generalized abdominal pain
        EXCLUDES 1   generalized abdominal pain associated with acute abdomen (R10.0)

R10.9 Unspecified abdominal pain

✓4ᵗʰ **R11 Nausea and vomiting**
     EXCLUDES 1   cyclical vomiting associated with migraine (G43.A-)
        excessive vomiting in pregnancy (O21.-)
        hematemesis (K92.0)
        neonatal hematemesis (P54.0)
        newborn vomiting (P92.0-)
        psychogenic vomiting (F50.89)
        vomiting associated with bulimia nervosa (F50.2)
        vomiting following gastrointestinal surgery (K91.0)
     AHA: 2017, 1Q, 28
     R11.0 Nausea
        Nausea NOS
        Nausea without vomiting
     ✓5ᵗʰ **R11.1 Vomiting**
        R11.10 Vomiting, unspecified
          Vomiting NOS
        R11.11 Vomiting without nausea
        R11.12 Projectile vomiting
        R11.13 Vomiting of fecal matter

Swallowing Function

Oral phase   Oropharyngeal phase

Pharyngeal phase   Pharyngoesophageal phase

        R11.14 Bilious vomiting
          Bilious emesis
     R11.2 Nausea with vomiting, unspecified
        Persistent nausea with vomiting NOS

R12 Heartburn
     EXCLUDES 1   dyspepsia NOS (R10.13)
        functional dyspepsia (K30)

✓4ᵗʰ **R13 Aphagia and dysphagia**
     R13.0 Aphagia
        Inability to swallow
        EXCLUDES 1   psychogenic aphagia (F50.9)
     ✓5ᵗʰ **R13.1 Dysphagia**
        Code first, if applicable, dysphagia following cerebrovascular disease (I69. with final characters -91)
        EXCLUDES 1   psychogenic dysphagia (F45.8)
        R13.10 Dysphagia, unspecified
          Difficulty in swallowing NOS
        R13.11 Dysphagia, oral phase
        R13.12 Dysphagia, oropharyngeal phase
        R13.13 Dysphagia, pharyngeal phase
        R13.14 Dysphagia, pharyngoesophageal phase
        R13.19 Other dysphagia
          Cervical dysphagia
          Neurogenic dysphagia

✓4ᵗʰ **R14 Flatulence and related conditions**
     EXCLUDES 1   psychogenic aerophagy (F45.8)
     R14.0 Abdominal distension (gaseous)
        Bloating
        Tympanites (abdominal) (intestinal)
     R14.1 Gas pain
     R14.2 Eructation
     R14.3 Flatulence

✓4ᵗʰ **R15 Fecal incontinence**
     INCLUDES   encopresis NOS
     EXCLUDES 1   fecal incontinence of nonorganic origin (F98.1)
     R15.0 Incomplete defecation
        EXCLUDES 1   constipation (K59.0-)
        fecal impaction (K56.41)
     R15.1 Fecal smearing
        Fecal soiling
     R15.2 Fecal urgency
     R15.9 Full incontinence of feces
        Fecal incontinence NOS

✓4ᵗʰ **R16 Hepatomegaly and splenomegaly, not elsewhere classified**
     R16.0 Hepatomegaly, not elsewhere classified
        Hepatomegaly NOS
     R16.1 Splenomegaly, not elsewhere classified
        Splenomegaly NOS
     R16.2 Hepatomegaly with splenomegaly, not elsewhere classified
        Hepatosplenomegaly NOS

☑ Additional Character Req   ☑x7ᵗʰ Placeholder Alert   Unacceptable PDx   Manifestation   H1-H14 HAC   HCC CMS-HCC Condition   EXCLUDES 1 Not Coded Here   EXCLUDES 2 Not Included Here

ICD-10-CM 2018   917

R17 Unspecified jaundice   CC
     EXCLUDES 1   *neonatal jaundice (P55, P57-P59)*
     CC Excl: PDX collection 1122

✓4th **R18 Ascites**
     INCLUDES   fluid in peritoneal cavity
     EXCLUDES 1   *ascites in alcoholic cirrhosis (K70.31)*
                ascites in alcoholic hepatitis (K70.11)
                ascites in toxic liver disease with chronic active hepatitis
                   (K71.51)

    R18.0 Malignant ascites   CC
        Code first malignancy, such as:
            malignant neoplasm of ovary (C56.-)
            secondary malignant neoplasm of retroperitoneum and
                peritoneum (C78.6)
        CC Excl: PDX collection 1123

    R18.8 Other ascites   CC
        Ascites NOS
        Peritoneal effusion (chronic)
        CC Excl: PDX collection 1123

✓4th **R19 Other symptoms and signs involving the digestive system and abdomen**
     EXCLUDES 1   *acute abdomen (R10.0)*

   ✓5th **R19.0 Intra-abdominal and pelvic swelling, mass and lump**
      EXCLUDES 1   *abdominal distension (gaseous) (R14.-)*
                ascites (R18.-)

     R19.00 Intra-abdominal and pelvic swelling, mass and lump, unspecified site
     R19.01 Right upper quadrant abdominal swelling, mass and lump
     R19.02 Left upper quadrant abdominal swelling, mass and lump
     R19.03 Right lower quadrant abdominal swelling, mass and lump
     R19.04 Left lower quadrant abdominal swelling, mass and lump
     R19.05 Periumbilic swelling, mass or lump
         Diffuse or generalized umbilical swelling or mass
     R19.06 Epigastric swelling, mass or lump
     R19.07 Generalized intra-abdominal and pelvic swelling, mass and lump
         Diffuse or generalized intra-abdominal swelling or mass NOS
         Diffuse or generalized pelvic swelling or mass NOS
     R19.09 Other intra-abdominal and pelvic swelling, mass and lump

   ✓5th **R19.1 Abnormal bowel sounds**
     R19.11 Absent bowel sounds
     R19.12 Hyperactive bowel sounds
     R19.15 Other abnormal bowel sounds
         Abnormal bowel sounds NOS

    R19.2 Visible peristalsis
        Hyperperistalsis
        DEF: Visible movements of muscular attempts to move food through the digestive tract; due to pyloric obstruction, stomach obstruction, or intestinal obstruction.

   ✓5th **R19.3 Abdominal rigidity**
      EXCLUDES 1   *abdominal rigidity with severe abdominal pain (R10.0)*
     R19.30 Abdominal rigidity, unspecified site
     R19.31 Right upper quadrant abdominal rigidity
     R19.32 Left upper quadrant abdominal rigidity
     R19.33 Right lower quadrant abdominal rigidity
     R19.34 Left lower quadrant abdominal rigidity
     R19.35 Periumbilic abdominal rigidity
     R19.36 Epigastric abdominal rigidity
     R19.37 Generalized abdominal rigidity

    R19.4 Change in bowel habit
      EXCLUDES 1   *constipation (K59.0-)*
                functional diarrhea (K59.1)

    R19.5 Other fecal abnormalities
        Abnormal stool color
        Bulky stools
        Mucus in stools
        Occult blood in feces
        Occult blood in stools
      EXCLUDES 1   *melena (K92.1)*
                neonatal melena (P54.1)

    R19.6 Halitosis
    R19.7 Diarrhea, unspecified
        Diarrhea NOS
      EXCLUDES 1   *functional diarrhea (K59.1)*
                neonatal diarrhea (P78.3)
                psychogenic diarrhea (F45.8)
    R19.8 Other specified symptoms and signs involving the digestive system and abdomen

Symptoms and signs involving the skin and subcutaneous tissue (R20-R23)
     EXCLUDES 2   *symptoms relating to breast (N64.4-N64.5)*

✓4th **R20 Disturbances of skin sensation**
     EXCLUDES 1   *dissociative anesthesia and sensory loss (F44.6)*
                psychogenic disturbances (F45.8)

    R20.0 Anesthesia of skin
    R20.1 Hypoesthesia of skin
    R20.2 Paresthesia of skin
        Formication
        Pins and needles
        Tingling skin
      EXCLUDES 1   *acroparesthesia (I73.8)*
    R20.3 Hyperesthesia
    R20.8 Other disturbances of skin sensation
    R20.9 Unspecified disturbances of skin sensation

   R21 Rash and other nonspecific skin eruption
     INCLUDES   rash NOS
     EXCLUDES 1   *specified type of rash—code to condition*
                vesicular eruption (R23.8)

✓4th **R22 Localized swelling, mass and lump of skin and subcutaneous tissue**
     INCLUDES   subcutaneous nodules (localized)(superficial)
     EXCLUDES 1   *abnormal findings on diagnostic imaging (R90-R93)*
                edema (R60.-)
                enlarged lymph nodes (R59.-)
                localized adiposity (E65)
                swelling of joint (M25.4-)

    R22.0 Localized swelling, mass and lump, head
    R22.1 Localized swelling, mass and lump, neck
    R22.2 Localized swelling, mass and lump, trunk
      EXCLUDES 1   *intra-abdominal or pelvic mass and lump (R19.0-)*
                intra-abdominal or pelvic swelling (R19.0-)
      EXCLUDES 2   *breast mass and lump (N63)*

   ✓5th **R22.3 Localized swelling, mass and lump, upper limb**
     R22.30 Localized swelling, mass and lump, unspecified upper limb
     R22.31 Localized swelling, mass and lump, right upper limb
     R22.32 Localized swelling, mass and lump, left upper limb
     R22.33 Localized swelling, mass and lump, upper limb, bilateral

   ✓5th **R22.4 Localized swelling, mass and lump, lower limb**
     R22.40 Localized swelling, mass and lump, unspecified lower limb
     R22.41 Localized swelling, mass and lump, right lower limb
     R22.42 Localized swelling, mass and lump, left lower limb
     R22.43 Localized swelling, mass and lump, lower limb, bilateral

    R22.9 Localized swelling, mass and lump, unspecified

✓4th **R23 Other skin changes**
    R23.0 Cyanosis
      EXCLUDES 1   *acrocyanosis (I73.8)*
                cyanotic attacks of newborn (P28.2)
        DEF: Bluish or purplish discoloration of the skin due to inadequate oxygen level of blood.

    R23.1 Pallor
        Clammy skin
    R23.2 Flushing
        Excessive blushing
        Code first, if applicable, menopausal and female climacteric states (N95.1)
    R23.3 Spontaneous ecchymoses
        Petechiae
      EXCLUDES 1   *ecchymoses of newborn (P54.5)*
                purpura (D69.-)

N Newborn: 0   P Pediatric: 0-17   M Maternity: 12-55   A Adult: 15-124   MCC Major CC Condition   PDx MCC PDx acts as own MCC   CC CC Condition   PDx CC PDx acts as own CC

918   ICD-10-CM 2018

R23.4   Changes in skin texture
Desquamation of skin
Induration of skin
Scaling of skin
EXCLUDES 1   epidermal thickening NOS (L85.9)

R23.8   Other skin changes

R23.9   Unspecified skin changes

Symptoms and signs involving the nervous and musculoskeletal systems (R25-R29)

✓4ᵗʰ R25   Abnormal involuntary movements
EXCLUDES 1   specific movement disorders (G20-G26)
stereotyped movement disorders (F98.4)
tic disorders (F95.-)

R25.0   Abnormal head movements

R25.1   Tremor, unspecified
EXCLUDES 1   chorea NOS (G25.5)
essential tremor (G25.0)
hysterical tremor (F44.4)
intention tremor (G25.2)

R25.2   Cramp and spasm
EXCLUDES 2   carpopedal spasm (R29.0)
charley-horse (M62.831)
infantile spasms (G40.4-)
muscle spasm of back (M62.830)
muscle spasm of calf (M62.831)

R25.3   Fasciculation
Twitching NOS

R25.8   Other abnormal involuntary movements

R25.9   Unspecified abnormal involuntary movements

✓4ᵗʰ R26   Abnormalities of gait and mobility
EXCLUDES 1   ataxia NOS (R27.0)
hereditary ataxia (G11.-)
locomotor (syphilitic) ataxia (A52.11)
immobility syndrome (paraplegic) (M62.3)

R26.0   Ataxic gait
Staggering gait

R26.1   Paralytic gait
Spastic gait

R26.2   Difficulty in walking, not elsewhere classified
EXCLUDES 1   falling (R29.6)
unsteadiness on feet (R26.81)
AHA: 2016, 2Q, 7

✓5ᵗʰ R26.8   Other abnormalities of gait and mobility
R26.81   Unsteadiness on feet
R26.89   Other abnormalities of gait and mobility

R26.9   Unspecified abnormalities of gait and mobility

✓4ᵗʰ R27   Other lack of coordination
EXCLUDES 1   ataxic gait (R26.0)
hereditary ataxia (G11.-)
vertigo NOS (R42)

R27.0   Ataxia, unspecified
EXCLUDES 1   ataxia following cerebrovascular disease (I69. with final characters -93)

R27.8   Other lack of coordination

R27.9   Unspecified lack of coordination

✓4ᵗʰ R29   Other symptoms and signs involving the nervous and musculoskeletal systems

R29.0   Tetany   `CC`
Carpopedal spasm
EXCLUDES 1   hysterical tetany (F44.5)
neonatal tetany (P71.3)
parathyroid tetany (E20.9)
post-thyroidectomy tetany (E89.2)
CC Excl: PDX collection 1124

R29.1   Meningismus   `CC`
CC Excl: PDX collection 1125

R29.2   Abnormal reflex
EXCLUDES 2   abnormal pupillary reflex (H57.0)
hyperactive gag reflex (J39.2)
vasovagal reaction or syncope (R55)

R29.3   Abnormal posture

R29.4   Clicking hip
EXCLUDES 1   congenital deformities of hip (Q65.-)

R29.5   Transient paralysis   `CC`
Code first any associated spinal cord injury (S14.0, S14.1-, S24.0, S24.1-, S34.0-, S34.1-)
EXCLUDES 1   transient ischemic attack (G45.9)
CC Excl: PDX collection 1126

R29.6   Repeated falls
Falling
Tendency to fall
EXCLUDES 2   at risk for falling (Z91.81)
history of falling (Z91.81)
AHA: 2016, 2Q, 6

✓5ᵗʰ R29.7   National Institutes of Health Stroke Scale (NIHSS) score
Code first the type of cerebral infarction (I63.-)

✓6ᵗʰ R29.70   NIHSS score 0-9
R29.700   NIHSS score 0
R29.701   NIHSS score 1
R29.702   NIHSS score 2
R29.703   NIHSS score 3
R29.704   NIHSS score 4
R29.705   NIHSS score 5
R29.706   NIHSS score 6
R29.707   NIHSS score 7
R29.708   NIHSS score 8
R29.709   NIHSS score 9

✓6ᵗʰ R29.71   NIHSS score 10-19
R29.710   NIHSS score 10
R29.711   NIHSS score 11
R29.712   NIHSS score 12
R29.713   NIHSS score 13
R29.714   NIHSS score 14
R29.715   NIHSS score 15
R29.716   NIHSS score 16
R29.717   NIHSS score 17
R29.718   NIHSS score 18
R29.719   NIHSS score 19

✓6ᵗʰ R29.72   NIHSS score 20-29
R29.720   NIHSS score 20
R29.721   NIHSS score 21
R29.722   NIHSS score 22
R29.723   NIHSS score 23
R29.724   NIHSS score 24
R29.725   NIHSS score 25
R29.726   NIHSS score 26
R29.727   NIHSS score 27
R29.728   NIHSS score 28
R29.729   NIHSS score 29

✓6ᵗʰ R29.73   NIHSS score 30-39
R29.730   NIHSS score 30
R29.731   NIHSS score 31
R29.732   NIHSS score 32
R29.733   NIHSS score 33
R29.734   NIHSS score 34
R29.735   NIHSS score 35
R29.736   NIHSS score 36
R29.737   NIHSS score 37
R29.738   NIHSS score 38
R29.739   NIHSS score 39

✓6ᵗʰ R29.74   NIHSS score 40-42
R29.740   NIHSS score 40
R29.741   NIHSS score 41
R29.742   NIHSS score 42

✓5ᵗʰ R29.8   Other symptoms and signs involving the nervous and musculoskeletal systems

✓6ᵗʰ R29.81   Other symptoms and signs involving the nervous system
R29.810   Facial weakness
Facial droop
EXCLUDES 1   Bell's palsy (G51.0)
facial weakness following cerebrovascular disease (I69. with final characters -92)

R29.818   Other symptoms and signs involving the nervous system

✓6th **R29.89   Other symptoms and signs involving the musculoskeletal system**
> EXCLUDES 2   *pain in limb (M79.6-)*

R29.890   Loss of height
> EXCLUDES 1   *osteoporosis (M80-M81)*

R29.891   Ocular torticollis
> EXCLUDES 1   *congenital (sternomastoid) torticollis Q68.0*
> *psychogenic torticollis (F45.8)*
> *spasmodic torticollis (G24.3)*
> *torticollis due to birth injury (P15.8)*
> *torticollis NOS M43.6*
>
> **DEF:** Abnormal head posture as a result of a contracted state of cervical muscles to correct a visual disturbance, either double vision or a visual field defect.

R29.898   Other symptoms and signs involving the musculoskeletal system

✓5th **R29.9   Unspecified symptoms and signs involving the nervous and musculoskeletal systems**

R29.90   Unspecified symptoms and signs involving the nervous system

R29.91   Unspecified symptoms and signs involving the musculoskeletal system

Symptoms and signs involving the genitourinary system (R30-R39)

✓4th **R30   Pain associated with micturition**
> EXCLUDES 1   *psychogenic pain associated with micturition (F45.8)*

R30.0   Dysuria
Strangury

R30.1   Vesical tenesmus

R30.9   Painful micturition, unspecified
Painful urination NOS

✓4th **R31   Hematuria**
> EXCLUDES 1   *hematuria included with underlying conditions, such as:*
> *acute cystitis with hematuria (N30.01)*
> *recurrent and persistent hematuria in glomerular diseases (N02.-)*
>
> **AHA:** 2017, 1Q, 17

R31.0   Gross hematuria

R31.1   Benign essential microscopic hematuria

✓5th **R31.2   Other microscopic hematuria**

R31.21   Asymptomatic microscopic hematuria
AMH

R31.29   Other microscopic hematuria

R31.9   Hematuria, unspecified

R32   Unspecified urinary incontinence
Enuresis NOS
> EXCLUDES 1   *functional urinary incontinence (R39.81)*
> *nonorganic enuresis (F98.0)*
> *stress incontinence and other specified urinary incontinence (N39.3-N39.4-)*
> *urinary incontinence associated with cognitive impairment (R39.81)*

✓4th **R33   Retention of urine**
> EXCLUDES 1   *psychogenic retention of urine (F45.8)*

R33.0   Drug induced retention of urine
Use additional code for adverse effect, if applicable, to identify drug (T36-T50 with fifth or sixth character 5)

R33.8   Other retention of urine
Code first, if applicable, any causal condition, such as:
enlarged prostate (N40.1)

R33.9   Retention of urine, unspecified

R34   Anuria and oliguria
> EXCLUDES 1   *anuria and oliguria complicating abortion or ectopic or molar pregnancy (O00-O07, O08.4)*
> *anuria and oliguria complicating pregnancy (O26.83-)*
> *anuria and oliguria complicating the puerperium (O90.4)*

✓4th **R35   Polyuria**
Code first, if applicable, any causal condition, such as:
enlarged prostate (N40.1)
> EXCLUDES 1   *psychogenic polyuria (F45.8)*

R35.0   Frequency of micturition

R35.1   Nocturia

R35.8   Other polyuria
Polyuria NOS

✓4th **R36   Urethral discharge**

R36.0   Urethral discharge without blood

R36.1   Hematospermia   ♂

R36.9   Urethral discharge, unspecified
Penile discharge NOS
Urethrorrhea

R37   Sexual dysfunction, unspecified

✓4th **R39   Other and unspecified symptoms and signs involving the genitourinary system**

R39.0   Extravasation of urine   CC
CC Excl: PDX collection 1127

✓5th **R39.1   Other difficulties with micturition**
Code first, if applicable, any causal condition, such as:
enlarged prostate (N40.1)

R39.11   Hesitancy of micturition

R39.12   Poor urinary stream
Weak urinary steam

R39.13   Splitting of urinary stream

R39.14   Feeling of incomplete bladder emptying

R39.15   Urgency of urination
> EXCLUDES 1   *urge incontinence (N39.41, N39.46)*

R39.16   Straining to void

✓6th **R39.19   Other difficulties with micturition**

R39.191   Need to immediately re-void

R39.192   Position dependent micturition

R39.198   Other difficulties with micturition

R39.2   Extrarenal uremia
Prerenal uremia
> EXCLUDES 1   *uremia NOS (N19)*

✓5th **R39.8   Other symptoms and signs involving the genitourinary system**

R39.81   Functional urinary incontinence
Urinary incontinence due to cognitive impairment, or severe physical disability or immobility
> EXCLUDES 1   *stress incontinence and other specified urinary incontinence (N39.3-N39.4-)*
> *urinary incontinence NOS (R32)*

R39.82   Chronic bladder pain

● **R39.83   Unilateral non-palpable testicle**   ♂

● **R39.84   Bilateral non-palpable testicles**   ♂

R39.89   Other symptoms and signs involving the genitourinary system

R39.9   Unspecified symptoms and signs involving the genitourinary system

Symptoms and signs involving cognition, perception, emotional state and behavior (R40-R46)

> EXCLUDES 2   *symptoms and signs constituting part of a pattern of mental disorder (F01-F99)*

✓4th **R40   Somnolence, stupor and coma**
> EXCLUDES 1   *neonatal coma (P91.5)*
> *somnolence, stupor and coma in diabetes (E08-E13)*
> *somnolence, stupor and coma in hepatic failure (K72.-)*
> *somnolence, stupor and coma in hypoglycemia (nondiabetic) (E15)*

R40.0   Somnolence
Drowsiness
> EXCLUDES 1   *coma (R40.2-)*

R40.1   Stupor
Catatonic stupor
Semicoma
> EXCLUDES 1   *catatonic schizophrenia (F20.2)*
> *coma (R40.2-)*
> *depressive stupor (F31-F33)*
> *dissociative stupor (F44.2)*
> *manic stupor (F30.2)*

✓5ᵗʰ **R40.2 Coma**
Code first any associated:
fracture of skull (S02.-)
intracranial injury (S06.-)
NOTE One code from each subcategory, R40.21-R40.23, is required to complete the coma scale
AHA: 2015, 2Q, 17; 2014, 1Q, 19

CC Excl: For MCC codes in subcategory R40.2: PDX collection 515

R40.20 Unspecified coma MCC HCC
Coma NOS
Unconsciousness NOS

✓6ᵗʰ **R40.21 Coma scale, eyes open**

The following appropriate 7th character is to be added to subcategories R40.21-, R40.22-, R40.23-, and R40.24-.
0   unspecified time
1   in the field [EMT or ambulance]
2   at arrival to emergency department
3   at hospital admission
4   24 hours or more after hospital admission

✓7ᵗʰ **R40.211 Coma scale, eyes open, never** MCC HCC
✓7ᵗʰ **R40.212 Coma scale, eyes open, to pain** MCC HCC
✓7ᵗʰ **R40.213 Coma scale, eyes open, to sound**
✓7ᵗʰ **R40.214 Coma scale, eyes open, spontaneous**

✓6ᵗʰ **R40.22 Coma scale, best verbal response**

✓7ᵗʰ **R40.221 Coma scale, best verbal response, none** MCC HCC

✓7ᵗʰ **R40.222 Coma scale, best verbal response, incomprehensible words** MCC HCC
▶Incomprehensible sounds (2-5 years of age)
Moans/grunts to pain; restless (< 2 years old)◀

✓7ᵗʰ **R40.223 Coma scale, best verbal response, inappropriate words**
▶Inappropriate crying or screaming (< 2 years of age)
Screaming (2-5 years of age)◀

✓7ᵗʰ **R40.224 Coma scale, best verbal response, confused conversation**
▶Inappropriate words (2-5 years of age)
Irritable cries (< 2 years of age)◀

✓7ᵗʰ **R40.225 Coma scale, best verbal response, oriented**
▶Cooing or babbling or crying appropriately (< 2 years of age)
Uses appropriate words (2- 5 years of age)◀

✓6ᵗʰ **R40.23 Coma scale, best motor response**

✓7ᵗʰ **R40.231 Coma scale, best motor response, none** MCC HCC

✓7ᵗʰ **R40.232 Coma scale, best motor response, extension** MCC HCC
▶Abnormal extensor posturing to pain or noxious stimuli (< 2 years of age)
Extensor posturing to pain or noxious stimuli (2-5 years of age)◀

✓7ᵗʰ **R40.233 Coma scale, best motor response, abnormal**
▶Abnormal flexure posturing to pain or noxious stimuli (0-5 years of age)
Flexion/decorticate posturing (< 2 years of age)◀

✓7ᵗʰ **R40.234 Coma scale, best motor response, flexion withdrawal** MCC HCC
▶Withdraws from pain or noxious stimuli (0-5 years of age)◀

✓7ᵗʰ **R40.235 Coma scale, best motor response, localizes pain**
▶Localizes pain (2-5 years of age)
Withdraws to touch (< 2 years of age)◀

✓7ᵗʰ **R40.236 Coma scale, best motor response, obeys commands**
▶Normal or spontaneous movement (< 2 years of age)
Obeys commands (2-5 years of age)◀

✓6ᵗʰ **R40.24 Glasgow coma scale, total score**
NOTE Assign a code from subcategory R40.24, when only the total coma score is documented

✓7ᵗʰ **R40.241 Glasgow coma scale score 13-15**
✓7ᵗʰ **R40.242 Glasgow coma scale score 9-12**
✓7ᵗʰ **R40.243 Glasgow coma scale score 3-8** HCC
✓7ᵗʰ **R40.244 Other coma, without documented Glasgow coma scale score, or with partial score reported** HCC

R40.3 Persistent vegetative state CC HCC
DEF: Persistent wakefulness without consciousness due to nonfunctioning cerebral cortex.
CC Excl: PDX collection 515

R40.4 Transient alteration of awareness

✓4ᵗʰ **R41 Other symptoms and signs involving cognitive functions and awareness**
EXCLUDES 1 dissociative [conversion] disorders (F44.-)
mild cognitive impairment, so stated (G31.84)

R41.0 Disorientation, unspecified
Confusion NOS
Delirium NOS

R41.1 Anterograde amnesia

R41.2 Retrograde amnesia

R41.3 Other amnesia
Amnesia NOS
Memory loss NOS
EXCLUDES 1 amnestic disorder due to known physiologic condition (F04)
amnestic syndrome due to psychoactive substance use (F10-F19 with 5th character .6)
mild memory disturbance due to known physiological condition (F06.8)
transient global amnesia (G45.4)

R41.4 Neurologic neglect syndrome CC
Asomatognosia
Hemi-akinesia
Hemi-inattention
Hemispatial neglect
Left-sided neglect
Sensory neglect
Visuospatial neglect
EXCLUDES 1 visuospatial deficit (R41.842)
CC Excl: PDX collection 1128

✓5ᵗʰ **R41.8 Other symptoms and signs involving cognitive functions and awareness**

R41.81 Age-related cognitive decline A
Senility NOS

R41.82 Altered mental status, unspecified
Change in mental status NOS
EXCLUDES 1 altered level of consciousness (R40.-)
altered mental status due to known condition—code to condition
delirium NOS (R41.0)
AHA: 2012, 4Q, 97

R41.83 Borderline intellectual functioning
IQ level 71 to 84
EXCLUDES 1 intellectual disabilities (F70-F79)

✓6ᵗʰ **R41.84 Other specified cognitive deficit**
EXCLUDES 1 cognitive deficits as sequelae of cerebrovascular disease (I69.01-, I69.11-, I69.21-, I69.31-, I69.81-, I69.91-)

R41.840 Attention and concentration deficit
EXCLUDES 1 attention-deficit hyperactivity disorders (F90.-)

R41.841 Cognitive communication deficit
R41.842 Visuospatial deficit
R41.843 Psychomotor deficit
R41.844 Frontal lobe and executive function deficit

R41.89 Other symptoms and signs involving cognitive functions and awareness
Anosognosia

R41.9 Unspecified symptoms and signs involving cognitive functions and awareness
▶Unspecified neurocognitive disorder◀

R42 Dizziness and giddiness
Light-headedness
Vertigo NOS
EXCLUDES 1   *vertiginous syndromes (H81.-)*
vertigo from infrasound (T75.23)

✓4ᵗʰ **R43 Disturbances of smell and taste**
R43.0 **Anosmia**
R43.1 **Parosmia**
R43.2 **Parageusia**
R43.8 **Other disturbances of smell and taste**
Mixed disturbance of smell and taste
R43.9 **Unspecified disturbances of smell and taste**

✓4ᵗʰ **R44 Other symptoms and signs involving general sensations and perceptions**
EXCLUDES 1   *alcoholic hallucinations (F1.5)*
hallucinations in drug psychosis (F11-F19 with .5)
hallucinations in mood disorders with psychotic symptoms (F30.2, F31.5, F32.3, F33.3)
hallucinations in schizophrenia, schizotypal and delusional disorders (F20-F29)
EXCLUDES 2   *disturbances of skin sensation (R20.-)*

CC Excl: For CC codes in category R44: PDX collection 1129

R44.0 **Auditory hallucinations**   CC
R44.1 **Visual hallucinations**
R44.2 **Other hallucinations**   CC
R44.3 **Hallucinations, unspecified**   CC
R44.8 **Other symptoms and signs involving general sensations and perceptions**
R44.9 **Unspecified symptoms and signs involving general sensations and perceptions**

✓4ᵗʰ **R45 Symptoms and signs involving emotional state**
R45.0 **Nervousness**
Nervous tension
R45.1 **Restlessness and agitation**
R45.2 **Unhappiness**
R45.3 **Demoralization and apathy**
EXCLUDES 1   *anhedonia (R45.84)*
R45.4 **Irritability and anger**
R45.5 **Hostility**
R45.6 **Violent behavior**
R45.7 **State of emotional shock and stress, unspecified**
✓5ᵗʰ R45.8 **Other symptoms and signs involving emotional state**
R45.81 **Low self-esteem**
R45.82 **Worries**
R45.83 **Excessive crying of child, adolescent or adult**
EXCLUDES 1   *excessive crying of infant (baby) R68.11*
R45.84 **Anhedonia**
✓6ᵗʰ R45.85 **Homicidal and suicidal ideations**
EXCLUDES 1   *suicide attempt (T14.91)*
R45.850 **Homicidal ideations**
R45.851 **Suicidal ideations**   CC
DEF: Thoughts of committing suicide; no actual attempt of suicide has been made.
CC Excl: PDX collection 1130
R45.86 **Emotional lability**
R45.87 **Impulsiveness**
R45.89 **Other symptoms and signs involving emotional state**

✓4ᵗʰ **R46 Symptoms and signs involving appearance and behavior**
EXCLUDES 1   *appearance and behavior in schizophrenia, schizotypal and delusional disorders (F20-F29)*
mental and behavioral disorders (F01-F99)
R46.0 **Very low level of personal hygiene**
R46.1 **Bizarre personal appearance**
R46.2 **Strange and inexplicable behavior**
R46.3 **Overactivity**
R46.4 **Slowness and poor responsiveness**
EXCLUDES 1   *stupor (R40.1)*
R46.5 **Suspiciousness and marked evasiveness**
R46.6 **Undue concern and preoccupation with stressful events**
R46.7 **Verbosity and circumstantial detail obscuring reason for contact**

✓5ᵗʰ R46.8 **Other symptoms and signs involving appearance and behavior**
R46.81 **Obsessive-compulsive behavior**
EXCLUDES 1   *obsessive-compulsive disorder (F42-)*
R46.89 **Other symptoms and signs involving appearance and behavior**

Symptoms and signs involving speech and voice (R47-R49)

✓4ᵗʰ **R47 Speech disturbances, not elsewhere classified**
EXCLUDES 1   *autism (F84.0)*
cluttering (F80.81)
specific developmental disorders of speech and language (F80.-)
stuttering (F80.81)

✓5ᵗʰ R47.0 **Dysphasia and aphasia**
R47.01 **Aphasia**   CC
EXCLUDES 1   *aphasia following cerebrovascular disease (I69. with final characters -20)*
progressive isolated aphasia (G31.01)
CC Excl: PDX collection 1131
R47.02 **Dysphasia**
EXCLUDES 1   *dysphasia following cerebrovascular disease (I69. with final characters -21)*
R47.1 **Dysarthria and anarthria**
EXCLUDES 1   *dysarthria following cerebrovascular disease (I69. with final characters -22)*

✓5ᵗʰ R47.8 **Other speech disturbances**
EXCLUDES 1   *dysarthria following cerebrovascular disease (I69. with final characters -28)*
R47.81 **Slurred speech**
R47.82 *Fluency disorder in conditions classified elsewhere*
Stuttering in conditions classified elsewhere
Code first underlying disease or condition, such as:
Parkinson's disease (G20)
EXCLUDES 1   *adult onset fluency disorder (F98.5)*
childhood onset fluency disorder (F80.81)
fluency disorder (stuttering) following cerebrovascular disease (I69. with final characters-23)
R47.89 **Other speech disturbances**
R47.9 **Unspecified speech disturbances**

✓4ᵗʰ **R48 Dyslexia and other symbolic dysfunctions, not elsewhere classified**
EXCLUDES 1   *specific developmental disorders of scholastic skills (F81.-)*
R48.0 **Dyslexia and alexia**
R48.1 **Agnosia**
Astereognosia (astereognosis)
Autotopagnosia
EXCLUDES 1   *visual object agnosia (R48.3)*
R48.2 **Apraxia**
EXCLUDES 1   *apraxia following cerebrovascular disease (I69. with final characters -90)*
R48.3 **Visual agnosia**
Prosopagnosia
Simultanagnosia (asimultagnosia)
R48.8 **Other symbolic dysfunctions**
Acalculia
Agraphia
AHA: 2017, 1Q, 27
R48.9 **Unspecified symbolic dysfunctions**

✓4ᵗʰ **R49 Voice and resonance disorders**
EXCLUDES 1   *psychogenic voice and resonance disorders (F44.4)*
R49.0 **Dysphonia**
Hoarseness
R49.1 **Aphonia**
Loss of voice
✓5ᵗʰ R49.2 **Hypernasality and hyponasality**
R49.21 **Hypernasality**
R49.22 **Hyponasality**
R49.8 **Other voice and resonance disorders**
R49.9 **Unspecified voice and resonance disorder**
Change in voice NOS
Resonance disorder NOS

General symptoms and signs (R50-R69)

✓4ᵗʰ R50   Fever of other and unknown origin
>   *EXCLUDES 1*   *chills without fever (R68.83)*
>   *febrile convulsions (R56.0-)*
>   *fever of unknown origin during labor (O75.2)*
>   *fever of unknown origin in newborn (P81.9)*
>   *hypothermia due to illness (R68.0)*
>   *malignant hyperthermia due to anesthesia (T88.3)*
>   *puerperal pyrexia NOS (O86.4)*

R50.2   Drug induced fever
>   Use additional code for adverse effect, if applicable, to identify drug (T36-T50 with fifth or sixth character 5)
>   *EXCLUDES 1*   *postvaccination (postimmunization) fever (R50.83)*

✓5ᵗʰ R50.8   Other specified fever

R50.81   *Fever presenting with conditions classified elsewhere*
>   Code first underlying condition when associated fever is present, such as with:
>   leukemia (C91-C95)
>   neutropenia (D70.-)
>   sickle-cell disease (D57.-)
>   **AHA:** 2014, 4Q, 22

R50.82   Postprocedural fever
>   *EXCLUDES 1*   *postprocedural infection (T81.4-)*
>   *posttransfusion fever (R50.84)*
>   *postvaccination (postimmunization) fever (R50.83)*

R50.83   Postvaccination fever
>   Postimmunization fever

R50.84   Febrile nonhemolytic transfusion reaction
>   FNHTR
>   Posttransfusion fever

R50.9   Fever, unspecified
Fever NOS	Hyperpyrexia NOS
Fever of unknown origin [FUO]	Persistent fever
Fever with chills	Pyrexia NOS
Fever with rigors	

R51   Headache
>   Facial pain NOS
>   *EXCLUDES 1*   *atypical face pain (G50.1)*
>   *migraine and other headache syndromes (G43-G44)*
>   *trigeminal neuralgia (G50.0)*

R52   Pain, unspecified
>   Acute pain NOS
>   Generalized pain NOS
>   Pain NOS
>   *EXCLUDES 1*   *acute and chronic pain, not elsewhere classified (G89.-)*
>   *localized pain, unspecified type—code to pain by site, such as:*
>   *abdomen pain (R10.-)*
>   *back pain (M54.9)*
>   *breast pain (N64.4)*
>   *chest pain (R07.1-R07.9)*
>   *ear pain (H92.0-)*
>   *eye pain (H57.1)*
>   *headache (R51)*
>   *joint pain (M25.5-)*
>   *limb pain (M79.6-)*
>   *lumbar region pain (M54.5)*
>   *pelvic and perineal pain (R10.2)*
>   *renal colic (N23)*
>   *shoulder pain (M25.51-)*
>   *spine pain (M54.-)*
>   *throat pain (R07.0)*
>   *tongue pain (K14.6)*
>   *tooth pain (K08.8)*
>   *pain disorders exclusively related to psychological factors (F45.41)*

✓4ᵗʰ R53   Malaise and fatigue

R53.0   Neoplastic (malignant) related fatigue
>   Code first associated neoplasm

R53.1   Weakness
>   Asthenia NOS
>   *EXCLUDES 1*   *age-related weakness (R54)*
>   *muscle weakness (M62.8-)*
>   *sarcopenia (M62.84)*
>   *senile asthenia (R54)*
>   **AHA:** 2017, 1Q, 7; 2015, 1Q, 25

R53.2   Functional quadriplegia   MCC HCC
>   Complete immobility due to severe physical disability or frailty
>   *EXCLUDES 1*   *frailty NOS (R54)*
>   *hysterical paralysis (F44.4)*
>   *immobility syndrome (M62.3)*
>   *neurologic quadriplegia (G82.5-)*
>   *quadriplegia (G82.50)*
>   **AHA:** 2016, 2Q, 6
>   **DEF:** Inability to move due to a nonphysiological condition, such as dementia; no mental ability to move independently; typically found in severely demented patients.
>   **CC Excl:** PDX collection 595

✓5ᵗʰ R53.8   Other malaise and fatigue
>   *EXCLUDES 1*   *combat exhaustion and fatigue (F43.0)*
>   *congenital debility (P96.9)*
>   ~~*exhaustion and fatigue due to depressive episode (F32.-)*~~
>   *exhaustion and fatigue due to excessive exertion (T73.3)*
>   *exhaustion and fatigue due to exposure (T73.2)*
>   *exhaustion and fatigue due to heat (T67.-)*
>   *exhaustion and fatigue due to pregnancy (O26.8-)*
>   *exhaustion and fatigue due to recurrent depressive episode (F33)*
>   *exhaustion and fatigue due to senile debility (R54)*

R53.81   Other malaise
Chronic debility	Malaise NOS
Debility NOS	Nervous debility
General physical deterioration	
>   *EXCLUDES 1*   *age-related physical debility (R54)*

R53.82   Chronic fatigue, unspecified
>   Chronic fatigue syndrome NOS
>   *EXCLUDES 1*   *postviral fatigue syndrome (G93.3)*

R53.83   Other fatigue
>   Fatigue NOS
>   Lack of energy
>   Lethargy
>   Tiredness
>   *EXCLUDES 2*   ▶*exhaustion and fatigue due to depressive episode (F32.-)*◀

R54   Age-related physical debility   Ⓐ
Frailty	Senile asthenia
Old age	Senile debility
Senescence	
>   *EXCLUDES 1*   *age-related cognitive decline (R41.81)*
>   *sarcopenia (M62.84)*
>   *senile psychosis (F03)*
>   *senility NOS (R41.81)*

R55   Syncope and collapse
Blackout	Vasovagal attack
Fainting	
>   *EXCLUDES 1*   *cardiogenic shock (R57.0)*
>   *carotid sinus syncope (G90.01)*
>   *heat syncope (T67.1)*
>   *neurocirculatory asthenia (F45.8)*
>   *neurogenic orthostatic hypotension (G90.3)*
>   *orthostatic hypotension (I95.1)*
>   *postprocedural shock (T81.1-)*
>   *psychogenic syncope (F48.8)*
>   *shock NOS (R57.9)*
>   *shock complicating or following abortion or ectopic or molar pregnancy (O00-O07, O08.3)*
>   *shock complicating or following labor and delivery (O75.1)*
>   *Stokes-Adams attack (I45.9)*
>   *unconsciousness NOS (R40.2-)*

✓4ᵗʰ R56   Convulsions, not elsewhere classified
>   *EXCLUDES 1*   *dissociative convulsions and seizures (F44.5)*
>   *epileptic convulsions and seizures (G40.-)*
>   *newborn convulsions and seizures (P90)*

✓5ᵗʰ R56.0   Febrile convulsions

R56.00   Simple febrile convulsions   CC HCC
>   Febrile convulsion NOS
>   Febrile seizure NOS
>   **CC Excl:** PDX collection 1132

R56.01   Complex febrile convulsions   CC HCC
>   Atypical febrile seizure
>   Complex febrile seizure
>   Complicated febrile seizure
>   *EXCLUDES 1*   *status epilepticus (G40.901)*
>   **CC Excl:** PDX collection 1132

R56.1 Post traumatic seizures `CC` `HCC`
> *EXCLUDES 1*   *post traumatic epilepsy (G40.-)*
> **CC Excl:** PDX collection 582

R56.9 Unspecified convulsions `HCC`
> Convulsion disorder
> Fit NOS
> Recurrent convulsions
> Seizure(s) (convulsive) NOS

✓4ᵗʰ **R57 Shock, not elsewhere classified**
> *EXCLUDES 1*   *anaphylactic shock NOS (T78.2)*
> *anaphylactic reaction or shock due to adverse food reaction (T78.0-)*
> *anaphylactic shock due to adverse effect of correct drug or medicament properly administered (T88.6)*
> *anaphylactic shock due to serum (T80.5-)*
> *anesthetic shock (T88.3)*
> *electric shock (T75.4)*
> *obstetric shock (O75.1)*
> *postprocedural shock (T81.1-)*
> *psychic shock (F43.0)*
> ~~septic shock (R65.21)~~
> *shock complicating or following ectopic or molar pregnancy (O00-O07, O08.3)*
> *shock due to lightning (T75.01)*
> *traumatic shock (T79.4)*
> *toxic shock syndrome (A48.3)*

> **CC Excl:** For CC/MCC codes in category R57: PDX collection 1133

[1] **R57.0 Cardiogenic shock** `MCC` `HCC`
> *EXCLUDES 2* ▶*septic shock (R65.21)*◀
> **DEF:** Associated with myocardial infarction, cardiac tamponade, and massive pulmonary embolism; symptoms include mental confusion, reduced blood pressure, tachycardia, pallor, and cold, clammy skin.

[1] **R57.1 Hypovolemic shock** `MCC` `HCC`
[1] **R57.8 Other shock** `MCC` `HCC`
R57.9 Shock, unspecified `CC` `HCC`
> Failure of peripheral circulation NOS

R58 Hemorrhage, not elsewhere classified
> Hemorrhage NOS
> *EXCLUDES 1* *hemorrhage included with underlying conditions, such as:*
>   *acute duodenal ulcer with hemorrhage (K26.0)*
>   *acute gastritis with bleeding (K29.01)*
>   *ulcerative enterocolitis with rectal bleeding (K51.01)*

✓4ᵗʰ **R59 Enlarged lymph nodes**
> *INCLUDES* swollen glands
> *EXCLUDES 1* *acute lymphadenitis (L04.-)*
> *chronic lymphadenitis (I88.1)*
> *lymphadenitis NOS (I88.9)*
> *mesenteric (acute) (chronic) lymphadenitis (I88.0)*

R59.0 Localized enlarged lymph nodes
R59.1 Generalized enlarged lymph nodes
> Lymphadenopathy NOS

R59.9 Enlarged lymph nodes, unspecified

✓4ᵗʰ **R60 Edema, not elsewhere classified**
> *EXCLUDES 1* *angioneurotic edema (T78.3)*
> *ascites (R18.-)*
> *cerebral edema (G93.6)*
> *cerebral edema due to birth injury (P11.0)*
> *edema of larynx (J38.4)*
> *edema of nasopharynx (J39.2)*
> *edema of pharynx (J39.2)*
> *gestational edema (O12.0-)*
> *hereditary edema (Q82.0)*
> *hydrops fetalis NOS (P83.2)*
> *hydrothorax (J94.8)*
> ~~nutritional edema (E40-E46)~~
> *hydrops fetalis NOS (P83.2)*
> *newborn edema (P83.3)*
> *pulmonary edema (J81.-)*

R60.0 Localized edema
R60.1 Generalized edema
> *EXCLUDES 2* ▶*nutritional edema (E40-E46)*◀

R60.9 Edema, unspecified
> Fluid retention NOS

R61 Generalized hyperhidrosis
> Excessive sweating
> Night sweats
> Secondary hyperhidrosis
> Code first, if applicable, menopausal and female climacteric states (N95.1)
> *EXCLUDES 1* *focal (primary) (secondary) hyperhidrosis (L74.5-)*
> *Frey's syndrome (L74.52)*
> *localized (primary) (secondary) hyperhidrosis (L74.5-)*

✓4ᵗʰ **R62 Lack of expected normal physiological development in childhood and adults**
> *EXCLUDES 1* *delayed puberty (E30.0)*
> *gonadal dysgenesis (Q99.1)*
> *hypopituitarism (E23.0)*

R62.0 Delayed milestone in childhood `P`
> Delayed attainment of expected physiological developmental stage
> Late talker
> Late walker

✓5ᵗʰ **R62.5 Other and unspecified lack of expected normal physiological development in childhood**
> *EXCLUDES 1* *HIV disease resulting in failure to thrive (B20)*
> *physical retardation due to malnutrition (E45)*

R62.50 Unspecified lack of expected normal physiological development in childhood
> Infantilism NOS

R62.51 Failure to thrive (child) `P`
> Failure to gain weight
> *EXCLUDES 1* *failure to thrive in child under 28 days old (P92.6)*
> **DEF:** Organic failure to thrive (FTT): Acute or chronic illness that interferes with nutritional intake, absorption, metabolism excretion, and energy requirements; nonorganic FTT is a symptom of neglect or abuse.

R62.52 Short stature (child)
> Lack of growth
> Physical retardation
> Short stature NOS
> *EXCLUDES 1* *short stature due to endocrine disorder (E34.3)*

R62.59 Other lack of expected normal physiological development in childhood

R62.7 Adult failure to thrive `A`

✓4ᵗʰ **R63 Symptoms and signs concerning food and fluid intake**
> *EXCLUDES 1* *bulimia NOS (F50.2)*
> *eating disorders of nonorganic origin (F50.-)*
> *malnutrition (E40-E46)*

R63.0 Anorexia
> Loss of appetite
> *EXCLUDES 1* *anorexia nervosa (F50.0-)*
> *loss of appetite of nonorganic origin (F50.89)*

R63.1 Polydipsia
> Excessive thirst

R63.2 Polyphagia
> Excessive eating
> Hyperalimentation NOS

R63.3 Feeding difficulties
> Feeding problem (elderly) (infant) NOS
> ▶Picky eater◀
> *EXCLUDES 1* ▶*eating disorders (F50.-)*◀
> *feeding problems of newborn (P92.-)*
> *infant feeding disorder of nonorganic origin (F98.2-)*
> **AHA:** 2017, 1Q, 28; 2016, 3Q, 19

R63.4 Abnormal weight loss
R63.5 Abnormal weight gain
> *EXCLUDES 1* *excessive weight gain in pregnancy (O26.0-)*
> *obesity (E66.-)*

R63.6 Underweight
> Use additional code to identify body mass index (BMI), if known (Z68.-)
> *EXCLUDES 1* *abnormal weight loss (R63.4)*
> *anorexia nervosa (F50.0-)*
> *malnutrition (E40-E46)*

R63.8 Other symptoms and signs concerning food and fluid intake

---

[1] MCC only if patient is discharged alive.

Ⓝ Newborn: 0   Ⓟ Pediatric: 0-17   Ⓜ Maternity: 12-55   Ⓐ Adult: 15-124   `MCC` Major CC Condition   `PDxMCC` PDx acts as own MCC   `CC` CC Condition   `PDxCC` PDx acts as own CC

924   ICD-10-CM 2018

R64　Cachexia　CC HCC
　　Wasting syndrome
　　Code first underlying condition, if known
　　　EXCLUDES 1　abnormal weight loss (R63.4)
　　　　　　　　　nutritional marasmus (E41)
　　CC Excl: PDX collection 1134

✓4th **R65　Symptoms and signs specifically associated with systemic inflammation and infection**

　　CC Excl: For CC/MCC codes in category R65, unless otherwise noted: PDX collection 71

✓5th **R65.1　Systemic inflammatory response syndrome [SIRS] of non-infectious origin**
　　　Code first underlying condition, such as:
　　　　heatstroke (T67.0)
　　　　injury and trauma (S00-T88)
　　　EXCLUDES 1　sepsis—code to infection
　　　　　　　　　severe sepsis (R65.2)

　　R65.10　Systemic inflammatory response syndrome [SIRS] of non-infectious origin without acute organ dysfunction　CC HCC
　　　Systemic inflammatory response syndrome (SIRS) NOS

　　R65.11　Systemic inflammatory response syndrome [SIRS] of non-infectious origin with acute organ dysfunction　MCC HCC
　　　Use additional code to identify specific acute organ dysfunction, such as:
　　　　acute kidney failure (N17.-)
　　　　acute respiratory failure (J96.0-)
　　　　critical illness myopathy (G72.81)
　　　　critical illness polyneuropathy (G62.81)
　　　　disseminated intravascular coagulopathy [DIC] (D65)
　　　　encephalopathy (metabolic) (septic) (G93.41)
　　　　hepatic failure (K72.0-)

✓5th **R65.2　Severe sepsis**
　　　Infection with associated acute organ dysfunction
　　　Sepsis with acute organ dysfunction
　　　Sepsis with multiple organ dysfunction
　　　Systemic inflammatory response syndrome due to infectious process with acute organ dysfunction
　　　Code first underlying infection, such as:
　　　　infection following a procedure (T81.4-)
　　　　infections following infusion, transfusion and therapeutic injection (T80.2-)
　　　　puerperal sepsis (O85)
　　　　sepsis following complete or unspecified spontaneous abortion (O03.87)
　　　　sepsis following ectopic and molar pregnancy (O08.82)
　　　　sepsis following incomplete spontaneous abortion (O03.37)
　　　　sepsis following (induced) termination of pregnancy (O04.87)
　　　　sepsis NOS (A41.9)
　　　Use additional code to identify specific acute organ dysfunction, such as:
　　　　acute kidney failure (N17.-)
　　　　acute respiratory failure (J96.0-)
　　　　critical illness myopathy (G72.81)
　　　　critical illness polyneuropathy (G62.81)
　　　　disseminated intravascular coagulopathy [DIC] (D65)
　　　　encephalopathy (metabolic) (septic) (G93.41)
　　　　hepatic failure (K72.0-)
　　　AHA: 2016, 3Q, 8

　　R65.20　Severe sepsis without septic shock　MCC HCC
　　　Severe sepsis NOS
　　　AHA: 2016, 3Q, 14; 2013, 4Q, 119

　　R65.21　Severe sepsis with septic shock　PDxMCC MCC HCC
　　　CC Excl: PDX collection 1133

✓4th **R68　Other general symptoms and signs**

　　R68.0　Hypothermia, not associated with low environmental temperature
　　　EXCLUDES 1　hypothermia due to anesthesia (T88.51)
　　　　　　　　　hypothermia due to low environmental temperature (T68)
　　　　　　　　　hypothermia NOS (accidental) (T68)
　　　　　　　　　newborn hypothermia (P80.-)

✓5th **R68.1　Nonspecific symptoms peculiar to infancy**
　　　EXCLUDES 1　colic, infantile (R10.83)
　　　　　　　　　neonatal cerebral irritability (P91.3)
　　　　　　　　　teething syndrome (K00.7)

　　R68.11　Excessive crying of infant (baby)　P
　　　EXCLUDES 1　excessive crying of child, adolescent, or adult (R45.83)

　　R68.12　Fussy infant (baby)　P
　　　Irritable infant

　　R68.13　Apparent life threatening event in infant (ALTE)　P
　　　Apparent life threatening event in newborn
　　　▶Brief resolved unexplained event (BRUE)◀
　　　Code first confirmed diagnosis, if known
　　　Use additional code(s) for associated signs and symptoms if no confirmed diagnosis established, or if signs and symptoms are not associated routinely with confirmed diagnosis, or provide additional information for cause of ALTE

　　R68.19　Other nonspecific symptoms peculiar to infancy　P

　　R68.2　Dry mouth, unspecified
　　　EXCLUDES 1　dry mouth due to dehydration (E86.0)
　　　　　　　　　dry mouth due to sicca syndrome [Sjögren] (M35.0-)
　　　　　　　　　salivary gland hyposecretion (K11.7)

　　R68.3　Clubbing of fingers
　　　Clubbing of nails
　　　EXCLUDES 1　congenital clubfinger (Q68.1)
　　　DEF: Enlarged soft tissue of distal fingers; usually occurs in heart and lung diseases.

✓5th **R68.8　Other general symptoms and signs**

　　R68.81　Early satiety
　　　DEF: The premature feeling of being full after eating only a small amount of food; mechanism of satiety is multifactorial.

　　R68.82　Decreased libido　A
　　　Decreased sexual desire

　　R68.83　Chills (without fever)
　　　Chills NOS
　　　EXCLUDES 1　chills with fever (R50.9)

　　R68.84　Jaw pain
　　　Mandibular pain
　　　Maxilla pain
　　　EXCLUDES 1　temporomandibular joint arthralgia (M26.62-)

　　R68.89　Other general symptoms and signs

R69　Illness, unspecified
　　Unknown and unspecified cases of morbidity

Abnormal findings on examination of blood, without diagnosis (R70-R79)

　EXCLUDES 2　abnormal findings on antenatal screening of mother (O28.-)
　　　　　　　abnormalities of lipids (E78.-)
　　　　　　　abnormalities of platelets and thrombocytes (D69.-)
　　　　　　　abnormalities of white blood cells classified elsewhere (D70-D72)
　　　　　　　coagulation hemorrhagic disorders (D65-D68)
　　　　　　　diagnostic abnormal findings classified elsewhere—see Alphabetical Index
　　　　　　　hemorrhagic and hematological disorders of newborn (P50-P61)

✓4th **R70　Elevated erythrocyte sedimentation rate and abnormality of plasma viscosity**

　　R70.0　Elevated erythrocyte sedimentation rate

　　R70.1　Abnormal plasma viscosity

✓4th **R71　Abnormality of red blood cells**
　　　EXCLUDES 1　anemias (D50-D64)
　　　　　　　　　anemia of premature infant (P61.2)
　　　　　　　　　benign (familial) polycythemia (D75.0)
　　　　　　　　　congenital anemias (P61.2-P61.4)
　　　　　　　　　newborn anemia due to isoimmunization (P55.-)
　　　　　　　　　polycythemia neonatorum (P61.1)
　　　　　　　　　polycythemia NOS (D75.1)
　　　　　　　　　polycythemia vera (D45)
　　　　　　　　　secondary polycythemia (D75.1)

　　R71.0　Precipitous drop in hematocrit　CC
　　　Drop (precipitous) in hemoglobin
　　　Drop in hematocrit
　　　CC Excl: PDX collection 1135

　　R71.8　Other abnormality of red blood cells
　　　Abnormal red-cell morphology NOS　　Anisocytosis
　　　Abnormal red-cell volume NOS　　　　Poikilocytosis

✓4th **R73 Elevated blood glucose level**
> *EXCLUDES 1*   diabetes mellitus (E08-E13)
> diabetes mellitus in pregnancy, childbirth and the puerperium (O24.-)
> neonatal disorders (P70.0-P70.2)
> postsurgical hypoinsulinemia (E89.1)

✓5th **R73.0 Abnormal glucose**
> *EXCLUDES 1*   abnormal glucose in pregnancy (O99.81-)
> diabetes mellitus (E08-E13)
> dysmetabolic syndrome X (E88.81)
> gestational diabetes (O24.4-)
> glycosuria (R81)
> hypoglycemia (E16.2)

    R73.01 Impaired fasting glucose
       Elevated fasting glucose

    R73.02 Impaired glucose tolerance (oral)
       Elevated glucose tolerance

    R73.03 Prediabetes
       Latent diabetes

    R73.09 Other abnormal glucose
       Abnormal glucose NOS
       Abnormal non-fasting glucose tolerance

    R73.9 Hyperglycemia, unspecified

✓4th **R74 Abnormal serum enzyme levels**

    R74.0 Nonspecific elevation of levels of transaminase and lactic acid dehydrogenase [LDH]

    R74.8 Abnormal levels of other serum enzymes
       Abnormal level of acid phosphatase
       Abnormal level of alkaline phosphatase
       Abnormal level of amylase
       Abnormal level of lipase [triacylglycerol lipase]

    R74.9 Abnormal serum enzyme level, unspecified

R75 Inconclusive laboratory evidence of human immunodeficiency virus [HIV]
    Nonconclusive HIV-test finding in infants
> *EXCLUDES 1*   asymptomatic human immunodeficiency virus [HIV] infection status (Z21)
> human immunodeficiency virus [HIV] disease (B20)

✓4th **R76 Other abnormal immunological findings in serum**

    R76.0 Raised antibody titer
> *EXCLUDES 1*   isoimmunization in pregnancy (O36.0-O36.1)
> isoimmunization affecting newborn (P55.-)

✓5th **R76.1 Nonspecific reaction to test for tuberculosis**

    R76.11 Nonspecific reaction to tuberculin skin test without active tuberculosis
       Abnormal result of Mantoux test
       PPD positive
       Tuberculin (skin test) positive
       Tuberculin (skin test) reactor
> *EXCLUDES 1*   nonspecific reaction to cell mediated immunity measurement of gamma interferon antigen response without active tuberculosis (R76.12)

    R76.12 Nonspecific reaction to cell mediated immunity measurement of gamma interferon antigen response without active tuberculosis
       Nonspecific reaction to QuantiFERON-TB test (QFT) without active tuberculosis
> *EXCLUDES 1*   nonspecific reaction to tuberculin skin test without active tuberculosis (R76.11)
> positive tuberculin skin test (R76.11)

    R76.8 Other specified abnormal immunological findings in serum
       Raised level of immunoglobulins NOS

    R76.9 Abnormal immunological finding in serum, unspecified

✓4th **R77 Other abnormalities of plasma proteins**
> *EXCLUDES 1*   disorders of plasma-protein metabolism (E88.0)

    R77.0 Abnormality of albumin

    R77.1 Abnormality of globulin
       Hyperglobulinemia NOS

    R77.2 Abnormality of alphafetoprotein

    R77.8 Other specified abnormalities of plasma proteins

    R77.9 Abnormality of plasma protein, unspecified

✓4th **R78 Findings of drugs and other substances, not normally found in blood**
    Use additional code to identify any retained foreign body, if applicable (Z18.-)
> *EXCLUDES 1*   mental or behavioral disorders due to psychoactive substance use (F10-F19)

    R78.0 Finding of alcohol in blood
       Use additional external cause code (Y90.-), for detail regarding alcohol level

    R78.1 Finding of opiate drug in blood

    R78.2 Finding of cocaine in blood

    R78.3 Finding of hallucinogen in blood

    R78.4 Finding of other drugs of addictive potential in blood

    R78.5 Finding of other psychotropic drug in blood

    R78.6 Finding of steroid agent in blood

✓5th **R78.7 Finding of abnormal level of heavy metals in blood**

    R78.71 Abnormal lead level in blood
> *EXCLUDES 1*   lead poisoning (T56.0-)

    R78.79 Finding of abnormal level of heavy metals in blood

✓5th **R78.8 Finding of other specified substances, not normally found in blood**

    R78.81 Bacteremia   **CC**
> *EXCLUDES 1*   sepsis—code to specified infection
> **DEF:** Laboratory finding of bacteria in the blood in the absence of two or more signs of sepsis; transient in nature, it progresses to septicemia with severe infectious process.
> **CC Excl:** PDX collection 1136

    R78.89 Finding of other specified substances, not normally found in blood
       Finding of abnormal level of lithium in blood

    R78.9 Finding of unspecified substance, not normally found in blood

✓4th **R79 Other abnormal findings of blood chemistry**
    Use additional code to identify any retained foreign body, if applicable (Z18.-)
> *EXCLUDES 1*   abnormality of fluid, electrolyte or acid-base balance (E86-E87)
> asymptomatic hyperuricemia (E79.0)
> hyperglycemia NOS (R73.9)
> hypoglycemia NOS (E16.2)
> neonatal hypoglycemia (P70.3-P70.4)
> specific findings indicating disorder of amino-acid metabolism (E70-E72)
> specific findings indicating disorder of carbohydrate metabolism (E73-E74)
> specific findings indicating disorder of lipid metabolism (E75.-)

    R79.0 Abnormal level of blood mineral
       Abnormal blood level of cobalt
       Abnormal blood level of copper
       Abnormal blood level of iron
       Abnormal blood level of magnesium
       Abnormal blood level of mineral NEC
       Abnormal blood level of zinc
> *EXCLUDES 1*   abnormal level of lithium (R78.89)
> disorders of mineral metabolism (E83.-)
> neonatal hypomagnesemia (P71.2)
> nutritional mineral deficiency (E58-E61)

    R79.1 Abnormal coagulation profile
       Abnormal or prolonged bleeding time
       Abnormal or prolonged coagulation time
       Abnormal or prolonged partial thromboplastin time [PTT]
       Abnormal or prolonged prothrombin time [PT]
> *EXCLUDES 1*   coagulation defects (D68.-)
> *EXCLUDES 2*   ▶abnormality of fluid, electrolyte or acid-base balance (E86-E87)◄

✓5th **R79.8 Other specified abnormal findings of blood chemistry**

    R79.81 Abnormal blood-gas level

    R79.82 Elevated C-reactive protein [CRP]

    R79.89 Other specified abnormal findings of blood chemistry

    R79.9 Abnormal finding of blood chemistry, unspecified

N Newborn: 0   P Pediatric: 0-17   M Maternity: 12-55   A Adult: 15-124   MCC Major CC Condition   PDx MCC PDx acts as own MCC   CC CC Condition   PDx CC PDx acts as own CC

Abnormal findings on examination of urine, without diagnosis (R80-R82)

> EXCLUDES 1   abnormal findings on antenatal screening of mother (O28.-)
> diagnostic abnormal findings classified elsewhere—see Alphabetical Index
> specific findings indicating disorder of amino-acid metabolism (E70-E72)

✓4th **R80 Proteinuria**
> EXCLUDES 1   gestational proteinuria (O12.1-)

R80.0 Isolated proteinuria
Idiopathic proteinuria
> EXCLUDES 1   isolated proteinuria with specific morphological lesion (N06.-)

R80.1 Persistent proteinuria, unspecified

R80.2 Orthostatic proteinuria, unspecified
Postural proteinuria

R80.3 Bence Jones proteinuria

R80.8 Other proteinuria

R80.9 Proteinuria, unspecified
Albuminuria NOS

R81 Glycosuria
> EXCLUDES 1   renal glycosuria (E74.8)

✓4th **R82 Other and unspecified abnormal findings in urine**
> INCLUDES   chromoabnormalities in urine
Use additional code to identify any retained foreign body, if applicable (Z18.-)
> EXCLUDES 2   hematuria (R31.-)

R82.0 Chyluria   CC
> EXCLUDES 1   filarial chyluria (B74.-)
CC Excl: PDX collection 1137

R82.1 Myoglobinuria   CC
CC Excl: PDX collection 1138

R82.2 Biliuria

R82.3 Hemoglobinuria
> EXCLUDES 1   hemoglobinuria due to hemolysis from external causes NEC (D59.6)
> hemoglobinuria due to paroxysmal nocturnal [Marchiafava-Micheli] (D59.5)
DEF: Free hemoglobin in blood due to rapid hemolysis of red blood cells; causes include burns, crushed injury, sickle cell anemia, thalassemia, parasitic infections, or kidney infections.

R82.4 Acetonuria
Ketonuria
DEF: Excessive excretion of acetone in urine; commonly occurs in diabetic acidosis.

R82.5 Elevated urine levels of drugs, medicaments and biological substances
Elevated urine levels of catecholamines
Elevated urine levels of indoleacetic acid
Elevated urine levels of 17-ketosteroids
Elevated urine levels of steroids

R82.6 Abnormal urine levels of substances chiefly nonmedicinal as to source
Abnormal urine level of heavy metals

✓5th **R82.7 Abnormal findings on microbiological examination of urine**
> EXCLUDES 1   colonization status (Z22.-)

R82.71 Bacteriuria

R82.79 Other abnormal findings on microbiological examination of urine
Positive culture findings of urine

R82.8 Abnormal findings on cytological and histological examination of urine

✓5th **R82.9 Other and unspecified abnormal findings in urine**

R82.90 Unspecified abnormal findings in urine

R82.91 Other chromoabnormalities of urine
Chromoconversion (dipstick)
Idiopathic dipstick converts positive for blood with no cellular forms in sediment
> EXCLUDES 1   hemoglobinuria (R82.3)
> myoglobinuria (R82.1)

R82.99 Other abnormal findings in urine
Cells and casts in urine
Crystalluria
Melanuria

Abnormal findings on examination of other body fluids, substances and tissues, without diagnosis (R83-R89)

> EXCLUDES 1   abnormal findings on antenatal screening of mother (O28.-)
> diagnostic abnormal findings classified elsewhere—see Alphabetical Index
> EXCLUDES 2   abnormal findings on examination of blood, without diagnosis (R70-R79)
> abnormal findings on examination of urine, without diagnosis (R80-R82)
> abnormal tumor markers (R97.-)

✓4th **R83 Abnormal findings in cerebrospinal fluid**

R83.0 Abnormal level of enzymes in cerebrospinal fluid

R83.1 Abnormal level of hormones in cerebrospinal fluid

R83.2 Abnormal level of other drugs, medicaments and biological substances in cerebrospinal fluid

R83.3 Abnormal level of substances chiefly nonmedicinal as to source in cerebrospinal fluid

R83.4 Abnormal immunological findings in cerebrospinal fluid

R83.5 Abnormal microbiological findings in cerebrospinal fluid
Positive culture findings in cerebrospinal fluid
> EXCLUDES 1   colonization status (Z22.-)

R83.6 Abnormal cytological findings in cerebrospinal fluid

R83.8 Other abnormal findings in cerebrospinal fluid
Abnormal chromosomal findings in cerebrospinal fluid

R83.9 Unspecified abnormal finding in cerebrospinal fluid

✓4th **R84 Abnormal findings in specimens from respiratory organs and thorax**
> INCLUDES   abnormal findings in bronchial washings
> abnormal findings in nasal secretions
> abnormal findings in pleural fluid
> abnormal findings in sputum
> abnormal findings in throat scrapings
> EXCLUDES 1   blood-stained sputum (R04.2)

R84.0 Abnormal level of enzymes in specimens from respiratory organs and thorax

R84.1 Abnormal level of hormones in specimens from respiratory organs and thorax

R84.2 Abnormal level of other drugs, medicaments and biological substances in specimens from respiratory organs and thorax

R84.3 Abnormal level of substances chiefly nonmedicinal as to source in specimens from respiratory organs and thorax

R84.4 Abnormal immunological findings in specimens from respiratory organs and thorax

Cerebrospinal Fluid

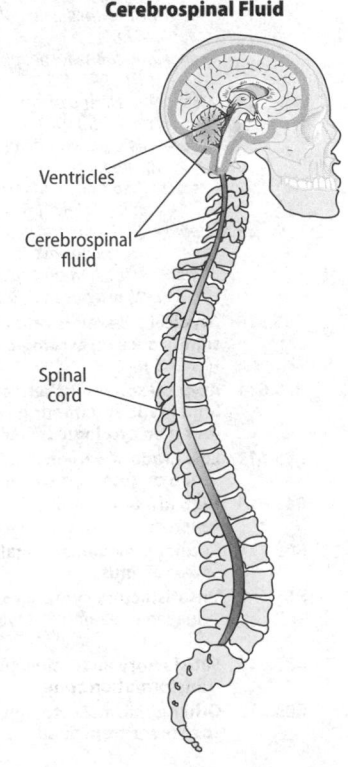

Ventricles

Cerebrospinal fluid

Spinal cord

R84.5   Abnormal microbiological findings in specimens from respiratory organs and thorax
Positive culture findings in specimens from respiratory organs and thorax
EXCLUDES 1   *colonization status (Z22.-)*

R84.6   Abnormal cytological findings in specimens from respiratory organs and thorax

R84.7   Abnormal histological findings in specimens from respiratory organs and thorax

R84.8   Other abnormal findings in specimens from respiratory organs and thorax
Abnormal chromosomal findings in specimens from respiratory organs and thorax

R84.9   Unspecified abnormal finding in specimens from respiratory organs and thorax

√4ᵗʰ **R85   Abnormal findings in specimens from digestive organs and abdominal cavity**
INCLUDES   abnormal findings in peritoneal fluid
abnormal findings in saliva
EXCLUDES 1   *cloudy peritoneal dialysis effluent (R88.0)*
fecal abnormalities (R19.5)

R85.0   Abnormal level of enzymes in specimens from digestive organs and abdominal cavity

R85.1   Abnormal level of hormones in specimens from digestive organs and abdominal cavity

R85.2   Abnormal level of other drugs, medicaments and biological substances in specimens from digestive organs and abdominal cavity

R85.3   Abnormal level of substances chiefly nonmedicinal as to source in specimens from digestive organs and abdominal cavity

R85.4   Abnormal immunological findings in specimens from digestive organs and abdominal cavity

R85.5   Abnormal microbiological findings in specimens from digestive organs and abdominal cavity
Positive culture findings in specimens from digestive organs and abdominal cavity
EXCLUDES 1   *colonization status (Z22.-)*

√5ᵗʰ **R85.6   Abnormal cytological findings in specimens from digestive organs and abdominal cavity**

√6ᵗʰ **R85.61   Abnormal cytologic smear of anus**
EXCLUDES 1   *abnormal cytological findings in specimens from other digestive organs and abdominal cavity (R85.69)*
anal intraepithelial neoplasia I [AIN I] (K62.82)
anal intraepithelial neoplasia II [AIN II] (K62.82)
anal intraepithelial neoplasia III [AIN III] (D01.3)
carcinoma in situ of anus (histologically confirmed) (D01.3)
dysplasia (mild) (moderate) of anus (histologically confirmed) (K62.82)
severe dysplasia of anus (histologically confirmed) (D01.3)
EXCLUDES 2   *anal high risk human papillomavirus (HPV) DNA test positive (R85.81)*
anal low risk human papillomavirus (HPV) DNA test positive (R85.82)

R85.610   Atypical squamous cells of undetermined significance on cytologic smear of anus [ASC-US]

R85.611   Atypical squamous cells cannot exclude high grade squamous intraepithelial lesion on cytologic smear of anus [ASC-H]

R85.612   Low grade squamous intraepithelial lesion on cytologic smear of anus [LGSIL]

R85.613   High grade squamous intraepithelial lesion on cytologic smear of anus [HGSIL]

R85.614   Cytologic evidence of malignancy on smear of anus

R85.615   Unsatisfactory cytologic smear of anus
Inadequate sample of cytologic smear of anus

R85.616   Satisfactory anal smear but lacking transformation zone

R85.618   Other abnormal cytological findings on specimens from anus

R85.619   Unspecified abnormal cytological findings in specimens from anus
Abnormal anal cytology NOS
Atypical glandular cells of anus NOS

R85.69   Abnormal cytological findings from specimens from other digestive organs and abdominal cavity

R85.7   Abnormal histological findings in specimens from digestive organs and abdominal cavity

√5ᵗʰ **R85.8   Other abnormal findings in specimens from digestive organs and abdominal cavity**

R85.81   Anal high risk human papillomavirus [HPV] DNA test positive
EXCLUDES 1   *anogenital warts due to human papillomavirus (HPV) (A63.0)*
condyloma acuminatum (A63.0)

R85.82   Anal low risk human papillomavirus [HPV] DNA test positive
Use additional code for associated human papillomavirus (B97.7)

R85.89   Other abnormal findings in specimens from digestive organs and abdominal cavity
Abnormal chromosomal findings in specimens from digestive organs and abdominal cavity

R85.9   Unspecified abnormal finding in specimens from digestive organs and abdominal cavity

√4ᵗʰ **R86   Abnormal findings in specimens from male genital organs**
INCLUDES   abnormal findings in prostatic secretions
abnormal findings in semen, seminal fluid
abnormal spermatozoa
EXCLUDES 1   *azoospermia (N46.0-)*
oligospermia (N46.1-)

R86.0   Abnormal level of enzymes in specimens from male genital organs   ♂

R86.1   Abnormal level of hormones in specimens from male genital organs   ♂

R86.2   Abnormal level of other drugs, medicaments and biological ♂ substances in specimens from male genital organs

R86.3   Abnormal level of substances chiefly nonmedicinal as to ♂ source in specimens from male genital organs

R86.4   Abnormal immunological findings in specimens from male ♂ genital organs

R86.5   Abnormal microbiological findings in specimens from male ♂ genital organs
Positive culture findings in specimens from male genital organs
EXCLUDES 1   *colonization status (Z22.-)*

R86.6   Abnormal cytological findings in specimens from male ♂ genital organs

R86.7   Abnormal histological findings in specimens from male ♂ genital organs

R86.8   Other abnormal findings in specimens from male genital ♂ organs
Abnormal chromosomal findings in specimens from male genital organs

R86.9   Unspecified abnormal finding in specimens from male ♂ genital organs

√4ᵗʰ **R87   Abnormal findings in specimens from female genital organs**
INCLUDES   abnormal findings in secretion and smears from cervix uteri
abnormal findings in secretion and smears from vagina
abnormal findings in secretion and smears from vulva

R87.0   Abnormal level of enzymes in specimens from female ♀ genital organs

R87.1   Abnormal level of hormones in specimens from female ♀ genital organs

R87.2   Abnormal level of other drugs, medicaments and ♀ biological substances in specimens from female genital organs

R87.3   Abnormal level of substances chiefly nonmedicinal as to ♀ source in specimens from female genital organs

R87.4   Abnormal immunological findings in specimens from ♀ female genital organs

R87.5   Abnormal microbiological findings in specimens from ♀ female genital organs
Positive culture findings in specimens from female genital organs
EXCLUDES 1   *colonization status (Z22.-)*

✓5th **R87.6** **Abnormal cytological findings in specimens from female genital organs**

✓6th **R87.61** **Abnormal cytological findings in specimens from cervix uteri**

EXCLUDES 1 *abnormal cytological findings in specimens from other female genital organs (R87.69)*

abnormal cytological findings in specimens from vagina (R87.62-)

carcinoma in situ of cervix uteri (histologically confirmed) (D06.-)

cervical intraepithelial neoplasia I [CIN I] (N87.0)

cervical intraepithelial neoplasia II [CIN II] (N87.1)

cervical intraepithelial neoplasia III [CIN III] (D06.-)

dysplasia (mild) (moderate) of cervix uteri (histologically confirmed) (N87.-)

severe dysplasia of cervix uteri (histologically confirmed) (D06.-)

EXCLUDES 2 *cervical high risk human papillomavirus (HPV) DNA test positive (R87.810)*

cervical low risk human papillomavirus (HPV) DNA test positive (R87.820)

R87.610 **Atypical squamous cells of undetermined significance on cytologic smear of cervix [ASC-US]** ♀

R87.611 **Atypical squamous cells cannot exclude high grade squamous intraepithelial lesion on cytologic smear of cervix [ASC-H]** ♀

R87.612 **Low grade squamous intraepithelial lesion on cytologic smear of cervix [LGSIL]** ♀

R87.613 **High grade squamous intraepithelial lesion on cytologic smear of cervix [HGSIL]** ♀

R87.614 **Cytologic evidence of malignancy on smear of cervix** ♀

R87.615 **Unsatisfactory cytologic smear of cervix** ♀

Inadequate sample of cytologic smear of cervix

R87.616 **Satisfactory cervical smear but lacking transformation zone** ♀

R87.618 **Other abnormal cytological findings on specimens from cervix uteri** ♀

R87.619 **Unspecified abnormal cytological findings in specimens from cervix uteri** ♀

Abnormal cervical cytology NOS

Abnormal Papanicolaou smear of cervix NOS

Abnormal thin preparation smear of cervix NOS

Atypical endocervial cells of cervix NOS

Atypical endometrial cells of cervix NOS

Atypical glandular cells of cervix NOS

✓6th **R87.62** **Abnormal cytological findings in specimens from vagina**

Use additional code to identify acquired absence of uterus and cervix, if applicable (Z90.71-)

EXCLUDES 1 *abnormal cytological findings in specimens from cervix uteri (R87.61-)*

abnormal cytological findings in specimens from other female genital organs (R87.69)

carcinoma in situ of vagina (histologically confirmed) (D07.2)

dysplasia (mild) (moderate) of vagina (histologically confirmed) (N89.-)

severe dysplasia of vagina (histologically confirmed) (D07.2)

vaginal intraepithelial neoplasia I [VAIN I] (N89.0)

vaginal intraepithelial neoplasia II [VAIN II] (N89.1)

vaginal intraepithelial neoplasia III [VAIN III] (D07.2)

EXCLUDES 2 *vaginal high risk human papillomavirus (HPV) DNA test positive (R87.811)*

vaginal low risk human papillomavirus (HPV) DNA test positive (R87.821)

R87.620 **Atypical squamous cells of undetermined significance on cytologic smear of vagina [ASC-US]** ♀

R87.621 **Atypical squamous cells cannot exclude high grade squamous intraepithelial lesion on cytologic smear of vagina [ASC-H]** ♀

R87.622 **Low grade squamous intraepithelial lesion on cytologic smear of vagina [LGSIL]** ♀

R87.623 **High grade squamous intraepithelial lesion on cytologic smear of vagina [HGSIL]** ♀

R87.624 **Cytologic evidence of malignancy on smear of vagina** ♀

R87.625 **Unsatisfactory cytologic smear of vagina** ♀

Inadequate sample of cytologic smear of vagina

R87.628 **Other abnormal cytological findings on specimens from vagina** ♀

R87.629 **Unspecified abnormal cytological findings in specimens from vagina** ♀

Abnormal Papanicolaou smear of vagina NOS

Abnormal thin preparation smear of vagina NOS

Abnormal vaginal cytology NOS

Atypical endocervical cells of vagina NOS

Atypical endometrial cells of vagina NOS

Atypical glandular cells of vagina NOS

R87.69 **Abnormal cytological findings in specimens from other female genital organs**

Abnormal cytological findings in specimens from female genital organs NOS

EXCLUDES 1 *dysplasia of vulva (histologically confirmed) (N90.0-N90.3)*

R87.7 **Abnormal histological findings in specimens from female genital organs** ♀

EXCLUDES 1 *carcinoma in situ (histologically confirmed) of female genital organs (D06-D07.3)*

cervical intraepithelial neoplasia I [CIN I] (N87.0)

cervical intraepithelial neoplasia II [CIN II] (N87.1)

cervical intraepithelial neoplasia III [CIN III] (D06.-)

dysplasia (mild) (moderate) of cervix uteri (histologically confirmed) (N87.-)

dysplasia (mild) (moderate) of vagina (histologically confirmed) (N89.-)

severe dysplasia of cervix uteri (histologically confirmed) (D06.-)

severe dysplasia of vagina (histologically confirmed) (D07.2)

vaginal intraepithelial neoplasia I [VAIN I] (N89.0)

vaginal intraepithelial neoplasia II [VAIN II] (N89.1)

vaginal intraepithelial neoplasia III [VAIN III] (D07.2)

✓5th **R87.8** **Other abnormal findings in specimens from female genital organs**

✓6th **R87.81** **High risk human papillomavirus [HPV] DNA test positive from female genital organs**

EXCLUDES 1 *anogenital warts due to human papillomavirus (HPV) (A63.0)*

condyloma acuminatum (A63.0)

R87.810 **Cervical high risk human papillomavirus [HPV] DNA test positive** ♀

R87.811 **Vaginal high risk human papillomavirus [HPV] DNA test positive** ♀

✓6th **R87.82** **Low risk human papillomavirus [HPV] DNA test positive from female genital organs**

Use additional code for associated human papillomavirus (B97.7)

R87.820 **Cervical low risk human papillomavirus [HPV] DNA test positive** ♀

R87.821 **Vaginal low risk human papillomavirus [HPV] DNA test positive** ♀

R87.89 **Other abnormal findings in specimens from female genital organs** ♀

Abnormal chromosomal findings in specimens from female genital organs

✔Additional Character Req ✔x7th Placeholder Alert Unacceptable PDx Manifestation H1 - H14 HAC HCC CMS-HCC Condition EXCLUDES 1 Not Coded Here EXCLUDES 2 Not Included Here

ICD-10-CM 2018 929

R87.9 Unspecified abnormal finding in specimens from female ♀ genital organs

✓4th **R88** **Abnormal findings in other body fluids and substances**

R88.0 Cloudy (hemodialysis) (peritoneal) dialysis effluent

R88.8 Abnormal findings in other body fluids and substances

✓4th **R89** **Abnormal findings in specimens from other organs, systems and tissues**

INCLUDES abnormal findings in nipple discharge
abnormal findings in synovial fluid
abnormal findings in wound secretions

R89.0 Abnormal level of enzymes in specimens from other organs, systems and tissues

R89.1 Abnormal level of hormones in specimens from other organs, systems and tissues

R89.2 Abnormal level of other drugs, medicaments and biological substances in specimens from other organs, systems and tissues

R89.3 Abnormal level of substances chiefly nonmedicinal as to source in specimens from other organs, systems and tissues

R89.4 Abnormal immunological findings in specimens from other organs, systems and tissues

R89.5 Abnormal microbiological findings in specimens from other organs, systems and tissues
Positive culture findings in specimens from other organs, systems and tissues
EXCLUDES 1 colonization status (Z22.-)

R89.6 Abnormal cytological findings in specimens from other organs, systems and tissues

R89.7 Abnormal histological findings in specimens from other organs, systems and tissues

R89.8 Other abnormal findings in specimens from other organs, systems and tissues
Abnormal chromosomal findings in specimens from other organs, systems and tissues

R89.9 Unspecified abnormal finding in specimens from other organs, systems and tissues

Abnormal findings on diagnostic imaging and in function studies, without diagnosis (R90-R94)

INCLUDES nonspecific abnormal findings on diagnostic imaging by computerized axial tomography [CAT scan]
nonspecific abnormal findings on diagnostic imaging by magnetic resonance imaging [MRI][NMR]
nonspecific abnormal findings on diagnostic imaging by positron emission tomography [PET scan]
nonspecific abnormal findings on diagnostic imaging by thermography
nonspecific abnormal findings on diagnostic imaging by ultrasound [echogram]
nonspecific abnormal findings on diagnostic imaging by X-ray examination
EXCLUDES 1 abnormal findings on antenatal screening of mother (O28.-)
diagnostic abnormal findings classified elsewhere—see Alphabetical Index

✓4th **R90** **Abnormal findings on diagnostic imaging of central nervous system**

R90.0 Intracranial space-occupying lesion found on diagnostic imaging of central nervous system

✓5th **R90.8** Other abnormal findings on diagnostic imaging of central nervous system

R90.81 Abnormal echoencephalogram

R90.82 White matter disease, unspecified

R90.89 Other abnormal findings on diagnostic imaging of central nervous system
Other cerebrovascular abnormality found on diagnostic imaging of central nervous system

✓4th **R91** **Abnormal findings on diagnostic imaging of lung**

R91.1 Solitary pulmonary nodule
Coin lesion lung
Solitary pulmonary nodule, subsegmental branch of the bronchial tree

R91.8 Other nonspecific abnormal finding of lung field
Lung mass NOS found on diagnostic imaging of lung
Pulmonary infiltrate NOS
Shadow, lung

✓4th **R92** **Abnormal and inconclusive findings on diagnostic imaging of breast**

R92.0 Mammographic microcalcification found on diagnostic imaging of breast
EXCLUDES 2 mammographic calcification (calculus) found on diagnostic imaging of breast (R92.1)
DEF: Calcium and cellular debris deposits in the breast that cannot be felt but can be detected on a mammogram; can be a sign of cancer, benign conditions, or changes in the breast tissue as a result of inflammation, injury, or obstructed duct.

R92.1 Mammographic calcification found on diagnostic imaging of breast
Mammographic calculus found on diagnostic imaging of breast

R92.2 Inconclusive mammogram
Dense breasts NOS
Inconclusive mammogram NEC
Inconclusive mammography due to dense breasts
Inconclusive mammography NEC
AHA: 2015, 1Q, 24

R92.8 Other abnormal and inconclusive findings on diagnostic imaging of breast

✓4th **R93** **Abnormal findings on diagnostic imaging of other body structures**

R93.0 Abnormal findings on diagnostic imaging of skull and head, not elsewhere classified
EXCLUDES 1 intracranial space-occupying lesion found on diagnostic imaging (R90.0)

R93.1 Abnormal findings on diagnostic imaging of heart and coronary circulation
Abnormal echocardiogram NOS
Abnormal heart shadow

R93.2 Abnormal findings on diagnostic imaging of liver and biliary tract
Nonvisualization of gallbladder

R93.3 Abnormal findings on diagnostic imaging of other parts of digestive tract

✓5th **R93.4** Abnormal findings on diagnostic imaging of urinary organs
EXCLUDES 2 hypertrophy of kidney (N28.81)

R93.41 Abnormal radiologic findings on diagnostic imaging of renal pelvis, ureter, or bladder
Filling defect of bladder found on diagnostic imaging
Filling defect of renal pelvis found on diagnostic imaging
Filling defect of ureter found on diagnostic imaging

✓6th **R93.42** Abnormal radiologic findings on diagnostic imaging of kidney

R93.421 Abnormal radiologic findings on diagnostic imaging of right kidney

R93.422 Abnormal radiologic findings on diagnostic imaging of left kidney

R93.429 Abnormal radiologic findings on diagnostic imaging of unspecified kidney

R93.49 Abnormal radiologic findings on diagnostic imaging of other urinary organs

R93.5 Abnormal findings on diagnostic imaging of other abdominal regions, including retroperitoneum

R93.6 Abnormal findings on diagnostic imaging of limbs
EXCLUDES 2 abnormal finding in skin and subcutaneous tissue (R93.8)

R93.7 Abnormal findings on diagnostic imaging of other parts of musculoskeletal system
EXCLUDES 2 abnormal findings on diagnostic imaging of skull (R93.0)

R93.8 Abnormal findings on diagnostic imaging of other specified body structures
Abnormal finding by radioisotope localization of placenta
Abnormal radiological finding in skin and subcutaneous tissue
Mediastinal shift

R93.9 Diagnostic imaging inconclusive due to excess body fat of patient

✓4th **R94** **Abnormal results of function studies**
INCLUDES abnormal results of radionuclide [radioisotope] uptake studies
abnormal results of scintigraphy

✓5th **R94.0** Abnormal results of function studies of central nervous system

R94.01 Abnormal electroencephalogram [EEG]

R94.02 Abnormal brain scan

N Newborn: 0 P Pediatric: 0-17 M Maternity: 12-55 A Adult: 15-124 MCC Major CC Condition PDxMCC PDx acts as own MCC CC CC Condition PDxCC PDx acts as own CC

930 ICD-10-CM 2018

R94.09   **Abnormal results of** other function studies **of central nervous system**

✓5ᵗʰ   R94.1   **Abnormal results of function studies of** peripheral nervous system and special senses

     ✓6ᵗʰ   R94.11   **Abnormal results of function studies of** eye

         R94.110   **Abnormal** electro-oculogram [EOG]

         R94.111   **Abnormal** electroretinogram [ERG]
                     Abnormal retinal function study

         R94.112   **Abnormal** visually evoked potential [VEP]

         R94.113   **Abnormal** oculomotor **study**

         R94.118   **Abnormal results of** other function studies of eye

     ✓6ᵗʰ   R94.12   **Abnormal results of function studies of** ear and other special senses
              AHA: 2016, 3Q, 17

         R94.120   **Abnormal** auditory **function study**

         R94.121   **Abnormal** vestibular **function study**

         R94.128   **Abnormal results of** other function studies of ear and other special senses

     ✓6ᵗʰ   R94.13   **Abnormal results of function studies of** peripheral nervous system

         R94.130   **Abnormal response to** nerve stimulation, **unspecified**

         R94.131   **Abnormal electromyogram [EMG]**
             EXCLUDES 1   electromyogram of eye (R94.113)

         R94.138   **Abnormal results of** other function studies of peripheral nervous system

R94.2   **Abnormal results of** pulmonary function **studies**
       Reduced ventilatory capacity
       Reduced vital capacity

✓5ᵗʰ   R94.3   **Abnormal results of** cardiovascular function **studies**

     R94.30   **Abnormal result of cardiovascular function study, unspecified**

     R94.31   **Abnormal** electrocardiogram [ECG] [EKG]
         EXCLUDES 1   long QT syndrome (I45.81)

     R94.39   **Abnormal result of** other **cardiovascular function study**
         Abnormal electrophysiological intracardiac studies
         Abnormal phonocardiogram
         Abnormal vectorcardiogram

R94.4   **Abnormal results of** kidney function **studies**
       Abnormal renal function test

R94.5   **Abnormal results of** liver function **studies**

R94.6   **Abnormal results of** thyroid function **studies**

R94.7   **Abnormal results of** other endocrine function **studies**
       EXCLUDES 2   abnormal glucose (R73.0-)

R94.8   **Abnormal results of function studies of** other organs and systems
       Abnormal basal metabolic rate [BMR]
       Abnormal bladder function test
       Abnormal splenic function test

Abnormal tumor markers (R97)

✓4ᵗʰ   **R97   Abnormal tumor markers**
       Elevated tumor associated antigens [TAA]
       Elevated tumor specific antigens [TSA]

R97.0   **Elevated carcinoembryonic antigen [CEA]**

R97.1   **Elevated cancer antigen 125 [CA 125]**

✓5ᵗʰ   R97.2   **Elevated prostate specific antigen [PSA]**

     [4]   R97.20   **Elevated prostate specific antigen [PSA]**   A ♂

     [4]   R97.21   **Rising PSA following treatment for malignant neoplasm of prostate**   A ♂

R97.8   **Other abnormal tumor markers**

Ill-defined and unknown cause of mortality (R99)

R99   Ill-defined and unknown cause of mortality
       Death (unexplained) NOS
       Unspecified cause of mortality

---

[4]   Questionable admission when used as PDx.

✓ Additional Character Req   ✓x7ᵗʰ Placeholder Alert   Unacceptable PDx   Manifestation   H1 - H14 HAC   HCC CMS-HCC Condition   *EXCLUDES 1* Not Coded Here   *EXCLUDES 2* Not Included Here

Chapter 19. Injury, Poisoning and Certain Other Consequences of External Causes (S00–T88)

Chapter Specific Guidelines with Coding Examples

The chapter specific guidelines from the ICD-10-CM Official Guidelines for Coding and Reporting have been provided below. Along with these guidelines are coding examples, contained in the shaded boxes, that have been developed to help illustrate the coding and/or sequencing guidance found in these guidelines.

a. Application of 7th characters in Chapter 19

Most categories in chapter 19 have a 7th character requirement for each applicable code. Most categories in this chapter have three 7th character values (with the exception of fractures): A, initial encounter, D, subsequent encounter and S, sequela. Categories for traumatic fractures have additional 7th character values. While the patient may be seen by a new or different provider over the course of treatment for an injury, assignment of the 7th character is based on whether the patient is undergoing active treatment and not whether the provider is seeing the patient for the first time.

For complication codes, active treatment refers to treatment for the condition described by the code, even though it may be related to an earlier precipitating problem. For example, code T84.50XA, Infection and inflammatory reaction due to unspecified internal joint prosthesis, initial encounter, is used when active treatment is provided for the infection, even though the condition relates to the prosthetic device, implant or graft that was placed at a previous encounter.

7th character "A", initial encounter is used for each encounter where the patient is receiving active treatment for the condition.

> Patient admitted after fall from a skateboard onto the sidewalk, x-rays identify a nondisplaced fracture to the distal pole of the right scaphoid bone. The patient is placed in a cast.
>
> **S62.014A**   **Nondisplaced fracture of distal pole of navicular [scaphoid] bone of right wrist, initial encounter for closed fracture**
>
> **V00.131A**   **Fall from skateboard, initial encounter**
>
> **Y92.480**   **Sidewalk as the place of occurrence of the external cause**
>
> **Y93.51**   **Activity, roller skating (inline) and skateboarding**
>
> **Y99.8**   **Other external cause status**
>
> *Explanation:* This fracture would be coded with a seventh character A for initial encounter because the patient received x-rays to identify the site of the fracture and treatment was rendered; this would be considered active treatment.

7th character "D" subsequent encounter is used for encounters after the patient has completed active treatment of the condition and is receiving routine care for the condition during the healing or recovery phase.

> Patient admitted after fall from a skateboard onto the sidewalk resulted in casting of the right arm. X-rays are taken to evaluate how well the nondisplaced fracture to the distal pole of the right scaphoid bone is healing. The physician feels the fracture is healing appropriately; no adjustments to the cast are made.
>
> **S62.014D**   **Nondisplaced fracture of distal pole of navicular [scaphoid] bone of right wrist, subsequent encounter for fracture with routine healing**
>
> **V00.131D**   **Fall from skateboard, subsequent encounter**
>
> *Explanation:* This fracture would be coded with a seventh character D for subsequent encounter, whether the same physician who provided the initial cast application or a different physician is now seeing the patient. Although the patient received x-rays, the intent of the x-rays was to assess how the fracture was healing. There was no active treatment rendered and the visit is therefore considered a subsequent encounter.

The aftercare Z codes should not be used for aftercare for conditions such as injuries or poisonings, where 7th characters are provided to identify subsequent care. For example, for aftercare of an injury, assign the acute injury code with the 7th character "D" (subsequent encounter).

7th character "S", sequela, is for use for complications or conditions that arise as a direct result of a condition, such as scar formation after a burn. The scars are sequelae of the burn. When using 7th character "S", it is

necessary to use both the injury code that precipitated the sequela and the code for the sequela itself. The "S" is added only to the injury code, not the sequela code. The 7th character "S" identifies the injury responsible for the sequela. The specific type of sequela (e.g. scar) is sequenced first, followed by the injury code.

See Section I.B.10 Sequelae, (Late Effects)

> Patient with a history of a nondisplaced fracture to the distal pole of the right scaphoid bone due to a fall from a skateboard is admitted for evaluation of arthritis to the right wrist that has developed as a consequence of the traumatic fracture.
>
> **M12.531**   **Traumatic arthropathy, right wrist**
>
> **S62.014S**   **Nondisplaced fracture of distal pole of navicular [scaphoid] bone of right wrist, sequela**
>
> **V00.131S**   **Fall from skateboard, sequela**
>
> *Explanation:* The code identifying the specific sequela condition (traumatic arthritis) should be coded first followed by the injury that instigated the development of the sequela (fracture). The scaphoid fracture injury code is given a 7th character S for sequela to represent its role as the inciting injury. The fracture has healed and is not being managed or treated on this admit and therefore is not applicable as a first listed or principal diagnosis. However, it is directly related to the development of the arthritis and should be appended as a secondary code to signify this cause and effect relationship.

b. Coding of injuries

When coding injuries, assign separate codes for each injury unless a combination code is provided, in which case the combination code is assigned. **Codes from category** T07, Unspecified multiple injuries should not be assigned in the inpatient setting unless information for a more specific code is not available. Traumatic injury codes (S00-T14.9) are not to be used for normal, healing surgical wounds or to identify complications of surgical wounds.

The code for the most serious injury, as determined by the provider and the focus of treatment, is sequenced first.

1) Superficial injuries

Superficial injuries such as abrasions or contusions are not coded when associated with more severe injuries of the same site.

2) Primary injury with damage to nerves/blood vessels

When a primary injury results in minor damage to peripheral nerves or blood vessels, the primary injury is sequenced first with additional code(s) for injuries to nerves and spinal cord (such as category S04), and/or injury to blood vessels (such as category S15). When the primary injury is to the blood vessels or nerves, that injury should be sequenced first.

c. Coding of traumatic fractures

The principles of multiple coding of injuries should be followed in coding fractures. Fractures of specified sites are coded individually by site in accordance with both the provisions within categories S02, S12, S22, S32, S42, S49, S52, S59, S62, S72, S79, S82, S89, S92 and the level of detail furnished by medical record content.

A fracture not indicated as open or closed should be coded to closed. A fracture not indicated whether displaced or not displaced should be coded to displaced.

More specific guidelines are as follows:

1) Initial vs. subsequent encounter for fractures

Traumatic fractures are coded using the appropriate 7th character for initial encounter (A, B, C) for each encounter where the patient is receiving active treatment for the fracture. The appropriate 7th character for initial encounter should also be assigned for a patient who delayed seeking treatment for the fracture or nonunion.

Fractures are coded using the appropriate 7th character for subsequent care for encounters after the patient has completed active treatment of the fracture and is receiving routine care for the fracture during the healing or recovery phase.

Care for complications of surgical treatment for fracture repairs during the healing or recovery phase should be coded with the appropriate complication codes.

Care of complications of fractures, such as malunion and nonunion, should be reported with the appropriate 7th character for subsequent care with nonunion (K, M, N,) or subsequent care with malunion (P, Q, R).

Malunion/nonunion: The appropriate 7th character for initial encounter should also be assigned for a patient who delayed seeking treatment for the fracture or nonunion.

> Female patient fell during a forest hiking excursion almost six months ago and until recently did not feel she needed to seek medical attention for her left ankle pain; x-rays show nonunion of lateral malleolus and surgery has been scheduled
>
> | | |
> |---|---|
> | S82.62XA | Displaced fracture of lateral malleolus of left fibula, initial encounter for closed fracture |
> | W01.0XXA | Fall on same level from slipping, tripping and stumbling without subsequent striking against object, initial encounter |
> | Y92.821 | Forest as place of occurrence of the external cause |
> | Y93.01 | Activity, walking, marching and hiking |
> | Y99.8 | Other external cause status |
>
> *Explanation:* A seventh character of A is used for the lateral malleolus nonunion fracture to signify that the fracture is receiving active treatment. The delayed care for the fracture has resulted in a nonunion, but capturing the nonunion in the seventh character is trumped by the provision of active care.

The open fracture designations in the assignment of the 7th character for fractures of the forearm, femur and lower leg, including ankle are based on the Gustilo open fracture classification. When the Gustilo classification type is not specified for an open fracture, the 7th character for open fracture type I or II should be assigned (B, E, H, M, Q).

> A 17-year-old arrives at the trauma center with open, displaced right forearm fracture with extensive soft tissue damage. He fell while being tackled playing football for his high school team. On-call orthopaedic specialist documents segmental type IIIA fracture of shaft radius with no need for plastic consult.
>
> | | |
> |---|---|
> | S52.361C | Displaced segmental fracture of shaft of radius, right arm, initial encounter for open fracture type IIIA, IIIB, or IIIC |
> | W03XXXA | Other fall on same level due to collision with another person, initial encounter |
> | Y92.321 | Football field as the place of occurrence of the external cause |
> | Y93.61 | Activity, American tackle football |
>
> *Explanation:* The seventh character for forearm fractures capture the type of encounter and whether the fracture is open or closed; open fractures are broken down further by the type of fracture based on the Gustilo classification. The Gustilo classification describes the severity of open fracture and soft tissue injury. Type IIIA describes an open fracture with extensive soft tissue injury but adequate soft tissue remaining for wound coverage. A segmental fracture means that the bone is broken in two places, leaving at least one segment unattached to the bone. There is no need to report an additional code for the soft tissue injury as it is captured in the fracture code.

A code from category M80, not a traumatic fracture code, should be used for any patient with known osteoporosis who suffers a fracture, even if the patient had a minor fall or trauma, if that fall or trauma would not usually break a normal, healthy bone.

See Section I.C.13. Osteoporosis.

The aftercare Z codes should not be used for aftercare for traumatic fractures. For aftercare of a traumatic fracture, assign the acute fracture code with the appropriate 7th character.

2) Multiple fractures sequencing

Multiple fractures are sequenced in accordance with the severity of the fracture.

d. Coding of burns and corrosions

The ICD-10-CM makes a distinction between burns and corrosions. The burn codes are for thermal burns, except sunburns, that come from a heat source, such as a fire or hot appliance. The burn codes are also for burns resulting from electricity and radiation. Corrosions are burns due to chemicals. The guidelines are the same for burns and corrosions.

Current burns (T20-T25) are classified by depth, extent and by agent (X code). Burns are classified by depth as first degree (erythema), second degree (blistering), and third degree (full-thickness involvement). Burns of the eye and internal organs (T26-T28) are classified by site, but not by degree.

1) Sequencing of burn and related condition codes

Sequence first the code that reflects the highest degree of burn when more than one burn is present.

a. When the reason for the admission or encounter is for treatment of external multiple burns, sequence first the code that reflects the burn of the highest degree.

b. When a patient has both internal and external burns, the circumstances of admission govern the selection of the principal diagnosis or first-listed diagnosis.

c. When a patient is admitted for burn injuries and other related conditions such as smoke inhalation and/or respiratory failure, the circumstances of admission govern the selection of the principal or first-listed diagnosis.

> Patient admitted with minor first-degree burns to multiple sites of her right and left hands as well as severe smoke inhalation. While she was sleeping at home, a candle on her dresser lit the bedroom curtains on fire.
>
> | | |
> |---|---|
> | T59.811A | Toxic effect of smoke, accidental (unintentional), initial encounter |
> | J70.5 | Respiratory conditions due to smoke inhalation |
> | T23.191A | Burn of first degree of multiple sites of right wrist and hand, initial encounter |
> | T23.192A | Burn of first degree of multiple sites of left wrist and hand, initial encounter |
> | X08.8XXA | Exposure to other specified smoke, fire and flames, initial encounter |
> | Y92.003 | Bedroom of unspecified non-institutional (private) residence as the place of occurrence of the external cause |
> | Y93.84 | Activity, sleeping |
>
> *Explanation:* Based on the documentation, the inhalation injury is more severe than the first-degree burns and is sequenced first. The burns to the hands are appended as secondary diagnoses.

2) Burns of the same local site

Classify burns of the same local site (three-character category level, T20-T28) but of different degrees to the subcategory identifying the highest degree recorded in the diagnosis.

> 10-year-old male patient is admitted for third-degree burns of his right palm and second-degree burns of multiple right fingers; right thumb not affected
>
> | | |
> |---|---|
> | T23.351A | Burn of third degree of right palm, initial encounter |
>
> *Explanation:* Although there is a code for second-degree burns of multiple fingers, not including the thumb (T23.131-), this code falls in the same three-digit category that the third-degree burn of the right palm falls under, category T23. Only the subcategory identifying the highest degree is captured when different burn degrees are classified to a single category.

> Patient is admitted with third-degree burns of the scalp as well as second-degree burns to the back of the right hand
>
> | | |
> |---|---|
> | T20.35XA | Burn of third degree of scalp [any part], initial encounter |
> | T23.261A | Burn of second degree of back of right hand, initial encounter |
>
> *Explanation:* Since burns to the hand and scalp are classified to two different three-digit categories, both burns may be reported as they represent distinct sites.

3) Non-healing burns

Non-healing burns are coded as acute burns.

Necrosis of burned skin should be coded as a non-healed burn.

4) Infected burn

For any documented infected burn site, use an additional code for the infection.

5) Assign separate codes for each burn site

When coding burns, assign separate codes for each burn site. Category T30, Burn and corrosion, body region unspecified is extremely vague and should rarely be used.

6) Burns and corrosions classified according to extent of body surface involved

Assign codes from category T31, Burns classified according to extent of body surface involved, or T32, Corrosions classified according to extent of body surface involved, when the site of the burn is not specified or when there is a need for additional data. It is advisable to use category T31 as additional coding when needed to provide data for evaluating burn mortality, such as that needed by burn units. It is also advisable to use category T31 as an additional code for reporting purposes when there is mention of a third-degree burn involving 20 percent or more of the body surface.

Categories T31 and T32 are based on the classic "rule of nines" in estimating body surface involved: head and neck are assigned nine percent, each arm nine percent, each leg 18 percent, the anterior trunk 18 percent, posterior trunk 18 percent, and genitalia one percent. Providers may change these percentage assignments where necessary to accommodate infants and children who have proportionately larger heads than adults, and patients who have large buttocks, thighs, or abdomen that involve burns.

Patient seen in burn unit for dressing change after he accidentally spilled acetic acid on himself two days ago. The second-degree burns to his right thigh, covering about 3 percent of his body surface, are healing appropriately.

T54.2X1D	Toxic effect of corrosive acids and acid-like substances, accidental (unintentional), subsequent encounter
T24.611D	Corrosion of second degree of right thigh, subsequent encounter
T32.0	Corrosions involving less than 10% of body surface

Explanation: Code T32.0 provides additional information as to how much of the patient's body was affected by the corrosive substance.

7) Encounters for treatment of sequela of burns

Encounters for the treatment of the late effects of burns or corrosions (i.e., scars or joint contractures) should be coded with a burn or corrosion code with the 7th character "S" for sequela.

8) Sequelae with a late effect code and current burn

When appropriate, both a code for a current burn or corrosion with 7th character "A" or "D" and a burn or corrosion code with 7th character "S" may be assigned on the same record (when both a current burn and sequelae of an old burn exist). Burns and corrosions do not heal at the same rate and a current healing wound may still exist with sequela of a healed burn or corrosion.

See Section I.B.10 Sequela (Late Effects)

Female patient seen in ED for second-degree burn to the left ear; she also has significant scarring on her left elbow from a third-degree burn from childhood

T20.212A	Burn of second degree of left ear [any part, except ear drum], initial encounter
L90.5	Scar conditions and fibrosis of skin
T22.322S	Burn of third degree of left elbow, sequela

Explanation: The patient is being seen for management of a current second-degree burn, which is reflected in the code by appending the seventh character of A, indicating active treatment or management of this burn. The elbow scarring is a sequela of a previous third-degree burn. The sequela condition precedes the original burn injury, which is appended with a seventh character of S.

9) Use of an external cause code with burns and corrosions

An external cause code should be used with burns and corrosions to identify the source and intent of the burn, as well as the place where it occurred.

e. Adverse effects, poisoning, underdosing and toxic effects

Codes in categories T36-T65 are combination codes that include the substance that was taken as well as the intent. No additional external cause code is required for poisonings, toxic effects, adverse effects and underdosing codes.

1) Do not code directly from the Table of Drugs

Do not code directly from the Table of Drugs and Chemicals. Always refer back to the Tabular List.

2) Use as many codes as necessary to describe

Use as many codes as necessary to describe completely all drugs, medicinal or biological substances.

3) If the same code would describe the causative agent

If the same code would describe the causative agent for more than one adverse reaction, poisoning, toxic effect or underdosing, assign the code only once.

4) If two or more drugs, medicinal or biological substances

If two or more drugs, medicinal or biological substances are reported, code each individually unless a combination code is listed in the Table of Drugs and Chemicals.

5) The occurrence of drug toxicity is classified in ICD-10-CM as follows:

(a) Adverse effect

When coding an adverse effect of a drug that has been correctly prescribed and properly administered, assign the appropriate code for the nature of the adverse effect followed by the appropriate code for the adverse effect of the drug (T36-T50). The code for the drug should have a 5th or 6th character "5" (for example T36.0X5-) Examples of the nature of an adverse effect are tachycardia, delirium, gastrointestinal hemorrhaging, vomiting, hypokalemia, hepatitis, renal failure, or respiratory failure.

Patient admitted for stomach pain and jaundice, indicated by physician as possible side-effects of Inderal, recently started for hypertension. Inderal was discontinued and the patient switched to Atenolol instead.

R10.9	Unspecified abdominal pain
R17	Unspecified jaundice
T44.7X5A	Adverse effect of beta-adrenoreceptor antagonists, initial encounter
I10	Essential (primary) hypertension

Explanation: The side-effects caused by the drug are listed first, followed by the code for the adverse effect of the drug to capture the specific drug that was used.

(b) Poisoning

When coding a poisoning or reaction to the improper use of a medication (e.g., overdose, wrong substance given or taken in error, wrong route of administration), first assign the appropriate code from categories T36-T50. The poisoning codes have an associated intent as their 5th or 6th character (accidental, intentional self-harm, assault and undetermined. If the intent of the poisoning is unknown or unspecified, code the intent as accidental intent. The undetermined intent is only for use if the documentation in the record specifies that the intent cannot be determined. Use additional code(s) for all manifestations of poisonings.

A 55-year-old female status post recent left knee replacement is admitted due to confusion, dizziness, and nausea. Her spouse brought in her prescribed Xanax, Ambien, and Percocet bottles but has no idea how many she took. It is suspected that her symptoms are due to an overdose of these medications.

T42.4X1A	Poisoning by benzodiazepines, accidental (unintentional), initial encounter
T42.6X1A	Poisoning by other antiepileptic and sedative-hypnotic drugs, accidental (unintentional), initial encounter
T40.2X1A	Poisoning by other opioids, accidental (unintentional), initial encounter
R41.0	Disorientation, unspecified
R42	Dizziness and giddiness
R11.0	Nausea

Explanation: It was not documented whether the overdose of the drugs was accidental or intentional; therefore the correct reporting of the poisoning codes is accidental intent. The poisoning codes are sequenced first, followed by manifestations of the poisoning.

If there is also a diagnosis of abuse or dependence of the substance, the abuse or dependence is assigned as an additional code.

Examples of poisoning include:

(i) Error was made in drug prescription

Errors made in drug prescription or in the administration of the drug by provider, nurse, patient, or other person.

(ii) Overdose of a drug intentionally taken

If an overdose of a drug was intentionally taken or administered and resulted in drug toxicity, it would be coded as a poisoning.

(iii) Nonprescribed drug taken with correctly prescribed and properly administered drug

If a nonprescribed drug or medicinal agent was taken in combination with a correctly prescribed and properly administered drug, any drug toxicity or other reaction resulting from the interaction of the two drugs would be classified as a poisoning.

(iv) Interaction of drug(s) and alcohol

When a reaction results from the interaction of a drug(s) and alcohol, this would be classified as poisoning.

See Section I.C.4. if poisoning is the result of insulin pump malfunctions.

(c) Underdosing

Underdosing refers to taking less of a medication than is prescribed by a provider or a manufacturer's instruction. For underdosing, assign the code from categories T36-T50 (fifth or sixth character "6").

Codes for underdosing should never be assigned as principal or first-listed codes. If a patient has a relapse or exacerbation of the medical condition for which the drug is prescribed because of the reduction in dose, then the medical condition itself should be coded.

Noncompliance (Z91.12-, Z91.13-) or complication of care (Y63.6-Y63.9) codes are to be used with an underdosing code to indicate intent, if known.

Patient admitted for atrial fibrillation with history of chronic atrial fibrillation for which she is prescribed amiodarone. Financial concerns have left the patient unable to pay for her prescriptions and she has been skipping her amiodarone dose every other day to offset the cost.

I48.2	Chronic atrial fibrillation
T46.2X6A	Underdosing of other antidysrhythmic drugs, initial encounter
Z91.120	Patient's intentional underdosing of medication regimen due to financial hardship

Explanation: By skipping her amiodarone pill every other day, the patient's atrial fibrillation returned. The condition for which the drug was being taken is reported first, followed by an underdosing code to show that the patient was not adhering to her prescription regiment. The Z code helps elaborate on the patient's social and/or economic circumstances that led to the patient taking less then what she was prescribed.

(d) Toxic effects

When a harmful substance is ingested or comes in contact with a person, this is classified as a toxic effect. The toxic effect codes are in categories T51-T65.

Toxic effect codes have an associated intent: accidental, intentional self-harm, assault and undetermined.

f. Adult and child abuse, neglect and other maltreatment

Sequence first the appropriate code from categories T74.- (Adult and child abuse, neglect and other maltreatment, confirmed) or T76.- (Adult and child abuse, neglect and other maltreatment, suspected) for abuse, neglect and other maltreatment, followed by any accompanying mental health or injury code(s).

If the documentation in the medical record states abuse or neglect it is coded as confirmed (T74.-). It is coded as suspected if it is documented as suspected (T76.-).

For cases of confirmed abuse or neglect an external cause code from the assault section (X92-Y09) should be added to identify the cause of any physical injuries. A perpetrator code (Y07) should be added when the perpetrator of the abuse is known. For suspected cases of abuse or neglect, do not report external cause or perpetrator code.

If a suspected case of abuse, neglect or mistreatment is ruled out during an encounter code Z04.71, Encounter for examination and observation following alleged physical adult abuse, ruled out, or code Z04.72, Encounter for examination and observation following alleged child physical abuse, ruled out, should be used, not a code from T76.

If a suspected case of alleged rape or sexual abuse is ruled out during an encounter code Z04.41, Encounter for examination and observation following alleged adult rape or code Z04.42, Encounter for examination and observation following alleged child rape, should be used, not a code from T76.

See Section I.C.15. Abuse in a pregnant patient.

g. Complications of care

1) General guidelines for complications of care

(a) Documentation of complications of care

See Section I.B.16. for information on documentation of complications of care.

2) Pain due to medical devices

Pain associated with devices, implants or grafts left in a surgical site (for example painful hip prosthesis) is assigned to the appropriate code(s) found in Chapter 19, Injury, poisoning, and certain other consequences of external causes. Specific codes for pain due to medical devices are found in the T code section of the ICD-10-CM. Use additional code(s) from category G89 to identify acute or chronic pain due to presence of the device, implant or graft (G89.18 or G89.28).

Chronic left breast pain secondary to breast implant

T85.848A   **Pain due to other internal prosthetic devices, implants and grafts, initial encounter**

N64.4   **Mastodynia**

G89.28   **Other chronic postprocedural pain**

Explanation: As the pain is a complication related to the breast implant, the complication code is sequenced first. The T code does not describe the site or type of pain, so additional codes may be appended to indicate that the patient is experiencing chronic pain in the breast.

3) Transplant complications

(a) Transplant complications other than kidney

Codes under category T86, Complications of transplanted organs and tissues, are for use for both complications and rejection of transplanted organs. A transplant complication code is only assigned if the complication affects the function of the transplanted organ. Two codes are required to fully describe a transplant complication: the appropriate code from category T86 and a secondary code that identifies the complication.

Pre-existing conditions or conditions that develop after the transplant are not coded as complications unless they affect the function of the transplanted organs.

See I.C.21. for transplant organ removal status

See I.C.2. for malignant neoplasm associated with transplanted organ.

(b) Kidney transplant complications

Patients who have undergone kidney transplant may still have some form of chronic kidney disease (CKD) because the kidney transplant may not fully restore kidney function. Code T86.1- should be assigned for documented complications of a kidney transplant, such as transplant failure or rejection or other transplant complication. Code T86.1- should not be assigned for post kidney transplant patients who have chronic kidney (CKD) unless a transplant complication such as transplant failure or rejection is documented. If the documentation is unclear as to whether the patient has a complication of the transplant, query the provider.

Conditions that affect the function of the transplanted kidney, other than CKD, should be assigned a code from subcategory T86.1, Complications of transplanted organ, Kidney, and a secondary code that identifies the complication.

For patients with CKD following a kidney transplant, but who do not have a complication such as failure or rejection, *see section I.C.14. Chronic kidney disease and kidney transplant status.*

Patient with chronic kidney disease stage 2; history of successful kidney transplant with no complications identified

N18.2   **Chronic kidney disease, stage 2 (mild)**

Z94.Ø   **Kidney transplant status**

Explanation: This patient's stage 2 CKD is not indicated as being due to the transplanted kidney but instead is just the residual disease the patient had prior to the transplant.

4) Complication codes that include the external cause

As with certain other T codes, some of the complications of care codes have the external cause included in the code. The code includes the nature of the complication as well as the type of procedure that caused the complication. No external cause code indicating the type of procedure is necessary for these codes.

5) Complications of care codes within the body system chapters

Intraoperative and postprocedural complication codes are found within the body system chapters with codes specific to the organs and structures of that body system. These codes should be sequenced first, followed by a code(s) for the specific complication, if applicable.

During a spinal fusion procedure, the surgeon inadvertently punctured the dura. The midline durotomy was repaired, and the fusion procedure was completed.

G97.41   **Accidental puncture or laceration of dura during a procedure**

Explanation: The accidental durotomy is not coded to an injury code in chapter 19 but instead is categorized to the nervous system chapter.

Muscle/Tendon Table

ICD-10-CM categorizes certain muscles and tendons in the upper and lower extremities by their action (e.g., extension, flexion), their anatomical location (e.g., posterior, anterior), and/or whether they are intrinsic or extrinsic to a certain anatomical area. The Muscle/Tendon Table is provided at the beginning of chapters 13 and 19 as a resource to help users when code selection depends on one or more of these characteristics. Please note that this table is not all-inclusive, and proper code assignment should be based on the provider's documentation.

Body Region	Muscle	Extensor Tendon	Flexor Tendon	Other Tendon
Shoulder				
	Deltoid	Posterior deltoid	Anterior deltoid	
	Rotator cuff			
	Infraspinatus			Infraspinatus
	Subscapularis			Subscapularis
	Supraspinatus			Supraspinatus
	Teres minor			Teres minor
	Teres major	Teres major		
Upper arm				
	Anterior muscles			
	Biceps brachii — long head		Biceps brachii — long head	
	Biceps brachii — short head		Biceps brachii — short head	
	Brachialis		Brachialis	
	Coracobrachialis		Coracobrachialis	
	Posterior muscles			
	Triceps brachii	Triceps brachii		
Forearm				
	Anterior muscles			
	Flexors			
	Deep			
	Flexor digitorum profundus		Flexor digitorum profundus	
	Flexor pollicis longus		Flexor pollicis longus	
	Intermediate			
	Flexor digitorum superficialis		Flexor digitorum superficialis	
	Superficial			
	Flexor carpi radialis		Flexor carpi radialis	
	Flexor carpi ulnaris		Flexor carpi ulnaris	
	Palmaris longus		Palmaris longus	
	Pronators			
	Pronator quadratus			Pronator quadratus
	Pronator teres			Pronator teres
	Posterior muscles			
	Extensors			
	Deep			
	Abductor pollicis longus			Abductor pollicis longus
	Extensor indicis	Extensor indicis		
	Extensor pollicis brevis	Extensor pollicis brevis		
	Extensor pollicis longus	Extensor pollicis longus		
	Superficial			
	Brachioradialis			Brachioradialis
	Extensor carpi radialis brevis	Extensor carpi radialis brevis		
	Extensor carpi radialis longus	Extensor carpi radialis longus		
	Extensor carpi ulnaris	Extensor carpi ulnaris		
	Extensor digiti minimi	Extensor digiti minimi		
	Extensor digitorum	Extensor digitorum		
	Anconeus	Anconeus		
	Supinator			Supinator

Body Region	Muscle	Extensor Tendon	Flexor Tendon	Other Tendon
Hand				
Extrinsic — attach to a site in the forearm as well as a site in the hand with action related to hand movement at the wrist				
	Extensor carpi radialis brevis	Extensor carpi radialis brevis		
	Extensor carpi radialis longus	Extensor carpie radialis longus		
	Extensor carpi ulnaris	Extensor carpi ulnaris		
	Flexor carpi radialis		Flexor carpi radialis	
	Flexor carpi ulnaris		Flexor carpi ulnaris	
	Flexor digitorum superficialis		Flexor digitorum superficialis	
	Palmaris longus		Palmaris longus	
Extrinsic — attach to a site in the forearm as well as a site in the hand with action in the hand related to finger movement				
	Adductor pollicis longus			Adductor pollicis longus
	Extensor digiti minimi	Extensor digiti minimi		
	Extensor digitorum	Extensor digitorum		
	Extensor indicis	Extensor indicis		
	Flexor digitorum profundus		Flexor digitorum profundus	
	Flexor digitorum superficialis		Flexor digitorum superficialis	
Extrinsic — attach to a site in the forearm as well as a site in the hand with action in the hand related to thumb movement				
	Extensor pollicis brevis	Extensor pollicis brevis		
	Extensor pollicis longus	Extensor pollicis longus		
	Flexor pollicis longus		Flexor pollicis longus	
Intrinsic — found within the hand only				
	Adductor pollicis			Adductor pollicis
	Dorsal interossei	Dorsal interossei	Dorsal interossei	
	Lumbricals	Lumbricals	Lumbricals	
	Palmaris brevis			Palmaris brevis
	Palmar interossei	Palmar interossei	Palmar interossei	
	Hypothenar muscles			
	Abductor digiti minimi			Abductor digiti minimi
	Flexor digiti minimi brevis		Flexor digiti minimi brevis	
	Oppenens digiti minimi		Oppenens digiti minimi	
	Thenar muscles			
	Abductor pollicis brevis			Abductor pollicis brevis
	Flexor pollicis brevis		Flexor pollicis brevis	
	Oppenens pollicis		Oppenens pollicis	
Thigh				
	Anterior muscles			
	Iliopsoas		Iliopsoas	
	Pectineus		Pectineus	
	Quadriceps	Quadriceps		
	Rectus femoris	Rectus femoris — Extends knee	Rectus femoris — Flexes hip	
	Vastus intermedius	Vastus intermedius		
	Vastus lateralis	Vastus lateralis		
	Vastus medialis	Vastus medialis		
	Sartorius		Sartorius	
	Medial muscles			
	Adductor brevis			Adductor brevis
	Adductor longus			Adductor longus
	Adductor magnus			Adductor magnus
	Gracilis			Gracilis
	Obturator externus			Obturator externus
	Posterior muscles			
	Hamstring	Hamstring — Extends hip	Hamstring — Flexes knee	
	Biceps femoris	Biceps femoris	Biceps femoris	
	Semimembranosus	Semimembranosus	Semimembranosus	
	Semitendinosus	Semitendinosus	Semitendinosus	

Chapter 19. Injury, Poisoning and Certain Other Consequences of External Causes

Body Region	Muscle	Extensor Tendon	Flexor Tendon	Other Tendon
Lower leg				
	Anterior muscles			
	Extensor digitorum longus	Extensor digitorum longus		
	Extensor hallucis longus	Extensor hallucis longus		
	Fibularis (peroneus) tertius	Fibularis (peroneus) tertius		
	Tibialis anterior	Tibialis anterior		Tibialis anterior
	Lateral muscles			
	Fibularis (peroneus) brevis		Fibularis (peroneus) brevis	
	Fibularis (peroneus) longus		Fibularis (peroneus) longus	
	Posterior muscles			
	Deep			
	Flexor digitorum longus		Flexor digitorum longus	
	Flexor hallucis longus		Flexor hallucis longus	
	Popliteus		Popliteus	
	Tibialis posterior		Tibialis posterior	
	Superficial			
	Gastrocnemius		Gastrocnemius	
	Plantaris		Plantaris	
	Soleus		Soleus	
				Calcaneal (Achilles)
Ankle/Foot				
Extrinsic — attach to a site in the lower leg as well as a site in the foot with action related to foot movement at the ankle				
	Plantaris		Plantaris	
	Soleus		Soleus	
	Tibialis anterior	Tibialis anterior		
	Tibialis posterior		Tibialis posterior	
Extrinsic — attach to a site in the lower leg as well as a site in the foot with action in the foot related to toe movement				
	Extensor digitorum longus	Extensor digitorum longus		
	Extensor hallicus longus	Extensor hallicus longus		
	Flexor digitorum longus		Flexor digitorum longus	
	Flexor hallucis longus		Flexor hallucis longus	
Intrinsic — found within the ankle/foot only				
	Dorsal muscles			
	Extensor digitorum brevis	Extensor digitorum brevis		
	Extensor hallucis brevis	Extensor hallucis brevis		
	Plantar muscles			
	Abductor digiti minimi		Abductor digiti minimi	
	Abductor hallucis		Abductor hallucis	
	Dorsal interossei	Dorsal interossei	Dorsal interossei	
	Flexor digiti minimi brevis		Flexor digiti minimi brevis	
	Flexor digitorum brevis		Flexor digitorum brevis	
	Flexor hallucis brevis		Flexor hallucis brevis	
	Lumbricals	Lumbricals	Lumbricals	
	Quadratus plantae		Quadratus plantae	
	Plantar interossei	Plantar interossei	Plantar interossei	

Chapter 19. Injury, Poisoning and Certain Other Consequences of External Causes (S00-T88)

NOTE   Use secondary code(s) from Chapter 20, External causes of morbidity, to indicate cause of injury. Codes within the T section that include the external cause do not require an additional external cause code.

Use additional code to identify any retained foreign body, if applicable (Z18.-)

EXCLUDES 1   *birth trauma (P10-P15)*
           obstetric trauma (O70-O71)

NOTE   The chapter uses the S-section for coding different types of injuries related to single body regions and the T-section to cover injuries to unspecified body regions as well as poisoning and certain other consequences of external causes.

AHA: 2016, 2Q, 3-7; 2015, 4Q, 35-38; 2015, 3Q, 37-39, 40; 2015, 2Q, 6; 2015, 1Q, 3-21

This chapter contains the following blocks:

S00-S09   Injuries to the head
S10-S19   Injuries to the neck
S20-S29   Injuries to the thorax
S30-S39   Injuries to the abdomen, lower back, lumbar spine, pelvis and external genitals
S40-S49   Injuries to the shoulder and upper arm
S50-S59   Injuries to the elbow and forearm
S60-S69   Injuries to the wrist, hand and fingers
S70-S79   Injuries to the hip and thigh
S80-S89   Injuries to the knee and lower leg
S90-S99   Injuries to the ankle and foot
T07   Injuries involving multiple body regions
T14   Injury of unspecified body region
T15-T19   Effects of foreign body entering through natural orifice
T20-T25   Burns and corrosions of external body surface, specified by site
T26-T28   Burns and corrosions confined to eye and internal organs
T30-T32   Burns and corrosions of multiple and unspecified body regions
T33-T34   Frostbite
T36-T50   Poisoning by, adverse effect of and underdosing of drugs, medicaments and biological substances
T51-T65   Toxic effects of substances chiefly nonmedicinal as to source
T66-T78   Other and unspecified effects of external causes
T79   Certain early complications of trauma
T80-T88   Complications of surgical and medical care, not elsewhere classified

Injuries to the head (S00-S09)

INCLUDES   injuries of ear
          injuries of eye
          injuries of face [any part]
          injuries of gum
          injuries of jaw
          injuries of oral cavity
          injuries of palate
          injuries of periocular area
          injuries of scalp
          injuries of temporomandibular joint area
          injuries of tongue
          injuries of tooth

Code also for any associated infection

EXCLUDES 2   *burns and corrosions (T20-T32)*
           effects of foreign body in ear (T16)
           effects of foreign body in larynx (T17.3)
           effects of foreign body in mouth NOS (T18.0)
           effects of foreign body in nose (T17.0-T17.1)
           effects of foreign body in pharynx (T17.2)
           effects of foreign body on external eye (T15.-)
           frostbite (T33-T34)
           insect bite or sting, venomous (T63.4)

✓4th **S00**   **Superficial injury of head**
     EXCLUDES 1   *diffuse cerebral contusion (S06.2-)*
             focal cerebral contusion (S06.3-)
             injury of eye and orbit (S05.-)
             open wound of head (S01.-)

> The appropriate 7th character is to be added to each code from category S00.
> A   initial encounter
> D   subsequent encounter
> S   sequela

✓5th **S00.0**   **Superficial injury of scalp**
     ✓x7th   **S00.00**   **Unspecified** superficial injury of scalp
     ✓x7th   **S00.01**   **Abrasion** of scalp
     ✓x7th   **S00.02**   **Blister (nonthermal)** of scalp

✓x7th   **S00.03**   **Contusion** of scalp
                  Bruise of scalp
                  Hematoma of scalp

✓x7th   **S00.04**   **External constriction** of part of scalp

✓x7th   **S00.05**   **Superficial foreign body** of scalp
                  Splinter in the scalp

✓x7th   **S00.06**   **Insect bite (nonvenomous)** of scalp

✓x7th   **S00.07**   **Other superficial bite** of scalp
         EXCLUDES 1   *open bite of scalp (S01.05)*

✓5th   **S00.1**   **Contusion of eyelid and periocular area**
        Black eye
        EXCLUDES 2   *contusion of eyeball and orbital tissues (S05.1)*

     ✓x7th   **S00.10**   **Contusion of unspecified** eyelid and periocular area
     ✓x7th   **S00.11**   **Contusion of right** eyelid and periocular area
     ✓x7th   **S00.12**   **Contusion of left** eyelid and periocular area

✓5th   **S00.2**   **Other and unspecified superficial injuries of eyelid and periocular area**
     EXCLUDES 2   *superficial injury of conjunctiva and cornea (S05.0-)*

     ✓6th   **S00.20**   **Unspecified superficial injury of eyelid and periocular area**
         ✓7th   **S00.201**   **Unspecified superficial injury of right** eyelid and periocular area
         ✓7th   **S00.202**   **Unspecified superficial injury of left** eyelid and periocular area
         ✓7th   **S00.209**   **Unspecified superficial injury of unspecified** eyelid and periocular area

     ✓6th   **S00.21**   **Abrasion of eyelid and periocular area**
         ✓7th   **S00.211**   **Abrasion of right** eyelid and periocular area
         ✓7th   **S00.212**   **Abrasion of left** eyelid and periocular area
         ✓7th   **S00.219**   **Abrasion of unspecified** eyelid and periocular area

     ✓6th   **S00.22**   **Blister (nonthermal) of eyelid and periocular area**
         ✓7th   **S00.221**   **Blister (nonthermal) of right** eyelid and periocular area
         ✓7th   **S00.222**   **Blister (nonthermal) of left** eyelid and periocular area
         ✓7th   **S00.229**   **Blister (nonthermal) of unspecified** eyelid and periocular area

     ✓6th   **S00.24**   **External constriction of eyelid and periocular area**
         ✓7th   **S00.241**   **External constriction of right** eyelid and periocular area
         ✓7th   **S00.242**   **External constriction of left** eyelid and periocular area
         ✓7th   **S00.249**   **External constriction of unspecified** eyelid and periocular area

     ✓6th   **S00.25**   **Superficial foreign body of eyelid and periocular area**
           Splinter of eyelid and periocular area
           EXCLUDES 2   *retained foreign body in eyelid (H02.81-)*
         ✓7th   **S00.251**   **Superficial foreign body of right** eyelid and periocular area
         ✓7th   **S00.252**   **Superficial foreign body of left** eyelid and periocular area
         ✓7th   **S00.259**   **Superficial foreign body of unspecified** eyelid and periocular area

     ✓6th   **S00.26**   **Insect bite (nonvenomous) of eyelid and periocular area**
         ✓7th   **S00.261**   **Insect bite (nonvenomous) of right** eyelid and periocular area
         ✓7th   **S00.262**   **Insect bite (nonvenomous) of left** eyelid and periocular area
         ✓7th   **S00.269**   **Insect bite (nonvenomous) of unspecified** eyelid and periocular area

     ✓6th   **S00.27**   **Other superficial bite of eyelid and periocular area**
         EXCLUDES 1   *open bite of eyelid and periocular area (S01.15)*
         ✓7th   **S00.271**   **Other superficial bite of right** eyelid and periocular area
         ✓7th   **S00.272**   **Other superficial bite of left** eyelid and periocular area
         ✓7th   **S00.279**   **Other superficial bite of unspecified** eyelid and periocular area

---

✓ Additional Character Req   ✓x7th Placeholder Alert   Unacceptable PDx   Manifestation   H1 - H14 HAC   HCC CMS-HCC Condition   EXCLUDES 1 Not Coded Here   EXCLUDES 2 Not Included Here

✓5ᵗʰ **S00.3** **Superficial injury of** nose

  √x7ᵗʰ **S00.30** **Unspecified superficial injury of nose**

  √x7ᵗʰ **S00.31** **Abrasion of nose**

  √x7ᵗʰ **S00.32** **Blister (nonthermal) of nose**

  √x7ᵗʰ **S00.33** **Contusion of nose**
       Bruise of nose
       Hematoma of nose

  √x7ᵗʰ **S00.34** **External constriction of nose**

  √x7ᵗʰ **S00.35** **Superficial** foreign body **of nose**
       Splinter in the nose

  √x7ᵗʰ **S00.36** **Insect bite (nonvenomous) of nose**

  √x7ᵗʰ **S00.37** **Other superficial bite of nose**
       EXCLUDES 1 *open bite of nose (S01.25)*

✓5ᵗʰ **S00.4** **Superficial injury of** ear

  ✓6ᵗʰ **S00.40** **Unspecified superficial injury of ear**

    √7ᵗʰ **S00.401** **Unspecified superficial injury of** right **ear**

    √7ᵗʰ **S00.402** **Unspecified superficial injury of** left **ear**

    √7ᵗʰ **S00.409** **Unspecified superficial injury of** unspecified **ear**

  ✓6ᵗʰ **S00.41** **Abrasion of ear**

    √7ᵗʰ **S00.411** **Abrasion of** right **ear**

    √7ᵗʰ **S00.412** **Abrasion of** left **ear**

    √7ᵗʰ **S00.419** **Abrasion of** unspecified **ear**

  ✓6ᵗʰ **S00.42** **Blister (nonthermal) of ear**

    √7ᵗʰ **S00.421** **Blister (nonthermal) of** right **ear**

    √7ᵗʰ **S00.422** **Blister (nonthermal) of** left **ear**

    √7ᵗʰ **S00.429** **Blister (nonthermal) of** unspecified **ear**

  ✓6ᵗʰ **S00.43** **Contusion of ear**
       Bruise of ear
       Hematoma of ear

    √7ᵗʰ **S00.431** **Contusion of** right **ear**

    √7ᵗʰ **S00.432** **Contusion of** left **ear**

    √7ᵗʰ **S00.439** **Contusion of** unspecified **ear**

  ✓6ᵗʰ **S00.44** **External constriction of ear**

    √7ᵗʰ **S00.441** **External constriction of** right **ear**

    √7ᵗʰ **S00.442** **External constriction of** left **ear**

    √7ᵗʰ **S00.449** **External constriction of** unspecified **ear**

  ✓6ᵗʰ **S00.45** **Superficial** foreign body **of ear**
       Splinter in the ear

    √7ᵗʰ **S00.451** **Superficial foreign body of** right **ear**

    √7ᵗʰ **S00.452** **Superficial foreign body of** left **ear**

    √7ᵗʰ **S00.459** **Superficial foreign body of** unspecified **ear**

  ✓6ᵗʰ **S00.46** **Insect bite (nonvenomous) of ear**

    √7ᵗʰ **S00.461** **Insect bite (nonvenomous) of** right **ear**

    √7ᵗʰ **S00.462** **Insect bite (nonvenomous) of** left **ear**

    √7ᵗʰ **S00.469** **Insect bite (nonvenomous) of** unspecified **ear**

  ✓6ᵗʰ **S00.47** **Other** superficial **bite of ear**
       EXCLUDES 1 *open bite of ear (S01.35)*

    √7ᵗʰ **S00.471** **Other superficial bite of** right **ear**

    √7ᵗʰ **S00.472** **Other superficial bite of** left **ear**

    √7ᵗʰ **S00.479** **Other superficial bite of** unspecified **ear**

✓5ᵗʰ **S00.5** **Superficial injury of** lip and oral cavity

  ✓6ᵗʰ **S00.50** **Unspecified superficial injury of lip and oral cavity**

    √7ᵗʰ **S00.501** **Unspecified superficial injury of** lip

    √7ᵗʰ **S00.502** **Unspecified superficial injury of** oral cavity

  ✓6ᵗʰ **S00.51** **Abrasion of lip and oral cavity**

    √7ᵗʰ **S00.511** **Abrasion of** lip

    √7ᵗʰ **S00.512** **Abrasion of** oral cavity

  ✓6ᵗʰ **S00.52** **Blister (nonthermal) of lip and oral cavity**

    √7ᵗʰ **S00.521** **Blister (nonthermal) of** lip

    √7ᵗʰ **S00.522** **Blister (nonthermal) of** oral cavity

  ✓6ᵗʰ **S00.53** **Contusion of lip and oral cavity**

    √7ᵗʰ **S00.531** **Contusion of** lip
       Bruise of lip
       ▶Hematoma of lip◀

    √7ᵗʰ **S00.532** **Contusion of** oral cavity
       ▶Bruise of oral cavity◀
       Hematoma of oral cavity

  ✓6ᵗʰ **S00.54** **External constriction of lip and oral cavity**

    √7ᵗʰ **S00.541** **External constriction of** lip

    √7ᵗʰ **S00.542** **External constriction of** oral cavity

  ✓6ᵗʰ **S00.55** **Superficial** foreign body **of lip and oral cavity**

    √7ᵗʰ **S00.551** **Superficial foreign body of** lip
       Splinter of lip and oral cavity

    √7ᵗʰ **S00.552** **Superficial foreign body of** oral cavity
       Splinter of lip and oral cavity

  ✓6ᵗʰ **S00.56** **Insect bite (nonvenomous) of lip and oral cavity**

    √7ᵗʰ **S00.561** **Insect bite (nonvenomous) of** lip

    √7ᵗʰ **S00.562** **Insect bite (nonvenomous) of** oral cavity

  ✓6ᵗʰ **S00.57** **Other** superficial **bite of lip and oral cavity**

    √7ᵗʰ **S00.571** **Other superficial bite of** lip
       EXCLUDES 1 *open bite of lip (S01.551)*

    √7ᵗʰ **S00.572** **Other superficial bite of** oral cavity
       EXCLUDES 1 *open bite of oral cavity (S01.552)*

✓5ᵗʰ **S00.8** **Superficial injury of** other parts of head
    Superfical injuries of face [any part]

  √x7ᵗʰ **S00.80** **Unspecified superficial injury of other part of head**

  √x7ᵗʰ **S00.81** **Abrasion of other part of head**

  √x7ᵗʰ **S00.82** **Blister (nonthermal) of other part of head**

  √x7ᵗʰ **S00.83** **Contusion of other part of head**
       Bruise of other part of head
       Hematoma of other part of head

  √x7ᵗʰ **S00.84** **External constriction of other part of head**

  √x7ᵗʰ **S00.85** **Superficial** foreign body **of other part of head**
       Splinter in other part of head

  √x7ᵗʰ **S00.86** **Insect bite (nonvenomous) of other part of head**

  √x7ᵗʰ **S00.87** **Other superficial bite of other part of head**
       EXCLUDES 1 *open bite of other part of head (S01.85)*

✓5ᵗʰ **S00.9** **Superficial injury of** unspecified part of head

  √x7ᵗʰ **S00.90** **Unspecified superficial injury of unspecified part of head**

  √x7ᵗʰ **S00.91** **Abrasion of unspecified part of head**

  √x7ᵗʰ **S00.92** **Blister (nonthermal) of unspecified part of head**

  √x7ᵗʰ **S00.93** **Contusion of unspecified part of head**
       Bruise of head
       Hematoma of head

  √x7ᵗʰ **S00.94** **External constriction of unspecified part of head**

  √x7ᵗʰ **S00.95** **Superficial** foreign body **of unspecified part of head**
       Splinter of head

  √x7ᵗʰ **S00.96** **Insect bite (nonvenomous) of unspecified part of head**

  √x7ᵗʰ **S00.97** **Other superficial bite of unspecified part of head**
       EXCLUDES 1 *open bite of head (S01.95)*

✓4ᵗʰ **S01** **Open wound of head**
    Code also any associated:
       injury of cranial nerve (S04.-)
       injury of muscle and tendon of head (S09.1-)
       intracranial injury (S06.-)
       wound infection
    EXCLUDES 1 *open skull fracture (S02- with 7th B)*
    EXCLUDES 2 *injury of eye and orbit (S05.-)*
        traumatic amputation of part of head (S08.-)

    The appropriate 7th character is to be added to each code from category S01.
    A   initial encounter
    D   subsequent encounter
    S   sequela

✓5ᵗʰ **S01.0** **Open wound of** scalp
    EXCLUDES 1 *avulsion of scalp (S08.0)*

  √x7ᵗʰ **S01.00** **Unspecified open wound of scalp**

  √x7ᵗʰ **S01.01** **Laceration without foreign body of scalp**

  √x7ᵗʰ **S01.02** **Laceration with foreign body of scalp**

  √x7ᵗʰ **S01.03** **Puncture wound without foreign body of scalp**

  √x7ᵗʰ **S01.04** **Puncture wound with foreign body of scalp**

  √x7ᵗʰ **S01.05** **Open bite of scalp**
       Bite of scalp NOS
       EXCLUDES 1 *superficial bite of scalp (S00.06, S00.07-)*

Ⓝ Newborn: 0   Ⓟ Pediatric: 0-17   Ⓜ Maternity: 12-55   Ⓐ Adult: 15-124   **MCC** Major CC Condition   **PDxMCC** PDx acts as own MCC   **CC** CC Condition   **PDxCC** PDx acts as own CC

942   ICD-10-CM 2018

S00.3–S01.05

✓5ᵗʰ **S01.1 Open wound of** eyelid and periocular area
Open wound of eyelid and periocular area with or without involvement of lacrimal passages

CC Excl: For codes in subcategory S01.1:
PDX collection 1139

✓6ᵗʰ **S01.10 Unspecified open wound of eyelid and periocular area**

✓7ᵗʰ **S01.101 Unspecified open wound of** right eyelid and periocular area **CC**

✓7ᵗʰ **S01.102 Unspecified open wound of** left eyelid and periocular area **CC**

✓7ᵗʰ **S01.109 Unspecified open wound of** unspecified eyelid and periocular area **CC**

✓6ᵗʰ **S01.11 Laceration without foreign body of eyelid and periocular area**

✓7ᵗʰ **S01.111 Laceration without foreign body of** right eyelid and periocular area

✓7ᵗʰ **S01.112 Laceration without foreign body of** left eyelid and periocular area

✓7ᵗʰ **S01.119 Laceration without foreign body of** unspecified eyelid and periocular area

✓6ᵗʰ **S01.12 Laceration with foreign body of eyelid and periocular area**

✓7ᵗʰ **S01.121 Laceration with foreign body of** right eyelid and periocular area

✓7ᵗʰ **S01.122 Laceration with foreign body of** left eyelid and periocular area

✓7ᵗʰ **S01.129 Laceration with foreign body of** unspecified eyelid and periocular area

✓6ᵗʰ **S01.13 Puncture wound without foreign body of eyelid and periocular area**

✓7ᵗʰ **S01.131 Puncture wound without foreign body of** right eyelid and periocular area

✓7ᵗʰ **S01.132 Puncture wound without foreign body of** left eyelid and periocular area

✓7ᵗʰ **S01.139 Puncture wound without foreign body of** unspecified eyelid and periocular area

✓6ᵗʰ **S01.14 Puncture wound with foreign body of eyelid and periocular area**

✓7ᵗʰ **S01.141 Puncture wound with foreign body of** right eyelid and periocular area

✓7ᵗʰ **S01.142 Puncture wound with foreign body of** left eyelid and periocular area

✓7ᵗʰ **S01.149 Puncture wound with foreign body of** unspecified eyelid and periocular area

✓6ᵗʰ **S01.15 Open bite of eyelid and periocular area**
Bite of eyelid and periocular area NOS
EXCLUDES 1 superficial bite of eyelid and periocular area (S00.26, S00.27)

✓7ᵗʰ **S01.151 Open bite of** right eyelid and periocular area

✓7ᵗʰ **S01.152 Open bite of** left eyelid and periocular area

✓7ᵗʰ **S01.159 Open bite of** unspecified eyelid and periocular area

✓5ᵗʰ **S01.2 Open wound of** nose

✓x7ᵗʰ **S01.20 Unspecified open wound of nose**

✓x7ᵗʰ **S01.21 Laceration without foreign body of nose**

✓x7ᵗʰ **S01.22 Laceration with foreign body of nose**

✓x7ᵗʰ **S01.23 Puncture wound without foreign body of nose**

✓x7ᵗʰ **S01.24 Puncture wound with foreign body of nose**

✓x7ᵗʰ **S01.25 Open bite of nose**
Bite of nose NOS
EXCLUDES 1 superficial bite of nose (S00.36, S00.37)

✓5ᵗʰ **S01.3 Open wound of** ear

✓6ᵗʰ **S01.30 Unspecified open wound of ear**

✓7ᵗʰ **S01.301 Unspecified open wound of** right ear

✓7ᵗʰ **S01.302 Unspecified open wound of** left ear

✓7ᵗʰ **S01.309 Unspecified open wound of** unspecified ear

✓6ᵗʰ **S01.31 Laceration without foreign body of ear**

✓7ᵗʰ **S01.311 Laceration without foreign body of** right ear

✓7ᵗʰ **S01.312 Laceration without foreign body of** left ear

✓7ᵗʰ **S01.319 Laceration without foreign body of** unspecified ear

✓6ᵗʰ **S01.32 Laceration with foreign body of ear**

✓7ᵗʰ **S01.321 Laceration with foreign body of** right ear

✓7ᵗʰ **S01.322 Laceration with foreign body of** left ear

✓7ᵗʰ **S01.329 Laceration with foreign body of** unspecified ear

✓6ᵗʰ **S01.33 Puncture wound without foreign body of ear**

✓7ᵗʰ **S01.331 Puncture wound without foreign body of** right ear

✓7ᵗʰ **S01.332 Puncture wound without foreign body of** left ear

✓7ᵗʰ **S01.339 Puncture wound without foreign body of** unspecified ear

✓6ᵗʰ **S01.34 Puncture wound with foreign body of ear**

✓7ᵗʰ **S01.341 Puncture wound with foreign body of** right ear

✓7ᵗʰ **S01.342 Puncture wound with foreign body of** left ear

✓7ᵗʰ **S01.349 Puncture wound with foreign body of** unspecified ear

✓6ᵗʰ **S01.35 Open bite of ear**
Bite of ear NOS
EXCLUDES 1 superficial bite of ear (S00.46, S00.47)

✓7ᵗʰ **S01.351 Open bite of** right ear

✓7ᵗʰ **S01.352 Open bite of** left ear

✓7ᵗʰ **S01.359 Open bite of** unspecified ear

✓5ᵗʰ **S01.4 Open wound of** cheek and temporomandibular area

✓6ᵗʰ **S01.40 Unspecified open wound of cheek and temporomandibular area**

✓7ᵗʰ **S01.401 Unspecified open wound of** right cheek and temporomandibular area

✓7ᵗʰ **S01.402 Unspecified open wound of** left cheek and temporomandibular area

✓7ᵗʰ **S01.409 Unspecified open wound of** unspecified cheek and temporomandibular area

✓6ᵗʰ **S01.41 Laceration without foreign body of cheek and temporomandibular area**

✓7ᵗʰ **S01.411 Laceration without foreign body of** right cheek and temporomandibular area

✓7ᵗʰ **S01.412 Laceration without foreign body of** left cheek and temporomandibular area

✓7ᵗʰ **S01.419 Laceration without foreign body of** unspecified cheek and temporomandibular area

✓6ᵗʰ **S01.42 Laceration with foreign body of cheek and temporomandibular area**

✓7ᵗʰ **S01.421 Laceration with foreign body of** right cheek and temporomandibular area

✓7ᵗʰ **S01.422 Laceration with foreign body of** left cheek and temporomandibular area

✓7ᵗʰ **S01.429 Laceration with foreign body of** unspecified cheek and temporomandibular area

✓6ᵗʰ **S01.43 Puncture wound without foreign body of cheek and temporomandibular area**

✓7ᵗʰ **S01.431 Puncture wound without foreign body of** right cheek and temporomandibular area

✓7ᵗʰ **S01.432 Puncture wound without foreign body of** left cheek and temporomandibular area

✓7ᵗʰ **S01.439 Puncture wound without foreign body of** unspecified cheek and temporomandibular area

✓6ᵗʰ **S01.44 Puncture wound with foreign body of cheek and temporomandibular area**

✓7ᵗʰ **S01.441 Puncture wound with foreign body of** right cheek and temporomandibular area

✓7ᵗʰ **S01.442 Puncture wound with foreign body of** left cheek and temporomandibular area

✓7ᵗʰ **S01.449 Puncture wound with foreign body of** unspecified cheek and temporomandibular area

---

☑6th **S01.45** **Open bite of cheek and temporomandibular area**
Bite of cheek and temporomandibular area NOS
EXCLUDES 2 *superficial bite of cheek and temporomandibular area (S00.86, S00.87)*

☑7th **S01.451** **Open bite of right cheek and temporomandibular area**

☑7th **S01.452** **Open bite of left cheek and temporomandibular area**

☑7th **S01.459** **Open bite of unspecified cheek and temporomandibular area**

☑5th **S01.5** **Open wound of lip and oral cavity**
EXCLUDES 2 *tooth dislocation (S03.2)*
tooth fracture (S02.5)

☑6th **S01.50** **Unspecified open wound of lip and oral cavity**

☑7th **S01.501** **Unspecified open wound of lip**

☑7th **S01.502** **Unspecified open wound of oral cavity**

☑6th **S01.51** **Laceration of lip and oral cavity without foreign body**

☑7th **S01.511** **Laceration without foreign body of lip**

☑7th **S01.512** **Laceration without foreign body of oral cavity**

☑6th **S01.52** **Laceration of lip and oral cavity with foreign body**

☑7th **S01.521** **Laceration with foreign body of lip**

☑7th **S01.522** **Laceration with foreign body of oral cavity**

☑6th **S01.53** **Puncture wound of lip and oral cavity without foreign body**

☑7th **S01.531** **Puncture wound without foreign body of lip**

☑7th **S01.532** **Puncture wound without foreign body of oral cavity**

☑6th **S01.54** **Puncture wound of lip and oral cavity with foreign body**

☑7th **S01.541** **Puncture wound with foreign body of lip**

☑7th **S01.542** **Puncture wound with foreign body of oral cavity**

☑6th **S01.55** **Open bite of lip and oral cavity**

☑7th **S01.551** **Open bite of lip**
Bite of lip NOS
EXCLUDES 1 *superficial bite of lip (S00.571)*

☑7th **S01.552** **Open bite of oral cavity**
Bite of oral cavity NOS
EXCLUDES 1 *superficial bite of oral cavity (S00.572)*

☑5th **S01.8** **Open wound of other parts of head**

☑×7th **S01.80** **Unspecified open wound of other part of head**

☑×7th **S01.81** **Laceration without foreign body of other part of head**

☑×7th **S01.82** **Laceration with foreign body of other part of head**

☑×7th **S01.83** **Puncture wound without foreign body of other part of head**

☑×7th **S01.84** **Puncture wound with foreign body of other part of head**

☑×7th **S01.85** **Open bite of other part of head**
Bite of other part of head NOS
EXCLUDES 1 *superficial bite of other part of head* ▶*(S00.87)*◄

☑5th **S01.9** **Open wound of unspecified part of head**

☑×7th **S01.90** **Unspecified open wound of unspecified part of head**

☑×7th **S01.91** **Laceration without foreign body of unspecified part of head**

☑×7th **S01.92** **Laceration with foreign body of unspecified part of head**

☑×7th **S01.93** **Puncture wound without foreign body of unspecified part of head**

☑×7th **S01.94** **Puncture wound with foreign body of unspecified part of head**

☑×7th **S01.95** **Open bite of unspecified part of head**
Bite of head NOS
EXCLUDES 1 *superficial bite of head NOS (S00.97)*

☑4th **S02** **Fracture of skull and facial bones**
NOTE   A fracture not indicated as open or closed should be coded to closed.
Code also any associated intracranial injury (S06.-)
AHA: 2017, 1Q, 42.

The appropriate 7th character is to be added to each code from category S02.
A   initial encounter for closed fracture
B   initial encounter for open fracture
D   subsequent encounter for fracture with routine healing
G   subsequent encounter for fracture with delayed healing
K   subsequent encounter for fracture with nonunion
S   sequela

6, 7, 11 ☑×7th **S02.0** **Fracture of vault of skull**   MCC CC H5 HCC
Fracture of frontal bone
Fracture of parietal bone

CC Excl: For codes in subcategory S02.0: CC with 7th character A or MCC with 7th character B:
PDX collection 1140
CC with 7th character K: PDX collection 897

☑5th **S02.1** **Fracture of base of skull**
EXCLUDES 1 *orbit NOS (S02.8)*
EXCLUDES 2 *orbital floor (S02.3-)*

CC Excl: For codes in subcategory S02.1:
CC with 7th character A or MCC with 7th character B:
PDX collection 1140
CC with 7th character K: PDX collection 897

☑6th **S02.10** **Unspecified fracture of base of skull**

6, 7, 11 ☑7th **S02.101** **Fracture of base of skull, right side**   MCC CC H5 HCC

6, 7, 11 ☑7th **S02.102** **Fracture of base of skull, left side**   MCC CC H5 HCC

6, 7, 11 ☑7th **S02.109** **Fracture of base of skull, unspecified side**   MCC CC H5 HCC

☑6th **S02.11** **Fracture of occiput**

6, 7, 11 ☑7th **S02.110** **Type I occipital condyle fracture, unspecified side**   MCC CC H5 HCC

6, 7, 11 ☑7th **S02.111** **Type II occipital condyle fracture, unspecified side**   MCC CC H5 HCC

6, 7, 11 ☑7th **S02.112** **Type III occipital condyle fracture, unspecified side**   MCC CC H5 HCC

6, 7, 11 ☑7th **S02.113** **Unspecified occipital condyle fracture**   MCC CC H5 HCC

6, 7, 11 ☑7th **S02.118** **Other fracture of occiput, unspecified side**   MCC CC H5 HCC

6, 7, 11 ☑7th **S02.119** **Unspecified fracture of occiput**   MCC CC H5 HCC

6, 7, 11 ☑7th **S02.11A** **Type I occipital condyle fracture, right side**   MCC CC H5 HCC

6, 7, 11 ☑7th **S02.11B** **Type I occipital condyle fracture, left side**   MCC CC H5 HCC

6, 7, 11 ☑7th **S02.11C** **Type II occipital condyle fracture, right side**   MCC CC H5 HCC

6, 7, 11 ☑7th **S02.11D** **Type II occipital condyle fracture, left side**   MCC CC H5 HCC

6, 7, 11 ☑7th **S02.11E** **Type III occipital condyle fracture, right side**   MCC CC H5 HCC

6, 7, 11 ☑7th **S02.11F** **Type III occipital condyle fracture, left side**   MCC CC H5 HCC

6, 7, 11 ☑7th **S02.11G** **Other fracture of occiput, right side**   MCC CC H5 HCC

6, 7, 11 ☑7th **S02.11H** **Other fracture of occiput, left side**   MCC CC H5 HCC

6,7,11 ☑×7th **S02.19** **Other fracture of base of skull**   MCC CC H5 HCC
Fracture of anterior fossa of base of skull
Fracture of ethmoid sinus
Fracture of frontal sinus
Fracture of middle fossa of base of skull
Fracture of orbital roof
Fracture of posterior fossa of base of skull
Fracture of sphenoid
Fracture of temporal bone

---

6   MCC when reported as an open fracture (7th character B or C – specific to category).
7   CC when reported as an initial encounter (7th character A, B, or C – specific to category) OR a subsequent encounter for nonunion or malunion (7th character K, M, N, P, Q, or R – specific to category).
11   HCC with 7th character indicating initial encounter (A or B - specific to category) OR sequela.

N Newborn: 0   P Pediatric: 0-17   M Maternity: 12-55   A Adult: 15-124   MCC Major CC Condition   PDxMCC PDx acts as own MCC   CC CC Condition   PDxCC PDx acts as own CC

S01.45–S02.19

944   ICD-10-CM 2018

⁷ ✓x7ᵗʰ S02.2 Fracture of nasal bones   CC H5
     CC Excl: CC with 7th character B: PDX collection 1141
     CC Excl: CC with 7th character K: PDX collection 897

✓5ᵗʰ S02.3 Fracture of orbital floor
     EXCLUDES 1   orbit NOS (S02.8)
     EXCLUDES 2   orbital roof (S02.1-)

     CC Excl: For codes in subcategory S02.3:
     CC with 7th character A or B: PDX collection 1142
     CC with 7th character K: PDX collection 897

7,11 ✓x7ᵗʰ S02.30 Fracture of orbital floor, unspecified side   CC H5 HCC
7,11 ✓x7ᵗʰ S02.31 Fracture of orbital floor, right side   CC H5 HCC
7,11 ✓x7ᵗʰ S02.32 Fracture of orbital floor, left side   CC H5 HCC

✓5ᵗʰ S02.4 Fracture of malar, maxillary and zygoma bones
     Fracture of superior maxilla
     Fracture of upper jaw (bone)
     Fracture of zygomatic process of temporal bone

     CC Excl: For codes in subcategory S02.4, unless otherwise noted:
     CC with 7th character A or B: PDX collection 1143
     CC with 7th character K: PDX collection 897

✓6ᵗʰ S02.40 Fracture of malar, maxillary and zygoma bones, unspecified
7,11 ✓7ᵗʰ S02.400 Malar fracture, unspecified side   CC H5 HCC
7,11 ✓7ᵗʰ S02.401 Maxillary fracture, unspecified side   CC H5 HCC
7,11 ✓7ᵗʰ S02.402 Zygomatic fracture, unspecified side   CC H5 HCC
7,11 ✓7ᵗʰ S02.40A Malar fracture, right side   CC H5 HCC
7,11 ✓7ᵗʰ S02.40B Malar fracture, left side   CC H5 HCC
7,11 ✓7ᵗʰ S02.40C Maxillary fracture, right side   CC H5 HCC
7,11 ✓7ᵗʰ S02.40D Maxillary fracture, left side   CC H5 HCC
7,11 ✓7ᵗʰ S02.40E Zygomatic fracture, right side   CC H5 HCC
7,11 ✓7ᵗʰ S02.40F Zygomatic fracture, left side   CC H5 HCC

✓6ᵗʰ S02.41 LeFort fracture
7,11 ✓7ᵗʰ S02.411 LeFort I fracture   CC H5 HCC
7,11 ✓7ᵗʰ S02.412 LeFort II fracture   CC H5 HCC
7,11 ✓7ᵗʰ S02.413 LeFort III fracture   CC H5 HCC

7,11 ✓x7ᵗʰ S02.42 Fracture of alveolus of maxilla   CC H5 HCC
     CC Excl: CC with 7th character B: PDX collection 1141
     CC Excl: CC with 7th character K: PDX collection 897

⁸ ✓x7ᵗʰ S02.5 Fracture of tooth (traumatic)   CC
     Broken tooth
     EXCLUDES 1   cracked tooth (nontraumatic) (K03.81)
     CC Excl: CC with 7th character K: PDX collection 897

LeFort Fracture Types

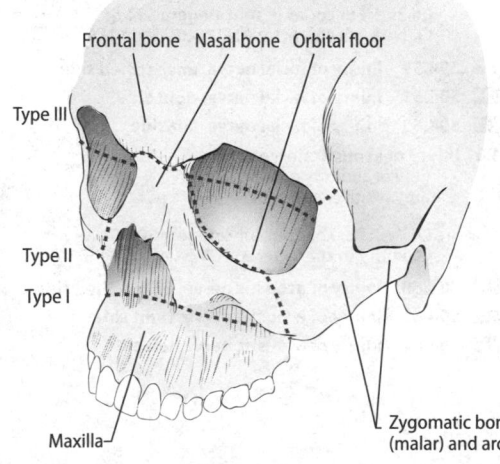

Frontal bone   Nasal bone   Orbital floor

Type III

Type II

Type I

Maxilla

Zygomatic bone (malar) and arch

✓5ᵗʰ S02.6 Fracture of mandible
     Fracture of lower jaw (bone)

     CC Excl: For codes in subcategory S02.6:
     CC with 7th character A or B: PDX collection 1143
     CC with 7th character K: PDX collection 897

✓6ᵗʰ S02.60 Fracture of mandible, unspecified
7,11 ✓7ᵗʰ S02.600 Fracture of unspecified part of body of mandible, unspecified side   CC H5 HCC
7,11 ✓7ᵗʰ S02.601 Fracture of unspecified part of body of right mandible   CC H5 HCC
7,11 ✓7ᵗʰ S02.602 Fracture of unspecified part of body of left mandible   CC H5 HCC
7,11 ✓7ᵗʰ S02.609 Fracture of mandible, unspecified   CC H5 HCC

✓6ᵗʰ S02.61 Fracture of condylar process of mandible
7,11 ✓7ᵗʰ S02.610 Fracture of condylar process of mandible, unspecified side   CC H5 HCC
7,11 ✓7ᵗʰ S02.611 Fracture of condylar process of right mandible   CC H5 HCC
7,11 ✓7ᵗʰ S02.612 Fracture of condylar process of left mandible   CC H5 HCC

✓6ᵗʰ S02.62 Fracture of subcondylar process of mandible
7,11 ✓7ᵗʰ S02.620 Fracture of subcondylar process of mandible, unspecified side   CC H5 HCC
7,11 ✓7ᵗʰ S02.621 Fracture of subcondylar process of right mandible   CC H5 HCC
7,11 ✓7ᵗʰ S02.622 Fracture of subcondylar process of left mandible   CC H5 HCC

✓6ᵗʰ S02.63 Fracture of coronoid process of mandible
7,11 ✓7ᵗʰ S02.630 Fracture of coronoid process of mandible, unspecified side   CC H5 HCC
7,11 ✓7ᵗʰ S02.631 Fracture of coronoid process of right mandible   CC H5 HCC
7,11 ✓7ᵗʰ S02.632 Fracture of coronoid process of left mandible   CC H5 HCC

✓6ᵗʰ S02.64 Fracture of ramus of mandible
7,11 ✓7ᵗʰ S02.640 Fracture of ramus of mandible, unspecified side   CC H5 HCC
7,11 ✓7ᵗʰ S02.641 Fracture of ramus of right mandible   CC H5 HCC
7,11 ✓7ᵗʰ S02.642 Fracture of ramus of left mandible   CC H5 HCC

✓6ᵗʰ S02.65 Fracture of angle of mandible
7,11 ✓7ᵗʰ S02.650 Fracture of angle of mandible, unspecified side   CC H5 HCC
7,11 ✓7ᵗʰ S02.651 Fracture of angle of right mandible   CC H5 HCC
7,11 ✓7ᵗʰ S02.652 Fracture of angle of left mandible   CC H5 HCC

7,11 ✓x7ᵗʰ S02.66 Fracture of symphysis of mandible   CC H5 HCC

✓6ᵗʰ S02.67 Fracture of alveolus of mandible
7,11 ✓7ᵗʰ S02.670 Fracture of alveolus of mandible, unspecified side   CC H5 HCC
7,11 ✓7ᵗʰ S02.671 Fracture of alveolus of right mandible   CC H5 HCC
7,11 ✓7ᵗʰ S02.672 Fracture of alveolus of left mandible   CC H5 HCC

7,11 ✓x7ᵗʰ S02.69 Fracture of mandible of other specified site   CC H5 HCC

✓5ᵗʰ S02.8 Fractures of other specified skull and facial bones
     Fracture of orbit NOS
     Fracture of palate
     EXCLUDES 1   fracture of orbital floor (S02.3-)
     fracture of orbital roof (S02.1-)

     CC Excl: For CC codes in subcategory S02.8:
     CC with 7th character A or B: PDX collection 1142
     CC with 7th character K: PDX collection 897

7,11 ✓x7ᵗʰ S02.80 Fracture of other specified skull and facial bones, unspecified side   CC H5 HCC

---

⁷ CC when reported as an initial encounter (7th character A, B, or C – specific to category) OR a subsequent encounter for nonunion or malunion (7th character K, M, N, P, Q, or R – specific to category).
⁸ CC when reported as a subsequent encounter for nonunion or malunion (7th character K, M, N, P, Q, or R – specific to category).
¹¹ HCC with 7th character indicating initial encounter (A or B - specific to category) OR sequela.

✓ Additional Character Req   ✓x7ᵗʰ Placeholder Alert   Unacceptable PDx   Manifestation   H1 -H14 HAC   HCC CMS-HCC Condition   *EXCLUDES 1* Not Coded Here   *EXCLUDES 2* Not Included Here

7,11   √x7ᵗʰ   **S02.81**   **Fracture of other specified skull and facial** CC H5 HCC **bones, right side**

7,11   √x7ᵗʰ   **S02.82**   **Fracture of other specified skull and facial** CC H5 HCC **bones, left side**

√5ᵗʰ   **S02.9**   **Fracture of unspecified skull and facial bones**

6, 7,11   √x7ᵗʰ   **S02.91**   **Unspecified fracture of skull**   MCC CC H5 HCC
     CC Excl: CC with 7th character A or MCC with 7th character B: PDX collection 1140
     CC with 7th character K: PDX collection 897

7,11   √x7ᵗʰ   **S02.92**   **Unspecified fracture of facial bones**   CC H5 HCC
     CC Excl: CC with 7th character A or B: PDX collection 1142
     CC with 7th character K: PDX collection 897

√4ᵗʰ   **S03**   **Dislocation and sprain of joints and ligaments of head**
    INCLUDES   avulsion of joint (capsule) or ligament of head
          laceration of cartilage, joint (capsule) or ligament of head
          sprain of cartilage, joint (capsule) or ligament of head
          traumatic hemarthrosis of joint or ligament of head
          traumatic rupture of joint or ligament of head
          traumatic subluxation of joint or ligament of head
          traumatic tear of joint or ligament of head

Code also any associated open wound
    EXCLUDES 2   *strain of muscle or tendon of head (S09.1)*

The appropriate 7th character is to be added to each code from category S03.
    A   initial encounter
    D   subsequent encounter
    S   sequela

√5ᵗʰ   **S03.0**   **Dislocation of jaw**
     Dislocation of jaw (cartilage) (meniscus)
     Dislocation of mandible
     Dislocation of temporomandibular (joint)

√x7ᵗʰ   **S03.00**   **Dislocation of jaw, unspecified side**

√x7ᵗʰ   **S03.01**   **Dislocation of jaw, right side**

√x7ᵗʰ   **S03.02**   **Dislocation of jaw, left side**

√x7ᵗʰ   **S03.03**   **Dislocation of jaw, bilateral**

√x7ᵗʰ   **S03.1**   **Dislocation of septal cartilage of nose**

√x7ᵗʰ   **S03.2**   **Dislocation of tooth**

√5ᵗʰ   **S03.4**   **Sprain of jaw**
     Sprain of temporomandibular (joint) (ligament)

√x7ᵗʰ   **S03.40**   **Sprain of jaw, unspecified side**

√x7ᵗʰ   **S03.41**   **Sprain of jaw, right side**

√x7ᵗʰ   **S03.42**   **Sprain of jaw, left side**

√x7ᵗʰ   **S03.43**   **Sprain of jaw, bilateral**

√x7ᵗʰ   **S03.8**   **Sprain of joints and ligaments of other parts of head**

√x7ᵗʰ   **S03.9**   **Sprain of joints and ligaments of unspecified parts of head**

√4ᵗʰ   **S04**   **Injury of cranial nerve**
    The selection of side should be based on the side of the body being affected
    Code first any associated intracranial injury (S06.-)
    Code also any associated:
      open wound of head (S01.-)
      skull fracture (S02.-)

The appropriate 7th character is to be added to each code from category S04.
    A   initial encounter
    D   subsequent encounter
    S   sequela

√5ᵗʰ   **S04.0**   **Injury of optic nerve and pathways**
     Use additional code to identify any visual field defect or blindness ▶(H53.4-, H54.-)◀

     CC Excl: For codes in subcategory S04.0:
     CC with 7th character A: PDX collection 1144

√6ᵗʰ   **S04.01**   **Injury of optic nerve**
     Injury of 2nd cranial nerve

√7ᵗʰ   **S04.011**   **Injury of optic nerve, right eye**   CC

√7ᵗʰ   **S04.012**   **Injury of optic nerve, left eye**   CC

√7ᵗʰ   **S04.019**   **Injury of optic nerve, unspecified eye**   CC
     Injury of optic nerve NOS

√7ᵗʰ   **S04.02**   **Injury of optic chiasm**   CC

√6ᵗʰ   **S04.03**   **Injury of optic tract and pathways**   CC
     Injury of optic radiation

▲   √7ᵗʰ   **S04.031**   **Injury of optic tract and pathways, right side**   CC

▲   √7ᵗʰ   **S04.032**   **Injury of optic tract and pathways, left side**   CC

▲   √7ᵗʰ   **S04.039**   **Injury of optic tract and pathways, unspecified side**   CC
     Injury of optic tract and pathways NOS

√6ᵗʰ   **S04.04**   **Injury of visual cortex**

▲   √7ᵗʰ   **S04.041**   **Injury of visual cortex, right side**   CC

▲   √7ᵗʰ   **S04.042**   **Injury of visual cortex, left side**   CC

▲   √7ᵗʰ   **S04.049**   **Injury of visual cortex, unspecified side**   CC
     Injury of visual cortex NOS

√5ᵗʰ   **S04.1**   **Injury of oculomotor nerve**
     Injury of 3rd cranial nerve

     CC Excl: For codes in subcategory S04.1:
     CC with 7th character A: PDX collection 1145

√x7ᵗʰ   **S04.10**   **Injury of oculomotor nerve, unspecified side**   CC

√x7ᵗʰ   **S04.11**   **Injury of oculomotor nerve, right side**   CC

√x7ᵗʰ   **S04.12**   **Injury of oculomotor nerve, left side**   CC

√5ᵗʰ   **S04.2**   **Injury of trochlear nerve**
     Injury of 4th cranial nerve

     CC Excl: For codes in subcategory S04.2:
     CC with 7th character A: PDX collection 1146

√x7ᵗʰ   **S04.20**   **Injury of trochlear nerve, unspecified side**   CC

√x7ᵗʰ   **S04.21**   **Injury of trochlear nerve, right side**   CC

√x7ᵗʰ   **S04.22**   **Injury of trochlear nerve, left side**   CC

√5ᵗʰ   **S04.3**   **Injury of trigeminal nerve**
     Injury of 5th cranial nerve

     CC Excl: For codes in subcategory S04.3:
     CC with 7th character A: PDX collection 1147

√x7ᵗʰ   **S04.30**   **Injury of trigeminal nerve, unspecified side**   CC

√x7ᵗʰ   **S04.31**   **Injury of trigeminal nerve, right side**   CC

√x7ᵗʰ   **S04.32**   **Injury of trigeminal nerve, left side**   CC

√5ᵗʰ   **S04.4**   **Injury of abducent nerve**
     Injury of 6th cranial nerve

     CC Excl: For codes in subcategory S04.4:
     CC with 7th character A: PDX collection 1148

√x7ᵗʰ   **S04.40**   **Injury of abducent nerve, unspecified side**   CC

√x7ᵗʰ   **S04.41**   **Injury of abducent nerve, right side**   CC

√x7ᵗʰ   **S04.42**   **Injury of abducent nerve, left side**   CC

√5ᵗʰ   **S04.5**   **Injury of facial nerve**
     Injury of 7th cranial nerve

     CC Excl: For codes in subcategory S04.5:
     CC with 7th character A: PDX collection 1149

√x7ᵗʰ   **S04.50**   **Injury of facial nerve, unspecified side**   CC

√x7ᵗʰ   **S04.51**   **Injury of facial nerve, right side**   CC

√x7ᵗʰ   **S04.52**   **Injury of facial nerve, left side**   CC

√5ᵗʰ   **S04.6**   **Injury of acoustic nerve**
     Injury of auditory nerve
     Injury of 8th cranial nerve

     CC Excl: For codes in subcategory S04.6:
     CC with 7th character A: PDX collection 1150

√x7ᵗʰ   **S04.60**   **Injury of acoustic nerve, unspecified side**   CC

√x7ᵗʰ   **S04.61**   **Injury of acoustic nerve, right side**   CC

√x7ᵗʰ   **S04.62**   **Injury of acoustic nerve, left side**   CC

---

[6]   MCC when reported as an open fracture (7th character B or C – specific to category).

[7]   CC when reported as an initial encounter (7th character A, B, or C – specific to category) OR a subsequent encounter for nonunion or malunion (7th character K, M, N, P, Q, or R – specific to category).

[11]   HCC with 7th character indicating initial encounter (A or B - specific to category) OR sequela.

N Newborn: 0   P Pediatric: 0-17   M Maternity: 12-55   A Adult: 15-124   MCC Major CC Condition   PDxMCC PDx acts as own MCC   CC CC Condition   PDxCC PDx acts as own CC

946   ICD-10-CM 2018

✓5ᵗʰ **S04.7** **Injury of** accessory nerve
Injury of 11th cranial nerve

> **CC Excl: For codes in subcategory S04.7:**
> **CC with 7th character A:** PDX collection 1151

✓x7ᵗʰ **S04.70** Injury of accessory nerve, unspecified side `CC`
✓x7ᵗʰ **S04.71** Injury of accessory nerve, right side `CC`
✓x7ᵗʰ **S04.72** Injury of accessory nerve, left side `CC`

✓5ᵗʰ **S04.8** **Injury of** other cranial nerves

> **CC Excl: For codes in subcategory S04.8: CC with 7th**
> **character A:** PDX collection 1152

✓6ᵗʰ **S04.81** **Injury of** olfactory [1st] nerve
✓7ᵗʰ **S04.811** Injury of olfactory [1st] nerve, right side `CC`
✓7ᵗʰ **S04.812** Injury of olfactory [1st] nerve, left side `CC`
✓7ᵗʰ **S04.819** Injury of olfactory [1st] nerve, unspecified side `CC`

✓6ᵗʰ **S04.89** **Injury of** other cranial nerves
Injury of vagus [10th] nerve
✓7ᵗʰ **S04.891** Injury of other cranial nerves, right side `CC`
✓7ᵗʰ **S04.892** Injury of other cranial nerves, left side `CC`
✓7ᵗʰ **S04.899** Injury of other cranial nerves, unspecified side `CC`

✓x7ᵗʰ **S04.9** **Injury of** unspecified cranial nerve `CC`
CC Excl: CC with 7th character A: PDX collection 1152

✓4ᵗʰ **S05** **Injury of eye and orbit**
INCLUDES   open wound of eye and orbit
EXCLUDES 2   2nd cranial [optic] nerve injury (S04.0-)
3rd cranial [oculomotor] nerve injury (S04.1-)
open wound of eyelid and periocular area (S01.1-)
orbital bone fracture (S02.1-, S02.3-, S02.8-)
superficial injury of eyelid (S00.1-S00.2)

> The appropriate 7th character is to be added to each code from
> category S05.
> A   initial encounter
> D   subsequent encounter
> S   sequela

> **CC Excl: For codes in category S05, unless otherwise noted:**
> **CC with 7th character A:** PDX collection 1139

✓5ᵗʰ **S05.0** **Injury of conjunctiva and corneal abrasion** without foreign body
EXCLUDES 1   foreign body in conjunctival sac (T15.1)
foreign body in cornea (T15.0)

✓x7ᵗʰ **S05.00** Injury of conjunctiva and corneal abrasion without foreign body, unspecified eye
✓x7ᵗʰ **S05.01** Injury of conjunctiva and corneal abrasion without foreign body, right eye
✓x7ᵗʰ **S05.02** Injury of conjunctiva and corneal abrasion without foreign body, left eye

✓5ᵗʰ **S05.1** **Contusion of eyeball and orbital tissues**
Traumatic hyphema
EXCLUDES 2   black eye NOS (S00.1)
contusion of eyelid and periocular area (S00.1)

✓x7ᵗʰ **S05.10** Contusion of eyeball and orbital tissues, unspecified eye
✓x7ᵗʰ **S05.11** Contusion of eyeball and orbital tissues, right eye
✓x7ᵗʰ **S05.12** Contusion of eyeball and orbital tissues, left eye

✓5ᵗʰ **S05.2** **Ocular laceration and rupture** with prolapse or loss of intraocular tissue
✓x7ᵗʰ **S05.20** Ocular laceration and rupture with prolapse or loss of intraocular tissue, unspecified eye `CC`
✓x7ᵗʰ **S05.21** Ocular laceration and rupture with prolapse or loss of intraocular tissue, right eye `CC`
✓x7ᵗʰ **S05.22** Ocular laceration and rupture with prolapse or loss of intraocular tissue, left eye `CC`

✓5ᵗʰ **S05.3** **Ocular laceration** without prolapse or loss of intraocular tissue
Laceration of eye NOS
DEF: Tear in ocular tissue without displacing structures; due to blunt trauma; characterized by pain, redness, and decreased vision.

✓x7ᵗʰ **S05.30** Ocular laceration without prolapse or loss of intraocular tissue, unspecified eye `CC`
✓x7ᵗʰ **S05.31** Ocular laceration without prolapse or loss of intraocular tissue, right eye `CC`
✓x7ᵗʰ **S05.32** Ocular laceration without prolapse or loss of intraocular tissue, left eye `CC`

✓5ᵗʰ **S05.4** **Penetrating wound of orbit** with or without foreign body
EXCLUDES 2   retained (old) foreign body following penetrating wound in orbit (H05.5-)

✓x7ᵗʰ **S05.40** Penetrating wound of orbit with or without foreign body, unspecified eye `CC`
✓x7ᵗʰ **S05.41** Penetrating wound of orbit with or without foreign body, right eye `CC`
✓x7ᵗʰ **S05.42** Penetrating wound of orbit with or without foreign body, left eye `CC`

✓5ᵗʰ **S05.5** **Penetrating wound with foreign body of eyeball**
EXCLUDES 2   retained (old) intraocular foreign body (H44.6-, H44.7)

> **CC Excl: For codes in subcategory S05.5:**
> **CC with 7th character A:** PDX collection 1153

✓x7ᵗʰ **S05.50** Penetrating wound with foreign body of unspecified eyeball `CC`
✓x7ᵗʰ **S05.51** Penetrating wound with foreign body of right eyeball `CC`
✓x7ᵗʰ **S05.52** Penetrating wound with foreign body of left eyeball `CC`

✓5ᵗʰ **S05.6** **Penetrating wound without foreign body of eyeball**
Ocular penetration NOS
✓x7ᵗʰ **S05.60** Penetrating wound without foreign body of unspecified eyeball
✓x7ᵗʰ **S05.61** Penetrating wound without foreign body of right eyeball
✓x7ᵗʰ **S05.62** Penetrating wound without foreign body of left eyeball

✓5ᵗʰ **S05.7** **Avulsion of eye**
Traumatic enucleation
✓x7ᵗʰ **S05.70** Avulsion of unspecified eye `CC`
✓x7ᵗʰ **S05.71** Avulsion of right eye `CC`
✓x7ᵗʰ **S05.72** Avulsion of left eye `CC`

✓5ᵗʰ **S05.8** **Other injuries of eye and orbit**
Lacrimal duct injury
✓6ᵗʰ **S05.8X** **Other injuries of eye and orbit**
✓7ᵗʰ **S05.8X1** Other injuries of right eye and orbit `CC`
✓7ᵗʰ **S05.8X2** Other injuries of left eye and orbit `CC`
✓7ᵗʰ **S05.8X9** Other injuries of unspecified eye and orbit `CC`

✓5ᵗʰ **S05.9** **Unspecified injury of eye and orbit**
Injury of eye NOS
✓x7ᵗʰ **S05.90** Unspecified injury of unspecified eye and orbit
✓x7ᵗʰ **S05.91** Unspecified injury of right eye and orbit `CC`
✓x7ᵗʰ **S05.92** Unspecified injury of left eye and orbit `CC`

✓ Additional Character Req   ✓x7ᵗʰ Placeholder Alert   Unacceptable PDx   Manifestation   H1-H14 HAC   HCC CMS-HCC Condition   EXCLUDES 1 Not Coded Here   EXCLUDES 2 Not Included Here

✓4ᵗʰ S06 Intracranial injury

NOTE ▶7th characters D and S do not apply to codes in category S06 with 6th character 7 – death due to brain injury prior to regaining consciousness, or 8 – death due to other cause prior to regaining consciousness◀

INCLUDES traumatic brain injury

Code also any associated:
open wound of head (S01.-)
skull fracture (S02.-)

EXCLUDES 1 head injury NOS (S09.90)

AHA: 2017, 1Q, 42; 2015, 3Q, 37

The appropriate 7th character is to be added to each code from category S06.
A   initial encounter
D   subsequent encounter
S   sequela

CC Excl: For codes in category S06, unless otherwise noted:
CC or MCC with 7th character A: PDX collection 1154

✓5ᵗʰ S06.0 Concussion
Commotio cerebri

EXCLUDES 1 concussion with other intracranial injuries classified in subcategories S06.1- to S06.6-, S06.81 and S06.82- code to specified intracranial injury

✓6ᵗʰ S06.0X Concussion

12 ✓7ᵗʰ **S06.0X0 Concussion** without loss of consciousness   **HCC**

12 ✓7ᵗʰ **S06.0X1 Concussion with loss of consciousness of** 30 minutes or less   **CC H5 HCC**

12 ✓7ᵗʰ **S06.0X9 Concussion with loss of consciousness of** unspecified duration   **CC H5 HCC**
Concussion NOS

✓5ᵗʰ S06.1 Traumatic cerebral edema
Diffuse traumatic cerebral edema
Focal traumatic cerebral edema

CC Excl: For codes in subcategory S06.1, unless otherwise noted:
MCC with 7th character A: PDX collection 1155

✓6ᵗʰ S06.1X Traumatic cerebral edema

11 ✓7ᵗʰ **S06.1X0 Traumatic cerebral edema** without loss of consciousness   **PDxMCC MCC HCC**
CC Excl: MCC with 7th character A: PDX collection 612

11 ✓7ᵗʰ **S06.1X1 Traumatic cerebral edema with loss of consciousness of** 30 minutes or less   **PDxMCC MCC H5 HCC**

11 ✓7ᵗʰ **S06.1X2 Traumatic cerebral edema with loss of consciousness of** 31 minutes to 59 minutes   **PDxMCC MCC H5 HCC**

11 ✓7ᵗʰ **S06.1X3 Traumatic cerebral edema with loss of consciousness of** 1 hour to 5 hours 59 minutes   **PDxMCC MCC H5 HCC**

11 ✓7ᵗʰ **S06.1X4 Traumatic cerebral edema with loss of consciousness of** 6 hours to 24 hours   **PDxMCC MCC H5 HCC**

11 ✓7ᵗʰ **S06.1X5 Traumatic cerebral edema with loss of consciousness** greater than 24 hours with return to pre-existing conscious level   **PDxMCC MCC H5 HCC**

11 ✓7ᵗʰ **S06.1X6 Traumatic cerebral edema with loss of consciousness** greater than 24 hours without return to pre-existing conscious level with patient surviving   **PDxMCC MCC H5 HCC**
CC Excl: MCC with 7th character A: PDX collection 1154

✓7ᵗʰ **S06.1X7 Traumatic cerebral edema with loss of consciousness of** any duration with death due to brain injury prior to regaining consciousness   **PDxMCC MCC H5**
CC Excl: MCC with 7th character A: PDX collection 1154

✓7ᵗʰ **S06.1X8 Traumatic cerebral edema with loss of consciousness of** any duration with death due to other cause prior to regaining consciousness   **PDxMCC MCC H5**
CC Excl: MCC with 7th character A: PDX collection 1154

11 ✓7ᵗʰ **S06.1X9 Traumatic cerebral edema with loss of consciousness of** unspecified duration   **PDxMCC MCC H5 HCC**
Traumatic cerebral edema NOS

✓5ᵗʰ S06.2 Diffuse traumatic brain injury
Diffuse axonal brain injury

EXCLUDES 1 traumatic diffuse cerebral edema (S06.1X-)

✓6ᵗʰ S06.2X Diffuse traumatic brain injury

11 ✓7ᵗʰ **S06.2X0 Diffuse traumatic brain injury** without loss of consciousness   **HCC**

11 ✓7ᵗʰ **S06.2X1 Diffuse traumatic brain injury with loss of consciousness of** 30 minutes or less   **CC H5 HCC**

11 ✓7ᵗʰ **S06.2X2 Diffuse traumatic brain injury with loss of consciousness of** 31 minutes to 59 minutes   **CC H5 HCC**

11 ✓7ᵗʰ **S06.2X3 Diffuse traumatic brain injury with loss of consciousness of** 1 hour to 5 hours 59 minutes   **CC H5 HCC**

11 ✓7ᵗʰ **S06.2X4 Diffuse traumatic brain injury with loss of consciousness of** 6 hours to 24 hours   **CC H5 HCC**

11 ✓7ᵗʰ **S06.2X5 Diffuse traumatic brain injury with loss of consciousness** greater than 24 hours with return to pre-existing conscious levels   **CC H5 HCC**

11 ✓7ᵗʰ **S06.2X6 Diffuse traumatic brain injury with loss of consciousness** greater than 24 hours without return to pre-existing conscious level with patient surviving   **MCC H5 HCC**

✓7ᵗʰ **S06.2X7 Diffuse traumatic brain injury with loss of consciousness of** any duration with death due to brain injury prior to regaining consciousness   **MCC H5**

✓7ᵗʰ **S06.2X8 Diffuse traumatic brain injury with loss of consciousness of** any duration with death due to other cause prior to regaining consciousness   **MCC H5**

11 ✓7ᵗʰ **S06.2X9 Diffuse traumatic brain injury with loss of consciousness of** unspecified duration   **CC H5 HCC**
Diffuse traumatic brain injury NOS

✓5ᵗʰ S06.3 Focal traumatic brain injury

EXCLUDES 1 any condition classifiable to S06.4-S06.6 focal cerebral edema (S06.1)

✓6ᵗʰ S06.30 Unspecified focal traumatic brain injury

11 ✓7ᵗʰ **S06.300 Unspecified focal traumatic brain injury** without loss of consciousness   **HCC**

11 ✓7ᵗʰ **S06.301 Unspecified focal traumatic brain injury with loss of consciousness of** 30 minutes or less   **CC H5 HCC**

11 ✓7ᵗʰ **S06.302 Unspecified focal traumatic brain injury with loss of consciousness of** 31 minutes to 59 minutes   **CC H5 HCC**

11 ✓7ᵗʰ **S06.303 Unspecified focal traumatic brain injury with loss of consciousness of** 1 hour to 5 hours 59 minutes   **CC H5 HCC**

11 ✓7ᵗʰ **S06.304 Unspecified focal traumatic brain injury with loss of consciousness of** 6 hours to 24 hours   **CC H5 HCC**

11 ✓7ᵗʰ **S06.305 Unspecified focal traumatic brain injury with loss of consciousness** greater than 24 hours with return to pre-existing conscious level   **CC H5 HCC**

11 ✓7ᵗʰ **S06.306 Unspecified focal traumatic brain injury with loss of consciousness** greater than 24 hours without return to pre-existing conscious level with patient surviving   **MCC H5 HCC**

---

11 HCC with 7th character indicating initial encounter (A or B - specific to category) OR sequela.
12 HCC with 7th character indicating sequela.

N Newborn: 0   **P** Pediatric: 0-17   **M** Maternity: 12-55   **A** Adult: 15-124   **MCC** Major CC Condition   **PDxMCC** PDx acts as own MCC   **CC** CC Condition   **PDxCC** PDx acts as own CC

948   ICD-10-CM 2018

√7ᵗʰ **S06.307** **Unspecified focal traumatic** `MCC` `H5`
brain injury with loss of consciousness of
any duration with death due to brain
injury prior to regaining consciousness

√7ᵗʰ **S06.308** **Unspecified focal traumatic brain** `MCC` `H5`
injury with loss of consciousness of
any duration with death due to other
cause prior to regaining consciousness

11 √7ᵗʰ **S06.309** **Unspecified focal traumatic** `CC` `H5` `HCC`
brain injury with loss of consciousness
of unspecified duration
> Unspecified focal traumatic brain injury
> NOS

√6ᵗʰ **S06.31** **Contusion and laceration of right cerebrum**

11 √7ᵗʰ **S06.310** **Contusion and laceration of** `MCC` `H5` `HCC`
rightcerebrum without loss of
consciousness

11 √7ᵗʰ **S06.311** **Contusion and laceration of** `MCC` `H5` `HCC`
right cerebrum with loss of
consciousness of 30 minutes or less

11 √7ᵗʰ **S06.312** **Contusion and laceration of** `MCC` `H5` `HCC`
right cerebrum with loss of
consciousness of 31 minutes
to 59 minutes

11 √7ᵗʰ **S06.313** **Contusion and laceration of** `MCC` `H5` `HCC`
right cerebrum with loss of
consciousness of 1 hour to
5 hours 59 minutes

11 √7ᵗʰ **S06.314** **Contusion and laceration of** `MCC` `H5` `HCC`
right cerebrum with loss of
consciousness of 6 hours to 24 hours

11 √7ᵗʰ **S06.315** **Contusion and laceration of** `MCC` `H5` `HCC`
right cerebrum with loss of consciousness
greater than 24 hours with return
to pre-existing conscious level

11 √7ᵗʰ **S06.316** **Contusion and laceration of** `MCC` `H5` `HCC`
right cerebrum with loss of
consciousness greater than 24 hours
without return to pre-existing
conscious level with patient surviving

√7ᵗʰ **S06.317** **Contusion and laceration of right** `MCC` `H5`
cerebrum with loss of consciousness
of any duration with death due to
brain injury prior to regaining
consciousness

√7ᵗʰ **S06.318** **Contusion and laceration of right** `MCC` `H5`
cerebrum with loss of consciousness
of any duration with death due to other
cause prior to regaining consciousness

11 √7ᵗʰ **S06.319** **Contusion and laceration of** `MCC` `H5` `HCC`
right cerebrum with loss of
consciousness of unspecified duration
> Contusion and laceration of right cerebrum
> NOS

√6ᵗʰ **S06.32** **Contusion and laceration of left cerebrum**

11 √7ᵗʰ **S06.320** **Contusion and laceration of** `MCC` `H5` `HCC`
left cerebrum without loss of
consciousness

11 √7ᵗʰ **S06.321** **Contusion and laceration of** `MCC` `H5` `HCC`
left cerebrum with loss of
consciousness of 30 minutes or less

11 √7ᵗʰ **S06.322** **Contusion and laceration of** `MCC` `H5` `HCC`
left cerebrum with loss of
consciousness of 31 minutes
to 59 minutes

11 √7ᵗʰ **S06.323** **Contusion and laceration of** `MCC` `H5` `HCC`
left cerebrum with loss of
consciousness of 1 hour to
5 hours 59 minutes

11 √7ᵗʰ **S06.324** **Contusion and laceration of** `MCC` `H5` `HCC`
left cerebrum with loss of
consciousness of 6 hours to 24 hours

11 √7ᵗʰ **S06.325** **Contusion and laceration of** `MCC` `H5` `HCC`
left cerebrum with loss of consciousness
greater than 24 hours with return to
pre-existing conscious level

11 √7ᵗʰ **S06.326** **Contusion and laceration of** `MCC` `H5` `HCC`
left cerebrum with loss of consciousness
greater than 24 hours without return
to pre-existing conscious level with
patient surviving

11 √7ᵗʰ **S06.327** **Contusion and laceration of left** `MCC` `H5`
cerebrum with loss of consciousness
of any duration with death due to brain
injury prior to regaining consciousness

√7ᵗʰ **S06.328** **Contusion and laceration of left** `MCC` `H5`
cerebrum with loss of consciousness
of any duration with death due to other
cause prior to regaining consciousness

11 √7ᵗʰ **S06.329** **Contusion and laceration of** `MCC` `H5` `HCC`
left cerebrum with loss of
consciousness of unspecified duration
> Contusion and laceration of left cerebrum
> NOS

√6ᵗʰ **S06.33** **Contusion and laceration of cerebrum, unspecified**

11 √7ᵗʰ **S06.330** **Contusion and laceration of** `MCC` `H5` `HCC`
cerebrum, unspecified, without loss
of consciousness

11 √7ᵗʰ **S06.331** **Contusion and laceration of** `MCC` `H5` `HCC`
cerebrum, unspecified, with loss of
consciousness of 30 minutes or less

11 √7ᵗʰ **S06.332** **Contusion and laceration of** `MCC` `H5` `HCC`
cerebrum, unspecified, with loss of
consciousness of 31 minutes to 59 minutes

11 √7ᵗʰ **S06.333** **Contusion and laceration of** `MCC` `H5` `HCC`
cerebrum, unspecified, with loss of
consciousness of 1 hour to 5 hours
59 minutes

11 √7ᵗʰ **S06.334** **Contusion and laceration of** `MCC` `H5` `HCC`
cerebrum, unspecified, with loss of
consciousness of 6 hours to 24 hours

11 √7ᵗʰ **S06.335** **Contusion and laceration of** `MCC` `H5` `HCC`
cerebrum, unspecified, with loss of
consciousness greater than 24 hours
with return to pre-existing conscious level

11 √7ᵗʰ **S06.336** **Contusion and laceration of** `MCC` `H5` `HCC`
cerebrum, unspecified, with loss of
consciousness greater than 24 hours
without return to pre-existing
conscious level with patient surviving

√7ᵗʰ **S06.337** **Contusion and laceration of** `MCC` `H5`
cerebrum, unspecified, with loss of
consciousness of any duration with
death due to brain injury prior to
regaining consciousness

√7ᵗʰ **S06.338** **Contusion and laceration of** `MCC` `H5`
cerebrum, unspecified, with loss of
consciousness of any duration with
death due to other cause prior to
regaining consciousness

11 √7ᵗʰ **S06.339** **Contusion and laceration of** `MCC` `H5` `HCC`
cerebrum, unspecified, with loss of
consciousness of unspecified duration
> Contusion and laceration of cerebrum NOS

√6ᵗʰ **S06.34** **Traumatic hemorrhage of right cerebrum**
> Traumatic intracerebral hemorrhage and hematoma
> of right cerebrum

11 √7ᵗʰ **S06.340** **Traumatic hemorrhage of** `MCC` `H5` `HCC`
right cerebrum without loss of
consciousness

11 √7ᵗʰ **S06.341** **Traumatic hemorrhage of** `MCC` `H5` `HCC`
right cerebrum with loss of
consciousness of 30 minutes or less

11 √7ᵗʰ **S06.342** **Traumatic hemorrhage of** `MCC` `H5` `HCC`
right cerebrum with loss of c
onsciousness of 31 minutes
to 59 minutes

11 √7ᵗʰ **S06.343** **Traumatic hemorrhage of** `MCC` `H5` `HCC`
right cerebrum with loss
of consciousness of 1 hours
to 5 hours 59 minutes

11 √7ᵗʰ **S06.344** **Traumatic hemorrhage of** `MCC` `H5` `HCC`
right cerebrum with loss of
consciousness of 6 hours to 24 hours

---

11   HCC with 7th character indicating initial encounter (A or B - specific to category) OR sequela.

✔ Additional Character Req   √x7ᵗʰ Placeholder Alert   Unacceptable PDx   Manifestation   H1 - H14 HAC   HCC CMS-HCC Condition   EXCLUDES 1 Not Coded Here   EXCLUDES 2 Not Included Here

ICD-10-CM 2018   **949**

11 ☑7ᵗʰ **S06.345** **Traumatic hemorrhage of** `MCC` `H5` `HCC`
right cerebrum with loss of consciousness greater than 24 hours with return to pre-existing conscious level

11 ☑7ᵗʰ **S06.346** **Traumatic hemorrhage of right** `MCC` `H5` `HCC`
cerebrum with loss of consciousness greater than 24 hours without return to pre-existing conscious level with patient surviving

☑7ᵗʰ **S06.347** **Traumatic hemorrhage of right** `MCC` `H5`
cerebrum with loss of consciousness of any duration with death due to brain injury prior to regaining consciousness

☑7ᵗʰ **S06.348** **Traumatic hemorrhage of right** `MCC` `H5`
cerebrum with loss of consciousness of any duration with death due to other cause prior to regaining consciousness

11 ☑7ᵗʰ **S06.349** **Traumatic hemorrhage of right** `MCC` `H5` `HCC`
cerebrum with loss of consciousness of unspecified duration
Traumatic hemorrhage of right cerebrum NOS

☑6ᵗʰ **S06.35** **Traumatic hemorrhage of left cerebrum**
Traumatic intracerebral hemorrhage and hematoma of left cerebrum

11 ☑7ᵗʰ **S06.350** **Traumatic hemorrhage of left** `MCC` `H5` `HCC`
cerebrum without loss of consciousness

11 ☑7ᵗʰ **S06.351** **Traumatic hemorrhage of left** `MCC` `H5` `HCC`
cerebrum with loss of consciousness of 30 minutes or less

11 ☑7ᵗʰ **S06.352** **Traumatic hemorrhage of left** `MCC` `H5` `HCC`
cerebrum with loss of consciousness of 31 minutes to 59 minutes

11 ☑7ᵗʰ **S06.353** **Traumatic hemorrhage of left** `MCC` `H5` `HCC`
cerebrum with loss of consciousness of 1 hours to 5 hours 59 minutes

11 ☑7ᵗʰ **S06.354** **Traumatic hemorrhage of left** `MCC` `H5` `HCC`
cerebrum with loss of consciousness of 6 hours to 24 hours

11 ☑7ᵗʰ **S06.355** **Traumatic hemorrhage of left** `MCC` `H5` `HCC`
cerebrum with loss of consciousness greater than 24 hours with return to pre-existing conscious level

11 ☑7ᵗʰ **S06.356** **Traumatic hemorrhage of left** `MCC` `H5` `HCC`
cerebrum with loss of consciousness greater than 24 hours without return to pre-existing conscious level with patient surviving

☑7ᵗʰ **S06.357** **Traumatic hemorrhage of left** `MCC` `H5`
cerebrum with loss of consciousness of any duration with death due to brain injury prior to regaining consciousness

☑7ᵗʰ **S06.358** **Traumatic hemorrhage of left** `MCC` `H5`
cerebrum with loss of consciousness of any duration with death due to other cause prior to regaining consciousness

11 ☑7ᵗʰ **S06.359** **Traumatic hemorrhage of left** `MCC` `H5` `HCC`
cerebrum with loss of consciousness of unspecified duration
Traumatic hemorrhage of left cerebrum NOS

☑6ᵗʰ **S06.36** **Traumatic hemorrhage of cerebrum, unspecified**
Traumatic intracerebral hemorrhage and hematoma, unspecified

11 ☑7ᵗʰ **S06.360** **Traumatic hemorrhage of** `MCC` `H5` `HCC`
cerebrum, unspecified, without loss of consciousness

11 ☑7ᵗʰ **S06.361** **Traumatic hemorrhage of** `MCC` `H5` `HCC`
cerebrum, unspecified, with loss of consciousness of 30 minutes or less

11 ☑7ᵗʰ **S06.362** **Traumatic hemorrhage of** `MCC` `H5` `HCC`
cerebrum, unspecified, with loss of consciousness of 31 minutes to 59 minutes

11 ☑7ᵗʰ **S06.363** **Traumatic hemorrhage of** `MCC` `H5` `HCC`
cerebrum, unspecified, with loss of consciousness of 1 hours to 5 hours 59 minutes

11 ☑7ᵗʰ **S06.364** **Traumatic hemorrhage of** `MCC` `H5` `HCC`
cerebrum, unspecified, with loss of consciousness of 6 hours to 24 hours

11 ☑7ᵗʰ **S06.365** **Traumatic hemorrhage of** `MCC` `H5` `HCC`
cerebrum, unspecified, with loss of consciousness greater than 24 hours with return to pre-existing conscious level

11 ☑7ᵗʰ **S06.366** **Traumatic hemorrhage of** `MCC` `H5` `HCC`
cerebrum, unspecified, with loss of consciousness greater than 24 hours without return to pre-existing conscious level with patient surviving

☑7ᵗʰ **S06.367** **Traumatic hemorrhage of** `MCC` `H5`
cerebrum, unspecified, with loss of consciousness of any duration with death due to brain injury prior to regaining consciousness

☑7ᵗʰ **S06.368** **Traumatic hemorrhage of** `MCC` `H5`
cerebrum, unspecified, with loss of consciousness of any duration with death due to other cause prior to regaining consciousness

11 ☑7ᵗʰ **S06.369** **Traumatic hemorrhage of** `MCC` `H5` `HCC`
cerebrum, unspecified, with loss of consciousness of unspecified duration
Traumatic hemorrhage of cerebrum NOS

☑6ᵗʰ **S06.37** **Contusion, laceration, and hemorrhage of cerebellum**

11 ☑7ᵗʰ **S06.370** **Contusion, laceration, and** `MCC` `H5` `HCC`
hemorrhage of cerebellum without loss of consciousness
CC Excl: No Excl

11 ☑7ᵗʰ **S06.371** **Contusion, laceration, and** `CC` `H5` `HCC`
hemorrhage of cerebellum with loss of consciousness of 30 minutes or less

11 ☑7ᵗʰ **S06.372** **Contusion, laceration, and** `CC` `H5` `HCC`
hemorrhage of cerebellum with loss of consciousness of 31 minutes to 59 minutes

11 ☑7ᵗʰ **S06.373** **Contusion, laceration, and** `CC` `H5` `HCC`
hemorrhage of cerebellum with loss of consciousness of 1 hour to 5 hours 59 minutes

11 ☑7ᵗʰ **S06.374** **Contusion, laceration, and** `CC` `H5` `HCC`
hemorrhage of cerebellum with loss of consciousness of 6 hours to 24 hours

11 ☑7ᵗʰ **S06.375** **Contusion, laceration, and** `CC` `H5` `HCC`
hemorrhage of cerebellum with loss of consciousness greater than 24 hours with return to pre-existing conscious level

11 ☑7ᵗʰ **S06.376** **Contusion, laceration, and** `MCC` `H5` `HCC`
hemorrhage of cerebellum with loss of consciousness greater than 24 hours without return to pre-existing conscious level with patient surviving

☑7ᵗʰ **S06.377** **Contusion, laceration, and** `MCC` `H5`
hemorrhage of cerebellum with loss of consciousness of any duration with death due to brain injury prior to regaining consciousness

☑7ᵗʰ **S06.378** **Contusion, laceration, and** `MCC` `H5`
hemorrhage of cerebellum with loss of consciousness of any duration with death due to other cause prior to regaining consciousness

11 ☑7ᵗʰ **S06.379** **Contusion, laceration, and** `CC` `H5` `HCC`
hemorrhage of cerebellum with loss of consciousness of unspecified duration
Contusion, laceration, and hemorrhage of cerebellum NOS

☑6ᵗʰ **S06.38** **Contusion, laceration, and hemorrhage of brainstem**

11 ☑7ᵗʰ **S06.380** **Contusion, laceration, and** `MCC` `H5` `HCC`
hemorrhage of brainstem without loss of consciousness
CC Excl: No Excl

---

11 HCC with 7th character indicating initial encounter (A or B - specific to category) OR sequela.

---

11 ✓7ᵗʰ **S06.381** Contusion, laceration, and `CC` `H5` `HCC`
hemorrhage of brainstem with loss of
consciousness of 30 minutes or less

11 ✓7ᵗʰ **S06.382** Contusion, laceration, and `H5` `HCC`
hemorrhage of brainstem with loss of
consciousness of 31 minutes to
59 minutes

11 ✓7ᵗʰ **S06.383** Contusion, laceration, and `CC` `H5` `HCC`
hemorrhage of brainstem with loss of
consciousness of 1 hour to 5 hours
59 minutes

11 ✓7ᵗʰ **S06.384** Contusion, laceration, and `CC` `H5` `HCC`
hemorrhage of brainstem with loss of
consciousness of 6 hours to 24 hours

11 ✓7ᵗʰ **S06.385** Contusion, laceration, and `CC` `H5` `HCC`
hemorrhage of brainstem with loss of
consciousness greater than 24 hours
with return to pre-existing conscious level

11 ✓7ᵗʰ **S06.386** Contusion, laceration, and `H5` `HCC`
hemorrhage of brainstem with loss of
consciousness greater than 24 hours
without return to pre-existing
conscious level with patient surviving

✓7ᵗʰ **S06.387** Contusion, laceration, and `MCC` `H5`
hemorrhage of brainstem with loss of
consciousness of any duration with
death due to brain injury prior to
regaining consciousness

✓7ᵗʰ **S06.388** Contusion, laceration, and `MCC` `H5`
hemorrhage of brainstem with loss
of consciousness of any duration with
death due to other cause prior to
regaining consciousness

11 ✓7ᵗʰ **S06.389** Contusion, laceration, and `CC` `H5` `HCC`
hemorrhage of brainstem with loss of
consciousness of unspecified duration
      Contusion, laceration, and hemorrhage of
      brainstem NOS

✓5ᵗʰ **S06.4** Epidural hemorrhage
      Extradural hemorrhage NOS
      Extradural hemorrhage (traumatic)

✓6ᵗʰ **S06.4X** Epidural hemorrhage

11 ✓7ᵗʰ **S06.4X0** Epidural hemorrhage without `MCC` `H5` `HCC`
loss of consciousness

11 ✓7ᵗʰ **S06.4X1** Epidural hemorrhage with `MCC` `H5` `HCC`
loss of consciousness of
30 minutes or less

11 ✓7ᵗʰ **S06.4X2** Epidural hemorrhage with `MCC` `H5` `HCC`
loss of consciousness of
31 minutes to 59 minutes

11 ✓7ᵗʰ **S06.4X3** Epidural hemorrhage with `MCC` `H5` `HCC`
loss of consciousness of
1 hour to 5 hours 59 minutes

11 ✓7ᵗʰ **S06.4X4** Epidural hemorrhage with `MCC` `H5` `HCC`
loss of consciousness of
6 hours to 24 hours

11 ✓7ᵗʰ **S06.4X5** Epidural hemorrhage with `MCC` `H5` `HCC`
loss of consciousness greater
than 24 hours with return to
pre-existing conscious level

11 ✓7ᵗʰ **S06.4X6** Epidural hemorrhage with `MCC` `H5` `HCC`
loss of consciousness greater than 24
hours without return to pre-existing
conscious level with patient surviving

✓7ᵗʰ **S06.4X7** Epidural hemorrhage with loss of `MCC` `H5`
consciousness of any duration with
death due to brain injury prior to
regaining consciousness

✓7ᵗʰ **S06.4X8** Epidural hemorrhage with loss of `MCC` `H5`
consciousness of any duration with
death due to other causes prior to
regaining consciousness

11 ✓7ᵗʰ **S06.4X9** Epidural hemorrhage with `MCC` `H5` `HCC`
loss of consciousness of
unspecified duration
      Epidural hemorrhage NOS

✓5ᵗʰ **S06.5** Traumatic subdural hemorrhage

✓6ᵗʰ **S06.5X** Traumatic subdural hemorrhage

11 ✓7ᵗʰ **S06.5X0** Traumatic subdural `MCC` `H5` `HCC`
hemorrhage without loss
of consciousness

11 ✓7ᵗʰ **S06.5X1** Traumatic subdural `MCC` `H5` `HCC`
hemorrhage with loss of
consciousness of 30 minutes or less

11 ✓7ᵗʰ **S06.5X2** Traumatic subdural `MCC` `H5` `HCC`
hemorrhage with loss of
consciousness of 31 minutes to 59 minutes

11 ✓7ᵗʰ **S06.5X3** Traumatic subdural `MCC` `H5` `HCC`
hemorrhagewith loss of consciousness
of 1 hour to 5 hours 59 minutes

11 ✓7ᵗʰ **S06.5X4** Traumatic subdural `MCC` `H5` `HCC`
hemorrhage with loss of consciousness
of 6 hours to 24 hours

11 ✓7ᵗʰ **S06.5X5** Traumatic subdural `MCC` `H5` `HCC`
hemorrhage with loss of consciousness
greater than 24 hours with return to
pre-existing conscious level

11 ✓7ᵗʰ **S06.5X6** Traumatic subdural `MCC` `H5` `HCC`
hemorrhage with loss of consciousness
greater than 24 hours without return
to pre-existing conscious level with
patient surviving

✓7ᵗʰ **S06.5X7** Traumatic subdural hemorrhage `MCC` `H5`
with loss of consciousness of any
duration with death due to brain
injury before regaining consciousness

✓7ᵗʰ **S06.5X8** Traumatic subdural hemorrhage `MCC` `H5`
with loss of consciousness of any
duration with death due to other
cause before regaining consciousness

11 ✓7ᵗʰ **S06.5X9** Traumatic subdural `MCC` `H5` `HCC`
hemorrhage with loss of consciousness
of unspecified duration
      Traumatic subdural hemorrhage NOS

✓5ᵗʰ **S06.6** Traumatic subarachnoid hemorrhage

✓6ᵗʰ **S06.6X** Traumatic subarachnoid hemorrhage

11 ✓7ᵗʰ **S06.6X0** Traumatic subarachnoid `MCC` `H5` `HCC`
hemorrhage without loss of consciousness

11 ✓7ᵗʰ **S06.6X1** Traumatic subarachnoid `MCC` `H5` `HCC`
hemorrhage with loss of consciousness
of 30 minutes or less

11 ✓7ᵗʰ **S06.6X2** Traumatic subarachnoid `MCC` `H5` `HCC`
hemorrhagewith loss of consciousness
of 31 minutes to 59 minutes

11 ✓7ᵗʰ **S06.6X3** Traumatic subarachnoid `MCC` `H5` `HCC`
hemorrhage with loss of consciousness
of 1 hour to 5 hours 59 minutes

11 ✓7ᵗʰ **S06.6X4** Traumatic subarachnoid `MCC` `H5` `HCC`
hemorrhage with loss of consciousness
of 6 hours to 24 hours

11 ✓7ᵗʰ **S06.6X5** Traumatic subarachnoid `MCC` `H5` `HCC`
hemorrhage with loss of consciousness
greater than 24 hours with return
to pre-existing conscious level

11 ✓7ᵗʰ **S06.6X6** Traumatic subarachnoid `MCC` `H5` `HCC`
hemorrhage with loss of consciousness
greater than 24 hours without return
to pre-existing conscious level with
patient surviving

✓7ᵗʰ **S06.6X7** Traumatic subarachnoid `MCC` `H5`
hemorrhage with loss of consciousness of
any duration with death due to brain
injury prior to regaining consciousness

✓7ᵗʰ **S06.6X8** Traumatic subarachnoid `MCC` `H5`
hemorrhage with loss of consciousness
of any duration with death due to other
cause prior to regaining consciousness

11 ✓7ᵗʰ **S06.6X9** Traumatic subarachnoid `MCC` `H5` `HCC`
hemorrhage with loss of consciousness
of unspecified duration
      Traumatic subarachnoid hemorrhage NOS

---

11 HCC with 7th character indicating initial encounter (A or B - specific to category) OR sequela.

☑ Additional Character Req   ✓x7ᵗʰ Placeholder Alert   Unacceptable PDx   Manifestation   `H1`-`H14` HAC   `HCC` CMS-HCC Condition   *EXCLUDES 1* Not Coded Here   *EXCLUDES 2* Not Included Here

Chapter 19. Injury, Poisoning and Certain Other Consequences of External Causes

✓5ᵗʰ **S06.8** **Other specified intracranial injuries**

  ✓6ᵗʰ **S06.81** **Injury of** right internal carotid artery, intracranial portion, not elsewhere classified

    11 ✓7ᵗʰ **S06.810** **Injury of right internal carotid artery, intracranial portion, not elsewhere classified** without loss of consciousness   `HCC`

    11 ✓7ᵗʰ **S06.811** **Injury of right internal carotid** `CC` `H5` `HCC` **artery, intracranial portion, not elsewhere classified with loss of consciousness of 30 minutes or less**

    11 ✓7ᵗʰ **S06.812** **Injury of right internal carotid** `CC` `H5` `HCC` **artery, intracranial portion, not elsewhere classified with loss of consciousness of 31 minutes to 59 minutes**

    11 ✓7ᵗʰ **S06.813** **Injury of right internal carotid** `CC` `H5` `HCC` **artery, intracranial portion, not elsewhere classified with loss of consciousness of 1 hour to 5 hours 59 minutes**

    11 ✓7ᵗʰ **S06.814** **Injury of right internal carotid** `CC` `H5` `HCC` **artery, intracranial portion, not elsewhere classified with loss of consciousness of 6 hours to 24 hours**

    11 ✓7ᵗʰ **S06.815** **Injury of right internal carotid** `CC` `H5` `HCC` **artery, intracranial portion, not elsewhere classified with loss of consciousness greater than 24 hours with return to pre-existing conscious level**

    11 ✓7ᵗʰ **S06.816** **Injury of right internal carotid** `MCC` `H5` `HCC` **artery, intracranial portion, not elsewhere classified with loss of consciousness greater than 24 hours without return to pre-existing conscious level with patient surviving**

    ✓7ᵗʰ **S06.817** **Injury of right internal carotid** `MCC` `H5` **artery, intracranial portion, not elsewhere classified with loss of consciousness of any duration with death due to brain injury prior to regaining consciousness**

    ✓7ᵗʰ **S06.818** **Injury of right internal carotid** `MCC` `H5` **artery, intracranial portion, not elsewhere classified with loss of consciousness of any duration with death due to other cause prior to regaining consciousness**

    11 ✓7ᵗʰ **S06.819** **Injury of right internal carotid** `CC` `H5` `HCC` **artery, intracranial portion, not elsewhere classified with loss of consciousness of unspecified duration**
        Injury of right internal carotid artery, intracranial portion, not elsewhere classified NOS

  ✓6ᵗʰ **S06.82** **Injury of** left internal carotid artery, intracranial portion, not elsewhere classified

    11 ✓7ᵗʰ **S06.820** **Injury of left internal carotid artery, intracranial portion, not elsewhere classified** without loss of consciousness   `HCC`

    11 ✓7ᵗʰ **S06.821** **Injury of left internal carotid** `CC` `H5` `HCC` **artery, intracranial portion, not elsewhere classified with loss of consciousness of 30 minutes or less**

    11 ✓7ᵗʰ **S06.822** **Injury of left internal carotid** `CC` `H5` `HCC` **artery, intracranial portion, not elsewhere classified with loss of consciousness of 31 minutes to 59 minutes**

    11 ✓7ᵗʰ **S06.823** **Injury of left internal carotid** `CC` `H5` `HCC` **artery, intracranial portion, not elsewhere classified with loss of consciousness of 1 hour to 5 hours 59 minutes**

    11 ✓7ᵗʰ **S06.824** **Injury of left internal carotid** `CC` `H5` `HCC` **artery, intracranial portion, not elsewhere classified with loss of consciousness of 6 hours to 24 hours**

    11 ✓7ᵗʰ **S06.825** **Injury of left internal carotid** `CC` `H5` `HCC` **artery, intracranial portion, not elsewhere classified with loss of consciousness greater than 24 hours with return to pre-existing conscious level**

    11 ✓7ᵗʰ **S06.826** **Injury of left internal carotid** `MCC` `H5` `HCC` **artery, intracranial portion, not elsewhere classified with loss of consciousness greater than 24 hours without return to pre-existing conscious level with patient surviving**

    ✓7ᵗʰ **S06.827** **Injury of left internal carotid** `MCC` `H5` **artery, intracranial portion, not elsewhere classified with loss of consciousness of any duration with death due to brain injury prior to regaining consciousness**

    ✓7ᵗʰ **S06.828** **Injury of left internal carotid** `MCC` `H5` **artery, intracranial portion, not elsewhere classified with loss of consciousness of any duration with death due to other cause prior to regaining consciousness**

    11 ✓7ᵗʰ **S06.829** **Injury of left internal carotid** `CC` `H5` `HCC` **artery, intracranial portion, not elsewhere classified with loss of consciousness of unspecified duration**
        Injury of left internal carotid artery, intracranial portion, not elsewhere classified NOS

  ✓6ᵗʰ **S06.89** **Other specified intracranial injury**
    EXCLUDES 1   concussion (S06.0X-)

    11 ✓7ᵗʰ **S06.890** **Other specified intracranial injury** `HCC` **without loss of consciousness**

    11 ✓7ᵗʰ **S06.891** **Other specified intracranial** `CC` `H5` `HCC` **injury with loss of consciousness of 30 minutes or less**

    11 ✓7ᵗʰ **S06.892** **Other specified intracranial** `CC` `H5` `HCC` **injury with loss of consciousness of 31 minutes to 59 minutes**

    11 ✓7ᵗʰ **S06.893** **Other specified intracranial** `CC` `H5` `HCC` **injury with loss of consciousness of 1 hour to 5 hours 59 minutes**

    11 ✓7ᵗʰ **S06.894** **Other specified intracranial** `CC` `H5` `HCC` **injury with loss of consciousness of 6 hours to 24 hours**

    11 ✓7ᵗʰ **S06.895** **Other specified intracranial** `CC` `H5` `HCC` **injury with loss of consciousness greater than 24 hours with return to pre-existing conscious level**

    11 ✓7ᵗʰ **S06.896** **Other specified intracranial** `MCC` `H5` `HCC` **injury with loss of consciousness greater than 24 hours without return to pre-existing conscious level with patient surviving**

    ✓7ᵗʰ **S06.897** **Other specified intracranial injury** `MCC` `H5` **with loss of consciousness of any duration with death due to brain injury prior to regaining consciousness**

    ✓7ᵗʰ **S06.898** **Other specified intracranial injury** `MCC` `H5` **with loss of consciousness of any duration with death due to other cause prior to regaining consciousness**

    11 ✓7ᵗʰ **S06.899** **Other specified intracranial** `CC` `H5` `HCC` **injury with loss of consciousness of unspecified duration**

✓5ᵗʰ **S06.9** **Unspecified intracranial injury**
    Brain injury NOS
    Head injury NOS with loss of consciousness
    Traumatic brain injury NOS
    EXCLUDES 1   conditions classifiable to S06.0- to S06.8- code to specified intracranial injury
        head injury NOS (S09.90)

  ✓6ᵗʰ **S06.9X** **Unspecified intracranial injury**

    11 ✓7ᵗʰ **S06.9X0** **Unspecified intracranial injury** `HCC` **without loss of consciousness**

    11 ✓7ᵗʰ **S06.9X1** **Unspecified intracranial injury** `CC` `H5` `HCC` **with loss of consciousness of 30 minutes or less**

    11 ✓7ᵗʰ **S06.9X2** **Unspecified intracranial injury** `CC` `H5` `HCC` **with loss of consciousness of 31 minutes to 59 minutes**

    11 ✓7ᵗʰ **S06.9X3** **Unspecified intracranial injury** `CC` `H5` `HCC` **with loss of consciousness of 1 hour to 5 hours 59 minutes**

---

11 HCC with 7th character indicating initial encounter (A or B - specific to category) OR sequela.

Ⓝ Newborn: 0   Ⓟ Pediatric: 0-17   Ⓜ Maternity: 12-55   Ⓐ Adult: 15-124   `MCC` Major CC Condition   `PDxMCC` PDx acts as own MCC   `CC` CC Condition   `PDxCC` PDx acts as own CC

952   ICD-10-CM 2018

11 **✓7ᵗʰ** **S06.9X4** **Unspecified intracranial injury** CC H5 HCC
**with loss of consciousness of
6 hours to 24 hours**

11 **✓7ᵗʰ** **S06.9X5** **Unspecified intracranial injury** CC H5 HCC
with loss of consciousness greater
**than 24 hours with return to
pre-existing conscious level**

11 **✓7ᵗʰ** **S06.9X6** **Unspecified intracranial injury** MCC H5 HCC
with loss of consciousness greater
**than 24 hours without return to
pre-existing conscious level with
patient surviving**

✓7ᵗʰ **S06.9X7** **Unspecified intracranial injury** MCC H5
with loss of consciousness of any duration
**with death due to brain injury prior
to regaining consciousness**

✓7ᵗʰ **S06.9X8** **Unspecified intracranial injury** MCC H5
with loss of consciousness of any duration
**with death due to other cause prior
to regaining consciousness**

11 **✓7ᵗʰ** **S06.9X9** **Unspecified intracranial injury** CC H5 HCC
**with loss of consciousness of
unspecified duration**

✓4ᵗʰ **S07** **Crushing injury of head**
Use additional code for all associated injuries, such as:
intracranial injuries (S06.-)
skull fractures (S02.-)

The appropriate 7th character is to be added to each code from
category S07.
A   initial encounter
D   subsequent encounter
S   sequela

CC Excl: For codes in category S07:
CC with 7th character A: PDX collection 1156

✓x7ᵗʰ **S07.0** **Crushing injury of** face   CC H5
✓x7ᵗʰ **S07.1** **Crushing injury of** skull   CC H5
✓x7ᵗʰ **S07.8** **Crushing injury of** other **parts of head**   CC H5
✓x7ᵗʰ **S07.9** **Crushing injury of** head, **part unspecified**   CC H5

✓4ᵗʰ **S08** **Avulsion and traumatic amputation of part of head**
An amputation not identified as partial or complete should be coded to
complete

The appropriate 7th character is to be added to each code from
category S08.
A   initial encounter
D   subsequent encounter
S   sequela

✓x7ᵗʰ **S08.0** **Avulsion of** scalp
✓5ᵗʰ **S08.1** **Traumatic amputation of** ear
     ✓6ᵗʰ **S08.11** **Complete traumatic amputation of ear**
         ✓7ᵗʰ **S08.111** **Complete traumatic amputation of** right
ear
         ✓7ᵗʰ **S08.112** **Complete traumatic amputation of** left **ear**
         ✓7ᵗʰ **S08.119** **Complete traumatic amputation of**
unspecified **ear**
     ✓6ᵗʰ **S08.12** **Partial traumatic amputation of ear**
         ✓7ᵗʰ **S08.121** **Partial traumatic amputation of** right **ear**
         ✓7ᵗʰ **S08.122** **Partial traumatic amputation of** left **ear**
         ✓7ᵗʰ **S08.129** **Partial traumatic amputation of**
unspecified **ear**
✓5ᵗʰ **S08.8** **Traumatic amputation of** other **parts of head**
     ✓6ᵗʰ **S08.81** **Traumatic amputation of** nose
         ✓7ᵗʰ **S08.811** **Complete** **traumatic amputation of nose**
         ✓7ᵗʰ **S08.812** **Partial** **traumatic amputation of nose**
     ✓x7ᵗʰ **S08.89** **Traumatic amputation of** other **parts of head**

✓4ᵗʰ **S09** **Other and unspecified injuries of head**

The appropriate 7th character is to be added to each code from
category S09.
A   initial encounter
D   subsequent encounter
S   sequela

CC Excl: For codes in category S09, unless otherwise noted:
CC with 7th character A: PDX collection 1158

✓x7ᵗʰ **S09.0** **Injury of** blood vessels **of head, not elsewhere classified** CC
EXCLUDES 1   injury of cerebral blood vessels (S06.-)
           injury of precerebral blood vessels (S15.-)
CC Excl: CC with 7th character A: PDX collection 1157

✓5ᵗʰ **S09.1** **Injury of** muscle and tendon **of head**
Code also any associated open wound (S01.-)
EXCLUDES 2   sprain to joints and ligament of head (S03.9)
     ✓x7ᵗʰ **S09.10** **Unspecified** **injury of muscle and tendon of head**
Injury of muscle and tendon of head NOS
     ✓x7ᵗʰ **S09.11** **Strain** **of muscle and tendon of head**
     ✓x7ᵗʰ **S09.12** **Laceration** **of muscle and tendon of head**
     ✓x7ᵗʰ **S09.19** **Other** **specified injury of muscle and tendon of head**
✓5ᵗʰ **S09.2** **Traumatic rupture of** ear drum
EXCLUDES 1   traumatic rupture of ear drum due to blast injury
           (S09.31-)
     ✓x7ᵗʰ **S09.20** **Traumatic rupture of** unspecified **ear drum** CC
     ✓x7ᵗʰ **S09.21** **Traumatic rupture of** right **ear drum** CC
     ✓x7ᵗʰ **S09.22** **Traumatic rupture of** left **ear drum** CC
✓5ᵗʰ **S09.3** **Other specified and unspecified injury of middle and inner
ear**
EXCLUDES 1   injury to ear NOS (S09.91-)
EXCLUDES 2   injury to external ear (S00.4-, S01.3-, S08.1-)
     ✓6ᵗʰ **S09.30** **Unspecified injury of** middle and inner ear
         ✓7ᵗʰ **S09.301** **Unspecified injury of** right **middle and** CC
inner ear
         ✓7ᵗʰ **S09.302** **Unspecified injury of** left **middle and** CC
inner ear
         ✓7ᵗʰ **S09.309** **Unspecified injury of** unspecified
middle and inner ear
     ✓6ᵗʰ **S09.31** **Primary** blast injury **of ear**
Blast injury of ear NOS
         ✓7ᵗʰ **S09.311** **Primary blast injury of** right **ear** CC
         ✓7ᵗʰ **S09.312** **Primary blast injury of** left **ear** CC
         ✓7ᵗʰ **S09.313** **Primary blast injury of ear,** bilateral CC
         ✓7ᵗʰ **S09.319** **Primary blast injury of** unspecified **ear** CC
     ✓6ᵗʰ **S09.39** **Other** **specified injury of middle and inner ear**
Secondary blast injury to ear
         ✓7ᵗʰ **S09.391** **Other specified injury of** right **middle** CC
and inner ear
         ✓7ᵗʰ **S09.392** **Other specified injury of** left **middle** CC
and inner ear
         ✓7ᵗʰ **S09.399** **Other specified injury of** unspecified CC
middle and inner ear
✓x7ᵗʰ **S09.8** **Other specified injuries of head**
✓5ᵗʰ **S09.9** **Unspecified injury of face and head**
     ✓x7ᵗʰ **S09.90** **Unspecified injury of** head
Head injury NOS
EXCLUDES 1   brain injury NOS (S06.9-)
           head injury NOS with loss of consciousness
           (S06.9-)
           intracranial injury NOS (S06.9-)
     ✓x7ᵗʰ **S09.91** **Unspecified injury of** ear
Injury of ear NOS
     ✓x7ᵗʰ **S09.92** **Unspecified injury of** nose
Injury of nose NOS
     ✓x7ᵗʰ **S09.93** **Unspecified injury of** face
Injury of face NOS

---

11 HCC with 7th character indicating initial encounter (A or B - specific to category) OR sequela.

✓ Additional Character Req   ✓x7ᵗʰ Placeholder Alert   Unacceptable PDx   Manifestation   H1-H14 HAC   HCC CMS-HCC Condition   EXCLUDES 1 Not Coded Here   EXCLUDES 2 Not Included Here

Injuries to the neck (S10-S19)

INCLUDES injuries of nape
injuries of supraclavicular region
injuries of throat
EXCLUDES 2 burns and corrosions (T20-T32)
effects of foreign body in esophagus (T18.1)
effects of foreign body in larynx (T17.3)
effects of foreign body in pharynx (T17.2)
effects of foreign body in trachea (T17.4)
frostbite (T33-T34)
insect bite or sting, venomous (T63.4)

√4th **S10 Superficial injury of neck**

> The appropriate 7th character is to be added to each code from category S10.
> A   initial encounter
> D   subsequent encounter
> S   sequela

√x7th **S10.0 Contusion of throat**
Contusion of cervical esophagus
Contusion of larynx
Contusion of pharynx
Contusion of trachea

√5th **S10.1 Other and unspecified superficial injuries of throat**
√x7th **S10.10** Unspecified superficial injuries of throat
√x7th **S10.11** Abrasion of throat
√x7th **S10.12** Blister (nonthermal) of throat
√x7th **S10.14** External constriction of part of throat
√x7th **S10.15** Superficial foreign body of throat
Splinter in the throat
√x7th **S10.16** Insect bite (nonvenomous) of throat
√x7th **S10.17** Other superficial bite of throat
EXCLUDES 1 open bite of throat (S11.85)

√5th **S10.8 Superficial injury of other specified parts of neck**
√x7th **S10.80** Unspecified superficial injury of other specified part of neck
√x7th **S10.81** Abrasion of other specified part of neck
√x7th **S10.82** Blister (nonthermal) of other specified part of neck
√x7th **S10.83** Contusion of other specified part of neck
√x7th **S10.84** External constriction of other specified part of neck
√x7th **S10.85** Superficial foreign body of other specified part of neck
Splinter in other specified part of neck
√x7th **S10.86** Insect bite of other specified part of neck
√x7th **S10.87** Other superficial bite of other specified part of neck
EXCLUDES 1 open bite of other specified parts of neck (S11.85)

√5th **S10.9 Superficial injury of unspecified part of neck**
√x7th **S10.90** Unspecified superficial injury of unspecified part of neck
√x7th **S10.91** Abrasion of unspecified part of neck
√x7th **S10.92** Blister (nonthermal) of unspecified part of neck
√x7th **S10.93** Contusion of unspecified part of neck
√x7th **S10.94** External constriction of unspecified part of neck
√x7th **S10.95** Superficial foreign body of unspecified part of neck
√x7th **S10.96** Insect bite of unspecified part of neck
√x7th **S10.97** Other superficial bite of unspecified part of neck

√4th **S11 Open wound of neck**
Code also any associated:
spinal cord injury (S14.0, S14.1-)
wound infection
EXCLUDES 2 open fracture of vertebra (S12- with 7th B)

> The appropriate 7th character is to be added to each code from category S11.
> A   initial encounter
> D   subsequent encounter
> S   sequela

√5th **S11.0 Open wound of larynx and trachea**

> **CC Excl:** For codes in subcategory S11.0, unless otherwise noted:
> **MCC with 7th character A:** PDX collection 1159

√6th **S11.01 Open wound of larynx**
EXCLUDES 2 open wound of vocal cord (S11.03)
√7th **S11.011** Laceration without foreign body of larynx   MCC
√7th **S11.012** Laceration with foreign body of larynx   MCC
√7th **S11.013** Puncture wound without foreign body of larynx   MCC
√7th **S11.014** Puncture wound with foreign body of larynx   MCC
√7th **S11.015** Open bite of larynx   MCC
Bite of larynx NOS
√7th **S11.019** Unspecified open wound of larynx   MCC

√6th **S11.02 Open wound of trachea**
Open wound of cervical trachea
Open wound of trachea NOS
EXCLUDES 2 open wound of thoracic trachea (S27.5-)
√7th **S11.021** Laceration without foreign body of trachea   MCC
√7th **S11.022** Laceration with foreign body of trachea   MCC
√7th **S11.023** Puncture wound without foreign body of trachea   MCC
√7th **S11.024** Puncture wound with foreign body of trachea   MCC
√7th **S11.025** Open bite of trachea   MCC
Bite of trachea NOS
√7th **S11.029** Unspecified open wound of trachea   MCC

√6th **S11.03 Open wound of vocal cord**
√7th **S11.031** Laceration without foreign body of vocal cord   MCC
√7th **S11.032** Laceration with foreign body of vocal cord   MCC
√7th **S11.033** Puncture wound without foreign body of vocal cord   MCC
√7th **S11.034** Puncture wound with foreign body of vocal cord   MCC
√7th **S11.035** Open bite of vocal cord   MCC
Bite of vocal cord NOS
√7th **S11.039** Unspecified open wound of vocal cord   MCC

√5th **S11.1 Open wound of thyroid gland**

> **CC Excl:** For codes in subcategory S11.1, unless otherwise noted:
> **CC with 7th character A:** PDX collection 1160

√x7th **S11.10** Unspecified open wound of thyroid gland   CC
√x7th **S11.11** Laceration without foreign body of thyroid gland   CC
√x7th **S11.12** Laceration with foreign body of thyroid gland   CC
CC Excl: CC with 7th character A: PDX collection 1161
√x7th **S11.13** Puncture wound without foreign body of thyroid gland   CC
√x7th **S11.14** Puncture wound with foreign body of thyroid gland   CC
CC Excl: CC with 7th character A: PDX collection 1161
√x7th **S11.15** Open bite of thyroid gland   CC
Bite of thyroid gland NOS

√5th **S11.2 Open wound of pharynx and cervical esophagus**
EXCLUDES 1 open wound of esophagus NOS (S27.8-)

> **CC Excl:** For codes in subcategory S11.2, unless otherwise noted:
> **CC with 7th character A:** PDX collection 1162

√x7th **S11.20** Unspecified open wound of pharynx and cervical esophagus   CC
√x7th **S11.21** Laceration without foreign body of pharynx and cervical esophagus   CC
√x7th **S11.22** Laceration with foreign body of pharynx and cervical esophagus   CC
CC Excl: CC with 7th character A: PDX collection 1163
√x7th **S11.23** Puncture wound without foreign body of pharynx and cervical esophagus   CC

Ⓝ Newborn: 0   Ⓟ Pediatric: 0-17   Ⓜ Maternity: 12-55   Ⓐ Adult: 15-124   **MCC** Major CC Condition   **PDxMCC** PDx acts as own MCC   **CC** CC Condition   **PDxCC** PDx acts as own CC

954   ICD-10-CM 2018

✓7ᵗʰ **S11.24 Puncture wound with foreign body** of pharynx **and cervical esophagus**   CC
      CC Excl: CC with 7th character A:
      PDX collection 1163

✓7ᵗʰ **S11.25 Open bite** of pharynx and cervical esophagus   CC
      Bite of pharynx and cervical esophagus NOS

✓5ᵗʰ **S11.8 Open wound of** other **specified parts of neck**

  ✓x7ᵗʰ **S11.80 Unspecified open wound of other specified part of** neck

  ✓x7ᵗʰ **S11.81 Laceration without foreign body of other specified part** of neck

  ✓x7ᵗʰ **S11.82 Laceration with foreign body of other specified part** of neck

  ✓x7ᵗʰ **S11.83 Puncture wound without foreign body of other specified part of neck**

  ✓x7ᵗʰ **S11.84 Puncture wound with foreign body of other specified part of neck**

  ✓x7ᵗʰ **S11.85 Open bite of other specified part of neck**
      Bite of other specified part of neck NOS
      EXCLUDES 1 superficial bite of other specified part of neck (S10.87)

  ✓x7ᵗʰ **S11.89 Other open wound of other specified part of neck**

✓5ᵗʰ **S11.9 Open wound of unspecified part of neck**

  ✓x7ᵗʰ **S11.90 Unspecified open wound of unspecified part of neck**

  ✓x7ᵗʰ **S11.91 Laceration without foreign body of unspecified part** of neck

  ✓x7ᵗʰ **S11.92 Laceration with foreign body of unspecified part of** neck

  ✓x7ᵗʰ **S11.93 Puncture wound without foreign body of unspecified part of neck**

  ✓x7ᵗʰ **S11.94 Puncture wound with foreign body of unspecified part of neck**

  ✓x7ᵗʰ **S11.95 Open bite of unspecified part of neck**
      Bite of neck NOS
      EXCLUDES 1 superficial bite of neck (S10.97)

✓4ᵗʰ **S12 Fracture of cervical vertebra and other parts of neck**

  NOTE A fracture not indicated as nondisplaced or displaced should be classified to displaced.
     A fracture not indicated as open or closed should be coded to closed.

  INCLUDES fracture of cervical neural arch
     fracture of cervical spine
     fracture of cervical spinous process
     fracture of cervical transverse process
     fracture of cervical vertebral arch
     fracture of neck

  Code first any associated cervical spinal cord injury (S14.0-, S14.1-)
  AHA: 2015, 3Q, 37-39

  The appropriate 7th character is to be added to all codes from subcategories S12.0-S12.6.
  A initial encounter for closed fracture
  B initial encounter for open fracture
  D subsequent encounter for fracture with routine healing
  G subsequent encounter for fracture with delayed healing
  K subsequent encounter for fracture with nonunion
  S sequela

  CC Excl: For codes in category S12, unless otherwise noted:
  CC with 7th character A or MCC with 7th character B:
  PDX collection 1164
  CC with 7th character K: PDX collection 897

✓5ᵗʰ **S12.0 Fracture of first cervical vertebra**
    Atlas

  ✓6ᵗʰ **S12.00 Unspecified fracture of first cervical vertebra**

  6,7,10 ✓7ᵗʰ **S12.000 Unspecified displaced fracture of first cervical vertebra**   MCC CC H5 HCC

  6,7,10 ✓7ᵗʰ **S12.001 Unspecified nondisplaced fracture of first cervical vertebra**   MCC CC H5 HCC

  6,7,10 ✓x7ᵗʰ **S12.01 Stable burst fracture of first cervical vertebra**   MCC CC H5 HCC

  6,7,10 ✓x7ᵗʰ **S12.02 Unstable burst fracture of first cervical vertebra**   MCC CC H5 HCC

  ✓6ᵗʰ **S12.03 Posterior arch fracture of first cervical vertebra**

  6,7,10 ✓7ᵗʰ **S12.030 Displaced posterior arch fracture of first cervical vertebra**   MCC CC H5 HCC

  6,7,10 ✓7ᵗʰ **S12.031 Nondisplaced posterior arch fracture of first cervical vertebra**   MCC CC H5 HCC

  ✓6ᵗʰ **S12.04 Lateral mass fracture of first cervical vertebra**

  6,7,10 ✓7ᵗʰ **S12.040 Displaced lateral mass fracture of first cervical vertebra**   MCC CC H5 HCC

  6,7,10 ✓7ᵗʰ **S12.041 Nondisplaced lateral mass fracture of first cervical vertebra**   MCC CC H5 HCC

  ✓6ᵗʰ **S12.09 Other fracture of first cervical vertebra**

  6,7,10 ✓7ᵗʰ **S12.090 Other displaced fracture of first cervical vertebra**   MCC CC H5 HCC

  6,7,10 ✓7ᵗʰ **S12.091 Other nondisplaced fracture of first cervical vertebra**   MCC CC H5 HCC

✓5ᵗʰ **S12.1 Fracture of second cervical vertebra**
    Axis

  ✓6ᵗʰ **S12.10 Unspecified fracture of second cervical vertebra**

  6,7,10 ✓7ᵗʰ **S12.100 Unspecified displaced fracture of second cervical vertebra**   MCC CC H5 HCC

  6,7,10 ✓7ᵗʰ **S12.101 Unspecified nondisplaced fracture of second cervical vertebra**   MCC CC H5 HCC

  ✓6ᵗʰ **S12.11 Type II dens fracture**

  6,7,10 ✓7ᵗʰ **S12.110 Anterior displaced Type II dens fracture**   MCC CC H5 HCC

  6,7,10 ✓7ᵗʰ **S12.111 Posterior displaced Type II dens fracture**   MCC CC H5 HCC

  6,7,10 ✓7ᵗʰ **S12.112 Nondisplaced Type II dens fracture**   MCC CC H5 HCC

  ✓6ᵗʰ **S12.12 Other dens fracture**

  6,7,10 ✓7ᵗʰ **S12.120 Other displaced dens fracture**   MCC CC H5 HCC

  6,7,10 ✓7ᵗʰ **S12.121 Other nondisplaced dens fracture**   MCC CC H5 HCC

  ✓6ᵗʰ **S12.13 Unspecified traumatic spondylolisthesis of second cervical vertebra**

  6,7,10 ✓7ᵗʰ **S12.130 Unspecified traumatic displaced spondylolisthesis of second cervical vertebra**   MCC CC H5 HCC

  6,7,10 ✓7ᵗʰ **S12.131 Unspecified traumatic nondisplaced spondylolisthesis of second cervical vertebra**   MCC CC H5 HCC

  6,7,10 ✓x7ᵗʰ **S12.14 Type III traumatic spondylolisthesis of second cervical vertebra**   MCC CC H5 HCC

  ✓6ᵗʰ **S12.15 Other traumatic spondylolisthesis of second cervical vertebra**

  6,7,10 ✓7ᵗʰ **S12.150 Other traumatic displaced spondylolisthesis of second cervical vertebra**   MCC CC H5 HCC

  6,7,10 ✓7ᵗʰ **S12.151 Other traumatic nondisplaced spondylolisthesis of second cervical vertebra**   MCC CC H5 HCC

  ✓6ᵗʰ **S12.19 Other fracture of second cervical vertebra**

  6,7,10 ✓7ᵗʰ **S12.190 Other displaced fracture of second cervical vertebra**   MCC CC H5 HCC

  6,7,10 ✓7ᵗʰ **S12.191 Other nondisplaced fracture of second cervical vertebra**   MCC CC H5 HCC

✓5ᵗʰ **S12.2 Fracture of third cervical vertebra**

  ✓6ᵗʰ **S12.20 Unspecified fracture of third cervical vertebra**

  6,7,10 ✓7ᵗʰ **S12.200 Unspecified displaced fracture of third cervical vertebra**   MCC CC H5 HCC

  6,7,10 ✓7ᵗʰ **S12.201 Unspecified nondisplaced fracture of third cervical vertebra**   MCC CC H5 HCC

  ✓6ᵗʰ **S12.23 Unspecified traumatic spondylolisthesis of third cervical vertebra**

  6,7,10 ✓7ᵗʰ **S12.230 Unspecified traumatic displaced spondylolisthesis of third cervical vertebra**   MCC CC H5 HCC

  6,7,10 ✓7ᵗʰ **S12.231 Unspecified traumatic nondisplaced spondylolisthesis of third cervical vertebra**   MCC CC H5 HCC

---

6 MCC when reported as an open fracture (7th character B or C – specific to category).

7 CC when reported as an initial encounter (7th character A, B, or C – specific to category) OR a subsequent encounter for nonunion or malunion (7th character K, M, N, P, Q, or R – specific to category).

10 HCC with 7th character indicating initial encounter (A, B or C - specific to category).

✔ Additional Character Req   ✓x7ᵗʰ Placeholder Alert   Unacceptable PDx   Manifestation   H1 - H14 HAC   HCC CMS-HCC Condition   EXCLUDES 1 Not Coded Here   EXCLUDES 2 Not Included Here

6,7,10   √x7ᵗʰ   **S12.24**   **Type III traumatic** spondylolisthesis **of third cervical vertebra**   MCC CC H5 HCC

√6ᵗʰ   **S12.25**   **Other traumatic spondylolisthesis of third cervical vertebra**

6,7,10   √7ᵗʰ   **S12.250**   **Other traumatic** displaced **spondylolisthesis of third cervical vertebra**   MCC CC H5 HCC

6,7,10   √7ᵗʰ   **S12.251**   **Other traumatic** nondisplaced **spondylolisthesis of third cervical vertebra**   MCC CC H5 HCC

√6ᵗʰ   **S12.29**   **Other fracture of third cervical vertebra**

6,7,10   √7ᵗʰ   **S12.290**   **Other** displaced **fracture of third cervical vertebra**   MCC CC H5 HCC

6,7,10   √7ᵗʰ   **S12.291**   **Other** nondisplaced **fracture of third cervical vertebra**   MCC CC H5 HCC

√5ᵗʰ   **S12.3**   **Fracture of fourth cervical vertebra**

√6ᵗʰ   **S12.30**   **Unspecified fracture of fourth cervical vertebra**

6,7,10   √7ᵗʰ   **S12.300**   **Unspecified** displaced **fracture of fourth cervical vertebra**   MCC CC H5 HCC

6,7,10   √7ᵗʰ   **S12.301**   **Unspecified** nondisplaced **fracture of fourth cervical vertebra**   MCC CC H5 HCC

√6ᵗʰ   **S12.33**   **Unspecified traumatic** spondylolisthesis **of fourth cervical vertebra**

6,7,10   √7ᵗʰ   **S12.330**   **Unspecified traumatic** displaced **spondylolisthesis of fourth cervical vertebra**   MCC CC H5 HCC

6,7,10   √7ᵗʰ   **S12.331**   **Unspecified traumatic** nondisplaced **spondylolisthesis of fourth cervical vertebra**   MCC CC H5 HCC

6,7,10   √x7ᵗʰ   **S12.34**   **Type III traumatic** spondylolisthesis **of fourth cervical vertebra**   MCC CC H5 HCC

√6ᵗʰ   **S12.35**   **Other traumatic spondylolisthesis of fourth cervical vertebra**

6,7,10   √7ᵗʰ   **S12.350**   **Other traumatic** displaced **spondylolisthesis of fourth cervical vertebra**   MCC CC H5 HCC

6,7,10   √7ᵗʰ   **S12.351**   **Other traumatic** nondisplaced **spondylolisthesis of fourth cervical vertebra**   MCC CC H5 HCC

√6ᵗʰ   **S12.39**   **Other fracture of fourth cervical vertebra**

6,7,10   √7ᵗʰ   **S12.390**   **Other** displaced **fracture of fourth cervical vertebra**   MCC CC H5 HCC

6,7,10   √7ᵗʰ   **S12.391**   **Other** nondisplaced **fracture of fourth cervical vertebra**   MCC CC H5 HCC

√5ᵗʰ   **S12.4**   **Fracture of fifth cervical vertebra**

√6ᵗʰ   **S12.40**   **Unspecified fracture of fifth cervical vertebra**

6,7,10   √7ᵗʰ   **S12.400**   **Unspecified** displaced **fracture of fifth cervical vertebra**   MCC CC H5 HCC

6,7,10   √7ᵗʰ   **S12.401**   **Unspecified** nondisplaced **fracture of fifth cervical vertebra**   MCC CC H5 HCC

√6ᵗʰ   **S12.43**   **Unspecified traumatic** spondylolisthesis **of fifth cervical vertebra**

6,7,10   √7ᵗʰ   **S12.430**   **Unspecified traumatic** displaced **spondylolisthesis of fifth cervical vertebra**   MCC CC H5 HCC

6,7,10   √7ᵗʰ   **S12.431**   **Unspecified traumatic** nondisplaced **spondylolisthesis of fifth cervical vertebra**   MCC CC H5 HCC

6,7,10   √x7ᵗʰ   **S12.44**   **Type III traumatic** spondylolisthesis **of fifth cervical vertebra**   MCC CC H5 HCC

√6ᵗʰ   **S12.45**   **Other traumatic spondylolisthesis of fifth cervical vertebra**

6,7,10   √7ᵗʰ   **S12.450**   **Other traumatic** displaced **spondylolisthesis of fifth cervical vertebra**   MCC CC H5 HCC

6,7,10   √7ᵗʰ   **S12.451**   **Other traumatic** nondisplaced **spondylolisthesis of fifth cervical vertebra**   MCC CC H5 HCC

√6ᵗʰ   **S12.49**   **Other fracture of fifth cervical vertebra**

6,7,10   √7ᵗʰ   **S12.490**   **Other** displaced **fracture of fifth cervical vertebra**   MCC CC H5 HCC

6,7,10   √7ᵗʰ   **S12.491**   **Other** nondisplaced **fracture of fifth cervical vertebra**   MCC CC H5 HCC

√5ᵗʰ   **S12.5**   **Fracture of sixth cervical vertebra**

√6ᵗʰ   **S12.50**   **Unspecified fracture of sixth cervical vertebra**

6,7,10   √7ᵗʰ   **S12.500**   **Unspecified** displaced **fracture of sixth cervical vertebra**   MCC CC H5 HCC

6,7,10   √7ᵗʰ   **S12.501**   **Unspecified** nondisplaced **fracture of sixth cervical vertebra**   MCC CC H5 HCC

√6ᵗʰ   **S12.53**   **Unspecified traumatic** spondylolisthesis **of sixth cervical vertebra**

6,7,10   √7ᵗʰ   **S12.530**   **Unspecified traumatic** displaced **spondylolisthesis of sixth cervical vertebra**   MCC CC H5 HCC

6,7,10   √7ᵗʰ   **S12.531**   **Unspecified traumatic** nondisplaced **spondylolisthesis of sixth cervical vertebra**   MCC CC H5 HCC

6,7,10   √x7ᵗʰ   **S12.54**   **Type III traumatic** spondylolisthesis **of sixth cervical vertebra**   MCC CC H5 HCC

√6ᵗʰ   **S12.55**   **Other traumatic spondylolisthesis of sixth cervical vertebra**

6,7,10   √7ᵗʰ   **S12.550**   **Other traumatic** displaced **spondylolisthesis of sixth cervical vertebra**   MCC CC H5 HCC

6,7,10   √7ᵗʰ   **S12.551**   **Other traumatic** nondisplaced **spondylolisthesis of sixth cervical vertebra**   MCC CC H5 HCC

√6ᵗʰ   **S12.59**   **Other fracture of sixth cervical vertebra**

6,7,10   √7ᵗʰ   **S12.590**   **Other** displaced **fracture of sixth cervical vertebra**   MCC CC H5 HCC

6,7,10   √7ᵗʰ   **S12.591**   **Other** nondisplaced **fracture of sixth cervical vertebra**   MCC CC H5 HCC

√5ᵗʰ   **S12.6**   **Fracture of seventh cervical vertebra**

√6ᵗʰ   **S12.60**   **Unspecified fracture of seventh cervical vertebra**

6,7,10   √7ᵗʰ   **S12.600**   **Unspecified** displaced **fracture of seventh cervical vertebra**   MCC CC H5 HCC

6,7,10   √7ᵗʰ   **S12.601**   **Unspecified** nondisplaced **fracture of seventh cervical vertebra**   MCC CC H5 HCC

√6ᵗʰ   **S12.63**   **Unspecified traumatic** spondylolisthesis **of seventh cervical vertebra**

6,7,10   √7ᵗʰ   **S12.630**   **Unspecified traumatic** displaced **spondylolisthesis of seventh cervical vertebra**   MCC CC H5 HCC

6,7,10   √7ᵗʰ   **S12.631**   **Unspecified traumatic** nondisplaced **spondylolisthesis of seventh cervical vertebra**   MCC CC H5 HCC

6,7,10   √x7ᵗʰ   **S12.64**   **Type III traumatic** spondylolisthesis **of seventh cervical vertebra**   MCC CC H5 HCC

√6ᵗʰ   **S12.65**   **Other traumatic** spondylolisthesis **of seventh cervical vertebra**

6,7,10   √7ᵗʰ   **S12.650**   **Other traumatic** displaced **spondylolisthesis of seventh cervical vertebra**   MCC CC H5 HCC

6,7,10   √7ᵗʰ   **S12.651**   **Other traumatic** nondisplaced **spondylolisthesis of seventh cervical vertebra**   MCC CC H5 HCC

√6ᵗʰ   **S12.69**   **Other** fracture **of seventh cervical vertebra**

6,7,10   √7ᵗʰ   **S12.690**   **Other** displaced **fracture of seventh cervical vertebra**   MCC CC H5 HCC

6,7,10   √7ᵗʰ   **S12.691**   **Other** nondisplaced **fracture of seventh cervical vertebra**   MCC CC H5 HCC

10   √x7ᵗʰ   **S12.8**   **Fracture of other parts of neck**   MCC H5 HCC

     Hyoid bone   Thyroid cartilage
     Larynx   Trachea

The appropriate 7th character is to be added to code S12.8.
A   initial encounter
D   subsequent encounter
S   sequela

CC Excl: MCC with 7th character A: PDX collection 1165

---

6   MCC when reported as an open fracture (7th character B or C – specific to category).
7   CC when reported as an initial encounter (7th character A, B, or C – specific to category) OR a subsequent encounter for nonunion or malunion (7th character K, M, N, P, Q, or R – specific to category).
10   HCC with 7th character indicating initial encounter (A, B or C - specific to category).

10   ✓x 7th   **S12.9   Fracture of neck, unspecified**   CC H5 HCC
Fracture of cervical spine NOS
Fracture of cervical vertebra NOS
Fracture of neck NOS

> The appropriate 7th character is to be added to code S12.9.
> A   initial encounter
> D   subsequent encounter
> S   sequela

CC Excl: CC with 7th character A: PDX collection 1164

✓4th   **S13   Dislocation and sprain of joints and ligaments at neck level**
   INCLUDES   avulsion of joint or ligament at neck level
   laceration of cartilage, joint or ligament at neck level
   sprain of cartilage, joint or ligament at neck level
   traumatic hemarthrosis of joint or ligament at neck level
   traumatic rupture of joint or ligament at neck level
   traumatic subluxation of joint or ligament at neck level
   traumatic tear of joint or ligament at neck level
Code also any associated open wound
   EXCLUDES 2   strain of muscle or tendon at neck level (S16.1)

> The appropriate 7th character is to be added to each code from
> category S13.
> A   initial encounter
> D   subsequent encounter
> S   sequela

CC Excl: For codes in category S13:
CC with 7th character A: PDX collection 913

✓x 7th   **S13.0   Traumatic rupture of cervical intervertebral disc**   CC H5
   EXCLUDES 1   rupture or displacement (nontraumatic) of cervical
   intervertebral disc NOS (M50.-)

✓5th   **S13.1   Subluxation and dislocation of cervical vertebrae**
Code also any associated:
   open wound of neck (S11.-)
   spinal cord injury (S14.1-)
   EXCLUDES 2   fracture of cervical vertebrae (S12.0--S12.3-)

✓6th   **S13.10   Subluxation and dislocation of unspecified cervical
vertebrae**
   ✓7th   **S13.100   Subluxation of unspecified cervical**   CC H5
   vertebrae
   ✓7th   **S13.101   Dislocation of unspecified cervical**   CC H5
   vertebrae

✓6th   **S13.11   Subluxation and dislocation of C0/C1 cervical
vertebrae**
   Subluxation and dislocation of atlantooccipital joint
   Subluxation and dislocation of atloidooccipital joint
   Subluxation and dislocation of occipitoatloid joint
   ✓7th   **S13.110   Subluxation of C0/C1 cervical**   CC H5
   vertebrae
   ✓7th   **S13.111   Dislocation of C0/C1 cervical**   CC H5
   vertebrae

✓6th   **S13.12   Subluxation and dislocation of C1/C2 cervical
vertebrae**
   Subluxation and dislocation of atlantoaxial joint
   ✓7th   **S13.120   Subluxation of C1/C2 cervical**   CC H5
   vertebrae
   ✓7th   **S13.121   Dislocation of C1/C2 cervical**   CC H5
   vertebrae

✓6th   **S13.13   Subluxation and dislocation of C2/C3 cervical
vertebrae**
   ✓7th   **S13.130   Subluxation of C2/C3 cervical**   CC H5
   vertebrae
   ✓7th   **S13.131   Dislocation of C2/C3 cervical**   CC H5
   vertebrae

✓6th   **S13.14   Subluxation and dislocation of C3/C4 cervical
vertebrae**
   ✓7th   **S13.140   Subluxation of C3/C4 cervical**   CC H5
   vertebrae
   ✓7th   **S13.141   Dislocation of C3/C4 cervical**   CC H5
   vertebrae

✓6th   **S13.15   Subluxation and dislocation of C4/C5 cervical
vertebrae**
   ✓7th   **S13.150   Subluxation of C4/C5 cervical**   CC H5
   vertebrae
   ✓7th   **S13.151   Dislocation of C4/C5 cervical**   CC H5
   vertebrae

✓6th   **S13.16   Subluxation and dislocation of C5/C6 cervical
vertebrae**
   ✓7th   **S13.160   Subluxation of C5/C6 cervical**   CC H5
   vertebrae
   ✓7th   **S13.161   Dislocation of C5/C6 cervical**   CC H5
   vertebrae

✓6th   **S13.17   Subluxation and dislocation of C6/C7 cervical
vertebrae**
   ✓7th   **S13.170   Subluxation of C6/C7 cervical**   CC H5
   vertebrae
   ✓7th   **S13.171   Dislocation of C6/C7 cervical**   CC H5
   vertebrae

✓6th   **S13.18   Subluxation and dislocation of C7/T1 cervical
vertebrae**
   ✓7th   **S13.180   Subluxation of C7/T1 cervical**   CC H5
   vertebrae
   ✓7th   **S13.181   Dislocation of C7/T1 cervical**   CC H5
   vertebrae

✓5th   **S13.2   Dislocation of other and unspecified parts of neck**
   S13.20   Dislocation of unspecified parts of neck   CC H5
   S13.29   Dislocation of other parts of neck   CC H5

✓x 7th   **S13.4   Sprain of ligaments of cervical spine**
   Sprain of anterior longitudinal (ligament), cervical
   Sprain of atlanto-axial (joints)
   Sprain of atlanto-occipital (joints)
   Whiplash injury of cervical spine

✓x 7th   **S13.5   Sprain of thyroid region**
   Sprain of cricoarytenoid (joint) (ligament)
   Sprain of cricothyroid (joint) (ligament)
   Sprain of thyroid cartilage

✓x 7th   **S13.8   Sprain of joints and ligaments of other parts of neck**
✓x 7th   **S13.9   Sprain of joints and ligaments of unspecified parts of neck**

✓4th   **S14   Injury of nerves and spinal cord at neck level**
   NOTE   Code to highest level of cervical cord injury.
Code also any associated:
   fracture of cervical vertebra (S12.0- – S12.6-)
   open wound of neck (S11.-)
   transient paralysis (R29.5)

> The appropriate 7th character is to be added to each code from
> category S14.
> A   initial encounter
> D   subsequent encounter
> S   sequela

CC Excl: For codes in category S14:
MCC with 7th character A: PDX collection 1166

✓x 7th   **S14.0   Concussion and edema of cervical spinal cord**   MCC HCC
✓5th   **S14.1   Other and unspecified injuries of cervical spinal cord**
   ✓6th   **S14.10   Unspecified injury of cervical spinal cord**
   ✓7th   **S14.101   Unspecified injury at C1 level**   MCC H5 HCC
   of cervical spinal cord
   ✓7th   **S14.102   Unspecified injury at C2 level**   MCC H5 HCC
   of cervical spinal cord
   ✓7th   **S14.103   Unspecified injury at C3 level**   MCC H5 HCC
   of cervical spinal cord
   ✓7th   **S14.104   Unspecified injury at C4 level**   MCC H5 HCC
   of cervical spinal cord
   ✓7th   **S14.105   Unspecified injury at C5 level**   MCC H5 HCC
   of cervical spinal cord
   ✓7th   **S14.106   Unspecified injury at C6 level**   MCC H5 HCC
   of cervical spinal cord
   ✓7th   **S14.107   Unspecified injury at C7 level**   MCC H5 HCC
   of cervical spinal cord
   ✓7th   **S14.108   Unspecified injury at C8 level**   MCC HCC
   of cervical spinal cord
   ✓7th   **S14.109   Unspecified injury at unspecified**   H5 HCC
   level of cervical spinal cord
   Injury of cervical spinal cord NOS
   ✓6th   **S14.11   Complete lesion of cervical spinal cord**
   ✓7th   **S14.111   Complete lesion at C1 level of**   MCC H5 HCC
   cervical spinal cord
   ✓7th   **S14.112   Complete lesion at C2 level of**   MCC H5 HCC
   cervical spinal cord

---

10   HCC with 7th character indicating initial encounter (A, B or C - specific to category).

√7th **S14.113 Complete lesion at C3 level of cervical spinal cord** `MCC` `H5` `HCC`

√7th **S14.114 Complete lesion at C4 level of cervical spinal cord** `MCC` `H5` `HCC`

√7th **S14.115 Complete lesion at C5 level of cervical spinal cord** `MCC` `H5` `HCC`

√7th **S14.116 Complete lesion at C6 level of cervical spinal cord** `MCC` `H5` `HCC`

√7th **S14.117 Complete lesion at C7 level of cervical spinal cord** `MCC` `H5` `HCC`

√7th **S14.118 Complete lesion at C8 level of cervical spinal cord** `MCC` `HCC`

√7th **S14.119 Complete lesion at unspecified level of cervical spinal cord** `HCC`

√6th **S14.12 Central cord syndrome of cervical spinal cord**

√7th **S14.121 Central cord syndrome at C1 level of cervical spinal cord** `MCC` `H5` `HCC`

√7th **S14.122 Central cord syndrome at C2 level of cervical spinal cord** `MCC` `H5` `HCC`

√7th **S14.123 Central cord syndrome at C3 level of cervical spinal cord** `MCC` `H5` `HCC`

√7th **S14.124 Central cord syndrome at C4 level of cervical spinal cord** `MCC` `H5` `HCC`

√7th **S14.125 Central cord syndrome at C5 level of cervical spinal cord** `MCC` `H5` `HCC`

√7th **S14.126 Central cord syndrome at C6 level of cervical spinal cord** `MCC` `H5` `HCC`

√7th **S14.127 Central cord syndrome at C7 level of cervical spinal cord** `MCC` `H5` `HCC`

√7th **S14.128 Central cord syndrome at C8 level of cervical spinal cord** `MCC` `HCC`

√7th **S14.129 Central cord syndrome at unspecified level of cervical spinal cord** `HCC`

√6th **S14.13 Anterior cord syndrome of cervical spinal cord**

√7th **S14.131 Anterior cord syndrome at C1 level of cervical spinal cord** `MCC` `H5` `HCC`

√7th **S14.132 Anterior cord syndrome at C2 level of cervical spinal cord** `MCC` `H5` `HCC`

√7th **S14.133 Anterior cord syndrome at C3 level of cervical spinal cord** `MCC` `H5` `HCC`

√7th **S14.134 Anterior cord syndrome at C4 level of cervical spinal cord** `MCC` `H5` `HCC`

√7th **S14.135 Anterior cord syndrome at C5 level of cervical spinal cord** `MCC` `H5` `HCC`

√7th **S14.136 Anterior cord syndrome at C6 level of cervical spinal cord** `MCC` `H5` `HCC`

√7th **S14.137 Anterior cord syndrome at C7 level of cervical spinal cord** `MCC` `H5` `HCC`

√7th **S14.138 Anterior cord syndrome at C8 level of cervical spinal cord** `MCC` `HCC`

√7th **S14.139 Anterior cord syndrome at unspecified level of cervical spinal cord** `HCC`

√6th **S14.14 Brown-Séquard syndrome of cervical spinal cord**

√7th **S14.141 Brown-Séquard syndrome at C1 level of cervical spinal cord** `MCC` `HCC`

√7th **S14.142 Brown-Séquard syndrome at C2 level of cervical spinal cord** `MCC` `HCC`

√7th **S14.143 Brown-Séquard syndrome at C3 level of cervical spinal cord** `MCC` `HCC`

√7th **S14.144 Brown-Séquard syndrome at C4 level of cervical spinal cord** `MCC` `HCC`

√7th **S14.145 Brown-Séquard syndrome at C5 level of cervical spinal cord** `MCC` `HCC`

√7th **S14.146 Brown-Séquard syndrome at C6 level of cervical spinal cord** `MCC` `HCC`

√7th **S14.147 Brown-Séquard syndrome at C7 level of cervical spinal cord** `MCC` `HCC`

√7th **S14.148 Brown-Séquard syndrome at C8 level of cervical spinal cord** `MCC` `HCC`

√7th **S14.149 Brown-Séquard syndrome at unspecified level of cervical spinal cord** `HCC`

√6th **S14.15 Other incomplete lesions of cervical spinal cord**
Incomplete lesion of cervical spinal cord NOS
Posterior cord syndrome of cervical spinal cord

√7th **S14.151 Other incomplete lesion at C1 level of cervical spinal cord** `MCC` `H5` `HCC`

√7th **S14.152 Other incomplete lesion at C2 level of cervical spinal cord** `MCC` `H5` `HCC`

√7th **S14.153 Other incomplete lesion at C3 level of cervical spinal cord** `MCC` `H5` `HCC`

√7th **S14.154 Other incomplete lesion at C4 level of cervical spinal cord** `MCC` `H5` `HCC`

√7th **S14.155 Other incomplete lesion at C5 level of cervical spinal cord** `MCC` `H5` `HCC`

√7th **S14.156 Other incomplete lesion at C6 level of cervical spinal cord** `MCC` `H5` `HCC`

√7th **S14.157 Other incomplete lesion at C7 level of cervical spinal cord** `MCC` `H5` `HCC`

√7th **S14.158 Other incomplete lesion at C8 level of cervical spinal cord** `MCC` `HCC`

√7th **S14.159 Other incomplete lesion at unspecified level of cervical spinal cord** `HCC`

√x7th **S14.2 Injury of nerve root of cervical spine**

√x7th **S14.3 Injury of brachial plexus**

√x7th **S14.4 Injury of peripheral nerves of neck**

√x7th **S14.5 Injury of cervical sympathetic nerves**

√x7th **S14.8 Injury of other specified nerves of neck**

√x7th **S14.9 Injury of unspecified nerves of neck**

√4th **S15 Injury of blood vessels at neck level**
Code also any associated open wound (S11.-)

> The appropriate 7th character is to be added to each code from category S15.
> A   initial encounter
> D   subsequent encounter
> S   sequela

> **CC Excl: For codes in category S15, unless otherwise noted:**
> **CC with 7th character A:** PDX collection 1157

√5th **S15.0 Injury of carotid artery of neck**
Injury of carotid artery (common) (external) (internal, extracranial portion)
Injury of carotid artery NOS
EXCLUDES 1   injury of internal carotid artery, intracranial portion (S06.8)

> **CC Excl: For codes in subcategory S15.0:**
> **CC with 7th character A:** PDX collection 1167

√6th **S15.00 Unspecified injury of carotid artery**

√7th **S15.001 Unspecified injury of right carotid artery** `CC`

√7th **S15.002 Unspecified injury of left carotid artery** `CC`

√7th **S15.009 Unspecified injury of unspecified carotid artery** `CC`

√6th **S15.01 Minor laceration of carotid artery**
Incomplete transection of carotid artery
Laceration of carotid artery NOS
Superficial laceration of carotid artery

√7th **S15.011 Minor laceration of right carotid artery** `CC`

√7th **S15.012 Minor laceration of left carotid artery** `CC`

√7th **S15.019 Minor laceration of unspecified carotid artery** `CC`

√6th **S15.02 Major laceration of carotid artery**
Complete transection of carotid artery
Traumatic rupture of carotid artery

√7th **S15.021 Major laceration of right carotid artery** `CC`

√7th **S15.022 Major laceration of left carotid artery** `CC`

√7th **S15.029 Major laceration of unspecified carotid artery** `CC`

√6th **S15.09 Other specified injury of carotid artery**

√7th **S15.091 Other specified injury of right carotid artery** `CC`

√7th **S15.092 Other specified injury of left carotid artery** `CC`

N Newborn: 0   P Pediatric: 0-17   M Maternity: 12-55   A Adult: 15-124   `MCC` Major CC Condition   `PDxMCC` PDx acts as own MCC   `CC` CC Condition   `PDxCC` PDx acts as own CC

958   ICD-10-CM 2018

S14.113–S15.092

✓7th **S15.Ø99 Other specified injury of** unspecified **carotid artery** CC

✓5th **S15.1 Injury of** vertebral artery
- ✓6th **S15.1Ø Unspecified injury of vertebral artery**
  - ✓7th **S15.1Ø1 Unspecified injury of** right **vertebral artery** CC
  - ✓7th **S15.1Ø2 Unspecified injury of** left **vertebral artery** CC
  - ✓7th **S15.1Ø9 Unspecified injury of** unspecified **vertebral artery** CC
- ✓6th **S15.11 Minor laceration of vertebral artery**
  Incomplete transection of vertebral artery
  Laceration of vertebral artery NOS
  Superficial laceration of vertebral artery
  - ✓7th **S15.111 Minor laceration of** right **vertebral artery** CC
  - ✓7th **S15.112 Minor laceration of** left **vertebral artery** CC
  - ✓7th **S15.119 Minor laceration of** unspecified **vertebral artery** CC
- ✓6th **S15.12 Major laceration of vertebral artery**
  Complete transection of vertebral artery
  Traumatic rupture of vertebral artery
  - ✓7th **S15.121 Major laceration of** right **vertebral artery** CC
  - ✓7th **S15.122 Major laceration of** left **vertebral artery** CC
  - ✓7th **S15.129 Major laceration of** unspecified **vertebral artery** CC
- ✓6th **S15.19 Other specified injury of vertebral artery**
  - ✓7th **S15.191 Other specified injury of** right **vertebral artery** CC
  - ✓7th **S15.192 Other specified injury of** left **vertebral artery** CC
  - ✓7th **S15.199 Other specified injury of** unspecified **vertebral artery** CC

✓5th **S15.2 Injury of** external jugular vein
- ✓6th **S15.2Ø Unspecified injury of external jugular vein**
  - ✓7th **S15.2Ø1 Unspecified injury of** right **external jugular vein** CC
  - ✓7th **S15.2Ø2 Unspecified injury of** left **external jugular vein** CC
  - ✓7th **S15.2Ø9 Unspecified injury of** unspecified **external jugular vein** CC
- ✓6th **S15.21 Minor laceration of external jugular vein**
  Incomplete transection of external jugular vein
  Laceration of external jugular vein NOS
  Superficial laceration of external jugular vein
  - ✓7th **S15.211 Minor laceration of** right **external jugular vein** CC
  - ✓7th **S15.212 Minor laceration of** left **external jugular vein** CC
  - ✓7th **S15.219 Minor laceration of** unspecified **external jugular vein** CC
- ✓6th **S15.22 Major laceration of external jugular vein**
  Complete transection of external jugular vein
  Traumatic rupture of external jugular vein
  - ✓7th **S15.221 Major laceration of** right **external jugular vein** CC
  - ✓7th **S15.222 Major laceration of** left **external jugular vein** CC
  - ✓7th **S15.229 Major laceration of** unspecified **external jugular vein** CC
- ✓6th **S15.29 Other specified injury of external jugular vein**
  - ✓7th **S15.291 Other specified injury of** right **external jugular vein** CC
  - ✓7th **S15.292 Other specified injury of** left **external jugular vein** CC
  - ✓7th **S15.299 Other specified injury of** unspecified **external jugular vein** CC

✓5th **S15.3 Injury of** internal jugular vein
- ✓6th **S15.3Ø Unspecified injury of internal jugular vein**
  - ✓7th **S15.3Ø1 Unspecified injury of** right **internal jugular vein** CC

✓7th **S15.3Ø2 Unspecified injury of** left **internal jugular vein** CC

✓7th **S15.3Ø9 Unspecified injury of** unspecified **internal jugular vein** CC

- ✓6th **S15.31 Minor laceration of internal jugular vein**
  Incomplete transection of internal jugular vein
  Laceration of internal jugular vein NOS
  Superficial laceration of internal jugular vein
  - ✓7th **S15.311 Minor laceration of** right **internal jugular vein** CC
  - ✓7th **S15.312 Minor laceration of** left **internal jugular vein** CC
  - ✓7th **S15.319 Minor laceration of** unspecified **internal jugular vein** CC
- ✓6th **S15.32 Major laceration of internal jugular vein**
  Complete transection of internal jugular vein
  Traumatic rupture of internal jugular vein
  - ✓7th **S15.321 Major laceration of** right **internal jugular vein** CC
  - ✓7th **S15.322 Major laceration of** left **internal jugular vein** CC
  - ✓7th **S15.329 Major laceration of** unspecified **internal jugular vein** CC
- ✓6th **S15.39 Other specified injury of internal jugular vein**
  - ✓7th **S15.391 Other specified injury of** right **internal jugular vein** CC
  - ✓7th **S15.392 Other specified injury of** left **internal jugular vein** CC
  - ✓7th **S15.399 Other specified injury of** unspecified **internal jugular vein** CC

✓x7th **S15.8 Injury of other specified blood vessels at neck level** CC

✓x7th **S15.9 Injury of unspecified blood vessel at neck level** CC

✓4th **S16 Injury of muscle, fascia and tendon at neck level**
Code also any associated open wound (S11.-)
EXCLUDES 2 *sprain of joint or ligament at neck level (S13.9)*

> The appropriate 7th character is to be added to each code from category S16.
> A initial encounter
> D subsequent encounter
> S sequela

✓x7th **S16.1 Strain of muscle, fascia and tendon at neck level**

✓x7th **S16.2 Laceration of muscle, fascia and tendon at neck level**

✓x7th **S16.8 Other specified injury of muscle, fascia and tendon at neck level**

✓x7th **S16.9 Unspecified injury of muscle, fascia and tendon at neck level**

✓4th **S17 Crushing injury of neck**
Use additional code for all associated injuries, such as:
injury of blood vessels (S15.-)
open wound of neck (S11.-)
spinal cord injury (S14.Ø, S14.1-)
vertebral fracture (S12.Ø- – S12.3-)

> The appropriate 7th character is to be added to each code from category S17.
> A initial encounter
> D subsequent encounter
> S sequela

> **CC Excl: For codes in category S17:**
> **CC with 7th character A:** PDX collection 1156

✓x7th **S17.Ø Crushing injury of larynx and trachea** CC H5

✓x7th **S17.8 Crushing injury of other specified parts of neck** CC H5

✓x7th **S17.9 Crushing injury of neck, part unspecified** CC H5

✓4th **S19 Other specified and unspecified injuries of neck**

> The appropriate 7th character is to be added to each code from category S19.
> A initial encounter
> D subsequent encounter
> S sequela

✓5th **S19.8 Other specified injuries of neck**
- ✓x7th **S19.8Ø Other specified injuries of** unspecified **part of neck**
- ✓x7th **S19.81 Other specified injuries of** larynx

√x7th **S19.82** Other specified injuries of cervical trachea
> EXCLUDES 2   other specified injury of thoracic trachea (S27.5-)

√x7th **S19.83** Other specified injuries of vocal cord

√x7th **S19.84** Other specified injuries of thyroid gland

√x7th **S19.85** Other specified injuries of pharynx and cervical esophagus

√x7th **S19.89** Other specified injuries of other specified part of neck

√x7th **S19.9** Unspecified injury of neck

Injuries to the thorax (S20-S29)

INCLUDES   injuries of breast
     injuries of chest (wall)
     injuries of interscapular area

EXCLUDES 2   burns and corrosions (T20-T32)
     effects of foreign body in bronchus (T17.5)
     effects of foreign body in esophagus (T18.1)
     effects of foreign body in lung (T17.8)
     effects of foreign body in trachea (T17.4)
     frostbite (T33-T34)
     injuries of axilla
     injuries of clavicle
     injuries of scapular region
     injuries of shoulder
     insect bite or sting, venomous (T63.4)

√4th **S20** **Superficial injury of thorax**

> The appropriate 7th character is to be added to each code from category S20.
> A   initial encounter
> D   subsequent encounter
> S   sequela

√5th **S20.0** Contusion of breast

√x7th **S20.00** Contusion of breast, unspecified breast

√x7th **S20.01** Contusion of right breast

√x7th **S20.02** Contusion of left breast

√5th **S20.1** Other and unspecified superficial injuries of breast

√6th **S20.10** Unspecified superficial injuries of breast

√7th **S20.101** Unspecified superficial injuries of breast, right breast

√7th **S20.102** Unspecified superficial injuries of breast, left breast

√7th **S20.109** Unspecified superficial injuries of breast, unspecified breast

√6th **S20.11** Abrasion of breast

√7th **S20.111** Abrasion of breast, right breast

√7th **S20.112** Abrasion of breast, left breast

√7th **S20.119** Abrasion of breast, unspecified breast

√6th **S20.12** Blister (nonthermal) of breast

√7th **S20.121** Blister (nonthermal) of breast, right breast

√7th **S20.122** Blister (nonthermal) of breast, left breast

√7th **S20.129** Blister (nonthermal) of breast, unspecified breast

√6th **S20.14** External constriction of part of breast

√7th **S20.141** External constriction of part of breast, right breast

√7th **S20.142** External constriction of part of breast, left breast

√7th **S20.149** External constriction of part of breast, unspecified breast

√6th **S20.15** Superficial foreign body of breast
> Splinter in the breast

√7th **S20.151** Superficial foreign body of breast, right breast

√7th **S20.152** Superficial foreign body of breast, left breast

√7th **S20.159** Superficial foreign body of breast, unspecified breast

√6th **S20.16** Insect bite (nonvenomous) of breast

√7th **S20.161** Insect bite (nonvenomous) of breast, right breast

√7th **S20.162** Insect bite (nonvenomous) of breast, left breast

√7th **S20.169** Insect bite (nonvenomous) of breast, unspecified breast

√6th **S20.17** Other superficial bite of breast
> EXCLUDES 1   open bite of breast (S21.05-)

√7th **S20.171** Other superficial bite of breast, right breast

√7th **S20.172** Other superficial bite of breast, left breast

√7th **S20.179** Other superficial bite of breast, unspecified breast

√5th **S20.2** Contusion of thorax

√x7th **S20.20** Contusion of thorax, unspecified

√6th **S20.21** Contusion of front wall of thorax

√7th **S20.211** Contusion of right front wall of thorax

√7th **S20.212** Contusion of left front wall of thorax

√7th **S20.219** Contusion of unspecified front wall of thorax

√6th **S20.22** Contusion of back wall of thorax

√7th **S20.221** Contusion of right back wall of thorax

√7th **S20.222** Contusion of left back wall of thorax

√7th **S20.229** Contusion of unspecified back wall of thorax

√5th **S20.3** Other and unspecified superficial injuries of front wall of thorax

√6th **S20.30** Unspecified superficial injuries of front wall of thorax

√7th **S20.301** Unspecified superficial injuries of right front wall of thorax

√7th **S20.302** Unspecified superficial injuries of left front wall of thorax

√7th **S20.309** Unspecified superficial injuries of unspecified front wall of thorax

√6th **S20.31** Abrasion of front wall of thorax

√7th **S20.311** Abrasion of right front wall of thorax

√7th **S20.312** Abrasion of left front wall of thorax

√7th **S20.319** Abrasion of unspecified front wall of thorax

√6th **S20.32** Blister (nonthermal) of front wall of thorax

√7th **S20.321** Blister (nonthermal) of right front wall of thorax

√7th **S20.322** Blister (nonthermal) of left front wall of thorax

√7th **S20.329** Blister (nonthermal) of unspecified front wall of thorax

√6th **S20.34** External constriction of front wall of thorax

√7th **S20.341** External constriction of right front wall of thorax

√7th **S20.342** External constriction of left front wall of thorax

√7th **S20.349** External constriction of unspecified front wall of thorax

√6th **S20.35** Superficial foreign body of front wall of thorax
> Splinter in front wall of thorax

√7th **S20.351** Superficial foreign body of right front wall of thorax

√7th **S20.352** Superficial foreign body of left front wall of thorax

√7th **S20.359** Superficial foreign body of unspecified front wall of thorax

√6th **S20.36** Insect bite (nonvenomous) of front wall of thorax

√7th **S20.361** Insect bite (nonvenomous) of right front wall of thorax

√7th **S20.362** Insect bite (nonvenomous) of left front wall of thorax

√7th **S20.369** Insect bite (nonvenomous) of unspecified front wall of thorax

√6th **S20.37** Other superficial bite of front wall of thorax
> EXCLUDES 1   open bite of front wall of thorax (S21.14)

√7th **S20.371** Other superficial bite of right front wall of thorax

√7th **S20.372** Other superficial bite of left front wall of thorax

√7th **S20.379** Other superficial bite of unspecified front wall of thorax

---

N Newborn: 0   P Pediatric: 0-17   M Maternity: 12-55   A Adult: 15-124   MCC Major CC Condition   PDx MCC PDx acts as own MCC   CC CC Condition   PDx CC PDx acts as own CC

✓5th **S20.4** **Other and unspecified superficial injuries of** back wall of thorax

  ✓6th **S20.40** Unspecified **superficial injuries of back wall of thorax**

    ✓7th **S20.401** **Unspecified superficial injuries of** right **back wall of thorax**

    ✓7th **S20.402** **Unspecified superficial injuries of** left **back wall of thorax**

    ✓7th **S20.409** **Unspecified superficial injuries of** unspecified **back wall of thorax**

  ✓6th **S20.41** Abrasion **of back wall of thorax**

    ✓7th **S20.411** **Abrasion of** right **back wall of thorax**

    ✓7th **S20.412** **Abrasion of** left **back wall of thorax**

    ✓7th **S20.419** **Abrasion of** unspecified **back wall of thorax**

  ✓6th **S20.42** Blister (nonthermal) **of back wall of thorax**

    ✓7th **S20.421** **Blister (nonthermal) of** right **back wall of thorax**

    ✓7th **S20.422** **Blister (nonthermal) of** left **back wall of thorax**

    ✓7th **S20.429** **Blister (nonthermal) of** unspecified **back wall of thorax**

  ✓6th **S20.44** External constriction **of back wall of thorax**

    ✓7th **S20.441** **External constriction of** right **back wall of thorax**

    ✓7th **S20.442** **External constriction of** left **back wall of thorax**

    ✓7th **S20.449** **External constriction of** unspecified **back wall of thorax**

  ✓6th **S20.45** Superficial foreign body **of back wall of thorax**
    Splinter of back wall of thorax

    ✓7th **S20.451** **Superficial foreign body of** right **back wall of thorax**

    ✓7th **S20.452** **Superficial foreign body of** left **back wall of thorax**

    ✓7th **S20.459** **Superficial foreign body of** unspecified **back wall of thorax**

  ✓6th **S20.46** Insect bite (nonvenomous) **of back wall of thorax**

    ✓7th **S20.461** **Insect bite (nonvenomous) of** right **back wall of thorax**

    ✓7th **S20.462** **Insect bite (nonvenomous) of** left **back wall of thorax**

    ✓7th **S20.469** **Insect bite (nonvenomous) of** unspecified **back wall of thorax**

  ✓6th **S20.47** Other superficial bite **of back wall of thorax**
    EXCLUDES 1   *open bite of back wall of thorax (S21.24)*

    ✓7th **S20.471** **Other superficial bite of** right **back wall of thorax**

    ✓7th **S20.472** **Other superficial bite of** left **back wall of thorax**

    ✓7th **S20.479** **Other superficial bite of** unspecified **back wall of thorax**

✓5th **S20.9** Superficial injury **of unspecified parts of thorax**
  EXCLUDES 1   *contusion of thorax NOS (S20.20)*

  ✓x7th **S20.90** **Unspecified superficial injury of** unspecified **parts of thorax**
    Superficial injury of thoracic wall NOS

  ✓x7th **S20.91** Abrasion **of unspecified parts of thorax**

  ✓x7th **S20.92** Blister (nonthermal) **of unspecified parts of thorax**

  ✓x7th **S20.94** External constriction **of unspecified parts of thorax**

  ✓x7th **S20.95** Superficial foreign body **of unspecified parts of thorax**
    Splinter in thorax NOS

  ✓x7th **S20.96** Insect bite (nonvenomous) **of unspecified parts of thorax**

  ✓x7th **S20.97** Other superficial bite **of unspecified parts of thorax**
    EXCLUDES 1   *open bite of thorax NOS (S21.95)*

✓4th **S21** **Open wound of thorax**
  Code also any associated injury, such as:
    injury of heart (S26.-)
    injury of intrathoracic organs (S27.-)
    rib fracture (S22.3-, S22.4-)
    spinal cord injury (S24.0-, S24.1-)
    traumatic hemopneumothorax (S27.3)
    traumatic hemothorax (S27.1)
    traumatic pneumothorax (S27.0)
    wound infection
  EXCLUDES 1   *traumatic amputation (partial) of thorax (S28.1)*

> The appropriate 7th character is to be added to each code from category S21.
> A   initial encounter
> D   subsequent encounter
> S   sequela

✓5th **S21.0** **Open wound of** breast

  ✓6th **S21.00** Unspecified **open wound of breast**

    ✓7th **S21.001** **Unspecified open wound of** right **breast**

    ✓7th **S21.002** **Unspecified open wound of** left **breast**

    ✓7th **S21.009** **Unspecified open wound of** unspecified **breast**

  ✓6th **S21.01** Laceration without foreign body **of breast**

    ✓7th **S21.011** **Laceration without foreign body of** right **breast**

    ✓7th **S21.012** **Laceration without foreign body of** left **breast**

    ✓7th **S21.019** **Laceration without foreign body of** unspecified **breast**

  ✓6th **S21.02** Laceration with foreign body **of breast**

    ✓7th **S21.021** **Laceration with foreign body of** right **breast**

    ✓7th **S21.022** **Laceration with foreign body of** left **breast**

    ✓7th **S21.029** **Laceration with foreign body of** unspecified **breast**

  ✓6th **S21.03** Puncture wound without foreign body **of breast**

    ✓7th **S21.031** **Puncture wound without foreign body of** right **breast**

    ✓7th **S21.032** **Puncture wound without foreign body of** left **breast**

    ✓7th **S21.039** **Puncture wound without foreign body of** unspecified **breast**

  ✓6th **S21.04** Puncture wound with foreign body **of breast**

    ✓7th **S21.041** **Puncture wound with foreign body of** right **breast**

    ✓7th **S21.042** **Puncture wound with foreign body of** left **breast**

    ✓7th **S21.049** **Puncture wound with foreign body of** unspecified **breast**

  ✓6th **S21.05** Open bite **of breast**
    Bite of breast NOS
    EXCLUDES 1   *superficial bite of breast (S20.17)*

    ✓7th **S21.051** **Open bite of** right **breast**

    ✓7th **S21.052** **Open bite of** left **breast**

    ✓7th **S21.059** **Open bite of** unspecified **breast**

✓5th **S21.1** **Open wound of** front wall of thorax without penetration **into thoracic cavity**
  Open wound of chest without penetration into thoracic cavity

> **CC Excl: For codes in subcategory S21.1:**
> **CC with 7th character A:** PDX collection 1168

  ✓6th **S21.10** Unspecified **open wound of front wall of thorax without penetration into thoracic cavity**

    ✓7th **S21.101** **Unspecified open wound of** right front **wall of thorax without penetration into thoracic cavity** `CC`

    ✓7th **S21.102** **Unspecified open wound of** left front **wall of thorax without penetration into thoracic cavity** `CC`

    ✓7th **S21.109** **Unspecified open wound of** unspecified **front wall of thorax without penetration into thoracic cavity** `CC`

✓ Additional Character Req   ✓x7th Placeholder Alert   Unacceptable PDx   Manifestation   H1-H14 HAC   HCC CMS-HCC Condition   *EXCLUDES 1* Not Coded Here   *EXCLUDES 2* Not Included Here

ICD-10-CM 2018   **961**

Chapter 19. Injury, Poisoning and Certain Other Consequences of External Causes

S21.11–S21.319

√6ᵗʰ **S21.11** Laceration without foreign body of front wall of thorax without penetration into thoracic cavity

     √7ᵗʰ **S21.111** Laceration without foreign body of right front wall of thorax without penetration into thoracic cavity   CC

     √7ᵗʰ **S21.112** Laceration without foreign body of left front wall of thorax without penetration into thoracic cavity   CC

     √7ᵗʰ **S21.119** Laceration without foreign body of unspecified front wall of thorax without penetration into thoracic cavity   CC

√6ᵗʰ **S21.12** Laceration with foreign body of front wall of thorax without penetration into thoracic cavity

     √7ᵗʰ **S21.121** Laceration with foreign body of right front wall of thorax without penetration into thoracic cavity   CC

     √7ᵗʰ **S21.122** Laceration with foreign body of left front wall of thorax without penetration into thoracic cavity   CC

     √7ᵗʰ **S21.129** Laceration with foreign body of unspecified front wall of thorax without penetration into thoracic cavity   CC

√6ᵗʰ **S21.13** Puncture wound without foreign body of front wall of thorax without penetration into thoracic cavity

     √7ᵗʰ **S21.131** Puncture wound without foreign body of right front wall of thorax without penetration into thoracic cavity   CC

     √7ᵗʰ **S21.132** Puncture wound without foreign body of left front wall of thorax without penetration into thoracic cavity   CC

     √7ᵗʰ **S21.139** Puncture wound without foreign body of unspecified front wall of thorax without penetration into thoracic cavity   CC

√6ᵗʰ **S21.14** Puncture wound with foreign body of front wall of thorax without penetration into thoracic cavity

     √7ᵗʰ **S21.141** Puncture wound with foreign body of right front wall of thorax without penetration into thoracic cavity   CC

     √7ᵗʰ **S21.142** Puncture wound with foreign body of left front wall of thorax without penetration into thoracic cavity   CC

     √7ᵗʰ **S21.149** Puncture wound with foreign body of unspecified front wall of thorax without penetration into thoracic cavity   CC

√6ᵗʰ **S21.15** Open bite of front wall of thorax without penetration into thoracic cavity
     Bite of front wall of thorax NOS
     EXCLUDES 1   *superficial bite of front wall of thorax (S20.37)*

     √7ᵗʰ **S21.151** Open bite of right front wall of thorax without penetration into thoracic cavity   CC

     √7ᵗʰ **S21.152** Open bite of left front wall of thorax without penetration into thoracic cavity   CC

     √7ᵗʰ **S21.159** Open bite of unspecified front wall of thorax without penetration into thoracic cavity   CC

√5ᵗʰ **S21.2** Open wound of back wall of thorax without penetration into thoracic cavity

√6ᵗʰ **S21.20** Unspecified open wound of back wall of thorax without penetration into thoracic cavity

     √7ᵗʰ **S21.201** Unspecified open wound of right back wall of thorax without penetration into thoracic cavity

     √7ᵗʰ **S21.202** Unspecified open wound of left back wall of thorax without penetration into thoracic cavity

     √7ᵗʰ **S21.209** Unspecified open wound of unspecified back wall of thorax without penetration into thoracic cavity

√6ᵗʰ **S21.21** Laceration without foreign body of back wall of thorax without penetration into thoracic cavity

     √7ᵗʰ **S21.211** Laceration without foreign body of right back wall of thorax without penetration into thoracic cavity

     √7ᵗʰ **S21.212** Laceration without foreign body of left back wall of thorax without penetration into thoracic cavity

     √7ᵗʰ **S21.219** Laceration without foreign body of unspecified back wall of thorax without penetration into thoracic cavity

√6ᵗʰ **S21.22** Laceration with foreign body of back wall of thorax without penetration into thoracic cavity

     √7ᵗʰ **S21.221** Laceration with foreign body of right back wall of thorax without penetration into thoracic cavity

     √7ᵗʰ **S21.222** Laceration with foreign body of left back wall of thorax without penetration into thoracic cavity

     √7ᵗʰ **S21.229** Laceration with foreign body of unspecified back wall of thorax without penetration into thoracic cavity

√6ᵗʰ **S21.23** Puncture wound without foreign body of back wall of thorax without penetration into thoracic cavity

     √7ᵗʰ **S21.231** Puncture wound without foreign body of right back wall of thorax without penetration into thoracic cavity

     √7ᵗʰ **S21.232** Puncture wound without foreign body of left back wall of thorax without penetration into thoracic cavity

     √7ᵗʰ **S21.239** Puncture wound without foreign body of unspecified back wall of thorax without penetration into thoracic cavity

√6ᵗʰ **S21.24** Puncture wound with foreign body of back wall of thorax without penetration into thoracic cavity

     √7ᵗʰ **S21.241** Puncture wound with foreign body of right back wall of thorax without penetration into thoracic cavity

     √7ᵗʰ **S21.242** Puncture wound with foreign body of left back wall of thorax without penetration into thoracic cavity

     √7ᵗʰ **S21.249** Puncture wound with foreign body of unspecified back wall of thorax without penetration into thoracic cavity

√6ᵗʰ **S21.25** Open bite of back wall of thorax without penetration into thoracic cavity
     Bite of back wall of thorax NOS
     EXCLUDES 1   *superficial bite of back wall of thorax (S20.47)*

     √7ᵗʰ **S21.251** Open bite of right back wall of thorax without penetration into thoracic cavity

     √7ᵗʰ **S21.252** Open bite of left back wall of thorax without penetration into thoracic cavity

     √7ᵗʰ **S21.259** Open bite of unspecified back wall of thorax without penetration into thoracic cavity

√5ᵗʰ **S21.3** Open wound of front wall of thorax with penetration into thoracic cavity
     Open wound of chest with penetration into thoracic cavity

> **CC Excl: For codes in subcategory S21.3, unless otherwise noted:**
> **MCC with 7th character A:** PDX collection 1169

√6ᵗʰ **S21.30** Unspecified open wound of front wall of thorax with penetration into thoracic cavity

     √7ᵗʰ **S21.301** Unspecified open wound of right front wall of thorax with penetration into thoracic cavity   MCC

     √7ᵗʰ **S21.302** Unspecified open wound of left front wall of thorax with penetration into thoracic cavity   MCC

     √7ᵗʰ **S21.309** Unspecified open wound of unspecified front wall of thorax with penetration into thoracic cavity   MCC
     CC Excl: MCC with 7th character A: PDX collection 1170

√6ᵗʰ **S21.31** Laceration without foreign body of front wall of thorax with penetration into thoracic cavity

     √7ᵗʰ **S21.311** Laceration without foreign body of right front wall of thorax with penetration into thoracic cavity   MCC

     √7ᵗʰ **S21.312** Laceration without foreign body of left front wall of thorax with penetration into thoracic cavity   MCC

     √7ᵗʰ **S21.319** Laceration without foreign body of unspecified front wall of thorax with penetration into thoracic cavity   MCC

N Newborn: 0   P Pediatric: 0-17   M Maternity: 12-55   A Adult: 15-124   MCC Major CC Condition   PDxMCC PDx acts as own MCC   CC CC Condition   PDxCC PDx acts as own CC

962   ICD-10-CM 2018

√6ᵗʰ **S21.32** Laceration with foreign body of front wall of thorax with penetration into thoracic cavity

    √7ᵗʰ **S21.321** Laceration with foreign body of right front wall of thorax with penetration into thoracic cavity   `MCC`

    √7ᵗʰ **S21.322** Laceration with foreign body of left front wall of thorax with penetration into thoracic cavity   `MCC`

    √7ᵗʰ **S21.329** Laceration with foreign body of unspecified front wall of thorax with penetration into thoracic cavity   `MCC`

√6ᵗʰ **S21.33** Puncture wound without foreign body of front wall of thorax with penetration into thoracic cavity

    √7ᵗʰ **S21.331** Puncture wound without foreign body of right front wall of thorax with penetration into thoracic cavity   `MCC`

    √7ᵗʰ **S21.332** Puncture wound without foreign body of left front wall of thorax with penetration into thoracic cavity   `MCC`

    √7ᵗʰ **S21.339** Puncture wound without foreign body of unspecified front wall of thorax with penetration into thoracic cavity   `MCC`

√6ᵗʰ **S21.34** Puncture wound with foreign body of front wall of thorax with penetration into thoracic cavity

    √7ᵗʰ **S21.341** Puncture wound with foreign body of right front wall of thorax with penetration into thoracic cavity   `MCC`

    √7ᵗʰ **S21.342** Puncture wound with foreign body of left front wall of thorax with penetration into thoracic cavity   `MCC`

    √7ᵗʰ **S21.349** Puncture wound with foreign body of unspecified front wall of thorax with penetration into thoracic cavity   `MCC`

√6ᵗʰ **S21.35** Open bite of front wall of thorax with penetration into thoracic cavity

    EXCLUDES 1   superficial bite of front wall of thorax (S20.37)

    √7ᵗʰ **S21.351** Open bite of right front wall of thorax with penetration into thoracic cavity   `MCC`

    √7ᵗʰ **S21.352** Open bite of left front wall of thorax with penetration into thoracic cavity   `MCC`

    √7ᵗʰ **S21.359** Open bite of unspecified front wall of thorax with penetration into thoracic cavity   `MCC`

√5ᵗʰ **S21.4** Open wound of back wall of thorax with penetration into thoracic cavity

> **CC Excl:** For codes in subcategory S21.4:
> MCC with 7th character A: PDX collection 1169

√6ᵗʰ **S21.40** Unspecified open wound of back wall of thorax with penetration into thoracic cavity

    √7ᵗʰ **S21.401** Unspecified open wound of right back wall of thorax with penetration into thoracic cavity   `MCC`

    √7ᵗʰ **S21.402** Unspecified open wound of left back wall of thorax with penetration into thoracic cavity   `MCC`

    √7ᵗʰ **S21.409** Unspecified open wound of unspecified back wall of thorax with penetration into thoracic cavity   `MCC`

√6ᵗʰ **S21.41** Laceration without foreign body of back wall of thorax with penetration into thoracic cavity

    √7ᵗʰ **S21.411** Laceration without foreign body of right back wall of thorax with penetration into thoracic cavity   `MCC`

    √7ᵗʰ **S21.412** Laceration without foreign body of left back wall of thorax with penetration into thoracic cavity   `MCC`

    √7ᵗʰ **S21.419** Laceration without foreign body of unspecified back wall of thorax with penetration into thoracic cavity   `MCC`

√6ᵗʰ **S21.42** Laceration with foreign body of back wall of thorax with penetration into thoracic cavity

    √7ᵗʰ **S21.421** Laceration with foreign body of right back wall of thorax with penetration into thoracic cavity   `MCC`

    √7ᵗʰ **S21.422** Laceration with foreign body of left back wall of thorax with penetration into thoracic cavity   `MCC`

    √7ᵗʰ **S21.429** Laceration with foreign body of unspecified back wall of thorax with penetration into thoracic cavity   `MCC`

√6ᵗʰ **S21.43** Puncture wound without foreign body of back wall of thorax with penetration into thoracic cavity

    √7ᵗʰ **S21.431** Puncture wound without foreign body of right back wall of thorax with penetration into thoracic cavity   `MCC`

    √7ᵗʰ **S21.432** Puncture wound without foreign body of left back wall of thorax with penetration into thoracic cavity   `MCC`

    √7ᵗʰ **S21.439** Puncture wound without foreign body of unspecified back wall of thorax with penetration into thoracic cavity   `MCC`

√6ᵗʰ **S21.44** Puncture wound with foreign body of back wall of thorax with penetration into thoracic cavity

    √7ᵗʰ **S21.441** Puncture wound with foreign body of right back wall of thorax with penetration into thoracic cavity   `MCC`

    √7ᵗʰ **S21.442** Puncture wound with foreign body of left back wall of thorax with penetration into thoracic cavity   `MCC`

    √7ᵗʰ **S21.449** Puncture wound with foreign body of unspecified back wall of thorax with penetration into thoracic cavity   `MCC`

√6ᵗʰ **S21.45** Open bite of back wall of thorax with penetration into thoracic cavity

    Bite of back wall of thorax NOS

    EXCLUDES 1   superficial bite of back wall of thorax (S20.47)

    √7ᵗʰ **S21.451** Open bite of right back wall of thorax with penetration into thoracic cavity   `MCC`

    √7ᵗʰ **S21.452** Open bite of left back wall of thorax with penetration into thoracic cavity   `MCC`

    √7ᵗʰ **S21.459** Open bite of unspecified back wall of thorax with penetration into thoracic cavity   `MCC`

√5ᵗʰ **S21.9** Open wound of unspecified part of thorax

    Open wound of thoracic wall NOS

> **CC Excl:** For codes in subcategory S21.9:
> CC with 7th character A: PDX collection 1168

√x7ᵗʰ **S21.90** Unspecified open wound of unspecified part of thorax   `CC`

√x7ᵗʰ **S21.91** Laceration without foreign body of unspecified part of thorax   `CC`

√x7ᵗʰ **S21.92** Laceration with foreign body of unspecified part of thorax   `CC`

√x7ᵗʰ **S21.93** Puncture wound without foreign body of unspecified part of thorax   `CC`

√x7ᵗʰ **S21.94** Puncture wound with foreign body of unspecified part of thorax   `CC`

√x7ᵗʰ **S21.95** Open bite of unspecified part of thorax   `CC`

    EXCLUDES 1   superficial bite of thorax (S20.97)

☑ Additional Character Req   √x7ᵗʰ Placeholder Alert   Unacceptable PDx   Manifestation   `H1`-`H14` HAC   `HCC` CMS-HCC Condition   *EXCLUDES 1* Not Coded Here   *EXCLUDES 2* Not Included Here

ICD-10-CM 2018   **963**

√4ᵗʰ **S22 Fracture of rib(s), sternum and thoracic spine**

NOTE A fracture not indicated as nondisplaced or displaced should be coded to displaced.
A fracture not indicated as open or closed should be coded to closed.

INCLUDES fracture of thoracic neural arch
fracture of thoracic spinous process
fracture of thoracic transverse process
fracture of thoracic vertebra
fracture of thoracic vertebral arch

Code first any associated:
injury of intrathoracic organ (S27.-)
spinal cord injury (S24.0-, S24.1-)

EXCLUDES 1 transection of thorax (S28.1)
EXCLUDES 2 fracture of clavicle (S42.0-)
fracture of scapula (S42.1-)

AHA: 2015, 3Q, 37-39

The appropriate 7th character is to be added to each code from category S22.
A initial encounter for closed fracture
B initial encounter for open fracture
D subsequent encounter for fracture with routine healing
G subsequent encounter for fracture with delayed healing
K subsequent encounter for fracture with nonunion
S sequela

√5ᵗʰ **S22.0 Fracture of thoracic vertebra**

CC Excl: For codes in subcategory S22.0:
CC with 7th character A or MCC with 7th character B:
PDX collection 1171
CC with 7th character K: PDX collection 897

√6ᵗʰ **S22.00 Fracture of unspecified thoracic vertebra**

6,7,10 √7ᵗʰ S22.000 Wedge compression fracture of unspecified thoracic vertebra   MCC CC H5 HCC

6,7,10 √7ᵗʰ S22.001 Stable burst fracture of unspecified thoracic vertebra   MCC CC H5 HCC

6,7,10 √7ᵗʰ S22.002 Unstable burst fracture of unspecified thoracic vertebra   MCC CC H5 HCC

6,7,10 √7ᵗʰ S22.008 Other fracture of unspecified thoracic vertebra   MCC CC H5 HCC

6,7,10 √7ᵗʰ S22.009 Unspecified fracture of unspecified thoracic vertebra   MCC CC H5 HCC

√6ᵗʰ **S22.01 Fracture of first thoracic vertebra**

6,7,10 √7ᵗʰ S22.010 Wedge compression fracture of first thoracic vertebra   MCC CC H5 HCC

6,7,10 √7ᵗʰ S22.011 Stable burst fracture of first thoracic vertebra   MCC CC H5 HCC

6,7,10 √7ᵗʰ S22.012 Unstable burst fracture of first thoracic vertebra   MCC CC H5 HCC

6,7,10 √7ᵗʰ S22.018 Other fracture of first thoracic vertebra   MCC CC H5 HCC

6,7,10 √7ᵗʰ S22.019 Unspecified fracture of first thoracic vertebra   MCC CC H5 HCC

√6ᵗʰ **S22.02 Fracture of second thoracic vertebra**

6,7,10 √7ᵗʰ S22.020 Wedge compression fracture of second thoracic vertebra   MCC CC H5 HCC

6,7,10 √7ᵗʰ S22.021 Stable burst fracture of second thoracic vertebra   MCC CC H5 HCC

6,7,10 √7ᵗʰ S22.022 Unstable burst fracture of second thoracic vertebra   MCC CC H5 HCC

6,7,10 √7ᵗʰ S22.028 Other fracture of second thoracic vertebra   MCC CC H5 HCC

6,7,10 √7ᵗʰ S22.029 Unspecified fracture of second thoracic vertebra   MCC CC H5 HCC

√6ᵗʰ **S22.03 Fracture of third thoracic vertebra**

6,7,10 √7ᵗʰ S22.030 Wedge compression fracture of third thoracic vertebra   MCC CC H5 HCC

6,7,10 √7ᵗʰ S22.031 Stable burst fracture of third thoracic vertebra   MCC CC H5 HCC

6,7,10 √7ᵗʰ S22.032 Unstable burst fracture of third thoracic vertebra   MCC CC H5 HCC

6,7,10 √7ᵗʰ S22.038 Other fracture of third thoracic vertebra   MCC CC H5 HCC

6,7,10 √7ᵗʰ S22.039 Unspecified fracture of third thoracic vertebra   MCC CC H5 HCC

√6ᵗʰ **S22.04 Fracture of fourth thoracic vertebra**

6,7,10 √7ᵗʰ S22.040 Wedge compression fracture of fourth thoracic vertebra   MCC CC H5 HCC

6,7,10 √7ᵗʰ S22.041 Stable burst fracture of fourth thoracic vertebra   MCC CC H5 HCC

6,7,10 √7ᵗʰ S22.042 Unstable burst fracture of fourth thoracic vertebra   MCC CC H5 HCC

6,7,10 √7ᵗʰ S22.048 Other fracture of fourth thoracic vertebra   MCC CC H5 HCC

6,7,10 √7ᵗʰ S22.049 Unspecified fracture of fourth thoracic vertebra   MCC CC H5 HCC

√6ᵗʰ **S22.05 Fracture of T5-T6 vertebra**

6,7,10 √7ᵗʰ S22.050 Wedge compression fracture of T5-T6 vertebra   MCC CC H5 HCC

6,7,10 √7ᵗʰ S22.051 Stable burst fracture of T5-T6 vertebra   MCC CC H5 HCC

6,7,10 √7ᵗʰ S22.052 Unstable burst fracture of T5-T6 vertebra   MCC CC H5 HCC

6,7,10 √7ᵗʰ S22.058 Other fracture of T5-T6 vertebra   MCC CC H5 HCC

6,7,10 √7ᵗʰ S22.059 Unspecified fracture of T5-T6 vertebra   MCC CC H5 HCC

√6ᵗʰ **S22.06 Fracture of T7-T8 vertebra**

6,7,10 √7ᵗʰ S22.060 Wedge compression fracture of T7-T8 vertebra   MCC CC H5 HCC

6,7,10 √7ᵗʰ S22.061 Stable burst fracture of T7-T8 vertebra   MCC CC H5 HCC

6,7,10 √7ᵗʰ S22.062 Unstable burst fracture of T7-T8 vertebra   MCC CC H5 HCC

6,7,10 √7ᵗʰ S22.068 Other fracture of T7-T8 thoracic vertebra   MCC CC H5 HCC

6,7,10 √7ᵗʰ S22.069 Unspecified fracture of T7-T8 vertebra   MCC CC H5 HCC

√6ᵗʰ **S22.07 Fracture of T9-T10 vertebra**

6,7,10 √7ᵗʰ S22.070 Wedge compression fracture of T9-T10 vertebra   MCC CC H5 HCC

6,7,10 √7ᵗʰ S22.071 Stable burst fracture of T9-T10 vertebra   MCC CC H5 HCC

6,7,10 √7ᵗʰ S22.072 Unstable burst fracture of T9-T10 vertebra   MCC CC H5 HCC

6,7,10 √7ᵗʰ S22.078 Other fracture of T9-T10 vertebra   MCC CC H5 HCC

6,7,10 √7ᵗʰ S22.079 Unspecified fracture of T9-T10 vertebra   MCC CC H5 HCC

√6ᵗʰ **S22.08 Fracture of T11-T12 vertebra**

6,7,10 √7ᵗʰ S22.080 Wedge compression fracture of T11-T12 vertebra   MCC CC H5 HCC

6,7,10 √7ᵗʰ S22.081 Stable burst fracture of T11-T12 vertebra   MCC CC H5 HCC

6,7,10 √7ᵗʰ S22.082 Unstable burst fracture of T11-T12 vertebra   MCC CC H5 HCC

6,7,10 √7ᵗʰ S22.088 Other fracture of T11-T12 vertebra   MCC CC H5 HCC

6,7,10 √7ᵗʰ S22.089 Unspecified fracture of T11-T12 vertebra   MCC CC H5 HCC

√5ᵗʰ **S22.2 Fracture of sternum**

DEF: Break in flat bone (breast bone) in anterior thorax; caused by blunt trauma to anterior chest.

CC Excl: For codes in subcategory S22.2:
CC with 7th character A or MCC with 7th character B:
PDX collection 1172
CC with 7th character K: PDX collection 897

6,7 √x7ᵗʰ S22.20 Unspecified fracture of sternum   MCC CC H5

6,7 √x7ᵗʰ S22.21 Fracture of manubrium   MCC CC H5

6,7 √x7ᵗʰ S22.22 Fracture of body of sternum   MCC CC H5

6,7 √x7ᵗʰ S22.23 Sternal manubrial dissociation   MCC CC H5

---

6   MCC when reported as an open fracture (7th character B or C – specific to category).
7   CC when reported as an initial encounter (7th character A, B, or C – specific to category) OR a subsequent encounter for nonunion or malunion (7th character K, M, N, P, Q, or R – specific to category).
10   HCC with 7th character indicating initial encounter (A, B or C - specific to category).

N Newborn: 0   P Pediatric: 0-17   M Maternity: 12-55   A Adult: 15-124   MCC Major CC Condition   PDxMCC PDx acts as own MCC   CC CC Condition   PDxCC PDx acts as own CC

6,7 √x7th **S22.24** **Fracture of** xiphoid process   `MCC` `CC` `H5`

√5th **S22.3** **Fracture of** one rib

> **CC Excl: For codes in subcategory S22.3:**
> **CC with 7th character A:** PDX collection 1173
> **MCC with 7th character B:** PDX collection 1174
> **CC with 7th character K:** PDX collection 897

6,7 √x7th **S22.31** **Fracture of one rib,** right **side**   `MCC` `CC` `H5`
6,7 √x7th **S22.32** **Fracture of one rib,** left **side**   `MCC` `CC` `H5`
6,7 √x7th **S22.39** **Fracture of one rib,** unspecified **side**   `MCC` `CC` `H5`

√5th **S22.4** **Multiple fractures of ribs**
Fractures of two or more ribs
EXCLUDES 1 flail chest (S22.5-)

> **CC Excl: For codes in subcategory S22.4, unless**
> **otherwise noted: CC with 7th character A or MCC with**
> **7th character B:** PDX collection 1174
> **CC with 7th character K:** PDX collection 897

6,7 √x7th **S22.41** **Multiple fractures of ribs,** right **side**   `MCC` `CC` `H5`
6,7 √x7th **S22.42** **Multiple fractures of ribs,** left **side**   `MCC` `CC` `H5`
6,7 √x7th **S22.43** **Multiple fractures of ribs,** bilateral   `MCC` `CC` `H5`
6,7 √x7th **S22.49** **Multiple fractures of ribs,** unspecified **side**   `MCC` `CC` `H5`
> **CC Excl: CC with 7th character A:** PDX collection 1174
> **MCC with 7th character B:** No Excl
> **CC with 7th character K:** PDX collection 897

8 √x7th **S22.5** **Flail chest**   `MCC` `CC` `H5`
> **CC Excl: CC with 7th character A or**
> **MCC with 7th character B:** PDX collection 1175
> **CC with 7th character K:** PDX collection 897

6,7 √x7th **S22.9** **Fracture of bony thorax, part unspecified**   `MCC` `CC` `H5`
> **CC Excl: CC with 7th character A or**
> **MCC with 7th character B:** PDX collection 1176
> **CC with 7th character K:** PDX collection 897

√4th **S23** **Dislocation and sprain of joints and ligaments of thorax**
INCLUDES avulsion of joint or ligament of thorax
laceration of cartilage, joint or ligament of thorax
sprain of cartilage, joint or ligament of thorax
traumatic hemarthrosis of joint or ligament of thorax
traumatic rupture of joint or ligament of thorax
traumatic subluxation of joint or ligament of thorax
traumatic tear of joint or ligament of thorax
Code also any associated open wound
EXCLUDES 2 dislocation, sprain of sternoclavicular joint (S43.2, S43.6)
strain of muscle or tendon of thorax (S29.01-)

> The appropriate 7th character is to be added to each code from
> category S23.
> A   initial encounter
> D   subsequent encounter
> S   sequela

√x7th **S23.0** **Traumatic rupture of thoracic intervertebral disc**
EXCLUDES 1 rupture or displacement (nontraumatic) of thoracic
intervertebral disc NOS (M51- with fifth
character 4)

√5th **S23.1** **Subluxation and dislocation of thoracic vertebra**
Code also any associated
open wound of thorax (S21.-)
spinal cord injury (S24.0-, S24.1-)
EXCLUDES 2 fracture of thoracic vertebrae (S22.0-)

√6th **S23.10** **Subluxation and dislocation of** unspecified **thoracic vertebra**
√7th **S23.100** **Subluxation** of unspecified thoracic **vertebra**
√7th **S23.101** **Dislocation** of unspecified thoracic **vertebra**

√6th **S23.11** **Subluxation and dislocation of** T1/T2 **thoracic vertebra**
√7th **S23.110** **Subluxation** of T1/T2 thoracic vertebra
√7th **S23.111** **Dislocation** of T1/T2 thoracic vertebra

√6th **S23.12** **Subluxation and dislocation of** T2/T3-T3/T4 **thoracic vertebra**
√7th **S23.120** **Subluxation** of T2/T3 thoracic vertebra
√7th **S23.121** **Dislocation** of T2/T3 thoracic vertebra
√7th **S23.122** **Subluxation** of T3/T4 thoracic vertebra

√7th **S23.123** **Dislocation** of T3/T4 thoracic vertebra

√6th **S23.13** **Subluxation and dislocation of** T4/T5-T5/T6 **thoracic vertebra**
√7th **S23.130** **Subluxation** of T4/T5 thoracic vertebra
√7th **S23.131** **Dislocation** of T4/T5 thoracic vertebra
√7th **S23.132** **Subluxation** of T5/T6 thoracic vertebra
√7th **S23.133** **Dislocation** of T5/T6 thoracic vertebra

√6th **S23.14** **Subluxation and dislocation of** T6/T7-T7/T8 **thoracic vertebra**
√7th **S23.140** **Subluxation** of T6/T7 thoracic vertebra
√7th **S23.141** **Dislocation** of T6/T7 thoracic vertebra
√7th **S23.142** **Subluxation** of T7/T8 thoracic vertebra
√7th **S23.143** **Dislocation** of T7/T8 thoracic vertebra

√6th **S23.15** **Subluxation and dislocation of** T8/T9-T9/T10 **thoracic vertebra**
√7th **S23.150** **Subluxation** of T8/T9 thoracic vertebra
√7th **S23.151** **Dislocation** of T8/T9 thoracic vertebra
√7th **S23.152** **Subluxation** of T9/T10 thoracic vertebra
√7th **S23.153** **Dislocation** of T9/T10 thoracic vertebra

√6th **S23.16** **Subluxation and dislocation of** T10/T11-T11/T12 **thoracic vertebra**
√7th **S23.160** **Subluxation** of T10/T11 thoracic vertebra
√7th **S23.161** **Dislocation** of T10/T11 thoracic vertebra
√7th **S23.162** **Subluxation** of T11/T12 thoracic vertebra
√7th **S23.163** **Dislocation** of T11/T12 thoracic vertebra

√6th **S23.17** **Subluxation and dislocation of** T12/L1 **thoracic vertebra**
√7th **S23.170** **Subluxation** of T12/L1 thoracic vertebra
√7th **S23.171** **Dislocation** of T12/L1 thoracic vertebra

√5th **S23.2** **Dislocation of other and unspecified parts of thorax**
√x7th **S23.20** **Dislocation of unspecified part of thorax**
√x7th **S23.29** **Dislocation of other parts of thorax**

√x7th **S23.3** **Sprain of ligaments of thoracic spine**

√5th **S23.4** **Sprain of ribs and sternum**
√x7th **S23.41** **Sprain of ribs**
√6th **S23.42** **Sprain of sternum**
√7th **S23.420** **Sprain of sternoclavicular (joint) (ligament)**
√7th **S23.421** **Sprain of chondrosternal joint**
√7th **S23.428** **Other sprain of sternum**
√7th **S23.429** **Unspecified sprain of sternum**

√x7th **S23.8** **Sprain of other specified parts of thorax**
√x7th **S23.9** **Sprain of unspecified parts of thorax**

√4th **S24** **Injury of nerves and spinal cord at thorax level**
NOTE Code to highest level of thoracic spinal cord injury.
Injuries to the spinal cord (S24.0 and S24.1) refer to the cord
level and not bone level injury, and can affect nerve roots at
and below the level given.
Code also any associated:
fracture of thoracic vertebra (S22.0-)
open wound of thorax (S21.-)
transient paralysis (R29.5)
EXCLUDES 2 injury of brachial plexus (S14.3)

> The appropriate 7th character is to be added to each code from
> category S24.
> A   initial encounter
> D   subsequent encounter
> S   sequela

> **CC Excl: For codes in category S24:**
> **MCC with 7th character A:** PDX collection 1177

√x7th **S24.0** **Concussion and edema of thoracic spinal cord**   `MCC` `HCC`
√5th **S24.1** **Other and unspecified injuries of thoracic spinal cord**
√6th **S24.10** **Unspecified injury of thoracic spinal cord**
√7th **S24.101** **Unspecified injury at T1 level** **of thoracic spinal cord**   `MCC` `H5` `HCC`

---

6 MCC when reported as an open fracture (7th character B or C – specific to category).
7 CC when reported as an initial encounter (7th character A, B, or C – specific to category) OR a subsequent encounter for nonunion or malunion
(7th character K, M, N, P, Q, or R – specific to category).
8 CC when reported as a subsequent encounter for nonunion or malunion (7th character K, M, N, P, Q, or R – specific to category).

✓ Additional Character Req   √x7th Placeholder Alert   Unacceptable PDx   Manifestation   `H1`-`H14` HAC   `HCC` CMS-HCC Condition   *EXCLUDES 1* Not Coded Here   *EXCLUDES 2* Not Included Here

✓7ᵗʰ S24.102 Unspecified injury at T2-T6 level of thoracic spinal cord `MCC` `H5` `HCC`

✓7ᵗʰ S24.103 Unspecified injury at T7-T10 level of thoracic spinal cord `MCC` `H5` `HCC`

✓7ᵗʰ S24.104 Unspecified injury at T11-T12 level thoracic spinal cord `MCC` `H5` `HCC`

✓7ᵗʰ S24.109 Unspecified injury at unspecified level of thoracic spinal cord `H5` `HCC`
Injury of thoracic spinal cord NOS

✓6ᵗʰ S24.11 Complete lesion of thoracic spinal cord

    ✓7ᵗʰ S24.111 Complete lesion at T1 level of thoracic spinal cord `MCC` `H5` `HCC`

    ✓7ᵗʰ S24.112 Complete lesion at T2-T6 level of thoracic spinal cord `MCC` `H5` `HCC`

    ✓7ᵗʰ S24.113 Complete lesion at T7-T10 level of thoracic spinal cord `MCC` `H5` `HCC`

    ✓7ᵗʰ S24.114 Complete lesion at T11-T12 level of thoracic spinal cord `MCC` `H5` `HCC`

    ✓7ᵗʰ S24.119 Complete lesion at unspecified level of thoracic spinal cord `HCC`

✓6ᵗʰ S24.13 Anterior cord syndrome of thoracic spinal cord

    ✓7ᵗʰ S24.131 Anterior cord syndrome at T1 level of thoracic spinal cord `MCC` `H5` `HCC`

    ✓7ᵗʰ S24.132 Anterior cord syndrome at T2-T6 level of thoracic spinal cord `MCC` `H5` `HCC`

    ✓7ᵗʰ S24.133 Anterior cord syndrome at T7-T10 level of thoracic spinal cord `MCC` `H5` `HCC`

    ✓7ᵗʰ S24.134 Anterior cord syndrome at T11-T12 level of thoracic spinal cord `MCC` `H5` `HCC`

    ✓7ᵗʰ S24.139 Anterior cord syndrome at unspecified level of thoracic spinal cord `HCC`

✓6ᵗʰ S24.14 Brown-Séquard syndrome of thoracic spinal cord

    ✓7ᵗʰ S24.141 Brown-Séquard syndrome at T1 level of thoracic spinal cord `MCC` `HCC`

    ✓7ᵗʰ S24.142 Brown-Séquard syndrome at T2-T6 level of thoracic spinal cord `MCC` `HCC`

    ✓7ᵗʰ S24.143 Brown-Séquard syndrome at T7-T10 level of thoracic spinal cord `MCC` `HCC`

    ✓7ᵗʰ S24.144 Brown-Séquard syndrome at T11-T12 level of thoracic spinal cord `MCC` `HCC`

    ✓7ᵗʰ S24.149 Brown-Séquard syndrome at unspecified level of thoracic spinal cord `HCC`

✓6ᵗʰ S24.15 Other incomplete lesions of thoracic spinal cord
Incomplete lesion of thoracic spinal cord NOS
Posterior cord syndrome of thoracic spinal cord

    ✓7ᵗʰ S24.151 Other incomplete lesion at T1 level of thoracic spinal cord `MCC` `H5` `HCC`

    ✓7ᵗʰ S24.152 Other incomplete lesion at T2-T6 level of thoracic spinal cord `MCC` `H5` `HCC`

    ✓7ᵗʰ S24.153 Other incomplete lesion at T7-T10 level of thoracic spinal cord `MCC` `H5` `HCC`

    ✓7ᵗʰ S24.154 Other incomplete lesion at T11-T12 level of thoracic spinal cord `MCC` `H5` `HCC`

    ✓7ᵗʰ S24.159 Other incomplete lesion at unspecified level of thoracic spinal cord `HCC`

✓x7ᵗʰ S24.2 Injury of nerve root of thoracic spine

✓x7ᵗʰ S24.3 Injury of peripheral nerves of thorax

✓x7ᵗʰ S24.4 Injury of thoracic sympathetic nervous system
Injury of cardiac plexus
Injury of esophageal plexus
Injury of pulmonary plexus
Injury of stellate ganglion
Injury of thoracic sympathetic ganglion

✓x7ᵗʰ S24.8 Injury of other specified nerves of thorax

✓x7ᵗʰ S24.9 Injury of unspecified nerve of thorax

✓4ᵗʰ S25 Injury of blood vessels of thorax
Code also any associated open wound (S21.-)

> The appropriate 7th character is to be added to each code from category S25.
> A   initial encounter
> D   subsequent encounter
> S   sequela

✓5ᵗʰ S25.0 Injury of thoracic aorta
Injury of aorta NOS

> **CC Excl: For codes in subcategory S25.0:**
> **MCC with 7th character A:** PDX collection 1178

✓x7ᵗʰ S25.00 Unspecified injury of thoracic aorta `MCC`

✓x7ᵗʰ S25.01 Minor laceration of thoracic aorta `MCC`
Incomplete transection of thoracic aorta
Laceration of thoracic aorta NOS
Superficial laceration of thoracic aorta

✓x7ᵗʰ S25.02 Major laceration of thoracic aorta `MCC`
Complete transection of thoracic aorta
Traumatic rupture of thoracic aorta

✓x7ᵗʰ S25.09 Other specified injury of thoracic aorta `MCC`

✓5ᵗʰ S25.1 Injury of innominate or subclavian artery

> **CC Excl: For codes in subcategory S25.1:**
> **MCC with 7th character A:** PDX collection 1179

✓6ᵗʰ S25.10 Unspecified injury of innominate or subclavian artery

    ✓7ᵗʰ S25.101 Unspecified injury of right innominate or subclavian artery `MCC`

    ✓7ᵗʰ S25.102 Unspecified injury of left innominate or subclavian artery `MCC`

    ✓7ᵗʰ S25.109 Unspecified injury of unspecified innominate or subclavian artery `MCC`

✓6ᵗʰ S25.11 Minor laceration of innominate or subclavian artery
Incomplete transection of innominate or subclavian artery
Laceration of innominate or subclavian artery NOS
Superficial laceration of innominate or subclavian artery

    ✓7ᵗʰ S25.111 Minor laceration of right innominate or subclavian artery `MCC`

    ✓7ᵗʰ S25.112 Minor laceration of left innominate or subclavian artery `MCC`

    ✓7ᵗʰ S25.119 Minor laceration of unspecified innominate or subclavian artery `MCC`

✓6ᵗʰ S25.12 Major laceration of innominate or subclavian artery
Complete transection of innominate or subclavian artery
Traumatic rupture of innominate or subclavian artery

    ✓7ᵗʰ S25.121 Major laceration of right innominate or subclavian artery `MCC`

    ✓7ᵗʰ S25.122 Major laceration of left innominate or subclavian artery `MCC`

    ✓7ᵗʰ S25.129 Major laceration of unspecified innominate or subclavian artery `MCC`

✓6ᵗʰ S25.19 Other specified injury of innominate or subclavian artery

    ✓7ᵗʰ S25.191 Other specified injury of right innominate or subclavian artery `MCC`

    ✓7ᵗʰ S25.192 Other specified injury of left innominate or subclavian artery `MCC`

    ✓7ᵗʰ S25.199 Other specified injury of unspecified innominate or subclavian artery `MCC`

✓5ᵗʰ S25.2 Injury of superior vena cava
Injury of vena cava NOS

> **CC Excl: For codes in subcategory S25.2:**
> **MCC with 7th character A:** PDX collection 1180

✓x7ᵗʰ S25.20 Unspecified injury of superior vena cava `MCC`

✓x7ᵗʰ S25.21 Minor laceration of superior vena cava `MCC`
Incomplete transection of superior vena cava
Laceration of superior vena cava NOS
Superficial laceration of superior vena cava

✓x7ᵗʰ S25.22 Major laceration of superior vena cava `MCC`
Complete transection of superior vena cava
Traumatic rupture of superior vena cava

✓x7ᵗʰ S25.29 Other specified injury of superior vena cava `MCC`

N Newborn: 0   **P** Pediatric: 0-17   **M** Maternity: 12-55   **A** Adult: 15-124   `MCC` Major CC Condition   `PDxMCC` PDx acts as own MCC   `CC` CC Condition   `PDxCC` PDx acts as own CC

966   ICD-10-CM 2018

√5th **S25.3** **Injury of** innominate or subclavian vein

> **CC Excl: For codes in subcategory S25.3:**
> **MCC with 7th character A:** PDX collection 1181

√6th **S25.30** **Unspecified** injury of innominate or subclavian vein

√7th **S25.301** **Unspecified injury of** right **MCC**
innominate or subclavian vein

√7th **S25.302** **Unspecified injury of** left innominate **MCC**
or subclavian vein

√7th **S25.309** **Unspecified injury of** unspecified **MCC**
innominate or subclavian vein

√6th **S25.31** **Minor laceration** of innominate or subclavian vein
Incomplete transection of innominate or subclavian vein
Laceration of innominate or subclavian vein NOS
Superficial laceration of innominate or subclavian vein

√7th **S25.311** **Minor laceration of** right innominate **MCC**
or subclavian vein

√7th **S25.312** **Minor laceration of** left innominate or **MCC**
subclavian vein

√7th **S25.319** **Minor laceration of** unspecified **MCC**
innominate or subclavian vein

√6th **S25.32** **Major laceration** of innominate or subclavian vein
Complete transection of innominate or subclavian vein
Traumatic rupture of innominate or subclavian vein

√7th **S25.321** **Major laceration of** right innominate **MCC**
or subclavian vein

√7th **S25.322** **Major laceration of** left innominate **MCC**
or subclavian vein

√7th **S25.329** **Major laceration of** unspecified **MCC**
innominate or subclavian vein

√6th **S25.39** **Other** specified injury of innominate or subclavian vein

√7th **S25.391** **Other specified injury of** right **MCC**
innominate or subclavian vein

√7th **S25.392** **Other specified injury of** left **MCC**
innominate or subclavian vein

√7th **S25.399** **Other specified injury of** unspecified **MCC**
innominate or subclavian vein

√5th **S25.4** **Injury of** pulmonary blood vessels

> **CC Excl: For codes in subcategory S25.4, unless**
> **otherwise noted:**
> **MCC with 7th character A:** PDX collection 1182

√6th **S25.40** **Unspecified** injury of pulmonary blood vessels

√7th **S25.401** **Unspecified injury of** right pulmonary **MCC**
blood vessels

√7th **S25.402** **Unspecified injury of** left pulmonary **MCC**
blood vessels

√7th **S25.409** **Unspecified injury of** unspecified **MCC**
pulmonary blood vessels

√6th **S25.41** **Minor laceration** of pulmonary blood vessels
Incomplete transection of pulmonary blood vessels
Laceration of pulmonary blood vessels NOS
Superficial laceration of pulmonary blood vessels

√7th **S25.411** **Minor laceration of** right pulmonary **MCC**
blood vessels

√7th **S25.412** **Minor laceration of** left pulmonary **MCC**
blood vessels

√7th **S25.419** **Minor laceration of** unspecified **MCC**
pulmonary blood vessels

√6th **S25.42** **Major laceration** of pulmonary blood vessels
Complete transection of pulmonary blood vessels
Traumatic rupture of pulmonary blood vessels

√7th **S25.421** **Major laceration of** right pulmonary **MCC**
blood vessels
> **CC Excl: MCC with 7th character A:**
> PDX collection 1183

√7th **S25.422** **Major laceration of** left pulmonary **MCC**
blood vessels

√7th **S25.429** **Major laceration of** unspecified **MCC**
pulmonary blood vessels

√6th **S25.49** **Other specified injury** of pulmonary blood vessels

√7th **S25.491** **Other specified injury of** right **MCC**
pulmonary blood vessels

√7th **S25.492** **Other specified injury of** left **MCC**
pulmonary blood vessels

√7th **S25.499** **Other specified injury of** unspecified **MCC**
pulmonary blood vessels

√5th **S25.5** **Injury of** intercostal blood vessels

> **CC Excl: For codes in subcategory S25.5:**
> **CC with 7th character A:** PDX collection 1184

√6th **S25.50** **Unspecified** injury of intercostal blood vessels

√7th **S25.501** **Unspecified injury of** intercostal **CC**
blood vessels, right side

√7th **S25.502** **Unspecified injury of** intercostal **CC**
blood vessels, left side

√7th **S25.509** **Unspecified injury of** intercostal **CC**
blood vessels, unspecified side

√6th **S25.51** **Laceration** of intercostal blood vessels

√7th **S25.511** **Laceration of** intercostal blood **CC**
vessels, right side

√7th **S25.512** **Laceration of** intercostal blood **CC**
vessels, left side

√7th **S25.519** **Laceration of** intercostal blood **CC**
vessels, unspecified side

√6th **S25.59** **Other** specified injury of intercostal blood vessels

√7th **S25.591** **Other specified injury of** intercostal **CC**
blood vessels, right side

√7th **S25.592** **Other specified injury of** intercostal **CC**
blood vessels, left side

√7th **S25.599** **Other specified injury of** intercostal **CC**
blood vessels, unspecified side

√5th **S25.8** **Injury of** other blood vessels of thorax
Injury of azygos vein
Injury of mammary artery or vein

> **CC Excl: For codes in subcategory S25.8:**
> **CC with 7th character A:** PDX collection 1185

√6th **S25.80** **Unspecified** injury of other blood vessels of thorax

√7th **S25.801** **Unspecified injury of** other blood **CC**
vessels of thorax, right side

√7th **S25.802** **Unspecified injury of** other blood **CC**
vessels of thorax, left side

√7th **S25.809** **Unspecified injury of** other blood **CC**
vessels of thorax, unspecified side

√6th **S25.81** **Laceration** of other blood vessels of thorax

√7th **S25.811** **Laceration of** other blood vessels of **CC**
thorax, right side

√7th **S25.812** **Laceration of** other blood vessels of **CC**
thorax, left side

√7th **S25.819** **Laceration of** other blood vessels of **CC**
thorax, unspecified side

√6th **S25.89** **Other** specified injury of other blood vessels of thorax

√7th **S25.891** **Other specified injury of** other blood **CC**
vessels of thorax, right side

√7th **S25.892** **Other specified injury of** other blood **CC**
vessels of thorax, left side

√7th **S25.899** **Other specified injury of** other blood **CC**
vessels of thorax, unspecified side

√5th **S25.9** **Injury of** unspecified blood vessel of thorax

> **CC Excl: For codes in subcategory S25.9:**
> **CC with 7th character A:** PDX collection 1185

√x7th **S25.90** **Unspecified injury of unspecified blood vessel** **CC**
of thorax

√x7th **S25.91** **Laceration of unspecified blood vessel of thorax** **CC**

√x7th **S25.99** **Other specified injury of unspecified blood** **CC**
vessel of thorax

✔ Additional Character Req   √x7th Placeholder Alert   Unacceptable PDx   Manifestation   H1-H14 HAC   HCC CMS-HCC Condition   *EXCLUDES 1* Not Coded Here   *EXCLUDES 2* Not Included Here

ICD-10-CM 2018   **967**

√4ᵗʰ **S26   Injury of heart**

Code also any associated:
   open wound of thorax (S21.-)
   traumatic hemopneumothorax (S27.2)
   traumatic hemothorax (S27.1)
   traumatic pneumothorax (S27.0)

> The appropriate 7th character is to be added to each code from
> category S26.
> A   initial encounter
> D   subsequent encounter
> S   sequela

> **CC Excl: For codes in category S26 unless otherwise noted:**
> **CC or MCC with 7th character A:** PDX collection 1187

√5ᵗʰ **S26.0   Injury of heart** with hemopericardium

√x7ᵗʰ **S26.00   Unspecified injury of heart with hemopericardium**   `CC`
   CC Excl: CC with 7th character A: PDX collection 1186

√x7ᵗʰ **S26.01   Contusion of heart with hemopericardium**   `CC`

√6ᵗʰ **S26.02   Laceration of heart with hemopericardium**

√7ᵗʰ **S26.020   Mild laceration of heart with hemopericardium**   `MCC`
   Laceration of heart without penetration of heart chamber

√7ᵗʰ **S26.021   Moderate laceration of heart with hemopericardium**   `MCC`
   Laceration of heart with penetration of heart chamber

√7ᵗʰ **S26.022   Major laceration of heart with hemopericardium**   `MCC`
   Laceration of heart with penetration of multiple heart chambers

√x7ᵗʰ **S26.09   Other injury of heart with hemopericardium**   `CC`
   CC Excl: CC with 7th character A: PDX collection 1186

√5ᵗʰ **S26.1   Injury of heart** without hemopericardium

√x7ᵗʰ **S26.10   Unspecified injury of heart without hemopericardium**   `CC`
   CC Excl: CC with 7th character A: PDX collection 1186

√x7ᵗʰ **S26.11   Contusion of heart without hemopericardium**   `CC`

√x7ᵗʰ **S26.12   Laceration of heart without hemopericardium**   `MCC`

√x7ᵗʰ **S26.19   Other injury of heart without hemopericardium**   `CC`
   CC Excl: CC with 7th character A: PDX collection 1186

√5ᵗʰ **S26.9   Injury of heart, unspecified with or without hemopericardium**

√x7ᵗʰ **S26.90   Unspecified injury of heart, unspecified with or without hemopericardium**   `CC`
   CC Excl: CC with 7th character A: PDX collection 1186

√x7ᵗʰ **S26.91   Contusion of heart, unspecified with or without hemopericardium**   `CC`
   DEF: Bruising within the heart muscle with no mention of open wound; usually caused by blunt chest trauma in motor vehicle accidents, falling from great heights, or receiving CPR.

√x7ᵗʰ **S26.92   Laceration of heart, unspecified with or without hemopericardium**   `MCC`
   Laceration of heart NOS

√x7ᵗʰ **S26.99   Other injury of heart, unspecified with or without hemopericardium**   `CC`
   CC Excl: CC with 7th character A: PDX collection 1186

√4ᵗʰ **S27   Injury of other and unspecified intrathoracic organs**

Code also any associated open wound of thorax (S21.-)
EXCLUDES 2 injury of cervical esophagus (S10-S19)
   injury of trachea (cervical) (S10-S19)

> The appropriate 7th character is to be added to each code from
> category S27.
> A   initial encounter
> D   subsequent encounter
> S   sequela

√x7ᵗʰ **S27.0   Traumatic pneumothorax**   `CC`
   EXCLUDES 1 spontaneous pneumothorax (J93.-)
   CC Excl: CC with 7th character A: PDX collection 1188

√x7ᵗʰ **S27.1   Traumatic hemothorax**   `MCC`
   CC Excl: MCC with 7th character A: PDX collection 1188

√x7ᵗʰ **S27.2   Traumatic hemopneumothorax**   `MCC`
   CC Excl: MCC with 7th character A: PDX collection 1188

√5ᵗʰ **S27.3   Other and unspecified injuries of lung**

> **CC Excl: For codes in subcategory S27.3, unless otherwise noted:**
> **CC with 7th character A:** PDX collection 1189

√6ᵗʰ **S27.30   Unspecified injury of lung**

√7ᵗʰ **S27.301   Unspecified injury of lung, unilateral**   `CC`

√7ᵗʰ **S27.302   Unspecified injury of lung, bilateral**   `CC`

√7ᵗʰ **S27.309   Unspecified injury of lung, unspecified**   `CC`

√6ᵗʰ **S27.31   Primary blast injury of lung**
   Blast injury of lung NOS

√7ᵗʰ **S27.311   Primary blast injury of lung, unilateral**   `CC`

√7ᵗʰ **S27.312   Primary blast injury of lung, bilateral**   `CC`

√7ᵗʰ **S27.319   Primary blast injury of lung, unspecified**   `CC`

√6ᵗʰ **S27.32   Contusion of lung**
   DEF: Bruising of lung without mention of open wound.

√7ᵗʰ **S27.321   Contusion of lung, unilateral**   `CC`

√7ᵗʰ **S27.322   Contusion of lung, bilateral**   `CC`

√7ᵗʰ **S27.329   Contusion of lung, unspecified**   `CC`

√6ᵗʰ **S27.33   Laceration of lung**

> **CC Excl: For codes in subcategory S27.33:**
> **MCC with 7th character A:** PDX collection 1190

√7ᵗʰ **S27.331   Laceration of lung, unilateral**   `MCC`

√7ᵗʰ **S27.332   Laceration of lung, bilateral**   `MCC`

√7ᵗʰ **S27.339   Laceration of lung, unspecified**   `MCC`

√6ᵗʰ **S27.39   Other injuries of lung**
   Secondary blast injury of lung

√7ᵗʰ **S27.391   Other injuries of lung, unilateral**   `CC`

√7ᵗʰ **S27.392   Other injuries of lung, bilateral**   `CC`

√7ᵗʰ **S27.399   Other injuries of lung, unspecified**   `CC`

√5ᵗʰ **S27.4   Injury of bronchus**

> **CC Excl: For codes in subcategory S27.4:**
> **MCC with 7th character A:** PDX collection 1191

√6ᵗʰ **S27.40   Unspecified injury of bronchus**

√7ᵗʰ **S27.401   Unspecified injury of bronchus, unilateral**   `MCC`

√7ᵗʰ **S27.402   Unspecified injury of bronchus, bilateral**   `MCC`

√7ᵗʰ **S27.409   Unspecified injury of bronchus, unspecified**   `MCC`

√6ᵗʰ **S27.41   Primary blast injury of bronchus**
   Blast injury of bronchus NOS

√7ᵗʰ **S27.411   Primary blast injury of bronchus, unilateral**   `MCC`

√7ᵗʰ **S27.412   Primary blast injury of bronchus, bilateral**   `MCC`

√7ᵗʰ **S27.419   Primary blast injury of bronchus, unspecified**   `MCC`

√6ᵗʰ **S27.42   Contusion of bronchus**

√7ᵗʰ **S27.421   Contusion of bronchus, unilateral**   `MCC`

√7ᵗʰ **S27.422   Contusion of bronchus, bilateral**   `MCC`

√7ᵗʰ **S27.429   Contusion of bronchus, unspecified**   `MCC`

√6ᵗʰ **S27.43   Laceration of bronchus**

√7ᵗʰ **S27.431   Laceration of bronchus, unilateral**   `MCC`

√7ᵗʰ **S27.432   Laceration of bronchus, bilateral**   `MCC`

√7ᵗʰ **S27.439   Laceration of bronchus, unspecified**   `MCC`

√6ᵗʰ **S27.49   Other injury of bronchus**
   Secondary blast injury of bronchus

√7ᵗʰ **S27.491   Other injury of bronchus, unilateral**   `MCC`

√7ᵗʰ **S27.492   Other injury of bronchus, bilateral**   `MCC`

√7ᵗʰ **S27.499   Other injury of bronchus, unspecified**   `MCC`

√5ᵗʰ **S27.5   Injury of thoracic trachea**

> **CC Excl: For codes in subcategory S27.5:**
> **CC with 7th character A:** PDX collection 1169

√x7ᵗʰ **S27.50   Unspecified injury of thoracic trachea**   `CC`

√x7ᵗʰ **S27.51   Primary blast injury of thoracic trachea**   `CC`
   Blast injury of thoracic trachea NOS

√x7ᵗʰ **S27.52   Contusion of thoracic trachea**   `CC`

√x7ᵗʰ **S27.53   Laceration of thoracic trachea**   `CC`

N Newborn: 0   **P** Pediatric: 0-17   **M** Maternity: 12-55   **A** Adult: 15-124   **MCC** Major CC Condition   **PDxMCC** PDx acts as own MCC   **CC** CC Condition   **PDxCC** PDx acts as own CC

✓x7ᵗʰ **S27.59**   Other **injury of thoracic trachea**   CC
Secondary blast injury of thoracic trachea

✓5ᵗʰ **S27.6**   **Injury of** pleura

> **CC Excl: For codes in subcategory S27.6:**
> **CC with 7th character A:** PDX collection 1169

✓x7ᵗʰ **S27.60**   Unspecified **injury of pleura**   CC

✓x7ᵗʰ **S27.63**   **Laceration of pleura**   CC

✓x7ᵗʰ **S27.69**   Other **injury of pleura**   CC

✓5ᵗʰ **S27.8**   **Injury of** other specified **intrathoracic organs**

✓6ᵗʰ **S27.80**   **Injury of** diaphragm

> **CC Excl: For codes in subcategory S27.80:**
> **CC with 7th character A:** PDX collection 1192

✓7ᵗʰ **S27.802**   **Contusion of diaphragm**   CC

✓7ᵗʰ **S27.803**   **Laceration of diaphragm**   CC

✓7ᵗʰ **S27.808**   Other **injury of diaphragm**   CC

✓7ᵗʰ **S27.809**   Unspecified **injury of diaphragm**   CC

✓6ᵗʰ **S27.81**   **Injury of** esophagus (thoracic part)

> **CC Excl: For codes in subcategory S27.81:**
> **MCC with 7th character A:** PDX collection 1193

✓7ᵗʰ **S27.812**   **Contusion of esophagus (thoracic part)**   MCC

✓7ᵗʰ **S27.813**   **Laceration of esophagus (thoracic part)**   MCC

✓7ᵗʰ **S27.818**   Other **injury of esophagus (thoracic part)**   MCC

✓7ᵗʰ **S27.819**   Unspecified **injury of esophagus (thoracic part)**   MCC

✓6ᵗʰ **S27.89**   **Injury of** other specified **intrathoracic organs**
Injury of lymphatic thoracic duct
Injury of thymus gland

> **CC Excl: For codes in subcategory S27.89:**
> **CC with 7th character A:** PDX collection 1169

✓7ᵗʰ **S27.892**   **Contusion of other specified intrathoracic organs**   CC

✓7ᵗʰ **S27.893**   **Laceration of other specified intrathoracic organs**   CC

✓7ᵗʰ **S27.898**   Other **injury of other specified intrathoracic organs**   CC

✓7ᵗʰ **S27.899**   Unspecified **injury of other specified intrathoracic organs**   CC

✓x7ᵗʰ **S27.9**   **Injury of** unspecified **intrathoracic organ**   CC
CC Excl: CC with 7th character A: PDX collection 1194

✓4ᵗʰ **S28**   **Crushing injury of thorax, and traumatic amputation of part of thorax**

> The appropriate 7th character is to be added to each code from category S28.
> A   initial encounter
> D   subsequent encounter
> S   sequela

✓x7ᵗʰ **S28.0**   **Crushed chest**
Use additional code for all associated injuries
> *EXCLUDES 1*   flail chest (S22.5)

✓x7ᵗʰ **S28.1**   **Traumatic amputation (partial) of** part of thorax, except breast   CC
CC Excl: CC with 7th character A: PDX collection 1168

✓5ᵗʰ **S28.2**   **Traumatic amputation of** breast

✓6ᵗʰ **S28.21**   Complete **traumatic amputation of breast**
Traumatic amputation of breast NOS

✓7ᵗʰ **S28.211**   Complete **traumatic amputation of** right **breast**

✓7ᵗʰ **S28.212**   Complete **traumatic amputation of** left **breast**

✓7ᵗʰ **S28.219**   Complete **traumatic amputation of** unspecified **breast**

✓6ᵗʰ **S28.22**   Partial **traumatic amputation of breast**

✓7ᵗʰ **S28.221**   Partial **traumatic amputation of** right **breast**

✓7ᵗʰ **S28.222**   Partial **traumatic amputation of** left **breast**

✓7ᵗʰ **S28.229**   Partial **traumatic amputation of** unspecified **breast**

✓4ᵗʰ **S29**   **Other and unspecified injuries of thorax**
Code also any associated open wound (S21.-)

> The appropriate 7th character is to be added to each code from category S29.
> A   initial encounter
> D   subsequent encounter
> S   sequela

✓5ᵗʰ **S29.0**   **Injury of muscle and tendon at thorax level**

✓6ᵗʰ **S29.00**   Unspecified **injury of muscle and tendon of thorax**

✓7ᵗʰ **S29.001**   Unspecified injury of muscle and tendon of front wall of thorax

✓7ᵗʰ **S29.002**   Unspecified injury of muscle and tendon of back wall of thorax

✓7ᵗʰ **S29.009**   Unspecified injury of muscle and tendon of unspecified wall of thorax

✓6ᵗʰ **S29.01**   Strain of muscle and tendon of thorax

✓7ᵗʰ **S29.011**   Strain of muscle and tendon of front wall of thorax

✓7ᵗʰ **S29.012**   Strain of muscle and tendon of back wall of thorax

✓7ᵗʰ **S29.019**   Strain of muscle and tendon of unspecified wall of thorax

✓6ᵗʰ **S29.02**   Laceration of muscle and tendon of thorax

✓7ᵗʰ **S29.021**   Laceration of muscle and tendon of front wall of thorax   CC
CC Excl: CC with 7th character A: PDX collection 1168

✓7ᵗʰ **S29.022**   Laceration of muscle and tendon of back wall of thorax

✓7ᵗʰ **S29.029**   Laceration of muscle and tendon of unspecified wall of thorax   CC
CC Excl: CC with 7th character A: PDX collection 1168

✓6ᵗʰ **S29.09**   Other injury of muscle and tendon of thorax

✓7ᵗʰ **S29.091**   Other injury of muscle and tendon of front wall of thorax

✓7ᵗʰ **S29.092**   Other injury of muscle and tendon of back wall of thorax

✓7ᵗʰ **S29.099**   Other injury of muscle and tendon of unspecified wall of thorax

✓x7ᵗʰ **S29.8**   **Other specified injuries of thorax**

✓x7ᵗʰ **S29.9**   **Unspecified injury of thorax**

Injuries to the abdomen, lower back, lumbar spine, pelvis and external genitals (S30-S39)

> *INCLUDES*   injuries to the abdominal wall
> injuries to the anus
> injuries to the buttock
> injuries to the external genitalia
> injuries to the flank
> injuries to the groin
> *EXCLUDES 2*   burns and corrosions (T20-T32)
> effects of foreign body in anus and rectum (T18.5)
> effects of foreign body in genitourinary tract (T19.-)
> effects of foreign body in stomach, small intestine and colon (T18.2-T18.4)
> frostbite (T33-T34)
> insect bite or sting, venomous (T63.4)

✓4ᵗʰ **S30**   **Superficial injury of abdomen, lower back, pelvis and external genitals**
> *EXCLUDES 2*   superficial injury of hip (S70.-)

> The appropriate 7th character is to be added to each code from category S30.
> A   initial encounter
> D   subsequent encounter
> S   sequela

✓x7ᵗʰ **S30.0**   **Contusion of lower back and pelvis**
Contusion of buttock

✓x7ᵗʰ **S30.1**   **Contusion of abdominal wall**
Contusion of flank
Contusion of groin

✓5ᵗʰ **S30.2**   **Contusion of** external genital organs

✓6ᵗʰ **S30.20**   Contusion of unspecified external genital organ

✓7ᵗʰ **S30.201**   Contusion of unspecified external genital organ, male   ♂

✓ Additional Character Req   ✓x7ᵗʰ Placeholder Alert   Unacceptable PDx   Manifestation   H1 - H14 HAC   HCC CMS-HCC Condition   *EXCLUDES 1* Not Coded Here   *EXCLUDES 2* Not Included Here

ICD-10-CM 2018   969

☑7ᵗʰ **S30.202** **Contusion of unspecified external genital organ, female** ♀

☑x7ᵗʰ **S30.21** **Contusion of** penis ♂

☑x7ᵗʰ **S30.22** **Contusion of** scrotum and testes ♂

☑x7ᵗʰ **S30.23** **Contusion of** vagina and vulva ♀

☑x7ᵗʰ **S30.3** **Contusion of anus**

☑5ᵗʰ **S30.8** **Other superficial injuries of abdomen, lower back, pelvis and external genitals**

  ☑6ᵗʰ **S30.81** **Abrasion of abdomen, lower back, pelvis and external genitals**

    ☑7ᵗʰ **S30.810** **Abrasion of** lower back and pelvis

    ☑7ᵗʰ **S30.811** **Abrasion of** abdominal wall

    ☑7ᵗʰ **S30.812** **Abrasion of** penis ♂

    ☑7ᵗʰ **S30.813** **Abrasion of** scrotum and testes ♂

    ☑7ᵗʰ **S30.814** **Abrasion of** vagina and vulva ♀

    ☑7ᵗʰ **S30.815** **Abrasion of** unspecified external genital organs, male ♂

    ☑7ᵗʰ **S30.816** **Abrasion of** unspecified external genital organs, female ♀

    ☑7ᵗʰ **S30.817** **Abrasion of** anus

  ☑6ᵗʰ **S30.82** **Blister (nonthermal) of abdomen, lower back, pelvis and external genitals**

    ☑7ᵗʰ **S30.820** **Blister (nonthermal) of** lower back and pelvis

    ☑7ᵗʰ **S30.821** **Blister (nonthermal) of** abdominal wall

    ☑7ᵗʰ **S30.822** **Blister (nonthermal) of** penis ♂

    ☑7ᵗʰ **S30.823** **Blister (nonthermal) of** scrotum and testes ♂

    ☑7ᵗʰ **S30.824** **Blister (nonthermal) of** vagina and vulva ♀

    ☑7ᵗʰ **S30.825** **Blister (nonthermal) of** unspecified external genital organs, male ♂

    ☑7ᵗʰ **S30.826** **Blister (nonthermal) of** unspecified external genital organs, female ♀

    ☑7ᵗʰ **S30.827** **Blister (nonthermal) of** anus

  ☑6ᵗʰ **S30.84** **External constriction of abdomen, lower back, pelvis and external genitals**

    ☑7ᵗʰ **S30.840** **External constriction of** lower back and pelvis

    ☑7ᵗʰ **S30.841** **External constriction of** abdominal wall

    ☑7ᵗʰ **S30.842** **External constriction of** penis ♂
        Hair tourniquet syndrome of penis
        Use additional cause code to identify the constricting item (W49.0-)

    ☑7ᵗʰ **S30.843** **External constriction of** scrotum and testes ♂

    ☑7ᵗʰ **S30.844** **External constriction of** vagina and vulva ♀

    ☑7ᵗʰ **S30.845** **External constriction of** unspecified external genital organs, male ♂

    ☑7ᵗʰ **S30.846** **External constriction of** unspecified external genital organs, female ♀

  ☑6ᵗʰ **S30.85** **Superficial foreign body of abdomen, lower back, pelvis and external genitals**
        Splinter in the abdomen, lower back, pelvis and external genitals

    ☑7ᵗʰ **S30.850** **Superficial foreign body of** lower back and pelvis

    ☑7ᵗʰ **S30.851** **Superficial foreign body of** abdominal wall

    ☑7ᵗʰ **S30.852** **Superficial foreign body of** penis ♂

    ☑7ᵗʰ **S30.853** **Superficial foreign body of** scrotum and testes ♂

    ☑7ᵗʰ **S30.854** **Superficial foreign body of** vagina and vulva ♀

    ☑7ᵗʰ **S30.855** **Superficial foreign body of** unspecified external genital organs, male ♂

    ☑7ᵗʰ **S30.856** **Superficial foreign body of** unspecified external genital organs, female ♀

    ☑7ᵗʰ **S30.857** **Superficial foreign body of** anus

  ☑6ᵗʰ **S30.86** **Insect bite (nonvenomous) of abdomen, lower back, pelvis and external genitals**

    ☑7ᵗʰ **S30.860** **Insect bite (nonvenomous) of** lower back and pelvis

    ☑7ᵗʰ **S30.861** **Insect bite (nonvenomous) of** abdominal wall

    ☑7ᵗʰ **S30.862** **Insect bite (nonvenomous) of** penis ♂

    ☑7ᵗʰ **S30.863** **Insect bite (nonvenomous) of** scrotum and testes ♂

    ☑7ᵗʰ **S30.864** **Insect bite (nonvenomous) of** vagina and vulva ♀

    ☑7ᵗʰ **S30.865** **Insect bite (nonvenomous) of** unspecified external genital organs, male ♂

    ☑7ᵗʰ **S30.866** **Insect bite (nonvenomous) of** unspecified external genital organs, female ♀

    ☑7ᵗʰ **S30.867** **Insect bite (nonvenomous) of** anus

  ☑6ᵗʰ **S30.87** **Other superficial bite of abdomen, lower back, pelvis and external genitals**
        EXCLUDES 1 *open bite of abdomen, lower back, pelvis and external genitals (S31.05, S31.15, S31.25, S31.35, S31.45, S31.55)*

    ☑7ᵗʰ **S30.870** **Other superficial bite of** lower back and pelvis

    ☑7ᵗʰ **S30.871** **Other superficial bite of** abdominal wall

    ☑7ᵗʰ **S30.872** **Other superficial bite of** penis ♂

    ☑7ᵗʰ **S30.873** **Other superficial bite of** scrotum and testes ♂

    ☑7ᵗʰ **S30.874** **Other superficial bite of** vagina and vulva ♀

    ☑7ᵗʰ **S30.875** **Other superficial bite of** unspecified external genital organs, male ♂

    ☑7ᵗʰ **S30.876** **Other superficial bite of** unspecified external genital organs, female ♀

    ☑7ᵗʰ **S30.877** **Other superficial bite of** anus

☑5ᵗʰ **S30.9** **Unspecified superficial injury of abdomen, lower back, pelvis and external genitals**

  ☑x7ᵗʰ **S30.91** **Unspecified superficial injury of** lower back and pelvis

  ☑x7ᵗʰ **S30.92** **Unspecified superficial injury of** abdominal wall

  ☑x7ᵗʰ **S30.93** **Unspecified superficial injury of** penis ♂

  ☑x7ᵗʰ **S30.94** **Unspecified superficial injury of** scrotum and testes ♂

  ☑x7ᵗʰ **S30.95** **Unspecified superficial injury of** vagina and vulva ♀

  ☑x7ᵗʰ **S30.96** **Unspecified superficial injury of** unspecified external genital organs, male ♂

  ☑x7ᵗʰ **S30.97** **Unspecified superficial injury of** unspecified external genital organs, female ♀

  ☑x7ᵗʰ **S30.98** **Unspecified superficial injury of** anus

☑4ᵗʰ **S31** **Open wound of abdomen, lower back, pelvis and external genitals**
    Code also any associated:
      spinal cord injury (S24.0, S24.1-, S34.0-, S34.1-)
      wound infection
    EXCLUDES 1 *traumatic amputation of part of abdomen, lower back and pelvis (S38.2-, S38.3)*
    EXCLUDES 2 *open wound of hip (S71.00-S71.02)*
                    open fracture of pelvis (S32.1- – S32.9 with 7th B)

> The appropriate 7th character is to be added to each code from category S31.
> A   initial encounter
> D   subsequent encounter
> S   sequela

> **CC Excl: For codes in category S31:**
> **MCC with 7th character A:** PDX collection 1195

☑5ᵗʰ **S31.0** **Open wound of lower back and pelvis**

  ☑6ᵗʰ **S31.00** **Unspecified open wound of lower back and pelvis**

    ☑7ᵗʰ **S31.000** **Unspecified open wound of lower back and pelvis** without penetration into retroperitoneum
        Unspecified open wound of lower back and pelvis NOS

    ☑7ᵗʰ **S31.001** **Unspecified open wound of lower back and pelvis** with penetration into retroperitoneum   ᴹᶜᶜ

ℕ Newborn: 0   ℙ Pediatric: 0-17   Ⓜ Maternity: 12-55   Ⓐ Adult: 15-124   **ᴹᶜᶜ** Major CC Condition   **ᴾᴰˣᴹᶜᶜ** PDx acts as own MCC   **ᶜᶜ** CC Condition   **ᴾᴰˣᶜᶜ** PDx acts as own CC

970   ICD-10-CM 2018

✓6ᵗʰ **S31.01** Laceration without foreign body of lower back and pelvis

     ✓7ᵗʰ **S31.010** **Laceration without foreign body of lower back and pelvis** without penetration into retroperitoneum

         Laceration without foreign body of lower back and pelvis NOS

     ✓7ᵗʰ **S31.011** **Laceration without foreign body of lower back and pelvis** with penetration into retroperitoneum   MCC

✓6ᵗʰ **S31.02** Laceration with foreign body of lower back and pelvis

     ✓7ᵗʰ **S31.020** **Laceration with foreign body of lower back and pelvis** without penetration into retroperitoneum

         Laceration with foreign body of lower back and pelvis NOS

     ✓7ᵗʰ **S31.021** **Laceration with foreign body of lower back and pelvis** with penetration into retroperitoneum   MCC

✓6ᵗʰ **S31.03** Puncture wound without foreign body of lower back and pelvis

     ✓7ᵗʰ **S31.030** **Puncture wound without foreign body of lower back and pelvis** without penetration into retroperitoneum

         Puncture wound without foreign body of lower back and pelvis NOS

     ✓7ᵗʰ **S31.031** **Puncture wound without foreign body of lower back and pelvis** with penetration into retroperitoneum   MCC

✓6ᵗʰ **S31.04** Puncture wound with foreign body of lower back and pelvis

     ✓7ᵗʰ **S31.040** **Puncture wound with foreign body of lower back and pelvis** without penetration into retroperitoneum

         Puncture wound with foreign body of lower back and pelvis NOS

     ✓7ᵗʰ **S31.041** **Puncture wound with foreign body of lower back and pelvis** with penetration into retroperitoneum   MCC

✓6ᵗʰ **S31.05** Open bite of lower back and pelvis

     Bite of lower back and pelvis NOS

     EXCLUDES 1   *superficial bite of lower back and pelvis (S30.860, S30.870)*

     ✓7ᵗʰ **S31.050** **Open bite of lower back and pelvis** without penetration into retroperitoneum

         Open bite of lower back and pelvis NOS

     ✓7ᵗʰ **S31.051** **Open bite of lower back and pelvis** with penetration into retroperitoneum   MCC

✓5ᵗʰ **S31.1** Open wound of abdominal wall without penetration into peritoneal cavity

     Open wound of abdominal wall NOS

     EXCLUDES 2   *open wound of abdominal wall with penetration into peritoneal cavity (S31.6-)*

✓6ᵗʰ **S31.10** Unspecified open wound of abdominal wall without penetration into peritoneal cavity

     ✓7ᵗʰ **S31.100** **Unspecified open wound of abdominal wall, right upper quadrant** without penetration into peritoneal cavity

     ✓7ᵗʰ **S31.101** **Unspecified open wound of abdominal wall, left upper quadrant** without penetration into peritoneal cavity

     ✓7ᵗʰ **S31.102** **Unspecified open wound of abdominal wall, epigastric region** without penetration into peritoneal cavity

     ✓7ᵗʰ **S31.103** **Unspecified open wound of abdominal wall, right lower quadrant** without penetration into peritoneal cavity

     ✓7ᵗʰ **S31.104** **Unspecified open wound of abdominal wall, left lower quadrant** without penetration into peritoneal cavity

     ✓7ᵗʰ **S31.105** **Unspecified open wound of abdominal wall, periumbilic region** without penetration into peritoneal cavity

     ✓7ᵗʰ **S31.109** **Unspecified open wound of abdominal wall, unspecified quadrant** without penetration into peritoneal cavity

         Unspecified open wound of abdominal wall NOS

✓6ᵗʰ **S31.11** Laceration without foreign body of abdominal wall without penetration into peritoneal cavity

     ✓7ᵗʰ **S31.110** **Laceration without foreign body of abdominal wall, right upper quadrant without penetration into peritoneal cavity**

     ✓7ᵗʰ **S31.111** **Laceration without foreign body of abdominal wall, left upper quadrant without penetration into peritoneal cavity**

     ✓7ᵗʰ **S31.112** **Laceration without foreign body of abdominal wall, epigastric region without penetration into peritoneal cavity**

     ✓7ᵗʰ **S31.113** **Laceration without foreign body of abdominal wall, right lower quadrant without penetration into peritoneal cavity**

     ✓7ᵗʰ **S31.114** **Laceration without foreign body of abdominal wall, left lower quadrant without penetration into peritoneal cavity**

     ✓7ᵗʰ **S31.115** **Laceration without foreign body of abdominal wall, periumbilic region without penetration into peritoneal cavity**

     ✓7ᵗʰ **S31.119** **Laceration without foreign body of abdominal wall, unspecified quadrant without penetration into peritoneal cavity**

✓6ᵗʰ **S31.12** Laceration with foreign body of abdominal wall without penetration into peritoneal cavity

     ✓7ᵗʰ **S31.120** **Laceration of abdominal wall with foreign body, right upper quadrant without penetration into peritoneal cavity**

     ✓7ᵗʰ **S31.121** **Laceration of abdominal wall with foreign body, left upper quadrant without penetration into peritoneal cavity**

     ✓7ᵗʰ **S31.122** **Laceration of abdominal wall with foreign body, epigastric region without penetration into peritoneal cavity**

     ✓7ᵗʰ **S31.123** **Laceration of abdominal wall with foreign body, right lower quadrant without penetration into peritoneal cavity**

     ✓7ᵗʰ **S31.124** **Laceration of abdominal wall with foreign body, left lower quadrant without penetration into peritoneal cavity**

     ✓7ᵗʰ **S31.125** **Laceration of abdominal wall with foreign body, periumbilic region without penetration into peritoneal cavity**

     ✓7ᵗʰ **S31.129** **Laceration of abdominal wall with foreign body, unspecified quadrant without penetration into peritoneal cavity**

✓6ᵗʰ **S31.13** Puncture wound of abdominal wall without foreign body without penetration into peritoneal cavity

     ✓7ᵗʰ **S31.130** **Puncture wound of abdominal wall without foreign body, right upper quadrant without penetration into peritoneal cavity**

     ✓7ᵗʰ **S31.131** **Puncture wound of abdominal wall without foreign body, left upper quadrant without penetration into peritoneal cavity**

     ✓7ᵗʰ **S31.132** **Puncture wound of abdominal wall without foreign body, epigastric region without penetration into peritoneal cavity**

     ✓7ᵗʰ **S31.133** **Puncture wound of abdominal wall without foreign body, right lower quadrant without penetration into peritoneal cavity**

     ✓7ᵗʰ **S31.134** **Puncture wound of abdominal wall without foreign body, left lower quadrant without penetration into peritoneal cavity**

     ✓7ᵗʰ **S31.135** **Puncture wound of abdominal wall without foreign body, periumbilic region without penetration into peritoneal cavity**

     ✓7ᵗʰ **S31.139** **Puncture wound of abdominal wall without foreign body, unspecified quadrant without penetration into peritoneal cavity**

✓6ᵗʰ **S31.14** Puncture wound of abdominal wall with foreign body without penetration into peritoneal cavity

     ✓7ᵗʰ **S31.140** **Puncture wound of abdominal wall with foreign body, right upper quadrant without penetration into peritoneal cavity**

✓ Additional Character Req   ✓x7ᵗʰ Placeholder Alert   Unacceptable PDx   Manifestation   **H1**-**H14** HAC   **HCC** CMS-HCC Condition   **EXCLUDES 1** Not Coded Here   **EXCLUDES 2** Not Included Here

ICD-10-CM 2018   **971**

✓7ᵗʰ **S31.141** Puncture wound of abdominal wall with foreign body, left upper quadrant without penetration into peritoneal cavity

✓7ᵗʰ **S31.142** Puncture wound of abdominal wall with foreign body, epigastric region without penetration into peritoneal cavity

✓7ᵗʰ **S31.143** Puncture wound of abdominal wall with foreign body, right lower quadrant without penetration into peritoneal cavity

✓7ᵗʰ **S31.144** Puncture wound of abdominal wall with foreign body, left lower quadrant without penetration into peritoneal cavity

✓7ᵗʰ **S31.145** Puncture wound of abdominal wall with foreign body, periumbilic region without penetration into peritoneal cavity

✓7ᵗʰ **S31.149** Puncture wound of abdominal wall with foreign body, unspecified quadrant without penetration into peritoneal cavity

✓6ᵗʰ **S31.15** Open bite of abdominal wall without penetration into peritoneal cavity
　Bite of abdominal wall NOS
　EXCLUDES 1　superficial bite of abdominal wall (S30.871)

✓7ᵗʰ **S31.150** Open bite of abdominal wall, right upper quadrant without penetration into peritoneal cavity

✓7ᵗʰ **S31.151** Open bite of abdominal wall, left upper quadrant without penetration into peritoneal cavity

✓7ᵗʰ **S31.152** Open bite of abdominal wall, epigastric region without penetration into peritoneal cavity

✓7ᵗʰ **S31.153** Open bite of abdominal wall, right lower quadrant without penetration into peritoneal cavity

✓7ᵗʰ **S31.154** Open bite of abdominal wall, left lower quadrant without penetration into peritoneal cavity

✓7ᵗʰ **S31.155** Open bite of abdominal wall, periumbilic region without penetration into peritoneal cavity

✓7ᵗʰ **S31.159** Open bite of abdominal wall, unspecified quadrant without penetration into peritoneal cavity

✓5ᵗʰ **S31.2** Open wound of penis

✓x7ᵗʰ **S31.20** Unspecified open wound of penis　♂

✓x7ᵗʰ **S31.21** Laceration without foreign body of penis　♂

✓x7ᵗʰ **S31.22** Laceration with foreign body of penis　♂

✓x7ᵗʰ **S31.23** Puncture wound without foreign body of penis　♂

✓x7ᵗʰ **S31.24** Puncture wound with foreign body of penis　♂

✓x7ᵗʰ **S31.25** Open bite of penis　♂
　Bite of penis NOS
　EXCLUDES 1　superficial bite of penis (S30.862, S30.872)

✓5ᵗʰ **S31.3** Open wound of scrotum and testes

✓x7ᵗʰ **S31.30** Unspecified open wound of scrotum and testes　♂

✓x7ᵗʰ **S31.31** Laceration without foreign body of scrotum and testes　♂

✓x7ᵗʰ **S31.32** Laceration with foreign body of scrotum and testes　♂

✓x7ᵗʰ **S31.33** Puncture wound without foreign body of scrotum and testes　♂

✓x7ᵗʰ **S31.34** Puncture wound with foreign body of scrotum and testes　♂

✓x7ᵗʰ **S31.35** Open bite of scrotum and testes　♂
　Bite of scrotum and testes NOS
　EXCLUDES 1　superficial bite of scrotum and testes (S30.863, S30.873)

✓5ᵗʰ **S31.4** Open wound of vagina and vulva
　EXCLUDES 1　injury to vagina and vulva during delivery (O70-, O71.4)

✓x7ᵗʰ **S31.40** Unspecified open wound of vagina and vulva　♀

✓x7ᵗʰ **S31.41** Laceration without foreign body of vagina and vulva　♀

✓x7ᵗʰ **S31.42** Laceration with foreign body of vagina and vulva　♀

✓x7ᵗʰ **S31.43** Puncture wound without foreign body of vagina and vulva　♀

✓x7ᵗʰ **S31.44** Puncture wound with foreign body of vagina and vulva　♀

✓x7ᵗʰ **S31.45** Open bite of vagina and vulva　♀
　Bite of vagina and vulva NOS
　EXCLUDES 1　superficial bite of vagina and vulva (S30.864, S30.874)

✓5ᵗʰ **S31.5** Open wound of unspecified external genital organs
　EXCLUDES 1　traumatic amputation of external genital organs (S38.21, S38.22)

✓6ᵗʰ **S31.50** Unspecified open wound of unspecified external genital organs

✓7ᵗʰ **S31.501** Unspecified open wound of unspecified external genital organs, male　♂

✓7ᵗʰ **S31.502** Unspecified open wound of unspecified external genital organs, female　♀

✓6ᵗʰ **S31.51** Laceration without foreign body of unspecified external genital organs

✓7ᵗʰ **S31.511** Laceration without foreign body of unspecified external genital organs, male　♂

✓7ᵗʰ **S31.512** Laceration without foreign body of unspecified external genital organs, female　♀

✓6ᵗʰ **S31.52** Laceration with foreign body of unspecified external genital organs

✓7ᵗʰ **S31.521** Laceration with foreign body of unspecified external genital organs, male　♂

✓7ᵗʰ **S31.522** Laceration with foreign body of unspecified external genital organs, female　♀

✓6ᵗʰ **S31.53** Puncture wound without foreign body of unspecified external genital organs

✓7ᵗʰ **S31.531** Puncture wound without foreign body of unspecified external genital organs, male　♂

✓7ᵗʰ **S31.532** Puncture wound without foreign body of unspecified external genital organs, female　♀

✓6ᵗʰ **S31.54** Puncture wound with foreign body of unspecified external genital organs

✓7ᵗʰ **S31.541** Puncture wound with foreign body of unspecified external genital organs, male　♂

✓7ᵗʰ **S31.542** Puncture wound with foreign body of unspecified external genital organs, female　♀

✓6ᵗʰ **S31.55** Open bite of unspecified external genital organs
　Bite of unspecified external genital organs NOS
　EXCLUDES 1　superficial bite of unspecified external genital organs (S30.865, S30.866, S30.875, S30.876)

✓7ᵗʰ **S31.551** Open bite of unspecified external genital organs, male　♂

✓7ᵗʰ **S31.552** Open bite of unspecified external genital organs, female　♀

✓5ᵗʰ **S31.6** Open wound of abdominal wall with penetration into peritoneal cavity

✓6ᵗʰ **S31.60** Unspecified open wound of abdominal wall with penetration into peritoneal cavity

✓7ᵗʰ **S31.600** Unspecified open wound of abdominal wall, right upper quadrant with penetration into peritoneal cavity　MCC

✓7ᵗʰ **S31.601** Unspecified open wound of abdominal wall, left upper quadrant with penetration into peritoneal cavity　MCC

✓7ᵗʰ **S31.602** Unspecified open wound of abdominal wall, epigastric region with penetration into peritoneal cavity　MCC

✓7ᵗʰ **S31.603** Unspecified open wound of abdominal wall, right lower quadrant with penetration into peritoneal cavity　MCC

✓7ᵗʰ **S31.604** Unspecified open wound of abdominal wall, left lower quadrant with penetration into peritoneal cavity　MCC

✓7ᵗʰ **S31.605** Unspecified open wound of abdominal wall, periumbilic region with penetration into peritoneal cavity　MCC

N Newborn: 0　P Pediatric: 0-17　M Maternity: 12-55　A Adult: 15-124　MCC Major CC Condition　PDx MCC PDx acts as own MCC　CC CC Condition　PDx CC PDx acts as own CC

972　　　　　ICD-10-CM 2018

√7ᵗʰ **S31.609** **Unspecified open wound of** `MCC` **abdominal wall,** unspecified quadrant **with penetration into peritoneal cavity**

√6ᵗʰ **S31.61** Laceration without foreign body **of abdominal wall with penetration into peritoneal cavity**

√7ᵗʰ **S31.610** **Laceration without foreign body of** `MCC` **abdominal wall,** right upper quadrant **with penetration into peritoneal cavity**

√7ᵗʰ **S31.611** **Laceration without foreign body of** `MCC` **abdominal wall,** left upper quadrant **with penetration into peritoneal cavity**

√7ᵗʰ **S31.612** **Laceration without foreign body of** `MCC` **abdominal wall,** epigastric region **with penetration into peritoneal cavity**

√7ᵗʰ **S31.613** **Laceration without foreign body of** `MCC` **abdominal wall,** right lower quadrant **with penetration into peritoneal cavity**

√7ᵗʰ **S31.614** **Laceration without foreign body of** `MCC` **abdominal wall,** left lower quadrant **with penetration into peritoneal cavity**

√7ᵗʰ **S31.615** **Laceration without foreign body of** `MCC` **abdominal wall,** periumbilic region **with penetration into peritoneal cavity**

√7ᵗʰ **S31.619** **Laceration without foreign body of** `MCC` **abdominal wall,** unspecified quadrant **with penetration into peritoneal cavity**

√6ᵗʰ **S31.62** Laceration with foreign body **of abdominal wall with penetration into peritoneal cavity**

√7ᵗʰ **S31.620** **Laceration with foreign body of** `MCC` **abdominal wall,** right upper quadrant **with penetration into peritoneal cavity**

√7ᵗʰ **S31.621** **Laceration with foreign body of** `MCC` **abdominal wall,** left upper quadrant **with penetration into peritoneal cavity**

√7ᵗʰ **S31.622** **Laceration with foreign body of** `MCC` **abdominal wall,** epigastric region **with penetration into peritoneal cavity**

√7ᵗʰ **S31.623** **Laceration with foreign body of** `MCC` **abdominal wall,** right lower quadrant **with penetration into peritoneal cavity**

√7ᵗʰ **S31.624** **Laceration with foreign body of** `MCC` **abdominal wall,** left lower quadrant **with penetration into peritoneal cavity**

√7ᵗʰ **S31.625** **Laceration with foreign body of** `MCC` **abdominal wall,** periumbilic region **with penetration into peritoneal cavity**

√7ᵗʰ **S31.629** **Laceration with foreign body of** `MCC` **abdominal wall,** unspecified quadrant **with penetration into peritoneal cavity**

√6ᵗʰ **S31.63** Puncture wound without foreign body **of abdominal wall with penetration into peritoneal cavity**

√7ᵗʰ **S31.630** **Puncture wound without foreign** `MCC` **body of abdominal wall,** right upper quadrant **with penetration into peritoneal cavity**

√7ᵗʰ **S31.631** **Puncture wound without foreign** `MCC` **body of abdominal wall,** left upper quadrant **with penetration into peritoneal cavity**

√7ᵗʰ **S31.632** **Puncture wound without foreign** `MCC` **body of abdominal wall,** epigastric region **with penetration into peritoneal cavity**

√7ᵗʰ **S31.633** **Puncture wound without foreign** `MCC` **body of abdominal wall,** right lower quadrant **with penetration into peritoneal cavity**

√7ᵗʰ **S31.634** **Puncture wound without foreign** `MCC` **body of abdominal wall,** left lower quadrant **with penetration into peritoneal cavity**

√7ᵗʰ **S31.635** **Puncture wound without foreign** `MCC` **body of abdominal wall,** periumbilic region **with penetration into peritoneal cavity**

√7ᵗʰ **S31.639** **Puncture wound without foreign** `MCC` **body of abdominal wall,** unspecified quadrant **with penetration into peritoneal cavity**

√6ᵗʰ **S31.64** Puncture wound with foreign body **of abdominal wall with penetration into peritoneal cavity**

√7ᵗʰ **S31.640** **Puncture wound with foreign body** `MCC` **of abdominal wall,** right upper quadrant **with penetration into peritoneal cavity**

√7ᵗʰ **S31.641** **Puncture wound with foreign body** `MCC` **of abdominal wall,** left upper quadrant **with penetration into peritoneal cavity**

√7ᵗʰ **S31.642** **Puncture wound with foreign body** `MCC` **of abdominal wall,** epigastric region **with penetration into peritoneal cavity**

√7ᵗʰ **S31.643** **Puncture wound with foreign body** `MCC` **of abdominal wall,** right lower quadrant **with penetration into peritoneal cavity**

√7ᵗʰ **S31.644** **Puncture wound with foreign body** `MCC` **of abdominal wall,** left lower quadrant **with penetration into peritoneal cavity**

√7ᵗʰ **S31.645** **Puncture wound with foreign body** `MCC` **of abdominal wall,** periumbilic region **with penetration into peritoneal cavity**

√7ᵗʰ **S31.649** **Puncture wound with foreign body** `MCC` **of abdominal wall,** unspecified quadrant **with penetration into peritoneal cavity**

√6ᵗʰ **S31.65** Open bite **of abdominal wall with penetration into peritoneal cavity**

> `EXCLUDES 1` *superficial bite of abdominal wall (S30.861, S30.871)*

√7ᵗʰ **S31.650** **Open bite of abdominal wall,** right `MCC` upper quadrant **with penetration into peritoneal cavity**

√7ᵗʰ **S31.651** **Open bite of abdominal wall,** left `MCC` upper quadrant **with penetration into peritoneal cavity**

√7ᵗʰ **S31.652** **Open bite of abdominal wall,** `MCC` epigastric region **with penetration into peritoneal cavity**

√7ᵗʰ **S31.653** **Open bite of abdominal wall,** right `MCC` lower quadrant **with penetration into peritoneal cavity**

√7ᵗʰ **S31.654** **Open bite of abdominal wall,** left `MCC` lower quadrant **with penetration into peritoneal cavity**

√7ᵗʰ **S31.655** **Open bite of abdominal wall,** `MCC` periumbilic region **with penetration into peritoneal cavity**

√7ᵗʰ **S31.659** **Open bite of abdominal wall,** `MCC` unspecified quadrant **with penetration into peritoneal cavity**

√5ᵗʰ **S31.8** **Open wound of other parts of abdomen, lower back and pelvis**

√6ᵗʰ **S31.80** **Open wound of** unspecified buttock

√7ᵗʰ **S31.801** Laceration without foreign body **of unspecified buttock**

√7ᵗʰ **S31.802** Laceration with foreign body **of unspecified buttock**

√7ᵗʰ **S31.803** Puncture wound without foreign body **of unspecified buttock**

√7ᵗʰ **S31.804** Puncture wound with foreign body **of unspecified buttock**

√7ᵗʰ **S31.805** Open bite **of unspecified buttock**
Bite of buttock NOS
> `EXCLUDES 1` *superficial bite of buttock (S30.870)*

√7ᵗʰ **S31.809** Unspecified **open wound of unspecified buttock**

√6ᵗʰ **S31.81** **Open wound of** right buttock

√7ᵗʰ **S31.811** Laceration without foreign body **of right buttock**

√7ᵗʰ **S31.812** Laceration with foreign body **of right buttock**

√7ᵗʰ **S31.813** Puncture wound without foreign body **of right buttock**

√7ᵗʰ **S31.814** Puncture wound with foreign body **of right buttock**

√7ᵗʰ **S31.815** Open bite **of right buttock**
Bite of right buttock NOS
> `EXCLUDES 1` *superficial bite of buttock (S30.870)*

☑Additional Character Req   √ₓ7ᵗʰ Placeholder Alert   Unacceptable PDx   Manifestation   **H1**-**H14** HAC   `HCC` CMS-HCC Condition   *EXCLUDES 1* Not Coded Here   *EXCLUDES 2* Not Included Here

Chapter 19. Injury, Poisoning and Certain Other Consequences of External Causes

☑7ᵗʰ **S31.819**   **Unspecified open wound of right buttock**

☑6ᵗʰ **S31.82**   **Open wound of** left buttock

☑7ᵗʰ **S31.821**   **Laceration without foreign body of left buttock**

☑7ᵗʰ **S31.822**   **Laceration with foreign body of left buttock**

☑7ᵗʰ **S31.823**   **Puncture wound without foreign body of left buttock**

☑7ᵗʰ **S31.824**   **Puncture wound with foreign body of left buttock**

☑7ᵗʰ **S31.825**   **Open bite of left buttock**
    Bite of left buttock NOS
    EXCLUDES 1   superficial bite of buttock (S30.870)

☑7ᵗʰ **S31.829**   **Unspecified open wound of left buttock**

☑6ᵗʰ **S31.83**   **Open wound of anus**

☑7ᵗʰ **S31.831**   **Laceration without foreign body of anus**

☑7ᵗʰ **S31.832**   **Laceration with foreign body of anus**

☑7ᵗʰ **S31.833**   **Puncture wound without foreign body of anus**

☑7ᵗʰ **S31.834**   **Puncture wound with foreign body of anus**

☑7ᵗʰ **S31.835**   **Open bite of anus**
    Bite of anus NOS
    EXCLUDES 1   superficial bite of anus (S30.877)

☑7ᵗʰ **S31.839**   **Unspecified open wound of anus**

☑4ᵗʰ **S32**   **Fracture of lumbar spine and pelvis**

NOTE   A fracture not indicated as displaced or nondisplaced should be coded to displaced.
A fracture not indicated as opened or closed should be coded to closed.

INCLUDES   fracture of lumbosacral neural arch
fracture of lumbosacral spinous process
fracture of lumbosacral transverse process
fracture of lumbosacral vertebra
fracture of lumbosacral vertebral arch

Code first any associated spinal cord and spinal nerve injury (S34.-)

EXCLUDES 1   transection of abdomen (S38.3)
EXCLUDES 2   fracture of hip NOS (S72.0-)
AHA: 2015, 3Q, 37-39; 2012, 4Q, 93

The appropriate 7th character is to be added to each code from category S32.
A   initial encounter for closed fracture
B   initial encounter for open fracture
D   subsequent encounter for fracture with routine healing
G   subsequent encounter for fracture with delayed healing
K   subsequent encounter for fracture with nonunion
S   sequela

☑5ᵗʰ **S32.0**   **Fracture of** lumbar vertebra
Fracture of lumbar spine NOS

CC Excl: For codes in subcategory S32.0:
CC with 7th character A or MCC with 7th character B:
PDX collection 1196
CC with 7th character K: PDX collection 897

☑6ᵗʰ **S32.00**   **Fracture of unspecified lumbar vertebra**

6,7,10 ☑7ᵗʰ **S32.000**   **Wedge compression fracture of unspecified lumbar vertebra**   MCC CC H5 HCC

6,7,10 ☑7ᵗʰ **S32.001**   **Stable burst fracture of unspecified lumbar vertebra**   MCC CC H5 HCC

6,7,10 ☑7ᵗʰ **S32.002**   **Unstable burst fracture of unspecified lumbar vertebra**   MCC CC H5 HCC

6,7,10 ☑7ᵗʰ **S32.008**   **Other fracture of unspecified lumbar vertebra**   MCC CC H5 HCC

6,7,10 ☑7ᵗʰ **S32.009**   **Unspecified fracture of unspecified lumbar vertebra**   MCC CC H5 HCC

☑6ᵗʰ **S32.01**   **Fracture of** first **lumbar vertebra**

6,7,10 ☑7ᵗʰ **S32.010**   **Wedge compression fracture of first lumbar vertebra**   MCC CC H5 HCC

6,7,10 ☑7ᵗʰ **S32.011**   **Stable burst fracture of first lumbar vertebra**   MCC CC H5 HCC

6,7,10 ☑7ᵗʰ **S32.012**   **Unstable burst fracture of first lumbar vertebra**   MCC CC H5 HCC

6,7,10 ☑7ᵗʰ **S32.018**   **Other fracture of first lumbar vertebra**   MCC CC H5 HCC

6,7,10 ☑7ᵗʰ **S32.019**   **Unspecified fracture of first lumbar vertebra**   MCC CC H5 HCC

☑6ᵗʰ **S32.02**   **Fracture of** second **lumbar vertebra**

6,7,10 ☑7ᵗʰ **S32.020**   **Wedge compression fracture of second lumbar vertebra**   MCC CC H5 HCC

6,7,10 ☑7ᵗʰ **S32.021**   **Stable burst fracture of second lumbar vertebra**   MCC CC H5 HCC

6,7,10 ☑7ᵗʰ **S32.022**   **Unstable burst fracture of second lumbar vertebra**   MCC CC H5 HCC

6,7,10 ☑7ᵗʰ **S32.028**   **Other fracture of second lumbar vertebra**   MCC CC H5 HCC

6,7,10 ☑7ᵗʰ **S32.029**   **Unspecified fracture of second lumbar vertebra**   MCC CC H5 HCC

☑6ᵗʰ **S32.03**   **Fracture of** third **lumbar vertebra**

6,7,10 ☑7ᵗʰ **S32.030**   **Wedge compression fracture of third lumbar vertebra**   MCC CC H5 HCC

6,7,10 ☑7ᵗʰ **S32.031**   **Stable burst fracture of third lumbar vertebra**   MCC CC H5 HCC

6,7,10 ☑7ᵗʰ **S32.032**   **Unstable burst fracture of third lumbar vertebra**   MCC CC H5 HCC

6,7,10 ☑7ᵗʰ **S32.038**   **Other fracture of third lumbar vertebra**   MCC CC H5 HCC

6,7,10 ☑7ᵗʰ **S32.039**   **Unspecified fracture of third lumbar vertebra**   MCC CC H5 HCC

☑6ᵗʰ **S32.04**   **Fracture of** fourth **lumbar vertebra**

6,7,10 ☑7ᵗʰ **S32.040**   **Wedge compression fracture of fourth lumbar vertebra**   MCC CC H5 HCC

6,7,10 ☑7ᵗʰ **S32.041**   **Stable burst fracture of fourth lumbar vertebra**   MCC CC H5 HCC

6,7,10 ☑7ᵗʰ **S32.042**   **Unstable burst fracture of fourth lumbar vertebra**   MCC CC H5 HCC

6,7,10 ☑7ᵗʰ **S32.048**   **Other fracture of fourth lumbar vertebra**   MCC CC H5 HCC

6,7,10 ☑7ᵗʰ **S32.049**   **Unspecified fracture of fourth lumbar vertebra**   MCC CC H5 HCC

☑6ᵗʰ **S32.05**   **Fracture of** fifth **lumbar vertebra**

6,7,10 ☑7ᵗʰ **S32.050**   **Wedge compression fracture of fifth lumbar vertebra**   MCC CC H5 HCC

6,7,10 ☑7ᵗʰ **S32.051**   **Stable burst fracture of fifth lumbar vertebra**   MCC CC H5 HCC

6,7,10 ☑7ᵗʰ **S32.052**   **Unstable burst fracture of fifth lumbar vertebra**   MCC CC H5 HCC

6,7,10 ☑7ᵗʰ **S32.058**   **Other fracture of fifth lumbar vertebra**   MCC CC H5 HCC

6,7,10 ☑7ᵗʰ **S32.059**   **Unspecified fracture of fifth lumbar vertebra**   MCC CC H5 HCC

☑5ᵗʰ **S32.1**   **Fracture of** sacrum
NOTE   For vertical fractures, code to most medial fracture extension.
Use two codes if both a vertical and transverse fracture are present.
Code also any associated fracture of pelvic ring (S32.8-)

CC Excl: For codes in subcategory S32.1:
CC with 7th character A or MCC with 7th character B:
PDX collection 1197
CC with 7th character K: PDX collection 897

6,7,10 ☑x7ᵗʰ **S32.10**   **Unspecified fracture of sacrum**   MCC CC H5 HCC

☑6ᵗʰ **S32.11**   **Zone I fracture of sacrum**
Vertical sacral ala fracture of sacrum

6,7,10 ☑7ᵗʰ **S32.110**   **Nondisplaced Zone I fracture of sacrum**   MCC CC H5 HCC

6,7,10 ☑7ᵗʰ **S32.111**   **Minimally displaced Zone I fracture of sacrum**   MCC CC H5 HCC

6,7,10 ☑7ᵗʰ **S32.112**   **Severely displaced Zone I fracture of sacrum**   MCC CC H5 HCC

---

6   MCC when reported as an open fracture (7th character B or C – specific to category).
7   CC when reported as an initial encounter (7th character A, B, or C – specific to category) OR a subsequent encounter for nonunion or malunion (7th character K, M, N, P, Q, or R – specific to category).
10   HCC with 7th character indicating initial encounter (A, B or C - specific to category).

N Newborn: 0   P Pediatric: 0-17   M Maternity: 12-55   A Adult: 15-124   MCC Major CC Condition   PDxMCC PDx acts as own MCC   CC CC Condition   PDxCC PDx acts as own CC

974   **ICD-10-CM 2018**

Vertical Sacral Fracture Zones

Zones: ① ② ③

Transverse Sacral Fracture Types

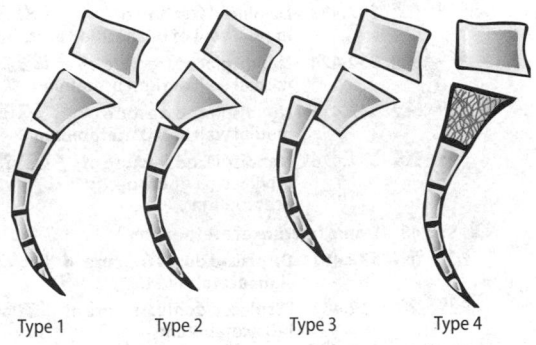

Type 1   Type 2   Type 3   Type 4

6,7,10 √7th **S32.119** Unspecified **Zone I fracture** MCC CC H5 HCC
of sacrum

√6th **S32.12** **Zone II fracture of sacrum**
Vertical foraminal region fracture of sacrum

6,7,10 √7th **S32.120** **Nondisplaced Zone II** MCC CC H5 HCC
fracture of sacrum

6,7,10 √7th **S32.121** **Minimally displaced Zone II** MCC CC H5 HCC
fracture of sacrum

6,7,10 √7th **S32.122** **Severely displaced Zone II** MCC CC H5 HCC
fracture of sacrum

6,7,10 √7th **S32.129** **Unspecified Zone II fracture** MCC CC H5 HCC
of sacrum

√6th **S32.13** **Zone III fracture of sacrum**
Vertical fracture into spinal canal region of sacrum

6,7,10 √7th **S32.130** **Nondisplaced Zone III** MCC CC H5 HCC
fracture of sacrum

6,7,10 √7th **S32.131** **Minimally displaced Zone III** MCC CC H5 HCC
fracture of sacrum

6,7,10 √7th **S32.132** **Severely displaced Zone III** MCC CC H5 HCC
fracture of sacrum

6,7,10 √7th **S32.139** **Unspecified Zone III** MCC CC H5 HCC
fracture of sacrum

6,7,10 √x7th **S32.14** **Type 1 fracture of sacrum** MCC CC H5 HCC
Transverse flexion fracture of sacrum without
displacement

6,7,10 √x7th **S32.15** **Type 2 fracture of sacrum** MCC CC H5 HCC
Transverse flexion fracture of sacrum with posterior
displacement

6,7,10 √x7th **S32.16** **Type 3 fracture of sacrum** MCC CC H5 HCC
Transverse extension fracture of sacrum with anterior
displacement

6,7,10 √x7th **S32.17** **Type 4 fracture of sacrum** MCC CC H5 HCC
Transverse segmental comminution of upper sacrum

6,7,10 √x7th **S32.19** **Other fracture of sacrum** MCC CC H5 HCC

6,7,10 √7th **S32.2** **Fracture of coccyx** MCC CC H5 HCC
CC Excl: See code S32.1

√5th **S32.3** **Fracture of ilium**
> *EXCLUDES 1*   fracture of ilium with associated disruption of pelvic
> ring (S32.8-)

> **CC Excl: For codes in subcategory S32.3:**
> **CC with 7th character A:** PDX collection 1176
> **MCC with 7th character B:** PDX collection 1198
> **CC with 7th character K:** PDX collection 897

√6th **S32.30** **Unspecified fracture of ilium**

6,7,10 √7th **S32.301** **Unspecified fracture of** MCC CC H5 HCC
right ilium

6,7,10 √7th **S32.302** **Unspecified fracture of** left MCC CC H5 HCC
ilium

6,7,10 √7th **S32.309** **Unspecified fracture of** MCC CC H5 HCC
unspecified ilium

√6th **S32.31** **Avulsion fracture of ilium**

6,7,10 √7th **S32.311** **Displaced avulsion fracture** MCC CC H5 HCC
of right ilium

6,7,10 √7th **S32.312** **Displaced avulsion fracture** MCC CC H5 HCC
of left **ilium**

6,7,10 √7th **S32.313** **Displaced avulsion fracture** MCC CC H5 HCC
of unspecified ilium

6,7,10 √7th **S32.314** **Nondisplaced avulsion** MCC CC H5 HCC
fracture of right ilium

6,7,10 √7th **S32.315** **Nondisplaced avulsion** MCC CC H5 HCC
fracture of left **ilium**

6,7,10 √7th **S32.316** **Nondisplaced avulsion** MCC CC H5 HCC
fracture of unspecified ilium

√6th **S32.39** **Other fracture of ilium**

6,7,10 √7th **S32.391** **Other fracture of right ilium** MCC CC H5 HCC

6,7,10 √7th **S32.392** **Other fracture of** left **ilium** MCC CC H5 HCC

6,7,10 √7th **S32.399** **Other fracture of** MCC CC H5 HCC
unspecified ilium

√5th **S32.4** **Fracture of acetabulum**
Code also any associated fracture of pelvic ring (S32.8-)
AHA: 2016, 3Q, 16

> **CC Excl: For codes in subcategory S32.4:**
> **MCC with 7th character A:** PDX collection 1199
> **MCC with 7th character B:** PDX collection 1200
> **CC with 7th character K:** PDX collection 897

√6th **S32.40** **Unspecified fracture of acetabulum**

8,10 √7th **S32.401** **Unspecified fracture of** MCC CC H5 HCC
right acetabulum

8,10 √7th **S32.402** **Unspecified fracture of** MCC CC H5 HCC
left acetabulum

8,10 √7th **S32.409** **Unspecified fracture of** MCC CC H5 HCC
unspecified acetabulum

√6th **S32.41** **Fracture of anterior wall of acetabulum**

8,10 √7th **S32.411** **Displaced fracture of** MCC CC H5 HCC
anterior wall of right
acetabulum

8,10 √7th **S32.412** **Displaced fracture of** MCC CC H5 HCC
anterior wall of left
acetabulum

8,10 √7th **S32.413** **Displaced fracture of** MCC CC H5 HCC
anterior wall of unspecified
acetabulum

8,10 √7th **S32.414** **Nondisplaced fracture of** MCC CC H5 HCC
anterior wall of right
acetabulum

8,10 √7th **S32.415** **Nondisplaced fracture of** MCC CC H5 HCC
anterior wall of left **acetabulum**

8,10 √7th **S32.416** **Nondisplaced fracture of** MCC CC H5 HCC
anterior wall of unspecified
acetabulum

√6th **S32.42** **Fracture of posterior wall of acetabulum**

8,10 √7th **S32.421** **Displaced fracture of** MCC CC H5 HCC
posterior wall of right
acetabulum

---

6   MCC when reported as an open fracture (7th character B or C – specific to category).
7   CC when reported as an initial encounter (7th character A, B, or C – specific to category) OR a subsequent encounter for nonunion or malunion
    (7th character K, M, N, P, Q, or R – specific to category).
8   CC when reported as a subsequent encounter for nonunion or malunion (7th character K, M, N, P, Q, or R – specific to category).
10   HCC with 7th character indicating initial encounter (A, B or C - specific to category).

✓ Additional Character Req   √x7th Placeholder Alert   Unacceptable PDx   Manifestation   H1-H14 HAC   HCC CMS-HCC Condition   *EXCLUDES 1* Not Coded Here   *EXCLUDES 2* Not Included Here

8,10 ✓7ᵗʰ **S32.422** Displaced **fracture** of **posteriorwall** of **left acetabulum** `MCC` `CC` `H5` `HCC`

8,10 ✓7ᵗʰ **S32.423** Displaced **fracture** of **posterior wall** of **unspecified acetabulum** `MCC` `CC` `H5` `HCC`

8,10 ✓7ᵗʰ **S32.424** Nondisplaced **fracture** of **posterior wall** of **right acetabulum** `MCC` `CC` `H5` `HCC`

8,10 ✓7ᵗʰ **S32.425** Nondisplaced **fracture** of **posterior wall** of **left acetabulum** `MCC` `CC` `H5` `HCC`

8,10 ✓7ᵗʰ **S32.426** Nondisplaced **fracture** of **posterior wall** of **unspecified acetabulum** `MCC` `CC` `H5` `HCC`

✓6ᵗʰ **S32.43** Fracture of **anterior column [iliopubic]** of **acetabulum**

8,10 ✓7ᵗʰ **S32.431** Displaced **fracture** of **anterior column [iliopubic]** of **right acetabulum** `MCC` `CC` `H5` `HCC`

8,10 ✓7ᵗʰ **S32.432** Displaced **fracture** of **anterior column [iliopubic]** of **left acetabulum** `MCC` `CC` `H5` `HCC`

8,10 ✓7ᵗʰ **S32.433** Displaced **fracture** of **anterior column [iliopubic]** of **unspecified acetabulum** `MCC` `CC` `H5` `HCC`

8,10 ✓7ᵗʰ **S32.434** Nondisplaced **fracture** of **anterior column [iliopubic]** of **right acetabulum** `MCC` `CC` `H5` `HCC`

8,10 ✓7ᵗʰ **S32.435** Nondisplaced **fracture** of **anterior column [iliopubic]** of **left acetabulum** `MCC` `CC` `H5` `HCC`

8,10 ✓7ᵗʰ **S32.436** Nondisplaced **fracture** of **anterior column [iliopubic]** of **unspecified acetabulum** `MCC` `CC` `H5` `HCC`

✓6ᵗʰ **S32.44** Fracture of **posterior column [ilioischial]** of **acetabulum**

8,10 ✓7ᵗʰ **S32.441** Displaced **fracture** of **posterior column [ilioischial]** of **right acetabulum** `MCC` `CC` `H5` `HCC`

8,10 ✓7ᵗʰ **S32.442** Displaced **fracture** of **posteriorcolumn [ilioischial]** of **left acetabulum** `MCC` `CC` `H5` `HCC`

8,10 ✓7ᵗʰ **S32.443** Displaced **fracture** of **posterior column [ilioischial]** of **unspecified acetabulum** `MCC` `CC` `H5` `HCC`

8,10 ✓7ᵗʰ **S32.444** Nondisplaced **fracture** of **posterior column [ilioischial]** of **right acetabulum** `MCC` `CC` `H5` `HCC`

8,10 ✓7ᵗʰ **S32.445** Nondisplaced **fracture** of **posterior column [ilioischial]** of **left acetabulum** `MCC` `CC` `H5` `HCC`

8,10 ✓7ᵗʰ **S32.446** Nondisplaced **fracture** of **posterior column [ilioischial]** of **unspecified acetabulum** `MCC` `CC` `H5` `HCC`

✓6ᵗʰ **S32.45** Transverse **fracture** of **acetabulum**

8,10 ✓7ᵗʰ **S32.451** Displaced **transverse fracture** of **right acetabulum** `MCC` `CC` `H5` `HCC`

8,10 ✓7ᵗʰ **S32.452** Displaced **transverse fractureof** **left acetabulum** `MCC` `CC` `H5` `HCC`

8,10 ✓7ᵗʰ **S32.453** Displaced **transverse fracture** of **unspecified acetabulum** `MCC` `CC` `H5` `HCC`

8,10 ✓7ᵗʰ **S32.454** Nondisplaced **transverse fracture** of **right acetabulum** `MCC` `CC` `H5` `HCC`

8,10 ✓7ᵗʰ **S32.455** Nondisplaced **transverse fracture** of **left acetabulum** `MCC` `CC` `H5` `HCC`

8,10 ✓7ᵗʰ **S32.456** Nondisplaced **transverse fracture** of **unspecified acetabulum** `MCC` `CC` `H5` `HCC`

✓6ᵗʰ **S32.46** Associated **transverse-posterior fracture** of **acetabulum**

8,10 ✓7ᵗʰ **S32.461** Displaced **associated transverse-posterior fracture** of **right acetabulum** `MCC` `CC` `H5` `HCC`

8,10 ✓7ᵗʰ **S32.462** Displaced **associated transverse-posterior fracture** of **left acetabulum** `MCC` `CC` `H5` `HCC`

8,10 ✓7ᵗʰ **S32.463** Displaced **associated transverse-posterior fracture** of **unspecified acetabulum** `MCC` `CC` `H5` `HCC`

8,10 ✓7ᵗʰ **S32.464** Nondisplaced **associated transverse-posterior fracture** of **right acetabulum** `MCC` `CC` `H5` `HCC`

8,10 ✓7ᵗʰ **S32.465** Nondisplaced **associated transverse-posterior fracture** of **left acetabulum** `MCC` `CC` `H5` `HCC`

8,10 ✓7ᵗʰ **S32.466** Nondisplaced **associated transverse-posterior fracture** of **unspecified acetabulum** `MCC` `CC` `H5` `HCC`

✓6ᵗʰ **S32.47** Fracture of **medial wall** of **acetabulum**

8,10 ✓7ᵗʰ **S32.471** Displaced **fracture** of **medial wall** of **right acetabulum** `MCC` `CC` `H5` `HCC`

8,10 ✓7ᵗʰ **S32.472** Displaced **fracture** of **medial wall** of **left acetabulum** `MCC` `CC` `H5` `HCC`

8,10 ✓7ᵗʰ **S32.473** Displaced **fracture** of **medial wall** of **unspecified acetabulum** `MCC` `CC` `H5` `HCC`

8,10 ✓7ᵗʰ **S32.474** Nondisplaced **fracture** of **medial wall** of **right acetabulum** `MCC` `CC` `H5` `HCC`

8,10 ✓7ᵗʰ **S32.475** Nondisplaced **fracture** of **medial wall** of **left acetabulum** `MCC` `CC` `H5` `HCC`

8,10 ✓7ᵗʰ **S32.476** Nondisplaced **fracture** of **medial wall** of **unspecified acetabulum** `MCC` `CC` `H5` `HCC`

✓6ᵗʰ **S32.48** Dome fracture of acetabulum

8,10 ✓7ᵗʰ **S32.481** Displaced **dome fracture** of **right acetabulum** `MCC` `CC` `H5` `HCC`

8,10 ✓7ᵗʰ **S32.482** Displaced **dome fracture** of **left acetabulum** `MCC` `CC` `H5` `HCC`

8,10 ✓7ᵗʰ **S32.483** Displaced **dome fracture** of **unspecified acetabulum** `MCC` `CC` `H5` `HCC`

8,10 ✓7ᵗʰ **S32.484** Nondisplaced **dome fracture** of **right acetabulum** `MCC` `CC` `H5` `HCC`

8,10 ✓7ᵗʰ **S32.485** Nondisplaced **dome fracture** of **left acetabulum** `MCC` `CC` `H5` `HCC`

8,10 ✓7ᵗʰ **S32.486** Nondisplaced **dome fracture** of **unspecified acetabulum** `MCC` `CC` `H5` `HCC`

✓6ᵗʰ **S32.49** Other specified fracture of acetabulum

8,10 ✓7ᵗʰ **S32.491** Other specified **fracture** of **right acetabulum** `MCC` `CC` `H5` `HCC`

8,10 ✓7ᵗʰ **S32.492** Other specified **fracture** of **left acetabulum** `MCC` `CC` `H5` `HCC`

8,10 ✓7ᵗʰ **S32.499** Other specified **fracture** of **unspecified acetabulum** `MCC` `CC` `H5` `HCC`

✓5ᵗʰ **S32.5** Fracture of **pubis**

EXCLUDES 1 *fracture of pubis with associated disruption of pelvic ring (S32.8-)*

CC Excl: For codes in subcategory S32.5:
CC with 7th character A or MCC with 7th character B: PDX collection 1201
CC with 7th character K: PDX collection 897

✓6ᵗʰ **S32.50** Unspecified **fracture of pubis**

6,7,10 ✓7ᵗʰ **S32.501** Unspecified **fracture** of **right pubis** `MCC` `CC` `HCC`

6,7,10 ✓7ᵗʰ **S32.502** Unspecified **fracture** of **left pubis** `MCC` `CC` `H5` `HCC`

6,7,10 ✓7ᵗʰ **S32.509** Unspecified **fracture** of **unspecified pubis** `MCC` `CC` `H5` `HCC`

✓6ᵗʰ **S32.51** Fracture of **superior rim** of **pubis**

6,7,10 ✓7ᵗʰ **S32.511** Fracture of **superior rim** of **right pubis** `MCC` `CC` `H5` `HCC`

6,7,10 ✓7ᵗʰ **S32.512** Fracture of **superior rim** of **left pubis** `MCC` `CC` `H5` `HCC`

6,7,10 ✓7ᵗʰ **S32.519** Fracture of **superior rim** of **unspecified pubis** `MCC` `CC` `H5` `HCC`

---

6 MCC when reported as an open fracture (7th character B or C – specific to category).

7 CC when reported as an initial encounter (7th character A, B, or C – specific to category) OR a subsequent encounter for nonunion or malunion (7th character K, M, N, P, Q, or R – specific to category).

8 CC when reported as a subsequent encounter for nonunion or malunion (7th character K, M, N, P, Q, or R – specific to category).

10 HCC with 7th character indicating initial encounter (A, B or C - specific to category).

`N` Newborn: 0 `P` Pediatric: 0-17 `M` Maternity: 12-55 `A` Adult: 15-124 `MCC` Major CC Condition `PDxMCC` PDx acts as own MCC `CC` CC Condition `PDxCC` PDx acts as own CC

√6ᵗʰ **S32.59** Other specified fracture of pubis

6,7,10 √7ᵗʰ **S32.591** Other specified fracture of right pubis `MCC` `CC` `H5` `HCC`

6,7,10 √7ᵗʰ **S32.592** Other specified fracture of left pubis `MCC` `CC` `H5` `HCC`

6,7,10 √7ᵗʰ **S32.599** Other specified fracture of unspecified pubis `MCC` `CC` `H5` `HCC`

√5ᵗʰ **S32.6** Fracture of ischium

> EXCLUDES 1   fracture of ischium with associated disruption of pelvic ring (S32.8-)

> CC Excl: For codes in subcategory S32.6:
> CC with 7th character A: PDX collection 1202
> MCC with 7th character B: PDX collection 1203
> CC with 7th character K: PDX collection 897

√6ᵗʰ **S32.60** Unspecified fracture of ischium

6,7,10 √7ᵗʰ **S32.601** Unspecified fracture of right ischium `MCC` `CC` `H5` `HCC`

6,7,10 √7ᵗʰ **S32.602** Unspecified fracture of left ischium `MCC` `CC` `H5` `HCC`

6,7,10 √7ᵗʰ **S32.609** Unspecified fracture of unspecified ischium `MCC` `CC` `H5` `HCC`

√6ᵗʰ **S32.61** Avulsion fracture of ischium

6,7,10 √7ᵗʰ **S32.611** Displaced avulsion fracture of right ischium `MCC` `CC` `H5` `HCC`

6,7,10 √7ᵗʰ **S32.612** Displaced avulsion fracture of left ischium `MCC` `CC` `H5` `HCC`

6,7,10 √7ᵗʰ **S32.613** Displaced avulsion fracture of unspecified ischium `MCC` `CC` `H5` `HCC`

6,7,10 √7ᵗʰ **S32.614** Nondisplaced avulsion fracture of right ischium `MCC` `CC` `H5` `HCC`

6,7,10 √7ᵗʰ **S32.615** Nondisplaced avulsion fracture of left ischium `MCC` `CC` `H5` `HCC`

6,7,10 √7ᵗʰ **S32.616** Nondisplaced avulsion fracture of unspecified ischium `MCC` `CC` `H5` `HCC`

√6ᵗʰ **S32.69** Other specified fracture of ischium

6,7,10 √7ᵗʰ **S32.691** Other specified fracture of right ischium `MCC` `CC` `H5` `HCC`

6,7,10 √7ᵗʰ **S32.692** Other specified fracture of left ischium `MCC` `CC` `H5` `HCC`

6,7,10 √7ᵗʰ **S32.699** Other specified fracture of unspecified ischium `MCC` `CC` `H5` `HCC`

√5ᵗʰ **S32.8** Fracture of other parts of pelvis

> Code also any associated:
> fracture of acetabulum (S32.4-)
> sacral fracture (S32.1-)

√6ᵗʰ **S32.81** Multiple fractures of pelvis with disruption of pelvic ring

> Multiple pelvic fractures with disruption of pelvic circle

> CC Excl: For codes in subcategory S32.81:
> CC with 7th character A or MCC with 7th character B: PDX collection 1204
> CC with 7th character K: PDX collection 897

6,7,10 √7ᵗʰ **S32.810** Multiple fractures of pelvis with stable disruption of pelvic ring `MCC` `CC` `H5` `HCC`

Fractures Disrupting Pelvic Circle

Stable

Unstable
(two-place fracture)

Iliac crest
Anterior superior iliac spine
Ischial spine
Acetabulum
Femur
Ischium
Pelvic circle
Ilium
L5
Sacrum
Coccyx
Pubis
Pubic symphysis
Pelvic Bones

6,7,10 √7ᵗʰ **S32.811** Multiple fractures of pelvis with unstable disruption of pelvic ring `MCC` `CC` `H5` `HCC`

6,7,10 √x7ᵗʰ **S32.82** Multiple fractures of pelvis without disruption of pelvic ring `MCC` `CC` `H5` `HCC`

> Multiple pelvic fractures without disruption of pelvic circle

> CC Excl: CC with 7th character A or MCC with 7th character B: PDX collection 1205
> CC with 7th character K: PDX collection 897

6,7,10 √x7ᵗʰ **S32.89** Fracture of other parts of pelvis `MCC` `CC` `H5` `HCC`

> CC Excl: CC with 7th character A or MCC with 7th character B: PDX collection 1206
> CC with 7th character K: PDX collection 897

6,7,10 √x7ᵗʰ **S32.9** Fracture of unspecified parts of lumbosacral spine and pelvis `MCC` `CC` `H5` `HCC`

> Fracture of lumbosacral spine NOS
> Fracture of pelvis NOS
> **AHA:** 2012, 4Q, 93
> CC Excl: CC with 7th character A or MCC with 7th character B: PDX collection 1204
> CC with 7th character K: PDX collection 897

√4ᵗʰ **S33** Dislocation and sprain of joints and ligaments of lumbar spine and pelvis

> INCLUDES   avulsion of joint or ligament of lumbar spine and pelvis
> laceration of cartilage, joint or ligament of lumbar spine and pelvis
> sprain of cartilage, joint or ligament of lumbar spine and pelvis
> traumatic hemarthrosis of joint or ligament of lumbar spine and pelvis
> traumatic rupture of joint or ligament of lumbar spine and pelvis
> traumatic subluxation of joint or ligament of lumbar spine and pelvis
> traumatic tear of joint or ligament of lumbar spine and pelvis

> Code also any associated open wound

> EXCLUDES 1   nontraumatic rupture or displacement of lumbar intervertebral disc NOS (M51.-)
> obstetric damage to pelvic joints and ligaments (O71.6)

> EXCLUDES 2   dislocation and sprain of joints and ligaments of hip (S73.-)
> strain of muscle of lower back and pelvis (S39.01-)

> The appropriate 7th character is to be added to each code from category S33.
> A   initial encounter
> D   subsequent encounter
> S   sequela

√x7ᵗʰ **S33.0** Traumatic rupture of lumbar intervertebral disc

> EXCLUDES 1   rupture or displacement (nontraumatic) of lumbar intervertebral disc NOS (M51- with fifth character 6)

√5ᵗʰ **S33.1** Subluxation and dislocation of lumbar vertebra

> Code also any associated:
> open wound of abdomen, lower back and pelvis (S31)
> spinal cord injury (S24.0, S24.1-, S34.0-, S34.1-)

> EXCLUDES 2   fracture of lumbar vertebrae (S32.0-)

√6ᵗʰ **S33.10** Subluxation and dislocation of unspecified lumbar vertebra

√7ᵗʰ **S33.100** Subluxation of unspecified lumbar vertebra

√7ᵗʰ **S33.101** Dislocation of unspecified lumbar vertebra

√6ᵗʰ **S33.11** Subluxation and dislocation of L1/L2 lumbar vertebra

√7ᵗʰ **S33.110** Subluxation of L1/L2 lumbar vertebra

√7ᵗʰ **S33.111** Dislocation of L1/L2 lumbar vertebra

√6ᵗʰ **S33.12** Subluxation and dislocation of L2/L3 lumbar vertebra

√7ᵗʰ **S33.120** Subluxation of L2/L3 lumbar vertebra

√7ᵗʰ **S33.121** Dislocation of L2/L3 lumbar vertebra

√6ᵗʰ **S33.13** Subluxation and dislocation of L3/L4 lumbar vertebra

√7ᵗʰ **S33.130** Subluxation of L3/L4 lumbar vertebra

√7ᵗʰ **S33.131** Dislocation of L3/L4 lumbar vertebra

---

6   MCC when reported as an open fracture (7th character B or C – specific to category).

7   CC when reported as an initial encounter (7th character A, B, or C – specific to category) OR a subsequent encounter for nonunion or malunion (7th character K, M, N, P, Q, or R – specific to category).

10   HCC with 7th character indicating initial encounter (A, B or C - specific to category).

✓ Additional Character Req   √x7ᵗʰ Placeholder Alert   Unacceptable PDx   Manifestation   `H1`–`H14` HAC   `HCC` CMS-HCC Condition   EXCLUDES 1 Not Coded Here   EXCLUDES 2 Not Included Here

√6ᵗʰ **S33.14** **Subluxation and dislocation of** L4/L5 **lumbar vertebra**

√7ᵗʰ **S33.140** Subluxation of L4/L5 lumbar vertebra

√7ᵗʰ **S33.141** Dislocation of L4/L5 lumbar vertebra

√x7ᵗʰ **S33.2** **Dislocation of** sacroiliac **and** sacrococcygeal **joint**

√5ᵗʰ **S33.3** **Dislocation of** other and unspecified parts **of lumbar spine and pelvis**

√x7ᵗʰ **S33.30** **Dislocation of** unspecified **parts of lumbar spine and pelvis**

√x7ᵗʰ **S33.39** **Dislocation of** other **parts of lumbar spine and pelvis**

√x7ᵗʰ **S33.4** **Traumatic rupture of** symphysis pubis

√x7ᵗʰ **S33.5** **Sprain of ligaments of** lumbar spine

√x7ᵗʰ **S33.6** **Sprain of** sacroiliac joint

√x7ᵗʰ **S33.8** **Sprain of** other **parts of lumbar spine and pelvis**

√x7ᵗʰ **S33.9** **Sprain of** unspecified **parts of lumbar spine and pelvis**

√4ᵗʰ **S34** **Injury of lumbar and sacral spinal cord and nerves at abdomen, lower back and pelvis level**

> **NOTE**   Code to highest level of lumbar cord injury.
> Injuries to the spinal cord (S34.0 and S34.1) refer to the cord level and not bone level injury, and can affect nerve roots at and below the level given.

Code also any associated:
   fracture of vertebra (S22.0-, S32.0-)
   open wound of abdomen, lower back and pelvis (S31.-)
   transient paralysis (R29.5)

The appropriate 7th character is to be added to each code from category S34.
A   initial encounter
D   subsequent encounter
S   sequela

CC Excl: For codes in category S34 unless otherwise noted: MCC with 7th character A: PDX collection 1207

√5ᵗʰ **S34.0** **Concussion and edema of lumbar and sacral spinal cord**

√x7ᵗʰ **S34.01** **Concussion and edema of** lumbar **spinal cord** `MCC` `HCC`

√x7ᵗʰ **S34.02** **Concussion and edema of** sacral **spinal cord** `MCC` `HCC`
Concussion and edema of conus medullaris
CC Excl: MCC with 7th character A: PDX collection 1208

√5ᵗʰ **S34.1** **Other and unspecified injury of lumbar and sacral spinal cord**

√6ᵗʰ **S34.10** **Unspecified injury to lumbar spinal cord**

√7ᵗʰ **S34.101** **Unspecified injury to** L1 level **of lumbar spinal cord** `MCC` `H5` `HCC`
Unspecified injury to lumbar spinal cord level 1

√7ᵗʰ **S34.102** **Unspecified injury to** L2 level **of lumbar spinal cord** `MCC` `H5` `HCC`
Unspecified injury to lumbar spinal cord level 2

√7ᵗʰ **S34.103** **Unspecified injury to** L3 level **of lumbar spinal cord** `MCC` `H5` `HCC`
Unspecified injury to lumbar spinal cord level 3

√7ᵗʰ **S34.104** **Unspecified injury to** L4 level **of lumbar spinal cord** `MCC` `H5` `HCC`
Unspecified injury to lumbar spinal cord level 4

√7ᵗʰ **S34.105** **Unspecified injury to** L5 level **of lumbar spinal cord** `MCC` `H5` `HCC`
Unspecified injury to lumbar spinal cord level 5

√7ᵗʰ **S34.109** **Unspecified injury to** unspecified level **of lumbar spinal cord** `MCC` `H5` `HCC`

√6ᵗʰ **S34.11** **Complete lesion of lumbar spinal cord**

√7ᵗʰ **S34.111** **Complete lesion of** L1 level **of lumbar spinal cord** `MCC` `H5` `HCC`
Complete lesion of lumbar spinal cord level 1

√7ᵗʰ **S34.112** **Complete lesion of** L2 level **of lumbar spinal cord** `MCC` `H5` `HCC`
Complete lesion of lumbar spinal cord level 2

√7ᵗʰ **S34.113** **Complete lesion of** L3 level **of lumbar spinal cord** `MCC` `H5` `HCC`
Complete lesion of lumbar spinal cord level 3

√7ᵗʰ **S34.114** **Complete lesion of** L4 level **of lumbar spinal cord** `MCC` `H5` `HCC`
Complete lesion of lumbar spinal cord level 4

√7ᵗʰ **S34.115** **Complete lesion of** L5 level **of lumbar spinal cord** `MCC` `H5` `HCC`
Complete lesion of lumbar spinal cord level 5

√7ᵗʰ **S34.119** **Complete lesion of** unspecified level **of lumbar spinal cord** `MCC` `H5` `HCC`

√6ᵗʰ **S34.12** **Incomplete lesion of lumbar spinal cord**

√7ᵗʰ **S34.121** **Incomplete lesion of** L1 level **of lumbar spinal cord** `MCC` `H5` `HCC`
Incomplete lesion of lumbar spinal cord level 1

√7ᵗʰ **S34.122** **Incomplete lesion of** L2 level **of lumbar spinal cord** `MCC` `H5` `HCC`
Incomplete lesion of lumbar spinal cord level 2

√7ᵗʰ **S34.123** **Incomplete lesion of** L3 level **of lumbar spinal cord** `MCC` `H5` `HCC`
Incomplete lesion of lumbar spinal cord level 3

√7ᵗʰ **S34.124** **Incomplete lesion of** L4 level **of lumbar spinal cord** `MCC` `H5` `HCC`
Incomplete lesion of lumbar spinal cord level 4

√7ᵗʰ **S34.125** **Incomplete lesion of** L5 level **of lumbar spinal cord** `MCC` `H5` `HCC`
Incomplete lesion of lumbar spinal cord level 5

√7ᵗʰ **S34.129** **Incomplete lesion of** unspecified level **of lumbar spinal cord** `MCC` `H5` `HCC`

√6ᵗʰ **S34.13** **Other and unspecified injury to** sacral **spinal cord**
Other injury to conus medullaris

CC Excl: For codes in subcategory S34.13: MCC with 7th character A: PDX collection 1208

√7ᵗʰ **S34.131** **Complete lesion of sacral spinal cord** `MCC` `H5` `HCC`
Complete lesion of conus medullaris

√7ᵗʰ **S34.132** **Incomplete lesion of sacral spinal cord** `MCC` `H5` `HCC`
Incomplete lesion of conus medullaris

√7ᵗʰ **S34.139** **Unspecified injury to sacral spinal cord** `MCC` `H5` `HCC`
Unspecified injury of conus medullaris

√5ᵗʰ **S34.2** **Injury of nerve root of lumbar and sacral spine**

√x7ᵗʰ **S34.21** **Injury of nerve root of** lumbar spine

√x7ᵗʰ **S34.22** **Injury of nerve root of** sacral spine

10 √x7ᵗʰ **S34.3** **Injury of cauda equina** `MCC` `H5` `HCC`
CC Excl: MCC with 7th character A: PDX collection 1208

√x7ᵗʰ **S34.4** **Injury of lumbosacral plexus**

√x7ᵗʰ **S34.5** **Injury of lumbar, sacral and pelvic sympathetic nerves**
Injury of celiac ganglion or plexus
Injury of hypogastric plexus
Injury of mesenteric plexus (inferior) (superior)
Injury of splanchnic nerve

√x7ᵗʰ **S34.6** **Injury of peripheral nerve(s) at abdomen, lower back and pelvis level**

√x7ᵗʰ **S34.8** **Injury of other nerves at abdomen, lower back and pelvis level**

√x7ᵗʰ **S34.9** **Injury of unspecified nerves at abdomen, lower back and pelvis level**

---

10 HCC with 7th character indicating initial encounter (A, B or C - specific to category).

Ⓝ Newborn: 0   Ⓟ Pediatric: 0-17   Ⓜ Maternity: 12-55   Ⓐ Adult: 15-124   `MCC` Major CC Condition   `PDxMCC` PDx acts as own MCC   `CC` CC Condition   `PDxCC` PDx acts as own CC

978   ICD-10-CM 2018

✓4ᵗʰ **S35**   **Injury of blood vessels at abdomen, lower back and pelvis level**
> Code also any associated open wound (S31.-)

> The appropriate 7th character is to be added to each code from category S35.
> A   initial encounter
> D   subsequent encounter
> S   sequela

✓5ᵗʰ **S35.0**   **Injury of** abdominal aorta
> *EXCLUDES 1*   injury of aorta NOS (S25.0)

> **CC Excl: For codes in subcategory S35.0:**
> MCC with 7th character A: PDX collection 1209

   ✓x7ᵗʰ **S35.00**   **Unspecified injury of** abdominal aorta   **MCC**

   ✓x7ᵗʰ **S35.01**   **Minor laceration of** abdominal aorta   **MCC**
> Incomplete transection of abdominal aorta
> Laceration of abdominal aorta NOS
> Superficial laceration of abdominal aorta

   ✓x7ᵗʰ **S35.02**   **Major laceration of** abdominal aorta   **MCC**
> Complete transection of abdominal aorta
> Traumatic rupture of abdominal aorta

   ✓x7ᵗʰ **S35.09**   **Other injury of** abdominal aorta   **MCC**

✓5ᵗʰ **S35.1**   **Injury of** inferior vena cava
> Injury of hepatic vein
> *EXCLUDES 1*   injury of vena cava NOS (S25.2)

> **CC Excl: For codes in subcategory S35.1:**
> MCC with 7th character A: PDX collection 1210

   ✓x7ᵗʰ **S35.10**   **Unspecified injury of** inferior vena cava   **MCC**

   ✓x7ᵗʰ **S35.11**   **Minor laceration of** inferior vena cava   **MCC**
> Incomplete transection of inferior vena cava
> Laceration of inferior vena cava NOS
> Superficial laceration of inferior vena cava

   ✓x7ᵗʰ **S35.12**   **Major laceration of** inferior vena cava   **MCC**
> Complete transection of inferior vena cava
> Traumatic rupture of inferior vena cava

   ✓x7ᵗʰ **S35.19**   **Other injury of** inferior vena cava   **MCC**

✓5ᵗʰ **S35.2**   **Injury of celiac or mesenteric artery and branches**

   ✓6ᵗʰ **S35.21**   **Injury of** celiac artery

> **CC Excl: For codes in subcategory S35.21:**
> MCC with 7th character A: PDX collection 1211

     ✓7ᵗʰ **S35.211**   **Minor laceration of** celiac artery   **MCC**
> Incomplete transection of celiac artery
> Laceration of celiac artery NOS
> Superficial laceration of celiac artery

     ✓7ᵗʰ **S35.212**   **Major laceration of** celiac artery   **MCC**
> Complete transection of celiac artery
> Traumatic rupture of celiac artery

     ✓7ᵗʰ **S35.218**   **Other injury of** celiac artery   **MCC**

     ✓7ᵗʰ **S35.219**   **Unspecified injury of** celiac artery   **MCC**

   ✓6ᵗʰ **S35.22**   **Injury of** superior mesenteric artery

> **CC Excl: For codes in subcategory S35.22:**
> MCC with 7th character A: PDX collection 1212

     ✓7ᵗʰ **S35.221**   **Minor laceration of** superior mesenteric artery   **MCC**
> Incomplete transection of superior mesenteric artery
> Laceration of superior mesenteric artery NOS
> Superficial laceration of superior mesenteric artery

     ✓7ᵗʰ **S35.222**   **Major laceration of** superior mesenteric artery   **MCC**
> Complete transection of superior mesenteric artery
> Traumatic rupture of superior mesenteric artery

     ✓7ᵗʰ **S35.228**   **Other injury of** superior mesenteric artery   **MCC**

     ✓7ᵗʰ **S35.229**   **Unspecified injury of** superior mesenteric artery   **MCC**

   ✓6ᵗʰ **S35.23**   **Injury of** inferior mesenteric artery

> **CC Excl: For codes in subcategory S35.23:**
> MCC with 7th character A: PDX collection 1213

     ✓7ᵗʰ **S35.231**   **Minor laceration of** inferior mesenteric artery   **MCC**
> Incomplete transection of inferior mesenteric artery
> Laceration of inferior mesenteric artery NOS
> Superficial laceration of inferior mesenteric artery

     ✓7ᵗʰ **S35.232**   **Major laceration of** inferior mesenteric artery   **MCC**
> Complete transection of inferior mesenteric artery
> Traumatic rupture of inferior mesenteric artery

     ✓7ᵗʰ **S35.238**   **Other injury of** inferior mesenteric artery   **MCC**

     ✓7ᵗʰ **S35.239**   **Unspecified injury of** inferior mesenteric artery   **MCC**

   ✓6ᵗʰ **S35.29**   **Injury of** branches of celiac and mesenteric artery
> Injury of gastric artery
> Injury of gastroduodenal artery
> Injury of hepatic artery
> Injury of splenic artery

     ✓7ᵗʰ **S35.291**   **Minor laceration of branches of celiac and mesenteric artery**   **MCC**
> Incomplete transection of branches of celiac and mesenteric artery
> Laceration of branches of celiac and mesenteric artery NOS
> Superficial laceration of branches of celiac and mesenteric artery
> **CC Excl: MCC with 7th character A:**
> PDX collection 1214

     ✓7ᵗʰ **S35.292**   **Major laceration of branches of celiac and mesenteric artery**   **MCC**
> Complete transection of branches of celiac and mesenteric artery
> Traumatic rupture of branches of celiac and mesenteric artery
> **CC Excl: MCC with 7th character A:**
> PDX collection 1215

     ✓7ᵗʰ **S35.298**   **Other injury of branches of celiac and mesenteric artery**   **MCC**
> **CC Excl: MCC with 7th character A:**
> PDX collection 1215

     ✓7ᵗʰ **S35.299**   **Unspecified injury of branches of celiac and mesenteric artery**   **MCC**
> **CC Excl: MCC with 7th character A:**
> PDX collection 1216

✓5ᵗʰ **S35.3**   **Injury of portal or splenic vein and branches**

   ✓6ᵗʰ **S35.31**   **Injury of** portal vein

> **CC Excl: For codes in subcategory S35.31:**
> MCC with 7th character A: PDX collection 1217

     ✓7ᵗʰ **S35.311**   **Laceration of** portal vein   **MCC**

     ✓7ᵗʰ **S35.318**   **Other specified injury of** portal vein   **MCC**

     ✓7ᵗʰ **S35.319**   **Unspecified injury of** portal vein   **MCC**

   ✓6ᵗʰ **S35.32**   **Injury of** splenic vein

> **CC Excl: For codes in subcategory S35.32:**
> MCC with 7th character A: PDX collection 1218

     ✓7ᵗʰ **S35.321**   **Laceration of** splenic vein   **MCC**

     ✓7ᵗʰ **S35.328**   **Other specified injury of** splenic vein   **MCC**

     ✓7ᵗʰ **S35.329**   **Unspecified injury of** splenic vein   **MCC**

   ✓6ᵗʰ **S35.33**   **Injury of** superior mesenteric vein

> **CC Excl: For codes in subcategory S35.33:**
> MCC with 7th character A: PDX collection 1219

     ✓7ᵗʰ **S35.331**   **Laceration of** superior mesenteric vein   **MCC**

     ✓7ᵗʰ **S35.338**   **Other specified injury of** superior mesenteric vein   **MCC**

     ✓7ᵗʰ **S35.339**   **Unspecified injury of** superior mesenteric vein   **MCC**

✓Additional Character Req   ✓x7ᵗʰ Placeholder Alert   Unacceptable PDx   Manifestation   H1-H14 HAC   HCC CMS-HCC Condition   *EXCLUDES 1* Not Coded Here   *EXCLUDES 2* Not Included Here

ICD-10-CM 2018   979

Chapter 19. Injury, Poisoning and Certain Other Consequences of External Causes

√6ᵗʰ **S35.34** Injury of inferior mesenteric vein

> CC Excl: For codes in subcategory S35.34: MCC with 7th character A: PDX collection 1220

√7ᵗʰ **S35.341** Laceration of inferior mesenteric vein `MCC`

√7ᵗʰ **S35.348** Other specified injury of inferior mesenteric vein `MCC`

√7ᵗʰ **S35.349** Unspecified injury of inferior mesenteric vein `MCC`

√5ᵗʰ **S35.4** Injury of renal blood vessels

> CC Excl: For codes in subcategory S35.4, unless otherwise noted: MCC with 7th character A: PDX collection 1221

√6ᵗʰ **S35.40** Unspecified injury of renal blood vessel

√7ᵗʰ **S35.401** Unspecified injury of right renal artery `MCC`

√7ᵗʰ **S35.402** Unspecified injury of left renal artery `MCC`

√7ᵗʰ **S35.403** Unspecified injury of unspecified renal artery `MCC`

√7ᵗʰ **S35.404** Unspecified injury of right renal vein `MCC`
> CC Excl: MCC with 7th character A: PDX collection 1222

√7ᵗʰ **S35.405** Unspecified injury of left renal vein `MCC`
> CC Excl: MCC with 7th character A: PDX collection 1222

√7ᵗʰ **S35.406** Unspecified injury of unspecified renal vein `MCC`
> CC Excl: MCC with 7th character A: PDX collection 1222

√6ᵗʰ **S35.41** Laceration of renal blood vessel

√7ᵗʰ **S35.411** Laceration of right renal artery `MCC`

√7ᵗʰ **S35.412** Laceration of left renal artery `MCC`

√7ᵗʰ **S35.413** Laceration of unspecified renal artery `MCC`

√7ᵗʰ **S35.414** Laceration of right renal vein `MCC`
> CC Excl: MCC with 7th character A: PDX collection 1222

√7ᵗʰ **S35.415** Laceration of left renal vein `MCC`
> CC Excl: MCC with 7th character A: PDX collection 1222

√7ᵗʰ **S35.416** Laceration of unspecified renal vein `MCC`
> CC Excl: MCC with 7th character A: PDX collection 1222

√6ᵗʰ **S35.49** Other specified injury of renal blood vessel

√7ᵗʰ **S35.491** Other specified injury of right renal artery `MCC`

√7ᵗʰ **S35.492** Other specified injury of left renal artery `MCC`

√7ᵗʰ **S35.493** Other specified injury of unspecified renal artery `MCC`

√7ᵗʰ **S35.494** Other specified injury of right renal vein `MCC`
> CC Excl: MCC with 7th character A: PDX collection 1222

√7ᵗʰ **S35.495** Other specified injury of left renal vein `MCC`
> CC Excl: MCC with 7th character A: PDX collection 1222

√7ᵗʰ **S35.496** Other specified injury of unspecified renal vein `MCC`
> CC Excl: MCC with 7th character A: PDX collection 1222

√5ᵗʰ **S35.5** Injury of iliac blood vessels

√x7ᵗʰ **S35.50** Injury of unspecified iliac blood vessel(s) `MCC`
> CC Excl: MCC with 7th character A: PDX collection 1223

√6ᵗʰ **S35.51** Injury of iliac artery or vein
> Injury of hypogastric artery or vein

√7ᵗʰ **S35.511** Injury of right iliac artery `MCC`
> CC Excl: MCC with 7th character A: PDX collection 1224

√7ᵗʰ **S35.512** Injury of left iliac artery `MCC`
> CC Excl: MCC with 7th character A: PDX collection 1224

√7ᵗʰ **S35.513** Injury of unspecified iliac artery `MCC`
> CCC Excl: MCC with 7th character A: PDX collection 1224

√7ᵗʰ **S35.514** Injury of right iliac vein `MCC`
> CC Excl: MCC with 7th character A: PDX collection 1225

√7ᵗʰ **S35.515** Injury of left iliac vein `MCC`
> CC Excl: MCC with 7th character A: PDX collection 1225

√7ᵗʰ **S35.516** Injury of unspecified iliac vein `MCC`
> CC Excl: MCC with 7th character A: PDX collection 1225

√6ᵗʰ **S35.53** Injury of uterine artery or vein

√7ᵗʰ **S35.531** Injury of right uterine artery `CC` ♀
> CC Excl: CC with 7th character A: PDX collection 1226

√7ᵗʰ **S35.532** Injury of left uterine artery `CC` ♀
> CC Excl: CC with 7th character A: PDX collection 1226

√7ᵗʰ **S35.533** Injury of unspecified uterine artery `CC` ♀
> CC Excl: CC with 7th character A: PDX collection 1226

√7ᵗʰ **S35.534** Injury of right uterine vein `CC` ♀
> CC Excl: CC with 7th character A: PDX collection 1227

√7ᵗʰ **S35.535** Injury of left uterine vein `CC` ♀
> CC Excl: CC with 7th character A: PDX collection 1227

√7ᵗʰ **S35.536** Injury of unspecified uterine vein `CC` ♀
> CC Excl: CC with 7th character A: PDX collection 1227

√x7ᵗʰ **S35.59** Injury of other iliac blood vessels `MCC`
> CC Excl: MCC with 7th character A: PDX collection 1223

√5ᵗʰ **S35.8** Injury of other blood vessels at abdomen, lower back and pelvis level
> Injury of ovarian artery or vein

√6ᵗʰ **S35.8X** Injury of other blood vessels at abdomen, lower back and pelvis level

> CC Excl: For codes in subcategory S35.8X: CC with 7th character A: PDX collection 1228

√7ᵗʰ **S35.8X1** Laceration of other blood vessels at abdomen, lower back and pelvis level `CC`

√7ᵗʰ **S35.8X8** Other specified injury of other blood vessels at abdomen, lower back and pelvis level `CC`

√7ᵗʰ **S35.8X9** Unspecified injury of other blood vessels at abdomen, lower back and pelvis level `CC`

√5ᵗʰ **S35.9** Injury of unspecified blood vessel at abdomen, lower back and pelvis level

> CC Excl: For codes in subcategory S35.9: CC with 7th character A: PDX collection 1229

√x7ᵗʰ **S35.90** Unspecified injury of unspecified blood vessel at abdomen, lower back and pelvis level `CC`

√x7ᵗʰ **S35.91** Laceration of unspecified blood vessel at abdomen, lower back and pelvis level `CC`

√x7ᵗʰ **S35.99** Other specified injury of unspecified blood vessel at abdomen, lower back and pelvis level `CC`

√4ᵗʰ **S36** Injury of intra-abdominal organs
> Code also any associated open wound (S31.-)

> The appropriate 7th character is to be added to each code from category S36.
> A   initial encounter
> D   subsequent encounter
> S   sequela

√5ᵗʰ **S36.0** Injury of spleen
> AHA: 2015, 2Q, 36; 2015, 1Q, 10

> CC Excl: For codes in subcategory S36.0: CC or MCC with 7th character A: PDX collection 1230

√x7ᵗʰ **S36.00** Unspecified injury of spleen `CC`

√6ᵗʰ **S36.02** Contusion of spleen

√7ᵗʰ **S36.020** Minor contusion of spleen `CC`
> Contusion of spleen less than 2 cm

√7ᵗʰ **S36.021** Major contusion of spleen `CC`
> Contusion of spleen greater than 2 cm

√7ᵗʰ **S36.029** Unspecified contusion of spleen `CC`

Ⓝ Newborn: 0   Ⓟ Pediatric: 0-17   Ⓜ Maternity: 12-55   Ⓐ Adult: 15-124   `MCC` Major CC Condition   `PDxMCC` PDx acts as own MCC   `CC` CC Condition   `PDxCC` PDx acts as own CC

980   ICD-10-CM 2018

✓6th **S36.03** Laceration of spleen

  ✓7th **S36.030** Superficial (capsular) laceration of spleen   `CC`
    Laceration of spleen less than 1cm
    Minor laceration of spleen

  ✓7th **S36.031** Moderate laceration of spleen   `MCC`
    Laceration of spleen 1 to 3 cm

  ✓7th **S36.032** Major laceration of spleen   `MCC`
    Avulsion of spleen
    Laceration of spleen greater than 3 cm
    Massive laceration of spleen
    Multiple moderate lacerations of spleen
    Stellate laceration of spleen

  ✓7th **S36.039** Unspecified laceration of spleen   `CC`

✓x7th **S36.09** Other injury of spleen   `CC`

✓5th **S36.1** Injury of liver and gallbladder and bile duct

  ✓6th **S36.11** Injury of liver

> **CC Excl:** For codes in subcategory S36.11:
> CC or MCC with 7th character A:
> PDX collection 1231

  ✓7th **S36.112** Contusion of liver   `CC`

  ✓7th **S36.113** Laceration of liver, unspecified degree   `CC`

  ✓7th **S36.114** Minor laceration of liver   `CC`
    Laceration involving capsule only, or, without significant involvement of hepatic parenchyma [i.e., less than 1cm deep]

  ✓7th **S36.115** Moderate laceration of liver   `MCC`
    Laceration involving parenchyma but without major disruption of parenchyma [i.e., less than 10 cm long and less than 3 cm deep]

  ✓7th **S36.116** Major laceration of liver   `MCC`
    Laceration with significant disruption of hepatic parenchyma [i.e., greater than 10 cm long and 3 cm deep]
    Multiple moderate lacerations, with or without hematoma
    Stellate laceration of liver

  ✓7th **S36.118** Other injury of liver   `CC`

  ✓7th **S36.119** Unspecified injury of liver   `CC`

  ✓6th **S36.12** Injury of gallbladder

> **CC Excl:** For codes in subcategory S36.12:
> CC with 7th character A: PDX collection 1232

  ✓7th **S36.122** Contusion of gallbladder   `CC`

  ✓7th **S36.123** Laceration of gallbladder   `CC`

  ✓7th **S36.128** Other injury of gallbladder   `CC`

  ✓7th **S36.129** Unspecified injury of gallbladder   `CC`

  ✓x7th **S36.13** Injury of bile duct   `CC`
    CC Excl: CC with 7th character A: PDX collection 1232

✓5th **S36.2** Injury of pancreas

> **CC Excl:** For codes in subcategory S36.2:
> CC with 7th character A: PDX collection 1233

  ✓6th **S36.20** Unspecified injury of pancreas

  ✓7th **S36.200** Unspecified injury of head of pancreas   `CC`

  ✓7th **S36.201** Unspecified injury of body of pancreas   `CC`

  ✓7th **S36.202** Unspecified injury of tail of pancreas   `CC`

  ✓7th **S36.209** Unspecified injury of unspecified part of pancreas   `CC`

  ✓6th **S36.22** Contusion of pancreas

  ✓7th **S36.220** Contusion of head of pancreas   `CC`

  ✓7th **S36.221** Contusion of body of pancreas   `CC`

  ✓7th **S36.222** Contusion of tail of pancreas   `CC`

  ✓7th **S36.229** Contusion of unspecified part of pancreas   `CC`

  ✓6th **S36.23** Laceration of pancreas, unspecified degree

  ✓7th **S36.230** Laceration of head of pancreas, unspecified degree   `CC`

  ✓7th **S36.231** Laceration of body of pancreas, unspecified degree   `CC`

  ✓7th **S36.232** Laceration of tail of pancreas, unspecified degree   `CC`

  ✓7th **S36.239** Laceration of unspecified part of pancreas, unspecified degree   `CC`

  ✓6th **S36.24** Minor laceration of pancreas

  ✓7th **S36.240** Minor laceration of head of pancreas   `CC`

  ✓7th **S36.241** Minor laceration of body of pancreas   `CC`

  ✓7th **S36.242** Minor laceration of tail of pancreas   `CC`

  ✓7th **S36.249** Minor laceration of unspecified part of pancreas   `CC`

  ✓6th **S36.25** Moderate laceration of pancreas

  ✓7th **S36.250** Moderate laceration of head of pancreas   `CC`

  ✓7th **S36.251** Moderate laceration of body of pancreas   `CC`

  ✓7th **S36.252** Moderate laceration of tail of pancreas   `CC`

  ✓7th **S36.259** Moderate laceration of unspecified part of pancreas   `CC`

  ✓6th **S36.26** Major laceration of pancreas

  ✓7th **S36.260** Major laceration of head of pancreas   `CC`

  ✓7th **S36.261** Major laceration of body of pancreas   `CC`

  ✓7th **S36.262** Major laceration of tail of pancreas   `CC`

  ✓7th **S36.269** Major laceration of unspecified part of pancreas   `CC`

  ✓6th **S36.29** Other injury of pancreas

  ✓7th **S36.290** Other injury of head of pancreas   `CC`

  ✓7th **S36.291** Other injury of body of pancreas   `CC`

  ✓7th **S36.292** Other injury of tail of pancreas   `CC`

  ✓7th **S36.299** Other injury of unspecified part of pancreas   `CC`

✓5th **S36.3** Injury of stomach

> **CC Excl:** For codes in subcategory S36.3:
> CC with 7th character A: PDX collection 1234

  ✓x7th **S36.30** Unspecified injury of stomach   `CC`

  ✓x7th **S36.32** Contusion of stomach   `CC`

  ✓x7th **S36.33** Laceration of stomach   `CC`

  ✓x7th **S36.39** Other injury of stomach   `CC`

✓5th **S36.4** Injury of small intestine

> **CC Excl:** For codes in subcategory S36.4:
> CC with 7th character A: PDX collection 1235

  ✓6th **S36.40** Unspecified injury of small intestine

  ✓7th **S36.400** Unspecified injury of duodenum   `CC`

  ✓7th **S36.408** Unspecified injury of other part of small intestine   `CC`

  ✓7th **S36.409** Unspecified injury of unspecified part of small intestine   `CC`

  ✓6th **S36.41** Primary blast injury of small intestine
    Blast injury of small intestine NOS

  ✓7th **S36.410** Primary blast injury of duodenum   `CC`

  ✓7th **S36.418** Primary blast injury of other part of small intestine   `CC`

  ✓7th **S36.419** Primary blast injury of unspecified part of small intestine   `CC`

  ✓6th **S36.42** Contusion of small intestine

  ✓7th **S36.420** Contusion of duodenum   `CC`

  ✓7th **S36.428** Contusion of other part of small intestine   `CC`

  ✓7th **S36.429** Contusion of unspecified part of small intestine   `CC`

  ✓6th **S36.43** Laceration of small intestine

  ✓7th **S36.430** Laceration of duodenum   `CC`

  ✓7th **S36.438** Laceration of other part of small intestine   `CC`

  ✓7th **S36.439** Laceration of unspecified part of small intestine   `CC`

  ✓6th **S36.49** Other injury of small intestine

  ✓7th **S36.490** Other injury of duodenum   `CC`

  ✓7th **S36.498** Other injury of other part of small intestine   `CC`

  ✓7th **S36.499** Other injury of unspecified part of small intestine   `CC`

✓ Additional Character Req   ✓x7th Placeholder Alert   Unacceptable PDx   Manifestation   `H1`-`H14` HAC   `HCC` CMS-HCC Condition   *EXCLUDES 1* Not Coded Here   *EXCLUDES 2* Not Included Here

Chapter 19. Injury, Poisoning and Certain Other Consequences of External Causes

S36.5–S37.062

√5ᵗʰ **S36.5 Injury of colon**

> EXCLUDES 2   injury of rectum (S36.6-)

> **CC Excl: For codes in subcategory S36.5:**
> **CC with 7th character A:** PDX collection 1236

√6ᵗʰ **S36.50 Unspecified injury of colon**

√7ᵗʰ **S36.500 Unspecified injury of ascending [right] colon** CC

√7ᵗʰ **S36.501 Unspecified injury of transverse colon** CC

√7ᵗʰ **S36.502 Unspecified injury of descending [left] colon** CC

√7ᵗʰ **S36.503 Unspecified injury of sigmoid colon** CC

√7ᵗʰ **S36.508 Unspecified injury of other part of colon** CC

√7ᵗʰ **S36.509 Unspecified injury of unspecified part of colon** CC

√6ᵗʰ **S36.51 Primary blast injury of colon**
Blast injury of colon NOS

√7ᵗʰ **S36.510 Primary blast injury of ascending [right] colon** CC

√7ᵗʰ **S36.511 Primary blast injury of transverse colon** CC

√7ᵗʰ **S36.512 Primary blast injury of descending [left] colon** CC

√7ᵗʰ **S36.513 Primary blast injury of sigmoid colon** CC

√7ᵗʰ **S36.518 Primary blast injury of other part of colon** CC

√7ᵗʰ **S36.519 Primary blast injury of unspecified part of colon** CC

√6ᵗʰ **S36.52 Contusion of colon**

√7ᵗʰ **S36.520 Contusion of ascending [right] colon** CC

√7ᵗʰ **S36.521 Contusion of transverse colon** CC

√7ᵗʰ **S36.522 Contusion of descending [left] colon** CC

√7ᵗʰ **S36.523 Contusion of sigmoid colon** CC

√7ᵗʰ **S36.528 Contusion of other part of colon** CC

√7ᵗʰ **S36.529 Contusion of unspecified part of colon** CC

√6ᵗʰ **S36.53 Laceration of colon**

√7ᵗʰ **S36.530 Laceration of ascending [right] colon** CC

√7ᵗʰ **S36.531 Laceration of transverse colon** CC

√7ᵗʰ **S36.532 Laceration of descending [left] colon** CC

√7ᵗʰ **S36.533 Laceration of sigmoid colon** CC

√7ᵗʰ **S36.538 Laceration of other part of colon** CC

√7ᵗʰ **S36.539 Laceration of unspecified part of colon** CC

√6ᵗʰ **S36.59 Other injury of colon**
Secondary blast injury of colon

√7ᵗʰ **S36.590 Other injury of ascending [right] colon** CC

√7ᵗʰ **S36.591 Other injury of transverse colon** CC

√7ᵗʰ **S36.592 Other injury of descending [left] colon** CC

√7ᵗʰ **S36.593 Other injury of sigmoid colon** CC

√7ᵗʰ **S36.598 Other injury of other part of colon** CC

√7ᵗʰ **S36.599 Other injury of unspecified part of colon** CC

√5ᵗʰ **S36.6 Injury of rectum**

> **CC Excl: For codes in subcategory S36.6:**
> **CC with 7th character A:** PDX collection 1236

√x7ᵗʰ **S36.60 Unspecified injury of rectum** CC

√x7ᵗʰ **S36.61 Primary blast injury of rectum** CC
Blast injury of rectum NOS

√x7ᵗʰ **S36.62 Contusion of rectum** CC

√x7ᵗʰ **S36.63 Laceration of rectum** CC

√x7ᵗʰ **S36.69 Other injury of rectum** CC
Secondary blast injury of rectum

√5ᵗʰ **S36.8 Injury of other intra-abdominal organs**

> **CC Excl: For codes in subcategory S36.8:**
> **CC with 7th character A:** PDX collection 1195

√x7ᵗʰ **S36.81 Injury of peritoneum** CC

√6ᵗʰ **S36.89 Injury of other intra-abdominal organs**
Injury of retroperitoneum

√7ᵗʰ **S36.892 Contusion of other intra-abdominal organs** CC

√7ᵗʰ **S36.893 Laceration of other intra-abdominal organs** CC

√7ᵗʰ **S36.898 Other injury of other intra-abdominal organs** CC

√7ᵗʰ **S36.899 Unspecified injury of other intra-abdominal organs** CC

√5ᵗʰ **S36.9 Injury of unspecified intra-abdominal organ**

> **CC Excl: For codes in subcategory S36.9:**
> **CC with 7th character A:** PDX collection 1195

√x7ᵗʰ **S36.90 Unspecified injury of unspecified intra-abdominal organ** CC

√x7ᵗʰ **S36.92 Contusion of unspecified intra-abdominal organ** CC

√x7ᵗʰ **S36.93 Laceration of unspecified intra-abdominal organ** CC

√x7ᵗʰ **S36.99 Other injury of unspecified intra-abdominal organ** CC

√4ᵗʰ **S37 Injury of urinary and pelvic organs**
Code also any associated open wound (S31.-)

> EXCLUDES 1   obstetric trauma to pelvic organs (O71.-)

> EXCLUDES 2   injury of peritoneum (S36.81)
>   injury of retroperitoneum (S36.89-)

> The appropriate 7th character is to be added to each code from category S37.
> A   initial encounter
> D   subsequent encounter
> S   sequela

√5ᵗʰ **S37.0 Injury of kidney**

> EXCLUDES 2   acute kidney injury (nontraumatic) (N17.9)

> **CC Excl: For codes in subcategory S37.0:**
> **CC or MCC with 7th character A:** PDX collection 1237

√6ᵗʰ **S37.00 Unspecified injury of kidney**

√7ᵗʰ **S37.001 Unspecified injury of right kidney** CC

√7ᵗʰ **S37.002 Unspecified injury of left kidney** CC

√7ᵗʰ **S37.009 Unspecified injury of unspecified kidney** CC

√6ᵗʰ **S37.01 Minor contusion of kidney**
Contusion of kidney less than 2 cm
Contusion of kidney NOS

√7ᵗʰ **S37.011 Minor contusion of right kidney** CC

√7ᵗʰ **S37.012 Minor contusion of left kidney** CC

√7ᵗʰ **S37.019 Minor contusion of unspecified kidney** CC

√6ᵗʰ **S37.02 Major contusion of kidney**
Contusion of kidney greater than 2 cm

√7ᵗʰ **S37.021 Major contusion of right kidney** CC

√7ᵗʰ **S37.022 Major contusion of left kidney** CC

√7ᵗʰ **S37.029 Major contusion of unspecified kidney** CC

√6ᵗʰ **S37.03 Laceration of kidney, unspecified degree**

√7ᵗʰ **S37.031 Laceration of right kidney, unspecified degree** CC

√7ᵗʰ **S37.032 Laceration of left kidney, unspecified degree** CC

√7ᵗʰ **S37.039 Laceration of unspecified kidney, unspecified degree** CC

√6ᵗʰ **S37.04 Minor laceration of kidney**
Laceration of kidney less than 1 cm

√7ᵗʰ **S37.041 Minor laceration of right kidney** CC

√7ᵗʰ **S37.042 Minor laceration of left kidney** CC

√7ᵗʰ **S37.049 Minor laceration of unspecified kidney** CC

√6ᵗʰ **S37.05 Moderate laceration of kidney**
Laceration of kidney 1 to 3 cm

√7ᵗʰ **S37.051 Moderate laceration of right kidney** CC

√7ᵗʰ **S37.052 Moderate laceration of left kidney** CC

√7ᵗʰ **S37.059 Moderate laceration of unspecified kidney** CC

√6ᵗʰ **S37.06 Major laceration of kidney**
Avulsion of kidney
Laceration of kidney greater than 3 cm
Massive laceration of kidney
Multiple moderate lacerations of kidney
Stellate laceration of kidney

√7ᵗʰ **S37.061 Major laceration of right kidney** MCC

√7ᵗʰ **S37.062 Major laceration of left kidney** MCC

N Newborn: 0   P Pediatric: 0-17   M Maternity: 12-55   A Adult: 15-124   MCC Major CC Condition   PDxMCC PDx acts as own MCC   CC CC Condition   PDxCC PDx acts as own CC

982   ICD-10-CM 2018

√7ᵗʰ **S37.069** Major laceration of unspecified kidney   `MCC`

√6ᵗʰ **S37.09** Other injury of kidney

    √7ᵗʰ **S37.091** Other injury of right kidney   `MCC`

    √7ᵗʰ **S37.092** Other injury of left kidney   `MCC`

    √7ᵗʰ **S37.099** Other injury of unspecified kidney   `MCC`

√5ᵗʰ **S37.1** Injury of ureter

> **CC Excl: For codes in subcategory S37.1:**
> CC with 7th character A: PDX collection 1238

√x7ᵗʰ **S37.10** Unspecified injury of ureter   `CC`

√x7ᵗʰ **S37.12** Contusion of ureter   `CC`

√x7ᵗʰ **S37.13** Laceration of ureter   `CC`

√x7ᵗʰ **S37.19** Other injury of ureter   `CC`

√5ᵗʰ **S37.2** Injury of bladder

> **CC Excl: For codes in subcategory S37.2:**
> CC with 7th character A: PDX collection 1239

√x7ᵗʰ **S37.20** Unspecified injury of bladder   `CC`

√x7ᵗʰ **S37.22** Contusion of bladder   `CC`

√x7ᵗʰ **S37.23** Laceration of bladder   `CC`

√x7ᵗʰ **S37.29** Other injury of bladder   `CC`

√5ᵗʰ **S37.3** Injury of urethra

> **CC Excl: For codes in subcategory S37.3:**
> CC with 7th character A: PDX collection 1239

√x7ᵗʰ **S37.30** Unspecified injury of urethra   `CC`

√x7ᵗʰ **S37.32** Contusion of urethra   `CC`

√x7ᵗʰ **S37.33** Laceration of urethra   `CC`

√x7ᵗʰ **S37.39** Other injury of urethra   `CC`

√5ᵗʰ **S37.4** Injury of ovary

√6ᵗʰ **S37.40** Unspecified injury of ovary

    √7ᵗʰ **S37.401** Unspecified injury of ovary, unilateral ♀

    √7ᵗʰ **S37.402** Unspecified injury of ovary, bilateral ♀

    √7ᵗʰ **S37.409** Unspecified injury of ovary, unspecified ♀

√6ᵗʰ **S37.42** Contusion of ovary

    √7ᵗʰ **S37.421** Contusion of ovary, unilateral ♀

    √7ᵗʰ **S37.422** Contusion of ovary, bilateral ♀

    √7ᵗʰ **S37.429** Contusion of ovary, unspecified ♀

√6ᵗʰ **S37.43** Laceration of ovary

    √7ᵗʰ **S37.431** Laceration of ovary, unilateral ♀

    √7ᵗʰ **S37.432** Laceration of ovary, bilateral ♀

    √7ᵗʰ **S37.439** Laceration of ovary, unspecified ♀

√6ᵗʰ **S37.49** Other injury of ovary

    √7ᵗʰ **S37.491** Other injury of ovary, unilateral ♀

    √7ᵗʰ **S37.492** Other injury of ovary, bilateral ♀

    √7ᵗʰ **S37.499** Other injury of ovary, unspecified ♀

√5ᵗʰ **S37.5** Injury of fallopian tube

√6ᵗʰ **S37.50** Unspecified injury of fallopian tube

    √7ᵗʰ **S37.501** Unspecified injury of fallopian tube, unilateral ♀

    √7ᵗʰ **S37.502** Unspecified injury of fallopian tube, bilateral ♀

    √7ᵗʰ **S37.509** Unspecified injury of fallopian tube, unspecified ♀

√6ᵗʰ **S37.51** Primary blast injury of fallopian tube
Blast injury of fallopian tube NOS

    √7ᵗʰ **S37.511** Primary blast injury of fallopian tube, unilateral ♀

    √7ᵗʰ **S37.512** Primary blast injury of fallopian tube, bilateral ♀

    √7ᵗʰ **S37.519** Primary blast injury of fallopian tube, unspecified ♀

√6ᵗʰ **S37.52** Contusion of fallopian tube

    √7ᵗʰ **S37.521** Contusion of fallopian tube, unilateral ♀

    √7ᵗʰ **S37.522** Contusion of fallopian tube, bilateral ♀

    √7ᵗʰ **S37.529** Contusion of fallopian tube, unspecified ♀

√6ᵗʰ **S37.53** Laceration of fallopian tube

    √7ᵗʰ **S37.531** Laceration of fallopian tube, unilateral ♀

    √7ᵗʰ **S37.532** Laceration of fallopian tube, bilateral ♀

    √7ᵗʰ **S37.539** Laceration of fallopian tube, unspecified ♀

√6ᵗʰ **S37.59** Other injury of fallopian tube
Secondary blast injury of fallopian tube

    √7ᵗʰ **S37.591** Other injury of fallopian tube, unilateral ♀

    √7ᵗʰ **S37.592** Other injury of fallopian tube, bilateral ♀

    √7ᵗʰ **S37.599** Other injury of fallopian tube, unspecified ♀

√5ᵗʰ **S37.6** Injury of uterus

> `EXCLUDES 1` injury to gravid uterus (O9A.2-)
> injury to uterus during delivery (O71.-)

> **CC Excl: For codes in subcategory S37.6:**
> CC with 7th character A: PDX collection 1240

√x7ᵗʰ **S37.60** Unspecified injury of uterus   `CC` ♀

√x7ᵗʰ **S37.62** Contusion of uterus   `CC` ♀

√x7ᵗʰ **S37.63** Laceration of uterus   `CC` ♀

√x7ᵗʰ **S37.69** Other injury of uterus   `CC` ♀

√5ᵗʰ **S37.8** Injury of other urinary and pelvic organs

√6ᵗʰ **S37.81** Injury of adrenal gland

> **CC Excl: For codes in subcategory S37.81:**
> CC with 7th character A: PDX collection 1241

    √7ᵗʰ **S37.812** Contusion of adrenal gland   `CC`

    √7ᵗʰ **S37.813** Laceration of adrenal gland   `CC`

    √7ᵗʰ **S37.818** Other injury of adrenal gland   `CC`

    √7ᵗʰ **S37.819** Unspecified injury of adrenal gland   `CC`

√6ᵗʰ **S37.82** Injury of prostate

    √7ᵗʰ **S37.822** Contusion of prostate ♂

    √7ᵗʰ **S37.823** Laceration of prostate ♂

    √7ᵗʰ **S37.828** Other injury of prostate ♂

    √7ᵗʰ **S37.829** Unspecified injury of prostate ♂

√6ᵗʰ **S37.89** Injury of other urinary and pelvic organ

> **CC Excl: For codes in subcategory S37.89:**
> CC with 7th character A: PDX collection 1242

    √7ᵗʰ **S37.892** Contusion of other urinary and pelvic organ   `CC`

    √7ᵗʰ **S37.893** Laceration of other urinary and pelvic organ   `CC`

    √7ᵗʰ **S37.898** Other injury of other urinary and pelvic organ   `CC`

    √7ᵗʰ **S37.899** Unspecified injury of other urinary and pelvic organ   `CC`

√5ᵗʰ **S37.9** Injury of unspecified urinary and pelvic organ

> **CC Excl: For codes in subcategory S37.9:**
> CC with 7th character A: PDX collection 1242

√x7ᵗʰ **S37.90** Unspecified injury of unspecified urinary and pelvic organ   `CC`

√x7ᵗʰ **S37.92** Contusion of unspecified urinary and pelvic organ   `CC`

√x7ᵗʰ **S37.93** Laceration of unspecified urinary and pelvic organ   `CC`

√x7ᵗʰ **S37.99** Other injury of unspecified urinary and pelvic organ   `CC`

√4ᵗʰ **S38** Crushing injury and traumatic amputation of abdomen, lower back, pelvis and external genitals
An amputation not identified as partial or complete should be coded to complete.

> The appropriate 7th character is to be added to each code from category S38.
> A   initial encounter
> D   subsequent encounter
> S   sequela

√5ᵗʰ **S38.0** Crushing injury of external genital organs
Use additional code for any associated injuries

√6ᵗʰ **S38.00** Crushing injury of unspecified external genital organs

    √7ᵗʰ **S38.001** Crushing injury of unspecified external genital organs, male ♂

☑ Additional Character Req   √x7ᵗʰ Placeholder Alert   Unacceptable PDx   Manifestation   `H1`-`H14` HAC   `HCC` CMS-HCC Condition   `EXCLUDES 1` Not Coded Here   `EXCLUDES 2` Not Included Here

√7ᵗʰ **S38.002** **Crushing injury of unspecified external genital organs, female** ♀

√x7ᵗʰ **S38.01** **Crushing injury of** penis ♂

√x7ᵗʰ **S38.02** **Crushing injury of** scrotum and testis ♂

√x7ᵗʰ **S38.03** **Crushing injury of** vulva ♀

√x7ᵗʰ **S38.1** **Crushing injury of abdomen, lower back, and pelvis**
Use additional code for all associated injuries, such as:
fracture of thoracic or lumbar spine and pelvis (S22.0-, S32-)
injury to intra-abdominal organs (S36.-)
injury to urinary and pelvic organs (S37.-)
open wound of abdominal wall (S31.-)
spinal cord injury (S34.0, S34.1-)
EXCLUDES 2 *crushing injury of external genital organs (S38.0-)*

√5ᵗʰ **S38.2** **Traumatic amputation of external genital organs**

√6ᵗʰ **S38.21** **Traumatic amputation of** female external genital organs
Traumatic amputation of clitoris
Traumatic amputation of labium (majus) (minus)
Traumatic amputation of vulva

√7ᵗʰ **S38.211** **Complete traumatic amputation of female external genital organs** ♀

√7ᵗʰ **S38.212** **Partial traumatic amputation of female external genital organs** ♀

√6ᵗʰ **S38.22** **Traumatic amputation of** penis

√7ᵗʰ **S38.221** **Complete traumatic amputation of penis** ♂

√7ᵗʰ **S38.222** **Partial traumatic amputation of penis** ♂

√6ᵗʰ **S38.23** **Traumatic amputation of** scrotum and testis

√7ᵗʰ **S38.231** **Complete traumatic amputation of scrotum and testis** ♂

√7ᵗʰ **S38.232** **Partial traumatic amputation of scrotum and testis** ♂

√x7ᵗʰ **S38.3** **Transection (partial) of abdomen**

√4ᵗʰ **S39** **Other and unspecified injuries of abdomen, lower back, pelvis and external genitals**
Code also any associated open wound (S31.-)
EXCLUDES 2 *sprain of joints and ligaments of lumbar spine and pelvis (S33.-)*

The appropriate 7th character is to be added to each code from category S39.
A   initial encounter
D   subsequent encounter
S   sequela

√5ᵗʰ **S39.0** **Injury of muscle, fascia and tendon of abdomen, lower back and pelvis**

√6ᵗʰ **S39.00** **Unspecified injury of muscle, fascia and tendon of abdomen, lower back and pelvis**

√7ᵗʰ **S39.001** **Unspecified injury of muscle, fascia and tendon of** abdomen

√7ᵗʰ **S39.002** **Unspecified injury of muscle, fascia and tendon of** lower back

√7ᵗʰ **S39.003** **Unspecified injury of muscle, fascia and tendon of** pelvis

√6ᵗʰ **S39.01** **Strain of muscle, fascia and tendon of abdomen, lower back and pelvis**

√7ᵗʰ **S39.011** **Strain of muscle, fascia and tendon of** abdomen

√7ᵗʰ **S39.012** **Strain of muscle, fascia and tendon of** lower back

√7ᵗʰ **S39.013** **Strain of muscle, fascia and tendon of** pelvis

√6ᵗʰ **S39.02** **Laceration of muscle, fascia and tendon of abdomen, lower back and pelvis**

√7ᵗʰ **S39.021** **Laceration of muscle, fascia and tendon of** abdomen

√7ᵗʰ **S39.022** **Laceration of muscle, fascia and tendon of** lower back

√7ᵗʰ **S39.023** **Laceration of muscle, fascia and tendon of** pelvis

√6ᵗʰ **S39.09** **Other injury of muscle, fascia and tendon of abdomen, lower back and pelvis**

√7ᵗʰ **S39.091** **Other injury of muscle, fascia and tendon of** abdomen

√7ᵗʰ **S39.092** **Other injury of muscle, fascia and tendon of** lower back

√7ᵗʰ **S39.093** **Other injury of muscle, fascia and tendon of** pelvis

√5ᵗʰ **S39.8** **Other specified injuries of abdomen, lower back, pelvis and external genitals**

√x7ᵗʰ **S39.81** **Other specified injuries of** abdomen

√x7ᵗʰ **S39.82** **Other specified injuries of** lower back

√x7ᵗʰ **S39.83** **Other specified injuries of** pelvis

√6ᵗʰ **S39.84** **Other specified injuries of** external genitals

√7ᵗʰ **S39.840** **Fracture of** corpus cavernosum penis ♂

√7ᵗʰ **S39.848** **Other specified injuries of external genitals**

√5ᵗʰ **S39.9** **Unspecified injury of abdomen, lower back, pelvis and external genitals**

√x7ᵗʰ **S39.91** **Unspecified injury of** abdomen

√x7ᵗʰ **S39.92** **Unspecified injury of** lower back

√x7ᵗʰ **S39.93** **Unspecified injury of** pelvis

√x7ᵗʰ **S39.94** **Unspecified injury of** external genitals

Injuries to the shoulder and upper arm (S40-S49)

INCLUDES   injuries of axilla
injuries of scapular region
EXCLUDES 2   *burns and corrosions (T20-T32)*
frostbite (T33-T34)
injuries of elbow (S50-S59)
insect bite or sting, venomous (T63.4)

√4ᵗʰ **S40** **Superficial injury of shoulder and upper arm**

The appropriate 7th character is to be added to each code from category S40.
A   initial encounter
D   subsequent encounter
S   sequela

√5ᵗʰ **S40.0** **Contusion of shoulder and upper arm**

√6ᵗʰ **S40.01** **Contusion of** shoulder

√7ᵗʰ **S40.011** **Contusion of** right shoulder

√7ᵗʰ **S40.012** **Contusion of** left shoulder

√7ᵗʰ **S40.019** **Contusion of** unspecified shoulder

√6ᵗʰ **S40.02** **Contusion of** upper arm

√7ᵗʰ **S40.021** **Contusion of** right upper arm

√7ᵗʰ **S40.022** **Contusion of** left upper arm

√7ᵗʰ **S40.029** **Contusion of** unspecified upper arm

√5ᵗʰ **S40.2** **Other superficial injuries of shoulder**

√6ᵗʰ **S40.21** **Abrasion of shoulder**

√7ᵗʰ **S40.211** **Abrasion of** right shoulder

√7ᵗʰ **S40.212** **Abrasion of** left shoulder

√7ᵗʰ **S40.219** **Abrasion of** unspecified shoulder

√6ᵗʰ **S40.22** **Blister (nonthermal) of shoulder**

√7ᵗʰ **S40.221** **Blister (nonthermal) of** right shoulder

√7ᵗʰ **S40.222** **Blister (nonthermal) of** left shoulder

√7ᵗʰ **S40.229** **Blister (nonthermal) of** unspecified shoulder

√6ᵗʰ **S40.24** **External constriction of shoulder**

√7ᵗʰ **S40.241** **External constriction of** right shoulder

√7ᵗʰ **S40.242** **External constriction of** left shoulder

√7ᵗʰ **S40.249** **External constriction of** unspecified shoulder

√6ᵗʰ **S40.25** **Superficial foreign body of shoulder**
Splinter in the shoulder

√7ᵗʰ **S40.251** **Superficial foreign body of** right shoulder

√7ᵗʰ **S40.252** **Superficial foreign body of** left shoulder

√7ᵗʰ **S40.259** **Superficial foreign body of** unspecified shoulder

√6ᵗʰ **S40.26** **Insect bite (nonvenomous) of shoulder**

√7ᵗʰ **S40.261** **Insect bite (nonvenomous) of** right shoulder

√7ᵗʰ **S40.262** **Insect bite (nonvenomous) of** left shoulder

√7ᵗʰ **S40.269** **Insect bite (nonvenomous) of** unspecified shoulder

√6ᵗʰ **S40.27** **Other superficial bite of shoulder**
EXCLUDES 1 *open bite of shoulder (S41.05)*

√7ᵗʰ **S40.271** **Other superficial bite of** right shoulder

Ⓝ Newborn: 0   Ⓟ Pediatric: 0-17   Ⓜ Maternity: 12-55   Ⓐ Adult: 15-124   MCC Major CC Condition   PDx MCC PDx acts as own MCC   CC CC Condition   PDx CC PDx acts as own CC

984   ICD-10-CM 2018

√7ᵗʰ **S40.272** Other superficial bite of left shoulder

√7ᵗʰ **S40.279** Other superficial bite of unspecified shoulder

√5ᵗʰ **S40.8** Other superficial injuries of upper arm

√6ᵗʰ **S40.81** Abrasion of upper arm

√7ᵗʰ **S40.811** Abrasion of right upper arm

√7ᵗʰ **S40.812** Abrasion of left upper arm

√7ᵗʰ **S40.819** Abrasion of unspecified upper arm

√6ᵗʰ **S40.82** Blister (nonthermal) of upper arm

√7ᵗʰ **S40.821** Blister (nonthermal) of right upper arm

√7ᵗʰ **S40.822** Blister (nonthermal) of left upper arm

√7ᵗʰ **S40.829** Blister (nonthermal) of unspecified upper arm

√6ᵗʰ **S40.84** External constriction of upper arm

√7ᵗʰ **S40.841** External constriction of right upper arm

√7ᵗʰ **S40.842** External constriction of left upper arm

√7ᵗʰ **S40.849** External constriction of unspecified upper arm

√6ᵗʰ **S40.85** Superficial foreign body of upper arm
Splinter in the upper arm

√7ᵗʰ **S40.851** Superficial foreign body of right upper arm

√7ᵗʰ **S40.852** Superficial foreign body of left upper arm

√7ᵗʰ **S40.859** Superficial foreign body of unspecified upper arm

√6ᵗʰ **S40.86** Insect bite (nonvenomous) of upper arm

√7ᵗʰ **S40.861** Insect bite (nonvenomous) of right upper arm

√7ᵗʰ **S40.862** Insect bite (nonvenomous) of left upper arm

√7ᵗʰ **S40.869** Insect bite (nonvenomous) of unspecified upper arm

√6ᵗʰ **S40.87** Other superficial bite of upper arm
EXCLUDES 1   *open bite of upper arm (S41.14)*
EXCLUDES 2   *other superficial bite of shoulder (S40.27-)*

√7ᵗʰ **S40.871** Other superficial bite of right upper arm

√7ᵗʰ **S40.872** Other superficial bite of left upper arm

√7ᵗʰ **S40.879** Other superficial bite of unspecified upper arm

√5ᵗʰ **S40.9** Unspecified superficial injury of shoulder and upper arm

√6ᵗʰ **S40.91** Unspecified superficial injury of shoulder

√7ᵗʰ **S40.911** Unspecified superficial injury of right shoulder

√7ᵗʰ **S40.912** Unspecified superficial injury of left shoulder

√7ᵗʰ **S40.919** Unspecified superficial injury of unspecified shoulder

√6ᵗʰ **S40.92** Unspecified superficial injury of upper arm

√7ᵗʰ **S40.921** Unspecified superficial injury of right upper arm

√7ᵗʰ **S40.922** Unspecified superficial injury of left upper arm

√7ᵗʰ **S40.929** Unspecified superficial injury of unspecified upper arm

√4ᵗʰ **S41** **Open wound of shoulder and upper arm**
Code also any associated wound infection
EXCLUDES 1   *traumatic amputation of shoulder and upper arm (S48.-)*
EXCLUDES 2   *open fracture of shoulder and upper arm (S42.- with 7th character B or C)*

The appropriate 7th character is to be added to each code from category S41.
A   initial encounter
D   subsequent encounter
S   sequela

√5ᵗʰ **S41.0** Open wound of shoulder

√6ᵗʰ **S41.00** Unspecified open wound of shoulder

√7ᵗʰ **S41.001** Unspecified open wound of right shoulder

√7ᵗʰ **S41.002** Unspecified open wound of left shoulder

√7ᵗʰ **S41.009** Unspecified open wound of unspecified shoulder

√6ᵗʰ **S41.01** Laceration without foreign body of shoulder

√7ᵗʰ **S41.011** Laceration without foreign body of right shoulder

√7ᵗʰ **S41.012** Laceration without foreign body of left shoulder

√7ᵗʰ **S41.019** Laceration without foreign body of unspecified shoulder

√6ᵗʰ **S41.02** Laceration with foreign body of shoulder

√7ᵗʰ **S41.021** Laceration with foreign body of right shoulder

√7ᵗʰ **S41.022** Laceration with foreign body of left shoulder

√7ᵗʰ **S41.029** Laceration with foreign body of unspecified shoulder

√6ᵗʰ **S41.03** Puncture wound without foreign body of shoulder

√7ᵗʰ **S41.031** Puncture wound without foreign body of right shoulder

√7ᵗʰ **S41.032** Puncture wound without foreign body of left shoulder

√7ᵗʰ **S41.039** Puncture wound without foreign body of unspecified shoulder

√6ᵗʰ **S41.04** Puncture wound with foreign body of shoulder

√7ᵗʰ **S41.041** Puncture wound with foreign body of right shoulder

√7ᵗʰ **S41.042** Puncture wound with foreign body of left shoulder

√7ᵗʰ **S41.049** Puncture wound with foreign body of unspecified shoulder

√6ᵗʰ **S41.05** Open bite of shoulder
Bite of shoulder NOS
EXCLUDES 1   *superficial bite of shoulder (S40.27)*

√7ᵗʰ **S41.051** Open bite of right shoulder

√7ᵗʰ **S41.052** Open bite of left shoulder

√7ᵗʰ **S41.059** Open bite of unspecified shoulder

√5ᵗʰ **S41.1** Open wound of upper arm

√6ᵗʰ **S41.10** Unspecified open wound of upper arm
AHA: 2016, 3Q, 24

√7ᵗʰ **S41.101** Unspecified open wound of right upper arm

√7ᵗʰ **S41.102** Unspecified open wound of left upper arm

√7ᵗʰ **S41.109** Unspecified open wound of unspecified upper arm

√6ᵗʰ **S41.11** Laceration without foreign body of upper arm

√7ᵗʰ **S41.111** Laceration without foreign body of right upper arm

√7ᵗʰ **S41.112** Laceration without foreign body of left upper arm

√7ᵗʰ **S41.119** Laceration without foreign body of unspecified upper arm

√6ᵗʰ **S41.12** Laceration with foreign body of upper arm

√7ᵗʰ **S41.121** Laceration with foreign body of right upper arm

√7ᵗʰ **S41.122** Laceration with foreign body of left upper arm

√7ᵗʰ **S41.129** Laceration with foreign body of unspecified upper arm

√6ᵗʰ **S41.13** Puncture wound without foreign body of upper arm
AHA: 2016, 3Q, 24

√7ᵗʰ **S41.131** Puncture wound without foreign body of right upper arm

√7ᵗʰ **S41.132** Puncture wound without foreign body of left upper arm

√7ᵗʰ **S41.139** Puncture wound without foreign body of unspecified upper arm

√6ᵗʰ **S41.14** Puncture wound with foreign body of upper arm
AHA: 2016, 3Q, 24

√7ᵗʰ **S41.141** Puncture wound with foreign body of right upper arm

√7ᵗʰ **S41.142** Puncture wound with foreign body of left upper arm

√7ᵗʰ **S41.149** Puncture wound with foreign body of unspecified upper arm

---

√6ᵗʰ **S41.15** **Open bite** of upper arm
Bite of upper arm NOS
EXCLUDES 1   *superficial bite of upper arm (S40.87)*

√7ᵗʰ **S41.151** Open bite of **right** upper arm
√7ᵗʰ **S41.152** Open bite of **left** upper arm
√7ᵗʰ **S41.159** Open bite of **unspecified** upper arm

√4ᵗʰ **S42** **Fracture of shoulder and upper arm**

NOTE   A fracture not indicated as displaced or nondisplaced should be coded to displaced.
A fracture not indicated as open or closed should be coded to closed.

EXCLUDES 1   *traumatic amputation of shoulder and upper arm (S48.-)*
AHA: 2015, 3Q, 37-39

The appropriate 7th character is to be added to all codes from category S42 [unless otherwise indicated].
A   initial encounter for closed fracture
B   initial encounter for open fracture
D   subsequent encounter for fracture with routine healing
G   subsequent encounter for fracture with delayed healing
K   subsequent encounter for fracture with nonunion
P   subsequent encounter for fracture with malunion
S   sequela

√5ᵗʰ **S42.0** **Fracture of** clavicle

CC Excl: For codes in subcategory S42.0:
CC with 7th character B: PDX collection 1243
CC with 7th character K or P: PDX collection 897

√6ᵗʰ **S42.00** **Fracture of unspecified** part of clavicle
7   √7ᵗʰ **S42.001** **Fracture of unspecified** part of **right clavicle** `CC` `H5`
7   √7ᵗʰ **S42.002** **Fracture of unspecified** part of **left clavicle** `CC` `H5`
7   √7ᵗʰ **S42.009** **Fracture of unspecified** part of **unspecified clavicle** `CC` `H5`
    AHA: 2012, 4Q, 93

√6ᵗʰ **S42.01** **Fracture of sternal end of clavicle**
7   √7ᵗʰ **S42.011** **Anterior displaced fracture of sternal end of right clavicle** `CC` `H5`
7   √7ᵗʰ **S42.012** **Anterior displaced fracture of sternal end of left clavicle** `CC` `H5`
7   √7ᵗʰ **S42.013** **Anterior displaced fracture of sternal end of unspecified clavicle** `CC` `H5`
    Displaced fracture of sternal end of clavicle NOS
7   √7ᵗʰ **S42.014** **Posterior displaced fracture of sternal end of right clavicle** `CC` `H5`
7   √7ᵗʰ **S42.015** **Posterior displaced fracture of sternal end of left clavicle** `CC` `H5`
7   √7ᵗʰ **S42.016** **Posterior displaced fracture of sternal end of unspecified clavicle** `CC` `H5`
7   √7ᵗʰ **S42.017** **Nondisplaced fracture of sternal end of right clavicle** `CC` `H5`
7   √7ᵗʰ **S42.018** **Nondisplaced fracture of sternal end of left clavicle** `CC` `H5`
7   √7ᵗʰ **S42.019** **Nondisplaced fracture of sternal end of unspecified clavicle** `CC` `H5`

√6ᵗʰ **S42.02** **Fracture of shaft of clavicle**
7   √7ᵗʰ **S42.021** **Displaced fracture of shaft of right clavicle** `CC` `H5`
7   √7ᵗʰ **S42.022** **Displaced fracture of shaft of left clavicle** `CC` `H5`
7   √7ᵗʰ **S42.023** **Displaced fracture of shaft of unspecified clavicle** `CC` `H5`
7   √7ᵗʰ **S42.024** **Nondisplaced fracture of shaft of right clavicle** `CC` `H5`
7   √7ᵗʰ **S42.025** **Nondisplaced fracture of shaft of left clavicle** `CC` `H5`
7   √7ᵗʰ **S42.026** **Nondisplaced fracture of shaft of unspecified clavicle** `CC` `H5`

√6ᵗʰ **S42.03** **Fracture of lateral end of clavicle**
    Fracture of acromial end of clavicle
7   √7ᵗʰ **S42.031** **Displaced fracture of lateral end of right clavicle** `CC` `H5`

7   √7ᵗʰ **S42.032** **Displaced fracture of lateral end of left clavicle** `CC` `H5`
7   √7ᵗʰ **S42.033** **Displaced fracture of lateral end of unspecified clavicle** `CC` `H5`
7   √7ᵗʰ **S42.034** **Nondisplaced fracture of lateral end of right clavicle** `CC` `H5`
7   √7ᵗʰ **S42.035** **Nondisplaced fracture of lateral end of left clavicle** `CC` `H5`
7   √7ᵗʰ **S42.036** **Nondisplaced fracture of lateral end of unspecified clavicle** `CC` `H5`

√5ᵗʰ **S42.1** **Fracture of** scapula

CC Excl: For codes in subcatagory S42.1:
CC with 7th character B: PDX collection 1244
CC with 7th character K or P: PDX collection 897

√6ᵗʰ **S42.10** **Fracture of unspecified** part of scapula
7   √7ᵗʰ **S42.101** **Fracture of unspecified part of scapula, right shoulder** `CC` `H5`
7   √7ᵗʰ **S42.102** **Fracture of unspecified part of scapula, left shoulder** `CC` `H5`
7   √7ᵗʰ **S42.109** **Fracture of unspecified part of scapula, unspecified shoulder** `CC` `H5`

√6ᵗʰ **S42.11** **Fracture of body of scapula**
7   √7ᵗʰ **S42.111** **Displaced fracture of body of scapula, right shoulder** `CC` `H5`
7   √7ᵗʰ **S42.112** **Displaced fracture of body of scapula, left shoulder** `CC` `H5`
7   √7ᵗʰ **S42.113** **Displaced fracture of body of scapula, unspecified shoulder** `CC` `H5`
7   √7ᵗʰ **S42.114** **Nondisplaced fracture of body of scapula, right shoulder** `CC` `H5`
7   √7ᵗʰ **S42.115** **Nondisplaced fracture of body of scapula, left shoulder** `CC` `H5`
7   √7ᵗʰ **S42.116** **Nondisplaced fracture of body of scapula, unspecified shoulder** `CC` `H5`

√6ᵗʰ **S42.12** **Fracture of** acromial process
7   √7ᵗʰ **S42.121** **Displaced fracture of acromial process, right shoulder** `CC` `H5`
7   √7ᵗʰ **S42.122** **Displaced fracture of acromial process, left shoulder** `CC` `H5`
7   √7ᵗʰ **S42.123** **Displaced fracture of acromial process, unspecified shoulder** `CC` `H5`
7   √7ᵗʰ **S42.124** **Nondisplaced fracture of acromial process, right shoulder** `CC` `H5`
7   √7ᵗʰ **S42.125** **Nondisplaced fracture of acromial process, left shoulder** `CC` `H5`
7   √7ᵗʰ **S42.126** **Nondisplaced fracture of acromial process, unspecified shoulder** `CC` `H5`

√6ᵗʰ **S42.13** **Fracture of** coracoid process
7   √7ᵗʰ **S42.131** **Displaced fracture of coracoid process, right shoulder** `CC` `H5`
7   √7ᵗʰ **S42.132** **Displaced fracture of coracoid process, left shoulder** `CC` `H5`
7   √7ᵗʰ **S42.133** **Displaced fracture of coracoid process, unspecified shoulder** `CC` `H5`
7   √7ᵗʰ **S42.134** **Nondisplaced fracture of coracoid process, right shoulder** `CC` `H5`
7   √7ᵗʰ **S42.135** **Nondisplaced fracture of coracoid process, left shoulder** `CC` `H5`
7   √7ᵗʰ **S42.136** **Nondisplaced fracture of coracoid process, unspecified shoulder** `CC` `H5`

√6ᵗʰ **S42.14** **Fracture of** glenoid cavity of scapula
7   √7ᵗʰ **S42.141** **Displaced fracture of glenoid cavity of scapula, right shoulder** `CC` `H5`
7   √7ᵗʰ **S42.142** **Displaced fracture of glenoid cavity of scapula, left shoulder** `CC` `H5`
7   √7ᵗʰ **S42.143** **Displaced fracture of glenoid cavity of scapula, unspecified shoulder** `CC` `H5`
7   √7ᵗʰ **S42.144** **Nondisplaced fracture of glenoid cavity of scapula, right shoulder** `CC` `H5`
7   √7ᵗʰ **S42.145** **Nondisplaced fracture of glenoid cavity of scapula, left shoulder** `CC` `H5`
7   √7ᵗʰ **S42.146** **Nondisplaced fracture of glenoid cavity of scapula, unspecified shoulder** `CC` `H5`

---

7   CC when reported as an initial encounter (7th character A, B, or C – specific to category) OR a subsequent encounter for nonunion or malunion (7th character K, M, N, P, Q, or R – specific to category).

✓6th **S42.15**   **Fracture of** neck **of scapula**

   7   ✓7th **S42.151**   **Displaced fracture of neck of scapula, right shoulder**   CC H5

   7   ✓7th **S42.152**   **Displaced fracture of neck of scapula, left shoulder**   CC H5

   7   ✓7th **S42.153**   **Displaced fracture of neck of scapula, unspecified shoulder**   CC H5

   7   ✓7th **S42.154**   **Nondisplaced fracture of neck of scapula, right shoulder**   CC H5

   7   ✓7th **S42.155**   **Nondisplaced fracture of neck of scapula, left shoulder**   CC H5

   7   ✓7th **S42.156**   **Nondisplaced fracture of neck of scapula, unspecified shoulder**   CC H5

✓6th **S42.19**   **Fracture of** other **part of scapula**

   7   ✓7th **S42.191**   **Fracture of other part of scapula, right shoulder**   CC H5

   7   ✓7th **S42.192**   **Fracture of other part of scapula, left shoulder**   CC H5

   7   ✓7th **S42.199**   **Fracture of other part of scapula, unspecified shoulder**   CC H5

✓5th **S42.2**   **Fracture of** upper end of humerus
Fracture of proximal end of humerus

> EXCLUDES 2   fracture of shaft of humerus (S42.3-)
> physeal fracture of upper end of humerus (S49.0-)

> **CC Excl: For CC/MCC codes in subcategory S42.2, unless otherwise noted:**
> **Right side:** See code S42.201
> **Left side:** See code S42.202
> **Unspecified side:** See code S42.209

✓6th **S42.20**   Unspecified **fracture of upper end of humerus**

   6,7   ✓7th **S42.201**   **Unspecified fracture of upper end of right humerus**   MCC CC H5
> **CC Excl: CC with 7th character A:**
> PDX collection 1245
> **MCC with 7th character B:**
> PDX collection 1246
> **CC with 7th character K or P:**
> PDX collection 897

   6,7   ✓7th **S42.202**   **Unspecified fracture of upper end of left humerus**   MCC CC H5
> **CC Excl: CC with 7th character A:**
> PDX collection 1247
> **MCC with 7th character B:**
> PDX collection 1246
> **CC with 7th character K or P:**
> PDX collection 897

   6,7   ✓7th **S42.209**   **Unspecified fracture of upper end of unspecified humerus**   MCC CC H5
> **CC Excl: CC with 7th character A:**
> PDX collection 1248
> **MCC with 7th character B:**
> PDX collection 1246
> **CC with 7th character K or P:**
> PDX collection 897

✓6th **S42.21**   Unspecified **fracture of surgical neck of humerus**
Fracture of neck of humerus NOS

   6,7   ✓7th **S42.211**   **Unspecified** displaced **fracture of surgical neck of right humerus**   MCC CC H5

   6,7   ✓7th **S42.212**   **Unspecified** displaced **fracture of surgical neck of** left **humerus**   MCC CC H5

   6,7   ✓7th **S42.213**   **Unspecified** displaced **fracture of surgical neck of** unspecified **humerus**   MCC CC H5

   6,7   ✓7th **S42.214**   **Unspecified** nondisplaced **fracture of surgical neck of right humerus**   MCC CC H5

   6,7   ✓7th **S42.215**   **Unspecified** nondisplaced **fracture of surgical neck of** left **humerus**   MCC CC H5

   6,7   ✓7th **S42.216**   **Unspecified** nondisplaced **fracture of surgical neck of** unspecified **humerus**   MCC CC H5

✓6th **S42.22**   2-part **fracture of surgical neck of humerus**

   6,7   ✓7th **S42.221**   **2-part** displaced **fracture of surgical neck of right humerus**   MCC CC H5

   6,7   ✓7th **S42.222**   **2-part** displaced **fracture of surgical neck of** left **humerus**   MCC CC H5

   6,7   ✓7th **S42.223**   **2-part** displaced **fracture of surgical neck of** unspecified **humerus**   MCC CC H5

   6,7   ✓7th **S42.224**   **2-part** nondisplaced **fracture of surgical neck of right humerus**   MCC CC H5

   6,7   ✓7th **S42.225**   **2-part** nondisplaced **fracture of surgical neck of** left **humerus**   MCC CC H5

   6,7   ✓7th **S42.226**   **2-part** nondisplaced **fracture of surgical neck of** unspecified **humerus**   MCC CC H5

✓6th **S42.23**   3-part **fracture of** surgical neck **of humerus**

   6,7   ✓7th **S42.231**   **3-part fracture of surgical neck of right humerus**   MCC CC H5

   6,7   ✓7th **S42.232**   **3-part fracture of surgical neck of** left **humerus**   MCC CC H5

   6,7   ✓7th **S42.239**   **3-part fracture of surgical neck of** unspecified **humerus**   MCC CC H5

✓6th **S42.24**   4-part **fracture of** surgical neck **of humerus**

   6,7   ✓7th **S42.241**   **4-part fracture of surgical neck of right humerus**   MCC CC H5

   6,7   ✓7th **S42.242**   **4-part fracture of surgical neck of** left **humerus**   MCC CC H5

   6,7   ✓7th **S42.249**   **4-part fracture of surgical neck of** unspecified **humerus**   MCC CC H5

✓6th **S42.25**   **Fracture of** greater tuberosity **of humerus**

   6,7   ✓7th **S42.251**   **Displaced fracture of greater tuberosity of right humerus**   MCC CC H5

   6,7   ✓7th **S42.252**   **Displaced fracture of greater tuberosity of** left **humerus**   MCC CC H5

   6,7   ✓7th **S42.253**   **Displaced fracture of greater tuberosity of** unspecified **humerus**   MCC CC H5

   6,7   ✓7th **S42.254**   **Nondisplaced fracture of greater tuberosity of right humerus**   MCC CC H5

   6,7   ✓7th **S42.255**   **Nondisplaced fracture of greater tuberosity of** left **humerus**   MCC CC H5

   6,7   ✓7th **S42.256**   **Nondisplaced fracture of greater tuberosity of** unspecified **humerus**   MCC CC H5

✓6th **S42.26**   **Fracture of** lesser tuberosity **of humerus**

   6,7   ✓7th **S42.261**   **Displaced fracture of lesser tuberosity of right humerus**   MCC CC H5

   6,7   ✓7th **S42.262**   **Displaced fracture of lesser tuberosity of** left **humerus**   MCC CC H5

   6,7   ✓7th **S42.263**   **Displaced fracture of lesser tuberosity of** unspecified **humerus**   MCC CC H5

   6,7   ✓7th **S42.264**   **Nondisplaced fracture of lesser tuberosity of right humerus**   MCC CC H5

   6,7   ✓7th **S42.265**   **Nondisplaced fracture of lesser tuberosity of** left **humerus**   MCC CC H5

   6,7   ✓7th **S42.266**   **Nondisplaced fracture of lesser tuberosity of** unspecified **humerus**   MCC CC H5

✓6th **S42.27**   Torus **fracture of upper end of humerus**

> The appropriate 7th character is to be added to all codes in subcategory S42.27.
> A   initial encounter for closed fracture
> D   subsequent encounter for fracture with routine healing
> G   subsequent encounter for fracture with delayed healing
> K   subsequent encounter for fracture with nonunion
> P   subsequent encounter for fracture with malunion
> S   sequela

   7   ✓7th **S42.271**   **Torus fracture of upper end of** right **humerus**   CC H5
> **CC Excl: CC with 7th character A:**
> PDX collection 1245
> **CC with 7th character K or P:**
> PDX collection 897

   7   ✓7th **S42.272**   **Torus fracture of upper end of** left **humerus**   CC H5
> **CC Excl: CC with 7th character A:**
> PDX collection 1247
> **CC with 7th character K or P:**
> PDX collection 897

---

6   MCC when reported as an open fracture (7th character B or C – specific to category).

7   CC when reported as an initial encounter (7th character A, B, or C – specific to category) OR a subsequent encounter for nonunion or malunion (7th character K, M, N, P, Q, or R – specific to category).

✓Additional Character Req   √x7th Placeholder Alert   Unacceptable PDx   Manifestation   H1-H14 HAC   HCC CMS-HCC Condition   EXCLUDES 1 Not Coded Here   EXCLUDES 2 Not Included Here

7 ✓7ᵗʰ **S42.279 Torus fracture of upper end of** `CC` `H5`
unspecified humerus
CC Excl: CC with 7th character A:
PDX collection 1248
CC with 7th character K or P:
PDX collection 897

✓6ᵗʰ **S42.29 Other fracture of upper end of humerus**
Fracture of anatomical neck of humerus
Fracture of articular head of humerus

6, 7 ✓7ᵗʰ **S42.291 Other displaced fracture of** `MCC` `CC` `H5`
upper end of right humerus

6, 7 ✓7ᵗʰ **S42.292 Other displaced fracture of** `MCC` `CC` `H5`
upper end of left humerus

6, 7 ✓7ᵗʰ **S42.293 Other displaced fracture of** `MCC` `CC` `H5`
upper end of unspecified humerus

6, 7 ✓7ᵗʰ **S42.294 Other nondisplaced fracture of** `MCC` `CC` `H5`
upper end of right humerus

6, 7 ✓7ᵗʰ **S42.295 Other nondisplaced fracture of** `MCC` `CC` `H5`
upper end of left humerus

6, 7 ✓7ᵗʰ **S42.296 Other nondisplaced fracture of** `MCC` `CC` `H5`
upper end of unspecified humerus

✓5ᵗʰ **S42.3 Fracture of shaft of humerus**
Fracture of humerus NOS
Fracture of upper arm NOS
EXCLUDES 2 *physeal fractures of upper end of humerus (S49.0-)*
physeal fractures of lower end of humerus (S49.1-)

CC Excl: For CC/MCC codes in subcategory S42.3, unless
otherwise noted:
Right side: See code S42.321
Left side: See code S42.322
Unspecified side: See code S42.323

✓6ᵗʰ **S42.30 Unspecified fracture of shaft of humerus**

6, 7 ✓7ᵗʰ **S42.301 Unspecified fracture of shaft of** `MCC` `CC` `H5`
humerus, right arm

6, 7 ✓7ᵗʰ **S42.302 Unspecified fracture of shaft of** `MCC` `CC` `H5`
humerus, left arm

6, 7 ✓7ᵗʰ **S42.309 Unspecified fracture of shaft of** `MCC` `CC` `H5`
humerus, unspecified arm

✓6ᵗʰ **S42.31 Greenstick fracture of shaft of humerus**

The appropriate 7th character is to be added to all
codes in subcategory S42.31.
A   initial encounter for closed fracture
D   subsequent encounter for fracture with
     routine healing
G   subsequent encounter for fracture with
     delayed healing
K   subsequent encounter for fracture with
     nonunion
P   subsequent encounter for fracture with
     malunion
S   sequela

7 ✓7ᵗʰ **S42.311 Greenstick fracture of shaft of** `CC` `H5`
humerus, right arm
CC Excl: CC with 7th character A:
PDX collection 1249
CC with 7th character K or P:
PDX collection 897

7 ✓7ᵗʰ **S42.312 Greenstick fracture of shaft of** `CC` `H5`
humerus, left arm
CC Excl: CC with 7th character A:
PDX collection 1250
CC with 7th character K or P:
PDX collection 897

7 ✓7ᵗʰ **S42.319 Greenstick fracture of shaft of** `CC` `H5`
humerus, unspecified arm
CC Excl: CC with 7th character A:
PDX collection 1251
CC with 7th character K or P:
PDX collection 897

✓6ᵗʰ **S42.32 Transverse fracture of shaft of humerus**

6, 7 ✓7ᵗʰ **S42.321 Displaced transverse fracture** `MCC` `CC` `H5`
of shaft of humerus, right arm
CC Excl: CC with 7th character A:
PDX collection 1249
MCC with 7th character B:
PDX collection 1246
CC with 7th character K or P:
PDX collection 897

6, 7 ✓7ᵗʰ **S42.322 Displaced transverse fracture** `MCC` `CC` `H5`
of shaft of humerus, left arm
CC Excl: CC with 7th character A:
PDX collection 1250
MCC with 7th character B:
PDX collection 1246
CC with 7th character K or P:
PDX collection 897

6, 7 ✓7ᵗʰ **S42.323 Displaced transverse fracture** `MCC` `CC` `H5`
of shaft of humerus, unspecified arm
CC Excl: CC with 7th character A:
PDX collection 1251
MCC with 7th character B:
PDX collection 1246
CC with 7th character K or P:
PDX collection 897

6, 7 ✓7ᵗʰ **S42.324 Nondisplaced transverse** `MCC` `CC` `H5`
fracture of shaft of humerus, right arm

6, 7 ✓7ᵗʰ **S42.325 Nondisplaced transverse** `MCC` `CC` `H5`
fracture of shaft of humerus, left arm

6, 7 ✓7ᵗʰ **S42.326 Nondisplaced transverse** `MCC` `CC` `H5`
fracture of shaft of humerus,
unspecified arm

✓6ᵗʰ **S42.33 Oblique fracture of shaft of humerus**

6, 7 ✓7ᵗʰ **S42.331 Displaced oblique fracture of** `MCC` `CC` `H5`
shaft of humerus, right arm

6, 7 ✓7ᵗʰ **S42.332 Displaced oblique fracture of** `MCC` `CC` `H5`
shaft of humerus, left arm

6, 7 ✓7ᵗʰ **S42.333 Displaced oblique fracture of** `MCC` `CC` `H5`
shaft of humerus, unspecified arm

6, 7 ✓7ᵗʰ **S42.334 Nondisplaced oblique fracture** `MCC` `CC` `H5`
of shaft of humerus, right arm

6, 7 ✓7ᵗʰ **S42.335 Nondisplaced oblique fracture** `MCC` `CC` `H5`
of shaft of humerus, left arm

6, 7 ✓7ᵗʰ **S42.336 Nondisplaced oblique fracture** `MCC` `CC` `H5`
of shaft of humerus, unspecified arm

✓6ᵗʰ **S42.34 Spiral fracture of shaft of humerus**

6, 7 ✓7ᵗʰ **S42.341 Displaced spiral fracture of** `MCC` `CC` `H5`
shaft of humerus, right arm

6, 7 ✓7ᵗʰ **S42.342 Displaced spiral fracture of** `MCC` `CC` `H5`
sharft of humerus, left arm

6, 7 ✓7ᵗʰ **S42.343 Displaced spiral fracture of** `MCC` `CC` `H5`
shaft of humerus, unspecified arm

6, 7 ✓7ᵗʰ **S42.344 Nondisplaced spiral fracture** `MCC` `CC` `H5`
of shaft of humerus, right arm

6, 7 ✓7ᵗʰ **S42.345 Nondisplaced spiral fracture** `MCC` `CC` `H5`
of shaft of humerus, left arm

6, 7 ✓7ᵗʰ **S42.346 Nondisplaced spiral fracture** `MCC` `CC` `H5`
of shaft of humerus, unspecified arm

✓6ᵗʰ **S42.35 Comminuted fracture of shaft of humerus**

6, 7 ✓7ᵗʰ **S42.351 Displaced comminuted fracture** `MCC` `CC` `H5`
of shaft of humerus, right arm

6, 7 ✓7ᵗʰ **S42.352 Displaced comminuted fracture** `MCC` `CC` `H5`
of shaft of humerus, left arm

6, 7 ✓7ᵗʰ **S42.353 Displaced comminuted fracture** `MCC` `CC` `H5`
of shaft of humerus, unspecified arm

6, 7 ✓7ᵗʰ **S42.354 Nondisplaced comminuted** `MCC` `CC` `H5`
fracture of shaft of humerus, right arm

6, 7 ✓7ᵗʰ **S42.355 Nondisplaced comminuted** `MCC` `CC` `H5`
fracture of shaft of humerus, left arm

6, 7 ✓7ᵗʰ **S42.356 Nondisplaced comminuted** `MCC` `CC` `H5`
fracture of shaft of humerus,
unspecified arm

✓6ᵗʰ **S42.36 Segmental fracture of shaft of humerus**

6, 7 ✓7ᵗʰ **S42.361 Displaced segmental fracture** `MCC` `CC` `H5`
of shaft of humerus, right arm

---

6   MCC when reported as an open fracture (7th character B or C – specific to category).
7   CC when reported as an initial encounter (7th character A, B, or C – specific to category) OR a subsequent encounter for nonunion or malunion
    (7th character K, M, N, P, Q, or R – specific to category).

`N` Newborn: 0   `P` Pediatric: 0-17   `M` Maternity: 12-55   `A` Adult: 15-124   `MCC` Major CC Condition   `PDxMCC` PDx acts as own MCC   `CC` CC Condition   `PDxCC` PDx acts as own CC

6, 7 ✓7ᵗʰ **S42.362** Displaced **segmental** fracture of shaft of humerus, **left arm** `MCC` `CC` `H5`

6, 7 ✓7ᵗʰ **S42.363** Displaced **segmental** fracture of shaft of humerus, **unspecified arm** `MCC` `CC` `H5`

6, 7 ✓7ᵗʰ **S42.364** Nondisplaced **segmental** fracture of shaft of humerus, **right arm** `MCC` `CC` `H5`

6, 7 ✓7ᵗʰ **S42.365** Nondisplaced **segmental** fracture of shaft of humerus, **left arm** `MCC` `CC` `H5`

6, 7 ✓7ᵗʰ **S42.366** Nondisplaced **segmental** fracture of shaft of humerus, **unspecified arm** `MCC` `CC` `H5`

✓6ᵗʰ **S42.39** Other fracture of shaft of humerus

6, 7 ✓7ᵗʰ **S42.391** Other fracture of shaft of **right** humerus `MCC` `CC` `H5`

6, 7 ✓7ᵗʰ **S42.392** Other fracture of shaft of **left** humerus `MCC` `CC` `H5`

6, 7 ✓7ᵗʰ **S42.399** Other fracture of shaft of **unspecified** humerus `MCC` `CC` `H5`

✓5ᵗʰ **S42.4** Fracture of **lower end** of humerus
Fracture of distal end of humerus

EXCLUDES 2   fracture of shaft of humerus (S42.3-)
physeal fracture of lower end of humerus (S49.1-)

> **CC Excl:** For CC/MCC codes in subcategory S42.4, unless otherwise noted:
> **Right side:** See code S42.201
> **Left side:** See code S42.202
> **Unspecified side:** See code S42.209

✓6ᵗʰ **S42.40** Unspecified fracture of lower end of humerus
Fracture of elbow NOS

6, 7 ✓7ᵗʰ **S42.401** Unspecified fracture of lower end of **right** humerus `MCC` `CC` `H5`

6, 7 ✓7ᵗʰ **S42.402** Unspecified fracture of lower end of **left** humerus `MCC` `CC` `H5`

6, 7 ✓7ᵗʰ **S42.409** Unspecified fracture of lower end of **unspecified** humerus `MCC` `CC` `H5`

✓6ᵗʰ **S42.41** Simple supracondylar fracture without intercondylar fracture of humerus

6, 7 ✓7ᵗʰ **S42.411** Displaced simple supracondylar fracture without intercondylar fracture of **right** humerus `MCC` `CC` `H5`

6, 7 ✓7ᵗʰ **S42.412** Displaced simple supracondylar fracture without intercondylar fracture of **left** humerus `MCC` `CC` `H5`

6, 7 ✓7ᵗʰ **S42.413** Displaced simple supracondylar fracture without intercondylar fracture of **unspecified** humerus `MCC` `CC` `H5`

6, 7 ✓7ᵗʰ **S42.414** Nondisplaced simple supracondylar fracture without intercondylar fracture of **right** humerus `MCC` `CC` `H5`

6, 7 ✓7ᵗʰ **S42.415** Nondisplaced simple supracondylar fracture without intercondylar fracture of **left** humerus `MCC` `CC` `H5`

6, 7 ✓7ᵗʰ **S42.416** Nondisplaced simple supracondylar fracture without intercondylar fracture of **unspecified** humerus `MCC` `CC` `H5`

✓6ᵗʰ **S42.42** Comminuted supracondylar fracture without intercondylar fracture of humerus

6, 7 ✓7ᵗʰ **S42.421** Displaced comminuted supracondylar fracture without intercondylar fracture of **right** humerus `MCC` `CC` `H5`

6, 7 ✓7ᵗʰ **S42.422** Displaced comminuted supracondylar fracture without intercondylar fracture of **left** humerus `MCC` `CC` `H5`

6, 7 ✓7ᵗʰ **S42.423** Displaced comminuted supracondylar fracture without intercondylar fracture of **unspecified** humerus `MCC` `CC` `H5`

6, 7 ✓7ᵗʰ **S42.424** Nondisplaced comminuted supracondylar fracture without intercondylar fracture of **right** humerus `MCC` `CC` `H5`

6, 7 ✓7ᵗʰ **S42.425** Nondisplaced comminuted supracondylar fracture without intercondylar fracture of **left** humerus `MCC` `CC` `H5`

6, 7 ✓7ᵗʰ **S42.426** Nondisplaced comminuted supracondylar fracture without intercondylar fracture of **unspecified** humerus `MCC` `CC` `H5`

✓6ᵗʰ **S42.43** Fracture (avulsion) of lateral epicondyle of humerus

6, 7 ✓7ᵗʰ **S42.431** Displaced fracture (avulsion) of lateral epicondyle of **right** humerus `MCC` `CC` `H5`

6, 7 ✓7ᵗʰ **S42.432** Displaced fracture (avulsion) of lateral epicondyle of **left** humerus `MCC` `CC` `H5`

6, 7 ✓7ᵗʰ **S42.433** Displaced fracture (avulsion) of lateral epicondyle of **unspecified** humerus `MCC` `CC` `H5`

6, 7 ✓7ᵗʰ **S42.434** Nondisplaced fracture (avulsion) of lateral epicondyle of **right** humerus `MCC` `CC` `H5`

6, 7 ✓7ᵗʰ **S42.435** Nondisplaced fracture (avulsion) of lateral epicondyle of **left** humerus `MCC` `CC` `H5`

6, 7 ✓7ᵗʰ **S42.436** Nondisplaced fracture (avulsion) of lateral epicondyle of **unspecified** humerus `MCC` `CC` `H5`

✓6ᵗʰ **S42.44** Fracture (avulsion) of medial epicondyle of humerus

6, 7 ✓7ᵗʰ **S42.441** Displaced fracture (avulsion) of medial epicondyle of **right** humerus `MCC` `CC` `H5`

6, 7 ✓7ᵗʰ **S42.442** Displaced fracture (avulsion) of medial epicondyle of **left** humerus `MCC` `CC` `H5`

6, 7 ✓7ᵗʰ **S42.443** Displaced fracture (avulsion) of medial epicondyle of **unspecified** humerus `MCC` `CC` `H5`

6, 7 ✓7ᵗʰ **S42.444** Nondisplaced fracture (avulsion) of medial epicondyle of **right** humerus `MCC` `CC` `H5`

6, 7 ✓7ᵗʰ **S42.445** Nondisplaced fracture (avulsion) of medial epicondyle of **left** humerus `MCC` `CC` `H5`

6, 7 ✓7ᵗʰ **S42.446** Nondisplaced fracture (avulsion) medial epicondyle of **unspecified** humerus `MCC` `CC` `H5`

6, 7 ✓7ᵗʰ **S42.447** Incarcerated fracture (avulsion) of medial epicondyle of **right** humerus `MCC` `CC` `H5`

6, 7 ✓7ᵗʰ **S42.448** Incarcerated fracture (avulsion) of medial epicondyle of **left** humerus `MCC` `CC` `H5`

6, 7 ✓7ᵗʰ **S42.449** Incarcerated fracture (avulsion) of medial epicondyle of **unspecified** humerus `MCC` `CC` `H5`

✓6ᵗʰ **S42.45** Fracture of lateral condyle of humerus
Fracture of capitellum of humerus

6, 7 ✓7ᵗʰ **S42.451** Displaced fracture of lateral condyle of **right** humerus `MCC` `CC` `H5`

6, 7 ✓7ᵗʰ **S42.452** Displaced fracture of lateral condyle of **left** humerus `MCC` `CC` `H5`

6, 7 ✓7ᵗʰ **S42.453** Displaced fracture of lateral condyle of **unspecified** humerus `MCC` `CC` `H5`

6, 7 ✓7ᵗʰ **S42.454** Nondisplaced fracture of lateral condyle of **right** humerus `MCC` `CC` `H5`

6, 7 ✓7ᵗʰ **S42.455** Nondisplaced fracture of lateral condyle of **left** humerus `MCC` `CC` `H5`

6, 7 ✓7ᵗʰ **S42.456** Nondisplaced fracture of lateral condyle of **unspecified** humerus `MCC` `CC` `H5`

✓6ᵗʰ **S42.46** Fracture of medial condyle of humerus
Trochlea fracture of humerus

6, 7 ✓7ᵗʰ **S42.461** Displaced fracture of medial condyle of **right** humerus `MCC` `CC` `H5`

6, 7 ✓7ᵗʰ **S42.462** Displaced fracture of medial condyle of **left** humerus `MCC` `CC` `H5`

6, 7 ✓7ᵗʰ **S42.463** Displaced fracture of medial condyle of **unspecified** humerus `MCC` `CC` `H5`

6, 7 ✓7ᵗʰ **S42.464** Nondisplaced fracture of medial condyle of **right** humerus `MCC` `CC` `H5`

---

6   MCC when reported as an open fracture (7th character B or C – specific to category).

7   CC when reported as an initial encounter (7th character A, B, or C – specific to category) OR a subsequent encounter for nonunion or malunion (7th character K, M, N, P, Q, or R – specific to category).

✓Additional Character Req   ✓ₓ7ᵗʰ Placeholder Alert   Unacceptable PDx   Manifestation   `H1`-`H14` HAC   `HCC` CMS-HCC Condition   *EXCLUDES 1* Not Coded Here   *EXCLUDES 2* Not Included Here

6, 7 ✓7th **S42.465** **Nondisplaced fracture of medial condyle of left humerus**   MCC CC H5

6, 7 ✓7th **S42.466** **Nondisplaced fracture of medial condyle of unspecified humerus**   MCC CC H5

✓6th **S42.47** **Transcondylar fracture of humerus**

6, 7 ✓7th **S42.471** **Displaced transcondylar fracture of right humerus**   MCC CC H5

6, 7 ✓7th **S42.472** **Displaced transcondylar fracture of left humerus**   MCC CC H5

6, 7 ✓7th **S42.473** **Displaced transcondylar fracture of unspecified humerus**   MCC CC H5

6, 7 ✓7th **S42.474** **Nondisplaced transcondylar fracture of right humerus**   MCC CC H5

6, 7 ✓7th **S42.475** **Nondisplaced transcondylar fracture of left humerus**   MCC CC H5

6, 7 ✓7th **S42.476** **Nondisplaced transcondylar fracture of unspecified humerus**   MCC CC H5

✓6th **S42.48** **Torus fracture of lower end of humerus**

> The appropriate 7th character is to be added to all codes in subcategory S42.48.
> A   initial encounter for closed fracture
> D   subsequent encounter for fracture with routine healing
> G   subsequent encounter for fracture with delayed healing
> K   subsequent encounter for fracture with nonunion
> P   subsequent encounter for fracture with malunion
> S   sequela

7 ✓7th **S42.481** **Torus fracture of lower end of right humerus**   CC H5
CC Excl: CC with 7th character A:
PDX collection 1245
CC with 7th character K or P:
PDX collection 897

7 ✓7th **S42.482** **Torus fracture of lower end of left humerus**   CC H5
CC Excl: CC with 7th character A:
PDX collection 1247
CC with 7th character K or P:
PDX collection 897

7 ✓7th **S42.489** **Torus fracture of lower end of unspecified humerus**   CC H5
CC Excl: CC with 7th character A:
PDX collection 1248
CC with 7th character K or P:
PDX collection 897

✓6th **S42.49** **Other fracture of lower end of humerus**

6, 7 ✓7th **S42.491** **Other displaced fracture of lower end of right humerus**   MCC CC H5

6, 7 ✓7th **S42.492** **Other displaced fracture of lower end of left humerus**   MCC CC H5

6, 7 ✓7th **S42.493** **Other displaced fracture of lower end of unspecified humerus**   MCC CC H5

6, 7 ✓7th **S42.494** **Other nondisplaced fracture of lower end of right humerus**   MCC CC H5

6, 7 ✓7th **S42.495** **Other nondisplaced fracture of lower end of left humerus**   MCC CC H5

6, 7 ✓7th **S42.496** **Other nondisplaced fracture of lower end of unspecified humerus**   MCC CC H5

✓5th **S42.9** **Fracture of shoulder girdle, part unspecified**
Fracture of shoulder NOS

CC Excl: For CC/MCC codes in subcategory S42.9:
See code S42.209

6, 7 ✓x7th **S42.90** **Fracture of unspecified shoulder girdle, part unspecified**   MCC CC H5

6, 7 ✓x7th **S42.91** **Fracture of right shoulder girdle, part unspecified**   MCC CC H5

6, 7 ✓x7th **S42.92** **Fracture of left shoulder girdle, part unspecified**   MCC CC H5

✓4th **S43** **Dislocation and sprain of joints and ligaments of shoulder girdle**
INCLUDES   avulsion of joint or ligament of shoulder girdle
laceration of cartilage, joint or ligament of shoulder girdle
sprain of cartilage, joint or ligament of shoulder girdle
traumatic hemarthrosis of joint or ligament of shoulder girdle
traumatic rupture of joint or ligament of shoulder girdle
traumatic subluxation of joint or ligament of shoulder girdle
traumatic tear of joint or ligament of shoulder girdle
Code also any associated open wound
EXCLUDES 2   strain of muscle, fascia and tendon of shoulder and upper arm (S46.-)

> The appropriate 7th character is to be added to each code from category S43.
> A   initial encounter
> D   subsequent encounter
> S   sequela

✓5th **S43.0** **Subluxation and dislocation of shoulder joint**
Dislocation of glenohumeral joint
Subluxation of glenohumeral joint

✓6th **S43.00** **Unspecified subluxation and dislocation of shoulder joint**
Dislocation of humerus NOS
Subluxation of humerus NOS

✓7th **S43.001** **Unspecified subluxation of right shoulder joint**

✓7th **S43.002** **Unspecified subluxation of left shoulder joint**

✓7th **S43.003** **Unspecified subluxation of unspecified shoulder joint**

✓7th **S43.004** **Unspecified dislocation of right shoulder joint**

✓7th **S43.005** **Unspecified dislocation of left shoulder joint**

✓7th **S43.006** **Unspecified dislocation of unspecified shoulder joint**

✓6th **S43.01** **Anterior subluxation and dislocation of humerus**

✓7th **S43.011** **Anterior subluxation of right humerus**

✓7th **S43.012** **Anterior subluxation of left humerus**

✓7th **S43.013** **Anterior subluxation of unspecified humerus**

✓7th **S43.014** **Anterior dislocation of right humerus**

✓7th **S43.015** **Anterior dislocation of left humerus**

✓7th **S43.016** **Anterior dislocation of unspecified humerus**

✓6th **S43.02** **Posterior subluxation and dislocation of humerus**

✓7th **S43.021** **Posterior subluxation of right humerus**

✓7th **S43.022** **Posterior subluxation of left humerus**

✓7th **S43.023** **Posterior subluxation of unspecified humerus**

✓7th **S43.024** **Posterior dislocation of right humerus**

✓7th **S43.025** **Posterior dislocation of left humerus**

✓7th **S43.026** **Posterior dislocation of unspecified humerus**

✓6th **S43.03** **Inferior subluxation and dislocation of humerus**

✓7th **S43.031** **Inferior subluxation of right humerus**

✓7th **S43.032** **Inferior subluxation of left humerus**

✓7th **S43.033** **Inferior subluxation of unspecified humerus**

✓7th **S43.034** **Inferior dislocation of right humerus**

✓7th **S43.035** **Inferior dislocation of left humerus**

✓7th **S43.036** **Inferior dislocation of unspecified humerus**

✓6th **S43.08** **Other subluxation and dislocation of shoulder joint**

✓7th **S43.081** **Other subluxation of right shoulder joint**

✓7th **S43.082** **Other subluxation of left shoulder joint**

✓7th **S43.083** **Other subluxation of unspecified shoulder joint**

✓7th **S43.084** **Other dislocation of right shoulder joint**

✓7th **S43.085** **Other dislocation of left shoulder joint**

✓7th **S43.086** **Other dislocation of unspecified shoulder joint**

---

6   MCC when reported as an open fracture (7th character B or C – specific to category).
7   CC when reported as an initial encounter (7th character A, B, or C – specific to category) OR a subsequent encounter for nonunion or malunion (7th character K, M, N, P, Q, or R – specific to category).

N Newborn: 0   P Pediatric: 0-17   M Maternity: 12-55   A Adult: 15-124   MCC Major CC Condition   PDxMCC PDx acts as own MCC   CC CC Condition   PDxCC PDx acts as own CC

990   ICD-10-CM 2018

√5ᵗʰ **S43.1** Subluxation and dislocation of acromioclavicular joint
- √6ᵗʰ **S43.10** Unspecified dislocation of acromioclavicular joint
  - √7ᵗʰ **S43.101** Unspecified dislocation of right acromioclavicular joint
  - √7ᵗʰ **S43.102** Unspecified dislocation of left acromioclavicular joint
  - √7ᵗʰ **S43.109** Unspecified dislocation of unspecified acromioclavicular joint
- √6ᵗʰ **S43.11** Subluxation of acromioclavicular joint
  - √7ᵗʰ **S43.111** Subluxation of right acromioclavicular joint
  - √7ᵗʰ **S43.112** Subluxation of left acromioclavicular joint
  - √7ᵗʰ **S43.119** Subluxation of unspecified acromioclavicular joint
- √6ᵗʰ **S43.12** Dislocation of acromioclavicular joint, 100%-200% displacement
  - √7ᵗʰ **S43.121** Dislocation of right acromioclavicular joint, 100%-200% displacement
  - √7ᵗʰ **S43.122** Dislocation of left acromioclavicular joint, 100%-200% displacement
  - √7ᵗʰ **S43.129** Dislocation of unspecified acromioclavicular joint, 100%-200% displacement
- √6ᵗʰ **S43.13** Dislocation of acromioclavicular joint, greater than 200% displacement
  - √7ᵗʰ **S43.131** Dislocation of right acromioclavicular joint, greater than 200% displacement
  - √7ᵗʰ **S43.132** Dislocation of left acromioclavicular joint, greater than 200% displacement
  - √7ᵗʰ **S43.139** Dislocation of unspecified acromioclavicular joint, greater than 200% displacement
- √6ᵗʰ **S43.14** Inferior dislocation of acromioclavicular joint
  - √7ᵗʰ **S43.141** Inferior dislocation of right acromioclavicular joint
  - √7ᵗʰ **S43.142** Inferior dislocation of left acromioclavicular joint
  - √7ᵗʰ **S43.149** Inferior dislocation of unspecified acromioclavicular joint
- √6ᵗʰ **S43.15** Posterior dislocation of acromioclavicular joint
  - √7ᵗʰ **S43.151** Posterior dislocation of right acromioclavicular joint
  - √7ᵗʰ **S43.152** Posterior dislocation of left acromioclavicular joint
  - √7ᵗʰ **S43.159** Posterior dislocation of unspecified acromioclavicular joint

√5ᵗʰ **S43.2** Subluxation and dislocation of sternoclavicular joint

> **CC Excl:** For CC codes in subcategory S43.2:
> **Right side:** PDX collection 1252
> **Left side:** PDX collection 1253
> **Unspecified side:** PDX collection 914

- √6ᵗʰ **S43.20** Unspecified subluxation and dislocation of sternoclavicular joint
  - √7ᵗʰ **S43.201** Unspecified subluxation of right sternoclavicular joint `CC` `H5`
  - √7ᵗʰ **S43.202** Unspecified subluxation of left sternoclavicular joint `CC` `H5`
  - √7ᵗʰ **S43.203** Unspecified subluxation of unspecified sternoclavicular joint `CC` `H5`
  - √7ᵗʰ **S43.204** Unspecified dislocation of right sternoclavicular joint `CC` `H5`
  - √7ᵗʰ **S43.205** Unspecified dislocation of left sternoclavicular joint `CC` `H5`
  - √7ᵗʰ **S43.206** Unspecified dislocation of unspecified sternoclavicular joint `CC` `H5`
- √6ᵗʰ **S43.21** Anterior subluxation and dislocation of sternoclavicular joint
  - √7ᵗʰ **S43.211** Anterior subluxation of right sternoclavicular joint `CC` `H5`
  - √7ᵗʰ **S43.212** Anterior subluxation of left sternoclavicular joint `CC` `H5`
  - √7ᵗʰ **S43.213** Anterior subluxation of unspecified sternoclavicular joint `CC` `H5`
  - √7ᵗʰ **S43.214** Anterior dislocation of right sternoclavicular joint `CC` `H5`
  - √7ᵗʰ **S43.215** Anterior dislocation of left sternoclavicular joint `CC` `H5`
  - √7ᵗʰ **S43.216** Anterior dislocation of unspecified sternoclavicular joint `CC` `H5`
- √6ᵗʰ **S43.22** Posterior subluxation and dislocation of sternoclavicular joint
  - √7ᵗʰ **S43.221** Posterior subluxation of right sternoclavicular joint `CC` `H5`
  - √7ᵗʰ **S43.222** Posterior subluxation of left sternoclavicular joint `CC` `H5`
  - √7ᵗʰ **S43.223** Posterior subluxation of unspecified sternoclavicular joint `CC` `H5`
  - √7ᵗʰ **S43.224** Posterior dislocation of right sternoclavicular joint `CC` `H5`
  - √7ᵗʰ **S43.225** Posterior dislocation of left sternoclavicular joint `CC` `H5`
  - √7ᵗʰ **S43.226** Posterior dislocation of unspecified sternoclavicular joint `CC` `H5`

√5ᵗʰ **S43.3** Subluxation and dislocation of other and unspecified parts of shoulder girdle
- √6ᵗʰ **S43.30** Subluxation and dislocation of unspecified parts of shoulder girdle
  - Dislocation of shoulder girdle NOS
  - Subluxation of shoulder girdle NOS
  - √7ᵗʰ **S43.301** Subluxation of unspecified parts of right shoulder girdle
  - √7ᵗʰ **S43.302** Subluxation of unspecified parts of left shoulder girdle
  - √7ᵗʰ **S43.303** Subluxation of unspecified parts of unspecified shoulder girdle
  - √7ᵗʰ **S43.304** Dislocation of unspecified parts of right shoulder girdle
  - √7ᵗʰ **S43.305** Dislocation of unspecified parts of left shoulder girdle
  - √7ᵗʰ **S43.306** Dislocation of unspecified parts of unspecified shoulder girdle
- √6ᵗʰ **S43.31** Subluxation and dislocation of scapula
  - √7ᵗʰ **S43.311** Subluxation of right scapula
  - √7ᵗʰ **S43.312** Subluxation of left scapula
  - √7ᵗʰ **S43.313** Subluxation of unspecified scapula
  - √7ᵗʰ **S43.314** Dislocation of right scapula
  - √7ᵗʰ **S43.315** Dislocation of left scapula
  - √7ᵗʰ **S43.316** Dislocation of unspecified scapula
- √6ᵗʰ **S43.39** Subluxation and dislocation of other parts of shoulder girdle
  - √7ᵗʰ **S43.391** Subluxation of other parts of right shoulder girdle
  - √7ᵗʰ **S43.392** Subluxation of other parts of left shoulder girdle
  - √7ᵗʰ **S43.393** Subluxation of other parts of unspecified shoulder girdle
  - √7ᵗʰ **S43.394** Dislocation of other parts of right shoulder girdle
  - √7ᵗʰ **S43.395** Dislocation of other parts of left shoulder girdle
  - √7ᵗʰ **S43.396** Dislocation of other parts of unspecified shoulder girdle

√5ᵗʰ **S43.4** Sprain of shoulder joint
- √6ᵗʰ **S43.40** Unspecified sprain of shoulder joint
  - √7ᵗʰ **S43.401** Unspecified sprain of right shoulder joint
  - √7ᵗʰ **S43.402** Unspecified sprain of left shoulder joint
  - √7ᵗʰ **S43.409** Unspecified sprain of unspecified shoulder joint
- √6ᵗʰ **S43.41** Sprain of coracohumeral (ligament)
  - √7ᵗʰ **S43.411** Sprain of right coracohumeral (ligament)
  - √7ᵗʰ **S43.412** Sprain of left coracohumeral (ligament)
  - √7ᵗʰ **S43.419** Sprain of unspecified coracohumeral (ligament)

☑ Additional Character Req   √x7ᵗʰ Placeholder Alert   Unacceptable PDx   Manifestation   **H1**-**H14** HAC   **HCC** CMS-HCC Condition   *EXCLUDES 1* Not Coded Here   *EXCLUDES 2* Not Included Here

ICD-10-CM 2018   991

√6ᵗʰ **S43.42** **Sprain of** rotator cuff capsule
> *EXCLUDES 1*   *rotator cuff syndrome (complete) (incomplete), not specified as traumatic (M75.1-)*
> *EXCLUDES 2*   *injury of tendon of rotator cuff (S46.Ø-)*

    √7ᵗʰ **S43.421** **Sprain of** right **rotator cuff capsule**
    √7ᵗʰ **S43.422** **Sprain of** left **rotator cuff capsule**
    √7ᵗʰ **S43.429** **Sprain of** unspecified **rotator cuff capsule**

√6ᵗʰ **S43.43** **Superior glenoid labrum** lesion
> SLAP lesion
> **DEF:** Detachment injury of the superior aspect of the glenoid labrum, which is the ring of fibrocartilage attached to the rim of the glenoid cavity of the scapula.

    √7ᵗʰ **S43.431** **Superior glenoid labrum lesion of** right **shoulder**
    √7ᵗʰ **S43.432** **Superior glenoid labrum lesion of** left **shoulder**
    √7ᵗʰ **S43.439** **Superior glenoid labrum lesion of** unspecified **shoulder**

√6ᵗʰ **S43.49** Other **sprain of shoulder joint**

    √7ᵗʰ **S43.491** **Other sprain of** right **shoulder joint**
    √7ᵗʰ **S43.492** **Other sprain of** left **shoulder joint**
    √7ᵗʰ **S43.499** **Other sprain of** unspecified **shoulder joint**

√5ᵗʰ **S43.5** **Sprain of** acromioclavicular **joint**
> Sprain of acromioclavicular ligament

   √x7ᵗʰ **S43.5Ø** **Sprain of** unspecified **acromioclavicular joint**
   √x7ᵗʰ **S43.51** **Sprain of** right **acromioclavicular joint**
   √x7ᵗʰ **S43.52** **Sprain of** left **acromioclavicular joint**

√5ᵗʰ **S43.6** **Sprain of** sternoclavicular **joint**

   √x7ᵗʰ **S43.6Ø** **Sprain of** unspecified **sternoclavicular joint**
   √x7ᵗʰ **S43.61** **Sprain of** right **sternoclavicular joint**
   √x7ᵗʰ **S43.62** **Sprain of** left **sternoclavicular joint**

√5ᵗʰ **S43.8** **Sprain of** other **specified parts of shoulder girdle**

   √x7ᵗʰ **S43.8Ø** **Sprain of other specified parts of** unspecified **shoulder girdle**
   √x7ᵗʰ **S43.81** **Sprain of other specified parts of** right **shoulder girdle**
   √x7ᵗʰ **S43.82** **Sprain of other specified parts of** left **shoulder girdle**

√5ᵗʰ **S43.9** **Sprain of** unspecified **parts of shoulder girdle**

   √x7ᵗʰ **S43.9Ø** **Sprain of unspecified parts of** unspecified **shoulder girdle**
> Sprain of shoulder girdle NOS

   √x7ᵗʰ **S43.91** **Sprain of unspecified parts of** right **shoulder girdle**
   √x7ᵗʰ **S43.92** **Sprain of unspecified parts of** left **shoulder girdle**

√4ᵗʰ **S44** **Injury of nerves at shoulder and upper arm level**
> Code also any associated open wound (S41.-)
> *EXCLUDES 2*   *injury of brachial plexus (S14.3-)*
>
> The appropriate 7th character is to be added to each code from category S44.
> A   initial encounter
> D   subsequent encounter
> S   sequela

√5ᵗʰ **S44.Ø** **Injury of** ulnar nerve **at upper arm level**
> *EXCLUDES 1*   *ulnar nerve NOS (S54.Ø)*

   √x7ᵗʰ **S44.ØØ** **Injury of ulnar nerve at upper arm level,** unspecified **arm**
   √x7ᵗʰ **S44.Ø1** **Injury of ulnar nerve at upper arm level,** right **arm**
   √x7ᵗʰ **S44.Ø2** **Injury of ulnar nerve at upper arm level,** left **arm**

√5ᵗʰ **S44.1** **Injury of** median nerve **at upper arm level**
> *EXCLUDES 1*   *median nerve NOS (S54.1)*

   √x7ᵗʰ **S44.1Ø** **Injury of median nerve at upper arm level,** unspecified **arm**
   √x7ᵗʰ **S44.11** **Injury of median nerve at upper arm level,** right **arm**
   √x7ᵗʰ **S44.12** **Injury of median nerve at upper arm level,** left **arm**

√5ᵗʰ **S44.2** **Injury of** radial nerve **at upper arm level**
> *EXCLUDES 1*   *radial nerve NOS (S54.2)*

   √x7ᵗʰ **S44.2Ø** **Injury of radial nerve at upper arm level,** unspecified **arm**
   √x7ᵗʰ **S44.21** **Injury of radial nerve at upper arm level,** right **arm**
   √x7ᵗʰ **S44.22** **Injury of radial nerve at upper arm level,** left **arm**

√5ᵗʰ **S44.3** **Injury of** axillary nerve

   √x7ᵗʰ **S44.3Ø** **Injury of axillary nerve,** unspecified **arm**
   √x7ᵗʰ **S44.31** **Injury of axillary nerve,** right **arm**
   √x7ᵗʰ **S44.32** **Injury of axillary nerve,** left **arm**

√5ᵗʰ **S44.4** **Injury of** musculocutaneous nerve

   √x7ᵗʰ **S44.4Ø** **Injury of musculocutaneous nerve,** unspecified **arm**
   √x7ᵗʰ **S44.41** **Injury of musculocutaneous nerve,** right **arm**
   √x7ᵗʰ **S44.42** **Injury of musculocutaneous nerve,** left **arm**

√5ᵗʰ **S44.5** **Injury of** cutaneous sensory nerve **at shoulder and upper arm level**

   √x7ᵗʰ **S44.5Ø** **Injury of cutaneous sensory nerve at shoulder and upper arm level,** unspecified **arm**
   √x7ᵗʰ **S44.51** **Injury of cutaneous sensory nerve at shoulder and upper arm level,** right **arm**
   √x7ᵗʰ **S44.52** **Injury of cutaneous sensory nerve at shoulder and upper arm level,** left **arm**

√5ᵗʰ **S44.8** **Injury of other nerves at shoulder and upper arm level**

   √6ᵗʰ **S44.8X** **Injury of** other nerves **at shoulder and upper arm level**

     √7ᵗʰ **S44.8X1** **Injury of other nerves at shoulder and upper arm level,** right **arm**
     √7ᵗʰ **S44.8X2** **Injury of other nerves at shoulder and upper arm level,** left **arm**
     √7ᵗʰ **S44.8X9** **Injury of other nerves at shoulder and upper arm level,** unspecified **arm**

√5ᵗʰ **S44.9** **Injury of** unspecified **nerve at shoulder and upper arm level**

   √x7ᵗʰ **S44.9Ø** **Injury of unspecified nerve at shoulder and upper arm level,** unspecified **arm**
   √x7ᵗʰ **S44.91** **Injury of unspecified nerve at shoulder and upper arm level,** right **arm**
   √x7ᵗʰ **S44.92** **Injury of unspecified nerve at shoulder and upper arm level,** left **arm**

√4ᵗʰ **S45** **Injury of blood vessels at shoulder and upper arm level**
> Code also any associated open wound (S41.-)
> *EXCLUDES 2*   *injury of subclavian artery (S25.1)*
>   *injury of subclavian vein (S25.3)*
>
> The appropriate 7th character is to be added to each code from category S45.
> A   initial encounter
> D   subsequent encounter
> S   sequela

√5ᵗʰ **S45.Ø** **Injury of** axillary artery

> **CC Excl: For MCC codes in subcategory S45.Ø:**
> **Right side:** PDX collection 1254
> **Left side:** PDX collection 1255
> **Unspecified side:** PDX collection 1256

   √6ᵗʰ **S45.ØØ** **Unspecified injury of axillary artery**

     √7ᵗʰ **S45.ØØ1** **Unspecified injury of axillary artery,** right **side** MCC
     √7ᵗʰ **S45.ØØ2** **Unspecified injury of axillary artery,** left **side** MCC
     √7ᵗʰ **S45.ØØ9** **Unspecified injury of axillary artery,** unspecified **side** MCC

   √6ᵗʰ **S45.Ø1** **Laceration of axillary artery**

     √7ᵗʰ **S45.Ø11** **Laceration of axillary artery,** right **side** MCC
     √7ᵗʰ **S45.Ø12** **Laceration of axillary artery,** left **side** MCC
     √7ᵗʰ **S45.Ø19** **Laceration of axillary artery,** unspecified **side** MCC

   √6ᵗʰ **S45.Ø9** **Other specified injury of axillary artery**

     √7ᵗʰ **S45.Ø91** **Other specified injury of axillary artery,** right **side** MCC
     √7ᵗʰ **S45.Ø92** **Other specified injury of axillary artery,** left **side** MCC
     √7ᵗʰ **S45.Ø99** **Other specified injury of axillary artery,** unspecified **side** MCC

☑5ᵗʰ **S45.1**   **Injury of** brachial artery

> **CC Excl: For CC codes in subcategory S45.1:**
> **Right side:** PDX collection 1257
> **Left side:** PDX collection 1258
> **Unspecified side:** PDX collection 1259

    ☑6ᵗʰ **S45.10**   **Unspecified** injury of brachial artery

       ☑7ᵗʰ **S45.101**   Unspecified injury of brachial artery, right **side**   CC

       ☑7ᵗʰ **S45.102**   Unspecified injury of brachial artery, left **side**   CC

       ☑7ᵗʰ **S45.109**   Unspecified injury of brachial artery, unspecified **side**   CC

    ☑6ᵗʰ **S45.11**   **Laceration** of brachial artery

       ☑7ᵗʰ **S45.111**   Laceration of brachial artery, right **side**   CC

       ☑7ᵗʰ **S45.112**   Laceration of brachial artery, left **side**   CC

       ☑7ᵗʰ **S45.119**   Laceration of brachial artery, unspecified **side**   CC

    ☑6ᵗʰ **S45.19**   **Other** specified injury of brachial artery

       ☑7ᵗʰ **S45.191**   Other specified injury of brachial artery, right **side**   CC

       ☑7ᵗʰ **S45.192**   Other specified injury of brachial artery, left **side**   CC

       ☑7ᵗʰ **S45.199**   Other specified injury of brachial artery, unspecified **side**   CC

☑5ᵗʰ **S45.2**   **Injury of** axillary or brachial vein

> **CC Excl: For CC codes in subcategory S45.2:**
> **Right side:** PDX collection 1257
> **Left side:** PDX collection 1258
> **Unspecified side:** PDX collection 1259

    ☑6ᵗʰ **S45.20**   **Unspecified** injury of axillary or brachial vein

       ☑7ᵗʰ **S45.201**   Unspecified injury of axillary or brachial vein, right **side**   CC

       ☑7ᵗʰ **S45.202**   Unspecified injury of axillary or brachial vein, left **side**   CC

       ☑7ᵗʰ **S45.209**   Unspecified injury of axillary or brachial vein, unspecified **side**   CC

    ☑6ᵗʰ **S45.21**   **Laceration** of axillary or brachial vein

       ☑7ᵗʰ **S45.211**   Laceration of axillary or brachial vein, right **side**   CC

       ☑7ᵗʰ **S45.212**   Laceration of axillary or brachial vein, left **side**   CC

       ☑7ᵗʰ **S45.219**   Laceration of axillary or brachial vein, unspecified **side**   CC

    ☑6ᵗʰ **S45.29**   **Other** specified injury of axillary or brachial vein

       ☑7ᵗʰ **S45.291**   Other specified injury of axillary or brachial vein, right **side**   CC

       ☑7ᵗʰ **S45.292**   Other specified injury of axillary or brachial vein, left **side**   CC

       ☑7ᵗʰ **S45.299**   Other specified injury of axillary or brachial vein, unspecified **side**   CC

☑5ᵗʰ **S45.3**   **Injury of** superficial vein **at shoulder and upper arm level**

> **CC Excl: For CC codes in subcategory S45.3:**
> **Right side:** PDX collection 1260
> **Left side:** PDX collection 1261
> **Unspecified side:** PDX collection 1262

    ☑6ᵗʰ **S45.30**   **Unspecified** injury of superficial vein at shoulder and upper arm level

       ☑7ᵗʰ **S45.301**   Unspecified injury of superficial vein at shoulder and upper arm level, right **arm**   CC

       ☑7ᵗʰ **S45.302**   Unspecified injury of superficial vein at shoulder and upper arm level, left **arm**   CC

       ☑7ᵗʰ **S45.309**   Unspecified injury of superficial vein at shoulder and upper arm level, unspecified **arm**   CC

    ☑6ᵗʰ **S45.31**   **Laceration** of superficial vein at shoulder and upper arm level

       ☑7ᵗʰ **S45.311**   Laceration of superficial vein at shoulder and upper arm level, right **arm**   CC

       ☑7ᵗʰ **S45.312**   Laceration of superficial vein at shoulder and upper arm level, left **arm**   CC

       ☑7ᵗʰ **S45.319**   Laceration of superficial vein at shoulder and upper arm level, unspecified **arm**   CC

    ☑6ᵗʰ **S45.39**   **Other** specified injury of superficial vein at shoulder and upper arm level

       ☑7ᵗʰ **S45.391**   Other specified injury of superficial vein at shoulder and upper arm level, right **arm**   CC

       ☑7ᵗʰ **S45.392**   Other specified injury of superficial vein at shoulder and upper arm level, left **arm**   CC

       ☑7ᵗʰ **S45.399**   Other specified injury of superficial vein at shoulder and upper arm level, unspecified **arm**   CC

☑5ᵗʰ **S45.8**   **Injury of** other specified blood vessels **at shoulder and upper arm level**

> **CC Excl: For CC codes in subcategory S45.8:**
> **Right side:** PDX collection 1260
> **Left side:** PDX collection 1261
> **Unspecified side:** PDX collection 1262

    ☑6ᵗʰ **S45.80**   **Unspecified** injury of other specified blood vessels at shoulder and upper arm level

       ☑7ᵗʰ **S45.801**   Unspecified injury of other specified blood vessels at shoulder and upper arm level, right **arm**   CC

       ☑7ᵗʰ **S45.802**   Unspecified injury of other specified blood vessels at shoulder and upper arm level, left **arm**   CC

       ☑7ᵗʰ **S45.809**   Unspecified injury of other specified blood vessels at shoulder and upper arm level, unspecified **arm**   CC

    ☑6ᵗʰ **S45.81**   **Laceration** of other specified blood vessels at shoulder and upper arm level

       ☑7ᵗʰ **S45.811**   Laceration of other specified blood vessels at shoulder and upper arm level, right **arm**   CC

       ☑7ᵗʰ **S45.812**   Laceration of other specified blood vessels at shoulder and upper arm level, left **arm**   CC

       ☑7ᵗʰ **S45.819**   Laceration of other specified blood vessels at shoulder and upper arm level, unspecified **arm**   CC

    ☑6ᵗʰ **S45.89**   **Other** specified injury of other specified blood vessels at shoulder and upper arm level

       ☑7ᵗʰ **S45.891**   Other specified injury of other specified blood vessels at shoulder and upper arm level, right **arm**   CC

       ☑7ᵗʰ **S45.892**   Other specified injury of other specified blood vessels at shoulder and upper arm level, left **arm**   CC

       ☑7ᵗʰ **S45.899**   Other specified injury of other specified blood vessels at shoulder and upper arm level, unspecified **arm**   CC

☑5ᵗʰ **S45.9**   **Injury of** unspecified blood vessel **at shoulder and upper arm level**

> **CC Excl: For CC codes in subcategory S45.9:**
> **Right side:** PDX collection 1260
> **Left side:** PDX collection 1261
> **Unspecified side:** PDX collection 1262

    ☑6ᵗʰ **S45.90**   **Unspecified** injury of unspecified blood vessel at shoulder and upper arm level

       ☑7ᵗʰ **S45.901**   Unspecified injury of unspecified blood vessel at shoulder and upper arm level, right **arm**   CC

       ☑7ᵗʰ **S45.902**   Unspecified injury of unspecified blood vessel at shoulder and upper arm level, left **arm**   CC

       ☑7ᵗʰ **S45.909**   Unspecified injury of unspecified blood vessel at shoulder and upper arm level, unspecified **arm**   CC

    ☑6ᵗʰ **S45.91**   **Laceration** of unspecified blood vessel at shoulder and upper arm level

       ☑7ᵗʰ **S45.911**   Laceration of unspecified blood vessel at shoulder and upper arm level, right **arm**   CC

☑ Additional Character Req   ☑ₓ7ᵗʰ Placeholder Alert   Unacceptable PDx   Manifestation   **H1**-**H14** HAC   **HCC** CMS-HCC Condition   *EXCLUDES 1* Not Coded Here   *EXCLUDES 2* Not Included Here

☑7ᵗʰ **S45.912** Laceration of unspecified blood vessel at shoulder and upper arm level, **left** arm   CC

☑7ᵗʰ **S45.919** Laceration of unspecified blood vessel at shoulder and upper arm level, **unspecified** arm   CC

☑6ᵗʰ **S45.99** Other specified injury of unspecified blood vessel at shoulder and upper arm level

☑7ᵗʰ **S45.991** Other specified injury of unspecified blood vessel at shoulder and upper arm level, **right** arm   CC

☑7ᵗʰ **S45.992** Other specified injury of unspecified blood vessel at shoulder and upper arm level, **left** arm   CC

☑7ᵗʰ **S45.999** Other specified injury of unspecified blood vessel at shoulder and upper arm level, **unspecified** arm   CC

☑4ᵗʰ **S46** **Injury of muscle, fascia and tendon at shoulder and upper arm level**

Code also any associated open wound (S41.-)

EXCLUDES 2   *injury of muscle, fascia and tendon at elbow (S56.-)*
sprain of joints and ligaments of shoulder girdle (S43.9)

TIP: Refer to the Muscle/Tendon table at the beginning of this chapter.

The appropriate 7th character is to be added to each code from category S46.
A   initial encounter
D   subsequent encounter
S   sequela

CC Excl: For CC codes in category S46:
Right side: PDX collection 1263
Left side: PDX collection 1264
Unspecified side: PDX collection 1265

☑5ᵗʰ **S46.0** **Injury of muscle(s) and tendon(s) of the rotator cuff of shoulder**

☑6ᵗʰ **S46.00** Unspecified injury of muscle(s) and tendon(s) of the rotator cuff of shoulder

☑7ᵗʰ **S46.001** Unspecified injury of muscle(s) and tendon(s) of the rotator cuff of **right** shoulder

☑7ᵗʰ **S46.002** Unspecified injury of muscle(s) and tendon(s) of the rotator cuff of **left** shoulder

☑7ᵗʰ **S46.009** Unspecified injury of muscle(s) and tendon(s) of the rotator cuff of **unspecified** shoulder

☑6ᵗʰ **S46.01** Strain of muscle(s) and tendon(s) of the rotator cuff of shoulder

☑7ᵗʰ **S46.011** Strain of muscle(s) and tendon(s) of the rotator cuff of **right** shoulder

☑7ᵗʰ **S46.012** Strain of muscle(s) and tendon(s) of the rotator cuff of **left** shoulder

☑7ᵗʰ **S46.019** Strain of muscle(s) and tendon(s) of the rotator cuff of **unspecified** shoulder

☑6ᵗʰ **S46.02** Laceration of muscle(s) and tendon(s) of the rotator cuff of shoulder

☑7ᵗʰ **S46.021** Laceration of muscle(s) and tendon(s) of the rotator cuff of **right** shoulder   CC

☑7ᵗʰ **S46.022** Laceration of muscle(s) and tendon(s) of the rotator cuff of **left** shoulder   CC

☑7ᵗʰ **S46.029** Laceration of muscle(s) and tendon(s) of the rotator cuff of **unspecified** shoulder   CC

☑6ᵗʰ **S46.09** Other injury of muscle(s) and tendon(s) of the rotator cuff of shoulder

☑7ᵗʰ **S46.091** Other injury of muscle(s) and tendon(s) of the rotator cuff of **right** shoulder

☑7ᵗʰ **S46.092** Other injury of muscle(s) and tendon(s) of the rotator cuff of **left** shoulder

☑7ᵗʰ **S46.099** Other injury of muscle(s) and tendon(s) of the rotator cuff of **unspecified** shoulder

☑5ᵗʰ **S46.1** Injury of muscle, fascia and tendon of long head of biceps

☑6ᵗʰ **S46.10** Unspecified injury of muscle, fascia and tendon of long head of biceps

☑7ᵗʰ **S46.101** Unspecified injury of muscle, fascia and tendon of long head of biceps, **right** arm

☑7ᵗʰ **S46.102** Unspecified injury of muscle, fascia and tendon of long head of biceps, **left** arm

☑7ᵗʰ **S46.109** Unspecified injury of muscle, fascia and tendon of long head of biceps, **unspecified** arm

☑6ᵗʰ **S46.11** Strain of muscle, fascia and tendon of long head of biceps

☑7ᵗʰ **S46.111** Strain of muscle, fascia and tendon of long head of biceps, **right** arm

☑7ᵗʰ **S46.112** Strain of muscle, fascia and tendon of long head of biceps, **left** arm

☑7ᵗʰ **S46.119** Strain of muscle, fascia and tendon of long head of biceps, **unspecified** arm

☑6ᵗʰ **S46.12** Laceration of muscle, fascia and tendon of long head of biceps

☑7ᵗʰ **S46.121** Laceration of muscle, fascia and tendon of long head of biceps, **right** arm   CC

☑7ᵗʰ **S46.122** Laceration of muscle, fascia and tendon of long head of biceps, **left** arm   CC

☑7ᵗʰ **S46.129** Laceration of muscle, fascia and tendon of long head of biceps, **unspecified** arm   CC

☑6ᵗʰ **S46.19** Other injury of muscle, fascia and tendon of long head of biceps

☑7ᵗʰ **S46.191** Other injury of muscle, fascia and tendon of long head of biceps, **right** arm

☑7ᵗʰ **S46.192** Other injury of muscle, fascia and tendon of long head of biceps, **left** arm

☑7ᵗʰ **S46.199** Other injury of muscle, fascia and tendon of long head of biceps, **unspecified** arm

☑5ᵗʰ **S46.2** Injury of muscle, fascia and tendon of **other parts** of biceps

☑6ᵗʰ **S46.20** Unspecified injury of muscle, fascia and tendon of other parts of biceps

☑7ᵗʰ **S46.201** Unspecified injury of muscle, fascia and tendon of other parts of biceps, **right** arm

☑7ᵗʰ **S46.202** Unspecified injury of muscle, fascia and tendon of other parts of biceps, **left** arm

☑7ᵗʰ **S46.209** Unspecified injury of muscle, fascia and tendon of other parts of biceps, **unspecified** arm

☑6ᵗʰ **S46.21** Strain of muscle, fascia and tendon of other parts of biceps

☑7ᵗʰ **S46.211** Strain of muscle, fascia and tendon of other parts of biceps, **right** arm

☑7ᵗʰ **S46.212** Strain of muscle, fascia and tendon of other parts of biceps, **left** arm

☑7ᵗʰ **S46.219** Strain of muscle, fascia and tendon of other parts of biceps, **unspecified** arm

☑6ᵗʰ **S46.22** Laceration of muscle, fascia and tendon of other parts of biceps

☑7ᵗʰ **S46.221** Laceration of muscle, fascia and tendon of other parts of biceps, **right** arm   CC

☑7ᵗʰ **S46.222** Laceration of muscle, fascia and tendon of other parts of biceps, **left** arm   CC

☑7ᵗʰ **S46.229** Laceration of muscle, fascia and tendon of other parts of biceps, **unspecified** arm   CC

☑6ᵗʰ **S46.29** Other injury of muscle, fascia and tendon of other parts of biceps

☑7ᵗʰ **S46.291** Other injury of muscle, fascia and tendon of other parts of biceps, **right** arm

☑7ᵗʰ **S46.292** Other injury of muscle, fascia and tendon of other parts of biceps, **left** arm

☑7ᵗʰ **S46.299** Other injury of muscle, fascia and tendon of other parts of biceps, **unspecified** arm

☑5ᵗʰ **S46.3** Injury of muscle, fascia and tendon of **triceps**

☑6ᵗʰ **S46.30** Unspecified injury of muscle, fascia and tendon of triceps

☑7ᵗʰ **S46.301** Unspecified injury of muscle, fascia and tendon of triceps, **right** arm

☑7ᵗʰ **S46.302** Unspecified injury of muscle, fascia and tendon of triceps, **left** arm

☑7ᵗʰ **S46.309** Unspecified injury of muscle, fascia and tendon of triceps, **unspecified** arm

N Newborn: 0   P Pediatric: 0-17   M Maternity: 12-55   A Adult: 15-124   MCC Major CC Condition   PDxMCC PDx acts as own MCC   CC CC Condition   PDxCC PDx acts as own CC

994   ICD-10-CM 2018

√6ᵗʰ **S46.31** Strain of muscle, fascia and tendon of triceps

√7ᵗʰ   **S46.311** Strain of muscle, fascia and tendon of triceps, **right arm**

√7ᵗʰ   **S46.312** Strain of muscle, fascia and tendon of triceps, **left arm**

√7ᵗʰ   **S46.319** Strain of muscle, fascia and tendon of triceps, **unspecified arm**

√6ᵗʰ **S46.32** Laceration of muscle, fascia and tendon of triceps

√7ᵗʰ   **S46.321** Laceration of muscle, fascia and tendon of triceps, **right arm** `CC`

√7ᵗʰ   **S46.322** Laceration of muscle, fascia and tendon of triceps, **left arm** `CC`

√7ᵗʰ   **S46.329** Laceration of muscle, fascia and tendon of triceps, **unspecified arm** `CC`

√6ᵗʰ **S46.39** Other injury of muscle, fascia and tendon of triceps

√7ᵗʰ   **S46.391** Other injury of muscle, fascia and tendon of triceps, **right arm**

√7ᵗʰ   **S46.392** Other injury of muscle, fascia and tendon of triceps, **left arm**

√7ᵗʰ   **S46.399** Other injury of muscle, fascia and tendon of triceps, **unspecified arm**

√5ᵗʰ **S46.8** Injury of other muscles, fascia and tendons at shoulder and upper arm level

√6ᵗʰ **S46.80** Unspecified injury of other muscles, fascia and tendons at shoulder and upper arm level

√7ᵗʰ   **S46.801** Unspecified injury of other muscles, fascia and tendons at shoulder and upper arm level, **right arm**

√7ᵗʰ   **S46.802** Unspecified injury of other muscles, fascia and tendons at shoulder and upper arm level, **left arm**

√7ᵗʰ   **S46.809** Unspecified injury of other muscles, fascia and tendons at shoulder and upper arm level, **unspecified arm**

√6ᵗʰ **S46.81** Strain of other muscles, fascia and tendons at shoulder and upper arm level

√7ᵗʰ   **S46.811** Strain of other muscles, fascia and tendons at shoulder and upper arm level, **right arm**

√7ᵗʰ   **S46.812** Strain of other muscles, fascia and tendons at shoulder and upper arm level, **left arm**

√7ᵗʰ   **S46.819** Strain of other muscles, fascia and tendons at shoulder and upper arm level, **unspecified arm**

√6ᵗʰ **S46.82** Laceration of other muscles, fascia and tendons at shoulder and upper arm level

√7ᵗʰ   **S46.821** Laceration of other muscles, fascia and tendons at shoulder and upper arm level, **right arm** `CC`

√7ᵗʰ   **S46.822** Laceration of other muscles, fascia and tendons at shoulder and upper arm level, **left arm** `CC`

√7ᵗʰ   **S46.829** Laceration of other muscles, fascia and tendons at shoulder and upper arm level, **unspecified arm** `CC`

√6ᵗʰ **S46.89** Other injury of other muscles, fascia and tendons at shoulder and upper arm level

√7ᵗʰ   **S46.891** Other injury of other muscles, fascia and tendons at shoulder and upper arm level, **right arm**

√7ᵗʰ   **S46.892** Other injury of other muscles, fascia and tendons at shoulder and upper arm level, **left arm**

√7ᵗʰ   **S46.899** Other injury of other muscles, fascia and tendons at shoulder and upper arm level, **unspecified arm**

√5ᵗʰ **S46.9** Injury of **unspecified** muscle, fascia and tendon at shoulder and upper arm level

√6ᵗʰ **S46.90** Unspecified injury of unspecified muscle, fascia and tendon at shoulder and upper arm level

√7ᵗʰ   **S46.901** Unspecified injury of unspecified muscle, fascia and tendon at shoulder and upper arm level, **right arm**

√7ᵗʰ   **S46.902** Unspecified injury of unspecified muscle, fascia and tendon at shoulder and upper arm level, **left arm**

√7ᵗʰ   **S46.909** Unspecified injury of unspecified muscle, fascia and tendon at shoulder and upper arm level, **unspecified arm**

√6ᵗʰ **S46.91** Strain of unspecified muscle, fascia and tendon at shoulder and upper arm level

√7ᵗʰ   **S46.911** Strain of unspecified muscle, fascia and tendon at shoulder and upper arm level, **right arm**

√7ᵗʰ   **S46.912** Strain of unspecified muscle, fascia and tendon at shoulder and upper arm level, **left arm**

√7ᵗʰ   **S46.919** Strain of unspecified muscle, fascia and tendon at shoulder and upper arm level, **unspecified arm**

√6ᵗʰ **S46.92** Laceration of unspecified muscle, fascia and tendon at shoulder and upper arm level

√7ᵗʰ   **S46.921** Laceration of unspecified muscle, fascia and tendon at shoulder and upper arm level, **right arm** `CC`

√7ᵗʰ   **S46.922** Laceration of unspecified muscle, fascia and tendon at shoulder and upper arm level, **left arm** `CC`

√7ᵗʰ   **S46.929** Laceration of unspecified muscle, fascia and tendon at shoulder and upper arm level, **unspecified arm** `CC`

√6ᵗʰ **S46.99** Other injury of unspecified muscle, fascia and tendon at shoulder and upper arm level

√7ᵗʰ   **S46.991** Other injury of unspecified muscle, fascia and tendon at shoulder and upper arm level, **right arm**

√7ᵗʰ   **S46.992** Other injury of unspecified muscle, fascia and tendon at shoulder and upper arm level, **left arm**

√7ᵗʰ   **S46.999** Other injury of unspecified muscle, fascia and tendon at shoulder and upper arm level, **unspecified arm**

√4ᵗʰ **S47** **Crushing injury of shoulder and upper arm**

Use additional code for all associated injuries

EXCLUDES 2   crushing injury of elbow (S57.0-)

> The appropriate 7th character is to be added to each code from category S47.
> A   initial encounter
> D   subsequent encounter
> S   sequela

√x7ᵗʰ **S47.1** Crushing injury of **right** shoulder and upper arm

√x7ᵗʰ **S47.2** Crushing injury of **left** shoulder and upper arm

√x7ᵗʰ **S47.9** Crushing injury of shoulder and upper arm, **unspecified** arm

√4ᵗʰ **S48** **Traumatic amputation of shoulder and upper arm**

An amputation not identified as partial or complete should be coded to complete.

EXCLUDES 1   traumatic amputation at elbow level (S58.0)

> The appropriate 7th character is to be added to each code from category S48.
> A   initial encounter
> D   subsequent encounter
> S   sequela

> **CC Excl: For CC codes in category S48:**
> **Right side:** PDX collection 1266
> **Left side:** PDX collection 1267
> **Unspecified side:** PDX collection 1268

√5ᵗʰ **S48.0** Traumatic amputation at **shoulder joint**

√6ᵗʰ **S48.01** Complete traumatic amputation at shoulder joint

[11] √7ᵗʰ   **S48.011** Complete traumatic amputation at **right** shoulder joint `CC` `HCC`

[11] √7ᵗʰ   **S48.012** Complete traumatic amputation at **left** shoulder joint `CC` `HCC`

[11] √7ᵗʰ   **S48.019** Complete traumatic amputation at **unspecified** shoulder joint `CC` `HCC`

---

[11] HCC with 7th character indicating initial encounter (A or B - specific to category) OR sequela.

✓ Additional Character Req   √x7ᵗʰ Placeholder Alert   Unacceptable PDx   Manifestation   H1-H14 HAC   HCC CMS-HCC Condition   *EXCLUDES 1* Not Coded Here   *EXCLUDES 2* Not Included Here

ICD-10-CM 2018   995

Chapter 19. Injury, Poisoning and Certain Other Consequences of External Causes

✓6ᵗʰ **S48.Ø2 Partial traumatic amputation at shoulder joint**

  11 ✓7ᵗʰ **S48.Ø21 Partial traumatic amputation at right shoulder joint** `CC` `HCC`

  11 ✓7ᵗʰ **S48.Ø22 Partial traumatic amputation at left shoulder joint** `CC` `HCC`

  11 ✓7ᵗʰ **S48.Ø29 Partial traumatic amputation at unspecified shoulder joint** `CC` `HCC`

✓5ᵗʰ **S48.1 Traumatic amputation at level between shoulder and elbow**

  ✓6ᵗʰ **S48.11 Complete traumatic amputation at level between shoulder and elbow**

    11 ✓7ᵗʰ **S48.111 Complete traumatic amputation at at level between right shoulder and elbow** `CC` `HCC`

    11 ✓7ᵗʰ **S48.112 Complete traumatic amputation at at level between left shoulder and elbow** `CC` `HCC`

    11 ✓7ᵗʰ **S48.119 Complete traumatic amputation at at level between unspecified shoulder and elbow** `CC` `HCC`

  ✓6ᵗʰ **S48.12 Partial traumatic amputation at level between shoulder and elbow**

    11 ✓7ᵗʰ **S48.121 Partial traumatic amputation at level between right shoulder and elbow** `CC` `HCC`

    11 ✓7ᵗʰ **S48.122 Partial traumatic amputation at level between left shoulder and elbow** `CC` `HCC`

    11 ✓7ᵗʰ **S48.129 Partial traumatic amputation at level between unspecified shoulder and elbow** `CC` `HCC`

✓5ᵗʰ **S48.9 Traumatic amputation of shoulder and upper arm, level unspecified**

  ✓6ᵗʰ **S48.91 Complete traumatic amputation of shoulder and upper arm, level unspecified**

    11 ✓7ᵗʰ **S48.911 Complete traumatic amputation of right shoulder and upper arm, level unspecified** `CC` `HCC`

    11 ✓7ᵗʰ **S48.912 Complete traumatic amputation of left shoulder and upper arm, level unspecified** `CC` `HCC`

    11 ✓7ᵗʰ **S48.919 Complete traumatic amputation of unspecified shoulder and upper arm, level unspecified** `CC` `HCC`

  ✓6ᵗʰ **S48.92 Partial traumatic amputation of shoulder and upper arm, level unspecified**

    11 ✓7ᵗʰ **S48.921 Partial traumatic amputation of right shoulder and upper arm, level unspecified** `CC` `HCC`

    11 ✓7ᵗʰ **S48.922 Partial traumatic amputation of left shoulder and upper arm, level unspecified** `CC` `HCC`

    11 ✓7ᵗʰ **S48.929 Partial traumatic amputation of unspecified shoulder and upper arm, level unspecified** `CC` `HCC`

✓4ᵗʰ **S49 Other and unspecified injuries of shoulder and upper arm**

> The appropriate 7th character is to be added to each code from subcategories S49.Ø and S49.1.
> A   initial encounter for closed fracture
> D   subsequent encounter for fracture with routine healing
> G   subsequent encounter for fracture with delayed healing
> K   subsequent encounter for fracture with nonunion
> P   subsequent encounter for fracture with malunion
> S   sequela
>
> **CC Excl: For CC codes in category S49:**
> **Right side:** See code S49.ØØ1
> **Left side:** See code S49.ØØ2
> **Unspecified side:** See code S49.ØØ9

✓5ᵗʰ **S49.Ø Physeal fracture of upper end of humerus**

  ✓6ᵗʰ **S49.ØØ Unspecified physeal fracture of upper end of humerus**

    7 ✓7ᵗʰ **S49.ØØ1 Unspecified physeal fracture of upper end of humerus, right arm** `CC` `H5`
        CC Excl: CC with 7th character A:
        PDX collection 1245
        CC with 7th character K or P:
        PDX collection 897

    7 ✓7ᵗʰ **S49.ØØ2 Unspecified physeal fracture of upper end of humerus, left arm** `CC` `H5`
        CC Excl: CC with 7th character A:
        PDX collection 1247
        CC with 7th character K or P:
        PDX collection 897

    7 ✓7ᵗʰ **S49.ØØ9 Unspecified physeal fracture of upper end of humerus, unspecified arm** `CC` `H5`
        CC Excl: CC with 7th character A:
        PDX collection 1248
        CC with 7th character K or P:
        PDX collection 897

  ✓6ᵗʰ **S49.Ø1 Salter-Harris Type I physeal fracture of upper end of humerus**

    7 ✓7ᵗʰ **S49.Ø11 Salter-Harris Type I physeal fracture of upper end of humerus, right arm** `CC` `H5`

    7 ✓7ᵗʰ **S49.Ø12 Salter-Harris Type I physeal fracture of upper end of humerus, left arm** `CC` `H5`

    7 ✓7ᵗʰ **S49.Ø19 Salter-Harris Type I physeal fracture of upper end of humerus, unspecified arm** `CC` `H5`

  ✓6ᵗʰ **S49.Ø2 Salter-Harris Type II physeal fracture of upper end of humerus**

    7 ✓7ᵗʰ **S49.Ø21 Salter-Harris Type II physeal fracture of upper end of humerus, right arm** `CC` `H5`

    7 ✓7ᵗʰ **S49.Ø22 Salter-Harris Type II physeal fracture of upper end of humerus, left arm** `CC` `H5`

    7 ✓7ᵗʰ **S49.Ø29 Salter-Harris Type II physeal fracture of upper end of humerus, unspecified arm** `CC` `H5`

  ✓6ᵗʰ **S49.Ø3 Salter-Harris Type III physeal fracture of upper end of humerus**

    7 ✓7ᵗʰ **S49.Ø31 Salter-Harris Type III physeal fracture of upper end of humerus, right arm** `CC` `H5`

    7 ✓7ᵗʰ **S49.Ø32 Salter-Harris Type III physeal fracture of upper end of humerus, left arm** `CC` `H5`

    7 ✓7ᵗʰ **S49.Ø39 Salter-Harris Type III physeal fracture of upper end of humerus, unspecified arm** `CC` `H5`

  ✓6ᵗʰ **S49.Ø4 Salter-Harris Type IV physeal fracture of upper end of humerus**

    7 ✓7ᵗʰ **S49.Ø41 Salter-Harris Type IV physeal fracture of upper end of humerus, right arm** `CC` `H5`

    7 ✓7ᵗʰ **S49.Ø42 Salter-Harris Type IV physeal fracture of upper end of humerus, left arm** `CC` `H5`

    7 ✓7ᵗʰ **S49.Ø49 Salter-Harris Type IV physeal fracture of upper end of humerus, unspecified arm** `CC` `H5`

  ✓6ᵗʰ **S49.Ø9 Other physeal fracture of upper end of humerus**

    7 ✓7ᵗʰ **S49.Ø91 Other physeal fracture of upper end of humerus, right arm** `CC` `H5`

    7 ✓7ᵗʰ **S49.Ø92 Other physeal fracture of upper end of humerus, left arm** `CC` `H5`

    7 ✓7ᵗʰ **S49.Ø99 Other physeal fracture of upper end of humerus, unspecified arm** `CC` `H5`

✓5ᵗʰ **S49.1 Physeal fracture of lower end of humerus**

  ✓6ᵗʰ **S49.1Ø Unspecified physeal fracture of lower end of humerus**

    7 ✓7ᵗʰ **S49.1Ø1 Unspecified physeal fracture of lower end of humerus, right arm** `CC` `H5`

    7 ✓7ᵗʰ **S49.1Ø2 Unspecified physeal fracture of lower end of humerus, left arm** `CC` `H5`

    7 ✓7ᵗʰ **S49.1Ø9 Unspecified physeal fracture of lower end of humerus, unspecified arm** `CC` `H5`

---

7   CC when reported as an initial encounter (7th character A, B, or C – specific to category) OR a subsequent encounter for nonunion or malunion (7th character K, M, N, P, Q, or R – specific to category).

11   HCC with 7th character indicating initial encounter (A or B - specific to category) OR sequela.

Ⓝ Newborn: 0   Ⓟ Pediatric: 0-17   Ⓜ Maternity: 12-55   Ⓐ Adult: 15-124   `MCC` Major CC Condition   `PDxMCC` PDx acts as own MCC   `CC` CC Condition   `PDxCC` PDx acts as own CC

996   ICD-10-CM 2018

✓6th **S49.11** Salter-Harris Type I physeal fracture of lower end of humerus

     7 ✓7th **S49.111** Salter-Harris Type I physeal fracture of lower end of humerus, **right** arm   `CC` `H5`

     7 ✓7th **S49.112** Salter-Harris Type I physeal fracture of lower end of humerus, **left** arm   `CC` `H5`

     7 ✓7th **S49.119** Salter-Harris Type I physeal fracture of lower end of humerus, **unspecified** arm   `CC` `H5`

✓6th **S49.12** Salter-Harris Type II physeal fracture of lower end of humerus

     7 ✓7th **S49.121** Salter-Harris Type II physeal fracture of lower end of humerus, **right** arm   `CC` `H5`

     7 ✓7th **S49.122** Salter-Harris Type II physeal fracture of lower end of humerus, **left** arm   `CC` `H5`

     7 ✓7th **S49.129** Salter-Harris Type II physeal fracture of lower end of humerus, **unspecified** arm   `CC` `H5`

✓6th **S49.13** Salter-Harris Type III physeal fracture of lower end of humerus

     7 ✓7th **S49.131** Salter-Harris Type III physeal fracture of lower end of humerus, **right** arm   `CC` `H5`

     7 ✓7th **S49.132** Salter-Harris Type III physeal fracture of lower end of humerus, **left** arm   `CC` `H5`

     7 ✓7th **S49.139** Salter-Harris Type III physeal fracture of lower end of humerus, **unspecified** arm   `CC` `H5`

✓6th **S49.14** Salter-Harris Type IV physeal fracture of lower end of humerus

     7 ✓7th **S49.141** Salter-Harris Type IV physeal fracture of lower end of humerus, **right** arm   `CC` `H5`

     7 ✓7th **S49.142** Salter-Harris Type IV physeal fracture of lower end of humerus, **left** arm   `CC` `H5`

     7 ✓7th **S49.149** Salter-Harris Type IV physeal fracture of lower end of humerus, **unspecified** arm   `CC` `H5`

✓6th **S49.19** Other physeal fracture of lower end of humerus

     7 ✓7th **S49.191** Other physeal fracture of lower end of humerus, **right** arm   `CC` `H5`

     7 ✓7th **S49.192** Other physeal fracture of lower end of humerus, **left** arm   `CC` `H5`

     7 ✓7th **S49.199** Other physeal fracture of lower end of humerus, **unspecified** arm   `CC` `H5`

✓5th **S49.8** Other specified injuries of shoulder and upper arm

> The appropriate 7th character is to be added to each code in subcategory S49.8.
> A   initial encounter
> D   subsequent encounter
> S   sequela

✓x7th **S49.80** Other specified injuries of shoulder and upper arm, **unspecified** arm

✓x7th **S49.81** Other specified injuries of **right** shoulder and upper arm

✓x7th **S49.82** Other specified injuries of **left** shoulder and upper arm

✓5th **S49.9** Unspecified injury of shoulder and upper arm

> The appropriate 7th character is to be added to each code in subcategory S49.9.
> A   initial encounter
> D   subsequent encounter
> S   sequela

✓x7th **S49.90** Unspecified injury of shoulder and upper arm, **unspecified** arm

✓x7th **S49.91** Unspecified injury of **right** shoulder and upper arm

✓x7th **S49.92** Unspecified injury of **left** shoulder and upper arm

Injuries to the elbow and forearm (S50-S59)

> `EXCLUDES 2` burns and corrosions (T20-T32)
> frostbite (T33-T34)
> injuries of wrist and hand (S60-S69)
> insect bite or sting, venomous (T63.4)

✓4th **S50** **Superficial injury of elbow and forearm**

> `EXCLUDES 2` superficial injury of wrist and hand (S60.-)

> The appropriate 7th character is to be added to each code from category S50.
> A   initial encounter
> D   subsequent encounter
> S   sequela

✓5th **S50.0** **Contusion of** elbow

     ✓x7th **S50.00** **Contusion of** unspecified **elbow**

     ✓x7th **S50.01** **Contusion of** right **elbow**

     ✓x7th **S50.02** **Contusion of** left **elbow**

✓5th **S50.1** **Contusion of** forearm

     ✓x7th **S50.10** **Contusion of** unspecified **forearm**

     ✓x7th **S50.11** **Contusion of** right **forearm**

     ✓x7th **S50.12** **Contusion of** left **forearm**

✓5th **S50.3** **Other superficial injuries of** elbow

     ✓6th **S50.31** **Abrasion** of elbow

         ✓7th **S50.311** **Abrasion of** right **elbow**

         ✓7th **S50.312** **Abrasion of** left **elbow**

         ✓7th **S50.319** **Abrasion of** unspecified **elbow**

     ✓6th **S50.32** **Blister (nonthermal) of** elbow

         ✓7th **S50.321** **Blister (nonthermal) of** right **elbow**

         ✓7th **S50.322** **Blister (nonthermal) of** left **elbow**

         ✓7th **S50.329** **Blister (nonthermal) of** unspecified **elbow**

     ✓6th **S50.34** **External constriction of** elbow

         ✓7th **S50.341** **External constriction of** right **elbow**

         ✓7th **S50.342** **External constriction of** left **elbow**

         ✓7th **S50.349** **External constriction of** unspecified **elbow**

     ✓6th **S50.35** **Superficial foreign body of** elbow
> Splinter in the elbow

         ✓7th **S50.351** **Superficial foreign body of** right **elbow**

         ✓7th **S50.352** **Superficial foreign body of** left **elbow**

         ✓7th **S50.359** **Superficial foreign body of** unspecified **elbow**

     ✓6th **S50.36** **Insect bite (nonvenomous) of** elbow

         ✓7th **S50.361** **Insect bite (nonvenomous) of** right **elbow**

         ✓7th **S50.362** **Insect bite (nonvenomous) of** left **elbow**

         ✓7th **S50.369** **Insect bite (nonvenomous) of** unspecified **elbow**

     ✓6th **S50.37** **Other superficial bite of** elbow
> `EXCLUDES 1` open bite of elbow (S51.04)

         ✓7th **S50.371** **Other superficial bite of** right **elbow**

         ✓7th **S50.372** **Other superficial bite of** left **elbow**

         ✓7th **S50.379** **Other superficial bite of** unspecified **elbow**

✓5th **S50.8** **Other superficial injuries of** forearm

     ✓6th **S50.81** **Abrasion of** forearm

         ✓7th **S50.811** **Abrasion of** right **forearm**

         ✓7th **S50.812** **Abrasion of** left **forearm**

         ✓7th **S50.819** **Abrasion of** unspecified **forearm**

     ✓6th **S50.82** **Blister (nonthermal) of** forearm

         ✓7th **S50.821** **Blister (nonthermal) of** right **forearm**

         ✓7th **S50.822** **Blister (nonthermal) of** left **forearm**

         ✓7th **S50.829** **Blister (nonthermal) of** unspecified **forearm**

     ✓6th **S50.84** **External constriction of** forearm

         ✓7th **S50.841** **External constriction of** right **forearm**

         ✓7th **S50.842** **External constriction of** left **forearm**

         ✓7th **S50.849** **External constriction of** unspecified **forearm**

     ✓6th **S50.85** **Superficial foreign body of** forearm
> Splinter in the forearm

         ✓7th **S50.851** **Superficial foreign body of** right **forearm**

---

7   CC when reported as an initial encounter (7th character A, B, or C – specific to category) OR a subsequent encounter for nonunion or malunion (7th character K, M, N, P, Q, or R – specific to category).

✓ Additional Character Req   ✓x7th Placeholder Alert   Unacceptable PDx   Manifestation   `H1`-`H14` HAC   `HCC` CMS-HCC Condition   `EXCLUDES 1` Not Coded Here   `EXCLUDES 2` Not Included Here

Chapter 19. Injury, Poisoning and Certain Other Consequences of External Causes

S50.852–S51.859

√7ᵗʰ **S50.852** Superficial foreign body of left forearm

√7ᵗʰ **S50.859** Superficial foreign body of unspecified forearm

√6ᵗʰ **S50.86** Insect bite (nonvenomous) of forearm

√7ᵗʰ **S50.861** Insect bite (nonvenomous) of right forearm

√7ᵗʰ **S50.862** Insect bite (nonvenomous) of left forearm

√7ᵗʰ **S50.869** Insect bite (nonvenomous) of unspecified forearm

√6ᵗʰ **S50.87** Other superficial bite of forearm
     EXCLUDES 1   *open bite of forearm (S51.84)*

√7ᵗʰ **S50.871** Other superficial bite of right forearm

√7ᵗʰ **S50.872** Other superficial bite of left forearm

√7ᵗʰ **S50.879** Other superficial bite of unspecified forearm

√5ᵗʰ **S50.9** Unspecified superficial injury of elbow and forearm

√6ᵗʰ **S50.90** Unspecified superficial injury of elbow

√7ᵗʰ **S50.901** Unspecified superficial injury of right elbow

√7ᵗʰ **S50.902** Unspecified superficial injury of left elbow

√7ᵗʰ **S50.909** Unspecified superficial injury of unspecified elbow

√6ᵗʰ **S50.91** Unspecified superficial injury of forearm

√7ᵗʰ **S50.911** Unspecified superficial injury of right forearm

√7ᵗʰ **S50.912** Unspecified superficial injury of left forearm

√7ᵗʰ **S50.919** Unspecified superficial injury of unspecified forearm

√4ᵗʰ **S51** **Open wound of elbow and forearm**
Code also any associated wound infection
     EXCLUDES 1   *open fracture of elbow and forearm (S52- with open fracture 7th character)*
             traumatic amputation of elbow and forearm (S58.-)
     EXCLUDES 2   *open wound of wrist and hand (S61.-)*

> The appropriate 7th character is to be added to each code from category S51.
> A   initial encounter
> D   subsequent encounter
> S   sequela

√5ᵗʰ **S51.0** Open wound of elbow

√6ᵗʰ **S51.00** Unspecified open wound of elbow

√7ᵗʰ **S51.001** Unspecified open wound of right elbow
     AHA: 2012, 4Q, 108

√7ᵗʰ **S51.002** Unspecified open wound of left elbow

√7ᵗʰ **S51.009** Unspecified open wound of unspecified elbow
     Open wound of elbow NOS

√6ᵗʰ **S51.01** Laceration without foreign body of elbow

√7ᵗʰ **S51.011** Laceration without foreign body of right elbow

√7ᵗʰ **S51.012** Laceration without foreign body of left elbow

√7ᵗʰ **S51.019** Laceration without foreign body of unspecified elbow

√6ᵗʰ **S51.02** Laceration with foreign body of elbow

√7ᵗʰ **S51.021** Laceration with foreign body of right elbow

√7ᵗʰ **S51.022** Laceration with foreign body of left elbow

√7ᵗʰ **S51.029** Laceration with foreign body of unspecified elbow

√6ᵗʰ **S51.03** Puncture wound without foreign body of elbow

√7ᵗʰ **S51.031** Puncture wound without foreign body of right elbow

√7ᵗʰ **S51.032** Puncture wound without foreign body of left elbow

√7ᵗʰ **S51.039** Puncture wound without foreign body of unspecified elbow

√6ᵗʰ **S51.04** Puncture wound with foreign body of elbow

√7ᵗʰ **S51.041** Puncture wound with foreign body of right elbow

√7ᵗʰ **S51.042** Puncture wound with foreign body of left elbow

√7ᵗʰ **S51.049** Puncture wound with foreign body of unspecified elbow

√6ᵗʰ **S51.05** Open bite of elbow
     Bite of elbow NOS
     EXCLUDES 1   *superficial bite of elbow (S50.36, S50.37)*

√7ᵗʰ **S51.051** Open bite, right elbow

√7ᵗʰ **S51.052** Open bite, left elbow

√7ᵗʰ **S51.059** Open bite, unspecified elbow

√5ᵗʰ **S51.8** Open wound of forearm
     EXCLUDES 2   *open wound of elbow (S51.0-)*

√6ᵗʰ **S51.80** Unspecified open wound of forearm
     AHA: 2016, 3Q, 24

√7ᵗʰ **S51.801** Unspecified open wound of right forearm

√7ᵗʰ **S51.802** Unspecified open wound of left forearm

√7ᵗʰ **S51.809** Unspecified open wound of unspecified forearm
     Open wound of forearm NOS

√6ᵗʰ **S51.81** Laceration without foreign body of forearm

√7ᵗʰ **S51.811** Laceration without foreign body of right forearm

√7ᵗʰ **S51.812** Laceration without foreign body of left forearm

√7ᵗʰ **S51.819** Laceration without foreign body of unspecified forearm

√6ᵗʰ **S51.82** Laceration with foreign body of forearm

√7ᵗʰ **S51.821** Laceration with foreign body of right forearm

√7ᵗʰ **S51.822** Laceration with foreign body of left forearm

√7ᵗʰ **S51.829** Laceration with foreign body of unspecified forearm

√6ᵗʰ **S51.83** Puncture wound without foreign body of forearm
     AHA: 2016, 3Q, 24

√7ᵗʰ **S51.831** Puncture wound without foreign body of right forearm

√7ᵗʰ **S51.832** Puncture wound without foreign body of left forearm

√7ᵗʰ **S51.839** Puncture wound without foreign body of unspecified forearm

√6ᵗʰ **S51.84** Puncture wound with foreign body of forearm
     AHA: 2016, 3Q, 24

√7ᵗʰ **S51.841** Puncture wound with foreign body of right forearm

√7ᵗʰ **S51.842** Puncture wound with foreign body of left forearm

√7ᵗʰ **S51.849** Puncture wound with foreign body of unspecified forearm

√6ᵗʰ **S51.85** Open bite of forearm
     Bite of forearm NOS
     EXCLUDES 1   *superficial bite of forearm (S50.86, S50.87)*

√7ᵗʰ **S51.851** Open bite of right forearm

√7ᵗʰ **S51.852** Open bite of left forearm

√7ᵗʰ **S51.859** Open bite of unspecified forearm

N Newborn: 0   P Pediatric: 0-17   M Maternity: 12-55   A Adult: 15-124   MCC Major CC Condition   PDxMCC PDx acts as own MCC   CC CC Condition   PDxCC PDx acts as own CC

998   ICD-10-CM 2018

✓4ᵗʰ S52   Fracture of forearm

NOTE
A fracture not indicated as displaced or nondisplaced should be coded to displaced.
A fracture not indicated as open or closed should be coded to closed.
The open fracture designations are based on the Gustilo open fracture classification.

EXCLUDES 1   *traumatic amputation of forearm (S58.-)*
EXCLUDES 2   *fracture at wrist and hand level (S62.-)*
AHA: 2016, 1Q, 33; 2015, 3Q, 37-39

The appropriate 7th character is to be added to all codes from category S52 [unless otherwise indicated].
A   initial encounter for closed fracture
B   initial encounter for open fracture type I or II
     initial encounter for open fracture NOS
C   initial encounter for open fracture type IIIA, IIIB, or IIIC
D   subsequent encounter for closed fracture with routine healing
E   subsequent encounter for open fracture type I or II with routine healing
F   subsequent encounter for open fracture type IIIA, IIIB, or IIIC with routine healing
G   subsequent encounter for closed fracture with delayed healing
H   subsequent encounter for open fracture type I or II with delayed healing
J   subsequent encounter for open fracture type IIIA, IIIB, or IIIC with delayed healing
K   subsequent encounter for closed fracture with nonunion
M   subsequent encounter for open fracture type I or II with nonunion
N   subsequent encounter for open fracture type IIIA, IIIB, or IIIC with nonunion
P   subsequent encounter for closed fracture with malunion
Q   subsequent encounter for open fracture type I or II with malunion
R   subsequent encounter for open fracture type IIIA, IIIB, or IIIC with malunion
S   sequela

✓5ᵗʰ S52.0   Fracture of upper end of ulna
Fracture of proximal end of ulna
EXCLUDES 2   *fracture of elbow NOS (S42.40-)*
         fractures of shaft of ulna (S52.2-)

✓6ᵗʰ S52.00   Unspecified fracture of upper end of ulna

CC Excl: For codes in subcatagory S52.00: MCC with 7th character B or C: PDX collection 1269
CC with 7th character K, M, N, P, Q, or R: PDX collection 897

6, 8   ✓7ᵗʰ S52.001   Unspecified fracture of upper end of **right** ulna   `MCC` `CC` `H5`

6, 8   ✓7ᵗʰ S52.002   Unspecified fracture of upper end of **left** ulna   `MCC` `CC` `H5`

6, 8   ✓7ᵗʰ S52.009   Unspecified fracture of upper end of **unspecified** ulna   `MCC` `CC` `H5`

✓6ᵗʰ S52.01   Torus fracture of upper end of ulna

The appropriate 7th character is to be added to all codes in subcategory S52.01.
A   initial encounter for closed fracture
D   subsequent encounter for fracture with routine healing
G   subsequent encounter for fracture with delayed healing
K   subsequent encounter for fracture with nonunion
P   subsequent encounter for fracture with malunion
S   sequela

7   ✓7ᵗʰ S52.011   Torus fracture of upper end of **right** ulna   `CC` `H5`
CC Excl: CC with 7th character A: PDX collection 1270
CC with 7th character K or P: PDX collection 897

7   ✓7ᵗʰ S52.012   Torus fracture of upper end of **left** ulna   `CC` `H5`
CC Excl: CC with 7th character A: PDX collection 1271
CC with 7th character K or P: PDX collection 897

7   ✓7ᵗʰ S52.019   Torus fracture of upper end of **unspecified** ulna   `CC` `H5`
CC Excl: CC with 7th character A: PDX collection 1272
CC with 7th character K or P: PDX collection 897

✓6ᵗʰ S52.02   Fracture of olecranon process without intraarticular extension of ulna

CC Excl: For codes in subcatagory S52.02:
MCC with 7th character B or C: PDX collection 1273
CC with 7th character K, M, N, P, Q, or R: PDX collection 897

6, 8   ✓7ᵗʰ S52.021   Displaced fracture of olecranon process without intraarticular extension of **right** ulna   `MCC` `CC` `H5`

6, 8   ✓7ᵗʰ S52.022   Displaced fracture of olecranon process without intraarticular extension of **left** ulna   `MCC` `CC` `H5`

6, 8   ✓7ᵗʰ S52.023   Displaced fracture of olecranon process without intraarticular extension of **unspecified** ulna   `MCC` `CC` `H5`

6, 8   ✓7ᵗʰ S52.024   Nondisplaced fracture of olecranon process without intraarticular extension of **right** ulna   `MCC` `CC` `H5`

6, 8   ✓7ᵗʰ S52.025   Nondisplaced fracture of olecranon process without intraarticular extension of **left** ulna   `MCC` `CC` `H5`

6, 8   ✓7ᵗʰ S52.026   Nondisplaced fracture of olecranon process without intra-articular extension of **unspecified** ulna   `MCC` `CC` `H5`

✓6ᵗʰ S52.03   Fracture of olecranon process with intraarticular extension of ulna

CC Excl: For codes in subcatagory S52.03:
MCC with 7th character B or C: PDX collection 1273
CC with 7th character K, M, N, P, Q, or R: PDX collection 897

6, 8   ✓7ᵗʰ S52.031   Displaced fracture of olecranon process with intraarticular extension of **right** ulna   `MCC` `CC` `H5`

6, 8   ✓7ᵗʰ S52.032   Displaced fracture of olecranon process with intraarticular extension of **left** ulna   `MCC` `CC` `H5`

6, 8   ✓7ᵗʰ S52.033   Displaced fracture of olecranon process with intraarticular extension of **unspecified** ulna   `MCC` `CC` `H5`

6, 8   ✓7ᵗʰ S52.034   Nondisplaced fracture of olecranon process with intraarticular extension of **right** ulna   `MCC` `CC` `H5`

6, 8   ✓7ᵗʰ S52.035   Nondisplaced fracture of olecranon process with intraarticular extension of **left** ulna   `MCC` `CC` `H5`

6, 8   ✓7ᵗʰ S52.036   Nondisplaced fracture of olecranon process with intraarticular extension of **unspecified** ulna   `MCC` `CC` `H5`

✓6ᵗʰ S52.04   Fracture of coronoid process of ulna

CC Excl: For codes in subcatagory S52.04:
MCC with 7th character B or C: PDX collection 1269
CC with 7th character K, M, N, P, Q, or R: PDX collection 897

6, 8   ✓7ᵗʰ S52.041   Displaced fracture of coronoid process of **right** ulna   `MCC` `CC` `H5`

6, 8   ✓7ᵗʰ S52.042   Displaced fracture of coronoid process of **left** ulna   `MCC` `CC` `H5`

6, 8   ✓7ᵗʰ S52.043   Displaced fracture of coronoid process of **unspecified** ulna   `MCC` `CC` `H5`

---

6   MCC when reported as an open fracture (7th character B or C – specific to category).

7   CC when reported as an initial encounter (7th character A, B, or C – specific to category) OR a subsequent encounter for nonunion or malunion (7th character K, M, N, P, Q, or R – specific to category).

8   CC when reported as a subsequent encounter for nonunion or malunion (7th character K, M, N, P, Q, or R – specific to category).

✔Additional Character Req   ✔ˣ7ᵗʰ Placeholder Alert   Unacceptable PDx   Manifestation   `H1`-`H14` HAC   `HCC` CMS-HCC Condition   *EXCLUDES 1* Not Coded Here   *EXCLUDES 2* Not Included Here

6, 8 ✓7th **S52.044** Nondisplaced **fracture of coronoid process of** right **ulna** `MCC` `CC` `H5`

6, 8 ✓7th **S52.045** Nondisplaced **fracture of coronoid process of** left **ulna** `MCC` `CC` `H5`

6, 8 ✓7th **S52.046** Nondisplaced **fracture of coronoid process of** unspecified **ulna** `MCC` `CC` `H5`

✓6th **S52.09** Other **fracture of upper end of ulna**

CC Excl: For codes in subcatagory S52.09:
MCC with 7th character B or C:
PDX collection 1269
CC with 7th character K, M, N, P, Q, or R:
PDX collection 897

6, 8 ✓7th **S52.091** Other **fracture of upper end of** right **ulna** `MCC` `CC` `H5`

6, 8 ✓7th **S52.092** Other **fracture of upper end of** left **ulna** `MCC` `CC` `H5`

6, 8 ✓7th **S52.099** Other **fracture of upper end of** unspecified **ulna** `MCC` `CC` `H5`

✓5th **S52.1** Fracture of **upper end of radius**
Fracture of proximal end of radius
EXCLUDES 2   *physeal fractures of upper end of radius (S59.2-)*
fracture of shaft of radius (S52.3-)

CC Excl: For CC/MCC codes in subcategory S52.1, unless otherwise noted:
MCC with 7th character B or C: PDX collection 1269
CC with 7th character K, M, N, P, Q, or R:
PDX collection 897

✓6th **S52.10** Unspecified **fracture of upper end of radius**

6, 8 ✓7th **S52.101** Unspecified **fracture of upper end of** right **radius** `MCC` `CC` `H5`

6, 8 ✓7th **S52.102** Unspecified **fracture of upper end of** left **radius** `MCC` `CC` `H5`

6, 8 ✓7th **S52.109** Unspecified **fracture of upper end of** unspecified **radius** `MCC` `CC` `H5`

✓6th **S52.11** Torus **fracture of upper end of radius**

The appropriate 7th character is to be added to all codes in subcategory S52.11.
A   initial encounter for closed fracture
D   subsequent encounter for fracture with routine healing
G   subsequent encounter for fracture with delayed healing
K   subsequent encounter for fracture with nonunion
P   subsequent encounter for fracture with malunion
S   sequela

7 ✓7th **S52.111** Torus **fracture of upper end of** right **radius** `CC` `H5`
CC Excl: CC with 7th character A:
PDX collection 1270
CC with 7th character K, P:
PDX collection 897

7 ✓7th **S52.112** Torus **fracture of upper end of** left **radius** `CC` `H5`
CC Excl: CC with 7th character A:
PDX collection 1271
CC with 7th character K or P:
PDX collection 897

7 ✓7th **S52.119** Torus **fracture of upper end of** unspecified **radius** `CC` `H5`
CC Excl: CC with 7th character A:
PDX collection 1272
CC Excl: CC with 7th character K or P:
PDX collection 897

✓6th **S52.12** Fracture of **head of radius**

6, 8 ✓7th **S52.121** Displaced **fracture of head of** right **radius** `MCC` `CC` `H5`

6, 8 ✓7th **S52.122** Displaced **fracture of head of** left **radius** `MCC` `CC` `H5`

6, 8 ✓7th **S52.123** Displaced **fracture of head of** unspecified **radius** `MCC` `CC` `H5`

6, 8 ✓7th **S52.124** Nondisplaced **fracture of head of** right **radius** `MCC` `CC` `H5`

6, 8 ✓7th **S52.125** Nondisplaced **fracture of head of** left **radius** `MCC` `CC` `H5`

6, 8 ✓7th **S52.126** Nondisplaced **fracture of head of** unspecified **radius** `MCC` `CC` `H5`

✓6th **S52.13** Fracture of **neck of radius**

6, 8 ✓7th **S52.131** Displaced **fracture of neck of** right **radius** `MCC` `CC` `H5`

6, 8 ✓7th **S52.132** Displaced **fracture of neck of** left **radius** `MCC` `CC` `H5`

6, 8 ✓7th **S52.133** Displaced **fracture of neck of** unspecified **radius** `MCC` `CC` `H5`

6, 8 ✓7th **S52.134** Nondisplaced **fracture of neck of** right **radius** `MCC` `CC` `H5`

6, 8 ✓7th **S52.135** Nondisplaced **fracture of neck of** left **radius** `MCC` `CC` `H5`

6, 8 ✓7th **S52.136** Nondisplaced **fracture of neck of** unspecified **radius** `MCC` `CC` `H5`

✓6th **S52.18** Other **fracture of upper end of radius**

6, 8 ✓7th **S52.181** Other **fracture of upper end of** right **radius** `MCC` `CC` `H5`

6, 8 ✓7th **S52.182** Other **fracture of upper end of** left **radius** `MCC` `CC` `H5`

6, 8 ✓7th **S52.189** Other **fracture of upper end of** unspecified **radius** `MCC` `CC` `H5`

✓5th **S52.2** Fracture of **shaft of ulna**

CC Excl: For CC/MCC codes in subcategory S52.2, unless otherwise noted:
Right side: See code S52.201
Left side: See code S52.202
Unspecified side: See code S52.209

✓6th **S52.20** Unspecified **fracture of shaft of ulna**
Fracture of ulna NOS

6, 7 ✓7th **S52.201** Unspecified **fracture of shaft of** right **ulna** `MCC` `CC` `H5`
CC Excl: CC with 7th character A:
PDX collection 1270
MCC with 7th character B or C:
PDX collection 1269
CC with 7th character K, M, N, P, Q or R:
PDX collection 897

6, 7 ✓7th **S52.202** Unspecified **fracture of shaft of** left **ulna** `MCC` `CC` `H5`
CC Excl: CC with 7th character A:
PDX collection 1271
MCC with 7th character B or C:
PDX collection 1269
CC with 7th character K, M, N, P, Q or R:
PDX collection 897

6, 7 ✓7th **S52.209** Unspecified **fracture of shaft of** unspecified **ulna** `MCC` `CC` `H5`
CC Excl: CC with 7th character A:
PDX collection 1272
MCC with 7th character B or C:
PDX collection 1269
CC with 7th character K, M, N, P, Q, or R:
PDX collection 897

---

6 MCC when reported as an open fracture (7th character B or C – specific to category).

7 CC when reported as an initial encounter (7th character A, B, or C – specific to category) OR a subsequent encounter for nonunion or malunion (7th character K, M, N, P, Q, or R – specific to category).

8 CC when reported as a subsequent encounter for nonunion or malunion (7th character K, M, N, P, Q, or R – specific to category).

N Newborn: 0 P Pediatric: 0-17 M Maternity: 12-55 A Adult: 15-124   `MCC` Major CC Condition   `PDxMCC` PDx acts as own MCC   `CC` CC Condition   `PDxCC` PDx acts as own CC

1000   ICD-10-CM 2018

✓6th **S52.21**   **Greenstick fracture of shaft of ulna**

> The appropriate 7th character is to be added to all codes in subcategory S52.21.
> A   initial encounter for closed fracture
> D   subsequent encounter for fracture with routine healing
> G   subsequent encounter for fracture with delayed healing
> K   subsequent encounter for fracture with nonunion
> P   subsequent encounter for fracture with malunion
> S   sequela

7   ✓7th **S52.211**   **Greenstick fracture of shaft of right ulna**   CC H5
> **CC Excl: CC with 7th character A:**
> PDX collection 1270
> **CC with 7th character K or P:**
> PDX collection 897

7   ✓7th **S52.212**   **Greenstick fracture of shaft of left ulna**   CC H5
> **CC Excl: CC with 7th character A:**
> PDX collection 1271
> **CC with 7th character K or P:**
> PDX collection 897

7   ✓7th **S52.219**   **Greenstick fracture of shaft of unspecified ulna**   CC H5
> **CC Excl: CC with 7th character A:**
> PDX collection 1272
> **CC with 7th character K or P:**
> PDX collection 897

✓6th **S52.22**   **Transverse fracture of shaft of ulna**

6, 7   ✓7th **S52.221**   **Displaced transverse fracture of shaft of right ulna**   MCC CC H5

6, 7   ✓7th **S52.222**   **Displaced transverse fracture of shaft of left ulna**   MCC CC H5

6, 7   ✓7th **S52.223**   **Displaced transverse fracture of shaft of unspecified ulna**   MCC CC H5

6, 7   ✓7th **S52.224**   **Nondisplaced transverse fracture of shaft of right ulna**   MCC CC H5

6, 7   ✓7th **S52.225**   **Nondisplaced transverse fracture of shaft of left ulna**   MCC CC H5

6, 7   ✓7th **S52.226**   **Nondisplaced transverse fracture of shaft of unspecified ulna**   MCC CC H5

✓6th **S52.23**   **Oblique fracture of shaft of ulna**

6, 7   ✓7th **S52.231**   **Displaced oblique fracture of shaft of right ulna**   MCC CC H5

6, 7   ✓7th **S52.232**   **Displaced oblique fracture of shaft of left ulna**   MCC CC H5

6, 7   ✓7th **S52.233**   **Displaced oblique fracture of shaft of unspecified ulna**   MCC CC H5

6, 7   ✓7th **S52.234**   **Nondisplaced oblique fracture of shaft of right ulna**   MCC CC H5

6, 7   ✓7th **S52.235**   **Nondisplaced oblique fracture of shaft of left ulna**   MCC CC H5

6, 7   ✓7th **S52.236**   **Nondisplaced oblique fracture of shaft of unspecified ulna**   MCC CC H5

✓6th **S52.24**   **Spiral fracture of shaft of ulna**

6, 7   ✓7th **S52.241**   **Displaced spiral fracture of shaft of ulna, right arm**   MCC CC H5

6, 7   ✓7th **S52.242**   **Displaced spiral fracture of shaft of ulna, left arm**   MCC CC H5

6, 7   ✓7th **S52.243**   **Displaced spiral fracture of shaft of ulna, unspecified arm**   MCC CC H5

6, 7   ✓7th **S52.244**   **Nondisplaced spiral fracture of of shaft of ulna, right arm**   MCC CC H5

6, 7   ✓7th **S52.245**   **Nondisplaced spiral fracture of of shaft of ulna, left arm**   MCC CC H5

6, 7   ✓7th **S52.246**   **Nondisplaced spiral fracture of of shaft of ulna, unspecified arm**   MCC CC H5

✓6th **S52.25**   **Comminuted fracture of shaft of ulna**

6, 7   ✓7th **S52.251**   **Displaced comminuted fracture of shaft of ulna, right arm**   MCC CC H5

6, 7   ✓7th **S52.252**   **Displaced comminuted fracture of shaft of ulna, left arm**   MCC CC H5

6, 7   ✓7th **S52.253**   **Displaced comminuted fracture of shaft of ulna, unspecified arm**   MCC CC H5

6, 7   ✓7th **S52.254**   **Nondisplaced comminuted fracture of shaft of ulna, right arm**   MCC CC H5

6, 7   ✓7th **S52.255**   **Nondisplaced comminuted fracture of shaft of ulna, left arm**   MCC CC H5

6, 7   ✓7th **S52.256**   **Nondisplaced comminuted fracture of shaft of ulna, unspecified arm**   MCC CC H5

✓6th **S52.26**   **Segmental fracture of shaft of ulna**

6, 7   ✓7th **S52.261**   **Displaced segmental fracture of shaft of ulna, right arm**   MCC CC H5

6, 7   ✓7th **S52.262**   **Displaced segmental fracture of shaft of ulna, left arm**   MCC CC H5

6, 7   ✓7th **S52.263**   **Displaced segmental fracture of shaft of ulna, unspecified arm**   MCC CC H5

6, 7   ✓7th **S52.264**   **Nondisplaced segmental fracture of shaft of ulna, right arm**   MCC CC H5

6, 7   ✓7th **S52.265**   **Nondisplaced segmental fracture of shaft of ulna, left arm**   MCC CC H5

6, 7   ✓7th **S52.266**   **Nondisplaced segmental fracture of shaft of ulna, unspecified arm**   MCC CC H5

✓6th **S52.27**   **Monteggia's fracture of ulna**
> Fracture of upper shaft of ulna with dislocation of radial head

> **CC Excl: For codes in subcategory S52.27:**
> **MCC with 7th character B or C:**
> PDX collection 1269
> **CC with 7th character K, M, N, P Q or R:**
> PDX collection 897

6, 8   ✓7th **S52.271**   **Monteggia's fracture of right ulna**   MCC CC H5

6, 8   ✓7th **S52.272**   **Monteggia's fracture of left ulna**   MCC CC H5

6, 8   ✓7th **S52.279**   **Monteggia's fracture of unspecified ulna**   MCC CC H5

✓6th **S52.28**   **Bent bone of ulna**

6, 7   ✓7th **S52.281**   **Bent bone of right ulna**   MCC CC H5

6, 7   ✓7th **S52.282**   **Bent bone of left ulna**   MCC CC H5

6, 7   ✓7th **S52.283**   **Bent bone of unspecified ulna**   MCC CC H5

✓6th **S52.29**   **Other fracture of shaft of ulna**

6, 7   ✓7th **S52.291**   **Other fracture of shaft of right ulna**   MCC CC H5

6, 7   ✓7th **S52.292**   **Other fracture of shaft of left ulna**   MCC CC H5

6, 7   ✓7th **S52.299**   **Other fracture of shaft of unspecified ulna**   MCC CC H5

✓5th **S52.3**   **Fracture of shaft of radius**

> **CC Excl: For CC/MCC codes in subcategory S52.3, unless otherwise noted:**
> **Right side:** See code S52.201
> **Left side:** See code S52.202
> **Unspecified side:** See code S52.209

✓6th **S52.30**   **Unspecified fracture of shaft of radius**

6, 7   ✓7th **S52.301**   **Unspecified fracture of shaft of right radius**   MCC CC H5

6, 7   ✓7th **S52.302**   **Unspecified fracture of shaft of left radius**   MCC CC H5

6, 7   ✓7th **S52.309**   **Unspecified fracture of shaft of unspecified radius**   MCC CC H5

---

6   MCC when reported as an open fracture (7th character B or C – specific to category).

7   CC when reported as an initial encounter (7th character A, B, or C – specific to category) OR a subsequent encounter for nonunion or malunion (7th character K, M, N, P, Q, or R – specific to category).

8   CC when reported as a subsequent encounter for nonunion or malunion (7th character K, M, N, P, Q, or R – specific to category).

✓ Additional Character Req   ✓x7th Placeholder Alert   Unacceptable PDx   Manifestation   H1-H14 HAC   HCC CMS-HCC Condition   EXCLUDES 1 Not Coded Here   EXCLUDES 2 Not Included Here

ICD-10-CM 2018   **1001**

√6ᵗʰ **S52.31** Greenstick **fracture of shaft of radius**

> The appropriate 7th character is to be added to all codes in subcategory S52.31.
> A   initial encounter for closed fracture
> D   subsequent encounter for fracture with routine healing
> G   subsequent encounter for fracture with delayed healing
> K   subsequent encounter for fracture with nonunion
> P   subsequent encounter for fracture with malunion
> S   sequela

7   √7ᵗʰ   **S52.311** Greenstick **fracture of shaft of radius, right arm**   `CC` `H5`
    CC Excl: See code: S52.211

7   √7ᵗʰ   **S52.312** Greenstick **fracture of shaft of radius, left arm**   `CC` `H5`
    CC Excl: See code: S52.212

7   √7ᵗʰ   **S52.319** Greenstick **fracture of shaft of radius, unspecified arm**   `CC` `H5`
    CC Excl: See code: S52.219

√6ᵗʰ **S52.32** Transverse **fracture of shaft of radius**

6, 7   √7ᵗʰ   **S52.321** Displaced **transverse fracture of shaft of right radius**   `MCC` `CC` `H5`

6, 7   √7ᵗʰ   **S52.322** Displaced **transverse fracture of shaft of left radius**   `MCC` `CC` `H5`

6, 7   √7ᵗʰ   **S52.323** Displaced **transverse fracture of shaft of unspecified radius**   `MCC` `CC` `H5`

6, 7   √7ᵗʰ   **S52.324** Nondisplaced **transverse fracture of shaft of right radius**   `MCC` `CC` `H5`

6, 7   √7ᵗʰ   **S52.325** Nondisplaced **transverse fracture of shaft of left radius**   `MCC` `CC` `H5`

6, 7   √7ᵗʰ   **S52.326** Nondisplaced **transverse fracture of shaft of unspecified radius**   `MCC` `CC` `H5`

√6ᵗʰ **S52.33** Oblique **fracture of shaft of radius**

6, 7   √7ᵗʰ   **S52.331** Displaced **oblique fracture of shaft of right radius**   `MCC` `CC` `H5`

6, 7   √7ᵗʰ   **S52.332** Displaced **oblique fracture of shaft of left radius**   `MCC` `CC` `H5`

6, 7   √7ᵗʰ   **S52.333** Displaced **oblique fracture of shaft of unspecified radius**   `MCC` `CC` `H5`

6, 7   √7ᵗʰ   **S52.334** Nondisplaced **oblique fracture of shaft of right radius**   `MCC` `CC` `H5`

6, 7   √7ᵗʰ   **S52.335** Nondisplaced **oblique fracture of shaft of left radius**   `MCC` `CC` `H5`

6, 7   √7ᵗʰ   **S52.336** Nondisplaced **oblique fracture of shaft of unspecified radius**   `MCC` `CC` `H5`

√6ᵗʰ **S52.34** Spiral **fracture of shaft of radius**

6, 7   √7ᵗʰ   **S52.341** Displaced **spiral fracture of shaft of radius, right arm**   `MCC` `CC` `H5`

6, 7   √7ᵗʰ   **S52.342** Displaced **spiral fracture of shaft of radius, left arm**   `MCC` `CC` `H5`

6, 7   √7ᵗʰ   **S52.343** Displaced **spiral fracture of shaft of radius, unspecified arm**   `MCC` `CC` `H5`

6, 7   √7ᵗʰ   **S52.344** Nondisplaced **spiral fracture of shaft of radius, right arm**   `MCC` `CC` `H5`

6, 7   √7ᵗʰ   **S52.345** Nondisplaced **spiral fracture of shaft of radius, left arm**   `MCC` `CC` `H5`

6, 7   √7ᵗʰ   **S52.346** Nondisplaced **spiral fracture of shaft of radius, unspecified arm**   `MCC` `CC` `H5`

√6ᵗʰ **S52.35** Comminuted **fracture of shaft of radius**

6, 7   √7ᵗʰ   **S52.351** Displaced **comminuted fracture of shaft of radius, right arm**   `MCC` `CC` `H5`

6, 7   √7ᵗʰ   **S52.352** Displaced **comminuted fracture of shaft of radius, left arm**   `MCC` `CC` `H5`

6, 7   √7ᵗʰ   **S52.353** Displaced **comminuted fracture of shaft of radius, unspecified arm**   `MCC` `CC` `H5`

6, 7   √7ᵗʰ   **S52.354** Nondisplaced **comminuted fracture of shaft of radius, right arm**   `MCC` `CC` `H5`

6, 7   √7ᵗʰ   **S52.355** Nondisplaced **comminuted fracture of shaft of radius, left arm**   `MCC` `CC` `H5`

6, 7   √7ᵗʰ   **S52.356** Nondisplaced **comminuted fracture of shaft of radius, unspecified arm**   `MCC` `CC` `H5`

√6ᵗʰ **S52.36** Segmental **fracture of shaft of radius**

6, 7   √7ᵗʰ   **S52.361** Displaced **segmental fracture of shaft of radius, right arm**   `MCC` `CC` `H5`

6, 7   √7ᵗʰ   **S52.362** Displaced **segmental fracture of shaft of radius, left arm**   `MCC` `CC` `H5`

6, 7   √7ᵗʰ   **S52.363** Displaced **segmental fracture of shaft of radius, unspecified arm**   `MCC` `CC` `H5`

6, 7   √7ᵗʰ   **S52.364** Nondisplaced **segmental fracture of shaft of radius, right arm**   `MCC` `CC` `H5`

6, 7   √7ᵗʰ   **S52.365** Nondisplaced **segmental fracture of shaft of radius, left arm**   `MCC` `CC` `H5`

6, 7   √7ᵗʰ   **S52.366** Nondisplaced **segmental fracture of shaft of radius, unspecified arm**   `MCC` `CC` `H5`

√6ᵗʰ **S52.37** Galeazzi's **fracture**
> Fracture of lower shaft of radius with radioulnar joint dislocation

6, 7   √7ᵗʰ   **S52.371** Galeazzi's **fracture of right radius**   `MCC` `CC` `H5`

6, 7   √7ᵗʰ   **S52.372** Galeazzi's **fracture of left radius**   `MCC` `CC` `H5`

6, 7   √7ᵗʰ   **S52.379** Galeazzi's **fracture of unspecified radius**   `MCC` `CC` `H5`

√6ᵗʰ **S52.38** Bent bone **of radius**

6, 7   √7ᵗʰ   **S52.381** Bent bone **of right radius**   `MCC` `CC` `H5`

6, 7   √7ᵗʰ   **S52.382** Bent bone **of left radius**   `MCC` `CC` `H5`

6, 7   √7ᵗʰ   **S52.389** Bent bone **of unspecified radius**   `MCC` `CC` `H5`

√6ᵗʰ **S52.39** Other **fracture of shaft of radius**

6, 7   √7ᵗʰ   **S52.391** Other **fracture of shaft of radius, right arm**   `MCC` `CC` `H5`

6, 7   √7ᵗʰ   **S52.392** Other **fracture of shaft of radius, left arm**   `MCC` `CC` `H5`

6, 7   √7ᵗʰ   **S52.399** Other **fracture of shaft of radius, unspecified arm**   `MCC` `CC` `H5`

√5ᵗʰ **S52.5** Fracture of **lower end of radius**
> Fracture of distal end of radius
> *EXCLUDES 2*   *physeal fractures of lower end of radius (S59.2-)*
> **DEF:** Fracture of distal end of radius above the wrist; most commonly caused by fall onto an outstretched hand.

> **CC Excl: For CC/MCC codes in subcategory S52.5, unless otherwise noted:**
> **Right side:** See code S52.201
> **Left side:** See code S52.202
> **Unspecified side:** See code S52.209

√6ᵗʰ **S52.50** Unspecified **fracture of the lower end of radius**

6, 7   √7ᵗʰ   **S52.501** Unspecified **fracture of the lower end of right radius**   `MCC` `CC` `H5`

6, 7   √7ᵗʰ   **S52.502** Unspecified **fracture of the lower end of left radius**   `MCC` `CC` `H5`

6, 7   √7ᵗʰ   **S52.509** Unspecified **fracture of the lower nd of unspecified radius**   `MCC` `CC` `H5`

√6ᵗʰ **S52.51** Fracture of **radial styloid process**

6, 7   √7ᵗʰ   **S52.511** Displaced **fracture of right radial styloid process**   `MCC` `CC` `H5`

6, 7   √7ᵗʰ   **S52.512** Displaced **fracture of left radial styloid process**   `MCC` `CC` `H5`

6, 7   √7ᵗʰ   **S52.513** Displaced **fracture of unspecified radial styloid process**   `MCC` `CC` `H5`

6, 7   √7ᵗʰ   **S52.514** Nondisplaced **fracture of right radial styloid process**   `MCC` `CC` `H5`

6, 7   √7ᵗʰ   **S52.515** Nondisplaced **fracture of left radial styloid process**   `MCC` `CC` `H5`

6, 7   √7ᵗʰ   **S52.516** Nondisplaced **fracture of unspecified radial styloid process**   `MCC` `CC` `H5`

---

6   MCC when reported as an open fracture (7th character B or C – specific to category).

7   CC when reported as an initial encounter (7th character A, B, or C – specific to category) OR a subsequent encounter for nonunion or malunion (7th character K, M, N, P, Q, or R – specific to category).

√6ᵗʰ **S52.52**   Torus **fracture of lower end of radius**

> The appropriate 7th character is to be added to all codes in subcategory S52.52.
> A   initial encounter for closed fracture
> D   subsequent encounter for fracture with routine healing
> G   subsequent encounter for fracture with delayed healing
> K   subsequent encounter for fracture with nonunion
> P   subsequent encounter for fracture with malunion
> S   sequela

7   √7ᵗʰ   **S52.521**   Torus **fracture of lower end of right radius**   CC H5
     CC Excl: See code: S52.211

7   √7ᵗʰ   **S52.522**   Torus **fracture of lower end of left radius**   CC H5
     CC Excl: See code: S52.212

7   √7ᵗʰ   **S52.529**   Torus **fracture of lower end of unspecified radius**   CC H5
     CC Excl: See code: S52.219

√6ᵗʰ **S52.53**   Colles' **fracture**

6, 7   √7ᵗʰ   **S52.531**   Colles' **fracture of right radius**   MCC CC H5
     AHA: 2016, 2Q, 4

6, 7   √7ᵗʰ   **S52.532**   Colles' **fracture of left radius**   MCC CC H5

6, 7   √7ᵗʰ   **S52.539**   Colles' **fracture of unspecified radius**   MCC CC H5

√6ᵗʰ **S52.54**   Smith's **fracture**

6, 7   √7ᵗʰ   **S52.541**   Smith's **fracture of right radius**   MCC CC H5

6, 7   √7ᵗʰ   **S52.542**   Smith's **fracture of left radius**   MCC CC H5

6, 7   √7ᵗʰ   **S52.549**   Smith's **fracture of unspecified radius**   MCC CC H5

√6ᵗʰ **S52.55**   Other extraarticular **fracture of lower end of radius**

6, 7   √7ᵗʰ   **S52.551**   Other extraarticular **fracture of lower end of right radius**   MCC CC H5

6, 7   √7ᵗʰ   **S52.552**   Other extraarticular **fracture of lower end of left radius**   MCC CC H5

6, 7   √7ᵗʰ   **S52.559**   Other extraarticular **fracture of lower end of unspecified radius**   MCC CC H5

√6ᵗʰ **S52.56**   Barton's **fracture**

6, 7   √7ᵗʰ   **S52.561**   Barton's **fracture of right radius**   MCC CC H5

6, 7   √7ᵗʰ   **S52.562**   Barton's **fracture of left radius**   MCC CC H5

6, 7   √7ᵗʰ   **S52.569**   Barton's **fracture of unspecified radius**   MCC CC H5

√6ᵗʰ **S52.57**   Other intraarticular **fracture of lower end of radius**

6, 7   √7ᵗʰ   **S52.571**   Other intraarticular **fracture of lower end of right radius**   MCC CC H5

6, 7   √7ᵗʰ   **S52.572**   Other intraarticular **fracture of lower end of left radius**   MCC CC H5

6, 7   √7ᵗʰ   **S52.579**   Other intraarticular **fracture of lower end of unspecified radius**   MCC CC H5

√6ᵗʰ **S52.59**   Other **fractures of lower end of radius**

6, 7   √7ᵗʰ   **S52.591**   Other **fractures of lower end of right radius**   MCC CC H5

6, 7   √7ᵗʰ   **S52.592**   Other **fractures of lower end of left radius**   MCC CC H5

6, 7   √7ᵗʰ   **S52.599**   Other **fractures of lower end of unspecified radius**   MCC CC H5

√5ᵗʰ **S52.6**   Fracture **of lower end of ulna**

> **CC Excl: For CC/MCC codes in subcategory S52.6, unless otherwise noted:**
> **Right side:** See code S52.201
> **Left side:** See code S52.202
> **Unspecified side:** See code S52.209

√6ᵗʰ **S52.60**   Unspecified **fracture of lower end of ulna**

6, 7   √7ᵗʰ   **S52.601**   Unspecified **fracture of lower end of right ulna**   MCC CC H5

6, 7   √7ᵗʰ   **S52.602**   Unspecified **fracture of lower end of left ulna**   MCC CC H5

6, 7   √7ᵗʰ   **S52.609**   Unspecified **fracture of lower end of unspecified ulna**   MCC CC H5

√6ᵗʰ **S52.61**   Fracture **of ulna styloid process**

6, 7   √7ᵗʰ   **S52.611**   Displaced **fracture of right ulna styloid process**   MCC CC H5

6, 7   √7ᵗʰ   **S52.612**   Displaced **fracture of left ulna styloid process**   MCC CC H5

6, 7   √7ᵗʰ   **S52.613**   Displaced **fracture of unspecified ulna styloid process**   MCC CC H5

6, 7   √7ᵗʰ   **S52.614**   Nondisplaced **fracture of right ulna styloid process**   MCC CC H5

6, 7   √7ᵗʰ   **S52.615**   Nondisplaced **fracture of left ulna styloid process**   MCC CC H5

6, 7   √7ᵗʰ   **S52.616**   Nondisplaced **fracture of unspecified ulna styloid process**   MCC CC H5

√6ᵗʰ **S52.62**   Torus **fracture of lower end of ulna**

> The appropriate 7th character is to be added to all codes in subcategory S52.62.
> A   initial encounter for closed fracture
> D   subsequent encounter for fracture with routine healing
> G   subsequent encounter for fracture with delayed healing
> K   subsequent encounter for fracture with nonunion
> P   subsequent encounter for fracture with malunion
> S   sequela

7   √7ᵗʰ   **S52.621**   Torus **fracture of lower end of right ulna**   CC H5
     CC Excl: See code: S52.211

7   √7ᵗʰ   **S52.622**   Torus **fracture of lower end of left ulna**   CC H5
     CC Excl: See code: S52.212

7   √7ᵗʰ   **S52.629**   Torus **fracture of lower end of unspecified ulna**   CC H5
     CC Excl: See code: S52.219

√6ᵗʰ **S52.69**   Other **fracture of lower end of ulna**

6, 7   √7ᵗʰ   **S52.691**   Other **fracture of lower end of right ulna**   MCC CC H5

6, 7   √7ᵗʰ   **S52.692**   Other **fracture of lower end of left ulna**   MCC CC H5

6, 7   √7ᵗʰ   **S52.699**   Other **fracture of lower end of unspecified ulna**   MCC CC H5

√5ᵗʰ **S52.9**   Unspecified **fracture of forearm**

> **CC Excl: For CC/MCC codes in subcategory S52.9:**
> See code S52.209

6, 7   √x7ᵗʰ   **S52.90**   Unspecified **fracture of unspecified forearm**   MCC CC H5

6, 7   √x7ᵗʰ   **S52.91**   Unspecified **fracture of right forearm**   MCC CC H5

6, 7   √x7ᵗʰ   **S52.92**   Unspecified **fracture of left forearm**   MCC CC H5

---

6   MCC when reported as an open fracture (7th character B or C – specific to category).

7   CC when reported as an initial encounter (7th character A, B, or C – specific to category) OR a subsequent encounter for nonunion or malunion (7th character K, M, N, P, Q, or R – specific to category).

✔ Additional Character Req   √x7ᵗʰ Placeholder Alert   Unacceptable PDx   Manifestation   H1-H14 HAC   HCC CMS-HCC Condition   *EXCLUDES 1* Not Coded Here   *EXCLUDES 2* Not Included Here

✓4ᵗʰ S53   Dislocation and sprain of joints and ligaments of elbow

INCLUDES   avulsion of joint or ligament of elbow
laceration of cartilage, joint or ligament of elbow
sprain of cartilage, joint or ligament of elbow
traumatic hemarthrosis of joint or ligament of elbow
traumatic rupture of joint or ligament of elbow
traumatic subluxation of joint or ligament of elbow
traumatic tear of joint or ligament of elbow

Code also any associated open wound

EXCLUDES 2   *strain of muscle, fascia and tendon at forearm level (S56.-)*

The appropriate 7th character is to be added to each code from category S53.
A   initial encounter
D   subsequent encounter
S   sequela

✓5ᵗʰ S53.0   Subluxation and dislocation of radial head
Dislocation of radiohumeral joint
Subluxation of radiohumeral joint

EXCLUDES 1   *Monteggia's fracture-dislocation (S52.27-)*

✓6ᵗʰ S53.00   Unspecified subluxation and dislocation of radial head

- **✓7ᵗʰ S53.001   Unspecified subluxation of right radial head**
- **✓7ᵗʰ S53.002   Unspecified subluxation of left radial head**
- **✓7ᵗʰ S53.003   Unspecified subluxation of unspecified radial head**
- **✓7ᵗʰ S53.004   Unspecified dislocation of right radial head**
- **✓7ᵗʰ S53.005   Unspecified dislocation of left radial head**
- **✓7ᵗʰ S53.006   Unspecified dislocation of unspecified radial head**

✓6ᵗʰ S53.01   Anterior subluxation and dislocation of radial head
Anteriomedial subluxation and dislocation of radial head

- **✓7ᵗʰ S53.011   Anterior subluxation of right radial head**
- **✓7ᵗʰ S53.012   Anterior subluxation of left radial head**
- **✓7ᵗʰ S53.013   Anterior subluxation of unspecified radial head**
- **✓7ᵗʰ S53.014   Anterior dislocation of right radial head**
- **✓7ᵗʰ S53.015   Anterior dislocation of left radial head**
- **✓7ᵗʰ S53.016   Anterior dislocation of unspecified radial head**

✓6ᵗʰ S53.02   Posterior subluxation and dislocation of radial head
Posteriolateral subluxation and dislocation of radial head

- **✓7ᵗʰ S53.021   Posterior subluxation of right radial head**
- **✓7ᵗʰ S53.022   Posterior subluxation of left radial head**
- **✓7ᵗʰ S53.023   Posterior subluxation of unspecified radial head**
- **✓7ᵗʰ S53.024   Posterior dislocation of right radial head**
- **✓7ᵗʰ S53.025   Posterior dislocation of left radial head**
- **✓7ᵗʰ S53.026   Posterior dislocation of unspecified radial head**

✓6ᵗʰ S53.03   Nursemaid's elbow

- **✓7ᵗʰ S53.031   Nursemaid's elbow, right elbow**
- **✓7ᵗʰ S53.032   Nursemaid's elbow, left elbow**
- **✓7ᵗʰ S53.033   Nursemaid's elbow, unspecified elbow**

✓6ᵗʰ S53.09   Other subluxation and dislocation of radial head

- **✓7ᵗʰ S53.091   Other subluxation of right radial head**
- **✓7ᵗʰ S53.092   Other subluxation of left radial head**
- **✓7ᵗʰ S53.093   Other subluxation of unspecified radial head**
- **✓7ᵗʰ S53.094   Other dislocation of right radial head**
- **✓7ᵗʰ S53.095   Other dislocation of left radial head**
- **✓7ᵗʰ S53.096   Other dislocation of unspecified radial head**

✓5ᵗʰ S53.1   Subluxation and dislocation of ulnohumeral joint
Subluxation and dislocation of elbow NOS

EXCLUDES 1   *dislocation of radial head alone (S53.0-)*

✓6ᵗʰ S53.10   Unspecified subluxation and dislocation of ulnohumeral joint

- **✓7ᵗʰ S53.101   Unspecified subluxation of right ulnohumeral joint**

- **✓7ᵗʰ S53.102   Unspecified subluxation of left ulnohumeral joint**
- **✓7ᵗʰ S53.103   Unspecified subluxation of unspecified ulnohumeral joint**
- **✓7ᵗʰ S53.104   Unspecified dislocation of right ulnohumeral joint**
- **✓7ᵗʰ S53.105   Unspecified dislocation of left ulnohumeral joint**
- **✓7ᵗʰ S53.106   Unspecified dislocation of unspecified ulnohumeral joint**

✓6ᵗʰ S53.11   Anterior subluxation and dislocation of ulnohumeral joint

- **✓7ᵗʰ S53.111   Anterior subluxation of right ulnohumeral joint**
- **✓7ᵗʰ S53.112   Anterior subluxation of left ulnohumeral joint**
- **✓7ᵗʰ S53.113   Anterior subluxation of unspecified ulnohumeral joint**
- **✓7ᵗʰ S53.114   Anterior dislocation of right ulnohumeral joint**
  AHA: 2012, 4Q, 108
- **✓7ᵗʰ S53.115   Anterior dislocation of left ulnohumeral joint**
- **✓7ᵗʰ S53.116   Anterior dislocation of unspecified ulnohumeral joint**

✓6ᵗʰ S53.12   Posterior subluxation and dislocation of ulnohumeral joint

- **✓7ᵗʰ S53.121   Posterior subluxation of right ulnohumeral joint**
- **✓7ᵗʰ S53.122   Posterior subluxation of left ulnohumeral joint**
- **✓7ᵗʰ S53.123   Posterior subluxation of unspecified ulnohumeral joint**
- **✓7ᵗʰ S53.124   Posterior dislocation of right ulnohumeral joint**
- **✓7ᵗʰ S53.125   Posterior dislocation of left ulnohumeral joint**
- **✓7ᵗʰ S53.126   Posterior dislocation of unspecified ulnohumeral joint**

✓6ᵗʰ S53.13   Medial subluxation and dislocation of ulnohumeral joint

- **✓7ᵗʰ S53.131   Medial subluxation of right ulnohumeral joint**
- **✓7ᵗʰ S53.132   Medial subluxation of left ulnohumeral joint**
- **✓7ᵗʰ S53.133   Medial subluxation of unspecified ulnohumeral joint**
- **✓7ᵗʰ S53.134   Medial dislocation of right ulnohumeral joint**
- **✓7ᵗʰ S53.135   Medial dislocation of left ulnohumeral joint**
- **✓7ᵗʰ S53.136   Medial dislocation of unspecified ulnohumeral joint**

✓6ᵗʰ S53.14   Lateral subluxation and dislocation of ulnohumeral joint

- **✓7ᵗʰ S53.141   Lateral subluxation of right ulnohumeral joint**
- **✓7ᵗʰ S53.142   Lateral subluxation of left ulnohumeral joint**
- **✓7ᵗʰ S53.143   Lateral subluxation of unspecified ulnohumeral joint**
- **✓7ᵗʰ S53.144   Lateral dislocation of right ulnohumeral joint**
- **✓7ᵗʰ S53.145   Lateral dislocation of left ulnohumeral joint**
- **✓7ᵗʰ S53.146   Lateral dislocation of unspecified ulnohumeral joint**

✓6ᵗʰ S53.19   Other subluxation and dislocation of ulnohumeral joint

- **✓7ᵗʰ S53.191   Other subluxation of right ulnohumeral joint**
- **✓7ᵗʰ S53.192   Other subluxation of left ulnohumeral joint**
- **✓7ᵗʰ S53.193   Other subluxation of unspecified ulnohumeral joint**

√7ᵗʰ **S53.194** **Other dislocation of right ulnohumeral joint**

√7ᵗʰ **S53.195** **Other dislocation of left ulnohumeral joint**

√7ᵗʰ **S53.196** **Other dislocation of unspecified ulnohumeral joint**

√5ᵗʰ **S53.2 Traumatic rupture of radial collateral ligament**

     EXCLUDES 1   *sprain of radial collateral ligament NOS (S53.43-)*

√x7ᵗʰ **S53.20** **Traumatic rupture of unspecified radial collateral ligament**

√x7ᵗʰ **S53.21** **Traumatic rupture of right radial collateral ligament**

√x7ᵗʰ **S53.22** **Traumatic rupture of left radial collateral ligament**

√5ᵗʰ **S53.3 Traumatic rupture of ulnar collateral ligament**

     EXCLUDES 1   *sprain of ulnar collateral ligament (S53.44-)*

√x7ᵗʰ **S53.30** **Traumatic rupture of unspecified ulnar collateral ligament**

√x7ᵗʰ **S53.31** **Traumatic rupture of right ulnar collateral ligament**

√x7ᵗʰ **S53.32** **Traumatic rupture of left ulnar collateral ligament**

√5ᵗʰ **S53.4 Sprain of elbow**

     EXCLUDES 2   *traumatic rupture of radial collateral ligament (S53.2-)*
               traumatic rupture of ulnar collateral ligament (S53.3-)

√6ᵗʰ **S53.40** **Unspecified sprain of elbow**

√7ᵗʰ **S53.401** **Unspecified sprain of right elbow**

√7ᵗʰ **S53.402** **Unspecified sprain of left elbow**

√7ᵗʰ **S53.409** **Unspecified sprain of unspecified elbow**
         Sprain of elbow NOS

√6ᵗʰ **S53.41** **Radiohumeral (joint) sprain**

√7ᵗʰ **S53.411** **Radiohumeral (joint) sprain of right elbow**

√7ᵗʰ **S53.412** **Radiohumeral (joint) sprain of left elbow**

√7ᵗʰ **S53.419** **Radiohumeral (joint) sprain of unspecified elbow**

√6ᵗʰ **S53.42** **Ulnohumeral (joint) sprain**

√7ᵗʰ **S53.421** **Ulnohumeral (joint) sprain of right elbow**

√7ᵗʰ **S53.422** **Ulnohumeral (joint) sprain of left elbow**

√7ᵗʰ **S53.429** **Ulnohumeral (joint) sprain of unspecified elbow**

√6ᵗʰ **S53.43** **Radial collateral ligament sprain**

√7ᵗʰ **S53.431** **Radial collateral ligament sprain of right elbow**

√7ᵗʰ **S53.432** **Radial collateral ligament sprain of left elbow**

√7ᵗʰ **S53.439** **Radial collateral ligament sprain of unspecified elbow**

√6ᵗʰ **S53.44** **Ulnar collateral ligament sprain**

√7ᵗʰ **S53.441** **Ulnar collateral ligament sprain of right elbow**

√7ᵗʰ **S53.442** **Ulnar collateral ligament sprain of left elbow**

√7ᵗʰ **S53.449** **Ulnar collateral ligament sprain of unspecified elbow**

√6ᵗʰ **S53.49** **Other sprain of elbow**

√7ᵗʰ **S53.491** **Other sprain of right elbow**

√7ᵗʰ **S53.492** **Other sprain of left elbow**

√7ᵗʰ **S53.499** **Other sprain of unspecified elbow**

√4ᵗʰ **S54 Injury of nerves at forearm level**

     Code also any associated open wound (S51.-)

     EXCLUDES 2   *injury of nerves at wrist and hand level (S64.-)*

     The appropriate 7th character is to be added to each code from category S54.
     A   initial encounter
     D   subsequent encounter
     S   sequela

√6ᵗʰ **S54.0 Injury of ulnar nerve at forearm level**
     Injury of ulnar nerve NOS

√x7ᵗʰ **S54.00** **Injury of ulnar nerve at forearm level, unspecified arm**

√x7ᵗʰ **S54.01** **Injury of ulnar nerve at forearm level, right arm**

√x7ᵗʰ **S54.02** **Injury of ulnar nerve at forearm level, left arm**

√5ᵗʰ **S54.1 Injury of median nerve at forearm level**
     Injury of median nerve NOS

√x7ᵗʰ **S54.10** **Injury of median nerve at forearm level, unspecified arm**

√x7ᵗʰ **S54.11** **Injury of median nerve at forearm level, right arm**

√x7ᵗʰ **S54.12** **Injury of median nerve at forearm level, left arm**

√5ᵗʰ **S54.2 Injury of radial nerve at forearm level**
     Injury of radial nerve NOS

√x7ᵗʰ **S54.20** **Injury of radial nerve at forearm level, unspecified arm**

√x7ᵗʰ **S54.21** **Injury of radial nerve at forearm level, right arm**

√x7ᵗʰ **S54.22** **Injury of radial nerve at forearm level, left arm**

√5ᵗʰ **S54.3 Injury of cutaneous sensory nerve at forearm level**

√x7ᵗʰ **S54.30** **Injury of cutaneous sensory nerve at forearm level, unspecified arm**

√x7ᵗʰ **S54.31** **Injury of cutaneous sensory nerve at forearm level, right arm**

√x7ᵗʰ **S54.32** **Injury of cutaneous sensory nerve at forearm level, left arm**

√5ᵗʰ **S54.8 Injury of other nerves at forearm level**

√6ᵗʰ **S54.8X** **Injury of other nerves at forearm level**

√7ᵗʰ **S54.8X1** **Injury of other nerves at forearm level, right arm**

√7ᵗʰ **S54.8X2** **Injury of other nerves at forearm level, left arm**

√7ᵗʰ **S54.8X9** **Injury of other nerves at forearm level, unspecified arm**

√5ᵗʰ **S54.9 Injury of unspecified nerve at forearm level**

√x7ᵗʰ **S54.90** **Injury of unspecified nerve at forearm level, unspecified arm**

√x7ᵗʰ **S54.91** **Injury of unspecified nerve at forearm level, right arm**

√x7ᵗʰ **S54.92** **Injury of unspecified nerve at forearm level, left arm**

√4ᵗʰ **S55 Injury of blood vessels at forearm level**

     Code also any associated open wound (S51.-)

     EXCLUDES 2   *injury of blood vessels at wrist and hand level (S65.-)*
               injury of brachial vessels (S45.1-S45.2)

     The appropriate 7th character is to be added to each code from category S55.
     A   initial encounter
     D   subsequent encounter
     S   sequela

√5ᵗʰ **S55.0 Injury of ulnar artery at forearm level**

     CC Excl: For CC codes in subcategory S55.0:
     Right side: PDX collection 1274
     Left side: PDX collection 1275
     Unspecified side: PDX collection 1276

√6ᵗʰ **S55.00** **Unspecified injury of ulnar artery at forearm level**

√7ᵗʰ **S55.001** **Unspecified injury of ulnar artery at forearm level, right arm**   CC

√7ᵗʰ **S55.002** **Unspecified injury of ulnar artery at forearm level, left arm**   CC

√7ᵗʰ **S55.009** **Unspecified injury of ulnar artery at forearm level, unspecified arm**   CC

√6ᵗʰ **S55.01** **Laceration of ulnar artery at forearm level**

√7ᵗʰ **S55.011** **Laceration of ulnar artery at forearm level, right arm**   CC

√7ᵗʰ **S55.012** **Laceration of ulnar artery at forearm level, left arm**   CC

√7ᵗʰ **S55.019** **Laceration of ulnar artery at forearm level, unspecified arm**   CC

√6ᵗʰ **S55.09** **Other specified injury of ulnar artery at forearm level**

√7ᵗʰ **S55.091** **Other specified injury of ulnar artery at forearm level, right arm**   CC

√7ᵗʰ **S55.092** **Other specified injury of ulnar artery at forearm level, left arm**   CC

√7ᵗʰ **S55.099** **Other specified injury of ulnar artery at forearm level, unspecified arm**   CC

☑ Additional Character Req   √x7ᵗʰ Placeholder Alert   Unacceptable PDx   Manifestation   H1-H14 HAC   HCC CMS-HCC Condition   EXCLUDES 1 Not Coded Here   EXCLUDES 2 Not Included Here

ICD-10-CM 2018   **1005**

√5ᵗʰ **S55.1** Injury of radial artery at forearm level

> **CC Excl:** For CC codes in subcategory S55.1:
> **Right side:** PDX collection 1277
> **Left side:** PDX collection 1278
> **Unspecified side:** PDX collection 1279

√6ᵗʰ **S55.10** Unspecified injury of radial artery at forearm level

√7ᵗʰ **S55.101** Unspecified injury of radial artery at forearm level, right arm `CC`

√7ᵗʰ **S55.102** Unspecified injury of radial artery at forearm level, left arm `CC`

√7ᵗʰ **S55.109** Unspecified injury of radial artery at forearm level, unspecified arm `CC`

√6ᵗʰ **S55.11** Laceration of radial artery at forearm level

√7ᵗʰ **S55.111** Laceration of radial artery at forearm level, right arm `CC`

√7ᵗʰ **S55.112** Laceration of radial artery at forearm level, left arm `CC`

√7ᵗʰ **S55.119** Laceration of radial artery at forearm level, unspecified arm `CC`

√6ᵗʰ **S55.19** Other specified injury of radial artery at forearm level

√7ᵗʰ **S55.191** Other specified injury of radial artery at forearm level, right arm `CC`

√7ᵗʰ **S55.192** Other specified injury of radial artery at forearm level, left arm `CC`

√7ᵗʰ **S55.199** Other specified injury of radial artery at forearm level, unspecified arm `CC`

√5ᵗʰ **S55.2** Injury of vein at forearm level

> **CC Excl:** For CC codes in subcategory S55.2:
> **Right side:** PDX collection 1260
> **Left side:** PDX collection 1261
> **Unspecified side:** PDX collection 1262

√6ᵗʰ **S55.20** Unspecified injury of vein at forearm level

√7ᵗʰ **S55.201** Unspecified injury of vein at forearm level, right arm `CC`

√7ᵗʰ **S55.202** Unspecified injury of vein at forearm level, left arm `CC`

√7ᵗʰ **S55.209** Unspecified injury of vein at forearm level, unspecified arm `CC`

√6ᵗʰ **S55.21** Laceration of vein at forearm level

√7ᵗʰ **S55.211** Laceration of vein at forearm level, right arm `CC`

√7ᵗʰ **S55.212** Laceration of vein at forearm level, left arm `CC`

√7ᵗʰ **S55.219** Laceration of vein at forearm level, unspecified arm `CC`

√6ᵗʰ **S55.29** Other specified injury of vein at forearm level

√7ᵗʰ **S55.291** Other specified injury of vein at forearm level, right arm `CC`

√7ᵗʰ **S55.292** Other specified injury of vein at forearm level, left arm `CC`

√7ᵗʰ **S55.299** Other specified injury of vein at forearm level, unspecified arm `CC`

√5ᵗʰ **S55.8** Injury of other blood vessels at forearm level

> **CC Excl:** For CC codes in subcategory S55.8:
> **Right side:** PDX collection 1260
> **Left side:** PDX collection 1261
> **Unspecified side:** PDX collection 1262

√6ᵗʰ **S55.80** Unspecified injury of other blood vessels at forearm level

√7ᵗʰ **S55.801** Unspecified injury of other blood vessels at forearm level, right arm `CC`

√7ᵗʰ **S55.802** Unspecified injury of other blood vessels at forearm level, left arm `CC`

√7ᵗʰ **S55.809** Unspecified injury of other blood vessels at forearm level, unspecified arm `CC`

√6ᵗʰ **S55.81** Laceration of other blood vessels at forearm level

√7ᵗʰ **S55.811** Laceration of other blood vessels at forearm level, right arm `CC`

√7ᵗʰ **S55.812** Laceration of other blood vessels at forearm level, left arm `CC`

√7ᵗʰ **S55.819** Laceration of other blood vessels at forearm level, unspecified arm `CC`

√6ᵗʰ **S55.89** Other specified injury of other blood vessels at forearm level

√7ᵗʰ **S55.891** Other specified injury of other blood vessels at forearm level, right arm `CC`

√7ᵗʰ **S55.892** Other specified injury of other blood vessels at forearm level, left arm `CC`

√7ᵗʰ **S55.899** Other specified injury of other blood vessels at forearm level, unspecified arm `CC`

√5ᵗʰ **S55.9** Injury of unspecified blood vessel at forearm level

> **CC Excl:** For CC codes in subcategory S55.9:
> **Right side:** PDX collection 1260
> **Left side:** PDX collection 1261
> **Unspecified side:** PDX collection 1262

√6ᵗʰ **S55.90** Unspecified injury of unspecified blood vessel at forearm level

√7ᵗʰ **S55.901** Unspecified injury of unspecified blood vessel at forearm level, right arm `CC`

√7ᵗʰ **S55.902** Unspecified injury of unspecified blood vessel at forearm level, left arm `CC`

√7ᵗʰ **S55.909** Unspecified injury of unspecified blood vessel at forearm level, unspecified arm `CC`

√6ᵗʰ **S55.91** Laceration of unspecified blood vessel at forearm level

√7ᵗʰ **S55.911** Laceration of unspecified blood vessel at forearm level, right arm `CC`

√7ᵗʰ **S55.912** Laceration of unspecified blood vessel at forearm level, left arm `CC`

√7ᵗʰ **S55.919** Laceration of unspecified blood vessel at forearm level, unspecified arm `CC`

√6ᵗʰ **S55.99** Other specified injury of unspecified blood vessel at forearm level

√7ᵗʰ **S55.991** Other specified injury of unspecified blood vessel at forearm level, right arm `CC`

√7ᵗʰ **S55.992** Other specified injury of unspecified blood vessel at forearm level, left arm `CC`

√7ᵗʰ **S55.999** Other specified injury of unspecified blood vessel at forearm level, unspecified arm `CC`

√4ᵗʰ **S56** Injury of muscle, fascia and tendon at forearm level

Code also any associated open wound (S51.-)

> *EXCLUDES 2*   injury of muscle, fascia and tendon at or below wrist (S66.-)
> sprain of joints and ligaments of elbow (S53.4-)

TIP: Refer to the Muscle/Tendon table at the beginning of this chapter.

> The appropriate 7th character is to be added to each code from category S56.
> A   initial encounter
> D   subsequent encounter
> S   sequela

> **CC Excl:** For CC codes in category S56:
> **Right side:** PDX collection 1280
> **Left side:** PDX collection 1281
> **Unspecified side:** PDX collection 1282

√5ᵗʰ **S56.0** Injury of flexor muscle, fascia and tendon of thumb at forearm level

√6ᵗʰ **S56.00** Unspecified injury of flexor muscle, fascia and tendon of thumb at forearm level

√7ᵗʰ **S56.001** Unspecified injury of flexor muscle, fascia and tendon of right thumb at forearm level

√7ᵗʰ **S56.002** Unspecified injury of flexor muscle, fascia and tendon of left thumb at forearm level

√7ᵗʰ **S56.009** Unspecified injury of flexor muscle, fascia and tendon of unspecified thumb at forearm level

√6ᵗʰ **S56.01** Strain of flexor muscle, fascia and tendon of thumb at forearm level

√7ᵗʰ **S56.011** Strain of flexor muscle, fascia and tendon of right thumb at forearm level

√7ᵗʰ **S56.012** Strain of flexor muscle, fascia and tendon of left thumb at forearm level

√7ᵗʰ **S56.019** Strain of flexor muscle, fascia and tendon of unspecified thumb at forearm level

✓6ᵗʰ **S56.02** Laceration of flexor muscle, fascia and tendon of thumb at forearm level

  ✓7ᵗʰ **S56.021** Laceration of flexor muscle, fascia and tendon of right thumb at forearm level CC

  ✓7ᵗʰ **S56.022** Laceration of flexor muscle, fascia and tendon of left thumb at forearm level CC

  ✓7ᵗʰ **S56.029** Laceration of flexor muscle, fascia and tendon of unspecified thumb at forearm level CC

✓6ᵗʰ **S56.09** Other injury of flexor muscle, fascia and tendon of thumb at forearm level

  ✓7ᵗʰ **S56.091** Other injury of flexor muscle, fascia and tendon of right thumb at forearm level

  ✓7ᵗʰ **S56.092** Other injury of flexor muscle, fascia and tendon of left thumb at forearm level

  ✓7ᵗʰ **S56.099** Other injury of flexor muscle, fascia and tendon of unspecified thumb at forearm level

✓5ᵗʰ **S56.1** Injury of flexor muscle, fascia and tendon of other and unspecified finger at forearm level

✓6ᵗʰ **S56.10** Unspecified injury of flexor muscle, fascia and tendon of other and unspecified finger at forearm level

  ✓7ᵗʰ **S56.101** Unspecified injury of flexor muscle, fascia and tendon of right index finger at forearm level

  ✓7ᵗʰ **S56.102** Unspecified injury of flexor muscle, fascia and tendon of left index finger at forearm level

  ✓7ᵗʰ **S56.103** Unspecified injury of flexor muscle, fascia and tendon of right middle finger at forearm level

  ✓7ᵗʰ **S56.104** Unspecified injury of flexor muscle, fascia and tendon of left middle finger at forearm level

  ✓7ᵗʰ **S56.105** Unspecified injury of flexor muscle, fascia and tendon of right ring finger at forearm level

  ✓7ᵗʰ **S56.106** Unspecified injury of flexor muscle, fascia and tendon of left ring finger at forearm level

  ✓7ᵗʰ **S56.107** Unspecified injury of flexor muscle, fascia and tendon of right little finger at forearm level

  ✓7ᵗʰ **S56.108** Unspecified injury of flexor muscle, fascia and tendon of left little finger at forearm level

  ✓7ᵗʰ **S56.109** Unspecified injury of flexor muscle, fascia and tendon of unspecified finger at forearm level

✓6ᵗʰ **S56.11** Strain of flexor muscle, fascia and tendon of other and unspecified finger at forearm level

  ✓7ᵗʰ **S56.111** Strain of flexor muscle, fascia and tendon of right index finger at forearm level

  ✓7ᵗʰ **S56.112** Strain of flexor muscle, fascia and tendon of left index finger at forearm level

  ✓7ᵗʰ **S56.113** Strain of flexor muscle, fascia and tendon of right middle finger at forearm level

  ✓7ᵗʰ **S56.114** Strain of flexor muscle, fascia and tendon of left middle finger at forearm level

  ✓7ᵗʰ **S56.115** Strain of flexor muscle, fascia and tendon of right ring finger at forearm level

  ✓7ᵗʰ **S56.116** Strain of flexor muscle, fascia and tendon of left ring finger at forearm level

  ✓7ᵗʰ **S56.117** Strain of flexor muscle, fascia and tendon of right little finger at forearm level

  ✓7ᵗʰ **S56.118** Strain of flexor muscle, fascia and tendon of left little finger at forearm level

  ✓7ᵗʰ **S56.119** Strain of flexor muscle, fascia and tendon of finger of unspecified finger at forearm level

✓6ᵗʰ **S56.12** Laceration of flexor muscle, fascia and tendon of other and unspecified finger at forearm level

  ✓7ᵗʰ **S56.121** Laceration of flexor muscle, fascia and tendon of right index finger at forearm level CC

✓7ᵗʰ **S56.122** Laceration of flexor muscle, fascia and tendon of left index finger at forearm level CC

✓7ᵗʰ **S56.123** Laceration of flexor muscle, fascia and tendon of right middle finger at forearm level CC

✓7ᵗʰ **S56.124** Laceration of flexor muscle, fascia and tendon of left middle finger at forearm level CC

✓7ᵗʰ **S56.125** Laceration of flexor muscle, fascia and tendon of right ring finger at forearm level CC

✓7ᵗʰ **S56.126** Laceration of flexor muscle, fascia and tendon of left ring finger at forearm level CC

✓7ᵗʰ **S56.127** Laceration of flexor muscle, fascia and tendon of right little finger at forearm level CC

✓7ᵗʰ **S56.128** Laceration of flexor muscle, fascia and tendon of left little finger at forearm level CC

✓7ᵗʰ **S56.129** Laceration of flexor muscle, fascia and tendon of unspecified finger at forearm level CC

✓6ᵗʰ **S56.19** Other injury of flexor muscle, fascia and tendon of other and unspecified finger at forearm level

  ✓7ᵗʰ **S56.191** Other injury of flexor muscle, fascia and tendon of right index finger at forearm level

  ✓7ᵗʰ **S56.192** Other injury of flexor muscle, fascia and tendon of left index finger at forearm level

  ✓7ᵗʰ **S56.193** Other injury of flexor muscle, fascia and tendon of right middle finger at forearm level

  ✓7ᵗʰ **S56.194** Other injury of flexor muscle, fascia and tendon of left middle finger at forearm level

  ✓7ᵗʰ **S56.195** Other injury of flexor muscle, fascia and tendon of right ring finger at forearm level

  ✓7ᵗʰ **S56.196** Other injury of flexor muscle, fascia and tendon of left ring finger at forearm level

  ✓7ᵗʰ **S56.197** Other injury of flexor muscle, fascia and tendon of right little finger at forearm level

  ✓7ᵗʰ **S56.198** Other injury of flexor muscle, fascia and tendon of left little finger at forearm level

  ✓7ᵗʰ **S56.199** Other injury of flexor muscle, fascia and tendon of unspecified finger at forearm level

✓5ᵗʰ **S56.2** Injury of other flexor muscle, fascia and tendon at forearm level

✓6ᵗʰ **S56.20** Unspecified injury of other flexor muscle, fascia and tendon at forearm level

  ✓7ᵗʰ **S56.201** Unspecified injury of other flexor muscle, fascia and tendon at forearm level, right arm

  ✓7ᵗʰ **S56.202** Unspecified injury of other flexor muscle, fascia and tendon at forearm level, left arm

  ✓7ᵗʰ **S56.209** Unspecified injury of other flexor muscle, fascia and tendon at forearm level, unspecified arm

✓6ᵗʰ **S56.21** Strain of other flexor muscle, fascia and tendon at forearm level

  ✓7ᵗʰ **S56.211** Strain of other flexor muscle, fascia and tendon at forearm level, right arm

  ✓7ᵗʰ **S56.212** Strain of other flexor muscle, fascia and tendon at forearm level, left arm

  ✓7ᵗʰ **S56.219** Strain of other flexor muscle, fascia and tendon at forearm level, unspecified arm

✓6ᵗʰ **S56.22** Laceration of other flexor muscle, fascia and tendon at forearm level

  ✓7ᵗʰ **S56.221** Laceration of other flexor muscle, fascia and tendon at forearm level, right arm CC

√7ᵗʰ **S56.222** **Laceration of other flexor muscle, fascia and tendon at forearm level, left arm** `CC`

√7ᵗʰ **S56.229** **Laceration of other flexor muscle, fascia and tendon at forearm level, unspecified arm** `CC`

√6ᵗʰ **S56.29** **Other injury of other flexor muscle, fascia and tendon at forearm level**

√7ᵗʰ **S56.291** **Other injury of other flexor muscle, fascia and tendon at forearm level, right arm**

√7ᵗʰ **S56.292** **Other injury of other flexor muscle, fascia and tendon at forearm level, left arm**

√7ᵗʰ **S56.299** **Other injury of other flexor muscle, fascia and tendon at forearm level, unspecified arm**

√5ᵗʰ **S56.3** **Injury of extensor or abductor muscles, fascia and tendons of thumb at forearm level**

√6ᵗʰ **S56.30** **Unspecified injury of extensor or abductor muscles, fascia and tendons of thumb at forearm level**

√7ᵗʰ **S56.301** **Unspecified injury of extensor or abductor muscles, fascia and tendons of right thumb at forearm level**

√7ᵗʰ **S56.302** **Unspecified injury of extensor or abductor muscles, fascia and tendons of left thumb at forearm level**

√7ᵗʰ **S56.309** **Unspecified injury of extensor or abductor muscles, fascia and tendons of unspecified thumb at forearm level**

√6ᵗʰ **S56.31** **Strain of extensor or abductor muscles, fascia and tendons of thumb at forearm level**

√7ᵗʰ **S56.311** **Strain of extensor or abductor muscles, fascia and tendons of right thumb at forearm level**

√7ᵗʰ **S56.312** **Strain of extensor or abductor muscles, fascia and tendons of left thumb at forearm level**

√7ᵗʰ **S56.319** **Strain of extensor or abductor muscles, fascia and tendons of unspecified thumb at forearm level**

√6ᵗʰ **S56.32** **Laceration of extensor or abductor muscles, fascia and tendons of thumb at forearm level**

√7ᵗʰ **S56.321** **Laceration of extensor or abductor muscles, fascia and tendons of right thumb at forearm level** `CC`

√7ᵗʰ **S56.322** **Laceration of extensor or abductor muscles, fascia and tendons of left thumb at forearm level** `CC`

√7ᵗʰ **S56.329** **Laceration of extensor or abductor muscles, fascia and tendons of unspecified thumb at forearm level** `CC`

√6ᵗʰ **S56.39** **Other injury of extensor or abductor muscles, fascia and tendons of thumb at forearm level**

√7ᵗʰ **S56.391** **Other injury of extensor or abductor muscles, fascia and tendons of right thumb at forearm level**

√7ᵗʰ **S56.392** **Other injury of extensor or abductor muscles, fascia and tendons of left thumb at forearm level**

√7ᵗʰ **S56.399** **Other injury of extensor or abductor muscles, fascia and tendons of unspecified thumb at forearm level**

√5ᵗʰ **S56.4** **Injury of extensor muscle, fascia and tendon of other and unspecified finger at forearm level**

√6ᵗʰ **S56.40** **Unspecified injury of extensor muscle, fascia and tendon of other and unspecified finger at forearm level**

√7ᵗʰ **S56.401** **Unspecified injury of extensor muscle, fascia and tendon of right index finger at forearm level**

√7ᵗʰ **S56.402** **Unspecified injury of extensor muscle, fascia and tendon of left index finger at forearm level**

√7ᵗʰ **S56.403** **Unspecified injury of extensor muscle, fascia and tendon of right middle finger at forearm level**

√7ᵗʰ **S56.404** **Unspecified injury of extensor muscle, fascia and tendon of left middle finger at forearm level**

√7ᵗʰ **S56.405** **Unspecified injury of extensor muscle, fascia and tendon of right ring finger at forearm level**

√7ᵗʰ **S56.406** **Unspecified injury of extensor muscle, fascia and tendon of left ring finger at forearm level**

√7ᵗʰ **S56.407** **Unspecified injury of extensor muscle, fascia and tendon of right little finger at forearm level**

√7ᵗʰ **S56.408** **Unspecified injury of extensor muscle, fascia and tendon of left little finger at forearm level**

√7ᵗʰ **S56.409** **Unspecified injury of extensor muscle, fascia and tendon of unspecified finger at forearm level**

√6ᵗʰ **S56.41** **Strain of extensor muscle, fascia and tendon of other and unspecified finger at forearm level**

√7ᵗʰ **S56.411** **Strain of extensor muscle, fascia and tendon of right index finger at forearm level**

√7ᵗʰ **S56.412** **Strain of extensor muscle, fascia and tendon of left index finger at forearm level**

√7ᵗʰ **S56.413** **Strain of extensor muscle, fascia and tendon of right middle finger at forearm level**

√7ᵗʰ **S56.414** **Strain of extensor muscle, fascia and tendon of left middle finger at forearm level**

√7ᵗʰ **S56.415** **Strain of extensor muscle, fascia and tendon of right ring finger at forearm level**

√7ᵗʰ **S56.416** **Strain of extensor muscle, fascia and tendon of left ring finger at forearm level**

√7ᵗʰ **S56.417** **Strain of extensor muscle, fascia and tendon of right little finger at forearm level**

√7ᵗʰ **S56.418** **Strain of extensor muscle, fascia and tendon of left little finger at forearm level**

√7ᵗʰ **S56.419** **Strain of extensor muscle, fascia and tendon of finger, unspecified finger at forearm level**

√6ᵗʰ **S56.42** **Laceration of extensor muscle, fascia and tendon of other and unspecified finger at forearm level**

√7ᵗʰ **S56.421** **Laceration of extensor muscle, fascia and tendon of right index finger at forearm level** `CC`

√7ᵗʰ **S56.422** **Laceration of extensor muscle, fascia and tendon of left index finger at forearm level** `CC`

√7ᵗʰ **S56.423** **Laceration of extensor muscle, fascia and tendon of right middle finger at forearm level** `CC`

√7ᵗʰ **S56.424** **Laceration of extensor muscle, fascia and tendon of left middle finger at forearm level** `CC`

√7ᵗʰ **S56.425** **Laceration of extensor muscle, fascia and tendon of right ring finger at forearm level** `CC`

√7ᵗʰ **S56.426** **Laceration of extensor muscle, fascia and tendon of left ring finger at forearm level** `CC`

√7ᵗʰ **S56.427** **Laceration of extensor muscle, fascia and tendon of right little finger at forearm level** `CC`

√7ᵗʰ **S56.428** **Laceration of extensor muscle, fascia and tendon of left little finger at forearm level** `CC`

√7ᵗʰ **S56.429** **Laceration of extensor muscle, fascia and tendon of unspecified finger at forearm level** `CC`

√6ᵗʰ **S56.49** **Other injury of extensor muscle, fascia and tendon of other and unspecified finger at forearm level**

√7ᵗʰ **S56.491** **Other injury of extensor muscle, fascia and tendon of right index finger at forearm level**

√7ᵗʰ **S56.492** **Other injury of extensor muscle, fascia and tendon of left index finger at forearm level**

N Newborn: 0   P Pediatric: 0-17   M Maternity: 12-55   A Adult: 15-124   MCC Major CC Condition   PDxMCC PDx acts as own MCC   CC CC Condition   PDxCC PDx acts as own CC

1008   ICD-10-CM 2018

✓7ᵗʰ **S56.493** Other injury of extensor muscle, fascia and tendon of right middle finger at forearm level

✓7ᵗʰ **S56.494** Other injury of extensor muscle, fascia and tendon of left middle finger at forearm level

✓7ᵗʰ **S56.495** Other injury of extensor muscle, fascia and tendon of right ring finger at forearm level

✓7ᵗʰ **S56.496** Other injury of extensor muscle, fascia and tendon of left ring finger at forearm level

✓7ᵗʰ **S56.497** Other injury of extensor muscle, fascia and tendon of right little finger at forearm level

✓7ᵗʰ **S56.498** Other injury of extensor muscle, fascia and tendon of left little finger at forearm level

✓7ᵗʰ **S56.499** Other injury of extensor muscle, fascia and tendon of unspecified finger at forearm level

✓5ᵗʰ **S56.5** Injury of other extensor muscle, fascia and tendon at forearm level

  ✓6ᵗʰ **S56.5Ø** Unspecified injury of other extensor muscle, fascia and tendon at forearm level

    ✓7ᵗʰ **S56.5Ø1** Unspecified injury of other extensor muscle, fascia and tendon at forearm level, right arm

    ✓7ᵗʰ **S56.5Ø2** Unspecified injury of other extensor muscle, fascia and tendon at forearm level, left arm

    ✓7ᵗʰ **S56.5Ø9** Unspecified injury of other extensor muscle, fascia and tendon at forearm level, unspecified arm

  ✓6ᵗʰ **S56.51** Strain of other extensor muscle, fascia and tendon at forearm level

    ✓7ᵗʰ **S56.511** Strain of other extensor muscle, fascia and tendon at forearm level, right arm

    ✓7ᵗʰ **S56.512** Strain of other extensor muscle, fascia and tendon at forearm level, left arm

    ✓7ᵗʰ **S56.519** Strain of other extensor muscle, fascia and tendon at forearm level, unspecified arm

  ✓6ᵗʰ **S56.52** Laceration of other extensor muscle, fascia and tendon at forearm level

    ✓7ᵗʰ **S56.521** Laceration of other extensor muscle, fascia and tendon at forearm level, right arm **CC**

    ✓7ᵗʰ **S56.522** Laceration of other extensor muscle, fascia and tendon at forearm level, left arm **CC**

    ✓7ᵗʰ **S56.529** Laceration of other extensor muscle, fascia and tendon at forearm level, unspecified arm **CC**

  ✓6ᵗʰ **S56.59** Other injury of other extensor muscle, fascia and tendon at forearm level

    ✓7ᵗʰ **S56.591** Other injury of other extensor muscle, fascia and tendon at forearm level, right arm

    ✓7ᵗʰ **S56.592** Other injury of other extensor muscle, fascia and tendon at forearm level, left arm

    ✓7ᵗʰ **S56.599** Other injury of other extensor muscle, fascia and tendon at forearm level, unspecified arm

✓5ᵗʰ **S56.8** Injury of other muscles, fascia and tendons at forearm level

  ✓6ᵗʰ **S56.8Ø** Unspecified injury of other muscles, fascia and tendons at forearm level

    ✓7ᵗʰ **S56.8Ø1** Unspecified injury of other muscles, fascia and tendons at forearm level, right arm

    ✓7ᵗʰ **S56.8Ø2** Unspecified injury of other muscles, fascia and tendons at forearm level, left arm

    ✓7ᵗʰ **S56.8Ø9** Unspecified injury of other muscles, fascia and tendons at forearm level, unspecified arm

  ✓6ᵗʰ **S56.81** Strain of other muscles, fascia and tendons at forearm level

    ✓7ᵗʰ **S56.811** Strain of other muscles, fascia and tendons at forearm level, right arm

    ✓7ᵗʰ **S56.812** Strain of other muscles, fascia and tendons at forearm level, left arm

    ✓7ᵗʰ **S56.819** Strain of other muscles, fascia and tendons at forearm level, unspecified arm

  ✓6ᵗʰ **S56.82** Laceration of other muscles, fascia and tendons at forearm level

    ✓7ᵗʰ **S56.821** Laceration of other muscles, fascia and tendons at forearm level, right arm **CC**

    ✓7ᵗʰ **S56.822** Laceration of other muscles, fascia and tendons at forearm level, left arm **CC**

    ✓7ᵗʰ **S56.829** Laceration of other muscles, fascia and tendons at forearm level, unspecified arm **CC**

  ✓6ᵗʰ **S56.89** Other injury of other muscles, fascia and tendons at forearm level

    ✓7ᵗʰ **S56.891** Other injury of other muscles, fascia and tendons at forearm level, right arm

    ✓7ᵗʰ **S56.892** Other injury of other muscles, fascia and tendons at forearm level, left arm

    ✓7ᵗʰ **S56.899** Other injury of other muscles, fascia and tendons at forearm level, unspecified arm

✓5ᵗʰ **S56.9** Injury of unspecified muscles, fascia and tendons at forearm level

  ✓6ᵗʰ **S56.9Ø** Unspecified injury of unspecified muscles, fascia and tendons at forearm level

    ✓7ᵗʰ **S56.9Ø1** Unspecified injury of unspecified muscles, fascia and tendons at forearm level, right arm

    ✓7ᵗʰ **S56.9Ø2** Unspecified injury of unspecified muscles, fascia and tendons at forearm level, left arm

    ✓7ᵗʰ **S56.9Ø9** Unspecified injury of unspecified muscles, fascia and tendons at forearm level, unspecified arm

  ✓6ᵗʰ **S56.91** Strain of unspecified muscles, fascia and tendons at forearm level

    ✓7ᵗʰ **S56.911** Strain of unspecified muscles, fascia and tendons at forearm level, right arm

    ✓7ᵗʰ **S56.912** Strain of unspecified muscles, fascia and tendons at forearm level, left arm

    ✓7ᵗʰ **S56.919** Strain of unspecified muscles, fascia and tendons at forearm level, unspecified arm

  ✓6ᵗʰ **S56.92** Laceration of unspecified muscles, fascia and tendons at forearm level

    ✓7ᵗʰ **S56.921** Laceration of unspecified muscles, fascia and tendons at forearm level, right arm **CC**

    ✓7ᵗʰ **S56.922** Laceration of unspecified muscles, fascia and tendons at forearm level, left arm **CC**

    ✓7ᵗʰ **S56.929** Laceration of unspecified muscles, fascia and tendons at forearm level, unspecified arm **CC**

  ✓6ᵗʰ **S56.99** Other injury of unspecified muscles, fascia and tendons at forearm level

    ✓7ᵗʰ **S56.991** Other injury of unspecified muscles, fascia and tendons at forearm level, right arm

    ✓7ᵗʰ **S56.992** Other injury of unspecified muscles, fascia and tendons at forearm level, left arm

    ✓7ᵗʰ **S56.999** Other injury of unspecified muscles, fascia and tendons at forearm level, unspecified arm

✓4ᵗʰ **S57** Crushing injury of elbow and forearm

Use additional code(s) for all associated injuries

EXCLUDES 2   crushing injury of wrist and hand (S67.-)

> The appropriate 7th character is to be added to each code from category S57.
> A   initial encounter
> D   subsequent encounter
> S   sequela

✓5ᵗʰ **S57.Ø** Crushing injury of elbow

  ✓x7ᵗʰ **S57.ØØ** Crushing injury of unspecified elbow

  ✓x7ᵗʰ **S57.Ø1** Crushing injury of right elbow

  ✓x7ᵗʰ **S57.Ø2** Crushing injury of left elbow

✓5ᵗʰ **S57.8** Crushing injury of forearm

  ✓x7ᵗʰ **S57.8Ø** Crushing injury of unspecified forearm

✓ Additional Character Req   ✓x7ᵗʰ Placeholder Alert   Unacceptable PDx   Manifestation   **H1**-**H14** HAC   **HCC** CMS-HCC Condition   *EXCLUDES 1* Not Coded Here   *EXCLUDES 2* Not Included Here

ICD-10-CM 2018   1009

√x 7ᵗʰ **S57.81**   **Crushing injury of right forearm**

√x 7ᵗʰ **S57.82**   **Crushing injury of left forearm**

√4ᵗʰ **S58**   **Traumatic amputation of elbow and forearm**

An amputation not identified as partial or complete should be coded to complete.

EXCLUDES 1   *traumatic amputation of wrist and hand (S68.-)*

The appropriate 7th character is to be added to each code from category S58.

A   initial encounter
D   subsequent encounter
S   sequela

CC Excl: For CC codes in category S58:
Right side: PDX collection 1266
Left side: PDX collection 1267
Unspecified side: PDX collection 1268

√5ᵗʰ **S58.0**   **Traumatic amputation at elbow level**

   √6ᵗʰ **S58.01**   **Complete traumatic amputation at elbow level**

     11 √7ᵗʰ **S58.011**   **Complete traumatic amputation at elbow level, right arm**   CC HCC

     11 √7ᵗʰ **S58.012**   **Complete traumatic amputation at elbow level, left arm**   CC HCC

     11 √7ᵗʰ **S58.019**   **Complete traumatic amputation at elbow level, unspecified arm**   CC HCC

   √6ᵗʰ **S58.02**   **Partial traumatic amputation at elbow level**

     11 √7ᵗʰ **S58.021**   **Partial traumatic amputation at elbow level, right arm**   CC HCC

     11 √7ᵗʰ **S58.022**   **Partial traumatic amputation at elbow level, left arm**   CC HCC

     11 √7ᵗʰ **S58.029**   **Partial traumatic amputation at elbow level, unspecified arm**   CC HCC

√5ᵗʰ **S58.1**   **Traumatic amputation at level between elbow and wrist**

   √6ᵗʰ **S58.11**   **Complete traumatic amputation at level between elbow and wrist**

     11 √7ᵗʰ **S58.111**   **Complete traumatic amputation at level between elbow and wrist, right arm**   CC HCC

     11 √7ᵗʰ **S58.112**   **Complete traumatic amputation at level between elbow and wrist, left arm**   CC HCC

     11 √7ᵗʰ **S58.119**   **Complete traumatic amputation at level between elbow and wrist, unspecified arm**   CC HCC

   √6ᵗʰ **S58.12**   **Partial traumatic amputation at level between elbow and wrist**

     11 √7ᵗʰ **S58.121**   **Partial traumatic amputation at level between elbow and wrist, right arm**   CC HCC

     11 √7ᵗʰ **S58.122**   **Partial traumatic amputation at level between elbow and wrist, left arm**   CC HCC

     11 √7ᵗʰ **S58.129**   **Partial traumatic amputation at level between elbow and wrist, unspecified arm**   CC HCC

√5ᵗʰ **S58.9**   **Traumatic amputation of forearm, level unspecified**

   EXCLUDES 1   *traumatic amputation of wrist (S68.-)*

   √6ᵗʰ **S58.91**   **Complete traumatic amputation of forearm, level unspecified**

     11 √7ᵗʰ **S58.911**   **Complete traumatic amputation of right forearm, level unspecified**   CC HCC

     11 √7ᵗʰ **S58.912**   **Complete traumatic amputation of left forearm, level unspecified**   CC HCC

     11 √7ᵗʰ **S58.919**   **Complete traumatic amputation of unspecified forearm, level unspecified**   CC HCC

   √6ᵗʰ **S58.92**   **Partial traumatic amputation of forearm, level unspecified**

     11 √7ᵗʰ **S58.921**   **Partial traumatic amputation of right forearm, level unspecified**   CC HCC

     11 √7ᵗʰ **S58.922**   **Partial traumatic amputation of left forearm, level unspecified**   CC HCC

     11 √7ᵗʰ **S58.929**   **Partial traumatic amputation of unspecified forearm, level unspecified**   CC HCC

√4ᵗʰ **S59**   **Other and unspecified injuries of elbow and forearm**

EXCLUDES 2   *other and unspecified injuries of wrist and hand (S69.-)*
AHA: 2015, 3Q, 37-39

The appropriate 7th character is to be added to each code from subcategories S59.0, S59.1, and S59.2.

A   initial encounter for closed fracture
D   subsequent encounter for fracture with routine healing
G   subsequent encounter for fracture with delayed healing
K   subsequent encounter for fracture with nonunion
P   subsequent encounter for fracture with malunion
S   sequela

√5ᵗʰ **S59.0**   **Physeal fracture of lower end of ulna**

CC Excl: For CC codes in subcategory S59.0:
Right side: See code S59.001
Left side: See code S59.002
Unspecified side: See code S59.009

   √6ᵗʰ **S59.00**   **Unspecified physeal fracture of lower end of ulna**

     7 √7ᵗʰ **S59.001**   **Unspecified physeal fracture of lower end of ulna, right arm**   CC H5
        CC Excl: CC with 7th character A:
        PDX collection 1270
        CC with 7th character K or P:
        PDX collection 897

     7 √7ᵗʰ **S59.002**   **Unspecified physeal fracture of lower end of ulna, left arm**   CC H5
        CC Excl: CC with 7th character A:
        PDX collection 1271
        CC with 7th character K or P:
        PDX collection 897

     7 √7ᵗʰ **S59.009**   **Unspecified physeal fracture of lower end of ulna, unspecified arm**   CC H5
        CC Excl: CC with 7th character A:
        PDX collection 1272
        CC with 7th character K or P:
        PDX collection 897

   √6ᵗʰ **S59.01**   **Salter-Harris Type I physeal fracture of lower end of ulna**

     7 √7ᵗʰ **S59.011**   **Salter-Harris Type I physeal fracture of lower end of ulna, right arm**   CC H5

     7 √7ᵗʰ **S59.012**   **Salter-Harris Type I physeal fracture of lower end of ulna, left arm**   CC H5

     7 √7ᵗʰ **S59.019**   **Salter-Harris Type I physeal fracture of lower end of ulna, unspecified arm**   CC H5

   √6ᵗʰ **S59.02**   **Salter-Harris Type II physeal fracture of lower end of ulna**

     7 √7ᵗʰ **S59.021**   **Salter-Harris Type II physeal fracture of lower end of ulna, right arm**   CC H5

     7 √7ᵗʰ **S59.022**   **Salter-Harris Type II physeal fracture of lower end of ulna, left arm**   CC H5

     7 √7ᵗʰ **S59.029**   **Salter-Harris Type II physeal fracture of lower end of ulna, unspecified arm**   CC H5

   √6ᵗʰ **S59.03**   **Salter-Harris Type III physeal fracture of lower end of ulna**

     7 √7ᵗʰ **S59.031**   **Salter-Harris Type III physeal fracture of lower end of ulna, right arm**   CC H5

     7 √7ᵗʰ **S59.032**   **Salter-Harris Type III physeal fracture of lower end of ulna, left arm**   CC H5

     7 √7ᵗʰ **S59.039**   **Salter-Harris Type III physeal fracture of lower end of ulna, unspecified arm**   CC H5

   √6ᵗʰ **S59.04**   **Salter-Harris Type IV physeal fracture of lower end of ulna**

     7 √7ᵗʰ **S59.041**   **Salter-Harris Type IV physeal fracture of lower end of ulna, right arm**   CC H5

     7 √7ᵗʰ **S59.042**   **Salter-Harris Type IV physeal fracture of lower end of ulna, left arm**   CC H5

     7 √7ᵗʰ **S59.049**   **Salter-Harris Type IV physeal fracture of lower end of ulna, unspecified arm**   CC H5

   √6ᵗʰ **S59.09**   **Other physeal fracture of lower end of ulna**

     7 √7ᵗʰ **S59.091**   **Other physeal fracture of lower end of ulna, right arm**   CC H5

     7 √7ᵗʰ **S59.092**   **Other physeal fracture of lower end of ulna, left arm**   CC H5

---

7   CC when reported as an initial encounter (7th character A, B or C - specific to category) OR a subsequent encounter for nonunion or malunion (7th character K, M, N, P, Q or R - specific to category).

11   HCC with 7th character indicating initial encounter (A or B - specific to category) OR sequela.

N Newborn: 0   P Pediatric: 0-17   M Maternity: 12-55   A Adult: 15-124   MCC Major CC Condition   PDxMCC PDx acts as own MCC   CC CC Condition   PDxCC PDx acts as own CC

7 ✓7ᵗʰ **S59.099** Other physeal fracture of lower end `CC` `H5` of ulna, **unspecified arm**

✓5ᵗʰ **S59.1** Physeal fracture of **upper end of radius**

> **CC Excl: For codes in subcategory S59.1:**
> **CC with 7th character K or P:** PDX collection 897

✓6ᵗʰ **S59.10** **Unspecified** physeal fracture of upper end of radius

   8 ✓7ᵗʰ **S59.101** Unspecified physeal fracture of upper `CC` end of radius, **right arm**

   8 ✓7ᵗʰ **S59.102** Unspecified physeal fracture of upper `CC` end of radius, **left arm**

   8 ✓7ᵗʰ **S59.109** Unspecified physeal fracture of upper `CC` end of radius, **unspecified arm**

✓6ᵗʰ **S59.11** Salter-Harris Type I physeal fracture of upper end of radius

   8 ✓7ᵗʰ **S59.111** Salter-Harris Type I physeal fracture `CC` of upper end of radius, **right arm**

   8 ✓7ᵗʰ **S59.112** Salter-Harris Type I physeal fracture `CC` of upper end of radius, **left arm**

   8 ✓7ᵗʰ **S59.119** Salter-Harris Type I physeal fracture `CC` of upper end of radius, **unspecified arm**

✓6ᵗʰ **S59.12** Salter-Harris Type II physeal fracture of upper end of radius

   8 ✓7ᵗʰ **S59.121** Salter-Harris Type II physeal fracture `CC` of upper end of radius, **right arm**

   8 ✓7ᵗʰ **S59.122** Salter-Harris Type II physeal fracture `CC` of upper end of radius, **left arm**

   8 ✓7ᵗʰ **S59.129** Salter-Harris Type II physeal fracture `CC` of upper end of radius, **unspecified arm**

✓6ᵗʰ **S59.13** Salter-Harris Type III physeal fracture of upper end of radius

   8 ✓7ᵗʰ **S59.131** Salter-Harris Type III physeal fracture `CC` of upper end of radius, **right arm**

   8 ✓7ᵗʰ **S59.132** Salter-Harris Type III physeal fracture `CC` of upper end of radius, **left arm**

   8 ✓7ᵗʰ **S59.139** Salter-Harris Type III physeal fracture `CC` of upper end of radius, **unspecified arm**

✓6ᵗʰ **S59.14** Salter-Harris Type IV physeal fracture of upper end of radius

   8 ✓7ᵗʰ **S59.141** Salter-Harris Type IV physeal fracture `CC` of upper end of radius, **right arm**

   8 ✓7ᵗʰ **S59.142** Salter-Harris Type IV physeal fracture `CC` of upper end of radius, **left arm**

   8 ✓7ᵗʰ **S59.149** Salter-Harris Type IV physeal fracture `CC` of upper end of radius, **unspecified arm**

✓6ᵗʰ **S59.19** Other physeal fracture of upper end of radius

   8 ✓7ᵗʰ **S59.191** Other physeal fracture of upper end `CC` of radius, **right arm**

   8 ✓7ᵗʰ **S59.192** Other physeal fracture of upper end of radius, **left arm**

   8 ✓7ᵗʰ **S59.199** Other physeal fracture of upper end `CC` of radius, **unspecified arm**

✓5ᵗʰ **S59.2** Physeal fracture of **lower end of radius**

> **CC Excl: For CC codes in subcategory S59.2:**
> **Right side:** See code S59.201
> **Left side:** See code S59.202
> **Unspecified side:** See code S59.209

✓6ᵗʰ **S59.20** **Unspecified** physeal fracture of lower end of radius

   7 ✓7ᵗʰ **S59.201** Unspecified physeal fracture of `CC` `H5` lower end of radius, **right arm**
     CC Excl: CC with 7th character A: PDX collection 1270
     CC with 7th character K or P: PDX collection 897

   7 ✓7ᵗʰ **S59.202** Unspecified physeal fracture of `CC` `H5` lower end of radius, **left arm**
     CC Excl: CC with 7th character A: PDX collection 1271
     CC with 7th character K or P: PDX collection 897

   7 ✓7ᵗʰ **S59.209** Unspecified physeal fracture of `CC` `H5` lower end of radius, **unspecified arm**
     CC Excl: CC with 7th character A: PDX collection 1272
     CC with 7th character K or P: PDX collection 897

✓6ᵗʰ **S59.21** Salter-Harris Type I physeal fracture of lower end of radius

   7 ✓7ᵗʰ **S59.211** Salter-Harris Type I physeal `CC` `H5` fracture of lower end of radius, **right arm**

   7 ✓7ᵗʰ **S59.212** Salter-Harris Type I physeal `CC` `H5` fracture of lower end of radius, **left arm**

   7 ✓7ᵗʰ **S59.219** Salter-Harris Type I physeal `CC` `H5` fracture of lower end of radius, **unspecified arm**

✓6ᵗʰ **S59.22** Salter-Harris Type II physeal fracture of lower end of radius

   7 ✓7ᵗʰ **S59.221** Salter-Harris Type II physeal `CC` `H5` fracture of lower end of radius, **right arm**

   7 ✓7ᵗʰ **S59.222** Salter-Harris Type II physeal `CC` fracture of lower end of radius, **left arm**

   7 ✓7ᵗʰ **S59.229** Salter-Harris Type II physeal `CC` `H5` fracture of lower end of radius, **unspecified arm**

✓6ᵗʰ **S59.23** Salter-Harris Type III physeal fracture of lower end of radius

   7 ✓7ᵗʰ **S59.231** Salter-Harris Type III physeal `CC` `H5` fracture of lower end of radius, **right arm**

   7 ✓7ᵗʰ **S59.232** Salter-Harris Type III physeal `CC` `H5` fracture of lower end of radius, **left arm**

   7 ✓7ᵗʰ **S59.239** Salter-Harris Type III physeal `CC` `H5` fracture of lower end of radius, **unspecified arm**

✓6ᵗʰ **S59.24** Salter-Harris Type IV physeal fracture of lower end of radius

   7 ✓7ᵗʰ **S59.241** Salter-Harris Type IV physeal `CC` `H5` fracture of lower end of radius, **right arm**

   7 ✓7ᵗʰ **S59.242** Salter-Harris Type IV physeal `CC` `H5` fracture of lower end of radius, **left arm**

   7 ✓7ᵗʰ **S59.249** Salter-Harris Type IV physeal `CC` `H5` fracture of lower end of radius, **unspecified arm**

✓6ᵗʰ **S59.29** Other physeal fracture of lower end of radius

   7 ✓7ᵗʰ **S59.291** Other physeal fracture of lower `CC` `H5` end of radius, **right arm**

   7 ✓7ᵗʰ **S59.292** Other physeal fracture of lower `CC` `H5` end of radius, **left arm**

   7 ✓7ᵗʰ **S59.299** Other physeal fracture of lower `CC` `H5` end of radius, **unspecified arm**

✓5ᵗʰ **S59.8** Other specified injuries of elbow and forearm

> The appropriate 7th character is to be added to each code in subcategory S59.8.
> A   initial encounter
> D   subsequent encounter
> S   sequela

✓6ᵗʰ **S59.80** Other specified injuries of **elbow**

   ✓7ᵗʰ **S59.801** Other specified injuries of **right elbow**

   ✓7ᵗʰ **S59.802** Other specified injuries of **left elbow**

   ✓7ᵗʰ **S59.809** Other specified injuries of **unspecified** elbow

✓6ᵗʰ **S59.81** Other specified injuries of **forearm**

   ✓7ᵗʰ **S59.811** Other specified injuries **right forearm**

   ✓7ᵗʰ **S59.812** Other specified injuries **left forearm**

   ✓7ᵗʰ **S59.819** Other specified injuries **unspecified forearm**

---

7   CC when reported as an initial encounter (7th character A, B, or C – specific to category) OR a subsequent encounter for nonunion or malunion (7th character K, M, N, P, Q, or R – specific to category).

8   CC when reported as a subsequent encounter for nonunion or malunion (7th character K, M, N, P, Q, or R – specific to category).

✔ Additional Character Req   ✓x7ᵗʰ Placeholder Alert   Unacceptable PDx   Manifestation   `H1`-`H14` HAC   `HCC` CMS-HCC Condition   *EXCLUDES 1* Not Coded Here   *EXCLUDES 2* Not Included Here

ICD-10-CM 2018   1011

√5th **S59.9** **Unspecified injury of elbow and forearm**

> The appropriate 7th character is to be added to each code
> in subcategory S59.9.
> A　initial encounter
> D　subsequent encounter
> S　sequela

√6th **S59.90** **Unspecified injury of elbow**
√7th **S59.901** Unspecified injury of right elbow
√7th **S59.902** Unspecified injury of left elbow
√7th **S59.909** Unspecified injury of unspecified elbow

√6th **S59.91** **Unspecified injury of forearm**
√7th **S59.911** Unspecified injury of right forearm
√7th **S59.912** Unspecified injury of left forearm
√7th **S59.919** Unspecified injury of unspecified forearm

Injuries to the wrist, hand and fingers (S60-S69)

EXCLUDES 2　*burns and corrosions (T20-T32)*
　　　　　　frostbite (T33-T34)
　　　　　　insect bite or sting, venomous (T63.4)

√4th **S60** **Superficial injury of wrist, hand and fingers**

> The appropriate 7th character is to be added to each code from
> category S60.
> A　initial encounter
> D　subsequent encounter
> S　sequela

√5th **S60.0** **Contusion of finger without damage to nail**
　EXCLUDES 1　*contusion involving nail (matrix) (S60.1)*

√x7th **S60.00** **Contusion of unspecified finger without damage to nail**
　　　Contusion of finger(s) NOS

√6th **S60.01** **Contusion of thumb without damage to nail**
√7th **S60.011** Contusion of right thumb without damage to nail
√7th **S60.012** Contusion of left thumb without damage to nail
√7th **S60.019** Contusion of unspecified thumb without damage to nail

√6th **S60.02** **Contusion of index finger without damage to nail**
√7th **S60.021** Contusion of right index finger without damage to nail
√7th **S60.022** Contusion of left index finger without damage to nail
√7th **S60.029** Contusion of unspecified index finger without damage to nail

√6th **S60.03** **Contusion of middle finger without damage to nail**
√7th **S60.031** Contusion of right middle finger without damage to nail
√7th **S60.032** Contusion of left middle finger without damage to nail
√7th **S60.039** Contusion of unspecified middle finger without damage to nail

√6th **S60.04** **Contusion of ring finger without damage to nail**
√7th **S60.041** Contusion of right ring finger without damage to nail
√7th **S60.042** Contusion of left ring finger without damage to nail
√7th **S60.049** Contusion of unspecified ring finger without damage to nail

√6th **S60.05** **Contusion of little finger without damage to nail**
√7th **S60.051** Contusion of right little finger without damage to nail
√7th **S60.052** Contusion of left little finger without damage to nail
√7th **S60.059** Contusion of unspecified little finger without damage to nail

√5th **S60.1** **Contusion of finger with damage to nail**
√x7th **S60.10** **Contusion of unspecified finger with damage to nail**
√6th **S60.11** **Contusion of thumb with damage to nail**
√7th **S60.111** Contusion of right thumb with damage to nail
√7th **S60.112** Contusion of left thumb with damage to nail

√7th **S60.119** Contusion of unspecified thumb with damage to nail

√6th **S60.12** **Contusion of index finger with damage to nail**
√7th **S60.121** Contusion of right index finger with damage to nail
√7th **S60.122** Contusion of left index finger with damage to nail
√7th **S60.129** Contusion of unspecified index finger with damage to nail

√6th **S60.13** **Contusion of middle finger with damage to nail**
√7th **S60.131** Contusion of right middle finger with damage to nail
√7th **S60.132** Contusion of left middle finger with damage to nail
√7th **S60.139** Contusion of unspecified middle finger with damage to nail

√6th **S60.14** **Contusion of ring finger with damage to nail**
√7th **S60.141** Contusion of right ring finger with damage to nail
√7th **S60.142** Contusion of left ring finger with damage to nail
√7th **S60.149** Contusion of unspecified ring finger with damage to nail

√6th **S60.15** **Contusion of little finger with damage to nail**
√7th **S60.151** Contusion of right little finger with damage to nail
√7th **S60.152** Contusion of left little finger with damage to nail
√7th **S60.159** Contusion of unspecified little finger with damage to nail

√5th **S60.2** **Contusion of wrist and hand**
　EXCLUDES 2　*contusion of fingers (S60.0-, S60.1-)*

√6th **S60.21** **Contusion of wrist**
√7th **S60.211** Contusion of right wrist
√7th **S60.212** Contusion of left wrist
√7th **S60.219** Contusion of unspecified wrist

√6th **S60.22** **Contusion of hand**
√7th **S60.221** Contusion of right hand
√7th **S60.222** Contusion of left hand
√7th **S60.229** Contusion of unspecified hand

√5th **S60.3** **Other superficial injuries of thumb**
√6th **S60.31** **Abrasion of thumb**
√7th **S60.311** Abrasion of right thumb
√7th **S60.312** Abrasion of left thumb
√7th **S60.319** Abrasion of unspecified thumb

√6th **S60.32** **Blister (nonthermal) of thumb**
√7th **S60.321** Blister (nonthermal) of right thumb
√7th **S60.322** Blister (nonthermal) of left thumb
√7th **S60.329** Blister (nonthermal) of unspecified thumb

√6th **S60.34** **External constriction of thumb**
　　　Hair tourniquet syndrome of thumb
　　　Use additional cause code to identify the constricting item (W49.0-)
√7th **S60.341** External constriction of right thumb
√7th **S60.342** External constriction of left thumb
√7th **S60.349** External constriction of unspecified thumb

√6th **S60.35** **Superficial foreign body of thumb**
　　　Splinter in the thumb
√7th **S60.351** Superficial foreign body of right thumb
√7th **S60.352** Superficial foreign body of left thumb
√7th **S60.359** Superficial foreign body of unspecified thumb

√6th **S60.36** **Insect bite (nonvenomous) of thumb**
√7th **S60.361** Insect bite (nonvenomous) of right thumb
√7th **S60.362** Insect bite (nonvenomous) of left thumb
√7th **S60.369** Insect bite (nonvenomous) of unspecified thumb

√6th **S60.37** **Other superficial bite of thumb**
　EXCLUDES 1　*open bite of thumb (S61.05-, S61.15-)*
√7th **S60.371** Other superficial bite of right thumb

N Newborn: 0　P Pediatric: 0-17　M Maternity: 12-55　A Adult: 15-124　MCC Major CC Condition　PDxMCC PDx acts as own MCC　CC CC Condition　PDxCC PDx acts as own CC

1012　　　　　　　　　　　　　　　　　　　　　　　　　　　　　　　　　　　　　　　ICD-10-CM 2018

√7ᵗʰ **S60.372** **Other superficial bite of left thumb**

√7ᵗʰ **S60.379** **Other superficial bite of unspecified thumb**

√6ᵗʰ **S60.39** Other superficial injuries of thumb

√7ᵗʰ **S60.391** **Other superficial injuries of right thumb**

√7ᵗʰ **S60.392** **Other superficial injuries of left thumb**

√7ᵗʰ **S60.399** **Other superficial injuries of unspecified thumb**

√5ᵗʰ **S60.4** **Other superficial injuries of other fingers**

√6ᵗʰ **S60.41** **Abrasion of fingers**

√7ᵗʰ **S60.410** **Abrasion of right index finger**

√7ᵗʰ **S60.411** **Abrasion of left index finger**

√7ᵗʰ **S60.412** **Abrasion of right middle finger**

√7ᵗʰ **S60.413** **Abrasion of left middle finger**

√7ᵗʰ **S60.414** **Abrasion of right ring finger**

√7ᵗʰ **S60.415** **Abrasion of left ring finger**

√7ᵗʰ **S60.416** **Abrasion of right little finger**

√7ᵗʰ **S60.417** **Abrasion of left little finger**

√7ᵗʰ **S60.418** **Abrasion of other finger**
Abrasion of specified finger with unspecified laterality

√7ᵗʰ **S60.419** **Abrasion of unspecified finger**

√6ᵗʰ **S60.42** Blister (nonthermal) of fingers

√7ᵗʰ **S60.420** **Blister (nonthermal) of right index finger**

√7ᵗʰ **S60.421** **Blister (nonthermal) of left index finger**

√7ᵗʰ **S60.422** **Blister (nonthermal) of right middle finger**

√7ᵗʰ **S60.423** **Blister (nonthermal) of left middle finger**

√7ᵗʰ **S60.424** **Blister (nonthermal) of right ring finger**

√7ᵗʰ **S60.425** **Blister (nonthermal) of left ring finger**

√7ᵗʰ **S60.426** **Blister (nonthermal) of right little finger**

√7ᵗʰ **S60.427** **Blister (nonthermal) of left little finger**

√7ᵗʰ **S60.428** **Blister (nonthermal) of other finger**
Blister (nonthermal) of specified finger with unspecified laterality

√7ᵗʰ **S60.429** **Blister (nonthermal) of unspecified finger**

√6ᵗʰ **S60.44** **External constriction of fingers**
Hair tourniquet syndrome of finger
Use additional cause code to identify the constricting item (W49.0-)

√7ᵗʰ **S60.440** **External constriction of right index finger**

√7ᵗʰ **S60.441** **External constriction of left index finger**

√7ᵗʰ **S60.442** **External constriction of right middle finger**

√7ᵗʰ **S60.443** **External constriction of left middle finger**

√7ᵗʰ **S60.444** **External constriction of right ring finger**

√7ᵗʰ **S60.445** **External constriction of left ring finger**

√7ᵗʰ **S60.446** **External constriction of right little finger**

√7ᵗʰ **S60.447** **External constriction of left little finger**

√7ᵗʰ **S60.448** **External constriction of other finger**
External constriction of specified finger with unspecified laterality

√7ᵗʰ **S60.449** **External constriction of unspecified finger**

√6ᵗʰ **S60.45** **Superficial foreign body of fingers**
Splinter in the finger(s)

√7ᵗʰ **S60.450** **Superficial foreign body of right index finger**

√7ᵗʰ **S60.451** **Superficial foreign body of left index finger**

√7ᵗʰ **S60.452** **Superficial foreign body of right middle finger**

√7ᵗʰ **S60.453** **Superficial foreign body of left middle finger**

√7ᵗʰ **S60.454** **Superficial foreign body of right ring finger**

√7ᵗʰ **S60.455** **Superficial foreign body of left ring finger**

√7ᵗʰ **S60.456** **Superficial foreign body of right little finger**

√7ᵗʰ **S60.457** **Superficial foreign body of left little finger**

√7ᵗʰ **S60.458** **Superficial foreign body of other finger**
Superficial foreign body of specified finger with unspecified laterality

√7ᵗʰ **S60.459** **Superficial foreign body of unspecified finger**

√6ᵗʰ **S60.46** Insect bite (nonvenomous) of fingers

√7ᵗʰ **S60.460** **Insect bite (nonvenomous) of right index finger**

√7ᵗʰ **S60.461** **Insect bite (nonvenomous) of left index finger**

√7ᵗʰ **S60.462** **Insect bite (nonvenomous) of right middle finger**

√7ᵗʰ **S60.463** **Insect bite (nonvenomous) of left middle finger**

√7ᵗʰ **S60.464** **Insect bite (nonvenomous) of right ring finger**

√7ᵗʰ **S60.465** **Insect bite (nonvenomous) of left ring finger**

√7ᵗʰ **S60.466** **Insect bite (nonvenomous) of right little finger**

√7ᵗʰ **S60.467** **Insect bite (nonvenomous) of left little finger**

√7ᵗʰ **S60.468** **Insect bite (nonvenomous) of other finger**
Insect bite (nonvenomous) of specified finger with unspecified laterality

√7ᵗʰ **S60.469** **Insect bite (nonvenomous) of unspecified finger**

√6ᵗʰ **S60.47** Other superficial bite of fingers
EXCLUDES 1 *open bite of fingers (S61.25-, S61.35-)*

√7ᵗʰ **S60.470** **Other superficial bite of right index finger**

√7ᵗʰ **S60.471** **Other superficial bite of left index finger**

√7ᵗʰ **S60.472** **Other superficial bite of right middle finger**

√7ᵗʰ **S60.473** **Other superficial bite of left middle finger**

√7ᵗʰ **S60.474** **Other superficial bite of right ring finger**

√7ᵗʰ **S60.475** **Other superficial bite of left ring finger**

√7ᵗʰ **S60.476** **Other superficial bite of right little finger**

√7ᵗʰ **S60.477** **Other superficial bite of left little finger**

√7ᵗʰ **S60.478** **Other superficial bite of other finger**
Other superficial bite of specified finger with unspecified laterality

√7ᵗʰ **S60.479** **Other superficial bite of unspecified finger**

√5ᵗʰ **S60.5** **Other superficial injuries of hand**
EXCLUDES 2 *superficial injuries of fingers (S60.3-, S60.4-)*

√6ᵗʰ **S60.51** Abrasion of hand

√7ᵗʰ **S60.511** **Abrasion of right hand**

√7ᵗʰ **S60.512** **Abrasion of left hand**

√7ᵗʰ **S60.519** **Abrasion of unspecified hand**

√6ᵗʰ **S60.52** Blister (nonthermal) of hand

√7ᵗʰ **S60.521** **Blister (nonthermal) of right hand**

√7ᵗʰ **S60.522** **Blister (nonthermal) of left hand**

√7ᵗʰ **S60.529** **Blister (nonthermal) of unspecified hand**

√6ᵗʰ **S60.54** External constriction of hand

√7ᵗʰ **S60.541** **External constriction of right hand**

√7ᵗʰ **S60.542** **External constriction of left hand**

√7ᵗʰ **S60.549** **External constriction of unspecified hand**

√6ᵗʰ **S60.55** Superficial foreign body of hand
Splinter in the hand

√7ᵗʰ **S60.551** **Superficial foreign body of right hand**

√7ᵗʰ **S60.552** **Superficial foreign body of left hand**

√7ᵗʰ **S60.559** **Superficial foreign body of unspecified hand**

√6ᵗʰ **S60.56** Insect bite (nonvenomous) of hand

√7ᵗʰ **S60.561** **Insect bite (nonvenomous) of right hand**

√7ᵗʰ **S60.562** **Insect bite (nonvenomous) of left hand**

√7ᵗʰ **S60.569** **Insect bite (nonvenomous) of unspecified hand**

√6ᵗʰ **S60.57** Other superficial bite of hand
EXCLUDES 1 *open bite of hand (S61.45-)*

√7ᵗʰ **S60.571** **Other superficial bite of hand of right hand**

√7ᵗʰ **S60.572** **Other superficial bite of hand of left hand**

√7ᵗʰ **S60.579** **Other superficial bite of hand of unspecified hand**

✓5th **S60.8 Other superficial injuries of wrist**

✓6th **S60.81 Abrasion of wrist**

✓7th **S60.811 Abrasion of right wrist**

✓7th **S60.812 Abrasion of left wrist**

✓7th **S60.819 Abrasion of unspecified wrist**

✓6th **S60.82 Blister (nonthermal) of wrist**

✓7th **S60.821 Blister (nonthermal) of right wrist**

✓7th **S60.822 Blister (nonthermal) of left wrist**

✓7th **S60.829 Blister (nonthermal) of unspecified wrist**

✓6th **S60.84 External constriction of wrist**

✓7th **S60.841 External constriction of right wrist**

✓7th **S60.842 External constriction of left wrist**

✓7th **S60.849 External constriction of unspecified wrist**

✓6th **S60.85 Superficial foreign body of wrist**
Splinter in the wrist

✓7th **S60.851 Superficial foreign body of right wrist**

✓7th **S60.852 Superficial foreign body of left wrist**

✓7th **S60.859 Superficial foreign body of unspecified wrist**

✓6th **S60.86 Insect bite (nonvenomous) of wrist**

✓7th **S60.861 Insect bite (nonvenomous) of right wrist**

✓7th **S60.862 Insect bite (nonvenomous) of left wrist**

✓7th **S60.869 Insect bite (nonvenomous) of unspecified wrist**

✓6th **S60.87 Other superficial bite of wrist**
EXCLUDES 1 *open bite of wrist (S61.55)*

✓7th **S60.871 Other superficial bite of right wrist**

✓7th **S60.872 Other superficial bite of left wrist**

✓7th **S60.879 Other superficial bite of unspecified wrist**

✓5th **S60.9 Unspecified superficial injury of wrist, hand and fingers**

✓6th **S60.91 Unspecified superficial injury of wrist**

✓7th **S60.911 Unspecified superficial injury of right wrist**

✓7th **S60.912 Unspecified superficial injury of left wrist**

✓7th **S60.919 Unspecified superficial injury of unspecified wrist**

✓6th **S60.92 Unspecified superficial injury of hand**

✓7th **S60.921 Unspecified superficial injury of right hand**

✓7th **S60.922 Unspecified superficial injury of left hand**

✓7th **S60.929 Unspecified superficial injury of unspecified hand**

✓6th **S60.93 Unspecified superficial injury of thumb**

✓7th **S60.931 Unspecified superficial injury of right thumb**

✓7th **S60.932 Unspecified superficial injury of left thumb**

✓7th **S60.939 Unspecified superficial injury of unspecified thumb**

✓6th **S60.94 Unspecified superficial injury of other fingers**

✓7th **S60.940 Unspecified superficial injury of right index finger**

✓7th **S60.941 Unspecified superficial injury of left index finger**

✓7th **S60.942 Unspecified superficial injury of right middle finger**

✓7th **S60.943 Unspecified superficial injury of left middle finger**

✓7th **S60.944 Unspecified superficial injury of right ring finger**

✓7th **S60.945 Unspecified superficial injury of left ring finger**

✓7th **S60.946 Unspecified superficial injury of right little finger**

✓7th **S60.947 Unspecified superficial injury of left little finger**

✓7th **S60.948 Unspecified superficial injury of other finger**
Unspecified superficial injury of specified finger with unspecified laterality

✓7th **S60.949 Unspecified superficial injury of unspecified finger**

✓4th **S61 Open wound of wrist, hand and fingers**
Code also any associated wound infection
EXCLUDES 1 *open fracture of wrist, hand and finger (S62- with 7th character B)*
traumatic amputation of wrist and hand (S68.-)

The appropriate 7th character is to be added to each code from category S61.
A   initial encounter
D   subsequent encounter
S   sequela

✓5th **S61.0 Open wound of thumb without damage to nail**
EXCLUDES 1 *open wound of thumb with damage to nail (S61.1-)*

✓6th **S61.00 Unspecified open wound of thumb without damage to nail**

✓7th **S61.001 Unspecified open wound of right thumb without damage to nail**

✓7th **S61.002 Unspecified open wound of left thumb without damage to nail**

✓7th **S61.009 Unspecified open wound of unspecified thumb without damage to nail**

✓6th **S61.01 Laceration without foreign body of thumb without damage to nail**

✓7th **S61.011 Laceration without foreign body of right thumb without damage to nail**

✓7th **S61.012 Laceration without foreign body of left thumb without damage to nail**

✓7th **S61.019 Laceration without foreign body of unspecified thumb without damage to nail**

✓6th **S61.02 Laceration with foreign body of thumb without damage to nail**

✓7th **S61.021 Laceration with foreign body of right thumb without damage to nail**

✓7th **S61.022 Laceration with foreign body of left thumb without damage to nail**

✓7th **S61.029 Laceration with foreign body of unspecified thumb without damage to nail**

✓6th **S61.03 Puncture wound without foreign body of thumb without damage to nail**

✓7th **S61.031 Puncture wound without foreign body of right thumb without damage to nail**

✓7th **S61.032 Puncture wound without foreign body of left thumb without damage to nail**

✓7th **S61.039 Puncture wound without foreign body of unspecified thumb without damage to nail**

✓6th **S61.04 Puncture wound with foreign body of thumb without damage to nail**

✓7th **S61.041 Puncture wound with foreign body of right thumb without damage to nail**

✓7th **S61.042 Puncture wound with foreign body of left thumb without damage to nail**

✓7th **S61.049 Puncture wound with foreign body of unspecified thumb without damage to nail**

✓6th **S61.05 Open bite of thumb without damage to nail**
Bite of thumb NOS
EXCLUDES 1 *superficial bite of thumb (S60.36-, S60.37-)*

✓7th **S61.051 Open bite of right thumb without damage to nail**

✓7th **S61.052 Open bite of left thumb without damage to nail**

✓7th **S61.059 Open bite of unspecified thumb without damage to nail**

✓5th **S61.1 Open wound of thumb with damage to nail**

✓6th **S61.10 Unspecified open wound of thumb with damage to nail**

✓7th **S61.101 Unspecified open wound of right thumb with damage to nail**

✓7th **S61.102 Unspecified open wound of left thumb with damage to nail**

✓7th **S61.109 Unspecified open wound of unspecified thumb with damage to nail**

N Newborn: 0   P Pediatric: 0-17   M Maternity: 12-55   A Adult: 15-124   MCC Major CC Condition   PDxMCC PDx acts as own MCC   CC CC Condition   PDxCC PDx acts as own CC

1014 ICD-10-CM 2018

☑6ᵗʰ **S61.11** Laceration without foreign body of thumb with damage to nail

   ☑7ᵗʰ **S61.111** Laceration without foreign body of right thumb with damage to nail

   ☑7ᵗʰ **S61.112** Laceration without foreign body of left thumb with damage to nail

   ☑7ᵗʰ **S61.119** Laceration without foreign body of unspecified thumb with damage to nail

☑6ᵗʰ **S61.12** Laceration with foreign body of thumb with damage to nail

   ☑7ᵗʰ **S61.121** Laceration with foreign body of right thumb with damage to nail

   ☑7ᵗʰ **S61.122** Laceration with foreign body of left thumb with damage to nail

   ☑7ᵗʰ **S61.129** Laceration with foreign body of unspecified thumb with damage to nail

☑6ᵗʰ **S61.13** Puncture wound without foreign body of thumb with damage to nail

   ☑7ᵗʰ **S61.131** Puncture wound without foreign body of right thumb with damage to nail

   ☑7ᵗʰ **S61.132** Puncture wound without foreign body of left thumb with damage to nail

   ☑7ᵗʰ **S61.139** Puncture wound without foreign body of unspecified thumb with damage to nail

☑6ᵗʰ **S61.14** Puncture wound with foreign body of thumb with damage to nail

   ☑7ᵗʰ **S61.141** Puncture wound with foreign body of right thumb with damage to nail

   ☑7ᵗʰ **S61.142** Puncture wound with foreign body of left thumb with damage to nail

   ☑7ᵗʰ **S61.149** Puncture wound with foreign body of unspecified thumb with damage to nail

☑6ᵗʰ **S61.15** Open bite of thumb with damage to nail
   Bite of thumb with damage to nail NOS
   EXCLUDES 1 superficial bite of thumb (S60.36-, S60.37-)

   ☑7ᵗʰ **S61.151** Open bite of right thumb with damage to nail

   ☑7ᵗʰ **S61.152** Open bite of left thumb with damage to nail

   ☑7ᵗʰ **S61.159** Open bite of unspecified thumb with damage to nail

☑5ᵗʰ **S61.2** Open wound of other finger without damage to nail
   EXCLUDES 1 open wound of finger involving nail (matrix) (S61.3-)
   EXCLUDES 2 open wound of thumb without damage to nail (S61.0-)

☑6ᵗʰ **S61.20** Unspecified open wound of other finger without damage to nail

   ☑7ᵗʰ **S61.200** Unspecified open wound of right index finger without damage to nail

   ☑7ᵗʰ **S61.201** Unspecified open wound of left index finger without damage to nail

   ☑7ᵗʰ **S61.202** Unspecified open wound of right middle finger without damage to nail

   ☑7ᵗʰ **S61.203** Unspecified open wound of left middle finger without damage to nail

   ☑7ᵗʰ **S61.204** Unspecified open wound of right ring finger without damage to nail

   ☑7ᵗʰ **S61.205** Unspecified open wound of left ring finger without damage to nail

   ☑7ᵗʰ **S61.206** Unspecified open wound of right little finger without damage to nail

   ☑7ᵗʰ **S61.207** Unspecified open wound of left little finger without damage to nail

   ☑7ᵗʰ **S61.208** Unspecified open wound of other finger without damage to nail
      Unspecified open wound of specified finger with unspecified laterality without damage to nail

   ☑7ᵗʰ **S61.209** Unspecified open wound of unspecified finger without damage to nail

☑6ᵗʰ **S61.21** Laceration without foreign body of finger without damage to nail

   ☑7ᵗʰ **S61.210** Laceration without foreign body of right index finger without damage to nail

   ☑7ᵗʰ **S61.211** Laceration without foreign body of left index finger without damage to nail

   ☑7ᵗʰ **S61.212** Laceration without foreign body of right middle finger without damage to nail

   ☑7ᵗʰ **S61.213** Laceration without foreign body of left middle finger without damage to nail

   ☑7ᵗʰ **S61.214** Laceration without foreign body of right ring finger without damage to nail

   ☑7ᵗʰ **S61.215** Laceration without foreign body of left ring finger without damage to nail

   ☑7ᵗʰ **S61.216** Laceration without foreign body of right little finger without damage to nail

   ☑7ᵗʰ **S61.217** Laceration without foreign body of left little finger without damage to nail

   ☑7ᵗʰ **S61.218** Laceration without foreign body of other finger without damage to nail
      Laceration without foreign body of specified finger with unspecified laterality without damage to nail

   ☑7ᵗʰ **S61.219** Laceration without foreign body of unspecified finger without damage to nail

☑6ᵗʰ **S61.22** Laceration with foreign body of finger without damage to nail

   ☑7ᵗʰ **S61.220** Laceration with foreign body of right index finger without damage to nail

   ☑7ᵗʰ **S61.221** Laceration with foreign body of left index finger without damage to nail

   ☑7ᵗʰ **S61.222** Laceration with foreign body of right middle finger without damage to nail

   ☑7ᵗʰ **S61.223** Laceration with foreign body of left middle finger without damage to nail

   ☑7ᵗʰ **S61.224** Laceration with foreign body of right ring finger without damage to nail

   ☑7ᵗʰ **S61.225** Laceration with foreign body of left ring finger without damage to nail

   ☑7ᵗʰ **S61.226** Laceration with foreign body of right little finger without damage to nail

   ☑7ᵗʰ **S61.227** Laceration with foreign body of left little finger without damage to nail

   ☑7ᵗʰ **S61.228** Laceration with foreign body of other finger without damage to nail
      Laceration with foreign body of specified finger with unspecified laterality without damage to nail

   ☑7ᵗʰ **S61.229** Laceration with foreign body of unspecified finger without damage to nail

☑6ᵗʰ **S61.23** Puncture wound without foreign body of finger without damage to nail

   ☑7ᵗʰ **S61.230** Puncture wound without foreign body of right index finger without damage to nail

   ☑7ᵗʰ **S61.231** Puncture wound without foreign body of left index finger without damage to nail

   ☑7ᵗʰ **S61.232** Puncture wound without foreign body of right middle finger without damage to nail

   ☑7ᵗʰ **S61.233** Puncture wound without foreign body of left middle finger without damage to nail

   ☑7ᵗʰ **S61.234** Puncture wound without foreign body of right ring finger without damage to nail

   ☑7ᵗʰ **S61.235** Puncture wound without foreign body of left ring finger without damage to nail

   ☑7ᵗʰ **S61.236** Puncture wound without foreign body of right little finger without damage to nail

   ☑7ᵗʰ **S61.237** Puncture wound without foreign body of left little finger without damage to nail

   ☑7ᵗʰ **S61.238** Puncture wound without foreign body of other finger without damage to nail
      Puncture wound without foreign body of specified finger with unspecified laterality without damage to nail

   ☑7ᵗʰ **S61.239** Puncture wound without foreign body of unspecified finger without damage to nail

☑6ᵗʰ **S61.24** Puncture wound with foreign body of finger without damage to nail

   ☑7ᵗʰ **S61.240** Puncture wound with foreign body of right index finger without damage to nail

   ☑7ᵗʰ **S61.241** Puncture wound with foreign body of left index finger without damage to nail

✓ Additional Character Req   **✓ˣ⁷ᵗʰ** Placeholder Alert   Unacceptable PDx   Manifestation   **H1** - **H14** HAC   **HCC** CMS-HCC Condition   *EXCLUDES 1* Not Coded Here   *EXCLUDES 2* Not Included Here

ICD-10-CM 2018   **1015**

√7ᵗʰ **S61.242** **Puncture wound with foreign body of right middle finger without damage to nail**

√7ᵗʰ **S61.243** **Puncture wound with foreign body of left middle finger without damage to nail**

√7ᵗʰ **S61.244** **Puncture wound with foreign body of right ring finger without damage to nail**

√7ᵗʰ **S61.245** **Puncture wound with foreign body of left ring finger without damage to nail**

√7ᵗʰ **S61.246** **Puncture wound with foreign body of right little finger without damage to nail**

√7ᵗʰ **S61.247** **Puncture wound with foreign body of left little finger without damage to nail**

√7ᵗʰ **S61.248** **Puncture wound with foreign body of other finger without damage to nail**
Puncture wound with foreign body of specified finger with unspecified laterality without damage to nail

√7ᵗʰ **S61.249** **Puncture wound with foreign body of unspecified finger without damage to nail**

√6ᵗʰ **S61.25** **Open bite of finger without damage to nail**
Bite of finger without damage to nail NOS
EXCLUDES 1   superficial bite of finger (S60.46-, S60.47-)

√7ᵗʰ **S61.250** **Open bite of right index finger without damage to nail**

√7ᵗʰ **S61.251** **Open bite of left index finger without damage to nail**

√7ᵗʰ **S61.252** **Open bite of right middle finger without damage to nail**

√7ᵗʰ **S61.253** **Open bite of left middle finger without damage to nail**

√7ᵗʰ **S61.254** **Open bite of right ring finger without damage to nail**

√7ᵗʰ **S61.255** **Open bite of left ring finger without damage to nail**

√7ᵗʰ **S61.256** **Open bite of right little finger without damage to nail**

√7ᵗʰ **S61.257** **Open bite of left little finger without damage to nail**

√7ᵗʰ **S61.258** **Open bite of other finger without damage to nail**
Open bite of specified finger with unspecified laterality without damage to nail

√7ᵗʰ **S61.259** **Open bite of unspecified finger without damage to nail**

√5ᵗʰ **S61.3** **Open wound of other finger with damage to nail**

√6ᵗʰ **S61.30** **Unspecified open wound of finger with damage to nail**

√7ᵗʰ **S61.300** **Unspecified open wound of right index finger with damage to nail**

√7ᵗʰ **S61.301** **Unspecified open wound of left index finger with damage to nail**

√7ᵗʰ **S61.302** **Unspecified open wound of right middle finger with damage to nail**

√7ᵗʰ **S61.303** **Unspecified open wound of left middle finger with damage to nail**

√7ᵗʰ **S61.304** **Unspecified open wound of right ring finger with damage to nail**

√7ᵗʰ **S61.305** **Unspecified open wound of left ring finger with damage to nail**

√7ᵗʰ **S61.306** **Unspecified open wound of right little finger with damage to nail**

√7ᵗʰ **S61.307** **Unspecified open wound of left little finger with damage to nail**

√7ᵗʰ **S61.308** **Unspecified open wound of other finger with damage to nail**
Unspecified open wound of specified finger with unspecified laterality with damage to nail

√7ᵗʰ **S61.309** **Unspecified open wound of unspecified finger with damage to nail**

√6ᵗʰ **S61.31** **Laceration without foreign body of finger with damage to nail**

√7ᵗʰ **S61.310** **Laceration without foreign body of right index finger with damage to nail**

√7ᵗʰ **S61.311** **Laceration without foreign body of left index finger with damage to nail**

√7ᵗʰ **S61.312** **Laceration without foreign body of right middle finger with damage to nail**

√7ᵗʰ **S61.313** **Laceration without foreign body of left middle finger with damage to nail**

√7ᵗʰ **S61.314** **Laceration without foreign body of right ring finger with damage to nail**

√7ᵗʰ **S61.315** **Laceration without foreign body of left ring finger with damage to nail**

√7ᵗʰ **S61.316** **Laceration without foreign body of right little finger with damage to nail**

√7ᵗʰ **S61.317** **Laceration without foreign body of left little finger with damage to nail**

√7ᵗʰ **S61.318** **Laceration without foreign body of other finger with damage to nail**
Laceration without foreign body of specified finger with unspecified laterality with damage to nail

√7ᵗʰ **S61.319** **Laceration without foreign body of unspecified finger with damage to nail**

√6ᵗʰ **S61.32** **Laceration with foreign body of finger with damage to nail**

√7ᵗʰ **S61.320** **Laceration with foreign body of right index finger with damage to nail**

√7ᵗʰ **S61.321** **Laceration with foreign body of left index finger with damage to nail**

√7ᵗʰ **S61.322** **Laceration with foreign body of right middle finger with damage to nail**

√7ᵗʰ **S61.323** **Laceration with foreign body of left middle finger with damage to nail**

√7ᵗʰ **S61.324** **Laceration with foreign body of right ring finger with damage to nail**

√7ᵗʰ **S61.325** **Laceration with foreign body of left ring finger with damage to nail**

√7ᵗʰ **S61.326** **Laceration with foreign body of right little finger with damage to nail**

√7ᵗʰ **S61.327** **Laceration with foreign body of left little finger with damage to nail**

√7ᵗʰ **S61.328** **Laceration with foreign body of other finger with damage to nail**
Laceration with foreign body of specified finger with unspecified laterality with damage to nail

√7ᵗʰ **S61.329** **Laceration with foreign body of unspecified finger with damage to nail**

√6ᵗʰ **S61.33** **Puncture wound without foreign body of finger with damage to nail**

√7ᵗʰ **S61.330** **Puncture wound without foreign body of right index finger with damage to nail**

√7ᵗʰ **S61.331** **Puncture wound without foreign body of left index finger with damage to nail**

√7ᵗʰ **S61.332** **Puncture wound without foreign body of right middle finger with damage to nail**

√7ᵗʰ **S61.333** **Puncture wound without foreign body of left middle finger with damage to nail**

√7ᵗʰ **S61.334** **Puncture wound without foreign body of right ring finger with damage to nail**

√7ᵗʰ **S61.335** **Puncture wound without foreign body of left ring finger with damage to nail**

√7ᵗʰ **S61.336** **Puncture wound without foreign body of right little finger with damage to nail**

√7ᵗʰ **S61.337** **Puncture wound without foreign body of left little finger with damage to nail**

√7ᵗʰ **S61.338** **Puncture wound without foreign body of other finger with damage to nail**
Puncture wound without foreign body of specified finger with unspecified laterality with damage to nail

√7ᵗʰ **S61.339** **Puncture wound without foreign body of unspecified finger with damage to nail**

N Newborn: 0   **P** Pediatric: 0-17   **M** Maternity: 12-55   **A** Adult: 15-124   **MCC** Major CC Condition   **PDxMCC** PDx acts as own MCC   **CC** CC Condition   **PDxCC** PDx acts as own CC

1016   ICD-10-CM 2018

√6ᵗʰ **S61.34** **Puncture wound with foreign body** of finger with damage to nail

  √7ᵗʰ **S61.340** **Puncture wound with foreign body of right index finger with damage to nail**

  √7ᵗʰ **S61.341** **Puncture wound with foreign body of left index finger with damage to nail**

  √7ᵗʰ **S61.342** **Puncture wound with foreign body of right middle finger with damage to nail**

  √7ᵗʰ **S61.343** **Puncture wound with foreign body of left middle finger with damage to nail**

  √7ᵗʰ **S61.344** **Puncture wound with foreign body of right ring finger with damage to nail**

  √7ᵗʰ **S61.345** **Puncture wound with foreign body of left ring finger with damage to nail**

  √7ᵗʰ **S61.346** **Puncture wound with foreign body of right little finger with damage to nail**

  √7ᵗʰ **S61.347** **Puncture wound with foreign body of left little finger with damage to nail**

  √7ᵗʰ **S61.348** **Puncture wound with foreign body of other finger with damage to nail**
      Puncture wound with foreign body of specified finger with unspecified laterality with damage to nail

  √7ᵗʰ **S61.349** **Puncture wound with foreign body of unspecified finger with damage to nail**

√6ᵗʰ **S61.35** **Open bite** of finger with damage to nail
    Bite of finger with damage to nail NOS
    EXCLUDES 1   superficial bite of finger (S60.46-, S60.47-)

  √7ᵗʰ **S61.350** **Open bite of right index finger with damage to nail**

  √7ᵗʰ **S61.351** **Open bite of left index finger with damage to nail**

  √7ᵗʰ **S61.352** **Open bite of right middle finger with damage to nail**

  √7ᵗʰ **S61.353** **Open bite of left middle finger with damage to nail**

  √7ᵗʰ **S61.354** **Open bite of right ring finger with damage to nail**

  √7ᵗʰ **S61.355** **Open bite of left ring finger with damage to nail**

  √7ᵗʰ **S61.356** **Open bite of right little finger with damage to nail**

  √7ᵗʰ **S61.357** **Open bite of left little finger with damage to nail**

  √7ᵗʰ **S61.358** **Open bite of other finger with damage to nail**
      Open bite of specified finger with unspecified laterality with damage to nail

  √7ᵗʰ **S61.359** **Open bite of unspecified finger with damage to nail**

√5ᵗʰ **S61.4** **Open wound of** hand

√6ᵗʰ **S61.40** **Unspecified** open wound of hand

  √7ᵗʰ **S61.401** **Unspecified open wound of right hand**

  √7ᵗʰ **S61.402** **Unspecified open wound of left hand**

  √7ᵗʰ **S61.409** **Unspecified open wound of unspecified hand**

√6ᵗʰ **S61.41** **Laceration without foreign body** of hand

  √7ᵗʰ **S61.411** **Laceration without foreign body of right hand**

  √7ᵗʰ **S61.412** **Laceration without foreign body of left hand**

  √7ᵗʰ **S61.419** **Laceration without foreign body of unspecified hand**

√6ᵗʰ **S61.42** **Laceration with foreign body** of hand

  √7ᵗʰ **S61.421** **Laceration with foreign body of right hand**

  √7ᵗʰ **S61.422** **Laceration with foreign body of left hand**

  √7ᵗʰ **S61.429** **Laceration with foreign body of unspecified hand**

√6ᵗʰ **S61.43** **Puncture wound without foreign body** of hand

  √7ᵗʰ **S61.431** **Puncture wound without foreign body of right hand**

  √7ᵗʰ **S61.432** **Puncture wound without foreign body of left hand**

  √7ᵗʰ **S61.439** **Puncture wound without foreign body of unspecified hand**

√6ᵗʰ **S61.44** **Puncture wound with foreign body** of hand

  √7ᵗʰ **S61.441** **Puncture wound with foreign body of right hand**

  √7ᵗʰ **S61.442** **Puncture wound with foreign body of left hand**

  √7ᵗʰ **S61.449** **Puncture wound with foreign body of unspecified hand**

√6ᵗʰ **S61.45** **Open bite** of hand
    Bite of hand NOS
    EXCLUDES 1   superficial bite of hand (S60.56-, S60.57-)

  √7ᵗʰ **S61.451** **Open bite of right hand**

  √7ᵗʰ **S61.452** **Open bite of left hand**

  √7ᵗʰ **S61.459** **Open bite of unspecified hand**

√5ᵗʰ **S61.5** **Open wound of wrist**

√6ᵗʰ **S61.50** **Unspecified** open wound of wrist

  √7ᵗʰ **S61.501** **Unspecified open wound of right wrist**

  √7ᵗʰ **S61.502** **Unspecified open wound of left wrist**

  √7ᵗʰ **S61.509** **Unspecified open wound of unspecified wrist**

√6ᵗʰ **S61.51** **Laceration without foreign body** of wrist

  √7ᵗʰ **S61.511** **Laceration without foreign body of right wrist**

  √7ᵗʰ **S61.512** **Laceration without foreign body of left wrist**

  √7ᵗʰ **S61.519** **Laceration without foreign body of unspecified wrist**

√6ᵗʰ **S61.52** **Laceration with foreign body** of wrist

  √7ᵗʰ **S61.521** **Laceration with foreign body of right wrist**

  √7ᵗʰ **S61.522** **Laceration with foreign body of left wrist**

  √7ᵗʰ **S61.529** **Laceration with foreign body of unspecified wrist**

√6ᵗʰ **S61.53** **Puncture wound without foreign body** of wrist

  √7ᵗʰ **S61.531** **Puncture wound without foreign body of right wrist**

  √7ᵗʰ **S61.532** **Puncture wound without foreign body of left wrist**

  √7ᵗʰ **S61.539** **Puncture wound without foreign body of unspecified wrist**

√6ᵗʰ **S61.54** **Puncture wound with foreign body** of wrist

  √7ᵗʰ **S61.541** **Puncture wound with foreign body of right wrist**

  √7ᵗʰ **S61.542** **Puncture wound with foreign body of left wrist**

  √7ᵗʰ **S61.549** **Puncture wound with foreign body of unspecified wrist**

√6ᵗʰ **S61.55** **Open bite** of wrist
    Bite of wrist NOS
    EXCLUDES 1   superficial bite of wrist (S60.86-, S60.87-)

  √7ᵗʰ **S61.551** **Open bite of right wrist**

  √7ᵗʰ **S61.552** **Open bite of left wrist**

  √7ᵗʰ **S61.559** **Open bite of unspecified wrist**

☑ Additional Character Req   √x7ᵗʰ Placeholder Alert   Unacceptable PDx   Manifestation   H1 - H14 HAC   HCC CMS-HCC Condition   *EXCLUDES 1* Not Coded Here   *EXCLUDES 2* Not Included Here

ICD-10-CM 2018   1017

✓4th **S62　Fracture at wrist and hand level**

NOTE　A fracture not indicated as displaced or nondisplaced should be coded to displaced.
A fracture not indicated as open or closed should be coded to closed.

EXCLUDES 1　*traumatic amputation of wrist and hand (S68.-)*
EXCLUDES 2　*fracture of distal parts of ulna and radius (S52.-)*
AHA: 2015, 3Q, 37-39

The appropriate 7th character is to be added to each code from category S62.
A　initial encounter for closed fracture
B　initial encounter for open fracture
D　subsequent encounter for fracture with routine healing
G　subsequent encounter for fracture with delayed healing
K　subsequent encounter for fracture with nonunion
P　subsequent encounter for fracture with malunion
S　sequela

✓5th **S62.0　Fracture of** navicular [scaphoid] **bone of wrist**

CC Excl: For codes in subcategory S62.0:
CC with 7th character B: PDX collection 1283
CC with 7th character K or P: PDX collection 897

✓6th **S62.00　Unspecified fracture of navicular [scaphoid] bone of wrist**

7　✓7th **S62.001　Unspecified fracture of navicular [scaphoid] bone of right wrist** CC H5

7　✓7th **S62.002　Unspecified fracture of navicular [scaphoid] bone of left wrist** CC H5
AHA: 2012, 4Q, 106

7　✓7th **S62.009　Unspecified fracture of navicular [scaphoid] bone of unspecified wrist** CC H5

✓6th **S62.01　Fracture of distal pole of navicular [scaphoid] bone of wrist**
Fracture of volar tuberosity of navicular [scaphoid] bone of wrist

7　✓7th **S62.011　Displaced fracture of distal pole of navicular [scaphoid] bone of right wrist** CC H5

7　✓7th **S62.012　Displaced fracture of distal pole of navicular [scaphoid] bone of left wrist** CC H5

7　✓7th **S62.013　Displaced fracture of distal pole of navicular [scaphoid] bone of unspecified wrist** CC H5

7　✓7th **S62.014　Nondisplaced fracture of distal pole of navicular [scaphoid] bone of right wrist** CC H5

7　✓7th **S62.015　Nondisplaced fracture of distal pole of navicular [scaphoid] bone of left wrist** CC H5

7　✓7th **S62.016　Nondisplaced fracture of distal pole of navicular [scaphoid] bone of unspecified wrist** CC H5

✓6th **S62.02　Fracture of middle third of navicular [scaphoid] bone of wrist**

7　✓7th **S62.021　Displaced fracture of middle third of navicular [scaphoid] bone of right wrist** CC H5

7　✓7th **S62.022　Displaced fracture of middle third of navicular [scaphoid] bone of left wrist** CC H5

7　✓7th **S62.023　Displaced fracture of middle third of navicular [scaphoid] bone of unspecified wrist** CC H5

7　✓7th **S62.024　Nondisplaced fracture of middle third of navicular [scaphoid] bone of right wrist** CC H5

7　✓7th **S62.025　Nondisplaced fracture of middle third of navicular [scaphoid] bone of left wrist** CC H5

7　✓7th **S62.026　Nondisplaced fracture of middle third of navicular [scaphoid] bone of unspecified wrist** CC H5

✓6th **S62.03　Fracture of proximal third of navicular [scaphoid] bone of wrist**

7　✓7th **S62.031　Displaced fracture of proximal third of navicular [scaphoid] bone of right wrist** CC H5

7　✓7th **S62.032　Displaced fracture of proximal third of navicular [scaphoid] bone of left wrist** CC H5

7　✓7th **S62.033　Displaced fracture of proximal third of navicular [scaphoid] bone of unspecified wrist** CC H5

7　✓7th **S62.034　Nondisplaced fracture of proximal third of navicular [scaphoid] bone of right wrist** CC H5

7　✓7th **S62.035　Nondisplaced fracture of proximal third of navicular [scaphoid] bone of left wrist** CC H5

7　✓7th **S62.036　Nondisplaced fracture of proximal third of navicular [scaphoid] bone of unspecified wrist** CC H5

✓5th **S62.1　Fracture of other and unspecified carpal bone(s)**
EXCLUDES 2　*fracture of scaphoid of wrist (S62.0-)*

CC Excl: For codes in subcategory S62.1:
CC with 7th character B: PDX collection 1283
CC with 7th character K or P: PDX collection 897

✓6th **S62.10　Fracture of unspecified carpal bone**
Fracture of wrist NOS

7　✓7th **S62.101　Fracture of unspecified carpal bone, right wrist** CC H5

7　✓7th **S62.102　Fracture of unspecified carpal bone, left wrist** CC H5
AHA: 2012, 4Q, 95

7　✓7th **S62.109　Fracture of unspecified carpal bone, unspecified wrist** CC H5

✓6th **S62.11　Fracture of triquetrum [cuneiform] bone of wrist**

7　✓7th **S62.111　Displaced fracture of triquetrum [cuneiform] bone, right wrist** CC H5

7　✓7th **S62.112　Displaced fracture of triquetrum [cuneiform] bone, left wrist** CC H5

7　✓7th **S62.113　Displaced fracture of triquetrum [cuneiform] bone, unspecified wrist** CC H5

7　✓7th **S62.114　Nondisplaced fracture of triquetrum [cuneiform] bone, right wrist** CC H5

7　✓7th **S62.115　Nondisplaced fracture of triquetrum [cuneiform] bone, left wrist** CC H5

7　✓7th **S62.116　Nondisplaced fracture of triquetrum [cuneiform] bone, unspecified wrist** CC H5

✓6th **S62.12　Fracture of lunate [semilunar]**

7　✓7th **S62.121　Displaced fracture of lunate [semilunar], right wrist** CC H5

7　✓7th **S62.122　Displaced fracture of lunate [semilunar], left wrist** CC H5

7　✓7th **S62.123　Displaced fracture of lunate [semilunar], unspecified wrist** CC H5

7　✓7th **S62.124　Nondisplaced fracture of lunate [semilunar], right wrist** CC H5

7　✓7th **S62.125　Nondisplaced fracture of lunate [semilunar], left wrist** CC H5

7　✓7th **S62.126　Nondisplaced fracture of lunate [semilunar], unspecified wrist** CC H5

✓6th **S62.13　Fracture of capitate [os magnum] bone**

7　✓7th **S62.131　Displaced fracture of capitate [os magnum] bone, right wrist** CC H5

7　✓7th **S62.132　Displaced fracture of capitate [os magnum] bone, left wrist** CC H5

7　✓7th **S62.133　Displaced fracture of capitate [os magnum] bone, unspecified wrist** CC H5

7　✓7th **S62.134　Nondisplaced fracture of capitate [os magnum] bone, right wrist** CC H5

7　✓7th **S62.135　Nondisplaced fracture of capitate [os magnum] bone, left wrist** CC H5

7　✓7th **S62.136　Nondisplaced fracture of capitate [os magnum] bone, unspecified wrist** CC H5

✓6th **S62.14　Fracture of body of hamate [unciform] bone**
Fracture of hamate [unciform] bone NOS

7　✓7th **S62.141　Displaced fracture of body of hamate [unciform] bone, right wrist** CC H5

7　CC when reported as an initial encounter (7th character A, B, or C – specific to category) OR a subsequent encounter for nonunion or malunion (7th character K, M, N, P, Q, or R – specific to category).

7 ✓7ᵗʰ **S62.142** Displaced fracture of body of hamate [unciform] bone, left wrist `CC` `H5`

7 ✓7ᵗʰ **S62.143** Displaced fracture of body of hamate [unciform] bone, unspecified wrist `CC` `H5`

7 ✓7ᵗʰ **S62.144** Nondisplaced fracture of body of hamate [unciform] bone, right wrist `CC` `H5`

7 ✓7ᵗʰ **S62.145** Nondisplaced fracture of body of hamate [unciform] bone, left wrist `CC` `H5`

7 ✓7ᵗʰ **S62.146** Nondisplaced fracture of body of hamate [unciform] bone, unspecified wrist `CC` `H5`

✓6ᵗʰ **S62.15** Fracture of hook process of hamate [unciform] bone
Fracture of unciform process of hamate [unciform] bone

7 ✓7ᵗʰ **S62.151** Displaced fracture of hook process of hamate [unciform] bone, right wrist `CC` `H5`

7 ✓7ᵗʰ **S62.152** Displaced fracture of hook process of hamate [unciform] bone, left wrist `CC` `H5`

7 ✓7ᵗʰ **S62.153** Displaced fracture of hook process of hamate [unciform] bone, unspecified wrist `CC` `H5`

7 ✓7ᵗʰ **S62.154** Nondisplaced fracture of hook process of hamate [unciform] bone, right wrist `CC` `H5`

7 ✓7ᵗʰ **S62.155** Nondisplaced fracture of hook process of hamate [unciform] bone, left wrist `CC` `H5`

7 ✓7ᵗʰ **S62.156** Nondisplaced fracture of hook process of hamate [unciform] bone, unspecified wrist `CC` `H5`

✓6ᵗʰ **S62.16** Fracture of pisiform

7 ✓7ᵗʰ **S62.161** Displaced fracture of pisiform, right wrist `CC` `H5`

7 ✓7ᵗʰ **S62.162** Displaced fracture of pisiform, left wrist `CC` `H5`

7 ✓7ᵗʰ **S62.163** Displaced fracture of pisiform, unspecified wrist `CC` `H5`

7 ✓7ᵗʰ **S62.164** Nondisplaced fracture of pisiform, right wrist `CC` `H5`

7 ✓7ᵗʰ **S62.165** Nondisplaced fracture of pisiform, left wrist `CC` `H5`

7 ✓7ᵗʰ **S62.166** Nondisplaced fracture of pisiform, unspecified wrist `CC` `H5`

✓6ᵗʰ **S62.17** Fracture of trapezium [larger multangular]

7 ✓7ᵗʰ **S62.171** Displaced fracture of trapezium [larger multangular], right wrist `CC` `H5`

7 ✓7ᵗʰ **S62.172** Displaced fracture of trapezium [larger multangular], left wrist `CC` `H5`

7 ✓7ᵗʰ **S62.173** Displaced fracture of trapezium [larger multangular], unspecified wrist `CC` `H5`

7 ✓7ᵗʰ **S62.174** Nondisplaced fracture of trapezium [larger multangular], right wrist `CC` `H5`

7 ✓7ᵗʰ **S62.175** Nondisplaced fracture of trapezium [larger multangular], left wrist `CC` `H5`

7 ✓7ᵗʰ **S62.176** Nondisplaced fracture of trapezium [larger multangular], unspecified wrist `CC` `H5`

✓6ᵗʰ **S62.18** Fracture of trapezoid [smaller multangular]

7 ✓7ᵗʰ **S62.181** Displaced fracture of trapezoid [smaller multangular], right wrist `CC` `H5`

7 ✓7ᵗʰ **S62.182** Displaced fracture of trapezoid [smaller multangular], left wrist `CC` `H5`

7 ✓7ᵗʰ **S62.183** Displaced fracture of trapezoid [smaller multangular], unspecified wrist `CC` `H5`

7 ✓7ᵗʰ **S62.184** Nondisplaced fracture of trapezoid [smaller multangular], right wrist `CC` `H5`

7 ✓7ᵗʰ **S62.185** Nondisplaced fracture of trapezoid [smaller multangular], left wrist `CC` `H5`

7 ✓7ᵗʰ **S62.186** Nondisplaced fracture of trapezoid [smaller multangular], unspecified wrist `CC` `H5`

✓5ᵗʰ **S62.2** Fracture of first metacarpal bone

> **CC Excl: For codes in subcategory S62.2:**
> **CC with 7th character B:** PDX collection 1284
> **CC with 7th character K or P:** PDX collection 897

✓6ᵗʰ **S62.20** Unspecified fracture of first metacarpal bone

7 ✓7ᵗʰ **S62.201** Unspecified fracture of first metacarpal bone, right hand `CC` `H5`

7 ✓7ᵗʰ **S62.202** Unspecified fracture of first metacarpal bone, left hand `CC` `H5`

7 ✓7ᵗʰ **S62.209** Unspecified fracture of first metacarpal bone, unspecified hand `CC` `H5`

✓6ᵗʰ **S62.21** Bennett's fracture

7 ✓7ᵗʰ **S62.211** Bennett's fracture, right hand `CC` `H5`

7 ✓7ᵗʰ **S62.212** Bennett's fracture, left hand `CC` `H5`

7 ✓7ᵗʰ **S62.213** Bennett's fracture, unspecified hand `CC` `H5`

✓6ᵗʰ **S62.22** Rolando's fracture

7 ✓7ᵗʰ **S62.221** Displaced Rolando's fracture, right hand `CC` `H5`

7 ✓7ᵗʰ **S62.222** Displaced Rolando's fracture, left hand `CC` `H5`

7 ✓7ᵗʰ **S62.223** Displaced Rolando's fracture, unspecified hand `CC` `H5`

7 ✓7ᵗʰ **S62.224** Nondisplaced Rolando's fracture, right hand `CC` `H5`

7 ✓7ᵗʰ **S62.225** Nondisplaced Rolando's fracture, left hand `CC` `H5`

7 ✓7ᵗʰ **S62.226** Nondisplaced Rolando's fracture, unspecified hand `CC` `H5`

✓6ᵗʰ **S62.23** Other fracture of base of first metacarpal bone

7 ✓7ᵗʰ **S62.231** Other displaced fracture of base of first metacarpal bone, right hand `CC` `H5`

7 ✓7ᵗʰ **S62.232** Other displaced fracture of base of first metacarpal bone, left hand `CC` `H5`

7 ✓7ᵗʰ **S62.233** Other displaced fracture of base of first metacarpal bone, unspecified hand `CC` `H5`

7 ✓7ᵗʰ **S62.234** Other nondisplaced fracture of base of first metacarpal bone, right hand `CC` `H5`

7 ✓7ᵗʰ **S62.235** Other nondisplaced fracture of base of first metacarpal bone, left hand `CC` `H5`

7 ✓7ᵗʰ **S62.236** Other nondisplaced fracture of base of first metacarpal bone, unspecified hand `CC` `H5`

✓6ᵗʰ **S62.24** Fracture of shaft of first metacarpal bone

7 ✓7ᵗʰ **S62.241** Displaced fracture of shaft of first metacarpal bone, right hand `CC` `H5`

7 ✓7ᵗʰ **S62.242** Displaced fracture of shaft of first metacarpal bone, left hand `CC` `H5`

7 ✓7ᵗʰ **S62.243** Displaced fracture of shaft of first metacarpal bone, unspecified hand `CC` `H5`

7 ✓7ᵗʰ **S62.244** Nondisplaced fracture of shaft of first metacarpal bone, right hand `CC` `H5`

7 ✓7ᵗʰ **S62.245** Nondisplaced fracture of shaft of first metacarpal bone, left hand `CC` `H5`

7 ✓7ᵗʰ **S62.246** Nondisplaced fracture of shaft of first metacarpal bone, unspecified hand `CC` `H5`

✓6ᵗʰ **S62.25** Fracture of neck of first metacarpal bone

7 ✓7ᵗʰ **S62.251** Displaced fracture of neck of first metacarpal bone, right hand `CC` `H5`

7 ✓7ᵗʰ **S62.252** Displaced fracture of neck of first metacarpal bone, left hand `CC` `H5`

7 ✓7ᵗʰ **S62.253** Displaced fracture of neck of first metacarpal bone, unspecified hand `CC` `H5`

7 ✓7ᵗʰ **S62.254** Nondisplaced fracture of neck of first metacarpal bone, right hand `CC` `H5`

7 ✓7ᵗʰ **S62.255** Nondisplaced fracture of neck of first metacarpal bone, left hand `CC` `H5`

7 ✓7ᵗʰ **S62.256** Nondisplaced fracture of neck of first metacarpal bone, unspecified hand `CC` `H5`

---

7 CC when reported as an initial encounter (7th character A, B, or C – specific to category) OR a subsequent encounter for nonunion or malunion (7th character K, M, N, P, Q, or R – specific to category).

✓Additional Character Req   ✓x7ᵗʰ Placeholder Alert   Unacceptable PDx   Manifestation   `H1`-`H14` HAC   `HCC` CMS-HCC Condition   *EXCLUDES1* Not Coded Here   *EXCLUDES2* Not Included Here

√6th **S62.29** Other fracture of first metacarpal bone
    7 √7th **S62.291** Other fracture of first metacarpal bone, **right hand** `CC` `H5`
    7 √7th **S62.292** Other fracture of first metacarpal bone, **left hand** `CC` `H5`
    7 √7th **S62.299** Other fracture of first metacarpal bone, **unspecified hand** `CC` `H5`

√5th **S62.3** Fracture of other and unspecified metacarpal **bone**
    EXCLUDES 2   *fracture of first metacarpal bone (S62.2-)*

> **CC Excl: For codes in subcategory S62.3:**
> **CC with 7th character B:** PDX collection 1284
> **CC with 7th character K or P:** PDX collection 897

√6th **S62.30** Unspecified **fracture of other metacarpal bone**
    7 √7th **S62.300** Unspecified fracture of second metacarpal bone, **right hand** `CC` `H5`
    7 √7th **S62.301** Unspecified fracture of second metacarpal bone, **left hand** `CC` `H5`
    7 √7th **S62.302** Unspecified fracture of third metacarpal bone, **right hand** `CC` `H5`
    7 √7th **S62.303** Unspecified fracture of third metacarpal bone, **left hand** `CC` `H5`
    7 √7th **S62.304** Unspecified fracture of fourth metacarpal bone, **right hand** `CC` `H5`
    7 √7th **S62.305** Unspecified fracture of fourth metacarpal bone, **left hand** `CC` `H5`
    7 √7th **S62.306** Unspecified fracture of fifth metacarpal bone, **right hand** `CC` `H5`
    7 √7th **S62.307** Unspecified fracture of fifth metacarpal bone, **left hand** `CC` `H5`
    7 √7th **S62.308** Unspecified fracture of other metacarpal bone `CC` `H5`
        Unspecified fracture of specified metacarpal bone with unspecified laterality
    7 √7th **S62.309** Unspecified fracture of unspecified metacarpal bone `CC` `H5`

√6th **S62.31** Displaced **fracture of base of other metacarpal bone**
    7 √7th **S62.37** Displaced fracture of base of second metacarpal bone, **right hand** `CC` `H5`
▲   7 √7th **S62.311** Displaced fracture of base of second metacarpal bone, **left hand** `CC` `H5`
    7 √7th **S62.312** Displaced fracture of base of third metacarpal bone, **right hand** `CC` `H5`
    7 √7th **S62.313** Displaced fracture of base of third metacarpal bone, **left hand** `CC` `H5`
    7 √7th **S62.314** Displaced fracture of base of fourth metacarpal bone, **right hand** `CC` `H5`
    7 √7th **S62.315** Displaced fracture of base of fourth metacarpal bone, **left hand** `CC` `H5`
    7 √7th **S62.316** Displaced fracture of base of fifth metacarpal bone, **right hand** `CC` `H5`
▲   7 √7th **S62.317** Displaced fracture of base of fifth metacarpal bone, **left hand** `CC` `H5`
    7 √7th **S62.318** Displaced fracture of base of other metacarpal bone `CC` `H5`
        Displaced fracture of base of specified metacarpal bone with unspecified laterality
    7 √7th **S62.319** Displaced fracture of base of unspecified metacarpal bone `CC` `H5`

√6th **S62.32** Displaced **fracture of shaft of other metacarpal bone**
    7 √7th **S62.320** Displaced fracture of shaft of second metacarpal bone, **right hand** `CC` `H5`
    7 √7th **S62.321** Displaced fracture of shaft of second metacarpal bone, **left hand** `CC` `H5`
    7 √7th **S62.322** Displaced fracture of shaft of third metacarpal bone, **right hand** `CC` `H5`
    7 √7th **S62.323** Displaced fracture of shaft of third metacarpal bone, **left hand** `CC` `H5`
    7 √7th **S62.324** Displaced fracture of shaft of fourth metacarpal bone, **right hand** `CC` `H5`
    7 √7th **S62.325** Displaced fracture of shaft of fourth metacarpal bone, **left hand** `CC` `H5`

    7 √7th **S62.326** Displaced fracture of shaft of fifth metacarpal bone, **right hand** `CC` `H5`
    7 √7th **S62.327** Displaced fracture of shaft of fifth metacarpal bone, **left hand** `CC` `H5`
    7 √7th **S62.328** Displaced fracture of shaft of other metacarpal bone `CC` `H5`
        Displaced fracture of shaft of specified metacarpal bone with unspecified laterality
    7 √7th **S62.329** Displaced fracture of shaft of unspecified metacarpal bone `CC` `H5`

√6th **S62.33** Displaced **fracture of neck of other metacarpal bone**
    7 √7th **S62.330** Displaced fracture of neck of second metacarpal bone, **right hand** `CC` `H5`
    7 √7th **S62.331** Displaced fracture of neck of second metacarpal bone, **left hand** `CC` `H5`
    7 √7th **S62.332** Displaced fracture of neck of third metacarpal bone, **right hand** `CC` `H5`
    7 √7th **S62.333** Displaced fracture of neck of third metacarpal bone, **left hand** `CC` `H5`
    7 √7th **S62.334** Displaced fracture of neck of fourth metacarpal bone, **right hand** `CC` `H5`
    7 √7th **S62.335** Displaced fracture of neck of fourth metacarpal bone, **left hand** `CC` `H5`
    7 √7th **S62.336** Displaced fracture of neck of fifth metacarpal bone, **right hand** `CC` `H5`
    7 √7th **S62.337** Displaced fracture of neck of fifth metacarpal bone, **left hand** `CC` `H5`
    7 √7th **S62.338** Displaced fracture of neck of other metacarpal bone `CC` `H5`
        Displaced fracture of neck of specified metacarpal bone with unspecified laterality
    7 √7th **S62.339** Displaced fracture of neck of unspecified metacarpal bone `CC` `H5`

√6th **S62.34** Nondisplaced **fracture of base of other metacarpal bone**
    7 √7th **S62.340** Nondisplaced fracture of base of second metacarpal bone, **right hand** `CC` `H5`
▲   7 √7th **S62.341** Nondisplaced fracture of base of second metacarpal bone, **left hand** `CC` `H5`
    7 √7th **S62.342** Nondisplaced fracture of base of third metacarpal bone, **right hand** `CC` `H5`
    7 √7th **S62.343** Nondisplaced fracture of base of third metacarpal bone, **left hand** `CC` `H5`
    7 √7th **S62.344** Nondisplaced fracture of base of fourth metacarpal bone, **right hand** `CC` `H5`
    7 √7th **S62.345** Nondisplaced fracture of base of fourth metacarpal bone, **left hand** `CC` `H5`
    7 √7th **S62.346** Nondisplaced fracture of base of fifth metacarpal bone, **right hand** `CC` `H5`
▲   7 √7th **S62.347** Nondisplaced fracture of base of fifth metacarpal bone, **left hand** `CC` `H5`
    7 √7th **S62.348** Nondisplaced fracture of base of other metacarpal bone `CC` `H5`
        Nondisplaced fracture of base of specified metacarpal bone with unspecified laterality
    7 √7th **S62.349** Nondisplaced fracture of base of unspecified metacarpal bone `CC` `H5`

√6th **S62.35** Nondisplaced **fracture of shaft of other metacarpal bone**
    7 √7th **S62.350** Nondisplaced fracture of shaft of second metacarpal bone, **right hand** `CC` `H5`
    7 √7th **S62.351** Nondisplaced fracture of shaft of second metacarpal bone, **left hand** `CC` `H5`
    7 √7th **S62.352** Nondisplaced fracture of shaft of third metacarpal bone, **right hand** `CC` `H5`
    7 √7th **S62.353** Nondisplaced fracture of shaft of third metacarpal bone, **left hand** `CC` `H5`
    7 √7th **S62.354** Nondisplaced fracture of shaft of fourth metacarpal bone, **right hand** `CC` `H5`
    7 √7th **S62.355** Nondisplaced fracture of shaft of fourth metacarpal bone, **left hand** `CC` `H5`

---

7 CC when reported as an initial encounter (7th character A, B, or C – specific to category) OR a subsequent encounter for nonunion or malunion (7th character K, M, N, P, Q, or R – specific to category).

7 ✓7ᵗʰ **S62.356** **Nondisplaced fracture of shaft of** fifth metacarpal bone, **right hand** `CC` `H5`

7 ✓7ᵗʰ **S62.357** **Nondisplaced fracture of shaft of** fifth metacarpal bone, **left hand** `CC` `H5`

7 ✓7ᵗʰ **S62.358** **Nondisplaced fracture of shaft of** other **metacarpal bone** `CC` `H5`
Nondisplaced fracture of shaft of specified metacarpal bone with unspecified laterality

7 ✓7ᵗʰ **S62.359** **Nondisplaced fracture of shaft of** unspecified **metacarpal bone** `CC` `H5`

✓6ᵗʰ **S62.36** **Nondisplaced fracture** of neck of other metacarpal **bone**

7 ✓7ᵗʰ **S62.360** **Nondisplaced fracture of neck of** second metacarpal bone, **right hand** `CC` `H5`

7 ✓7ᵗʰ **S62.361** **Nondisplaced fracture of neck of** second metacarpal bone, **left hand** `CC` `H5`

7 ✓7ᵗʰ **S62.362** **Nondisplaced fracture of neck of** third metacarpal bone, **right hand** `CC` `H5`

7 ✓7ᵗʰ **S62.363** **Nondisplaced fracture of neck of** third metacarpal bone, **left hand** `CC` `H5`

7 ✓7ᵗʰ **S62.364** **Nondisplaced fracture of neck of** fourth metacarpal bone, **right hand** `CC` `H5`

7 ✓7ᵗʰ **S62.365** **Nondisplaced fracture of neck of** fourth metacarpal bone, **left hand** `CC` `H5`

7 ✓7ᵗʰ **S62.366** **Nondisplaced fracture of neck of** fifth metacarpal bone, **right hand** `CC` `H5`

7 ✓7ᵗʰ **S62.367** **Nondisplaced fracture of neck of** fifth metacarpal bone, **left hand** `CC` `H5`

7 ✓7ᵗʰ **S62.368** **Nondisplaced fracture of neck of** other **metacarpal bone** `CC` `H5`
Nondisplaced fracture of neck of specified metacarpal bone with unspecified laterality

7 ✓7ᵗʰ **S62.369** **Nondisplaced fracture of neck of** unspecified **metacarpal bone** `CC` `H5`

✓6ᵗʰ **S62.39** **Other fracture of** other **metacarpal bone**

7 ✓7ᵗʰ **S62.390** **Other fracture of** second **metacarpal bone, right hand** `CC` `H5`

7 ✓7ᵗʰ **S62.391** **Other fracture of** second **metacarpal bone, left hand** `CC` `H5`

7 ✓7ᵗʰ **S62.392** **Other fracture of** third **metacarpal bone, right hand** `CC` `H5`

7 ✓7ᵗʰ **S62.393** **Other fracture of** third **metacarpal bone, left hand** `CC` `H5`

7 ✓7ᵗʰ **S62.394** **Other fracture of** fourth **metacarpal bone, right hand** `CC` `H5`

7 ✓7ᵗʰ **S62.395** **Other fracture of** fourth **metacarpal bone, left hand** `CC` `H5`

7 ✓7ᵗʰ **S62.396** **Other fracture of** fifth **metacarpal bone, right hand** `CC` `H5`

7 ✓7ᵗʰ **S62.397** **Other fracture of** fifth **metacarpal bone, left hand** `CC` `H5`

7 ✓7ᵗʰ **S62.398** **Other fracture of** other **metacarpal bone** `CC` `H5`
Other fracture of specified metacarpal bone with unspecified laterality

7 ✓7ᵗʰ **S62.399** **Other fracture of** unspecified **metacarpal bone** `CC` `H5`

✓5ᵗʰ **S62.5** **Fracture of** thumb

CC Excl: For codes in subcategory S62.5:
CC with 7th character B: PDX collection 1285
CC with 7th character K or P: PDX collection 897

✓6ᵗʰ **S62.50** **Fracture of** unspecified **phalanx of thumb**

7 ✓7ᵗʰ **S62.501** **Fracture of unspecified phalanx of** right **thumb** `CC` `H5`

7 ✓7ᵗʰ **S62.502** **Fracture of unspecified phalanx of** left **thumb** `CC` `H5`

7 ✓7ᵗʰ **S62.509** **Fracture of unspecified phalanx of** unspecified **thumb** `CC` `H5`

✓6ᵗʰ **S62.51** **Fracture of** proximal phalanx **of thumb**

7 ✓7ᵗʰ **S62.511** **Displaced fracture of proximal** phalanx of **right thumb** `CC` `H5`

7 ✓7ᵗʰ **S62.512** **Displaced fracture of proximal** phalanx of **left thumb** `CC` `H5`

7 ✓7ᵗʰ **S62.513** **Displaced fracture of proximal** phalanx of **unspecified thumb** `CC` `H5`

7 ✓7ᵗʰ **S62.514** **Nondisplaced fracture of proximal** phalanx of **right thumb** `CC` `H5`

7 ✓7ᵗʰ **S62.515** **Nondisplaced fracture of proximal** phalanx of **left thumb** `CC` `H5`

7 ✓7ᵗʰ **S62.516** **Nondisplaced fracture of proximal** phalanx of **unspecified thumb** `CC` `H5`

✓6ᵗʰ **S62.52** **Fracture of distal phalanx of thumb**

7 ✓7ᵗʰ **S62.521** **Displaced fracture of distal phalanx** of **right thumb** `CC` `H5`

7 ✓7ᵗʰ **S62.522** **Displaced fracture of distal phalanx** of **left thumb** `CC` `H5`

7 ✓7ᵗʰ **S62.523** **Displaced fracture of distal phalanx** of **unspecified thumb** `CC` `H5`

7 ✓7ᵗʰ **S62.524** **Nondisplaced fracture of distal** phalanx of **right thumb** `CC` `H5`

7 ✓7ᵗʰ **S62.525** **Nondisplaced fracture of distal** phalanx of **left thumb** `CC` `H5`

7 ✓7ᵗʰ **S62.526** **Nondisplaced fracture of distal** phalanx of **unspecified thumb** `CC` `H5`

✓5ᵗʰ **S62.6** **Fracture of other and unspecified** finger(s)
EXCLUDES 2   *fracture of thumb (S62.5-)*

CC Excl: For codes in subcategory S62.6:
CC with 7th character B: PDX collection 1285
CC with 7th character K or P: PDX collection 897

✓6ᵗʰ **S62.60** **Fracture of** unspecified phalanx **of finger**

7 ✓7ᵗʰ **S62.600** **Fracture of unspecified phalanx** of **right index finger** `CC` `H5`

7 ✓7ᵗʰ **S62.601** **Fracture of unspecified phalanx** of **left index finger** `CC` `H5`

7 ✓7ᵗʰ **S62.602** **Fracture of unspecified phalanx** of **right middle finger** `CC` `H5`

7 ✓7ᵗʰ **S62.603** **Fracture of unspecified phalanx** of **left middle finger** `CC` `H5`

7 ✓7ᵗʰ **S62.604** **Fracture of unspecified phalanx** of **right ring finger** `CC` `H5`

7 ✓7ᵗʰ **S62.605** **Fracture of unspecified phalanx** of **left ring finger** `CC` `H5`

7 ✓7ᵗʰ **S62.606** **Fracture of unspecified phalanx** of **right little finger** `CC` `H5`

7 ✓7ᵗʰ **S62.607** **Fracture of unspecified phalanx** of **left little finger** `CC` `H5`

7 ✓7ᵗʰ **S62.608** **Fracture of unspecified phalanx** of other **finger** `CC` `H5`
Fracture of unspecified phalanx of specified finger with unspecified laterality

7 ✓7ᵗʰ **S62.609** **Fracture of unspecified phalanx of** unspecified **finger** `CC` `H5`

✓6ᵗʰ **S62.61** **Displaced fracture of** proximal phalanx **of finger**

7 ✓7ᵗʰ **S62.610** **Displaced fracture of proximal** phalanx of **right index finger** `CC` `H5`

7 ✓7ᵗʰ **S62.611** **Displaced fracture of proximal** phalanx of **left index finger** `CC` `H5`

7 ✓7ᵗʰ **S62.612** **Displaced fracture of proximal** phalanx of **right middle finger** `CC` `H5`

7 ✓7ᵗʰ **S62.613** **Displaced fracture of proximal** phalanx of **left middle finger** `CC` `H5`

7 ✓7ᵗʰ **S62.614** **Displaced fracture of proximal** phalanx of **right ring finger** `CC` `H5`

7 ✓7ᵗʰ **S62.615** **Displaced fracture of proximal** phalanx of **left ring finger** `CC` `H5`

7 ✓7ᵗʰ **S62.616** **Displaced fracture of proximal** phalanx of **right little finger** `CC` `H5`

7 ✓7ᵗʰ **S62.617** **Displaced fracture of proximal** phalanx of **left little finger** `CC` `H5`

7 ✓7ᵗʰ **S62.618** **Displaced fracture of proximal** phalanx of **other finger** `CC` `H5`
Displaced fracture of proximal phalanx of specified finger with unspecified laterality

---

7   CC when reported as an initial encounter (7th character A, B, or C – specific to category) OR a subsequent encounter for nonunion or malunion (7th character K, M, N, P, Q, or R – specific to category).

✓Additional Character Req   ✓x7ᵗʰ Placeholder Alert   Unacceptable PDx   Manifestation   `H1`-`H14` HAC   `HCC` CMS-HCC Condition   *EXCLUDES 1* Not Coded Here   *EXCLUDES 2* Not Included Here

Chapter 19. Injury, Poisoning and Certain Other Consequences of External Causes

7 ✓7ᵗʰ **S62.619** **Displaced fracture of proximal phalanx of unspecified finger** `CC` `H5`

▲ ✓6ᵗʰ **S62.62** Displaced **fracture of middle phalanx of finger**

▲ 7 ✓7ᵗʰ **S62.620** **Displaced fracture of middle phalanx of right index finger** `CC` `H5`

▲ 7 ✓7ᵗʰ **S62.621** **Displaced fracture of middle phalanx of left index finger** `CC` `H5`

▲ 7 ✓7ᵗʰ **S62.622** **Displaced fracture of middle phalanx of right middle finger** `CC` `H5`

▲ 7 ✓7ᵗʰ **S62.623** **Displaced fracture of middle phalanx of left middle finger** `CC` `H5`

▲ 7 ✓7ᵗʰ **S62.624** **Displaced fracture of middle phalanx of right ring finger** `CC` `H5`

▲ 7 ✓7ᵗʰ **S62.625** **Displaced fracture of middle phalanx of left ring finger** `CC` `H5`

7 ✓7ᵗʰ **S62.626** **Displaced fracture of medial phalanx of right little finger** `CC` `H5`

7 ✓7ᵗʰ **S62.627** **Displaced fracture of medial phalanx of left little finger** `CC` `H5`

7 ✓7ᵗʰ **S62.628** **Displaced fracture of medial phalanx of other finger** `CC` `H5`
Displaced fracture of medial phalanx of specified finger with unspecified laterality

7 ✓7ᵗʰ **S62.629** **Displaced fracture of medial phalanx of unspecified finger** `CC` `H5`

✓6ᵗʰ **S62.63** Displaced **fracture of distal phalanx of finger**

7 ✓7ᵗʰ **S62.630** **Displaced fracture of distal phalanx of right index finger** `CC` `H5`

7 ✓7ᵗʰ **S62.631** **Displaced fracture of distal phalanx of left index finger** `CC` `H5`

7 ✓7ᵗʰ **S62.632** **Displaced fracture of distal phalanx of right middle finger** `CC` `H5`

7 ✓7ᵗʰ **S62.633** **Displaced fracture of distal phalanx of left middle finger** `CC` `H5`

7 ✓7ᵗʰ **S62.634** **Displaced fracture of distal phalanx of right ring finger** `CC` `H5`

7 ✓7ᵗʰ **S62.635** **Displaced fracture of distal phalanx of left ring finger** `CC` `H5`

7 ✓7ᵗʰ **S62.636** **Displaced fracture of distal phalanx of right little finger** `CC` `H5`

7 ✓7ᵗʰ **S62.637** **Displaced fracture of distal phalanx of left little finger** `CC` `H5`

7 ✓7ᵗʰ **S62.638** **Displaced fracture of distal phalanx of other finger** `CC` `H5`
Displaced fracture of distal phalanx of specified finger with unspecified laterality

7 ✓7ᵗʰ **S62.639** **Displaced fracture of distal phalanx of unspecified finger** `CC` `H5`

✓6ᵗʰ **S62.64** Nondisplaced **fracture of proximal phalanx of finger**

7 ✓7ᵗʰ **S62.640** **Nondisplaced fracture of proximal phalanx of right index finger** `CC` `H5`

7 ✓7ᵗʰ **S62.641** **Nondisplaced fracture of proximal phalanx of left index finger** `CC` `H5`

7 ✓7ᵗʰ **S62.642** **Nondisplaced fracture of proximal phalanx of right middle finger** `CC` `H5`

7 ✓7ᵗʰ **S62.643** **Nondisplaced fracture of proximal phalanx of left middle finger** `CC` `H5`

7 ✓7ᵗʰ **S62.644** **Nondisplaced fracture of proximal phalanx of right ring finger** `CC` `H5`

7 ✓7ᵗʰ **S62.645** **Nondisplaced fracture of proximal phalanx of left ring finger** `CC` `H5`

7 ✓7ᵗʰ **S62.646** **Nondisplaced fracture of proximal phalanx of right little finger** `CC` `H5`

7 ✓7ᵗʰ **S62.647** **Nondisplaced fracture of proximal phalanx of left little finger** `CC` `H5`

7 ✓7ᵗʰ **S62.648** **Nondisplaced fracture of proximal phalanx of other finger** `CC` `H5`
Nondisplaced fracture of proximal phalanx of specified finger with unspecified laterality

7 ✓7ᵗʰ **S62.649** **Nondisplaced fracture of proximal phalanx of unspecified finger** `CC` `H5`

▲ ✓6ᵗʰ **S62.65** Nondisplaced **fracture of middle phalanx of finger**

7 ✓7ᵗʰ **S62.650** **Nondisplaced fracture of middle phalanx of right index finger** `CC` `H5`

▲ 7 ✓7ᵗʰ **S62.651** **Nondisplaced fracture of middle phalanx of left index finger** `CC` `H5`

▲ 7 ✓7ᵗʰ **S62.652** **Nondisplaced fracture of middle phalanx of right middle finger** `CC` `H5`

▲ 7 ✓7ᵗʰ **S62.653** **Nondisplaced fracture of middle phalanx of left middle finger** `CC` `H5`

7 ✓7ᵗʰ **S62.654** **Nondisplaced fracture of medial phalanx of right ring finger** `CC` `H5`

7 ✓7ᵗʰ **S62.655** **Nondisplaced fracture of medial phalanx of left ring finger** `CC` `H5`

7 ✓7ᵗʰ **S62.656** **Nondisplaced fracture of medial phalanx of right little finger** `CC` `H5`

7 ✓7ᵗʰ **S62.657** **Nondisplaced fracture of medial phalanx of left little finger** `CC` `H5`

7 ✓7ᵗʰ **S62.658** **Nondisplaced fracture of medial phalanx of other finger** `CC` `H5`
Nondisplaced fracture of medial phalanx of specified finger with unspecified laterality

7 ✓7ᵗʰ **S62.659** **Nondisplaced fracture of medial phalanx of unspecified finger** `CC` `H5`

✓6ᵗʰ **S62.66** Nondisplaced **fracture of distal phalanx of finger**

7 ✓7ᵗʰ **S62.660** **Nondisplaced fracture of distal phalanx of right index finger** `CC` `H5`

7 ✓7ᵗʰ **S62.661** **Nondisplaced fracture of distal phalanx of left index finger** `CC` `H5`

7 ✓7ᵗʰ **S62.662** **Nondisplaced fracture of distal phalanx of right middle finger** `CC` `H5`

7 ✓7ᵗʰ **S62.663** **Nondisplaced fracture of distal phalanx of left middle finger** `CC` `H5`

7 ✓7ᵗʰ **S62.664** **Nondisplaced fracture of distal phalanx of right ring finger** `CC` `H5`

7 ✓7ᵗʰ **S62.665** **Nondisplaced fracture of distal phalanx of left ring finger** `CC` `H5`

7 ✓7ᵗʰ **S62.666** **Nondisplaced fracture of distal phalanx of right little finger** `CC` `H5`

7 ✓7ᵗʰ **S62.667** **Nondisplaced fracture of distal phalanx of left little finger** `CC` `H5`

7 ✓7ᵗʰ **S62.668** **Nondisplaced fracture of distal phalanx of other finger** `CC` `H5`
Nondisplaced fracture of distal phalanx of specified finger with unspecified laterality

7 ✓7ᵗʰ **S62.669** **Nondisplaced fracture of distal phalanx of unspecified finger** `CC` `H5`

✓5ᵗʰ **S62.9** Unspecified **fracture of wrist and hand**

7 ✓x7ᵗʰ **S62.90** **Unspecified fracture of unspecified wrist and hand** `CC` `H5`
CC Excl: CC with 7th character B: PDX collection 1286
CC with 7th character K or P: PDX collection 897

7 ✓x7ᵗʰ **S62.91** **Unspecified fracture of right wrist and hand** `CC` `H5`
CC Excl: CC with 7th character B: PDX collection 1287
CC with 7th character K or P: PDX collection 897

7 ✓x7ᵗʰ **S62.92** **Unspecified fracture of left wrist and hand** `CC` `H5`
CC Excl: CC with 7th character B: PDX collection 1287
CC with 7th character K or P: PDX collection 897

---

7 CC when reported as an initial encounter (7th character A, B, or C – specific to category) OR a subsequent encounter for nonunion or malunion (7th character K, M, N, P, Q, or R – specific to category).

Ⓝ Newborn: 0   Ⓟ Pediatric: 0-17   Ⓜ Maternity: 12-55   Ⓐ Adult: 15-124   `MCC` Major CC Condition   `PDxMCC` PDx acts as own MCC   `CC` CC Condition   `PDxCC` PDx acts as own CC

1022   ICD-10-CM 2018

√4ᵗʰ **S63**   **Dislocation and sprain of joints and ligaments at wrist and hand level**

> INCLUDES   avulsion of joint or ligament at wrist and hand level
> laceration of cartilage, joint or ligament at wrist and hand level
> sprain of cartilage, joint or ligament at wrist and hand level
> traumatic hemarthrosis of joint or ligament at wrist and hand level
> traumatic rupture of joint or ligament at wrist and hand level
> traumatic subluxation of joint or ligament at wrist and hand level
> traumatic tear of joint or ligament at wrist and hand level

> Code also any associated open wound
> EXCLUDES 2   *strain of muscle, fascia and tendon of wrist and hand (S66.-)*

> The appropriate 7th character is to be added to each code from category S63.
> A   initial encounter
> D   subsequent encounter
> S   sequela

√5ᵗʰ   **S63.0**   **Subluxation and dislocation of** wrist and hand joints

  √6ᵗʰ   **S63.00**   **Unspecified subluxation and dislocation of wrist and hand**
     Dislocation of carpal bone NOS
     Dislocation of distal end of radius NOS
     Subluxation of carpal bone NOS
     Subluxation of distal end of radius NOS

    √7ᵗʰ   **S63.001**   **Unspecified subluxation of** right **wrist and hand**
    √7ᵗʰ   **S63.002**   **Unspecified subluxation of** left **wrist and hand**
    √7ᵗʰ   **S63.003**   **Unspecified subluxation of** unspecified **wrist and hand**
    √7ᵗʰ   **S63.004**   **Unspecified dislocation of** right **wrist and hand**
    √7ᵗʰ   **S63.005**   **Unspecified dislocation of** left **wrist and hand**
    √7ᵗʰ   **S63.006**   **Unspecified dislocation of** unspecified **wrist and hand**

  √6ᵗʰ   **S63.01**   **Subluxation and dislocation of** distal radioulnar **joint**

    √7ᵗʰ   **S63.011**   **Subluxation of distal radioulnar joint of right wrist**
    √7ᵗʰ   **S63.012**   **Subluxation of distal radioulnar joint of left wrist**
    √7ᵗʰ   **S63.013**   **Subluxation of distal radioulnar joint of unspecified wrist**
    √7ᵗʰ   **S63.014**   **Dislocation of distal radioulnar joint of right wrist**
    √7ᵗʰ   **S63.015**   **Dislocation of distal radioulnar joint of** left **wrist**
    √7ᵗʰ   **S63.016**   **Dislocation of distal radioulnar joint of unspecified wrist**

  √6ᵗʰ   **S63.02**   **Subluxation and dislocation of** radiocarpal **joint**

    √7ᵗʰ   **S63.021**   **Subluxation of radiocarpal joint of** right **wrist**
    √7ᵗʰ   **S63.022**   **Subluxation of radiocarpal joint of** left **wrist**
    √7ᵗʰ   **S63.023**   **Subluxation of radiocarpal joint of** unspecified **wrist**
    √7ᵗʰ   **S63.024**   **Dislocation of radiocarpal joint of** right **wrist**
    √7ᵗʰ   **S63.025**   **Dislocation of radiocarpal joint of** left **wrist**
    √7ᵗʰ   **S63.026**   **Dislocation of radiocarpal joint of** unspecified **wrist**

  √6ᵗʰ   **S63.03**   **Subluxation and dislocation of** midcarpal **joint**

    √7ᵗʰ   **S63.031**   **Subluxation of midcarpal joint of** right **wrist**
    √7ᵗʰ   **S63.032**   **Subluxation of midcarpal joint of** left **wrist**
    √7ᵗʰ   **S63.033**   **Subluxation of midcarpal joint of** unspecified **wrist**
    √7ᵗʰ   **S63.034**   **Dislocation of midcarpal joint of** right **wrist**
    √7ᵗʰ   **S63.035**   **Dislocation of midcarpal joint of** left **wrist**
    √7ᵗʰ   **S63.036**   **Dislocation of midcarpal joint of** unspecified **wrist**

  √6ᵗʰ   **S63.04**   **Subluxation and dislocation of** carpometacarpal **joint of** thumb

> EXCLUDES 2   *interphalangeal subluxation and dislocation of thumb (S63.1-)*

    √7ᵗʰ   **S63.041**   **Subluxation of carpometacarpal joint of right thumb**
    √7ᵗʰ   **S63.042**   **Subluxation of carpometacarpal joint of left thumb**
    √7ᵗʰ   **S63.043**   **Subluxation of carpometacarpal joint of unspecified thumb**
    √7ᵗʰ   **S63.044**   **Dislocation of carpometacarpal joint of right thumb**
    √7ᵗʰ   **S63.045**   **Dislocation of carpometacarpal joint of left thumb**
    √7ᵗʰ   **S63.046**   **Dislocation of carpometacarpal joint of unspecified thumb**

  √6ᵗʰ   **S63.05**   **Subluxation and dislocation of** other carpometacarpal **joint**

> EXCLUDES 2   *subluxation and dislocation of carpometacarpal joint of thumb (S63.04-)*

    √7ᵗʰ   **S63.051**   **Subluxation of other carpometacarpal joint of** right **hand**
    √7ᵗʰ   **S63.052**   **Subluxation of other carpometacarpal joint of** left **hand**
    √7ᵗʰ   **S63.053**   **Subluxation of other carpometacarpal joint of** unspecified **hand**
    √7ᵗʰ   **S63.054**   **Dislocation of other carpometacarpal joint of** right **hand**
    √7ᵗʰ   **S63.055**   **Dislocation of other carpometacarpal joint of** left **hand**
    √7ᵗʰ   **S63.056**   **Dislocation of other carpometacarpal joint of** unspecified **hand**

  √6ᵗʰ   **S63.06**   **Subluxation and dislocation of** metacarpal (bone), proximal end

    √7ᵗʰ   **S63.061**   **Subluxation of metacarpal (bone), proximal end of** right **hand**
    √7ᵗʰ   **S63.062**   **Subluxation of metacarpal (bone), proximal end of** left **hand**
    √7ᵗʰ   **S63.063**   **Subluxation of metacarpal (bone), proximal end of** unspecified **hand**
    √7ᵗʰ   **S63.064**   **Dislocation of metacarpal (bone), proximal end of** right **hand**
    √7ᵗʰ   **S63.065**   **Dislocation of metacarpal (bone), proximal end of** left **hand**
    √7ᵗʰ   **S63.066**   **Dislocation of metacarpal (bone), proximal end of** unspecified **hand**

  √6ᵗʰ   **S63.07**   **Subluxation and dislocation of** distal end of ulna

    √7ᵗʰ   **S63.071**   **Subluxation of distal end of** right **ulna**
    √7ᵗʰ   **S63.072**   **Subluxation of distal end of** left **ulna**
    √7ᵗʰ   **S63.073**   **Subluxation of distal end of** unspecified **ulna**
    √7ᵗʰ   **S63.074**   **Dislocation of distal end of** right **ulna**
    √7ᵗʰ   **S63.075**   **Dislocation of distal end of** left **ulna**
    √7ᵗʰ   **S63.076**   **Dislocation of distal end of** unspecified **ulna**

  √6ᵗʰ   **S63.09**   **Other subluxation and dislocation of** wrist and hand

    √7ᵗʰ   **S63.091**   **Other subluxation of** right **wrist and hand**
    √7ᵗʰ   **S63.092**   **Other subluxation of** left **wrist and hand**
    √7ᵗʰ   **S63.093**   **Other subluxation of** unspecified **wrist and hand**
    √7ᵗʰ   **S63.094**   **Other dislocation of** right **wrist and hand**
    √7ᵗʰ   **S63.095**   **Other dislocation of** left **wrist and hand**
    √7ᵗʰ   **S63.096**   **Other dislocation of** unspecified **wrist and hand**

√5ᵗʰ   **S63.1**   **Subluxation and dislocation of** thumb

  √6ᵗʰ   **S63.10**   **Unspecified subluxation and dislocation of thumb**

    √7ᵗʰ   **S63.101**   **Unspecified subluxation of** right **thumb**
    √7ᵗʰ   **S63.102**   **Unspecified subluxation of** left **thumb**
    √7ᵗʰ   **S63.103**   **Unspecified subluxation of** unspecified **thumb**
    √7ᵗʰ   **S63.104**   **Unspecified dislocation of** right **thumb**
    √7ᵗʰ   **S63.105**   **Unspecified dislocation of** left **thumb**

✔ Additional Character Req   √7ᵗʰ Placeholder Alert   Unacceptable PDx   Manifestation   H1 - H14 HAC   HCC CMS-HCC Condition   EXCLUDES 1 Not Coded Here   EXCLUDES 2 Not Included Here

ICD-10-CM 2018   **1023**

☑7ᵗʰ **S63.106** Unspecified dislocation of unspecified thumb

☑6ᵗʰ **S63.11** Subluxation and dislocation of metacarpophalangeal joint of thumb

☑7ᵗʰ **S63.111** Subluxation of metacarpophalangeal joint of right thumb

☑7ᵗʰ **S63.112** Subluxation of metacarpophalangeal joint of left thumb

☑7ᵗʰ **S63.113** Subluxation of metacarpophalangeal joint of unspecified thumb

☑7ᵗʰ **S63.114** Dislocation of metacarpophalangeal joint of right thumb

☑7ᵗʰ **S63.115** Dislocation of metacarpophalangeal joint of left thumb

☑7ᵗʰ **S63.116** Dislocation of metacarpophalangeal joint of unspecified thumb

▲ ☑6ᵗʰ **S63.12** Subluxation and dislocation of interphalangeal joint of thumb

▲ ☑7ᵗʰ **S63.121** Subluxation of interphalangeal joint of right thumb

▲ ☑7ᵗʰ **S63.122** Subluxation of interphalangeal joint of left thumb

▲ ☑7ᵗʰ **S63.123** Subluxation of interphalangeal joint of unspecified thumb

▲ ☑7ᵗʰ **S63.124** Dislocation of interphalangeal joint of right thumb

▲ ☑7ᵗʰ **S63.125** Dislocation of interphalangeal joint of left thumb

▲ ☑7ᵗʰ **S63.126** Dislocation of interphalangeal joint of unspecified thumb

☑6ᵗʰ ~~**S63.13** Subluxation and dislocation of proximal interphalangeal joint of thumb~~

☑7ᵗʰ ~~**S63.131** Subluxation of proximal interphalangeal joint of right thumb~~

☑7ᵗʰ ~~**S63.132** Subluxation of proximal interphalangeal joint of left thumb~~

☑7ᵗʰ ~~**S63.133** Subluxation of proximal interphalangeal joint of unspecified thumb~~

☑7ᵗʰ ~~**S63.134** Dislocation of proximal interphalangeal joint of right thumb~~

☑7ᵗʰ ~~**S63.135** Dislocation of proximal interphalangeal joint of left thumb~~

☑7ᵗʰ ~~**S63.136** Dislocation of proximal interphalangeal joint of unspecified thumb~~

☑6ᵗʰ ~~**S63.14** Subluxation and dislocation of distal interphalangeal joint of thumb~~

☑7ᵗʰ ~~**S63.141** Subluxation of distal interphalangeal joint of right thumb~~

☑7ᵗʰ ~~**S63.142** Subluxation of distal interphalangeal joint of left thumb~~

☑7ᵗʰ ~~**S63.143** Subluxation of distal interphalangeal joint of unspecified thumb~~

☑7ᵗʰ ~~**S63.144** Dislocation of distal interphalangeal joint of right thumb~~

☑7ᵗʰ ~~**S63.145** Dislocation of distal interphalangeal joint of left thumb~~

☑7ᵗʰ ~~**S63.146** Dislocation of distal interphalangeal joint of unspecified thumb~~

☑5ᵗʰ **S63.2** Subluxation and dislocation of other finger(s)

> EXCLUDES 2   subluxation and dislocation of thumb (S63.1-)

☑6ᵗʰ **S63.20** Unspecified subluxation of other finger

☑7ᵗʰ **S63.200** Unspecified subluxation of right index finger

☑7ᵗʰ **S63.201** Unspecified subluxation of left index finger

☑7ᵗʰ **S63.202** Unspecified subluxation of right middle finger

☑7ᵗʰ **S63.203** Unspecified subluxation of left middle finger

☑7ᵗʰ **S63.204** Unspecified subluxation of right ring finger

☑7ᵗʰ **S63.205** Unspecified subluxation of left ring finger

☑7ᵗʰ **S63.206** Unspecified subluxation of right little finger

☑7ᵗʰ **S63.207** Unspecified subluxation of left little finger

☑7ᵗʰ **S63.208** Unspecified subluxation of other finger

> Unspecified subluxation of specified finger with unspecified laterality

☑7ᵗʰ **S63.209** Unspecified subluxation of unspecified finger

☑6ᵗʰ **S63.21** Subluxation of metacarpophalangeal joint of finger

☑7ᵗʰ **S63.210** Subluxation of metacarpophalangeal joint of right index finger

☑7ᵗʰ **S63.211** Subluxation of metacarpophalangeal joint of left index finger

☑7ᵗʰ **S63.212** Subluxation of metacarpophalangeal joint of right middle finger

☑7ᵗʰ **S63.213** Subluxation of metacarpophalangeal joint of left middle finger

☑7ᵗʰ **S63.214** Subluxation of metacarpophalangeal joint of right ring finger

☑7ᵗʰ **S63.215** Subluxation of metacarpophalangeal joint of left ring finger

☑7ᵗʰ **S63.216** Subluxation of metacarpophalangeal joint of right little finger

☑7ᵗʰ **S63.217** Subluxation of metacarpophalangeal joint of left little finger

☑7ᵗʰ **S63.218** Subluxation of metacarpophalangeal joint of other finger

> Subluxation of metacarpophalangeal joint of specified finger with unspecified laterality

☑7ᵗʰ **S63.219** Subluxation of metacarpophalangeal joint of unspecified finger

☑6ᵗʰ **S63.22** Subluxation of unspecified interphalangeal joint of finger

☑7ᵗʰ **S63.220** Subluxation of unspecified interphalangeal joint of right index finger

☑7ᵗʰ **S63.221** Subluxation of unspecified interphalangeal joint of left index finger

☑7ᵗʰ **S63.222** Subluxation of unspecified interphalangeal joint of right middle finger

☑7ᵗʰ **S63.223** Subluxation of unspecified interphalangeal joint of left middle finger

☑7ᵗʰ **S63.224** Subluxation of unspecified interphalangeal joint of right ring finger

☑7ᵗʰ **S63.225** Subluxation of unspecified interphalangeal joint of left ring finger

☑7ᵗʰ **S63.226** Subluxation of unspecified interphalangeal joint of right little finger

☑7ᵗʰ **S63.227** Subluxation of unspecified interphalangeal joint of left little finger

☑7ᵗʰ **S63.228** Subluxation of unspecified interphalangeal joint of other finger

> Subluxation of unspecified interphalangeal joint of specified finger with unspecified laterality

☑7ᵗʰ **S63.229** Subluxation of unspecified interphalangeal joint of unspecified finger

☑6ᵗʰ **S63.23** Subluxation of proximal interphalangeal joint of finger

☑7ᵗʰ **S63.230** Subluxation of proximal interphalangeal joint of right index finger

☑7ᵗʰ **S63.231** Subluxation of proximal interphalangeal joint of left index finger

☑7ᵗʰ **S63.232** Subluxation of proximal interphalangeal joint of right middle finger

☑7ᵗʰ **S63.233** Subluxation of proximal interphalangeal joint of left middle finger

☑7ᵗʰ **S63.234** Subluxation of proximal interphalangeal joint of right ring finger

☑7ᵗʰ **S63.235** Subluxation of proximal interphalangeal joint of left ring finger

☑7ᵗʰ **S63.236** Subluxation of proximal interphalangeal joint of right little finger

☑7ᵗʰ **S63.237** Subluxation of proximal interphalangeal joint of left little finger

Ⓝ Newborn: 0   Ⓟ Pediatric: 0-17   Ⓜ Maternity: 12-55   Ⓐ Adult: 15-124   **MCC** Major CC Condition   **PDx MCC** PDx acts as own MCC   **CC** CC Condition   **PDx CC** PDx acts as own CC

1024   ICD-10-CM 2018

✓7ᵗʰ **S63.238** **Subluxation of proximal interphalangeal joint of other finger**
     Subluxation of proximal interphalangeal joint of specified finger with unspecified laterality

✓7ᵗʰ **S63.239** **Subluxation of proximal interphalangeal joint of unspecified finger**

✓6ᵗʰ **S63.24** **Subluxation of distal interphalangeal joint of finger**

✓7ᵗʰ **S63.240** **Subluxation of distal interphalangeal joint of right index finger**

✓7ᵗʰ **S63.241** **Subluxation of distal interphalangeal joint of left index finger**

✓7ᵗʰ **S63.242** **Subluxation of distal interphalangeal joint of right middle finger**

✓7ᵗʰ **S63.243** **Subluxation of distal interphalangeal joint of left middle finger**

✓7ᵗʰ **S63.244** **Subluxation of distal interphalangeal joint of right ring finger**

✓7ᵗʰ **S63.245** **Subluxation of distal interphalangeal joint of left ring finger**

✓7ᵗʰ **S63.246** **Subluxation of distal interphalangeal joint of right little finger**

✓7ᵗʰ **S63.247** **Subluxation of distal interphalangeal joint of left little finger**

✓7ᵗʰ **S63.248** **Subluxation of distal interphalangeal joint of other finger**
     Subluxation of distal interphalangeal joint of specified finger with unspecified laterality

✓7ᵗʰ **S63.249** **Subluxation of distal interphalangeal joint of unspecified finger**

✓6ᵗʰ **S63.25** **Unspecified dislocation of other finger**

✓7ᵗʰ **S63.250** **Unspecified dislocation of right index finger**

✓7ᵗʰ **S63.251** **Unspecified dislocation of left index finger**

✓7ᵗʰ **S63.252** **Unspecified dislocation of right middle finger**

✓7ᵗʰ **S63.253** **Unspecified dislocation of left middle finger**

✓7ᵗʰ **S63.254** **Unspecified dislocation of right ring finger**

✓7ᵗʰ **S63.255** **Unspecified dislocation of left ring finger**

✓7ᵗʰ **S63.256** **Unspecified dislocation of right little finger**

✓7ᵗʰ **S63.257** **Unspecified dislocation of left little finger**

✓7ᵗʰ **S63.258** **Unspecified dislocation of other finger**
     Unspecified dislocation of specified finger with unspecified laterality

✓7ᵗʰ **S63.259** **Unspecified dislocation of unspecified finger**
     ►Unspecified dislocation of unspecified finger with unspecified laterality◄

✓6ᵗʰ **S63.26** **Dislocation of metacarpophalangeal joint of finger**

✓7ᵗʰ **S63.260** **Dislocation of metacarpophalangeal joint of right index finger**

✓7ᵗʰ **S63.261** **Dislocation of metacarpophalangeal joint of left index finger**

✓7ᵗʰ **S63.262** **Dislocation of metacarpophalangeal joint of right middle finger**

✓7ᵗʰ **S63.263** **Dislocation of metacarpophalangeal joint of left middle finger**

✓7ᵗʰ **S63.264** **Dislocation of metacarpophalangeal joint of right ring finger**

✓7ᵗʰ **S63.265** **Dislocation of metacarpophalangeal joint of left ring finger**

✓7ᵗʰ **S63.266** **Dislocation of metacarpophalangeal joint of right little finger**

✓7ᵗʰ **S63.267** **Dislocation of metacarpophalangeal joint of left little finger**

✓7ᵗʰ **S63.268** **Dislocation of metacarpophalangeal joint of other finger**
     Dislocation of metacarpophalangeal joint of specified finger with unspecified laterality

✓7ᵗʰ **S63.269** **Dislocation of metacarpophalangeal joint of unspecified finger**

✓6ᵗʰ **S63.27** **Dislocation of unspecified interphalangeal joint of finger**

✓7ᵗʰ **S63.270** **Dislocation of unspecified interphalangeal joint of right index finger**

✓7ᵗʰ **S63.271** **Dislocation of unspecified interphalangeal joint of left index finger**

✓7ᵗʰ **S63.272** **Dislocation of unspecified interphalangeal joint of right middle finger**

✓7ᵗʰ **S63.273** **Dislocation of unspecified interphalangeal joint of left middle finger**

✓7ᵗʰ **S63.274** **Dislocation of unspecified interphalangeal joint of right ring finger**

✓7ᵗʰ **S63.275** **Dislocation of unspecified interphalangeal joint of left ring finger**

✓7ᵗʰ **S63.276** **Dislocation of unspecified interphalangeal joint of right little finger**

✓7ᵗʰ **S63.277** **Dislocation of unspecified interphalangeal joint of left little finger**

✓7ᵗʰ **S63.278** **Dislocation of unspecified interphalangeal joint of other finger**
     Dislocation of unspecified interphalangeal joint of specified finger with unspecified laterality

✓7ᵗʰ **S63.279** **Dislocation of unspecified interphalangeal joint of unspecified finger**
     ►Dislocation of unspecified interphalangeal joint of unspecified finger without specified laterality◄

✓6ᵗʰ **S63.28** **Dislocation of proximal interphalangeal joint of finger**

✓7ᵗʰ **S63.280** **Dislocation of proximal interphalangeal joint of right index finger**

✓7ᵗʰ **S63.281** **Dislocation of proximal interphalangeal joint of left index finger**

✓7ᵗʰ **S63.282** **Dislocation of proximal interphalangeal joint of right middle finger**

✓7ᵗʰ **S63.283** **Dislocation of proximal interphalangeal joint of left middle finger**

✓7ᵗʰ **S63.284** **Dislocation of proximal interphalangeal joint of right ring finger**

✓7ᵗʰ **S63.285** **Dislocation of proximal interphalangeal joint of left ring finger**

✓7ᵗʰ **S63.286** **Dislocation of proximal interphalangeal joint of right little finger**

✓7ᵗʰ **S63.287** **Dislocation of proximal interphalangeal joint of left little finger**

✓7ᵗʰ **S63.288** **Dislocation of proximal interphalangeal joint of other finger**
     Dislocation of proximal interphalangeal joint of specified finger with unspecified laterality

✓7ᵗʰ **S63.289** **Dislocation of proximal interphalangeal joint of unspecified finger**

✓6ᵗʰ **S63.29** **Dislocation of distal interphalangeal joint of finger**

✓7ᵗʰ **S63.290** **Dislocation of distal interphalangeal joint of right index finger**

✓7ᵗʰ **S63.291** **Dislocation of distal interphalangeal joint of left index finger**

✓7ᵗʰ **S63.292** **Dislocation of distal interphalangeal joint of right middle finger**

✓7ᵗʰ **S63.293** **Dislocation of distal interphalangeal joint of left middle finger**

✓7ᵗʰ **S63.294** **Dislocation of distal interphalangeal joint of right ring finger**

✓7ᵗʰ **S63.295** **Dislocation of distal interphalangeal joint of left ring finger**

✓7ᵗʰ **S63.296** **Dislocation of distal interphalangeal joint of right little finger**

✓7ᵗʰ **S63.297** **Dislocation of distal interphalangeal joint of left little finger**

✓7ᵗʰ **S63.298** **Dislocation of distal interphalangeal joint of other finger**
     Dislocation of distal interphalangeal joint of specified finger with unspecified laterality

✓Additional Character Req   ✓x7ᵗʰ Placeholder Alert   Unacceptable PDx   Manifestation   H1-H14 HAC   HCC CMS-HCC Condition   *EXCLUDES 1* Not Coded Here   *EXCLUDES 2* Not Included Here

ICD-10-CM 2018   1025

√7ᵗʰ **S63.299** Dislocation of distal interphalangeal joint of unspecified finger

√5ᵗʰ **S63.3** Traumatic rupture of ligament of wrist

√6ᵗʰ **S63.30** Traumatic rupture of unspecified ligament of wrist

√7ᵗʰ **S63.301** Traumatic rupture of unspecified ligament of right wrist

√7ᵗʰ **S63.302** Traumatic rupture of unspecified ligament of left wrist

√7ᵗʰ **S63.309** Traumatic rupture of unspecified ligament of unspecified wrist

√6ᵗʰ **S63.31** Traumatic rupture of collateral ligament of wrist

√7ᵗʰ **S63.311** Traumatic rupture of collateral ligament of right wrist

√7ᵗʰ **S63.312** Traumatic rupture of collateral ligament of left wrist

√7ᵗʰ **S63.319** Traumatic rupture of collateral ligament of unspecified wrist

√6ᵗʰ **S63.32** Traumatic rupture of radiocarpal ligament

√7ᵗʰ **S63.321** Traumatic rupture of right radiocarpal ligament

√7ᵗʰ **S63.322** Traumatic rupture of left radiocarpal ligament

√7ᵗʰ **S63.329** Traumatic rupture of unspecified radiocarpal ligament

√6ᵗʰ **S63.33** Traumatic rupture of ulnocarpal (palmar) ligament

√7ᵗʰ **S63.331** Traumatic rupture of right ulnocarpal (palmar) ligament

√7ᵗʰ **S63.332** Traumatic rupture of left ulnocarpal (palmar) ligament

√7ᵗʰ **S63.339** Traumatic rupture of unspecified ulnocarpal (palmar) ligament

√6ᵗʰ **S63.39** Traumatic rupture of other ligament of wrist

√7ᵗʰ **S63.391** Traumatic rupture of other ligament of right wrist

√7ᵗʰ **S63.392** Traumatic rupture of other ligament of left wrist

√7ᵗʰ **S63.399** Traumatic rupture of other ligament of unspecified wrist

√5ᵗʰ **S63.4** Traumatic rupture of ligament of finger at metacarpophalangeal and interphalangeal joint(s)

√6ᵗʰ **S63.40** Traumatic rupture of unspecified ligament of finger at metacarpophalangeal and interphalangeal joint

√7ᵗʰ **S63.400** Traumatic rupture of unspecified ligament of right index finger at metacarpophalangeal and interphalangeal joint

√7ᵗʰ **S63.401** Traumatic rupture of unspecified ligament of left index finger at metacarpophalangeal and interphalangeal joint

√7ᵗʰ **S63.402** Traumatic rupture of unspecified ligament of right middle finger at metacarpophalangeal and interphalangeal joint

√7ᵗʰ **S63.403** Traumatic rupture of unspecified ligament of left middle finger at metacarpophalangeal and interphalangeal joint

√7ᵗʰ **S63.404** Traumatic rupture of unspecified ligament of right ring finger at metacarpophalangeal and interphalangeal joint

√7ᵗʰ **S63.405** Traumatic rupture of unspecified ligament of left ring finger at metacarpophalangeal and interphalangeal joint

√7ᵗʰ **S63.406** Traumatic rupture of unspecified ligament of right little finger at metacarpophalangeal and interphalangeal joint

√7ᵗʰ **S63.407** Traumatic rupture of unspecified ligament of left little finger at metacarpophalangeal and interphalangeal joint

√7ᵗʰ **S63.408** Traumatic rupture of unspecified ligament of other finger at metacarpophalangeal and interphalangeal joint

Traumatic rupture of unspecified ligament of specified finger with unspecified laterality at metacarpophalangeal and interphalangeal joint

√7ᵗʰ **S63.409** Traumatic rupture of unspecified ligament of unspecified finger at metacarpophalangeal and interphalangeal joint

√6ᵗʰ **S63.41** Traumatic rupture of collateral ligament of finger at metacarpophalangeal and interphalangeal joint

√7ᵗʰ **S63.410** Traumatic rupture of collateral ligament of right index finger at metacarpophalangeal and interphalangeal joint

√7ᵗʰ **S63.411** Traumatic rupture of collateral ligament of left index finger at metacarpophalangeal and interphalangeal joint

√7ᵗʰ **S63.412** Traumatic rupture of collateral ligament of right middle finger at metacarpophalangeal and interphalangeal joint

√7ᵗʰ **S63.413** Traumatic rupture of collateral ligament of left middle finger at metacarpophalangeal and interphalangeal joint

√7ᵗʰ **S63.414** Traumatic rupture of collateral ligament of right ring finger at metacarpophalangeal and interphalangeal joint

√7ᵗʰ **S63.415** Traumatic rupture of collateral ligament of left ring finger at metacarpophalangeal and interphalangeal joint

√7ᵗʰ **S63.416** Traumatic rupture of collateral ligament of right little finger at metacarpophalangeal and interphalangeal joint

√7ᵗʰ **S63.417** Traumatic rupture of collateral ligament of left little finger at metacarpophalangeal and interphalangeal joint

√7ᵗʰ **S63.418** Traumatic rupture of collateral ligament of other finger at metacarpophalangeal and interphalangeal joint

Traumatic rupture of collateral ligament of specified finger with unspecified laterality at metacarpophalangeal and interphalangeal joint

√7ᵗʰ **S63.419** Traumatic rupture of collateral ligament of unspecified finger at metacarpophalangeal and interphalangeal joint

√6ᵗʰ **S63.42** Traumatic rupture of palmar ligament of finger at metacarpophalangeal and interphalangeal joint

√7ᵗʰ **S63.420** Traumatic rupture of palmar ligament of right index finger at metacarpophalangeal and interphalangeal joint

√7ᵗʰ **S63.421** Traumatic rupture of palmar ligament of left index finger at metacarpophalangeal and interphalangeal joint

√7ᵗʰ **S63.422** Traumatic rupture of palmar ligament of right middle finger at metacarpophalangeal and interphalangeal joint

√7ᵗʰ **S63.423** Traumatic rupture of palmar ligament of left middle finger at metacarpophalangeal and interphalangeal joint

√7ᵗʰ **S63.424** Traumatic rupture of palmar ligament of right ring finger at metacarpophalangeal and interphalangeal joint

√7ᵗʰ **S63.425** Traumatic rupture of palmar ligament of left ring finger at metacarpophalangeal and interphalangeal joint

√7ᵗʰ **S63.426** Traumatic rupture of palmar ligament of right little finger at metacarpophalangeal and interphalangeal joint

Ⓝ Newborn: 0 Ⓟ Pediatric: 0-17 Ⓜ Maternity: 12-55 Ⓐ Adult: 15-124 **MCC** Major CC Condition **PDxMCC** PDx acts as own MCC **CC** CC Condition **PDxCC** PDx acts as own CC

1026 ICD-10-CM 2018

√7ᵗʰ **S63.427** Traumatic rupture of palmar ligament of left little finger at metacarpophalangeal and interphalangeal joint

√7ᵗʰ **S63.428** Traumatic rupture of palmar ligament of other finger at metacarpophalangeal and interphalangeal joint

Traumatic rupture of palmar ligament of specified finger with unspecified laterality at metacarpophalangeal and interphalangeal joint

√7ᵗʰ **S63.429** Traumatic rupture of palmar ligament of unspecified finger at metacarpophalangeal and interphalangeal joint

√6ᵗʰ **S63.43** Traumatic rupture of volar plate of finger at metacarpophalangeal and interphalangeal joint

√7ᵗʰ **S63.430** Traumatic rupture of volar plate of right index finger at metacarpophalangeal and interphalangeal joint

√7ᵗʰ **S63.431** Traumatic rupture of volar plate of left index finger at metacarpophalangeal and interphalangeal joint

√7ᵗʰ **S63.432** Traumatic rupture of volar plate of right middle finger at metacarpophalangeal and interphalangeal joint

√7ᵗʰ **S63.433** Traumatic rupture of volar plate of left middle finger at metacarpophalangeal and interphalangeal joint

√7ᵗʰ **S63.434** Traumatic rupture of volar plate of right ring finger at metacarpophalangeal and interphalangeal joint

√7ᵗʰ **S63.435** Traumatic rupture of volar plate of left ring finger at metacarpophalangeal and interphalangeal joint

√7ᵗʰ **S63.436** Traumatic rupture of volar plate of right little finger at metacarpophalangeal and interphalangeal joint

√7ᵗʰ **S63.437** Traumatic rupture of volar plate of left little finger at metacarpophalangeal and interphalangeal joint

√7ᵗʰ **S63.438** Traumatic rupture of volar plate of other finger at metacarpophalangeal and interphalangeal joint

Traumatic rupture of volar plate of specified finger with unspecified laterality at metacarpophalangeal and interphalangeal joint

√7ᵗʰ **S63.439** Traumatic rupture of volar plate of unspecified finger at metacarpophalangeal and interphalangeal joint

√6ᵗʰ **S63.49** Traumatic rupture of other ligament of finger at metacarpophalangeal and interphalangeal joint

√7ᵗʰ **S63.490** Traumatic rupture of other ligament of right index finger at metacarpophalangeal and interphalangeal joint

√7ᵗʰ **S63.491** Traumatic rupture of other ligament of left index finger at metacarpophalangeal and interphalangeal joint

√7ᵗʰ **S63.492** Traumatic rupture of other ligament of right middle finger at metacarpophalangeal and interphalangeal joint

√7ᵗʰ **S63.493** Traumatic rupture of other ligament of left middle finger at metacarpophalangeal and interphalangeal joint

√7ᵗʰ **S63.494** Traumatic rupture of other ligament of right ring finger at metacarpophalangeal and interphalangeal joint

√7ᵗʰ **S63.495** Traumatic rupture of other ligament of left ring finger at metacarpophalangeal and interphalangeal joint

√7ᵗʰ **S63.496** Traumatic rupture of other ligament of right little finger at metacarpophalangeal and interphalangeal joint

√7ᵗʰ **S63.497** Traumatic rupture of other ligament of left little finger at metacarpophalangeal and interphalangeal joint

√7ᵗʰ **S63.498** Traumatic rupture of other ligament of other finger at metacarpophalangeal and interphalangeal joint

Traumatic rupture of ligament of specified finger with unspecified laterality at metacarpophalangeal and interphalangeal joint

√7ᵗʰ **S63.499** Traumatic rupture of other ligament of unspecified finger at metacarpophalangeal and interphalangeal joint

√5ᵗʰ **S63.5** Other and unspecified sprain of wrist

√6ᵗʰ **S63.50** Unspecified sprain of wrist

√7ᵗʰ **S63.501** Unspecified sprain of right wrist

√7ᵗʰ **S63.502** Unspecified sprain of left wrist

√7ᵗʰ **S63.509** Unspecified sprain of unspecified wrist

√6ᵗʰ **S63.51** Sprain of carpal (joint)

√7ᵗʰ **S63.511** Sprain of carpal joint of right wrist

√7ᵗʰ **S63.512** Sprain of carpal joint of left wrist

√7ᵗʰ **S63.519** Sprain of carpal joint of unspecified wrist

√6ᵗʰ **S63.52** Sprain of radiocarpal joint

EXCLUDES 1   *traumatic rupture of radiocarpal ligament (S63.32-)*

√7ᵗʰ **S63.521** Sprain of radiocarpal joint of right wrist

√7ᵗʰ **S63.522** Sprain of radiocarpal joint of left wrist

√7ᵗʰ **S63.529** Sprain of radiocarpal joint of unspecified wrist

√6ᵗʰ **S63.59** Other specified sprain of wrist

√7ᵗʰ **S63.591** Other specified sprain of right wrist

√7ᵗʰ **S63.592** Other specified sprain of left wrist

√7ᵗʰ **S63.599** Other specified sprain of unspecified wrist

√5ᵗʰ **S63.6** Other and unspecified sprain of finger(s)

EXCLUDES 1   *traumatic rupture of ligament of finger at metacarpophalangeal and interphalangeal joint(s) (S63.4-)*

√6ᵗʰ **S63.60** Unspecified sprain of thumb

√7ᵗʰ **S63.601** Unspecified sprain of right thumb

√7ᵗʰ **S63.602** Unspecified sprain of left thumb

√7ᵗʰ **S63.609** Unspecified sprain of unspecified thumb

√6ᵗʰ **S63.61** Unspecified sprain of other and unspecified finger(s)

√7ᵗʰ **S63.610** Unspecified sprain of right index finger

√7ᵗʰ **S63.611** Unspecified sprain of left index finger

√7ᵗʰ **S63.612** Unspecified sprain of right middle finger

√7ᵗʰ **S63.613** Unspecified sprain of left middle finger

√7ᵗʰ **S63.614** Unspecified sprain of right ring finger

√7ᵗʰ **S63.615** Unspecified sprain of left ring finger

√7ᵗʰ **S63.616** Unspecified sprain of right little finger

√7ᵗʰ **S63.617** Unspecified sprain of left little finger

√7ᵗʰ **S63.618** Unspecified sprain of other finger

Unspecified sprain of specified finger with unspecified laterality

√7ᵗʰ **S63.619** Unspecified sprain of unspecified finger

√6ᵗʰ **S63.62** Sprain of interphalangeal joint of thumb

√7ᵗʰ **S63.621** Sprain of interphalangeal joint of right thumb

√7ᵗʰ **S63.622** Sprain of interphalangeal joint of left thumb

√7ᵗʰ **S63.629** Sprain of interphalangeal joint of unspecified thumb

√6ᵗʰ **S63.63** Sprain of interphalangeal joint of other and unspecified finger(s)

√7ᵗʰ **S63.630** Sprain of interphalangeal joint of right index finger

√7ᵗʰ **S63.631** Sprain of interphalangeal joint of left index finger

√7ᵗʰ **S63.632** Sprain of interphalangeal joint of right middle finger

√7ᵗʰ **S63.633** Sprain of interphalangeal joint of left middle finger

√7ᵗʰ **S63.634** Sprain of interphalangeal joint of right ring finger

√7ᵗʰ **S63.635** Sprain of interphalangeal joint of left ring finger

---

√7th **S63.636** Sprain of interphalangeal joint of right little finger

√7th **S63.637** Sprain of interphalangeal joint of left little finger

√7th **S63.638** Sprain of interphalangeal joint of other finger

√7th **S63.639** Sprain of interphalangeal joint of unspecified finger

√6th **S63.64** Sprain of metacarpophalangeal joint of thumb

√7th **S63.641** Sprain of metacarpophalangeal joint of right thumb

√7th **S63.642** Sprain of metacarpophalangeal joint of left thumb

√7th **S63.649** Sprain of metacarpophalangeal joint of unspecified thumb

√6th **S63.65** Sprain of metacarpophalangeal joint of other and unspecified finger(s)

√7th **S63.650** Sprain of metacarpophalangeal joint of right index finger

√7th **S63.651** Sprain of metacarpophalangeal joint of left index finger

√7th **S63.652** Sprain of metacarpophalangeal joint of right middle finger

√7th **S63.653** Sprain of metacarpophalangeal joint of left middle finger

√7th **S63.654** Sprain of metacarpophalangeal joint of right ring finger

√7th **S63.655** Sprain of metacarpophalangeal joint of left ring finger

√7th **S63.656** Sprain of metacarpophalangeal joint of right little finger

√7th **S63.657** Sprain of metacarpophalangeal joint of left little finger

√7th **S63.658** Sprain of metacarpophalangeal joint of other finger
Sprain of metacarpophalangeal joint of specified finger with unspecified laterality

√7th **S63.659** Sprain of metacarpophalangeal joint of unspecified finger

√6th **S63.68** Other sprain of thumb

√7th **S63.681** Other sprain of right thumb

√7th **S63.682** Other sprain of left thumb

√7th **S63.689** Other sprain of unspecified thumb

√6th **S63.69** Other sprain of other and unspecified finger(s)

√7th **S63.690** Other sprain of right index finger

√7th **S63.691** Other sprain of left index finger

√7th **S63.692** Other sprain of right middle finger

√7th **S63.693** Other sprain of left middle finger

√7th **S63.694** Other sprain of right ring finger

√7th **S63.695** Other sprain of left ring finger

√7th **S63.696** Other sprain of right little finger

√7th **S63.697** Other sprain of left little finger

√7th **S63.698** Other sprain of other finger
Other sprain of specified finger with unspecified laterality

√7th **S63.699** Other sprain of unspecified finger

√5th **S63.8** Sprain of other part of wrist and hand

√6th **S63.8X** Sprain of other part of wrist and hand

√7th **S63.8X1** Sprain of other part of right wrist and hand

√7th **S63.8X2** Sprain of other part of left wrist and hand

√7th **S63.8X9** Sprain of other part of unspecified wrist and hand

√5th **S63.9** Sprain of unspecified part of wrist and hand

√x7th **S63.90** Sprain of unspecified part of unspecified wrist and hand

√x7th **S63.91** Sprain of unspecified part of right wrist and hand

√x7th **S63.92** Sprain of unspecified part of left wrist and hand

√4th **S64** Injury of nerves at wrist and hand level
Code also any associated open wound (S61.-)

> The appropriate 7th character is to be added to each code from category S64.
> A   initial encounter
> D   subsequent encounter
> S   sequela

√5th **S64.0** Injury of ulnar nerve at wrist and hand level

√x7th **S64.00** Injury of ulnar nerve at wrist and hand level of unspecified arm

√x7th **S64.01** Injury of ulnar nerve at wrist and hand level of right arm

√x7th **S64.02** Injury of ulnar nerve at wrist and hand level of left arm

√5th **S64.1** Injury of median nerve at wrist and hand level

√x7th **S64.10** Injury of median nerve at wrist and hand level of unspecified arm

√x7th **S64.11** Injury of median nerve at wrist and hand level of right arm

√x7th **S64.12** Injury of median nerve at wrist and hand level of left arm

√5th **S64.2** Injury of radial nerve at wrist and hand level

√x7th **S64.20** Injury of radial nerve at wrist and hand level of unspecified arm

√x7th **S64.21** Injury of radial nerve at wrist and hand level of right arm

√x7th **S64.22** Injury of radial nerve at wrist and hand level of left arm

√5th **S64.3** Injury of digital nerve of thumb

√x7th **S64.30** Injury of digital nerve of unspecified thumb

√x7th **S64.31** Injury of digital nerve of right thumb

√x7th **S64.32** Injury of digital nerve of left thumb

√5th **S64.4** Injury of digital nerve of other and unspecified finger

√x7th **S64.40** Injury of digital nerve of unspecified finger

√6th **S64.49** Injury of digital nerve of other finger

√7th **S64.490** Injury of digital nerve of right index finger

√7th **S64.491** Injury of digital nerve of left index finger

√7th **S64.492** Injury of digital nerve of right middle finger

√7th **S64.493** Injury of digital nerve of left middle finger

√7th **S64.494** Injury of digital nerve of right ring finger

√7th **S64.495** Injury of digital nerve of left ring finger

√7th **S64.496** Injury of digital nerve of right little finger

√7th **S64.497** Injury of digital nerve of left little finger

√7th **S64.498** Injury of digital nerve of other finger
Injury of digital nerve of specified finger with unspecified laterality

√5th **S64.8** Injury of other nerves at wrist and hand level

√6th **S64.8X** Injury of other nerves at wrist and hand level

√7th **S64.8X1** Injury of other nerves at wrist and hand level of right arm

√7th **S64.8X2** Injury of other nerves at wrist and hand level of left arm

√7th **S64.8X9** Injury of other nerves at wrist and hand level of unspecified arm

√5th **S64.9** Injury of unspecified nerve at wrist and hand level

√x7th **S64.90** Injury of unspecified nerve at wrist and hand level of unspecified arm

√x7th **S64.91** Injury of unspecified nerve at wrist and hand level of right arm

√x7th **S64.92** Injury of unspecified nerve at wrist and hand level of left arm

✓4th S65   Injury of blood vessels at wrist and hand level

Code also any associated open wound (S61.-)

The appropriate 7th character is to be added to each code from category S65.
- A   initial encounter
- D   subsequent encounter
- S   sequela

✓5th S65.0   Injury of ulnar artery at wrist and hand level

CC Excl: For CC codes in subcategory S65.0:
Right side: PDX collection 1274
Left side: PDX collection 1275
Unspecified side: PDX collection 1276

✓6th S65.00   Unspecified injury of ulnar artery at wrist and hand level

   ✓7th **S65.001**   Unspecified injury of ulnar artery at wrist and hand level of right arm   CC

   ✓7th **S65.002**   Unspecified injury of ulnar artery at wrist and hand level of left arm   CC

   ✓7th **S65.009**   Unspecified injury of ulnar artery at wrist and hand level of unspecified arm   CC

✓6th S65.01   Laceration of ulnar artery at wrist and hand level

   ✓7th **S65.011**   Laceration of ulnar artery at wrist and hand level of right arm   CC

   ✓7th **S65.012**   Laceration of ulnar artery at wrist and hand level of left arm   CC

   ✓7th **S65.019**   Laceration of ulnar artery at wrist and hand level of unspecified arm   CC

✓6th S65.09   Other specified injury of ulnar artery at wrist and hand level

   ✓7th **S65.091**   Other specified injury of ulnar artery at wrist and hand level of right arm   CC

   ✓7th **S65.092**   Other specified injury of ulnar artery at wrist and hand level of left arm   CC

   ✓7th **S65.099**   Other specified injury of ulnar artery at wrist and hand level of unspecified arm   CC

✓5th S65.1   Injury of radial artery at wrist and hand level

CC Excl: For CC codes in subcategory S65.1:
Right side: PDX collection 1277
Left side: PDX collection 1278
Unspecified side: PDX collection 1279

✓6th S65.10   Unspecified injury of radial artery at wrist and hand level

   ✓7th **S65.101**   Unspecified injury of radial artery at wrist and hand level of right arm   CC

   ✓7th **S65.102**   Unspecified injury of radial artery at wrist and hand level of left arm   CC

   ✓7th **S65.109**   Unspecified injury of radial artery at wrist and hand level of unspecified arm   CC

✓6th S65.11   Laceration of radial artery at wrist and hand level

   ✓7th **S65.111**   Laceration of radial artery at wrist and hand level of right arm   CC

   ✓7th **S65.112**   Laceration of radial artery at wrist and hand level of left arm   CC

   ✓7th **S65.119**   Laceration of radial artery at wrist and hand level of unspecified arm   CC

✓6th S65.19   Other specified injury of radial artery at wrist and hand level

   ✓7th **S65.191**   Other specified injury of radial artery at wrist and hand level of right arm   CC

   ✓7th **S65.192**   Other specified injury of radial artery at wrist and hand level of left arm   CC

   ✓7th **S65.199**   Other specified injury of radial artery at wrist and hand level of unspecified arm   CC

✓5th S65.2   Injury of superficial palmar arch

CC Excl: For CC codes in subcategory S65.2:
Right side: PDX collection 1288
Left side: PDX collection 1289
Unspecified side: PDX collection 1290

✓6th S65.20   Unspecified injury of superficial palmar arch

   ✓7th **S65.201**   Unspecified injury of superficial palmar arch of right hand   CC

   ✓7th **S65.202**   Unspecified injury of superficial palmar arch of left hand   CC

   ✓7th **S65.209**   Unspecified injury of superficial palmar arch of unspecified hand   CC

✓6th S65.21   Laceration of superficial palmar arch

   ✓7th **S65.211**   Laceration of superficial palmar arch of right hand   CC

   ✓7th **S65.212**   Laceration of superficial palmar arch of left hand   CC

   ✓7th **S65.219**   Laceration of superficial palmar arch of unspecified hand   CC

✓6th S65.29   Other specified injury of superficial palmar arch

   ✓7th **S65.291**   Other specified injury of superficial palmar arch of right hand   CC

   ✓7th **S65.292**   Other specified injury of superficial palmar arch of left hand   CC

   ✓7th **S65.299**   Other specified injury of superficial palmar arch of unspecified hand   CC

✓5th S65.3   Injury of deep palmar arch

CC Excl: For CC codes in subcategory S65.3:
Right side: PDX collection 1288
Left side: PDX collection 1289
Unspecified side: PDX collection 1290

✓6th S65.30   Unspecified injury of deep palmar arch

   ✓7th **S65.301**   Unspecified injury of deep palmar arch of right hand   CC

   ✓7th **S65.302**   Unspecified injury of deep palmar arch of left hand   CC

   ✓7th **S65.309**   Unspecified injury of deep palmar arch of unspecified hand   CC

✓6th S65.31   Laceration of deep palmar arch

   ✓7th **S65.311**   Laceration of deep palmar arch of right hand   CC

   ✓7th **S65.312**   Laceration of deep palmar arch of left hand   CC

   ✓7th **S65.319**   Laceration of deep palmar arch of unspecified hand   CC

✓6th S65.39   Other specified injury of deep palmar arch

   ✓7th **S65.391**   Other specified injury of deep palmar arch of right hand   CC

   ✓7th **S65.392**   Other specified injury of deep palmar arch of left hand   CC

   ✓7th **S65.399**   Other specified injury of deep palmar arch of unspecified hand   CC

✓5th S65.4   Injury of blood vessel of thumb

CC Excl: For CC codes in subcategory S65.4:
Right side: PDX collection 1291
Left side: PDX collection 1292
Unspecified side: PDX collection 1293

✓6th S65.40   Unspecified injury of blood vessel of thumb

   ✓7th **S65.401**   Unspecified injury of blood vessel of right thumb   CC

   ✓7th **S65.402**   Unspecified injury of blood vessel of left thumb   CC

   ✓7th **S65.409**   Unspecified injury of blood vessel of unspecified thumb   CC

✓6th S65.41   Laceration of blood vessel of thumb

   ✓7th **S65.411**   Laceration of blood vessel of right thumb   CC

   ✓7th **S65.412**   Laceration of blood vessel of left thumb   CC

   ✓7th **S65.419**   Laceration of blood vessel of unspecified thumb   CC

✓6th S65.49   Other specified injury of blood vessel of thumb

   ✓7th **S65.491**   Other specified injury of blood vessel of right thumb   CC

   ✓7th **S65.492**   Other specified injury of blood vessel of left thumb   CC

   ✓7th **S65.499**   Other specified injury of blood vessel of unspecified thumb   CC

✓ Additional Character Req   ✓x7th Placeholder Alert   Unacceptable PDx   Manifestation   H1–H14 HAC   HCC CMS-HCC Condition   EXCLUDES 1 Not Coded Here   EXCLUDES 2 Not Included Here

Chapter 19. Injury, Poisoning and Certain Other Consequences of External Causes *(left margin)*

S65.5–S65.991 *(left margin)*

√5ᵗʰ **S65.5**　Injury of blood vessel of other and unspecified finger

> **CC Excl: For CC codes in subcategory S65.5:**
> **Right side:** PDX collection 1291
> **Left side:** PDX collection 1292
> **Other or unspecified side:** PDX collection 1293

√6ᵗʰ **S65.50**　Unspecified injury of blood vessel of other and unspecified finger

√7ᵗʰ **S65.500**　Unspecified injury of blood vessel of right index finger　CC

√7ᵗʰ **S65.501**　Unspecified injury of blood vessel of left index finger　CC

√7ᵗʰ **S65.502**　Unspecified injury of blood vessel of right middle finger　CC

√7ᵗʰ **S65.503**　Unspecified injury of blood vessel of left middle finger　CC

√7ᵗʰ **S65.504**　Unspecified injury of blood vessel of right ring finger　CC

√7ᵗʰ **S65.505**　Unspecified injury of blood vessel of left ring finger　CC

√7ᵗʰ **S65.506**　Unspecified injury of blood vessel of right little finger　CC

√7ᵗʰ **S65.507**　Unspecified injury of blood vessel of left little finger　CC

√7ᵗʰ **S65.508**　Unspecified injury of blood vessel of other finger　CC
> Unspecified injury of blood vessel of specified finger with unspecified laterality

√7ᵗʰ **S65.509**　Unspecified injury of blood vessel of unspecified finger　CC

√6ᵗʰ **S65.51**　Laceration of blood vessel of other and unspecified finger

√7ᵗʰ **S65.510**　Laceration of blood vessel of right index finger　CC

√7ᵗʰ **S65.511**　Laceration of blood vessel of left index finger　CC

√7ᵗʰ **S65.512**　Laceration of blood vessel of right middle finger　CC

√7ᵗʰ **S65.513**　Laceration of blood vessel of left middle finger　CC

√7ᵗʰ **S65.514**　Laceration of blood vessel of right ring finger　CC

√7ᵗʰ **S65.515**　Laceration of blood vessel of left ring finger　CC

√7ᵗʰ **S65.516**　Laceration of blood vessel of right little finger　CC

√7ᵗʰ **S65.517**　Laceration of blood vessel of left little finger　CC

√7ᵗʰ **S65.518**　Laceration of blood vessel of other finger　CC
> Laceration of blood vessel of specified finger with unspecified laterality

√7ᵗʰ **S65.519**　Laceration of blood vessel of unspecified finger　CC

√6ᵗʰ **S65.59**　Other specified injury of blood vessel of other and unspecified finger

√7ᵗʰ **S65.590**　Other specified injury of blood vessel of right index finger　CC

√7ᵗʰ **S65.591**　Other specified injury of blood vessel of left index finger　CC

√7ᵗʰ **S65.592**　Other specified injury of blood vessel of right middle finger　CC

√7ᵗʰ **S65.593**　Other specified injury of blood vessel of left middle finger　CC

√7ᵗʰ **S65.594**　Other specified injury of blood vessel of right ring finger　CC

√7ᵗʰ **S65.595**　Other specified injury of blood vessel of left ring finger　CC

√7ᵗʰ **S65.596**　Other specified injury of blood vessel of right little finger　CC

√7ᵗʰ **S65.597**　Other specified injury of blood vessel of left little finger　CC

√7ᵗʰ **S65.598**　Other specified injury of blood vessel of other finger　CC
> Other specified injury of blood vessel of specified finger with unspecified laterality

√7ᵗʰ **S65.599**　Other specified injury of blood vessel of unspecified finger　CC

√5ᵗʰ **S65.8**　Injury of other blood vessels at wrist and hand level

> **CC Excl: For CC codes in subcategory S65.8:**
> **Right side:** PDX collection 1260
> **Left side:** PDX collection 1261
> **Unspecified side:** PDX collection 1262

√6ᵗʰ **S65.80**　Unspecified injury of other blood vessels at wrist and hand level

√7ᵗʰ **S65.801**　Unspecified injury of other blood vessels at wrist and hand level of right arm　CC

√7ᵗʰ **S65.802**　Unspecified injury of other blood vessels at wrist and hand level of left arm　CC

√7ᵗʰ **S65.809**　Unspecified injury of other blood vessels at wrist and hand level of unspecified arm　CC

√6ᵗʰ **S65.81**　Laceration of other blood vessels at wrist and hand level

√7ᵗʰ **S65.811**　Laceration of other blood vessels at wrist and hand level of right arm　CC

√7ᵗʰ **S65.812**　Laceration of other blood vessels at wrist and hand level of left arm　CC

√7ᵗʰ **S65.819**　Laceration of other blood vessels at wrist and hand level of unspecified arm　CC

√6ᵗʰ **S65.89**　Other specified injury of other blood vessels at wrist and hand level

√7ᵗʰ **S65.891**　Other specified injury of other blood vessels at wrist and hand level of right arm　CC

√7ᵗʰ **S65.892**　Other specified injury of other blood vessels at wrist and hand level of left arm　CC

√7ᵗʰ **S65.899**　Other specified injury of other blood vessels at wrist and hand level of unspecified arm　CC

√5ᵗʰ **S65.9**　Injury of unspecified blood vessel at wrist and hand level

> **CC Excl: For CC codes in subcategory S65.9:**
> **Right side:** PDX collection 1260
> **Left side:** PDX collection 1261
> **Unspecified side:** PDX collection 1262

√6ᵗʰ **S65.90**　Unspecified injury of unspecified blood vessel at wrist and hand level

√7ᵗʰ **S65.901**　Unspecified injury of unspecified blood vessel at wrist and hand level of right arm　CC

√7ᵗʰ **S65.902**　Unspecified injury of unspecified blood vessel at wrist and hand level of left arm　CC

√7ᵗʰ **S65.909**　Unspecified injury of unspecified blood vessel at wrist and hand level of unspecified arm　CC

√6ᵗʰ **S65.91**　Laceration of unspecified blood vessel at wrist and hand level

√7ᵗʰ **S65.911**　Laceration of unspecified blood vessel at wrist and hand level of right arm　CC

√7ᵗʰ **S65.912**　Laceration of unspecified blood vessel at wrist and hand level of left arm　CC

√7ᵗʰ **S65.919**　Laceration of unspecified blood vessel at wrist and hand level of unspecified arm　CC

√6ᵗʰ **S65.99**　Other specified injury of unspecified blood vessel at wrist and hand level

√7ᵗʰ **S65.991**　Other specified injury of unspecified blood vessel at wrist and hand of right arm　CC

√7ᵗʰ **S65.992** Other specified injury of unspecified blood vessel at wrist and hand of left arm　**CC**

√7ᵗʰ **S65.999** Other specified injury of unspecified blood vessel at wrist and hand of unspecified arm　**CC**

√4ᵗʰ **S66 Injury of muscle, fascia and tendon at wrist and hand level**
Code also any associated open wound (S61.-)
EXCLUDES 2 sprain of joints and ligaments of wrist and hand (S63.-)
TIP: Refer to the Muscle/Tendon table at the beginning of this chapter.

The appropriate 7th character is to be added to each code from category S66.
A　initial encounter
D　subsequent encounter
S　sequela

CC Excl: For CC codes in category S66:
Right side: PDX collection 1294
Left side: PDX collection 1295
Other or unspecified side: PDX collection 1296

√5ᵗʰ **S66.0 Injury of long flexor muscle, fascia and tendon of thumb at wrist and hand level**

√6ᵗʰ **S66.00** Unspecified injury of long flexor muscle, fascia and tendon of thumb at wrist and hand level

√7ᵗʰ **S66.001** Unspecified injury of long flexor muscle, fascia and tendon of right thumb at wrist and hand level

√7ᵗʰ **S66.002** Unspecified injury of long flexor muscle, fascia and tendon of left thumb at wrist and hand level

√7ᵗʰ **S66.009** Unspecified injury of long flexor muscle, fascia and tendon of unspecified thumb at wrist and hand level

√6ᵗʰ **S66.01** Strain of long flexor muscle, fascia and tendon of thumb at wrist and hand level

√7ᵗʰ **S66.011** Strain of long flexor muscle, fascia and tendon of right thumb at wrist and hand level

√7ᵗʰ **S66.012** Strain of long flexor muscle, fascia and tendon of left thumb at wrist and hand level

√7ᵗʰ **S66.019** Strain of long flexor muscle, fascia and tendon of unspecified thumb at wrist and hand level

√6ᵗʰ **S66.02** Laceration of long flexor muscle, fascia and tendon of thumb at wrist and hand level

√7ᵗʰ **S66.021** Laceration of long flexor muscle, fascia and tendon of right thumb at wrist and hand level　**CC**

√7ᵗʰ **S66.022** Laceration of long flexor muscle, fascia and tendon of left thumb at wrist and hand level　**CC**

√7ᵗʰ **S66.029** Laceration of long flexor muscle, fascia and tendon of unspecified thumb at wrist and hand level　**CC**

√6ᵗʰ **S66.09** Other specified injury of long flexor muscle, fascia and tendon of thumb at wrist and hand level

√7ᵗʰ **S66.091** Other specified injury of long flexor muscle, fascia and tendon of right thumb at wrist and hand level

√7ᵗʰ **S66.092** Other specified injury of long flexor muscle, fascia and tendon of left thumb at wrist and hand level

√7ᵗʰ **S66.099** Other specified injury of long flexor muscle, fascia and tendon of unspecified thumb at wrist and hand level

√5ᵗʰ **S66.1 Injury of flexor muscle, fascia and tendon of other and unspecified finger at wrist and hand level**
EXCLUDES 2 Injury of long flexor muscle, fascia and tendon of thumb at wrist and hand level (S66.0-)

√6ᵗʰ **S66.10** Unspecified injury of flexor muscle, fascia and tendon of other and unspecified finger at wrist and hand level

√7ᵗʰ **S66.100** Unspecified injury of flexor muscle, fascia and tendon of right index finger at wrist and hand level

√7ᵗʰ **S66.101** Unspecified injury of flexor muscle, fascia and tendon of left index finger at wrist and hand level

√7ᵗʰ **S66.102** Unspecified injury of flexor muscle, fascia and tendon of right middle finger at wrist and hand level

√7ᵗʰ **S66.103** Unspecified injury of flexor muscle, fascia and tendon of left middle finger at wrist and hand level

√7ᵗʰ **S66.104** Unspecified injury of flexor muscle, fascia and tendon of right ring finger at wrist and hand level

√7ᵗʰ **S66.105** Unspecified injury of flexor muscle, fascia and tendon of left ring finger at wrist and hand level

√7ᵗʰ **S66.106** Unspecified injury of flexor muscle, fascia and tendon of right little finger at wrist and hand level

√7ᵗʰ **S66.107** Unspecified injury of flexor muscle, fascia and tendon of left little finger at wrist and hand level

√7ᵗʰ **S66.108** Unspecified injury of flexor muscle, fascia and tendon of other finger at wrist and hand level
Unspecified injury of flexor muscle, fascia and tendon of specified finger with unspecified laterality at wrist and hand level

√7ᵗʰ **S66.109** Unspecified injury of flexor muscle, fascia and tendon of unspecified finger at wrist and hand level

√6ᵗʰ **S66.11** Strain of flexor muscle, fascia and tendon of other and unspecified finger at wrist and hand level

√7ᵗʰ **S66.110** Strain of flexor muscle, fascia and tendon of right index finger at wrist and hand level

√7ᵗʰ **S66.111** Strain of flexor muscle, fascia and tendon of left index finger at wrist and hand level

√7ᵗʰ **S66.112** Strain of flexor muscle, fascia and tendon of right middle finger at wrist and hand level

√7ᵗʰ **S66.113** Strain of flexor muscle, fascia and tendon of left middle finger at wrist and hand level

√7ᵗʰ **S66.114** Strain of flexor muscle, fascia and tendon of right ring finger at wrist and hand level

√7ᵗʰ **S66.115** Strain of flexor muscle, fascia and tendon of left ring finger at wrist and hand level

√7ᵗʰ **S66.116** Strain of flexor muscle, fascia and tendon of right little finger at wrist and hand level

√7ᵗʰ **S66.117** Strain of flexor muscle, fascia and tendon of left little finger at wrist and hand level

√7ᵗʰ **S66.118** Strain of flexor muscle, fascia and tendon of other finger at wrist and hand level
Strain of flexor muscle, fascia and tendon of specified finger with unspecified laterality at wrist and hand level

√7ᵗʰ **S66.119** Strain of flexor muscle, fascia and tendon of unspecified finger at wrist and hand level

√6ᵗʰ **S66.12** Laceration of flexor muscle, fascia and tendon of other and unspecified finger at wrist and hand level

√7ᵗʰ **S66.120** Laceration of flexor muscle, fascia and tendon of right index finger at wrist and hand level　**CC**

√7ᵗʰ **S66.121** Laceration of flexor muscle, fascia and tendon of left index finger at wrist and hand level　**CC**

√7ᵗʰ **S66.122** Laceration of flexor muscle, fascia and tendon of right middle finger at wrist and hand level　**CC**

√7ᵗʰ **S66.123** Laceration of flexor muscle, fascia and tendon of left middle finger at wrist and hand level　**CC**

√7ᵗʰ **S66.124** Laceration of flexor muscle, fascia and tendon of right ring finger at wrist and hand level　**CC**

✓7ᵗʰ **S66.125** Laceration of flexor muscle, fascia and tendon of left ring finger at wrist and hand level `CC`

✓7ᵗʰ **S66.126** Laceration of flexor muscle, fascia and tendon of right little finger at wrist and hand level `CC`

✓7ᵗʰ **S66.127** Laceration of flexor muscle, fascia and tendon of left little finger at wrist and hand level `CC`

✓7ᵗʰ **S66.128** Laceration of flexor muscle, fascia and tendon of other finger at wrist and hand level `CC`

     Laceration of flexor muscle, fascia and tendon of specified finger with unspecified laterality at wrist and hand level

✓7ᵗʰ **S66.129** Laceration of flexor muscle, fascia and tendon of unspecified finger at wrist and hand level `CC`

✓6ᵗʰ **S66.19** Other injury of flexor muscle, fascia and tendon of other and unspecified finger at wrist and hand level

✓7ᵗʰ **S66.190** Other injury of flexor muscle, fascia and tendon of right index finger at wrist and hand level

✓7ᵗʰ **S66.191** Other injury of flexor muscle, fascia and tendon of left index finger at wrist and hand level

✓7ᵗʰ **S66.192** Other injury of flexor muscle, fascia and tendon of right middle finger at wrist and hand level

✓7ᵗʰ **S66.193** Other injury of flexor muscle, fascia and tendon of left middle finger at wrist and hand level

✓7ᵗʰ **S66.194** Other injury of flexor muscle, fascia and tendon of right ring finger at wrist and hand level

✓7ᵗʰ **S66.195** Other injury of flexor muscle, fascia and tendon of left ring finger at wrist and hand level

✓7ᵗʰ **S66.196** Other injury of flexor muscle, fascia and tendon of right little finger at wrist and hand level

✓7ᵗʰ **S66.197** Other injury of flexor muscle, fascia and tendon of left little finger at wrist and hand level

✓7ᵗʰ **S66.198** Other injury of flexor muscle, fascia and tendon of other finger at wrist and hand level

     Other injury of flexor muscle, fascia and tendon of specified finger with unspecified laterality at wrist and hand level

✓7ᵗʰ **S66.199** Other injury of flexor muscle, fascia and tendon of unspecified finger at wrist and hand level

✓5ᵗʰ **S66.2** Injury of extensor muscle, fascia and tendon of thumb at wrist and hand level

✓6ᵗʰ **S66.20** Unspecified injury of extensor muscle, fascia and tendon of thumb at wrist and hand level

✓7ᵗʰ **S66.201** Unspecified injury of extensor muscle, fascia and tendon of right thumb at wrist and hand level

✓7ᵗʰ **S66.202** Unspecified injury of extensor muscle, fascia and tendon of left thumb at wrist and hand level

✓7ᵗʰ **S66.209** Unspecified injury of extensor muscle, fascia and tendon of unspecified thumb at wrist and hand level

✓6ᵗʰ **S66.21** Strain of extensor muscle, fascia and tendon of thumb at wrist and hand level

✓7ᵗʰ **S66.211** Strain of extensor muscle, fascia and tendon of right thumb at wrist and hand level

✓7ᵗʰ **S66.212** Strain of extensor muscle, fascia and tendon of left thumb at wrist and hand level

✓7ᵗʰ **S66.219** Strain of extensor muscle, fascia and tendon of unspecified thumb at wrist and hand level

✓6ᵗʰ **S66.22** Laceration of extensor muscle, fascia and tendon of thumb at wrist and hand level

✓7ᵗʰ **S66.221** Laceration of extensor muscle, fascia and tendon of right thumb at wrist and hand level `CC`

✓7ᵗʰ **S66.222** Laceration of extensor muscle, fascia and tendon of left thumb at wrist and hand level `CC`

✓7ᵗʰ **S66.229** Laceration of extensor muscle, fascia and tendon of unspecified thumb at wrist and hand level `CC`

✓6ᵗʰ **S66.29** Other specified injury of extensor muscle, fascia and tendon of thumb at wrist and hand level

✓7ᵗʰ **S66.291** Other specified injury of extensor muscle, fascia and tendon of right thumb at wrist and hand level

✓7ᵗʰ **S66.292** Other specified injury of extensor muscle, fascia and tendon of left thumb at wrist and hand level

✓7ᵗʰ **S66.299** Other specified injury of extensor muscle, fascia and tendon of unspecified thumb at wrist and hand level

✓5ᵗʰ **S66.3** Injury of extensor muscle, fascia and tendon of other and unspecified finger at wrist and hand level

     EXCLUDES 2 *Injury of extensor muscle, fascia and tendon of thumb at wrist and hand level (S66.2-)*

✓6ᵗʰ **S66.30** Unspecified injury of extensor muscle, fascia and tendon of other and unspecified finger at wrist and hand level

✓7ᵗʰ **S66.300** Unspecified injury of extensor muscle, fascia and tendon of right index finger at wrist and hand level

✓7ᵗʰ **S66.301** Unspecified injury of extensor muscle, fascia and tendon of left index finger at wrist and hand level

✓7ᵗʰ **S66.302** Unspecified injury of extensor muscle, fascia and tendon of right middle finger at wrist and hand level

✓7ᵗʰ **S66.303** Unspecified injury of extensor muscle, fascia and tendon of left middle finger at wrist and hand level

✓7ᵗʰ **S66.304** Unspecified injury of extensor muscle, fascia and tendon of right ring finger at wrist and hand level

✓7ᵗʰ **S66.305** Unspecified injury of extensor muscle, fascia and tendon of left ring finger at wrist and hand level

✓7ᵗʰ **S66.306** Unspecified injury of extensor muscle, fascia and tendon of right little finger at wrist and hand level

✓7ᵗʰ **S66.307** Unspecified injury of extensor muscle, fascia and tendon of left little finger at wrist and hand level

✓7ᵗʰ **S66.308** Unspecified injury of extensor muscle, fascia and tendon of other finger at wrist and hand level

     Unspecified injury of extensor muscle, fascia and tendon of specified finger with unspecified laterality at wrist and hand level

✓7ᵗʰ **S66.309** Unspecified injury of extensor muscle, fascia and tendon of unspecified finger at wrist and hand level

✓6ᵗʰ **S66.31** Strain of extensor muscle, fascia and tendon of other and unspecified finger at wrist and hand level

✓7ᵗʰ **S66.310** Strain of extensor muscle, fascia and tendon of right index finger at wrist and hand level

✓7ᵗʰ **S66.311** Strain of extensor muscle, fascia and tendon of left index finger at wrist and hand level

✓7ᵗʰ **S66.312** Strain of extensor muscle, fascia and tendon of right middle finger at wrist and hand level

✓7ᵗʰ **S66.313** Strain of extensor muscle, fascia and tendon of left middle finger at wrist and hand level

N Newborn: 0   P Pediatric: 0-17   M Maternity: 12-55   A Adult: 15-124   MCC Major CC Condition   PDxMCC PDx acts as own MCC   CC CC Condition   PDxCC PDx acts as own CC

1032   ICD-10-CM 2018

✓7ᵗʰ **S66.314** Strain of extensor muscle, fascia and tendon of **right ring** finger at wrist and hand level

✓7ᵗʰ **S66.315** Strain of extensor muscle, fascia and tendon of **left ring** finger at wrist and hand level

✓7ᵗʰ **S66.316** Strain of extensor muscle, fascia and tendon of **right little** finger at wrist and hand level

✓7ᵗʰ **S66.317** Strain of extensor muscle, fascia and tendon of **left little** finger at wrist and hand level

✓7ᵗʰ **S66.318** Strain of extensor muscle, fascia and tendon of **other** finger at wrist and hand level

> Strain of extensor muscle, fascia and tendon of specified finger with unspecified laterality at wrist and hand level

✓7ᵗʰ **S66.319** Strain of extensor muscle, fascia and tendon of **unspecified** finger at wrist and hand level

✓6ᵗʰ **S66.32** Laceration of extensor muscle, fascia and tendon of **other and unspecified** finger at wrist and hand level

✓7ᵗʰ **S66.320** Laceration of extensor muscle, fascia and tendon of **right index** finger at wrist and hand level **CC**

✓7ᵗʰ **S66.321** Laceration of extensor muscle, fascia and tendon of **left index** finger at wrist and hand level **CC**

✓7ᵗʰ **S66.322** Laceration of extensor muscle, fascia and tendon of **right middle** finger at wrist and hand level **CC**

✓7ᵗʰ **S66.323** Laceration of extensor muscle, fascia and tendon of **left middle** finger at wrist and hand level **CC**

✓7ᵗʰ **S66.324** Laceration of extensor muscle, fascia and tendon of **right ring** finger at wrist and hand level **CC**

✓7ᵗʰ **S66.325** Laceration of extensor muscle, fascia and tendon of **left ring** finger at wrist and hand level **CC**

✓7ᵗʰ **S66.326** Laceration of extensor muscle, fascia and tendon of **right little** finger at wrist and hand level **CC**

✓7ᵗʰ **S66.327** Laceration of extensor muscle, fascia and tendon of **left little** finger at wrist and hand level **CC**

✓7ᵗʰ **S66.328** Laceration of extensor muscle, fascia and tendon of **other** finger at wrist and hand level **CC**

> Laceration of extensor muscle, fascia and tendon of specified finger with unspecified laterality at wrist and hand level

✓7ᵗʰ **S66.329** Laceration of extensor muscle, fascia and tendon of **unspecified** finger at wrist and hand level **CC**

✓6ᵗʰ **S66.39** **Other** injury of extensor muscle, fascia and tendon of **other and unspecified** finger at wrist and hand level

✓7ᵗʰ **S66.390** Other injury of extensor muscle, fascia and tendon of **right index** finger at wrist and hand level

✓7ᵗʰ **S66.391** Other injury of extensor muscle, fascia and tendon of **left index** finger at wrist and hand level

✓7ᵗʰ **S66.392** Other injury of extensor muscle, fascia and tendon of **right middle** finger at wrist and hand level

✓7ᵗʰ **S66.393** Other injury of extensor muscle, fascia and tendon of **left middle** finger at wrist and hand level

✓7ᵗʰ **S66.394** Other injury of extensor muscle, fascia and tendon of **right ring** finger at wrist and hand level

✓7ᵗʰ **S66.395** Other injury of extensor muscle, fascia and tendon of **left ring** finger at wrist and hand level

✓7ᵗʰ **S66.396** Other injury of extensor muscle, fascia and tendon of **right little** finger at wrist and hand level

✓7ᵗʰ **S66.397** Other injury of extensor muscle, fascia and tendon of **left little** finger at wrist and hand level

✓7ᵗʰ **S66.398** Other injury of extensor muscle, fascia and tendon of **other** finger at wrist and hand level

> Other injury of extensor muscle, fascia and tendon of specified finger with unspecified laterality at wrist and hand level

✓7ᵗʰ **S66.399** Other injury of extensor muscle, fascia and tendon of **unspecified** finger at wrist and hand level

✓5ᵗʰ **S66.4** **Injury of intrinsic muscle, fascia and tendon of thumb at wrist and hand level**

✓6ᵗʰ **S66.40** **Unspecified** injury of intrinsic muscle, fascia and tendon of thumb at wrist and hand level

✓7ᵗʰ **S66.401** Unspecified injury of intrinsic muscle, fascia and tendon of **right** thumb at wrist and hand level

✓7ᵗʰ **S66.402** Unspecified injury of intrinsic muscle, fascia and tendon of **left** thumb at wrist and hand level

✓7ᵗʰ **S66.409** Unspecified injury of intrinsic muscle, fascia and tendon of **unspecified** thumb at wrist and hand level

✓6ᵗʰ **S66.41** **Strain** of intrinsic muscle, fascia and tendon of thumb at wrist and hand level

✓7ᵗʰ **S66.411** Strain of intrinsic muscle, fascia and tendon of **right** thumb at wrist and hand level

✓7ᵗʰ **S66.412** Strain of intrinsic muscle, fascia and tendon of **left** thumb at wrist and hand level

✓7ᵗʰ **S66.419** Strain of intrinsic muscle, fascia and tendon of **unspecified** thumb at wrist and hand level

✓6ᵗʰ **S66.42** **Laceration** of intrinsic muscle, fascia and tendon of thumb at wrist and hand level

✓7ᵗʰ **S66.421** Laceration of intrinsic muscle, fascia and tendon of **right** thumb at wrist and hand level **CC**

✓7ᵗʰ **S66.422** Laceration of intrinsic muscle, fascia and tendon of **left** thumb at wrist and hand level **CC**

✓7ᵗʰ **S66.429** Laceration of intrinsic muscle, fascia and tendon of **unspecified** thumb at wrist and hand level **CC**

✓6ᵗʰ **S66.49** **Other specified** injury of intrinsic muscle, fascia and tendon of thumb at wrist and hand level

✓7ᵗʰ **S66.491** Other specified injury of intrinsic muscle, fascia and tendon of **right** thumb at wrist and hand level

✓7ᵗʰ **S66.492** Other specified injury of intrinsic muscle, fascia and tendon of **left** thumb at wrist and hand level

✓7ᵗʰ **S66.499** Other specified injury of intrinsic muscle, fascia and tendon of **unspecified** thumb at wrist and hand level

✓5ᵗʰ **S66.5** **Injury of intrinsic muscle, fascia and tendon of other and unspecified finger at wrist and hand level**

> **EXCLUDES 2** *injury of intrinsic muscle, fascia and tendon of thumb at wrist and hand level (S66.4-)*

✓6ᵗʰ **S66.50** **Unspecified** injury of intrinsic muscle, fascia and tendon of other and unspecified finger at wrist and hand level

✓7ᵗʰ **S66.500** Unspecified injury of intrinsic muscle, fascia and tendon of **right index** finger at wrist and hand level

✓7ᵗʰ **S66.501** Unspecified injury of intrinsic muscle, fascia and tendon of **left index** finger at wrist and hand level

✓7ᵗʰ **S66.502** Unspecified injury of intrinsic muscle, fascia and tendon of **right middle** finger at wrist and hand level

✓ Additional Character Req ✓ᵡ7ᵗʰ Placeholder Alert Unacceptable PDx Manifestation **H1**-**H14** HAC **HCC** CMS-HCC Condition *EXCLUDES 1* Not Coded Here *EXCLUDES 2* Not Included Here

ICD-10-CM 2018   1033

√7ᵗʰ **S66.503** Unspecified injury of intrinsic muscle, fascia and tendon of left middle finger at wrist and hand level

√7ᵗʰ **S66.504** Unspecified injury of intrinsic muscle, fascia and tendon of right ring finger at wrist and hand level

√7ᵗʰ **S66.505** Unspecified injury of intrinsic muscle, fascia and tendon of left ring finger at wrist and hand level

√7ᵗʰ **S66.506** Unspecified injury of intrinsic muscle, fascia and tendon of right little finger at wrist and hand level

√7ᵗʰ **S66.507** Unspecified injury of intrinsic muscle, fascia and tendon of left little finger at wrist and hand level

√7ᵗʰ **S66.508** Unspecified injury of intrinsic muscle, fascia and tendon of other finger at wrist and hand level
> Unspecified injury of intrinsic muscle, fascia and tendon of specified finger with unspecified laterality at wrist and hand level

√7ᵗʰ **S66.509** Unspecified injury of intrinsic muscle, fascia and tendon of unspecified finger at wrist and hand level

√6ᵗʰ **S66.51** Strain of intrinsic muscle, fascia and tendon of other and unspecified finger at wrist and hand level

√7ᵗʰ **S66.510** Strain of intrinsic muscle, fascia and tendon of right index finger at wrist and hand level

√7ᵗʰ **S66.511** Strain of intrinsic muscle, fascia and tendon of left index finger at wrist and hand level

√7ᵗʰ **S66.512** Strain of intrinsic muscle, fascia and tendon of right middle finger at wrist and hand level

√7ᵗʰ **S66.513** Strain of intrinsic muscle, fascia and tendon of left middle finger at wrist and hand level

√7ᵗʰ **S66.514** Strain of intrinsic muscle, fascia and tendon of right ring finger at wrist and hand level

√7ᵗʰ **S66.515** Strain of intrinsic muscle, fascia and tendon of left ring finger at wrist and hand level

√7ᵗʰ **S66.516** Strain of intrinsic muscle, fascia and tendon of right little finger at wrist and hand level

√7ᵗʰ **S66.517** Strain of intrinsic muscle, fascia and tendon of left little finger at wrist and hand level

√7ᵗʰ **S66.518** Strain of intrinsic muscle, fascia and tendon of other finger at wrist and hand level
> Strain of intrinsic muscle, fascia and tendon of specified finger with unspecified laterality at wrist and hand level

√7ᵗʰ **S66.519** Strain of intrinsic muscle, fascia and tendon of unspecified finger at wrist and hand level

√6ᵗʰ **S66.52** Laceration of intrinsic muscle, fascia and tendon of other and unspecified finger at wrist and hand level

√7ᵗʰ **S66.520** Laceration of intrinsic muscle, fascia and tendon of right index finger at wrist and hand level   CC

√7ᵗʰ **S66.521** Laceration of intrinsic muscle, fascia and tendon of left index finger at wrist and hand level   CC

√7ᵗʰ **S66.522** Laceration of intrinsic muscle, fascia and tendon of right middle finger at wrist and hand level   CC

√7ᵗʰ **S66.523** Laceration of intrinsic muscle, fascia and tendon of left middle finger at wrist and hand level   CC

√7ᵗʰ **S66.524** Laceration of intrinsic muscle, fascia and tendon of right ring finger at wrist and hand level   CC

√7ᵗʰ **S66.525** Laceration of intrinsic muscle, fascia and tendon of left ring finger at wrist and hand level   CC

√7ᵗʰ **S66.526** Laceration of intrinsic muscle, fascia and tendon of right little finger at wrist and hand level   CC

√7ᵗʰ **S66.527** Laceration of intrinsic muscle, fascia and tendon of left little finger at wrist and hand level   CC

√7ᵗʰ **S66.528** Laceration of intrinsic muscle, fascia and tendon of other finger at wrist and hand level   CC
> Laceration of intrinsic muscle, fascia and tendon of specified finger with unspecified laterality at wrist and hand level

√7ᵗʰ **S66.529** Laceration of intrinsic muscle, fascia and tendon of unspecified finger at wrist and hand level   CC

√6ᵗʰ **S66.59** Other injury of intrinsic muscle, fascia and tendon of other and unspecified finger at wrist and hand level

√7ᵗʰ **S66.590** Other injury of intrinsic muscle, fascia and tendon of right index finger at wrist and hand level

√7ᵗʰ **S66.591** Other injury of intrinsic muscle, fascia and tendon of left index finger at wrist and hand level

√7ᵗʰ **S66.592** Other injury of intrinsic muscle, fascia and tendon of right middle finger at wrist and hand level

√7ᵗʰ **S66.593** Other injury of intrinsic muscle, fascia and tendon of left middle finger at wrist and hand level

√7ᵗʰ **S66.594** Other injury of intrinsic muscle, fascia and tendon of right ring finger at wrist and hand level

√7ᵗʰ **S66.595** Other injury of intrinsic muscle, fascia and tendon of left ring finger at wrist and hand level

√7ᵗʰ **S66.596** Other injury of intrinsic muscle, fascia and tendon of right little finger at wrist and hand level

√7ᵗʰ **S66.597** Other injury of intrinsic muscle, fascia and tendon of left little finger at wrist and hand level

√7ᵗʰ **S66.598** Other injury of intrinsic muscle, fascia and tendon of other finger at wrist and hand level
> Other injury of intrinsic muscle, fascia and tendon of specified finger with unspecified laterality at wrist and hand level

√7ᵗʰ **S66.599** Other injury of intrinsic muscle, fascia and tendon of unspecified finger at wrist and hand level

√5ᵗʰ **S66.8** Injury of other specified muscles, fascia and tendons at wrist and hand level

√6ᵗʰ **S66.80** Unspecified injury of other specified muscles, fascia and tendons at wrist and hand level

√7ᵗʰ **S66.801** Unspecified injury of other specified muscles, fascia and tendons at wrist and hand level, right hand

√7ᵗʰ **S66.802** Unspecified injury of other specified muscles, fascia and tendons at wrist and hand level, left hand

√7ᵗʰ **S66.809** Unspecified injury of other specified muscles, fascia and tendons at wrist and hand level, unspecified hand

√6ᵗʰ **S66.81** Strain of other specified muscles, fascia and tendons at wrist and hand level

√7ᵗʰ **S66.811** Strain of other specified muscles, fascia and tendons at wrist and hand level, right hand

√7ᵗʰ **S66.812** Strain of other specified muscles, fascia and tendons at wrist and hand level, left hand

√7ᵗʰ **S66.819** Strain of other specified muscles, fascia and tendons at wrist and hand level, unspecified hand

---

N Newborn: 0   P Pediatric: 0-17   M Maternity: 12-55   A Adult: 15-124   MCC Major CC Condition   PDxMCC PDx acts as own MCC   CC CC Condition   PDxCC PDx acts as own CC

1034   ICD-10-CM 2018

√6ᵗʰ **S66.82** Laceration of other specified muscles, fascia and tendons at wrist and hand level

    √7ᵗʰ **S66.821** Laceration of other specified muscles, fascia and tendons at wrist and hand level, right hand   cc

    √7ᵗʰ **S66.822** Laceration of other specified muscles, fascia and tendons at wrist and hand level, left hand   cc

    √7ᵗʰ **S66.829** Laceration of other specified muscles, fascia and tendons at wrist and hand level, unspecified hand   cc

√6ᵗʰ **S66.89** Other injury of other specified muscles, fascia and tendons at wrist and hand level

    √7ᵗʰ **S66.891** Other injury of other specified muscles, fascia and tendons at wrist and hand level, right hand

    √7ᵗʰ **S66.892** Other injury of other specified muscles, fascia and tendons at wrist and hand level, left hand

    √7ᵗʰ **S66.899** Other injury of other specified muscles, fascia and tendons at wrist and hand level, unspecified hand

√5ᵗʰ **S66.9** Injury of unspecified muscle, fascia and tendon at wrist and hand level

  √6ᵗʰ **S66.90** Unspecified injury of unspecified muscle, fascia and tendon at wrist and hand level

    √7ᵗʰ **S66.901** Unspecified injury of unspecified muscle, fascia and tendon at wrist and hand level, right hand

    √7ᵗʰ **S66.902** Unspecified injury of unspecified muscle, fascia and tendon at wrist and hand level, left hand

    √7ᵗʰ **S66.909** Unspecified injury of unspecified muscle, fascia and tendon at wrist and hand level, unspecified hand

  √6ᵗʰ **S66.91** Strain of unspecified muscle, fascia and tendon at wrist and hand level

    √7ᵗʰ **S66.911** Strain of unspecified muscle, fascia and tendon at wrist and hand level, right hand

    √7ᵗʰ **S66.912** Strain of unspecified muscle, fascia and tendon at wrist and hand level, left hand

    √7ᵗʰ **S66.919** Strain of unspecified muscle, fascia and tendon at wrist and hand level, unspecified hand

  √6ᵗʰ **S66.92** Laceration of unspecified muscle, fascia and tendon at wrist and hand level

    √7ᵗʰ **S66.921** Laceration of unspecified muscle, fascia and tendon at wrist and hand level, right hand   cc

    √7ᵗʰ **S66.922** Laceration of unspecified muscle, fascia and tendon at wrist and hand level, left hand   cc

    √7ᵗʰ **S66.929** Laceration of unspecified muscle, fascia and tendon at wrist and hand level, unspecified hand   cc

  √6ᵗʰ **S66.99** Other injury of unspecified muscle, fascia and tendon at wrist and hand level

    √7ᵗʰ **S66.991** Other injury of unspecified muscle, fascia and tendon at wrist and hand level, right hand

    √7ᵗʰ **S66.992** Other injury of unspecified muscle, fascia and tendon at wrist and hand level, left hand

    √7ᵗʰ **S66.999** Other injury of unspecified muscle, fascia and tendon at wrist and hand level, unspecified hand

√4ᵗʰ **S67** Crushing injury of wrist, hand and fingers

Use additional code for all associated injuries, such as:
  fracture of wrist and hand (S62.-)
  open wound of wrist and hand (S61.-)

> The appropriate 7th character is to be added to each code from category S67.
> A   initial encounter
> D   subsequent encounter
> S   sequela

√5ᵗʰ **S67.0** Crushing injury of thumb

  √x7ᵗʰ **S67.00** Crushing injury of unspecified thumb

  √x7ᵗʰ **S67.01** Crushing injury of right thumb

  √x7ᵗʰ **S67.02** Crushing injury of left thumb

√5ᵗʰ **S67.1** Crushing injury of other and unspecified finger(s)

    EXCLUDES 2   crushing injury of thumb (S67.0-)

  √x7ᵗʰ **S67.10** Crushing injury of unspecified finger(s)

  √6ᵗʰ **S67.19** Crushing injury of other finger(s)

    √7ᵗʰ **S67.190** Crushing injury of right index finger

    √7ᵗʰ **S67.191** Crushing injury of left index finger

    √7ᵗʰ **S67.192** Crushing injury of right middle finger

    √7ᵗʰ **S67.193** Crushing injury of left middle finger

    √7ᵗʰ **S67.194** Crushing injury of right ring finger

    √7ᵗʰ **S67.195** Crushing injury of left ring finger

    √7ᵗʰ **S67.196** Crushing injury of right little finger

    √7ᵗʰ **S67.197** Crushing injury of left little finger

    √7ᵗʰ **S67.198** Crushing injury of other finger
       Crushing injury of specified finger with unspecified laterality

√5ᵗʰ **S67.2** Crushing injury of hand

    EXCLUDES 2   crushing injury of fingers (S67.1-)
                   crushing injury of thumb (S67.0-)

  √x7ᵗʰ **S67.20** Crushing injury of unspecified hand

  √x7ᵗʰ **S67.21** Crushing injury of right hand

  √x7ᵗʰ **S67.22** Crushing injury of left hand

√5ᵗʰ **S67.3** Crushing injury of wrist

  √x7ᵗʰ **S67.30** Crushing injury of unspecified wrist

  √x7ᵗʰ **S67.31** Crushing injury of right wrist

  √x7ᵗʰ **S67.32** Crushing injury of left wrist

√5ᵗʰ **S67.4** Crushing injury of wrist and hand

    EXCLUDES 1   crushing injury of hand alone (S67.2-)
                   crushing injury of wrist alone (S67.3-)
    EXCLUDES 2   crushing injury of fingers (S67.1-)
                   crushing injury of thumb (S67.0-)

  √x7ᵗʰ **S67.40** Crushing injury of unspecified wrist and hand

  √x7ᵗʰ **S67.41** Crushing injury of right wrist and hand

  √x7ᵗʰ **S67.42** Crushing injury of left wrist and hand

√5ᵗʰ **S67.9** Crushing injury of unspecified part(s) of wrist, hand and fingers

  √x7ᵗʰ **S67.90** Crushing injury of unspecified part(s) of unspecified wrist, hand and fingers

  √x7ᵗʰ **S67.91** Crushing injury of unspecified part(s) of right wrist, hand and fingers

  √x7ᵗʰ **S67.92** Crushing injury of unspecified part(s) of left wrist, hand and fingers

√ Additional Character Req   √x7ᵗʰ Placeholder Alert   Unacceptable PDx   Manifestation   H1 - H14 HAC   HCC CMS-HCC Condition   *EXCLUDES 1* Not Coded Here   *EXCLUDES 2* Not Included Here

ICD-10-CM 2018   1035

☑4ᵗʰ S68 Traumatic amputation of wrist, hand and fingers
An amputation not identified as partial or complete should be coded to complete.

The appropriate 7th character is to be added to each code from category S68.
A   initial encounter
D   subsequent encounter
S   sequela

CC Excl: For CC codes in category S68:
Right side: PDX collection 1266
Left side: PDX collection 1267
Unspecified side: PDX collection 1268

☑5ᵗʰ S68.0 Traumatic metacarpophalangeal amputation of thumb
Traumatic amputation of thumb NOS

  ☑6ᵗʰ S68.01 Complete traumatic metacarpophalangeal amputation of thumb

    12 ☑7ᵗʰ **S68.011 Complete traumatic metacarpophalangeal amputation of right thumb** HCC

    12 ☑7ᵗʰ **S68.012 Complete traumatic metacarpophalangeal amputation of left thumb** HCC

    12 ☑7ᵗʰ **S68.019 Complete traumatic metacarpophalangeal amputation of unspecified thumb** HCC

  ☑6ᵗʰ S68.02 Partial traumatic metacarpophalangeal amputation of thumb

    12 ☑7ᵗʰ **S68.021 Partial traumatic metacarpophalangeal amputation of right thumb** HCC

    12 ☑7ᵗʰ **S68.022 Partial traumatic metacarpophalangeal amputation of left thumb** HCC

    12 ☑7ᵗʰ **S68.029 Partial traumatic metacarpophalangeal amputation of unspecified thumb** HCC

☑5ᵗʰ S68.1 Traumatic metacarpophalangeal amputation of other and unspecified finger
Traumatic amputation of finger NOS
    EXCLUDES 2   *traumatic metacarpophalangeal amputation of thumb (S68.0-)*

  ☑6ᵗʰ S68.11 Complete traumatic metacarpophalangeal amputation of other and unspecified finger

    12 ☑7ᵗʰ **S68.110 Complete traumatic metacarpophalangeal amputation of right index finger** HCC

    12 ☑7ᵗʰ **S68.111 Complete traumatic metacarpophalangeal amputation of left index finger** HCC

    12 ☑7ᵗʰ **S68.112 Complete traumatic metacarpophalangeal amputation of right middle finger** HCC

    12 ☑7ᵗʰ **S68.113 Complete traumatic metacarpophalangeal amputation of left middle finger** HCC

    12 ☑7ᵗʰ **S68.114 Complete traumatic metacarpophalangeal amputation of right ring finger** HCC

    12 ☑7ᵗʰ **S68.115 Complete traumatic metacarpophalangeal amputation of left ring finger** HCC

    12 ☑7ᵗʰ **S68.116 Complete traumatic metacarpophalangeal amputation of right little finger** HCC

    12 ☑7ᵗʰ **S68.117 Complete traumatic metacarpophalangeal amputation of left little finger** HCC

    12 ☑7ᵗʰ **S68.118 Complete traumatic metacarpophalangeal amputation of other finger** HCC
        Complete traumatic metacarpophalangeal amputation of specified finger with unspecified laterality

    12 ☑7ᵗʰ **S68.119 Complete traumatic metacarpophalangeal amputation of unspecified finger** HCC

☑6ᵗʰ S68.12 Partial traumatic metacarpophalangeal amputation of other and unspecified finger

    12 ☑7ᵗʰ **S68.120 Partial traumatic metacarpophalangeal amputation of right index finger** HCC

    12 ☑7ᵗʰ **S68.121 Partial traumatic metacarpophalangeal amputation of left index finger** HCC

    12 ☑7ᵗʰ **S68.122 Partial traumatic metacarpophalangeal amputation of right middle finger** HCC

    12 ☑7ᵗʰ **S68.123 Partial traumatic metacarpophalangeal amputation of left middle finger** HCC

    12 ☑7ᵗʰ **S68.124 Partial traumatic metacarpophalangeal amputation of right ring finger** HCC

    12 ☑7ᵗʰ **S68.125 Partial traumatic metacarpophalangeal amputation of left ring finger** HCC

    12 ☑7ᵗʰ **S68.126 Partial traumatic metacarpophalangeal amputation of right little finger** HCC

    12 ☑7ᵗʰ **S68.127 Partial traumatic metacarpophalangeal amputation of left little finger** HCC

    12 ☑7ᵗʰ **S68.128 Partial traumatic metacarpophalangeal amputation of other finger** HCC
        Partial traumatic metacarpophalangeal amputation of specified finger with unspecified laterality

    12 ☑7ᵗʰ **S68.129 Partial traumatic metacarpophalangeal amputation of unspecified finger** HCC

☑5ᵗʰ S68.4 Traumatic amputation of hand at wrist level
Traumatic amputation of hand NOS
Traumatic amputation of wrist

  ☑6ᵗʰ S68.41 Complete traumatic amputation of hand at wrist level

    11 ☑7ᵗʰ **S68.411 Complete traumatic amputation of right hand at wrist level** CC HCC

    11 ☑7ᵗʰ **S68.412 Complete traumatic amputation of left hand at wrist level** CC HCC

    11 ☑7ᵗʰ **S68.419 Complete traumatic amputation of unspecified hand at wrist level** CC HCC

  ☑6ᵗʰ S68.42 Partial traumatic amputation of hand at wrist level

    11 ☑7ᵗʰ **S68.421 Partial traumatic amputation of right hand at wrist level** CC HCC

    11 ☑7ᵗʰ **S68.422 Partial traumatic amputation of left hand at wrist level** CC HCC

    11 ☑7ᵗʰ **S68.429 Partial traumatic amputation of unspecified hand at wrist level** CC HCC

☑5ᵗʰ S68.5 Traumatic transphalangeal amputation of thumb
Traumatic interphalangeal joint amputation of thumb

  ☑6ᵗʰ S68.51 Complete traumatic transphalangeal amputation of thumb

    12 ☑7ᵗʰ **S68.511 Complete traumatic transphalangeal amputation of right thumb** HCC

    12 ☑7ᵗʰ **S68.512 Complete traumatic transphalangeal amputation of left thumb** HCC

    12 ☑7ᵗʰ **S68.519 Complete traumatic transphalangeal amputation of unspecified thumb** HCC

  ☑6ᵗʰ S68.52 Partial traumatic transphalangeal amputation of thumb

    12 ☑7ᵗʰ **S68.521 Partial traumatic transphalangeal amputation of right thumb** HCC

    12 ☑7ᵗʰ **S68.522 Partial traumatic transphalangeal amputation of left thumb** HCC

    12 ☑7ᵗʰ **S68.529 Partial traumatic transphalangeal amputation of unspecified thumb** HCC

---

11 HCC with 7th character indicating initial encounter (A or B - specific to category) OR sequela.
12 HCC with 7th character indicating sequela.

✓5th **S68.6 Traumatic transphalangeal amputation of other and unspecified finger**

  ✓6th **S68.61 Complete traumatic transphalangeal amputation of other and unspecified finger(s)**

    12 ✓7th **S68.610 Complete traumatic transphalangeal amputation of right index finger** HCC

    12 ✓7th **S68.611 Complete traumatic transphalangeal amputation of left index finger** HCC

    12 ✓7th **S68.612 Complete traumatic transphalangeal amputation of right middle finger** HCC

    12 ✓7th **S68.613 Complete traumatic transphalangeal amputation of left middle finger** HCC

    12 ✓7th **S68.614 Complete traumatic transphalangeal amputation of right ring finger** HCC

    12 ✓7th **S68.615 Complete traumatic transphalangeal amputation of left ring finger** HCC

    12 ✓7th **S68.616 Complete traumatic transphalangeal amputation of right little finger** HCC

    12 ✓7th **S68.617 Complete traumatic transphalangeal amputation of left little finger** HCC

    12 ✓7th **S68.618 Complete traumatic transphalangeal amputation of other finger** HCC
      Complete traumatic transphalangeal amputation of specified finger with unspecified laterality

    12 ✓7th **S68.619 Complete traumatic transphalangeal amputation of unspecified finger** HCC

  ✓6th **S68.62 Partial traumatic transphalangeal amputation of other and unspecified finger**

    12 ✓7th **S68.620 Partial traumatic transphalangeal amputation of right index finger** HCC

    12 ✓7th **S68.621 Partial traumatic transphalangeal amputation of left index finger** HCC

    12 ✓7th **S68.622 Partial traumatic transphalangeal amputation of right middle finger** HCC

    12 ✓7th **S68.623 Partial traumatic transphalangeal amputation of left middle finger** HCC

    12 ✓7th **S68.624 Partial traumatic transphalangeal amputation of right ring finger** HCC

    12 ✓7th **S68.625 Partial traumatic transphalangeal amputation of left ring finger** HCC

    12 ✓7th **S68.626 Partial traumatic transphalangeal amputation of right little finger** HCC

    12 ✓7th **S68.627 Partial traumatic transphalangeal amputation of left little finger** HCC

    12 ✓7th **S68.628 Partial traumatic transphalangeal amputation of other finger** HCC
      Partial traumatic transphalangeal amputation of specified finger with unspecified laterality

    12 ✓7th **S68.629 Partial traumatic transphalangeal amputation of unspecified finger** HCC

✓5th **S68.7 Traumatic transmetacarpal amputation of hand**

  ✓6th **S68.71 Complete traumatic transmetacarpal amputation of hand**

    11 ✓7th **S68.711 Complete traumatic transmetacarpal amputation of right hand** CC HCC

    11 ✓7th **S68.712 Complete traumatic transmetacarpal amputation of left hand** CC HCC

    11 ✓7th **S68.719 Complete traumatic transmetacarpal amputation of unspecified hand** CC HCC

  ✓6th **S68.72 Partial traumatic transmetacarpal amputation of hand**

    11 ✓7th **S68.721 Partial traumatic transmetacarpal amputation of right hand** CC HCC

    11 ✓7th **S68.722 Partial traumatic transmetacarpal amputation of left hand** CC HCC

    11 ✓7th **S68.729 Partial traumatic transmetacarpal amputation of unspecified hand** CC HCC

✓4th **S69 Other and unspecified injuries of wrist, hand and finger(s)**

  The appropriate 7th character is to be added to each code from category S69.
  A   initial encounter
  D   subsequent encounter
  S   sequela

  ✓5th **S69.8 Other specified injuries of wrist, hand and finger(s)**

    ✓x7th **S69.80 Other specified injuries of unspecified wrist, hand and finger(s)**

    ✓x7th **S69.81 Other specified injuries of right wrist, hand and finger(s)**

    ✓x7th **S69.82 Other specified injuries of left wrist, hand and finger(s)**

  ✓5th **S69.9 Unspecified injury of wrist, hand and finger(s)**

    ✓x7th **S69.90 Unspecified injury of unspecified wrist, hand and finger(s)**

    ✓x7th **S69.91 Unspecified injury of right wrist, hand and finger(s)**

    ✓x7th **S69.92 Unspecified injury of left wrist, hand and finger(s)**

Injuries to the hip and thigh (S70-S79)

EXCLUDES 2   *burns and corrosions (T20-T32)*
    frostbite (T33-T34)
    snake bite (T63.0-)
    venomous insect bite or sting (T63.4-)

✓4th **S70 Superficial injury of hip and thigh**

  The appropriate 7th character is to be added to each code from category S70.
  A   initial encounter
  D   subsequent encounter
  S   sequela

  ✓5th **S70.0 Contusion of hip**

    ✓x7th **S70.00 Contusion of unspecified hip**

    ✓x7th **S70.01 Contusion of right hip**

    ✓x7th **S70.02 Contusion of left hip**

  ✓5th **S70.1 Contusion of thigh**

    ✓x7th **S70.10 Contusion of unspecified thigh**

    ✓x7th **S70.11 Contusion of right thigh**

    ✓x7th **S70.12 Contusion of left thigh**

  ✓5th **S70.2 Other superficial injuries of hip**

    ✓6th **S70.21 Abrasion of hip**

      ✓7th **S70.211 Abrasion, right hip**

      ✓7th **S70.212 Abrasion, left hip**

      ✓7th **S70.219 Abrasion, unspecified hip**

    ✓6th **S70.22 Blister (nonthermal) of hip**

      ✓7th **S70.221 Blister (nonthermal), right hip**

      ✓7th **S70.222 Blister (nonthermal), left hip**

      ✓7th **S70.229 Blister (nonthermal), unspecified hip**

    ✓6th **S70.24 External constriction of hip**

      ✓7th **S70.241 External constriction, right hip**

      ✓7th **S70.242 External constriction, left hip**

      ✓7th **S70.249 External constriction, unspecified hip**

    ✓6th **S70.25 Superficial foreign body of hip**
      Splinter in the hip

      ✓7th **S70.251 Superficial foreign body, right hip**

      ✓7th **S70.252 Superficial foreign body, left hip**

      ✓7th **S70.259 Superficial foreign body, unspecified hip**

    ✓6th **S70.26 Insect bite (nonvenomous) of hip**

      ✓7th **S70.261 Insect bite (nonvenomous), right hip**

      ✓7th **S70.262 Insect bite (nonvenomous), left hip**

      ✓7th **S70.269 Insect bite (nonvenomous), unspecified hip**

    ✓6th **S70.27 Other superficial bite of hip**
      EXCLUDES 1   *open bite of hip (S71.05-)*

      ✓7th **S70.271 Other superficial bite of hip, right hip**

      ✓7th **S70.272 Other superficial bite of hip, left hip**

      ✓7th **S70.279 Other superficial bite of hip, unspecified hip**

---

11 HCC with 7th character indicating initial encounter (A or B - specific to category) OR sequela.
12 HCC with 7th character indicating sequela.

✓ Additional Character Req   ✓x7th Placeholder Alert   Unacceptable PDx   Manifestation   H1 - H14 HAC   HCC CMS-HCC Condition   EXCLUDES 1 Not Coded Here   EXCLUDES 2 Not Included Here

Chapter 19. Injury, Poisoning and Certain Other Consequences of External Causes

☑5ᵗʰ **S70.3** **Other superficial injuries of** thigh

   ☑6ᵗʰ **S70.31** **Abrasion of thigh**

     ☑7ᵗʰ **S70.311** **Abrasion, right thigh**

     ☑7ᵗʰ **S70.312** **Abrasion, left thigh**

     ☑7ᵗʰ **S70.319** **Abrasion, unspecified thigh**

   ☑6ᵗʰ **S70.32** **Blister (nonthermal) of thigh**

     ☑7ᵗʰ **S70.321** **Blister (nonthermal), right thigh**

     ☑7ᵗʰ **S70.322** **Blister (nonthermal), left thigh**

     ☑7ᵗʰ **S70.329** **Blister (nonthermal), unspecified thigh**

   ☑6ᵗʰ **S70.34** **External constriction of thigh**

     ☑7ᵗʰ **S70.341** **External constriction, right thigh**

     ☑7ᵗʰ **S70.342** **External constriction, left thigh**

     ☑7ᵗʰ **S70.349** **External constriction, unspecified thigh**

   ☑6ᵗʰ **S70.35** **Superficial foreign body of thigh**

     Splinter in the thigh

     ☑7ᵗʰ **S70.351** **Superficial foreign body, right thigh**

     ☑7ᵗʰ **S70.352** **Superficial foreign body, left thigh**

     ☑7ᵗʰ **S70.359** **Superficial foreign body, unspecified thigh**

   ☑6ᵗʰ **S70.36** **Insect bite (nonvenomous) of thigh**

     ☑7ᵗʰ **S70.361** **Insect bite (nonvenomous), right thigh**

     ☑7ᵗʰ **S70.362** **Insect bite (nonvenomous), left thigh**

     ☑7ᵗʰ **S70.369** **Insect bite (nonvenomous), unspecified thigh**

   ☑6ᵗʰ **S70.37** **Other superficial bite of thigh**

     EXCLUDES 1   *open bite of thigh (S71.15)*

     ☑7ᵗʰ **S70.371** **Other superficial bite of right thigh**

     ☑7ᵗʰ **S70.372** **Other superficial bite of left thigh**

     ☑7ᵗʰ **S70.379** **Other superficial bite of unspecified thigh**

☑5ᵗʰ **S70.9** **Unspecified superficial injury of hip and thigh**

   ☑6ᵗʰ **S70.91** **Unspecified superficial injury of hip**

     ☑7ᵗʰ **S70.911** **Unspecified superficial injury of right hip**

     ☑7ᵗʰ **S70.912** **Unspecified superficial injury of left hip**

     ☑7ᵗʰ **S70.919** **Unspecified superficial injury of unspecified hip**

   ☑6ᵗʰ **S70.92** **Unspecified superficial injury of thigh**

     ☑7ᵗʰ **S70.921** **Unspecified superficial injury of right thigh**

     ☑7ᵗʰ **S70.922** **Unspecified superficial injury of left thigh**

     ☑7ᵗʰ **S70.929** **Unspecified superficial injury of unspecified thigh**

☑4ᵗʰ **S71** **Open wound of hip and thigh**

   Code also any associated wound infection

   EXCLUDES 1   *open fracture of hip and thigh (S72.-)*

             traumatic amputation of hip and thigh (S78.-)

   EXCLUDES 2   *bite of venomous animal (T63.-)*

             open wound of ankle, foot and toes (S91.-)

             open wound of knee and lower leg (S81.-)

> The appropriate 7th character is to be added to each code from category S71.
> A   initial encounter
> D   subsequent encounter
> S   sequela

☑5ᵗʰ **S71.0** **Open wound of hip**

   ☑6ᵗʰ **S71.00** **Unspecified open wound of hip**

     ☑7ᵗʰ **S71.001** **Unspecified open wound, right hip**

     ☑7ᵗʰ **S71.002** **Unspecified open wound, left hip**

     ☑7ᵗʰ **S71.009** **Unspecified open wound, unspecified hip**

   ☑6ᵗʰ **S71.01** **Laceration without foreign body of hip**

     ☑7ᵗʰ **S71.011** **Laceration without foreign body, right hip**

     ☑7ᵗʰ **S71.012** **Laceration without foreign body, left hip**

     ☑7ᵗʰ **S71.019** **Laceration without foreign body, unspecified hip**

   ☑6ᵗʰ **S71.02** **Laceration with foreign body of hip**

     ☑7ᵗʰ **S71.021** **Laceration with foreign body, right hip**

     ☑7ᵗʰ **S71.022** **Laceration with foreign body, left hip**

     ☑7ᵗʰ **S71.029** **Laceration with foreign body, unspecified hip**

   ☑6ᵗʰ **S71.03** **Puncture wound without foreign body of hip**

     ☑7ᵗʰ **S71.031** **Puncture wound without foreign body, right hip**

     ☑7ᵗʰ **S71.032** **Puncture wound without foreign body, left hip**

     ☑7ᵗʰ **S71.039** **Puncture wound without foreign body, unspecified hip**

   ☑6ᵗʰ **S71.04** **Puncture wound with foreign body of hip**

     ☑7ᵗʰ **S71.041** **Puncture wound with foreign body, right hip**

     ☑7ᵗʰ **S71.042** **Puncture wound with foreign body, left hip**

     ☑7ᵗʰ **S71.049** **Puncture wound with foreign body, unspecified hip**

   ☑6ᵗʰ **S71.05** **Open bite of hip**

     Bite of hip NOS

     EXCLUDES 1   *superficial bite of hip (S70.26, S70.27)*

     ☑7ᵗʰ **S71.051** **Open bite, right hip**

     ☑7ᵗʰ **S71.052** **Open bite, left hip**

     ☑7ᵗʰ **S71.059** **Open bite, unspecified hip**

☑5ᵗʰ **S71.1** **Open wound of thigh**

   ☑6ᵗʰ **S71.10** **Unspecified open wound of thigh**

     AHA: 2016, 3Q, 24

     ☑7ᵗʰ **S71.101** **Unspecified open wound, right thigh**

     ☑7ᵗʰ **S71.102** **Unspecified open wound, left thigh**

     ☑7ᵗʰ **S71.109** **Unspecified open wound, unspecified thigh**

   ☑6ᵗʰ **S71.11** **Laceration without foreign body of thigh**

     ☑7ᵗʰ **S71.111** **Laceration without foreign body, right thigh**

     ☑7ᵗʰ **S71.112** **Laceration without foreign body, left thigh**

     ☑7ᵗʰ **S71.119** **Laceration without foreign body, unspecified thigh**

   ☑6ᵗʰ **S71.12** **Laceration with foreign body of thigh**

     ☑7ᵗʰ **S71.121** **Laceration with foreign body, right thigh**

     ☑7ᵗʰ **S71.122** **Laceration with foreign body, left thigh**

     ☑7ᵗʰ **S71.129** **Laceration with foreign body, unspecified thigh**

   ☑6ᵗʰ **S71.13** **Puncture wound without foreign body of thigh**

     AHA: 2016, 3Q, 24

     ☑7ᵗʰ **S71.131** **Puncture wound without foreign body, right thigh**

     ☑7ᵗʰ **S71.132** **Puncture wound without foreign body, left thigh**

     ☑7ᵗʰ **S71.139** **Puncture wound without foreign body, unspecified thigh**

   ☑6ᵗʰ **S71.14** **Puncture wound with foreign body of thigh**

     AHA: 2016, 3Q, 24

     ☑7ᵗʰ **S71.141** **Puncture wound with foreign body, right thigh**

     ☑7ᵗʰ **S71.142** **Puncture wound with foreign body, left thigh**

     ☑7ᵗʰ **S71.149** **Puncture wound with foreign body, unspecified thigh**

   ☑6ᵗʰ **S71.15** **Open bite of thigh**

     Bite of thigh NOS

     EXCLUDES 1   *superficial bite of thigh (S70.37-)*

     ☑7ᵗʰ **S71.151** **Open bite, right thigh**

     ☑7ᵗʰ **S71.152** **Open bite, left thigh**

     ☑7ᵗʰ **S71.159** **Open bite, unspecified thigh**

Ⓝ Newborn: 0   Ⓟ Pediatric: 0-17   Ⓜ Maternity: 12-55   Ⓐ Adult: 15-124   **MCC** Major CC Condition   **PDxMCC** PDx acts as own MCC   **CC** CC Condition   **PDxCC** PDx acts as own CC

1038   ICD-10-CM 2018

☑4ᵗʰ **S72 Fracture of femur**

NOTE A fracture not indicated as displaced or nondisplaced should be coded to displaced.

The open fracture designations are based on the Gustilo open fracture classification A fracture not indicated as open or closed should be coded to closed.

EXCLUDES 1 traumatic amputation of hip and thigh (S78.-)
EXCLUDES 2 fracture of lower leg and ankle (S82.-)
fracture of foot (S92.-)
periprosthetic fracture of prosthetic implant of hip ▶(M97.0-)◀
AHA: 2016, 1Q, 33; 2015, 3Q, 37-39; 2015, 1Q, 17; 2013, 4Q, 128

The appropriate 7th character is to be added to all codes from category S72 [unless otherwise indicated].
A initial encounter for closed fracture
B initial encounter for open fracture type I or II
   initial encounter for open fracture NOS
C initial encounter for open fracture type IIIA, IIIB, or IIIC
D subsequent encounter for closed fracture with routine healing
E subsequent encounter for open fracture type I or II with routine healing
F subsequent encounter for open fracture type IIIA, IIIB, or IIIC with routine healing
G subsequent encounter for closed fracture with delayed healing
H subsequent encounter for open fracture type I or II with delayed healing
J subsequent encounter for open fracture type IIIA, IIIB, or IIIC with delayed healing
K subsequent encounter for closed fracture with nonunion
M subsequent encounter for open fracture type I or II with nonunion
N subsequent encounter for open fracture type IIIA, IIIB, or IIIC with nonunion
P subsequent encounter for closed fracture with malunion
Q subsequent encounter for open fracture type I or II with malunion
R subsequent encounter for open fracture type IIIA, IIIB, or IIIC with malunion
S sequela

☑5ᵗʰ **S72.0 Fracture of head and neck of femur**
EXCLUDES 2 physeal fracture of upper end of femur (S79.0-)
AHA: 2016, 3Q, 16

CC Excl: For CC/MCC codes in subcategory S72.0:
Right side: See code S72.001
Left side: See code S72.002
Unspecified side: See code S72.009

☑6ᵗʰ **S72.00 Fracture of unspecified part of neck of femur**
Fracture of hip NOS
Fracture of neck of femur NOS

8,10 ☑7ᵗʰ **S72.001 Fracture of unspecified part** `MCC` `CC` `H5` `HCC`
of neck of right femur
CC Excl: MCC with 7th character A:
PDX collection 1297
MCC with 7th character B or C:
PDX collection 1298
CC with 7th character K, M, N, P, Q or R:
PDX collection 897

8,10 ☑7ᵗʰ **S72.002 Fracture of unspecified part** `MCC` `CC` `H5` `HCC`
of neck of left femur
CC Excl: MCC with 7th character A:
PDX collection 1299
MCC with 7th character B or C:
PDX collection 1298
CC with 7th character K, M, N, P, Q or R:
PDX collection 897

8,10 ☑7ᵗʰ **S72.009 Fracture of unspecified part** `MCC` `CC` `H5` `HCC`
of neck of unspecified femur
CC Excl: MCC with 7th character A, B or C:
PDX collection 1298
CC with 7th character K, M, N, P, Q or R:
PDX collection 897

☑6ᵗʰ **S72.01 Unspecified intracapsular fracture of femur**
Subcapital fracture of femur

8,10 ☑7ᵗʰ **S72.011 Unspecified intracapsular** `MCC` `CC` `H5` `HCC`
fracture of right femur

8,10 ☑7ᵗʰ **S72.012 Unspecified intracapsular** `MCC` `CC` `H5` `HCC`
fracture of left femur

8,10 ☑7ᵗʰ **S72.019 Unspecified intracapsular** `MCC` `CC` `H5` `HCC`
fracture of unspecified femur

☑6ᵗʰ **S72.02 Fracture of epiphysis (separation) (upper) of femur**
Transepiphyseal fracture of femur
EXCLUDES 1 capital femoral epiphyseal fracture (pediatric) of femur (S79.01-)
Salter-Harris Type I physeal fracture of upper end of femur (S79.01-)

8,10 ☑7ᵗʰ **S72.021 Displaced fracture of** `MCC` `CC` `H5` `HCC`
epiphysis (separation) (upper) of right femur

8,10 ☑7ᵗʰ **S72.022 Displaced fracture of** `MCC` `CC` `H5` `HCC`
epiphysis (separation) (upper) of left femur

8,10 ☑7ᵗʰ **S72.023 Displaced fracture of** `MCC` `CC` `H5` `HCC`
epiphysis (separation) (upper) of unspecified femur

8,10 ☑7ᵗʰ **S72.024 Nondisplaced fracture of** `MCC` `CC` `H5` `HCC`
epiphysis (separation) (upper) of right femur

8,10 ☑7ᵗʰ **S72.025 Nondisplaced fracture of** `MCC` `CC` `H5` `HCC`
epiphysis (separation) (upper) of left femur

8,10 ☑7ᵗʰ **S72.026 Nondisplaced fracture of** `MCC` `CC` `H5` `HCC`
epiphysis (separation) (upper) of unspecified femur

☑6ᵗʰ **S72.03 Midcervical fracture of femur**
Transcervical fracture of femur NOS

8,10 ☑7ᵗʰ **S72.031 Displaced midcervical** `MCC` `CC` `H5` `HCC`
fracture of right femur

8,10 ☑7ᵗʰ **S72.032 Displaced midcervical** `MCC` `CC` `H5` `HCC`
fracture of left femur

8,10 ☑7ᵗʰ **S72.033 Displaced midcervical** `MCC` `CC` `H5` `HCC`
fracture of unspecified femur

8,10 ☑7ᵗʰ **S72.034 Nondisplaced midcervical** `MCC` `CC` `H5` `HCC`
fracture of right femur

8,10 ☑7ᵗʰ **S72.035 Nondisplaced midcervical** `MCC` `CC` `H5` `HCC`
fracture of left femur

8,10 ☑7ᵗʰ **S72.036 Nondisplaced midcervical** `MCC` `CC` `H5` `HCC`
fracture of unspecified femur

☑6ᵗʰ **S72.04 Fracture of base of neck of femur**
Cervicotrochanteric fracture of femur

8,10 ☑7ᵗʰ **S72.041 Displaced fracture of base** `MCC` `CC` `H5` `HCC`
of neck of right femur

8,10 ☑7ᵗʰ **S72.042 Displaced fracture of base** `MCC` `CC` `H5` `HCC`
of neck of left femur

8,10 ☑7ᵗʰ **S72.043 Displaced fracture of base** `MCC` `CC` `H5` `HCC`
of neck of unspecified femur

8,10 ☑7ᵗʰ **S72.044 Nondisplaced fracture of** `MCC` `CC` `H5` `HCC`
base of neck of right femur

8,10 ☑7ᵗʰ **S72.045 Nondisplaced fracture of** `MCC` `CC` `H5` `HCC`
base of neck of left femur

8,10 ☑7ᵗʰ **S72.046 Nondisplaced fracture of** `MCC` `CC` `H5` `HCC`
base of neck of unspecified femur

☑6ᵗʰ **S72.05 Unspecified fracture of head of femur**
Fracture of head of femur NOS

8,10 ☑7ᵗʰ **S72.051 Unspecified fracture of** `MCC` `CC` `H5` `HCC`
head of right femur

8,10 ☑7ᵗʰ **S72.052 Unspecified fracture of** `MCC` `CC` `H5` `HCC`
head of left femur

8,10 ☑7ᵗʰ **S72.059 Unspecified fracture of** `MCC` `CC` `H5` `HCC`
head of unspecified femur

☑6ᵗʰ **S72.06 Articular fracture of head of femur**

8,10 ☑7ᵗʰ **S72.061 Displaced articular fracture** `MCC` `CC` `H5` `HCC`
of head of right femur

8,10 ☑7ᵗʰ **S72.062 Displaced articular fracture** `MCC` `CC` `H5` `HCC`
of head of left femur

8,10 ☑7ᵗʰ **S72.063 Displaced articular** `MCC` `CC` `H5` `HCC`
fracture of head of unspecified femur

8,10 ☑7ᵗʰ **S72.064 Nondisplaced articular** `MCC` `CC` `H5` `HCC`
fracture of head of right femur

8,10 ☑7ᵗʰ **S72.065 Nondisplaced articular** `MCC` `CC` `H5` `HCC`
fracture of head of left femur

8,10 ☑7ᵗʰ **S72.066 Nondisplaced articular** `MCC` `CC` `H5` `HCC`
fracture of head of unspecified femur

---

8 CC when reported as a subsequent encounter for nonunion or malunion (7th character K, M, N, P, Q, or R).
10 HCC with 7th character indicating initial encounter (A, B or C - specific to category).

☑ Additional Character Req   ☑ˣ7ᵗʰ Placeholder Alert   Unacceptable PDx   Manifestation   `H1`–`H14` HAC   `HCC` CMS-HCC Condition   *EXCLUDES 1* Not Coded Here   *EXCLUDES 2* Not Included Here

Chapter 19. Injury, Poisoning and Certain Other Consequences of External Causes

√6th **S72.09** Other fracture of head and neck of femur

8,10 √7th **S72.091** Other fracture of head and neck of right femur `MCC` `CC` `H5` `HCC`

8,10 √7th **S72.092** Other fracture of head and neck of left femur `MCC` `CC` `H5` `HCC`

8,10 √7th **S72.099** Other fracture of head and neck of unspecified femur `MCC` `CC` `H5` `HCC`

√5th **S72.1** Pertrochanteric fracture
AHA: 2016, 3Q, 16

> **CC Excl: For CC/MCC codes in subcategory S72.1:**
> **Right side:** See code S72.001
> **Left side:** See code S72.002
> **Unspecified side:** See code S72.009

√6th **S72.10** Unspecified trochanteric fracture of femur
Fracture of trochanter NOS

8,10 √7th **S72.101** Unspecified trochanteric fracture of right femur `MCC` `CC` `H5` `HCC`

8,10 √7th **S72.102** Unspecified trochanteric fracture of left femur `MCC` `CC` `H5` `HCC`

8,10 √7th **S72.109** Unspecified trochanteric fracture of unspecified femur `MCC` `CC` `H5` `HCC`

√6th **S72.11** Fracture of greater trochanter of femur

8,10 √7th **S72.111** Displaced fracture of greater trochanter of right femur `MCC` `CC` `H5` `HCC`

8,10 √7th **S72.112** Displaced fracture of greater trochanter of left femur `MCC` `CC` `H5` `HCC`

8,10 √7th **S72.113** Displaced fracture of greatertrochanter of unspecified femur `MCC` `CC` `H5` `HCC`

8,10 √7th **S72.114** Nondisplaced fracture of greater trochanter of right femur `MCC` `CC` `H5` `HCC`

8,10 √7th **S72.115** Nondisplaced fracture of greater trochanter of left femur `MCC` `CC` `H5` `HCC`

8,10 √7th **S72.116** Nondisplaced fracture of greater trochanter of unspecified femur `MCC` `CC` `H5` `HCC`

√6th **S72.12** Fracture of lesser trochanter of femur

8,10 √7th **S72.121** Displaced fracture of lesser trochanter of right femur `MCC` `CC` `H5` `HCC`

8,10 √7th **S72.122** Displaced fracture of lesser trochanter of left femur `MCC` `CC` `H5` `HCC`

8,10 √7th **S72.123** Displaced fracture of lesser trochanter of unspecified femur `MCC` `CC` `H5` `HCC`

8,10 √7th **S72.124** Nondisplaced fracture of lesser trochanter of right femur `MCC` `CC` `H5` `HCC`

8,10 √7th **S72.125** Nondisplaced fracture of lesser trochanter of left femur `MCC` `CC` `H5` `HCC`

8,10 √7th **S72.126** Nondisplaced fracture of lesser trochanter of unspecified femur `MCC` `CC` `H5` `HCC`

√6th **S72.13** Apophyseal fracture of femur
EXCLUDES 1   chronic (nontraumatic) slipped upper femoral epiphysis (M93.0-)

8,10 √7th **S72.131** Displaced apophyseal fracture of right femur `MCC` `CC` `H5` `HCC`

8,10 √7th **S72.132** Displaced apophyseal fracture of left femur `MCC` `CC` `H5` `HCC`

8,10 √7th **S72.133** Displaced apophyseal fracture of unspecified femur `MCC` `CC` `H5` `HCC`

8,10 √7th **S72.134** Nondisplaced apophyseal fracture of right femur `MCC` `CC` `H5` `HCC`

8,10 √7th **S72.135** Nondisplaced apophyseal fractureof left femur `MCC` `CC` `H5` `HCC`

8,10 √7th **S72.136** Nondisplaced apophyseal fracture of unspecified femur `MCC` `CC` `H5` `HCC`

√6th **S72.14** Intertrochanteric fracture of femur

8,10 √7th **S72.141** Displaced intertrochanteric fracture of right femur `MCC` `CC` `H5` `HCC`

8,10 √7th **S72.142** Displaced intertrochanteric fracture of left femur `MCC` `CC` `H5` `HCC`

8,10 √7th **S72.143** Displaced intertrochanteric fracture of unspecified femur `MCC` `CC` `H5` `HCC`

8,10 √7th **S72.144** Nondisplaced intertrochanteric fracture of right femur `MCC` `CC` `H5` `HCC`

8,10 √7th **S72.145** Nondisplaced intertrochanteric fracture of left femur `MCC` `CC` `H5` `HCC`

8,10 √7th **S72.146** Nondisplaced intertrochanteric fracture of unspecified femur `MCC` `CC` `H5` `HCC`

√5th **S72.2** Subtrochanteric fracture of femur

> **CC Excl: For CC/MCC codes in subcategory S72.2:**
> **Right side:** See code S72.009
> **Left side:** See code S72.009
> **Unspecified side:** See code S72.009

8,10 √x7th **S72.21** Displaced subtrochanteric fracture of right femur `MCC` `CC` `H5` `HCC`

8,10 √x7th **S72.22** Displaced subtrochanteric fracture of left femur `MCC` `CC` `H5` `HCC`

8,10 √x7th **S72.23** Displaced subtrochanteric fracture of unspecified femur `MCC` `CC` `H5` `HCC`

8,10 √x7th **S72.24** Nondisplaced subtrochanteric fracture of right femur `MCC` `CC` `H5` `HCC`

8,10 √x7th **S72.25** Nondisplaced subtrochanteric fracture of left femur `MCC` `CC` `H5` `HCC`

8,10 √x7th **S72.26** Nondisplaced subtrochanteric fracture of unspecified femur `MCC` `CC` `H5` `HCC`

√5th **S72.3** Fracture of shaft of femur

> **CC Excl: For CC/MCC codes in subcategory S72.3:**
> **Right side:** See code S72.001
> **Left side:** See code S72.002
> **Unspecified side:** See code S72.009

√6th **S72.30** Unspecified fracture of shaft of femur

8,10 √7th **S72.301** Unspecified fracture of shaft of right femur `MCC` `CC` `H5` `HCC`

8,10 √7th **S72.302** Unspecified fracture of shaft of left femur `MCC` `CC` `H5` `HCC`

8,10 √7th **S72.309** Unspecified fracture of shaft of unspecified femur `MCC` `CC` `H5` `HCC`

√6th **S72.32** Transverse fracture of shaft of femur

8,10 √7th **S72.321** Displaced transverse fracture of shaft of right femur `MCC` `CC` `H5` `HCC`

8,10 √7th **S72.322** Displaced transverse fracture of shaft of left femur `MCC` `CC` `H5` `HCC`

8,10 √7th **S72.323** Displaced transverse fracture of shaft of unspecified femur `MCC` `CC` `H5` `HCC`

8,10 √7th **S72.324** Nondisplaced transverse fracture of shaft of right femur `MCC` `CC` `H5` `HCC`

8,10 √7th **S72.325** Nondisplaced transverse fracture of shaft of left femur `MCC` `CC` `H5` `HCC`

8,10 √7th **S72.326** Nondisplaced transverse fracture of shaft of unspecified femur `MCC` `CC` `H5` `HCC`

√6th **S72.33** Oblique fracture of shaft of femur

8,10 √7th **S72.331** Displaced oblique fracture of shaft of right femur `MCC` `CC` `H5` `HCC`

8,10 √7th **S72.332** Displaced oblique fracture of shaft of left femur `MCC` `CC` `H5` `HCC`

8,10 √7th **S72.333** Displaced oblique fracture of shaft of unspecified femur `MCC` `CC` `H5` `HCC`

8,10 √7th **S72.334** Nondisplaced oblique fracture of shaft of right femur `MCC` `CC` `H5` `HCC`

8,10 √7th **S72.335** Nondisplaced oblique fracture of shaft of left femur `MCC` `CC` `H5` `HCC`

8,10 √7th **S72.336** Nondisplaced oblique fracture of shaft of unspecified femur `MCC` `CC` `H5` `HCC`

√6th **S72.34** Spiral fracture of shaft of femur

8,10 √7th **S72.341** Displaced spiral fracture of shaft of right femur `MCC` `CC` `H5` `HCC`

8,10 √7th **S72.342** Displaced spiral fracture of shaft of left femur `MCC` `CC` `H5` `HCC`

8,10 √7th **S72.343** Displaced spiral fracture of shaft of unspecified femur `MCC` `CC` `H5` `HCC`

8,10 √7th **S72.344** Nondisplaced spiral fracture of shaft of right femur `MCC` `CC` `H5` `HCC`

---

8   CC when reported as a subsequent encounter for nonunion or malunion (7th character K, M, N, P, Q, or R).
10   HCC with 7th character indicating initial encounter (A, B or C - specific to category).

`N` Newborn: 0   `P` Pediatric: 0-17   `M` Maternity: 12-55   `A` Adult: 15-124   `MCC` Major CC Condition   `PDxMCC` PDx acts as own MCC   `CC` CC Condition   `PDxCC` PDx acts as own CC

8,10 ✓7ᵗʰ **S72.345** **Nondisplaced spiral fracture of left femur** `MCC` `CC` `H5` `HCC`

8,10 ✓7ᵗʰ **S72.346** **Nondisplaced spiral fracture of shaft of unspecified femur** `MCC` `CC` `H5` `HCC`

✓6ᵗʰ **S72.35** **Comminuted fracture of shaft of femur**

8,10 ✓7ᵗʰ **S72.351** **Displaced comminuted fracture of shaft of right femur** `MCC` `CC` `H5` `HCC`

8,10 ✓7ᵗʰ **S72.352** **Displaced comminuted fracture of shaft of left femur** `MCC` `CC` `H5` `HCC`

8,10 ✓7ᵗʰ **S72.353** **Displaced comminuted fracture of shaft of unspecified femur** `MCC` `CC` `H5` `HCC`

8,10 ✓7ᵗʰ **S72.354** **Nondisplaced comminuted fracture of shaft of right femur** `MCC` `CC` `H5` `HCC`

8,10 ✓7ᵗʰ **S72.355** **Nondisplaced comminuted fracture of shaft of left femur** `MCC` `CC` `H5` `HCC`

8,10 ✓7ᵗʰ **S72.356** **Nondisplaced comminuted fracture of shaft of unspecified femur** `MCC` `CC` `H5` `HCC`

✓6ᵗʰ **S72.36** **Segmental fracture of shaft of femur**

8,10 ✓7ᵗʰ **S72.361** **Displaced segmental fracture of shaft of right femur** `MCC` `CC` `H5` `HCC`

8,10 ✓7ᵗʰ **S72.362** **Displaced segmental fracture of shaft of left femur** `MCC` `CC` `H5` `HCC`

8,10 ✓7ᵗʰ **S72.363** **Displaced segmental fracture of shaft of unspecified femur** `MCC` `CC` `H5` `HCC`

8,10 ✓7ᵗʰ **S72.364** **Nondisplaced segmental fracture of shaft of right femur** `MCC` `CC` `H5` `HCC`

8,10 ✓7ᵗʰ **S72.365** **Nondisplaced segmental fracture of shaft of left femur** `MCC` `CC` `H5` `HCC`

8,10 ✓7ᵗʰ **S72.366** **Nondisplaced segmental fracture of shaft of unspecified femur** `MCC` `CC` `H5` `HCC`

✓6ᵗʰ **S72.39** **Other fracture of shaft of femur**

8,10 ✓7ᵗʰ **S72.391** **Other fracture of shaft of right femur** `MCC` `CC` `H5` `HCC`

8,10 ✓7ᵗʰ **S72.392** **Other fracture of shaft of left femur** `MCC` `CC` `H5` `HCC`

8,10 ✓7ᵗʰ **S72.399** **Other fracture of shaft of unspecified femur** `MCC` `CC` `H5` `HCC`

✓5ᵗʰ **S72.4** **Fracture of lower end of femur**
Fracture of distal end of femur
EXCLUDES 2   *fracture of shaft of femur (S72.3-)*
     physeal fracture of lower end of femur (S79.1-)

> **CC Excl: For CC/MCC codes in subcategory S72.4, unless otherwise noted:**
> **Right side:** See code S72.401
> **Left side:** See code S72.402
> **Unspecified side:** See code S72.409

✓6ᵗʰ **S72.40** **Unspecified fracture of lower end of femur**

6,7,10 ✓7ᵗʰ **S72.401** **Unspecified fracture of lower end of right femur** `MCC` `CC` `H5` `HCC`
     CC Excl: MCC with 7th character A:
     PDX collection 1300
     MCC with 7th character B or C:
     PDX collection 1301
     CC with 7th character K, M, N, P, Q or R:
     PDX collection 897

6,7,10 ✓7ᵗʰ **S72.402** **Unspecified fracture of lower end of left femur** `MCC` `CC` `H5` `HCC`
     CC Excl: MCC with 7th character A:
     PDX collection 1302
     MCC with 7th character B or C:
     PDX collection 1301
     CC with 7th character K, M, N, P, Q or R:
     PDX collection 897

6,7,10 ✓7ᵗʰ **S72.409** **Unspecified fracture of lower end of unspecified femur** `MCC` `CC` `H5` `HCC`
     CC Excl: MCC with 7th character A, B or C:
     PDX collection 1301
     CC with 7th character K, M, N, P, Q or R:
     PDX collection 897

✓6ᵗʰ **S72.41** **Unspecified condyle fracture of lower end of femur**
Condyle fracture of femur NOS

6,7,10 ✓7ᵗʰ **S72.411** **Displaced unspecified condyle fracture of lower end of right femur** `MCC` `CC` `H5` `HCC`

6,7,10 ✓7ᵗʰ **S72.412** **Displaced unspecified condyle fracture of lower end of left femur** `MCC` `CC` `H5` `HCC`

6,7,10 ✓7ᵗʰ **S72.413** **Displaced unspecified condyle fracture of lower end of unspecified femur** `MCC` `CC` `H5` `HCC`

6,7,10 ✓7ᵗʰ **S72.414** **Nondisplaced unspecified condyle fracture of lower end of right femur** `MCC` `CC` `H5` `HCC`

6,7,10 ✓7ᵗʰ **S72.415** **Nondisplaced unspecified condyle fracture of lower end of left femur** `MCC` `CC` `H5` `HCC`

6,7,10 ✓7ᵗʰ **S72.416** **Nondisplaced unspecified condyle fracture of lower end of unspecified femur** `MCC` `CC` `H5` `HCC`

✓6ᵗʰ **S72.42** **Fracture of lateral condyle of femur**

6,7,10 ✓7ᵗʰ **S72.421** **Displaced fracture of lateral condyle of right femur** `MCC` `CC` `H5` `HCC`

6,7,10 ✓7ᵗʰ **S72.422** **Displaced fracture of lateral condyle of left femur** `MCC` `CC` `H5` `HCC`

6,7,10 ✓7ᵗʰ **S72.423** **Displaced fracture of lateral condyle of unspecified femur** `MCC` `CC` `H5` `HCC`

6,7,10 ✓7ᵗʰ **S72.424** **Nondisplaced fracture of lateral condyle of right femur** `MCC` `CC` `H5` `HCC`

6,7,10 ✓7ᵗʰ **S72.425** **Nondisplaced fracture of lateral condyle of left femur** `MCC` `CC` `H5` `HCC`

6,7,10 ✓7ᵗʰ **S72.426** **Nondisplaced fracture of lateral condyle of unspecified femur** `MCC` `CC` `H5` `HCC`

✓6ᵗʰ **S72.43** **Fracture of medial condyle of femur**

6,7,10 ✓7ᵗʰ **S72.431** **Displaced fracture of medial condyle of right femur** `MCC` `CC` `H5` `HCC`

6,7,10 ✓7ᵗʰ **S72.432** **Displaced fracture of medial condyle of left femur** `MCC` `CC` `H5` `HCC`

6,7,10 ✓7ᵗʰ **S72.433** **Displaced fracture of medial condyle of unspecified femur** `MCC` `CC` `H5` `HCC`

6,7,10 ✓7ᵗʰ **S72.434** **Nondisplaced fracture of medial condyle of right femur** `MCC` `CC` `H5` `HCC`

6,7,10 ✓7ᵗʰ **S72.435** **Nondisplaced fracture of medial condyle of left femur** `MCC` `CC` `H5` `HCC`

6,7,10 ✓7ᵗʰ **S72.436** **Nondisplaced fracture of medial condyle of unspecified femur** `MCC` `CC` `H5` `HCC`

✓6ᵗʰ **S72.44** **Fracture of lower epiphysis (separation) of femur**
EXCLUDES 1   *Salter-Harris Type I physeal fracture of lower end of femur (S79.11-)*

6,7,10 ✓7ᵗʰ **S72.441** **Displaced fracture of lower epiphysis (separation) of right femur** `MCC` `CC` `H5` `HCC`

6,7,10 ✓7ᵗʰ **S72.442** **Displaced fracture of lower epiphysis (separation) of left femur** `MCC` `CC` `H5` `HCC`

6,7,10 ✓7ᵗʰ **S72.443** **Displaced fracture of lower epiphysis (separation) of unspecified femur** `MCC` `CC` `H5` `HCC`

6,7,10 ✓7ᵗʰ **S72.444** **Nondisplaced fracture of lowerepiphysis (separation) of right femur** `MCC` `CC` `H5` `HCC`

6,7,10 ✓7ᵗʰ **S72.445** **Nondisplaced fracture of lower epiphysis (separation) of left femur** `MCC` `CC` `H5` `HCC`

6,7,10 ✓7ᵗʰ **S72.446** **Nondisplaced fracture of lower epiphysis (separation) of unspecified femur** `MCC` `CC` `H5` `HCC`

---

⁶   MCC when reported as an open fracture (7th character B or C).
⁷   CC when reported as an initial encounter (7th character A, B, or C – specific to category) OR a subsequent encounter for nonunion or malunion (7th character K, M, N, P, Q, or R – specific to category).
⁸   CC when reported as a subsequent encounter for nonunion or malunion (7th character K, M, N, P, Q, or R).
¹⁰   HCC with 7th character indicating initial encounter (A, B or C - specific to category).

✓ Additional Character Req   ✓ₓ7ᵗʰ Placeholder Alert   Unacceptable PDx   Manifestation   `H1`-`H14` HAC   `HCC` CMS-HCC Condition   *EXCLUDES 1* Not Coded Here   *EXCLUDES 2* Not Included Here

Chapter 19. Injury, Poisoning and Certain Other Consequences of External Causes

√6ᵗʰ **S72.45** **Supracondylar fracture without intracondylar extension of lower end of femur**
    Supracondylar fracture of lower end of femur NOS
    EXCLUDES 1   *supracondylar fracture with intracondylar extension of lower end of femur (S72.46-)*

6,7,10 √7ᵗʰ **S72.451** **Displaced supracondylar fracture without intracondylar extension of lower end of right femur** `MCC` `CC` `H5` `HCC`

6,7,10 √7ᵗʰ **S72.452** **Displaced supracondylar fracture without intracondylar extension of lower end of left femur** `MCC` `CC` `H5` `HCC`

6,7,10 √7ᵗʰ **S72.453** **Displaced supracondylar fracture without intracondylar extension of lower end of unspecified femur** `MCC` `CC` `H5` `HCC`

6,7,10 √7ᵗʰ **S72.454** **Nondisplaced supracondylar fracture without intracondylar extension of lower end of right femur** `MCC` `CC` `H5` `HCC`

6,7,10 √7ᵗʰ **S72.455** **Nondisplaced supracondylar fracture without intracondylar extension of lower end of left femur** `MCC` `CC` `H5` `HCC`

6,7,10 √7ᵗʰ **S72.456** **Nondisplaced supracondylar fracture without intracondylar extension of lower end of unspecified femur** `MCC` `CC` `H5` `HCC`

√6ᵗʰ **S72.46** **Supracondylar fracture with intracondylar extension of lower end of femur**
    EXCLUDES 1   *supracondylar fracture without intracondylar extension of lower end of femur (S72.45-)*

6,7,10 √7ᵗʰ **S72.461** **Displaced supracondylar fracture with intracondylar extension of lower end of right femur** `MCC` `CC` `H5` `HCC`

6,7,10 √7ᵗʰ **S72.462** **Displaced supracondylar fracture with intracondylar extension of lower end of left femur** `MCC` `CC` `H5` `HCC`

6,7,10 √7ᵗʰ **S72.463** **Displaced supracondylar fracture with intracondylar extension of lower end of unspecified femur** `MCC` `CC` `H5` `HCC`

6,7,10 √7ᵗʰ **S72.464** **Nondisplaced supracondylar fracture with intracondylar extension of lower end of right femur** `MCC` `CC` `H5` `HCC`

6,7,10 √7ᵗʰ **S72.465** **Nondisplaced supracondylar fracture with intracondylar extension of lower end of left femur** `MCC` `CC` `H5` `HCC`

6,7,10 √7ᵗʰ **S72.466** **Nondisplaced supracondylar fracture with intracondylar extension of lower end of unspecified femur** `MCC` `CC` `H5` `HCC`

√6ᵗʰ **S72.47** **Torus fracture of lower end of femur**

The appropriate 7th character is to be added to all codes in subcategory S72.47.
A   initial encounter for closed fracture
D   subsequent encounter for fracture with routine healing
G   subsequent encounter for fracture with delayed healing
K   subsequent encounter for fracture with nonunion
P   subsequent encounter for fracture with malunion
S   sequela

7,10 √7ᵗʰ **S72.471** **Torus fracture of lower end of right femur** `CC` `H5` `HCC`
    CC Excl: CC with 7th character A:
    PDX collection 1300
    CC Excl: CC with 7th character K or P:
    PDX collection 897

7,10 √7ᵗʰ **S72.472** **Torus fracture of lower end of left femur** `CC` `H5` `HCC`
    CC Excl: CC with 7th character A:
    PDX collection 1302
    CC Excl: CC with 7th character K or P:
    PDX collection 897

7,10 √7ᵗʰ **S72.479** **Torus fracture of lower end of unspecified femur** `CC` `H5` `HCC`
    CC Excl: CC with 7th character A:
    PDX collection 1301
    CC Excl: CC with 7th character K or P:
    PDX collection 897

√6ᵗʰ **S72.49** **Other fracture of lower end of femur**

6,7,10 √7ᵗʰ **S72.491** **Other fracture of lower end of right femur** `MCC` `CC` `H5` `HCC`
    CC Excl: MCC with 7th character A:
    PDX collection 1300
    MCC with 7th character B or C:
    PDX collection 1303
    CC with 7th character K, M, N, P, Q or R:
    PDX collection 897

6,7,10 √7ᵗʰ **S72.492** **Other fracture of lower end of left femur** `MCC` `CC` `H5` `HCC`
    CC Excl: MCC with 7th character A:
    PDX collection 1302
    MCC with 7th character B or C:
    PDX collection 1303
    CC with 7th character K, M, N, P, Q or R:
    PDX collection 897

6,7,10 √7ᵗʰ **S72.499** **Other fracture of lower end of unspecified femur** `MCC` `CC` `H5` `HCC`
    CC Excl: MCC with 7th character A:
    PDX collection 1301
    MCC with 7th character B or C:
    PDX collection 1303
    CC with 7th character K, M, N, P, Q or R:
    PDX collection 897

√5ᵗʰ **S72.8** **Other fracture of femur**

√6ᵗʰ **S72.8X** **Other fracture of femur**

CC Excl: For codes in subcategory S72.8X:
MCC with 7th character A, B or C:
PDX collection 1298
CC with 7th character K, M, N, P, Q or R:
PDX collection 897

8,10 √7ᵗʰ **S72.8X1** **Other fracture of right femur** `MCC` `CC` `H5` `HCC`

8,10 √7ᵗʰ **S72.8X2** **Other fracture of left femur** `MCC` `CC` `H5` `HCC`

8,10 √7ᵗʰ **S72.8X9** **Other fracture of unspecified femur** `MCC` `CC` `H5` `HCC`

√5ᵗʰ **S72.9** **Unspecified fracture of femur**
    Fracture of thigh NOS
    Fracture of upper leg NOS
    EXCLUDES 1   *fracture of hip NOS (S72.00-, S72.01-)*

CC Excl: For codes in subcategory S72.9:
MCC with 7th character A, B or C:
PDX collection 1298
CC with 7th character K, M, N, P, Q or R:
PDX collection 897

8,10 √x7ᵗʰ **S72.90** **Unspecified fracture of unspecified femur** `MCC` `CC` `H5` `HCC`
    AHA: 2012, 4Q, 93

8,10 √x7ᵗʰ **S72.91** **Unspecified fracture of right femur** `MCC` `CC` `H5` `HCC`

8,10 √x7ᵗʰ **S72.92** **Unspecified fracture of left femur** `MCC` `CC` `H5` `HCC`

---

6   MCC when reported as an open fracture (7th character B or C).

7   CC when reported as an initial encounter (7th character A, B, or C – specific to category) OR a subsequent encounter for nonunion or malunion (7th character K, M, N, P, Q, or R – specific to category).

8   CC when reported as a subsequent encounter for nonunion or malunion (7th character K, M, N, P, Q, or R).

10   HCC with 7th character indicating initial encounter (A, B or C - specific to category).

`N` Newborn: 0   `P` Pediatric: 0-17   `M` Maternity: 12-55   `A` Adult: 15-124   `MCC` Major CC Condition   `PDxMCC` PDx acts as own MCC   `CC` CC Condition   `PDxCC` PDx acts as own CC

✓4ᵗʰ **S73　Dislocation and sprain of joint and ligaments of hip**
　　INCLUDES　avulsion of joint or ligament of hip
　　　　　　laceration of cartilage, joint or ligament of hip
　　　　　　sprain of cartilage, joint or ligament of hip
　　　　　　traumatic hemarthrosis of joint or ligament of hip
　　　　　　traumatic rupture of joint or ligament of hip
　　　　　　traumatic subluxation of joint or ligament of hip
　　　　　　traumatic tear of joint or ligament of hip
　　Code also any associated open wound
　　EXCLUDES 2　strain of muscle, fascia and tendon of hip and thigh (S76.-)

The appropriate 7th character is to be added to each code from category S73.
A　initial encounter
D　subsequent encounter
S　sequela

✓5ᵗʰ **S73.0　Subluxation and dislocation of hip**
　　EXCLUDES 2　dislocation and subluxation of hip prosthesis (T84.020, T84.021)

　✓6ᵗʰ **S73.00　Unspecified subluxation and dislocation of hip**
　　　　Dislocation of hip NOS
　　　　Subluxation of hip NOS
　　　10 ✓7ᵗʰ **S73.001　Unspecified subluxation of right hip** CC H5 HCC
　　　　　　CC Excl: CC with 7th character A:
　　　　　　PDX collection 1304
　　　10 ✓7ᵗʰ **S73.002　Unspecified subluxation of left hip** CC H5 HCC
　　　　　　CC Excl: CC with 7th character A:
　　　　　　PDX collection 1305
　　　10 ✓7ᵗʰ **S73.003　Unspecified subluxation of unspecified hip** CC H5 HCC
　　　　　　CC Excl: CC with 7th character A:
　　　　　　PDX collection 1306
　　　10 ✓7ᵗʰ **S73.004　Unspecified dislocation of right hip** CC H5 HCC
　　　　　　CC Excl: CC with 7th character A:
　　　　　　PDX collection 1304
　　　10 ✓7ᵗʰ **S73.005　Unspecified dislocation of left hip** CC H5 HCC
　　　　　　CC Excl: CC with 7th character A:
　　　　　　PDX collection 1305
　　　10 ✓7ᵗʰ **S73.006　Unspecified dislocation of unspecified hip** CC H5 HCC
　　　　　　CC Excl: CC with 7th character A:
　　　　　　PDX collection 1306

　✓6ᵗʰ **S73.01　Posterior subluxation and dislocation of hip**
　　　10 ✓7ᵗʰ **S73.011　Posterior subluxation of right hip** CC H5 HCC
　　　　　　CC Excl: CC with 7th character A:
　　　　　　PDX collection 1307
　　　10 ✓7ᵗʰ **S73.012　Posterior subluxation of left hip** CC H5 HCC
　　　　　　CC Excl: CC with 7th character A:
　　　　　　PDX collection 1308
　　　10 ✓7ᵗʰ **S73.013　Posterior subluxation of unspecified hip** CC H5 HCC
　　　　　　CC Excl: CC with 7th character A:
　　　　　　PDX collection 1309
　　　10 ✓7ᵗʰ **S73.014　Posterior dislocation of right hip** CC H5 HCC
　　　　　　CC Excl: CC with 7th character A:
　　　　　　PDX collection 1307
　　　10 ✓7ᵗʰ **S73.015　Posterior dislocation of left hip** CC H5 HCC
　　　　　　CC Excl: CC with 7th character A:
　　　　　　PDX collection 1308
　　　10 ✓7ᵗʰ **S73.016　Posterior dislocation of unspecified hip** CC H5 HCC
　　　　　　CC Excl: CC with 7th character A:
　　　　　　PDX collection 1309

　✓6ᵗʰ **S73.02　Obturator subluxation and dislocation of hip**
　　　10 ✓7ᵗʰ **S73.021　Obturator subluxation of right hip** CC H5 HCC
　　　　　　CC Excl: CC with 7th character A:
　　　　　　PDX collection 1310
　　　10 ✓7ᵗʰ **S73.022　Obturator subluxation of left hip** CC H5 HCC
　　　　　　CC Excl: CC with 7th character A:
　　　　　　PDX collection 1311
　　　10 ✓7ᵗʰ **S73.023　Obturator subluxation of unspecified hip** CC H5 HCC
　　　　　　CC Excl: CC with 7th character A:
　　　　　　PDX collection 1312

　　　10 ✓7ᵗʰ **S73.024　Obturator dislocation of right hip** CC H5 HCC
　　　　　　CC Excl: CC with 7th character A:
　　　　　　PDX collection 1310
　　　10 ✓7ᵗʰ **S73.025　Obturator dislocation of left hip** CC H5 HCC
　　　　　　CC Excl: CC with 7th character A:
　　　　　　PDX collection 1311
　　　10 ✓7ᵗʰ **S73.026　Obturator dislocation of unspecified hip** CC H5 HCC
　　　　　　CC Excl: CC with 7th character A:
　　　　　　PDX collection 1312

▲　✓6ᵗʰ **S73.03　Other anterior subluxation and dislocation of hip**
　　　10 ✓7ᵗʰ **S73.031　Other anterior subluxation of right hip** CC H5 HCC
　　　　　　CC Excl: CC with 7th character A:
　　　　　　PDX collection 1313
　　　10 ✓7ᵗʰ **S73.032　Other anterior subluxation of left hip** CC H5 HCC
　　　　　　CC Excl: CC with 7th character A:
　　　　　　PDX collection 1314
　　　10 ✓7ᵗʰ **S73.033　Other anterior subluxation of unspecified hip** CC H5 HCC
　　　　　　CC Excl: CC with 7th character A:
　　　　　　PDX collection 1315
　　　10 ✓7ᵗʰ **S73.034　Other anterior dislocation of right hip** CC H5 HCC
　　　　　　CC Excl: CC with 7th character A:
　　　　　　PDX collection 1313
　　　10 ✓7ᵗʰ **S73.035　Other anterior dislocation of left hip** CC H5 HCC
　　　　　　CC Excl: CC with 7th character A:
　　　　　　PDX collection 1314
　　　10 ✓7ᵗʰ **S73.036　Other anterior dislocation of unspecified hip** CC H5 HCC
　　　　　　CC Excl: CC with 7th character A:
　　　　　　PDX collection 1315

▲　✓6ᵗʰ **S73.04　Central subluxation and dislocation of hip**
　　　10 ✓7ᵗʰ **S73.041　Central subluxation of right hip** CC H5 HCC
　　　　　　CC Excl: CC with 7th character A:
　　　　　　PDX collection 1304
　　　10 ✓7ᵗʰ **S73.042　Central subluxation of left hip** CC H5 HCC
　　　　　　CC Excl: CC with 7th character A:
　　　　　　PDX collection 1305
　　　10 ✓7ᵗʰ **S73.043　Central subluxation of unspecified hip** CC H5 HCC
　　　　　　CC Excl: CC with 7th character A:
　　　　　　PDX collection 1306
　　　10 ✓7ᵗʰ **S73.044　Central dislocation of right hip** CC H5 HCC
　　　　　　CC Excl: CC with 7th character A:
　　　　　　PDX collection 1304
　　　10 ✓7ᵗʰ **S73.045　Central dislocation of left hip** CC H5 HCC
　　　　　　CC Excl: CC with 7th character A:
　　　　　　PDX collection 1305
　　　10 ✓7ᵗʰ **S73.046　Central dislocation of unspecified hip** CC H5 HCC
　　　　　　CC Excl: CC with 7th character A:
　　　　　　PDX collection 1306

✓5ᵗʰ **S73.1　Sprain of hip**
　　AHA: 2014, 4Q, 25
　✓6ᵗʰ **S73.10　Unspecified sprain of hip**
　　　✓7ᵗʰ **S73.101　Unspecified sprain of right hip**
　　　✓7ᵗʰ **S73.102　Unspecified sprain of left hip**
　　　✓7ᵗʰ **S73.109　Unspecified sprain of unspecified hip**
　✓6ᵗʰ **S73.11　Iliofemoral ligament sprain of hip**
　　　✓7ᵗʰ **S73.111　Iliofemoral ligament sprain of right hip**
　　　✓7ᵗʰ **S73.112　Iliofemoral ligament sprain of left hip**
　　　✓7ᵗʰ **S73.119　Iliofemoral ligament sprain of unspecified hip**
　✓6ᵗʰ **S73.12　Ischiocapsular (ligament) sprain of hip**
　　　✓7ᵗʰ **S73.121　Ischiocapsular ligament sprain of right hip**
　　　✓7ᵗʰ **S73.122　Ischiocapsular ligament sprain of left hip**
　　　✓7ᵗʰ **S73.129　Ischiocapsular ligament sprain of unspecified hip**
　✓6ᵗʰ **S73.19　Other sprain of hip**
　　　✓7ᵗʰ **S73.191　Other sprain of right hip**
　　　✓7ᵗʰ **S73.192　Other sprain of left hip**
　　　✓7ᵗʰ **S73.199　Other sprain of unspecified hip**

---

10 HCC with 7th character indicating initial encounter (A, B or C - specific to category).

Chapter 19. Injury, Poisoning and Certain Other Consequences of External Causes

S74–S75.201

✓4ᵗʰ S74 Injury of nerves at hip and thigh level

Code also any associated open wound (S71.-)

EXCLUDES 2   injury of nerves at ankle and foot level (S94.-)
injury of nerves at lower leg level (S84.-)

The appropriate 7th character is to be added to each code from category S74.
A   initial encounter
D   subsequent encounter
S   sequela

✓5ᵗʰ S74.0 Injury of sciatic nerve at hip and thigh level

✓x7ᵗʰ **S74.00**   Injury of sciatic nerve at hip and thigh level, unspecified leg

✓x7ᵗʰ **S74.01**   Injury of sciatic nerve at hip and thigh level, right leg

✓x7ᵗʰ **S74.02**   Injury of sciatic nerve at hip and thigh level, left leg

✓5ᵗʰ S74.1 Injury of femoral nerve at hip and thigh level

✓x7ᵗʰ **S74.10**   Injury of femoral nerve at hip and thigh level, unspecified leg

✓x7ᵗʰ **S74.11**   Injury of femoral nerve at hip and thigh level, right leg

✓x7ᵗʰ **S74.12**   Injury of femoral nerve at hip and thigh level, left leg

✓5ᵗʰ S74.2 Injury of cutaneous sensory nerve at hip and thigh level

✓x7ᵗʰ **S74.20**   Injury of cutaneous sensory nerve at hip and thigh level, unspecified leg

✓x7ᵗʰ **S74.21**   Injury of cutaneous sensory nerve at hip and high level, right leg

✓x7ᵗʰ **S74.22**   Injury of cutaneous sensory nerve at hip and thigh level, left leg

✓5ᵗʰ S74.8 Injury of other nerves at hip and thigh level

✓6ᵗʰ **S74.8X**   Injury of other nerves at hip and thigh level

✓7ᵗʰ **S74.8X1**   Injury of other nerves at hip and thigh level, right leg

✓7ᵗʰ **S74.8X2**   Injury of other nerves at hip and thigh level, left leg

✓7ᵗʰ **S74.8X9**   Injury of other nerves at hip and thigh level, unspecified leg

✓5ᵗʰ S74.9 Injury of unspecified nerve at hip and thigh level

✓x7ᵗʰ **S74.90**   Injury of unspecified nerve at hip and thigh level, unspecified leg

✓x7ᵗʰ **S74.91**   Injury of unspecified nerve at hip and thigh level, right leg

✓x7ᵗʰ **S74.92**   Injury of unspecified nerve at hip and thigh level, left leg

✓4ᵗʰ S75 Injury of blood vessels at hip and thigh level

Code also any associated open wound (S71.-)

EXCLUDES 2   injury of blood vessels at lower leg level (S85.-)
injury of popliteal artery (S85.0)

The appropriate 7th character is to be added to each code from category S75.
A   initial encounter
D   subsequent encounter
S   sequela

✓5ᵗʰ S75.0 Injury of femoral artery

CC Excl: For CC codes in subcategory S75.0:
Right side: PDX collection 1316
Left side: PDX collection 1317
Unspecified side: PDX collection 1318

✓6ᵗʰ **S75.00**   Unspecified injury of femoral artery

✓7ᵗʰ **S75.001**   Unspecified injury of femoral artery, right leg   MCC

✓7ᵗʰ **S75.002**   Unspecified injury of femoral artery, left leg   MCC

✓7ᵗʰ **S75.009**   Unspecified injury of femoral artery, unspecified leg   MCC

✓6ᵗʰ **S75.01**   Minor laceration of femoral artery
Incomplete transection of femoral artery
Laceration of femoral artery NOS
Superficial laceration of femoral artery

✓7ᵗʰ **S75.011**   Minor laceration of femoral artery, right leg   MCC

✓7ᵗʰ **S75.012**   Minor laceration of femoral artery, left leg   MCC

✓7ᵗʰ **S75.019**   Minor laceration of femoral artery, unspecified leg   MCC

✓6ᵗʰ **S75.02**   Major laceration of femoral artery
Complete transection of femoral artery
Traumatic rupture of femoral artery

✓7ᵗʰ **S75.021**   Major laceration of femoral artery, right leg   MCC

✓7ᵗʰ **S75.022**   Major laceration of femoral artery, left leg   MCC

✓7ᵗʰ **S75.029**   Major laceration of femoral artery, unspecified leg   MCC

✓6ᵗʰ **S75.09**   Other specified injury of femoral artery

✓7ᵗʰ **S75.091**   Other specified injury of femoral artery, right leg   MCC

✓7ᵗʰ **S75.092**   Other specified injury of femoral artery, left leg   MCC

✓7ᵗʰ **S75.099**   Other specified injury of femoral artery, unspecified leg   MCC

✓5ᵗʰ S75.1 Injury of femoral vein at hip and thigh level

CC Excl: For CC codes in subcategory S75.1:
Right side: PDX collection 1319
Left side: PDX collection 1320
Unspecified side: PDX collection 1321

✓6ᵗʰ **S75.10**   Unspecified injury of femoral vein at hip and thigh level

✓7ᵗʰ **S75.101**   Unspecified injury of femoral vein at hip and thigh level, right leg   MCC

✓7ᵗʰ **S75.102**   Unspecified injury of femoral vein at hip and thigh level, left leg   MCC

✓7ᵗʰ **S75.109**   Unspecified injury of femoral vein at hip and thigh level, unspecified leg   MCC

✓6ᵗʰ **S75.11**   Minor laceration of femoral vein at hip and thigh level
Incomplete transection of femoral vein at hip and thigh level
Laceration of femoral vein at hip and thigh level NOS
Superficial laceration of femoral vein at hip and thigh level

✓7ᵗʰ **S75.111**   Minor laceration of femoral vein at hip and thigh level, right leg   MCC

✓7ᵗʰ **S75.112**   Minor laceration of femoral vein at hip and thigh level, left leg   MCC

✓7ᵗʰ **S75.119**   Minor laceration of femoral vein at hip and thigh level, unspecified leg   MCC

✓6ᵗʰ **S75.12**   Major laceration of femoral vein at hip and thigh level
Complete transection of femoral vein at hip and thigh level
Traumatic rupture of femoral vein at hip and thigh level

✓7ᵗʰ **S75.121**   Major laceration of femoral vein at hip and thigh level, right leg   MCC

✓7ᵗʰ **S75.122**   Major laceration of femoral vein at hip and thigh level, left leg   MCC

✓7ᵗʰ **S75.129**   Major laceration of femoral vein at hip and thigh level, unspecified leg   MCC

✓6ᵗʰ **S75.19**   Other specified injury of femoral vein at hip and thigh level

✓7ᵗʰ **S75.191**   Other specified injury of femoral vein at hip and thigh level, right leg   MCC

✓7ᵗʰ **S75.192**   Other specified injury of femoral vein at hip and thigh level, left leg   MCC

✓7ᵗʰ **S75.199**   Other specified injury of femoral vein at hip and thigh level, unspecified leg   MCC

✓5ᵗʰ S75.2 Injury of greater saphenous vein at hip and thigh level

EXCLUDES 1   greater saphenous vein NOS (S85.3)

CC Excl: For CC codes in subcategory S75.2:
Right side: PDX collection 1322
Left side: PDX collection 1323
Unspecified side: PDX collection 1324

✓6ᵗʰ **S75.20**   Unspecified injury of greater saphenous vein at hip and thigh level

✓7ᵗʰ **S75.201**   Unspecified injury of greater saphenous vein at hip and thigh level, right leg   CC

N Newborn: 0   P Pediatric: 0-17   M Maternity: 12-55   A Adult: 15-124   MCC Major CC Condition   PDxMCC PDx acts as own MCC   CC CC Condition   PDxCC PDx acts as own CC

1044   ICD-10-CM 2018

✓7ᵗʰ S75.202 Unspecified injury of greater saphenous vein at hip and thigh level, **left leg**   CC

✓7ᵗʰ S75.209 Unspecified injury of greater saphenous vein at hip and thigh level, **unspecified leg**   CC

✓6ᵗʰ S75.21 Minor laceration of greater saphenous vein at hip and thigh level
Incomplete transection of greater saphenous vein at hip and thigh level
Laceration of greater saphenous vein at hip and thigh level NOS
Superficial laceration of greater saphenous vein at hip and thigh level

✓7ᵗʰ S75.211 Minor laceration of greater saphenous vein at hip and thigh level, **right leg**   CC

✓7ᵗʰ S75.212 Minor laceration of greater saphenous vein at hip and thigh level, **left leg**   CC

✓7ᵗʰ S75.219 Minor laceration of greater saphenous vein at hip and thigh level, **unspecified leg**   CC

✓6ᵗʰ S75.22 Major laceration of greater saphenous vein at hip and thigh level
Complete transection of greater saphenous vein at hip and thigh level
Traumatic rupture of greater saphenous vein at hip and thigh level

✓7ᵗʰ S75.221 Major laceration of greater saphenous vein at hip and thigh level, **right leg**   CC

✓7ᵗʰ S75.222 Major laceration of greater saphenous vein at hip and thigh level, **left leg**   CC

✓7ᵗʰ S75.229 Major laceration of greater saphenous vein at hip and thigh level, **unspecified leg**   CC

✓6ᵗʰ S75.29 Other specified injury of greater saphenous vein at hip and thigh level

✓7ᵗʰ S75.291 Other specified injury of greater saphenous vein at hip and thigh level, **right leg**   CC

✓7ᵗʰ S75.292 Other specified injury of greater saphenous vein at hip and thigh level, **left leg**   CC

✓7ᵗʰ S75.299 Other specified injury of greater saphenous vein at hip and thigh level, **unspecified leg**   CC

✓5ᵗʰ S75.8 Injury of other blood vessels at hip and thigh level

CC Excl: For CC codes in subcategory S75.8:
Right side: PDX collection 1325
Left side: PDX collection 1326
Unspecified side: PDX collection 1327

✓6ᵗʰ S75.80 Unspecified injury of other blood vessels at hip and thigh level

✓7ᵗʰ S75.801 Unspecified injury of other blood vessels at hip and thigh level, **right leg**   CC

✓7ᵗʰ S75.802 Unspecified injury of other blood vessels at hip and thigh level, **left leg**   CC

✓7ᵗʰ S75.809 Unspecified injury of other blood vessels at hip and thigh level, **unspecified leg**   CC

✓6ᵗʰ S75.81 Laceration of other blood vessels at hip and thigh level

✓7ᵗʰ S75.811 Laceration of other blood vessels at hip and thigh level, **right leg**   CC

✓7ᵗʰ S75.812 Laceration of other blood vessels at hip and thigh level, **left leg**   CC

✓7ᵗʰ S75.819 Laceration of other blood vessels at hip and thigh level, **unspecified leg**   CC

✓6ᵗʰ S75.89 Other specified injury of other blood vessels at hip and thigh level

✓7ᵗʰ S75.891 Other specified injury of other blood vessels at hip and thigh level, **right leg**   CC

✓7ᵗʰ S75.892 Other specified injury of other blood vessels at hip and thigh level, **left leg**   CC

✓7ᵗʰ S75.899 Other specified injury of other blood vessels at hip and thigh level, **unspecified leg**   CC

✓5ᵗʰ S75.9 Injury of unspecified blood vessel at hip and thigh level

CC Excl: For CC codes in subcategory S75.9:
Right side: PDX collection 1325
Left side: PDX collection 1326
Unspecified side: PDX collection 1327

✓6ᵗʰ S75.90 Unspecified injury of unspecified blood vessel at hip and thigh level

✓7ᵗʰ S75.901 Unspecified injury of unspecified blood vessel at hip and thigh level, **right leg**   CC

✓7ᵗʰ S75.902 Unspecified injury of unspecified blood vessel at hip and thigh level, **left leg**   CC

✓7ᵗʰ S75.909 Unspecified injury of unspecified blood vessel at hip and thigh level, **unspecified leg**   CC

✓6ᵗʰ S75.91 Laceration of unspecified blood vessel at hip and thigh level

✓7ᵗʰ S75.911 Laceration of unspecified blood vessel at hip and thigh level, **right leg**   CC

✓7ᵗʰ S75.912 Laceration of unspecified blood vessel at hip and thigh level, **left leg**   CC

✓7ᵗʰ S75.919 Laceration of unspecified blood vessel at hip and thigh level, **unspecified leg**   CC

✓6ᵗʰ S75.99 Other specified injury of unspecified blood vessel at hip and thigh level

✓7ᵗʰ S75.991 Other specified injury of unspecified blood vessel at hip and thigh level, **right leg**   CC

✓7ᵗʰ S75.992 Other specified injury of unspecified blood vessel at hip and thigh level, **left leg**   CC

✓7ᵗʰ S75.999 Other specified injury of unspecified blood vessel at hip and thigh level, **unspecified leg**   CC

✓4ᵗʰ S76 Injury of muscle, fascia and tendon at hip and thigh level
Code also any associated open wound (S71.-)
EXCLUDES 2   injury of muscle, fascia and tendon at lower leg level (S86)
sprain of joint and ligament of hip (S73.1)
TIP: Refer to the Muscle/Tendon table at the beginning of this chapter.

The appropriate 7th character is to be added to each code from category S76.
A   initial encounter
D   subsequent encounter
S   sequela

CC Excl: For CC codes in category S76:
Right side: PDX collection 1328
Left side: PDX collection 1329
Unspecified side: PDX collection 1330

✓5ᵗʰ S76.0 Injury of muscle, fascia and tendon of hip

✓6ᵗʰ S76.00 Unspecified injury of muscle, fascia and tendon of hip

✓7ᵗʰ S76.001 Unspecified injury of muscle, fascia and tendon of **right** hip

✓7ᵗʰ S76.002 Unspecified injury of muscle, fascia and tendon of **left** hip

✓7ᵗʰ S76.009 Unspecified injury of muscle, fascia and tendon of **unspecified** hip

✓6ᵗʰ S76.01 Strain of muscle, fascia and tendon of hip

✓7ᵗʰ S76.011 Strain of muscle, fascia and tendon of **right** hip

✓7ᵗʰ S76.012 Strain of muscle, fascia and tendon of **left** hip

✓7ᵗʰ S76.019 Strain of muscle, fascia and tendon of **unspecified** hip

✓6ᵗʰ S76.02 Laceration of muscle, fascia and tendon of hip

✓7ᵗʰ S76.021 Laceration of muscle, fascia and tendon of **right** hip   CC

✓7ᵗʰ S76.022 Laceration of muscle, fascia and tendon of **left** hip   CC

✓7ᵗʰ S76.029 Laceration of muscle, fascia and tendon of **unspecified** hip   CC

√6ᵗʰ **S76.09** Other specified injury of muscle, fascia and tendon of hip

√7ᵗʰ **S76.091** Other specified injury of muscle, fascia and tendon of right hip

√7ᵗʰ **S76.092** Other specified injury of muscle, fascia and tendon of left hip

√7ᵗʰ **S76.099** Other specified injury of muscle, fascia and tendon of unspecified hip

√5ᵗʰ **S76.1** Injury of quadriceps muscle, fascia and tendon
Injury of patellar ligament (tendon)

√6ᵗʰ **S76.10** Unspecified injury of quadriceps muscle, fascia and tendon

√7ᵗʰ **S76.101** Unspecified injury of right quadriceps muscle, fascia and tendon

√7ᵗʰ **S76.102** Unspecified injury of left quadriceps muscle, fascia and tendon

√7ᵗʰ **S76.109** Unspecified injury of unspecified quadriceps muscle, fascia and tendon

√6ᵗʰ **S76.11** Strain of quadriceps muscle, fascia and tendon

√7ᵗʰ **S76.111** Strain of right quadriceps muscle, fascia and tendon

√7ᵗʰ **S76.112** Strain of left quadriceps muscle, fascia and tendon

√7ᵗʰ **S76.119** Strain of unspecified quadriceps muscle, fascia and tendon

√6ᵗʰ **S76.12** Laceration of quadriceps muscle, fascia and tendon

√7ᵗʰ **S76.121** Laceration of right quadriceps muscle, fascia and tendon `CC`

√7ᵗʰ **S76.122** Laceration of left quadriceps muscle, fascia and tendon `CC`

√7ᵗʰ **S76.129** Laceration of unspecified quadriceps muscle, fascia and tendon `CC`

√6ᵗʰ **S76.19** Other specified injury of quadriceps muscle, fascia and tendon

√7ᵗʰ **S76.191** Other specified injury of right quadriceps muscle, fascia and tendon

√7ᵗʰ **S76.192** Other specified injury of left quadriceps muscle, fascia and tendon

√7ᵗʰ **S76.199** Other specified injury of unspecified quadriceps muscle, fascia and tendon

√5ᵗʰ **S76.2** Injury of adductor muscle, fascia and tendon of thigh

√6ᵗʰ **S76.20** Unspecified injury of adductor muscle, fascia and tendon of thigh

√7ᵗʰ **S76.201** Unspecified injury of adductor muscle, fascia and tendon of right thigh

√7ᵗʰ **S76.202** Unspecified injury of adductor muscle, fascia and tendon of left thigh

√7ᵗʰ **S76.209** Unspecified injury of adductor muscle, fascia and tendon of unspecified thigh

√6ᵗʰ **S76.21** Strain of adductor muscle, fascia and tendon of thigh

√7ᵗʰ **S76.211** Strain of adductor muscle, fascia and tendon of right thigh

√7ᵗʰ **S76.212** Strain of adductor muscle, fascia and tendon of left thigh

√7ᵗʰ **S76.219** Strain of adductor muscle, fascia and tendon of unspecified thigh

√6ᵗʰ **S76.22** Laceration of adductor muscle, fascia and tendon of thigh

√7ᵗʰ **S76.221** Laceration of adductor muscle, fascia and tendon of right thigh `CC`

√7ᵗʰ **S76.222** Laceration of adductor muscle, fascia and tendon of left thigh `CC`

√7ᵗʰ **S76.229** Laceration of adductor muscle, fascia and tendon of unspecified thigh `CC`

√6ᵗʰ **S76.29** Other injury of adductor muscle, fascia and tendon of thigh

√7ᵗʰ **S76.291** Other injury of adductor muscle, fascia and tendon of right thigh

√7ᵗʰ **S76.292** Other injury of adductor muscle, fascia and tendon of left thigh

√7ᵗʰ **S76.299** Other injury of adductor muscle, fascia and tendon of unspecified thigh

√5ᵗʰ **S76.3** Injury of muscle, fascia and tendon of the posterior muscle group at thigh level

√6ᵗʰ **S76.30** Unspecified injury of muscle, fascia and tendon of the posterior muscle group at thigh level

√7ᵗʰ **S76.301** Unspecified injury of muscle, fascia and tendon of the posterior muscle group at thigh level, right thigh

√7ᵗʰ **S76.302** Unspecified injury of muscle, fascia and tendon of the posterior muscle group at thigh level, left thigh

√7ᵗʰ **S76.309** Unspecified injury of muscle, fascia and tendon of the posterior muscle group at thigh level, unspecified thigh

√6ᵗʰ **S76.31** Strain of muscle, fascia and tendon of the posterior muscle group at thigh level

√7ᵗʰ **S76.311** Strain of muscle, fascia and tendon of the posterior muscle group at thigh level, right thigh

√7ᵗʰ **S76.312** Strain of muscle, fascia and tendon of the posterior muscle group at thigh level, left thigh

√7ᵗʰ **S76.319** Strain of muscle, fascia and tendon of the posterior muscle group at thigh level, unspecified thigh

√6ᵗʰ **S76.32** Laceration of muscle, fascia and tendon of the posterior muscle group at thigh level

√7ᵗʰ **S76.321** Laceration of muscle, fascia and tendon of the posterior muscle group at thigh level, right thigh `CC`

√7ᵗʰ **S76.322** Laceration of muscle, fascia and tendon of the posterior muscle group at thigh level, left thigh `CC`

√7ᵗʰ **S76.329** Laceration of muscle, fascia and tendon of the posterior muscle group at thigh level, unspecified thigh `CC`

√6ᵗʰ **S76.39** Other specified injury of muscle, fascia and tendon of the posterior muscle group at thigh level

√7ᵗʰ **S76.391** Other specified injury of muscle, fascia and tendon of the posterior muscle group at thigh level, right thigh

√7ᵗʰ **S76.392** Other specified injury of muscle, fascia and tendon of the posterior muscle group at thigh level, left thigh

√7ᵗʰ **S76.399** Other specified injury of muscle, fascia and tendon of the posterior muscle group at thigh level, unspecified thigh

√5ᵗʰ **S76.8** Injury of other specified muscles, fascia and tendons at thigh level

√6ᵗʰ **S76.80** Unspecified injury of other specified muscles, fascia and tendons at thigh level

√7ᵗʰ **S76.801** Unspecified injury of other specified muscles, fascia and tendons at thigh level, right thigh

√7ᵗʰ **S76.802** Unspecified injury of other specified muscles, fascia and tendons at thigh level, left thigh

√7ᵗʰ **S76.809** Unspecified injury of other specified muscles, fascia and tendons at thigh level, unspecified thigh

√6ᵗʰ **S76.81** Strain of other specified muscles, fascia and tendons at thigh level

√7ᵗʰ **S76.811** Strain of other specified muscles, fascia and tendons at thigh level, right thigh

√7ᵗʰ **S76.812** Strain of other specified muscles, fascia and tendons at thigh level, left thigh

√7ᵗʰ **S76.819** Strain of other specified muscles, fascia and tendons at thigh level, unspecified thigh

√6ᵗʰ **S76.82** Laceration of other specified muscles, fascia and tendons at thigh level

√7ᵗʰ **S76.821** Laceration of other specified muscles, fascia and tendons at thigh level, right thigh `CC`

√7ᵗʰ **S76.822** Laceration of other specified muscles, fascia and tendons at thigh level, left thigh `CC`

N Newborn: 0   P Pediatric: 0-17   M Maternity: 12-55   A Adult: 15-124   MCC Major CC Condition   PDxMCC PDx acts as own MCC   CC CC Condition   PDxCC PDx acts as own CC

1046   ICD-10-CM 2018

✓7th **S76.829** Laceration of other specified muscles, `CC` fascia and tendons at thigh level, unspecified thigh

✓6th **S76.89** Other injury of other specified muscles, fascia and tendons at thigh level

   ✓7th **S76.891** Other injury of other specified muscles, fascia and tendons at thigh level, right thigh

   ✓7th **S76.892** Other injury of other specified muscles, fascia and tendons at thigh level, left thigh

   ✓7th **S76.899** Other injury of other specified muscles, fascia and tendons at thigh level, unspecified thigh

✓5th **S76.9** Injury of unspecified muscles, fascia and tendons at thigh level

   ✓6th **S76.90** Unspecified injury of unspecified muscles, fascia and tendons at thigh level

      ✓7th **S76.901** Unspecified injury of unspecified muscles, fascia and tendons at thigh level, right thigh

      ✓7th **S76.902** Unspecified injury of unspecified muscles, fascia and tendons at thigh level, left thigh

      ✓7th **S76.909** Unspecified injury of unspecified muscles, fascia and tendons at thigh level, unspecified thigh

   ✓6th **S76.91** Strain of unspecified muscles, fascia and tendons at thigh level

      ✓7th **S76.911** Strain of unspecified muscles, fascia and tendons at thigh level, right thigh

      ✓7th **S76.912** Strain of unspecified muscles, fascia and tendons at thigh level, left thigh

      ✓7th **S76.919** Strain of unspecified muscles, fascia and tendons at thigh level, unspecified thigh

   ✓6th **S76.92** Laceration of unspecified muscles, fascia and tendons at thigh level

      ✓7th **S76.921** Laceration of unspecified muscles, `CC` fascia and tendons at thigh level, right thigh

      ✓7th **S76.922** Laceration of unspecified muscles, `CC` fascia and tendons at thigh level, left thigh

      ✓7th **S76.929** Laceration of unspecified muscles, `CC` fascia and tendons at thigh level, unspecified thigh

   ✓6th **S76.99** Other specified injury of unspecified muscles, fascia and tendons at thigh level

      ✓7th **S76.991** Other specified injury of unspecified muscles, fascia and tendons at thigh level, right thigh

      ✓7th **S76.992** Other specified injury of unspecified muscles, fascia and tendons at thigh level, left thigh

      ✓7th **S76.999** Other specified injury of unspecified muscles, fascia and tendons at thigh level, unspecified thigh

✓4th **S77** Crushing injury of hip and thigh

   Use additional code(s) for all associated injuries
   EXCLUDES 2 *crushing injury of ankle and foot (S97.-)*
   crushing injury of lower leg (S87.-)

   The appropriate 7th character is to be added to each code from category S77.
   A   initial encounter
   D   subsequent encounter
   S   sequela

✓5th **S77.0** Crushing injury of hip

   CC Excl: For CC codes in subcategory S77.0:
   PDX collection 1331

   ✓x7th **S77.00** Crushing injury of unspecified hip   `CC` `H5`
   ✓x7th **S77.01** Crushing injury of right hip   `CC` `H5`
   ✓x7th **S77.02** Crushing injury of left hip   `CC` `H5`

✓5th **S77.1** Crushing injury of thigh

   CC Excl: For CC codes in subcategory S77.1:
   PDX collection 1332

   ✓x7th **S77.10** Crushing injury of unspecified thigh   `CC` `H5`
   ✓x7th **S77.11** Crushing injury of right thigh   `CC` `H5`
   ✓x7th **S77.12** Crushing injury of left thigh   `CC` `H5`

✓5th **S77.2** Crushing injury of hip with thigh

   ✓x7th **S77.20** Crushing injury of unspecified hip with thigh
   ✓x7th **S77.21** Crushing injury of right hip with thigh
   ✓x7th **S77.22** Crushing injury of left hip with thigh

✓4th **S78** Traumatic amputation of hip and thigh

   An amputation not identified as partial or complete should be coded to complete.
   EXCLUDES 1 *traumatic amputation of knee (S88.0-)*

   The appropriate 7th character is to be added to each code from category S78.
   A   initial encounter
   D   subsequent encounter
   S   sequela

   CC Excl: For CC codes in category S78:
   Right side: PDX collection 1333
   Left side: PDX collection 1334
   Unspecified side: PDX collection 1335

✓5th **S78.0** Traumatic amputation at hip joint

   ✓6th **S78.01** Complete traumatic amputation at hip joint

      ✓7th **S78.011** Complete traumatic amputation at `CC` `HCC` right hip joint

      ✓7th **S78.012** Complete traumatic amputation at `CC` `HCC` left hip joint

      ✓7th **S78.019** Complete traumatic amputation at unspecified hip joint `CC` `HCC`

   ✓6th **S78.02** Partial traumatic amputation at hip joint

      ✓7th **S78.021** Partial traumatic amputation at `CC` `HCC` right hip joint

      ✓7th **S78.022** Partial traumatic amputation at `CC` `HCC` left hip joint

      ✓7th **S78.029** Partial traumatic amputation at `CC` `HCC` unspecified hip joint

✓5th **S78.1** Traumatic amputation at level between hip and knee
   EXCLUDES 1 *traumatic amputation of knee (S88.0-)*

   ✓6th **S78.11** Complete traumatic amputation at level between hip and knee

      ✓7th **S78.111** Complete traumatic amputation at `CC` `HCC` level between right hip and knee

      ✓7th **S78.112** Complete traumatic amputation at `CC` `HCC` level between left hip and knee

      ✓7th **S78.119** Complete traumatic amputation at `CC` `HCC` level between unspecified hip and knee

   ✓6th **S78.12** Partial traumatic amputation at level between hip and knee

      ✓7th **S78.121** Partial traumatic amputation at `CC` `HCC` level between right hip and knee

      ✓7th **S78.122** Partial traumatic amputation at `CC` `HCC` level between left hip and knee

      ✓7th **S78.129** Partial traumatic amputation at `CC` `HCC` level between unspecified hip and knee

✓5th **S78.9** Traumatic amputation of hip and thigh, level unspecified

   ✓6th **S78.91** Complete traumatic amputation of hip and thigh, level unspecified

      ✓7th **S78.911** Complete traumatic amputation `CC` `HCC` of right hip and thigh, level unspecified

      ✓7th **S78.912** Complete traumatic amputation `CC` `HCC` of left hip and thigh, level unspecified

      ✓7th **S78.919** Complete traumatic amputation `CC` `HCC` of unspecified hip and thigh, level unspecified

   ✓6th **S78.92** Partial traumatic amputation of hip and thigh, level unspecified

      ✓7th **S78.921** Partial traumatic amputation of `CC` `HCC` right hip and thigh, level unspecified

      ✓7th **S78.922** Partial traumatic amputation of `CC` `HCC` left hip and thigh, level unspecified

✓ Additional Character Req   ✓x7th Placeholder Alert   Unacceptable PDx   Manifestation   `H1`-`H14` HAC   `HCC` CMS-HCC Condition   *EXCLUDES 1* Not Coded Here   *EXCLUDES 2* Not Included Here

ICD-10-CM 2018   1047

Chapter 19. Injury, Poisoning and Certain Other Consequences of External Causes

S76.829–S78.922

☑7th **S78.929** **Partial traumatic amputation of** CC HCC
unspecified hip and thigh, level
unspecified

☑4th **S79** **Other and unspecified injuries of hip and thigh**
NOTE   A fracture not indicated as open or closed should
be coded to closed.
AHA: 2015, 3Q, 37-39

The appropriate 7th character is to be added to each code from
subcategory S79.0 and S79.1
A   initial encounter for closed fracture
D   subsequent encounter for fracture with routine healing
G   subsequent encounter for fracture with delayed healing
K   subsequent encounter for fracture with nonunion
P   subsequent encounter for fracture with malunion
S   sequela

☑5th **S79.0** **Physeal fracture of upper end of femur**
EXCLUDES 1   apophyseal fracture of upper end of femur (S72.13-)
nontraumatic slipped upper femoral epiphysis
(M93.0-)

CC Excl: For CC/MCC codes in subcategory S79.0:
Right side: See code S79.001
Left side: See code S79.002
Unspecified side: See code S79.009

☑6th **S79.00** **Unspecified physeal fracture of upper end of femur**
8,10 ☑7th **S79.001** **Unspecified physeal** MCC CC H5 HCC
fracture of upper end
of right femur
CC Excl: MCC with 7th character A:
PDX collection 1297
CC with 7th character K or P:
PDX collection 897

8,10 ☑7th **S79.002** **Unspecified physeal** MCC CC H5 HCC
fracture of upper end
of left femur
CC Excl: MCC with 7th character A:
PDX collection 1299
CC with 7th character K or P:
PDX collection 897

8,10 ☑7th **S79.009** **Unspecified physeal** MCC CC H5 HCC
fracture of upper end of
unspecified femur
CC Excl: MCC with 7th character A:
PDX collection 1298
CC with 7th character K or P:
PDX collection 897

☑6th **S79.01** **Salter-Harris Type I physeal fracture of upper end of**
femur
Acute on chronic slipped capital femoral epiphysis
(traumatic)
Acute slipped capital femoral epiphysis (traumatic)
Capital femoral epiphyseal fracture
EXCLUDES 1   chronic slipped upper femoral epiphysis
(nontraumatic) (M93.02-)
8,10 ☑7th **S79.011** **Salter-Harris Type I physeal** MCC CC H5 HCC
fracture of upper end of
right femur
8,10 ☑7th **S79.012** **Salter-Harris Type I physeal** MCC CC H5 HCC
fracture of upper end of
left femur
8,10 ☑7th **S79.019** **Salter-Harris Type I physeal** MCC CC H5 HCC
fracture of upper end of
unspecified femur

☑6th **S79.09** **Other physeal fracture of upper end of femur**
8,10 ☑7th **S79.091** **Other physeal fracture of** MCC CC H5 HCC
upper end of right femur
8,10 ☑7th **S79.092** **Other physeal fracture of** MCC CC H5 HCC
upper end of left femur
8,10 ☑7th **S79.099** **Other physeal fracture of** MCC CC H5 HCC
upper end of unspecified femur

☑5th **S79.1** **Physeal fracture of lower end of femur**

CC Excl: For CC/MCC codes in subcategory S79.1:
Right side: See code S79.101
Left side: See code S79.102
Unspecified side: See code S79.109

☑6th **S79.10** **Unspecified physeal fracture of lower end of femur**
7,10 ☑7th **S79.101** **Unspecified physeal fracture of** CC H5 HCC
lower end of right femur
CC Excl: CC with 7th character A:
PDX collection 1300
CC with 7th character K or P:
PDX collection 897

7,10 ☑7th **S79.102** **Unspecified physeal fracture of** CC H5 HCC
lower end of left femur
CC Excl: CC with 7th character A:
PDX collection 1302
CC with 7th character K or P:
PDX collection 897

7,10 ☑7th **S79.109** **Unspecified physeal fracture of** CC H5 HCC
lower end of unspecified femur
CC Excl: CC with 7th character A:
PDX collection 1301
CC with 7th character K or P:
PDX collection 897

☑6th **S79.11** **Salter-Harris Type I physeal fracture of lower end of**
femur
7,10 ☑7th **S79.111** **Salter-Harris Type I physeal** CC H5 HCC
fracture of lower end of right femur
7,10 ☑7th **S79.112** **Salter-Harris Type I physeal** CC H5 HCC
fracture of lower end of left femur
7,10 ☑7th **S79.119** **Salter-Harris Type I physeal** CC H5 HCC
fracture of lower end of unspecified femur

☑6th **S79.12** **Salter-Harris Type II physeal fracture of lower end of**
femur
7,10 ☑7th **S79.121** **Salter-Harris Type II physeal** CC H5 HCC
fracture of lower end of right femur
7,10 ☑7th **S79.122** **Salter-Harris Type II physeal** CC H5 HCC
fracture of lower end of left femur
7,10 ☑7th **S79.129** **Salter-Harris Type II physeal** CC H5 HCC
fracture of lower end of unspecified femur

☑6th **S79.13** **Salter-Harris Type III physeal fracture of lower end of**
femur
7,10 ☑7th **S79.131** **Salter-Harris Type III physeal** CC H5 HCC
fracture of lower end of right femur
7,10 ☑7th **S79.132** **Salter-Harris Type III physeal** CC H5 HCC
fracture of lower end of left femur
7,10 ☑7th **S79.139** **Salter-Harris Type III physeal** CC H5 HCC
fracture of lower end of unspecified femur

☑6th **S79.14** **Salter-Harris Type IV physeal fracture of lower end of**
femur
7,10 ☑7th **S79.141** **Salter-Harris Type IV physeal** CC H5 HCC
fracture of lower end of right femur
7,10 ☑7th **S79.142** **Salter-Harris Type IV physeal** CC H5 HCC
fracture of lower end of left femur
7,10 ☑7th **S79.149** **Salter-Harris Type IV physeal** CC H5 HCC
fracture of lower end of unspecified femur

☑6th **S79.19** **Other physeal fracture of lower end of femur**
7,10 ☑7th **S79.191** **Other physeal fracture of lower** CC H5 HCC
end of right femur
7,10 ☑7th **S79.192** **Other physeal fracture of lower** CC H5 HCC
end of left femur
7,10 ☑7th **S79.199** **Other physeal fracture of lower** CC H5 HCC
end of unspecified femur

☑5th **S79.8** **Other specified injuries of hip and thigh**

The appropriate 7th character is to be added to each code
in subcategory S79.8.
A   initial encounter
D   subsequent encounter
S   sequela

☑6th **S79.81** **Other specified injuries of hip**
☑7th **S79.811** **Other specified injuries of right hip**
☑7th **S79.812** **Other specified injuries of left hip**

---

7   CC when reported as an initial encounter (7th character A, B, or C – specific to category) OR a subsequent encounter for nonunion or malunion
(7th character K, M, N, P, Q, or R – specific to category).
8   CC when reported as a subsequent encounter for nonunion or malunion (7th character K, M, N, P, Q, or R – specific to category).
10   HCC with 7th character indicating initial encounter (A, B or C - specific to category).

N Newborn: 0   P Pediatric: 0-17   M Maternity: 12-55   A Adult: 15-124   MCC Major CC Condition   PDxMCC PDx acts as own MCC   CC CC Condition   PDxCC PDx acts as own CC

✓7ᵗʰ   **S79.819**   Other specified injuries of unspecified hip

✓6ᵗʰ   **S79.82**   Other specified injuries of thigh

    ✓7ᵗʰ   **S79.821**   Other specified injuries of right thigh

    ✓7ᵗʰ   **S79.822**   Other specified injuries of left thigh

    ✓7ᵗʰ   **S79.829**   Other specified injuries of unspecified thigh

✓5ᵗʰ   **S79.9**   Unspecified injury of hip and thigh

> The appropriate 7th character is to be added to each code in subcategory S79.9.
> A   initial encounter
> D   subsequent encounter
> S   sequela

✓6ᵗʰ   **S79.91**   Unspecified injury of hip

    ✓7ᵗʰ   **S79.911**   Unspecified injury of right hip

    ✓7ᵗʰ   **S79.912**   Unspecified injury of left hip

    ✓7ᵗʰ   **S79.919**   Unspecified injury of unspecified hip

✓6ᵗʰ   **S79.92**   Unspecified injury of thigh

    ✓7ᵗʰ   **S79.921**   Unspecified injury of right thigh

    ✓7ᵗʰ   **S79.922**   Unspecified injury of left thigh

    ✓7ᵗʰ   **S79.929**   Unspecified injury of unspecified thigh

Injuries to the knee and lower leg (S80-S89)

EXCLUDES 2   burns and corrosions (T20-T32)
frostbite (T33-T34)
injuries of ankle and foot, except fracture of ankle and malleolus (S90-S99)
insect bite or sting, venomous (T63.4)

✓4ᵗʰ   **S80**   **Superficial injury of knee and lower leg**

    EXCLUDES 2   superficial injury of ankle and foot (S90.-)

> The appropriate 7th character is to be added to each code from category S80.
> A   initial encounter
> D   subsequent encounter
> S   sequela

✓5ᵗʰ   **S80.0**   Contusion of knee

    ✓x7ᵗʰ   **S80.00**   Contusion of unspecified knee

    ✓x7ᵗʰ   **S80.01**   Contusion of right knee

    ✓x7ᵗʰ   **S80.02**   Contusion of left knee

✓5ᵗʰ   **S80.1**   Contusion of lower leg

    ✓x7ᵗʰ   **S80.10**   Contusion of unspecified lower leg

    ✓x7ᵗʰ   **S80.11**   Contusion of right lower leg

    ✓x7ᵗʰ   **S80.12**   Contusion of left lower leg

✓5ᵗʰ   **S80.2**   Other superficial injuries of knee

    ✓6ᵗʰ   **S80.21**   Abrasion of knee

       ✓7ᵗʰ   **S80.211**   Abrasion, right knee

       ✓7ᵗʰ   **S80.212**   Abrasion, left knee

       ✓7ᵗʰ   **S80.219**   Abrasion, unspecified knee

    ✓6ᵗʰ   **S80.22**   Blister (nonthermal) of knee

       ✓7ᵗʰ   **S80.221**   Blister (nonthermal), right knee

       ✓7ᵗʰ   **S80.222**   Blister (nonthermal), left knee

       ✓7ᵗʰ   **S80.229**   Blister (nonthermal), unspecified knee

    ✓6ᵗʰ   **S80.24**   External constriction of knee

       ✓7ᵗʰ   **S80.241**   External constriction, right knee

       ✓7ᵗʰ   **S80.242**   External constriction, left knee

       ✓7ᵗʰ   **S80.249**   External constriction, unspecified knee

    ✓6ᵗʰ   **S80.25**   Superficial foreign body of knee
       Splinter in the knee

       ✓7ᵗʰ   **S80.251**   Superficial foreign body, right knee

       ✓7ᵗʰ   **S80.252**   Superficial foreign body, left knee

       ✓7ᵗʰ   **S80.259**   Superficial foreign body, unspecified knee

    ✓6ᵗʰ   **S80.26**   Insect bite (nonvenomous) of knee

       ✓7ᵗʰ   **S80.261**   Insect bite (nonvenomous), right knee

       ✓7ᵗʰ   **S80.262**   Insect bite (nonvenomous), left knee

       ✓7ᵗʰ   **S80.269**   Insect bite (nonvenomous), unspecified knee

    ✓6ᵗʰ   **S80.27**   Other superficial bite of knee

       EXCLUDES 1   open bite of knee (S81.05-)

       ✓7ᵗʰ   **S80.271**   Other superficial bite of right knee

       ✓7ᵗʰ   **S80.272**   Other superficial bite of left knee

---

       ✓7ᵗʰ   **S80.279**   Other superficial bite of unspecified knee

✓5ᵗʰ   **S80.8**   Other superficial injuries of lower leg

    ✓6ᵗʰ   **S80.81**   Abrasion of lower leg

       ✓7ᵗʰ   **S80.811**   Abrasion, right lower leg

       ✓7ᵗʰ   **S80.812**   Abrasion, left lower leg

       ✓7ᵗʰ   **S80.819**   Abrasion, unspecified lower leg

    ✓6ᵗʰ   **S80.82**   Blister (nonthermal) of lower leg

       ✓7ᵗʰ   **S80.821**   Blister (nonthermal), right lower leg

       ✓7ᵗʰ   **S80.822**   Blister (nonthermal), left lower leg

       ✓7ᵗʰ   **S80.829**   Blister (nonthermal), unspecified lower leg

    ✓6ᵗʰ   **S80.84**   External constriction of lower leg

       ✓7ᵗʰ   **S80.841**   External constriction, right lower leg

       ✓7ᵗʰ   **S80.842**   External constriction, left lower leg

       ✓7ᵗʰ   **S80.849**   External constriction, unspecified lower leg

    ✓6ᵗʰ   **S80.85**   Superficial foreign body of lower leg
       Splinter in the lower leg

       ✓7ᵗʰ   **S80.851**   Superficial foreign body, right lower leg

       ✓7ᵗʰ   **S80.852**   Superficial foreign body, left lower leg

       ✓7ᵗʰ   **S80.859**   Superficial foreign body, unspecified lower leg

    ✓6ᵗʰ   **S80.86**   Insect bite (nonvenomous) of lower leg

       ✓7ᵗʰ   **S80.861**   Insect bite (nonvenomous), right lower leg

       ✓7ᵗʰ   **S80.862**   Insect bite (nonvenomous), left lower leg

       ✓7ᵗʰ   **S80.869**   Insect bite (nonvenomous), unspecified lower leg

    ✓6ᵗʰ   **S80.87**   Other superficial bite of lower leg

       EXCLUDES 1   open bite of lower leg (S81.85-)

       ✓7ᵗʰ   **S80.871**   Other superficial bite, right lower leg

       ✓7ᵗʰ   **S80.872**   Other superficial bite, left lower leg

       ✓7ᵗʰ   **S80.879**   Other superficial bite, unspecified lower leg

✓5ᵗʰ   **S80.9**   Unspecified superficial injury of knee and lower leg

    ✓6ᵗʰ   **S80.91**   Unspecified superficial injury of knee

       ✓7ᵗʰ   **S80.911**   Unspecified superficial injury of right knee

       ✓7ᵗʰ   **S80.912**   Unspecified superficial injury of left knee

       ✓7ᵗʰ   **S80.919**   Unspecified superficial injury of unspecified knee

    ✓6ᵗʰ   **S80.92**   Unspecified superficial injury of lower leg

       ✓7ᵗʰ   **S80.921**   Unspecified superficial injury of right lower leg

       ✓7ᵗʰ   **S80.922**   Unspecified superficial injury of left lower leg

       ✓7ᵗʰ   **S80.929**   Unspecified superficial injury of unspecified lower leg

✓4ᵗʰ   **S81**   **Open wound of knee and lower leg**

    Code also any associated wound infection

    EXCLUDES 1   open fracture of knee and lower leg (S82.-)
                  traumatic amputation of lower leg (S88.-)

    EXCLUDES 2   open wound of ankle and foot (S91.-)

> The appropriate 7th character is to be added to each code from category S81.
> A   initial encounter
> D   subsequent encounter
> S   sequela

✓5ᵗʰ   **S81.0**   Open wound of knee

    ✓6ᵗʰ   **S81.00**   Unspecified open wound of knee

       ✓7ᵗʰ   **S81.001**   Unspecified open wound, right knee

       ✓7ᵗʰ   **S81.002**   Unspecified open wound, left knee

       ✓7ᵗʰ   **S81.009**   Unspecified open wound, unspecified knee

    ✓6ᵗʰ   **S81.01**   Laceration without foreign body of knee

       ✓7ᵗʰ   **S81.011**   Laceration without foreign body, right knee

       ✓7ᵗʰ   **S81.012**   Laceration without foreign body, left knee

       ✓7ᵗʰ   **S81.019**   Laceration without foreign body, unspecified knee

    ✓6ᵗʰ   **S81.02**   Laceration with foreign body of knee

       ✓7ᵗʰ   **S81.021**   Laceration with foreign body, right knee

---

✓ Additional Character Req   ✓x7ᵗʰ Placeholder Alert   Unacceptable PDx   Manifestation   H1 - H14 HAC   HCC CMS-HCC Condition   EXCLUDES 1 Not Coded Here   EXCLUDES 2 Not Included Here

ICD-10-CM 2018   **1049**

√7ᵗʰ **S81.022 Laceration with foreign body,** left **knee**

√7ᵗʰ **S81.029 Laceration with foreign body,** unspecified **knee**

√6ᵗʰ **S81.03 Puncture wound without foreign body** of knee

√7ᵗʰ **S81.031 Puncture wound without foreign body,** right **knee**

√7ᵗʰ **S81.032 Puncture wound without foreign body,** left **knee**

√7ᵗʰ **S81.039 Puncture wound without foreign body,** unspecified **knee**

√6ᵗʰ **S81.04 Puncture wound with foreign body** of knee

√7ᵗʰ **S81.041 Puncture wound with foreign body,** right **knee**

√7ᵗʰ **S81.042 Puncture wound with foreign body,** left **knee**

√7ᵗʰ **S81.049 Puncture wound with foreign body,** unspecified **knee**

√6ᵗʰ **S81.05 Open bite** of knee
Bite of knee NOS
EXCLUDES 1 *superficial bite of knee (S80.27-)*

√7ᵗʰ **S81.051 Open bite,** right **knee**

√7ᵗʰ **S81.052 Open bite,** left **knee**

√7ᵗʰ **S81.059 Open bite,** unspecified **knee**

√5ᵗʰ **S81.8 Open wound of lower leg**

√6ᵗʰ **S81.80 Unspecified open wound of lower leg**
AHA: 2016, 3Q, 24

√7ᵗʰ **S81.801 Unspecified open wound,** right **lower leg**

√7ᵗʰ **S81.802 Unspecified open wound,** left **lower leg**

√7ᵗʰ **S81.809 Unspecified open wound,** unspecified **lower leg**

√6ᵗʰ **S81.81 Laceration without foreign body** of lower leg

√7ᵗʰ **S81.811 Laceration without foreign body,** right **lower leg**

√7ᵗʰ **S81.812 Laceration without foreign body,** left **lower leg**

√7ᵗʰ **S81.819 Laceration without foreign body,** unspecified **lower leg**

√6ᵗʰ **S81.82 Laceration with foreign body** of lower leg

√7ᵗʰ **S81.821 Laceration with foreign body,** right **lower leg**

√7ᵗʰ **S81.822 Laceration with foreign body,** left **lower leg**

√7ᵗʰ **S81.829 Laceration with foreign body,** unspecified **lower leg**

√6ᵗʰ **S81.83 Puncture wound without foreign body** of lower leg
AHA: 2016, 3Q, 24

√7ᵗʰ **S81.831 Puncture wound without foreign body,** right **lower leg**

√7ᵗʰ **S81.832 Puncture wound without foreign body,** left **lower leg**

√7ᵗʰ **S81.839 Puncture wound without foreign body,** unspecified **lower leg**

√6ᵗʰ **S81.84 Puncture wound with foreign body** of lower leg
AHA: 2016, 3Q, 24

√7ᵗʰ **S81.841 Puncture wound with foreign body,** right **lower leg**

√7ᵗʰ **S81.842 Puncture wound with foreign body,** left **lower leg**

√7ᵗʰ **S81.849 Puncture wound with foreign body,** unspecified **lower leg**

√6ᵗʰ **S81.85 Open bite** of lower leg
Bite of lower leg NOS
EXCLUDES 1 *superficial bite of lower leg (S80.86-, S80.87-)*

√7ᵗʰ **S81.851 Open bite,** right **lower leg**

√7ᵗʰ **S81.852 Open bite,** left **lower leg**

√7ᵗʰ **S81.859 Open bite,** unspecified **lower leg**

√4ᵗʰ **S82 Fracture of lower leg, including ankle**
NOTE A fracture not indicated as displaced or nondisplaced should be coded to displaced.
A fracture not designated as open or closed should be coded to closed.
The open fracture designations are based on the Gustilo open fracture classification.
INCLUDES fracture of malleolus
EXCLUDES 1 *traumatic amputation of lower leg (S88.-)*
EXCLUDES 2 *fracture of foot, except ankle (S92.-)*
periprosthetic fracture of prosthetic implant of knee ▶(M97.0-)◀
AHA: 2016, 1Q, 33; 2015, 3Q, 37-39; 2015, 3Q, 37-39

The appropriate 7th character is to be added to all codes from category S82 [unless otherwise indicated].
A   initial encounter for closed fracture
B   initial encounter for open fracture type I or II
    initial encounter for open fracture NOS
C   initial encounter for open fracture type IIIA, IIIB, or IIIC
D   subsequent encounter for closed fracture with routine healing
E   subsequent encounter for open fracture type I or II with routine healing
F   subsequent encounter for open fracture type IIIA, IIIB, or IIIC with routine healing
G   subsequent encounter for closed fracture with delayed healing
H   subsequent encounter for open fracture type I or II with delayed healing
J   subsequent encounter for open fracture type IIIA, IIIB or IIIC with delayed healing
K   subsequent encounter for closed fracture with nonunion
M   subsequent encounter for open fracture type I or II with nonunion
N   subsequent encounter for open fracture type IIIA, IIIB or IIIC with nonunion
P   subsequent encounter for closed fracture with malunion
Q   subsequent encounter for open fracture type I or II with malunion
R   subsequent encounter for open fracture type IIIA, IIIB or IIIC with malunion
S   sequela

√5ᵗʰ **S82.0 Fracture of** patella
Knee cap

CC Excl: For CC codes in subcategory S82.0:
Right side: See code S82.001
Left side: See code S82.002
Unspecified side: See code S82.009

√6ᵗʰ **S82.00 Unspecified fracture of patella**

7 √7ᵗʰ **S82.001 Unspecified fracture of** right **patella** CC H5
CC Excl: CC with 7th character A:
PDX collection 1336
CC with 7th character B or C:
PDX collection 1337
CC with 7th character K, M, N, P, Q or R:
PDX collection 897

7 √7ᵗʰ **S82.002 Unspecified fracture of** left **patella** CC H5
CC Excl: CC with 7th character A:
PDX collection 1338
CC with 7th character B or C:
PDX collection 1337
CC with 7th character K, M, N, P, Q or R:
PDX collection 897

7 √7ᵗʰ **S82.009 Unspecified fracture of** unspecified **patella**
CC Excl: CC with 7th character A:
PDX collection 1339
CC with 7th character B or C:
PDX collection 1337
CC with 7th character K, M, N, P, Q or R:
PDX collection 897

√6ᵗʰ **S82.01 Osteochondral fracture of patella**

7 √7ᵗʰ **S82.011 Displaced osteochondral fracture of** right **patella** CC H5

7 √7ᵗʰ **S82.012 Displaced osteochondral fracture of** left **patella** CC H5

7 √7ᵗʰ **S82.013 Displaced osteochondral fracture of** unspecified **patella** CC H5

7 √7ᵗʰ **S82.014 Nondisplaced osteochondral fracture of** right **patella** CC H5

---

7 CC when reported as an initial encounter (7th character A, B, or C – specific to category) OR a subsequent encounter for nonunion or malunion (7th character K, M, N, P, Q, or R – specific to category).

7 √7ᵗʰ **S82.015** **Nondisplaced** osteochondral CC H5
fracture of left **patella**

7 √7ᵗʰ **S82.016** **Nondisplaced** osteochondral CC H5
fracture of unspecified **patella**

√6ᵗʰ **S82.02** **Longitudinal** fracture of patella

7 √7ᵗʰ **S82.021** **Displaced** longitudinal fracture of CC H5
right **patella**

7 √7ᵗʰ **S82.022** **Displaced** longitudinal fracture of CC H5
left **patella**

7 √7ᵗʰ **S82.023** **Displaced** longitudinal fracture of CC H5
unspecified **patella**

7 √7ᵗʰ **S82.024** **Nondisplaced** longitudinal fracture CC H5
of right **patella**

7 √7ᵗʰ **S82.025** **Nondisplaced** longitudinal fracture CC H5
of left **patella**

7 √7ᵗʰ **S82.026** **Nondisplaced** longitudinal fracture CC H5
of unspecified **patella**

√6ᵗʰ **S82.03** **Transverse** fracture of patella

7 √7ᵗʰ **S82.031** **Displaced** transverse fracture of CC H5
right **patella**

7 √7ᵗʰ **S82.032** **Displaced** transverse fracture of CC H5
left **patella**

7 √7ᵗʰ **S82.033** **Displaced** transverse fracture of CC H5
unspecified **patella**

7 √7ᵗʰ **S82.034** **Nondisplaced** transverse fracture CC H5
of right **patella**

7 √7ᵗʰ **S82.035** **Nondisplaced** transverse fracture CC H5
of left **patella**

7 √7ᵗʰ **S82.036** **Nondisplaced** transverse fracture CC H5
of unspecified **patella**

√6ᵗʰ **S82.04** **Comminuted** fracture of patella

7 √7ᵗʰ **S82.041** **Displaced** comminuted fracture CC H5
of right **patella**

7 √7ᵗʰ **S82.042** **Displaced** comminuted fracture of CC H5
left **patella**

7 √7ᵗʰ **S82.043** **Displaced** comminuted fracture of CC H5
unspecified **patella**

7 √7ᵗʰ **S82.044** **Nondisplaced** comminuted fracture CC H5
of right **patella**

7 √7ᵗʰ **S82.045** **Nondisplaced** comminuted fracture CC H5
of left **patella**

7 √7ᵗʰ **S82.046** **Nondisplaced** comminuted fracture CC H5
of unspecified **patella**

√6ᵗʰ **S82.09** **Other** fracture of patella

7 √7ᵗʰ **S82.091** **Other** fracture of right **patella** CC H5

7 √7ᵗʰ **S82.092** **Other** fracture of left **patella** CC H5

7 √7ᵗʰ **S82.099** **Other** fracture of unspecified CC H5
patella

√5ᵗʰ **S82.1** **Fracture of** upper end of tibia
Fracture of proximal end of tibia

EXCLUDES 2 fracture of shaft of tibia (S82.2-)
physeal fracture of upper end of tibia (S89.0-)

**CC Excl: For CC/MCC codes in subcategory S82.1,
unless otherwise noted:
Right side:** See code S82.101
Left side: See code S82.102
Unspecified side: See code S82.109

√6ᵗʰ **S82.10** **Unspecified** fracture of upper end of tibia

6, 7 √7ᵗʰ **S82.101** **Unspecified** fracture of upper MCC CC H5
end of right **tibia**
CC Excl: CC with 7th character A:
PDX collection 1340
MCC with 7th character B or C:
PDX collection 1341
CC with 7th character K, M, N, P, Q or R:
PDX collection 897

6, 7 √7ᵗʰ **S82.102** **Unspecified** fracture of upper MCC CC H5
end of left **tibia**
CC Excl: CC with 7th character A:
PDX collection 1342
MCC with 7th character B or C:
PDX collection 1341
CC with 7th character K, M, N, P, Q or R:
PDX collection 897

6, 7 √7ᵗʰ **S82.109** **Unspecified** fracture of upper MCC CC H5
end of unspecified **tibia**
**CC Excl:
CC or MCC with 7th character A, B or C:**
PDX collection 1341
CC with 7th character K, M, N, P, Q or R:
PDX collection 897

√6ᵗʰ **S82.11** **Fracture of** tibial spine

6, 7 √7ᵗʰ **S82.111** **Displaced** fracture of right MCC CC H5
tibial **spine**

6, 7 √7ᵗʰ **S82.112** **Displaced** fracture of left MCC CC H5
tibial **spine**

6, 7 √7ᵗʰ **S82.113** **Displaced** fracture of MCC CC H5
unspecified tibial **spine**

6, 7 √7ᵗʰ **S82.114** **Nondisplaced** fracture of MCC CC H5
right tibial **spine**

6, 7 √7ᵗʰ **S82.115** **Nondisplaced** fracture of left MCC CC H5
tibial **spine**

6, 7 √7ᵗʰ **S82.116** **Nondisplaced** fracture of MCC CC H5
unspecified tibial **spine**

√6ᵗʰ **S82.12** **Fracture of** lateral condyle of tibia

6, 7 √7ᵗʰ **S82.121** **Displaced** fracture of lateral MCC CC H5
condyle of right **tibia**

6, 7 √7ᵗʰ **S82.122** **Displaced** fracture of lateral MCC CC H5
condyle of left **tibia**

6, 7 √7ᵗʰ **S82.123** **Displaced** fracture of lateral MCC CC H5
condyle of unspecified **tibia**

6, 7 √7ᵗʰ **S82.124** **Nondisplaced** fracture of MCC CC H5
lateral condyle of right **tibia**

6, 7 √7ᵗʰ **S82.125** **Nondisplaced** fracture of MCC CC H5
lateral condyle of left **tibia**

6, 7 √7ᵗʰ **S82.126** **Nondisplaced** fracture of MCC CC H5
lateral condyle of unspecified **tibia**

√6ᵗʰ **S82.13** **Fracture of** medial condyle of tibia

6, 7 √7ᵗʰ **S82.131** **Displaced** fracture of medial MCC CC H5
condyle of right **tibia**

6, 7 √7ᵗʰ **S82.132** **Displaced** fracture of medial MCC CC H5
condyle of left **tibia**

6, 7 √7ᵗʰ **S82.133** **Displaced** fracture of medial MCC CC H5
condyle of unspecified **tibia**

6, 7 √7ᵗʰ **S82.134** **Nondisplaced** fracture of MCC CC H5
medial condyle of right **tibia**

6, 7 √7ᵗʰ **S82.135** **Nondisplaced** fracture of MCC CC H5
medial condyle of left **tibia**

6, 7 √7ᵗʰ **S82.136** **Nondisplaced** fracture of MCC CC H5
medial condyle of unspecified **tibia**

√6ᵗʰ **S82.14** **Bicondylar** fracture of tibia
Fracture of tibial plateau NOS

6, 7 √7ᵗʰ **S82.141** **Displaced** bicondylar fracture MCC CC H5
of right **tibia**

6, 7 √7ᵗʰ **S82.142** **Displaced** bicondylar fracture MCC CC H5
of left **tibia**

6, 7 √7ᵗʰ **S82.143** **Displaced** bicondylar fracture MCC CC H5
of unspecified **tibia**

6, 7 √7ᵗʰ **S82.144** **Nondisplaced** bicondylar MCC CC H5
fracture of right **tibia**

6, 7 √7ᵗʰ **S82.145** **Nondisplaced** bicondylar MCC CC H5
fracture of left **tibia**

6, 7 √7ᵗʰ **S82.146** **Nondisplaced** bicondylar MCC CC H5
fracture of unspecified **tibia**

√6ᵗʰ **S82.15** **Fracture of** tibial tuberosity

6, 7 √7ᵗʰ **S82.151** **Displaced** fracture of right MCC CC H5
tibial **tuberosity**

6, 7 √7ᵗʰ **S82.152** **Displaced** fracture of left MCC CC H5
tibial **tuberosity**

6, 7 √7ᵗʰ **S82.153** **Displaced** fracture of MCC CC H5
unspecified tibial **tuberosity**

6, 7 √7ᵗʰ **S82.154** **Nondisplaced** fracture of MCC CC H5
right tibial **tuberosity**

6, 7 √7ᵗʰ **S82.155** **Nondisplaced** fracture of left MCC CC H5
tibial **tuberosity**

6, 7 √7ᵗʰ **S82.156** **Nondisplaced** fracture of MCC CC H5
unspecified tibial **tuberosity**

---

6   MCC when reported as an open fracture (7th character B or C).
7   CC when reported as an initial encounter (7th character A, B, or C – specific to category) OR a subsequent encounter for nonunion or malunion
(7th character K, M, N, P, Q, or R – specific to category).

☑ Additional Character Req   √x7ᵗʰ Placeholder Alert   Unacceptable PDx   Manifestation   H1 - H14 HAC   HCC CMS-HCC Condition   EXCLUDES 1 Not Coded Here   EXCLUDES 2 Not Included Here

ICD-10-CM 2018   **1051**

√6ᵗʰ **S82.16** **Torus** fracture of upper end of tibia

> The appropriate 7th character is to be added to all codes in subcategory S82.16.
> A   initial encounter for closed fracture
> D   subsequent encounter for fracture with routine healing
> G   subsequent encounter for fracture with delayed healing
> K   subsequent encounter for fracture with nonunion
> P   subsequent encounter for fracture with malunion
> S   sequela

7   √7ᵗʰ **S82.161** **Torus** fracture of upper end of **right tibia**   CC H5
> **CC Excl:** CC with 7th character A:
> PDX collection 1343
> **CC with 7th character K or P:**
> PDX collection 897

7   √7ᵗʰ **S82.162** **Torus** fracture of upper end of **left tibia**   CC H5
> **CC Excl:** CC with 7th character A:
> PDX collection 1344
> **CC with 7th character K or P:**
> PDX collection 897

7   √7ᵗʰ **S82.169** **Torus** fracture of upper end of **unspecified tibia**   CC H5
> **CC Excl:** CC with 7th character A:
> PDX collection 1345
> **CC with 7th character K or P:**
> PDX collection 897

√6ᵗʰ **S82.19** Other fracture of upper end of tibia

6,7   √7ᵗʰ **S82.191** Other fracture of upper end of right tibia   MCC CC H5

6,7   √7ᵗʰ **S82.192** Other fracture of upper end of left tibia   MCC CC H5

6,7   √7ᵗʰ **S82.199** Other fracture of upper end of unspecified tibia   MCC CC H5

√5ᵗʰ **S82.2** Fracture of shaft of tibia

> **CC Excl: For CC/MCC codes in subcategory S82.2, unless otherwise noted:**
> **Right side:** See code S82.101
> **Left side:** See code S82.102
> **Unspecified side:** See code S82.109

√6ᵗʰ **S82.20** **Unspecified** fracture of shaft of tibia
> Fracture of tibia NOS

6,7   √7ᵗʰ **S82.201** **Unspecified** fracture of shaft of **right tibia**   MCC CC H5
> **CC Excl:** CC with 7th character A:
> PDX collection 1346
> **MCC with 7th character B or C:**
> PDX collection 1341
> **CC with 7th character K, M, N, P, Q or R:**
> PDX collection 897

6,7   √7ᵗʰ **S82.202** **Unspecified** fracture of shaft of **left tibia**   MCC CC H5
> **CC Excl:** CC with 7th character A:
> PDX collection 1342
> **MCC with 7th character B or C:**
> PDX collection 1341
> **CC with 7th character K, M, N, P, Q or R:**
> PDX collection 897

6,7   √7ᵗʰ **S82.209** **Unspecified** fracture of shaft of **unspecified tibia**   MCC CC H5
> **CC Excl:**
> **CC or MCC with 7th character A, B or C:**
> PDX collection 1341
> **CC with 7th character K, M, N, P, Q or R:**
> PDX collection 897

√6ᵗʰ **S82.22** **Transverse** fracture of shaft of tibia

6,7   √7ᵗʰ **S82.221** **Displaced transverse** fracture of shaft of **right tibia**   MCC CC H5

6,7   √7ᵗʰ **S82.222** **Displaced transverse** fracture of shaft of **left tibia**   MCC CC H5

6,7   √7ᵗʰ **S82.223** **Displaced transverse** fracture of shaft of **unspecified tibia**   MCC CC H5

6,7   √7ᵗʰ **S82.224** **Nondisplaced transverse** fracture of shaft of **right tibia**   MCC CC H5

6,7   √7ᵗʰ **S82.225** **Nondisplaced transverse** fracture of shaft of **left tibia**   MCC CC H5

6,7   √7ᵗʰ **S82.226** **Nondisplaced transverse** fracture of shaft of **unspecified tibia**   MCC CC H5

√6ᵗʰ **S82.23** **Oblique** fracture of shaft of tibia

6,7   √7ᵗʰ **S82.231** **Displaced oblique** fracture of shaft of **right tibia**   MCC CC H5

6,7   √7ᵗʰ **S82.232** **Displaced oblique** fracture of shaft of **left tibia**   MCC CC H5

6,7   √7ᵗʰ **S82.233** **Displaced oblique** fracture of shaft of **unspecified tibia**   MCC CC H5

6,7   √7ᵗʰ **S82.234** **Nondisplaced oblique** fracture of shaft of **right tibia**   MCC CC H5

6,7   √7ᵗʰ **S82.235** **Nondisplaced oblique** fracture of shaft of **left tibia**   MCC CC H5

6,7   √7ᵗʰ **S82.236** **Nondisplaced oblique** fracture of shaft of **unspecified tibia**   MCC CC H5

√6ᵗʰ **S82.24** **Spiral** fracture of shaft of tibia
> Toddler fracture

6,7   √7ᵗʰ **S82.241** **Displaced spiral** fracture of shaft of **right tibia**   MCC CC H5

6,7   √7ᵗʰ **S82.242** **Displaced spiral** fracture of shaft of **left tibia**   MCC CC H5

6,7   √7ᵗʰ **S82.243** **Displaced spiral** fracture of shaft of **unspecified tibia**   MCC CC H5

6,7   √7ᵗʰ **S82.244** **Nondisplaced spiral** fracture of shaft of **right tibia**   MCC CC H5

6,7   √7ᵗʰ **S82.245** **Nondisplaced spiral** fracture of shaft of **left tibia**   MCC CC H5

6,7   √7ᵗʰ **S82.246** **Nondisplaced spiral** fracture of shaft of **unspecified tibia**   MCC CC H5

√6ᵗʰ **S82.25** **Comminuted** fracture of shaft of tibia

6,7   √7ᵗʰ **S82.251** **Displaced comminuted** fracture of shaft of **right tibia**   MCC CC H5

6,7   √7ᵗʰ **S82.252** **Displaced comminuted** fracture of shaft of **left tibia**   MCC CC H5

6,7   √7ᵗʰ **S82.253** **Displaced comminuted** fracture of shaft of **unspecified tibia**   MCC CC H5

6,7   √7ᵗʰ **S82.254** **Nondisplaced comminuted** fracture of shaft of **right tibia**   MCC CC H5

6,7   √7ᵗʰ **S82.255** **Nondisplaced comminuted** fracture of shaft of **left tibia**   MCC CC H5

6,7   √7ᵗʰ **S82.256** **Nondisplaced comminuted** fracture of shaft of **unspecified tibia**   MCC CC H5

√6ᵗʰ **S82.26** **Segmental** fracture of shaft of tibia

6,7   √7ᵗʰ **S82.261** **Displaced segmental** fracture of shaft of **right tibia**   MCC CC H5

6,7   √7ᵗʰ **S82.262** **Displaced segmental** fracture of shaft of **left tibia**   MCC CC H5

6,7   √7ᵗʰ **S82.263** **Displaced segmental** fracture of shaft of **unspecified tibia**   MCC CC H5

6,7   √7ᵗʰ **S82.264** **Nondisplaced segmental** fracture of shaft of **right tibia**   MCC CC H5

6,7   √7ᵗʰ **S82.265** **Nondisplaced segmental** fracture of shaft of **left tibia**   MCC CC H5

6,7   √7ᵗʰ **S82.266** **Nondisplaced segmental** fracture of shaft of **unspecified tibia**   MCC CC H5

√6ᵗʰ **S82.29** Other fracture of shaft of tibia

6,7   √7ᵗʰ **S82.291** Other fracture of shaft of **right tibia**   MCC CC H5

6,7   √7ᵗʰ **S82.292** Other fracture of shaft of **left tibia**   MCC CC H5

6,7   √7ᵗʰ **S82.299** Other fracture of shaft of **unspecified tibia**   MCC CC H5

---

6   MCC when reported as an open fracture (7th character B or C).

7   CC when reported as an initial encounter (7th character A, B, or C – specific to category) OR a subsequent encounter for nonunion or malunion (7th character K, M, N, P, Q, or R – specific to category).

N Newborn: 0   **P** Pediatric: 0-17   **M** Maternity: 12-55   **A** Adult: 15-124   **MCC** Major CC Condition   **PDxMCC** PDx acts as own MCC   **CC** CC Condition   **PDxCC** PDx acts as own CC

1052   ICD-10-CM 2018

✓5ᵗʰ **S82.3 Fracture of** lower end of tibia

> EXCLUDES 1   bimalleolar fracture of lower leg (S82.84-)
> fracture of medial malleolus alone (S82.5-)
> Maisonneuve's fracture (S82.86-)
> pilon fracture of distal tibia (S82.87-)
> trimalleolar fractures of lower leg (S82.85-)

✓6ᵗʰ **S82.30 Unspecified fracture of lower end of tibia**

> **CC Excl: For codes in subcategory S82.30:**
> **CC with 7th character B or C:** PDX collection 1347
> **CC with 7th character K, M, N, P, Q or R:**
> PDX collection 897

7   ✓7ᵗʰ **S82.301 Unspecified fracture of lower end** CC H5
of right **tibia**

7   ✓7ᵗʰ **S82.302 Unspecified fracture of lower end** CC H5
of left **tibia**

7   ✓7ᵗʰ **S82.309 Unspecified fracture of lower end** CC H5
of unspecified **tibia**

✓6ᵗʰ **S82.31 Torus fracture of lower end of tibia**

> The appropriate 7th character is to be added to
> all codes in subcategory S82.31.
> A   initial encounter for closed fracture
> D   subsequent encounter for fracture with
>   routine healing
> G   subsequent encounter for fracture with
>   delayed healing
> K   subsequent encounter for fracture with
>   nonunion
> P   subsequent encounter for fracture with
>   malunion
> S   sequela

7   ✓7ᵗʰ **S82.311 Torus fracture of lower end of** right CC H5
tibia
> **CC Excl: CC with 7th character A:**
> PDX collection 1343
> **CC with 7th character K or P:**
> PDX collection 897

7   ✓7ᵗʰ **S82.312 Torus fracture of lower end of** left CC H5
tibia
> **CC Excl: CC with 7th character A:**
> PDX collection 1344
> **CC with 7th character K or P:**
> PDX collection 897

7   ✓7ᵗʰ **S82.319 Torus fracture of lower end of** CC H5
unspecified **tibia**
> **CC Excl: CC with 7th character A:**
> PDX collection 1345
> **CC with 7th character K or P:**
> PDX collection 897

✓6ᵗʰ **S82.39 Other fracture of lower end of tibia**
AHA: 2015, 1Q, 25

> **CC Excl: For codes in subcategory S82.39:**
> **CC for codes with 7th character B or C:**
> PDX collection 1347
> **CC with 7th character K, M, N, P, Q or R:**
> PDX collection 897

7   ✓7ᵗʰ **S82.391 Other fracture of lower end of** right CC H5
tibia

7   ✓7ᵗʰ **S82.392 Other fracture of lower end of** left CC H5
tibia

7   ✓7ᵗʰ **S82.399 Other fracture of lower end of** CC H5
unspecified **tibia**

✓5ᵗʰ **S82.4 Fracture of** shaft of fibula

> EXCLUDES 2   fracture of lateral malleolus alone (S82.6-)

> **CC Excl: For codes in subcategory S82.4:**
> **MCC for codes with 7th character B or C:**
> PDX collection 1341
> **CC with 7th character K, M, N, P, Q or R:** PDX collection 897

✓6ᵗʰ **S82.40 Unspecified fracture of shaft of fibula**

6, 8   ✓7ᵗʰ **S82.401 Unspecified fracture of shaft of** MCC CC H5
right **fibula**

6, 8   ✓7ᵗʰ **S82.402 Unspecified fracture of shaft of** MCC CC H5
left **fibula**

6, 8   ✓7ᵗʰ **S82.409 Unspecified fracture of shaft of** MCC CC H5
unspecified **fibula**

✓6ᵗʰ **S82.42 Transverse fracture of shaft of fibula**

6, 8   ✓7ᵗʰ **S82.421 Displaced transverse fracture** MCC CC H5
of shaft of right **fibula**

6, 8   ✓7ᵗʰ **S82.422 Displaced transverse fracture** MCC CC H5
of shaft of left **fibula**

6, 8   ✓7ᵗʰ **S82.423 Displaced transverse fracture** MCC CC H5
of shaft of unspecified **fibula**

6, 8   ✓7ᵗʰ **S82.424 Nondisplaced transverse** MCC CC H5
fracture of shaft of right **fibula**

6, 8   ✓7ᵗʰ **S82.425 Nondisplaced transverse** MCC CC H5
fracture of shaft of left **fibula**

6, 8   ✓7ᵗʰ **S82.426 Nondisplaced transverse** MCC CC H5
fracture of shaft of unspecified
fibula

✓6ᵗʰ **S82.43 Oblique fracture of shaft of fibula**

6, 8   ✓7ᵗʰ **S82.431 Displaced oblique fracture of** MCC CC H5
shaft of right **fibula**

6, 8   ✓7ᵗʰ **S82.432 Displaced oblique fracture of** MCC CC H5
shaft of left **fibula**

6, 8   ✓7ᵗʰ **S82.433 Displaced oblique fracture of** MCC CC H5
shaft of unspecified **fibula**

6, 8   ✓7ᵗʰ **S82.434 Nondisplaced oblique fracture** MCC CC H5
of shaft of right **fibula**

6, 8   ✓7ᵗʰ **S82.435 Nondisplaced oblique fracture** MCC CC H5
of shaft of left **fibula**

6, 8   ✓7ᵗʰ **S82.436 Nondisplaced oblique fracture** MCC CC H5
of shaft of unspecified **fibula**

✓6ᵗʰ **S82.44 Spiral fracture of shaft of fibula**

6, 8   ✓7ᵗʰ **S82.441 Displaced spiral fracture of** MCC CC H5
shaft of right **fibula**

6, 8   ✓7ᵗʰ **S82.442 Displaced spiral fracture of** MCC CC H5
shaft of left **fibula**

6, 8   ✓7ᵗʰ **S82.443 Displaced spiral fracture of** MCC CC H5
shaft of unspecified **fibula**

6, 8   ✓7ᵗʰ **S82.444 Nondisplaced spiral fracture** MCC CC H5
of shaft of right **fibula**

6, 8   ✓7ᵗʰ **S82.445 Nondisplaced spiral fracture of** MCC CC H5
shaft of left **fibula**

6, 8   ✓7ᵗʰ **S82.446 Nondisplaced spiral fracture of** MCC CC H5
sahft of unspecified **fibula**

✓6ᵗʰ **S82.45 Comminuted fracture of shaft of fibula**

6, 8   ✓7ᵗʰ **S82.451 Displaced comminuted fracture** MCC CC H5
of shaft of right **fibula**

6, 8   ✓7ᵗʰ **S82.452 Displaced comminuted fracture** MCC CC H5
of shaft of left **fibula**

6, 8   ✓7ᵗʰ **S82.453 Displaced comminuted fracture** MCC CC H5
of shaft of unspecified **fibula**

6, 8   ✓7ᵗʰ **S82.454 Nondisplaced comminuted** MCC CC H5
fracture of shaft of right **fibula**

6, 8   ✓7ᵗʰ **S82.455 Nondisplaced comminuted** MCC CC H5
fracture of shaft of left **fibula**

6, 8   ✓7ᵗʰ **S82.456 Nondisplaced comminuted** MCC CC H5
fracture of shaft of unspecified
fibula

✓6ᵗʰ **S82.46 Segmental fracture of shaft of fibula**

6, 8   ✓7ᵗʰ **S82.461 Displaced segmental fracture** MCC CC H5
of shaft of right **fibula**

6, 8   ✓7ᵗʰ **S82.462 Displaced segmental fracture** MCC CC H5
of shaft of left **fibula**

6, 8   ✓7ᵗʰ **S82.463 Displaced segmental fracture** MCC CC H5
of shaft of unspecified **fibula**

6, 8   ✓7ᵗʰ **S82.464 Nondisplaced segmental** MCC CC H5
fracture of shaft of right **fibula**

6, 8   ✓7ᵗʰ **S82.465 Nondisplaced segmental** MCC CC H5
fracture of shaft of left **fibula**

6, 8   ✓7ᵗʰ **S82.466 Nondisplaced segmental** MCC CC H5
fracture of shaft of unspecified
fibula

---

6   MCC when reported as an open fracture (7th character B or C).

7   CC when reported as an initial encounter (7th character A, B, or C – specific to category) OR a subsequent encounter for nonunion or malunion
(7th character K, M, N, P, Q, or R – specific to category).

8   CC when reported as a subsequent encounter for nonunion or malunion (7th character K, M, N, P, Q, or R).

✓ Additional Character Req   ✓ₓ7ᵗʰ Placeholder Alert   Unacceptable PDx   Manifestation   H1-H14 HAC   HCC CMS-HCC Condition   EXCLUDES 1 Not Coded Here   EXCLUDES 2 Not Included Here

✓6th S82.49 Other fracture of shaft of fibula

  6, 8   ✓7th   **S82.491 Other fracture of shaft of right fibula** `MCC` `CC` `H5`

  6, 8   ✓7th   **S82.492 Other fracture of shaft of left fibula** `MCC` `CC` `H5`

  6, 8   ✓7th   **S82.499 Other fracture of shaft of unspecified fibula** `MCC` `CC` `H5`

✓5th S82.5 Fracture of medial malleolus

    EXCLUDES 1   pilon fracture of distal tibia (S82.87-)
             Salter-Harris type III of lower end of tibia (S89.13-)
             Salter-Harris type IV of lower end of tibia (S89.14-)

    CC Excl: For codes in subcategory S82.5:
    CC with 7th character B or C: PDX collection 1347
    CC with 7th character K, M, N, P, Q or R: PDX collection 897

  7   ✓x7th   **S82.51 Displaced fracture of medial malleolus of right tibia** `CC` `H5`

  7   ✓x7th   **S82.52 Displaced fracture of medial malleolus of left tibia** `CC` `H5`

  7   ✓x7th   **S82.53 Displaced fracture of medial malleolus of unspecified tibia** `CC` `H5`

  7   ✓x7th   **S82.54 Nondisplaced fracture of medial malleolus of right tibia** `CC` `H5`

  7   ✓x7th   **S82.55 Nondisplaced fracture of medial malleolus of left tibia** `CC` `H5`

  7   ✓x7th   **S82.56 Nondisplaced fracture of medial malleolus of unspecified tibia** `CC` `H5`

✓5th S82.6 Fracture of lateral malleolus

    EXCLUDES 1   pilon fracture of distal tibia (S82.87-)

    CC Excl: For codes in subcategory S82.6:
    CC with 7th character B or C: PDX collection 1347
    CC with 7th character K, M, N, P, Q or R: PDX collection 897

  7   ✓x7th   **S82.61 Displaced fracture of lateral malleolus of right fibula** `CC` `H5`

  7   ✓x7th   **S82.62 Displaced fracture of lateral malleolus of left fibula** `CC` `H5`

  7   ✓x7th   **S82.63 Displaced fracture of lateral malleolus of unspecified fibula** `CC` `H5`

  7   ✓x7th   **S82.64 Nondisplaced fracture of lateral malleolus of right fibula** `CC` `H5`

  7   ✓x7th   **S82.65 Nondisplaced fracture of lateral malleolus of left fibula** `CC` `H5`

  7   ✓x7th   **S82.66 Nondisplaced fracture of lateral malleolus of unspecified fibula** `CC` `H5`

✓5th S82.8 Other fractures of lower leg

   ✓6th S82.81 Torus fracture of upper end of fibula

    The appropriate 7th character is to be added to all codes in subcategory S82.81.
    A   initial encounter for closed fracture
    D   subsequent encounter for fracture with routine healing
    G   subsequent encounter for fracture with delayed healing
    K   subsequent encounter for fracture wit nonunion
    P   subsequent encounter for fracture with malunion
    S   sequela

    CC Excl: For codes in subcatgory S82.81:
    CC with 7th character K or P: PDX collection 897

  8   ✓7th   **S82.811 Torus fracture of upper end of right fibula** `CC`

  8   ✓7th   **S82.812 Torus fracture of upper end of left fibula** `CC`

  8   ✓7th   **S82.819 Torus fracture of upper end of unspecified fibula** `CC`

✓6th S82.82 Torus fracture of lower end of fibula

    The appropriate 7th character is to be added to all codes in subcategory S82.82.
    A   initial encounter for closed fracture
    D   subsequent encounter for fracture with routine healing
    G   subsequent encounter for fracture with delayed healing
    K   subsequent encounter for fracture with nonunion
    P   subsequent encounter for fracture with malunion
    S   sequela

    CC Excl: For codes in subcatgory S82.82:
    CC with 7th character K or P: PDX collection 897

  8   ✓7th   **S82.821 Torus fracture of lower end of right fibula** `CC`

  8   ✓7th   **S82.822 Torus fracture of lower end of left fibula** `CC`

  8   ✓7th   **S82.829 Torus fracture of lower end of unspecified fibula** `CC`

✓6th S82.83 Other fracture of upper and lower end of fibula
    AHA: 2015, 1Q, 25

    CC Excl: For codes in subcatgory S82.83:
    MCC with 7th B or C: PDX collection 1341
    CC with 7th character K, M, N, P, Q or R: PDX collection 897

  6, 8   ✓7th   **S82.831 Other fracture of upper and lower end of right fibula** `MCC` `CC` `H5`

  6, 8   ✓7th   **S82.832 Other fracture of upper and lower end of left fibula** `MCC` `CC` `H5`

  6, 8   ✓7th   **S82.839 Other fracture of upper and lower end of unspecified fibula** `MCC` `CC` `H5`

✓6th S82.84 Bimalleolar fracture of lower leg

    CC Excl: For codes in subcatgory S82.84:
    CC with 7th character B or C: PDX collection 1347
    CC with 7th character K, M, N, P, Q or R: PDX collection 897

  7   ✓7th   **S82.841 Displaced bimalleolar fracture of right lower leg** `CC` `H5`

  7   ✓7th   **S82.842 Displaced bimalleolar fracture of left lower leg** `CC` `H5`

  7   ✓7th   **S82.843 Displaced bimalleolar fracture of unspecified lower leg** `CC` `H5`

Right Bimalleolar Fracture

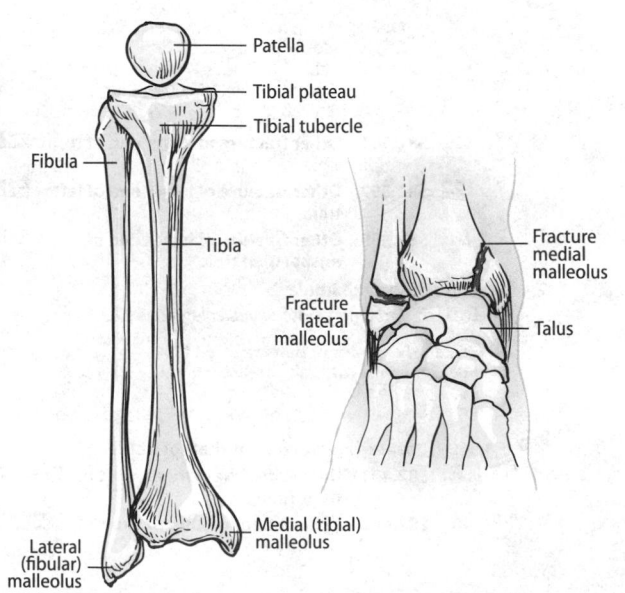

Patella
Tibial plateau
Tibial tubercle
Fibula
Tibia
Fracture medial malleolus
Fracture lateral malleolus
Talus
Medial (tibial) malleolus
Lateral (fibular) malleolus

---

6   MCC when reported as an open fracture (7th character B or C).
7   CC when reported as an initial encounter (7th character A, B, or C – specific to category) OR a subsequent encounter for nonunion or malunion (7th character K, M, N, P, Q, or R – specific to category).
8   CC when reported as a subsequent encounter for nonunion or malunion (7th character K, M, N, P, Q, or R).

`N` Newborn: 0   `P` Pediatric: 0-17   `M` Maternity: 12-55   `A` Adult: 15-124   `MCC` Major CC Condition   `PDxMCC` PDx acts as own MCC   `CC` CC Condition   `PDxCC` PDx acts as own CC

1054   ICD-10-CM 2018

7 ✓7ᵗʰ **S82.844** Nondisplaced **bimalleolar** fracture of right **lower leg** `CC` `H5`

7 ✓7ᵗʰ **S82.845** Nondisplaced **bimalleolar** fracture of left **lower leg** `CC` `H5`

7 ✓7ᵗʰ **S82.846** Nondisplaced **bimalleolar** fracture of unspecified **lower leg** `CC` `H5`

✓6ᵗʰ **S82.85** Trimalleolar **fracture of lower leg**

> **CC Excl: For codes in subcatgory S82.85:**
> **CC with 7th character B or C:** PDX collection 1347
> **CC with 7th character K, M, N, P, Q or R:**
> PDX collection 897

7 ✓7ᵗʰ **S82.851** Displaced **trimalleolar** fracture of right **lower leg** `CC` `H5`

7 ✓7ᵗʰ **S82.852** Displaced **trimalleolar** fracture of left **lower leg** `CC` `H5`

7 ✓7ᵗʰ **S82.853** Displaced **trimalleolar** fracture of unspecified **lower leg** `CC` `H5`

7 ✓7ᵗʰ **S82.854** Nondisplaced **trimalleolar** fracture of right **lower leg** `CC` `H5`

7 ✓7ᵗʰ **S82.855** Nondisplaced **trimalleolar** fracture of left **lower leg** `CC` `H5`

7 ✓7ᵗʰ **S82.856** Nondisplaced **trimalleolar** fracture of unspecified **lower leg** `CC` `H5`

✓6ᵗʰ **S82.86** Maisonneuve's **fracture**

> **CC Excl: For codes in subcatgory S82.86:**
> **MCC with 7th character B or C:** PDX collection 1341
> **CC with 7th character K, M, N, P, Q or R:**
> PDX collection 897

6, 8 ✓7ᵗʰ **S82.861** Displaced **Maisonneuve's fracture of** right **leg** `MCC` `CC` `H5`

6, 8 ✓7ᵗʰ **S82.862** Displaced **Maisonneuve's fracture of** left **leg** `MCC` `CC` `H5`

6, 8 ✓7ᵗʰ **S82.863** Displaced **Maisonneuve's fracture of** unspecified **leg** `MCC` `CC` `H5`

6, 8 ✓7ᵗʰ **S82.864** Nondisplaced **Maisonneuve's fracture of** right **leg** `MCC` `CC` `H5`

6, 8 ✓7ᵗʰ **S82.865** Nondisplaced **Maisonneuve's fracture of** left **leg** `MCC` `CC` `H5`

6, 8 ✓7ᵗʰ **S82.866** Nondisplaced **Maisonneuve's fracture of** unspecified **leg** `MCC` `CC` `H5`

✓6ᵗʰ **S82.87** Pilon **fracture of tibia**

> **CC Excl: For codes in subcatgory S82.87:**
> **CC with 7th character B or C:** PDX collection 1347
> **CC with 7th character K, M, N, P, Q or R:**
> PDX collection 897

7 ✓7ᵗʰ **S82.871** Displaced **pilon fracture of** right **tibia** `CC` `H5`

7 ✓7ᵗʰ **S82.872** Displaced **pilon fracture of** left **tibia** `CC` `H5`

7 ✓7ᵗʰ **S82.873** Displaced **pilon fracture of** unspecified **tibia** `CC` `H5`

7 ✓7ᵗʰ **S82.874** Nondisplaced **pilon fracture of** right **tibia** `CC` `H5`

7 ✓7ᵗʰ **S82.875** Nondisplaced **pilon fracture of** left **tibia** `CC` `H5`

7 ✓7ᵗʰ **S82.876** Nondisplaced **pilon fracture of** unspecified **tibia** `CC` `H5`

✓6ᵗʰ **S82.89** Other **fractures of lower leg**
Fracture of ankle NOS

> **CC Excl: For codes in subcatgory S82.89:**
> **CC with 7th character B or C:** PDX collection 1347
> **CC with 7th character K, M, N, P, Q or R:**
> PDX collection 897

7 ✓7ᵗʰ **S82.891** Other fracture of right **lower leg** `CC` `H5`

7 ✓7ᵗʰ **S82.892** Other fracture of left **lower leg** `CC` `H5`

7 ✓7ᵗʰ **S82.899** Other fracture of unspecified **lower leg** `CC` `H5`

✓5ᵗʰ **S82.9** Unspecified **fracture of lower leg**

> **CC Excl: For codes in subcatgory S82.9:**
> **CC with 7th character B or C:** PDX collection 1348
> **CC with 7th character K, M, N, P, Q or R:**
> PDX collection 897

7 ✓x7ᵗʰ **S82.90** Unspecified fracture of unspecified **lower leg** `CC` `H5`

7 ✓x7ᵗʰ **S82.91** Unspecified fracture of right **lower leg** `CC` `H5`

7 ✓x7ᵗʰ **S82.92** Unspecified fracture of left **lower leg** `CC` `H5`

✓4ᵗʰ **S83** **Dislocation and sprain of joints and ligaments of knee**

`INCLUDES` avulsion of joint or ligament of knee
laceration of cartilage, joint or ligament of knee
sprain of cartilage, joint or ligament of knee
traumatic hemarthrosis of joint or ligament of knee
traumatic rupture of joint or ligament of knee
traumatic subluxation of joint or ligament of knee
traumatic tear of joint or ligament of knee

Code also any associated open wound

`EXCLUDES 1` derangement of patella (M22.0-M22.3)
injury of patellar ligament (tendon) (S76.1-)
internal derangement of knee (M23.-)
old dislocation of knee (M24.36)
pathological dislocation of knee (M24.36)
recurrent dislocation of knee (M22.0)

`EXCLUDES 2` strain of muscle, fascia and tendon of lower leg (S86.-)

> The appropriate 7th character is to be added to each code from
> category S83.
> A   initial encounter
> D   subsequent encounter
> S   sequela

✓5ᵗʰ **S83.0** Subluxation and dislocation of patella

✓6ᵗʰ **S83.00** Unspecified **subluxation and dislocation of patella**

✓7ᵗʰ **S83.001** Unspecified **subluxation of** right **patella**

✓7ᵗʰ **S83.002** Unspecified **subluxation of** left **patella**

✓7ᵗʰ **S83.003** Unspecified **subluxation of** unspecified **patella**

✓7ᵗʰ **S83.004** Unspecified **dislocation of** right **patella**

✓7ᵗʰ **S83.005** Unspecified **dislocation of** left **patella**

✓7ᵗʰ **S83.006** Unspecified **dislocation of** unspecified **patella**

✓6ᵗʰ **S83.01** Lateral **subluxation and dislocation of patella**

✓7ᵗʰ **S83.011** Lateral **subluxation of** right **patella**

✓7ᵗʰ **S83.012** Lateral **subluxation of** left **patella**

✓7ᵗʰ **S83.013** Lateral **subluxation of** unspecified **patella**

✓7ᵗʰ **S83.014** Lateral **dislocation of** right **patella**

✓7ᵗʰ **S83.015** Lateral **dislocation of** left **patella**

✓7ᵗʰ **S83.016** Lateral **dislocation of** unspecified **patella**

✓6ᵗʰ **S83.09** Other **subluxation and dislocation of patella**

✓7ᵗʰ **S83.091** Other **subluxation of** right **patella**

✓7ᵗʰ **S83.092** Other **subluxation of** left **patella**

✓7ᵗʰ **S83.093** Other **subluxation of** unspecified **patella**

✓7ᵗʰ **S83.094** Other **dislocation of** right **patella**

✓7ᵗʰ **S83.095** Other **dislocation of** left **patella**

✓7ᵗʰ **S83.096** Other **dislocation of** unspecified **patella**

✓5ᵗʰ **S83.1** Subluxation and dislocation of knee

`EXCLUDES 2` instability of knee prosthesis (T84.022, T84.023)

✓6ᵗʰ **S83.10** Unspecified **subluxation and dislocation of knee**

✓7ᵗʰ **S83.101** Unspecified **subluxation of** right **knee**

✓7ᵗʰ **S83.102** Unspecified **subluxation of** left **knee**

✓7ᵗʰ **S83.103** Unspecified **subluxation of** unspecified **knee**

✓7ᵗʰ **S83.104** Unspecified **dislocation of** right **knee**

✓7ᵗʰ **S83.105** Unspecified **dislocation of** left **knee**

✓7ᵗʰ **S83.106** Unspecified **dislocation of** unspecified **knee**

---

6   MCC when reported as an open fracture (7th character B or C).

7   CC when reported as an initial encounter (7th character A, B, or C – specific to category) OR a subsequent encounter for nonunion or malunion
(7th character K, M, N, P, Q, or R – specific to category).

8   CC when reported as a subsequent encounter for nonunion or malunion (7th character K, M, N, P, Q, or R).

☑ Additional Character Req   ✓x7ᵗʰ Placeholder Alert   Unacceptable PDx   Manifestation   `H1`-`H14` HAC   `HCC` CMS-HCC Condition   `EXCLUDES 1` Not Coded Here   `EXCLUDES 2` Not Included Here

√6ᵗʰ **S83.11** **Anterior** subluxation and dislocation of proximal end of tibia
Posterior subluxation and dislocation of distal end of femur

√7ᵗʰ **S83.111** **Anterior** subluxation of proximal end of tibia, **right knee**

√7ᵗʰ **S83.112** **Anterior** subluxation of proximal end of tibia, **left knee**

√7ᵗʰ **S83.113** **Anterior** subluxation of proximal end of tibia, **unspecified knee**

√7ᵗʰ **S83.114** **Anterior** dislocation of proximal end of tibia, **right knee**

√7ᵗʰ **S83.115** **Anterior** dislocation of proximal end of tibia, **left knee**

√7ᵗʰ **S83.116** **Anterior** dislocation of proximal end of tibia, **unspecified knee**

√6ᵗʰ **S83.12** **Posterior** subluxation and dislocation of proximal end of tibia
Anterior dislocation of distal end of femur

√7ᵗʰ **S83.121** **Posterior** subluxation of proximal end of tibia, **right knee**

√7ᵗʰ **S83.122** **Posterior** subluxation of proximal end of tibia, **left knee**

√7ᵗʰ **S83.123** **Posterior** subluxation of proximal end of tibia, **unspecified knee**

√7ᵗʰ **S83.124** **Posterior** dislocation of proximal end of tibia, **right knee**

√7ᵗʰ **S83.125** **Posterior** dislocation of proximal end of tibia, **left knee**

√7ᵗʰ **S83.126** **Posterior** dislocation of proximal end of tibia, **unspecified knee**

√6ᵗʰ **S83.13** **Medial** subluxation and dislocation of proximal end of tibia

√7ᵗʰ **S83.131** **Medial** subluxation of proximal end of tibia, **right knee**

√7ᵗʰ **S83.132** **Medial** subluxation of proximal end of tibia, **left knee**

√7ᵗʰ **S83.133** **Medial** subluxation of proximal end of tibia, **unspecified knee**

√7ᵗʰ **S83.134** **Medial** dislocation of proximal end of tibia, **right knee**

√7ᵗʰ **S83.135** **Medial** dislocation of proximal end of tibia, **left knee**

√7ᵗʰ **S83.136** **Medial** dislocation of proximal end of tibia, **unspecified knee**

√6ᵗʰ **S83.14** **Lateral** subluxation and dislocation of proximal end of tibia

√7ᵗʰ **S83.141** **Lateral** subluxation of proximal end of tibia, **right knee**

√7ᵗʰ **S83.142** **Lateral** subluxation of proximal end of tibia, **left knee**

√7ᵗʰ **S83.143** **Lateral** subluxation of proximal end of tibia, **unspecified knee**

√7ᵗʰ **S83.144** **Lateral** dislocation of proximal end of tibia, **right knee**

√7ᵗʰ **S83.145** **Lateral** dislocation of proximal end of tibia, **left knee**

√7ᵗʰ **S83.146** **Lateral** dislocation of proximal end of tibia, **unspecified knee**

√6ᵗʰ **S83.19** **Other** subluxation and dislocation of knee

√7ᵗʰ **S83.191** **Other** subluxation of **right knee**

√7ᵗʰ **S83.192** **Other** subluxation of **left knee**

√7ᵗʰ **S83.193** **Other** subluxation of **unspecified knee**

√7ᵗʰ **S83.194** **Other** dislocation of **right knee**

√7ᵗʰ **S83.195** **Other** dislocation of **left knee**

√7ᵗʰ **S83.196** **Other** dislocation of **unspecified knee**

√5ᵗʰ **S83.2** **Tear of meniscus, current injury**
EXCLUDES 1 *old bucket-handle tear (M23.2)*

√6ᵗʰ **S83.20** **Tear of unspecified meniscus, current injury**
Tear of meniscus of knee NOS

√7ᵗʰ **S83.200** **Bucket-handle** tear of unspecified meniscus, current injury, **right knee**

√7ᵗʰ **S83.201** **Bucket-handle** tear of unspecified meniscus, current injury, **left knee**

√7ᵗʰ **S83.202** **Bucket-handle** tear of unspecified meniscus, current injury, **unspecified knee**

√7ᵗʰ **S83.203** **Other** tear of unspecified meniscus, current injury, **right knee**

√7ᵗʰ **S83.204** **Other** tear of unspecified meniscus, current injury, **left knee**

√7ᵗʰ **S83.205** **Other** tear of unspecified meniscus, current injury, **unspecified knee**

√7ᵗʰ **S83.206** **Unspecified** tear of unspecified meniscus, current injury, **right knee**

√7ᵗʰ **S83.207** **Unspecified** tear of unspecified meniscus, current injury, **left knee**

√7ᵗʰ **S83.209** **Unspecified** tear of unspecified meniscus, current injury, **unspecified knee**

√6ᵗʰ **S83.21** **Bucket-handle** tear of **medial** meniscus, current injury

√7ᵗʰ **S83.211** **Bucket-handle** tear of medial meniscus, current injury, **right knee**

√7ᵗʰ **S83.212** **Bucket-handle** tear of medial meniscus, current injury, **left knee**

√7ᵗʰ **S83.219** **Bucket-handle** tear of medial meniscus, current injury, **unspecified knee**

√6ᵗʰ **S83.22** **Peripheral** tear of **medial** meniscus, current injury

√7ᵗʰ **S83.221** **Peripheral** tear of medial meniscus, current injury, **right knee**

√7ᵗʰ **S83.222** **Peripheral** tear of medial meniscus, current injury, **left knee**

√7ᵗʰ **S83.229** **Peripheral** tear of medial meniscus, current injury, **unspecified knee**

√6ᵗʰ **S83.23** **Complex** tear of **medial** meniscus, current injury

√7ᵗʰ **S83.231** **Complex** tear of medial meniscus, current injury, **right knee**

√7ᵗʰ **S83.232** **Complex** tear of medial meniscus, current injury, **left knee**

√7ᵗʰ **S83.239** **Complex** tear of medial meniscus, current injury, **unspecified knee**

√6ᵗʰ **S83.24** **Other** tear of **medial** meniscus, current injury

√7ᵗʰ **S83.241** **Other** tear of medial meniscus, current injury, **right knee**

√7ᵗʰ **S83.242** **Other** tear of medial meniscus, current injury, **left knee**

√7ᵗʰ **S83.249** **Other** tear of medial meniscus, current injury, **unspecified knee**

√6ᵗʰ **S83.25** **Bucket-handle** tear of **lateral** meniscus, current injury

√7ᵗʰ **S83.251** **Bucket-handle** tear of lateral meniscus, current injury, **right knee**

√7ᵗʰ **S83.252** **Bucket-handle** tear of lateral meniscus, current injury, **left knee**

√7ᵗʰ **S83.259** **Bucket-handle** tear of lateral meniscus, current injury, **unspecified knee**

√6ᵗʰ **S83.26** **Peripheral** tear of **lateral** meniscus, current injury

√7ᵗʰ **S83.261** **Peripheral** tear of lateral meniscus, current injury, **right knee**

√7ᵗʰ **S83.262** **Peripheral** tear of lateral meniscus, current injury, **left knee**

√7ᵗʰ **S83.269** **Peripheral** tear of lateral meniscus, current injury, **unspecified knee**

√6ᵗʰ **S83.27** **Complex** tear of **lateral** meniscus, current injury

√7ᵗʰ **S83.271** **Complex** tear of lateral meniscus, current injury, **right knee**

√7ᵗʰ **S83.272** **Complex** tear of lateral meniscus, current injury, **left knee**

√7ᵗʰ **S83.279** **Complex** tear of lateral meniscus, current injury, **unspecified knee**

√6ᵗʰ **S83.28** **Other** tear of **lateral** meniscus, current injury

√7ᵗʰ **S83.281** **Other** tear of lateral meniscus, current injury, **right knee**

√7ᵗʰ **S83.282** **Other** tear of lateral meniscus, current injury, **left knee**

√7ᵗʰ **S83.289** **Other** tear of lateral meniscus, current injury, **unspecified knee**

√5ᵗʰ **S83.3** Tear of articular cartilage of knee, current

   √x7ᵗʰ **S83.30** Tear of articular cartilage of unspecified knee, current

   √x7ᵗʰ **S83.31** Tear of articular cartilage of right knee, current

   √x7ᵗʰ **S83.32** Tear of articular cartilage of left knee, current

√5ᵗʰ **S83.4** Sprain of collateral ligament of knee

   √6ᵗʰ **S83.40** Sprain of unspecified collateral ligament of knee

      √7ᵗʰ **S83.401** Sprain of unspecified collateral ligament of right knee

      √7ᵗʰ **S83.402** Sprain of unspecified collateral ligament of left knee

      √7ᵗʰ **S83.409** Sprain of unspecified collateral ligament of unspecified knee

   √6ᵗʰ **S83.41** Sprain of medial collateral ligament of knee
      Sprain of tibial collateral ligament

      √7ᵗʰ **S83.411** Sprain of medial collateral ligament of right knee

      √7ᵗʰ **S83.412** Sprain of medial collateral ligament of left knee

      √7ᵗʰ **S83.419** Sprain of medial collateral ligament of unspecified knee

   √6ᵗʰ **S83.42** Sprain of lateral collateral ligament of knee
      Sprain of fibular collateral ligament

      √7ᵗʰ **S83.421** Sprain of lateral collateral ligament of right knee

      √7ᵗʰ **S83.422** Sprain of lateral collateral ligament of left knee

      √7ᵗʰ **S83.429** Sprain of lateral collateral ligament of unspecified knee

√5ᵗʰ **S83.5** Sprain of cruciate ligament of knee
   AHA: 2016, 2Q, 3

   √6ᵗʰ **S83.50** Sprain of unspecified cruciate ligament of knee

      √7ᵗʰ **S83.501** Sprain of unspecified cruciate ligament of right knee

      √7ᵗʰ **S83.502** Sprain of unspecified cruciate ligament of left knee

      √7ᵗʰ **S83.509** Sprain of unspecified cruciate ligament of unspecified knee

   √6ᵗʰ **S83.51** Sprain of anterior cruciate ligament of knee

      √7ᵗʰ **S83.511** Sprain of anterior cruciate ligament of right knee

      √7ᵗʰ **S83.512** Sprain of anterior cruciate ligament of left knee

      √7ᵗʰ **S83.519** Sprain of anterior cruciate ligament of unspecified knee

   √6ᵗʰ **S83.52** Sprain of posterior cruciate ligament of knee

      √7ᵗʰ **S83.521** Sprain of posterior cruciate ligament of right knee

      √7ᵗʰ **S83.522** Sprain of posterior cruciate ligament of left knee

      √7ᵗʰ **S83.529** Sprain of posterior cruciate ligament of unspecified knee

√5ᵗʰ **S83.6** Sprain of the superior tibiofibular joint and ligament

   √x7ᵗʰ **S83.60** Sprain of the superior tibiofibular joint and ligament, unspecified knee

   √x7ᵗʰ **S83.61** Sprain of the superior tibiofibular joint and ligament, right knee

   √x7ᵗʰ **S83.62** Sprain of the superior tibiofibular joint and ligament, left knee

√5ᵗʰ **S83.8** Sprain of other specified parts of knee

   √6ᵗʰ **S83.8X** Sprain of other specified parts of knee

      √7ᵗʰ **S83.8X1** Sprain of other specified parts of right knee

      √7ᵗʰ **S83.8X2** Sprain of other specified parts of left knee

      √7ᵗʰ **S83.8X9** Sprain of other specified parts of unspecified knee

√5ᵗʰ **S83.9** Sprain of unspecified site of knee

   √x7ᵗʰ **S83.90** Sprain of unspecified site of unspecified knee

   √x7ᵗʰ **S83.91** Sprain of unspecified site of right knee

   √x7ᵗʰ **S83.92** Sprain of unspecified site of left knee

√4ᵗʰ **S84** Injury of nerves at lower leg level
   Code also any associated open wound (S81.-)
   EXCLUDES 2 injury of nerves at ankle and foot level (S94.-)

> The appropriate 7th character is to be added to each code from category S84.
> A initial encounter
> D subsequent encounter
> S sequela

√5ᵗʰ **S84.0** Injury of tibial nerve at lower leg level

   √x7ᵗʰ **S84.00** Injury of tibial nerve at lower leg level, unspecified leg

   √x7ᵗʰ **S84.01** Injury of tibial nerve at lower leg level, right leg

   √x7ᵗʰ **S84.02** Injury of tibial nerve at lower leg level, left leg

√5ᵗʰ **S84.1** Injury of peroneal nerve at lower leg level

   √x7ᵗʰ **S84.10** Injury of peroneal nerve at lower leg level, unspecified leg

   √x7ᵗʰ **S84.11** Injury of peroneal nerve at lower leg level, right leg

   √x7ᵗʰ **S84.12** Injury of peroneal nerve at lower leg level, left leg

√5ᵗʰ **S84.2** Injury of cutaneous sensory nerve at lower leg level

   √x7ᵗʰ **S84.20** Injury of cutaneous sensory nerve at lower leg level, unspecified leg

   √x7ᵗʰ **S84.21** Injury of cutaneous sensory nerve at lower leg level, right leg

   √x7ᵗʰ **S84.22** Injury of cutaneous sensory nerve at lower leg level, left leg

√5ᵗʰ **S84.8** Injury of other nerves at lower leg level

   √6ᵗʰ **S84.80** Injury of other nerves at lower leg level

      √7ᵗʰ **S84.801** Injury of other nerves at lower leg level, right leg

      √7ᵗʰ **S84.802** Injury of other nerves at lower leg level, left leg

      √7ᵗʰ **S84.809** Injury of other nerves at lower leg level, unspecified leg

√5ᵗʰ **S84.9** Injury of unspecified nerve at lower leg level

   √x7ᵗʰ **S84.90** Injury of unspecified nerve at lower leg level, unspecified leg

   √x7ᵗʰ **S84.91** Injury of unspecified nerve at lower leg level, right leg

   √x7ᵗʰ **S84.92** Injury of unspecified nerve at lower leg level, left leg

√4ᵗʰ **S85** Injury of blood vessels at lower leg level
   Code also any associated open wound (S81.-)
   EXCLUDES 2 injury of blood vessels at ankle and foot level (S95.-)

> The appropriate 7th character is to be added to each code from category S85.
> A initial encounter
> D subsequent encounter
> S sequela

√5ᵗʰ **S85.0** Injury of popliteal artery

> **CC Excl: For MCC codes in subcategory S85.0:**
> **Right side:** PDX collection 1349
> **Left side:** PDX collection 1350
> **Unspecified side:** PDX collection 1351

   √6ᵗʰ **S85.00** Unspecified injury of popliteal artery

      √7ᵗʰ **S85.001** Unspecified injury of popliteal artery, right leg **MCC**

      √7ᵗʰ **S85.002** Unspecified injury of popliteal artery, left leg **MCC**

      √7ᵗʰ **S85.009** Unspecified injury of popliteal artery, unspecified leg **MCC**

   √6ᵗʰ **S85.01** Laceration of popliteal artery

      √7ᵗʰ **S85.011** Laceration of popliteal artery, right leg **MCC**

      √7ᵗʰ **S85.012** Laceration of popliteal artery, left leg **MCC**

      √7ᵗʰ **S85.019** Laceration of popliteal artery, unspecified leg **MCC**

   √6ᵗʰ **S85.09** Other specified injury of popliteal artery

      √7ᵗʰ **S85.091** Other specified injury of popliteal artery, right leg **MCC**

      √7ᵗʰ **S85.092** Other specified injury of popliteal artery, left leg **MCC**

✔ Additional Character Req   √x7ᵗʰ Placeholder Alert   Unacceptable PDx   Manifestation   **H1**-**H14** HAC   **HCC** CMS-HCC Condition   *EXCLUDES 1* Not Coded Here   *EXCLUDES 2* Not Included Here

ICD-10-CM 2018   **1057**

☑7ᵗʰ **S85.099** Other specified injury of popliteal artery, **unspecified** leg　`MCC`

☑5ᵗʰ **S85.1** Injury of tibial artery

☑6ᵗʰ **S85.10** Unspecified injury of unspecified tibial artery
Injury of tibial artery NOS

☑7ᵗʰ **S85.101** Unspecified injury of unspecified tibial artery, **right** leg　`CC`

☑7ᵗʰ **S85.102** Unspecified injury of unspecified tibial artery, **left** leg　`CC`

☑7ᵗʰ **S85.109** Unspecified injury of unspecified tibial artery, **unspecified** leg　`CC`

☑6ᵗʰ **S85.11** Laceration of unspecified tibial artery

☑7ᵗʰ **S85.111** Laceration of unspecified tibial artery, **right** leg　`CC`
CC Excl: PDX collection 1352

☑7ᵗʰ **S85.112** Laceration of unspecified tibial artery, **left** leg　`CC`
CC Excl: PDX collection 1353

☑7ᵗʰ **S85.119** Laceration of unspecified tibial artery, **unspecified** leg　`CC`
CC Excl: PDX collection 1354

☑6ᵗʰ **S85.12** Other specified injury of unspecified tibial artery

☑7ᵗʰ **S85.121** Other specified injury of unspecified tibial artery, **right** leg　`CC`
CC Excl: PDX collection 1352

☑7ᵗʰ **S85.122** Other specified injury of unspecified tibial artery, **left** leg　`CC`
CC Excl: PDX collection 1353

☑7ᵗʰ **S85.129** Other specified injury of unspecified tibial artery, **unspecified** leg　`CC`
CC Excl: PDX collection 1354

☑6ᵗʰ **S85.13** Unspecified injury of anterior tibial artery

☑7ᵗʰ **S85.131** Unspecified injury of anterior tibial artery, **right** leg　`CC`
CC Excl: PDX collection 1355

☑7ᵗʰ **S85.132** Unspecified injury of anterior tibial artery, **left** leg　`CC`
CC Excl: PDX collection 1356

☑7ᵗʰ **S85.139** Unspecified injury of anterior tibial artery, **unspecified** leg　`CC`
CC Excl: PDX collection 1357

☑6ᵗʰ **S85.14** Laceration of anterior tibial artery

☑7ᵗʰ **S85.141** Laceration of anterior tibial artery, **right** leg　`CC`
CC Excl: PDX collection 1355

☑7ᵗʰ **S85.142** Laceration of anterior tibial artery, **left** leg　`CC`
CC Excl: PDX collection 1356

☑7ᵗʰ **S85.149** Laceration of anterior tibial artery, **unspecified** leg　`CC`
CC Excl: PDX collection 1357

☑6ᵗʰ **S85.15** Other specified injury of anterior tibial artery

☑7ᵗʰ **S85.151** Other specified injury of anterior tibial artery, **right** leg　`CC`
CC Excl: PDX collection 1355

☑7ᵗʰ **S85.152** Other specified injury of anterior tibial artery, **left** leg　`CC`
CC Excl: PDX collection 1356

☑7ᵗʰ **S85.159** Other specified injury of anterior tibial artery, **unspecified** leg　`CC`
CC Excl: PDX collection 1357

☑6ᵗʰ **S85.16** Unspecified injury of posterior tibial artery

☑7ᵗʰ **S85.161** Unspecified injury of posterior tibial artery, **right** leg　`CC`
CC Excl: PDX collection 1358

☑7ᵗʰ **S85.162** Unspecified injury of posterior tibial artery, **left** leg　`CC`
CC Excl: PDX collection 1359

☑7ᵗʰ **S85.169** Unspecified injury of posterior tibial artery, **unspecified** leg　`CC`
CC Excl: PDX collection 1360

☑6ᵗʰ **S85.17** Laceration of posterior tibial artery

☑7ᵗʰ **S85.171** Laceration of posterior tibial artery, **right** leg　`CC`
CC Excl: PDX collection 1358

☑7ᵗʰ **S85.172** Laceration of posterior tibial artery, **left** leg　`CC`
CC Excl: PDX collection 1359

☑7ᵗʰ **S85.179** Laceration of posterior tibial artery, **unspecified** leg　`CC`
CC Excl: PDX collection 1360

☑6ᵗʰ **S85.18** Other specified injury of posterior tibial artery

☑7ᵗʰ **S85.181** Other specified injury of posterior tibial artery, **right** leg　`CC`
CC Excl: PDX collection 1358

☑7ᵗʰ **S85.182** Other specified injury of posterior tibial artery, **left** leg　`CC`
CC Excl: PDX collection 1359

☑7ᵗʰ **S85.189** Other specified injury of posterior tibial artery, **unspecified** leg　`CC`
CC Excl: PDX collection 1360

☑5ᵗʰ **S85.2** Injury of peroneal artery

> **CC Excl: For CC codes in subcategory S85.2:**
> **Right side:** PDX collection 1325
> **Left side:** PDX collection 1326
> **Unspecified side:** PDX collection 1327

☑6ᵗʰ **S85.20** Unspecified injury of peroneal artery

☑7ᵗʰ **S85.201** Unspecified injury of peroneal artery, **right** leg　`CC`

☑7ᵗʰ **S85.202** Unspecified injury of peroneal artery, **left** leg　`CC`

☑7ᵗʰ **S85.209** Unspecified injury of peroneal artery, **unspecified** leg　`CC`

☑6ᵗʰ **S85.21** Laceration of peroneal artery

☑7ᵗʰ **S85.211** Laceration of peroneal artery, **right** leg　`CC`

☑7ᵗʰ **S85.212** Laceration of peroneal artery, **left** leg　`CC`

☑7ᵗʰ **S85.219** Laceration of peroneal artery, **unspecified** leg　`CC`

☑6ᵗʰ **S85.29** Other specified injury of peroneal artery

☑7ᵗʰ **S85.291** Other specified injury of peroneal artery, **right** leg　`CC`

☑7ᵗʰ **S85.292** Other specified injury of peroneal artery, **left** leg　`CC`

☑7ᵗʰ **S85.299** Other specified injury of peroneal artery, **unspecified** leg　`CC`

☑5ᵗʰ **S85.3** Injury of greater saphenous vein at lower leg level
Injury of greater saphenous vein NOS
Injury of saphenous vein NOS

> **CC Excl: For CC codes in subcategory S85.3:**
> **Right side:** PDX collection 1322
> **Left side:** PDX collection 1323
> **Unspecified side:** PDX collection 1324

☑6ᵗʰ **S85.30** Unspecified injury of greater saphenous vein at lower leg level

☑7ᵗʰ **S85.301** Unspecified injury of greater saphenous vein at lower leg level, **right** leg　`CC`

☑7ᵗʰ **S85.302** Unspecified injury of greater saphenous vein at lower leg level, **left** leg　`CC`

☑7ᵗʰ **S85.309** Unspecified injury of greater saphenous vein at lower leg level, **unspecified** leg　`CC`

☑6ᵗʰ **S85.31** Laceration of greater saphenous vein at lower leg level

☑7ᵗʰ **S85.311** Laceration of greater saphenous vein at lower leg level, **right** leg　`CC`

☑7ᵗʰ **S85.312** Laceration of greater saphenous vein at lower leg level, **left** leg　`CC`

☑7ᵗʰ **S85.319** Laceration of greater saphenous vein at lower leg level, **unspecified** leg　`CC`

☑6ᵗʰ **S85.39** Other specified injury of greater saphenous vein at lower leg level

☑7ᵗʰ **S85.391** Other specified injury of greater saphenous vein at lower leg level, **right** leg　`CC`

☑7ᵗʰ **S85.392** Other specified injury of greater saphenous vein at lower leg level, **left** leg　`CC`

Ⓝ Newborn: 0　　Ⓟ Pediatric: 0-17　　Ⓜ Maternity: 12-55　　Ⓐ Adult: 15-124　　`MCC` Major CC Condition　　`PDx MCC` PDx acts as own MCC　　`CC` CC Condition　　`PDx CC` PDx acts as own CC

1058　　　　　　　　　　　　　　　　　　　　　　　　　　　　　　　　　　　　ICD-10-CM 2018

√7ᵗʰ **S85.399** Other specified injury of greater saphenous vein at lower leg level, unspecified leg   CC

√5ᵗʰ **S85.4** Injury of lesser saphenous vein at lower leg level

> **CC Excl: For CC codes in subcategory S85.4:**
> **Right side:** PDX collection 1322
> **Left side:** PDX collection 1323
> **Unspecified side:** PDX collection 1324

√6ᵗʰ **S85.40** Unspecified injury of lesser saphenous vein at lower leg level

√7ᵗʰ **S85.401** Unspecified injury of lesser saphenous vein at lower leg level, right leg   CC

√7ᵗʰ **S85.402** Unspecified injury of lesser saphenous vein at lower leg level, left leg   CC

√7ᵗʰ **S85.409** Unspecified injury of lesser saphenous vein at lower leg level, unspecified leg   CC

√6ᵗʰ **S85.41** Laceration of lesser saphenous vein at lower leg level

√7ᵗʰ **S85.411** Laceration of lesser saphenous vein at lower leg level, right leg   CC

√7ᵗʰ **S85.412** Laceration of lesser saphenous vein at lower leg level, left leg   CC

√7ᵗʰ **S85.419** Laceration of lesser saphenous vein at lower leg level, unspecified leg   CC

√6ᵗʰ **S85.49** Other specified injury of lesser saphenous vein at lower leg level

√7ᵗʰ **S85.491** Other specified injury of lesser saphenous vein at lower leg level, right leg   CC

√7ᵗʰ **S85.492** Other specified injury of lesser saphenous vein at lower leg level, left leg   CC

√7ᵗʰ **S85.499** Other specified injury of lesser saphenous vein at lower leg level, unspecified leg   CC

√5ᵗʰ **S85.5** Injury of popliteal vein

> **CC Excl: For MCC codes in subcategory S85.5:**
> **Right side:** PDX collection 1361
> **Left side:** PDX collection 1362
> **Unspecified side:** PDX collection 1363

√6ᵗʰ **S85.50** Unspecified injury of popliteal vein

√7ᵗʰ **S85.501** Unspecified injury of popliteal vein, right leg   MCC

√7ᵗʰ **S85.502** Unspecified injury of popliteal vein, left leg   MCC

√7ᵗʰ **S85.509** Unspecified injury of popliteal vein, unspecified leg   MCC

√6ᵗʰ **S85.51** Laceration of popliteal vein

√7ᵗʰ **S85.511** Laceration of popliteal vein, right leg   MCC

√7ᵗʰ **S85.512** Laceration of popliteal vein, left leg   MCC

√7ᵗʰ **S85.519** Laceration of popliteal vein, unspecified leg   MCC

√6ᵗʰ **S85.59** Other specified injury of popliteal vein

√7ᵗʰ **S85.591** Other specified injury of popliteal vein, right leg   MCC

√7ᵗʰ **S85.592** Other specified injury of popliteal vein, left leg   MCC

√7ᵗʰ **S85.599** Other specified injury of popliteal vein, unspecified leg   MCC

√5ᵗʰ **S85.8** Injury of other blood vessels at lower leg level

> **CC Excl: For CC codes in subcategory S85.8:**
> **Right side:** PDX collection 1325
> **Left side:** PDX collection 1326
> **Unspecified side:** PDX collection 1327

√6ᵗʰ **S85.80** Unspecified injury of other blood vessels at lower leg level

√7ᵗʰ **S85.801** Unspecified injury of other blood vessels at lower leg level, right leg   CC

√7ᵗʰ **S85.802** Unspecified injury of other blood vessels at lower leg level, left leg   CC

√7ᵗʰ **S85.809** Unspecified injury of other blood vessels at lower leg level, unspecified leg   CC

√6ᵗʰ **S85.81** Laceration of other blood vessels at lower leg level

√7ᵗʰ **S85.811** Laceration of other blood vessels at lower leg level, right leg   CC

√7ᵗʰ **S85.812** Laceration of other blood vessels at lower leg level, left leg   CC

√7ᵗʰ **S85.819** Laceration of other blood vessels at lower leg level, unspecified leg   CC

√6ᵗʰ **S85.89** Other specified injury of other blood vessels at lower leg level

√7ᵗʰ **S85.891** Other specified injury of other blood vessels at lower leg level, right leg   CC

√7ᵗʰ **S85.892** Other specified injury of other blood vessels at lower leg level, left leg   CC

√7ᵗʰ **S85.899** Other specified injury of other blood vessels at lower leg level, unspecified leg   CC

√5ᵗʰ **S85.9** Injury of unspecified blood vessel at lower leg level

> **CC Excl: For CC codes in subcategory S85.9:**
> **Right side:** PDX collection 1325
> **Left side:** PDX collection 1326
> **Unspecified side:** PDX collection 1327

√6ᵗʰ **S85.90** Unspecified injury of unspecified blood vessel at lower leg level

√7ᵗʰ **S85.901** Unspecified injury of unspecified blood vessel at lower leg level, right leg   CC

√7ᵗʰ **S85.902** Unspecified injury of unspecified blood vessel at lower leg level, left leg   CC

√7ᵗʰ **S85.909** Unspecified injury of unspecified blood vessel at lower leg level, unspecified leg   CC

√6ᵗʰ **S85.91** Laceration of unspecified blood vessel at lower leg level

√7ᵗʰ **S85.911** Laceration of unspecified blood vessel at lower leg level, right leg   CC

√7ᵗʰ **S85.912** Laceration of unspecified blood vessel at lower leg level, left leg   CC

√7ᵗʰ **S85.919** Laceration of unspecified blood vessel at lower leg level, unspecified leg   CC

√6ᵗʰ **S85.99** Other specified injury of unspecified blood vessel at lower leg level

√7ᵗʰ **S85.991** Other specified injury of unspecified blood vessel at lower leg level, right leg   CC

√7ᵗʰ **S85.992** Other specified injury of unspecified blood vessel at lower leg level, left leg   CC

√7ᵗʰ **S85.999** Other specified injury of unspecified blood vessel at lower leg level, unspecified leg   CC

√4ᵗʰ **S86** **Injury of muscle, fascia and tendon at lower leg level**

Code also any associated open wound (S81.-)

EXCLUDES 2   injury of muscle, fascia and tendon at ankle (S96.-)
injury of patellar ligament (tendon) (S76.1-)
sprain of joints and ligaments of knee (S83.-)

TIP: Refer to the Muscle/Tendon table at the beginning of this chapter

> The appropriate 7th character is to be added to each code from category S86.
> A   initial encounter
> D   subsequent encounter
> S   sequela

> **CC Excl: For CC codes in category S86:**
> **Right side:** PDX collection 1364
> **Left side:** PDX collection 1365
> **Unspecified side:** PDX collection 1366

√5ᵗʰ **S86.0** Injury of Achilles tendon

√6ᵗʰ **S86.00** Unspecified injury of Achilles tendon

√7ᵗʰ **S86.001** Unspecified injury of right Achilles tendon

√7ᵗʰ **S86.002** Unspecified injury of left Achilles tendon

✓ Additional Character Req   √x 7ᵗʰ Placeholder Alert   Unacceptable PDx   Manifestation   H1-H14 HAC   HCC CMS-HCC Condition   *EXCLUDES 1* Not Coded Here   *EXCLUDES 2* Not Included Here

ICD-10-CM 2018   1059

√7ᵗʰ **S86.009** Unspecified injury of unspecified Achilles tendon

√6ᵗʰ **S86.01** Strain of Achilles tendon

√7ᵗʰ **S86.011** Strain of right Achilles tendon

√7ᵗʰ **S86.012** Strain of left Achilles tendon

√7ᵗʰ **S86.019** Strain of unspecified Achilles tendon

√6ᵗʰ **S86.02** Laceration of Achilles tendon

√7ᵗʰ **S86.021** Laceration of right Achilles tendon `CC`

√7ᵗʰ **S86.022** Laceration of left Achilles tendon `CC`

√7ᵗʰ **S86.029** Laceration of unspecified Achilles tendon `CC`

√6ᵗʰ **S86.09** Other specified injury of Achilles tendon

√7ᵗʰ **S86.091** Other specified injury of right Achilles tendon

√7ᵗʰ **S86.092** Other specified injury of left Achilles tendon

√7ᵗʰ **S86.099** Other specified injury of unspecified Achilles tendon

√5ᵗʰ **S86.1** Injury of other muscle(s) and tendon(s) of posterior muscle group at lower leg level

√6ᵗʰ **S86.10** Unspecified injury of other muscle(s) and tendon(s) of posterior muscle group at lower leg level

√7ᵗʰ **S86.101** Unspecified injury of other muscle(s) and tendon(s) of posterior muscle group at lower leg level, right leg

√7ᵗʰ **S86.102** Unspecified injury of other muscle(s) and tendon(s) of posterior muscle group at lower leg level, left leg

√7ᵗʰ **S86.109** Unspecified injury of other muscle(s) and tendon(s) of posterior muscle group at lower leg level, unspecified leg

√6ᵗʰ **S86.11** Strain of other muscle(s) and tendon(s) of posterior muscle group at lower leg level

√7ᵗʰ **S86.111** Strain of other muscle(s) and tendon(s) of posterior muscle group at lower leg level, right leg

√7ᵗʰ **S86.112** Strain of other muscle(s) and tendon(s) of posterior muscle group at lower leg level, left leg

√7ᵗʰ **S86.119** Strain of other muscle(s) and tendon(s) of posterior muscle group at lower leg level, unspecified leg

√6ᵗʰ **S86.12** Laceration of other muscle(s) and tendon(s) of posterior muscle group at lower leg level

√7ᵗʰ **S86.121** Laceration of other muscle(s) and tendon(s) of posterior muscle group at lower leg level, right leg `CC`

√7ᵗʰ **S86.122** Laceration of other muscle(s) and tendon(s) of posterior muscle group at lower leg level, left leg `CC`

√7ᵗʰ **S86.129** Laceration of other muscle(s) and tendon(s) of posterior muscle group at lower leg level, unspecified leg `CC`

√6ᵗʰ **S86.19** Other injury of other muscle(s) and tendon(s) of posterior muscle group at lower leg level

√7ᵗʰ **S86.191** Other injury of other muscle(s) and tendon(s) of posterior muscle group at lower leg level, right leg

√7ᵗʰ **S86.192** Other injury of other muscle(s) and tendon(s) of posterior muscle group at lower leg level, left leg

√7ᵗʰ **S86.199** Other injury of other muscle(s) and tendon(s) of posterior muscle group at lower leg level, unspecified leg

√5ᵗʰ **S86.2** Injury of muscle(s) and tendon(s) of anterior muscle group at lower leg level

√6ᵗʰ **S86.20** Unspecified injury of muscle(s) and tendon(s) of anterior muscle group at lower leg level

√7ᵗʰ **S86.201** Unspecified injury of muscle(s) and tendon(s) of anterior muscle group at lower leg level, right leg

√7ᵗʰ **S86.202** Unspecified injury of muscle(s) and tendon(s) of anterior muscle group at lower leg level, left leg

√7ᵗʰ **S86.209** Unspecified injury of muscle(s) and tendon(s) of anterior muscle group at lower leg level, unspecified leg

√6ᵗʰ **S86.21** Strain of muscle(s) and tendon(s) of anterior muscle group at lower leg level

√7ᵗʰ **S86.211** Strain of muscle(s) and tendon(s) of anterior muscle group at lower leg level, right leg

√7ᵗʰ **S86.212** Strain of muscle(s) and tendon(s) of anterior muscle group at lower leg level, left leg

√7ᵗʰ **S86.219** Strain of muscle(s) and tendon(s) of anterior muscle group at lower leg level, unspecified leg

√6ᵗʰ **S86.22** Laceration of muscle(s) and tendon(s) of anterior muscle group at lower leg level

√7ᵗʰ **S86.221** Laceration of muscle(s) and tendon(s) of anterior muscle group at lower leg level, right leg `CC`

√7ᵗʰ **S86.222** Laceration of muscle(s) and tendon(s) of anterior muscle group at lower leg level, left leg `CC`

√7ᵗʰ **S86.229** Laceration of muscle(s) and tendon(s) of anterior muscle group at lower leg level, unspecified leg `CC`

√6ᵗʰ **S86.29** Other injury of muscle(s) and tendon(s) of anterior muscle group at lower leg level

√7ᵗʰ **S86.291** Other injury of muscle(s) and tendon(s) of anterior muscle group at lower leg level, right leg

√7ᵗʰ **S86.292** Other injury of muscle(s) and tendon(s) of anterior muscle group at lower leg level, left leg

√7ᵗʰ **S86.299** Other injury of muscle(s) and tendon(s) of anterior muscle group at lower leg level, unspecified leg

√5ᵗʰ **S86.3** Injury of muscle(s) and tendon(s) of peroneal muscle group at lower leg level

√6ᵗʰ **S86.30** Unspecified injury of muscle(s) and tendon(s) of peroneal muscle group at lower leg level

√7ᵗʰ **S86.301** Unspecified injury of muscle(s) and tendon(s) of peroneal muscle group at lower leg level, right leg

√7ᵗʰ **S86.302** Unspecified injury of muscle(s) and tendon(s) of peroneal muscle group at lower leg level, left leg

√7ᵗʰ **S86.309** Unspecified injury of muscle(s) and tendon(s) of peroneal muscle group at lower leg level, unspecified leg

√6ᵗʰ **S86.31** Strain of muscle(s) and tendon(s) of peroneal muscle group at lower leg level

√7ᵗʰ **S86.311** Strain of muscle(s) and tendon(s) of peroneal muscle group at lower leg level, right leg

√7ᵗʰ **S86.312** Strain of muscle(s) and tendon(s) of peroneal muscle group at lower leg level, left leg

√7ᵗʰ **S86.319** Strain of muscle(s) and tendon(s) of peroneal muscle group at lower leg level, unspecified leg

√6ᵗʰ **S86.32** Laceration of muscle(s) and tendon(s) of peroneal muscle group at lower leg level

√7ᵗʰ **S86.321** Laceration of muscle(s) and tendon(s) of peroneal muscle group at lower leg level, right leg `CC`

√7ᵗʰ **S86.322** Laceration of muscle(s) and tendon(s) of peroneal muscle group at lower leg level, left leg `CC`

√7ᵗʰ **S86.329** Laceration of muscle(s) and tendon(s) of peroneal muscle group at lower leg level, unspecified leg `CC`

√6ᵗʰ **S86.39** Other injury of muscle(s) and tendon(s) of peroneal muscle group at lower leg level

√7ᵗʰ **S86.391** Other injury of muscle(s) and tendon(s) of peroneal muscle group at lower leg level, right leg

N Newborn: 0   P Pediatric: 0-17   M Maternity: 12-55   A Adult: 15-124   MCC Major CC Condition   PDxMCC PDx acts as own MCC   CC CC Condition   PDxCC PDx acts as own CC

1060   ICD-10-CM 2018

√7ᵗʰ **S86.392** Other injury of muscle(s) and tendon(s) of peroneal muscle group at lower leg level, left leg

√7ᵗʰ **S86.399** Other injury of muscle(s) and tendon(s) of peroneal muscle group at lower leg level, unspecified leg

√5ᵗʰ **S86.8 Injury of other muscles and tendons at lower leg level**

√6ᵗʰ **S86.80** Unspecified injury of other muscles and tendons at lower leg level

√7ᵗʰ **S86.801** Unspecified injury of other muscle(s) and tendon(s) at lower leg level, right leg

√7ᵗʰ **S86.802** Unspecified injury of other muscle(s) and tendon(s) at lower leg level, left leg

√7ᵗʰ **S86.809** Unspecified injury of other muscle(s) and tendon(s) at lower leg level, unspecified leg

√6ᵗʰ **S86.81** Strain of other muscles and tendons at lower leg level

√7ᵗʰ **S86.811** Strain of other muscle(s) and tendon(s) at lower leg level, right leg

√7ᵗʰ **S86.812** Strain of other muscle(s) and tendon(s) at lower leg level, left leg

√7ᵗʰ **S86.819** Strain of other muscle(s) and tendon(s) at lower leg level, unspecified leg

√6ᵗʰ **S86.82** Laceration of other muscles and tendons at lower leg level

√7ᵗʰ **S86.821** Laceration of other muscle(s) and tendon(s) at lower leg level, right leg   CC

√7ᵗʰ **S86.822** Laceration of other muscle(s) and tendon(s) at lower leg level, left leg   CC

√7ᵗʰ **S86.829** Laceration of other muscle(s) and tendon(s) at lower leg level, unspecified leg   CC

√6ᵗʰ **S86.89** Other injury of other muscles and tendons at lower leg level

√7ᵗʰ **S86.891** Other injury of other muscle(s) and tendon(s) at lower leg level, right leg

√7ᵗʰ **S86.892** Other injury of other muscle(s) and tendon(s) at lower leg level, left leg

√7ᵗʰ **S86.899** Other injury of other muscle(s) and tendon(s) at lower leg level, unspecified leg

√5ᵗʰ **S86.9 Injury of unspecified muscle and tendon at lower leg level**

√6ᵗʰ **S86.90** Unspecified injury of unspecified muscle and tendon at lower leg level

√7ᵗʰ **S86.901** Unspecified injury of unspecified muscle(s) and tendon(s) at lower leg level, right leg

√7ᵗʰ **S86.902** Unspecified injury of unspecified muscle(s) and tendon(s) at lower leg level, left leg

√7ᵗʰ **S86.909** Unspecified injury of unspecified muscle(s) and tendon(s) at lower leg level, unspecified leg

√6ᵗʰ **S86.91** Strain of unspecified muscle and tendon at lower leg level

√7ᵗʰ **S86.911** Strain of unspecified muscle(s) and tendon(s) at lower leg level, right leg

√7ᵗʰ **S86.912** Strain of unspecified muscle(s) and tendon(s) at lower leg level, left leg

√7ᵗʰ **S86.919** Strain of unspecified muscle(s) and tendon(s) at lower leg level, unspecified leg

√6ᵗʰ **S86.92** Laceration of unspecified muscle and tendon at lower leg level

√7ᵗʰ **S86.921** Laceration of unspecified muscle(s) and tendon(s) at lower leg level, right leg   CC

√7ᵗʰ **S86.922** Laceration of unspecified muscle(s) and tendon(s) at lower leg level, left leg   CC

√7ᵗʰ **S86.929** Laceration of unspecified muscle(s) and tendon(s) at lower leg level, unspecified leg   CC

√6ᵗʰ **S86.99** Other injury of unspecified muscle and tendon at lower leg level

√7ᵗʰ **S86.991** Other injury of unspecified muscle(s) and tendon(s) at lower leg level, right leg

√7ᵗʰ **S86.992** Other injury of unspecified muscle(s) and tendon(s) at lower leg level, left leg

√7ᵗʰ **S86.999** Other injury of unspecified muscle(s) and tendon(s) at lower leg level, unspecified leg

√4ᵗʰ **S87 Crushing injury of lower leg**

Use additional code(s) for all associated injuries

EXCLUDES 2   crushing injury of ankle and foot (S97.-)

> The appropriate 7th character is to be added to each code from category S87.
> A   initial encounter
> D   subsequent encounter
> S   sequela

√5ᵗʰ **S87.0 Crushing injury of knee**

√x7ᵗʰ **S87.00** Crushing injury of unspecified knee

√x7ᵗʰ **S87.01** Crushing injury of right knee

√x7ᵗʰ **S87.02** Crushing injury of left knee

√5ᵗʰ **S87.8 Crushing injury of lower leg**

√x7ᵗʰ **S87.80** Crushing injury of unspecified lower leg

√x7ᵗʰ **S87.81** Crushing injury of right lower leg

√x7ᵗʰ **S87.82** Crushing injury of left lower leg

√4ᵗʰ **S88 Traumatic amputation of lower leg**

An amputation not identified as partial or complete should be coded to complete.

EXCLUDES 1   traumatic amputation of ankle and foot (S98.-)

> The appropriate 7th character is to be added to each code from category S88.
> A   initial encounter
> D   subsequent encounter
> S   sequela

> **CC Excl: For CC codes in category S88:**
> **Right side:** PDX collection 1333
> **Left side:** PDX collection 1334
> **Unspecified side:** PDX collection 1335

√5ᵗʰ **S88.0 Traumatic amputation at knee level**

√6ᵗʰ **S88.01** Complete traumatic amputation at knee level

√7ᵗʰ **S88.011** Complete traumatic amputation at knee level, right lower leg   CC HCC

√7ᵗʰ **S88.012** Complete traumatic amputation at knee level, left lower leg   CC HCC

√7ᵗʰ **S88.019** Complete traumatic amputation at knee level, unspecified lower leg   CC HCC

√6ᵗʰ **S88.02** Partial traumatic amputation at knee level

√7ᵗʰ **S88.021** Partial traumatic amputation at knee level, right lower leg   CC HCC

√7ᵗʰ **S88.022** Partial traumatic amputation at knee level, left lower leg   CC HCC

√7ᵗʰ **S88.029** Partial traumatic amputation at knee level, unspecified lower leg   CC HCC

√5ᵗʰ **S88.1 Traumatic amputation at level between knee and ankle**

√6ᵗʰ **S88.11** Complete traumatic amputation at level between knee and ankle

√7ᵗʰ **S88.111** Complete traumatic amputation at level between knee and ankle, right lower leg   CC HCC

√7ᵗʰ **S88.112** Complete traumatic amputation at level between knee and ankle, left lower leg   CC HCC

√7ᵗʰ **S88.119** Complete traumatic amputation at level between knee and ankle, unspecified lower leg   CC HCC

√6ᵗʰ **S88.12** Partial traumatic amputation at level between knee and ankle

√7ᵗʰ **S88.121** Partial traumatic amputation at level between knee and ankle, right lower leg   CC HCC

√7ᵗʰ **S88.122** Partial traumatic amputation at levelbetween knee and ankle, left lower leg   CC HCC

✔ Additional Character Req   √x7ᵗʰ Placeholder Alert   Unacceptable PDx   Manifestation   H1 -H14 HAC   HCC CMS-HCC Condition   *EXCLUDES 1* Not Coded Here   *EXCLUDES 2* Not Included Here

ICD-10-CM 2018   1061

√7th **S88.129**   **Partial traumatic amputation at level between knee and ankle, unspecified lower leg** `CC` `HCC`

√5th **S88.9**   **Traumatic amputation of lower leg, level unspecified**

√6th **S88.91**   **Complete traumatic amputation of lower leg, level unspecified**

√7th **S88.911**   **Complete traumatic amputation of right lower leg, level unspecified** `CC` `HCC`

√7th **S88.912**   **Complete traumatic amputation of left lower leg, level unspecified** `CC` `HCC`

√7th **S88.919**   **Complete traumatic amputation of unspecified lower leg, level unspecified** `CC` `HCC`

√6th **S88.92**   **Partial traumatic amputation of lower leg, level unspecified**

√7th **S88.921**   **Partial traumatic amputation of right lower leg, level unspecified** `CC` `HCC`

√7th **S88.922**   **Partial traumatic amputation of left lower leg, level unspecified** `CC` `HCC`

√7th **S88.929**   **Partial traumatic amputation of unspecified lower leg, level unspecified** `CC` `HCC`

√4th **S89**   **Other and unspecified injuries of lower leg**

> **NOTE**   A fracture not indicated as open or closed should be coded to closed.
>
> *EXCLUDES 2*   other and unspecified injuries of ankle and foot (S99.-)
>
> **AHA:** 2015, 3Q, 37-39

> The appropriate 7th character is to be added to each code from subcategories S89.0, S89.1, S89.2, and S89.3.
> - A   initial encounter for closed fracture
> - D   subsequent encounter for fracture with routine healing
> - G   subsequent encounter for fracture with delayed healing
> - K   subsequent encounter for fracture with nonunion
> - P   subsequent encounter for fracture with malunion
> - S   sequela

√5th **S89.0**   **Physeal fracture of upper end of tibia**

> **CC Excl: For CC codes in subcategory S89.0:**
> **Right side:** See code S89.001
> **Left side:** See code S89.002
> **Unspecified side:** See code S89.009

√6th **S89.00**   **Unspecified physeal fracture of upper end of tibia**

7 √7th **S89.001**   **Unspecified physeal fracture of upper end of right tibia** `CC` `H5`
> **CC Excl: CC with 7th character A:** PDX collection 1340
> **CC with 7th character K or P:** PDX collection 897

7 √7th **S89.002**   **Unspecified physeal fracture of upper end of left tibia** `CC` `H5`
> **CC Excl: CC with 7th character A:** PDX collection 1342
> **CC with 7th character K or P:** PDX collection 897

7 √7th **S89.009**   **Unspecified physeal fracture of upper end of unspecified tibia** `CC` `H5`
> **CC Excl: CC with 7th character A:** PDX collection 1341
> **CC with 7th character K or P:** PDX collection 897

√6th **S89.01**   **Salter-Harris Type I physeal fracture of upper end of tibia**

7 √7th **S89.011**   **Salter-Harris Type I physeal fracture of upper end of right tibia** `CC` `H5`

7 √7th **S89.012**   **Salter-Harris Type I physeal fracture of upper end of left tibia** `CC` `H5`

7 √7th **S89.019**   **Salter-Harris Type I physeal fracture of upper end of unspecified tibia** `CC` `H5`

√6th **S89.02**   **Salter-Harris Type II physeal fracture of upper end of tibia**

7 √7th **S89.021**   **Salter-Harris Type II physeal fracture of upper end of right tibia** `CC` `H5`

7 √7th **S89.022**   **Salter-Harris Type II physeal fracture of upper end of left tibia** `CC` `H5`

7 √7th **S89.029**   **Salter-Harris Type II physeal fracture of upper end of unspecified tibia** `CC` `H5`

√6th **S89.03**   **Salter-Harris Type III physeal fracture of upper end of tibia**

7 √7th **S89.031**   **Salter-Harris Type III physeal fracture of upper end of right tibia** `CC` `H5`

7 √7th **S89.032**   **Salter-Harris Type III physeal fracture of upper end of left tibia** `CC` `H5`

7 √7th **S89.039**   **Salter-Harris Type III physeal fracture of upper end of unspecified tibia** `CC` `H5`

√6th **S89.04**   **Salter-Harris Type IV physeal fracture of upper end of tibia**

7 √7th **S89.041**   **Salter-Harris Type IV physeal fracture of upper end of right tibia** `CC` `H5`

7 √7th **S89.042**   **Salter-Harris Type IV physeal fracture of upper end of left tibia** `CC` `H5`

7 √7th **S89.049**   **Salter-Harris Type IV physeal fracture of upper end of unspecified tibia** `CC` `H5`

√6th **S89.09**   **Other physeal fracture of upper end of tibia**

7 √7th **S89.091**   **Other physeal fracture of upper end of right tibia** `CC` `H5`

7 √7th **S89.092**   **Other physeal fracture of upper end of left tibia** `CC` `H5`

7 √7th **S89.099**   **Other physeal fracture of upper end of unspecified tibia** `CC` `H5`

√5th **S89.1**   **Physeal fracture of lower end of tibia**

> **CC Excl: For codes in subcategory S89.1:**
> **CC with 7th character K or P:** PDX collection 897

√6th **S89.10**   **Unspecified physeal fracture of lower end of tibia**

8 √7th **S89.101**   **Unspecified physeal fracture of lower end of right tibia** `CC`

8 √7th **S89.102**   **Unspecified physeal fracture of lower end of left tibia** `CC`

8 √7th **S89.109**   **Unspecified physeal fracture of lower end of unspecified tibia** `CC`

√6th **S89.11**   **Salter-Harris Type I physeal fracture of ower end of tibia**

8 √7th **S89.111**   **Salter-Harris Type I physeal fracture of lower end of right tibia** `CC`

8 √7th **S89.112**   **Salter-Harris Type I physeal fracture oflower end of left tibia** `CC`

8 √7th **S89.119**   **Salter-Harris Type I physeal fracture of lower end of unspecified tibia** `CC`

√6th **S89.12**   **Salter-Harris Type II physeal fracture of lower end of tibia**

8 √7th **S89.121**   **Salter-Harris Type II physeal fracture of lower end of right tibia** `CC`

8 √7th **S89.122**   **Salter-Harris Type II physeal fracture of lower end of left tibia** `CC`

8 √7th **S89.129**   **Salter-Harris Type II physeal fracture of lower end of unspecified tibia** `CC`

√6th **S89.13**   **Salter-Harris Type III physeal fracture of lower end of tibia**

> *EXCLUDES 1*   fracture of medial malleolus (adult) (S82.5-)

8 √7th **S89.131**   **Salter-Harris Type III physeal fracture of lower end of right tibia** `CC`

8 √7th **S89.132**   **Salter-Harris Type III physeal fracture of lower end of left tibia** `CC`

8 √7th **S89.139**   **Salter-Harris Type III physeal fracture of lower end of unspecified tibia** `CC`

√6th **S89.14**   **Salter-Harris Type IV physeal fracture of lower end of tibia**

> *EXCLUDES 1*   fracture of medial malleolus (adult) (S82.5-)

8 √7th **S89.141**   **Salter-Harris Type IV physeal fracture oflower end of right tibia** `CC`

8 √7th **S89.142**   **Salter-Harris Type IV physeal fracture of lower end of left tibia** `CC`

8 √7th **S89.149**   **Salter-Harris Type IV physeal fracture of lower end of unspecified tibia** `CC`

√6th **S89.19**   **Other physeal fracture of lower end of tibia**

8 √7th **S89.191**   **Other physeal fracture of lower end of right tibia** `CC`

8 √7th **S89.192**   **Other physeal fracture of lower end of left tibia** `CC`

---

7   CC when reported as an initial encounter (7th character A, B, or C – specific to category) OR a subsequent encounter for nonunion or malunion (7th character K, M, N, P, Q, or R – specific to category).

8   CC when reported as a subsequent encounter for nonunion or malunion (7th character K, M, N, P, Q, or R – specific to category).

`N` Newborn: 0   `P` Pediatric: 0-17   `M` Maternity: 12-55   `A` Adult: 15-124   `MCC` Major CC Condition   `PDxMCC` PDx acts as own MCC   `CC` CC Condition   `PDxCC` PDx acts as own CC

1062   ICD-10-CM 2018

8 ✓7ᵗʰ **S89.199** Other physeal fracture of lower end of unspecified tibia ⚞CC⚟

✓5ᵗʰ **S89.2** Physeal fracture of upper end of fibula

> **CC Excl:** For codes in subcategory S89.2:
> CC with 7th character K or P: PDX collection 897

✓6ᵗʰ **S89.20** Unspecified physeal fracture of upper end of fibula

8 ✓7ᵗʰ **S89.201** Unspecified physeal fracture of upper end of right fibula ⚞CC⚟

8 ✓7ᵗʰ **S89.202** Unspecified physeal fracture of upper end of left fibula ⚞CC⚟

8 ✓7ᵗʰ **S89.209** Unspecified physeal fracture of upper end of unspecified fibula ⚞CC⚟

✓6ᵗʰ **S89.21** Salter-Harris Type I physeal fracture of upper end of fibula

8 ✓7ᵗʰ **S89.211** Salter-Harris Type I physeal fracture of upper end of right fibula ⚞CC⚟

8 ✓7ᵗʰ **S89.212** Salter-Harris Type I physeal fracture of upper end of left fibula ⚞CC⚟

8 ✓7ᵗʰ **S89.219** Salter-Harris Type I physeal fracture of upper end of unspecified fibula ⚞CC⚟

✓6ᵗʰ **S89.22** Salter-Harris Type II physeal fracture of upper end of fibula

8 ✓7ᵗʰ **S89.221** Salter-Harris Type II physeal fracture of upper end of right fibula ⚞CC⚟

8 ✓7ᵗʰ **S89.222** Salter-Harris Type II physeal fracture of upper end of left fibula ⚞CC⚟

8 ✓7ᵗʰ **S89.229** Salter-Harris Type II physeal fracture of upper end of unspecified fibula ⚞CC⚟

✓6ᵗʰ **S89.29** Other physeal fracture of upper end of fibula

8 ✓7ᵗʰ **S89.291** Other physeal fracture of upper end of right fibula ⚞CC⚟

8 ✓7ᵗʰ **S89.292** Other physeal fracture of upper end of left fibula ⚞CC⚟

8 ✓7ᵗʰ **S89.299** Other physeal fracture of upper end of unspecified fibula ⚞CC⚟

✓5ᵗʰ **S89.3** Physeal fracture of lower end of fibula

> **CC Excl:** For codes in subcategory S89.3:
> CC with 7th character K or P: PDX collection 897

✓6ᵗʰ **S89.30** Unspecified physeal fracture of lower end of fibula

8 ✓7ᵗʰ **S89.301** Unspecified physeal fracture of lower end of right fibula ⚞CC⚟

8 ✓7ᵗʰ **S89.302** Unspecified physeal fracture of lower end of left fibula ⚞CC⚟

8 ✓7ᵗʰ **S89.309** Unspecified physeal fracture of lower end of unspecified fibula ⚞CC⚟

✓6ᵗʰ **S89.31** Salter-Harris Type I physeal fracture of lower end of fibula

8 ✓7ᵗʰ **S89.311** Salter-Harris Type I physeal fracture of lower end of right fibula ⚞CC⚟

8 ✓7ᵗʰ **S89.312** Salter-Harris Type I physeal fracture of lower end of left fibula ⚞CC⚟

8 ✓7ᵗʰ **S89.319** Salter-Harris Type I physeal fracture of lower end of unspecified fibula ⚞CC⚟

✓6ᵗʰ **S89.32** Salter-Harris Type II physeal fracture of lower end of fibula

8 ✓7ᵗʰ **S89.321** Salter-Harris Type II physeal fracture of lower end of right fibula ⚞CC⚟

8 ✓7ᵗʰ **S89.322** Salter-Harris Type II physeal fracture of lower end of left fibula ⚞CC⚟

8 ✓7ᵗʰ **S89.329** Salter-Harris Type II physeal fracture of lower end of unspecified fibula ⚞CC⚟

✓6ᵗʰ **S89.39** Other physeal fracture of lower end of fibula

8 ✓7ᵗʰ **S89.391** Other physeal fracture of lower end of right fibula ⚞CC⚟

8 ✓7ᵗʰ **S89.392** Other physeal fracture of lower end of left fibula ⚞CC⚟

8 ✓7ᵗʰ **S89.399** Other physeal fracture of lower end of unspecified fibula ⚞CC⚟

✓5ᵗʰ **S89.8** Other specified injuries of lower leg

> The appropriate 7th character is to be added to each code in subcategory S89.8.
> A   initial encounter
> D   subsequent encounter
> S   sequela

✓x7ᵗʰ **S89.80** Other specified injuries of unspecified lower leg

✓x7ᵗʰ **S89.81** Other specified injuries of right lower leg

✓x7ᵗʰ **S89.82** Other specified injuries of left lower leg

✓5ᵗʰ **S89.9** Unspecified injury of lower leg

> The appropriate 7th character is to be added to each code in subcategory S89.9.
> A   initial encounter
> D   subsequent encounter
> S   sequela

✓x7ᵗʰ **S89.90** Unspecified injury of unspecified lower leg

✓x7ᵗʰ **S89.91** Unspecified injury of right lower leg

✓x7ᵗʰ **S89.92** Unspecified injury of left lower leg

Injuries to the ankle and foot (S90-S99)

EXCLUDES 2   burns and corrosions (T20-T32)
fracture of ankle and malleolus (S82.-)
frostbite (T33-T34)
insect bite or sting, venomous (T63.4)

✓4ᵗʰ **S90** Superficial injury of ankle, foot and toes

> The appropriate 7th character is to be added to each code from category S90.
> A   initial encounter
> D   subsequent encounter
> S   sequela

✓5ᵗʰ **S90.0** Contusion of ankle

✓x7ᵗʰ **S90.00** Contusion of unspecified ankle

✓x7ᵗʰ **S90.01** Contusion of right ankle

✓x7ᵗʰ **S90.02** Contusion of left ankle

✓5ᵗʰ **S90.1** Contusion of toe without damage to nail

✓6ᵗʰ **S90.11** Contusion of great toe without damage to nail

✓7ᵗʰ **S90.111** Contusion of right great toe without damage to nail

✓7ᵗʰ **S90.112** Contusion of left great toe without damage to nail

✓7ᵗʰ **S90.119** Contusion of unspecified great toe without damage to nail

✓6ᵗʰ **S90.12** Contusion of lesser toe without damage to nail

✓7ᵗʰ **S90.121** Contusion of right lesser toe(s) without damage to nail

✓7ᵗʰ **S90.122** Contusion of left lesser toe(s) without damage to nail

✓7ᵗʰ **S90.129** Contusion of unspecified lesser toe(s) without damage to nail
Contusion of toe NOS

✓5ᵗʰ **S90.2** Contusion of toe with damage to nail

✓6ᵗʰ **S90.21** Contusion of great toe with damage to nail

✓7ᵗʰ **S90.211** Contusion of right great toe with damage to nail

✓7ᵗʰ **S90.212** Contusion of left great toe with damage to nail

✓7ᵗʰ **S90.219** Contusion of unspecified great toe with damage to nail

✓6ᵗʰ **S90.22** Contusion of lesser toe with damage to nail

✓7ᵗʰ **S90.221** Contusion of right lesser toe(s) with damage to nail

✓7ᵗʰ **S90.222** Contusion of left lesser toe(s) with damage to nail

✓7ᵗʰ **S90.229** Contusion of unspecified lesser toe(s) with damage to nail

✓5ᵗʰ **S90.3** Contusion of foot

EXCLUDES 2   contusion of toes (S90.1-, S90.2-)

✓x7ᵗʰ **S90.30** Contusion of unspecified foot
Contusion of foot NOS

✓x7ᵗʰ **S90.31** Contusion of right foot

---

8   CC when reported as a subsequent encounter for nonunion or malunion (7th character K, M, N, P, Q, or R – specific to category).

☑ Additional Character Req   ✓x7ᵗʰ Placeholder Alert   Unacceptable PDx   Manifestation   ⚞H1⚟-⚞H14⚟ HAC   ⚞HCC⚟ CMS-HCC Condition   *EXCLUDES 1* Not Coded Here   *EXCLUDES 2* Not Included Here

Chapter 19. Injury, Poisoning and Certain Other Consequences of External Causes

S90.32–S90.935

√x7th **S90.32**   Contusion of left foot

√5th **S90.4**   Other superficial injuries of toe

√6th **S90.41**   Abrasion of toe
- √7th **S90.411**   Abrasion, right great toe
- √7th **S90.412**   Abrasion, left great toe
- √7th **S90.413**   Abrasion, unspecified great toe
- √7th **S90.414**   Abrasion, right lesser toe(s)
- √7th **S90.415**   Abrasion, left lesser toe(s)
- √7th **S90.416**   Abrasion, unspecified lesser toe(s)

√6th **S90.42**   Blister (nonthermal) of toe
- √7th **S90.421**   Blister (nonthermal), right great toe
- √7th **S90.422**   Blister (nonthermal), left great toe
- √7th **S90.423**   Blister (nonthermal), unspecified great toe
- √7th **S90.424**   Blister (nonthermal), right lesser toe(s)
- √7th **S90.425**   Blister (nonthermal), left lesser toe(s)
- √7th **S90.426**   Blister (nonthermal), unspecified lesser toe(s)

√6th **S90.44**   External constriction of toe
Hair tourniquet syndrome of toe
- √7th **S90.441**   External constriction, right great toe
- √7th **S90.442**   External constriction, left great toe
- √7th **S90.443**   External constriction, unspecified great toe
- √7th **S90.444**   External constriction, right lesser toe(s)
- √7th **S90.445**   External constriction, left lesser toe(s)
- √7th **S90.446**   External constriction, unspecified lesser toe(s)

√6th **S90.45**   Superficial foreign body of toe
Splinter in the toe
- √7th **S90.451**   Superficial foreign body, right great toe
- √7th **S90.452**   Superficial foreign body, left great toe
- √7th **S90.453**   Superficial foreign body, unspecified great toe
- √7th **S90.454**   Superficial foreign body, right lesser toe(s)
- √7th **S90.455**   Superficial foreign body, left lesser toe(s)
- √7th **S90.456**   Superficial foreign body, unspecified lesser toe(s)

√6th **S90.46**   Insect bite (nonvenomous) of toe
- √7th **S90.461**   Insect bite (nonvenomous), right great toe
- √7th **S90.462**   Insect bite (nonvenomous), left great toe
- √7th **S90.463**   Insect bite (nonvenomous), unspecified great toe
- √7th **S90.464**   Insect bite (nonvenomous), right lesser toe(s)
- √7th **S90.465**   Insect bite (nonvenomous), left lesser toe(s)
- √7th **S90.466**   Insect bite (nonvenomous), unspecified lesser toe(s)

√6th **S90.47**   Other superficial bite of toe
EXCLUDES 1   *open bite of toe (S91.15-, S91.25-)*
- √7th **S90.471**   Other superficial bite of right great toe
- √7th **S90.472**   Other superficial bite of left great toe
- √7th **S90.473**   Other superficial bite of unspecified great toe
- √7th **S90.474**   Other superficial bite of right lesser toe(s)
- √7th **S90.475**   Other superficial bite of left lesser toe(s)
- √7th **S90.476**   Other superficial bite of unspecified lesser toe(s)

√5th **S90.5**   Other superficial injuries of ankle

√6th **S90.51**   Abrasion of ankle
- √7th **S90.511**   Abrasion, right ankle
- √7th **S90.512**   Abrasion, left ankle
- √7th **S90.519**   Abrasion, unspecified ankle

√6th **S90.52**   Blister (nonthermal) of ankle
- √7th **S90.521**   Blister (nonthermal), right ankle
- √7th **S90.522**   Blister (nonthermal), left ankle
- √7th **S90.529**   Blister (nonthermal), unspecified ankle

√6th **S90.54**   External constriction of ankle
- √7th **S90.541**   External constriction, right ankle

- √7th **S90.542**   External constriction, left ankle
- √7th **S90.549**   External constriction, unspecified ankle

√6th **S90.55**   Superficial foreign body of ankle
Splinter in the ankle
- √7th **S90.551**   Superficial foreign body, right ankle
- √7th **S90.552**   Superficial foreign body, left ankle
- √7th **S90.559**   Superficial foreign body, unspecified ankle

√6th **S90.56**   Insect bite (nonvenomous) of ankle
- √7th **S90.561**   Insect bite (nonvenomous), right ankle
- √7th **S90.562**   Insect bite (nonvenomous), left ankle
- √7th **S90.569**   Insect bite (nonvenomous), unspecified ankle

√6th **S90.57**   Other superficial bite of ankle
EXCLUDES 1   *open bite of ankle (S91.05-)*
- √7th **S90.571**   Other superficial bite of ankle, right ankle
- √7th **S90.572**   Other superficial bite of ankle, left ankle
- √7th **S90.579**   Other superficial bite of ankle, unspecified ankle

√5th **S90.8**   Other superficial injuries of foot

√6th **S90.81**   Abrasion of foot
- √7th **S90.811**   Abrasion, right foot
- √7th **S90.812**   Abrasion, left foot
- √7th **S90.819**   Abrasion, unspecified foot

√6th **S90.82**   Blister (nonthermal) of foot
- √7th **S90.821**   Blister (nonthermal), right foot
- √7th **S90.822**   Blister (nonthermal), left foot
- √7th **S90.829**   Blister (nonthermal), unspecified foot

√6th **S90.84**   External constriction of foot
- √7th **S90.841**   External constriction, right foot
- √7th **S90.842**   External constriction, left foot
- √7th **S90.849**   External constriction, unspecified foot

√6th **S90.85**   Superficial foreign body of foot
Splinter in the foot
- √7th **S90.851**   Superficial foreign body, right foot
- √7th **S90.852**   Superficial foreign body, left foot
- √7th **S90.859**   Superficial foreign body, unspecified foot

√6th **S90.86**   Insect bite (nonvenomous) of foot
- √7th **S90.861**   Insect bite (nonvenomous), right foot
- √7th **S90.862**   Insect bite (nonvenomous), left foot
- √7th **S90.869**   Insect bite (nonvenomous), unspecified foot

√6th **S90.87**   Other superficial bite of foot
EXCLUDES 1   *open bite of foot (S91.35-)*
- √7th **S90.871**   Other superficial bite of right foot
- √7th **S90.872**   Other superficial bite of left foot
- √7th **S90.879**   Other superficial bite of unspecified foot

√5th **S90.9**   Unspecified superficial injury of ankle, foot and toe

√6th **S90.91**   Unspecified superficial injury of ankle
- √7th **S90.911**   Unspecified superficial injury of right ankle
- √7th **S90.912**   Unspecified superficial injury of left ankle
- √7th **S90.919**   Unspecified superficial injury of unspecified ankle

√6th **S90.92**   Unspecified superficial injury of foot
- √7th **S90.921**   Unspecified superficial injury of right foot
- √7th **S90.922**   Unspecified superficial injury of left foot
- √7th **S90.929**   Unspecified superficial injury of unspecified foot

√6th **S90.93**   Unspecified superficial injury of toes
- √7th **S90.931**   Unspecified superficial injury of right great toe
- √7th **S90.932**   Unspecified superficial injury of left great toe
- √7th **S90.933**   Unspecified superficial injury of unspecified great toe
- √7th **S90.934**   Unspecified superficial injury of right lesser toe(s)
- √7th **S90.935**   Unspecified superficial injury of left lesser toe(s)

N Newborn: 0   P Pediatric: 0-17   M Maternity: 12-55   A Adult: 15-124   MCC Major CC Condition   PDxMCC PDx acts as own MCC   CC CC Condition   PDxCC PDx acts as own CC

1064   ICD-10-CM 2018

☑7ᵗʰ **S90.936** **Unspecified superficial injury of unspecified lesser toe(s)**

☑4ᵗʰ **S91** **Open wound of ankle, foot and toes**
Code also any associated wound infection
EXCLUDES 1   open fracture of ankle, foot and toes (S92-with 7th B)
traumatic amputation of ankle and foot (S98.-)

The appropriate 7th character is to be added to each code from category S91.
A   initial encounter
D   subsequent encounter
S   sequela

☑5ᵗʰ **S91.0** **Open wound of ankle**
☑6ᵗʰ **S91.00** **Unspecified open wound of ankle**
☑7ᵗʰ **S91.001** **Unspecified open wound, right ankle**
☑7ᵗʰ **S91.002** **Unspecified open wound, left ankle**
☑7ᵗʰ **S91.009** **Unspecified open wound, unspecified ankle**
☑6ᵗʰ **S91.01** **Laceration without foreign body of ankle**
☑7ᵗʰ **S91.011** **Laceration without foreign body, right ankle**
☑7ᵗʰ **S91.012** **Laceration without foreign body, left ankle**
☑7ᵗʰ **S91.019** **Laceration without foreign body, unspecified ankle**
☑6ᵗʰ **S91.02** **Laceration with foreign body of ankle**
☑7ᵗʰ **S91.021** **Laceration with foreign body, right ankle**
☑7ᵗʰ **S91.022** **Laceration with foreign body, left ankle**
☑7ᵗʰ **S91.029** **Laceration with foreign body, unspecified ankle**
☑6ᵗʰ **S91.03** **Puncture wound without foreign body of ankle**
☑7ᵗʰ **S91.031** **Puncture wound without foreign body, right ankle**
☑7ᵗʰ **S91.032** **Puncture wound without foreign body, left ankle**
☑7ᵗʰ **S91.039** **Puncture wound without foreign body, unspecified ankle**
☑6ᵗʰ **S91.04** **Puncture wound with foreign body of ankle**
☑7ᵗʰ **S91.041** **Puncture wound with foreign body, right ankle**
☑7ᵗʰ **S91.042** **Puncture wound with foreign body, left ankle**
☑7ᵗʰ **S91.049** **Puncture wound with foreign body, unspecified ankle**
☑6ᵗʰ **S91.05** **Open bite of ankle**
EXCLUDES 1   superficial bite of ankle (S90.56-, S90.57-)
☑7ᵗʰ **S91.051** **Open bite, right ankle**
☑7ᵗʰ **S91.052** **Open bite, left ankle**
☑7ᵗʰ **S91.059** **Open bite, unspecified ankle**
☑5ᵗʰ **S91.1** **Open wound of toe without damage to nail**
☑6ᵗʰ **S91.10** **Unspecified open wound of toe without damage to nail**
☑7ᵗʰ **S91.101** **Unspecified open wound of right great toe without damage to nail**
☑7ᵗʰ **S91.102** **Unspecified open wound of left great toe without damage to nail**
☑7ᵗʰ **S91.103** **Unspecified open wound of unspecified great toe without damage to nail**
☑7ᵗʰ **S91.104** **Unspecified open wound of right lesser toe(s) without damage to nail**
☑7ᵗʰ **S91.105** **Unspecified open wound of left lesser toe(s) without damage to nail**
☑7ᵗʰ **S91.106** **Unspecified open wound of unspecified lesser toe(s) without damage to nail**
☑7ᵗʰ **S91.109** **Unspecified open wound of unspecified toe(s) without damage to nail**
☑6ᵗʰ **S91.11** **Laceration without foreign body of toe without damage to nail**
☑7ᵗʰ **S91.111** **Laceration without foreign body of right great toe without damage to nail**
☑7ᵗʰ **S91.112** **Laceration without foreign body of left great toe without damage to nail**

☑7ᵗʰ **S91.113** **Laceration without foreign body of unspecified great toe without damage to nail**
☑7ᵗʰ **S91.114** **Laceration without foreign body of right lesser toe(s) without damage to nail**
☑7ᵗʰ **S91.115** **Laceration without foreign body of left lesser toe(s) without damage to nail**
☑7ᵗʰ **S91.116** **Laceration without foreign body of unspecified lesser toe(s) without damage to nail**
☑7ᵗʰ **S91.119** **Laceration without foreign body of unspecified toe without damage to nail**
☑6ᵗʰ **S91.12** **Laceration with foreign body of toe without damage to nail**
☑7ᵗʰ **S91.121** **Laceration with foreign body of right great toe without damage to nail**
☑7ᵗʰ **S91.122** **Laceration with foreign body of left great toe without damage to nail**
☑7ᵗʰ **S91.123** **Laceration with foreign body of unspecified great toe without damage to nail**
☑7ᵗʰ **S91.124** **Laceration with foreign body of right lesser toe(s) without damage to nail**
☑7ᵗʰ **S91.125** **Laceration with foreign body of left lesser toe(s) without damage to nail**
☑7ᵗʰ **S91.126** **Laceration with foreign body of unspecified lesser toe(s) without damage to nail**
☑7ᵗʰ **S91.129** **Laceration with foreign body of unspecified toe(s) without damage to nail**
☑6ᵗʰ **S91.13** **Puncture wound without foreign body of toe without damage to nail**
☑7ᵗʰ **S91.131** **Puncture wound without foreign body of right great toe without damage to nail**
☑7ᵗʰ **S91.132** **Puncture wound without foreign body of left great toe without damage to nail**
☑7ᵗʰ **S91.133** **Puncture wound without foreign body of unspecified great toe without damage to nail**
☑7ᵗʰ **S91.134** **Puncture wound without foreign body of right lesser toe(s) without damage to nail**
☑7ᵗʰ **S91.135** **Puncture wound without foreign body of left lesser toe(s) without damage to nail**
☑7ᵗʰ **S91.136** **Puncture wound without foreign body of unspecified lesser toe(s) without damage to nail**
☑7ᵗʰ **S91.139** **Puncture wound without foreign body of unspecified toe(s) without damage to nail**
☑6ᵗʰ **S91.14** **Puncture wound with foreign body of toe without damage to nail**
☑7ᵗʰ **S91.141** **Puncture wound with foreign body of right great toe without damage to nail**
☑7ᵗʰ **S91.142** **Puncture wound with foreign body of left great toe without damage to nail**
☑7ᵗʰ **S91.143** **Puncture wound with foreign body of unspecified great toe without damage to nail**
☑7ᵗʰ **S91.144** **Puncture wound with foreign body of right lesser toe(s) without damage to nail**
☑7ᵗʰ **S91.145** **Puncture wound with foreign body of left lesser toe(s) without damage to nail**
☑7ᵗʰ **S91.146** **Puncture wound with foreign body of unspecified lesser toe(s) without damage to nail**
☑7ᵗʰ **S91.149** **Puncture wound with foreign body of unspecified toe(s) without damage to nail**
☑6ᵗʰ **S91.15** **Open bite of toe without damage to nail**
Bite of toe NOS
EXCLUDES 1   superficial bite of toe (S90.46-, S90.47-)
☑7ᵗʰ **S91.151** **Open bite of right great toe without damage to nail**
☑7ᵗʰ **S91.152** **Open bite of left great toe without damage to nail**
☑7ᵗʰ **S91.153** **Open bite of unspecified great toe without damage to nail**
☑7ᵗʰ **S91.154** **Open bite of right lesser toe(s) without damage to nail**

✓7ᵗʰ **S91.155** Open bite of left lesser toe(s) without damage to nail

✓7ᵗʰ **S91.156** Open bite of unspecified lesser toe(s) without damage to nail

✓7ᵗʰ **S91.159** Open bite of unspecified toe(s) without damage to nail

✓5ᵗʰ **S91.2 Open wound of toe with damage to nail**

✓6ᵗʰ **S91.20 Unspecified open wound of toe with damage to nail**

✓7ᵗʰ **S91.201** Unspecified open wound of right great toe with damage to nail

✓7ᵗʰ **S91.202** Unspecified open wound of left great toe with damage to nail

✓7ᵗʰ **S91.203** Unspecified open wound of unspecified great toe with damage to nail

✓7ᵗʰ **S91.204** Unspecified open wound of right lesser toe(s) with damage to nail

✓7ᵗʰ **S91.205** Unspecified open wound of left lesser toe(s) with damage to nail

✓7ᵗʰ **S91.206** Unspecified open wound of unspecified lesser toe(s) with damage to nail

✓7ᵗʰ **S91.209** Unspecified open wound of unspecified toe(s) with damage to nail

✓6ᵗʰ **S91.21 Laceration without foreign body of toe with damage to nail**

✓7ᵗʰ **S91.211** Laceration without foreign body of right great toe with damage to nail

✓7ᵗʰ **S91.212** Laceration without foreign body of left great toe with damage to nail

✓7ᵗʰ **S91.213** Laceration without foreign body of unspecified great toe with damage to nail

✓7ᵗʰ **S91.214** Laceration without foreign body of right lesser toe(s) with damage to nail

✓7ᵗʰ **S91.215** Laceration without foreign body of left lesser toe(s) with damage to nail

✓7ᵗʰ **S91.216** Laceration without foreign body of unspecified lesser toe(s) with damage to nail

✓7ᵗʰ **S91.219** Laceration without foreign body of unspecified toe(s) with damage to nail

✓6ᵗʰ **S91.22 Laceration with foreign body of toe with damage to nail**

✓7ᵗʰ **S91.221** Laceration with foreign body of right great toe with damage to nail

✓7ᵗʰ **S91.222** Laceration with foreign body of left great toe with damage to nail

✓7ᵗʰ **S91.223** Laceration with foreign body of unspecified great toe with damage to nail

✓7ᵗʰ **S91.224** Laceration with foreign body of right lesser toe(s) with damage to nail

✓7ᵗʰ **S91.225** Laceration with foreign body of left lesser toe(s) with damage to nail

✓7ᵗʰ **S91.226** Laceration with foreign body of unspecified lesser toe(s) with damage to nail

✓7ᵗʰ **S91.229** Laceration with foreign body of unspecified toe(s) with damage to nail

✓6ᵗʰ **S91.23 Puncture wound without foreign body of toe with damage to nail**

✓7ᵗʰ **S91.231** Puncture wound without foreign body of right great toe with damage to nail

✓7ᵗʰ **S91.232** Puncture wound without foreign body of left great toe with damage to nail

✓7ᵗʰ **S91.233** Puncture wound without foreign body of unspecified great toe with damage to nail

✓7ᵗʰ **S91.234** Puncture wound without foreign body of right lesser toe(s) with damage to nail

✓7ᵗʰ **S91.235** Puncture wound without foreign body of left lesser toe(s) with damage to nail

✓7ᵗʰ **S91.236** Puncture wound without foreign body of unspecified lesser toe(s) with damage to nail

✓7ᵗʰ **S91.239** Puncture wound without foreign body of unspecified toe(s) with damage to nail

✓6ᵗʰ **S91.24 Puncture wound with foreign body of toe with damage to nail**

✓7ᵗʰ **S91.241** Puncture wound with foreign body of right great toe with damage to nail

✓7ᵗʰ **S91.242** Puncture wound with foreign body of left great toe with damage to nail

✓7ᵗʰ **S91.243** Puncture wound with foreign body of unspecified great toe with damage to nail

✓7ᵗʰ **S91.244** Puncture wound with foreign body of right lesser toe(s) with damage to nail

✓7ᵗʰ **S91.245** Puncture wound with foreign body of left lesser toe(s) with damage to nail

✓7ᵗʰ **S91.246** Puncture wound with foreign body of unspecified lesser toe(s) with damage to nail

✓7ᵗʰ **S91.249** Puncture wound with foreign body of unspecified toe(s) with damage to nail

✓6ᵗʰ **S91.25 Open bite of toe with damage to nail**
Bite of toe with damage to nail NOS
EXCLUDES 1 *superficial bite of toe (S90.46-, S90.47-)*

✓7ᵗʰ **S91.251** Open bite of right great toe with damage to nail

✓7ᵗʰ **S91.252** Open bite of left great toe with damage to nail

✓7ᵗʰ **S91.253** Open bite of unspecified great toe with damage to nail

✓7ᵗʰ **S91.254** Open bite of right lesser toe(s) with damage to nail

✓7ᵗʰ **S91.255** Open bite of left lesser toe(s) with damage to nail

✓7ᵗʰ **S91.256** Open bite of unspecified lesser toe(s) with damage to nail

✓7ᵗʰ **S91.259** Open bite of unspecified toe(s) with damage to nail

✓5ᵗʰ **S91.3 Open wound of foot**

✓6ᵗʰ **S91.30 Unspecified open wound of foot**

✓7ᵗʰ **S91.301** Unspecified open wound, right foot

✓7ᵗʰ **S91.302** Unspecified open wound, left foot

✓7ᵗʰ **S91.309** Unspecified open wound, unspecified foot

✓6ᵗʰ **S91.31 Laceration without foreign body of foot**

✓7ᵗʰ **S91.311** Laceration without foreign body, right foot

✓7ᵗʰ **S91.312** Laceration without foreign body, left foot

✓7ᵗʰ **S91.319** Laceration without foreign body, unspecified foot

✓6ᵗʰ **S91.32 Laceration with foreign body of foot**

✓7ᵗʰ **S91.321** Laceration with foreign body, right foot

✓7ᵗʰ **S91.322** Laceration with foreign body, left foot

✓7ᵗʰ **S91.329** Laceration with foreign body, unspecified foot

✓6ᵗʰ **S91.33 Puncture wound without foreign body of foot**

✓7ᵗʰ **S91.331** Puncture wound without foreign body, right foot

✓7ᵗʰ **S91.332** Puncture wound without foreign body, left foot

✓7ᵗʰ **S91.339** Puncture wound without foreign body, unspecified foot

✓6ᵗʰ **S91.34 Puncture wound with foreign body of foot**

✓7ᵗʰ **S91.341** Puncture wound with foreign body, right foot

✓7ᵗʰ **S91.342** Puncture wound with foreign body, left foot

✓7ᵗʰ **S91.349** Puncture wound with foreign body, unspecified foot

✓6ᵗʰ **S91.35 Open bite of foot**
EXCLUDES 1 *superficial bite of foot (S90.86-, S90.87-)*

✓7ᵗʰ **S91.351** Open bite, right foot

✓7ᵗʰ **S91.352** Open bite, left foot

✓7ᵗʰ **S91.359** Open bite, unspecified foot

ℕ Newborn: 0   ℙ Pediatric: 0-17   Ⓜ Maternity: 12-55   Ⓐ Adult: 15-124   **MCC** Major CC Condition   **PDxMCC** PDx acts as own MCC   **CC** CC Condition   **PDxCC** PDx acts as own CC

1066   ICD-10-CM 2018

✓4ᵗʰ **S92   Fracture of foot and toe, except ankle**

NOTE   A fracture not indicated as displaced or nondisplaced should be coded to displaced.
A fracture not indicated as open or closed should be coded to closed.

EXCLUDES 1   traumatic amputation of ankle and foot (S98.-)
EXCLUDES 2   fracture of ankle (S82.-)
fracture of malleolus (S82.-)

AHA: 2015, 3Q, 37-39

The appropriate 7th character is to be added to each code from category S92.
A   initial encounter for closed fracture
B   initial encounter for open fracture
D   subsequent encounter for fracture with routine healing
G   subsequent encounter for fracture with delayed healing
K   subsequent encounter for fracture with nonunion
P   subsequent encounter for fracture with malunion
S   sequela

✓5ᵗʰ **S92.0   Fracture of** calcaneus
Heel bone
Os calcis

EXCLUDES 2   physeal fracture of calcaneus (S99.0-)

CC Excl: For codes in subcategory S92.0:
CC with 7th character B: PDX collection 1367
CC with 7th character K or P: PDX collection 897

✓6ᵗʰ **S92.00   Unspecified fracture of calcaneus**
7   ✓7ᵗʰ   S92.001   Unspecified fracture of right calcaneus   CC H5
7   ✓7ᵗʰ   S92.002   Unspecified fracture of left calcaneus   CC H5
7   ✓7ᵗʰ   S92.009   Unspecified fracture of unspecified calcaneus   CC H5

✓6ᵗʰ **S92.01   Fracture of** body of calcaneus
7   ✓7ᵗʰ   S92.011   Displaced fracture of body of right calcaneus   CC H5
7   ✓7ᵗʰ   S92.012   Displaced fracture of body of left calcaneus   CC H5
7   ✓7ᵗʰ   S92.013   Displaced fracture of body of unspecified calcaneus   CC H5
7   ✓7ᵗʰ   S92.014   Nondisplaced fracture of body of right calcaneus   CC H5
7   ✓7ᵗʰ   S92.015   Nondisplaced fracture of body of left calcaneus   CC H5
7   ✓7ᵗʰ   S92.016   Nondisplaced fracture of body of unspecified calcaneus   CC H5

✓6ᵗʰ **S92.02   Fracture of** anterior process of calcaneus
7   ✓7ᵗʰ   S92.021   Displaced fracture of anterior process of right calcaneus   CC H5
7   ✓7ᵗʰ   S92.022   Displaced fracture of anterior process of left calcaneus   CC H5
7   ✓7ᵗʰ   S92.023   Displaced fracture of anterior process of unspecified calcaneus   CC H5
7   ✓7ᵗʰ   S92.024   Nondisplaced fracture of anterior process of right calcaneus   CC H5
7   ✓7ᵗʰ   S92.025   Nondisplaced fracture of anterior process of left calcaneus   CC H5
7   ✓7ᵗʰ   S92.026   Nondisplaced fracture of anterior process of unspecified calcaneus   CC H5

✓6ᵗʰ **S92.03   Avulsion fracture of** tuberosity of calcaneus
7   ✓7ᵗʰ   S92.031   Displaced avulsion fracture of tuberosity of right calcaneus   CC H5
7   ✓7ᵗʰ   S92.032   Displaced avulsion fracture of tuberosity of left calcaneus   CC H5
7   ✓7ᵗʰ   S92.033   Displaced avulsion fracture of tuberosity of unspecified calcaneus   CC H5
7   ✓7ᵗʰ   S92.034   Nondisplaced avulsion fracture of tuberosity of right calcaneus   CC H5
7   ✓7ᵗʰ   S92.035   Nondisplaced avulsion fracture of tuberosity of left calcaneus   CC H5
7   ✓7ᵗʰ   S92.036   Nondisplaced avulsion fracture of tuberosity of unspecified calcaneus   CC H5

✓6ᵗʰ **S92.04   Other fracture of** tuberosity of calcaneus
7   ✓7ᵗʰ   S92.041   Displaced other fracture of tuberosity of right calcaneus   CC H5

7   ✓7ᵗʰ   S92.042   Displaced other fracture of tuberosity of left calcaneus   CC H5
7   ✓7ᵗʰ   S92.043   Displaced other fracture of tuberosity of unspecified calcaneus   CC H5
7   ✓7ᵗʰ   S92.044   Nondisplaced other fracture of tuberosity of right calcaneus   CC H5
7   ✓7ᵗʰ   S92.045   Nondisplaced other fracture of tuberosity of left calcaneus   CC H5
7   ✓7ᵗʰ   S92.046   Nondisplaced other fracture of tuberosity of unspecified calcaneus   CC H5

✓6ᵗʰ **S92.05   Other extraarticular fracture of calcaneus**
7   ✓7ᵗʰ   S92.051   Displaced other extraarticular fracture of right calcaneus   CC H5
7   ✓7ᵗʰ   S92.052   Displaced other extraarticular fracture of left calcaneus   CC H5
7   ✓7ᵗʰ   S92.053   Displaced other extraarticular fracture of unspecified calcaneus   CC H5
7   ✓7ᵗʰ   S92.054   Nondisplaced other extraarticular fracture of right calcaneus   CC H5
7   ✓7ᵗʰ   S92.055   Nondisplaced other extraarticular fracture of left calcaneus   CC H5
7   ✓7ᵗʰ   S92.056   Nondisplaced other extraarticular fracture of unspecified calcaneus   CC H5

✓6ᵗʰ **S92.06   Intraarticular fracture of calcaneus**
7   ✓7ᵗʰ   S92.061   Displaced intraarticular fracture of right calcaneus   CC H5
7   ✓7ᵗʰ   S92.062   Displaced intraarticular fracture of left calcaneus   CC H5
7   ✓7ᵗʰ   S92.063   Displaced intraarticular fracture of unspecified calcaneus   CC H5
7   ✓7ᵗʰ   S92.064   Nondisplaced intraarticular fracture of right calcaneus   CC H5
7   ✓7ᵗʰ   S92.065   Nondisplaced intraarticular fracture of left calcaneus   CC H5
7   ✓7ᵗʰ   S92.066   Nondisplaced intraarticular fracture of unspecified calcaneus   CC H5

✓5ᵗʰ **S92.1   Fracture of talus**
Astragalus

CC Excl: For codes in subcategory S92.1:
CC with 7th character B: PDX collection 1368
CC with 7th character K or P: PDX collection 897

✓6ᵗʰ **S92.10   Unspecified fracture of talus**
7   ✓7ᵗʰ   S92.101   Unspecified fracture of right talus   CC H5
7   ✓7ᵗʰ   S92.102   Unspecified fracture of left talus   CC H5
7   ✓7ᵗʰ   S92.109   Unspecified fracture of unspecified talus   CC H5

✓6ᵗʰ **S92.11   Fracture of neck of talus**
7   ✓7ᵗʰ   S92.111   Displaced fracture of neck of right talus   CC H5
7   ✓7ᵗʰ   S92.112   Displaced fracture of neck of left talus   CC H5
7   ✓7ᵗʰ   S92.113   Displaced fracture of neck of unspecified talus   CC H5
7   ✓7ᵗʰ   S92.114   Nondisplaced fracture of neck of right talus   CC H5
7   ✓7ᵗʰ   S92.115   Nondisplaced fracture of neck of left talus   CC H5
7   ✓7ᵗʰ   S92.116   Nondisplaced fracture of neck of unspecified talus   CC H5

✓6ᵗʰ **S92.12   Fracture of body of talus**
7   ✓7ᵗʰ   S92.121   Displaced fracture of body of right talus   CC H5
7   ✓7ᵗʰ   S92.122   Displaced fracture of body of left talus   CC H5
7   ✓7ᵗʰ   S92.123   Displaced fracture of body of unspecified talus   CC H5
7   ✓7ᵗʰ   S92.124   Nondisplaced fracture of body of right talus   CC H5
7   ✓7ᵗʰ   S92.125   Nondisplaced fracture of body of left talus   CC H5
7   ✓7ᵗʰ   S92.126   Nondisplaced fracture of body of unspecified talus   CC H5

---

7   CC when reported as an initial encounter (7th character A, B, or C – specific to category) OR a subsequent encounter for nonunion or malunion (7th character K, M, N, P, Q, or R – specific to category).

✓ Additional Character Req   ✓x7ᵗʰ Placeholder Alert   Unacceptable PDx   ◆ Manifestation   H1-H14 HAC   HCC CMS-HCC Condition   *EXCLUDES 1* Not Coded Here   *EXCLUDES 2* Not Included Here

✓6ᵗʰ S92.13 Fracture of posterior process of talus

- 7   ✓7ᵗʰ **S92.131** Displaced **fracture of posterior process of right talus**   CC H5
- 7   ✓7ᵗʰ **S92.132** Displaced **fracture of posterior process of left talus**   CC H5
- 7   ✓7ᵗʰ **S92.133** Displaced **fracture of posterior process of unspecified talus**   CC H5
- 7   ✓7ᵗʰ **S92.134** Nondisplaced **fracture of posterior process of right talus**   CC H5
- 7   ✓7ᵗʰ **S92.135** Nondisplaced **fracture of posterior process of left talus**   CC H5
- 7   ✓7ᵗʰ **S92.136** Nondisplaced **fracture of posterior process of unspecified talus**   CC H5

✓6ᵗʰ S92.14 Dome fracture of talus

EXCLUDES 1   *osteochondritis dissecans (M93.2)*

- 7   ✓7ᵗʰ **S92.141** Displaced **dome fracture of right talus**   CC H5
- 7   ✓7ᵗʰ **S92.142** Displaced **dome fracture of left talus**   CC H5
- 7   ✓7ᵗʰ **S92.143** Displaced **dome fracture of unspecified talus**   CC H5
- 7   ✓7ᵗʰ **S92.144** Nondisplaced **dome fracture of right talus**   CC H5
- 7   ✓7ᵗʰ **S92.145** Nondisplaced **dome fracture of left talus**   CC H5
- 7   ✓7ᵗʰ **S92.146** Nondisplaced **dome fracture of unspecified talus**   CC H5

✓6ᵗʰ S92.15 Avulsion fracture (chip fracture) of talus

- 7   ✓7ᵗʰ **S92.151** Displaced **avulsion fracture (chip fracture) of right talus**   CC H5
- 7   ✓7ᵗʰ **S92.152** Displaced **avulsion fracture (chip fracture) of left talus**   CC H5
- 7   ✓7ᵗʰ **S92.153** Displaced **avulsion fracture (chip fracture) of unspecified talus**   CC H5
- 7   ✓7ᵗʰ **S92.154** Nondisplaced **avulsion fracture (chip fracture) of right talus**   CC H5
- 7   ✓7ᵗʰ **S92.155** Nondisplaced **avulsion fracture (chip fracture) of left talus**   CC H5
- 7   ✓7ᵗʰ **S92.156** Nondisplaced **avulsion fracture (chip fracture) of unspecified talus**   CC H5

✓6ᵗʰ S92.19 Other fracture of talus

- 7   ✓7ᵗʰ **S92.191** Other **fracture of right talus**   CC H5
- 7   ✓7ᵗʰ **S92.192** Other **fracture of left talus**   CC H5
- 7   ✓7ᵗʰ **S92.199** Other **fracture of unspecified talus**   CC H5

✓5ᵗʰ S92.2 Fracture of other and unspecified tarsal bone(s)

> **CC Excl: For codes in subcategory S92.2, unless otherwise noted:**
> **CC with 7th character B:** PDX collection 1368
> **CC with 7th character K or P:** PDX collection 897

✓6ᵗʰ S92.20 Fracture of unspecified tarsal bone(s)

> **CC Excl: For codes in subcategory S92.20:**
> **CC with 7th character B:** PDX collection 1369
> **CC with 7th character K or P:** PDX collection 897

- 7   ✓7ᵗʰ **S92.201** Fracture of unspecified tarsal **bone(s) of right foot**   CC H5
- 7   ✓7ᵗʰ **S92.202** Fracture of unspecified tarsal **bone(s) of left foot**   CC H5
- 7   ✓7ᵗʰ **S92.209** Fracture of unspecified tarsal **bone(s) of unspecified foot**   CC H5

✓6ᵗʰ S92.21 Fracture of cuboid bone

- 7   ✓7ᵗʰ **S92.211** Displaced **fracture of cuboid bone of right foot**   CC H5
- 7   ✓7ᵗʰ **S92.212** Displaced **fracture of cuboid bone of left foot**   CC H5
- 7   ✓7ᵗʰ **S92.213** Displaced **fracture of cuboid bone of unspecified foot**   CC H5
- 7   ✓7ᵗʰ **S92.214** Nondisplaced **fracture of cuboid bone of right foot**   CC H5
- 7   ✓7ᵗʰ **S92.215** Nondisplaced **fracture of cuboid bone of left foot**   CC H5
- 7   ✓7ᵗʰ **S92.216** Nondisplaced **fracture of cuboid bone of unspecified foot**   CC H5

✓6ᵗʰ S92.22 Fracture of lateral cuneiform

- 7   ✓7ᵗʰ **S92.221** Displaced **fracture of lateral cuneiform of right foot**   CC H5
- 7   ✓7ᵗʰ **S92.222** Displaced **fracture of lateral cuneiform of left foot**   CC H5
- 7   ✓7ᵗʰ **S92.223** Displaced **fracture of lateral cuneiform of unspecified foot**   CC H5
- 7   ✓7ᵗʰ **S92.224** Nondisplaced **fracture of lateral cuneiform of right foot**   CC H5
- 7   ✓7ᵗʰ **S92.225** Nondisplaced **fracture of lateral cuneiform of left foot**   CC H5
- 7   ✓7ᵗʰ **S92.226** Nondisplaced **fracture of lateral cuneiform of unspecified foot**   CC H5

✓6ᵗʰ S92.23 Fracture of intermediate cuneiform

- 7   ✓7ᵗʰ **S92.231** Displaced **fracture of intermediate cuneiform of right foot**   CC H5
- 7   ✓7ᵗʰ **S92.232** Displaced **fracture of intermediate cuneiform of left foot**   CC H5
- 7   ✓7ᵗʰ **S92.233** Displaced **fracture of intermediate cuneiform of unspecified foot**   CC H5
- 7   ✓7ᵗʰ **S92.234** Nondisplaced **fracture of intermediate cuneiform of right foot**   CC H5
- 7   ✓7ᵗʰ **S92.235** Nondisplaced **fracture of intermediate cuneiform of left foot**   CC H5
- 7   ✓7ᵗʰ **S92.236** Nondisplaced **fracture of intermediate cuneiform of unspecified foot**   CC H5

✓6ᵗʰ S92.24 Fracture of medial cuneiform

- 7   ✓7ᵗʰ **S92.241** Displaced **fracture of medial cuneiform of right foot**   CC H5
- 7   ✓7ᵗʰ **S92.242** Displaced **fracture of medial cuneiform of left foot**   CC H5
- 7   ✓7ᵗʰ **S92.243** Displaced **fracture of medial cuneiform of unspecified foot**   CC H5
- 7   ✓7ᵗʰ **S92.244** Nondisplaced **fracture of medial cuneiform of right foot**   CC H5
- 7   ✓7ᵗʰ **S92.245** Nondisplaced **fracture of medial cuneiform of left foot**   CC H5
- 7   ✓7ᵗʰ **S92.246** Nondisplaced **fracture of medial cuneiform of unspecified foot**   CC H5

✓6ᵗʰ S92.25 Fracture of navicular [scaphoid] of foot

- 7   ✓7ᵗʰ **S92.251** Displaced **fracture of navicular [scaphoid] of right foot**   CC H5
- 7   ✓7ᵗʰ **S92.252** Displaced **fracture of navicular [scaphoid] of left foot**   CC H5
- 7   ✓7ᵗʰ **S92.253** Displaced **fracture of navicular [scaphoid] of unspecified foot**   CC H5
- 7   ✓7ᵗʰ **S92.254** Nondisplaced **fracture of navicular [scaphoid] of right foot**   CC H5
- 7   ✓7ᵗʰ **S92.255** Nondisplaced **fracture of navicular [scaphoid] of left foot**   CC H5
- 7   ✓7ᵗʰ **S92.256** Nondisplaced **fracture of navicular [scaphoid] of unspecified foot**   CC H5

✓5ᵗʰ S92.3 Fracture of metatarsal bone(s)

EXCLUDES 2   *physeal fracture of metatarsal (S99.1-)*

> **CC Excl: For codes in subcategory S92.3:**
> **CC with 7th character B:** PDX collection 1368
> **CC with 7th character K or P:** PDX collection 897

✓6ᵗʰ S92.30 Fracture of unspecified metatarsal bone(s)

- 7   ✓7ᵗʰ **S92.301** Fracture of unspecified metatarsal **bone(s), right foot**   CC H5
- 7   ✓7ᵗʰ **S92.302** Fracture of unspecified metatarsal **bone(s), left foot**   CC H5
- 7   ✓7ᵗʰ **S92.309** Fracture of unspecified metatarsal **bone(s), unspecified foot**   CC H5

✓6ᵗʰ S92.31 Fracture of first metatarsal bone

- 7   ✓7ᵗʰ **S92.311** Displaced **fracture of first metatarsal bone, right foot**   CC H5
- 7   ✓7ᵗʰ **S92.312** Displaced **fracture of first metatarsal bone, left foot**   CC H5
- 7   ✓7ᵗʰ **S92.313** Displaced **fracture of first metatarsal bone, unspecified foot**   CC H5

---

7   CC when reported as an initial encounter (7th character A, B, or C – specific to category) OR a subsequent encounter for nonunion or malunion (7th character K, M, N, P, Q, or R – specific to category).

N Newborn: 0   P Pediatric: 0-17   M Maternity: 12-55   A Adult: 15-124   MCC Major CC Condition   PDxMCC PDx acts as own MCC   CC CC Condition   PDxCC PDx acts as own CC

1068   ICD-10-CM 2018

7 ✓7ᵗʰ **S92.314** Nondisplaced **fracture of first metatarsal bone, right** foot   `CC` `H5`

7 ✓7ᵗʰ **S92.315** Nondisplaced **fracture of first metatarsal bone, left** foot   `CC` `H5`

7 ✓7ᵗʰ **S92.316** Nondisplaced **fracture of first metatarsal bone, unspecified** foot   `CC` `H5`

✓6ᵗʰ **S92.32** Fracture of second **metatarsal bone**

7 ✓7ᵗʰ **S92.321** Displaced **fracture of second metatarsal bone, right** foot   `CC` `H5`

7 ✓7ᵗʰ **S92.322** Displaced **fracture of second metatarsal bone, left** foot   `CC` `H5`

7 ✓7ᵗʰ **S92.323** Displaced **fracture of second metatarsal bone, unspecified** foot   `CC` `H5`

7 ✓7ᵗʰ **S92.324** Nondisplaced **fracture of second metatarsal bone, right** foot   `CC` `H5`

7 ✓7ᵗʰ **S92.325** Nondisplaced **fracture of second metatarsal bone, left** foot   `CC` `H5`

7 ✓7ᵗʰ **S92.326** Nondisplaced **fracture of second metatarsal bone, unspecified** foot   `CC` `H5`

✓6ᵗʰ **S92.33** Fracture of third **metatarsal bone**

7 ✓7ᵗʰ **S92.331** Displaced **fracture of third metatarsal bone, right** foot   `CC` `H5`

7 ✓7ᵗʰ **S92.332** Displaced **fracture of third metatarsal bone, left** foot   `CC` `H5`

7 ✓7ᵗʰ **S92.333** Displaced **fracture of third metatarsal bone, unspecified** foot   `CC` `H5`

7 ✓7ᵗʰ **S92.334** Nondisplaced **fracture of third metatarsal bone, right** foot   `CC` `H5`

7 ✓7ᵗʰ **S92.335** Nondisplaced **fracture of third metatarsal bone, left** foot   `CC` `H5`

7 ✓7ᵗʰ **S92.336** Nondisplaced **fracture of third metatarsal bone, unspecified** foot   `CC` `H5`

✓6ᵗʰ **S92.34** Fracture of fourth **metatarsal bone**

7 ✓7ᵗʰ **S92.341** Displaced **fracture of fourth metatarsal bone, right** foot   `CC` `H5`

7 ✓7ᵗʰ **S92.342** Displaced **fracture of fourth metatarsal bone, left** foot   `CC` `H5`

7 ✓7ᵗʰ **S92.343** Displaced **fracture of fourth metatarsal bone, unspecified** foot   `CC` `H5`

7 ✓7ᵗʰ **S92.344** Nondisplaced **fracture of fourth metatarsal bone, right** foot   `CC` `H5`

7 ✓7ᵗʰ **S92.345** Nondisplaced **fracture of fourth metatarsal bone, left** foot   `CC` `H5`

7 ✓7ᵗʰ **S92.346** Nondisplaced **fracture of fourth metatarsal bone, unspecified** foot   `CC` `H5`

✓6ᵗʰ **S92.35** Fracture of fifth **metatarsal bone**

7 ✓7ᵗʰ **S92.351** Displaced **fracture of fifth metatarsal bone, right** foot   `CC` `H5`

7 ✓7ᵗʰ **S92.352** Displaced **fracture of fifth metatarsal bone, left** foot   `CC` `H5`

7 ✓7ᵗʰ **S92.353** Displaced **fracture of fifth metatarsal bone, unspecified** foot   `CC` `H5`

7 ✓7ᵗʰ **S92.354** Nondisplaced **fracture of fifth metatarsal bone, right** foot   `CC` `H5`

7 ✓7ᵗʰ **S92.355** Nondisplaced **fracture of fifth metatarsal bone, left** foot   `CC` `H5`

7 ✓7ᵗʰ **S92.356** Nondisplaced **fracture of fifth metatarsal bone, unspecified** foot   `CC` `H5`

✓5ᵗʰ **S92.4** Fracture of great **toe**

EXCLUDES 2   physeal fracture of phalanx of toe (S99.2-)

CC Excl: For codes in subcategory S92.4:
CC with 7th character K or P: PDX collection 897

✓6ᵗʰ **S92.40** Unspecified **fracture of great toe**

8 ✓7ᵗʰ **S92.401** Displaced **unspecified fracture of right great** toe   `CC`

8 ✓7ᵗʰ **S92.402** Displaced **unspecified fracture of left great** toe   `CC`

8 ✓7ᵗʰ **S92.403** Displaced **unspecified fracture of unspecified great** toe   `CC`

8 ✓7ᵗʰ **S92.404** Nondisplaced **unspecified fracture of right great** toe   `CC`

8 ✓7ᵗʰ **S92.405** Nondisplaced **unspecified fracture of left great** toe   `CC`

8 ✓7ᵗʰ **S92.406** Nondisplaced **unspecified fracture of unspecified great** toe   `CC`

✓6ᵗʰ **S92.41** Fracture of proximal phalanx **of great toe**

8 ✓7ᵗʰ **S92.411** Displaced **fracture of proximal phalanx of right great** toe   `CC`

8 ✓7ᵗʰ **S92.412** Displaced **fracture of proximal phalanx of left great** toe   `CC`

8 ✓7ᵗʰ **S92.413** Displaced **fracture of proximal phalanx of unspecified great** toe   `CC`

8 ✓7ᵗʰ **S92.414** Nondisplaced **fracture of proximal phalanx of right great** toe   `CC`

8 ✓7ᵗʰ **S92.415** Nondisplaced **fracture of proximal phalanx of left great** toe   `CC`

8 ✓7ᵗʰ **S92.416** Nondisplaced **fracture of proximal phalanx of unspecified great** toe   `CC`

✓6ᵗʰ **S92.42** Fracture of distal phalanx **of great toe**

8 ✓7ᵗʰ **S92.421** Displaced **fracture of distal phalanx of right great** toe   `CC`

8 ✓7ᵗʰ **S92.422** Displaced **fracture of distal phalanx of left great** toe   `CC`

8 ✓7ᵗʰ **S92.423** Displaced **fracture of distal phalanx of unspecified great** toe   `CC`

8 ✓7ᵗʰ **S92.424** Nondisplaced **fracture of distal phalanx of right great** toe   `CC`

8 ✓7ᵗʰ **S92.425** Nondisplaced **fracture of distal phalanx of left great** toe   `CC`

8 ✓7ᵗʰ **S92.426** Nondisplaced **fracture of distal phalanx of unspecified great** toe   `CC`

✓6ᵗʰ **S92.49** Other **fracture of great toe**

8 ✓7ᵗʰ **S92.491** Other **fracture of right great** toe   `CC`

8 ✓7ᵗʰ **S92.492** Other **fracture of left great** toe   `CC`

8 ✓7ᵗʰ **S92.499** Other **fracture of unspecified great** toe   `CC`

✓5ᵗʰ **S92.5** Fracture of lesser **toe(s)**

EXCLUDES 2   physeal fracture of phalanx of toe (S99.2-)

CC Excl: For codes in subcategory S92.5:
CC with 7th character K or P: PDX collection 897

✓6ᵗʰ **S92.50** Unspecified **fracture of lesser toe(s)**

8 ✓7ᵗʰ **S92.501** Displaced **unspecified fracture of right lesser** toe(s)   `CC`

8 ✓7ᵗʰ **S92.502** Displaced **unspecified fracture of left lesser** toe(s)   `CC`

8 ✓7ᵗʰ **S92.503** Displaced **unspecified fracture of unspecified lesser** toe(s)   `CC`

8 ✓7ᵗʰ **S92.504** Nondisplaced **unspecified fracture of right lesser** toe(s)   `CC`

8 ✓7ᵗʰ **S92.505** Nondisplaced **unspecified fracture of left lesser** toe(s)   `CC`

8 ✓7ᵗʰ **S92.506** Nondisplaced **unspecified fracture of unspecified lesser** toe(s)   `CC`

✓6ᵗʰ **S92.51** Fracture of proximal phalanx **of lesser toe(s)**

8 ✓7ᵗʰ **S92.511** Displaced **fracture of proximal phalanx of right lesser** toe(s)   `CC`

8 ✓7ᵗʰ **S92.512** Displaced **fracture of proximal phalanx of left lesser** toe(s)   `CC`

8 ✓7ᵗʰ **S92.513** Displaced **fracture of proximal phalanx of unspecified lesser** toe(s)   `CC`

8 ✓7ᵗʰ **S92.514** Nondisplaced **fracture of proximal phalanx of right lesser** toe(s)   `CC`

8 ✓7ᵗʰ **S92.515** Nondisplaced **fracture of proximal phalanx of left lesser** toe(s)   `CC`

8 ✓7ᵗʰ **S92.516** Nondisplaced **fracture of proximal phalanx of unspecified lesser** toe(s)   `CC`

✓6ᵗʰ **S92.52** Fracture of middle phalanx **of lesser toe(s)**

8 ✓7ᵗʰ **S92.521** Displaced **fracture of middle phalanx of right lesser** toe(s)   `CC` ▲

8 ✓7ᵗʰ **S92.522** Displaced **fracture of middle phalanx of left lesser** toe(s)   `CC` ▲

8 ✓7ᵗʰ **S92.523** Displaced **fracture of middle phalanx of unspecified lesser** toe(s)   `CC` ▲

---

7   CC when reported as an initial encounter (7th character A, B, or C – specific to category) OR a subsequent encounter for nonunion or malunion (7th character K, M, N, P, Q, or R – specific to category).

8   CC when reported as a subsequent encounter for nonunion or malunion (7th character K, M, N, P, Q, or R – specific to category).

☑ Additional Character Req   ✓ₓ7ᵗʰ Placeholder Alert   Unacceptable PDx   Manifestation   `H1`-`H14` HAC   `HCC` CMS-HCC Condition   *EXCLUDES 1* Not Coded Here   *EXCLUDES 2* Not Included Here

▲   8   ✓7ᵗʰ **S92.524** **Nondisplaced fracture of middle phalanx of right lesser toe(s)**   CC

▲   8   ✓7ᵗʰ **S92.525** **Nondisplaced fracture of middle phalanx of left lesser toe(s)**   CC

▲   8   ✓7ᵗʰ **S92.526** **Nondisplaced fracture of middle phalanx of unspecified lesser toe(s)**   CC

✓6ᵗʰ **S92.53** **Fracture of distal phalanx of lesser toe(s)**

   8   ✓7ᵗʰ **S92.531** **Displaced fracture of distal phalanx of right lesser toe(s)**   CC

   8   ✓7ᵗʰ **S92.532** **Displaced fracture of distal phalanx of left lesser toe(s)**   CC

   8   ✓7ᵗʰ **S92.533** **Displaced fracture of distal phalanx of unspecified lesser toe(s)**   CC

   8   ✓7ᵗʰ **S92.534** **Nondisplaced fracture of distal phalanx of right lesser toe(s)**   CC

   8   ✓7ᵗʰ **S92.535** **Nondisplaced fracture of distal phalanx of left lesser toe(s)**   CC

   8   ✓7ᵗʰ **S92.536** **Nondisplaced fracture of distal phalanx of unspecified lesser toe(s)**   CC

✓6ᵗʰ **S92.59** **Other fracture of lesser toe(s)**

   8   ✓7ᵗʰ **S92.591** **Other fracture of right lesser toe(s)**   CC

   8   ✓7ᵗʰ **S92.592** **Other fracture of left lesser toe(s)**   CC

   8   ✓7ᵗʰ **S92.599** **Other fracture of unspecified lesser toe(s)**   CC

✓5ᵗʰ **S92.8** **Other fracture of foot, except ankle**

   ✓6ᵗʰ **S92.81** **Other fracture of foot**
       Sesamoid fracture of foot

> **CC Excl: For codes in subcategory S92.81:**
> **CC with 7th character B:** PDX collection 1369
> **CC with 7th character K or P:** PDX collection 897

   7   ✓7ᵗʰ **S92.811** **Other fracture of right foot**   CC H5

   7   ✓7ᵗʰ **S92.812** **Other fracture of left foot**   CC H5

   7   ✓7ᵗʰ **S92.819** **Other fracture of unspecified foot**   CC H5

✓5ᵗʰ **S92.9** **Unspecified fracture of foot and toe**

   ✓6ᵗʰ **S92.90** **Unspecified fracture of foot**

> **CC Excl: For codes in subcategory S92.90:**
> **CC with 7th character B:** PDX collection 1369
> **CC with 7th character K or P:** PDX collection 897

   7   ✓7ᵗʰ **S92.901** **Unspecified fracture of right foot**   CC H5

   7   ✓7ᵗʰ **S92.902** **Unspecified fracture of left foot**   CC H5

   7   ✓7ᵗʰ **S92.909** **Unspecified fracture of unspecified foot**   CC H5

   ✓6ᵗʰ **S92.91** **Unspecified fracture of toe**

> **CC Excl: For codes in subcategory S92.91:**
> **CC with 7th character K or P:** PDX collection 897

   8   ✓7ᵗʰ **S92.911** **Unspecified fracture of right toe(s)**   CC

   8   ✓7ᵗʰ **S92.912** **Unspecified fracture of left toe(s)**   CC

   8   ✓7ᵗʰ **S92.919** **Unspecified fracture of unspecified toe(s)**   CC

✓4ᵗʰ **S93** **Dislocation and sprain of joints and ligaments at ankle, foot and toe level**

   INCLUDES   avulsion of joint or ligament of ankle, foot and toe
        laceration of cartilage, joint or ligament of ankle, foot and toe
        sprain of cartilage, joint or ligament of ankle, foot and toe
        traumatic hemarthrosis of joint or ligament of ankle, foot and toe
        traumatic rupture of joint or ligament of ankle, foot and toe
        traumatic subluxation of joint or ligament of ankle, foot and toe
        traumatic tear of joint or ligament of ankle, foot and toe

   Code also any associated open wound
   EXCLUDES 2   *strain of muscle and tendon of ankle and foot (S96.-)*

> The appropriate 7th character is to be added to each code from category S93.
> A   initial encounter
> D   subsequent encounter
> S   sequela

✓5ᵗʰ **S93.0** **Subluxation and dislocation of ankle joint**
     Subluxation and dislocation of astragalus
     Subluxation and dislocation of fibula, lower end
     Subluxation and dislocation of talus
     Subluxation and dislocation of tibia, lower end

   ✓x7ᵗʰ **S93.01** **Subluxation of right ankle joint**

   ✓x7ᵗʰ **S93.02** **Subluxation of left ankle joint**

   ✓x7ᵗʰ **S93.03** **Subluxation of unspecified ankle joint**

   ✓x7ᵗʰ **S93.04** **Dislocation of right ankle joint**

   ✓x7ᵗʰ **S93.05** **Dislocation of left ankle joint**

   ✓x7ᵗʰ **S93.06** **Dislocation of unspecified ankle joint**

✓5ᵗʰ **S93.1** **Subluxation and dislocation of toe**

   ✓6ᵗʰ **S93.10** **Unspecified subluxation and dislocation of toe**
       Dislocation of toe NOS
       Subluxation of toe NOS

     ✓7ᵗʰ **S93.101** **Unspecified subluxation of right toe(s)**

     ✓7ᵗʰ **S93.102** **Unspecified subluxation of left toe(s)**

     ✓7ᵗʰ **S93.103** **Unspecified subluxation of unspecified toe(s)**

     ✓7ᵗʰ **S93.104** **Unspecified dislocation of right toe(s)**

     ✓7ᵗʰ **S93.105** **Unspecified dislocation of left toe(s)**

     ✓7ᵗʰ **S93.106** **Unspecified dislocation of unspecified toe(s)**

   ✓6ᵗʰ **S93.11** **Dislocation of interphalangeal joint**

     ✓7ᵗʰ **S93.111** **Dislocation of interphalangeal joint of right great toe**

     ✓7ᵗʰ **S93.112** **Dislocation of interphalangeal joint of left great toe**

     ✓7ᵗʰ **S93.113** **Dislocation of interphalangeal joint of unspecified great toe**

     ✓7ᵗʰ **S93.114** **Dislocation of interphalangeal joint of right lesser toe(s)**

     ✓7ᵗʰ **S93.115** **Dislocation of interphalangeal joint of left lesser toe(s)**

     ✓7ᵗʰ **S93.116** **Dislocation of interphalangeal joint of unspecified lesser toe(s)**

     ✓7ᵗʰ **S93.119** **Dislocation of interphalangeal joint of unspecified toe(s)**

   ✓6ᵗʰ **S93.12** **Dislocation of metatarsophalangeal joint**

     ✓7ᵗʰ **S93.121** **Dislocation of metatarsophalangeal joint of right great toe**

     ✓7ᵗʰ **S93.122** **Dislocation of metatarsophalangeal joint of left great toe**

     ✓7ᵗʰ **S93.123** **Dislocation of metatarsophalangeal joint of unspecified great toe**

     ✓7ᵗʰ **S93.124** **Dislocation of metatarsophalangeal joint of right lesser toe(s)**

     ✓7ᵗʰ **S93.125** **Dislocation of metatarsophalangeal joint of left lesser toe(s)**

     ✓7ᵗʰ **S93.126** **Dislocation of metatarsophalangeal joint of unspecified lesser toe(s)**

     ✓7ᵗʰ **S93.129** **Dislocation of metatarsophalangeal joint of unspecified toe(s)**

   ✓6ᵗʰ **S93.13** **Subluxation of interphalangeal joint**

     ✓7ᵗʰ **S93.131** **Subluxation of interphalangeal joint of right great toe**

     ✓7ᵗʰ **S93.132** **Subluxation of interphalangeal joint of left great toe**

     ✓7ᵗʰ **S93.133** **Subluxation of interphalangeal joint of unspecified great toe**

     ✓7ᵗʰ **S93.134** **Subluxation of interphalangeal joint of right lesser toe(s)**

     ✓7ᵗʰ **S93.135** **Subluxation of interphalangeal joint of left lesser toe(s)**

     ✓7ᵗʰ **S93.136** **Subluxation of interphalangeal joint of unspecified lesser toe(s)**

     ✓7ᵗʰ **S93.139** **Subluxation of interphalangeal joint of unspecified toe(s)**

---

7   CC when reported as an initial encounter (7th character A, B, or C – specific to category) OR a subsequent encounter for nonunion or malunion (7th character K, M, N, P, Q, or R – specific to category).

8   CC when reported as a subsequent encounter for nonunion or malunion (7th character K, M, N, P, Q, or R – specific to category).

✓6ᵗʰ **S93.14** Subluxation of **metatarsophalangeal joint**

  ✓7ᵗʰ **S93.141** **Subluxation of metatarsophalangeal joint of** right great **toe**

  ✓7ᵗʰ **S93.142** **Subluxation of metatarsophalangeal joint of** left great **toe**

  ✓7ᵗʰ **S93.143** **Subluxation of metatarsophalangeal joint of** unspecified great **toe**

  ✓7ᵗʰ **S93.144** **Subluxation of metatarsophalangeal joint of** right lesser **toe(s)**

  ✓7ᵗʰ **S93.145** **Subluxation of metatarsophalangeal joint of** left lesser **toe(s)**

  ✓7ᵗʰ **S93.146** **Subluxation of metatarsophalangeal joint of** unspecified lesser **toe(s)**

  ✓7ᵗʰ **S93.149** **Subluxation of metatarsophalangeal joint of** unspecified **toe(s)**

✓5ᵗʰ **S93.3** **Subluxation and dislocation of** foot

  EXCLUDES 2   *dislocation of toe (S93.1-)*

  ✓6ᵗʰ **S93.30** **Unspecified** subluxation and dislocation of foot

    Dislocation of foot NOS

    Subluxation of foot NOS

    ✓7ᵗʰ **S93.301** **Unspecified** subluxation **of** right **foot**

    ✓7ᵗʰ **S93.302** **Unspecified** subluxation **of** left **foot**

    ✓7ᵗʰ **S93.303** **Unspecified** subluxation **of** unspecified **foot**

    ✓7ᵗʰ **S93.304** **Unspecified** dislocation **of** right **foot**

    ✓7ᵗʰ **S93.305** **Unspecified** dislocation **of** left **foot**

    ✓7ᵗʰ **S93.306** **Unspecified** dislocation **of** unspecified **foot**

  ✓6ᵗʰ **S93.31** **Subluxation and dislocation of** tarsal joint

    ✓7ᵗʰ **S93.311** **Subluxation of tarsal joint of** right **foot**

    ✓7ᵗʰ **S93.312** **Subluxation of tarsal joint of** left **foot**

    ✓7ᵗʰ **S93.313** **Subluxation of tarsal joint of** unspecified **foot**

    ✓7ᵗʰ **S93.314** **Dislocation of tarsal joint of** right **foot**

    ✓7ᵗʰ **S93.315** **Dislocation of tarsal joint of** left **foot**

    ✓7ᵗʰ **S93.316** **Dislocation of tarsal joint of** unspecified **foot**

  ✓6ᵗʰ **S93.32** **Subluxation and dislocation of** tarsometatarsal **joint**

    ✓7ᵗʰ **S93.321** **Subluxation of tarsometatarsal joint of** right **foot**

    ✓7ᵗʰ **S93.322** **Subluxation of tarsometatarsal joint of** left **foot**

    ✓7ᵗʰ **S93.323** **Subluxation of tarsometatarsal joint of** unspecified **foot**

    ✓7ᵗʰ **S93.324** **Dislocation of tarsometatarsal joint of** right **foot**

    ✓7ᵗʰ **S93.325** **Dislocation of tarsometatarsal joint of** left **foot**

    ✓7ᵗʰ **S93.326** **Dislocation of tarsometatarsal joint of** unspecified **foot**

  ✓6ᵗʰ **S93.33** **Other subluxation and dislocation of** foot

    ✓7ᵗʰ **S93.331** **Other** subluxation **of** right **foot**

    ✓7ᵗʰ **S93.332** **Other** subluxation **of** left **foot**

    ✓7ᵗʰ **S93.333** **Other** subluxation **of** unspecified **foot**

    ✓7ᵗʰ **S93.334** **Other** dislocation **of** right **foot**

    ✓7ᵗʰ **S93.335** **Other** dislocation **of** left **foot**

    ✓7ᵗʰ **S93.336** **Other** dislocation **of** unspecified **foot**

✓5ᵗʰ **S93.4** **Sprain of** ankle

  EXCLUDES 2   *injury of Achilles tendon (S86.0-)*

  ✓6ᵗʰ **S93.40** **Sprain of** unspecified **ligament of ankle**

    Sprain of ankle NOS

    Sprained ankle NOS

    ✓7ᵗʰ **S93.401** **Sprain of unspecified ligament of** right **ankle**

    ✓7ᵗʰ **S93.402** **Sprain of unspecified ligament of** left **ankle**

    ✓7ᵗʰ **S93.409** **Sprain of unspecified ligament of** unspecified **ankle**

  ✓6ᵗʰ **S93.41** **Sprain of** calcaneofibular **ligament**

    ✓7ᵗʰ **S93.411** **Sprain of calcaneofibular ligament of** right **ankle**

    ✓7ᵗʰ **S93.412** **Sprain of calcaneofibular ligament of** left **ankle**

    ✓7ᵗʰ **S93.419** **Sprain of calcaneofibular ligament of** unspecified **ankle**

  ✓6ᵗʰ **S93.42** **Sprain of** deltoid **ligament**

    ✓7ᵗʰ **S93.421** **Sprain of deltoid ligament of** right **ankle**

    ✓7ᵗʰ **S93.422** **Sprain of deltoid ligament of** left **ankle**

    ✓7ᵗʰ **S93.429** **Sprain of deltoid ligament of** unspecified **ankle**

  ✓6ᵗʰ **S93.43** **Sprain of** tibiofibular **ligament**

    ✓7ᵗʰ **S93.431** **Sprain of tibiofibular ligament of** right **ankle**

    ✓7ᵗʰ **S93.432** **Sprain of tibiofibular ligament of** left **ankle**

    ✓7ᵗʰ **S93.439** **Sprain of tibiofibular ligament of** unspecified **ankle**

  ✓6ᵗʰ **S93.49** **Sprain of** other **ligament of ankle**

    Sprain of internal collateral ligament

    Sprain of talofibular ligament

    ✓7ᵗʰ **S93.491** **Sprain of other ligament of** right **ankle**

    ✓7ᵗʰ **S93.492** **Sprain of other ligament of** left **ankle**

    ✓7ᵗʰ **S93.499** **Sprain of other ligament of** unspecified **ankle**

✓5ᵗʰ **S93.5** **Sprain of** toe

  ✓6ᵗʰ **S93.50** **Unspecified** sprain of toe

    ✓7ᵗʰ **S93.501** **Unspecified sprain of** right great **toe**

    ✓7ᵗʰ **S93.502** **Unspecified sprain of** left great **toe**

    ✓7ᵗʰ **S93.503** **Unspecified sprain of** unspecified great **toe**

    ✓7ᵗʰ **S93.504** **Unspecified sprain of** right lesser **toe(s)**

    ✓7ᵗʰ **S93.505** **Unspecified sprain of** left lesser **toe(s)**

    ✓7ᵗʰ **S93.506** **Unspecified sprain of** unspecified lesser **toe(s)**

    ✓7ᵗʰ **S93.509** **Unspecified sprain of** unspecified **toe(s)**

  ✓6ᵗʰ **S93.51** **Sprain of** interphalangeal joint **of toe**

    ✓7ᵗʰ **S93.511** **Sprain of interphalangeal joint of** right great **toe**

    ✓7ᵗʰ **S93.512** **Sprain of interphalangeal joint of** left great **toe**

    ✓7ᵗʰ **S93.513** **Sprain of interphalangeal joint of** unspecified great **toe**

    ✓7ᵗʰ **S93.514** **Sprain of interphalangeal joint of** right lesser **toe(s)**

    ✓7ᵗʰ **S93.515** **Sprain of interphalangeal joint of** left lesser **toe(s)**

    ✓7ᵗʰ **S93.516** **Sprain of interphalangeal joint of** unspecified lesser **toe(s)**

    ✓7ᵗʰ **S93.519** **Sprain of interphalangeal joint of** unspecified **toe(s)**

  ✓6ᵗʰ **S93.52** **Sprain of** metatarsophalangeal joint **of toe**

    ✓7ᵗʰ **S93.521** **Sprain of metatarsophalangeal joint of** right great **toe**

    ✓7ᵗʰ **S93.522** **Sprain of metatarsophalangeal joint of** left great **toe**

    ✓7ᵗʰ **S93.523** **Sprain of metatarsophalangeal joint of** unspecified great **toe**

    ✓7ᵗʰ **S93.524** **Sprain of metatarsophalangeal joint of** right lesser **toe(s)**

    ✓7ᵗʰ **S93.525** **Sprain of metatarsophalangeal joint of** left lesser **toe(s)**

    ✓7ᵗʰ **S93.526** **Sprain of metatarsophalangeal joint of** unspecified lesser **toe(s)**

    ✓7ᵗʰ **S93.529** **Sprain of metatarsophalangeal joint of** unspecified **toe(s)**

✓5ᵗʰ **S93.6** **Sprain of** foot

  EXCLUDES 2   *sprain of metatarsophalangeal joint of toe (S93.52-)*

            sprain of toe (S93.5-)

  ✓6ᵗʰ **S93.60** **Unspecified** sprain of foot

    ✓7ᵗʰ **S93.601** **Unspecified sprain of** right **foot**

    ✓7ᵗʰ **S93.602** **Unspecified sprain of** left **foot**

    ✓7ᵗʰ **S93.609** **Unspecified sprain of** unspecified **foot**

  ✓6ᵗʰ **S93.61** **Sprain of** tarsal ligament **of foot**

    ✓7ᵗʰ **S93.611** **Sprain of tarsal ligament of** right **foot**

    ✓7ᵗʰ **S93.612** **Sprain of tarsal ligament of** left **foot**

✓ Additional Character Req   ✓ₓ7ᵗʰ Placeholder Alert   Unacceptable PDx   Manifestation   **H1**-**H14** HAC   **HCC** CMS-HCC Condition   *EXCLUDES 1* Not Coded Here   *EXCLUDES 2* Not Included Here

√7ᵗʰ **S93.619** **Sprain of tarsal ligament of** unspecified **foot**

√6ᵗʰ **S93.62** **Sprain of** tarsometatarsal ligament **of foot**

    √7ᵗʰ **S93.621** **Sprain of tarsometatarsal ligament of** right **foot**

    √7ᵗʰ **S93.622** **Sprain of tarsometatarsal ligament of** left **foot**

    √7ᵗʰ **S93.629** **Sprain of tarsometatarsal ligament of** unspecified **foot**

√6ᵗʰ **S93.69** **Other sprain of foot**

    √7ᵗʰ **S93.691** **Other sprain of** right **foot**

    √7ᵗʰ **S93.692** **Other sprain of** left **foot**

    √7ᵗʰ **S93.699** **Other sprain of** unspecified **foot**

√4ᵗʰ **S94** **Injury of nerves at ankle and foot level**

Code also any associated open wound (S91.-)

The appropriate 7th character is to be added to each code from category S94.
A   initial encounter
D   subsequent encounter
S   sequela

√5ᵗʰ **S94.0** **Injury of** lateral plantar **nerve**

    √x7ᵗʰ **S94.00** **Injury of lateral plantar nerve,** unspecified **leg**

    √x7ᵗʰ **S94.01** **Injury of lateral plantar nerve,** right **leg**

    √x7ᵗʰ **S94.02** **Injury of lateral plantar nerve,** left **leg**

√5ᵗʰ **S94.1** **Injury of** medial plantar **nerve**

    √x7ᵗʰ **S94.10** **Injury of medial plantar nerve,** unspecified **leg**

    √x7ᵗʰ **S94.11** **Injury of medial plantar nerve,** right **leg**

    √x7ᵗʰ **S94.12** **Injury of medial plantar nerve,** left **leg**

√5ᵗʰ **S94.2** **Injury of** deep peroneal nerve at ankle and foot level
    Injury of terminal, lateral branch of deep peroneal nerve

    √x7ᵗʰ **S94.20** **Injury of deep peroneal nerve at ankle and foot level,** unspecified **leg**

    √x7ᵗʰ **S94.21** **Injury of deep peroneal nerve at ankle and foot level,** right **leg**

    √x7ᵗʰ **S94.22** **Injury of deep peroneal nerve at ankle and foot level,** left **leg**

√5ᵗʰ **S94.3** **Injury of** cutaneous sensory **nerve at ankle and foot level**

    √x7ᵗʰ **S94.30** **Injury of cutaneous sensory nerve at ankle and foot level,** unspecified **leg**

    √x7ᵗʰ **S94.31** **Injury of cutaneous sensory nerve at ankle and foot level,** right **leg**

    √x7ᵗʰ **S94.32** **Injury of cutaneous sensory nerve at ankle and foot level,** left **leg**

√5ᵗʰ **S94.8** **Injury of** other **nerves at ankle and foot level**

    √6ᵗʰ **S94.8X** **Injury of other nerves at ankle and foot level**

        √7ᵗʰ **S94.8X1** **Injury of other nerves at ankle and foot level,** right **leg**

        √7ᵗʰ **S94.8X2** **Injury of other nerves at ankle and foot level,** left **leg**

        √7ᵗʰ **S94.8X9** **Injury of other nerves at ankle and foot level,** unspecified **leg**

√5ᵗʰ **S94.9** **Injury of** unspecified **nerve at ankle and foot level**

    √x7ᵗʰ **S94.90** **Injury of unspecified nerve at ankle and foot level,** unspecified **leg**

    √x7ᵗʰ **S94.91** **Injury of unspecified nerve at ankle and foot level,** right **leg**

    √x7ᵗʰ **S94.92** **Injury of unspecified nerve at ankle and foot level,** left **leg**

√4ᵗʰ **S95** **Injury of blood vessels at ankle and foot level**

Code also any associated open wound (S91.-)
EXCLUDES 2   injury of posterior tibial artery and vein (S85.1-, S85.8-)

The appropriate 7th character is to be added to each code from category S95.
A   initial encounter
D   subsequent encounter
S   sequela

CC Excl: For CC codes in category S95, unless otherwise noted:
Right side: PDX collection 1325
Left side: PDX collection 1326
Unspecified side: PDX collection 1327

√5ᵗʰ **S95.0** **Injury of** dorsal artery **of foot**

    √6ᵗʰ **S95.00** **Unspecified injury of dorsal artery of foot**

        √7ᵗʰ **S95.001** **Unspecified injury of dorsal artery of** right **foot**   CC

        √7ᵗʰ **S95.002** **Unspecified injury of dorsal artery of** left **foot**   CC

        √7ᵗʰ **S95.009** **Unspecified injury of dorsal artery of** unspecified **foot**   CC

    √6ᵗʰ **S95.01** **Laceration of dorsal artery of foot**

        √7ᵗʰ **S95.011** **Laceration of dorsal artery of** left **foot**   CC

        √7ᵗʰ **S95.012** **Laceration of dorsal artery of** left **foot**   CC

        √7ᵗʰ **S95.019** **Laceration of dorsal artery of** unspecified **foot**   CC

    √6ᵗʰ **S95.09** **Other** specified **injury of dorsal artery of foot**

        √7ᵗʰ **S95.091** **Other specified injury of dorsal artery of** right **foot**   CC

        √7ᵗʰ **S95.092** **Other specified injury of dorsal artery of** left **foot**   CC

        √7ᵗʰ **S95.099** **Other specified injury of dorsal artery of** unspecified **foot**   CC

√5ᵗʰ **S95.1** **Injury of** plantar artery **of foot**

CC Excl: For CC codes in subcategory S95.1:
Right side: PDX collection 1370
Left side: PDX collection 1371
Unspecified side: PDX collection 1372

    √6ᵗʰ **S95.10** **Unspecified injury of plantar artery of foot**

        √7ᵗʰ **S95.101** **Unspecified injury of plantar artery of** right **foot**   CC

        √7ᵗʰ **S95.102** **Unspecified injury of plantar artery of** left **foot**   CC

        √7ᵗʰ **S95.109** **Unspecified injury of plantar artery of** unspecified **foot**   CC

    √6ᵗʰ **S95.11** **Laceration of plantar artery of foot**

        √7ᵗʰ **S95.111** **Laceration of plantar artery of** right **foot**   CC

        √7ᵗʰ **S95.112** **Laceration of plantar artery of** left **foot**   CC

        √7ᵗʰ **S95.119** **Laceration of plantar artery of** unspecified **foot**   CC

    √6ᵗʰ **S95.19** **Other** specified **injury of plantar artery of foot**

        √7ᵗʰ **S95.191** **Other specified injury of plantar artery of** right **foot**   CC

        √7ᵗʰ **S95.192** **Other specified injury of plantar artery of** left **foot**   CC

        √7ᵗʰ **S95.199** **Other specified injury of plantar artery of** unspecified **foot**   CC

√5ᵗʰ **S95.2** **Injury of** dorsal vein **of foot**

    √6ᵗʰ **S95.20** **Unspecified injury of dorsal vein of foot**

        √7ᵗʰ **S95.201** **Unspecified injury of dorsal vein of** right **foot**   CC

        √7ᵗʰ **S95.202** **Unspecified injury of dorsal vein of** left **foot**   CC

        √7ᵗʰ **S95.209** **Unspecified injury of dorsal vein of** unspecified **foot**   CC

    √6ᵗʰ **S95.21** **Laceration of dorsal vein of foot**

        √7ᵗʰ **S95.211** **Laceration of dorsal vein of** right **foot**   CC

        √7ᵗʰ **S95.212** **Laceration of dorsal vein of** left **foot**   CC

        √7ᵗʰ **S95.219** **Laceration of dorsal vein of** unspecified **foot**   CC

N Newborn: 0   P Pediatric: 0-17   M Maternity: 12-55   A Adult: 15-124   MCC Major CC Condition   PDxMCC PDx acts as own MCC   CC CC Condition   PDxCC PDx acts as own CC

1072   ICD-10-CM 2018

√6ᵗʰ **S95.29** Other specified injury of dorsal vein of foot

  √7ᵗʰ **S95.291** Other specified injury of dorsal vein of right foot   CC

  √7ᵗʰ **S95.292** Other specified injury of dorsal vein of left foot   CC

  √7ᵗʰ **S95.299** Other specified injury of dorsal vein of unspecified foot   CC

√5ᵗʰ **S95.8** Injury of other blood vessels at ankle and foot level

 √6ᵗʰ **S95.80** Unspecified injury of other blood vessels at ankle and foot level

  √7ᵗʰ **S95.801** Unspecified injury of other blood vessels at ankle and foot level, right leg   CC

  √7ᵗʰ **S95.802** Unspecified injury of other blood vessels at ankle and foot level, left leg   CC

  √7ᵗʰ **S95.809** Unspecified injury of other blood vessels at ankle and foot level, unspecified leg   CC

 √6ᵗʰ **S95.81** Laceration of other blood vessels at ankle and foot level

  √7ᵗʰ **S95.811** Laceration of other blood vessels at ankle and foot level, right leg   CC

  √7ᵗʰ **S95.812** Laceration of other blood vessels at ankle and foot level, left leg   CC

  √7ᵗʰ **S95.819** Laceration of other blood vessels at ankle and foot level, unspecified leg   CC

 √6ᵗʰ **S95.89** Other specified injury of other blood vessels at ankle and foot level

  √7ᵗʰ **S95.891** Other specified injury of other blood vessels at ankle and foot level, right leg   CC

  √7ᵗʰ **S95.892** Other specified injury of other blood vessels at ankle and foot level, left leg   CC

  √7ᵗʰ **S95.899** Other specified injury of other blood vessels at ankle and foot level, unspecified leg   CC

√5ᵗʰ **S95.9** Injury of unspecified blood vessel at ankle and foot level

 √6ᵗʰ **S95.90** Unspecified injury of unspecified blood vessel at ankle and foot level

  √7ᵗʰ **S95.901** Unspecified injury of unspecified blood vessel at ankle and foot level, right leg   CC

  √7ᵗʰ **S95.902** Unspecified injury of unspecified blood vessel at ankle and foot level, left leg   CC

  √7ᵗʰ **S95.909** Unspecified injury of unspecified blood vessel at ankle and foot level, unspecified leg   CC

 √6ᵗʰ **S95.91** Laceration of unspecified blood vessel at ankle and foot level

  √7ᵗʰ **S95.911** Laceration of unspecified blood vessel at ankle and foot level, right leg   CC

  √7ᵗʰ **S95.912** Laceration of unspecified blood vessel at ankle and foot level, left leg   CC

  √7ᵗʰ **S95.919** Laceration of unspecified blood vessel at ankle and foot level, unspecified leg   CC

 √6ᵗʰ **S95.99** Other specified injury of unspecified blood vessel at ankle and foot level

  √7ᵗʰ **S95.991** Other specified injury of unspecified blood vessel at ankle and foot level, right leg   CC

  √7ᵗʰ **S95.992** Other specified injury of unspecified blood vessel at ankle and foot level, left leg   CC

  √7ᵗʰ **S95.999** Other specified injury of unspecified blood vessel at ankle and foot level, unspecified leg   CC

√4ᵗʰ **S96** **Injury of muscle and tendon at ankle and foot level**

Code also any associated open wound (S91.-)

EXCLUDES 2   injury of Achilles tendon (S86.0-)

         sprain of joints and ligaments of ankle and foot (S93.-)

TIP: Refer to the Muscle/Tendon table at the beginning of this chapter

The appropriate 7th character is to be added to each code from category S96.

A   initial encounter
D   subsequent encounter
S   sequela

CC Excl: For CC codes in category S96:
Right side: PDX collection 1364
Left side: PDX collection 1365
Unspecified side: PDX collection 1366

√5ᵗʰ **S96.0** Injury of muscle and tendon of long flexor muscle of toe at ankle and foot level

 √6ᵗʰ **S96.00** Unspecified injury of muscle and tendon of long flexor muscle of toe at ankle and foot level

  √7ᵗʰ **S96.001** Unspecified injury of muscle and tendon of long flexor muscle of toe at ankle and foot level, right foot

  √7ᵗʰ **S96.002** Unspecified injury of muscle and tendon of long flexor muscle of toe at ankle and foot level, left foot

  √7ᵗʰ **S96.009** Unspecified injury of muscle and tendon of long flexor muscle of toe at ankle and foot level, unspecified foot

 √6ᵗʰ **S96.01** Strain of muscle and tendon of long flexor muscle of toe at ankle and foot level

  √7ᵗʰ **S96.011** Strain of muscle and tendon of long flexor muscle of toe at ankle and foot level, right foot

  √7ᵗʰ **S96.012** Strain of muscle and tendon of long flexor muscle of toe at ankle and foot level, left foot

  √7ᵗʰ **S96.019** Strain of muscle and tendon of long flexor muscle of toe at ankle and foot level, unspecified foot

 √6ᵗʰ **S96.02** Laceration of muscle and tendon of long flexor muscle of toe at ankle and foot level

  √7ᵗʰ **S96.021** Laceration of muscle and tendon of long flexor muscle of toe at ankle and foot level, right foot   CC

  √7ᵗʰ **S96.022** Laceration of muscle and tendon of long flexor muscle of toe at ankle and foot level, left foot   CC

  √7ᵗʰ **S96.029** Laceration of muscle and tendon of long flexor muscle of toe at ankle and foot level, unspecified foot   CC

 √6ᵗʰ **S96.09** Other injury of muscle and tendon of long flexor muscle of toe at ankle and foot level

  √7ᵗʰ **S96.091** Other injury of muscle and tendon of long flexor muscle of toe at ankle and foot level, right foot

  √7ᵗʰ **S96.092** Other injury of muscle and tendon of long flexor muscle of toe at ankle and foot level, left foot

  √7ᵗʰ **S96.099** Other injury of muscle and tendon of long flexor muscle of toe at ankle and foot level, unspecified foot

√5ᵗʰ **S96.1** Injury of muscle and tendon of long extensor muscle of toe at ankle and foot level

 √6ᵗʰ **S96.10** Unspecified injury of muscle and tendon of long extensor muscle of toe at ankle and foot level

  √7ᵗʰ **S96.101** Unspecified injury of muscle and tendon of long extensor muscle of toe at ankle and foot level, right foot

  √7ᵗʰ **S96.102** Unspecified injury of muscle and tendon of long extensor muscle of toe at ankle and foot level, left foot

  √7ᵗʰ **S96.109** Unspecified injury of muscle and tendon of long extensor muscle of toe at ankle and foot level, unspecified foot

Chapter 19. Injury, Poisoning and Certain Other Consequences of External Causes

√6th **S96.11** Strain of muscle and tendon of long extensor muscle of toe at ankle and foot level

     √7th **S96.111** Strain of muscle and tendon of long extensor muscle of toe at ankle and foot level, right foot

     √7th **S96.112** Strain of muscle and tendon of long extensor muscle of toe at ankle and foot level, left foot

     √7th **S96.119** Strain of muscle and tendon of long extensor muscle of toe at ankle and foot level, unspecified foot

√6th **S96.12** Laceration of muscle and tendon of long extensor muscle of toe at ankle and foot level

     √7th **S96.121** Laceration of muscle and tendon of long extensor muscle of toe at ankle and foot level, right foot   CC

     √7th **S96.122** Laceration of muscle and tendon of long extensor muscle of toe at ankle and foot level, left foot   CC

     √7th **S96.129** Laceration of muscle and tendon of long extensor muscle of toe at ankle and foot level, unspecified foot   CC

√6th **S96.19** Other specified injury of muscle and tendon of long extensor muscle of toe at ankle and foot level

     √7th **S96.191** Other specified injury of muscle and tendon of long extensor muscle of toe at ankle and foot level, right foot

     √7th **S96.192** Other specified injury of muscle and tendon of long extensor muscle of toe at ankle and foot level, left foot

     √7th **S96.199** Other specified injury of muscle and tendon of long extensor muscle of toe at ankle and foot level, unspecified foot

√5th **S96.2** Injury of intrinsic muscle and tendon at ankle and foot level

√6th **S96.20** Unspecified injury of intrinsic muscle and tendon at ankle and foot level

     √7th **S96.201** Unspecified injury of intrinsic muscle and tendon at ankle and foot level, right foot

     √7th **S96.202** Unspecified injury of intrinsic muscle and tendon at ankle and foot level, left foot

     √7th **S96.209** Unspecified injury of intrinsic muscle and tendon at ankle and foot level, unspecified foot

√6th **S96.21** Strain of intrinsic muscle and tendon at ankle and foot level

     √7th **S96.211** Strain of intrinsic muscle and tendon at ankle and foot level, right foot

     √7th **S96.212** Strain of intrinsic muscle and tendon at ankle and foot level, left foot

     √7th **S96.219** Strain of intrinsic muscle and tendon at ankle and foot level, unspecified foot

√6th **S96.22** Laceration of intrinsic muscle and tendon at ankle and foot level

     √7th **S96.221** Laceration of intrinsic muscle and tendon at ankle and foot level, right foot   CC

     √7th **S96.222** Laceration of intrinsic muscle and tendon at ankle and foot level, left foot   CC

     √7th **S96.229** Laceration of intrinsic muscle and tendon at ankle and foot level, unspecified foot   CC

√6th **S96.29** Other specified injury of intrinsic muscle and tendon at ankle and foot level

     √7th **S96.291** Other specified injury of intrinsic muscle and tendon at ankle and foot level, right foot

     √7th **S96.292** Other specified injury of intrinsic muscle and tendon at ankle and foot level, left foot

     √7th **S96.299** Other specified injury of intrinsic muscle and tendon at ankle and foot level, unspecified foot

√5th **S96.8** Injury of other specified muscles and tendons at ankle and foot level

√6th **S96.80** Unspecified injury of other specified muscles and tendons at ankle and foot level

     √7th **S96.801** Unspecified injury of other specified muscles and tendons at ankle and foot level, right foot

     √7th **S96.802** Unspecified injury of other specified muscles and tendons at ankle and foot level, left foot

     √7th **S96.809** Unspecified injury of other specified muscles and tendons at ankle and foot level, unspecified foot

√6th **S96.81** Strain of other specified muscles and tendons at ankle and foot level

     √7th **S96.811** Strain of other specified muscles and tendons at ankle and foot level, right foot

     √7th **S96.812** Strain of other specified muscles and tendons at ankle and foot level, left foot

     √7th **S96.819** Strain of other specified muscles and tendons at ankle and foot level, unspecified foot

√6th **S96.82** Laceration of other specified muscles and tendons at ankle and foot level

     √7th **S96.821** Laceration of other specified muscles and tendons at ankle and foot level, right foot   CC

     √7th **S96.822** Laceration of other specified muscles and tendons at ankle and foot level, left foot   CC

     √7th **S96.829** Laceration of other specified muscles and tendons at ankle and foot level, unspecified foot   CC

√6th **S96.89** Other specified injury of other specified muscles and tendons at ankle and foot level

     √7th **S96.891** Other specified injury of other specified muscles and tendons at ankle and foot level, right foot

     √7th **S96.892** Other specified injury of other specified muscles and tendons at ankle and foot level, left foot

     √7th **S96.899** Other specified injury of other specified muscles and tendons at ankle and foot level, unspecified foot

√5th **S96.9** Injury of unspecified muscle and tendon at ankle and foot level

√6th **S96.90** Unspecified injury of unspecified muscle and tendon at ankle and foot level

     √7th **S96.901** Unspecified injury of unspecified muscle and tendon at ankle and foot level, right foot

     √7th **S96.902** Unspecified injury of unspecified muscle and tendon at ankle and foot level, left foot

     √7th **S96.909** Unspecified injury of unspecified muscle and tendon at ankle and foot level, unspecified foot

√6th **S96.91** Strain of unspecified muscle and tendon at ankle and foot level

     √7th **S96.911** Strain of unspecified muscle and tendon at ankle and foot level, right foot

     √7th **S96.912** Strain of unspecified muscle and tendon at ankle and foot level, left foot

     √7th **S96.919** Strain of unspecified muscle and tendon at ankle and foot level, unspecified foot

√6th **S96.92** Laceration of unspecified muscle and tendon at ankle and foot level

     √7th **S96.921** Laceration of unspecified muscle and tendon at ankle and foot level, right foot   CC

     √7th **S96.922** Laceration of unspecified muscle and tendon at ankle and foot level, left foot   CC

     √7th **S96.929** Laceration of unspecified muscle and tendon at ankle and foot level, unspecified foot   CC

N Newborn: 0   P Pediatric: 0-17   M Maternity: 12-55   A Adult: 15-124   MCC Major CC Condition   PDxMCC PDx acts as own MCC   CC CC Condition   PDxCC PDx acts as own CC

1074   ICD-10-CM 2018

√6ᵗʰ **S96.99** Other specified injury of unspecified muscle and tendon at ankle and foot level

     √7ᵗʰ **S96.991** Other specified injury of unspecified muscle and tendon at ankle and foot level, right foot

     √7ᵗʰ **S96.992** Other specified injury of unspecified muscle and tendon at ankle and foot level, left foot

     √7ᵗʰ **S96.999** Other specified injury of unspecified muscle and tendon at ankle and foot level, unspecified foot

√4ᵗʰ **S97** Crushing injury of ankle and foot

     Use additional code(s) for all associated injuries

     The appropriate 7th character is to be added to each code from category S97.
     A   initial encounter
     D   subsequent encounter
     S   sequela

√5ᵗʰ **S97.0** Crushing injury of ankle

     √x7ᵗʰ **S97.00** Crushing injury of unspecified ankle

     √x7ᵗʰ **S97.01** Crushing injury of right ankle

     √x7ᵗʰ **S97.02** Crushing injury of left ankle

√5ᵗʰ **S97.1** Crushing injury of toe

     √6ᵗʰ **S97.10** Crushing injury of unspecified toe(s)

         √7ᵗʰ **S97.101** Crushing injury of unspecified right toe(s)

         √7ᵗʰ **S97.102** Crushing injury of unspecified left toe(s)

         √7ᵗʰ **S97.109** Crushing injury of unspecified toe(s)
            Crushing injury of toe NOS

     √6ᵗʰ **S97.11** Crushing injury of great toe

         √7ᵗʰ **S97.111** Crushing injury of right great toe

         √7ᵗʰ **S97.112** Crushing injury of left great toe

         √7ᵗʰ **S97.119** Crushing injury of unspecified great toe

     √6ᵗʰ **S97.12** Crushing injury of lesser toe(s)

         √7ᵗʰ **S97.121** Crushing injury of right lesser toe(s)

         √7ᵗʰ **S97.122** Crushing injury of left lesser toe(s)

         √7ᵗʰ **S97.129** Crushing injury of unspecified lesser toe(s)

√5ᵗʰ **S97.8** Crushing injury of foot

     √x7ᵗʰ **S97.80** Crushing injury of unspecified foot
         Crushing injury of foot NOS

     √x7ᵗʰ **S97.81** Crushing injury of right foot

     √x7ᵗʰ **S97.82** Crushing injury of left foot

√4ᵗʰ **S98** Traumatic amputation of ankle and foot

     An amputation not identified as partial or complete should be coded to complete

     The appropriate 7th character is to be added to each code from category S98.
     A   initial encounter
     D   subsequent encounter
     S   sequela

     CC Excl: For CC codes in category S98:
     Right side: PDX collection 1333
     Left side: PDX collection 1334
     Unspecified side: PDX collection 1335

√5ᵗʰ **S98.0** Traumatic amputation of foot at ankle level

     √6ᵗʰ **S98.01** Complete traumatic amputation of foot at ankle level

         √7ᵗʰ **S98.011** Complete traumatic amputation of right foot at ankle level   CC HCC

         √7ᵗʰ **S98.012** Complete traumatic amputation of left foot at ankle level   CC HCC

         √7ᵗʰ **S98.019** Complete traumatic amputation of unspecified foot at ankle level   CC HCC

     √6ᵗʰ **S98.02** Partial traumatic amputation of foot at ankle level

         √7ᵗʰ **S98.021** Partial traumatic amputation of right foot at ankle level   CC HCC

         √7ᵗʰ **S98.022** Partial traumatic amputation of left foot at ankle level   CC HCC

         √7ᵗʰ **S98.029** Partial traumatic amputation of unspecified foot at ankle level   CC HCC

√5ᵗʰ **S98.1** Traumatic amputation of one toe

     √6ᵗʰ **S98.11** Complete traumatic amputation of great toe

         √7ᵗʰ **S98.111** Complete traumatic amputation of right great toe   HCC

         √7ᵗʰ **S98.112** Complete traumatic amputation of left great toe   HCC

         √7ᵗʰ **S98.119** Complete traumatic amputation of unspecified great toe   HCC

     √6ᵗʰ **S98.12** Partial traumatic amputation of great toe

         √7ᵗʰ **S98.121** Partial traumatic amputation of right great toe   HCC

         √7ᵗʰ **S98.122** Partial traumatic amputation of left great toe   HCC

         √7ᵗʰ **S98.129** Partial traumatic amputation of unspecified great toe   HCC

     √6ᵗʰ **S98.13** Complete traumatic amputation of one lesser toe
         Traumatic amputation of toe NOS

         √7ᵗʰ **S98.131** Complete traumatic amputation of one right lesser toe   HCC

         √7ᵗʰ **S98.132** Complete traumatic amputation of one left lesser toe   HCC

         √7ᵗʰ **S98.139** Complete traumatic amputation of one unspecified lesser toe   HCC

     √6ᵗʰ **S98.14** Partial traumatic amputation of one lesser toe

         √7ᵗʰ **S98.141** Partial traumatic amputation of one right lesser toe   HCC

         √7ᵗʰ **S98.142** Partial traumatic amputation of one left lesser toe   HCC

         √7ᵗʰ **S98.149** Partial traumatic amputation of one unspecified lesser toe   HCC

√5ᵗʰ **S98.2** Traumatic amputation of two or more lesser toes

     √6ᵗʰ **S98.21** Complete traumatic amputation of two or more lesser toes

         √7ᵗʰ **S98.211** Complete traumatic amputation of two or more right lesser toes   HCC

         √7ᵗʰ **S98.212** Complete traumatic amputation of two or more left lesser toes   HCC

         √7ᵗʰ **S98.219** Complete traumatic amputation of two or more unspecified lesser toes   HCC

     √6ᵗʰ **S98.22** Partial traumatic amputation of two or more lesser toes

         √7ᵗʰ **S98.221** Partial traumatic amputation of two or more right lesser toes   HCC

         √7ᵗʰ **S98.222** Partial traumatic amputation of two or more left lesser toes   HCC

         √7ᵗʰ **S98.229** Partial traumatic amputation of two or more unspecified lesser toes   HCC

√5ᵗʰ **S98.3** Traumatic amputation of midfoot

     √6ᵗʰ **S98.31** Complete traumatic amputation of midfoot

         √7ᵗʰ **S98.311** Complete traumatic amputation of right midfoot   CC HCC

         √7ᵗʰ **S98.312** Complete traumatic amputation of left midfoot   CC HCC

         √7ᵗʰ **S98.319** Complete traumatic amputation of unspecified midfoot   CC HCC

     √6ᵗʰ **S98.32** Partial traumatic amputation of midfoot

         √7ᵗʰ **S98.321** Partial traumatic amputation of right midfoot   CC HCC

         √7ᵗʰ **S98.322** Partial traumatic amputation of left midfoot   CC HCC

         √7ᵗʰ **S98.329** Partial traumatic amputation of unspecified midfoot   CC HCC

√5ᵗʰ **S98.9** Traumatic amputation of foot, level unspecified

     √6ᵗʰ **S98.91** Complete traumatic amputation of foot, level unspecified

         √7ᵗʰ **S98.911** Complete traumatic amputation of right foot, level unspecified   CC HCC

         √7ᵗʰ **S98.912** Complete traumatic amputation of left foot, level unspecified   CC HCC

         √7ᵗʰ **S98.919** Complete traumatic amputation of unspecified foot, level unspecified   CC HCC

✔Additional Character Req   √x7ᵗʰ Placeholder Alert   Unacceptable PDx   Manifestation   H1 - H14 HAC   HCC CMS-HCC Condition   *EXCLUDES 1* Not Coded Here   *EXCLUDES 2* Not Included Here

ICD-10-CM 2018   **1075**

✓6ᵗʰ **S98.92　Partial** traumatic amputation of foot, level unspecified

 ✓7ᵗʰ **S98.921　Partial** traumatic amputation of **right** foot, level unspecified　CC HCC

 ✓7ᵗʰ **S98.922　Partial** traumatic amputation of **left** foot, level unspecified　CC HCC

 ✓7ᵗʰ **S98.929　Partial** traumatic amputation of **unspecified** foot, level unspecified　CC HCC

✓4ᵗʰ **S99　Other and unspecified injuries of ankle and foot**

 ✓5ᵗʰ **S99.0　Physeal fracture of** calcaneus

> The appropriate 7th character is to be added to each code from subcategories S99.0.
> A initial encounter for closed fracture
> B initial encounter for open fracture
> D subsequent encounter for fracture with routine healing
> G subsequent encounter for fracture with delayed healing
> K subsequent encounter for fracture with nonunion
> P subsequent encounter for fracture with malunion
> S sequela

 ✓6ᵗʰ **S99.00　Unspecified** physeal fracture of calcaneus

  ✓7ᵗʰ **S99.001　Unspecified** physeal fracture of **right** calcaneus

  ✓7ᵗʰ **S99.002　Unspecified** physeal fracture of **left** calcaneus

  ✓7ᵗʰ **S99.009　Unspecified** physeal fracture of **unspecified** calcaneus

 ✓6ᵗʰ **S99.01　Salter-Harris Type I** physeal fracture of calcaneus

  ✓7ᵗʰ **S99.011　Salter-Harris Type I** physeal fracture of **right** calcaneus

  ✓7ᵗʰ **S99.012　Salter-Harris Type I** physeal fracture of **left** calcaneus

  ✓7ᵗʰ **S99.019　Salter-Harris Type I** physeal fracture of **unspecified** calcaneus

 ✓6ᵗʰ **S99.02　Salter-Harris Type II** physeal fracture of calcaneus

  ✓7ᵗʰ **S99.021　Salter-Harris Type II** physeal fracture of **right** calcaneus

  ✓7ᵗʰ **S99.022　Salter-Harris Type II** physeal fracture of **left** calcaneus

  ✓7ᵗʰ **S99.029　Salter-Harris Type II** physeal fracture of **unspecified** calcaneus

 ✓6ᵗʰ **S99.03　Salter-Harris Type III** physeal fracture of calcaneus

  ✓7ᵗʰ **S99.031　Salter-Harris Type III** physeal fracture of **right** calcaneus

  ✓7ᵗʰ **S99.032　Salter-Harris Type III** physeal fracture of **left** calcaneus

  ✓7ᵗʰ **S99.039　Salter-Harris Type III** physeal fracture of **unspecified** calcaneus

 ✓6ᵗʰ **S99.04　Salter-Harris Type IV** physeal fracture of calcaneus

  ✓7ᵗʰ **S99.041　Salter-Harris Type IV** physeal fracture of **right** calcaneus

  ✓7ᵗʰ **S99.042　Salter-Harris Type IV** physeal fracture of **left** calcaneus

  ✓7ᵗʰ **S99.049　Salter-Harris Type IV** physeal fracture of **unspecified** calcaneus

 ✓6ᵗʰ **S99.09　Other** physeal fracture of calcaneus

  ✓7ᵗʰ **S99.091　Other** physeal fracture of **right** calcaneus

  ✓7ᵗʰ **S99.092　Other** physeal fracture of **left** calcaneus

  ✓7ᵗʰ **S99.099　Other** physeal fracture of **unspecified** calcaneus

 ✓5ᵗʰ **S99.1　Physeal fracture of** metatarsal

> The appropriate 7th character is to be added to each code from subcategories S99.1.
> A initial encounter for closed fracture
> B initial encounter for open fracture
> D subsequent encounter for fracture with routine healing
> G subsequent encounter for fracture with delayed healing
> K subsequent encounter for fracture with nonunion
> P subsequent encounter for fracture with malunion
> S sequela

 ✓6ᵗʰ **S99.10　Unspecified** physeal fracture of metatarsal

  ✓7ᵗʰ **S99.101　Unspecified** physeal fracture of **right** metatarsal

  ✓7ᵗʰ **S99.102　Unspecified** physeal fracture of **left** metatarsal

  ✓7ᵗʰ **S99.109　Unspecified** physeal fracture of **unspecified** metatarsal

 ✓6ᵗʰ **S99.11　Salter-Harris Type I** physeal fracture of metatarsal

  ✓7ᵗʰ **S99.111　Salter-Harris Type I** physeal fracture of **right** metatarsal

  ✓7ᵗʰ **S99.112　Salter-Harris Type I** physeal fracture of **left** metatarsal

  ✓7ᵗʰ **S99.119　Salter-Harris Type I** physeal fracture of **unspecified** metatarsal

 ✓6ᵗʰ **S99.12　Salter-Harris Type II** physeal fracture of metatarsal

  ✓7ᵗʰ **S99.121　Salter-Harris Type II** physeal fracture of **right** metatarsal

  ✓7ᵗʰ **S99.122　Salter-Harris Type II** physeal fracture of **left** metatarsal

  ✓7ᵗʰ **S99.129　Salter-Harris Type II** physeal fracture of **unspecified** metatarsal

 ✓6ᵗʰ **S99.13　Salter-Harris Type III** physeal fracture of metatarsal

  ✓7ᵗʰ **S99.131　Salter-Harris Type III** physeal fracture of **right** metatarsal

  ✓7ᵗʰ **S99.132　Salter-Harris Type III** physeal fracture of **left** metatarsal

  ✓7ᵗʰ **S99.139　Salter-Harris Type III** physeal fracture of **unspecified** metatarsal

 ✓6ᵗʰ **S99.14　Salter-Harris Type IV** physeal fracture of metatarsal

  ✓7ᵗʰ **S99.141　Salter-Harris Type IV** physeal fracture of **right** metatarsal

  ✓7ᵗʰ **S99.142　Salter-Harris Type IV** physeal fracture of **left** metatarsal

  ✓7ᵗʰ **S99.149　Salter-Harris Type IV** physeal fracture of **unspecified** metatarsal

 ✓6ᵗʰ **S99.19　Other** physeal fracture of metatarsal

  ✓7ᵗʰ **S99.191　Other** physeal fracture of **right** metatarsal

  ✓7ᵗʰ **S99.192　Other** physeal fracture of **left** metatarsal

  ✓7ᵗʰ **S99.199　Other** physeal fracture of **unspecified** metatarsal

 ✓5ᵗʰ **S99.2　Physeal fracture of** phalanx of toe

> The appropriate 7th character is to be added to each code from subcategories S99.2.
> A initial encounter for closed fracture
> B initial encounter for open fracture
> D subsequent encounter for fracture with routine healing
> G subsequent encounter for fracture with delayed healing
> K subsequent encounter for fracture with nonunion
> P subsequent encounter for fracture with malunion
> S sequela

 ✓6ᵗʰ **S99.20　Unspecified** physeal fracture of phalanx of toe

  ✓7ᵗʰ **S99.201　Unspecified** physeal fracture of phalanx of **right** toe

  ✓7ᵗʰ **S99.202　Unspecified** physeal fracture of phalanx of **left** toe

  ✓7ᵗʰ **S99.209　Unspecified** physeal fracture of phalanx of **unspecified** toe

 ✓6ᵗʰ **S99.21　Salter-Harris Type I** physeal fracture of phalanx of toe

  ✓7ᵗʰ **S99.211　Salter-Harris Type I** physeal fracture of phalanx of **right** toe

  ✓7ᵗʰ **S99.212　Salter-Harris Type I** physeal fracture of phalanx of **left** toe

  ✓7ᵗʰ **S99.219　Salter-Harris Type I** physeal fracture of phalanx of **unspecified** toe

 ✓6ᵗʰ **S99.22　Salter-Harris Type II** physeal fracture of phalanx of toe

  ✓7ᵗʰ **S99.221　Salter-Harris Type II** physeal fracture of phalanx of **right** toe

  ✓7ᵗʰ **S99.222　Salter-Harris Type II** physeal fracture of phalanx of **left** toe

  ✓7ᵗʰ **S99.229　Salter-Harris Type II** physeal fracture of phalanx of **unspecified** toe

 ✓6ᵗʰ **S99.23　Salter-Harris Type III** physeal fracture of phalanx of toe

  ✓7ᵗʰ **S99.231　Salter-Harris Type III** physeal fracture of phalanx of **right** toe

  ✓7ᵗʰ **S99.232　Salter-Harris Type III** physeal fracture of phalanx of **left** toe

---

N Newborn: 0　P Pediatric: 0-17　M Maternity: 12-55　A Adult: 15-124　MCC Major CC Condition　PDxMCC PDx acts as own MCC　CC CC Condition　PDxCC PDx acts as own CC

1076

ICD-10-CM 2018

✓7ᵗʰ **S99.239** Salter-Harris Type III physeal fracture of phalanx of unspecified toe

✓6ᵗʰ **S99.24** Salter-Harris Type IV physeal fracture of phalanx of toe

     ✓7ᵗʰ **S99.241** Salter-Harris Type IV physeal fracture of phalanx of right toe

     ✓7ᵗʰ **S99.242** Salter-Harris Type IV physeal fracture of phalanx of left toe

     ✓7ᵗʰ **S99.249** Salter-Harris Type IV physeal fracture of phalanx of unspecified toe

✓6ᵗʰ **S99.29** Other physeal fracture of phalanx of toe

     ✓7ᵗʰ **S99.291** Other physeal fracture of phalanx of right toe

     ✓7ᵗʰ **S99.292** Other physeal fracture of phalanx of left toe

     ✓7ᵗʰ **S99.299** Other physeal fracture of phalanx of unspecified toe

✓5ᵗʰ **S99.8** Other specified injuries of ankle and foot

The appropriate 7th character is to be added to each code from subcategory S99.8.
A   initial encounter
D   subsequent encounter
S   sequela

✓6ᵗʰ **S99.81** Other specified injuries of ankle

     ✓7ᵗʰ **S99.811** Other specified injuries of right ankle

     ✓7ᵗʰ **S99.812** Other specified injuries of left ankle

     ✓7ᵗʰ **S99.819** Other specified injuries of unspecified ankle

✓6ᵗʰ **S99.82** Other specified injuries of foot

     ✓7ᵗʰ **S99.821** Other specified injuries of right foot

     ✓7ᵗʰ **S99.822** Other specified injuries of left foot

     ✓7ᵗʰ **S99.829** Other specified injuries of unspecified foot

✓5ᵗʰ **S99.9** Unspecified injury of ankle and foot

The appropriate 7th character is to be added to each code from subcategory S99.9.
A   initial encounter
D   subsequent encounter
S   sequela

✓6ᵗʰ **S99.91** Unspecified injury of ankle

     ✓7ᵗʰ **S99.911** Unspecified injury of right ankle

     ✓7ᵗʰ **S99.912** Unspecified injury of left ankle

     ✓7ᵗʰ **S99.919** Unspecified injury of unspecified ankle

✓6ᵗʰ **S99.92** Unspecified injury of foot

     ✓7ᵗʰ **S99.921** Unspecified injury of right foot

     ✓7ᵗʰ **S99.922** Unspecified injury of left foot

     ✓7ᵗʰ **S99.929** Unspecified injury of unspecified foot

Injury, Poisoning And Certain Other Consequences Of External Causes (T07-T88)

Injuries involving multiple body regions (T07)

EXCLUDES 1   burns and corrosions (T20-T32)
frostbite (T33-T34)
insect bite or sting, venomous (T63.4)
sunburn (L55.-)

✓x7ᵗʰ **T07** Unspecified multiple injuries

EXCLUDES 1   injury NOS ▶(T14.90)◀

The appropriate 7th character is to be added to code T07.
A   initial encounter
D   subsequent encounter
S   sequela

Injury of unspecified body region (T14)

✓4ᵗʰ **T14** Injury of unspecified body region

EXCLUDES 1   multiple unspecified injuries (T07)

The appropriate 7th character is to be added to each code from category T14.
A   initial encounter
D   subsequent encounter
S   sequela

✓x7ᵗʰ **T14.8** Other injury of unspecified body region
Abrasion NOS
Contusion NOS
Crush injury NOS
Fracture NOS
Skin injury NOS
Vascular injury NOS
▶Wound NOS◀

✓5ᵗʰ **T14.9** Unspecified injury

     ✓x7ᵗʰ **T14.90** Injury, unspecified
Injury NOS

     ✓x7ᵗʰ **T14.91** Suicide attempt   HCC
Attempted suicide NOS

Effects of foreign body entering through natural orifice (T15-T19)

EXCLUDES 2   foreign body accidentally left in operation wound (T81.5-)
foreign body in penetrating wound—See open wound by body region
residual foreign body in soft tissue (M79.5)
splinter, without open wound—See superficial injury by body region

✓4ᵗʰ **T15** Foreign body on external eye

EXCLUDES 2   foreign body in penetrating wound of orbit and eye ball (S05.4-, S05.5-)
open wound of eyelid and periocular area (S01.1-)
retained foreign body in eyelid (H02.8-)
retained (old) foreign body in penetrating wound of orbit and eye ball (H05.5-, H44.6-, H44.7-)
superficial foreign body of eyelid and periocular area (S00.25-)

The appropriate 7th character is to be added to each code from category T15.
A   initial encounter
D   subsequent encounter
S   sequela

✓5ᵗʰ **T15.0** Foreign body in cornea

     ✓x7ᵗʰ **T15.00** Foreign body in cornea, unspecified eye

     ✓x7ᵗʰ **T15.01** Foreign body in cornea, right eye

     ✓x7ᵗʰ **T15.02** Foreign body in cornea, left eye

✓5ᵗʰ **T15.1** Foreign body in conjunctival sac

     ✓x7ᵗʰ **T15.10** Foreign body in conjunctival sac, unspecified eye

     ✓x7ᵗʰ **T15.11** Foreign body in conjunctival sac, right eye

     ✓x7ᵗʰ **T15.12** Foreign body in conjunctival sac, left eye

✓5ᵗʰ **T15.8** Foreign body in other and multiple parts of external eye
Foreign body in lacrimal punctum

     ✓x7ᵗʰ **T15.80** Foreign body in other and multiple parts of external eye, unspecified eye

     ✓x7ᵗʰ **T15.81** Foreign body in other and multiple parts of external eye, right eye

     ✓x7ᵗʰ **T15.82** Foreign body in other and multiple parts of external eye, left eye

✓5ᵗʰ **T15.9** Foreign body on external eye, part unspecified

     ✓x7ᵗʰ **T15.90** Foreign body on external eye, part unspecified, unspecified eye

     ✓x7ᵗʰ **T15.91** Foreign body on external eye, part unspecified, right eye

     ✓x7ᵗʰ **T15.92** Foreign body on external eye, part unspecified, left eye

✓4ᵗʰ **T16** Foreign body in ear

INCLUDES   foreign body in auditory canal

The appropriate 7th character is to be added to each code from category T16.
A   initial encounter
D   subsequent encounter
S   sequela

✓x7ᵗʰ **T16.1** Foreign body in right ear

✓x7ᵗʰ **T16.2** Foreign body in left ear

✓x7ᵗʰ **T16.9** Foreign body in ear, unspecified ear

✓ Additional Character Req   ✓x7ᵗʰ Placeholder Alert   Unacceptable PDx   Manifestation   H1-H14 HAC   HCC CMS-HCC Condition   EXCLUDES 1 Not Coded Here   EXCLUDES 2 Not Included Here

ICD-10-CM 2018   **1077**

✓4ᵗʰ **T17**   **Foreign body in respiratory tract**

> The appropriate 7th character is to be added to each code from category T17.
> A   initial encounter
> D   subsequent encounter
> S   sequela

✓x7ᵗʰ **T17.0**   **Foreign body in** nasal sinus

✓x7ᵗʰ **T17.1**   **Foreign body in** nostril
     Foreign body in nose NOS

✓5ᵗʰ **T17.2**   **Foreign body in** pharynx
     Foreign body in nasopharynx
     Foreign body in throat NOS

   ✓6ᵗʰ **T17.20**   **Unspecified foreign body in pharynx**
     ✓7ᵗʰ **T17.200**   **Unspecified foreign body in pharynx causing asphyxiation**
     ✓7ᵗʰ **T17.208**   **Unspecified foreign body in pharynx causing other injury**

   ✓6ᵗʰ **T17.21**   **Gastric contents in pharynx**
     Aspiration of gastric contents into pharynx
     Vomitus in pharynx
     ✓7ᵗʰ **T17.210**   **Gastric contents in pharynx causing asphyxiation**
     ✓7ᵗʰ **T17.218**   **Gastric contents in pharynx causing other injury**

   ✓6ᵗʰ **T17.22**   **Food in pharynx**
     Bones in pharynx
     Seeds in pharynx
     ✓7ᵗʰ **T17.220**   **Food in pharynx causing asphyxiation**
     ✓7ᵗʰ **T17.228**   **Food in pharynx causing other injury**

   ✓6ᵗʰ **T17.29**   **Other foreign object in pharynx**
     ✓7ᵗʰ **T17.290**   **Other foreign object in pharynx causing asphyxiation**
     ✓7ᵗʰ **T17.298**   **Other foreign object in pharynx causing other injury**

✓5ᵗʰ **T17.3**   **Foreign body in** larynx

   ✓6ᵗʰ **T17.30**   **Unspecified foreign body in larynx**
     ✓7ᵗʰ **T17.300**   **Unspecified foreign body in larynx causing asphyxiation**
     ✓7ᵗʰ **T17.308**   **Unspecified foreign body in larynx causing other injury**

   ✓6ᵗʰ **T17.31**   **Gastric contents in larynx**
     Aspiration of gastric contents into larynx
     Vomitus in larynx
     ✓7ᵗʰ **T17.310**   **Gastric contents in larynx causing asphyxiation**
     ✓7ᵗʰ **T17.318**   **Gastric contents in larynx causing other injury**

   ✓6ᵗʰ **T17.32**   **Food in larynx**
     Bones in larynx
     Seeds in larynx
     ✓7ᵗʰ **T17.320**   **Food in larynx causing asphyxiation**
     ✓7ᵗʰ **T17.328**   **Food in larynx causing other injury**

   ✓6ᵗʰ **T17.39**   **Other foreign object in larynx**
     ✓7ᵗʰ **T17.390**   **Other foreign object in larynx causing asphyxiation**
     ✓7ᵗʰ **T17.398**   **Other foreign object in larynx causing other injury**

✓5ᵗʰ **T17.4**   **Foreign body in** trachea

> **CC Excl: For codes in subcategory T17.4:**
> PDX collection 1373

   ✓6ᵗʰ **T17.40**   **Unspecified foreign body in trachea**
     ✓7ᵗʰ **T17.400**   **Unspecified foreign body in trachea causing asphyxiation** `CC`
     ✓7ᵗʰ **T17.408**   **Unspecified foreign body in trachea causing other injury** `CC`

   ✓6ᵗʰ **T17.41**   **Gastric contents in trachea**
     Aspiration of gastric contents into trachea
     Vomitus in trachea
     ✓7ᵗʰ **T17.410**   **Gastric contents in trachea causing asphyxiation** `CC`
     ✓7ᵗʰ **T17.418**   **Gastric contents in trachea causing other injury** `CC`

   ✓6ᵗʰ **T17.42**   **Food in trachea**
     Bones in trachea   Seeds in trachea
     ✓7ᵗʰ **T17.420**   **Food in trachea causing asphyxiation** `CC`
     ✓7ᵗʰ **T17.428**   **Food in trachea causing other injury** `CC`

   ✓6ᵗʰ **T17.49**   **Other foreign object in trachea**
     ✓7ᵗʰ **T17.490**   **Other foreign object in trachea causing asphyxiation**
     ✓7ᵗʰ **T17.498**   **Other foreign object in trachea causing other injury**

✓5ᵗʰ **T17.5**   **Foreign body in** bronchus

> **CC Excl: For codes in subcategory T17.5:**
> PDX collection 1374

   ✓6ᵗʰ **T17.50**   **Unspecified foreign body in bronchus**
     ✓7ᵗʰ **T17.500**   **Unspecified foreign body in bronchus causing asphyxiation** `CC`
     ✓7ᵗʰ **T17.508**   **Unspecified foreign body in bronchus causing other injury** `CC`

   ✓6ᵗʰ **T17.51**   **Gastric contents in bronchus**
     Aspiration of gastric contents into bronchus
     Vomitus in bronchus
     ✓7ᵗʰ **T17.510**   **Gastric contents in bronchus causing asphyxiation** `CC`
     ✓7ᵗʰ **T17.518**   **Gastric contents in bronchus causing other injury** `CC`

   ✓6ᵗʰ **T17.52**   **Food in bronchus**
     Bones in bronchus
     Seeds in bronchus
     ✓7ᵗʰ **T17.520**   **Food in bronchus causing asphyxiation** `CC`
     ✓7ᵗʰ **T17.528**   **Food in bronchus causing other injury** `CC`

   ✓6ᵗʰ **T17.59**   **Other foreign object in bronchus**
     ✓7ᵗʰ **T17.590**   **Other foreign object in bronchus causing asphyxiation** `CC`
     ✓7ᵗʰ **T17.598**   **Other foreign object in bronchus causing other injury** `CC`

✓5ᵗʰ **T17.8**   **Foreign body in** other parts **of respiratory tract**
     Foreign body in bronchioles
     Foreign body in lung

> **CC Excl: For codes in subcategory T17.8, unless otherwise noted:** PDX collection 1374

   ✓6ᵗʰ **T17.80**   **Unspecified foreign body in other parts of respiratory tract**
     ✓7ᵗʰ **T17.800**   **Unspecified foreign body in other parts of respiratory tract causing asphyxiation** `CC`
     ✓7ᵗʰ **T17.808**   **Unspecified foreign body in other parts of respiratory tract causing other injury** `CC`

   ✓6ᵗʰ **T17.81**   **Gastric contents in other parts of respiratory tract**
     Aspiration of gastric contents into other parts of respiratory tract
     Vomitus in other parts of respiratory tract
     ✓7ᵗʰ **T17.810**   **Gastric contents in other parts of respiratory tract causing asphyxiation** `CC`
     ✓7ᵗʰ **T17.818**   **Gastric contents in other parts of respiratory tract causing other injury** `CC`

   ✓6ᵗʰ **T17.82**   **Food in other parts of respiratory tract**
     Bones in other parts of respiratory tract
     Seeds in other parts of respiratory tract
     ✓7ᵗʰ **T17.820**   **Food in other parts of respiratory tract causing asphyxiation** `CC`
     ✓7ᵗʰ **T17.828**   **Food in other parts of respiratory tract causing other injury** `CC`

   ✓6ᵗʰ **T17.89**   **Other foreign object in other parts of respiratory tract**
     ✓7ᵗʰ **T17.890**   **Other foreign object in other parts of respiratory tract causing asphyxiation** `CC`
     ✓7ᵗʰ **T17.898**   **Other foreign object in other parts of respiratory tract causing other injury** `CC`

✓5ᵗʰ **T17.9**   **Foreign body in respiratory tract, part unspecified**
   ✓6ᵗʰ **T17.90**   **Unspecified foreign body in respiratory tract, part unspecified**

☑7ᵗʰ **T17.900** Unspecified foreign body in respiratory tract, part unspecified causing asphyxiation

☑7ᵗʰ **T17.908** Unspecified foreign body in respiratory tract, part unspecified causing other injury

☑6ᵗʰ **T17.91** Gastric contents in respiratory tract, part unspecified
Aspiration of gastric contents into respiratory tract, part unspecified
Vomitus in trachea respiratory tract, part unspecified

☑7ᵗʰ **T17.910** Gastric contents in respiratory tract, part unspecified causing asphyxiation

☑7ᵗʰ **T17.918** Gastric contents in respiratory tract, part unspecified causing other injury

☑6ᵗʰ **T17.92** Food in respiratory tract, part unspecified
Bones in respiratory tract, part unspecified
Seeds in respiratory tract, part unspecified

☑7ᵗʰ **T17.920** Food in respiratory tract, part unspecified causing asphyxiation

☑7ᵗʰ **T17.928** Food in respiratory tract, part unspecified causing other injury

☑6ᵗʰ **T17.99** Other foreign object in respiratory tract, part unspecified

☑7ᵗʰ **T17.990** Other foreign object in respiratory tract, part unspecified in causing asphyxiation

☑7ᵗʰ **T17.998** Other foreign object in respiratory tract, part unspecified causing other injury

☑4ᵗʰ **T18 Foreign body in alimentary tract**
EXCLUDES 2 foreign body in pharynx (T17.2-)

The appropriate 7th character is to be added to each code from category T18.
A   initial encounter
D   subsequent encounter
S   sequela

☑x7ᵗʰ **T18.0 Foreign body in mouth**

☑5ᵗʰ **T18.1 Foreign body in esophagus**
EXCLUDES 2 foreign body in respiratory tract (T17.-)

☑6ᵗʰ **T18.10** Unspecified foreign body in esophagus

☑7ᵗʰ **T18.100** Unspecified foreign body in esophagus causing compression of trachea
Unspecified foreign body in esophagus causing obstruction of respiration

☑7ᵗʰ **T18.108** Unspecified foreign body in esophagus causing other injury

☑6ᵗʰ **T18.11** Gastric contents in esophagus
Vomitus in esophagus

☑7ᵗʰ **T18.110** Gastric contents in esophagus causing compression of trachea
Gastric contents in esophagus causing obstruction of respiration

☑7ᵗʰ **T18.118** Gastric contents in esophagus causing other injury

☑6ᵗʰ **T18.12** Food in esophagus
Bones in esophagus
Seeds in esophagus

☑7ᵗʰ **T18.120** Food in esophagus causing compression of trachea
Food in esophagus causing obstruction of respiration

☑7ᵗʰ **T18.128** Food in esophagus causing other injury

☑6ᵗʰ **T18.19** Other foreign object in esophagus
AHA: 2015, 1Q, 23

☑7ᵗʰ **T18.190** Other foreign object in esophagus causing compression of trachea
Other foreign body in esophagus causing obstruction of respiration

☑7ᵗʰ **T18.198** Other foreign object in esophagus causing other injury

☑x7ᵗʰ **T18.2 Foreign body in stomach**

☑x7ᵗʰ **T18.3 Foreign body in small intestine**

☑x7ᵗʰ **T18.4 Foreign body in colon**

☑x7ᵗʰ **T18.5 Foreign body in anus and rectum**
Foreign body in rectosigmoid (junction)

☑x7ᵗʰ **T18.8 Foreign body in other parts of alimentary tract**

☑x7ᵗʰ **T18.9 Foreign body of alimentary tract, part unspecified**
Foreign body in digestive system NOS
Swallowed foreign body NOS

☑4ᵗʰ **T19 Foreign body in genitourinary tract**
EXCLUDES 2 complications due to implanted mesh (T83.7-)
mechanical complications of contraceptive device (intrauterine) (vaginal) (T83.3-)
presence of contraceptive device (intrauterine) (vaginal) (Z97.5)

The appropriate 7th character is to be added to each code from category T19.
A   initial encounter
D   subsequent encounter
S   sequela

☑x7ᵗʰ **T19.0 Foreign body in urethra**

☑x7ᵗʰ **T19.1 Foreign body in bladder**

☑x7ᵗʰ **T19.2 Foreign body in vulva and vagina** ♀

☑x7ᵗʰ **T19.3 Foreign body in uterus** ♀

☑x7ᵗʰ **T19.4 Foreign body in penis** ♂

☑x7ᵗʰ **T19.8 Foreign body in other parts of genitourinary tract**

☑x7ᵗʰ **T19.9 Foreign body in genitourinary tract, part unspecified**

Burns and corrosions (T20-T32)

INCLUDES burns (thermal) from electrical heating appliances
burns (thermal) from electricity
burns (thermal) from flame
burns (thermal) from friction
burns (thermal) from hot air and hot gases
burns (thermal) from hot objects
burns (thermal) from lightning
burns (thermal) from radiation
chemical burn [corrosion] (external) (internal)
scalds
EXCLUDES 2 erythema [dermatitis] ab igne (L59.0)
radiation-related disorders of the skin and subcutaneous tissue (L55-L59)
sunburn (L55.-)
AHA: 2016, 2Q, 4

Burns and corrosions of external body surface, specified by site (T20-T25)

INCLUDES burns and corrosions of first degree [erythema]
burns and corrosions of second degree [blisters] [epidermal loss]
burns and corrosions of third degree [deep necrosis of underlying tissue] [full-thickness skin loss]
Use additional code from category T31 or T32 to identify extent of body surface involved

☑4ᵗʰ **T20 Burn and corrosion of head, face, and neck**
EXCLUDES 2 burn and corrosion of ear drum (T28.41, T28.91)
burn and corrosion of eye and adnexa (T26.-)
burn and corrosion of mouth and pharynx (T28.0)
AHA: 2015, 1Q, 18-19

The appropriate 7th character is to be added to each code from category T20.
A   initial encounter
D   subsequent encounter
S   sequela

☑5ᵗʰ **T20.0 Burn of unspecified degree of head, face, and neck**
Use additional external cause code to identify the source, place and intent of the burn (X00-X19, X75-X77, X96-X98, Y92)

☑x7ᵗʰ **T20.00** Burn of unspecified degree of head, face, and neck, unspecified site

☑6ᵗʰ **T20.01** Burn of unspecified degree of ear [any part, except ear drum]
EXCLUDES 2 burn of ear drum (T28.41-)

☑7ᵗʰ **T20.011** Burn of unspecified degree of right ear [any part, except ear drum]

☑7ᵗʰ **T20.012** Burn of unspecified degree of left ear [any part, except ear drum]

☑7ᵗʰ **T20.019** Burn of unspecified degree of unspecified ear [any part, except ear drum]

☑x7ᵗʰ **T20.02** Burn of unspecified degree of lip(s)

☑x7ᵗʰ **T20.03** Burn of unspecified degree of chin

☑x7ᵗʰ **T20.04** Burn of unspecified degree of nose (septum)

☑x7ᵗʰ **T20.05** Burn of unspecified degree of scalp [any part]

☑x7ᵗʰ **T20.06** Burn of unspecified degree of forehead and cheek

Rule of Nines Estimation of Total Body Surface Burned

Head and neck 9%

Each arm 9%

Anterior trunk 18%

Posterior trunk 18%

Genitalia 1%

Anterior leg 9%

Posterior leg 9%

Degree of Burns

Epidermis
Dermis
Subcutaneous

Normal   First Degree Burn

Epidermis
Dermis
Subcutaneous

Second Degree Burn   Third Degree Burn

√x7ᵗʰ **T20.07**   Burn of unspecified degree of neck

√x7ᵗʰ **T20.09**   Burn of unspecified degree of multiple sites of head, face, and neck

√5ᵗʰ **T20.1**   **Burn of first degree of head, face, and neck**
   Use additional external cause code to identify the source, place and intent of the burn (X00-X19, X75-X77, X96-X98, Y92)

√x7ᵗʰ **T20.10**   Burn of first degree of head, face, and neck, unspecified site

√6ᵗʰ **T20.11**   Burn of first degree of ear [any part, except ear drum]
   EXCLUDES 2   burn of ear drum (T28.41-)

√7ᵗʰ **T20.111**   Burn of first degree of right ear [any part, except ear drum]

√7ᵗʰ **T20.112**   Burn of first degree of left ear [any part, except ear drum]

√7ᵗʰ **T20.119**   Burn of first degree of unspecified ear [any part, except ear drum]

√x7ᵗʰ **T20.12**   Burn of first degree of lip(s)

√x7ᵗʰ **T20.13**   Burn of first degree of chin

√x7ᵗʰ **T20.14**   Burn of first degree of nose (septum)

√x7ᵗʰ **T20.15**   Burn of first degree of scalp [any part]

√x7ᵗʰ **T20.16**   Burn of first degree of forehead and cheek

√x7ᵗʰ **T20.17**   Burn of first degree of neck

√x7ᵗʰ **T20.19**   Burn of first degree of multiple sites of head, face, and neck

√5ᵗʰ **T20.2**   **Burn of second degree of head, face, and neck**
   Use additional external cause code to identify the source, place and intent of the burn (X00-X19, X75-X77, X96-X98, Y92)

√x7ᵗʰ **T20.20**   Burn of second degree of head, face, and neck, unspecified site

√6ᵗʰ **T20.21**   Burn of second degree of ear [any part, except ear drum]
   EXCLUDES 2   burn of ear drum (T28.41-)

√7ᵗʰ **T20.211**   Burn of second degree of right ear [any part, except ear drum]

√7ᵗʰ **T20.212**   Burn of second degree of left ear [any part, except ear drum]

√7ᵗʰ **T20.219**   Burn of second degree of unspecified ear [any part, except ear drum]

√x7ᵗʰ **T20.22**   Burn of second degree of lip(s)

√x7ᵗʰ **T20.23**   Burn of second degree of chin

√x7ᵗʰ **T20.24**   Burn of second degree of nose (septum)

√x7ᵗʰ **T20.25**   Burn of second degree of scalp [any part]

√x7ᵗʰ **T20.26**   Burn of second degree of forehead and cheek

√x7ᵗʰ **T20.27**   Burn of second degree of neck

√x7ᵗʰ **T20.29**   Burn of second degree of multiple sites of head, face, and neck

√5ᵗʰ **T20.3**   **Burn of third degree of head, face, and neck**
   Use additional external cause code to identify the source, place and intent of the burn (X00-X19, X75-X77, X96-X98, Y92)

√x7ᵗʰ **T20.30**   Burn of third degree of head, face, and neck, unspecified site   **CC H5**
   CC Excl: PDX collection 1375

√6ᵗʰ **T20.31**   Burn of third degree of ear [any part, except ear drum]
   EXCLUDES 2   burn of ear drum (T28.41-)
   AHA: 2015, 1Q, 18

   CC Excl: For codes in subcategory T20.31:
   PDX collection 1376

√7ᵗʰ **T20.311**   Burn of third degree of right ear [any part, except ear drum]   **CC H5**

√7ᵗʰ **T20.312**   Burn of third degree of left ear [any part, except ear drum]   **CC H5**

√7ᵗʰ **T20.319**   Burn of third degree of unspecified ear [any part, except ear drum]   **CC H5**

√x7ᵗʰ **T20.32**   Burn of third degree of lip(s)   **CC H5**
   CC Excl: PDX collection 1377

√x7ᵗʰ **T20.33**   Burn of third degree of chin   **CC H5**
   CC Excl: PDX collection 1378

√x7ᵗʰ **T20.34**   Burn of third degree of nose (septum)   **CC H5**
   CC Excl: PDX collection 1379

√x7ᵗʰ **T20.35**   Burn of third degree of scalp [any part]   **CC H5**
   CC Excl: PDX collection 1380

√x7ᵗʰ **T20.36**   Burn of third degree of forehead and cheek   **CC H5**
   CC Excl: PDX collection 1381

√x7ᵗʰ **T20.37**   Burn of third degree of neck   **CC H5**
   CC Excl: PDX collection 1382

√x7ᵗʰ **T20.39**   Burn of third degree of multiple sites of head, face, and neck   **CC H5**
   CC Excl: PDX collection 1383

√5ᵗʰ **T20.4**   **Corrosion of unspecified degree of head, face, and neck**
   Code first (T51-T65) to identify chemical and intent
   Use additional external cause code to identify place (Y92)

√x7ᵗʰ **T20.40**   Corrosion of unspecified degree of head, face, and neck, unspecified site

√6ᵗʰ **T20.41**   Corrosion of unspecified degree of ear [any part, except ear drum]
   EXCLUDES 2   corrosion of ear drum (T28.91-)

√7ᵗʰ **T20.411**   Corrosion of unspecified degree of right ear [any part, except ear drum]

√7ᵗʰ **T20.412**   Corrosion of unspecified degree of left ear [any part, except ear drum]

√7ᵗʰ **T20.419**   Corrosion of unspecified degree of unspecified ear [any part, except ear drum]

√x7ᵗʰ **T20.42**   Corrosion of unspecified degree of lip(s)

√x7ᵗʰ **T20.43**   Corrosion of unspecified degree of chin

N Newborn: 0   **P** Pediatric: 0-17   **M** Maternity: 12-55   **A** Adult: 15-124   **MCC** Major CC Condition   **PDxMCC** PDx acts as own MCC   **CC** CC Condition   **PDxCC** PDx acts as own CC

√7ᵗʰ **T20.44** Corrosion of unspecified degree of nose (septum)

√7ᵗʰ **T20.45** Corrosion of unspecified degree of scalp [any part]

√7ᵗʰ **T20.46** Corrosion of unspecified degree of forehead and cheek

√7ᵗʰ **T20.47** Corrosion of unspecified degree of neck

√7ᵗʰ **T20.49** Corrosion of unspecified degree of multiple sites of head, face, and neck

√5ᵗʰ **T20.5** Corrosion of first degree of head, face, and neck
Code first (T51-T65) to identify chemical and intent
Use additional external cause code to identify place (Y92)

√7ᵗʰ **T20.50** Corrosion of first degree of head, face, and neck, unspecified site

√6ᵗʰ **T20.51** Corrosion of first degree of ear [any part, except ear drum]
EXCLUDES 2 corrosion of ear drum (T28.91-)

√7ᵗʰ **T20.511** Corrosion of first degree of right ear [any part, except ear drum]

√7ᵗʰ **T20.512** Corrosion of first degree of left ear [any part, except ear drum]

√7ᵗʰ **T20.519** Corrosion of first degree of unspecified ear [any part, except ear drum]

√7ᵗʰ **T20.52** Corrosion of first degree of lip(s)

√7ᵗʰ **T20.53** Corrosion of first degree of chin

√7ᵗʰ **T20.54** Corrosion of first degree of nose (septum)

√7ᵗʰ **T20.55** Corrosion of first degree of scalp [any part]

√7ᵗʰ **T20.56** Corrosion of first degree of forehead and cheek

√7ᵗʰ **T20.57** Corrosion of first degree of neck

√7ᵗʰ **T20.59** Corrosion of first degree of multiple sites of head, face, and neck

√5ᵗʰ **T20.6** Corrosion of second degree of head, face, and neck
Code first (T51-T65) to identify chemical and intent
Use additional external cause code to identify place (Y92)

√7ᵗʰ **T20.60** Corrosion of second degree of head, face, and neck, unspecified site

√6ᵗʰ **T20.61** Corrosion of second degree of ear [any part, except ear drum]
EXCLUDES 2 corrosion of ear drum (T28.91-)

√7ᵗʰ **T20.611** Corrosion of second degree of right ear [any part, except ear drum]

√7ᵗʰ **T20.612** Corrosion of second degree of left ear [any part, except ear drum]

√7ᵗʰ **T20.619** Corrosion of second degree of unspecified ear [any part, except ear drum]

√7ᵗʰ **T20.62** Corrosion of second degree of lip(s)

√7ᵗʰ **T20.63** Corrosion of second degree of chin

√7ᵗʰ **T20.64** Corrosion of second degree of nose (septum)

√7ᵗʰ **T20.65** Corrosion of second degree of scalp [any part]

√7ᵗʰ **T20.66** Corrosion of second degree of forehead and cheek

√7ᵗʰ **T20.67** Corrosion of second degree of neck

√7ᵗʰ **T20.69** Corrosion of second degree of multiple sites of head, face, and neck

√5ᵗʰ **T20.7** Corrosion of third degree of head, face, and neck
Code first (T51-T65) to identify chemical and intent
Use additional external cause code to identify place (Y92)

√7ᵗʰ **T20.70** Corrosion of third degree of head, face, and neck, unspecified site **CC H5**
CC Excl: PDX collection 1375

√6ᵗʰ **T20.71** Corrosion of third degree of ear [any part, except ear drum]
EXCLUDES 2 corrosion of ear drum (T28.91-)
CC Excl: For codes in subcategory T20.71: PDX collection 1376

√7ᵗʰ **T20.711** Corrosion of third degree of right ear [any part, except ear drum] **CC H5**

√7ᵗʰ **T20.712** Corrosion of third degree of left ear [any part, except ear drum] **CC H5**

√7ᵗʰ **T20.719** Corrosion of third degree of unspecified ear [any part, except ear drum] **CC H5**

√7ᵗʰ **T20.72** Corrosion of third degree of lip(s) **CC H5**
CC Excl: PDX collection 1377

√7ᵗʰ **T20.73** Corrosion of third degree of chin **CC H5**
CC Excl: PDX collection 1378

√7ᵗʰ **T20.74** Corrosion of third degree of nose (septum) **CC H5**
CC Excl: PDX collection 1379

√7ᵗʰ **T20.75** Corrosion of third degree of scalp [any part] **CC H5**
CC Excl: PDX collection 1380

√7ᵗʰ **T20.76** Corrosion of third degree of forehead and cheek **CC H5**
CC Excl: PDX collection 1381

√7ᵗʰ **T20.77** Corrosion of third degree of neck **CC H5**
CC Excl: PDX collection 1382

√7ᵗʰ **T20.79** Corrosion of third degree of multiple sites of head, face, and neck **CC H5**
CC Excl: PDX collection 1383

√4ᵗʰ **T21** Burn and corrosion of trunk
INCLUDES burns and corrosion of hip region
EXCLUDES 2 burns and corrosion of axilla (T22.- with fifth character 4)
burns and corrosion of scapular region (T22.- with fifth character 6)
burns and corrosion of shoulder (T22.- with fifth character 5)

The appropriate 7th character is to be added to each code from category T21.
A   initial encounter
D   subsequent encounter
S   sequela

√5ᵗʰ **T21.0** Burn of unspecified degree of trunk
Use additional external cause code to identify the source, place and intent of the burn (X00-X19, X75-X77, X96-X98, Y92)

√7ᵗʰ **T21.00** Burn of unspecified degree of trunk, unspecified site

√7ᵗʰ **T21.01** Burn of unspecified degree of chest wall
Burn of of unspecified degree of breast

√7ᵗʰ **T21.02** Burn of unspecified degree of abdominal wall
Burn of unspecified degree of flank
Burn of unspecified degree of groin

√7ᵗʰ **T21.03** Burn of unspecified degree of upper back
Burn of unspecified degree of interscapular region

√7ᵗʰ **T21.04** Burn of unspecified degree of lower back

√7ᵗʰ **T21.05** Burn of unspecified degree of buttock
Burn of unspecified degree of anus

√7ᵗʰ **T21.06** Burn of unspecified degree of male genital region ♂
Burn of unspecified degree of penis
Burn of unspecified degree of scrotum
Burn of unspecified degree of testis

√7ᵗʰ **T21.07** Burn of unspecified degree of female genital region ♀
Burn of unspecified degree of labium (majus) (minus)
Burn of unspecified degree of perineum
Burn of unspecified degree of vulva
EXCLUDES 2 burn of vagina (T28.3)

√7ᵗʰ **T21.09** Burn of unspecified degree of other site of trunk

√5ᵗʰ **T21.1** Burn of first degree of trunk
Use additional external cause code to identify the source, place and intent of the burn (X00-X19, X75-X77, X96-X98, Y92)

√7ᵗʰ **T21.10** Burn of first degree of trunk, unspecified site

√7ᵗʰ **T21.11** Burn of first degree of chest wall
Burn of first degree of breast

√7ᵗʰ **T21.12** Burn of first degree of abdominal wall
Burn of first degree of flank
Burn of first degree of groin

√7ᵗʰ **T21.13** Burn of first degree of upper back
Burn of first degree of interscapular region

√7ᵗʰ **T21.14** Burn of first degree of lower back

√7ᵗʰ **T21.15** Burn of first degree of buttock
Burn of first degree of anus

√7ᵗʰ **T21.16** Burn of first degree of male genital region ♂
Burn of first degree of penis
Burn of first degree of scrotum
Burn of first degree of testis

√7ᵗʰ **T21.17** Burn of first degree of female genital region ♀
Burn of first degree of labium (majus) (minus)
Burn of first degree of perineum
Burn of first degree of vulva
EXCLUDES 2 burn of vagina (T28.3)

√7ᵗʰ **T21.19** Burn of first degree of other site of trunk

✓5ᵗʰ **T21.2　Burn of second degree of trunk**
Use additional external cause code to identify the source, place and intent of the burn (X00-X19, X75-X77, X96-X98, Y92)

✓x7ᵗʰ **T21.20　Burn of second degree of trunk, unspecified site**

✓x7ᵗʰ **T21.21　Burn of second degree of chest wall**
Burn of second degree of breast

✓x7ᵗʰ **T21.22　Burn of second degree of abdominal wall**
Burn of second degree of flank
Burn of second degree of groin

✓x7ᵗʰ **T21.23　Burn of second degree of upper back**
Burn of second degree of interscapular region

✓x7ᵗʰ **T21.24　Burn of second degree of lower back**

✓x7ᵗʰ **T21.25　Burn of second degree of buttock**
Burn of second degree of anus

✓x7ᵗʰ **T21.26　Burn of second degree of male genital region**　♂
Burn of second degree of penis
Burn of second degree of scrotum
Burn of second degree of testis

✓x7ᵗʰ **T21.27　Burn of second degree of female genital region**　♀
Burn of second degree of labium (majus) (minus)
Burn of second degree of perineum
Burn of second degree of vulva
EXCLUDES 2　*burn of vagina (T28.3)*

✓x7ᵗʰ **T21.29　Burn of second degree of other site of trunk**

✓5ᵗʰ **T21.3　Burn of third degree of trunk**
Use additional external cause code to identify the source, place and intent of the burn (X00-X19, X75-X77, X96-X98, Y92)

✓x7ᵗʰ **T21.30　Burn of third degree of trunk, unspecified site**　CC H5
CC Excl: PDX collection 1384

✓x7ᵗʰ **T21.31　Burn of third degree of chest wall**　CC H5
Burn of third degree of breast
AHA: 2016, 2Q, 5
CC Excl: PDX collection 1385

✓x7ᵗʰ **T21.32　Burn of third degree of abdominal wall**　CC H5
Burn of third degree of flank
Burn of third degree of groin
CC Excl: PDX collection 1386

✓x7ᵗʰ **T21.33　Burn of third degree of upper back**　CC H5
Burn of third degree of interscapular region
CC Excl: PDX collection 1387

✓x7ᵗʰ **T21.34　Burn of third degree of lower back**　CC H5
CC Excl: PDX collection 1387

✓x7ᵗʰ **T21.35　Burn of third degree of buttock**　CC H5
Burn of third degree of anus
CC Excl: PDX collection 1387

✓x7ᵗʰ **T21.36　Burn of third degree of male genital region**　CC H5 ♂
Burn of third degree of penis
Burn of third degree of scrotum
Burn of third degree of testis
CC Excl: PDX collection 1388

✓x7ᵗʰ **T21.37　Burn of third degree of female genital region**　CC H5 ♀
Burn of third degree of labium (majus) (minus)
Burn of third degree of perineum
Burn of third degree of vulva
EXCLUDES 2　*burn of vagina (T28.3)*
CC Excl: PDX collection 1388

✓x7ᵗʰ **T21.39　Burn of third degree of other site of trunk**　CC H5
CC Excl: PDX collection 1384

✓5ᵗʰ **T21.4　Corrosion of unspecified degree of trunk**
Code first (T51-T65) to identify chemical and intent
Use additional external cause code to identify place (Y92)

✓x7ᵗʰ **T21.40　Corrosion of unspecified degree of trunk, unspecified site**

✓x7ᵗʰ **T21.41　Corrosion of unspecified degree of chest wall**
Corrosion of unspecified degree of breast

✓x7ᵗʰ **T21.42　Corrosion of unspecified degree of abdominal wall**
Corrosion of unspecified degree of flank
Corrosion of unspecified degree of groin

✓x7ᵗʰ **T21.43　Corrosion of unspecified degree of upper back**
Corrosion of unspecified degree of interscapular region

✓x7ᵗʰ **T21.44　Corrosion of unspecified degree of lower back**

✓x7ᵗʰ **T21.45　Corrosion of unspecified degree of buttock**
Corrosion of unspecified degree of anus

✓x7ᵗʰ **T21.46　Corrosion of unspecified degree of male genital region**　♂
Corrosion of unspecified degree of penis
Corrosion of unspecified degree of scrotum
Corrosion of unspecified degree of testis

✓x7ᵗʰ **T21.47　Corrosion of unspecified degree of female genital region**　♀
Corrosion of unspecified degree of labium (majus) (minus)
Corrosion of unspecified degree of perineum
Corrosion of unspecified degree of vulva
EXCLUDES 2　*corrosion of vagina (T28.8)*

✓x7ᵗʰ **T21.49　Corrosion of unspecified degree of other site of trunk**

✓5ᵗʰ **T21.5　Corrosion of first degree of trunk**
Code first (T51-T65) to identify chemical and intent
Use additional external cause code to identify place (Y92)

✓x7ᵗʰ **T21.50　Corrosion of first degree of trunk, unspecified site**

✓x7ᵗʰ **T21.51　Corrosion of first degree of chest wall**
Corrosion of first degree of breast

✓x7ᵗʰ **T21.52　Corrosion of first degree of abdominal wall**
Corrosion of first degree of flank
Corrosion of first degree of groin

✓x7ᵗʰ **T21.53　Corrosion of first degree of upper back**
Corrosion of first degree of interscapular region

✓x7ᵗʰ **T21.54　Corrosion of first degree of lower back**

✓x7ᵗʰ **T21.55　Corrosion of first degree of buttock**
Corrosion of first degree of anus

✓x7ᵗʰ **T21.56　Corrosion of first degree of male genital region**　♂
Corrosion of first degree of penis
Corrosion of first degree of scrotum
Corrosion of first degree of testis

✓x7ᵗʰ **T21.57　Corrosion of first degree of female genital region**　♀
Corrosion of first degree of labium (majus) (minus)
Corrosion of first degree of perineum
Corrosion of first degree of vulva
EXCLUDES 2　*corrosion of vagina (T28.8)*

✓x7ᵗʰ **T21.59　Corrosion of first degree of other site of trunk**

✓5ᵗʰ **T21.6　Corrosion of second degree of trunk**
Code first (T51-T65) to identify chemical and intent
Use additional external cause code to identify place (Y92)

✓x7ᵗʰ **T21.60　Corrosion of second degree of trunk, unspecified site**

✓x7ᵗʰ **T21.61　Corrosion of second degree of chest wall**
Corrosion of second degree of breast

✓x7ᵗʰ **T21.62　Corrosion of second degree of abdominal wall**
Corrosion of second degree of flank
Corrosion of second degree of groin

✓x7ᵗʰ **T21.63　Corrosion of second degree of upper back**
Corrosion of second degree of interscapular region

✓x7ᵗʰ **T21.64　Corrosion of second degree of lower back**

✓x7ᵗʰ **T21.65　Corrosion of second degree of buttock**
Corrosion of second degree of anus

✓x7ᵗʰ **T21.66　Corrosion of second degree of male genital region**　♂
Corrosion of second degree of penis
Corrosion of second degree of scrotum
Corrosion of second degree of testis

✓x7ᵗʰ **T21.67　Corrosion of second degree of female genital region**　♀
Corrosion of second degree of labium (majus) (minus)
Corrosion of second degree of perineum
Corrosion of second degree of vulva
EXCLUDES 2　*corrosion of vagina (T28.8)*

✓x7ᵗʰ **T21.69　Corrosion of second degree of other site of trunk**

✓5ᵗʰ **T21.7　Corrosion of third degree of trunk**
Code first (T51-T65) to identify chemical and intent
Use additional external cause code to identify place (Y92)

✓x7ᵗʰ **T21.70　Corrosion of third degree of trunk, unspecified site**　CC H5
CC Excl: PDX collection 1384

✓x7ᵗʰ **T21.71　Corrosion of third degree of chest wall**　CC H5
Corrosion of third degree of breast
CC Excl: PDX collection 1385

✓x7ᵗʰ **T21.72　Corrosion of third degree of abdominal wall**　CC H5
Corrosion of third degree of flank
Corrosion of third degree of groin
CC Excl: PDX collection 1386

√x7ᵗʰ **T21.73** **Corrosion of third degree of** upper back   **CC** **H5**
 Corrosion of third degree of interscapular region
 CC Excl: PDX collection 1387

√x7ᵗʰ **T21.74** **Corrosion of third degree of** lower back   **CC** **H5**
 CC Excl: PDX collection 1387

√x7ᵗʰ **T21.75** **Corrosion of third degree of** buttock   **CC** **H5**
 Corrosion of third degree of anus
 CC Excl: PDX collection 1387

√x7ᵗʰ **T21.76** **Corrosion of third degree of** male genital   **CC** **H5** ♂
 region
 Corrosion of third degree of penis
 Corrosion of third degree of scrotum
 Corrosion of third degree of testis
 CC Excl: PDX collection 1388

√x7ᵗʰ **T21.77** **Corrosion of third degree of** female genital   **CC** **H5** ♀
 region
 Corrosion of third degree of labium (majus) (minus)
 Corrosion of third degree of perineum
 Corrosion of third degree of vulva
 EXCLUDES 2 corrosion of vagina (T28.8)
 CC Excl: PDX collection 1388

√x7ᵗʰ **T21.79** **Corrosion of third degree of** other site of   **CC** **H5**
 trunk
 CC Excl: PDX collection 1384

√4ᵗʰ **T22** **Burn and corrosion of shoulder and upper limb, except wrist and hand**
 EXCLUDES 2 burn and corrosion of interscapular region (T21.-)
 burn and corrosion of wrist and hand (T23.-)

 The appropriate 7th character is to be added to each code from category T22.
 A initial encounter
 D subsequent encounter
 S sequela

√5ᵗʰ **T22.0** **Burn of** unspecified degree **of shoulder and upper limb, except wrist and hand**
 Use additional external cause code to identify the source, place and intent of the burn (X00-X19, X75-X77, X96-X98, Y92)

√x7ᵗʰ **T22.00** **Burn of unspecified degree of shoulder and upper limb, except wrist and hand,** unspecified site

√6ᵗʰ **T22.01** **Burn of unspecified degree of** forearm

 √7ᵗʰ **T22.011** **Burn of unspecified degree of** right forearm

 √7ᵗʰ **T22.012** **Burn of unspecified degree of** left forearm

 √7ᵗʰ **T22.019** **Burn of unspecified degree of** unspecified forearm

√6ᵗʰ **T22.02** **Burn of unspecified degree of** elbow

 √7ᵗʰ **T22.021** **Burn of unspecified degree of** right elbow

 √7ᵗʰ **T22.022** **Burn of unspecified degree of** left elbow

 √7ᵗʰ **T22.029** **Burn of unspecified degree of** unspecified elbow

√6ᵗʰ **T22.03** **Burn of unspecified degree of** upper arm

 √7ᵗʰ **T22.031** **Burn of unspecified degree of** right upper arm

 √7ᵗʰ **T22.032** **Burn of unspecified degree of** left upper arm

 √7ᵗʰ **T22.039** **Burn of unspecified degree of** unspecified upper arm

√6ᵗʰ **T22.04** **Burn of unspecified degree of** axilla

 √7ᵗʰ **T22.041** **Burn of unspecified degree of** right axilla

 √7ᵗʰ **T22.042** **Burn of unspecified degree of** left axilla

 √7ᵗʰ **T22.049** **Burn of unspecified degree of** unspecified axilla

√6ᵗʰ **T22.05** **Burn of unspecified degree of** shoulder

 √7ᵗʰ **T22.051** **Burn of unspecified degree of** right shoulder

 √7ᵗʰ **T22.052** **Burn of unspecified degree of** left shoulder

 √7ᵗʰ **T22.059** **Burn of unspecified degree of** unspecified shoulder

√6ᵗʰ **T22.06** **Burn of unspecified degree of** scapular region

 √7ᵗʰ **T22.061** **Burn of unspecified degree of** right scapular region

 √7ᵗʰ **T22.062** **Burn of unspecified degree of** left scapular region

 √7ᵗʰ **T22.069** **Burn of unspecified degree of** unspecified scapular region

√6ᵗʰ **T22.09** **Burn of unspecified degree of** multiple sites of shoulder and upper limb, except wrist and hand

 √7ᵗʰ **T22.091** **Burn of unspecified degree of multiple sites of** right shoulder and upper limb, except wrist and hand

 √7ᵗʰ **T22.092** **Burn of unspecified degree of multiple sites of** left shoulder and upper limb, except wrist and hand

 √7ᵗʰ **T22.099** **Burn of unspecified degree of multiple sites of** unspecified shoulder and upper limb, except wrist and hand

√5ᵗʰ **T22.1** **Burn of** first degree **of shoulder and upper limb, except wrist and hand**
 Use additional external cause code to identify the source, place and intent of the burn (X00-X19, X75-X77, X96-X98, Y92)

√x7ᵗʰ **T22.10** **Burn of first degree of shoulder and upper limb, except wrist and hand,** unspecified site

√6ᵗʰ **T22.11** **Burn of first degree of** forearm

 √7ᵗʰ **T22.111** **Burn of first degree of** right forearm

 √7ᵗʰ **T22.112** **Burn of first degree of** left forearm

 √7ᵗʰ **T22.119** **Burn of first degree of** unspecified forearm

√6ᵗʰ **T22.12** **Burn of first degree of** elbow

 √7ᵗʰ **T22.121** **Burn of first degree of** right elbow

 √7ᵗʰ **T22.122** **Burn of first degree of** left elbow

 √7ᵗʰ **T22.129** **Burn of first degree of** unspecified elbow

√6ᵗʰ **T22.13** **Burn of first degree of** upper arm

 √7ᵗʰ **T22.131** **Burn of first degree of** right upper arm

 √7ᵗʰ **T22.132** **Burn of first degree of** left upper arm

 √7ᵗʰ **T22.139** **Burn of first degree of** unspecified upper arm

√6ᵗʰ **T22.14** **Burn of first degree of** axilla

 √7ᵗʰ **T22.141** **Burn of first degree of** right axilla

 √7ᵗʰ **T22.142** **Burn of first degree of** left axilla

 √7ᵗʰ **T22.149** **Burn of first degree of** unspecified axilla

√6ᵗʰ **T22.15** **Burn of first degree of** shoulder

 √7ᵗʰ **T22.151** **Burn of first degree of** right shoulder

 √7ᵗʰ **T22.152** **Burn of first degree of** left shoulder

 √7ᵗʰ **T22.159** **Burn of first degree of** unspecified shoulder

√6ᵗʰ **T22.16** **Burn of first degree of** scapular region

 √7ᵗʰ **T22.161** **Burn of first degree of** right scapular region

 √7ᵗʰ **T22.162** **Burn of first degree of** left scapular region

 √7ᵗʰ **T22.169** **Burn of first degree of** unspecified scapular region

√6ᵗʰ **T22.19** **Burn of first degree of** multiple sites of shoulder and upper limb, except wrist and hand

 √7ᵗʰ **T22.191** **Burn of first degree of multiple sites of** right shoulder and upper limb, except wrist and hand

 √7ᵗʰ **T22.192** **Burn of first degree of multiple sites of** left shoulder and upper limb, except wrist and hand

 √7ᵗʰ **T22.199** **Burn of first degree of multiple sites of** unspecified shoulder and upper limb, except wrist and hand

√5ᵗʰ **T22.2** **Burn of** second degree **of shoulder and upper limb, except wrist and hand**
 Use additional external cause code to identify the source, place and intent of the burn (X00-X19, X75-X77, X96-X98, Y92)

√x7ᵗʰ **T22.20** **Burn of second degree of shoulder and upper limb, except wrist and hand,** unspecified site

√6ᵗʰ **T22.21** **Burn of second degree of** forearm

 √7ᵗʰ **T22.211** **Burn of second degree of** right forearm

 √7ᵗʰ **T22.212** **Burn of second degree of** left forearm

 √7ᵗʰ **T22.219** **Burn of second degree of** unspecified forearm

√6ᵗʰ **T22.22** **Burn of second degree of** elbow

 √7ᵗʰ **T22.221** **Burn of second degree of** right elbow

 √7ᵗʰ **T22.222** **Burn of second degree of** left elbow

√7th **T22.229** Burn of second degree of unspecified elbow

√6th **T22.23** Burn of second degree of upper arm

√7th **T22.231** Burn of second degree of right upper arm

√7th **T22.232** Burn of second degree of left upper arm

√7th **T22.239** Burn of second degree of unspecified upper arm

√6th **T22.24** Burn of second degree of axilla

√7th **T22.241** Burn of second degree of right axilla

√7th **T22.242** Burn of second degree of left axilla

√7th **T22.249** Burn of second degree of unspecified axilla

√6th **T22.25** Burn of second degree of shoulder

√7th **T22.251** Burn of second degree of right shoulder

√7th **T22.252** Burn of second degree of left shoulder

√7th **T22.259** Burn of second degree of unspecified shoulder

√6th **T22.26** Burn of second degree of scapular region

√7th **T22.261** Burn of second degree of right scapular region

√7th **T22.262** Burn of second degree of left scapular region

√7th **T22.269** Burn of second degree of unspecified scapular region

√6th **T22.29** Burn of second degree of multiple sites of shoulder and upper limb, except wrist and hand

√7th **T22.291** Burn of second degree of multiple sites of right shoulder and upper limb, except wrist and hand

√7th **T22.292** Burn of second degree of multiple sites of left shoulder and upper limb, except wrist and hand

√7th **T22.299** Burn of second degree of multiple sites of unspecified shoulder and upper limb, except wrist and hand

√5th **T22.3** Burn of third degree of shoulder and upper limb, except wrist and hand

Use additional external cause code to identify the source, place and intent of the burn (X00-X19, X75-X77, X96-X98, Y92)

√x7th **T22.30** Burn of third degree of shoulder and upper limb, except wrist and hand, unspecified site   CC H5
CC Excl: PDX collection 1389

√6th **T22.31** Burn of third degree of forearm

CC Excl: For codes in subcategory T22.31:
PDX collection 1390

√7th **T22.311** Burn of third degree of right forearm   CC H5

√7th **T22.312** Burn of third degree of left forearm   CC H5

√7th **T22.319** Burn of third degree of unspecified forearm   CC H5

√6th **T22.32** Burn of third degree of elbow

CC Excl: For codes in subcategory T22.32:
PDX collection 1391

√7th **T22.321** Burn of third degree of right elbow   CC H5

√7th **T22.322** Burn of third degree of left elbow   CC H5

√7th **T22.329** Burn of third degree of unspecified elbow   CC H5

√6th **T22.33** Burn of third degree of upper arm

CC Excl: For codes in subcategory T22.33:
PDX collection 1392

√7th **T22.331** Burn of third degree of right upper arm   CC H5

√7th **T22.332** Burn of third degree of left upper arm   CC H5

√7th **T22.339** Burn of third degree of unspecified upper arm   CC H5

√6th **T22.34** Burn of third degree of axilla

CC Excl: For codes in subcategory T22.34:
PDX collection 1393

√7th **T22.341** Burn of third degree of right axilla   CC H5

√7th **T22.342** Burn of third degree of left axilla   CC H5

√7th **T22.349** Burn of third degree of unspecified axilla   CC H5

√6th **T22.35** Burn of third degree of shoulder

CC Excl: For codes in subcategory T22.35:
PDX collection 1394

√7th **T22.351** Burn of third degree of right shoulder   CC H5

√7th **T22.352** Burn of third degree of left shoulder   CC H5

√7th **T22.359** Burn of third degree of unspecified shoulder   CC H5

√6th **T22.36** Burn of third degree of scapular region

CC Excl: For codes in subcategory T22.36:
PDX collection 1395

√7th **T22.361** Burn of third degree of right scapular region   CC H5

√7th **T22.362** Burn of third degree of left scapular region   CC H5

√7th **T22.369** Burn of third degree of unspecified scapular region   CC H5

√6th **T22.39** Burn of third degree of multiple sites of shoulder and upper limb, except wrist and hand

CC Excl: For codes in subcategory T22.39:
PDX collection 1389

√7th **T22.391** Burn of third degree of multiple sites of right shoulder and upper limb, except wrist and hand   CC H5

√7th **T22.392** Burn of third degree of multiple sites of left shoulder and upper limb, except wrist and hand   CC H5

√7th **T22.399** Burn of third degree of multiple sites of unspecified shoulder and upper limb, except wrist and hand   CC H5

√5th **T22.4** Corrosion of unspecified degree of shoulder and upper limb, except wrist and hand

Code first (T51-T65) to identify chemical and intent
Use additional external cause code to identify place (Y92)

√x7th **T22.40** Corrosion of unspecified degree of shoulder and upper limb, except wrist and hand, unspecified site

√6th **T22.41** Corrosion of unspecified degree of forearm

√7th **T22.411** Corrosion of unspecified degree of right forearm

√7th **T22.412** Corrosion of unspecified degree of left forearm

√7th **T22.419** Corrosion of unspecified degree of unspecified forearm

√6th **T22.42** Corrosion of unspecified degree of elbow

√7th **T22.421** Corrosion of unspecified degree of right elbow

√7th **T22.422** Corrosion of unspecified degree of left elbow

√7th **T22.429** Corrosion of unspecified degree of unspecified elbow

√6th **T22.43** Corrosion of unspecified degree of upper arm

√7th **T22.431** Corrosion of unspecified degree of right upper arm

√7th **T22.432** Corrosion of unspecified degree of left upper arm

√7th **T22.439** Corrosion of unspecified degree of unspecified upper arm

√6th **T22.44** Corrosion of unspecified degree of axilla

√7th **T22.441** Corrosion of unspecified degree of right axilla

√7th **T22.442** Corrosion of unspecified degree of left axilla

√7th **T22.449** Corrosion of unspecified degree of unspecified axilla

√6th **T22.45** Corrosion of unspecified degree of shoulder

√7th **T22.451** Corrosion of unspecified degree of right shoulder

√7th **T22.452** Corrosion of unspecified degree of left shoulder

√7th **T22.459** Corrosion of unspecified degree of unspecified shoulder

N Newborn: 0   P Pediatric: 0-17   M Maternity: 12-55   A Adult: 15-124   MCC Major CC Condition   PDxMCC PDx acts as own MCC   CC CC Condition   PDxCC PDx acts as own CC

1084   ICD-10-CM 2018

√6ᵗʰ **T22.46** Corrosion of unspecified degree of scapular region

  √7ᵗʰ **T22.461** Corrosion of unspecified degree of right scapular region

  √7ᵗʰ **T22.462** Corrosion of unspecified degree of left scapular region

  √7ᵗʰ **T22.469** Corrosion of unspecified degree of unspecified scapular region

√6ᵗʰ **T22.49** Corrosion of unspecified degree of multiple sites of shoulder and upper limb, except wrist and hand

  √7ᵗʰ **T22.491** Corrosion of unspecified degree of multiple sites of right shoulder and upper limb, except wrist and hand

  √7ᵗʰ **T22.492** Corrosion of unspecified degree of multiple sites of left shoulder and upper limb, except wrist and hand

  √7ᵗʰ **T22.499** Corrosion of unspecified degree of multiple sites of unspecified shoulder and upper limb, except wrist and hand

√5ᵗʰ **T22.5** Corrosion of first degree of shoulder and upper limb, except wrist and hand

    Code first (T51-T65) to identify chemical and intent
    Use additional external cause code to identify place (Y92)

√x7ᵗʰ **T22.50** Corrosion of first degree of shoulder and upper limb, except wrist and hand unspecified site

√6ᵗʰ **T22.51** Corrosion of first degree of forearm

  √7ᵗʰ **T22.511** Corrosion of first degree of right forearm

  √7ᵗʰ **T22.512** Corrosion of first degree of left forearm

  √7ᵗʰ **T22.519** Corrosion of first degree of unspecified forearm

√6ᵗʰ **T22.52** Corrosion of first degree of elbow

  √7ᵗʰ **T22.521** Corrosion of first degree of right elbow

  √7ᵗʰ **T22.522** Corrosion of first degree of left elbow

  √7ᵗʰ **T22.529** Corrosion of first degree of unspecified elbow

√6ᵗʰ **T22.53** Corrosion of first degree of upper arm

  √7ᵗʰ **T22.531** Corrosion of first degree of right upper arm

  √7ᵗʰ **T22.532** Corrosion of first degree of left upper arm

  √7ᵗʰ **T22.539** Corrosion of first degree of unspecified upper arm

√6ᵗʰ **T22.54** Corrosion of first degree of axilla

  √7ᵗʰ **T22.541** Corrosion of first degree of right axilla

  √7ᵗʰ **T22.542** Corrosion of first degree of left axilla

  √7ᵗʰ **T22.549** Corrosion of first degree of unspecified axilla

√6ᵗʰ **T22.55** Corrosion of first degree of shoulder

  √7ᵗʰ **T22.551** Corrosion of first degree of right shoulder

  √7ᵗʰ **T22.552** Corrosion of first degree of left shoulder

  √7ᵗʰ **T22.559** Corrosion of first degree of unspecified shoulder

√6ᵗʰ **T22.56** Corrosion of first degree of scapular region

  √7ᵗʰ **T22.561** Corrosion of first degree of right scapular region

  √7ᵗʰ **T22.562** Corrosion of first degree of left scapular region

  √7ᵗʰ **T22.569** Corrosion of first degree of unspecified scapular region

√6ᵗʰ **T22.59** Corrosion of first degree of multiple sites of shoulder and upper limb, except wrist and hand

  √7ᵗʰ **T22.591** Corrosion of first degree of multiple sites of right shoulder and upper limb, except wrist and hand

  √7ᵗʰ **T22.592** Corrosion of first degree of multiple sites of left shoulder and upper limb, except wrist and hand

  √7ᵗʰ **T22.599** Corrosion of first degree of multiple sites of unspecified shoulder and upper limb, except wrist and hand

√5ᵗʰ **T22.6** Corrosion of second degree of shoulder and upper limb, except wrist and hand

    Code first (T51-T65) to identify chemical and intent
    Use additional external cause code to identify place (Y92)

√x7ᵗʰ **T22.60** Corrosion of second degree of shoulder and upper limb, except wrist and hand, unspecified site

√6ᵗʰ **T22.61** Corrosion of second degree of forearm

  √7ᵗʰ **T22.611** Corrosion of second degree of right forearm

  √7ᵗʰ **T22.612** Corrosion of second degree of left forearm

  √7ᵗʰ **T22.619** Corrosion of second degree of unspecified forearm

√6ᵗʰ **T22.62** Corrosion of second degree of elbow

  √7ᵗʰ **T22.621** Corrosion of second degree of right elbow

  √7ᵗʰ **T22.622** Corrosion of second degree of left elbow

  √7ᵗʰ **T22.629** Corrosion of second degree of unspecified elbow

√6ᵗʰ **T22.63** Corrosion of second degree of upper arm

  √7ᵗʰ **T22.631** Corrosion of second degree of right upper arm

  √7ᵗʰ **T22.632** Corrosion of second degree of left upper arm

  √7ᵗʰ **T22.639** Corrosion of second degree of unspecified upper arm

√6ᵗʰ **T22.64** Corrosion of second degree of axilla

  √7ᵗʰ **T22.641** Corrosion of second degree of right axilla

  √7ᵗʰ **T22.642** Corrosion of second degree of left axilla

  √7ᵗʰ **T22.649** Corrosion of second degree of unspecified axilla

√6ᵗʰ **T22.65** Corrosion of second degree of shoulder

  √7ᵗʰ **T22.651** Corrosion of second degree of right shoulder

  √7ᵗʰ **T22.652** Corrosion of second degree of left shoulder

  √7ᵗʰ **T22.659** Corrosion of second degree of unspecified shoulder

√6ᵗʰ **T22.66** Corrosion of second degree of scapular region

  √7ᵗʰ **T22.661** Corrosion of second degree of right scapular region

  √7ᵗʰ **T22.662** Corrosion of second degree of left scapular region

  √7ᵗʰ **T22.669** Corrosion of second degree of unspecified scapular region

√6ᵗʰ **T22.69** Corrosion of second degree of multiple sites of shoulder and upper limb, except wrist and hand

  √7ᵗʰ **T22.691** Corrosion of second degree of multiple sites of right shoulder and upper limb, except wrist and hand

  √7ᵗʰ **T22.692** Corrosion of second degree of multiple sites of left shoulder and upper limb, except wrist and hand

  √7ᵗʰ **T22.699** Corrosion of second degree of multiple sites of unspecified shoulder and upper limb, except wrist and hand

√5ᵗʰ **T22.7** Corrosion of third degree of shoulder and upper limb, except wrist and hand

    Code first (T51-T65) to identify chemical and intent
    Use additional external cause code to identify place (Y92)

√x7ᵗʰ **T22.70** Corrosion of third degree of shoulder and upper limb, except wrist and hand, unspecified site   CC H5
    CC Excl: PDX collection 1389

√6ᵗʰ **T22.71** Corrosion of third degree of forearm

    CC Excl: For codes in subcategory T22.71: PDX collection 1390

  √7ᵗʰ **T22.711** Corrosion of third degree of right forearm   CC H5

  √7ᵗʰ **T22.712** Corrosion of third degree of left forearm   CC H5

  √7ᵗʰ **T22.719** Corrosion of third degree of unspecified forearm   CC H5

√6ᵗʰ **T22.72** Corrosion of third degree of elbow

    CC Excl: For codes in subcategory T22.72: PDX collection 1391

  √7ᵗʰ **T22.721** Corrosion of third degree of right elbow   CC H5

  √7ᵗʰ **T22.722** Corrosion of third degree of left elbow   CC H5

  √7ᵗʰ **T22.729** Corrosion of third degree of unspecified elbow   CC H5

√6ᵗʰ **T22.73** **Corrosion of third degree of** upper arm

> **CC Excl: For codes in subcategory T22.73:** PDX collection 1392

     √7ᵗʰ **T22.731** **Corrosion of third degree of** right upper arm   `CC` `H5`

     √7ᵗʰ **T22.732** **Corrosion of third degree of** left upper arm   `CC` `H5`

     √7ᵗʰ **T22.739** **Corrosion of third degree of** unspecified upper arm   `CC` `H5`

√6ᵗʰ **T22.74** **Corrosion of third degree of** axilla

> **CC Excl: For codes in subcategory T22.74:** PDX collection 1393

     √7ᵗʰ **T22.741** **Corrosion of third degree of** right axilla   `CC` `H5`

     √7ᵗʰ **T22.742** **Corrosion of third degree of** left axilla   `CC` `H5`

     √7ᵗʰ **T22.749** **Corrosion of third degree of** unspecified axilla   `CC` `H5`

√6ᵗʰ **T22.75** **Corrosion of third degree of** shoulder

> **CC Excl: For codes in subcategory T22.75:** PDX collection 1394

     √7ᵗʰ **T22.751** **Corrosion of third degree of** right shoulder   `CC` `H5`

     √7ᵗʰ **T22.752** **Corrosion of third degree of** left shoulder   `CC` `H5`

     √7ᵗʰ **T22.759** **Corrosion of third degree of** unspecified shoulder   `CC` `H5`

√6ᵗʰ **T22.76** **Corrosion of third degree of** scapular region

> **CC Excl: For codes in subcategory T22.76:** PDX collection 1395

     √7ᵗʰ **T22.761** **Corrosion of third degree of** right scapular region   `CC` `H5`

     √7ᵗʰ **T22.762** **Corrosion of third degree of** left scapular region   `CC` `H5`

     √7ᵗʰ **T22.769** **Corrosion of third degree of** unspecified scapular region   `CC` `H5`

√6ᵗʰ **T22.79** **Corrosion of third degree of** multiple sites of shoulder and upper limb, except wrist and hand

> **CC Excl: For codes in subcategory T22.79:** PDX collection 1389

     √7ᵗʰ **T22.791** **Corrosion of third degree of** multiple sites of right shoulder and upper limb, except wrist and hand   `CC` `H5`

     √7ᵗʰ **T22.792** **Corrosion of third degree of** multiple sites of left shoulder and upper limb, except wrist and hand   `CC` `H5`

     √7ᵗʰ **T22.799** **Corrosion of third degree of** multiple sites of unspecified shoulder and upper limb, except wrist and hand   `CC` `H5`

√4ᵗʰ **T23** **Burn and corrosion of wrist and hand**
AHA: 2015, 1Q, 19

> The appropriate 7th character is to be added to each code from category T23.
> A   initial encounter
> D   subsequent encounter
> S   sequela

√5ᵗʰ **T23.0** **Burn of** unspecified degree of wrist and hand
Use additional external cause code to identify the source, place and intent of the burn (X00-X19, X75-X77, X96-X98, Y92)

   √6ᵗʰ **T23.00** **Burn of unspecified degree of hand,** unspecified site

     √7ᵗʰ **T23.001** **Burn of unspecified degree of** right hand, unspecified site

     √7ᵗʰ **T23.002** **Burn of unspecified degree of** left hand, unspecified site

     √7ᵗʰ **T23.009** **Burn of unspecified degree of** unspecified hand, unspecified site

   √6ᵗʰ **T23.01** **Burn of unspecified degree of** thumb (nail)

     √7ᵗʰ **T23.011** **Burn of unspecified degree of** right thumb (nail)

     √7ᵗʰ **T23.012** **Burn of unspecified degree of** left thumb (nail)

     √7ᵗʰ **T23.019** **Burn of unspecified degree of** unspecified thumb (nail)

√6ᵗʰ **T23.02** **Burn of unspecified degree of** single finger (nail) except thumb

     √7ᵗʰ **T23.021** **Burn of unspecified degree of** single right finger (nail) except thumb

     √7ᵗʰ **T23.022** **Burn of unspecified degree of** single left finger (nail) except thumb

     √7ᵗʰ **T23.029** **Burn of unspecified degree of** unspecified single finger (nail) except thumb

√6ᵗʰ **T23.03** **Burn of unspecified degree of** multiple fingers (nail), not including thumb

     √7ᵗʰ **T23.031** **Burn of unspecified degree of multiple** right fingers (nail), not including thumb

     √7ᵗʰ **T23.032** **Burn of unspecified degree of multiple** left fingers (nail), not including thumb

     √7ᵗʰ **T23.039** **Burn of unspecified degree of** unspecified multiple fingers (nail), not including thumb

√6ᵗʰ **T23.04** **Burn of unspecified degree of** multiple fingers (nail), including thumb

     √7ᵗʰ **T23.041** **Burn of unspecified degree of multiple** right fingers (nail), including thumb

     √7ᵗʰ **T23.042** **Burn of unspecified degree of multiple** left fingers (nail), including thumb

     √7ᵗʰ **T23.049** **Burn of unspecified degree of** unspecified multiple fingers (nail), including thumb

√6ᵗʰ **T23.05** **Burn of unspecified degree of** palm

     √7ᵗʰ **T23.051** **Burn of unspecified degree of** right palm

     √7ᵗʰ **T23.052** **Burn of unspecified degree of** left palm

     √7ᵗʰ **T23.059** **Burn of unspecified degree of** unspecified palm

√6ᵗʰ **T23.06** **Burn of unspecified degree of** back of hand

     √7ᵗʰ **T23.061** **Burn of unspecified degree of back of** right hand

     √7ᵗʰ **T23.062** **Burn of unspecified degree of back of** left hand

     √7ᵗʰ **T23.069** **Burn of unspecified degree of back of** unspecified hand

√6ᵗʰ **T23.07** **Burn of unspecified degree of** wrist

     √7ᵗʰ **T23.071** **Burn of unspecified degree of** right wrist

     √7ᵗʰ **T23.072** **Burn of unspecified degree of** left wrist

     √7ᵗʰ **T23.079** **Burn of unspecified degree of** unspecified wrist

√6ᵗʰ **T23.09** **Burn of unspecified degree of** multiple sites of wrist and hand

     √7ᵗʰ **T23.091** **Burn of unspecified degree of multiple** sites of right wrist and hand

     √7ᵗʰ **T23.092** **Burn of unspecified degree of multiple** sites of left wrist and hand

     √7ᵗʰ **T23.099** **Burn of unspecified degree of multiple** sites of unspecified wrist and hand

√5ᵗʰ **T23.1** **Burn of** first degree of wrist and hand
Use additional external cause code to identify the source, place and intent of the burn (X00-X19, X75-X77, X96-X98, Y92)

   √6ᵗʰ **T23.10** **Burn of first degree of hand,** unspecified site

     √7ᵗʰ **T23.101** **Burn of first degree of** right hand, unspecified site

     √7ᵗʰ **T23.102** **Burn of first degree of** left hand, unspecified site

     √7ᵗʰ **T23.109** **Burn of first degree of** unspecified hand, unspecified site

   √6ᵗʰ **T23.11** **Burn of first degree of** thumb (nail)

     √7ᵗʰ **T23.111** **Burn of first degree of** right thumb (nail)

     √7ᵗʰ **T23.112** **Burn of first degree of** left thumb (nail)

     √7ᵗʰ **T23.119** **Burn of first degree of** unspecified thumb (nail)

   √6ᵗʰ **T23.12** **Burn of first degree of** single finger (nail) except thumb

     √7ᵗʰ **T23.121** **Burn of first degree of single** right finger (nail) except thumb

     √7ᵗʰ **T23.122** **Burn of first degree of single** left finger (nail) except thumb

N Newborn: 0   P Pediatric: 0-17   M Maternity: 12-55   A Adult: 15-124   MCC Major CC Condition   PDx MCC PDx acts as own MCC   CC CC Condition   PDx CC PDx acts as own CC

1086   ICD-10-CM 2018

√7ᵗʰ **T23.129** Burn of first degree of unspecified single finger (nail) except thumb

√6ᵗʰ **T23.13** Burn of first degree of multiple fingers (nail), not including thumb

  √7ᵗʰ **T23.131** Burn of first degree of multiple right fingers (nail), not including thumb

  √7ᵗʰ **T23.132** Burn of first degree of multiple left fingers (nail), not including thumb

  √7ᵗʰ **T23.139** Burn of first degree of unspecified multiple fingers (nail), not including thumb

√6ᵗʰ **T23.14** Burn of first degree of multiple fingers (nail), including thumb

  √7ᵗʰ **T23.141** Burn of first degree of multiple right fingers (nail), including thumb

  √7ᵗʰ **T23.142** Burn of first degree of multiple left fingers (nail), including thumb

  √7ᵗʰ **T23.149** Burn of first degree of unspecified multiple fingers (nail), including thumb

√6ᵗʰ **T23.15** Burn of first degree of palm

  √7ᵗʰ **T23.151** Burn of first degree of right palm

  √7ᵗʰ **T23.152** Burn of first degree of left palm

  √7ᵗʰ **T23.159** Burn of first degree of unspecified palm

√6ᵗʰ **T23.16** Burn of first degree of back of hand

  √7ᵗʰ **T23.161** Burn of first degree of back of right hand

  √7ᵗʰ **T23.162** Burn of first degree of back of left hand

  √7ᵗʰ **T23.169** Burn of first degree of back of unspecified hand

√6ᵗʰ **T23.17** Burn of first degree of wrist

  √7ᵗʰ **T23.171** Burn of first degree of right wrist

  √7ᵗʰ **T23.172** Burn of first degree of left wrist

  √7ᵗʰ **T23.179** Burn of first degree of unspecified wrist

√6ᵗʰ **T23.19** Burn of first degree of multiple sites of wrist and hand

  √7ᵗʰ **T23.191** Burn of first degree of multiple sites of right wrist and hand

  √7ᵗʰ **T23.192** Burn of first degree of multiple sites of left wrist and hand

  √7ᵗʰ **T23.199** Burn of first degree of multiple sites of unspecified wrist and hand

√5ᵗʰ **T23.2** Burn of second degree of wrist and hand
Use additional external cause code to identify the source, place and intent of the burn (X00-X19, X75-X77, X96-X98, Y92)

√6ᵗʰ **T23.20** Burn of second degree of hand, unspecified site

  √7ᵗʰ **T23.201** Burn of second degree of right hand, unspecified site

  √7ᵗʰ **T23.202** Burn of second degree of left hand, unspecified site

  √7ᵗʰ **T23.209** Burn of second degree of unspecified hand, unspecified site

√6ᵗʰ **T23.21** Burn of second degree of thumb (nail)

  √7ᵗʰ **T23.211** Burn of second degree of right thumb (nail)

  √7ᵗʰ **T23.212** Burn of second degree of left thumb (nail)

  √7ᵗʰ **T23.219** Burn of second degree of unspecified thumb (nail)

√6ᵗʰ **T23.22** Burn of second degree of single finger (nail) except thumb

  √7ᵗʰ **T23.221** Burn of second degree of single right finger (nail) except thumb

  √7ᵗʰ **T23.222** Burn of second degree of single left finger (nail) except thumb

  √7ᵗʰ **T23.229** Burn of second degree of unspecified single finger (nail) except thumb

√6ᵗʰ **T23.23** Burn of second degree of multiple fingers (nail), not including thumb

  √7ᵗʰ **T23.231** Burn of second degree of multiple right fingers (nail), not including thumb

  √7ᵗʰ **T23.232** Burn of second degree of multiple left fingers (nail), not including thumb

  √7ᵗʰ **T23.239** Burn of second degree of unspecified multiple fingers (nail), not including thumb

√6ᵗʰ **T23.24** Burn of second degree of multiple fingers (nail), including thumb

  √7ᵗʰ **T23.241** Burn of second degree of multiple right fingers (nail), including thumb

  √7ᵗʰ **T23.242** Burn of second degree of multiple left fingers (nail), including thumb

  √7ᵗʰ **T23.249** Burn of second degree of unspecified multiple fingers (nail), including thumb

√6ᵗʰ **T23.25** Burn of second degree of palm

  √7ᵗʰ **T23.251** Burn of second degree of right palm

  √7ᵗʰ **T23.252** Burn of second degree of left palm

  √7ᵗʰ **T23.259** Burn of second degree of unspecified palm

√6ᵗʰ **T23.26** Burn of second degree of back of hand

  √7ᵗʰ **T23.261** Burn of second degree of back of right hand

  √7ᵗʰ **T23.262** Burn of second degree of back of left hand

  √7ᵗʰ **T23.269** Burn of second degree of back of unspecified hand

√6ᵗʰ **T23.27** Burn of second degree of wrist

  √7ᵗʰ **T23.271** Burn of second degree of right wrist

  √7ᵗʰ **T23.272** Burn of second degree of left wrist

  √7ᵗʰ **T23.279** Burn of second degree of unspecified wrist

√6ᵗʰ **T23.29** Burn of second degree of multiple sites of wrist and hand

  √7ᵗʰ **T23.291** Burn of second degree of multiple sites of right wrist and hand

  √7ᵗʰ **T23.292** Burn of second degree of multiple sites of left wrist and hand

  √7ᵗʰ **T23.299** Burn of second degree of multiple sites of unspecified wrist and hand

√5ᵗʰ **T23.3** Burn of third degree of wrist and hand
Use additional external cause code to identify the source, place and intent of the burn (X00-X19, X75-X77, X96-X98, Y92)

√6ᵗʰ **T23.30** Burn of third degree of hand, unspecified site
AHA: 2016, 2Q, 5

CC Excl: For codes in subcategory T23.30:
PDX collection 1396

  √7ᵗʰ **T23.301** Burn of third degree of right hand, unspecified site CC H5

  √7ᵗʰ **T23.302** Burn of third degree of left hand, unspecified site CC H5

  √7ᵗʰ **T23.309** Burn of third degree of unspecified hand, unspecified site CC H5

√6ᵗʰ **T23.31** Burn of third degree of thumb (nail)

CC Excl: For codes in subcategory T23.31:
PDX collection 1397

  √7ᵗʰ **T23.311** Burn of third degree of right thumb (nail) CC H5

  √7ᵗʰ **T23.312** Burn of third degree of left thumb (nail) CC H5

  √7ᵗʰ **T23.319** Burn of third degree of unspecified thumb (nail) CC H5

√6ᵗʰ **T23.32** Burn of third degree of single finger (nail) except thumb

CC Excl: For codes in subcategory T23.32:
PDX collection 1398

  √7ᵗʰ **T23.321** Burn of third degree of single right finger (nail) except thumb CC H5

  √7ᵗʰ **T23.322** Burn of third degree of single left finger (nail) except thumb CC H5

  √7ᵗʰ **T23.329** Burn of third degree of unspecified single finger (nail) except thumb CC H5

√6ᵗʰ **T23.33** Burn of third degree of multiple fingers (nail), not including thumb

CC Excl: For codes in subcategory T23.33:
PDX collection 1399

  √7ᵗʰ **T23.331** Burn of third degree of multiple right fingers (nail), not including thumb CC H5

  √7ᵗʰ **T23.332** Burn of third degree of multiple left fingers (nail), not including thumb CC H5

✓7ᵗʰ **T23.339** Burn of third degree of unspecified `CC` `H5` multiple fingers (nail), not including thumb

✓6ᵗʰ **T23.34** Burn of third degree of multiple fingers (nail), including thumb

> **CC Excl:** For codes in subcategory T23.34:
> PDX collection 1400

✓7ᵗʰ **T23.341** Burn of third degree of multiple `CC` `H5` right fingers (nail), including thumb

✓7ᵗʰ **T23.342** Burn of third degree of multiple `CC` `H5` left fingers (nail), including thumb

✓7ᵗʰ **T23.349** Burn of third degree of unspecified `CC` `H5` multiple fingers (nail), including thumb

✓6ᵗʰ **T23.35** Burn of third degree of palm

> **CC Excl:** For codes in subcategory T23.35:
> PDX collection 1401

✓7ᵗʰ **T23.351** Burn of third degree of right palm `CC` `H5`

✓7ᵗʰ **T23.352** Burn of third degree of left palm `CC` `H5`

✓7ᵗʰ **T23.359** Burn of third degree of unspecified `CC` `H5` palm

✓6ᵗʰ **T23.36** Burn of third degree of back of hand

> **CC Excl:** For codes in subcategory T23.36:
> PDX collection 1402

✓7ᵗʰ **T23.361** Burn of third degree of back of `CC` `H5` right hand

✓7ᵗʰ **T23.362** Burn of third degree of back of left `CC` `H5` hand

✓7ᵗʰ **T23.369** Burn of third degree of back of `CC` `H5` unspecified hand

✓6ᵗʰ **T23.37** Burn of third degree of wrist

> **CC Excl:** For codes in subcategory T23.37:
> PDX collection 1403

✓7ᵗʰ **T23.371** Burn of third degree of right wrist `CC` `H5`

✓7ᵗʰ **T23.372** Burn of third degree of left wrist `CC` `H5`

✓7ᵗʰ **T23.379** Burn of third degree of unspecified `CC` `H5` wrist

✓6ᵗʰ **T23.39** Burn of third degree of multiple sites of wrist and hand

> **CC Excl:** For codes in subcategory T23.39:
> PDX collection 1396

✓7ᵗʰ **T23.391** Burn of third degree of multiple `CC` `H5` sites of right wrist and hand

✓7ᵗʰ **T23.392** Burn of third degree of multiple `CC` `H5` sites of left wrist and hand

✓7ᵗʰ **T23.399** Burn of third degree of multiple `CC` `H5` sites of unspecified wrist and hand

✓5ᵗʰ **T23.4** Corrosion of unspecified degree of wrist and hand
Code first (T51-T65) to identify chemical and intent
Use additional external cause code to identify place (Y92)

✓6ᵗʰ **T23.40** Corrosion of unspecified degree of hand, unspecified site

✓7ᵗʰ **T23.401** Corrosion of unspecified degree of right hand, unspecified site

✓7ᵗʰ **T23.402** Corrosion of unspecified degree of left hand, unspecified site

✓7ᵗʰ **T23.409** Corrosion of unspecified degree of unspecified hand, unspecified site

✓6ᵗʰ **T23.41** Corrosion of unspecified degree of thumb (nail)

✓7ᵗʰ **T23.411** Corrosion of unspecified degree of right thumb (nail)

✓7ᵗʰ **T23.412** Corrosion of unspecified degree of left thumb (nail)

✓7ᵗʰ **T23.419** Corrosion of unspecified degree of unspecified thumb (nail)

✓6ᵗʰ **T23.42** Corrosion of unspecified degree of single finger (nail) except thumb

✓7ᵗʰ **T23.421** Corrosion of unspecified degree of single right finger (nail) except thumb

✓7ᵗʰ **T23.422** Corrosion of unspecified degree of single left finger (nail) except thumb

✓7ᵗʰ **T23.429** Corrosion of unspecified degree of unspecified single finger (nail) except thumb

✓6ᵗʰ **T23.43** Corrosion of unspecified degree of multiple fingers (nail), not including thumb

✓7ᵗʰ **T23.431** Corrosion of unspecified degree of multiple right fingers (nail), not including thumb

✓7ᵗʰ **T23.432** Corrosion of unspecified degree of multiple left fingers (nail), not including thumb

✓7ᵗʰ **T23.439** Corrosion of unspecified degree of unspecified multiple fingers (nail), not including thumb

✓6ᵗʰ **T23.44** Corrosion of unspecified degree of multiple fingers (nail), including thumb

✓7ᵗʰ **T23.441** Corrosion of unspecified degree of multiple right fingers (nail), including thumb

✓7ᵗʰ **T23.442** Corrosion of unspecified degree of multiple left fingers (nail), including thumb

✓7ᵗʰ **T23.449** Corrosion of unspecified degree of unspecified multiple fingers (nail), including thumb

✓6ᵗʰ **T23.45** Corrosion of unspecified degree of palm

✓7ᵗʰ **T23.451** Corrosion of unspecified degree of right palm

✓7ᵗʰ **T23.452** Corrosion of unspecified degree of left palm

✓7ᵗʰ **T23.459** Corrosion of unspecified degree of unspecified palm

✓6ᵗʰ **T23.46** Corrosion of unspecified degree of back of hand

✓7ᵗʰ **T23.461** Corrosion of unspecified degree of back of right hand

✓7ᵗʰ **T23.462** Corrosion of unspecified degree of back of left hand

✓7ᵗʰ **T23.469** Corrosion of unspecified degree of back of unspecified hand

✓6ᵗʰ **T23.47** Corrosion of unspecified degree of wrist

✓7ᵗʰ **T23.471** Corrosion of unspecified degree of right wrist

✓7ᵗʰ **T23.472** Corrosion of unspecified degree of left wrist

✓7ᵗʰ **T23.479** Corrosion of unspecified degree of unspecified wrist

✓6ᵗʰ **T23.49** Corrosion of unspecified degree of multiple sites of wrist and hand

✓7ᵗʰ **T23.491** Corrosion of unspecified degree of multiple sites of right wrist and hand

✓7ᵗʰ **T23.492** Corrosion of unspecified degree of multiple sites of left wrist and hand

✓7ᵗʰ **T23.499** Corrosion of unspecified degree of multiple sites of unspecified wrist and hand

✓5ᵗʰ **T23.5** Corrosion of first degree of wrist and hand
Code first (T51-T65) to identify chemical and intent
Use additional external cause code to identify place (Y92)

✓6ᵗʰ **T23.50** Corrosion of first degree of hand, unspecified site

✓7ᵗʰ **T23.501** Corrosion of first degree of right hand, unspecified site

✓7ᵗʰ **T23.502** Corrosion of first degree of left hand, unspecified site

✓7ᵗʰ **T23.509** Corrosion of first degree of unspecified hand, unspecified site

✓6ᵗʰ **T23.51** Corrosion of first degree of thumb (nail)

✓7ᵗʰ **T23.511** Corrosion of first degree of right thumb (nail)

✓7ᵗʰ **T23.512** Corrosion of first degree of left thumb (nail)

✓7ᵗʰ **T23.519** Corrosion of first degree of unspecified thumb (nail)

✓6ᵗʰ **T23.52** Corrosion of first degree of single finger (nail) except thumb

✓7ᵗʰ **T23.521** Corrosion of first degree of single right finger (nail) except thumb

√7ᵗʰ **T23.522** Corrosion of first degree of single left finger (nail) except thumb

√7ᵗʰ **T23.529** Corrosion of first degree of unspecified single finger (nail) except thumb

√6ᵗʰ **T23.53** Corrosion of first degree of multiple fingers (nail), not including thumb

√7ᵗʰ **T23.531** Corrosion of first degree of multiple right fingers (nail), not including thumb

√7ᵗʰ **T23.532** Corrosion of first degree of multiple left fingers (nail), not including thumb

√7ᵗʰ **T23.539** Corrosion of first degree of unspecified multiple fingers (nail), not including thumb

√6ᵗʰ **T23.54** Corrosion of first degree of multiple fingers (nail), including thumb

√7ᵗʰ **T23.541** Corrosion of first degree of multiple right fingers (nail), including thumb

√7ᵗʰ **T23.542** Corrosion of first degree of multiple left fingers (nail), including thumb

√7ᵗʰ **T23.549** Corrosion of first degree of unspecified multiple fingers (nail), including thumb

√6ᵗʰ **T23.55** Corrosion of first degree of palm

√7ᵗʰ **T23.551** Corrosion of first degree of right palm

√7ᵗʰ **T23.552** Corrosion of first degree of left palm

√7ᵗʰ **T23.559** Corrosion of first degree of unspecified palm

√6ᵗʰ **T23.56** Corrosion of first degree of back of hand

√7ᵗʰ **T23.561** Corrosion of first degree of back of right hand

√7ᵗʰ **T23.562** Corrosion of first degree of back of left hand

√7ᵗʰ **T23.569** Corrosion of first degree of back of unspecified hand

√6ᵗʰ **T23.57** Corrosion of first degree of wrist

√7ᵗʰ **T23.571** Corrosion of first degree of right wrist

√7ᵗʰ **T23.572** Corrosion of first degree of left wrist

√7ᵗʰ **T23.579** Corrosion of first degree of unspecified wrist

√6ᵗʰ **T23.59** Corrosion of first degree of multiple sites of wrist and hand

√7ᵗʰ **T23.591** Corrosion of first degree of multiple sites of right wrist and hand

√7ᵗʰ **T23.592** Corrosion of first degree of multiple sites of left wrist and hand

√7ᵗʰ **T23.599** Corrosion of first degree of multiple sites of unspecified wrist and hand

√5ᵗʰ **T23.6** Corrosion of second degree of wrist and hand

Code first (T51-T65) to identify chemical and intent

Use additional external cause code to identify place (Y92)

√6ᵗʰ **T23.60** Corrosion of second degree of hand, unspecified site

√7ᵗʰ **T23.601** Corrosion of second degree of right hand, unspecified site

√7ᵗʰ **T23.602** Corrosion of second degree of left hand, unspecified site

√7ᵗʰ **T23.609** Corrosion of second degree of unspecified hand, unspecified site

√6ᵗʰ **T23.61** Corrosion of second degree of thumb (nail)

√7ᵗʰ **T23.611** Corrosion of second degree of right thumb (nail)

√7ᵗʰ **T23.612** Corrosion of second degree of left thumb (nail)

√7ᵗʰ **T23.619** Corrosion of second degree of unspecified thumb (nail)

√6ᵗʰ **T23.62** Corrosion of second degree of single finger (nail) except thumb

√7ᵗʰ **T23.621** Corrosion of second degree of single right finger (nail) except thumb

√7ᵗʰ **T23.622** Corrosion of second degree of single left finger (nail) except thumb

√7ᵗʰ **T23.629** Corrosion of second degree of unspecified single finger (nail) except thumb

√6ᵗʰ **T23.63** Corrosion of second degree of multiple fingers (nail), not including thumb

√7ᵗʰ **T23.631** Corrosion of second degree of multiple right fingers (nail), not including thumb

√7ᵗʰ **T23.632** Corrosion of second degree of multiple left fingers (nail), not including thumb

√7ᵗʰ **T23.639** Corrosion of second degree of unspecified multiple fingers (nail), not including thumb

√6ᵗʰ **T23.64** Corrosion of second degree of multiple fingers (nail), including thumb

√7ᵗʰ **T23.641** Corrosion of second degree of multiple right fingers (nail), including thumb

√7ᵗʰ **T23.642** Corrosion of second degree of multiple left fingers (nail), including thumb

√7ᵗʰ **T23.649** Corrosion of second degree of unspecified multiple fingers (nail), including thumb

√6ᵗʰ **T23.65** Corrosion of second degree of palm

√7ᵗʰ **T23.651** Corrosion of second degree of right palm

√7ᵗʰ **T23.652** Corrosion of second degree of left palm

√7ᵗʰ **T23.659** Corrosion of second degree of unspecified palm

√6ᵗʰ **T23.66** Corrosion of second degree of back of hand

√7ᵗʰ **T23.661** Corrosion of second degree back of right hand

√7ᵗʰ **T23.662** Corrosion of second degree back of left hand

√7ᵗʰ **T23.669** Corrosion of second degree back of unspecified hand

√6ᵗʰ **T23.67** Corrosion of second degree of wrist

√7ᵗʰ **T23.671** Corrosion of second degree of right wrist

√7ᵗʰ **T23.672** Corrosion of second degree of left wrist

√7ᵗʰ **T23.679** Corrosion of second degree of unspecified wrist

√6ᵗʰ **T23.69** Corrosion of second degree of multiple sites of wrist and hand

√7ᵗʰ **T23.691** Corrosion of second degree of multiple sites of right wrist and hand

√7ᵗʰ **T23.692** Corrosion of second degree of multiple sites of left wrist and hand

√7ᵗʰ **T23.699** Corrosion of second degree of multiple sites of unspecified wrist and hand

√5ᵗʰ **T23.7** Corrosion of third degree of wrist and hand

Code first (T51-T65) to identify chemical and intent

Use additional external cause code to identify place (Y92)

√6ᵗʰ **T23.70** Corrosion of third degree of hand, unspecified site

> **CC Excl: For codes in subcategory T23.70:**
> PDX collection 1396

√7ᵗʰ **T23.701** Corrosion of third degree of right hand, unspecified site   **CC H5**

√7ᵗʰ **T23.702** Corrosion of third degree of left hand, unspecified site   **CC H5**

√7ᵗʰ **T23.709** Corrosion of third degree of unspecified hand, unspecified site   **CC H5**

√6ᵗʰ **T23.71** Corrosion of third degree of thumb (nail)

> **CC Excl: For codes in subcategory T23.71:**
> PDX collection 1397

√7ᵗʰ **T23.711** Corrosion of third degree of right thumb (nail)   **CC H5**

√7ᵗʰ **T23.712** Corrosion of third degree of left thumb (nail)   **CC H5**

√7ᵗʰ **T23.719** Corrosion of third degree of unspecified thumb (nail)   **CC H5**

√6ᵗʰ **T23.72** Corrosion of third degree of single finger (nail) except thumb

> **CC Excl: For codes in subcategory T23.72:**
> PDX collection 1398

√7ᵗʰ **T23.721** Corrosion of third degree of single right finger (nail) except thumb   **CC H5**

√7ᵗʰ **T23.722** Corrosion of third degree of single left finger (nail) except thumb   **CC H5**

✔ Additional Character Req   √x7ᵗʰ Placeholder Alert   Unacceptable PDx   Manifestation   **H1**-**H14** HAC   **HCC** CMS-HCC Condition   *EXCLUDES 1* Not Coded Here   *EXCLUDES 2* Not Included Here

ICD-10-CM 2018   1089

√7ᵗʰ **T23.729** Corrosion of third degree of unspecified single finger (nail) except thumb   CC H5

√6ᵗʰ **T23.73** Corrosion of third degree of multiple fingers (nail), not including thumb

> **CC Excl: For codes in subcategory T23.73:**
> PDX collection 1399

√7ᵗʰ **T23.731** Corrosion of third degree of multiple right fingers (nail), not including thumb   CC H5

√7ᵗʰ **T23.732** Corrosion of third degree of multiple left fingers (nail), not including thumb   CC H5

√7ᵗʰ **T23.739** Corrosion of third degree of unspecified multiple fingers (nail), not including thumb   CC H5

√6ᵗʰ **T23.74** Corrosion of third degree of multiple fingers (nail), including thumb

> **CC Excl: For codes in subcategory T23.74:**
> PDX collection 1400

√7ᵗʰ **T23.741** Corrosion of third degree of multiple right fingers (nail), including thumb   CC H5

√7ᵗʰ **T23.742** Corrosion of third degree of multiple left fingers (nail), including thumb   CC H5

√7ᵗʰ **T23.749** Corrosion of third degree of unspecified multiple fingers (nail), including thumb   CC H5

√6ᵗʰ **T23.75** Corrosion of third degree of palm

> **CC Excl: For codes in subcategory T23.75:**
> PDX collection 1401

√7ᵗʰ **T23.751** Corrosion of third degree of right palm   CC H5

√7ᵗʰ **T23.752** Corrosion of third degree of left palm   CC H5

√7ᵗʰ **T23.759** Corrosion of third degree of unspecified palm   CC H5

√6ᵗʰ **T23.76** Corrosion of third degree of back of hand

> **CC Excl: For codes in subcategory T23.76:**
> PDX collection 1402

√7ᵗʰ **T23.761** Corrosion of third degree of back of right hand   CC H5

√7ᵗʰ **T23.762** Corrosion of third degree of back of left hand   CC H5

√7ᵗʰ **T23.769** Corrosion of third degree back of unspecified hand   CC H5

√6ᵗʰ **T23.77** Corrosion of third degree of wrist

> **CC Excl: For codes in subcategory T23.77:**
> PDX collection 1403

√7ᵗʰ **T23.771** Corrosion of third degree of right wrist   CC H5

√7ᵗʰ **T23.772** Corrosion of third degree of left wrist   CC H5

√7ᵗʰ **T23.779** Corrosion of third degree of unspecified wrist   CC H5

√6ᵗʰ **T23.79** Corrosion of third degree of multiple sites of wrist and hand

> **CC Excl: For codes in subcategory T23.79:**
> PDX collection 1396

√7ᵗʰ **T23.791** Corrosion of third degree of multiple sites of right wrist and hand   CC H5

√7ᵗʰ **T23.792** Corrosion of third degree of multiple sites of left wrist and hand   CC H5

√7ᵗʰ **T23.799** Corrosion of third degree of multiple sites of unspecified wrist and hand   CC H5

√4ᵗʰ **T24** **Burn and corrosion of lower limb, except ankle and foot**

> **EXCLUDES 2** burn and corrosion of ankle and foot (T25.-)
> burn and corrosion of hip region (T21.-)

> The appropriate 7th character is to be added to each code from category T24.
> A   initial encounter
> D   subsequent encounter
> S   sequela

√5ᵗʰ **T24.0** Burn of unspecified degree of lower limb, except ankle and foot

> Use additional external cause code to identify the source, place and intent of the burn (X00-X19, X75-X77, X96-X98, Y92)

√6ᵗʰ **T24.00** Burn of unspecified degree of unspecified site of lower limb, except ankle and foot

√7ᵗʰ **T24.001** Burn of unspecified degree of unspecified site of right lower limb, except ankle and foot

√7ᵗʰ **T24.002** Burn of unspecified degree of unspecified site of left lower limb, except ankle and foot

√7ᵗʰ **T24.009** Burn of unspecified degree of unspecified site of unspecified lower limb, except ankle and foot

√6ᵗʰ **T24.01** Burn of unspecified degree of thigh

√7ᵗʰ **T24.011** Burn of unspecified degree of right thigh

√7ᵗʰ **T24.012** Burn of unspecified degree of left thigh

√7ᵗʰ **T24.019** Burn of unspecified degree of unspecified thigh

√6ᵗʰ **T24.02** Burn of unspecified degree of knee

√7ᵗʰ **T24.021** Burn of unspecified degree of right knee

√7ᵗʰ **T24.022** Burn of unspecified degree of left knee

√7ᵗʰ **T24.029** Burn of unspecified degree of unspecified knee

√6ᵗʰ **T24.03** Burn of unspecified degree of lower leg

√7ᵗʰ **T24.031** Burn of unspecified degree of right lower leg

√7ᵗʰ **T24.032** Burn of unspecified degree of left lower leg

√7ᵗʰ **T24.039** Burn of unspecified degree of unspecified lower leg

√6ᵗʰ **T24.09** Burn of unspecified degree of multiple sites of lower limb, except ankle and foot

√7ᵗʰ **T24.091** Burn of unspecified degree of multiple sites of right lower limb, except ankle and foot

√7ᵗʰ **T24.092** Burn of unspecified degree of multiple sites of left lower limb, except ankle and foot

√7ᵗʰ **T24.099** Burn of unspecified degree of multiple sites of unspecified lower limb, except ankle and foot

√5ᵗʰ **T24.1** Burn of first degree of lower limb, except ankle and foot

> Use additional external cause code to identify the source, place and intent of the burn (X00-X19, X75-X77, X96-X98, Y92)

√6ᵗʰ **T24.10** Burn of first degree of unspecified site of lower limb, except ankle and foot

√7ᵗʰ **T24.101** Burn of first degree of unspecified site of right lower limb, except ankle and foot

√7ᵗʰ **T24.102** Burn of first degree of unspecified site of left lower limb, except ankle and foot

√7ᵗʰ **T24.109** Burn of first degree of unspecified site of unspecified lower limb, except ankle and foot

√6ᵗʰ **T24.11** Burn of first degree of thigh

√7ᵗʰ **T24.111** Burn of first degree of right thigh

√7ᵗʰ **T24.112** Burn of first degree of left thigh

√7ᵗʰ **T24.119** Burn of first degree of unspecified thigh

√6ᵗʰ **T24.12** Burn of first degree of knee

√7ᵗʰ **T24.121** Burn of first degree of right knee

√7ᵗʰ **T24.122** Burn of first degree of left knee

√7ᵗʰ **T24.129** Burn of first degree of unspecified knee

√6ᵗʰ **T24.13** Burn of first degree of lower leg

√7ᵗʰ **T24.131** Burn of first degree of right lower leg

√7ᵗʰ **T24.132** Burn of first degree of left lower leg

✓7ᵗʰ **T24.139** Burn of first degree of unspecified lower leg

✓6ᵗʰ **T24.19** Burn of first degree of multiple sites of lower limb, except ankle and foot

   ✓7ᵗʰ **T24.191** Burn of first degree of multiple sites of right lower limb, except ankle and foot

   ✓7ᵗʰ **T24.192** Burn of first degree of multiple sites of left lower limb, except ankle and foot

   ✓7ᵗʰ **T24.199** Burn of first degree of multiple sites of unspecified lower limb, except ankle and foot

✓5ᵗʰ **T24.2** Burn of second degree of lower limb, except ankle and foot
Use additional external cause code to identify the source, place and intent of the burn (X00-X19, X75-X77, X96-X98, Y92)

 ✓6ᵗʰ **T24.20** Burn of second degree of unspecified site of lower limb, except ankle and foot

   ✓7ᵗʰ **T24.201** Burn of second degree of unspecified site of right lower limb, except ankle and foot

   ✓7ᵗʰ **T24.202** Burn of second degree of unspecified site of left lower limb, except ankle and foot

   ✓7ᵗʰ **T24.209** Burn of second degree of unspecified site of unspecified lower limb, except ankle and foot

 ✓6ᵗʰ **T24.21** Burn of second degree of thigh

   ✓7ᵗʰ **T24.211** Burn of second degree of right thigh

   ✓7ᵗʰ **T24.212** Burn of second degree of left thigh

   ✓7ᵗʰ **T24.219** Burn of second degree of unspecified thigh

 ✓6ᵗʰ **T24.22** Burn of second degree of knee

   ✓7ᵗʰ **T24.221** Burn of second degree of right knee

   ✓7ᵗʰ **T24.222** Burn of second degree of left knee

   ✓7ᵗʰ **T24.229** Burn of second degree of unspecified knee

 ✓6ᵗʰ **T24.23** Burn of second degree of lower leg

   ✓7ᵗʰ **T24.231** Burn of second degree of right lower leg

   ✓7ᵗʰ **T24.232** Burn of second degree of left lower leg

   ✓7ᵗʰ **T24.239** Burn of second degree of unspecified lower leg

 ✓6ᵗʰ **T24.29** Burn of second degree of multiple sites of lower limb, except ankle and foot

   ✓7ᵗʰ **T24.291** Burn of second degree of multiple sites of right lower limb, except ankle and foot

   ✓7ᵗʰ **T24.292** Burn of second degree of multiple sites of left lower limb, except ankle and foot

   ✓7ᵗʰ **T24.299** Burn of second degree of multiple sites of unspecified lower limb, except ankle and foot

✓5ᵗʰ **T24.3** Burn of third degree of lower limb, except ankle and foot
Use additional external cause code to identify the source, place and intent of the burn (X00-X19, X75-X77, X96-X98, Y92)

 ✓6ᵗʰ **T24.30** Burn of third degree of unspecified site of lower limb, except ankle and foot

> **CC Excl: For codes in subcategory T24.30:**
> PDX collection 1404

   ✓7ᵗʰ **T24.301** Burn of third degree of unspecified site of right lower limb, except ankle and foot **CC H5**

   ✓7ᵗʰ **T24.302** Burn of third degree of unspecified site of left lower limb, except ankle and foot **CC H5**

   ✓7ᵗʰ **T24.309** Burn of third degree of unspecified site of unspecified lower limb, except ankle and foot **CC H5**

 ✓6ᵗʰ **T24.31** Burn of third degree of thigh

> **CC Excl: For codes in subcategory T24.31:**
> PDX collection 1405

   ✓7ᵗʰ **T24.311** Burn of third degree of right thigh **CC H5**

   ✓7ᵗʰ **T24.312** Burn of third degree of left thigh **CC H5**

   ✓7ᵗʰ **T24.319** Burn of third degree of unspecified thigh **CC H5**

 ✓6ᵗʰ **T24.32** Burn of third degree of knee

> **CC Excl: For codes in subcategory T24.32:**
> PDX collection 1406

   ✓7ᵗʰ **T24.321** Burn of third degree of right knee **CC H5**

   ✓7ᵗʰ **T24.322** Burn of third degree of left knee **CC H5**

   ✓7ᵗʰ **T24.329** Burn of third degree of unspecified knee **CC H5**

 ✓6ᵗʰ **T24.33** Burn of third degree of lower leg

> **CC Excl: For codes in subcategory T24.33:**
> PDX collection 1407

   ✓7ᵗʰ **T24.331** Burn of third degree of right lower leg **CC H5**

   ✓7ᵗʰ **T24.332** Burn of third degree of left lower leg **CC H5**

   ✓7ᵗʰ **T24.339** Burn of third degree of unspecified lower leg **CC H5**

 ✓6ᵗʰ **T24.39** Burn of third degree of multiple sites of lower limb, except ankle and foot
AHA: 2016, 2Q, 4

> **CC Excl: For codes in subcategory T24.39:**
> PDX collection 1404

   ✓7ᵗʰ **T24.391** Burn of third degree of multiple sites of right lower limb, except ankle and foot **CC H5**

   ✓7ᵗʰ **T24.392** Burn of third degree of multiple sites of left lower limb, except ankle and foot **CC H5**

   ✓7ᵗʰ **T24.399** Burn of third degree of multiple sites of unspecified lower limb, except ankle and foot **CC H5**

✓5ᵗʰ **T24.4** Corrosion of unspecified degree of lower limb, except ankle and foot
Code first (T51-T65) to identify chemical and intent
Use additional external cause code to identify place (Y92)

 ✓6ᵗʰ **T24.40** Corrosion of unspecified degree of unspecified site of lower limb, except ankle and foot

   ✓7ᵗʰ **T24.401** Corrosion of unspecified degree of unspecified site of right lower limb, except ankle and foot

   ✓7ᵗʰ **T24.402** Corrosion of unspecified degree of unspecified site of left lower limb, except ankle and foot

   ✓7ᵗʰ **T24.409** Corrosion of unspecified degree of unspecified site of unspecified lower limb, except ankle and foot

 ✓6ᵗʰ **T24.41** Corrosion of unspecified degree of thigh

   ✓7ᵗʰ **T24.411** Corrosion of unspecified degree of right thigh

   ✓7ᵗʰ **T24.412** Corrosion of unspecified degree of left thigh

   ✓7ᵗʰ **T24.419** Corrosion of unspecified degree of unspecified thigh

 ✓6ᵗʰ **T24.42** Corrosion of unspecified degree of knee

   ✓7ᵗʰ **T24.421** Corrosion of unspecified degree of right knee

   ✓7ᵗʰ **T24.422** Corrosion of unspecified degree of left knee

   ✓7ᵗʰ **T24.429** Corrosion of unspecified degree of unspecified knee

 ✓6ᵗʰ **T24.43** Corrosion of unspecified degree of lower leg

   ✓7ᵗʰ **T24.431** Corrosion of unspecified degree of right lower leg

   ✓7ᵗʰ **T24.432** Corrosion of unspecified degree of left lower leg

   ✓7ᵗʰ **T24.439** Corrosion of unspecified degree of unspecified lower leg

 ✓6ᵗʰ **T24.49** Corrosion of unspecified degree of multiple sites of lower limb, except ankle and foot

   ✓7ᵗʰ **T24.491** Corrosion of unspecified degree of multiple sites of right lower limb, except ankle and foot

   ✓7ᵗʰ **T24.492** Corrosion of unspecified degree of multiple sites of left lower limb, except ankle and foot

✓7ᵗʰ **T24.499** Corrosion of unspecified degree of multiple sites of unspecified lower limb, except ankle and foot

✓5ᵗʰ **T24.5** Corrosion of first degree of lower limb, except ankle and foot
> Code first (T51-T65) to identify chemical and intent
> Use additional external cause code to identify place (Y92)

  ✓6ᵗʰ **T24.50** Corrosion of first degree of unspecified site of lower limb, except ankle and foot

    ✓7ᵗʰ **T24.501** Corrosion of first degree of unspecified site of right lower limb, except ankle and foot

    ✓7ᵗʰ **T24.502** Corrosion of first degree of unspecified site of left lower limb, except ankle and foot

    ✓7ᵗʰ **T24.509** Corrosion of first degree of unspecified site of unspecified lower limb, except ankle and foot

  ✓6ᵗʰ **T24.51** Corrosion of first degree of thigh

    ✓7ᵗʰ **T24.511** Corrosion of first degree of right thigh

    ✓7ᵗʰ **T24.512** Corrosion of first degree of left thigh

    ✓7ᵗʰ **T24.519** Corrosion of first degree of unspecified thigh

  ✓6ᵗʰ **T24.52** Corrosion of first degree of knee

    ✓7ᵗʰ **T24.521** Corrosion of first degree of right knee

    ✓7ᵗʰ **T24.522** Corrosion of first degree of left knee

    ✓7ᵗʰ **T24.529** Corrosion of first degree of unspecified knee

  ✓6ᵗʰ **T24.53** Corrosion of first degree of lower leg

    ✓7ᵗʰ **T24.531** Corrosion of first degree of right lower leg

    ✓7ᵗʰ **T24.532** Corrosion of first degree of left lower leg

    ✓7ᵗʰ **T24.539** Corrosion of first degree of unspecified lower leg

  ✓6ᵗʰ **T24.59** Corrosion of first degree of multiple sites of lower limb, except ankle and foot

    ✓7ᵗʰ **T24.591** Corrosion of first degree of multiple sites of right lower limb, except ankle and foot

    ✓7ᵗʰ **T24.592** Corrosion of first degree of multiple sites of left lower limb, except ankle and foot

    ✓7ᵗʰ **T24.599** Corrosion of first degree of multiple sites of unspecified lower limb, except ankle and foot

✓5ᵗʰ **T24.6** Corrosion of second degree of lower limb, except ankle and foot
> Code first (T51-T65) to identify chemical and intent
> Use additional external cause code to identify place (Y92)

  ✓6ᵗʰ **T24.60** Corrosion of second degree of unspecified site of lower limb, except ankle and foot

    ✓7ᵗʰ **T24.601** Corrosion of second degree of unspecified site of right lower limb, except ankle and foot

    ✓7ᵗʰ **T24.602** Corrosion of second degree of unspecified site of left lower limb, except ankle and foot

    ✓7ᵗʰ **T24.609** Corrosion of second degree of unspecified site of unspecified lower limb, except ankle and foot

  ✓6ᵗʰ **T24.61** Corrosion of second degree of thigh

    ✓7ᵗʰ **T24.611** Corrosion of second degree of right thigh

    ✓7ᵗʰ **T24.612** Corrosion of second degree of left thigh

    ✓7ᵗʰ **T24.619** Corrosion of second degree of unspecified thigh

  ✓6ᵗʰ **T24.62** Corrosion of second degree of knee

    ✓7ᵗʰ **T24.621** Corrosion of second degree of right knee

    ✓7ᵗʰ **T24.622** Corrosion of second degree of left knee

    ✓7ᵗʰ **T24.629** Corrosion of second degree of unspecified knee

  ✓6ᵗʰ **T24.63** Corrosion of second degree of lower leg

    ✓7ᵗʰ **T24.631** Corrosion of second degree of right lower leg

    ✓7ᵗʰ **T24.632** Corrosion of second degree of left lower leg

    ✓7ᵗʰ **T24.639** Corrosion of second degree of unspecified lower leg

  ✓6ᵗʰ **T24.69** Corrosion of second degree of multiple sites of lower limb, except ankle and foot

    ✓7ᵗʰ **T24.691** Corrosion of second degree of multiple sites of right lower limb, except ankle and foot

    ✓7ᵗʰ **T24.692** Corrosion of second degree of multiple sites of left lower limb, except ankle and foot

    ✓7ᵗʰ **T24.699** Corrosion of second degree of multiple sites of unspecified lower limb, except ankle and foot

✓5ᵗʰ **T24.7** Corrosion of third degree of lower limb, except ankle and foot
> Code first (T51-T65) to identify chemical and intent
> Use additional external cause code to identify place (Y92)

  ✓6ᵗʰ **T24.70** Corrosion of third degree of unspecified site of lower limb, except ankle and foot

> **CC Excl: For codes in subcategory T24.70:**
> PDX collection 1404

    ✓7ᵗʰ **T24.701** Corrosion of third degree of unspecified site of right lower limb, except ankle and foot `CC` `H5`

    ✓7ᵗʰ **T24.702** Corrosion of third degree of unspecified site of left lower limb, except ankle and foot `CC` `H5`

    ✓7ᵗʰ **T24.709** Corrosion of third degree of unspecified site of unspecified lower limb, except ankle and foot `CC` `H5`

  ✓6ᵗʰ **T24.71** Corrosion of third degree of thigh

> **CC Excl: For codes in subcategory T24.71:**
> PDX collection 1405

    ✓7ᵗʰ **T24.711** Corrosion of third degree of right thigh `CC` `H5`

    ✓7ᵗʰ **T24.712** Corrosion of third degree of left thigh `CC` `H5`

    ✓7ᵗʰ **T24.719** Corrosion of third degree of unspecified thigh `CC` `H5`

  ✓6ᵗʰ **T24.72** Corrosion of third degree of knee

> **CC Excl: For codes in subcategory T24.72:**
> PDX collection 1406

    ✓7ᵗʰ **T24.721** Corrosion of third degree of right knee `CC` `H5`

    ✓7ᵗʰ **T24.722** Corrosion of third degree of left knee `CC` `H5`

    ✓7ᵗʰ **T24.729** Corrosion of third degree of unspecified knee `CC` `H5`

  ✓6ᵗʰ **T24.73** Corrosion of third degree of lower leg

> **CC Excl: For codes in subcategory T24.73:**
> PDX collection 1407

    ✓7ᵗʰ **T24.731** Corrosion of third degree of right lower leg `CC` `H5`

    ✓7ᵗʰ **T24.732** Corrosion of third degree of left lower leg `CC` `H5`

    ✓7ᵗʰ **T24.739** Corrosion of third degree of unspecified lower leg `CC` `H5`

  ✓6ᵗʰ **T24.79** Corrosion of third degree of multiple sites of lower limb, except ankle and foot

> **CC Excl: For codes in subcategory T24.79:**
> PDX collection 1404

    ✓7ᵗʰ **T24.791** Corrosion of third degree of multiple sites of right lower limb, except ankle and foot `CC` `H5`

    ✓7ᵗʰ **T24.792** Corrosion of third degree of multiple sites of left lower limb, except ankle and foot `CC` `H5`

    ✓7ᵗʰ **T24.799** Corrosion of third degree of multiple sites of unspecified lower limb, except ankle and foot `CC` `H5`

N Newborn: 0   P Pediatric: 0-17   M Maternity: 12-55   A Adult: 15-124   **MCC** Major CC Condition   **PDxMCC** PDx acts as own MCC   **CC** CC Condition   **PDxCC** PDx acts as own CC

1092   ICD-10-CM 2018

√4ᵗʰ **T25**   **Burn and corrosion of ankle and foot**

> The appropriate 7th character is to be added to each code from category T25.
> A   initial encounter
> D   subsequent encounter
> S   sequela

√5ᵗʰ **T25.0**   **Burn of unspecified degree of ankle and foot**

> Use additional external cause code to identify the source, place and intent of the burn (X00–X19, X75–X77, X96–X98, Y92)

   √6ᵗʰ **T25.01**   **Burn of unspecified degree of ankle**

     √7ᵗʰ **T25.011**   **Burn of unspecified degree of right ankle**

     √7ᵗʰ **T25.012**   **Burn of unspecified degree of left ankle**

     √7ᵗʰ **T25.019**   **Burn of unspecified degree of unspecified ankle**

   √6ᵗʰ **T25.02**   **Burn of unspecified degree of foot**

> EXCLUDES 2   burn of unspecified degree of toe(s) (nail) (T25.03-)

     √7ᵗʰ **T25.021**   **Burn of unspecified degree of right foot**

     √7ᵗʰ **T25.022**   **Burn of unspecified degree of left foot**

     √7ᵗʰ **T25.029**   **Burn of unspecified degree of unspecified foot**

   √6ᵗʰ **T25.03**   **Burn of unspecified degree of toe(s) (nail)**

     √7ᵗʰ **T25.031**   **Burn of unspecified degree of right toe(s) (nail)**

     √7ᵗʰ **T25.032**   **Burn of unspecified degree of left toe(s) (nail)**

     √7ᵗʰ **T25.039**   **Burn of unspecified degree of unspecified toe(s) (nail)**

   √6ᵗʰ **T25.09**   **Burn of unspecified degree of multiple sites of ankle and foot**

     √7ᵗʰ **T25.091**   **Burn of unspecified degree of multiple sites of right ankle and foot**

     √7ᵗʰ **T25.092**   **Burn of unspecified degree of multiple sites of left ankle and foot**

     √7ᵗʰ **T25.099**   **Burn of unspecified degree of multiple sites of unspecified ankle and foot**

√5ᵗʰ **T25.1**   **Burn of first degree of ankle and foot**

> Use additional external cause code to identify the source, place and intent of the burn (X00–X19, X75–X77, X96–X98, Y92)

   √6ᵗʰ **T25.11**   **Burn of first degree of ankle**

     √7ᵗʰ **T25.111**   **Burn of first degree of right ankle**

     √7ᵗʰ **T25.112**   **Burn of first degree of left ankle**

     √7ᵗʰ **T25.119**   **Burn of first degree of unspecified ankle**

   √6ᵗʰ **T25.12**   **Burn of first degree of foot**

> EXCLUDES 2   burn of first degree of toe(s) (nail) (T25.13-)

     √7ᵗʰ **T25.121**   **Burn of first degree of right foot**

     √7ᵗʰ **T25.122**   **Burn of first degree of left foot**

     √7ᵗʰ **T25.129**   **Burn of first degree of unspecified foot**

   √6ᵗʰ **T25.13**   **Burn of first degree of toe(s) (nail)**

     √7ᵗʰ **T25.131**   **Burn of first degree of right toe(s) (nail)**

     √7ᵗʰ **T25.132**   **Burn of first degree of left toe(s) (nail)**

     √7ᵗʰ **T25.139**   **Burn of first degree of unspecified toe(s) (nail)**

   √6ᵗʰ **T25.19**   **Burn of first degree of multiple sites of ankle and foot**

     √7ᵗʰ **T25.191**   **Burn of first degree of multiple sites of right ankle and foot**

     √7ᵗʰ **T25.192**   **Burn of first degree of multiple sites of left ankle and foot**

     √7ᵗʰ **T25.199**   **Burn of first degree of multiple sites of unspecified ankle and foot**

√5ᵗʰ **T25.2**   **Burn of second degree of ankle and foot**

> Use additional external cause code to identify the source, place and intent of the burn (X00–X19, X75–X77, X96–X98, Y92)

   √6ᵗʰ **T25.21**   **Burn of second degree of ankle**

     √7ᵗʰ **T25.211**   **Burn of second degree of right ankle**

     √7ᵗʰ **T25.212**   **Burn of second degree of left ankle**

     √7ᵗʰ **T25.219**   **Burn of second degree of unspecified ankle**

   √6ᵗʰ **T25.22**   **Burn of second degree of foot**

> EXCLUDES 2   burn of second degree of toe(s) (nail) (T25.23-)

     √7ᵗʰ **T25.221**   **Burn of second degree of right foot**

     √7ᵗʰ **T25.222**   **Burn of second degree of left foot**

     √7ᵗʰ **T25.229**   **Burn of second degree of unspecified foot**

   √6ᵗʰ **T25.23**   **Burn of second degree of toe(s) (nail)**

     √7ᵗʰ **T25.231**   **Burn of second degree of right toe(s) (nail)**

     √7ᵗʰ **T25.232**   **Burn of second degree of left toe(s) (nail)**

     √7ᵗʰ **T25.239**   **Burn of second degree of unspecified toe(s) (nail)**

   √6ᵗʰ **T25.29**   **Burn of second degree of multiple sites of ankle and foot**

     √7ᵗʰ **T25.291**   **Burn of second degree of multiple sites of right ankle and foot**

     √7ᵗʰ **T25.292**   **Burn of second degree of multiple sites of left ankle and foot**

     √7ᵗʰ **T25.299**   **Burn of second degree of multiple sites of unspecified ankle and foot**

√5ᵗʰ **T25.3**   **Burn of third degree of ankle and foot**

> Use additional external cause code to identify the source, place and intent of the burn (X00–X19, X75–X77, X96–X98, Y92)

   √6ᵗʰ **T25.31**   **Burn of third degree of ankle**

> **CC Excl: For codes in subcategory T25.31:** PDX collection 1408

     √7ᵗʰ **T25.311**   **Burn of third degree of right ankle**   CC H5

     √7ᵗʰ **T25.312**   **Burn of third degree of left ankle**   CC H5

     √7ᵗʰ **T25.319**   **Burn of third degree of unspecified ankle**   CC H5

   √6ᵗʰ **T25.32**   **Burn of third degree of foot**

> EXCLUDES 2   burn of third degree of toe(s) (nail) (T25.33-)

> **CC Excl: For codes in subcategory T25.32:** PDX collection 1409

     √7ᵗʰ **T25.321**   **Burn of third degree of right foot**   CC H5

     √7ᵗʰ **T25.322**   **Burn of third degree of left foot**   CC H5

     √7ᵗʰ **T25.329**   **Burn of third degree of unspecified foot**   CC H5

   √6ᵗʰ **T25.33**   **Burn of third degree of toe(s) (nail)**

> **CC Excl: For codes in subcategory T25.33:** PDX collection 1410

     √7ᵗʰ **T25.331**   **Burn of third degree of right toe(s) (nail)**   CC H5

     √7ᵗʰ **T25.332**   **Burn of third degree of left toe(s) (nail)**   CC H5

     √7ᵗʰ **T25.339**   **Burn of third degree of unspecified toe(s) (nail)**   CC H5

   √6ᵗʰ **T25.39**   **Burn of third degree of multiple sites of ankle and foot**

> **CC Excl: For codes in subcategory T25.39:** PDX collection 1404

     √7ᵗʰ **T25.391**   **Burn of third degree of multiple sites of right ankle and foot**   CC H5

     √7ᵗʰ **T25.392**   **Burn of third degree of multiple sites of left ankle and foot**   CC H5

     √7ᵗʰ **T25.399**   **Burn of third degree of multiple sites of unspecified ankle and foot**   CC H5

√5ᵗʰ **T25.4**   **Corrosion of unspecified degree of ankle and foot**

> Code first (T51-T65) to identify chemical and intent
> Use additional external cause code to identify place (Y92)

   √6ᵗʰ **T25.41**   **Corrosion of unspecified degree of ankle**

     √7ᵗʰ **T25.411**   **Corrosion of unspecified degree of right ankle**

     √7ᵗʰ **T25.412**   **Corrosion of unspecified degree of left ankle**

     √7ᵗʰ **T25.419**   **Corrosion of unspecified degree of unspecified ankle**

   √6ᵗʰ **T25.42**   **Corrosion of unspecified degree of foot**

> EXCLUDES 2   corrosion of unspecified degree of toe(s) (nail) (T25.43-)

     √7ᵗʰ **T25.421**   **Corrosion of unspecified degree of right foot**

     √7ᵗʰ **T25.422**   **Corrosion of unspecified degree of left foot**

     √7ᵗʰ **T25.429**   **Corrosion of unspecified degree of unspecified foot**

✔Additional Character Req   √x7ᵗʰ Placeholder Alert   Unacceptable PDx   Manifestation   H1–H14 HAC   HCC CMS-HCC Condition   EXCLUDES 1 Not Coded Here   EXCLUDES 2 Not Included Here

ICD-10-CM 2018   **1093**

√6th **T25.43** Corrosion of unspecified degree of toe(s) (nail)
- √7th **T25.431** Corrosion of unspecified degree of right toe(s) (nail)
- √7th **T25.432** Corrosion of unspecified degree of left toe(s) (nail)
- √7th **T25.439** Corrosion of unspecified degree of unspecified toe(s) (nail)

√6th **T25.49** Corrosion of unspecified degree of multiple sites of ankle and foot
- √7th **T25.491** Corrosion of unspecified degree of multiple sites of right ankle and foot
- √7th **T25.492** Corrosion of unspecified degree of multiple sites of left ankle and foot
- √7th **T25.499** Corrosion of unspecified degree of multiple sites of unspecified ankle and foot

√5th **T25.5** Corrosion of first degree of ankle and foot
Code first (T51-T65) to identify chemical and intent
Use additional external cause code to identify place (Y92)

√6th **T25.51** Corrosion of first degree of ankle
- √7th **T25.511** Corrosion of first degree of right ankle
- √7th **T25.512** Corrosion of first degree of left ankle
- √7th **T25.519** Corrosion of first degree of unspecified ankle

√6th **T25.52** Corrosion of first degree of foot
EXCLUDES 2 corrosion of first degree of toe(s) (nail) (T25.53-)
- √7th **T25.521** Corrosion of first degree of right foot
- √7th **T25.522** Corrosion of first degree of left foot
- √7th **T25.529** Corrosion of first degree of unspecified foot

√6th **T25.53** Corrosion of first degree of toe(s) (nail)
- √7th **T25.531** Corrosion of first degree of right toe(s) (nail)
- √7th **T25.532** Corrosion of first degree of left toe(s) (nail)
- √7th **T25.539** Corrosion of first degree of unspecified toe(s) (nail)

√6th **T25.59** Corrosion of first degree of multiple sites of ankle and foot
- √7th **T25.591** Corrosion of first degree of multiple sites of right ankle and foot
- √7th **T25.592** Corrosion of first degree of multiple sites of left ankle and foot
- √7th **T25.599** Corrosion of first degree of multiple sites of unspecified ankle and foot

√5th **T25.6** Corrosion of second degree of ankle and foot
Code first (T51-T65) to identify chemical and intent
Use additional external cause code to identify place (Y92)

√6th **T25.61** Corrosion of second degree of ankle
- √7th **T25.611** Corrosion of second degree of right ankle
- √7th **T25.612** Corrosion of second degree of left ankle
- √7th **T25.619** Corrosion of second degree of unspecified ankle

√6th **T25.62** Corrosion of second degree of foot
EXCLUDES 2 corrosion of second degree of toe(s) (nail) (T25.63-)
- √7th **T25.621** Corrosion of second degree of right foot
- √7th **T25.622** Corrosion of second degree of left foot
- √7th **T25.629** Corrosion of second degree of unspecified foot

√6th **T25.63** Corrosion of second degree of toe(s) (nail)
- √7th **T25.631** Corrosion of second degree of right toe(s) (nail)
- √7th **T25.632** Corrosion of second degree of left toe(s) (nail)
- √7th **T25.639** Corrosion of second degree of unspecified toe(s) (nail)

√6th **T25.69** Corrosion of second degree of multiple sites of ankle and foot
- √7th **T25.691** Corrosion of second degree of right ankle and foot
- √7th **T25.692** Corrosion of second degree of left ankle and foot

√7th **T25.699** Corrosion of second degree of unspecified ankle and foot

√5th **T25.7** Corrosion of third degree of ankle and foot
Code first (T51-T65) to identify chemical and intent
Use additional external cause code to identify place (Y92)

√6th **T25.71** Corrosion of third degree of ankle
CC Excl: For codes in subcategory T25.71: PDX collection 1408
- √7th **T25.711** Corrosion of third degree of right ankle CC H5
- √7th **T25.712** Corrosion of third degree of left ankle CC H5
- √7th **T25.719** Corrosion of third degree of unspecified ankle CC H5

√6th **T25.72** Corrosion of third degree of foot
EXCLUDES 2 corrosion of third degree of toe(s) (nail) (T25.73-)
CC Excl: For codes in subcategory T25.72: PDX collection 1409
- √7th **T25.721** Corrosion of third degree of right foot CC H5
- √7th **T25.722** Corrosion of third degree of left foot CC H5
- √7th **T25.729** Corrosion of third degree of unspecified foot CC H5

√6th **T25.73** Corrosion of third degree of toe(s) (nail)
CC Excl: For codes in subcategory T25.73: PDX collection 1410
- √7th **T25.731** Corrosion of third degree of right toe(s) (nail) CC H5
- √7th **T25.732** Corrosion of third degree of left toe(s) (nail) CC H5
- √7th **T25.739** Corrosion of third degree of unspecified toe(s) (nail) CC H5

√6th **T25.79** Corrosion of third degree of multiple sites of ankle and foot
CC Excl: For codes in subcategory T25.79: PDX collection 1404
- √7th **T25.791** Corrosion of third degree of multiple sites of right ankle and foot CC H5
- √7th **T25.792** Corrosion of third degree of multiple sites of left ankle and foot CC H5
- √7th **T25.799** Corrosion of third degree of multiple sites of unspecified ankle and foot CC H5

Burns and corrosions confined to eye and internal organs (T26-T28)

√4th **T26** Burn and corrosion confined to eye and adnexa

The appropriate 7th character is to be added to each code from category T26.
A   initial encounter
D   subsequent encounter
S   sequela

√5th **T26.0** Burn of eyelid and periocular area
Use additional external cause code to identify the source, place and intent of the burn (X00-X19, X75-X77, X96-X98, Y92)
- √x7th **T26.00** Burn of unspecified eyelid and periocular area
- √x7th **T26.01** Burn of right eyelid and periocular area
- √x7th **T26.02** Burn of left eyelid and periocular area

√5th **T26.1** Burn of cornea and conjunctival sac
Use additional external cause code to identify the source, place and intent of the burn (X00-X19, X75-X77, X96-X98, Y92)
- √x7th **T26.10** Burn of cornea and conjunctival sac, unspecified eye
- √x7th **T26.11** Burn of cornea and conjunctival sac, right eye
- √x7th **T26.12** Burn of cornea and conjunctival sac, left eye

✓5th **T26.2** **Burn with resulting rupture and destruction of eyeball**
Use additional external cause code to identify the source, place and intent of the burn (X00-X19, X75-X77, X96-X98, Y92)

✓x7th **T26.20** **Burn with resulting rupture and destruction of unspecified eyeball** `CC` `H5`
CC Excl: No Excl

✓x7th **T26.21** **Burn with resulting rupture and destruction of right eyeball** `CC` `H5`
CC Excl: No Excl

✓x7th **T26.22** **Burn with resulting rupture and destruction of left eyeball** `CC` `H5`
CC Excl: No Excl

✓5th **T26.3** **Burns of other specified parts of eye and adnexa**
Use additional external cause code to identify the source, place and intent of the burn (X00-X19, X75-X77, X96-X98, Y92)

✓x7th **T26.30** **Burns of other specified parts of unspecified eye and adnexa**

✓x7th **T26.31** **Burns of other specified parts of right eye and adnexa**

✓x7th **T26.32** **Burns of other specified parts of left eye and adnexa**

✓5th **T26.4** **Burn of eye and adnexa, part unspecified**
Use additional external cause code to identify the source, place and intent of the burn (X00-X19, X75-X77, X96-X98, Y92)

✓x7th **T26.40** **Burn of unspecified eye and adnexa, part unspecified**

✓x7th **T26.41** **Burn of right eye and adnexa, part unspecified**

✓x7th **T26.42** **Burn of left eye and adnexa, part unspecified**

✓5th **T26.5** **Corrosion of eyelid and periocular area**
Code first (T51-T65) to identify chemical and intent
Use additional external cause code to identify place (Y92)

✓x7th **T26.50** **Corrosion of unspecified eyelid and periocular area**

✓x7th **T26.51** **Corrosion of right eyelid and periocular area**

✓x7th **T26.52** **Corrosion of left eyelid and periocular area**

✓5th **T26.6** **Corrosion of cornea and conjunctival sac**
Code first (T51-T65) to identify chemical and intent
Use additional external cause code to identify place (Y92)

✓x7th **T26.60** **Corrosion of cornea and conjunctival sac, unspecified eye**

✓x7th **T26.61** **Corrosion of cornea and conjunctival sac, right eye**

✓x7th **T26.62** **Corrosion of cornea and conjunctival sac, left eye**

✓5th **T26.7** **Corrosion with resulting rupture and destruction of eyeball**
Code first (T51-T65) to identify chemical and intent
Use additional external cause code to identify place (Y92)

✓x7th **T26.70** **Corrosion with resulting rupture and destruction of unspecified eyeball** `CC` `H5`
CC Excl: No Excl

✓x7th **T26.71** **Corrosion with resulting rupture and destruction of right eyeball** `CC` `H5`
CC Excl: No Excl

✓x7th **T26.72** **Corrosion with resulting rupture and destruction of left eyeball** `CC` `H5`
CC Excl: No Excl

✓5th **T26.8** **Corrosions of other specified parts of eye and adnexa**
Code first (T51-T65) to identify chemical and intent
Use additional external cause code to identify place (Y92)

✓x7th **T26.80** **Corrosions of other specified parts of unspecified eye and adnexa**

✓x7th **T26.81** **Corrosions of other specified parts of right eye and adnexa**

✓x7th **T26.82** **Corrosions of other specified parts of left eye and adnexa**

✓5th **T26.9** **Corrosion of eye and adnexa, part unspecified**
Code first (T51-T65) to identify chemical and intent
Use additional external cause code to identify place (Y92)

✓x7th **T26.90** **Corrosion of unspecified eye and adnexa, part unspecified**

✓x7th **T26.91** **Corrosion of right eye and adnexa, part unspecified**

✓x7th **T26.92** **Corrosion of left eye and adnexa, part unspecified**

✓4th **T27** **Burn and corrosion of respiratory tract**
Use additional external cause code to identify the source and intent of the burn (X00-X19, X75-X77, X96-X98)
Use additional external cause code to identify place (Y92)

The appropriate 7th character is to be added to each code from category T27.
A initial encounter
D subsequent encounter
S sequela

CC Excl: For codes in subcategory T27: PDX collection 1411

✓x7th **T27.0** **Burn of larynx and trachea** `CC` `H5`

✓x7th **T27.1** **Burn involving larynx and trachea with lung** `CC` `H5`

✓x7th **T27.2** **Burn of other parts of respiratory tract** `CC` `H5`
Burn of thoracic cavity

✓x7th **T27.3** **Burn of respiratory tract, part unspecified** `CC` `H5`
~~Code first (T51-T65) to identify chemical and intent for codes T27.4-T27.7~~

✓x7th **T27.4** **Corrosion of larynx and trachea** `CC` `H5`
►Code first (T51-T65) to identify chemical and intent◄

✓x7th **T27.5** **Corrosion involving larynx and trachea with lung** `CC` `H5`

✓x7th **T27.6** **Corrosion of other parts of respiratory tract** `CC` `H5`
►Code first (T51-T65) to identify chemical and intent◄

✓x7th **T27.7** **Corrosion of respiratory tract, part unspecified** `CC` `H5`
►Code first (T51-T65) to identify chemical and intent◄

✓4th **T28** **Burn and corrosion of other internal organs**
Use additional external cause code to identify the source and intent of the burn (X00- X19, X75-X77, X96-X98)
Use additional external cause code to identify place (Y92)

The appropriate 7th character is to be added to each code from category T28.
A initial encounter
D subsequent encounter
S sequela

✓x7th **T28.0** **Burn of mouth and pharynx**

✓x7th **T28.1** **Burn of esophagus** `CC` `H5`
CC Excl: CC with 7th character A: PDX collection 1412

✓x7th **T28.2** **Burn of other parts of alimentary tract** `CC` `H5`
CC Excl: CC with 7th character A: PDX collection 1413

✓x7th **T28.3** **Burn of internal genitourinary organs**

✓5th **T28.4** **Burns of other and unspecified internal organs**
►Code first (T51-T65) to identify chemical and intent◄

✓x7th **T28.40** **Burn of unspecified internal organ**

✓6th **T28.41** **Burn of ear drum**

✓7th **T28.411** **Burn of right ear drum**

✓7th **T28.412** **Burn of left ear drum**

✓7th **T28.419** **Burn of unspecified ear drum**

✓x7th **T28.49** **Burn of other internal organ**
~~Code first (T51-T65) to identify chemical and intent for T28.5-T28.9~~

✓x7th **T28.5** **Corrosion of mouth and pharynx**
►Code first (T51-T65) to identify chemical and intent◄

✓x7th **T28.6** **Corrosion of esophagus** `CC` `H5`
►Code first (T51-T65) to identify chemical and intent◄
CC Excl: CC with 7th character A: PDX collection 1412

✓x7th **T28.7** **Corrosion of other parts of alimentary tract** `CC` `H5`
►Code first (T51-T65) to identify chemical and intent◄
CC Excl: CC with 7th character A: PDX collection 1413

✓x7th **T28.8** **Corrosion of internal genitourinary organs**
►Code first (T51-T65) to identify chemical and intent◄

✓5th **T28.9** **Corrosions of other and unspecified internal organs**
►Code first (T51-T65) to identify chemical and intent◄

✓x7th **T28.90** **Corrosions of unspecified internal organs**

✓6th **T28.91** **Corrosions of ear drum**

✓7th **T28.911** **Corrosions of right ear drum**

✓7th **T28.912** **Corrosions of left ear drum**

✓7th **T28.919** **Corrosions of unspecified ear drum**

✓x7th **T28.99** **Corrosions of other internal organs**

☑ Additional Character Req　✓x7th Placeholder Alert　Unacceptable PDx　Manifestation　`H1`-`H14` HAC　`HCC` CMS-HCC Condition　*EXCLUDES 1* Not Coded Here　*EXCLUDES 2* Not Included Here

Burns and corrosions of multiple and unspecified body regions (T30-T32)

✓4ᵗʰ **T30** **Burn and corrosion, body region unspecified**

T30.0 Burn of unspecified body region, unspecified degree
This code is not for inpatient use. Code to specified site and degree of burns.
Burn NOS
Multiple burns NOS

T30.4 Corrosion of unspecified body region, unspecified degree
This code is not for inpatient use. Code to specified site and degree of corrosion.
Corrosion NOS
Multiple corrosion NOS

✓4ᵗʰ **T31** **Burns classified according to extent of body surface involved**

NOTE This category is to be used as the primary code only when the site of the burn is unspecified. It should be used as a supplementary code with categories T20-T25 when the site is specified.

CC Excl: For CC/MCC codes in category T31: PDX collection 1414

T31.0 Burns involving less than 10% of body surface

✓5ᵗʰ **T31.1** Burns involving 10-19% of body surface

    T31.10 Burns involving 10-19% of body surface with 0% to 9% third degree burns `CC` `H5`
        Burns involving 10-19% of body surface NOS

    T31.11 Burns involving 10-19% of body surface with 10-19% third degree burns `CC` `H5` `HCC`

✓5ᵗʰ **T31.2** Burns involving 20-29% of body surface

    T31.20 Burns involving 20-29% of body surface with 0% to 9% third degree burns `CC` `H5`
        Burns involving 20-29% of body surface NOS

    T31.21 Burns involving 20-29% of body surface with 10-19% third degree burns `MCC` `H5` `HCC`

    T31.22 Burns involving 20-29% of body surface with 20-29% third degree burns `MCC` `H5` `HCC`

✓5ᵗʰ **T31.3** Burns involving 30-39% of body surface

    T31.30 Burns involving 30-39% of body surface with 0% to 9% third degree burns `CC` `H5`
        Burns involving 30-39% of body surface NOS

    T31.31 Burns involving 30-39% of body surface with 10-19% third degree burns `MCC` `H5` `HCC`

    T31.32 Burns involving 30-39% of body surface with 20-29% third degree burns `MCC` `H5` `HCC`

    T31.33 Burns involving 30-39% of body surface 30-39% third degree burns `MCC` `H5` `HCC`

✓5ᵗʰ **T31.4** Burns involving 40-49% of body surface

    T31.40 Burns involving 40-49% of body surface with 0% to 9% third degree burns `CC` `H5`
        Burns involving 40-49% of body surface NOS

    T31.41 Burns involving 40-49% of body surface with 10-19% third degree burns `MCC` `H5` `HCC`

    T31.42 Burns involving 40-49% of body surface with 20-29% third degree burns `MCC` `H5` `HCC`

    T31.43 Burns involving 40-49% of body surface with 30-39% third degree burns `MCC` `H5` `HCC`

    T31.44 Burns involving 40-49% of body surface with 40-49% third degree burns `MCC` `H5` `HCC`

✓5ᵗʰ **T31.5** Burns involving 50-59% of body surface

    T31.50 Burns involving 50-59% of body surface with 0% to 9% third degree burns `CC` `H5`
        Burns involving 50-59% of body surface NOS

    T31.51 Burns involving 50-59% of body surface with 10-19% third degree burns `MCC` `H5` `HCC`

    T31.52 Burns involving 50-59% of body surface with 20-29% third degree burns `MCC` `H5` `HCC`

    T31.53 Burns involving 50-59% of body surface with 30-39% third degree burns `MCC` `H5` `HCC`

    T31.54 Burns involving 50-59% of body surface with 40-49% third degree burns `MCC` `H5` `HCC`

    T31.55 Burns involving 50-59% of body surface with 50-59% third degree burns `MCC` `H5` `HCC`

✓5ᵗʰ **T31.6** Burns involving 60-69% of body surface

    T31.60 Burns involving 60-69% of body surface with 0% to 9% third degree burns `CC` `H5`
        Burns involving 60-69% of body surface NOS

    T31.61 Burns involving 60-69% of body surface with 10-19% third degree burns `MCC` `H5` `HCC`

    T31.62 Burns involving 60-69% of body surface with 20-29% third degree burns `MCC` `H5` `HCC`

    T31.63 Burns involving 60-69% of body surface with 30-39% third degree burns `MCC` `H5` `HCC`

    T31.64 Burns involving 60-69% of body surface with 40-49% third degree burns `MCC` `H5` `HCC`

    T31.65 Burns involving 60-69% of body surface with 50-59% third degree burns `MCC` `H5` `HCC`

    T31.66 Burns involving 60-69% of body surface with 60-69% third degree burns `MCC` `H5` `HCC`

✓5ᵗʰ **T31.7** Burns involving 70-79% of body surface

    T31.70 Burns involving 70-79% of body surface with 0% to 9% third degree burns `CC` `H5`
        Burns involving 70-79% of body surface NOS

    T31.71 Burns involving 70-79% of body surface with 10-19% third degree burns `MCC` `H5` `HCC`

    T31.72 Burns involving 70-79% of body surface with 20-29% third degree burns `MCC` `H5` `HCC`

    T31.73 Burns involving 70-79% of body surface with 30-39% third degree burns `MCC` `H5` `HCC`

    T31.74 Burns involving 70-79% of body surface with 40-49% third degree burns `MCC` `H5` `HCC`

    T31.75 Burns involving 70-79% of body surface with 50-59% third degree burns `MCC` `H5` `HCC`

    T31.76 Burns involving 70-79% of body surface with 60-69% third degree burns `MCC` `H5` `HCC`

    T31.77 Burns involving 70-79% of body surface with 70-79% third degree burns `MCC` `H5` `HCC`

✓5ᵗʰ **T31.8** Burns involving 80-89% of body surface

    T31.80 Burns involving 80-89% of body surface with 0% to 9% third degree burns `CC` `H5`
        Burns involving 80-89% of body surface NOS

    T31.81 Burns involving 80-89% of body surface with 10-19% third degree burns `MCC` `H5` `HCC`

    T31.82 Burns involving 80-89% of body surface with 20-29% third degree burns `MCC` `H5` `HCC`

    T31.83 Burns involving 80-89% of body surface with 30-39% third degree burns `MCC` `H5` `HCC`

    T31.84 Burns involving 80-89% of body surface with 40-49% third degree burns `MCC` `H5` `HCC`

    T31.85 Burns involving 80-89% of body surface with 50-59% third degree burns `MCC` `H5` `HCC`

    T31.86 Burns involving 80-89% of body surface with 60-69% third degree burns `MCC` `H5` `HCC`

    T31.87 Burns involving 80-89% of body surface with 70-79% third degree burns `MCC` `H5` `HCC`

    T31.88 Burns involving 80-89% of body surface with 80-89% third degree burns `MCC` `H5` `HCC`

✓5ᵗʰ **T31.9** Burns involving 90% or more of body surface

    T31.90 Burns involving 90% or more of body surface with 0% to 9% third degree burns `CC` `H5`
        Burns involving 90% or more of body surface NOS

    T31.91 Burns involving 90% or more of body surface with 10-19% third degree burns `MCC` `H5` `HCC`

    T31.92 Burns involving 90% or more of body surface with 20-29% third degree burns `MCC` `H5` `HCC`

    T31.93 Burns involving 90% or more of body surface with 30-39% third degree burns `MCC` `H5` `HCC`

    T31.94 Burns involving 90% or more of body surface with 40-49% third degree burns `MCC` `H5` `HCC`

    T31.95 Burns involving 90% or more of body surface with 50-59% third degree burns `MCC` `H5` `HCC`

    T31.96 Burns involving 90% or more of body surface with 60-69% third degree burns `MCC` `H5` `HCC`

    T31.97 Burns involving 90% or more of body surface with 70-79% third degree burns `MCC` `H5` `HCC`

    T31.98 Burns involving 90% or more of body surface with 80-89% third degree burns `MCC` `H5` `HCC`

    T31.99 Burns involving 90% or more of body surface with 90% or more third degree burns `MCC` `H5` `HCC`

☑4ᵗʰ **T32** **Corrosions classified according to extent of body surface involved**

> **NOTE**   This category is to be used as the primary code only when the site of the corrosion is unspecified. It may be used as a supplementary code with categories T20-T25 when the site is specified.

> **CC Excl: For CC/MCC codes in category T32:** PDX collection 1414

   T32.0 **Corrosions involving** less than 10% **of body surface**

☑5ᵗʰ **T32.1** **Corrosions involving** 10-19% **of body surface**

     T32.10 **Corrosions involving 10-19% of body surface** `CC` `H5`
       with 0% to 9% **third degree corrosion**
       Corrosions involving 10-19% of body surface NOS

     T32.11 **Corrosions involving 10-19% of body** `CC` `H5` `HCC`
       surface with 10-19% **third degree corrosion**

☑5ᵗʰ **T32.2** **Corrosions involving** 20-29% **of body surface**

     T32.20 **Corrosions involving 20-29% of body surface** `CC` `H5`
       with 0% to 9% **third degree corrosion**

     T32.21 **Corrosions involving 20-29% of body** `MCC` `H5` `HCC`
       surface with 10-19% **third degree corrosion**

     T32.22 **Corrosions involving 20-29% of body** `MCC` `H5` `HCC`
       surface with 20-29% **third degree corrosion**

☑5ᵗʰ **T32.3** **Corrosions involving** 30-39% **of body surface**

     T32.30 **Corrosions involving 30-39% of body surface** `CC` `H5`
       with 0% to 9% **third degree corrosion**

     T32.31 **Corrosions involving 30-39% of body** `MCC` `H5` `HCC`
       surface with 10-19% **third degree corrosion**

     T32.32 **Corrosions involving 30-39% of body** `MCC` `H5` `HCC`
       surface with 20-29% **third degree corrosion**

     T32.33 **Corrosions involving 30-39% of body** `MCC` `H5` `HCC`
       surface with 30-39% **third degree corrosion**

☑5ᵗʰ **T32.4** **Corrosions involving** 40-49% **of body surface**

     T32.40 **Corrosions involving 40-49% of body** `CC` `H5`
       surface with 0% to 9% **third degree corrosion**

     T32.41 **Corrosions involving 40-49% of body** `MCC` `H5` `HCC`
       surface with 10-19% **third degree corrosion**

     T32.42 **Corrosions involving 40-49% of body** `MCC` `H5` `HCC`
       surface with 20-29% **third degree corrosion**

     T32.43 **Corrosions involving 40-49% of body** `MCC` `H5` `HCC`
       surface with 30-39% **third degree corrosion**

     T32.44 **Corrosions involving 40-49% of body** `MCC` `H5` `HCC`
       surface with 40-49% **third degree corrosion**

☑5ᵗʰ **T32.5** **Corrosions involving** 50-59% **of body surface**

     T32.50 **Corrosions involving 50-59% of body surface** `CC` `H5`
       with 0% to 9% **third degree corrosion**

     T32.51 **Corrosions involving 50-59% of body** `MCC` `H5` `HCC`
       surface with 10-19% **third degree corrosion**

     T32.52 **Corrosions involving 50-59% of body** `MCC` `H5` `HCC`
       surface with 20-29% **third degree corrosion**

     T32.53 **Corrosions involving 50-59% of body** `MCC` `H5` `HCC`
       surface with 30-39% **third degree corrosion**

     T32.54 **Corrosions involving 50-59% of body** `MCC` `H5` `HCC`
       surface with 40-49% **third degree corrosion**

     T32.55 **Corrosions involving 50-59% of body** `MCC` `H5` `HCC`
       surface with 50-59% **third degree corrosion**

☑5ᵗʰ **T32.6** **Corrosions involving** 60-69% **of body surface**

     T32.60 **Corrosions involving 60-69% of body surface** `CC` `H5`
       with 0% to 9% **third degree corrosion**

     T32.61 **Corrosions involving 60-69% of body** `MCC` `H5` `HCC`
       surface with 10-19% **third degree corrosion**

     T32.62 **Corrosions involving 60-69% of body** `MCC` `H5` `HCC`
       surface with 20-29% **third degree corrosion**

     T32.63 **Corrosions involving 60-69% of body** `MCC` `H5` `HCC`
       surface with 30-39% **third degree corrosion**

     T32.64 **Corrosions involving 60-69% of body** `MCC` `H5` `HCC`
       surface with 40-49% **third degree corrosion**

     T32.65 **Corrosions involving 60-69% of body** `MCC` `H5` `HCC`
       surface with 50-59% **third degree corrosion**

     T32.66 **Corrosions involving 60-69% of body** `MCC` `H5` `HCC`
       surface with 60-69% **third degree corrosion**

☑5ᵗʰ **T32.7** **Corrosions involving** 70-79% **of body surface**

     T32.70 **Corrosions involving 70-79% of body surface** `CC` `H5`
       with 0% to 9% **third degree corrosion**

     T32.71 **Corrosions involving 70-79% of body** `MCC` `H5` `HCC`
       surface with 10-19% **third degree corrosion**

     T32.72 **Corrosions involving 70-79% of body** `MCC` `H5` `HCC`
       surface with 20-29% **third degree corrosion**

     T32.73 **Corrosions involving 70-79% of body** `MCC` `H5` `HCC`
       surface with 30-39% **third degree corrosion**

     T32.74 **Corrosions involving 70-79% of body** `MCC` `H5` `HCC`
       surface with 40-49% **third degree corrosion**

     T32.75 **Corrosions involving 70-79% of body** `MCC` `H5` `HCC`
       surface with 50-59% **third degree corrosion**

     T32.76 **Corrosions involving 70-79% of body** `MCC` `H5` `HCC`
       surface with 60-69% **third degree corrosion**

     T32.77 **Corrosions involving 70-79% of body** `MCC` `H5` `HCC`
       surface with 70-79% **third degree corrosion**

☑5ᵗʰ **T32.8** **Corrosions involving** 80-89% **of body surface**

     T32.80 **Corrosions involving 80-89% of body surface** `CC` `H5`
       with 0% to 9% **third degree corrosion**

     T32.81 **Corrosions involving 80-89% of body** `MCC` `H5` `HCC`
       surface with 10-19% **third degree corrosion**

     T32.82 **Corrosions involving 80-89% of body** `MCC` `H5` `HCC`
       surface with 20-29% **third degree corrosion**

     T32.83 **Corrosions involving 80-89% of body** `MCC` `H5` `HCC`
       surface with 30-39% **third degree corrosion**

     T32.84 **Corrosions involving 80-89% of body** `MCC` `H5` `HCC`
       surface with 40-49% **third degree corrosion**

     T32.85 **Corrosions involving 80-89% of body** `MCC` `H5` `HCC`
       surface with 50-59% **third degree corrosion**

     T32.86 **Corrosions involving 80-89% of body** `MCC` `H5` `HCC`
       surface with 60-69% **third degree corrosion**

     T32.87 **Corrosions involving 80-89% of body** `MCC` `H5` `HCC`
       surface with 70-79% **third degree corrosion**

     T32.88 **Corrosions involving 80-89% of body** `MCC` `H5` `HCC`
       surface with 80-89% **third degree corrosion**

☑5ᵗʰ **T32.9** **Corrosions involving** 90% or more **of body surface**

     T32.90 **Corrosions involving 90% or more of body** `CC` `H5`
       surface with 0% to 9% **third degree corrosion**

     T32.91 **Corrosions involving 90% or more of** `MCC` `H5` `HCC`
       body surface with 10-19% **third degree corrosion**

     T32.92 **Corrosions involving 90% or more of** `MCC` `H5` `HCC`
       body surface with 20-29% **third degree corrosion**

     T32.93 **Corrosions involving 90% or more of** `MCC` `H5` `HCC`
       body surface with 30-39% **third degree corrosion**

     T32.94 **Corrosions involving 90% or more of** `MCC` `H5` `HCC`
       body surface with 40-49% **third degree corrosion**

     T32.95 **Corrosions involving 90% or more of** `MCC` `H5` `HCC`
       body surface with 50-59% **third degree corrosion**

     T32.96 **Corrosions involving 90% or more of** `MCC` `H5` `HCC`
       body surface with 60-69% **third degree corrosion**

     T32.97 **Corrosions involving 90% or more of** `MCC` `H5` `HCC`
       body surface with 70-79% **third degree corrosion**

     T32.98 **Corrosions involving 90% or more of** `MCC` `H5` `HCC`
       body surface with 80-89% **third degree corrosion**

     T32.99 **Corrosions involving 90% or more of** `MCC` `H5` `HCC`
       body surface with 90% or more **third degree corrosion**

Frostbite (T33-T34)

> **EXCLUDES 2**   *hypothermia and other effects of reduced temperature (T68, T69-)*

☑4ᵗʰ **T33** **Superficial frostbite**

> **INCLUDES**   frostbite with partial thickness skin loss

> The appropriate 7th character is to be added to each code from category T33.
> A   initial encounter
> D   subsequent encounter
> S   sequela

> **CC Excl: For CC codes in category T33, unless otherwise noted:** PDX collection 1416

☑5ᵗʰ **T33.0** **Superficial frostbite of** head

> **CC Excl: For CC codes in subcategory T33.0:** PDX collection 1415

     ☑6ᵗʰ **T33.01** **Superficial frostbite of** ear

       ☑7ᵗʰ **T33.011** **Superficial frostbite of** right ear   `CC` `H5`

       ☑7ᵗʰ **T33.012** **Superficial frostbite of** left ear   `CC` `H5`

       ☑7ᵗʰ **T33.019** **Superficial frostbite of** unspecified   `CC` `H5`
         ear

     ☑x7ᵗʰ **T33.02** **Superficial frostbite of** nose   `CC` `H5`

     ☑x7ᵗʰ **T33.09** **Superficial frostbite of** other part **of head**   `CC` `H5`

☑ Additional Character Req   ☑x7ᵗʰ Placeholder Alert   Unacceptable PDx   Manifestation   `H1`-`H14` HAC   `HCC` CMS-HCC Condition   *EXCLUDES 1* Not Coded Here   *EXCLUDES 2* Not Included Here

ICD-10-CM 2018   **1097**

Chapter 19. Injury, Poisoning and Certain Other Consequences of External Causes

√x7ᵗʰ **T33.1** **Superficial frostbite of** neck   CC H5
     CC Excl: CC with 7th character A: PDX collection 1415

√x7ᵗʰ **T33.2** **Superficial frostbite of** thorax   CC H5

√x7ᵗʰ **T33.3** **Superficial frostbite of** abdominal wall, lower back and pelvis   CC H5

√5ᵗʰ **T33.4** **Superficial frostbite of** arm
     EXCLUDES 2   superficial frostbite of wrist and hand (T33.5-)

   √x7ᵗʰ **T33.40** **Superficial frostbite of** unspecified arm   CC H5

   √x7ᵗʰ **T33.41** **Superficial frostbite of** right arm   CC H5

   √x7ᵗʰ **T33.42** **Superficial frostbite of** left arm   CC H5

√5ᵗʰ **T33.5** **Superficial frostbite of** wrist, hand, and fingers

   CC Excl: For codes in subcategory T33.5:
   PDX collection 1417

   √6ᵗʰ **T33.51** **Superficial frostbite of** wrist

     √7ᵗʰ **T33.511** **Superficial frostbite of** right wrist   CC H5

     √7ᵗʰ **T33.512** **Superficial frostbite of** left wrist   CC H5

     √7ᵗʰ **T33.519** **Superficial frostbite of** unspecified wrist   CC H5

   √6ᵗʰ **T33.52** **Superficial frostbite of** hand
     EXCLUDES 2   superficial frostbite of fingers (T33.53-)

     √7ᵗʰ **T33.521** **Superficial frostbite of** right hand   CC H5

     √7ᵗʰ **T33.522** **Superficial frostbite of** left hand   CC H5

     √7ᵗʰ **T33.529** **Superficial frostbite of** unspecified hand   CC H5

   √6ᵗʰ **T33.53** **Superficial frostbite of** finger(s)

     √7ᵗʰ **T33.531** **Superficial frostbite of** right finger(s)   CC H5

     √7ᵗʰ **T33.532** **Superficial frostbite of** left finger(s)   CC H5

     √7ᵗʰ **T33.539** **Superficial frostbite of** unspecified finger(s)   CC H5

√5ᵗʰ **T33.6** **Superficial frostbite of** hip and thigh

   √x7ᵗʰ **T33.60** **Superficial frostbite of** unspecified hip and thigh   CC H5

   √x7ᵗʰ **T33.61** **Superficial frostbite of** right hip and thigh   CC H5

   √x7ᵗʰ **T33.62** **Superficial frostbite of** left hip and thigh   CC H5

√5ᵗʰ **T33.7** **Superficial frostbite of** knee and lower leg
     EXCLUDES 2   superficial frostbite of ankle and foot (T33.8-)

   √x7ᵗʰ **T33.70** **Superficial frostbite of** unspecified knee and lower leg   CC H5

   √x7ᵗʰ **T33.71** **Superficial frostbite of** right knee and lower leg   CC H5

   √x7ᵗʰ **T33.72** **Superficial frostbite of** left knee and lower leg   CC H5

√5ᵗʰ **T33.8** **Superficial frostbite of** ankle, foot, and toe(s)

   CC Excl: For codes in subcategory T33.8:
   PDX collection 1418

   √6ᵗʰ **T33.81** **Superficial frostbite of** ankle

     √7ᵗʰ **T33.811** **Superficial frostbite of** right ankle   CC H5

     √7ᵗʰ **T33.812** **Superficial frostbite of** left ankle   CC H5

     √7ᵗʰ **T33.819** **Superficial frostbite of** unspecified ankle   CC H5

   √6ᵗʰ **T33.82** **Superficial frostbite of** foot

     √7ᵗʰ **T33.821** **Superficial frostbite of** right foot   CC H5

     √7ᵗʰ **T33.822** **Superficial frostbite of** left foot   CC H5

     √7ᵗʰ **T33.829** **Superficial frostbite of** unspecified foot   CC H5

   √6ᵗʰ **T33.83** **Superficial frostbite of** toe(s)

     √7ᵗʰ **T33.831** **Superficial frostbite of** right toe(s)   CC H5

     √7ᵗʰ **T33.832** **Superficial frostbite of** left toe(s)   CC H5

     √7ᵗʰ **T33.839** **Superficial frostbite of** unspecified toe(s)   CC H5

√5ᵗʰ **T33.9** **Superficial frostbite of** other and unspecified sites

   √x7ᵗʰ **T33.90** **Superficial frostbite of** unspecified sites   CC H5
     Superficial frostbite NOS

   √x7ᵗʰ **T33.99** **Superficial frostbite of** other sites   CC H5
     Superficial frostbite of leg NOS
     Superficial frostbite of trunk NOS

√4ᵗʰ **T34** **Frostbite** with tissue necrosis

   The appropriate 7th character is to be added to each code from category T34.
   A   initial encounter
   D   subsequent encounter
   S   sequela

   CC Excl: For CC codes in category T34, unless otherwise noted:
   PDX collection 1416

√5ᵗʰ **T34.0** **Frostbite with tissue necrosis of** head

   CC Excl: For CC codes in subcategory T34.0:
   PDX collection 1415

   √6ᵗʰ **T34.01** **Frostbite with tissue necrosis of** ear

     √7ᵗʰ **T34.011** **Frostbite with tissue necrosis of** right ear   CC H5

     √7ᵗʰ **T34.012** **Frostbite with tissue necrosis of** left ear   CC H5

     √7ᵗʰ **T34.019** **Frostbite with tissue necrosis of** unspecified ear   CC H5

   √x7ᵗʰ **T34.02** **Frostbite with tissue necrosis of** nose   CC H5

   √x7ᵗʰ **T34.09** **Frostbite with tissue necrosis of** other part of head   CC H5

√x7ᵗʰ **T34.1** **Frostbite with tissue necrosis of** neck   CC H5
     CC Excl: PDX collection 1415

√x7ᵗʰ **T34.2** **Frostbite with tissue necrosis of** thorax   CC H5

√x7ᵗʰ **T34.3** **Frostbite with tissue necrosis of** abdominal wall, lower back and pelvis   CC H5

√5ᵗʰ **T34.4** **Frostbite with tissue necrosis of** arm
     EXCLUDES 2   frostbite with tissue necrosis of wrist and hand (T34.5-)

   √x7ᵗʰ **T34.40** **Frostbite with tissue necrosis of** unspecified arm   CC H5

   √x7ᵗʰ **T34.41** **Frostbite with tissue necrosis of** right arm   CC H5

   √x7ᵗʰ **T34.42** **Frostbite with tissue necrosis of** left arm   CC H5

√5ᵗʰ **T34.5** **Frostbite with tissue necrosis of** wrist, hand, and finger(s)

   CC Excl: For CC codes in subcategory T34.5: PDX collection 1417

   √6ᵗʰ **T34.51** **Frostbite with tissue necrosis of** wrist

     √7ᵗʰ **T34.511** **Frostbite with tissue necrosis of** right wrist   CC H5

     √7ᵗʰ **T34.512** **Frostbite with tissue necrosis of** left wrist   CC H5

     √7ᵗʰ **T34.519** **Frostbite with tissue necrosis of** unspecified wrist   CC H5

   √6ᵗʰ **T34.52** **Frostbite with tissue necrosis of** hand
     EXCLUDES 2   frostbite with tissue necrosis of finger(s) (T34.53-)

     √7ᵗʰ **T34.521** **Frostbite with tissue necrosis of** right hand   CC H5

     √7ᵗʰ **T34.522** **Frostbite with tissue necrosis of** left hand   CC H5

     √7ᵗʰ **T34.529** **Frostbite with tissue necrosis of** unspecified hand   CC H5

   √6ᵗʰ **T34.53** **Frostbite with tissue necrosis of** finger(s)

     √7ᵗʰ **T34.531** **Frostbite with tissue necrosis of** right finger(s)   CC H5

     √7ᵗʰ **T34.532** **Frostbite with tissue necrosis of** left finger(s)   CC H5

     √7ᵗʰ **T34.539** **Frostbite with tissue necrosis of** unspecified finger(s)   CC H5

√5ᵗʰ **T34.6** **Frostbite with tissue necrosis of** hip and thigh

   √x7ᵗʰ **T34.60** **Frostbite with tissue necrosis of** unspecified hip and thigh   CC H5

   √x7ᵗʰ **T34.61** **Frostbite with tissue necrosis of** right hip and thigh   CC H5

   √x7ᵗʰ **T34.62** **Frostbite with tissue necrosis of** left hip and thigh   CC H5

√5ᵗʰ **T34.7** **Frostbite with tissue necrosis of** knee and lower leg
     EXCLUDES 2   frostbite with tissue necrosis of ankle and foot (T34.8-)

   √x7ᵗʰ **T34.70** **Frostbite with tissue necrosis of** unspecified knee and lower leg   CC H5

   √x7ᵗʰ **T34.71** **Frostbite with tissue necrosis of** right knee and lower leg   CC H5

N Newborn: 0   P Pediatric: 0-17   M Maternity: 12-55   A Adult: 15-124   MCC Major CC Condition   PDx MCC PDx acts as own MCC   CC CC Condition   PDx CC PDx acts as own CC

1098   ICD-10-CM 2018

√x7ᵗʰ **T34.72** Frostbite with tissue necrosis of left knee and lower leg   CC H5

√5ᵗʰ **T34.8** Frostbite with tissue necrosis of ankle, foot, and toe(s)

> **CC Excl: For CC codes in subcategory T34.8:**
> PDX collection 1418

√6ᵗʰ **T34.81** Frostbite with tissue necrosis of ankle

√7ᵗʰ **T34.811** Frostbite with tissue necrosis of right ankle   CC H5

√7ᵗʰ **T34.812** Frostbite with tissue necrosis of left ankle   CC H5

√7ᵗʰ **T34.819** Frostbite with tissue necrosis of unspecified ankle   CC H5

√6ᵗʰ **T34.82** Frostbite with tissue necrosis of foot

√7ᵗʰ **T34.821** Frostbite with tissue necrosis of right foot   CC H5

√7ᵗʰ **T34.822** Frostbite with tissue necrosis of left foot   CC H5

√7ᵗʰ **T34.829** Frostbite with tissue necrosis of unspecified foot   CC H5

√6ᵗʰ **T34.83** Frostbite with tissue necrosis of toe(s)

√7ᵗʰ **T34.831** Frostbite with tissue necrosis of right toe(s)   CC H5

√7ᵗʰ **T34.832** Frostbite with tissue necrosis of left toe(s)   CC H5

√7ᵗʰ **T34.839** Frostbite with tissue necrosis of unspecified toe(s)   CC H5

√5ᵗʰ **T34.9** Frostbite with tissue necrosis of other and unspecified sites

√x7ᵗʰ **T34.90** Frostbite with tissue necrosis of unspecified sites   CC H5
Frostbite with tissue necrosis NOS

√x7ᵗʰ **T34.99** Frostbite with tissue necrosis of other sites   CC H5
Frostbite with tissue necrosis of leg NOS
Frostbite with tissue necrosis of trunk NOS

Poisoning by, adverse effects of and underdosing of drugs, medicaments and biological substances (T36-T50)

INCLUDES   adverse effect of correct substance properly administered
poisoning by overdose of substance
poisoning by wrong substance given or taken in error
underdosing by (inadvertently) (deliberately) taking less substance than prescribed or instructed

Code first, for adverse effects, the nature of the adverse effect, such as:
adverse effect NOS (T88.7)
aspirin gastritis (K29.-)
blood disorders (D56-D76)
contact dermatitis (L23-L25)
dermatitis due to substances taken internally (L27.-)
nephropathy (N14.0-N14.2)

NOTE   The drug giving rise to the adverse effect should be identified by use of codes from categories T36-T50 with fifth or sixth character 5.

Use additional code(s) to specify:
manifestations of poisoning
underdosing or failure in dosage during medical and surgical care (Y63.6, Y63.8-Y63.9)
underdosing of medication regimen (Z91.12-, Z91.13-)

EXCLUDES 1   *toxic reaction to local anesthesia in pregnancy (O29.3-)*
EXCLUDES 2   *abuse and dependence of psychoactive substances (F10-F19)*
abuse of non-dependence-producing substances (F55.-)
drug reaction and poisoning affecting newborn (P00-P96)
pathological drug intoxication (inebriation) (F10-F19)

AHA: 2016, 2Q, 8; 2015, 3Q, 22

√4ᵗʰ **T36** **Poisoning by, adverse effect of and underdosing of systemic antibiotics**

EXCLUDES 1   *antineoplastic antibiotics (T45.1-)*
locally applied antibiotic NEC (T49.0)
topically used antibiotic for ear, nose and throat (T49.6)
topically used antibiotic for eye (T49.5)

> The appropriate 7th character is to be added to each code from category T36.
> A   initial encounter
> D   subsequent encounter
> S   sequela

√5ᵗʰ **T36.0** Poisoning by, adverse effect of and underdosing of penicillins

√6ᵗʰ **T36.0X** Poisoning by, adverse effect of and underdosing of penicillins

√7ᵗʰ **T36.0X1** Poisoning by penicillins, accidental (unintentional)
Poisoning by penicillins NOS

11 √7ᵗʰ **T36.0X2** Poisoning by penicillins, intentional self-harm   HCC

√7ᵗʰ **T36.0X3** Poisoning by penicillins, assault

√7ᵗʰ **T36.0X4** Poisoning by penicillins, undetermined

√7ᵗʰ **T36.0X5** Adverse effect of penicillins

√7ᵗʰ **T36.0X6** Underdosing of penicillins

√5ᵗʰ **T36.1** Poisoning by, adverse effect of and underdosing of cephalosporins and other beta-lactam antibiotics

√6ᵗʰ **T36.1X** Poisoning by, adverse effect of and underdosing of cephalosporins and other beta-lactam antibiotics

√7ᵗʰ **T36.1X1** Poisoning by cephalosporins and other beta-lactam antibiotics, accidental (unintentional)
Poisoning by cephalosporins and other beta-lactam antibiotics NOS

11 √7ᵗʰ **T36.1X2** Poisoning by cephalosporins and other beta-lactam antibiotics, intentional self-harm   HCC

√7ᵗʰ **T36.1X3** Poisoning by cephalosporins and other beta-lactam antibiotics, assault

√7ᵗʰ **T36.1X4** Poisoning by cephalosporins and other beta-lactam antibiotics, undetermined

√7ᵗʰ **T36.1X5** Adverse effect of cephalosporins and other beta-lactam antibiotics

√7ᵗʰ **T36.1X6** Underdosing of cephalosporins and other beta-lactam antibiotics

√5ᵗʰ **T36.2** Poisoning by, adverse effect of and underdosing of chloramphenicol group

√6ᵗʰ **T36.2X** Poisoning by, adverse effect of and underdosing of chloramphenicol group

√7ᵗʰ **T36.2X1** Poisoning by chloramphenicol group, accidental (unintentional)
Poisoning by chloramphenicol group NOS

11 √7ᵗʰ **T36.2X2** Poisoning by chloramphenicol group, intentional self-harm   HCC

√7ᵗʰ **T36.2X3** Poisoning by chloramphenicol group, assault

√7ᵗʰ **T36.2X4** Poisoning by chloramphenicol group, undetermined

√7ᵗʰ **T36.2X5** Adverse effect of chloramphenicol group

√7ᵗʰ **T36.2X6** Underdosing of chloramphenicol group

√5ᵗʰ **T36.3** Poisoning by, adverse effect of and underdosing of macrolides

√6ᵗʰ **T36.3X** Poisoning by, adverse effect of and underdosing of macrolides

√7ᵗʰ **T36.3X1** Poisoning by macrolides, accidental (unintentional)
Poisoning by macrolides NOS

11 √7ᵗʰ **T36.3X2** Poisoning by macrolides, intentional self-harm   HCC

√7ᵗʰ **T36.3X3** Poisoning by macrolides, assault

√7ᵗʰ **T36.3X4** Poisoning by macrolides, undetermined

√7ᵗʰ **T36.3X5** Adverse effect of macrolides

√7ᵗʰ **T36.3X6** Underdosing of macrolides

√5ᵗʰ **T36.4** Poisoning by, adverse effect of and underdosing of tetracyclines

√6ᵗʰ **T36.4X** Poisoning by, adverse effect of and underdosing of tetracyclines

√7ᵗʰ **T36.4X1** Poisoning by tetracyclines, accidental (unintentional)
Poisoning by tetracyclines NOS

11 √7ᵗʰ **T36.4X2** Poisoning by tetracyclines, intentional self-harm   HCC

√7ᵗʰ **T36.4X3** Poisoning by tetracyclines, assault

√7ᵗʰ **T36.4X4** Poisoning by tetracyclines, undetermined

√7ᵗʰ **T36.4X5** Adverse effect of tetracyclines

√7ᵗʰ **T36.4X6** Underdosing of tetracyclines

---

11   HCC with 7th character indicating initial encounter (A or B - specific to category) OR sequela.

☑ Additional Character Req   √x7ᵗʰ Placeholder Alert   Unacceptable PDx   Manifestation   H1-H14 HAC   HCC CMS-HCC Condition   EXCLUDES 1 Not Coded Here   EXCLUDES 2 Not Included Here

ICD-10-CM 2018   1099

✓5ᵗʰ T36.5 Poisoning by, adverse effect of and underdosing of aminoglycosides
Poisoning by, adverse effect of and underdosing of streptomycin

  ✓6ᵗʰ T36.5X Poisoning by, adverse effect of and underdosing of aminoglycosides

    ✓7ᵗʰ T36.5X1 Poisoning by aminoglycosides, accidental (unintentional)
Poisoning by aminoglycosides NOS

    11 **✓7ᵗʰ T36.5X2 Poisoning by aminoglycosides, intentional self-harm** [HCC]

    ✓7ᵗʰ T36.5X3 Poisoning by aminoglycosides, assault

    ✓7ᵗʰ T36.5X4 Poisoning by aminoglycosides, undetermined

    ✓7ᵗʰ T36.5X5 Adverse effect of aminoglycosides

    ✓7ᵗʰ T36.5X6 Underdosing of aminoglycosides

✓5ᵗʰ T36.6 Poisoning by, adverse effect of and underdosing of rifampicins

  ✓6ᵗʰ T36.6X Poisoning by, adverse effect of and underdosing of rifampicins

    ✓7ᵗʰ T36.6X1 Poisoning by rifampicins, accidental (unintentional)
Poisoning by rifampicins NOS

    11 **✓7ᵗʰ T36.6X2 Poisoning by rifampicins, intentional self-harm** [HCC]

    ✓7ᵗʰ T36.6X3 Poisoning by rifampicins, assault

    ✓7ᵗʰ T36.6X4 Poisoning by rifampicins, undetermined

    ✓7ᵗʰ T36.6X5 Adverse effect of rifampicins

    ✓7ᵗʰ T36.6X6 Underdosing of rifampicins

✓5ᵗʰ T36.7 Poisoning by, adverse effect of and underdosing of antifungal antibiotics, systemically used

  ✓6ᵗʰ T36.7X Poisoning by, adverse effect of and underdosing of antifungal antibiotics, systemically used

    ✓7ᵗʰ T36.7X1 Poisoning by antifungal antibiotics, systemically used, accidental (unintentional)
Poisoning by antifungal antibiotics, systemically used NOS

    11 **✓7ᵗʰ T36.7X2 Poisoning by antifungal antibiotics, systemically used, intentional self-harm** [HCC]

    ✓7ᵗʰ T36.7X3 Poisoning by antifungal antibiotics, systemically used, assault

    ✓7ᵗʰ T36.7X4 Poisoning by antifungal antibiotics, systemically used, undetermined

    ✓7ᵗʰ T36.7X5 Adverse effect of antifungal antibiotics, systemically used

    ✓7ᵗʰ T36.7X6 Underdosing of antifungal antibiotics, systemically used

✓5ᵗʰ T36.8 Poisoning by, adverse effect of and underdosing of other systemic antibiotics

  ✓6ᵗʰ T36.8X Poisoning by, adverse effect of and underdosing of other systemic antibiotics
AHA: 2017, 1Q, 39

    ✓7ᵗʰ T36.8X1 Poisoning by other systemic antibiotics, accidental (unintentional)
Poisoning by other systemic antibiotics NOS

    11 **✓7ᵗʰ T36.8X2 Poisoning by other systemic antibiotics, intentional self-harm** [HCC]

    ✓7ᵗʰ T36.8X3 Poisoning by other systemic antibiotics, assault

    ✓7ᵗʰ T36.8X4 Poisoning by other systemic antibiotics, undetermined

    ✓7ᵗʰ T36.8X5 Adverse effect of other systemic antibiotics

    ✓7ᵗʰ T36.8X6 Underdosing of other systemic antibiotics

✓5ᵗʰ T36.9 Poisoning by, adverse effect of and underdosing of unspecified systemic antibiotic

  ✓x7ᵗʰ T36.91 Poisoning by unspecified systemic antibiotic, accidental (unintentional)
Poisoning by systemic antibiotic NOS

  11 **✓x7ᵗʰ T36.92 Poisoning by unspecified systemic antibiotic, intentional self-harm** [HCC]

  ✓x7ᵗʰ T36.93 Poisoning by unspecified systemic antibiotic, assault

  ✓x7ᵗʰ T36.94 Poisoning by unspecified systemic antibiotic, undetermined

  ✓x7ᵗʰ T36.95 Adverse effect of unspecified systemic antibiotic

  ✓x7ᵗʰ T36.96 Underdosing of unspecified systemic antibiotic

✓4ᵗʰ T37 Poisoning by, adverse effect of and underdosing of other systemic anti-infectives and antiparasitics
> **EXCLUDES 1**   anti-infectives topically used for ear, nose and throat (T49.6-)
> anti-infectives topically used for eye (T49.5-)
> locally applied anti-infectives NEC (T49.0-)

> The appropriate 7th character is to be added to each code from category T37.
> A   initial encounter
> D   subsequent encounter
> S   sequela

✓5ᵗʰ T37.0 Poisoning by, adverse effect of and underdosing of sulfonamides

  ✓6ᵗʰ T37.0X Poisoning by, adverse effect of and underdosing of sulfonamides

    ✓7ᵗʰ T37.0X1 Poisoning by sulfonamides, accidental (unintentional)
Poisoning by sulfonamides NOS

    11 **✓7ᵗʰ T37.0X2 Poisoning by sulfonamides, intentional self-harm** [HCC]

    ✓7ᵗʰ T37.0X3 Poisoning by sulfonamides, assault

    ✓7ᵗʰ T37.0X4 Poisoning by sulfonamides, undetermined

    ✓7ᵗʰ T37.0X5 Adverse effect of sulfonamides

    ✓7ᵗʰ T37.0X6 Underdosing of sulfonamides

✓5ᵗʰ T37.1 Poisoning by, adverse effect of and underdosing of antimycobacterial drugs
> **EXCLUDES 1**   rifampicins (T36.6-)
> streptomycin (T36.5-)

  ✓6ᵗʰ T37.1X Poisoning by, adverse effect of and underdosing of antimycobacterial drugs

    ✓7ᵗʰ T37.1X1 Poisoning by antimycobacterial drugs, accidental (unintentional)
Poisoning by antimycobacterial drugs NOS

    11 **✓7ᵗʰ T37.1X2 Poisoning by antimycobacterial drugs, intentional self-harm** [HCC]

    ✓7ᵗʰ T37.1X3 Poisoning by antimycobacterial drugs, assault

    ✓7ᵗʰ T37.1X4 Poisoning by antimycobacterial drugs, undetermined

    ✓7ᵗʰ T37.1X5 Adverse effect of antimycobacterial drugs

    ✓7ᵗʰ T37.1X6 Underdosing of antimycobacterial drugs

✓5ᵗʰ T37.2 Poisoning by, adverse effect of and underdosing of antimalarials and drugs acting on other blood protozoa
> **EXCLUDES 1**   hydroxyquinoline derivatives (T37.8-)

  ✓6ᵗʰ T37.2X Poisoning by, adverse effect of and underdosing of antimalarials and drugs acting on other blood protozoa

    ✓7ᵗʰ T37.2X1 Poisoning by antimalarials and drugs acting on other blood protozoa, accidental (unintentional)
Poisoning by antimalarials and drugs acting on other blood protozoa NOS

    11 **✓7ᵗʰ T37.2X2 Poisoning by antimalarials and drugs acting on other blood protozoa, intentional self-harm** [HCC]

    ✓7ᵗʰ T37.2X3 Poisoning by antimalarials and drugs acting on other blood protozoa, assault

    ✓7ᵗʰ T37.2X4 Poisoning by antimalarials and drugs acting on other blood protozoa, undetermined

    ✓7ᵗʰ T37.2X5 Adverse effect of antimalarials and drugs acting on other blood protozoa

    ✓7ᵗʰ T37.2X6 Underdosing of antimalarials and drugs acting on other blood protozoa

---

11 HCC with 7th character indicating initial encounter (A or B - specific to category) OR sequela.

Chapter 19. Injury, Poisoning and Certain Other Consequences of External Causes

✓5th **T37.3 Poisoning by, adverse effect of and underdosing of other antiprotozoal drugs**

✓6th   **T37.3X Poisoning by, adverse effect of and underdosing of other antiprotozoal drugs**

✓7th   **T37.3X1 Poisoning by other antiprotozoal drugs, accidental (unintentional)**
Poisoning by other antiprotozoal drugs NOS

11 ✓7th   **T37.3X2 Poisoning by other antiprotozoal drugs, intentional self-harm** HCC

✓7th   **T37.3X3 Poisoning by other antiprotozoal drugs, assault**

✓7th   **T37.3X4 Poisoning by other antiprotozoal drugs, undetermined**

✓7th   **T37.3X5 Adverse effect of other antiprotozoal drugs**

✓7th   **T37.3X6 Underdosing of other antiprotozoal drugs**

✓5th **T37.4 Poisoning by, adverse effect of and underdosing of anthelminthics**

✓6th   **T37.4X Poisoning by, adverse effect of and underdosing of anthelminthics**

✓7th   **T37.4X1 Poisoning by anthelminthics, accidental (unintentional)**
Poisoning by anthelminthics NOS

11 ✓7th   **T37.4X2 Poisoning by anthelminthics, intentional self-harm** HCC

✓7th   **T37.4X3 Poisoning by anthelminthics, assault**

✓7th   **T37.4X4 Poisoning by anthelminthics, undetermined**

✓7th   **T37.4X5 Adverse effect of anthelminthics**

✓7th   **T37.4X6 Underdosing of anthelminthics**

✓5th **T37.5 Poisoning by, adverse effect of and underdosing of antiviral drugs**

EXCLUDES 1   amantadine (T42.8-)
cytarabine (T45.1-)

✓6th   **T37.5X Poisoning by, adverse effect of and underdosing of antiviral drugs**

✓7th   **T37.5X1 Poisoning by antiviral drugs, accidental (unintentional)**
Poisoning by antiviral drugs NOS

11 ✓7th   **T37.5X2 Poisoning by antiviral drugs, intentional self-harm** HCC

✓7th   **T37.5X3 Poisoning by antiviral drugs, assault**

✓7th   **T37.5X4 Poisoning by antiviral drugs, undetermined**

✓7th   **T37.5X5 Adverse effect of antiviral drugs**

✓7th   **T37.5X6 Underdosing of antiviral drugs**

✓5th **T37.8 Poisoning by, adverse effect of and underdosing of other specified systemic anti-infectives and antiparasitics**
Poisoning by, adverse effect of and underdosing of hydroxyquinoline derivatives

EXCLUDES 1   antimalarial drugs (T37.2-)

✓6th   **T37.8X Poisoning by, adverse effect of and underdosing of other specified systemic anti-infectives and antiparasitics**

✓7th   **T37.8X1 Poisoning by other specified systemic anti-infectives and antiparasitics, accidental (unintentional)**
Poisoning by other specified systemic anti-infectives and antiparasitics NOS

11 ✓7th   **T37.8X2 Poisoning by other specified systemic anti-infectives and antiparasitics, intentional self-harm** HCC

✓7th   **T37.8X3 Poisoning by other specified systemic anti-infectives and antiparasitics, assault**

✓7th   **T37.8X4 Poisoning by other specified systemic anti-infectives and antiparasitics, undetermined**

✓7th   **T37.8X5 Adverse effect of other specified systemic anti-infectives and antiparasitics**

✓7th   **T37.8X6 Underdosing of other specified systemic anti-infectives and antiparasitics**

✓5th **T37.9 Poisoning by, adverse effect of and underdosing of unspecified systemic anti-infective and antiparasitics**

✓x7th   **T37.91 Poisoning by unspecified systemic anti-infective and antiparasitics, accidental (unintentional)**
Poisoning by, adverse effect of and underdosing of systemic anti-infective and antiparasitics NOS

11 ✓x7th   **T37.92 Poisoning by unspecified systemic anti-infective and antiparasitics, intentional self-harm** HCC

✓x7th   **T37.93 Poisoning by unspecified systemic anti-infective and antiparasitics, assault**

✓x7th   **T37.94 Poisoning by unspecified systemic anti-infective and antiparasitics, undetermined**

✓x7th   **T37.95 Adverse effect of unspecified systemic anti-infective and antiparasitic**

✓x7th   **T37.96 Underdosing of unspecified systemic anti-infectives and antiparasitics**

✓4th **T38 Poisoning by, adverse effect of and underdosing of hormones and their synthetic substitutes and antagonists, not elsewhere classified**

EXCLUDES 1   mineralocorticoids and their antagonists (T50.0-)
oxytocic hormones (T48.0-)
parathyroid hormones and derivatives (T50.9-)

> The appropriate 7th character is to be added to each code from category T38.
> A   initial encounter
> D   subsequent encounter
> S   sequela

✓5th **T38.0 Poisoning by, adverse effect of and underdosing of glucocorticoids and synthetic analogues**

EXCLUDES 1   glucocorticoids, topically used (T49.-)

✓6th   **T38.0X Poisoning by, adverse effect of and underdosing of glucocorticoids and synthetic analogues**

✓7th   **T38.0X1 Poisoning by glucocorticoids and synthetic analogues, accidental (unintentional)**
Poisoning by glucocorticoids and synthetic analogues NOS

11 ✓7th   **T38.0X2 Poisoning by glucocorticoids and synthetic analogues, intentional self-harm** HCC

✓7th   **T38.0X3 Poisoning by glucocorticoids and synthetic analogues, assault**

✓7th   **T38.0X4 Poisoning by glucocorticoids and synthetic analogues, undetermined**

✓7th   **T38.0X5 Adverse effect of glucocorticoids and synthetic analogues**

✓7th   **T38.0X6 Underdosing of glucocorticoids and synthetic analogues**

✓5th **T38.1 Poisoning by, adverse effect of and underdosing of thyroid hormones and substitutes**

✓6th   **T38.1X Poisoning by, adverse effect of and underdosing of thyroid hormones and substitutes**

✓7th   **T38.1X1 Poisoning by thyroid hormones and substitutes, accidental (unintentional)**
Poisoning by thyroid hormones and substitutes NOS

11 ✓7th   **T38.1X2 Poisoning by thyroid hormones and substitutes, intentional self-harm** HCC

✓7th   **T38.1X3 Poisoning by thyroid hormones and substitutes, assault**

✓7th   **T38.1X4 Poisoning by thyroid hormones and substitutes, undetermined**

✓7th   **T38.1X5 Adverse effect of thyroid hormones and substitutes**

✓7th   **T38.1X6 Underdosing of thyroid hormones and substitutes**

✓5th **T38.2 Poisoning by, adverse effect of and underdosing of antithyroid drugs**

✓6th   **T38.2X Poisoning by, adverse effect of and underdosing of antithyroid drugs**

✓7th   **T38.2X1 Poisoning by antithyroid drugs, accidental (unintentional)**
Poisoning by antithyroid drugs NOS

11 ✓7th   **T38.2X2 Poisoning by antithyroid drugs, intentional self-harm** HCC

---

11 HCC with 7th character indicating initial encounter (A or B - specific to category) OR sequela.

✓ Additional Character Req   ✓x7th Placeholder Alert   Unacceptable PDx   Manifestation   H1 - H14 HAC   HCC CMS-HCC Condition   *EXCLUDES 1* Not Coded Here   *EXCLUDES 2* Not Included Here

✓7th **T38.2X3** Poisoning by antithyroid drugs, assault
✓7th **T38.2X4** Poisoning by antithyroid drugs, undetermined
✓7th **T38.2X5** Adverse effect of antithyroid drugs
✓7th **T38.2X6** Underdosing of antithyroid drugs

✓5th **T38.3** Poisoning by, adverse effect of and underdosing of insulin and oral hypoglycemic [antidiabetic] drugs
 ✓6th **T38.3X** Poisoning by, adverse effect of and underdosing of insulin and oral hypoglycemic [antidiabetic] drugs
  ✓7th **T38.3X1** Poisoning by insulin and oral hypoglycemic [antidiabetic] drugs, accidental (unintentional)
   Poisoning by insulin and oral hypoglycemic [antidiabetic] drugs NOS
  11 ✓7th **T38.3X2** Poisoning by insulin and oral hypoglycemic [antidiabetic] drugs, intentional self-harm   HCC
  ✓7th **T38.3X3** Poisoning by insulin and oral hypoglycemic [antidiabetic] drugs, assault
  ✓7th **T38.3X4** Poisoning by insulin and oral hypoglycemic [antidiabetic] drugs, undetermined
  ✓7th **T38.3X5** Adverse effect of insulin and oral hypoglycemic [antidiabetic] drugs
  ✓7th **T38.3X6** Underdosing of insulin and oral hypoglycemic [antidiabetic] drugs

✓5th **T38.4** Poisoning by, adverse effect of and underdosing of oral contraceptives
  Poisoning by, adverse effect of and underdosing of multiple- and single-ingredient oral contraceptive preparations
 ✓6th **T38.4X** Poisoning by, adverse effect of and underdosing of oral contraceptives
  ✓7th **T38.4X1** Poisoning by oral contraceptives, accidental (unintentional)
   Poisoning by oral contraceptives NOS
  11 ✓7th **T38.4X2** Poisoning by oral contraceptives, intentional self-harm   HCC
  ✓7th **T38.4X3** Poisoning by oral contraceptives, assault
  ✓7th **T38.4X4** Poisoning by oral contraceptives, undetermined
  ✓7th **T38.4X5** Adverse effect of oral contraceptives
  ✓7th **T38.4X6** Underdosing of oral contraceptives

✓5th **T38.5** Poisoning by, adverse effect of and underdosing of other estrogens and progestogens
  Poisoning by, adverse effect of and underdosing of estrogens and progestogens mixtures and substitutes
 ✓6th **T38.5X** Poisoning by, adverse effect of and underdosing of other estrogens and progestogens
  ✓7th **T38.5X1** Poisoning by other estrogens and progestogens, accidental (unintentional)
   Poisoning by other estrogens and progestogens NOS
  11 ✓7th **T38.5X2** Poisoning by other estrogens and progestogens, intentional self-harm   HCC
  ✓7th **T38.5X3** Poisoning by other estrogens and progestogens, assault
  ✓7th **T38.5X4** Poisoning by other estrogens and progestogens, undetermined
  ✓7th **T38.5X5** Adverse effect of other estrogens and progestogens
  ✓7th **T38.5X6** Underdosing of other estrogens and progestogens

✓5th **T38.6** Poisoning by, adverse effect of and underdosing of antigonadotrophins, antiestrogens, antiandrogens, not elsewhere classified
  Poisoning by, adverse effect of and underdosing of tamoxifen
 ✓6th **T38.6X** Poisoning by, adverse effect of and underdosing of antigonadotrophins, antiestrogens, antiandrogens, not elsewhere classified
  ✓7th **T38.6X1** Poisoning by antigonadotrophins, antiestrogens, antiandrogens, not elsewhere classified, accidental (unintentional)
   Poisoning by antigonadotrophins, antiestrogens, antiandrogens, not elsewhere classified NOS

11 ✓7th **T38.6X2** Poisoning by antigonadotrophins, antiestrogens, antiandrogens, not elsewhere classified, intentional self-harm   HCC
✓7th **T38.6X3** Poisoning by antigonadotrophins, antiestrogens, antiandrogens, not elsewhere classified, assault
✓7th **T38.6X4** Poisoning by antigonadotrophins, antiestrogens, antiandrogens, not elsewhere classified, undetermined
✓7th **T38.6X5** Adverse effect of antigonadotrophins, antiestrogens, antiandrogens, not elsewhere classified
✓7th **T38.6X6** Underdosing of antigonadotrophins, antiestrogens, antiandrogens, not elsewhere classified

✓5th **T38.7** Poisoning by, adverse effect of and underdosing of androgens and anabolic congeners
 ✓6th **T38.7X** Poisoning by, adverse effect of and underdosing of androgens and anabolic congeners
  ✓7th **T38.7X1** Poisoning by androgens and anabolic congeners, accidental (unintentional)
   Poisoning by androgens and anabolic congeners NOS
  11 ✓7th **T38.7X2** Poisoning by androgens and anabolic congeners, intentional self-harm   HCC
  ✓7th **T38.7X3** Poisoning by androgens and anabolic congeners, assault
  ✓7th **T38.7X4** Poisoning by androgens and anabolic congeners, undetermined
  ✓7th **T38.7X5** Adverse effect of androgens and anabolic congeners
  ✓7th **T38.7X6** Underdosing of androgens and anabolic congeners

✓5th **T38.8** Poisoning by, adverse effect of and underdosing of other and unspecified hormones and synthetic substitutes
 ✓6th **T38.80** Poisoning by, adverse effect of and underdosing of unspecified hormones and synthetic substitutes
  ✓7th **T38.801** Poisoning by unspecified hormones and synthetic substitutes, accidental (unintentional)
   Poisoning by unspecified hormones and synthetic substitutes NOS
  11 ✓7th **T38.802** Poisoning by unspecified hormones and synthetic substitutes, intentional self-harm   HCC
  ✓7th **T38.803** Poisoning by unspecified hormones and synthetic substitutes, assault
  ✓7th **T38.804** Poisoning by unspecified hormones and synthetic substitutes, undetermined
  ✓7th **T38.805** Adverse effect of unspecified hormones and synthetic substitutes
  ✓7th **T38.806** Underdosing of unspecified hormones and synthetic substitutes
 ✓6th **T38.81** Poisoning by, adverse effect of and underdosing of anterior pituitary [adenohypophyseal] hormones
  ✓7th **T38.811** Poisoning by anterior pituitary [adenohypophyseal] hormones, accidental (unintentional)
   Poisoning by anterior pituitary [adenohypophyseal] hormones NOS
  11 ✓7th **T38.812** Poisoning by anterior pituitary [adenohypophyseal] hormones, intentional self-harm   HCC
  ✓7th **T38.813** Poisoning by anterior pituitary [adenohypophyseal] hormones, assault
  ✓7th **T38.814** Poisoning by anterior pituitary [adenohypophyseal] hormones, undetermined
  ✓7th **T38.815** Adverse effect of anterior pituitary [adenohypophyseal] hormones
  ✓7th **T38.816** Underdosing of anterior pituitary [adenohypophyseal] hormones

11 HCC with 7th character indicating initial encounter (A or B - specific to category) OR sequela.

√6ᵗʰ **T38.89 Poisoning by, adverse effect of and underdosing of other hormones and synthetic substitutes**

     √7ᵗʰ **T38.891 Poisoning by other hormones and synthetic substitutes, accidental (unintentional)**
         Poisoning by other hormones and synthetic substitutes NOS

     11 √7ᵗʰ **T38.892 Poisoning by other hormones and synthetic substitutes, intentional self-harm** HCC

     √7ᵗʰ **T38.893 Poisoning by other hormones and synthetic substitutes, assault**

     √7ᵗʰ **T38.894 Poisoning by other hormones and synthetic substitutes, undetermined**

     √7ᵗʰ **T38.895 Adverse effect of other hormones and synthetic substitutes**

     √7ᵗʰ **T38.896 Underdosing of other hormones and synthetic substitutes**

√5ᵗʰ **T38.9 Poisoning by, adverse effect of and underdosing of other and unspecified hormone antagonists**

     √6ᵗʰ **T38.90 Poisoning by, adverse effect of and underdosing of unspecified hormone antagonists**

         √7ᵗʰ **T38.901 Poisoning by unspecified hormone antagonists, accidental (unintentional)**
           Poisoning by unspecified hormone antagonists NOS

         11 √7ᵗʰ **T38.902 Poisoning by unspecified hormone antagonists, intentional self-harm** HCC

         √7ᵗʰ **T38.903 Poisoning by unspecified hormone antagonists, assault**

         √7ᵗʰ **T38.904 Poisoning by unspecified hormone antagonists, undetermined**

         √7ᵗʰ **T38.905 Adverse effect of unspecified hormone antagonists**

         √7ᵗʰ **T38.906 Underdosing of unspecified hormone antagonists**

     √6ᵗʰ **T38.99 Poisoning by, adverse effect of and underdosing of other hormone antagonists**

         √7ᵗʰ **T38.991 Poisoning by other hormone antagonists, accidental (unintentional)**
           Poisoning by other hormone antagonists NOS

         11 √7ᵗʰ **T38.992 Poisoning by other hormone antagonists, intentional self-harm** HCC

         √7ᵗʰ **T38.993 Poisoning by other hormone antagonists, assault**

         √7ᵗʰ **T38.994 Poisoning by other hormone antagonists, undetermined**

         √7ᵗʰ **T38.995 Adverse effect of other hormone antagonists**

         √7ᵗʰ **T38.996 Underdosing of other hormone antagonists**

√4ᵗʰ **T39 Poisoning by, adverse effect of and underdosing of nonopioid analgesics, antipyretics and antirheumatics**

> The appropriate 7th character is to be added to each code from category T39.
> A   initial encounter
> D   subsequent encounter
> S   sequela

√5ᵗʰ **T39.0 Poisoning by, adverse effect of and underdosing of salicylates**

     √6ᵗʰ **T39.01 Poisoning by, adverse effect of and underdosing of aspirin**
         Poisoning by, adverse effect of and underdosing of acetylsalicylic acid

         √7ᵗʰ **T39.011 Poisoning by aspirin, accidental (unintentional)**

         11 √7ᵗʰ **T39.012 Poisoning by aspirin, intentional self-harm** HCC

         √7ᵗʰ **T39.013 Poisoning by aspirin, assault**

         √7ᵗʰ **T39.014 Poisoning by aspirin, undetermined**

         √7ᵗʰ **T39.015 Adverse effect of aspirin**
           AHA: 2016, 1Q, 15

         √7ᵗʰ **T39.016 Underdosing of aspirin**

√6ᵗʰ **T39.09 Poisoning by, adverse effect of and underdosing of other salicylates**

     √7ᵗʰ **T39.091 Poisoning by salicylates, accidental (unintentional)**
         Poisoning by salicylates NOS

     11 √7ᵗʰ **T39.092 Poisoning by salicylates, intentional self-harm** HCC

     √7ᵗʰ **T39.093 Poisoning by salicylates, assault**

     √7ᵗʰ **T39.094 Poisoning by salicylates, undetermined**

     √7ᵗʰ **T39.095 Adverse effect of salicylates**

     √7ᵗʰ **T39.096 Underdosing of salicylates**

√5ᵗʰ **T39.1 Poisoning by, adverse effect of and underdosing of 4-Aminophenol derivatives**

     √6ᵗʰ **T39.1X Poisoning by, adverse effect of and underdosing of 4-Aminophenol derivatives**

         √7ᵗʰ **T39.1X1 Poisoning by 4-Aminophenol derivatives, accidental (unintentional)**
           Poisoning by 4-Aminophenol derivatives NOS

         11 √7ᵗʰ **T39.1X2 Poisoning by 4-Aminophenol derivatives, intentional self-harm** HCC

         √7ᵗʰ **T39.1X3 Poisoning by 4-Aminophenol derivatives, assault**

         √7ᵗʰ **T39.1X4 Poisoning by 4-Aminophenol derivatives, undetermined**

         √7ᵗʰ **T39.1X5 Adverse effect of 4-Aminophenol derivatives**

         √7ᵗʰ **T39.1X6 Underdosing of 4-Aminophenol derivatives**

√5ᵗʰ **T39.2 Poisoning by, adverse effect of and underdosing of pyrazolone derivatives**

     √6ᵗʰ **T39.2X Poisoning by, adverse effect of and underdosing of pyrazolone derivatives**

         √7ᵗʰ **T39.2X1 Poisoning by pyrazolone derivatives, accidental (unintentional)**
           Poisoning by pyrazolone derivatives NOS

         11 √7ᵗʰ **T39.2X2 Poisoning by pyrazolone derivatives, intentional self-harm** HCC

         √7ᵗʰ **T39.2X3 Poisoning by pyrazolone derivatives, assault**

         √7ᵗʰ **T39.2X4 Poisoning by pyrazolone derivatives, undetermined**

         √7ᵗʰ **T39.2X5 Adverse effect of pyrazolone derivatives**

         √7ᵗʰ **T39.2X6 Underdosing of pyrazolone derivatives**

√5ᵗʰ **T39.3 Poisoning by, adverse effect of and underdosing of other nonsteroidal anti-inflammatory drugs [NSAID]**

     √6ᵗʰ **T39.31 Poisoning by, adverse effect of and underdosing of propionic acid derivatives**
         Poisoning by, adverse effect of and underdosing of fenoprofen
         Poisoning by, adverse effect of and underdosing of flurbiprofen
         Poisoning by, adverse effect of and underdosing of ibuprofen
         Poisoning by, adverse effect of and underdosing of ketoprofen
         Poisoning by, adverse effect of and underdosing of naproxen
         Poisoning by, adverse effect of and underdosing of oxaprozin

         √7ᵗʰ **T39.311 Poisoning by propionic acid derivatives, accidental (unintentional)**

         11 √7ᵗʰ **T39.312 Poisoning by propionic acid derivatives, intentional self-harm** HCC

         √7ᵗʰ **T39.313 Poisoning by propionic acid derivatives, assault**

         √7ᵗʰ **T39.314 Poisoning by propionic acid derivatives, undetermined**

         √7ᵗʰ **T39.315 Adverse effect of propionic acid derivatives**

         √7ᵗʰ **T39.316 Underdosing of propionic acid derivatives**

---

11   HCC with 7th character indicating initial encounter (A or B - specific to category) OR sequela.

✔Additional Character Req   √ˣ7ᵗʰ Placeholder Alert   Unacceptable PDx   Manifestation   H1 - H14 HAC   HCC CMS-HCC Condition   *EXCLUDES 1* Not Coded Here   *EXCLUDES 2* Not Included Here

✓6ᵗʰ **T39.39 Poisoning by, adverse effect of and underdosing of** other nonsteroidal anti-inflammatory drugs [NSAID]

    ✓7ᵗʰ **T39.391 Poisoning by other nonsteroidal anti-inflammatory drugs [NSAID], accidental (unintentional)**
        Poisoning by other nonsteroidal anti-inflammatory drugs NOS

    11 ✓7ᵗʰ **T39.392 Poisoning by other nonsteroidal anti-inflammatory drugs [NSAID], intentional self-harm**   HCC

    ✓7ᵗʰ **T39.393 Poisoning by other nonsteroidal anti-inflammatory drugs [NSAID], assault**

    ✓7ᵗʰ **T39.394 Poisoning by other nonsteroidal anti-inflammatory drugs [NSAID], undetermined**

    ✓7ᵗʰ **T39.395 Adverse effect of other nonsteroidal anti-inflammatory drugs [NSAID]**

    ✓7ᵗʰ **T39.396 Underdosing of other nonsteroidal anti-inflammatory drugs [NSAID]**

✓5ᵗʰ **T39.4 Poisoning by, adverse effect of and underdosing of antirheumatics, not elsewhere classified**
    EXCLUDES 1   *poisoning by, adverse effect of and underdosing of glucocorticoids (T38.0-)*
                  poisoning by, adverse effect of and underdosing of salicylates (T39.0-)

  ✓6ᵗʰ **T39.4X Poisoning by, adverse effect of and underdosing of** antirheumatics, not elsewhere classified

    ✓7ᵗʰ **T39.4X1 Poisoning by antirheumatics, not elsewhere classified, accidental (unintentional)**
        Poisoning by antirheumatics, not elsewhere classified NOS

    11 ✓7ᵗʰ **T39.4X2 Poisoning by antirheumatics, not elsewhere classified, intentional self-harm**   HCC

    ✓7ᵗʰ **T39.4X3 Poisoning by antirheumatics, not elsewhere classified, assault**

    ✓7ᵗʰ **T39.4X4 Poisoning by antirheumatics, not elsewhere classified, undetermined**

    ✓7ᵗʰ **T39.4X5 Adverse effect of antirheumatics, not elsewhere classified**

    ✓7ᵗʰ **T39.4X6 Underdosing of antirheumatics, not elsewhere classified**

✓5ᵗʰ **T39.8 Poisoning by, adverse effect of and underdosing of other nonopioid analgesics and antipyretics, not elsewhere classified**

  ✓6ᵗʰ **T39.8X Poisoning by, adverse effect of and underdosing of** other nonopioid analgesics and antipyretics, **not elsewhere classified**

    ✓7ᵗʰ **T39.8X1 Poisoning by other nonopioid analgesics and antipyretics, not elsewhere classified, accidental (unintentional)**
        Poisoning by other nonopioid analgesics and antipyretics, not elsewhere classified NOS

    11 ✓7ᵗʰ **T39.8X2 Poisoning by other nonopioid analgesics and antipyretics, not elsewhere classified, intentional self-harm**   HCC

    ✓7ᵗʰ **T39.8X3 Poisoning by other nonopioid analgesics and antipyretics, not elsewhere classified, assault**

    ✓7ᵗʰ **T39.8X4 Poisoning by other nonopioid analgesics and antipyretics, not elsewhere classified, undetermined**

    ✓7ᵗʰ **T39.8X5 Adverse effect of other nonopioid analgesics and antipyretics, not elsewhere classified**

    ✓7ᵗʰ **T39.8X6 Underdosing of other nonopioid analgesics and antipyretics, not elsewhere classified**

✓5ᵗʰ **T39.9 Poisoning by, adverse effect of and underdosing of** unspecified nonopioid analgesic, antipyretic and antirheumatic

  ✓x7ᵗʰ **T39.91 Poisoning by unspecified nonopioid analgesic, antipyretic and antirheumatic, accidental (unintentional)**
    Poisoning by nonopioid analgesic, antipyretic and antirheumatic NOS

---

  11 ✓x7ᵗʰ **T39.92 Poisoning by unspecified nonopioid analgesic, antipyretic and antirheumatic, intentional self-harm**   HCC

  ✓x7ᵗʰ **T39.93 Poisoning by unspecified nonopioid analgesic, antipyretic and antirheumatic, assault**

  ✓x7ᵗʰ **T39.94 Poisoning by unspecified nonopioid analgesic, antipyretic and antirheumatic, undetermined**

  ✓x7ᵗʰ **T39.95 Adverse effect of unspecified nonopioid analgesic, antipyretic and antirheumatic**

  ✓x7ᵗʰ **T39.96 Underdosing of unspecified nonopioid analgesic, antipyretic and antirheumatic**

✓4ᵗʰ **T40 Poisoning by, adverse effect of and underdosing of narcotics and psychodysleptics [hallucinogens]**
    EXCLUDES 2   *drug dependence and related mental and behavioral disorders due to psychoactive substance use (F10-F19-)*

    The appropriate 7th character is to be added to each code from category T40.
    A   initial encounter
    D   subsequent encounter
    S   sequela

✓5ᵗʰ **T40.0 Poisoning by, adverse effect of and underdosing of opium**

  ✓6ᵗʰ **T40.0X Poisoning by, adverse effect of and underdosing of** opium

    ✓7ᵗʰ **T40.0X1 Poisoning by opium, accidental (unintentional)**
        Poisoning by opium NOS

    11 ✓7ᵗʰ **T40.0X2 Poisoning by opium, intentional self-harm**   HCC

    ✓7ᵗʰ **T40.0X3 Poisoning by opium, assault**

    ✓7ᵗʰ **T40.0X4 Poisoning by opium, undetermined**

    ✓7ᵗʰ **T40.0X5 Adverse effect of opium**

    ✓7ᵗʰ **T40.0X6 Underdosing of opium**

✓5ᵗʰ **T40.1 Poisoning by and adverse effect of heroin**

  ✓6ᵗʰ **T40.1X Poisoning by and adverse effect of heroin**

    ✓7ᵗʰ **T40.1X1 Poisoning by heroin, accidental (unintentional)**
        Poisoning by heroin NOS

    11 ✓7ᵗʰ **T40.1X2 Poisoning by heroin, intentional self-harm**   HCC

    ✓7ᵗʰ **T40.1X3 Poisoning by heroin, assault**

    ✓7ᵗʰ **T40.1X4 Poisoning by heroin, undetermined**

✓5ᵗʰ **T40.2 Poisoning by, adverse effect of and underdosing of other opioids**

  ✓6ᵗʰ **T40.2X Poisoning by, adverse effect of and underdosing of** other opioids

    ✓7ᵗʰ **T40.2X1 Poisoning by other opioids, accidental (unintentional)**
        Poisoning by other opioids NOS

    11 ✓7ᵗʰ **T40.2X2 Poisoning by other opioids, intentional self-harm**   HCC

    ✓7ᵗʰ **T40.2X3 Poisoning by other opioids, assault**

    ✓7ᵗʰ **T40.2X4 Poisoning by other opioids, undetermined**

    ✓7ᵗʰ **T40.2X5 Adverse effect of other opioids**

    ✓7ᵗʰ **T40.2X6 Underdosing of other opioids**

✓5ᵗʰ **T40.3 Poisoning by, adverse effect of and underdosing of methadone**

  ✓6ᵗʰ **T40.3X Poisoning by, adverse effect of and underdosing of** methadone

    ✓7ᵗʰ **T40.3X1 Poisoning by methadone, accidental (unintentional)**
        Poisoning by methadone NOS

    11 ✓7ᵗʰ **T40.3X2 Poisoning by methadone, intentional self-harm**   HCC

    ✓7ᵗʰ **T40.3X3 Poisoning by methadone, assault**

    ✓7ᵗʰ **T40.3X4 Poisoning by methadone, undetermined**

    ✓7ᵗʰ **T40.3X5 Adverse effect of methadone**

    ✓7ᵗʰ **T40.3X6 Underdosing of methadone**

---

11   HCC with 7th character indicating initial encounter (A or B - specific to category) OR sequela.

Ⓝ Newborn: 0   Ⓟ Pediatric: 0-17   Ⓜ Maternity: 12-55   Ⓐ Adult: 15-124   **MCC** Major CC Condition   **PDxMCC** PDx acts as own MCC   **CC** CC Condition   **PDxCC** PDx acts as own CC

1104   ICD-10-CM 2018

☑5ᵗʰ **T40.4** **Poisoning by, adverse effect of and underdosing of other synthetic narcotics**

     ☑6ᵗʰ **T40.4X** **Poisoning by, adverse effect of and underdosing of** other synthetic narcotics

       ☑7ᵗʰ **T40.4X1** **Poisoning by other synthetic narcotics,** accidental **(unintentional)**
         Poisoning by other synthetic narcotics NOS

       11 ☑7ᵗʰ **T40.4X2** **Poisoning by other synthetic narcotics, intentional self-harm**   HCC

       ☑7ᵗʰ **T40.4X3** **Poisoning by other synthetic narcotics, assault**

       ☑7ᵗʰ **T40.4X4** **Poisoning by other synthetic narcotics, undetermined**

       ☑7ᵗʰ **T40.4X5** Adverse effect **of other synthetic narcotics**

       ☑7ᵗʰ **T40.4X6** Underdosing **of other synthetic narcotics**

☑5ᵗʰ **T40.5** **Poisoning by, adverse effect of and underdosing of cocaine**

     ☑6ᵗʰ **T40.5X** **Poisoning by, adverse effect of and underdosing of** cocaine

       ☑7ᵗʰ **T40.5X1** **Poisoning by cocaine,** accidental **(unintentional)**
         Poisoning by cocaine NOS
         AHA: 2016, 2Q, 8

       11 ☑7ᵗʰ **T40.5X2** **Poisoning by cocaine,** intentional self-harm   HCC

       ☑7ᵗʰ **T40.5X3** **Poisoning by cocaine,** assault

       ☑7ᵗʰ **T40.5X4** **Poisoning by cocaine,** undetermined

       ☑7ᵗʰ **T40.5X5** Adverse effect **of cocaine**

       ☑7ᵗʰ **T40.5X6** Underdosing **of cocaine**

☑5ᵗʰ **T40.6** **Poisoning by, adverse effect of and underdosing of other and unspecified narcotics**

     ☑6ᵗʰ **T40.60** **Poisoning by, adverse effect of and underdosing of** unspecified narcotics

       ☑7ᵗʰ **T40.601** **Poisoning by unspecified narcotics, accidental (unintentional)**
         Poisoning by narcotics NOS

       11 ☑7ᵗʰ **T40.602** **Poisoning by unspecified narcotics, intentional self-harm**   HCC

       ☑7ᵗʰ **T40.603** **Poisoning by unspecified narcotics, assault**

       ☑7ᵗʰ **T40.604** **Poisoning by unspecified narcotics, undetermined**

       ☑7ᵗʰ **T40.605** Adverse effect **of unspecified narcotics**

       ☑7ᵗʰ **T40.606** Underdosing **of unspecified narcotics**

     ☑6ᵗʰ **T40.69** **Poisoning by, adverse effect of and underdosing of** other narcotics

       ☑7ᵗʰ **T40.691** **Poisoning by other narcotics,** accidental **(unintentional)**
         Poisoning by other narcotics NOS

       11 ☑7ᵗʰ **T40.692** **Poisoning by other narcotics, intentional self-harm**   HCC

       ☑7ᵗʰ **T40.693** **Poisoning by other narcotics,** assault

       ☑7ᵗʰ **T40.694** **Poisoning by other narcotics, undetermined**

       ☑7ᵗʰ **T40.695** Adverse effect **of other narcotics**

       ☑7ᵗʰ **T40.696** Underdosing **of other narcotics**

☑5ᵗʰ **T40.7** **Poisoning by, adverse effect of and underdosing of cannabis (derivatives)**

     ☑6ᵗʰ **T40.7X** **Poisoning by, adverse effect of and underdosing of** cannabis **(derivatives)**

       ☑7ᵗʰ **T40.7X1** **Poisoning by cannabis (derivatives),** accidental **(unintentional)**
         Poisoning by cannabis NOS

       11 ☑7ᵗʰ **T40.7X2** **Poisoning by cannabis (derivatives),** intentional self-harm   HCC

       ☑7ᵗʰ **T40.7X3** **Poisoning by cannabis (derivatives), assault**

       ☑7ᵗʰ **T40.7X4** **Poisoning by cannabis (derivatives), undetermined**

       ☑7ᵗʰ **T40.7X5** Adverse effect **of cannabis (derivatives)**

       ☑7ᵗʰ **T40.7X6** Underdosing **of cannabis (derivatives)**

☑5ᵗʰ **T40.8** **Poisoning by and adverse effect of** lysergide [LSD]

     ☑6ᵗʰ **T40.8X** **Poisoning by and adverse effect of lysergide [LSD]**

       ☑7ᵗʰ **T40.8X1** **Poisoning by lysergide [LSD],** accidental **(unintentional)**
         Poisoning by lysergide [LSD]NOS

       11 ☑7ᵗʰ **T40.8X2** **Poisoning by lysergide [LSD], intentional self-harm**   HCC

       ☑7ᵗʰ **T40.8X3** **Poisoning by lysergide [LSD],** assault

       ☑7ᵗʰ **T40.8X4** **Poisoning by lysergide [LSD],** undetermined

☑5ᵗʰ **T40.9** **Poisoning by, adverse effect of and underdosing of other and unspecified psychodysleptics [hallucinogens]**

     ☑6ᵗʰ **T40.90** **Poisoning by, adverse effect of and underdosing of** unspecified psychodysleptics [hallucinogens]

       ☑7ᵗʰ **T40.901** **Poisoning by unspecified psychodysleptics [hallucinogens], accidental (unintentional)**

       11 ☑7ᵗʰ **T40.902** **Poisoning by unspecified psychodysleptics [hallucinogens], intentional self-harm**   HCC

       ☑7ᵗʰ **T40.903** **Poisoning by unspecified psychodysleptics [hallucinogens],** assault

       ☑7ᵗʰ **T40.904** **Poisoning by unspecified psychodysleptics [hallucinogens], undetermined**

       ☑7ᵗʰ **T40.905** Adverse effect **of unspecified psychodysleptics [hallucinogens]**

       ☑7ᵗʰ **T40.906** Underdosing **of unspecified psychodysleptics**

     ☑6ᵗʰ **T40.99** **Poisoning by, adverse effect of and underdosing of** other psychodysleptics [hallucinogens]

       ☑7ᵗʰ **T40.991** **Poisoning by other psychodysleptics [hallucinogens],** accidental **(unintentional)**
         Poisoning by other psychodysleptics [hallucinogens] NOS

       11 ☑7ᵗʰ **T40.992** **Poisoning by other psychodysleptics [hallucinogens],** intentional self-harm   HCC

       ☑7ᵗʰ **T40.993** **Poisoning by other psychodysleptics [hallucinogens],** assault

       ☑7ᵗʰ **T40.994** **Poisoning by other psychodysleptics [hallucinogens],** undetermined

       ☑7ᵗʰ **T40.995** Adverse effect **of other psychodysleptics [hallucinogens]**

       ☑7ᵗʰ **T40.996** Underdosing **of other psychodysleptics**

☑4ᵗʰ **T41** **Poisoning by, adverse effect of and underdosing of anesthetics and therapeutic gases**

     EXCLUDES 1   *benzodiazepines (T42.4-)*
         cocaine (T40.5-)
         complications of anesthesia during labor and delivery (O74.-)
         complications of anesthesia during pregnancy (O29.-)
         complications of anesthesia during the puerperium (O89.-)
         opioids (T40.0-T40.2-)

     The appropriate 7th character is to be added to each code from category T41.
     A   initial encounter
     D   subsequent encounter
     S   sequela

     ☑5ᵗʰ **T41.0** **Poisoning by, adverse effect of and underdosing of inhaled anesthetics**

       EXCLUDES 1   *oxygen (T41.5-)*

       ☑6ᵗʰ **T41.0X** **Poisoning by, adverse effect of and underdosing of** inhaled anesthetics

         ☑7ᵗʰ **T41.0X1** **Poisoning by inhaled anesthetics,** accidental **(unintentional)**
           Poisoning by inhaled anesthetics NOS

         11 ☑7ᵗʰ **T41.0X2** **Poisoning by inhaled anesthetics, intentional self-harm**   HCC

         ☑7ᵗʰ **T41.0X3** **Poisoning by inhaled anesthetics,** assault

         ☑7ᵗʰ **T41.0X4** **Poisoning by inhaled anesthetics, undetermined**

         ☑7ᵗʰ **T41.0X5** Adverse effect **of inhaled anesthetics**

         ☑7ᵗʰ **T41.0X6** Underdosing **of inhaled anesthetics**

---

11 HCC with 7th character indicating initial encounter (A or B - specific to category) OR sequela.

☑ Additional Character Req   ☑7ᵗʰ Placeholder Alert   Unacceptable PDx   Manifestation   H1-H14 HAC   HCC CMS-HCC Condition   EXCLUDES 1 Not Coded Here   EXCLUDES 2 Not Included Here

ICD-10-CM 2018   **1105**

Chapter 19. Injury, Poisoning and Certain Other Consequences of External Causes

T41.1–T42.2X5

✓5ᵗʰ **T41.1 Poisoning by, adverse effect of and underdosing of intravenous anesthetics**
Poisoning by, adverse effect of and underdosing of thiobarbiturates

✓6ᵗʰ **T41.1X Poisoning by, adverse effect of and underdosing of intravenous anesthetics**

     ✓7ᵗʰ **T41.1X1 Poisoning by intravenous anesthetics, accidental (unintentional)**
Poisoning by intravenous anesthetics NOS

     11 ✓7ᵗʰ **T41.1X2 Poisoning by intravenous anesthetics, intentional self-harm** HCC

     ✓7ᵗʰ **T41.1X3 Poisoning by intravenous anesthetics, assault**

     ✓7ᵗʰ **T41.1X4 Poisoning by intravenous anesthetics, undetermined**

     ✓7ᵗʰ **T41.1X5 Adverse effect of intravenous anesthetics**

     ✓7ᵗʰ **T41.1X6 Underdosing of intravenous anesthetics**

✓5ᵗʰ **T41.2 Poisoning by, adverse effect of and underdosing of other and unspecified general anesthetics**

✓6ᵗʰ **T41.20 Poisoning by, adverse effect of and underdosing of unspecified general anesthetics**

     ✓7ᵗʰ **T41.201 Poisoning by unspecified general anesthetics, accidental (unintentional)**
Poisoning by general anesthetics NOS

     11 ✓7ᵗʰ **T41.202 Poisoning by unspecified general anesthetics, intentional self-harm** HCC

     ✓7ᵗʰ **T41.203 Poisoning by unspecified general anesthetics, assault**

     ✓7ᵗʰ **T41.204 Poisoning by unspecified general anesthetics, undetermined**

     ✓7ᵗʰ **T41.205 Adverse effect of unspecified general anesthetics**

     ✓7ᵗʰ **T41.206 Underdosing of unspecified general anesthetics**

✓6ᵗʰ **T41.29 Poisoning by, adverse effect of and underdosing of other general anesthetics**

     ✓7ᵗʰ **T41.291 Poisoning by other general anesthetics, accidental (unintentional)**
Poisoning by other general anesthetics NOS

     11 ✓7ᵗʰ **T41.292 Poisoning by other general anesthetics, intentional self-harm** HCC

     ✓7ᵗʰ **T41.293 Poisoning by other general anesthetics, assault**

     ✓7ᵗʰ **T41.294 Poisoning by other general anesthetics, undetermined**

     ✓7ᵗʰ **T41.295 Adverse effect of other general anesthetics**

     ✓7ᵗʰ **T41.296 Underdosing of other general anesthetics**

✓5ᵗʰ **T41.3 Poisoning by, adverse effect of and underdosing of local anesthetics**
Cocaine (topical)

     EXCLUDES 2   *poisoning by cocaine used as a central nervous system stimulant (T40.5X1-T40.5X4)*

✓6ᵗʰ **T41.3X Poisoning by, adverse effect of and underdosing of local anesthetics**

     ✓7ᵗʰ **T41.3X1 Poisoning by local anesthetics, accidental (unintentional)**
Poisoning by local anesthetics NOS

     11 ✓7ᵗʰ **T41.3X2 Poisoning by local anesthetics, intentional self-harm** HCC

     ✓7ᵗʰ **T41.3X3 Poisoning by local anesthetics, assault**

     ✓7ᵗʰ **T41.3X4 Poisoning by local anesthetics, undetermined**

     ✓7ᵗʰ **T41.3X5 Adverse effect of local anesthetics**

     ✓7ᵗʰ **T41.3X6 Underdosing of local anesthetics**

✓5ᵗʰ **T41.4 Poisoning by, adverse effect of and underdosing of unspecified anesthetic**

     ✓x7ᵗʰ **T41.41 Poisoning by unspecified anesthetic, accidental (unintentional)**
Poisoning by anesthetic NOS

     11 ✓x7ᵗʰ **T41.42 Poisoning by unspecified anesthetic, intentional self-harm** HCC

     ✓x7ᵗʰ **T41.43 Poisoning by unspecified anesthetic, assault**

     ✓x7ᵗʰ **T41.44 Poisoning by unspecified anesthetic, undetermined**

     ✓x7ᵗʰ **T41.45 Adverse effect of unspecified anesthetic**

     ✓x7ᵗʰ **T41.46 Underdosing of unspecified anesthetics**

✓5ᵗʰ **T41.5 Poisoning by, adverse effect of and underdosing of therapeutic gases**

✓6ᵗʰ **T41.5X Poisoning by, adverse effect of and underdosing of therapeutic gases**

     ✓7ᵗʰ **T41.5X1 Poisoning by therapeutic gases, accidental (unintentional)**
Poisoning by therapeutic gases NOS

     11 ✓7ᵗʰ **T41.5X2 Poisoning by therapeutic gases, intentional self-harm** HCC

     ✓7ᵗʰ **T41.5X3 Poisoning by therapeutic gases, assault**

     ✓7ᵗʰ **T41.5X4 Poisoning by therapeutic gases, undetermined**

     ✓7ᵗʰ **T41.5X5 Adverse effect of therapeutic gases**

     ✓7ᵗʰ **T41.5X6 Underdosing of therapeutic gases**

✓4ᵗʰ **T42 Poisoning by, adverse effect of and underdosing of antiepileptic, sedative- hypnotic and antiparkinsonism drugs**

     EXCLUDES 2   *drug dependence and related mental and behavioral disorders due to psychoactive substance use (F10- – F19-)*

The appropriate 7th character is to be added to each code from category T42.
A   initial encounter
D   subsequent encounter
S   sequela

✓5ᵗʰ **T42.0 Poisoning by, adverse effect of and underdosing of hydantoin derivatives**

✓6ᵗʰ **T42.0X Poisoning by, adverse effect of and underdosing of hydantoin derivatives**

     ✓7ᵗʰ **T42.0X1 Poisoning by hydantoin derivatives, accidental (unintentional)**
Poisoning by hydantoin derivatives NOS

     11 ✓7ᵗʰ **T42.0X2 Poisoning by hydantoin derivatives, intentional self-harm** HCC

     ✓7ᵗʰ **T42.0X3 Poisoning by hydantoin derivatives, assault**

     ✓7ᵗʰ **T42.0X4 Poisoning by hydantoin derivatives, undetermined**

     ✓7ᵗʰ **T42.0X5 Adverse effect of hydantoin derivatives**

     ✓7ᵗʰ **T42.0X6 Underdosing of hydantoin derivatives**

✓5ᵗʰ **T42.1 Poisoning by, adverse effect of and underdosing of iminostilbenes**
Poisoning by, adverse effect of and underdosing of carbamazepine

✓6ᵗʰ **T42.1X Poisoning by, adverse effect of and underdosing of iminostilbenes**

     ✓7ᵗʰ **T42.1X1 Poisoning by iminostilbenes, accidental (unintentional)**
Poisoning by iminostilbenes NOS

     11 ✓7ᵗʰ **T42.1X2 Poisoning by iminostilbenes, intentional self-harm** HCC

     ✓7ᵗʰ **T42.1X3 Poisoning by iminostilbenes, assault**

     ✓7ᵗʰ **T42.1X4 Poisoning by iminostilbenes, undetermined**

     ✓7ᵗʰ **T42.1X5 Adverse effect of iminostilbenes**

     ✓7ᵗʰ **T42.1X6 Underdosing of iminostilbenes**

✓5ᵗʰ **T42.2 Poisoning by, adverse effect of and underdosing of succinimides and oxazolidinediones**

✓6ᵗʰ **T42.2X Poisoning by, adverse effect of and underdosing of succinimides and oxazolidinediones**

     ✓7ᵗʰ **T42.2X1 Poisoning by succinimides and oxazolidinediones, accidental (unintentional)**
Poisoning by succinimides and oxazolidinediones NOS

     11 ✓7ᵗʰ **T42.2X2 Poisoning by succinimides and oxazolidinediones, intentional self-harm** HCC

     ✓7ᵗʰ **T42.2X3 Poisoning by succinimides and oxazolidinediones, assault**

     ✓7ᵗʰ **T42.2X4 Poisoning by succinimides and oxazolidinediones, undetermined**

     ✓7ᵗʰ **T42.2X5 Adverse effect of succinimides and oxazolidinediones**

---

11 HCC with 7th character indicating initial encounter (A or B - specific to category) OR sequela.

N Newborn: 0   P Pediatric: 0-17   M Maternity: 12-55   A Adult: 15-124   MCC Major CC Condition   PDxMCC PDx acts as own MCC   CC CC Condition   PDxCC PDx acts as own CC

1106   ICD-10-CM 2018

✓7ᵗʰ **T42.2X6** Underdosing of succinimides and oxazolidinediones

✓5ᵗʰ **T42.3** Poisoning by, adverse effect of and underdosing of barbiturates

     EXCLUDES 1   poisoning by, adverse effect of and underdosing of thiobarbiturates (T41.1-)

     ✓6ᵗʰ **T42.3X** Poisoning by, adverse effect of and underdosing of barbiturates

         ✓7ᵗʰ **T42.3X1** Poisoning by barbiturates, accidental (unintentional)

             Poisoning by barbiturates NOS

         11 ✓7ᵗʰ **T42.3X2** Poisoning by barbiturates, intentional self-harm   HCC

         ✓7ᵗʰ **T42.3X3** Poisoning by barbiturates, assault

         ✓7ᵗʰ **T42.3X4** Poisoning by barbiturates, undetermined

         ✓7ᵗʰ **T42.3X5** Adverse effect of barbiturates

         ✓7ᵗʰ **T42.3X6** Underdosing of barbiturates

✓5ᵗʰ **T42.4** Poisoning by, adverse effect of and underdosing of benzodiazepines

     ✓6ᵗʰ **T42.4X** Poisoning by, adverse effect of and underdosing of benzodiazepines

         ✓7ᵗʰ **T42.4X1** Poisoning by benzodiazepines, accidental (unintentional)

             Poisoning by benzodiazepines NOS

         11 ✓7ᵗʰ **T42.4X2** Poisoning by benzodiazepines, intentional self-harm   HCC

         ✓7ᵗʰ **T42.4X3** Poisoning by benzodiazepines, assault

         ✓7ᵗʰ **T42.4X4** Poisoning by benzodiazepines, undetermined

         ✓7ᵗʰ **T42.4X5** Adverse effect of benzodiazepines

         ✓7ᵗʰ **T42.4X6** Underdosing of benzodiazepines

✓5ᵗʰ **T42.5** Poisoning by, adverse effect of and underdosing of mixed antiepileptics

     ✓6ᵗʰ **T42.5X** Poisoning by, adverse effect of and underdosing of antiepileptics

         ✓7ᵗʰ **T42.5X1** Poisoning by mixed antiepileptics, accidental (unintentional)

             Poisoning by mixed antiepileptics NOS

         11 ✓7ᵗʰ **T42.5X2** Poisoning by mixed antiepileptics, intentional self-harm   HCC

         ✓7ᵗʰ **T42.5X3** Poisoning by mixed antiepileptics, assault

         ✓7ᵗʰ **T42.5X4** Poisoning by mixed antiepileptics, undetermined

         ✓7ᵗʰ **T42.5X5** Adverse effect of mixed antiepileptics

         ✓7ᵗʰ **T42.5X6** Underdosing of mixed antiepileptics

✓5ᵗʰ **T42.6** Poisoning by, adverse effect of and underdosing of other antiepileptic and sedative-hypnotic drugs

     Poisoning by, adverse effect of and underdosing of methaqualone

     Poisoning by, adverse effect of and underdosing of valproic acid

     EXCLUDES 1   poisoning by, adverse effect of and underdosing of carbamazepine (T42.1-)

     ✓6ᵗʰ **T42.6X** Poisoning by, adverse effect of and underdosing of other antiepileptic and sedative-hypnotic drugs

         ✓7ᵗʰ **T42.6X1** Poisoning by other antiepileptic and sedative-hypnotic drugs, accidental (unintentional)

             Poisoning by other antiepileptic and sedative-hypnotic drugs NOS

         11 ✓7ᵗʰ **T42.6X2** Poisoning by other antiepileptic and sedative-hypnotic drugs, intentional self-harm   HCC

         ✓7ᵗʰ **T42.6X3** Poisoning by other antiepileptic and sedative-hypnotic drugs, assault

         ✓7ᵗʰ **T42.6X4** Poisoning by other antiepileptic and sedative-hypnotic drugs, undetermined

         ✓7ᵗʰ **T42.6X5** Adverse effect of other antiepileptic and sedative-hypnotic drugs

         ✓7ᵗʰ **T42.6X6** Underdosing of other antiepileptic and sedative-hypnotic drugs

✓5ᵗʰ **T42.7** Poisoning by, adverse effect of and underdosing of unspecified antiepileptic and sedative-hypnotic drugs

     ✓x7ᵗʰ **T42.71** Poisoning by unspecified antiepileptic and sedative-hypnotic drugs, accidental (unintentional)

         Poisoning by antiepileptic and sedative-hypnotic drugs NOS

     11 ✓x7ᵗʰ **T42.72** Poisoning by unspecified antiepileptic and sedative-hypnotic drugs, intentional self-harm   HCC

     ✓x7ᵗʰ **T42.73** Poisoning by unspecified antiepileptic and sedative-hypnotic drugs, assault

     ✓x7ᵗʰ **T42.74** Poisoning by unspecified antiepileptic and sedative-hypnotic drugs, undetermined

     ✓x7ᵗʰ **T42.75** Adverse effect of unspecified antiepileptic and sedative-hypnotic drugs

     ✓x7ᵗʰ **T42.76** Underdosing of unspecified antiepileptic and sedative-hypnotic drugs

✓5ᵗʰ **T42.8** Poisoning by, adverse effect of and underdosing of antiparkinsonism drugs and other central muscle-tone depressants

     Poisoning by, adverse effect of and underdosing of amantadine

     ✓6ᵗʰ **T42.8X** Poisoning by, adverse effect of and underdosing of antiparkinsonism drugs and other central muscle-tone depressants

         ✓7ᵗʰ **T42.8X1** Poisoning by antiparkinsonism drugs and other central muscle-tone depressants, accidental (unintentional)

             Poisoning by antiparkinsonism drugs and other central muscle-tone depressants NOS

         11 ✓7ᵗʰ **T42.8X2** Poisoning by antiparkinsonism drugs and other central muscle-tone depressants, intentional self-harm   HCC

         ✓7ᵗʰ **T42.8X3** Poisoning by antiparkinsonism drugs and other central muscle-tone depressants, assault

         ✓7ᵗʰ **T42.8X4** Poisoning by antiparkinsonism drugs and other central muscle-tone depressants, undetermined

         ✓7ᵗʰ **T42.8X5** Adverse effect of antiparkinsonism drugs and other central muscle-tone depressants

         ✓7ᵗʰ **T42.8X6** Underdosing of antiparkinsonism drugs and other central muscle-tone depressants

✓4ᵗʰ **T43** Poisoning by, adverse effect of and underdosing of psychotropic drugs, not elsewhere classified

     EXCLUDES 1   appetite depressants (T50.5-)
               barbiturates (T42.3-)
               benzodiazepines (T42.4-)
               methaqualone (T42.6-)
               psychodysleptics [hallucinogens] (T40.7-T40.9-)

     EXCLUDES 2   drug dependence and related mental and behavioral disorders due to psychoactive substance use (F10.- – F19.-)

     The appropriate 7th character is to be added to each code from category T43.
     A   initial encounter
     D   subsequent encounter
     S   sequela

✓5ᵗʰ **T43.0** Poisoning by, adverse effect of and underdosing of tricyclic and tetracyclic antidepressants

     ✓6ᵗʰ **T43.01** Poisoning by, adverse effect of and underdosing of tricyclic antidepressants

         ✓7ᵗʰ **T43.011** Poisoning by tricyclic antidepressants, accidental (unintentional)

             Poisoning by tricyclic antidepressants NOS

         11 ✓7ᵗʰ **T43.012** Poisoning by tricyclic antidepressants, intentional self-harm   HCC

         ✓7ᵗʰ **T43.013** Poisoning by tricyclic antidepressants, assault

         ✓7ᵗʰ **T43.014** Poisoning by tricyclic antidepressants, undetermined

         ✓7ᵗʰ **T43.015** Adverse effect of tricyclic antidepressants

         ✓7ᵗʰ **T43.016** Underdosing of tricyclic antidepressants

---

11 HCC with 7th character indicating initial encounter (A or B - specific to category) OR sequela.

✓ Additional Character Req   ✓x7ᵗʰ Placeholder Alert   Unacceptable PDx   Manifestation   H1 - H14 HAC   HCC CMS-HCC Condition   EXCLUDES 1 Not Coded Here   EXCLUDES 2 Not Included Here

ICD-10-CM 2018   1107

✓6th T43.02 Poisoning by, adverse effect of and underdosing of tetracyclic antidepressants

    ✓7th T43.021 Poisoning by tetracyclic antidepressants, accidental (unintentional)
         Poisoning by tetracyclic antidepressants NOS

    11 **✓7th T43.022 Poisoning by tetracyclic antidepressants, intentional self-harm** `HCC`

    ✓7th T43.023 Poisoning by tetracyclic antidepressants, assault

    ✓7th T43.024 Poisoning by tetracyclic antidepressants, undetermined

    ✓7th T43.025 Adverse effect of tetracyclic antidepressants

    ✓7th T43.026 Underdosing of tetracyclic antidepressants

✓5th T43.1 Poisoning by, adverse effect of and underdosing of monoamine-oxidase-inhibitor antidepressants

    ✓6th T43.1X Poisoning by, adverse effect of and underdosing of monoamine-oxidase-inhibitor antidepressants

        ✓7th T43.1X1 Poisoning by monoamine-oxidase-inhibitor antidepressants, accidental (unintentional)
             Poisoning by monoamine-oxidase-inhibitor antidepressants NOS

        11 **✓7th T43.1X2 Poisoning by monoamine-oxidase-inhibitor antidepressants, intentional self-harm** `HCC`

        ✓7th T43.1X3 Poisoning by monoamine-oxidase-inhibitor antidepressants, assault

        ✓7th T43.1X4 Poisoning by monoamine-oxidase-inhibitor antidepressants, undetermined

        ✓7th T43.1X5 Adverse effect of monoamine-oxidase-inhibitor antidepressants

        ✓7th T43.1X6 Underdosing of monoamine-oxidase-inhibitor antidepressants

✓5th T43.2 Poisoning by, adverse effect of and underdosing of other and unspecified antidepressants

    ✓6th T43.20 Poisoning by, adverse effect of and underdosing of unspecified antidepressants

        ✓7th T43.201 Poisoning by unspecified antidepressants, accidental (unintentional)
             Poisoning by antidepressants NOS

        11 **✓7th T43.202 Poisoning by unspecified antidepressants, intentional self-harm** `HCC`

        ✓7th T43.203 Poisoning by unspecified antidepressants, assault

        ✓7th T43.204 Poisoning by unspecified antidepressants, undetermined

        ✓7th T43.205 Adverse effect of unspecified antidepressants
             ▶Antidepressant discontinuation syndrome◀

        ✓7th T43.206 Underdosing of unspecified antidepressants

    ✓6th T43.21 Poisoning by, adverse effect of and underdosing of selective serotonin and norepinephrine reuptake inhibitors
         Poisoning by, adverse effect of and underdosing of SSNRI antidepressants

        ✓7th T43.211 Poisoning by selective serotonin and norepinephrine reuptake inhibitors, accidental (unintentional)

        11 **✓7th T43.212 Poisoning by selective serotonin and norepinephrine reuptake inhibitors, intentional self-harm** `HCC`

        ✓7th T43.213 Poisoning by selective serotonin and norepinephrine reuptake inhibitors, assault

        ✓7th T43.214 Poisoning by selective serotonin and norepinephrine reuptake inhibitors, undetermined

        ✓7th T43.215 Adverse effect of selective serotonin and norepinephrine reuptake inhibitors

        ✓7th T43.216 Underdosing of selective serotonin and norepinephrine reuptake inhibitors

✓6th T43.22 Poisoning by, adverse effect of and underdosing of selective serotonin reuptake inhibitors
     Poisoning by, adverse effect of and underdosing of SSRI antidepressants

    ✓7th T43.221 Poisoning by selective serotonin reuptake inhibitors, accidental (unintentional)

    11 **✓7th T43.222 Poisoning by selective serotonin reuptake inhibitors, intentional self-harm** `HCC`

    ✓7th T43.223 Poisoning by selective serotonin reuptake inhibitors, assault

    ✓7th T43.224 Poisoning by selective serotonin reuptake inhibitors, undetermined

    ✓7th T43.225 Adverse effect of selective serotonin reuptake inhibitors

    ✓7th T43.226 Underdosing of selective serotonin reuptake inhibitors

✓6th T43.29 Poisoning by, adverse effect of and underdosing of other antidepressants

    ✓7th T43.291 Poisoning by other antidepressants, accidental (unintentional)
         Poisoning by other antidepressants NOS

    11 **✓7th T43.292 Poisoning by other antidepressants, intentional self-harm** `HCC`

    ✓7th T43.293 Poisoning by other antidepressants, assault

    ✓7th T43.294 Poisoning by other antidepressants, undetermined

    ✓7th T43.295 Adverse effect of other antidepressants

    ✓7th T43.296 Underdosing of other antidepressants

✓5th T43.3 Poisoning by, adverse effect of and underdosing of phenothiazine antipsychotics and neuroleptics

    ✓6th T43.3X Poisoning by, adverse effect of and underdosing of phenothiazine antipsychotics and neuroleptics

        ✓7th T43.3X1 Poisoning by phenothiazine antipsychotics and neuroleptics, accidental (unintentional)
             Poisoning by phenothiazine antipsychotics and neuroleptics NOS

        11 **✓7th T43.3X2 Poisoning by phenothiazine antipsychotics and neuroleptics, intentional self-harm** `HCC`

        ✓7th T43.3X3 Poisoning by phenothiazine antipsychotics and neuroleptics, assault

        ✓7th T43.3X4 Poisoning by phenothiazine antipsychotics and neuroleptics, undetermined

        ✓7th T43.3X5 Adverse effect of phenothiazine antipsychotics and neuroleptics

        ✓7th T43.3X6 Underdosing of phenothiazine antipsychotics and neuroleptics

✓5th T43.4 Poisoning by, adverse effect of and underdosing of butyrophenone and thiothixene neuroleptics

    ✓6th T43.4X Poisoning by, adverse effect of and underdosing of butyrophenone and thiothixene neuroleptics

        ✓7th T43.4X1 Poisoning by butyrophenone and thiothixene neuroleptics, accidental (unintentional)
             Poisoning by butyrophenone and thiothixene neuroleptics NOS

        11 **✓7th T43.4X2 Poisoning by butyrophenone and thiothixene neuroleptics, intentional self-harm** `HCC`

        ✓7th T43.4X3 Poisoning by butyrophenone and thiothixene neuroleptics, assault

        ✓7th T43.4X4 Poisoning by butyrophenone and thiothixene neuroleptics, undetermined

        ✓7th T43.4X5 Adverse effect of butyrophenone and thiothixene neuroleptics

        ✓7th T43.4X6 Underdosing of butyrophenone and thiothixene neuroleptics

---

11 HCC with 7th character indicating initial encounter (A or B - specific to category) OR sequela.

N Newborn: 0   P Pediatric: 0-17   M Maternity: 12-55   A Adult: 15-124   MCC Major CC Condition   PDxMCC PDx acts as own MCC   CC CC Condition   PDxCC PDx acts as own CC

1108   ICD-10-CM 2018

✓5th **T43.5** **Poisoning by, adverse effect of and underdosing of other and unspecified antipsychotics and neuroleptics**

> EXCLUDES 1 *poisoning by, adverse effect of and underdosing of rauwolfia (T46.5-)*

✓6th **T43.50** **Poisoning by, adverse effect of and underdosing of unspecified antipsychotics and neuroleptics**

✓7th **T43.501** **Poisoning by unspecified antipsychotics and neuroleptics, accidental (unintentional)**
Poisoning by antipsychotics and neuroleptics NOS

11 ✓7th **T43.502** **Poisoning by unspecified antipsychotics and neuroleptics, intentional self-harm** HCC

✓7th **T43.503** **Poisoning by unspecified antipsychotics and neuroleptics, assault**

✓7th **T43.504** **Poisoning by unspecified antipsychotics and neuroleptics, undetermined**

✓7th **T43.505** **Adverse effect of unspecified antipsychotics and neuroleptics**

✓7th **T43.506** **Underdosing of unspecified antipsychotics and neuroleptics**

✓6th **T43.59** **Poisoning by, adverse effect of and underdosing of other antipsychotics and neuroleptics**
AHA: 2017, 1Q, 40

✓7th **T43.591** **Poisoning by other antipsychotics and neuroleptics, accidental (unintentional)**
Poisoning by other antipsychotics and neuroleptics NOS

11 ✓7th **T43.592** **Poisoning by other antipsychotics and neuroleptics, intentional self-harm** HCC

✓7th **T43.593** **Poisoning by other antipsychotics and neuroleptics, assault**

✓7th **T43.594** **Poisoning by other antipsychotics and neuroleptics, undetermined**

✓7th **T43.595** **Adverse effect of other antipsychotics and neuroleptics**

✓7th **T43.596** **Underdosing of other antipsychotics and neuroleptics**

✓5th **T43.6** **Poisoning by, adverse effect of and underdosing of psychostimulants**

> EXCLUDES 1 *poisoning by, adverse effect of and underdosing of cocaine (T40.5-)*

✓6th **T43.60** **Poisoning by, adverse effect of and underdosing of unspecified psychostimulant**

✓7th **T43.601** **Poisoning by unspecified psychostimulants, accidental (unintentional)**
Poisoning by psychostimulants NOS

11 ✓7th **T43.602** **Poisoning by unspecified psychostimulants, intentional self-harm** HCC

✓7th **T43.603** **Poisoning by unspecified psychostimulants, assault**

✓7th **T43.604** **Poisoning by unspecified psychostimulants, undetermined**

✓7th **T43.605** **Adverse effect of unspecified psychostimulants**

✓7th **T43.606** **Underdosing of unspecified psychostimulants**

✓6th **T43.61** **Poisoning by, adverse effect of and underdosing of caffeine**

✓7th **T43.611** **Poisoning by caffeine, accidental (unintentional)**
Poisoning by caffeine NOS

11 ✓7th **T43.612** **Poisoning by caffeine, intentional self-harm** HCC

✓7th **T43.613** **Poisoning by caffeine, assault**

✓7th **T43.614** **Poisoning by caffeine, undetermined**

✓7th **T43.615** **Adverse effect of caffeine**

✓7th **T43.616** **Underdosing of caffeine**

✓6th **T43.62** **Poisoning by, adverse effect of and underdosing of amphetamines**
Poisoning by, adverse effect of and underdosing of methamphetamines

✓7th **T43.621** **Poisoning by amphetamines, accidental (unintentional)**
Poisoning by amphetamines NOS

11 ✓7th **T43.622** **Poisoning by amphetamines, intentional self-harm** HCC

✓7th **T43.623** **Poisoning by amphetamines, assault**

✓7th **T43.624** **Poisoning by amphetamines, undetermined**

✓7th **T43.625** **Adverse effect of amphetamines**

✓7th **T43.626** **Underdosing of amphetamines**

✓6th **T43.63** **Poisoning by, adverse effect of and underdosing of methylphenidate**

✓7th **T43.631** **Poisoning by methylphenidate, accidental (unintentional)**
Poisoning by methylphenidate NOS

11 ✓7th **T43.632** **Poisoning by methylphenidate, intentional self-harm** HCC

✓7th **T43.633** **Poisoning by methylphenidate, assault**

✓7th **T43.634** **Poisoning by methylphenidate, undetermined**

✓7th **T43.635** **Adverse effect of methylphenidate**

✓7th **T43.636** **Underdosing of methylphenidate**

✓6th **T43.69** **Poisoning by, adverse effect of and underdosing of other psychostimulants**

✓7th **T43.691** **Poisoning by other psychostimulants, accidental (unintentional)**
Poisoning by other psychostimulants NOS

11 ✓7th **T43.692** **Poisoning by other psychostimulants, intentional self-harm** HCC

✓7th **T43.693** **Poisoning by other psychostimulants, assault**

✓7th **T43.694** **Poisoning by other psychostimulants, undetermined**

✓7th **T43.695** **Adverse effect of other psychostimulants**

✓7th **T43.696** **Underdosing of other psychostimulants**

✓5th **T43.8** **Poisoning by, adverse effect of and underdosing of other psychotropic drugs**

✓6th **T43.8X** **Poisoning by, adverse effect of and underdosing of other psychotropic drugs**

✓7th **T43.8X1** **Poisoning by other psychotropic drugs, accidental (unintentional)**
Poisoning by other psychotropic drugs NOS

11 ✓7th **T43.8X2** **Poisoning by other psychotropic drugs, intentional self-harm** HCC

✓7th **T43.8X3** **Poisoning by other psychotropic drugs, assault**

✓7th **T43.8X4** **Poisoning by other psychotropic drugs, undetermined**

✓7th **T43.8X5** **Adverse effect of other psychotropic drugs**

✓7th **T43.8X6** **Underdosing of other psychotropic drugs**

✓5th **T43.9** **Poisoning by, adverse effect of and underdosing of unspecified psychotropic drug**

✓x7th **T43.91** **Poisoning by unspecified psychotropic drug, accidental (unintentional)**
Poisoning by psychotropic drug NOS

11 ✓x7th **T43.92** **Poisoning by unspecified psychotropic drug, intentional self-harm** HCC

✓x7th **T43.93** **Poisoning by unspecified psychotropic drug, assault**

✓x7th **T43.94** **Poisoning by unspecified psychotropic drug, undetermined**

✓x7th **T43.95** **Adverse effect of unspecified psychotropic drug**

✓x7th **T43.96** **Underdosing of unspecified psychotropic drug**

---

11 HCC with 7th character indicating initial encounter (A or B - specific to category) OR sequela.

✓ Additional Character Req   ✓x7th Placeholder Alert   Unacceptable PDx   Manifestation   H1 - H14 HAC   HCC CMS-HCC Condition   EXCLUDES 1 Not Coded Here   EXCLUDES 2 Not Included Here

√4ᵗʰ T44 Poisoning by, adverse effect of and underdosing of drugs primarily affecting the autonomic nervous system

> The appropriate 7th character is to be added to each code from category T44.
> A   initial encounter
> D   subsequent encounter
> S   sequela

√5ᵗʰ T44.0 Poisoning by, adverse effect of and underdosing of anticholinesterase agents

  √6ᵗʰ T44.0X Poisoning by, adverse effect of and underdosing of anticholinesterase agents

  √7ᵗʰ T44.0X1 Poisoning by anticholinesterase agents, accidental (unintentional)
  Poisoning by anticholinesterase agents NOS

  11 **√7ᵗʰ T44.0X2 Poisoning by anticholinesterase agents, intentional self-harm**   HCC

  √7ᵗʰ T44.0X3 Poisoning by anticholinesterase agents, assault

  √7ᵗʰ T44.0X4 Poisoning by anticholinesterase agents, undetermined

  √7ᵗʰ T44.0X5 Adverse effect of anticholinesterase agents

  √7ᵗʰ T44.0X6 Underdosing of anticholinesterase agents

√5ᵗʰ T44.1 Poisoning by, adverse effect of and underdosing of other parasympathomimetics [cholinergics]

  √6ᵗʰ T44.1X Poisoning by, adverse effect of and underdosing of other parasympathomimetics [cholinergics]

  √7ᵗʰ T44.1X1 Poisoning by other parasympathomimetics [cholinergics], accidental (unintentional)
  Poisoning by other parasympathomimetics [cholinergics] NOS

  11 **√7ᵗʰ T44.1X2 Poisoning by other parasympathomimetics [cholinergics], intentional self-harm**   HCC

  √7ᵗʰ T44.1X3 Poisoning by other parasympathomimetics [cholinergics], assault

  √7ᵗʰ T44.1X4 Poisoning by other parasympathomimetics [cholinergics], undetermined

  √7ᵗʰ T44.1X5 Adverse effect of other parasympathomimetics [cholinergics]

  √7ᵗʰ T44.1X6 Underdosing of other parasympathomimetics

√5ᵗʰ T44.2 Poisoning by, adverse effect of and underdosing of ganglionic blocking drugs

  √6ᵗʰ T44.2X Poisoning by, adverse effect of and underdosing of ganglionic blocking drugs

  √7ᵗʰ T44.2X1 Poisoning by ganglionic blocking drugs, accidental (unintentional)
  Poisoning by ganglionic blocking drugs NOS

  11 **√7ᵗʰ T44.2X2 Poisoning by ganglionic blocking drugs, intentional self-harm**   HCC

  √7ᵗʰ T44.2X3 Poisoning by ganglionic blocking drugs, assault

  √7ᵗʰ T44.2X4 Poisoning by ganglionic blocking drugs, undetermined

  √7ᵗʰ T44.2X5 Adverse effect of ganglionic blocking drugs

  √7ᵗʰ T44.2X6 Underdosing of ganglionic blocking drugs

√5ᵗʰ T44.3 Poisoning by, adverse effect of and underdosing of other parasympatholytics [anticholinergics and antimuscarinics] and spasmolytics
  Poisoning by, adverse effect of and underdosing of papaverine

  √6ᵗʰ T44.3X Poisoning by, adverse effect of and underdosing of other parasympatholytics [anticholinergics and antimuscarinics] and spasmolytics

  √7ᵗʰ T44.3X1 Poisoning by other parasympatholytics [anticholinergics and antimuscarinics] and spasmolytics, accidental (unintentional)
  Poisoning by other parasympatholytics [anticholinergics and antimuscarinics] and spasmolytics NOS

  11 **√7ᵗʰ T44.3X2 Poisoning by other parasympatholytics [anticholinergics and antimuscarinics] and spasmolytics, intentional self-harm**   HCC

  √7ᵗʰ T44.3X3 Poisoning by other parasympatholytics [anticholinergics and antimuscarinics] and spasmolytics, assault

  √7ᵗʰ T44.3X4 Poisoning by other parasympatholytics [anticholinergics and antimuscarinics] and spasmolytics, undetermined

  √7ᵗʰ T44.3X5 Adverse effect of other parasympatholytics [anticholinergics and antimuscarinics] and spasmolytics

  √7ᵗʰ T44.3X6 Underdosing of other parasympatholytics [anticholinergics and antimuscarinics] and spasmolytics

√5ᵗʰ T44.4 Poisoning by, adverse effect of and underdosing of predominantly alpha-adrenoreceptor agonists
  Poisoning by, adverse effect of and underdosing of metaraminol

  √6ᵗʰ T44.4X Poisoning by, adverse effect of and underdosing of predominantly alpha-adrenoreceptor agonists

  √7ᵗʰ T44.4X1 Poisoning by predominantly alpha-adrenoreceptor agonists, accidental (unintentional)
  Poisoning by predominantly alpha-adrenoreceptor agonists NOS

  11 **√7ᵗʰ T44.4X2 Poisoning by predominantly alpha-adrenoreceptor agonists, intentional self-harm**   HCC

  √7ᵗʰ T44.4X3 Poisoning by predominantly alpha-adrenoreceptor agonists, assault

  √7ᵗʰ T44.4X4 Poisoning by predominantly alpha-adrenoreceptor agonists, undetermined

  √7ᵗʰ T44.4X5 Adverse effect of predominantly alpha-adrenoreceptor agonists

  √7ᵗʰ T44.4X6 Underdosing of predominantly alpha-adrenoreceptor agonists

√5ᵗʰ T44.5 Poisoning by, adverse effect of and underdosing of predominantly beta-adrenoreceptor agonists

  EXCLUDES 1   *poisoning by, adverse effect of and underdosing of beta-adrenoreceptor agonists used in asthma therapy (T48.6-)*

  √6ᵗʰ T44.5X Poisoning by, adverse effect of and underdosing of predominantly beta-adrenoreceptor agonists

  √7ᵗʰ T44.5X1 Poisoning by predominantly beta-adrenoreceptor agonists, accidental (unintentional)
  Poisoning by predominantly beta-adrenoreceptor agonists NOS

  11 **√7ᵗʰ T44.5X2 Poisoning by predominantly beta-adrenoreceptor agonists, intentional self-harm**   HCC

  √7ᵗʰ T44.5X3 Poisoning by predominantly beta-adrenoreceptor agonists, assault

  √7ᵗʰ T44.5X4 Poisoning by predominantly beta-adrenoreceptor agonists, undetermined

  √7ᵗʰ T44.5X5 Adverse effect of predominantly beta-adrenoreceptor agonists

  √7ᵗʰ T44.5X6 Underdosing of predominantly beta-adrenoreceptor agonists

√5ᵗʰ T44.6 Poisoning by, adverse effect of and underdosing of alpha-adrenoreceptor antagonists

  EXCLUDES 1   *poisoning by, adverse effect of and underdosing of ergot alkaloids (T48.0)*

  √6ᵗʰ T44.6X Poisoning by, adverse effect of and underdosing of alpha-adrenoreceptor antagonists

  √7ᵗʰ T44.6X1 Poisoning by alpha-adrenoreceptor antagonists, accidental (unintentional)
  Poisoning by alpha-adrenoreceptor antagonists NOS

  11 **√7ᵗʰ T44.6X2 Poisoning by alpha-adrenoreceptor antagonists, intentional self-harm**   HCC

  √7ᵗʰ T44.6X3 Poisoning by alpha-adrenoreceptor antagonists, assault

  √7ᵗʰ T44.6X4 Poisoning by alpha-adrenoreceptor antagonists, undetermined

---

11 HCC with 7th character indicating initial encounter (A or B - specific to category) OR sequela.

N Newborn: 0   P Pediatric: 0-17   M Maternity: 12-55   A Adult: 15-124   MCC Major CC Condition   PDxMCC PDx acts as own MCC   CC CC Condition   PDxCC PDx acts as own CC

1110   ICD-10-CM 2018

✓7ᵗʰ **T44.6X5** Adverse effect of alpha-adrenoreceptor antagonists

✓7ᵗʰ **T44.6X6** Underdosing of alpha-adrenoreceptor antagonists

✓5ᵗʰ **T44.7** Poisoning by, adverse effect of and underdosing of beta-adrenoreceptor antagonists

  ✓6ᵗʰ **T44.7X** Poisoning by, adverse effect of and underdosing of beta-adrenoreceptor antagonists

    ✓7ᵗʰ **T44.7X1** Poisoning by beta-adrenoreceptor antagonists, accidental (unintentional)
      Poisoning by beta-adrenoreceptor antagonists NOS

    11 ✓7ᵗʰ **T44.7X2** Poisoning by beta-adrenoreceptor antagonists, intentional self-harm   **HCC**

    ✓7ᵗʰ **T44.7X3** Poisoning by beta-adrenoreceptor antagonists, assault

    ✓7ᵗʰ **T44.7X4** Poisoning by beta-adrenoreceptor antagonists, undetermined

    ✓7ᵗʰ **T44.7X5** Adverse effect of beta-adrenoreceptor antagonists

    ✓7ᵗʰ **T44.7X6** Underdosing of beta-adrenoreceptor antagonists

✓5ᵗʰ **T44.8** Poisoning by, adverse effect of and underdosing of centrally-acting and adrenergic-neuron- blocking agents
    EXCLUDES 1   poisoning by, adverse effect of and underdosing of clonidine (T46.5)
        poisoning by, adverse effect of and underdosing of guanethidine (T46.5)

  ✓6ᵗʰ **T44.8X** Poisoning by, adverse effect of and underdosing of centrally-acting and adrenergic-neuron-blocking agents

    ✓7ᵗʰ **T44.8X1** Poisoning by centrally-acting and adrenergic-neuron-blocking agents, accidental (unintentional)
      Poisoning by centrally-acting and adrenergic-neuron-blocking agents NOS

    11 ✓7ᵗʰ **T44.8X2** Poisoning by centrally-acting and adrenergic-neuron-blocking agents, intentional self-harm   **HCC**

    ✓7ᵗʰ **T44.8X3** Poisoning by centrally-acting and adrenergic-neuron-blocking agents, assault

    ✓7ᵗʰ **T44.8X4** Poisoning by centrally-acting and adrenergic-neuron-blocking agents, undetermined

    ✓7ᵗʰ **T44.8X5** Adverse effect of centrally-acting and adrenergic-neuron-blocking agents

    ✓7ᵗʰ **T44.8X6** Underdosing of centrally-acting and adrenergic-neuron-blocking agents

✓5ᵗʰ **T44.9** Poisoning by, adverse effect of and underdosing of other and unspecified drugs primarily affecting the autonomic nervous system
    Poisoning by, adverse effect of and underdosing of drug stimulating both alpha and beta-adrenoreceptors

  ✓6ᵗʰ **T44.90** Poisoning by, adverse effect of and underdosing of unspecified drugs primarily affecting the autonomic nervous system

    ✓7ᵗʰ **T44.901** Poisoning by unspecified drugs primarily affecting the autonomic nervous system, accidental (unintentional)
      Poisoning by unspecified drugs primarily affecting the autonomic nervous system NOS

    11 ✓7ᵗʰ **T44.902** Poisoning by unspecified drugs primarily affecting the autonomic nervous system, intentional self-harm   **HCC**

    ✓7ᵗʰ **T44.903** Poisoning by unspecified drugs primarily affecting the autonomic nervous system, assault

    ✓7ᵗʰ **T44.904** Poisoning by unspecified drugs primarily affecting the autonomic nervous system, undetermined

    ✓7ᵗʰ **T44.905** Adverse effect of unspecified drugs primarily affecting the autonomic nervous system

    ✓7ᵗʰ **T44.906** Underdosing of unspecified drugs primarily affecting the autonomic nervous system

  ✓6ᵗʰ **T44.99** Poisoning by, adverse effect of and underdosing of other drugs primarily affecting the autonomic nervous system

    ✓7ᵗʰ **T44.991** Poisoning by other drug primarily affecting the autonomic nervous system, accidental (unintentional)
      Poisoning by other drugs primarily affecting the autonomic nervous system NOS

    11 ✓7ᵗʰ **T44.992** Poisoning by other drug primarily affecting the autonomic nervous system, intentional self-harm   **HCC**

    ✓7ᵗʰ **T44.993** Poisoning by other drug primarily affecting the autonomic nervous system, assault

    ✓7ᵗʰ **T44.994** Poisoning by other drug primarily affecting the autonomic nervous system, undetermined

    ✓7ᵗʰ **T44.995** Adverse effect of other drug primarily affecting the autonomic nervous system

    ✓7ᵗʰ **T44.996** Underdosing of other drug primarily affecting the autonomic nervous system

✓4ᵗʰ **T45** Poisoning by, adverse effect of and underdosing of primarily systemic and hematological agents, not elsewhere classified

    The appropriate 7th character is to be added to each code from category T45.
    A   initial encounter
    D   subsequent encounter
    S   sequela

✓5ᵗʰ **T45.0** Poisoning by, adverse effect of and underdosing of antiallergic and antiemetic drugs
    EXCLUDES 1   poisoning by, adverse effect of and underdosing of phenothiazine-based neuroleptics (T43.3)

  ✓6ᵗʰ **T45.0X** Poisoning by, adverse effect of and underdosing of antiallergic and antiemetic drugs

    ✓7ᵗʰ **T45.0X1** Poisoning by antiallergic and antiemetic drugs, accidental (unintentional)
      Poisoning by antiallergic and antiemetic drugs NOS

    11 ✓7ᵗʰ **T45.0X2** Poisoning by antiallergic and antiemetic drugs, intentional self-harm   **HCC**

    ✓7ᵗʰ **T45.0X3** Poisoning by antiallergic and antiemetic drugs, assault

    ✓7ᵗʰ **T45.0X4** Poisoning by antiallergic and antiemetic drugs, undetermined

    ✓7ᵗʰ **T45.0X5** Adverse effect of antiallergic and antiemetic drugs

    ✓7ᵗʰ **T45.0X6** Underdosing of antiallergic and antiemetic drugs

✓5ᵗʰ **T45.1** Poisoning by, adverse effect of and underdosing of antineoplastic and immunosuppressive drugs
    EXCLUDES 1   poisoning by, adverse effect of and underdosing of tamoxifen (T38.6)
    AHA: 2014, 4Q, 22

  ✓6ᵗʰ **T45.1X** Poisoning by, adverse effect of and underdosing of antineoplastic and immunosuppressive drugs

    ✓7ᵗʰ **T45.1X1** Poisoning by antineoplastic and immunosuppressive drugs, accidental (unintentional)
      Poisoning by antineoplastic and immunosuppressive drugs NOS

    11 ✓7ᵗʰ **T45.1X2** Poisoning by antineoplastic and immunosuppressive drugs, intentional self-harm   **HCC**

    ✓7ᵗʰ **T45.1X3** Poisoning by antineoplastic and immunosuppressive drugs, assault

    ✓7ᵗʰ **T45.1X4** Poisoning by antineoplastic and immunosuppressive drugs, undetermined

    ✓7ᵗʰ **T45.1X5** Adverse effect of antineoplastic and immunosuppressive drugs

    ✓7ᵗʰ **T45.1X6** Underdosing of antineoplastic and immunosuppressive drugs

---

11 HCC with 7th character indicating initial encounter (A or B - specific to category) OR sequela.

✓ Additional Character Req   ✓x7ᵗʰ Placeholder Alert   Unacceptable PDx   Manifestation   **H1**-**H14** HAC   **HCC** CMS-HCC Condition   **EXCLUDES 1** Not Coded Here   **EXCLUDES 2** Not Included Here

ICD-10-CM 2018   **1111**

✓5th **T45.2 Poisoning by, adverse effect of and underdosing of vitamins**

> EXCLUDES 2   *poisoning by, adverse effect of and underdosing of iron (T45.4)*
> *poisoning by, adverse effect of and underdosing of nicotinic acid (derivatives) (T46.7)*
> *poisoning by, adverse effect of and underdosing of vitamin K (T45.7)*

✓6th **T45.2X Poisoning by, adverse effect of and underdosing of vitamins**

    ✓7th **T45.2X1 Poisoning by vitamins, accidental (unintentional)**
       Poisoning by vitamins NOS

    11 ✓7th **T45.2X2 Poisoning by vitamins, intentional self-harm** `HCC`

    ✓7th **T45.2X3 Poisoning by vitamins, assault**

    ✓7th **T45.2X4 Poisoning by vitamins, undetermined**

    ✓7th **T45.2X5 Adverse effect of vitamins**

    ✓7th **T45.2X6 Underdosing of vitamins**
       EXCLUDES 1   *vitamin deficiencies (E50-E56)*

✓5th **T45.3 Poisoning by, adverse effect of and underdosing of enzymes**

✓6th **T45.3X Poisoning by, adverse effect of and underdosing of enzymes**

    ✓7th **T45.3X1 Poisoning by enzymes, accidental (unintentional)**
       Poisoning by enzymes NOS

    11 ✓7th **T45.3X2 Poisoning by enzymes, intentional self-harm** `HCC`

    ✓7th **T45.3X3 Poisoning by enzymes, assault**

    ✓7th **T45.3X4 Poisoning by enzymes, undetermined**

    ✓7th **T45.3X5 Adverse effect of enzymes**

    ✓7th **T45.3X6 Underdosing of enzymes**

✓5th **T45.4 Poisoning by, adverse effect of and underdosing of iron and its compounds**

✓6th **T45.4X Poisoning by, adverse effect of and underdosing of iron and its compounds**

    ✓7th **T45.4X1 Poisoning by iron and its compounds, accidental (unintentional)**
       Poisoning by iron and its compounds NOS

    11 ✓7th **T45.4X2 Poisoning by iron and its compounds, intentional self-harm** `HCC`

    ✓7th **T45.4X3 Poisoning by iron and its compounds, assault**

    ✓7th **T45.4X4 Poisoning by iron and its compounds, undetermined**

    ✓7th **T45.4X5 Adverse effect of iron and its compounds**

    ✓7th **T45.4X6 Underdosing of iron and its compounds**
       EXCLUDES 1   *iron deficiency (E61.1)*

✓5th **T45.5 Poisoning by, adverse effect of and underdosing of anticoagulants and antithrombotic drugs**

✓6th **T45.51 Poisoning by, adverse effect of and underdosing of anticoagulants**

    ✓7th **T45.511 Poisoning by anticoagulants, accidental (unintentional)**
       Poisoning by anticoagulants NOS

    11 ✓7th **T45.512 Poisoning by anticoagulants, intentional self-harm** `HCC`

    ✓7th **T45.513 Poisoning by anticoagulants, assault**

    ✓7th **T45.514 Poisoning by anticoagulants, undetermined**

    ✓7th **T45.515 Adverse effect of anticoagulants**
       AHA: 2016, 1Q, 14; 2013, 2Q, 34

    ✓7th **T45.516 Underdosing of anticoagulants**

✓6th **T45.52 Poisoning by, adverse effect of and underdosing of antithrombotic drugs**
       Poisoning by, adverse effect of and underdosing of antiplatelet drugs

       EXCLUDES 2   *poisoning by, adverse effect of and underdosing of aspirin (T39.01-)*
          poisoning by, adverse effect of and underdosing of acetylsalicylic acid (T39.01-)

    ✓7th **T45.521 Poisoning by antithrombotic drugs, accidental (unintentional)**
       Poisoning by antithrombotic drug NOS

    11 ✓7th **T45.522 Poisoning by antithrombotic drugs, intentional self-harm** `HCC`

    ✓7th **T45.523 Poisoning by antithrombotic drugs, assault**

    ✓7th **T45.524 Poisoning by antithrombotic drugs, undetermined**

    ✓7th **T45.525 Adverse effect of antithrombotic drugs**
       AHA: 2016, 1Q, 15

    ✓7th **T45.526 Underdosing of antithrombotic drugs**

✓5th **T45.6 Poisoning by, adverse effect of and underdosing of fibrinolysis-affecting drugs**

✓6th **T45.60 Poisoning by, adverse effect of and underdosing of unspecified fibrinolysis-affecting drugs**

    ✓7th **T45.601 Poisoning by unspecified fibrinolysis-affecting drugs, accidental (unintentional)**
       Poisoning by fibrinolysis-affecting drug NOS

    11 ✓7th **T45.602 Poisoning by unspecified fibrinolysis-affecting drugs, intentional self-harm** `HCC`

    ✓7th **T45.603 Poisoning by unspecified fibrinolysis-affecting drugs, assault**

    ✓7th **T45.604 Poisoning by unspecified fibrinolysis-affecting drugs, undetermined**

    ✓7th **T45.605 Adverse effect of unspecified fibrinolysis-affecting drugs**

    ✓7th **T45.606 Underdosing of unspecified fibrinolysis-affecting drugs**

✓6th **T45.61 Poisoning by, adverse effect of and underdosing of thrombolytic drugs**

    ✓7th **T45.611 Poisoning by thrombolytic drug, accidental (unintentional)**
       Poisoning by thrombolytic drug NOS

    11 ✓7th **T45.612 Poisoning by thrombolytic drug, intentional self-harm** `HCC`

    ✓7th **T45.613 Poisoning by thrombolytic drug, assault**

    ✓7th **T45.614 Poisoning by thrombolytic drug, undetermined**

    ✓7th **T45.615 Adverse effect of thrombolytic drugs**
       AHA: 2017, 2Q, 9

    ✓7th **T45.616 Underdosing of thrombolytic drugs**

✓6th **T45.62 Poisoning by, adverse effect of and underdosing of hemostatic drugs**

    ✓7th **T45.621 Poisoning by hemostatic drug, accidental (unintentional)**
       Poisoning by hemostatic drug NOS

    11 ✓7th **T45.622 Poisoning by hemostatic drug, intentional self-harm** `HCC`

    ✓7th **T45.623 Poisoning by hemostatic drug, assault**

    ✓7th **T45.624 Poisoning by hemostatic drug, undetermined**

    ✓7th **T45.625 Adverse effect of hemostatic drug**

    ✓7th **T45.626 Underdosing of hemostatic drugs**

✓6th **T45.69 Poisoning by, adverse effect of and underdosing of other fibrinolysis-affecting drugs**

    ✓7th **T45.691 Poisoning by other fibrinolysis-affecting drugs, accidental (unintentional)**
       Poisoning by other fibrinolysis-affecting drug NOS

    11 ✓7th **T45.692 Poisoning by other fibrinolysis-affecting drugs, intentional self-harm** `HCC`

    ✓7th **T45.693 Poisoning by other fibrinolysis-affecting drugs, assault**

    ✓7th **T45.694 Poisoning by other fibrinolysis-affecting drugs, undetermined**

    ✓7th **T45.695 Adverse effect of other fibrinolysis-affecting drugs**

    ✓7th **T45.696 Underdosing of other fibrinolysis-affecting drugs**

---

11   HCC with 7th character indicating initial encounter (A or B - specific to category) OR sequela.

`N` Newborn: 0   `P` Pediatric: 0-17   `M` Maternity: 12-55   `A` Adult: 15-124   `MCC` Major CC Condition   `PDxMCC` PDx acts as own MCC   `CC` CC Condition   `PDxCC` PDx acts as own CC

☑5th **T45.7** **Poisoning by, adverse effect of and underdosing of anticoagulant antagonists, vitamin K and other coagulants**

    ☑6th **T45.7X** **Poisoning by, adverse effect of and underdosing of anticoagulant antagonists, vitamin K and other coagulants**

        ☑7th **T45.7X1** **Poisoning by anticoagulant antagonists, vitamin K and other coagulants, accidental (unintentional)**

             Poisoning by anticoagulant antagonists, vitamin K and other coagulants NOS

       11 ☑7th **T45.7X2** **Poisoning by anticoagulant antagonists, vitamin K and other coagulants, intentional self-harm** [HCC]

        ☑7th **T45.7X3** **Poisoning by anticoagulant antagonists, vitamin K and other coagulants, assault**

        ☑7th **T45.7X4** **Poisoning by anticoagulant antagonists, vitamin K and other coagulants, undetermined**

        ☑7th **T45.7X5** **Adverse effect of anticoagulant antagonists, vitamin K and other coagulants**

        ☑7th **T45.7X6** **Underdosing of anticoagulant antagonist, vitamin K and other coagulants**

             EXCLUDES 1 *vitamin K deficiency (E56.1)*

☑5th **T45.8** **Poisoning by, adverse effect of and underdosing of other primarily systemic and hematological agents**

     Poisoning by, adverse effect of and underdosing of liver preparations and other antianemic agents

     Poisoning by, adverse effect of and underdosing of natural blood and blood products

     Poisoning by, adverse effect of and underdosing of plasma substitute

     EXCLUDES 2 *poisoning by, adverse effect of and underdosing of immunoglobulin (T50.Z1)*

             poisoning by, adverse effect of and underdosing of iron (T45.4)

             transfusion reactions (T80.-)

    ☑6th **T45.8X** **Poisoning by, adverse effect of and underdosing of other primarily systemic and hematological agents**

        ☑7th **T45.8X1** **Poisoning by other primarily systemic and hematological agents, accidental (unintentional)**

             Poisoning by other primarily systemic and hematological agents NOS

       11 ☑7th **T45.8X2** **Poisoning by other primarily systemic and hematological agents, intentional self-harm** [HCC]

        ☑7th **T45.8X3** **Poisoning by other primarily systemic and hematological agents, assault**

        ☑7th **T45.8X4** **Poisoning by other primarily systemic and hematological agents, undetermined**

        ☑7th **T45.8X5** **Adverse effect of other primarily systemic and hematological agents**

        ☑7th **T45.8X6** **Underdosing of other primarily systemic and hematological agents**

☑5th **T45.9** **Poisoning by, adverse effect of and underdosing of unspecified primarily systemic and hematological agent**

    ☑x7th **T45.91** **Poisoning by unspecified primarily systemic and hematological agent, accidental (unintentional)**

         Poisoning by primarily systemic and hematological agent NOS

   11 ☑x7th **T45.92** **Poisoning by unspecified primarily systemic and hematological agent, intentional self-harm** [HCC]

    ☑x7th **T45.93** **Poisoning by unspecified primarily systemic and hematological agent, assault**

    ☑x7th **T45.94** **Poisoning by unspecified primarily systemic and hematological agent, undetermined**

    ☑x7th **T45.95** **Adverse effect of unspecified primarily systemic and hematological agent**

    ☑x7th **T45.96** **Underdosing of unspecified primarily systemic and hematological agent**

☑4th **T46** **Poisoning by, adverse effect of and underdosing of agents primarily affecting the cardiovascular system**

     EXCLUDES 1 *poisoning by, adverse effect of and underdosing of metaraminol (T44.4)*

     The appropriate 7th character is to be added to each code from category T46.
     A   initial encounter
     D   subsequent encounter
     S   sequela

☑5th **T46.0** **Poisoning by, adverse effect of and underdosing of cardiac-stimulant glycosides and drugs of similar action**

    ☑6th **T46.0X** **Poisoning by, adverse effect of and underdosing of cardiac-stimulant glycosides and drugs of similar action**

        ☑7th **T46.0X1** **Poisoning by cardiac-stimulant glycosides and drugs of similar action, accidental (unintentional)**

             Poisoning by cardiac-stimulant glycosides and drugs of similar action NOS

       11 ☑7th **T46.0X2** **Poisoning by cardiac-stimulant glycosides and drugs of similar action, intentional self-harm** [HCC]

        ☑7th **T46.0X3** **Poisoning by cardiac-stimulant glycosides and drugs of similar action, assault**

        ☑7th **T46.0X4** **Poisoning by cardiac-stimulant glycosides and drugs of similar action, undetermined**

        ☑7th **T46.0X5** **Adverse effect of cardiac-stimulant glycosides and drugs of similar action**

        ☑7th **T46.0X6** **Underdosing of cardiac-stimulant glycosides and drugs of similar action**

☑5th **T46.1** **Poisoning by, adverse effect of and underdosing of calcium-channel blockers**

    ☑6th **T46.1X** **Poisoning by, adverse effect of and underdosing of calcium-channel blockers**

        ☑7th **T46.1X1** **Poisoning by calcium-channel blockers, accidental (unintentional)**

             Poisoning by calcium-channel blockers NOS

       11 ☑7th **T46.1X2** **Poisoning by calcium-channel blockers, intentional self-harm** [HCC]

        ☑7th **T46.1X3** **Poisoning by calcium-channel blockers, assault**

        ☑7th **T46.1X4** **Poisoning by calcium-channel blockers, undetermined**

        ☑7th **T46.1X5** **Adverse effect of calcium-channel blockers**

        ☑7th **T46.1X6** **Underdosing of calcium-channel blockers**

☑5th **T46.2** **Poisoning by, adverse effect of and underdosing of other antidysrhythmic drugs, not elsewhere classified**

     EXCLUDES 1 *poisoning by, adverse effect of and underdosing of beta-adrenoreceptor antagonists (T44.7-)*

    ☑6th **T46.2X** **Poisoning by, adverse effect of and underdosing of other antidysrhythmic drugs**

        ☑7th **T46.2X1** **Poisoning by other antidysrhythmic drugs, accidental (unintentional)**

             Poisoning by other antidysrhythmic drugs NOS

       11 ☑7th **T46.2X2** **Poisoning by other antidysrhythmic drugs, intentional self-harm** [HCC]

        ☑7th **T46.2X3** **Poisoning by other antidysrhythmic drugs, assault**

        ☑7th **T46.2X4** **Poisoning by other antidysrhythmic drugs, undetermined**

        ☑7th **T46.2X5** **Adverse effect of other antidysrhythmic drugs**

        ☑7th **T46.2X6** **Underdosing of other antidysrhythmic drugs**

---

11 HCC with 7th character indicating initial encounter (A or B - specific to category) OR sequela.

☑ Additional Character Req   ☑x7th Placeholder Alert   Unacceptable PDx   Manifestation   H1 - H14 HAC   HCC CMS-HCC Condition   EXCLUDES 1 Not Coded Here   EXCLUDES 2 Not Included Here

ICD-10-CM 2018   1113

✓5ᵗʰ **T46.3** **Poisoning by, adverse effect of and underdosing of coronary vasodilators**
Poisoning by, adverse effect of and underdosing of dipyridamole
> EXCLUDES 1   *poisoning by, adverse effect of and underdosing of calcium-channel blockers (T46.1)*

✓6ᵗʰ **T46.3X** **Poisoning by, adverse effect of and underdosing of coronary vasodilators**

     ✓7ᵗʰ **T46.3X1** **Poisoning by coronary vasodilators, accidental (unintentional)**
Poisoning by coronary vasodilators NOS

     11 ✓7ᵗʰ **T46.3X2** **Poisoning by coronary vasodilators, intentional self-harm** ᴴᶜᶜ

     ✓7ᵗʰ **T46.3X3** **Poisoning by coronary vasodilators, assault**

     ✓7ᵗʰ **T46.3X4** **Poisoning by coronary vasodilators, undetermined**

     ✓7ᵗʰ **T46.3X5** **Adverse effect of coronary vasodilators**

     ✓7ᵗʰ **T46.3X6** **Underdosing of coronary vasodilators**

✓5ᵗʰ **T46.4** **Poisoning by, adverse effect of and underdosing of angiotensin-converting-enzyme inhibitors**

✓6ᵗʰ **T46.4X** **Poisoning by, adverse effect of and underdosing of angiotensin-converting-enzyme inhibitors**

     ✓7ᵗʰ **T46.4X1** **Poisoning by angiotensin-converting-enzyme inhibitors, accidental (unintentional)**
Poisoning by angiotensin-converting-enzyme inhibitors NOS

     11 ✓7ᵗʰ **T46.4X2** **Poisoning by angiotensin-converting-enzyme inhibitors, intentional self-harm** ᴴᶜᶜ

     ✓7ᵗʰ **T46.4X3** **Poisoning by angiotensin-converting-enzyme inhibitors, assault**

     ✓7ᵗʰ **T46.4X4** **Poisoning by angiotensin-converting-enzyme inhibitors, undetermined**

     ✓7ᵗʰ **T46.4X5** **Adverse effect of angiotensin-converting-enzyme inhibitors**

     ✓7ᵗʰ **T46.4X6** **Underdosing of angiotensin-converting-enzyme inhibitors**

✓5ᵗʰ **T46.5** **Poisoning by, adverse effect of and underdosing of other antihypertensive drugs**
> EXCLUDES 2   *poisoning by, adverse effect of and underdosing of beta-adrenoreceptor antagonists (T44.7)*
> *poisoning by, adverse effect of and underdosing of calcium-channel blockers (T46.1)*
> *poisoning by, adverse effect of and underdosing of diuretics (T50.0-T50.2)*

✓6ᵗʰ **T46.5X** **Poisoning by, adverse effect of and underdosing of other antihypertensive drugs**

     ✓7ᵗʰ **T46.5X1** **Poisoning by other antihypertensive drugs, accidental (unintentional)**
Poisoning by other antihypertensive drugs NOS

     11 ✓7ᵗʰ **T46.5X2** **Poisoning by other antihypertensive drugs, intentional self-harm** ᴴᶜᶜ

     ✓7ᵗʰ **T46.5X3** **Poisoning by other antihypertensive drugs, assault**

     ✓7ᵗʰ **T46.5X4** **Poisoning by other antihypertensive drugs, undetermined**

     ✓7ᵗʰ **T46.5X5** **Adverse effect of other antihypertensive drugs**

     ✓7ᵗʰ **T46.5X6** **Underdosing of other antihypertensive drugs**

✓5ᵗʰ **T46.6** **Poisoning by, adverse effect of and underdosing of antihyperlipidemic and antiarteriosclerotic drugs**

✓6ᵗʰ **T46.6X** **Poisoning by, adverse effect of and underdosing of antihyperlipidemic and antiarteriosclerotic drugs**

     ✓7ᵗʰ **T46.6X1** **Poisoning by antihyperlipidemic and antiarteriosclerotic drugs, accidental (unintentional)**
Poisoning by antihyperlipidemic and antiarteriosclerotic drugs NOS

     11 ✓7ᵗʰ **T46.6X2** **Poisoning by antihyperlipidemic and antiarteriosclerotic drugs, intentional self-harm** ᴴᶜᶜ

     ✓7ᵗʰ **T46.6X3** **Poisoning by antihyperlipidemic and antiarteriosclerotic drugs, assault**

     ✓7ᵗʰ **T46.6X4** **Poisoning by antihyperlipidemic and antiarteriosclerotic drugs, undetermined**

     ✓7ᵗʰ **T46.6X5** **Adverse effect of antihyperlipidemic and antiarteriosclerotic drugs**

     ✓7ᵗʰ **T46.6X6** **Underdosing of antihyperlipidemic and antiarteriosclerotic drugs**

✓5ᵗʰ **T46.7** **Poisoning by, adverse effect of and underdosing of peripheral vasodilators**
Poisoning by, adverse effect of and underdosing of nicotinic acid (derivatives)
> EXCLUDES 1   *poisoning by, adverse effect of and underdosing of papaverine (T44.3)*

✓6ᵗʰ **T46.7X** **Poisoning by, adverse effect of and underdosing of peripheral vasodilators**

     ✓7ᵗʰ **T46.7X1** **Poisoning by peripheral vasodilators, accidental (unintentional)**
Poisoning by peripheral vasodilators NOS

     11 ✓7ᵗʰ **T46.7X2** **Poisoning by peripheral vasodilators, intentional self-harm** ᴴᶜᶜ

     ✓7ᵗʰ **T46.7X3** **Poisoning by peripheral vasodilators, assault**

     ✓7ᵗʰ **T46.7X4** **Poisoning by peripheral vasodilators, undetermined**

     ✓7ᵗʰ **T46.7X5** **Adverse effect of peripheral vasodilators**

     ✓7ᵗʰ **T46.7X6** **Underdosing of peripheral vasodilators**

✓5ᵗʰ **T46.8** **Poisoning by, adverse effect of and underdosing of antivaricose drugs, including sclerosing agents**

✓6ᵗʰ **T46.8X** **Poisoning by, adverse effect of and underdosing of antivaricose drugs, including sclerosing agents**

     ✓7ᵗʰ **T46.8X1** **Poisoning by antivaricose drugs, including sclerosing agents, accidental (unintentional)**
Poisoning by antivaricose drugs, including sclerosing agents NOS

     11 ✓7ᵗʰ **T46.8X2** **Poisoning by antivaricose drugs, including sclerosing agents, intentional self-harm** ᴴᶜᶜ

     ✓7ᵗʰ **T46.8X3** **Poisoning by antivaricose drugs, including sclerosing agents, assault**

     ✓7ᵗʰ **T46.8X4** **Poisoning by antivaricose drugs, including sclerosing agents, undetermined**

     ✓7ᵗʰ **T46.8X5** **Adverse effect of antivaricose drugs, including sclerosing agents**

     ✓7ᵗʰ **T46.8X6** **Underdosing of antivaricose drugs, including sclerosing agents**

✓5ᵗʰ **T46.9** **Poisoning by, adverse effect of and underdosing of other and unspecified agents primarily affecting the cardiovascular system**

✓6ᵗʰ **T46.90** **Poisoning by, adverse effect of and underdosing of unspecified agents primarily affecting the cardiovascular system**

     ✓7ᵗʰ **T46.901** **Poisoning by unspecified agents primarily affecting the cardiovascular system, accidental (unintentional)**

     11 ✓7ᵗʰ **T46.902** **Poisoning by unspecified agents primarily affecting the cardiovascular system, intentional self-harm** ᴴᶜᶜ

     ✓7ᵗʰ **T46.903** **Poisoning by unspecified agents primarily affecting the cardiovascular system, assault**

     ✓7ᵗʰ **T46.904** **Poisoning by unspecified agents primarily affecting the cardiovascular system, undetermined**

     ✓7ᵗʰ **T46.905** **Adverse effect of unspecified agents primarily affecting the cardiovascular system**

     ✓7ᵗʰ **T46.906** **Underdosing of unspecified agents primarily affecting the cardiovascular system**

✓6ᵗʰ **T46.99** **Poisoning by, adverse effect of and underdosing of other agents primarily affecting the cardiovascular system**

     ✓7ᵗʰ **T46.991** **Poisoning by other agents primarily affecting the cardiovascular system, accidental (unintentional)**

---

¹¹ HCC with 7th character indicating initial encounter (A or B - specific to category) OR sequela.

Ⓝ Newborn: 0   Ⓟ Pediatric: 0-17   Ⓜ Maternity: 12-55   Ⓐ Adult: 15-124   **MCC** Major CC Condition   **PDx MCC** PDx acts as own MCC   **CC** CC Condition   **PDx CC** PDx acts as own CC

1114   ICD-10-CM 2018

[11] ✓7ᵗʰ **T46.992** Poisoning by other agents primarily affecting the cardiovascular system, intentional self-harm **HCC**

✓7ᵗʰ **T46.993** Poisoning by other agents primarily affecting the cardiovascular system, assault

✓7ᵗʰ **T46.994** Poisoning by other agents primarily affecting the cardiovascular system, undetermined

✓7ᵗʰ **T46.995** Adverse effect of other agents primarily affecting the cardiovascular system

✓7ᵗʰ **T46.996** Underdosing of other agents primarily affecting the cardiovascular system

✓4ᵗʰ **T47** Poisoning by, adverse effect of and underdosing of agents primarily affecting the gastrointestinal system

> The appropriate 7th character is to be added to each code from category T47.
> A   initial encounter
> D   subsequent encounter
> S   sequela

✓5ᵗʰ **T47.0** Poisoning by, adverse effect of and underdosing of histamine H2-receptor blockers

     ✓6ᵗʰ **T47.0X** Poisoning by, adverse effect of and underdosing of histamine H2-receptor blockers

         ✓7ᵗʰ **T47.0X1** Poisoning by histamine H2-receptor blockers, accidental (unintentional)
             Poisoning by histamine H2-receptor blockers NOS

         [11] ✓7ᵗʰ **T47.0X2** Poisoning by histamine H2-receptor blockers, intentional self-harm **HCC**

         ✓7ᵗʰ **T47.0X3** Poisoning by histamine H2-receptor blockers, assault

         ✓7ᵗʰ **T47.0X4** Poisoning by histamine H2-receptor blockers, undetermined

         ✓7ᵗʰ **T47.0X5** Adverse effect of histamine H2-receptor blockers

         ✓7ᵗʰ **T47.0X6** Underdosing of histamine H2-receptor blockers

✓5ᵗʰ **T47.1** Poisoning by, adverse effect of and underdosing of other antacids and anti-gastric-secretion drugs

     ✓6ᵗʰ **T47.1X** Poisoning by, adverse effect of and underdosing of other antacids and anti-gastric-secretion drugs

         ✓7ᵗʰ **T47.1X1** Poisoning by other antacids and anti-gastric-secretion drugs, accidental (unintentional)
             Poisoning by other antacids and anti-gastric-secretion drugs NOS

         [11] ✓7ᵗʰ **T47.1X2** Poisoning by other antacids and anti-gastric-secretion drugs, intentional self-harm **HCC**

         ✓7ᵗʰ **T47.1X3** Poisoning by other antacids and anti-gastric-secretion drugs, assault

         ✓7ᵗʰ **T47.1X4** Poisoning by other antacids and anti-gastric-secretion drugs, undetermined

         ✓7ᵗʰ **T47.1X5** Adverse effect of other antacids and anti-gastric-secretion drugs

         ✓7ᵗʰ **T47.1X6** Underdosing of other antacids and anti-gastric-secretion drugs

✓5ᵗʰ **T47.2** Poisoning by, adverse effect of and underdosing of stimulant laxatives

     ✓6ᵗʰ **T47.2X** Poisoning by, adverse effect of and underdosing of stimulant laxatives

         ✓7ᵗʰ **T47.2X1** Poisoning by stimulant laxatives, accidental (unintentional)
             Poisoning by stimulant laxatives NOS

         [11] ✓7ᵗʰ **T47.2X2** Poisoning by stimulant laxatives, intentional self-harm **HCC**

         ✓7ᵗʰ **T47.2X3** Poisoning by stimulant laxatives, assault

         ✓7ᵗʰ **T47.2X4** Poisoning by stimulant laxatives, undetermined

         ✓7ᵗʰ **T47.2X5** Adverse effect of stimulant laxatives

         ✓7ᵗʰ **T47.2X6** Underdosing of stimulant laxatives

✓5ᵗʰ **T47.3** Poisoning by, adverse effect of and underdosing of saline and osmotic laxatives

     ✓6ᵗʰ **T47.3X** Poisoning by and adverse effect of saline and osmotic laxatives

         ✓7ᵗʰ **T47.3X1** Poisoning by saline and osmotic laxatives, accidental (unintentional)
             Poisoning by saline and osmotic laxatives NOS

         [11] ✓7ᵗʰ **T47.3X2** Poisoning by saline and osmotic laxatives, intentional self-harm **HCC**

         ✓7ᵗʰ **T47.3X3** Poisoning by saline and osmotic laxatives, assault

         ✓7ᵗʰ **T47.3X4** Poisoning by saline and osmotic laxatives, undetermined

         ✓7ᵗʰ **T47.3X5** Adverse effect of saline and osmotic laxatives

         ✓7ᵗʰ **T47.3X6** Underdosing of saline and osmotic laxatives

✓5ᵗʰ **T47.4** Poisoning by, adverse effect of and underdosing of other laxatives

     ✓6ᵗʰ **T47.4X** Poisoning by, adverse effect of and underdosing of other laxatives

         ✓7ᵗʰ **T47.4X1** Poisoning by other laxatives, accidental (unintentional)
             Poisoning by other laxatives NOS

         [11] ✓7ᵗʰ **T47.4X2** Poisoning by other laxatives, intentional self-harm **HCC**

         ✓7ᵗʰ **T47.4X3** Poisoning by other laxatives, assault

         ✓7ᵗʰ **T47.4X4** Poisoning by other laxatives, undetermined

         ✓7ᵗʰ **T47.4X5** Adverse effect of other laxatives

         ✓7ᵗʰ **T47.4X6** Underdosing of other laxatives

✓5ᵗʰ **T47.5** Poisoning by, adverse effect of and underdosing of digestants

     ✓6ᵗʰ **T47.5X** Poisoning by, adverse effect of and underdosing of digestants

         ✓7ᵗʰ **T47.5X1** Poisoning by digestants, accidental (unintentional)
             Poisoning by digestants NOS

         [11] ✓7ᵗʰ **T47.5X2** Poisoning by digestants, intentional self-harm **HCC**

         ✓7ᵗʰ **T47.5X3** Poisoning by digestants, assault

         ✓7ᵗʰ **T47.5X4** Poisoning by digestants, undetermined

         ✓7ᵗʰ **T47.5X5** Adverse effect of digestants

         ✓7ᵗʰ **T47.5X6** Underdosing of digestants

✓5ᵗʰ **T47.6** Poisoning by, adverse effect of and underdosing of antidiarrheal drugs

> **EXCLUDES 2** poisoning by, adverse effect of and underdosing of systemic antibiotics and other anti-infectives (T36-T37)

     ✓6ᵗʰ **T47.6X** Poisoning by, adverse effect of and underdosing of antidiarrheal drugs

         ✓7ᵗʰ **T47.6X1** Poisoning by antidiarrheal drugs, accidental (unintentional)
             Poisoning by antidiarrheal drugs NOS

         [11] ✓7ᵗʰ **T47.6X2** Poisoning by antidiarrheal drugs, intentional self-harm **HCC**

         ✓7ᵗʰ **T47.6X3** Poisoning by antidiarrheal drugs, assault

         ✓7ᵗʰ **T47.6X4** Poisoning by antidiarrheal drugs, undetermined

         ✓7ᵗʰ **T47.6X5** Adverse effect of antidiarrheal drugs

         ✓7ᵗʰ **T47.6X6** Underdosing of antidiarrheal drugs

✓5ᵗʰ **T47.7** Poisoning by, adverse effect of and underdosing of emetics

     ✓6ᵗʰ **T47.7X** Poisoning by, adverse effect of and underdosing of emetics

         ✓7ᵗʰ **T47.7X1** Poisoning by emetics, accidental (unintentional)
             Poisoning by emetics NOS

         [11] ✓7ᵗʰ **T47.7X2** Poisoning by emetics, intentional self-harm **HCC**

         ✓7ᵗʰ **T47.7X3** Poisoning by emetics, assault

         ✓7ᵗʰ **T47.7X4** Poisoning by emetics, undetermined

         ✓7ᵗʰ **T47.7X5** Adverse effect of emetics

---

[11] HCC with 7th character indicating initial encounter (A or B - specific to category) OR sequela.

✔ Additional Character Req   ✓x7ᵗʰ Placeholder Alert   Unacceptable PDx   Manifestation   **H1**-**H14** HAC   **HCC** CMS-HCC Condition   **EXCLUDES 1** Not Coded Here   **EXCLUDES 2** Not Included Here

√7ᵗʰ **T47.7X6** Underdosing of emetics

√5ᵗʰ **T47.8 Poisoning by, adverse effect of and underdosing of other agents primarily affecting gastrointestinal system**

　√6ᵗʰ **T47.8X Poisoning by, adverse effect of and underdosing of other agents primarily affecting gastrointestinal system**

　　√7ᵗʰ **T47.8X1 Poisoning by other agents primarily affecting gastrointestinal system, accidental (unintentional)**
　　　　Poisoning by other agents primarily affecting gastrointestinal system NOS

　　11 √7ᵗʰ **T47.8X2 Poisoning by other agents primarily affecting gastrointestinal system, intentional self-harm** HCC

　　√7ᵗʰ **T47.8X3 Poisoning by other agents primarily affecting gastrointestinal system, assault**

　　√7ᵗʰ **T47.8X4 Poisoning by other agents primarily affecting gastrointestinal system, undetermined**

　　√7ᵗʰ **T47.8X5 Adverse effect of other agents primarily affecting gastrointestinal system**

　　√7ᵗʰ **T47.8X6 Underdosing of other agents primarily affecting gastrointestinal system**

√5ᵗʰ **T47.9 Poisoning by, adverse effect of and underdosing of unspecified agents primarily affecting the gastrointestinal system**

　√x7ᵗʰ **T47.91 Poisoning by unspecified agents primarily affecting the gastrointestinal system, accidental (unintentional)**
　　　Poisoning by agents primarily affecting the gastrointestinal system NOS

　11 √x7ᵗʰ **T47.92 Poisoning by unspecified agents primarily affecting the gastrointestinal system, intentional self-harm** HCC

　√x7ᵗʰ **T47.93 Poisoning by unspecified agents primarily affecting the gastrointestinal system, assault**

　√x7ᵗʰ **T47.94 Poisoning by unspecified agents primarily affecting the gastrointestinal system, undetermined**

　√x7ᵗʰ **T47.95 Adverse effect of unspecified agents primarily affecting the gastrointestinal system**

　√x7ᵗʰ **T47.96 Underdosing of unspecified agents primarily affecting the gastrointestinal system**

√4ᵗʰ **T48 Poisoning by, adverse effect of and underdosing of agents primarily acting on smooth and skeletal muscles and the respiratory system**

> The appropriate 7th character is to be added to each code from category T48.
> A　initial encounter
> D　subsequent encounter
> S　sequela

√5ᵗʰ **T48.0 Poisoning by, adverse effect of and underdosing of oxytocic drugs**

　　EXCLUDES 1　*poisoning by, adverse effect of and underdosing of estrogens, progestogens and antagonists (T38.4-T38.6)*

　√6ᵗʰ **T48.0X Poisoning by, adverse effect of and underdosing of oxytocic drugs**

　　√7ᵗʰ **T48.0X1 Poisoning by oxytocic drugs, accidental (unintentional)**
　　　　Poisoning by oxytocic drugs NOS

　　11 √7ᵗʰ **T48.0X2 Poisoning by oxytocic drugs, intentional self-harm** HCC

　　√7ᵗʰ **T48.0X3 Poisoning by oxytocic drugs, assault**

　　√7ᵗʰ **T48.0X4 Poisoning by oxytocic drugs, undetermined**

　　√7ᵗʰ **T48.0X5 Adverse effect of oxytocic drugs**

　　√7ᵗʰ **T48.0X6 Underdosing of oxytocic drugs**

√5ᵗʰ **T48.1 Poisoning by, adverse effect of and underdosing of skeletal muscle relaxants [neuromuscular blocking agents]**

　√6ᵗʰ **T48.1X Poisoning by, adverse effect of and underdosing of skeletal muscle relaxants [neuromuscular blocking agents]**

　　√7ᵗʰ **T48.1X1 Poisoning by skeletal muscle relaxants [neuromuscular blocking agents], accidental (unintentional)**
　　　　Poisoning by skeletal muscle relaxants [neuromuscular blocking agents] NOS

　　11 √7ᵗʰ **T48.1X2 Poisoning by skeletal muscle relaxants [neuromuscular blocking agents], intentional self-harm** HCC

　　√7ᵗʰ **T48.1X3 Poisoning by skeletal muscle relaxants [neuromuscular blocking agents], assault**

　　√7ᵗʰ **T48.1X4 Poisoning by skeletal muscle relaxants [neuromuscular blocking agents], undetermined**

　　√7ᵗʰ **T48.1X5 Adverse effect of skeletal muscle relaxants [neuromuscular blocking agents]**

　　√7ᵗʰ **T48.1X6 Underdosing of skeletal muscle relaxants [neuromuscular blocking agents]**

√5ᵗʰ **T48.2 Poisoning by, adverse effect of and underdosing of other and unspecified drugs acting on muscles**

　√6ᵗʰ **T48.20 Poisoning by, adverse effect of and underdosing of unspecified drugs acting on muscles**

　　√7ᵗʰ **T48.201 Poisoning by unspecified drugs acting on muscles, accidental (unintentional)**
　　　　Poisoning by unspecified drugs acting on muscles NOS

　　11 √7ᵗʰ **T48.202 Poisoning by unspecified drugs acting on muscles, intentional self-harm** HCC

　　√7ᵗʰ **T48.203 Poisoning by unspecified drugs acting on muscles, assault**

　　√7ᵗʰ **T48.204 Poisoning by unspecified drugs acting on muscles, undetermined**

　　√7ᵗʰ **T48.205 Adverse effect of unspecified drugs acting on muscles**

　　√7ᵗʰ **T48.206 Underdosing of unspecified drugs acting on muscles**

　√6ᵗʰ **T48.29 Poisoning by, adverse effect of and underdosing of other drugs acting on muscles**

　　√7ᵗʰ **T48.291 Poisoning by other drugs acting on muscles, accidental (unintentional)**
　　　　Poisoning by other drugs acting on muscles NOS

　　11 √7ᵗʰ **T48.292 Poisoning by other drugs acting on muscles, intentional self-harm** HCC

　　√7ᵗʰ **T48.293 Poisoning by other drugs acting on muscles, assault**

　　√7ᵗʰ **T48.294 Poisoning by other drugs acting on muscles, undetermined**

　　√7ᵗʰ **T48.295 Adverse effect of other drugs acting on muscles**

　　√7ᵗʰ **T48.296 Underdosing of other drugs acting on muscles**

√5ᵗʰ **T48.3 Poisoning by, adverse effect of and underdosing of antitussives**

　√6ᵗʰ **T48.3X Poisoning by, adverse effect of and underdosing of antitussives**

　　√7ᵗʰ **T48.3X1 Poisoning by antitussives, accidental (unintentional)**
　　　　Poisoning by antitussives NOS

　　11 √7ᵗʰ **T48.3X2 Poisoning by antitussives, intentional self-harm** HCC

　　√7ᵗʰ **T48.3X3 Poisoning by antitussives, assault**

　　√7ᵗʰ **T48.3X4 Poisoning by antitussives, undetermined**

　　√7ᵗʰ **T48.3X5 Adverse effect of antitussives**

　　√7ᵗʰ **T48.3X6 Underdosing of antitussives**

---

11 HCC with 7th character indicating initial encounter (A or B - specific to category) OR sequela.

N Newborn: 0　P Pediatric: 0-17　M Maternity: 12-55　A Adult: 15-124　MCC Major CC Condition　PDxMCC PDx acts as own MCC　CC CC Condition　PDxCC PDx acts as own CC

1116　　　　　　　　　　　　　　　　　　　　　　　　　　　　　　　ICD-10-CM 2018

✓5ᵗʰ T48.4 Poisoning by, adverse effect of and underdosing of expectorants

✓6ᵗʰ T48.4X Poisoning by, adverse effect of and underdosing of expectorants

✓7ᵗʰ **T48.4X1 Poisoning by expectorants, accidental (unintentional)**
Poisoning by expectorants NOS

11 ✓7ᵗʰ **T48.4X2 Poisoning by expectorants, intentional self-harm** HCC

✓7ᵗʰ **T48.4X3 Poisoning by expectorants, assault**

✓7ᵗʰ **T48.4X4 Poisoning by expectorants, undetermined**

✓7ᵗʰ **T48.4X5 Adverse effect of expectorants**

✓7ᵗʰ **T48.4X6 Underdosing of expectorants**

✓5ᵗʰ T48.5 Poisoning by, adverse effect of and underdosing of other anti-common-cold drugs
Poisoning by, adverse effect of and underdosing of decongestants

EXCLUDES 2 poisoning by, adverse effect of and underdosing of antipyretics, NEC (T39.9-)
poisoning by, adverse effect of and underdosing of non-steroidal antiinflammatory drugs (T39.3-)
poisoning by, adverse effect of and underdosing of salicylates (T39.0-)

✓6ᵗʰ T48.5X Poisoning by, adverse effect of and underdosing of other anti-common-cold drugs

✓7ᵗʰ **T48.5X1 Poisoning by other anti-common-cold drugs, accidental (unintentional)**
Poisoning by other anti-common-cold drugs NOS

11 ✓7ᵗʰ **T48.5X2 Poisoning by other anti-common-cold drugs, intentional self-harm** HCC

✓7ᵗʰ **T48.5X3 Poisoning by other anti-common-cold drugs, assault**

✓7ᵗʰ **T48.5X4 Poisoning by other anti-common-cold drugs, undetermined**

✓7ᵗʰ **T48.5X5 Adverse effect of other anti-common-cold drugs**

✓7ᵗʰ **T48.5X6 Underdosing of other anti-common-cold drugs**

✓5ᵗʰ T48.6 Poisoning by, adverse effect of and underdosing of antiasthmatics, not elsewhere classified
Poisoning by, adverse effect of and underdosing of beta-adrenoreceptor agonists used in asthma therapy

EXCLUDES 1 poisoning by, adverse effect of and underdosing of anterior pituitary [adenohypophyseal] hormones (T38.8)
poisoning by, adverse effect of and underdosing of beta-adrenoreceptor agonists not used in asthma therapy (T44.5)

✓6ᵗʰ T48.6X Poisoning by, adverse effect of and underdosing of antiasthmatics

✓7ᵗʰ **T48.6X1 Poisoning by antiasthmatics, accidental (unintentional)**
Poisoning by antiasthmatics NOS

11 ✓7ᵗʰ **T48.6X2 Poisoning by antiasthmatics, intentional self-harm** HCC

✓7ᵗʰ **T48.6X3 Poisoning by antiasthmatics, assault**

✓7ᵗʰ **T48.6X4 Poisoning by antiasthmatics, undetermined**

✓7ᵗʰ **T48.6X5 Adverse effect of antiasthmatics**

✓7ᵗʰ **T48.6X6 Underdosing of antiasthmatics**

✓5ᵗʰ T48.9 Poisoning by, adverse effect of and underdosing of other and unspecified agents primarily acting on the respiratory system

✓6ᵗʰ T48.90 Poisoning by, adverse effect of and underdosing of unspecified agents primarily acting on the respiratory system

✓7ᵗʰ **T48.901 Poisoning by unspecified agents primarily acting on the respiratory system, accidental (unintentional)**

11 ✓7ᵗʰ **T48.902 Poisoning by unspecified agents primarily acting on the respiratory system, intentional self-harm** HCC

✓7ᵗʰ **T48.903 Poisoning by unspecified agents primarily acting on the respiratory system, assault**

✓7ᵗʰ **T48.904 Poisoning by unspecified agents primarily acting on the respiratory system, undetermined**

✓7ᵗʰ **T48.905 Adverse effect of unspecified agents primarily acting on the respiratory system**

✓7ᵗʰ **T48.906 Underdosing of unspecified agents primarily acting on the respiratory system**

✓6ᵗʰ T48.99 Poisoning by, adverse effect of and underdosing of other agents primarily acting on the respiratory system

✓7ᵗʰ **T48.991 Poisoning by other agents primarily acting on the respiratory system, accidental (unintentional)**

11 ✓7ᵗʰ **T48.992 Poisoning by other agents primarily acting on the respiratory system, intentional self-harm** HCC

✓7ᵗʰ **T48.993 Poisoning by other agents primarily acting on the respiratory system, assault**

✓7ᵗʰ **T48.994 Poisoning by other agents primarily acting on the respiratory system, undetermined**

✓7ᵗʰ **T48.995 Adverse effect of other agents primarily acting on the respiratory system**

✓7ᵗʰ **T48.996 Underdosing of other agents primarily acting on the respiratory system**

✓4ᵗʰ T49 Poisoning by, adverse effect of and underdosing of topical agents primarily affecting skin and mucous membrane and by ophthalmological, otorhinolaryngological and dental drugs

INCLUDES poisoning by, adverse effect of and underdosing of glucocorticoids, topically used

The appropriate 7th character is to be added to each code from category T49.
A initial encounter
D subsequent encounter
S sequela

✓5ᵗʰ T49.0 Poisoning by, adverse effect of and underdosing of local antifungal, anti-infective and anti-inflammatory drugs

✓6ᵗʰ T49.0X Poisoning by, adverse effect of and underdosing of local antifungal, anti-infective and anti-inflammatory drugs

✓7ᵗʰ **T49.0X1 Poisoning by local antifungal, anti-infective and anti-inflammatory drugs, accidental (unintentional)**
Poisoning by local antifungal, anti-infective and anti-inflammatory drugs NOS

11 ✓7ᵗʰ **T49.0X2 Poisoning by local antifungal, anti-infective and anti-inflammatory drugs, intentional self-harm** HCC

✓7ᵗʰ **T49.0X3 Poisoning by local antifungal, anti-infective and anti-inflammatory drugs, assault**

✓7ᵗʰ **T49.0X4 Poisoning by local antifungal, anti-infective and anti-inflammatory drugs, undetermined**

✓7ᵗʰ **T49.0X5 Adverse effect of local antifungal, anti-infective and anti-inflammatory drugs**

✓7ᵗʰ **T49.0X6 Underdosing of local antifungal, anti-infective and anti-inflammatory drugs**

✓5ᵗʰ T49.1 Poisoning by, adverse effect of and underdosing of antipruritics

✓6ᵗʰ T49.1X Poisoning by, adverse effect of and underdosing of antipruritics

✓7ᵗʰ **T49.1X1 Poisoning by antipruritics, accidental (unintentional)**
Poisoning by antipruritics NOS

11 ✓7ᵗʰ **T49.1X2 Poisoning by antipruritics, intentional self-harm** HCC

✓7ᵗʰ **T49.1X3 Poisoning by antipruritics, assault**

✓7ᵗʰ **T49.1X4 Poisoning by antipruritics, undetermined**

✓7ᵗʰ **T49.1X5 Adverse effect of antipruritics**

✓7ᵗʰ **T49.1X6 Underdosing of antipruritics**

---

11 HCC with 7th character indicating initial encounter (A or B - specific to category) OR sequela.

☑5ᵗʰ **T49.2** **Poisoning by, adverse effect of and underdosing of local astringents and local detergents**

    ☑6ᵗʰ **T49.2X** **Poisoning by, adverse effect of and underdosing of local astringents and local detergents**

        ☑7ᵗʰ **T49.2X1** **Poisoning by local astringents and local detergents, accidental (unintentional)**
            Poisoning by local astringents and local detergents NOS

        11 ☑7ᵗʰ **T49.2X2** **Poisoning by local astringents and local detergents, intentional self-harm** HCC

        ☑7ᵗʰ **T49.2X3** **Poisoning by local astringents and local detergents, assault**

        ☑7ᵗʰ **T49.2X4** **Poisoning by local astringents and local detergents, undetermined**

        ☑7ᵗʰ **T49.2X5** **Adverse effect of local astringents and local detergents**

        ☑7ᵗʰ **T49.2X6** **Underdosing of local astringents and local detergents**

☑5ᵗʰ **T49.3** **Poisoning by, adverse effect of and underdosing of emollients, demulcents and protectants**

    ☑6ᵗʰ **T49.3X** **Poisoning by, adverse effect of and underdosing of emollients, demulcents and protectants**

        ☑7ᵗʰ **T49.3X1** **Poisoning by emollients, demulcents and protectants, accidental (unintentional)**
            Poisoning by emollients, demulcents and protectants NOS

        11 ☑7ᵗʰ **T49.3X2** **Poisoning by emollients, demulcents and protectants, intentional self-harm** HCC

        ☑7ᵗʰ **T49.3X3** **Poisoning by emollients, demulcents and protectants, assault**

        ☑7ᵗʰ **T49.3X4** **Poisoning by emollients, demulcents and protectants, undetermined**

        ☑7ᵗʰ **T49.3X5** **Adverse effect of emollients, demulcents and protectants**

        ☑7ᵗʰ **T49.3X6** **Underdosing of emollients, demulcents and protectants**

☑5ᵗʰ **T49.4** **Poisoning by, adverse effect of and underdosing of keratolytics, keratoplastics, and other hair treatment drugs and preparations**

    ☑6ᵗʰ **T49.4X** **Poisoning by, adverse effect of and underdosing of keratolytics, keratoplastics, and other hair treatment drugs and preparations**

        ☑7ᵗʰ **T49.4X1** **Poisoning by keratolytics, keratoplastics, and other hair treatment drugs and preparations, accidental (unintentional)**
            Poisoning by keratolytics, keratoplastics, and other hair treatment drugs and preparations NOS

        11 ☑7ᵗʰ **T49.4X2** **Poisoning by keratolytics, keratoplastics, and other hair treatment drugs and preparations, intentional self-harm** HCC

        ☑7ᵗʰ **T49.4X3** **Poisoning by keratolytics, keratoplastics, and other hair treatment drugs and preparations, assault**

        ☑7ᵗʰ **T49.4X4** **Poisoning by keratolytics, keratoplastics, and other hair treatment drugs and preparations, undetermined**

        ☑7ᵗʰ **T49.4X5** **Adverse effect of keratolytics, keratoplastics, and other hair treatment drugs and preparations**

        ☑7ᵗʰ **T49.4X6** **Underdosing of keratolytics, keratoplastics, and other hair treatment drugs and preparations**

☑5ᵗʰ **T49.5** **Poisoning by, adverse effect of and underdosing of ophthalmological drugs and preparations**

    ☑6ᵗʰ **T49.5X** **Poisoning by, adverse effect of and underdosing of ophthalmological drugs and preparations**

        ☑7ᵗʰ **T49.5X1** **Poisoning by ophthalmological drugs and preparations, accidental (unintentional)**
            Poisoning by ophthalmological drugs and preparations NOS

        11 ☑7ᵗʰ **T49.5X2** **Poisoning by ophthalmological drugs and preparations, intentional self-harm** HCC

        ☑7ᵗʰ **T49.5X3** **Poisoning by ophthalmological drugs and preparations, assault**

        ☑7ᵗʰ **T49.5X4** **Poisoning by ophthalmological drugs and preparations, undetermined**

        ☑7ᵗʰ **T49.5X5** **Adverse effect of ophthalmological drugs and preparations**

        ☑7ᵗʰ **T49.5X6** **Underdosing of ophthalmological drugs and preparations**

☑5ᵗʰ **T49.6** **Poisoning by, adverse effect of and underdosing of otorhinolaryngological drugs and preparations**

    ☑6ᵗʰ **T49.6X** **Poisoning by, adverse effect of and underdosing of otorhinolaryngological drugs and preparations**

        ☑7ᵗʰ **T49.6X1** **Poisoning by otorhinolaryngological drugs and preparations, accidental (unintentional)**
            Poisoning by otorhinolaryngological drugs and preparations NOS

        11 ☑7ᵗʰ **T49.6X2** **Poisoning by otorhinolaryngological drugs and preparations, intentional self-harm** HCC

        ☑7ᵗʰ **T49.6X3** **Poisoning by otorhinolaryngological drugs and preparations, assault**

        ☑7ᵗʰ **T49.6X4** **Poisoning by otorhinolaryngological drugs and preparations, undetermined**

        ☑7ᵗʰ **T49.6X5** **Adverse effect of otorhinolaryngological drugs and preparations**

        ☑7ᵗʰ **T49.6X6** **Underdosing of otorhinolaryngological drugs and preparations**

☑5ᵗʰ **T49.7** **Poisoning by, adverse effect of and underdosing of dental drugs, topically applied**

    ☑6ᵗʰ **T49.7X** **Poisoning by, adverse effect of and underdosing of dental drugs, topically applied**

        ☑7ᵗʰ **T49.7X1** **Poisoning by dental drugs, topically applied, accidental (unintentional)**
            Poisoning by dental drugs, topically applied NOS

        11 ☑7ᵗʰ **T49.7X2** **Poisoning by dental drugs, topically applied, intentional self-harm** HCC

        ☑7ᵗʰ **T49.7X3** **Poisoning by dental drugs, topically applied, assault**

        ☑7ᵗʰ **T49.7X4** **Poisoning by dental drugs, topically applied, undetermined**

        ☑7ᵗʰ **T49.7X5** **Adverse effect of dental drugs, topically applied**

        ☑7ᵗʰ **T49.7X6** **Underdosing of dental drugs, topically applied**

☑5ᵗʰ **T49.8** **Poisoning by, adverse effect of and underdosing of other topical agents**
    Poisoning by, adverse effect of and underdosing of spermicides

    ☑6ᵗʰ **T49.8X** **Poisoning by, adverse effect of and underdosing of other topical agents**

        ☑7ᵗʰ **T49.8X1** **Poisoning by other topical agents, accidental (unintentional)**
            Poisoning by other topical agents NOS

        11 ☑7ᵗʰ **T49.8X2** **Poisoning by other topical agents, intentional self-harm** HCC

        ☑7ᵗʰ **T49.8X3** **Poisoning by other topical agents, assault**

        ☑7ᵗʰ **T49.8X4** **Poisoning by other topical agents, undetermined**

        ☑7ᵗʰ **T49.8X5** **Adverse effect of other topical agents**

        ☑7ᵗʰ **T49.8X6** **Underdosing of other topical agents**

☑5ᵗʰ **T49.9** **Poisoning by, adverse effect of and underdosing of unspecified topical agent**

    ☑x7ᵗʰ **T49.91** **Poisoning by unspecified topical agent, accidental (unintentional)**

    11 ☑x7ᵗʰ **T49.92** **Poisoning by unspecified topical agent, intentional self-harm** HCC

    ☑x7ᵗʰ **T49.93** **Poisoning by unspecified topical agent, assault**

    ☑x7ᵗʰ **T49.94** **Poisoning by unspecified topical agent, undetermined**

    ☑x7ᵗʰ **T49.95** **Adverse effect of unspecified topical agent**

    ☑x7ᵗʰ **T49.96** **Underdosing of unspecified topical agent**

---

11 HCC with 7th character indicating initial encounter (A or B - specific to category) OR sequela.

N Newborn: 0   **P** Pediatric: 0-17   **M** Maternity: 12-55   **A** Adult: 15-124   **MCC** Major CC Condition   **PDxMCC** PDx acts as own MCC   **CC** CC Condition   **PDxCC** PDx acts as own CC

1118   ICD-10-CM 2018

✓4ᵗʰ **T50** **Poisoning by, adverse effect of and underdosing of diuretics and other and unspecified drugs, medicaments and biological substances**

> The appropriate 7th character is to be added to each code from category T50.
> A   initial encounter
> D   subsequent encounter
> S   sequela

✓5ᵗʰ **T50.0** **Poisoning by, adverse effect of and underdosing of mineralocorticoids and their antagonists**

  ✓6ᵗʰ **T50.0X** **Poisoning by, adverse effect of and underdosing of mineralocorticoids and their antagonists**

    ✓7ᵗʰ **T50.0X1** **Poisoning by mineralocorticoids and their antagonists, accidental (unintentional)**
       Poisoning by mineralocorticoids and their antagonists NOS

    11 ✓7ᵗʰ **T50.0X2** **Poisoning by mineralocorticoids and their antagonists, intentional self-harm** HCC

    ✓7ᵗʰ **T50.0X3** **Poisoning by mineralocorticoids and their antagonists, assault**

    ✓7ᵗʰ **T50.0X4** **Poisoning by mineralocorticoids and their antagonists, undetermined**

    ✓7ᵗʰ **T50.0X5** **Adverse effect of mineralocorticoids and their antagonists**

    ✓7ᵗʰ **T50.0X6** **Underdosing of mineralocorticoids and their antagonists**

✓5ᵗʰ **T50.1** **Poisoning by, adverse effect of and underdosing of loop [high-ceiling] diuretics**

  ✓6ᵗʰ **T50.1X** **Poisoning by, adverse effect of and underdosing of loop [high-ceiling] diuretics**

    ✓7ᵗʰ **T50.1X1** **Poisoning by loop [high-ceiling] diuretics, accidental (unintentional)**
       Poisoning by loop [high-ceiling] diuretics NOS

    11 ✓7ᵗʰ **T50.1X2** **Poisoning by loop [high-ceiling] diuretics, intentional self-harm** HCC

    ✓7ᵗʰ **T50.1X3** **Poisoning by loop [high-ceiling] diuretics, assault**

    ✓7ᵗʰ **T50.1X4** **Poisoning by loop [high-ceiling] diuretics, undetermined**

    ✓7ᵗʰ **T50.1X5** **Adverse effect of loop [high-ceiling] diuretics**

    ✓7ᵗʰ **T50.1X6** **Underdosing of loop [high-ceiling] diuretics**

✓5ᵗʰ **T50.2** **Poisoning by, adverse effect of and underdosing of carbonic-anhydrase inhibitors, benzothiadiazides and other diuretics**
   Poisoning by, adverse effect of and underdosing of acetazolamide

  ✓6ᵗʰ **T50.2X** **Poisoning by, adverse effect of and underdosing of carbonic-anhydrase inhibitors, benzothiadiazides and other diuretics**

    ✓7ᵗʰ **T50.2X1** **Poisoning by carbonic-anhydrase inhibitors, benzothiadiazides and other diuretics, accidental (unintentional)**
       Poisoning by carbonic-anhydrase inhibitors, benzothiadiazides and other diuretics NOS

    11 ✓7ᵗʰ **T50.2X2** **Poisoning by carbonic-anhydrase inhibitors, benzothiadiazides and other diuretics, intentional self-harm** HCC

    ✓7ᵗʰ **T50.2X3** **Poisoning by carbonic-anhydrase inhibitors, benzothiadiazides and other diuretics, assault**

    ✓7ᵗʰ **T50.2X4** **Poisoning by carbonic-anhydrase inhibitors, benzothiadiazides and other diuretics, undetermined**

    ✓7ᵗʰ **T50.2X5** **Adverse effect of carbonic-anhydrase inhibitors, benzothiadiazides and other diuretics**

    ✓7ᵗʰ **T50.2X6** **Underdosing of carbonic-anhydrase inhibitors, benzothiadiazides and other diuretics**

✓5ᵗʰ **T50.3** **Poisoning by, adverse effect of and underdosing of electrolytic, caloric and water-balance agents**
   Poisoning by, adverse effect of and underdosing of oral rehydration salts

  ✓6ᵗʰ **T50.3X** **Poisoning by, adverse effect of and underdosing of electrolytic, caloric and water-balance agents**

    ✓7ᵗʰ **T50.3X1** **Poisoning by electrolytic, caloric and water-balance agents, accidental (unintentional)**
       Poisoning by electrolytic, caloric and water-balance agents NOS

    11 ✓7ᵗʰ **T50.3X2** **Poisoning by electrolytic, caloric and water-balance agents, intentional self-harm** HCC

    ✓7ᵗʰ **T50.3X3** **Poisoning by electrolytic, caloric and water-balance agents, assault**

    ✓7ᵗʰ **T50.3X4** **Poisoning by electrolytic, caloric and water-balance agents, undetermined**

    ✓7ᵗʰ **T50.3X5** **Adverse effect of electrolytic, caloric and water-balance agents**

    ✓7ᵗʰ **T50.3X6** **Underdosing of electrolytic, caloric and water-balance agents**

✓5ᵗʰ **T50.4** **Poisoning by, adverse effect of and underdosing of drugs affecting uric acid metabolism**

  ✓6ᵗʰ **T50.4X** **Poisoning by, adverse effect of and underdosing of drugs affecting uric acid metabolism**

    ✓7ᵗʰ **T50.4X1** **Poisoning by drugs affecting uric acid metabolism, accidental (unintentional)**
       Poisoning by drugs affecting uric acid metabolism NOS

    11 ✓7ᵗʰ **T50.4X2** **Poisoning by drugs affecting uric acid metabolism, intentional self-harm** HCC

    ✓7ᵗʰ **T50.4X3** **Poisoning by drugs affecting uric acid metabolism, assault**

    ✓7ᵗʰ **T50.4X4** **Poisoning by drugs affecting uric acid metabolism, undetermined**

    ✓7ᵗʰ **T50.4X5** **Adverse effect of drugs affecting uric acid metabolism**

    ✓7ᵗʰ **T50.4X6** **Underdosing of drugs affecting uric acid metabolism**

✓5ᵗʰ **T50.5** **Poisoning by, adverse effect of and underdosing of appetite depressants**

  ✓6ᵗʰ **T50.5X** **Poisoning by, adverse effect of and underdosing of appetite depressants**

    ✓7ᵗʰ **T50.5X1** **Poisoning by appetite depressants, accidental (unintentional)**
       Poisoning by appetite depressants NOS

    11 ✓7ᵗʰ **T50.5X2** **Poisoning by appetite depressants, intentional self-harm** HCC

    ✓7ᵗʰ **T50.5X3** **Poisoning by appetite depressants, assault**

    ✓7ᵗʰ **T50.5X4** **Poisoning by appetite depressants, undetermined**

    ✓7ᵗʰ **T50.5X5** **Adverse effect of appetite depressants**

    ✓7ᵗʰ **T50.5X6** **Underdosing of appetite depressants**

✓5ᵗʰ **T50.6** **Poisoning by, adverse effect of and underdosing of antidotes and chelating agents**
   Poisoning by, adverse effect of and underdosing of alcohol deterrents

  ✓6ᵗʰ **T50.6X** **Poisoning by, adverse effect of and underdosing of antidotes and chelating agents**

    ✓7ᵗʰ **T50.6X1** **Poisoning by antidotes and chelating agents, accidental (unintentional)**
       Poisoning by antidotes and chelating agents NOS

    11 ✓7ᵗʰ **T50.6X2** **Poisoning by antidotes and chelating agents, intentional self-harm** HCC

    ✓7ᵗʰ **T50.6X3** **Poisoning by antidotes and chelating agents, assault**

    ✓7ᵗʰ **T50.6X4** **Poisoning by antidotes and chelating agents, undetermined**

    ✓7ᵗʰ **T50.6X5** **Adverse effect of antidotes and chelating agents**

    ✓7ᵗʰ **T50.6X6** **Underdosing of antidotes and chelating agents**

---

11 HCC with 7th character indicating initial encounter (A or B - specific to category) OR sequela.

✓ Additional Character Req   ✓x7ᵗʰ Placeholder Alert   Unacceptable PDx   Manifestation   H1–H14 HAC   HCC CMS-HCC Condition   *EXCLUDES 1* Not Coded Here   *EXCLUDES 2* Not Included Here

✓5ᵗʰ **T50.7** **Poisoning by, adverse effect of and underdosing of analeptics and opioid receptor antagonists**

    ✓6ᵗʰ **T50.7X** **Poisoning by, adverse effect of and underdosing of analeptics and opioid receptor antagonists**

       ✓7ᵗʰ **T50.7X1** **Poisoning by analeptics and opioid receptor antagonists, accidental (unintentional)**
           Poisoning by analeptics and opioid receptor antagonists NOS

       11 ✓7ᵗʰ **T50.7X2** **Poisoning by analeptics and opioid** HCC **receptor antagonists, intentional self-harm**

       ✓7ᵗʰ **T50.7X3** **Poisoning by analeptics and opioid receptor antagonists, assault**

       ✓7ᵗʰ **T50.7X4** **Poisoning by analeptics and opioid receptor antagonists, undetermined**

       ✓7ᵗʰ **T50.7X5** **Adverse effect of analeptics and opioid receptor antagonists**

       ✓7ᵗʰ **T50.7X6** **Underdosing of analeptics and opioid receptor antagonists**

✓5ᵗʰ **T50.8** **Poisoning by, adverse effect of and underdosing of diagnostic agents**

    ✓6ᵗʰ **T50.8X** **Poisoning by, adverse effect of and underdosing of diagnostic agents**

       ✓7ᵗʰ **T50.8X1** **Poisoning by diagnostic agents, accidental (unintentional)**
           Poisoning by diagnostic agents NOS

       11 ✓7ᵗʰ **T50.8X2** **Poisoning by diagnostic agents,** HCC **intentional self-harm**

       ✓7ᵗʰ **T50.8X3** **Poisoning by diagnostic agents, assault**

       ✓7ᵗʰ **T50.8X4** **Poisoning by diagnostic agents, undetermined**

       ✓7ᵗʰ **T50.8X5** **Adverse effect of diagnostic agents**

       ✓7ᵗʰ **T50.8X6** **Underdosing of diagnostic agents**

✓5ᵗʰ **T50.A** **Poisoning by, adverse effect of and underdosing of bacterial vaccines**

    ✓6ᵗʰ **T50.A1** **Poisoning by, adverse effect of and underdosing of pertussis vaccine, including combinations with a pertussis component**

       ✓7ᵗʰ **T50.A11** **Poisoning by pertussis vaccine, including combinations with a pertussis component, accidental (unintentional)**

       11 ✓7ᵗʰ **T50.A12** **Poisoning by pertussis vaccine,** HCC **including combinations with a pertussis component, intentional self-harm**

       ✓7ᵗʰ **T50.A13** **Poisoning by pertussis vaccine, including combinations with a pertussis component, assault**

       ✓7ᵗʰ **T50.A14** **Poisoning by pertussis vaccine, including combinations with a pertussis component, undetermined**

       ✓7ᵗʰ **T50.A15** **Adverse effect of pertussis vaccine, including combinations with a pertussis component**

       ✓7ᵗʰ **T50.A16** **Underdosing of pertussis vaccine, including combinations with a pertussis component**

    ✓6ᵗʰ **T50.A2** **Poisoning by, adverse effect of and underdosing of mixed bacterial vaccines without a pertussis component**

       ✓7ᵗʰ **T50.A21** **Poisoning by mixed bacterial vaccines without a pertussis component, accidental (unintentional)**

       11 ✓7ᵗʰ **T50.A22** **Poisoning by mixed bacterial vaccines** HCC **without a pertussis component, intentional self-harm**

       ✓7ᵗʰ **T50.A23** **Poisoning by mixed bacterial vaccines without a pertussis component, assault**

       ✓7ᵗʰ **T50.A24** **Poisoning by mixed bacterial vaccines without a pertussis component, undetermined**

       ✓7ᵗʰ **T50.A25** **Adverse effect of mixed bacterial vaccines without a pertussis component**

       ✓7ᵗʰ **T50.A26** **Underdosing of mixed bacterial vaccines without a pertussis component**

    ✓6ᵗʰ **T50.A9** **Poisoning by, adverse effect of and underdosing of other bacterial vaccines**

       ✓7ᵗʰ **T50.A91** **Poisoning by other bacterial vaccines, accidental (unintentional)**

       11 ✓7ᵗʰ **T50.A92** **Poisoning by other bacterial vaccines,** HCC **intentional self-harm**

       ✓7ᵗʰ **T50.A93** **Poisoning by other bacterial vaccines, assault**

       ✓7ᵗʰ **T50.A94** **Poisoning by other bacterial vaccines, undetermined**

       ✓7ᵗʰ **T50.A95** **Adverse effect of other bacterial vaccines**

       ✓7ᵗʰ **T50.A96** **Underdosing of other bacterial vaccines**

✓5ᵗʰ **T50.B** **Poisoning by, adverse effect of and underdosing of viral vaccines**

    ✓6ᵗʰ **T50.B1** **Poisoning by, adverse effect of and underdosing of smallpox vaccines**

       ✓7ᵗʰ **T50.B11** **Poisoning by smallpox vaccines, accidental (unintentional)**

       11 ✓7ᵗʰ **T50.B12** **Poisoning by smallpox vaccines,** HCC **intentional self-harm**

       ✓7ᵗʰ **T50.B13** **Poisoning by smallpox vaccines, assault**

       ✓7ᵗʰ **T50.B14** **Poisoning by smallpox vaccines, undetermined**

       ✓7ᵗʰ **T50.B15** **Adverse effect of smallpox vaccines**

       ✓7ᵗʰ **T50.B16** **Underdosing of smallpox vaccines**

    ✓6ᵗʰ **T50.B9** **Poisoning by, adverse effect of and underdosing of other viral vaccines**

       ✓7ᵗʰ **T50.B91** **Poisoning by other viral vaccines, accidental (unintentional)**

       11 ✓7ᵗʰ **T50.B92** **Poisoning by other viral vaccines,** HCC **intentional self-harm**

       ✓7ᵗʰ **T50.B93** **Poisoning by other viral vaccines, assault**

       ✓7ᵗʰ **T50.B94** **Poisoning by other viral vaccines, undetermined**

       ✓7ᵗʰ **T50.B95** **Adverse effect of other viral vaccines**

       ✓7ᵗʰ **T50.B96** **Underdosing of other viral vaccines**

✓5ᵗʰ **T50.Z** **Poisoning by, adverse effect of and underdosing of other vaccines and biological substances**

    ✓6ᵗʰ **T50.Z1** **Poisoning by, adverse effect of and underdosing of immunoglobulin**

       ✓7ᵗʰ **T50.Z11** **Poisoning by immunoglobulin, accidental (unintentional)**

       11 ✓7ᵗʰ **T50.Z12** **Poisoning by immunoglobulin,** HCC **intentional self-harm**

       ✓7ᵗʰ **T50.Z13** **Poisoning by immunoglobulin, assault**

       ✓7ᵗʰ **T50.Z14** **Poisoning by immunoglobulin, undetermined**

       ✓7ᵗʰ **T50.Z15** **Adverse effect of immunoglobulin**

       ✓7ᵗʰ **T50.Z16** **Underdosing of immunoglobulin**

    ✓6ᵗʰ **T50.Z9** **Poisoning by, adverse effect of and underdosing of other vaccines and biological substances**

       ✓7ᵗʰ **T50.Z91** **Poisoning by other vaccines and biological substances, accidental (unintentional)**

       11 ✓7ᵗʰ **T50.Z92** **Poisoning by other vaccines and** HCC **biological substances, intentional self-harm**

       ✓7ᵗʰ **T50.Z93** **Poisoning by other vaccines and biological substances, assault**

       ✓7ᵗʰ **T50.Z94** **Poisoning by other vaccines and biological substances, undetermined**

       ✓7ᵗʰ **T50.Z95** **Adverse effect of other vaccines and biological substances**

       ✓7ᵗʰ **T50.Z96** **Underdosing of other vaccines and biological substances**

✓5ᵗʰ **T50.9** **Poisoning by, adverse effect of and underdosing of other and unspecified drugs, medicaments and biological substances**
      AHA: 2016, 1Q, 38; 2015, 1Q, 21

    ✓6ᵗʰ **T50.90** **Poisoning by, adverse effect of and underdosing of unspecified drugs, medicaments and biological substances**

       ✓7ᵗʰ **T50.901** **Poisoning by unspecified drugs, medicaments and biological substances, accidental (unintentional)**

---

11 HCC with 7th character indicating initial encounter (A or B - specific to category) OR sequela.

N Newborn: 0   P Pediatric: 0-17   M Maternity: 12-55   A Adult: 15-124   MCC Major CC Condition   PDxMCC PDx acts as own MCC   CC CC Condition   PDxCC PDx acts as own CC

1120   ICD-10-CM 2018

11 ✓7ᵗʰ **T50.902** **Poisoning by unspecified drugs, medicaments and biological substances, intentional self-harm** `HCC`

✓7ᵗʰ **T50.903** **Poisoning by unspecified drugs, medicaments and biological substances, assault**

✓7ᵗʰ **T50.904** **Poisoning by unspecified drugs, medicaments and biological substances, undetermined**

✓7ᵗʰ **T50.905** Adverse effect of unspecified drugs, medicaments and biological substances

✓7ᵗʰ **T50.906** Underdosing of unspecified drugs, medicaments and biological substances

✓6ᵗʰ **T50.99** **Poisoning by, adverse effect of and underdosing of other drugs, medicaments and biological substances**

✓7ᵗʰ **T50.991** **Poisoning by other drugs, medicaments and biological substances, accidental (unintentional)**

11 ✓7ᵗʰ **T50.992** **Poisoning by other drugs, medicaments and biological substances, intentional self-harm** `HCC`

✓7ᵗʰ **T50.993** **Poisoning by other drugs, medicaments and biological substances, assault**

✓7ᵗʰ **T50.994** **Poisoning by other drugs, medicaments and biological substances, undetermined**

✓7ᵗʰ **T50.995** Adverse effect of other drugs, medicaments and biological substances

✓7ᵗʰ **T50.996** Underdosing of other drugs, medicaments and biological substances

Toxic effects of substances chiefly nonmedicinal as to source (T51-T65)

`NOTE` When no intent is indicated code to accidental. Undetermined intent is only for use when there is specific documentation in the record that the intent of the toxic effect cannot be determined.

Use additional code(s) for all associated manifestations of toxic effect, such as:
personal history of foreign body fully removed (Z87.821)
respiratory conditions due to external agents (J60-J70)
to identify any retained foreign body, if applicable (Z18.-)

`EXCLUDES 1` contact with and (suspected) exposure to toxic substances (Z77.-)
AHA: 2017, 1Q, 39-40

✓4ᵗʰ **T51** **Toxic effect of alcohol**

The appropriate 7th character is to be added to each code from category T51.
A   initial encounter
D   subsequent encounter
S   sequela

✓5ᵗʰ **T51.0** **Toxic effect of ethanol**
Toxic effect of ethyl alcohol

`EXCLUDES 2` acute alcohol intoxication or 'hangover' effects (F10.129, F10.229, F10.929)
drunkenness (F10.129, F10.229, F10.929)
pathological alcohol intoxication (F10.129, F10.229, F10.929)

✓6ᵗʰ **T51.0X** **Toxic effect of ethanol**

✓7ᵗʰ **T51.0X1** **Toxic effect of ethanol, accidental (unintentional)**
Toxic effect of ethanol NOS

11 ✓7ᵗʰ **T51.0X2** **Toxic effect of ethanol, intentional self-harm** `HCC`

✓7ᵗʰ **T51.0X3** **Toxic effect of ethanol, assault**

✓7ᵗʰ **T51.0X4** **Toxic effect of ethanol, undetermined**

✓5ᵗʰ **T51.1** **Toxic effect of methanol**
Toxic effect of methyl alcohol

✓6ᵗʰ **T51.1X** **Toxic effect of methanol**

✓7ᵗʰ **T51.1X1** **Toxic effect of methanol, accidental (unintentional)**
Toxic effect of methanol NOS

11 ✓7ᵗʰ **T51.1X2** **Toxic effect of methanol, intentional self-harm** `HCC`

✓7ᵗʰ **T51.1X3** **Toxic effect of methanol, assault**

✓7ᵗʰ **T51.1X4** **Toxic effect of methanol, undetermined**

✓5ᵗʰ **T51.2** **Toxic effect of 2-Propanol**
Toxic effect of isopropyl alcohol

✓6ᵗʰ **T51.2X** **Toxic effect of 2-Propanol**

✓7ᵗʰ **T51.2X1** **Toxic effect of 2-Propanol, accidental (unintentional)**
Toxic effect of 2-Propanol NOS

11 ✓7ᵗʰ **T51.2X2** **Toxic effect of 2-Propanol, intentional self-harm** `HCC`

✓7ᵗʰ **T51.2X3** **Toxic effect of 2-Propanol, assault**

✓7ᵗʰ **T51.2X4** **Toxic effect of 2-Propanol, undetermined**

✓5ᵗʰ **T51.3** **Toxic effect of fusel oil**
Toxic effect of amyl alcohol
Toxic effect of butyl [1-butanol] alcohol
Toxic effect of propyl [1-propanol] alcohol

✓6ᵗʰ **T51.3X** **Toxic effect of fusel oil**

✓7ᵗʰ **T51.3X1** **Toxic effect of fusel oil, accidental (unintentional)**
Toxic effect of fusel oil NOS

11 ✓7ᵗʰ **T51.3X2** **Toxic effect of fusel oil, intentional self-harm** `HCC`

✓7ᵗʰ **T51.3X3** **Toxic effect of fusel oil, assault**

✓7ᵗʰ **T51.3X4** **Toxic effect of fusel oil, undetermined**

✓5ᵗʰ **T51.8** **Toxic effect of other alcohols**

✓6ᵗʰ **T51.8X** **Toxic effect of other alcohols**

✓7ᵗʰ **T51.8X1** **Toxic effect of other alcohols, accidental (unintentional)**
Toxic effect of other alcohols NOS

11 ✓7ᵗʰ **T51.8X2** **Toxic effect of other alcohols, intentional self-harm** `HCC`

✓7ᵗʰ **T51.8X3** **Toxic effect of other alcohols, assault**

✓7ᵗʰ **T51.8X4** **Toxic effect of other alcohols, undetermined**

✓5ᵗʰ **T51.9** **Toxic effect of unspecified alcohol**

✓x7ᵗʰ **T51.91** **Toxic effect of unspecified alcohol, accidental (unintentional)**

11 ✓x7ᵗʰ **T51.92** **Toxic effect of unspecified alcohol, intentional self-harm** `HCC`

✓x7ᵗʰ **T51.93** **Toxic effect of unspecified alcohol, assault**

✓x7ᵗʰ **T51.94** **Toxic effect of unspecified alcohol, undetermined**

✓4ᵗʰ **T52** **Toxic effect of organic solvents**

`EXCLUDES 1` halogen derivatives of aliphatic and aromatic hydrocarbons (T53.-)

The appropriate 7th character is to be added to each code from category T52.
A   initial encounter
D   subsequent encounter
S   sequela

✓5ᵗʰ **T52.0** **Toxic effects of petroleum products**
Toxic effects of ether petroleum
Toxic effects of gasoline [petrol]
Toxic effects of kerosene [paraffin oil]
Toxic effects of naphtha petroleum
Toxic effects of paraffin wax
Toxic effects of spirit petroleum

✓6ᵗʰ **T52.0X** **Toxic effects of petroleum products**

✓7ᵗʰ **T52.0X1** **Toxic effect of petroleum products, accidental (unintentional)**
Toxic effects of petroleum products NOS

11 ✓7ᵗʰ **T52.0X2** **Toxic effect of petroleum products, intentional self-harm** `HCC`

✓7ᵗʰ **T52.0X3** **Toxic effect of petroleum products, assault**

✓7ᵗʰ **T52.0X4** **Toxic effect of petroleum products, undetermined**

✓5ᵗʰ **T52.1** **Toxic effects of benzene**

`EXCLUDES 1` homologues of benzene (T52.2)
nitroderivatives and aminoderivatives of benzene and its homologues (T65.3)

✓6ᵗʰ **T52.1X** **Toxic effects of benzene**

✓7ᵗʰ **T52.1X1** **Toxic effect of benzene, accidental (unintentional)**
Toxic effects of benzene NOS

---

11 HCC with 7th character indicating initial encounter (A or B - specific to category) OR sequela.

✓ Additional Character Req   ✓x7ᵗʰ Placeholder Alert   Unacceptable PDx   Manifestation   `H1`-`H14` HAC   `HCC` CMS-HCC Condition   `EXCLUDES 1` Not Coded Here   `EXCLUDES 2` Not Included Here

¹¹ √7ᵗʰ T52.1X2 Toxic effect of benzene, intentional self-harm   **HCC**

√7ᵗʰ T52.1X3 Toxic effect of benzene, assault

√7ᵗʰ T52.1X4 Toxic effect of benzene, undetermined

√5ᵗʰ T52.2 Toxic effects of homologues of benzene
Toxic effects of toluene [methylbenzene]
Toxic effects of xylene [dimethylbenzene]

√6ᵗʰ T52.2X Toxic effects of homologues of benzene

√7ᵗʰ T52.2X1 Toxic effect of homologues of benzene, accidental (unintentional)
Toxic effects of homologues of benzene NOS

¹¹ √7ᵗʰ T52.2X2 Toxic effect of homologues of benzene, intentional self-harm   **HCC**

√7ᵗʰ T52.2X3 Toxic effect of homologues of benzene, assault

√7ᵗʰ T52.2X4 Toxic effect of homologues of benzene, undetermined

√5ᵗʰ T52.3 Toxic effects of glycols

√6ᵗʰ T52.3X Toxic effects of glycols

√7ᵗʰ T52.3X1 Toxic effect of glycols, accidental (unintentional)
Toxic effects of glycols NOS

¹¹ √7ᵗʰ T52.3X2 Toxic effect of glycols, intentional self-harm   **HCC**

√7ᵗʰ T52.3X3 Toxic effect of glycols, assault

√7ᵗʰ T52.3X4 Toxic effect of glycols, undetermined

√5ᵗʰ T52.4 Toxic effects of ketones

√6ᵗʰ T52.4X Toxic effects of ketones

√7ᵗʰ T52.4X1 Toxic effect of ketones, accidental (unintentional)
Toxic effects of ketones NOS

¹¹ √7ᵗʰ T52.4X2 Toxic effect of ketones, intentional self-harm   **HCC**

√7ᵗʰ T52.4X3 Toxic effect of ketones, assault

√7ᵗʰ T52.4X4 Toxic effect of ketones, undetermined

√5ᵗʰ T52.8 Toxic effects of other organic solvents

√6ᵗʰ T52.8X Toxic effects of other organic solvents

√7ᵗʰ T52.8X1 Toxic effect of other organic solvents, accidental (unintentional)
Toxic effects of other organic solvents NOS

¹¹ √7ᵗʰ T52.8X2 Toxic effect of other organic solvents, intentional self-harm   **HCC**

√7ᵗʰ T52.8X3 Toxic effect of other organic solvents, assault

√7ᵗʰ T52.8X4 Toxic effect of other organic solvents, undetermined

√5ᵗʰ T52.9 Toxic effects of unspecified organic solvent

√ₓ7ᵗʰ T52.91 Toxic effect of unspecified organic solvent, accidental (unintentional)

¹¹ √ₓ7ᵗʰ T52.92 Toxic effect of unspecified organic solvent, intentional self-harm   **HCC**

√ₓ7ᵗʰ T52.93 Toxic effect of unspecified organic solvent, assault

√ₓ7ᵗʰ T52.94 Toxic effect of unspecified organic solvent, undetermined

√4ᵗʰ T53 Toxic effect of halogen derivatives of aliphatic and aromatic hydrocarbons

The appropriate 7th character is to be added to each code from category T53.
A   initial encounter
D   subsequent encounter
S   sequela

√5ᵗʰ T53.0 Toxic effects of carbon tetrachloride
Toxic effects of tetrachloromethane

√6ᵗʰ T53.0X Toxic effects of carbon tetrachloride

√7ᵗʰ T53.0X1 Toxic effect of carbon tetrachloride, accidental (unintentional)
Toxic effects of carbon tetrachloride NOS

¹¹ √7ᵗʰ T53.0X2 Toxic effect of carbon tetrachloride, intentional self-harm   **HCC**

√7ᵗʰ T53.0X3 Toxic effect of carbon tetrachloride, assault

√7ᵗʰ T53.0X4 Toxic effect of carbon tetrachloride, undetermined

√5ᵗʰ T53.1 Toxic effects of chloroform
Toxic effects of trichloromethane

√6ᵗʰ T53.1X Toxic effects of chloroform

√7ᵗʰ T53.1X1 Toxic effect of chloroform, accidental (unintentional)
Toxic effects of chloroform NOS

¹¹ √7ᵗʰ T53.1X2 Toxic effect of chloroform, intentional self-harm   **HCC**

√7ᵗʰ T53.1X3 Toxic effect of chloroform, assault

√7ᵗʰ T53.1X4 Toxic effect of chloroform, undetermined

√5ᵗʰ T53.2 Toxic effects of trichloroethylene
Toxic effects of trichloroethene

√6ᵗʰ T53.2X Toxic effects of trichloroethylene

√7ᵗʰ T53.2X1 Toxic effect of trichloroethylene, accidental (unintentional)
Toxic effects of trichloroethylene NOS

¹¹ √7ᵗʰ T53.2X2 Toxic effect of trichloroethylene, intentional self-harm   **HCC**

√7ᵗʰ T53.2X3 Toxic effect of trichloroethylene, assault

√7ᵗʰ T53.2X4 Toxic effect of trichloroethylene, undetermined

√5ᵗʰ T53.3 Toxic effects of tetrachloroethylene
Toxic effects of perchloroethylene
Toxic effect of tetrachloroethene

√6ᵗʰ T53.3X Toxic effects of tetrachloroethylene

√7ᵗʰ T53.3X1 Toxic effect of tetrachloroethylene, accidental (unintentional)
Toxic effects of tetrachloroethylene NOS

¹¹ √7ᵗʰ T53.3X2 Toxic effect of tetrachloroethylene, intentional self-harm   **HCC**

√7ᵗʰ T53.3X3 Toxic effect of tetrachloroethylene, assault

√7ᵗʰ T53.3X4 Toxic effect of tetrachloroethylene, undetermined

√5ᵗʰ T53.4 Toxic effects of dichloromethane
Toxic effects of methylene chloride

√6ᵗʰ T53.4X Toxic effects of dichloromethane

√7ᵗʰ T53.4X1 Toxic effect of dichloromethane, accidental (unintentional)
Toxic effects of dichloromethane NOS

¹¹ √7ᵗʰ T53.4X2 Toxic effect of dichloromethane, intentional self-harm   **HCC**

√7ᵗʰ T53.4X3 Toxic effect of dichloromethane, assault

√7ᵗʰ T53.4X4 Toxic effect of dichloromethane, undetermined

√5ᵗʰ T53.5 Toxic effects of chlorofluorocarbons

√6ᵗʰ T53.5X Toxic effects of chlorofluorocarbons

√7ᵗʰ T53.5X1 Toxic effect of chlorofluorocarbons, accidental (unintentional)
Toxic effects of chlorofluorocarbons NOS

¹¹ √7ᵗʰ T53.5X2 Toxic effect of chlorofluorocarbons, intentional self-harm   **HCC**

√7ᵗʰ T53.5X3 Toxic effect of chlorofluorocarbons, assault

√7ᵗʰ T53.5X4 Toxic effect of chlorofluorocarbons, undetermined

√5ᵗʰ T53.6 Toxic effects of other halogen derivatives of aliphatic hydrocarbons

√6ᵗʰ T53.6X Toxic effects of other halogen derivatives of aliphatic hydrocarbons

√7ᵗʰ T53.6X1 Toxic effect of other halogen derivatives of aliphatic hydrocarbons, accidental (unintentional)
Toxic effects of other halogen derivatives of aliphatic hydrocarbons NOS

¹¹ √7ᵗʰ T53.6X2 Toxic effect of other halogen derivatives of aliphatic hydrocarbons, intentional self-harm   **HCC**

√7ᵗʰ T53.6X3 Toxic effect of other halogen derivatives of aliphatic hydrocarbons, assault

√7ᵗʰ T53.6X4 Toxic effect of other halogen derivatives of aliphatic hydrocarbons, undetermined

---

¹¹ HCC with 7th character indicating initial encounter (A or B - specific to category) OR sequela.

Ⓝ Newborn: 0   Ⓟ Pediatric: 0-17   Ⓜ Maternity: 12-55   Ⓐ Adult: 15-124   **MCC** Major CC Condition   **PDxMCC** PDx acts as own MCC   **CC** CC Condition   **PDxCC** PDx acts as own CC

1122   ICD-10-CM 2018

✓5th **T53.7** **Toxic effects of other halogen derivatives of aromatic hydrocarbons**

    ✓6th **T53.7X** **Toxic effects of other** halogen derivatives of aromatic hydrocarbons

       ✓7th **T53.7X1** **Toxic effect of other halogen derivatives of aromatic hydrocarbons,** accidental (unintentional)
          Toxic effects of other halogen derivatives of aromatic hydrocarbons NOS

      11 ✓7th **T53.7X2** **Toxic effect of other halogen derivatives of aromatic hydrocarbons, intentional self-harm**   HCC

       ✓7th **T53.7X3** **Toxic effect of other halogen derivatives of aromatic hydrocarbons, assault**

       ✓7th **T53.7X4** **Toxic effect of other halogen derivatives of aromatic hydrocarbons, undetermined**

✓5th **T53.9** **Toxic effects of** unspecified halogen derivatives of aliphatic and aromatic hydrocarbons

    ✓x7th **T53.91** **Toxic effect of unspecified halogen derivatives of aliphatic and aromatic hydrocarbons, accidental (unintentional)**

   11 ✓x7th **T53.92** **Toxic effect of unspecified halogen derivatives of aliphatic and aromatic hydrocarbons, intentional self-harm**   HCC

    ✓x7th **T53.93** **Toxic effect of unspecified halogen derivatives of aliphatic and aromatic hydrocarbons, assault**

    ✓x7th **T53.94** **Toxic effect of unspecified halogen derivatives of aliphatic and aromatic hydrocarbons, undetermined**

✓4th **T54** **Toxic effect of corrosive substances**

> The appropriate 7th character is to be added to each code from category T54.
> A   initial encounter
> D   subsequent encounter
> S   sequela

   ✓5th **T54.0** **Toxic effects of phenol and phenol homologues**

    ✓6th **T54.0X** **Toxic effects of** phenol and phenol homologues

       ✓7th **T54.0X1** **Toxic effect of phenol and phenol homologues, accidental (unintentional)**
          Toxic effects of phenol and phenol homologues NOS

      11 ✓7th **T54.0X2** **Toxic effect of phenol and phenol homologues, intentional self-harm**   HCC

       ✓7th **T54.0X3** **Toxic effect of phenol and phenol homologues, assault**

       ✓7th **T54.0X4** **Toxic effect of phenol and phenol homologues, undetermined**

   ✓5th **T54.1** **Toxic effects of other corrosive organic compounds**

    ✓6th **T54.1X** **Toxic effects of** other corrosive organic compounds

       ✓7th **T54.1X1** **Toxic effect of other corrosive organic compounds, accidental (unintentional)**
          Toxic effects of other corrosive organic compounds NOS

      11 ✓7th **T54.1X2** **Toxic effect of other corrosive organic compounds, intentional self-harm**   HCC

       ✓7th **T54.1X3** **Toxic effect of other corrosive organic compounds, assault**

       ✓7th **T54.1X4** **Toxic effect of other corrosive organic compounds, undetermined**

   ✓5th **T54.2** **Toxic effects of corrosive acids and acid-like substances**
      Toxic effects of hydrochloric acid
      Toxic effects of sulfuric acid

    ✓6th **T54.2X** **Toxic effects of corrosive** acids and acid-like substances

       ✓7th **T54.2X1** **Toxic effect of corrosive acids and acid-like substances, accidental (unintentional)**
          Toxic effects of corrosive acids and acid-like substances NOS

      11 ✓7th **T54.2X2** **Toxic effect of corrosive acids and acid-like substances, intentional self-harm**   HCC

       ✓7th **T54.2X3** **Toxic effect of corrosive acids and acid-like substances, assault**

       ✓7th **T54.2X4** **Toxic effect of corrosive acids and acid-like substances, undetermined**

✓5th **T54.3** **Toxic effects of corrosive alkalis and alkali-like substances**
      Toxic effects of potassium hydroxide
      Toxic effects of sodium hydroxide

    ✓6th **T54.3X** **Toxic effects of corrosive** alkalis and alkali-like substances

       ✓7th **T54.3X1** **Toxic effect of corrosive alkalis and alkali-like substances, accidental (unintentional)**
          Toxic effects of corrosive alkalis and alkali-like substances NOS

      11 ✓7th **T54.3X2** **Toxic effect of corrosive alkalis and alkali-like substances, intentional self-harm**   HCC

       ✓7th **T54.3X3** **Toxic effect of corrosive alkalis and alkali-like substances, assault**

       ✓7th **T54.3X4** **Toxic effect of corrosive alkalis and alkali-like substances, undetermined**

✓5th **T54.9** **Toxic effects of** unspecified corrosive substance

    ✓x7th **T54.91** **Toxic effect of unspecified corrosive substance, accidental (unintentional)**

   11 ✓x7th **T54.92** **Toxic effect of unspecified corrosive substance, intentional self-harm**   HCC

    ✓x7th **T54.93** **Toxic effect of unspecified corrosive substance, assault**

    ✓x7th **T54.94** **Toxic effect of unspecified corrosive substance, undetermined**

✓4th **T55** **Toxic effect of soaps and detergents**

> The appropriate 7th character is to be added to each code from category T55.
> A   initial encounter
> D   subsequent encounter
> S   sequela

   ✓5th **T55.0** **Toxic effect of soaps**

    ✓6th **T55.0X** **Toxic effect of** soaps

       ✓7th **T55.0X1** **Toxic effect of soaps, accidental (unintentional)**
          Toxic effect of soaps NOS

      11 ✓7th **T55.0X2** **Toxic effect of soaps, intentional self-harm**   HCC

       ✓7th **T55.0X3** **Toxic effect of soaps, assault**

       ✓7th **T55.0X4** **Toxic effect of soaps, undetermined**

   ✓5th **T55.1** **Toxic effect of detergents**

    ✓6th **T55.1X** **Toxic effect of** detergents

       ✓7th **T55.1X1** **Toxic effect of detergents, accidental (unintentional)**
          Toxic effect of detergents NOS

      11 ✓7th **T55.1X2** **Toxic effect of detergents, intentional self-harm**   HCC

       ✓7th **T55.1X3** **Toxic effect of detergents, assault**

       ✓7th **T55.1X4** **Toxic effect of detergents, undetermined**

✓4th **T56** **Toxic effect of metals**
    INCLUDES   toxic effects of fumes and vapors of metals
          toxic effects of metals from all sources, except medicinal substances
   Use additional code to identify any retained metal foreign body, if applicable (Z18.0-, T18.1-)
    EXCLUDES 1   arsenic and its compounds (T57.0)
          manganese and its compounds (T57.2)

> The appropriate 7th character is to be added to each code from category T56.
> A   initial encounter
> D   subsequent encounter
> S   sequela

   ✓5th **T56.0** **Toxic effects of lead and its compounds**

    ✓6th **T56.0X** **Toxic effects of** lead and its compounds

       ✓7th **T56.0X1** **Toxic effect of lead and its compounds, accidental (unintentional)**
          Toxic effects of lead and its compounds NOS

      11 ✓7th **T56.0X2** **Toxic effect of lead and its compounds, intentional self-harm**   HCC

       ✓7th **T56.0X3** **Toxic effect of lead and its compounds, assault**

---

11   HCC with 7th character indicating initial encounter (A or B - specific to category) OR sequela.

✓ Additional Character Req   ✓x7th Placeholder Alert   Unacceptable PDx   Manifestation   H1 - H14 HAC   HCC CMS-HCC Condition   EXCLUDES 1 Not Coded Here   EXCLUDES 2 Not Included Here

ICD-10-CM 2018   1123

T53.7–T56.0X3

✓7th **T56.0X4** **Toxic effect of lead and its compounds, undetermined**

✓5th **T56.1** **Toxic effects of mercury and its compounds**

    ✓6th **T56.1X** **Toxic effects of mercury and its compounds**

       ✓7th **T56.1X1** **Toxic effect of mercury and its compounds, accidental (unintentional)**
          Toxic effects of mercury and its compounds NOS

       11 ✓7th **T56.1X2** **Toxic effect of mercury and its compounds, intentional self-harm** `HCC`

       ✓7th **T56.1X3** **Toxic effect of mercury and its compounds, assault**

       ✓7th **T56.1X4** **Toxic effect of mercury and its compounds, undetermined**

✓5th **T56.2** **Toxic effects of chromium and its compounds**

    ✓6th **T56.2X** **Toxic effects of chromium and its compounds**

       ✓7th **T56.2X1** **Toxic effect of chromium and its compounds, accidental (unintentional)**
          Toxic effects of chromium and its compounds NOS

       11 ✓7th **T56.2X2** **Toxic effect of chromium and its compounds, intentional self-harm** `HCC`

       ✓7th **T56.2X3** **Toxic effect of chromium and its compounds, assault**

       ✓7th **T56.2X4** **Toxic effect of chromium and its compounds, undetermined**

✓5th **T56.3** **Toxic effects of cadmium and its compounds**

    ✓6th **T56.3X** **Toxic effects of cadmium and its compounds**

       ✓7th **T56.3X1** **Toxic effect of cadmium and its compounds, accidental (unintentional)**
          Toxic effects of cadmium and its compounds NOS

       11 ✓7th **T56.3X2** **Toxic effect of cadmium and its compounds, intentional self-harm** `HCC`

       ✓7th **T56.3X3** **Toxic effect of cadmium and its compounds, assault**

       ✓7th **T56.3X4** **Toxic effect of cadmium and its compounds, undetermined**

✓5th **T56.4** **Toxic effects of copper and its compounds**

    ✓6th **T56.4X** **Toxic effects of copper and its compounds**

       ✓7th **T56.4X1** **Toxic effect of copper and its compounds, accidental (unintentional)**
          Toxic effect of copper and its compounds NOS

       11 ✓7th **T56.4X2** **Toxic effect of copper and its compounds, intentional self-harm** `HCC`

       ✓7th **T56.4X3** **Toxic effect of copper and its compounds, assault**

       ✓7th **T56.4X4** **Toxic effect of copper and its compounds, undetermined**

✓5th **T56.5** **Toxic effects of zinc and its compounds**

    ✓6th **T56.5X** **Toxic effects of zinc and its compounds**

       ✓7th **T56.5X1** **Toxic effect of zinc and its compounds, accidental (unintentional)**
          Toxic effect of zinc and its compounds NOS

       11 ✓7th **T56.5X2** **Toxic effect of zinc and its compounds, intentional self-harm** `HCC`

       ✓7th **T56.5X3** **Toxic effect of zinc and its compounds, assault**

       ✓7th **T56.5X4** **Toxic effect of zinc and its compounds, undetermined**

✓5th **T56.6** **Toxic effects of tin and its compounds**

    ✓6th **T56.6X** **Toxic effects of tin and its compounds**

       ✓7th **T56.6X1** **Toxic effect of tin and its compounds, accidental (unintentional)**
          Toxic effects of tin and its compounds NOS

       11 ✓7th **T56.6X2** **Toxic effect of tin and its compounds, intentional self-harm** `HCC`

       ✓7th **T56.6X3** **Toxic effect of tin and its compounds, assault**

       ✓7th **T56.6X4** **Toxic effect of tin and its compounds, undetermined**

✓5th **T56.7** **Toxic effects of beryllium and its compounds**

    ✓6th **T56.7X** **Toxic effects of beryllium and its compounds**

       ✓7th **T56.7X1** **Toxic effect of beryllium and its compounds, accidental (unintentional)**
          Toxic effects of beryllium and its compounds NOS

       11 ✓7th **T56.7X2** **Toxic effect of beryllium and its compounds, intentional self-harm** `HCC`

       ✓7th **T56.7X3** **Toxic effect of beryllium and its compounds, assault**

       ✓7th **T56.7X4** **Toxic effect of beryllium and its compounds, undetermined**

✓5th **T56.8** **Toxic effects of other metals**

    ✓6th **T56.81** **Toxic effect of thallium**

       ✓7th **T56.811** **Toxic effect of thallium, accidental (unintentional)**
          Toxic effect of thallium NOS

       11 ✓7th **T56.812** **Toxic effect of thallium, intentional self-harm** `HCC`

       ✓7th **T56.813** **Toxic effect of thallium, assault**

       ✓7th **T56.814** **Toxic effect of thallium, undetermined**

    ✓6th **T56.89** **Toxic effects of other metals**

       ✓7th **T56.891** **Toxic effect of other metals, accidental (unintentional)**
          Toxic effects of other metals NOS

       11 ✓7th **T56.892** **Toxic effect of other metals, intentional self-harm** `HCC`

       ✓7th **T56.893** **Toxic effect of other metals, assault**

       ✓7th **T56.894** **Toxic effect of other metals, undetermined**

✓5th **T56.9** **Toxic effects of unspecified metal**

    ✓x7th **T56.91** **Toxic effect of unspecified metal, accidental (unintentional)**

    11 ✓x7th **T56.92** **Toxic effect of unspecified metal, intentional self-harm** `HCC`

    ✓x7th **T56.93** **Toxic effect of unspecified metal, assault**

    ✓x7th **T56.94** **Toxic effect of unspecified metal, undetermined**

✓4th **T57** **Toxic effect of other inorganic substances**

> The appropriate 7th character is to be added to each code from category T57.
> A   initial encounter
> D   subsequent encounter
> S   sequela

✓5th **T57.0** **Toxic effect of arsenic and its compounds**

    ✓6th **T57.0X** **Toxic effect of arsenic and its compounds**

       ✓7th **T57.0X1** **Toxic effect of arsenic and its compounds, accidental (unintentional)**
          Toxic effect of arsenic and its compounds NOS

       11 ✓7th **T57.0X2** **Toxic effect of arsenic and its compounds, intentional self-harm** `HCC`

       ✓7th **T57.0X3** **Toxic effect of arsenic and its compounds, assault**

       ✓7th **T57.0X4** **Toxic effect of arsenic and its compounds, undetermined**

✓5th **T57.1** **Toxic effect of phosphorus and its compounds**

    EXCLUDES 1   *organophosphate insecticides (T60.0)*

    ✓6th **T57.1X** **Toxic effect of phosphorus and its compounds**

       ✓7th **T57.1X1** **Toxic effect of phosphorus and its compounds, accidental (unintentional)**
          Toxic effect of phosphorus and its compounds NOS

       11 ✓7th **T57.1X2** **Toxic effect of phosphorus and its compounds, intentional self-harm** `HCC`

       ✓7th **T57.1X3** **Toxic effect of phosphorus and its compounds, assault**

       ✓7th **T57.1X4** **Toxic effect of phosphorus and its compounds, undetermined**

---

11 HCC with 7th character indicating initial encounter (A or B - specific to category) OR sequela.

N Newborn: 0   P Pediatric: 0-17   M Maternity: 12-55   A Adult: 15-124   `MCC` Major CC Condition   `PDxMCC` PDx acts as own MCC   `CC` CC Condition   `PDxCC` PDx acts as own CC

1124   ICD-10-CM 2018

✓5th **T57.2** **Toxic effect of manganese and its compounds**

     ✓6th **T57.2X** **Toxic effect of manganese and its compounds**

         ✓7th **T57.2X1** **Toxic effect of manganese and its compounds, accidental (unintentional)**
             Toxic effect of manganese and its compounds NOS

         11 ✓7th **T57.2X2** **Toxic effect of manganese and its compounds, intentional self-harm** HCC

         ✓7th **T57.2X3** **Toxic effect of manganese and its compounds, assault**

         ✓7th **T57.2X4** **Toxic effect of manganese and its compounds, undetermined**

✓5th **T57.3** **Toxic effect of hydrogen cyanide**

     ✓6th **T57.3X** **Toxic effect of hydrogen cyanide**

         ✓7th **T57.3X1** **Toxic effect of hydrogen cyanide, accidental (unintentional)**
             Toxic effect of hydrogen cyanide NOS

         11 ✓7th **T57.3X2** **Toxic effect of hydrogen cyanide, intentional self-harm** HCC

         ✓7th **T57.3X3** **Toxic effect of hydrogen cyanide, assault**

         ✓7th **T57.3X4** **Toxic effect of hydrogen cyanide, undetermined**

✓5th **T57.8** **Toxic effect of other specified inorganic substances**

     ✓6th **T57.8X** **Toxic effect of other specified inorganic substances**

         ✓7th **T57.8X1** **Toxic effect of other specified inorganic substances, accidental (unintentional)**
             Toxic effect of other specified inorganic substances NOS

         11 ✓7th **T57.8X2** **Toxic effect of other specified inorganic substances, intentional self-harm** HCC

         ✓7th **T57.8X3** **Toxic effect of other specified inorganic substances, assault**

         ✓7th **T57.8X4** **Toxic effect of other specified inorganic substances, undetermined**

✓5th **T57.9** **Toxic effect of unspecified inorganic substance**

     ✓x7th **T57.91** **Toxic effect of unspecified inorganic substance, accidental (unintentional)**

     11 ✓x7th **T57.92** **Toxic effect of unspecified inorganic substance, intentional self-harm** HCC

     ✓x7th **T57.93** **Toxic effect of unspecified inorganic substance, assault**

     ✓x7th **T57.94** **Toxic effect of unspecified inorganic substance, undetermined**

✓4th **T58** **Toxic effect of carbon monoxide**

     INCLUDES   asphyxiation from carbon monoxide
              toxic effect of carbon monoxide from all sources

     The appropriate 7th character is to be added to each code from category T58.
     A   initial encounter
     D   subsequent encounter
     S   sequela

     ✓5th **T58.0** **Toxic effect of carbon monoxide from motor vehicle exhaust**
         Toxic effect of exhaust gas from gas engine
         Toxic effect of exhaust gas from motor pump

         ✓x7th **T58.01** **Toxic effect of carbon monoxide from motor vehicle exhaust, accidental (unintentional)**

         11 ✓x7th **T58.02** **Toxic effect of carbon monoxide from motor vehicle exhaust, intentional self-harm** HCC

         ✓x7th **T58.03** **Toxic effect of carbon monoxide from motor vehicle exhaust, assault**

         ✓x7th **T58.04** **Toxic effect of carbon monoxide from motor vehicle exhaust, undetermined**

     ✓5th **T58.1** **Toxic effect of carbon monoxide from utility gas**
         Toxic effect of acetylene
         Toxic effect of gas NOS used for lighting, heating, cooking
         Toxic effect of water gas

         ✓x7th **T58.11** **Toxic effect of carbon monoxide from utility gas, accidental (unintentional)**

         11 ✓x7th **T58.12** **Toxic effect of carbon monoxide from utility gas, intentional self-harm** HCC

         ✓x7th **T58.13** **Toxic effect of carbon monoxide from utility gas, assault**

         ✓x7th **T58.14** **Toxic effect of carbon monoxide from utility gas, undetermined**

     ✓5th **T58.2** **Toxic effect of carbon monoxide from incomplete combustion of other domestic fuels**
         Toxic effect of carbon monoxide from incomplete combustion of coal, coke, kerosene, wood

         ✓6th **T58.2X** **Toxic effect of carbon monoxide from incomplete combustion of other domestic fuels**

             ✓7th **T58.2X1** **Toxic effect of carbon monoxide from incomplete combustion of other domestic fuels, accidental (unintentional)**

             11 ✓7th **T58.2X2** **Toxic effect of carbon monoxide from incomplete combustion of other domestic fuels, intentional self-harm** HCC

             ✓7th **T58.2X3** **Toxic effect of carbon monoxide from incomplete combustion of other domestic fuels, assault**

             ✓7th **T58.2X4** **Toxic effect of carbon monoxide from incomplete combustion of other domestic fuels, undetermined**

     ✓5th **T58.8** **Toxic effect of carbon monoxide from other source**
         Toxic effect of carbon monoxide from blast furnace gas
         Toxic effect of carbon monoxide from fuels in industrial use
         Toxic effect of carbon monoxide from kiln vapor

         ✓6th **T58.8X** **Toxic effect of carbon monoxide from other source**

             ✓7th **T58.8X1** **Toxic effect of carbon monoxide from other source, accidental (unintentional)**

             11 ✓7th **T58.8X2** **Toxic effect of carbon monoxide from other source, intentional self-harm** HCC

             ✓7th **T58.8X3** **Toxic effect of carbon monoxide from other source, assault**

             ✓7th **T58.8X4** **Toxic effect of carbon monoxide from other source, undetermined**

     ✓5th **T58.9** **Toxic effect of carbon monoxide from unspecified source**

         ✓x7th **T58.91** **Toxic effect of carbon monoxide from unspecified source, accidental (unintentional)**

         11 ✓x7th **T58.92** **Toxic effect of carbon monoxide from unspecified source, intentional self-harm** HCC

         ✓x7th **T58.93** **Toxic effect of carbon monoxide from unspecified source, assault**

         ✓x7th **T58.94** **Toxic effect of carbon monoxide from unspecified source, undetermined**

✓4th **T59** **Toxic effect of other gases, fumes and vapors**

     INCLUDES   aerosol propellants
     EXCLUDES 1   *chlorofluorocarbons (T53.5)*

     The appropriate 7th character is to be added to each code from category T59.
     A   initial encounter
     D   subsequent encounter
     S   sequela

     ✓5th **T59.0** **Toxic effect of nitrogen oxides**

         ✓6th **T59.0X** **Toxic effect of nitrogen oxides**

             ✓7th **T59.0X1** **Toxic effect of nitrogen oxides, accidental (unintentional)**
                 Toxic effect of nitrogen oxides NOS

             11 ✓7th **T59.0X2** **Toxic effect of nitrogen oxides, intentional self-harm** HCC

             ✓7th **T59.0X3** **Toxic effect of nitrogen oxides, assault**

             ✓7th **T59.0X4** **Toxic effect of nitrogen oxides, undetermined**

     ✓5th **T59.1** **Toxic effect of sulfur dioxide**

         ✓6th **T59.1X** **Toxic effect of sulfur dioxide**

             ✓7th **T59.1X1** **Toxic effect of sulfur dioxide, accidental (unintentional)**
                 Toxic effect of sulfur dioxide NOS

             11 ✓7th **T59.1X2** **Toxic effect of sulfur dioxide, intentional self-harm** HCC

             ✓7th **T59.1X3** **Toxic effect of sulfur dioxide, assault**

             ✓7th **T59.1X4** **Toxic effect of sulfur dioxide, undetermined**

---

11   HCC with 7th character indicating initial encounter (A or B - specific to category) OR sequela.

✓ Additional Character Req   ✓x7th Placeholder Alert   Unacceptable PDx   Manifestation   H1 - H14 HAC   HCC CMS-HCC Condition   EXCLUDES 1 Not Coded Here   EXCLUDES 2 Not Included Here

T59.2 Toxic effect of formaldehyde

  T59.2X Toxic effect of formaldehyde

    T59.2X1 Toxic effect of formaldehyde, accidental (unintentional)
Toxic effect of formaldehyde NOS

    11 **T59.2X2 Toxic effect of formaldehyde, intentional self-harm** HCC

    T59.2X3 Toxic effect of formaldehyde, assault

    T59.2X4 Toxic effect of formaldehyde, undetermined

T59.3 Toxic effect of lacrimogenic gas
Toxic effect of tear gas

  T59.3X Toxic effect of lacrimogenic gas

    T59.3X1 Toxic effect of lacrimogenic gas, accidental (unintentional)
Toxic effect of lacrimogenic gas NOS

    11 **T59.3X2 Toxic effect of lacrimogenic gas, intentional self-harm** HCC

    T59.3X3 Toxic effect of lacrimogenic gas, assault

    T59.3X4 Toxic effect of lacrimogenic gas, undetermined

T59.4 Toxic effect of chlorine gas

  T59.4X Toxic effect of chlorine gas

    T59.4X1 Toxic effect of chlorine gas, accidental (unintentional)
Toxic effect of chlorine gas NOS

    11 **T59.4X2 Toxic effect of chlorine gas, intentional self-harm** HCC

    T59.4X3 Toxic effect of chlorine gas, assault

    T59.4X4 Toxic effect of chlorine gas, undetermined

T59.5 Toxic effect of fluorine gas and hydrogen fluoride

  T59.5X Toxic effect of fluorine gas and hydrogen fluoride

    T59.5X1 Toxic effect of fluorine gas and hydrogen fluoride, accidental (unintentional)
Toxic effect of fluorine gas and hydrogen fluoride NOS

    11 **T59.5X2 Toxic effect of fluorine gas and hydrogen fluoride, intentional self-harm** HCC

    T59.5X3 Toxic effect of fluorine gas and hydrogen fluoride, assault

    T59.5X4 Toxic effect of fluorine gas and hydrogen fluoride, undetermined

T59.6 Toxic effect of hydrogen sulfide

  T59.6X Toxic effect of hydrogen sulfide

    T59.6X1 Toxic effect of hydrogen sulfide, accidental (unintentional)
Toxic effect of hydrogen sulfide NOS

    11 **T59.6X2 Toxic effect of hydrogen sulfide, intentional self-harm** HCC

    T59.6X3 Toxic effect of hydrogen sulfide, assault

    T59.6X4 Toxic effect of hydrogen sulfide, undetermined

T59.7 Toxic effect of carbon dioxide

  T59.7X Toxic effect of carbon dioxide

    T59.7X1 Toxic effect of carbon dioxide, accidental (unintentional)
Toxic effect of carbon dioxide NOS

    11 **T59.7X2 Toxic effect of carbon dioxide, intentional self-harm** HCC

    T59.7X3 Toxic effect of carbon dioxide, assault

    T59.7X4 Toxic effect of carbon dioxide, undetermined

T59.8 Toxic effect of other specified gases, fumes and vapors

  T59.81 Toxic effect of smoke
Smoke inhalation

    EXCLUDES 2 *toxic effect of cigarette (tobacco) smoke (T65.22-)*

    T59.811 Toxic effect of smoke, accidental (unintentional)
Toxic effect of smoke NOS
AHA: 2013, 4Q, 121

    11 **T59.812 Toxic effect of smoke, intentional self-harm** HCC

    T59.813 Toxic effect of smoke, assault

    T59.814 Toxic effect of smoke, undetermined

  T59.89 Toxic effect of other specified gases, fumes and vapors

    T59.891 Toxic effect of other specified gases, fumes and vapors, accidental (unintentional)

    11 **T59.892 Toxic effect of other specified gases, fumes and vapors, intentional self-harm** HCC

    T59.893 Toxic effect of other specified gases, fumes and vapors, assault

    T59.894 Toxic effect of other specified gases, fumes and vapors, undetermined

T59.9 Toxic effect of unspecified gases, fumes and vapors

  T59.91 Toxic effect of unspecified gases, fumes and vapors, accidental (unintentional)

  11 **T59.92 Toxic effect of unspecified gases, fumes and vapors, intentional self-harm** HCC

  T59.93 Toxic effect of unspecified gases, fumes and vapors, assault

  T59.94 Toxic effect of unspecified gases, fumes and vapors, undetermined

T60 Toxic effect of pesticides

  INCLUDES toxic effect of wood preservatives

> The appropriate 7th character is to be added to each code from category T60.
> A   initial encounter
> D   subsequent encounter
> S   sequela

T60.0 Toxic effect of organophosphate and carbamate insecticides

  T60.0X Toxic effect of organophosphate and carbamate insecticides

    T60.0X1 Toxic effect of organophosphate and carbamate insecticides, accidental (unintentional)
Toxic effect of organophosphate and carbamate insecticides NOS

    11 **T60.0X2 Toxic effect of organophosphate and carbamate insecticides, intentional self-harm** HCC

    T60.0X3 Toxic effect of organophosphate and carbamate insecticides, assault

    T60.0X4 Toxic effect of organophosphate and carbamate insecticides, undetermined

T60.1 Toxic effect of halogenated insecticides

  EXCLUDES 1 *chlorinated hydrocarbon (T53.-)*

  T60.1X Toxic effect of halogenated insecticides

    T60.1X1 Toxic effect of halogenated insecticides, accidental (unintentional)
Toxic effect of halogenated insecticides NOS

    11 **T60.1X2 Toxic effect of halogenated insecticides, intentional self-harm** HCC

    T60.1X3 Toxic effect of halogenated insecticides, assault

    T60.1X4 Toxic effect of halogenated insecticides, undetermined

T60.2 Toxic effect of other insecticides

  T60.2X Toxic effect of other insecticides

    T60.2X1 Toxic effect of other insecticides, accidental (unintentional)
Toxic effect of other insecticides NOS

    11 **T60.2X2 Toxic effect of other insecticides, intentional self-harm** HCC

    T60.2X3 Toxic effect of other insecticides, assault

    T60.2X4 Toxic effect of other insecticides, undetermined

T60.3 Toxic effect of herbicides and fungicides

  T60.3X Toxic effect of herbicides and fungicides

    T60.3X1 Toxic effect of herbicides and fungicides, accidental (unintentional)
Toxic effect of herbicides and fungicides NOS

---

11 HCC with 7th character indicating initial encounter (A or B - specific to category) OR sequela.

N Newborn: 0   P Pediatric: 0-17   M Maternity: 12-55   A Adult: 15-124   MCC Major CC Condition   PDx MCC PDx acts as own MCC   CC CC Condition   PDx CC PDx acts as own CC

1126   ICD-10-CM 2018

     11   ✓7ᵗʰ   **T60.3X2**   **Toxic effect of herbicides and**   HCC
                              fungicides, intentional self-harm

      ✓7ᵗʰ   **T60.3X3**   **Toxic effect of herbicides and fungicides,** **assault**

      ✓7ᵗʰ   **T60.3X4**   **Toxic effect of herbicides and fungicides,** **undetermined**

✓5ᵗʰ   **T60.4**   **Toxic effect of rodenticides**
        EXCLUDES 1   strychnine and its salts (T65.1)
                   thallium (T56.81-)

   ✓6ᵗʰ   **T60.4X**   **Toxic effect of** rodenticides

      ✓7ᵗʰ   **T60.4X1**   **Toxic effect of rodenticides, accidental** **(unintentional)**
                             Toxic effect of rodenticides NOS

     11   ✓7ᵗʰ   **T60.4X2**   **Toxic effect of rodenticides,**   HCC
                              intentional self-harm

      ✓7ᵗʰ   **T60.4X3**   **Toxic effect of rodenticides, assault**

      ✓7ᵗʰ   **T60.4X4**   **Toxic effect of rodenticides,** **undetermined**

✓5ᵗʰ   **T60.8**   **Toxic effect of other pesticides**

   ✓6ᵗʰ   **T60.8X**   **Toxic effect of** other pesticides

      ✓7ᵗʰ   **T60.8X1**   **Toxic effect of other pesticides, accidental** **(unintentional)**
                              Toxic effect of other pesticides NOS

     11   ✓7ᵗʰ   **T60.8X2**   **Toxic effect of other pesticides,**   HCC
                              intentional self-harm

      ✓7ᵗʰ   **T60.8X3**   **Toxic effect of other pesticides, assault**

      ✓7ᵗʰ   **T60.8X4**   **Toxic effect of other pesticides,** **undetermined**

✓5ᵗʰ   **T60.9**   **Toxic effect of** unspecified pesticide

   ✓x7ᵗʰ   **T60.91**   **Toxic effect of unspecified pesticide, accidental** **(unintentional)**

   11   ✓x7ᵗʰ   **T60.92**   **Toxic effect of unspecified pesticide,**   HCC
                         intentional self-harm

   ✓x7ᵗʰ   **T60.93**   **Toxic effect of unspecified pesticide, assault**

   ✓x7ᵗʰ   **T60.94**   **Toxic effect of unspecified pesticide, undetermined**

✓4ᵗʰ   **T61**   **Toxic effect of noxious substances eaten as seafood**
      EXCLUDES 1   allergic reaction to food, such as:
                 anaphylactic reaction or shock due to adverse food reaction
                    (T78.0-)
                 bacterial foodborne intoxications (A05.-)
                 dermatitis (L23.6, L25.4, L27.2)
         food protein-induced enterocolitis syndrome (K52.21)
                 food protein-induced enteropathy (K52.22)
                 gastroenteritis (noninfective) (K52.29)
         toxic effect of aflatoxin and other mycotoxins (T64)
         toxic effect of cyanides (T65.0-)
         toxic effect of harmful algae bloom (T65.82-)
         toxic effect of hydrogen cyanide (T57.3-)
         toxic effect of mercury (T56.1-)
         toxic effect of red tide (T65.82-)

     The appropriate 7th character is to be added to each code from
     category T61.
     A   initial encounter
     D   subsequent encounter
     S   sequela

   ✓5ᵗʰ   **T61.0**   **Ciguatera fish poisoning**

     ✓x7ᵗʰ   **T61.01**   **Ciguatera fish poisoning, accidental (unintentional)**

   11   ✓x7ᵗʰ   **T61.02**   **Ciguatera fish poisoning, intentional self-harm**   HCC

     ✓x7ᵗʰ   **T61.03**   **Ciguatera fish poisoning, assault**

     ✓x7ᵗʰ   **T61.04**   **Ciguatera fish poisoning, undetermined**

   ✓5ᵗʰ   **T61.1**   **Scombroid fish poisoning**
           Histamine-like syndrome

     ✓x7ᵗʰ   **T61.11**   **Scombroid fish poisoning, accidental (unintentional)**

   11   ✓x7ᵗʰ   **T61.12**   **Scombroid fish poisoning, intentional self-harm**   HCC

     ✓x7ᵗʰ   **T61.13**   **Scombroid fish poisoning, assault**

     ✓x7ᵗʰ   **T61.14**   **Scombroid fish poisoning, undetermined**

   ✓5ᵗʰ   **T61.7**   **Other fish and shellfish poisoning**

     ✓6ᵗʰ   **T61.77**   **Other fish poisoning**

       ✓7ᵗʰ   **T61.771**   **Other fish poisoning, accidental** **(unintentional)**

     11   ✓7ᵗʰ   **T61.772**   **Other fish poisoning, intentional**   HCC
                            self-harm

       ✓7ᵗʰ   **T61.773**   **Other fish poisoning, assault**

       ✓7ᵗʰ   **T61.774**   **Other fish poisoning, undetermined**

     ✓6ᵗʰ   **T61.78**   **Other shellfish poisoning**

       ✓7ᵗʰ   **T61.781**   **Other shellfish poisoning, accidental** **(unintentional)**

     11   ✓7ᵗʰ   **T61.782**   **Other shellfish poisoning, intentional**   HCC
                            self-harm

       ✓7ᵗʰ   **T61.783**   **Other shellfish poisoning, assault**

       ✓7ᵗʰ   **T61.784**   **Other shellfish poisoning, undetermined**

   ✓5ᵗʰ   **T61.8**   **Toxic effect of other seafood**

     ✓6ᵗʰ   **T61.8X**   **Toxic effect of** other seafood

       ✓7ᵗʰ   **T61.8X1**   **Toxic effect of other seafood, accidental** **(unintentional)**

     11   ✓7ᵗʰ   **T61.8X2**   **Toxic effect of other seafood,**   HCC
                            intentional self-harm

       ✓7ᵗʰ   **T61.8X3**   **Toxic effect of other seafood, assault**

       ✓7ᵗʰ   **T61.8X4**   **Toxic effect of other seafood,** **undetermined**

   ✓5ᵗʰ   **T61.9**   **Toxic effect of** unspecified seafood

     ✓x7ᵗʰ   **T61.91**   **Toxic effect of unspecified seafood, accidental** **(unintentional)**

   11   ✓x7ᵗʰ   **T61.92**   **Toxic effect of unspecified seafood, intentional**   HCC
                         self-harm

     ✓x7ᵗʰ   **T61.93**   **Toxic effect of unspecified seafood, assault**

     ✓x7ᵗʰ   **T61.94**   **Toxic effect of unspecified seafood, undetermined**

✓4ᵗʰ   **T62**   **Toxic effect of other noxious substances eaten as food**
      EXCLUDES 1   allergic reaction to food, such as:
                 anaphylactic shock (reaction) due to adverse food reaction
                    (T78.0-)
                 bacterial food borne intoxications (A05.-)
                 dermatitis (L23.6, L25.4, L27.2)
         food protein-induced enterocolitis syndrome (K52.21)
                 food protein-induced enteropathy (K52.22)
                 gastroenteritis (noninfective) (K52.29)
         toxic effect of aflatoxin and other mycotoxins (T64)
         toxic effect of cyanides (T65.0-)
         toxic effect of hydrogen cyanide (T57.3-)
         toxic effect of mercury (T56.1-)

     The appropriate 7th character is to be added to each code from
     category T62.
     A   initial encounter
     D   subsequent encounter
     S   sequela

   ✓5ᵗʰ   **T62.0**   **Toxic effect of ingested mushrooms**

     ✓6ᵗʰ   **T62.0X**   **Toxic effect of** ingested mushrooms

       ✓7ᵗʰ   **T62.0X1**   **Toxic effect of ingested mushrooms,** **accidental (unintentional)**
                            Toxic effect of ingested mushrooms NOS

     11   ✓7ᵗʰ   **T62.0X2**   **Toxic effect of ingested mushrooms,**   HCC
                            intentional self-harm

       ✓7ᵗʰ   **T62.0X3**   **Toxic effect of ingested mushrooms,** **assault**

       ✓7ᵗʰ   **T62.0X4**   **Toxic effect of ingested mushrooms,** **undetermined**

   ✓5ᵗʰ   **T62.1**   **Toxic effect of ingested berries**

     ✓6ᵗʰ   **T62.1X**   **Toxic effect of** ingested berries

       ✓7ᵗʰ   **T62.1X1**   **Toxic effect of ingested berries, accidental** **(unintentional)**
                            Toxic effect of ingested berries NOS

     11   ✓7ᵗʰ   **T62.1X2**   **Toxic effect of ingested berries,**   HCC
                            intentional self-harm

       ✓7ᵗʰ   **T62.1X3**   **Toxic effect of ingested berries, assault**

       ✓7ᵗʰ   **T62.1X4**   **Toxic effect of ingested berries,** **undetermined**

   ✓5ᵗʰ   **T62.2**   **Toxic effect of other ingested (parts of) plant(s)**

     ✓6ᵗʰ   **T62.2X**   **Toxic effect of** other ingested (parts of) plant(s)

       ✓7ᵗʰ   **T62.2X1**   **Toxic effect of other ingested (parts of)** **plant(s), accidental (unintentional)**
                            Toxic effect of other ingested (parts of)
                            plant(s) NOS

     11   ✓7ᵗʰ   **T62.2X2**   **Toxic effect of other ingested**   HCC
                            (parts of) plant(s), intentional self-harm

---

11 HCC with 7th character indicating initial encounter (A or B - specific to category) OR sequela.

✓ Additional Character Req   ✓x7ᵗʰ Placeholder Alert   Unacceptable PDx   Manifestation   H1 - H14 HAC   HCC CMS-HCC Condition   EXCLUDES 1 Not Coded Here   EXCLUDES 2 Not Included Here

ICD-10-CM 2018   1127

√7ᵗʰ **T62.2X3** **Toxic effect of other ingested (parts of) plant(s)**, assault

√7ᵗʰ **T62.2X4** **Toxic effect of other ingested (parts of) plant(s)**, undetermined

√5ᵗʰ **T62.8** **Toxic effect of other specified** noxious substances eaten as food

√6ᵗʰ **T62.8X** **Toxic effect of** other specified noxious substances eaten as food

√7ᵗʰ **T62.8X1** **Toxic effect of other specified noxious substances eaten as food**, accidental (unintentional)

Toxic effect of other specified noxious substances eaten as food NOS

11 √7ᵗʰ **T62.8X2** **Toxic effect of other specified** HCC **noxious substances eaten as food, intentional self-harm**

√7ᵗʰ **T62.8X3** **Toxic effect of other specified noxious substances eaten as food**, assault

√7ᵗʰ **T62.8X4** **Toxic effect of other specified noxious substances eaten as food**, undetermined

√5ᵗʰ **T62.9** **Toxic effect of** unspecified **noxious substance eaten as food**

√x7ᵗʰ **T62.91** **Toxic effect of unspecified noxious substance eaten as food**, accidental (unintentional)

Toxic effect of unspecified noxious substance eaten as food NOS

11 √x7ᵗʰ **T62.92** **Toxic effect of unspecified noxious substance** HCC **eaten as food**, intentional self-harm

√x7ᵗʰ **T62.93** **Toxic effect of unspecified noxious substance eaten as food**, assault

√x7ᵗʰ **T62.94** **Toxic effect of unspecified noxious substance eaten as food**, undetermined

√4ᵗʰ **T63** **Toxic effect of contact with venomous animals and plants**

INCLUDES   bite or touch of venomous animal
pricked or stuck by thorn or leaf

EXCLUDES 2   *ingestion of toxic animal or plant (T61.-, T62.-)*

The appropriate 7th character is to be added to each code from category T63.
A   initial encounter
D   subsequent encounter
S   sequela

√5ᵗʰ **T63.0** **Toxic effect of** snake venom

√6ᵗʰ **T63.00** **Toxic effect of** unspecified **snake venom**

√7ᵗʰ **T63.001** **Toxic effect of unspecified snake venom**, accidental (unintentional)

Toxic effect of unspecified snake venom NOS

11 √7ᵗʰ **T63.002** **Toxic effect of unspecified snake** HCC **venom**, intentional self-harm

√7ᵗʰ **T63.003** **Toxic effect of unspecified snake venom**, assault

√7ᵗʰ **T63.004** **Toxic effect of unspecified snake venom**, undetermined

√6ᵗʰ **T63.01** **Toxic effect of** rattlesnake **venom**

√7ᵗʰ **T63.011** **Toxic effect of rattlesnake venom**, accidental (unintentional)

Toxic effect of rattlesnake venom NOS

11 √7ᵗʰ **T63.012** **Toxic effect of rattlesnake venom**, HCC **intentional self-harm**

√7ᵗʰ **T63.013** **Toxic effect of rattlesnake venom**, assault

√7ᵗʰ **T63.014** **Toxic effect of rattlesnake venom**, undetermined

√6ᵗʰ **T63.02** **Toxic effect of** coral snake **venom**

√7ᵗʰ **T63.021** **Toxic effect of coral snake venom**, accidental (unintentional)

Toxic effect of coral snake venom NOS

11 √7ᵗʰ **T63.022** **Toxic effect of coral snake venom**, HCC **intentional self-harm**

√7ᵗʰ **T63.023** **Toxic effect of coral snake venom**, assault

√7ᵗʰ **T63.024** **Toxic effect of coral snake venom**, undetermined

√6ᵗʰ **T63.03** **Toxic effect of** taipan **venom**

√7ᵗʰ **T63.031** **Toxic effect of taipan venom**, accidental (unintentional)

Toxic effect of taipan venom NOS

11 √7ᵗʰ **T63.032** **Toxic effect of taipan venom**, HCC **intentional self-harm**

√7ᵗʰ **T63.033** **Toxic effect of taipan venom**, assault

√7ᵗʰ **T63.034** **Toxic effect of taipan venom**, undetermined

√6ᵗʰ **T63.04** **Toxic effect of** cobra **venom**

√7ᵗʰ **T63.041** **Toxic effect of cobra venom**, accidental (unintentional)

Toxic effect of cobra venom NOS

11 √7ᵗʰ **T63.042** **Toxic effect of cobra venom**, HCC **intentional self-harm**

√7ᵗʰ **T63.043** **Toxic effect of cobra venom**, assault

√7ᵗʰ **T63.044** **Toxic effect of cobra venom**, undetermined

√6ᵗʰ **T63.06** **Toxic effect of venom of** other North and South American snake

√7ᵗʰ **T63.061** **Toxic effect of venom of other North and South American snake**, accidental (unintentional)

Toxic effect of venom of other North and South American snake NOS

11 √7ᵗʰ **T63.062** **Toxic effect of venom of other North** HCC **and South American snake**, intentional self-harm

√7ᵗʰ **T63.063** **Toxic effect of venom of other North and South American snake**, assault

√7ᵗʰ **T63.064** **Toxic effect of venom of other North and South American snake**, undetermined

√6ᵗʰ **T63.07** **Toxic effect of venom of** other Australian snake

√7ᵗʰ **T63.071** **Toxic effect of venom of other Australian snake**, accidental (unintentional)

Toxic effect of venom of other Australian snake NOS

11 √7ᵗʰ **T63.072** **Toxic effect of venom of other** HCC **Australian snake**, intentional self-harm

√7ᵗʰ **T63.073** **Toxic effect of venom of other Australian snake**, assault

√7ᵗʰ **T63.074** **Toxic effect of venom of other Australian snake**, undetermined

√6ᵗʰ **T63.08** **Toxic effect of venom of** other African and Asian snake

√7ᵗʰ **T63.081** **Toxic effect of venom of other African and Asian snake**, accidental (unintentional)

Toxic effect of venom of other African and Asian snake NOS

11 √7ᵗʰ **T63.082** **Toxic effect of venom of other African** HCC **and Asian snake**, intentional self-harm

√7ᵗʰ **T63.083** **Toxic effect of venom of other African and Asian snake**, assault

√7ᵗʰ **T63.084** **Toxic effect of venom of other African and Asian snake**, undetermined

√6ᵗʰ **T63.09** **Toxic effect of venom of** other snake

√7ᵗʰ **T63.091** **Toxic effect of venom of other snake**, accidental (unintentional)

Toxic effect of venom of other snake NOS

11 √7ᵗʰ **T63.092** **Toxic effect of venom of other snake**, HCC **intentional self-harm**

√7ᵗʰ **T63.093** **Toxic effect of venom of other snake**, assault

√7ᵗʰ **T63.094** **Toxic effect of venom of other snake**, undetermined

√5ᵗʰ **T63.1** **Toxic effect of venom of** other reptiles

√6ᵗʰ **T63.11** **Toxic effect of venom of** gila monster

√7ᵗʰ **T63.111** **Toxic effect of venom of gila monster**, accidental (unintentional)

Toxic effect of venom of gila monster NOS

11 √7ᵗʰ **T63.112** **Toxic effect of venom of gila monster**, HCC **intentional self-harm**

√7ᵗʰ **T63.113** **Toxic effect of venom of gila monster**, assault

√7ᵗʰ **T63.114** **Toxic effect of venom of gila monster**, undetermined

---

11 HCC with 7th character indicating initial encounter (A or B - specific to category) OR sequela.

N Newborn: 0   P Pediatric: 0-17   M Maternity: 12-55   A Adult: 15-124   MCC Major CC Condition   PDxMCC PDx acts as own MCC   CC CC Condition   PDxCC PDx acts as own CC

1128   ICD-10-CM 2018

✓6th **T63.12** **Toxic effect of venom of** other venomous lizard

    ✓7th **T63.121** **Toxic effect of venom of other venomous lizard,** accidental **(unintentional)**
         Toxic effect of venom of other venomous lizard NOS

    11 ✓7th **T63.122** **Toxic effect of venom of other venomous lizard,** intentional self-harm   HCC

    ✓7th **T63.123** **Toxic effect of venom of other venomous lizard,** assault

    ✓7th **T63.124** **Toxic effect of venom of other venomous lizard,** undetermined

✓6th **T63.19** **Toxic effect of venom of** other reptiles

    ✓7th **T63.191** **Toxic effect of venom of other reptiles,** accidental **(unintentional)**
         Toxic effect of venom of other reptiles NOS

    11 ✓7th **T63.192** **Toxic effect of venom of other reptiles,** intentional self-harm   HCC

    ✓7th **T63.193** **Toxic effect of venom of other reptiles,** assault

    ✓7th **T63.194** **Toxic effect of venom of other reptiles,** undetermined

✓5th **T63.2** **Toxic effect of venom of** scorpion

  ✓6th **T63.2X** **Toxic effect of venom of scorpion**

    ✓7th **T63.2X1** **Toxic effect of venom of scorpion,** accidental **(unintentional)**
         Toxic effect of venom of scorpion NOS

    11 ✓7th **T63.2X2** **Toxic effect of venom of scorpion,** intentional self-harm   HCC

    ✓7th **T63.2X3** **Toxic effect of venom of scorpion,** assault

    ✓7th **T63.2X4** **Toxic effect of venom of scorpion,** undetermined

✓5th **T63.3** **Toxic effect of venom of** spider

  ✓6th **T63.30** **Toxic effect of** unspecified **spider venom**

    ✓7th **T63.301** **Toxic effect of unspecified spider venom,** accidental **(unintentional)**

    11 ✓7th **T63.302** **Toxic effect of unspecified spider venom,** intentional self-harm   HCC

    ✓7th **T63.303** **Toxic effect of unspecified spider venom,** assault

    ✓7th **T63.304** **Toxic effect of unspecified spider venom,** undetermined

  ✓6th **T63.31** **Toxic effect of venom of** black widow **spider**

    ✓7th **T63.311** **Toxic effect of venom of black widow spider,** accidental **(unintentional)**

    11 ✓7th **T63.312** **Toxic effect of venom of black widow spider,** intentional self-harm   HCC

    ✓7th **T63.313** **Toxic effect of venom of black widow spider,** assault

    ✓7th **T63.314** **Toxic effect of venom of black widow spider,** undetermined

  ✓6th **T63.32** **Toxic effect of venom of** tarantula

    ✓7th **T63.321** **Toxic effect of venom of tarantula,** accidental **(unintentional)**

    11 ✓7th **T63.322** **Toxic effect of venom of tarantula,** intentional self-harm   HCC

    ✓7th **T63.323** **Toxic effect of venom of tarantula,** assault

    ✓7th **T63.324** **Toxic effect of venom of tarantula,** undetermined

  ✓6th **T63.33** **Toxic effect of venom of** brown recluse **spider**

    ✓7th **T63.331** **Toxic effect of venom of brown recluse spider,** accidental **(unintentional)**

    11 ✓7th **T63.332** **Toxic effect of venom of brown recluse spider,** intentional self-harm   HCC

    ✓7th **T63.333** **Toxic effect of venom of brown recluse spider,** assault

    ✓7th **T63.334** **Toxic effect of venom of brown recluse spider,** undetermined

  ✓6th **T63.39** **Toxic effect of venom of** other **spider**

    ✓7th **T63.391** **Toxic effect of venom of other spider,** accidental **(unintentional)**

    11 ✓7th **T63.392** **Toxic effect of venom of other spider,** intentional self-harm   HCC

    ✓7th **T63.393** **Toxic effect of venom of other spider,** assault

    ✓7th **T63.394** **Toxic effect of venom of other spider,** undetermined

✓5th **T63.4** **Toxic effect of venom of** other arthropods

  ✓6th **T63.41** **Toxic effect of venom of** centipedes and venomous millipedes

    ✓7th **T63.411** **Toxic effect of venom of centipedes and venomous millipedes,** accidental **(unintentional)**

    11 ✓7th **T63.412** **Toxic effect of venom of centipedes and venomous millipedes,** intentional self-harm   HCC

    ✓7th **T63.413** **Toxic effect of venom of centipedes and venomous millipedes,** assault

    ✓7th **T63.414** **Toxic effect of venom of centipedes and venomous millipedes,** undetermined

  ✓6th **T63.42** **Toxic effect of venom of** ants

    ✓7th **T63.421** **Toxic effect of venom of ants,** accidental **(unintentional)**

    11 ✓7th **T63.422** **Toxic effect of venom of ants,** intentional self-harm   HCC

    ✓7th **T63.423** **Toxic effect of venom of ants,** assault

    ✓7th **T63.424** **Toxic effect of venom of ants,** undetermined

  ✓6th **T63.43** **Toxic effect of venom of** caterpillars

    ✓7th **T63.431** **Toxic effect of venom of caterpillars,** accidental **(unintentional)**

    11 ✓7th **T63.432** **Toxic effect of venom of caterpillars,** intentional self-harm   HCC

    ✓7th **T63.433** **Toxic effect of venom of caterpillars,** assault

    ✓7th **T63.434** **Toxic effect of venom of caterpillars,** undetermined

  ✓6th **T63.44** **Toxic effect of venom of** bees

    ✓7th **T63.441** **Toxic effect of venom of bees,** accidental **(unintentional)**

    11 ✓7th **T63.442** **Toxic effect of venom of bees,** intentional self-harm   HCC

    ✓7th **T63.443** **Toxic effect of venom of bees,** assault

    ✓7th **T63.444** **Toxic effect of venom of bees,** undetermined

  ✓6th **T63.45** **Toxic effect of venom of** hornets

    ✓7th **T63.451** **Toxic effect of venom of hornets,** accidental **(unintentional)**

    11 ✓7th **T63.452** **Toxic effect of venom of hornets,** intentional self-harm   HCC

    ✓7th **T63.453** **Toxic effect of venom of hornets,** assault

    ✓7th **T63.454** **Toxic effect of venom of hornets,** undetermined

  ✓6th **T63.46** **Toxic effect of venom of** wasps
       Toxic effect of yellow jacket

    ✓7th **T63.461** **Toxic effect of venom of wasps,** accidental **(unintentional)**

    11 ✓7th **T63.462** **Toxic effect of venom of wasps,** intentional self-harm   HCC

    ✓7th **T63.463** **Toxic effect of venom of wasps,** assault

    ✓7th **T63.464** **Toxic effect of venom of wasps,** undetermined

  ✓6th **T63.48** **Toxic effect of venom of** other arthropod

    ✓7th **T63.481** **Toxic effect of venom of other arthropod,** accidental **(unintentional)**

    11 ✓7th **T63.482** **Toxic effect of venom of other arthropod,** intentional self-harm   HCC

    ✓7th **T63.483** **Toxic effect of venom of other arthropod,** assault

    ✓7th **T63.484** **Toxic effect of venom of other arthropod,** undetermined

✓5th **T63.5** **Toxic effect of contact with** venomous fish
     EXCLUDES 2   *poisoning by ingestion of fish (T61.-)*

  ✓6th **T63.51** **Toxic effect of contact with** stingray

    ✓7th **T63.511** **Toxic effect of contact with stingray,** accidental **(unintentional)**

---

11 HCC with 7th character indicating initial encounter (A or B - specific to category) OR sequela.

✓Additional Character Req   ✓x7th Placeholder Alert   Unacceptable PDx   Manifestation   H1 - H14 HAC   HCC CMS-HCC Condition   EXCLUDES 1 Not Coded Here   EXCLUDES 2 Not Included Here

ICD-10-CM 2018   1129

Chapter 19. Injury, Poisoning and Certain Other Consequences of External Causes

T63.12–T63.511

11 ✓7ᵗʰ **T63.512** Toxic effect of contact with stingray, HCC
intentional self-harm

✓7ᵗʰ **T63.513** Toxic effect of contact with stingray,
assault

✓7ᵗʰ **T63.514** Toxic effect of contact with stingray,
undetermined

✓6ᵗʰ **T63.59** Toxic effect of contact with other venomous fish

✓7ᵗʰ **T63.591** Toxic effect of contact with other
venomous fish, accidental (unintentional)

11 ✓7ᵗʰ **T63.592** Toxic effect of contact with other HCC
venomous fish, intentional self-harm

✓7ᵗʰ **T63.593** Toxic effect of contact with other
venomous fish, assault

✓7ᵗʰ **T63.594** Toxic effect of contact with other
venomous fish, undetermined

✓5ᵗʰ **T63.6** Toxic effect of contact with other venomous marine animals

    EXCLUDES 1   sea-snake venom (T63.Ø9)

    EXCLUDES 2   poisoning by ingestion of shellfish (T61.78-)

✓6ᵗʰ **T63.61** Toxic effect of contact with Portugese Man-o-war
Toxic effect of contact with bluebottle

✓7ᵗʰ **T63.611** Toxic effect of contact with Portugese
Man-o-war, accidental (unintentional)

11 ✓7ᵗʰ **T63.612** Toxic effect of contact with Portugese HCC
Man-o-war, intentional self-harm

✓7ᵗʰ **T63.613** Toxic effect of contact with Portugese
Man-o-war, assault

✓7ᵗʰ **T63.614** Toxic effect of contact with Portugese
Man-o-war, undetermined

✓6ᵗʰ **T63.62** Toxic effect of contact with other jellyfish

✓7ᵗʰ **T63.621** Toxic effect of contact with other jellyfish,
accidental (unintentional)

11 ✓7ᵗʰ **T63.622** Toxic effect of contact with other HCC
jellyfish, intentional self-harm

✓7ᵗʰ **T63.623** Toxic effect of contact with other jellyfish,
assault

✓7ᵗʰ **T63.624** Toxic effect of contact with other jellyfish,
undetermined

✓6ᵗʰ **T63.63** Toxic effect of contact with sea anemone

✓7ᵗʰ **T63.631** Toxic effect of contact with sea anemone,
accidental (unintentional)

11 ✓7ᵗʰ **T63.632** Toxic effect of contact with sea HCC
anemone, intentional self-harm

✓7ᵗʰ **T63.633** Toxic effect of contact with sea anemone,
assault

✓7ᵗʰ **T63.634** Toxic effect of contact with sea anemone,
undetermined

✓6ᵗʰ **T63.69** Toxic effect of contact with other venomous marine animals

✓7ᵗʰ **T63.691** Toxic effect of contact with other
venomous marine animals, accidental
(unintentional)

11 ✓7ᵗʰ **T63.692** Toxic effect of contact with other HCC
venomous marine animals, intentional
self-harm

✓7ᵗʰ **T63.693** Toxic effect of contact with other
venomous marine animals, assault

✓7ᵗʰ **T63.694** Toxic effect of contact with other
venomous marine animals, undetermined

✓5ᵗʰ **T63.7** Toxic effect of contact with venomous plant

✓6ᵗʰ **T63.71** Toxic effect of contact with venomous marine plant

✓7ᵗʰ **T63.711** Toxic effect of contact with venomous
marine plant, accidental (unintentional)

11 ✓7ᵗʰ **T63.712** Toxic effect of contact with venomous HCC
marine plant, intentional self-harm

✓7ᵗʰ **T63.713** Toxic effect of contact with venomous
marine plant, assault

✓7ᵗʰ **T63.714** Toxic effect of contact with venomous
marine plant, undetermined

✓6ᵗʰ **T63.79** Toxic effect of contact with other venomous plant

✓7ᵗʰ **T63.791** Toxic effect of contact with other
venomous plant, accidental
(unintentional)

11 ✓7ᵗʰ **T63.792** Toxic effect of contact with other HCC
venomous plant, intentional self-harm

✓7ᵗʰ **T63.793** Toxic effect of contact with other
venomous plant, assault

✓7ᵗʰ **T63.794** Toxic effect of contact with other
venomous plant, undetermined

✓5ᵗʰ **T63.8** Toxic effect of contact with other venomous animals

✓6ᵗʰ **T63.81** Toxic effect of contact with venomous frog

    EXCLUDES 1   contact with nonvenomous frog (W62.Ø)

✓7ᵗʰ **T63.811** Toxic effect of contact with venomous
frog, accidental (unintentional)

11 ✓7ᵗʰ **T63.812** Toxic effect of contact with venomous HCC
frog, intentional self-harm

✓7ᵗʰ **T63.813** Toxic effect of contact with venomous
frog, assault

✓7ᵗʰ **T63.814** Toxic effect of contact with venomous
frog, undetermined

✓6ᵗʰ **T63.82** Toxic effect of contact with venomous toad

    EXCLUDES 1   contact with nonvenomous toad (W62.1)

✓7ᵗʰ **T63.821** Toxic effect of contact with venomous
toad, accidental (unintentional)

11 ✓7ᵗʰ **T63.822** Toxic effect of contact with venomous HCC
toad, intentional self-harm

✓7ᵗʰ **T63.823** Toxic effect of contact with venomous
toad, assault

✓7ᵗʰ **T63.824** Toxic effect of contact with venomous
toad, undetermined

✓6ᵗʰ **T63.83** Toxic effect of contact with other venomous
amphibian

    EXCLUDES 1   contact with nonvenomous amphibian
(W62.9)

✓7ᵗʰ **T63.831** Toxic effect of contact with other
venomous amphibian, accidental
(unintentional)

11 ✓7ᵗʰ **T63.832** Toxic effect of contact with other HCC
venomous amphibian, intentional
self-harm

✓7ᵗʰ **T63.833** Toxic effect of contact with other
venomous amphibian, assault

✓7ᵗʰ **T63.834** Toxic effect of contact with other
venomous amphibian, undetermined

✓6ᵗʰ **T63.89** Toxic effect of contact with other venomous animals

✓7ᵗʰ **T63.891** Toxic effect of contact with other
venomous animals, accidental
(unintentional)

11 ✓7ᵗʰ **T63.892** Toxic effect of contact with other HCC
venomous animals, intentional self-harm

✓7ᵗʰ **T63.893** Toxic effect of contact with other
venomous animals, assault

✓7ᵗʰ **T63.894** Toxic effect of contact with other
venomous animals, undetermined

✓5ᵗʰ **T63.9** Toxic effect of contact with unspecified venomous animal

✓x7ᵗʰ **T63.91** Toxic effect of contact with unspecified venomous
animal, accidental (unintentional)

11 ✓x7ᵗʰ **T63.92** Toxic effect of contact with unspecified HCC
venomous animal, intentional self-harm

✓x7ᵗʰ **T63.93** Toxic effect of contact with unspecified venomous
animal, assault

✓x7ᵗʰ **T63.94** Toxic effect of contact with unspecified venomous
animal, undetermined

✓4ᵗʰ **T64**   **Toxic effect of aflatoxin and other mycotoxin food contaminants**

> The appropriate 7th character is to be added to each code from
> category T64.
> A   initial encounter
> D   subsequent encounter
> S   sequela

✓5ᵗʰ **T64.Ø** Toxic effect of aflatoxin

✓x7ᵗʰ **T64.Ø1** Toxic effect of aflatoxin, accidental (unintentional)

11 ✓x7ᵗʰ **T64.Ø2** Toxic effect of aflatoxin, intentional self-harm HCC

✓x7ᵗʰ **T64.Ø3** Toxic effect of aflatoxin, assault

✓x7ᵗʰ **T64.Ø4** Toxic effect of aflatoxin, undetermined

---

11 HCC with 7th character indicating initial encounter (A or B - specific to category) OR sequela.

Ⓝ Newborn: 0   Ⓟ Pediatric: 0-17   Ⓜ Maternity: 12-55   Ⓐ Adult: 15-124   **MCC** Major CC Condition   **PDxMCC** PDx acts as own MCC   **CC** CC Condition   **PDxCC** PDx acts as own CC

1130   ICD-10-CM 2018

✓5ᵗʰ **T64.8 Toxic effect of** other mycotoxin **food contaminants**

     ✓x7ᵗʰ **T64.81 Toxic effect of other mycotoxin food contaminants,** accidental **(unintentional)**

     11 ✓x7ᵗʰ **T64.82 Toxic effect of other mycotoxin food**   HCC
     contaminants, intentional self-harm

     ✓x7ᵗʰ **T64.83 Toxic effect of other mycotoxin food contaminants,** assault

     ✓x7ᵗʰ **T64.84 Toxic effect of other mycotoxin food contaminants,** undetermined

✓4ᵗʰ **T65 Toxic effect of other and unspecified substances**

> The appropriate 7th character is to be added to each code from category T65.
> A   initial encounter
> D   subsequent encounter
> S   sequela

✓5ᵗʰ **T65.0 Toxic effect of** cyanides

     EXCLUDES 1   hydrogen cyanide (T57.3-)

     ✓6ᵗʰ **T65.0X Toxic effect of cyanides**

         ✓7ᵗʰ **T65.0X1 Toxic effect of cyanides,** accidental **(unintentional)**
             Toxic effect of cyanides NOS

       11 ✓7ᵗʰ **T65.0X2 Toxic effect of cyanides,** intentional   HCC
         self-harm

         ✓7ᵗʰ **T65.0X3 Toxic effect of cyanides,** assault

         ✓7ᵗʰ **T65.0X4 Toxic effect of cyanides,** undetermined

✓5ᵗʰ **T65.1 Toxic effect of** strychnine and its salts

     ✓6ᵗʰ **T65.1X Toxic effect of strychnine and its salts**

         ✓7ᵗʰ **T65.1X1 Toxic effect of strychnine and its salts,** accidental **(unintentional)**
             Toxic effect of strychnine and its salts NOS

       11 ✓7ᵗʰ **T65.1X2 Toxic effect of strychnine and its salts,** HCC
         intentional self-harm

         ✓7ᵗʰ **T65.1X3 Toxic effect of strychnine and its salts,** assault

         ✓7ᵗʰ **T65.1X4 Toxic effect of strychnine and its salts,** undetermined

✓5ᵗʰ **T65.2 Toxic effect of** tobacco and nicotine

     EXCLUDES 2   nicotine dependence (F17.-)

     ✓6ᵗʰ **T65.21 Toxic effect of** chewing tobacco

         ✓7ᵗʰ **T65.211 Toxic effect of chewing tobacco,** accidental **(unintentional)**
             Toxic effect of chewing tobacco NOS

       11 ✓7ᵗʰ **T65.212 Toxic effect of chewing tobacco,**   HCC
         intentional self-harm

         ✓7ᵗʰ **T65.213 Toxic effect of chewing tobacco,** assault

         ✓7ᵗʰ **T65.214 Toxic effect of chewing tobacco,** undetermined

     ✓6ᵗʰ **T65.22 Toxic effect of** tobacco cigarettes
         Toxic effect of tobacco smoke
         Use additional code for exposure to second hand tobacco smoke (Z57.31, Z77.22)

         ✓7ᵗʰ **T65.221 Toxic effect of tobacco cigarettes,** accidental **(unintentional)**
             Toxic effect of tobacco cigarettes NOS

       11 ✓7ᵗʰ **T65.222 Toxic effect of tobacco cigarettes,** HCC
         intentional self-harm

         ✓7ᵗʰ **T65.223 Toxic effect of tobacco cigarettes,** assault

         ✓7ᵗʰ **T65.224 Toxic effect of tobacco cigarettes,** undetermined

     ✓6ᵗʰ **T65.29 Toxic effect of** other tobacco and nicotine

         ✓7ᵗʰ **T65.291 Toxic effect of other tobacco and nicotine,** accidental **(unintentional)**
             Toxic effect of other tobacco and nicotine NOS

       11 ✓7ᵗʰ **T65.292 Toxic effect of other tobacco and**   HCC
         nicotine, intentional self-harm

         ✓7ᵗʰ **T65.293 Toxic effect of other tobacco and nicotine,** assault

         ✓7ᵗʰ **T65.294 Toxic effect of other tobacco and nicotine,** undetermined

✓5ᵗʰ **T65.3 Toxic effect of** nitroderivatives and aminoderivatives of benzene and its homologues
     Toxic effect of anilin [benzenamine]
     Toxic effect of nitrobenzene
     Toxic effect of trinitrotoluene

     ✓6ᵗʰ **T65.3X Toxic effect of nitroderivatives and aminoderivatives of benzene and its homologues**

         ✓7ᵗʰ **T65.3X1 Toxic effect of nitroderivatives and aminoderivatives of benzene and its homologues,** accidental **(unintentional)**
             Toxic effect of nitroderivatives and aminoderivatives of benzene and its homologues NOS

       11 ✓7ᵗʰ **T65.3X2 Toxic effect of nitroderivatives and**   HCC
         aminoderivatives of benzene and its homologues, intentional self-harm

         ✓7ᵗʰ **T65.3X3 Toxic effect of nitroderivatives and aminoderivatives of benzene and its homologues,** assault

         ✓7ᵗʰ **T65.3X4 Toxic effect of nitroderivatives and aminoderivatives of benzene and its homologues,** undetermined

✓5ᵗʰ **T65.4 Toxic effect of** carbon disulfide

     ✓6ᵗʰ **T65.4X Toxic effect of carbon disulfide**

         ✓7ᵗʰ **T65.4X1 Toxic effect of carbon disulfide,** accidental **(unintentional)**
             Toxic effect of carbon disulfide NOS

       11 ✓7ᵗʰ **T65.4X2 Toxic effect of carbon disulfide,**   HCC
         intentional self-harm

         ✓7ᵗʰ **T65.4X3 Toxic effect of carbon disulfide,** assault

         ✓7ᵗʰ **T65.4X4 Toxic effect of carbon disulfide,** undetermined

✓5ᵗʰ **T65.5 Toxic effect of** nitroglycerin and other nitric acids and esters
     Toxic effect of 1,2,3-Propanetriol trinitrate

     ✓6ᵗʰ **T65.5X Toxic effect of nitroglycerin and other nitric acids and esters**

         ✓7ᵗʰ **T65.5X1 Toxic effect of nitroglycerin and other nitric acids and esters,** accidental **(unintentional)**
             Toxic effect of nitroglycerin and other nitric acids and esters NOS

       11 ✓7ᵗʰ **T65.5X2 Toxic effect of nitroglycerin and**   HCC
         other nitric acids and esters, intentional self-harm

         ✓7ᵗʰ **T65.5X3 Toxic effect of nitroglycerin and other nitric acids and esters,** assault

         ✓7ᵗʰ **T65.5X4 Toxic effect of nitroglycerin and other nitric acids and esters,** undetermined

✓5ᵗʰ **T65.6 Toxic effect of** paints and dyes, not elsewhere classified

     ✓6ᵗʰ **T65.6X Toxic effect of paints and dyes, not elsewhere classified**

         ✓7ᵗʰ **T65.6X1 Toxic effect of paints and dyes, not elsewhere classified,** accidental **(unintentional)**
             Toxic effect of paints and dyes NOS

       11 ✓7ᵗʰ **T65.6X2 Toxic effect of paints and dyes, not**   HCC
         elsewhere classified, intentional self-harm

         ✓7ᵗʰ **T65.6X3 Toxic effect of paints and dyes, not elsewhere classified,** assault

         ✓7ᵗʰ **T65.6X4 Toxic effect of paints and dyes, not elsewhere classified,** undetermined

✓5ᵗʰ **T65.8 Toxic effect of** other specified substances

     ✓6ᵗʰ **T65.81 Toxic effect of latex**

         ✓7ᵗʰ **T65.811 Toxic effect of latex,** accidental **(unintentional)**
             Toxic effect of latex NOS

       11 ✓7ᵗʰ **T65.812 Toxic effect of latex,** intentional   HCC
         self-harm

         ✓7ᵗʰ **T65.813 Toxic effect of latex,** assault

         ✓7ᵗʰ **T65.814 Toxic effect of latex,** undetermined

---

11 HCC with 7th character indicating initial encounter (A or B - specific to category) OR sequela.

✓ Additional Character Req   ✓x7ᵗʰ Placeholder Alert   Unacceptable PDx   Manifestation   H1-H14 HAC   HCC CMS-HCC Condition   EXCLUDES 1 Not Coded Here   EXCLUDES 2 Not Included Here

Chapter 19. Injury, Poisoning and Certain Other Consequences of External Causes *(side margin)*

T65.82–T69.9 *(side margin)*

√6ᵗʰ **T65.82 Toxic effect of harmful algae and algae toxins**
Toxic effect of (harmful) algae bloom NOS
Toxic effect of blue-green algae bloom
Toxic effect of brown tide
Toxic effect of cyanobacteria bloom
Toxic effect of Florida red tide
Toxic effect of pfiesteria piscicida
Toxic effect of red tide

    √7ᵗʰ **T65.821 Toxic effect of harmful algae and algae toxins, accidental (unintentional)**
Toxic effect of harmful algae and algae toxins NOS

    11 √7ᵗʰ **T65.822 Toxic effect of harmful algae and algae toxins, intentional self-harm** `HCC`

    √7ᵗʰ **T65.823 Toxic effect of harmful algae and algae toxins, assault**

    √7ᵗʰ **T65.824 Toxic effect of harmful algae and algae toxins, undetermined**

√6ᵗʰ **T65.83 Toxic effect of fiberglass**

    √7ᵗʰ **T65.831 Toxic effect of fiberglass, accidental (unintentional)**
Toxic effect of fiberglass NOS

    11 √7ᵗʰ **T65.832 Toxic effect of fiberglass, intentional self-harm** `HCC`

    √7ᵗʰ **T65.833 Toxic effect of fiberglass, assault**

    √7ᵗʰ **T65.834 Toxic effect of fiberglass, undetermined**

√6ᵗʰ **T65.89 Toxic effect of other specified substances**

    √7ᵗʰ **T65.891 Toxic effect of other specified substances, accidental (unintentional)**
Toxic effect of other specified substances NOS

    11 √7ᵗʰ **T65.892 Toxic effect of other specified substances, intentional self-harm** `HCC`

    √7ᵗʰ **T65.893 Toxic effect of other specified substances, assault**

    √7ᵗʰ **T65.894 Toxic effect of other specified substances, undetermined**

√5ᵗʰ **T65.9 Toxic effect of unspecified substance**

    √x7ᵗʰ **T65.91 Toxic effect of unspecified substance, accidental (unintentional)**
Poisoning NOS

    11 √x7ᵗʰ **T65.92 Toxic effect of unspecified substance, intentional self-harm** `HCC`

    √x7ᵗʰ **T65.93 Toxic effect of unspecified substance, assault**

    √x7ᵗʰ **T65.94 Toxic effect of unspecified substance, undetermined**

Other and unspecified effects of external causes (T66-T78)

√x7ᵗʰ **T66 Radiation sickness, unspecified**
EXCLUDES 1 specified adverse effects of radiation, such as:
    burns (T20-T31)
    leukemia (C91-C95)
    radiation gastroenteritis and colitis (K52.0)
    radiation pneumonitis (J70.0)
    radiation related disorders of the skin and subcutaneous tissue (L55-L59)
    radiation sunburn (L55.-)

The appropriate 7th character is to be added to code T66.
A   initial encounter
D   subsequent encounter
S   sequela

√4ᵗʰ **T67 Effects of heat and light**
EXCLUDES 1 erythema [dermatitis] ab igne (L59.0)
    malignant hyperpyrexia due to anesthesia (T88.3)
    radiation-related disorders of the skin and subcutaneous tissue (L55-L59)
EXCLUDES 2 burns (T20-T31)
    sunburn (L55.-)
    sweat disorder due to heat (L74-L75)

The appropriate 7th character is to be added to each code from category T67.
A   initial encounter
D   subsequent encounter
S   sequela

√x7ᵗʰ **T67.0 Heatstroke and sunstroke** `CC` `H5`
Heat apoplexy   Siriasis
Heat pyrexia   Thermoplegia
Use additional code(s) to identify any associated complications of heatstroke, such as:
    coma and stupor (R40.-)
    systemic inflammatory response syndrome (R65.1-)
DEF: Headache, vertigo, cramps, and elevated body temperature due to prolonged exposure to high environmental temperatures; requires emergency intervention.
CC Excl: PDX collection 1419

√x7ᵗʰ **T67.1 Heat syncope**
Heat collapse

√x7ᵗʰ **T67.2 Heat cramp**

√x7ᵗʰ **T67.3 Heat exhaustion, anhydrotic**
Heat prostration due to water depletion
EXCLUDES 1 heat exhaustion due to salt depletion (T67.4)

√x7ᵗʰ **T67.4 Heat exhaustion due to salt depletion**
Heat prostration due to salt (and water) depletion

√x7ᵗʰ **T67.5 Heat exhaustion, unspecified**
Heat prostration NOS

√x7ᵗʰ **T67.6 Heat fatigue, transient**

√x7ᵗʰ **T67.7 Heat edema**

√x7ᵗʰ **T67.8 Other effects of heat and light**

√x7ᵗʰ **T67.9 Effect of heat and light, unspecified**

√x7ᵗʰ **T68 Hypothermia**
Accidental hypothermia
Hypothermia NOS
Use additional code to identify source of exposure:
    exposure to excessive cold of man-made origin (W93)
    exposure to excessive cold of natural origin (X31)
EXCLUDES 1 hypothermia following anesthesia (T88.51)
    hypothermia not associated with low environmental temperature (R68.0)
    hypothermia of newborn (P80.-)
EXCLUDES 2 frostbite (T33-T34)

The appropriate 7th character is to be added to code T68.
A   initial encounter
D   subsequent encounter
S   sequela

√4ᵗʰ **T69 Other effects of reduced temperature**
Use additional code to identify source of exposure:
    exposure to excessive cold of man-made origin (W93)
    exposure to excessive cold of natural origin (X31)
EXCLUDES 2 frostbite (T33-T34)

The appropriate 7th character is to be added to each code from category T69.
A   initial encounter
D   subsequent encounter
S   sequela

√5ᵗʰ **T69.0 Immersion hand and foot**

    √6ᵗʰ **T69.01 Immersion hand**

      √7ᵗʰ **T69.011 Immersion hand, right hand**

      √7ᵗʰ **T69.012 Immersion hand, left hand**

      √7ᵗʰ **T69.019 Immersion hand, unspecified hand**

    √6ᵗʰ **T69.02 Immersion foot**
Trench foot

      CC Excl: For codes in subcategory T69.02:
PDX collection 1420

      √7ᵗʰ **T69.021 Immersion foot, right foot** `CC` `H5`

      √7ᵗʰ **T69.022 Immersion foot, left foot** `CC` `H5`

      √7ᵗʰ **T69.029 Immersion foot, unspecified foot** `CC` `H5`

√x7ᵗʰ **T69.1 Chilblains**
DEF: Red, swollen, itchy skin primarily affecting the fingers and toes, nose and ears, and legs; follows damp-cold exposure; can also be associated with pruritus and a burning feeling.

√x7ᵗʰ **T69.8 Other specified effects of reduced temperature**

√x7ᵗʰ **T69.9 Effect of reduced temperature, unspecified**

---

11 HCC with 7th character indicating initial encounter (A or B - specific to category) OR sequela.

Ⓝ Newborn: 0   Ⓟ Pediatric: 0-17   Ⓜ Maternity: 12-55   Ⓐ Adult: 15-124   `MCC` Major CC Condition   `PDxMCC` PDx acts as own MCC   `CC` CC Condition   `PDxCC` PDx acts as own CC

1132   ICD-10-CM 2018

√4ᵗʰ **T70 Effects of air pressure and water pressure**

> The appropriate 7th character is to be added to each code from category T70.
> A   initial encounter
> D   subsequent encounter
> S   sequela

√x7ᵗʰ **T70.0 Otitic barotrauma**
Aero-otitis media
Effects of change in ambient atmospheric pressure or water pressure on ears

√x7ᵗʰ **T70.1 Sinus barotrauma**
Aerosinusitis
Effects of change in ambient atmospheric pressure on sinuses

√5ᵗʰ **T70.2 Other and unspecified effects of high altitude**
> EXCLUDES 2   polycythemia due to high altitude (D75.1)

√x7ᵗʰ **T70.20 Unspecified effects of high altitude**

√x7ᵗʰ **T70.29 Other effects of high altitude**
Alpine sickness   Hypobaropathy
Anoxia due to high altitude   Mountain sickness
Barotrauma NOS

√x7ᵗʰ **T70.3 Caisson disease [decompression sickness]**   CC H5
Compressed-air disease
Diver's palsy or paralysis
DEF: Rapid reduction in air pressure while breathing compressed air; symptoms include skin lesions, joint pains, and respiratory and neurological problems.
CC Excl: PDX collection 1421

√x7ᵗʰ **T70.4 Effects of high-pressure fluids**
Hydraulic jet injection (industrial)
Pneumatic jet injection (industrial)
Traumatic jet injection (industrial)

√x7ᵗʰ **T70.8 Other effects of air pressure and water pressure**

√x7ᵗʰ **T70.9 Effect of air pressure and water pressure, unspecified**

√4ᵗʰ **T71 Asphyxiation**
Mechanical suffocation
Traumatic suffocation
> EXCLUDES 1   acute respiratory distress (syndrome) (J80)
> anoxia due to high altitude (T70.2)
> asphyxia NOS (R09.01)
> asphyxia from carbon monoxide (T58.-)
> asphyxia from inhalation of food or foreign body (T17.-)
> asphyxia from other gases, fumes and vapors (T59.-)
> respiratory distress (syndrome) in newborn (P22.-)

> The appropriate 7th character is to be added to each code from category T71.
> A   initial encounter
> D   subsequent encounter
> S   sequela

> CC Excl: For codes in category T71: PDX collection 1422

√5ᵗʰ **T71.1 Asphyxiation due to mechanical threat to breathing**
Suffocation due to mechanical threat to breathing

√6ᵗʰ **T71.11 Asphyxiation due to smothering under pillow**

√7ᵗʰ **T71.111 Asphyxiation due to smothering under pillow, accidental**   CC H5
Asphyxiation due to smothering under pillow NOS

11 √7ᵗʰ **T71.112 Asphyxiation due to smothering under pillow, intentional self-harm**   CC H5 HCC

√7ᵗʰ **T71.113 Asphyxiation due to smothering under pillow, assault**   CC H5

√7ᵗʰ **T71.114 Asphyxiation due to smothering under pillow, undetermined**   CC H5

√6ᵗʰ **T71.12 Asphyxiation due to plastic bag**

√7ᵗʰ **T71.121 Asphyxiation due to plastic bag, accidental**   CC H5
Asphyxiation due to plastic bag NOS

11 √7ᵗʰ **T71.122 Asphyxiation due to plastic bag, intentional self-harm**   CC H5 HCC

√7ᵗʰ **T71.123 Asphyxiation due to plastic bag, assault**   CC H5

√7ᵗʰ **T71.124 Asphyxiation due to plastic bag, undetermined**   CC H5

√6ᵗʰ **T71.13 Asphyxiation due to being trapped in bed linens**

√7ᵗʰ **T71.131 Asphyxiation due to being trapped in bed linens, accidental**   CC H5
Asphyxiation due to being trapped in bed linens NOS

11 √7ᵗʰ **T71.132 Asphyxiation due to being trapped in bed linens, intentional self-harm**   CC H5 HCC

√7ᵗʰ **T71.133 Asphyxiation due to being trapped in bed linens, assault**   CC H5

√7ᵗʰ **T71.134 Asphyxiation due to being trapped in bed linens, undetermined**   CC H5

√6ᵗʰ **T71.14 Asphyxiation due to smothering under another person's body (in bed)**

√7ᵗʰ **T71.141 Asphyxiation due to smothering under another person's body (in bed), accidental**   CC H5
Asphyxiation due to smothering under another person's body (in bed) NOS

√7ᵗʰ **T71.143 Asphyxiation due to smothering under another person's body (in bed), assault**   CC H5

√7ᵗʰ **T71.144 Asphyxiation due to smothering under another person's body (in bed), undetermined**   CC H5

√6ᵗʰ **T71.15 Asphyxiation due to smothering in furniture**

√7ᵗʰ **T71.151 Asphyxiation due to smothering in furniture, accidental**   CC H5
Asphyxiation due to smothering in furniture NOS

11 √7ᵗʰ **T71.152 Asphyxiation due to smothering in furniture, intentional self-harm**   CC H5 HCC

√7ᵗʰ **T71.153 Asphyxiation due to smothering in furniture, assault**   CC H5

√7ᵗʰ **T71.154 Asphyxiation due to smothering in furniture, undetermined**   CC H5

√6ᵗʰ **T71.16 Asphyxiation due to hanging**
Hanging by window shade cord
Use additional code for any associated injuries, such as:
crushing injury of neck (S17.-)
fracture of cervical vertebrae (S12.0-S12.2-)
open wound of neck (S11.-)

√7ᵗʰ **T71.161 Asphyxiation due to hanging, accidental**   CC H5
Asphyxiation due to hanging NOS
Hanging NOS

11 √7ᵗʰ **T71.162 Asphyxiation due to hanging, intentional self-harm**   CC H5 HCC

√7ᵗʰ **T71.163 Asphyxiation due to hanging, assault**   CC H5

√7ᵗʰ **T71.164 Asphyxiation due to hanging, undetermined**   CC H5

√6ᵗʰ **T71.19 Asphyxiation due to mechanical threat to breathing due to other causes**

√7ᵗʰ **T71.191 Asphyxiation due to mechanical threat to breathing due to other causes, accidental**   CC H5
Asphyxiation due to other causes NOS

11 √7ᵗʰ **T71.192 Asphyxiation due to mechanical threat to breathing due to other causes, intentional self-harm**   CC H5 HCC

√7ᵗʰ **T71.193 Asphyxiation due to mechanical threat to breathing due to other causes, assault**   CC H5

√7ᵗʰ **T71.194 Asphyxiation due to mechanical threat to breathing due to other causes, undetermined**   CC H5

√5ᵗʰ **T71.2 Asphyxiation due to systemic oxygen deficiency due to low oxygen content in ambient air**
Suffocation due to systemic oxygen deficiency due to low oxygen content in ambient air

√x7ᵗʰ **T71.20 Asphyxiation due to systemic oxygen deficiency due to low oxygen content in ambient air due to unspecified cause**   CC H5

---

11 HCC with 7th character indicating initial encounter (A or B - specific to category) OR sequela.

✓ Additional Character Req   √x7ᵗʰ Placeholder Alert   Unacceptable PDx   Manifestation   H1 - H14 HAC   HCC CMS-HCC Condition   EXCLUDES1 Not Coded Here   EXCLUDES2 Not Included Here

√x7ᵗʰ **T71.21** **Asphyxiation due to** cave-in or falling earth   CC H5
Use additional code for any associated cataclysm
(X34-X38)

√6ᵗʰ **T71.22** **Asphyxiation due to** being trapped in a car trunk

√7ᵗʰ **T71.221** **Asphyxiation due to being trapped in**   CC
a car trunk, accidental

11 √7ᵗʰ **T71.222** **Asphyxiation due to being trapped** CC HCC
in a car trunk, intentional self-harm

√7ᵗʰ **T71.223** **Asphyxiation due to being trapped in**   CC
a car trunk, assault

√7ᵗʰ **T71.224** **Asphyxiation due to being trapped in**   CC
a car trunk, undetermined

√6ᵗʰ **T71.23** **Asphyxiation due to being** trapped in a (discarded)
refrigerator

√7ᵗʰ **T71.231** **Asphyxiation due to being trapped in**   CC
a (discarded) refrigerator, accidental

11 √7ᵗʰ **T71.232** **Asphyxiation due to being trapped** CC HCC
in a (discarded) refrigerator, intentional
self-harm

√7ᵗʰ **T71.233** **Asphyxiation due to being trapped**   CC
in a (discarded) refrigerator, assault

√7ᵗʰ **T71.234** **Asphyxiation due to being trapped**   CC
in a (discarded) refrigerator,
undetermined

√x7ᵗʰ **T71.29** **Asphyxiation due to being trapped in** other   CC H5
low oxygen environment

√x7ᵗʰ **T71.9** **Asphyxiation due to** unspecified cause   CC H5
Suffocation (by strangulation) due to unspecified cause
Suffocation NOS
Systemic oxygen deficiency due to low oxygen content in
ambient air due to unspecified cause
Systemic oxygen deficiency due to mechanical threat to
breathing due to unspecified cause
Traumatic asphyxia NOS

√4ᵗʰ **T73** **Effects of other deprivation**

The appropriate 7th character is to be added to each code from
category T73.
A   initial encounter
D   subsequent encounter
S   sequela

√x7ᵗʰ **T73.0** **Starvation**
Deprivation of food

√x7ᵗʰ **T73.1** **Deprivation of water**

√x7ᵗʰ **T73.2** **Exhaustion due to exposure**

√x7ᵗʰ **T73.3** **Exhaustion due to excessive exertion**
Exhaustion due to overexertion

√x7ᵗʰ **T73.8** **Other effects of deprivation**

√x7ᵗʰ **T73.9** **Effect of deprivation, unspecified**

√4ᵗʰ **T74** **Adult and child abuse, neglect and other maltreatment,
confirmed**
Use additional code, if applicable, to identify any associated current
injury
Use additional external cause code to identify perpetrator, if known
(Y07.-)
EXCLUDES 1   *abuse and maltreatment in pregnancy (O9A.3-, O9A.4-, O9A.5-)*
adult and child maltreatment, suspected (T76.-)

The appropriate 7th character is to be added to each code from
category T74.
A   initial encounter
D   subsequent encounter
S   sequela

CC Excl: For codes in category T74, unless otherwise noted:
PDX collection 1423

√5ᵗʰ **T74.0** **Neglect or abandonment, confirmed**

√x7ᵗʰ **T74.01** **Adult neglect or abandonment, confirmed**   CC A

√x7ᵗʰ **T74.02** **Child neglect or abandonment, confirmed**   CC P

√5ᵗʰ **T74.1** **Physical abuse, confirmed**
EXCLUDES 2   *sexual abuse (T74.2-)*

√x7ᵗʰ **T74.11** **Adult physical abuse, confirmed**   CC A

√x7ᵗʰ **T74.12** **Child physical abuse, confirmed**   CC P
EXCLUDES 2   *shaken infant syndrome (T74.4)*

√5ᵗʰ **T74.2** **Sexual abuse, confirmed**
Rape, confirmed
Sexual assault, confirmed

√x7ᵗʰ **T74.21** **Adult sexual abuse, confirmed**   CC A

√x7ᵗʰ **T74.22** **Child sexual abuse, confirmed**   CC P

√5ᵗʰ **T74.3** **Psychological abuse, confirmed**

√x7ᵗʰ **T74.31** **Adult psychological abuse, confirmed**   A

√x7ᵗʰ **T74.32** **Child psychological abuse, confirmed**   CC P

√x7ᵗʰ **T74.4** **Shaken infant syndrome**   CC P

√5ᵗʰ **T74.9** **Unspecified maltreatment, confirmed**

√x7ᵗʰ **T74.91** **Unspecified adult maltreatment, confirmed**   CC A
CC Excl: CC with 7th character A: PDX collection 1424

√x7ᵗʰ **T74.92** **Unspecified child maltreatment, confirmed**   CC P

√4ᵗʰ **T75** **Other and unspecified effects of other external causes**
EXCLUDES 1   *adverse effects NEC (T78.-)*
EXCLUDES 2   *burns (electric) (T20-T31)*

The appropriate 7th character is to be added to each code from
category T75.
A   initial encounter
D   subsequent encounter
S   sequela

√5ᵗʰ **T75.0** **Effects of lightning**
Struck by lightning

√x7ᵗʰ **T75.00** **Unspecified effects of lightning**
Struck by lightning NOS

√x7ᵗʰ **T75.01** **Shock due to being struck by lightning**

√x7ᵗʰ **T75.09** **Other effects of lightning**
Use additional code for other effects of lightning

√x7ᵗʰ **T75.1** **Unspecified effects of drowning and nonfatal**   CC H5
submersion
Immersion
EXCLUDES 1   *specified effects of drowning—code to effects*
CC Excl: PDX collection 1425

√5ᵗʰ **T75.2** **Effects of vibration**

√x7ᵗʰ **T75.20** **Unspecified effects of vibration**

√x7ᵗʰ **T75.21** **Pneumatic hammer syndrome**

√x7ᵗʰ **T75.22** **Traumatic vasospastic syndrome**

√x7ᵗʰ **T75.23** **Vertigo from infrasound**
EXCLUDES 1   *vertigo NOS (R42)*

T75.29 **Other effects of vibration**

√x7ᵗʰ **T75.3** **Motion sickness**
Airsickness
Seasickness
Travel sickness
Use additional external cause code to identify vehicle or type of
motion (Y92.81-, Y93.5-)

√x7ᵗʰ **T75.4** **Electrocution**
Shock from electric current
Shock from electroshock gun (taser)

√5ᵗʰ **T75.8** **Other specified effects of external causes**

√x7ᵗʰ **T75.81** **Effects of abnormal gravitation [G] forces**

√x7ᵗʰ **T75.82** **Effects of weightlessness**

√x7ᵗʰ **T75.89** **Other specified effects of external causes**

---

11 HCC with 7th character indicating initial encounter (A or B - specific to category) OR sequela.

N Newborn: 0   P Pediatric: 0-17   M Maternity: 12-55   A Adult: 15-124   MCC Major CC Condition   PDx MCC PDx acts as own MCC   CC CC Condition   PDx CC PDx acts as own CC

1134   **ICD-10-CM 2018**

☑4ᵗʰ **T76 Adult and child abuse, neglect and other maltreatment, suspected**

Use additional code, if applicable, to identify any associated current injury

EXCLUDES 1   adult and child maltreatment, confirmed (T74.-)
suspected abuse and maltreatment in pregnancy (O9A.3-, O9A.4-, O9A.5-)
suspected adult physical and sexual abuse, ruled out (Z04.71)
suspected adult sexual abused, ruled out (Z04.41)
suspected child physical abuse, ruled out (Z04.72)
suspected child sexual abuse, ruled out (Z04.42)

The appropriate 7th character is to be added to each code from category T76.
A   initial encounter
D   subsequent encounter
S   sequela

CC Excl: For codes in category T76, unless otherwise noted: PDX collection 1423

☑5ᵗʰ **T76.0 Neglect or abandonment, suspected**
  ✓x7ᵗʰ **T76.01** Adult **neglect or abandonment, suspected** CC A
  ✓x7ᵗʰ **T76.02** Child **neglect or abandonment, suspected** CC P

☑5ᵗʰ **T76.1 Physical abuse, suspected**
  ✓x7ᵗʰ **T76.11** Adult **physical abuse, suspected** CC A
  ✓x7ᵗʰ **T76.12** Child **physical abuse, suspected** CC P

☑5ᵗʰ **T76.2 Sexual abuse, suspected**
Rape, suspected
~~Sexual abuse, suspected~~
EXCLUDES 1   alleged abuse, ruled out (Z04.7)
  ✓x7ᵗʰ **T76.21** Adult **sexual abuse, suspected** CC A
  ✓x7ᵗʰ **T76.22** Child **sexual abuse, suspected** CC P

☑5ᵗʰ **T76.3 Psychological abuse, suspected**
  ✓x7ᵗʰ **T76.31** Adult **psychological abuse, suspected** A
  ✓x7ᵗʰ **T76.32** Child **psychological abuse, suspected** CC P

☑5ᵗʰ **T76.9 Unspecified maltreatment, suspected**
  ✓x7ᵗʰ **T76.91** Unspecified adult **maltreatment, suspected** CC A
      CC Excl: CC with 7th character A: PDX collection 1424
  ✓x7ᵗʰ **T76.92** Unspecified child **maltreatment, suspected** CC P

☑4ᵗʰ **T78 Adverse effects, not elsewhere classified**
EXCLUDES 2   complications of surgical and medical care NEC (T80-T88)

The appropriate 7th character is to be added to each code from category T78.
A   initial encounter
D   subsequent encounter
S   sequela

CC Excl: For CC codes in category T78: PDX collection 1426

☑5ᵗʰ **T78.0 Anaphylactic reaction due to food**
Anaphylactic reaction due to adverse food reaction
Anaphylactic shock or reaction due to nonpoisonous foods
Anaphylactoid reaction due to food
  ✓x7ᵗʰ **T78.00 Anaphylactic reaction due to** unspecified **food** CC
  ✓x7ᵗʰ **T78.01 Anaphylactic reaction due to** peanuts CC
  ✓x7ᵗʰ **T78.02 Anaphylactic reaction due to** shellfish (crustaceans) CC
  ✓x7ᵗʰ **T78.03 Anaphylactic reaction due to** other fish CC
  ✓x7ᵗʰ **T78.04 Anaphylactic reaction due to** fruits and vegetables CC
  ✓x7ᵗʰ **T78.05 Anaphylactic reaction due to** tree nuts and seeds CC
    EXCLUDES 2   anaphylactic reaction due to peanuts (T78.01)
  ✓x7ᵗʰ **T78.06 Anaphylactic reaction due to** food additives CC
  ✓x7ᵗʰ **T78.07 Anaphylactic reaction due to** milk and dairy products CC
  ✓x7ᵗʰ **T78.08 Anaphylactic reaction due to** eggs CC
  ✓x7ᵗʰ **T78.09 Anaphylactic reaction due to** other food products CC

✓x7ᵗʰ **T78.1 Other adverse food reactions, not elsewhere classified**
Use additional code to identify the type of reaction, if applicable
EXCLUDES 1   anaphylactic reaction or shock due to adverse food reaction (T78.0-)
anaphylactic reaction due to food (T78.0-)
bacterial food borne intoxications (A05.-)
EXCLUDES 2   allergic and dietetic gastroenteritis and colitis (K52.29)
allergic rhinitis due to food (J30.5)
dermatitis due to food in contact with skin (L23.6, L24.6, L25.4)
dermatitis due to ingested food (L27.2)
food protein-induced enterocolitis syndrome (K52.21)
food protein-induced enteropathy (K52.22)

✓x7ᵗʰ **T78.2 Anaphylactic shock, unspecified** CC
Allergic shock   Anaphylaxis
Anaphylactic reaction
EXCLUDES 1   anaphylactic reaction or shock due to adverse effect of correct medicinal substance properly administered (T88.6)
anaphylactic reaction or shock due to adverse food reaction (T78.0-)
anaphylactic reaction or shock due to serum (T80.5-)

✓x7ᵗʰ **T78.3 Angioneurotic edema**
Allergic angioedema
Giant urticaria
Quincke's edema
EXCLUDES 1   serum urticaria (T80.6-)
urticaria (L50.-)

☑5ᵗʰ **T78.4 Other and unspecified allergy**
EXCLUDES 1   specified types of allergic reaction such as:
allergic diarrhea (K52.29)
allergic gastroenteritis and colitis (K52.29)
dermatitis (L23-L25, L27-)
food protein-induced enterocolitis syndrome (K52.21)
food protein-induced enteropathy (K52.22)
hay fever (J30.1)
  ✓x7ᵗʰ **T78.40 Allergy, unspecified**
Allergic reaction NOS
Hypersensitivity NOS
  ✓x7ᵗʰ **T78.41 Arthus phenomenon**
Arthus reaction
  ✓x7ᵗʰ **T78.49 Other allergy**

✓x7ᵗʰ **T78.8 Other adverse effects, not elsewhere classified**

Certain early complications of trauma (T79)

☑4ᵗʰ **T79 Certain early complications of trauma, not elsewhere classified**
EXCLUDES 2   acute respiratory distress syndrome (J80)
complications occurring during or following medical procedures (T80-T88)
complications of surgical and medical care NEC (T80-T88)
newborn respiratory distress syndrome (P22.0)

The appropriate 7th character is to be added to each code from category T79.
A   initial encounter
D   subsequent encounter
S   sequela

10 ✓x7ᵗʰ **T79.0 Air embolism (traumatic)** MCC HCC
EXCLUDES 1   air embolism complicating abortion or ectopic or molar pregnancy (O00-O07, O08.2)
air embolism complicating pregnancy, childbirth and the puerperium (O88.0)
air embolism following infusion, transfusion, and therapeutic injection (T80.0)
air embolism following procedure NEC (T81.7-)
DEF: Arterial or venous obstruction due to introduction of air bubbles into the blood vessels following surgery or trauma.
CC Excl: PDX collection 1427

10 ✓x7ᵗʰ **T79.1 Fat embolism (traumatic)** MCC HCC
EXCLUDES 1   fat embolism complicating:
abortion or ectopic or molar pregnancy (O00-O07, O08.2)
pregnancy, childbirth and the puerperium (O88.8)
DEF: Arterial blockage due to the entrance of fat into the circulatory system after fracture of large bones or administration of corticosteroids.
CC Excl: PDX collection 1428

10 ✓x7ᵗʰ **T79.2 Traumatic secondary and recurrent hemorrhage and seroma** CC HCC
CC Excl: PDX collection 1429

---

10   HCC with 7th character indicating initial encounter (A, B or C - specific to category).

☑Additional Character Req   ✓x7ᵗʰ Placeholder Alert   <u>Unacceptable PDx</u>   Manifestation   H1-H14 HAC   HCC CMS-HCC Condition   *EXCLUDES 1* Not Coded Here   *EXCLUDES 2* Not Included Here

10 ✓x 7th **T79.4 Traumatic shock** `MCC` `HCC`
Shock (immediate) (delayed) following injury
EXCLUDES 1 *anaphylactic shock due to adverse food reaction*
(T78.0-)
anaphylactic shock due to correct medicinal substance
properly administered (T88.6)
anaphylactic shock due to serum (T80.5-)
anaphylactic shock NOS (T78.2)
anesthetic shock (T88.2)
electric shock (T75.4)
nontraumatic shock NEC (R57.-)
obstetric shock (O75.1)
postprocedural shock (T81.1-)
septic shock (R65.21)
shock complicating abortion or ectopic or molar
pregnancy (O00-O07, O08.3)
shock due to lightning (T75.01)
shock NOS (R57.9)
CC Excl: PDX collection 1430

10 ✓x 7th **T79.5 Traumatic anuria** `MCC` `HCC`
Crush syndrome
Renal failure following crushing
CC Excl: PDX collection 1431

10 ✓x 7th **T79.6 Traumatic ischemia of muscle** `HCC`
Traumatic rhabdomyolysis
Volkmann's ischemic contracture
EXCLUDES 2 *anterior tibial syndrome (M76.8)*
compartment syndrome (traumatic) (T79.A-)
nontraumatic ischemia of muscle (M62.2-)

10 ✓x 7th **T79.7 Traumatic subcutaneous emphysema** `CC` `HCC`
EXCLUDES 1 *emphysema NOS (J43)*
emphysema (subcutaneous) resulting from a
procedure (T81.82)
CC Excl: PDX collection 1432

✓5th **T79.A Traumatic compartment syndrome**
EXCLUDES 1 *fibromyalgia (M79.7)*
nontraumatic compartment syndrome (M79.A-)
traumatic ischemic infarction of muscle (T79.6)
DEF: Compression of nerves and blood vessels within an enclosed
muscle space due to previous trauma, which leads to impaired
blood flow and muscle and nerve damage.

10 ✓x 7th **T79.A0 Compartment syndrome, unspecified** `CC` `HCC`
Compartment syndrome NOS
CC Excl: PDX collection 896

✓6th **T79.A1 Traumatic compartment syndrome of upper**
extremity
Traumatic compartment syndrome of shoulder, arm,
forearm, wrist, hand, and fingers

CC Excl: For codes in category T79.A1:
PDX collection 1433

10 ✓7th **T79.A11 Traumatic compartment syndrome** `CC` `HCC`
of right upper extremity

10 ✓7th **T79.A12 Traumatic compartment syndrome** `CC` `HCC`
of left upper extremity

10 ✓7th **T79.A19 Traumatic compartment syndrome** `CC` `HCC`
of unspecified upper extremity

✓6th **T79.A2 Traumatic compartment syndrome of lower**
extremity
Traumatic compartment syndrome of hip, buttock,
thigh, leg, foot, and toes

CC Excl: For codes in category T79.A2:
PDX collection 1433

10 ✓7th **T79.A21 Traumatic compartment syndrome** `CC` `HCC`
of right lower extremity

10 ✓7th **T79.A22 Traumatic compartment syndrome** `CC` `HCC`
of left lower extremity

10 ✓7th **T79.A29 Traumatic compartment syndrome** `CC` `HCC`
of unspecified lower extremity

10 ✓x 7th **T79.A3 Traumatic compartment syndrome of** `CC` `HCC`
abdomen
CC Excl: PDX collection 1434

10 ✓x 7th **T79.A9 Traumatic compartment syndrome of other** `CC` `HCC`
sites
CC Excl: PDX collection 896

10 ✓x 7th **T79.8 Other early complications of trauma** `HCC`

10 ✓x 7th **T79.9 Unspecified early complication of trauma** `HCC`

Complications of surgical and medical care, not elsewhere classified (T80-T88)

Use additional code for adverse effect, if applicable, to identify drug (T36-T50
with fifth or sixth character 5)
Use additional code(s) to identify the specified condition resulting from the
complication
Use additional code to identify devices involved and details of circumstances
(Y62-Y82)
EXCLUDES 2 *any encounters with medical care for postprocedural conditions in*
which no complications are present, such as:
artificial opening status (Z93.-)
closure of external stoma (Z43.-)
fitting and adjustment of external prosthetic device (Z44.-)
burns and corrosions from local applications and irradiation (T20-T32)
complications of surgical procedures during pregnancy, childbirth and
the puerperium (O00-O9A)
mechanical complication of respirator [ventilator] (J95.850)
poisoning and toxic effects of drugs and chemicals (T36-T65 with fifth
or sixth character 1-4 or 6)
postprocedural fever (R50.82)
specified complications classified elsewhere, such as:
cerebrospinal fluid leak from spinal puncture (G97.0)
colostomy malfunction (K94.0-)
disorders of fluid and electrolyte imbalance (E86-E87)
functional disturbances following cardiac surgery (I97.0-I97.1)
intraoperative and postprocedural complications of specified body
systems (D78.-, E36.-, E89.-, G97.3-, G97.4, H59.3-, H59.-,
H95.2-, H95.3, I97.4-, I97.5, J95.6-, J95.7, K91.6-, L76.-,
M96.-, N99.-)
ostomy complications (J95.0-, K94-, N99.5-)
postgastric surgery syndromes (K91.1)
postlaminectomy syndrome NEC (M96.1)
postmastectomy lymphedema syndrome (I97.2)
postsurgical blind-loop syndrome (K91.2)
ventilator associated pneumonia (J95.851)
AHA: 2015, 1Q, 15

✓4th **T80 Complications following infusion, transfusion and therapeutic**
injection
`INCLUDES` complications following perfusion
EXCLUDES 2 *bone marrow transplant rejection (T86.01)*
febrile nonhemolytic transfusion reaction (R50.84)
fluid overload due to transfusion (E87.71)
posttransfusion purpura (D69.51)
transfusion associated circulatory overload (TACO) (E87.71)
transfusion (red blood cell) associated hemochromatosis
(E83.111)
transfusion related acute lung injury (TRALI) (J95.84)

The appropriate 7th character is to be added to each code from
category T80.
A   initial encounter
D   subsequent encounter
S   sequela

✓x 7th **T80.0 Air embolism following infusion, transfusion and** `MCC` `H2`
therapeutic injection
CC Excl: PDX collection 1435

✓x 7th **T80.1 Vascular complications following infusion, transfusion** `CC`
and therapeutic injection
Use additional code to identify the vascular complication
EXCLUDES 2 *extravasation of vesicant agent (T80.81-)*
infiltration of vesicant agent (T80.81-)
postprocedural vascular complications (T81.7-)
vascular complications specified as due to prosthetic
devices, implants and grafts (T82.8-, T83.8-,
T84.8-, T85.8-)
CC Excl: PDX collection 1436

✓5th **T80.2 Infections following infusion, transfusion and therapeutic**
injection
Use additional code to identify the specific infection, such as:
sepsis (A41.9)
Use additional code (R65.2-) to identify severe sepsis, if
applicable
EXCLUDES 2 *infections specified as due to prosthetic devices,*
implants and grafts (T82.6-T82.7, T83.5-T83.6,
T84.5-T84.7, T85.7)
postprocedural infections (T81.4-)

CC Excl: For codes in subcategory T80.2:
PDX collection 948

---

10 HCC with 7th character indicating initial encounter (A, B or C - specific to category).

√6ᵗʰ **T80.21** **Infection** due to central venous catheter
Infection due to pulmonary artery catheter (Swan-Ganz catheter)

√7ᵗʰ **T80.211** **Bloodstream infection** due to   `CC` `H7`
central venous catheter
Catheter-related bloodstream infection (CRBSI) NOS
Central line-associated bloodstream infection (CLABSI)
Bloodstream infection due to Hickman catheter
Bloodstream infection due to peripherally inserted central catheter (PICC)
Bloodstream infection due to portacath (port-a-cath)
Bloodstream infection due to pulmonary artery catheter
Bloodstream infection due to triple lumen catheter
Bloodstream infection due to umbilical venous catheter

√7ᵗʰ **T80.212** **Local infection** due to central   `CC` `H7`
venous catheter
Exit or insertion site infection
Local infection due to Hickman catheter
Local infection due to peripherally inserted central catheter (PICC)
Local infection due to portacath (port-a-cath)
Local infection due to pulmonary artery catheter
Local infection due to triple lumen catheter
Local infection due to umbilical venous catheter
Port or reservoir infection
Tunnel infection

√7ᵗʰ **T80.218** **Other infection** due to central   `CC` `H7`
venous catheter
Other central line-associated infection
Other infection due to Hickman catheter
Other infection due to peripherally inserted central catheter (PICC)
Other infection due to portacath (port-a-cath)
Other infection due to pulmonary artery catheter
Other infection due to triple lumen catheter
Other infection due to umbilical venous catheter

√7ᵗʰ **T80.219** **Unspecified** infection due to   `CC` `H7`
central venous catheter
Central line-associated infection NOS
Unspecified infection due to Hickman catheter
Unspecified infection due to peripherally inserted central catheter (PICC)
Unspecified infection due to portacath (port-a-cath)
Unspecified infection due to pulmonary artery catheter
Unspecified infection due to triple lumen catheter
Unspecified infection due to umbilical venous catheter

√x7ᵗʰ **T80.22** **Acute infection following transfusion, infusion,**   `CC`
or injection of blood and blood products

√x7ᵗʰ **T80.29** **Infection following other infusion, transfusion**   `CC`
and therapeutic injection

√5ᵗʰ **T80.3** **ABO incompatibility** reaction due to transfusion of blood or
blood products
EXCLUDES 1   *minor blood group antigens reactions (Duffy) (E)*
(K(ell)) (Kidd) (Lewis) (M) (N) (P) (S) (T80.A)

CC Excl: For codes in subcategory T80.3:
PDX collection 1437

√x7ᵗʰ **T80.30** **ABO incompatibility reaction due to**   `CC` `H3`
transfusion of blood or blood products,
unspecified
ABO incompatibility blood transfusion NOS
Reaction to ABO incompatibility from transfusion NOS

√6ᵗʰ **T80.31** **ABO incompatibility** with hemolytic transfusion
reaction

√7ᵗʰ **T80.310** **ABO incompatibility** with acute   `CC` `H3`
hemolytic transfusion reaction
ABO incompatibility with hemolytic transfusion reaction less than 24 hours after transfusion
Acute hemolytic transfusion reaction (AHTR) due to ABO incompatibility

√7ᵗʰ **T80.311** **ABO incompatibility** with delayed   `CC` `H3`
hemolytic transfusion reaction
ABO incompatibility with hemolytic transfusion reaction 24 hours or more after transfusion
Delayed hemolytic transfusion reaction (DHTR) due to ABO incompatibility

√7ᵗʰ **T80.319** **ABO incompatibility** with hemolytic   `CC` `H3`
transfusion reaction, unspecified
ABO incompatibility with hemolytic transfusion reaction at unspecified time after transfusion
Hemolytic transfusion reaction (HTR) due to ABO incompatibility NOS

√x7ᵗʰ **T80.39** **Other ABO incompatibility reaction due to**   `CC` `H3`
transfusion of blood or blood products
Delayed serologic transfusion reaction (DSTR) from ABO incompatibility
Other ABO incompatible blood transfusion
Other reaction to ABO incompatible blood transfusion

√5ᵗʰ **T80.4** **Rh incompatibility** reaction due to transfusion of blood or
blood products
Reaction due to incompatibility of Rh antigens (C) (c) (D) (E) (e)

CC Excl: For codes in subcategory T80.4, unless
otherwise noted: PDX collection 1437

√7ᵗʰ **T80.40** **Rh incompatibility reaction due to transfusion**   `CC`
of blood or blood products, unspecified
Reaction due to Rh factor in transfusion NOS
Rh incompatible blood transfusion NOS

√6ᵗʰ **T80.41** **Rh incompatibility** with hemolytic transfusion
reaction

√7ᵗʰ **T80.410** **Rh incompatibility** with acute   `CC`
hemolytic transfusion reaction
Acute hemolytic transfusion reaction (AHTR) due to Rh incompatibility
Rh incompatibility with hemolytic transfusion reaction less than 24 hours after transfusion

√7ᵗʰ **T80.411** **Rh incompatibility** with delayed   `CC`
hemolytic transfusion reaction
Delayed hemolytic transfusion reaction (DHTR) due to Rh incompatibility
Rh incompatibility with hemolytic transfusion reaction 24 hours or more after transfusion

√7ᵗʰ **T80.419** **Rh incompatibility** with hemolytic   `CC`
transfusion reaction, unspecified
Hemolytic transfusion reaction (HTR) due to Rh incompatibility NOS
Rh incompatibility with hemolytic transfusion reaction at unspecified time after transfusion

√x7ᵗʰ **T80.49** **Other Rh incompatibility reaction due to**   `CC`
transfusion of blood or blood products
Delayed serologic transfusion reaction (DSTR) from Rh incompatibility
Other reaction to Rh incompatible blood transfusion
CC Excl: PDX collection 1438

√5ᵗʰ **T80.A** **Non-ABO incompatibility** reaction due to transfusion of blood
or blood products
Reaction due to incompatibility of minor antigens (Duffy) (Kell) (Kidd) (Lewis) (M) (N) (P) (S)

CC Excl: For codes in subcategory T80.A, unless
otherwise noted: PDX collection 1438

√x7ᵗʰ **T80.A0** **Non-ABO incompatibility reaction due to**   `CC`
transfusion of blood or blood products,
unspecified
Non-ABO antigen incompatibility reaction from transfusion NOS

✔Additional Character Req   √x7ᵗʰ Placeholder Alert   Unacceptable PDx   Manifestation   `H1`-`H14` HAC   `HCC` CMS-HCC Condition   *EXCLUDES 1* Not Coded Here   *EXCLUDES 2* Not Included Here

√6ᵗʰ **T80.A1**   **Non-ABO incompatibility** with hemolytic transfusion reaction

√7ᵗʰ **T80.A10**   **Non-ABO incompatibility with** acute **hemolytic transfusion reaction**   `CC`

Acute hemolytic transfusion reaction (AHTR) due to non-ABO incompatibility

Non-ABO incompatibility with hemolytic transfusion reaction less than 24 hours after transfusion

√7ᵗʰ **T80.A11**   **Non-ABO incompatibility with** delayed **hemolytic transfusion reaction**   `CC`

Delayed hemolytic transfusion reaction (DHTR) due to non-ABO incompatibility

Non-ABO incompatibility with hemolytic transfusion reaction 24 or more hours after transfusion

√7ᵗʰ **T80.A19**   **Non-ABO incompatibility with hemolytic transfusion reaction, unspecified**   `CC`

Hemolytic transfusion reaction (HTR) due to non-ABO incompatibility NOS

Non-ABO incompatibility with hemolytic transfusion reaction at unspecified time after transfusion

√x7ᵗʰ **T80.A9**   **Other** non-ABO incompatibility reaction due to transfusion of blood or blood products   `CC`

Delayed serologic transfusion reaction (DSTR) from non-ABO incompatibility

Other reaction to non-ABO incompatible blood transfusion

CC Excl: PDX collection 1437

√5ᵗʰ **T80.5**   **Anaphylactic reaction due to serum**

Allergic shock due to serum

Anaphylactic shock due to serum

Anaphylactoid reaction due to serum

Anaphylaxis due to serum

EXCLUDES 1   *ABO incompatibility reaction due to transfusion of blood or blood products (T80.3-)*

allergic reaction or shock NOS (T78.2)

anaphylactic reaction or shock NOS (T78.2)

anaphylactic reaction or shock due to adverse effect of correct medicinal substance properly administered (T88.6)

other serum reaction (T80.6-)

DEF: Life-threatening hypersensitivity to foreign serum; causes respiratory distress, vascular collapse, and shock.

CC Excl: For codes in subcategory T80.5: PDX collection 1439

√x7ᵗʰ **T80.51**   **Anaphylactic reaction due to** administration of blood and blood products   `CC`

√x7ᵗʰ **T80.52**   **Anaphylactic reaction due to** vaccination   `CC`

√x7ᵗʰ **T80.59**   **Anaphylactic reaction due to** other serum   `CC`

√5ᵗʰ **T80.6**   **Other serum reactions**

Intoxication by serum   Serum sickness

Protein sickness   Serum urticaria

Serum rash

EXCLUDES 2   *serum hepatitis (B16-B19)*

DEF: Serum sickness: Hypersensitivity to foreign serum; causes fever, hives, swelling, and lymphadenopathy.

CC Excl: For codes in subcategory T80.6, unless otherwise noted: CC with 7th character A: PDX collection 1439

√x7ᵗʰ **T80.61**   **Other serum reaction** due to administration of blood and blood products   `CC`

√x7ᵗʰ **T80.62**   **Other serum reaction** due to vaccination   `CC`

√x7ᵗʰ **T80.69**   **Other serum reaction** due to other serum   `CC`

▶Code also, if applicable, arthropathy in hypersensitivity reactions classified elsewhere (M36.4)◀

CC Excl: PDX collection 1440

√5ᵗʰ **T80.8**   **Other complications following infusion, transfusion and therapeutic injection**

√6ᵗʰ **T80.81**   **Extravasation of vesicant agent**

Infiltration of vesicant agent

√7ᵗʰ **T80.810**   **Extravasation of vesicant antineoplastic chemotherapy**   `CC`

Infiltration of vesicant antineoplastic chemotherapy

CC Excl: PDX collection 1436

√7ᵗʰ **T80.818**   **Extravasation of other vesicant agent**   `CC`

Infiltration of other vesicant agent

CC Excl: PDX collection 1436

√x7ᵗʰ **T80.89**   **Other complications following infusion, transfusion and therapeutic injection**

Delayed serologic transfusion reaction (DSTR), unspecified incompatibility

Use additional code to identify graft-versus-host reaction, if applicable, (D89.81-)

√5ᵗʰ **T80.9**   **Unspecified complication following infusion, transfusion and therapeutic injection**

√x7ᵗʰ **T80.90**   **Unspecified complication** following infusion and therapeutic injection

√6ᵗʰ **T80.91**   **Hemolytic transfusion reaction,** unspecified **incompatibility**

EXCLUDES 1   *ABO incompatibility with hemolytic transfusion reaction (T80.31-)*

Non-ABO incompatibility with hemolytic transfusion reaction (T80.A1-)

Rh incompatibility with hemolytic transfusion reaction (T80.41-)

CC Excl: For codes in subcategory T80.91: PDX collection 1437

√7ᵗʰ **T80.910**   Acute **hemolytic transfusion reaction, unspecified incompatibility**   `CC`

√7ᵗʰ **T80.911**   Delayed **hemolytic transfusion reaction, unspecified incompatibility**   `CC`

√7ᵗʰ **T80.919**   **Hemolytic transfusion reaction,** unspecified **incompatibility, unspecified as acute or delayed**   `CC`

Hemolytic transfusion reaction NOS

√x7ᵗʰ **T80.92**   **Unspecified transfusion reaction**

Transfusion reaction NOS

√4ᵗʰ **T81**   **Complications of procedures, not elsewhere classified**

Use additional code for adverse effect, if applicable, to identify drug (T36-T50 with fifth or sixth character 5)

EXCLUDES 2   *complications following immunization (T88.0-T88.1)*

complications following infusion, transfusion and therapeutic injection (T80.-)

complications of transplanted organs and tissue (T86.-)

specified complications classified elsewhere, such as:

complication of prosthetic devices, implants and grafts (T82-T85)

dermatitis due to drugs and medicaments (L23.3, L24.4, L25.1, L27.0-L27.1)

endosseous dental implant failure (M27.6-)

floppy iris syndrome (IFIS) (intraoperative) (H21.81)

intraoperative and postprocedural complications of specific body system (D78.-, E36.-, E89.-, G97.3-, G97.4, H59.3-, H59.-, H95.2-, H95.3, I97.4-, I97.5, J95., K91.-, L76.-, M96.-, N99.-)

ostomy complications (J95.0-, K94.-, N99.5-)

plateau iris syndrome (post-iridectomy) (postprocedural) (H21.82)

poisoning and toxic effects of drugs and chemicals (T36-T65 with fifth or sixth character 1-4 or 6)

The appropriate 7th character is to be added to each code from category T81.

A   initial encounter

D   subsequent encounter

S   sequela

Ⓝ Newborn: 0   Ⓟ Pediatric: 0-17   Ⓜ Maternity: 12-55   Ⓐ Adult: 15-124   `MCC` Major CC Condition   `PDxMCC` PDx acts as own MCC   `CC` CC Condition   `PDxCC` PDx acts as own CC

1138   ICD-10-CM 2018

☑5ᵗʰ **T81.1** **Postprocedural shock**
Shock during or resulting from a procedure, not elsewhere classified
EXCLUDES 1   *anaphylactic shock due to correct substance properly administered (T88.6)*
anaphylactic shock due to serum (T80.5-)
anaphylactic shock NOS (T78.2)
anesthetic shock (T88.2)
electric shock (T75.4)
obstetric shock (O75.1)
septic shock (R65.21)
shock following abortion or ectopic or molar pregnancy (O00-O07, O08.3)
traumatic shock (T79.4)

CC Excl: For codes in subcategory T81.1:
PDX collection 1441

☑x7ᵗʰ **T81.10** **Postprocedural shock unspecified**   `CC`
Collapse NOS during or resulting from a procedure, not elsewhere classified
Postprocedural failure of peripheral circulation
Postprocedural shock NOS

¹⁰ ☑x7ᵗʰ **T81.11** **Postprocedural cardiogenic shock**   `MCC` `HCC`

³,¹⁰ ☑x7ᵗʰ **T81.12** **Postprocedural septic shock**   `MCC` `HCC`
Postprocedural endotoxic shock resulting from a procedure, not elsewhere classified
Postprocedural gram-negative shock resulting from a procedure, not elsewhere classified
Code first underlying infection
Use additional code, to identify any associated acute organ dysfunction, if applicable

☑x7ᵗʰ **T81.19** **Other postprocedural shock**   `MCC`
Postprocedural hypovolemic shock

☑5ᵗʰ **T81.3** **Disruption of wound, not elsewhere classified**
Disruption of any suture materials or other closure methods
EXCLUDES 1   *breakdown (mechanical) of permanent sutures (T85.612)*
displacement of permanent sutures (T85.622)
disruption of cesarean delivery wound (O90.0)
disruption of perineal obstetric wound (O90.1)
mechanical complication of permanent sutures NEC (T85.692)

AHA: 2014, 1Q, 23

CC Excl: For codes in subcategory T81.3:
PDX collection 1442

☑x7ᵗʰ **T81.30** **Disruption of wound, unspecified**   `CC`
Disruption of wound NOS

☑x7ᵗʰ **T81.31** **Disruption of external operation (surgical) wound, not elsewhere classified**   `CC`
Dehiscence of operation wound NOS
Disruption of operation wound NOS
Disruption or dehiscence of closure of cornea
Disruption or dehiscence of closure of mucosa
Disruption or dehiscence of closure of skin and subcutaneous tissue
Full-thickness skin disruption or dehiscence
Superficial disruption or dehiscence of operation wound
EXCLUDES 1   *dehiscence of amputation stump (T87.81)*

☑x7ᵗʰ **T81.32** **Disruption of internal operation (surgical) wound, not elsewhere classified**   `CC`
Deep disruption or dehiscence of operation wound NOS
Disruption or dehiscence of closure of internal organ or other internal tissue
Disruption or dehiscence of closure of muscle or muscle flap
Disruption or dehiscence of closure of ribs or rib cage
Disruption or dehiscence of closure of skull or craniotomy
Disruption or dehiscence of closure of sternum or sternotomy
Disruption or dehiscence of closure of tendon or ligament
Disruption or dehiscence of closure of superficial or muscular fascia

☑x7ᵗʰ **T81.33** **Disruption of traumatic injury wound repair**   `CC`
Disruption or dehiscence of closure of traumatic laceration (external) (internal)

☑x7ᵗʰ **T81.4** **Infection following a procedure**   `CC` `H11` `H12` `H13`
Intra-abdominal abscess following a procedure
Postprocedural infection, not elsewhere classified
Sepsis following a procedure
Stitch abscess following a procedure
Subphrenic abscess following a procedure
Wound abscess following a procedure
Use additional code to identify infection
Use additional code (R65.2-) to identify severe sepsis, if applicable
EXCLUDES 1   *obstetric surgical wound infection (O86.0)*
postprocedural fever NOS (R50.82)
postprocedural retroperitoneal abscess (K68.11)
EXCLUDES 2   *bleb associated endophthalmitis (H59.4-)*
infection due to infusion, transfusion and therapeutic injection (T80.2-)
infection due to prosthetic devices, implants and grafts (T82.6-T82.7, T83.5-T83.6, T84.5-T84.7, T85.7)

AHA: 2014, 1Q, 23
CC Excl: PDX collection 805

☑5ᵗʰ **T81.5** **Complications of foreign body accidentally left in body following procedure**
AHA: 2014, 4Q, 24

CC Excl: For codes in subcategory T81.5:
PDX collection 1443

☑6ᵗʰ **T81.50** **Unspecified complication of foreign body accidentally left in body following procedure**

☑7ᵗʰ **T81.500** **Unspecified complication of foreign body accidentally left in body following surgical operation**   `CC` `H1`

☑7ᵗʰ **T81.501** **Unspecified complication of foreign body accidentally left in body following infusion or transfusion**   `CC` `H1`

☑7ᵗʰ **T81.502** **Unspecified complication of foreign body accidentally left in body following kidney dialysis**   `CC` `H1` `HCC`

☑7ᵗʰ **T81.503** **Unspecified complication of foreign body accidentally left in body following injection or immunization**   `CC` `H1`

☑7ᵗʰ **T81.504** **Unspecified complication of foreign body accidentally left in body following endoscopic examination**   `CC` `H1`

☑7ᵗʰ **T81.505** **Unspecified complication of foreign body accidentally left in body following heart catheterization**   `CC` `H1`

☑7ᵗʰ **T81.506** **Unspecified complication of foreign body accidentally left in body following aspiration, puncture or other catheterization**   `CC` `H1`

☑7ᵗʰ **T81.507** **Unspecified complication of foreign body accidentally left in body following removal of catheter or packing**   `CC` `H1`

☑7ᵗʰ **T81.508** **Unspecified complication of foreign body accidentally left in body following other procedure**   `CC` `H1`

☑7ᵗʰ **T81.509** **Unspecified complication of foreign body accidentally left in body following unspecified procedure**   `CC` `H1`

☑6ᵗʰ **T81.51** **Adhesions due to foreign body accidentally left in body following procedure**

☑7ᵗʰ **T81.510** **Adhesions due to foreign body accidentally left in body following surgical operation**   `CC` `H1`

☑7ᵗʰ **T81.511** **Adhesions due to foreign body accidentally left in body following infusion or transfusion**   `CC` `H1`

☑7ᵗʰ **T81.512** **Adhesions due to foreign body accidentally left in body following kidney dialysis**   `CC` `H1` `HCC`

☑7ᵗʰ **T81.513** **Adhesions due to foreign body accidentally left in body following injection or immunization**   `CC` `H1`

☑7ᵗʰ **T81.514** **Adhesions due to foreign body accidentally left in body following endoscopic examination**   `CC` `H1`

---

³   Unacceptable PDx for all encounters (7th character A, D, OR S).
¹⁰   HCC with 7th character indicating initial encounter (A, B or C - specific to category).

☑ Additional Character Req   ☑x7ᵗʰ Placeholder Alert   Unacceptable PDx   Manifestation   `H1`-`H14` HAC   `HCC` CMS-HCC Condition   *EXCLUDES 1* Not Coded Here   *EXCLUDES 2* Not Included Here

ICD-10-CM 2018   **1139**

✓7ᵗʰ T81.515 **Adhesions due to foreign body accidentally left in body following heart catheterization** `CC` `H1`

✓7ᵗʰ T81.516 **Adhesions due to foreign body accidentally left in body following aspiration, puncture or other catheterization** `CC` `H1`

✓7ᵗʰ T81.517 **Adhesions due to foreign body accidentally left in body following removal of catheter or packing** `CC` `H1`

✓7ᵗʰ T81.518 **Adhesions due to foreign body accidentally left in body following other procedure** `CC` `H1`

✓7ᵗʰ T81.519 **Adhesions due to foreign body accidentally left in body following unspecified procedure** `CC` `H1`

✓6ᵗʰ T81.52 **Obstruction due to foreign body accidentally left in body following procedure**

✓7ᵗʰ T81.520 **Obstruction due to foreign body accidentally left in body following surgical operation** `CC` `H1`

✓7ᵗʰ T81.521 **Obstruction due to foreign body accidentally left in body following infusion or transfusion** `CC` `H1`

✓7ᵗʰ T81.522 **Obstruction due to foreign body accidentally left in body following kidney dialysis** `CC` `H1` `HCC`

✓7ᵗʰ T81.523 **Obstruction due to foreign body accidentally left in body following injection or immunization** `CC` `H1`

✓7ᵗʰ T81.524 **Obstruction due to foreign body accidentally left in body following endoscopic examination** `CC` `H1`

✓7ᵗʰ T81.525 **Obstruction due to foreign body accidentally left in body following heart catheterization** `CC` `H1`

✓7ᵗʰ T81.526 **Obstruction due to foreign body accidentally left in body following aspiration, puncture or other catheterization** `CC` `H1`

✓7ᵗʰ T81.527 **Obstruction due to foreign body accidentally left in body following removal of catheter or packing** `CC` `H1`

✓7ᵗʰ T81.528 **Obstruction due to foreign body accidentally left in body following other procedure** `CC` `H1`

✓7ᵗʰ T81.529 **Obstruction due to foreign body accidentally left in body following unspecified procedure** `CC` `H1`

✓6ᵗʰ T81.53 **Perforation due to foreign body accidentally left in body following procedure**

✓7ᵗʰ T81.530 **Perforation due to foreign body accidentally left in body following surgical operation** `CC` `H1`

✓7ᵗʰ T81.531 **Perforation due to foreign body accidentally left in body following infusion or transfusion** `CC` `H1`

✓7ᵗʰ T81.532 **Perforation due to foreign body accidentally left in body following kidney dialysis** `CC` `H1` `HCC`

✓7ᵗʰ T81.533 **Perforation due to foreign body accidentally left in body following injection or immunization** `CC` `H1`

✓7ᵗʰ T81.534 **Perforation due to foreign body accidentally left in body following endoscopic examination** `CC` `H1`

✓7ᵗʰ T81.535 **Perforation due to foreign body accidentally left in body following heart catheterization** `CC` `H1`

✓7ᵗʰ T81.536 **Perforation due to foreign body accidentally left in body following aspiration, puncture or other catheterization** `CC` `H1`

✓7ᵗʰ T81.537 **Perforation due to foreign body accidentally left in body following removal of catheter or packing** `CC` `H1`

✓7ᵗʰ T81.538 **Perforation due to foreign body accidentally left in body following other procedure**

✓7ᵗʰ T81.539 **Perforation due to foreign body accidentally left in body following unspecified procedure** `CC` `H1`

✓6ᵗʰ T81.59 **Other complications of foreign body accidentally left in body following procedure**
> *EXCLUDES 2*   obstruction or perforation due to prosthetic devices and implants intentionally left in body (T82.0-T82.5, T83.0-T83.4, T83.7, T84.0-T84.4, T85.0-T85.6)

✓7ᵗʰ T81.590 **Other complications of foreign body accidentally left in body following surgical operation** `CC` `H1`

✓7ᵗʰ T81.591 **Other complications of foreign body accidentally left in body following infusion or transfusion** `CC` `H1`

✓7ᵗʰ T81.592 **Other complications of foreign body accidentally left in body following kidney dialysis** `CC` `H1` `HCC`

✓7ᵗʰ T81.593 **Other complications of foreign body accidentally left in body following injection or immunization** `CC` `H1`

✓7ᵗʰ T81.594 **Other complications of foreign body accidentally left in body following endoscopic examination** `CC` `H1`

✓7ᵗʰ T81.595 **Other complications of foreign body accidentally left in body following heart catheterization** `CC` `H1`

✓7ᵗʰ T81.596 **Other complications of foreign body accidentally left in body following aspiration, puncture or other catheterization** `CC` `H1`

✓7ᵗʰ T81.597 **Other complications of foreign body accidentally left in body following removal of catheter or packing** `CC` `H1`

✓7ᵗʰ T81.598 **Other complications of foreign body accidentally left in body following other procedure** `CC` `H1`

✓7ᵗʰ T81.599 **Other complications of foreign body accidentally left in body following unspecified procedure** `CC` `H1`

✓5ᵗʰ T81.6 **Acute reaction to foreign substance accidentally left during a procedure**
> *EXCLUDES 2*   complications of foreign body accidentally left in body cavity or operation wound following procedure (T81.5-)

> **CC Excl: For codes in subcategory T81.6:** PDX collection 1444

✓x7ᵗʰ T81.60 **Unspecified acute reaction to foreign substance accidentally left during a procedure** `CC` `H1`

✓x7ᵗʰ T81.61 **Aseptic peritonitis due to foreign substance accidentally left during a procedure** `CC` `H1`
Chemical peritonitis

✓x7ᵗʰ T81.69 **Other acute reaction to foreign substance accidentally left during a procedure** `CC` `H1`

✓5ᵗʰ T81.7 **Vascular complications following a procedure, not elsewhere classified**
Air embolism following procedure NEC
Phlebitis or thrombophlebitis resulting from a procedure
> *EXCLUDES 1*   embolism complicating abortion or ectopic or molar pregnancy (O00-O07, O08.2)
> embolism complicating pregnancy, childbirth and the puerperium (O88.-)
> traumatic embolism (T79.0)
> *EXCLUDES 2*   embolism due to prosthetic devices, implants and grafts (T82.8-, T83.81, T84.8-, T85.81-)
> embolism following infusion, transfusion and therapeutic injection (T80.0)

✓6ᵗʰ T81.71 **Complication of artery following a procedure, not elsewhere classified**

✓7ᵗʰ T81.710 **Complication of mesenteric artery following a procedure, not elsewhere classified** `CC`
CC Excl: PDX collection 1445

✓7ᵗʰ T81.711 **Complication of renal artery following a procedure, not elsewhere classified** `CC`
CC Excl: PDX collection 1445

`N` Newborn: 0   `P` Pediatric: 0-17   `M` Maternity: 12-55   `A` Adult: 15-124   `MCC` Major CC Condition   `PDx MCC` PDx acts as own MCC   `CC` CC Condition   `PDx CC` PDx acts as own CC

✓7ᵗʰ **T81.718** **Complication of** other **artery following a procedure, not elsewhere classified** `CC`
     CC Excl: PDX collection 1446

✓7ᵗʰ **T81.719** **Complication of** unspecified **artery following a procedure, not elsewhere classified** `CC`
     CC Excl: PDX collection 1446

✓x7ᵗʰ **T81.72** **Complication of** vein **following a procedure, not elsewhere classified** `CC`
     CC Excl: PDX collection 1446

✓5ᵗʰ **T81.8** **Other complications of procedures, not elsewhere classified**
     EXCLUDES 2   *hypothermia following anesthesia (T88.51)*
                 malignant hyperpyrexia due to anesthesia (T88.3)

✓x7ᵗʰ **T81.81** **Complication of inhalation therapy**

✓x7ᵗʰ **T81.82** **Emphysema (subcutaneous) resulting from a procedure**

✓x7ᵗʰ **T81.83** **Persistent postprocedural fistula** `CC`
     CC Excl: PDX collection 1447

✓x7ᵗʰ **T81.89** **Other complications of procedures, not elsewhere classified**
     Use additional code to specify complication, such as:
         postprocedural delirium (F05)
     AHA: 2014, 1Q, 23

✓x7ᵗʰ **T81.9** **Unspecified complication of procedure**

✓4ᵗʰ **T82** **Complications of cardiac and vascular prosthetic devices, implants and grafts**
     EXCLUDES 2   *failure and rejection of transplanted organs and tissue (T86.-)*

> The appropriate 7th character is to be added to each code from category T82.
> A   initial encounter
> D   subsequent encounter
> S   sequela

✓5ᵗʰ **T82.0** **Mechanical complication of** heart valve prosthesis
     Mechanical complication of artificial heart valve
     EXCLUDES 1   *mechanical complication of biological heart valve graft (T82.22-)*

> **CC Excl: For codes in subcategory T82.0:**
> PDX collection 1448

✓x7ᵗʰ **T82.01** **Breakdown (mechanical) of heart valve prosthesis** `CC`

✓x7ᵗʰ **T82.02** **Displacement of heart valve prosthesis** `CC`
     Malposition of heart valve prosthesis

✓x7ᵗʰ **T82.03** **Leakage of heart valve prosthesis** `CC`

✓x7ᵗʰ **T82.09** **Other mechanical complication of heart valve prosthesis** `CC`
     Obstruction (mechanical) of heart valve prosthesis
     Perforation of heart valve prosthesis
     Protrusion of heart valve prosthesis

✓5ᵗʰ **T82.1** **Mechanical complication of** cardiac electronic device

> **CC Excl: For codes in subcategory T82.1, unless otherwise noted:** PDX collection 1449

✓6ᵗʰ **T82.11** **Breakdown (mechanical) of cardiac electronic device**

     ✓7ᵗʰ **T82.110** **Breakdown (mechanical) of cardiac electrode** `CC`

     ✓7ᵗʰ **T82.111** **Breakdown (mechanical) of cardiac pulse generator (battery)** `CC`

     ✓7ᵗʰ **T82.118** **Breakdown (mechanical) of other cardiac electronic device** `CC`
         CC Excl: PDX collection 1450

     ✓7ᵗʰ **T82.119** **Breakdown (mechanical) of** unspecified **cardiac electronic device** `CC`
         CC Excl: No Excl

✓6ᵗʰ **T82.12** **Displacement of cardiac electronic device**
     Malposition of cardiac electronic device

     ✓7ᵗʰ **T82.120** **Displacement of** cardiac electrode `CC`

     ✓7ᵗʰ **T82.121** **Displacement of cardiac** pulse generator (battery) `CC`

     ✓7ᵗʰ **T82.128** **Displacement of other cardiac electronic device** `CC`
         CC Excl: PDX collection 1450

     ✓7ᵗʰ **T82.129** **Displacement of** unspecified **cardiac electronic device** `CC`
         CC Excl: No Excl

✓6ᵗʰ **T82.19** **Other mechanical complication of cardiac electronic device**
     Leakage of cardiac electronic device
     Obstruction of cardiac electronic device
     Perforation of cardiac electronic device
     Protrusion of cardiac electronic device

     ✓7ᵗʰ **T82.190** **Other mechanical complication of cardiac electrode** `CC`

     ✓7ᵗʰ **T82.191** **Other mechanical complication of cardiac** pulse generator (battery) `CC`

     ✓7ᵗʰ **T82.198** **Other mechanical complication of other cardiac** electronic device `CC`
         CC Excl: PDX collection 1450

     ✓7ᵗʰ **T82.199** **Other mechanical complication of** unspecified **cardiac device** `CC`
         CC Excl: No Excl

✓5ᵗʰ **T82.2** **Mechanical complication of** coronary artery bypass graft **and** biological heart valve graft
     EXCLUDES 1   *mechanical complication of artificial heart valve prosthesis (T82.0-)*

✓6ᵗʰ **T82.21** **Mechanical complication of** coronary artery bypass graft

> **CC Excl: For codes in subcategory T82.21:**
> PDX collection 1451

     ✓7ᵗʰ **T82.211** **Breakdown (mechanical) of coronary artery bypass graft** `CC`

     ✓7ᵗʰ **T82.212** **Displacement of coronary artery bypass graft** `CC`
         Malposition of coronary artery bypass graft

     ✓7ᵗʰ **T82.213** **Leakage of coronary artery bypass graft** `CC`

     ✓7ᵗʰ **T82.218** **Other mechanical complication of coronary artery bypass graft** `CC`
         Obstruction, mechanical of coronary artery bypass graft
         Perforation of coronary artery bypass graft
         Protrusion of coronary artery bypass graft

✓6ᵗʰ **T82.22** **Mechanical complication of** biological heart valve graft

> **CC Excl: For codes in subcategory T82.22:**
> PDX collection 1450

     ✓7ᵗʰ **T82.221** **Breakdown (mechanical) of biological heart valve graft** `CC`

     ✓7ᵗʰ **T82.222** **Displacement of biological heart valve graft** `CC`
         Malposition of biological heart valve graft

     ✓7ᵗʰ **T82.223** **Leakage of biological heart valve graft** `CC`

     ✓7ᵗʰ **T82.228** **Other mechanical complication of biological heart valve graft** `CC`
         Obstruction of biological heart valve graft
         Perforation of biological heart valve graft
         Protrusion of biological heart valve graft

✓5ᵗʰ **T82.3** **Mechanical complication of** other vascular grafts

> **CC Excl: For codes in subcategory T82.3:**
> PDX collection 1452

✓6ᵗʰ **T82.31** **Breakdown (mechanical) of other vascular grafts**

     10 ✓7ᵗʰ **T82.310** **Breakdown (mechanical) of** aortic (bifurcation) graft (replacement) `CC` `HCC`

     10 ✓7ᵗʰ **T82.311** **Breakdown (mechanical) of** carotid arterial graft (bypass) `CC` `HCC`

     10 ✓7ᵗʰ **T82.312** **Breakdown (mechanical) of** femoral arterial graft (bypass) `CC` `HCC`

     10 ✓7ᵗʰ **T82.318** **Breakdown (mechanical) of** other vascular grafts `CC` `HCC`

     10 ✓7ᵗʰ **T82.319** **Breakdown (mechanical) of** unspecified **vascular grafts** `CC` `HCC`

✓6ᵗʰ **T82.32** **Displacement of other vascular grafts**
     Malposition of other vascular grafts

     10 ✓7ᵗʰ **T82.320** **Displacement of** aortic (bifurcation) graft (replacement) `CC` `HCC`

     10 ✓7ᵗʰ **T82.321** **Displacement of** carotid arterial graft (bypass) `CC` `HCC`

     10 ✓7ᵗʰ **T82.322** **Displacement of** femoral arterial graft (bypass) `CC` `HCC`

---

[10] HCC with 7th character indicating initial encounter (A, B or C - specific to category).

✓ Additional Character Req   ✓x7ᵗʰ Placeholder Alert   Unacceptable PDx   Manifestation   **H1** - **H14** HAC   **HCC** CMS-HCC Condition   *EXCLUDES 1* Not Coded Here   *EXCLUDES 2* Not Included Here

ICD-10-CM 2018   **1141**

Chapter 19. Injury, Poisoning and Certain Other Consequences of External Causes   **T82.328–T82.7**

10 √7ʰ **T82.328 Displacement of** other **vascular graft** CC HCC

10 √7ʰ **T82.329 Displacement of** unspecified **vascular grafts** CC HCC

√6ʰ **T82.33 Leakage of other vascular grafts**

10 √7ʰ **T82.330 Leakage of** aortic (bifurcation) **graft (replacement)** CC HCC

10 √7ʰ **T82.331 Leakage of** carotid arterial graft **(bypass)** CC HCC

10 √7ʰ **T82.332 Leakage of** femoral arterial graft **(bypass)** CC HCC

10 √7ʰ **T82.338 Leakage of** other **vascular grafts** CC HCC

10 √7ʰ **T82.339 Leakage of** unspecified **vascular graft** CC HCC

√6ʰ **T82.39 Other mechanical complication of other vascular grafts**

     Obstruction (mechanical) of other vascular grafts
     Perforation of other vascular grafts
     Protrusion of other vascular grafts

10 √7ʰ **T82.390 Other mechanical complication of** aortic (bifurcation) graft (replacement) CC HCC

10 √7ʰ **T82.391 Other mechanical complication of** carotid arterial graft (bypass) CC HCC

10 √7ʰ **T82.392 Other mechanical complication of** femoral arterial graft (bypass) CC HCC

10 √7ʰ **T82.398 Other mechanical complication of** other vascular grafts CC HCC

10 √7ʰ **T82.399 Other mechanical complication of** unspecified vascular grafts CC HCC

√5ʰ **T82.4 Mechanical complication of vascular dialysis catheter**
     Mechanical complication of hemodialysis catheter
     EXCLUDES 1   *mechanical complication of intraperitoneal dialysis catheter (T85.62)*

     CC Excl: For codes in subcategory T82.4:
     PDX collection 1452

√x7ʰ **T82.41 Breakdown (mechanical) of vascular dialysis catheter** CC HCC

√x7ʰ **T82.42 Displacement of vascular dialysis catheter** CC HCC
     Malposition of vascular dialysis catheter

√x7ʰ **T82.43 Leakage of vascular dialysis catheter** CC HCC

√x7ʰ **T82.49 Other complication of vascular dialysis catheter** CC HCC
     Obstruction (mechanical) of vascular dialysis catheter
     Perforation of vascular dialysis catheter
     Protrusion of vascular dialysis catheter

√5ʰ **T82.5 Mechanical complication of other cardiac and vascular devices and implants**
     EXCLUDES 2   *mechanical complication of epidural and subdural infusion catheter (T85.61)*

     CC Excl: For codes in subcategory T82.5, unless otherwise noted: PDX collection 1452

√6ʰ **T82.51 Breakdown (mechanical) of other cardiac and vascular devices and implants**

10 √7ʰ **T82.510 Breakdown (mechanical) of** surgically created arteriovenous fistula CC HCC

10 √7ʰ **T82.511 Breakdown (mechanical) of** surgically created arteriovenous shunt CC HCC

√7ʰ **T82.512 Breakdown (mechanical) of** artificial heart CC
     CC Excl: PDX collection 1450

10 √7ʰ **T82.513 Breakdown (mechanical) of** balloon (counterpulsation) device CC HCC

10 √7ʰ **T82.514 Breakdown (mechanical) of** infusion catheter CC HCC

10 √7ʰ **T82.515 Breakdown (mechanical) of** umbrella device CC HCC

10 √7ʰ **T82.518 Breakdown (mechanical) of** other cardiac and vascular devices and implants CC HCC

√7ʰ **T82.519 Breakdown (mechanical) of** unspecified cardiac and vascular devices and implants CC
     CC Excl: PDX collection 1453

√6ʰ **T82.52 Displacement of other cardiac and vascular devices and implants**
     Malposition of other cardiac and vascular devices and implants

10 √7ʰ **T82.520 Displacement of** surgically created arteriovenous fistula CC HCC

10 √7ʰ **T82.521 Displacement of** surgically created arteriovenous shunt CC HCC

√7ʰ **T82.522 Displacement of** artificial heart CC
     CC Excl: PDX collection 1450

10 √7ʰ **T82.523 Displacement of** balloon (counterpulsation) device CC HCC

10 √7ʰ **T82.524 Displacement of** infusion catheter CC HCC

10 √7ʰ **T82.525 Displacement of** umbrella device CC HCC

10 √7ʰ **T82.528 Displacement of** other cardiac and vascular devices and implants CC HCC

√7ʰ **T82.529 Displacement of** unspecified cardiac and vascular devices and implants CC

√6ʰ **T82.53 Leakage of other cardiac and vascular devices and implants**

10 √7ʰ **T82.530 Leakage of** surgically created arteriovenous fistula CC HCC

10 √7ʰ **T82.531 Leakage of** surgically created arteriovenous shunt CC HCC

√7ʰ **T82.532 Leakage of** artificial heart CC
     CC Excl: PDX collection 1450

10 √7ʰ **T82.533 Leakage of** balloon (counterpulsation) device CC HCC

10 √7ʰ **T82.534 Leakage of** infusion catheter CC HCC

10 √7ʰ **T82.535 Leakage of** umbrella device CC HCC

√7ʰ **T82.538 Leakage of** other cardiac and vascular devices and implants CC HCC

√7ʰ **T82.539 Leakage of** unspecified cardiac and vascular devices and implants CC
     CC Excl: PDX collection 1453

√6ʰ **T82.59 Other mechanical complication of other cardiac and vascular devices and implants**
     Obstruction (mechanical) of other cardiac and vascular devices and implants
     Perforation of other cardiac and vascular devices and implants
     Protrusion of other cardiac and vascular devices and implants

10 √7ʰ **T82.590 Other mechanical complication of** surgically created arteriovenous fistula CC HCC

10 √7ʰ **T82.591 Other mechanical complication of** surgically created arteriovenous shunt CC HCC

√7ʰ **T82.592 Other mechanical complication of** artificial heart CC
     CC Excl: PDX collection 1450

10 √7ʰ **T82.593 Other mechanical complication of** balloon (counterpulsation) device CC HCC

10 √7ʰ **T82.594 Other mechanical complication of** infusion catheter CC HCC
     CC Excl: PDX collection 1450

10 √7ʰ **T82.595 Other mechanical complication of** umbrella device CC HCC

10 √7ʰ **T82.598 Other mechanical complication of** other cardiac and vascular devices and implants CC HCC
     CC Excl: PDX collection 1450

√7ʰ **T82.599 Other mechanical complication of** unspecified cardiac and vascular devices and implants CC
     CC Excl: PDX collection 1453

10 √x7ʰ **T82.6 Infection and inflammatory reaction due to cardiac valveprosthesis** CC H13 HCC
     Use additional code to identify infection
     CC Excl: PDX collection 1454

10 √x7ʰ **T82.7 Infection and inflammatory reaction due to** other **cardiac and vascular devices, implants and grafts** CC H13 HCC
     Use additional code to identify infection
     CC Excl: PDX collection 1454

---

10 HCC with 7th character indicating initial encounter (A, B or C - specific to category).

N Newborn: 0   P Pediatric: 0-17   M Maternity: 12-55   A Adult: 15-124   **MCC** Major CC Condition   **PDxMCC** PDx acts as own MCC   **CC** CC Condition   **PDxCC** PDx acts as own CC

1142   ICD-10-CM 2018

✓5ᵗʰ **T82.8** Other specified complications of cardiac and vascular prosthetic devices, implants and grafts

✓6ᵗʰ   **T82.81** Embolism due to cardiac and vascular prosthetic devices, implants and grafts

✓7ᵗʰ   **T82.817** Embolism due to cardiac prosthetic devices, implants and grafts   CC
        CC Excl: PDX collection 1455

10 ✓7ᵗʰ   **T82.818** Embolism due to vascular prosthetic devices, implants and grafts   CC HCC
        CC Excl: PDX collection 1454

✓6ᵗʰ   **T82.82** Fibrosis due to cardiac and vascular prosthetic devices, implants and grafts

✓7ᵗʰ   **T82.827** Fibrosis due to cardiac prosthetic devices, implants and grafts   CC
        CC Excl: PDX collection 1455

10 ✓7ᵗʰ   **T82.828** Fibrosis due to vascular prosthetic devices, implants and grafts   CC HCC
        CC Excl: PDX collection 1454

✓6ᵗʰ   **T82.83** Hemorrhage due to cardiac and vascular prosthetic devices, implants and grafts

✓7ᵗʰ   **T82.837** Hemorrhage due to cardiac prosthetic devices, implants and grafts   CC
        CC Excl: PDX collection 1455

10 ✓7ᵗʰ   **T82.838** Hemorrhage due to vascular prosthetic devices, implants and grafts   CC HCC
        CC Excl: PDX collection 1454

✓6ᵗʰ   **T82.84** Pain due to cardiac and vascular prosthetic devices, implants and grafts

✓7ᵗʰ   **T82.847** Pain due to cardiac prosthetic devices, implants and grafts   CC
        CC Excl: PDX collection 1455

10 ✓7ᵗʰ   **T82.848** Pain due to vascular prosthetic devices, implants and grafts   CC HCC
        CC Excl: PDX collection 1454

✓6ᵗʰ   **T82.85** Stenosis due to cardiac and vascular prosthetic devices, implants and grafts

✓7ᵗʰ   **T82.855** Stenosis of coronary artery stent   CC
        In-stent stenosis (restenosis) of coronary artery stent
        Restenosis of coronary artery stent
        CC Excl: PDX collection 1455

10 ✓7ᵗʰ   **T82.856** Stenosis of peripheral vascular stent   CC HCC
        In-stent stenosis (restenosis) of peripheral vascular stent
        Restenosis of peripheral vascular stent
        CC Excl: PDX collection 1454

✓7ᵗʰ   **T82.857** Stenosis of other cardiac prosthetic devices, implants and grafts   CC
        CC Excl: PDX collection 1455

10 ✓7ᵗʰ   **T82.858** Stenosis of other vascular prostheticdevices, implants and grafts   CC HCC
        CC Excl: PDX collection 1454

✓6ᵗʰ   **T82.86** Thrombosis of cardiac and vascular prosthetic devices, implants and grafts

✓7ᵗʰ   **T82.867** Thrombosis due to cardiac prosthetic devices, implants and grafts   CC
        CC Excl: PDX collection 1455

10 ✓7ᵗʰ   **T82.868** Thrombosis due to vascular prosthetic devices, implants and grafts   CC HCC
        CC Excl: PDX collection 1454

✓6ᵗʰ   **T82.89** Other specified complication of cardiac and vascular prosthetic devices, implants and grafts

✓7ᵗʰ   **T82.897** Other specified complication of cardiac prosthetic devices, implants and grafts   CC
        CC Excl: PDX collection 1455

10 ✓7ᵗʰ   **T82.898** Other specified complication of vascular prosthetic devices, implants and grafts   CC HCC
        CC Excl: PDX collection 1454

✓x7ᵗʰ **T82.9** Unspecified complication of cardiac and vascular prosthetic device, implant and graft   CC
    CC Excl: PDX collection 1455

✓4ᵗʰ **T83** Complications of genitourinary prosthetic devices, implants and grafts

EXCLUDES 2   failure and rejection of transplanted organs and tissue (T86.-)

> The appropriate 7th character is to be added to each code from category T83.
> A   initial encounter
> D   subsequent encounter
> S   sequela

> CC Excl: For CC codes in category T83, unless otherwise noted:
>   PDX collection 1456

✓5ᵗʰ **T83.Ø** Mechanical complication of urinary catheter

EXCLUDES 2   complications of stoma of urinary tract (N99.5-)

✓6ᵗʰ   **T83.Ø1** Breakdown (mechanical) of urinary catheter

10 ✓7ᵗʰ   **T83.Ø1Ø** Breakdown (mechanical) of cystostomy catheter   CC HCC

10 ✓7ᵗʰ   **T83.Ø11** Breakdown (mechanical) of indwelling urethral catheter   HCC

10 ✓7ᵗʰ   **T83.Ø12** Breakdown (mechanical) of nephrostomy catheter   HCC

10 ✓7ᵗʰ   **T83.Ø18** Breakdown (mechanical) of other urinary catheter   HCC
        Breakdown (mechanical) of Hopkins catheter
        Breakdown (mechanical) of ileostomy catheter
        Breakdown (mechanical) urostomy catheter

✓6ᵗʰ   **T83.Ø2** Displacement of urinary catheter
      Malposition of urinary catheter

10 ✓7ᵗʰ   **T83.Ø2Ø** Displacement of cystostomy catheter   CC HCC

10 ✓7ᵗʰ   **T83.Ø21** Displacement of indwelling urethral catheter   HCC

10 ✓7ᵗʰ   **T83.Ø22** Displacement of nephrostomy catheter   HCC

10 ✓7ᵗʰ   **T83.Ø28** Displacement of other urinary catheter   HCC
        Displacement of Hopkins catheter
        Displacement of ileostomy catheter
        Displacement of urostomy catheter

✓6ᵗʰ   **T83.Ø3** Leakage of urinary catheter

10 ✓7ᵗʰ   **T83.Ø3Ø** Leakage of cystostomy catheter   CC HCC

10 ✓7ᵗʰ   **T83.Ø31** Leakage of indwelling urethral catheter   HCC

10 ✓7ᵗʰ   **T83.Ø32** Leakage of nephrostomy catheter   HCC

10 ✓7ᵗʰ   **T83.Ø38** Leakage of other urinary catheter   HCC
        Leakage of Hopkins catheter
        Leakage of ileostomy catheter
        Leakage of urostomy catheter

✓6ᵗʰ   **T83.Ø9** Other mechanical complication of urinary catheter
      Obstruction (mechanical) of urinary catheter
      Perforation of urinary catheter
      Protrusion of urinary catheter

10 ✓7ᵗʰ   **T83.Ø9Ø** Other mechanical complication of cystostomy catheter   CC HCC

10 ✓7ᵗʰ   **T83.Ø91** Other mechanical complication of indwelling urethral catheter   HCC

10 ✓7ᵗʰ   **T83.Ø92** Other mechanical complication of nephrostomy catheter   HCC

10 ✓7ᵗʰ   **T83.Ø98** Other mechanical complication of other urinary catheter   HCC
        Other mechanical complication of Hopkins catheter
        Other mechanical complication of ileostomy catheter
        Other mechanical complication of urostomy catheter

---

10 HCC with 7th character indicating initial encounter (A, B or C - specific to category).

✓ Additional Character Req   ✓x7ᵗʰ Placeholder Alert   Unacceptable PDx   Manifestation   H1 - H14 HAC   HCC CMS-HCC Condition   *EXCLUDES 1* Not Coded Here   *EXCLUDES 2* Not Included Here

ICD-10-CM 2018   1143

√5ᵗʰ **T83.1** **Mechanical complication of** other urinary devices and implants

   √6ᵗʰ **T83.11** **Breakdown (mechanical) of** other urinary devices and implants

      10 √7ᵗʰ **T83.110** **Breakdown (mechanical) of urinary** CC HCC **electronic stimulator device**

         EXCLUDES 2   *breakdown (mechanical) of electrode (lead) for sacral nerve neurostimulator (T85.111)*
                breakdown (mechanical) of implanted electronic sacral neurostimulator, pulse generator or receiver (T85.113)

      10 √7ᵗʰ **T83.111** **Breakdown (mechanical) of** CC HCC **implanted urinary sphincter**

      10 √7ᵗʰ **T83.112** **Breakdown (mechanical) of** CC HCC **indwelling ureteral stent**

      10 √7ᵗʰ **T83.113** **Breakdown (mechanical) of** other CC HCC **urinary stents**

         Breakdown (mechanical) of ileal conduit stent
         Breakdown (mechanical) of nephroureteral stent

      10 √7ᵗʰ **T83.118** **Breakdown (mechanical) of** other CC HCC **urinary devices and implants**

   √6ᵗʰ **T83.12** **Displacement of other urinary devices and implants**
      Malposition of other urinary devices and implants

      10 √7ᵗʰ **T83.120** **Displacement of urinary electronic** CC HCC **stimulator device**

         EXCLUDES 2   *displacement of electrode (lead) for sacral nerve neurostimulator (T85.121)*
                displacement of implanted electronic sacral neurostimulator, pulse generator or receiver (T85.123)

      10 √7ᵗʰ **T83.121** **Displacement of implanted** CC HCC **urinary sphincter**

      10 √7ᵗʰ **T83.122** **Displacement of indwelling** CC HCC **ureteral stent**

      10 √7ᵗʰ **T83.123** **Displacement of other urinary** CC HCC **stents**

         Displacement of ileal conduit stent
         Displacement of nephroureteral stent

      10 √7ᵗʰ **T83.128** **Displacement of** other urinary CC HCC **devices and implants**

   √6ᵗʰ **T83.19** **Other mechanical complication of other urinary devices and implants**
      Leakage of other urinary devices and implants
      Obstruction (mechanical) of other urinary devices and implants
      Perforation of other urinary devices and implants
      Protrusion of other urinary devices and implants

      10 √7ᵗʰ **T83.190** **Other mechanical complication of** CC HCC **urinary electronic stimulator device**

         EXCLUDES 2   *other mechanical complication of electrode (lead) for sacral nerve neurostimulator (T85.191)*
                other mechanical complication of implanted electronic sacral neurostimulator, pulse generator or receiver (T85.193)

      10 √7ᵗʰ **T83.191** **Other mechanical complication of** CC HCC **implanted urinary sphincter**

      10 √7ᵗʰ **T83.192** **Other mechanical complication of** CC HCC **indwelling ureteral stent**

      10 √7ᵗʰ **T83.193** **Other mechanical complication of** CC HCC **other urinary stent**

         Other mechanical complication of ileal conduit stent
         Other mechanical complication of nephroureteral stent

      10 √7ᵗʰ **T83.198** **Other mechanical complication of** CC HCC **other urinary devices and implants**

√5ᵗʰ **T83.2** **Mechanical complication of** graft of urinary organ

   10 √x7ᵗʰ **T83.21** **Breakdown (mechanical) of graft of urinary** CC HCC **organ**

   10 √x7ᵗʰ **T83.22** **Displacement of graft of urinary organ** CC HCC
      Malposition of graft of urinary organ

   10 √x7ᵗʰ **T83.23** **Leakage of graft of urinary organ** CC HCC

   10 √x7ᵗʰ **T83.24** **Erosion of graft of urinary organ** CC HCC

   10 √x7ᵗʰ **T83.25** **Exposure of graft of urinary organ** CC HCC

   10 √x7ᵗʰ **T83.29** **Other mechanical complication of graft of** CC HCC **urinary organ**
      Obstruction (mechanical) of graft of urinary organ
      Perforation of graft of urinary organ
      Protrusion of graft of urinary organ

√5ᵗʰ **T83.3** **Mechanical complication of** intrauterine contraceptive device

   √x7ᵗʰ **T83.31** **Breakdown (mechanical) of intrauterine** ♀ **contraceptive device**

   √x7ᵗʰ **T83.32** **Displacement of intrauterine contraceptive** ♀ **device**
      Malposition of intrauterine contraceptive device
      Missing string of intrauterine contraceptive device

   √x7ᵗʰ **T83.39** **Other mechanical complication of intrauterine** ♀ **contraceptive device**
      Leakage of intrauterine contraceptive device
      Obstruction (mechanical) of intrauterine contraceptive device
      Perforation of intrauterine contraceptive device
      Protrusion of intrauterine contraceptive device

√5ᵗʰ **T83.4** **Mechanical complication of** other prosthetic devices, implants and grafts of genital tract

   √6ᵗʰ **T83.41** **Breakdown (mechanical) of other prosthetic devices, implants and grafts of genital tract**

      10 √7ᵗʰ **T83.410** **Breakdown (mechanical) of** CC HCC ♂ **implanted penile prosthesis**
         Breakdown (mechanical) of penile prosthesis cylinder
         Breakdown (mechanical) of penile prosthesis pump
         Breakdown (mechanical) of penile prosthesis reservoir

      10 √7ᵗʰ **T83.411** **Breakdown (mechanical) of** CC HCC **implanted testicular prosthesis**

      10 √7ᵗʰ **T83.418** **Breakdown (mechanical) of** other CC HCC **prosthetic devices, implants and grafts of genital tract**

   √6ᵗʰ **T83.42** **Displacement of other prosthetic devices, implants and grafts of genital tract**
      Malposition of other prosthetic devices, implants and grafts of genital tract

      10 √7ᵗʰ **T83.420** **Displacement of** implanted penile CC HCC ♂ **prosthesis**
         Displacement of penile prosthesis cylinder
         Displacement of penile prosthesis pump
         Displacement of penile prosthesis reservoir

      10 √7ᵗʰ **T83.421** **Displacement of** implanted CC HCC **testicular prosthesis**

      10 √7ᵗʰ **T83.428** **Displacement of** other prosthetic CC HCC **devices, implants and grafts of genital tract**

   √6ᵗʰ **T83.49** **Other mechanical complication of other prosthetic devices, implants and grafts of genital tract**
      Leakage of other prosthetic devices, implants and grafts of genital tract
      Obstruction, mechanical of other prosthetic devices, implants and grafts of genital tract
      Perforation of other prosthetic devices, implants and grafts of genital tract
      Protrusion of other prosthetic devices, implants and grafts of genital tract

      10 √7ᵗʰ **T83.490** **Other mechanical complication** CC HCC ♂ **of implanted penile prosthesis**
         Other mechanical complication of penile prosthesis cylinder
         Other mechanical complication of penile prosthesis pump
         Other mechanical complication of penile prosthesis reservoir

---

10 HCC with 7th character indicating initial encounter (A, B or C - specific to category).

N Newborn: 0   P Pediatric: 0-17   M Maternity: 12-55   A Adult: 15-124   MCC Major CC Condition   PDxMCC PDx acts as own MCC   CC CC Condition   PDxCC PDx acts as own CC

1144   ICD-10-CM 2018

10 ✓7ᵗʰ **T83.491** **Other mechanical complication of** `CC` `HCC`
implanted testicular prosthesis

10 ✓7ᵗʰ **T83.498** **Other mechanical complication of** `CC` `HCC`
**other prosthetic devices, implants and
grafts of genital tract**

✓5ᵗʰ **T83.5** **Infection and inflammatory reaction due to prosthetic device,
implant and graft in urinary system**
Use additional code to identify infection

> **CC Excl: For codes in subcategory T83.5, unless
> otherwise noted:** PDX collection 1458

✓6ᵗʰ **T83.51** **Infection and inflammatory reaction due to urinary
catheter**
EXCLUDES 2   *complications of stoma of urinary tract
(N99.5-)*

10 ✓7ᵗʰ **T83.510** **Infection and inflammatory** `CC` `HCC`
reaction due to cystostomy catheter

10 ✓7ᵗʰ **T83.511** **Infection and inflammatory** `CC` `H5` `HCC`
**reaction due to indwelling urethral
catheter**
CC Excl: PDX collection 1457

10 ✓7ᵗʰ **T83.512** **Infection and inflammatory** `CC` `HCC`
reaction due to nephrostomy catheter

10 ✓7ᵗʰ **T83.518** **Infection and inflammatory** `CC` `H5` `HCC`
reaction due to other urinary catheter
Infection and inflammatory reaction due to
Hopkins catheter
Infection and inflammatory reaction due to
ileostomy catheter
Infection and inflammatory reaction due to
urostomy catheter

✓6ᵗʰ **T83.59** **Infection and inflammatory reaction due to
prosthetic device, implant and graft in urinary
system**

10 ✓7ᵗʰ **T83.590** **Infection and inflammatory** `CC` `HCC`
**reaction due to implanted urinary
neurostimulation device**
EXCLUDES 2   *infection and inflammatory
reaction due to electrode
lead of sacral nerve
neurostimulator (T85.732)
infection and inflammatory
reaction due to pulse
generator or receiver of
sacral nerve neurostimulator
(T85.734)*

10 ✓7ᵗʰ **T83.591** **Infection and inflammatory** `CC` `HCC`
**reaction due to implanted urinary
sphincter**

10 ✓7ᵗʰ **T83.592** **Infection and inflammatory** `CC` `HCC`
reaction due to indwelling ureteral stent

10 ✓7ᵗʰ **T83.593** **Infection and inflammatory** `CC` `HCC`
reaction due to other urinary stents
Infection and inflammatory reaction due to
ileal conduit stents
Infection and inflammatory reaction due to
nephroureteral stent

10 ✓7ᵗʰ **T83.598** **Infection and inflammatory** `CC` `HCC`
**reaction due to other prosthetic device,
implant and graft in urinary system**

✓5ᵗʰ **T83.6** **Infection and inflammatory reaction due to prosthetic device,
implant and graft in genital tract**
Use additional code to identify infection

> **CC Excl: For codes in subcategory T83.6:**
> PDX collection 1458

10 ✓x7ᵗʰ **T83.61** **Infection and inflammatory reaction due to** `CC` `HCC`
implanted penile prosthesis
Infection and inflammatory reaction due to penile
prosthesis cylinder
Infection and inflammatory reaction due to penile
prosthesis pump
Infection and inflammatory reaction due to penile
prosthesis reservoir

10 ✓x7ᵗʰ **T83.62** **Infection and inflammatory reaction due to** `CC` `HCC`
implanted testicular prosthesis

10 ✓x7ᵗʰ **T83.69** **Infection and inflammatory reaction due to** `CC` `HCC`
**other prosthetic device, implant and graft in
genital tract**

✓5ᵗʰ **T83.7** **Complications due to implanted mesh and other prosthetic
materials**

✓6ᵗʰ **T83.71** **Erosion of implanted mesh and other prosthetic
materials to surrounding organ or tissue**

10 ✓7ᵗʰ **T83.711** **Erosion of implanted vaginal mesh** `HCC` ♀
to surrounding organ or tissue
Erosion of implanted vaginal mesh into
pelvic floor muscles

10 ✓7ᵗʰ **T83.712** **Erosion of implanted urethral** `CC` `HCC`
mesh to surrounding organ or tissue
Erosion of implanted female urethral sling
Erosion of implanted male urethral sling
Erosion of implanted urethral mesh into
pelvic floor muscles

10 ✓7ᵗʰ **T83.713** **Erosion of implanted urethral** `CC` `HCC`
**bulking agent to surrounding
organ or tissue**

10 ✓7ᵗʰ **T83.714** **Erosion of implanted ureteral** `CC` `HCC`
**bulking agent to surrounding
organ or tissue**

10 ✓7ᵗʰ **T83.718** **Erosion of other implanted mesh** `CC` `HCC`
to organ or tissue

10 ✓7ᵗʰ **T83.719** **Erosion of other prosthetic** `CC` `HCC`
materials to surrounding organ or tissue

✓6ᵗʰ **T83.72** **Exposure of implanted mesh and other prosthetic
materials into surrounding organ or tissue**
Extrusion of implanted mesh

10 ✓7ᵗʰ **T83.721** **Exposure of implanted vaginal mesh** `HCC` ♀
into vagina
Exposure of implanted vaginal mesh
through vaginal wall

10 ✓7ᵗʰ **T83.722** **Exposure of implanted urethral** `CC` `HCC`
mesh into urethra
Exposure of implanted female urethral
sling
Exposure of implanted male urethral sling
Exposure of implanted urethral mesh
through urethral wall

10 ✓7ᵗʰ **T83.723** **Exposure of implanted urethral** `CC` `HCC`
bulking agent into urethra

10 ✓7ᵗʰ **T83.724** **Exposure of implanted ureteral** `CC` `HCC`
bulking agent into ureter

10 ✓7ᵗʰ **T83.728** **Exposure of other implanted mesh** `CC` `HCC`
into organ or tissue

10 ✓7ᵗʰ **T83.729** **Exposure of other prosthetic** `CC` `HCC`
materials into organ or tissue

10 ✓x7ᵗʰ **T83.79** **Other specified complications due to other** `CC` `HCC`
genitourinary prosthetic materials
CC Excl: PDX collection 1458

✓5ᵗʰ **T83.8** **Other specified complications of genitourinary prosthetic
devices, implants and grafts**

> **CC Excl: For codes in subcategory T83.8:**
> PDX collection 1458

10 ✓x7ᵗʰ **T83.81** **Embolism due to genitourinary prosthetic** `CC` `HCC`
devices, implants and grafts

10 ✓x7ᵗʰ **T83.82** **Fibrosis due to genitourinary prosthetic** `CC` `HCC`
devices, implants and grafts

10 ✓x7ᵗʰ **T83.83** **Hemorrhage due to genitourinary prosthetic** `CC` `HCC`
devices, implants and grafts

10 ✓x7ᵗʰ **T83.84** **Pain due to genitourinary prosthetic devices,** `CC` `HCC`
implants and grafts

10 ✓x7ᵗʰ **T83.85** **Stenosis due to genitourinary prosthetic** `CC` `HCC`
devices, implants and grafts

10 ✓x7ᵗʰ **T83.86** **Thrombosis due to genitourinary prosthetic** `CC` `HCC`
devices, implants and grafts

10 ✓x7ᵗʰ **T83.89** **Other specified complication of genitourinary** `CC` `HCC`
prosthetic devices, implants and grafts

10 ✓x7ᵗʰ **T83.9** **Unspecified complication of genitourinary prosthetic** `CC` `HCC`
device, implant and graft
CC Excl: PDX collection 1458

---

10 HCC with 7th character indicating initial encounter (A, B or C - specific to category).

✓ Additional Character Req   ✓x7ᵗʰ Placeholder Alert   Unacceptable PDx   Manifestation   `H1`–`H14` HAC   `HCC` CMS-HCC Condition   EXCLUDES 1 Not Coded Here   EXCLUDES 2 Not Included Here

✓4ᵗʰ T84 Complications of internal orthopedic prosthetic devices, implants and grafts

> EXCLUDES 2   *failure and rejection of transplanted organs and tissues (T86.-)*
> *fracture of bone following insertion of orthopedic implant, joint prosthesis or bone plate (M96.6)*

> The appropriate 7th character is to be added to each code from category T84.
> A   initial encounter
> D   subsequent encounter
> S   sequela

> **CC Excl: For codes in category T84, unless otherwise noted:**
> PDX collection 911

✓5ᵗʰ T84.0 Mechanical complication of internal joint prosthesis

  ✓6ᵗʰ T84.01 Broken internal joint prosthesis
    Breakage (fracture) of prosthetic joint
    Broken prosthetic joint implant
>   EXCLUDES 1   *periprosthetic joint implant fracture ▶(M97-)◀*

    10 ✓7ᵗʰ **T84.010 Broken internal right hip prosthesis** CC HCC
    10 ✓7ᵗʰ **T84.011 Broken internal left hip prosthesis** CC HCC
    10 ✓7ᵗʰ **T84.012 Broken internal right knee prosthesis** CC HCC
    10 ✓7ᵗʰ **T84.013 Broken internal left knee prosthesis** CC HCC
    10 ✓7ᵗʰ **T84.018 Broken internal joint prosthesis, other site** CC HCC
        Use additional code to identify the joint (Z96.6-)
    10 ✓7ᵗʰ **T84.019 Broken internal joint prosthesis, unspecified site** CC HCC

  ✓6ᵗʰ T84.02 Dislocation of internal joint prosthesis
    Instability of internal joint prosthesis
    Subluxation of internal joint prosthesis

    10 ✓7ᵗʰ **T84.020 Dislocation of internal right hip prosthesis** CC HCC
    10 ✓7ᵗʰ **T84.021 Dislocation of internal left hip prosthesis** CC HCC
    10 ✓7ᵗʰ **T84.022 Instability of internal right knee prosthesis** CC HCC
    10 ✓7ᵗʰ **T84.023 Instability of internal left knee prosthesis** CC HCC
    10 ✓7ᵗʰ **T84.028 Dislocation of other internal joint prosthesis** CC HCC
        Use additional code to identify the joint (Z96.6-)
    10 ✓7ᵗʰ **T84.029 Dislocation of unspecified internal joint prosthesis** CC HCC

  ✓6ᵗʰ T84.03 Mechanical loosening of internal prosthetic joint
    Aseptic loosening of prosthetic joint

    10 ✓7ᵗʰ **T84.030 Mechanical loosening of internal right hip prosthetic joint** CC HCC
    10 ✓7ᵗʰ **T84.031 Mechanical loosening of internal left hip prosthetic joint** CC HCC
    10 ✓7ᵗʰ **T84.032 Mechanical loosening of internal right knee prosthetic joint** CC HCC
    10 ✓7ᵗʰ **T84.033 Mechanical loosening of internal left knee prosthetic joint** CC HCC
    10 ✓7ᵗʰ **T84.038 Mechanical loosening of other internal prosthetic joint** CC HCC
        Use additional code to identify the joint (Z96.6-)
    10 ✓7ᵗʰ **T84.039 Mechanical loosening of unspecified internal prosthetic joint** CC HCC

  ✓6ᵗʰ T84.05 Periprosthetic osteolysis of internal prosthetic joint
    Use additional code to identify major osseous defect, if applicable (M89.7-)

    10 ✓7ᵗʰ **T84.050 Periprosthetic osteolysis of internal prosthetic right hip joint** CC HCC
    10 ✓7ᵗʰ **T84.051 Periprosthetic osteolysis of internal prosthetic left hip joint** CC HCC
    10 ✓7ᵗʰ **T84.052 Periprosthetic osteolysis of internal prosthetic right knee joint** CC HCC
    10 ✓7ᵗʰ **T84.053 Periprosthetic osteolysis of internal prosthetic left knee joint** CC HCC

    10 ✓7ᵗʰ **T84.058 Periprosthetic osteolysis of other internal prosthetic joint** CC HCC
        Use additional code to identify the joint (Z96.6-)
    10 ✓7ᵗʰ **T84.059 Periprosthetic osteolysis of unspecified internal prosthetic joint** CC HCC

  ✓6ᵗʰ T84.06 Wear of articular bearing surface of internal prosthetic joint

    10 ✓7ᵗʰ **T84.060 Wear of articular bearing surface of internal prosthetic right hip joint** CC HCC
    10 ✓7ᵗʰ **T84.061 Wear of articular bearing surface of internal prosthetic left hip joint** CC HCC
    10 ✓7ᵗʰ **T84.062 Wear of articular bearing surface of internal prosthetic right knee joint** CC HCC
    10 ✓7ᵗʰ **T84.063 Wear of articular bearing surface of internal prosthetic left knee joint** CC HCC
    10 ✓7ᵗʰ **T84.068 Wear of articular bearing surface of other internal prosthetic joint** CC HCC
        Use additional code to identify the joint (Z96.6-)
    10 ✓7ᵗʰ **T84.069 Wear of articular bearing surface of unspecified internal prosthetic joint** CC HCC

  ✓6ᵗʰ T84.09 Other mechanical complication of internal joint prosthesis
    Prosthetic joint implant failure NOS

    10 ✓7ᵗʰ **T84.090 Other mechanical complication of internal right hip prosthesis** CC HCC
    10 ✓7ᵗʰ **T84.091 Other mechanical complication of internal left hip prosthesis** CC HCC
    10 ✓7ᵗʰ **T84.092 Other mechanical complication of internal right knee prosthesis** CC HCC
    10 ✓7ᵗʰ **T84.093 Other mechanical complication of internal left knee prosthesis** CC HCC
    10 ✓7ᵗʰ **T84.098 Other mechanical complication of other internal joint prosthesis** CC HCC
        Use additional code to identify the joint (Z96.6-)
    10 ✓7ᵗʰ **T84.099 Other mechanical complication of unspecified internal joint prosthesis** CC HCC

✓5ᵗʰ T84.1 Mechanical complication of internal fixation device of bones of limb

> EXCLUDES 2   *mechanical complication of internal fixation device of bones of feet (T84.2-)*
> *mechanical complication of internal fixation device of bones of fingers (T84.2-)*
> *mechanical complication of internal fixation device of bones of hands (T84.2-)*
> *mechanical complication of internal fixation device of bones of toes (T84.2-)*

  ✓6ᵗʰ T84.11 Breakdown (mechanical) of internal fixation device of bones of limb

    10 ✓7ᵗʰ **T84.110 Breakdown (mechanical) of internal fixation device of right humerus** CC HCC
    10 ✓7ᵗʰ **T84.111 Breakdown (mechanical) of internal fixation device of left humerus** CC HCC
    10 ✓7ᵗʰ **T84.112 Breakdown (mechanical) of internal fixation device of bone of right forearm** CC HCC
    10 ✓7ᵗʰ **T84.113 Breakdown (mechanical) of internal fixation device of bone of left forearm** CC HCC
    10 ✓7ᵗʰ **T84.114 Breakdown (mechanical) of internal fixation device of right femur** CC HCC
    10 ✓7ᵗʰ **T84.115 Breakdown (mechanical) of internal fixation device of left femur** CC HCC
    10 ✓7ᵗʰ **T84.116 Breakdown (mechanical) of internal fixation device of bone of right lower leg** CC HCC
    10 ✓7ᵗʰ **T84.117 Breakdown (mechanical) of internal fixation device of bone of left lower leg** CC HCC
    10 ✓7ᵗʰ **T84.119 Breakdown (mechanical) of internal fixation device of unspecified bone of limb** CC HCC

---

10 HCC with 7th character indicating initial encounter (A, B or C - specific to category).

N Newborn: 0   P Pediatric: 0-17   M Maternity: 12-55   A Adult: 15-124   MCC Major CC Condition   PDxMCC PDx acts as own MCC   CC CC Condition   PDxCC PDx acts as own CC

1146   ICD-10-CM 2018

√6ᵗʰ **T84.12** Displacement of internal fixation device of bones of limb

     Malposition of internal fixation device of bones of limb

10 √7ᵗʰ **T84.120** Displacement of internal fixation device of **right humerus** `CC` `HCC`

10 √7ᵗʰ **T84.121** Displacement of internal fixation device of **left humerus** `CC` `HCC`

10 √7ᵗʰ **T84.122** Displacement of internal fixation device of bone of **right forearm** `CC` `HCC`

10 √7ᵗʰ **T84.123** Displacement of internal fixation device of bone of **left forearm** `CC` `HCC`

10 √7ᵗʰ **T84.124** Displacement of internal fixation device of **right femur** `CC` `HCC`

10 √7ᵗʰ **T84.125** Displacement of internal fixation device of **left femur** `CC` `HCC`

10 √7ᵗʰ **T84.126** Displacement of internal fixation device of bone of **right lower leg** `CC` `HCC`

10 √7ᵗʰ **T84.127** Displacement of internal fixation device of bone of **left lower leg** `CC` `HCC`

10 √7ᵗʰ **T84.129** Displacement of internal fixation device of **unspecified bone** of limb `CC` `HCC`

√6ᵗʰ **T84.19** Other mechanical complication of internal fixation device of bones of limb

     Obstruction (mechanical) of internal fixation device of bones of limb

     Perforation of internal fixation device of bones of limb

     Protrusion of internal fixation device of bones of limb

10 √7ᵗʰ **T84.190** Other mechanical complication of internal fixation device of **right humerus** `CC` `HCC`

10 √7ᵗʰ **T84.191** Other mechanical complication of internal fixation device of **left humerus** `CC` `HCC`

10 √7ᵗʰ **T84.192** Other mechanical complication of internal fixation device of bone of **right forearm** `CC` `HCC`

10 √7ᵗʰ **T84.193** Other mechanical complication of internal fixation device of bone of **left forearm** `CC` `HCC`

10 √7ᵗʰ **T84.194** Other mechanical complication of internal fixation device of **right femur** `CC` `HCC`

10 √7ᵗʰ **T84.195** Other mechanical complication of internal fixation device of **left femur** `CC` `HCC`

10 √7ᵗʰ **T84.196** Other mechanical complication of internal fixation device of bone of **right lower leg** `CC` `HCC`

10 √7ᵗʰ **T84.197** Other mechanical complication of internal fixation device of bone of **left lower leg** `CC` `HCC`

10 √7ᵗʰ **T84.199** Other mechanical complication of internal fixation device of **unspecified bone** of limb `CC` `HCC`

√5ᵗʰ **T84.2** Mechanical complication of internal fixation device of other bones

√6ᵗʰ **T84.21** Breakdown (mechanical) of internal fixation device of other bones

10 √7ᵗʰ **T84.210** Breakdown (mechanical) of internal fixation device of bones of **hand and fingers** `CC` `HCC`

10 √7ᵗʰ **T84.213** Breakdown (mechanical) of internal fixation device of bones of **foot and toes** `CC` `HCC`

10 √7ᵗʰ **T84.216** Breakdown (mechanical) of internal fixation device of **vertebrae** `CC` `HCC`

10 √7ᵗʰ **T84.218** Breakdown (mechanical) of internal fixation device of **other bones** `CC` `HCC`

√6ᵗʰ **T84.22** Displacement of internal fixation device of other bones

     Malposition of internal fixation device of other bones

10 √7ᵗʰ **T84.220** Displacement of internal fixation device of bones of **hand and fingers** `CC` `HCC`

10 √7ᵗʰ **T84.223** Displacement of internal fixation device of bones of **foot and toes** `CC` `HCC`

10 √7ᵗʰ **T84.226** Displacement of internal fixation device of **vertebrae** `CC` `HCC`

10 √7ᵗʰ **T84.228** Displacement of internal fixation device of **other bones** `CC` `HCC`

√6ᵗʰ **T84.29** Other mechanical complication of internal fixation device of other bones

     Obstruction (mechanical) of internal fixation device of other bones

     Perforation of internal fixation device of other bones

     Protrusion of internal fixation device of other bones

10 √7ᵗʰ **T84.290** Other mechanical complication of internal fixation device of bones of **hand and fingers** `CC` `HCC`

10 √7ᵗʰ **T84.293** Other mechanical complication of internal fixation device of bones of **foot and toes** `CC` `HCC`

10 √7ᵗʰ **T84.296** Other mechanical complication of internal fixation device of **vertebrae** `CC` `HCC`

10 √7ᵗʰ **T84.298** Other mechanical complication of internal fixation device of **other bones** `CC` `HCC`

√5ᵗʰ **T84.3** Mechanical complication of other bone devices, implants and grafts

     EXCLUDES 2   other complications of bone graft (T86.83-)

√6ᵗʰ **T84.31** Breakdown (mechanical) of other bone devices, implants and grafts

10 √7ᵗʰ **T84.310** Breakdown (mechanical) of **electronic bone stimulator** `CC` `HCC`

10 √7ᵗʰ **T84.318** Breakdown (mechanical) of **other bone devices, implants and grafts** `CC` `HCC`

√6ᵗʰ **T84.32** Displacement of other bone devices, implants and grafts

     Malposition of other bone devices, implants and grafts

10 √7ᵗʰ **T84.320** Displacement of **electronic bone stimulator** `CC` `HCC`

10 √7ᵗʰ **T84.328** Displacement of **other bone devices, implants and grafts** `CC` `HCC`

         AHA: 2014, 4Q, 28

√6ᵗʰ **T84.39** Other mechanical complication of other bone devices, implants and grafts

     Obstruction (mechanical) of other bone devices, implants and grafts

     Perforation of other bone devices, implants and grafts

     Protrusion of other bone devices, implants and grafts

10 √7ᵗʰ **T84.390** Other mechanical complication of **electronic bone stimulator** `CC` `HCC`

10 √7ᵗʰ **T84.398** Other mechanical complication of **other bone devices, implants and grafts** `CC` `HCC`

√5ᵗʰ **T84.4** Mechanical complication of other internal orthopedic devices, implants and grafts

√6ᵗʰ **T84.41** Breakdown (mechanical) of other internal orthopedic devices, implants and grafts

10 √7ᵗʰ **T84.410** Breakdown (mechanical) of **muscle and tendon graft** `CC` `HCC`

10 √7ᵗʰ **T84.418** Breakdown (mechanical) of **other internal orthopedic devices, implants and grafts** `CC` `HCC`

√6ᵗʰ **T84.42** Displacement of other internal orthopedic devices, implants and grafts

     Malposition of other internal orthopedic devices, implants and grafts

10 √7ᵗʰ **T84.420** Displacement of **muscle and tendon graft** `CC` `HCC`

10 √7ᵗʰ **T84.428** Displacement of **other internal orthopedic devices, implants and grafts** `CC` `HCC`

√6ᵗʰ **T84.49** Other mechanical complication of other internal orthopedic devices, implants and grafts

     Mechanical complication of other internal orthopedic devices, implants and grafts NOS

     Obstruction (mechanical) of other internal orthopedic devices, implants and grafts

     Perforation of other internal orthopedic devices, implants and grafts

     Protrusion of other internal orthopedic devices, implants and grafts

10 √7ᵗʰ **T84.490** Other mechanical complication of **muscle and tendon graft** `CC` `HCC`

10 √7ᵗʰ **T84.498** Other mechanical complication of **other internal orthopedic devices, implants and grafts** `CC` `HCC`

---

10 HCC with 7th character indicating initial encounter (A, B or C - specific to category).

✔Additional Character Req   √ₓ7ᵗʰ Placeholder Alert   Unacceptable PDx   Manifestation   **H1**-**H14** HAC   `HCC` CMS-HCC Condition   *EXCLUDES 1* Not Coded Here   *EXCLUDES 2* Not Included Here

√5ᵗʰ T84.5 Infection and inflammatory reaction due to internal joint prosthesis

Use additional code to identify infection
AHA: 2015, 1Q, 16

> **CC Excl: For codes in subcategory T84.5:**
> PDX collection 1459

10 √x7ᵗʰ **T84.50 Infection and inflammatory reaction due to unspecified internal joint prosthesis** `CC` `HCC`

10 √x7ᵗʰ **T84.51 Infection and inflammatory reaction due to internal right hip prosthesis** `CC` `HCC`

10 √x7ᵗʰ **T84.52 Infection and inflammatory reaction due to internal left hip prosthesis** `CC` `HCC`

10 √x7ᵗʰ **T84.53 Infection and inflammatory reaction due to internal right knee prosthesis** `CC` `HCC`

10 √x7ᵗʰ **T84.54 Infection and inflammatory reaction due to internal left knee prosthesis** `CC` `HCC`

10 √x7ᵗʰ **T84.59 Infection and inflammatory reaction due to other internal joint prosthesis** `CC` `HCC`

√5ᵗʰ T84.6 Infection and inflammatory reaction due to internal fixation device

Use additional code to identify infection

> **CC Excl: For codes in subcategory T84.6:**
> PDX collection 1459

10 √x7ᵗʰ **T84.60 Infection and inflammatory reaction due to internal fixation device of unspecified site** `CC` `H12` `HCC`

√6ᵗʰ **T84.61 Infection and inflammatory reaction due to internal fixation device of arm**

     10 √7ᵗʰ **T84.610 Infection and inflammatory reaction due to internal fixation device of right humerus** `CC` `H12` `HCC`

     10 √7ᵗʰ **T84.611 Infection and inflammatory reaction due to internal fixation device of left humerus** `CC` `H12` `HCC`

     10 √7ᵗʰ **T84.612 Infection and inflammatory reaction due to internal fixation device of right radius** `CC` `H12` `HCC`

     10 √7ᵗʰ **T84.613 Infection and inflammatory reaction due to internal fixation device of left radius** `CC` `H12` `HCC`

     10 √7ᵗʰ **T84.614 Infection and inflammatory reaction due to internal fixation device of right ulna** `CC` `H12` `HCC`

     10 √7ᵗʰ **T84.615 Infection and inflammatory reaction due to internal fixation device of left ulna** `CC` `H12` `HCC`

     10 √7ᵗʰ **T84.619 Infection and inflammatory reaction due to internal fixation device of unspecified bone of arm** `CC` `H12` `HCC`

√6ᵗʰ **T84.62 Infection and inflammatory reaction due to internal fixation device of leg**

     10 √7ᵗʰ **T84.620 Infection and inflammatory reaction due to internal fixation device of right femur** `CC` `HCC`

     10 √7ᵗʰ **T84.621 Infection and inflammatory reaction due to internal fixation device of left femur** `CC` `HCC`

     10 √7ᵗʰ **T84.622 Infection and inflammatory reaction due to internal fixation device of right tibia** `CC` `HCC`

     10 √7ᵗʰ **T84.623 Infection and inflammatory reaction due to internal fixation device of left tibia** `CC` `HCC`

     10 √7ᵗʰ **T84.624 Infection and inflammatory reaction due to internal fixation device of right fibula** `CC` `HCC`

     10 √7ᵗʰ **T84.625 Infection and inflammatory reaction due to internal fixation device of left fibula** `CC` `HCC`

     10 √7ᵗʰ **T84.629 Infection and inflammatory reaction due to internal fixation device of unspecified bone of leg** `CC` `HCC`

10 √x7ᵗʰ **T84.63 Infection and inflammatory reaction due to internal fixation device of spine** `CC` `H12` `HCC`

10 √x7ᵗʰ **T84.69 Infection and inflammatory reaction due to internal fixation device of other site** `CC` `H12` `HCC`

10 √x7ᵗʰ **T84.7 Infection and inflammatory reaction due to other internal orthopedic prosthetic devices, implants and grafts** `CC` `H12` `HCC`

Use additional code to identify infection
CC Excl: PDX collection 1459

√5ᵗʰ T84.8 Other specified complications of internal orthopedic prosthetic devices, implants and grafts

> **CC Excl: For codes in subcategory T84.8:**
> PDX collection 1459

10 √x7ᵗʰ **T84.81 Embolism due to internal orthopedic prosthetic devices, implants and grafts** `CC` `HCC`

10 √x7ᵗʰ **T84.82 Fibrosis due to internal orthopedic prosthetic devices, implants and grafts** `CC` `HCC`

10 √x7ᵗʰ **T84.83 Hemorrhage due to internal orthopedic prosthetic devices, implants and grafts** `CC` `HCC`

10 √x7ᵗʰ **T84.84 Pain due to internal orthopedic prosthetic devices, implants and grafts** `CC` `HCC`

10 √x7ᵗʰ **T84.85 Stenosis due to internal orthopedic prosthetic devices, implants and grafts** `CC` `HCC`

10 √x7ᵗʰ **T84.86 Thrombosis due to internal orthopedic prosthetic devices, implants and grafts** `CC` `HCC`

10 √x7ᵗʰ **T84.89 Other specified complication of internal orthopedic prosthetic devices, implants and grafts** `CC` `HCC`

10 √x7ᵗʰ **T84.9 Unspecified complication of internal orthopedic prosthetic device, implant and graft** `CC` `HCC`
CC Excl: PDX collection 1459

√4ᵗʰ T85 Complications of other internal prosthetic devices, implants and grafts

> **EXCLUDES 2** failure and rejection of transplanted organs and tissue (T86.-)

> The appropriate 7th character is to be added to each code from category T85.
> A   initial encounter
> D   subsequent encounter
> S   sequela

√5ᵗʰ T85.0 Mechanical complication of ventricular intracranial (communicating) shunt

> **CC Excl: For codes in subcategory T85.0:**
> PDX collection 1460

10 √x7ᵗʰ **T85.01 Breakdown (mechanical) of ventricular intracranial (communicating) shunt** `CC` `HCC`

10 √x7ᵗʰ **T85.02 Displacement of ventricular intracranial (communicating) shunt** `CC` `HCC`

     Malposition of ventricular intracranial (communicating) shunt

10 √x7ᵗʰ **T85.03 Leakage of ventricular intracranial (communicating) shunt** `CC` `HCC`

10 √x7ᵗʰ **T85.09 Other mechanical complication of ventricular intracranial (communicating) shunt** `CC` `HCC`

     Obstruction (mechanical) of ventricular intracranial (communicating) shunt
     Perforation of ventricular intracranial (communicating) shunt
     Protrusion of ventricular intracranial (communicating) shunt

√5ᵗʰ T85.1 Mechanical complication of implanted electronic stimulator of nervous system

> **CC Excl: For codes in subcategory T85.1:**
> PDX collection 1460

√6ᵗʰ **T85.11 Breakdown (mechanical) of implanted electronic stimulator of nervous system**

     10 √7ᵗʰ **T85.110 Breakdown (mechanical) of implanted electronic neurostimulator of brain electrode (lead)** `CC` `HCC`

     10 √7ᵗʰ **T85.111 Breakdown (mechanical) of implanted electronic neurostimulator of peripheral nerve electrode (lead)** `CC` `HCC`

       Breakdown of electrode (lead) for cranial nerve neurostimulators
       Breakdown of electrode (lead) for gastric neurostimulator
       Breakdown of electrode (lead) for sacral nerve neurostimulator
       Breakdown of electrode (lead) for vagal nerve neurostimulators

---

10 HCC with 7th character indicating initial encounter (A, B or C - specific to category).

N Newborn: 0   P Pediatric: 0-17   M Maternity: 12-55   A Adult: 15-124   MCC Major CC Condition   PDxMCC PDx acts as own MCC   CC CC Condition   PDxCC PDx acts as own CC

1148   ICD-10-CM 2018

10 ✓7ᵗʰ **T85.112** **Breakdown (mechanical) of** CC HCC
implanted electronic neurostimulator
of spinal cord electrode (lead)

10 ✓7ᵗʰ **T85.113** **Breakdown (mechanical) of** CC HCC
implanted electronic neurostimulator,
generator
Breakdown (mechanical) of implanted
electronic neurostimuator generator,
brain, peripheral, gastric, spinal
Breakdown (mechanical) of implanted
electronic sacral neurostimulator,
pulse generator or receiver

10 ✓7ᵗʰ **T85.118** **Breakdown (mechanical) of other** CC HCC
implanted electronic stimulator
of nervous system

✓6ᵗʰ **T85.12** **Displacement of implanted electronic stimulator of**
nervous system
Malposition of implanted electronic stimulator of
nervous system

10 ✓7ᵗʰ **T85.120** **Displacement of implanted** CC HCC
electronic neurostimulator
of brain electrode (lead)

10 ✓7ᵗʰ **T85.121** **Displacement of implanted** CC HCC
electronic neurostimulator of
peripheral nerve electrode (lead)
Displacement of electrode (lead) for cranial
nerve neurostimulators
Displacement of electrode (lead) for gastric
neurostimulator
Displacement of electrode (lead) for sacral
nerve neurostimulator
Displacement of electrode (lead) for vagal
nerve neurostimulators

10 ✓7ᵗʰ **T85.122** **Displacement of implanted** CC HCC
electronic neurostimulator of
spinal cord electrode (lead)

10 ✓7ᵗʰ **T85.123** **Displacement of implanted** CC HCC
electronic neurostimulator, *generator*
Displacement of implanted electronic
neurostimulator generator, brain,
peripheral, gastric, spinal
Displacement of implanted electronic
sacral neurostimulator, pulse
generator or receiver

10 ✓7ᵗʰ **T85.128** **Displacement of other implanted** CC HCC
electronic stimulator of *nervous system*

✓6ᵗʰ **T85.19** **Other mechanical complication of implanted**
electronic stimulator of nervous system
Leakage of implanted electronic stimulator of nervous
system
Obstruction (mechanical) of implanted electronic
stimulator of nervous system
Perforation of implanted electronic stimulator of
nervous system
Protrusion of implanted electronic stimulator of
nervous system

10 ✓7ᵗʰ **T85.190** **Other mechanical complication of** CC HCC
implanted electronic neurostimulator
of brain electrode (lead)

10 ✓7ᵗʰ **T85.191** **Other mechanical complication of** CC HCC
implanted electronic neurostimulator
of peripheral nerve electrode (lead)
Other mechanical complication of
electrode (lead) for cranial nerve
neurostimulators
Other mechanical complication of
electrode (lead) for gastric
neurostimulator
Other mechanical complication of
electrode (lead) for sacral nerve
neurostimulator
Other mechanical complication of
electrode (lead) for vagal nerve
neurostimulators

10 ✓7ᵗʰ **T85.192** **Other mechanical complication of** CC HCC
implanted electronic neurostimulator
of spinal cord electrode (lead)

10 ✓7ᵗʰ **T85.193** **Other mechanical complication of** CC HCC
implanted electronic neurostimulator,
generator
Other mechanical complication of
implanted electronic neurostimulator
generator, brain, peripheral, gastric,
spinal
Other mechanical complication of
implanted electronic sacral
neurostimulator, pulse generator or
receiver

10 ✓7ᵗʰ **T85.199** **Other mechanical complication of** CC HCC
other implanted electronic stimulator
of nervous system

✓5ᵗʰ **T85.2** **Mechanical complication of** *intraocular lens*

CC Excl: For codes in subcategory T85.2:
PDX collection 1461

✓x7ᵗʰ **T85.21** **Breakdown (mechanical) of intraocular lens** CC

✓x7ᵗʰ **T85.22** **Displacement of intraocular lens** CC
Malposition of intraocular lens

✓x7ᵗʰ **T85.29** **Other mechanical complication of intraocular** CC
lens
Obstruction (mechanical) of intraocular lens
Perforation of intraocular lens
Protrusion of intraocular lens

✓5ᵗʰ **T85.3** **Mechanical complication of** *other ocular prosthetic devices,*
implants and grafts
EXCLUDES 2 *other complications of corneal graft (T86.84-)*

CC Excl: For codes in subcategory T85.3:
PDX collection 1462

✓6ᵗʰ **T85.31** **Breakdown (mechanical) of other ocular prosthetic**
devices, implants and grafts

✓7ᵗʰ **T85.310** **Breakdown (mechanical) of prosthetic** CC
orbit of *right eye*

✓7ᵗʰ **T85.311** **Breakdown (mechanical) of prosthetic** CC
orbit of *left eye*

✓7ᵗʰ **T85.318** **Breakdown (mechanical) of** *other* ocular
prosthetic devices, implants and grafts

✓6ᵗʰ **T85.32** **Displacement of other ocular prosthetic devices,**
implants and grafts
Malposition of other ocular prosthetic devices,
implants and grafts

✓7ᵗʰ **T85.320** **Displacement of prosthetic orbit of** CC
right eye

✓7ᵗʰ **T85.321** **Displacement of prosthetic orbit of** CC
left eye

✓7ᵗʰ **T85.328** **Displacement of** *other ocular prosthetic*
devices, implants and grafts

✓6ᵗʰ **T85.39** **Other mechanical complication of other ocular**
prosthetic devices, implants and grafts
Obstruction (mechanical) of other ocular prosthetic
devices, implants and grafts
Perforation of other ocular prosthetic devices,
implants and grafts
Protrusion of other ocular prosthetic devices, implants
and grafts

✓7ᵗʰ **T85.390** **Other mechanical complication of** CC
prosthetic orbit of *right eye*

✓7ᵗʰ **T85.391** **Other mechanical complication of** CC
prosthetic orbit of *left eye*

✓7ᵗʰ **T85.398** **Other mechanical complication of** *other*
ocular prosthetic devices, implants and
grafts

✓6ᵗʰ **T85.4** **Mechanical complication of** *breast prosthesis and implant*

CC Excl: For codes in subcategory T85.4:
PDX collection 1463

✓x7ᵗʰ **T85.41** **Breakdown (mechanical) of breast prosthesis** CC
and implant

✓x7ᵗʰ **T85.42** **Displacement of breast prosthesis and implant** CC
Malposition of breast prosthesis and implant

✓x7ᵗʰ **T85.43** **Leakage of breast prosthesis and implant** CC

✓x7ᵗʰ **T85.44** **Capsular contracture of breast implant** CC

---

10 HCC with 7th character indicating initial encounter (A, B or C - specific to category).

☑Additional Character Req   ✓x7ᵗʰ Placeholder Alert   Unacceptable PDx   Manifestation   H1-H14 HAC   HCC CMS-HCC Condition   EXCLUDES 1 Not Coded Here   EXCLUDES 2 Not Included Here

ICD-10-CM 2018   1149

Chapter 19. Injury, Poisoning and Certain Other Consequences of External Causes

T85.112–T85.44

✓x7ᵗʰ T85.49 Other mechanical complication of breast prosthesis and implant   CC
     Obstruction (mechanical) of breast prosthesis and implant
     Perforation of breast prosthesis and implant
     Protrusion of breast prosthesis and implant

✓5ᵗʰ T85.5 Mechanical complication of gastrointestinal prosthetic devices, implants and grafts

> **CC Excl: For codes in subcategory T85.5:**
> PDX collection 1464

✓6ᵗʰ T85.51 Breakdown (mechanical) of gastrointestinal prosthetic devices, implants and grafts

     ✓7ᵗʰ T85.510 Breakdown (mechanical) of bile duct prosthesis   CC

     ✓7ᵗʰ T85.511 Breakdown (mechanical) of esophageal anti-reflux device   CC

     ✓7ᵗʰ T85.518 Breakdown (mechanical) of other gastrointestinal prosthetic devices, implants and grafts   CC

✓6ᵗʰ T85.52 Displacement of gastrointestinal prosthetic devices, implants and grafts
     Malposition of gastrointestinal prosthetic devices, implants and grafts

     ✓7ᵗʰ T85.520 Displacement of bile duct prosthesis   CC

     ✓7ᵗʰ T85.521 Displacement of esophageal anti-reflux device   CC

     ✓7ᵗʰ T85.528 Displacement of other gastrointestinal prosthetic devices, implants and grafts   CC

✓6ᵗʰ T85.59 Other mechanical complication of gastrointestinal prosthetic devices, implants and grafts
     Obstruction, mechanical of gastrointestinal prosthetic devices, implants and grafts
     Perforation of gastrointestinal prosthetic devices, implants and grafts
     Protrusion of gastrointestinal prosthetic devices, implants and grafts

     ✓7ᵗʰ T85.590 Other mechanical complication of bile duct prosthesis   CC

     ✓7ᵗʰ T85.591 Other mechanical complication of esophageal anti-reflux device   CC

     ✓7ᵗʰ T85.598 Other mechanical complication of other gastrointestinal prosthetic devices, implants and grafts   CC

✓5ᵗʰ T85.6 Mechanical complication of other specified internal and external prosthetic devices, implants and grafts

✓6ᵗʰ T85.61 Breakdown (mechanical) of other specified internal prosthetic devices, implants and grafts

     ✓7ᵗʰ T85.610 Breakdown (mechanical) of cranial or spinal infusion catheter   CC
         Breakdown (mechanical) of epidural infusion catheter
         Breakdown (mechanical) of intrathecal infusion catheter
         Breakdown (mechanical) of subarachnoid infusion catheter
         Breakdown (mechanical) of subdural infusion catheter
         CC Excl: PDX collection 1465

     ✓7ᵗʰ T85.611 Breakdown (mechanical) of intraperitoneal dialysis catheter   CC HCC
         EXCLUDES 1   mechanical complication of vascular dialysis catheter (T82.4-)
         CC Excl: PDX collection 1466

     ✓7ᵗʰ T85.612 Breakdown (mechanical) of permanent sutures   CC
         EXCLUDES 1   mechanical complication of permanent (wire) suture used in bone repair (T84.1-T84.2)
         CC Excl: PDX collection 1467

✓7ᵗʰ T85.613 Breakdown (mechanical) of artificial skin graft and decellularized allodermis   CC
     Failure of artificial skin graft and decellularized allodermis
     Non-adherence of artificial skin graft and decellularized allodermis
     Poor incorporation of artificial skin graft and decellularized allodermis
     Shearing of artificial skin graft and decellularized allodermis
     CC Excl: PDX collection 1468

✓7ᵗʰ T85.614 Breakdown (mechanical) of insulin pump   CC
     CC Excl: PDX collection 1469

10 ✓7ᵗʰ T85.615 Breakdown (mechanical) of other nervous system device, implant or graft   CC HCC
     Breakdown (mechanical) of intrathecal infusion pump
     CC Excl: PDX collection 1467

✓7ᵗʰ T85.618 Breakdown (mechanical) of other specified internal prosthetic devices, implants and grafts   CC
     CC Excl: PDX collection 1467

✓6ᵗʰ T85.62 Displacement of other specified internal prosthetic devices, implants and grafts
     Malposition of other specified internal prosthetic devices, implants and grafts

     ✓7ᵗʰ T85.620 Displacement of cranial or spinal infusion catheter   CC
         Displacement of epidural infusion catheter
         Displacement of intrathecal infusion catheter
         Displacement of subarachnoid infusion catheter
         Displacement of subdural infusion catheter
         CC Excl: PDX collection 1465

     ✓7ᵗʰ T85.621 Displacement of intraperitoneal dialysis catheter   CC HCC
         EXCLUDES 1   mechanical complication of vascular dialysis catheter (T82.4-)
         CC Excl: PDX collection 1466

     ✓7ᵗʰ T85.622 Displacement of permanent sutures   CC
         EXCLUDES 1   mechanical complication of permanent (wire) suture used in bone repair (T84.1-T84.2)
         CC Excl: PDX collection 1467

     ✓7ᵗʰ T85.623 Displacement of artificial skin graft and decellularized allodermis   CC
         Dislodgement of artificial skin graft and decellularized allodermis
         ~~Displacement of artificial skin graft and decellularized allodermis~~
         CC Excl: PDX collection 1468

     ✓7ᵗʰ T85.624 Displacement of insulin pump   CC
         CC Excl: PDX collection 1469

     10 ✓7ᵗʰ T85.625 Displacement of other nervous system device, implant or graft   CC HCC
         Displacement of intrathecal infusion pump
         CC Excl: PDX collection 1467

     ✓7ᵗʰ T85.628 Displacement of other specified internal prosthetic devices, implants and grafts   CC
         CC Excl: PDX collection 1467

✓6ᵗʰ T85.63 Leakage of other specified internal prosthetic devices, implants and grafts

     ✓7ᵗʰ T85.630 Leakage of cranial or spinal infusion catheter   CC
         Leakage of epidural infusion catheter
         Leakage of intrathecal infusion catheter infusion catheter
         Leakage of subdural infusion catheter
         Leakage of subarachnoid infusion catheter
         CC Excl: PDX collection 1465

     ✓7ᵗʰ T85.631 Leakage of intraperitoneal dialysis catheter   CC HCC
         EXCLUDES 1   mechanical complication of vascular dialysis catheter (T82.4)
         CC Excl: PDX collection 1466

---

10   HCC with 7th character indicating initial encounter (A, B or C - specific to category).

Ⓝ Newborn: 0   Ⓟ Pediatric: 0-17   Ⓜ Maternity: 12-55   Ⓐ Adult: 15-124   **MCC** Major CC Condition   **PDxMCC** PDx acts as own MCC   **CC** CC Condition   **PDxCC** PDx acts as own CC

✓7ᵗʰ **T85.633** **Leakage of insulin pump**   `CC`
CC Excl: PDX collection 1469

10 ✓7ᵗʰ **T85.635** **Leakage of other nervous system**   `CC` `HCC`
device, implant or graft
Leakage of intrathecal infusion pump
CC Excl: PDX collection 1467

✓7ᵗʰ **T85.638** **Leakage of other specified internal**   `CC`
prosthetic devices, implants and grafts
CC Excl: PDX collection 1467

✓6ᵗʰ **T85.69** **Other mechanical complication of other specified**
internal prosthetic devices, implants and grafts
Obstruction, mechanical of other specified internal
prosthetic devices, implants and grafts
Perforation of other specified internal prosthetic
devices, implants and grafts
Protrusion of other specified internal prosthetic
devices, implants and grafts

✓7ᵗʰ **T85.690** **Other mechanical complication of**   `CC`
cranial or spinal infusion catheter
Other mechanical complication of epidural
infusion catheter
Other mechanical complication of
intrathecal infusion catheter
Other mechanical complication of
subarachnoid infusion catheter
Other mechanical complication of subdural
infusion catheter
CC Excl: PDX collection 1465

✓7ᵗʰ **T85.691** **Other mechanical complication of**   `CC` `HCC`
intraperitoneal dialysis catheter
EXCLUDES 1 *mechanical complication of*
vascular dialysis catheter
(T82.4)
CC Excl: PDX collection 1466

✓7ᵗʰ **T85.692** **Other mechanical complication of**   `CC`
permanent sutures
EXCLUDES 1 *mechanical complication of*
permanent (wire) suture
used in bone repair
(T84.1-T84.2)
CC Excl: PDX collection 1467

✓7ᵗʰ **T85.693** **Other mechanical complication of**   `CC`
artificial skin graft and decellularized
allodermis
CC Excl: PDX collection 1468

✓7ᵗʰ **T85.694** **Other mechanical complication of**   `CC`
insulin pump
CC Excl: PDX collection 1469

10 ✓7ᵗʰ **T85.695** **Other mechanical complication of**   `CC` `HCC`
other nervous system device, implant
or graft
Other mechanical complication of
intrathecal infusion pump
CC Excl: PDX collection 1467

✓7ᵗʰ **T85.698** **Other mechanical complication of**   `CC`
other specified internal prosthetic
devices, implants and grafts
Mechanical complication of nonabsorbable
surgical material NOS
CC Excl: PDX collection 1467

✓5ᵗʰ **T85.7** **Infection and inflammatory reaction due to other internal**
prosthetic devices, implants and grafts
Use additional code to identify infection

CC Excl: For codes in subcategory T85.7, unless
otherwise noted: PDX collection 1470

✓x7ᵗʰ **T85.71** **Infection and inflammatory reaction due to**   `CC` `HCC`
peritoneal dialysis catheter
CC Excl: PDX collection 1467

10 ✓x7ᵗʰ **T85.72** **Infection and inflammatory reaction due to**   `CC` `HCC`
insulin pump
CC Excl: PDX collection 1470

✓6ᵗʰ **T85.73** **Infection and inflammatory reaction due to nervous**
system devices, implants and graft

10 ✓7ᵗʰ **T85.730** **Infection and inflammatory**   `CC` `HCC`
reaction due to ventricular intracranial
(communicating) shunt

10 ✓7ᵗʰ **T85.731** **Infection and inflammatory**   `CC` `HCC`
reaction due to implanted electronic
neurostimulator of brain, electrode (lead)

10 ✓7ᵗʰ **T85.732** **Infection and inflammatory**   `CC` `HCC`
reaction due to implanted electronic
neurostimulator of peripheral nerve,
electrode (lead)
Infection and inflammatory reaction due to
electrode (lead) for cranial nerve
neurostimulators
Infection and inflammatory reaction due to
electrode (lead) for gastric
neurostimulator
Infection and inflammatory reaction due to
electrode (lead) for sacral nerve
neurostimulator
Infection and inflammatory reaction due to
electrode (lead) for vagal nerve
neurostimulators

10 ✓7ᵗʰ **T85.733** **Infection and inflammatory**   `CC` `HCC`
reaction due to implanted electronic
neurostimulator of spinal cord, electrode
(lead)

10 ✓7ᵗʰ **T85.734** **Infection and inflammatory**   `CC` `HCC`
reaction due to implanted electronic
neurostimulator, generator
Generator pocket infection

10 ✓7ᵗʰ **T85.735** **Infection and inflammatory**   `CC` `HCC`
reaction due to cranial or spinal infusion
catheter
Infection and inflammatory reaction due to
epidural catheter
Infection and inflammatory reaction due to
intrathecal infusion catheter
Infection and inflammatory reaction due to
subarachnoid catheter
Infection and inflammatory reaction due to
subdural catheter

10 ✓7ᵗʰ **T85.738** **Infection and inflammatory**   `CC` `HCC`
reaction due to other nervous system
device, implant or graft
Infection and inflammatory reaction due to
intrathecal infusion pump

10 ✓x7ᵗʰ **T85.79** **Infection and inflammatory reaction due to**   `CC` `HCC`
other internal prosthetic devices, implants and
grafts
CC Excl: PDX collection 1470

✓5ᵗʰ **T85.8** **Other specified complications of internal prosthetic devices,**
implants and grafts, not elsewhere classified

CC Excl: For CC codes in subcategory T85.8:
CC with 7th character A or D: PDX collection 1470

✓6ᵗʰ **T85.81** **Embolism due to internal prosthetic devices,**
implants and grafts, not elsewhere classified

9,10 ✓7ᵗʰ **T85.810** **Embolism due to nervous system**   `CC` `HCC`
prosthetic devices, implants and grafts

✓7ᵗʰ **T85.818** **Embolism due to other internal prosthetic**
devices, implants and grafts

✓6ᵗʰ **T85.82** **Fibrosis due to internal prosthetic devices, implants**
and grafts, not elsewhere classified

9,10 ✓7ᵗʰ **T85.820** **Fibrosis due to nervous system**   `CC` `HCC`
prosthetic devices, implants and grafts

✓7ᵗʰ **T85.828** **Fibrosis due to other internal prosthetic**
devices, implants and grafts

✓6ᵗʰ **T85.83** **Hemorrhage due to internal prosthetic devices,**
implants and grafts, not elsewhere classified

9,10 ✓7ᵗʰ **T85.830** **Hemorrhage due to nervous**   `CC` `HCC`
system prosthetic devices, implants and
grafts

✓7ᵗʰ **T85.838** **Hemorrhage due to other internal**
prosthetic devices, implants and grafts

✓6ᵗʰ **T85.84** **Pain due to internal prosthetic devices, implants and**
grafts, not elsewhere classified

9,10 ✓7ᵗʰ **T85.840** **Pain due to nervous system**   `CC` `HCC`
prosthetic devices, implants and grafts

✓7ᵗʰ **T85.848** **Pain due to other internal prosthetic**
devices, implants and grafts

✓6ᵗʰ **T85.85** **Stenosis due to internal prosthetic devices, implants**
and grafts, not elsewhere classified

9,10 ✓7ᵗʰ **T85.850** **Stenosis due to nervous system**   `CC` `HCC`
prosthetic devices, implants and grafts

---

9 CC when reported as an initial or subsequent encounter (7th character A or D).
10 HCC with 7th character indicating initial encounter (A, B or C - specific to category).

☑Additional Character Req   ✓x7ᵗʰ Placeholder Alert   Unacceptable PDx   Manifestation   `H1`-`H14` HAC   `HCC` CMS-HCC Condition   EXCLUDES 1 Not Coded Here   EXCLUDES 2 Not Included Here

☑7ᵗʰ **T85.858** Stenosis due to other internal prosthetic devices, implants and grafts

☑6ᵗʰ **T85.86** Thrombosis due to internal prosthetic devices, implants and grafts, not elsewhere classified

9,10 ☑7ᵗʰ **T85.860** Thrombosis due to nervous system prosthetic devices, implants and grafts `CC` `HCC`

☑7ᵗʰ **T85.868** Thrombosis due to other internal prosthetic devices, implants and grafts

☑6ᵗʰ **T85.89** Other specified complication of internal prosthetic devices, implants and grafts, not elsewhere classified

Erosion or breakdown of subcutaneous device pocket

9,10 ☑7ᵗʰ **T85.890** Other specified complication of nervous system prosthetic devices, implants and grafts `CC` `HCC`

☑7ᵗʰ **T85.898** Other specified complication of other internal prosthetic devices, implants and grafts

☑x7ᵗʰ **T85.9** Unspecified complication of internal prosthetic device, implant and graft

Complication of internal prosthetic device, implant and graft NOS

☑4ᵗʰ **T86** Complications of transplanted organs and tissue

Use additional code to identify other transplant complications, such as:
graft-versus-host disease (D89.81-)
malignancy associated with organ transplant (C80.2)
post-transplant lymphoproliferative disorders (PTLD) (D47.Z1)

☑5ᵗʰ **T86.0** Complications of bone marrow transplant

CC Excl: For codes in subcategory T86.0:
PDX collection 514

T86.00 Unspecified complication of bone marrow transplant `CC` `HCC`

T86.01 Bone marrow transplant rejection `CC` `HCC`

T86.02 Bone marrow transplant failure `CC` `HCC`

T86.03 Bone marrow transplant infection `CC` `HCC`

T86.09 Other complications of bone marrow transplant `CC` `HCC`

☑5ᵗʰ **T86.1** Complications of kidney transplant

CC Excl: For codes in subcategory T86.1:
PDX collection 1471

T86.10 Unspecified complication of kidney transplant `CC`

T86.11 Kidney transplant rejection `CC`

T86.12 Kidney transplant failure `CC`
AHA: 2013, 1Q, 24

T86.13 Kidney transplant infection `CC`
Use additional code to specify infection

T86.19 Other complication of kidney transplant `CC`

☑5ᵗʰ **T86.2** Complications of heart transplant

EXCLUDES 1 complication of:
artificial heart device (T82.5)
heart-lung transplant (T86.3)

CC Excl: For codes in subcategory T86.2:
PDX collection 1472

T86.20 Unspecified complication of heart transplant `CC` `HCC`

T86.21 Heart transplant rejection `CC` `HCC`

T86.22 Heart transplant failure `CC` `HCC`

T86.23 Heart transplant infection `CC` `HCC`
Use additional code to specify infection

☑6ᵗʰ **T86.29** Other complications of heart transplant

T86.290 Cardiac allograft vasculopathy `CC` `HCC`
EXCLUDES 1 atherosclerosis of coronary arteries (I25.75-, I25.76-, I25.81-)

T86.298 Other complications of heart transplant `CC` `HCC`

☑5ᵗʰ **T86.3** Complications of heart-lung transplant

CC Excl: For codes in subcategory T86.3:
PDX collection 1472

T86.30 Unspecified complication of heart-lung transplant `PDxCC` `CC` `HCC`

T86.31 Heart-lung transplant rejection `PDxCC` `CC` `HCC`

T86.32 Heart-lung transplant failure `PDxCC` `CC` `HCC`

T86.33 Heart-lung transplant infection `PDxCC` `CC` `HCC`
Use additional code to specify infection

T86.39 Other complications of heart-lung transplant `PDxCC` `CC` `HCC`

☑5ᵗʰ **T86.4** Complications of liver transplant

CC Excl: For codes in subcategory T86.4:
PDX collection 1473

T86.40 Unspecified complication of liver transplant `CC` `HCC`

T86.41 Liver transplant rejection `CC` `HCC`

T86.42 Liver transplant failure `CC` `HCC`

T86.43 Liver transplant infection `CC` `HCC`
Use additional code to identify infection, such as:
cytomegalovirus (CMV) infection (B25.-)

T86.49 Other complications of liver transplant `CC` `HCC`

T86.5 Complications of stem cell transplant `CC` `HCC`
Complications from stem cells from peripheral blood
Complications from stem cells from umbilical cord
CC Excl: PDX collection 1474

☑5ᵗʰ **T86.8** Complications of other transplanted organs and tissues

☑6ᵗʰ **T86.81** Complications of lung transplant
EXCLUDES 1 complication of heart-lung transplant (T86.3-)

CC Excl: For codes in subcategory T86.81:
PDX collection 1475

T86.810 Lung transplant rejection `CC` `HCC`

T86.811 Lung transplant failure `CC` `HCC`

T86.812 Lung transplant infection `CC` `HCC`
Use additional code to specify infection

T86.818 Other complications of lung transplant `CC` `HCC`

T86.819 Unspecified complication of lung transplant `CC` `HCC`

☑6ᵗʰ **T86.82** Complications of skin graft (allograft) (autograft)
EXCLUDES 2 complication of artificial skin graft (T85.693)

CC Excl: For codes in subcategory T86.82:
PDX collection 1476

T86.820 Skin graft (allograft) rejection `CC`

T86.821 Skin graft (allograft) (autograft) failure `CC`

T86.822 Skin graft (allograft) (autograft) infection `CC`
Use additional code to specify infection

T86.828 Other complications of skin graft (allograft) (autograft) `CC`

T86.829 Unspecified complication of skin graft (allograft) (autograft) `CC`

☑6ᵗʰ **T86.83** Complications of bone graft
EXCLUDES 2 mechanical complications of bone graft (T84.3-)

CC Excl: For codes in subcategory T86.83:
PDX collection 1477

T86.830 Bone graft rejection `CC`

T86.831 Bone graft failure `CC`

T86.832 Bone graft infection `CC`
Use additional code to specify infection

T86.838 Other complications of bone graft `CC`

T86.839 Unspecified complication of bone graft `CC`

☑6ᵗʰ **T86.84** Complications of corneal transplant
EXCLUDES 2 mechanical complications of corneal graft (T85.3-)

T86.840 Corneal transplant rejection `CC`
CC Excl: PDX collection 1478

T86.841 Corneal transplant failure `CC`
CC Excl: PDX collection 1478

T86.842 Corneal transplant infection `CC` `HCC`
Use additional code to specify infection
CC Excl: PDX collection 1479

T86.848 Other complications of corneal transplant `CC`
CC Excl: PDX collection 1479

---

9 CC when reported as an initial or subsequent encounter (7th character A or D).
10 HCC with 7th character indicating initial encounter (A, B or C - specific to category).

`N` Newborn: 0   `P` Pediatric: 0-17   `M` Maternity: 12-55   `A` Adult: 15-124   `MCC` Major CC Condition   `PDxMCC` PDx acts as own MCC   `CC` CC Condition   `PDxCC` PDx acts as own CC

T86.849   Unspecified **complication** of **corneal transplant**   `CC`
     CC Excl: PDX collection 1479

✓6ᵗʰ **T86.85**   **Complication** of **intestine transplant**

> **CC Excl: For codes in subcategory T86.85:** PDX collection 495

     T86.850   **Intestine transplant** rejection   `CC` `HCC`
     T86.851   **Intestine transplant** failure   `CC` `HCC`
     T86.852   **Intestine transplant** infection   `CC` `HCC`
         Use additional code to specify infection
     T86.858   Other **complications of intestine transplant**   `CC` `HCC`
     T86.859   Unspecified **complication of intestine transplant**   `CC` `HCC`

✓6ᵗʰ **T86.89**   **Complications of** other **transplanted tissue**
     Transplant failure or rejection of pancreas

> **CC Excl: For codes in subcategory T86.89:** PDX collection 1480

     T86.890   **Other transplanted tissue** rejection   `CC`
     T86.891   **Other transplanted tissue** failure   `CC`
     T86.892   **Other transplanted tissue** infection   `CC`
         Use additional code to specify infection
     T86.898   Other **complications of** other **transplanted tissue**
     T86.899   Unspecified **complication of** other **transplanted tissue**   `CC`

✓5ᵗʰ **T86.9**   **Complication of** unspecified **transplanted organ and tissue**

> **CC Excl: For codes in subcategory T86.9:** PDX collection 495

     T86.90   Unspecified **complication of** unspecified **transplanted organ and tissue**   `CC`
     T86.91   Unspecified **transplanted organ and tissue** rejection   `CC`
     T86.92   Unspecified **transplanted organ and tissue** failure   `CC`
     T86.93   Unspecified **transplanted organ and tissue** infection   `CC`
         Use additional code to specify infection
     T86.99   Other **complications of** unspecified **transplanted organ and tissue**   `CC`

✓4ᵗʰ **T87**   **Complications peculiar to reattachment and amputation**

✓5ᵗʰ **T87.0**   **Complications of reattached (part of)** upper extremity

✓6ᵗʰ **T87.0X**   **Complications of reattached (part of) upper extremity**

> **CC Excl: For codes in subcategory T87.0X:** PDX collection 1481

     T87.0X1   **Complications of reattached (part of)** right **upper extremity**   `CC` `HCC`
     T87.0X2   **Complications of reattached (part of)** left **upper extremity**   `CC` `HCC`
     T87.0X9   **Complications of reattached (part of)** unspecified **upper extremity**   `CC` `HCC`

✓5ᵗʰ **T87.1**   **Complications of reattached (part of)** lower extremity

✓6ᵗʰ **T87.1X**   **Complications of reattached (part of) lower extremity**

> **CC Excl: For codes in subcategory T87.1X:** PDX collection 1482

     T87.1X1   **Complications of reattached (part of)** right **lower extremity**   `CC` `HCC`
     T87.1X2   **Complications of reattached (part of)** left **lower extremity**   `CC` `HCC`
     T87.1X9   **Complications of reattached (part of)** unspecified **lower extremity**   `CC` `HCC`

T87.2   **Complications of** other **reattached** body part   `CC` `HCC`
     CC Excl: PDX collection 1483

✓5ᵗʰ **T87.3**   **Neuroma of amputation stump**
     DEF: Non-neoplastic tumor generated at the proximal end of severed, partially transected, or injured nerve following amputation.
     T87.30   **Neuroma of amputation stump,** unspecified **extremity**   `HCC`
     T87.31   **Neuroma of amputation stump,** right upper **extremity**   `HCC`

     T87.32   **Neuroma of amputation stump,** left upper **extremity**   `HCC`
     T87.33   **Neuroma of amputation stump,** right lower **extremity**   `HCC`
     T87.34   **Neuroma of amputation stump,** left lower **extremity**   `HCC`

✓5ᵗʰ **T87.4**   **Infection of amputation stump**

> **CC Excl: For codes in subcategory T87.4:** PDX collection 1484

     T87.40   **Infection of amputation stump,** unspecified **extremity**   `CC` `HCC`
     T87.41   **Infection of amputation stump,** right upper **extremity**   `CC` `HCC`
     T87.42   **Infection of amputation stump,** left upper **extremity**   `CC` `HCC`
     T87.43   **Infection of amputation stump,** right lower **extremity**   `CC` `HCC`
     T87.44   **Infection of amputation stump,** left lower **extremity**   `CC` `HCC`

✓5ᵗʰ **T87.5**   **Necrosis of amputation stump**
     T87.50   **Necrosis of amputation stump,** unspecified **extremity**   `HCC`
     T87.51   **Necrosis of amputation stump,** right upper **extremity**   `HCC`
     T87.52   **Necrosis of amputation stump,** left upper **extremity**   `HCC`
     T87.53   **Necrosis of amputation stump,** right lower **extremity**   `HCC`
     T87.54   **Necrosis of amputation stump,** left lower **extremity**   `HCC`

✓5ᵗʰ **T87.8**   **Other complications of amputation stump**
     T87.81   **Dehiscence of amputation stump**   `HCC`
     T87.89   Other **complications of amputation stump**   `HCC`
         Amputation stump contracture
         Amputation stump contracture of next proximal joint
         Amputation stump flexion
         Amputation stump edema
         Amputation stump hematoma
         EXCLUDES 2   *phantom limb syndrome (G54.6-G54.7)*

T87.9   Unspecified **complications of amputation stump**   `HCC`

✓4ᵗʰ **T88**   **Other complications of surgical and medical care, not elsewhere classified**
     EXCLUDES 2   *complication following infusion, transfusion and therapeutic injection (T80.-)*
         complication following procedure NEC (T81.-)
         complications of anesthesia in labor and delivery (O74.-)
         complications of anesthesia in pregnancy (O29.-)
         complications of anesthesia in puerperium (O89.-)
         complications of devices, implants and grafts (T82-T85)
         complications of obstetric surgery and procedure (O75.4)
         dermatitis due to drugs and medicaments (L23.3, L24.4, L25.1, L27.0-L27.1)
         poisoning and toxic effects of drugs and chemicals (T36-T65 with fifth or sixth character 1-4 or 6)
         specified complications classified elsewhere

> The appropriate 7th character is to be added to each code from category T88.
> A   initial encounter
> D   subsequent encounter
> S   sequela

✓x7ᵗʰ **T88.0**   **Infection following immunization**   `CC`
     Sepsis following immunization
     CC Excl: PDX collection 948

✓x7ᵗʰ **T88.1**   **Other complications following immunization, not elsewhere classified**   `CC`
     Generalized vaccinia
     Rash following immunization
     EXCLUDES 1   *vaccinia not from vaccine (B08.011)*
     EXCLUDES 2   *anaphylactic shock due to serum (T80.5-)*
         other serum reactions (T80.6-)
         postimmunization arthropathy (M02.2)
         postimmunization encephalitis (G04.02)
         postimmunization fever (R50.83)
     CC Excl: PDX collection 1485

✔ Additional Character Req   ✓x7ᵗʰ Placeholder Alert   Unacceptable PDx   Manifestation   `H1`-`H14` HAC   `HCC` CMS-HCC Condition   *EXCLUDES 1* Not Coded Here   *EXCLUDES 2* Not Included Here

ICD-10-CM 2018   **1153**

√x 7ᵗʰ **T88.2　Shock due to anesthesia**　　`CC`
Use additional code for adverse effect, if applicable, to identify drug (T41.- with fifth or sixth character 5)
> EXCLUDES 1　*complications of anesthesia (in):*
> *labor and delivery (O74.-)*
> *postprocedural shock NOS (T81.1-)*
> *pregnancy (O29.-)*
> *puerperium (O89.-)*

CC Excl: PDX collection 1441

√x 7ᵗʰ **T88.3　Malignant hyperthermia due to anesthesia**　　`CC`
Use additional code for adverse effect, if applicable, to identify drug (T41.- with fifth or sixth character 5)
CC Excl: PDX collection 1486

√x 7ᵗʰ **T88.4　Failed or difficult intubation**

√ 5ᵗʰ **T88.5　Other complications of anesthesia**
Use additional code for adverse effect, if applicable, to identify drug (T41.- with fifth or sixth character 5)

√x 7ᵗʰ **T88.51　Hypothermia following anesthesia**

√x 7ᵗʰ **T88.52　Failed moderate sedation during procedure**
Failed conscious sedation during procedure
> EXCLUDES 2　*personal history of failed moderate sedation (Z92.83)*

√x 7ᵗʰ **T88.53　Unintended awareness under general anesthesia during procedure**
> EXCLUDES 2　*personal history of unintended awareness under general anesthesia (Z92.84)*

√x 7ᵗʰ **T88.59　Other complications of anesthesia**

√x 7ᵗʰ **T88.6　Anaphylactic reaction due to adverse effect of correct drug or medicament properly administered**　　`CC`
Anaphylactic shock due to adverse effect of correct drug or medicament properly administered
Anaphylactoid reaction NOS
Use additional code for adverse effect, if applicable, to identify drug (T41.- with fifth or sixth character 5)
> EXCLUDES 1　*anaphylactic reaction due to serum (T80.5-)*
> *anaphylactic shock or reaction due to adverse food reaction (T78.0-)*

CC Excl: PDX collection 1426

√x 7ᵗʰ **T88.7　Unspecified adverse effect of drug or medicament**
Drug hypersensitivity NOS
Drug reaction NOS
Use additional code for adverse effect, if applicable, to identify drug (T41.- with fifth or sixth character 5)
> EXCLUDES 1　*specified adverse effects of drugs and medicaments (A00-R94 and T80-T88.6, T88.8)*

√x 7ᵗʰ **T88.8　Other specified complications of surgical and medical care, not elsewhere classified**
Use additional code to identify the complication

√x 7ᵗʰ **T88.9　Complication of surgical and medical care, unspecified**

Ⓝ Newborn: 0　Ⓟ Pediatric: 0-17　Ⓜ Maternity: 12-55　Ⓐ Adult: 15-124　`MCC` Major CC Condition　`PDxMCC` PDx acts as own MCC　`CC` CC Condition　`PDxCC` PDx acts as own CC

1154　　ICD-10-CM 2018

Chapter 20. External Causes of Morbidity (V00–Y99)

Chapter Specific Guidelines with Coding Examples

The chapter specific guidelines from the ICD-10-CM Official Guidelines for Coding and Reporting have been provided below. Along with these guidelines are coding examples, contained in the shaded boxes, that have been developed to help illustrate the coding and/or sequencing guidance found in these guidelines.

The external causes of morbidity codes should never be sequenced as the first-listed or principal diagnosis.

External cause codes are intended to provide data for injury research and evaluation of injury prevention strategies. These codes capture how the injury or health condition happened (cause), the intent (unintentional or accidental; or intentional, such as suicide or assault), the place where the event occurred the activity of the patient at the time of the event, and the person's status (e.g., civilian, military).

There is no national requirement for mandatory ICD-10-CM external cause code reporting. Unless a provider is subject to a state-based external cause code reporting mandate or these codes are required by a particular payer, reporting of ICD-10-CM codes in Chapter 20, External Causes of Morbidity, is not required. In the absence of a mandatory reporting requirement, providers are encouraged to voluntarily report external cause codes, as they provide valuable data for injury research and evaluation of injury prevention strategies.

a. General external cause coding guidelines

1) Used with any code in the range of A00.0–T88.9, Z00–Z99

An external cause code may be used with any code in the range of A00.0-T88.9, Z00–Z99, classification that **represents** a health condition due to an external cause. Though they are most applicable to injuries, they are also valid for use with such things as infections or diseases due to an external source, and other health conditions, such as a heart attack that occurs during strenuous physical activity.

> Actinic reticuloid due to tanning bed use
>
> **L57.1**   **Actinic reticuloid**
>
> **W89.1XXA**   **Exposure to tanning bed, initial encounter**
>
> *Explanation:* An external cause code may be used with any code in the range of A00.0–T88.9, Z00–Z99, classifications that describe health conditions due to an external cause. Code W89.1 Exposure to tanning bed requires a seventh character of A to report this initial encounter, with a placeholder X for the fifth and sixth characters.

2) External cause code used for length of treatment

Assign the external cause code, with the appropriate 7th character (initial encounter, subsequent encounter or sequela) for each encounter for which the injury or condition is being treated.

Most categories in chapter 20 have a 7th character requirement for each applicable code. Most categories in this chapter have three 7th character values: A, initial encounter, D, subsequent encounter and S, sequela. While the patient may be seen by a new or different provider over the course of treatment for an injury or condition, assignment of the 7th character for external cause should match the 7th character of the code assigned for the associated injury or condition for the encounter.

3) Use the full range of external cause codes

Use the full range of external cause codes to completely describe the cause, the intent, the place of occurrence, and if applicable, the activity of the patient at the time of the event, and the patient's status, for all injuries, and other health conditions due to an external cause.

4) Assign as many external cause codes as necessary

Assign as many external cause codes as necessary to fully explain each cause. If only one external code can be recorded, assign the code most related to the principal diagnosis.

5) The selection of the appropriate external cause code

The selection of the appropriate external cause code is guided by the Alphabetic Index of External Causes and by Inclusion and Exclusion notes in the Tabular List.

6) External cause code can never be a principal diagnosis

An external cause code can never be a principal (first-listed) diagnosis.

7) Combination external cause codes

Certain of the external cause codes are combination codes that identify sequential events that result in an injury, such as a fall which results in striking against an object. The injury may be due to either event or both.

The combination external cause code used should correspond to the sequence of events regardless of which caused the most serious injury.

> Toddler tripped and fell while walking and struck his head on an end table, sustaining a scalp contusion
>
> **S00.03XA**   **Contusion of scalp, initial encounter**
>
> **W01.190A**   **Fall on same level from slipping, tripping and stumbling with subsequent striking against furniture, initial encounter**
>
> *Explanation:* Combination external cause codes identify sequential events that result in an injury, such as a fall resulting in striking against an object. The injury may be due to either or both events.

8) No external cause code needed in certain circumstances

No external cause code from Chapter 20 is needed if the external cause and intent are included in a code from another chapter (e.g. T36.0X1-Poisoning by penicillins, accidental (unintentional)).

b. Place of occurrence guideline

Codes from category Y92, Place of occurrence of the external cause, are secondary codes for use after other external cause codes to identify the location of the patient at the time of injury or other condition.

Generally, a place of occurrence code is assigned only once, at the initial encounter for treatment. However, in the rare instance that a new injury occurs during hospitalization, an additional place of occurrence code may be assigned. No 7th characters are used for Y92.

Do not use place of occurrence code Y92.9 if the place is not stated or is not applicable.

> A farmer was working in his barn and sustained a foot contusion when the horse stepped on his left foot
>
> **S90.32XA**   **Contusion of left foot, initial encounter**
>
> **W55.19XA**   **Other contact with horse, initial encounter**
>
> **Y92.71**   **Barn as the place of occurrence of the external cause**
>
> *Explanation:* A place-of-occurrence code from category Y92 is assigned at the initial encounter to identify the location of the patient at the time the injury occurred.

c. Activity code

Assign a code from category Y93, Activity code, to describe the activity of the patient at the time the injury or other health condition occurred.

An activity code is used only once, at the initial encounter for treatment. Only one code from Y93 should be recorded on a medical record.

The activity codes are not applicable to poisonings, adverse effects, misadventures or sequela.

Do not assign Y93.9, Unspecified activity, if the activity is not stated.

A code from category Y93 is appropriate for use with external cause and intent codes if identifying the activity provides additional information about the event.

> Ranch hand who was grooming a horse sustained a foot contusion when the horse stepped on his left foot
>
> **S90.32XA**   **Contusion of left foot, initial encounter**
>
> **W55.19XA**   **Other contact with horse, initial encounter**
>
> **Y93.K3**   **Activity, grooming and shearing an animal**
>
> *Explanation:* One activity code from category Y93 is assigned at the initial encounter only to describe the activity of the patient at the time the injury occurred.

d. Place of occurrence, activity, and status codes used with other external cause code

When applicable, place of occurrence, activity, and external cause status codes are sequenced after the main external cause code(s). Regardless of the number of external cause codes assigned, generally there should be only one place of occurrence code, one activity code, and one external cause status code assigned to an encounter. However, in the rare instance that a new injury occurs during hospitalization, an additional place of occurrence code may be assigned.

e. If the reporting format limits the number of external cause codes

If the reporting format limits the number of external cause codes that can be used in reporting clinical data, report the code for the cause/intent most related to the principal diagnosis. If the format permits capture of additional external cause codes, the cause/intent, including medical misadventures, of the additional events should be reported rather than the codes for place, activity, or external status.

f. Multiple external cause coding guidelines

More than one external cause code is required to fully describe the external cause of an illness or injury. The assignment of external cause codes should be sequenced in the following priority:

If two or more events cause separate injuries, an external cause code should be assigned for each cause. The first-listed external cause code will be selected in the following order:

External codes for child and adult abuse take priority over all other external cause codes.

See Section I.C.19., Child and Adult abuse guidelines.

External cause codes for terrorism events take priority over all other external cause codes except child and adult abuse.

External cause codes for cataclysmic events take priority over all other external cause codes except child and adult abuse and terrorism.

External cause codes for transport accidents take priority over all other external cause codes except cataclysmic events, child and adult abuse and terrorism.

Activity and external cause status codes are assigned following all causal (intent) external cause codes.

The first-listed external cause code should correspond to the cause of the most serious diagnosis due to an assault, accident, or self-harm, following the order of hierarchy listed above..

30-year-old man accidentally discharged his hunting rifle, sustaining an open gunshot wound to the right thigh, which caused him to fall down the stairs, resulting in closed displaced comminuted fracture of his left radial shaft

S71.101A	**Unspecified open wound, right thigh, initial encounter**
W33.02XA	**Accidental discharge of hunting rifle, initial encounter**
S52.352A	**Displaced comminuted fracture of shaft of radius, left arm, initial encounter for closed fracture**
W10.9XXA	**Fall (on) (from) unspecified stairs and steps, initial encounter**

Explanation: If two or more events cause separate injuries, an external cause code should be assigned for each cause.

---

g. Child and adult abuse guideline

Adult and child abuse, neglect and maltreatment are classified as assault. Any of the assault codes may be used to indicate the external cause of any injury resulting from the confirmed abuse.

For confirmed cases of abuse, neglect and maltreatment, when the perpetrator is known, a code from Y07, Perpetrator of maltreatment and neglect, should accompany any other assault codes.

See Section I.C.19. Adult and child abuse, neglect and other maltreatment

h. Unknown or undetermined intent guideline

If the intent (accident, self-harm, assault) of the cause of an injury or other condition is unknown or unspecified, code the intent as accidental intent. All transport accident categories assume accidental intent.

1) Use of undetermined intent

External cause codes for events of undetermined intent are only for use if the documentation in the record specifies that the intent cannot be determined.

i. Sequelae (late effects) of external cause guidelines

1) Sequelae external cause codes

Sequelae are reported using the external cause code with the 7th character "S" for sequela. These codes should be used with any report of a late effect or sequela resulting from a previous injury.

See Section I.B.10 Sequela (Late Effects)

2) Sequela external cause code with a related current injury

A sequela external cause code should never be used with a related current nature of injury code.

3) Use of sequela external cause codes for subsequent visits

Use a late effect external cause code for subsequent visits when a late effect of the initial injury is being treated. Do not use a late effect external cause code for subsequent visits for follow-up care (e.g., to assess healing, to receive rehabilitative therapy) of the injury when no late effect of the injury has been documented.

j. Terrorism guidelines

1) Cause of injury identified by the Federal Government (FBI) as terrorism

When the cause of an injury is identified by the Federal Government (FBI) as terrorism, the first-listed external cause code should be a code from category Y38, Terrorism. The definition of terrorism employed by the FBI is found at the inclusion note at the beginning of category Y38. Use additional code for place of occurrence (Y92.-). More than one Y38 code may be assigned if the injury is the result of more than one mechanism of terrorism.

2) Cause of an injury is suspected to be the result of terrorism

When the cause of an injury is suspected to be the result of terrorism a code from category Y38 should not be assigned. Suspected cases should be classified as assault.

3) Code Y38.9, Terrorism, secondary effects

Assign code Y38.9, Terrorism, secondary effects, for conditions occurring subsequent to the terrorist event. This code should not be assigned for conditions that are due to the initial terrorist act.

It is acceptable to assign code Y38.9 with another code from Y38 if there is an injury due to the initial terrorist event and an injury that is a subsequent result of the terrorist event.

k. External cause status

A code from category Y99, External cause status, should be assigned whenever any other external cause code is assigned for an encounter, including an Activity code, except for the events noted below. Assign a code from category Y99, External cause status, to indicate the work status of the person at the time the event occurred. The status code indicates whether the event occurred during military activity, whether a non-military person was at work, whether an individual including a student or volunteer was involved in a non-work activity at the time of the causal event.

A code from Y99, External cause status, should be assigned, when applicable, with other external cause codes, such as transport accidents and falls. The external cause status codes are not applicable to poisonings, adverse effects, misadventures or late effects.

Do not assign a code from category Y99 if no other external cause codes (cause, activity) are applicable for the encounter.

An external cause status code is used only once, at the initial encounter for treatment. Only one code from Y99 should be recorded on a medical record.

Do not assign code Y99.9, Unspecified external cause status, if the status is not stated.

Chapter 20. External Causes of Morbidity (V00-Y99)

NOTE This chapter permits the classification of environmental events and circumstances as the cause of injury, and other adverse effects. Where a code from this section is applicable, it is intended that it shall be used secondary to a code from another chapter of the Classification indicating the nature of the condition. Most often, the condition will be classifiable to Chapter 19, Injury, poisoning and certain other consequences of external causes (S00-T88). Other conditions that may be stated to be due to external causes are classified in Chapters I to XVIII. For these conditions, codes from Chapter 20 should be used to provide additional information as to the cause of the condition.

This chapter contains the following blocks:

V00-X58	Accidents
V00-V99	Transport accidents
V00-V09	Pedestrian injured in transport accident
V10-V19	Pedal cycle rider injured in transport accident
V20-V29	Motorcycle rider injured in transport accident
V30-V39	Occupant of three-wheeled motor vehicle injured in transport accident
V40-V49	Car occupant injured in transport accident
V50-V59	Occupant of pick-up truck or van injured in transport accident
V60-V69	Occupant of heavy transport vehicle injured in transport accident
V70-V79	Bus occupant injured in transport accident
V80-V89	Other land transport accidents
V90-V94	Water transport accidents
V95-V97	Air and space transport accidents
V98-V99	Other and unspecified transport accidents
W00-X58	Other external causes of accidental injury
W00-W19	Slipping, tripping, stumbling and falls
W20-W49	Exposure to inanimate mechanical forces
W50-W64	Exposure to animate mechanical forces
W65-W74	Accidental non-transport drowning and submersion
W85-W99	Exposure to electric current, radiation and extreme ambient air temperature and pressure
X00-X08	Exposure to smoke, fire and flames
X10-X19	Contact with heat and hot substances
X30-X39	Exposure to forces of nature
~~X50~~	~~Overexertion and strenuous or repetitive movements~~
X52-X58	Accidental exposure to other specified factors
X71-X83	Intentional self-harm
X92-Y09	Assault
Y21-Y33	Event of undetermined intent
Y35-Y38	Legal intervention, operations of war, military operations, and terrorism
Y62-Y84	Complications of medical and surgical care
Y62-Y69	Misadventures to patients during surgical and medical care
Y70-Y82	Medical devices associated with adverse incidents in diagnostic and therapeutic use
Y83-Y84	Surgical and other medical procedures as the cause of abnormal reaction of the patient, or of later complication, without mention of misadventure at the time of the procedure
Y90-Y99	Supplementary factors related to causes of morbidity classified elsewhere

Accidents (V00-X58)

Transport accidents (V00-V99)

NOTE This section is structured in 12 groups. Those relating to land transport accidents (V00-V89) reflect the victim's mode of transport and are subdivided to identify the victim's 'counterpart' or the type of event. The vehicle of which the injured person is an occupant is identified in the first two characters since it is seen as the most important factor to identify for prevention purposes. A transport accident is one in which the vehicle involved must be moving or running or in use for transport purposes at the time of the accident.

Use additional code to identify:
  airbag injury (W22.1)
  type of street or road (Y92.4-)
  use of cellular telephone and other electronic equipment at the time of the transport accident (Y93.C-)

EXCLUDES 1 *agricultural vehicles in stationary use or maintenance (W31.-)*
assault by crashing of motor vehicle (Y03.-)
automobile or motor cycle in stationary use or maintenance—code to type of accident
crashing of motor vehicle, undetermined intent (Y32)
intentional self-harm by crashing of motor vehicle (X82)

EXCLUDES 2 *transport accidents due to cataclysm (X34-X38)*

NOTE Definitions related to transport accidents:

(a) A transport accident (V00-V99) is any accident involving a device designed primarily for, or used at the time primarily for, conveying persons or good from one place to another.

(b) A public highway [trafficway] or street is the entire width between property lines (or other boundary lines) of land open to the public as a matter of right or custom for purposes of moving persons or property from one place to another. A roadway is that part of the public highway designed, improved and customarily used for vehicular traffic.

(c) A traffic accident is any vehicle accident occurring on the public highway [i.e. originating on, terminating on, or involving a vehicle partially on the highway]. A vehicle accident is assumed to have occurred on the public highway unless another place is specified, except in the case of accidents involving only off-road motor vehicles, which are classified as nontraffic accidents unless the contrary is stated.

(d) A nontraffic accident is any vehicle accident that occurs entirely in any place other than a public highway.

(e) A pedestrian is any person involved in an accident who was not at the time of the accident riding in or on a motor vehicle, railway train, streetcar or animal-drawn or other vehicle, or on a pedal cycle or animal. This includes, a person changing a tire, working on a parked car, or a person on foot. It also includes the user of a pedestrian conveyance such as a babystroller, ice-skates, skis, sled, roller skates, a skateboard, nonmotorized or motorized wheelchair, motorized mobility scooter, or nonmotorized scooter.

(f) A driver is an occupant of a transport vehicle who is operating or intending to operate it.

(g) A passenger is any occupant of a transport vehicle other than the driver, except a person traveling on the outside of the vehicle.

(h) A person on the outside of a vehicle is any person being transported by a vehicle but not occupying the space normally reserved for the driver or passengers, or the space intended for the transport of property. This includes a person travelling on the bodywork, bumper, fender, roof, running board or step of a vehicle, as well as, hanging on the outside of the vehicle.

(i) A pedal cycle is any land transport vehicle operated solely by nonmotorized pedals including a bicycle or tricycle.

(j) A pedal cyclist is any person riding a pedal cycle or in a sidecar or trailer attached to a pedal cycle.

(k) A motorcycle is a two-wheeled motor vehicle with one or two riding saddles and sometimes with a third wheel for the support of a sidecar. The sidecar is considered part of the motorcycle. This includes a moped, motor scooter, or motorized bicycle.

(l) A motorcycle rider is any person riding a motorcycle or in a sidecar or trailer attached to the motorcycle.

(m) A three-wheeled motor vehicle is a motorized tricycle designed primarily for on-road use. This includes a motor-driven tricycle, a motorized rickshaw, or a three-wheeled motor car.

(n) A car [automobile] is a four-wheeled motor vehicle designed primarily for carrying up to 7 persons. A trailer being towed by the car is considered part of the car. It does not include a van or minivan - see definition (o).

(o) A pick-up truck or van is a four or six-wheeled motor vehicle designed for carrying passengers as well as property or cargo weighing less than the local limit for classification as a heavy goods vehicle, and not requiring a special driver's license. This includes a minivan and a sport-utility vehicle (SUV).

(p) A heavy transport vehicle is a motor vehicle designed primarily for carrying property, meeting local criteria for classification as a heavy goods vehicle in terms of weight and requiring a special driver's license.

(q) A bus (coach) is a motor vehicle designed or adapted primarily for carrying more than 10 passengers, and requiring a special driver's license.

(r) A railway train or railway vehicle is any device, with or without freight or passenger cars couple to it, designed for traffic on a railway track. This includes subterranean (subways) or elevated trains.

(s) A streetcar, is a device designed and used primarily for transporting passengers within a municipality, running on rails, usually subject to normal traffic control signals, and operated principally on a right-of-way that forms part of the roadway. This includes a tram or trolley that runs on rails. A trailer being towed by a streetcar is considered part of the streetcar.

(t) A special vehicle mainly used on industrial premises is a motor vehicle designed primarily for use within the buildings and premises of industrial or commercial establishments. This includes battery-powered airport passenger vehicles or baggage/mail trucks, forklifts, coal-cars in a coal mine, logging cars and trucks used in mines or quarries.

✓ Additional Character Req   ✓x7ᵗʰ Placeholder Alert   Unacceptable PDx   Manifestation   H1 - H14 HAC   HCC CMS-HCC Condition   EXCLUDES 1 Not Coded Here   EXCLUDES 2 Not Included Here

ICD-10-CM 2018   1157

(u) A special vehicle mainly used in agriculture is a motor vehicle designed specifically for use in farming and agriculture (horticulture), to work the land, tend and harvest crops and transport materials on the farm. This includes harvesters, farm machinery and tractor and trailers.

(v) A special construction vehicle is a motor vehicle designed specifically for use on construction and demolition sites. This includes bulldozers, diggers, earth levellers, dump trucks. backhoes, front-end loaders, pavers, and mechanical shovels.

(w) A special all-terrain vehicle is a motor vehicle of special design to enable it to negotiate over rough or soft terrain, snow or sand. Examples of special design are high construction, special wheels and tires, tracks, and support on a cushion of air. This includes snow mobiles, All-terrain vehicles (ATV), and dune buggies. It does not include passenger vehicle designated as Sport Utility Vehicles. (SUV)

(x) A watercraft is any device designed for transporting passengers or goods on water. This includes motor or sailboats, ships, and hovercraft.

(y) An aircraft is any device for transporting passengers or goods in the air. This includes hot-air balloons, gliders, helicopters and airplanes.

(z) A military vehicle is any motorized vehicle operating on a public roadway owned by the military and being operated by a member of the military

Pedestrian injured in transport accident (V00–V09)

INCLUDES person changing tire on transport vehicle
person examining engine of vehicle broken down in (on side of) road

EXCLUDES1 *fall due to non-transport collision with other person (W03)*
pedestrian on foot falling (slipping) on ice and snow (W00.-)
struck or bumped by another person (W51)

> The appropriate 7th character is to be added to each code from categories V00-V09.
> A   initial encounter
> D   subsequent encounter
> S   sequela

√4th V00 Pedestrian conveyance accident

Use additional place of occurrence and activity external cause codes, if known (Y92-, Y93-)

EXCLUDES1 *collision with another person without fall (W51)*
fall due to person on foot colliding with another person on foot (W03)
fall from non-moving wheelchair, nonmotorized scooter and motorized mobility scooter without collision (W05.-)
pedestrian (conveyance) collision with other land transport vehicle (V01-V09)
pedestrian on foot falling (slipping) on ice and snow (W00.-)

√5th V00.0 Pedestrian on foot injured in collision with pedestrian conveyance

√x7th V00.01 Pedestrian on foot injured in collision with roller-skater

√x7th V00.02 Pedestrian on foot injured in collision with skateboarder

√x7th V00.09 Pedestrian on foot injured in collision with other pedestrian conveyance

√5th V00.1 Rolling-type pedestrian conveyance accident

EXCLUDES1 *accident with babystroller (V00.82-)*
accident with motorized mobility scooter (V00.83-)
accident with wheelchair (powered) (V00.81-)

√6th V00.11 In-line roller-skate accident

√7th V00.111 Fall from in-line roller-skates

√7th V00.112 In-line roller-skater colliding with stationary object

√7th V00.118 Other in-line roller-skate accident
EXCLUDES1 *roller-skater collision with other land transport vehicle (V01-V09 with 5th character 1)*

√6th V00.12 Non-in-line roller-skate accident

√7th V00.121 Fall from non-in-line roller-skates

√7th V00.122 Non-in-line roller-skater colliding with stationary object

√7th V00.128 Other non-in-line roller-skating accident
EXCLUDES1 *roller-skater collision with other land transport vehicle (V01-V09 with 5th character 1)*

√6th V00.13 Skateboard accident

√7th V00.131 Fall from skateboard

√7th V00.132 Skateboarder colliding with stationary object

√7th V00.138 Other skateboard accident
EXCLUDES1 *skateboarder collision with other land transport vehicle (V01-V09 with 5th character 2)*

√6th V00.14 Scooter (nonmotorized) accident
EXCLUDES1 *motorscooter accident (V20-V29)*

√7th V00.141 Fall from scooter (nonmotorized)

√7th V00.142 Scooter (nonmotorized) colliding with stationary object

√7th V00.148 Other scooter (nonmotorized) accident
EXCLUDES1 *scooter (nonmotorized) collision with other land transport vehicle (V01-V09 with fifth character 9)*

√6th V00.15 Heelies accident
Rolling shoe
Wheeled shoe
Wheelies accident

√7th V00.151 Fall from heelies

√7th V00.152 Heelies colliding with stationary object

√7th V00.158 Other heelies accident

√6th V00.18 Accident on other rolling-type pedestrian conveyance

√7th V00.181 Fall from other rolling-type pedestrian conveyance

√7th V00.182 Pedestrian on other rolling-type pedestrian conveyance colliding with stationary object

√7th V00.188 Other accident on other rolling-type pedestrian conveyance

√5th V00.2 Gliding-type pedestrian conveyance accident

√6th V00.21 Ice-skates accident

√7th V00.211 Fall from ice-skates

√7th V00.212 Ice-skater colliding with stationary object

√7th V00.218 Other ice-skates accident
EXCLUDES1 *ice-skater collision with other land transport vehicle (V01-V09 with 5th digit 9)*

√6th V00.22 Sled accident

√7th V00.221 Fall from sled

√7th V00.222 Sledder colliding with stationary object

√7th V00.228 Other sled accident
EXCLUDES1 *sled collision with other land transport vehicle (V01-V09 with 5th digit 9)*

√6th V00.28 Other gliding-type pedestrian conveyance accident

√7th V00.281 Fall from other gliding-type pedestrian conveyance

√7th V00.282 Pedestrian on other gliding-type pedestrian conveyance colliding with stationary object

√7th V00.288 Other accident on other gliding-type pedestrian conveyance
EXCLUDES1 *gliding-type pedestrian conveyance collision with other land transport vehicle (V01-V09 with 5th digit 9)*

√5th V00.3 Flat-bottomed pedestrian conveyance accident

√6th V00.31 Snowboard accident

√7th V00.311 Fall from snowboard

√7th V00.312 Snowboarder colliding with stationary object

√7th V00.318 Other snowboard accident
EXCLUDES1 *snowboarder collision with other land transport vehicle (V01-V09 with 5th digit 9)*

√6th V00.32 Snow-ski accident

√7th V00.321 Fall from snow-skis

√7th V00.322 Snow-skier colliding with stationary object

√7th V00.328 Other snow-ski accident
EXCLUDES1 *snow-skier collision with other land transport vehicle (V01-V09 with 5th digit 9)*

N Newborn: 0   P Pediatric: 0-17   M Maternity: 12-55   A Adult: 15-124   MCC Major CC Condition   PDxMCC PDx acts as own MCC   CC CC Condition   PDxCC PDx acts as own CC

1158   ICD-10-CM 2018

Chapter 20. External Causes of Morbidity

☑6ᵗʰ **V00.38** Other flat-bottomed pedestrian conveyance accident

    ☑7ᵗʰ **V00.381** Fall from other flat-bottomed pedestrian conveyance

    ☑7ᵗʰ **V00.382** Pedestrian on other flat-bottomed pedestrian conveyance colliding with stationary object

    ☑7ᵗʰ **V00.388** Other accident on other flat-bottomed pedestrian conveyance

☑5ᵗʰ **V00.8** Accident on other pedestrian conveyance

   ☑6ᵗʰ **V00.81** Accident with wheelchair (powered)

    ☑7ᵗʰ **V00.811** Fall from moving wheelchair (powered)
      EXCLUDES 1   fall from non-moving wheelchair (W05.0)

    ☑7ᵗʰ **V00.812** Wheelchair (powered) colliding with stationary object

    ☑7ᵗʰ **V00.818** Other accident with wheelchair (powered)

   ☑6ᵗʰ **V00.82** Accident with babystroller

    ☑7ᵗʰ **V00.821** Fall from babystroller

    ☑7ᵗʰ **V00.822** Babystroller colliding with stationary object

    ☑7ᵗʰ **V00.828** Other accident with babystroller

   ☑6ᵗʰ **V00.83** Accident with motorized mobility scooter

    ☑7ᵗʰ **V00.831** Fall from motorized mobility scooter
      EXCLUDES 1   fall from non-moving motorized mobility scooter (W05.2)

    ☑7ᵗʰ **V00.832** Motorized mobility scooter colliding with stationary object

    ☑7ᵗʰ **V00.838** Other accident with motorized mobility scooter

   ☑6ᵗʰ **V00.89** Accident on other pedestrian conveyance

    ☑7ᵗʰ **V00.891** Fall from other pedestrian conveyance

    ☑7ᵗʰ **V00.892** Pedestrian on other pedestrian conveyance colliding with stationary object

    ☑7ᵗʰ **V00.898** Other accident on other pedestrian conveyance
      EXCLUDES 1   other pedestrian (conveyance) collision with other land transport vehicle (V01-V09 with 5th digit 9)

☑4ᵗʰ **V01** Pedestrian injured in collision with pedal cycle

☑5ᵗʰ **V01.0** Pedestrian injured in collision with pedal cycle in nontraffic accident

   ☑x7ᵗʰ **V01.00** Pedestrian on foot injured in collision with pedal cycle in nontraffic accident
     Pedestrian NOS injured in collision with pedal cycle in nontraffic accident

   ☑x7ᵗʰ **V01.01** Pedestrian on roller-skates injured in collision with pedal cycle in nontraffic accident

   ☑x7ᵗʰ **V01.02** Pedestrian on skateboard injured in collision with pedal cycle in nontraffic accident

   ☑x7ᵗʰ **V01.09** Pedestrian with other conveyance injured in collision with pedal cycle in nontraffic accident
     Pedestrian with babystroller injured in collision with pedal cycle in nontraffic accident
     Pedestrian on ice-skates injured in collision with pedal cycle in nontraffic accident
     Pedestrian on nonmotorized scooter injured in collision with pedal cycle in nontraffic accident
     Pedestrian on sled injured in collision with pedal cycle in nontraffic accident
     Pedestrian on snowboard injured in collision with pedal cycle in nontraffic accident
     Pedestrian on snow-skis injured in collision with pedal cycle in nontraffic accident
     Pedestrian in wheelchair (powered) injured in collision with pedal cycle in nontraffic accident
     Pedestrian in motorized mobility scooter injured in collision with pedal cycle in nontraffic accident

☑5ᵗʰ **V01.1** Pedestrian injured in collision with pedal cycle in traffic accident

   ☑x7ᵗʰ **V01.10** Pedestrian on foot injured in collision with pedal cycle in traffic accident
     Pedestrian NOS injured in collision with pedal cycle in traffic accident

   ☑x7ᵗʰ **V01.11** Pedestrian on roller-skates injured in collision with pedal cycle in traffic accident

   ☑x7ᵗʰ **V01.12** Pedestrian on skateboard injured in collision with pedal cycle in traffic accident

   ☑x7ᵗʰ **V01.19** Pedestrian with other conveyance injured in collision with pedal cycle in traffic accident
     Pedestrian with babystroller injured in collision with pedal cycle in traffic accident
     Pedestrian on ice-skates injured in collision with pedal cycle in traffic accident
     Pedestrian on nonmotorized scooter injured in collision with pedal cycle in traffic accident
     Pedestrian on sled injured in collision with pedal cycle in traffic accident
     Pedestrian on snowboard injured in collision with pedal cycle in traffic accident
     Pedestrian on snow-skis injured in collision with pedal cycle in traffic accident
     Pedestrian in wheelchair (powered) injured in collision with pedal cycle in traffic accident
     Pedestrian in motorized mobility scooter injured in collision with pedal cycle in traffic accident

☑5ᵗʰ **V01.9** Pedestrian injured in collision with pedal cycle, unspecified whether traffic or nontraffic accident

   ☑x7ᵗʰ **V01.90** Pedestrian on foot injured in collision with pedal cycle, unspecified whether traffic or nontraffic accident
     Pedestrian NOS injured in collision with pedal cycle, unspecified whether traffic or nontraffic accident

   ☑x7ᵗʰ **V01.91** Pedestrian on roller-skates injured in collision with pedal cycle, unspecified whether traffic or nontraffic accident

   ☑x7ᵗʰ **V01.92** Pedestrian on skateboard injured in collision with pedal cycle, unspecified whether traffic or nontraffic accident

   ☑x7ᵗʰ **V01.99** Pedestrian with other conveyance injured in collision with pedal cycle, unspecified whether traffic or nontraffic accident
     Pedestrian with babystroller injured in collision with pedal cycle, unspecified whether traffic or nontraffic accident
     Pedestrian on ice-skates injured in collision with pedal cycle unspecified, whether traffic or nontraffic accident
     Pedestrian on nonmotorized scooter injured in collision with pedal cycle, unspecified whether traffic or nontraffic accident
     Pedestrian on sled injured in collision with pedal cycle unspecified, whether traffic or nontraffic accident
     Pedestrian on snowboard injured in collision with pedal cycle, unspecified whether traffic or nontraffic accident
     Pedestrian on snow-skis injured in collision with pedal cycle, unspecified whether traffic or nontraffic accident
     Pedestrian in wheelchair (powered) injured in collision with pedal cycle, unspecified whether traffic or nontraffic accident
     Pedestrian in motorized mobility scooter injured in collision with pedal cycle, unspecified whether traffic or nontraffic accident

☑4ᵗʰ **V02** Pedestrian injured in collision with two- or three-wheeled motor vehicle

☑5ᵗʰ **V02.0** Pedestrian injured in collision with two- or three-wheeled motor vehicle in nontraffic accident

   ☑x7ᵗʰ **V02.00** Pedestrian on foot injured in collision with two- or three-wheeled motor vehicle in nontraffic accident
     Pedestrian NOS injured in collision with two- or three-wheeled motor vehicle in nontraffic accident

   ☑x7ᵗʰ **V02.01** Pedestrian on roller-skates injured in collision with two- or three-wheeled motor vehicle in nontraffic accident

   ☑x7ᵗʰ **V02.02** Pedestrian on skateboard injured in collision with two- or three-wheeled motor vehicle in nontraffic accident

☑ Additional Character Req   ☑x7ᵗʰ Placeholder Alert   Unacceptable PDx   Manifestation   **H1**-**H14** HAC   **HCC** CMS-HCC Condition   *EXCLUDES 1* Not Coded Here   *EXCLUDES 2* Not Included Here

ICD-10-CM 2018   1159

Chapter 20. External Causes of Morbidity

√x 7th **V02.09 Pedestrian with other conveyance injured in collision with two- or three-wheeled motor vehicle in nontraffic accident**
Pedestrian with babystroller injured in collision with two- or three-wheeled motor vehicle in nontraffic accident
Pedestrian on ice-skates injured in collision with two- or three-wheeled motor vehicle in nontraffic accident
Pedestrian on nonmotorized scooter injured in collision with two- or three-wheeled motor vehicle in nontraffic accident
Pedestrian on sled injured in collision with two- or three-wheeled motor vehicle in nontraffic accident
Pedestrian on snowboard injured in collision with two- or three-wheeled motor vehicle in nontraffic accident
Pedestrian on snow-skis injured in collision with two- or three-wheeled motor vehicle in nontraffic accident
Pedestrian in wheelchair (powered) injured in collision with two- or three-wheeled motor vehicle in nontraffic accident
Pedestrian in motorized mobility scooter injured in collision with two- or three-wheeled motor vehicle in nontraffic accident

√5th **V02.1 Pedestrian injured in collision with two- or three-wheeled motor vehicle in traffic accident**

√x 7th **V02.10 Pedestrian on foot injured in collision with two- or three-wheeled motor vehicle in traffic accident**
Pedestrian NOS injured in collision with two- or three-wheeled motor vehicle in traffic accident

√x 7th **V02.11 Pedestrian on roller-skates injured in collision with two- or three-wheeled motor vehicle in traffic accident**

√x 7th **V02.12 Pedestrian on skateboard injured in collision with two- or three-wheeled motor vehicle in traffic accident**

√x 7th **V02.19 Pedestrian with other conveyance injured in collision with two- or three-wheeled motor vehicle in traffic accident**
Pedestrian with babystroller injured in collision with two- or three-wheeled motor vehicle in traffic accident
Pedestrian on ice-skates injured in collision with two- or three-wheeled motor vehicle in traffic accident
Pedestrian on nonmotorized scooter injured in collision with two- or three-wheeled motor vehicle in traffic accident
Pedestrian on sled injured in collision with two- or three-wheeled motor vehicle in traffic accident
Pedestrian on snowboard injured in collision with two- or three-wheeled motor vehicle in traffic accident
Pedestrian on snow-skis injured in collision with two- or three-wheeled motor vehicle in traffic accident
Pedestrian in wheelchair (powered) injured in collision with two- or three-wheeled motor vehicle in traffic accident
Pedestrian in motorized mobility scooter injured in collision with two- or three-wheeled motor vehicle in traffic accident

√5th **V02.9 Pedestrian injured in collision with two- or three-wheeled motor vehicle, unspecified whether traffic or nontraffic accident**

√x 7th **V02.90 Pedestrian on foot injured in collision with two- or three-wheeled motor vehicle, unspecified whether traffic or nontraffic accident**
Pedestrian NOS injured in collision with two- or three-wheeled motor vehicle, unspecified whether traffic or nontraffic accident

√x 7th **V02.91 Pedestrian on roller-skates injured in collision with two- or three-wheeled motor vehicle, unspecified whether traffic or nontraffic accident**

√x 7th **V02.92 Pedestrian on skateboard injured in collision with two- or three-wheeled motor vehicle, unspecified whether traffic or nontraffic accident**

√x 7th **V02.99 Pedestrian with other conveyance injured in collision with two- or three-wheeled motor vehicle, unspecified whether traffic or nontraffic accident**
Pedestrian with babystroller injured in collision with two- or three-wheeled motor vehicle, unspecified whether traffic or nontraffic accident
Pedestrian on ice-skates injured in collision with two- or three-wheeled motor vehicle, unspecified whether traffic or nontraffic accident
Pedestrian on nonmotorized scooter injured in collision with two- or three-wheeled motor vehicle, unspecified whether traffic or nontraffic accident
Pedestrian on sled injured in collision with two- or three-wheeled motor vehicle, unspecified whether traffic or nontraffic accident
Pedestrian on snowboard injured in collision with two- or three-wheeled motor vehicle, unspecified whether traffic or nontraffic accident
Pedestrian on snow-skis injured in collision with two- or three-wheeled motor vehicle, unspecified whether traffic or nontraffic accident
Pedestrian in wheelchair (powered) injured in collision with two- or three-wheeled motor vehicle, unspecified whether traffic or nontraffic accident
Pedestrian in motorized mobility scooter injured in collision with two- or three-wheeled motor vehicle, unspecified whether traffic or nontraffic accident

√4th **V03 Pedestrian injured in collision with car, pick-up truck or van**

√5th **V03.0 Pedestrian injured in collision with car, pick-up truck or van in nontraffic accident**

√x 7th **V03.00 Pedestrian on foot injured in collision with car, pick-up truck or van in nontraffic accident**
Pedestrian NOS injured in collision with car, pick-up truck or van in nontraffic accident

√x 7th **V03.01 Pedestrian on roller-skates injured in collision with car, pick-up truck or van in nontraffic accident**

√x 7th **V03.02 Pedestrian on skateboard injured in collision with car, pick-up truck or van in nontraffic accident**

√x 7th **V03.09 Pedestrian with other conveyance injured in collision with car, pick-up truck or van in nontraffic accident**
Pedestrian with babystroller injured in collision with car, pick-up truck or van in nontraffic accident
Pedestrian on ice-skates injured in collision with car, pick-up truck or van in nontraffic accident
Pedestrian on nonmotorized scooter injured in collision with car, pick-up truck or van in nontraffic accident
Pedestrian on sled injured in collision with car, pick-up truck or van in nontraffic accident
Pedestrian on snowboard injured in collision with car, pick-up truck or van in nontraffic accident
Pedestrian on snow-skis injured in collision with car, pick-up truck or van in nontraffic accident
Pedestrian in wheelchair (powered) injured in collision with car, pick-up truck or van in nontraffic accident
Pedestrian in motorized mobility scooter injured in collision with car, pick-up truck or van in nontraffic accident

√5th **V03.1 Pedestrian injured in collision with car, pick-up truck or van in traffic accident**

√x 7th **V03.10 Pedestrian on foot injured in collision with car, pick-up truck or van in traffic accident**
Pedestrian NOS injured in collision with car, pick-up truck or van in traffic accident

√x 7th **V03.11 Pedestrian on roller-skates injured in collision with car, pick-up truck or van in traffic accident**

√x 7th **V03.12 Pedestrian on skateboard injured in collision with car, pick-up truck or van in traffic accident**

N Newborn: 0   P Pediatric: 0-17   M Maternity: 12-55   A Adult: 15-124   MCC Major CC Condition   PDx MCC PDx acts as own MCC   CC CC Condition   PDx CC PDx acts as own CC
1160   ICD-10-CM 2018

V02.09–V03.12

✓x7ᵗʰ **V03.19** **Pedestrian with other conveyance injured in collision with car, pick-up truck or van in traffic accident**
　Pedestrian with babystroller injured in collision with car, pick-up truck or van in traffic accident
　Pedestrian on ice-skates injured in collision with car, pick-up truck or van in traffic accident
　Pedestrian on nonmotorized scooter injured in collision with car, pick-up truck or van in traffic accident
　Pedestrian on sled injured in collision with car, pick-up truck or van in traffic accident
　Pedestrian on snowboard injured in collision with car, pick-up truck or van in traffic accident
　Pedestrian on snow-skis injured in collision with car, pick-up truck or van in traffic accident
　Pedestrian in wheelchair (powered) injured in collision with car, pick-up truck or van in traffic accident
　Pedestrian in motorized mobility scooter injured in collision with car, pick-up truck or van in traffic accident

✓5ᵗʰ **V03.9** **Pedestrian injured in collision with car, pick-up truck or van, unspecified whether traffic or nontraffic accident**

✓x7ᵗʰ **V03.90** **Pedestrian on foot injured in collision with car, pick-up truck or van, unspecified whether traffic or nontraffic accident**
　Pedestrian NOS injured in collision with car, pick-up truck or van, unspecified whether traffic or nontraffic accident

✓x7ᵗʰ **V03.91** **Pedestrian on roller-skates injured in collision with car, pick-up truck or van, unspecified whether traffic or nontraffic accident**

✓x7ᵗʰ **V03.92** **Pedestrian on skateboard injured in collision with car, pick-up truck or van, unspecified whether traffic or nontraffic accident**

✓x7ᵗʰ **V03.99** **Pedestrian with other conveyance injured in collision with car, pick-up truck or van, unspecified whether traffic or nontraffic accident**
　Pedestrian with babystroller injured in collision with car, pick-up truck or van, unspecified whether traffic or nontraffic accident
　Pedestrian on ice-skates injured in collision with car, pick-up truck or van, unspecified whether traffic or nontraffic accident
　Pedestrian on nonmotorized scooter injured in collision with car, pick-up truck or van, unspecified whether traffic or nontraffic accident
　Pedestrian on sled injured in collision with car, pick-up truck or van in nontraffic accident
　Pedestrian on snowboard injured in collision with car, pick-up truck or van, unspecified whether traffic or nontraffic accident
　Pedestrian on snow-skis injured in collision with car, pick-up truck or van, unspecified whether traffic or nontraffic accident
　Pedestrian in wheelchair (powered) injured in collision with car, pick-up truck or van, unspecified whether traffic or nontraffic accident
　Pedestrian in motorized mobility scooter injured in collision with car, pick-up truck or van, unspecified whether traffic or nontraffic accident

✓4ᵗʰ **V04** **Pedestrian injured in collision with heavy transport vehicle or bus**
　EXCLUDES 1　pedestrian injured in collision with military vehicle (V09.01, V09.21)

✓5ᵗʰ **V04.0** **Pedestrian injured in collision with heavy transport vehicle or bus in nontraffic accident**

✓x7ᵗʰ **V04.00** **Pedestrian on foot injured in collision with heavy transport vehicle or bus in nontraffic accident**
　Pedestrian NOS injured in collision with heavy transport vehicle or bus in nontraffic accident

✓x7ᵗʰ **V04.01** **Pedestrian on roller-skates injured in collision with heavy transport vehicle or bus in nontraffic accident**

✓x7ᵗʰ **V04.02** **Pedestrian on skateboard injured in collision with heavy transport vehicle or bus in nontraffic accident**

✓x7ᵗʰ **V04.09** **Pedestrian with other conveyance injured in collision with heavy transport vehicle or bus in nontraffic accident**
　Pedestrian with babystroller injured in collision with heavy transport vehicle or bus in nontraffic accident
　Pedestrian on ice-skates injured in collision with heavy transport vehicle or bus in nontraffic accident
　Pedestrian on nonmotorized scooter injured in collision with heavy transport vehicle or bus in nontraffic accident
　Pedestrian on sled injured in collision with heavy transport vehicle or bus in nontraffic accident
　Pedestrian on snowboard injured in collision with heavy transport vehicle or bus in nontraffic accident
　Pedestrian on snow-skis injured in collision with heavy transport vehicle or bus in nontraffic accident
　Pedestrian in wheelchair (powered) injured in collision with heavy transport vehicle or bus in nontraffic accident
　Pedestrian in motorized mobility scooter injured in collision with heavy transport vehicle or bus in nontraffic accident

✓5ᵗʰ **V04.1** **Pedestrian injured in collision with heavy transport vehicle or bus in traffic accident**

✓x7ᵗʰ **V04.10** **Pedestrian on foot injured in collision with heavy transport vehicle or bus in traffic accident**
　Pedestrian NOS injured in collision with heavy transport vehicle or bus in traffic accident

✓x7ᵗʰ **V04.11** **Pedestrian on roller-skates injured in collision with heavy transport vehicle or bus in traffic accident**

✓x7ᵗʰ **V04.12** **Pedestrian on skateboard injured in collision with heavy transport vehicle or bus in traffic accident**

✓x7ᵗʰ **V04.19** **Pedestrian with other conveyance injured in collision with heavy transport vehicle or bus in traffic accident**
　Pedestrian with babystroller injured in collision with heavy transport vehicle or bus in traffic accident
　Pedestrian on ice-skates injured in collision with heavy transport vehicle or bus in traffic accident
　Pedestrian on nonmotorized scooter injured in collision with heavy transport vehicle or bus in traffic accident
　Pedestrian on sled injured in collision with heavy transport vehicle or bus in traffic accident
　Pedestrian on snowboard injured in collision with heavy transport vehicle or bus in traffic accident
　Pedestrian on snow-skis injured in collision with heavy transport vehicle or bus in traffic accident
　Pedestrian in wheelchair (powered) injured in collision with heavy transport vehicle or bus in traffic accident
　Pedestrian in motorized mobility scooter injured in collision with heavy transport vehicle or bus in traffic accident

✓5ᵗʰ **V04.9** **Pedestrian injured in collision with heavy transport vehicle or bus, unspecified whether traffic or nontraffic accident**

✓x7ᵗʰ **V04.90** **Pedestrian on foot injured in collision with heavy transport vehicle or bus, unspecified whether traffic or nontraffic accident**
　Pedestrian NOS injured in collision with heavy transport vehicle or bus, unspecified whether traffic or nontraffic accident

✓x7ᵗʰ **V04.91** **Pedestrian on roller-skates injured in collision with heavy transport vehicle or bus, unspecified whether traffic or nontraffic accident**

✓x7ᵗʰ **V04.92** **Pedestrian on skateboard injured in collision with heavy transport vehicle or bus, unspecified whether traffic or nontraffic accident**

✓ Additional Character Req　✓x7ᵗʰ Placeholder Alert　Unacceptable PDx　Manifestation　H1-H14 HAC　HCC CMS-HCC Condition　*EXCLUDES 1* Not Coded Here　*EXCLUDES 2* Not Included Here

ICD-10-CM 2018　　　　　　　　　　　　　　　　　　　　　　　　　　　　　　　　　　1161

√x7ᵗʰ **V04.99** **Pedestrian with other conveyance injured in collision with heavy transport vehicle or bus, unspecified whether traffic or nontraffic accident**
Pedestrian with babystroller injured in collision with heavy transport vehicle or bus, unspecified whether traffic or nontraffic accident
Pedestrian on ice-skates injured in collision with heavy transport vehicle or bus, unspecified whether traffic or nontraffic accident
Pedestrian on nonmotorized scooter injured in collision with heavy transport vehicle or bus, unspecified whether traffic or nontraffic accident
Pedestrian on sled injured in collision with heavy transport vehicle or bus, unspecified whether traffic or nontraffic accident
Pedestrian on snowboard injured in collision with heavy transport vehicle or bus, unspecified whether traffic or nontraffic accident
Pedestrian on snow-skis injured in collision with heavy transport vehicle or bus, unspecified whether traffic or nontraffic accident
Pedestrian in wheelchair (powered) injured in collision with heavy transport vehicle or bus, unspecified whether traffic or nontraffic accident
Pedestrian in motorized mobility scooter injured in collision with heavy transport vehicle or bus, unspecified whether traffic or nontraffic accident

√4ᵗʰ **V05** **Pedestrian injured in collision with railway train or railway vehicle**

√5ᵗʰ **V05.0** **Pedestrian injured in collision with railway train or railway vehicle in nontraffic accident**

√x7ᵗʰ **V05.00** **Pedestrian on foot injured in collision with railway train or railway vehicle in nontraffic accident**
Pedestrian NOS injured in collision with railway train or railway vehicle in nontraffic accident

√x7ᵗʰ **V05.01** **Pedestrian on roller-skates injured in collision with railway train or railway vehicle in nontraffic accident**

√x7ᵗʰ **V05.02** **Pedestrian on skateboard injured in collision with railway train or railway vehicle in nontraffic accident**

√x7ᵗʰ **V05.09** **Pedestrian with other conveyance injured in collision with railway train or railway vehicle in nontraffic accident**
Pedestrian with babystroller injured in collision with railway train or railway vehicle in nontraffic accident
Pedestrian on ice-skates injured in collision with railway train or railway vehicle in nontraffic accident
Pedestrian on nonmotorized scooter injured in collision with railway train or railway vehicle in nontraffic accident
Pedestrian on sled injured in collision with railway train or railway vehicle in nontraffic accident
Pedestrian on snowboard injured in collision with railway train or railway vehicle in nontraffic accident
Pedestrian on snow-skis injured in collision with railway train or railway vehicle in nontraffic accident
Pedestrian in wheelchair (powered) injured in collision with railway train or railway vehicle in nontraffic accident
Pedestrian in motorized mobility scooter injured in collision with railway train or railway vehicle in nontraffic accident

√5ᵗʰ **V05.1** **Pedestrian injured in collision with railway train or railway vehicle in traffic accident**

√x7ᵗʰ **V05.10** **Pedestrian on foot injured in collision with railway train or railway vehicle in traffic accident**
Pedestrian NOS injured in collision with railway train or railway vehicle in traffic accident

√x7ᵗʰ **V05.11** **Pedestrian on roller-skates injured in collision with railway train or railway vehicle in traffic accident**

√x7ᵗʰ **V05.12** **Pedestrian on skateboard injured in collision with railway train or railway vehicle in traffic accident**

√x7ᵗʰ **V05.19** **Pedestrian with other conveyance injured in collision with railway train or railway vehicle in traffic accident**
Pedestrian with babystroller injured in collision with railway train or railway vehicle in traffic accident
Pedestrian on ice-skates injured in collision with railway train or railway vehicle in traffic accident
Pedestrian on nonmotorized scooter injured in collision with railway train or railway vehicle in traffic accident
Pedestrian on sled injured in collision with railway train or railway vehicle in traffic accident
Pedestrian on snowboard injured in collision with railway train or railway vehicle in traffic accident
Pedestrian on snow-skis injured in collision with railway train or railway vehicle in traffic accident
Pedestrian in wheelchair (powered) injured in collision with railway train or railway vehicle in traffic accident
Pedestrian in motorized mobility scooter injured in collision with railway train or railway vehicle in traffic accident

√5ᵗʰ **V05.9** **Pedestrian injured in collision with railway train or railway vehicle, unspecified whether traffic or nontraffic accident**

√x7ᵗʰ **V05.90** **Pedestrian on foot injured in collision with railway train or railway vehicle, unspecified whether traffic or nontraffic accident**
Pedestrian NOS injured in collision with railway train or railway vehicle, unspecified whether traffic or nontraffic accident

√x7ᵗʰ **V05.91** **Pedestrian on roller-skates injured in collision with railway train or railway vehicle, unspecified whether traffic or nontraffic accident**

√x7ᵗʰ **V05.92** **Pedestrian on skateboard injured in collision with railway train or railway vehicle, unspecified whether traffic or nontraffic accident**

√x7ᵗʰ **V05.99** **Pedestrian with other conveyance injured in collision with railway train or railway vehicle, unspecified whether traffic or nontraffic accident**
Pedestrian with babystroller injured in collision with railway train or railway vehicle, unspecified whether traffic or nontraffic
Pedestrian on ice-skates injured in collision with railway train or railway vehicle, unspecified whether traffic or nontraffic
Pedestrian on nonmotorized scooter injured in collision with railway train or railway vehicle, unspecified whether traffic or nontraffic
Pedestrian on sled injured in collision with railway train or railway vehicle, unspecified whether traffic or nontraffic
Pedestrian on snowboard injured in collision with railway train or railway vehicle, unspecified whether traffic or nontraffic
Pedestrian on snow-skis injured in collision with railway train or railway vehicle, unspecified whether traffic or nontraffic
Pedestrian in wheelchair (powered) injured in collision with railway train or railway vehicle, unspecified whether traffic or nontraffic
Pedestrian in motorized mobility scooter injured in collision with railway train or railway vehicle, unspecified whether traffic or nontraffic

√4ᵗʰ **V06** **Pedestrian injured in collision with other nonmotor vehicle**
INCLUDES collision with animal-drawn vehicle, animal being ridden, nonpowered streetcar
EXCLUDES 1 pedestrian injured in collision with pedestrian conveyance (V00.0-)

√5ᵗʰ **V06.0** **Pedestrian injured in collision with other nonmotor vehicle in nontraffic accident**

√x7ᵗʰ **V06.00** **Pedestrian on foot injured in collision with other nonmotor vehicle in nontraffic accident**
Pedestrian NOS injured in collision with other nonmotor vehicle in nontraffic accident

√x7ᵗʰ **V06.01** **Pedestrian on roller-skates injured in collision with other nonmotor vehicle in nontraffic accident**

√x7ᵗʰ **V06.02** **Pedestrian on skateboard injured in collision with other nonmotor vehicle in nontraffic accident**

N Newborn: 0   **P** Pediatric: 0-17   **M** Maternity: 12-55   **A** Adult: 15-124   **MCC** Major CC Condition   **PDxMCC** PDx acts as own MCC   **CC** CC Condition   **PDxCC** PDx acts as own CC

1162   ICD-10-CM 2018

☑x7ʰ **V06.09** **Pedestrian** with other conveyance **injured in collision with other nonmotor vehicle in nontraffic accident**

  Pedestrian with babystroller injured in collision with other nonmotor vehicle in nontraffic accident

  Pedestrian on ice-skates injured in collision with other nonmotor vehicle in nontraffic accident

  Pedestrian on nonmotorized scooter injured in collision with other nonmotor vehicle in nontraffic accident

  Pedestrian on sled injured in collision with other nonmotor vehicle in nontraffic accident

  Pedestrian on snowboard injured in collision with other nonmotor vehicle in nontraffic accident

  Pedestrian on snow-skis injured in collision with other nonmotor vehicle in nontraffic accident

  Pedestrian in wheelchair (powered) injured in collision with other nonmotor vehicle in nontraffic accident

  Pedestrian in motorized mobility scooter injured in collision with other nonmotor vehicle in nontraffic accident

☑5ʰ **V06.1** **Pedestrian injured in collision with other nonmotor vehicle** in **traffic accident**

  ☑x7ʰ **V06.10** **Pedestrian** on foot **injured in collision with other nonmotor vehicle in traffic accident**

   Pedestrian NOS injured in collision with other nonmotor vehicle in traffic accident

  ☑x7ʰ **V06.11** **Pedestrian** on roller-skates **injured in collision with other nonmotor vehicle in traffic accident**

  ☑x7ʰ **V06.12** **Pedestrian** on skateboard **injured in collision with other nonmotor vehicle in traffic accident**

  ☑x7ʰ **V06.19** **Pedestrian** with other conveyance **injured in collision with other nonmotor vehicle in traffic accident**

   Pedestrian with babystroller injured in collision with other nonmotor vehicle in nontraffic accident

   Pedestrian on ice-skates injured in collision with other nonmotor vehicle in traffic accident

   Pedestrian on nonmotorized scooter injured in collision with other nonmotor vehicle in traffic accident

   Pedestrian on sled injured in collision with other nonmotor vehicle in traffic accident

   Pedestrian on snowboard injured in collision with other nonmotor vehicle in traffic accident

   Pedestrian on snow-skis injured in collision with other nonmotor vehicle in traffic accident

   Pedestrian in wheelchair (powered) injured in collision with other nonmotor vehicle in traffic accident

   Pedestrian in motorized mobility scooter injured in collision with other nonmotor vehicle in traffic accident

☑5ʰ **V06.9** **Pedestrian injured in collision with other nonmotor vehicle, unspecified whether traffic or nontraffic accident**

  ☑x7ʰ **V06.90** **Pedestrian** on foot **injured in collision with other nonmotor vehicle, unspecified whether traffic or nontraffic accident**

   Pedestrian NOS injured in collision with other nonmotor vehicle, unspecified whether traffic or nontraffic accident

  ☑x7ʰ **V06.91** **Pedestrian** on roller-skates **injured in collision with other nonmotor vehicle, unspecified whether traffic or nontraffic accident**

  ☑x7ʰ **V06.92** **Pedestrian** on skateboard **injured in collision with other nonmotor vehicle, unspecified whether traffic or nontraffic accident**

☑x7ʰ **V06.99** **Pedestrian** with other conveyance **injured in collision with other nonmotor vehicle, unspecified whether traffic or nontraffic accident**

  Pedestrian with babystroller injured in collision with other nonmotor vehicle, unspecified whether traffic or nontraffic accident

  Pedestrian on ice-skates injured in collision with other nonmotor vehicle, unspecified whether traffic or nontraffic accident

  Pedestrian on nonmotorized scooter injured in collision with other nonmotor vehicle, unspecified whether traffic or nontraffic accident

  Pedestrian on sled injured in collision with other nonmotor vehicle, unspecified whether traffic or nontraffic accident

  Pedestrian on snowboard injured in collision with other nonmotor vehicle, unspecified whether traffic or nontraffic accident

  Pedestrian on snow-skis injured in collision with other nonmotor vehicle, unspecified whether traffic or nontraffic accident

  Pedestrian in wheelchair (powered) injured in collision with other nonmotor vehicle, unspecified whether traffic or nontraffic accident

  Pedestrian in motorized mobility scooter injured in collision with other nonmotor vehicle, unspecified whether traffic or nontraffic accident

☑4ʰ **V09** **Pedestrian injured in other and unspecified transport accidents**

☑5ʰ **V09.0** **Pedestrian injured in** nontraffic **accident involving** other **and unspecified motor vehicles**

  ☑x7ʰ **V09.00** **Pedestrian injured in nontraffic accident involving** unspecified **motor vehicles**

  ☑x7ʰ **V09.01** **Pedestrian injured in nontraffic accident involving** military **vehicle**

  ☑x7ʰ **V09.09** **Pedestrian injured in nontraffic accident involving** other **motor vehicles**

   Pedestrian injured in nontraffic accident by special vehicle

☑x7ʰ **V09.1** **Pedestrian injured in** unspecified nontraffic **accident**

☑5ʰ **V09.2** **Pedestrian injured in** traffic accident **involving other and unspecified motor vehicles**

  ☑x7ʰ **V09.20** **Pedestrian injured in traffic accident involving** unspecified **motor vehicles**

  ☑x7ʰ **V09.21** **Pedestrian injured in traffic accident involving** military **vehicle**

  ☑x7ʰ **V09.29** **Pedestrian injured in traffic accident involving** other **motor vehicles**

☑x7ʰ **V09.3** **Pedestrian injured in** unspecified traffic **accident**

☑x7ʰ **V09.9** **Pedestrian injured in** unspecified transport **accident**

Pedal cycle rider injured in transport accident (V10–V19)

INCLUDES   any non-motorized vehicle, excluding an animal-drawn vehicle, or a sidecar or trailer attached to the pedal cycle

EXCLUDES 2   rupture of pedal cycle tire (W37.0)

> The appropriate 7th character is to be added to each code from categories V10–V19.
> A   initial encounter
> D   subsequent encounter
> S   sequela

☑4ʰ **V10** **Pedal cycle rider injured in collision with pedestrian or animal**

  EXCLUDES 1   pedal cycle rider collision with animal-drawn vehicle or animal being ridden (V16.-)

☑x7ʰ **V10.0** **Pedal cycle** driver **injured in collision with pedestrian or animal** in nontraffic accident

☑x7ʰ **V10.1** **Pedal cycle** passenger **injured in collision with pedestrian or animal** in nontraffic accident

☑x7ʰ **V10.2** Unspecified **pedal cyclist injured in collision with pedestrian or animal in** nontraffic accident

☑x7ʰ **V10.3** Person boarding or alighting **a pedal cycle injured in collision with pedestrian or animal**

☑x7ʰ **V10.4** **Pedal cycle** driver **injured in collision with pedestrian or animal** in traffic accident

☑x7ʰ **V10.5** **Pedal cycle** passenger **injured in collision with pedestrian or animal** in traffic accident

☑x7ʰ **V10.9** Unspecified **pedal cyclist injured in collision with pedestrian or animal in** traffic accident

☑ Additional Character Req   ☑x7ʰ Placeholder Alert   Unacceptable PDx   Manifestation   H1-H14 HAC   HCC CMS-HCC Condition   EXCLUDES 1 Not Coded Here   EXCLUDES 2 Not Included Here

ICD-10-CM 2018   1163

Chapter 20. External Causes of Morbidity *(side tab)*

V11–V19.19 *(side tab)*

✓4ᵗʰ **V11 Pedal cycle rider injured in collision with other pedal cycle**

✓x7ᵗʰ **V11.0 Pedal cycle driver injured in collision with other pedal cycle in nontraffic accident**

✓x7ᵗʰ **V11.1 Pedal cycle passenger injured in collision with other pedal cycle in nontraffic accident**

✓x7ᵗʰ **V11.2 Unspecified pedal cyclist injured in collision with other pedal cycle in nontraffic accident**

✓x7ᵗʰ **V11.3 Person boarding or alighting a pedal cycle injured in collision with other pedal cycle**

✓x7ᵗʰ **V11.4 Pedal cycle driver injured in collision with other pedal cycle in traffic accident**

✓x7ᵗʰ **V11.5 Pedal cycle passenger injured in collision with other pedal cycle in traffic accident**

✓x7ᵗʰ **V11.9 Unspecified pedal cyclist injured in collision with other pedal cycle in traffic accident**

✓4ᵗʰ **V12 Pedal cycle rider injured in collision with two- or three-wheeled motor vehicle**

✓x7ᵗʰ **V12.0 Pedal cycle driver injured in collision with two- or three-wheeled motor vehicle in nontraffic accident**

✓x7ᵗʰ **V12.1 Pedal cycle passenger injured in collision with two- or three-wheeled motor vehicle in nontraffic accident**

✓x7ᵗʰ **V12.2 Unspecified pedal cyclist injured in collision with two- or three-wheeled motor vehicle in nontraffic accident**

✓x7ᵗʰ **V12.3 Person boarding or alighting a pedal cycle injured in collision with two- or three-wheeled motor vehicle**

✓x7ᵗʰ **V12.4 Pedal cycle driver injured in collision with two- or three-wheeled motor vehicle in traffic accident**

✓x7ᵗʰ **V12.5 Pedal cycle passenger injured in collision with two- or three-wheeled motor vehicle in traffic accident**

✓x7ᵗʰ **V12.9 Unspecified pedal cyclist injured in collision with two- or three-wheeled motor vehicle in traffic accident**

✓4ᵗʰ **V13 Pedal cycle rider injured in collision with car, pick-up truck or van**

✓x7ᵗʰ **V13.0 Pedal cycle driver injured in collision with car, pick-up truck or van in nontraffic accident**

✓x7ᵗʰ **V13.1 Pedal cycle passenger injured in collision with car, pick-up truck or van in nontraffic accident**

✓x7ᵗʰ **V13.2 Unspecified pedal cyclist injured in collision with car, pick-up truck or van in nontraffic accident**

✓x7ᵗʰ **V13.3 Person boarding or alighting a pedal cycle injured in collision with car, pick-up truck or van**

✓x7ᵗʰ **V13.4 Pedal cycle driver injured in collision with car, pick-up truck or van in traffic accident**

✓x7ᵗʰ **V13.5 Pedal cycle passenger injured in collision with car, pick-up truck or van in traffic accident**

✓x7ᵗʰ **V13.9 Unspecified pedal cyclist injured in collision with car, pick-up truck or van in traffic accident**

✓4ᵗʰ **V14 Pedal cycle rider injured in collision with heavy transport vehicle or bus**

> **EXCLUDES 1** *pedal cycle rider injured in collision with military vehicle (V19.81)*

✓x7ᵗʰ **V14.0 Pedal cycle driver injured in collision with heavy transport vehicle or bus in nontraffic accident**

✓x7ᵗʰ **V14.1 Pedal cycle passenger injured in collision with heavy transport vehicle or bus in nontraffic accident**

✓x7ᵗʰ **V14.2 Unspecified pedal cyclist injured in collision with heavy transport vehicle or bus in nontraffic accident**

✓x7ᵗʰ **V14.3 Person boarding or alighting a pedal cycle injured in collision with heavy transport vehicle or bus**

✓x7ᵗʰ **V14.4 Pedal cycle driver injured in collision with heavy transport vehicle or bus in traffic accident**

✓x7ᵗʰ **V14.5 Pedal cycle passenger injured in collision with heavy transport vehicle or bus in traffic accident**

✓x7ᵗʰ **V14.9 Unspecified pedal cyclist injured in collision with heavy transport vehicle or bus in traffic accident**

✓4ᵗʰ **V15 Pedal cycle rider injured in collision with railway train or railway vehicle**

✓x7ᵗʰ **V15.0 Pedal cycle driver injured in collision with railway train or railway vehicle in nontraffic accident**

✓x7ᵗʰ **V15.1 Pedal cycle passenger injured in collision with railway train or railway vehicle in nontraffic accident**

✓x7ᵗʰ **V15.2 Unspecified pedal cyclist injured in collision with railway train or railway vehicle in nontraffic accident**

✓x7ᵗʰ **V15.3 Person boarding or alighting a pedal cycle injured in collision with railway train or railway vehicle**

✓x7ᵗʰ **V15.4 Pedal cycle driver injured in collision with railway train or railway vehicle in traffic accident**

✓x7ᵗʰ **V15.5 Pedal cycle passenger injured in collision with railway train or railway vehicle in traffic accident**

✓x7ᵗʰ **V15.9 Unspecified pedal cyclist injured in collision with railway train or railway vehicle in traffic accident**

✓4ᵗʰ **V16 Pedal cycle rider injured in collision with other nonmotor vehicle**

> **INCLUDES** collision with animal-drawn vehicle, animal being ridden, streetcar

✓x7ᵗʰ **V16.0 Pedal cycle driver injured in collision with other nonmotor vehicle in nontraffic accident**

✓x7ᵗʰ **V16.1 Pedal cycle passenger injured in collision with other nonmotor vehicle in nontraffic accident**

✓x7ᵗʰ **V16.2 Unspecified pedal cyclist injured in collision with other nonmotor vehicle in nontraffic accident**

✓x7ᵗʰ **V16.3 Person boarding or alighting a pedal cycle injured in collision with other nonmotor vehicle in nontraffic accident**

✓x7ᵗʰ **V16.4 Pedal cycle driver injured in collision with other nonmotor vehicle in traffic accident**

✓x7ᵗʰ **V16.5 Pedal cycle passenger injured in collision with other nonmotor vehicle in traffic accident**

✓x7ᵗʰ **V16.9 Unspecified pedal cyclist injured in collision with other nonmotor vehicle in traffic accident**

✓4ᵗʰ **V17 Pedal cycle rider injured in collision with fixed or stationary object**

✓x7ᵗʰ **V17.0 Pedal cycle driver injured in collision with fixed or stationary object in nontraffic accident**

✓x7ᵗʰ **V17.1 Pedal cycle passenger injured in collision with fixed or stationary object in nontraffic accident**

✓x7ᵗʰ **V17.2 Unspecified pedal cyclist injured in collision with fixed or stationary object in nontraffic accident**

✓x7ᵗʰ **V17.3 Person boarding or alighting a pedal cycle injured in collision with fixed or stationary object**

✓x7ᵗʰ **V17.4 Pedal cycle driver injured in collision with fixed or stationary object in traffic accident**

✓x7ᵗʰ **V17.5 Pedal cycle passenger injured in collision with fixed or stationary object in traffic accident**

✓x7ᵗʰ **V17.9 Unspecified pedal cyclist injured in collision with fixed or stationary object in traffic accident**

✓4ᵗʰ **V18 Pedal cycle rider injured in noncollision transport accident**

> **INCLUDES** fall or thrown from pedal cycle (without antecedent collision)
> overturning pedal cycle NOS
> overturning pedal cycle without collision

✓x7ᵗʰ **V18.0 Pedal cycle driver injured in noncollision transport accident in nontraffic accident**

✓x7ᵗʰ **V18.1 Pedal cycle passenger injured in noncollision transport accident in nontraffic accident**

✓x7ᵗʰ **V18.2 Unspecified pedal cyclist injured in noncollision transport accident in nontraffic accident**

✓x7ᵗʰ **V18.3 Person boarding or alighting a pedal cycle injured in noncollision transport accident**

✓x7ᵗʰ **V18.4 Pedal cycle driver injured in noncollision transport accident in traffic accident**

✓x7ᵗʰ **V18.5 Pedal cycle passenger injured in noncollision transport accident in traffic accident**

✓x7ᵗʰ **V18.9 Unspecified pedal cyclist injured in noncollision transport accident in traffic accident**

✓4ᵗʰ **V19 Pedal cycle rider injured in other and unspecified transport accidents**

✓5ᵗʰ **V19.0 Pedal cycle driver injured in collision with other and unspecified motor vehicles in nontraffic accident**

✓x7ᵗʰ **V19.00 Pedal cycle driver injured in collision with unspecified motor vehicles in nontraffic accident**

✓x7ᵗʰ **V19.09 Pedal cycle driver injured in collision with other motor vehicles in nontraffic accident**

✓5ᵗʰ **V19.1 Pedal cycle passenger injured in collision with other and unspecified motor vehicles in nontraffic accident**

✓x7ᵗʰ **V19.10 Pedal cycle passenger injured in collision with unspecified motor vehicles in nontraffic accident**

✓x7ᵗʰ **V19.19 Pedal cycle passenger injured in collision with other motor vehicles in nontraffic accident**

N Newborn: 0   P Pediatric: 0-17   M Maternity: 12-55   A Adult: 15-124   MCC Major CC Condition   PDxMCC PDx acts as own MCC   CC CC Condition   PDxCC PDx acts as own CC

1164   ICD-10-CM 2018

☑5ᵗʰ **V19.2 Unspecified pedal cyclist injured in collision with** other and unspecified motor vehicles in nontraffic accident

  ☑x7ᵗʰ **V19.20 Unspecified pedal cyclist injured in collision with** unspecified **motor vehicles in nontraffic accident**
    Pedal cycle collision NOS, nontraffic

  ☑x7ᵗʰ **V19.29 Unspecified pedal cyclist injured in collision with** other **motor vehicles in nontraffic accident**

☑7ᵗʰ **V19.3 Pedal cyclist (driver) (passenger) injured in unspecified nontraffic accident**
  Pedal cycle accident NOS, nontraffic
  Pedal cyclist injured in nontraffic accident NOS

☑5ᵗʰ **V19.4 Pedal cycle** driver **injured in collision with other and unspecified motor vehicles in traffic accident**

  ☑x7ᵗʰ **V19.40 Pedal cycle driver injured in collision with** unspecified **motor vehicles in traffic accident**

  ☑x7ᵗʰ **V19.49 Pedal cycle driver injured in collision with** other **motor vehicles in traffic accident**

☑5ᵗʰ **V19.5 Pedal cycle** passenger **injured in collision with other and unspecified motor vehicles in traffic accident**

  ☑x7ᵗʰ **V19.50 Pedal cycle passenger injured in collision with** unspecified **motor vehicles in traffic accident**

  ☑x7ᵗʰ **V19.59 Pedal cycle passenger injured in collision with** other **motor vehicles in traffic accident**

☑5ᵗʰ **V19.6** Unspecified **pedal cyclist injured in collision with** other and unspecified motor vehicles in traffic accident

  ☑x7ᵗʰ **V19.60 Unspecified pedal cyclist injured in collision with** unspecified **motor vehicles in traffic accident**
    Pedal cycle collision NOS (traffic)

  ☑x7ᵗʰ **V19.69 Unspecified pedal cyclist injured in collision with** other **motor vehicles in traffic accident**

☑5ᵗʰ **V19.8 Pedal cyclist (driver) (passenger) injured in** other specified transport accidents

  ☑x7ᵗʰ **V19.81 Pedal cyclist (driver) (passenger) injured in transport accident with** military vehicle

  ☑x7ᵗʰ **V19.88 Pedal cyclist (driver) (passenger) injured in** other specified transport accidents

☑x7ᵗʰ **V19.9 Pedal cyclist (driver) (passenger) injured in unspecified traffic accident**
  Pedal cycle accident NOS

Motorcycle rider injured in transport accident (V20-V29)

INCLUDES   moped
    motorcycle with sidecar
    motorized bicycle
    motor scooter
EXCLUDES 1   *three-wheeled motor vehicle (V30-V39)*

The appropriate 7th character is to be added to each code from categories V20-V29.
A   initial encounter
D   subsequent encounter
S   sequela

☑4ᵗʰ **V20 Motorcycle rider injured in collision with pedestrian or animal**
  EXCLUDES 1   *motorcycle rider collision with animal-drawn vehicle or animal being ridden (V26.-)*

  ☑x7ᵗʰ **V20.0 Motorcycle** driver **injured in collision with pedestrian or animal** in nontraffic accident

  ☑x7ᵗʰ **V20.1 Motorcycle** passenger **injured in collision with pedestrian or animal** in nontraffic accident

  ☑x7ᵗʰ **V20.2** Unspecified **motorcycle rider injured in collision with pedestrian or animal** in nontraffic accident

  ☑x7ᵗʰ **V20.3** Person boarding or alighting **a motorcycle injured in collision with pedestrian or animal**

  ☑x7ᵗʰ **V20.4 Motorcycle** driver **injured in collision with pedestrian or animal** in traffic accident

  ☑x7ᵗʰ **V20.5 Motorcycle** passenger **injured in collision with pedestrian or animal** in traffic accident

  ☑x7ᵗʰ **V20.9** Unspecified **motorcycle rider injured in collision with pedestrian or animal** in traffic accident

☑4ᵗʰ **V21 Motorcycle rider injured in collision with pedal cycle**

  ☑x7ᵗʰ **V21.0 Motorcycle** driver **injured in collision with pedal cycle in** nontraffic accident

  ☑x7ᵗʰ **V21.1 Motorcycle** passenger **injured in collision with pedal cycle in** nontraffic accident

  ☑x7ᵗʰ **V21.2** Unspecified **motorcycle rider injured in collision with pedal cycle** in nontraffic accident

  ☑x7ᵗʰ **V21.3** Person boarding or alighting **a motorcycle injured in collision with pedal cycle**

  ☑x7ᵗʰ **V21.4 Motorcycle** driver **injured in collision with pedal cycle in** traffic accident

  ☑x7ᵗʰ **V21.5 Motorcycle** passenger **injured in collision with pedal cycle in** traffic accident

  ☑x7ᵗʰ **V21.9** Unspecified **motorcycle rider injured in collision with pedal cycle** in traffic accident

☑4ᵗʰ **V22 Motorcycle rider injured in collision with two- or three-wheeled motor vehicle**

  ☑x7ᵗʰ **V22.0 Motorcycle** driver **injured in collision with two- or three-wheeled motor vehicle** in nontraffic accident

  ☑x7ᵗʰ **V22.1 Motorcycle** passenger **injured in collision with two- or three-wheeled motor vehicle** in nontraffic accident

  ☑x7ᵗʰ **V22.2** Unspecified **motorcycle rider injured in collision with two- or three-wheeled motor vehicle** in nontraffic accident

  ☑x7ᵗʰ **V22.3** Person boarding or alighting **a motorcycle injured in collision with two- or three-wheeled motor vehicle**

  ☑x7ᵗʰ **V22.4 Motorcycle** driver **injured in collision with two- or three-wheeled motor vehicle** in traffic accident

  ☑x7ᵗʰ **V22.5 Motorcycle** passenger **injured in collision with two- or three-wheeled motor vehicle** in traffic accident

  ☑x7ᵗʰ **V22.9** Unspecified **motorcycle rider injured in collision with two- or three-wheeled motor vehicle** in traffic accident

☑4ᵗʰ **V23 Motorcycle rider injured in collision with car, pick-up truck or van**

  ☑x7ᵗʰ **V23.0 Motorcycle** driver **injured in collision with car, pick-up truck or van** in nontraffic accident

  ☑x7ᵗʰ **V23.1 Motorcycle** passenger **injured in collision with car, pick-up truck or van** in nontraffic accident

  ☑x7ᵗʰ **V23.2** Unspecified **motorcycle rider injured in collision with car, pick-up truck or van** in nontraffic accident

  ☑x7ᵗʰ **V23.3** Person boarding or alighting **a motorcycle injured in collision with car, pick-up truck or van**

  ☑x7ᵗʰ **V23.4 Motorcycle** driver **injured in collision with car, pick-up truck or van** in traffic accident

  ☑x7ᵗʰ **V23.5 Motorcycle** passenger **injured in collision with car, pick-up truck or van** in traffic accident

  ☑x7ᵗʰ **V23.9** Unspecified **motorcycle rider injured in collision with car, pick-up truck or van** in traffic accident

☑4ᵗʰ **V24 Motorcycle rider injured in collision with heavy transport vehicle or bus**
  EXCLUDES 1   *motorcycle rider injured in collision with military vehicle (V29.81)*

  ☑x7ᵗʰ **V24.0 Motorcycle** driver **injured in collision with heavy transport vehicle or bus** in nontraffic accident

  ☑x7ᵗʰ **V24.1 Motorcycle** passenger **injured in collision with heavy transport vehicle or bus** in nontraffic accident

  ☑x7ᵗʰ **V24.2** Unspecified **motorcycle rider injured in collision with heavy transport vehicle or bus** in nontraffic accident

  ☑x7ᵗʰ **V24.3** Person boarding or alighting **a motorcycle injured in collision with heavy transport vehicle or bus**

  ☑x7ᵗʰ **V24.4 Motorcycle** driver **injured in collision with heavy transport vehicle or bus** in traffic accident

  ☑x7ᵗʰ **V24.5 Motorcycle** passenger **injured in collision with heavy transport vehicle or bus** in traffic accident

  ☑x7ᵗʰ **V24.9** Unspecified **motorcycle rider injured in collision with heavy transport vehicle or bus** in traffic accident

☑4ᵗʰ **V25 Motorcycle rider injured in collision with railway train or railway vehicle**

  ☑x7ᵗʰ **V25.0 Motorcycle** driver **injured in collision with railway train or railway vehicle** in nontraffic accident

  ☑x7ᵗʰ **V25.1 Motorcycle** passenger **injured in collision with railway train or railway vehicle** in nontraffic accident

  ☑x7ᵗʰ **V25.2** Unspecified **motorcycle rider injured in collision with railway train or railway vehicle** in nontraffic accident

  ☑x7ᵗʰ **V25.3** Person boarding or alighting **a motorcycle injured in collision with railway train or railway vehicle**

  ☑x7ᵗʰ **V25.4 Motorcycle** driver **injured in collision with railway train or railway vehicle** in traffic accident

  ☑x7ᵗʰ **V25.5 Motorcycle** passenger **injured in collision with railway train or railway vehicle** in traffic accident

✓x7th **V25.9** Unspecified motorcycle rider injured in collision with railway train or railway vehicle in traffic accident

✓4th **V26 Motorcycle rider injured in collision with other nonmotor vehicle**
    INCLUDES collision with animal-drawn vehicle, animal being ridden, streetcar

✓x7th **V26.0** Motorcycle driver injured in collision with other nonmotor vehicle in nontraffic accident

✓x7th **V26.1** Motorcycle passenger injured in collision with other nonmotor vehicle in nontraffic accident

✓x7th **V26.2** Unspecified motorcycle rider injured in collision with other nonmotor vehicle in nontraffic accident

✓x7th **V26.3** Person boarding or alighting a motorcycle injured in collision with other nonmotor vehicle

✓x7th **V26.4** Motorcycle driver injured in collision with other nonmotor vehicle in traffic accident

✓x7th **V26.5** Motorcycle passenger injured in collision with other nonmotor vehicle in traffic accident

✓x7th **V26.9** Unspecified motorcycle rider injured in collision with other nonmotor vehicle in traffic accident

✓4th **V27 Motorcycle rider injured in collision with fixed or stationary object**

✓x7th **V27.0** Motorcycle driver injured in collision with fixed or stationary object in nontraffic accident

✓x7th **V27.1** Motorcycle passenger injured in collision with fixed or stationary object in nontraffic accident

✓x7th **V27.2** Unspecified motorcycle rider injured in collision with fixed or stationary object in nontraffic accident

✓x7th **V27.3** Person boarding or alighting a motorcycle injured in collision with fixed or stationary object

✓x7th **V27.4** Motorcycle driver injured in collision with fixed or stationary object in traffic accident

✓x7th **V27.5** Motorcycle passenger injured in collision with fixed or stationary object in traffic accident

✓x7th **V27.9** Unspecified motorcycle rider injured in collision with fixed or stationary object in traffic accident

✓4th **V28 Motorcycle rider injured in noncollision transport accident**
    INCLUDES fall or thrown from motorcycle (without antecedent collision)
        overturning motorcycle NOS
        overturning motorcycle without collision

✓x7th **V28.0** Motorcycle driver injured in noncollision transport accident in nontraffic accident

✓x7th **V28.1** Motorcycle passenger injured in noncollision transport accident in nontraffic accident

✓x7th **V28.2** Unspecified motorcycle rider injured in noncollision transport accident in nontraffic accident

✓x7th **V28.3** Person boarding or alighting a motorcycle injured in noncollision transport accident

✓x7th **V28.4** Motorcycle driver injured in noncollision transport accident in traffic accident

✓x7th **V28.5** Motorcycle passenger injured in noncollision transport accident in traffic accident

✓x7th **V28.9** Unspecified motorcycle rider injured in noncollision transport accident in traffic accident

✓4th **V29 Motorcycle rider injured in other and unspecified transport accidents**

✓5th **V29.0** Motorcycle driver injured in collision with other and unspecified motor vehicles in nontraffic accident

  ✓x7th **V29.00** Motorcycle driver injured in collision with unspecified motor vehicles in nontraffic accident

  ✓x7th **V29.09** Motorcycle driver injured in collision with other motor vehicles in nontraffic accident

✓5th **V29.1** Motorcycle passenger injured in collision with other and unspecified motor vehicles in nontraffic accident

  ✓x7th **V29.10** Motorcycle passenger injured in collision with unspecified motor vehicles in nontraffic accident

  ✓x7th **V29.19** Motorcycle passenger injured in collision with other motor vehicles in nontraffic accident

✓5th **V29.2** Unspecified motorcycle rider injured in collision with other and unspecified motor vehicles in nontraffic accident

  ✓x7th **V29.20** Unspecified motorcycle rider injured in collision with unspecified motor vehicles in nontraffic accident
      Motorcycle collision NOS, nontraffic

✓x7th **V29.29** Unspecified motorcycle rider injured in collision with other motor vehicles in nontraffic accident

✓x7th **V29.3** Motorcycle rider (driver) (passenger) injured in unspecified nontraffic accident
    Motorcycle accident NOS, nontraffic
    Motorcycle rider injured in nontraffic accident NOS

✓5th **V29.4** Motorcycle driver injured in collision with other and unspecified motor vehicles in traffic accident

  ✓x7th **V29.40** Motorcycle driver injured in collision with unspecified motor vehicles in traffic accident

  ✓x7th **V29.49** Motorcycle driver injured in collision with other motor vehicles in traffic accident

✓5th **V29.5** Motorcycle passenger injured in collision with other and unspecified motor vehicles in traffic accident

  ✓x7th **V29.50** Motorcycle passenger injured in collision with unspecified motor vehicles in traffic accident

  ✓x7th **V29.59** Motorcycle passenger injured in collision with other motor vehicles in traffic accident

✓5th **V29.6** Unspecified motorcycle rider injured in collision with other and unspecified motor vehicles in traffic accident

  ✓x7th **V29.60** Unspecified motorcycle rider injured in collision with unspecified motor vehicles in traffic accident
      Motorcycle collision NOS (traffic)

  ✓x7th **V29.69** Unspecified motorcycle rider injured in collision with other motor vehicles in traffic accident

✓5th **V29.8** Motorcycle rider (driver) (passenger) injured in other specified transport accidents

  ✓x7th **V29.81** Motorcycle rider (driver) (passenger) injured in transport accident with military vehicle

  ✓x7th **V29.88** Motorcycle rider (driver) (passenger) injured in other specified transport accidents

✓x7th **V29.9** Motorcycle rider (driver) (passenger) injured in unspecified traffic accident
    Motorcycle accident NOS

Occupant of three-wheeled motor vehicle injured in transport accident (V30-V39)

    INCLUDES motorized tricycle
        motorized rickshaw
        three-wheeled motor car
    EXCLUDES 1 all-terrain vehicles (V86.-)
        motorcycle with sidecar (V20-V29)
        vehicle designed primarily for off-road use (V86.-)

> The appropriate 7th character is to be added to each code from categories V30-V39.
> A   initial encounter
> D   subsequent encounter
> S   sequela

✓4th **V30 Occupant of three-wheeled motor vehicle injured in collision with pedestrian or animal**
    EXCLUDES 1 three-wheeled motor vehicle collision with animal-drawn vehicle or animal being ridden (V36.-)

✓x7th **V30.0** Driver of three-wheeled motor vehicle injured in collision with pedestrian or animal in nontraffic accident

✓x7th **V30.1** Passenger in three-wheeled motor vehicle injured in collision with pedestrian or animal in nontraffic accident

✓x7th **V30.2** Person on outside of three-wheeled motor vehicle injured in collision with pedestrian or animal in nontraffic accident

✓x7th **V30.3** Unspecified occupant of three-wheeled motor vehicle injured in collision with pedestrian or animal in nontraffic accident

✓x7th **V30.4** Person boarding or alighting a three-wheeled motor vehicle injured in collision with pedestrian or animal

✓x7th **V30.5** Driver of three-wheeled motor vehicle injured in collision with pedestrian or animal in traffic accident

✓x7th **V30.6** Passenger in three-wheeled motor vehicle injured in collision with pedestrian or animal in traffic accident

✓x7th **V30.7** Person on outside of three-wheeled motor vehicle injured in collision with pedestrian or animal in traffic accident

✓x7th **V30.9** Unspecified occupant of three-wheeled motor vehicle injured in collision with pedestrian or animal in traffic accident

✓4th **V31 Occupant of three-wheeled motor vehicle injured in collision with pedal cycle**

✓x7th **V31.0** Driver of three-wheeled motor vehicle injured in collision with pedal cycle in nontraffic accident

N Newborn: 0 P Pediatric: 0-17 M Maternity: 12-55 A Adult: 15-124 MCC Major CC Condition PDx MCC PDx acts as own MCC CC CC Condition PDx CC PDx acts as own CC

1166   ICD-10-CM 2018

√x7ᵗʰ **V31.1** Passenger in three-wheeled motor vehicle injured in collision with pedal cycle in nontraffic accident

√x7ᵗʰ **V31.2** Person on outside of three-wheeled motor vehicle injured in collision with pedal cycle in nontraffic accident

√x7ᵗʰ **V31.3** Unspecified occupant of three-wheeled motor vehicle injured in collision with pedal cycle in nontraffic accident

√x7ᵗʰ **V31.4** Person boarding or alighting a three-wheeled motor vehicle injured in collision with pedal cycle

√x7ᵗʰ **V31.5** Driver of three-wheeled motor vehicle injured in collision with pedal cycle in traffic accident

√x7ᵗʰ **V31.6** Passenger in three-wheeled motor vehicle injured in collision with pedal cycle in traffic accident

√x7ᵗʰ **V31.7** Person on outside of three-wheeled motor vehicle injured in collision with pedal cycle in traffic accident

√x7ᵗʰ **V31.9** Unspecified occupant of three-wheeled motor vehicle injured in collision with pedal cycle in traffic accident

√4ᵗʰ **V32 Occupant of three-wheeled motor vehicle injured in collision with two- or three-wheeled motor vehicle**

√x7ᵗʰ **V32.0** Driver of three-wheeled motor vehicle injured in collision with two- or three-wheeled motor vehicle in nontraffic accident

√x7ᵗʰ **V32.1** Passenger in three-wheeled motor vehicle injured in collision with two- or three-wheeled motor vehicle in nontraffic accident

√x7ᵗʰ **V32.2** Person on outside of three-wheeled motor vehicle injured in collision with two- or three-wheeled motor vehicle in nontraffic accident

√x7ᵗʰ **V32.3** Unspecified occupant of three-wheeled motor vehicle injured in collision with two- or three-wheeled motor vehicle in nontraffic accident

√x7ᵗʰ **V32.4** Person boarding or alighting a three-wheeled motor vehicle injured in collision with two- or three-wheeled motor vehicle

√x7ᵗʰ **V32.5** Driver of three-wheeled motor vehicle injured in collision with two- or three-wheeled motor vehicle in traffic accident

√x7ᵗʰ **V32.6** Passenger in three-wheeled motor vehicle injured in collision with two- or three-wheeled motor vehicle in traffic accident

√x7ᵗʰ **V32.7** Person on outside of three-wheeled motor vehicle injured in collision with two- or three-wheeled motor vehicle in traffic accident

√x7ᵗʰ **V32.9** Unspecified occupant of three-wheeled motor vehicle injured in collision with two- or three-wheeled motor vehicle in traffic accident

√4ᵗʰ **V33 Occupant of three-wheeled motor vehicle injured in collision with car, pick-up truck or van**

√x7ᵗʰ **V33.0** Driver of three-wheeled motor vehicle injured in collision with car, pick-up truck or van in nontraffic accident

√x7ᵗʰ **V33.1** Passenger in three-wheeled motor vehicle injured in collision with car, pick-up truck or van in nontraffic accident

√x7ᵗʰ **V33.2** Person on outside of three-wheeled motor vehicle injured in collision with car, pick-up truck or van in nontraffic accident

√x7ᵗʰ **V33.3** Unspecified occupant of three-wheeled motor vehicle injured in collision with car, pick-up truck or van in nontraffic accident

√x7ᵗʰ **V33.4** Person boarding or alighting a three-wheeled motor vehicle injured in collision with car, pick-up truck or van

√x7ᵗʰ **V33.5** Driver of three-wheeled motor vehicle injured in collision with car, pick-up truck or van in traffic accident

√x7ᵗʰ **V33.6** Passenger in three-wheeled motor vehicle injured in collision with car, pick-up truck or van in traffic accident

√x7ᵗʰ **V33.7** Person on outside of three-wheeled motor vehicle injured in collision with car, pick-up truck or van in traffic accident

√x7ᵗʰ **V33.9** Unspecified occupant of three-wheeled motor vehicle injured in collision with car, pick-up truck or van in traffic accident

√4ᵗʰ **V34 Occupant of three-wheeled motor vehicle injured in collision with heavy transport vehicle or bus**

EXCLUDES 1 *occupant of three-wheeled motor vehicle injured in collision with military vehicle (V39.81)*

√x7ᵗʰ **V34.0** Driver of three-wheeled motor vehicle injured in collision with heavy transport vehicle or bus in nontraffic accident

√x7ᵗʰ **V34.1** Passenger in three-wheeled motor vehicle injured in collision with heavy transport vehicle or bus in nontraffic accident

√x7ᵗʰ **V34.2** Person on outside of three-wheeled motor vehicle injured in collision with heavy transport vehicle or bus in nontraffic accident

√x7ᵗʰ **V34.3** Unspecified occupant of three-wheeled motor vehicle injured in collision with heavy transport vehicle or bus in nontraffic accident

√x7ᵗʰ **V34.4** Person boarding or alighting a three-wheeled motor vehicle injured in collision with heavy transport vehicle or bus

√x7ᵗʰ **V34.5** Driver of three-wheeled motor vehicle injured in collision with heavy transport vehicle or bus in traffic accident

√x7ᵗʰ **V34.6** Passenger in three-wheeled motor vehicle injured in collision with heavy transport vehicle or bus in traffic accident

√x7ᵗʰ **V34.7** Person on outside of three-wheeled motor vehicle injured in collision with heavy transport vehicle or bus in traffic accident

√x7ᵗʰ **V34.9** Unspecified occupant of three-wheeled motor vehicle injured in collision with heavy transport vehicle or bus in traffic accident

√4ᵗʰ **V35 Occupant of three-wheeled motor vehicle injured in collision with railway train or railway vehicle**

√x7ᵗʰ **V35.0** Driver of three-wheeled motor vehicle injured in collision with railway train or railway vehicle in nontraffic accident

√x7ᵗʰ **V35.1** Passenger in three-wheeled motor vehicle injured in collision with railway train or railway vehicle in nontraffic accident

√x7ᵗʰ **V35.2** Person on outside of three-wheeled motor vehicle injured in collision with railway train or railway vehicle in nontraffic accident

√x7ᵗʰ **V35.3** Unspecified occupant of three-wheeled motor vehicle injured in collision with railway train or railway vehicle in nontraffic accident

√x7ᵗʰ **V35.4** Person boarding or alighting a three-wheeled motor vehicle injured in collision with railway train or railway vehicle

√x7ᵗʰ **V35.5** Driver of three-wheeled motor vehicle injured in collision with railway train or railway vehicle in traffic accident

√x7ᵗʰ **V35.6** Passenger in three-wheeled motor vehicle injured in collision with railway train or railway vehicle in traffic accident

√x7ᵗʰ **V35.7** Person on outside of three-wheeled motor vehicle injured in collision with railway train or railway vehicle in traffic accident

√x7ᵗʰ **V35.9** Unspecified occupant of three-wheeled motor vehicle injured in collision with railway train or railway vehicle in traffic accident

√4ᵗʰ **V36 Occupant of three-wheeled motor vehicle injured in collision with other nonmotor vehicle**

INCLUDES collision with animal-drawn vehicle, animal being ridden, streetcar

√x7ᵗʰ **V36.0** Driver of three-wheeled motor vehicle injured in collision with other nonmotor vehicle in nontraffic accident

√x7ᵗʰ **V36.1** Passenger in three-wheeled motor vehicle injured in collision with other nonmotor vehicle in nontraffic accident

√x7ᵗʰ **V36.2** Person on outside of three-wheeled motor vehicle injured in collision with other nonmotor vehicle in nontraffic accident

√x7ᵗʰ **V36.3** Unspecified occupant of three-wheeled motor vehicle injured in collision with other nonmotor vehicle in nontraffic accident

√x7ᵗʰ **V36.4** Person boarding or alighting a three-wheeled motor vehicle injured in collision with other nonmotor vehicle

√x7ᵗʰ **V36.5** Driver of three-wheeled motor vehicle injured in collision with other nonmotor vehicle in traffic accident

√x7ᵗʰ **V36.6** Passenger in three-wheeled motor vehicle injured in collision with other nonmotor vehicle in traffic accident

√x7ᵗʰ **V36.7** Person on outside of three-wheeled motor vehicle injured in collision with other nonmotor vehicle in traffic accident

√x7ᵗʰ **V36.9** Unspecified occupant of three-wheeled motor vehicle injured in collision with other nonmotor vehicle in traffic accident

√4ᵗʰ **V37 Occupant of three-wheeled motor vehicle injured in collision with fixed or stationary object**

√x7ᵗʰ **V37.0** Driver of three-wheeled motor vehicle injured in collision with fixed or stationary object in nontraffic accident

√x7ᵗʰ **V37.1** Passenger in three-wheeled motor vehicle injured in collision with fixed or stationary object in nontraffic accident

√x7ᵗʰ **V37.2** Person on outside of three-wheeled motor vehicle injured in collision with fixed or stationary object in nontraffic accident

√x7ᵗʰ **V37.3** Unspecified occupant of three-wheeled motor vehicle injured in collision with fixed or stationary object in nontraffic accident

√x7ᵗʰ **V37.4** Person boarding or alighting a three-wheeled motor vehicle injured in collision with fixed or stationary object

✔ Additional Character Req   √x7ᵗʰ Placeholder Alert   Unacceptable PDx   Manifestation   **H1**-**H14** HAC   **HCC** CMS-HCC Condition   **EXCLUDES 1** Not Coded Here   **EXCLUDES 2** Not Included Here

ICD-10-CM 2018   **1167**

✓x7th **V37.5** **Driver** of three-wheeled motor vehicle injured in collision with **fixed or stationary object** in **traffic accident**

✓x7th **V37.6** **Passenger** in three-wheeled motor vehicle injured in collision with **fixed or stationary object** in **traffic accident**

✓x7th **V37.7** **Person on outside** of three-wheeled motor vehicle injured in collision with fixed or stationary object in **traffic accident**

✓x7th **V37.9** **Unspecified** occupant of three-wheeled motor vehicle injured in collision with fixed or stationary object in **traffic accident**

✓4th **V38** **Occupant of three-wheeled motor vehicle injured in noncollision transport accident**
> INCLUDES   fall or thrown from three-wheeled motor vehicle
> overturning of three-wheeled motor vehicle NOS
> overturning of three-wheeled motor vehicle without collision

✓x7th **V38.0** **Driver** of three-wheeled motor vehicle injured in noncollision transport accident in **nontraffic accident**

✓x7th **V38.1** **Passenger** in three-wheeled motor vehicle injured in noncollision transport accident in **nontraffic accident**

✓x7th **V38.2** **Person on outside** of three-wheeled motor vehicle injured in noncollision transport accident in **nontraffic accident**

✓x7th **V38.3** **Unspecified** occupant of three-wheeled motor vehicle injured in noncollision transport accident in **nontraffic accident**

✓x7th **V38.4** **Person boarding or alighting** a three-wheeled motor vehicle injured in noncollision transport accident

✓x7th **V38.5** **Driver** of three-wheeled motor vehicle injured in noncollision transport accident in **traffic accident**

✓x7th **V38.6** **Passenger** in three-wheeled motor vehicle injured in noncollision transport accident in **traffic accident**

✓x7th **V38.7** **Person on outside** of three-wheeled motor vehicle injured in noncollision transport accident in **traffic accident**

✓x7th **V38.9** **Unspecified** occupant of three-wheeled motor vehicle injured in noncollision transport accident in **traffic accident**

✓4th **V39** **Occupant of three-wheeled motor vehicle injured in other and unspecified transport accidents**

✓5th **V39.0** **Driver** of three-wheeled motor vehicle injured in collision with other and unspecified motor vehicles in **nontraffic accident**

✓x7th **V39.00** Driver of three-wheeled motor vehicle injured in collision with **unspecified** motor vehicles in **nontraffic accident**

✓x7th **V39.09** Driver of three-wheeled motor vehicle injured in collision with **other** motor vehicles in **nontraffic accident**

✓5th **V39.1** **Passenger** in three-wheeled motor vehicle injured in collision with other and unspecified motor vehicles in **nontraffic accident**

✓x7th **V39.10** Passenger in three-wheeled motor vehicle injured in collision with **unspecified** motor vehicles in **nontraffic accident**

✓x7th **V39.19** Passenger in three-wheeled motor vehicle injured in collision with **other** motor vehicles in **nontraffic accident**

✓5th **V39.2** **Unspecified** occupant of three-wheeled motor vehicle injured in collision with other and unspecified motor vehicles in **nontraffic accident**

✓x7th **V39.20** Unspecified occupant of three-wheeled motor vehicle injured in collision with **unspecified** motor vehicles in **nontraffic accident**
> Collision NOS involving three-wheeled motor vehicle, nontraffic

✓x7th **V39.29** Unspecified occupant of three-wheeled motor vehicle injured in collision with **other** motor vehicles in **nontraffic accident**

✓x7th **V39.3** **Occupant (driver) (passenger)** of three-wheeled motor vehicle injured in unspecified **nontraffic accident**
> Accident NOS involving three-wheeled motor vehicle, nontraffic
> Occupant of three-wheeled motor vehicle injured in nontraffic accident NOS

✓5th **V39.4** **Driver** of three-wheeled motor vehicle injured in collision with other and unspecified motor vehicles in **traffic accident**

✓x7th **V39.40** Driver of three-wheeled motor vehicle injured in collision with **unspecified** motor vehicles in **traffic accident**

✓x7th **V39.49** Driver of three-wheeled motor vehicle injured in collision with **other** motor vehicles in **traffic accident**

✓5th **V39.5** **Passenger** in three-wheeled motor vehicle injured in collision with **other and unspecified** motor vehicles in **traffic accident**

✓x7th **V39.50** Passenger in three-wheeled motor vehicle injured in collision with **unspecified** motor vehicles in traffic accident

✓x7th **V39.59** Passenger in three-wheeled motor vehicle injured in collision with **other** motor vehicles in traffic accident

✓5th **V39.6** **Unspecified** occupant of three-wheeled motor vehicle injured in collision with other and unspecified motor vehicles in **traffic accident**

✓x7th **V39.60** Unspecified occupant of three-wheeled motor vehicle injured in collision with **unspecified** motor vehicles in traffic accident
> Collision NOS involving three-wheeled motor vehicle (traffic)

✓x7th **V39.69** Unspecified occupant of three-wheeled motor vehicle injured in collision with **other** motor vehicles in traffic accident

✓5th **V39.8** **Occupant (driver) (passenger)** of three-wheeled motor vehicle injured in **other specified transport accidents**

✓x7th **V39.81** Occupant (driver) (passenger) of three-wheeled motor vehicle injured in transport accident with **military vehicle**

✓x7th **V39.89** Occupant (driver) (passenger) of three-wheeled motor vehicle injured in **other specified** transport accidents

✓x7th **V39.9** **Occupant (driver) (passenger)** of three-wheeled motor vehicle injured in **unspecified traffic accident**
> Accident NOS involving three-wheeled motor vehicle

Car occupant injured in transport accident (V40-V49)

> INCLUDES   a four-wheeled motor vehicle designed primarily for carrying passengers
> automobile (pulling a trailer or camper)
>
> EXCLUDES 1   bus (V50-V59)
> minibus (V50-V59)
> minivan (V50-V59)
> motorcoach (V70-V79)
> pick-up truck (V50-V59)
> sport utility vehicle (SUV) (V50-V59)

> The appropriate 7th character is to be added to each code from categories V40-V49.
> A   initial encounter
> D   subsequent encounter
> S   sequela

✓4th **V40** **Car occupant injured in collision with pedestrian or animal**
> EXCLUDES 1   car collision with animal-drawn vehicle or animal being ridden (V46.-)

✓x7th **V40.0** **Car driver** injured in collision with pedestrian or animal in **nontraffic accident**

✓x7th **V40.1** **Car passenger** injured in collision with pedestrian or animal in **nontraffic accident**

✓x7th **V40.2** **Person on outside** of car injured in collision with pedestrian or animal in **nontraffic accident**

✓x7th **V40.3** **Unspecified** car occupant injured in collision with pedestrian or animal in **nontraffic accident**

✓x7th **V40.4** **Person boarding or alighting** a car injured in collision with **pedestrian or animal**

✓x7th **V40.5** **Car driver** injured in collision with pedestrian or animal in **traffic accident**

✓x7th **V40.6** **Car passenger** injured in collision with pedestrian or animal in **traffic accident**

✓x7th **V40.7** **Person on outside** of car injured in collision with pedestrian or animal in **traffic accident**

✓x7th **V40.9** **Unspecified** car occupant injured in collision with pedestrian or animal in **traffic accident**

✓4th **V41** **Car occupant injured in collision with pedal cycle**

✓x7th **V41.0** **Car driver** injured in collision with pedal cycle in **nontraffic accident**

✓x7th **V41.1** **Car passenger** injured in collision with pedal cycle in **nontraffic accident**

✓x7th **V41.2** **Person on outside** of car injured in collision with pedal cycle in **nontraffic accident**

✓x7th **V41.3** **Unspecified** car occupant injured in collision with pedal cycle in **nontraffic accident**

N Newborn: 0   P Pediatric: 0-17   M Maternity: 12-55   A Adult: 15-124   MCC Major CC Condition   PDxMCC PDx acts as own MCC   CC CC Condition   PDxCC PDx acts as own CC

1168

ICD-10-CM 2018

☑x7ᵗʰ **V41.4** Person boarding or alighting a car injured in collision with pedal cycle

☑x7ᵗʰ **V41.5** Car driver injured in collision with pedal cycle in traffic accident

☑x7ᵗʰ **V41.6** Car passenger injured in collision with pedal cycle in traffic accident

☑x7ᵗʰ **V41.7** Person on outside of car injured in collision with pedal cycle in traffic accident

☑x7ᵗʰ **V41.9** Unspecified car occupant injured in collision with pedal cycle in traffic accident

☑4ᵗʰ **V42** Car occupant injured in collision with two- or three-wheeled motor vehicle

☑x7ᵗʰ **V42.0** Car driver injured in collision with two- or three-wheeled motor vehicle in nontraffic accident

☑x7ᵗʰ **V42.1** Car passenger injured in collision with two- or three-wheeled motor vehicle in nontraffic accident

☑x7ᵗʰ **V42.2** Person on outside of car injured in collision with two- or three-wheeled motor vehicle in nontraffic accident

☑x7ᵗʰ **V42.3** Unspecified car occupant injured in collision with two- or three-wheeled motor vehicle in nontraffic accident

☑x7ᵗʰ **V42.4** Person boarding or alighting a car injured in collision with two- or three-wheeled motor vehicle

☑x7ᵗʰ **V42.5** Car driver injured in collision with two- or three-wheeled motor vehicle in traffic accident

☑x7ᵗʰ **V42.6** Car passenger injured in collision with two- or three-wheeled motor vehicle in traffic accident

☑x7ᵗʰ **V42.7** Person on outside of car injured in collision with two- or three-wheeled motor vehicle in traffic accident

☑x7ᵗʰ **V42.9** Unspecified car occupant injured in collision with two- or three-wheeled motor vehicle in traffic accident

☑4ᵗʰ **V43** Car occupant injured in collision with car, pick-up truck or van

☑5ᵗʰ **V43.0** Car driver injured in collision with car, pick-up truck or van in nontraffic accident

☑x7ᵗʰ **V43.01** Car driver injured in collision with sport utility vehicle in nontraffic accident

☑x7ᵗʰ **V43.02** Car driver injured in collision with other type car in nontraffic accident

☑x7ᵗʰ **V43.03** Car driver injured in collision with pick-up truck in nontraffic accident

☑x7ᵗʰ **V43.04** Car driver injured in collision with van in nontraffic accident

☑5ᵗʰ **V43.1** Car passenger injured in collision with car, pick-up truck or van in nontraffic accident

☑x7ᵗʰ **V43.11** Car passenger injured in collision with sport utility vehicle in nontraffic accident

☑x7ᵗʰ **V43.12** Car passenger injured in collision with other type car in nontraffic accident

☑x7ᵗʰ **V43.13** Car passenger injured in collision with pick-up in nontraffic accident

☑x7ᵗʰ **V43.14** Car passenger injured in collision with van in nontraffic accident

☑5ᵗʰ **V43.2** Person on outside of car injured in collision with car, pick-up truck or van in nontraffic accident

☑x7ᵗʰ **V43.21** Person on outside of car injured in collision with sport utility vehicle in nontraffic accident

☑x7ᵗʰ **V43.22** Person on outside of car injured in collision with other type car in nontraffic accident

☑x7ᵗʰ **V43.23** Person on outside of car injured in collision with pick-up truck in nontraffic accident

☑x7ᵗʰ **V43.24** Person on outside of car injured in collision with van in nontraffic accident

☑5ᵗʰ **V43.3** Unspecified car occupant injured in collision with car, pick-up truck or van in nontraffic accident

☑x7ᵗʰ **V43.31** Unspecified car occupant injured in collision with sport utility vehicle in nontraffic accident

☑x7ᵗʰ **V43.32** Unspecified car occupant injured in collision with other type car in nontraffic accident

☑x7ᵗʰ **V43.33** Unspecified car occupant injured in collision with pick-up truck in nontraffic accident

☑x7ᵗʰ **V43.34** Unspecified car occupant injured in collision with van in nontraffic accident

☑5ᵗʰ **V43.4** Person boarding or alighting a car injured in collision with car, pick-up truck or van

☑x7ᵗʰ **V43.41** Person boarding or alighting a car injured in collision with sport utility vehicle

☑x7ᵗʰ **V43.42** Person boarding or alighting a car injured in collision with other type car

☑x7ᵗʰ **V43.43** Person boarding or alighting a car injured in collision with pick-up truck

☑x7ᵗʰ **V43.44** Person boarding or alighting a car injured in collision with van

☑5ᵗʰ **V43.5** Car driver injured in collision with car, pick-up truck or van in traffic accident

☑x7ᵗʰ **V43.51** Car driver injured in collision with sport utility vehicle in traffic accident

☑x7ᵗʰ **V43.52** Car driver injured in collision with other type car in traffic accident

☑x7ᵗʰ **V43.53** Car driver injured in collision with pick-up truck in traffic accident

☑x7ᵗʰ **V43.54** Car driver injured in collision with van in traffic accident

☑5ᵗʰ **V43.6** Car passenger injured in collision with car, pick-up truck or van in traffic accident

☑x7ᵗʰ **V43.61** Car passenger injured in collision with sport utility vehicle in traffic accident

☑x7ᵗʰ **V43.62** Car passenger injured in collision with other type car in traffic accident

☑x7ᵗʰ **V43.63** Car passenger injured in collision with pick-up truck in traffic accident

☑x7ᵗʰ **V43.64** Car passenger injured in collision with van in traffic accident

☑5ᵗʰ **V43.7** Person on outside of car injured in collision with car, pick-up truck or van in traffic accident

☑x7ᵗʰ **V43.71** Person on outside of car injured in collision with sport utility vehicle in traffic accident

☑x7ᵗʰ **V43.72** Person on outside of car injured in collision with other type car in traffic accident

☑x7ᵗʰ **V43.73** Person on outside of car injured in collision with pick-up truck in traffic accident

☑x7ᵗʰ **V43.74** Person on outside of car injured in collision with van in traffic accident

☑5ᵗʰ **V43.9** Unspecified car occupant injured in collision with car, pick-up truck or van in traffic accident

☑x7ᵗʰ **V43.91** Unspecified car occupant injured in collision with sport utility vehicle in traffic accident

☑x7ᵗʰ **V43.92** Unspecified car occupant injured in collision with other type car in traffic accident

☑x7ᵗʰ **V43.93** Unspecified car occupant injured in collision with pick-up truck in traffic accident

☑x7ᵗʰ **V43.94** Unspecified car occupant injured in collision with van in traffic accident

☑4ᵗʰ **V44** Car occupant injured in collision with heavy transport vehicle or bus

EXCLUDES 1　car occupant injured in collision with military vehicle (V49.81)

☑x7ᵗʰ **V44.0** Car driver injured in collision with heavy transport vehicle or bus in nontraffic accident

☑x7ᵗʰ **V44.1** Car passenger injured in collision with heavy transport vehicle or bus in nontraffic accident

☑x7ᵗʰ **V44.2** Person on outside of car injured in collision with heavy transport vehicle or bus in nontraffic accident

☑x7ᵗʰ **V44.3** Unspecified car occupant injured in collision with heavy transport vehicle or bus in nontraffic accident

☑x7ᵗʰ **V44.4** Person boarding or alighting a car injured in collision with heavy transport vehicle or bus

☑x7ᵗʰ **V44.5** Car driver injured in collision with heavy transport vehicle or bus in traffic accident

☑x7ᵗʰ **V44.6** Car passenger injured in collision with heavy transport vehicle or bus in traffic accident

☑x7ᵗʰ **V44.7** Person on outside of car injured in collision with heavy transport vehicle or bus in traffic accident

☑x7ᵗʰ **V44.9** Unspecified car occupant injured in collision with heavy transport vehicle or bus in traffic accident

✔Additional Character Req　☑x7ᵗʰ Placeholder Alert　Unacceptable PDx　Manifestation　H1 - H14 HAC　HCC CMS-HCC Condition　*EXCLUDES 1* Not Coded Here　*EXCLUDES 2* Not Included Here

ICD-10-CM 2018　　　　　　　　　　　　　　　　　　　　　　　　　　　　　　　　　　　　　1169

Chapter 20. External Causes of Morbidity　　V41.4–V44.9

√4th **V45** **Car occupant injured in collision with railway train or railway vehicle**

  √x7th **V45.0** Car driver injured in collision with railway train or railway vehicle in nontraffic accident

  √x7th **V45.1** Car passenger injured in collision with railway train or railway vehicle in nontraffic accident

  √x7th **V45.2** Person on outside of car injured in collision with railway train or railway vehicle in nontraffic accident

  √x7th **V45.3** Unspecified car occupant injured in collision with railway train or railway vehicle in nontraffic accident

  √x7th **V45.4** Person boarding or alighting a car injured in collision with railway train or railway vehicle

  √x7th **V45.5** Car driver injured in collision with railway train or railway vehicle in traffic accident

  √x7th **V45.6** Car passenger injured in collision with railway train or railway vehicle in traffic accident

  √x7th **V45.7** Person on outside of car injured in collision with railway train or railway vehicle in traffic accident

  √x7th **V45.9** Unspecified car occupant injured in collision with railway train or railway vehicle in traffic accident

√4th **V46** **Car occupant injured in collision with other nonmotor vehicle**
    INCLUDES collision with animal-drawn vehicle, animal being ridden, streetcar

  √x7th **V46.0** Car driver injured in collision with other nonmotor vehicle in nontraffic accident

  √x7th **V46.1** Car passenger injured in collision with other nonmotor vehicle in nontraffic accident

  √x7th **V46.2** Person on outside of car injured in collision with other nonmotor vehicle in nontraffic accident

  √x7th **V46.3** Unspecified car occupant injured in collision with other nonmotor vehicle in nontraffic accident

  √x7th **V46.4** Person boarding or alighting a car injured in collision with other nonmotor vehicle

  √x7th **V46.5** Car driver injured in collision with other nonmotor vehicle in traffic accident

  √x7th **V46.6** Car passenger injured in collision with other nonmotor vehicle in traffic accident

  √x7th **V46.7** Person on outside of car injured in collision with other nonmotor vehicle in traffic accident

  √x7th **V46.9** Unspecified car occupant injured in collision with other nonmotor vehicle in traffic accident

√4th **V47** **Car occupant injured in collision with fixed or stationary object**

  √x7th **V47.0** Car driver injured in collision with fixed or stationary object in nontraffic accident

  √x7th **V47.1** Car passenger injured in collision with fixed or stationary object in nontraffic accident

  √x7th **V47.2** Person on outside of car injured in collision with fixed or stationary object in nontraffic accident

  √x7th **V47.3** Unspecified car occupant injured in collision with fixed or stationary object in nontraffic accident

  √x7th **V47.4** Person boarding or alighting a car injured in collision with fixed or stationary object

  √x7th **V47.5** Car driver injured in collision with fixed or stationary object in traffic accident

  √x7th **V47.6** Car passenger injured in collision with fixed or stationary object in traffic accident

  √x7th **V47.7** Person on outside of car injured in collision with fixed or stationary object in traffic accident

  √x7th **V47.9** Unspecified car occupant injured in collision with fixed or stationary object in traffic accident

√4th **V48** **Car occupant injured in noncollision transport accident**
    INCLUDES overturning car NOS
             overturning car without collision

  √x7th **V48.0** Car driver injured in noncollision transport accident in nontraffic accident

  √x7th **V48.1** Car passenger injured in noncollision transport accident in nontraffic accident

  √x7th **V48.2** Person on outside of car injured in noncollision transport accident in nontraffic accident

  √x7th **V48.3** Unspecified car occupant injured in noncollision transport accident in nontraffic accident

  √x7th **V48.4** Person boarding or alighting a car injured in noncollision transport accident

  √x7th **V48.5** Car driver injured in noncollision transport accident in traffic accident

  √x7th **V48.6** Car passenger injured in noncollision transport accident in traffic accident

  √x7th **V48.7** Person on outside of car injured in noncollision transport accident in traffic accident

  √x7th **V48.9** Unspecified car occupant injured in noncollision transport accident in traffic accident

√4th **V49** **Car occupant injured in other and unspecified transport accidents**

  √5th **V49.0** Driver injured in collision with other and unspecified motor vehicles in nontraffic accident

    √x7th **V49.00** Driver injured in collision with unspecified motor vehicles in nontraffic accident

    √x7th **V49.09** Driver injured in collision with other motor vehicles in nontraffic accident

  √5th **V49.1** Passenger injured in collision with other and unspecified motor vehicles in nontraffic accident

    √x7th **V49.10** Passenger injured in collision with unspecified motor vehicles in nontraffic accident

    √x7th **V49.19** Passenger injured in collision with other motor vehicles in nontraffic accident

  √5th **V49.2** Unspecified car occupant injured in collision with other and unspecified motor vehicles in nontraffic accident

    √x7th **V49.20** Unspecified car occupant injured in collision with unspecified motor vehicles in nontraffic accident
           Car collision NOS, nontraffic

    √x7th **V49.29** Unspecified car occupant injured in collision with other motor vehicles in nontraffic accident

  √x7th **V49.3** Car occupant (driver) (passenger) injured in unspecified nontraffic accident
       Car accident NOS, nontraffic
       Car occupant injured in nontraffic accident NOS

  √5th **V49.4** Driver injured in collision with other and unspecified motor vehicles in traffic accident

    √x7th **V49.40** Driver injured in collision with unspecified motor vehicles in traffic accident

    √x7th **V49.49** Driver injured in collision with other motor vehicles in traffic accident

  √5th **V49.5** Passenger injured in collision with other and unspecified motor vehicles in traffic accident

    √x7th **V49.50** Passenger injured in collision with unspecified motor vehicles in traffic accident

    √x7th **V49.59** Passenger injured in collision with other motor vehicles in traffic accident

  √5th **V49.6** Unspecified car occupant injured in collision with other and unspecified motor vehicles in traffic accident

    √x7th **V49.60** Unspecified car occupant injured in collision with unspecified motor vehicles in traffic accident
           Car collision NOS (traffic)

    √x7th **V49.69** Unspecified car occupant injured in collision with other motor vehicles in traffic accident

  √5th **V49.8** Car occupant (driver) (passenger) injured in other specified transport accidents

    √x7th **V49.81** Car occupant (driver) (passenger) injured in transport accident with military vehicle

    √x7th **V49.88** Car occupant (driver) (passenger) injured in other specified transport accidents

  √x7th **V49.9** Car occupant (driver) (passenger) injured in unspecified traffic accident
       Car accident NOS

N Newborn: 0   P Pediatric: 0-17   M Maternity: 12-55   A Adult: 15-124   **MCC** Major CC Condition   **PDxMCC** PDx acts as own MCC   **CC** CC Condition   **PDxCC** PDx acts as own CC

1170   ICD-10-CM 2018

Occupant of pick-up truck or van injured in transport accident (V50-V59)

INCLUDES   a four or six wheel motor vehicle designed primarily for carrying passengers and property but weighing less than the local limit for classification as a heavy goods vehicle

     minibus
     minivan
     sport utility vehicle (SUV)
     truck
     van

EXCLUDES 1   *heavy transport vehicle (V60-V69)*

> The appropriate 7th character is to be added to each code from categories V50-V59.
> A   initial encounter
> D   subsequent encounter
> S   sequela

✓4th V50 Occupant of pick-up truck or van injured in collision with pedestrian or animal

EXCLUDES 1   *pick-up truck or van collision with animal-drawn vehicle or animal being ridden (V56.-)*

- ✓x7th **V50.0** Driver of pick-up truck or van injured in collision with pedestrian or animal in nontraffic accident
- ✓x7th **V50.1** Passenger in pick-up truck or van injured in collision with pedestrian or animal in nontraffic accident
- ✓x7th **V50.2** Person on outside of pick-up truck or van injured in collision with pedestrian or animal in nontraffic accident
- ✓x7th **V50.3** Unspecified occupant of pick-up truck or van injured in collision with pedestrian or animal in nontraffic accident
- ✓x7th **V50.4** Person boarding or alighting a pick-up truck or van injured in collision with pedestrian or animal
- ✓x7th **V50.5** Driver of pick-up truck or van injured in collision with pedestrian or animal in traffic accident
- ✓x7th **V50.6** Passenger in pick-up truck or van injured in collision with pedestrian or animal in traffic accident
- ✓x7th **V50.7** Person on outside of pick-up truck or van injured in collision with pedestrian or animal in traffic accident
- ✓x7th **V50.9** Unspecified occupant of pick-up truck or van injured in collision with pedestrian or animal in traffic accident

✓4th V51 Occupant of pick-up truck or van injured in collision with pedal cycle

- ✓x7th **V51.0** Driver of pick-up truck or van injured in collision with pedal cycle in nontraffic accident
- ✓x7th **V51.1** Passenger in pick-up truck or van injured in collision with pedal cycle in nontraffic accident
- ✓x7th **V51.2** Person on outside of pick-up truck or van injured in collision with pedal cycle in nontraffic accident
- ✓x7th **V51.3** Unspecified occupant of pick-up truck or van injured in collision with pedal cycle in nontraffic accident
- ✓x7th **V51.4** Person boarding or alighting a pick-up truck or van injured in collision with pedal cycle
- ✓x7th **V51.5** Driver of pick-up truck or van injured in collision with pedal cycle in traffic accident
- ✓x7th **V51.6** Passenger in pick-up truck or van injured in collision with pedal cycle in traffic accident
- ✓x7th **V51.7** Person on outside of pick-up truck or van injured in collision with pedal cycle in traffic accident
- ✓x7th **V51.9** Unspecified occupant of pick-up truck or van injured in collision with pedal cycle in traffic accident

✓4th V52 Occupant of pick-up truck or van injured in collision with two- or three-wheeled motor vehicle

- ✓x7th **V52.0** Driver of pick-up truck or van injured in collision with two- or three-wheeled motor vehicle in nontraffic accident
- ✓x7th **V52.1** Passenger in pick-up truck or van injured in collision with two- or three-wheeled motor vehicle in nontraffic accident
- ✓x7th **V52.2** Person on outside of pick-up truck or van injured in collision with two- or three-wheeled motor vehicle in nontraffic accident
- ✓x7th **V52.3** Unspecified occupant of pick-up truck or van injured in collision with two- or three-wheeled motor vehicle in nontraffic accident
- ✓x7th **V52.4** Person boarding or alighting a pick-up truck or van injured in collision with two- or three-wheeled motor vehicle
- ✓x7th **V52.5** Driver of pick-up truck or van injured in collision with two- or three-wheeled motor vehicle in traffic accident

- ✓x7th **V52.6** Passenger in pick-up truck or van injured in collision with two- or three-wheeled motor vehicle in traffic accident
- ✓x7th **V52.7** Person on outside of pick-up truck or van injured in collision with two- or three-wheeled motor vehicle in traffic accident
- ✓x7th **V52.9** Unspecified occupant of pick-up truck or van injured in collision with two- or three-wheeled motor vehicle in traffic accident

✓4th V53 Occupant of pick-up truck or van injured in collision with car, pick-up truck or van

- ✓x7th **V53.0** Driver of pick-up truck or van injured in collision with car, pick-up truck or van in nontraffic accident
- ✓x7th **V53.1** Passenger in pick-up truck or van injured in collision with car, pick-up truck or van in nontraffic accident
- ✓x7th **V53.2** Person on outside of pick-up truck or van injured in collision with car, pick-up truck or van in nontraffic accident
- ✓x7th **V53.3** Unspecified occupant of pick-up truck or van injured in collision with car, pick-up truck or van in nontraffic accident
- ✓x7th **V53.4** Person boarding or alighting a pick-up truck or van injured in collision with car, pick-up truck or van
- ✓x7th **V53.5** Driver of pick-up truck or van injured in collision with car, pick-up truck or van in traffic accident
- ✓x7th **V53.6** Passenger in pick-up truck or van injured in collision with car, pick-up truck or van in traffic accident
- ✓x7th **V53.7** Person on outside of pick-up truck or van injured in collision with car, pick-up truck or van in traffic accident
- ✓x7th **V53.9** Unspecified occupant of pick-up truck or van injured in collision with car, pick-up truck or van in traffic accident

✓4th V54 Occupant of pick-up truck or van injured in collision with heavy transport vehicle or bus

EXCLUDES 1   *occupant of pick-up truck or van injured in collision with military vehicle (V59.81)*

- ✓x7th **V54.0** Driver of pick-up truck or van injured in collision with heavy transport vehicle or bus in nontraffic accident
- ✓x7th **V54.1** Passenger in pick-up truck or van injured in collision with heavy transport vehicle or bus in nontraffic accident
- ✓x7th **V54.2** Person on outside of pick-up truck or van injured in collision with heavy transport vehicle or bus in nontraffic accident
- ✓x7th **V54.3** Unspecified occupant of pick-up truck or van injured in collision with heavy transport vehicle or bus in nontraffic accident
- ✓x7th **V54.4** Person boarding or alighting a pick-up truck or van injured in collision with heavy transport vehicle or bus
- ✓x7th **V54.5** Driver of pick-up truck or van injured in collision with heavy transport vehicle or bus in traffic accident
- ✓x7th **V54.6** Passenger in pick-up truck or van injured in collision with heavy transport vehicle or bus in traffic accident
- ✓x7th **V54.7** Person on outside of pick-up truck or van injured in collision with heavy transport vehicle or bus in traffic accident
- ✓x7th **V54.9** Unspecified occupant of pick-up truck or van injured in collision with heavy transport vehicle or bus in traffic accident

✓4th V55 Occupant of pick-up truck or van injured in collision with railway train or railway vehicle

- ✓x7th **V55.0** Driver of pick-up truck or van injured in collision with railway train or railway vehicle in nontraffic accident
- ✓x7th **V55.1** Passenger in pick-up truck or van injured in collision with railway train or railway vehicle in nontraffic accident
- ✓x7th **V55.2** Person on outside of pick-up truck or van injured in collision with railway train or railway vehicle in nontraffic accident
- ✓x7th **V55.3** Unspecified occupant of pick-up truck or van injured in collision with railway train or railway vehicle in nontraffic accident
- ✓x7th **V55.4** Person boarding or alighting a pick-up truck or van injured in collision with railway train or railway vehicle
- ✓x7th **V55.5** Driver of pick-up truck or van injured in collision with railway train or railway vehicle in traffic accident
- ✓x7th **V55.6** Passenger in pick-up truck or van injured in collision with railway train or railway vehicle in traffic accident
- ✓x7th **V55.7** Person on outside of pick-up truck or van injured in collision with railway train or railway vehicle in traffic accident
- ✓x7th **V55.9** Unspecified occupant of pick-up truck or van injured in collision with railway train or railway vehicle in traffic accident

---

✓ Additional Character Req   ✓x7th Placeholder Alert   Unacceptable PDx   Manifestation   H1-H14 HAC   HCC CMS-HCC Condition   EXCLUDES 1 Not Coded Here   EXCLUDES 2 Not Included Here

ICD-10-CM 2018   1171

Chapter 20. External Causes of Morbidity

√4ᵗʰ **V56** **Occupant of pick-up truck or van injured in collision with other nonmotor vehicle**
    INCLUDES   collision with animal-drawn vehicle, animal being ridden, streetcar

√x7ᵗʰ **V56.0** Driver of pick-up truck or van injured in collision with other nonmotor vehicle in nontraffic accident

√x7ᵗʰ **V56.1** Passenger in pick-up truck or van injured in collision with other nonmotor vehicle in nontraffic accident

√x7ᵗʰ **V56.2** Person on outside of pick-up truck or van injured in collision with other nonmotor vehicle in nontraffic accident

√x7ᵗʰ **V56.3** Unspecified occupant of pick-up truck or van injured in collision with other nonmotor vehicle in nontraffic accident

√x7ᵗʰ **V56.4** Person boarding or alighting a pick-up truck or van injured in collision with other nonmotor vehicle

√x7ᵗʰ **V56.5** Driver of pick-up truck or van injured in collision with other nonmotor vehicle in traffic accident

√x7ᵗʰ **V56.6** Passenger in pick-up truck or van injured in collision with other nonmotor vehicle in traffic accident

√x7ᵗʰ **V56.7** Person on outside of pick-up truck or van injured in collision with other nonmotor vehicle in traffic accident

√x7ᵗʰ **V56.9** Unspecified occupant of pick-up truck or van injured in collision with other nonmotor vehicle in traffic accident

√4ᵗʰ **V57** **Occupant of pick-up truck or van injured in collision with fixed or stationary object**

√x7ᵗʰ **V57.0** Driver of pick-up truck or van injured in collision with fixed or stationary object in nontraffic accident

√x7ᵗʰ **V57.1** Passenger in pick-up truck or van injured in collision with fixed or stationary object in nontraffic accident

√x7ᵗʰ **V57.2** Person on outside of pick-up truck or van injured in collision with fixed or stationary object in nontraffic accident

√x7ᵗʰ **V57.3** Unspecified occupant of pick-up truck or van injured in collision with fixed or stationary object in nontraffic accident

√x7ᵗʰ **V57.4** Person boarding or alighting a pick-up truck or van injured in collision with fixed or stationary object

√x7ᵗʰ **V57.5** Driver of pick-up truck or van injured in collision with fixed or stationary object in traffic accident

√x7ᵗʰ **V57.6** Passenger in pick-up truck or van injured in collision with fixed or stationary object in traffic accident

√x7ᵗʰ **V57.7** Person on outside of pick-up truck or van injured in collision with fixed or stationary object in traffic accident

√x7ᵗʰ **V57.9** Unspecified occupant of pick-up truck or van injured in collision with fixed or stationary object in traffic accident

√4ᵗʰ **V58** **Occupant of pick-up truck or van injured in noncollision transport accident**
    INCLUDES   overturning pick-up truck or van NOS
                overturning pick-up truck or van without collision

√x7ᵗʰ **V58.0** Driver of pick-up truck or van injured in noncollision transport accident in nontraffic accident

√x7ᵗʰ **V58.1** Passenger in pick-up truck or van injured in noncollision transport accident in nontraffic accident

√x7ᵗʰ **V58.2** Person on outside of pick-up truck or van injured in noncollision transport accident in nontraffic accident

√x7ᵗʰ **V58.3** Unspecified occupant of pick-up truck or van injured in noncollision transport accident in nontraffic accident

√x7ᵗʰ **V58.4** Person boarding or alighting a pick-up truck or van injured in noncollision transport accident

√x7ᵗʰ **V58.5** Driver of pick-up truck or van injured in noncollision transport accident in traffic accident

√x7ᵗʰ **V58.6** Passenger in pick-up truck or van injured in noncollision transport accident in traffic accident

√x7ᵗʰ **V58.7** Person on outside of pick-up truck or van injured in noncollision transport accident in traffic accident

√x7ᵗʰ **V58.9** Unspecified occupant of pick-up truck or van injured in noncollision transport accident in traffic accident

√4ᵗʰ **V59** **Occupant of pick-up truck or van injured in other and unspecified transport accidents**

√5ᵗʰ **V59.0** Driver of pick-up truck or van injured in collision with other and unspecified motor vehicles in nontraffic accident

√x7ᵗʰ **V59.00** Driver of pick-up truck or van injured in collision with unspecified motor vehicles in nontraffic accident

√x7ᵗʰ **V59.09** Driver of pick-up truck or van injured in collision with other motor vehicles in nontraffic accident

√5ᵗʰ **V59.1** Passenger in pick-up truck or van injured in collision with other and unspecified motor vehicles in nontraffic accident

√x7ᵗʰ **V59.10** Passenger in pick-up truck or van injured in collision with unspecified motor vehicles in nontraffic accident

√x7ᵗʰ **V59.19** Passenger in pick-up truck or van injured in collision with other motor vehicles in nontraffic accident

√5ᵗʰ **V59.2** Unspecified occupant of pick-up truck or van injured in collision with other and unspecified motor vehicles in nontraffic accident

√x7ᵗʰ **V59.20** Unspecified occupant of pick-up truck or van injured in collision with unspecified motor vehicles in nontraffic accident
       Collision NOS involving pick-up truck or van, nontraffic

√x7ᵗʰ **V59.29** Unspecified occupant of pick-up truck or van injured in collision with other motor vehicles in nontraffic accident

√x7ᵗʰ **V59.3** Occupant (driver) (passenger) of pick-up truck or van injured in unspecified nontraffic accident
       Accident NOS involving pick-up truck or van, nontraffic
       Occupant of pick-up truck or van injured in nontraffic accident NOS

√5ᵗʰ **V59.4** Driver of pick-up truck or van injured in collision with other and unspecified motor vehicles in traffic accident

√x7ᵗʰ **V59.40** Driver of pick-up truck or van injured in collision with unspecified motor vehicles in traffic accident

√x7ᵗʰ **V59.49** Driver of pick-up truck or van injured in collision with other motor vehicles in traffic accident

√5ᵗʰ **V59.5** Passenger in pick-up truck or van injured in collision with other and unspecified motor vehicles in traffic accident

√x7ᵗʰ **V59.50** Passenger in pick-up truck or van injured in collision with unspecified motor vehicles in traffic accident

√x7ᵗʰ **V59.59** Passenger in pick-up truck or van injured in collision with other motor vehicles in traffic accident

√5ᵗʰ **V59.6** Unspecified occupant of pick-up truck or van injured in collision with other and unspecified motor vehicles in traffic accident

√x7ᵗʰ **V59.60** Unspecified occupant of pick-up truck or van injured in collision with unspecified motor vehicles in traffic accident
       Collision NOS involving pick-up truck or van (traffic)

√x7ᵗʰ **V59.69** Unspecified occupant of pick-up truck or van injured in collision with other motor vehicles in traffic accident

√5ᵗʰ **V59.8** Occupant (driver) (passenger) of pick-up truck or van injured in other specified transport accidents

√x7ᵗʰ **V59.81** Occupant (driver) (passenger) of pick-up truck or van injured in transport accident with military vehicle

√x7ᵗʰ **V59.88** Occupant (driver) (passenger) of pick-up truck or van injured in other specified transport accidents

√x7ᵗʰ **V59.9** Occupant (driver) (passenger) of pick-up truck or van injured in unspecified traffic accident
       Accident NOS involving pick-up truck or van

Occupant of heavy transport vehicle injured in transport accident (V60–V69)

    INCLUDES   18 wheeler
                armored car
                panel truck
    EXCLUDES 1   bus
                motorcoach

The appropriate 7th character is to be added to each code from categories V60-V69.
A   initial encounter
D   subsequent encounter
S   sequela

√4ᵗʰ **V60** **Occupant of heavy transport vehicle injured in collision with pedestrian or animal**
    EXCLUDES 1   heavy transport vehicle collision with animal-drawn vehicle or animal being ridden (V66.-)

√x7ᵗʰ **V60.0** Driver of heavy transport vehicle injured in collision with pedestrian or animal in nontraffic accident

√x7ᵗʰ **V60.1** Passenger in heavy transport vehicle injured in collision with pedestrian or animal in nontraffic accident

√x7ᵗʰ **V60.2** Person on outside of heavy transport vehicle injured in collision with pedestrian or animal in nontraffic accident

N Newborn: 0   P Pediatric: 0-17   M Maternity: 12-55   A Adult: 15-124   MCC Major CC Condition   PDxMCC PDx acts as own MCC   CC CC Condition   PDxCC PDx acts as own CC

1172   ICD-10-CM 2018

✓x7th **V60.3** Unspecified occupant of heavy transport vehicle injured in collision with pedestrian or animal in nontraffic accident

✓x7th **V60.4** Person boarding or alighting a heavy transport vehicle injured in collision with pedestrian or animal

✓x7th **V60.5** Driver of heavy transport vehicle injured in collision with pedestrian or animal in traffic accident

✓x7th **V60.6** Passenger in heavy transport vehicle injured in collision with pedestrian or animal in traffic accident

✓x7th **V60.7** Person on outside of heavy transport vehicle injured in collision with pedestrian or animal in traffic accident

✓x7th **V60.9** Unspecified occupant of heavy transport vehicle injured in collision with pedestrian or animal in traffic accident

✓4th **V61 Occupant of heavy transport vehicle injured in collision with pedal cycle**

✓x7th **V61.0** Driver of heavy transport vehicle injured in collision with pedal cycle in nontraffic accident

✓x7th **V61.1** Passenger in heavy transport vehicle injured in collision with pedal cycle in nontraffic accident

✓x7th **V61.2** Person on outside of heavy transport vehicle injured in collision with pedal cycle in nontraffic accident

✓x7th **V61.3** Unspecified occupant of heavy transport vehicle injured in collision with pedal cycle in nontraffic accident

✓x7th **V61.4** Person boarding or alighting a heavy transport vehicle injured in collision with pedal cycle while boarding or alighting

✓x7th **V61.5** Driver of heavy transport vehicle injured in collision with pedal cycle in traffic accident

✓x7th **V61.6** Passenger in heavy transport vehicle injured in collision with pedal cycle in traffic accident

✓x7th **V61.7** Person on outside of heavy transport vehicle injured in collision with pedal cycle in traffic accident

✓x7th **V61.9** Unspecified occupant of heavy transport vehicle injured in collision with pedal cycle in traffic accident

✓4th **V62 Occupant of heavy transport vehicle injured in collision with two- or three-wheeled motor vehicle**

✓x7th **V62.0** Driver of heavy transport vehicle injured in collision with two- or three-wheeled motor vehicle in nontraffic accident

✓x7th **V62.1** Passenger in heavy transport vehicle injured in collision with two- or three-wheeled motor vehicle in nontraffic accident

✓x7th **V62.2** Person on outside of heavy transport vehicle injured in collision with two- or three-wheeled motor vehicle in nontraffic accident

✓x7th **V62.3** Unspecified occupant of heavy transport vehicle injured in collision with two- or three-wheeled motor vehicle in nontraffic accident

✓x7th **V62.4** Person boarding or alighting a heavy transport vehicle injured in collision with two- or three-wheeled motor vehicle

✓x7th **V62.5** Driver of heavy transport vehicle injured in collision with two- or three-wheeled motor vehicle in traffic accident

✓x7th **V62.6** Passenger in heavy transport vehicle injured in collision with two- or three-wheeled motor vehicle in traffic accident

✓x7th **V62.7** Person on outside of heavy transport vehicle injured in collision with two- or three-wheeled motor vehicle in traffic accident

✓x7th **V62.9** Unspecified occupant of heavy transport vehicle injured in collision with two- or three-wheeled motor vehicle in traffic accident

✓4th **V63 Occupant of heavy transport vehicle injured in collision with car, pick-up truck or van**

✓x7th **V63.0** Driver of heavy transport vehicle injured in collision with car, pick-up truck or van in nontraffic accident

✓x7th **V63.1** Passenger in heavy transport vehicle injured in collision with car, pick-up truck or van in nontraffic accident

✓x7th **V63.2** Person on outside of heavy transport vehicle injured in collision with car, pick-up truck or van in nontraffic accident

✓x7th **V63.3** Unspecified occupant of heavy transport vehicle injured in collision with car, pick-up truck or van in nontraffic accident

✓x7th **V63.4** Person boarding or alighting a heavy transport vehicle injured in collision with car, pick-up truck or van

✓x7th **V63.5** Driver of heavy transport vehicle injured in collision with car, pick-up truck or van in traffic accident

✓x7th **V63.6** Passenger in heavy transport vehicle injured in collision with car, pick-up truck or van in traffic accident

✓x7th **V63.7** Person on outside of heavy transport vehicle injured in collision with car, pick-up truck or van in traffic accident

✓x7th **V63.9** Unspecified occupant of heavy transport vehicle injured in collision with car, pick-up truck or van in traffic accident

✓4th **V64 Occupant of heavy transport vehicle injured in collision with heavy transport vehicle or bus**

> EXCLUDES 1   occupant of heavy transport vehicle injured in collision with military vehicle (V69.81)

✓x7th **V64.0** Driver of heavy transport vehicle injured in collision with heavy transport vehicle or bus in nontraffic accident

✓x7th **V64.1** Passenger in heavy transport vehicle injured in collision with heavy transport vehicle or bus in nontraffic accident

✓x7th **V64.2** Person on outside of heavy transport vehicle injured in collision with heavy transport vehicle or bus in nontraffic accident

✓x7th **V64.3** Unspecified occupant of heavy transport vehicle injured in collision with heavy transport vehicle or bus in nontraffic accident

✓x7th **V64.4** Person boarding or alighting a heavy transport vehicle injured in collision with heavy transport vehicle or bus while boarding or alighting

✓x7th **V64.5** Driver of heavy transport vehicle injured in collision with heavy transport vehicle or bus in traffic accident

✓x7th **V64.6** Passenger in heavy transport vehicle injured in collision with heavy transport vehicle or bus in traffic accident

✓x7th **V64.7** Person on outside of heavy transport vehicle injured in collision with heavy transport vehicle or bus in traffic accident

✓x7th **V64.9** Unspecified occupant of heavy transport vehicle injured in collision with heavy transport vehicle or bus in traffic accident

✓4th **V65 Occupant of heavy transport vehicle injured in collision with railway train or railway vehicle**

✓x7th **V65.0** Driver of heavy transport vehicle injured in collision with railway train or railway vehicle in nontraffic accident

✓x7th **V65.1** Passenger in heavy transport vehicle injured in collision with railway train or railway vehicle in nontraffic accident

✓x7th **V65.2** Person on outside of heavy transport vehicle injured in collision with railway train or railway vehicle in nontraffic accident

✓x7th **V65.3** Unspecified occupant of heavy transport vehicle injured in collision with railway train or railway vehicle in nontraffic accident

✓x7th **V65.4** Person boarding or alighting a heavy transport vehicle injured in collision with railway train or railway vehicle

✓x7th **V65.5** Driver of heavy transport vehicle injured in collision with railway train or railway vehicle in traffic accident

✓x7th **V65.6** Passenger in heavy transport vehicle injured in collision with railway train or railway vehicle in traffic accident

✓x7th **V65.7** Person on outside of heavy transport vehicle injured in collision with railway train or railway vehicle in traffic accident

✓x7th **V65.9** Unspecified occupant of heavy transport vehicle injured in collision with railway train or railway vehicle in traffic accident

✓4th **V66 Occupant of heavy transport vehicle injured in collision with other nonmotor vehicle**

> INCLUDES   collision with animal-drawn vehicle, animal being ridden, streetcar

✓x7th **V66.0** Driver of heavy transport vehicle injured in collision with other nonmotor vehicle in nontraffic accident

✓x7th **V66.1** Passenger in heavy transport vehicle injured in collision with other nonmotor vehicle in nontraffic accident

✓x7th **V66.2** Person on outside of heavy transport vehicle injured in collision with other nonmotor vehicle in nontraffic accident

✓x7th **V66.3** Unspecified occupant of heavy transport vehicle injured in collision with other nonmotor vehicle in nontraffic accident

✓x7th **V66.4** Person boarding or alighting a heavy transport vehicle injured in collision with other nonmotor vehicle

✓x7th **V66.5** Driver of heavy transport vehicle injured in collision with other nonmotor vehicle in traffic accident

✓x7th **V66.6** Passenger in heavy transport vehicle injured in collision with other nonmotor vehicle in traffic accident

✓x7th **V66.7** Person on outside of heavy transport vehicle injured in collision with other nonmotor vehicle in traffic accident

---

✓ Additional Character Req   ✓x7th Placeholder Alert   Unacceptable PDx   Manifestation   H1–H14 HAC   HCC CMS-HCC Condition   EXCLUDES 1 Not Coded Here   EXCLUDES 2 Not Included Here

Chapter 20. External Causes of Morbidity

✓x7ᵗʰ **V66.9** Unspecified occupant of heavy transport vehicle injured in collision with other nonmotor vehicle in traffic accident

✓4ᵗʰ **V67** **Occupant of heavy transport vehicle injured in collision with fixed or stationary object**

✓x7ᵗʰ **V67.0** Driver of heavy transport vehicle injured in collision with fixed or stationary object in nontraffic accident

✓x7ᵗʰ **V67.1** Passenger in heavy transport vehicle injured in collision with fixed or stationary object in nontraffic accident

✓x7ᵗʰ **V67.2** Person on outside of heavy transport vehicle injured in collision with fixed or stationary object in nontraffic accident

✓x7ᵗʰ **V67.3** Unspecified occupant of heavy transport vehicle injured in collision with fixed or stationary object in nontraffic accident

✓x7ᵗʰ **V67.4** Person boarding or alighting a heavy transport vehicle injured in collision with fixed or stationary object

✓x7ᵗʰ **V67.5** Driver of heavy transport vehicle injured in collision with fixed or stationary object in traffic accident

✓x7ᵗʰ **V67.6** Passenger in heavy transport vehicle injured in collision with fixed or stationary object in traffic accident

✓x7ᵗʰ **V67.7** Person on outside of heavy transport vehicle injured in collision with fixed or stationary object in traffic accident

✓x7ᵗʰ **V67.9** Unspecified occupant of heavy transport vehicle injured in collision with fixed or stationary object in traffic accident

✓4ᵗʰ **V68** **Occupant of heavy transport vehicle injured in noncollision transport accident**

     INCLUDES   overturning heavy transport vehicle NOS
                overturning heavy transport vehicle without collision

✓x7ᵗʰ **V68.0** Driver of heavy transport vehicle injured in noncollision transport accident in nontraffic accident

✓x7ᵗʰ **V68.1** Passenger in heavy transport vehicle injured in noncollision transport accident in nontraffic accident

✓x7ᵗʰ **V68.2** Person on outside of heavy transport vehicle injured in noncollision transport accident in nontraffic accident

✓x7ᵗʰ **V68.3** Unspecified occupant of heavy transport vehicle injured in noncollision transport accident in nontraffic accident

✓x7ᵗʰ **V68.4** Person boarding or alighting a heavy transport vehicle injured in noncollision transport accident

✓x7ᵗʰ **V68.5** Driver of heavy transport vehicle injured in noncollision transport accident in traffic accident

✓x7ᵗʰ **V68.6** Passenger in heavy transport vehicle injured in noncollision transport accident in traffic accident

✓x7ᵗʰ **V68.7** Person on outside of heavy transport vehicle injured in noncollision transport accident in traffic accident

✓x7ᵗʰ **V68.9** Unspecified occupant of heavy transport vehicle injured in noncollision transport accident in traffic accident

✓4ᵗʰ **V69** **Occupant of heavy transport vehicle injured in other and unspecified transport accidents**

✓5ᵗʰ **V69.0** Driver of heavy transport vehicle injured in collision with other and unspecified motor vehicles in nontraffic accident

✓x7ᵗʰ **V69.00** Driver of heavy transport vehicle injured in collision with unspecified motor vehicles in nontraffic accident

✓x7ᵗʰ **V69.09** Driver of heavy transport vehicle injured in collision with other motor vehicles in nontraffic accident

✓5ᵗʰ **V69.1** Passenger in heavy transport vehicle injured in collision with other and unspecified motor vehicles in nontraffic accident

✓x7ᵗʰ **V69.10** Passenger in heavy transport vehicle injured in collision with unspecified motor vehicles in nontraffic accident

✓x7ᵗʰ **V69.19** Passenger in heavy transport vehicle injured in collision with other motor vehicles in nontraffic accident

✓5ᵗʰ **V69.2** Unspecified occupant of heavy transport vehicle injured in collision with other and unspecified motor vehicles in nontraffic accident

✓x7ᵗʰ **V69.20** Unspecified occupant of heavy transport vehicle injured in collision with unspecified motor vehicles in nontraffic accident
     Collision NOS involving heavy transport vehicle, nontraffic

✓x7ᵗʰ **V69.29** Unspecified occupant of heavy transport vehicle injured in collision with other motor vehicles in nontraffic accident

✓x7ᵗʰ **V69.3** Occupant (driver) (passenger) of heavy transport vehicle injured in unspecified nontraffic accident
     Accident NOS involving heavy transport vehicle, nontraffic
     Occupant of heavy transport vehicle injured in nontraffic accident NOS

✓5ᵗʰ **V69.4** Driver of heavy transport vehicle injured in collision with other and unspecified motor vehicles in traffic accident

✓x7ᵗʰ **V69.40** Driver of heavy transport vehicle injured in collision with unspecified motor vehicles in traffic accident

✓x7ᵗʰ **V69.49** Driver of heavy transport vehicle injured in collision with other motor vehicles in traffic accident

✓5ᵗʰ **V69.5** Passenger in heavy transport vehicle injured in collision with other and unspecified motor vehicles in traffic accident

✓x7ᵗʰ **V69.50** Passenger in heavy transport vehicle injured in collision with unspecified motor vehicles in traffic accident

✓x7ᵗʰ **V69.59** Passenger in heavy transport vehicle injured in collision with other motor vehicles in traffic accident

✓5ᵗʰ **V69.6** Unspecified occupant of heavy transport vehicle injured in collision with other and unspecified motor vehicles in traffic accident

✓x7ᵗʰ **V69.60** Unspecified occupant of heavy transport vehicle injured in collision with unspecified motor vehicles in traffic accident
     Collision NOS involving heavy transport vehicle (traffic)

✓x7ᵗʰ **V69.69** Unspecified occupant of heavy transport vehicle injured in collision with other motor vehicles in traffic accident

✓5ᵗʰ **V69.8** Occupant (driver) (passenger) of heavy transport vehicle injured in other specified transport accidents

✓x7ᵗʰ **V69.81** Occupant (driver) (passenger) of heavy transport vehicle injured in transport accidents with military vehicle

✓x7ᵗʰ **V69.88** Occupant (driver) (passenger) of heavy transport vehicle injured in other specified transport accidents

✓x7ᵗʰ **V69.9** Occupant (driver) (passenger) of heavy transport vehicle injured in unspecified traffic accident
     Accident NOS involving heavy transport vehicle

Bus occupant injured in transport accident (V70-V79)

INCLUDES   motorcoach
EXCLUDES 1   minibus (V50-V59)

The appropriate 7th character is to be added to each code from categories V70-V79.
A   initial encounter
D   subsequent encounter
S   sequela

✓4ᵗʰ **V70** **Bus occupant injured in collision with pedestrian or animal**
     EXCLUDES 1   bus collision with animal-drawn vehicle or animal being ridden (V76.-)

✓x7ᵗʰ **V70.0** Driver of bus injured in collision with pedestrian or animal in nontraffic accident

✓x7ᵗʰ **V70.1** Passenger on bus injured in collision with pedestrian or animal in nontraffic accident

✓x7ᵗʰ **V70.2** Person on outside of bus injured in collision with pedestrian or animal in nontraffic accident

✓x7ᵗʰ **V70.3** Unspecified occupant of bus injured in collision with pedestrian or animal in nontraffic accident

✓x7ᵗʰ **V70.4** Person boarding or alighting from bus injured in collision with pedestrian or animal

✓x7ᵗʰ **V70.5** Driver of bus injured in collision with pedestrian or animal in traffic accident

✓x7ᵗʰ **V70.6** Passenger on bus injured in collision with pedestrian or animal in traffic accident

✓x7ᵗʰ **V70.7** Person on outside of bus injured in collision with pedestrian or animal in traffic accident

✓x7ᵗʰ **V70.9** Unspecified occupant of bus injured in collision with pedestrian or animal in traffic accident

✓4ᵗʰ **V71** **Bus occupant injured in collision with pedal cycle**

✓x7ᵗʰ **V71.0** Driver of bus injured in collision with pedal cycle in nontraffic accident

✓x7ᵗʰ **V71.1** Passenger on bus injured in collision with pedal cycle in nontraffic accident

N Newborn: 0   P Pediatric: 0-17   M Maternity: 12-55   A Adult: 15-124   MCC Major CC Condition   PDx MCC PDx acts as own MCC   CC CC Condition   PDx CC PDx acts as own CC

1174   ICD-10-CM 2018

√x7ᵗʰ **V71.2** Person on outside of bus injured in collision with pedal cycle in nontraffic accident

√x7ᵗʰ **V71.3** Unspecified occupant of bus injured in collision with pedal cycle in nontraffic accident

√x7ᵗʰ **V71.4** Person boarding or alighting from bus injured in collision with pedal cycle

√x7ᵗʰ **V71.5** Driver of bus injured in collision with pedal cycle in traffic accident

√x7ᵗʰ **V71.6** Passenger on bus injured in collision with pedal cycle in traffic accident

√x7ᵗʰ **V71.7** Person on outside of bus injured in collision with pedal cycle in traffic accident

√x7ᵗʰ **V71.9** Unspecified occupant of bus injured in collision with pedal cycle in traffic accident

√4ᵗʰ **V72 Bus occupant injured in collision with two- or three-wheeled motor vehicle**

√x7ᵗʰ **V72.0** Driver of bus injured in collision with two- or three-wheeled motor vehicle in nontraffic accident

√x7ᵗʰ **V72.1** Passenger on bus injured in collision with two- or three-wheeled motor vehicle in nontraffic accident

√x7ᵗʰ **V72.2** Person on outside of bus injured in collision with two- or three-wheeled motor vehicle in nontraffic accident

√x7ᵗʰ **V72.3** Unspecified occupant of bus injured in collision with two- or three-wheeled motor vehicle in nontraffic accident

√x7ᵗʰ **V72.4** Person boarding or alighting from bus injured in collision with two- or three-wheeled motor vehicle

√x7ᵗʰ **V72.5** Driver of bus injured in collision with two- or three-wheeled motor vehicle in traffic accident

√x7ᵗʰ **V72.6** Passenger on bus injured in collision with two- or three-wheeled motor vehicle in traffic accident

√x7ᵗʰ **V72.7** Person on outside of bus injured in collision with two- or three-wheeled motor vehicle in traffic accident

√x7ᵗʰ **V72.9** Unspecified occupant of bus injured in collision with two- or three-wheeled motor vehicle in traffic accident

√4ᵗʰ **V73 Bus occupant injured in collision with car, pick-up truck or van**

√x7ᵗʰ **V73.0** Driver of bus injured in collision with car, pick-up truck or van in nontraffic accident

√x7ᵗʰ **V73.1** Passenger on bus injured in collision with car, pick-up truck or van in nontraffic accident

√x7ᵗʰ **V73.2** Person on outside of bus injured in collision with car, pick-up truck or van in nontraffic accident

√x7ᵗʰ **V73.3** Unspecified occupant of bus injured in collision with car, pick-up truck or van in nontraffic accident

√x7ᵗʰ **V73.4** Person boarding or alighting from bus injured in collision with car, pick-up truck or van

√x7ᵗʰ **V73.5** Driver of bus injured in collision with car, pick-up truck or van in traffic accident

√x7ᵗʰ **V73.6** Passenger on bus injured in collision with car, pick-up truck or van in traffic accident

√x7ᵗʰ **V73.7** Person on outside of bus injured in collision with car, pick-up truck or van in traffic accident

√x7ᵗʰ **V73.9** Unspecified occupant of bus injured in collision with car, pick-up truck or van in traffic accident

√4ᵗʰ **V74 Bus occupant injured in collision with heavy transport vehicle or bus**

> EXCLUDES 1   *bus occupant injured in collision with military vehicle (V79.81)*

√x7ᵗʰ **V74.0** Driver of bus injured in collision with heavy transport vehicle or bus in nontraffic accident

√x7ᵗʰ **V74.1** Passenger on bus injured in collision with heavy transport vehicle or bus in nontraffic accident

√x7ᵗʰ **V74.2** Person on outside of bus injured in collision with heavy transport vehicle or bus in nontraffic accident

√x7ᵗʰ **V74.3** Unspecified occupant of bus injured in collision with heavy transport vehicle or bus in nontraffic accident

√x7ᵗʰ **V74.4** Person boarding or alighting from bus injured in collision with heavy transport vehicle or bus

√x7ᵗʰ **V74.5** Driver of bus injured in collision with heavy transport vehicle or bus in traffic accident

√x7ᵗʰ **V74.6** Passenger on bus injured in collision with heavy transport vehicle or bus in traffic accident

√x7ᵗʰ **V74.7** Person on outside of bus injured in collision with heavy transport vehicle or bus in traffic accident

√x7ᵗʰ **V74.9** Unspecified occupant of bus injured in collision with heavy transport vehicle or bus in traffic accident

√4ᵗʰ **V75 Bus occupant injured in collision with railway train or railway vehicle**

√x7ᵗʰ **V75.0** Driver of bus injured in collision with railway train or railway vehicle in nontraffic accident

√x7ᵗʰ **V75.1** Passenger on bus injured in collision with railway train or railway vehicle in nontraffic accident

√x7ᵗʰ **V75.2** Person on outside of bus injured in collision with railway train or railway vehicle in nontraffic accident

√x7ᵗʰ **V75.3** Unspecified occupant of bus injured in collision with railway train or railway vehicle in nontraffic accident

√x7ᵗʰ **V75.4** Person boarding or alighting from bus injured in collision with railway train or railway vehicle

√x7ᵗʰ **V75.5** Driver of bus injured in collision with railway train or railway vehicle in traffic accident

√x7ᵗʰ **V75.6** Passenger on bus injured in collision with railway train or railway vehicle in traffic accident

√x7ᵗʰ **V75.7** Person on outside of bus injured in collision with railway train or railway vehicle in traffic accident

√x7ᵗʰ **V75.9** Unspecified occupant of bus injured in collision with railway train or railway vehicle in traffic accident

√4ᵗʰ **V76 Bus occupant injured in collision with other nonmotor vehicle**

> INCLUDES   collision with animal-drawn vehicle, animal being ridden, streetcar

√x7ᵗʰ **V76.0** Driver of bus injured in collision with other nonmotor vehicle in nontraffic accident

√x7ᵗʰ **V76.1** Passenger on bus injured in collision with other nonmotor vehicle in nontraffic accident

√x7ᵗʰ **V76.2** Person on outside of bus injured in collision with other nonmotor vehicle in nontraffic accident

√x7ᵗʰ **V76.3** Unspecified occupant of bus injured in collision with other nonmotor vehicle in nontraffic accident

√x7ᵗʰ **V76.4** Person boarding or alighting from bus injured in collision with other nonmotor vehicle

√x7ᵗʰ **V76.5** Driver of bus injured in collision with other nonmotor vehicle in traffic accident

√x7ᵗʰ **V76.6** Passenger on bus injured in collision with other nonmotor vehicle in traffic accident

√x7ᵗʰ **V76.7** Person on outside of bus injured in collision with other nonmotor vehicle in traffic accident

√x7ᵗʰ **V76.9** Unspecified occupant of bus injured in collision with other nonmotor vehicle in traffic accident

√4ᵗʰ **V77 Bus occupant injured in collision with fixed or stationary object**

√x7ᵗʰ **V77.0** Driver of bus injured in collision with fixed or stationary object in nontraffic accident

√x7ᵗʰ **V77.1** Passenger on bus injured in collision with fixed or stationary object in nontraffic accident

√x7ᵗʰ **V77.2** Person on outside of bus injured in collision with fixed or stationary object in nontraffic accident

√x7ᵗʰ **V77.3** Unspecified occupant of bus injured in collision with fixed or stationary object in nontraffic accident

√x7ᵗʰ **V77.4** Person boarding or alighting from bus injured in collision with fixed or stationary object

√x7ᵗʰ **V77.5** Driver of bus injured in collision with fixed or stationary object in traffic accident

√x7ᵗʰ **V77.6** Passenger on bus injured in collision with fixed or stationary object in traffic accident

√x7ᵗʰ **V77.7** Person on outside of bus injured in collision with fixed or stationary object in traffic accident

√x7ᵗʰ **V77.9** Unspecified occupant of bus injured in collision with fixed or stationary object in traffic accident

√4ᵗʰ **V78 Bus occupant injured in noncollision transport accident**

> INCLUDES   overturning bus NOS
> overturning bus without collision

√x7ᵗʰ **V78.0** Driver of bus injured in noncollision transport accident in nontraffic accident

√x7ᵗʰ **V78.1** Passenger on bus injured in noncollision transport accident in nontraffic accident

√x7ᵗʰ **V78.2** Person on outside of bus injured in noncollision transport accident in nontraffic accident

√x7ᵗʰ **V78.3** Unspecified occupant of bus injured in noncollision transport accident in nontraffic accident

☑ Additional Character Req   √x7ᵗʰ Placeholder Alert   Unacceptable PDx   Manifestation   H1-H14 HAC   HCC CMS-HCC Condition   EXCLUDES 1 Not Coded Here   EXCLUDES 2 Not Included Here

ICD-10-CM 2018   1175

√x7ᵗʰ **V78.4** Person boarding or alighting from bus injured in noncollision transport accident

√x7ᵗʰ **V78.5** Driver of bus injured in noncollision transport accident in traffic accident

√x7ᵗʰ **V78.6** Passenger on bus injured in noncollision transport accident in traffic accident

√x7ᵗʰ **V78.7** Person on outside of bus injured in noncollision transport accident in traffic accident

√x7ᵗʰ **V78.9** Unspecified occupant of bus injured in noncollision transport accident in traffic accident

√4ᵗʰ **V79** Bus occupant injured in other and unspecified transport accidents

√5ᵗʰ **V79.0** Driver of bus injured in collision with other and unspecified motor vehicles in nontraffic accident

     √x7ᵗʰ **V79.00** Driver of bus injured in collision with unspecified motor vehicles in nontraffic accident

     √x7ᵗʰ **V79.09** Driver of bus injured in collision with other motor vehicles in nontraffic accident

√5ᵗʰ **V79.1** Passenger on bus injured in collision with other and unspecified motor vehicles in nontraffic accident

     √x7ᵗʰ **V79.10** Passenger on bus injured in collision with unspecified motor vehicles in nontraffic accident

     √x7ᵗʰ **V79.19** Passenger on bus injured in collision with other motor vehicles in nontraffic accident

√5ᵗʰ **V79.2** Unspecified bus occupant injured in collision with other and unspecified motor vehicles in nontraffic accident

     √x7ᵗʰ **V79.20** Unspecified bus occupant injured in collision with unspecified motor vehicles in nontraffic accident
         Bus collision NOS, nontraffic

     √x7ᵗʰ **V79.29** Unspecified bus occupant injured in collision with other motor vehicles in nontraffic accident

√x7ᵗʰ **V79.3** Bus occupant (driver) (passenger) injured in unspecified nontraffic accident
     Bus accident NOS, nontraffic
     Bus occupant injured in nontraffic accident NOS

√5ᵗʰ **V79.4** Driver of bus injured in collision with other and unspecified motor vehicles in traffic accident

     √x7ᵗʰ **V79.40** Driver of bus injured in collision with unspecified motor vehicles in traffic accident

     √x7ᵗʰ **V79.49** Driver of bus injured in collision with other motor vehicles in traffic accident

√5ᵗʰ **V79.5** Passenger on bus injured in collision with other and unspecified motor vehicles in traffic accident

     √x7ᵗʰ **V79.50** Passenger on bus injured in collision with unspecified motor vehicles in traffic accident

     √x7ᵗʰ **V79.59** Passenger on bus injured in collision with other motor vehicles in traffic accident

√5ᵗʰ **V79.6** Unspecified bus occupant injured in collision with other and unspecified motor vehicles in traffic accident

     √x7ᵗʰ **V79.60** Unspecified bus occupant injured in collision with unspecified motor vehicles in traffic accident
         Bus collision NOS (traffic)

     √x7ᵗʰ **V79.69** Unspecified bus occupant injured in collision with other motor vehicles in traffic accident

√5ᵗʰ **V79.8** Bus occupant (driver) (passenger) injured in other specified transport accidents

     √x7ᵗʰ **V79.81** Bus occupant (driver) (passenger) injured in transport accidents with military vehicle

     √x7ᵗʰ **V79.88** Bus occupant (driver) (passenger) injured in other specified transport accidents

√x7ᵗʰ **V79.9** Bus occupant (driver) (passenger) injured in unspecified traffic accident
     Bus accident NOS

Other land transport accidents (V80-V89)

The appropriate 7th character is to be added to each code from categories V80-V89.
A   initial encounter
D   subsequent encounter
S   sequela

√4ᵗʰ **V80** Animal-rider or occupant of animal-drawn vehicle injured in transport accident

√5ᵗʰ **V80.0** Animal-rider or occupant of animal drawn vehicle injured by fall from or being thrown from animal or animal-drawn vehicle in noncollision accident

     √6ᵗʰ **V80.01** Animal-rider injured by fall from or being thrown from animal in noncollision accident

         √7ᵗʰ **V80.010** Animal-rider injured by fall from or being thrown from horse in noncollision accident

         √7ᵗʰ **V80.018** Animal-rider injured by fall from or being thrown from other animal in noncollision accident

     √x7ᵗʰ **V80.02** Occupant of animal-drawn vehicle injured by fall from or being thrown from animal-drawn vehicle in noncollision accident
         Overturning animal-drawn vehicle NOS
         Overturning animal-drawn vehicle without collision

√5ᵗʰ **V80.1** Animal-rider or occupant of animal-drawn vehicle injured in collision with pedestrian or animal
     EXCLUDES 1   animal-rider or animal-drawn vehicle collision with animal-drawn vehicle or animal being ridden (V80.7)

     √x7ᵗʰ **V80.11** Animal-rider injured in collision with pedestrian or animal

     √x7ᵗʰ **V80.12** Occupant of animal-drawn vehicle injured in collision with pedestrian or animal

√5ᵗʰ **V80.2** Animal-rider or occupant of animal-drawn vehicle injured in collision with pedal cycle

     √x7ᵗʰ **V80.21** Animal-rider injured in collision with pedal cycle

     √x7ᵗʰ **V80.22** Occupant of animal-drawn vehicle injured in collision with pedal cycle

√5ᵗʰ **V80.3** Animal-rider or occupant of animal-drawn vehicle injured in collision with two- or three-wheeled motor vehicle

     √x7ᵗʰ **V80.31** Animal-rider injured in collision with two- or three-wheeled motor vehicle

     √x7ᵗʰ **V80.32** Occupant of animal-drawn vehicle injured in collision with two- or three-wheeled motor vehicle

√5ᵗʰ **V80.4** Animal-rider or occupant of animal-drawn vehicle injured in collision with car, pick-up truck, van, heavy transport vehicle or bus
     EXCLUDES 1   animal-rider injured in collision with military vehicle (V80.910)
         occupant of animal-drawn vehicle injured in collision with military vehicle (V80.920)

     √x7ᵗʰ **V80.41** Animal-rider injured in collision with car, pick-up truck, van, heavy transport vehicle or bus

     √x7ᵗʰ **V80.42** Occupant of animal-drawn vehicle injured in collision with car, pick-up truck, van, heavy transport vehicle or bus

√5ᵗʰ **V80.5** Animal-rider or occupant of animal-drawn vehicle injured in collision with other specified motor vehicle

     √x7ᵗʰ **V80.51** Animal-rider injured in collision with other specified motor vehicle

     √x7ᵗʰ **V80.52** Occupant of animal-drawn vehicle injured in collision with other specified motor vehicle

√5ᵗʰ **V80.6** Animal-rider or occupant of animal-drawn vehicle injured in collision with railway train or railway vehicle

     √x7ᵗʰ **V80.61** Animal-rider injured in collision with railway train or railway vehicle

     √x7ᵗʰ **V80.62** Occupant of animal-drawn vehicle injured in collision with railway train or railway vehicle

√5ᵗʰ **V80.7** Animal-rider or occupant of animal-drawn vehicle injured in collision with other nonmotor vehicles

     √6ᵗʰ **V80.71** Animal-rider or occupant of animal-drawn vehicle injured in collision with animal being ridden

         √7ᵗʰ **V80.710** Animal-rider injured in collision with other animal being ridden

N Newborn: 0   P Pediatric: 0-17   M Maternity: 12-55   A Adult: 15-124   **MCC** Major CC Condition   **PDxMCC** PDx acts as own MCC   **CC** CC Condition   **PDxCC** PDx acts as own CC

1176   ICD-10-CM 2018

☑7ᵗʰ **V80.711** Occupant of animal-drawn vehicle injured in collision with animal being ridden

☑6ᵗʰ **V80.72** Animal-rider or occupant of animal-drawn vehicle injured in collision with other animal-drawn vehicle

    ☑7ᵗʰ **V80.720** Animal-rider injured in collision with animal-drawn vehicle

    ☑7ᵗʰ **V80.721** Occupant of animal-drawn vehicle injured in collision with other animal-drawn vehicle

☑6ᵗʰ **V80.73** Animal-rider or occupant of animal-drawn vehicle injured in collision with streetcar

    ☑7ᵗʰ **V80.730** Animal-rider injured in collision with streetcar

    ☑7ᵗʰ **V80.731** Occupant of animal-drawn vehicle injured in collision with streetcar

☑6ᵗʰ **V80.79** Animal-rider or occupant of animal-drawn vehicle injured in collision with other nonmotor vehicles

    ☑7ᵗʰ **V80.790** Animal-rider injured in collision with other nonmotor vehicles

    ☑7ᵗʰ **V80.791** Occupant of animal-drawn vehicle injured in collision with other nonmotor vehicles

☑5ᵗʰ **V80.8** Animal-rider or occupant of animal-drawn vehicle injured in collision with fixed or stationary object

    ☑x7ᵗʰ **V80.81** Animal-rider injured in collision with fixed or stationary object

    ☑x7ᵗʰ **V80.82** Occupant of animal-drawn vehicle injured in collision with fixed or stationary object

☑5ᵗʰ **V80.9** Animal-rider or occupant of animal-drawn vehicle injured in other and unspecified transport accidents

☑6ᵗʰ **V80.91** Animal-rider injured in other and unspecified transport accidents

    ☑7ᵗʰ **V80.910** Animal-rider injured in transport accident with military vehicle

    ☑7ᵗʰ **V80.918** Animal-rider injured in other transport accident

    ☑7ᵗʰ **V80.919** Animal-rider injured in unspecified transport accident
        Animal rider accident NOS

☑6ᵗʰ **V80.92** Occupant of animal-drawn vehicle injured in other and unspecified transport accidents

    ☑7ᵗʰ **V80.920** Occupant of animal-drawn vehicle injured in transport accident with military vehicle

    ☑7ᵗʰ **V80.928** Occupant of animal-drawn vehicle injured in other transport accident

    ☑7ᵗʰ **V80.929** Occupant of animal-drawn vehicle injured in unspecified transport accident
        Animal-drawn vehicle accident NOS

☑4ᵗʰ **V81** Occupant of railway train or railway vehicle injured in transport accident
    INCLUDES derailment of railway train or railway vehicle
        person on outside of train
    EXCLUDES 1 streetcar (V82.-)

☑x7ᵗʰ **V81.0** Occupant of railway train or railway vehicle injured in collision with motor vehicle in nontraffic accident
    EXCLUDES 1 occupant of railway train or railway vehicle injured due to collision with military vehicle (V81.83)

☑x7ᵗʰ **V81.1** Occupant of railway train or railway vehicle injured in collision with motor vehicle in traffic accident
    EXCLUDES 1 occupant of railway train or railway vehicle injured due to collision with military vehicle (V81.83)

☑x7ᵗʰ **V81.2** Occupant of railway train or railway vehicle injured in collision with or hit by rolling stock

☑x7ᵗʰ **V81.3** Occupant of railway train or railway vehicle injured in collision with other object
    Railway collision NOS

☑x7ᵗʰ **V81.4** Person injured while boarding or alighting from railway train or railway vehicle

☑x7ᵗʰ **V81.5** Occupant of railway train or railway vehicle injured by fall in railway train or railway vehicle

☑x7ᵗʰ **V81.6** Occupant of railway train or railway vehicle injured by fall from railway train or railway vehicle

☑x7ᵗʰ **V81.7** Occupant of railway train or railway vehicle injured in derailment without antecedent collision

☑5ᵗʰ **V81.8** Occupant of railway train or railway vehicle injured in other specified railway accidents

☑x7ᵗʰ **V81.81** Occupant of railway train or railway vehicle injured due to explosion or fire on train

☑x7ᵗʰ **V81.82** Occupant of railway train or railway vehicle injured due to object falling onto train
    Occupant of railway train or railway vehicle injured due to falling earth onto train
    Occupant of railway train or railway vehicle injured due to falling rocks onto train
    Occupant of railway train or railway vehicle injured due to falling snow onto train
    Occupant of railway train or railway vehicle injured due to falling trees onto train

☑x7ᵗʰ **V81.83** Occupant of railway train or railway vehicle injured due to collision with military vehicle

☑x7ᵗʰ **V81.89** Occupant of railway train or railway vehicle injured due to other specified railway accident

☑x7ᵗʰ **V81.9** Occupant of railway train or railway vehicle injured in unspecified railway accident
    Railway accident NOS

☑4ᵗʰ **V82** Occupant of powered streetcar injured in transport accident
    INCLUDES interurban electric car
        person on outside of streetcar
        tram (car)
        trolley (car)
    EXCLUDES 1 bus (V70-V79)
        motorcoach (V70-V79)
        nonpowered streetcar (V76.-)
        train (V81.-)

☑x7ᵗʰ **V82.0** Occupant of streetcar injured in collision with motor vehicle in nontraffic accident

☑x7ᵗʰ **V82.1** Occupant of streetcar injured in collision with motor vehicle in traffic accident

☑x7ᵗʰ **V82.2** Occupant of streetcar injured in collision with or hit by rolling stock

☑x7ᵗʰ **V82.3** Occupant of streetcar injured in collision with other object
    EXCLUDES 1 collision with animal-drawn vehicle or animal being ridden (V82.8)

☑x7ᵗʰ **V82.4** Person injured while boarding or alighting from streetcar

☑x7ᵗʰ **V82.5** Occupant of streetcar injured by fall in streetcar
    EXCLUDES 1 fall in streetcar:
        while boarding or alighting (V82.4)
        with antecedent collision (V82.0-V82.3)

☑x7ᵗʰ **V82.6** Occupant of streetcar injured by fall from streetcar
    EXCLUDES 1 fall from streetcar:
        while boarding or alighting (V82.4)
        with antecedent collision (V82.0-V82.3)

☑x7ᵗʰ **V82.7** Occupant of streetcar injured in derailment without antecedent collision
    EXCLUDES 1 occupant of streetcar injured in derailment with antecedent collision (V82.0-V82.3)

☑x7ᵗʰ **V82.8** Occupant of streetcar injured in other specified transport accidents
    Streetcar collision with military vehicle
    Streetcar collision with train or nonmotor vehicles

☑x7ᵗʰ **V82.9** Occupant of streetcar injured in unspecified traffic accident
    Streetcar accident NOS

☑4ᵗʰ **V83** Occupant of special vehicle mainly used on industrial premises injured in transport accident
    INCLUDES battery-powered airport passenger vehicle
        battery-powered truck (baggage) (mail)
        coal-car in mine
        forklift (truck)
        logging car
        self-propelled industrial truck
        station baggage truck (powered)
        tram, truck, or tub (powered) in mine or quarry
    EXCLUDES 1 special construction vehicles (V85.-)
        special industrial vehicle in stationary use or maintenance (W31.-)

☑x7ᵗʰ **V83.0** Driver of special industrial vehicle injured in traffic accident

☑x7ᵗʰ **V83.1** Passenger of special industrial vehicle injured in traffic accident

☑x7ᵗʰ **V83.2** Person on outside of special industrial vehicle injured in traffic accident

☑x7ᵗʰ **V83.3** Unspecified occupant of special industrial vehicle injured in traffic accident

---

☑ Additional Character Req   ☑x7ᵗʰ Placeholder Alert   Unacceptable PDx   Manifestation   H1 - H14 HAC   HCC CMS-HCC Condition   EXCLUDES 1 Not Coded Here   EXCLUDES 2 Not Included Here

Chapter 20. External Causes of Morbidity

√x7ᵗʰ **V83.4** Person injured while boarding or alighting from special industrial vehicle

√x7ᵗʰ **V83.5** Driver of special industrial vehicle injured in nontraffic accident

√x7ᵗʰ **V83.6** Passenger of special industrial vehicle injured in nontraffic accident

√x7ᵗʰ **V83.7** Person on outside of special industrial vehicle injured in nontraffic accident

√x7ᵗʰ **V83.9** Unspecified occupant of special industrial vehicle injured in nontraffic accident
Special-industrial-vehicle accident NOS

√4ᵗʰ **V84** Occupant of special vehicle mainly used in agriculture injured in transport accident
INCLUDES   self-propelled farm machinery
tractor (and trailer)
EXCLUDES 1   animal-powered farm machinery accident (W30.8-)
contact with combine harvester (W30.0)
special agricultural vehicle in stationary use or maintenance (W30.-)

√x7ᵗʰ **V84.0** Driver of special agricultural vehicle injured in traffic accident

√x7ᵗʰ **V84.1** Passenger of special agricultural vehicle injured in traffic accident

√x7ᵗʰ **V84.2** Person on outside of special agricultural vehicle injured in traffic accident

√x7ᵗʰ **V84.3** Unspecified occupant of special agricultural vehicle injured in traffic accident

√x7ᵗʰ **V84.4** Person injured while boarding or alighting from special agricultural vehicle

√x7ᵗʰ **V84.5** Driver of special agricultural vehicle injured in nontraffic accident

√x7ᵗʰ **V84.6** Passenger of special agricultural vehicle injured in nontraffic accident

√x7ᵗʰ **V84.7** Person on outside of special agricultural vehicle injured in nontraffic accident

√x7ᵗʰ **V84.9** Unspecified occupant of special agricultural vehicle injured in nontraffic accident
Special-agricultural vehicle accident NOS

√4ᵗʰ **V85** Occupant of special construction vehicle injured in transport accident
INCLUDES   bulldozer
digger
dump truck
earth-leveller
mechanical shovel
road-roller
EXCLUDES 1   special industrial vehicle (V83.-)
special construction vehicle in stationary use or maintenance (W31.-)

√x7ᵗʰ **V85.0** Driver of special construction vehicle injured in traffic accident

√x7ᵗʰ **V85.1** Passenger of special construction vehicle injured in traffic accident

√x7ᵗʰ **V85.2** Person on outside of special construction vehicle injured in traffic accident

√x7ᵗʰ **V85.3** Unspecified occupant of special construction vehicle injured in traffic accident

√x7ᵗʰ **V85.4** Person injured while boarding or alighting from special construction vehicle

√x7ᵗʰ **V85.5** Driver of special construction vehicle injured in nontraffic accident

√x7ᵗʰ **V85.6** Passenger of special construction vehicle injured in nontraffic accident

√x7ᵗʰ **V85.7** Person on outside of special construction vehicle injured in nontraffic accident

√x7ᵗʰ **V85.9** Unspecified occupant of special construction vehicle injured in nontraffic accident
Special-construction-vehicle accident NOS

√4ᵗʰ **V86** Occupant of special all-terrain or other off-road motor vehicle, injured in transport accident
EXCLUDES 1   special all-terrain vehicle in stationary use or maintenance (W31.-)
sport-utility vehicle (V50-V59)
three-wheeled motor vehicle designed for on-road use (V30-V39)

√5ᵗʰ **V86.0** Driver of special all-terrain or other off-road motor vehicle injured in traffic accident

√x7ᵗʰ **V86.01** Driver of ambulance or fire engine injured in traffic accident

√x7ᵗʰ **V86.02** Driver of snowmobile injured in traffic accident

√x7ᵗʰ **V86.03** Driver of dune buggy injured in traffic accident

√x7ᵗʰ **V86.04** Driver of military vehicle injured in traffic accident

● √x7ᵗʰ **V86.05** Driver of 3- or 4- wheeled all-terrain vehicle (ATV) injured in traffic accident

● √x7ᵗʰ **V86.06** Driver of dirt bike or motor/cross bike injured in traffic accident

√x7ᵗʰ **V86.09** Driver of other special all-terrain or other off-road motor vehicle injured in traffic accident
Driver of dirt bike injured in traffic accident
Driver of go cart injured in traffic accident
Driver of golf cart injured in traffic accident

√5ᵗʰ **V86.1** Passenger of special all-terrain or other off-road motor vehicle injured in traffic accident

√x7ᵗʰ **V86.11** Passenger of ambulance or fire engine injured in traffic accident

√x7ᵗʰ **V86.12** Passenger of snowmobile injured in traffic accident

√x7ᵗʰ **V86.13** Passenger of dune buggy injured in traffic accident

√x7ᵗʰ **V86.14** Passenger of military vehicle injured in traffic accident

● √x7ᵗʰ **V86.15** Passenger of 3- or 4- wheeled all-terrain vehicle (ATV) injured in traffic accident

● √x7ᵗʰ **V86.16** Passenger of dirt bike or motor/cross bike injured in traffic accident

√x7ᵗʰ **V86.19** Passenger of other special all-terrain or other off-road motor vehicle injured in traffic accident
Passenger of dirt bike injured in traffic accident
Passenger of go cart injured in traffic accident
Passenger of golf cart injured in traffic accident

√5ᵗʰ **V86.2** Person on outside of special all-terrain or other off-road motor vehicle injured in traffic accident

√x7ᵗʰ **V86.21** Person on outside of ambulance or fire engine injured in traffic accident

√x7ᵗʰ **V86.22** Person on outside of snowmobile injured in traffic accident

√x7ᵗʰ **V86.23** Person on outside of dune buggy injured in traffic accident

√x7ᵗʰ **V86.24** Person on outside of military vehicle injured in traffic accident

● √x7ᵗʰ **V86.25** Person on outside of 3- or 4- wheeled all-terrain vehicle (ATV) injured in traffic accident

● √x7ᵗʰ **V86.26** Person on outside of dirt bike or motor/cross bike injured in traffic accident

√x7ᵗʰ **V86.29** Person on outside of other special all-terrain or other off-road motor vehicle injured in traffic accident
Person on outside of dirt bike injured in traffic accident
Person on outside of go cart in traffic accident
Person on outside of golf cart injured in traffic accident

√5ᵗʰ **V86.3** Unspecified occupant of special all-terrain or other off-road motor vehicle injured in traffic accident

√x7ᵗʰ **V86.31** Unspecified occupant of ambulance or fire engine injured in traffic accident

√x7ᵗʰ **V86.32** Unspecified occupant of snowmobile injured in traffic accident

√x7ᵗʰ **V86.33** Unspecified occupant of dune buggy injured in traffic accident

√x7ᵗʰ **V86.34** Unspecified occupant of military vehicle injured in traffic accident

● √x7ᵗʰ **V86.35** Unspecified occupant of 3- or 4- wheeled all-terrain vehicle (ATV) injured in traffic accident

● √x7ᵗʰ **V86.36** Unspecified occupant of dirt bike or motor/cross bike injured in traffic accident

V86.39   Unspecified occupant of other special all-terrain or other off-road motor vehicle injured in traffic accident

     Unspecified occupant of dirt bike injured in traffic accident

     Unspecified occupant of go cart injured in traffic accident

     Unspecified occupant of golf cart injured in traffic accident

✓5ᵗʰ V86.4   Person injured while boarding or alighting from special all-terrain or other off-road motor vehicle

V86.41   Person injured while boarding or alighting from ambulance or fire engine

V86.42   Person injured while boarding or alighting from snowmobile

V86.43   Person injured while boarding or alighting from dune buggy

V86.44   Person injured while boarding or alighting from military vehicle

● **V86.45**   Person injured while boarding or alighting from a 3- or 4- wheeled all-terrain vehicle (ATV)

● **V86.46**   Person injured while boarding or alighting from a dirt bike or motor/cross bike

V86.49   Person injured while boarding or alighting from other special all-terrain or other off-road motor vehicle

     Person injured while boarding or alighting from dirt bike

     Person injured while boarding or alighting from go cart

     Person injured while boarding or alighting from golf cart

✓5ᵗʰ V86.5   Driver of special all-terrain or other off-road motor vehicle injured in nontraffic accident

V86.51   Driver of ambulance or fire engine injured in nontraffic accident

V86.52   Driver of snowmobile injured in nontraffic accident

V86.53   Driver of dune buggy injured in nontraffic accident

V86.54   Driver of military vehicle injured in nontraffic accident

● **V86.55**   Driver of 3- or 4- wheeled all-terrain vehicle (ATV) injured in nontraffic accident

● **V86.56**   Driver of dirt bike or motor/cross bike injured in nontraffic accident

V86.59   Driver of other special all-terrain or other off-road motor vehicle injured in nontraffic accident

     Driver of dirt bike injured in nontraffic accident

     Driver of go cart injured in nontraffic accident

     Driver of golf cart injured in nontraffic accident

✓5ᵗʰ V86.6   Passenger of special all-terrain or other off-road motor vehicle injured in nontraffic accident

V86.61   Passenger of ambulance or fire engine injured in nontraffic accident

V86.62   Passenger of snowmobile injured in nontraffic accident

V86.63   Passenger of dune buggy injured in nontraffic accident

V86.64   Passenger of military vehicle injured in nontraffic accident

● **V86.65**   Passenger of 3- or 4- wheeled all-terrain vehicle (ATV) injured in nontraffic accident

● **V86.66**   Passenger of dirt bike or motor/cross bike injured in nontraffic accident

V86.69   Passenger of other special all-terrain or other off-road motor vehicle injured in nontraffic accident

     Passenger of dirt bike injured in nontraffic accident

     Passenger of go cart injured in nontraffic accident

     Passenger of golf cart injured in nontraffic accident

✓5ᵗʰ V86.7   Person on outside of special all-terrain or other off-road motor vehicle injured in nontraffic accident

V86.71   Person on outside of ambulance or fire engine injured in nontraffic accident

V86.72   Person on outside of snowmobile injured in nontraffic accident

V86.73   Person on outside of dune buggy injured in nontraffic accident

V86.74   Person on outside of military vehicle injured in nontraffic accident

● **V86.75**   Person on outside of 3- or 4- wheeled all-terrain vehicle (ATV) injured in nontraffic accident

● **V86.76**   Person on outside of dirt bike or motor/cross bike injured in nontraffic accident

V86.79   Person on outside of other special all-terrain or other off-road motor vehicles injured in nontraffic accident

     Person on outside of dirt bike injured in nontraffic accident

     Person on outside of go cart injured in nontraffic accident

     Person on outside of golf cart injured in nontraffic accident

✓5ᵗʰ V86.9   Unspecified occupant of special all-terrain or other off-road motor vehicle injured in nontraffic accident

V86.91   Unspecified occupant of ambulance or fire engine injured in nontraffic accident

V86.92   Unspecified occupant of snowmobile injured in nontraffic accident

V86.93   Unspecified occupant of dune buggy injured in nontraffic accident

V86.94   Unspecified occupant of military vehicle injured in nontraffic accident

● **V86.95**   Unspecified occupant of 3- or 4- wheeled all-terrain vehicle (ATV) injured in nontraffic accident

● **V86.96**   Unspecified occupant of dirt bike or motor/cross bike injured in nontraffic accident

V86.99   Unspecified occupant of other special all-terrain or other off-road motor vehicle injured in nontraffic accident

     All-terrain motor-vehicle accident NOS

     Off-road motor-vehicle accident NOS

     Other motor-vehicle accident NOS

     ~~Unspecified occupant of dirt bike injured in nontraffic accident~~

     Unspecified occupant of go cart injured in nontraffic accident

     Unspecified occupant of golf cart injured in nontraffic accident

✓4ᵗʰ V87   **Traffic accident of specified type but victim's mode of transport unknown**

     EXCLUDES 1   collision involving:
       pedal cycle (V10-V19)
       pedestrian (V01-V09)

V87.0   Person injured in collision between car and two- or three-wheeled powered vehicle (traffic)

V87.1   Person injured in collision between other motor vehicle and two- or three-wheeled motor vehicle (traffic)

V87.2   Person injured in collision between car and pick-up truck or van (traffic)

V87.3   Person injured in collision between car and bus (traffic)

V87.4   Person injured in collision between car and heavy transport vehicle (traffic)

V87.5   Person injured in collision between heavy transport vehicle and bus (traffic)

V87.6   Person injured in collision between railway train or railway vehicle and car (traffic)

V87.7   Person injured in collision between other specified motor vehicles (traffic)

V87.8   Person injured in other specified noncollision transport accidents involving motor vehicle (traffic)

V87.9   Person injured in other specified (collision)(noncollision) transport accidents involving nonmotor vehicle (traffic)

✓4ᵗʰ V88   **Nontraffic accident of specified type but victim's mode of transport unknown**

     EXCLUDES 1   collision involving:
       pedal cycle (V10-V19)
       pedestrian (V01-V09)

V88.0   Person injured in collision between car and two- or three-wheeled motor vehicle, nontraffic

V88.1   Person injured in collision between other motor vehicle and two- or three-wheeled motor vehicle, nontraffic

V88.2   Person injured in collision between car and pick-up truck or van, nontraffic

V88.3   Person injured in collision between car and bus, nontraffic

---

✓ Additional Character Req   ✓x7ᵗʰ Placeholder Alert   Unacceptable PDx   Manifestation   H1-H14 HAC   HCC CMS-HCC Condition   *EXCLUDES 1* Not Coded Here   *EXCLUDES 2* Not Included Here

ICD-10-CM 2018   1179

Chapter 20. External Causes of Morbidity

✓x7ᵗʰ **V88.4** **Person injured in collision between** car and heavy transport vehicle, **nontraffic**

✓x7ᵗʰ **V88.5** **Person injured in collision between** heavy transport vehicle and bus, **nontraffic**

✓x7ᵗʰ **V88.6** **Person injured in collision between** railway train or railway vehicle and car, **nontraffic**

✓x7ᵗʰ **V88.7** **Person injured in collision between** other specified motor vehicle, **nontraffic**

✓x7ᵗʰ **V88.8** **Person injured in** other specified noncollision transport accidents **involving** motor vehicle, **nontraffic**

✓x7ᵗʰ **V88.9** **Person injured in** other specified (collision)(noncollision) transport accidents **involving** nonmotor vehicle, **nontraffic**

✓4ᵗʰ **V89** **Motor- or nonmotor-vehicle accident, type of vehicle unspecified**

✓x7ᵗʰ **V89.0** **Person injured in unspecified** motor-vehicle **accident,** nontraffic
  Motor-vehicle accident NOS, nontraffic

✓x7ᵗʰ **V89.1** **Person injured in unspecified** nonmotor-vehicle **accident,** nontraffic
  Nonmotor-vehicle accident NOS (nontraffic)

✓x7ᵗʰ **V89.2** **Person injured in** unspecified motor-vehicle **accident,** traffic
  Motor-vehicle accident [MVA] NOS
  Road (traffic) accident [RTA] NOS

✓x7ᵗʰ **V89.3** **Person injured in** unspecified nonmotor-vehicle **accident,** traffic
  Nonmotor-vehicle traffic accident NOS

✓x7ᵗʰ **V89.9** **Person injured in** unspecified vehicle accident
  Collision NOS

Water transport accidents (V90-V94)

> The appropriate 7th character is to be added to each code from categories V90-V94.
> A   initial encounter
> D   subsequent encounter
> S   sequela

✓4ᵗʰ **V90** **Drowning and submersion due to accident to watercraft**

EXCLUDES 1   *civilian water transport accident involving military watercraft (V94.81-)*
  fall into water not from watercraft (W16.-)
  military watercraft accident in military or war operations (Y36.0-, Y37.0-)
  water-transport-related drowning or submersion without accident to watercraft (V92.-)

✓5ᵗʰ **V90.0** **Drowning and submersion due to** watercraft overturning

✓x7ᵗʰ **V90.00** **Drowning and submersion due to** merchant ship overturning

✓x7ᵗʰ **V90.01** **Drowning and submersion due to** passenger ship overturning
  Drowning and submersion due to Ferry-boat overturning
  Drowning and submersion due to Liner overturning

✓x7ᵗʰ **V90.02** **Drowning and submersion due to** fishing boat overturning

✓x7ᵗʰ **V90.03** **Drowning and submersion due to** other powered watercraft overturning
  Drowning and submersion due to Hovercraft (on open water) overturning
  Drowning and submersion due to Jet ski overturning

✓x7ᵗʰ **V90.04** **Drowning and submersion due to** sailboat overturning

✓x7ᵗʰ **V90.05** **Drowning and submersion due to** canoe or kayak overturning

✓x7ᵗʰ **V90.06** **Drowning and submersion due to** (nonpowered) inflatable craft overturning

✓x7ᵗʰ **V90.08** **Drowning and submersion due to** other unpowered watercraft overturning
  Drowning and submersion due to windsurfer overturning

✓x7ᵗʰ **V90.09** **Drowning and submersion due to** unspecified watercraft overturning
  Drowning and submersion due to boat NOS overturning
  Drowning and submersion due to ship NOS overturning
  Drowning and submersion due to watercraft NOS overturning

✓5ᵗʰ **V90.1** **Drowning and submersion due to** watercraft sinking

✓x7ᵗʰ **V90.10** **Drowning and submersion due to** merchant ship sinking

✓x7ᵗʰ **V90.11** **Drowning and submersion due to** passenger ship sinking
  Drowning and submersion due to Ferry-boat sinking
  Drowning and submersion due to Liner sinking

✓x7ᵗʰ **V90.12** **Drowning and submersion due to** fishing boat sinking

✓x7ᵗʰ **V90.13** **Drowning and submersion due to** other powered watercraft sinking
  Drowning and submersion due to Hovercraft (on open water) sinking
  Drowning and submersion due to Jet ski sinking

✓x7ᵗʰ **V90.14** **Drowning and submersion due to** sailboat sinking

✓x7ᵗʰ **V90.15** **Drowning and submersion due to** canoe or kayak sinking

✓x7ᵗʰ **V90.16** **Drowning and submersion due to** (nonpowered) inflatable craft sinking

✓x7ᵗʰ **V90.18** **Drowning and submersion due to** other unpowered watercraft sinking

✓x7ᵗʰ **V90.19** **Drowning and submersion due to** unspecified watercraft sinking
  Drowning and submersion due to boat NOS sinking
  Drowning and submersion due to ship NOS sinking
  Drowning and submersion due to watercraft NOS sinking

✓5ᵗʰ **V90.2** **Drowning and submersion due to** falling or jumping from burning **watercraft**

✓x7ᵗʰ **V90.20** **Drowning and submersion due to falling or jumping from burning** merchant ship

✓x7ᵗʰ **V90.21** **Drowning and submersion due to falling or jumping from burning** passenger ship
  Drowning and submersion due to falling or jumping from burning Ferry-boat
  Drowning and submersion due to falling or jumping from burning Liner

✓x7ᵗʰ **V90.22** **Drowning and submersion due to falling or jumping from burning** fishing boat

✓x7ᵗʰ **V90.23** **Drowning and submersion due to falling or jumping from** other burning powered **watercraft**
  Drowning and submersion due to falling and jumping from burning Hovercraft (on open water)
  Drowning and submersion due to falling and jumping from burning Jet ski

✓x7ᵗʰ **V90.24** **Drowning and submersion due to falling or jumping from burning** sailboat

✓x7ᵗʰ **V90.25** **Drowning and submersion due to falling or jumping from burning** canoe or kayak

✓x7ᵗʰ **V90.26** **Drowning and submersion due to falling or jumping from burning** (nonpowered) inflatable craft

✓x7ᵗʰ **V90.27** **Drowning and submersion due to falling or jumping from burning** water-skis

✓x7ᵗʰ **V90.28** **Drowning and submersion due to falling or jumping from** other burning unpowered **watercraft**
  Drowning and submersion due to falling and jumping from burning surf-board
  Drowning and submersion due to falling and jumping from burning windsurfer

✓x7ᵗʰ **V90.29** **Drowning and submersion due to falling or jumping from** unspecified burning watercraft
  Drowning and submersion due to falling or jumping from burning boat NOS
  Drowning and submersion due to falling or jumping from burning ship NOS
  Drowning and submersion due to falling or jumping from burning watercraft NOS

✓5ᵗʰ **V90.3** **Drowning and submersion due to** falling or jumping from crushed watercraft

✓x7ᵗʰ **V90.30** **Drowning and submersion due to falling or jumping from crushed** merchant ship

✓x7ᵗʰ **V90.31** **Drowning and submersion due to falling or jumping from crushed** passenger ship
  Drowning and submersion due to falling and jumping from crushed Ferry boat
  Drowning and submersion due to falling and jumping from crushed Liner

Ⓝ Newborn: 0   Ⓟ Pediatric: 0-17   Ⓜ Maternity: 12-55   Ⓐ Adult: 15-124   **MCC** Major CC Condition   **PDxMCC** PDx acts as own MCC   **CC** CC Condition   **PDxCC** PDx acts as own CC

1180   ICD-10-CM 2018

✓x7th **V90.32** **Drowning and submersion due to falling or jumping from crushed** fishing boat

✓x7th **V90.33** **Drowning and submersion due to falling or jumping from** other crushed powered **watercraft**
     Drowning and submersion due to falling and jumping from crushed Hovercraft
     Drowning and submersion due to falling and jumping from crushed Jet ski

✓x7th **V90.34** **Drowning and submersion due to falling or jumping from crushed** sailboat

✓x7th **V90.35** **Drowning and submersion due to falling or jumping from crushed** canoe or kayak

✓x7th **V90.36** **Drowning and submersion due to falling or jumping from crushed (nonpowered)** inflatable craft

✓x7th **V90.37** **Drowning and submersion due to falling or jumping from crushed** water-skis

✓x7th **V90.38** **Drowning and submersion due to falling or jumping from** other crushed unpowered **watercraft**
     Drowning and submersion due to falling and jumping from crushed surf-board
     Drowning and submersion due to falling and jumping from crushed windsurfer

✓x7th **V90.39** **Drowning and submersion due to falling or jumping from crushed** unspecified **watercraft**
     Drowning and submersion due to falling and jumping from crushed boat NOS
     Drowning and submersion due to falling and jumping from crushed ship NOS
     Drowning and submersion due to falling and jumping from crushed watercraft NOS

✓5th **V90.8** **Drowning and submersion due to** other accident to **watercraft**

✓x7th **V90.80** **Drowning and submersion due to other accident to** merchant ship

✓x7th **V90.81** **Drowning and submersion due to other accident to** passenger ship
     Drowning and submersion due to other accident to Ferry-boat
     Drowning and submersion due to other accident to Liner

✓x7th **V90.82** **Drowning and submersion due to other accident to** fishing boat

✓x7th **V90.83** **Drowning and submersion due to other accident to** other powered **watercraft**
     Drowning and submersion due to other accident to Hovercraft (on open water)
     Drowning and submersion due to other accident to Jet ski

✓x7th **V90.84** **Drowning and submersion due to other accident to** sailboat

✓x7th **V90.85** **Drowning and submersion due to other accident to** canoe or kayak

✓x7th **V90.86** **Drowning and submersion due to other accident to (nonpowered)** inflatable craft

✓x7th **V90.87** **Drowning and submersion due to other accident to** water-skis

✓x7th **V90.88** **Drowning and submersion due to other accident to** other unpowered **watercraft**
     Drowning and submersion due to other accident to surf-board
     Drowning and submersion due to other accident to windsurfer

✓x7th **V90.89** **Drowning and submersion due to other accident to** unspecified **watercraft**
     Drowning and submersion due to other accident to boat NOS
     Drowning and submersion due to other accident to ship NOS
     Drowning and submersion due to other accident to watercraft NOS

✓4th **V91** **Other injury due to accident to watercraft**
     INCLUDES   any injury except drowning and submersion as a result of an accident to watercraft
     EXCLUDES 1   *civilian water transport accident involving military watercraft (V94.81-)*
     military watercraft accident in military or war operations (Y36, Y37.-)
     EXCLUDES 2   *drowning and submersion due to accident to watercraft (V90.-)*

✓5th **V91.0** **Burn due to watercraft on fire**
     EXCLUDES 1   *burn from localized fire or explosion on board ship without accident to watercraft (V93.-)*

✓x7th **V91.00** **Burn due to merchant ship on fire**

✓x7th **V91.01** **Burn due to passenger ship on fire**
     Burn due to Ferry-boat on fire
     Burn due to Liner on fire

✓x7th **V91.02** **Burn due to fishing boat on fire**

✓x7th **V91.03** **Burn due to other powered watercraft on fire**
     Burn due to Hovercraft (on open water) on fire
     Burn due to Jet ski on fire

✓x7th **V91.04** **Burn due to sailboat on fire**

✓x7th **V91.05** **Burn due to canoe or kayak on fire**

✓x7th **V91.06** **Burn due to (nonpowered) inflatable craft on fire**

✓x7th **V91.07** **Burn due to water-skis on fire**

✓x7th **V91.08** **Burn due to other unpowered watercraft on fire**

✓x7th **V91.09** **Burn due to unspecified watercraft on fire**
     Burn due to boat NOS on fire
     Burn due to ship NOS on fire
     Burn due to watercraft NOS on fire

✓5th **V91.1** **Crushed between watercraft and other watercraft or other object due to collision**
     Crushed by lifeboat after abandoning ship in a collision
     NOTE   Select the specified type of watercraft that the victim was on at the time of the collision

✓x7th **V91.10** **Crushed between merchant ship and other watercraft or other object due to collision**

✓x7th **V91.11** **Crushed between passenger ship and other watercraft or other object due to collision**
     Crushed between Ferry-boat and other watercraft or other object due to collision
     Crushed between Liner and other watercraft or other object due to collision

✓x7th **V91.12** **Crushed between fishing boat and other watercraft or other object due to collision**

✓x7th **V91.13** **Crushed between other powered watercraft and other watercraft or other object due to collision**
     Crushed between Hovercraft (on open water) and other watercraft or other object due to collision
     Crushed between Jet ski and other watercraft or other object due to collision

✓x7th **V91.14** **Crushed between sailboat and other watercraft or other object due to collision**

✓x7th **V91.15** **Crushed between canoe or kayak and other watercraft or other object due to collision**

✓x7th **V91.16** **Crushed between (nonpowered) inflatable craft and other watercraft or other object due to collision**

✓x7th **V91.18** **Crushed between other unpowered watercraft and other watercraft or other object due to collision**
     Crushed between surfboard and other watercraft or other object due to collision
     Crushed between windsurfer and other watercraft or other object due to collision

✓x7th **V91.19** **Crushed between unspecified watercraft and other watercraft or other object due to collision**
     Crushed between boat NOS and other watercraft or other object due to collision
     Crushed between ship NOS and other watercraft or other object due to collision
     Crushed between watercraft NOS and other watercraft or other object due to collision

✓ Additional Character Req   ✓x7th Placeholder Alert   Unacceptable PDx   Manifestation   H1-H14 HAC   HCC CMS-HCC Condition   EXCLUDES 1 Not Coded Here   EXCLUDES 2 Not Included Here

ICD-10-CM 2018   1181

V90.32–V91.19

✓5ᵗʰ V91.2 Fall due to collision between watercraft and other watercraft or other object

Fall while remaining on watercraft after collision

> **NOTE** Select the specified type of watercraft that the victim was on at the time of the collision.

> **EXCLUDES 1** crushed between watercraft and other watercraft and other object due to collision (V91.1-)
> drowning and submersion due to falling from crushed watercraft (V90.3-)

✓x 7ᵗʰ V91.20 Fall due to collision between merchant ship and other watercraft or other object

✓x 7ᵗʰ V91.21 Fall due to collision between passenger ship and other watercraft or other object

Fall due to collision between Ferry-boat and other watercraft or other object
Fall due to collision between Liner and other watercraft or other object

✓x 7ᵗʰ V91.22 Fall due to collision between fishing boat and other watercraft or other object

✓x 7ᵗʰ V91.23 Fall due to collision between other powered watercraft and other watercraft or other object

Fall due to collision between Hovercraft (on open water) and other watercraft or other object
Fall due to collision between Jet ski and other watercraft or other object

✓x 7ᵗʰ V91.24 Fall due to collision between sailboat and other watercraft or other object

✓x 7ᵗʰ V91.25 Fall due to collision between canoe or kayak and other watercraft or other object

✓x 7ᵗʰ V91.26 Fall due to collision between (nonpowered) inflatable craft and other watercraft or other object

✓x 7ᵗʰ V91.29 Fall due to collision between unspecified watercraft and other watercraft or other object

Fall due to collision between boat NOS and other watercraft or other object
Fall due to collision between ship NOS and other watercraft or other object
Fall due to collision between watercraft NOS and other watercraft or other object

✓5ᵗʰ V91.3 Hit or struck by falling object due to accident to watercraft

Hit or struck by falling object (part of damaged watercraft or other object) after falling or jumping from damaged watercraft

> **EXCLUDES 2** drowning or submersion due to fall or jumping from damaged watercraft (V90.2-, V90.3-)

✓x 7ᵗʰ V91.30 Hit or struck by falling object due to accident to merchant ship

✓x 7ᵗʰ V91.31 Hit or struck by falling object due to accident to passenger ship

Hit or struck by falling object due to accident to Ferry-boat
Hit or struck by falling object due to accident to Liner

✓x 7ᵗʰ V91.32 Hit or struck by falling object due to accident to fishing boat

✓x 7ᵗʰ V91.33 Hit or struck by falling object due to accident to other powered watercraft

Hit or struck by falling object due to accident to Hovercraft (on open water)
Hit or struck by falling object due to accident to Jet ski

✓x 7ᵗʰ V91.34 Hit or struck by falling object due to accident to sailboat

✓x 7ᵗʰ V91.35 Hit or struck by falling object due to accident to canoe or kayak

✓x 7ᵗʰ V91.36 Hit or struck by falling object due to accident to (nonpowered) inflatable craft

✓x 7ᵗʰ V91.37 Hit or struck by falling object due to accident to water-skis

Hit by water-skis after jumping off of waterskis

✓x 7ᵗʰ V91.38 Hit or struck by falling object due to accident to other unpowered watercraft

Hit or struck by surf-board after falling off damaged surf-board
Hit or struck by object after falling off damaged windsurfer

✓x 7ᵗʰ V91.39 Hit or struck by falling object due to accident to unspecified watercraft

Hit or struck by falling object due to accident to boat NOS
Hit or struck by falling object due to accident to ship NOS
Hit or struck by falling object due to accident to watercraft NOS

✓5ᵗʰ V91.8 Other injury due to other accident to watercraft

✓x 7ᵗʰ V91.80 Other injury due to other accident to merchant ship

✓x 7ᵗʰ V91.81 Other injury due to other accident to passenger ship

Other injury due to other accident to Ferry-boat
Other injury due to other accident to Liner

✓x 7ᵗʰ V91.82 Other injury due to other accident to fishing boat

✓x 7ᵗʰ V91.83 Other injury due to other accident to other powered watercraft

Other injury due to other accident to Hovercraft (on open water)
Other injury due to other accident to Jet ski

✓x 7ᵗʰ V91.84 Other injury due to other accident to sailboat

✓x 7ᵗʰ V91.85 Other injury due to other accident to canoe or kayak

✓x 7ᵗʰ V91.86 Other injury due to other accident to (nonpowered) inflatable craft

✓x 7ᵗʰ V91.87 Other injury due to other accident to water-skis

✓x 7ᵗʰ V91.88 Other injury due to other accident to other unpowered watercraft

Other injury due to other accident to surf-board
Other injury due to other accident to windsurfer

✓x 7ᵗʰ V91.89 Other injury due to other accident to unspecified watercraft

Other injury due to other accident to boat NOS
Other injury due to other accident to ship NOS
Other injury due to other accident to watercraft NOS

✓4ᵗʰ V92 Drowning and submersion due to accident on board watercraft, without accident to watercraft

> **EXCLUDES 1** civilian water transport accident involving military watercraft (V94.81-)
> drowning or submersion due to accident to watercraft (V90-V91)
> drowning or submersion of diver who voluntarily jumps from boat not involved in an accident (W16.711, W16.721)
> fall into water without watercraft (W16.-)
> military watercraft accident in military or war operations (Y36, Y37)

✓5ᵗʰ V92.0 Drowning and submersion due to fall off watercraft

Drowning and submersion due to fall from gangplank of watercraft
Drowning and submersion due to fall overboard watercraft

> **EXCLUDES 2** hitting head on object or bottom of body of water due to fall from watercraft (V94.0-)

✓x 7ᵗʰ V92.00 Drowning and submersion due to fall off merchant ship

✓x 7ᵗʰ V92.01 Drowning and submersion due to fall off passenger ship

Drowning and submersion due to fall off Ferry-boat
Drowning and submersion due to fall off Liner

✓x 7ᵗʰ V92.02 Drowning and submersion due to fall off fishing boat

✓x 7ᵗʰ V92.03 Drowning and submersion due to fall off other powered watercraft

Drowning and submersion due to fall off Hovercraft (on open water)
Drowning and submersion due to fall off Jet ski

✓x 7ᵗʰ V92.04 Drowning and submersion due to fall off sailboat

✓x 7ᵗʰ V92.05 Drowning and submersion due to fall off canoe or kayak

✓x 7ᵗʰ V92.06 Drowning and submersion due to fall off (nonpowered) inflatable craft

✓x 7ᵗʰ V92.07 Drowning and submersion due to fall off water-skis

> **EXCLUDES 1** drowning and submersion due to falling off burning water-skis (V90.27)
> drowning and submersion due to falling off crushed water-skis (V90.37)
> hit by boat while water-skiing NOS (V94.X)

Ⓝ Newborn: 0 Ⓟ Pediatric: 0-17 Ⓜ Maternity: 12-55 Ⓐ Adult: 15-124 MCC Major CC Condition PDxMCC PDx acts as own MCC CC CC Condition PDxCC PDx acts as own CC

1182   ICD-10-CM 2018

✓x7ᵗʰ V92.08 Drowning and submersion due to fall off other unpowered **watercraft**
    Drowning and submersion due to fall off surf-board
    Drowning and submersion due to fall off windsurfer
    EXCLUDES 1 *drowning and submersion due to fall off burning unpowered watercraft (V90.28)*
        drowning and submersion due to fall off crushed unpowered watercraft (V90.38)
        drowning and submersion due to fall off damaged unpowered watercraft (V90.88)
        drowning and submersion due to rider of nonpowered watercraft being hit by other watercraft (V94.-)
        other injury due to rider of nonpowered watercraft being hit by other watercraft (V94.-)

✓x7ᵗʰ V92.09 Drowning and submersion due to fall off unspecified **watercraft**
    Drowning and submersion due to fall off boat NOS
    Drowning and submersion due to fall off ship
    Drowning and submersion due to fall off watercraft NOS

✓5ᵗʰ V92.1 Drowning and submersion due to being thrown overboard **by motion of watercraft**
    EXCLUDES 1 *drowning and submersion due to fall off surf-board (V92.08)*
        drowning and submersion due to fall off water-skis (V92.07)
        drowning and submersion due to fall off windsurfer (V92.08)

✓x7ᵗʰ V92.10 Drowning and submersion due to being thrown overboard by motion of merchant ship

✓x7ᵗʰ V92.11 Drowning and submersion due to being thrown overboard by motion of passenger ship
    Drowning and submersion due to being thrown overboard by motion of Ferry-boat
    Drowning and submersion due to being thrown overboard by motion of Liner

✓x7ᵗʰ V92.12 Drowning and submersion due to being thrown overboard by motion of fishing boat

✓x7ᵗʰ V92.13 Drowning and submersion due to being thrown overboard by motion of other powered **watercraft**
    Drowning and submersion due to being thrown overboard by motion of Hovercraft

✓x7ᵗʰ V92.14 Drowning and submersion due to being thrown overboard by motion of sailboat

✓x7ᵗʰ V92.15 Drowning and submersion due to being thrown overboard by motion of canoe or kayak

✓x7ᵗʰ V92.16 Drowning and submersion due to being thrown overboard by motion of (nonpowered) inflatable **craft**

✓x7ᵗʰ V92.19 Drowning and submersion due to being thrown overboard by motion of unspecified **watercraft**
    Drowning and submersion due to being thrown overboard by motion of boat NOS
    Drowning and submersion due to being thrown overboard by motion of ship NOS
    Drowning and submersion due to being thrown overboard by motion of watercraft NOS

✓5ᵗʰ V92.2 Drowning and submersion due to being washed overboard **from watercraft**
    Code first any associated cataclysm (X37.0-)

✓x7ᵗʰ V92.20 Drowning and submersion due to being washed overboard from merchant ship

✓x7ᵗʰ V92.21 Drowning and submersion due to being washed overboard from passenger ship
    Drowning and submersion due to being washed overboard from Ferry-boat
    Drowning and submersion due to being washed overboard from Liner

✓x7ᵗʰ V92.22 Drowning and submersion due to being washed overboard from fishing boat

✓x7ᵗʰ V92.23 Drowning and submersion due to being washed overboard from other powered **watercraft**
    Drowning and submersion due to being washed overboard from Hovercraft (on open water)
    Drowning and submersion due to being washed overboard from Jet ski

✓x7ᵗʰ V92.24 Drowning and submersion due to being washed overboard from sailboat

✓x7ᵗʰ V92.25 Drowning and submersion due to being washed overboard from canoe or kayak

✓x7ᵗʰ V92.26 Drowning and submersion due to being washed overboard from (nonpowered) inflatable craft

✓x7ᵗʰ V92.27 Drowning and submersion due to being washed overboard from water-skis
    EXCLUDES 1 *drowning and submersion due to fall off water-skis (V92.07)*

✓x7ᵗʰ V92.28 Drowning and submersion due to being washed overboard from other unpowered **watercraft**
    Drowning and submersion due to being washed overboard from surf-board
    Drowning and submersion due to being washed overboard from windsurfer

✓x7ᵗʰ V92.29 Drowning and submersion due to being washed overboard from unspecified **watercraft**
    Drowning and submersion due to being washed overboard from boat NOS
    Drowning and submersion due to being washed overboard from ship NOS
    Drowning and submersion due to being washed overboard from watercraft NOS

✓4ᵗʰ V93 Other injury due to accident on board watercraft, without accident to watercraft
    EXCLUDES 1 *civilian water transport accident involving military watercraft (V94.81-)*
        other injury due to accident to watercraft (V91.-)
        military watercraft accident in military or war operations (Y36, Y37.-)
    EXCLUDES 2 *drowning and submersion due to accident on board watercraft, without accident to watercraft (V92.-)*

✓5ᵗʰ V93.0 Burn due to localized fire on board watercraft
    EXCLUDES 1 *burn due to watercraft on fire (V91.0-)*

✓x7ᵗʰ V93.00 Burn due to localized fire on board merchant vessel

✓x7ᵗʰ V93.01 Burn due to localized fire on board passenger vessel
    Burn due to localized fire on board Ferry-boat
    Burn due to localized fire on board Liner

✓x7ᵗʰ V93.02 Burn due to localized fire on board fishing boat

✓x7ᵗʰ V93.03 Burn due to localized fire on board other powered **watercraft**
    Burn due to localized fire on board Hovercraft
    Burn due to localized fire on board Jet ski

✓x7ᵗʰ V93.04 Burn due to localized fire on board sailboat

✓x7ᵗʰ V93.09 Burn due to localized fire on board unspecified **watercraft**
    Burn due to localized fire on board boat NOS
    Burn due to localized fire on board ship NOS
    Burn due to localized fire on board watercraft NOS

✓5ᵗʰ V93.1 Other burn on board watercraft
    Burn due to source other than fire on board watercraft
    EXCLUDES 1 *burn due to watercraft on fire (V91.0-)*

✓x7ᵗʰ V93.10 Other burn on board merchant vessel

✓x7ᵗʰ V93.11 Other burn on board passenger vessel
    Other burn on board Ferry-boat
    Other burn on board Liner

✓x7ᵗʰ V93.12 Other burn on board fishing boat

✓x7ᵗʰ V93.13 Other burn on board other powered **watercraft**
    Other burn on board Hovercraft
    Other burn on board Jet ski

✓x7ᵗʰ V93.14 Other burn on board sailboat

✓x7ᵗʰ V93.19 Other burn on board unspecified **watercraft**
    Other burn on board boat NOS
    Other burn on board ship NOS
    Other burn on board watercraft NOS

✓5ᵗʰ V93.2 Heat exposure on board watercraft
    EXCLUDES 1 *exposure to man-made heat not aboard watercraft (W92)*
        exposure to natural heat while on board watercraft (X30)
        exposure to sunlight while on board watercraft (X32)
    EXCLUDES 2 *burn due to fire on board watercraft (V93.0-)*

✓x7ᵗʰ V93.20 Heat exposure on board merchant ship

✓x7ᵗʰ V93.21 Heat exposure on board passenger ship
    Heat exposure on board Ferry-boat
    Heat exposure on board Liner

✓x7ᵗʰ V93.22 Heat exposure on board fishing boat

✔Additional Character Req   ✓x7ᵗʰ Placeholder Alert   Unacceptable PDx   Manifestation   **H1**-**H14** HAC   **HCC** CMS-HCC Condition   **EXCLUDES 1** Not Coded Here   **EXCLUDES 2** Not Included Here

Chapter 20. External Causes of Morbidity

V93.23–V94.81Ø

√x7ᵗʰ **V93.23 Heat exposure on board** other powered **watercraft**
Heat exposure on board hovercraft

√x7ᵗʰ **V93.24 Heat exposure on board** sailboat

√x7ᵗʰ **V93.29 Heat exposure on board** unspecified **watercraft**
Heat exposure on board boat NOS
Heat exposure on board ship NOS
Heat exposure on board watercraft NOS

√5ᵗʰ **V93.3 Fall on board watercraft**
EXCLUDES 1   *fall due to collision of watercraft (V91.2-)*

√x7ᵗʰ **V93.3Ø Fall on board** merchant ship

√x7ᵗʰ **V93.31 Fall on board** passenger ship
Fall on board Ferry-boat
Fall on board Liner

√x7ᵗʰ **V93.32 Fall on board** fishing boat

√x7ᵗʰ **V93.33 Fall on board** other powered **watercraft**
Fall on board Hovercraft (on open water)
Fall on board Jet ski

√x7ᵗʰ **V93.34 Fall on board** sailboat

√x7ᵗʰ **V93.35 Fall on board** canoe or kayak

√x7ᵗʰ **V93.36 Fall on board (nonpowered)** inflatable craft

√x7ᵗʰ **V93.38 Fall on board** other unpowered **watercraft**

√x7ᵗʰ **V93.39 Fall on board** unspecified **watercraft**
Fall on board boat NOS
Fall on board ship NOS
Fall on board watercraft NOS

√5ᵗʰ **V93.4 Struck by falling object on board watercraft**
Hit by falling object on board watercraft
EXCLUDES 1   *struck by falling object due to accident to watercraft (V91.3)*

√x7ᵗʰ **V93.4Ø Struck by falling object on** merchant ship

√x7ᵗʰ **V93.41 Struck by falling object on** passenger ship
Struck by falling object on Ferry-boat
Struck by falling object on Liner

√x7ᵗʰ **V93.42 Struck by falling object on** fishing boat

√x7ᵗʰ **V93.43 Struck by falling object on** other powered **watercraft**
Struck by falling object on Hovercraft

√x7ᵗʰ **V93.44 Struck by falling object on** sailboat

√x7ᵗʰ **V93.48 Struck by falling object on** other unpowered **watercraft**

√x7ᵗʰ **V93.49 Struck by falling object on** unspecified **watercraft**

√5ᵗʰ **V93.5 Explosion on board watercraft**
Boiler explosion on steamship
EXCLUDES 2   *fire on board watercraft (V93.Ø-)*

√x7ᵗʰ **V93.5Ø Explosion on board** merchant ship

√x7ᵗʰ **V93.51 Explosion on board** passenger ship
Explosion on board Ferry-boat
Explosion on board Liner

√x7ᵗʰ **V93.52 Explosion on board** fishing boat

√x7ᵗʰ **V93.53 Explosion on board** other powered **watercraft**
Explosion on board Hovercraft
Explosion on board Jet ski

√x7ᵗʰ **V93.54 Explosion on board** sailboat

√x7ᵗʰ **V93.59 Explosion on board** unspecified **watercraft**
Explosion on board boat NOS
Explosion on board ship NOS
Explosion on board watercraft NOS

√5ᵗʰ **V93.6 Machinery accident on board watercraft**
EXCLUDES 1   *machinery explosion on board watercraft (V93.4-)*
machinery fire on board watercraft (V93.Ø-)

√x7ᵗʰ **V93.6Ø Machinery accident on board** merchant ship

√x7ᵗʰ **V93.61 Machinery accident on board** passenger ship
Machinery accident on board Ferry-boat
Machinery accident on board Liner

√x7ᵗʰ **V93.62 Machinery accident on board** fishing boat

√x7ᵗʰ **V93.63 Machinery accident on board** other powered **watercraft**
Machinery accident on board Hovercraft

√x7ᵗʰ **V93.64 Machinery accident on board** sailboat

√x7ᵗʰ **V93.69 Machinery accident on board** unspecified **watercraft**
Machinery accident on board boat NOS
Machinery accident on board ship NOS
Machinery accident on board watercraft NOS

√5ᵗʰ **V93.8 Other injury due to other accident on board watercraft**
Accidental poisoning by gases or fumes on watercraft

√x7ᵗʰ **V93.8Ø Other injury due to other accident on board** merchant ship

√x7ᵗʰ **V93.81 Other injury due to other accident on board** passenger ship
Other injury due to other accident on board Ferry-boat
Other injury due to other accident on board Liner

√x7ᵗʰ **V93.82 Other injury due to other accident on board** fishing boat

√x7ᵗʰ **V93.83 Other injury due to other accident on board** other powered **watercraft**
Other injury due to other accident on board Hovercraft
Other injury due to other accident on board Jet ski

√x7ᵗʰ **V93.84 Other injury due to other accident on board** sailboat

√x7ᵗʰ **V93.85 Other injury due to other accident on board** canoe or kayak

√x7ᵗʰ **V93.86 Other injury due to other accident on board (nonpowered)** inflatable craft

√x7ᵗʰ **V93.87 Other injury due to other accident on board** water-skis
Hit or struck by object while waterskiing

√x7ᵗʰ **V93.88 Other injury due to other accident on board** other unpowered **watercraft**
Hit or struck by object while surfing
Hit or struck by object while on board windsurfer

√x7ᵗʰ **V93.89 Other injury due to other accident on board** unspecified **watercraft**
Other injury due to other accident on board boat NOS
Other injury due to other accident on board ship NOS
Other injury due to other accident on board watercraft NOS

√4ᵗʰ **V94 Other and unspecified water transport accidents**
EXCLUDES 1   *military watercraft accidents in military or war operations (Y36, Y37)*

√x7ᵗʰ **V94.Ø Hitting object or bottom of body of water due to fall from watercraft**
EXCLUDES 2   *drowning and submersion due to fall from watercraft (V92.Ø-)*

√5ᵗʰ **V94.1 Bather struck by watercraft**
Swimmer hit by watercraft

√x7ᵗʰ **V94.11 Bather struck by** powered **watercraft**

√x7ᵗʰ **V94.12 Bather struck by** nonpowered **watercraft**

√5ᵗʰ **V94.2 Rider of nonpowered watercraft struck by other watercraft**

√x7ᵗʰ **V94.21 Rider of nonpowered watercraft struck by** other nonpowered **watercraft**
Canoer hit by other nonpowered watercraft
Surfer hit by other nonpowered watercraft
Windsurfer hit by other nonpowered watercraft

√x7ᵗʰ **V94.22 Rider of nonpowered watercraft struck by** powered **watercraft**
Canoer hit by motorboat
Surfer hit by motorboat
Windsurfer hit by motorboat

√5ᵗʰ **V94.3 Injury to rider of (inflatable) watercraft being pulled behind other watercraft**

√x7ᵗʰ **V94.31 Injury to rider of (inflatable)** recreational **watercraft being pulled behind other watercraft**
Injury to rider of inner-tube pulled behind motor boat

√x7ᵗʰ **V94.32 Injury to rider of** non-recreational **watercraft being pulled behind other watercraft**
Injury to occupant of dingy being pulled behind boat or ship
Injury to occupant of life-raft being pulled behind boat or ship

√x7ᵗʰ **V94.4 Injury to barefoot water-skier**
Injury to person being pulled behind boat or ship

√5ᵗʰ **V94.8 Other water transport accident**

√6ᵗʰ **V94.81 Water transport accident involving military watercraft**

√7ᵗʰ **V94.81Ø Civilian watercraft involved in water transport accident with military watercraft**
Passenger on civilian watercraft injured due to accident with military watercraft

---

N Newborn: 0   P Pediatric: 0-17   M Maternity: 12-55   A Adult: 15-124   MCC Major CC Condition   PDxMCC PDx acts as own MCC   CC CC Condition   PDxCC PDx acts as own CC

1184   ICD-10-CM 2018

✓7ᵗʰ **V94.811** Civilian in water injured by military watercraft

✓7ᵗʰ **V94.818** Other water transport accident involving military watercraft

✓x7ᵗʰ **V94.89** Other water transport accident

✓x7ᵗʰ **V94.9** Unspecified water transport accident
Water transport accident NOS

Air and space transport accidents (V95-V97)

EXCLUDES 1 *military aircraft accidents in military or war operations (Y36, Y37)*

The appropriate 7th character is to be added to each code from categories V95-V97.
A   initial encounter
D   subsequent encounter
S   sequela

✓4ᵗʰ **V95** Accident to powered aircraft causing injury to occupant

✓5ᵗʰ **V95.0** Helicopter accident injuring occupant

✓x7ᵗʰ **V95.00** Unspecified helicopter accident injuring occupant

✓x7ᵗʰ **V95.01** Helicopter crash injuring occupant

✓x7ᵗʰ **V95.02** Forced landing of helicopter injuring occupant

✓x7ᵗʰ **V95.03** Helicopter collision injuring occupant
Helicopter collision with any object, fixed, movable or moving

✓x7ᵗʰ **V95.04** Helicopter fire injuring occupant

✓x7ᵗʰ **V95.05** Helicopter explosion injuring occupant

✓x7ᵗʰ **V95.09** Other helicopter accident injuring occupant

✓5ᵗʰ **V95.1** Ultralight, microlight or powered-glider accident injuring occupant

✓x7ᵗʰ **V95.10** Unspecified ultralight, microlight or powered-glider accident injuring occupant

✓x7ᵗʰ **V95.11** Ultralight, microlight or powered-glider crash injuring occupant

✓x7ᵗʰ **V95.12** Forced landing of ultralight, microlight or powered-glider injuring occupant

✓x7ᵗʰ **V95.13** Ultralight, microlight or powered-glider collision injuring occupant
Ultralight, microlight or powered-glider collision with any object, fixed, movable or moving

✓x7ᵗʰ **V95.14** Ultralight, microlight or powered-glider fire injuring occupant

✓x7ᵗʰ **V95.15** Ultralight, microlight or powered-glider explosion injuring occupant

✓x7ᵗʰ **V95.19** Other ultralight, microlight or powered-glider accident injuring occupant

✓5ᵗʰ **V95.2** Other private fixed-wing aircraft accident injuring occupant

✓x7ᵗʰ **V95.20** Unspecified accident to other private fixed-wing aircraft, injuring occupant

✓x7ᵗʰ **V95.21** Other private fixed-wing aircraft crash injuring occupant

✓x7ᵗʰ **V95.22** Forced landing of other private fixed-wing aircraft injuring occupant

✓x7ᵗʰ **V95.23** Other private fixed-wing aircraft collision injuring occupant
Other private fixed-wing aircraft collision with any object, fixed, movable or moving

✓x7ᵗʰ **V95.24** Other private fixed-wing aircraft fire injuring occupant

✓x7ᵗʰ **V95.25** Other private fixed-wing aircraft explosion injuring occupant

✓x7ᵗʰ **V95.29** Other accident to other private fixed-wing aircraft injuring occupant

✓5ᵗʰ **V95.3** Commercial fixed-wing aircraft accident injuring occupant

✓x7ᵗʰ **V95.30** Unspecified accident to commercial fixed-wing aircraft injuring occupant

✓x7ᵗʰ **V95.31** Commercial fixed-wing aircraft crash injuring occupant

✓x7ᵗʰ **V95.32** Forced landing of commercial fixed-wing aircraft injuring occupant

✓x7ᵗʰ **V95.33** Commercial fixed-wing aircraft collision injuring occupant
Commercial fixed-wing aircraft collision with any object, fixed, movable or moving

✓x7ᵗʰ **V95.34** Commercial fixed-wing aircraft fire injuring occupant

✓x7ᵗʰ **V95.35** Commercial fixed-wing aircraft explosion injuring occupant

✓x7ᵗʰ **V95.39** Other accident to commercial fixed-wing aircraft injuring occupant

✓5ᵗʰ **V95.4** Spacecraft accident injuring occupant

✓x7ᵗʰ **V95.40** Unspecified spacecraft accident injuring occupant

✓x7ᵗʰ **V95.41** Spacecraft crash injuring occupant

✓x7ᵗʰ **V95.42** Forced landing of spacecraft injuring occupant

✓x7ᵗʰ **V95.43** Spacecraft collision injuring occupant
Spacecraft collision with any object, fixed, moveable or moving

✓x7ᵗʰ **V95.44** Spacecraft fire injuring occupant

✓x7ᵗʰ **V95.45** Spacecraft explosion injuring occupant

✓x7ᵗʰ **V95.49** Other spacecraft accident injuring occupant

✓x7ᵗʰ **V95.8** Other powered aircraft accidents injuring occupant

✓x7ᵗʰ **V95.9** Unspecified aircraft accident injuring occupant
Aircraft accident NOS
Air transport accident NOS

✓4ᵗʰ **V96** Accident to nonpowered aircraft causing injury to occupant

✓5ᵗʰ **V96.0** Balloon accident injuring occupant

✓x7ᵗʰ **V96.00** Unspecified balloon accident injuring occupant

✓x7ᵗʰ **V96.01** Balloon crash injuring occupant

✓x7ᵗʰ **V96.02** Forced landing of balloon injuring occupant

✓x7ᵗʰ **V96.03** Balloon collision injuring occupant
Balloon collision with any object, fixed, moveable or moving

✓x7ᵗʰ **V96.04** Balloon fire injuring occupant

✓x7ᵗʰ **V96.05** Balloon explosion injuring occupant

✓x7ᵗʰ **V96.09** Other balloon accident injuring occupant

✓5ᵗʰ **V96.1** Hang-glider accident injuring occupant

✓x7ᵗʰ **V96.10** Unspecified hang-glider accident injuring occupant

✓x7ᵗʰ **V96.11** Hang-glider crash injuring occupant

✓x7ᵗʰ **V96.12** Forced landing of hang-glider injuring occupant

✓x7ᵗʰ **V96.13** Hang-glider collision injuring occupant
Hang-glider collision with any object, fixed, moveable or moving

✓x7ᵗʰ **V96.14** Hang-glider fire injuring occupant

✓x7ᵗʰ **V96.15** Hang-glider explosion injuring occupant

✓x7ᵗʰ **V96.19** Other hang-glider accident injuring occupant

✓5ᵗʰ **V96.2** Glider (nonpowered) accident injuring occupant

✓x7ᵗʰ **V96.20** Unspecified glider (nonpowered) accident injuring occupant

✓x7ᵗʰ **V96.21** Glider (nonpowered) crash injuring occupant

✓x7ᵗʰ **V96.22** Forced landing of glider (nonpowered) injuring occupant

✓x7ᵗʰ **V96.23** Glider (nonpowered) collision injuring occupant
Glider (nonpowered) collision with any object, fixed, moveable or moving

✓x7ᵗʰ **V96.24** Glider (nonpowered) fire injuring occupant

✓x7ᵗʰ **V96.25** Glider (nonpowered) explosion injuring occupant

✓x7ᵗʰ **V96.29** Other glider (nonpowered) accident injuring occupant

✓x7ᵗʰ **V96.8** Other nonpowered-aircraft accidents injuring occupant
Kite carrying a person accident injuring occupant

✓x7ᵗʰ **V96.9** Unspecified nonpowered-aircraft accident injuring occupant
Nonpowered-aircraft accident NOS

✓4ᵗʰ **V97** Other specified air transport accidents

✓x7ᵗʰ **V97.0** Occupant of aircraft injured in other specified air transport accidents
Fall in, on or from aircraft in air transport accident
EXCLUDES 1 *accident while boarding or alighting aircraft (V97.1)*

✓x7ᵗʰ **V97.1** Person injured while boarding or alighting from aircraft

✓5ᵗʰ **V97.2** Parachutist accident

✓x7ᵗʰ **V97.21** Parachutist entangled in object
Parachutist landing in tree

✓x7ᵗʰ **V97.22** Parachutist injured on landing

✓x7ᵗʰ **V97.29** Other parachutist accident

✓Additional Character Req   ✓x7ᵗʰ Placeholder Alert   Unacceptable PDx   Manifestation   H1 - H14 HAC   HCC CMS-HCC Condition   EXCLUDES 1 Not Coded Here   EXCLUDES 2 Not Included Here

☑5ᵗʰ V97.3 Person on ground injured in air transport accident

    ☑x7ᵗʰ **V97.31 Hit by object falling from aircraft**
        Hit by crashing aircraft
        Injured by aircraft hitting house
        Injured by aircraft hitting car

    ☑x7ᵗʰ **V97.32 Injured by rotating propeller**

    ☑x7ᵗʰ **V97.33 Sucked into jet engine**

    ☑x7ᵗʰ **V97.39 Other injury to person on ground due to air transport accident**

☑5ᵗʰ V97.8 Other air transport accidents, not elsewhere classified
    EXCLUDES 1   *aircraft accident NOS (V95.9)*
        exposure to changes in air pressure during ascent or descent (W94.-)

    ☑6ᵗʰ **V97.81 Air transport accident involving military aircraft**

        ☑7ᵗʰ **V97.810 Civilian aircraft involved in air transport accident with military aircraft**
            Passenger in civilian aircraft injured due to accident with military aircraft

        ☑7ᵗʰ **V97.811 Civilian injured by military aircraft**

        ☑7ᵗʰ **V97.818 Other air transport accident involving military aircraft**

    ☑x7ᵗʰ **V97.89 Other air transport accidents, not elsewhere classified**
        Injury from machinery on aircraft

Other and unspecified transport accidents (V98-V99)

EXCLUDES 1   *vehicle accident, type of vehicle unspecified (V89.-)*

The appropriate 7th character is to be added to each code from categories V98-V99.
A   initial encounter
D   subsequent encounter
S   sequela

☑4ᵗʰ V98 Other specified transport accidents

    ☑x7ᵗʰ **V98.0 Accident to, on or involving cable-car, not on rails**
        Caught or dragged by cable-car, not on rails
        Fall or jump from cable-car, not on rails
        Object thrown from or in cable-car, not on rails

    ☑x7ᵗʰ **V98.1 Accident to, on or involving land-yacht**

    ☑x7ᵗʰ **V98.2 Accident to, on or involving ice yacht**

    ☑x7ᵗʰ **V98.3 Accident to, on or involving ski lift**
        Accident to, on or involving ski chair-lift
        Accident to, on or involving ski-lift with gondola

    ☑x7ᵗʰ **V98.8 Other specified transport accidents**

☑x7ᵗʰ V99 Unspecified transport accident

OTHER EXTERNAL CAUSES OF ACCIDENTAL INJURY (W00-X58)

Slipping, tripping, stumbling and falls (W00-W19)

EXCLUDES 1   *assault involving a fall (Y01-Y02)*
        fall from animal (V80.-)
        fall (in) (from) machinery (in operation) (W28-W31)
        fall (in) (from) transport vehicle (V01-V99)
        intentional self-harm involving a fall (X80-X81)
EXCLUDES 2   *at risk for fall (history of fall) (Z91.81)*
        fall (in) (from) burning building (X00.-)
        fall into fire ▶(X00-X04, X08)◄

The appropriate 7th character is to be added to each code from category W00-W19.
A   initial encounter
D   subsequent encounter
S   sequela

☑4ᵗʰ W00 Fall due to ice and snow
    INCLUDES   pedestrian on foot falling (slipping) on ice and snow
    EXCLUDES 1   *fall on (from) ice and snow involving pedestrian conveyance (V00.-)*
        fall from stairs and steps not due to ice and snow (W10.-)
    AHA: 2016, 2Q, 4

    ☑x7ᵗʰ **W00.0 Fall on same level due to ice and snow**

    ☑x7ᵗʰ **W00.1 Fall from stairs and steps due to ice and snow**

    ☑x7ᵗʰ **W00.2 Other fall from one level to another due to ice and snow**

    ☑x7ᵗʰ **W00.9 Unspecified fall due to ice and snow**

☑4ᵗʰ W01 Fall on same level from slipping, tripping and stumbling
    INCLUDES   fall on moving sidewalk
    EXCLUDES 1   *fall due to bumping (striking) against object (W18.0-)*
        fall in shower or bathtub (W18.2-)
        fall on same level NOS (W18.30)
        fall on same level from slipping, tripping and stumbling due to ice or snow (W00.0)
        fall off or from toilet (W18.1-)
        slipping, tripping and stumbling NOS (W18.40)
        slipping, tripping and stumbling without falling (W18.4-)

    ☑7ᵗʰ **W01.0 Fall on same level from slipping, tripping and stumbling without subsequent striking against object**
        Falling over animal

    ☑5ᵗʰ **W01.1 Fall on same level from slipping, tripping and stumbling with subsequent striking against object**

        ☑x7ᵗʰ **W01.10 Fall on same level from slipping, tripping and stumbling with subsequent striking against unspecified object**

        ☑6ᵗʰ **W01.11 Fall on same level from slipping, tripping and stumbling with subsequent striking against sharp object**

            ☑7ᵗʰ **W01.110 Fall on same level from slipping, tripping and stumbling with subsequent striking against sharp glass**

            ☑7ᵗʰ **W01.111 Fall on same level from slipping, tripping and stumbling with subsequent striking against power tool or machine**

            ☑7ᵗʰ **W01.118 Fall on same level from slipping, tripping and stumbling with subsequent striking against other sharp object**

            ☑7ᵗʰ **W01.119 Fall on same level from slipping, tripping and stumbling with subsequent striking against unspecified sharp object**

        ☑6ᵗʰ **W01.19 Fall on same level from slipping, tripping and stumbling with subsequent striking against other object**

            ☑7ᵗʰ **W01.190 Fall on same level from slipping, tripping and stumbling with subsequent striking against furniture**

            ☑7ᵗʰ **W01.198 Fall on same level from slipping, tripping and stumbling with subsequent striking against other object**

☑x7ᵗʰ W03 Other fall on same level due to collision with another person
    Fall due to non-transport collision with other person
    EXCLUDES 1   *collision with another person without fall (W51)*
        crushed or pushed by a crowd or human stampede (W52)
        fall involving pedestrian conveyance (V00-V09)
        fall due to ice or snow (W00)
        fall on same level NOS (W18.30)
    AHA: 2012, 4Q, 108

☑x7ᵗʰ W04 Fall while being carried or supported by other persons
    Accidentally dropped while being carried

☑4ᵗʰ W05 Fall from non-moving wheelchair, nonmotorized scooter and motorized mobility scooter
    EXCLUDES 1   *fall from moving motorized mobility scooter (V00.831)*
        fall from moving wheelchair (powered) (V00.811)
        fall from nonmotorized scooter (V00.141)

    ☑x7ᵗʰ **W05.0 Fall from non-moving wheelchair**

    ☑x7ᵗʰ **W05.1 Fall from non-moving nonmotorized scooter**

    ☑x7ᵗʰ **W05.2 Fall from non-moving motorized mobility scooter**

☑x7ᵗʰ W06 Fall from bed

☑x7ᵗʰ W07 Fall from chair

☑x7ᵗʰ W08 Fall from other furniture

☑4ᵗʰ W09 Fall on and from playground equipment
    EXCLUDES 1   *fall involving recreational machinery (W31)*

    ☑x7ᵗʰ **W09.0 Fall on or from playground slide**

    ☑x7ᵗʰ **W09.1 Fall from playground swing**

    ☑x7ᵗʰ **W09.2 Fall on or from jungle gym**

    ☑x7ᵗʰ **W09.8 Fall on or from other playground equipment**

☑4ᵗʰ W10 Fall on and from stairs and steps
    EXCLUDES 1   *Fall from stairs and steps due to ice and snow (W00.1)*

    ☑x7ᵗʰ **W10.0 Fall (on)(from) escalator**

    ☑x7ᵗʰ **W10.1 Fall (on)(from) sidewalk curb**

    ☑x7ᵗʰ **W10.2 Fall (on)(from) incline**
        Fall (on) (from) ramp

N Newborn: 0   P Pediatric: 0-17   M Maternity: 12-55   A Adult: 15-124   MCC Major CC Condition   PDxMCC PDx acts as own MCC   CC CC Condition   PDxCC PDx acts as own CC

1186   ICD-10-CM 2018

√x7th W10.8 Fall (on) (from) other stairs and steps

√x7th W10.9 Fall (on) (from) unspecified stairs and steps

√x7th W11 Fall on and from ladder

√x7th W12 Fall on and from scaffolding

√4th W13 Fall from, out of or through building or structure

> **√x7th W13.0 Fall from, out of or through balcony**
> Fall from, out of or through railing

> **√x7th W13.1 Fall from, out of or through bridge**

> **√x7th W13.2 Fall from, out of or through roof**

> **√x7th W13.3 Fall through floor**

> **√x7th W13.4 Fall from, out of or through window**
> > *EXCLUDES 2*   *fall with subsequent striking against sharp glass (W01.110)*

> **√x7th W13.8 Fall from, out of or through other building or structure**
> Fall from, out of or through viaduct
> Fall from, out of or through wall
> Fall from, out of or through flag-pole

> **√x7th W13.9 Fall from, out of or through building, not otherwise specified**
> > *EXCLUDES 1*   *collapse of a building or structure (W20.-)*
> > *fall or jump from burning building or structure (X00.-)*

√x7th W14 Fall from tree

√x7th W15 Fall from cliff

√4th W16 Fall, jump or diving into water
> *EXCLUDES 1*   *accidental non-watercraft drowning and submersion not involving fall (W65-W74)*
> *effects of air pressure from diving (W94.-)*
> *fall into water from watercraft (V90-V94)*
> *hitting an object or against bottom when falling from watercraft (V94.0)*
> *EXCLUDES 2*   *striking or hitting diving board (W21.4)*

> **√5th W16.0 Fall into swimming pool**
> Fall into swimming pool NOS
> > *EXCLUDES 1*   *fall into empty swimming pool (W17.3)*

> > **√6th W16.01 Fall into swimming pool striking water surface**
> > > **√7th W16.011 Fall into swimming pool striking water surface causing drowning and submersion**
> > > > *EXCLUDES 1*   *drowning and submersion while in swimming pool without fall (W67)*

> > > **√7th W16.012 Fall into swimming pool striking water surface causing other injury**

> > **√6th W16.02 Fall into swimming pool striking bottom**
> > > **√7th W16.021 Fall into swimming pool striking bottom causing drowning and submersion**
> > > > *EXCLUDES 1*   *drowning and submersion while in swimming pool without fall (W67)*

> > > **√7th W16.022 Fall into swimming pool striking bottom causing other injury**

> > **√6th W16.03 Fall into swimming pool striking wall**
> > > **√7th W16.031 Fall into swimming pool striking wall causing drowning and submersion**
> > > > *EXCLUDES 1*   *drowning and submersion while in swimming pool without fall (W67)*

> > > **√7th W16.032 Fall into swimming pool striking wall causing other injury**

> **√5th W16.1 Fall into natural body of water**
> Fall into laker
> Fall into open sea
> Fall into river
> Fall into stream

> > **√6th W16.11 Fall into natural body of water striking water surface**
> > > **√7th W16.111 Fall into natural body of water striking water surface causing drowning and submersion**
> > > > *EXCLUDES 1*   *drowning and submersion while in natural body of water without fall (W69)*

> > > **√7th W16.112 Fall into natural body of water striking water surface causing other injury**

> > **√6th W16.12 Fall into natural body of water striking bottom**
> > > **√7th W16.121 Fall into natural body of water striking bottom causing drowning and submersion**
> > > > *EXCLUDES 1*   *drowning and submersion while in natural body of water without fall (W69)*

> > > **√7th W16.122 Fall into natural body of water striking bottom causing other injury**

> > **√6th W16.13 Fall into natural body of water striking side**
> > > **√7th W16.131 Fall into natural body of water striking side causing drowning and submersion**
> > > > *EXCLUDES 1*   *drowning and submersion while in natural body of water without fall (W69)*

> > > **√7th W16.132 Fall into natural body of water striking side causing other injury**

> **√5th W16.2 Fall in (into) filled bathtub or bucket of water**

> > **√6th W16.21 Fall in (into) filled bathtub**
> > > *EXCLUDES 1*   *fall into empty bathtub (W18.2)*

> > > **√7th W16.211 Fall in (into) filled bathtub causing drowning and submersion**
> > > > *EXCLUDES 1*   *drowning and submersion while in filled bathtub without fall (W65)*

> > > **√7th W16.212 Fall in (into) filled bathtub causing other injury**

> > **√6th W16.22 Fall in (into) bucket of water**
> > > **√7th W16.221 Fall in (into) bucket of water causing drowning and submersion**

> > > **√7th W16.222 Fall in (into) bucket of water causing other injury**

> **√5th W16.3 Fall into other water**
> Fall into fountain
> Fall into reservoir

> > **√6th W16.31 Fall into other water striking water surface**
> > > **√7th W16.311 Fall into other water striking water surface causing drowning and submersion**
> > > > *EXCLUDES 1*   *drowning and submersion while in other water without fall (W73)*

> > > **√7th W16.312 Fall into other water striking water surface causing other injury**

> > **√6th W16.32 Fall into other water striking bottom**
> > > **√7th W16.321 Fall into other water striking bottom causing drowning and submersion**
> > > > *EXCLUDES 1*   *drowning and submersion while in other water without fall (W73)*

> > > **√7th W16.322 Fall into other water striking bottom causing other injury**

> > **√6th W16.33 Fall into other water striking wall**
> > > **√7th W16.331 Fall into other water striking wall causing drowning and submersion**
> > > > *EXCLUDES 1*   *drowning and submersion while in other water without fall (W73)*

> > > **√7th W16.332 Fall into other water striking wall causing other injury**

> **√5th W16.4 Fall into unspecified water**

> > **√x7th W16.41 Fall into unspecified water causing drowning and submersion**

> > **√x7th W16.42 Fall into unspecified water causing other injury**

> **√5th W16.5 Jumping or diving into swimming pool**

> > **√6th W16.51 Jumping or diving into swimming pool striking water surface**
> > > **√7th W16.511 Jumping or diving into swimming pool striking water surface causing drowning and submersion**
> > > > *EXCLUDES 1*   *drowning and submersion while in swimming pool without jumping or diving (W67)*

> > > **√7th W16.512 Jumping or diving into swimming pool striking water surface causing other injury**

✓ Additional Character Req   √x7th Placeholder Alert   Unacceptable PDx   Manifestation   H1 - H14 HAC   HCC CMS-HCC Condition   *EXCLUDES 1* Not Coded Here   *EXCLUDES 2* Not Included Here

ICD-10-CM 2018   1187

Chapter 20. External Causes of Morbidity

☑6ᵗʰ **W16.52 Jumping or diving into swimming pool striking bottom**
- ☑7ᵗʰ **W16.521 Jumping or diving into swimming pool striking bottom causing drowning and submersion**
  - EXCLUDES 1   *drowning and submersion while in swimming pool without jumping or diving (W67)*
- ☑7ᵗʰ **W16.522 Jumping or diving into swimming pool striking bottom causing other injury**

☑6ᵗʰ **W16.53 Jumping or diving into swimming pool striking wall**
- ☑7ᵗʰ **W16.531 Jumping or diving into swimming pool striking wall causing drowning and submersion**
  - EXCLUDES 1   *drowning and submersion while in swimming pool without jumping or diving (W67)*
- ☑7ᵗʰ **W16.532 Jumping or diving into swimming pool striking wall causing other injury**

☑5ᵗʰ **W16.6 Jumping or diving into natural body of water**
    Jumping or diving into lake
    Jumping or diving into open sea
    Jumping or diving into river
    Jumping or diving into stream

☑6ᵗʰ **W16.61 Jumping or diving into natural body of water striking water surface**
- ☑7ᵗʰ **W16.611 Jumping or diving into natural body of water striking water surface causing drowning and submersion**
  - EXCLUDES 1   *drowning and submersion while in natural body of water without jumping or diving (W69)*
- ☑7ᵗʰ **W16.612 Jumping or diving into natural body of water striking water surface causing other injury**

☑6ᵗʰ **W16.62 Jumping or diving into natural body of water striking bottom**
- ☑7ᵗʰ **W16.621 Jumping or diving into natural body of water striking bottom causing drowning and submersion**
  - EXCLUDES 1   *drowning and submersion while in natural body of water without jumping or diving (W69)*
- ☑7ᵗʰ **W16.622 Jumping or diving into natural body of water striking bottom causing other injury**

☑5ᵗʰ **W16.7 Jumping or diving from boat**
- EXCLUDES 1   *fall from boat into water—see watercraft accident (V90-V94)*

☑6ᵗʰ **W16.71 Jumping or diving from boat striking water surface**
- ☑7ᵗʰ **W16.711 Jumping or diving from boat striking water surface causing drowning and submersion**
- ☑7ᵗʰ **W16.712 Jumping or diving from boat striking water surface causing other injury**

☑6ᵗʰ **W16.72 Jumping or diving from boat striking bottom**
- ☑7ᵗʰ **W16.721 Jumping or diving from boat striking bottom causing drowning and submersion**
- ☑7ᵗʰ **W16.722 Jumping or diving from boat striking bottom causing other injury**

☑5ᵗʰ **W16.8 Jumping or diving into other water**
    Jumping or diving into fountain
    Jumping or diving into reservoir

☑6ᵗʰ **W16.81 Jumping or diving into other water striking water surface**
- ☑7ᵗʰ **W16.811 Jumping or diving into other water striking water surface causing drowning and submersion**
  - EXCLUDES 1   *drowning and submersion while in other water without jumping or diving (W73)*
- ☑7ᵗʰ **W16.812 Jumping or diving into other water striking water surface causing other injury**

☑6ᵗʰ **W16.82 Jumping or diving into other water striking bottom**
- ☑7ᵗʰ **W16.821 Jumping or diving into other water striking bottom causing drowning and submersion**
  - EXCLUDES 1   *drowning and submersion while in other water without jumping or diving (W73)*
- ☑7ᵗʰ **W16.822 Jumping or diving into other water striking bottom causing other injury**

☑6ᵗʰ **W16.83 Jumping or diving into other water striking wall**
- ☑7ᵗʰ **W16.831 Jumping or diving into other water striking wall causing drowning and submersion**
  - EXCLUDES 1   *drowning and submersion while in other water without jumping or diving (W73)*
- ☑7ᵗʰ **W16.832 Jumping or diving into other water striking wall causing other injury**

☑5ᵗʰ **W16.9 Jumping or diving into unspecified water**
- ☑×7ᵗʰ **W16.91 Jumping or diving into unspecified water causing drowning and submersion**
- ☑×7ᵗʰ **W16.92 Jumping or diving into unspecified water causing other injury**

☑4ᵗʰ **W17 Other fall from one level to another**

☑×7ᵗʰ **W17.0 Fall into well**

☑×7ᵗʰ **W17.1 Fall into storm drain or manhole**

☑×7ᵗʰ **W17.2 Fall into hole**
    Fall into pit

☑×7ᵗʰ **W17.3 Fall into empty swimming pool**
- EXCLUDES 1   *fall into filled swimming pool (W16.0-)*

☑×7ᵗʰ **W17.4 Fall from dock**

☑5ᵗʰ **W17.8 Other fall from one level to another**
- ☑×7ᵗʰ **W17.81 Fall down embankment (hill)**
- ☑×7ᵗʰ **W17.82 Fall from (out of) grocery cart**
  - Fall due to grocery cart tipping over
- ☑×7ᵗʰ **W17.89 Other fall from one level to another**
  - Fall from cherry picker
  - Fall from lifting device
  - Fall from mobile elevated work platform [MEWP]
  - Fall from sky lift
  - **AHA:** 2015, 2Q, 6

☑4ᵗʰ **W18 Other slipping, tripping and stumbling and falls**

☑5ᵗʰ **W18.0 Fall due to bumping against object**
    Striking against object with subsequent fall
- EXCLUDES 1   *fall on same level due to slipping, tripping, or stumbling with subsequent striking against object (W01.1-)*

- ☑×7ᵗʰ **W18.00 Striking against unspecified object with subsequent fall**
- ☑×7ᵗʰ **W18.01 Striking against sports equipment with subsequent fall**
- ☑×7ᵗʰ **W18.02 Striking against glass with subsequent fall**
- ☑×7ᵗʰ **W18.09 Striking against other object with subsequent fall**

☑5ᵗʰ **W18.1 Fall from or off toilet**
- ☑×7ᵗʰ **W18.11 Fall from or off toilet without subsequent striking against object**
  - Fall from (off) toilet NOS
- ☑×7ᵗʰ **W18.12 Fall from or off toilet with subsequent striking against object**

☑×7ᵗʰ **W18.2 Fall in (into) shower or empty bathtub**
- EXCLUDES 1   *fall in full bathtub causing drowning or submersion (W16.21-)*

☑5ᵗʰ **W18.3 Other and unspecified fall on same level**
- ☑×7ᵗʰ **W18.30 Fall on same level, unspecified**
- ☑×7ᵗʰ **W18.31 Fall on same level due to stepping on an object**
  - Fall on same level due to stepping on an animal
  - EXCLUDES 1   *slipping, tripping and stumbling without fall due to stepping on animal (W18.41)*
- ☑×7ᵗʰ **W18.39 Other fall on same level**

☑5ᵗʰ **W18.4 Slipping, tripping and stumbling without falling**
- EXCLUDES 1   *collision with another person without fall (W51)*
- ☑×7ᵗʰ **W18.40 Slipping, tripping and stumbling without falling, unspecified**

N Newborn: 0   P Pediatric: 0-17   M Maternity: 12-55   A Adult: 15-124   MCC Major CC Condition   PDx MCC PDx acts as own MCC   CC CC Condition   PDx CC PDx acts as own CC

√x7ᵗʰ **W18.41 Slipping, tripping and stumbling without falling due to stepping on object**
     Slipping, tripping and stumbling without falling due to stepping on animal
        EXCLUDES 1   *slipping, tripping and stumbling with fall due to stepping on animal (W18.31)*

√x7ᵗʰ **W18.42 Slipping, tripping and stumbling without falling due to stepping into hole or opening**

√x7ᵗʰ **W18.43 Slipping, tripping and stumbling without falling due to stepping from one level to another**

√x7ᵗʰ **W18.49 Other slipping, tripping and stumbling without falling**

√x7ᵗʰ **W19 Unspecified fall**
     Accidental fall NOS
     AHA: 2012, 4Q, 95

Exposure to inanimate mechanical forces (W20-W49)

EXCLUDES 1   *assault (X92-Y09)*
        contact or collision with animals or persons (W50-W64)
        exposure to inanimate mechanical forces involving military or war operations (Y36.-, Y37.-)
        intentional self-harm (X71-X83)

> The appropriate 7th character is to be added to each code from categories W20-W49.
> A   initial encounter
> D   subsequent encounter
> S   sequela

√4ᵗʰ **W20 Struck by thrown, projected or falling object**
     Code first any associated:
     cataclysm (X34-X39)
     lightning strike (T75.00)
        EXCLUDES 1   *falling object in machinery accident (W24, W28-W31)*
            falling object in transport accident (V01-V99)
            object set in motion by explosion (W35-W40)
            object set in motion by firearm (W32-W34)
            struck by thrown sports equipment (W21.-)

√x7ᵗʰ **W20.0 Struck by falling object in cave-in**
        EXCLUDES 2   *asphyxiation due to cave-in (T71.21)*

√x7ᵗʰ **W20.1 Struck by object due to collapse of building**
        EXCLUDES 1   *struck by object due to collapse of burning building (X00.2, X02.2)*

√x7ᵗʰ **W20.8 Other cause of strike by thrown, projected or falling object**
        EXCLUDES 1   *struck by thrown sports equipment (W21.-)*

√4ᵗʰ **W21 Striking against or struck by sports equipment**
        EXCLUDES 1   *assault with sports equipment (Y08.0-)*
            striking against or struck by sports equipment with subsequent fall (W18.01)

√5ᵗʰ **W21.0 Struck by hit or thrown ball**

√x7ᵗʰ **W21.00 Struck by hit or thrown ball, unspecified type**

√x7ᵗʰ **W21.01 Struck by football**

√x7ᵗʰ **W21.02 Struck by soccer ball**

√x7ᵗʰ **W21.03 Struck by baseball**

√x7ᵗʰ **W21.04 Struck by golf ball**

√x7ᵗʰ **W21.05 Struck by basketball**

√x7ᵗʰ **W21.06 Struck by volleyball**

√x7ᵗʰ **W21.07 Struck by softball**

√x7ᵗʰ **W21.09 Struck by other hit or thrown ball**

√5ᵗʰ **W21.1 Struck by bat, racquet or club**

√x7ᵗʰ **W21.11 Struck by baseball bat**

√x7ᵗʰ **W21.12 Struck by tennis racquet**

√x7ᵗʰ **W21.13 Struck by golf club**

√x7ᵗʰ **W21.19 Struck by other bat, racquet or club**

√5ᵗʰ **W21.2 Struck by hockey stick or puck**

√6ᵗʰ **W21.21 Struck by hockey stick**

√7ᵗʰ **W21.210 Struck by ice hockey stick**

√7ᵗʰ **W21.211 Struck by field hockey stick**

√6ᵗʰ **W21.22 Struck by hockey puck**

√7ᵗʰ **W21.220 Struck by ice hockey puck**

√7ᵗʰ **W21.221 Struck by field hockey puck**

√5ᵗʰ **W21.3 Struck by sports foot wear**

√x7ᵗʰ **W21.31 Struck by shoe cleats**
     Stepped on by shoe cleats

√x7ᵗʰ **W21.32 Struck by skate blades**
     Skated over by skate blades

√x7ᵗʰ **W21.39 Struck by other sports foot wear**

√x7ᵗʰ **W21.4 Striking against diving board**
     Use additional code for subsequent falling into water, if applicable (W16.-)

√5ᵗʰ **W21.8 Striking against or struck by other sports equipment**

√x7ᵗʰ **W21.81 Striking against or struck by football helmet**

√x7ᵗʰ **W21.89 Striking against or struck by other sports equipment**

√x7ᵗʰ **W21.9 Striking against or struck by unspecified sports equipment**

√4ᵗʰ **W22 Striking against or struck by other objects**
        EXCLUDES 1   *striking against or struck by object with subsequent fall (W18.09)*

√5ᵗʰ **W22.0 Striking against stationary object**
        EXCLUDES 1   *striking against stationary sports equipment (W21.8)*

√x7ᵗʰ **W22.01 Walked into wall**

√x7ᵗʰ **W22.02 Walked into lamppost**

√x7ᵗʰ **W22.03 Walked into furniture**

√6ᵗʰ **W22.04 Striking against wall of swimming pool**

√7ᵗʰ **W22.041 Striking against wall of swimming pool causing drowning and submersion**
        EXCLUDES 1   *drowning and submersion while swimming without striking against wall (W67)*

√7ᵗʰ **W22.042 Striking against wall of swimming pool causing other injury**

√x7ᵗʰ **W22.09 Striking against other stationary object**

√5ᵗʰ **W22.1 Striking against or struck by automobile airbag**

√x7ᵗʰ **W22.10 Striking against or struck by unspecified automobile airbag**

√x7ᵗʰ **W22.11 Striking against or struck by driver side automobile airbag**

√x7ᵗʰ **W22.12 Striking against or struck by front passenger side automobile airbag**

√x7ᵗʰ **W22.19 Striking against or struck by other automobile airbag**

√x7ᵗʰ **W22.8 Striking against or struck by other objects**
     Striking against or struck by object NOS
        EXCLUDES 1   *struck by thrown, projected or falling object (W20.-)*

√4ᵗʰ **W23 Caught, crushed, jammed or pinched in or between objects**
        EXCLUDES 1   *injury caused by cutting or piercing instruments (W25-W27)*
            injury caused by firearms malfunction (W32.1, W33.1-, W34.1-)
            injury caused by lifting and transmission devices (W24.-)
            injury caused by machinery (W28-W31)
            injury caused by nonpowered hand tools (W27.-)
            injury caused by transport vehicle being used as a means of transportation (V01-V99)
            injury caused by struck by thrown, projected or falling object (W20.-)

√x7ᵗʰ **W23.0 Caught, crushed, jammed, or pinched between moving objects**

√x7ᵗʰ **W23.1 Caught, crushed, jammed, or pinched between stationary objects**

√4ᵗʰ **W24 Contact with lifting and transmission devices, not elsewhere classified**
        EXCLUDES 1   *transport accidents (V01-V99)*

√x7ᵗʰ **W24.0 Contact with lifting devices, not elsewhere classified**
     Contact with chain hoist
     Contact with drive belt
     Contact with pulley (block)

√x7ᵗʰ **W24.1 Contact with transmission devices, not elsewhere classified**
     Contact with transmission belt or cable

√x7ᵗʰ **W25 Contact with sharp glass**
     Code first any associated:
     injury due to flying glass from explosion or firearm discharge (W32-W40)
     transport accident (V00-V99)
        EXCLUDES 1   *fall on same level due to slipping, tripping and stumbling with subsequent striking against sharp glass (W01.10)*
            striking against sharp glass with subsequent fall (W18.02)
        EXCLUDES 2   *glass embedded in skin (W45)*

√ Additional Character Req   √x7ᵗʰ Placeholder Alert   Unacceptable PDx   Manifestation   **H1**-**H14** HAC   **HCC** CMS-HCC Condition   *EXCLUDES 1* Not Coded Here   *EXCLUDES 2* Not Included Here

Chapter 20. External Causes of Morbidity

☑4ᵗʰ **W26 Contact with other sharp objects**
     EXCLUDES 2   *sharp object(s) embedded in skin (W45)*

√x7ᵗʰ **W26.0 Contact with knife**
     EXCLUDES 1   *contact with electric knife (W29.1)*

√x7ᵗʰ **W26.1 Contact with sword or dagger**

√x7ᵗʰ **W26.2 Contact with edge of stiff paper**
     Paper cut

√x7ᵗʰ **W26.8 Contact with other sharp object(s), not elsewhere classified**
     Contact with tin can lid

√x7ᵗʰ **W26.9 Contact with unspecified sharp object(s)**

☑4ᵗʰ **W27 Contact with nonpowered hand tool**

√x7ᵗʰ **W27.0 Contact with workbench tool**
     Contact with auger   Contact with handsaw
     Contact with axe   Contact with screwdriver
     Contact with chisel

√x7ᵗʰ **W27.1 Contact with garden tool**
     Contact with hoe
     Contact with nonpowered lawn mower
     Contact with pitchfork
     Contact with rake

√x7ᵗʰ **W27.2 Contact with scissors**

√x7ᵗʰ **W27.3 Contact with needle (sewing)**
     EXCLUDES 1   *contact with hypodermic needle (W46.-)*

√x7ᵗʰ **W27.4 Contact with kitchen utensil**
     Contact with fork
     Contact with ice-pick
     Contact with can-opener NOS

√x7ᵗʰ **W27.5 Contact with paper-cutter**

√x7ᵗʰ **W27.8 Contact with other nonpowered hand tool**
     Contact with nonpowered sewing machine
     Contact with shovel

☑7ᵗʰ **W28 Contact with powered lawn mower**
     Powered lawn mower (commercial) (residential)
     EXCLUDES 1   *contact with nonpowered lawn mower (W27.1)*
     EXCLUDES 2   *exposure to electric current (W86.-)*

☑4ᵗʰ **W29 Contact with other powered hand tools and household machinery**
     EXCLUDES 1   *contact with commercial machinery (W31.82)*
          contact with hot household appliance (X15)
          contact with nonpowered hand tool (W27.-)
          exposure to electric current (W86)

√x7ᵗʰ **W29.0 Contact with powered kitchen appliance**
     Contact with blender   Contact with garbage disposal
     Contact with can-opener   Contact with mixer

√x7ᵗʰ **W29.1 Contact with electric knife**

√x7ᵗʰ **W29.2 Contact with other powered household machinery**
     Contact with electric fan
     Contact with powered dryer (clothes) (powered) (spin)
     Contact with washing-machine
     Contact with sewing machine

√x7ᵗʰ **W29.3 Contact with powered garden and outdoor hand tools and machinery**
     Contact with chainsaw
     Contact with edger
     Contact with garden cultivator (tiller)
     Contact with hedge trimmer
     Contact with other powered garden tool
     EXCLUDES 1   *contact with powered lawn mower (W28)*

√x7ᵗʰ **W29.4 Contact with nail gun**

▲ √x7ᵗʰ **W29.8 Contact with other powered hand tools and household machinery**
     Contact with do-it-yourself tool NOS

☑4ᵗʰ **W30 Contact with agricultural machinery**
     INCLUDES   animal-powered farm machine
     EXCLUDES 1   *agricultural transport vehicle accident (V01-V99)*
          explosion of grain store (W40.8)
          exposure to electric current (W86.-)

√x7ᵗʰ **W30.0 Contact with combine harvester**
     Contact with reaper   Contact with thresher

√x7ᵗʰ **W30.1 Contact with power take-off devices (PTO)**

√x7ᵗʰ **W30.2 Contact with hay derrick**

√x7ᵗʰ **W30.3 Contact with grain storage elevator**
     EXCLUDES 1   *explosion of grain store (W40.8)*

√x7ᵗʰ **W30.8 Contact with other specified agricultural machinery**

√x7ᵗʰ **W30.81 Contact with agricultural transport vehicle in stationary use**
     Contact with agricultural transport vehicle under repair, not on public roadway
     EXCLUDES 1   *agricultural transport vehicle accident (V01-V99)*

√x7ᵗʰ **W30.89 Contact with other specified agricultural machinery**

√x7ᵗʰ **W30.9 Contact with unspecified agricultural machinery**
     Contact with farm machinery NOS

☑4ᵗʰ **W31 Contact with other and unspecified machinery**
     EXCLUDES 1   *contact with agricultural machinery (W30.-)*
          contact with machinery in transport under own power or being towed by a vehicle (V01-V99)
          exposure to electric current (W86)

√x7ᵗʰ **W31.0 Contact with mining and earth-drilling machinery**
     Contact with bore or drill (land) (seabed)
     Contact with shaft hoist
     Contact with shaft lift
     Contact with undercutter

√x7ᵗʰ **W31.1 Contact with metalworking machines**
     Contact with abrasive wheel
     Contact with forging machine
     Contact with lathe
     Contact with mechanical shears
     Contact with metal drilling machine
     Contact with milling machine
     Contact with power press
     Contact with rolling-mill
     Contact with metal sawing machine

√x7ᵗʰ **W31.2 Contact with powered woodworking and forming machines**
     Contact with band saw   Contact with overhead plane
     Contact with bench saw   Contact with powered saw
     Contact with circular saw   Contact with radial saw
     Contact with molding machine   Contact with sander
     EXCLUDES 1   *nonpowered woodworking tools (W27.0)*

√x7ᵗʰ **W31.3 Contact with prime movers**
     Contact with gas turbine
     Contact with internal combustion engine
     Contact with steam engine
     Contact with water driven turbine

√5ᵗʰ **W31.8 Contact with other specified machinery**

√x7ᵗʰ **W31.81 Contact with recreational machinery**
     Contact with roller coaster

√x7ᵗʰ **W31.82 Contact with other commercial machinery**
     Contact with commercial electric fan
     Contact with commercial kitchen appliances
     Contact with commercial powered dryer (clothes) (powered) (spin)
     Contact with commercial washing-machine
     Contact with commercial sewing machine
     EXCLUDES 1   *contact with household machinery (W29.-)*
          contact with powered lawn mower (W28)

√x7ᵗʰ **W31.83 Contact with special construction vehicle in stationary use**
     Contact with special construction vehicle under repair, not on public roadway
     EXCLUDES 1   *special construction vehicle accident (V01-V99)*

√x7ᵗʰ **W31.89 Contact with other specified machinery**

√x7ᵗʰ **W31.9 Contact with unspecified machinery**
     Contact with machinery NOS

Ⓝ Newborn: 0   Ⓟ Pediatric: 0-17   Ⓜ Maternity: 12-55   Ⓐ Adult: 15-124   MCC Major CC Condition   PDxMCC PDx acts as own MCC   CC CC Condition   PDxCC PDx acts as own CC

1190   ICD-10-CM 2018

☑4th **W32 Accidental handgun discharge and malfunction**
- INCLUDES   accidental discharge and malfunction of gun for single hand use
  - accidental discharge and malfunction of pistol
  - accidental discharge and malfunction of revolver
  - handgun discharge and malfunction NOS
- EXCLUDES 1   *accidental airgun discharge and malfunction (W34.010, W34.110)*
  - *accidental BB gun discharge and malfunction (W34.010, W34.110)*
  - *accidental pellet gun discharge and malfunction (W34.010, W34.110)*
  - *accidental shotgun discharge and malfunction (W33.01, W33.11)*
  - *assault by handgun discharge (X93)*
  - *handgun discharge involving legal intervention (Y35.0-)*
  - *handgun discharge involving military or war operations (Y36.4-)*
  - *intentional self-harm by handgun discharge (X72)*
  - *Very pistol discharge and malfunction (W34.09, W34.19)*

☑x7th **W32.0 Accidental handgun discharge**

☑x7th **W32.1 Accidental handgun malfunction**
- Injury due to explosion of handgun (parts)
- Injury due to malfunction of mechanism or component of handgun
- Injury due to recoil of handgun
- Powder burn from handgun

☑4th **W33 Accidental rifle, shotgun and larger firearm discharge and malfunction**
- INCLUDES   rifle, shotgun and larger firearm discharge and malfunction NOS
- EXCLUDES 1   *accidental airgun discharge and malfunction (W34.010, W34.110)*
  - *accidental BB gun discharge and malfunction (W34.010, W34.110)*
  - *accidental handgun discharge and malfunction (W32.-)*
  - *accidental pellet gun discharge and malfunction (W34.010, W34.110)*
  - *assault by rifle, shotgun and larger firearm discharge (X94)*
  - *firearm discharge involving legal intervention (Y35.0-)*
  - *firearm discharge involving military or war operations (Y36.4-)*
  - *intentional self-harm by rifle, shotgun and larger firearm discharge (X73)*

☑5th **W33.0 Accidental rifle, shotgun and larger firearm discharge**

☑x7th **W33.00 Accidental discharge of unspecified larger firearm**
- Discharge of unspecified larger firearm NOS

☑x7th **W33.01 Accidental discharge of shotgun**
- Discharge of shotgun NOS

☑x7th **W33.02 Accidental discharge of hunting rifle**
- Discharge of hunting rifle NOS

☑x7th **W33.03 Accidental discharge of machine gun**
- Discharge of machine gun NOS

☑x7th **W33.09 Accidental discharge of other larger firearm**
- Discharge of other larger firearm NOS

☑5th **W33.1 Accidental rifle, shotgun and larger firearm malfunction**
- Injury due to explosion of rifle, shotgun and larger firearm (parts)
- Injury due to malfunction of mechanism or component of rifle, shotgun and larger firearm
- Injury due to piercing, cutting, crushing or pinching due to (by) slide trigger mechanism, scope or other gun part
- Injury due to recoil of rifle, shotgun and larger firearm
- Powder burn from rifle, shotgun and larger firearm

☑x7th **W33.10 Accidental malfunction of unspecified larger firearm**
- Malfunction of unspecified larger firearm NOS

☑x7th **W33.11 Accidental malfunction of shotgun**
- Malfunction of shotgun NOS

☑x7th **W33.12 Accidental malfunction of hunting rifle**
- Malfunction of hunting rifle NOS

☑x7th **W33.13 Accidental malfunction of machine gun**
- Malfunction of machine gun NOS

☑x7th **W33.19 Accidental malfunction of other larger firearm**
- Malfunction of other larger firearm NOS

☑4th **W34 Accidental discharge and malfunction from other and unspecified firearms and guns**

☑5th **W34.0 Accidental discharge from other and unspecified firearms and guns**

☑x7th **W34.00 Accidental discharge from unspecified firearms or gun**
- Discharge from firearm NOS
- Gunshot wound NOS
- Shot NOS

☑6th **W34.01 Accidental discharge of gas, air or spring-operated guns**

☑x7th **W34.010 Accidental discharge of airgun**
- Accidental discharge of BB gun
- Accidental discharge of pellet gun

☑x7th **W34.011 Accidental discharge of paintball gun**
- Accidental injury due to paintball discharge

☑x7th **W34.018 Accidental discharge of other gas, air or spring-operated gun**

☑x7th **W34.09 Accidental discharge from other specified firearms**
- Accidental discharge from Very pistol [flare]

☑5th **W34.1 Accidental malfunction from other and unspecified firearms and guns**

☑x7th **W34.10 Accidental malfunction from unspecified firearms or gun**
- Firearm malfunction NOS

☑6th **W34.11 Accidental malfunction of gas, air or spring-operated guns**

☑x7th **W34.110 Accidental malfunction of airgun**
- Accidental malfunction of BB gun
- Accidental malfunction of pellet gun

☑x7th **W34.111 Accidental malfunction of paintball gun**
- Accidental injury due to paintball gun malfunction

☑x7th **W34.118 Accidental malfunction of other gas, air or spring-operated gun**

☑x7th **W34.19 Accidental malfunction from other specified firearms**
- Accidental malfunction from Very pistol [flare]

☑x7th **W35 Explosion and rupture of boiler**
- EXCLUDES 1   *explosion and rupture of boiler on watercraft (V93.4)*

☑4th **W36 Explosion and rupture of gas cylinder**

☑x7th **W36.1 Explosion and rupture of aerosol can**

☑x7th **W36.2 Explosion and rupture of air tank**

☑x7th **W36.3 Explosion and rupture of pressurized-gas tank**

☑x7th **W36.8 Explosion and rupture of other gas cylinder**

☑x7th **W36.9 Explosion and rupture of unspecified gas cylinder**

☑4th **W37 Explosion and rupture of pressurized tire, pipe or hose**

☑x7th **W37.0 Explosion of bicycle tire**

☑x7th **W37.8 Explosion and rupture of other pressurized tire, pipe or hose**

☑x7th **W38 Explosion and rupture of other specified pressurized devices**

☑x7th **W39 Discharge of firework**

☑4th **W40 Explosion of other materials**
- EXCLUDES 1   *assault by explosive material (X96)*
  - *explosion involving legal intervention (Y35.1-)*
  - *explosion involving military or war operations (Y36.0-, Y36.2-)*
  - *intentional self-harm by explosive material (X75)*

☑x7th **W40.0 Explosion of blasting material**
- Explosion of blasting cap
- Explosion of detonator
- Explosion of dynamite
- Explosion of explosive (any) used in blasting operations

☑x7th **W40.1 Explosion of explosive gases**
- Explosion of acetylene   Explosion of fire damp
- Explosion of butane   Explosion of gasoline fumes
- Explosion of coal gas   Explosion of methane
- Explosion in mine NOS   Explosion of propane
- Explosion of explosive gas

☑x7th **W40.8 Explosion of other specified explosive materials**
- Explosion in dump NOS   Explosion in grain store
- Explosion in factory NOS   Explosion in munitions
- EXCLUDES 1   *explosion involving legal intervention (Y35.1-)*
  - *explosion involving military or war operations (Y36.0-, Y36.2-)*

☑ Additional Character Req   ☑x7th Placeholder Alert   Unacceptable PDx   Manifestation   H1 - H14 HAC   HCC CMS-HCC Condition   EXCLUDES 1 Not Coded Here   EXCLUDES 2 Not Included Here

ICD-10-CM 2018   1191

W32–W40.8

√x7ᵗʰ **W40.9 Explosion of** unspecified **explosive materials**
Explosion NOS

√4ᵗʰ **W42 Exposure to noise**

√x7ᵗʰ **W42.0 Exposure to supersonic waves**

√x7ᵗʰ **W42.9 Exposure to other noise**
Exposure to sound waves NOS

√4ᵗʰ **W45 Foreign body or object entering through skin**
INCLUDES   foreign body or object embedded in skin
nail embedded in skin
EXCLUDES 2   *contact with hand tools (nonpowered) (powered) (W27-W29)*
contact with other sharp object(s) (W26.-)
contact with sharp glass (W25.-)
struck by objects (W20-W22)

√x7ᵗʰ **W45.0 Nail entering through skin**

√x7ᵗʰ **W45.8 Other foreign body or object entering through skin**
Splinter in skin NOS

√4ᵗʰ **W46 Contact with hypodermic needle**

√x7ᵗʰ **W46.0 Contact with hypodermic needle**
Hypodermic needle stick NOS

√x7ᵗʰ **W46.1 Contact with** contaminated **hypodermic needle**

√4ᵗʰ **W49 Exposure to other inanimate mechanical forces**
INCLUDES   exposure to abnormal gravitational [G] forces
exposure to inanimate mechanical forces NEC
EXCLUDES 1   *exposure to inanimate mechanical forces involving military or war operations (Y36.-, Y37.-)*

√5ᵗʰ **W49.0 Item causing** external constriction

√x7ᵗʰ **W49.01 Hair causing external constriction**

√x7ᵗʰ **W49.02 String or thread causing external constriction**

√x7ᵗʰ **W49.03 Rubber band causing external constriction**

√x7ᵗʰ **W49.04 Ring or other jewelry causing external constriction**

√x7ᵗʰ **W49.09 Other specified item causing external constriction**

√x7ᵗʰ **W49.9 Exposure to other inanimate mechanical forces**

Exposure to animate mechanical forces (W50-W64)

EXCLUDES 1   *Toxic effect of contact with venomous animals and plants (T63.-)*

The appropriate 7th character is to be added to each code from categories W50-W64.
A   initial encounter
D   subsequent encounter
S   sequela

√4ᵗʰ **W50 Accidental hit, strike, kick, twist, bite or scratch by another person**
INCLUDES   hit, strike, kick, twist, bite, or scratch by another person NOS
EXCLUDES 1   *assault by bodily force (Y04)*
struck by objects (W20-W22)

√x7ᵗʰ **W50.0 Accidental** hit or strike **by another person**
Hit or strike by another person NOS

√x7ᵗʰ **W50.1 Accidental** kick **by another person**
Kick by another person NOS

√x7ᵗʰ **W50.2 Accidental** twist **by another person**
Twist by another person NOS

√x7ᵗʰ **W50.3 Accidental** bite **by another person**
Human bite   Bite by another person NOS

√x7ᵗʰ **W50.4 Accidental** scratch **by another person**
Scratch by another person NOS

√x7ᵗʰ **W51 Accidental striking against or bumped into by another person**
EXCLUDES 1   *assault by striking against or bumping into by another person (Y04.2)*
fall due to collision with another person (W03)

√x7ᵗʰ **W52 Crushed, pushed or stepped on by crowd or human stampede**
Crushed, pushed or stepped on by crowd or human stampede with or without fall

√4ᵗʰ **W53 Contact with rodent**
INCLUDES   contact with saliva, feces or urine of rodent

√5ᵗʰ **W53.0 Contact with** mouse

√x7ᵗʰ **W53.01 Bitten by mouse**

√x7ᵗʰ **W53.09 Other contact with mouse**

√5ᵗʰ **W53.1 Contact with** rat

√x7ᵗʰ **W53.11 Bitten by rat**

√x7ᵗʰ **W53.19 Other contact with rat**

√5ᵗʰ **W53.2 Contact with** squirrel

√x7ᵗʰ **W53.21 Bitten by squirrel**

√x7ᵗʰ **W53.29 Other contact with squirrel**

√5ᵗʰ **W53.8 Contact with other rodent**

√x7ᵗʰ **W53.81 Bitten by other rodent**

√x7ᵗʰ **W53.89 Other contact with other rodent**

√4ᵗʰ **W54 Contact with dog**
INCLUDES   contact with saliva, feces or urine of dog

√x7ᵗʰ **W54.0 Bitten by dog**

√x7ᵗʰ **W54.1 Struck by dog**
Knocked over by dog

√x7ᵗʰ **W54.8 Other contact with dog**

√4ᵗʰ **W55 Contact with other mammals**
INCLUDES   contact with saliva, feces or urine of mammal
EXCLUDES 1   *animal being ridden—see transport accidents*
bitten or struck by dog (W54)
bitten or struck by rodent (W53.-)
contact with marine mammals (W56.-)

√5ᵗʰ **W55.0 Contact with** cat

√x7ᵗʰ **W55.01 Bitten by cat**

√x7ᵗʰ **W55.03 Scratched by cat**

√x7ᵗʰ **W55.09 Other contact with cat**

√5ᵗʰ **W55.1 Contact with** horse

√x7ᵗʰ **W55.11 Bitten by horse**

√x7ᵗʰ **W55.12 Struck by horse**

√x7ᵗʰ **W55.19 Other contact with horse**

√5ᵗʰ **W55.2 Contact with** cow
Contact with bull

√x7ᵗʰ **W55.21 Bitten by cow**

√x7ᵗʰ **W55.22 Struck by cow**
Gored by bull

√x7ᵗʰ **W55.29 Other contact with cow**

√5ᵗʰ **W55.3 Contact with other** hoof stock
Contact with goats
Contact with sheep

√x7ᵗʰ **W55.31 Bitten by other hoof stock**

√x7ᵗʰ **W55.32 Struck by other hoof stock**
Gored by goat
Gored by ram

√x7ᵗʰ **W55.39 Other contact with other hoof stock**

√5ᵗʰ **W55.4 Contact with** pig

√x7ᵗʰ **W55.41 Bitten by pig**

√x7ᵗʰ **W55.42 Struck by pig**

√x7ᵗʰ **W55.49 Other contact with pig**

√5ᵗʰ **W55.5 Contact with** raccoon

√x7ᵗʰ **W55.51 Bitten by raccoon**

√x7ᵗʰ **W55.52 Struck by raccoon**

√x7ᵗʰ **W55.59 Other contact with raccoon**

√5ᵗʰ **W55.8 Contact with other** mammals

√x7ᵗʰ **W55.81 Bitten by other mammals**

√x7ᵗʰ **W55.82 Struck by other mammals**

√x7ᵗʰ **W55.89 Other contact with other mammals**

√4ᵗʰ **W56 Contact with nonvenomous marine animal**
EXCLUDES 1   *contact with venomous marine animal (T63.-)*

√5ᵗʰ **W56.0 Contact with** dolphin

√x7ᵗʰ **W56.01 Bitten by dolphin**

√x7ᵗʰ **W56.02 Struck by dolphin**

√x7ᵗʰ **W56.09 Other contact with dolphin**

√5ᵗʰ **W56.1 Contact with** sea lion

√x7ᵗʰ **W56.11 Bitten by sea lion**

√x7ᵗʰ **W56.12 Struck by sea lion**

√x7ᵗʰ **W56.19 Other contact with sea lion**

√5ᵗʰ **W56.2 Contact with** orca
Contact with killer whale

√x7ᵗʰ **W56.21 Bitten by orca**

√x7ᵗʰ **W56.22 Struck by orca**

√x7ᵗʰ **W56.29 Other contact with orca**

N Newborn: 0   P Pediatric: 0-17   M Maternity: 12-55   A Adult: 15-124   MCC Major CC Condition   PDx MCC PDx acts as own MCC   CC CC Condition   PDx CC PDx acts as own CC

1192   ICD-10-CM 2018

✓5ᵗʰ **W56.3 Contact with** other marine mammals

   ✓x7ᵗʰ **W56.31 Bitten by other marine mammals**

   ✓x7ᵗʰ **W56.32 Struck by other marine mammals**

   ✓x7ᵗʰ **W56.39 Other contact with other marine mammals**

✓5ᵗʰ **W56.4 Contact with** shark

   ✓x7ᵗʰ **W56.41 Bitten by shark**

   ✓x7ᵗʰ **W56.42 Struck by shark**

   ✓x7ᵗʰ **W56.49 Other contact with shark**

✓5ᵗʰ **W56.5 Contact with** other fish

   ✓x7ᵗʰ **W56.51 Bitten by other fish**

   ✓x7ᵗʰ **W56.52 Struck by other fish**

   ✓x7ᵗʰ **W56.59 Other contact with other fish**

✓5ᵗʰ **W56.8 Contact with** other nonvenomous marine animals

   ✓x7ᵗʰ **W56.81 Bitten by other nonvenomous marine animals**

   ✓x7ᵗʰ **W56.82 Struck by other nonvenomous marine animals**

   ✓x7ᵗʰ **W56.89 Other contact with other nonvenomous marine animals**

✓x7ᵗʰ **W57 Bitten or stung by nonvenomous insect and other nonvenomous arthropods**

   EXCLUDES 1   contact with venomous insects and arthropods (T63.2-, T63.3-, T63.4-)

✓4ᵗʰ **W58 Contact with crocodile or alligator**

✓5ᵗʰ **W58.0 Contact with** alligator

   ✓x7ᵗʰ **W58.01 Bitten by alligator**

   ✓x7ᵗʰ **W58.02 Struck by alligator**

   ✓x7ᵗʰ **W58.03 Crushed by alligator**

   ✓x7ᵗʰ **W58.09 Other contact with alligator**

✓5ᵗʰ **W58.1 Contact with** crocodile

   ✓x7ᵗʰ **W58.11 Bitten by crocodile**

   ✓x7ᵗʰ **W58.12 Struck by crocodile**

   ✓x7ᵗʰ **W58.13 Crushed by crocodile**

   ✓x7ᵗʰ **W58.19 Other contact with crocodile**

✓4ᵗʰ **W59 Contact with other nonvenomous reptiles**

   EXCLUDES 1   contact with venomous reptile (T63.0-, T63.1-)

✓5ᵗʰ **W59.0 Contact with nonvenomous** lizards

   ✓x7ᵗʰ **W59.01 Bitten by nonvenomous lizards**

   ✓x7ᵗʰ **W59.02 Struck by nonvenomous lizards**

   ✓x7ᵗʰ **W59.09 Other contact with nonvenomous lizards**
       Exposure to nonvenomous lizards

✓5ᵗʰ **W59.1 Contact with nonvenomous** snakes

   ✓x7ᵗʰ **W59.11 Bitten by nonvenomous snake**

   ✓x7ᵗʰ **W59.12 Struck by nonvenomous snake**

   ✓x7ᵗʰ **W59.13 Crushed by nonvenomous snake**

   ✓x7ᵗʰ **W59.19 Other contact with nonvenomous snake**

✓5ᵗʰ **W59.2 Contact with** turtles

    EXCLUDES 1   contact with tortoises (W59.8-)

   ✓x7ᵗʰ **W59.21 Bitten by turtle**

   ✓x7ᵗʰ **W59.22 Struck by turtle**

   ✓x7ᵗʰ **W59.29 Other contact with turtle**
       Exposure to turtles

✓5ᵗʰ **W59.8 Contact with** other nonvenomous reptiles

   ✓x7ᵗʰ **W59.81 Bitten by other nonvenomous reptiles**

   ✓x7ᵗʰ **W59.82 Struck by other nonvenomous reptiles**

   ✓x7ᵗʰ **W59.83 Crushed by other nonvenomous reptiles**

   ✓x7ᵗʰ **W59.89 Other contact with other nonvenomous reptiles**

✓x7ᵗʰ **W60 Contact with nonvenomous plant thorns and spines and sharp leaves**

   EXCLUDES 1   contact with venomous plants (T63.7-)

✓4ᵗʰ **W61 Contact with birds (domestic) (wild)**

   INCLUDES   contact with excreta of birds

✓5ᵗʰ **W61.0 Contact with** parrot

   ✓x7ᵗʰ **W61.01 Bitten by parrot**

   ✓x7ᵗʰ **W61.02 Struck by parrot**

   ✓x7ᵗʰ **W61.09 Other contact with parrot**
       Exposure to parrots

✓5ᵗʰ **W61.1 Contact with** macaw

   ✓x7ᵗʰ **W61.11 Bitten by macaw**

   ✓x7ᵗʰ **W61.12 Struck by macaw**

   ✓x7ᵗʰ **W61.19 Other contact with macaw**
       Exposure to macaws

✓5ᵗʰ **W61.2 Contact with other** psittacines

   ✓x7ᵗʰ **W61.21 Bitten by other psittacines**

   ✓x7ᵗʰ **W61.22 Struck by other psittacines**

   ✓x7ᵗʰ **W61.29 Other contact with other psittacines**
       Exposure to other psittacines

✓5ᵗʰ **W61.3 Contact with** chicken

   ✓x7ᵗʰ **W61.32 Struck by chicken**

   ✓x7ᵗʰ **W61.33 Pecked by chicken**

   ✓x7ᵗʰ **W61.39 Other contact with chicken**
       Exposure to chickens

✓5ᵗʰ **W61.4 Contact with** turkey

   ✓x7ᵗʰ **W61.42 Struck by turkey**

   ✓x7ᵗʰ **W61.43 Pecked by turkey**

   ✓x7ᵗʰ **W61.49 Other contact with turkey**

✓5ᵗʰ **W61.5 Contact with** goose

   ✓x7ᵗʰ **W61.51 Bitten by goose**

   ✓x7ᵗʰ **W61.52 Struck by goose**

   ✓x7ᵗʰ **W61.59 Other contact with goose**

✓5ᵗʰ **W61.6 Contact with** duck

   ✓x7ᵗʰ **W61.61 Bitten by duck**

   ✓x7ᵗʰ **W61.62 Struck by duck**

   ✓x7ᵗʰ **W61.69 Other contact with duck**

✓5ᵗʰ **W61.9 Contact with** other birds

   ✓x7ᵗʰ **W61.91 Bitten by other birds**

   ✓x7ᵗʰ **W61.92 Struck by other birds**

   ✓x7ᵗʰ **W61.99 Other contact with other birds**
       Contact with bird NOS

✓4ᵗʰ **W62 Contact with nonvenomous amphibians**

   EXCLUDES 1   contact with venomous amphibians (T63.81-R63.83)

   ✓x7ᵗʰ **W62.0 Contact with nonvenomous** frogs

   ✓x7ᵗʰ **W62.1 Contact with nonvenomous** toads

   ✓x7ᵗʰ **W62.9 Contact with other nonvenomous** amphibians

✓x7ᵗʰ **W64 Exposure to other animate mechanical forces**

   INCLUDES   exposure to nonvenomous animal NOS

   EXCLUDES 1   contact with venomous animal (T63.-)

Accidental non-transport drowning and submersion (W65-W74)

   EXCLUDES 1   accidental drowning and submersion due to fall into water (W16.-)
        accidental drowning and submersion due to water transport accident (V90.-, V92.-)

   EXCLUDES 2   accidental drowning and submersion due to cataclysm (X34-X39)

> The appropriate 7th character is to be added to each code from categories W65-W74.
> A   initial encounter
> D   subsequent encounter
> S   sequela

✓x7ᵗʰ **W65 Accidental drowning and submersion while in** bath-tub

   EXCLUDES 1   accidental drowning and submersion due to fall in (into) bathtub (W16.211)

✓x7ᵗʰ **W67 Accidental drowning and submersion while in** swimming-pool

   EXCLUDES 1   accidental drowning and submersion due to fall into swimming pool (W16.011, W16.021, W16.031)
        accidental drowning and submersion due to striking into wall of swimming pool (W22.041)

✓x7ᵗʰ **W69 Accidental drowning and submersion while in** natural water
   Accidental drowning and submersion while in lake
   Accidental drowning and submersion while in open sea
   Accidental drowning and submersion while in river
   Accidental drowning and submersion while in stream

   EXCLUDES 1   accidental drowning and submersion due to fall into natural body of water (W16.111, W16.121, W16.131)

✓ Additional Character Req   ✓x7ᵗʰ Placeholder Alert   Unacceptable PDx   Manifestation   H1 - H14 HAC   HCC CMS-HCC Condition   EXCLUDES 1 Not Coded Here   EXCLUDES 2 Not Included Here

ICD-10-CM 2018   1193

√x7ᵗʰ **W73 Other specified cause of accidental non-transport drowning and submersion**
    Accidental drowning and submersion while in quenching tank
    Accidental drowning and submersion while in reservoir
    EXCLUDES 1   *accidental drowning and submersion due to fall into other water (W16.311, W16.321, W16.331)*

√x7ᵗʰ **W74 Unspecified cause of accidental drowning and submersion**
    Drowning NOS

Exposure to electric current, radiation and extreme ambient air temperature and pressure (W85-W99)

    EXCLUDES 1   exposure to:
         failure in dosage of radiation or temperature during surgical and medical care (Y63.2-Y63.5)
         lightning (T75.0-)
         natural cold (X31)
         natural heat (X30)
         natural radiation NOS (X39)
         radiological procedure and radiotherapy (Y84.2)
         sunlight (X32)

> The appropriate 7th character is to be added to each code from categories W85-W99.
> A   initial encounter
> D   subsequent encounter
> S   sequela

√x7ᵗʰ **W85 Exposure to electric transmission lines**
    Broken power line

√4ᵗʰ **W86 Exposure to other specified electric current**

  √x7ᵗʰ **W86.0 Exposure to domestic wiring and appliances**

  √x7ᵗʰ **W86.1 Exposure to industrial wiring, appliances and electrical machinery**
      Exposure to conductors
      Exposure to control apparatus
      Exposure to electrical equipment and machinery
      Exposure to transformers

  √x7ᵗʰ **W86.8 Exposure to other electric current**
      Exposure to wiring and appliances in or on farm (not farmhouse)
      Exposure to wiring and appliances outdoors
      Exposure to wiring and appliances in or on public building
      Exposure to wiring and appliances in or on residential institutions
      Exposure to wiring and appliances in or on schools

√4ᵗʰ **W88 Exposure to ionizing radiation**
    EXCLUDES 1   *exposure to sunlight (X32)*

  √x7ᵗʰ **W88.0 Exposure to X-rays**

  √x7ᵗʰ **W88.1 Exposure to radioactive isotopes**

  √x7ᵗʰ **W88.8 Exposure to other ionizing radiation**

√4ᵗʰ **W89 Exposure to man-made visible and ultraviolet light**
    INCLUDES   exposure to welding light (arc)
    EXCLUDES 1   *exposure to sunlight (X32)*

  √x7ᵗʰ **W89.0 Exposure to welding light (arc)**

  √x7ᵗʰ **W89.1 Exposure to tanning bed**

  √x7ᵗʰ **W89.8 Exposure to other man-made visible and ultraviolet light**

  √x7ᵗʰ **W89.9 Exposure to unspecified man-made visible and ultraviolet light**

√4ᵗʰ **W90 Exposure to other nonionizing radiation**
    EXCLUDES 1   *exposure to sunlight (X32)*

  √x7ᵗʰ **W90.0 Exposure to radiofrequency**

  √x7ᵗʰ **W90.1 Exposure to infrared radiation**

  √x7ᵗʰ **W90.2 Exposure to laser radiation**

  √x7ᵗʰ **W90.8 Exposure to other nonionizing radiation**

√x7ᵗʰ **W92 Exposure to excessive heat of man-made origin**

√4ᵗʰ **W93 Exposure to excessive cold of man-made origin**

  √5ᵗʰ **W93.0 Contact with or inhalation of dry ice**

    √x7ᵗʰ **W93.01 Contact with dry ice**

    √x7ᵗʰ **W93.02 Inhalation of dry ice**

  √5ᵗʰ **W93.1 Contact with or inhalation of liquid air**

    √x7ᵗʰ **W93.11 Contact with liquid air**
        Contact with liquid hydrogen
        Contact with liquid nitrogen

    √x7ᵗʰ **W93.12 Inhalation of liquid air**
        Inhalation of liquid hydrogen
        Inhalation of liquid nitrogen

  √x7ᵗʰ **W93.2 Prolonged exposure in deep freeze unit or refrigerator**

  √x7ᵗʰ **W93.8 Exposure to other excessive cold of man-made origin**

√4ᵗʰ **W94 Exposure to high and low air pressure and changes in air pressure**

  √x7ᵗʰ **W94.0 Exposure to prolonged high air pressure**

  √5ᵗʰ **W94.1 Exposure to prolonged low air pressure**

    √x7ᵗʰ **W94.11 Exposure to residence or prolonged visit at high altitude**

    √x7ᵗʰ **W94.12 Exposure to other prolonged low air pressure**

  √5ᵗʰ **W94.2 Exposure to rapid changes in air pressure during ascent**

    √x7ᵗʰ **W94.21 Exposure to reduction in atmospheric pressure while surfacing from deep-water diving**

    √x7ᵗʰ **W94.22 Exposure to reduction in atmospheric pressure while surfacing from underground**

    √x7ᵗʰ **W94.23 Exposure to sudden change in air pressure in aircraft during ascent**

    √x7ᵗʰ **W94.29 Exposure to other rapid changes in air pressure during ascent**

  √5ᵗʰ **W94.3 Exposure to rapid changes in air pressure during descent**

    √x7ᵗʰ **W94.31 Exposure to sudden change in air pressure in aircraft during descent**

    √x7ᵗʰ **W94.32 Exposure to high air pressure from rapid descent in water**

    √x7ᵗʰ **W94.39 Exposure to other rapid changes in air pressure during descent**

√x7ᵗʰ **W99 Exposure to other man-made environmental factors**

Exposure to smoke, fire and flames (X00-X08)

    EXCLUDES 1   *arson (X97)*
    EXCLUDES 2   *explosions (W35-W40)*
           lightning (T75.0-)
           transport accident (V01-V99)

> The appropriate 7th character is to be added to each code from categories X00-X08.
> A   initial encounter
> D   subsequent encounter
> S   sequela

√4ᵗʰ **X00 Exposure to uncontrolled fire in building or structure**
    INCLUDES   conflagration in building or structure
    Code first any associated cataclysm
    EXCLUDES 2   *exposure to ignition or melting of nightwear (X05)*
           exposure to ignition or melting of other clothing and apparel (X06.-)
           exposure to other specified smoke, fire and flames (X08.-)
    AHA: 2016, 2Q, 5

  √x7ᵗʰ **X00.0 Exposure to flames in uncontrolled fire in building or structure**

  √x7ᵗʰ **X00.1 Exposure to smoke in uncontrolled fire in building or structure**

  √x7ᵗʰ **X00.2 Injury due to collapse of burning building or structure in uncontrolled fire**
    EXCLUDES 1   *injury due to collapse of building not on fire (W20.1)*

  √x7ᵗʰ **X00.3 Fall from burning building or structure in uncontrolled fire**

  √x7ᵗʰ **X00.4 Hit by object from burning building or structure in uncontrolled fire**
    AHA: 2016, 2Q, 4

  √x7ᵗʰ **X00.5 Jump from burning building or structure in uncontrolled fire**

  √x7ᵗʰ **X00.8 Other exposure to uncontrolled fire in building or structure**

√4ᵗʰ **X01 Exposure to uncontrolled fire, not in building or structure**
    INCLUDES   exposure to forest fire

  √x7ᵗʰ **X01.0 Exposure to flames in uncontrolled fire, not in building or structure**

  √x7ᵗʰ **X01.1 Exposure to smoke in uncontrolled fire, not in building or structure**

  √x7ᵗʰ **X01.3 Fall due to uncontrolled fire, not in building or structure**

  √x7ᵗʰ **X01.4 Hit by object due to uncontrolled fire, not in building or structure**

  √x7ᵗʰ **X01.8 Other exposure to uncontrolled fire, not in building or structure**

Ⓝ Newborn: 0   Ⓟ Pediatric: 0-17   Ⓜ Maternity: 12-55   Ⓐ Adult: 15-124   ᴹᶜᶜ Major CC Condition   ᴾᴰˣᴹᶜᶜ PDx acts as own MCC   ᶜᶜ CC Condition   ᴾᴰˣᶜᶜ PDx acts as own CC

1194   ICD-10-CM 2018

✓4th **X02**   **Exposure to controlled fire in building or structure**
     INCLUDES   exposure to fire in fireplace
                exposure to fire in stove

    ✓x7th **X02.0**   **Exposure to flames in controlled fire in building or structure**

    ✓x7th **X02.1**   **Exposure to smoke in controlled fire in building or structure**

    ✓x7th **X02.2**   **Injury due to collapse of burning building or structure in controlled fire**
         EXCLUDES 1   *injury due to collapse of building not on fire (W20.1)*

    ✓x7th **X02.3**   **Fall from burning building or structure in controlled fire**

    ✓x7th **X02.4**   **Hit by object from burning building or structure in controlled fire**

    ✓x7th **X02.5**   **Jump from burning building or structure in controlled fire**

    ✓x7th **X02.8**   **Other exposure to controlled fire in building or structure**

✓4th **X03**   **Exposure to controlled fire, not in building or structure**
     INCLUDES   exposure to bon fire
                exposure to camp-fire
                exposure to trash fire

    ✓x7th **X03.0**   **Exposure to flames in controlled fire, not in building or structure**

    ✓x7th **X03.1**   **Exposure to smoke in controlled fire, not in building or structure**

    ✓x7th **X03.3**   **Fall due to controlled fire, not in building or structure**

    ✓x7th **X03.4**   **Hit by object due to controlled fire, not in building or structure**

    ✓x7th **X03.8**   **Other exposure to controlled fire, not in building or structure**

✓x7th **X04**   **Exposure to ignition of highly flammable material**
     Exposure to ignition of gasoline
     Exposure to ignition of kerosene
     Exposure to ignition of petrol
     EXCLUDES 2   *exposure to ignition or melting of nightwear (X05)*
                   exposure to ignition or melting of other clothing and apparel (X06)
     AHA: 2016, 2Q, 4

✓x7th **X05**   **Exposure to ignition or melting of nightwear**
     EXCLUDES 2   *exposure to uncontrolled fire in building or structure (X00.-)*
                   exposure to uncontrolled fire, not in building or structure (X01.-)
                   exposure to controlled fire in building or structure (X02.-)
                   exposure to controlled fire, not in building or structure (X03.-)
                   exposure to ignition of highly flammable materials (X04.-)

✓4th **X06**   **Exposure to ignition or melting of other clothing and apparel**
     EXCLUDES 2   *exposure to uncontrolled fire in building or structure (X00.-)*
                   exposure to uncontrolled fire, not in building or structure (X01.-)
                   exposure to controlled fire in building or structure (X02.-)
                   exposure to controlled fire, not in building or structure (X03.-)
                   exposure to ignition of highly flammable materials (X04.-)

    ✓x7th **X06.0**   **Exposure to ignition of plastic jewelry**

    ✓x7th **X06.1**   **Exposure to melting of plastic jewelry**

    ✓x7th **X06.2**   **Exposure to ignition of other clothing and apparel**

    ✓x7th **X06.3**   **Exposure to melting of other clothing and apparel**

✓4th **X08**   **Exposure to other specified smoke, fire and flames**

    ✓5th **X08.0**   **Exposure to bed fire**
         Exposure to mattress fire

       ✓x7th **X08.00**   **Exposure to bed fire due to unspecified burning material**

       ✓x7th **X08.01**   **Exposure to bed fire due to burning cigarette**

       ✓x7th **X08.09**   **Exposure to bed fire due to other burning material**

    ✓5th **X08.1**   **Exposure to sofa fire**

       ✓x7th **X08.10**   **Exposure to sofa fire due to unspecified burning material**

       ✓x7th **X08.11**   **Exposure to sofa fire due to burning cigarette**

       ✓x7th **X08.19**   **Exposure to sofa fire due to other burning material**

    ✓5th **X08.2**   **Exposure to other furniture fire**

       ✓x7th **X08.20**   **Exposure to other furniture fire due to unspecified burning material**

       ✓x7th **X08.21**   **Exposure to other furniture fire due to burning cigarette**

       ✓x7th **X08.29**   **Exposure to other furniture fire due to other burning material**

    ✓x7th **X08.8**   **Exposure to other specified smoke, fire and flames**

Contact with heat and hot substances (X10-X19)

     EXCLUDES 1   *exposure to excessive natural heat (X30)*
                   exposure to fire and flames ▶(X00-X08)◀

> The appropriate 7th character is to be added to each code from categories X10-X19.
> A   initial encounter
> D   subsequent encounter
> S   sequela

✓4th **X10**   **Contact with hot drinks, food, fats and cooking oils**

    ✓x7th **X10.0**   **Contact with hot drinks**

    ✓x7th **X10.1**   **Contact with hot food**

    ✓x7th **X10.2**   **Contact with fats and cooking oils**

✓4th **X11**   **Contact with hot tap-water**
     INCLUDES   contact with boiling tap-water
                contact with boiling water NOS
     EXCLUDES 1   *contact with water heated on stove (X12)*

    ✓x7th **X11.0**   **Contact with hot water in bath or tub**
         EXCLUDES 1   *contact with running hot water in bath or tub (X11.1)*

    ✓x7th **X11.1**   **Contact with running hot water**
         Contact with hot water running out of hose
         Contact with hot water running out of tap

    ✓x7th **X11.8**   **Contact with other hot tap-water**
         Contact with hot water in bucket
         Contact with hot tap-water NOS

✓x7th **X12**   **Contact with other hot fluids**
     Contact with water heated on stove
     EXCLUDES 1   *hot (liquid) metals (X18)*

✓4th **X13**   **Contact with steam and other hot vapors**

    ✓x7th **X13.0**   **Inhalation of steam and other hot vapors**

    ✓x7th **X13.1**   **Other contact with steam and other hot vapors**

✓4th **X14**   **Contact with hot air and other hot gases**

    ✓x7th **X14.0**   **Inhalation of hot air and gases**

    ✓x7th **X14.1**   **Other contact with hot air and other hot gases**

✓4th **X15**   **Contact with hot household appliances**
     EXCLUDES 1   *contact with heating appliances (X16)*
                   contact with powered household appliances (W29.-)
                   exposure to controlled fire in building or structure due to household appliance (X02.8)
                   exposure to household appliances electrical current (W86.0)

    ✓x7th **X15.0**   **Contact with hot stove (kitchen)**

    ✓x7th **X15.1**   **Contact with hot toaster**

    ✓x7th **X15.2**   **Contact with hotplate**

    ✓x7th **X15.3**   **Contact with hot saucepan or skillet**

    ✓x7th **X15.8**   **Contact with other hot household appliances**
         Contact with cooker
         Contact with kettle
         Contact with light bulbs

✓x7th **X16**   **Contact with hot heating appliances, radiators and pipes**
     EXCLUDES 1   *contact with powered appliances (W29.-)*
                   exposure to controlled fire in building or structure due to appliance (X02.8)
                   exposure to industrial appliances electrical current (W86.1)

✓x7th **X17**   **Contact with hot engines, machinery and tools**
     EXCLUDES 1   *contact with hot heating appliances, radiators and pipes (X16)*
                   contact with hot household appliances (X15)

✓x7th **X18**   **Contact with other hot metals**
     Contact with liquid metal

✓x7th **X19**   **Contact with other heat and hot substances**
     EXCLUDES 1   *objects that are not normally hot, e.g., an object made hot by a house fire ▶(X00-X08)◀*

☑ Additional Character Req   ✓x7th Placeholder Alert   Unacceptable PDx   Manifestation   H1 - H14 HAC   HCC CMS-HCC Condition   EXCLUDES 1 Not Coded Here   EXCLUDES 2 Not Included Here

ICD-10-CM 2018   **1195**

Chapter 20. External Causes of Morbidity

Exposure to forces of nature (X30-X39)

> The appropriate 7th character is to be added to each code from categories X30-X39.
> A   initial encounter
> D   subsequent encounter
> S   sequela

√x7th **X30 Exposure to excessive natural heat**
Exposure to excessive heat as the cause of sunstroke
Exposure to heat NOS
EXCLUDES 1   *excessive heat of man-made origin (W92)*
exposure to man-made radiation (W89)
exposure to sunlight (X32)
exposure to tanning bed (W89)

√x7th **X31 Exposure to excessive natural cold**
Excessive cold as the cause of chilblains NOS
Excessive cold as the cause of immersion foot or hand
Exposure to cold NOS
Exposure to weather conditions
EXCLUDES 1   *cold of man-made origin (W93.-)*
contact with or inhalation of dry ice (W93.-)
contact with or inhalation of liquefied gas (W93.-)

√x7th **X32 Exposure to sunlight**
EXCLUDES 1   *man-made radiation (tanning bed) (W89)*
EXCLUDES 2   ▶*radiation-related disorders of the skin and subcutaneous tissue (L55-L59)*◀

√x7th **X34 Earthquake**
EXCLUDES 2   *tidal wave (tsunami) due to earthquake (X37.41)*

√x7th **X35 Volcanic eruption**
EXCLUDES 2   *tidal wave (tsunami) due to volcanic eruption (X37.41)*

√4th **X36 Avalanche, landslide and other earth movements**
INCLUDES   victim of mudslide of cataclysmic nature
EXCLUDES 1   *earthquake (X34)*
EXCLUDES 2   *transport accident involving collision with avalanche or landslide not in motion (V01-V99)*

√x7th **X36.0 Collapse of dam or man-made structure causing earth movement**

√x7th **X36.1 Avalanche, landslide, or mudslide**

√4th **X37 Cataclysmic storm**

√x7th **X37.0 Hurricane**
Storm surge
Typhoon

√x7th **X37.1 Tornado**
Cyclone
Twister

√x7th **X37.2 Blizzard (snow)(ice)**

√x7th **X37.3 Dust storm**

√5th **X37.4 Tidalwave**

√x7th **X37.41 Tidal wave due to earthquake or volcanic eruption**
Tidal wave NOS
Tsunami

√x7th **X37.42 Tidal wave due to storm**

√x7th **X37.43 Tidal wave due to landslide**

√x7th **X37.8 Other cataclysmic storms**
Cloudburst
Torrential rain
EXCLUDES 2   *flood (X38)*

√x7th **X37.9 Unspecified cataclysmic storm**
Storm NOS
EXCLUDES 1   *collapse of dam or man-made structure causing earth movement (X39.0)*

√x7th **X38 Flood**
Flood arising from remote storm
Flood of cataclysmic nature arising from melting snow
Flood resulting directly from storm
EXCLUDES 1   *collapse of dam or man-made structure causing earth movement (X39.0)*
tidal wave NOS (X37.41)
tidal wave caused by storm (X37.2)

√4th **X39 Exposure to other forces of nature**

√5th **X39.0 Exposure to natural radiation**
EXCLUDES 1   *contact with and (suspected) exposure to radon and other naturally occuring radiation (Z77.123)*
exposure to man-made radiation (W88-W90)
exposure to sunlight (X32)

√x7th **X39.01 Exposure to radon**

√x7th **X39.08 Exposure to other natural radiation**

√x7th **X39.8 Other exposure to forces of nature**

Overexertion and strenuous or repetitive movements (X50)

√4th **X50 Overexertion and strenuous or repetitive movements**

> The appropriate 7th character is to be added to each code from category X50.
> A   initial encounter
> D   subsequent encounter
> S   sequela

√x7th **X50.0 Overexertion from strenuous movement or load**
Lifting heavy objects
Lifting weights

√x7th **X50.1 Overexertion from prolonged static or awkward postures**
Prolonged bending
Prolonged kneeling
Prolonged reaching
Prolonged sitting
Prolonged standing
Prolonged twisting
Static bending
Static kneeling
Static reaching
Static sitting
Static standing
Static twisting

√x7th **X50.3 Overexertion from repetitive movements**
Use of hand as hammer
EXCLUDES 2   *overuse from prolonged static or awkward postures (X50.1)*

√x7th **X50.9 Other and unspecified overexertion or strenuous movements or postures**
Contact pressure
Contact stress

Accidental exposure to other specified factors (X52-X58)

> The appropriate 7th character is to be added to each code from categories X52 and X58.
> A   initial encounter
> D   subsequent encounter
> S   sequela

√x7th **X52 Prolonged stay in weightless environment**
Weightlessness in spacecraft (simulator)

√x7th **X58 Exposure to other specified factors**
Accident NOS   Exposure NOS

Intentional self-harm (X71-X83)

Purposely self-inflicted injury
Suicide (attempted)

> The appropriate 7th character is to be added to each code from categories X71-X83.
> A   initial encounter
> D   subsequent encounter
> S   sequela

√4th **X71 Intentional self-harm by drowning and submersion**

√x7th **X71.0 Intentional self-harm by drowning and submersion while in bathtub**   HCC

√x7th **X71.1 Intentional self-harm by drowning and submersion while in swimming pool**   HCC

√x7th **X71.2 Intentional self-harm by drowning and submersion after jump into swimming pool**   HCC

√x7th **X71.3 Intentional self-harm by drowning and submersion in natural water**   HCC

√x7th **X71.8 Other intentional self-harm by drowning and submersion**   HCC

√x7th **X71.9 Intentional self-harm by drowning and submersion, unspecified**   HCC

N Newborn: 0   P Pediatric: 0-17   M Maternity: 12-55   A Adult: 15-124   MCC Major CC Condition   PDxMCC PDx acts as own MCC   CC CC Condition   PDxCC PDx acts as own CC

☑x7ᵗʰ **X72** **Intentional self-harm by handgun discharge** `HCC`
    Intentional self-harm by gun for single hand use
    Intentional self-harm by pistol
    Intentional self-harm by revolver
    `EXCLUDES 1`   Very pistol (X74.8)

☑4ᵗʰ **X73** **Intentional self-harm by rifle, shotgun and larger firearm discharge**
    `EXCLUDES 1`   airgun (X74.01)

    ☑x7ᵗʰ **X73.0** Intentional self-harm by shotgun discharge `HCC`
    ☑x7ᵗʰ **X73.1** Intentional self-harm by hunting rifle discharge `HCC`
    ☑x7ᵗʰ **X73.2** Intentional self-harm by machine gun discharge `HCC`
    ☑x7ᵗʰ **X73.8** Intentional self-harm by other larger firearm discharge `HCC`
    ☑x7ᵗʰ **X73.9** Intentional self-harm by unspecified larger firearm discharge `HCC`

☑4ᵗʰ **X74** **Intentional self-harm by other and unspecified firearm and gun discharge**

    ☑5ᵗʰ **X74.0** Intentional self-harm by gas, air or spring-operated guns

        ☑x7ᵗʰ **X74.01** Intentional self-harm by airgun `HCC`
            Intentional self-harm by BB gun discharge
            Intentional self-harm by pellet gun discharge

        ☑x7ᵗʰ **X74.02** Intentional self-harm by paintball gun `HCC`
        ☑x7ᵗʰ **X74.09** Intentional self-harm by other gas, air or spring-operated gun `HCC`

    ☑x7ᵗʰ **X74.8** Intentional self-harm by other firearm discharge `HCC`
        Intentional self-harm by Very pistol [flare] discharge

    ☑x7ᵗʰ **X74.9** Intentional self-harm by unspecified firearm discharge `HCC`

☑x7ᵗʰ **X75** **Intentional self-harm by explosive material** `HCC`

☑x7ᵗʰ **X76** **Intentional self-harm by smoke, fire and flames** `HCC`

☑4ᵗʰ **X77** **Intentional self-harm by steam, hot vapors and hot objects**

    ☑x7ᵗʰ **X77.0** Intentional self-harm by steam or hot vapors `HCC`
    ☑x7ᵗʰ **X77.1** Intentional self-harm by hot tap water `HCC`
    ☑x7ᵗʰ **X77.2** Intentional self-harm by other hot fluids `HCC`
    ☑x7ᵗʰ **X77.3** Intentional self-harm by hot household appliances `HCC`
    ☑x7ᵗʰ **X77.8** Intentional self-harm by other hot objects `HCC`
    ☑x7ᵗʰ **X77.9** Intentional self-harm by unspecified hot objects `HCC`

☑4ᵗʰ **X78** **Intentional self-harm by sharp object**

    ☑x7ᵗʰ **X78.0** Intentional self-harm by sharp glass `HCC`
    ☑x7ᵗʰ **X78.1** Intentional self-harm by knife `HCC`
    ☑x7ᵗʰ **X78.2** Intentional self-harm by sword or dagger `HCC`
    ☑x7ᵗʰ **X78.8** Intentional self-harm by other sharp object `HCC`
    ☑x7ᵗʰ **X78.9** Intentional self-harm by unspecified sharp object `HCC`

☑x7ᵗʰ **X79** **Intentional self-harm by blunt object** `HCC`

☑x7ᵗʰ **X80** **Intentional self-harm by jumping from a high place** `HCC`
    Intentional fall from one level to another

☑4ᵗʰ **X81** **Intentional self-harm by jumping or lying in front of moving object**

    ☑x7ᵗʰ **X81.0** Intentional self-harm by jumping or lying in front of motor vehicle `HCC`
    ☑x7ᵗʰ **X81.1** Intentional self-harm by jumping or lying in front of (subway) train `HCC`
    ☑x7ᵗʰ **X81.8** Intentional self-harm by jumping or lying in front of other moving object `HCC`

☑4ᵗʰ **X82** **Intentional self-harm by crashing of motor vehicle**

    ☑x7ᵗʰ **X82.0** Intentional collision of motor vehicle with other motor vehicle `HCC`
    ☑x7ᵗʰ **X82.1** Intentional collision of motor vehicle with train `HCC`
    ☑x7ᵗʰ **X82.2** Intentional collision of motor vehicle with tree `HCC`
    ☑x7ᵗʰ **X82.8** Other intentional self-harm by crashing of motor vehicle `HCC`

☑4ᵗʰ **X83** **Intentional self-harm by other specified means**
    `EXCLUDES 1`   intentional self-harm by poisoning or contact with toxic substance—see Table of Drugs and Chemicals

    ☑x7ᵗʰ **X83.0** Intentional self-harm by crashing of aircraft `HCC`
    ☑x7ᵗʰ **X83.1** Intentional self-harm by electrocution `HCC`
    ☑x7ᵗʰ **X83.2** Intentional self-harm by exposure to extremes of cold `HCC`
    ☑x7ᵗʰ **X83.8** Intentional self-harm by other specified means `HCC`

Assault (X92-Y09)

`INCLUDES`   homicide
           injuries inflicted by another person with intent to injure or kill, by any means
`EXCLUDES 1`   injuries due to legal intervention (Y35.-)
           injuries due to operations of war (Y36.-)
           injuries due to terrorism (Y38.-)

The appropriate 7th character is to be added to each code from categories X92-Y04 and Y08.
  A   initial encounter
  D   subsequent encounter
  S   sequela

☑4ᵗʰ **X92** **Assault by drowning and submersion**

    ☑x7ᵗʰ **X92.0** Assault by drowning and submersion while in bathtub
    ☑x7ᵗʰ **X92.1** Assault by drowning and submersion while in swimming pool
    ☑x7ᵗʰ **X92.2** Assault by drowning and submersion after push into swimming pool
    ☑x7ᵗʰ **X92.3** Assault by drowning and submersion in natural water
    ☑x7ᵗʰ **X92.8** Other assault by drowning and submersion
    ☑x7ᵗʰ **X92.9** Assault by drowning and submersion, unspecified

☑x7ᵗʰ **X93** **Assault by handgun discharge**
    Assault by discharge of gun for single hand use
    Assault by discharge of pistol
    Assault by discharge of revolver
    `EXCLUDES 1`   Very pistol (X95.8)

☑4ᵗʰ **X94** **Assault by rifle, shotgun and larger firearm discharge**
    `EXCLUDES 1`   airgun (X95.01)

    ☑x7ᵗʰ **X94.0** Assault by shotgun
    ☑x7ᵗʰ **X94.1** Assault by hunting rifle
    ☑x7ᵗʰ **X94.2** Assault by machine gun
    ☑x7ᵗʰ **X94.8** Assault by other larger firearm discharge
    ☑x7ᵗʰ **X94.9** Assault by unspecified larger firearm discharge

☑4ᵗʰ **X95** **Assault by other and unspecified firearm and gun discharge**

    ☑5ᵗʰ **X95.0** Assault by gas, air or spring-operated guns

        ☑x7ᵗʰ **X95.01** Assault by airgun discharge
            Assault by BB gun discharge
            Assault by pellet gun discharge

        ☑x7ᵗʰ **X95.02** Assault by paintball gun discharge
        ☑x7ᵗʰ **X95.09** Assault by other gas, air or spring-operated gun

    ☑x7ᵗʰ **X95.8** Assault by other firearm discharge
        Assault by Very pistol [flare] discharge

    ☑x7ᵗʰ **X95.9** Assault by unspecified firearm discharge

☑4ᵗʰ **X96** **Assault by explosive material**
    `EXCLUDES 1`   incendiary device (X97)
           terrorism involving explosive material (Y38.2-)

    ☑x7ᵗʰ **X96.0** Assault by antipersonnel bomb
        `EXCLUDES 1`   antipersonnel bomb use in military or war (Y36.2-)

    ☑x7ᵗʰ **X96.1** Assault by gasoline bomb
    ☑x7ᵗʰ **X96.2** Assault by letter bomb
    ☑x7ᵗʰ **X96.3** Assault by fertilizer bomb
    ☑x7ᵗʰ **X96.4** Assault by pipe bomb
    ☑x7ᵗʰ **X96.8** Assault by other specified explosive
    ☑x7ᵗʰ **X96.9** Assault by unspecified explosive

☑x7ᵗʰ **X97** **Assault by smoke, fire and flames**
    Assault by arson
    Assault by cigarettes
    Assault by incendiary device

☑4ᵗʰ **X98** **Assault by steam, hot vapors and hot objects**

    ☑x7ᵗʰ **X98.0** Assault by steam or hot vapors
    ☑x7ᵗʰ **X98.1** Assault by hot tap water
    ☑x7ᵗʰ **X98.2** Assault by hot fluids
    ☑x7ᵗʰ **X98.3** Assault by hot household appliances
    ☑x7ᵗʰ **X98.8** Assault by other hot objects
    ☑x7ᵗʰ **X98.9** Assault by unspecified hot objects

☑4ᵗʰ **X99** **Assault by sharp object**
    `EXCLUDES 1`   assault by strike by sports equipment (Y08.0-)

    ☑x7ᵗʰ **X99.0** Assault by sharp glass
    ☑x7ᵗʰ **X99.1** Assault by knife
    ☑x7ᵗʰ **X99.2** Assault by sword or dagger

☑Additional Character Req   ☑x7ᵗʰ Placeholder Alert   Unacceptable PDx   Manifestation   H1 - H14 HAC   HCC CMS-HCC Condition   EXCLUDES 1 Not Coded Here   EXCLUDES 2 Not Included Here

ICD-10-CM 2018   1197

Chapter 20. External Causes of Morbidity

√x7ᵗʰ **X99.8 Assault by other sharp object**

√x7ᵗʰ **X99.9 Assault by unspecified sharp object**
Assault by stabbing NOS

√x7ᵗʰ **Y00 Assault by blunt object**
EXCLUDES 1   *assault by strike by sports equipment (Y08.0-)*

√x7ᵗʰ **Y01 Assault by pushing from high place**

√4ᵗʰ **Y02 Assault by pushing or placing victim in front of moving object**

√x7ᵗʰ **Y02.0 Assault by pushing or placing victim in front of motor vehicle**

√x7ᵗʰ **Y02.1 Assault by pushing or placing victim in front of (subway) train**

√x7ᵗʰ **Y02.8 Assault by pushing or placing victim in front of other moving object**

√4ᵗʰ **Y03 Assault by crashing of motor vehicle**

√x7ᵗʰ **Y03.0 Assault by being hit or run over by motor vehicle**

√x7ᵗʰ **Y03.8 Other assault by crashing of motor vehicle**

√4ᵗʰ **Y04 Assault by bodily force**
EXCLUDES 1   *assault by:*
    submersion (X92.-)
    use of weapon (X93-X95, X99, Y00)

√x7ᵗʰ **Y04.0 Assault by unarmed brawl or fight**

√x7ᵗʰ **Y04.1 Assault by human bite**

√x7ᵗʰ **Y04.2 Assault by strike against or bumped into by another person**

√x7ᵗʰ **Y04.8 Assault by other bodily force**
Assault by bodily force NOS

√4ᵗʰ **Y07 Perpetrator of assault, maltreatment and neglect**
NOTE   Codes from this category are for use only in cases of confirmed abuse (T74.-)
Selection of the correct perpetrator code is based on the relationship between the perpetrator and the victim
INCLUDES   perpetrator of abandonment
perpetrator of emotional neglect
perpetrator of mental cruelty
perpetrator of physical abuse
perpetrator of physical neglect
perpetrator of sexual abuse
perpetrator of torture

√5ᵗʰ **Y07.0 Spouse or partner, perpetrator of maltreatment and neglect**
Spouse or partner, perpetrator of maltreatment and neglect against spouse or partner

Y07.01 Husband, perpetrator of maltreatment and neglect

Y07.02 Wife, perpetrator of maltreatment and neglect

Y07.03 Male partner, perpetrator of maltreatment and neglect

Y07.04 Female partner, perpetrator of maltreatment and neglect

√5ᵗʰ **Y07.1 Parent (adoptive) (biological), perpetrator of maltreatment and neglect**

Y07.11 Biological father, perpetrator of maltreatment and neglect

Y07.12 Biological mother, perpetrator of maltreatment and neglect

Y07.13 Adoptive father, perpetrator of maltreatment and neglect

Y07.14 Adoptive mother, perpetrator of maltreatment and neglect

√5ᵗʰ **Y07.4 Other family member, perpetrator of maltreatment and neglect**

√6ᵗʰ **Y07.41 Sibling, perpetrator of maltreatment and neglect**
EXCLUDES 1   *stepsibling, perpetrator of maltreatment and neglect (Y07.435, Y07.436)*

Y07.410 Brother, perpetrator of maltreatment and neglect

Y07.411 Sister, perpetrator of maltreatment and neglect

√6ᵗʰ **Y07.42 Foster parent, perpetrator of maltreatment and neglect**

Y07.420 Foster father, perpetrator of maltreatment and neglect

Y07.421 Foster mother, perpetrator of maltreatment and neglect

√6ᵗʰ **Y07.43 Stepparent or stepsibling, perpetrator of maltreatment and neglect**

Y07.430 Stepfather, perpetrator of maltreatment and neglect

Y07.432 Male friend of parent (co-residing in household), perpetrator of maltreatment and neglect

Y07.433 Stepmother, perpetrator of maltreatment and neglect

Y07.434 Female friend of parent (co-residing in household), perpetrator of maltreatment and neglect

Y07.435 Stepbrother, perpetrator or maltreatment and neglect

Y07.436 Stepsister, perpetrator of maltreatment and neglect

√6ᵗʰ **Y07.49 Other family member, perpetrator of maltreatment and neglect**

Y07.490 Male cousin, perpetrator of maltreatment and neglect

Y07.491 Female cousin, perpetrator of maltreatment and neglect

Y07.499 Other family member, perpetrator of maltreatment and neglect

√5ᵗʰ **Y07.5 Non-family member, perpetrator of maltreatment and neglect**

Y07.50 Unspecified non-family member, perpetrator of maltreatment and neglect

√6ᵗʰ **Y07.51 Daycare provider, perpetrator of maltreatment and neglect**

Y07.510 At-home childcare provider, perpetrator of maltreatment and neglect

Y07.511 Daycare center childcare provider, perpetrator of maltreatment and neglect

Y07.512 At-home adultcare provider, perpetrator of maltreatment and neglect

Y07.513 Adultcare center provider, perpetrator of maltreatment and neglect

Y07.519 Unspecified daycare provider, perpetrator of maltreatment and neglect

√6ᵗʰ **Y07.52 Healthcare provider, perpetrator of maltreatment and neglect**

Y07.521 Mental health provider, perpetrator of maltreatment and neglect

Y07.528 Other therapist or healthcare provider, perpetrator of maltreatment and neglect
Nurse, perpetrator of maltreatment and neglect
Occupational therapist, perpetrator of maltreatment and neglect
Physical therapist, perpetrator of maltreatment and neglect
Speech therapist, perpetrator of maltreatment and neglect

Y07.529 Unspecified healthcare provider, perpetrator of maltreatment and neglect

Y07.53 Teacher or instructor, perpetrator of maltreatment and neglect
Coach, perpetrator of maltreatment and neglect

Y07.59 Other non-family member, perpetrator of maltreatment and neglect

Y07.9 Unspecified perpetrator of maltreatment and neglect

√4ᵗʰ **Y08 Assault by other specified means**

√5ᵗʰ **Y08.0 Assault by strike by sport equipment**

√x7ᵗʰ **Y08.01 Assault by strike by hockey stick**

√x7ᵗʰ **Y08.02 Assault by strike by baseball bat**

√x7ᵗʰ **Y08.09 Assault by strike by other specified type of sport equipment**

√5ᵗʰ **Y08.8 Assault by other specified means**

√x7ᵗʰ **Y08.81 Assault by crashing of aircraft**

√x7ᵗʰ **Y08.89 Assault by other specified means**

Y09 Assault by unspecified means
Assassination (attempted) NOS
Homicide (attempted) NOS
Manslaughter (attempted) NOS
Murder (attempted) NOS

N Newborn: 0   P Pediatric: 0-17   M Maternity: 12-55   A Adult: 15-124   MCC Major CC Condition   PDxMCC PDx acts as own MCC   CC CC Condition   PDxCC PDx acts as own CC

Event of undetermined intent (Y21-Y33)

Undetermined intent is only for use when there is specific documentation in the record that the intent of the injury cannot be determined. If no such documentation is present, code to accidental (unintentional)

✓4th **Y21   Drowning and submersion, undetermined intent**

> The appropriate 7th character is to be added to each code from categories Y21-Y33.
> A   initial encounter
> D   subsequent encounter
> S   sequela

✓x7th **Y21.0   Drowning and submersion** while in bathtub**, undetermined intent**

✓x7th **Y21.1   Drowning and submersion** after fall into bathtub**, undetermined intent**

✓x7th **Y21.2   Drowning and submersion** while in swimming pool**, undetermined intent**

✓x7th **Y21.3   Drowning and submersion** after fall into swimming pool**, undetermined intent**

✓x7th **Y21.4   Drowning and submersion** in natural water**, undetermined intent**

✓x7th **Y21.8   Other** drowning and submersion, undetermined intent

✓x7th **Y21.9   Unspecified** drowning and submersion, undetermined intent

✓x7th **Y22   Handgun** discharge, undetermined intent
> Discharge of gun for single hand use, undetermined intent
> Discharge of pistol, undetermined intent
> Discharge of revolver, undetermined intent
> EXCLUDES 2   *Very pistol (Y24.8)*

✓4th **Y23   Rifle, shotgun and larger firearm** discharge, undetermined intent
> EXCLUDES 2   *airgun (Y24.0)*

✓x7th **Y23.0   Shotgun** discharge, undetermined intent

✓x7th **Y23.1   Hunting rifle** discharge, undetermined intent

✓x7th **Y23.2   Military firearm** discharge, undetermined intent

✓x7th **Y23.3   Machine gun** discharge, undetermined intent

✓x7th **Y23.8   Other** larger firearm discharge, undetermined intent

✓x7th **Y23.9   Unspecified** larger firearm discharge, undetermined intent

✓4th **Y24   Other and unspecified firearm discharge, undetermined intent**

✓x7th **Y24.0   Airgun** discharge, undetermined intent
> BB gun discharge, undetermined intent
> Pellet gun discharge, undetermined intent

✓x7th **Y24.8   Other** firearm discharge, undetermined intent
> Paintball gun discharge, undetermined intent
> Very pistol [flare] discharge, undetermined intent

✓x7th **Y24.9   Unspecified** firearm discharge, undetermined intent

✓x7th **Y25   Contact with explosive material, undetermined intent**

✓x7th **Y26   Exposure to smoke, fire and flames, undetermined intent**

✓4th **Y27   Contact with steam, hot vapors and hot objects, undetermined intent**

✓x7th **Y27.0   Contact with steam and hot** vapors**, undetermined intent**

✓x7th **Y27.1   Contact with hot** tap water**, undetermined intent**

✓x7th **Y27.2   Contact with hot** fluids**, undetermined intent**

✓x7th **Y27.3   Contact with hot household** appliance**, undetermined intent**

✓x7th **Y27.8   Contact with** other **hot objects, undetermined intent**

✓x7th **Y27.9   Contact with** unspecified **hot objects, undetermined intent**

✓4th **Y28   Contact with sharp object, undetermined intent**

✓x7th **Y28.0   Contact with sharp** glass**, undetermined intent**

✓x7th **Y28.1   Contact with** knife**, undetermined intent**

✓x7th **Y28.2   Contact with** sword or dagger**, undetermined intent**

✓x7th **Y28.8   Contact with** other **sharp object, undetermined intent**

✓x7th **Y28.9   Contact with** unspecified **sharp object, undetermined intent**

✓x7th **Y29   Contact with blunt object, undetermined intent**

✓x7th **Y30   Falling, jumping or pushed from a high place, undetermined intent**
> Victim falling from one level to another, undetermined intent

✓x7th **Y31   Falling, lying or running before or into moving object, undetermined intent**

✓x7th **Y32   Crashing of motor vehicle, undetermined intent**

✓x7th **Y33   Other specified events, undetermined intent**

Legal intervention, operations of war, military operations, and terrorism (Y35-Y38)

> The appropriate 7th character is to be added to each code from categories Y35-Y38.
> A   initial encounter
> D   subsequent encounter
> S   sequela

✓4th **Y35   Legal intervention**
> INCLUDES   any injury sustained as a result of an encounter with any law enforcement official, serving in any capacity at the time of the encounter, whether on-duty or off-duty.
> Includes: injury to law enforcement official, suspect and bystander

✓5th **Y35.0   Legal intervention involving** firearm discharge

✓6th **Y35.00   Legal intervention involving** unspecified firearm discharge
> Legal intervention involving gunshot wound
> Legal intervention involving shot NOS

✓7th **Y35.001   Legal intervention involving unspecified firearm discharge,** law enforcement official **injured**

✓7th **Y35.002   Legal intervention involving unspecified firearm discharge,** bystander **injured**

✓7th **Y35.003   Legal intervention involving unspecified firearm discharge,** suspect **injured**

✓6th **Y35.01   Legal intervention involving injury by** machine gun

✓7th **Y35.011   Legal intervention involving injury by machine gun,** law enforcement **official injured**

✓7th **Y35.012   Legal intervention involving injury by machine gun,** bystander **injured**

✓7th **Y35.013   Legal intervention involving injury by machine gun,** suspect **injured**

✓6th **Y35.02   Legal intervention involving injury by** handgun

✓7th **Y35.021   Legal intervention involving injury by handgun,** law enforcement **official injured**

✓7th **Y35.022   Legal intervention involving injury by handgun,** bystander **injured**

✓7th **Y35.023   Legal intervention involving injury by handgun,** suspect **injured**

✓6th **Y35.03   Legal intervention involving injury by** rifle pellet

✓7th **Y35.031   Legal intervention involving injury by rifle pellet,** law enforcement **official injured**

✓7th **Y35.032   Legal intervention involving injury by rifle pellet,** bystander **injured**

✓7th **Y35.033   Legal intervention involving injury by rifle pellet,** suspect **injured**

✓6th **Y35.04   Legal intervention involving injury by** rubber bullet

✓7th **Y35.041   Legal intervention involving injury by rubber bullet,** law enforcement **official injured**

✓7th **Y35.042   Legal intervention involving injury by rubber bullet,** bystander **injured**

✓7th **Y35.043   Legal intervention involving injury by rubber bullet,** suspect **injured**

✓6th **Y35.09   Legal intervention involving** other firearm discharge

✓7th **Y35.091   Legal intervention involving other firearm discharge,** law enforcement **official injured**

✓7th **Y35.092   Legal intervention involving other firearm discharge,** bystander **injured**

✓7th **Y35.093   Legal intervention involving other firearm discharge,** suspect **injured**

Chapter 20. External Causes of Morbidity

√5ᵗʰ **Y35.1 Legal intervention involving** explosives

√6ᵗʰ **Y35.10 Legal intervention involving** unspecified **explosives**

√7ᵗʰ **Y35.101 Legal intervention involving unspecified explosives,** law enforcement official **injured**

√7ᵗʰ **Y35.102 Legal intervention involving unspecified explosives,** bystander **injured**

√7ᵗʰ **Y35.103 Legal intervention involving unspecified explosives,** suspect **injured**

√6ᵗʰ **Y35.11 Legal intervention involving injury by** dynamite

√7ᵗʰ **Y35.111 Legal intervention involving injury by dynamite,** law enforcement official **injured**

√7ᵗʰ **Y35.112 Legal intervention involving injury by dynamite,** bystander **injured**

√7ᵗʰ **Y35.113 Legal intervention involving injury by dynamite,** suspect **injured**

√6ᵗʰ **Y35.12 Legal intervention involving injury by** explosive shell

√7ᵗʰ **Y35.121 Legal intervention involving injury by explosive shell,** law enforcement official **injured**

√7ᵗʰ **Y35.122 Legal intervention involving injury by explosive shell,** bystander **injured**

√7ᵗʰ **Y35.123 Legal intervention involving injury by explosive shell,** suspect **injured**

√6ᵗʰ **Y35.19 Legal intervention involving** other explosives
Legal intervention involving injury by grenade
Legal intervention involving injury by mortar bomb

√7ᵗʰ **Y35.191 Legal intervention involving other explosives,** law enforcement official **injured**

√7ᵗʰ **Y35.192 Legal intervention involving other explosives,** bystander **injured**

√7ᵗʰ **Y35.193 Legal intervention involving other explosives,** suspect **injured**

√5ᵗʰ **Y35.2 Legal intervention involving** gas
Legal intervention involving asphyxiation by gas
Legal intervention involving poisoning by gas

√6ᵗʰ **Y35.20 Legal intervention involving** unspecified **gas**

√7ᵗʰ **Y35.201 Legal intervention involving unspecified gas,** law enforcement official **injured**

√7ᵗʰ **Y35.202 Legal intervention involving unspecified gas,** bystander **injured**

√7ᵗʰ **Y35.203 Legal intervention involving unspecified gas,** suspect **injured**

√6ᵗʰ **Y35.21 Legal intervention involving injury by** tear gas

√7ᵗʰ **Y35.211 Legal intervention involving injury by tear gas,** law enforcement official **injured**

√7ᵗʰ **Y35.212 Legal intervention involving injury by tear gas,** bystander **injured**

√7ᵗʰ **Y35.213 Legal intervention involving injury by tear gas,** suspect **injured**

√6ᵗʰ **Y35.29 Legal intervention involving** other gas

√7ᵗʰ **Y35.291 Legal intervention involving other gas,** law enforcement **official injured**

√7ᵗʰ **Y35.292 Legal intervention involving other gas,** bystander **injured**

√7ᵗʰ **Y35.293 Legal intervention involving other gas,** suspect **injured**

√5ᵗʰ **Y35.3 Legal intervention involving** blunt objects
Legal intervention involving being hit or struck by blunt object

√6ᵗʰ **Y35.30 Legal intervention involving** unspecified blunt **objects**

√7ᵗʰ **Y35.301 Legal intervention involving unspecified blunt objects,** law enforcement official **injured**

√7ᵗʰ **Y35.302 Legal intervention involving unspecified blunt objects,** bystander **injured**

√7ᵗʰ **Y35.303 Legal intervention involving unspecified blunt objects,** suspect **injured**

√6ᵗʰ **Y35.31 Legal intervention involving** baton

√7ᵗʰ **Y35.311 Legal intervention involving baton,** law enforcement official **injured**

√7ᵗʰ **Y35.312 Legal intervention involving baton,** bystander **injured**

√7ᵗʰ **Y35.313 Legal intervention involving baton,** suspect **injured**

√6ᵗʰ **Y35.39 Legal intervention involving** other blunt objects

√7ᵗʰ **Y35.391 Legal intervention involving other blunt objects,** law enforcement official **injured**

√7ᵗʰ **Y35.392 Legal intervention involving other blunt objects,** bystander **injured**

√7ᵗʰ **Y35.393 Legal intervention involving other blunt objects,** suspect **injured**

√5ᵗʰ **Y35.4 Legal intervention involving** sharp objects
Legal intervention involving being cut by sharp objects
Legal intervention involving being stabbed by sharp objects

√6ᵗʰ **Y35.40 Legal intervention involving** unspecified sharp **objects**

√7ᵗʰ **Y35.401 Legal intervention involving unspecified sharp objects,** law enforcement official **injured**

√7ᵗʰ **Y35.402 Legal intervention involving unspecified sharp objects,** bystander **injured**

√7ᵗʰ **Y35.403 Legal intervention involving unspecified sharp objects,** suspect **injured**

√6ᵗʰ **Y35.41 Legal intervention involving** bayonet

√7ᵗʰ **Y35.411 Legal intervention involving bayonet,** law enforcement official injured

√7ᵗʰ **Y35.412 Legal intervention involving bayonet,** bystander **injured**

√7ᵗʰ **Y35.413 Legal intervention involving bayonet,** suspect **injured**

√6ᵗʰ **Y35.49 Legal intervention involving** other sharp objects

√7ᵗʰ **Y35.491 Legal intervention involving other sharp objects,** law enforcement official injured

√7ᵗʰ **Y35.492 Legal intervention involving other sharp objects,** bystander **injured**

√7ᵗʰ **Y35.493 Legal intervention involving other sharp objects,** suspect **injured**

√5ᵗʰ **Y35.8 Legal intervention involving** other **specified** means

√6ᵗʰ **Y35.81 Legal intervention involving** manhandling

√7ᵗʰ **Y35.811 Legal intervention involving manhandling,** law enforcement official **injured**

√7ᵗʰ **Y35.812 Legal intervention involving manhandling,** bystander **injured**

√7ᵗʰ **Y35.813 Legal intervention involving manhandling,** suspect **injured**

√6ᵗʰ **Y35.89 Legal intervention involving** other specified means

√7ᵗʰ **Y35.891 Legal intervention involving other specified means,** law enforcement official **injured**

√7ᵗʰ **Y35.892 Legal intervention involving other specified means,** bystander **injured**

√7ᵗʰ **Y35.893 Legal intervention involving other specified means,** suspect **injured**

√5ᵗʰ **Y35.9 Legal intervention, means** unspecified

√x7ᵗʰ **Y35.91 Legal intervention, means unspecified,** law enforcement official injured

√x7ᵗʰ **Y35.92 Legal intervention, means unspecified,** bystander injured

√x7ᵗʰ **Y35.93 Legal intervention, means unspecified,** suspect injured

Ⓝ Newborn: 0   Ⓟ Pediatric: 0-17   Ⓜ Maternity: 12-55   Ⓐ Adult: 15-124   MCC Major CC Condition   PDxMCC PDx acts as own MCC   CC CC Condition   PDxCC PDx acts as own CC

1200   ICD-10-CM 2018

☑️4th **Y36** **Operations of war**

INCLUDES injuries to military personnel and civilians caused by war, civil insurrection, and peacekeeping missions

EXCLUDES 1 *injury to military personnel occurring during peacetime military operations (Y37.-)*

military vehicles involved in transport accidents with non-military vehicle during peacetime (V09.01, V09.21, V19.81, V29.81, V39.81, V49.81, V59.81, V69.81, V79.81)

AHA: 2014, 3Q, 4

☑️5th **Y36.0** **War operations involving** explosion of marine weapons

  ☑️6th **Y36.00** **War operations involving explosion of** unspecified marine weapon

    War operations involving underwater blast NOS

    ☑️7th **Y36.000** **War operations involving explosion of unspecified marine weapon,** military personnel

    ☑️7th **Y36.001** **War operations involving explosion of unspecified marine weapon,** civilian

  ☑️6th **Y36.01** **War operations involving explosion of** depth-charge

    ☑️7th **Y36.010** **War operations involving explosion of depth-charge,** military personnel

    ☑️7th **Y36.011** **War operations involving explosion of depth-charge,** civilian

  ☑️6th **Y36.02** **War operations involving explosion of** marine mine

    War operations involving explosion of marine mine, at sea or in harbor

    ☑️7th **Y36.020** **War operations involving explosion of marine mine,** military personnel

    ☑️7th **Y36.021** **War operations involving explosion of marine mine,** civilian

  ☑️6th **Y36.03** **War operations involving explosion of** sea-based artillery shell

    ☑️7th **Y36.030** **War operations involving explosion of sea-based artillery shell,** military personnel

    ☑️7th **Y36.031** **War operations involving explosion of sea-based artillery shell,** civilian

  ☑️6th **Y36.04** **War operations involving explosion of** torpedo

    ☑️7th **Y36.040** **War operations involving explosion of torpedo,** military personnel

    ☑️7th **Y36.041** **War operations involving explosion of torpedo,** civilian

  ☑️6th **Y36.05** **War operations involving** accidental detonation of onboard marine weapons

    ☑️7th **Y36.050** **War operations involving accidental detonation of onboard marine weapons,** military personnel

    ☑️7th **Y36.051** **War operations involving accidental detonation of onboard marine weapons,** civilian

  ☑️6th **Y36.09** **War operations involving explosion of** other marine weapons

    ☑️7th **Y36.090** **War operations involving explosion of other marine weapons,** military personnel

    ☑️7th **Y36.091** **War operations involving explosion of other marine weapons,** civilian

☑️5th **Y36.1** **War operations involving** destruction of aircraft

  ☑️6th **Y36.10** **War operations involving** unspecified destruction of aircraft

    ☑️7th **Y36.100** **War operations involving unspecified destruction of aircraft,** military personnel

    ☑️7th **Y36.101** **War operations involving unspecified destruction of aircraft,** civilian

  ☑️6th **Y36.11** **War operations involving destruction of aircraft due** to enemy fire or explosives

    War operations involving destruction of aircraft due to air to air missile

    War operations involving destruction of aircraft due to explosive placed on aircraft

    War operations involving destruction of aircraft due to rocket propelled grenade [RPG]

    War operations involving destruction of aircraft due to small arms fire

    War operations involving destruction of aircraft due to surface to air missile

    ☑️7th **Y36.110** **War operations involving destruction of aircraft due to enemy fire or explosives,** military personnel

    ☑️7th **Y36.111** **War operations involving destruction of aircraft due to enemy fire or explosives,** civilian

  ☑️6th **Y36.12** **War operations involving destruction of aircraft due to** collision with other aircraft

    ☑️7th **Y36.120** **War operations involving destruction of aircraft due to collision with other aircraft,** military personnel

    ☑️7th **Y36.121** **War operations involving destruction of aircraft due to collision with other aircraft,** civilian

  ☑️6th **Y36.13** **War operations involving destruction of aircraft due to** onboard fire

    ☑️7th **Y36.130** **War operations involving destruction of aircraft due to onboard fire,** military personnel

    ☑️7th **Y36.131** **War operations involving destruction of aircraft due to onboard fire,** civilian

  ☑️6th **Y36.14** **War operations involving destruction of aircraft due to** accidental detonation of onboard munitions and explosives

    ☑️7th **Y36.140** **War operations involving destruction of aircraft due to accidental detonation of onboard munitions and explosives,** military personnel

    ☑️7th **Y36.141** **War operations involving destruction of aircraft due to accidental detonation of onboard munitions and explosives,** civilian

  ☑️6th **Y36.19** **War operations involving** other destruction of aircraft

    ☑️7th **Y36.190** **War operations involving other destruction of aircraft,** military personnel

    ☑️7th **Y36.191** **War operations involving other destruction of aircraft,** civilian

☑️5th **Y36.2** **War operations involving** other explosions and fragments

EXCLUDES 1 *war operations involving explosion of aircraft (Y36.1-)*

war operations involving explosion of marine weapons (Y36.0-)

war operations involving explosion of nuclear weapons (Y36.5-)

war operations involving explosion occurring after cessation of hostilities (Y36.8-)

  ☑️6th **Y36.20** **War operations involving** unspecified explosion and fragments

    War operations involving air blast NOS

    War operations involving blast NOS

    War operations involving blast fragments NOS

    War operations involving blast wave NOS

    War operations involving blast wind NOS

    War operations involving explosion NOS

    War operations involving explosion of bomb NOS

    ☑️7th **Y36.200** **War operations involving unspecified explosion and fragments,** military personnel

    ☑️7th **Y36.201** **War operations involving unspecified explosion and fragments,** civilian

  ☑️6th **Y36.21** **War operations involving explosion of** aerial bomb

    ☑️7th **Y36.210** **War operations involving explosion of aerial bomb,** military personnel

    ☑️7th **Y36.211** **War operations involving explosion of aerial bomb,** civilian

  ☑️6th **Y36.22** **War operations involving explosion of** guided missile

    ☑️7th **Y36.220** **War operations involving explosion of guided missile,** military personnel

    ☑️7th **Y36.221** **War operations involving explosion of guided missile,** civilian

---

☑️Additional Character Req   vx7th Placeholder Alert   Unacceptable PDx   Manifestation   H1 - H14 HAC   HCC CMS-HCC Condition   EXCLUDES 1 Not Coded Here   EXCLUDES 2 Not Included Here

√6th **Y36.23** War operations involving explosion of improvised explosive device [IED]

War operations involving explosion of person-borne improvised explosive device [IED]

War operations involving explosion of vehicle-borne improvised explosive device [IED]

War operations involving explosion of roadside improvised explosive device [IED]

√7th **Y36.230** War operations involving explosion of improvised explosive device [IED], military personnel

√7th **Y36.231** War operations involving explosion of improvised explosive device [IED], civilian

√6th **Y36.24** War operations involving explosion due to accidental detonation and discharge of own munitions or munitions launch device

√7th **Y36.240** War operations involving explosion due to accidental detonation and discharge of own munitions or munitions launch device, military personnel

√7th **Y36.241** War operations involving explosion due to accidental detonation and discharge of own munitions or munitions launch device, civilian

√6th **Y36.25** War operations involving fragments from munitions

√7th **Y36.250** War operations involving fragments from munitions, military personnel

√7th **Y36.251** War operations involving fragments from munitions, civilian

√6th **Y36.26** War operations involving fragments of improvised explosive device [IED]

War operations involving fragments of person-borne improvised explosive device [IED]

War operations involving fragments of vehicle-borne improvised explosive device [IED]

War operations involving fragments of roadside improvised explosive device [IED]

√7th **Y36.260** War operations involving fragments of improvised explosive device [IED], military personnel

√7th **Y36.261** War operations involving fragments of improvised explosive device [IED], civilian

√6th **Y36.27** War operations involving fragments from weapons

√7th **Y36.270** War operations involving fragments from weapons, military personnel

√7th **Y36.271** War operations involving fragments from weapons, civilian

√6th **Y36.29** War operations involving other explosions and fragments

War operations involving explosion of grenade

War operations involving explosions of land mine

War operations involving shrapnel NOS

√7th **Y36.290** War operations involving other explosions and fragments, military personnel

√7th **Y36.291** War operations involving other explosions and fragments, civilian

√5th **Y36.3** War operations involving fires, conflagrations and hot substances

War operations involving smoke, fumes, and heat from fires, conflagrations and hot substances

EXCLUDES 1   *war operations involving fires and conflagrations aboard military aircraft (Y36.1-)*

war operations involving fires and conflagrations aboard military watercraft (Y36.0-)

war operations involving fires and conflagrations caused indirectly by conventional weapons (Y36.2-)

war operations involving fires and thermal effects of nuclear weapons (Y36.53-)

√6th **Y36.30** War operations involving unspecified fire, conflagration and hot substance

√7th **Y36.300** War operations involving unspecified fire, conflagration and hot substance, military personnel

√7th **Y36.301** War operations involving unspecified fire, conflagration and hot substance, civilian

√6th **Y36.31** War operations involving gasoline bomb

War operations involving incendiary bomb

War operations involving petrol bomb

√7th **Y36.310** War operations involving gasoline bomb, military personnel

√7th **Y36.311** War operations involving gasoline bomb, civilian

√6th **Y36.32** War operations involving incendiary bullet

√7th **Y36.320** War operations involving incendiary bullet, military personnel

√7th **Y36.321** War operations involving incendiary bullet, civilian

√6th **Y36.33** War operations involving flamethrower

√7th **Y36.330** War operations involving flamethrower, military personnel

√7th **Y36.331** War operations involving flamethrower, civilian

√6th **Y36.39** War operations involving other fires, conflagrations and hot substances

√7th **Y36.390** War operations involving other fires, conflagrations and hot substances, military personnel

√7th **Y36.391** War operations involving other fires, conflagrations and hot substances, civilian

√5th **Y36.4** War operations involving firearm discharge and other forms of conventional warfare

√6th **Y36.41** War operations involving rubber bullets

√7th **Y36.410** War operations involving rubber bullets, military personnel

√7th **Y36.411** War operations involving rubber bullets, civilian

√6th **Y36.42** War operations involving firearms pellets

√7th **Y36.420** War operations involving firearms pellets, military personnel

√7th **Y36.421** War operations involving firearms pellets, civilian

√6th **Y36.43** War operations involving other firearms discharge

War operations involving bullets NOS

EXCLUDES 1   *war operations involving munitions fragments (Y36.25-)*

war operations involving incendiary bullets (Y36.32-)

√7th **Y36.430** War operations involving other firearms discharge, military personnel

√7th **Y36.431** War operations involving other firearms discharge, civilian

√6th **Y36.44** War operations involving unarmed hand to hand combat

EXCLUDES 1   *war operations involving combat using blunt or piercing object (Y36.45-)*

war operations involving intentional restriction of air and airway (Y36.46-)

war operations involving unintentional restriction of air and airway (Y36.47-)

√7th **Y36.440** War operations involving unarmed hand to hand combat, military personnel

√7th **Y36.441** War operations involving unarmed hand to hand combat, civilian

√6th **Y36.45** War operations involving combat using blunt or piercing object

√7th **Y36.450** War operations involving combat using blunt or piercing object, military personnel

√7th **Y36.451** War operations involving combat using blunt or piercing object, civilian

√6th **Y36.46** War operations involving intentional restriction of air and airway

√7th **Y36.460** War operations involving intentional restriction of air and airway, military personnel

√7th **Y36.461** War operations involving intentional restriction of air and airway, civilian

N Newborn: 0   P Pediatric: 0-17   M Maternity: 12-55   A Adult: 15-124   MCC Major CC Condition   PDxMCC PDx acts as own MCC   CC CC Condition   PDxCC PDx acts as own CC

1202   ICD-10-CM 2018

✓6ᵗʰ **Y36.47** **War operations involving** unintentional restriction of air and airway

     ✓7ᵗʰ **Y36.470** **War operations involving unintentional restriction of air and airway,** military personnel

     ✓7ᵗʰ **Y36.471** **War operations involving unintentional restriction of air and airway,** civilian

✓6ᵗʰ **Y36.49** **War operations involving** other forms of conventional warfare

     ✓7ᵗʰ **Y36.490** **War operations involving other forms of conventional warfare,** military personnel

     ✓7ᵗʰ **Y36.491** **War operations involving other forms of conventional warfare,** civilian

✓5ᵗʰ **Y36.5** **War operations involving** nuclear weapons
War operations involving dirty bomb NOS

✓6ᵗʰ **Y36.50** **War operations involving** unspecified **effect of nuclear weapon**

     ✓7ᵗʰ **Y36.500** **War operations involving unspecified effect of nuclear weapon,** military personnel

     ✓7ᵗʰ **Y36.501** **War operations involving unspecified effect of nuclear weapon,** civilian

✓6ᵗʰ **Y36.51** **War operations involving** direct blast **effect of nuclear weapon**
War operations involving blast pressure of nuclear weapon

     ✓7ᵗʰ **Y36.510** **War operations involving direct blast effect of nuclear weapon,** military personnel

     ✓7ᵗʰ **Y36.511** **War operations involving direct blast effect of nuclear weapon,** civilian

✓6ᵗʰ **Y36.52** **War operations involving** indirect blast **effect of nuclear weapon**
War operations involving being thrown by blast of nuclear weapon
War operations involving being struck or crushed by blast debris of nuclear weapon

     ✓7ᵗʰ **Y36.520** **War operations involving indirect blast effect of nuclear weapon,** military personnel

     ✓7ᵗʰ **Y36.521** **War operations involving indirect blast effect of nuclear weapon,** civilian

✓6ᵗʰ **Y36.53** **War operations involving** thermal radiation **effect of nuclear weapon**
War operations involving direct heat from nuclear weapon
War operation involving fireball effects from nuclear weapon

     ✓7ᵗʰ **Y36.530** **War operations involving thermal radiation effect of nuclear weapon,** military personnel

     ✓7ᵗʰ **Y36.531** **War operations involving thermal radiation effect of nuclear weapon,** civilian

✓6ᵗʰ **Y36.54** **War operation involving** nuclear radiation **effects of nuclear weapon**
War operation involving acute radiation exposure from nuclear weapon
War operation involving exposure to immediate ionizing radiation from nuclear weapon
War operation involving fallout exposure from nuclear weapon
War operation involving secondary effects of nuclear weapons

     ✓7ᵗʰ **Y36.540** **War operation involving nuclear radiation effects of nuclear weapon,** military personnel

     ✓7ᵗʰ **Y36.541** **War operation involving nuclear radiation effects of nuclear weapon,** civilian

✓6ᵗʰ **Y36.59** **War operation involving** other **effects of nuclear weapons**

     ✓7ᵗʰ **Y36.590** **War operation involving other effects of nuclear weapons,** military personnel

     ✓7ᵗʰ **Y36.591** **War operation involving other effects of nuclear weapons,** civilian

✓5ᵗʰ **Y36.6** **War operations involving biological weapons**

✓6ᵗʰ **Y36.6X** **War operations involving** biological weapons

     ✓7ᵗʰ **Y36.6X0** **War operations involving biological weapons,** military personnel

     ✓7ᵗʰ **Y36.6X1** **War operations involving biological weapons,** civilian

✓5ᵗʰ **Y36.7** **War operations involving chemical weapons and other forms of unconventional warfare**
     EXCLUDES 1   *war operations involving incendiary devices (Y36.3-, Y36.5-)*

✓6ᵗʰ **Y36.7X** **War operations involving** chemical weapons **and** other **forms of** unconventional warfare

     ✓7ᵗʰ **Y36.7X0** **War operations involving chemical weapons and other forms of unconventional warfare,** military personnel

     ✓7ᵗʰ **Y36.7X1** **War operations involving chemical weapons and other forms of unconventional warfare,** civilian

✓5ᵗʰ **Y36.8** **War operations occurring** after cessation of hostilities
War operations classifiable to categories Y36.0-Y36.8 but occurring after cessation of hostilities

✓6ᵗʰ **Y36.81** **Explosion of** mine **placed during war operations but exploding after cessation of hostilities**

     ✓7ᵗʰ **Y36.810** **Explosion of mine placed during war operations but exploding after cessation of hostilities,** military personnel

     ✓7ᵗʰ **Y36.811** **Explosion of mine placed during war operations but exploding after cessation of hostilities,** civilian

✓6ᵗʰ **Y36.82** **Explosion of** bomb **placed during war operations but exploding after cessation of hostilities**

     ✓7ᵗʰ **Y36.820** **Explosion of bomb placed during war operations but exploding after cessation of hostilities,** military personnel

     ✓7ᵗʰ **Y36.821** **Explosion of bomb placed during war operations but exploding after cessation of hostilities,** civilian

✓6ᵗʰ **Y36.88** Other **war operations occurring after cessation of hostilities**

     ✓7ᵗʰ **Y36.880** **Other war operations occurring after cessation of hostilities,** military personnel

     ✓7ᵗʰ **Y36.881** **Other war operations occurring after cessation of hostilities,** civilian

✓6ᵗʰ **Y36.89** Unspecified **war operations occurring after cessation of hostilities**

     ✓7ᵗʰ **Y36.890** **Unspecified war operations occurring after cessation of hostilities,** military personnel

     ✓7ᵗʰ **Y36.891** **Unspecified war operations occurring after cessation of hostilities,** civilian

✓5ᵗʰ **Y36.9** **Other and unspecified war operations**

     ✓x7ᵗʰ **Y36.90** **War operations,** unspecified

     ✓x7ᵗʰ **Y36.91** **War operations** involving unspecified weapon of mass destruction [WMD]

     ✓x7ᵗʰ **Y36.92** **War operations** involving friendly fire

✓4ᵗʰ **Y37** **Military operations**
     INCLUDES   injuries to military personnel and civilians occurring during peacetime on military property and during routine military exercises and operations
     EXCLUDES 1   *military aircraft involved in aircraft accident with civilian aircraft (V97.81-)*
           military vehicles involved in transport accident with civilian vehicle (V09.01, V09.21, V19.81, V29.81, V39.81, V49.81, V59.81, V69.81, V79.81)
           military watercraft involved in water transport accident with civilian watercraft (V94.81-)
           war operations (Y36.-)

✓5ᵗʰ **Y37.0** **Military operations involving** explosion of marine weapons

✓6ᵗʰ **Y37.00** **Military operations involving explosion of** unspecified **marine weapon**
Military operations involving underwater blast NOS

     ✓7ᵗʰ **Y37.000** **Military operations involving explosion of unspecified marine weapon,** military personnel

     ✓7ᵗʰ **Y37.001** **Military operations involving explosion of unspecified marine weapon,** civilian

---

✓ Additional Character Req   ✓x7ᵗʰ Placeholder Alert   Unacceptable PDx   Manifestation   H1 - H14 HAC   HCC CMS-HCC Condition   EXCLUDES 1 Not Coded Here   EXCLUDES 2 Not Included Here

✓6ᵗʰ **Y37.01** **Military operations involving explosion of** depth-charge

  ✓7ᵗʰ **Y37.010** **Military operations involving explosion of depth-charge,** military personnel

  ✓7ᵗʰ **Y37.011** **Military operations involving explosion of depth-charge,** civilian

✓6ᵗʰ **Y37.02** **Military operations involving explosion of** marine mine

    Military operations involving explosion of marine mine, at sea or in harbor

  ✓7ᵗʰ **Y37.020** **Military operations involving explosion of marine mine,** military personnel

  ✓7ᵗʰ **Y37.021** **Military operations involving explosion of marine mine,** civilian

✓6ᵗʰ **Y37.03** **Military operations involving explosion of** sea-based artillery shell

  ✓7ᵗʰ **Y37.030** **Military operations involving explosion of sea-based artillery shell,** military personnel

  ✓7ᵗʰ **Y37.031** **Military operations involving explosion of sea-based artillery shell,** civilian

✓6ᵗʰ **Y37.04** **Military operations involving explosion of** torpedo

  ✓7ᵗʰ **Y37.040** **Military operations involving explosion of torpedo,** military personnel

  ✓7ᵗʰ **Y37.041** **Military operations involving explosion of torpedo,** civilian

✓6ᵗʰ **Y37.05** **Military operations involving accidental detonation of** onboard marine weapons

  ✓7ᵗʰ **Y37.050** **Military operations involving accidental detonation of onboard marine weapons,** military personnel

  ✓7ᵗʰ **Y37.051** **Military operations involving accidental detonation of onboard marine weapons,** civilian

✓6ᵗʰ **Y37.09** **Military operations involving explosion of** other marine weapons

  ✓7ᵗʰ **Y37.090** **Military operations involving explosion of other marine weapons,** military personnel

  ✓7ᵗʰ **Y37.091** **Military operations involving explosion of other marine weapons,** civilian

✓5ᵗʰ **Y37.1** **Military operations involving** destruction of aircraft

✓6ᵗʰ **Y37.10** **Military operations involving** unspecified destruction of aircraft

  ✓7ᵗʰ **Y37.100** **Military operations involving unspecified destruction of aircraft,** military personnel

  ✓7ᵗʰ **Y37.101** **Military operations involving unspecified destruction of aircraft,** civilian

✓6ᵗʰ **Y37.11** **Military operations involving destruction of aircraft due to enemy fire or explosives**

    Military operations involving destruction of aircraft due to air to air missile

    Military operations involving destruction of aircraft due to explosive placed on aircraft

    Military operations involving destruction of aircraft due to rocket propelled grenade [RPG]

    Military operations involving destruction of aircraft due to small arms fire

    Military operations involving destruction of aircraft due to surface to air missile

  ✓7ᵗʰ **Y37.110** **Military operations involving destruction of aircraft due to enemy fire or explosives,** military personnel

  ✓7ᵗʰ **Y37.111** **Military operations involving destruction of aircraft due to enemy fire or explosives,** civilian

✓6ᵗʰ **Y37.12** **Military operations involving destruction of aircraft due to collision with other aircraft**

  ✓7ᵗʰ **Y37.120** **Military operations involving destruction of aircraft due to collision with other aircraft,** military personnel

  ✓7ᵗʰ **Y37.121** **Military operations involving destruction of aircraft due to collision with other aircraft,** civilian

✓6ᵗʰ **Y37.13** **Military operations involving destruction of aircraft due to onboard fire**

  ✓7ᵗʰ **Y37.130** **Military operations involving destruction of aircraft due to onboard fire,** military personnel

✓7ᵗʰ **Y37.131** **Military operations involving destruction of aircraft due to onboard fire,** civilian

✓6ᵗʰ **Y37.14** **Military operations involving destruction of aircraft due to** accidental detonation of onboard munitions and explosives

  ✓7ᵗʰ **Y37.140** **Military operations involving destruction of aircraft due to accidental detonation of onboard munitions and explosives,** military personnel

  ✓7ᵗʰ **Y37.141** **Military operations involving destruction of aircraft due to accidental detonation of onboard munitions and explosives,** civilian

✓6ᵗʰ **Y37.19** **Military operations involving other** destruction of aircraft

  ✓7ᵗʰ **Y37.190** **Military operations involving other destruction of aircraft,** military personnel

  ✓7ᵗʰ **Y37.191** **Military operations involving other destruction of aircraft,** civilian

✓5ᵗʰ **Y37.2** **Military operations involving** other explosions and fragments

    EXCLUDES 1   *military operations involving explosion of aircraft (Y37.1-)*

    military operations involving explosion of marine weapons (Y37.0-)

    military operations involving explosion of nuclear weapons (Y37.5-)

✓6ᵗʰ **Y37.20** **Military operations involving** unspecified **explosion and fragments**

    Military operations involving air blast NOS

    Military operations involving blast NOS

    Military operations involving blast fragments NOS

    Military operations involving blast wave NOS

    Military operations involving blast wind NOS

    Military operations involving explosion NOS

    Military operations involving explosion of bomb NOS

  ✓7ᵗʰ **Y37.200** **Military operations involving unspecified explosion and fragments,** military personnel

  ✓7ᵗʰ **Y37.201** **Military operations involving unspecified explosion and fragments,** civilian

✓6ᵗʰ **Y37.21** **Military operations involving explosion of** aerial bomb

  ✓7ᵗʰ **Y37.210** **Military operations involving explosion of aerial bomb,** military personnel

  ✓7ᵗʰ **Y37.211** **Military operations involving explosion of aerial bomb,** civilian

✓6ᵗʰ **Y37.22** **Military operations involving explosion of** guided missile

  ✓7ᵗʰ **Y37.220** **Military operations involving explosion of guided missile,** military personnel

  ✓7ᵗʰ **Y37.221** **Military operations involving explosion of guided missile,** civilian

✓6ᵗʰ **Y37.23** **Military operations involving explosion of** improvised explosive device [IED]

    Military operations involving explosion of person-borne improvised explosive device [IED]

    Military operations involving explosion of vehicle-borne improvised explosive device [IED]

    Military operations involving explosion of roadside improvised explosive device [IED]

  ✓7ᵗʰ **Y37.230** **Military operations involving explosion of improvised explosive device [IED],** military personnel

  ✓7ᵗʰ **Y37.231** **Military operations involving explosion of improvised explosive device [IED],** civilian

✓6ᵗʰ **Y37.24** **Military operations involving explosion** due to accidental detonation and discharge of own munitions or munitions launch device

  ✓7ᵗʰ **Y37.240** **Military operations involving explosion due to accidental detonation and discharge of own munitions or munitions launch device,** military personnel

  ✓7ᵗʰ **Y37.241** **Military operations involving explosion due to accidental detonation and discharge of own munitions or munitions launch device,** civilian

N Newborn: 0   P Pediatric: 0-17   M Maternity: 12-55   A Adult: 15-124   **MCC** Major CC Condition   **PDxMCC** PDx acts as own MCC   **CC** CC Condition   **PDxCC** PDx acts as own CC

1204   ICD-10-CM 2018

✓6ᵗʰ **Y37.25 Military operations involving** fragments from munitions

    ✓7ᵗʰ **Y37.250 Military operations involving fragments from munitions,** military personnel

    ✓7ᵗʰ **Y37.251 Military operations involving fragments from munitions,** civilian

✓6ᵗʰ **Y37.26 Military operations involving** fragments of improvised explosive device [IED]

    Military operations involving fragments of person-borne improvised explosive device [IED]

    Military operations involving fragments of vehicle-borne improvised explosive device [IED]

    Military operations involving fragments of roadside improvised explosive device [IED]

    ✓7ᵗʰ **Y37.260 Military operations involving fragments of improvised explosive device [IED],** military personnel

    ✓7ᵗʰ **Y37.261 Military operations involving fragments of improvised explosive device [IED],** civilian

✓6ᵗʰ **Y37.27 Military operations involving** fragments from weapons

    ✓7ᵗʰ **Y37.270 Military operations involving fragments from weapons,** military personnel

    ✓7ᵗʰ **Y37.271 Military operations involving fragments from weapons,** civilian

✓6ᵗʰ **Y37.29 Military operations involving** other explosions and fragments

    Military operations involving explosion of grenade

    Military operations involving explosions of land mine

    Military operations involving shrapnel NOS

    ✓7ᵗʰ **Y37.290 Military operations involving other explosions and fragments,** military personnel

    ✓7ᵗʰ **Y37.291 Military operations involving other explosions and fragments,** civilian

✓5ᵗʰ **Y37.3 Military operations involving** fires, conflagrations and hot substances

    Military operations involving smoke, fumes, and heat from fires, conflagrations and hot substances

    EXCLUDES 1   *military operations involving fires and conflagrations aboard military aircraft (Y37.1-)*

        military operations involving fires and conflagrations aboard military watercraft (Y37.0-)

        military operations involving fires and conflagrations caused indirectly by conventional weapons (Y37.2-)

        military operations involving fires and thermal effects of nuclear weapons (Y36.53-)

✓6ᵗʰ **Y37.30 Military operations involving** unspecified fire, conflagration and hot substance

    ✓7ᵗʰ **Y37.300 Military operations involving unspecified fire, conflagration and hot substance,** military personnel

    ✓7ᵗʰ **Y37.301 Military operations involving unspecified fire, conflagration and hot substance,** civilian

✓6ᵗʰ **Y37.31 Military operations involving** gasoline bomb

    Military operations involving incendiary bomb

    Military operations involving petrol bomb

    ✓7ᵗʰ **Y37.310 Military operations involving gasoline bomb,** military personnel

    ✓7ᵗʰ **Y37.311 Military operations involving gasoline bomb,** civilian

✓6ᵗʰ **Y37.32 Military operations involving** incendiary bullet

    ✓7ᵗʰ **Y37.320 Military operations involving incendiary bullet,** military personnel

    ✓7ᵗʰ **Y37.321 Military operations involving incendiary bullet,** civilian

✓6ᵗʰ **Y37.33 Military operations involving** flamethrower

    ✓7ᵗʰ **Y37.330 Military operations involving flamethrower,** military personnel

    ✓7ᵗʰ **Y37.331 Military operations involving flamethrower,** civilian

✓6ᵗʰ **Y37.39 Military operations involving** other fires, conflagrations and hot substances

    ✓7ᵗʰ **Y37.390 Military operations involving other fires, conflagrations and hot substances,** military personnel

    ✓7ᵗʰ **Y37.391 Military operations involving other fires, conflagrations and hot substances,** civilian

✓5ᵗʰ **Y37.4 Military operations involving firearm discharge and other forms of conventional warfare**

✓6ᵗʰ **Y37.41 Military operations involving** rubber bullets

    ✓7ᵗʰ **Y37.410 Military operations involving rubber bullets,** military personnel

    ✓7ᵗʰ **Y37.411 Military operations involving rubber bullets,** civilian

✓6ᵗʰ **Y37.42 Military operations involving** firearms pellets

    ✓7ᵗʰ **Y37.420 Military operations involving firearms pellets,** military personnel

    ✓7ᵗʰ **Y37.421 Military operations involving firearms pellets,** civilian

✓6ᵗʰ **Y37.43 Military operations involving** other firearms discharge

    Military operations involving bullets NOS

    EXCLUDES 1   *military operations involving munitions fragments (Y37.25-)*

        military operations involving incendiary bullets (Y37.32-)

    ✓7ᵗʰ **Y37.430 Military operations involving other firearms discharge,** military personnel

    ✓7ᵗʰ **Y37.431 Military operations involving other firearms discharge,** civilian

✓6ᵗʰ **Y37.44 Military operations involving** unarmed hand to hand combat

    EXCLUDES 1   *military operations involving combat using blunt or piercing object (Y37.45-)*

        military operations involving intentional restriction of air and airway (Y37.46-)

        military operations involving unintentional restriction of air and airway (Y37.47-)

    ✓7ᵗʰ **Y37.440 Military operations involving unarmed hand to hand combat,** military personnel

    ✓7ᵗʰ **Y37.441 Military operations involving unarmed hand to hand combat,** civilian

✓6ᵗʰ **Y37.45 Military operations involving** combat using blunt or piercing object

    ✓7ᵗʰ **Y37.450 Military operations involving combat using blunt or piercing object,** military personnel

    ✓7ᵗʰ **Y37.451 Military operations involving combat using blunt or piercing object,** civilian

✓6ᵗʰ **Y37.46 Military operations involving** intentional restriction of air and airway

    ✓7ᵗʰ **Y37.460 Military operations involving intentional restriction of air and airway,** military personnel

    ✓7ᵗʰ **Y37.461 Military operations involving intentional restriction of air and airway,** civilian

✓6ᵗʰ **Y37.47 Military operations involving** unintentional restriction of air and airway

    ✓7ᵗʰ **Y37.470 Military operations involving unintentional restriction of air and airway,** military personnel

    ✓7ᵗʰ **Y37.471 Military operations involving unintentional restriction of air and airway,** civilian

✓6ᵗʰ **Y37.49 Military operations involving** other forms of conventional warfare

    ✓7ᵗʰ **Y37.490 Military operations involving other forms of conventional warfare,** military personnel

    ✓7ᵗʰ **Y37.491 Military operations involving other forms of conventional warfare,** civilian

✔ Additional Character Req   ✓x7ᵗʰ Placeholder Alert   Unacceptable PDx   ■ Manifestation   H1-H14 HAC   HCC CMS-HCC Condition   *EXCLUDES 1* Not Coded Here   *EXCLUDES 2* Not Included Here

ICD-10-CM 2018   1205

Chapter 20. External Causes of Morbidity *(left margin)*

Y37.5–Y38.2X3 *(left margin)*

✓5th **Y37.5 Military operations involving** nuclear weapons
Military operation involving dirty bomb NOS

  ✓6th **Y37.50 Military operations involving** unspecified effect of nuclear weapon

    ✓7th **Y37.500 Military operations involving unspecified effect of nuclear weapon,** military personnel

    ✓7th **Y37.501 Military operations involving unspecified effect of nuclear weapon,** civilian

  ✓6th **Y37.51 Military operations involving** direct blast effect of nuclear weapon
Military operations involving blast pressure of nuclear weapon

    ✓7th **Y37.510 Military operations involving direct blast effect of nuclear weapon,** military personnel

    ✓7th **Y37.511 Military operations involving direct blast effect of nuclear weapon,** civilian

  ✓6th **Y37.52 Military operations involving** indirect blast effect of nuclear weapon
Military operations involving being thrown by blast of nuclear weapon
Military operations involving being struck or crushed by blast debris of nuclear weapon

    ✓7th **Y37.520 Military operations involving indirect blast effect of nuclear weapon,** military personnel

    ✓7th **Y37.521 Military operations involving indirect blast effect of nuclear weapon,** civilian

  ✓6th **Y37.53 Military operations involving** thermal radiation effect of nuclear weapon
Military operations involving direct heat from nuclear weapon
Military operation involving fireball effects from nuclear weapon

    ✓7th **Y37.530 Military operations involving thermal radiation effect of nuclear weapon,** military personnel

    ✓7th **Y37.531 Military operations involving thermal radiation effect of nuclear weapon,** civilian

  ✓6th **Y37.54 Military operation involving** nuclear radiation effects of nuclear weapon
Military operation involving acute radiation exposure from nuclear weapon
Military operation involving exposure to immediate ionizing radiation from nuclear weapon
Military operation involving fallout exposure from nuclear weapon
Military operation involving secondary effects of nuclear weapons

    ✓7th **Y37.540 Military operation involving nuclear radiation effects of nuclear weapon,** military personnel

    ✓7th **Y37.541 Military operation involving nuclear radiation effects of nuclear weapon,** civilian

  ✓6th **Y37.59 Military operation involving** other effects of nuclear weapons

    ✓7th **Y37.590 Military operation involving other effects of nuclear weapons,** military personnel

    ✓7th **Y37.591 Military operation involving other effects of nuclear weapons,** civilian

✓5th **Y37.6 Military operations involving** biological weapons

  ✓6th **Y37.6X Military operations involving biological weapons**

    ✓7th **Y37.6X0 Military operations involving biological weapons,** military personnel

    ✓7th **Y37.6X1 Military operations involving biological weapons,** civilian

✓5th **Y37.7 Military operations involving** chemical weapons and other forms of unconventional warfare
  EXCLUDES 1 *military operations involving incendiary devices (Y36.3-, Y36.5-)*

  ✓6th **Y37.7X Military operations involving** chemical weapons and other forms of unconventional warfare

    ✓7th **Y37.7X0 Military operations involving chemical weapons and other forms of unconventional warfare,** military personnel

    ✓7th **Y37.7X1 Military operations involving chemical weapons and other forms of unconventional warfare,** civilian

✓5th **Y37.9 Other and unspecified military operations**

  ✓x7th **Y37.90 Military operations,** unspecified

  ✓x7th **Y37.91 Military operations** involving unspecified weapon of mass destruction [WMD]

  ✓x7th **Y37.92 Military operations involving** friendly fire

✓4th **Y38 Terrorism**
  NOTE   These codes are for use to identify injuries resulting from the unlawful use of force or violence against persons or property to intimidate or coerce a Government, the civilian population, or any segment thereof, in furtherance of political or social objective.
  Use additional code for place of occurrence (Y92.-)

✓5th **Y38.0 Terrorism involving explosion of marine weapons**
Terrorism involving depth-charge
Terrorism involving marine mine
Terrorism involving mine NOS, at sea or in harbor
Terrorism involving sea-based artillery shell
Terrorism involving torpedo
Terrorism involving underwater blast

  ✓6th **Y38.0X Terrorism involving explosion of** marine weapons

    ✓7th **Y38.0X1 Terrorism involving explosion of marine weapons,** public safety official injured

    ✓7th **Y38.0X2 Terrorism involving explosion of marine weapons,** civilian injured

    ✓7th **Y38.0X3 Terrorism involving explosion of marine weapons,** terrorist injured

✓5th **Y38.1 Terrorism involving destruction of aircraft**
Terrorism involving aircraft burned
Terrorism involving aircraft exploded
Terrorism involving aircraft being shot down
Terrorism involving aircraft used as a weapon

  ✓6th **Y38.1X Terrorism involving** destruction of aircraft

    ✓7th **Y38.1X1 Terrorism involving destruction of aircraft,** public safety official injured

    ✓7th **Y38.1X2 Terrorism involving destruction of aircraft,** civilian injured

    ✓7th **Y38.1X3 Terrorism involving destruction of aircraft,** terrorist injured

✓5th **Y38.2 Terrorism involving other explosions and fragments**
Terrorism involving antipersonnel (fragments) bomb
Terrorism involving blast NOS
Terrorism involving explosion NOS
Terrorism involving explosion of breech block
Terrorism involving explosion of cannon block
Terrorism involving explosion (fragments) of artillery shell
Terrorism involving explosion (fragments) of bomb
Terrorism involving explosion (fragments) of grenade
Terrorism involving explosion (fragments) of guided missile
Terrorism involving explosion (fragments) of land mine
Terrorism involving explosion of mortar bomb
Terrorism involving explosion of munitions
Terrorism involving explosion (fragments) of rocket
Terrorism involving explosion (fragments) of shell
Terrorism involving shrapnel
Terrorism involving mine NOS, on land
  EXCLUDES 1 *terrorism involving explosion of nuclear weapon (Y38.5)*
              terrorism involving suicide bomber (Y38.81)

  ✓6th **Y38.2X Terrorism involving** other explosions and fragments

    ✓7th **Y38.2X1 Terrorism involving other explosions and fragments,** public safety official injured

    ✓7th **Y38.2X2 Terrorism involving other explosions and fragments,** civilian injured

    ✓7th **Y38.2X3 Terrorism involving other explosions and fragments,** terrorist injured

N Newborn: 0   P Pediatric: 0-17   M Maternity: 12-55   A Adult: 15-124   MCC Major CC Condition   PDxMCC PDx acts as own MCC   CC CC Condition   PDxCC PDx acts as own CC

1206   ICD-10-CM 2018

☑5ᵗʰ **Y38.3 Terrorism involving fires, conflagration and hot substances**
Terrorism involving conflagration NOS
Terrorism involving fire NOS
Terrorism involving petrol bomb
EXCLUDES 1   *terrorism involving fire or heat of nuclear weapon (Y38.5)*

☑6ᵗʰ **Y38.3X Terrorism involving fires, conflagration and hot substances**

☑7ᵗʰ **Y38.3X1 Terrorism involving fires, conflagration and hot substances, public safety official injured**

☑7ᵗʰ **Y38.3X2 Terrorism involving fires, conflagration and hot substances, civilian injured**

☑7ᵗʰ **Y38.3X3 Terrorism involving fires, conflagration and hot substances, terrorist injured**

☑5ᵗʰ **Y38.4 Terrorism involving firearms**
Terrorism involving carbine bullet
Terrorism involving machine gun bullet
Terrorism involving pellets (shotgun)
Terrorism involving pistol bullet
Terrorism involving rifle bullet
Terrorism involving rubber (rifle) bullet

☑6ᵗʰ **Y38.4X Terrorism involving firearms**

☑7ᵗʰ **Y38.4X1 Terrorism involving firearms, public safety official injured**

☑7ᵗʰ **Y38.4X2 Terrorism involving firearms, civilian injured**

☑7ᵗʰ **Y38.4X3 Terrorism involving firearms, terrorist injured**

☑5ᵗʰ **Y38.5 Terrorism involving nuclear weapons**
Terrorism involving blast effects of nuclear weapon
Terrorism involving exposure to ionizing radiation from nuclear weapon
Terrorism involving fireball effect of nuclear weapon
Terrorism involving heat from nuclear weapon

☑6ᵗʰ **Y38.5X Terrorism involving nuclear weapons**

☑7ᵗʰ **Y38.5X1 Terrorism involving nuclear weapons, public safety official injured**

☑7ᵗʰ **Y38.5X2 Terrorism involving nuclear weapons, civilian injured**

☑7ᵗʰ **Y38.5X3 Terrorism involving nuclear weapons, terrorist injured**

☑5ᵗʰ **Y38.6 Terrorism involving biological weapons**
Terrorism involving anthrax
Terrorism involving cholera
Terrorism involving smallpox

☑6ᵗʰ **Y38.6X Terrorism involving biological weapons**

☑7ᵗʰ **Y38.6X1 Terrorism involving biological weapons, public safety official injured**

☑7ᵗʰ **Y38.6X2 Terrorism involving biological weapons, civilian injured**

☑7ᵗʰ **Y38.6X3 Terrorism involving biological weapons, terrorist injured**

☑5ᵗʰ **Y38.7 Terrorism involving chemical weapons**
Terrorism involving gases, fumes, chemicals
Terrorism involving hydrogen cyanide
Terrorism involving phosgene
Terrorism involving sarin

☑6ᵗʰ **Y38.7X Terrorism involving chemical weapons**

☑7ᵗʰ **Y38.7X1 Terrorism involving chemical weapons, public safety official injured**

☑7ᵗʰ **Y38.7X2 Terrorism involving chemical weapons, civilian injured**

☑7ᵗʰ **Y38.7X3 Terrorism involving chemical weapons, terrorist injured**

☑5ᵗʰ **Y38.8 Terrorism involving other and unspecified means**

☑x7ᵗʰ **Y38.80 Terrorism involving unspecified means**
Terrorism NOS

☑6ᵗʰ **Y38.81 Terrorism involving suicide bomber**

☑7ᵗʰ **Y38.811 Terrorism involving suicide bomber, public safety official injured**

☑7ᵗʰ **Y38.812 Terrorism involving suicide bomber, civilian injured**

☑6ᵗʰ **Y38.89 Terrorism involving other means**
Terrorism involving drowning and submersion
Terrorism involving lasers
Terrorism involving piercing or stabbing instruments

☑7ᵗʰ **Y38.891 Terrorism involving other means, public safety official injured**

☑7ᵗʰ **Y38.892 Terrorism involving other means, civilian injured**

☑7ᵗʰ **Y38.893 Terrorism involving other means, terrorist injured**

☑5ᵗʰ **Y38.9 Terrorism, secondary effects**
NOTE   This code is for use to identify injuries occurring subsequent to a terrorist attack, not those that are due to the initial terrorist attack.

☑6ᵗʰ **Y38.9X Terrorism, secondary effects**

☑7ᵗʰ **Y38.9X1 Terrorism, secondary effects, public safety official injured**

☑7ᵗʰ **Y38.9X2 Terrorism, secondary effects, civilian injured**

Complications of medical and surgical care (Y62-Y84)

INCLUDES   complications of medical devices
surgical and medical procedures as the cause of abnormal reaction of the patient, or of later complication, without mention of misadventure at the time of the procedure

Misadventures to patients during surgical and medical care (Y62-Y69)

EXCLUDES 1   *surgical and medical procedures as the cause of abnormal reaction of the patient, without mention of misadventure at the time of the procedure (Y83-Y84)*
EXCLUDES 2   *breakdown or malfunctioning of medical device (during procedure) (after implantation) (ongoing use) (Y70-Y82)*

☑4ᵗʰ **Y62 Failure of sterile precautions during surgical and medical care**

Y62.0 Failure of sterile precautions during surgical operation

Y62.1 Failure of sterile precautions during infusion or transfusion

Y62.2 Failure of sterile precautions during kidney dialysis **HCC** **and other perfusion**

Y62.3 Failure of sterile precautions during injection or immunization

Y62.4 Failure of sterile precautions during endoscopic examination

Y62.5 Failure of sterile precautions during heart catheterization

Y62.6 Failure of sterile precautions during aspiration, puncture and other catheterization

Y62.8 Failure of sterile precautions during other surgical and medical care

Y62.9 Failure of sterile precautions during unspecified surgical and medical care

☑4ᵗʰ **Y63 Failure in dosage during surgical and medical care**
EXCLUDES 2   *accidental overdose of drug or wrong drug given in error (T36-T50)*

Y63.0 Excessive amount of blood or other fluid given during transfusion or infusion

Y63.1 Incorrect dilution of fluid used during infusion

Y63.2 Overdose of radiation given during therapy

Y63.3 Inadvertent exposure of patient to radiation during medical care

Y63.4 Failure in dosage in electroshock or insulin-shock therapy

Y63.5 Inappropriate temperature in local application and packing

Y63.6 Underdosing and nonadministration of necessary drug, medicament or biological substance

Y63.8 Failure in dosage during other surgical and medical care

Y63.9 Failure in dosage during unspecified surgical and medical care

☑4ᵗʰ **Y64 Contaminated medical or biological substances**

Y64.0 Contaminated medical or biological substance, transfused or infused

Y64.1 Contaminated medical or biological substance, injected or used for immunization

Y64.8 Contaminated medical or biological substance administered by other means

Y64.9 Contaminated medical or biological substance administered by unspecified means
Administered contaminated medical or biological substance NOS

☑ Additional Character Req   ☑x7ᵗʰ Placeholder Alert   Unacceptable PDx   Manifestation   **H1**-**H14** HAC   **HCC** CMS-HCC Condition   *EXCLUDES 1* Not Coded Here   *EXCLUDES 2* Not Included Here

☑4ᵗʰ Y65 Other misadventures during surgical and medical care

- **Y65.0 Mismatched blood in transfusion**
- **Y65.1 Wrong fluid used in infusion**
- **Y65.2 Failure in suture or ligature during surgical operation**
- **Y65.3 Endotracheal tube wrongly placed during anesthetic procedure**
- **Y65.4 Failure to introduce or to remove other tube or instrument**
- **☑5ᵗʰ Y65.5 Performance of wrong procedure (operation)**
    - **² Y65.51 Performance of wrong procedure (operation) on correct patient**
        Wrong device implanted into correct surgical site
        EXCLUDES 1 *performance of correct procedure (operation) on wrong side or body part (Y65.53)*
    - **² Y65.52 Performance of procedure (operation) on patient not scheduled for surgery**
        Performance of procedure (operation) intended for another patient
        Performance of procedure (operation) on wrong patient
    - **² Y65.53 Performance of correct procedure (operation) on wrong side or body part**
        Performance of correct procedure (operation) on wrong side
        Performance of correct procedure (operation) on wrong site
- **Y65.8 Other specified misadventures during surgical and medical care**

Y66 Nonadministration of surgical and medical care
    Premature cessation of surgical and medical care
    EXCLUDES 1 *DNR status (Z66)*
    palliative care (Z51.5)

Y69 Unspecified misadventure during surgical and medical care

Medical devices associated with adverse incidents in diagnostic and therapeutic use (Y70-Y82)

INCLUDES breakdown or malfunction of medical devices (during use) (after implantation) (ongoing use)

EXCLUDES 2 *breakdown or malfunctioning of medical device (after implantation) (during procedure) (ongoing use) (Y70-Y82)*
    later complications following use of medical devices without breakdown or malfunctioning of device (Y83-Y84)
    misadventure to patients during surgical and medical care, classifiable to (Y62-Y69)
    surgical and other medical procedures as the cause of abnormal reaction of the patient, or of later complication, without mention of misadventure at the time of the procedure (Y83-Y84)

☑4ᵗʰ Y70 Anesthesiology devices associated with adverse incidents

- **Y70.0 Diagnostic and monitoring anesthesiology devices associated with adverse incidents**
- **Y70.1 Therapeutic (nonsurgical) and rehabilitative anesthesiology devices associated with adverse incidents**
- **Y70.2 Prosthetic and other implants, materials and accessory anesthesiology devices associated with adverse incidents**
- **Y70.3 Surgical instruments, materials and anesthesiology devices (including sutures) associated with adverse incidents**
- **Y70.8 Miscellaneous anesthesiology devices associated with adverse incidents, not elsewhere classified**

☑4ᵗʰ Y71 Cardiovascular devices associated with adverse incidents

- **Y71.0 Diagnostic and monitoring cardiovascular devices associated with adverse incidents**
- **Y71.1 Therapeutic (nonsurgical) and rehabilitative cardiovascular devices associated with adverse incidents**
- **Y71.2 Prosthetic and other implants, materials and accessory cardiovascular devices associated with adverse incidents**
- **Y71.3 Surgical instruments, materials and cardiovascular devices (including sutures) associated with adverse incidents**
- **Y71.8 Miscellaneous cardiovascular devices associated with adverse incidents, not elsewhere classified**

☑4ᵗʰ Y72 Otorhinolaryngological devices associated with adverse incidents

- **Y72.0 Diagnostic and monitoring otorhinolaryngological devices associated with adverse incidents**
- **Y72.1 Therapeutic (nonsurgical) and rehabilitative otorhinolaryngological devices associated with adverse incidents**
- **Y72.2 Prosthetic and other implants, materials and accessory otorhinolaryngological devices associated with adverse incidents**
- **Y72.3 Surgical instruments, materials and otorhinolaryngological devices (including sutures) associated with adverse incidents**
- **Y72.8 Miscellaneous otorhinolaryngological devices associated with adverse incidents, not elsewhere classified**

☑4ᵗʰ Y73 Gastroenterology and urology devices associated with adverse incidents

- **Y73.0 Diagnostic and monitoring gastroenterology and urology devices associated with adverse incidents**
- **Y73.1 Therapeutic (nonsurgical) and rehabilitative gastroenterology and urology devices associated with adverse incidents**
- **Y73.2 Prosthetic and other implants, materials and accessory gastroenterology and urology devices associated with adverse incidents**
- **Y73.3 Surgical instruments, materials and gastroenterology and urology devices (including sutures) associated with adverse incidents**
- **Y73.8 Miscellaneous gastroenterology and urology devices associated with adverse incidents, not elsewhere classified**

☑4ᵗʰ Y74 General hospital and personal-use devices associated with adverse incidents

- **Y74.0 Diagnostic and monitoring general hospital and personal-use devices associated with adverse incidents**
- **Y74.1 Therapeutic (nonsurgical) and rehabilitative general hospital and personal-use devices associated with adverse incidents**
- **Y74.2 Prosthetic and other implants, materials and accessory general hospital and personal-use devices associated with adverse incidents**
- **Y74.3 Surgical instruments, materials and general hospital and personal-use devices (including sutures) associated with adverse incidents**
- **Y74.8 Miscellaneous general hospital and personal-use devices associated with adverse incidents, not elsewhere classified**

☑4ᵗʰ Y75 Neurological devices associated with adverse incidents

- **Y75.0 Diagnostic and monitoring neurological devices associated with adverse incidents**
- **Y75.1 Therapeutic (nonsurgical) and rehabilitative neurological devices associated with adverse incidents**
- **Y75.2 Prosthetic and other implants, materials and neurological devices associated with adverse incidents**
- **Y75.3 Surgical instruments, materials and neurological devices (including sutures) associated with adverse incidents**
- **Y75.8 Miscellaneous neurological devices associated with adverse incidents, not elsewhere classified**

☑4ᵗʰ Y76 Obstetric and gynecological devices associated with adverse incidents

- **Y76.0 Diagnostic and monitoring obstetric and gynecological devices associated with adverse incidents** ♀
- **Y76.1 Therapeutic (nonsurgical) and rehabilitative obstetric and gynecological devices associated with adverse incidents** ♀
- **Y76.2 Prosthetic and other implants, materials and accessory obstetric and gynecological devices associated with adverse incidents** ♀
- **Y76.3 Surgical instruments, materials and obstetric and gynecological devices (including sutures) associated with adverse incidents** ♀
- **Y76.8 Miscellaneous obstetric and gynecological devices associated with adverse incidents, not elsewhere classified** ♀

☑4ᵗʰ Y77 Ophthalmic devices associated with adverse incidents

- **Y77.0 Diagnostic and monitoring ophthalmic devices associated with adverse incidents**
- **Y77.1 Therapeutic (nonsurgical) and rehabilitative ophthalmic devices associated with adverse incidents**
- **Y77.2 Prosthetic and other implants, materials and accessory ophthalmic devices associated with adverse incidents**
- **Y77.3 Surgical instruments, materials and ophthalmic devices (including sutures) associated with adverse incidents**
- **Y77.8 Miscellaneous ophthalmic devices associated with adverse incidents, not elsewhere classified**

---

² Wrong procedure performed edit applies.

Ⓝ Newborn: 0   Ⓟ Pediatric: 0-17   Ⓜ Maternity: 12-55   Ⓐ Adult: 15-124   MCC Major CC Condition   PDxMCC PDx acts as own MCC   CC CC Condition   PDxCC PDx acts as own CC

1208   ICD-10-CM 2018

✓4ᵗʰ Y78 Radiological devices associated with adverse incidents

- **Y78.0** Diagnostic and monitoring radiological devices associated with adverse incidents
- **Y78.1** Therapeutic (nonsurgical) and rehabilitative radiological devices associated with adverse incidents
- **Y78.2** Prosthetic and other implants, materials and accessory radiological devices associated with adverse incidents
- **Y78.3** Surgical instruments, materials and radiological devices (including sutures) associated with adverse incidents
- **Y78.8** Miscellaneous radiological devices associated with adverse incidents, not elsewhere classified

✓4ᵗʰ Y79 Orthopedic devices associated with adverse incidents

- **Y79.0** Diagnostic and monitoring orthopedic devices associated with adverse incidents
- **Y79.1** Therapeutic (nonsurgical) and rehabilitative orthopedic devices associated with adverse incidents
- **Y79.2** Prosthetic and other implants, materials and accessory orthopedic devices associated with adverse incidents
- **Y79.3** Surgical instruments, materials and orthopedic devices (including sutures) associated with adverse incidents
- **Y79.8** Miscellaneous orthopedic devices associated with adverse incidents, not elsewhere classified

✓4ᵗʰ Y80 Physical medicine devices associated with adverse incidents

- **Y80.0** Diagnostic and monitoring physical medicine devices associated with adverse incidents
- **Y80.1** Therapeutic (nonsurgical) and rehabilitative physical medicine devices associated with adverse incidents
- **Y80.2** Prosthetic and other implants, materials and accessory physical medicine devices associated with adverse incidents
- **Y80.3** Surgical instruments, materials and physical medicine devices (including sutures) associated with adverse incidents
- **Y80.8** Miscellaneous physical medicine devices associated with adverse incidents, not elsewhere classified

✓4ᵗʰ Y81 General- and plastic-surgery devices associated with adverse incidents

- **Y81.0** Diagnostic and monitoring general- and plastic-surgery devices associated with adverse incidents
- **Y81.1** Therapeutic (nonsurgical) and rehabilitative general- and plastic-surgery devices associated with adverse incidents
- **Y81.2** Prosthetic and other implants, materials and accessory general- and plastic-surgery devices associated with adverse incidents
- **Y81.3** Surgical instruments, materials and general- and plastic-surgery devices (including sutures) associated with adverse incidents
- **Y81.8** Miscellaneous general- and plastic-surgery devices associated with adverse incidents, not elsewhere classified

✓4ᵗʰ Y82 Other and unspecified medical devices associated with adverse incidents

- **Y82.8** Other medical devices associated with adverse incidents
- **Y82.9** Unspecified medical devices associated with adverse incidents

Surgical and other medical procedures as the cause of abnormal reaction of the patient, or of later complication, without mention of misadventure at the time of the procedure (Y83-Y84)

EXCLUDES 1   misadventures to patients during surgical and medical care, classifiable to (Y62-Y69)

EXCLUDES 2   breakdown or malfunctioning of medical device (after implantation) (during procedure) (ongoing use) (Y70-Y82)

✓4ᵗʰ Y83 Surgical operation and other surgical procedures as the cause of abnormal reaction of the patient, or of later complication, without mention of misadventure at the time of the procedure

- **Y83.0** Surgical operation with transplant of whole organ as the cause of abnormal reaction of the patient, or of later complication, without mention of misadventure at the time of the procedure
- **Y83.1** Surgical operation with implant of artificial internal device as the cause of abnormal reaction of the patient, or of later complication, without mention of misadventure at the time of the procedure
- **Y83.2** Surgical operation with anastomosis, bypass or graft as the cause of abnormal reaction of the patient, or of later complication, without mention of misadventure at the time of the procedure
- **Y83.3** Surgical operation with formation of external stoma as the cause of abnormal reaction of the patient, or of later complication, without mention of misadventure at the time of the procedure
- **Y83.4** Other reconstructive surgery as the cause of abnormal reaction of the patient, or of later complication, without mention of misadventure at the time of the procedure
- **Y83.5** Amputation of limb(s) as the cause of abnormal reaction of the patient, or of later complication, without mention of misadventure at the time of the procedure
- **Y83.6** Removal of other organ (partial) (total) as the cause of abnormal reaction of the patient, or of later complication, without mention of misadventure at the time of the procedure
- **Y83.8** Other surgical procedures as the cause of abnormal reaction of the patient, or of later complication, without mention of misadventure at the time of the procedure
- **Y83.9** Surgical procedure, unspecified as the cause of abnormal reaction of the patient, or of later complication, without mention of misadventure at the time of the procedure

✓4ᵗʰ Y84 Other medical procedures as the cause of abnormal reaction of the patient, or of later complication, without mention of misadventure at the time of the procedure

- **Y84.0** Cardiac catheterization as the cause of abnormal reaction of the patient, or of later complication, without mention of misadventure at the time of the procedure
- **Y84.1** Kidney dialysis as the cause of abnormal reaction of the patient, or of later complication, without mention of misadventure at the time of the procedure
- **Y84.2** Radiological procedure and radiotherapy as the cause of abnormal reaction of the patient, or of later complication, without mention of misadventure at the time of the procedure
  AHA: 2017, 1Q, 33
- **Y84.3** Shock therapy as the cause of abnormal reaction of the patient, or of later complication, without mention of misadventure at the time of the procedure
- **Y84.4** Aspiration of fluid as the cause of abnormal reaction of the patient, or of later complication, without mention of misadventure at the time of the procedure
- **Y84.5** Insertion of gastric or duodenal sound as the cause of abnormal reaction of the patient, or of later complication, without mention of misadventure at the time of the procedure
- **Y84.6** Urinary catheterization as the cause of abnormal reaction of the patient, or of later complication, without mention of misadventure at the time of the procedure
- **Y84.7** Blood-sampling as the cause of abnormal reaction of the patient, or of later complication, without mention of misadventure at the time of the procedure
- **Y84.8** Other medical procedures as the cause of abnormal reaction of the patient, or of later complication, without mention of misadventure at the time of the procedure
  AHA: 2014, 4Q, 24
- **Y84.9** Medical procedure, unspecified as the cause of abnormal reaction of the patient, or of later complication, without mention of misadventure at the time of the procedure

Supplementary factors related to causes of morbidity classified elsewhere (Y90-Y99)

NOTE   These categories may be used to provide supplementary information concerning causes of morbidity. They are not to be used for single-condition coding.

✓4ᵗʰ Y90 Evidence of alcohol involvement determined by blood alcohol level

Code first any associated alcohol related disorders (F10)

- **Y90.0** Blood alcohol level of less than 20 mg/100 ml
- **Y90.1** Blood alcohol level of 20-39 mg/100 ml
- **Y90.2** Blood alcohol level of 40-59 mg/100 ml
- **Y90.3** Blood alcohol level of 60-79 mg/100 ml
- **Y90.4** Blood alcohol level of 80-99 mg/100 ml
- **Y90.5** Blood alcohol level of 100-119 mg/100 ml
- **Y90.6** Blood alcohol level of 120-199 mg/100 ml
- **Y90.7** Blood alcohol level of 200-239 mg/100 ml
- **Y90.8** Blood alcohol level of 240 mg/100 ml or more
- **Y90.9** Presence of alcohol in blood, level not specified

✔ Additional Character Req   ✓×7ᵗʰ Placeholder Alert   Unacceptable PDx   Manifestation   H1-H14 HAC   HCC CMS-HCC Condition   EXCLUDES 1 Not Coded Here   EXCLUDES 2 Not Included Here

ICD-10-CM 2018   1209

✓4th **Y92** **Place of occurrence of the external cause**

The following category is for use, when relevant, to identify the place of occurrence of the external cause. Use in conjunction with an activity code.

Place of occurrence should be recorded only at the initial encounter for treatment

✓5th **Y92.0** **Non-institutional (private) residence as the place of occurrence of the external cause**

EXCLUDES 1 *abandoned or derelict house (Y92.89)*
home under construction but not yet occupied (Y92.6-)
institutional place of residence (Y92.1-)

✓6th **Y92.00** **Unspecified** non-institutional (private) residence as the place of occurrence of the external cause

Y92.000 **Kitchen** of unspecified non-institutional (private) residence as the place of occurrence of the external cause

Y92.001 **Dining room** of unspecified non-institutional (private) residence as the place of occurrence of the external cause

Y92.002 **Bathroom** of unspecified non-institutional (private) residence single-family (private) house as the place of occurrence of the external cause

Y92.003 **Bedroom** of unspecified non-institutional (private) residence as the place of occurrence of the external cause

Y92.007 **Garden or yard** of unspecified non-institutional (private) residence as the place of occurrence of the external cause

Y92.008 **Other** place in unspecified non-institutional (private) residence as the place of occurrence of the external cause

Y92.009 **Unspecified** place in unspecified non-institutional (private) residence as the place of occurrence of the external cause
Home (NOS) as the place of occurrence of the external cause

✓6th **Y92.01** **Single-family** non-institutional (private) house as the place of occurrence of the external cause
Farmhouse as the place of occurrence of the external cause

EXCLUDES 1 *barn (Y92.71)*
chicken coop or hen house (Y92.72)
farm field (Y92.73)
orchard (Y92.74)
single family mobile home or trailer (Y92.02-)
slaughter house (Y92.86)

Y92.010 **Kitchen** of single-family (private) house as the place of occurrence of the external cause

Y92.011 **Dining room** of single-family (private) house as the place of occurrence of the external cause

Y92.012 **Bathroom** of single-family (private) house as the place of occurrence of the external cause

Y92.013 **Bedroom** of single-family (private) house as the place of occurrence of the external cause

Y92.014 **Private driveway** to single-family (private) house as the place of occurrence of the external cause

Y92.015 **Private garage** of single-family (private) house as the place of occurrence of the external cause

Y92.016 **Swimming-pool** in single-family (private) house or garden as the place of occurrence of the external cause

Y92.017 **Garden or yard** in single-family (private) house as the place of occurrence of the external cause

Y92.018 **Other** place in single-family (private) house as the place of occurrence of the external cause

Y92.019 **Unspecified** place in single-family (private) house as the place of occurrence of the external cause

✓6th **Y92.02** **Mobile home** as the place of occurrence of the external cause

Y92.020 **Kitchen** in mobile home as the place of occurrence of the external cause

Y92.021 **Dining room** in mobile home as the place of occurrence of the external cause

Y92.022 **Bathroom** in mobile home as the place of occurrence of the external cause

Y92.023 **Bedroom** in mobile home as the place of occurrence of the external cause

Y92.024 **Driveway** of mobile home as the place of occurrence of the external cause

Y92.025 **Garage** of mobile home as the place of occurrence of the external cause

Y92.026 **Swimming-pool** of mobile home as the place of occurrence of the external cause

Y92.027 **Garden or yard** of mobile home as the place of occurrence of the external cause

Y92.028 **Other** place in mobile home as the place of occurrence of the external cause

Y92.029 **Unspecified** place in mobile home as the place of occurrence of the external cause

✓6th **Y92.03** **Apartment** as the place of occurrence of the external cause
Condominium as the place of occurrence of the external cause
Co-op apartment as the place of occurrence of the external cause

Y92.030 **Kitchen** in apartment as the place of occurrence of the external cause

Y92.031 **Bathroom** in apartment as the place of occurrence of the external cause

Y92.032 **Bedroom** in apartment as the place of occurrence of the external cause

Y92.038 **Other** place in apartment as the place of occurrence of the external cause

Y92.039 **Unspecified** place in apartment as the place of occurrence of the external cause

✓6th **Y92.04** **Boarding-house** as the place of occurrence of the external cause

Y92.040 **Kitchen** in boarding-house as the place of occurrence of the external cause

Y92.041 **Bathroom** in boarding-house as the place of occurrence of the external cause

Y92.042 **Bedroom** in boarding-house as the place of occurrence of the external cause

Y92.043 **Driveway** of boarding-house as the place of occurrence of the external cause

Y92.044 **Garage** of boarding-house as the place of occurrence of the external cause

Y92.045 **Swimming-pool** of boarding-house as the place of occurrence of the external cause

Y92.046 **Garden or yard** of boarding-house as the place of occurrence of the external cause

Y92.048 **Other** place in boarding-house as the place of occurrence of the external cause

Y92.049 **Unspecified** place in boarding-house as the place of occurrence of the external cause

✓6th **Y92.09** **Other** non-institutional residence as the place of occurrence of the external cause
AHA: 2017, 2Q, 10

Y92.090 **Kitchen** in other non-institutional residence as the place of occurrence of the external cause

Y92.091 **Bathroom** in other non-institutional residence as the place of occurrence of the external cause

Y92.092 **Bedroom** in other non-institutional residence as the place of occurrence of the external cause

Y92.093 **Driveway** of other non-institutional residence as the place of occurrence of the external cause

Y92.094 **Garage** of other non-institutional residence as the place of occurrence of the external cause

Y92.095 **Swimming-pool** of other non-institutional residence as the place of occurrence of the external cause

Y92.096 **Garden or yard** of other non-institutional residence as the place of occurrence of the external cause

Y92.Ø98   Other place in other non-institutional residence as the place of occurrence of the external cause

Y92.Ø99   Unspecified place in other non-institutional residence as the place of occurrence of the external cause

√5ᵗʰ   **Y92.1**   Institutional (nonprivate) residence as the place of occurrence of the external cause

Y92.1Ø   Unspecified residential institution as the place of occurrence of the external cause

√6ᵗʰ   **Y92.11**   Children's home and orphanage as the place of occurrence of the external cause

Y92.11Ø   Kitchen in children's home and orphanage as the place of occurrence of the external cause

Y92.111   Bathroom in children's home and orphanage as the place of occurrence of the external cause

Y92.112   Bedroom in children's home and orphanage as the place of occurrence of the external cause

Y92.113   Driveway of children's home and orphanage as the place of occurrence of the external cause

Y92.114   Garage of children's home and orphanage as the place of occurrence of the external cause

Y92.115   Swimming-pool of children's home and orphanage as the place of occurrence of the external cause

Y92.116   Garden or yard of children's home and orphanage as the place of occurrence of the external cause

Y92.118   Other place in children's home and orphanage as the place of occurrence of the external cause

Y92.119   Unspecified place in children's home and orphanage as the place of occurrence of the external cause

√6ᵗʰ   **Y92.12**   Nursing home as the place of occurrence of the external cause

Home for the sick as the place of occurrence of the external cause

Hospice as the place of occurrence of the external cause

AHA: 2017, 2Q, 10

Y92.12Ø   Kitchen in nursing home as the place of occurrence of the external cause

Y92.121   Bathroom in nursing home as the place of occurrence of the external cause

Y92.122   Bedroom in nursing home as the place of occurrence of the external cause

Y92.123   Driveway of nursing home as the place of occurrence of the external cause

Y92.124   Garage of nursing home as the place of occurrence of the external cause

Y92.125   Swimming-pool of nursing home as the place of occurrence of the external cause

Y92.126   Garden or yard of nursing home as the place of occurrence of the external cause

Y92.128   Other place in nursing home as the place of occurrence of the external cause

Y92.129   Unspecified place in nursing home as the place of occurrence of the external cause

√6ᵗʰ   **Y92.13**   Military base as the place of occurrence of the external cause

EXCLUDES 1   *military training grounds (Y92.83)*

Y92.13Ø   Kitchen on military base as the place of occurrence of the external cause

Y92.131   Mess hall on military base as the place of occurrence of the external cause

Y92.133   Barracks on military base as the place of occurrence of the external cause

Y92.135   Garage on military base as the place of occurrence of the external cause

Y92.136   Swimming-pool on military base as the place of occurrence of the external cause

Y92.137   Garden or yard on military base as the place of occurrence of the external cause

Y92.138   Other place on military base as the place of occurrence of the external cause

Y92.139   Unspecified place military base as the place of occurrence of the external cause

√6ᵗʰ   **Y92.14**   Prison as the place of occurrence of the external cause

Y92.14Ø   Kitchen in prison as the place of occurrence of the external cause

Y92.141   Dining room in prison as the place of occurrence of the external cause

Y92.142   Bathroom in prison as the place of occurrence of the external cause

Y92.143   Cell of prison as the place of occurrence of the external cause

Y92.146   Swimming-pool of prison as the place of occurrence of the external cause

Y92.147   Courtyard of prison as the place of occurrence of the external cause

Y92.148   Other place in prison as the place of occurrence of the external cause

Y92.149   Unspecified place in prison as the place of occurrence of the external cause

√6ᵗʰ   **Y92.15**   Reform school as the place of occurrence of the external cause

Y92.15Ø   Kitchen in reform school as the place of occurrence of the external cause

Y92.151   Dining room in reform school as the place of occurrence of the external cause

Y92.152   Bathroom in reform school as the place of occurrence of the external cause

Y92.153   Bedroom in reform school as the place of occurrence of the external cause

Y92.154   Driveway of reform school as the place of occurrence of the external cause

Y92.155   Garage of reform school as the place of occurrence of the external cause

Y92.156   Swimming-pool of reform school as the place of occurrence of the external cause

Y92.157   Garden or yard of reform school as the place of occurrence of the external cause

Y92.158   Other place in reform school as the place of occurrence of the external cause

Y92.159   Unspecified place in reform school as the place of occurrence of the external cause

√6ᵗʰ   **Y92.16**   School dormitory as the place of occurrence of the external cause

EXCLUDES 1   *reform school as the place of occurrence of the external cause (Y92.15-)*
school buildings and grounds as the place of occurrence of the external cause (Y92.2-)
school sports and athletic areas as the place of occurrence of the external cause (Y92.3-)

Y92.16Ø   Kitchen in school dormitory as the place of occurrence of the external cause

Y92.161   Dining room in school dormitory as the place of occurrence of the external cause

Y92.162   Bathroom in school dormitory as the place of occurrence of the external cause

Y92.163   Bedroom in school dormitory as the place of occurrence of the external cause

Y92.168   Other place in school dormitory as the place of occurrence of the external cause

Y92.169   Unspecified place in school dormitory as the place of occurrence of the external cause

√6ᵗʰ   **Y92.19**   Other specified residential institution as the place of occurrence of the external cause

AHA: 2017, 2Q, 10

Y92.19Ø   Kitchen in other specified residential institution as the place of occurrence of the external cause

Y92.191   Dining room in other specified residential institution as the place of occurrence of the external cause

Y92.192   Bathroom in other specified residential institution as the place of occurrence of the external cause

☑ Additional Character Req   √x7ᵗʰ Placeholder Alert   Unacceptable PDx   Manifestation   **H1**-**H14** HAC   **HCC** CMS-HCC Condition   *EXCLUDES 1* Not Coded Here   *EXCLUDES 2* Not Included Here

ICD-10-CM 2018   1211

Y92.193 Bedroom in other specified residential institution as the place of occurrence of the external cause

Y92.194 Driveway of other specified residential institution as the place of occurrence of the external cause

Y92.195 Garage of other specified residential institution as the place of occurrence of the external cause

Y92.196 Pool of other specified residential institution as the place of occurrence of the external cause

Y92.197 Garden or yard of other specified residential institution as the place of occurrence of the external cause

Y92.198 Other place in other specified residential institution as the place of occurrence of the external cause

Y92.199 Unspecified place in other specified residential institution as the place of occurrence of the external cause

✓5th **Y92.2** School, other institution and public administrative area as the place of occurrence of the external cause

Building and adjacent grounds used by the general public or by a particular group of the public

EXCLUDES 1   *building under construction as the place of occurrence of the external cause (Y92.6)*
residential institution as the place of occurrence of the external cause (Y92.1)
school dormitory as the place of occurrence of the external cause (Y92.16-)
sports and athletics area of schools as the place of occurrence of the external cause (Y92.3-)

✓6th **Y92.21** School (private) (public) (state) as the place of occurrence of the external cause

Y92.210 Daycare center as the place of occurrence of the external cause

Y92.211 Elementary school as the place of occurrence of the external cause
Kindergarten as the place of occurrence of the external cause

Y92.212 Middle school as the place of occurrence of the external cause

Y92.213 High school as the place of occurrence of the external cause
AHA: 2012, 4Q, 108

Y92.214 College as the place of occurrence of the external cause
University as the place of occurrence of the external cause

Y92.215 Trade school as the place of occurrence of the external cause

Y92.218 Other school as the place of occurrence of the external cause

Y92.219 Unspecified school as the place of occurrence of the external cause

Y92.22 Religious institution as the place of occurrence of the external cause
Church as the place of occurrence of the external cause
Mosque as the place of occurrence of the external cause
Synagogue as the place of occurrence of the external cause

✓6th **Y92.23** Hospital as the place of occurrence of the external cause

EXCLUDES 1   *ambulatory (outpatient) health services establishments (Y92.53-)*
home for the sick as the place of occurrence of the external cause (Y92.12-)
hospice as the place of occurrence of the external cause (Y92.12-)
nursing home as the place of occurrence of the external cause (Y92.12-)

Y92.230 Patient room in hospital as the place of occurrence of the external cause

Y92.231 Patient bathroom in hospital as the place of occurrence of the external cause

Y92.232 Corridor of hospital as the place of occurrence of the external cause

Y92.233 Cafeteria of hospital as the place of occurrence of the external cause

Y92.234 Operating room of hospital as the place of occurrence of the external cause

Y92.238 Other place in hospital as the place of occurrence of the external cause

Y92.239 Unspecified place in hospital as the place of occurrence of the external cause

✓6th **Y92.24** Public administrative building as the place of occurrence of the external cause

Y92.240 Courthouse as the place of occurrence of the external cause

Y92.241 Library as the place of occurrence of the external cause

Y92.242 Post office as the place of occurrence of the external cause

Y92.243 City hall as the place of occurrence of the external cause

Y92.248 Other public administrative building as the place of occurrence of the external cause

✓6th **Y92.25** Cultural building as the place of occurrence of the external cause

Y92.250 Art Gallery as the place of occurrence of the external cause

Y92.251 Museum as the place of occurrence of the external cause

Y92.252 Music hall as the place of occurrence of the external cause

Y92.253 Opera house as the place of occurrence of the external cause

Y92.254 Theater (live) as the place of occurrence of the external cause

Y92.258 Other cultural public building as the place of occurrence of the external cause

Y92.26 Movie house or cinema as the place of occurrence of the external cause

Y92.29 Other specified public building as the place of occurrence of the external cause
Assembly hall as the place of occurrence of the external cause
Clubhouse as the place of occurrence of the external cause

✓5th **Y92.3** Sports and athletics area as the place of occurrence of the external cause

✓6th **Y92.31** Athletic court as the place of occurrence of the external cause

EXCLUDES 1   *tennis court in private home or garden (Y92.09)*

Y92.310 Basketball court as the place of occurrence of the external cause

Y92.311 Squash court as the place of occurrence of the external cause

Y92.312 Tennis court as the place of occurrence of the external cause

Y92.318 Other athletic court as the place of occurrence of the external cause

✓6th **Y92.32** Athletic field as the place of occurrence of the external cause

Y92.320 Baseball field as the place of occurrence of the external cause

Y92.321 Football field as the place of occurrence of the external cause

Y92.322 Soccer field as the place of occurrence of the external cause

Y92.328 Other athletic field as the place of occurrence of the external cause
Cricket field as the place of occurrence of the external cause
Hockey field as the place of occurrence of the external cause

✓6th **Y92.33** Skating rink as the place of occurrence of the external cause

Y92.330 Ice skating rink (indoor) (outdoor) as the place of occurrence of the external cause

Y92.331 Roller skating rink as the place of occurrence of the external cause

Y92.34 Swimming pool (public) as the place of occurrence of the external cause

EXCLUDES 1   *swimming pool in private home or garden (Y92.016)*

N Newborn: 0   P Pediatric: 0-17   M Maternity: 12-55   A Adult: 15-124   MCC Major CC Condition   PDxMCC PDx acts as own MCC   CC CC Condition   PDxCC PDx acts as own CC

1212   ICD-10-CM 2018

Y92.39   **Other specified sports and athletic area as the place of occurrence of the external cause**
- Golf-course as the place of occurrence of the external cause
- Gymnasium as the place of occurrence of the external cause
- Riding-school as the place of occurrence of the external cause
- Stadium as the place of occurrence of the external cause

✓5ᵗʰ **Y92.4**   **Street, highway and other paved roadways as the place of occurrence of the external cause**

     EXCLUDES 1   *private driveway of residence (Y92.014, Y92.024, Y92.043, Y92.093, Y92.113, Y92.123, Y92.154, Y92.194)*

✓6ᵗʰ **Y92.41**   **Street and highway as the place of occurrence of the external cause**

   Y92.410   **Unspecified street and highway as the place of occurrence of the external cause**
- Road NOS as the place of occurrence of the external cause

   Y92.411   **Interstate highway as the place of occurrence of the external cause**
- Freeway as the place of occurrence of the external cause
- Motorway as the place of occurrence of the external cause

   Y92.412   **Parkway as the place of occurrence of the external cause**

   Y92.413   **State road as the place of occurrence of the external cause**

   Y92.414   **Local residential or business street as the place of occurrence of the external cause**

   Y92.415   **Exit ramp or entrance ramp of street or highway as the place of occurrence of the external cause**

✓6ᵗʰ **Y92.48**   **Other paved roadways as the place of occurrence of the external cause**

   Y92.480   **Sidewalk as the place of occurrence of the external cause**

   Y92.481   **Parking lot as the place of occurrence of the external cause**

   Y92.482   **Bike path as the place of occurrence of the external cause**

   Y92.488   **Other paved roadways as the place of occurrence of the external cause**

✓5ᵗʰ **Y92.5**   **Trade and service area as the place of occurrence of the external cause**

     EXCLUDES 1   *garage in private home (Y92.015)*
              schools and other public administration buildings (Y92.2-)

✓6ᵗʰ **Y92.51**   **Private commercial establishments as the place of occurrence of the external cause**

   Y92.510   **Bank as the place of occurrence of the external cause**

   Y92.511   **Restaurant or café as the place of occurrence of the external cause**

   Y92.512   **Supermarket, store or market as the place of occurrence of the external cause**

   Y92.513   **Shop (commercial) as the place of occurrence of the external cause**

✓6ᵗʰ **Y92.52**   **Service areas as the place of occurrence of the external cause**

   Y92.520   **Airport as the place of occurrence of the external cause**

   Y92.521   **Bus station as the place of occurrence of the external cause**

   Y92.522   **Railway station as the place of occurrence of the external cause**

   Y92.523   **Highway rest stop as the place of occurrence of the external cause**

   Y92.524   **Gas station as the place of occurrence of the external cause**
- Petroleum station as the place of occurrence of the external cause
- Service station as the place of occurrence of the external cause

✓6ᵗʰ **Y92.53**   **Ambulatory health services establishments as the place of occurrence of the external cause**

   Y92.530   **Ambulatory surgery center as the place of occurrence of the external cause**
- Outpatient surgery center, including that connected with a hospital as the place of occurrence of the external cause
- Same day surgery center, including that connected with a hospital as the place of occurrence of the external cause

   Y92.531   **Health care provider office as the place of occurrence of the external cause**
- Physician office as the place of occurrence of the external cause

   Y92.532   **Urgent care center as the place of occurrence of the external cause**

   Y92.538   **Other ambulatory health services establishments as the place of occurrence of the external cause**

Y92.59   **Other trade areas as the place of occurrence of the external cause**
- Office building as the place of occurrence of the external cause
- Casino as the place of occurrence of the external cause
- Garage (commercial) as the place of occurrence of the external cause
- Hotel as the place of occurrence of the external cause
- Radio or television station as the place of occurrence of the external cause
- Shopping mall as the place of occurrence of the external cause
- Warehouse as the place of occurrence of the external cause

✓5ᵗʰ **Y92.6**   **Industrial and construction area as the place of occurrence of the external cause**

   Y92.61   **Building [any] under construction as the place of occurrence of the external cause**

   Y92.62   **Dock or shipyard as the place of occurrence of the external cause**
- Dockyard as the place of occurrence of the external cause
- Dry dock as the place of occurrence of the external cause
- Shipyard as the place of occurrence of the external cause

   Y92.63   **Factory as the place of occurrence of the external cause**
- Factory building as the place of occurrence of the external cause
- Factory premises as the place of occurrence of the external cause
- Industrial yard as the place of occurrence of the external cause

   Y92.64   **Mine or pit as the place of occurrence of the external cause**
- Mine as the place of occurrence of the external cause

   Y92.65   **Oil rig as the place of occurrence of the external cause**
- Pit (coal) (gravel) (sand) as the place of occurrence of the external cause

   Y92.69   **Other specified industrial and construction area as the place of occurrence of the external cause**
- Gasworks as the place of occurrence of the external cause
- Power-station (coal) (nuclear) (oil) as the place of occurrence of the external cause
- Tunnel under construction as the place of occurrence of the external cause
- Workshop as the place of occurrence of the external cause

✓5ᵗʰ **Y92.7**   **Farm as the place of occurrence of the external cause**
- Ranch as the place of occurrence of the external cause

     EXCLUDES 1   *farmhouse and home premises of farm (Y92.01-)*

   Y92.71   **Barn as the place of occurrence of the external cause**

   Y92.72   **Chicken coop as the place of occurrence of the external cause**
- Hen house as the place of occurrence of the external cause

   Y92.73   **Farm field as the place of occurrence of the external cause**

   Y92.74   **Orchard as the place of occurrence of the external cause**

✓Additional Character Req   ✓x7ᵗʰ Placeholder Alert   Unacceptable PDx   Manifestation   H1-H14 HAC   HCC CMS-HCC Condition   *EXCLUDES 1* Not Coded Here   *EXCLUDES 2* Not Included Here

ICD-10-CM 2018   1213

Y92.79   Other farm location as the place of occurrence of the external cause

✓5ᵗʰ **Y92.8**   Other places as the place of occurrence of the external cause

✓6ᵗʰ **Y92.81**   Transport vehicle as the place of occurrence of the external cause

     EXCLUDES 1   transport accidents (V00-V99)

Y92.810   Car as the place of occurrence of the external cause

Y92.811   Bus as the place of occurrence of the external cause

Y92.812   Truck as the place of occurrence of the external cause

Y92.813   Airplane as the place of occurrence of the external cause

Y92.814   Boat as the place of occurrence of the external cause

Y92.815   Train as the place of occurrence of the external cause

Y92.816   Subway car as the place of occurrence of the external cause

Y92.818   Other transport vehicle as the place of occurrence of the external cause

✓6ᵗʰ **Y92.82**   Wilderness area

Y92.820   Desert as the place of occurrence of the external cause

Y92.821   Forest as the place of occurrence of the external cause

Y92.828   Other wilderness area as the place of occurrence of the external cause

     Swamp as the place of occurrence of the external cause

     Mountain as the place of occurrence of the external cause

     Marsh as the place of occurrence of the external cause

     Prairie as the place of occurrence of the external cause

✓6ᵗʰ **Y92.83**   Recreation area as the place of occurrence of the external cause

Y92.830   Public park as the place of occurrence of the external cause

Y92.831   Amusement park as the place of occurrence of the external cause

Y92.832   Beach as the place of occurrence of the external cause

     Seashore as the place of occurrence of the external cause

Y92.833   Campsite as the place of occurrence of the external cause

Y92.834   Zoological garden (Zoo) as the place of occurrence of the external cause

Y92.838   Other recreation area as the place of occurrence of the external cause

Y92.84   Military training ground as the place of occurrence of the external cause

Y92.85   Railroad track as the place of occurrence of the external cause

Y92.86   Slaughter house as the place of occurrence of the external cause

Y92.89   Other specified places as the place of occurrence of the external cause

     Derelict house as the place of occurrence of the external cause

Y92.9   Unspecified place or not applicable

✓4ᵗʰ **Y93**   Activity codes

NOTE   Category Y93 is provided for use to indicate the activity of the person seeking healthcare for an injury or health condition, such as a heart attack while shoveling snow, which resulted from, or was contributed to, by the activity. These codes are appropriate for use for both acute injuries, such as those from chapter 19, and conditions that are due to the long-term, cumulative effects of an activity, such as those from chapter 13. They are also appropriate for use with external cause codes for cause and intent if identifying the activity provides additional information on the event. These codes should be used in conjunction with codes for external cause status (Y99) and place of occurrence (Y92).

This section contains the following broad activity categories:

Y93.0   Activities involving walking and running
Y93.1   Activities involving water and water craft
Y93.2   Activities involving ice and snow
Y93.3   Activities involving climbing, rappelling, and jumping off
Y93.4   Activities involving dancing and other rhythmic movement
Y93.5   Activities involving other sports and athletics played individually
Y93.6   Activities involving other sports and athletics played as a team or group
Y93.7   Activities involving other specified sports and athletics
Y93.A   Activities involving other cardiorespiratory exercise
Y93.B   Activities involving other muscle strengthening exercises
Y93.C   Activities involving computer technology and electronic devices
Y93.D   Activities involving arts and handcrafts
Y93.E   Activities involving personal hygiene and interior property and clothing maintenance
Y93.F   Activities involving caregiving
Y93.G   Activities involving food preparation, cooking and grilling
Y93.H   Activities involving exterior property and land maintenance, building and construction
Y93.I   Activities involving roller coasters and other types of external motion
Y93.J   Activities involving playing musical instrument
Y93.K   Activities involving animal care
Y93.8   Activities, other specified
Y93.9   Activity, unspecified

✓5ᵗʰ **Y93.0**   Activities involving walking and running

     EXCLUDES 1   activity, walking an animal (Y93.K1)
         activity, walking or running on a treadmill (Y93.A1)

Y93.01   Activity, walking, marching and hiking

     Activity, walking, marching and hiking on level or elevated terrain

     EXCLUDES 1   activity, mountain climbing (Y93.31)

Y93.02   Activity, running

✓5ᵗʰ **Y93.1**   Activities involving water and water craft

     EXCLUDES 1   activities involving ice (Y93.2-)

Y93.11   Activity, swimming

Y93.12   Activity, springboard and platform diving

Y93.13   Activity, water polo

Y93.14   Activity, water aerobics and water exercise

Y93.15   Activity, underwater diving and snorkeling

     Activity, SCUBA diving

Y93.16   Activity, rowing, canoeing, kayaking, rafting and tubing

     Activity, canoeing, kayaking, rafting and tubing in calm and turbulent water

Y93.17   Activity, water skiing and wake boarding

Y93.18   Activity, surfing, windsurfing and boogie boarding

     Activity, water sliding

Y93.19   Activity, other involving water and watercraft

     Activity involving water NOS
     Activity, parasailing
     Activity, water survival training and testing

✓5ᵗʰ **Y93.2**   Activities involving ice and snow

     EXCLUDES 1   activity, shoveling ice and snow (Y93.H1)

Y93.21   Activity, ice skating

     Activity, figure skating (singles) (pairs)
     Activity, ice dancing
     EXCLUDES 1   activity, ice hockey (Y93.22)

Y93.22   Activity, ice hockey

Y93.23   Activity, snow (alpine) (downhill) skiing, snow boarding, sledding, tobogganing and snow tubing

     EXCLUDES 1   activity, cross country skiing (Y93.24)

Y93.24   Activity, cross country skiing

     Activity, nordic skiing

N Newborn: 0   **P** Pediatric: 0-17   **M** Maternity: 12-55   **A** Adult: 15-124   **MCC** Major CC Condition   **PDxMCC** PDx acts as own MCC   **CC** CC Condition   **PDxCC** PDx acts as own CC

1214   ICD-10-CM 2018

Y93.29 Activity, other involving ice and snow
Activity involving ice and snow NOS

✓5ᵗʰ **Y93.3 Activities involving climbing, rappelling and jumping off**
EXCLUDES 1   activity, hiking on level or elevated terrain (Y93.Ø1)
activity, jumping rope (Y93.56)
activity, trampoline jumping (Y93.44)

Y93.31 Activity, mountain climbing, rock climbing and wall climbing

Y93.32 Activity, rappelling

Y93.33 Activity, BASE jumping
Activity, Building, Antenna, Span, Earth jumping

Y93.34 Activity, bungee jumping

Y93.35 Activity, hang gliding

Y93.39 Activity, other involving climbing, rappelling and jumping off

✓5ᵗʰ **Y93.4 Activities involving dancing and other rhythmic movement**
EXCLUDES 1   activity, martial arts (Y93.75)

Y93.41 Activity, dancing
AHA: 2012, 4Q, 108

Y93.42 Activity, yoga

Y93.43 Activity, gymnastics
Activity, rhythmic gymnastics
EXCLUDES 1   activity, trampolining (Y93.44)

Y93.44 Activity, trampolining

Y93.45 Activity, cheerleading

Y93.49 Activity, other involving dancing and other rhythmic movements

✓5ᵗʰ **Y93.5 Activities involving other sports and athletics played individually**
EXCLUDES 1   activity, dancing (Y93.41)
activity, gymnastic (Y93.43)
activity, trampolining (Y93.44)
activity, yoga (Y93.42)

Y93.51 Activity, roller skating (inline) and skateboarding

Y93.52 Activity, horseback riding

Y93.53 Activity, golf

Y93.54 Activity, bowling

Y93.55 Activity, bike riding

Y93.56 Activity, jumping rope

Y93.57 Activity, non-running track and field events
EXCLUDES 1   activity, running (any form) (Y93.Ø2)

Y93.59 Activity, other involving other sports and athletics played individually
EXCLUDES 1   activities involving climbing, rappelling, and jumping (Y93.3-)
activities involving ice and snow (Y93.2-)
activities involving walking and running (Y93.Ø-)
activities involving water and watercraft (Y93.1-)

✓5ᵗʰ **Y93.6 Activities involving other sports and athletics played as a team or group**
EXCLUDES 1   activity, ice hockey (Y93.22)
activity, water polo (Y93.13)

Y93.61 Activity, American tackle football
Activity, football NOS

Y93.62 Activity, American flag or touch football

Y93.63 Activity, rugby

Y93.64 Activity, baseball
Activity, softball

Y93.65 Activity, lacrosse and field hockey

Y93.66 Activity, soccer

Y93.67 Activity, basketball

Y93.68 Activity, volleyball (beach) (court)

Y93.6A Activity, physical games generally associated with school recess, summer camp and children
Activity, capture the flag   Activity, four square
Activity, dodge ball   Activity, kickball

Y93.69 Activity, other involving other sports and athletics played as a team or group
Activity, cricket

✓5ᵗʰ **Y93.7 Activities involving other specified sports and athletics**

Y93.71 Activity, boxing

Y93.72 Activity, wrestling

Y93.73 Activity, racquet and hand sports
Activity, handball   Activity, squash
Activity, racquetball   Activity, tennis

Y93.74 Activity, frisbee
Activity, ultimate frisbee

Y93.75 Activity, martial arts
Activity, combatives

Y93.79 Activity, other specified sports and athletics
EXCLUDES 1   sports and athletics activities specified in categories Y93.Ø-Y93.6

✓5ᵗʰ **Y93.A Activities involving other cardiorespiratory exercise**
Activities involving physical training

Y93.A1 Activity, exercise machines primarily for cardiorespiratory conditioning
Activity, elliptical and stepper machines
Activity, stationary bike
Activity, treadmill

Y93.A2 Activity, calisthenics
Activity, jumping jacks
Activity, warm up and cool down

Y93.A3 Activity, aerobic and step exercise

Y93.A4 Activity, circuit training

Y93.A5 Activity, obstacle course
Activity, challenge course
Activity, confidence course

Y93.A6 Activity, grass drills
Activity, guerilla drills

Y93.A9 Activity, other involving cardiorespiratory exercise
EXCLUDES 1   activities involving cardiorespiratory exercise specified in categories Y93.Ø-Y93.7

✓5ᵗʰ **Y93.B Activities involving other muscle strengthening exercises**

Y93.B1 Activity, exercise machines primarily for muscle strengthening

Y93.B2 Activity, push-ups, pull-ups, sit-ups

Y93.B3 Activity, free weights
Activity, barbells   Activity, dumbbells

Y93.B4 Activity, pilates

Y93.B9 Activity, other involving muscle strengthening exercises
EXCLUDES 1   activities involving muscle strengthening specified in categories Y93.Ø-Y93.A

✓5ᵗʰ **Y93.C Activities involving computer technology and electronic devices**
EXCLUDES 1   activity, electronic musical keyboard or instruments (Y93.J-)

Y93.C1 Activity, computer keyboarding
Activity, electronic game playing using keyboard or other stationary device

Y93.C2 Activity, hand held interactive electronic device
Activity, cellular telephone and communication device
Activity, electronic game playing using interactive device
EXCLUDES 1   activity, electronic game playing using keyboard or other stationary device (Y93.C1)

Y93.C9 Activity, other involving computer technology and electronic devices

✓5ᵗʰ **Y93.D Activities involving arts and handcrafts**
EXCLUDES 1   activities involving playing musical instrument (Y93.J-)

Y93.D1 Activity, knitting and crocheting

Y93.D2 Activity, sewing

Y93.D3 Activity, furniture building and finishing
Activity, furniture repair

Y93.D9 Activity, other involving arts and handcrafts

✓5ᵗʰ **Y93.E Activities involving personal hygiene and interior property and clothing maintenance**
EXCLUDES 1   activities involving cooking and grilling (Y93.G-)
activities involving exterior property and land maintenance, building and construction (Y93.H-)
activities involving caregiving (Y93.F-)
activity, dishwashing (Y93.G1)
activity, food preparation (Y93.G1)
activity, gardening (Y93.H2)

Y93.E1 Activity, personal bathing and showering

Y93.E2 Activity, laundry

Y93.E3 Activity, vacuuming

Y93.E4 Activity, ironing

✓ Additional Character Req   ✓x7ᵗʰ Placeholder Alert   Unacceptable PDx   Manifestation   H1 - H14 HAC   HCC CMS-HCC Condition   *EXCLUDES 1* Not Coded Here   *EXCLUDES 2* Not Included Here

Chapter 20. External Causes of Morbidity

Y93.E5   **Activity,** floor mopping and cleaning

Y93.E6   **Activity,** residential relocation
Activity, packing up and unpacking involved in moving to a new residence

Y93.E8   **Activity,** other personal hygiene

Y93.E9   **Activity,** other interior property and clothing maintenance

✓5ᵗʰ **Y93.F**   **Activities involving** caregiving
Activity involving the provider of caregiving

Y93.F1   **Activity, caregiving,** bathing

Y93.F2   **Activity, caregiving,** lifting

Y93.F9   **Activity,** other **caregiving**

✓5ᵗʰ **Y93.G**   **Activities involving food preparation, cooking and grilling**

Y93.G1   **Activity, food** preparation and clean up
Activity, dishwashing

Y93.G2   **Activity,** grilling and smoking food

Y93.G3   **Activity,** cooking and baking
Activity, use of stove, oven and microwave oven

Y93.G9   **Activity,** other **involving cooking and grilling**

✓5ᵗʰ **Y93.H**   **Activities involving exterior property and land maintenance, building and construction**

Y93.H1   **Activity,** digging, shoveling and raking
Activity, dirt digging
Activity, raking leaves
Activity, snow shoveling

Y93.H2   **Activity,** gardening and landscaping
Activity, pruning, trimming shrubs, weeding

Y93.H3   **Activity,** building and construction

Y93.H9   **Activity,** other **involving exterior property and land maintenance, building and construction**

✓5ᵗʰ **Y93.I**   **Activities involving roller coasters and other types of external motion**

Y93.I1   **Activity,** rollercoaster riding

Y93.I9   **Activity,** other **involving external motion**

✓5ᵗʰ **Y93.J**   **Activities involving playing musical instrument**
Activity involving playing electric musical instrument

Y93.J1   **Activity,** piano **playing**
Activity, musical keyboard (electronic) playing

Y93.J2   **Activity,** drum and other percussion instrument **playing**

Y93.J3   **Activity,** string instrument **playing**

Y93.J4   **Activity,** winds and brass instrument **playing**

✓5ᵗʰ **Y93.K**   **Activities involving** animal care

    EXCLUDES 1   *activity, horseback riding (Y93.52)*

Y93.K1   **Activity,** walking **an animal**

Y93.K2   **Activity,** milking **an animal**

Y93.K3   **Activity,** grooming and shearing **an animal**

Y93.K9   **Activity,** other **involving animal care**

✓5ᵗʰ **Y93.8**   **Activities,** other specified

Y93.81   **Activity,** refereeing **a sports activity**

Y93.82   **Activity,** spectator **at an event**

Y93.83   **Activity,** rough housing and horseplay

Y93.84   **Activity,** sleeping

Y93.85   **Activity,** choking game
Activity, blackout game
Activity, fainting game
Activity, pass out game

Y93.89   **Activity,** other specified

Y93.9   **Activity,** unspecified

Y95   **Nosocomial condition**
    AHA: 2013, 4Q, 119

✓4ᵗʰ **Y99**   **External cause status**

    NOTE   A single code from category Y99 should be used in conjunction with the external cause code(s) assigned to a record to indicate the status of the person at the time the event occurred.

Y99.0   **Civilian** activity done for income or pay
Civilian activity done for financial or other compensation

    EXCLUDES 1   *military activity (Y99.1)*
               volunteer activity (Y99.2)

Y99.1   **Military** activity

    EXCLUDES 1   *activity of off duty military personnel (Y99.8)*

Y99.2   **Volunteer** activity

    EXCLUDES 1   *activity of child or other family member assisting in compensated work of other family member (Y99.8)*

Y99.8   Other external cause status
Activity NEC
Activity of child or other family member assisting in compensated work of other family member
Hobby not done for income
Leisure activity
Off-duty activity of military personnel
Recreation or sport not for income or while a student
Student activity

    EXCLUDES 1   *civilian activity done for income or compensation (Y99.0)*
               military activity (Y99.1)

    AHA: 2012, 4Q, 108

Y99.9   **Unspecified external cause status**

N Newborn: 0   P Pediatric: 0-17   M Maternity: 12-55   A Adult: 15-124   MCC Major CC Condition   PDxMCC PDx acts as own MCC   CC CC Condition   PDxCC PDx acts as own CC

1216   ICD-10-CM 2018

Chapter 21. Factors Influencing Health Status and Contact with Health Services (Z00–Z99)

Chapter Specific Guidelines with Coding Examples

The chapter specific guidelines from the ICD-10-CM Official Guidelines for Coding and Reporting have been provided below. Along with these guidelines are coding examples, contained in the shaded boxes, that have been developed to help illustrate the coding and/or sequencing guidance found in these guidelines.

Note: The chapter specific guidelines provide additional information about the use of Z codes for specified encounters.

a. Use of Z codes in any healthcare setting

Z codes are for use in any healthcare setting. Z codes may be used as either a first-listed (principal diagnosis code in the inpatient setting) or secondary code, depending on the circumstances of the encounter. Certain Z codes may only be used as first-listed or principal diagnosis.

> Patient with middle lobe lung cancer admitted for initiation of chemotherapy
>
> **Z51.11**   **Encounter for antineoplastic chemotherapy**
>
> **C34.2**   **Malignant neoplasm of middle lobe, bronchus or lung**
>
> *Explanation:* A Z code can be used as first-listed in this situation based on guidelines in this chapter as well as chapter 2, "Neoplasms."

> Patient has chronic lymphocytic leukemia for which the patient had previous chemotherapy and is now in remission
>
> **C91.11**   **Chronic lymphocytic leukemia of B-cell type in remission**
>
> **Z92.21**   **Personal history of antineoplastic chemotherapy**
>
> *Explanation:*The personal history Z code is used to describe a secondary (supplementary) diagnosis to identify that this patient has had chemotherapy in the past.

b. Z codes indicate a reason for an encounter

Z codes are not procedure codes. A corresponding procedure code must accompany a Z code to describe any procedure performed.

c. Categories of Z codes

1) Contact/exposure

Category Z20 indicates contact with, and suspected exposure to, communicable diseases. These codes are for patients who do not show any sign or symptom of a disease but are suspected to have been exposed to it by close personal contact with an infected individual or are in an area where a disease is epidemic.

Category Z77, Other contact with and (suspected) exposures hazardous to health, indicates contact with and suspected exposures hazardous to health.

Contact/exposure codes may be used as a first-listed code to explain an encounter for testing, or, more commonly, as a secondary code to identify a potential risk.

2) Inoculations and vaccinations

Code Z23 is for encounters for inoculations and vaccinations. It indicates that a patient is being seen to receive a prophylactic inoculation against a disease. Procedure codes are required to identify the actual administration of the injection and the type(s) of immunizations given. Code Z23 may be used as a secondary code if the inoculation is given as a routine part of preventive health care, such as a well-baby visit.

3) Status

Status codes indicate that a patient is either a carrier of a disease or has the sequelae or residual of a past disease or condition. This includes such things as the presence of prosthetic or mechanical devices resulting from past treatment. A status code is informative, because the status may affect the course of treatment and its outcome. A status code is distinct from a history code. The history code indicates that the patient no longer has the condition.

A status code should not be used with a diagnosis code from one of the body system chapters, if the diagnosis code includes the information provided by the status code. For example, code Z94.1, Heart transplant status, should not be used with a code from subcategory T86.2, Complications of heart transplant. The status code does not provide

additional information. The complication code indicates that the patient is a heart transplant patient.

For encounters for weaning from a mechanical ventilator, assign a code from subcategory J96.1, Chronic respiratory failure, followed by code Z99.11, Dependence on respirator [ventilator] status.

The status Z codes/categories are:

Z14	Genetic carrier

Genetic carrier status indicates that a person carries a gene, associated with a particular disease, which may be passed to offspring who may develop that disease. The person does not have the disease and is not at risk of developing the disease.

Z15	Genetic susceptibility to disease

Genetic susceptibility indicates that a person has a gene that increases the risk of that person developing the disease.

Codes from category Z15 should not be used as principal or first-listed codes. If the patient has the condition to which he/she is susceptible, and that condition is the reason for the encounter, the code for the current condition should be sequenced first. If the patient is being seen for follow-up after completed treatment for this condition, and the condition no longer exists, a follow-up code should be sequenced first, followed by the appropriate personal history and genetic susceptibility codes. If the purpose of the encounter is genetic counseling associated with procreative management, code Z31.5, Encounter for genetic counseling, should be assigned as the first-listed code, followed by a code from category Z15. Additional codes should be assigned for any applicable family or personal history.

Z16	Resistance to antimicrobial drugs

This code indicates that a patient has a condition that is resistant to antimicrobial drug treatment. Sequence the infection code first.

Z17	Estrogen receptor status
Z18	Retained foreign body fragments
Z19	Hormone sensitivity malignancy status
Z21	Asymptomatic HIV infection status

This code indicates that a patient has tested positive for HIV but has manifested no signs or symptoms of the disease.

Z22	Carrier of infectious disease

Carrier status indicates that a person harbors the specific organisms of a disease without manifest symptoms and is capable of transmitting the infection.

Z28.3	Underimmunization status
Z33.1	Pregnant state, incidental

This code is a secondary code only for use when the pregnancy is in no way complicating the reason for visit. Otherwise, a code from the obstetric chapter is required.

Z66	Do not resuscitate

This code may be used when it is documented by the provider that a patient is on do not resuscitate status at any time during the stay.

Z67	Blood type
Z68	Body mass index (BMI)

As with all other secondary diagnosis codes, the BMI codes should only be assigned when they meet the definition of a reportable diagnosis (see Section III, Reporting Additional Diagnoses).

Z74.01	Bed confinement status
Z76.82	Awaiting organ transplant status
Z78	Other specified health status

Code Z78.1, Physical restraint status, may be used when it is documented by the provider that a patient has been put in restraints during the current encounter. Please note that this code should not be reported when it is documented by the provider that a patient is temporarily restrained during a procedure.

Z79	Long-term (current) drug therapy

Codes from this category indicate a patient's continuous use of a prescribed drug (including such things as aspirin therapy) for the long-term treatment of a condition or for prophylactic use. It is not for use for patients who have addictions to drugs. This subcategory is not for use of medications for detoxification or maintenance programs to prevent withdrawal symptoms in patients with drug dependence (e.g., methadone maintenance for opiate dependence). Assign the appropriate code for the drug dependence instead.

Assign a code from Z79 if the patient is receiving a medication for an extended period as a prophylactic measure (such as for the prevention of deep vein thrombosis) or as treatment of a chronic condition (such as arthritis) or a disease requiring a lengthy course of treatment (such as cancer). Do not assign a code from category Z79 for medication being administered for a brief period of time to treat an acute illness or injury (such as a course of antibiotics to treat acute bronchitis).

Z88   Allergy status to drugs, medicaments and biological substances

Except: Z88.9, Allergy status to unspecified drugs, medicaments and biological substances status

Z89   Acquired absence of limb

Z9Ø   Acquired absence of organs, not elsewhere classified

Z91.Ø-   Allergy status, other than to drugs and biological substances

Z92.82   Status post administration of tPA (rtPA) in a different facility within the last 24 hours prior to admission to a current facility

Assign code Z92.82, Status post administration of tPA (rtPA) in a different facility within the last 24 hours prior to admission to current facility, as a secondary diagnosis when a patient is received by transfer into a facility and documentation indicates they were administered tissue plasminogen activator (tPA) within the last 24 hours prior to admission to the current facility.

This guideline applies even if the patient is still receiving the tPA at the time they are received into the current facility.

The appropriate code for the condition for which the tPA was administered (such as cerebrovascular disease or myocardial infarction) should be assigned first.

Code Z92.82 is only applicable to the receiving facility record and not to the transferring facility record.

Z93   Artificial opening status

Z94   Transplanted organ and tissue status

Z95   Presence of cardiac and vascular implants and grafts

Z96   Presence of other functional implants

Z97   Presence of other devices

Z98   Other postprocedural states

Assign code Z98.85, Transplanted organ removal status, to indicate that a transplanted organ has been previously removed. This code should not be assigned for the encounter in which the transplanted organ is removed. The complication necessitating removal of the transplant organ should be assigned for that encounter.

See section I.C19. for information on the coding of organ transplant complications.

Z99   Dependence on enabling machines and devices, not elsewhere classified

Note: Categories Z89-Z9Ø and Z93-Z99 are for use only if there are no complications or malfunctions of the organ or tissue replaced, the amputation site or the equipment on which the patient is dependent.

4) History (of)

There are two types of history Z codes, personal and family. Personal history codes explain a patient's past medical condition that no longer exists and is not receiving any treatment, but that has the potential for recurrence, and therefore may require continued monitoring.

Family history codes are for use when a patient has a family member(s) who has had a particular disease that causes the patient to be at higher risk of also contracting the disease.

Personal history codes may be used in conjunction with follow-up codes and family history codes may be used in conjunction with screening codes to explain the need for a test or procedure. History codes are also acceptable on any medical record regardless of the reason for visit. A history of an illness, even if no longer present, is important information that may alter the type of treatment ordered.

The history Z code categories are:

Z8Ø   Family history of primary malignant neoplasm

Z81   Family history of mental and behavioral disorders

Z82   Family history of certain disabilities and chronic diseases (leading to disablement)

Z83   Family history of other specific disorders

Z84   Family history of other conditions

Z85   Personal history of malignant neoplasm

Z86   Personal history of certain other diseases

Z87   Personal history of other diseases and conditions

Z91.4-   Personal history of psychological trauma, not elsewhere classified

Z91.5   Personal history of self-harm

Z91.81   History of falling

Z91.82   Personal history of military deployment

Z92   Personal history of medical treatment

Except: Z92.Ø, Personal history of contraception

Except: Z92.82, Status post administration of tPA (rtPA) in a different facility within the last 24 hours prior to admission to a current facility

5) Screening

Screening is the testing for disease or disease precursors in seemingly well individuals so that early detection and treatment can be provided for those who test positive for the disease (e.g., screening mammogram).

The testing of a person to rule out or confirm a suspected diagnosis because the patient has some sign or symptom is a diagnostic examination, not a screening. In these cases, the sign or symptom is used to explain the reason for the test.

A screening code may be a first-listed code if the reason for the visit is specifically the screening exam. It may also be used as an additional code if the screening is done during an office visit for other health problems. A screening code is not necessary if the screening is inherent to a routine examination, such as a pap smear done during a routine pelvic examination.

Should a condition be discovered during the screening then the code for the condition may be assigned as an additional diagnosis.

The Z code indicates that a screening exam is planned. A procedure code is required to confirm that the screening was performed.

The screening Z codes/categories:

Z11   Encounter for screening for infectious and parasitic diseases

Z12   Encounter for screening for malignant neoplasms

Z13   Encounter for screening for other diseases and disorders

Except: Z13.9, Encounter for screening, unspecified

Z36   Encounter for antenatal screening for mother

6) Observation

There are three observation Z code categories. They are for use in very limited circumstances when a person is being observed for a suspected condition that is ruled out. The observation codes are not for use if an injury or illness or any signs or symptoms related to the suspected condition are present. In such cases the diagnosis/symptom code is used with the corresponding external cause code.

The observation codes are to be used as principal diagnosis only. The only exception to this is when the principal diagnosis is required to be a code from category Z38, Liveborn infants according to place of birth and type of delivery. Then a code from category ZØ5, Encounter for observation and evaluation of newborn for suspected diseases and conditions ruled out, is sequenced after the Z38 code. Additional codes may be used in addition to the observation code but only if they are unrelated to the suspected condition being observed.

Codes from subcategory ZØ3.7, Encounter for suspected maternal and fetal conditions ruled out, may either be used as a first-listed or as an additional code assignment depending on the case. They are for use in very limited circumstances on a maternal record when an encounter is for a suspected maternal or fetal condition that is ruled out during that encounter (for example, a maternal or fetal condition may be suspected due to an abnormal test result). These codes should not be used when the condition is confirmed. In those cases, the confirmed condition should be coded. In addition, these codes are not for use if an illness or any signs or symptoms related to the suspected condition or problem are present. In such cases the diagnosis/symptom code is used.

Additional codes may be used in addition to the code from subcategory ZØ3.7, but only if they are unrelated to the suspected condition being evaluated.

Codes from subcategory ZØ3.7 may not be used for encounters for antenatal screening of mother. *See Section I.C.21. Screening.*

For encounters for suspected fetal condition that are inconclusive following testing and evaluation, assign the appropriate code from category O35, O36, O40 or O41.

The observation Z code categories:

Z03   Encounter for medical observation for suspected diseases and conditions ruled out

Z04   Encounter for examination and observation for other reasons

Except: Z04.9, Encounter for examination and observation for unspecified reason

Z05   Encounter for observation and evaluation of newborn for suspected diseases and conditions ruled out

---

Upon initial examination, a heart murmur was heard in a newborn infant delivered vaginally in the hospital; however, after further observation, any serious cardiac conditions were ruled out.

Z38.00   **Single liveborn infant, delivered vaginally**

Z05.0   **Observation and evaluation of newborn for suspected cardiac condition ruled out**

Explanation: Normally an observation code is used as the principal diagnosis except when the patient is a newborn. A code from category Z38 Liveborn infants according to place of birth and type of delivery code would be sequenced first, followed by the encounter for observation and evaluation of newborn for suspected diseases and conditions ruled out.

---

7) Aftercare

Aftercare visit codes cover situations when the initial treatment of a disease has been performed and the patient requires continued care during the healing or recovery phase, or for the long-term consequences of the disease. The aftercare Z code should not be used if treatment is directed at a current, acute disease. The diagnosis code is to be used in these cases. Exceptions to this rule are codes Z51.0, Encounter for antineoplastic radiation therapy, and codes from subcategory Z51.1, Encounter for antineoplastic chemotherapy and immunotherapy. These codes are to be first-listed, followed by the diagnosis code when a patient's encounter is solely to receive radiation therapy, chemotherapy, or immunotherapy for the treatment of a neoplasm. If the reason for the encounter is more than one type of antineoplastic therapy, code Z51.0 and a code from subcategory Z51.1 may be assigned together, in which case one of these codes would be reported as a secondary diagnosis.

The aftercare Z codes should also not be used for aftercare for injuries. For aftercare of an injury, assign the acute injury code with the appropriate 7th character (for subsequent encounter).

The aftercare codes are generally first-listed to explain the specific reason for the encounter. An aftercare code may be used as an additional code when some type of aftercare is provided in addition to the reason for admission and no diagnosis code is applicable. An example of this would be the closure of a colostomy during an encounter for treatment of another condition.

Aftercare codes should be used in conjunction with other aftercare codes or diagnosis codes to provide better detail on the specifics of an aftercare encounter visit, unless otherwise directed by the classification. Should a patient receive multiple types of antineoplastic therapy during the same encounter, code Z51.0, Encounter for antineoplastic radiation therapy, and codes from subcategory Z51.1, Encounter for antineoplastic chemotherapy and immunotherapy, may be used together on a record. The sequencing of multiple aftercare codes depends on the circumstances of the encounter.

Certain aftercare Z code categories need a secondary diagnosis code to describe the resolving condition or sequelae. For others, the condition is included in the code title.

Additional Z code aftercare category terms include fitting and adjustment, and attention to artificial openings.

Status Z codes may be used with aftercare Z codes to indicate the nature of the aftercare. For example code Z95.1, Presence of aortocoronary bypass graft, may be used with code Z48.812, Encounter for surgical aftercare following surgery on the circulatory system, to indicate the surgery for which the aftercare is being performed. A status code should not be used when the aftercare code indicates the type of status, such as using Z43.0, Encounter for attention to tracheostomy, with Z93.0, Tracheostomy status.

The aftercare Z category/codes:

Z42   Encounter for plastic and reconstructive surgery following medical procedure or healed injury

Z43   Encounter for attention to artificial openings

Z44   Encounter for fitting and adjustment of external prosthetic device

Z45   Encounter for adjustment and management of implanted device

Z46   Encounter for fitting and adjustment of other devices

Z47   Orthopedic aftercare

Z48   Encounter for other postprocedural aftercare

Z49   Encounter for care involving renal dialysis

Z51   Encounter for other aftercare and medical care

8) Follow-up

The follow-up codes are used to explain continuing surveillance following completed treatment of a disease, condition, or injury. They imply that the condition has been fully treated and no longer exists. They should not be confused with aftercare codes, or injury codes with a 7th character for subsequent encounter, that explain ongoing care of a healing condition or its sequelae. Follow-up codes may be used in conjunction with history codes to provide the full picture of the healed condition and its treatment. The follow-up code is sequenced first, followed by the history code.

A follow-up code may be used to explain multiple visits. Should a condition be found to have recurred on the follow-up visit, then the diagnosis code for the condition should be assigned in place of the follow-up code.

The follow-up Z code categories:

Z08   Encounter for follow-up examination after completed treatment for malignant neoplasm

Z09   Encounter for follow-up examination after completed treatment for conditions other than malignant neoplasm

Z39   Encounter for maternal postpartum care and examination

9) Donor

Codes in category Z52, Donors of organs and tissues, are used for living individuals who are donating blood or other body tissue. These codes are only for individuals donating for others, not for self-donations. They are not used to identify cadaveric donations.

10) Counseling

Counseling Z codes are used when a patient or family member receives assistance in the aftermath of an illness or injury, or when support is required in coping with family or social problems.

The counseling Z codes/categories:

Z30.0-   Encounter for general counseling and advice on contraception

Z31.5   Encounter for **procreative** genetic counseling

Z31.6-   Encounter for general counseling and advice on procreation

Z32.2   Encounter for childbirth instruction

Z32.3   Encounter for childcare instruction

Z69   Encounter for mental health services for victim and perpetrator of abuse

Z70   Counseling related to sexual attitude, behavior and orientation

Z71   Persons encountering health services for other counseling and medical advice, not elsewhere classified

Z76.81   Expectant mother prebirth pediatrician visit

11) Encounters for obstetrical and reproductive services

See Section I.C.15. Pregnancy, Childbirth, and the Puerperium, for further instruction on the use of these codes.

Z codes for pregnancy are for use in those circumstances when none of the problems or complications included in the codes from the Obstetrics chapter exist (a routine prenatal visit or postpartum care). Codes in category Z34, Encounter for supervision of normal pregnancy, are always first-listed and are not to be used with any other code from the OB chapter.

Codes in category Z3A, Weeks of gestation, may be assigned to provide additional information about the pregnancy. Category Z3A codes should not be assigned for pregnancies with abortive outcomes (categories O00-O08), elective termination of pregnancy (code **Z33.2**), nor for postpartum conditions, as category Z3A is not applicable to these conditions. The date of the admission should be used to determine weeks of gestation for inpatient admissions that encompass more than one gestational week.

The outcome of delivery, category Z37, should be included on all maternal delivery records. It is always a secondary code. Codes in category Z37 should not be used on the newborn record.

Z codes for family planning (contraceptive) or procreative management and counseling should be included on an obstetric record either during the pregnancy or the postpartum stage, if applicable.

Z codes/categories for obstetrical and reproductive services:

Z30   Encounter for contraceptive management

Z31   Encounter for procreative management

Z32.2   Encounter for childbirth instruction

Z32.3	Encounter for childcare instruction
Z33	Pregnant state
Z34	Encounter for supervision of normal pregnancy
Z36	Encounter for antenatal screening of mother
Z3A	Weeks of gestation
Z37	Outcome of delivery
Z39	Encounter for maternal postpartum care and examination
Z76.81	Expectant mother prebirth pediatrician visit

12)Newborns and infants

See Section I.C.16. Newborn (Perinatal) Guidelines, for further instruction on the use of these codes.

Newborn Z codes/categories:

Z76.1	Encounter for health supervision and care of foundling
Z00.1-	Encounter for routine child health examination
Z38	Liveborn infants according to place of birth and type of delivery

13)Routine and administrative examinations

The Z codes allow for the description of encounters for routine examinations, such as, a general check-up, or, examinations for administrative purposes, such as, a pre-employment physical. The codes are not to be used if the examination is for diagnosis of a suspected condition or for treatment purposes. In such cases the diagnosis code is used. During a routine exam, should a diagnosis or condition be discovered, it should be coded as an additional code. Pre-existing and chronic conditions and history codes may also be included as additional codes as long as the examination is for administrative purposes and not focused on any particular condition.

Some of the codes for routine health examinations distinguish between "with" and "without" abnormal findings. Code assignment depends on the information that is known at the time the encounter is being coded. For example, if no abnormal findings were found during the examination, but the encounter is being coded before test results are back, it is acceptable to assign the code for "without abnormal findings." When assigning a code for "with abnormal findings," additional code(s) should be assigned to identify the specific abnormal finding(s).

Pre-operative examination and pre-procedural laboratory examination Z codes are for use only in those situations when a patient is being cleared for a procedure or surgery and no treatment is given.

The Z codes/categories for routine and administrative examinations:

Z00	Encounter for general examination without complaint, suspected or reported diagnosis
Z01	Encounter for other special examination without complaint, suspected or reported diagnosis
Z02	Encounter for administrative examination
	Except: Z02.9, Encounter for administrative examinations, unspecified
Z32.0-	Encounter for pregnancy test

14)Miscellaneous Z codes

The miscellaneous Z codes capture a number of other health care encounters that do not fall into one of the other categories. Certain of these codes identify the reason for the encounter; others are for use as additional codes that provide useful information on circumstances that may affect a patient's care and treatment.

Prophylactic organ removal

For encounters specifically for prophylactic removal of an organ (such as prophylactic removal of breasts due to a genetic susceptibility to cancer or a family history of cancer), the principal or first-listed code should be a code from category Z40, Encounter for prophylactic surgery, followed by the appropriate codes to identify the associated risk factor (such as genetic susceptibility or family history).

If the patient has a malignancy of one site and is having prophylactic removal at another site to prevent either a new primary malignancy or metastatic disease, a code for the malignancy should also be assigned in addition to a code from subcategory Z40.0, Encounter for prophylactic surgery for risk factors related to malignant neoplasms. A Z40.0 code should not be assigned if the patient is having organ removal for treatment of a malignancy, such as the removal of the testes for the treatment of prostate cancer.

Miscellaneous Z codes/categories:

Z28	Immunization not carried out
	Except: Z28.3, Underimmunization status
Z29	Encounter for other prophylactic measures
Z40	Encounter for prophylactic surgery

Z41	Encounter for procedures for purposes other than remedying health state
	Except: Z41.9, Encounter for procedure for purposes other than remedying health state, unspecified
Z53	Persons encountering health services for specific procedures and treatment, not carried out
Z55	Problems related to education and literacy
Z56	Problems related to employment and unemployment
Z57	Occupational exposure to risk factors
Z58	Problems related to physical environment
Z59	Problems related to housing and economic circumstances
Z60	Problems related to social environment
Z62	Problems related to upbringing
Z63	Other problems related to primary support group, including family circumstances
Z64	Problems related to certain psychosocial circumstances
Z65	Problems related to other psychosocial circumstances
Z72	Problems related to lifestyle
	Note: These codes should be assigned only when the documentation specifies that the patient has an associated problem
Z73	Problems related to life management difficulty
Z74	Problems related to care provider dependency
	Except: Z74.01, Bed confinement status
Z75	Problems related to medical facilities and other health care
Z76.0	Encounter for issue of repeat prescription
Z76.3	Healthy person accompanying sick person
Z76.4	Other boarder to healthcare facility
Z76.5	Malingerer [conscious simulation]
Z91.1-	Patient's noncompliance with medical treatment and regimen
Z91.83	Wandering in diseases classified elsewhere
Z91.84-	**Oral health risk factors**
Z91.89	Other specified personal risk factors, not elsewhere classified

15)Nonspecific Z codes

Certain Z codes are so non-specific, or potentially redundant with other codes in the classification, that there can be little justification for their use in the inpatient setting. Their use in the outpatient setting should be limited to those instances when there is no further documentation to permit more precise coding. Otherwise, any sign or symptom or any other reason for visit that is captured in another code should be used.

Nonspecific Z codes/categories:

Z02.9	Encounter for administrative examinations, unspecified
Z04.9	Encounter for examination and observation for unspecified reason
Z13.9	Encounter for screening, unspecified
Z41.9	Encounter for procedure for purposes other than remedying health state, unspecified
Z52.9	Donor of unspecified organ or tissue
Z86.59	Personal history of other mental and behavioral disorders
Z88.9	Allergy status to unspecified drugs, medicaments and biological substances status
Z92.0	Personal history of contraception

16)Z codes that may only be principal/first-listed diagnosis

The following Z codes/categories may only be reported as the principal/first-listed diagnosis, except when there are multiple encounters on the same day and the medical records for the encounters are combined:

Z00	Encounter for general examination without complaint, suspected or reported diagnosis
	Except: Z00.6
Z01	Encounter for other special examination without complaint, suspected or reported diagnosis
Z02	Encounter for administrative examination
Z03	Encounter for medical observation for suspected diseases and conditions ruled out
Z04	Encounter for examination and observation for other reasons
Z33.2	Encounter for elective termination of pregnancy
Z31.81	Encounter for male factor infertility in female patient
Z31.83	Encounter for assisted reproductive fertility procedure cycle
Z31.84	Encounter for fertility preservation procedure

Z34	Encounter for supervision of normal pregnancy
Z39	Encounter for maternal postpartum care and examination
Z38	Liveborn infants according to place of birth and type of delivery
Z40	**Encounter for prophylactic surgery**
Z42	Encounter for plastic and reconstructive surgery following medical procedure or healed injury
Z51.Ø	Encounter for antineoplastic radiation therapy
Z51.1-	Encounter for antineoplastic chemotherapy and immunotherapy
Z52	Donors of organs and tissues
	Except: Z52.9, Donor of unspecified organ or tissue
Z76.1	Encounter for health supervision and care of foundling
Z76.2	Encounter for health supervision and care of other healthy infant and child
Z99.12	Encounter for respirator [ventilator] dependence during power failure

Chapter 21. Factors Influencing Health Status and Contact With Health Services (Z00-Z99)

NOTE   Z codes represent reasons for encounters. A corresponding procedure code must accompany a Z code if a procedure is performed. Categories Z00-Z99 are provided for occasions when circumstances other than a disease, injury or external cause classifiable to categories A00-Y89 are recorded as "diagnoses" or "problems". This can arise in two main ways:

(a) When a person who may or may not be sick encounters the health services for some specific purpose, such as to receive limited care or service for a current condition, to donate an organ or tissue, to receive prophylactic vaccination (immunization), or to discuss a problem which is in itself not a disease or injury.

(b) When some circumstance or problem is present which influences the person's health status but is not in itself a current illness or injury.

This chapter contains the following blocks:

Z00-Z13   Persons encountering health services for examinations
Z14-Z15   Genetic carrier and genetic susceptibility to disease
Z16   Resistance to antimicrobial drugs
Z17   Estrogen receptor status
Z18   Retained foreign body fragments
~~Z19~~   ~~Hormone sensitivity malignancy status~~
Z20-Z29   Persons with potential health hazards related to communicable diseases
Z30-Z39   Persons encountering health services in circumstances related to reproduction
Z40-Z53   Encounters for other specific health care
Z55-Z65   Persons with potential health hazards related to socioeconomic and psychosocial circumstances
Z66   Do not resuscitate status
Z67   Blood type
Z68   Body mass index (BMI)
Z69-Z76   Persons encountering health services in other circumstances
Z77-Z99   Persons with potential health hazards related to family and personal history and certain conditions influencing health status

Persons encountering health services for examinations (Z00-Z13)

NOTE   Nonspecific abnormal findings disclosed at the time of these examinations are classified to categories R70-R94.

EXCLUDES 1   *examinations related to pregnancy and reproduction (Z30-Z36, Z39-)*

✓4ᵗʰ **Z00**   **Encounter for general examination without complaint, suspected or reported diagnosis**

   EXCLUDES 1   *encounter for examination for administrative purposes (Z02.-)*

   EXCLUDES 2   *encounter for pre-procedural examinations (Z01.81-)*
     special screening examinations (Z11-Z13)

✓5ᵗʰ **Z00.0**   **Encounter for general adult medical examination**
   Encounter for adult periodic examination (annual) (physical) and any associated laboratory and radiologic examinations

     EXCLUDES 1   *encounter for examination of sign or symptom—code to sign or symptom*
       general health check-up of infant or child (Z00.12-)

   Z00.00   **Encounter for general adult medical examination** *without abnormal findings*   A
     Encounter for adult health check-up NOS
     AHA: 2016, 1Q, 36

   Z00.01   **Encounter for general adult medical examination** *with abnormal findings*   A
     Use additional code to identify abnormal findings
     AHA: 2016, 1Q, 35-36

✓5ᵗʰ **Z00.1**   **Encounter for** *newborn, infant and child health* **examinations**

   ✓6ᵗʰ **Z00.11**   **Newborn health examination**
     Health check for child under 29 days old
     Use additional code to identify any abnormal findings
     EXCLUDES 1   *health check for child over 28 days old (Z00.12-)*

     Z00.110   **Health examination for newborn under 8 days old**   N
       Health check for newborn under 8 days old

     Z00.111   **Health examination for newborn 8 to 28 days old**   N
       Health check for newborn 8 to 28 days old
       Newborn weight check

   ✓6ᵗʰ **Z00.12**   **Encounter for** *routine child* **health examination**
     Encounter for development testing of infant or child
     Health check (routine) for child over 28 days old
     EXCLUDES 1   *health check for child under 29 days old (Z00.11-)*
       health supervision of foundling or other healthy infant or child (Z76.1-Z76.2)
       newborn health examination (Z00.11-)

     Z00.121   **Encounter for routine child health examination** *with abnormal findings*   P
       Use additional code to identify abnormal findings
       AHA: 2016, 1Q, 34-35

     Z00.129   **Encounter for routine child health examination** *without abnormal findings*   P
       Encounter for routine child health examination NOS
       AHA: 2016, 1Q, 34

Z00.2   **Encounter for examination for** *period of rapid growth in childhood*   P

Z00.3   **Encounter for examination for** *adolescent development state*   P
   Encounter for puberty development state

Z00.5   **Encounter for examination of** *potential donor of organ and tissue*

Z00.6   **Encounter for examination for** *normal comparison and control in clinical research program*
   Examination of participant or control in clinical research program

✓5ᵗʰ **Z00.7**   **Encounter for examination for period of** *delayed growth in childhood*

   Z00.70   **Encounter for examination for period of delayed growth in childhood** *without abnormal findings*   P

   Z00.71   **Encounter for examination for period of delayed growth in childhood** *with abnormal findings*   P
     Use additional code to identify abnormal findings

Z00.8   **Encounter for** *other* **general examination**
   Encounter for health examination in population surveys

✓4ᵗʰ **Z01**   **Encounter for other** *special examination* **without complaint, suspected or reported diagnosis**

   INCLUDES   routine examination of specific system
   NOTE   Codes from category Z01 represent the reason for the encounter. A separate procedure code is required to identify any examinations or procedures performed.

   EXCLUDES 1   *encounter for examination for administrative purposes (Z02.-)*
     encounter for examination for suspected conditions, proven not to exist (Z03.-)
     encounter for laboratory and radiologic examinations as a component of general medical examinations (Z00.0-)
     encounter for laboratory, radiologic and imaging examinations for sign(s) and symptom(s)—code to the sign(s) or symptom(s)

   EXCLUDES 2   *screening examinations (Z11-Z13)*

✓5ᵗʰ **Z01.0**   **Encounter for examination of** *eyes and vision*
   EXCLUDES 1   *examination for driving license (Z02.4)*

   Z01.00   **Encounter for examination of eyes and vision** *without abnormal findings*
     Encounter for examination of eyes and vision NOS

   Z01.01   **Encounter for examination of eyes and vision** *with abnormal findings*
     Use additional code to identify abnormal findings

✓5ᵗʰ **Z01.1**   **Encounter for examination of** *ears and hearing*

   Z01.10   **Encounter for examination of ears and hearing** *without abnormal findings*
     Encounter for examination of ears and hearing NOS
     AHA: 2016, 4Q, 24

   ✓6ᵗʰ **Z01.11**   **Encounter for examination of ears and hearing** *with abnormal findings*
     AHA: 2016, 3Q, 17-18

     Z01.110   **Encounter for hearing examination following** *failed hearing screening*

     Z01.118   **Encounter for examination of ears and hearing with** *other abnormal findings*
       Use additional code to identify abnormal findings

   Z01.12   **Encounter for** *hearing conservation and treatment*

✓5ᵗʰ **Z01.2**   **Encounter for** *dental examination and cleaning*

   Z01.20   **Encounter for dental examination and cleaning** *without abnormal findings*
     Encounter for dental examination and cleaning NOS

N Newborn: 0   P Pediatric: 0-17   M Maternity: 12-55   A Adult: 15-124   **MCC** Major CC Condition   **PDxMCC** PDx acts as own MCC   **CC** CC Condition   **PDxCC** PDx acts as own CC

1222   ICD-10-CM 2018

Z01.21 **Encounter for dental examination and cleaning with abnormal findings**
Use additional code to identify abnormal findings

✓5ᵗʰ **Z01.3** **Encounter for examination of blood pressure**

Z01.30 **Encounter for examination of blood pressure without abnormal findings**
Encounter for examination of blood pressure NOS

Z01.31 **Encounter for examination of blood pressure with abnormal findings**
Use additional code to identify abnormal findings

✓5ᵗʰ **Z01.4** **Encounter for gynecological examination**
EXCLUDES 2   *pregnancy examination or test (Z32.0-)*
routine examination for contraceptive maintenance (Z30.4-)

✓6ᵗʰ **Z01.41** **Encounter for routine gynecological examination**
Encounter for general gynecological examination with or without cervical smear
Encounter for gynecological examination (general) (routine) NOS
Encounter for pelvic examination (annual) (periodic)
Use additional code:
for screening for human papillomavirus, if applicable, (Z11.51)
for screening vaginal pap smear, if applicable (Z12.72)
to identify acquired absence of uterus, if applicable (Z90.71-)
EXCLUDES 1   *gynecologic examination status-post hysterectomy for malignant condition (Z08)*
screening cervical pap smear not a part of a routine gynecological examination (Z12.4)

Z01.411 **Encounter for gynecological examination (general) (routine) with abnormal findings** ♀
Use additional code to identify abnormal findings

Z01.419 **Encounter for gynecological examination (general) (routine) without abnormal findings** ♀

Z01.42 **Encounter for cervical smear to confirm findings of recent normal smear following initial abnormal smear** ♀

✓5ᵗʰ **Z01.8** **Encounter for other specified special examinations**

✓6ᵗʰ **Z01.81** **Encounter for preprocedural examinations**
Encounter for preoperative examinations
Encounter for radiological and imaging examinations as part of preprocedural examination

Z01.810 **Encounter for preprocedural cardiovascular examination**

Z01.811 **Encounter for preprocedural respiratory examination**

Z01.812 **Encounter for preprocedural laboratory examination**
Blood and urine tests prior to treatment or procedure

Z01.818 **Encounter for other preprocedural examination**
Encounter for preprocedural examination NOS
Encounter for examinations prior to antineoplastic chemotherapy

Z01.82 **Encounter for allergy testing**
EXCLUDES 1   *encounter for antibody response examination (Z01.84)*

Z01.83 **Encounter for blood typing**
Encounter for Rh typing

Z01.84 **Encounter for antibody response examination**
Encounter for immunity status testing
EXCLUDES 1   *encounter for allergy testing (Z01.82)*

Z01.89 **Encounter for other specified special examinations**

✓4ᵗʰ **Z02** **Encounter for administrative examination**

Z02.0 **Encounter for examination for admission to educational institution**
Encounter for examination for admission to preschool (education)
Encounter for examination for re-admission to school following illness or medical treatment

Z02.1 **Encounter for pre-employment examination**

Z02.2 **Encounter for examination for admission to residential institution**
EXCLUDES 1   *examination for admission to prison (Z02.89)*

Z02.3 **Encounter for examination for recruitment to armed forces**

Z02.4 **Encounter for examination for driving license**

Z02.5 **Encounter for examination for participation in sport**
EXCLUDES 1   *blood-alcohol and blood-drug test (Z02.83)*

Z02.6 **Encounter for examination for insurance purposes**

✓5ᵗʰ **Z02.7** **Encounter for issue of medical certificate**
EXCLUDES 1   *encounter for general medical examination (Z00-Z01, Z02.0-Z02.6, Z02.8-Z02.9)*

Z02.71 **Encounter for disability determination**
Encounter for issue of medical certificate of incapacity
Encounter for issue of medical certificate of invalidity

Z02.79 **Encounter for issue of other medical certificate**

✓5ᵗʰ **Z02.8** **Encounter for other administrative examinations**

Z02.81 **Encounter for paternity testing**

Z02.82 **Encounter for adoption services**

Z02.83 **Encounter for blood-alcohol and blood-drug test**
Use additional code for findings of alcohol or drugs in blood (R78.-)

Z02.89 **Encounter for other administrative examinations**
Encounter for examination for admission to prison
Encounter for examination for admission to summer camp
Encounter for immigration examination
Encounter for naturalization examination
Encounter for premarital examination
EXCLUDES 1   *health supervision of foundling or other healthy infant or child (Z76.1-Z76.2)*

Z02.9 **Encounter for administrative examinations, unspecified**

✓4ᵗʰ **Z03** **Encounter for medical observation for suspected diseases and conditions ruled out**
NOTE This category is to be used when a person without a diagnosis is suspected of having an abnormal condition, without signs or symptoms, which requires study, but after examination and observation, is ruled out. This category is also for use for administrative and legal observation status.
EXCLUDES 1   *contact with and (suspected) exposures hazardous to health (Z77.-)*
▶*encounter for observation and evaluation of newborn for suspected diseases and conditions ruled out (Z05.0-)*◀
newborn observation for suspected condition, ruled out (P00-P04)
person with feared complaint in whom no diagnosis is made (Z71.1)
signs or symptoms under study—code to signs or symptoms

Z03.6 **Encounter for observation for suspected toxic effect from ingested substance ruled out**
Encounter for observation for suspected adverse effect from drug
Encounter for observation for suspected poisoning

✓5ᵗʰ **Z03.7** **Encounter for suspected maternal and fetal conditions ruled out**
Encounter for suspected maternal and fetal conditions not found
EXCLUDES 1   *known or suspected fetal anomalies affecting management of mother, not ruled out (O26-, O35-, O36-, O40-, O41-)*

Z03.71 **Encounter for suspected problem with amniotic cavity and membrane ruled out** Ⓜ♀
Encounter for suspected oligohydramnios ruled out
Encounter for suspected polyhydramnios ruled out

Z03.72 **Encounter for suspected placental problem ruled out** Ⓜ♀

Z03.73 **Encounter for suspected fetal anomaly ruled out** Ⓜ♀

Z03.74 **Encounter for suspected problem with fetal growth ruled out** Ⓜ♀

Z03.75 **Encounter for suspected cervical shortening ruled out** Ⓜ♀

Z03.79 **Encounter for other suspected maternal and fetal conditions ruled out** Ⓜ♀

✓5ᵗʰ **Z03.8** **Encounter for observation for other suspected diseases and conditions ruled out**

✓6ᵗʰ **Z03.81** **Encounter for observation for suspected exposure to biological agents ruled out**

Z03.810 **Encounter for observation for suspected exposure to anthrax ruled out**

Z03.818 Encounter for observation for suspected exposure to **other** biological agents ruled out

Z03.89 Encounter for observation for **other** suspected diseases and conditions ruled out

✓4ᵗʰ **Z04** **Encounter for examination and observation for other reasons**

INCLUDES encounter for examination for medicolegal reasons

This category is to be used when a person without a diagnosis is suspected of having an abnormal condition, without signs or symptoms, which requires study, but after examination and observation, is ruled-out. This category is also for use for administrative and legal observation status.

Z04.1 Encounter for examination and observation following **transport** accident

EXCLUDES 1 encounter for examination and observation following work accident (Z04.2)

Z04.2 Encounter for examination and observation following **work** accident

Z04.3 Encounter for examination and observation following **other** accident

✓5ᵗʰ **Z04.4** Encounter for examination and observation following **alleged rape**

Encounter for examination and observation of victim following alleged rape

Encounter for examination and observation of victim following alleged sexual abuse

Z04.41 Encounter for examination and observation following alleged **adult** rape [A]

Suspected adult rape, ruled out

Suspected adult sexual abuse, ruled out

Z04.42 Encounter for examination and observation following alleged **child** rape [P]

Suspected child rape, ruled out

Suspected child sexual abuse, ruled out

Z04.6 Encounter for **general psychiatric examination, requested by authority**

✓5ᵗʰ **Z04.7** Encounter for examination and observation following **alleged physical abuse**

Z04.71 Encounter for examination and observation following alleged **adult** physical abuse [A]

Suspected adult physical abuse, ruled out

EXCLUDES 1 confirmed case of adult physical abuse (T74.-)

encounter for examination and observation following alleged adult sexual abuse (Z04.41)

suspected case of adult physical abuse, not ruled out (T76.-)

Z04.72 Encounter for examination and observation following alleged **child** physical abuse [P]

Suspected child physical abuse, ruled out

EXCLUDES 1 confirmed case of child physical abuse (T74.-)

encounter for examination and observation following alleged child sexual abuse (Z04.42)

suspected case of child physical abuse, not ruled out (T76.-)

Z04.8 Encounter for examination and observation for **other** specified reasons

Encounter for examination and observation for request for expert evidence

Z04.9 Encounter for examination and observation for **unspecified** reason

Encounter for observation NOS

✓4ᵗʰ **Z05** **Encounter for observation of newborn for suspected diseases and conditions ruled out**

▶This category is to be used for newborns, within the neonatal period (the first 28 days of life), who are suspected of having an abnormal condition, but without signs or symptoms, and which, after examination and observation, is ruled out.◄

EXCLUDES 2 ~~newborn observation for suspected condition, related to exposure from the mother or birth process (P00-P04)~~

Z05.0 Observation and evaluation of newborn for suspected **cardiac** condition ruled out

Z05.1 Observation and evaluation of newborn for suspected **infectious** condition ruled out

Z05.2 Observation and evaluation of newborn for suspected **neurological** condition ruled out

Z05.3 Observation and evaluation of newborn for suspected **respiratory** condition ruled out

✓5ᵗʰ **Z05.4** Observation and evaluation of newborn for suspected **genetic, metabolic or immunologic** condition ruled out

Z05.41 Observation and evaluation of newborn for suspected **genetic** condition ruled out

Z05.42 Observation and evaluation of newborn for suspected **metabolic** condition ruled out

Z05.43 Observation and evaluation of newborn for suspected **immunologic** condition ruled out

Z05.5 Observation and evaluation of newborn for suspected **gastrointestinal** condition ruled out

Z05.6 Observation and evaluation of newborn for suspected **genitourinary** condition ruled out

✓5ᵗʰ **Z05.7** Observation and evaluation of newborn for suspected **skin, subcutaneous, musculoskeletal and connective tissue** condition ruled out

Z05.71 Observation and evaluation of newborn for suspected **skin and subcutaneous** tissue condition ruled out

Z05.72 Observation and evaluation of newborn for suspected **musculoskeletal** condition ruled out

Z05.73 Observation and evaluation of newborn for suspected **connective tissue** condition ruled out

Z05.8 Observation and evaluation of newborn for **other** specified suspected condition ruled out

Z05.9 Observation and evaluation of newborn for **unspecified** suspected condition ruled out

Z08 **Encounter for follow-up examination after completed treatment for malignant neoplasm**

Medical surveillance following completed treatment

Use additional code to identify any acquired absence of organs (Z90.-)

Use additional code to identify the personal history of malignant neoplasm (Z85.-)

EXCLUDES 1 aftercare following medical care (Z43-Z49, Z51)

Z09 **Encounter for follow-up examination after completed treatment for conditions other than malignant neoplasm**

Medical surveillance following completed treatment

Use additional code to identify any applicable history of disease code (Z86.-. Z87.-)

EXCLUDES 1 aftercare following medical care (Z43-Z49, Z51)

surveillance of contraception (Z30.4-)

surveillance of prosthetic and other medical devices (Z44-Z46)

AHA: 2017, 1Q, 9; 2015, 1Q, 8

✓4ᵗʰ **Z11** **Encounter for screening for infectious and parasitic diseases**

Screening is the testing for disease or disease precursors in asymptomatic individuals so that early detection and treatment can be provided for those who test positive for the disease.

EXCLUDES 1 encounter for diagnostic examination—code to sign or symptom

Z11.0 **Encounter for screening for intestinal infectious diseases**

Z11.1 **Encounter for screening for respiratory tuberculosis**

Z11.2 **Encounter for screening for other bacterial diseases**

Z11.3 **Encounter for screening for infections with a predominantly sexual mode of transmission**

EXCLUDES 2 encounter for screening for human immunodeficiency virus [HIV] (Z11.4)

encounter for screening for human papillomavirus (Z11.51)

Z11.4 **Encounter for screening for human immunodeficiency virus [HIV]**

✓5ᵗʰ **Z11.5** **Encounter for screening for other viral diseases**

EXCLUDES 2 encounter for screening for viral intestinal disease (Z11.0)

Z11.51 **Encounter for screening for human papillomavirus (HPV)**

Z11.59 **Encounter for screening for other viral diseases**

Z11.6 **Encounter for screening for other protozoal diseases and helminthiases**

EXCLUDES 2 encounter for screening for protozoal intestinal disease (Z11.0)

Z11.8 **Encounter for screening for other infectious and parasitic diseases**

Encounter for screening for chlamydia

Encounter for screening for rickettsial

Encounter for screening for spirochetal

Encounter for screening for mycoses

Z11.9 **Encounter for screening for infectious and parasitic diseases, unspecified**

[N] Newborn: 0   [P] Pediatric: 0-17   [M] Maternity: 12-55   [A] Adult: 15-124   [MCC] Major CC Condition   [PDxMCC] PDx acts as own MCC   [CC] CC Condition   [PDxCC] PDx acts as own CC

1224   ICD-10-CM 2018

✓4ᵗʰ Z12 Encounter for screening for malignant neoplasms

Screening is the testing for disease or disease precursors in asymptomatic individuals so that early detection and treatment can be provided for those who test positive for the disease.

Use additional code to identify any family history of malignant neoplasm (Z80.-)

EXCLUDES 1   *encounter for diagnostic examination—code to sign or symptom*

Z12.0 Encounter for screening for malignant neoplasm of stomach

✓5ᵗʰ Z12.1 Encounter for screening for malignant neoplasm of intestinal tract

AHA: 2017, 1Q, 8, 9

Z12.10 Encounter for screening for malignant neoplasm of intestinal tract, unspecified

Z12.11 Encounter for screening for malignant neoplasm of colon

Encounter for screening colonoscopy NOS

Z12.12 Encounter for screening for malignant neoplasm of rectum

Z12.13 Encounter for screening for malignant neoplasm of small intestine

Z12.2 Encounter for screening for malignant neoplasm of respiratory organs

✓5ᵗʰ Z12.3 Encounter for screening for malignant neoplasm of breast

Z12.31 Encounter for screening mammogram for malignant neoplasm of breast

EXCLUDES 1   *inconclusive mammogram (R92.2)*

AHA: 2015, 1Q, 24

Z12.39 Encounter for other screening for malignant neoplasm of breast

Z12.4 Encounter for screening for malignant neoplasm of cervix ♀

Encounter for screening pap smear for malignant neoplasm of cervix

EXCLUDES 1   *when screening is part of general gynecological examination (Z01.4-)*

EXCLUDES 2   *encounter for screening for human papillomavirus (Z11.51)*

Z12.5 Encounter for screening for malignant neoplasm of prostate ♂

Z12.6 Encounter for screening for malignant neoplasm of bladder

✓5ᵗʰ Z12.7 Encounter for screening for malignant neoplasm of other genitourinary organs

Z12.71 Encounter for screening for malignant neoplasm of testis ♂

Z12.72 Encounter for screening for malignant neoplasm of vagina ♀

Vaginal pap smear status-post hysterectomy for non-malignant condition

Use additional code to identify acquired absence of uterus (Z90.71-)

EXCLUDES 1   *vaginal pap smear status-post hysterectomy for malignant conditions (Z08)*

Z12.73 Encounter for screening for malignant neoplasm of ovary ♀

Z12.79 Encounter for screening for malignant neoplasm of other genitourinary organs

✓5ᵗʰ Z12.8 Encounter for screening for malignant neoplasm of other sites

Z12.81 Encounter for screening for malignant neoplasm of oral cavity

Z12.82 Encounter for screening for malignant neoplasm of nervous system

Z12.83 Encounter for screening for malignant neoplasm of skin

Z12.89 Encounter for screening for malignant neoplasm of other sites

Z12.9 Encounter for screening for malignant neoplasm, site unspecified

✓4ᵗʰ Z13 Encounter for screening for other diseases and disorders

Screening is the testing for disease or disease precursors in asymptomatic individuals so that early detection and treatment can be provided for those who test positive for the disease.

EXCLUDES 1   *encounter for diagnostic examination—code to sign or symptom*

Z13.0 Encounter for screening for diseases of the blood and blood-forming organs and certain disorders involving the immune mechanism

Z13.1 Encounter for screening for diabetes mellitus

✓5ᵗʰ Z13.2 Encounter for screening for nutritional, metabolic and other endocrine disorders

Z13.21 Encounter for screening for nutritional disorder

✓6ᵗʰ Z13.22 Encounter for screening for metabolic disorder

Z13.220 Encounter for screening for lipoid disorders

Encounter for screening for cholesterol level

Encounter for screening for hypercholesterolemia

Encounter for screening for hyperlipidemia

Z13.228 Encounter for screening for other metabolic disorders

Z13.29 Encounter for screening for other suspected endocrine disorder

EXCLUDES 1   *encounter for screening for diabetes mellitus (Z13.1)*

Z13.4 Encounter for screening for certain developmental disorders in childhood   **P**

Encounter for screening for developmental handicaps in early childhood

EXCLUDES 1   *routine development testing of infant or child (Z00.1-)*

Z13.5 Encounter for screening for eye and ear disorders

EXCLUDES 2   *encounter for general hearing examination (Z01.1-)*
encounter for general vision examination (Z01.0-)

AHA: 2016, 3Q, 17

Z13.6 Encounter for screening for cardiovascular disorders

✓5ᵗʰ Z13.7 Encounter for screening for genetic and chromosomal anomalies

EXCLUDES 1   *genetic testing for procreative management (Z31.4-)*

Z13.71 Encounter for nonprocreative screening for genetic disease carrier status

Z13.79 Encounter for other screening for genetic and chromosomal anomalies

✓5ᵗʰ Z13.8 Encounter for screening for other specified diseases and disorders

EXCLUDES 2   *screening for malignant neoplasms (Z12.-)*

✓6ᵗʰ Z13.81 Encounter for screening for digestive system disorders

Z13.810 Encounter for screening for upper gastrointestinal disorder

Z13.811 Encounter for screening for lower gastrointestinal disorder

EXCLUDES 1   *encounter for screening for intestinal infectious disease (Z11.0)*

Z13.818 Encounter for screening for other digestive system disorders

✓6ᵗʰ Z13.82 Encounter for screening for musculoskeletal disorder

Z13.820 Encounter for screening for osteoporosis

Z13.828 Encounter for screening for other musculoskeletal disorder

Z13.83 Encounter for screening for respiratory disorder NEC

EXCLUDES 1   *encounter for screening for respiratory tuberculosis (Z11.1)*

Z13.84 Encounter for screening for dental disorders

✓6ᵗʰ Z13.85 Encounter for screening for nervous system disorders

Z13.850 Encounter for screening for traumatic brain injury

Z13.858 Encounter for screening for other nervous system disorders

Z13.88 Encounter for screening for disorder due to exposure to contaminants

EXCLUDES 1   *those exposed to contaminants without suspected disorders (Z57-Z77-)*

Z13.89 Encounter for screening for other disorder

Encounter for screening for genitourinary disorders

Z13.9 Encounter for screening, unspecified

✓ Additional Character Req   ✓x7ᵗʰ Placeholder Alert   Unacceptable PDx   Manifestation   **H1-H14** HAC   **HCC** CMS-HCC Condition   *EXCLUDES 1* Not Coded Here   *EXCLUDES 2* Not Included Here

Genetic carrier and genetic susceptibility to disease (Z14-Z15)

✓4th Z14 Genetic carrier
> **DEF:** Individuals carrying a gene mutation associated with a certain disease who typically do not develop the disease but are able to pass mutated gene to offspring.

   ✓5th Z14.0 Hemophilia A carrier
      Z14.01 Asymptomatic hemophilia A carrier
      Z14.02 Symptomatic hemophilia A carrier
   Z14.1 Cystic fibrosis carrier
   Z14.8 Genetic carrier of other disease

✓4th Z15 Genetic susceptibility to disease
> **INCLUDES** confirmed abnormal gene
> Use additional code, if applicable, for any associated family history of the disease (Z80-Z84)
> **EXCLUDES 1** chromosomal anomalies (Q90-Q99)

   ✓5th Z15.0 Genetic susceptibility to malignant neoplasm
> Code first, if applicable, any current malignant neoplasm (C00-C75, C81-C96)
> Use additional code, if applicable, for any personal history of malignant neoplasm (Z85.-)

      Z15.01 Genetic susceptibility to malignant neoplasm of breast
      Z15.02 Genetic susceptibility to malignant neoplasm of ovary ♀
      Z15.03 Genetic susceptibility to malignant neoplasm of prostate ♂
      Z15.04 Genetic susceptibility to malignant neoplasm of endometrium ♀
      Z15.09 Genetic susceptibility to other malignant neoplasm

   ✓5th Z15.8 Genetic susceptibility to other disease
      Z15.81 Genetic susceptibility to multiple endocrine neoplasia [MEN]
> **EXCLUDES 1** multiple endocrine neoplasia [MEN] syndromes (E31.2-)

      Z15.89 Genetic susceptibility to other disease

Resistance to antimicrobial drugs (Z16)

✓4th Z16 Resistance to antimicrobial drugs
> **NOTE** The codes in this category are provided for use as additional codes to identify the resistance and non-responsiveness of a condition to antimicrobial drugs.
> Code first the infection
> **EXCLUDES 1** Methicillin resistant Staphylococcus aureus infection (A49.02)
> ~~Methicillin resistant Staphylococcus aureus infection in diseases classified elsewhere (B95.62)~~
> Methicillin resistant Staphylococcus aureus pneumonia (J15.212)
> sepsis due to Methicillin resistant Staphylococcus aureus (A41.02)

   ✓5th Z16.1 Resistance to beta lactam antibiotics
      Z16.10 Resistance to unspecified beta lactam antibiotics
      Z16.11 Resistance to penicillins
> Resistance to amoxicillin
> Resistance to ampicillin

      Z16.12 Extended spectrum beta lactamase (ESBL) resistance
> **EXCLUDES 2** ►Methicillin resistant Staphylococcus aureus infection in diseases classified elsewhere (B95.62)◄

      Z16.19 Resistance to other specified beta lactam antibiotics
> Resistance to cephalosporins

   ✓5th Z16.2 Resistance to other antibiotics
      Z16.20 Resistance to unspecified antibiotic
> Resistance to antibiotics NOS

      Z16.21 Resistance to vancomycin
      Z16.22 Resistance to vancomycin related antibiotics
      Z16.23 Resistance to quinolones and fluoroquinolones
      Z16.24 Resistance to multiple antibiotics
      Z16.29 Resistance to other single specified antibiotic
> Resistance to aminoglycosides
> Resistance to macrolides
> Resistance to sulfonamides
> Resistance to tetracyclines

   ✓5th Z16.3 Resistance to other antimicrobial drugs
> **EXCLUDES 1** resistance to antibiotics (Z16.1-, Z16.2-)

      Z16.30 Resistance to unspecified antimicrobial drugs
> Drug resistance NOS

      Z16.31 Resistance to antiparasitic drug(s)
> Resistance to quinine and related compounds

      Z16.32 Resistance to antifungal drug(s)
      Z16.33 Resistance to antiviral drug(s)
      ✓6th Z16.34 Resistance to antimycobacterial drug(s)
> Resistance to tuberculostatics

         Z16.341 Resistance to single antimycobacterial drug
> Resistance to antimycobacterial drug NOS

         Z16.342 Resistance to multiple antimycobacterial drugs

      Z16.35 Resistance to multiple antimicrobial drugs
> **EXCLUDES 1** Resistance to multiple antibiotics only (Z16.24)

      Z16.39 Resistance to other specified antimicrobial drug

Estrogen receptor status (Z17)

✓4th Z17 Estrogen receptor status
> Code first malignant neoplasm of breast (C50.-)

   Z17.0 Estrogen receptor positive status [ER+]
   Z17.1 Estrogen receptor negative status [ER-]

Retained foreign body fragment (Z18)

✓4th Z18 Retained foreign body fragments
> **INCLUDES** embedded fragment (status)
> embedded splinter (status)
> retained foreign body status
> **EXCLUDES 1** artificial joint prosthesis status (Z96.6-)
> foreign body accidentally left during a procedure (T81.5-)
> foreign body entering through orifice (T15-T19)
> in situ cardiac device (Z95.-)
> organ or tissue replaced by means other than transplant (Z96.-, Z97.-)
> organ or tissue replaced by transplant (Z94.-)
> personal history of retained foreign body fully removed (Z87.821)
> superficial foreign body (non-embedded splinter)—code to superficial foreign body, by site
> **DEF:** Embedded or retained fragment, splinter, or foreign body; natural or synthetic; can cause infection.

   ✓5th Z18.0 Retained radioactive fragments
      Z18.01 Retained depleted uranium fragments
      Z18.09 Other retained radioactive fragments
> Other retained depleted isotope fragments
> Retained nontherapeutic radioactive fragments

   ✓5th Z18.1 Retained metal fragments
> **EXCLUDES 1** retained radioactive metal fragments (Z18.01-Z18.09)

      Z18.10 Retained metal fragments, unspecified
> Retained metal fragment NOS

      Z18.11 Retained magnetic metal fragments
      Z18.12 Retained nonmagnetic metal fragments
   Z18.2 Retained plastic fragments
> Acrylics fragments
> Diethylhexylphthalates fragments
> Isocyanate fragments

   ✓5th Z18.3 Retained organic fragments
      Z18.31 Retained animal quills or spines
      Z18.32 Retained tooth
      Z18.33 Retained wood fragments
      Z18.39 Other retained organic fragments

   ✓5th Z18.8 Other specified retained foreign body
      Z18.81 Retained glass fragments
      Z18.83 Retained stone or crystalline fragments
> Retained concrete or cement fragments

      Z18.89 Other specified retained foreign body fragments
   Z18.9 Retained foreign body fragments, unspecified material

---

N Newborn: 0   P Pediatric: 0-17   M Maternity: 12-55   A Adult: 15-124   **MCC** Major CC Condition   **PDxMCC** PDx acts as own MCC   **CC** CC Condition   **PDxCC** PDx acts as own CC

Hormone sensitivity malignancy status (Z19)

☑4ᵗʰ Z19   Hormone sensitivity malignancy status
> Code first malignant neoplasm — see Table of Neoplasms, by site, malignant

Z19.1   Hormone sensitive malignancy status

Z19.2   Hormone resistant malignancy status
> Castrate resistant prostate malignancy status

Persons with potential health hazards related to communicable diseases (Z20-Z29)

☑4ᵗʰ Z20   Contact with and (suspected) exposure to communicable diseases
> EXCLUDES 1   carrier of infectious disease (Z22.-)
> diagnosed current infectious or parasitic disease—see Alphabetic Index
> EXCLUDES 2   personal history of infectious and parasitic diseases (Z86.1-)

☑5ᵗʰ Z20.0   Contact with and (suspected) exposure to intestinal infectious diseases

Z20.01   Contact with and (suspected) exposure to intestinal infectious diseases due to Escherichia coli (E. coli)

Z20.09   Contact with and (suspected) exposure to other intestinal infectious diseases

Z20.1   Contact with and (suspected) exposure to tuberculosis

Z20.2   Contact with and (suspected) exposure to infections with a predominantly sexual mode of transmission

Z20.3   Contact with and (suspected) exposure to rabies

Z20.4   Contact with and (suspected) exposure to rubella

Z20.5   Contact with and (suspected) exposure to viral hepatitis

Z20.6   Contact with and (suspected) exposure to human immunodeficiency virus [HIV]
> EXCLUDES 1   asymptomatic human immunodeficiency virus [HIV] HIV infection status (Z21)

Z20.7   Contact with and (suspected) exposure to pediculosis, acariasis and other infestations

☑5ᵗʰ Z20.8   Contact with and (suspected) exposure to other communicable diseases

☑6ᵗʰ Z20.81   Contact with and (suspected) exposure to other bacterial communicable diseases

Z20.810   Contact with and (suspected) exposure to anthrax

Z20.811   Contact with and (suspected) exposure to meningococcus

Z20.818   Contact with and (suspected) exposure to other bacterial communicable diseases

☑6ᵗʰ Z20.82   Contact with and (suspected) exposure to other viral communicable diseases

Z20.820   Contact with and (suspected) exposure to varicella

Z20.828   Contact with and (suspected) exposure to other viral communicable diseases

Z20.89   Contact with and (suspected) exposure to other communicable diseases

Z20.9   Contact with and (suspected) exposure to unspecified communicable disease

⁴ Z21   Asymptomatic human immunodeficiency virus [HIV] infection status   **HCC**
> HIV positive NOS
> Code first human immunodeficiency virus [HIV] disease complicating pregnancy, childbirth and the puerperium, if applicable (O98.7-)
> EXCLUDES 1   acquired immunodeficiency syndrome (B20)
> contact with human immunodeficiency virus [HIV] (Z20.6)
> exposure to human immunodeficiency virus [HIV] (Z20.6)
> human immunodeficiency virus [HIV] disease (B20)
> inconclusive laboratory evidence of human immunodeficiency virus [HIV] (R75)
> **DEF:** Phase of human immunodeficiency virus (HIV) infection with no clinical symptoms; may last for 10 years or more.

☑4ᵗʰ Z22   Carrier of infectious disease
> INCLUDES   colonization status
> suspected carrier
> EXCLUDES 2   carrier of viral hepatitis (B18.-)

Z22.0   Carrier of typhoid

Z22.1   Carrier of other intestinal infectious diseases

Z22.2   Carrier of diphtheria

☑5ᵗʰ Z22.3   Carrier of other specified bacterial diseases

Z22.31   Carrier of bacterial disease due to meningococci

☑6ᵗʰ Z22.32   Carrier of bacterial disease due to staphylococci

Z22.321   Carrier or suspected carrier of Methicillin susceptible Staphylococcus aureus
> MSSA colonization

Z22.322   Carrier or suspected carrier of Methicillin resistant Staphylococcus aureus
> MRSA colonization

☑6ᵗʰ Z22.33   Carrier of bacterial disease due to streptococci

Z22.330   Carrier of Group B streptococcus
> EXCLUDES 1   carrier of streptococcus group B (GBS) complicating pregnancy, childbirth and the puerperium (O99.82-)

Z22.338   Carrier of other streptococcus

Z22.39   Carrier of other specified bacterial diseases

Z22.4   Carrier of infections with a predominantly sexual mode of transmission

Z22.6   Carrier of human T-lymphotropic virus type-1 [HTLV-1] infection

Z22.8   Carrier of other infectious diseases

Z22.9   Carrier of infectious disease, unspecified

Z23   Encounter for immunization
> Code first any routine childhood examination
> NOTE   Procedure codes are required to identify the types of immunizations given

☑4ᵗʰ Z28   Immunization not carried out and underimmunization status
> INCLUDES   vaccination not carried out

☑5ᵗʰ Z28.0   Immunization not carried out because of contraindication

Z28.01   Immunization not carried out because of acute illness of patient

Z28.02   Immunization not carried out because of chronic illness or condition of patient

Z28.03   Immunization not carried out because of immune compromised state of patient

Z28.04   Immunization not carried out because of patient allergy to vaccine or component

Z28.09   Immunization not carried out because of other contraindication

Z28.1   Immunization not carried out because of patient decision for reasons of belief or group pressure
> Immunization not carried out because of religious belief

☑5ᵗʰ Z28.2   Immunization not carried out because of patient decision for other and unspecified reason

Z28.20   Immunization not carried out because of patient decision for unspecified reason

Z28.21   Immunization not carried out because of patient refusal

Z28.29   Immunization not carried out because of patient decision for other reason

Z28.3   Underimmunization status
> Delinquent immunization status
> Lapsed immunization schedule status

☑5ᵗʰ Z28.8   Immunization not carried out for other reason

Z28.81   Immunization not carried out due to patient having had the disease

Z28.82   Immunization not carried out because of caregiver refusal
> Immunization not carried out because of guardian refusal
> Immunization not carried out because of parent refusal
> EXCLUDES 1   immunization not carried out because of caregiver refusal because of religious belief (Z28.1)

Z28.89   Immunization not carried out for other reason

Z28.9   Immunization not carried out for unspecified reason

☑4ᵗʰ Z29   Encounter for other prophylactic measures
> EXCLUDES 1   desensitization to allergens (Z51.6)
> prophylactic surgery (Z40.-)

☑5ᵗʰ Z29.1   Encounter for prophylactic immunotherapy
> Encounter for administration of immunoglobulin

Z29.11   Encounter for prophylactic immunotherapy for respiratory syncytial virus (RSV)

---

⁴   Questionable admission when used as PDx.

☑ Additional Character Req   ☑x7ᵗʰ Placeholder Alert   Unacceptable PDx   Manifestation   **H1 - H14** HAC   **HCC** CMS-HCC Condition   *EXCLUDES 1* Not Coded Here   *EXCLUDES 2* Not Included Here

Z29.12   **Encounter for prophylactic antivenin**

Z29.13   **Encounter for prophylactic Rho(D) immune globulin**

Z29.14   **Encounter for prophylactic rabies immune globin**

Z29.3   **Encounter for prophylactic fluoride administration**

Z29.8   **Encounter for other specified prophylactic measures**

Z29.9   **Encounter for prophylactic measures, unspecified**

Persons encountering health services in circumstances related to reproduction (Z30-Z39)

√4th **Z30**   **Encounter for contraceptive management**
>DEF: Contraceptive management to prevent pregnancy; methods include oral medications, intrauterine devices, and surgical procedures for males and females (sterilization).

√5th   **Z30.0**   **Encounter for general counseling and advice on contraception**

√6th   **Z30.01**   **Encounter for initial prescription of contraceptives**
>EXCLUDES 1   encounter for surveillance of contraceptives (Z30.4-)

Z30.011   **Encounter for initial prescription of contraceptive pills** ♀

Z30.012   **Encounter for prescription of emergency contraception** ♀
>Encounter for postcoital contraception

Z30.013   **Encounter for initial prescription of injectable contraceptive** ♀

Z30.014   **Encounter for initial prescription of intrauterine contraceptive device** ♀
>EXCLUDES 1   encounter for insertion of intrauterine contraceptive device (Z30.430, Z30.432)

Z30.015   **Encounter for initial prescription of vaginal ring hormonal contraceptive**

Z30.016   **Encounter for initial prescription of transdermal patch hormonal contraceptive device**

Z30.017   **Encounter for initial prescription of implantable subdermal contraceptive**

Z30.018   **Encounter for initial prescription of other contraceptives** ♀
>Encounter for initial prescription of barrier contraception
>Encounter for initial prescription of diaphragm

Z30.019   **Encounter for initial prescription of contraceptives, unspecified** ♀

Z30.02   **Counseling and instruction in natural family planning to avoid pregnancy**

Z30.09   **Encounter for other general counseling and advice on contraception**
>Encounter for family planning advice NOS

Z30.2   **Encounter for sterilization**

√5th   **Z30.4**   **Encounter for surveillance of contraceptives**

Z30.40   **Encounter for surveillance of contraceptives, unspecified**

Z30.41   **Encounter for surveillance of contraceptive pills** ♀
>Encounter for repeat prescription for contraceptive pill

Z30.42   **Encounter for surveillance of injectable contraceptive** ♀

√6th   **Z30.43**   **Encounter for surveillance of intrauterine contraceptive device**

Z30.430   **Encounter for insertion of intrauterine contraceptive device** ♀

Z30.431   **Encounter for routine checking of intrauterine contraceptive device** ♀

Z30.432   **Encounter for removal of intrauterine contraceptive device** ♀

Z30.433   **Encounter for removal and reinsertion of intrauterine contraceptive device** ♀
>Encounter for replacement of intrauterine contraceptive device

Z30.44   **Encounter for surveillance of vaginal ring hormonal contraceptive device** ♀

Z30.45   **Encounter for surveillance of transdermal patch hormonal contraceptive device** ♀

Z30.46   **Encounter for surveillance of implantable subdermal contraceptive** ♀
>Encounter for checking, reinsertion or removal of implantable subdermal contraceptive

Z30.49   **Encounter for surveillance of other contraceptives** ♀
>Encounter for surveillance of barrier contraception
>Encounter for surveillance of diaphragm

Z30.8   **Encounter for other contraceptive management**
>Encounter for postvasectomy sperm count
>Encounter for routine examination for contraceptive maintenance
>>EXCLUDES 1   sperm count following sterilization reversal (Z31.42)
>>sperm count for fertility testing (Z31.41)

Z30.9   **Encounter for contraceptive management, unspecified**

√4th **Z31**   **Encounter for procreative management**
>EXCLUDES 1   complications associated with artificial fertilization (N98.-)
>female infertility (N97.-)
>male infertility (N46.-)

Z31.0   **Encounter for reversal of previous sterilization**

√5th   **Z31.4**   **Encounter for procreative investigation and testing**
>EXCLUDES 1   postvasectomy sperm count (Z30.8)

Z31.41   **Encounter for fertility testing**
>Encounter for fallopian tube patency testing
>Encounter for sperm count for fertility testing

Z31.42   **Aftercare following sterilization reversal**
>Sperm count following sterilization reversal

√6th   **Z31.43**   **Encounter for genetic testing of female for procreative management**
>Use additional code for recurrent pregnancy loss, if applicable (N96, O26.2-)
>>EXCLUDES 1   nonprocreative genetic testing (Z13.7-)

Z31.430   **Encounter of female for testing for genetic disease carrier status for procreative management** ♀

Z31.438   **Encounter for other genetic testing of female for procreative management** ♀

√6th   **Z31.44**   **Encounter for genetic testing of male for procreative management**
>EXCLUDES 1   nonprocreative genetic testing (Z13.7-)

Z31.440   **Encounter of male for testing for genetic disease carrier status for procreative management** ♂

Z31.441   **Encounter for testing of male partner of patient with recurrent pregnancy loss** A♂

Z31.448   **Encounter for other genetic testing of male for procreative management** A♂

Z31.49   **Encounter for other procreative investigation and testing**

▲   **Z31.5**   **Encounter for procreative genetic counseling**

√5th   **Z31.6**   **Encounter for general counseling and advice on procreation**

Z31.61   **Procreative counseling and advice using natural family planning**

Z31.62   **Encounter for fertility preservation counseling**
>Encounter for fertility preservation counseling prior to cancer therapy
>Encounter for fertility preservation counseling prior to surgical removal of gonads

Z31.69   **Encounter for other general counseling and advice on procreation**

Z31.7   **Encounter for procreative management and counseling for gestational carrier**
>EXCLUDES 1   pregnant state, gestational carrier (Z33.3)

√5th   **Z31.8**   **Encounter for other procreative management**

Z31.81   **Encounter for male factor infertility in female patient** ♀

Z31.82   **Encounter for Rh incompatibility status** ♀
>AHA: 2015, 3Q, 40; 2014, 4Q, 17

Z31.83   **Encounter for assisted reproductive fertility procedure cycle** ♀
>Patient undergoing in vitro fertilization cycle
>Use additional code to identify the type of infertility
>>EXCLUDES 1   pre-cycle diagnosis and testing—code to reason for encounter

Z31.84   **Encounter for fertility preservation procedure**
>Encounter for fertility preservation procedure prior to cancer therapy
>Encounter for fertility preservation procedure prior to surgical removal of gonads

Z31.89   **Encounter for other procreative management**

Z31.9   **Encounter for procreative management, unspecified**

N Newborn: 0   P Pediatric: 0-17   M Maternity: 12-55   A Adult: 15-124   MCC Major CC Condition   PDxMCC PDx acts as own MCC   CC CC Condition   PDxCC PDx acts as own CC

1228   ICD-10-CM 2018

✓4ᵗʰ **Z32 Encounter for pregnancy test and childbirth and childcare instruction**

  ✓5ᵗʰ **Z32.0 Encounter for** pregnancy test

    Z32.00 Encounter for pregnancy test, result unknown ♀
      Encounter for pregnancy test NOS

    Z32.01 Encounter for pregnancy test, result positive Ⓜ♀

    Z32.02 Encounter for pregnancy test, result negative ♀

  Z32.2 Encounter for childbirth instruction

  Z32.3 Encounter for childcare instruction
    Encounter for prenatal or postpartum childcare instruction

✓4ᵗʰ **Z33 Pregnant state**

  Z33.1 Pregnant state, incidental Ⓜ♀
    Pregnant state NOS
    EXCLUDES 1   complications of pregnancy (O00-O9A)
           pregnant state, gestational carrier (Z33.3)

  Z33.2 Encounter for elective termination of pregnancy Ⓜ♀
    EXCLUDES 1   early fetal death with retention of dead fetus (O02.1)
           late fetal death (O36.4)
           spontaneous abortion (O03)

  Z33.3 Pregnant state, gestational carrier Ⓜ♀
    EXCLUDES 1   encounter for procreative management and
           counseling for gestational carrier (Z31.7)

✓4ᵗʰ **Z34 Encounter for supervision of normal pregnancy**
  EXCLUDES 1   any complication of pregnancy (O00-O9A)
           encounter for pregnancy test (Z32.0-)
           encounter for supervision of high risk pregnancy (O09.-)
  AHA: 2014, 4Q, 17

  ✓5ᵗʰ **Z34.0 Encounter for supervision of normal** first **pregnancy**

    Z34.00 Encounter for supervision of normal first pregnancy, unspecified **trimester** Ⓜ♀

    Z34.01 Encounter for supervision of normal first pregnancy, first **trimester** Ⓜ♀

    Z34.02 Encounter for supervision of normal first pregnancy, second **trimester** Ⓜ♀

    Z34.03 Encounter for supervision of normal first pregnancy, third **trimester** Ⓜ♀

  ✓5ᵗʰ **Z34.8 Encounter for supervision of** other **normal pregnancy**

    Z34.80 Encounter for supervision of other normal pregnancy, unspecified **trimester** Ⓜ♀

    Z34.81 Encounter for supervision of other normal pregnancy, first **trimester** Ⓜ♀

    Z34.82 Encounter for supervision of other normal pregnancy, second **trimester** Ⓜ♀

    Z34.83 Encounter for supervision of other normal pregnancy, third **trimester** Ⓜ♀

  ✓5ᵗʰ **Z34.9 Encounter for supervision of normal pregnancy,** unspecified

    Z34.90 Encounter for supervision of normal pregnancy, unspecified, unspecified **trimester** Ⓜ♀

    Z34.91 Encounter for supervision of normal pregnancy, unspecified, first **trimester** Ⓜ♀

    Z34.92 Encounter for supervision of normal pregnancy, unspecified, second **trimester** Ⓜ♀

    Z34.93 Encounter for supervision of normal pregnancy, unspecified, third **trimester** Ⓜ♀

✓4ᵗʰ **Z36 Encounter for** antenatal screening **of mother**
  INCLUDES ▶encounter for placental sample (taken vaginally)
     screening is the testing for disease or disease precursors in
     asymptomatic individuals so that early detection and
     treatment can be provided for those who test positive
     for the disease◀
  EXCLUDES 1 abnormal findings on antenatal screening of mother (O28.-)
     diagnostic examination—code to sign or symptom
     encounter for suspected maternal and fetal conditions ruled out
         (Z03.7-)
     suspected fetal condition affecting management of
         pregnancy—code to condition in Chapter 15
  EXCLUDES 2 ▶abnormal findings on antenatal screening of mother (O28.-)◀
     genetic counseling and testing (Z31.43-, Z31.5)
     routine prenatal care (Z34)

 ● **Z36.0 Encounter for antenatal screening for** chromosomal anomalies

 ● **Z36.1 Encounter for antenatal screening for** raised alphafetoprotein level
    Encounter for antenatal screening for elevated maternal serum alphafetoprotein level

 ● **Z36.2 Encounter for other antenatal screening follow-up**
    Non-visualized anatomy on a previous scan

 ● **Z36.3 Encounter for antenatal screening for** malformations
    Screening for a suspected anomaly

 ● **Z36.4 Encounter for antenatal screening for** fetal growth retardation
    Intrauterine growth restriction (IUGR)/small-for-dates

 ● **Z36.5 Encounter for antenatal screening for** isoimmunization

 ● ✓5ᵗʰ **Z36.8 Encounter for other antenatal screening**

 ● **Z36.81 Encounter for antenatal screening for** hydrops fetalis

 ● **Z36.82 Encounter for antenatal screening for** nuchal translucency

 ● **Z36.83 Encounter for fetal screening for** congenital cardiac abnormalities

 ● **Z36.84 Encounter for antenatal screening for** fetal lung maturity

 ● **Z36.85 Encounter for antenatal screening for** Streptococcus B

 ● **Z36.86 Encounter for antenatal screening for** cervical length
    Screening for risk of pre-term labor

 ● **Z36.87 Encounter for antenatal screening for** uncertain dates

 ● **Z36.88 Encounter for antenatal screening for** fetal macrosomia
    Screening for large-for-dates

 ● **Z36.89 Encounter for other specified antenatal screening**

 ● **Z36.8A Encounter for antenatal screening for other** genetic defects

 ● **Z36.9 Encounter for antenatal screening,** unspecified

✓4ᵗʰ **Z3A Weeks of gestation**
  NOTE   Codes from category Z3A are for use, only on the maternal
     record, to indicate the weeks of gestation of the pregnancy, if
     known.
  Code first complications of pregnancy, childbirth and the puerperium
     ▶(O00-O9A)◀
  AHA: 2016, 2Q, 34; 2014, 3Q, 17; 2014, 2Q, 9; 2013, 2Q, 33

  ✓5ᵗʰ **Z3A.0 Weeks of gestation of pregnancy,** unspecified or less than 10 weeks

    Z3A.00 Weeks of gestation of pregnancy not specified Ⓜ♀
    Z3A.01 Less than 8 weeks gestation of pregnancy Ⓜ♀
    Z3A.08 8 weeks gestation of pregnancy Ⓜ♀
    Z3A.09 9 weeks gestation of pregnancy Ⓜ♀

  ✓5ᵗʰ **Z3A.1 Weeks of gestation of pregnancy, weeks** 10-19

    Z3A.10 10 weeks gestation of pregnancy Ⓜ♀
    Z3A.11 11 weeks gestation of pregnancy Ⓜ♀
    Z3A.12 12 weeks gestation of pregnancy Ⓜ♀
    Z3A.13 13 weeks gestation of pregnancy Ⓜ♀
    Z3A.14 14 weeks gestation of pregnancy Ⓜ♀
    Z3A.15 15 weeks gestation of pregnancy Ⓜ♀
    Z3A.16 16 weeks gestation of pregnancy Ⓜ♀
    Z3A.17 17 weeks gestation of pregnancy Ⓜ♀
    Z3A.18 18 weeks gestation of pregnancy Ⓜ♀
    Z3A.19 19 weeks gestation of pregnancy Ⓜ♀

  ✓5ᵗʰ **Z3A.2 Weeks of gestation of pregnancy, weeks** 20-29

    Z3A.20 20 weeks gestation of pregnancy Ⓜ♀
    Z3A.21 21 weeks gestation of pregnancy Ⓜ♀
    Z3A.22 22 weeks gestation of pregnancy Ⓜ♀
    Z3A.23 23 weeks gestation of pregnancy Ⓜ♀
    Z3A.24 24 weeks gestation of pregnancy Ⓜ♀
    Z3A.25 25 weeks gestation of pregnancy Ⓜ♀
    Z3A.26 26 weeks gestation of pregnancy Ⓜ♀
    Z3A.27 27 weeks gestation of pregnancy Ⓜ♀
    Z3A.28 28 weeks gestation of pregnancy Ⓜ♀
    Z3A.29 29 weeks gestation of pregnancy Ⓜ♀

  ✓5ᵗʰ **Z3A.3 Weeks of gestation of pregnancy, weeks** 30-39

    Z3A.30 30 weeks gestation of pregnancy Ⓜ♀
    Z3A.31 31 weeks gestation of pregnancy Ⓜ♀
    Z3A.32 32 weeks gestation of pregnancy Ⓜ♀
    Z3A.33 33 weeks gestation of pregnancy Ⓜ♀
    Z3A.34 34 weeks gestation of pregnancy Ⓜ♀
    Z3A.35 35 weeks gestation of pregnancy Ⓜ♀
    Z3A.36 36 weeks gestation of pregnancy Ⓜ♀
    Z3A.37 37 weeks gestation of pregnancy Ⓜ♀

✓ Additional Character Req   ✓x7ᵗʰ Placeholder Alert   Unacceptable PDx   Manifestation   H1-H14 HAC   HCC CMS-HCC Condition   EXCLUDES 1 Not Coded Here   EXCLUDES 2 Not Included Here

Z3A.38 **38 weeks** gestation of pregnancy Ⓜ♀
Z3A.39 **39 weeks** gestation of pregnancy Ⓜ♀

✓5ᵗʰ **Z3A.4 Weeks of gestation of pregnancy, weeks 40 or greater**
AHA: 2014, 4Q, 23

Z3A.40 **40 weeks** gestation of pregnancy Ⓜ♀
Z3A.41 **41 weeks** gestation of pregnancy Ⓜ♀
Z3A.42 **42 weeks** gestation of pregnancy Ⓜ♀
Z3A.49 **Greater than 42 weeks** gestation of pregnancy Ⓜ♀

✓4ᵗʰ **Z37 Outcome of delivery**
This category is intended for use as an additional code to identify the outcome of delivery on the mother's record. It is not for use on the newborn record.
EXCLUDES 1   stillbirth (P95)

Z37.0 **Single live birth** Ⓜ♀
AHA: 2016, 2Q, 34; 2014, 2Q, 9
Z37.1 **Single stillbirth** Ⓜ♀
Z37.2 **Twins, both liveborn** Ⓜ♀
Z37.3 **Twins, one liveborn and one stillborn** Ⓜ♀
Z37.4 **Twins, both stillborn** Ⓜ♀

✓5ᵗʰ **Z37.5 Other multiple births, all liveborn**
Z37.50 **Multiple births, unspecified, all liveborn** Ⓜ♀
Z37.51 **Triplets, all liveborn** Ⓜ♀
Z37.52 **Quadruplets, all liveborn** Ⓜ♀
Z37.53 **Quintuplets, all liveborn** Ⓜ♀
Z37.54 **Sextuplets, all liveborn** Ⓜ♀
Z37.59 **Other multiple births, all liveborn** Ⓜ♀

✓5ᵗʰ **Z37.6 Other multiple births, some liveborn**
Z37.60 **Multiple births, unspecified, some liveborn** Ⓜ♀
Z37.61 **Triplets, some liveborn** Ⓜ♀
Z37.62 **Quadruplets, some liveborn** Ⓜ♀
Z37.63 **Quintuplets, some liveborn** Ⓜ♀
Z37.64 **Sextuplets, some liveborn** Ⓜ♀
Z37.69 **Other multiple births, some liveborn** Ⓜ♀

Z37.7 **Other multiple births, all stillborn** Ⓜ♀
Z37.9 **Outcome of delivery, unspecified** Ⓜ♀
Multiple birth NOS
Single birth NOS

✓4ᵗʰ **Z38 Liveborn infants according to place of birth and type of delivery**
This category is for use as the principal code on the initial record of a newborn baby. It is to be used for the initial birth record only. It is not to be used on the mother's record.
AHA: 2017, 2Q, 5-7; 2016, 3Q, 18; 2015, 2Q, 15

✓5ᵗʰ **Z38.0 Single liveborn infant, born in hospital**
Single liveborn infant, born in birthing center or other health care facility
Z38.00 **Single liveborn infant, delivered vaginally** Ⓝ
Z38.01 **Single liveborn infant, delivered by cesarean** Ⓝ

Z38.1 **Single liveborn infant, born outside hospital** Ⓝ
Z38.2 **Single liveborn infant, unspecified as to place of birth** Ⓝ
Single liveborn infant NOS

✓5ᵗʰ **Z38.3 Twin liveborn infant, born in hospital**
Z38.30 **Twin liveborn infant, delivered vaginally** Ⓝ
Z38.31 **Twin liveborn infant, delivered by cesarean** Ⓝ

Z38.4 **Twin liveborn infant, born outside hospital** Ⓝ
Z38.5 **Twin liveborn infant, unspecified as to place of birth** Ⓝ

✓5ᵗʰ **Z38.6 Other multiple liveborn infant, born in hospital**
Z38.61 **Triplet liveborn infant, delivered vaginally** Ⓝ
Z38.62 **Triplet liveborn infant, delivered by cesarean** Ⓝ
Z38.63 **Quadruplet liveborn infant, delivered vaginally** Ⓝ
Z38.64 **Quadruplet liveborn infant, delivered by cesarean** Ⓝ
Z38.65 **Quintuplet liveborn infant, delivered vaginally** Ⓝ
Z38.66 **Quintuplet liveborn infant, delivered by cesarean** Ⓝ
Z38.68 **Other multiple liveborn infant, delivered vaginally** Ⓝ
Z38.69 **Other multiple liveborn infant, delivered by cesarean** Ⓝ

Z38.7 **Other multiple liveborn infant, born outside hospital** Ⓝ
Z38.8 **Other multiple liveborn infant, unspecified as to place of birth** Ⓝ

✓4ᵗʰ **Z39 Encounter for maternal postpartum care and examination**

Z39.0 **Encounter for care and examination of mother immediately after delivery** Ⓜ♀
Care and observation in uncomplicated cases when the delivery occurs outside a healthcare facility
EXCLUDES 1   care for postpartum complication—see Alphabetic index

Z39.1 **Encounter for care and examination of lactating mother** Ⓜ♀
Encounter for supervision of lactation
EXCLUDES 1   disorders of lactation (O92.-)

Z39.2 **Encounter for routine postpartum follow-up** Ⓜ♀

Encounters for other specific health care (Z40-Z53)

Categories Z40-Z53 are intended for use to indicate a reason for care. They may be used for patients who have already been treated for a disease or injury, but who are receiving aftercare or prophylactic care, or care to consolidate the treatment, or to deal with a residual state.
EXCLUDES 2   follow-up examination for medical surveillance after treatment (Z08-Z09)

✓4ᵗʰ **Z40 Encounter for prophylactic surgery**
EXCLUDES 1   organ donations (Z52.-)
therapeutic organ removal—code to condition

✓5ᵗʰ **Z40.0 Encounter for prophylactic surgery for risk factors related to malignant neoplasms**
Admission for prophylactic organ removal
Use additional code to identify risk factor
Z40.00 **Encounter for prophylactic removal of unspecified organ**
Z40.01 **Encounter for prophylactic removal of breast**
▲ Z40.02 **Encounter for prophylactic removal of ovary(s)** ♀
▶Encounter for prophylactic removal of ovary(s) and fallopian tube(s)◀
● Z40.03 **Encounter for prophylactic removal of fallopian tube(s)** ♀
Z40.09 **Encounter for prophylactic removal of other organ**

Z40.8 **Encounter for other prophylactic surgery**
Z40.9 **Encounter for prophylactic surgery, unspecified**

✓4ᵗʰ **Z41 Encounter for procedures for purposes other than remedying health state**

Z41.1 **Encounter for cosmetic surgery**
Encounter for cosmetic breast implant
Encounter for cosmetic procedure
EXCLUDES 1   encounter for plastic and reconstructive surgery following medical procedure or healed injury (Z42.-)
encounter for post-mastectomy breast implantation (Z42.1)

Z41.2 **Encounter for routine and ritual male circumcision** ♂
Z41.3 **Encounter for ear piercing**
Z41.8 **Encounter for other procedures for purposes other than remedying health state**
Z41.9 **Encounter for procedure for purposes other than remedying health state, unspecified**

✓4ᵗʰ **Z42 Encounter for plastic and reconstructive surgery following medical procedure or healed injury**
EXCLUDES 1   encounter for cosmetic plastic surgery (Z41.1)
encounter for plastic surgery for treatment of current injury—code to relevant injury

Z42.1 **Encounter for breast reconstruction following mastectomy** Ⓐ
EXCLUDES 1   deformity and disproportion of reconstructed breast (N65.1-)

Z42.8 **Encounter for other plastic and reconstructive surgery following medical procedure or healed injury**
AHA: 2017, 1Q, 42

✓4ᵗʰ **Z43 Encounter for attention to artificial openings**
INCLUDES   closure of artificial openings
passage of sounds or bougies through artificial openings
reforming artificial openings
removal of catheter from artificial openings
toilet or cleansing of artificial openings
EXCLUDES 1   artificial opening status only, without need for care (Z93.-)
complications of external stoma (J95.0-, K94.-, N99.5-)
EXCLUDES 2   fitting and adjustment of prosthetic and other devices (Z44-Z46)

Z43.0 **Encounter for attention to tracheostomy** HCC

Z43.1   **Encounter for attention to** gastrostomy   `CC` `HCC`

> `EXCLUDES 2` ▶*artificial opening status only, without need for care (Z93.-)*◀
>
> **CC Excl:** PDX collection 1487

Z43.2   **Encounter for attention to** ileostomy   `HCC`

Z43.3   **Encounter for attention to** colostomy   `HCC`

Z43.4   **Encounter for attention to other artificial** openings of digestive tract   `HCC`

Z43.5   **Encounter for attention to** cystostomy   `HCC`

Z43.6   **Encounter for attention to other artificial** openings of urinary tract   `HCC`

> Encounter for attention to nephrostomy
> Encounter for attention to ureterostomy
> Encounter for attention to urethrostomy

Z43.7   **Encounter for attention to artificial** vagina

Z43.8   **Encounter for attention to other artificial openings**   `HCC`

Z43.9   **Encounter for attention to** unspecified **artificial opening**   `HCC`

`✓4ᵗʰ` **Z44**   **Encounter for fitting and adjustment of external prosthetic device**

> `INCLUDES` removal or replacement of external prosthetic device
> `EXCLUDES 1` *malfunction or other complications of device—see Alphabetical Index*
> *presence of prosthetic device (Z97.-)*

`✓5ᵗʰ` **Z44.0**   **Encounter for fitting and adjustment of** artificial arm

   `✓6ᵗʰ` **Z44.00**   **Encounter for fitting and adjustment of** unspecified **artificial arm**

     Z44.001   **Encounter for fitting and adjustment of unspecified** right **artificial arm**

     Z44.002   **Encounter for fitting and adjustment of unspecified** left **artificial arm**

     Z44.009   **Encounter for fitting and adjustment of unspecified artificial arm,** unspecified **arm**

   `✓6ᵗʰ` **Z44.01**   **Encounter for fitting and adjustment of** complete **artificial arm**

     Z44.011   **Encounter for fitting and adjustment of complete** right **artificial arm**

     Z44.012   **Encounter for fitting and adjustment of complete** left **artificial arm**

     Z44.019   **Encounter for fitting and adjustment of complete artificial arm,** unspecified **arm**

   `✓6ᵗʰ` **Z44.02**   **Encounter for fitting and adjustment of** partial **artificial arm**

     Z44.021   **Encounter for fitting and adjustment of partial artificial** right **arm**

     Z44.022   **Encounter for fitting and adjustment of partial artificial** left **arm**

     Z44.029   **Encounter for fitting and adjustment of partial artificial arm,** unspecified **arm**

`✓5ᵗʰ` **Z44.1**   **Encounter for fitting and adjustment of** artificial leg

   `✓6ᵗʰ` **Z44.10**   **Encounter for fitting and adjustment of** unspecified **artificial leg**

     Z44.101   **Encounter for fitting and adjustment of unspecified** right **artificial leg**   `HCC`

     Z44.102   **Encounter for fitting and adjustment of unspecified** left **artificial leg**   `HCC`

     Z44.109   **Encounter for fitting and adjustment of unspecified artificial leg,** unspecified **leg**   `HCC`

   `✓6ᵗʰ` **Z44.11**   **Encounter for fitting and adjustment of** complete **artificial leg**

     Z44.111   **Encounter for fitting and adjustment of complete** right **artificial leg**   `HCC`

     Z44.112   **Encounter for fitting and adjustment of complete** left **artificial leg**   `HCC`

     Z44.119   **Encounter for fitting and adjustment of complete artificial leg,** unspecified **leg**   `HCC`

   `✓6ᵗʰ` **Z44.12**   **Encounter for fitting and adjustment of** partial **artificial leg**

     Z44.121   **Encounter for fitting and adjustment of partial artificial** right **leg**   `HCC`

     Z44.122   **Encounter for fitting and adjustment of partial artificial** left **leg**   `HCC`

     Z44.129   **Encounter for fitting and adjustment of partial artificial leg,** unspecified **leg**   `HCC`

`✓5ᵗʰ` **Z44.2**   **Encounter for fitting and adjustment of** artificial eye

> `EXCLUDES 1` *mechanical complication of ocular prosthesis (T85.3)*

   Z44.20   **Encounter for fitting and adjustment of artificial eye,** unspecified

   Z44.21   **Encounter for fitting and adjustment of artificial** right **eye**

   Z44.22   **Encounter for fitting and adjustment of artificial** left **eye**

`✓5ᵗʰ` **Z44.3**   **Encounter for fitting and adjustment of** external breast prosthesis

> `EXCLUDES 1` *complications of breast implant (T85.4-)*
> *encounter for adjustment or removal of breast implant (Z45.81-)*
> *encounter for initial breast implant insertion for cosmetic breast augmentation (Z41.1)*
> *encounter for breast reconstruction following mastectomy (Z42.1)*

   Z44.30   **Encounter for fitting and adjustment of external breast prosthesis,** unspecified **breast**

   Z44.31   **Encounter for fitting and adjustment of external** right **breast prosthesis**

   Z44.32   **Encounter for fitting and adjustment of external** left **breast prosthesis**

Z44.8   **Encounter for fitting and adjustment of** other external prosthetic devices

Z44.9   **Encounter for fitting and adjustment of** unspecified **external prosthetic device**

`✓4ᵗʰ` **Z45**   **Encounter for adjustment and management of implanted device**

> `INCLUDES` removal or replacement of implanted device
> `EXCLUDES 1` *malfunction or other complications of device – see Alphabetical Index*
> ~~*presence of prosthetic and other devices (Z95-Z97)*~~
> `EXCLUDES 2` *encounter for fitting and adjustment of non-implanted device (Z46.-)*

`✓5ᵗʰ` **Z45.0**   **Encounter for adjustment and management of** cardiac device

   `✓6ᵗʰ` **Z45.01**   **Encounter for adjustment and management of cardiac** pacemaker

> Encounter for adjustment and management of cardiac resynchronization therapy pacemaker (CRT-P)
> `EXCLUDES 1` *encounter for adjustment and management of automatic implantable cardiac defibrillator with synchronous cardiac pacemaker (Z45.02)*

     ⁴ **Z45.010**   **Encounter for checking and testing of cardiac pacemaker pulse generator [battery]**

> Encounter for replacing cardiac pacemaker pulse generator [battery]

     ⁴ **Z45.018**   **Encounter for adjustment and management of other part of cardiac pacemaker**

> `EXCLUDES 2` ▶*presence of prosthetic and other devices (Z95-Z97)*◀

   ⁴ **Z45.02**   **Encounter for adjustment and management of automatic implantable cardiac defibrillator**

> Encounter for adjustment and management of automatic implantable cardiac defibrillator with synchronous cardiac pacemaker
> Encounter for adjustment and management of cardiac resynchronization therapy defibrillator (CRT-D)

   ⁴ **Z45.09**   **Encounter for adjustment and management of other cardiac device**

Z45.1   **Encounter for adjustment and management of** infusion pump

Z45.2   **Encounter for adjustment and management of** vascular access device

> Encounter for adjustment and management of vascular catheters
> `EXCLUDES 1` *encounter for adjustment and management of renal dialysis catheter (Z49.01)*

`✓5ᵗʰ` **Z45.3**   **Encounter for adjustment and management of** implanted devices of the special senses

   Z45.31   **Encounter for adjustment and management of implanted** visual **substitution device**

---

⁴   Questionable admission when used as PDx.

☑Additional Character Req   `✓x7ᵗʰ` ▶Placeholder Alert   Unacceptable PDx   Manifestation   `H1`-`H14` HAC   `HCC` CMS-HCC Condition   `EXCLUDES 1` Not Coded Here   `EXCLUDES 2` Not Included Here

ICD-10-CM 2018   **1231**

√6th **Z45.32 Encounter for adjustment and management of implanted hearing device**

EXCLUDES 1 *encounter for fitting and adjustment of hearing aide (Z46.1)*

Z45.320 Encounter for adjustment and management of bone conduction device

Z45.321 Encounter for adjustment and management of cochlear device

Z45.328 Encounter for adjustment and management of other implanted hearing device

√5th **Z45.4 Encounter for adjustment and management of implanted nervous system device**

Z45.41 Encounter for adjustment and management of cerebrospinal fluid drainage device

Encounter for adjustment and management of cerebral ventricular (communicating) shunt

Z45.42 Encounter for adjustment and management of neuropacemaker (brain) (peripheral nerve) (spinal cord)

Z45.49 Encounter for adjustment and management of other implanted nervous system device

AHA: 2014, 3Q, 19

√5th **Z45.8 Encounter for adjustment and management of other implanted devices**

√6th **Z45.81 Encounter for adjustment or removal of breast implant**

Encounter for elective implant exchange (different material) (different size)

Encounter removal of tissue expander without synchronous insertion of permanent implant

EXCLUDES 1 *complications of breast implant (T85.4-)*

encounter for initial breast implant insertion for cosmetic breast augmentation (Z41.1)

encounter for breast reconstruction following mastectomy (Z42.1)

Z45.811 Encounter for adjustment or removal of right breast implant

Z45.812 Encounter for adjustment or removal of left breast implant

Z45.819 Encounter for adjustment or removal of unspecified breast implant

Z45.82 Encounter for adjustment or removal of myringotomy device (stent) (tube)

Z45.89 Encounter for adjustment and management of other implanted devices

AHA: 2014, 4Q, 26-28

Z45.9 Encounter for adjustment and management of unspecified implanted device

√4th **Z46 Encounter for fitting and adjustment of other devices**

INCLUDES removal or replacement of other device

EXCLUDES 1 *malfunction or other complications of device—see Alphabetical Index*

EXCLUDES 2 *encounter for fitting and management of implanted devices (Z45.-)*

issue of repeat prescription only (Z76.0)

presence of prosthetic and other devices (Z95-Z97)

Z46.0 Encounter for fitting and adjustment of spectacles and contact lenses

Z46.1 Encounter for fitting and adjustment of hearing aid

EXCLUDES 1 *encounter for adjustment and management of implanted hearing device (Z45.32-)*

Z46.2 Encounter for fitting and adjustment of other devices related to nervous system and special senses

EXCLUDES 2 *encounter for adjustment and management of implanted nervous system device (Z45.4-)*

encounter for adjustment and management of implanted visual substitution device (Z45.31)

Z46.3 Encounter for fitting and adjustment of dental prosthetic device

Encounter for fitting and adjustment of dentures

Z46.4 Encounter for fitting and adjustment of orthodontic device

√5th **Z46.5 Encounter for fitting and adjustment of other gastrointestinal appliance and device**

EXCLUDES 1 *encounter for attention to artificial openings of digestive tract (Z43.1-Z43.4)*

Z46.51 Encounter for fitting and adjustment of gastric lap band

Z46.59 Encounter for fitting and adjustment of other gastrointestinal appliance and device

Z46.6 Encounter for fitting and adjustment of urinary device

EXCLUDES 2 *attention to artificial openings of urinary tract (Z43.5, Z43.6)*

√5th **Z46.8 Encounter for fitting and adjustment of other specified devices**

Z46.81 Encounter for fitting and adjustment of insulin pump

Encounter for insulin pump instruction and training

Encounter for insulin pump titration

Z46.82 Encounter for fitting and adjustment of non-vascular catheter

Z46.89 Encounter for fitting and adjustment of other specified devices

Encounter for fitting and adjustment of wheelchair

AHA: 2014, 4Q, 26-28

Z46.9 Encounter for fitting and adjustment of unspecified device

√4th **Z47 Orthopedic aftercare**

EXCLUDES 1 *aftercare for healing fracture—code to fracture with 7th character D*

Z47.1 Aftercare following joint replacement surgery

Use additional code to identify the joint (Z96.6-)

Z47.2 Encounter for removal of internal fixation device

EXCLUDES 1 *encounter for adjustment of internal fixation device for fracture treatment—code to fracture with appropriate 7th character*

encounter for removal of external fixation device—code to fracture with 7th character D

infection or inflammatory reaction to internal fixation device (T84.6-)

mechanical complication of internal fixation device (T84.1-)

√5th **Z47.3 Aftercare following explanation of joint prosthesis**

Aftercare following explanation of joint prosthesis, staged procedure

Encounter for joint prosthesis insertion following prior explanation of joint prosthesis

AHA: 2015, 1Q, 16

Z47.31 Aftercare following explanation of shoulder joint prosthesis

EXCLUDES 1 *acquired absence of shoulder joint following prior explanation of shoulder joint prosthesis (Z89.23-)*

shoulder joint prosthesis explanation status (Z89.23-)

Z47.32 Aftercare following explanation of hip joint prosthesis

EXCLUDES 1 *acquired absence of hip joint following prior explanation of hip joint prosthesis (Z89.62-)*

hip joint prosthesis explanation status (Z89.62-)

Z47.33 Aftercare following explanation of knee joint prosthesis

EXCLUDES 1 *acquired absence of knee joint following prior explanation of knee prosthesis (Z89.52-)*

knee joint prosthesis explanation status (Z89.52-)

√5th **Z47.8 Encounter for other orthopedic aftercare**

Z47.81 Encounter for orthopedic aftercare following surgical amputation

Use additional code to identify the limb amputated (Z89.-)

Z47.82 Encounter for orthopedic aftercare following scoliosis surgery

Z47.89 Encounter for other orthopedic aftercare

AHA: 2015, 1Q, 8

N Newborn: 0   P Pediatric: 0-17   M Maternity: 12-55   A Adult: 15-124   MCC Major CC Condition   PDx MCC PDx acts as own MCC   CC CC Condition   PDx CC PDx acts as own CC

1232   ICD-10-CM 2018

Chapter 21. Factors Influencing Health Status and Contact with Health Services

✓4ᵗʰ Z48 Encounter for other postprocedural aftercare

> *EXCLUDES 1* ►*encounter for aftercare following injury – code to Injury, by site, with appropriate 7th character for subsequent encounter*◄
> *encounter for follow-up examination after completed treatment (Z08-Z09)*
>
> *EXCLUDES 2* *encounter for attention to artificial openings (Z43.-)*
> *encounter for fitting and adjustment of prosthetic and other devices (Z44-Z46)*
>
> **AHA:** 2015, 4Q, 38; 2015, 1Q, 6-7

✓5ᵗʰ Z48.0 Encounter for attention to dressings, sutures and drains

> *EXCLUDES 1* *encounter for planned postprocedural wound closure (Z48.1)*

  Z48.00 Encounter for change or removal of nonsurgical wound dressing
Encounter for change or removal of wound dressing NOS

  Z48.01 Encounter for change or removal of surgical wound dressing

  Z48.02 Encounter for removal of sutures
Encounter for removal of staples

  Z48.03 Encounter for change or removal of drains

Z48.1 Encounter for planned postprocedural wound closure

> *EXCLUDES 1* *encounter for attention to dressings and sutures (Z48.0-)*

✓5ᵗʰ Z48.2 Encounter for aftercare following organ transplant

  Z48.21 Encounter for aftercare following heart transplant PDxCC CC HCC
CC Excl: PDX collection 1488

  Z48.22 Encounter for aftercare following kidney transplant PDxCC CC
CC Excl: PDX collection 1489

  Z48.23 Encounter for aftercare following liver transplant PDxCC CC HCC
CC Excl: PDX collection 1490

  Z48.24 Encounter for aftercare following lung transplant PDxCC CC HCC
CC Excl: PDX collection 1491

  ✓6ᵗʰ Z48.28 Encounter for aftercare following multiple organ transplant

    Z48.280 Encounter for aftercare following heart-lung transplant PDxCC CC HCC
CC Excl: PDX collection 1488

    Z48.288 Encounter for aftercare following multiple organ transplant

  ✓6ᵗʰ Z48.29 Encounter for aftercare following other organ transplant

    Z48.290 Encounter for aftercare following bone marrow transplant PDxCC CC HCC
CC Excl: PDX collection 1492

    Z48.298 Encounter for aftercare following other organ transplant

Z48.3 Aftercare following surgery for neoplasm
Use additional code to identify the neoplasm

✓5ᵗʰ Z48.8 Encounter for other specified postprocedural aftercare

  ✓6ᵗʰ Z48.81 Encounter for surgical aftercare following surgery on specified body systems

> **NOTE** These codes identify the body system requiring aftercare. They are for use in conjunction with other aftercare codes to fully explain the aftercare encounter. The condition treated should also be coded if still present.
>
> *EXCLUDES 1* *aftercare for injury—code the injury with 7th character D*
> *aftercare following surgery for neoplasm (Z48.3)*
>
> *EXCLUDES 2* *aftercare following organ transplant (Z48.2-)*
> *orthopedic aftercare (Z47.-)*
>
> **AHA:** 2015, 4Q, 38

    Z48.810 Encounter for surgical aftercare following surgery on the sense organs

    Z48.811 Encounter for surgical aftercare following surgery on the nervous system

> *EXCLUDES 2* *encounter for surgical aftercare following surgery on the sense organs (Z48.810)*

    Z48.812 Encounter for surgical aftercare following surgery on the circulatory system
AHA: 2012, 4Q, 96

    Z48.813 Encounter for surgical aftercare following surgery on the respiratory system

    Z48.814 Encounter for surgical aftercare following surgery on the teeth or oral cavity

    Z48.815 Encounter for surgical aftercare following surgery on the digestive system

    Z48.816 Encounter for surgical aftercare following surgery on the genitourinary system

> *EXCLUDES 1* *encounter for aftercare following sterilization reversal (Z31.42)*

    Z48.817 Encounter for surgical aftercare following surgery on the skin and subcutaneous tissue

  Z48.89 Encounter for other specified surgical aftercare

✓4ᵗʰ Z49 Encounter for care involving renal dialysis

Code also associated end stage renal disease (N18.6)

✓5ᵗʰ Z49.0 Preparatory care for renal dialysis
Encounter for dialysis instruction and training

  Z49.01 Encounter for fitting and adjustment of extracorporeal dialysis catheter HCC
Removal or replacement of renal dialysis catheter
Toilet or cleansing of renal dialysis catheter

  Z49.02 Encounter for fitting and adjustment of peritoneal dialysis catheter HCC

✓5ᵗʰ Z49.3 Encounter for adequacy testing for dialysis

  Z49.31 Encounter for adequacy testing for hemodialysis HCC

  Z49.32 Encounter for adequacy testing for peritoneal dialysis HCC
Encounter for peritoneal equilibration test

✓4ᵗʰ Z51 Encounter for other aftercare and medical care

Code also condition requiring care

> *EXCLUDES 1* *follow-up examination after treatment (Z08-Z09)*

Z51.0 Encounter for antineoplastic radiation therapy

✓5ᵗʰ Z51.1 Encounter for antineoplastic chemotherapy and immunotherapy

> *EXCLUDES 2* *encounter for chemotherapy and immunotherapy for nonneoplastic condition—code to condition*

  Z51.11 Encounter for antineoplastic chemotherapy
AHA: 2015, 3Q, 19

  Z51.12 Encounter for antineoplastic immunotherapy

Z51.5 Encounter for palliative care
AHA: 2017, 1Q, 48

Z51.6 Encounter for desensitization to allergens

✓5ᵗʰ Z51.8 Encounter for other specified aftercare

> *EXCLUDES 1* *holiday relief care (Z75.5)*

  Z51.81 Encounter for therapeutic drug level monitoring
Code also any long-term (current) drug therapy (Z79.-)

> *EXCLUDES 1* *encounter for blood-drug test for administrative or medicolegal reasons (Z02.83)*

> **DEF:** Drug monitoring: Measurement of the level of a specific medication in the body or measurement of a specific function to assess effectiveness of a drug.

  ⁵ **Z51.89 Encounter for other specified aftercare**
AHA: 2012, 4Q, 95-97

✓4ᵗʰ Z52 Donors of organs and tissues

> **INCLUDES** autologous and other living donors
>
> *EXCLUDES 1* *cadaveric donor—omit code*
> *examination of potential donor (Z00.5)*
>
> **AHA:** 2012, 4Q, 99

✓5ᵗʰ Z52.0 Blood donor

  ✓6ᵗʰ Z52.00 Unspecified blood donor

    Z52.000 Unspecified donor, whole blood

    Z52.001 Unspecified donor, stem cells

    Z52.008 Unspecified donor, other blood

  ✓6ᵗʰ Z52.01 Autologous blood donor

    Z52.010 Autologous donor, whole blood

    Z52.011 Autologous donor, stem cells

    Z52.018 Autologous donor, other blood

  ✓6ᵗʰ Z52.09 Other blood donor
Volunteer donor

    Z52.090 Other blood donor, whole blood

    Z52.091 Other blood donor, stem cells

    Z52.098 Other blood donor, other blood

---

⁵ Unacceptable PDx unless a secondary diagnosis is present.

✓ Additional Character Req   vx7ᵗʰ Placeholder Alert   Unacceptable PDx   Manifestation   **H1**-**H14** HAC   **HCC** CMS-HCC Condition   *EXCLUDES 1* Not Coded Here   *EXCLUDES 2* Not Included Here

Chapter 21. Factors Influencing Health Status and Contact with Health Services

☑5ᵗʰ **Z52.1** Skin donor

Z52.10 Skin donor, unspecified

Z52.11 Skin donor, autologous

Z52.19 Skin donor, other

☑5ᵗʰ **Z52.2** Bone donor

Z52.20 Bone donor, unspecified

Z52.21 Bone donor, autologous

Z52.29 Bone donor, other

Z52.3 Bone marrow donor

Z52.4 Kidney donor

Z52.5 Cornea donor

Z52.6 Liver donor

☑5ᵗʰ **Z52.8** Donor of other specified organs or tissues

☑6ᵗʰ **Z52.81** Egg (Oocyte) donor

Z52.810 Egg (Oocyte) donor under age 35, anonymous recipient   ♀
Egg donor under age 35 NOS

Z52.811 Egg (Oocyte) donor under age 35, designated recipient   ♀

Z52.812 Egg (Oocyte) donor age 35 and over, anonymous recipient   ♀
Egg donor age 35 and over NOS

Z52.813 Egg (Oocyte) donor age 35 and over, designated recipient   ♀

Z52.819 Egg (Oocyte) donor, unspecified   ♀

Z52.89 Donor of other specified organs or tissues

Z52.9 Donor of unspecified organ or tissue
Donor NOS

☑4ᵗʰ **Z53** Persons encountering health services for specific procedures and treatment, not carried out

☑5ᵗʰ **Z53.0** Procedure and treatment not carried out because of contraindication

Z53.01 Procedure and treatment not carried out due to patient smoking

Z53.09 Procedure and treatment not carried out because of other contraindication

Z53.1 Procedure and treatment not carried out because of patient's decision for reasons of belief and group pressure

☑5ᵗʰ **Z53.2** Procedure and treatment not carried out because of patient's decision for other and unspecified reasons

Z53.20 Procedure and treatment not carried out because of patient's decision for unspecified reasons

Z53.21 Procedure and treatment not carried out due to patient leaving prior to being seen by health care provider

Z53.29 Procedure and treatment not carried out because of patient's decision for other reasons

☑5ᵗʰ **Z53.3** Procedure converted to open procedure

Z53.31 Laparoscopic surgical procedure converted to open procedure

Z53.32 Thoracoscopic surgical procedure converted to open procedure

Z53.33 Arthroscopic surgical procedure converted to open procedure

Z53.39 Other specified procedure converted to open procedure

Z53.8 Procedure and treatment not carried out for other reasons

Z53.9 Procedure and treatment not carried out, unspecified reason

Persons with potential health hazards related to socioeconomic and psychosocial circumstances (Z55-Z65)

☑4ᵗʰ **Z55** Problems related to education and literacy
EXCLUDES 1   disorders of psychological development (F80-F89)

Z55.0 Illiteracy and low-level literacy

Z55.1 Schooling unavailable and unattainable

Z55.2 Failed school examinations

Z55.3 Underachievement in school

Z55.4 Educational maladjustment and discord with teachers and classmates

Z55.8 Other problems related to education and literacy
Problems related to inadequate teaching

Z55.9 Problems related to education and literacy, unspecified
Academic problems NOS

☑4ᵗʰ **Z56** Problems related to employment and unemployment
EXCLUDES 2   occupational exposure to risk factors (Z57.-)
problems related to housing and economic circumstances (Z59.-)

Z56.0 Unemployment, unspecified

Z56.1 Change of job   A

Z56.2 Threat of job loss

Z56.3 Stressful work schedule

Z56.4 Discord with boss and workmates

Z56.5 Uncongenial work environment
Difficult conditions at work

Z56.6 Other physical and mental strain related to work

☑5ᵗʰ **Z56.8** Other problems related to employment

Z56.81 Sexual harassment on the job

Z56.82 Military deployment status
Individual (civilian or military) currently deployed in theater or in support of military war, peacekeeping and humanitarian operations

Z56.89 Other problems related to employment

Z56.9 Unspecified problems related to employment
Occupational problems NOS

☑4ᵗʰ **Z57** Occupational exposure to risk factors

Z57.0 Occupational exposure to noise

Z57.1 Occupational exposure to radiation

Z57.2 Occupational exposure to dust

☑5ᵗʰ **Z57.3** Occupational exposure to other air contaminants

Z57.31 Occupational exposure to environmental tobacco smoke
EXCLUDES 2   exposure to environmental tobacco smoke (Z77.22)

Z57.39 Occupational exposure to other air contaminants

Z57.4 Occupational exposure to toxic agents in agriculture
Occupational exposure to solids, liquids, gases or vapors in agriculture

Z57.5 Occupational exposure to toxic agents in other industries
Occupational exposure to solids, liquids, gases or vapors in other industries

Z57.6 Occupational exposure to extreme temperature

Z57.7 Occupational exposure to vibration

Z57.8 Occupational exposure to other risk factors

Z57.9 Occupational exposure to unspecified risk factor

☑4ᵗʰ **Z59** Problems related to housing and economic circumstances
EXCLUDES 2   problems related to upbringing (Z62.-)

Z59.0 Homelessness

Z59.1 Inadequate housing
Lack of heating
Restriction of space
Technical defects in home preventing adequate care
Unsatisfactory surroundings
EXCLUDES 1   problems related to the natural and physical environment (Z77.1-)

Z59.2 Discord with neighbors, lodgers and landlord

Z59.3 Problems related to living in residential institution
Boarding-school resident
EXCLUDES 1   institutional upbringing (Z62.2)

Z59.4 Lack of adequate food and safe drinking water
Inadequate drinking water supply
EXCLUDES 1   effects of hunger (T73.0)
inappropriate diet or eating habits (Z72.4)
malnutrition (E40-E46)

Z59.5 Extreme poverty

Z59.6 Low income

Z59.7 Insufficient social insurance and welfare support

Z59.8 Other problems related to housing and economic circumstances
Foreclosure on loan   Problems with creditors
Isolated dwelling

Z59.9 Problem related to housing and economic circumstances, unspecified

☑4ᵗʰ **Z60** Problems related to social environment

Z60.0 Problems of adjustment to life-cycle transitions
Empty nest syndrome   Problem with adjustment
Phase of life problem   to retirement [pension]

Z60.2 Problems related to living alone

N Newborn: 0   P Pediatric: 0-17   M Maternity: 12-55   A Adult: 15-124   MCC Major CC Condition   PDxMCC PDx acts as own MCC   CC CC Condition   PDxCC PDx acts as own CC

1234   ICD-10-CM 2018

Z60.3   **Acculturation difficulty**
Problem with migration
Problem with social transplantation
DEF: A problem in adapting to a different culture or environment not based on any coexisting mental disorder.

Z60.4   **Social exclusion and rejection**
Exclusion and rejection on the basis of personal characteristics, such as unusual physical appearance, illness or behavior.
EXCLUDES 1   *target of adverse discrimination such as for racial or religious reasons (Z60.5)*

Z60.5   **Target of (perceived) adverse discrimination and persecution**
EXCLUDES 1   *social exclusion and rejection (Z60.4)*

Z60.8   **Other problems related to social environment**

Z60.9   **Problem related to social environment, unspecified**

✓4th **Z62**   **Problems related to upbringing**
INCLUDES   current and past negative life events in childhood
current and past problems of a child related to upbringing
EXCLUDES 2   *maltreatment syndrome (T74.-)*
problems related to housing and economic circumstances (Z59.-)

Z62.0   **Inadequate parental supervision and control**

Z62.1   **Parental overprotection**

✓5th **Z62.2**   **Upbringing away from parents**
EXCLUDES 1   *problems with boarding school (Z59.3)*

     Z62.21   **Child in welfare custody**   ℗
Child in care of non-parental family member
Child in foster care
EXCLUDES 2   *problem for parent due to child in welfare custody (Z63.5)*

     Z62.22   **Institutional upbringing**
Child living in orphanage or group home

     Z62.29   **Other upbringing away from parents**

Z62.3   **Hostility towards and scapegoating of child**   ℗

Z62.6   **Inappropriate (excessive) parental pressure**

✓5th **Z62.8**   **Other specified problems related to upbringing**

     ✓6th **Z62.81**   **Personal history of abuse in childhood**

         Z62.810   **Personal history of physical and sexual abuse in childhood**
EXCLUDES 1   *current child physical abuse (T74.12, T76.12)*
current child sexual abuse (T74.22, T76.22)

         Z62.811   **Personal history of psychological abuse in childhood**
EXCLUDES 1   *current child psychological abuse (T74.32, T76.32)*

         Z62.812   **Personal history of neglect in childhood**
EXCLUDES 1   *current child neglect (T74.02, T76.02)*

         Z62.819   **Personal history of unspecified abuse in childhood**
EXCLUDES 1   *current child abuse NOS (T74.92, T76.92)*

     ✓6th **Z62.82**   **Parent-child conflict**

         Z62.820   **Parent-biological child conflict**
Parent-child problem NOS

         Z62.821   **Parent-adopted child conflict**

         Z62.822   **Parent-foster child conflict**

     ✓6th **Z62.89**   **Other specified problems related to upbringing**

         Z62.890   **Parent-child estrangement NEC**

         Z62.891   **Sibling rivalry**

         Z62.898   **Other specified problems related to upbringing**

Z62.9   **Problem related to upbringing, unspecified**

✓4th **Z63**   **Other problems related to primary support group, including family circumstances**
EXCLUDES 2   *maltreatment syndrome (T74-, T76)*
parent-child problems (Z62.-)
problems related to negative life events in childhood (Z62.-)
problems related to upbringing (Z62.-)

Z63.0   **Problems in relationship with spouse or partner**
▶Relationship distress with spouse or intimate partner◀
EXCLUDES 1   *counseling for spousal or partner abuse problems (Z69.1)*
counseling related to sexual attitude, behavior, and orientation (Z70.-)

Z63.1   **Problems in relationship with in-laws**

✓5th **Z63.3**   **Absence of family member**
EXCLUDES 1   *absence of family member due to disappearance and death (Z63.4)*
absence of family member due to separation and divorce (Z63.5)

     Z63.31   **Absence of family member due to military deployment**
Individual or family affected by other family member being on military deployment
EXCLUDES 1   *family disruption due to return of family member from military deployment (Z63.71)*

     Z63.32   **Other absence of family member**

Z63.4   **Disappearance and death of family member**
Assumed death of family member
Bereavement
AHA: 2014, 1Q, 25

Z63.5   **Disruption of family by separation and divorce**
Marital estrangement

Z63.6   **Dependent relative needing care at home**

✓5th **Z63.7**   **Other stressful life events affecting family and household**

     Z63.71   **Stress on family due to return of family member from military deployment**
Individual or family affected by family member having returned from military deployment (current or past conflict)

     Z63.72   **Alcoholism and drug addiction in family**

     Z63.79   **Other stressful life events affecting family and household**
Anxiety (normal) about sick person in family
Health problems within family
Ill or disturbed family member
Isolated family

Z63.8   **Other specified problems related to primary support group**
Family discord NOS
Family estrangement NOS
High expressed emotional level within family
Inadequate family support NOS
Inadequate or distorted communication within family

Z63.9   **Problem related to primary support group, unspecified**
Relationship disorder NOS

✓4th **Z64**   **Problems related to certain psychosocial circumstances**

Z64.0   **Problems related to unwanted pregnancy**   ♀

Z64.1   **Problems related to multiparity**   ♀

Z64.4   **Discord with counselors**
Discord with probation officer
Discord with social worker

✓4th **Z65**   **Problems related to other psychosocial circumstances**

Z65.0   **Conviction in civil and criminal proceedings without imprisonment**

Z65.1   **Imprisonment and other incarceration**

Z65.2   **Problems related to release from prison**

Z65.3   **Problems related to other legal circumstances**
Arrest
Child custody or support proceedings
Litigation
Prosecution

Z65.4   **Victim of crime and terrorism**
Victim of torture

Z65.5   **Exposure to disaster, war and other hostilities**
EXCLUDES 1   *target of perceived discrimination or persecution (Z60.5)*

Z65.8   **Other specified problems related to psychosocial circumstances**
▶Religious or spiritual problem◀

Z65.9   **Problem related to unspecified psychosocial circumstances**

Do not resuscitate status (Z66)

Z66   **Do not resuscitate**
DNR status
DEF: Medical order written by a physician that instructs others not to perform cardiopulmonary resuscitation (CPR), intubation, or advanced life support (ACLS); prevents unnecessary invasive treatment to prolong life should breathing stop or cardiac arrest occur.

✔ Additional Character Req   ✓x7th Placeholder Alert   Unacceptable PDx   Manifestation   H1-H14 HAC   HCC CMS-HCC Condition   *EXCLUDES 1* Not Coded Here   *EXCLUDES 2* Not Included Here

ICD-10-CM 2018   1235

Chapter 21. Factors Influencing Health Status and Contact with Health Services *(left margin)*

Blood Types

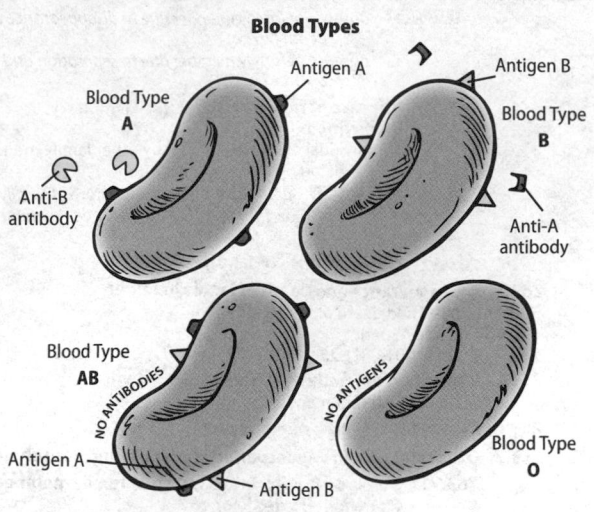

Blood Type A — Antigen A — Anti-B antibody

Blood Type B — Antigen B — Anti-A antibody

Blood Type AB — NO ANTIBODIES — Antigen A — Antigen B

Blood Type O — NO ANTIGENS

Blood type (Z67)

✓4th **Z67** **Blood type**
AHA: 2015, 3Q, 40

  ✓5th **Z67.1** **Type A blood**
    Z67.10   **Type A blood, Rh positive**
    Z67.11   **Type A blood, Rh negative**

  ✓5th **Z67.2** **Type B blood**
    Z67.20   **Type B blood, Rh positive**
    Z67.21   **Type B blood, Rh negative**

  ✓5th **Z67.3** **Type AB blood**
    Z67.30   **Type AB blood, Rh positive**
    Z67.31   **Type AB blood, Rh negative**

  ✓5th **Z67.4** **Type O blood**
    Z67.40   **Type O blood, Rh positive**
    Z67.41   **Type O blood, Rh negative**

  ✓5th **Z67.9** **Unspecified blood type**
    Z67.90   **Unspecified blood type, Rh positive**
    Z67.91   **Unspecified blood type, Rh negative**

Body mass index [BMI] (Z68)

✓4th **Z68** **Body mass index [BMI]**
Kilograms per meters squared
NOTE   BMI adult codes are for use for persons 21 years of age or older.
      BMI pediatric codes are for use for persons 2-20 years of age. These percentiles are based on the growth charts published by the Centers for Disease Control and Prevention (CDC)
AHA: 2017, 1Q, 39
DEF: Index used to help determine whether an individual is underweight, a healthy weight, overweight, or obese.

▲   **Z68.1**   **Body mass index [BMI] 19.9 or less, adult**   CC A
    CC Excl: PDX collection 1493

  ✓5th **Z68.2** **Body mass index [BMI] 20-29, adult**
    Z68.20   **Body mass index [BMI] 20.0-20.9, adult**   A
    Z68.21   **Body mass index [BMI] 21.0-21.9, adult**   A
    Z68.22   **Body mass index [BMI] 22.0-22.9, adult**   A
    Z68.23   **Body mass index [BMI] 23.0-23.9, adult**   A
    Z68.24   **Body mass index [BMI] 24.0-24.9, adult**   A
    Z68.25   **Body mass index [BMI] 25.0-25.9, adult**   A
    Z68.26   **Body mass index [BMI] 26.0-26.9, adult**   A
    Z68.27   **Body mass index [BMI] 27.0-27.9, adult**   A
    Z68.28   **Body mass index [BMI] 28.0-28.9, adult**   A
    Z68.29   **Body mass index [BMI] 29.0-29.9, adult**   A

  ✓5th **Z68.3** **Body mass index [BMI] 30-39, adult**
    Z68.30   **Body mass index [BMI] 30.0-30.9, adult**   A
    Z68.31   **Body mass index [BMI] 31.0-31.9, adult**   A
    Z68.32   **Body mass index [BMI] 32.0-32.9, adult**   A
    Z68.33   **Body mass index [BMI] 33.0-33.9, adult**   A
    Z68.34   **Body mass index [BMI] 34.0-34.9, adult**   A

    Z68.35   **Body mass index [BMI] 35.0-35.9, adult**   A
    Z68.36   **Body mass index [BMI] 36.0-36.9, adult**   A
    Z68.37   **Body mass index [BMI] 37.0-37.9, adult**   A
    Z68.38   **Body mass index [BMI] 38.0-38.9, adult**   A
    Z68.39   **Body mass index [BMI] 39.0-39.9, adult**   A

  ✓5th **Z68.4** **Body mass index [BMI] 40 or greater, adult**

    CC Excl: For CC codes in subcategory Z68.4, unless otherwise noted: PDX collection 1494

    Z68.41   **Body mass index [BMI] 40.0-44.9, adult**   CC HCC A
    Z68.42   **Body mass index [BMI] 45.0-49.9, adult**   CC HCC A
    Z68.43   **Body mass index [BMI] 50-59.9, adult**   CC HCC A
    Z68.44   **Body mass index [BMI] 60.0-69.9, adult**   CC HCC A
    Z68.45   **Body mass index [BMI] 70 or greater, adult**   CC HCC A

  ✓5th **Z68.5** **Body mass index [BMI] pediatric**
    Z68.51   **Body mass index [BMI] pediatric, less than 5th percentile for age**
    Z68.52   **Body mass index [BMI] pediatric, 5th percentile to less than 85th percentile for age**
    Z68.53   **Body mass index [BMI] pediatric, 85th percentile to less than 95th percentile for age**
    Z68.54   **Body mass index [BMI] pediatric, greater than or equal to 95th percentile for age**

Persons encountering health services in other circumstances (Z69-Z76)

✓4th **Z69** **Encounter for mental health services for victim and perpetrator of abuse**
    INCLUDES   counseling for victims and perpetrators of abuse

  ✓5th **Z69.0** **Encounter for mental health services for child abuse problems**

    ✓6th **Z69.01** **Encounter for mental health services for parental child abuse**

      Z69.010   **Encounter for mental health services for victim of parental child abuse**   P
         ▶Encounter for mental health services for victim of child abuse by parent
         Encounter for mental health services for victim of child neglect by parent
         Encounter for mental health services for victim of child psychological abuse by parent
         Encounter for mental health services for victim of child sexual abuse by parent◀

      Z69.011   **Encounter for mental health services for perpetrator of parental child abuse**
         ▶Encounter for mental health services for perpetrator of parental child neglect
         Encounter for mental health services for perpetrator of parental child psychological abuse
         Encounter for mental health services for perpetrator of parental child sexual abuse◀
         EXCLUDES 1   encounter for mental health services for non-parental child abuse (Z69.02-)

    ✓6th **Z69.02** **Encounter for mental health services for non-parental child abuse**

      Z69.020   **Encounter for mental health services for victim of non-parental child abuse**   P
         ▶Encounter for mental health services for victim of non-parental child neglect
         Encounter for mental health services for victim of non-parental child psychological abuse
         Encounter for mental health services for victim of non-parental child sexual abuse◀

N Newborn: 0   P Pediatric: 0-17   M Maternity: 12-55   A Adult: 15-124   MCC Major CC Condition   PDxMCC PDx acts as own MCC   CC CC Condition   PDxCC PDx acts as own CC

1236   ICD-10-CM 2018

Z67–Z69.020 *(left margin bottom)*

Z69.021 **Encounter for mental health services for perpetrator of non-parental child abuse**
▶Encounter for mental health services for perpetrator of non-parental child neglect
Encounter for mental health services for perpetrator of non-parental child psychological abuse
Encounter for mental health services for perpetrator of non-parental child sexual abuse◀

✓5ᵗʰ **Z69.1** **Encounter for mental health services for spousal or partner abuse problems**

Z69.11 **Encounter for mental health services for victim of spousal or partner abuse**
▶Encounter for mental health services for victim of spouse or partner neglect
Encounter for mental health services for victim of spouse or partner psychological abuse
Encounter for mental health services for victim of spouse or partner violence, physical◀

Z69.12 **Encounter for mental health services for perpetrator of spousal or partner abuse**
▶Encounter for mental health services for perpetrator of spouse or partner neglect
Encounter for mental health services for perpetrator of spouse or partner psychological abuse
Encounter for mental health services for perpetrator of spouse or partner violence, physical
Encounter for mental health services for perpetrator of spouse or partner violence, sexual◀

✓5ᵗʰ **Z69.8** **Encounter for mental health services for victim or perpetrator of other abuse**

Z69.81 **Encounter for mental health services for victim of other abuse**
▶Encounter for mental health services for perpetrator of non-spousal adult abuse
Encounter for mental health services for victim of non-spousal adult abuse
Encounter for mental health services for victim of spouse or partner violence, sexual◀
Encounter for rape victim counseling

Z69.82 **Encounter for mental health services for perpetrator of other abuse**

✓4ᵗʰ **Z70** **Counseling related to sexual attitude, behavior and orientation**
INCLUDES encounter for mental health services for sexual attitude, behavior and orientation
EXCLUDES 2 contraceptive or procreative counseling (Z30-Z31)

Z70.0 **Counseling related to sexual attitude**

Z70.1 **Counseling related to patient's sexual behavior and orientation**
Patient concerned regarding impotence
Patient concerned regarding non-responsiveness
Patient concerned regarding promiscuity
Patient concerned regarding sexual orientation

Z70.2 **Counseling related to sexual behavior and orientation of third party**
Advice sought regarding sexual behavior and orientation of child
Advice sought regarding sexual behavior and orientation of partner
Advice sought regarding sexual behavior and orientation of spouse

Z70.3 **Counseling related to combined concerns regarding sexual attitude, behavior and orientation**

Z70.8 **Other sex counseling**
Encounter for sex education

Z70.9 **Sex counseling, unspecified**

✓4ᵗʰ **Z71** **Persons encountering health services for other counseling and medical advice, not elsewhere classified**
EXCLUDES 2 contraceptive or procreation counseling (Z30-Z31)
sex counseling (Z70.-)

Z71.0 **Person encountering health services to consult on behalf of another person**
Person encountering health services to seek advice or treatment for non-attending third party
EXCLUDES 2 anxiety (normal) about sick person in family (Z63.7)
expectant (adoptive) parent(s) pre-birth pediatrician visit (Z76.81)

Z71.1 **Person with feared health complaint in whom no diagnosis is made**
Person encountering health services with feared condition which was not demonstrated
Person encountering health services in which problem was normal state
"Worried well"
EXCLUDES 1 medical observation for suspected diseases and conditions proven not to exist (Z03.-)

Z71.2 **Person consulting for explanation of examination or test findings**

Z71.3 **Dietary counseling and surveillance**
Use additional code for any associated underlying medical condition
Use additional code to identify body mass index (BMI), if known (Z68.-)

✓5ᵗʰ **Z71.4** **Alcohol abuse counseling and surveillance**
Use additional code for alcohol abuse or dependence (F10.-)

Z71.41 **Alcohol abuse counseling and surveillance of alcoholic**

Z71.42 **Counseling for family member of alcoholic**
Counseling for significant other, partner, or friend of alcoholic

✓5ᵗʰ **Z71.5** **Drug abuse counseling and surveillance**
Use additional code for drug abuse or dependence (F11-F16, F18-F19)

Z71.51 **Drug abuse counseling and surveillance of drug abuser**

Z71.52 **Counseling for family member of drug abuser**
Counseling for significant other, partner, or friend of drug abuser

Z71.6 **Tobacco abuse counseling**
Use additional code for nicotine dependence (F17.-)

Z71.7 **Human immunodeficiency virus [HIV] counseling**

✓5ᵗʰ **Z71.8** **Other specified counseling**
EXCLUDES 2 counseling for contraception (Z30.0-)
~~counseling for genetics (Z31.5)~~
~~counseling for procreative management (Z31.6-)~~

Z71.81 **Spiritual or religious counseling**

● **Z71.82** **Exercise counseling**

● **Z71.83** **Encounter for nonprocreative genetic counseling**
EXCLUDES 1 counseling for procreative genetics (Z31.5)
counseling for procreative management (Z31.6)

Z71.89 **Other specified counseling**

Z71.9 **Counseling, unspecified**
Encounter for medical advice NOS

✓4ᵗʰ **Z72** **Problems related to lifestyle**
EXCLUDES 2 problems related to life-management difficulty (Z73.-)
problems related to socioeconomic and psychosocial circumstances (Z55-Z65)

Z72.0 **Tobacco use**
Tobacco use NOS
EXCLUDES 1 history of tobacco dependence (Z87.891)
nicotine dependence (F17.2-)
tobacco dependence (F17.2-)
tobacco use during pregnancy (O99.33-)

Z72.3 **Lack of physical exercise**

Z72.4 **Inappropriate diet and eating habits**
EXCLUDES 1 behavioral eating disorders of infancy or childhood (F98.2- F98.3)
eating disorders (F50.-)
lack of adequate food (Z59.4)
malnutrition and other nutritional deficiencies (E40-E64)

✓5ᵗʰ **Z72.5** **High risk sexual behavior**
Promiscuity
EXCLUDES 1 paraphilias (F65)

Z72.51 **High risk heterosexual behavior**

Z72.52 **High risk homosexual behavior**

Z72.53 **High risk bisexual behavior**

Z72.6 **Gambling and betting**
EXCLUDES 1 compulsive or pathological gambling (F63.0)

✓ Additional Character Req　✓x7ᵗʰ Placeholder Alert　Unacceptable PDx　Manifestation　H1-H14 HAC　HCC CMS-HCC Condition　EXCLUDES 1 Not Coded Here　EXCLUDES 2 Not Included Here

ICD-10-CM 2018　　**1237**

Z72.8   Other problems related to lifestyle

✓6th **Z72.81   Antisocial behavior**
    EXCLUDES 1   *conduct disorders (F91.-)*

    Z72.810   Child and adolescent antisocial P
        behavior
        Antisocial behavior (child) (adolescent)
            without manifest psychiatric disorder
        Delinquency NOS
        Group delinquency
        Offenses in the context of gang
            membership
        Stealing in company with others
        Truancy from school

    Z72.811   Adult antisocial behavior A
        Adult antisocial behavior without manifest
            psychiatric disorder

✓6th **Z72.82   Problems related to sleep**
    Z72.820   Sleep deprivation
        Lack of adequate sleep
        EXCLUDES 1   *insomnia (G47.0-)*

    Z72.821   Inadequate sleep hygiene
        Bad sleep habits
        Irregular sleep habits
        Unhealthy sleep wake schedule
        EXCLUDES 1   *insomnia (F51.0-, G47.0-)*

    Z72.89   Other problems related to lifestyle
        Self-damaging behavior

Z72.9   Problem related to lifestyle, unspecified

✓4th **Z73   Problems related to life management difficulty**
    EXCLUDES 2   *problems related to socioeconomic and psychosocial*
            circumstances (Z55-Z65)
    DEF: State of emotional, mental, and physical exhaustion; causing
    difficulties in managing personal, school, or work circumstances; usually
    due to prolonged stress; poor interpersonal relationship skills, or parenting
    skills.

Z73.0   Burn-out

Z73.1   Type A behavior pattern

Z73.2   Lack of relaxation and leisure

Z73.3   Stress, not elsewhere classified
    Physical and mental strain NOS
    EXCLUDES 1   *stress related to employment or unemployment (Z56.-)*

Z73.4   Inadequate social skills, not elsewhere classified

Z73.5   Social role conflict, not elsewhere classified

Z73.6   Limitation of activities due to disability
    EXCLUDES 1   *care-provider dependency (Z74.-)*

✓5th **Z73.8   Other problems related to life management difficulty**
    ✓6th **Z73.81   Behavioral insomnia of childhood**
        DEF: Behaviors on the part of the child or caregivers that
        cause negative compliance with a child's sleep schedule;
        results in lack of adequate sleep.

        Z73.810   Behavioral insomnia of childhood, P
            sleep-onset association type

        Z73.811   Behavioral insomnia of childhood, P
            limit setting type

        Z73.812   Behavioral insomnia of childhood, P
            combined type

        Z73.819   Behavioral insomnia of childhood, P
            unspecified type

    Z73.82   Dual sensory impairment

    Z73.89   Other problems related to life management
        difficulty

Z73.9   Problem related to life management difficulty, unspecified

✓4th **Z74   Problems related to care provider dependency**
    EXCLUDES 2   *dependence on enabling machines or devices NEC (Z99.-)*

✓5th **Z74.0   Reduced mobility**
    Z74.01   Bed confinement status
        Bedridden

    Z74.09   Other reduced mobility
        Chair ridden
        Reduced mobility NOS
        EXCLUDES 2   *wheelchair dependence (Z99.3)*

Z74.1   Need for assistance with personal care

Z74.2   Need for assistance at home and no other household member able to render care

Z74.3   Need for continuous supervision

Z74.8   Other problems related to care provider dependency

Z74.9   Problem related to care provider dependency, unspecified

✓4th **Z75   Problems related to medical facilities and other health care**
    Z75.0   Medical services not available in home
        EXCLUDES 1   *no other household member able to render care (Z74.2)*

    Z75.1   Person awaiting admission to adequate facility elsewhere

    Z75.2   Other waiting period for investigation and treatment

    Z75.3   Unavailability and inaccessibility of health-care facilities
        EXCLUDES 1   *bed unavailable (Z75.1)*

    Z75.4   Unavailability and inaccessibility of other helping agencies

    Z75.5   Holiday relief care

    Z75.8   Other problems related to medical facilities and other health care

    Z75.9   Unspecified problem related to medical facilities and other health care

✓4th **Z76   Persons encountering health services in other circumstances**
    Z76.0   Encounter for issue of repeat prescription
        Encounter for issue of repeat prescription for appliance
        Encounter for issue of repeat prescription for medicaments
        Encounter for issue of repeat prescription for spectacles
        EXCLUDES 2   *issue of medical certificate (Z02.7)*
            repeat prescription for contraceptive (Z30.4-)

    Z76.1   Encounter for health supervision and care of foundling

    Z76.2   Encounter for health supervision and care of other P
        healthy infant and child
        Encounter for medical or nursing care or supervision of healthy
            infant under circumstances such as adverse socioeconomic
            conditions at home
        Encounter for medical or nursing care or supervision of healthy
            infant under circumstances such as awaiting foster or
            adoptive placement
        Encounter for medical or nursing care or supervision of healthy
            infant under circumstances such as maternal illness
        Encounter for medical or nursing care or supervision of healthy
            infant under circumstances such as number of children at
            home preventing or interfering with normal care

    Z76.3   Healthy person accompanying sick person

    Z76.4   Other boarder to healthcare facility
        EXCLUDES 1   *homelessness (Z59.0)*

    Z76.5   Malingerer [conscious simulation]
        Person feigning illness (with obvious motivation)
        EXCLUDES 1   *factitious disorder (F68.1-)*
            peregrinating patient (F68.1-)
        DEF: Act of intentionally exaggerating an illness or disability in
        order to receive personal gain; or to avoid punishment or
        responsibility.

✓5th **Z76.8   Persons encountering health services in other specified circumstances**
    Z76.81   Expectant parent(s) prebirth pediatrician visit
        Pre-adoption pediatrician visit for adoptive parent(s)

    Z76.82   Awaiting organ transplant status
        Patient waiting for organ availability

    Z76.89   Persons encountering health services in other specified circumstances
        Persons encountering health services NOS
        AHA: 2014, 2Q, 10

N Newborn: 0   P Pediatric: 0-17   M Maternity: 12-55   A Adult: 15-124   MCC Major CC Condition   PDx MCC PDx acts as own MCC   CC CC Condition   PDx CC PDx acts as own CC

1238

ICD-10-CM 2018

Persons with potential health hazards related to family and personal history and certain conditions influencing health status (Z77-Z99)

Code also any follow-up examination (Z08-Z09)

✓4th Z77 Other contact with and (suspected) exposures hazardous to health

> **INCLUDES** contact with and (suspected) exposures to potential hazards to health
>
> **EXCLUDES 2** contact with and (suspected) exposure to communicable diseases (Z20.-)
> exposure to (parental) (environmental) tobacco smoke in the perinatal period (P96.81)
> newborn affected by noxious substances transmitted via placenta or breast milk (P04.-)
> occupational exposure to risk factors (Z57.-)
> retained foreign body (Z18.-)
> retained foreign body fully removed (Z87.821)
> toxic effects of substances chiefly nonmedicinal as to source (T51-T65)

✓5th Z77.0 Contact with and (suspected) exposure to hazardous, chiefly nonmedicinal, chemicals

> **✓6th Z77.01 Contact with and (suspected) exposure to hazardous metals**
>
> **Z77.010 Contact with and (suspected) exposure to arsenic**
>
> **Z77.011 Contact with and (suspected) exposure to lead**
>
> **Z77.012 Contact with and (suspected) exposure to uranium**
>> **EXCLUDES 1** retained depleted uranium fragments (Z18.01)
>
> **Z77.018 Contact with and (suspected) exposure to other hazardous metals**
>> Contact with and (suspected) exposure to chromium compounds
>> Contact with and (suspected) exposure to nickel dust
>
> **✓6th Z77.02 Contact with and (suspected) exposure to hazardous aromatic compounds**
>
> **Z77.020 Contact with and (suspected) exposure to aromatic amines**
>
> **Z77.021 Contact with and (suspected) exposure to benzene**
>
> **Z77.028 Contact with and (suspected) exposure to other hazardous aromatic compounds**
>> Aromatic dyes NOS
>> Polycyclic aromatic hydrocarbons
>
> **✓6th Z77.09 Contact with and (suspected) exposure to other hazardous, chiefly nonmedicinal, chemicals**
>
> **Z77.090 Contact with and (suspected) exposure to asbestos**
>
> **Z77.098 Contact with and (suspected) exposure to other hazardous, chiefly nonmedicinal, chemicals**
>> Dyes NOS

✓5th Z77.1 Contact with and (suspected) exposure to environmental pollution and hazards in the physical environment

> **✓6th Z77.11 Contact with and (suspected) exposure to environmental pollution**
>
> **Z77.110 Contact with and (suspected) exposure to air pollution**
>
> **Z77.111 Contact with and (suspected) exposure to water pollution**
>
> **Z77.112 Contact with and (suspected) exposure to soil pollution**
>
> **Z77.118 Contact with and (suspected) exposure to other environmental pollution**
>
> **✓6th Z77.12 Contact with and (suspected) exposure to hazards in the physical environment**
>
> **Z77.120 Contact with and (suspected) exposure to mold (toxic)**

> **Z77.121 Contact with and (suspected) exposure to harmful algae and algae toxins**
>> Contact with and (suspected) exposure to (harmful) algae bloom NOS
>> Contact with and (suspected) exposure to blue-green algae bloom
>> Contact with and (suspected) exposure to brown tide
>> Contact with and (suspected) exposure to cyanobacteria bloom
>> Contact with and (suspected) exposure to Florida red tide
>> Contact with and (suspected) exposure to pfiesteria piscicida
>> Contact with and (suspected) exposure to red tide
>
> **Z77.122 Contact with and (suspected) exposure to noise**
>
> **Z77.123 Contact with and (suspected) exposure to radon and other naturally occuring radiation**
>> **EXCLUDES 2** radiation exposure as the cause of a confirmed condition (W88-W90, X39.0-)
>> radiation sickness NOS (T66)
>
> **Z77.128 Contact with and (suspected) exposure to other hazards in the physical environment**

✓5th Z77.2 Contact with and (suspected) exposure to other hazardous substances

> **Z77.21 Contact with and (suspected) exposure to potentially hazardous body fluids**
>
> **Z77.22 Contact with and (suspected) exposure to environmental tobacco smoke (acute) (chronic)**
>> Exposure to second hand tobacco smoke (acute) (chronic)
>> Passive smoking (acute) (chronic)
>> **EXCLUDES 1** nicotine dependence (F17.-)
>> tobacco use (Z72.0)
>> **EXCLUDES 2** occupational exposure to environmental tobacco smoke (Z57.31)
>
> **Z77.29 Contact with and (suspected) exposure to other hazardous substances**
>> **AHA:** 2016, 2Q, 33

Z77.9 Other contact with and (suspected) exposures hazardous to health

✓4th Z78 Other specified health status

> **EXCLUDES 2** asymptomatic human immunodeficiency virus [HIV] infection status (Z21)
> postprocedural status (Z93- Z99)
> sex reassignment status (Z87.890)

Z78.0 Asymptomatic menopausal state   A ♀
> Menopausal state NOS
> Postmenopausal status NOS
> **EXCLUDES 2** symptomatic menopausal state (N95.1)

Z78.1 Physical restraint status
> **EXCLUDES 1** physical restraint due to a procedure - omit code
> **DEF:** Application of mechanical restraining devices or manual restraints; used to limit physical mobility of a patient.

Z78.9 Other specified health status

✓4th Z79 Long term (current) drug therapy
> **INCLUDES** long term (current) drug use for prophylactic purposes
> Code also any therapeutic drug level monitoring (Z51.81)
> **EXCLUDES 2** drug abuse and dependence (F11-F19)
> drug use complicating pregnancy, childbirth, and the puerperium (O99.32-)
> long term (current) use of oral antidiabetic drugs (Z79.84)
> long term (current) use of oral hypoglycemic drugs (Z79.84)

✓5th Z79.0 Long term (current) use of anticoagulants and antithrombotics/antiplatelets
> **EXCLUDES 2** long term (current) use of aspirin (Z79.82)
>
> **Z79.01 Long term (current) use of anticoagulants**
>
> **Z79.02 Long term (current) use of antithrombotics/antiplatelets**

Z79.1 Long term (current) use of non-steroidal anti-inflammatories (NSAID)
> **EXCLUDES 2** long term (current) use of aspirin (Z79.82)

Z79.2 Long term (current) use of antibiotics

Z79.3 Long term (current) use of hormonal contraceptives
> Long term (current) use of birth control pill or patch

Z79.4 Long term (current) use of insulin   HCC

✓ Additional Character Req   ✓x7th Placeholder Alert   Unacceptable PDx   Manifestation   H1 - H14 HAC   HCC CMS-HCC Condition   EXCLUDES 1 Not Coded Here   EXCLUDES 2 Not Included Here

Chapter 21. Factors Influencing Health Status and Contact with Health Services

√5ᵗʰ **Z79.5 Long term (current) use of steroids**

     Z79.51 Long term (current) use of inhaled steroids

     Z79.52 Long term (current) use of systemic steroids

√5ᵗʰ **Z79.8 Other long term (current) drug therapy**

     √6ᵗʰ **Z79.81 Long term (current) use of agents affecting estrogen receptors and estrogen levels**

         Code first, if applicable:

         malignant neoplasm of breast (C50.-)

         malignant neoplasm of prostate (C61)

         Use additional code, if applicable, to identify:

         estrogen receptor positive status (Z17.0)

         family history of breast cancer (Z80.3)

         genetic susceptibility to malignant neoplasm (cancer) (Z15.0-)

         personal history of breast cancer (Z85.3)

         personal history of prostate cancer (Z85.46)

         postmenopausal status (Z78.0)

         EXCLUDES 1 ▶hormone replacement therapy◀ (Z79.890)

         Z79.810 Long term (current) use of selective estrogen receptor modulators (SERMs)

             Long term (current) use of raloxifene (Evista)

             Long term (current) use of tamoxifen (Nolvadex)

             Long term (current) use of toremifene (Fareston)

         Z79.811 Long term (current) use of aromatase inhibitors

             Long term (current) use of anastrozole (Arimidex)

             Long term (current) use of exemestane (Aromasin)

             Long term (current) use of letrozole (Femara)

         Z79.818 Long term (current) use of other agents affecting estrogen receptors and estrogen levels

             Long term (current) use of estrogen receptor downregulators

             Long term (current) use of fulvestrant (Faslodex)

             Long term (current) use of gonadotropin-releasing hormone (GnRH) agonist

             Long term (current) use of goserelin acetate (Zoladex)

             Long term (current) use of leuprolide acetate (leuprorelin) (Lupron)

             Long term (current) use of megestrol acetate (Megace)

     Z79.82 Long term (current) use of aspirin

     Z79.83 Long term (current) use of bisphosphonates

     Z79.84 Long term (current) use of oral hypoglycemic drugs

         Long term (current) use of oral antidiabetic drugs

         EXCLUDES 2 long term (current) use of insulin (Z79.4)

     √6ᵗʰ **Z79.89 Other long term (current) drug therapy**

▲   **Z79.890 Hormone replacement therapy**

     Z79.891 Long term (current) use of opiate analgesic

         Long term (current) use of methadone for pain management

         EXCLUDES 1 methadone use NOS (F11.9-)

             use of methadone for treatment of heroin addiction (F11.2-)

     Z79.899 Other long term (current) drug therapy

         AHA: 2015, 4Q, 34; 2015, 3Q, 21

√4ᵗʰ **Z80 Family history of primary malignant neoplasm**

     Z80.0 Family history of malignant neoplasm of digestive organs

         Conditions classifiable to C15-C26

     Z80.1 Family history of malignant neoplasm of trachea, bronchus and lung

         Conditions classifiable to C33-C34

     Z80.2 Family history of malignant neoplasm of other respiratory and intrathoracic organs

         Conditions classifiable to C30-C32, C37-C39

     Z80.3 Family history of malignant neoplasm of breast

         Conditions classifiable to C50-

√5ᵗʰ **Z80.4 Family history of malignant neoplasm of genital organs**

         Conditions classifiable to C51-C63

     Z80.41 Family history of malignant neoplasm of ovary

     Z80.42 Family history of malignant neoplasm of prostate

     Z80.43 Family history of malignant neoplasm of testis

     Z80.49 Family history of malignant neoplasm of other genital organs

√5ᵗʰ **Z80.5 Family history of malignant neoplasm of urinary tract**

         Conditions classifiable to C64-C68

     Z80.51 Family history of malignant neoplasm of kidney

     Z80.52 Family history of malignant neoplasm of bladder

     Z80.59 Family history of malignant neoplasm of other urinary tract organ

     Z80.6 Family history of leukemia

         Conditions classifiable to C91-C95

     Z80.7 Family history of other malignant neoplasms of lymphoid, hematopoietic and related tissues

         Conditions classifiable to C81-C90, C96-

     Z80.8 Family history of malignant neoplasm of other organs or systems

         Conditions classifiable to C00-C14, C40-C49, C69-C79

     Z80.9 Family history of malignant neoplasm, unspecified

         Conditions classifiable to C80.1

√4ᵗʰ **Z81 Family history of mental and behavioral disorders**

     Z81.0 Family history of intellectual disabilities

         Conditions classifiable to F70-F79

     Z81.1 Family history of alcohol abuse and dependence

         Conditions classifiable to F10-

     Z81.2 Family history of tobacco abuse and dependence

         Conditions classifiable to F17-

     Z81.3 Family history of other psychoactive substance abuse and dependence

         Conditions classifiable to F11-F16, F18-F19

     Z81.4 Family history of other substance abuse and dependence

         Conditions classifiable to F55

     Z81.8 Family history of other mental and behavioral disorders

         Conditions classifiable elsewhere in F01-F99

√4ᵗʰ **Z82 Family history of certain disabilities and chronic diseases (leading to disablement)**

     Z82.0 Family history of epilepsy and other diseases of the nervous system

         Conditions classifiable to G00-G99

     Z82.1 Family history of blindness and visual loss

         Conditions classifiable to H54-

     Z82.2 Family history of deafness and hearing loss

         Conditions classifiable to H90-H91

     Z82.3 Family history of stroke

         Conditions classifiable to I60-I64

√5ᵗʰ **Z82.4 Family history of ischemic heart disease and other diseases of the circulatory system**

         Conditions classifiable to I00-I52, I65-I99

     Z82.41 Family history of sudden cardiac death

     Z82.49 Family history of ischemic heart disease and other diseases of the circulatory system

     Z82.5 Family history of asthma and other chronic lower respiratory diseases

         Conditions classifiable to J40-J47

         EXCLUDES 2 family history of other diseases of the respiratory system (Z83.6)

√5ᵗʰ **Z82.6 Family history of arthritis and other diseases of the musculoskeletal system and connective tissue**

         Conditions classifiable to M00-M99

     Z82.61 Family history of arthritis

     Z82.62 Family history of osteoporosis

     Z82.69 Family history of other diseases of the musculoskeletal system and connective tissue

√5ᵗʰ **Z82.7 Family history of congenital malformations, deformations and chromosomal abnormalities**

         Conditions classifiable to Q00-Q99

     Z82.71 Family history of polycystic kidney

     Z82.79 Family history of other congenital malformations, deformations and chromosomal abnormalities

     Z82.8 Family history of other disabilities and chronic diseases leading to disablement, not elsewhere classified

N Newborn: 0   **P** Pediatric: 0-17   **M** Maternity: 12-55   **A** Adult: 15-124   **MCC** Major CC Condition   **PDxMCC** PDx acts as own MCC   **CC** CC Condition   **PDxCC** PDx acts as own CC

1240

ICD-10-CM 2018

☑4ᵗʰ Z83 Family history of other specific disorders

    EXCLUDES 2   contact with and (suspected) exposure to communicable disease in the family (Z20.-)

   Z83.0 Family history of human immunodeficiency virus [HIV] disease
     Conditions classifiable to B20

   Z83.1 Family history of other infectious and parasitic diseases
     Conditions classifiable to A00-B19, B25-B94, B99

   Z83.2 Family history of diseases of the blood and blood-forming organs and certain disorders involving the immune mechanism
     Conditions classifiable to D50-D89

   Z83.3 Family history of diabetes mellitus
     Conditions classifiable to E08-E13

   ☑5ᵗʰ Z83.4 Family history of other endocrine, nutritional and metabolic diseases
     Conditions classifiable to E00-E07, E15-E88

     Z83.41 Family history of multiple endocrine neoplasia [MEN] syndrome

     Z83.42 Family history of familial hypercholesterolemia

     Z83.49 Family history of other endocrine, nutritional and metabolic diseases

   ☑5ᵗʰ Z83.5 Family history of eye and ear disorders

     ✓6ᵗʰ Z83.51 Family history of eye disorders
       Conditions classifiable to H00-H53, H55-H59
       EXCLUDES 2   family history of blindness and visual loss (Z82.1)

       Z83.511 Family history of glaucoma
       Z83.518 Family history of other specified eye disorder

     Z83.52 Family history of ear disorders
       Conditions classifiable to H60-H83, H92-H95
       EXCLUDES 2   family history of deafness and hearing loss (Z82.2)

   Z83.6 Family history of other diseases of the respiratory system
     Conditions classifiable to J00-J39, J60-J99
     EXCLUDES 2   family history of asthma and other chronic lower respiratory diseases (Z82.5)

   ☑5ᵗʰ Z83.7 Family history of diseases of the digestive system
     Conditions classifiable to K00-K93

     Z83.71 Family history of colonic polyps
       EXCLUDES 1   family history of malignant neoplasm of digestive organs (Z80.0)
       EXCLUDES 2   ▶family history of malignant neoplasm of digestive organs (Z80.0)◀

     Z83.79 Family history of other diseases of the digestive system

☑4ᵗʰ Z84 Family history of other conditions

   Z84.0 Family history of diseases of the skin and subcutaneous tissue
     Conditions classifiable to L00-L99

   Z84.1 Family history of disorders of kidney and ureter
     Conditions classifiable to N00-N29

   Z84.2 Family history of other diseases of the genitourinary system
     Conditions classifiable to N30-N99

   Z84.3 Family history of consanguinity

   ☑5ᵗʰ Z84.8 Family history of other specified conditions

     Z84.81 Family history of carrier of genetic disease

     Z84.82 Family history of sudden infant death syndrome
       Family history of SIDS

     Z84.89 Family history of other specified conditions

☑4ᵗʰ Z85 Personal history of malignant neoplasm
     Code first any follow-up examination after treatment of malignant neoplasm (Z08)
     Use additional code to identify:
       alcohol use and dependence (F10.-)
       exposure to environmental tobacco smoke (Z77.22)
       history of tobacco dependence (Z87.891)
       occupational exposure to environmental tobacco smoke (Z57.31)
       tobacco dependence (F17.-)
       tobacco use (Z72.0)
     EXCLUDES 2   personal history of benign neoplasm (Z86.01-)
                personal history of carcinoma-in-situ (Z86.00-)

   ☑5ᵗʰ Z85.0 Personal history of malignant neoplasm of digestive organs
     AHA: 2017, 1Q, 9

     Z85.00 Personal history of malignant neoplasm of unspecified digestive organ

     Z85.01 Personal history of malignant neoplasm of esophagus
       Conditions classifiable to C15

   ☑6ᵗʰ Z85.02 Personal history of malignant neoplasm of stomach

     Z85.020 Personal history of malignant carcinoid tumor of stomach
       Conditions classifiable to C7A.092

     Z85.028 Personal history of other malignant neoplasm of stomach
       Conditions classifiable to C16

   ☑6ᵗʰ Z85.03 Personal history of malignant neoplasm of large intestine

     Z85.030 Personal history of malignant carcinoid tumor of large intestine
       Conditions classifiable to C7A.022-C7A.025, C7A.029

     Z85.038 Personal history of other malignant neoplasm of large intestine
       Conditions classifiable to C18

   ☑6ᵗʰ Z85.04 Personal history of malignant neoplasm of rectum, rectosigmoid junction, and anus

     Z85.040 Personal history of malignant carcinoid tumor of rectum
       Conditions classifiable to C7A.026

     Z85.048 Personal history of other malignant neoplasm of rectum, rectosigmoid junction, and anus
       Conditions classifiable to C19-C21

     Z85.05 Personal history of malignant neoplasm of liver
       Conditions classifiable to C22

   ☑6ᵗʰ Z85.06 Personal history of malignant neoplasm of small intestine

     Z85.060 Personal history of malignant carcinoid tumor of small intestine
       Conditions classifiable to C7A.01-

     Z85.068 Personal history of other malignant neoplasm of small intestine
       Conditions classifiable to C17

     Z85.07 Personal history of malignant neoplasm of pancreas
       Conditions classifiable to C25

     Z85.09 Personal history of malignant neoplasm of other digestive organs

   ☑5ᵗʰ Z85.1 Personal history of malignant neoplasm of trachea, bronchus and lung

   ☑6ᵗʰ Z85.11 Personal history of malignant neoplasm of bronchus and lung

     Z85.110 Personal history of malignant carcinoid tumor of bronchus and lung
       Conditions classifiable to C7A.090

     Z85.118 Personal history of other malignant neoplasm of bronchus and lung
       Conditions classifiable to C34

     Z85.12 Personal history of malignant neoplasm of trachea
       Conditions classifiable to C33

   ☑5ᵗʰ Z85.2 Personal history of malignant neoplasm of other respiratory and intrathoracic organs

     Z85.20 Personal history of malignant neoplasm of unspecified respiratory organ

     Z85.21 Personal history of malignant neoplasm of larynx
       Conditions classifiable to C32

     Z85.22 Personal history of malignant neoplasm of nasal cavities, middle ear, and accessory sinuses
       Conditions classifiable to C30-C31

   ☑6ᵗʰ Z85.23 Personal history of malignant neoplasm of thymus

     Z85.230 Personal history of malignant carcinoid tumor of thymus
       Conditions classifiable to C7A.091

     Z85.238 Personal history of other malignant neoplasm of thymus
       Conditions classifiable to C37

     Z85.29 Personal history of malignant neoplasm of other respiratory and intrathoracic organs

   Z85.3 Personal history of malignant neoplasm of breast
     Conditions classifiable to C50.-

   ☑5ᵗʰ Z85.4 Personal history of malignant neoplasm of genital organs
     Conditions classifiable to C51-C63

     Z85.40 Personal history of malignant neoplasm of unspecified female genital organ   ♀

☑ Additional Character Req   ☑x7ᵗʰ Placeholder Alert   Unacceptable PDx   Manifestation   **H1 - H14** HAC   **HCC** CMS-HCC Condition   *EXCLUDES 1* Not Coded Here   *EXCLUDES 2* Not Included Here

Z85.41 Personal history of malignant neoplasm of **cervix uteri** ♀

Z85.42 Personal history of malignant neoplasm of **other parts of uterus** ♀

Z85.43 Personal history of malignant neoplasm of **ovary** ♀

Z85.44 Personal history of malignant neoplasm of **other female genital organs** ♀

Z85.45 Personal history of malignant neoplasm of **unspecified male genital organ** ♂

Z85.46 Personal history of malignant neoplasm of **prostate** ♂

Z85.47 Personal history of malignant neoplasm of **testis** ♂

Z85.48 Personal history of malignant neoplasm of **epididymis** ♂

Z85.49 Personal history of malignant neoplasm of **other male genital organs** ♂

✓5th **Z85.5** Personal history of malignant neoplasm of **urinary tract**
Conditions classifiable to C64-C68

Z85.50 Personal history of malignant neoplasm of **unspecified urinary tract organ**

Z85.51 Personal history of malignant neoplasm of **bladder**

✓6th **Z85.52** Personal history of malignant neoplasm of **kidney**
EXCLUDES 1   personal history of malignant neoplasm of renal pelvis (Z85.53)

    Z85.520 Personal history of malignant **carcinoid tumor of kidney**
Conditions classifiable to C7A.093

    Z85.528 Personal history of **other malignant neoplasm of kidney**
Conditions classifiable to C64

Z85.53 Personal history of malignant neoplasm of **renal pelvis**

Z85.54 Personal history of malignant neoplasm of **ureter**

Z85.59 Personal history of malignant neoplasm of **other urinary tract organ**

Z85.6 Personal history of **leukemia**
Conditions classifiable to C91-C95
EXCLUDES 1   leukemia in remission C91.0-C95.9 with 5th character 1

✓5th **Z85.7** Personal history of other malignant neoplasms of lymphoid, hematopoietic and related tissues

    Z85.71 Personal history of **Hodgkin lymphoma**
Conditions classifiable to C81

    Z85.72 Personal history of **non-Hodgkin lymphomas**
Conditions classifiable to C82-C85

    Z85.79 Personal history of **other malignant neoplasms of lymphoid, hematopoietic and related tissues**
Conditions classifiable to C88-C90, C96
EXCLUDES 1   multiple myeloma in remission (C90.01)
plasma cell leukemia in remission (C90.11)
plasmacytoma in remission (C90.21)

✓5th **Z85.8** Personal history of malignant neoplasms of other organs and systems
Conditions classifiable to C00-C14, C40-C49, C69-C75, C7A.098, C76-C79

✓6th **Z85.81** Personal history of malignant neoplasm of **lip, oral cavity, and pharynx**

    Z85.810 Personal history of malignant neoplasm of **tongue**

    Z85.818 Personal history of malignant neoplasm of **other sites of lip, oral cavity, and pharynx**

    Z85.819 Personal history of malignant neoplasm of **unspecified site of lip, oral cavity, and pharynx**

✓6th **Z85.82** Personal history of malignant neoplasm of **skin**

    Z85.820 Personal history of malignant **melanoma of skin**
Conditions classifiable to C43

    Z85.821 Personal history of **Merkel cell carcinoma**
Conditions classifiable to C4A

    Z85.828 Personal history of **other malignant neoplasm of skin**
Conditions classifiable to C44

✓6th **Z85.83** Personal history of malignant neoplasm of **bone and soft tissue**

    Z85.830 Personal history of malignant neoplasm of **bone**

    Z85.831 Personal history of malignant neoplasm of **soft tissue**
EXCLUDES 2   personal history of malignant neoplasm of skin (Z85.82-)

✓6th **Z85.84** Personal history of malignant neoplasm of **eye and nervous tissue**

    Z85.840 Personal history of malignant neoplasm of **eye**

    Z85.841 Personal history of malignant neoplasm of **brain**

    Z85.848 Personal history of malignant neoplasm of **other parts of nervous tissue**

✓6th **Z85.85** Personal history of malignant neoplasm of **endocrine glands**

    Z85.850 Personal history of malignant neoplasm of **thyroid**

    Z85.858 Personal history of malignant neoplasm of **other endocrine glands**

Z85.89 Personal history of malignant neoplasm of **other organs and systems**

Z85.9 Personal history of malignant neoplasm, **unspecified**
Conditions classifiable to C7A.00, C80.1

✓4th **Z86** Personal history of certain other diseases
Code first any follow-up examination after treatment (Z09)

✓5th **Z86.0** Personal history of in-situ and benign neoplasms and neoplasms of uncertain behavior
EXCLUDES 2   personal history of malignant neoplasms (Z85.-)
AHA: 2017, 1Q, 9

✓6th **Z86.00** Personal history of **in-situ neoplasm**
Conditions classifiable to D00-D09

    Z86.000 Personal history of in-situ neoplasm of **breast**

    Z86.001 Personal history of in-situ neoplasm of **cervix uteri** ♀
Personal history of cervical intraepithelial neoplasia III [CIN III]

    Z86.008 Personal history of in-situ neoplasm of **other site**
Personal history of vaginal intraepithelial neoplasia III [VAIN III]
Personal history of vulvar intraepithelial neoplasia III [VIN III]

✓6th **Z86.01** Personal history of **benign neoplasm**

    Z86.010 Personal history of **colonic polyps**
AHA: 2017, 1Q, 14

    Z86.011 Personal history of benign neoplasm of **the brain**

    Z86.012 Personal history of benign **carcinoid tumor**

    Z86.018 Personal history of **other benign neoplasm**
AHA: 2017, 1Q, 14

Z86.03 Personal history of **neoplasm of uncertain behavior**

✓5th **Z86.1** Personal history of infectious and parasitic diseases
Conditions classifiable to A00-B89, B99
EXCLUDES 1   personal history of infectious diseases specific to a body system
sequelae of infectious and parasitic diseases (B90-B94)

Z86.11 Personal history of **tuberculosis**

Z86.12 Personal history of **poliomyelitis**

Z86.13 Personal history of **malaria**

Z86.14 Personal history of **Methicillin resistant Staphylococcus aureus infection**
Personal history of MRSA infection

Z86.19 Personal history of **other infectious and parasitic diseases**

Z86.2 Personal history of diseases of the **blood and blood-forming organs and certain disorders involving the immune mechanism**
Conditions classifiable to D50-D89

✓5th **Z86.3** Personal history of **endocrine, nutritional and metabolic diseases**
Conditions classifiable to E00-E88

Z86.31 Personal history of **diabetic foot ulcer**
EXCLUDES 2   current diabetic foot ulcer (E08.621, E09.621, E10.621, E11.621, E13.621)

N Newborn: 0   P Pediatric: 0-17   M Maternity: 12-55   A Adult: 15-124   **MCC** Major CC Condition   **PDx MCC** PDx acts as own MCC   **CC** CC Condition   **PDx CC** PDx acts as own CC

Z86.32   **Personal history of gestational diabetes**   ♀
Personal history of conditions classifiable to O24.4-
EXCLUDES 1   *gestational diabetes mellitus in current pregnancy (O24.4-)*

Z86.39   **Personal history of other endocrine, nutritional and metabolic disease**

✓5ᵗʰ **Z86.5**   **Personal history of mental and behavioral disorders**
Conditions classifiable to F40-F59

Z86.51   **Personal history of combat and operational stress reaction**   A

Z86.59   **Personal history of other mental and behavioral disorders**

✓5ᵗʰ **Z86.6**   **Personal history of diseases of the nervous system and sense organs**
Conditions classifiable to G00-G99, H00-H95
EXCLUDES 2   *personal history of anaphylactic shock (Z87.892)*

Z86.61   **Personal history of infections of the central nervous system**
Personal history of encephalitis
Personal history of meningitis

Z86.69   **Personal history of other diseases of the nervous system and sense organs**

✓5ᵗʰ **Z86.7**   **Personal history of diseases of the circulatory system**
Conditions classifiable to I00-I99
EXCLUDES 2   *old myocardial infarction (I25.2)*
personal history of anaphylactic shock (Z87.892)
postmyocardial infarction syndrome (I24.1)

✓6ᵗʰ **Z86.71**   **Personal history of venous thrombosis and embolism**

Z86.711   **Personal history of pulmonary embolism**

Z86.718   **Personal history of other venous thrombosis and embolism**

Z86.72   **Personal history of thrombophlebitis**

Z86.73   **Personal history of transient ischemic attack (TIA), and cerebral infarction without residual deficits**
Personal history of prolonged reversible ischemic neurological deficit (PRIND)
Personal history of stroke NOS without residual deficits
EXCLUDES 1   *personal history of traumatic brain injury (Z87.820)*
sequelae of cerebrovascular disease (I69.-)
AHA: 2012, 4Q, 92

Z86.74   **Personal history of sudden cardiac arrest**
Personal history of sudden cardiac death successfully resuscitated

Z86.79   **Personal history of other diseases of the circulatory system**

✓4ᵗʰ **Z87**   **Personal history of other diseases and conditions**
Code first any follow-up examination after treatment (Z09)

✓5ᵗʰ **Z87.0**   **Personal history of diseases of the respiratory system**
Conditions classifiable to J00-J99

Z87.01   **Personal history of pneumonia (recurrent)**

Z87.09   **Personal history of other diseases of the respiratory system**

✓5ᵗʰ **Z87.1**   **Personal history of diseases of the digestive system**
Conditions classifiable to K00-K93

Z87.11   **Personal history of peptic ulcer disease**

Z87.19   **Personal history of other diseases of the digestive system**
AHA: 2017, 1Q, 14

Z87.2   **Personal history of diseases of the skin and subcutaneous tissue**
Conditions classifiable to L00-L99
EXCLUDES 2   *personal history of diabetic foot ulcer (Z86.31)*

✓5ᵗʰ **Z87.3**   **Personal history of diseases of the musculoskeletal system and connective tissue**
Conditions classifiable to M00-M99
EXCLUDES 2   *personal history of (healed) traumatic fracture (Z87.81)*

✓6ᵗʰ **Z87.31**   **Personal history of (healed) nontraumatic fracture**

Z87.310   **Personal history of (healed) osteoporosis fracture**
Personal history of (healed) fragility fracture
Personal history of (healed) collapsed vertebra due to osteoporosis

Z87.311   **Personal history of (healed) other pathological fracture**
Personal history of (healed) collapsed vertebra NOS
EXCLUDES 2   *personal history of osteoporosis fracture (Z87.310)*

Z87.312   **Personal history of (healed) stress fracture**
Personal history of (healed) fatigue fracture

Z87.39   **Personal history of other diseases of the musculoskeletal system and connective tissue**

✓5ᵗʰ **Z87.4**   **Personal history of diseases of genitourinary system**
Conditions classifiable to N00-N99

✓6ᵗʰ **Z87.41**   **Personal history of dysplasia of the female genital tract**
EXCLUDES 1   *personal history of intraepithelial neoplasia III of female genital tract ▶(Z86.001, Z86.008)◀*
personal history of malignant neoplasm of female genital tract (Z85.40-Z85.44)

Z87.410   **Personal history of cervical dysplasia**   ♀

Z87.411   **Personal history of vaginal dysplasia**   ♀

Z87.412   **Personal history of vulvar dysplasia**   ♀

Z87.42   **Personal history of other diseases of the female genital tract**   ♀

✓6ᵗʰ **Z87.43**   **Personal history of diseases of the male genital organs**

Z87.430   **Personal history of prostatic dysplasia**   ♂
EXCLUDES 1   *personal history of malignant neoplasm of prostate (Z85.46)*

Z87.438   **Personal history of other diseases of male genital organs**   ♂

✓6ᵗʰ **Z87.44**   **Personal history of diseases of the urinary system**
EXCLUDES 1   *personal history of malignant neoplasm of cervix uteri (Z85.41)*

Z87.440   **Personal history of urinary (tract) infections**

Z87.441   **Personal history of nephrotic syndrome**

Z87.442   **Personal history of urinary calculi**
Personal history of kidney stones

Z87.448   **Personal history of other diseases of urinary system**

✓5ᵗʰ **Z87.5**   **Personal history of complications of pregnancy, childbirth and the puerperium**
Conditions classifiable to O00-O9A
EXCLUDES 2   *recurrent pregnancy loss (N96)*

Z87.51   **Personal history of pre-term labor**   ♀
EXCLUDES 1   *current pregnancy with history of pre-term labor (O09.21-)*

Z87.59   **Personal history of other complications of pregnancy, childbirth and the puerperium**   ♀
Personal history of trophoblastic disease

✓5th Z87.7 Personal history of (corrected) congenital malformations
Conditions classifiable to Q00-Q89 that have been repaired or corrected

> EXCLUDES 1   congenital malformations that have been partially corrected or repaired but which still require medical treatment—code to condition

> EXCLUDES 2   other postprocedural states (Z98.-)
> personal history of medical treatment (Z92.-)
> presence of cardiac and vascular implants and grafts (Z95.-)
> presence of other devices (Z97.-)
> presence of other functional implants (Z96.-)
> transplanted organ and tissue status (Z94.-)

✓6th Z87.71 Personal history of (corrected) congenital malformations of genitourinary system

     Z87.710 Personal history of (corrected) hypospadias ♂

     Z87.718 Personal history of other specified (corrected) congenital malformations of genitourinary system

✓6th Z87.72 Personal history of (corrected) congenital malformations of nervous system and sense organs

     Z87.720 Personal history of (corrected) congenital malformations of eye

     Z87.721 Personal history of (corrected) congenital malformations of ear

     Z87.728 Personal history of other specified (corrected) congenital malformations of nervous system and sense organs

✓6th Z87.73 Personal history of (corrected) congenital malformations of digestive system

     Z87.730 Personal history of (corrected) cleft lip and palate

     Z87.738 Personal history of other specified (corrected) congenital malformations of digestive system

Z87.74 Personal history of (corrected) congenital malformations of heart and circulatory system

Z87.75 Personal history of (corrected) congenital malformations of respiratory system

Z87.76 Personal history of (corrected) congenital malformations of integument, limbs and musculoskeletal system

✓6th Z87.79 Personal history of other (corrected) congenital malformations

     Z87.790 Personal history of (corrected) congenital malformations of face and neck

     Z87.798 Personal history of other (corrected) congenital malformations

✓5th Z87.8 Personal history of other specified conditions

> EXCLUDES 2   personal history of self harm (Z91.5)

Z87.81 Personal history of (healed) traumatic fracture

> EXCLUDES 2   personal history of (healed) nontraumatic fracture (Z87.31-)

✓6th Z87.82 Personal history of other (healed) physical injury and trauma
Conditions classifiable to S00-T88, except traumatic fractures

     Z87.820 Personal history of traumatic brain injury

> EXCLUDES 1   personal history of transient ischemic attack (TIA), and cerebral infarction without residual deficits (Z86.73)

     Z87.821 Personal history of retained foreign body fully removed

     Z87.828 Personal history of other (healed) physical injury and trauma

✓6th Z87.89 Personal history of other specified conditions

     Z87.890 Personal history of sex reassignment

     Z87.891 Personal history of nicotine dependence

> EXCLUDES 1   current nicotine dependence (F17.2-)

> AHA: 2017, 2Q, 27

     Z87.892 Personal history of anaphylaxis
Code also allergy status such as:
allergy status to drugs, medicaments and biological substances (Z88.-)
allergy status, other than to drugs and biological substances (Z91.0-)

Z87.898 Personal history of other specified conditions

> AHA: 2013, 1Q, 21

✓4th Z88 Allergy status to drugs, medicaments and biological substances

> EXCLUDES 2   allergy status, other than to drugs and biological substances (Z91.0-)

> AHA: 2015, 3Q, 23

Z88.0 Allergy status to penicillin

Z88.1 Allergy status to other antibiotic agents status

Z88.2 Allergy status to sulfonamides status

Z88.3 Allergy status to other anti-infective agents status

Z88.4 Allergy status to anesthetic agent status

Z88.5 Allergy status to narcotic agent status

Z88.6 Allergy status to analgesic agent status

Z88.7 Allergy status to serum and vaccine status

Z88.8 Allergy status to other drugs, medicaments and biological substances status

Z88.9 Allergy status to unspecified drugs, medicaments and biological substances status

✓4th Z89 Acquired absence of limb

> INCLUDES   amputation status
> postprocedural loss of limb
> post-traumatic loss of limb

> EXCLUDES 1   acquired deformities of limbs (M20-M21)
> congenital absence of limbs (Q71-Q73)

✓5th Z89.0 Acquired absence of thumb and other finger(s)

✓6th Z89.01 Acquired absence of thumb

     Z89.011 Acquired absence of right thumb

     Z89.012 Acquired absence of left thumb

     Z89.019 Acquired absence of unspecified thumb

✓6th Z89.02 Acquired absence of other finger(s)

> EXCLUDES 2   acquired absence of thumb (Z89.01-)

     Z89.021 Acquired absence of right finger(s)

     Z89.022 Acquired absence of left finger(s)

     Z89.029 Acquired absence of unspecified finger(s)

✓5th Z89.1 Acquired absence of hand and wrist

✓6th Z89.11 Acquired absence of hand

     Z89.111 Acquired absence of right hand

     Z89.112 Acquired absence of left hand

     Z89.119 Acquired absence of unspecified hand

✓6th Z89.12 Acquired absence of wrist
Disarticulation at wrist

     Z89.121 Acquired absence of right wrist

     Z89.122 Acquired absence of left wrist

     Z89.129 Acquired absence of unspecified wrist

✓5th Z89.2 Acquired absence of upper limb above wrist

✓6th Z89.20 Acquired absence of upper limb, unspecified level

     Z89.201 Acquired absence of right upper limb, unspecified level

     Z89.202 Acquired absence of left upper limb, unspecified level

     Z89.209 Acquired absence of unspecified upper limb, unspecified level
Acquired absence of arm NOS

✓6th Z89.21 Acquired absence of upper limb below elbow

     Z89.211 Acquired absence of right upper limb below elbow

     Z89.212 Acquired absence of left upper limb below elbow

     Z89.219 Acquired absence of unspecified upper limb below elbow

✓6th Z89.22 Acquired absence of upper limb above elbow
Disarticulation at elbow

     Z89.221 Acquired absence of right upper limb above elbow

     Z89.222 Acquired absence of left upper limb above elbow

     Z89.229 Acquired absence of unspecified upper limb above elbow

✓6th Z89.23 Acquired absence of shoulder
Acquired absence of shoulder joint following explantation of shoulder joint prosthesis, with or without presence of antibiotic-impregnated cement spacer

     Z89.231 Acquired absence of right shoulder

     Z89.232   **Acquired absence of** left shoulder

     Z89.239   **Acquired absence of** unspecified **shoulder**

✓5ᵗʰ **Z89.4   Acquired absence of** toe(s), foot, and ankle

   ✓6ᵗʰ **Z89.41   Acquired absence of** great toe

     Z89.411   **Acquired absence of** right great toe   HCC

     Z89.412   **Acquired absence of** left great toe   HCC

     Z89.419   **Acquired absence of** unspecified great toe   HCC

   ✓6ᵗʰ **Z89.42   Acquired absence of** other toe(s)

     EXCLUDES 2   *acquired absence of great toe (Z89.41-)*

     Z89.421   **Acquired absence of other right toe(s)** HCC

     Z89.422   **Acquired absence of other left toe(s)** HCC

     Z89.429   **Acquired absence of other toe(s), unspecified side** HCC

   ✓6ᵗʰ **Z89.43   Acquired absence of** foot

     Z89.431   **Acquired absence of** right foot   HCC

     Z89.432   **Acquired absence of** left foot   HCC

     Z89.439   **Acquired absence of** unspecified foot   HCC

   ✓6ᵗʰ **Z89.44   Acquired absence of** ankle

     Disarticulation of ankle

     Z89.441   **Acquired absence of** right ankle   HCC

     Z89.442   **Acquired absence of** left ankle   HCC

     Z89.449   **Acquired absence of** unspecified ankle HCC

✓5ᵗʰ **Z89.5   Acquired absence of leg below knee**

   ✓6ᵗʰ **Z89.51   Acquired absence of** leg below knee

     Z89.511   **Acquired absence of** right leg below knee   HCC

     Z89.512   **Acquired absence of** left leg below knee   HCC

     Z89.519   **Acquired absence of** unspecified leg below knee   HCC

   ✓6ᵗʰ **Z89.52   Acquired absence of** knee

     Acquired absence of knee joint following explantation of knee joint prosthesis, with or without presence of antibiotic-impregnated cement spacer

     Z89.521   **Acquired absence of** right **knee**

     Z89.522   **Acquired absence of** left **knee**

     Z89.529   **Acquired absence of** unspecified **knee**

✓5ᵗʰ **Z89.6   Acquired absence of leg above knee**

   ✓6ᵗʰ **Z89.61   Acquired absence of** leg above knee

     Acquired absence of leg NOS

     Disarticulation at knee

     Z89.611   **Acquired absence of** right leg above knee   HCC

     Z89.612   **Acquired absence of** left leg above knee   HCC

     Z89.619   **Acquired absence of** unspecified leg above knee   HCC

   ✓6ᵗʰ **Z89.62   Acquired absence of** hip

     Acquired absence of hip joint following explantation of hip joint prosthesis, with or without presence of antibiotic-impregnated cement spacer

     Disarticulation at hip

     Z89.621   **Acquired absence of** right hip joint

     Z89.622   **Acquired absence of** left hip joint

     Z89.629   **Acquired absence of** unspecified hip joint

  Z89.9   Acquired absence of limb, unspecified

✓4ᵗʰ **Z90   Acquired absence of organs, not elsewhere classified**

   INCLUDES   postprocedural or post-traumatic loss of body part NEC

   EXCLUDES 1   *congenital absence—see Alphabetical Index*

   EXCLUDES 2   *postprocedural absence of endocrine glands (E89.-)*

   ✓5ᵗʰ **Z90.0   Acquired absence of part of** head and neck

     Z90.01   **Acquired absence of** eye

     Z90.02   **Acquired absence of** larynx

     Z90.09   **Acquired absence of** other **part of head and neck**

      Acquired absence of nose

      EXCLUDES 2   *teeth (K08.1)*

   ✓5ᵗʰ **Z90.1   Acquired absence of** breast and nipple

     Z90.10   **Acquired absence of** unspecified **breast and nipple**

     Z90.11   **Acquired absence of** right **breast and nipple**

     Z90.12   **Acquired absence of** left **breast and nipple**

     Z90.13   **Acquired absence of** bilateral **breasts and nipples**

  Z90.2   Acquired absence of lung [part of]

  Z90.3   Acquired absence of stomach [part of]

   ✓5ᵗʰ **Z90.4   Acquired absence of** other specified parts of digestive tract

   ✓6ᵗʰ **Z90.41   Acquired absence of** pancreas

     Code also exocrine pancreatic insufficiency (K86.81)

     Use additional code to identify any associated:

      insulin use (Z79.4)

      diabetes mellitus, postpancreatectomy (E13.-)

     Z90.410   **Acquired total absence of pancreas**

      Acquired absence of pancreas NOS

     Z90.411   **Acquired partial absence of pancreas**

     Z90.49   **Acquired absence of** other specified parts of digestive tract

  Z90.5   Acquired absence of kidney

  Z90.6   Acquired absence of other parts of urinary tract

     Acquired absence of bladder

   ✓5ᵗʰ **Z90.7   Acquired absence of** genital organ(s)

     EXCLUDES 1   *personal history of sex reassignment (Z87.890)*

     EXCLUDES 2   *female genital mutilation status (N90.81-)*

   ✓6ᵗʰ **Z90.71   Acquired absence of** cervix and uterus

     Z90.710   **Acquired absence of** both **cervix and uterus** ♀

      Acquired absence of uterus NOS

      Status post total hysterectomy

     Z90.711   **Acquired absence of uterus with remaining cervical stump** ♀

      Status post partial hysterectomy with remaining cervical stump

     Z90.712   **Acquired absence of cervix with remaining uterus** ♀

   ✓6ᵗʰ **Z90.72   Acquired absence of** ovaries

     Z90.721   **Acquired absence of ovaries,** unilateral ♀

     Z90.722   **Acquired absence of ovaries,** bilateral ♀

     Z90.79   **Acquired absence of** other genital organ(s)

   ✓5ᵗʰ **Z90.8   Acquired absence of** other organs

     Z90.81   **Acquired absence of** spleen

     Z90.89   **Acquired absence of** other organs

✓4ᵗʰ **Z91   Personal risk factors, not elsewhere classified**

   EXCLUDES 2   *contact with and (suspected) exposures hazardous to health (Z77.-)*

     exposure to pollution and other problems related to physical environment (Z77.1-)

     ▶*female genital mutilation status (N90.81-)*◀

     personal history of physical injury and trauma (Z87.81, Z87.82-)

     occupational exposure to risk factors (Z57.-)

   ✓5ᵗʰ **Z91.0   Allergy status, other than to drugs and biological substances**

     EXCLUDES 2   *allergy status to drugs, medicaments, and biological substances (Z88.-)*

   ✓6ᵗʰ **Z91.01   Food allergy status**

     EXCLUDES 2   *food additives allergy status (Z91.02)*

     Z91.010   **Allergy to** peanuts

     Z91.011   **Allergy to** milk products

      EXCLUDES 1   *lactose intolerance (E73.-)*

     Z91.012   **Allergy to** eggs

     Z91.013   **Allergy to** seafood

      Allergy to shellfish

      Allergy to octopus or squid ink

     Z91.018   **Allergy to** other **foods**

      Allergy to nuts other than peanuts

     Z91.02   **Food additives allergy status**

   ✓6ᵗʰ **Z91.03   Insect allergy status**

     Z91.030   **Bee allergy status**

     Z91.038   **Other insect allergy status**

   ✓6ᵗʰ **Z91.04   Nonmedicinal substance allergy status**

     Z91.040   **Latex allergy status**

      Latex sensitivity status

     Z91.041   **Radiographic dye allergy status**

      Allergy status to contrast media used for diagnostic X-ray procedure

     Z91.048   **Other nonmedicinal substance allergy status**

     Z91.09   **Other allergy status, other than to drugs and biological substances**

   ✓5ᵗʰ **Z91.1   Patient's noncompliance with medical treatment and regimen**

     Z91.11   **Patient's noncompliance with** dietary regimen

---

✓ Additional Character Req   ✓x7ᵗʰ Placeholder Alert   Unacceptable PDx   Manifestation   H1 - H14 HAC   HCC CMS-HCC Condition   EXCLUDES 1 Not Coded Here   EXCLUDES 2 Not Included Here

ICD-10-CM 2018   1245

Chapter 21. Factors Influencing Health Status and Contact with Health Services

✓6ᵗʰ **Z91.12 Patient's intentional underdosing of medication regimen**
Code first underdosing of medication (T36-T50) with fifth or sixth character 6
EXCLUDES 1   *adverse effect of prescribed drug taken as directed—code to adverse effect*
poisoning (overdose)—code to poisoning

Z91.120 Patient's intentional underdosing of medication regimen due to financial hardship

Z91.128 Patient's intentional underdosing of medication regimen for other reason

✓6ᵗʰ **Z91.13 Patient's unintentional underdosing of medication regimen**
Code first underdosing of medication (T36-T50) with fifth or sixth character 6
EXCLUDES 1   *adverse effect of prescribed drug taken as directed—code to adverse effect*
poisoning (overdose)—code to poisoning

Z91.130 Patient's unintentional underdosing of medication regimen due to age-related debility

Z91.138 Patient's unintentional underdosing of medication regimen for other reason

Z91.14 Patient's other noncompliance with medication regimen
Patient's underdosing of medication NOS

Z91.15 Patient's noncompliance with renal dialysis   HCC

Z91.19 Patient's noncompliance with other medical treatment and regimen
▶Nonadherence to medical treatment◀

✓5ᵗʰ **Z91.4 Personal history of psychological trauma, not elsewhere classified**

✓6ᵗʰ **Z91.41 Personal history of adult abuse**
EXCLUDES 2   *personal history of abuse in childhood (Z62.81-)*

Z91.410 Personal history of adult physical and sexual abuse   A
EXCLUDES 1   *current adult physical abuse (T74.11, T76.11)*
current adult sexual abuse (T74.21, T76.11)

Z91.411 Personal history of adult psychological abuse   A

Z91.412 Personal history of adult neglect   A
EXCLUDES 1   *current adult neglect (T74.01, T76.01)*

Z91.419 Personal history of unspecified adult abuse   A

Z91.49 Other personal history of psychological trauma, not elsewhere classified

Z91.5 Personal history of self-harm
Personal history of parasuicide
Personal history of self-poisoning
Personal history of suicide attempt

✓5ᵗʰ **Z91.8 Other specified personal risk factors, not elsewhere classified**

Z91.81 History of falling
At risk for falling

Z91.82 Personal history of military deployment   A
Individual (civilian or military) with past history of military war, peacekeeping and humanitarian deployment (current or past conflict)
Returned from military deployment

Z91.83 Wandering in diseases classified elsewhere
Code first underlying disorder such as:
Alzheimer's disease (G30.-)
autism or pervasive developmental disorder (F84.-)
intellectual disabilities (F70-F79)
unspecified dementia with behavioral disturbance (F03.9-)

✓6ᵗʰ **Z91.84 Oral health risk factors**

Z91.841 Risk for dental caries, low

Z91.842 Risk for dental caries, moderate

Z91.843 Risk for dental caries, high

Z91.849 Unspecified risk for dental caries

Z91.89 Other specified personal risk factors, not elsewhere classified
AHA: 2017, 1Q, 45

✓4ᵗʰ **Z92 Personal history of medical treatment**
EXCLUDES 2   *postprocedural states (Z98.-)*

Z92.0 Personal history of contraception
EXCLUDES 1   *counseling or management of current contraceptive practices (Z30.-)*
long term (current) use of contraception (Z79.3)
presence of (intrauterine) contraceptive device (Z97.5)

✓5ᵗʰ **Z92.2 Personal history of drug therapy**
EXCLUDES 2   *long term (current) drug therapy (Z79.-)*

Z92.21 Personal history of antineoplastic chemotherapy

Z92.22 Personal history of monoclonal drug therapy

Z92.23 Personal history of estrogen therapy

✓6ᵗʰ **Z92.24 Personal history of steroid therapy**

Z92.240 Personal history of inhaled steroid therapy

Z92.241 Personal history of systemic steroid therapy
Personal history of steroid therapy NOS

Z92.25 Personal history of immunosupression therapy
EXCLUDES 2   *personal history of steroid therapy (Z92.24)*

Z92.29 Personal history of other drug therapy

Z92.3 Personal history of irradiation
Personal history of exposure to therapeutic radiation
EXCLUDES 1   *exposure to radiation in the physical environment (Z77.12)*
occupational exposure to radiation (Z57.1)

✓5ᵗʰ **Z92.8 Personal history of other medical treatment**

Z92.81 Personal history of extracorporeal membrane oxygenation (ECMO)

Z92.82 Status post administration of tPA (rtPA) in a different facility within the last 24 hours prior to admission to current facility
Code first condition requiring tPA administration, such as:
acute cerebral infarction (I63.-)
acute myocardial infarction (I21-, I22-)
AHA: 2013, 4Q, 124

Z92.83 Personal history of failed moderate sedation
Personal history of failed conscious sedation
EXCLUDES 2   *failed moderate sedation during procedure (T88.52)*

Z92.84 Personal history of unintended awareness under general anesthesia
EXCLUDES 2   *unintended awareness under general anesthesia during procedure (T88.53)*

Z92.89 Personal history of other medical treatment

✓4ᵗʰ **Z93 Artificial opening status**
EXCLUDES 1   *artificial openings requiring attention or management (Z43.-)*
complications of external stoma (J95.0-, K94.-, N99.5-)

Z93.0 Tracheostomy status   HCC
AHA: 2013, 4Q, 129

Z93.1 Gastrostomy status   HCC

Z93.2 Ileostomy status   HCC

Z93.3 Colostomy status   HCC

Z93.4 Other artificial openings of gastrointestinal tract status   HCC

✓5ᵗʰ **Z93.5 Cystostomy status**

Z93.50 Unspecified cystostomy status   HCC

Z93.51 Cutaneous-vesicostomy status   HCC

Z93.52 Appendico-vesicostomy status   HCC

Z93.59 Other cystostomy status   HCC

Z93.6 Other artificial openings of urinary tract status   HCC
Nephrostomy status
Ureterostomy status
Urethrostomy status

Z93.8 Other artificial opening status   HCC

Z93.9 Artificial opening status, unspecified   HCC

✓4ᵗʰ **Z94 Transplanted organ and tissue status**
INCLUDES   organ or tissue replaced by heterogenous or homogenous transplant
EXCLUDES 1   *complications of transplanted organ or tissue—see Alphabetical Index*
EXCLUDES 2   *presence of vascular grafts (Z95.-)*

Z94.0 Kidney transplant status   CC
CC Excl: PDX collection 1489

N Newborn: 0   P Pediatric: 0-17   M Maternity: 12-55   A Adult: 15-124   MCC Major CC Condition   PDxMCC PDx acts as own MCC   CC CC Condition   PDxCC PDx acts as own CC

Z94.1 Heart transplant status   `CC` `HCC`
> *EXCLUDES 1*   *artificial heart status (Z95.812)*
> *heart-valve replacement status (Z95.2-Z95.4)*
> **CC Excl:** PDX collection 1488

Z94.2 Lung transplant status   `CC` `HCC`
> **CC Excl:** PDX collection 1491

Z94.3 Heart and lungs transplant status   `PDxCC` `CC` `HCC`
> **CC Excl:** PDX collection 1488

Z94.4 Liver transplant status   `CC` `HCC`
> **CC Excl:** PDX collection 1490

Z94.5 Skin transplant status
> Autogenous skin transplant status

Z94.6 Bone transplant status

Z94.7 Corneal transplant status

√5ᵗʰ **Z94.8** Other transplanted organ and tissue status

> **Z94.81** Bone marrow transplant status   `CC` `HCC`
> > **CC Excl:** PDX collection 1492

> **Z94.82** Intestine transplant status   `CC` `HCC`
> > **CC Excl:** PDX collection 1495

> **Z94.83** Pancreas transplant status   `CC` `HCC`
> > **CC Excl:** PDX collection 1496

> **Z94.84** Stem cells transplant status   `CC` `HCC`
> > **CC Excl:** PDX collection 1497

> **Z94.89** Other transplanted organ and tissue status

Z94.9 Transplanted organ and tissue status, unspecified

√4ᵗʰ **Z95** Presence of cardiac and vascular implants and grafts
> *EXCLUDES 1* ~~complications of cardiac and vascular devices, implants and grafts (T82.-)~~
> *EXCLUDES 2* ▶complications of cardiac and vascular devices, implants and grafts (T82.-)◀

Z95.0 Presence of cardiac pacemaker
> Presence of cardiac resynchronization therapy (CRT-P) pacemaker
> *EXCLUDES 1*   *adjustment or management of cardiac device (Z45.0-)*
> *adjustment or management of cardiac pacemaker (Z45.0)*
> *presence of automatic (implantable) cardiac defibrillator with synchronous cardiac pacemaker (Z95.810)*

Z95.1 Presence of aortocoronary bypass graft
> Presence of coronary artery bypass graft

Z95.2 Presence of prosthetic heart valve
> Presence of heart valve NOS

Z95.3 Presence of xenogenic heart valve

Z95.4 Presence of other heart-valve replacement

Z95.5 Presence of coronary angioplasty implant and graft
> *EXCLUDES 1*   *coronary angioplasty status without implant and graft (Z98.61)*

√5ᵗʰ **Z95.8** Presence of other cardiac and vascular implants and grafts

> √6ᵗʰ **Z95.81** Presence of other cardiac implants and grafts

> > **Z95.810** Presence of automatic (implantable) cardiac defibrillator
> > > Presence of automatic (implantable) cardiac defibrillator with synchronous cardiac pacemaker
> > > Presence of cardiac resynchronization therapy defibrillator (CRT-D)
> > > Presence of cardioverter-defibrillator (ICD)

> > **Z95.811** Presence of heart assist device   `CC` `HCC`
> > > **CC Excl:** PDX collection 1498

> > **Z95.812** Presence of fully implantable artificial heart   `CC` `HCC`
> > > **CC Excl:** PDX collection 1498

> > **Z95.818** Presence of other cardiac implants and grafts

> √6ᵗʰ **Z95.82** Presence of other vascular implants and grafts

> > **Z95.820** Peripheral vascular angioplasty status with implants and grafts
> > > *EXCLUDES 1*   *peripheral vascular angioplasty without implant and graft (Z98.62)*

> > **Z95.828** Presence of other vascular implants and grafts
> > > Presence of intravascular prosthesis NEC

Z95.9 Presence of cardiac and vascular implant and graft, unspecified

---

√4ᵗʰ **Z96** Presence of other functional implants
> *EXCLUDES 2*   *complications of internal prosthetic devices, implants and grafts (T82-T85)*
> *fitting and adjustment of prosthetic and other devices (Z44-Z46)*

Z96.0 Presence of urogenital implants

Z96.1 Presence of intraocular lens
> Presence of pseudophakia

√5ᵗʰ **Z96.2** Presence of otological and audiological implants

> **Z96.20** Presence of otological and audiological implant, unspecified

> **Z96.21** Cochlear implant status

> **Z96.22** Myringotomy tube(s) status

> **Z96.29** Presence of other otological and audiological implants
> > Presence of bone-conduction hearing device
> > Presence of eustachian tube stent
> > Stapes replacement

Z96.3 Presence of artificial larynx

√5ᵗʰ **Z96.4** Presence of endocrine implants

> **Z96.41** Presence of insulin pump (external) (internal)

> **Z96.49** Presence of other endocrine implants

Z96.5 Presence of tooth-root and mandibular implants

√5ᵗʰ **Z96.6** Presence of orthopedic joint implants

> **Z96.60** Presence of unspecified orthopedic joint implant

> √6ᵗʰ **Z96.61** Presence of artificial shoulder joint
> > **Z96.611** Presence of right artificial shoulder joint
> > **Z96.612** Presence of left artificial shoulder joint
> > **Z96.619** Presence of unspecified artificial shoulder joint

> √6ᵗʰ **Z96.62** Presence of artificial elbow joint
> > **Z96.621** Presence of right artificial elbow joint
> > **Z96.622** Presence of left artificial elbow joint
> > **Z96.629** Presence of unspecified artificial elbow joint

> √6ᵗʰ **Z96.63** Presence of artificial wrist joint
> > **Z96.631** Presence of right artificial wrist joint
> > **Z96.632** Presence of left artificial wrist joint
> > **Z96.639** Presence of unspecified artificial wrist joint

> √6ᵗʰ **Z96.64** Presence of artificial hip joint
> > Hip-joint replacement (partial) (total)
> > **Z96.641** Presence of right artificial hip joint
> > **Z96.642** Presence of left artificial hip joint
> > **Z96.643** Presence of artificial hip joint, bilateral
> > **Z96.649** Presence of unspecified artificial hip joint

> √6ᵗʰ **Z96.65** Presence of artificial knee joint
> > **Z96.651** Presence of right artificial knee joint
> > **Z96.652** Presence of left artificial knee joint
> > **Z96.653** Presence of artificial knee joint, bilateral
> > **Z96.659** Presence of unspecified artificial knee joint

> √6ᵗʰ **Z96.66** Presence of artificial ankle joint
> > **Z96.661** Presence of right artificial ankle joint
> > **Z96.662** Presence of left artificial ankle joint
> > **Z96.669** Presence of unspecified artificial ankle joint

> √6ᵗʰ **Z96.69** Presence of other orthopedic joint implants
> > **Z96.691** Finger-joint replacement of right hand
> > **Z96.692** Finger-joint replacement of left hand
> > **Z96.693** Finger-joint replacement, bilateral
> > **Z96.698** Presence of other orthopedic joint implants

Z96.7 Presence of other bone and tendon implants
> Presence of skull plate

√5ᵗʰ **Z96.8** Presence of other specified functional implants

> **Z96.81** Presence of artificial skin

> **Z96.89** Presence of other specified functional implants

Z96.9 Presence of functional implant, unspecified

√ Additional Character Req   √ˣ7ᵗʰ Placeholder Alert   Unacceptable PDx   Manifestation   `H1`-`H14` HAC   `HCC` CMS-HCC Condition   *EXCLUDES 1* Not Coded Here   *EXCLUDES 2* Not Included Here

Chapter 21. Factors Influencing Health Status and Contact with Health Services

Z97–Z99.89

✓4ᵗʰ **Z97 Presence of other devices**
    EXCLUDES 1 *complications of internal prosthetic devices, implants and grafts (T82-T85)*
        fitting and adjustment of prosthetic and other devices (Z44-Z46)
    EXCLUDES 2 *presence of cerebrospinal fluid drainage device (Z98.2)*

    Z97.0 Presence of artificial eye

✓5ᵗʰ   **Z97.1 Presence of artificial limb (complete) (partial)**
    Z97.10 Presence of artificial limb (complete) (partial), unspecified
    Z97.11 Presence of artificial right arm (complete) (partial)
    Z97.12 Presence of artificial left arm (complete) (partial)
    Z97.13 Presence of artificial right leg (complete) (partial)
    Z97.14 Presence of artificial left leg (complete) (partial)
    Z97.15 Presence of artificial arms, bilateral (complete) (partial)
    Z97.16 Presence of artificial legs, bilateral (complete) (partial)

    Z97.2 Presence of dental prosthetic device (complete) (partial)
      Presence of dentures (complete) (partial)

    Z97.3 Presence of spectacles and contact lenses

    Z97.4 Presence of external hearing-aid

    Z97.5 Presence of (intrauterine) contraceptive device ♀
    EXCLUDES 1 *checking, reinsertion or removal of implantable subdermal contraceptive (Z30.46)*
        checking, reinsertion or removal of intrauterine contraceptive device (Z30.43-)

    Z97.8 Presence of other specified devices

✓4ᵗʰ **Z98 Other postprocedural states**
    EXCLUDES 2 *aftercare (Z43-Z49, Z51)*
        follow-up medical care (Z08- Z09)
        postprocedural complication—see Alphabetical Index

    Z98.0 Intestinal bypass and anastomosis status
    EXCLUDES 2 *bariatric surgery status (Z98.84)*
        gastric bypass status (Z98.84)
        obesity surgery status (Z98.84)

    Z98.1 Arthrodesis status

    Z98.2 Presence of cerebrospinal fluid drainage device
      Presence of CSF shunt

    Z98.3 Post therapeutic collapse of lung status
      Code first underlying disease

✓5ᵗʰ   **Z98.4 Cataract extraction status**
    Use additional code to identify intraocular lens implant status (Z96.1)
    EXCLUDES 1 *aphakia (H27.0)*
    Z98.41 Cataract extraction status, right eye
    Z98.42 Cataract extraction status, left eye
    Z98.49 Cataract extraction status, unspecified eye

✓5ᵗʰ   **Z98.5 Sterilization status**
    EXCLUDES 1 *female infertility (N97.-)*
        male infertility (N46.-)
    Z98.51 Tubal ligation status ♀
    Z98.52 Vasectomy status Ⓐ♂

✓5ᵗʰ   **Z98.6 Angioplasty status**
    Z98.61 Coronary angioplasty status
    EXCLUDES 1 *coronary angioplasty status with implant and graft (Z95.5)*
    Z98.62 Peripheral vascular angioplasty status
    EXCLUDES 1 *peripheral vascular angioplasty status with implant and graft (Z95.820)*

✓5ᵗʰ   **Z98.8 Other specified postprocedural states**
✓6ᵗʰ   **Z98.81 Dental procedure status**
      Z98.810 Dental sealant status
      Z98.811 Dental restoration status
        Dental crown status
        Dental fillings status
      Z98.818 Other dental procedure status
    Z98.82 Breast implant status
    EXCLUDES 1 *breast implant removal status (Z98.86)*
    Z98.83 Filtering (vitreous) bleb after glaucoma surgery status
    EXCLUDES 1 *inflammation (infection) of postprocedural bleb (H59.4-)*

    Z98.84 Bariatric surgery status
      Gastric banding status
      Gastric bypass status for obesity
      Obesity surgery status
    EXCLUDES 1 *bariatric surgery status complicating pregnancy, childbirth, or the puerperium (O99.84)*
    EXCLUDES 2 *intestinal bypass and anastomosis status (Z98.0)*

    Z98.85 Transplanted organ removal status
      Transplanted organ previously removed due to complication, failure, rejection or infection
    EXCLUDES 1 *encounter for removal of transplanted organ—code to complication of transplanted organ (T86.-)*

    Z98.86 Personal history of breast implant removal

✓6ᵗʰ   **Z98.87 Personal history of in utero procedure**
    Z98.870 Personal history of in utero procedure during pregnancy ♀
    EXCLUDES 2 *complications from in utero procedure for current pregnancy (O35.7)*
        supervision of current pregnancy with history of in utero procedure during previous pregnancy (O09.82-)
    Z98.871 Personal history of in utero procedure while a fetus

✓6ᵗʰ   **Z98.89 Other specified postprocedural states**
    Z98.890 Other specified postprocedural states
      Personal history of surgery, not elsewhere classified
    Z98.891 History of uterine scar from previous surgery
    EXCLUDES 1 *maternal care due to uterine scar from previous surgery (O34.2-)*

✓4ᵗʰ **Z99 Dependence on enabling machines and devices, not elsewhere classified**
    EXCLUDES 1 *cardiac pacemaker status (Z95.0)*

    Z99.0 Dependence on aspirator

✓5ᵗʰ   **Z99.1 Dependence on respirator**
    Dependence on ventilator

    CC Excl: For CC codes in subcategory Z99.1, unless otherwise noted: PDX collection 759

    Z99.11 Dependence on respirator [ventilator] status CC HCC
      AHA: 2015, 1Q, 21
    Z99.12 Encounter for respirator [ventilator] dependence during power failure CC HCC
    EXCLUDES 1 *mechanical complication of respirator [ventilator] (J95.850)*

    Z99.2 Dependence on renal dialysis HCC
      Hemodialysis status
      Peritoneal dialysis status
      Presence of arteriovenous shunt for dialysis
      Renal dialysis status NOS
    EXCLUDES 1 *encounter for fitting and adjustment of dialysis catheter (Z49.0-)*
    EXCLUDES 2 *noncompliance with renal dialysis (Z91.15)*
    AHA: 2016, 1Q, 12; 2013, 4Q, 125

    Z99.3 Dependence on wheelchair
      Wheelchair confinement status
      Code first cause of dependence, such as:
        muscular dystrophy (G71.0)
        obesity (E66.-)

✓5ᵗʰ   **Z99.8 Dependence on other enabling machines and devices**
    Z99.81 Dependence on supplemental oxygen
      Dependence on long-term oxygen
      AHA: 2013, 4Q, 129
    Z99.89 Dependence on other enabling machines and devices
      Dependence on machine or device NOS

Ⓝ Newborn: 0   Ⓟ Pediatric: 0-17   Ⓜ Maternity: 12-55   Ⓐ Adult: 15-124   **MCC** Major CC Condition   **PDxMCC** PDx acts as own MCC   **CC** CC Condition   **PDxCC** PDx acts as own CC

1248   ICD-10-CM 2018

Appendixes

Appendix A: 10 Steps to Correct Coding

Follow the 10 steps below to correctly code encounters for health care services.

Step 1: Identify the reason for the visit or encounter (i.e., a sign, symptom, diagnosis and/or condition).

The medical record documentation should accurately reflect the patient's condition, using terminology that includes specific diagnoses and symptoms or clearly states the reasons for the encounter.

Choosing the main term that best describes the reason chiefly responsible for the service provided is the most important step in coding. If symptoms are present and documented but a definitive diagnosis has not yet been determined, code the symptoms. **For outpatient cases, do not code conditions that are referred to as "rule out," "suspected," "probable," or "questionable."** Diagnoses often are not established at the time of the initial encounter/visit and may require two or more visits to be established. Code only what is documented in the available records and only to the highest degree of certainty known at the time of the patient's visit, unless it is an inpatient medical record, in which case uncertain diagnoses may be reported if documented at the time of discharge.

Step 2: After selecting the reason for the encounter, always consult the alphabetic index before verifying code selection in the tabular section.

The most critical rule is to begin code selection in the *alphabetic index.* Never turn first to the tabular list. The index provides cross-references, essential and nonessential modifiers, and inclusion terms not found in the tabular list. To prevent coding errors, always use both the alphabetic index (to identify a code) and the tabular list (to verify a code), as the index does not include the important instructional notes found in the tabular list. An added benefit of using the tabular list, which groups like things together, is that while looking at one code in the list, a coder might see a more specific one that would have been missed had the coder relied solely on the alphabetic index. Additionally, many of the codes require a fourth, fifth, sixth, or seventh, character to be valid, and many of these characters can be found only in the tabular list.

Step 3: Locate the main term entry.

The alphabetic index is a listing of conditions, which may be expressed as nouns or eponyms, with critical use of adjectives. Some conditions known by several names have multiple main entries. Reasons for encounters may be located under general terms such as admission, encounter, and examination. Other general terms such as history of, status post, or presence (of) are used to locate factors influencing health.

Step 4: Read cross-references listed with the main term or the subterm.

Cross-references such as *"see"* and *"see also"* are identified by italicized type and should always be checked to ensure that all alternative terms are researched.

Step 5: Review entries for modifiers.

Nonessential modifiers are the terms in parentheses following the main term entry. These parenthetical terms are supplementary words or explanatory information that may or may not appear in the diagnostic statement and do not affect code selection. The subterms listed under the main term are essential modifiers that do affect coding assignment. Each line of indent represents a more specific code entry. The nonessential modifiers apply to the subterms following a main term except when they are mutually exclusive, in which case the subterm takes precedence. For example, if "acute" is listed as a nonessential modifier but there is a subentry for "chronic," then the nonessential modifier of "acute" does not apply.

Step 6: Interpret abbreviations, cross-references, default codes, additional characters, and brackets.

The abbreviation NEC (not elsewhere classified) that follows some main terms or subterms indicates that there is no specific code for the condition even though the medical documentation may be very specific. The code next to the main term is called the default code. It represents the condition most commonly associated with the main term or the unspecified code for the main term. Additional characters may be required to construct the code; the tabular list must be referenced to determine what those specific characters should be. The alphabetic index uses brackets [ ] to enclose manifestation codes that can be

used only as secondary codes to the underlying condition code immediately preceding it. Both codes must be reported in this multiple-coding situation.

Step 7: Choose a potential code and locate it in the tabular list.

The coder must follow any Includes, Excludes 1 and Excludes 2 notes, and other instructional notes, such as "Code first" and "Use additional code," listed in the tabular list for the chapter, category, subcategory, and subclassification level of code selection that direct the coder to use a different or additional code. Any codes in the tabular range, A00.0- through T88.9-, may be used to identify the diagnostic reason for the encounter. The tabular list encompasses many codes describing disease and injury classifications (e.g., infectious and parasitic diseases, neoplasms, symptoms, nervous and circulatory system etc.).

Codes that describe symptoms and signs, as opposed to definitive diagnoses, should be reported when an established diagnosis has not been made (confirmed) by the physician. Chapter 18 of the ICD-10-CM code book, "Symptoms, Signs, and Abnormal Clinical and Laboratory Findings, Not Elsewhere Classified" (codes R00.--R99), contains many, but not all, codes for symptoms.

ICD-10-CM classifies encounters with health care providers for circumstances other than a disease or injury using codes in chapter 21, "Factors Influencing Health Status and Contact with Health Services" (codes Z00–Z99). Circumstances other than a disease or injury often are recorded as chiefly responsible for the encounter.

Step 8: Determine whether the code is at the highest level of specificity.

A code is invalid if it has not been coded to the full number of characters (greatest level of specificity) required. Codes in ICD-10-CM can contain from three up to seven alphanumeric characters. A three-character code is to be used only if the category is not further subdivided into four-, five-, six-, or seven-character codes. Placeholder character X is used both to allow for future expansion and as a placeholder for empty characters in a code that requires a seventh character but has no fourth, fifth, or sixth character. Certain categories require seventh characters that apply to all codes in that category. Always check the category level for applicable seventh characters for that category.

Step 9: Assign the code.

Having reviewed all relevant information concerning the possible code choices, assign the code that most completely describes the condition.

Repeat steps one through nine for all additional documented conditions that meet the following criteria:

- Conditions that currently exist at the time of the visit
- Conditions that require or affect patient care, treatment, or management

Step 10: Sequence codes correctly.

Sequencing is the order in which the codes are listed on the claim. List first the ICD-10-CM code for the diagnosis, condition, problem, or other reason for the encounter/visit, which is shown in the medical record to be chiefly responsible for the services provided. List additional codes that describe any coexisting conditions. Follow the official coding guidelines (see section II, "Selection of Principal Diagnosis"; section III, "Reporting Additional Diagnoses"; and section IV, "Diagnostic Coding and Reporting Guidelines for Outpatient Services") on proper sequencing of codes.

Coding Examples

Diagnosis: Anorexia

Step 1: The reason for the encounter was the condition, anorexia.

Step 2: Consult the alphabetic index.

Step 3: Locate the main term "Anorexia."

Step 4: There are no cross-references to check.

Step 5: Note that there are two possible subterms (essential modifiers), "hysterical" and "nervosa," neither of which is documented in this instance and therefore cannot be used in code selection. The code listed next to the main term is called the default code selection.

Step 6: There are no abbreviations, cross-references, additional character icons, or brackets.

Step 7: Turn to code R63.0 in the tabular list and read the instructional notes. In this case the Excludes 1 note indicates that anorexia nervosa and loss of appetite determined to be of nonorganic origin should be coded to a code from chapter 5. The diagnostic statement does not indicate nonorganic origin.

Step 8: There is no further division of the category past the fourth character subcategory. Therefore, the subcategory code level is the highest level of specificity.

Step 9: The default code, R63.0 Anorexia, is the correct code selection.

Step 10: Since anorexia is listed as the chief reason for the health care encounter, the first-listed, or principal, diagnosis is R63.0. Note that this is a chapter 18 symptom code but can be assigned since the provider did not establish a more definitive diagnosis.

Diagnosis: Acute bronchitis

Step 1: The reason for the encounter was the condition, acute bronchitis.

Step 2: Consult the alphabetic index.

Step 3: Locate the main term "Bronchitis."

Step 4: There are cross-references to interpret.

Step 5: Review entries for modifiers. Since "acute" is not listed as a nonessential modifier, read past the "with" modifier until you find the subterm "acute or subacute" with a nonessential modifier of "with bronchospasm or obstruction," code J20.9.

Step 6: There are no abbreviations, cross-references, additional character icons, or brackets.

Step 7: Since there are no more appropriate subterms, turn to code J20.9 in the tabular list. The Includes note under category J20 does refer to other alternative terms for acute bronchitis. Note that the inclusion term list is not exhaustive but is only a representative selection of diagnoses that are included in the subcategory. The Excludes 1 note refers bronchitis and tracheobronchitis NOS to category J40. There are several Excludes 2 notes that, if applicable, can be coded in addition to this code.

Step 8: Note that the subcategories included in J20 represent acute bronchitis due to various infectious organisms that would be selected if identified in the documentation. In this case, the organism was not identified and there is no further division of the category past the fourth character subcategory. Therefore, the subcategory code level is the highest level of specificity.

Step 9: Assign code J20.9 Acute bronchitis, unspecified.

Step 10: Repeat steps 1-9 for any additional code assignments.

Diagnosis: Infectious diarrhea

Step 1: The reason for the encounter was the condition, infectious diarrhea.

Step 2: Consult the alphabetic index.

Step 3: Locate the main term "Diarrhea" in the alphabetic index.

Step 4: There are no cross-references to check.

Step 5: Review entries for modifiers. Note that the nonessential modifiers (in parentheses) after the main term do not include the term "infectious," which means that the coder should search the subterms for the term "infectious." The subterm "infectious" refers to code A09.

Step 6: There are no abbreviations, cross-references, additional character icons, or brackets.

Step 7: Locate code A09 in the tabular list, and read all instructional notes under the main category and subcategories. The Includes notes does not list the term "infectious diarrhea" under code A09; however, as instructed by the alphabetic index, you should code the condition to A09. The ICD-10-CM code book implies that infectious diarrhea is the same as infectious gastroenteritis, enteritis, and colitis.

Step 8: There is no further division of the category past the third-character category level. Therefore, the category code level is the highest level of specificity. The final code assignment would be A09.

Step 9: Assign code A09 Infectious gastroenteritis and colitis, unspecified.

Step 10: Since infectious diarrhea is listed as the chief reason for the health care encounter, the first-listed, or principal, diagnosis is A09.

Diagnosis: Decubitus ulcer of right elbow with skin loss and necrosis of subcutaneous tissue

Step 1: The reason for the encounter was the condition, decubitus ulcer.

Step 2: Consult the alphabetic index.

Step 3: Locate the main term "Ulcer" in the alphabetic index.

Step 4: There are no cross-references to check.

Step 5: This entry does not have any important nonessential modifiers; however, there are other terms such as ulcerated, ulcerating, etc., that are included as main terms. Locate the subterm "decubitus" and note that there is an italicized cross-reference to "*see* Ulcer, pressure, by site." Go to the subterm "pressure" and locate "elbow," which refers to code L89.0-.

Step 6: Note that the code L89.0 is followed by a dash and an additional character icon, which indicate that more characters are required. From here, the tabular list can be consulted at code L89.0-.

Step 7: Locate code L89.0 in the tabular list, and check the category level L89 for any instructional, Includes, and Excludes 1 and 2 notes. Note that "decubitus" is an Includes note under L89 Pressure ulcer. Excludes 2 notes indicate that if this were documented as a diabetic pressure ulcer, it would be necessary to use a code from chapter 4.

Step 8: Read through the subcategory codes under L89.0 and note that the fifth character describes laterality. Locate the right elbow at subcategory L89.01. See that an additional sixth character is now needed to complete the code. The sixth character specifies the stage of the ulcer, which can be determined either by the specific documentation of the stage (e.g., stage 1, stage 2) or in this case, a description that matches one of the Includes notes that follow each stage code. For example, the description in this case of "skin loss and necrosis of the subcutaneous tissue" matches the Includes notes under L89.013 Pressure ulcer of right elbow, stage 3.

Step 9: Assign code L89.013 Pressure ulcer of right elbow, stage 3

Step 10: Since the decubitus ulcer is listed as the chief reason for the health care encounter, the first-listed, or principal, diagnosis is L89.013. However, according to the Code first instructional note at the L89 category level, gangrene would be sequenced before the pressure ulcer if it were documented.

Diagnosis: First visit for bimalleolar fracture of the right ankle due to trauma

Step 1: The reason for the encounter was the condition, bimalleolar fracture of the right ankle.

Step 2: Consult the alphabetic index.

Step 3: Locate the main term "Fracture" in the alphabetic index.

Step 4: Note that the first main term for Fracture is pathological with cross-reference to "*see also* Fracture, traumatic." Locate the main term "Fracture, traumatic."

Step 5: Review entries for nonessential modifiers. Locate the subterms "ankle," "bimalleolar." Note that "displaced" is a nonessential modifier following "bimalleolar," indicating that S82.84- is the default code unless the fracture is specified as nondisplaced.

Step 6: Note that code S82.84- is followed by a dash and an additional character icon, both of which indicate that more characters are required. From here, the tabular list can be consulted at code S82.84.

Step 7: Locate code S82.84 Bimalleolar fracture of lower leg, in the tabular list and check the category level S82 for any instructional, Includes, and Excludes 1 and 2 notes. See the instructional notes indicating that fractures not specified as displaced or nondisplaced default to displaced, and fractures not designated as open or closed default to closed. See also the list of appropriate seventh characters to be added to all codes from category S82.

Step 8: Read through the subcategory codes under S82.84, and note that the sixth character specifies displaced or nondisplaced and laterality. Locate the displaced bimalleolar fracture of the right lower leg at code S82.841. See that an additional seventh character is still needed to complete the code. The seventh character specifies the type of encounter and whether the fracture is open or closed. Use character A listed in the box at the category level to describe initial encounter, closed fracture.

Step 9: Assign code S82.841A Displaced bimalleolar fracture of right lower leg, initial encounter for closed fracture.

Step 10: Since this is an injury code, code additionally any external cause, place of occurrence, and activity codes, with the injury (fracture) sequenced first.

Appendix B: Valid 3-character ICD-10-CM Codes

A09	Infectious gastroenteritis and colitis, unspecified
A33	Tetanus neonatorum
A34	Obstetrical tetanus
A35	Other tetanus
A46	Erysipelas
A55	Chlamydial lymphogranuloma (venereum)
A57	Chancroid
A58	Granuloma inguinale
A64	Unspecified sexually transmitted disease
A65	Nonvenereal syphilis
A70	Chlamydia psittaci infections
A78	Q fever
A86	Unspecified viral encephalitis
A89	Unspecified viral infection of central nervous system
A90	Dengue fever [classical dengue]
A91	Dengue hemorrhagic fever
A94	Unspecified arthropod-borne viral fever
A99	Unspecified viral hemorrhagic fever
B03	Smallpox
B04	Monkeypox
B09	Unspecified viral infection characterized by skin and mucous membrane lesions
B20	Human immunodeficiency virus [HIV] disease
B49	Unspecified mycosis
B54	Unspecified malaria
B59	Pneumocystosis
B64	Unspecified protozoal disease
B72	Dracunculiasis
B75	Trichinellosis
B79	Trichuriasis
B80	Enterobiasis
B86	Scabies
B89	Unspecified parasitic disease
B91	Sequelae of poliomyelitis
B92	Sequelae of leprosy
C01	Malignant neoplasm of base of tongue
C07	Malignant neoplasm of parotid gland
C12	Malignant neoplasm of pyriform sinus
C19	Malignant neoplasm of rectosigmoid junction
C20	Malignant neoplasm of rectum
C23	Malignant neoplasm of gallbladder
C33	Malignant neoplasm of trachea
C37	Malignant neoplasm of thymus
C52	Malignant neoplasm of vagina
C55	Malignant neoplasm of uterus, part unspecified
C58	Malignant neoplasm of placenta
C61	Malignant neoplasm of prostate
C73	Malignant neoplasm of thyroid gland
D34	Benign neoplasm of thyroid gland
D45	Polycythemia vera
D62	Acute posthemorrhagic anemia
D65	Disseminated intravascular coagulation [defibrination A syndrome]
D66	Hereditary factor VIII deficiency
D67	Hereditary factor IX deficiency
D71	Functional disorders of polymorphonuclear neutrophils
D77	Other disorders of blood and blood-forming organs in diseases classified elsewhere
E02	Subclinical iodine-deficiency hypothyroidism
E15	Nondiabetic hypoglycemic coma
E35	Disorders of endocrine glands in diseases classified elsewhere
E40	Kwashiorkor
E41	Nutritional marasmus
E42	Marasmic kwashiorkor
E43	Unspecified severe protein-calorie malnutrition
E45	Retarded development following protein-calorie malnutrition
E46	Unspecified protein-calorie malnutrition
E52	Niacin deficiency [pellagra]
E54	Ascorbic acid deficiency
E58	Dietary calcium deficiency
E59	Dietary selenium deficiency
E60	Dietary zinc deficiency
E65	Localized adiposity
E68	Sequelae of hyperalimentation
F04	Amnestic disorder due to known physiological condition
F05	Delirium due to known physiological condition
F09	Unspecified mental disorder due to known physiological condition
F21	Schizotypal disorder
F22	Delusional disorders
F23	Brief psychotic disorder
F24	Shared psychotic disorder
F28	Other psychotic disorder not due to a substance or known physiological condition
F29	Unspecified psychosis not due to a substance or known physiological condition
F39	Unspecified mood [affective] disorder
F53	Puerperal psychosis
F54	Psychological and behavioral factors associated with disorders or diseases classified elsewhere
F59	Unspecified behavioral syndromes associated with physiological disturbances and physical factors
F66	Other sexual disorders
F69	Unspecified disorder of adult personality and behavior
F70	Mild intellectual disabilities
F71	Moderate intellectual disabilities
F72	Severe intellectual disabilities
F73	Profound intellectual disabilities
F78	Other intellectual disabilities
F79	Unspecified intellectual disabilities
F82	Specific developmental disorder of motor function
F88	Other disorders of psychological development
F89	Unspecified disorder of psychological development
F99	Mental disorder, not otherwise specified
G01	Meningitis in bacterial diseases classified elsewhere
G02	Meningitis in other infectious and parasitic diseases classified elsewhere
G07	Intracranial and intraspinal abscess and granuloma in diseases classified elsewhere
G08	Intracranial and intraspinal phlebitis and thrombophlebitis
G09	Sequelae of inflammatory diseases of central nervous system
G10	Huntington's disease
G14	Postpolio syndrome
G20	Parkinson's disease
G26	Extrapyramidal and movement disorders in diseases classified elsewhere
G35	Multiple sclerosis
G53	Cranial nerve disorders in diseases classified elsewhere
G55	Nerve root and plexus compressions in diseases classified elsewhere
G59	Mononeuropathy in diseases classified elsewhere
G63	Polyneuropathy in diseases classified elsewhere
G64	Other disorders of peripheral nervous system
G92	Toxic encephalopathy
G94	Other disorders of brain in diseases classified elsewhere
H22	Disorders of iris and ciliary body in diseases classified elsewhere
H28	Cataract in diseases classified elsewhere
H32	Chorioretinal disorders in diseases classified elsewhere
H36	Retinal disorders in diseases classified elsewhere
H42	Glaucoma in diseases classified elsewhere
I00	Rheumatic fever without heart involvement
I10	Essential (primary) hypertension
I32	Pericarditis in diseases classified elsewhere
I38	Endocarditis, valve unspecified

I39	Endocarditis and heart valve disorders in diseases classified elsewhere
I41	Myocarditis in diseases classified elsewhere
I43	Cardiomyopathy in diseases classified elsewhere
I52	Other heart disorders in diseases classified elsewhere
I76	Septic arterial embolism
I81	Portal vein thrombosis
I96	Gangrene, not elsewhere classified
J00	Acute nasopharyngitis (common cold)
J13	Pneumonia due to Streptococcus pneumoniae
J14	Pneumonia due to Hemophilus influenzae
J17	Pneumonia in diseases classified elsewhere
J22	Unspecified acute lower respiratory infection
J36	Peritonsillar abscess
J40	Bronchitis, not specified as acute or chronic
J42	Unspecified chronic bronchitis
J60	Coalworker's pneumoconiosis
J61	Pneumoconiosis due to asbestos and other mineral fibers
J64	Unspecified pneumoconiosis
J65	Pneumoconiosis associated with tuberculosis
J80	Acute respiratory distress syndrome
J82	Pulmonary eosinophilia, not elsewhere classified
J90	Pleural effusion, not elsewhere classified
J99	Respiratory disorders in diseases classified elsewhere
K23	Disorders of esophagus in diseases classified elsewhere
K30	Functional dyspepsia
K36	Other appendicitis
K37	Unspecified appendicitis
K67	Disorders of peritoneum in infectious diseases classified elsewhere
K77	Liver disorders in diseases classified elsewhere
K87	Disorders of gallbladder, biliary tract and pancreas in diseases classified elsewhere
L00	Staphylococcal scalded skin syndrome
L14	Bullous disorders in diseases classified elsewhere
L22	Diaper dermatitis
L26	Exfoliative dermatitis
L42	Pityriasis rosea
L45	Papulosquamous disorders in diseases classified elsewhere
L52	Erythema nodosum
L54	Erythema in diseases classified elsewhere
L62	Nail disorders in diseases classified elsewhere
L80	Vitiligo
L83	Acanthosis nigricans
L84	Corns and callosities
L86	Keratoderma in diseases classified elsewhere
L88	Pyoderma gangrenosum
L99	Other disorders of skin and subcutaneous tissue in diseases classified elsewhere
N08	Glomerular disorders in diseases classified elsewhere
N10	Acute tubulo-interstitial nephritis
N12	Tubulo-interstitial nephritis, not specified as acute or chronic
N16	Renal tubulo-interstitial disorders in diseases classified elsewhere
N19	Unspecified kidney failure
N22	Calculus of urinary tract in diseases classified elsewhere
N23	Unspecified renal colic
N29	Other disorders of kidney and ureter in diseases classified elsewhere
N33	Bladder disorders in diseases classified elsewhere
N37	Urethral disorders in diseases classified elsewhere
N51	Disorders of male genital organs in diseases classified elsewhere
N62	Hypertrophy of breast
N72	Inflammatory disease of cervix uteri
N74	Female pelvic inflammatory disorders in diseases classified elsewhere
N86	Erosion and ectropion of cervix uteri
N96	Recurrent pregnancy loss
O68	Labor and delivery complicated by abnormality of fetal acid-base balance
O76	Abnormality in fetal heart rate and rhythm complicating labor and delivery
O80	Encounter for full-term uncomplicated delivery
O82	Encounter for cesarean delivery without indication
O85	Puerperal sepsis
O94	Sequelae of complication of pregnancy, childbirth, and the puerperium
P09	Abnormal findings on neonatal screening
P53	Hemorrhagic disease of newborn
P60	Disseminated intravascular coagulation of newborn
P84	Other problems with newborn
P90	Convulsions of newborn
P95	Stillbirth
Q02	Microcephaly
R05	Cough
R12	Heartburn
R17	Unspecified jaundice
R21	Rash and other nonspecific skin eruption
R32	Unspecified urinary incontinence
R34	Anuria and oliguria
R37	Sexual dysfunction, unspecified
R42	Dizziness and giddiness
R51	Headache
R52	Pain, unspecified
R54	Age-related physical debility
R55	Syncope and collapse
R58	Hemorrhage, not elsewhere classified
R61	Generalized hyperhidrosis
R64	Cachexia
R69	Illness, unspecified
R75	Inconclusive laboratory evidence of human immunodeficiency virus [HIV]
R81	Glycosuria
R99	Ill-defined and unknown cause of mortality
Y09	Assault by unspecified means
Y66	Nonadministration of surgical and medical care
Y69	Unspecified misadventure during surgical and medical care
Y95	Nosocomial condition
Z08	Encounter for follow-up examination after completed treatment for malignant neoplasm
Z09	Encounter for follow-up examination after completed treatment for conditions other than malignant neoplasm
Z21	Asymptomatic human immunodeficiency virus [HIV] infection status
Z23	Encounter for immunization
Z66	Do not resuscitate

Appendix C: Pharmacology List 2018

This section enables the coder to quickly review drugs, drug actions, and indications that are often associated with overlooked or undocumented diagnoses. The coder should review the patient's medication record and know what condition the physician is treating with the prescribed medication based on documentation in the medical record. When documentation is lacking, the coder can reference this section to locate the drug, determine the drug action, confirm drug indications, and when necessary query the physician.

Drug	Z Code	Drug Action	Indications
Abilify [aripiprazole]		Antipsychotic	Depression, bipolar disorder, schizophrenia, autism symptoms
Acarbose [acarbose]	Z79.84	Blood glucose regulator	Diabetes mellitus
Accupril [quinapril hydrochloride]		ACE inhibitor; antihypertensive	Congestive heart failure; essential hypertension
Acetaminophen with codeine [acetominophen/codeine phosphate]	Z79.891	Analgesic, general; analgesic-narcotic	Pain, moderate to severe
Actemra [tocilizumab]		Antirheumatic	Rheumatoid arthritis
Actimmune [interferon gamma-1b]	Z79.899	Antineoplastic interferons; antiviral interferons	Chronic granulomatous disease; malignant osteopetrosis
Activella [estradiol/norethindrone acetate]	Z79.890	Estrogen therapy	Menopause symptoms; vaginal and vulvar atrophy; osteoporosis prevention
Actonel [risedronate sodium]	Z79.83	Electrolytic and renal agent; bone resorption inhibitor	Decrease in bone loss in multiple myeloma patients; Paget's disease; hyperparathyroidism; osteoporosis
Actoplus Met [metformin hydrochloride/pioglitazone hydrochloride]	Z79.84	Blood glucose regulator	Diabetes mellitus
Actos [pioglitazone hydrochloride]	Z79.84	Blood glucose regulator	Diabetes mellitus
Adalat CC [nifedipine]		Calcium channel blocker	Vasospastic angina; chronic stable angina; essential hypertension
Advair [fluticasone propionate/salmeterol xinafoate]	Z79.51	Corticosteroids--inhaled; antiasthmatic	Prophylaxis and treatment of asthma and COPD
Advil [ibuprofen]	Z79.1	Nonsteroidal anti-inflammatory drug (NSAID)	Pain or fever relief
Aerospan [flunisolide]	Z79.51	Corticosteroids--inhaled; antiasthmatic	Prophylaxis and treatment of asthma
Afrezza [human insulin recombinant]	Z79.4	Blood glucose regulator	Diabetes mellitus
Aggrastat [tirofiban hydrochloride]	Z79.02	Antithrombotic platelet aggregation inhibitor	Unstable angina or heart attacks
Aggrenox [aspirin/dipyridamole]	Z79.02	Antithrombotic platelet aggregation inhibitor	Lessening of the chance of heart attack or stroke
Akne-Mycin [erythromycin]	Z79.2	Antibacterial	Severe acne treatment
Aldactone [spironolactone]		Cardiovascular agent; antihypertensive agent; diuretic; electrolytic and renal agent	Severe heart failure; ascites associated with cirrhosis; hypokalemia
Aleve [naproxen sodium]	Z79.1	Nonsteroidal anti-inflammatory drug (NSAID)	Reduction of temporary aches and pains
Allegra [fexofenadine hydrochloride]		Antihistamine	Seasonal allergic rhinitis
Allopurinol [allopurinol]		Antigout	Gouty arthritis, renal calculus, hyperuricemia, hyperuricemia secondary to leukemia, hyperuricemia secondary to lymphoma
Alora [estradiol]	Z79.890	Estrogen therapy	Menopause symptoms
Alphagan P [brimonidine tartrate]		Antiglaucoma agent (ophthalmic) antihypertensive, ocular	Open angle glaucoma or another condition in which pressure in the eye is too high (ocular hypertension)
Alprazolam [alprazolam]		Antianxiety; sedative/hypnotic	
Altabax [retapamulin]	Z79.2	Antibacterial	Skin infections
Altace [ramipril]		ACE inhibitor; antihypertensive	Congestive heart failure, essential hypertension
Altavera [ethinyl estradiol/levonorgestrel]	Z79.3	Contraceptive	Contraception
Alvesco [ciclesonide]	Z79.51	Corticosteroids--inhaled; antiasthmatic	Prophylaxis and treatment of asthma
Alyacen [ethinyl estradiol/norethindrone]	Z79.3	Contraceptive	Contraception
Amaryl [glimepiride]	Z79.84	Blood glucose regulator	Diabetes mellitus
Ambien [zolpidem tartrate]		Sedative/hypnotic	Insomnia
A-Methapred [methylprednisolone sodium succinate]	Z79.52	Corticosteroids	Severe inflammation
Amikacin [amikacin sulfate]		Aminoglycoside antibiotic	Active in treatment of gram-negative bacterial infections such as *Pseudomonas, Escherichia coli (E. coli), Proteus, Klebsiella-Enterobacter-Serratia*

Drug	Z Code	Drug Action	Indications
Aminophylline [aminophylline]		Bronchodilator, pulmonary vasodilator, smooth muscle relaxant	Relief and/or prevention of symptoms from asthma and reversible bronchospasms in bronchitis and emphysema
Amitriptyline hydrochloride [amitriptyline hydrochloride]		Anorexiant/CNS stimulant; antidepressant	Depression
Amoxicillin [amoxicillin]	Z79.2	Penicillin	Effective for infections with a broad spectrum of bactericidal activity against many gram-positive and gram-negative micro-organisms; otitis media, gonorrhea, skin, respiratory, gastrointestinal, and genitourinary infections
Ampicillin [ampicillin sodium]	Z79.2	Antibacterial	Bacterial infections
Amrix [cyclobenzaprine hydrochloride]		Muscle relaxant	Adjunct to rest and physical therapy for muscle spasms
Anaprox [naproxen sodium]	Z79.1	Nonsteroidal anti-inflammatory drug (NSAID)	Pain, inflammation, or fever relief
Anastrozole [anastrozole]	Z79.811	Aromatase inhibitor	Postmenopausal breast cancer
Ancef [cefazolin sodium]	Z79.2	Semisynthetic cephalosporin antibiotic	Respiratory tract infections due to *Streptococcus pneumoniae, Klebsiella* species, *Haemophilus influenzae* (*H. influenzae*), *Staphylococcus aureus,* and group A betahemolytic streptococci; urinary tract infections due to *E. coli, Proteus mirabilis, Klebsiella* species and some strains of *Enterobacter* and enterococci; skin and skin structure infections, biliary tract infections, bone and joint infections, genital infections, septicemia, and endocarditis
Angeliq [drospirenone/estradiol]	Z79.89	Estrogen therapy	Menopause symptoms
Angiomax [bivalirudin]	Z79.02	Antithrombotic platelet aggregation inhibitor	Prevention of blood clots
Antabuse [disulfiram]		Alcohol treatment	Alcoholism
Antineoplastic/chemotherapy	Z79.899	Antineoplastic	Cancer
Anzemet [dolasetron mesylate]		Antiemetic/antinauseant	Management of nausea/vomiting following surgery or from effects of chemotherapy or cancer
Apidra [insulin glulisine recombinant]	Z79.4	Blood glucose regulator	Diabetes mellitus
Aranelle [ethinyl estradiol/norethindrone]	Z79.3	Contraceptive	Contraception; acne
Aranesp [darbepoetin alfa]		Erythropoiesis-stimulating agent (ESA)	Lower than normal blood cell count (anemia) from disorders such as CKD and neoplasms
Argatroban [argatroban]	Z79.2	Antithrombotic platelet aggregation inhibitor	Prophylaxis and treatment of venous thrombosis in thrombocytopenia patients
Aricept [donepezil hydrochloride]		Acetylcholine sterase inhibitor	Symptoms of mild to moderate Alzheimer's disease; can improve thinking ability in some patients
Arimidex [anastrozole]	Z79.811	Aromatase inhibitor	Postmenopausal breast cancer
Aristospan [triamcinolone hexacetonide]	Z79.52	Corticosteroids	Severe inflammation
Arixtra [fondaparinux sodium]	Z79.01	Anticoagulant	Venous thrombosis and pulmonary embolism
Arnuity Ellipta [fluticasone furoate]	Z79.51	Corticosteroids--inhaled; antiasthmatic	Prophylaxis and treatment of asthma
Aromasin [exemestane]	Z79.811	Aromatase inhibitor	Postmenopausal breast cancer
Arthrotec [diclofenac sodium/misoprostol]	Z79.1	Analgesic	Arthritis in patients who may develop stomach ulcers from taking nonsteroidal anti-inflammatory drugs (NSAIDs) alone; used to help relieve some symptoms of arthritis, such as inflammation, swelling, stiffness, and joint pain
Ashlyna [ethinyl estradiol/levonorgestrel]	Z79.3	Contraceptive	Contraception
Asmanex [mometasone furoate]	Z79.51	Corticosteroids--inhaled; antiasthmatic	Prophylaxis and treatment of asthma
Astagraf XL [tacrolimus]	Z79.899	Immunosuppressant	Prophylaxis of organ transplant rejection
Astramorph [morphine sulfate]	Z79.891	Narcotic analgesic	Pain
Atelvia [risedronate sodium]	Z79.83	Bisphosphonates	Prevention of thinning of the bones (osteoporosis)
Atenolol [atenolol]		Antianginal; antihypertensive; beta blocker	Chronic stable angina pectoris; essential hypertension; reduces cardiovascular mortality in those with definite or suspected acute myocardial infarction
Ativan [lorazepam]		Antianxiety; sedative/hypnotic	Anxiety disorder associated with depressive symptoms; controls tension, agitation, irritability, and insomnia
Atrovent [ipratropium bromide]		Antiasthmatic/bronchodilator	Chronic bronchitis, emphysema; bronchial asthma
Augmentin [amoxicillin/clavulanate potassium]	Z79.2	Antibacterial	Middle ear, lower respiratory, sinus, skin and skin structures, and urinary tract infections
Avandia [rosiglitazone maleate]	Z79.84	Blood glucose regulator	Diabetes mellitus

Drug	Z Code	Drug Action	Indications
Avapro [irbesartan]		Antihypertensive	Hypertension
Aviane [ethinyl estradiol/levonorgestrel]	Z79.3	Contraceptive	Contraception
Avonex [interferon beta-1a]	Z79.899	Antiviral interferon	Relapsing multiple sclerosis
Axid AR [nizatidine]		Histamine H2-receptor antagonist	Acid/peptic disorder; gastroesophageal reflux; duodenal, gastric, and peptic ulcers
Aygestin [norethindrone acetate]	Z79.3	Contraceptive	Contraception; menstrual disorders
Azactam [aztreonam]	Z79.2	Antibacterial	Severe or life-threatening bacterial infections
Azithromycin [azithromycin]	Z79.2	Antibacterial	Treatment of bacterial infections
Bactrim [sulfamethoxazole/trimethoprim]	Z79.2	Antibacterial	Urinary tract infections, acute otitis media, acute exacerbation of chronic bronchitis, shigellosis, and *Pneumocystis carinii*
Bactroban [mupirocin]	Z79.2	Dermatologic; topical anti-infective	Topical treatment of impetigo
Balziva [ethinyl estradiol/norethindrone]	Z79.3	Contraceptive	Contraception
Basaglar [insulin glargine]	Z79.4	Blood glucose regulator	Diabetes mellitus
Bayer [acetylsalicylic acid]	Z79.82	Aspirin	Prophylaxis and treatment of heart attacks, angina, or strokes; reduction of fever, pain, and inflammation
Beconase AQ [beclomethasone dipropionate monohydrate]		Corticosteroids; antiasthmatic	Bronchial asthma, prevention of nasal polyps, perennial allergies, seasonal allergies, and vasomotor rhinitis
Bekyree [desogestrel/ethinyl estradiol]	Z79.3	Contraceptive	Contraception
Betoptic [betaxolol hydrochloride]		Cardioselective beta-adrenergic receptor blocking agent	Lowering of intraocular pressure; also used for treatment of ocular hypertension and chronic open-angle glaucoma
Beyaz [drospirenone/ethinyl estradiol/levomefolate calcium]	Z79.3	Contraceptive	Contraception; acne
Biaxin [clarithromycin]		Macrolide	Acid/peptic disorder or ulcer, acute exacerbation chronic bronchitis, HIV, lower and upper respiratory tract infections, sinus infection, prophylaxis mycobacterium avium complex, pharyngitis, pneumonia, tonsillitis
Binosto [alendronate sodium]	Z79.83	Bisphosphonates	Prevention of thinning of the bones (osteoporosis)
Boniva [ibandronate sodium]	Z79.83	Bisphosphonates	Prevention of thinning of the bones (osteoporosis)
Brevicon [ethinyl estradiol/norethindrone]	Z79.3	Contraceptive	Contraception; acne
Briellyn [ethinyl estradiol/norethindrone]	Z79.3	Contraceptive	Contraception
Brilinta [ticagrelor]	Z79.02	Antithrombotic platelet aggregation inhibitor	Unstable angina or heart attacks and prevention of blood clots
Bufferin [acetylsalicylic acid]	Z79.82	Aspirin	Prophylaxis and treatment of heart attacks, angina or strokes; reduction of fever, pain, and inflammation
Buprenex [buprenorphine hydrochloride]	Z79.891	Narcotic analgesic	Moderate to severe pain
Buprenorphine HCl [buprenorphine hydrochloride]	Z79.891	Narcotic analgesic	Moderate to severe pain
Buspirone [buspirone hydrochloride]		Antianxiety agent	Generalized anxiety disorder
Butorphanol Tartrate [butorphanol tartrate]		Narcotic analgesic	Moderate to severe postsurgical pain
Butrans [buprenorphine]	Z79.891	Narcotic analgesic	Chronic pain
Calan [verapamil hydrochloride]		Antianginal; antiarrhythmic, antiarthritic, antihypertensive, calcium channel blocker	Angina pectoris at rest and chronic stable, arrhythmia, atrial fibrillation, atrial flutter, paroxysmal supraventricular tachycardia, ventricular arrhythmia, essential hypertension
Caldolor [ibuprofen]	Z79.1	Nonsteroidal anti-inflammatory drug (NSAID)	Pain or fever relief
Cambia [diclofenac potassium]	Z79.1	Nonsteroidal anti-inflammatory drug (NSAID)	Migraine headaches
Camila [norethindrone]	Z79.3	Contraceptive	Contraception; menstrual disorders
Cardizem CD [diltiazem hydrochloride]		Antianginal, antiarrhythmic, antihypertensive, channel blocker, coronary vasodilator	Chronic stable angina, atrial fibrillation, atrial flutter, essential hypertension, paroxysmal supraventricular tachycardia
Cardura [doxazosin mesylate]		Antihypertensive	Benign prostatic hyperplasia, essential hypertension
Catapres [clonidine hydrochloride]		Antihypertensive	Hypertension
Cefprozil [cefprozil]		Antibiotic: second generation cephalosporins	Acute exacerbation and chronic bronchitis, lower and upper respiratory tract infections, pharyngitis, tonsillitis

Drug	Z Code	Drug Action	Indications
Ceftin [cefuroxime axetil]		Antibiotic: second generation cephalosporins	Acute exacerbation and chronic bronchitis, middle ear infection, sexually transmitted gonorrhea infection, upper respiratory tract infection, urinary tract infection, pharyngitis, tonsillitis
Ceftriaxone [ceftriaxone sodium]	Z79.2	Antibacterial	Bacterial infections
Celebrex [celecoxib]	Z79.1	Antirheumatic, nonsteroidal anti-inflammatory	Relief of some symptoms caused by arthritis, such as inflammation, swelling, stiffness, and joint pain
Celestone Soluspan [betamethasone acetate/ betamethasone sodium phosphate]	Z79.52	Corticosteroids; antiasthmatic	Asthma; severe inflammation
Celexa [citalopram hydrobromide]		Antidepressant	Depression
Cellcept [mycophenolate mofetil]	Z79.899	Immunosuppressant	Prophylaxis of organ transplant rejection
Centany [mupirocin]	Z79.2	Antibacterial	Topical treatment of skin infections
Cephalexin [cephalexin]	Z79.2	Antibacterial	Bacterial infections
Chantix [varenicline tartrate]		Smoking cessation aid	Nicotine addiction, smoking
Cipro [ciprofloxacin hydrochloride]	Z79.2	Anti-infective; quinolone	Cystitis, infectious diarrhea, gonorrhea, bone and joint infection, gastrointestinal tract infection, lower and upper respiratory tract infections, sinus infection, urinary tract infection, nosocomial pneumonia, chronic prostatitis
Ciprofloxacin [ciprofloxacin]	Z79.2	Antibacterial	Bacterial infections
Clarithromycin [clarithromycin]	Z79.2	Antibacterial	Skin and respiratory bacterial infections
Claritin [loratadine]		Antihistamine	Seasonal allergic rhinitis, chronic idiopathic urticaria
Cleocin [clindamycin phosphate]	Z79.2	Antibacterial	Bacterial infections
Climara [estradiol]	Z79.890	Estrogen therapy	Osteoporosis prevention and menopausal symptoms; vaginal and vulvar atrophy; hypoestrogenism; ovarian failure
Clindamycin [clindamycin phosphate]	Z79.2	Antibacterial	Bacterial infections
Clonazepam [clonazepam]		Anticonvulsant	Absence, akinetic, and myoclonic epilepsy, Lennox-Gastaut syndrome
Clonidine [clonidine hydrochloride]		Antihypertensive	Hypertension
Clopidogrel bisulfate [clopidogrel bisulfate]	Z79.02	Antithrombotic platelet aggregation inhibitor	Treatment of unstable angina or heart attacks and prevention of blood clots
Codeine [codeine sulfate]	Z79.891	Narcotic analgesic	Mild to moderate pain
Cogentin [benztropine mesylate]		Antiparkinsonism	Parkinson's disease
Colace [docusate sodium]		Gastrointestinal agent; laxative, stool softener	Constipation
Colocort [hydrocortisone]	Z79.52	Corticosteroids	Inflammation of the colon
CombiPatch [ethinyl estradiol/norethindrone acetate]	Z79.890	Estrogen therapy	Menopause symptoms; vaginal and vulvar atrophy; osteoporosis prevention
Combivent [ipratropium bromide/albuterol sulfate]		Antiasthmatic/bronchodilator	Chronic bronchitis, emphysema; bronchial asthma
Compro [prochlorperazine]		Antiemetic, antipsychotic	Nausea, vomiting, and manic phase of bipolar syndrome or schizophrenia
Cortef [hydrocortisone]	Z79.52	Corticosteroids	Severe inflammation
Cortenema [hydrocortisone]	Z79.52	Corticosteroids	Inflammation of the colon
Cortifoam [hydrocortisone acetate]	Z79.52	Corticosteroids	Colon and rectum inflammation
Cortisone acetate [cortisone acetate]	Z79.52	Corticosteroids	Inflammation
Cortisporin [hydrocortisone acetate/neomycin sulfate/polymyxin B sulfate]		Topical anti-infective, topical steroid	Dermatosis
Coumadin [warfarin sodium]	Z79.01	Anticoagulant	Prophylaxis and treatment of venous thrombosis, treatment of atrial fibrillation with embolization (pulmonary embolism), arrhythmias, myocardial infarction, and stroke prevention
Cozaar [losartan potassium]		Antihypertensive	Essential hypertension
Crestor [rosuvastatin calcium]		HMG-CoA reductase inhibitor (statin)	Hypercholesterolemia, hyperlipidemia, hyperproteinemia
Crixivan [indinavir sulfate]		HIV inhibitor	HIV, asymptomatic HIV
Cryselle [ethinyl estradiol/norgestrel]	Z79.3	Contraceptive	Contraception
Cyclafem [ethinyl estradiol/norethindrone]	Z79.3	Contraceptive	Contraception
Cyclessa [desogestrel/ethinyl estradiol]	Z79.3	Contraceptive	Contraception

Drug	Z Code	Drug Action	Indications
Cyclosporine [cyclosporine]	Z79.899	Immunosuppressant	Prophylaxis of organ transplant rejection
Cytomel [liothyronine sodium]		Thyroid hormone	Treatment of hypothyroidism or prevention of euthyroid goiters
Daptomycin [daptomycin]	Z79.2	Antibacterial	Skin and underlying tissue bacterial infections
Dasetta [ethinyl estradiol/norethindrone]	Z79.3	Contraceptive	Contraception
Daypro [oxaprozin]	Z79.1	Nonsteroidal anti-inflammatory drug (NSAID)	Osteoarthritis and rheumatoid arthritis
Daysee [ethinyl estradiol/levonorgestrel]	Z79.3	Contraceptive	Contraception
Delestrogen [estradiol valerate]	Z79.890	Estrogen therapy	Menopause symptoms
Demerol [meperidine hydrochloride]	Z79.891	Narcotic analgesic	Moderate to severe pain
Depakote [divalproex sodium]		Anticonvulsant	Bipolar affective disorder; complex absence, complex partial, and mixed pattern epilepsy; migraine headache
Depo-Medrol [methylprednisolone acetate]	Z79.52	Corticosteroids	Arthritis and joint disorders
Depo-Provera [medroxyprogesterone acetate]	Z79.3, Z79.890	Antineoplastic; contraceptive; progestin	Amenorrhea; carcinoma, endometrium, adjunct; carcinoma, renal; contraception; hemorrhage
Depo-SubQ Provera [medroxyprogesterone acetate]	Z79.3	Contraceptive	Contraception; menstrual disorder pain
Desogen [desogestrel/ethinyl estradiol]	Z79.3	Contraceptive; estrogen/progestin	Contraception
Detrol [tolterodine tartrate]		Muscarinic receptor antagonist	Overactive bladders in patients with urinary frequency, urgency, or urge incontinence
Dexamethasone Intensol [dexamethasone]	Z79.52	Corticosteroids	Arthritis; allergic disorders; breathing disorders; lupus
Didronel [etidronate disodium]	Z79.83	Bisphosphonates	Paget's disease and irregular bone growth
Dificid [fidaxomicin]	Z79.2	Antibacterial	*Clostridium difficile*
Diflucan [fluconazole]		Antifungal agent	Oropharyngeal and esophageal candidiasis and cryptococcal meningitis in AIDS patients
Digoxin [digoxin]		Cardiotonic glycoside	Heart failure, atrial flutter, atrial fibrillation, and supraventricular tachycardia
Dilantin [phenytoin sodium]		Anticonvulsant	Control of grand mal and psychomotor seizures
Dilaudid [hydromorphone hydrochloride]	Z79.891	Narcotic analgesic	Moderate to severe pain
Diovan [valsartan]		ACE inhibitor	Essential hypertension
Divigel [estradiol]	Z79.890	Estrogen therapy	Menopause symptoms
Dolophine HCl [methadone hydrochloride]	Z79.891	Narcotic analgesic	Pain; treatment of opioid addiction
Doxycycline [doxycycline]	Z79.2	Antibacterial	Treatment of bacterial infections; acne
Duavee [bazedoxifene acetate/conjugated estrogens]	Z79.890	Estrogen therapy	Treatment of menopause symptoms; osteoporosis prevention
Duetact [glimepiride/pioglitazone hydrochloride]	Z79.84	Blood glucose regulator	Diabetes mellitus
Duexis [famotidine/ibuprofen]	Z79.1	Nonsteroidal anti-inflammatory drug (NSAID)	Symptomatic treatment of osteoarthritis and rheumatoid arthritis; reduction of risk of ulcers
Dulera [formoterol fumarate/mometasone furoate]	Z79.51	Corticosteroids -inhaled; antiasthmatic	Prophylaxis and treatment of asthma
Duragesic [fentanyl]	Z79.891	Narcotic analgesic	Chronic pain
Duramorph [morphine sulfate]	Z79.891	Narcotic analgesic	Moderate to severe pain
Dyloject [diclofenac sodium]	Z79.1	Nonsteroidal anti-inflammatory drug (NSAID)	Pain relief
Dynacin [minocycline hydrochloride]	Z79.2	Antibacterial	Severe acne treatment
E.E.S. [erythromycin ethylsuccinate]	Z79.2	Antibacterial	Bacterial infections
Ecotrin [acetylsalicylic acid]	Z79.82	Aspirin	Prophylaxis and treatment of heart attacks, angina or strokes; reduction of fever, pain and inflammation
Effexor XR [venlafaxine hydrochloride]		Antidepressant	Depression
Effient [prasugrel hydrochloride]	Z79.02	Antithrombotic platelet aggregation inhibitor	Lessening of the chance of heart attack or stroke
Elestrin [estradiol]	Z79.890	Estrogen therapy	Menopause symptoms
Eligard [leuprolide acetate]	Z79.818	Agents affecting estrogen receptors and estrogen levels	Endometriosis; uterine fibroids; symptoms of prostate cancer

Drug	Z Code	Drug Action	Indications
Elinest [norgestrel/ethinyl estradiol]	Z79.3	Contraceptive	Contraception
Eliquis [apixaban]	Z79.Ø1	Anticoagulant	Venous thrombosis
Embeda [morphine sulfate/naltrexone hydrochloride]	Z79.891	Narcotic analgesic	Moderate to severe pain
Emoquette [ethinyl estradiol/desogestrel]	Z79.3	Contraceptive	Contraception
Enjuvia [conjugated synthetic b estrogens]	Z79.89Ø	Estrogen therapy	Osteoporosis prevention and to treat menopausal symptoms; vaginal and vulvar atrophy; hypoestrogenism; ovarian failure
Enpresse [ethinyl estradiol/levonorgestrel]	Z79.3	Contraceptive	Contraception
Enskyce [desogestrel/ethinyl estradiol]	Z79.3	Contraceptive	Contraception
Entocort EC [budesonide]	Z79.52	Corticosteroids	Crohn's disease; ulcerative colitis
Envarsus XR [tacrolimus]	Z79.899	Immunosuppressant	Prophylaxis of organ transplant rejection
Epinephrine [epinephrine]		Bronchodilator, cardiotonic	Most commonly, relief of respiratory distress due to bronchospasm and restoration of cardiac rhythm in cardiac arrest
Epivir, Epivir-HBV [lamivudine]		HIV and HBV inhibitor	HIV, hepatitis B (HBV), asymptomatic HIV
Errin [norethindrone]	Z79.3	Contraceptive	Contraception
Ertapenem [ertapenem sodium]	Z79.2	Antibacterial	Stomach, urinary tract, pelvis, skin and lung infections
ERYC [erythromycin]	Z79.2	Antibacterial	Lower respiratory tract infections
Erygel [erythromycin]	Z79.2	Antibacterial	Treatment of bacterial infections; rheumatic fever attacks
EryPed [erythromycin ethylsuccinate]	Z79.2	Antibacterial	Treatment of bacterial infections; rheumatic fever attacks
Ery-Tab [erythromycin]	Z79.2	Acne product; macrolide; ocular anti-infective; topical anti-infective	Acne vulgaris, intestinal amebiasis, infectious conjunctivitis, diphtheria, endocarditis, prevention, treatment of erythrasma infections: endocervical, gynecologic, lower and upper respiratory tract, ophthalmic, and rectal; skin and skin structures, and urethral; Legionnaires' disease, pelvic inflammatory disease, pertussis, pneumonia, rheumatic fever, prophylaxis, syphilis
Erythrocin [erythromycin lactobionate]	Z79.2	Antibacterial	Bacterial infections
Erythromycin [erythromycin]	Z79.2	Antibacterial	Respiratory tract infections
Estarylla [ethinyl estradiol/norgestimate]	Z79.3	Contraceptive	Contraception
Estrace [estradiol]	Z79.89Ø	Estrogen therapy	Vaginal cream used to treat vaginal and vulvar atrophy
Estraderm [estradiol]	Z79.89Ø	Estrogen therapy	Osteoporosis prevention and to treat menopausal symptoms, vaginal and vulvar atrophy, hypoestrogenism, ovarian failure
Estrasorb [estradiol hemihydrate]	Z79.89Ø	Estrogen therapy	Menopause symptoms
EstroGel [estradiol]	Z79.89Ø	Estrogen therapy	Menopause symptoms
Estrostep Fe [ethinyl estradiol/norethindrone acetate]	Z79.3	Contraceptive	Contraception
Evista [raloxifene hydrochloride]	Z79.81Ø	Estrogen receptor modulator, selective osteoporosis prophylactic	Prevention of thinning of the bones (osteoporosis) only in postmenopausal women
Exalgo [hydromorphone hydrochloride]	Z79.891	Narcotic analgesic	Moderate to severe pain
Exemestane [exemestane]	Z79.811	Aromatase inhibitor	Postmenopausal breast cancer
Factive [gemifloxacin mesylate]	Z79.2	Antibacterial	Bacterial lung infections
Falmina [ethinyl estradiol/levonorgestrel]	Z79.3	Contraceptive	Contraception
Fareston [toremifene citrate]	Z79.81Ø	Selective estrogen receptor modulator (SERM)	Metastatic breast cancer in postmenopausal women
Faslodex [fulvestrant]	Z79.818	Agents affecting estrogen receptors and estrogen levels	Metastatic breast cancer in postmenopausal women
Feldene [piroxicam]	Z79.1	Nonsteroidal anti-inflammatory drug (NSAID)	Treatment of pain and inflammation due to arthritis
Femara [letrozole]	Z79.811	Aromatase inhibitor	Postmenopausal breast cancer
Femcon Fe [ethinyl estradiol/norethindrone]	Z79.3	Contraceptive	Contraception; acne
Femhrt [ethinyl estradiol/norethindrone acetate]	Z79.3, Z79.89Ø	Contraceptive; estrogen therapy	Contraception; menopause symptoms; osteoporosis prevention
Femring [estradiol acetate]	Z79.89Ø	Estrogen therapy	Osteoporosis prevention and to treat menopausal symptoms; hypoestrogenism; ovarian failure
Femtrace [estradiol acetate]	Z79.89Ø	Estrogen therapy	Menopause symptoms

Drug	Z Code	Drug Action	Indications
Fentanyl [fentanyl]	Z79.891	Narcotic analgesic	Postprocedural or chronic pain
Fentora [fentanyl citrate]	Z79.891	Narcotic analgesic	Breakthrough cancer pain
Fioricet with codeine [acetaminophen/butalbital/caffeine/codeine phosphate]	Z79.891	Narcotic analgesic	Tension headaches
Flagyl [metronidazole]	Z79.2	Antibacterial	Treatment of bacterial infections
Flavoxate hydrochloride [flavoxate hydrochloride]		Urinary tract spasmolytic	Relief of dysuria, urgency, nocturia, suprapubic pain, frequency, and incontinence associated with cystitis, prostatitis, urethritis, and urethrocystitis/urethrotrigonitis
Flomax [tamsulosin hydrochloride]		Alpha-adrenergic blocker, benign prostatic hypertrophy therapy agent	Signs and symptoms of benign enlargement of the prostate (benign prostatic hyperplasia, or BPH)
Flonase [fluticasone propionate]		Corticosteroid-inhalation/nasal; topical steroid	Corticosteroid-responsive dermatosis; perennial allergic and seasonal allergic rhinitis
Flovent HFA [fluticasone propionate]	Z79.51	Corticosteroid-inhaled/nasal; topical steroid	Corticosteroid-responsive dermatosis, perennial allergic and seasonal allergic rhinitis
Fortamet [metformin hydrochloride]	Z79.84	Blood glucose regulator	Diabetes mellitus
Fortaz [ceftazidime]	Z79.2	Antibacterial	Pneumonia and lower respiratory infections
Fosamax [alendronate sodium]	Z79.83	Calcium metabolism	Osteoporosis; Paget's disease
Fosinopril sodium [fosinopril sodium]		ACE inhibitor; antihypertensive	Essential hypertension
Fragmin [dalteparin sodium]	Z79.01	Anticoagulant	Prophylaxis and treatment of blood clots
Fulvestrant [fulvestrant]	Z79.818	Agents affecting estrogen receptors and estrogen levels	Treatment of metastatic breast cancer in postmenopausal women
Gengraf [cyclosporine]	Z79.899	Immunosuppressant	Prophylaxis of organ transplant rejection
Gentamicin sulfate [gentamicin sulfate]	Z79.2	Antibacterial	Severe bacterial infections
Gildagia [ethinyl estradiol/norethindrone]	Z79.3	Contraceptive	Contraception
Gildess [ethinyl estradiol/norethindrone acetate]	Z79.3	Contraceptive	Contraception
Glimepiride [glimepiride]	Z79.84	Blood glucose regulator	Diabetes mellitus
Glucophage [metformin hydrochloride]	Z79.84	Blood glucose regulator	Diabetes mellitus
Glucotrol [glipizide]	Z79.84	Oral blood-glucose-lowering agent	Diabetes mellitus
Glucovance [glyburide/metformin hydrochloride]	Z79.84	Blood glucose regulator	Diabetes mellitus
Glumetza [metformin hydrochloride]	Z79.84	Blood glucose regulator	Diabetes mellitus
Glyburide (micronized) [glyburide]	Z79.84	Blood glucose regulator	Diabetes mellitus
Heparin sodium [heparin sodium]	Z79.01	Anticoagulant	Prophylaxis and treatment of venous thrombosis, pulmonary embolism; prevention of cerebral thrombosis, and treatment of consumptive coagulopathies
Humalog [insulin lispro recombinant]	Z79.4	Blood glucose regulator	Diabetes mellitus
Humulin [insulin recombinant]	Z79.4	Blood glucose regulator	Diabetes mellitus
Hydrochlorothiazide [hydrochlorothiazide]		Diuretic, antihypertensive	Management of hypertension and in adjunctive therapy for edema associated with congestive heart failure, hepatic cirrhosis, corticosteroid, and estrogen therapy
Hydrocodone [acetaminophen/hydrocodone bitartrate]	Z79.891	Narcotic analgesic	Moderate to severe pain
Hydrocodone bitartrate and acetaminophen [acetaminophen/hydrocodone bitartrate]	Z79.891	Analgesic, general; analgesic-narcotic; antitussive/expectorant	Pain, moderate to severe
Hydrocortisone [hydrocortisone]	Z79.52	Corticosteroids	Addison's disease; arthritis; immune disorders; allergies; breathing problems
Hydromorphone HCl [hydromorphone hydrochloride]	Z79.891	Narcotic analgesic	Moderate to severe pain
Hyzaar [hydrochlorothiazide/ losartan potassium]		Antihypertensive	Hypertension
Ibuprofen [ibuprofen]	Z79.1	Nonsteroidal anti-inflammatory drug (NSAID)	Pain or fever relief
Imitrex [sumatriptan succinate]		Antimigraine	Migraine headache
Imuran [azathioprine]	Z79.899	Immunosuppressant	Rheumatoid arthritis

Drug	Z Code	Drug Action	Indications
Inderal [propranolol hydrochloride]		Beta-adrenergic blocking agent	Management of hypertension, long-term management of angina pectoris due to coronary atherosclerosis, cardiac arrhythmias
Indocin [indomethacin]	Z79.1	Nonsteroidal anti-inflammatory drug (NSAID)	Treatment of pain and inflammation
Integrilin [eptifibatide]	Z79.02	Antithrombotic platelet aggregation inhibitor	Treatment of unstable angina or heart attacks and prevention of blood clots
Intron [interferon alfa 2-b]	Z79.899	Antineoplastic interferons; antiviral interferons	Cancer; hepatitis
Introvale [levonorgestrel/ethinyl estradiol]	Z79.3	Contraceptive	Contraception
Invanz [ertapeneum sodium]	Z79.2	Antibacterial	Stomach, urinary tract, pelvis, skin and lung infections
Invokamet [canagliflozin/metformin hydrochloride]	Z79.84	Blood glucose regulator	Diabetes mellitus
Iprivask [desirudin recombinant]	Z79.02	Antithrombotic platelet aggregation inhibitor	Prophylaxis and treatment of venous thrombosis and pulmonary embolism
Isoniazid [isoniazid]	Z79.2	Antibacterial	Prophylaxis and treatment of tuberculosis
Isordil [isosorbide dinitrate]		Smooth muscle relaxant	Acute anginal attacks
Isuprel [isoproterenol hydrochloride]		Adrenergic agent	Bronchodilator for asthma, chronic pulmonary emphysema, bronchitis, and other conditions accompanied by bronchospasm; can be used in cardiogenic shock cases
Jantoven [warfarin sodium]	Z79.01	Anticoagulant	Prophylaxis and treatment of venous thrombosis, pulmonary embolism; prevention of cerebral thrombosis, and treatment of consumptive coagulopathies
Janumet [metformin hydrochloride/sitagliptin phosphate]	Z79.84	Blood glucose regulator	Diabetes mellitus
Januvia [sitagliptin phosphate]	Z79.84	Blood glucose regulator	Diabetes mellitus
Jencycla [norethindrone]	Z79.3	Contraceptive	Contraception
Jentadueto [linagliptin/metformin hydrochloride]	Z79.84	Blood glucose regulator	Diabetes mellitus
Junel [ethinyl estradiol/norethindrone acetate]	Z79.3	Contraceptive	Contraception
Kadian [morphine sulfate]	Z79.891	Narcotic analgesic	Moderate to severe pain
Kariva [desogestrel/ethinyl estradiol]	Z79.3	Contraceptive	Contraception
Kazano [alogliptin benzoate/metformin hydrochloride]	Z79.84	Blood glucose regulator	Diabetes mellitus
Keflex [cephalexin]	Z79.2	Antibacterial	Bone, middle ear, skin and skin structures, upper respiratory tract and urinary tract infections; acute prostatitis
Kefzol [cefazolin sodium]	Z79.2	Antibacterial	Skin, ear, urinary tract, and upper respiratory bacterial infections
Kelnor [ethynodiol diacetate/ethinyl estradiol]	Z79.3	Contraceptive	Contraception
Kenalog [triamcinolone acetonide]	Z79.52	Corticosteroids	Eczema; allergic reactions; psoriasis
Kimidess [ethinyl estradiol/desogestrel]	Z79.3	Contraceptive	Contraception
Klaron [sulfacetamide sodium]	Z79.2	Antibacterial	Acne
Klonopin [clonazepam]		Anticonvulsant, anxiolytic - benzodiazepine	Epilepsy, seizures, panic disorder
Klor-Con [potassium chloride]		Replaces potassium and maintains potassium level	Hypokalemia
Kombiglyze [metformin hydrochloride/saxagliptin hydrochloride]	Z79.84	Blood glucose regulator	Diabetes mellitus
K-Tab [potassium chloride]		Replaces potassium and maintains potassium level	Hypokalemia
Kurvelo [ethinyl estradiol/levonorgestrel]	Z79.3	Contraceptive	Contraception; menstrual disorders
Lamisil [terbinafine hydrochloride]		Antifungal	*Tinea cruris* (jock itch), *T. pedis* (athlete's foot), *T. corporis* (ringworm)
Lanoxin [digoxin]		Cardiotonic glycoside	Congestive heart failure
Lantus [insulin glargine recombinant]	Z79.4	Blood glucose regulator	Diabetes mellitus
Larin [ethinyl estradiol/norethindrone acetate]	Z79.3	Contraceptive	Contraception
Lasix [furosemide]		Antihypertensive; diuretic	Management of edema associated with congestive heart failure, renal disease, including nephrotic syndrome and hypertension

Drug	Z Code	Drug Action	Indications
Lescol [fluvastatin sodium]		HMG-CoA reductase inhibitor (statin)	Hypercholesterolemia; hyperlipidemia; hyperlipoproteinemia
Lessina [ethinyl estradiol/levonorgestrel]	Z79.3	Contraceptive	Contraception
Letrozole [letrozole]	Z79.811	Aromatase inhibitor	Postmenopausal breast cancer
Levaquin [levofloxacin]	Z79.2	Fluoroquinolone antibacterial	Acute exacerbation chronic bronchitis; cellulitis; furuncle; impetigo; infections of the lower and upper respiratory tracts, sinus, skin and skin structures, and urinary tract; pneumonia, community-acquired; pyoderma
Levemir [insulin detemir recombinant]	Z79.4	Blood glucose regulator	Diabetes mellitus
Levonest [levonorgestrel/ethinyl estradiol]	Z79.3	Contraceptive	Contraception; menstrual disorders; acne
Levora [levonorgestrel/ethinyl estradiol]	Z79.3	Contraceptive	Contraception
Levothroid [levothyroxine sodium]		Thyroid hormone	Treatment of hypothyroidism
Levoxyl [levothyroxine sodium]		Synthetic thyroid hormone	Euthyroid goiter; hypothyroidism
Lexapro [escitalopram oxalate]		Antidepressant—selective serotonin reuptake inhibitor (SSRI)	Depression, anxiety
Librium [chlordiazepoxide hydrochloride]		Antianxiety agent	Acute withdrawal symptoms, especially from alcohol, or for other anxiety-producing conditions
Lidocaine hydrochloride [lidocaine hydrochloride]		Antiarrhythmic	Management of ventricular arrhythmias or during cardiac manipulation, such as cardiac surgery
Liletta [levonorgestrel]	Z79.3	Contraceptive	Intrauterine device for contraception
Lincocin [lincocin hydrochloride]	Z79.2	Antibacterial	Serious bacterial infections
Lipitor [atorvastatin calcium]		HMG-CoA reductase inhibitor (statin)	Hypercholesterolemia, hyperlipidemia, hyperproteinemia
Lithium [lithium carbonate]		Antimanic	Control of manic episodes in bipolar disorders
Lo Loestrin Fe [ethinyl estradiol/norethindrone acetate]	Z79.3	Contraceptive	Contraception
Lo Minastrin Fe [ethinyl estradiol/norethindrone acetate]	Z79.3	Contraceptive	Contraception
Loestrin [ethinyl estradiol/norethindrone acetate]	Z79.3	Contraceptive	Contraception
Lomotil [diphenoxylate hydrochloride/atropine sulfate]		Antidiarrheal	Treatment of symptoms of chronic and functional diarrhea
Lopid [gemfibrozil]		Lipid regulating agent	Hypercholesterolemia, hyperlipidemia, hyperlipoproteinemia, hypertriglyceridemia
Lopressor [metoprolol tartrate]		Antihypertensive, betablocker antianginal; antihypertensive; betablocker	Essential hypertension therapy, angina pectoris, and myocardial infarction
Lorazepam [lorazepam]		Antianxiety; sedative/hypnotic	Anxiety disorder associated with depressive symptoms; controls tension, agitation, irritability, and insomnia
Loryna [drospirenone/ethinyl estradiol]	Z79.3	Contraceptive	Contraception
LoSeasonique [ethinyl estradiol/levonorgestrel]	Z79.3	Contraceptive	Contraception
Lotensin [benazepril hydrochloride]		ACE inhibitor; antihypertensive	Essential hypertension
Lotrel [amlodipine besylate/benazepril hydrochloride]		Antihypertensive	Hypertension
Lotrisone [clotrimazole/ betamethasone dipropionate]		Antifungal-corticosteroid	Relief of redness, swelling, itching, and other discomfort of fungus infections
Lovastatin [lovastatin]		HMG-CoA reductase inhibitor (statin)	Hypercholesterolemia; hyperlipidemia, hyperlipoproteinemia
Lovenox [enoxaparin sodium]	Z79.Ø1	Anticoagulant	Prophylaxis and treatment of venous thrombosis and pulmonary embolism
Low-Ogestrel [norgestrel/ethinyl estradiol]	Z79.3	Contraceptive	Contraception
Lupron [leuprolide acetate]	Z79.818	Agents affecting estrogen receptors and estrogen levels	Treatment of metastatic breast cancer in postmenopausal women; prostate cancer symptoms
Macrobid [nitrofuantoin]	Z79.2	Antibacterial	Bacterial urinary tract infections
Macrodantin [nitrofurantoin]		Antibacterial	Urinary tract infection; prophylaxis
Marlissa [ethinyl estradiol/levonorgestrel]	Z79.3	Contraceptive	Contraception
Maxipime [cefepime hydrochloride]	Z79.2	Antibacterial	Treatment of bacterial infections
Meclizine hydrochloride [meclizine hydrochloride]		Antihistamine	Management of nausea and vomiting, and dizziness associated with motion sickness

Drug	Z Code	Drug Action	Indications
Medrol [methylprednisolone]	Z79.52	Glucocorticoid; anti-inflammatory	Acute/chronic adrenal insufficiency, congenital adrenal hyperplasia, adrenal insufficiency secondary to pituitary insufficiency; nonendocrine disorders, including arthritis, rheumatic carditis, bronchial asthma, cerebral edema, and allergic, collagen, intestinal tract, liver, ocular, renal, and skin diseases
Mefoxin [cefoxitin sodium]	Z79.2	Antibacterial	Bacterial infections
Megace ES [megestrol acetate]	Z79.818	Agents affecting estrogen receptors and estrogen levels	Endometrial or advanced breast cancers; weight loss due to AIDS
Menest [esteriefied estrogens]	Z79.890	Estrogen therapy	Menopause symptoms; ovarian failure
Menostar [estradiol]	Z79.890	Estrogen therapy	Menopause symptoms; osteoporosis prevention
Mepron [atovaquone]	Z79.2	Antibacterial	Pneumonia
Merrem [meropenem]	Z79.2	Antibacterial	Bacterial infections of skin or stomach; bacterial meningitis
Metformin [metformin hydrochloride]	Z79.84	Blood glucose regulator	Diabetes mellitus
Methadone HCl [methadone hydrochloride]	Z79.891	Narcotic analgesic	Pain; treatment of opoid addiction
Methadose [methadone hydrochloride]	Z79.891	Narcotic analgesic	Acute and chronic pain
Methergine [methylergonovine maleate]		Oxytocic agent	Routine management of postpartum hemorrhage after delivery of placenta
Methylprednisolone [methylprednisolone]	Z79.52	Corticosteroids	Inflammatory disorders
Metro [metronidazole]	Z79.2	Antibacterial	Bacterial infections
Metronidazole [metronidazole]	Z79.2	Antibacterial	Bacterial infections
Miacalcin [calcitonin salmon]		Calcitonin; a peptide hormone	Hypercalcemia, osteoporosis, postmenopausal symptoms, Paget's disease
Microgestin [ethinyl estradiol/norethindrone acetate]	Z79.3	Contraceptive	Contraception
Micronor [norethindrone]	Z79.3	Contraceptive	Contraception
Minastrin [ethinyl estradiol/norethindrone acetate]	Z79.3	Contraceptive	Contraception
Minivelle [estradiol]	Z79.890	Estrogen therapy	Menopause symptoms; osteoporosis prevention
Minocin [minocycline hydrochloride]	Z79.2	Antibacterial	Bacterial infections; acne
Mirena [levonorgestrel]	Z79.3	Contraceptive	Intrauterine device for contraception; menstrual disorders
Mobic [meloxicam]	Z79.1	Nonsteroidal anti-inflammatory drug (NSAID)	Pain and inflammation due to osteoarthritis and rheumatoid arthritis
Modicon [ethinyl estradiol/norethindrone]	Z79.3	Contraceptive	Contraception
Monoclonal antibodies	Z79.899	Monoclonal antibodies	Cancer; prophylaxis of organ transplant rejection
Monodox [doxycycline]	Z79.2	Antibacterial	Bacterial infections; acne
Monoket [isosorbide mononitrate]		Antianginal; coronary vasodilator, nitrate	Angina pectoris
Mono-Linyah [norgestimate/ethinyl estradiol]	Z79.3	Contraceptive	Contraception; menstrual disorders; acne
Monurol [fosfomycin tromethamine]	Z79.2	Antibacterial	Bacterial bladder infections
Morphine [morphine sulfate]	Z79.891	Narcotic analgesic	Moderate to severe pain
Motrin [ibuprofen]	Z79.1	Analgesic, general; analgesic, non-narcotic; antiarthritic; antigout; antipyretic; NSAID	Osteoarthritis and rheumatoid arthritis, dysmenorrhea, fever; pain, mild to moderate
Moxatag [amoxicillin]	Z79.2	Antibacterial	Bacterial tonsillitis and pharyngitis
MS Contin [morphine sulfate]	Z79.891	Narcotic analgesic	Moderate to severe pain
Multaq [dronedarone hydrochloride]		Cardiac rhythm regulator	Treatment of patients with recent episodes of atrial fibrillation or atrial flutter
Mycobutin [rifabutin]	Z79.2	Antibacterial	Mycobacterium avium complex (MAC) prophylactic
Myzilra [ethinyl estradiol/levonorgestrel]	Z79.3	Contraceptive	Contraception
Nabumetone [nabumetone]	Z79.1	Non-steroidal anti-inflammatory drug (NSAID)	Osteoarthritis and rheumatoid arthritis
Nalfon [fenoprofen calcium]	Z79.1	Nonsteroidal anti-inflammatory drug (NSAID)	Pain or inflammation relief
Naprelan [naproxen sodium]	Z79.1	Nonsteroidal anti-inflammatory drug (NSAID)	Pain or inflammation relief

Drug	Z Code	Drug Action	Indications
Naprosyn [naproxen]	Z79.1	Anti-inflammatory analgesic, general; analgesic, non-narcotic; antiarthritic; antigout; NSAID	Rheumatoid, gouty arthritis and osteoarthritis; ankylosing spondylitis; bursitis; dysmenorrhea; pain, mild to moderate; tendonitis
Natazia [estradiol valerate/dienogest]	Z79.3	Contraceptive	Contraception; menstrual disorders
Nebupent [pentamidine isethionate]	Z79.2	Antibacterial	Serious bacterial lung infection in high-risk patients with HIV
Nefazodone hydrochloride [nefazodone hydrochloride]		Antidepressant	Depression
Nembutal sodium [pentobarbital sodium]		Sedative; hypnotic	Adjunct medication in diagnostic procedures or for emergency use with convulsive disorders
NeoProfen [ibuprofen lysine]	Z79.1	Nonsteroidal anti-inflammatory drug (NSAID)	Pain or fever relief
Neoral [cyclosporine]	Z79.899	Immunosuppressant	Prophylaxis of organ transplant rejection
Neurontin [gabapentin]		Anticonvulsant	Epilepsy, partial
Nexium [esomeprazole magnesium]		Proton pump inhibitor	Gastroesophageal reflux disease (GERD), erosive esophagitis
Nexplanon [etonogestrel]	Z79.3	Contraceptive	Implantable contraception
Nitrofurantoin [nitrofurantoin]	Z79.2	Antibacterial	Bacterial urinary tract infections
Nitropress [sodium nitroprusside]		Vasodilator	Potent, rapid action in reducing blood pressure in hypertensive crisis or for controlling bleeding during anesthesia by producing controlled hypotension
Nitrostat [nitroglycerin]		Muscle relaxant antianginal; antihypertensive; coronary vasodilator	Prophylaxis and treatment of angina pectoris; heart failure associated with myocardial infarction; hypertension, perioperative; surgery, adjunct
Norco [acetaminophen/hydrocodone bitartrate]	Z79.891	Narcotic analgesic	Moderate to severe pain
Norinyl [mestranol/norethisterone]	Z79.3	Contraceptive	Contraception
Norpace [disopyramide phosphate]		Antiarrhythmic	Coronary artery disease, for prevention, recurrence, and control of unifocal, multifocal, and paired PVCs
Nor-QD [norethindrone]	Z79.3	Contraceptive	Contraception
Nortrel [ethinyl estradiol/norethindrone]	Z79.3	Contraceptive	Contraception
Norvasc [amlodipine besylate]		Calcium channel blocker	Hypertension, chronic stable angina, and vasospastic angina
Novolin [insulin recombinant]	Z79.4	Blood glucose regulator	Diabetes mellitus
NovoLog [insulin recombinant]	Z79.4	Blood glucose regulator	Diabetes mellitus
Nucynta [tapentadol hydrochloride]	Z79.891	Narcotic analgesic	Moderate to severe pain
NuvaRing [etonogestrel/ethinyl estradiol]	Z79.3	Contraceptive	Vaginal ring for contraception
Ogestrel [norgestrel/ethinyl estradiol]	Z79.3	Contraceptive	Contraception
Onglyza [saxagliptin hydrochloride]	Z79.84	Blood glucose regulator	Diabetes mellitus
Opana [oxymorphone hydrochloride]	Z79.891	Narcotic analgesic	Moderate to severe pain
Oracea [doxycycline]	Z79.2	Antibacterial	Rosacea
OraprED ODT [prednisolone sodium phosphate]	Z79.52	Corticosteroids	Inflammatory disorders
Orbactiv [oritavancin diphosphate]	Z79.2	Antibacterial	Bacterial skin infections
Orphenadrine citrate [orphenadrine citrate]		Muscle relaxant	Acute spasms, tension, and post-trauma cases
Orsythia [ethinyl estradiol/levonorgestrel]	Z79.3	Contraceptive	Contraception
Ortho Cyclen [ethinyl estradiol/norgestimate]	Z79.3	Contraceptive	Contraception
Ortho-Novum [norethindrone/ethinyl estradiol]	Z79.3	Contraceptive	Contraception
Ortho-Tri-Cyclen [ethinyl estradiol/norgestimate]	Z79.3	Contraceptive	Contraception
Oseni [alogliptin benzoate/pioglitazone hydrochloride]	Z79.84	Blood glucose regulator	Diabetes mellitus
Osphena [ospemifene]	Z79.810, Z79.890	Selective estrogen receptor modulator (SERM)	Postmenopausal dyspareunia due to vaginal atrophy; osteoporosis prevention and treatment of menopause symptoms
Oxazepam [oxazepam]		Antianxiety agent	Anxiety, tension, and alcohol withdrawal
Oxycodone HCl [oxycodone hydrochloride]	Z79.891	Narcotic analgesic	Moderate to severe pain

Drug	Z Code	Drug Action	Indications
OxyContin [oxycodone hydrochloride]	Z79.891	Narcotic analgesic	Moderate to severe pain
Pavabid [papaverine hydrochloride]		Vasodilator	Relief of cerebral and peripheral ischemia
Paxil [paroxetine hydrochloride]		Antidepressant	Anxiety with panic disorder and depression; obsessive-compulsive disorder
PCE [erythromycin]	Z79.2	Antibacterial	Bacterial infections
PediaPred [prednisolone sodium phosphate]	Z79.52	Corticosteroids	Inflammatory disorders
Pegintron [peginterferon alfa-2b]	Z79.899	Antiviral interferon	Hepatitis C
Penicillin-VK [penicillin V potassium]	Z79.2	Natural penicillin	Chorea prevention; endocarditis prevention, secondary to tooth extraction; erysipelas; infections of the skin and skin structures, upper respiratory tract; rheumatic fever, prophylaxis; scarlet fever; Vincent's gingivitis; Vincent's pharyngitis
Pentam [pentamidine isethionate]	Z79.2	Antibacterial	Serious bacterial lung infections
Pepcid [famotidine]		Histamine H2-receptor inhibitor	Acid/peptic disorder; adenoma, secretory; gastroesophageal reflux; duodenal and gastric ulcer; Zollinger-Ellison syndrome
Percocet [oxycodone hydrochloride/acetaminophen]	Z79.891	Analgesic, general; analgesic-narcotic	Pain, moderate to severe
Persantine [dipyridamole]	Z79.02	Platelet inhibitor	Therapy for chronic angina pectoris, preventing clots post heart valve surgery
Pfizerpen [penicillin g potassium]	Z79.2	Antibacterial	Severe bacterial infections
Phenobarbital [phenobarbital sodium]		Barbiturate	Grand mal epilepsy
Philith [ethinyl estradiol/norethindrone]	Z79.3	Contraceptive	Contraception
Pimtrea [desogestrel/ethinyl estradiol]	Z79.3	Contraceptive	Contraception
Pirmella [ethinyl estradiol/norethindrone]	Z79.3	Contraceptive	Contraception
Pitocin [oxytocin]		Synthetic oxytocin	Induction or stimulation of labor at term
Plan B One-Step [levonorgestrel]	Z79.3	Contraceptive	Contraception
Plasmanate [plasma, plasma protein fraction]		Blood volume expander	Hypovolemic shock, burn patients, and hemorrhages when whole blood is unavailable
Plavix [clopidogrel bisulfate]	Z79.02	Antithrombotic platelet aggregation inhibitor	Lessening of the chance of heart attack or stroke
Ponstel [mefenamic acid]	Z79.1	Nonsteroidal anti-inflammatory drug (NSAID)	Pain
Portia [ethinyl estradiol/levonorgestrel]	Z79.3	Contraceptive	Contraception
Pradaxa [dabigatran etexilate mesylate]	Z79.01	Anticoagulant	Prophylaxis and treatment of blood clots in patients with atrial fibrillation
Prandimet [metformin hydrochloride/repaglinide]	Z79.84	Blood glucose regulator	Diabetes mellitus
Prandin [repaglinide]	Z79.84	Blood glucose regulator	Diabetes mellitus
Pravachol [pravastatin sodium]		HMG-CoA reductase inhibitor (statin)	Hypercholesterolemia, hyperlipidemia, hyperlipoproteinemia
Precose [acarbose]	Z79.84	Blood glucose regulator	Diabetes mellitus
Prednisolone [prednisolone]	Z79.52	Corticosteroids	Inflammatory disorders
Prednisone [prednisone]	Z79.52	Adrenocorticoid, corticosteroid	Used for its immunosuppressant effects and for relief of inflammations; used in arthritis, polymyositis and other systemic diseases
Pregnyl [chorionic gonadotropin]		Gonadotropic hormone	Prepubertal cryptorchidism, hypogonadism, corpus luteum insufficiency and infertility
Prelone [prednisolone]	Z79.52	Corticosteroids; antiasthmatic	Inflammatory disorders
Premarin [conjugated estrogens]	Z79.890	Antineoplastic; estrogen	Vasomotor symptoms associated with menopause; atrophic vaginitis; kraurosis vulvae, female hypogonadism; primary ovarian failure
Prempro [conjugated estrogens/medroxyprogesterone acetate]	Z79.890	Estrogen/progestin	Menopause, osteoporosis, atrophic vaginitis
Prevacid [lansoprazole]		Proton pump inhibitor (PPI)	Acid/peptic disorder, erosive esophagitis, duodenal ulcer, Zollinger-Ellison syndrome
Previfem [ethinyl estradiol/norgestimate]	Z79.3	Contraceptive	Contraception
Priftin [rifapentine]	Z79.2	Antibacterial	Prophylaxis and treatment of tuberculosis

Drug	Z Code	Drug Action	Indications
Prilosec [omeprazole magnesium]		Proton pump inhibitor	Acid/peptic disorder; endocrine adenoma; erosive esophagitis; systemic mastocytosis; gastroesophageal reflux; duodenal, peptic and gastric ulcer; Zollinger-Ellison syndrome
Primaxin [cilastatin sodium/imipenem]	Z79.2	Antibacterial	Skin, stomach, female reproductive organs or lower respiratory tract infections
Prinivil [lisinopril]		Synthetic peptide derivative, long-acting angiotensin converting enzyme inhibitor	Congestive heart failure, essential hypertension
Procardia [nifedipine]		Antianginal agent; calcium channel blocker	Management of vasospastic angina and chronic stable angina, essential hypertension
Prograf [tacrolimus]	Z79.899	Immunosuppressant	Prophylaxis of organ transplant rejection
Promethazine hydrochloride [promethazine hydrochloride]		Anesthesia, adjunct to; antiemetic; antihistamine; antitussive/expectorant; sedative/hypnotic; vertigo/motion sickness/vomiting	Anesthesia; adjunct; angioedema; conjunctivitis; dermographism; hypersensitivity, motion sickness; pain; perennial, seasonal, and allergic rhinitis; sedation, obstetrical; urticaria
Protonix [pantoprazole]		Proton pump inhibitor (PPI)	Short-term treatment and maintenance therapy of erosive esophagitis associated with gastroesophageal reflux disease (GERD)
Protopic [tacrolimus]	Z79.899	Immunosuppressant	Atomic dermatitis (eczema)
Proventil-HFA [albuterol sulfate]		Antiasthmatic/bronchodilator	Asthma
Provera [medroxyprogesterone acetate]	Z79.3, Z79.890	Antineoplastic; contraceptive; progestin	Amenorrhea; carcinoma, endometrium, adjunct; carcinoma, renal; contraception; hemorrhage
Prozac [fluoxetine hydrochloride]		Serotonin reuptake inhibitor	Bulimia nervosa; depression; obsessive-compulsive disorder
Pulmicort [budesonide]	Z79.51	Corticosteroids -inhaled; antiasthmatic	Prophylaxis and treatment of asthma
Qnasl [beclomethasone dipropionate]		Corticosteroid	Perennial allergies, seasonal allergies, and vasomotor rhinitis
Qtern [dapagliflozin propanediol/saxagliptin hydrochloride]	Z79.84	Blood glucose regulator	Diabetes mellitus
Quartette [levonorgestrel/ethinyl estradiol]	Z79.3	Contraceptive	Contraception
Quasense [ethinyl estradiol/levonorgestrel]	Z79.3	Contraceptive	Contraception
Quinidine gluconate [quinidine gluconate]		Antiarrhythmic	Management of cardiac arrhythmias
Qvar [beclomethasone dipropionate]	Z79.51	Corticosteroids -inhaled; antiasthmatic	Prevention and control of symptoms related to asthma
Raloxifene [raloxifene hydrochloride]	Z79.810	Selective estrogen receptor modulator (SERM)	Prevention of thinning of the bones (osteoporosis) only in postmenopausal women
Rapamune [sirolimus]	Z79.899	Immunosuppressant	Prophylaxis of organ transplant rejection
Rayos [prednisone]	Z79.52	Corticosteroids; antiasthmatic	Arthritis, blood disorders, allergies, asthma
Rebif [interferon beta-1a]	Z79.899	Antiviral interferon	Relapsing multiple sclerosis
Reclast [zoledronic acid]	Z79.83	Bisphosphonates	Prevention of thinning of the bones (osteoporosis); Paget's disease; bone cancer
Repaglinide [repaglinide]	Z79.84	Blood glucose regulator	Diabetes mellitus
Reprexain [hydrocodone bitartrate/ibuprofen]	Z79.891	Opioid analgesic/Nonsteroidal anti-inflammatory drug (NSAID)	Pain, inflammation, or fever relief
Restoril [temazepam]		Sedative/hypnotic	Insomnia
Retrovir [zidovudine]		Antiretroviral agent	Indicated in symptomatic HIV infection
Rifadin [rifampin]	Z79.2	Antibacterial	Prophylaxis and treatment of tuberculosis
Rimactane [rifampin]	Z79.2	Antibacterial	Prophylaxis and treatment of tuberculosis
Riomet [metformin hydrochloride]	Z79.84	Blood glucose regulator	Diabetes mellitus
Risperdal [risperidone]		Antipsychotic/antimanic	Schizophrenia; bipolar I disorder
Ritalin [methylphenidate hydrochloride]		Central nervous system (CNS) stimulant	Treatment of depression and hyperkinetic activity in children
Roxicet [oxycodone hydrochloride/acetaminophen]	Z79.891	Analgesic, general; analgesic-narcotic	Pain, moderate to severe
Roxicodone [oxycodone hydrochloride]	Z79.891	Narcotic analgesic	Pain relief
Ryzodeg [insulin aspart/insulin degludec]	Z79.4	Blood glucose regulator	Diabetes mellitus
Sabril [vigabatrin]		Anticonvulsant	Refractory complex partial seizures
Safyral [drospirenone/ethinyl estradiol/levomefolate calcium]	Z79.3	Contraceptive	Contraception
Sandimmune [cyclosporine]	Z79.899	Immunosuppressant	Prophylaxis of organ transplant rejection

Drug	Z Code	Drug Action	Indications
Savaysa [edoxaban tosylate]	Z79.01	Anticoagulant	Prophylaxis and treatment of venous thrombosis, pulmonary embolism; prevention of blood clots due to atrial fibrillation
Seasonale [levonorgestrel/ethinyl estradiol]	Z79.3	Contraceptive	Contraception
Seasonique [ethinyl estradiol/levonorgestrel]	Z79.3	Contraceptive	Contraception
Septra [sulfamethoxazole trimethoprim]	Z79.2	Antibacterial	Treatment of urinary tract infections, acute otitis media, acute exacerbations of chronic bronchitis, and shigellosis
Serevent [salmeterol xinafoate]		Bronchodilator	Asthma
Seromycin [cycloserine]	Z79.2	Antibacterial	Tuberculosis; urinary tract infections
Setlakin [ethinyl estradiol/levonorgestrel]	Z79.3	Contraceptive	Contraception
Simulect [basiliximab]	Z79.899	Immunosuppressant	Prophylaxis of organ transplant rejection
Sinemet [carbidopa/levodopa]		Antiparkinsonian	Parkinson's disease
Singulair [montelukast sodium]		Antiasthmatic, leukotriene receptor antagonist	Treatment of mild to moderate asthma to decrease the symptoms of asthma and the number of acute asthma attacks
Sirolimus [sirolimus]	Z79.899	Immunosuppressant	Prophylaxis of organ transplant rejection
Sitagliptin [sitagliptin/metformin hydrochloride]	Z79.84	Blood glucose regulator	Diabetes mellitus
Sivextro [tedizolid phosphate]	Z79.2	Antibacterial	Skin infections including MRSA
Skyla [levonorgestrel]	Z79.3	Contraceptive	Intrauterine device for contraception
Solodyn [minocycline hydrochloride]	Z79.2	Antibacterial	Bacterial infections
Soltamox [tamoxifen citrate]	Z79.810	Selective estrogen receptor modulator (SERM)	Breast cancer
Solu-Cortef [hydrocortisone sodium succinate]	Z79.52	Corticosteroids; antiasthmatic	Asthma; severe inflammation; allergic reactions
Solu-Medrol [methylprednisolone sodium succinate]	Z79.52	Adrenocorticosteroid	Anti-inflammatory and antiallergenic for shock and ulcerative colitis
Sprintec [norgestimate/ethinyl estradiol]	Z79.3	Contraceptive	Contraception
Streptomycin sulfate [streptomycin sulfate]	Z79.2	Antibacterial	Severe bacterial infections
Sublimaze [fentanyl citrate]	Z79.891	Narcotic analgesic	Pain relief
Supprelin LA [histrelin acetate]	Z79.818	Agents affecting estrogen receptors and estrogen levels	Precocious puberty; prostate cancer symptoms
Suprax [cefixime]	Z79.2	Antibacterial	Bacterial infections
Syeda [drospirenone/ethinyl estradiol]	Z79.3	Contraceptive	Contraception
Sylatron [peginterferon alfa-2b]	Z79.899	Antineoplastic interferons; antiviral interferons	Prevention of recurrent malignant melanoma
Symbicort [budesonide/formoterol fumarate dihydrate]	Z79.51	Corticosteroids -inhaled; antiasthmatic	Prophylaxis and treatment of asthma and COPD
Synarel [nafarelin acetate]	Z79.818	Agents affecting estrogen receptors and estrogen levels	Endometriosis symptoms; precocious puberty
Synercid [dalfopristin/quinupristin]	Z79.2	Antibacterial	Severe blood infections
Synjardy [empagliflozin/metformin hydrochloride]	Z79.84	Blood glucose regulator	Diabetes mellitus
Synthroid [levothyroxine sodium]		Thyroid hormone	Treatment of hypothyroidism
Tacrolimus [tacrolimus]	Z79.899	Immunosuppressant	Prophylaxis of organ transplant rejection
Tagamet HB [cimetidine]		Acid reducer	Treatment of active duodenal ulcer, short-term treatment of active, benign gastric ulcer, and treatment of pathological hypersecretory conditions
Tamoxifen [tamoxifen citrate]	Z79.810	Selective estrogen receptor modulator (SERM)	Metastatic breast cancer in postmenopausal women
Tazicef [ceftazidime]	Z79.2	Antibacterial	Confirmed or suspected bacterial infections
Teflaro [ceftaroline fosamil]	Z79.2	Antibacterial	Bacterial skin infections; pneumonia
Tegretol [carbamazepine]		Anticonvulsant; analgesic	Epilepsy, especially with complex symptomatology; specific analgesic for trigeminal neuralgia
Tenormin [atenolol]		Antianginal; antihypertensive; beta blocker	Treatment of hypertension; lowering blood pressure lowers the risk of fatal and nonfatal cardiovascular events, primarily strokes and myocardial infarctions

Drug	Z Code	Drug Action	Indications
Terazosin hydrochloride [terazosin hydrochloride]		Alpha-blocker; antihypertensive; diuretic	Benign prostatic hypertrophy; essential hypertension
Tetracycline HCl [tetracycline hydrochloride]	Z79.2	Antibacterial	Bacterial infections
Tiazac [diltiazem hydrochloride]		Antianginal, antiarrhythmic, antihypertensive, channel blocker, coronary vasodilator	Chronic stable angina, atrial fibrillation, atrial flutter, essential hypertension, paroxysmal supraventricular tachycardia
Tivorbex [indomethacin]	Z79.1	Nonsteroidal anti-inflammatory drug (NSAID)	Pain, inflammation and joint stiffness
Tobradex [tobramycin/dexamethasone]		Aminoglycoside ocular anti-infective; anti-inflammatory	Infectious conjunctivitis; dermatosis, corticosteroid-responsive with secondary infection; foreign body in eye; corneal inflammation; uveitis
Tobramycin [dexamethasone/tobramycin]	Z79.2	Antibacterial	Bacterial eye infections
Toprol-XL [metoprolol succinate]		Antianginal antihypertensive beta blocker	Angina pectoris, essential hypertension
Toremifene [toremifene citrate]	Z79.810	Selective estrogen receptor modulator (SERM)	Metastatic breast cancer in postmenopausal women
Torisel [temsirolimus]	Z79.899	Antineoplastic	Renal cell carcinoma
Toujeo Solostar [insulin glargine recombinant]	Z79.4	Blood glucose regulator	Diabetes mellitus
Trazodone hydrochloride [trazodone hydrochloride]		Antidepressant	Depression
Trelstar [triptorelin pamoate]	Z79.818	Agents affecting estrogen receptors and estrogen levels	Prophylaxis of chemo-induced menopause; prostate cancer symptoms
Tresiba [insulin degludec]	Z79.4	Blood glucose regulator	Diabetes mellitus
Triamterene and hydrochlorothiazide [triamterene/ hydrochlorothiazide]		Antihypertensive, diuretic	Edema; essential hypertension
Tri-Estarylla [ethinyl estradiol/norgestimate]	Z79.3	Contraceptive	Contraception; acne
Tri-Legest [ethinyl estradiol/norethindrone acetate]	Z79.3	Contraceptive	Contraception
Tri-Linyah [ethinyl estradiol/norgestimate]	Z79.3	Contraceptive	Contraception
Tri-Lo-Estarylla [ethinyl estradiol/norgestimate]	Z79.3	Contraceptive	Contraception
Tri-Lo-Sprintec [ethinyl estradiol/norgestimate]	Z79.3	Contraceptive	Contraception
Trimethoprim [trimethoprim]	Z79.2	Antibacterial	Acute exacerbation chronic bronchitis; travelers' diarrhea; infections of the middle and lower respiratory tracts, and urinary tract; pneumonia, pneumocystis; shigellosis
Tri-Norinyl [ethinyl estradiol/norethindrone]	Z79.3	Contraceptive	Contraception
Tri-Previfem [ethinyl estradiol/norgestimate]	Z79.3	Contraceptive	Contraception
Tri-Sprintec [ethinyl estradiol/norgestimate]	Z79.3	Contraceptive	Contraception; acne
Trivora [ethinyl estradiol/ levonorgestrel]	Z79.3	Contraceptive	Contraception
Tygacil [tigecycline]	Z79.2	Antibacterial	Bacterial skin or digestive system infections; pneumonia
Tylenol with codeine [acetaminophen/codeine phosphate]	Z79.891	Narcotic analgesic	Pain and cough
Ultram [tramadol hydrochloride]	Z79.891	Analgesic, non-narcotic (opiate, narcotic-like)	Pain, moderate to moderately severe
Unasyn [ampicillin sodium/sulbactam sodium]	Z79.2	Antibacterial	Bacterial infections
Vagifem [estradiol]	Z79.890	Estrogen therapy	Menopause symptoms
Valium [diazepam]		Antianxiety, muscle relaxant, anticonvulsant	Anxiety, tension, withdrawal from alcohol, muscle spasms and anticonvulsant therapy; epilepsy, generalized tonic-clonic; status epilepticus; stiff-man syndrome; tetanus
Vancocin HCl [vancomycin hydrochloride]	Z79.2	Antibacterial	Serious bacterial infections
Vancomycin HCl [vancomycin hydrochloride]	Z79.2	Antibacterial	Serious bacterial infections

Drug	Z Code	Drug Action	Indications
Vantas [histrelin acetate]	Z79.818	Agents affecting estrogen receptors and estrogen levels	Prostate cancer symptoms; breast cancer; endometriosis
Vasotec [enalaprilat maleate]		ACE inhibitor; antihypertensive	Congestive heart failure; essential hypertension
Velivet [desogestrel/ethinyl estradiol]	Z79.3	Contraceptive	Contraception
Ventolin HFA [albuterol sulfate]		Antiasthmatic/bronchodilator	Asthma
Verapamil HCL [verapamil hydrochloride]		Antianginal, antiarrhythmic, antiarthritic, antihypertensive, calcium channel blocker	Angina pectoris, chronic stable angina, atrial fibrillation, atrial flutter, paroxysmal supraventricular tachycardia, ventricular arrhythmia, essential hypertension
Viagra [sildenafil citrate]		Phosphodiesterase-5 (PDE5) inhibitor	Erectile dysfunction
Vibativ [telavancin hydrochloride]	Z79.2	Antibacterial	Pneumonia; severe bacterial skin infections
Vibramycin [doxycycline calcium]	Z79.2	Antibacterial	Bacterial infections
Vicoprofen [hydrocodone bitartrate/ibuprofen]	Z79.891	Opioid analgesic/ Nonsteroidal anti-inflammatory drug (NSAID)	Pain, inflammation, or fever relief
Victoza [liraglutide (rDNA) injection]		Glucagon-like peptide-1 (GLP-1) receptor agonist	Diabetes mellitus
Vienva [ethinyl estradiol/levonorgestrel]	Z79.3	Contraceptive	Contraception
Viorele [desogestrel/ethinyl estradiol]	Z79.3	Contraceptive	Contraception
Virazole [ribavirin]		Antiviral	Respiratory syncytial virus (RSV)
Vistaril [hydroxyzine pamoate]		Antianxiety agent, antiemetic	Treatment of nausea and vomiting, for reducing narcotic requirement in surgery and as tranquilizer for tension, anxiety, or agitation states
Vivelle [estradiol]	Z79.89Ø	Estrogen therapy	Menopause symptoms; osteoporosis prevention
Voltaren [diclofenac sodium]	Z79.1	Nonsteroidal anti-inflammatory drug (NSAID)	Treatment of pain, inflammation, and joint stiffness due to arthritis
Warfarin [warfarin sodium]	Z79.Ø1	Anticoagulant	Prophylaxis and treatment of venous thrombosis, treatment of atrial fibrillation with embolization (pulmonary embolism), arrhythmias, myocardial infarction, and stroke prevention
Wellbutrin SR, Wellbutrin XL [bupropion hydrochloride]		Antidepressant; CNS	Depression; smoking cessation
Wera [ethinyl estradiol/norethindrone]	Z79.3	Contraceptive	Contraception
Xalatan [latanoprost]		Prostaglandin F2α analogue	Glaucoma, open-angle; ocular hypertension
Xanax, Xanax XR [alprazolam]		Antianxiety; sedative/hypnotic	Anxiety disorders with panic disorder and depression
Xarelto [rivaraxaban]	Z79.Ø1	Anticoagulant	Prophylaxis and treatment of venous thrombosis, pulmonary embolism; prevention of blood clots due to atrial fibrillation
Xifaxan [rifaximin]	Z79.2	Antibacterial	*E. coli* diarrhea
Xigduo [dapagliflozin propanediol/metformin hydrochloride]	Z79.84	Blood glucose regulator	Diabetes mellitus
Xigris [drotrecogin alfa]		Biologic response modifier	Severe sepsis
Yasmin [drospirenone/ethinyl estradiol]	Z79.3	Contraceptive	Contraception
Yaz [drospirenone/ethinyl estradiol]	Z79.3	Contraceptive	Contraception; menstrual disorders
Zantac [ranitidine hydrochloride]		Histamine H2-receptors inhibitor	Acid/peptic disorder, erosive esophagitis, gastrointestinal hypersecretion, mastocytosis, gastroesophageal reflux, peptic ulcer, Zollinger-Ellison syndrome
Zerbaxa [ceftolozane sulfate/tazobactam sodium]	Z79.2	Antibacterial	Complicated urinary tract and intra-abdominal infections
Zestoretic [lisinopril/hydrochlorothiazide]		ACE inhibitor; antihypertensive	Congestive heart failure; essential hypertension
Zestril [lisinopril]		ACE inhibitor; antihypertensive	Congestive heart failure; essential hypertension
Ziac [bisoprolol fumarate/hydrochlorothiazide]		Antihypertensive	Essential hypertension
Zinacef [cefuroxime sodium]	Z79.2	Antibacterial	Bacterial infections
Zipsor [diclofenac potassium]	Z79.1	Nonsteroidal anti-inflammatory drug (NSAID)	Pain and inflammation relief
Zithromax [azithromycin]	Z79.2	Macrolide	Infections of the cervix, lower respiratory tract, skin and skin structures, urethra, nongonococcal; mycobacterium avium complex; pharyngitis, streptococcal pneumonia; tonsillitis
Zmax [azithromycin]	Z79.2	Antibacterial	Pneumonia; sinusitis
Zocor [simvastatin]		HMG-CoA reductase inhibitor (statin)	Hypercholesterolemia, hyperlipidemia, hyperlipoproteinemia, hypertriglyceridemia

Drug	Z Code	Drug Action	Indications
Zoladex [goserelin acetate]	Z79.818	Agents affecting estrogen receptors and estrogen levels	Prostate cancer symptoms and advanced breast cancer
Zoloft [sertraline hydrochloride]		Antidepressant	Anxiety with panic disorder and depression; obsessive-compulsive disorder
Zometa [zoledronic acid]	Z79.83	Bisphosphonates	Multiple myeloma; Paget's disease
Zorvolex [diclofenac]	Z79.1	Nonsteroidal anti-inflammatory drug (NSAID)	Pain, inflammation or fever relief
Zosyn [piperacillin sodium/tazobactam sodium]	Z79.2	Antibacterial	Bacterial infections
Zovia [ethynodiol diacetate/ethinyl estradiol]	Z79.3	Contraceptive	Contraception
Zovirax [acyclovir]		Antiviral	Genital herpes and herpes zoster infections
Zyloprim [allopurinol]		Antigout	Gouty arthritis, renal calculus, hyperuricemia, hyperuricemia secondary to leukemia, hyperuricemia secondary to lymphoma
Zyprexa [olanzapine]		Antipsychotic/antimanic	Psychotic disorders; schizophrenia
Zyrtec [cetirizine hydrochloride]		Antihistamine	Perennial allergic and seasonal allergic rhinitis; chronic urticaria
Zyvox [linezolid]	Z79.2	Antibacterial	Serious bacterial infections

Z79.01 Long term (current) use of anticoagulants
Arixtra
Coumadin
Eliquis
Fragmin
Heparin
Jantoven
Lovenox
Pradaxa
Savaysa
Warfarin
Xarelto

Z79.02 Long term (current) use of antithrombotics/antiplatelets
Aggrastat
Aggrenox
Angiomax
Argatroban
Brilinta
Clopidogrel bisulfate
Effient
Integrilin
Iprivask
Persantine
Plavix

Z79.1 Long term (current) use of non-steroidal anti-inflammatories (NSAID)
Advil
Aleve
Anaprox
Arthrotec
Caldolor
Cambia
Celebrex
Daypro
Duexis
Dyloject
Feldene
Ibuprofen
Indocin
Mobic
Motrin
Nabumetone
Nalfon
Naprelan
Naprosyn
NeoProfen
Ponstel
Tivorbex
Voltaren
Zipsor
Zorvolex

Z79.2 Long term (current) use of antibiotics
Akne-Mycin
Altabax
Amoxicillin
Ampicillin
Ancef
Augmentin
Azactam
Azithromycin
Bactrim
Bactroban
Ceftriaxone
Centany
Cephalexin
Cipro
Ciprofloxacin
Clarithromycin
Cleocin
Clindamycin
Daptomycin
Dificid

Doxycycline
Dynacin
E.E.S.
Ertapenem
ERYC
Erygel
EryPed
Ery-Tab
Erythrocin
Erythromycin
Factive
Flagyl
Fortaz
Gentamicin sulfate
Invanz
Isoniazid
Keflex
Kefzol
Klaron
Levaquin
Lincocin
Macrobid
Maxipime
Mefoxin
Mepron
Merrem
Metro
Metronidazole
Minocin
Monodox
Monurol
Moxatag
Mycobutin
Nebupent
Nitrofurantoin
Oracea
Orbactiv
PCE
Penicillin-VK
Pentam
Pfizerpen
Priftin
Primaxin
Rifadin
Rimactane
Septra
Seromycin
Sivextro
Solodyn
Streptomycin sulfate
Suprax
Synercid
Tazicef
Teflaro
Tetracycline HCl
Tobramycin
Trimethoprim
Tygacil
Unasyn
Vancocin HCl
Vancomycin HCl
Vibativ
Vibramycin
Xifaxan
Zerbaxa
Zinacef
Zithromax
Zmax
Zosyn
Zyvox

Z79.3 Long term (current) use of hormonal contraceptives
Altavera
Alyacen
Aranelle

Ashlyna
Aviane
Aygestin
Balziva
Bekyree
Beyaz
Brevicon
Briellyn
Camila
Cryselle
Cyclafem
Cyclessa
Dasetta
Daysee
Depo-Provera
Depo-SubQ Provera
Desogen
Elinest
Emoquette
Enpresse
Enskyce
Errin
Estarylla
Estrostep Fe
Falmina
Femcon Fe
Femhrt
Gildagia
Gildess
Introvale
Jencycla
Junel
Kariva
Kelnor
Kimidess
Kurvelo
Larin
Lessina
Levonest
Levora
Liletta
Lo Loestrin Fe
Lo Minastrin Fe
Loestrin
Loryna
LoSeasonique
Low-Ogestrel
Marlissa
Microgestin
Micronor
Minastrin
Mirena
Modicon
Mono-Linyah
Myzilra
Natazia
Nexplanon
Norinyl
Nor-QD
Nortrel
NuvaRing
Ogestrel
Orsythia
Ortho Cyclen
Ortho-Novum
Ortho-Tri-Cyclen
Philith
Pimtrea
Pirmella
Plan B One-Step
Portia
Previfem
Provera
Quartette
Quasense

Appendix D: Z Codes for Long-Term Drug Use with Associated Drugs

Safyral
Seasonale
Seasonique
Setlakin
Skyla
Sprintec
Syeda
Tri-Estarylla
Tri-Legest
Tri-Linyah
Tri-Lo-Estarylla
Tri-Lo-Sprintec
Tri-Norinyl
Tri-Previfem
Tri-Sprintec
Trivora
Velivet
Vienva
Viorele
Wera
Yasmin
Yaz
Zovia

Z79.4   Long term (current) use of insulin
Afrezza
Apidra
Basaglar
Humalog
Humulin
Lantus
Levemir
Novolin
NovoLog
Ryzodeg
Toujeo Solostar
Tresiba

Z79.51   Long term (current) use of inhaled steroids
Advair
Aerospan
Alvesco
Arnuity Ellipta
Asmanex
Dulera
Flovent
Pulmicort
Qvar
Symbicort

Z79.52   Long term (current) use of systemic steroids
A-Methapred
Aristospan
Celestone Soluspan
Colocort
Cortef
Cortenema
Cortifoam
Cortisone acetate
Depo-Medrol
Dexamethasone Intensol
Entocort EC
Hydrocortisone
Kenalog
Medrol
Methylprednisolone
Orapred ODT
PediaPred
Prednisolone
Prednisone
Prelone
Rayos
Solu-Cortef
Solu-Medrol

Z79.810 Long term (current) use of selective estrogen receptor modulators (SERMs)
Evista
Fareston
Osphena
Raloxifene
Soltamox
Tamoxifen
Toremifene

Z79.811 Long term (current) use of aromatase inhibitors
Anastrozole
Arimidex
Aromasin
Exemestane
Femara
Letrozole

Z79.818 Long term (current) use of other agents affecting estrogen receptors and estrogen levels
Eligard
Faslodex
Fulvestrant
Lupron
Megace ES
Supprelin LA
Synarel
Trelstar
Vantas
Zoladex

Z79.82   Long term (current) use of aspirin
Bayer
Bufferin
Ecotrin

Z79.83   Long term (current) use of bisphosphonates
Actonel
Atelvia
Binosto
Boniva
Didronel
Fosamax
Reclast
Zometa

Z79.84   Long term (current) use of oral hypoglycemic drugs
Acarbose
Actoplus Met
Actos
Amaryl
Avandia
Duetact
Fortamet
Glimepiride
Glucophage
Glucotrol
Glucovance
Glumetza
Glyburide
Invokamet
Janumet
Januvia
Jentadueto
Kazano
Kombiglyze
Metformin
Onglyza
Oseni
PrandiMet
Prandin
Precose
Qtern
Repaglinide
Riomet
Sitagliptin

Synjardy
Xigduo

Z79.890 Hormone replacement therapy
Activella
Alora
Angeliq
Climara
CombiPatch
Delestrogen
Divigel
Duavee
Elestrin
Enjuvia
Estrace
Estraderm
Estrasorb
EstroGel
Femhrt
Femring
Femtrace
Menest
Menostar
Minivelle
Osphena
Premarin
Prempro
Provera
Vagifem
Vivelle

Z79.891 Long term (current) use of opiate analgesic
Acetaminophen with codeine
Astramorph
Buprenex
Buprenorphine HCl
Butrans
Codeine
Demerol
Dilaudid
Dolophine HCl
Duragesic
Duramorph
Embeda
Exalgo
Fentanyl
Fentora
Fioricet with codeine
Hydrocodone
Hydrocodone bitartrate and acetaminophen
Hydromorphone HCl
Kadian
Methadone HCl
Methadose
Morphine
MS Contin
Norco
Nucynta
Opana
Oxycodone HCl
OxyContin
Percocet
Reprexain
Roxicet
Roxicodone
Sublimaze
Tylenol with codeine
Ultram
Vicoprofen

Z79.899 Other long term (current) drug therapy
Actimmune
Antineoplastic/chemotherapy
Astagraf XL
Avonex
Cellcept
Cyclosporine
Envarsus XR
Gengraf
Imuran
Intron
Monoclonal antibodies
Neoral
Pegintron
Prograf
Protopic
Rapamune
Rebif
Sandimmune
Simulect
Sirolimus
Sylatron
Tacrolimus
Torisel

Z79.899 Other long term (current) drug therapy

Appendix E: Major Complication and Comorbidity (MCC) Code List

Note: The following list of MCCs are based on the *Federal Register,* volume 82, number 81, April 28, 2017 ("Hospital Inpatient Prospective Payment Systems for Acute Care Hospitals and the Long-Term Care Hospital Prospective Payment System and Proposed Policy Changes and Fiscal Year 2018 Rates; Proposed Rule"). The most current version, v35, of the ICD-10 MS-DRG Definitions Manual was not available at the time this book was printed. For the most current files related to IPPS please refer to the following: https://www.cms.gov/Medicare/Medicare-Fee-for-Service-Payment/AcuteInpatientPPS/IPPS-Regulations-and-Notices.html.

A02.1	A48.1	B45.1	E13.00	I21.09	I61.9	I63.432	J12.3	K25.5
A02.21	A48.3	B46.0	E13.01	I21.11	I62.00	I63.433	J12.81	K25.6
A02.22	A50.41	B46.1	E13.10	I21.19	I62.01	I63.439	J12.89	K26.0
A06.4	A50.42	B46.2	E13.11	I21.21	I62.02	I63.441	J12.9	K26.1
A06.5	A51.41	B46.3	E13.641	I21.29	I62.03	I63.442	J13	K26.2
A06.6	A52.13	B46.4	E40	I21.3	I62.1	I63.443	J14	K26.4
A17.0	A52.14	B46.5	E41	I21.4	I63.00	I63.449	J15.0	K26.5
A17.1	A54.81	B46.8	E42	I22.0	I63.011	I63.49	J15.1	K26.6
A17.81	A54.86	B46.9	E43	I22.1	I63.012	I63.50	J15.20	K27.0
A17.82	A80.0	B50.9	E84.0	I22.2	I63.013	I63.511	J15.211	K27.1
A17.83	A80.1	B58.2	E84.11	I22.8	I63.019	I63.512	J15.212	K27.2
A17.89	A80.2	B58.3	E88.3	I22.9	I63.02	I63.513	J15.29	K27.4
A18.31	A80.30	B58.81	G00.0	I23.4	I63.031	I63.519	J15.3	K27.5
A19.0	A80.39	B59	G00.1	I23.5	I63.032	I63.521	J15.4	K27.6
A19.1	A83.0	B77.81	G00.2	I25.42	I63.033	I63.522	J15.5	K28.0
A19.2	A83.1	D57.00	G00.3	I26.01	I63.039	I63.523	J15.6	K28.1
A19.8	A83.2	D57.01	G00.8	I26.02	I63.09	I63.529	J15.7	K28.2
A19.9	A83.3	D57.02	G00.9	I26.09	I63.10	I63.531	J15.8	K28.4
A20.0	A83.4	D57.211	G01	I26.90	I63.111	I63.532	J15.9	K28.5
A20.1	A83.5	D57.212	G02	I26.92	I63.112	I63.533	J16.0	K28.6
A20.2	A83.6	D57.219	G03.0	I26.99	I63.113	I63.539	J16.8	K29.01
A20.3	A83.8	D57.411	G03.8	I33.0	I63.119	I63.541	J17	K29.21
A20.7	A83.9	D57.412	G03.9	I33.9	I63.12	I63.542	J18.0	K29.31
A20.8	A84.0	D57.419	G04.00	I40.0	I63.131	I63.543	J18.1	K29.41
A20.9	A84.1	D57.811	G04.01	I40.1	I63.132	I63.549	J18.8	K29.51
A22.1	A84.8	D57.812	G04.02	I40.8	I63.133	I63.59	J18.9	K29.61
A22.7	A84.9	D57.819	G04.2	I40.9	I63.139	I63.6	J68.1	K29.71
A26.7	A85.2	D59.3	G04.30	I41	I63.19	I63.8	J69.0	K29.81
A27.81	A92.30	D60.0	G04.31	I46.2	I63.20	I63.9	J69.1	K29.91
A32.7	A92.31	D60.1	G04.32	I46.8	I63.211	I67.0	J69.8	K31.811
A33	A92.32	D60.8	G04.39	I46.9	I63.212	I67.83	J81.0	K31.82
A35	A92.39	D60.9	G04.81	I49.01	I63.213	I71.00	J84.81	K35.2
A37.01	B00.3	D61.1	G04.89	I49.02	I63.219	I71.01	J84.83	K35.3
A37.11	B00.4	D61.2	G04.90	I50.21	I63.22	I71.02	J84.841	K40.10
A37.81	B00.7	D61.3	G04.91	I50.23	I63.231	I71.03	J84.842	K40.11
A37.91	B00.82	D61.810	G05.3	I50.31	I63.232	I71.1	J84.843	K40.40
A39.0	B01.11	D61.811	G05.4	I50.33	I63.233	I71.3	J84.848	K40.41
A39.1	B01.12	D61.89	G06.0	I50.41	I63.239	I71.5	J85.0	K41.10
A39.2	B01.2	D65	G06.1	I50.43	I63.29	I71.8	J85.1	K41.11
A39.3	B02.1	D66	G06.2	I51.1	I63.30	I74.01	J85.2	K41.40
A39.4	B02.24	D67	G07	I51.2	I63.311	I77.70	J85.3	K41.41
A39.50	B05.0	E03.5	G08	I60.00	I63.312	I77.71	J86.0	K42.1
A39.51	B05.2	E05.01	G21.0	I60.01	I63.313	I77.72	J86.9	K43.1
A39.52	B06.01	E05.11	G37.4	I60.02	I63.319	I77.73	J93.0	K43.4
A39.53	B10.01	E05.21	G40.301	I60.10	I63.321	I77.74	J95.1	K43.7
A39.81	B10.09	E05.31	G40.311	I60.11	I63.322	I77.75	J95.2	K44.1
A40.0	B15.0	E05.41	G40.319	I60.12	I63.323	I77.76	J95.3	K45.1
A40.1	B16.0	E05.81	G70.01	I60.2	I63.329	I77.77	J95.821	K46.1
A40.3	B16.2	E05.91	G80.0	I60.30	I63.331	I77.79	J95.822	K55.011
A40.8	B17.11	E08.00	G82.50	I60.31	I63.332	I81	J96.00	K55.012
A40.9	B19.0	E08.01	G82.51	I60.32	I63.333	I82.0	J96.01	K55.019
A41.01	B19.11	E08.10	G82.52	I60.4	I63.339	I82.220	J96.02	K55.021
A41.02	B19.21	E08.11	G82.53	I60.50	I63.341	I82.221	J96.20	K55.022
A41.1	B20	E08.641	G82.54	I60.51	I63.342	I85.01	J96.21	K55.029
A41.2	B25.0	E09.00	G83.5	I60.52	I63.343	I85.11	J96.22	K55.031
A41.3	B25.2	E09.01	G92	I60.6	I63.349	J04.11	J96.90	K55.032
A41.4	B26.1	E09.10	G93.40	I60.7	I63.39	J04.31	J96.91	K55.039
A41.50	B26.2	E09.11	G93.41	I60.8	I63.40	J05.11	J96.92	K55.041
A41.51	B37.1	E09.641	G93.49	I60.9	I63.411	J09.X1	J98.51	K55.042
A41.52	B37.5	E10.10	G93.5	I61.0	I63.412	J10.00	J98.59	K55.049
A41.53	B37.6	E10.11	G93.6	I61.1	I63.413	J10.01	K22.11	K55.051
A41.59	B37.7	E10.641	G93.7	I61.2	I63.419	J10.08	K22.3	K55.052
A41.81	B38.4	E11.00	G93.82	I61.3	I63.421	J11.00	K22.6	K55.059
A41.89	B39.0	E11.01	G95.11	I61.4	I63.422	J11.08	K25.0	K55.061
A41.9	B39.1	E11.10	G95.19	I61.5	I63.423	J12.0	K25.1	K55.062
A42.7	B39.2	E11.11	I21.01	I61.6	I63.429	J12.1	K25.2	K55.069
A48.0	B44.0	E11.641	I21.02	I61.8	I63.431	J12.2	K25.4	K55.21

Appendix E: Major Complication and Comorbidity (MCC) Code List

K55.30	L89.143	O08.4	O41.1425	O60.22X9	P26.8	Q04.3	R40.2342	S06.341A
K55.31	L89.144	O10.42	O41.1429	O60.23X0	P26.9	Q20.0	R40.2343	S06.342A
K55.32	L89.153	O11.1	O41.1430	O60.23X1	P27.0	Q20.1	R40.2344	S06.343A
K55.33	L89.154	O11.2	O41.1431	O60.23X2	P27.1	Q20.2	R53.2	S06.344A
K56.2	L89.203	O11.3	O41.1432	O60.23X3	P27.8	Q20.3	R57.0	S06.345A
K57.01	L89.204	O14.12	O41.1433	O60.23X4	P27.9	Q20.4	R57.1	S06.346A
K57.11	L89.213	O14.13	O41.1434	O60.23X5	P28.5	Q21.3	R57.8	S06.347A
K57.13	L89.214	O14.22	O41.1435	O60.23X9	P28.81	Q22.0	R65.11	S06.348A
K57.21	L89.223	O14.23	O41.1439	O67.0	P29.30	Q22.4	R65.20	S06.349A
K57.31	L89.224	O15.02	O44.11	O71.02	P29.38	Q22.5	R65.21	S06.350A
K57.33	L89.303	O15.03	O44.12	O71.03	P29.81	Q22.6	S02.0XXB	S06.351A
K57.41	L89.304	O15.1	O44.13	O71.1	P35.1	Q22.8	S02.101B	S06.352A
K57.51	L89.313	O15.2	O44.31	O75.1	P35.2	Q22.9	S02.102B	S06.353A
K57.53	L89.314	O22.31	O44.32	O75.3	P35.3	Q23.4	S02.109B	S06.354A
K57.81	L89.323	O22.32	O44.33	O85	P35.8	Q24.2	S02.110B	S06.355A
K57.91	L89.324	O22.33	O44.51	O86.81	P35.9	Q24.4	S02.111B	S06.356A
K57.93	L89.43	O24.02	O44.52	O86.89	P36.0	Q24.6	S02.112B	S06.357A
K63.1	L89.44	O24.12	O44.53	O87.1	P36.10	Q25.5	S02.113B	S06.358A
K63.81	L89.503	O24.32	O45.001	O88.011	P36.19	Q25.6	S02.118B	S06.359A
K65.0	L89.504	O24.82	O45.002	O88.012	P36.2	Q25.71	S02.119B	S06.360A
K65.1	L89.513	O34.31	O45.003	O88.013	P36.30	Q25.72	S02.11AB	S06.361A
K65.2	L89.514	O34.32	O45.011	O88.02	P36.39	Q25.79	S02.11BB	S06.362A
K65.3	L89.523	O34.33	O45.012	O88.03	P36.4	Q28.2	S02.11CB	S06.363A
K65.8	L89.524	O41.1010	O45.013	O88.111	P36.5	Q28.3	S02.11DB	S06.364A
K65.9	L89.603	O41.1011	O45.021	O88.112	P36.8	Q33.2	S02.11EB	S06.365A
K66.1	L89.604	O41.1012	O45.022	O88.113	P36.9	Q33.3	S02.11FB	S06.366A
K67	L89.613	O41.1013	O45.023	O88.12	P37.0	Q33.6	S02.11GB	S06.367A
K68.12	L89.614	O41.1014	O45.091	O88.13	P37.1	Q39.0	S02.11HB	S06.368A
K68.19	L89.623	O41.1015	O45.092	O88.211	P37.2	Q39.1	S02.19XB	S06.369A
K68.9	L89.624	O41.1019	O45.093	O88.212	P37.3	Q39.2	S02.91XB	S06.370A
K70.41	L89.813	O41.1020	O45.8X1	O88.213	P37.4	Q39.3	S06.1X0A	S06.376A
K71.11	L89.814	O41.1021	O45.8X2	O88.22	P37.8	Q39.4	S06.1X1A	S06.377A
K72.00	L89.893	O41.1022	O45.8X3	O88.23	P37.9	Q44.2	S06.1X2A	S06.378A
K72.01	L89.894	O41.1023	O45.91	O88.311	P52.21	Q44.3	S06.1X3A	S06.380A
K72.11	L89.93	O41.1024	O45.92	O88.312	P52.22	Q79.0	S06.1X4A	S06.386A
K72.91	L89.94	O41.1025	O45.93	O88.313	P52.4	Q79.1	S06.1X5A	S06.387A
K75.0	M31.1	O41.1029	O46.001	O88.32	P52.5	Q79.2	S06.1X6A	S06.388A
K75.1	M72.6	O41.1030	O46.002	O88.33	P52.6	Q79.3	S06.1X7A	S06.4X0A
K76.2	N00.0	O41.1031	O46.003	O88.811	P52.8	Q79.4	S06.1X8A	S06.4X1A
K76.3	N00.1	O41.1032	O46.011	O88.812	P52.9	Q79.51	S06.1X9A	S06.4X2A
K76.7	N00.2	O41.1033	O46.012	O88.813	P54.1	Q79.59	S06.2X6A	S06.4X3A
K80.67	N00.3	O41.1034	O46.013	O88.82	P54.2	Q89.4	S06.2X7A	S06.4X4A
K82.2	N00.4	O41.1035	O46.021	O88.83	P54.3	Q93.81	S06.2X8A	S06.4X5A
K83.1	N00.5	O41.1039	O46.022	O90.3	P56.0	R09.2	S06.306A	S06.4X6A
K83.2	N00.6	O41.1210	O46.023	O90.4	P56.90	R40.20	S06.307A	S06.4X7A
K85.00	N00.7	O41.1211	O46.091	O99.42	P56.99	R40.2110	S06.308A	S06.4X8A
K85.01	N00.8	O41.1212	O46.092	P10.0	P57.0	R40.2111	S06.310A	S06.4X9A
K85.02	N00.9	O41.1213	O46.093	P10.1	P57.8	R40.2112	S06.311A	S06.5X0A
K85.10	N01.0	O41.1214	O60.02	P10.3	P57.9	R40.2113	S06.312A	S06.5X1A
K85.11	N01.1	O41.1215	O60.03	P10.4	P59.1	R40.2114	S06.313A	S06.5X2A
K85.12	N01.2	O41.1219	O60.12X0	P10.8	P59.20	R40.2120	S06.314A	S06.5X3A
K85.20	N01.3	O41.1220	O60.12X1	P10.9	P59.29	R40.2121	S06.315A	S06.5X4A
K85.21	N01.4	O41.1221	O60.12X2	P11.0	P60	R40.2122	S06.316A	S06.5X5A
K85.22	N01.5	O41.1222	O60.12X3	P11.2	P61.0	R40.2123	S06.317A	S06.5X6A
K85.30	N01.6	O41.1223	O60.12X4	P11.9	P61.5	R40.2124	S06.318A	S06.5X7A
K85.31	N01.7	O41.1224	O60.12X5	P22.0	P74.0	R40.2210	S06.319A	S06.5X8A
K85.32	N01.8	O41.1225	O60.12X9	P23.0	P77.1	R40.2211	S06.320A	S06.5X9A
K85.80	N01.9	O41.1229	O60.13X0	P23.1	P77.2	R40.2212	S06.321A	S06.6X0A
K85.81	N15.1	O41.1230	O60.13X1	P23.2	P77.3	R40.2213	S06.322A	S06.6X1A
K85.82	N17.0	O41.1231	O60.13X2	P23.3	P77.9	R40.2214	S06.323A	S06.6X2A
K85.90	N17.1	O41.1232	O60.13X3	P23.4	P78.0	R40.2220	S06.324A	S06.6X3A
K85.91	N17.2	O41.1233	O60.13X4	P23.5	P83.2	R40.2221	S06.325A	S06.6X4A
K85.92	N18.6	O41.1234	O60.13X5	P23.6	P90	R40.2222	S06.326A	S06.6X5A
L89.003	N73.3	O41.1235	O60.13X9	P23.8	P91.0	R40.2223	S06.327A	S06.6X6A
L89.004	O03.2	O41.1239	O60.14X0	P23.9	P91.1	R40.2224	S06.328A	S06.6X7A
L89.013	O03.31	O41.1410	O60.14X1	P24.01	P91.2	R40.2310	S06.329A	S06.6X8A
L89.014	O03.32	O41.1411	O60.14X2	P24.11	P91.3	R40.2311	S06.330A	S06.6X9A
L89.023	O03.81	O41.1412	O60.14X3	P24.21	P91.4	R40.2312	S06.331A	S06.816A
L89.024	O03.82	O41.1413	O60.14X4	P24.31	P91.5	R40.2313	S06.332A	S06.817A
L89.103	O04.7	O41.1414	O60.14X5	P24.81	P91.63	R40.2314	S06.333A	S06.818A
L89.104	O04.81	O41.1415	O60.14X9	P25.0	P92.01	R40.2320	S06.334A	S06.826A
L89.113	O04.82	O41.1419	O60.22X0	P25.1	Q00.0	R40.2321	S06.335A	S06.827A
L89.114	O07.2	O41.1420	O60.22X1	P25.2	Q00.1	R40.2322	S06.336A	S06.828A
L89.123	O07.31	O41.1421	O60.22X2	P25.3	Q00.2	R40.2323	S06.337A	S06.896A
L89.124	O07.32	O41.1422	O60.22X3	P25.8	Q04.0	R40.2324	S06.338A	S06.897A
L89.133	O08.2	O41.1423	O60.22X4	P26.0	Q04.1	R40.2340	S06.339A	S06.898A
L89.134	O08.3	O41.1424	O60.22X5	P26.1	Q04.2	R40.2341	S06.340A	S06.9X6A

S06.9X7A	S12.551B	S21.351A	S22.49XB	S27.332A	S32.018B	S32.424A	S32.486B	S35.291A
S06.9X8A	S12.590B	S21.352A	S22.5XXA	S27.339A	S32.019B	S32.424B	S32.491A	S35.292A
S11.011A	S12.591B	S21.359A	S22.5XXB	S27.401A	S32.020B	S32.425A	S32.491B	S35.298A
S11.012A	S12.600B	S21.401A	S22.9XXB	S27.402A	S32.021B	S32.425B	S32.492A	S35.299A
S11.013A	S12.601B	S21.402A	S24.0XXA	S27.409A	S32.022B	S32.426A	S32.492B	S35.311A
S11.014A	S12.630B	S21.409A	S24.101A	S27.411A	S32.028B	S32.426B	S32.499A	S35.318A
S11.015A	S12.631B	S21.411A	S24.102A	S27.412A	S32.029B	S32.431A	S32.499B	S35.319A
S11.019A	S12.64XB	S21.412A	S24.103A	S27.419A	S32.030B	S32.431B	S32.501B	S35.321A
S11.021A	S12.650B	S21.419A	S24.104A	S27.421A	S32.031B	S32.432A	S32.502B	S35.328A
S11.022A	S12.651B	S21.421A	S24.111A	S27.422A	S32.032B	S32.432B	S32.509B	S35.329A
S11.023A	S12.690B	S21.422A	S24.112A	S27.429A	S32.038B	S32.433A	S32.511B	S35.331A
S11.024A	S12.691B	S21.429A	S24.113A	S27.431A	S32.039B	S32.433B	S32.512B	S35.338A
S11.025A	S12.8XXB	S21.431A	S24.114A	S27.432A	S32.040B	S32.434A	S32.519B	S35.339A
S11.029A	S14.0XXA	S21.432A	S24.131A	S27.439A	S32.041B	S32.434B	S32.591B	S35.341A
S11.031A	S14.101A	S21.439A	S24.132A	S27.491A	S32.042B	S32.435A	S32.592B	S35.348A
S11.032A	S14.102A	S21.441A	S24.133A	S27.492A	S32.048B	S32.435B	S32.599B	S35.349A
S11.033A	S14.103A	S21.442A	S24.134A	S27.499A	S32.049B	S32.436A	S32.601B	S35.401A
S11.034A	S14.104A	S21.449A	S24.141A	S27.812A	S32.050B	S32.436B	S32.602B	S35.402A
S11.035A	S14.105A	S21.451A	S24.142A	S27.813A	S32.051B	S32.441A	S32.609B	S35.403A
S11.039A	S14.106A	S21.452A	S24.143A	S27.818A	S32.052B	S32.441B	S32.611B	S35.404A
S12.000B	S14.107A	S21.459A	S24.144A	S27.819A	S32.058B	S32.442A	S32.612B	S35.405A
S12.001B	S14.108A	S22.000B	S24.151A	S31.001A	S32.059B	S32.442B	S32.613B	S35.406A
S12.01XB	S14.111A	S22.001B	S24.152A	S31.011A	S32.10XB	S32.443A	S32.614B	S35.411A
S12.02XB	S14.112A	S22.002B	S24.153A	S31.021A	S32.110B	S32.443B	S32.615B	S35.412A
S12.030B	S14.113A	S22.008B	S24.154A	S31.031A	S32.111B	S32.444A	S32.616B	S35.413A
S12.031B	S14.114A	S22.009B	S25.00XA	S31.041A	S32.112B	S32.444B	S32.691B	S35.414A
S12.040B	S14.115A	S22.010B	S25.01XA	S31.051A	S32.119B	S32.445A	S32.692B	S35.415A
S12.041B	S14.116A	S22.011B	S25.02XA	S31.600A	S32.120B	S32.445B	S32.699B	S35.416A
S12.090B	S14.117A	S22.012B	S25.09XA	S31.601A	S32.121B	S32.446A	S32.810B	S35.491A
S12.091B	S14.118A	S22.018B	S25.101A	S31.602A	S32.122B	S32.446B	S32.811B	S35.492A
S12.100B	S14.121A	S22.019B	S25.102A	S31.603A	S32.129B	S32.451A	S32.82XB	S35.493A
S12.101B	S14.122A	S22.020B	S25.109A	S31.604A	S32.130B	S32.451B	S32.89XB	S35.494A
S12.110B	S14.123A	S22.021B	S25.111A	S31.605A	S32.131B	S32.452A	S32.9XXB	S35.495A
S12.111B	S14.124A	S22.022B	S25.112A	S31.609A	S32.132B	S32.452B	S34.01XA	S35.496A
S12.112B	S14.125A	S22.028B	S25.119A	S31.610A	S32.139B	S32.453A	S34.02XA	S35.50XA
S12.120B	S14.126A	S22.029B	S25.121A	S31.611A	S32.14XB	S32.453B	S34.101A	S35.511A
S12.121B	S14.127A	S22.030B	S25.122A	S31.612A	S32.15XB	S32.454A	S34.102A	S35.512A
S12.130B	S14.128A	S22.031B	S25.129A	S31.613A	S32.16XB	S32.454B	S34.103A	S35.513A
S12.131B	S14.131A	S22.032B	S25.191A	S31.614A	S32.17XB	S32.455A	S34.104A	S35.514A
S12.14XB	S14.132A	S22.038B	S25.192A	S31.615A	S32.19XB	S32.455B	S34.105A	S35.515A
S12.150B	S14.133A	S22.039B	S25.199A	S31.619A	S32.2XXB	S32.456A	S34.109A	S35.516A
S12.151B	S14.134A	S22.040B	S25.20XA	S31.620A	S32.301B	S32.456B	S34.111A	S35.59XA
S12.190B	S14.135A	S22.041B	S25.21XA	S31.621A	S32.302B	S32.461A	S34.112A	S36.031A
S12.191B	S14.136A	S22.042B	S25.22XA	S31.622A	S32.309B	S32.461B	S34.113A	S36.032A
S12.200B	S14.137A	S22.048B	S25.29XA	S31.623A	S32.311B	S32.462A	S34.114A	S36.115A
S12.201B	S14.138A	S22.049B	S25.301A	S31.624A	S32.312B	S32.462B	S34.115A	S36.116A
S12.230B	S14.141A	S22.050B	S25.302A	S31.625A	S32.313B	S32.463A	S34.119A	S37.061A
S12.231B	S14.142A	S22.051B	S25.309A	S31.629A	S32.314B	S32.463B	S34.121A	S37.062A
S12.24XB	S14.143A	S22.052B	S25.311A	S31.630A	S32.315B	S32.464A	S34.122A	S37.069A
S12.250B	S14.144A	S22.058B	S25.312A	S31.631A	S32.316B	S32.464B	S34.123A	S37.091A
S12.251B	S14.145A	S22.059B	S25.319A	S31.632A	S32.391B	S32.465A	S34.124A	S37.092A
S12.290B	S14.146A	S22.060B	S25.321A	S31.633A	S32.392B	S32.465B	S34.125A	S37.099A
S12.291B	S14.147A	S22.061B	S25.322A	S31.634A	S32.399B	S32.466A	S34.129A	S42.201B
S12.300B	S14.148A	S22.062B	S25.329A	S31.635A	S32.401A	S32.466B	S34.131A	S42.202B
S12.301B	S14.151A	S22.068B	S25.391A	S31.639A	S32.401B	S32.471A	S34.132A	S42.209B
S12.330B	S14.152A	S22.069B	S25.392A	S31.640A	S32.402A	S32.471B	S34.139A	S42.211B
S12.331B	S14.153A	S22.070B	S25.399A	S31.641A	S32.402B	S32.472A	S34.3XXA	S42.212B
S12.34XB	S14.154A	S22.071B	S25.401A	S31.642A	S32.409A	S32.472B	S35.00XA	S42.213B
S12.350B	S14.155A	S22.072B	S25.402A	S31.643A	S32.409B	S32.473A	S35.01XA	S42.214B
S12.351B	S14.156A	S22.078B	S25.409A	S31.644A	S32.411A	S32.473B	S35.02XA	S42.215B
S12.390B	S14.157A	S22.079B	S25.411A	S31.645A	S32.411B	S32.474A	S35.09XA	S42.216B
S12.391B	S14.158A	S22.080B	S25.412A	S31.649A	S32.412A	S32.474B	S35.10XA	S42.221B
S12.400B	S21.301A	S22.081B	S25.419A	S31.650A	S32.412B	S32.475A	S35.11XA	S42.222B
S12.401B	S21.302A	S22.082B	S25.421A	S31.651A	S32.413A	S32.475B	S35.12XA	S42.223B
S12.430B	S21.309A	S22.088B	S25.422A	S31.652A	S32.413B	S32.476A	S35.19XA	S42.224B
S12.431B	S21.311A	S22.089B	S25.429A	S31.653A	S32.414A	S32.476B	S35.211A	S42.225B
S12.44XB	S21.312A	S22.20XB	S25.491A	S31.654A	S32.414B	S32.481A	S35.212A	S42.226B
S12.450B	S21.319A	S22.21XB	S25.492A	S31.655A	S32.415A	S32.481B	S35.218A	S42.231B
S12.451B	S21.321A	S22.22XB	S25.499A	S31.659A	S32.415B	S32.482A	S35.219A	S42.232B
S12.490B	S21.322A	S22.23XB	S26.020A	S32.000B	S32.416A	S32.482B	S35.221A	S42.239B
S12.491B	S21.329A	S22.24XB	S26.021A	S32.001B	S32.416B	S32.483A	S35.222A	S42.241B
S12.500B	S21.331A	S22.31XB	S26.022A	S32.002B	S32.421A	S32.483B	S35.228A	S42.242B
S12.501B	S21.332A	S22.32XB	S26.12XA	S32.008B	S32.421B	S32.484A	S35.229A	S42.249B
S12.530B	S21.339A	S22.39XB	S26.92XA	S32.009B	S32.422A	S32.484B	S35.231A	S42.251B
S12.531B	S21.341A	S22.41XB	S27.1XXA	S32.010B	S32.422B	S32.485A	S35.232A	S42.252B
S12.54XB	S21.342A	S22.42XB	S27.2XXA	S32.011B	S32.423A	S32.485B	S35.238A	S42.253B
S12.550B	S21.349A	S22.43XB	S27.331A	S32.012B	S32.423B	S32.486A	S35.239A	S42.254B

Appendix E: Major Complication and Comorbidity (MCC) Code List

S42.255B	S42.447B	S52.045B	S52.241C	S52.334B	S52.516C	S72.011B	S72.063A	S72.134C
S42.256B	S42.448B	S52.045C	S52.242B	S52.334C	S52.531B	S72.011C	S72.063B	S72.135A
S42.261B	S42.449B	S52.046B	S52.242C	S52.335B	S52.531C	S72.012A	S72.063C	S72.135B
S42.262B	S42.451B	S52.046C	S52.243B	S52.335C	S52.532B	S72.012B	S72.064A	S72.135C
S42.263B	S42.452B	S52.091B	S52.243C	S52.336B	S52.532C	S72.012C	S72.064B	S72.136A
S42.264B	S42.453B	S52.091C	S52.244B	S52.336C	S52.539B	S72.019A	S72.064C	S72.136B
S42.265B	S42.454B	S52.092B	S52.244C	S52.341B	S52.539C	S72.019B	S72.065A	S72.136C
S42.266B	S42.455B	S52.092C	S52.245B	S52.341C	S52.541B	S72.019C	S72.065B	S72.141A
S42.291B	S42.456B	S52.099B	S52.245C	S52.342B	S52.541C	S72.021A	S72.066A	S72.141B
S42.292B	S42.461B	S52.099C	S52.246B	S52.342C	S52.542B	S72.021B	S72.066B	S72.141C
S42.293B	S42.462B	S52.101B	S52.246C	S52.343B	S52.542C	S72.021C	S72.066C	S72.142A
S42.294B	S42.463B	S52.101C	S52.251B	S52.343C	S52.549B	S72.022A	S72.091B	S72.142B
S42.295B	S42.464B	S52.102B	S52.251C	S52.344B	S52.549C	S72.022B	S72.091C	S72.142C
S42.296B	S42.465B	S52.102C	S52.252B	S52.344C	S52.551B	S72.022C	S72.092A	S72.143A
S42.301B	S42.466B	S52.109B	S52.252C	S52.345B	S52.551C	S72.023A	S72.092B	S72.143B
S42.302B	S42.471B	S52.109C	S52.253B	S52.345C	S52.552B	S72.023B	S72.092C	S72.143C
S42.309B	S42.472B	S52.121B	S52.253C	S52.346B	S52.552C	S72.023C	S72.099A	S72.144A
S42.321B	S42.473B	S52.121C	S52.254B	S52.346C	S52.559B	S72.024A	S72.099B	S72.144B
S42.322B	S42.474B	S52.122B	S52.254C	S52.351B	S52.559C	S72.024B	S72.099C	S72.144C
S42.323B	S42.475B	S52.122C	S52.255B	S52.351C	S52.561B	S72.024C	S72.101A	S72.145A
S42.324B	S42.476B	S52.123B	S52.255C	S52.352B	S52.561C	S72.025A	S72.101B	S72.145B
S42.325B	S42.491B	S52.123C	S52.256B	S52.352C	S52.562B	S72.025B	S72.101C	S72.145C
S42.326B	S42.492B	S52.124B	S52.256C	S52.353B	S52.562C	S72.025C	S72.102A	S72.146A
S42.331B	S42.493B	S52.124C	S52.261B	S52.353C	S52.569B	S72.026A	S72.102B	S72.146B
S42.332B	S42.494B	S52.125B	S52.261C	S52.354B	S52.569C	S72.026B	S72.102C	S72.146C
S42.333B	S42.495B	S52.125C	S52.262B	S52.354C	S52.571B	S72.026C	S72.109A	S72.21XA
S42.334B	S42.496B	S52.126B	S52.262C	S52.355B	S52.571C	S72.031A	S72.109B	S72.21XB
S42.335B	S42.90XB	S52.126C	S52.263B	S52.355C	S52.572B	S72.031B	S72.109C	S72.21XC
S42.336B	S42.91XB	S52.131B	S52.263C	S52.356B	S52.572C	S72.031C	S72.111A	S72.22XA
S42.341B	S42.92XB	S52.131C	S52.264B	S52.356C	S52.579B	S72.032A	S72.111B	S72.22XB
S42.342B	S45.001A	S52.132B	S52.264C	S52.361B	S52.579C	S72.032B	S72.111C	S72.22XC
S42.343B	S45.002A	S52.132C	S52.265B	S52.361C	S52.591B	S72.032C	S72.112A	S72.23XA
S42.344B	S45.009A	S52.133B	S52.265C	S52.362B	S52.591C	S72.033A	S72.112B	S72.23XB
S42.345B	S45.011A	S52.133C	S52.266B	S52.362C	S52.592B	S72.033B	S72.112C	S72.23XC
S42.346B	S45.012A	S52.134B	S52.266C	S52.363B	S52.592C	S72.033C	S72.113A	S72.24XA
S42.351B	S45.019A	S52.134C	S52.271B	S52.363C	S52.599B	S72.034A	S72.113B	S72.24XB
S42.352B	S45.091A	S52.135B	S52.271C	S52.364B	S52.599C	S72.034B	S72.113C	S72.24XC
S42.353B	S45.092A	S52.135C	S52.272B	S52.364C	S52.601B	S72.034C	S72.114A	S72.25XA
S42.354B	S45.099A	S52.136B	S52.272C	S52.365B	S52.601C	S72.035A	S72.114B	S72.25XB
S42.355B	S52.001B	S52.136C	S52.279B	S52.365C	S52.602B	S72.035B	S72.114C	S72.25XC
S42.356B	S52.001C	S52.181B	S52.279C	S52.366B	S52.602C	S72.035C	S72.115A	S72.26XA
S42.361B	S52.002B	S52.181C	S52.281B	S52.366C	S52.609B	S72.036A	S72.115B	S72.26XB
S42.362B	S52.002C	S52.182B	S52.281C	S52.371B	S52.609C	S72.036B	S72.115C	S72.26XC
S42.363B	S52.009B	S52.182C	S52.282B	S52.371C	S52.611B	S72.036C	S72.116A	S72.301A
S42.364B	S52.009C	S52.189B	S52.282C	S52.372B	S52.611C	S72.041A	S72.116B	S72.301B
S42.365B	S52.021B	S52.189C	S52.283B	S52.372C	S52.612B	S72.041B	S72.116C	S72.301C
S42.366B	S52.021C	S52.201B	S52.283C	S52.379B	S52.612C	S72.041C	S72.121A	S72.302A
S42.391B	S52.022B	S52.201C	S52.291B	S52.379C	S52.613B	S72.042A	S72.121B	S72.302B
S42.392B	S52.022C	S52.202B	S52.291C	S52.381B	S52.613C	S72.042B	S72.121C	S72.302C
S42.399B	S52.023B	S52.202C	S52.292B	S52.381C	S52.614B	S72.042C	S72.122A	S72.309A
S42.401B	S52.023C	S52.209B	S52.292C	S52.382B	S52.614C	S72.043A	S72.122B	S72.309B
S42.402B	S52.024B	S52.209C	S52.299B	S52.382C	S52.615B	S72.043B	S72.122C	S72.309C
S42.409B	S52.024C	S52.221B	S52.299C	S52.389B	S52.615C	S72.043C	S72.123A	S72.321A
S42.411B	S52.025B	S52.221C	S52.301B	S52.389C	S52.616B	S72.044A	S72.123B	S72.321B
S42.412B	S52.025C	S52.222B	S52.301C	S52.391B	S52.616C	S72.044B	S72.123C	S72.321C
S42.413B	S52.026B	S52.222C	S52.302B	S52.391C	S52.691B	S72.044C	S72.124A	S72.322A
S42.414B	S52.026C	S52.223B	S52.302C	S52.392B	S52.691C	S72.045A	S72.124B	S72.322B
S42.415B	S52.031B	S52.223C	S52.309B	S52.392C	S52.692B	S72.045B	S72.124C	S72.322C
S42.416B	S52.031C	S52.224B	S52.309C	S52.399B	S52.692C	S72.045C	S72.125A	S72.323A
S42.421B	S52.032B	S52.224C	S52.321B	S52.399C	S52.699B	S72.046A	S72.125B	S72.323B
S42.422B	S52.032C	S52.225B	S52.321C	S52.501B	S52.699C	S72.046B	S72.125C	S72.323C
S42.423B	S52.033B	S52.225C	S52.322B	S52.501C	S52.90XB	S72.046C	S72.126A	S72.324A
S42.424B	S52.033C	S52.226B	S52.322C	S52.502B	S52.90XC	S72.051A	S72.126B	S72.324B
S42.425B	S52.034B	S52.226C	S52.323B	S52.502C	S52.91XB	S72.051B	S72.126C	S72.324C
S42.426B	S52.034C	S52.231B	S52.323C	S52.509B	S52.91XC	S72.051C	S72.131A	S72.325A
S42.431B	S52.035B	S52.231C	S52.324B	S52.509C	S52.92XB	S72.052A	S72.131B	S72.325B
S42.432B	S52.035C	S52.232B	S52.324C	S52.511B	S52.92XC	S72.052B	S72.131C	S72.325C
S42.433B	S52.036B	S52.232C	S52.325B	S52.511C	S72.001A	S72.052C	S72.132A	S72.326A
S42.434B	S52.036C	S52.233B	S52.325C	S52.512B	S72.001B	S72.059A	S72.132B	S72.326B
S42.435B	S52.041B	S52.233C	S52.326B	S52.512C	S72.001C	S72.059B	S72.132C	S72.326C
S42.436B	S52.041C	S52.234B	S52.326C	S52.513B	S72.002A	S72.059C	S72.133A	S72.331A
S42.441B	S52.042B	S52.234C	S52.331B	S52.513C	S72.002B	S72.061A	S72.133B	S72.331B
S42.442B	S52.042C	S52.235B	S52.331C	S52.514B	S72.002C	S72.061B	S72.133C	S72.331C
S42.443B	S52.043B	S52.235C	S52.332B	S52.514C	S72.009A	S72.061C	S72.133C	S72.332A
S42.444B	S52.043C	S52.236B	S52.332C	S52.515B	S72.009B	S72.062A	S72.134A	S72.332B
S42.445B	S52.044B	S52.236C	S52.333B	S52.515C	S72.009C	S72.062B	S72.134A	ICD.332C
S42.446B	S52.044C	S52.241B	S52.333C	S52.516B	S72.011A	S72.062C	S72.134B	S72.333A

S72.333B	S72.366A	S72.445B	S75.092A	S82.135C	S82.236C	S82.431C	S82.862C	T31.91
S72.333C	S72.366B	S72.445C	S75.099A	S82.136B	S82.241B	S82.432B	S82.863B	T31.92
S72.334A	S72.366C	S72.446B	S75.101A	S82.136C	S82.241C	S82.432C	S82.863C	T31.93
S72.334B	S72.391A	S72.446B	S75.102A	S82.141B	S82.242B	S82.433B	S82.864B	T31.94
S72.334C	S72.391B	S72.451B	S75.109A	S82.141C	S82.242C	S82.433C	S82.864C	T31.95
S72.335A	S72.391C	S72.451C	S75.111A	S82.142B	S82.243B	S82.434B	S82.865B	T31.96
S72.335B	S72.392A	S72.452B	S75.112A	S82.142C	S82.243C	S82.434C	S82.865C	T31.97
S72.335C	S72.392B	S72.452C	S75.119A	S82.143B	S82.244B	S82.435B	S82.866B	T31.98
S72.336A	S72.392C	S72.453B	S75.121A	S82.143C	S82.244C	S82.435C	S82.866C	T31.99
S72.336B	S72.399A	S72.453C	S75.122A	S82.144B	S82.245B	S82.436B	S85.001A	T32.21
S72.336C	S72.399B	S72.454B	S75.129A	S82.144C	S82.245C	S82.436C	S85.002A	T32.22
S72.341A	S72.399C	S72.454C	S75.191A	S82.145B	S82.246B	S82.441B	S85.009A	T32.31
S72.341B	S72.401B	S72.455B	S75.192A	S82.145C	S82.246C	S82.441C	S85.011A	T32.32
S72.341C	S72.401C	S72.455C	S75.199A	S82.146B	S82.251B	S82.442B	S85.012A	T32.33
S72.342A	S72.402B	S72.456B	S79.001A	S82.146C	S82.251C	S82.442C	S85.019A	T32.41
S72.342B	S72.402C	S72.456C	S79.002A	S82.151B	S82.252B	S82.443B	S85.091A	T32.42
S72.342C	S72.409B	S72.461B	S79.009A	S82.151C	S82.252C	S82.443C	S85.092A	T32.43
S72.343A	S72.409C	S72.461C	S79.011A	S82.152B	S82.253B	S82.444B	S85.099A	T32.44
S72.343B	S72.411B	S72.462B	S79.012A	S82.152C	S82.253C	S82.444C	S85.501A	T32.51
S72.343C	S72.411C	S72.462C	S79.019A	S82.153B	S82.254B	S82.445B	S85.502A	T32.52
S72.344A	S72.412B	S72.463B	S79.091A	S82.153C	S82.254C	S82.445C	S85.509A	T32.53
S72.344B	S72.412C	S72.463C	S79.092A	S82.154B	S82.255B	S82.446B	S85.511A	T32.54
S72.344C	S72.413B	S72.464B	S79.099A	S82.154C	S82.255C	S82.446C	S85.512A	T32.55
S72.345A	S72.413C	S72.464C	S82.101B	S82.155B	S82.256B	S82.451B	S85.519A	T32.61
S72.345B	S72.414B	S72.465B	S82.101C	S82.155C	S82.256C	S82.451C	S85.591A	T32.62
S72.345C	S72.414C	S72.465C	S82.102B	S82.156B	S82.261B	S82.452B	S85.592A	T32.63
S72.346A	S72.415B	S72.466B	S82.102C	S82.156C	S82.261C	S82.452C	S85.599A	T32.64
S72.346B	S72.415C	S72.466C	S82.109B	S82.191B	S82.262B	S82.453B	T31.21	T32.65
S72.346C	S72.416B	S72.491B	S82.109C	S82.191C	S82.262C	S82.453C	T31.22	T32.66
S72.351A	S72.416C	S72.491C	S82.111B	S82.192B	S82.263B	S82.454B	T31.31	T32.71
S72.351B	S72.421B	S72.492B	S82.111C	S82.192C	S82.263C	S82.454C	T31.32	T32.72
S72.351C	S72.421C	S72.492C	S82.112B	S82.199B	S82.264B	S82.455B	T31.33	T32.73
S72.352A	S72.422B	S72.499B	S82.112C	S82.199C	S82.264C	S82.455C	T31.41	T32.74
S72.352B	S72.422C	S72.499C	S82.113B	S82.201B	S82.265B	S82.456B	T31.42	T32.75
S72.352C	S72.423B	S72.8X1A	S82.113C	S82.201C	S82.265C	S82.456C	T31.43	T32.76
S72.353A	S72.423C	S72.8X1B	S82.114B	S82.202B	S82.266B	S82.461B	T31.44	T32.77
S72.353B	S72.424B	S72.8X1C	S82.114C	S82.202C	S82.266C	S82.461C	T31.51	T32.81
S72.353C	S72.424C	S72.8X2A	S82.115B	S82.209B	S82.291B	S82.462B	T31.52	T32.82
S72.354A	S72.425B	S72.8X2B	S82.115C	S82.209C	S82.291C	S82.462C	T31.53	T32.83
S72.354B	S72.425C	S72.8X2C	S82.116B	S82.221B	S82.292B	S82.463B	T31.54	T32.84
S72.354C	S72.426B	S72.8X9A	S82.116C	S82.221C	S82.292C	S82.463C	T31.55	T32.85
S72.355A	S72.426C	S72.8X9B	S82.121B	S82.222B	S82.299B	S82.464B	T31.61	T32.86
S72.355B	S72.431B	S72.8X9C	S82.121C	S82.222C	S82.299C	S82.464C	T31.62	T32.87
S72.355C	S72.431C	S72.90XA	S82.122B	S82.223B	S82.401B	S82.465B	T31.63	T32.88
S72.356A	S72.432B	S72.90XB	S82.122C	S82.223C	S82.401C	S82.465C	T31.64	T32.91
S72.356B	S72.432C	S72.90XC	S82.123B	S82.224B	S82.402B	S82.466B	T31.65	T32.92
S72.356C	S72.433B	S72.91XA	S82.123C	S82.224C	S82.402C	S82.466C	T31.66	T32.93
S72.361A	S72.433C	S72.91XB	S82.124B	S82.225B	S82.409B	S82.491B	T31.71	T32.94
S72.361B	S72.434B	S72.91XC	S82.124C	S82.225C	S82.409C	S82.491C	T31.72	T32.95
S72.361C	S72.434C	S72.92XA	S82.125B	S82.226B	S82.421B	S82.492B	T31.73	T32.96
S72.362A	S72.435B	S72.92XB	S82.125C	S82.226C	S82.421C	S82.492C	T31.74	T32.97
S72.362B	S72.435C	S72.92XC	S82.126B	S82.231B	S82.422B	S82.499B	T31.75	T32.98
S72.362C	S72.436B	S75.001A	S82.126C	S82.231C	S82.422C	S82.499C	T31.76	T32.99
S72.363A	S72.436C	S75.002A	S82.131B	S82.232B	S82.423B	S82.831B	T31.77	T79.0XXA
S72.363B	S72.441B	S75.009A	S82.131C	S82.232C	S82.423C	S82.831C	T31.81	T79.1XXA
S72.363C	S72.441C	S75.011A	S82.132B	S82.233B	S82.424B	S82.832B	T31.82	T79.4XXA
S72.364A	S72.442B	S75.012A	S82.132C	S82.233C	S82.424C	S82.832C	T31.83	T79.5XXA
S72.364B	S72.442C	S75.019A	S82.133B	S82.234B	S82.425B	S82.839B	T31.84	T80.0XXA
S72.364C	S72.443B	S75.021A	S82.133C	S82.234C	S82.425C	S82.839C	T31.85	T81.11XA
S72.365A	S72.443C	S75.022A	S82.134B	S82.235B	S82.426B	S82.861B	T31.86	T81.12XA
S72.365B	S72.444B	S75.029A	S82.134C	S82.235C	S82.426C	S82.861C	T31.87	T81.19XA
S72.365C	S72.444C	S75.091A	S82.135B	S82.236B	S82.431B	S82.862B	T31.88	

Appendix F: Complication and Comorbidity (CC) Code List

Note: The following list of CCs are based on the *Federal Register,* volume 82, number 81, April 28, 2017 ("Hospital Inpatient Prospective Payment Systems for Acute Care Hospitals and the Long-Term Care Hospital Prospective Payment System and Proposed Policy Changes and Fiscal Year 2018 Rates; Proposed Rule"). The most current version, v35, of the ICD-10 MS-DRG Definitions Manual was not available at the time this book was printed. For the most current files related to IPPS please refer to the following:
https://www.cms.gov/Medicare/Medicare-Fee-for-Service-Payment/AcuteInpatientPPS/IPPS-Regulations-and-Notices.html.

A00.0	A15.9	A30.5	A50.2	A54.33	A89	B15.9	B45.0	B66.4
A00.1	A17.9	A30.8	A50.30	A54.39	A90	B16.1	B45.2	B66.5
A00.9	A18.01	A30.9	A50.31	A54.40	A91	B16.9	B45.3	B66.8
A01.00	A18.02	A31.0	A50.32	A54.41	A92.0	B17.0	B45.7	B67.0
A01.01	A18.03	A31.1	A50.39	A54.42	A92.1	B17.10	B45.8	B67.1
A01.02	A18.09	A31.2	A50.40	A54.43	A92.2	B17.2	B45.9	B67.2
A01.03	A18.10	A31.8	A50.43	A54.49	A92.4	B17.8	B47.0	B67.31
A01.04	A18.11	A31.9	A50.44	A54.82	A92.5	B17.9	B47.1	B67.32
A01.05	A18.12	A32.0	A50.45	A54.83	A92.8	B18.0	B47.9	B67.39
A01.09	A18.13	A32.11	A50.49	A54.84	A92.9	B18.1	B48.2	B67.4
A01.1	A18.14	A32.12	A50.51	A54.85	A93.0	B18.8	B48.3	B67.5
A01.2	A18.15	A32.81	A50.52	A54.89	A93.1	B18.9	B48.4	B67.61
A01.3	A18.16	A32.82	A50.53	A54.9	A93.2	B19.10	B48.8	B67.69
A01.4	A18.17	A32.89	A50.54	A68.0	A93.8	B19.9	B49	B67.7
A02.0	A18.18	A32.9	A50.55	A68.1	A94	B25.1	B50.0	B67.8
A02.23	A18.2	A34	A50.56	A68.9	A95.0	B25.8	B50.8	B67.90
A02.24	A18.32	A36.0	A50.57	A69.1	A95.1	B25.9	B51.0	B67.99
A02.25	A18.39	A36.1	A50.59	A69.20	A95.9	B26.0	B51.8	B68.0
A02.29	A18.4	A36.2	A51.31	A69.21	A96.0	B26.3	B51.9	B68.1
A02.8	A18.50	A36.3	A51.32	A69.22	A96.1	B26.81	B52.0	B68.9
A02.9	A18.51	A36.81	A51.39	A69.23	A96.8	B26.82	B52.8	B69.0
A03.0	A18.52	A36.82	A51.42	A69.29	A96.9	B26.83	B52.9	B69.1
A04.0	A18.53	A36.83	A51.43	A70	A98.0	B26.84	B53.0	B69.81
A04.1	A18.54	A36.84	A51.44	A75.0	A98.1	B26.85	B53.1	B69.89
A04.2	A18.59	A36.85	A51.45	A75.1	A98.2	B26.89	B53.8	B69.9
A04.3	A18.6	A36.86	A51.46	A75.2	A98.5	B33.1	B54	B70.0
A04.4	A18.7	A36.89	A51.49	A75.3	A98.8	B33.20	B55.0	B70.1
A04.5	A18.81	A36.9	A52.00	A75.9	A99	B33.21	B55.1	B71.0
A04.6	A18.82	A37.00	A52.01	A77.0	B00.2	B33.22	B55.2	B71.1
A04.71	A18.83	A37.10	A52.02	A77.1	B00.50	B33.23	B55.9	B71.8
A04.72	A18.84	A37.80	A52.03	A77.2	B00.51	B33.4	B56.0	B72
A04.8	A18.85	A37.90	A52.04	A77.3	B00.52	B34.3	B56.1	B73.00
A04.9	A18.89	A38.0	A52.05	A77.40	B00.53	B37.0	B56.9	B73.01
A05.0	A21.0	A38.1	A52.06	A77.41	B00.59	B37.41	B57.0	B73.02
A05.1	A21.1	A38.8	A52.09	A77.49	B00.81	B37.49	B57.1	B73.09
A05.2	A21.2	A38.9	A52.10	A77.8	B00.89	B37.81	B57.2	B73.1
A05.3	A21.3	A39.82	A52.11	A77.9	B01.0	B37.82	B57.30	B74.0
A05.4	A21.7	A39.83	A52.12	A78	B01.81	B37.83	B57.31	B74.1
A05.5	A21.8	A39.84	A52.15	A79.0	B01.89	B37.84	B57.32	B74.2
A05.8	A21.9	A39.89	A52.16	A79.1	B01.9	B37.89	B57.39	B74.3
A06.0	A22.0	A39.9	A52.17	A79.81	B02.0	B38.0	B57.40	B74.4
A06.1	A22.2	A42.0	A52.19	A79.89	B02.21	B38.1	B57.41	B74.8
A06.2	A22.8	A42.1	A52.2	A79.9	B02.22	B38.2	B57.42	B74.9
A06.3	A22.9	A42.2	A52.3	A81.00	B02.23	B38.3	B57.49	B75
A06.81	A23.8	A42.81	A52.71	A81.01	B02.29	B38.7	B57.5	B76.0
A06.82	A23.9	A42.82	A52.72	A81.09	B02.30	B38.81	B58.00	B76.1
A06.89	A24.0	A42.89	A52.73	A81.1	B02.31	B38.89	B58.01	B76.8
A07.1	A24.1	A42.9	A52.74	A81.2	B02.32	B38.9	B58.09	B76.9
A07.2	A24.2	A43.0	A52.75	A81.81	B02.33	B39.3	B58.1	B77.0
A07.3	A24.3	A43.1	A52.76	A81.82	B02.34	B40.0	B58.82	B77.89
A07.4	A24.9	A43.8	A52.77	A81.83	B02.39	B40.1	B58.83	B77.9
A07.8	A25.0	A43.9	A52.78	A81.89	B02.7	B40.2	B58.89	B78.0
A07.9	A25.1	A44.0	A52.79	A81.9	B02.8	B40.3	B58.9	B78.7
A08.0	A25.9	A44.1	A54.00	A82.0	B03	B40.7	B60.0	B78.9
A08.11	A27.0	A44.8	A54.01	A82.1	B04	B40.81	B60.10	B79
A08.19	A27.89	A44.9	A54.02	A82.9	B05.1	B40.89	B60.19	B80
A08.2	A27.9	A48.51	A54.03	A85.0	B05.4	B40.9	B60.2	B81.0
A08.31	A28.0	A48.52	A54.09	A85.1	B05.81	B41.0	B65.0	B81.1
A08.32	A28.1	A50.01	A54.1	A85.8	B05.89	B41.7	B65.1	B81.2
A08.39	A28.2	A50.02	A54.21	A86	B06.00	B41.8	B65.2	B81.3
A09	A28.8	A50.03	A54.22	A87.0	B06.02	B41.9	B65.3	B81.4
A15.0	A28.9	A50.04	A54.23	A87.1	B06.09	B44.1	B65.8	B81.8
A15.4	A30.0	A50.05	A54.24	A87.2	B06.81	B44.2	B65.9	B82.0
A15.5	A30.1	A50.06	A54.29	A87.8	B06.82	B44.7	B66.0	B97.21
A15.6	A30.2	A50.07	A54.30	A87.9	B06.89	B44.81	B66.1	B97.33
A15.7	A30.3	A50.08	A54.31	A88.0	B08.3	B44.89	B66.2	B97.34
A15.8	A30.4	A50.09	A54.32	A88.8	B08.71	B44.9	B66.3	B97.35

Appendix F: Complication and Comorbidity (CC) Code List

C15.3	C38.2	C49.A9	C78.5	C81.18	C82.25	C83.12	C84.19	C85.26
C15.4	C38.3	C56.1	C78.6	C81.19	C82.26	C83.13	C84.40	C85.27
C15.5	C38.4	C56.2	C78.7	C81.20	C82.27	C83.14	C84.41	C85.28
C15.8	C38.8	C56.9	C78.80	C81.21	C82.28	C83.15	C84.42	C85.29
C15.9	C40.00	C64.1	C78.89	C81.22	C82.29	C83.16	C84.43	C85.80
C16.0	C40.01	C64.2	C79.00	C81.23	C82.30	C83.17	C84.44	C85.81
C16.1	C40.02	C64.9	C79.01	C81.24	C82.31	C83.18	C84.45	C85.82
C16.2	C40.10	C65.1	C79.02	C81.25	C82.32	C83.19	C84.46	C85.83
C16.3	C40.11	C65.2	C79.10	C81.26	C82.33	C83.30	C84.47	C85.84
C16.4	C40.12	C65.9	C79.11	C81.27	C82.34	C83.31	C84.48	C85.85
C16.5	C40.20	C66.1	C79.19	C81.28	C82.35	C83.32	C84.49	C85.86
C16.6	C40.21	C66.2	C79.2	C81.29	C82.36	C83.33	C84.60	C85.87
C16.8	C40.22	C66.9	C79.31	C81.30	C82.37	C83.34	C84.61	C85.88
C16.9	C40.30	C68.0	C79.32	C81.31	C82.38	C83.35	C84.62	C85.89
C17.0	C40.31	C68.1	C79.40	C81.32	C82.39	C83.36	C84.63	C85.90
C17.1	C40.32	C68.8	C79.49	C81.33	C82.40	C83.37	C84.64	C85.91
C17.2	C40.80	C68.9	C79.51	C81.34	C82.41	C83.38	C84.65	C85.92
C17.3	C40.81	C70.0	C79.52	C81.35	C82.42	C83.39	C84.66	C85.93
C17.8	C40.82	C70.1	C79.60	C81.36	C82.43	C83.50	C84.67	C85.94
C17.9	C40.90	C70.9	C79.61	C81.37	C82.44	C83.51	C84.68	C85.95
C18.0	C40.91	C71.0	C79.62	C81.38	C82.45	C83.52	C84.69	C85.96
C18.1	C40.92	C71.1	C79.70	C81.39	C82.46	C83.53	C84.70	C85.97
C18.2	C41.0	C71.2	C79.71	C81.40	C82.47	C83.54	C84.71	C85.98
C18.3	C41.1	C71.3	C79.72	C81.41	C82.48	C83.55	C84.72	C85.99
C18.4	C41.2	C71.4	C79.81	C81.42	C82.49	C83.56	C84.73	C86.0
C18.5	C41.3	C71.5	C79.82	C81.43	C82.50	C83.57	C84.74	C86.1
C18.6	C41.4	C71.6	C79.89	C81.44	C82.51	C83.58	C84.75	C86.2
C18.7	C41.9	C71.7	C79.9	C81.45	C82.52	C83.59	C84.76	C86.3
C18.8	C45.0	C71.8	C7A.00	C81.46	C82.53	C83.70	C84.77	C86.4
C18.9	C45.1	C71.9	C7A.010	C81.47	C82.54	C83.71	C84.78	C86.5
C19	C45.2	C72.0	C7A.011	C81.48	C82.55	C83.72	C84.79	C86.6
C20	C46.0	C72.1	C7A.012	C81.49	C82.56	C83.73	C84.90	C88.2
C21.0	C46.1	C72.20	C7A.019	C81.70	C82.57	C83.74	C84.91	C88.3
C21.1	C46.2	C72.21	C7A.020	C81.71	C82.58	C83.75	C84.92	C88.4
C21.2	C46.3	C72.22	C7A.021	C81.72	C82.59	C83.76	C84.93	C88.8
C21.8	C46.4	C72.30	C7A.022	C81.73	C82.60	C83.78	C84.94	C88.9
C22.0	C46.50	C72.31	C7A.023	C81.74	C82.61	C83.79	C84.95	C90.00
C22.1	C46.51	C72.32	C7A.024	C81.75	C82.62	C83.80	C84.96	C90.01
C22.2	C46.52	C72.40	C7A.025	C81.76	C82.63	C83.81	C84.97	C90.02
C22.3	C46.7	C72.41	C7A.026	C81.77	C82.64	C83.82	C84.98	C90.10
C22.4	C46.9	C72.42	C7A.029	C81.78	C82.65	C83.83	C84.99	C90.11
C22.7	C47.0	C72.50	C7A.090	C81.79	C82.66	C83.84	C84.A0	C90.12
C22.8	C47.10	C72.59	C7A.091	C81.90	C82.67	C83.85	C84.A1	C90.20
C22.9	C47.11	C72.9	C7A.092	C81.91	C82.68	C83.86	C84.A2	C90.21
C23	C47.12	C74.00	C7A.093	C81.92	C82.69	C83.87	C84.A3	C90.22
C24.0	C47.20	C74.01	C7A.094	C81.93	C82.80	C83.88	C84.A4	C90.30
C24.1	C47.21	C74.02	C7A.095	C81.94	C82.81	C83.89	C84.A5	C90.31
C24.8	C47.22	C74.10	C7A.096	C81.95	C82.82	C83.90	C84.A6	C90.32
C24.9	C47.3	C74.11	C7A.098	C81.96	C82.83	C83.91	C84.A7	C91.00
C25.0	C47.4	C74.12	C7A.1	C81.97	C82.84	C83.92	C84.A8	C91.01
C25.1	C47.5	C74.90	C7A.8	C81.98	C82.85	C83.93	C84.A9	C91.02
C25.2	C47.6	C74.91	C7B.01	C81.99	C82.86	C83.94	C84.Z0	C91.10
C25.3	C47.8	C74.92	C7B.02	C82.00	C82.87	C83.95	C84.Z1	C91.11
C25.4	C47.9	C75.0	C7B.03	C82.01	C82.88	C83.96	C84.Z2	C91.12
C25.7	C48.0	C75.1	C7B.04	C82.02	C82.89	C83.97	C84.Z3	C91.30
C25.8	C48.1	C75.2	C7B.09	C82.03	C82.90	C83.98	C84.Z4	C91.31
C25.9	C48.2	C75.3	C7B.8	C82.04	C82.91	C83.99	C84.Z5	C91.32
C33	C48.8	C75.4	C80.0	C82.05	C82.92	C84.00	C84.Z6	C91.40
C34.00	C49.0	C75.5	C80.2	C82.06	C82.93	C84.01	C84.Z7	C91.41
C34.01	C49.10	C75.8	C81.00	C82.07	C82.94	C84.02	C84.Z8	C91.42
C34.02	C49.11	C75.9	C81.01	C82.08	C82.95	C84.03	C84.Z9	C91.50
C34.10	C49.12	C77.0	C81.02	C82.09	C82.96	C84.04	C85.10	C91.51
C34.11	C49.20	C77.1	C81.03	C82.10	C82.97	C84.05	C85.11	C91.52
C34.12	C49.21	C77.2	C81.04	C82.11	C82.98	C84.06	C85.12	C91.60
C34.2	C49.22	C77.3	C81.05	C82.12	C82.99	C84.07	C85.13	C91.61
C34.30	C49.3	C77.4	C81.06	C82.13	C83.00	C84.08	C85.14	C91.62
C34.31	C49.4	C77.5	C81.07	C82.14	C83.01	C84.09	C85.15	C91.90
C34.32	C49.5	C77.8	C81.08	C82.15	C83.02	C84.10	C85.16	C91.91
C34.80	C49.6	C77.9	C81.09	C82.16	C83.03	C84.11	C85.17	C91.92
C34.81	C49.8	C78.00	C81.10	C82.17	C83.04	C84.12	C85.18	C91.A0
C34.82	C49.9	C78.01	C81.11	C82.18	C83.05	C84.13	C85.19	C91.A1
C34.90	C49.A0	C78.02	C81.12	C82.19	C83.06	C84.14	C85.20	C91.A2
C34.91	C49.A1	C78.1	C81.13	C82.20	C83.07	C84.15	C85.21	C91.Z0
C34.92	C49.A2	C78.2	C81.14	C82.21	C83.08	C84.16	C85.22	C91.Z1
C37	C49.A3	C78.30	C81.15	C82.22	C83.09	C84.17	C85.23	C91.Z2
C38.0	C49.A4	C78.39	C81.16	C82.23	C83.10	C84.18	C85.24	C92.00
C38.1	C49.A5	C78.4	C81.17	C82.24	C83.11		C85.25	C92.01

C92.02	C96.A	D81.3	E70.328	E74.4	F10.180	F14.121	F19.230	F84.5
C92.10	C96.Z	D81.4	E70.329	E74.8	F10.181	F14.150	F19.231	F84.8
C92.11	D46.22	D81.5	E70.330	E75.00	F10.188	F14.151	F19.232	F84.9
C92.12	D46.C	D81.6	E70.331	E75.01	F10.19	F14.20	F19.239	G03.1
C92.20	D47.01	D81.7	E70.338	E75.02	F10.221	F14.221	F19.250	G03.2
C92.21	D47.02	D81.89	E70.339	E75.09	F10.230	F14.222	F19.251	G04.1
C92.22	D47.09	D81.9	E70.39	E75.10	F10.231	F14.229	F19.259	G10
C92.30	D47.1	D82.0	E70.40	E75.11	F10.232	F14.23	F19.26	G11.0
C92.31	D47.9	D82.1	E70.41	E75.19	F10.239	F14.250	F19.27	G11.1
C92.32	D47.Z1	D83.0	E70.49	E75.23	F10.24	F14.251	F19.280	G11.2
C92.40	D47.Z2	D83.1	E70.5	E75.25	F10.251	F14.259	F19.281	G11.3
C92.41	D47.Z9	D83.2	E70.8	E75.29	F10.259	F14.280	F19.282	G11.4
C92.42	D58.8	D83.8	E70.9	E75.4	F10.27	F14.281	F19.288	G11.8
C92.50	D58.9	D83.9	E71.0	E76.01	F10.280	F14.282	F19.921	G11.9
C92.51	D59.0	D84.8	E71.110	E76.02	F10.281	F14.288	F19.930	G12.0
C92.52	D59.1	D84.9	E71.111	E76.03	F10.288	F14.921	F19.931	G12.1
C92.60	D59.2	D89.810	E71.118	E76.1	F10.29	F14.950	F19.932	G12.20
C92.61	D59.4	D89.811	E71.120	E76.210	F10.921	F14.951	F19.939	G12.21
C92.62	D59.9	D89.812	E71.121	E76.211	F10.94	F15.121	F19.950	G12.22
C92.90	D61.01	D89.813	E71.128	E76.219	F10.951	F15.150	F19.951	G12.23
C92.91	D61.09	E06.0	E71.19	E76.22	F10.959	F15.151	F19.97	G12.24
C92.92	D61.818	E08.52	E71.2	E76.29	F10.980	F15.20	F20.0	G12.25
C92.A0	D61.82	E09.52	E71.310	E76.3	F10.981	F15.221	F20.1	G12.29
C92.A1	D61.9	E10.52	E71.311	E76.8	F10.988	F15.222	F20.2	G12.8
C92.A2	D62	E11.52	E71.312	E76.9	F10.99	F15.23	F20.5	G12.9
C92.Z0	D68.0	E13.52	E71.313	E78.71	F11.121	F15.250	F20.81	G21.11
C92.Z1	D68.1	E15	E71.314	E78.72	F11.150	F15.251	F20.89	G21.19
C92.Z2	D68.2	E22.1	E71.318	E79.1	F11.151	F15.259	F23	G21.2
C93.00	D68.311	E22.2	E71.32	E79.2	F11.20	F15.280	F30.10	G21.3
C93.01	D68.312	E22.8	E71.39	E79.8	F11.221	F15.281	F30.11	G21.8
C93.02	D68.318	E22.9	E71.50	E79.9	F11.222	F15.282	F30.12	G21.9
C93.10	D68.32	E23.0	E71.510	E80.0	F11.23	F15.288	F30.13	G23.0
C93.11	D68.4	E23.2	E71.511	E80.1	F11.250	F15.921	F30.2	G23.1
C93.12	D68.51	E24.0	E71.518	E80.20	F11.251	F15.93	F30.9	G23.2
C93.30	D68.52	E24.2	E71.520	E80.21	F11.259	F15.950	F31.0	G23.8
C93.31	D68.59	E24.3	E71.521	E80.29	F11.281	F15.951	F31.10	G23.9
C93.32	D68.61	E24.4	E71.522	E80.3	F11.282	F16.121	F31.11	G24.02
C93.90	D68.62	E24.8	E71.528	E84.19	F11.288	F16.150	F31.12	G24.09
C93.91	D68.69	E24.9	E71.529	E84.8	F11.921	F16.151	F31.13	G24.2
C93.92	D68.8	E27.0	E71.53	E84.9	F11.93	F16.20	F31.2	G24.8
C93.Z0	D68.9	E27.1	E71.540	E85.0	F11.950	F16.221	F31.30	G25.82
C93.Z1	D69.0	E27.2	E71.541	E85.1	F11.951	F16.250	F31.31	G25.9
C93.Z2	D69.3	E27.3	E71.542	E85.2	F12.121	F16.251	F31.32	G31.81
C94.00	D69.41	E27.40	E71.548	E85.3	F12.150	F16.259	F31.4	G31.82
C94.01	D69.42	E27.49	E72.00	E85.4	F12.151	F16.280	F31.5	G32.0
C94.02	D74.0	E27.5	E72.01	E85.81	F12.221	F16.283	F31.60	G32.81
C94.20	D74.8	E32.1	E72.02	E85.82	F12.250	F16.288	F31.61	G36.0
C94.21	D74.9	E34.0	E72.03	E85.89	F12.251	F16.921	F31.62	G36.1
C94.22	D75.81	E36.01	E72.04	E85.9	F12.921	F16.950	F31.63	G36.8
C94.30	D76.1	E36.02	E72.09	E87.0	F12.950	F16.951	F31.64	G36.9
C94.31	D76.2	E36.11	E72.10	E87.1	F12.951	F17.203	F31.81	G37.0
C94.32	D76.3	E36.12	E72.11	E87.2	F13.121	F17.213	F31.89	G37.1
C94.40	D78.01	E44.0	E72.12	E87.3	F13.150	F17.293	F32.0	G37.2
C94.41	D78.02	E44.1	E72.19	E87.4	F13.151	F18.121	F32.1	G37.3
C94.42	D78.11	E45	E72.20	E88.40	F13.20	F18.150	F32.2	G37.5
C94.6	D78.12	E46	E72.21	E88.41	F13.221	F18.151	F32.3	G37.8
C94.80	D78.21	E51.11	E72.22	E88.42	F13.230	F18.17	F33.0	G37.9
C94.81	D78.22	E51.12	E72.23	E88.49	F13.231	F18.20	F33.1	G40.001
C94.82	D78.31	E51.2	E72.29	E89.1	F13.232	F18.221	F33.2	G40.009
C95.00	D78.32	E51.8	E72.3	E89.6	F13.239	F18.250	F33.3	G40.011
C95.01	D78.33	E51.9	E72.4	E89.810	F13.250	F18.251	F33.40	G40.019
C95.02	D78.34	E53.0	E72.50	E89.811	F13.251	F18.259	F33.8	G40.101
C95.10	D78.81	E55.0	E72.51	E89.820	F13.259	F18.27	F33.9	G40.109
C95.11	D78.89	E64.0	E72.52	E89.821	F13.26	F18.280	F34.81	G40.111
C95.12	D80.0	E66.2	E72.53	E89.822	F13.27	F18.288	F34.89	G40.119
C95.90	D80.1	E70.0	E72.59	E89.823	F13.280	F18.921	F34.9	G40.201
C95.91	D80.2	E70.1	E72.8	E89.89	F13.281	F18.950	F50.00	G40.209
C95.92	D80.3	E70.20	E72.9	F01.51	F13.282	F18.951	F50.01	G40.219
C96.0	D80.4	E70.21	E74.00	F02.81	F13.288	F18.97	F50.02	G40.411
C96.20	D80.5	E70.29	E74.01	F03.91	F13.921	F19.121	F50.2	G40.419
C96.21	D80.6	E70.30	E74.02	F05	F13.930	F19.150	F68.10	G40.501
C96.22	D80.7	E70.310	E74.03	F06.0	F13.931	F19.151	F68.12	G40.509
C96.29	D80.8	E70.311	E74.04	F06.2	F13.932	F19.17	F72	G40.801
C96.4	D80.9	E70.318	E74.09	F10.121	F13.939	F19.20	F73	G40.802
C96.5	D81.0	E70.319	E74.20	F10.14	F13.950	F19.221	F84.0	G40.803
C96.6	D81.1	E70.320	E74.21	F10.151	F13.951	F19.222	F84.2	G40.804
C96.9	D81.2	E70.321	E74.29	F10.159	F13.97		F84.3	

Appendix F: Complication and Comorbidity (CC) Code List

G40.811	G90.59	H30.133	H35.731	H53.132	H95.21	I27.82	I69.352	I70.642	
G40.812	G91.0	H30.139	H35.732	H53.133	H95.22	I28.0	I69.353	I70.643	
G40.813	G91.1	H30.141	H35.733	H53.139	H95.31	I28.1	I69.354	I70.644	
G40.814	G91.2	H30.142	H35.739	H59.011	H95.32	I30.0	I69.359	I70.648	
G40.821	G91.3	H30.143	H35.82	H59.012	H95.41	I30.1	I69.851	I70.649	
G40.822	G91.8	H30.149	H40.211	H59.013	H95.42	I30.8	I69.852	I70.661	
G40.823	G91.9	H30.891	H40.212	H59.019	H95.51	I30.9	I69.853	I70.662	
G40.824	G93.1	H30.892	H40.213	H59.031	H95.52	I31.0	I69.854	I70.663	
G40.89	G95.0	H30.893	H40.219	H59.032	H95.53	I31.1	I69.859	I70.668	
G40.911	G95.20	H30.899	H44.001	H59.033	H95.54	I31.2	I69.951	I70.669	
G40.919	G95.29	H30.90	H44.002	H59.039	H95.811	I31.3	I69.952	I70.731	
G40.A11	G95.81	H30.91	H44.003	H59.091	H95.812	I31.4	I69.953	I70.732	
G40.A19	G95.89	H30.92	H44.009	H59.092	H95.813	I31.8	I69.954	I70.733	
G40.B01	G95.9	H30.93	H44.011	H59.093	H95.819	I31.9	I69.959	I70.734	
G40.B09	G96.0	H31.321	H44.012	H59.099	H95.88	I32	I70.261	I70.738	
G40.B11	G96.11	H31.322	H44.013	H59.111	H95.89	I38	I70.262	I70.739	
G40.B19	G97.0	H31.323	H44.019	H59.112	I01.0	I39	I70.263	I70.741	
G43.601	G97.2	H31.329	H44.021	H59.113	I01.1	I42.0	I70.268	I70.742	
G43.609	G97.31	H31.401	H44.022	H59.119	I01.2	I42.1	I70.269	I70.743	
G43.611	G97.32	H31.402	H44.023	H59.121	I01.8	I42.2	I70.331	I70.744	
G43.619	G97.41	H31.403	H44.029	H59.122	I01.9	I42.3	I70.332	I70.748	
G45.0	G97.48	H31.409	H44.111	H59.123	I02.0	I42.4	I70.333	I70.749	
G45.1	G97.49	H31.411	H44.112	H59.129	I02.9	I42.5	I70.334	I70.761	
G45.2	G97.51	H31.412	H44.113	H59.211	I09.0	I42.6	I70.338	I70.762	
G45.3	G97.52	H31.413	H44.119	H59.212	I09.2	I42.7	I70.339	I70.763	
G45.8	G97.61	H31.419	H44.121	H59.213	I09.81	I42.8	I70.341	I70.768	
G45.9	G97.62	H31.421	H44.122	H59.219	I12.0	I42.9	I70.342	I70.769	
G46.0	G97.63	H31.422	H44.123	H59.221	I13.0	I43	I70.343	I70.92	
G46.1	G97.64	H31.423	H44.129	H59.222	I13.11	I44.2	I70.344	I73.01	
G46.2	G97.81	H31.429	H44.131	H59.223	I13.2	I45.2	I70.348	I74.09	
G60.1	G97.82	H33.121	H44.132	H59.229	I16.1	I45.3	I70.349	I74.10	
G61.0	G99.0	H33.122	H44.133	H59.311	I16.9	I45.89	I70.361	I74.11	
G61.81	G99.2	H33.123	H44.139	H59.312	I20.0	I47.0	I70.362	I74.19	
G62.81	H05.011	H33.129	H44.19	H59.313	I20.1	I47.1	I70.363	I74.2	
G70.80	H05.012	H33.20	H46.00	H59.319	I23.0	I47.2	I70.368	I74.3	
G70.81	H05.013	H33.21	H46.01	H59.321	I23.1	I48.1	I70.369	I74.4	
G71.0	H05.019	H33.22	H46.02	H59.322	I23.2	I48.3	I70.431	I74.5	
G71.2	H05.021	H33.23	H46.03	H59.323	I23.3	I48.4	I70.432	I74.8	
G72.0	H05.022	H33.40	H46.10	H59.329	I23.6	I48.92	I70.433	I74.9	
G72.1	H05.023	H33.41	H46.11	H59.331	I23.7	I49.2	I70.434	I75.011	
G72.2	H05.029	H33.42	H46.12	H59.332	I23.8	I50.1	I70.438	I75.012	
G72.81	H05.031	H33.43	H46.13	H59.333	I24.0	I50.20	I70.439	I75.013	
G73.1	H05.032	H33.8	H46.8	H59.339	I24.1	I50.22	I70.441	I75.019	
G73.3	H05.033	H34.00	H46.9	H59.341	I24.8	I50.30	I70.442	I75.021	
G80.1	H05.039	H34.01	H47.10	H59.342	I24.9	I50.32	I70.443	I75.022	
G80.2	H20.00	H34.02	H47.11	H59.343	I25.110	I50.40	I70.444	I75.023	
G80.3	H20.011	H34.03	H47.41	H59.349	I25.3	I50.42	I70.448	I75.029	
G81.00	H20.012	H34.10	H47.42	H59.351	I25.700	I51.0	I70.449	I75.81	
G81.01	H20.013	H34.11	H47.43	H59.352	I25.710	I51.81	I70.461	I75.89	
G81.02	H20.019	H34.12	H47.49	H59.353	I25.711	I62.9	I70.462	I76	
G81.03	H20.021	H34.13	H47.511	H59.359	I25.718	I67.3	I70.463	I77.2	
G81.04	H20.022	H34.211	H47.512	H59.361	I25.719	I67.4	I70.468	I77.4	
G81.10	H20.023	H34.212	H47.519	H59.362	I25.720	I67.5	I70.469	I77.5	
G81.11	H20.029	H34.213	H47.521	H59.363	I25.721	I67.6	I70.531	I80.10	
G81.12	H20.031	H34.219	H47.522	H59.369	I25.728	I67.7	I70.532	I80.11	
G81.13	H20.032	H34.231	H47.529	H59.811	I25.729	I67.81	I70.533	I80.12	
G81.14	H20.033	H34.232	H47.531	H59.812	I25.730	I67.82	I70.534	I80.13	
G81.90	H20.039	H34.233	H47.532	H59.813	I25.731	I67.841	I70.538	I80.201	
G81.91	H20.9	H34.239	H47.539	H59.819	I25.738	I67.848	I70.539	I80.202	
G81.92	H21.331	H34.8110	H47.621	H59.88	I25.739	I67.89	I70.541	I80.203	
G81.93	H21.332	H34.8111	H47.622	H59.89	I25.750	I68.2	I70.542	I80.209	
G81.94	H21.333	H34.8112	H47.629	H60.20	I25.751	I69.051	I70.543	I80.211	
G82.20	H21.339	H34.8120	H47.631	H60.21	I25.758	I69.052	I70.544	I80.212	
G82.21	H30.101	H34.8121	H47.632	H60.22	I25.759	I69.053	I70.548	I80.213	
G82.22	H30.102	H34.8122	H47.639	H60.23	I25.760	I69.054	I70.549	I80.219	
G83.0	H30.103	H34.8130	H47.641	H70.001	I25.761	I69.059	I70.561	I80.221	
G83.4	H30.109	H34.8131	H47.642	H70.002	I25.768	I69.151	I70.562	I80.222	
G90.3	H30.111	H34.8132	H47.649	H70.009	I25.769	I69.152	I70.563	I80.223	
G90.50	H30.112	H34.8190	H49.811	H70.011	I25.790	I69.153	I70.568	I80.229	
G90.511	H30.113	H34.8191	H49.812	H70.012	I25.791	I69.154	I70.569	I80.231	
G90.512	H30.119	H34.8192	H49.813	H70.013	I25.798	I69.159	I70.631	I80.232	
G90.513	H30.121	H34.9	H49.819	H70.019	I25.799	I69.251	I70.632	I80.233	
G90.519	H30.122	H35.70	H53.121	H70.091	I25.810	I69.252	I70.633	I80.239	
G90.521	H30.123	H35.721	H53.122	H70.092	I25.811	I69.253	I70.634	I80.291	
G90.522	H30.129	H35.722	H53.123	H70.093	I25.812	I69.254	I70.638	I80.292	
G90.523	H30.131	H35.723	H53.129	H70.099	I27.0	I69.259	I70.639	I80.293	
G90.529	H30.132	H35.729	H53.131		I27.1	I69.351	I70.641	I80.299	

I82.1	I82.619	I87.032	J70.1	K40.31	K51.812	K80.44	L02.01	L10.89
I82.210	I82.621	I87.033	J80	K41.00	K51.813	K80.45	L02.11	L10.9
I82.211	I82.622	I87.039	J81.1	K41.01	K51.814	K80.46	L02.211	L12.0
I82.290	I82.623	I87.1	J82	K41.30	K51.818	K80.47	L02.212	L12.30
I82.291	I82.629	I87.311	J84.01	K41.31	K51.819	K80.51	L02.213	L12.31
I82.3	I82.701	I87.312	J84.02	K42.0	K51.90	K80.60	L02.214	L12.35
I82.401	I82.702	I87.313	J84.03	K43.0	K51.911	K80.61	L02.215	L12.8
I82.402	I82.703	I87.319	J84.09	K43.3	K51.912	K80.62	L02.216	L12.9
I82.403	I82.709	I87.331	J84.114	K43.6	K51.913	K80.63	L02.219	L49.3
I82.409	I82.711	I87.332	J84.116	K44.0	K51.914	K80.64	L02.31	L49.4
I82.411	I82.712	I87.333	J84.117	K45.0	K51.918	K80.65	L02.411	L49.5
I82.412	I82.713	I87.339	J84.2	K46.0	K51.919	K80.66	L02.412	L49.6
I82.413	I82.719	I96	J84.82	K50.00	K52.0	K80.71	L02.413	L49.7
I82.419	I82.721	I97.110	J84.9	K50.011	K52.1	K80.81	L02.414	L49.8
I82.421	I82.722	I97.111	J90	K50.012	K55.1	K81.0	L02.415	L49.9
I82.422	I82.723	I97.120	J91.0	K50.013	K55.8	K81.2	L02.416	L51.1
I82.423	I82.729	I97.121	J91.8	K50.014	K55.9	K82.0	L02.419	L51.2
I82.429	I82.811	I97.130	J93.11	K50.018	K56.0	K82.1	L02.511	L51.3
I82.431	I82.812	I97.131	J93.12	K50.019	K56.1	K82.3	L02.512	L53.0
I82.432	I82.813	I97.190	J93.81	K50.10	K56.3	K83.0	L02.519	L53.1
I82.433	I82.819	I97.191	J93.82	K50.111	K56.49	K83.3	L02.611	L53.2
I82.439	I82.890	I97.410	J93.83	K50.112	K56.50	K86.0	L02.612	L53.3
I82.441	I82.891	I97.411	J93.9	K50.113	K56.51	K86.1	L02.619	L76.01
I82.442	I82.90	I97.418	J94.0	K50.114	K56.52	K86.2	L02.811	L76.02
I82.443	I82.91	I97.42	J94.2	K50.118	K56.600	K86.3	L02.818	L76.11
I82.449	I82.A11	I97.51	J94.8	K50.119	K56.601	K90.1	L02.91	L76.12
I82.491	I82.A12	I97.52	J95.00	K50.80	K56.609	K90.2	L03.111	L76.21
I82.492	I82.A13	I97.610	J95.01	K50.811	K56.690	K90.3	L03.112	L76.22
I82.493	I82.A19	I97.611	J95.02	K50.812	K56.691	K90.41	L03.113	L76.31
I82.499	I82.A21	I97.618	J95.03	K50.813	K56.699	K90.49	L03.114	L76.32
I82.4Y1	I82.A22	I97.620	J95.04	K50.814	K56.7	K90.81	L03.115	L76.33
I82.4Y2	I82.A23	I97.621	J95.09	K50.818	K57.00	K90.89	L03.116	L76.34
I82.4Y3	I82.A29	I97.622	J95.4	K50.819	K57.12	K90.9	L03.119	L88
I82.4Y9	I82.B11	I97.630	J95.5	K50.90	K57.20	K91.2	L03.121	L97.101
I82.4Z1	I82.B12	I97.631	J95.61	K50.911	K57.32	K91.30	L03.122	L97.102
I82.4Z2	I82.B13	I97.638	J95.62	K50.912	K57.40	K91.31	L03.123	L97.103
I82.4Z3	I82.B19	I97.640	J95.71	K50.913	K57.52	K91.32	L03.124	L97.104
I82.4Z9	I82.B21	I97.641	J95.72	K50.914	K57.80	K91.61	L03.125	L97.105
I82.501	I82.B22	I97.648	J95.811	K50.918	K57.92	K91.62	L03.126	L97.106
I82.502	I82.B23	I97.710	J95.812	K50.919	K59.2	K91.71	L03.129	L97.108
I82.503	I82.B29	I97.711	J95.830	K51.00	K59.31	K91.72	L03.211	L97.109
I82.509	I82.C11	I97.790	J95.831	K51.011	K59.39	K91.81	L03.212	L97.111
I82.511	I82.C12	I97.791	J95.84	K51.012	K61.0	K91.82	L03.213	L97.112
I82.512	I82.C13	I97.810	J95.850	K51.013	K61.1	K91.83	L03.221	L97.113
I82.513	I82.C19	I97.811	J95.851	K51.014	K61.2	K91.840	L03.222	L97.114
I82.519	I82.C21	I97.820	J95.859	K51.018	K61.3	K91.841	L03.311	L97.115
I82.521	I82.C22	I97.821	J95.860	K51.019	K61.4	K91.850	L03.312	L97.116
I82.522	I82.C23	I97.88	J95.861	K51.20	K62.5	K91.858	L03.313	L97.118
I82.523	I82.C29	I97.89	J95.862	K51.211	K62.6	K91.86	L03.314	L97.119
I82.529	I83.201	J05.10	J95.863	K51.212	K63.0	K91.870	L03.315	L97.121
I82.531	I83.202	J18.2	J95.88	K51.213	K63.2	K91.871	L03.316	L97.122
I82.532	I83.203	J21.0	J95.89	K51.214	K63.3	K91.872	L03.317	L97.123
I82.533	I83.204	J21.1	J96.10	K51.218	K65.4	K91.873	L03.319	L97.124
I82.539	I83.205	J21.8	J96.11	K51.219	K68.11	K91.89	L03.321	L97.125
I82.541	I83.208	J21.9	J96.12	K51.30	K76.6	K92.0	L03.322	L97.126
I82.542	I83.209	J36	J98.11	K51.311	K77	K92.1	L03.323	L97.128
I82.543	I83.211	J39.0	J98.19	K51.312	K80.00	K92.2	L03.324	L97.129
I82.549	I83.212	J39.1	K04.01	K51.313	K80.01	K92.81	L03.325	L97.201
I82.591	I83.213	J44.0	K04.02	K51.314	K80.10	K94.01	L03.326	L97.202
I82.592	I83.214	J44.1	K04.4	K51.318	K80.11	K94.02	L03.327	L97.203
I82.593	I83.215	J45.21	K11.3	K51.319	K80.12	K94.03	L03.329	L97.204
I82.599	I83.218	J45.22	K11.4	K51.40	K80.13	K94.09	L03.811	L97.205
I82.5Y1	I83.219	J45.31	K12.2	K51.411	K80.18	K94.11	L03.818	L97.206
I82.5Y2	I83.221	J45.32	K22.10	K51.412	K80.19	K94.12	L03.891	L97.208
I82.5Y3	I83.222	J45.41	K25.3	K51.413	K80.21	K94.13	L03.898	L97.209
I82.5Y9	I83.223	J45.42	K26.3	K51.414	K80.30	K94.19	L03.90	L97.211
I82.5Z1	I83.224	J45.51	K27.3	K51.418	K80.31	K94.22	L03.91	L97.212
I82.5Z2	I83.225	J45.52	K28.3	K51.419	K80.32	K94.23	L05.01	L97.213
I82.5Z3	I83.228	J45.901	K31.0	K51.50	K80.33	K94.30	L05.02	L97.214
I82.5Z9	I83.229	J45.902	K31.1	K51.511	K80.34	K94.31	L08.1	L97.215
I82.601	I85.00	J47.0	K31.5	K51.512	K80.35	K94.32	L10.0	L97.216
I82.602	I85.10	J47.1	K31.6	K51.513	K80.36	K94.33	L10.1	L97.218
I82.603	I87.011	J67.7	K35.80	K51.514	K80.37	K94.39	L10.2	L97.219
I82.609	I87.012	J67.8	K35.89	K51.518	K80.40	K95.01	L10.3	L97.221
I82.611	I87.013	J67.9	K40.00	K51.519	K80.41	K95.09	L10.4	L97.222
I82.612	I87.019	J68.0	K40.01	K51.80	K80.42	K95.81	L10.5	L97.223
I82.613	I87.031	J70.0	K40.30	K51.811	K80.43	K95.89	L10.81	L97.224

L97.225	L97.821	M00.142	M01.X59	M02.872	M33.19	M50.023	M80.032A	M80.841P
L97.226	L97.822	M00.149	M01.X61	M02.879	M33.20	M50.03	M80.032K	M80.842A
L97.228	L97.823	M00.151	M01.X62	M02.88	M33.21	M51.04	M80.032P	M80.842K
L97.229	L97.824	M00.152	M01.X69	M02.89	M33.22	M51.05	M80.039A	M80.842P
L97.301	L97.825	M00.159	M01.X71	M05.40	M33.29	M51.06	M80.039K	M80.849A
L97.302	L97.826	M00.161	M01.X72	M05.411	M33.90	M60.000	M80.039P	M80.849K
L97.303	L97.828	M00.162	M01.X79	M05.412	M33.91	M60.001	M80.041A	M80.849P
L97.304	L97.829	M00.169	M01.X8	M05.419	M33.92	M60.002	M80.041K	M80.851A
L97.305	L97.901	M00.171	M01.X9	M05.421	M33.93	M60.003	M80.041P	M80.851K
L97.306	L97.902	M00.172	M02.10	M05.422	M33.99	M60.004	M80.042A	M80.851P
L97.308	L97.903	M00.179	M02.111	M05.429	M34.81	M60.005	M80.042K	M80.852A
L97.309	L97.904	M00.18	M02.112	M05.431	M34.82	M60.009	M80.042P	M80.852K
L97.311	L97.905	M00.19	M02.119	M05.432	M35.03	M60.011	M80.049A	M80.852P
L97.312	L97.906	M00.20	M02.121	M05.439	M35.1	M60.012	M80.049K	M80.859A
L97.313	L97.908	M00.211	M02.122	M05.441	M35.2	M60.019	M80.049P	M80.859K
L97.314	L97.909	M00.212	M02.129	M05.442	M35.5	M60.021	M80.051A	M80.859P
L97.315	L97.911	M00.219	M02.131	M05.449	M35.8	M60.022	M80.051K	M80.861A
L97.316	L97.912	M00.221	M02.132	M05.451	M36.0	M60.029	M80.051P	M80.861K
L97.318	L97.913	M00.222	M02.139	M05.452	M46.20	M60.031	M80.052A	M80.861P
L97.319	L97.914	M00.229	M02.141	M05.459	M46.21	M60.032	M80.052K	M80.862A
L97.321	L97.915	M00.231	M02.142	M05.461	M46.22	M60.039	M80.052P	M80.862K
L97.322	L97.916	M00.232	M02.149	M05.462	M46.23	M60.041	M80.059A	M80.862P
L97.323	L97.918	M00.239	M02.151	M05.469	M46.24	M60.042	M80.059K	M80.869A
L97.324	L97.919	M00.241	M02.152	M05.471	M46.25	M60.043	M80.059P	M80.869K
L97.325	L97.921	M00.242	M02.159	M05.472	M46.26	M60.044	M80.061A	M80.869P
L97.326	L97.922	M00.249	M02.161	M05.479	M46.27	M60.045	M80.061K	M80.871A
L97.328	L97.923	M00.251	M02.162	M05.49	M46.28	M60.046	M80.061P	M80.871K
L97.329	L97.924	M00.252	M02.169	M25.00	M46.30	M60.051	M80.062A	M80.871P
L97.401	L97.925	M00.259	M02.171	M25.011	M46.31	M60.052	M80.062K	M80.872A
L97.402	L97.926	M00.261	M02.172	M25.012	M46.32	M60.059	M80.062P	M80.872K
L97.403	L97.928	M00.262	M02.179	M25.019	M46.33	M60.061	M80.069A	M80.872P
L97.404	L97.929	M00.269	M02.18	M25.021	M46.34	M60.062	M80.069K	M80.879A
L97.405	L98.3	M00.271	M02.19	M25.022	M46.35	M60.069	M80.069P	M80.879K
L97.406	L98.415	M00.272	M02.30	M25.029	M46.36	M60.070	M80.071A	M80.879P
L97.408	L98.416	M00.279	M02.311	M25.031	M46.37	M60.071	M80.071K	M80.88XA
L97.409	L98.418	M00.28	M02.312	M25.032	M46.38	M60.072	M80.071P	M80.88XK
L97.411	L98.425	M00.29	M02.319	M25.039	M46.39	M60.073	M80.072A	M80.88XP
L97.412	L98.426	M00.80	M02.321	M25.041	M47.011	M60.074	M80.072K	M84.30XK
L97.413	L98.428	M00.811	M02.322	M25.042	M47.012	M60.075	M80.072P	M84.30XP
L97.414	L98.495	M00.812	M02.329	M25.049	M47.013	M60.076	M80.079A	M84.311K
L97.415	L98.496	M00.819	M02.331	M25.051	M47.014	M60.077	M80.079K	M84.311P
L97.416	L98.498	M00.821	M02.332	M25.052	M47.015	M60.078	M80.079P	M84.312K
L97.418	M00.00	M00.822	M02.339	M25.059	M47.016	M60.08	M80.08XA	M84.312P
L97.419	M00.011	M00.829	M02.341	M25.061	M47.019	M60.09	M80.08XK	M84.319K
L97.421	M00.012	M00.831	M02.342	M25.062	M47.021	M62.82	M80.08XP	M84.319P
L97.422	M00.019	M00.832	M02.349	M25.069	M47.022	M79.A11	M80.80XA	M84.321K
L97.423	M00.021	M00.839	M02.351	M25.071	M47.029	M79.A12	M80.80XK	M84.321P
L97.424	M00.022	M00.841	M02.352	M25.072	M47.10	M79.A19	M80.80XP	M84.322K
L97.425	M00.029	M00.842	M02.359	M25.073	M47.11	M79.A21	M80.811A	M84.322P
L97.426	M00.031	M00.849	M02.361	M25.074	M47.12	M79.A22	M80.811K	M84.329K
L97.428	M00.032	M00.851	M02.362	M25.075	M47.13	M79.A29	M80.811P	M84.329P
L97.429	M00.039	M00.852	M02.369	M25.076	M47.14	M79.A3	M80.812A	M84.331K
L97.505	M00.041	M00.859	M02.371	M25.08	M47.15	M79.A9	M80.812K	M84.331P
L97.506	M00.042	M00.861	M02.372	M30.0	M47.16	M80.00XA	M80.812P	M84.332K
L97.508	M00.049	M00.862	M02.379	M30.1	M48.30	M80.00XK	M80.819A	M84.332P
L97.515	M00.051	M00.869	M02.38	M30.2	M48.31	M80.00XP	M80.819K	M84.333K
L97.516	M00.052	M00.871	M02.39	M30.3	M48.32	M80.011A	M80.819P	M84.333P
L97.518	M00.059	M00.872	M02.80	M30.8	M48.33	M80.011K	M80.821A	M84.334K
L97.525	M00.061	M00.879	M02.811	M31.0	M48.34	M80.011P	M80.821K	M84.334P
L97.526	M00.062	M00.88	M02.812	M31.2	M48.35	M80.012A	M80.821P	M84.339K
L97.528	M00.069	M00.89	M02.819	M31.30	M48.36	M80.012K	M80.822A	M84.339P
L97.801	M00.071	M00.9	M02.821	M31.31	M48.37	M80.012P	M80.822K	M84.341K
L97.802	M00.072	M01.X0	M02.822	M31.4	M48.38	M80.019A	M80.822P	M84.341P
L97.803	M00.079	M01.X11	M02.829	M31.7	M48.50XA	M80.019K	M80.829A	M84.342K
L97.804	M00.08	M01.X12	M02.831	M31.8	M48.51XA	M80.019P	M80.829K	M84.342P
L97.805	M00.09	M01.X19	M02.832	M31.9	M48.52XA	M80.021A	M80.829P	M84.343K
L97.806	M00.10	M01.X21	M02.839	M32.11	M48.53XA	M80.021K	M80.831A	M84.343P
L97.808	M00.111	M01.X22	M02.841	M32.12	M48.54XA	M80.021P	M80.831K	M84.344K
L97.809	M00.112	M01.X29	M02.842	M33.00	M48.55XA	M80.022A	M80.831P	M84.344P
L97.811	M00.119	M01.X31	M02.849	M33.01	M48.56XA	M80.022K	M80.832A	M84.345K
L97.812	M00.121	M01.X32	M02.851	M33.02	M48.57XA	M80.022P	M80.832K	M84.345P
L97.813	M00.122	M01.X39	M02.852	M33.03	M48.58XA	M80.029A	M80.832P	M84.346K
L97.814	M00.129	M01.X41	M02.859	M33.09	M50.00	M80.029K	M80.839A	M84.346P
L97.815	M00.131	M01.X42	M02.861	M33.10	M50.01	M80.029P	M80.839K	M84.350K
L97.816	M00.132	M01.X49	M02.862	M33.11	M50.020	M80.031A	M80.839P	M84.350P
L97.818	M00.139	M01.X51	M02.869	M33.12	M50.021	M80.031K	M80.841A	ICD.84.351K
L97.819	M00.141	M01.X52	M02.871	M33.13	M50.022	M80.031P	M80.841K	M84.351P

M84.352K	M84.442P	M84.511K	M84.573A	M84.661P	M86.051	M86.369	M86.69	M87.150
M84.352P	M84.443A	M84.511P	M84.573K	M84.662A	M86.052	M86.371	M86.8X0	M87.151
M84.353K	M84.443K	M84.512A	M84.573P	M84.662K	M86.059	M86.372	M86.8X1	M87.152
M84.353P	M84.443P	M84.512K	M84.574A	M84.662P	M86.061	M86.379	M86.8X2	M87.159
M84.359K	M84.444A	M84.512P	M84.574K	M84.663A	M86.062	M86.38	M86.8X3	M87.161
M84.359P	M84.444K	M84.519A	M84.574P	M84.663K	M86.069	M86.39	M86.8X4	M87.162
M84.361K	M84.444P	M84.519K	M84.575A	M84.663P	M86.071	M86.40	M86.8X5	M87.163
M84.361P	M84.445A	M84.519P	M84.575K	M84.664A	M86.072	M86.411	M86.8X6	M87.164
M84.362K	M84.445K	M84.521A	M84.575P	M84.664K	M86.079	M86.412	M86.8X7	M87.165
M84.362P	M84.445P	M84.521K	M84.576A	M84.664P	M86.08	M86.419	M86.8X8	M87.166
M84.363K	M84.446A	M84.521P	M84.576K	M84.669A	M86.09	M86.421	M86.8X9	M87.171
M84.363P	M84.446K	M84.522A	M84.576P	M84.669K	M86.10	M86.422	M86.9	M87.172
M84.364K	M84.446P	M84.522K	M84.58XA	M84.669P	M86.111	M86.429	M87.00	M87.173
M84.364P	M84.451A	M84.522P	M84.58XK	M84.671A	M86.112	M86.431	M87.011	M87.174
M84.369K	M84.451K	M84.529A	M84.58XP	M84.671K	M86.119	M86.432	M87.012	M87.175
M84.369P	M84.451P	M84.529K	M84.60XA	M84.671P	M86.121	M86.439	M87.019	M87.176
M84.371K	M84.452A	M84.529P	M84.60XK	M84.672A	M86.122	M86.441	M87.021	M87.177
M84.371P	M84.452K	M84.531A	M84.60XP	M84.672K	M86.129	M86.442	M87.022	M87.178
M84.372K	M84.452P	M84.531K	M84.611A	M84.672P	M86.131	M86.449	M87.029	M87.179
M84.372P	M84.453A	M84.531P	M84.611K	M84.673A	M86.132	M86.451	M87.031	M87.180
M84.373K	M84.453K	M84.532A	M84.611P	M84.673K	M86.139	M86.452	M87.032	M87.188
M84.373P	M84.453P	M84.532K	M84.612A	M84.673P	M86.141	M86.459	M87.033	M87.19
M84.374K	M84.454A	M84.532P	M84.612K	M84.674A	M86.142	M86.461	M87.034	M87.20
M84.374P	M84.454K	M84.533A	M84.612P	M84.674K	M86.149	M86.462	M87.035	M87.211
M84.375K	M84.454P	M84.533K	M84.619A	M84.674P	M86.151	M86.469	M87.036	M87.212
M84.375P	M84.459A	M84.533P	M84.619K	M84.675A	M86.152	M86.471	M87.037	M87.219
M84.376K	M84.459K	M84.534A	M84.619P	M84.675K	M86.159	M86.472	M87.038	M87.221
M84.376P	M84.459P	M84.534K	M84.621A	M84.675P	M86.161	M86.479	M87.039	M87.222
M84.377K	M84.461A	M84.534P	M84.621K	M84.676A	M86.162	M86.48	M87.041	M87.229
M84.377P	M84.461K	M84.539A	M84.621P	M84.676K	M86.169	M86.49	M87.042	M87.231
M84.378K	M84.461P	M84.539K	M84.622A	M84.676P	M86.171	M86.50	M87.043	M87.232
M84.378P	M84.462A	M84.539P	M84.622K	M84.68XA	M86.172	M86.511	M87.044	M87.233
M84.379K	M84.462K	M84.541A	M84.622P	M84.68XK	M86.179	M86.512	M87.045	M87.234
M84.379P	M84.462P	M84.541K	M84.629A	M84.68XP	M86.18	M86.519	M87.046	M87.235
M84.38XK	M84.463A	M84.541P	M84.629K	M84.750A	M86.19	M86.521	M87.050	M87.236
M84.38XP	M84.463K	M84.542A	M84.629P	M84.750K	M86.20	M86.522	M87.051	M87.237
M84.40XA	M84.463P	M84.542K	M84.631A	M84.750P	M86.211	M86.529	M87.052	M87.238
M84.40XK	M84.464A	M84.542P	M84.631K	M84.751A	M86.212	M86.531	M87.059	M87.239
M84.40XP	M84.464K	M84.549A	M84.631P	M84.751K	M86.219	M86.532	M87.061	M87.241
M84.411A	M84.464P	M84.549K	M84.632A	M84.751P	M86.221	M86.539	M87.062	M87.242
M84.411K	M84.469A	M84.549P	M84.632K	M84.752A	M86.222	M86.541	M87.063	M87.243
M84.411P	M84.469K	M84.550A	M84.632P	M84.752K	M86.229	M86.542	M87.064	M87.244
M84.412A	M84.469P	M84.550K	M84.633A	M84.752P	M86.231	M86.549	M87.065	M87.245
M84.412K	M84.471A	M84.550P	M84.633K	M84.753A	M86.232	M86.551	M87.066	M87.246
M84.412P	M84.471K	M84.551A	M84.633P	M84.753K	M86.239	M86.552	M87.071	M87.250
M84.419A	M84.471P	M84.551K	M84.634A	M84.753P	M86.241	M86.559	M87.072	M87.251
M84.419K	M84.472A	M84.551P	M84.634K	M84.754A	M86.242	M86.561	M87.073	M87.252
M84.419P	M84.472K	M84.552A	M84.634P	M84.754K	M86.249	M86.562	M87.074	M87.256
M84.421A	M84.472P	M84.552K	M84.639A	M84.754P	M86.251	M86.569	M87.075	M87.261
M84.421K	M84.473A	M84.552P	M84.639K	M84.755A	M86.252	M86.571	M87.076	M87.262
M84.421P	M84.473K	M84.553A	M84.639P	M84.755K	M86.259	M86.572	M87.077	M87.263
M84.422A	M84.473P	M84.553K	M84.641A	M84.755P	M86.261	M86.579	M87.078	M87.264
M84.422K	M84.474A	M84.553P	M84.641K	M84.756A	M86.262	M86.58	M87.079	M87.265
M84.422P	M84.474K	M84.559A	M84.641P	M84.756K	M86.269	M86.59	M87.08	M87.266
M84.429A	M84.474P	M84.559K	M84.642A	M84.756P	M86.271	M86.60	M87.09	M87.271
M84.429K	M84.475A	M84.559P	M84.642K	M84.757A	M86.272	M86.611	M87.10	M87.272
M84.429P	M84.475K	M84.561A	M84.642P	M84.757K	M86.279	M86.612	M87.111	M87.273
M84.431A	M84.475P	M84.561K	M84.649A	M84.757P	M86.28	M86.619	M87.112	M87.274
M84.431K	M84.476A	M84.561P	M84.649K	M84.758A	M86.29	M86.621	M87.119	M87.275
M84.431P	M84.476K	M84.562A	M84.649P	M84.758K	M86.30	M86.622	M87.121	M87.276
M84.432A	M84.476P	M84.562K	M84.650A	M84.758P	M86.311	M86.629	M87.122	M87.277
M84.432K	M84.477A	M84.562P	M84.650K	M84.759A	M86.312	M86.631	M87.129	M87.278
M84.432P	M84.477K	M84.563A	M84.650P	M84.759K	M86.319	M86.632	M87.131	M87.279
M84.433A	M84.477P	M84.563K	M84.651A	M84.759P	M86.321	M86.639	M87.132	M87.28
M84.433K	M84.478A	M84.563P	M84.651K	M86.00	M86.322	M86.641	M87.133	M87.29
M84.433P	M84.478K	M84.564A	M84.651P	M86.011	M86.329	M86.642	M87.134	M87.30
M84.434A	M84.478P	M84.564K	M84.652A	M86.012	M86.331	M86.649	M87.135	M87.311
M84.434K	M84.479A	M84.564P	M84.652K	M86.019	M86.339	M86.651	M87.136	M87.312
M84.434P	M84.479K	M84.569A	M84.652P	M86.021	M86.341	M86.652	M87.137	M87.319
M84.439A	M84.479P	M84.569K	M84.653A	M86.022	M86.342	M86.659	M87.138	M87.321
M84.439K	M84.48XA	M84.569P	M84.653K	M86.029	M86.349	M86.661	M87.139	M87.322
M84.439P	M84.48XK	M84.571A	M84.653P	M86.031	M86.351	M86.662	M87.141	M87.329
M84.441A	M84.48XP	M84.571K	M84.659A	M86.032	M86.352	M86.669	M87.142	M87.331
M84.441K	M84.50XA	M84.571P	M84.659K	M86.039	M86.359	M86.671	M87.143	M87.332
M84.441P	M84.50XK	M84.572A	M84.659P	M86.041	M86.361	M86.672	M87.144	M87.333
M84.442A	M84.50XP	M84.572K	M84.661A	M86.042	M86.362	M86.679	M87.145	M87.334
M84.442K	M84.511A	M84.572P	M84.661K	M86.049	M86.362	M86.68	M87.146	M87.335

Appendix F: Complication and Comorbidity (CC) Code List

M87.336	M90.512	N03.4	N70.02	O03.87	O23.01	O30.211	O36.0929	O72.1
M87.337	M90.519	N03.5	N70.03	O03.88	O23.02	O30.212	O36.0930	O72.2
M87.338	M90.521	N03.6	N71.0	O03.89	O23.03	O30.213	O36.0931	O75.2
M87.339	M90.522	N03.7	N73.0	O04.5	O23.11	O30.221	O36.0932	O86.11
M87.341	M90.529	N03.8	N73.4	O04.80	O23.12	O30.222	O36.0933	O86.12
M87.342	M90.531	N03.9	N75.1	O04.83	O23.13	O30.223	O36.0934	O86.13
M87.343	M90.532	N04.0	N76.4	O04.84	O23.21	O30.291	O36.0935	O86.19
M87.344	M90.539	N04.1	N76.81	O04.85	O23.22	O30.292	O36.0939	O86.20
M87.345	M90.541	N04.2	N82.0	O04.86	O23.23	O30.293	O36.4XX0	O86.21
M87.346	M90.542	N04.3	N82.1	O04.87	O23.31	O30.801	O36.4XX1	O86.22
M87.350	M90.549	N04.4	N82.2	O04.88	O23.32	O30.802	O36.4XX2	O86.29
M87.351	M90.551	N04.5	N82.3	O04.89	O23.33	O30.803	O36.4XX3	O86.4
M87.352	M90.552	N04.6	N82.4	O07.0	O23.41	O30.811	O36.4XX4	O87.0
M87.353	M90.559	N04.7	N82.5	O07.1	O23.42	O30.812	O36.4XX5	O87.2
M87.361	M90.561	N04.8	N82.8	O07.30	O23.43	O30.813	O36.4XX9	O87.3
M87.362	M90.562	N04.9	N82.9	O07.33	O23.511	O30.821	O41.01X0	O87.8
M87.363	M90.569	N05.2	N83.511	O07.34	O23.512	O30.822	O41.01X1	O88.319
M87.364	M90.571	N05.3	N83.512	O07.35	O23.513	O30.823	O41.01X2	O98.011
M87.365	M90.572	N05.4	N83.519	O07.36	O23.521	O30.891	O41.01X3	O98.012
M87.366	M90.579	N05.5	N83.521	O07.37	O23.522	O30.892	O41.01X4	O98.013
M87.371	M90.58	N06.2	N83.522	O07.38	O23.523	O30.893	O41.01X5	O98.02
M87.372	M90.59	N06.3	N83.529	O07.39	O23.591	O31.8X10	O41.01X9	O98.03
M87.373	M96.0	N06.4	N83.53	O08.0	O23.592	O31.8X11	O41.02X0	O98.111
M87.374	M96.621	N06.5	N98.0	O08.1	O23.593	O31.8X12	O41.02X1	O98.112
M87.375	M96.622	N07.2	N98.1	O08.5	O23.91	O31.8X13	O41.02X2	O98.113
M87.376	M96.629	N07.3	N98.2	O08.6	O23.92	O31.8X14	O41.02X3	O98.12
M87.377	M96.631	N07.4	N98.3	O08.7	O23.93	O31.8X15	O41.02X4	O98.13
M87.378	M96.632	N07.5	N98.8	O08.81	O24.011	O31.8X19	O41.02X5	O98.211
M87.379	M96.639	N10	N98.9	O08.82	O24.012	O31.8X20	O41.02X9	O98.212
M87.38	M96.65	N11.1	N99.510	O08.83	O24.013	O31.8X21	O41.03X0	O98.213
M87.39	M96.661	N11.8	N99.511	O08.89	O24.019	O31.8X22	O41.03X1	O98.22
M87.80	M96.662	N11.9	N99.512	O08.9	O24.03	O31.8X23	O41.03X2	O98.23
M87.811	M96.669	N12	N99.518	O10.011	O24.111	O31.8X24	O41.03X3	O98.311
M87.812	M96.671	N13.0	N99.61	O10.012	O24.112	O31.8X25	O41.03X4	O98.312
M87.819	M96.672	N13.1	N99.62	O10.013	O24.113	O31.8X29	O41.03X5	O98.313
M87.821	M96.679	N13.2	N99.71	O10.02	O24.119	O31.8X30	O41.03X9	O98.32
M87.822	M96.69	N13.30	N99.72	O10.411	O24.13	O31.8X31	O44.01	O98.33
M87.829	M96.810	N13.39	N99.820	O10.412	O24.311	O31.8X32	O44.02	O98.411
M87.831	M96.811	N13.4	N99.821	O10.413	O24.312	O31.8X33	O44.03	O98.412
M87.832	M96.820	N13.6	N99.840	O10.911	O24.313	O31.8X34	O44.21	O98.413
M87.833	M96.821	N13.8	N99.841	O10.912	O24.319	O31.8X35	O44.22	O98.42
M87.834	M96.830	N17.8	N99.842	O10.913	O24.33	O31.8X39	O44.23	O98.43
M87.835	M96.831	N17.9	N99.843	O10.92	O24.811	O33.0	O44.41	O98.511
M87.836	M96.840	N18.4	O00.00	O12.11	O24.812	O36.0110	O44.42	O98.512
M87.837	M96.841	N18.5	O00.01	O12.12	O24.813	O36.0111	O44.43	O98.513
M87.838	M96.842	N20.1	O00.101	O12.13	O24.819	O36.0112	O47.02	O98.52
M87.839	M96.843	N20.2	O00.102	O12.21	O24.83	O36.0113	O47.03	O98.53
M87.841	M96.89	N25.1	O00.109	O12.22	O24.911	O36.0114	O47.1	O98.611
M87.842	M97.01XA	N25.81	O00.111	O12.23	O24.912	O36.0115	O60.10X0	O98.612
M87.843	M97.02XA	N28.0	O00.112	O14.02	O24.913	O36.0119	O60.10X1	O98.613
M87.844	M97.11XA	N28.84	O00.119	O14.03	O24.919	O36.0120	O60.10X2	O98.62
M87.845	M97.12XA	N28.85	O00.201	O14.92	O24.93	O36.0121	O60.10X3	O98.63
M87.849	M97.21XA	N28.86	O00.202	O14.93	O26.611	O36.0122	O60.10X4	O98.711
M87.850	M97.22XA	N30.00	O00.209	O16.1	O26.612	O36.0123	O60.10X5	O98.712
M87.851	M97.31XA	N30.01	O00.211	O16.2	O26.613	O36.0124	O60.10X9	O98.713
M87.852	M97.32XA	N30.40	O00.212	O16.3	O26.62	O36.0125	O60.20X0	O98.72
M87.859	M97.41XA	N30.41	O00.219	O20.0	O26.831	O36.0129	O60.20X1	O98.73
M87.861	M97.42XA	N32.1	O00.80	O20.9	O26.832	O36.0130	O60.20X2	O98.811
M87.862	M97.8XXA	N32.2	O00.81	O22.20	O26.833	O36.0131	O60.20X3	O98.812
M87.863	M97.9XXA	N34.0	O00.90	O22.21	O26.872	O36.0132	O60.20X4	O98.813
M87.864	M99.10	N36.0	O00.91	O22.22	O26.873	O36.0133	O60.20X5	O98.82
M87.865	M99.11	N39.0	O03.0	O22.23	O26.879	O36.0134	O60.20X9	O98.83
M87.869	M99.18	N41.0	O03.30	O22.30	O30.101	O36.0135	O63.9	O98.911
M87.871	N02.0	N41.2	O03.33	O22.40	O30.102	O36.0139	O68	O98.912
M87.872	N02.1	N43.1	O03.34	O22.41	O30.103	O36.0910	O70.20	O98.913
M87.873	N02.2	N44.00	O03.35	O22.42	O30.111	O36.0911	O70.21	O98.92
M87.874	N02.3	N44.01	O03.36	O22.43	O30.112	O36.0912	O70.22	O98.93
M87.875	N02.4	N44.02	O03.37	O22.50	O30.113	O36.0913	O70.23	O99.111
M87.876	N02.5	N44.03	O03.38	O22.51	O30.121	O36.0914	O70.3	O99.112
M87.877	N02.6	N44.04	O03.39	O22.52	O30.122	O36.0915	O70.4	O99.113
M87.878	N02.7	N45.4	O03.5	O22.53	O30.123	O36.0919	O71.2	O99.119
M87.879	N02.8	N48.30	O03.7	O22.8X1	O30.191	O36.0920	O71.3	O99.12
M87.88	N02.9	N48.31	O03.80	O22.8X2	O30.192	O36.0921	O71.4	O99.13
M87.89	N03.0	N48.32	O03.83	O22.8X3	O30.193	O36.0922	O71.5	O99.321
M87.9	N03.1	N48.33	O03.84	O22.8X9	O30.201	O36.0923	O71.6	O99.322
M90.50	N03.2	N48.39	O03.85	O22.90	O30.202	O36.0924	O71.7	O99.323
M90.511	N03.3	N70.01	O03.86		O30.203	O36.0925	O72.0	O99.324

O99.325	Q05.3	Q43.1	Q87.3	S02.113A	S02.600K	S02.81XB	S06.302A	S12.02XA
O99.354	Q05.4	Q43.2	Q87.40	S02.113K	S02.601A	S02.81XK	S06.303A	S12.02XK
O99.355	Q07.02	Q43.3	Q87.410	S02.118A	S02.601B	S02.82XA	S06.304A	S12.030A
O99.411	Q07.03	Q43.4	Q87.418	S02.118K	S02.601K	S02.82XB	S06.305A	S12.030K
O99.412	Q20.5	Q43.5	Q87.42	S02.119A	S02.602A	S02.82XK	S06.309A	S12.031A
O99.413	Q21.0	Q43.6	Q87.43	S02.119K	S02.602B	S02.91XA	S06.371A	S12.031K
O99.43	Q21.1	Q43.7	Q87.5	S02.11AA	S02.602K	S02.91XK	S06.372A	S12.040A
O99.830	Q21.2	Q43.8	Q87.81	S02.11AK	S02.609A	S02.92XA	S06.373A	S12.040K
O99.834	Q22.1	Q43.9	Q87.82	S02.11BA	S02.609B	S02.92XB	S06.374A	S12.041A
O99.835	Q22.2	Q44.0	Q87.89	S02.11BK	S02.609K	S02.92XK	S06.375A	S12.041K
P10.2	Q22.3	Q44.1	Q89.01	S02.11CA	S02.610A	S04.011A	S06.379A	S12.090A
P12.2	Q23.0	Q44.4	Q89.09	S02.11CK	S02.610B	S04.012A	S06.381A	S12.090K
P28.0	Q23.1	Q44.5	Q89.3	S02.11DA	S02.610K	S04.019A	S06.382A	S12.091A
P28.10	Q23.2	Q44.6	Q89.7	S02.11DK	S02.611A	S04.02XA	S06.383A	S12.091K
P28.11	Q23.3	Q44.7	Q89.8	S02.11EA	S02.611B	S04.031A	S06.384A	S12.100A
P28.19	Q24.0	Q45.0	Q91.0	S02.11EK	S02.611K	S04.032A	S06.385A	S12.100K
P28.2	Q24.1	Q45.1	Q91.1	S02.11FA	S02.612A	S04.039A	S06.389A	S12.101A
P28.3	Q24.3	Q45.2	Q91.2	S02.11FK	S02.612B	S04.041A	S06.811A	S12.101K
P28.4	Q24.5	Q45.3	Q91.3	S02.11GA	S02.612K	S04.042A	S06.812A	S12.110A
P35.0	Q25.0	Q60.0	Q91.4	S02.11GK	S02.620A	S04.049A	S06.813A	S12.110K
P38.1	Q25.1	Q60.1	Q91.5	S02.11HA	S02.620B	S04.10XA	S06.814A	S12.111A
P38.9	Q25.21	Q60.2	Q91.6	S02.11HK	S02.620K	S04.11XA	S06.815A	S12.111K
P39.0	Q25.29	Q60.3	Q91.7	S02.19XA	S02.621A	S04.12XA	S06.819A	S12.112A
P39.2	Q25.3	Q60.4	Q93.3	S02.19XK	S02.621B	S04.20XA	S06.821A	S12.120A
P39.3	Q25.40	Q60.5	Q93.4	S02.2XXB	S02.621K	S04.21XA	S06.822A	S12.120K
P39.4	Q25.41	Q60.6	Q93.5	S02.2XXK	S02.622A	S04.22XA	S06.823A	S12.121A
P39.8	Q25.42	Q61.00	Q93.7	S02.30XA	S02.622B	S04.30XA	S06.824A	S12.121K
P39.9	Q25.43	Q61.01	Q93.88	S02.30XB	S02.622K	S04.31XA	S06.825A	S12.130A
P52.0	Q25.44	Q61.02	Q93.89	S02.30XK	S02.630A	S04.32XA	S06.829A	S12.130K
P52.1	Q25.45	Q61.11	Q93.9	S02.31XA	S02.630B	S04.40XA	S06.891A	S12.131A
P52.3	Q25.46	Q61.19	R04.2	S02.31XB	S02.630K	S04.41XA	S06.892A	S12.131K
P53	Q25.47	Q61.2	R04.81	S02.31XK	S02.631A	S04.42XA	S06.893A	S12.14XA
P54.4	Q25.48	Q61.3	R04.89	S02.32XA	S02.631B	S04.50XA	S06.894A	S12.14XK
P61.2	Q25.49	Q61.4	R04.9	S02.32XB	S02.631K	S04.51XA	S06.895A	S12.150A
P61.3	Q25.8	Q61.5	R06.3	S02.32XK	S02.632A	S04.52XA	S06.899A	S12.150K
P61.4	Q25.9	Q61.8	R09.01	S02.400A	S02.632B	S04.60XA	S06.9X1A	S12.151A
P61.6	Q26.0	Q61.9	R17	S02.400B	S02.632K	S04.61XA	S06.9X2A	S12.151K
P70.2	Q26.1	Q62.0	R18.0	S02.400K	S02.63XA	S04.62XA	S06.9X3A	S12.190A
P70.8	Q26.2	Q62.10	R18.8	S02.401A	S02.63XB	S04.70XA	S06.9X4A	S12.190K
P71.0	Q26.3	Q62.11	R29.0	S02.401B	S02.63XK	S04.71XA	S06.9X5A	S12.191A
P71.1	Q26.4	Q62.12	R29.1	S02.401K	S02.640A	S04.72XA	S06.9X9A	S12.191K
P71.2	Q26.8	Q62.2	R29.5	S02.402A	S02.640B	S04.811A	S07.0XXA	S12.200A
P71.3	Q26.9	Q62.31	R39.0	S02.402B	S02.640K	S04.812A	S07.1XXA	S12.200K
P71.4	Q27.30	Q62.32	R40.3	S02.402K	S02.641A	S04.819A	S07.8XXA	S12.201A
P71.8	Q27.4	Q62.39	R41.4	S02.40AA	S02.641B	S04.891A	S07.9XXA	S12.201K
P71.9	Q28.0	Q64.10	R44.0	S02.40AB	S02.641K	S04.892A	S09.0XXA	S12.230A
P72.0	Q28.1	Q64.11	R44.2	S02.40AK	S02.642A	S04.899A	S09.20XA	S12.230K
P72.1	Q28.8	Q64.12	R44.3	S02.40BA	S02.642B	S04.9XXA	S09.21XA	S12.231A
P72.2	Q28.9	Q64.19	R45.851	S02.40BB	S02.642K	S05.20XA	S09.22XA	S12.231K
P72.8	Q31.1	Q64.2	R47.01	S02.40BK	S02.650A	S05.21XA	S09.301A	S12.24XA
P74.5	Q31.2	Q64.31	R56.00	S02.40CA	S02.650B	S05.22XA	S09.302A	S12.24XK
P74.6	Q31.3	Q64.32	R56.01	S02.40CB	S02.650K	S05.30XA	S09.309A	S12.250A
P74.8	Q31.5	Q64.33	R56.1	S02.40CK	S02.651A	S05.31XA	S09.311A	S12.250K
P76.1	Q31.8	Q64.39	R57.9	S02.40DA	S02.651B	S05.32XA	S09.312A	S12.251A
P83.0	Q31.9	Q67.5	R64	S02.40DB	S02.651K	S05.40XA	S09.313A	S12.251K
P83.30	Q32.0	Q67.8	R65.10	S02.40DK	S02.652A	S05.41XA	S09.319A	S12.290A
P83.39	Q32.1	Q68.1	R71.0	S02.40EA	S02.652B	S05.42XA	S09.391A	S12.290K
P91.60	Q32.2	Q74.3	R78.81	S02.40EB	S02.652K	S05.50XA	S09.392A	S12.291A
P91.61	Q32.3	Q76.3	R82.0	S02.40EK	S02.66XA	S05.51XA	S09.399A	S12.291K
P91.62	Q32.4	Q76.425	R82.1	S02.40FA	S02.66XB	S05.52XA	S11.10XA	S12.300A
P93.0	Q33.0	Q76.426	S01.101A	S02.40FB	S02.66XK	S05.70XA	S11.11XA	S12.300K
P93.8	Q33.4	Q76.427	S01.102A	S02.40FK	S02.670A	S05.71XA	S11.12XA	S12.301A
P94.0	Q39.5	Q76.428	S01.109A	S02.411A	S02.670B	S05.72XA	S11.13XA	S12.301K
P96.1	Q39.6	Q76.429	S02.0XXA	S02.411B	S02.670K	S05.8X1A	S11.14XA	S12.330A
P96.2	Q39.8	Q76.6	S02.0XXK	S02.411K	S02.671A	S05.8X2A	S11.15XA	S12.330K
Q01.0	Q39.9	Q76.7	S02.101A	S02.412A	S02.671B	S05.8X9A	S11.20XA	S12.331A
Q01.1	Q41.0	Q76.8	S02.101K	S02.412B	S02.671K	S05.91XA	S11.21XA	S12.331K
Q01.2	Q41.1	Q76.9	S02.102A	S02.412K	S02.672A	S05.92XA	S11.22XA	S12.34XA
Q01.8	Q41.2	Q77.2	S02.102K	S02.413A	S02.672B	S06.0X1A	S11.23XA	S12.34XK
Q01.9	Q41.8	Q78.0	S02.109A	S02.413B	S02.672K	S06.0X9A	S11.24XA	S12.350A
Q04.4	Q41.9	Q78.2	S02.109K	S02.413K	S02.69XA	S06.2X1A	S11.25XA	S12.350K
Q04.5	Q42.0	Q79.6	S02.110A	S02.42XA	S02.69XB	S06.2X2A	S12.000A	S12.351A
Q04.6	Q42.1	Q85.1	S02.110K	S02.42XB	S02.69XK	S06.2X3A	S12.000K	S12.351K
Q04.8	Q42.2	Q85.8	S02.111A	S02.42XK	S02.80XA	S06.2X4A	S12.001A	S12.390A
Q05.0	Q42.3	Q85.9	S02.111K	S02.5XXK	S02.80XB	S06.2X5A	S12.001K	S12.390K
Q05.1	Q42.8	Q87.1	S02.112A	S02.600A	S02.80XK	S06.2X9A	S12.01XA	S12.391A
Q05.2	Q42.9	Q87.2	S02.112K	S02.600B	S02.81XA	S06.301A	S12.01XK	

S12.391K	S15.001A	S22.000A	S22.078K	S27.321A	S32.050K	S32.414K	S32.613K	S36.291A
S12.400A	S15.002A	S22.000K	S22.079A	S27.322A	S32.051A	S32.415K	S32.614A	S36.292A
S12.400K	S15.009A	S22.001A	S22.079K	S27.329A	S32.051K	S32.416K	S32.614K	S36.299A
S12.401A	S15.011A	S22.001K	S22.080A	S27.391A	S32.052A	S32.421K	S32.615A	S36.30XA
S12.401K	S15.012A	S22.002A	S22.080K	S27.392A	S32.052K	S32.422K	S32.615K	S36.32XA
S12.430A	S15.019A	S22.002K	S22.081A	S27.399A	S32.058A	S32.423K	S32.616A	S36.33XA
S12.430K	S15.021A	S22.008A	S22.081K	S27.50XA	S32.058K	S32.424K	S32.616K	S36.39XA
S12.431A	S15.022A	S22.008K	S22.082A	S27.51XA	S32.059A	S32.425K	S32.691A	S36.400A
S12.431K	S15.029A	S22.009A	S22.082K	S27.52XA	S32.059K	S32.426K	S32.691K	S36.408A
S12.44XA	S15.091A	S22.009K	S22.088A	S27.53XA	S32.10XA	S32.431K	S32.692A	S36.409A
S12.44XK	S15.092A	S22.010A	S22.088K	S27.59XA	S32.10XK	S32.432K	S32.692K	S36.410A
S12.450A	S15.099A	S22.010K	S22.089A	S27.60XA	S32.110A	S32.433K	S32.699A	S36.418A
S12.450K	S15.101A	S22.011A	S22.089K	S27.63XA	S32.110K	S32.434K	S32.699K	S36.419A
S12.451A	S15.102A	S22.011K	S22.20XA	S27.69XA	S32.111A	S32.435K	S32.810A	S36.420A
S12.451K	S15.109A	S22.012A	S22.20XK	S27.802A	S32.111K	S32.436K	S32.810K	S36.428A
S12.490A	S15.111A	S22.012K	S22.21XA	S27.803A	S32.112A	S32.441K	S32.811A	S36.429A
S12.490K	S15.112A	S22.018A	S22.21XK	S27.808A	S32.112K	S32.442K	S32.811K	S36.430A
S12.491A	S15.119A	S22.018K	S22.22XA	S27.809A	S32.119A	S32.443K	S32.82XA	S36.438A
S12.491K	S15.121A	S22.019A	S22.22XK	S27.892A	S32.119K	S32.444K	S32.82XK	S36.439A
S12.500A	S15.122A	S22.019K	S22.23XA	S27.893A	S32.120A	S32.445K	S32.89XA	S36.490A
S12.500K	S15.129A	S22.020A	S22.23XK	S27.898A	S32.120K	S32.446K	S32.89XK	S36.498A
S12.501A	S15.191A	S22.020K	S22.24XA	S27.899A	S32.121A	S32.451K	S32.9XXA	S36.499A
S12.501K	S15.192A	S22.021A	S22.24XK	S27.9XXA	S32.121K	S32.452K	S32.9XXK	S36.500A
S12.530A	S15.199A	S22.021K	S22.31XA	S28.1XXA	S32.122A	S32.453K	S35.531A	S36.501A
S12.530K	S15.201A	S22.022A	S22.31XK	S29.021A	S32.122K	S32.454K	S35.532A	S36.502A
S12.531A	S15.202A	S22.022K	S22.32XA	S29.029A	S32.129A	S32.455K	S35.533A	S36.503A
S12.531K	S15.209A	S22.028A	S22.32XK	S32.000A	S32.129K	S32.456K	S35.534A	S36.508A
S12.54XA	S15.211A	S22.028K	S22.39XA	S32.000K	S32.130A	S32.461K	S35.535A	S36.509A
S12.54XK	S15.212A	S22.029A	S22.39XK	S32.001A	S32.130K	S32.462K	S35.536A	S36.510A
S12.550A	S15.219A	S22.029K	S22.41XA	S32.001K	S32.131A	S32.463K	S35.8X1A	S36.511A
S12.550K	S15.221A	S22.030A	S22.41XK	S32.002A	S32.131K	S32.464K	S35.8X8A	S36.512A
S12.551A	S15.222A	S22.030K	S22.42XA	S32.002K	S32.132A	S32.465K	S35.8X9A	S36.513A
S12.551K	S15.229A	S22.031A	S22.42XK	S32.008A	S32.132K	S32.466K	S35.90XA	S36.518A
S12.590A	S15.291A	S22.031K	S22.43XA	S32.008K	S32.139A	S32.471K	S35.91XA	S36.519A
S12.590K	S15.292A	S22.032A	S22.43XK	S32.009A	S32.139K	S32.472K	S35.99XA	S36.520A
S12.591A	S15.299A	S22.032K	S22.49XA	S32.009K	S32.14XA	S32.473K	S36.00XA	S36.521A
S12.591K	S15.301A	S22.038A	S22.49XK	S32.010A	S32.14XK	S32.474K	S36.020A	S36.522A
S12.600A	S15.302A	S22.038K	S22.5XXK	S32.010K	S32.15XA	S32.475K	S36.021A	S36.523A
S12.600K	S15.309A	S22.039A	S22.9XXA	S32.011A	S32.15XK	S32.476K	S36.029A	S36.528A
S12.601A	S15.311A	S22.039K	S22.9XXK	S32.011K	S32.16XA	S32.481K	S36.030A	S36.529A
S12.601K	S15.312A	S22.040A	S25.501A	S32.012A	S32.16XK	S32.482K	S36.039A	S36.530A
S12.630A	S15.319A	S22.040K	S25.502A	S32.012K	S32.17XA	S32.483K	S36.09XA	S36.531A
S12.630K	S15.321A	S22.041A	S25.509A	S32.018A	S32.17XK	S32.484K	S36.112A	S36.532A
S12.631A	S15.322A	S22.041K	S25.511A	S32.018K	S32.19XA	S32.485K	S36.113A	S36.533A
S12.631K	S15.329A	S22.042A	S25.512A	S32.019A	S32.19XK	S32.486K	S36.114A	S36.538A
S12.64XA	S15.391A	S22.042K	S25.519A	S32.019K	S32.2XXA	S32.491K	S36.118A	S36.539A
S12.64XK	S15.392A	S22.048A	S25.591A	S32.020A	S32.2XXK	S32.492K	S36.119A	S36.590A
S12.650A	S15.399A	S22.048K	S25.592A	S32.020K	S32.301A	S32.499K	S36.122A	S36.591A
S12.650K	S15.8XXA	S22.049A	S25.599A	S32.021A	S32.301K	S32.501A	S36.123A	S36.592A
S12.651A	S15.9XXA	S22.049K	S25.801A	S32.021K	S32.302A	S32.501K	S36.128A	S36.593A
S12.651K	S17.0XXA	S22.050A	S25.802A	S32.022A	S32.309A	S32.502A	S36.129A	S36.598A
S12.690A	S17.8XXA	S22.050K	S25.809A	S32.022K	S32.309K	S32.502K	S36.13XA	S36.599A
S12.690K	S17.9XXA	S22.051A	S25.811A	S32.028A	S32.311A	S32.509A	S36.200A	S36.60XA
S12.691A	S21.101A	S22.051K	S25.812A	S32.028K	S32.311K	S32.509K	S36.201A	S36.61XA
S12.691K	S21.102A	S22.052A	S25.819A	S32.029A	S32.312A	S32.511A	S36.202A	S36.62XA
S12.9XXA	S21.109A	S22.052K	S25.891A	S32.029K	S32.312K	S32.511K	S36.209A	S36.63XA
S13.0XXA	S21.111A	S22.058A	S25.892A	S32.030A	S32.313A	S32.512A	S36.220A	S36.69XA
S13.100A	S21.112A	S22.058K	S25.899A	S32.030K	S32.313K	S32.512K	S36.221A	S36.81XA
S13.101A	S21.119A	S22.059A	S25.90XA	S32.031A	S32.314A	S32.519A	S36.222A	S36.892A
S13.110A	S21.121A	S22.059K	S25.91XA	S32.031K	S32.314K	S32.519K	S36.229A	S36.893A
S13.111A	S21.122A	S22.060A	S25.99XA	S32.032A	S32.315A	S32.591A	S36.230A	S36.898A
S13.120A	S21.129A	S22.060K	S26.00XA	S32.032K	S32.315K	S32.591K	S36.231A	S36.899A
S13.121A	S21.131A	S22.061A	S26.01XA	S32.038A	S32.316A	S32.592A	S36.232A	S36.90XA
S13.130A	S21.132A	S22.061K	S26.09XA	S32.038K	S32.316K	S32.592K	S36.239A	S36.92XA
S13.131A	S21.139A	S22.062A	S26.10XA	S32.039A	S32.391A	S32.599A	S36.240A	S36.93XA
S13.140A	S21.141A	S22.062K	S26.11XA	S32.039K	S32.391K	S32.599K	S36.241A	S37.001A
S13.141A	S21.142A	S22.068A	S26.19XA	S32.040A	S32.392A	S32.601A	S36.242A	S37.002A
S13.150A	S21.149A	S22.068K	S26.90XA	S32.040K	S32.392K	S32.601K	S36.249A	S37.009A
S13.151A	S21.151A	S22.069A	S26.91XA	S32.041A	S32.399A	S32.602A	S36.250A	S37.011A
S13.160A	S21.152A	S22.069K	S26.99XA	S32.041K	S32.399K	S32.602K	S36.251A	S37.012A
S13.161A	S21.159A	S22.070A	S27.0XXA	S32.042A	S32.401A	S32.609A	S36.252A	S37.019A
S13.170A	S21.90XA	S22.070K	S27.301A	S32.042K	S32.402K	S32.609K	S36.259A	S37.021A
S13.171A	S21.91XA	S22.071A	S27.302A	S32.048A	S32.409K	S32.611A	S36.260A	S37.022A
S13.180A	S21.92XA	S22.071K	S27.309A	S32.048K	S32.411K	S32.611K	S36.261A	S37.029A
S13.181A	S21.93XA	S22.072A	S27.311A	S32.049A	S32.412K	S32.612A	S36.262A	S37.031A
S13.20XA	S21.94XA	S22.072K	S27.312A	S32.049K	S32.413K	S32.612K	S36.269A	S37.032A
S13.29XA	S21.95XA	S22.078A	S27.319A	S32.050A		S32.613A	S36.290A	

S37.039A	S42.023B	S42.131P	S42.213K	S42.265A	S42.333P	S42.402K	S42.447A	S42.492P
S37.041A	S42.023K	S42.132B	S42.213P	S42.265K	S42.334A	S42.402P	S42.447K	S42.493A
S37.042A	S42.023P	S42.132K	S42.214A	S42.265P	S42.334K	S42.409A	S42.447P	S42.493K
S37.049A	S42.024B	S42.132P	S42.214K	S42.266A	S42.334P	S42.409K	S42.448A	S42.493P
S37.051A	S42.024K	S42.133B	S42.214P	S42.266K	S42.335A	S42.409P	S42.448K	S42.494A
S37.052A	S42.024P	S42.133K	S42.215A	S42.266P	S42.335K	S42.411A	S42.448P	S42.494K
S37.059A	S42.025B	S42.133P	S42.215K	S42.271A	S42.335P	S42.411K	S42.449A	S42.494P
S37.10XA	S42.025K	S42.134B	S42.215P	S42.271K	S42.336A	S42.411P	S42.449K	S42.495A
S37.12XA	S42.025P	S42.134K	S42.216A	S42.271P	S42.336K	S42.412A	S42.449P	S42.495K
S37.13XA	S42.026B	S42.134P	S42.216K	S42.272A	S42.336P	S42.412K	S42.451A	S42.495P
S37.19XA	S42.026K	S42.135B	S42.216P	S42.272K	S42.341A	S42.412P	S42.451K	S42.496A
S37.20XA	S42.026P	S42.135K	S42.221A	S42.272P	S42.341K	S42.413A	S42.451P	S42.496K
S37.22XA	S42.031B	S42.135P	S42.221K	S42.279A	S42.341P	S42.413K	S42.452A	S42.496P
S37.23XA	S42.031K	S42.136B	S42.221P	S42.279K	S42.342A	S42.413P	S42.452K	S42.90XA
S37.29XA	S42.031P	S42.136K	S42.222A	S42.279P	S42.342K	S42.414A	S42.452P	S42.90XK
S37.30XA	S42.032B	S42.136P	S42.222K	S42.291A	S42.342P	S42.414K	S42.453A	S42.90XP
S37.32XA	S42.032K	S42.141B	S42.222P	S42.291K	S42.343A	S42.414P	S42.453K	S42.91XA
S37.33XA	S42.032P	S42.141K	S42.223A	S42.291P	S42.343K	S42.415A	S42.453P	S42.91XK
S37.39XA	S42.033B	S42.141P	S42.223K	S42.292A	S42.343P	S42.415K	S42.454A	S42.91XP
S37.60XA	S42.033K	S42.142B	S42.223P	S42.292K	S42.344A	S42.415P	S42.454K	S42.92XA
S37.62XA	S42.033P	S42.142K	S42.224A	S42.292P	S42.344K	S42.416A	S42.454P	S42.92XK
S37.63XA	S42.034B	S42.142P	S42.224K	S42.293A	S42.344P	S42.416K	S42.455A	S42.92XP
S37.69XA	S42.034K	S42.143B	S42.224P	S42.293K	S42.345A	S42.416P	S42.455K	S43.201A
S37.812A	S42.034P	S42.143K	S42.225A	S42.293P	S42.345K	S42.421A	S42.455P	S43.202A
S37.813A	S42.035B	S42.143P	S42.225K	S42.294A	S42.345P	S42.421K	S42.456A	S43.203A
S37.818A	S42.035K	S42.144B	S42.225P	S42.294K	S42.346A	S42.421P	S42.456K	S43.204A
S37.819A	S42.035P	S42.144K	S42.226A	S42.294P	S42.346K	S42.422A	S42.456P	S43.205A
S37.892A	S42.036B	S42.144P	S42.226K	S42.295A	S42.346P	S42.422K	S42.461A	S43.206A
S37.893A	S42.036K	S42.145B	S42.226P	S42.295K	S42.351A	S42.422P	S42.461K	S43.211A
S37.898A	S42.036P	S42.145K	S42.231A	S42.295P	S42.351K	S42.423A	S42.461P	S43.212A
S37.899A	S42.101B	S42.145P	S42.231K	S42.296A	S42.351P	S42.423K	S42.462A	S43.213A
S37.90XA	S42.101K	S42.146B	S42.231P	S42.296K	S42.352A	S42.423P	S42.462K	S43.214A
S37.92XA	S42.101P	S42.146K	S42.232A	S42.296P	S42.352K	S42.424A	S42.462P	S43.215A
S37.93XA	S42.102B	S42.146P	S42.232K	S42.301A	S42.352P	S42.424K	S42.463A	S43.216A
S37.99XA	S42.102K	S42.151B	S42.232P	S42.301K	S42.353A	S42.424P	S42.463K	S43.221A
S42.001B	S42.102P	S42.151K	S42.239A	S42.301P	S42.353K	S42.425A	S42.463P	S43.222A
S42.001K	S42.109B	S42.151P	S42.239K	S42.302A	S42.353P	S42.425K	S42.464A	S43.223A
S42.001P	S42.109K	S42.152B	S42.239P	S42.302K	S42.354A	S42.425P	S42.464K	S43.224A
S42.002B	S42.109P	S42.152K	S42.241A	S42.302P	S42.354K	S42.426A	S42.464P	S43.225A
S42.002K	S42.111B	S42.152P	S42.241K	S42.309A	S42.354P	S42.426K	S42.465A	S43.226A
S42.002P	S42.111K	S42.153B	S42.241P	S42.309K	S42.355A	S42.426P	S42.465K	S45.101A
S42.009B	S42.111P	S42.153K	S42.242A	S42.309P	S42.355K	S42.431A	S42.465P	S45.102A
S42.009K	S42.112B	S42.153P	S42.242K	S42.311A	S42.355P	S42.431K	S42.466A	S45.109A
S42.009P	S42.112K	S42.154B	S42.242P	S42.311K	S42.356A	S42.431P	S42.466K	S45.111A
S42.011B	S42.112P	S42.154K	S42.249A	S42.311P	S42.356K	S42.432A	S42.466P	S45.112A
S42.011K	S42.113B	S42.154P	S42.249K	S42.312A	S42.356P	S42.432K	S42.471A	S45.119A
S42.011P	S42.113K	S42.155B	S42.249P	S42.312K	S42.361A	S42.432P	S42.471K	S45.191A
S42.012B	S42.113P	S42.155K	S42.251A	S42.312P	S42.361K	S42.433A	S42.471P	S45.192A
S42.012K	S42.114B	S42.155P	S42.251K	S42.319A	S42.361P	S42.433K	S42.472A	S45.199A
S42.012P	S42.114K	S42.156B	S42.251P	S42.319K	S42.362A	S42.433P	S42.472K	S45.201A
S42.013B	S42.114P	S42.156K	S42.252A	S42.319P	S42.362K	S42.434A	S42.472P	S45.202A
S42.013K	S42.115B	S42.156P	S42.252K	S42.321A	S42.362P	S42.434K	S42.473A	S45.209A
S42.013P	S42.115K	S42.191B	S42.252P	S42.321K	S42.363A	S42.434P	S42.473K	S45.211A
S42.014B	S42.115P	S42.191K	S42.253A	S42.321P	S42.363K	S42.435A	S42.473P	S45.212A
S42.014K	S42.116B	S42.191P	S42.253K	S42.322A	S42.363P	S42.435K	S42.474A	S45.219A
S42.014P	S42.116K	S42.192B	S42.253P	S42.322K	S42.364A	S42.435P	S42.474K	S45.291A
S42.015B	S42.116P	S42.192K	S42.254A	S42.322P	S42.364K	S42.436A	S42.474P	S45.292A
S42.015K	S42.121B	S42.192P	S42.254K	S42.323A	S42.364P	S42.436K	S42.475A	S45.299A
S42.015P	S42.121K	S42.199B	S42.254P	S42.323K	S42.365A	S42.436P	S42.475K	S45.301A
S42.016B	S42.121P	S42.199K	S42.255A	S42.323P	S42.365K	S42.441A	S42.475P	S45.302A
S42.016K	S42.122B	S42.199P	S42.255K	S42.324A	S42.365P	S42.441K	S42.476A	S45.309A
S42.016P	S42.122K	S42.201A	S42.255P	S42.324K	S42.366A	S42.441P	S42.476K	S45.311A
S42.017B	S42.122P	S42.201K	S42.256A	S42.324P	S42.366K	S42.442A	S42.476P	S45.312A
S42.017K	S42.123B	S42.201P	S42.256K	S42.325A	S42.366P	S42.442K	S42.481A	S45.319A
S42.017P	S42.123K	S42.202A	S42.256P	S42.325K	S42.391A	S42.442P	S42.481K	S45.391A
S42.018B	S42.123P	S42.202K	S42.261A	S42.325P	S42.391K	S42.443A	S42.481P	S45.392A
S42.018K	S42.124B	S42.202P	S42.261K	S42.326A	S42.391P	S42.443K	S42.482A	S45.399A
S42.018P	S42.124K	S42.209A	S42.261P	S42.326K	S42.392A	S42.443P	S42.482K	S45.801A
S42.019B	S42.124P	S42.209K	S42.262A	S42.326P	S42.392K	S42.444A	S42.482P	S45.802A
S42.019K	S42.125B	S42.209P	S42.262K	S42.331A	S42.392P	S42.444K	S42.489A	S45.809A
S42.019P	S42.125K	S42.211A	S42.262P	S42.331K	S42.399A	S42.444P	S42.489K	S45.811A
S42.021B	S42.125P	S42.211K	S42.263A	S42.331P	S42.399K	S42.445A	S42.489P	S45.812A
S42.021K	S42.126B	S42.211P	S42.263K	S42.332A	S42.399P	S42.445K	S42.491A	S45.819A
S42.021P	S42.126K	S42.212A	S42.263P	S42.332K	S42.401A	S42.445P	S42.491K	S45.891A
S42.022B	S42.126P	S42.212K	S42.264A	S42.332P	S42.401K	S42.446A	S42.491P	S45.892A
S42.022K	S42.131B	S42.212P	S42.264K	S42.333A	S42.401P	S42.446K	S42.492A	S45.899A
S42.022P	S42.131K	S42.213A	S42.264P	S42.333K	S42.402A	S42.446P	S42.492K	S45.901A

Appendix F: Complication and Comorbidity (CC) Code List

S45.902A	S49.039A	S52.001N	S52.033Q	S52.101P	S52.133R	S52.222N	S52.241N	S52.256N
S45.909A	S49.039K	S52.001P	S52.033R	S52.101Q	S52.134K	S52.222P	S52.241P	S52.256P
S45.911A	S49.039P	S52.001Q	S52.034K	S52.101R	S52.134M	S52.222Q	S52.241Q	S52.256Q
S45.912A	S49.041A	S52.001R	S52.034M	S52.102K	S52.134N	S52.222R	S52.241R	S52.256R
S45.919A	S49.041K	S52.002K	S52.034N	S52.102M	S52.134P	S52.223A	S52.242A	S52.261A
S45.991A	S49.041P	S52.002M	S52.034P	S52.102N	S52.134Q	S52.223K	S52.242K	S52.261K
S45.992A	S49.042A	S52.002N	S52.034Q	S52.102P	S52.134R	S52.223M	S52.242M	S52.261M
S45.999A	S49.042K	S52.002P	S52.034R	S52.102Q	S52.135K	S52.223N	S52.242N	S52.261N
S46.021A	S49.042P	S52.002Q	S52.035K	S52.102R	S52.135M	S52.223P	S52.242P	S52.261P
S46.022A	S49.049A	S52.002R	S52.035M	S52.109K	S52.135N	S52.223Q	S52.242Q	S52.261Q
S46.029A	S49.049K	S52.009K	S52.035N	S52.109M	S52.135P	S52.223R	S52.242R	S52.261R
S46.121A	S49.049P	S52.009M	S52.035P	S52.109N	S52.135Q	S52.224A	S52.243A	S52.262A
S46.122A	S49.091A	S52.009N	S52.035Q	S52.109P	S52.135R	S52.224K	S52.243K	S52.262K
S46.129A	S49.091K	S52.009P	S52.035R	S52.109Q	S52.136K	S52.224M	S52.243M	S52.262M
S46.221A	S49.091P	S52.009Q	S52.036K	S52.109R	S52.136M	S52.224N	S52.243N	S52.262N
S46.222A	S49.092A	S52.009R	S52.036M	S52.111A	S52.136N	S52.224P	S52.243P	S52.262P
S46.229A	S49.092K	S52.011A	S52.036N	S52.111K	S52.136P	S52.224Q	S52.243Q	S52.262Q
S46.321A	S49.092P	S52.011K	S52.036P	S52.111P	S52.136Q	S52.224R	S52.243R	S52.262R
S46.322A	S49.099A	S52.011P	S52.036Q	S52.112A	S52.136R	S52.225A	S52.244A	S52.263A
S46.329A	S49.099K	S52.012A	S52.036R	S52.112K	S52.181K	S52.225K	S52.244K	S52.263K
S46.821A	S49.099P	S52.012K	S52.041K	S52.112P	S52.181M	S52.225M	S52.244M	S52.263M
S46.822A	S49.101A	S52.012P	S52.041M	S52.119A	S52.181N	S52.225N	S52.244N	S52.263N
S46.829A	S49.101K	S52.019A	S52.041N	S52.119K	S52.181P	S52.225P	S52.244P	S52.263P
S46.921A	S49.101P	S52.019K	S52.041P	S52.119P	S52.181Q	S52.225Q	S52.244Q	S52.263Q
S46.922A	S49.102A	S52.019P	S52.041Q	S52.121K	S52.181R	S52.225R	S52.244R	S52.263R
S46.929A	S49.102K	S52.021K	S52.041R	S52.121M	S52.182K	S52.226A	S52.245A	S52.264A
S48.011A	S49.102P	S52.021M	S52.042K	S52.121N	S52.182M	S52.226K	S52.245K	S52.264K
S48.012A	S49.109A	S52.021N	S52.042M	S52.121P	S52.182N	S52.226M	S52.245M	S52.264M
S48.019A	S49.109K	S52.021P	S52.042N	S52.121Q	S52.182P	S52.226N	S52.245N	S52.264P
S48.021A	S49.109P	S52.021Q	S52.042P	S52.121R	S52.182Q	S52.226P	S52.245P	S52.264Q
S48.022A	S49.111A	S52.021R	S52.042Q	S52.122K	S52.182R	S52.226Q	S52.245Q	S52.264R
S48.029A	S49.111K	S52.022K	S52.042R	S52.122M	S52.189K	S52.226R	S52.245R	S52.265A
S48.111A	S49.111P	S52.022M	S52.043K	S52.122N	S52.189M	S52.231A	S52.246A	S52.265K
S48.112A	S49.112A	S52.022N	S52.043M	S52.122P	S52.189N	S52.231K	S52.246K	S52.265M
S48.119A	S49.112K	S52.022P	S52.043N	S52.122Q	S52.189P	S52.231M	S52.246M	S52.265P
S48.121A	S49.112P	S52.022Q	S52.043P	S52.122R	S52.189Q	S52.231N	S52.246N	S52.265Q
S48.122A	S49.119A	S52.022R	S52.043Q	S52.123K	S52.189R	S52.231P	S52.246P	S52.265R
S48.129A	S49.119K	S52.023K	S52.043R	S52.123M	S52.201A	S52.231Q	S52.246Q	S52.266A
S48.911A	S49.119P	S52.023M	S52.044K	S52.123N	S52.201K	S52.231R	S52.246R	S52.266K
S48.912A	S49.121A	S52.023N	S52.044M	S52.123P	S52.201M	S52.232A	S52.251A	S52.266M
S48.919A	S49.121K	S52.023P	S52.044N	S52.123Q	S52.201N	S52.232K	S52.251K	S52.266P
S48.921A	S49.121P	S52.023Q	S52.044P	S52.123R	S52.201P	S52.232M	S52.251M	S52.266Q
S48.922A	S49.122A	S52.023R	S52.044Q	S52.124K	S52.201Q	S52.232N	S52.251N	S52.266R
S48.929A	S49.122K	S52.024K	S52.044R	S52.124M	S52.201R	S52.232P	S52.251P	S52.271K
S49.001A	S49.122P	S52.024M	S52.045K	S52.124N	S52.202A	S52.232Q	S52.251Q	S52.271M
S49.001K	S49.129A	S52.024N	S52.045M	S52.124P	S52.202K	S52.232R	S52.251R	S52.271N
S49.001P	S49.129K	S52.024P	S52.045N	S52.124Q	S52.202M	S52.233A	S52.252A	S52.271P
S49.002A	S49.129P	S52.024Q	S52.045P	S52.124R	S52.202N	S52.233K	S52.252K	S52.271Q
S49.002K	S49.131A	S52.024R	S52.045Q	S52.125K	S52.202P	S52.233M	S52.252M	S52.271R
S49.002P	S49.131K	S52.025K	S52.045R	S52.125M	S52.202Q	S52.233N	S52.252N	S52.272K
S49.009A	S49.131P	S52.025M	S52.046K	S52.125N	S52.202R	S52.233P	S52.252P	S52.272M
S49.009K	S49.132A	S52.025P	S52.046M	S52.125P	S52.209A	S52.233Q	S52.252Q	S52.272N
S49.009P	S49.132K	S52.025Q	S52.046N	S52.125Q	S52.209K	S52.233R	S52.252R	S52.272P
S49.011A	S49.132P	S52.025R	S52.046P	S52.125R	S52.209M	S52.234A	S52.253A	S52.272R
S49.011K	S49.139A	S52.026K	S52.046Q	S52.126K	S52.209N	S52.234K	S52.253K	S52.279K
S49.011P	S49.139K	S52.026M	S52.046R	S52.126M	S52.209P	S52.234M	S52.253M	S52.279M
S49.012A	S49.139P	S52.026N	S52.091K	S52.126N	S52.209Q	S52.234N	S52.253N	S52.279N
S49.012K	S49.141A	S52.026P	S52.091M	S52.126P	S52.209R	S52.234P	S52.253P	S52.279P
S49.012P	S49.141K	S52.026Q	S52.091N	S52.126Q	S52.211A	S52.234Q	S52.253Q	S52.279Q
S49.019A	S49.141P	S52.026R	S52.091P	S52.126R	S52.211K	S52.234R	S52.253R	S52.279R
S49.019K	S49.142A	S52.031K	S52.091Q	S52.131K	S52.211P	S52.235A	S52.254A	S52.281A
S49.019P	S49.142K	S52.031M	S52.091R	S52.131M	S52.212A	S52.235K	S52.254K	S52.281K
S49.021A	S49.142P	S52.031N	S52.092K	S52.131N	S52.212K	S52.235M	S52.254M	S52.281M
S49.021K	S49.149A	S52.031P	S52.092M	S52.131P	S52.212P	S52.235N	S52.254N	S52.281N
S49.021P	S49.149K	S52.031Q	S52.092N	S52.131Q	S52.219A	S52.235P	S52.254P	S52.281P
S49.022A	S49.149P	S52.031R	S52.092P	S52.131R	S52.219K	S52.235Q	S52.254Q	S52.281Q
S49.022K	S49.191A	S52.032K	S52.092Q	S52.132K	S52.219P	S52.235R	S52.254R	S52.281R
S49.022P	S49.191K	S52.032M	S52.092R	S52.132M	S52.221A	S52.236A	S52.255A	S52.282A
S49.029A	S49.191P	S52.032N	S52.099K	S52.132N	S52.221K	S52.236K	S52.255K	S52.282K
S49.029K	S49.192A	S52.032P	S52.099M	S52.132P	S52.221M	S52.236M	S52.255M	S52.282M
S49.029P	S49.192K	S52.032Q	S52.099N	S52.132Q	S52.221N	S52.236N	S52.255N	S52.282N
S49.031A	S49.192P	S52.032R	S52.099P	S52.132R	S52.221P	S52.236P	S52.255P	S52.282P
S49.031K	S49.199A	S52.033K	S52.099Q	S52.133K	S52.221Q	S52.236Q	S52.255Q	S52.282Q
S49.031P	S49.199K	S52.033M	S52.099R	S52.133M	S52.221R	S52.236R	S52.255R	
S49.032A	S49.199P	S52.033N	S52.101K	S52.133N	S52.222A	S52.241A	S52.256A	
S49.032K	S52.001K	S52.033P	S52.101M	S52.133P	S52.222K	S52.241K	S52.256K	
S49.032P	S52.001M		S52.101N	S52.133Q	S52.222M	S52.241M	S52.256M	

S52.282R	S52.323P	S52.342P	S52.361P	S52.389P	S52.515P	S52.559M	S52.602M	S52.699A
S52.283A	S52.323Q	S52.342Q	S52.361Q	S52.389Q	S52.515Q	S52.559N	S52.602N	S52.699K
S52.283K	S52.323R	S52.342R	S52.361R	S52.389R	S52.515R	S52.559P	S52.602P	S52.699M
S52.283M	S52.324A	S52.343A	S52.362A	S52.391A	S52.516A	S52.559Q	S52.602Q	S52.699N
S52.283N	S52.324K	S52.343K	S52.362K	S52.391K	S52.516K	S52.559R	S52.602R	S52.699P
S52.283P	S52.324M	S52.343M	S52.362M	S52.391M	S52.516M	S52.561A	S52.609A	S52.699Q
S52.283Q	S52.324N	S52.343N	S52.362N	S52.391N	S52.516N	S52.561K	S52.609K	S52.699R
S52.283R	S52.324P	S52.343P	S52.362P	S52.391P	S52.516P	S52.561M	S52.609M	S52.90XA
S52.291A	S52.324Q	S52.343Q	S52.362Q	S52.391Q	S52.516Q	S52.561N	S52.609N	S52.90XK
S52.291K	S52.324R	S52.343R	S52.362R	S52.391R	S52.516R	S52.561P	S52.609P	S52.90XM
S52.291M	S52.325A	S52.344A	S52.363A	S52.392A	S52.521A	S52.561Q	S52.609Q	S52.90XN
S52.291N	S52.325K	S52.344K	S52.363K	S52.392K	S52.521K	S52.561R	S52.609R	S52.90XP
S52.291P	S52.325M	S52.344M	S52.363M	S52.392M	S52.521P	S52.562A	S52.611A	S52.90XQ
S52.291Q	S52.325N	S52.344N	S52.363N	S52.392N	S52.522A	S52.562K	S52.611K	S52.90XR
S52.291R	S52.325P	S52.344P	S52.363P	S52.392P	S52.522K	S52.562M	S52.611M	S52.91XA
S52.292A	S52.325Q	S52.344Q	S52.363Q	S52.392Q	S52.522P	S52.562N	S52.611N	S52.91XK
S52.292K	S52.325R	S52.344R	S52.363R	S52.392R	S52.529A	S52.562P	S52.611P	S52.91XM
S52.292M	S52.326A	S52.345A	S52.364A	S52.399A	S52.529K	S52.562Q	S52.611Q	S52.91XN
S52.292N	S52.326K	S52.345K	S52.364K	S52.399K	S52.529P	S52.562R	S52.611R	S52.91XP
S52.292P	S52.326M	S52.345M	S52.364M	S52.399M	S52.531A	S52.569A	S52.612A	S52.91XQ
S52.292Q	S52.326N	S52.345N	S52.364N	S52.399N	S52.531K	S52.569K	S52.612K	S52.91XR
S52.292R	S52.326P	S52.345P	S52.364P	S52.399P	S52.531M	S52.569M	S52.612M	S52.92XA
S52.299A	S52.326Q	S52.345Q	S52.364Q	S52.399Q	S52.531N	S52.569N	S52.612N	S52.92XK
S52.299K	S52.326R	S52.345R	S52.364R	S52.399R	S52.531P	S52.569P	S52.612P	S52.92XM
S52.299M	S52.331A	S52.346A	S52.365A	S52.501A	S52.531Q	S52.569Q	S52.612Q	S52.92XN
S52.299N	S52.331K	S52.346K	S52.365K	S52.501K	S52.531R	S52.569R	S52.612R	S52.92XP
S52.299P	S52.331M	S52.346M	S52.365M	S52.501M	S52.532A	S52.571A	S52.613A	S52.92XQ
S52.299Q	S52.331N	S52.346N	S52.365N	S52.501N	S52.532K	S52.571K	S52.613K	S52.92XR
S52.299R	S52.331P	S52.346P	S52.365P	S52.501P	S52.532M	S52.571M	S52.613M	S55.001A
S52.301A	S52.331Q	S52.346Q	S52.365Q	S52.501Q	S52.532N	S52.571N	S52.613N	S55.002A
S52.301K	S52.331R	S52.346R	S52.365R	S52.501R	S52.532P	S52.571P	S52.613P	S55.009A
S52.301M	S52.332A	S52.351A	S52.366A	S52.502A	S52.532Q	S52.571Q	S52.613Q	S55.011A
S52.301N	S52.332K	S52.351K	S52.366K	S52.502K	S52.532R	S52.571R	S52.613R	S55.012A
S52.301P	S52.332M	S52.351M	S52.366M	S52.502M	S52.539A	S52.572A	S52.614A	S55.019A
S52.301Q	S52.332N	S52.351N	S52.366N	S52.502N	S52.539K	S52.572K	S52.614K	S55.091A
S52.301R	S52.332P	S52.351P	S52.366P	S52.502P	S52.539M	S52.572M	S52.614M	S55.092A
S52.302A	S52.332Q	S52.351Q	S52.366Q	S52.502Q	S52.539N	S52.572N	S52.614N	S55.099A
S52.302K	S52.332R	S52.351R	S52.366R	S52.502R	S52.539P	S52.572P	S52.614P	S55.101A
S52.302M	S52.333A	S52.352A	S52.371A	S52.509A	S52.539Q	S52.572Q	S52.614Q	S55.102A
S52.302N	S52.333K	S52.352K	S52.371K	S52.509K	S52.539R	S52.572R	S52.614R	S55.109A
S52.302P	S52.333M	S52.352M	S52.371M	S52.509M	S52.541A	S52.579A	S52.615A	S55.111A
S52.302Q	S52.333N	S52.352N	S52.371N	S52.509N	S52.541K	S52.579K	S52.615K	S55.112A
S52.302R	S52.333P	S52.352P	S52.371P	S52.509P	S52.541M	S52.579M	S52.615M	S55.119A
S52.309A	S52.333Q	S52.352Q	S52.371Q	S52.509Q	S52.541N	S52.579N	S52.615N	S55.191A
S52.309K	S52.333R	S52.352R	S52.371R	S52.509R	S52.541P	S52.579P	S52.615P	S55.192A
S52.309M	S52.334A	S52.353A	S52.372A	S52.511A	S52.541Q	S52.579Q	S52.615Q	S55.199A
S52.309N	S52.334K	S52.353K	S52.372K	S52.511K	S52.541R	S52.579R	S52.615R	S55.201A
S52.309P	S52.334M	S52.353M	S52.372M	S52.511M	S52.542A	S52.591A	S52.616A	S55.202A
S52.309Q	S52.334N	S52.353N	S52.372N	S52.511N	S52.542K	S52.591K	S52.616K	S55.209A
S52.309R	S52.334P	S52.353P	S52.372P	S52.511P	S52.542M	S52.591M	S52.616M	S55.211A
S52.311A	S52.334Q	S52.353Q	S52.372Q	S52.511Q	S52.542N	S52.591N	S52.616N	S55.212A
S52.311K	S52.334R	S52.353R	S52.372R	S52.511R	S52.542P	S52.591P	S52.616Q	S55.219A
S52.311P	S52.335A	S52.354A	S52.379A	S52.512A	S52.542Q	S52.591Q	S52.616R	S55.291A
S52.312A	S52.335K	S52.354K	S52.379K	S52.512K	S52.542R	S52.591R	S52.621A	S55.292A
S52.312K	S52.335M	S52.354M	S52.379M	S52.512M	S52.549A	S52.592A	S52.621K	S55.299A
S52.312P	S52.335N	S52.354N	S52.379N	S52.512N	S52.549K	S52.592K	S52.621P	S55.801A
S52.319A	S52.335P	S52.354P	S52.379P	S52.512P	S52.549M	S52.592M	S52.622A	S55.802A
S52.319K	S52.335Q	S52.354Q	S52.379Q	S52.512Q	S52.549N	S52.592N	S52.622K	S55.809A
S52.319P	S52.335R	S52.354R	S52.379R	S52.512R	S52.549P	S52.592P	S52.622P	S55.811A
S52.321A	S52.336A	S52.355A	S52.381A	S52.513A	S52.549Q	S52.592Q	S52.629A	S55.812A
S52.321K	S52.336K	S52.355K	S52.381K	S52.513K	S52.549R	S52.592R	S52.629K	S55.819A
S52.321M	S52.336M	S52.355M	S52.381M	S52.513M	S52.551A	S52.599A	S52.629P	S55.891A
S52.321N	S52.336N	S52.355N	S52.381N	S52.513N	S52.551K	S52.599K	S52.691A	S55.892A
S52.321P	S52.336P	S52.355P	S52.381P	S52.513P	S52.551M	S52.599M	S52.691K	S55.899A
S52.321Q	S52.336Q	S52.355Q	S52.381Q	S52.513Q	S52.551N	S52.599N	S52.691M	S55.901A
S52.321R	S52.336R	S52.355R	S52.381R	S52.513R	S52.551P	S52.599P	S52.691N	S55.902A
S52.322A	S52.341A	S52.356A	S52.382A	S52.514A	S52.551Q	S52.599Q	S52.691P	S55.909A
S52.322K	S52.341K	S52.356K	S52.382K	S52.514K	S52.551R	S52.599R	S52.691Q	S55.911A
S52.322M	S52.341M	S52.356M	S52.382M	S52.514M	S52.552A	S52.601A	S52.691R	S55.912A
S52.322N	S52.341N	S52.356N	S52.382N	S52.514N	S52.552K	S52.601K	S52.692A	S55.919A
S52.322P	S52.341P	S52.356P	S52.382P	S52.514P	S52.552M	S52.601M	S52.692K	S55.991A
S52.322Q	S52.341Q	S52.356Q	S52.382Q	S52.514Q	S52.552N	S52.601N	S52.692M	S55.992A
S52.322R	S52.341R	S52.356R	S52.382R	S52.514R	S52.552P	S52.601P	S52.692N	S55.999A
S52.323A	S52.342A	S52.361A	S52.389A	S52.515A	S52.552Q	S52.601Q	S52.692P	S56.021A
S52.323K	S52.342K	S52.361K	S52.389K	S52.515K	S52.552R	S52.601R	S52.692Q	S56.022A
S52.323M	S52.342M	S52.361M	S52.389M	S52.515M	S52.559A	S52.602A	S52.692R	S56.029A
S52.323N	S52.342N	S52.361N	S52.389N	S52.515N	S52.559K	S52.602K		S56.121A

Appendix F: Complication and Comorbidity (CC) Code List

S56.122A	S59.031A	S59.212P	S62.024K	S62.133B	S62.174P	S62.236K	S62.310B	S62.335P
S56.123A	S59.031K	S59.219A	S62.024P	S62.133K	S62.175B	S62.236P	S62.310K	S62.336B
S56.124A	S59.031P	S59.219K	S62.025B	S62.133P	S62.175K	S62.241B	S62.310P	S62.336K
S56.125A	S59.032A	S59.219P	S62.025K	S62.134B	S62.175P	S62.241K	S62.311B	S62.336P
S56.126A	S59.032K	S59.221A	S62.025P	S62.134K	S62.176B	S62.241P	S62.311K	S62.337B
S56.127A	S59.032P	S59.221K	S62.026B	S62.134P	S62.176K	S62.242B	S62.311P	S62.337K
S56.128A	S59.039A	S59.221P	S62.026K	S62.135B	S62.176P	S62.242K	S62.312B	S62.337P
S56.129A	S59.039K	S59.222A	S62.026P	S62.135K	S62.181B	S62.242P	S62.312K	S62.338B
S56.221A	S59.039P	S59.222K	S62.031B	S62.135P	S62.181K	S62.243B	S62.312P	S62.338K
S56.222A	S59.041A	S59.222P	S62.031K	S62.136B	S62.181P	S62.243K	S62.313B	S62.338P
S56.229A	S59.041K	S59.229A	S62.031P	S62.136K	S62.182B	S62.243P	S62.313K	S62.339B
S56.321A	S59.041P	S59.229K	S62.032B	S62.136P	S62.182K	S62.244B	S62.313P	S62.339K
S56.322A	S59.042A	S59.229P	S62.032K	S62.141B	S62.182P	S62.244K	S62.314B	S62.339P
S56.329A	S59.042K	S59.231A	S62.032P	S62.141K	S62.183B	S62.244P	S62.314K	S62.340B
S56.421A	S59.042P	S59.231K	S62.033B	S62.141P	S62.183K	S62.245B	S62.314P	S62.340K
S56.422A	S59.049A	S59.231P	S62.033K	S62.142B	S62.183P	S62.245K	S62.315B	S62.340P
S56.423A	S59.049K	S59.232A	S62.033P	S62.142K	S62.184B	S62.245P	S62.315K	S62.341B
S56.424A	S59.049P	S59.232K	S62.034B	S62.142P	S62.184K	S62.246B	S62.315P	S62.341K
S56.425A	S59.091A	S59.232P	S62.034K	S62.143B	S62.184P	S62.246K	S62.316B	S62.341P
S56.426A	S59.091K	S59.239A	S62.034P	S62.143K	S62.185B	S62.246P	S62.316K	S62.342B
S56.427A	S59.091P	S59.239K	S62.035B	S62.143P	S62.185K	S62.251B	S62.316P	S62.342P
S56.428A	S59.092A	S59.239P	S62.035K	S62.144B	S62.185P	S62.251K	S62.317B	S62.343B
S56.429A	S59.092K	S59.241A	S62.035P	S62.144K	S62.186B	S62.251P	S62.317K	S62.343K
S56.521A	S59.092P	S59.241K	S62.036B	S62.144P	S62.186K	S62.252B	S62.317P	S62.343P
S56.522A	S59.099A	S59.241P	S62.036K	S62.145B	S62.186P	S62.252K	S62.318B	S62.344B
S56.529A	S59.099K	S59.242A	S62.036P	S62.145K	S62.201B	S62.252P	S62.318K	S62.344K
S56.821A	S59.099P	S59.242K	S62.101B	S62.145P	S62.201K	S62.253B	S62.318P	S62.344P
S56.822A	S59.101K	S59.242P	S62.101K	S62.146B	S62.201P	S62.253K	S62.319B	S62.345B
S56.829A	S59.101P	S59.249A	S62.101P	S62.146K	S62.202B	S62.253P	S62.319K	S62.345K
S56.921A	S59.102K	S59.249K	S62.102B	S62.146P	S62.202K	S62.254B	S62.319P	S62.345P
S56.922A	S59.102P	S59.249P	S62.102K	S62.151B	S62.202P	S62.254K	S62.320B	S62.346B
S56.929A	S59.109K	S59.291A	S62.102P	S62.151K	S62.209B	S62.254P	S62.320K	S62.346K
S58.011A	S59.109P	S59.291K	S62.109B	S62.151P	S62.209K	S62.255B	S62.320P	S62.346P
S58.012A	S59.111K	S59.291P	S62.109K	S62.152B	S62.209P	S62.255K	S62.321B	S62.347B
S58.019A	S59.111P	S59.292A	S62.109P	S62.152K	S62.211B	S62.255P	S62.321K	S62.347K
S58.021A	S59.112K	S59.292K	S62.111B	S62.152P	S62.211K	S62.256B	S62.321P	S62.347P
S58.022A	S59.112P	S59.292P	S62.111K	S62.153B	S62.211P	S62.256K	S62.322B	S62.348B
S58.029A	S59.119K	S59.299A	S62.111P	S62.153K	S62.212B	S62.256P	S62.322K	S62.348K
S58.111A	S59.119P	S59.299K	S62.112B	S62.153P	S62.212K	S62.291B	S62.322P	S62.348P
S58.112A	S59.121K	S59.299P	S62.112K	S62.154B	S62.212P	S62.291K	S62.323B	S62.349B
S58.119A	S59.121P	S62.001B	S62.112P	S62.154K	S62.213B	S62.291P	S62.323K	S62.349K
S58.121A	S59.122K	S62.001K	S62.113B	S62.154P	S62.213K	S62.292B	S62.323P	S62.349P
S58.122A	S59.122P	S62.001P	S62.113K	S62.155B	S62.213P	S62.292K	S62.324B	S62.350B
S58.129A	S59.129K	S62.002B	S62.113P	S62.155K	S62.221B	S62.292P	S62.324K	S62.350K
S58.911A	S59.129P	S62.002K	S62.114B	S62.155P	S62.221K	S62.299B	S62.324P	S62.350P
S58.912A	S59.131K	S62.002P	S62.114K	S62.156B	S62.221P	S62.299K	S62.325B	S62.351B
S58.919A	S59.131P	S62.009B	S62.114P	S62.156K	S62.222B	S62.299P	S62.325K	S62.351K
S58.921A	S59.132K	S62.009K	S62.115B	S62.156P	S62.222K	S62.300B	S62.325P	S62.351P
S58.922A	S59.132P	S62.009P	S62.115K	S62.161B	S62.222P	S62.300K	S62.326B	S62.352B
S58.929A	S59.139K	S62.011B	S62.115P	S62.161K	S62.223B	S62.300P	S62.326K	S62.352K
S59.001A	S59.139P	S62.011K	S62.116B	S62.161P	S62.223K	S62.301B	S62.326P	S62.352P
S59.001K	S59.141K	S62.011P	S62.116K	S62.162B	S62.223P	S62.301K	S62.327B	S62.353B
S59.001P	S59.141P	S62.012B	S62.116P	S62.162K	S62.224B	S62.301P	S62.327K	S62.353K
S59.002A	S59.142K	S62.012K	S62.121B	S62.162P	S62.224K	S62.302B	S62.327P	S62.353P
S59.002K	S59.142P	S62.012P	S62.121K	S62.163B	S62.224P	S62.302K	S62.328B	S62.354B
S59.002P	S59.149K	S62.013B	S62.121P	S62.163K	S62.225B	S62.302P	S62.328K	S62.354K
S59.009A	S59.149P	S62.013K	S62.122B	S62.163P	S62.225K	S62.303B	S62.328P	S62.354P
S59.009K	S59.191K	S62.013P	S62.122K	S62.164B	S62.225P	S62.303K	S62.329B	S62.355B
S59.009P	S59.191P	S62.014B	S62.122P	S62.164P	S62.226B	S62.303P	S62.329K	S62.355K
S59.011A	S59.192K	S62.014K	S62.123B	S62.165B	S62.226K	S62.304B	S62.329P	S62.355P
S59.011K	S59.192P	S62.014P	S62.123K	S62.165K	S62.226P	S62.304K	S62.330B	S62.356B
S59.011P	S59.199K	S62.015B	S62.123P	S62.165P	S62.231B	S62.304P	S62.330K	S62.356K
S59.012A	S59.199P	S62.015K	S62.124B	S62.166B	S62.231K	S62.305B	S62.330P	S62.356P
S59.012K	S59.201A	S62.015P	S62.124K	S62.166K	S62.231P	S62.305P	S62.331B	S62.357B
S59.012P	S59.201K	S62.016B	S62.124P	S62.166P	S62.232B	S62.306B	S62.331K	S62.357K
S59.019A	S59.201P	S62.016K	S62.125B	S62.171B	S62.232K	S62.306K	S62.331P	S62.357P
S59.019K	S59.202A	S62.016P	S62.125K	S62.171K	S62.232P	S62.306P	S62.332B	S62.358B
S59.019P	S59.202K	S62.021B	S62.125P	S62.171P	S62.233B	S62.307B	S62.332K	S62.358K
S59.021A	S59.202P	S62.021K	S62.126B	S62.172B	S62.233K	S62.307K	S62.332P	S62.358P
S59.021K	S59.209A	S62.021P	S62.126K	S62.172K	S62.233P	S62.307P	S62.333B	S62.359B
S59.021P	S59.209K	S62.022B	S62.126P	S62.172P	S62.234B	S62.308B	S62.333K	S62.359K
S59.022A	S59.209P	S62.022K	S62.131B	S62.173B	S62.234K	S62.308K	S62.333P	S62.359P
S59.022K	S59.211A	S62.022P	S62.131K	S62.173K	S62.234P	S62.308P	S62.334B	S62.360B
S59.022P	S59.211K	S62.023B	S62.131P	S62.173P	S62.235B	S62.309B	S62.334K	S62.360K
S59.029A	S59.211P	S62.023K	S62.132B	S62.174B	S62.235K	S62.309K	S62.334P	S62.360P
S59.029K	S59.212A	S62.023P	S62.132K	S62.174K	S62.235P	S62.309P	S62.335B	S62.361B
S59.029P	S59.212K	S62.024B	S62.132P		S62.236B		S62.335K	

S62.361K	S62.515B	S62.617P	S62.643K	S62.669B	S65.590A	S68.422A	S72.026P	S72.051N
S62.361P	S62.515K	S62.618B	S62.643P	S62.669K	S65.591A	S68.429A	S72.026Q	S72.051P
S62.362B	S62.515P	S62.618K	S62.644B	S62.669P	S65.592A	S68.711A	S72.026R	S72.051Q
S62.362K	S62.516B	S62.618P	S62.644K	S62.90XB	S65.593A	S68.712A	S72.031K	S72.051R
S62.362P	S62.516K	S62.619B	S62.644P	S62.90XK	S65.594A	S68.719A	S72.031M	S72.052K
S62.363B	S62.516P	S62.619K	S62.645B	S62.90XP	S65.595A	S68.721A	S72.031N	S72.052M
S62.363K	S62.521B	S62.619P	S62.645K	S62.91XB	S65.596A	S68.722A	S72.031P	S72.052N
S62.363P	S62.521K	S62.620B	S62.645P	S62.91XK	S65.597A	S68.729A	S72.031Q	S72.052P
S62.364B	S62.521P	S62.620K	S62.646B	S62.91XP	S65.598A	S72.001K	S72.031R	S72.052Q
S62.364K	S62.522B	S62.620P	S62.646K	S62.92XB	S65.599A	S72.001M	S72.032K	S72.052R
S62.364P	S62.522K	S62.621B	S62.646P	S62.92XK	S65.801A	S72.001N	S72.032M	S72.059K
S62.365B	S62.522P	S62.621K	S62.647B	S62.92XP	S65.802A	S72.001P	S72.032N	S72.059N
S62.365K	S62.523B	S62.621P	S62.647K	S65.001A	S65.809A	S72.001Q	S72.032P	S72.059P
S62.365P	S62.523K	S62.622B	S62.647P	S65.002A	S65.811A	S72.001R	S72.032Q	S72.059Q
S62.366B	S62.523P	S62.622K	S62.648B	S65.009A	S65.812A	S72.002K	S72.032R	S72.059R
S62.366K	S62.524B	S62.622P	S62.648K	S65.011A	S65.819A	S72.002M	S72.033K	S72.061K
S62.366P	S62.524K	S62.623B	S62.648P	S65.012A	S65.891A	S72.002N	S72.033M	S72.061M
S62.367B	S62.524P	S62.623K	S62.649B	S65.019A	S65.892A	S72.002P	S72.033N	S72.061N
S62.367K	S62.525B	S62.623P	S62.649K	S65.091A	S65.899A	S72.002Q	S72.033P	S72.061P
S62.367P	S62.525K	S62.624B	S62.649P	S65.092A	S65.901A	S72.002R	S72.033Q	S72.061Q
S62.368B	S62.525P	S62.624K	S62.650B	S65.099A	S65.902A	S72.009K	S72.033R	S72.061R
S62.368K	S62.526B	S62.624P	S62.650K	S65.101A	S65.909A	S72.009M	S72.034K	S72.062K
S62.368P	S62.526K	S62.625B	S62.650P	S65.102A	S65.911A	S72.009N	S72.034M	S72.062M
S62.369B	S62.526P	S62.625K	S62.651B	S65.109A	S65.912A	S72.009P	S72.034N	S72.062N
S62.369K	S62.600B	S62.625P	S62.651K	S65.111A	S65.919A	S72.009Q	S72.034P	S72.062P
S62.369P	S62.600K	S62.626B	S62.651P	S65.112A	S65.991A	S72.009R	S72.034Q	S72.062Q
S62.390B	S62.600P	S62.626K	S62.652B	S65.119A	S65.992A	S72.011K	S72.034R	S72.062R
S62.390K	S62.601B	S62.626P	S62.652K	S65.191A	S65.999A	S72.011M	S72.035K	S72.063K
S62.390P	S62.601K	S62.627B	S62.652P	S65.192A	S66.021A	S72.011N	S72.035M	S72.063M
S62.391B	S62.601P	S62.627K	S62.653B	S65.199A	S66.022A	S72.011P	S72.035N	S72.063N
S62.391K	S62.602B	S62.627P	S62.653K	S65.201A	S66.029A	S72.011Q	S72.035P	S72.063P
S62.391P	S62.602K	S62.628B	S62.653P	S65.202A	S66.120A	S72.011R	S72.035Q	S72.063Q
S62.392B	S62.602P	S62.628K	S62.654B	S65.209A	S66.121A	S72.012K	S72.035R	S72.063R
S62.392K	S62.603B	S62.628P	S62.654K	S65.211A	S66.122A	S72.012M	S72.036K	S72.064K
S62.392P	S62.603K	S62.629B	S62.654P	S65.212A	S66.123A	S72.012N	S72.036M	S72.064M
S62.393B	S62.603P	S62.629K	S62.655B	S65.219A	S66.124A	S72.012P	S72.036N	S72.064N
S62.393K	S62.604B	S62.629P	S62.655K	S65.291A	S66.125A	S72.012Q	S72.036P	S72.064P
S62.393P	S62.604K	S62.630B	S62.655P	S65.292A	S66.126A	S72.012R	S72.036Q	S72.064Q
S62.394B	S62.604P	S62.630K	S62.656B	S65.299A	S66.127A	S72.019K	S72.036R	S72.064R
S62.394K	S62.605B	S62.630P	S62.656K	S65.301A	S66.128A	S72.019M	S72.041K	S72.065K
S62.394P	S62.605K	S62.631B	S62.656P	S65.302A	S66.129A	S72.019N	S72.041N	S72.065M
S62.395B	S62.605P	S62.631K	S62.657B	S65.309A	S66.221A	S72.019P	S72.041P	S72.065N
S62.395K	S62.606B	S62.631P	S62.657K	S65.311A	S66.222A	S72.019Q	S72.041Q	S72.065P
S62.395P	S62.606K	S62.632B	S62.657P	S65.312A	S66.229A	S72.019R	S72.041R	S72.065Q
S62.396B	S62.606P	S62.632K	S62.658B	S65.319A	S66.320A	S72.021K	S72.042K	S72.065R
S62.396K	S62.607B	S62.632P	S62.658K	S65.391A	S66.321A	S72.021M	S72.042M	S72.066K
S62.396P	S62.607K	S62.633B	S62.658P	S65.392A	S66.322A	S72.021N	S72.042N	S72.066M
S62.397B	S62.607P	S62.633K	S62.659B	S65.399A	S66.323A	S72.021P	S72.042Q	S72.066N
S62.397K	S62.608B	S62.633P	S62.659K	S65.401A	S66.324A	S72.021R	S72.042R	S72.066P
S62.397P	S62.608K	S62.634B	S62.659P	S65.402A	S66.325A	S72.022K	S72.043K	S72.066Q
S62.398B	S62.608P	S62.634K	S62.660B	S65.409A	S66.326A	S72.022M	S72.043M	S72.066R
S62.398K	S62.609B	S62.634P	S62.660K	S65.411A	S66.327A	S72.022N	S72.043N	S72.091K
S62.398P	S62.609K	S62.635B	S62.660P	S65.412A	S66.328A	S72.022P	S72.043P	S72.091M
S62.399B	S62.609P	S62.635K	S62.661B	S65.419A	S66.329A	S72.022Q	S72.043Q	S72.091N
S62.399K	S62.610B	S62.635P	S62.661K	S65.491A	S66.421A	S72.022R	S72.043R	S72.091P
S62.399P	S62.610K	S62.636B	S62.661P	S65.492A	S66.422A	S72.023K	S72.044K	S72.091Q
S62.501B	S62.610P	S62.636K	S62.662B	S65.499A	S66.429A	S72.023M	S72.044M	S72.091R
S62.501K	S62.611B	S62.636P	S62.662K	S65.500A	S66.520A	S72.023N	S72.044N	S72.092K
S62.501P	S62.611K	S62.637B	S62.662P	S65.501A	S66.521A	S72.023P	S72.044P	S72.092M
S62.502B	S62.611P	S62.637K	S62.663B	S65.502A	S66.522A	S72.023Q	S72.044Q	S72.092N
S62.502K	S62.612B	S62.637P	S62.663K	S65.503A	S66.523A	S72.023R	S72.044R	S72.092P
S62.502P	S62.612K	S62.638B	S62.663P	S65.504A	S66.524A	S72.024K	S72.045K	S72.092Q
S62.509B	S62.612P	S62.638K	S62.664B	S65.505A	S66.525A	S72.024M	S72.045M	S72.092R
S62.509K	S62.613B	S62.638P	S62.664K	S65.506A	S66.526A	S72.024N	S72.045N	S72.099K
S62.509P	S62.613K	S62.639B	S62.664P	S65.507A	S66.527A	S72.024P	S72.045P	S72.099M
S62.511B	S62.613P	S62.639K	S62.665B	S65.508A	S66.528A	S72.024Q	S72.045Q	S72.099N
S62.511K	S62.614B	S62.639P	S62.665K	S65.509A	S66.529A	S72.024R	S72.045R	S72.099P
S62.511P	S62.614K	S62.640B	S62.665P	S65.510A	S66.821A	S72.025K	S72.046K	S72.099Q
S62.512B	S62.614P	S62.640K	S62.666B	S65.511A	S66.822A	S72.025M	S72.046M	S72.099R
S62.512K	S62.615B	S62.640P	S62.666K	S65.512A	S66.829A	S72.025N	S72.046N	S72.101K
S62.512P	S62.615K	S62.641B	S62.666P	S65.513A	S66.921A	S72.025P	S72.046P	S72.101M
S62.513B	S62.615P	S62.641K	S62.667B	S65.514A	S66.922A	S72.025Q	S72.046Q	S72.101N
S62.513K	S62.616B	S62.641P	S62.667K	S65.515A	S66.929A	S72.025R	S72.046R	S72.101P
S62.513P	S62.616K	S62.642B	S62.667P	S65.516A	S68.411A	S72.026K	S72.051K	S72.101Q
S62.514B	S62.616P	S62.642K	S62.668B	S65.517A	S68.412A	S72.026M	S72.051M	S72.101R
S62.514K	S62.617B	S62.642P	S62.668K	S65.518A	S68.419A	S72.026N		S72.102K
S62.514P	S62.617K	S62.643B	S62.668P	S65.519A	S68.421A			

S72.102M	S72.126K	S72.146R	S72.324Q	S72.345P	S72.366N	S72.415R	S72.434R	S72.453R
S72.102N	S72.126M	S72.21XK	S72.324R	S72.345Q	S72.366P	S72.416A	S72.435A	S72.454A
S72.102P	S72.126N	S72.21XM	S72.325K	S72.345R	S72.366Q	S72.416K	S72.435K	S72.454K
S72.102Q	S72.126P	S72.21XN	S72.325M	S72.346K	S72.366R	S72.416M	S72.435M	S72.454M
S72.102R	S72.126Q	S72.21XP	S72.325P	S72.346M	S72.391K	S72.416N	S72.435N	S72.454N
S72.109K	S72.126R	S72.21XQ	S72.325Q	S72.346P	S72.391M	S72.416P	S72.435P	S72.454P
S72.109M	S72.131K	S72.21XR	S72.325R	S72.346Q	S72.391N	S72.416Q	S72.435Q	S72.454Q
S72.109N	S72.131M	S72.22XK	S72.326K	S72.346R	S72.391P	S72.416R	S72.435R	S72.454R
S72.109P	S72.131N	S72.22XM	S72.326M	S72.351K	S72.391Q	S72.421A	S72.436A	S72.455A
S72.109Q	S72.131P	S72.22XN	S72.326N	S72.351M	S72.391R	S72.421K	S72.436K	S72.455K
S72.109R	S72.131Q	S72.22XP	S72.326P	S72.351N	S72.392K	S72.421M	S72.436M	S72.455M
S72.111K	S72.131R	S72.22XQ	S72.326Q	S72.351P	S72.392M	S72.421N	S72.436N	S72.455N
S72.111M	S72.132K	S72.22XR	S72.326R	S72.351Q	S72.392N	S72.421P	S72.436P	S72.455P
S72.111N	S72.132M	S72.23XK	S72.331K	S72.351R	S72.392P	S72.421Q	S72.436Q	S72.455Q
S72.111P	S72.132N	S72.23XM	S72.331M	S72.352K	S72.392Q	S72.421R	S72.436R	S72.455R
S72.111Q	S72.132P	S72.23XN	S72.331N	S72.352M	S72.392R	S72.422A	S72.441A	S72.456A
S72.111R	S72.132Q	S72.23XP	S72.331P	S72.352N	S72.399K	S72.422K	S72.441K	S72.456K
S72.112K	S72.132R	S72.23XQ	S72.331Q	S72.352P	S72.399M	S72.422M	S72.441M	S72.456M
S72.112M	S72.133K	S72.23XR	S72.331R	S72.352Q	S72.399N	S72.422N	S72.441N	S72.456N
S72.112N	S72.133M	S72.24XK	S72.332K	S72.352R	S72.399P	S72.422P	S72.441P	S72.456P
S72.112P	S72.133N	S72.24XM	S72.332M	S72.353K	S72.399Q	S72.422Q	S72.441Q	S72.456Q
S72.112Q	S72.133P	S72.24XN	S72.332N	S72.353M	S72.399R	S72.422R	S72.441R	S72.456R
S72.112R	S72.133Q	S72.24XP	S72.332P	S72.353N	S72.401A	S72.423A	S72.442A	S72.461A
S72.113K	S72.133R	S72.24XQ	S72.332Q	S72.353P	S72.401K	S72.423K	S72.442K	S72.461K
S72.113M	S72.134K	S72.24XR	S72.332R	S72.353Q	S72.401M	S72.423M	S72.442M	S72.461M
S72.113N	S72.134M	S72.25XK	S72.333K	S72.353R	S72.401N	S72.423N	S72.442N	S72.461N
S72.113P	S72.134N	S72.25XM	S72.333M	S72.354K	S72.401P	S72.423P	S72.442P	S72.461P
S72.113Q	S72.134P	S72.25XN	S72.333N	S72.354M	S72.401Q	S72.423Q	S72.442Q	S72.461Q
S72.113R	S72.134Q	S72.25XP	S72.333P	S72.354N	S72.401R	S72.423R	S72.442R	S72.461R
S72.114K	S72.134R	S72.25XQ	S72.333Q	S72.354P	S72.402A	S72.424A	S72.443A	S72.462A
S72.114M	S72.135K	S72.25XR	S72.333R	S72.354Q	S72.402K	S72.424K	S72.443K	S72.462K
S72.114N	S72.135M	S72.26XK	S72.334K	S72.354R	S72.402M	S72.424M	S72.443M	S72.462M
S72.114P	S72.135N	S72.26XM	S72.334M	S72.355K	S72.402N	S72.424N	S72.443N	S72.462N
S72.114Q	S72.135P	S72.26XN	S72.334N	S72.355M	S72.402P	S72.424P	S72.443P	S72.462P
S72.114R	S72.135Q	S72.26XP	S72.334P	S72.355N	S72.402Q	S72.424Q	S72.443Q	S72.462Q
S72.115K	S72.135R	S72.26XQ	S72.334Q	S72.355P	S72.402R	S72.424R	S72.443R	S72.462R
S72.115M	S72.136K	S72.26XR	S72.334R	S72.355Q	S72.409A	S72.425A	S72.444A	S72.463A
S72.115N	S72.136M	S72.301K	S72.335K	S72.355R	S72.409K	S72.425K	S72.444K	S72.463K
S72.115P	S72.136N	S72.301M	S72.335M	S72.356K	S72.409M	S72.425M	S72.444M	S72.463M
S72.115Q	S72.136P	S72.301N	S72.335N	S72.356M	S72.409N	S72.425N	S72.444N	S72.463N
S72.115R	S72.136Q	S72.301P	S72.335P	S72.356N	S72.409P	S72.425P	S72.444P	S72.463P
S72.116K	S72.136R	S72.301Q	S72.335Q	S72.356P	S72.409Q	S72.425Q	S72.444Q	S72.463Q
S72.116M	S72.141K	S72.301R	S72.335R	S72.356Q	S72.409R	S72.425R	S72.444R	S72.463R
S72.116N	S72.141M	S72.302K	S72.336K	S72.356R	S72.411A	S72.426A	S72.445A	S72.464A
S72.116P	S72.141N	S72.302M	S72.336M	S72.361K	S72.411K	S72.426K	S72.445K	S72.464K
S72.116Q	S72.141P	S72.302N	S72.336N	S72.361M	S72.411M	S72.426M	S72.445M	S72.464M
S72.116R	S72.141Q	S72.302P	S72.336P	S72.361N	S72.411N	S72.426N	S72.445N	S72.464N
S72.121K	S72.141R	S72.302Q	S72.336Q	S72.361P	S72.411P	S72.426P	S72.445P	S72.464P
S72.121M	S72.142K	S72.302R	S72.336R	S72.361Q	S72.411Q	S72.426Q	S72.445Q	S72.464Q
S72.121N	S72.142M	S72.309K	S72.341K	S72.361R	S72.411R	S72.426R	S72.445R	S72.464R
S72.121P	S72.142N	S72.309M	S72.341M	S72.362K	S72.412A	S72.431A	S72.446A	S72.465A
S72.121Q	S72.142P	S72.309N	S72.341N	S72.362M	S72.412K	S72.431K	S72.446K	S72.465K
S72.121R	S72.142Q	S72.309P	S72.341P	S72.362N	S72.412M	S72.431M	S72.446M	S72.465M
S72.122K	S72.142R	S72.309Q	S72.341Q	S72.362P	S72.412N	S72.431N	S72.446N	S72.465N
S72.122M	S72.143K	S72.309R	S72.341R	S72.362Q	S72.412P	S72.431P	S72.446P	S72.465P
S72.122N	S72.143M	S72.321K	S72.342K	S72.362R	S72.412Q	S72.431Q	S72.446Q	S72.465Q
S72.122P	S72.143N	S72.321M	S72.342M	S72.363K	S72.412R	S72.431R	S72.446R	S72.465R
S72.122Q	S72.143P	S72.321N	S72.342N	S72.363M	S72.413A	S72.432A	S72.451A	S72.466A
S72.122R	S72.143Q	S72.321P	S72.342P	S72.363N	S72.413K	S72.432K	S72.451K	S72.466K
S72.123K	S72.143R	S72.321Q	S72.342Q	S72.363P	S72.413M	S72.432M	S72.451M	S72.466M
S72.123M	S72.144K	S72.321R	S72.342R	S72.363Q	S72.413N	S72.432N	S72.451N	S72.466N
S72.123N	S72.144M	S72.322K	S72.343K	S72.363R	S72.413P	S72.432P	S72.451P	S72.466P
S72.123P	S72.144N	S72.322M	S72.343M	S72.364K	S72.413Q	S72.432Q	S72.451Q	S72.466Q
S72.123Q	S72.144P	S72.322N	S72.343N	S72.364M	S72.413R	S72.432R	S72.451R	S72.466R
S72.123R	S72.144Q	S72.322P	S72.343P	S72.364N	S72.414A	S72.433A	S72.452A	S72.471A
S72.124K	S72.144R	S72.322Q	S72.343Q	S72.364P	S72.414K	S72.433K	S72.452K	S72.471K
S72.124M	S72.145K	S72.322R	S72.343R	S72.364Q	S72.414M	S72.433M	S72.452M	S72.471P
S72.124N	S72.145M	S72.323K	S72.344K	S72.364R	S72.414N	S72.433N	S72.452N	S72.472A
S72.124P	S72.145N	S72.323M	S72.344M	S72.365K	S72.414P	S72.433P	S72.452P	S72.472K
S72.124Q	S72.145P	S72.323N	S72.344N	S72.365M	S72.414Q	S72.433Q	S72.452Q	S72.472P
S72.124R	S72.145Q	S72.323P	S72.344P	S72.365N	S72.414R	S72.433R	S72.452R	S72.479A
S72.125K	S72.145R	S72.323Q	S72.344Q	S72.365P	S72.415A	S72.434A	S72.453A	S72.479K
S72.125M	S72.146K	S72.323R	S72.344R	S72.365Q	S72.415K	S72.434K	S72.453K	S72.479P
S72.125N	S72.146M	S72.324K	S72.345K	S72.365R	S72.415M	S72.434M	S72.453M	S72.491A
S72.125P	S72.146N	S72.324M	S72.345M	S72.366K	S72.415N	S72.434N	S72.453N	S72.491K
S72.125Q	S72.146P	S72.324N	S72.345N	S72.366M	S72.415P	S72.434P	S72.453P	ICD-10-CM 2018
S72.125R	S72.146Q	S72.324P	S72.345N	S72.366M	S72.415Q	S72.434Q	S72.453Q	S72.491M
								S72.491N

S72.491P	S73.041A	S78.929A	S82.001M	S82.021A	S82.033N	S82.046B	S82.114A	S82.133A
S72.491Q	S73.042A	S79.001K	S82.001N	S82.021B	S82.033P	S82.046C	S82.114K	S82.133K
S72.491R	S73.043A	S79.001P	S82.001P	S82.021C	S82.033Q	S82.046K	S82.114M	S82.133M
S72.492A	S73.044A	S79.002K	S82.001Q	S82.021K	S82.033R	S82.046M	S82.114N	S82.133N
S72.492K	S73.045A	S79.002P	S82.001R	S82.021M	S82.034A	S82.046N	S82.114P	S82.133P
S72.492M	S73.046A	S79.009K	S82.002A	S82.021N	S82.034B	S82.046P	S82.114Q	S82.133Q
S72.492N	S75.201A	S79.009P	S82.002B	S82.021P	S82.034C	S82.046Q	S82.114R	S82.133R
S72.492P	S75.202A	S79.011K	S82.002C	S82.021Q	S82.034K	S82.046R	S82.115A	S82.134A
S72.492Q	S75.209A	S79.011P	S82.002K	S82.021R	S82.034M	S82.091A	S82.115K	S82.134K
S72.492R	S75.211A	S79.012K	S82.002M	S82.022A	S82.034N	S82.091B	S82.115M	S82.134M
S72.499A	S75.212A	S79.012P	S82.002N	S82.022B	S82.034Q	S82.091C	S82.115N	S82.134N
S72.499K	S75.219A	S79.019K	S82.002P	S82.022C	S82.034R	S82.091K	S82.115P	S82.134P
S72.499M	S75.221A	S79.019P	S82.002Q	S82.022K	S82.035A	S82.091M	S82.115Q	S82.134Q
S72.499N	S75.222A	S79.091K	S82.002R	S82.022M	S82.035B	S82.091N	S82.115R	S82.134R
S72.499P	S75.229A	S79.091P	S82.009A	S82.022N	S82.035C	S82.091P	S82.116A	S82.135A
S72.499Q	S75.291A	S79.092K	S82.009B	S82.022P	S82.035K	S82.091Q	S82.116K	S82.135K
S72.499R	S75.292A	S79.092P	S82.009C	S82.022Q	S82.035M	S82.091R	S82.116M	S82.135M
S72.8X1K	S75.299A	S79.099K	S82.009K	S82.022R	S82.035N	S82.092A	S82.116N	S82.135N
S72.8X1M	S75.801A	S79.099P	S82.009M	S82.023A	S82.035P	S82.092B	S82.116P	S82.135P
S72.8X1N	S75.802A	S79.101A	S82.009N	S82.023B	S82.035Q	S82.092C	S82.116Q	S82.135Q
S72.8X1P	S75.809A	S79.101K	S82.009P	S82.023C	S82.035R	S82.092K	S82.116R	S82.135R
S72.8X1Q	S75.811A	S79.101P	S82.009Q	S82.023K	S82.036A	S82.092M	S82.121A	S82.136A
S72.8X1R	S75.812A	S79.102A	S82.009R	S82.023M	S82.036B	S82.092N	S82.121K	S82.136K
S72.8X2K	S75.819A	S79.102K	S82.011A	S82.023N	S82.036C	S82.092P	S82.121M	S82.136M
S72.8X2M	S75.891A	S79.102P	S82.011B	S82.023P	S82.036K	S82.092Q	S82.121N	S82.136N
S72.8X2N	S75.892A	S79.109A	S82.011C	S82.023Q	S82.036M	S82.092R	S82.121P	S82.136P
S72.8X2P	S75.899A	S79.109K	S82.011K	S82.023R	S82.036N	S82.099A	S82.121Q	S82.136Q
S72.8X2Q	S75.901A	S79.109P	S82.011M	S82.024A	S82.036P	S82.099B	S82.121R	S82.136R
S72.8X2R	S75.902A	S79.111A	S82.011N	S82.024B	S82.036Q	S82.099C	S82.122A	S82.141A
S72.8X9K	S75.909A	S79.111K	S82.011P	S82.024C	S82.036R	S82.099K	S82.122K	S82.141K
S72.8X9M	S75.911A	S79.111P	S82.011Q	S82.024K	S82.041A	S82.099M	S82.122M	S82.141M
S72.8X9N	S75.912A	S79.112A	S82.011R	S82.024M	S82.041B	S82.099N	S82.122N	S82.141N
S72.8X9P	S75.919A	S79.112K	S82.012A	S82.024N	S82.041C	S82.099P	S82.122P	S82.141P
S72.8X9Q	S75.991A	S79.112P	S82.012B	S82.024P	S82.041K	S82.099Q	S82.122Q	S82.141Q
S72.8X9R	S75.992A	S79.119A	S82.012C	S82.024Q	S82.041M	S82.099R	S82.122R	S82.141R
S72.90XK	S75.999A	S79.119K	S82.012K	S82.024R	S82.041N	S82.101A	S82.123A	S82.142A
S72.90XM	S76.021A	S79.119P	S82.012M	S82.025A	S82.041P	S82.101K	S82.123K	S82.142K
S72.90XN	S76.022A	S79.121A	S82.012N	S82.025B	S82.041Q	S82.101M	S82.123M	S82.142M
S72.90XP	S76.029A	S79.121K	S82.012P	S82.025C	S82.041R	S82.101N	S82.123N	S82.142N
S72.90XQ	S76.121A	S79.121P	S82.012Q	S82.025K	S82.042A	S82.101P	S82.123P	S82.142P
S72.90XR	S76.122A	S79.122A	S82.012R	S82.025M	S82.042B	S82.101Q	S82.123Q	S82.142Q
S72.91XK	S76.129A	S79.122K	S82.013A	S82.025N	S82.042C	S82.101R	S82.123R	S82.142R
S72.91XM	S76.221A	S79.122P	S82.013B	S82.025P	S82.042K	S82.102A	S82.124A	S82.143A
S72.91XN	S76.222A	S79.129A	S82.013C	S82.025Q	S82.042M	S82.102K	S82.124K	S82.143K
S72.91XP	S76.229A	S79.129K	S82.013K	S82.025R	S82.042N	S82.102M	S82.124M	S82.143M
S72.91XQ	S76.321A	S79.129P	S82.013M	S82.026A	S82.042P	S82.102N	S82.124N	S82.143N
S72.91XR	S76.322A	S79.131A	S82.013N	S82.026B	S82.042Q	S82.102P	S82.124P	S82.143P
S72.92XK	S76.329A	S79.131K	S82.013P	S82.026C	S82.042R	S82.102Q	S82.124Q	S82.143Q
S72.92XM	S76.821A	S79.131P	S82.013Q	S82.026K	S82.043A	S82.102R	S82.124R	S82.143R
S72.92XN	S76.822A	S79.132A	S82.013R	S82.026M	S82.043B	S82.109A	S82.125A	S82.144A
S72.92XP	S76.829A	S79.132K	S82.014A	S82.026N	S82.043C	S82.109K	S82.125K	S82.144K
S72.92XQ	S76.921A	S79.132P	S82.014B	S82.026P	S82.043K	S82.109M	S82.125M	S82.144M
S72.92XR	S76.922A	S79.139A	S82.014C	S82.026Q	S82.043M	S82.109N	S82.125N	S82.144N
S73.001A	S76.929A	S79.139K	S82.014K	S82.026R	S82.043N	S82.109P	S82.125P	S82.144P
S73.002A	S77.00XA	S79.139P	S82.014M	S82.031A	S82.043P	S82.109Q	S82.125Q	S82.144Q
S73.003A	S77.01XA	S79.141A	S82.014N	S82.031B	S82.043Q	S82.109R	S82.125R	S82.144R
S73.004A	S77.02XA	S79.141K	S82.014P	S82.031C	S82.043R	S82.111A	S82.126A	S82.145A
S73.005A	S77.10XA	S79.141P	S82.014Q	S82.031K	S82.044A	S82.111K	S82.126K	S82.145K
S73.006A	S77.11XA	S79.142A	S82.014R	S82.031M	S82.044B	S82.111M	S82.126M	S82.145M
S73.011A	S77.12XA	S79.142K	S82.015A	S82.031N	S82.044C	S82.111N	S82.126N	S82.145N
S73.012A	S78.011A	S79.142P	S82.015B	S82.031P	S82.044K	S82.111P	S82.126P	S82.145P
S73.013A	S78.012A	S79.149A	S82.015C	S82.031Q	S82.044M	S82.111Q	S82.126Q	S82.145Q
S73.014A	S78.019A	S79.149K	S82.015K	S82.031R	S82.044N	S82.111R	S82.126R	S82.145R
S73.015A	S78.021A	S79.149P	S82.015M	S82.032A	S82.044P	S82.112A	S82.131A	S82.146A
S73.016A	S78.022A	S79.191A	S82.015N	S82.032B	S82.044Q	S82.112K	S82.131K	S82.146K
S73.021A	S78.029A	S79.191K	S82.015P	S82.032C	S82.044R	S82.112M	S82.131M	S82.146M
S73.022A	S78.111A	S79.191P	S82.015Q	S82.032K	S82.045A	S82.112N	S82.131N	S82.146N
S73.023A	S78.112A	S79.192A	S82.015R	S82.032M	S82.045B	S82.112P	S82.131P	S82.146P
S73.024A	S78.119A	S79.192K	S82.016A	S82.032N	S82.045C	S82.112Q	S82.131Q	S82.146Q
S73.025A	S78.121A	S79.192P	S82.016B	S82.032P	S82.045K	S82.112R	S82.131R	S82.146R
S73.026A	S78.122A	S79.199A	S82.016C	S82.032Q	S82.045M	S82.113A	S82.132A	S82.151A
S73.031A	S78.129A	S79.199K	S82.016K	S82.032R	S82.045N	S82.113K	S82.132K	S82.151K
S73.032A	S78.911A	S79.199P	S82.016M	S82.033A	S82.045P	S82.113M	S82.132M	S82.151M
S73.033A	S78.912A	S82.001A	S82.016N	S82.033B	S82.045Q	S82.113N	S82.132N	S82.151N
S73.034A	S78.919A	S82.001B	S82.016P	S82.033C	S82.045R	S82.113P	S82.132P	S82.151P
S73.035A	S78.921A	S82.001C	S82.016Q	S82.033K	S82.046A	S82.113Q	S82.132Q	S82.151Q
S73.036A	S78.922A	S82.001K	S82.016R	S82.033M	S82.046A	S82.113R	S82.132R	S82.151R

Appendix F: Complication and Comorbidity (CC) Code List

S82.152A	S82.202Q	S82.234Q	S82.253Q	S82.292Q	S82.402R	S82.436Q	S82.461P	S82.54XK
S82.152K	S82.202R	S82.234R	S82.253R	S82.292R	S82.409K	S82.436R	S82.461Q	S82.54XM
S82.152M	S82.209A	S82.235A	S82.254A	S82.299A	S82.409M	S82.441K	S82.461R	S82.54XN
S82.152N	S82.209K	S82.235K	S82.254K	S82.299K	S82.409N	S82.441M	S82.462K	S82.54XP
S82.152P	S82.209M	S82.235M	S82.254M	S82.299M	S82.409P	S82.441N	S82.462M	S82.54XQ
S82.152Q	S82.209N	S82.235N	S82.254N	S82.299N	S82.409Q	S82.441P	S82.462N	S82.54XR
S82.152R	S82.209P	S82.235P	S82.254P	S82.299P	S82.409R	S82.441Q	S82.462P	S82.55XB
S82.153A	S82.209Q	S82.235Q	S82.254Q	S82.299Q	S82.421K	S82.441R	S82.462Q	S82.55XC
S82.153K	S82.209R	S82.235R	S82.254R	S82.299R	S82.421M	S82.442K	S82.462R	S82.55XK
S82.153M	S82.221A	S82.236A	S82.255A	S82.301B	S82.421N	S82.442M	S82.463K	S82.55XM
S82.153N	S82.221K	S82.236K	S82.255K	S82.301C	S82.421P	S82.442N	S82.463N	S82.55XN
S82.153Q	S82.221M	S82.236M	S82.255M	S82.301K	S82.421Q	S82.442P	S82.463P	S82.55XP
S82.153R	S82.221N	S82.236N	S82.255N	S82.301M	S82.421R	S82.442Q	S82.463Q	S82.55XQ
S82.154A	S82.221P	S82.236P	S82.255P	S82.301N	S82.422K	S82.442R	S82.463R	S82.55XR
S82.154K	S82.221Q	S82.236Q	S82.255Q	S82.301P	S82.422M	S82.443K	S82.464K	S82.56XB
S82.154M	S82.221R	S82.236R	S82.255R	S82.301Q	S82.422N	S82.443M	S82.464M	S82.56XC
S82.154N	S82.222A	S82.241A	S82.256A	S82.301R	S82.422P	S82.443N	S82.464N	S82.56XM
S82.154P	S82.222K	S82.241K	S82.256K	S82.302B	S82.422Q	S82.443P	S82.464P	S82.56XN
S82.154Q	S82.222M	S82.241M	S82.256M	S82.302C	S82.422R	S82.443R	S82.464Q	S82.56XP
S82.154R	S82.222N	S82.241N	S82.256N	S82.302K	S82.423K	S82.444K	S82.464R	S82.56XQ
S82.155A	S82.222P	S82.241P	S82.256P	S82.302M	S82.423M	S82.444M	S82.465K	S82.56XR
S82.155K	S82.222Q	S82.241Q	S82.256Q	S82.302N	S82.423N	S82.444N	S82.465M	S82.61XB
S82.155M	S82.222R	S82.241R	S82.256R	S82.302P	S82.423P	S82.444P	S82.465N	S82.61XC
S82.155N	S82.223A	S82.242A	S82.261A	S82.302Q	S82.423Q	S82.444Q	S82.465P	S82.61XK
S82.155P	S82.223K	S82.242K	S82.261K	S82.302R	S82.423R	S82.445K	S82.465R	S82.61XM
S82.155Q	S82.223M	S82.242M	S82.261M	S82.309B	S82.424K	S82.445M	S82.466K	S82.61XN
S82.155R	S82.223N	S82.242N	S82.261N	S82.309C	S82.424M	S82.445N	S82.466M	S82.61XP
S82.156A	S82.223P	S82.242P	S82.261P	S82.309K	S82.424N	S82.445P	S82.466N	S82.61XQ
S82.156K	S82.223Q	S82.242Q	S82.261Q	S82.309M	S82.424P	S82.445Q	S82.466P	S82.61XR
S82.156M	S82.223R	S82.242R	S82.261R	S82.309N	S82.424Q	S82.445R	S82.466Q	S82.62XB
S82.156N	S82.224A	S82.243A	S82.262A	S82.309P	S82.424R	S82.446K	S82.466R	S82.62XC
S82.156P	S82.224K	S82.243K	S82.262K	S82.309Q	S82.425K	S82.446M	S82.491K	S82.62XK
S82.156Q	S82.224M	S82.243M	S82.262M	S82.309R	S82.425M	S82.446N	S82.491M	S82.62XM
S82.156R	S82.224N	S82.243N	S82.262N	S82.311A	S82.425N	S82.446P	S82.491N	S82.62XN
S82.161A	S82.224P	S82.243P	S82.262P	S82.311K	S82.425P	S82.446Q	S82.491P	S82.62XP
S82.161K	S82.224Q	S82.243Q	S82.262Q	S82.311P	S82.425Q	S82.446R	S82.491Q	S82.62XQ
S82.161P	S82.224R	S82.243R	S82.262R	S82.312A	S82.425R	S82.451K	S82.491R	S82.62XR
S82.162A	S82.225A	S82.244A	S82.263A	S82.312K	S82.426K	S82.451M	S82.492K	S82.63XB
S82.162K	S82.225K	S82.244K	S82.263K	S82.312P	S82.426M	S82.451N	S82.492M	S82.63XC
S82.162P	S82.225M	S82.244M	S82.263M	S82.319A	S82.426N	S82.451P	S82.492N	S82.63XK
S82.169A	S82.225N	S82.244N	S82.263N	S82.319K	S82.426P	S82.451Q	S82.492P	S82.63XM
S82.169K	S82.225P	S82.244P	S82.263P	S82.319P	S82.426Q	S82.451R	S82.492Q	S82.63XN
S82.169P	S82.225Q	S82.244Q	S82.263Q	S82.391B	S82.426R	S82.452K	S82.492R	S82.63XP
S82.191A	S82.225R	S82.244R	S82.263R	S82.391C	S82.431K	S82.452M	S82.499K	S82.63XQ
S82.191K	S82.226A	S82.245A	S82.264A	S82.391K	S82.431M	S82.452N	S82.499M	S82.63XR
S82.191M	S82.226K	S82.245K	S82.264K	S82.391M	S82.431N	S82.452Q	S82.499N	S82.64XB
S82.191N	S82.226M	S82.245M	S82.264M	S82.391N	S82.431P	S82.452R	S82.499P	S82.64XC
S82.191P	S82.226N	S82.245N	S82.264N	S82.391Q	S82.431Q	S82.453K	S82.499Q	S82.64XK
S82.191Q	S82.226P	S82.245P	S82.264P	S82.391R	S82.431R	S82.453M	S82.499R	S82.64XM
S82.191R	S82.226Q	S82.245Q	S82.264Q	S82.392B	S82.432K	S82.453N	S82.51XB	S82.64XN
S82.192A	S82.226R	S82.245R	S82.264R	S82.392C	S82.432M	S82.453P	S82.51XC	S82.64XP
S82.192K	S82.231A	S82.246A	S82.265A	S82.392K	S82.432N	S82.453Q	S82.51XK	S82.64XQ
S82.192M	S82.231K	S82.246K	S82.265K	S82.392M	S82.432P	S82.453R	S82.51XN	S82.64XR
S82.192N	S82.231M	S82.246M	S82.265M	S82.392N	S82.432Q	S82.454K	S82.51XP	S82.65XB
S82.192P	S82.231N	S82.246N	S82.265N	S82.392P	S82.432R	S82.454M	S82.51XQ	S82.65XC
S82.192Q	S82.231P	S82.246P	S82.265P	S82.392R	S82.433K	S82.454N	S82.51XR	S82.65XK
S82.192R	S82.231Q	S82.246Q	S82.265Q	S82.399B	S82.433M	S82.454P	S82.52XB	S82.65XM
S82.199A	S82.231R	S82.246R	S82.265R	S82.399C	S82.433N	S82.454Q	S82.52XC	S82.65XN
S82.199K	S82.232A	S82.251A	S82.266A	S82.399K	S82.433P	S82.454R	S82.52XK	S82.65XP
S82.199M	S82.232K	S82.251K	S82.266K	S82.399M	S82.433Q	S82.455K	S82.52XM	S82.65XQ
S82.199N	S82.232M	S82.251M	S82.266M	S82.399P	S82.433R	S82.455M	S82.52XN	S82.65XR
S82.199P	S82.232N	S82.251N	S82.266N	S82.399Q	S82.434K	S82.455N	S82.52XP	S82.66XB
S82.199Q	S82.232P	S82.251P	S82.266P	S82.399R	S82.434N	S82.455P	S82.52XQ	S82.66XC
S82.199R	S82.232Q	S82.251Q	S82.266Q	S82.401K	S82.434P	S82.455Q	S82.52XR	S82.66XK
S82.201A	S82.232R	S82.251R	S82.266R	S82.401M	S82.434Q	S82.455R	S82.53XB	S82.66XM
S82.201K	S82.233A	S82.252A	S82.291A	S82.401N	S82.434R	S82.456K	S82.53XC	S82.66XN
S82.201M	S82.233K	S82.252K	S82.291K	S82.401P	S82.435K	S82.456M	S82.53XK	S82.66XP
S82.201N	S82.233M	S82.252M	S82.291M	S82.401Q	S82.435M	S82.456N	S82.53XM	S82.66XQ
S82.201P	S82.233N	S82.252N	S82.291N	S82.401R	S82.435N	S82.456P	S82.53XN	S82.66XR
S82.201Q	S82.233P	S82.252P	S82.291P	S82.402K	S82.435P	S82.456Q	S82.53XP	S82.811K
S82.201R	S82.233Q	S82.252Q	S82.291Q	S82.402M	S82.435Q	S82.456R	S82.53XQ	S82.811P
S82.202A	S82.233R	S82.252R	S82.291R	S82.402N	S82.435R	S82.461K	S82.53XR	S82.812K
S82.202K	S82.234A	S82.253A	S82.292A	S82.402P	S82.436K	S82.461M	S82.54XB	S82.812P
S82.202M	S82.234K	S82.253K	S82.292K	S82.402Q	S82.436M	S82.461N	S82.54XC	S82.819K
S82.202N	S82.234M	S82.253M	S82.292M		S82.436N			S82.819P
S82.202P	S82.234N	S82.253N	S82.292N		S82.436P			S82.821K
	S82.234P	S82.253P	S82.292P					

S82.821P	S82.851Q	S82.866R	S82.90XN	S85.811A	S89.029P	S89.221P	S92.026B	S92.101P
S82.822K	S82.851R	S82.871B	S82.90XP	S85.812A	S89.031A	S89.222K	S92.026K	S92.102B
S82.822P	S82.852B	S82.871C	S82.90XQ	S85.819A	S89.031K	S89.222P	S92.026P	S92.102K
S82.829K	S82.852C	S82.871K	S82.90XR	S85.891A	S89.031P	S89.229K	S92.031B	S92.102P
S82.829P	S82.852K	S82.871M	S82.91XB	S85.892A	S89.032A	S89.229P	S92.031K	S92.109B
S82.831K	S82.852M	S82.871N	S82.91XC	S85.899A	S89.032K	S89.291K	S92.031P	S92.109K
S82.831M	S82.852N	S82.871P	S82.91XK	S85.901A	S89.032P	S89.291P	S92.032B	S92.109P
S82.831N	S82.852P	S82.871Q	S82.91XM	S85.902A	S89.039A	S89.292K	S92.032K	S92.111B
S82.831P	S82.852Q	S82.871R	S82.91XN	S85.909A	S89.039K	S89.292P	S92.032P	S92.111K
S82.831Q	S82.852R	S82.872B	S82.91XP	S85.911A	S89.039P	S89.299K	S92.033B	S92.111P
S82.831R	S82.853B	S82.872C	S82.91XQ	S85.912A	S89.041A	S89.299P	S92.033K	S92.112B
S82.832K	S82.853C	S82.872K	S82.91XR	S85.919A	S89.041K	S89.301K	S92.033P	S92.112K
S82.832M	S82.853K	S82.872M	S82.92XB	S85.991A	S89.041P	S89.301P	S92.034B	S92.112P
S82.832N	S82.853M	S82.872N	S82.92XC	S85.992A	S89.042A	S89.302K	S92.034K	S92.113B
S82.832P	S82.853N	S82.872P	S82.92XK	S85.999A	S89.042K	S89.302P	S92.034P	S92.113K
S82.832Q	S82.853P	S82.872Q	S82.92XM	S86.021A	S89.042P	S89.309K	S92.035B	S92.113P
S82.832R	S82.853Q	S82.872R	S82.92XN	S86.022A	S89.049A	S89.309P	S92.035K	S92.114B
S82.839K	S82.853R	S82.873B	S82.92XP	S86.029A	S89.049K	S89.311K	S92.035P	S92.114K
S82.839M	S82.854B	S82.873C	S82.92XQ	S86.121A	S89.049P	S89.311P	S92.036B	S92.114P
S82.839N	S82.854C	S82.873K	S82.92XR	S86.122A	S89.091A	S89.312K	S92.036K	S92.115B
S82.839P	S82.854K	S82.873M	S85.101A	S86.129A	S89.091K	S89.312P	S92.036P	S92.115K
S82.839Q	S82.854M	S82.873N	S85.102A	S86.221A	S89.091P	S89.319K	S92.041B	S92.115P
S82.839R	S82.854N	S82.873P	S85.109A	S86.222A	S89.092A	S89.319P	S92.041K	S92.116B
S82.841B	S82.854P	S82.873Q	S85.111A	S86.229A	S89.092K	S89.321K	S92.041P	S92.116K
S82.841C	S82.854Q	S82.873R	S85.112A	S86.321A	S89.092P	S89.321P	S92.042B	S92.116P
S82.841K	S82.854R	S82.874B	S85.119A	S86.322A	S89.099A	S89.322K	S92.042K	S92.121B
S82.841M	S82.855B	S82.874C	S85.121A	S86.329A	S89.099K	S89.322P	S92.042P	S92.121K
S82.841N	S82.855C	S82.874K	S85.122A	S86.821A	S89.099P	S89.329K	S92.043B	S92.121P
S82.841P	S82.855K	S82.874M	S85.129A	S86.822A	S89.101K	S89.329P	S92.043K	S92.122B
S82.841Q	S82.855M	S82.874N	S85.131A	S86.829A	S89.101P	S89.391K	S92.043P	S92.122K
S82.841R	S82.855N	S82.874P	S85.132A	S86.921A	S89.102K	S89.391P	S92.044B	S92.122P
S82.842B	S82.855P	S82.874Q	S85.139A	S86.922A	S89.102P	S89.392K	S92.044K	S92.123B
S82.842C	S82.855Q	S82.874R	S85.141A	S86.929A	S89.109K	S89.392P	S92.044P	S92.123K
S82.842K	S82.855R	S82.875B	S85.142A	S88.011A	S89.109P	S89.399K	S92.045B	S92.123P
S82.842M	S82.856B	S82.875C	S85.149A	S88.012A	S89.111K	S89.399P	S92.045K	S92.124B
S82.842N	S82.856C	S82.875K	S85.151A	S88.019A	S89.111P	S92.001B	S92.045P	S92.124K
S82.842P	S82.856K	S82.875M	S85.152A	S88.021A	S89.112K	S92.001P	S92.046B	S92.124P
S82.842Q	S82.856M	S82.875N	S85.159A	S88.022A	S89.112P	S92.002B	S92.046K	S92.125B
S82.842R	S82.856N	S82.875P	S85.161A	S88.029A	S89.119K	S92.002K	S92.046P	S92.125K
S82.843B	S82.856P	S82.875Q	S85.162A	S88.111A	S89.119P	S92.002P	S92.051B	S92.125P
S82.843C	S82.856Q	S82.875R	S85.169A	S88.112A	S89.121K	S92.009B	S92.051K	S92.126B
S82.843K	S82.856R	S82.876B	S85.171A	S88.119A	S89.121P	S92.009K	S92.051P	S92.126K
S82.843M	S82.861K	S82.876C	S85.172A	S88.121A	S89.122K	S92.009P	S92.052B	S92.126P
S82.843N	S82.861M	S82.876M	S85.179A	S88.122A	S89.122P	S92.011B	S92.052K	S92.131B
S82.843P	S82.861N	S82.876N	S85.181A	S88.129A	S89.129K	S92.011K	S92.052P	S92.131K
S82.843Q	S82.861P	S82.876P	S85.182A	S88.911A	S89.129P	S92.011P	S92.053B	S92.131P
S82.843R	S82.861Q	S82.876Q	S85.189A	S88.912A	S89.131K	S92.012B	S92.053K	S92.132B
S82.844B	S82.861R	S82.876R	S85.201A	S88.919A	S89.131P	S92.012K	S92.053P	S92.132K
S82.844C	S82.862K	S82.891B	S85.202A	S88.921A	S89.132K	S92.012P	S92.054B	S92.132P
S82.844K	S82.862M	S82.891C	S85.209A	S88.922A	S89.132P	S92.013B	S92.054K	S92.133B
S82.844M	S82.862N	S82.891K	S85.211A	S88.929A	S89.139K	S92.013K	S92.054P	S92.133K
S82.844N	S82.862P	S82.891M	S85.212A	S89.001A	S89.139P	S92.013P	S92.055B	S92.133P
S82.844P	S82.862Q	S82.891N	S85.219A	S89.001K	S89.141K	S92.014B	S92.055K	S92.134B
S82.844Q	S82.862R	S82.891P	S85.291A	S89.001P	S89.141P	S92.014K	S92.055P	S92.134K
S82.844R	S82.863K	S82.891Q	S85.292A	S89.002A	S89.142K	S92.014P	S92.056B	S92.134P
S82.845B	S82.863M	S82.891R	S85.299A	S89.002K	S89.142P	S92.015B	S92.056K	S92.135B
S82.845C	S82.863N	S82.892B	S85.301A	S89.002P	S89.149K	S92.015K	S92.056P	S92.135K
S82.845K	S82.863P	S82.892C	S85.302A	S89.009A	S89.149P	S92.015P	S92.061B	S92.135P
S82.845M	S82.863Q	S82.892K	S85.309A	S89.009K	S89.191K	S92.016B	S92.061K	S92.136B
S82.845N	S82.863R	S82.892M	S85.311A	S89.009P	S89.191P	S92.016K	S92.061P	S92.136K
S82.845P	S82.864K	S82.892N	S85.312A	S89.011A	S89.192K	S92.016P	S92.062B	S92.136P
S82.845Q	S82.864M	S82.892P	S85.319A	S89.011K	S89.192P	S92.021B	S92.062K	S92.141B
S82.845R	S82.864N	S82.892Q	S85.391A	S89.011P	S89.199K	S92.021K	S92.062P	S92.141K
S82.846B	S82.864P	S82.892R	S85.392A	S89.012A	S89.199P	S92.021P	S92.063B	S92.141P
S82.846C	S82.864Q	S82.899B	S85.399A	S89.012K	S89.201K	S92.022B	S92.063K	S92.142B
S82.846K	S82.864R	S82.899C	S85.401A	S89.012P	S89.201P	S92.022K	S92.063P	S92.142K
S82.846M	S82.865K	S82.899K	S85.402A	S89.019A	S89.202K	S92.022P	S92.064B	S92.142P
S82.846N	S82.865M	S82.899M	S85.409A	S89.019K	S89.202P	S92.023B	S92.064K	S92.143B
S82.846P	S82.865N	S82.899N	S85.411A	S89.019P	S89.209K	S92.023K	S92.064P	S92.143K
S82.846Q	S82.865P	S82.899P	S85.412A	S89.021A	S89.209P	S92.023P	S92.065B	S92.143P
S82.846R	S82.865Q	S82.899Q	S85.419A	S89.021K	S89.211K	S92.024B	S92.065K	S92.144B
S82.851B	S82.865R	S82.899R	S85.491A	S89.021P	S89.211P	S92.024K	S92.065P	S92.144K
S82.851C	S82.866K	S82.90XB	S85.492A	S89.022A	S89.212K	S92.024P	S92.066B	S92.144P
S82.851K	S82.866M	S82.90XC	S85.499A	S89.022K	S89.212P	S92.025B	S92.066K	S92.145B
S82.851M	S82.866N	S82.90XK	S85.801A	S89.022P	S89.219K	S92.025K	S92.066P	S92.145K
S82.851N	S82.866P	S82.90XM	S85.802A	S89.029A	S89.219P	S92.025P	S92.101B	S92.145P
S82.851P	S82.866Q	S82.90XM	S85.809A	S89.029K	S89.221K		S92.101K	S92.146B

S92.146K	S92.232B	S92.316P	S92.403K	S92.532P	S95.909A	T20.712A	T23.321A	T24.799A
S92.146P	S92.232K	S92.321B	S92.403P	S92.533K	S95.911A	T20.719A	T23.322A	T25.311A
S92.151B	S92.232P	S92.321K	S92.404K	S92.533P	S95.912A	T20.72XA	T23.329A	T25.312A
S92.151K	S92.233B	S92.321K	S92.404P	S92.534K	S95.919A	T20.73XA	T23.331A	T25.319A
S92.151P	S92.233K	S92.321P	S92.405K	S92.534P	S95.991A	T20.74XA	T23.332A	T25.321A
S92.152B	S92.233P	S92.322B	S92.405P	S92.535K	S95.992A	T20.75XA	T23.339A	T25.322A
S92.152K	S92.234B	S92.322K	S92.406K	S92.535P	S95.999A	T20.76XA	T23.341A	T25.329A
S92.152P	S92.234K	S92.322P	S92.406P	S92.536K	S96.021A	T20.77XA	T23.342A	T25.331A
S92.153B	S92.234P	S92.323B	S92.411K	S92.536P	S96.022A	T20.79XA	T23.349A	T25.332A
S92.153K	S92.235B	S92.323K	S92.411P	S92.591K	S96.029A	T21.30XA	T23.351A	T25.339A
S92.153P	S92.235K	S92.323P	S92.412K	S92.591P	S96.121A	T21.31XA	T23.352A	T25.391A
S92.154B	S92.235P	S92.324B	S92.412P	S92.592K	S96.122A	T21.32XA	T23.359A	T25.392A
S92.154K	S92.236B	S92.324K	S92.413K	S92.592P	S96.129A	T21.33XA	T23.361A	T25.399A
S92.154P	S92.236K	S92.324P	S92.413P	S92.599K	S96.221A	T21.34XA	T23.362A	T25.711A
S92.155B	S92.236P	S92.325B	S92.414K	S92.599P	S96.222A	T21.35XA	T23.369A	T25.712A
S92.155K	S92.241B	S92.325K	S92.414P	S92.811B	S96.229A	T21.36XA	T23.371A	T25.719A
S92.155P	S92.241K	S92.325P	S92.415K	S92.811K	S96.821A	T21.37XA	T23.372A	T25.721A
S92.156B	S92.241P	S92.326B	S92.415P	S92.811P	S96.822A	T21.39XA	T23.379A	T25.722A
S92.156K	S92.242B	S92.326K	S92.416K	S92.812B	S96.829A	T21.70XA	T23.391A	T25.729A
S92.156P	S92.242K	S92.326P	S92.416P	S92.812K	S96.921A	T21.71XA	T23.392A	T25.731A
S92.191B	S92.242P	S92.331B	S92.421K	S92.812P	S96.922A	T21.72XA	T23.399A	T25.732A
S92.191K	S92.243B	S92.331K	S92.421P	S92.819B	S96.929A	T21.73XA	T23.701A	T25.739A
S92.191P	S92.243K	S92.331P	S92.422K	S92.819K	S98.011A	T21.74XA	T23.702A	T25.791A
S92.192B	S92.243P	S92.332B	S92.422P	S92.819P	S98.012A	T21.75XA	T23.709A	T25.792A
S92.192K	S92.244B	S92.332K	S92.423K	S92.901B	S98.019A	T21.76XA	T23.711A	T25.799A
S92.192P	S92.244K	S92.332P	S92.423P	S92.901K	S98.021A	T21.77XA	T23.712A	T26.20XA
S92.199B	S92.244P	S92.333B	S92.424K	S92.901P	S98.022A	T21.79XA	T23.719A	T26.21XA
S92.199K	S92.245B	S92.333K	S92.424P	S92.902B	S98.029A	T22.30XA	T23.721A	T26.22XA
S92.199P	S92.245K	S92.333P	S92.425K	S92.902K	S98.311A	T22.311A	T23.722A	T26.70XA
S92.201B	S92.245P	S92.334B	S92.425P	S92.902P	S98.312A	T22.312A	T23.729A	T26.71XA
S92.201K	S92.246B	S92.334K	S92.426K	S92.909B	S98.319A	T22.319A	T23.731A	T26.72XA
S92.201P	S92.246K	S92.334P	S92.426P	S92.909K	S98.321A	T22.321A	T23.732A	T27.0XXA
S92.202B	S92.246P	S92.335B	S92.491K	S92.909P	S98.322A	T22.322A	T23.739A	T27.1XXA
S92.202K	S92.251B	S92.335K	S92.491P	S92.911K	S98.329A	T22.329A	T23.741A	T27.2XXA
S92.202P	S92.251K	S92.335P	S92.492K	S92.911P	S98.911A	T22.331A	T23.742A	T27.3XXA
S92.209B	S92.251P	S92.336B	S92.492P	S92.912K	S98.912A	T22.332A	T23.749A	T27.4XXA
S92.209K	S92.252B	S92.336K	S92.499K	S92.912P	S98.919A	T22.339A	T23.751A	T27.5XXA
S92.209P	S92.252K	S92.336P	S92.499P	S92.919K	S98.921A	T22.341A	T23.752A	T27.6XXA
S92.211B	S92.252P	S92.341B	S92.501K	S92.919P	S98.922A	T22.342A	T23.759A	T27.7XXA
S92.211K	S92.253B	S92.341K	S92.501P	S95.001A	S98.929A	T22.349A	T23.761A	T28.1XXA
S92.211P	S92.253K	S92.341P	S92.502K	S95.002A	T17.400A	T22.351A	T23.762A	T28.2XXA
S92.212B	S92.253P	S92.342B	S92.502P	S95.009A	T17.408A	T22.352A	T23.769A	T28.6XXA
S92.212K	S92.254B	S92.342K	S92.503K	S95.011A	T17.410A	T22.359A	T23.771A	T28.7XXA
S92.212P	S92.254K	S92.342P	S92.503P	S95.012A	T17.418A	T22.361A	T23.772A	T31.10
S92.213B	S92.254P	S92.343B	S92.504K	S95.019A	T17.420A	T22.362A	T23.779A	T31.11
S92.213K	S92.255B	S92.343K	S92.504P	S95.091A	T17.428A	T22.369A	T23.791A	T31.20
S92.213P	S92.255K	S92.343P	S92.505K	S95.092A	T17.490A	T22.391A	T23.792A	T31.30
S92.214B	S92.255P	S92.344B	S92.505P	S95.099A	T17.498A	T22.392A	T23.799A	T31.40
S92.214K	S92.256B	S92.344K	S92.506K	S95.101A	T17.500A	T22.399A	T24.301A	T31.50
S92.214P	S92.256K	S92.344P	S92.506P	S95.102A	T17.508A	T22.70XA	T24.302A	T31.60
S92.215B	S92.256P	S92.345B	S92.511K	S95.109A	T17.510A	T22.711A	T24.309A	T31.70
S92.215K	S92.301B	S92.345K	S92.511P	S95.111A	T17.518A	T22.712A	T24.311A	T31.80
S92.215P	S92.301K	S92.345P	S92.512K	S95.112A	T17.520A	T22.719A	T24.312A	T31.90
S92.216B	S92.301P	S92.346B	S92.512P	S95.119A	T17.528A	T22.721A	T24.319A	T32.10
S92.216K	S92.302B	S92.346K	S92.513K	S95.191A	T17.590A	T22.722A	T24.321A	T32.11
S92.216P	S92.302K	S92.346P	S92.513P	S95.192A	T17.598A	T22.729A	T24.322A	T32.20
S92.221B	S92.302P	S92.351B	S92.514K	S95.199A	T17.800A	T22.731A	T24.329A	T32.30
S92.221K	S92.309B	S92.351K	S92.514P	S95.201A	T17.808A	T22.732A	T24.331A	T32.40
S92.221P	S92.309K	S92.351P	S92.515K	S95.202A	T17.810A	T22.739A	T24.332A	T32.50
S92.222B	S92.309P	S92.352B	S92.515P	S95.209A	T17.818A	T22.741A	T24.339A	T32.60
S92.222K	S92.311B	S92.352K	S92.516K	S95.211A	T17.820A	T22.742A	T24.391A	T32.70
S92.222P	S92.311K	S92.352P	S92.516P	S95.212A	T17.828A	T22.749A	T24.392A	T32.80
S92.223B	S92.311P	S92.353B	S92.521K	S95.219A	T17.890A	T22.751A	T24.399A	T32.90
S92.223K	S92.312B	S92.353K	S92.521P	S95.291A	T17.898A	T22.752A	T24.701A	T33.011A
S92.223P	S92.312K	S92.353P	S92.522K	S95.292A	T20.30XA	T22.759A	T24.702A	T33.012A
S92.224B	S92.312P	S92.354B	S92.522P	S95.299A	T20.311A	T22.761A	T24.709A	T33.019A
S92.224K	S92.313B	S92.354K	S92.523K	S95.801A	T20.312A	T22.762A	T24.711A	T33.02XA
S92.224P	S92.313K	S92.354P	S92.523P	S95.802A	T20.319A	T22.769A	T24.712A	T33.09XA
S92.225B	S92.313P	S92.355B	S92.524K	S95.809A	T20.32XA	T22.791A	T24.719A	T33.1XXA
S92.225K	S92.314B	S92.355K	S92.524P	S95.811A	T20.33XA	T22.792A	T24.721A	T33.2XXA
S92.225P	S92.314K	S92.355P	S92.525K	S95.812A	T20.34XA	T22.799A	T24.722A	T33.3XXA
S92.226B	S92.314P	S92.356B	S92.525P	S95.819A	T20.35XA	T23.301A	T24.729A	T33.40XA
S92.226K	S92.315B	S92.356K	S92.526K	S95.891A	T20.36XA	T23.302A	T24.731A	T33.41XA
S92.226P	S92.315K	S92.356P	S92.526P	S95.892A	T20.37XA	T23.309A	T24.732A	T33.42XA
S92.231B	S92.315P	S92.401K	S92.531K	S95.899A	T20.39XA	T23.311A	T24.739A	T33.511A
S92.231K	S92.316B	S92.401P	S92.531P	S95.901A	T20.70XA	T23.312A	T24.791A	ICD33.512A
S92.231P	S92.316K	S92.402K	S92.532K	S95.902A	T20.711A	T23.319A	T24.792A	T33.519A

T33.521A	T71.141A	T80.310A	T81.596A	T82.530A	T83.598A	T84.190A	T85.123A	T85.860D
T33.522A	T71.143A	T80.311A	T81.597A	T82.531A	T83.61XA	T84.191A	T85.128A	T85.890A
T33.529A	T71.144A	T80.319A	T81.598A	T82.532A	T83.62XA	T84.192A	T85.190A	T85.890D
T33.531A	T71.151A	T80.39XA	T81.599A	T82.533A	T83.69XA	T84.193A	T85.191A	T86.00
T33.532A	T71.152A	T80.40XA	T81.60XA	T82.534A	T83.712A	T84.194A	T85.192A	T86.01
T33.539A	T71.153A	T80.410A	T81.61XA	T82.535A	T83.713A	T84.195A	T85.193A	T86.02
T33.60XA	T71.154A	T80.411A	T81.69XA	T82.538A	T83.714A	T84.196A	T85.199A	T86.03
T33.61XA	T71.161A	T80.419A	T81.710A	T82.539A	T83.718A	T84.197A	T85.21XA	T86.09
T33.62XA	T71.162A	T80.49XA	T81.711A	T82.590A	T83.719A	T84.199A	T85.22XA	T86.10
T33.70XA	T71.163A	T80.51XA	T81.718A	T82.591A	T83.722A	T84.210A	T85.29XA	T86.11
T33.71XA	T71.164A	T80.52XA	T81.719A	T82.592A	T83.723A	T84.213A	T85.310A	T86.12
T33.72XA	T71.191A	T80.59XA	T81.72XA	T82.593A	T83.724A	T84.216A	T85.311A	T86.13
T33.811A	T71.192A	T80.61XA	T81.83XA	T82.594A	T83.728A	T84.218A	T85.320A	T86.19
T33.812A	T71.193A	T80.62XA	T82.01XA	T82.595A	T83.729A	T84.220A	T85.321A	T86.20
T33.819A	T71.194A	T80.69XA	T82.02XA	T82.598A	T83.79XA	T84.223A	T85.390A	T86.21
T33.821A	T71.20XA	T80.810A	T82.03XA	T82.599A	T83.81XA	T84.226A	T85.391A	T86.22
T33.822A	T71.21XA	T80.818A	T82.09XA	T82.6XXA	T83.82XA	T84.228A	T85.41XA	T86.23
T33.829A	T71.221A	T80.910A	T82.110A	T82.7XXA	T83.83XA	T84.290A	T85.42XA	T86.290
T33.831A	T71.222A	T80.911A	T82.111A	T82.817A	T83.84XA	T84.293A	T85.43XA	T86.298
T33.832A	T71.223A	T80.919A	T82.118A	T82.818A	T83.85XA	T84.296A	T85.44XA	T86.30
T33.839A	T71.224A	T80.A0XA	T82.119A	T82.819A	T83.86XA	T84.298A	T85.49XA	T86.31
T33.90XA	T71.231A	T80.A10A	T82.120A	T82.827A	T83.89XA	T84.310A	T85.510A	T86.32
T33.99XA	T71.232A	T80.A11A	T82.121A	T82.828A	T83.9XXA	T84.318A	T85.511A	T86.33
T34.011A	T71.233A	T80.A19A	T82.128A	T82.837A	T84.010A	T84.320A	T85.518A	T86.39
T34.012A	T71.234A	T80.A9XA	T82.129A	T82.838A	T84.011A	T84.328A	T85.520A	T86.40
T34.019A	T71.29XA	T81.10XA	T82.190A	T82.847A	T84.012A	T84.390A	T85.521A	T86.41
T34.02XA	T71.9XXA	T81.30XA	T82.191A	T82.848A	T84.013A	T84.398A	T85.528A	T86.42
T34.09XA	T74.01XA	T81.31XA	T82.198A	T82.855A	T84.018A	T84.410A	T85.590A	T86.43
T34.1XXA	T74.02XA	T81.32XA	T82.199A	T82.856A	T84.019A	T84.418A	T85.591A	T86.49
T34.2XXA	T74.11XA	T81.33XA	T82.211A	T82.857A	T84.020A	T84.420A	T85.598A	T86.5
T34.3XXA	T74.12XA	T81.4XXA	T82.212A	T82.858A	T84.021A	T84.428A	T85.610A	T86.810
T34.40XA	T74.21XA	T81.500A	T82.213A	T82.867A	T84.022A	T84.490A	T85.611A	T86.811
T34.41XA	T74.22XA	T81.501A	T82.218A	T82.868A	T84.023A	T84.498A	T85.612A	T86.812
T34.42XA	T74.32XA	T81.502A	T82.221A	T82.897A	T84.028A	T84.50XA	T85.613A	T86.818
T34.511A	T74.4XXA	T81.503A	T82.222A	T82.898A	T84.029A	T84.51XA	T85.614A	T86.819
T34.512A	T74.91XA	T81.504A	T82.223A	T82.9XXA	T84.030A	T84.52XA	T85.615A	T86.820
T34.519A	T74.92XA	T81.505A	T82.228A	T83.010A	T84.031A	T84.53XA	T85.618A	T86.821
T34.521A	T75.1XXA	T81.506A	T82.310A	T83.020A	T84.032A	T84.54XA	T85.620A	T86.822
T34.522A	T76.01XA	T81.507A	T82.311A	T83.030A	T84.033A	T84.59XA	T85.621A	T86.828
T34.529A	T76.02XA	T81.508A	T82.312A	T83.090A	T84.038A	T84.60XA	T85.622A	T86.829
T34.531A	T76.11XA	T81.509A	T82.318A	T83.110A	T84.039A	T84.610A	T85.623A	T86.830
T34.532A	T76.12XA	T81.510A	T82.319A	T83.111A	T84.050A	T84.611A	T85.624A	T86.831
T34.539A	T76.21XA	T81.511A	T82.320A	T83.112A	T84.051A	T84.612A	T85.625A	T86.832
T34.60XA	T76.22XA	T81.512A	T82.321A	T83.113A	T84.052A	T84.613A	T85.628A	T86.838
T34.61XA	T76.32XA	T81.513A	T82.322A	T83.118A	T84.053A	T84.614A	T85.630A	T86.839
T34.62XA	T76.91XA	T81.514A	T82.328A	T83.120A	T84.058A	T84.615A	T85.631A	T86.840
T34.70XA	T76.92XA	T81.515A	T82.329A	T83.121A	T84.059A	T84.619A	T85.633A	T86.841
T34.71XA	T78.00XA	T81.516A	T82.330A	T83.122A	T84.060A	T84.620A	T85.635A	T86.842
T34.72XA	T78.01XA	T81.517A	T82.331A	T83.123A	T84.061A	T84.621A	T85.638A	T86.848
T34.811A	T78.02XA	T81.518A	T82.332A	T83.128A	T84.062A	T84.622A	T85.690A	T86.849
T34.812A	T78.03XA	T81.519A	T82.338A	T83.190A	T84.063A	T84.623A	T85.691A	T86.850
T34.819A	T78.04XA	T81.520A	T82.339A	T83.191A	T84.068A	T84.624A	T85.692A	T86.851
T34.821A	T78.05XA	T81.521A	T82.390A	T83.192A	T84.069A	T84.625A	T85.693A	T86.852
T34.822A	T78.06XA	T81.522A	T82.391A	T83.193A	T84.090A	T84.629A	T85.694A	T86.858
T34.829A	T78.07XA	T81.523A	T82.392A	T83.198A	T84.091A	T84.63XA	T85.695A	T86.859
T34.831A	T78.08XA	T81.524A	T82.398A	T83.21XA	T84.092A	T84.69XA	T85.698A	T86.890
T34.832A	T78.09XA	T81.525A	T82.399A	T83.22XA	T84.093A	T84.7XXA	T85.71XA	T86.891
T34.839A	T78.2XXA	T81.526A	T82.41XA	T83.23XA	T84.098A	T84.81XA	T85.72XA	T86.892
T34.90XA	T79.2XXA	T81.527A	T82.42XA	T83.24XA	T84.099A	T84.82XA	T85.730A	T86.898
T34.99XA	T79.7XXA	T81.528A	T82.43XA	T83.25XA	T84.110A	T84.83XA	T85.731A	T86.899
T67.0XXA	T79.A0XA	T81.529A	T82.49XA	T83.29XA	T84.111A	T84.84XA	T85.732A	T86.90
T69.021A	T79.A11A	T81.530A	T82.510A	T83.410A	T84.112A	T84.85XA	T85.733A	T86.91
T69.022A	T79.A12A	T81.531A	T82.511A	T83.411A	T84.113A	T84.86XA	T85.734A	T86.92
T69.029A	T79.A19A	T81.532A	T82.512A	T83.418A	T84.114A	T84.89XA	T85.735A	T86.93
T70.3XXA	T79.A21A	T81.533A	T82.513A	T83.420A	T84.115A	T84.9XXA	T85.738A	T86.99
T71.111A	T79.A22A	T81.534A	T82.514A	T83.421A	T84.116A	T85.01XA	T85.79XA	T87.0X1
T71.112A	T79.A29A	T81.535A	T82.515A	T83.428A	T84.117A	T85.02XA	T85.810A	T87.0X2
T71.113A	T79.A3XA	T81.536A	T82.518A	T83.490A	T84.119A	T85.03XA	T85.810D	T87.0X9
T71.114A	T79.A9XA	T81.537A	T82.519A	T83.491A	T84.120A	T85.09XA	T85.820A	T87.1X1
T71.121A	T80.1XXA	T81.538A	T82.520A	T83.498A	T84.121A	T85.110A	T85.820D	T87.1X2
T71.122A	T80.211A	T81.539A	T82.521A	T83.510A	T84.122A	T85.111A	T85.830A	T87.1X9
T71.123A	T80.212A	T81.590A	T82.522A	T83.511A	T84.123A	T85.112A	T85.830D	T87.2
T71.124A	T80.218A	T81.591A	T82.523A	T83.512A	T84.124A	T85.113A	T85.840A	T87.40
T71.131A	T80.219A	T81.592A	T82.524A	T83.518A	T84.125A	T85.118A	T85.840D	T87.41
T71.132A	T80.22XA	T81.593A	T82.525A	T83.590A	T84.126A	T85.120A	T85.850A	T87.42
T71.133A	T80.29XA	T81.594A	T82.528A	T83.591A	T84.127A	T85.121A	T85.850D	T87.43
T71.134A	T80.30XA	T81.595A	T82.529A	T83.593A	T84.129A	T85.122A	T85.860A	T87.44

Appendix F: Complication and Comorbidity (CC) Code List

T88.ØXXA	Z48.21	Z68.1	Z94.Ø	Z94.82	Z99.12
T88.1XXA	Z48.22	Z68.41	Z94.1	Z94.83	
T88.2XXA	Z48.23	Z68.42	Z94.2	Z94.84	
T88.3XXA	Z48.24	Z68.43	Z94.3	Z95.811	
T88.6XXA	Z48.28Ø	Z68.44	Z94.4	Z95.812	
Z43.1	Z48.29Ø	Z68.45	Z94.81	Z99.11	

Appendix G: Lists of Principal Diagnoses That Are Their Own CC and Their Own MCC

Note: The following lists are based on the *Federal Register,* volume 82, number 81, April 28, 2017 ("Hospital Inpatient Prospective Payment Systems for Acute Care Hospitals and the Long-Term Care Hospital Prospective Payment System and Proposed Policy Changes and Fiscal Year 2018 Rates; Proposed Rule"). The most current version, v35, of the ICD-10 MS-DRG Definitions Manual was not available at the time this book was printed. For the most current files related to IPPS please refer to the following:
https://www.cms.gov/Medicare/Medicare-Fee-for-Service-Payment/AcuteInpatientPPS/IPPS-Regulations-and-Notices.html.

Principal Diagnoses That Are Their Own CC

B25.1	I70.368	I70.562	I70.749	K51.513	M02.331	M05.459	M90.559
B52.0	I70.369	I70.563	I70.761	K51.514	M02.332	M05.461	M90.561
D57.211	I70.431	I70.568	I70.762	K51.812	M02.339	M05.462	M90.562
D57.411	I70.432	I70.569	I70.763	K51.813	M02.341	M05.469	M90.569
E08.52	I70.433	I70.631	I70.768	K51.814	M02.342	M05.471	M90.571
E09.52	I70.434	I70.632	I70.769	K51.912	M02.349	M05.472	M90.572
E10.52	I70.438	I70.633	I73.01	K51.913	M02.351	M05.479	M90.579
E11.52	I70.439	I70.634	K50.012	K51.914	M02.352	M05.49	M90.58
E13.52	I70.441	I70.638	K50.013	K57.00	M02.359	M32.11	M90.59
I25.110	I70.442	I70.639	K50.014	K57.01	M02.361	M32.12	N11.1
I25.700	I70.443	I70.641	K50.112	K57.20	M02.362	M33.02	N13.0
I25.710	I70.444	I70.642	K50.113	K57.21	M02.369	M33.12	N13.1
I25.720	I70.448	I70.643	K50.114	K57.40	M02.371	M33.22	N13.2
I25.730	I70.449	I70.644	K50.812	K57.41	M02.372	M33.92	O12.21
I25.750	I70.461	I70.648	K50.813	K57.52	M02.379	M34.81	O12.22
I25.760	I70.462	I70.649	K50.814	K57.80	M02.38	M34.82	O12.23
I25.790	I70.463	I70.661	K50.912	K57.81	M02.39	M35.03	T86.30
I70.331	I70.468	I70.662	K50.913	K80.30	M05.40	M90.50	T86.31
I70.332	I70.469	I70.663	K50.914	K80.31	M05.411	M90.511	T86.32
I70.333	I70.531	I70.668	K51.012	K80.32	M05.412	M90.512	T86.33
I70.334	I70.532	I70.669	K51.013	K80.33	M05.419	M90.519	T86.39
I70.338	I70.533	I70.731	K51.014	K80.34	M05.421	M90.521	Z48.21
I70.339	I70.534	I70.732	K51.212	K80.35	M05.422	M90.522	Z48.22
I70.341	I70.538	I70.733	K51.213	K80.36	M05.429	M90.529	Z48.23
I70.342	I70.539	I70.734	K51.214	K80.37	M05.431	M90.531	Z48.24
I70.343	I70.541	I70.738	K51.312	M02.30	M05.432	M90.532	Z48.280
I70.344	I70.542	I70.739	K51.313	M02.311	M05.439	M90.539	Z48.290
I70.348	I70.543	I70.741	K51.314	M02.312	M05.441	M90.541	Z94.3
I70.349	I70.544	I70.742	K51.412	M02.319	M05.442	M90.542	
I70.361	I70.548	I70.743	K51.413	M02.321	M05.449	M90.549	
I70.362	I70.549	I70.744	K51.414	M02.322	M05.451	M90.551	
I70.363	I70.561	I70.748	K51.512	M02.329	M05.452	M90.552	

Principal Diagnoses That Are Their Own MCC

A22.7	B44.0	L89.004	L89.133	L89.224	L89.513	L89.814	S06.1X5A
A26.7	B45.1	L89.013	L89.134	L89.303	L89.514	L89.893	S06.1X6A
A32.7	B77.81	L89.014	L89.143	L89.304	L89.523	L89.894	S06.1X7A
A37.01	I26.01	L89.023	L89.144	L89.313	L89.524	L89.93	S06.1X8A
A37.11	I26.02	L89.024	L89.153	L89.314	L89.603	L89.94	S06.1X9A
A37.81	I26.09	L89.103	L89.154	L89.323	L89.604	R65.21	
A37.91	K70.41	L89.104	L89.203	L89.324	L89.613	S06.1X0A	
A54.86	K71.11	L89.113	L89.204	L89.43	L89.614	S06.1X1A	
B25.0	K72.01	L89.114	L89.213	L89.44	L89.623	S06.1X2A	
B25.2	K72.11	L89.123	L89.214	L89.503	L89.624	S06.1X3A	
B37.7	L89.003	L89.124	L89.223	L89.504	L89.813	S06.1X4A	

Appendix H: Present on Admission (POA) Tutorial

Present-on-admission (POA) indicators are required on all diagnoses and external cause-of-injury codes for all inpatient acute care hospital discharges, according to the requirement outlined in the Deficit Reduction Act of 2005, section 5001(c). The only exception is for a select group of codes that have been designated as exempt from the POA regulations. Certain facilities are also exempt from this reporting requirement and include the following:

- Critical access hospitals
- Long-term care hospitals
- Cancer hospitals
- Inpatient psychiatric hospitals
- Inpatient rehabilitation facilities
- Veterans Administration/Department of Defense Hospitals
- Children's inpatient facilities

The POA indicator guidelines are not intended to replace the official *ICD-10-CM Official Guidelines for Coding and Reporting*. Nor will the POA guidelines supersede the Uniform Hospital Discharge Data Set (UHDDS) definition of principal diagnosis, defined as the condition established after study to be chiefly responsible for occasioning the admission of the patient to the hospital. The definition of "additional diagnoses" also remains the same. Coders must report all conditions that coexist at the time of admission, develop subsequently, or that affect the treatment received and/or the length of stay. This significantly affects assignment of the POA indicators. Because the POA indicator should accurately reflect the patient's conditions upon admission, review of POA guidelines as well as the *ICD-10-CM Official Guidelines for Coding and Reporting* is required.

The following is a summary of the POA guidelines:

- A POA condition is defined not only as one that is clearly present at the time of admission, but also one that was clearly present but not diagnosed until after the time of admission.

- Present on admission is defined as present at the time the order for an inpatient admission is made, whether or not the patient's episode of care originated in the emergency department, ambulatory surgery area, or other outpatient area. Conditions that develop during an outpatient encounter are considered present on admission.

- A POA indicator is assigned to the principal diagnosis, secondary diagnoses, and the external cause-of-injury codes.

- The POA guidelines are not intended to replace any of the other *ICD-10-CM Official Guidelines for Coding and Reporting*.

- The intent of the POA guidelines is not to determine whether or not a condition should be coded, but rather how to apply the POA indicator.

The following reporting options, with definitions, should be used to indicate whether a condition was POA:

Y   *Yes: Present at the time of inpatient admission*

N   *No: Not present at the time of inpatient admission*

U   *Unknown: Documentation is insufficient to determine if condition is present at the time of inpatient admission*

W   *Clinically undetermined: Provider is unable to clinically determine whether condition was or was not present at the time of inpatient admission*

Unreported/not used—(exempt from POA reporting)—Most ICD-10-CM codes require the assignment of a POA indicator. However, there are some diagnoses that are considered exempt from the POA reporting. For these exempt conditions the POA field should be left blank.

Note: A data file of all POA exempt codes can be accessed at the following: http://www.optum360coding.com/ProdcutUpdates/ Title: "2018 ICD-10-CM for Hospitals POA Exemption Data File" Password: OptumPOAExempt18

Timeframe for POA identification and documentation

There is no timeframe during the encounter in which a condition must be diagnosed to be considered present on admission. In many cases, it is not clinically possible for the provider to determine a definitive diagnosis until well into the admission, after labs, imaging, and other tests have been performed and results examined. In these cases the condition is still considered to be present on admission, indicated with Y.

Examples

- A patient was admitted for diagnostic work-up for cachexia. The final diagnosis was malignant neoplasm of lung with metastasis.

  Assign Y in the POA field for the malignant neoplasm, which was clearly present on admission, although it was not diagnosed until after the admission occurred.

- A patient with severe cough and difficulty breathing was diagnosed during his hospitalization to have lung cancer.

  Assign Y in the POA field for the lung cancer. Even though the cancer was not diagnosed until after admission, it is a chronic condition that was clearly present before the patient's admission.

- A urine culture was obtained on admission. The provider documented urinary tract infection when the culture results became available a few days later.

  Assign Y to the urinary tract infection since the diagnosis is based on test results from a specimen obtained on admission. It may not be possible for a provider to make a definitive diagnosis for a period of time after admission. There is no required timeframe as to when a provider must identify or document a condition for it to be considered present on admission.

Condition is on the "Exempt from Reporting" list

Several codes are exempt from POA reporting. A detailed list of codes can be found as an official download at http://www.cms.gov/Medicare/Coding/ICD10/Downloads/2017-POA-Exempt-List.zip. The POA field is left blank for codes excluded from POA reporting.

Examples

- A patient was admitted for inpatient surgery on a burn contracture from scar tissue from a burn five years ago.

  Assign Y for the principal condition of the scar; however, the secondary code for the specifics of the burn injury with a seventh character for sequela is left blank since it is excluded from POA reporting.

- A patient was admitted to inpatient for a PEG tube insertion because of residual dysphagia due to a recent CVA.

  No POA indicator is assigned for the dysphagia following a CVA. Codes under I69.- are defined as sequela of cerebrovascular disease and are exempt from POA reporting.

- A patient was admitted to inpatient for corrective surgery for a malunion of a closed femur fracture.

  No POA indicator is assigned for the malunion of a closed fracture because the seventh character for malunion of fractures is considered a subsequent encounter and is exempt from POA reporting.

- A patient was admitted for breast reconstruction following mastectomy.

  The POA indicator field is left blank as this Z code is exempt from POA reporting.

- A patient was admitted for changing the battery in his AICD as it is at the end of its useful life.

  The POA indicator field is left blank as this Z code is exempt from POA reporting.

POA explicitly documented

If the provider explicitly documents a condition as being present on admission or not present on admission, assign the appropriate Y or N POA indicator based on that documentation. If there is conflicting documentation by different providers, query the attending physician.

Examples

- Even though sepsis is not diagnosed in the ED, the discharge summary states that the patient presented with sepsis at the time of admission.

  The provider explicitly stated that the sepsis was present on admission and therefore the Y POA indicator should be used.

- The patient was admitted with chills and cough and two days later diagnosed with pneumonia. The discharge summary documents that the pneumonia was not present on admission.

  Although the patient showed some symptoms of pneumonia on admission, the provider may have clinical evidence (e.g., chest x-rays, cultures) that indicates that pneumonia did not develop until after admission. Since this was explicitly stated in the discharge summary, the appropriate POA indicator is N.

- A consult note states that a patient came in with renal failure while the discharge summary states that the renal failure was not present on admission.

When in doubt and there is conflicting documentation, query the attending physician.

Conditions diagnosed prior to inpatient admission

Conditions that were diagnosed prior to admission—for example, chronic conditions such as hypertension, diabetes, and asthma—are assigned the POA indicator of Y. A tip to help establish that a condition was POA is to check the patient's medication history for drugs that are routinely prescribed for these types of chronic conditions.

Examples

- The history and physical states that the patient has a history of hypertension and seizure disorder, and it is noted that the patient is currently on Atenolol and Dilantin.

  The hypertension and seizure disorder existed prior to admission; therefore, the appropriate POA indicator is Y. Verification that the patient is on long-term use of Atenolol and Dilantin can help solidify that these conditions are currently being treated.

- A 56-year-old male was admitted as an inpatient for multi-trauma wounds. Because the patient was unconscious on admission, his medical history was unknown. A progress note two days into the stay noted that the patient was on Metformin for history of type 2 diabetes.

  The timeframe of the diagnosis is irrelevant to POA. Even though it was not discovered until two days into the encounter that the patient had a history of DM2, the DM2 was still present prior to this admission and would be identified as such with the Y POA indicator.

- A patient was admitted to an inpatient facility from the ED. The admitting provider indicated that the patient had a current history of lung cancer and chronic kidney disease.

  Both of these conditions are indicated with Y, present on admission.

- During the course of an eight-day inpatient stay with surgery, a patient was diagnosed postoperatively with hypertension and discharged on Metoprolol.

  The hypertension was not diagnosed prior to admission and would be reported with an N POA indicator.

Conditions diagnosed during the admission but clearly present before admission

The POA indicator Y is assigned for conditions that clearly presented with applicable signs and symptoms but may have not been definitively diagnosed until later on, or even at the end of the encounter. Even if the presenting diagnosis was documented on admission as suspected, possible, or rule out, or written as a differential diagnosis and later confirmed, it is still considered present on admission.

Examples

- A patient was admitted with jaundice, fatigue, and mental confusion. Differential diagnosis on admission lists possible liver failure. The definitive diagnosis of liver failure is not made until two days after admission.

  Assign Y to the liver failure since the symptoms were present on admission and the differential diagnosis listed "possible" liver failure on admission even though the final diagnosis was two days later.

- An aid worker recently returned from Afghanistan presents to the ED with hematemesis, chest pain, and fever. Patient is put into inpatient isolation with suspected TB documented on the H & P. TB is confirmed the next day.

  The POA indicator Y is assigned because, even though the TB was only "suspected" on admission, it was confirmed the next day.

Condition develops during outpatient encounter prior to inpatient admission

Assign Y for any condition that develops during an outpatient encounter such as same-day surgery, observation, or extended recovery prior to a written order for inpatient admission. This also pertains to conditions that develop in facilities such as transitional care units, skilled nursing homes, long-term care, hospice, or rehabilitation facilities with the patient transferring to inpatient hospital admission.

Examples

- A patient underwent outpatient surgery. During the recovery period, the patient developed atrial fibrillation and was subsequently admitted to the hospital as an inpatient.

Assign Y on the POA field for the atrial fibrillation since it developed prior to a written order for inpatient admission.

- A patient was treated in observation and while in observation fell out of bed and broke a hip. The patient was subsequently admitted as an inpatient to treat the hip fracture.

  Assign Y on the POA field for the hip fracture since it developed prior to a written order for inpatient admission.

- An elderly patient underwent outpatient surgery with plans to go home after the surgery. In recovery, the patient developed shortness of breath, chest pain, and fever. A sputum sample was taken, and the surgeon decided to admit the patient to inpatient. The next day the patient was diagnosed with staphylococcal pneumonia based on sputum results and admitting chest x-ray.

  Assign Y to the staphylococcal pneumonia even though it was not diagnosed until the day following the admission. Even though the patient had undergone outpatient surgery, the sputum sample, signs, and symptoms were evident prior to the inpatient admission.

Documentation does not indicate whether condition was present on admission

If the documentation in the medical record is unclear as to the presence of a condition on admission, assign a U for unknown. This should be used sparingly and, if possible, the physician should be queried for further clarification.

Example

- A wheelchair-bound patient was admitted in respiratory failure from a long-term care facility to an inpatient hospital with severe aspiration pneumonia. A progress note three days into the admission listed a pressure ulcer stage 2 on the lower back.

  Assign U for the stage 2 pressure ulcer if unknown whether it was present on admission. Since the patient was wheelchair-bound and critically ill on admission, it is possible that the ulcer was present and not immediately addressed. The admitting physician can be queried to clarify, or a U is assigned if that is not possible.

Documentation states it cannot be determined whether the condition was or was not present on admission

A W is assigned when the documentation states that it cannot be clinically determined whether the condition was POA or not.

Examples

- An elderly patient was admitted with multi-trauma injuries from a motor vehicle accident. Two days into the admission, a urinary tract infection was diagnosed. No labs or urine cultures had been taken on admission as focus was stabilization from traumatic wounds. Documentation from the provider in a progress note stated that it was not clinically possible to determine whether the UTI was present on admission.

  Assign W for the UTI as it was specifically stated that it was not clinically possible to determine whether it was present on admission.

- A patient was admitted with high fever and pneumonia. The patient rapidly deteriorated and became septic. The discharge diagnosis listed sepsis and pneumonia. The documentation was unclear as to whether the sepsis was present on admission or developed shortly after admission.

  Query the physician as to whether the sepsis was present on admission, developed shortly after admission, or it cannot be clinically determined as to whether it was or was not present on admission.

Chronic condition with acute exacerbation during the admission

If a single code identifies only the chronic condition and not the acute exacerbation, assign Y. For instance, when there is no code for the acute exacerbation of a chronic condition as in acute exacerbation of chronic leukemia, the Y is assigned for the chronic leukemia.

For a single combination code that identifies both the chronic and acute exacerbation, see the combination code instructions.

Example

- Documentation on admission stated that the patient had chronic myelomonocytic leukemia. A progress note three days into the stay stated that the patient had, since admission, developed an acute exacerbation of his myelomonocytic leukemia.

  There is no code for an acute exacerbation of chronic myelomonocytic leukemia; therefore, assign Y since the chronic leukemia (either not specified as in remission, or in relapse) is represented by a single code and was present on admission.

Acute and chronic conditions

Assign Y to acute conditions present on admission and N to acute conditions not present at the time of admission.

Assign Y to conditions specified as chronic, even though they may not be diagnosed until after admission.

See the POA guideline "Codes that contain multiple clinical concepts" for a single code that identifies both the acute and chronic condition.

Examples

- A patient was admitted to the hospital for coronary artery bypass surgery. Postoperatively he developed a pulmonary embolism.

  Assign N in the POA field for the pulmonary embolism. This is an acute condition that was not present on admission.
- A patient admitted with sepsis due to pneumonia with acute respiratory failure, developed acute renal failure on day three.

  Assign Y for the sepsis, pneumonia, and acute respiratory failure, which were all acute conditions, present on admission. Assign N for the acute renal failure; even though it is an acute condition, it was not present until after the patient was admitted.
- A patient admitted with hypoglycemia, weakness, confusion, and slurred speech was diagnosed the next day with type 2 diabetes.

  Assign Y to the type 2 diabetes since it is a chronic condition that was present on admission, even though it was not diagnosed until the next day.

Codes that contain multiple clinical concepts

If at least one of the clinical concepts included in a code was not present on admission, assign N. If all the clinical concepts included in a code are present on admission, assign Y.

Examples

- Patient has history of gastrojejunal ulcer which started bleeding two days into the encounter.

  Assign a POA indicator of N to chronic gastrojejunal ulcer with bleeding; although the gastrojejunal ulcer is a chronic condition that was present at the time of admission, the bleeding did not occur until after the admission.
- A patient with chronic diastolic heart failure decompensated after admission.

  Assign N to the code for acute on chronic diastolic (congestive) heart failure. Although the heart failure was present on admission, the acute decompensation of the failure was not.
- A patient with viral hepatitis B progressed to hepatic coma after admission.

  Assign N for the viral hepatitis B with hepatic coma because a condition described by part of the code description did not develop until after admission.
- A patient with known systolic congestive heart failure was admitted to the hospital with decompensated systolic heart failure.

  Assign Y in the POA field for the acute on chronic systolic (congestive) heart failure as both the chronic and acute parts of the condition were present on admission.

Assign Y for infection codes that include the organism if the infection was present on admission even though the culture results are not available until after admission.

Example

- A patient was septic on admission with blood, sputum, and urine cultures taken. Two days later, *E. coli* was determined to be the causal organism.

  Assign Y even though the test results were not confirmed until after admission.

Conditions documented as possible, probable, suspected, or rule out at the time of discharge or conditions documented as impending or threatened at the time of discharge

If the final diagnosis contains language identifying a condition as possible, probable, suspected, or rule out, or as an impending or threatened diagnosis but the diagnosis is based on signs and symptoms that were present on admission, the POA indicator is Y. If those signs and symptoms were not present on admission, the appropriate POA indicator is N.

Examples

- A patient underwent inpatient surgery, after which the patient developed fever and was treated aggressively. The physician's final diagnosis documented "possible postoperative infection following surgery."

  Assign N on the POA field for the postoperative infection since final diagnoses that contain the terms "possible," "probable," "suspected," or "rule out" and that are based on symptoms or clinical findings that were not present on admission should be reported as N.
- A patient with prior cardiac intervention history was admitted with chest pain. After two days, the chest pain diminished with no underlying cause found. The discharge summary stated, "Suspected costochondritis or coronary artery spasm. Pain resolved. Follow up at regular cardiology office visit."

  Since the chest pain was present on admission, both suspected conditions of costochondritis and coronary artery spasm are represented by the POA indicator of Y.
- A patient was admitted with a known history of coronary atherosclerosis, status post myocardial infarction five years ago, and was then admitted for treatment of impending myocardial infarction. The patient was transferred to a larger facility with a cath lab. The final diagnosis was documented as "impending myocardial infarction."

  Assign Y to the impending myocardial infarction because the condition is present on admission.

Same diagnosis code for two or more conditions

When two or more separate conditions are classified to the same diagnosis code in the same encounter, assign Y if all conditions represented by the single code were present on admission and N if any of the conditions were not present on admission.

Examples

- A patient was admitted with diabetes type 2 with ketoacidosis.

  Assign Y since both the diabetes and ketoacidosis were present on admission.
- A patient involved in a car accident was admitted with hemorrhage to the abdomen secondary to the trauma; shortly after being admitted the patient also developed a seroma as a result of the trauma.

  The secondary traumatic hemorrhage was present on admission, and the traumatic seroma did not develop until after admission. Both of these conditions are classified to one code, but because both conditions were not present when the patient was admitted, a POA of N should be assigned.

Obstetrical conditions

The POA assignment for obstetrical conditions is not affected by whether the patient delivers during the encounter but rather by whether the pregnancy complication was or was not present at the time of admission. If two or more conditions are classified to a single code, all conditions represented by that single code must be present on admission to correctly assign a Y. If all conditions are not present at the time of admission, the appropriate POA indicator is N. Several obstetrics codes are listed in the POA exclusion list; for obstetrics codes that are not on the exclusion list, all applicable POA guidelines apply.

Examples

- A female patient was admitted to the hospital and underwent a normal delivery.

  Leave the "present on admission" (POA) field blank. Code O80 Normal delivery, is on the "exempt from reporting" list.
- A patient was admitted in late pregnancy due to excessive vomiting and dehydration. During admission, the patient went into premature labor.

  Assign Y for the excessive vomiting and the dehydration. Assign N for the premature labor.

- A patient was admitted in active labor. During the stay, a breast abscess was noted when the mother attempted to breastfeed. The provider was unable to clinically determine whether the abscess was present on admission.

  Assign W for the breast abscess since the provider was unable to clinically determine whether the abscess was present on admission.

- A patient was admitted in active labor. After 12 hours of labor, it was noted that the infant was in fetal distress, and a cesarean section was performed.

  Assign N for the fetal distress even if it is used for the principal diagnosis, since it did not develop until later in the admission. In obstetrics cases, the principal diagnosis may have a POA indicator of N.

Perinatal and congenital conditions

Newborns are not considered admitted until after birth; therefore all conditions that develop in utero, occur during delivery, or are present at birth are represented by the POA indicator Y. Any conditions that develop after birth and admission are represented by N.

All congenital conditions and anomalies not found in chapter 17 should have a POA indicator of Y assigned. Chapter 17 codes in categories Q00–Q99 are exempt from POA reporting. All congenital conditions, regardless of the coding chapter to which they are assigned, are considered present on admission.

Examples

- A single liveborn infant was delivered in the hospital via cesarean section. The physician documented fetal bradycardia during labor as the final diagnosis in the newborn record.

  Assign Y because the bradycardia developed prior to the newborn admission (birth).

- A newborn developed diarrhea, which was believed to be due to the hospital baby formula.

  Assign N because the diarrhea developed after admission.

- A newborn was diagnosed with cephalhematoma due to birth injury.

  Assign Y because the injury occurred during delivery.

- A newborn was diagnosed with congenital pneumonia.

  Assign Y for the congenital pneumonia. Congenital conditions from chapter 16 are always considered present on admission and require the POA indicator.

- A newborn was diagnosed with congenital hydrocephalus.

  There should be no POA indicator assigned. This condition is coded in chapter 17 and is excluded from POA reporting.

- A 10-year-old boy was admitted for complications of spina bifida with hydrocephalus.

  No POA indicator is assigned. This condition is coded in chapter 17 and is excluded from POA reporting.

External cause and injury codes

If an injury or poisoning occurred prior to or at the time of admission and the seventh character indicates an initial encounter or active treatment, the code for the injury/poisoning is reported with POA indicator Y. Injury and poisoning codes S00–T88 with the seventh character indicating subsequent or sequela are exempt from POA indicators since, in order to be a subsequent or sequela encounter, the condition must have occurred before the admission. Many of the external causes of morbidity codes from chapters V, W, and X are also exempt from POA reporting when the seventh character of S or D, representing subsequent or sequela encounters, are used.

Coders should be extremely careful in assigning the appropriate POA indicator if a patient suffers an injury while an inpatient. For example, if a patient falls from the hospital bed and fractures a hip, the codes representing that injury (along with the appropriate initial-encounter seventh character) should be assigned N for the corresponding POA indicator.

Examples

- A 12-year-old was admitted for treatment of fractured arm from falling out of a tree house.

  The injury itself and the cause of the injury are both assigned a Y POA indicator. **Note:** *The injury code and external cause code POA indicators should always match.*

- A patient admitted for pneumonia sustained a laceration of the right arm after falling and hitting his arm against a cart in the hospital room, requiring stitches.

  Assign N for the laceration for the right arm because it was not present on admission. The external cause code POA indicator should also be N.

- A patient was admitted for manipulation of a knee contracture due to a scar from a burn injury 10 years ago.

  Assign Y for the code for the scar, but leave blank the POA indicator for the burn injury with the seventh character of S for sequela. Sequela and subsequent-encounter codes in chapter 19 are exempt from POA reporting.

Appendix I: Hospital Acquired Conditions

Hospital-acquired conditions (HACs) are conditions considered reasonably preventable through the application of evidence-based guidelines. These conditions, in and of themselves, are either a complication or comorbidity (CC) or major complication or comorbidity (MCC) that as a secondary diagnosis will move the MS-DRG assignment from a lower-paying MS-DRG to a higher-paying MS-DRG. However, if these conditions are not present on admission (meaning they developed during the hospital stay), the CC or MCC designation is nullified and the case will not group to the higher-paying MS-DRG based solely upon the reporting of the HAC code.

HACs are grouped into 14 categories. ICD-10-CM codes in the tabular section of this book that are grouped to one of these HAC categories are identified by an icon specific to that category. As many of these HACs are conditional, this resource provides any additional stipulations that may be required before the code can be considered a HAC. For example, code I26.02 has an **H10** indicating it falls in the HAC 10 category for Deep Vein Thrombosis (DVT) or Pulmonary Embolism (PE) with Total Knee or Hip Replacement. However I26.02 is not, by itself, a HAC there must also be a specific ICD-10-PCS code, such as ØSR9Ø19 Replacement of Right Hip Joint with Metal Synthetic Substitute, Cemented, Open Approach, applied in order for I26.02 to act as a HAC.

Note: The resource used to compile this list is the fiscal 2017 ICD-10 MS-DRG Definitions Manual Files v34. The most current version, v35, of ICD-10 MS-DRG Definitions Manual was not available at the time this book was printed. For the most current files related to IPPS please refer to the following: https://www.cms.gov/Medicare/Medicare-Fee-for-Service-Payment/AcuteInpatientPPS/IPPS-Regulations-and-Notices.html.

HAC 01: Foreign Object Retained After Surgery
Secondary diagnosis not POA:

- T81.500A
- T81.501A
- T81.502A
- T81.503A
- T81.504A
- T81.505A
- T81.506A
- T81.507A
- T81.508A
- T81.509A
- T81.510A
- T81.511A
- T81.512A
- T81.513A
- T81.514A
- T81.515A
- T81.516A
- T81.517A
- T81.518A
- T81.519A
- T81.520A
- T81.521A
- T81.522A
- T81.523A
- T81.524A
- T81.525A
- T81.526A
- T81.527A
- T81.528A
- T81.529A
- T81.530A
- T81.531A
- T81.532A
- T81.533A
- T81.534A
- T81.535A
- T81.536A
- T81.537A
- T81.538A
- T81.539A
- T81.590A
- T81.591A
- T81.592A
- T81.593A
- T81.594A
- T81.595A
- T81.596A
- T81.597A
- T81.598A
- T81.599A
- T81.60XA
- T81.61XA
- T81.69XA

HAC 02: Air Embolism
Secondary diagnosis not POA:

- T80.0XXA

HAC 03: Blood Incompatibility
Secondary diagnosis not POA:

- T80.30XA
- T80.310A
- T80.311A
- T80.319A
- T80.39XA

HAC 04: Stage III and IV Pressure Ulcers
Secondary diagnosis not POA:

- L89.003
- L89.004
- L89.013
- L89.014
- L89.023
- L89.024
- L89.103
- L89.104
- L89.113
- L89.114
- L89.123
- L89.124
- L89.133
- L89.134
- L89.143
- L89.144
- L89.153
- L89.154
- L89.203
- L89.204
- L89.213
- L89.214
- L89.223
- L89.224
- L89.303
- L89.304
- L89.313
- L89.314
- L89.323
- L89.324
- L89.43
- L89.44
- L89.503
- L89.504
- L89.513
- L89.514
- L89.523
- L89.524
- L89.603
- L89.604
- L89.613
- L89.614
- L89.623
- L89.624
- L89.813
- L89.814
- L89.893
- L89.894
- L89.93
- L89.94

HAC 05: Falls and Trauma
Secondary diagnosis not POA:

- M99.10
- M99.11
- M99.18
- S02.0XXA
- S02.0XXB
- S02.101A
- S02.101B
- S02.102A
- S02.102B
- S02.109A
- S02.109B
- S02.110A
- S02.110B
- S02.111A
- S02.111B
- S02.112A
- S02.112B
- S02.113A
- S02.113B
- S02.118A
- S02.118B
- S02.119A
- S02.119B
- S02.11AA
- S02.11AB
- S02.11BA
- S02.11BB
- S02.11CA
- S02.11CB
- S02.11DA
- S02.11DB
- S02.11EA
- S02.11EB
- S02.11FA
- S02.11FB
- S02.11GA
- S02.11GB
- S02.11HA
- S02.11HB
- S02.19XA
- S02.19XB
- S02.2XXB
- S02.30XA
- S02.30XB
- S02.31XA
- S02.31XB
- S02.32XA
- S02.32XB
- S02.400A
- S02.400B
- S02.401A
- S02.401B
- S02.402A
- S02.402B
- S02.40AA
- S02.40AB
- S02.40BA
- S02.40BB
- S02.40CA
- S02.40CB
- S02.40DA
- S02.40DB
- S02.40EA
- S02.40EB
- S02.40FA
- S02.40FB
- S02.411A
- S02.411B
- S02.412A
- S02.412B
- S02.413A
- S02.413B
- S02.42XA
- S02.42XB
- S02.600A
- S02.600B
- S02.601A
- S02.601B
- S02.602A
- S02.602B
- S02.609A
- S02.609B
- S02.610A
- S02.610B
- S02.611A
- S02.611B
- S02.612A
- S02.612B
- S02.620A
- S02.620B
- S02.621A
- S02.621B
- S02.622A
- S02.622B
- S02.630A
- S02.630B
- S02.631A
- S02.631B
- S02.632A
- S02.632B
- S02.640A
- S02.640B
- S02.641A
- S02.641B
- S02.642A
- S02.642B
- S02.650A
- S02.650B
- S02.651A
- S02.651B
- S02.652A
- S02.652B
- S02.66XA
- S02.66XB
- S02.670A
- S02.670B
- S02.671A
- S02.671B
- S02.672A
- S02.672B
- S02.69XA
- S02.69XB
- S02.80XA
- S02.80XB
- S02.81XA
- S02.81XB
- S02.82XA
- S02.82XB
- S02.91XA
- S02.91XB
- S02.92XA
- S02.92XB
- S06.0X1A
- S06.0X9A
- S06.1X1A
- S06.1X2A
- S06.1X3A
- S06.1X4A
- S06.1X5A
- S06.1X6A
- S06.1X7A
- S06.1X8A
- S06.1X9A
- S06.2X1A
- S06.2X2A
- S06.2X3A
- S06.2X4A
- S06.2X5A
- S06.2X6A
- S06.2X7A
- S06.2X8A
- S06.2X9A
- S06.301A
- S06.302A
- S06.303A
- S06.304A
- S06.305A
- S06.306A
- S06.307A
- S06.308A
- S06.309A
- S06.310A
- S06.311A
- S06.312A
- S06.313A
- S06.314A
- S06.315A
- S06.316A
- S06.317A
- S06.318A
- S06.319A
- S06.320A
- S06.321A
- S06.322A
- S06.323A
- S06.324A
- S06.325A
- S06.326A
- S06.327A
- S06.328A
- S06.329A
- S06.330A
- S06.331A
- S06.332A
- S06.333A
- S06.334A
- S06.335A
- S06.336A
- S06.337A
- S06.338A
- S06.339A
- S06.340A
- S06.341A
- S06.342A
- S06.343A
- S06.344A
- S06.345A
- S06.346A
- S06.347A
- S06.348A
- S06.349A
- S06.350A
- S06.351A
- S06.352A
- S06.353A
- S06.354A
- S06.355A
- S06.356A
- S06.357A
- S06.358A
- S06.359A
- S06.360A
- S06.361A

Appendix I: Hospital Acquired Conditions

HAC 05: Falls and Trauma (continued)					
S06.362A	S06.829A	S12.231A	S12.650B	S22.009A	S22.082B
S06.363A	S06.891A	S12.231B	S12.651A	S22.009B	S22.088A
S06.364A	S06.892A	S12.24XA	S12.651B	S22.010A	S22.088B
S06.365A	S06.893A	S12.24XB	S12.690A	S22.010B	S22.089A
S06.366A	S06.894A	S12.250A	S12.690B	S22.011A	S22.089B
S06.367A	S06.895A	S12.250B	S12.691A	S22.011B	S22.20XA
S06.368A	S06.896A	S12.251A	S12.691B	S22.012A	S22.20XB
S06.369A	S06.897A	S12.251B	S12.8XXA	S22.012B	S22.21XA
S06.370A	S06.898A	S12.290A	S12.9XXA	S22.018A	S22.21XB
S06.371A	S06.899A	S12.290B	S13.0XXA	S22.018B	S22.22XA
S06.372A	S06.9X1A	S12.291A	S13.100A	S22.019A	S22.22XB
S06.373A	S06.9X2A	S12.291B	S13.101A	S22.019B	S22.23XA
S06.374A	S06.9X3A	S12.300A	S13.110A	S22.020A	S22.23XB
S06.375A	S06.9X4A	S12.300B	S13.111A	S22.020B	S22.24XA
S06.376A	S06.9X5A	S12.301A	S13.120A	S22.021A	S22.24XB
S06.377A	S06.9X6A	S12.301B	S13.121A	S22.021B	S22.31XA
S06.378A	S06.9X7A	S12.330A	S13.130A	S22.022A	S22.31XB
S06.379A	S06.9X8A	S12.330B	S13.131A	S22.022B	S22.32XA
S06.380A	S06.9X9A	S12.331A	S13.140A	S22.028A	S22.32XB
S06.381A	S07.0XXA	S12.331B	S13.141A	S22.028B	S22.39XA
S06.382A	S07.1XXA	S12.34XA	S13.150A	S22.029A	S22.39XB
S06.383A	S07.8XXA	S12.34XB	S13.151A	S22.029B	S22.41XA
S06.384A	S07.9XXA	S12.350A	S13.160A	S22.030A	S22.41XB
S06.385A	S12.000A	S12.350B	S13.161A	S22.030B	S22.42XA
S06.386A	S12.000B	S12.351A	S13.170A	S22.031A	S22.42XB
S06.387A	S12.001A	S12.351B	S13.171A	S22.031B	S22.43XA
S06.388A	S12.001B	S12.390A	S13.180A	S22.032A	S22.43XB
S06.389A	S12.01XA	S12.390B	S13.181A	S22.032B	S22.49XA
S06.4X0A	S12.01XB	S12.391A	S13.20XA	S22.038A	S22.49XB
S06.4X1A	S12.02XA	S12.391B	S13.29XA	S22.038B	S22.5XXA
S06.4X2A	S12.02XB	S12.400A	S14.101A	S22.039A	S22.5XXB
S06.4X3A	S12.030A	S12.400B	S14.102A	S22.039B	S22.9XXA
S06.4X4A	S12.030B	S12.401A	S14.103A	S22.040A	S22.9XXB
S06.4X5A	S12.031A	S12.401B	S14.104A	S22.040B	S24.101A
S06.4X6A	S12.031B	S12.430A	S14.105A	S22.041A	S24.102A
S06.4X7A	S12.040A	S12.430B	S14.106A	S22.041B	S24.103A
S06.4X8A	S12.040B	S12.431A	S14.107A	S22.042A	S24.104A
S06.4X9A	S12.041A	S12.431B	S14.109A	S22.042B	S24.109A
S06.5X0A	S12.041B	S12.44XA	S14.111A	S22.048A	S24.111A
S06.5X1A	S12.090A	S12.44XB	S14.112A	S22.048B	S24.112A
S06.5X2A	S12.090B	S12.450A	S14.113A	S22.049A	S24.113A
S06.5X3A	S12.091A	S12.450B	S14.114A	S22.049B	S24.114A
S06.5X4A	S12.091B	S12.451A	S14.115A	S22.050A	S24.131A
S06.5X5A	S12.100A	S12.451B	S14.116A	S22.050B	S24.132A
S06.5X6A	S12.100B	S12.490A	S14.117A	S22.051A	S24.133A
S06.5X7A	S12.101A	S12.490B	S14.121A	S22.051B	S24.134A
S06.5X8A	S12.101B	S12.491A	S14.122A	S22.052A	S24.151A
S06.5X9A	S12.110A	S12.491B	S14.123A	S22.052B	S24.152A
S06.6X0A	S12.110B	S12.500A	S14.124A	S22.058A	S24.153A
S06.6X1A	S12.111A	S12.500B	S14.125A	S22.058B	S24.154A
S06.6X2A	S12.111B	S12.501A	S14.126A	S22.059A	S32.000A
S06.6X3A	S12.112A	S12.501B	S14.127A	S22.059B	S32.000B
S06.6X4A	S12.112B	S12.530A	S14.131A	S22.060A	S32.001A
S06.6X5A	S12.120A	S12.530B	S14.132A	S22.060B	S32.001B
S06.6X6A	S12.120B	S12.531A	S14.133A	S22.061A	S32.002A
S06.6X7A	S12.121A	S12.531B	S14.134A	S22.061B	S32.002B
S06.6X8A	S12.121B	S12.54XA	S14.135A	S22.062A	S32.008A
S06.6X9A	S12.130A	S12.54XB	S14.136A	S22.062B	S32.008B
S06.811A	S12.130B	S12.550A	S14.137A	S22.068A	S32.009A
S06.812A	S12.131A	S12.550B	S14.151A	S22.068B	S32.009B
S06.813A	S12.131B	S12.551A	S14.152A	S22.069A	S32.010A
S06.814A	S12.14XA	S12.551B	S14.153A	S22.069B	S32.010B
S06.815A	S12.14XB	S12.590A	S14.154A	S22.070A	S32.011A
S06.816A	S12.150A	S12.590B	S14.155A	S22.070B	S32.011B
S06.817A	S12.150B	S12.591A	S14.156A	S22.071A	S32.012A
S06.818A	S12.151A	S12.591B	S14.157A	S22.071B	S32.012B
S06.819A	S12.151B	S12.600A	S17.0XXA	S22.072A	S32.018A
S06.821A	S12.190A	S12.600B	S17.8XXA	S22.072B	S32.018B
S06.822A	S12.190B	S12.601A	S17.9XXA	S22.078A	S32.019A
S06.823A	S12.191A	S12.601B	S22.000A	S22.078B	S32.019B
S06.824A	S12.191B	S12.630A	S22.000B	S22.079A	S32.020A
S06.825A	S12.200A	S12.630B	S22.001A	S22.079B	S32.020B
S06.826A	S12.200B	S12.631A	S22.001B	S22.080A	S32.021A
S06.827A	S12.201A	S12.631B	S22.002A	S22.080B	S32.021B
S06.828A	S12.201B	S12.64XA	S22.002B	S22.081A	S32.022A
	S12.230A	S12.64XB	S22.008A	S22.081B	S32.022B
	S12.230B	S12.650A	S22.008B	S22.082A	S32.028A

HAC 05: Falls and Trauma (continued)

S32.028B	S32.309A	S32.452B	S32.612A	S42.113B
S32.029A	S32.309B	S32.453A	S32.612B	S42.114B
S32.029B	S32.311A	S32.453B	S32.613A	S42.115B
S32.030A	S32.311B	S32.454A	S32.613B	S42.116B
S32.030B	S32.312A	S32.454B	S32.614A	S42.121B
S32.031A	S32.312B	S32.455A	S32.614B	S42.122B
S32.031B	S32.313A	S32.455B	S32.615A	S42.123B
S32.032A	S32.313B	S32.456A	S32.615B	S42.124B
S32.032B	S32.314A	S32.456B	S32.616A	S42.125B
S32.038A	S32.314B	S32.461A	S32.616B	S42.126B
S32.038B	S32.315A	S32.461B	S32.691A	S42.131B
S32.039A	S32.315B	S32.462A	S32.691B	S42.132B
S32.039B	S32.316A	S32.462B	S32.692A	S42.133B
S32.040A	S32.316B	S32.463A	S32.692B	S42.134B
S32.040B	S32.391A	S32.463B	S32.699A	S42.135B
S32.041A	S32.391B	S32.464A	S32.699B	S42.136B
S32.041B	S32.392A	S32.464B	S32.810A	S42.141B
S32.042A	S32.392B	S32.465A	S32.810B	S42.142B
S32.042B	S32.399A	S32.465B	S32.811A	S42.143B
S32.048A	S32.399B	S32.466A	S32.811B	S42.144B
S32.048B	S32.401A	S32.466B	S32.82XA	S42.145B
S32.049A	S32.401B	S32.471A	S32.82XB	S42.146B
S32.049B	S32.402A	S32.471B	S32.89XA	S42.151B
S32.050A	S32.402B	S32.472A	S32.89XB	S42.152B
S32.050B	S32.409A	S32.472B	S32.9XXA	S42.153B
S32.051A	S32.409B	S32.473A	S32.9XXB	S42.154B
S32.051B	S32.411A	S32.473B	S34.101A	S42.155B
S32.052A	S32.411B	S32.474A	S34.102A	S42.156B
S32.052B	S32.412A	S32.474B	S34.103A	S42.191B
S32.058A	S32.412B	S32.475A	S34.104A	S42.192B
S32.058B	S32.413A	S32.475B	S34.105A	S42.199B
S32.059A	S32.413B	S32.476A	S34.109A	S42.201A
S32.059B	S32.414A	S32.476B	S34.111A	S42.201B
S32.10XA	S32.414B	S32.481A	S34.112A	S42.202A
S32.10XB	S32.415A	S32.481B	S34.113A	S42.202B
S32.110A	S32.415B	S32.482A	S34.114A	S42.209A
S32.110B	S32.416A	S32.482B	S34.115A	S42.209B
S32.111A	S32.416B	S32.483A	S34.119A	S42.211A
S32.111B	S32.421A	S32.483B	S34.121A	S42.211B
S32.112A	S32.421B	S32.484A	S34.122A	S42.212A
S32.112B	S32.422A	S32.484B	S34.123A	S42.212B
S32.119A	S32.422B	S32.485A	S34.124A	S42.213A
S32.119B	S32.423A	S32.485B	S34.125A	S42.213B
S32.120A	S32.423B	S32.486A	S34.129A	S42.214A
S32.120B	S32.424A	S32.486B	S34.131A	S42.214B
S32.121A	S32.424B	S32.491A	S34.132A	S42.215A
S32.121B	S32.425A	S32.491B	S34.139A	S42.215B
S32.122A	S32.425B	S32.492A	S34.3XXA	S42.216A
S32.122B	S32.426A	S32.492B	S42.001B	S42.216B
S32.129A	S32.426B	S32.499A	S42.002B	S42.221A
S32.129B	S32.431A	S32.499B	S42.009B	S42.221B
S32.130A	S32.431B	S32.501A	S42.011B	S42.222A
S32.130B	S32.432A	S32.501B	S42.012B	S42.222B
S32.131A	S32.432B	S32.502A	S42.013B	S42.223A
S32.131B	S32.433A	S32.502B	S42.014B	S42.223B
S32.132A	S32.433B	S32.509A	S42.015B	S42.224A
S32.132B	S32.434A	S32.509B	S42.016B	S42.224B
S32.139A	S32.434B	S32.511A	S42.017B	S42.225A
S32.139B	S32.435A	S32.511B	S42.018B	S42.225B
S32.14XA	S32.435B	S32.512A	S42.019B	S42.226A
S32.14XB	S32.436A	S32.512B	S42.021B	S42.226B
S32.15XA	S32.436B	S32.519A	S42.022B	S42.231A
S32.15XB	S32.441A	S32.519B	S42.023B	S42.231B
S32.16XA	S32.441B	S32.591A	S42.024B	S42.232A
S32.16XB	S32.442A	S32.591B	S42.025B	S42.232B
S32.17XA	S32.442B	S32.592A	S42.026B	S42.239A
S32.17XB	S32.443A	S32.592B	S42.031B	S42.239B
S32.19XA	S32.443B	S32.599A	S42.032B	S42.241A
S32.19XB	S32.444A	S32.599B	S42.033B	S42.241B
S32.2XXA	S32.444B	S32.601A	S42.034B	S42.242A
S32.2XXB	S32.445A	S32.601B	S42.035B	S42.242B
S32.301A	S32.445B	S32.602A	S42.036B	S42.249A
S32.301B	S32.446A	S32.602B	S42.101B	S42.249B
S32.302A	S32.446B	S32.609A	S42.102B	S42.251A
S32.302B	S32.451A	S32.609B	S42.109B	S42.251B
	S32.451B	S32.611A	S42.111B	S42.252A
	S32.452A	S32.611B	S42.112B	S42.252B

S42.253A
S42.253B
S42.254A
S42.254B
S42.255A
S42.255B
S42.256A
S42.256B
S42.261A
S42.261B
S42.262A
S42.262B
S42.263A
S42.263B
S42.264A
S42.264B
S42.265A
S42.265B
S42.266A
S42.266B
S42.271A
S42.272A
S42.279A
S42.291A
S42.291B
S42.292A
S42.292B
S42.293A
S42.293B
S42.294A
S42.294B
S42.295A
S42.295B
S42.296A
S42.296B
S42.301A
S42.301B
S42.302A
S42.302B
S42.309A
S42.309B
S42.311A
S42.312A
S42.319A
S42.321A
S42.321B
S42.322A
S42.322B
S42.323A
S42.323B
S42.324A
S42.324B
S42.325A
S42.325B
S42.326A
S42.326B
S42.331A
S42.331B
S42.332A
S42.332B
S42.333A
S42.333B
S42.334A
S42.334B
S42.335A
S42.335B
S42.336A
S42.336B
S42.341A
S42.341B
S42.342A
S42.342B
S42.343A
S42.343B
S42.344A
S42.344B
S42.345A

HAC 05: Falls and Trauma (continued)

S42.345B	S42.441A	S43.203A	S52.033B	S52.221A	S52.262C
S42.346A	S42.441B	S43.204A	S52.033C	S52.221B	S52.263A
S42.346B	S42.442A	S43.205A	S52.034B	S52.221C	S52.263B
S42.351A	S42.442B	S43.206A	S52.034C	S52.222A	S52.263C
S42.351B	S42.443A	S43.211A	S52.035B	S52.222B	S52.264A
S42.352A	S42.443B	S43.212A	S52.035C	S52.222C	S52.264B
S42.352B	S42.444A	S43.213A	S52.036B	S52.223A	S52.264C
S42.353A	S42.444B	S43.214A	S52.036C	S52.223B	S52.265A
S42.353B	S42.445A	S43.215A	S52.041B	S52.223C	S52.265B
S42.354A	S42.445B	S43.216A	S52.041C	S52.224A	S52.265C
S42.354B	S42.446A	S43.221A	S52.042B	S52.224B	S52.266A
S42.355A	S42.446B	S43.222A	S52.042C	S52.224C	S52.266B
S42.355B	S42.447A	S43.223A	S52.043B	S52.225A	S52.266C
S42.356A	S42.447B	S43.224A	S52.043C	S52.225B	S52.271B
S42.356B	S42.448A	S43.225A	S52.044B	S52.225C	S52.271C
S42.361A	S42.448B	S43.226A	S52.044C	S52.226A	S52.272B
S42.361B	S42.449A	S49.001A	S52.045B	S52.226B	S52.272C
S42.362A	S42.449B	S49.002A	S52.045C	S52.226C	S52.279B
S42.362B	S42.451A	S49.009A	S52.046B	S52.231A	S52.279C
S42.363A	S42.451B	S49.011A	S52.046C	S52.231B	S52.281A
S42.363B	S42.452A	S49.012A	S52.091B	S52.231C	S52.281B
S42.364A	S42.452B	S49.019A	S52.091C	S52.232A	S52.281C
S42.364B	S42.453A	S49.021A	S52.092B	S52.232B	S52.282A
S42.365A	S42.453B	S49.022A	S52.092C	S52.232C	S52.282B
S42.365B	S42.454A	S49.029A	S52.099B	S52.233A	S52.282C
S42.366A	S42.454B	S49.031A	S52.099C	S52.233B	S52.283A
S42.366B	S42.455A	S49.032A	S52.101B	S52.233C	S52.283B
S42.391A	S42.455B	S49.039A	S52.101C	S52.234A	S52.283C
S42.391B	S42.456A	S49.041A	S52.102B	S52.234B	S52.291A
S42.392A	S42.456B	S49.042A	S52.102C	S52.234C	S52.291B
S42.392B	S42.461A	S49.049A	S52.109B	S52.235A	S52.291C
S42.399A	S42.461B	S49.091A	S52.109C	S52.235B	S52.292A
S42.399B	S42.462A	S49.092A	S52.111A	S52.235C	S52.292B
S42.401A	S42.462B	S49.099A	S52.112A	S52.236A	S52.292C
S42.401B	S42.463A	S49.101A	S52.119A	S52.236B	S52.299A
S42.402A	S42.463B	S49.102A	S52.121B	S52.236C	S52.299B
S42.402B	S42.464A	S49.109A	S52.121C	S52.241A	S52.299C
S42.409A	S42.464B	S49.111A	S52.122B	S52.241B	S52.301A
S42.409B	S42.465A	S49.112A	S52.122C	S52.241C	S52.301B
S42.411A	S42.465B	S49.119A	S52.123B	S52.242A	S52.301C
S42.411B	S42.466A	S49.121A	S52.123C	S52.242B	S52.302A
S42.412A	S42.466B	S49.122A	S52.124B	S52.242C	S52.302B
S42.412B	S42.471A	S49.129A	S52.124C	S52.243A	S52.302C
S42.413A	S42.471B	S49.131A	S52.125B	S52.243B	S52.309A
S42.413B	S42.472A	S49.132A	S52.125C	S52.243C	S52.309B
S42.414A	S42.472B	S49.139A	S52.126B	S52.244A	S52.309C
S42.414B	S42.473A	S49.141A	S52.126C	S52.244B	S52.311A
S42.415A	S42.473B	S49.142A	S52.131B	S52.244C	S52.312A
S42.415B	S42.474A	S49.149A	S52.131C	S52.245A	S52.319A
S42.416A	S42.474B	S49.191A	S52.132B	S52.245B	S52.321A
S42.416B	S42.475A	S49.192A	S52.132C	S52.245C	S52.321B
S42.421A	S42.475B	S49.199A	S52.133B	S52.246A	S52.321C
S42.421B	S42.476A	S52.001B	S52.133C	S52.246B	S52.322A
S42.422A	S42.476B	S52.001C	S52.134B	S52.246C	S52.322B
S42.422B	S42.481A	S52.002B	S52.134C	S52.251A	S52.322C
S42.423A	S42.482A	S52.002C	S52.135B	S52.251B	S52.323A
S42.423B	S42.489A	S52.009B	S52.135C	S52.251C	S52.323B
S42.424A	S42.491A	S52.009C	S52.136B	S52.252A	S52.323C
S42.424B	S42.491B	S52.011A	S52.136C	S52.252B	S52.324A
S42.425A	S42.492A	S52.012A	S52.181B	S52.252C	S52.324B
S42.425B	S42.492B	S52.019A	S52.181C	S52.253A	S52.324C
S42.426A	S42.493A	S52.021B	S52.182B	S52.253B	S52.325A
S42.426B	S42.493B	S52.021C	S52.182C	S52.253C	S52.325B
S42.431A	S42.494A	S52.022B	S52.189B	S52.254A	S52.325C
S42.431B	S42.494B	S52.022C	S52.189C	S52.254B	S52.326A
S42.432A	S42.495A	S52.023B	S52.201A	S52.254C	S52.326B
S42.432B	S42.495B	S52.023C	S52.201B	S52.255A	S52.326C
S42.433A	S42.496A	S52.024B	S52.201C	S52.255B	S52.331A
S42.433B	S42.496B	S52.024C	S52.202A	S52.255C	S52.331B
S42.434A	S42.90XA	S52.025B	S52.202B	S52.256A	S52.331C
S42.434B	S42.90XB	S52.025C	S52.202C	S52.256B	S52.332A
S42.435A	S42.91XA	S52.026B	S52.209A	S52.256C	S52.332B
S42.435B	S42.91XB	S52.026C	S52.209B	S52.261A	S52.332C
S42.436A	S42.92XA	S52.031B	S52.209C	S52.261B	S52.333A
S42.436B	S42.92XB	S52.031C	S52.211A	S52.261C	S52.333B
	S43.201A	S52.032B	S52.212A	S52.262A	S52.333C
	S43.202A	S52.032C	S52.219A	S52.262B	S52.334A

HAC 05: Falls and Trauma (continued)

S52.334B	S52.382B	S52.569A	S59.029A	S62.152B	S62.321B
S52.334C	S52.382C	S52.569B	S59.031A	S62.153B	S62.322B
S52.335A	S52.389A	S52.569C	S59.032A	S62.154B	S62.323B
S52.335B	S52.389B	S52.571A	S59.039A	S62.155B	S62.324B
S52.335C	S52.389C	S52.571B	S59.041A	S62.156B	S62.325B
S52.336A	S52.391A	S52.571C	S59.042A	S62.161B	S62.326B
S52.336B	S52.391B	S52.572A	S59.049A	S62.162B	S62.327B
S52.336C	S52.391C	S52.572B	S59.091A	S62.163B	S62.328B
S52.341A	S52.392A	S52.572C	S59.092A	S62.164B	S62.329B
S52.341B	S52.392B	S52.579A	S59.099A	S62.165B	S62.330B
S52.341C	S52.392C	S52.579B	S59.201A	S62.166B	S62.331B
S52.342A	S52.399A	S52.579C	S59.202A	S62.171B	S62.332B
S52.342B	S52.399B	S52.591A	S59.209A	S62.172B	S62.333B
S52.342C	S52.399C	S52.591B	S59.211A	S62.173B	S62.334B
S52.343A	S52.501A	S52.591C	S59.212A	S62.174B	S62.335B
S52.343B	S52.501B	S52.592A	S59.219A	S62.175B	S62.336B
S52.343C	S52.501C	S52.592B	S59.221A	S62.176B	S62.337B
S52.344A	S52.502A	S52.592C	S59.222A	S62.181B	S62.338B
S52.344B	S52.502B	S52.599A	S59.229A	S62.182B	S62.339B
S52.344C	S52.502C	S52.599B	S59.231A	S62.183B	S62.340B
S52.345A	S52.509A	S52.599C	S59.232A	S62.184B	S62.341B
S52.345B	S52.509B	S52.601A	S59.239A	S62.185B	S62.342B
S52.345C	S52.509C	S52.601B	S59.241A	S62.186B	S62.343B
S52.346A	S52.511A	S52.601C	S59.242A	S62.201B	S62.344B
S52.346B	S52.511B	S52.602A	S59.249A	S62.202B	S62.345B
S52.346C	S52.511C	S52.602B	S59.291A	S62.209B	S62.346B
S52.351A	S52.512A	S52.602C	S59.292A	S62.211B	S62.347B
S52.351B	S52.512B	S52.609A	S59.299A	S62.212B	S62.348B
S52.351C	S52.512C	S52.609B	S62.001B	S62.213B	S62.349B
S52.352A	S52.513A	S52.609C	S62.002B	S62.221B	S62.350B
S52.352B	S52.513B	S52.611A	S62.009B	S62.222B	S62.351B
S52.352C	S52.513C	S52.611B	S62.011B	S62.223B	S62.352B
S52.353A	S52.514A	S52.611C	S62.012B	S62.224B	S62.353B
S52.353B	S52.514B	S52.612A	S62.013B	S62.225B	S62.354B
S52.353C	S52.514C	S52.612B	S62.014B	S62.226B	S62.355B
S52.354A	S52.515A	S52.612C	S62.015B	S62.231B	S62.356B
S52.354B	S52.515B	S52.613A	S62.016B	S62.232B	S62.357B
S52.354C	S52.515C	S52.613B	S62.021B	S62.233B	S62.358B
S52.355A	S52.516A	S52.613C	S62.022B	S62.234B	S62.359B
S52.355B	S52.516B	S52.614A	S62.023B	S62.235B	S62.360B
S52.355C	S52.516C	S52.614B	S62.024B	S62.236B	S62.361B
S52.356A	S52.521A	S52.614C	S62.025B	S62.241B	S62.362B
S52.356B	S52.522A	S52.615A	S62.026B	S62.242B	S62.363B
S52.356C	S52.529A	S52.615B	S62.031B	S62.243B	S62.364B
S52.361A	S52.531A	S52.615C	S62.032B	S62.244B	S62.365B
S52.361B	S52.531B	S52.616A	S62.033B	S62.245B	S62.366B
S52.361C	S52.531C	S52.616B	S62.034B	S62.246B	S62.367B
S52.362A	S52.532A	S52.616C	S62.035B	S62.251B	S62.368B
S52.362B	S52.532B	S52.621A	S62.036B	S62.252B	S62.369B
S52.362C	S52.532C	S52.622A	S62.101B	S62.253B	S62.390B
S52.363A	S52.539A	S52.629A	S62.102B	S62.254B	S62.391B
S52.363B	S52.539B	S52.691A	S62.109B	S62.255B	S62.392B
S52.363C	S52.539C	S52.691B	S62.111B	S62.256B	S62.393B
S52.364A	S52.541A	S52.691C	S62.112B	S62.291B	S62.394B
S52.364B	S52.541B	S52.692A	S62.113B	S62.292B	S62.395B
S52.364C	S52.541C	S52.692B	S62.114B	S62.299B	S62.396B
S52.365A	S52.542A	S52.692C	S62.115B	S62.300B	S62.397B
S52.365B	S52.542B	S52.699A	S62.116B	S62.301B	S62.398B
S52.365C	S52.542C	S52.699B	S62.121B	S62.302B	S62.399B
S52.366A	S52.549A	S52.699C	S62.122B	S62.303B	S62.501B
S52.366B	S52.549B	S52.90XA	S62.123B	S62.304B	S62.502B
S52.366C	S52.549C	S52.90XB	S62.124B	S62.305B	S62.509B
S52.371A	S52.551A	S52.90XC	S62.125B	S62.306B	S62.511B
S52.371B	S52.551B	S52.91XA	S62.126B	S62.307B	S62.512B
S52.371C	S52.551C	S52.91XB	S62.131B	S62.308B	S62.513B
S52.372A	S52.552A	S52.91XC	S62.132B	S62.309B	S62.514B
S52.372B	S52.552B	S52.92XA	S62.133B	S62.310B	S62.515B
S52.372C	S52.552C	S52.92XB	S62.134B	S62.311B	S62.516B
S52.379A	S52.559A	S52.92XC	S62.135B	S62.312B	S62.521B
S52.379B	S52.559B	S59.001A	S62.136B	S62.313B	S62.522B
S52.379C	S52.559C	S59.002A	S62.141B	S62.314B	S62.523B
S52.381A	S52.561A	S59.009A	S62.142B	S62.315B	S62.524B
S52.381B	S52.561B	S59.011A	S62.143B	S62.316B	S62.525B
S52.381C	S52.561C	S59.012A	S62.144B	S62.317B	S62.526B
S52.382A	S52.562A	S59.019A	S62.145B	S62.318B	S62.600B
	S52.562B	S59.021A	S62.146B	S62.319B	S62.601B
	S52.562C	S59.022A	S62.151B	S62.320B	S62.602B

HAC 05: Falls and Trauma (continued)

S62.603B	S72.002C	S72.061B	S72.133A	S72.331C	S72.399B
S62.604B	S72.009A	S72.061C	S72.133B	S72.332A	S72.399C
S62.605B	S72.009B	S72.062A	S72.133C	S72.332B	S72.401A
S62.606B	S72.009C	S72.062B	S72.134A	S72.332C	S72.401B
S62.607B	S72.011A	S72.062C	S72.134B	S72.333A	S72.401C
S62.608B	S72.011B	S72.063A	S72.134C	S72.333B	S72.402A
S62.609B	S72.011C	S72.063B	S72.135A	S72.333C	S72.402B
S62.610B	S72.012A	S72.063C	S72.135B	S72.334A	S72.402C
S62.611B	S72.012B	S72.064A	S72.135C	S72.334B	S72.409A
S62.612B	S72.012C	S72.064B	S72.136A	S72.334C	S72.409B
S62.613B	S72.019A	S72.064C	S72.136B	S72.335A	S72.409C
S62.614B	S72.019B	S72.065A	S72.136C	S72.335B	S72.411A
S62.615B	S72.019C	S72.065B	S72.141A	S72.335C	S72.411B
S62.616B	S72.021A	S72.065C	S72.141B	S72.336A	S72.411C
S62.617B	S72.021B	S72.066A	S72.141C	S72.336B	S72.412A
S62.618B	S72.021C	S72.066B	S72.142A	S72.336C	S72.412B
S62.619B	S72.022A	S72.066C	S72.142B	S72.341A	S72.412C
S62.620B	S72.022B	S72.091A	S72.142C	S72.341B	S72.413A
S62.621B	S72.022C	S72.091B	S72.143A	S72.341C	S72.413B
S62.622B	S72.023A	S72.091C	S72.143B	S72.342A	S72.413C
S62.623B	S72.023B	S72.092A	S72.143C	S72.342B	S72.414A
S62.624B	S72.023C	S72.092B	S72.144A	S72.342C	S72.414B
S62.625B	S72.024A	S72.092C	S72.144B	S72.343A	S72.414C
S62.626B	S72.024B	S72.099A	S72.144C	S72.343B	S72.415A
S62.627B	S72.024C	S72.099B	S72.145A	S72.343C	S72.415B
S62.628B	S72.025A	S72.099C	S72.145B	S72.344A	S72.415C
S62.629B	S72.025B	S72.101A	S72.145C	S72.344B	S72.416A
S62.630B	S72.025C	S72.101B	S72.146A	S72.344C	S72.416B
S62.631B	S72.026A	S72.101C	S72.146B	S72.345A	S72.416C
S62.632B	S72.026B	S72.102A	S72.146C	S72.345B	S72.421A
S62.633B	S72.026C	S72.102B	S72.21XA	S72.345C	S72.421B
S62.634B	S72.031A	S72.102C	S72.21XB	S72.346A	S72.421C
S62.635B	S72.031B	S72.109A	S72.21XC	S72.346B	S72.422A
S62.636B	S72.031C	S72.109B	S72.22XA	S72.346C	S72.422B
S62.637B	S72.032A	S72.109C	S72.22XB	S72.351A	S72.422C
S62.638B	S72.032B	S72.111A	S72.22XC	S72.351B	S72.423A
S62.639B	S72.032C	S72.111B	S72.23XA	S72.351C	S72.423B
S62.640B	S72.033A	S72.111C	S72.23XB	S72.352A	S72.423C
S62.641B	S72.033B	S72.112A	S72.23XC	S72.352B	S72.424A
S62.642B	S72.033C	S72.112B	S72.24XA	S72.352C	S72.424B
S62.643B	S72.034A	S72.112C	S72.24XB	S72.353A	S72.424C
S62.644B	S72.034B	S72.113A	S72.24XC	S72.353B	S72.425A
S62.645B	S72.034C	S72.113B	S72.25XA	S72.353C	S72.425B
S62.646B	S72.035A	S72.113C	S72.25XB	S72.354A	S72.425C
S62.647B	S72.035B	S72.114A	S72.25XC	S72.354B	S72.426A
S62.648B	S72.035C	S72.114B	S72.26XA	S72.354C	S72.426B
S62.649B	S72.036A	S72.114C	S72.26XB	S72.355A	S72.426C
S62.650B	S72.036B	S72.115A	S72.26XC	S72.355B	S72.431A
S62.651B	S72.036C	S72.115B	S72.301A	S72.355C	S72.431B
S62.652B	S72.041A	S72.115C	S72.301B	S72.356A	S72.431C
S62.653B	S72.041B	S72.116A	S72.301C	S72.356B	S72.432A
S62.654B	S72.041C	S72.116B	S72.302A	S72.356C	S72.432B
S62.655B	S72.042A	S72.116C	S72.302B	S72.361A	S72.432C
S62.656B	S72.042B	S72.121A	S72.302C	S72.361B	S72.433A
S62.657B	S72.042C	S72.121B	S72.309A	S72.361C	S72.433B
S62.658B	S72.043A	S72.121C	S72.309B	S72.362A	S72.433C
S62.659B	S72.043B	S72.122A	S72.309C	S72.362B	S72.434A
S62.660B	S72.043C	S72.122B	S72.321A	S72.362C	S72.434B
S62.661B	S72.044A	S72.122C	S72.321B	S72.363A	S72.434C
S62.662B	S72.044B	S72.123A	S72.321C	S72.363B	S72.435A
S62.663B	S72.044C	S72.123B	S72.322A	S72.363C	S72.435B
S62.664B	S72.045A	S72.123C	S72.322B	S72.364A	S72.435C
S62.665B	S72.045B	S72.124A	S72.322C	S72.364B	S72.436A
S62.666B	S72.045C	S72.124B	S72.323A	S72.364C	S72.436B
S62.667B	S72.046A	S72.124C	S72.323B	S72.365A	S72.436C
S62.668B	S72.046B	S72.125A	S72.323C	S72.365B	S72.441A
S62.669B	S72.046C	S72.125B	S72.324A	S72.365C	S72.441B
S62.90XB	S72.051A	S72.125C	S72.324B	S72.366A	S72.441C
S62.91XB	S72.051B	S72.126A	S72.324C	S72.366B	S72.442A
S62.92XB	S72.051C	S72.126B	S72.325A	S72.366C	S72.442B
S72.001A	S72.052A	S72.126C	S72.325B	S72.391A	S72.442C
S72.001B	S72.052B	S72.131A	S72.325C	S72.391B	S72.443A
S72.001C	S72.052C	S72.131B	S72.326A	S72.391C	S72.443B
S72.002A	S72.059A	S72.131C	S72.326B	S72.392A	S72.443C
S72.002B	S72.059B	S72.132A	S72.326C	S72.392B	S72.444A
	S72.059C	S72.132B	S72.331A	S72.392C	S72.444B
	S72.061A	S72.132C	S72.331B	S72.399A	S72.444C

HAC 05: Falls and Trauma (continued)	S73.004A	S82.013C	S82.102B	S82.151A	S82.241C
S72.445A	S73.005A	S82.014A	S82.102C	S82.151B	S82.242A
S72.445B	S73.006A	S82.014B	S82.109A	S82.151C	S82.242B
S72.445C	S73.011A	S82.014C	S82.109B	S82.152A	S82.242C
S72.446A	S73.012A	S82.015A	S82.109C	S82.152B	S82.243A
S72.446B	S73.013A	S82.015B	S82.111A	S82.152C	S82.243B
S72.446C	S73.014A	S82.015C	S82.111B	S82.153A	S82.243C
S72.451A	S73.015A	S82.016A	S82.111C	S82.153B	S82.244A
S72.451B	S73.016A	S82.016B	S82.112A	S82.153C	S82.244B
S72.451C	S73.021A	S82.016C	S82.112B	S82.154A	S82.244C
S72.452A	S73.022A	S82.021A	S82.112C	S82.154B	S82.245A
S72.452B	S73.023A	S82.021B	S82.113A	S82.154C	S82.245B
S72.452C	S73.024A	S82.021C	S82.113B	S82.155A	S82.245C
S72.453A	S73.025A	S82.022A	S82.113C	S82.155B	S82.246A
S72.453B	S73.026A	S82.022B	S82.114A	S82.155C	S82.246B
S72.453C	S73.031A	S82.022C	S82.114B	S82.156A	S82.246C
S72.454A	S73.032A	S82.023A	S82.114C	S82.156B	S82.251A
S72.454B	S73.033A	S82.023B	S82.115A	S82.156C	S82.251B
S72.454C	S73.034A	S82.023C	S82.115B	S82.161A	S82.251C
S72.455A	S73.035A	S82.024A	S82.115C	S82.162A	S82.252A
S72.455B	S73.036A	S82.024B	S82.116A	S82.169A	S82.252B
S72.455C	S73.041A	S82.024C	S82.116B	S82.191A	S82.252C
S72.456A	S73.042A	S82.025A	S82.116C	S82.191B	S82.253A
S72.456B	S73.043A	S82.025B	S82.121A	S82.191C	S82.253B
S72.456C	S73.044A	S82.025C	S82.121B	S82.192A	S82.253C
S72.461A	S73.045A	S82.026A	S82.121C	S82.192B	S82.254A
S72.461B	S73.046A	S82.026B	S82.122A	S82.192C	S82.254B
S72.461C	S77.00XA	S82.026C	S82.122B	S82.199A	S82.254C
S72.462A	S77.01XA	S82.031A	S82.122C	S82.199B	S82.255A
S72.462B	S77.02XA	S82.031B	S82.123A	S82.199C	S82.255B
S72.462C	S77.10XA	S82.031C	S82.123B	S82.201A	S82.255C
S72.463A	S77.11XA	S82.032A	S82.123C	S82.201B	S82.256A
S72.463B	S77.12XA	S82.032B	S82.124A	S82.201C	S82.256B
S72.463C	S79.001A	S82.032C	S82.124B	S82.202A	S82.256C
S72.464A	S79.002A	S82.033A	S82.124C	S82.202B	S82.261A
S72.464B	S79.009A	S82.033B	S82.125A	S82.202C	S82.261B
S72.464C	S79.011A	S82.033C	S82.125B	S82.209A	S82.261C
S72.465A	S79.012A	S82.034A	S82.125C	S82.209B	S82.262A
S72.465B	S79.019A	S82.034B	S82.126A	S82.209C	S82.262B
S72.465C	S79.091A	S82.034C	S82.126B	S82.221A	S82.262C
S72.466A	S79.092A	S82.035A	S82.126C	S82.221B	S82.263A
S72.466B	S79.099A	S82.035B	S82.131A	S82.221C	S82.263B
S72.466C	S79.101A	S82.035C	S82.131B	S82.222A	S82.263C
S72.471A	S79.102A	S82.036A	S82.131C	S82.222B	S82.264A
S72.472A	S79.109A	S82.036B	S82.132A	S82.222C	S82.264B
S72.479A	S79.111A	S82.036C	S82.132B	S82.223A	S82.264C
S72.491A	S79.112A	S82.041A	S82.132C	S82.223B	S82.265A
S72.491B	S79.119A	S82.041B	S82.133A	S82.223C	S82.265B
S72.491C	S79.121A	S82.041C	S82.133B	S82.224A	S82.265C
S72.492A	S79.122A	S82.042A	S82.133C	S82.224B	S82.266A
S72.492B	S79.129A	S82.042B	S82.134A	S82.224C	S82.266B
S72.492C	S79.131A	S82.042C	S82.134B	S82.225A	S82.266C
S72.499A	S79.132A	S82.043A	S82.134C	S82.225B	S82.291A
S72.499B	S79.139A	S82.043B	S82.135A	S82.225C	S82.291B
S72.499C	S79.141A	S82.043C	S82.135B	S82.226A	S82.291C
S72.8X1A	S79.142A	S82.044A	S82.135C	S82.226B	S82.292A
S72.8X1B	S79.149A	S82.044B	S82.136A	S82.226C	S82.292B
S72.8X1C	S79.191A	S82.044C	S82.136B	S82.231A	S82.292C
S72.8X2A	S79.192A	S82.045A	S82.136C	S82.231B	S82.299A
S72.8X2B	S79.199A	S82.045B	S82.141A	S82.231C	S82.299B
S72.8X2C	S82.001A	S82.045C	S82.141B	S82.232A	S82.299C
S72.8X9A	S82.001B	S82.046A	S82.141C	S82.232B	S82.301B
S72.8X9B	S82.001C	S82.046B	S82.142A	S82.232C	S82.301C
S72.8X9C	S82.002A	S82.046C	S82.142B	S82.233A	S82.302B
S72.90XA	S82.002B	S82.091A	S82.142C	S82.233B	S82.302C
S72.90XB	S82.002C	S82.091B	S82.143A	S82.233C	S82.309B
S72.90XC	S82.009A	S82.091C	S82.143B	S82.234A	S82.309C
S72.91XA	S82.009B	S82.092A	S82.143C	S82.234B	S82.311A
S72.91XB	S82.009C	S82.092B	S82.144A	S82.234C	S82.312A
S72.91XC	S82.011A	S82.092C	S82.144B	S82.235A	S82.319A
S72.92XA	S82.011B	S82.099A	S82.144C	S82.235B	S82.391B
S72.92XB	S82.011C	S82.099B	S82.145A	S82.235C	S82.391C
S72.92XC	S82.012A	S82.099C	S82.145B	S82.236A	S82.392B
S73.001A	S82.012B	S82.101A	S82.145C	S82.236B	S82.392C
S73.002A	S82.012C	S82.101B	S82.146A	S82.236C	S82.399B
S73.003A	S82.013A	S82.101C	S82.146B	S82.241A	S82.399C
	S82.013B	S82.102A	S82.146C	S82.241B	S82.401B

Appendix I: Hospital Acquired Conditions

HAC 05: Falls and Trauma (continued)				
S82.401C	S82.53XB	S82.892C	S92.123B	S92.335B	T22.362A
S82.402B	S82.53XC	S82.899B	S92.124B	S92.336B	T22.369A
S82.402C	S82.54XB	S82.899C	S92.125B	S92.341B	T22.391A
S82.409B	S82.54XC	S82.90XB	S92.126B	S92.342B	T22.392A
S82.409C	S82.55XB	S82.90XC	S92.131B	S92.343B	T22.399A
S82.421B	S82.55XC	S82.91XB	S92.132B	S92.344B	T22.70XA
S82.421C	S82.56XB	S82.91XC	S92.133B	S92.345B	T22.711A
S82.422B	S82.56XC	S82.92XB	S92.134B	S92.346B	T22.712A
S82.422C	S82.61XB	S82.92XC	S92.135B	S92.351B	T22.719A
S82.423B	S82.61XC	S89.001A	S92.136B	S92.352B	T22.721A
S82.423C	S82.62XB	S89.002A	S92.141B	S92.353B	T22.722A
S82.424B	S82.62XC	S89.009A	S92.142B	S92.354B	T22.729A
S82.424C	S82.63XB	S89.011A	S92.143B	S92.355B	T22.731A
S82.425B	S82.63XC	S89.012A	S92.144B	S92.356B	T22.732A
S82.425C	S82.64XB	S89.019A	S92.145B	S92.811B	T22.739A
S82.426B	S82.64XC	S89.021A	S92.146B	S92.812B	T22.741A
S82.426C	S82.65XB	S89.022A	S92.151B	S92.819B	T22.742A
S82.431B	S82.65XC	S89.029A	S92.152B	S92.901B	T22.749A
S82.431C	S82.66XB	S89.031A	S92.153B	S92.902B	T22.751A
S82.432B	S82.66XC	S89.032A	S92.154B	S92.909B	T22.752A
S82.432C	S82.831B	S89.039A	S92.155B	T20.30XA	T22.759A
S82.433B	S82.831C	S89.041A	S92.156B	T20.311A	T22.761A
S82.433C	S82.832B	S89.042A	S92.191B	T20.312A	T22.762A
S82.434B	S82.832C	S89.049A	S92.192B	T20.319A	T22.769A
S82.434C	S82.839B	S89.091A	S92.199B	T20.32XA	T22.791A
S82.435B	S82.839C	S89.092A	S92.201B	T20.33XA	T22.792A
S82.435C	S82.841B	S89.099A	S92.202B	T20.34XA	T22.799A
S82.436B	S82.841C	S92.001B	S92.209B	T20.35XA	T23.301A
S82.436C	S82.842B	S92.002B	S92.211B	T20.36XA	T23.302A
S82.441B	S82.842C	S92.009B	S92.212B	T20.37XA	T23.309A
S82.441C	S82.843B	S92.011B	S92.213B	T20.39XA	T23.311A
S82.442B	S82.843C	S92.012B	S92.214B	T20.70XA	T23.312A
S82.442C	S82.844B	S92.013B	S92.215B	T20.711A	T23.319A
S82.443B	S82.844C	S92.014B	S92.216B	T20.712A	T23.321A
S82.443C	S82.845B	S92.015B	S92.221B	T20.719A	T23.322A
S82.444B	S82.845C	S92.016B	S92.222B	T20.72XA	T23.329A
S82.444C	S82.846B	S92.021B	S92.223B	T20.73XA	T23.331A
S82.445B	S82.846C	S92.022B	S92.224B	T20.74XA	T23.332A
S82.445C	S82.851B	S92.023B	S92.225B	T20.75XA	T23.339A
S82.446B	S82.851C	S92.024B	S92.226B	T20.76XA	T23.341A
S82.446C	S82.852B	S92.025B	S92.231B	T20.77XA	T23.342A
S82.451B	S82.852C	S92.026B	S92.232B	T20.79XA	T23.349A
S82.451C	S82.853B	S92.031B	S92.233B	T21.30XA	T23.351A
S82.452B	S82.853C	S92.032B	S92.234B	T21.31XA	T23.352A
S82.452C	S82.854B	S92.033B	S92.235B	T21.32XA	T23.359A
S82.453B	S82.854C	S92.034B	S92.236B	T21.33XA	T23.361A
S82.453C	S82.855B	S92.035B	S92.241B	T21.34XA	T23.362A
S82.454B	S82.855C	S92.036B	S92.242B	T21.35XA	T23.369A
S82.454C	S82.856B	S92.041B	S92.243B	T21.36XA	T23.371A
S82.455B	S82.856C	S92.042B	S92.244B	T21.37XA	T23.372A
S82.455C	S82.861B	S92.043B	S92.245B	T21.39XA	T23.379A
S82.456B	S82.861C	S92.044B	S92.246B	T21.70XA	T23.391A
S82.456C	S82.862B	S92.045B	S92.251B	T21.71XA	T23.392A
S82.461B	S82.862C	S92.046B	S92.252B	T21.72XA	T23.399A
S82.461C	S82.863B	S92.051B	S92.253B	T21.73XA	T23.701A
S82.462B	S82.863C	S92.052B	S92.254B	T21.74XA	T23.702A
S82.462C	S82.864B	S92.053B	S92.255B	T21.75XA	T23.709A
S82.463B	S82.864C	S92.054B	S92.256B	T21.76XA	T23.711A
S82.463C	S82.865B	S92.055B	S92.301B	T21.77XA	T23.712A
S82.464B	S82.865C	S92.056B	S92.302B	T21.79XA	T23.719A
S82.464C	S82.866B	S92.061B	S92.309B	T22.30XA	T23.721A
S82.465B	S82.866C	S92.062B	S92.311B	T22.311A	T23.722A
S82.465C	S82.871B	S92.063B	S92.312B	T22.312A	T23.729A
S82.466B	S82.871C	S92.064B	S92.313B	T22.319A	T23.731A
S82.466C	S82.872B	S92.065B	S92.314B	T22.321A	T23.732A
S82.491B	S82.872C	S92.066B	S92.315B	T22.322A	T23.739A
S82.491C	S82.873B	S92.101B	S92.316B	T22.329A	T23.741A
S82.492B	S82.873C	S92.102B	S92.321B	T22.331A	T23.742A
S82.492C	S82.874B	S92.109B	S92.322B	T22.332A	T23.749A
S82.499B	S82.874C	S92.111B	S92.323B	T22.339A	T23.751A
S82.499C	S82.875B	S92.112B	S92.324B	T22.341A	T23.752A
S82.51XB	S82.875C	S92.113B	S92.325B	T22.342A	T23.759A
S82.51XC	S82.876B	S92.114B	S92.326B	T22.349A	T23.761A
S82.52XB	S82.876C	S92.115B	S92.331B	T22.351A	T23.762A
S82.52XC	S82.891B	S92.116B	S92.332B	T22.352A	T23.769A
	S82.891C	S92.121B	S92.333B	T22.359A	T23.771A
	S82.892B	S92.122B	S92.334B	T22.361A	T23.772A

HAC 05: Falls and Trauma (continued)	T25.791A	T31.81	T32.84	T34.1XXA	T71.162A
T23.779A	T25.792A	T31.82	T32.85	T34.2XXA	T71.163A
T23.791A	T25.799A	T31.83	T32.86	T34.3XXA	T71.164A
T23.792A	T26.20XA	T31.84	T32.87	T34.40XA	T71.191A
T23.799A	T26.21XA	T31.85	T32.88	T34.41XA	T71.192A
T24.301A	T26.22XA	T31.86	T32.90	T34.42XA	T71.193A
T24.302A	T26.70XA	T31.87	T32.91	T34.511A	T71.194A
T24.309A	T26.71XA	T31.88	T32.92	T34.512A	T71.20XA
T24.311A	T26.72XA	T31.90	T32.93	T34.519A	T71.21XA
T24.312A	T27.0XXA	T31.91	T32.94	T34.521A	T71.29XA
T24.319A	T27.1XXA	T31.92	T32.95	T34.522A	T71.9XXA
T24.321A	T27.2XXA	T31.93	T32.96	T34.529A	T75.1XXA
T24.322A	T27.3XXA	T31.94	T32.97	T34.531A	
T24.329A	T27.4XXA	T31.95	T32.98	T34.532A	**HAC 06: Catheter Associated Urinary Tract Infection (UTI)**
T24.331A	T27.5XXA	T31.96	T32.99	T34.539A	
T24.332A	T27.6XXA	T31.97	T33.011A	T34.60XA	Secondary diagnosis not POA:
T24.339A	T27.7XXA	T31.98	T33.012A	T34.61XA	T83.511A
T24.391A	T28.1XXA	T31.99	T33.019A	T34.62XA	T83.518A
T24.392A	T28.2XXA	T32.10	T33.02XA	T34.70XA	
T24.399A	T28.6XXA	T32.11	T33.09XA	T34.71XA	**With or Without**
T24.701A	T28.7XXA	T32.20	T33.1XXA	T34.72XA	Secondary diagnosis (also not POA) of:
T24.702A	T31.10	T32.21	T33.2XXA	T34.811A	B37.41
T24.709A	T31.11	T32.22	T33.3XXA	T34.812A	B37.49
T24.711A	T31.20	T32.30	T33.40XA	T34.819A	N10
T24.712A	T31.21	T32.31	T33.41XA	T34.821A	N11.9
T24.719A	T31.22	T32.32	T33.42XA	T34.822A	N12
T24.721A	T31.30	T32.33	T33.511A	T34.829A	N13.6
T24.722A	T31.31	T32.40	T33.512A	T34.831A	N15.1
T24.729A	T31.32	T32.41	T33.519A	T34.832A	N28.84
T24.731A	T31.33	T32.42	T33.521A	T34.839A	N28.85
T24.732A	T31.40	T32.43	T33.522A	T34.90XA	N28.86
T24.739A	T31.41	T32.44	T33.529A	T34.99XA	N30.00
T24.791A	T31.42	T32.50	T33.531A	T67.0XXA	N30.01
T24.792A	T31.43	T32.51	T33.532A	T69.021A	N34.0
T24.799A	T31.44	T32.52	T33.539A	T69.022A	N39.0
T25.311A	T31.50	T32.53	T33.60XA	T69.029A	
T25.312A	T31.51	T32.54	T33.61XA	T70.3XXA	**HAC 07: Vascular Catheter Associated Infection**
T25.319A	T31.52	T32.55	T33.62XA	T71.111A	
T25.321A	T31.53	T32.60	T33.70XA	T71.112A	Secondary diagnosis not POA:
T25.322A	T31.54	T32.61	T33.71XA	T71.113A	T80.211A
T25.329A	T31.55	T32.62	T33.72XA	T71.114A	T80.212A
T25.331A	T31.60	T32.63	T33.811A	T71.121A	T80.218A
T25.332A	T31.61	T32.64	T33.812A	T71.122A	T80.219A
T25.339A	T31.62	T32.65	T33.819A	T71.123A	
T25.391A	T31.63	T32.66	T33.821A	T71.124A	
T25.392A	T31.64	T32.70	T33.822A	T71.131A	
T25.399A	T31.65	T32.71	T33.829A	T71.132A	
T25.711A	T31.66	T32.72	T33.831A	T71.133A	
T25.712A	T31.70	T32.73	T33.832A	T71.134A	
T25.719A	T31.71	T32.74	T33.839A	T71.141A	
T25.721A	T31.72	T32.75	T33.90XA	T71.143A	
T25.722A	T31.73	T32.76	T33.99XA	T71.144A	
T25.729A	T31.74	T32.77	T34.011A	T71.151A	
T25.731A	T31.75	T32.80	T34.012A	T71.152A	
T25.732A	T31.76	T32.81	T34.019A	T71.153A	
T25.739A	T31.77	T32.82	T34.02XA	T71.154A	
	T31.80	T32.83	T34.09XA	T71.161A	

HAC 08: Surgical Site Infection of Mediastinitis Following Coronary Bypass Graft (CABG) Procedures

Secondary diagnosis not POA:

J98.51

J98.59

AND

Any of the following procedures:

0210083 Bypass Coronary Artery, One Artery from Coronary Artery with Zooplastic Tissue, Open Approach

0210088 Bypass Coronary Artery, One Artery from Right Internal Mammary with Zooplastic Tissue, Open Approach

0210089 Bypass Coronary Artery, One Artery from Left Internal Mammary with Zooplastic Tissue, Open Approach

021008C Bypass Coronary Artery, One Artery from Thoracic Artery with Zooplastic Tissue, Open Approach

021008F Bypass Coronary Artery, One Artery from Abdominal Artery with Zooplastic Tissue, Open Approach

021008W Bypass Coronary Artery, One Artery from Aorta with Zooplastic Tissue, Open Approach

0210093 Bypass Coronary Artery, One Artery from Coronary Artery with Autologous Venous Tissue, Open Approach

0210098 Bypass Coronary Artery, One Artery from Right Internal Mammary with Autologous Venous Tissue, Open Approach

0210099 Bypass Coronary Artery, One Artery from Left Internal Mammary with Autologous Venous Tissue, Open Approach

021009C Bypass Coronary Artery, One Artery from Thoracic Artery with Autologous Venous Tissue, Open Approach

021009F Bypass Coronary Artery, One Artery from Abdominal Artery with Autologous Venous Tissue, Open Approach

021009W Bypass Coronary Artery, One Artery from Aorta with Autologous Venous Tissue, Open Approach

02100A3 Bypass Coronary Artery, One Artery from Coronary Artery with Autologous Arterial Tissue, Open Approach

02100A8 Bypass Coronary Artery, One Artery from Right Internal Mammary with Autologous Arterial Tissue, Open Approach

02100A9 Bypass Coronary Artery, One Artery from Left Internal Mammary with Autologous Arterial Tissue, Open Approach

02100AC Bypass Coronary Artery, One Artery from Thoracic Artery with Autologous Arterial Tissue, Open Approach

02100AF Bypass Coronary Artery, One Artery from Abdominal Artery with Autologous Arterial Tissue, Open Approach

02100AW Bypass Coronary Artery, One Artery from Aorta with Autologous Arterial Tissue, Open Approach

02100J3 Bypass Coronary Artery, One Artery from Coronary Artery with Synthetic Substitute, Open Approach

02100J8 Bypass Coronary Artery, One Artery from Right Internal Mammary with Synthetic Substitute, Open Approach

02100J9 Bypass Coronary Artery, One Artery from Left Internal Mammary with Synthetic Substitute, Open Approach

02100JC Bypass Coronary Artery, One Artery from Thoracic Artery with Synthetic Substitute, Open Approach

02100JF Bypass Coronary Artery, One Artery from Abdominal Artery with Synthetic Substitute, Open Approach

02100JW Bypass Coronary Artery, One Artery from Aorta with Synthetic Substitute, Open Approach

02100K3 Bypass Coronary Artery, One Artery from Coronary Artery with Nonautologous Tissue Substitute, Open Approach

02100K8 Bypass Coronary Artery, One Artery from Right Internal Mammary with Nonautologous Tissue Substitute, Open Approach

02100K9 Bypass Coronary Artery, One Artery from Left Internal Mammary with Nonautologous Tissue Substitute, Open Approach

02100KC Bypass Coronary Artery, One Artery from Thoracic Artery with Nonautologous Tissue Substitute, Open Approach

02100KF Bypass Coronary Artery, One Artery from Abdominal Artery with Nonautologous Tissue Substitute, Open Approach

02100KW Bypass Coronary Artery, One Artery from Aorta with Nonautologous Tissue Substitute, Open Approach

02100Z3 Bypass Coronary Artery, One Artery from Coronary Artery, Open Approach

02100Z8 Bypass Coronary Artery, One Artery from Right Internal Mammary, Open Approach

02100Z9 Bypass Coronary Artery, One Artery from Left Internal Mammary, Open Approach

02100ZC Bypass Coronary Artery, One Artery from Thoracic Artery, Open Approach

02100ZF Bypass Coronary Artery, One Artery from Abdominal Artery, Open Approach

0210483 Bypass Coronary Artery, One Artery from Coronary Artery with Zooplastic Tissue, Percutaneous Endoscopic Approach

0210488 Bypass Coronary Artery, One Artery from Right Internal Mammary with Zooplastic Tissue, Percutaneous Endoscopic Approach

0210489 Bypass Coronary Artery, One Artery from Left Internal Mammary with Zooplastic Tissue, Percutaneous Endoscopic Approach

021048C Bypass Coronary Artery, One Artery from Thoracic Artery with Zooplastic Tissue, Percutaneous Endoscopic Approach

021048F Bypass Coronary Artery, One Artery from Abdominal Artery with Zooplastic Tissue, Percutaneous Endoscopic Approach

021048W Bypass Coronary Artery, One Artery from Aorta with Zooplastic Tissue, Percutaneous Endoscopic Approach

0210493 Bypass Coronary Artery, One Artery from Coronary Artery with Autologous Venous Tissue, Percutaneous Endoscopic Approach

0210498 Bypass Coronary Artery, One Artery from Right Internal Mammary with Autologous Venous Tissue, Percutaneous Endoscopic Approach

0210499 Bypass Coronary Artery, One Artery from Left Internal Mammary with Autologous Venous Tissue, Percutaneous Endoscopic Approach

021049C Bypass Coronary Artery, One Artery from Thoracic Artery with Autologous Venous Tissue, Percutaneous Endoscopic Approach

021049F Bypass Coronary Artery, One Artery from Abdominal Artery with Autologous Venous Tissue, Percutaneous Endoscopic Approach

021049W Bypass Coronary Artery, One Artery from Aorta with Autologous Venous Tissue, Percutaneous Endoscopic Approach

02104A3 Bypass Coronary Artery, One Artery from Coronary Artery with Autologous Arterial Tissue, Percutaneous Endoscopic Approach

02104A8 Bypass Coronary Artery, One Artery from Right Internal Mammary with Autologous Arterial Tissue, Percutaneous Endoscopic Approach

02104A9 Bypass Coronary Artery, One Artery from Left Internal Mammary with Autologous Arterial Tissue, Percutaneous Endoscopic Approach

02104AC Bypass Coronary Artery, One Artery from Thoracic Artery with Autologous Arterial Tissue, Percutaneous Endoscopic Approach

02104AF Bypass Coronary Artery, One Artery from Abdominal Artery with Autologous Arterial Tissue, Percutaneous Endoscopic Approach

02104AW Bypass Coronary Artery, One Artery from Aorta with Autologous Arterial Tissue, Percutaneous Endoscopic Approach

02104J3 Bypass Coronary Artery, One Artery from Coronary Artery with Synthetic Substitute, Percutaneous Endoscopic Approach

02104J8 Bypass Coronary Artery, One Artery from Right Internal Mammary with Synthetic Substitute, Percutaneous Endoscopic Approach

02104J9 Bypass Coronary Artery, One Artery from Left Internal Mammary with Synthetic Substitute, Percutaneous Endoscopic Approach

02104JC Bypass Coronary Artery, One Artery from Thoracic Artery with Synthetic Substitute, Percutaneous Endoscopic Approach

02104JF Bypass Coronary Artery, One Artery from Abdominal Artery with Synthetic Substitute, Percutaneous Endoscopic Approach

02104JW Bypass Coronary Artery, One Artery from Aorta with Synthetic Substitute, Percutaneous Endoscopic Approach

02104K3 Bypass Coronary Artery, One Artery from Coronary Artery with Nonautologous Tissue Substitute, Percutaneous Endoscopic Approach

02104K8 Bypass Coronary Artery, One Artery from Right Internal Mammary with Nonautologous Tissue Substitute, Percutaneous Endoscopic Approach

02104K9 Bypass Coronary Artery, One Artery from Left Internal Mammary with Nonautologous Tissue Substitute, Percutaneous Endoscopic Approach

02104KC Bypass Coronary Artery, One Artery from Thoracic Artery with Nonautologous Tissue Substitute, Percutaneous Endoscopic Approach

02104KF Bypass Coronary Artery, One Artery from Abdominal Artery with Nonautologous Tissue Substitute, Percutaneous Endoscopic Approach

02104KW Bypass Coronary Artery, One Artery from Aorta with Nonautologous Tissue Substitute, Percutaneous Endoscopic Approach

02104Z3 Bypass Coronary Artery, One Artery from Coronary Artery, Percutaneous Endoscopic Approach

HAC 08: Surgical Artery Infection of Mediastinitis Following Coronary Bypass Graft (CABG) Procedures (continued)

0210478   Bypass Coronary Artery, One Artery from Right Internal Mammary, Percutaneous Endoscopic Approach

0210479   Bypass Coronary Artery, One Artery from Left Internal Mammary, Percutaneous Endoscopic Approach

02104ZC   Bypass Coronary Artery, One Artery from Thoracic Artery, Percutaneous Endoscopic Approach

02104ZF   Bypass Coronary Artery, One Artery from Abdominal Artery, Percutaneous Endoscopic Approach

0211083   Bypass Coronary Artery, Two Arteries from Coronary Artery with Zooplastic Tissue, Open Approach

0211088   Bypass Coronary Artery, Two Arteries from Right Internal Mammary with Zooplastic Tissue, Open Approach

0211089   Bypass Coronary Artery, Two Arteries from Left Internal Mammary with Zooplastic Tissue, Open Approach

021108C   Bypass Coronary Artery, Two Arteries from Thoracic Artery with Zooplastic Tissue, Open Approach

021108F   Bypass Coronary Artery, Two Arteries from Abdominal Artery with Zooplastic Tissue, Open Approach

021108W   Bypass Coronary Artery, Two Arteries from Aorta with Zooplastic Tissue, Open Approach

0211093   Bypass Coronary Artery, Two Arteries from Coronary Artery with Autologous Venous Tissue, Open Approach

0211098   Bypass Coronary Artery, Two Arteries from Right Internal Mammary with Autologous Venous Tissue, Open Approach

0211099   Bypass Coronary Artery, Two Arteries from Left Internal Mammary with Autologous Venous Tissue, Open Approach

021109C   Bypass Coronary Artery, Two Arteries from Thoracic Artery with Autologous Venous Tissue, Open Approach

021109F   Bypass Coronary Artery, Two Arteries from Abdominal Artery with Autologous Venous Tissue, Open Approach

021109W   Bypass Coronary Artery, Two Arteries from Aorta with Autologous Venous Tissue, Open Approach

02110A3   Bypass Coronary Artery, Two Arteries from Coronary Artery with Autologous Arterial Tissue, Open Approach

02110A8   Bypass Coronary Artery, Two Arteries from Right Internal Mammary with Autologous Arterial Tissue, Open Approach

02110A9   Bypass Coronary Artery, Two Arteries from Left Internal Mammary with Autologous Arterial Tissue, Open Approach

02110AC   Bypass Coronary Artery, Two Arteries from Thoracic Artery with Autologous Arterial Tissue, Open Approach

02110AF   Bypass Coronary Artery, Two Arteries from Abdominal Artery with Autologous Arterial Tissue, Open Approach

02110AW   Bypass Coronary Artery, Two Arteries from Aorta with Autologous Arterial Tissue, Open Approach

02110J3   Bypass Coronary Artery, Two Arteries from Coronary Artery with Synthetic Substitute, Open Approach

02110J8   Bypass Coronary Artery, Two Arteries from Right Internal Mammary with Synthetic Substitute, Open Approach

02110J9   Bypass Coronary Artery, Two Arteries from Left Internal Mammary with Synthetic Substitute, Open Approach

02110JC   Bypass Coronary Artery, Two Arteries from Thoracic Artery with Synthetic Substitute, Open Approach

02110JF   Bypass Coronary Artery, Two Arteries from Abdominal Artery with Synthetic Substitute, Open Approach

02110JW   Bypass Coronary Artery, Two Arteries from Aorta with Synthetic Substitute, Open Approach

02110K3   Bypass Coronary Artery, Two Arteries from Coronary Artery with Nonautologous Tissue Substitute, Open Approach

02110K8   Bypass Coronary Artery, Two Arteries from Right Internal Mammary with Nonautologous Tissue Substitute, Open Approach

02110K9   Bypass Coronary Artery, Two Arteries from Left Internal Mammary with Nonautologous Tissue Substitute, Open Approach

02110KC   Bypass Coronary Artery, Two Arteries from Thoracic Artery with Nonautologous Tissue Substitute, Open Approach

02110KF   Bypass Coronary Artery, Two Arteries from Abdominal Artery with Nonautologous Tissue Substitute, Open Approach

02110KW   Bypass Coronary Artery, Two Arteries from Aorta with Nonautologous Tissue Substitute, Open Approach

02110Z3   Bypass Coronary Artery, Two Arteries from Coronary Artery, Open Approach

02110Z8   Bypass Coronary Artery, Two Arteries from Right Internal Mammary, Open Approach

02110Z9   Bypass Coronary Artery, Two Arteries from Left Internal Mammary, Open Approach

02110ZC   Bypass Coronary Artery, Two Arteries from Thoracic Artery, Open Approach

02110ZF   Bypass Coronary Artery, Two Arteries from Abdominal Artery, Open Approach

0211483   Bypass Coronary Artery, Two Arteries from Coronary Artery with Zooplastic Tissue, Percutaneous Endoscopic Approach

0211488   Bypass Coronary Artery, Two Arteries from Right Internal Mammary with Zooplastic Tissue, Percutaneous Endoscopic Approach

0211489   Bypass Coronary Artery, Two Arteries from Left Internal Mammary with Zooplastic Tissue, Percutaneous Endoscopic Approach

021148C   Bypass Coronary Artery, Two Arteries from Thoracic Artery with Zooplastic Tissue, Percutaneous Endoscopic Approach

021148F   Bypass Coronary Artery, Two Arteries from Abdominal Artery with Zooplastic Tissue, Percutaneous Endoscopic Approach

021148W   Bypass Coronary Artery, Two Arteries from Aorta with Zooplastic Tissue, Percutaneous Endoscopic Approach

0211493   Bypass Coronary Artery, Two Arteries from Coronary Artery with Autologous Venous Tissue, Percutaneous Endoscopic Approach

0211498   Bypass Coronary Artery, Two Arteries from Right Internal Mammary with Autologous Venous Tissue, Percutaneous Endoscopic Approach

0211499   Bypass Coronary Artery, Two Arteries from Left Internal Mammary with Autologous Venous Tissue, Percutaneous Endoscopic Approach

021149C   Bypass Coronary Artery, Two Arteries from Thoracic Artery with Autologous Venous Tissue, Percutaneous Endoscopic Approach

021149F   Bypass Coronary Artery, Two Arteries from Abdominal Artery with Autologous Venous Tissue, Percutaneous Endoscopic Approach

021149W   Bypass Coronary Artery, Two Arteries from Aorta with Autologous Venous Tissue, Percutaneous Endoscopic Approach

02114A3   Bypass Coronary Artery, Two Arteries from Coronary Artery with Autologous Arterial Tissue, Percutaneous Endoscopic Approach

02114A8   Bypass Coronary Artery, Two Arteries from Right Internal Mammary with Autologous Arterial Tissue, Percutaneous Endoscopic Approach

02114A9   Bypass Coronary Artery, Two Arteries from Left Internal Mammary with Autologous Arterial Tissue, Percutaneous Endoscopic Approach

02114AC   Bypass Coronary Artery, Two Arteries from Thoracic Artery with Autologous Arterial Tissue, Percutaneous Endoscopic Approach

02114AF   Bypass Coronary Artery, Two Arteries from Abdominal Artery with Autologous Arterial Tissue, Percutaneous Endoscopic Approach

02114AW   Bypass Coronary Artery, Two Arteries from Aorta with Autologous Arterial Tissue, Percutaneous Endoscopic Approach

02114J3   Bypass Coronary Artery, Two Arteries from Coronary Artery with Synthetic Substitute, Percutaneous Endoscopic Approach

02114J8   Bypass Coronary Artery, Two Arteries from Right Internal Mammary with Synthetic Substitute, Percutaneous Endoscopic Approach

02114J9   Bypass Coronary Artery, Two Arteries from Left Internal Mammary with Synthetic Substitute, Percutaneous Endoscopic Approach

02114JC   Bypass Coronary Artery, Two Arteries from Thoracic Artery with Synthetic Substitute, Percutaneous Endoscopic Approach

02114JF   Bypass Coronary Artery, Two Arteries from Abdominal Artery with Synthetic Substitute, Percutaneous Endoscopic Approach

02114JW   Bypass Coronary Artery, Two Arteries from Aorta with Synthetic Substitute, Percutaneous Endoscopic Approach

02114K3   Bypass Coronary Artery, Two Arteries from Coronary Artery with Nonautologous Tissue Substitute, Percutaneous Endoscopic Approach

02114K8   Bypass Coronary Artery, Two Arteries from Right Internal Mammary with Nonautologous Tissue Substitute, Percutaneous Endoscopic Approach

HAC 08: Surgical Site Infection of Mediastinitis Following Coronary Bypass Graft (CABG) Procedures (continued)

0211 4K9 Bypass Coronary Artery, Two Arteries from Left Internal Mammary with Nonautologous Tissue Substitute, Percutaneous Endoscopic Approach

0211 4KC Bypass Coronary Artery, Two Arteries from Thoracic Artery with Nonautologous Tissue Substitute, Percutaneous Endoscopic Approach

0211 4KF Bypass Coronary Artery, Two Arteries from Abdominal Artery with Nonautologous Tissue Substitute, Percutaneous Endoscopic Approach

0211 4KW Bypass Coronary Artery, Two Arteries from Aorta with Nonautologous Tissue Substitute, Percutaneous Endoscopic Approach

0211 4Z3 Bypass Coronary Artery, Two Arteries from Coronary Artery, Percutaneous Endoscopic Approach

0211 4Z8 Bypass Coronary Artery, Two Arteries from Right Internal Mammary, Percutaneous Endoscopic Approach

0211 4Z9 Bypass Coronary Artery, Two Arteries from Left Internal Mammary, Percutaneous Endoscopic Approach

0211 4ZC Bypass Coronary Artery, Two Arteries from Thoracic Artery, Percutaneous Endoscopic Approach

0211 4ZF Bypass Coronary Artery, Two Arteries from Abdominal Artery, Percutaneous Endoscopic Approach

0212 083 Bypass Coronary Artery, Three Arteries from Coronary Artery with Zooplastic Tissue, Open Approach

0212 088 Bypass Coronary Artery, Three Arteries from Right Internal Mammary with Zooplastic Tissue, Open Approach

0212 089 Bypass Coronary Artery, Three Arteries from Left Internal Mammary with Zooplastic Tissue, Open Approach

0212 08C Bypass Coronary Artery, Three Arteries from Thoracic Artery with Zooplastic Tissue, Open Approach

0212 08F Bypass Coronary Artery, Three Arteries from Abdominal Artery with Zooplastic Tissue, Open Approach

0212 08W Bypass Coronary Artery, Three Arteries from Aorta with Zooplastic Tissue, Open Approach

0212 093 Bypass Coronary Artery, Three Arteries from Coronary Artery with Autologous Venous Tissue, Open Approach

0212 098 Bypass Coronary Artery, Three Arteries from Right Internal Mammary with Autologous Venous Tissue, Open Approach

0212 099 Bypass Coronary Artery, Three Arteries from Left Internal Mammary with Autologous Venous Tissue, Open Approach

0212 09C Bypass Coronary Artery, Three Arteries from Thoracic Artery with Autologous Venous Tissue, Open Approach

0212 09F Bypass Coronary Artery, Three Arteries from Abdominal Artery with Autologous Venous Tissue, Open Approach

0212 09W Bypass Coronary Artery, Three Arteries from Aorta with Autologous Venous Tissue, Open Approach

0212 0A3 Bypass Coronary Artery, Three Arteries from Coronary Artery with Autologous Arterial Tissue, Open Approach

0212 0A8 Bypass Coronary Artery, Three Arteries from Right Internal Mammary with Autologous Arterial Tissue, Open Approach

0212 0A9 Bypass Coronary Artery, Three Arteries from Left Internal Mammary with Autologous Arterial Tissue, Open Approach

0212 0AC Bypass Coronary Artery, Three Arteries from Thoracic Artery with Autologous Arterial Tissue, Open Approach

0212 0AF Bypass Coronary Artery, Three Arteries from Abdominal Artery with Autologous Arterial Tissue, Open Approach

0212 0AW Bypass Coronary Artery, Three Arteries from Aorta with Autologous Arterial Tissue, Open Approach

0212 0J3 Bypass Coronary Artery, Three Arteries from Coronary Artery with Synthetic Substitute, Open Approach

0212 0J8 Bypass Coronary Artery, Three Arteries from Right Internal Mammary with Synthetic Substitute, Open Approach

0212 0J9 Bypass Coronary Artery, Three Arteries from Left Internal Mammary with Synthetic Substitute, Open Approach

0212 0JC Bypass Coronary Artery, Three Arteries from Thoracic Artery with Synthetic Substitute, Open Approach

0212 0JF Bypass Coronary Artery, Three Arteries from Abdominal Artery with Synthetic Substitute, Open Approach

0212 0JW Bypass Coronary Artery, Three Arteries from Aorta with Synthetic Substitute, Open Approach

0212 0K3 Bypass Coronary Artery, Three Arteries from Coronary Artery with Nonautologous Tissue Substitute, Open Approach

0212 0K8 Bypass Coronary Artery, Three Arteries from Right Internal Mammary with Nonautologous Tissue Substitute, Open Approach

0212 0K9 Bypass Coronary Artery, Three Arteries from Left Internal Mammary with Nonautologous Tissue Substitute, Open Approach

0212 0KC Bypass Coronary Artery, Three Arteries from Thoracic Artery with Nonautologous Tissue Substitute, Open Approach

0212 0KF Bypass Coronary Artery, Three Arteries from Abdominal Artery with Nonautologous Tissue Substitute, Open Approach

0212 0KW Bypass Coronary Artery, Three Arteries from Aorta with Nonautologous Tissue Substitute, Open Approach

0212 0Z3 Bypass Coronary Artery, Three Arteries from Coronary Artery, Open Approach

0212 0Z8 Bypass Coronary Artery, Three Arteries from Right Internal Mammary, Open Approach

0212 0Z9 Bypass Coronary Artery, Three Arteries from Left Internal Mammary, Open Approach

0212 0ZC Bypass Coronary Artery, Three Arteries from Thoracic Artery, Open Approach

0212 0ZF Bypass Coronary Artery, Three Arteries from Abdominal Artery, Open Approach

0212 483 Bypass Coronary Artery, Three Arteries from Coronary Artery with Zooplastic Tissue, Percutaneous Endoscopic Approach

0212 488 Bypass Coronary Artery, Three Arteries from Right Internal Mammary with Zooplastic Tissue, Percutaneous Endoscopic Approach

0212 489 Bypass Coronary Artery, Three Arteries from Left Internal Mammary with Zooplastic Tissue, Percutaneous Endoscopic Approach

0212 48C Bypass Coronary Artery, Three Arteries from Thoracic Artery with Zooplastic Tissue, Percutaneous Endoscopic Approach

0212 48F Bypass Coronary Artery, Three Arteries from Abdominal Artery with Zooplastic Tissue, Percutaneous Endoscopic Approach

0212 48W Bypass Coronary Artery, Three Arteries from Aorta with Zooplastic Tissue, Percutaneous Endoscopic Approach

0212 493 Bypass Coronary Artery, Three Arteries from Coronary Artery with Autologous Venous Tissue, Percutaneous Endoscopic Approach

0212 498 Bypass Coronary Artery, Three Arteries from Right Internal Mammary with Autologous Venous Tissue, Percutaneous Endoscopic Approach

0212 499 Bypass Coronary Artery, Three Arteries from Left Internal Mammary with Autologous Venous Tissue, Percutaneous Endoscopic Approach

0212 49C Bypass Coronary Artery, Three Arteries from Thoracic Artery with Autologous Venous Tissue, Percutaneous Endoscopic Approach

0212 49F Bypass Coronary Artery, Three Arteries from Abdominal Artery with Autologous Venous Tissue, Percutaneous Endoscopic Approach

0212 49W Bypass Coronary Artery, Three Arteries from Aorta with Autologous Venous Tissue, Percutaneous Endoscopic Approach

0212 4A3 Bypass Coronary Artery, Three Arteries from Coronary Artery with Autologous Arterial Tissue, Percutaneous Endoscopic Approach

0212 4A8 Bypass Coronary Artery, Three Arteries from Right Internal Mammary with Autologous Arterial Tissue, Percutaneous Endoscopic Approach

0212 4A9 Bypass Coronary Artery, Three Arteries from Left Internal Mammary with Autologous Arterial Tissue, Percutaneous Endoscopic Approach

0212 4AC Bypass Coronary Artery, Three Arteries from Thoracic Artery with Autologous Arterial Tissue, Percutaneous Endoscopic Approach

0212 4AF Bypass Coronary Artery, Three Arteries from Abdominal Artery with Autologous Arterial Tissue, Percutaneous Endoscopic Approach

0212 4AW Bypass Coronary Artery, Three Arteries from Aorta with Autologous Arterial Tissue, Percutaneous Endoscopic Approach

0212 4J3 Bypass Coronary Artery, Three Arteries from Coronary Artery with Synthetic Substitute, Percutaneous Endoscopic Approach

0212 4J8 Bypass Coronary Artery, Three Arteries from Right Internal Mammary with Synthetic Substitute, Percutaneous Endoscopic Approach

HAC 08: Surgical Site Infection of Mediastinitis Following Coronary Bypass Graft (CABG) Procedures (continued)

Ø2124J9 Bypass Coronary Artery, Three Arteries from Left Internal Mammary with Synthetic Substitute, Percutaneous Endoscopic Approach

Ø2124JC Bypass Coronary Artery, Three Arteries from Thoracic Artery with Synthetic Substitute, Percutaneous Endoscopic Approach

Ø2124JF Bypass Coronary Artery, Three Arteries from Abdominal Artery with Synthetic Substitute, Percutaneous Endoscopic Approach

Ø2124JW Bypass Coronary Artery, Three Arteries from Aorta with Synthetic Substitute, Percutaneous Endoscopic Approach

Ø2124K3 Bypass Coronary Artery, Three Arteries from Coronary Artery with Nonautologous Tissue Substitute, Percutaneous Endoscopic Approach

Ø2124K8 Bypass Coronary Artery, Three Arteries from Right Internal Mammary with Nonautologous Tissue Substitute, Percutaneous Endoscopic Approach

Ø2124K9 Bypass Coronary Artery, Three Arteries from Left Internal Mammary with Nonautologous Tissue Substitute, Percutaneous Endoscopic Approach

Ø2124KC Bypass Coronary Artery, Three Arteries from Thoracic Artery with Nonautologous Tissue Substitute, Percutaneous Endoscopic Approach

Ø2124KF Bypass Coronary Artery, Three Arteries from Abdominal Artery with Nonautologous Tissue Substitute, Percutaneous Endoscopic Approach

Ø2124KW Bypass Coronary Artery, Three Arteries from Aorta with Nonautologous Tissue Substitute, Percutaneous Endoscopic Approach

Ø2124Z3 Bypass Coronary Artery, Three Arteries from Coronary Artery, Percutaneous Endoscopic Approach

Ø2124Z8 Bypass Coronary Artery, Three Arteries from Right Internal Mammary, Percutaneous Endoscopic Approach

Ø2124Z9 Bypass Coronary Artery, Three Arteries from Left Internal Mammary, Percutaneous Endoscopic Approach

Ø2124ZC Bypass Coronary Artery, Three Arteries from Thoracic Artery, Percutaneous Endoscopic Approach

Ø2124ZF Bypass Coronary Artery, Three Arteries from Abdominal Artery, Percutaneous Endoscopic Approach

Ø213Ø83 Bypass Coronary Artery, Four or More Arteries from Coronary Artery with Zooplastic Tissue, Open Approach

Ø213Ø88 Bypass Coronary Artery, Four or More Arteries from Right Internal Mammary with Zooplastic Tissue, Open Approach

Ø213Ø89 Bypass Coronary Artery, Four or More Arteries from Left Internal Mammary with Zooplastic Tissue, Open Approach

Ø213Ø8C Bypass Coronary Artery, Four or More Arteries from Thoracic Artery with Zooplastic Tissue, Open Approach

Ø213Ø8F Bypass Coronary Artery, Four or More Arteries from Abdominal Artery with Zooplastic Tissue, Open Approach

Ø213Ø8W Bypass Coronary Artery, Four or More Arteries from Aorta with Zooplastic Tissue, Open Approach

Ø213Ø93 Bypass Coronary Artery, Four or More Arteries from Coronary Artery with Autologous Venous Tissue, Open Approach

Ø213Ø98 Bypass Coronary Artery, Four or More Arteries from Right Internal Mammary with Autologous Venous Tissue, Open Approach

Ø213Ø99 Bypass Coronary Artery, Four or More Arteries from Left Internal Mammary with Autologous Venous Tissue, Open Approach

Ø21309C Bypass Coronary Artery, Four or More Arteries from Thoracic Artery with Autologous Venous Tissue, Open Approach

Ø21309F Bypass Coronary Artery, Four or More Arteries from Abdominal Artery with Autologous Venous Tissue, Open Approach

Ø21309W Bypass Coronary Artery, Four or More Arteries from Aorta with Autologous Venous Tissue, Open Approach

Ø2130A3 Bypass Coronary Artery, Four or More Arteries from Coronary Artery with Autologous Arterial Tissue, Open Approach

Ø2130A8 Bypass Coronary Artery, Four or More Arteries from Right Internal Mammary with Autologous Arterial Tissue, Open Approach

Ø2130A9 Bypass Coronary Artery, Four or More Arteries from Left Internal Mammary with Autologous Arterial Tissue, Open Approach

Ø2130AC Bypass Coronary Artery, Four or More Arteries from Thoracic Artery with Autologous Arterial Tissue, Open Approach

Ø2130AF Bypass Coronary Artery, Four or More Arteries from Abdominal Artery with Autologous Arterial Tissue, Open Approach

Ø2130AW Bypass Coronary Artery, Four or More Arteries from Aorta with Autologous Arterial Tissue, Open Approach

Ø2130J3 Bypass Coronary Artery, Four or More Arteries from Coronary Artery with Synthetic Substitute, Open Approach

Ø2130J8 Bypass Coronary Artery, Four or More Arteries from Right Internal Mammary with Synthetic Substitute, Open Approach

Ø2130J9 Bypass Coronary Artery, Four or More Arteries from Left Internal Mammary with Synthetic Substitute, Open Approach

Ø2130JC Bypass Coronary Artery, Four or More Arteries from Thoracic Artery with Synthetic Substitute, Open Approach

Ø2130JF Bypass Coronary Artery, Four or More Arteries from Abdominal Artery with Synthetic Substitute, Open Approach

Ø2130JW Bypass Coronary Artery, Four or More Arteries from Aorta with Synthetic Substitute, Open Approach

Ø2130K3 Bypass Coronary Artery, Four or More Arteries from Coronary Artery with Nonautologous Tissue Substitute, Open Approach

Ø2130K8 Bypass Coronary Artery, Four or More Arteries from Right Internal Mammary with Nonautologous Tissue Substitute, Open Approach

Ø2130K9 Bypass Coronary Artery, Four or More Arteries from Left Internal Mammary with Nonautologous Tissue Substitute, Open Approach

Ø2130KC Bypass Coronary Artery, Four or More Arteries from Thoracic Artery with Nonautologous Tissue Substitute, Open Approach

Ø2130KF Bypass Coronary Artery, Four or More Arteries from Abdominal Artery with Nonautologous Tissue Substitute, Open Approach

Ø2130KW Bypass Coronary Artery, Four or More Arteries from Aorta with Nonautologous Tissue Substitute, Open Approach

Ø2130Z3 Bypass Coronary Artery, Four or More Arteries from Coronary Artery, Open Approach

Ø2130Z8 Bypass Coronary Artery, Four or More Arteries from Right Internal Mammary, Open Approach

Ø2130Z9 Bypass Coronary Artery, Four or More Arteries from Left Internal Mammary, Open Approach

Ø2130ZC Bypass Coronary Artery, Four or More Arteries from Thoracic Artery, Open Approach

Ø2130ZF Bypass Coronary Artery, Four or More Arteries from Abdominal Artery, Open Approach

Ø213483 Bypass Coronary Artery, Four or More Arteries from Coronary Artery with Zooplastic Tissue, Percutaneous Endoscopic Approach

Ø213488 Bypass Coronary Artery, Four or More Arteries from Right Internal Mammary with Zooplastic Tissue, Percutaneous Endoscopic Approach

Ø213489 Bypass Coronary Artery, Four or More Arteries from Left Internal Mammary with Zooplastic Tissue, Percutaneous Endoscopic Approach

Ø21348C Bypass Coronary Artery, Four or More Arteries from Thoracic Artery with Zooplastic Tissue, Percutaneous Endoscopic Approach

Ø21348F Bypass Coronary Artery, Four or More Arteries from Abdominal Artery with Zooplastic Tissue, Percutaneous Endoscopic Approach

Ø21348W Bypass Coronary Artery, Four or More Arteries from Aorta with Zooplastic Tissue, Percutaneous Endoscopic Approach

Ø213493 Bypass Coronary Artery, Four or More Arteries from Coronary Artery with Autologous Venous Tissue, Percutaneous Endoscopic Approach

Ø213498 Bypass Coronary Artery, Four or More Arteries from Right Internal Mammary with Autologous Venous Tissue, Percutaneous Endoscopic Approach

Ø213499 Bypass Coronary Artery, Four or More Arteries from Left Internal Mammary with Autologous Venous Tissue, Percutaneous Endoscopic Approach

Ø21349C Bypass Coronary Artery, Four or More Arteries from Thoracic Artery with Autologous Venous Tissue, Percutaneous Endoscopic Approach

Ø21349F Bypass Coronary Artery, Four or More Arteries from Abdominal Artery with Autologous Venous Tissue, Percutaneous Endoscopic Approach

Ø21349W Bypass Coronary Artery, Four or More Arteries from Aorta with Autologous Venous Tissue, Percutaneous Endoscopic Approach

HAC 08: Surgical Site Infection of Mediastinitis Following Coronary Bypass Graft (CABG) Procedures (continued)

02134A3 Bypass Coronary Artery, Four or More Arteries from Coronary Artery with Autologous Arterial Tissue, Percutaneous Endoscopic Approach

02134A8 Bypass Coronary Artery, Four or More Arteries from Right Internal Mammary with Autologous Arterial Tissue, Percutaneous Endoscopic Approach

02134A9 Bypass Coronary Artery, Four or More Arteries from Left Internal Mammary with Autologous Arterial Tissue, Percutaneous Endoscopic Approach

02134AC Bypass Coronary Artery, Four or More Arteries from Thoracic Artery with Autologous Arterial Tissue, Percutaneous Endoscopic Approach

02134AF Bypass Coronary Artery, Four or More Arteries from Abdominal Artery with Autologous Arterial Tissue, Percutaneous Endoscopic Approach

02134AW Bypass Coronary Artery, Four or More Arteries from Aorta with Autologous Arterial Tissue, Percutaneous Endoscopic Approach

02134J3 Bypass Coronary Artery, Four or More Arteries from Coronary Artery with Synthetic Substitute, Percutaneous Endoscopic Approach

02134J8 Bypass Coronary Artery, Four or More Arteries from Right Internal Mammary with Synthetic Substitute, Percutaneous Endoscopic Approach

02134J9 Bypass Coronary Artery, Four or More Arteries from Left Internal Mammary with Synthetic Substitute, Percutaneous Endoscopic Approach

02134JC Bypass Coronary Artery, Four or More Arteries from Thoracic Artery with Synthetic Substitute, Percutaneous Endoscopic Approach

02134JF Bypass Coronary Artery, Four or More Arteries from Abdominal Artery with Synthetic Substitute, Percutaneous Endoscopic Approach

02134JW Bypass Coronary Artery, Four or More Arteries from Aorta with Synthetic Substitute, Percutaneous Endoscopic Approach

02134K3 Bypass Coronary Artery, Four or More Arteries from Coronary Artery with Nonautologous Tissue Substitute, Percutaneous Endoscopic Approach

02134K8 Bypass Coronary Artery, Four or More Arteries from Right Internal Mammary with Nonautologous Tissue Substitute, Percutaneous Endoscopic Approach

02134K9 Bypass Coronary Artery, Four or More Arteries from Left Internal Mammary with Nonautologous Tissue Substitute, Percutaneous Endoscopic Approach

02134KC Bypass Coronary Artery, Four or More Arteries from Thoracic Artery with Nonautologous Tissue Substitute, Percutaneous Endoscopic Approach

02134KF Bypass Coronary Artery, Four or More Arteries from Abdominal Artery with Nonautologous Tissue Substitute, Percutaneous Endoscopic Approach

02134KW Bypass Coronary Artery, Four or More Arteries from Aorta with Nonautologous Tissue Substitute, Percutaneous Endoscopic Approach

02134Z3 Bypass Coronary Artery, Four or More Arteries from Coronary Artery, Percutaneous Endoscopic Approach

02134Z8 Bypass Coronary Artery, Four or More Arteries from Right Internal Mammary, Percutaneous Endoscopic Approach

02134Z9 Bypass Coronary Artery, Four or More Arteries from Left Internal Mammary, Percutaneous Endoscopic Approach

02134ZC Bypass Coronary Artery, Four or More Arteries from Thoracic Artery, Percutaneous Endoscopic Approach

02134ZF Bypass Coronary Artery, Four or More Arteries from Abdominal Artery, Percutaneous Endoscopic Approach

HAC 09: Manifestations of Poor Glycemic Control

Secondary diagnosis not POA:

E08.00
E08.01
E08.10
E09.00
E09.01
E09.10
E10.10
E11.00
E11.01
E13.00
E13.01
E13.10
E15

HAC 10: Deep Vein Thrombosis (DVT) or Pulmonary Embolism (PE) with Total Knee or Hip Replacement

Secondary diagnosis not POA:

I26.02
I26.09
I26.92
I26.99
I82.401
I82.402
I82.403
I82.409
I82.411
I82.412
I82.413
I82.419
I82.421
I82.422
I82.423
I82.429
I82.431
I82.432
I82.433
I82.439
I82.441
I82.442
I82.443
I82.449
I82.491
I82.492
I82.493
I82.499
I82.4Y1
I82.4Y2
I82.4Y3
I82.4Y9
I82.4Z1
I82.4Z2
I82.4Z3
I82.4Z9

AND

Any of the following procedures:

0SR9019 Replacement of Right Hip Joint with Metal Synthetic Substitute, Cemented, Open Approach

0SR901A Replacement of Right Hip Joint with Metal Synthetic Substitute, Uncemented, Open Approach

0SR901Z Replacement of Right Hip Joint with Metal Synthetic Substitute, Open Approach

0SR9029 Replacement of Right Hip Joint with Metal on Polyethylene Synthetic Substitute, Cemented, Open Approach

0SR902A Replacement of Right Hip Joint with Metal on Polyethylene Synthetic Substitute, Uncemented, Open Approach

0SR902Z Replacement of Right Hip Joint with Metal on Polyethylene Synthetic Substitute, Open Approach

0SR9039 Replacement of Right Hip Joint with Ceramic Synthetic Substitute, Cemented, Open Approach

0SR903A Replacement of Right Hip Joint with Ceramic Synthetic Substitute, Uncemented, Open Approach

0SR903Z Replacement of Right Hip Joint with Ceramic Synthetic Substitute, Open Approach

0SR9049 Replacement of Right Hip Joint with Ceramic on Polyethylene Synthetic Substitute, Cemented, Open Approach

0SR904A Replacement of Right Hip Joint with Ceramic on Polyethylene Synthetic Substitute, Uncemented, Open Approach

0SR904Z Replacement of Right Hip Joint with Ceramic on Polyethylene Synthetic Substitute, Open Approach

0SR907Z Replacement of Right Hip Joint with Autologous Tissue Substitute, Open Approach

0SR90J9 Replacement of Right Hip Joint with Synthetic Substitute, Cemented, Open Approach

0SR90JA Replacement of Right Hip Joint with Synthetic Substitute, Uncemented, Open Approach

0SR90JZ Replacement of Right Hip Joint with Synthetic Substitute, Open Approach

0SR90KZ Replacement of Right Hip Joint with Nonautologous Tissue Substitute, Open Approach

0SRA009 Replacement of Right Hip Joint, Acetabular Surface with Polyethylene Synthetic Substitute, Cemented, Open Approach

0SRA00A Replacement of Right Hip Joint, Acetabular Surface with Polyethylene Synthetic Substitute, Uncemented, Open Approach

0SRA00Z Replacement of Right Hip Joint, Acetabular Surface with Polyethylene Synthetic Substitute, Open Approach

0SRA019 Replacement of Right Hip Joint, Acetabular Surface with Metal Synthetic Substitute, Cemented, Open Approach

0SRA01A Replacement of Right Hip Joint, Acetabular Surface with Metal Synthetic Substitute, Uncemented, Open Approach

0SRA01Z Replacement of Right Hip Joint, Acetabular Surface with Metal Synthetic Substitute, Open Approach

0SRA039 Replacement of Right Hip Joint, Acetabular Surface with Ceramic Synthetic Substitute, Cemented, Open Approach

0SRA03A Replacement of Right Hip Joint, Acetabular Surface with Ceramic Synthetic Substitute, Uncemented, Open Approach

HAC 10: Deep Vein Thrombosis (DVT) or Pulmonary Embolism (PE) with Total Knee or Hip Replacement (continued)

ØSRAØ3Z   Replacement of Right Hip Joint, Acetabular Surface with Ceramic Synthetic Substitute, Open Approach

ØSRAØ7Z   Replacement of Right Hip Joint, Acetabular Surface with Autologous Tissue Substitute, Open Approach

ØSRAØJ9   Replacement of Right Hip Joint, Acetabular Surface with Synthetic Substitute, Cemented, Open Approach

ØSRAØJA   Replacement of Right Hip Joint, Acetabular Surface with Synthetic Substitute, Uncemented, Open Approach

ØSRAØJZ   Replacement of Right Hip Joint, Acetabular Surface with Synthetic Substitute, Open Approach

ØSRAØKZ   Replacement of Right Hip Joint, Acetabular Surface with Nonautologous Tissue Substitute, Open Approach

ØSRBØ19   Replacement of Left Hip Joint with Metal Synthetic Substitute, Cemented, Open Approach

ØSRBØ1A   Replacement of Left Hip Joint with Metal Synthetic Substitute, Uncemented, Open Approach

ØSRBØ1Z   Replacement of Left Hip Joint with Metal Synthetic Substitute, Open Approach

ØSRBØ29   Replacement of Left Hip Joint with Metal on Polyethylene Synthetic Substitute, Cemented, Open Approach

ØSRBØ2A   Replacement of Left Hip Joint with Metal on Polyethylene Synthetic Substitute, Uncemented, Open Approach

ØSRBØ2Z   Replacement of Left Hip Joint with Metal on Polyethylene Synthetic Substitute, Open Approach

ØSRBØ39   Replacement of Left Hip Joint with Ceramic Synthetic Substitute, Cemented, Open Approach

ØSRBØ3A   Replacement of Left Hip Joint with Ceramic Synthetic Substitute, Uncemented, Open Approach

ØSRBØ3Z   Replacement of Left Hip Joint with Ceramic Synthetic Substitute, Open Approach

ØSRBØ49   Replacement of Left Hip Joint with Ceramic on Polyethylene Synthetic Substitute, Cemented, Open Approach

ØSRBØ4A   Replacement of Left Hip Joint with Ceramic on Polyethylene Synthetic Substitute, Uncemented, Open Approach

ØSRBØ4Z   Replacement of Left Hip Joint with Ceramic on Polyethylene Synthetic Substitute, Open Approach

ØSRBØ7Z   Replacement of Left Hip Joint with Autologous Tissue Substitute, Open Approach

ØSRBØJ9   Replacement of Left Hip Joint with Synthetic Substitute, Cemented, Open Approach

ØSRBØJA   Replacement of Left Hip Joint with Synthetic Substitute, Uncemented, Open Approach

ØSRBØJZ   Replacement of Left Hip Joint with Synthetic Substitute, Open Approach

ØSRBØKZ   Replacement of Left Hip Joint with Nonautologous Tissue Substitute, Open Approach

ØSRCØ7Z   Replacement of Right Knee Joint with Autologous Tissue Substitute, Open Approach

ØSRCØJ9   Replacement of Right Knee Joint with Synthetic Substitute, Cemented, Open Approach

ØSRCØJA   Replacement of Right Knee Joint with Synthetic Substitute, Uncemented, Open Approach

ØSRCØJZ   Replacement of Right Knee Joint with Synthetic Substitute, Open Approach

ØSRCØKZ   Replacement of Right Knee Joint with Nonautologous Tissue Substitute, Open Approach

ØSRCØL9   Replacement of Right Knee Joint with Unicondylar Synthetic Substitute, Cemented, Open Approach

ØSRCØLA   Replacement of Right Knee Joint with Unicondylar Synthetic Substitute, Uncemented, Open Approach

ØSRCØLZ   Replacement of Right Knee Joint with Unicondylar Synthetic Substitute, Open Approach

ØSRDØ7Z   Replacement of Left Knee Joint with Autologous Tissue Substitute, Open Approach

ØSRDØJ9   Replacement of Left Knee Joint with Synthetic Substitute, Cemented, Open Approach

ØSRDØJA   Replacement of Left Knee Joint with Synthetic Substitute, Uncemented, Open Approach

ØSRDØJZ   Replacement of Left Knee Joint with Synthetic Substitute, Open Approach

ØSRDØKZ   Replacement of Left Knee Joint with Nonautologous Tissue Substitute, Open Approach

ØSRDØL9   Replacement of Left Knee Joint with Unicondylar Synthetic Substitute, Cemented, Open Approach

ØSRDØLA   Replacement of Left Knee Joint with Unicondylar Synthetic Substitute, Uncemented, Open Approach

ØSRDØLZ   Replacement of Left Knee Joint with Unicondylar Synthetic Substitute, Open Approach

ØSREØØ9   Replacement of Left Hip Joint, Acetabular Surface with Polyethylene Synthetic Substitute, Cemented, Open Approach

ØSREØØA   Replacement of Left Hip Joint, Acetabular Surface with Polyethylene Synthetic Substitute, Uncemented, Open Approach

ØSREØØZ   Replacement of Left Hip Joint, Acetabular Surface with Polyethylene Synthetic Substitute, Open Approach

ØSREØ19   Replacement of Left Hip Joint, Acetabular Surface with Metal Synthetic Substitute, Cemented, Open Approach

ØSREØ1A   Replacement of Left Hip Joint, Acetabular Surface with Metal Synthetic Substitute, Uncemented, Open Approach

ØSREØ1Z   Replacement of Left Hip Joint, Acetabular Surface with Metal Synthetic Substitute, Open Approach

ØSREØ39   Replacement of Left Hip Joint, Acetabular Surface with Ceramic Synthetic Substitute, Cemented, Open Approach

ØSREØ3A   Replacement of Left Hip Joint, Acetabular Surface with Ceramic Synthetic Substitute, Uncemented, Open Approach

ØSREØ3Z   Replacement of Left Hip Joint, Acetabular Surface with Ceramic Synthetic Substitute, Open Approach

ØSREØ7Z   Replacement of Left Hip Joint, Acetabular Surface with Autologous Tissue Substitute, Open Approach

ØSREØJ9   Replacement of Left Hip Joint, Acetabular Surface with Synthetic Substitute, Cemented, Open Approach

ØSREØJA   Replacement of Left Hip Joint, Acetabular Surface with Synthetic Substitute, Uncemented, Open Approach

ØSREØJZ   Replacement of Left Hip Joint, Acetabular Surface with Synthetic Substitute, Open Approach

ØSREØKZ   Replacement of Left Hip Joint, Acetabular Surface with Nonautologous Tissue Substitute, Open Approach

ØSRRØ19   Replacement of Right Hip Joint, Femoral Surface with Metal Synthetic Substitute, Cemented, Open Approach

ØSRRØ1A   Replacement of Right Hip Joint, Femoral Surface with Metal Synthetic Substitute, Uncemented, Open Approach

ØSRRØ1Z   Replacement of Right Hip Joint, Femoral Surface with Metal Synthetic Substitute, Open Approach

ØSRRØ39   Replacement of Right Hip Joint, Femoral Surface with Ceramic Synthetic Substitute, Cemented, Open Approach

ØSRRØ3A   Replacement of Right Hip Joint, Femoral Surface with Ceramic Synthetic Substitute, Uncemented, Open Approach

ØSRRØ3Z   Replacement of Right Hip Joint, Femoral Surface with Ceramic Synthetic Substitute, Open Approach

ØSRRØ7Z   Replacement of Right Hip Joint, Femoral Surface with Autologous Tissue Substitute, Open Approach

ØSRRØJ9   Replacement of Right Hip Joint, Femoral Surface with Synthetic Substitute, Cemented, Open Approach

ØSRRØJA   Replacement of Right Hip Joint, Femoral Surface with Synthetic Substitute, Uncemented, Open Approach

ØSRRØJZ   Replacement of Right Hip Joint, Femoral Surface with Synthetic Substitute, Open Approach

ØSRRØKZ   Replacement of Right Hip Joint, Femoral Surface with Nonautologous Tissue Substitute, Open Approach

ØSRSØ19   Replacement of Left Hip Joint, Femoral Surface with Metal Synthetic Substitute, Cemented, Open Approach

ØSRSØ1A   Replacement of Left Hip Joint, Femoral Surface with Metal Synthetic Substitute, Uncemented, Open Approach

ØSRSØ1Z   Replacement of Left Hip Joint, Femoral Surface with Metal Synthetic Substitute, Open Approach

ØSRSØ39   Replacement of Left Hip Joint, Femoral Surface with Ceramic Synthetic Substitute, Cemented, Open Approach

ØSRSØ3A   Replacement of Left Hip Joint, Femoral Surface with Ceramic Synthetic Substitute, Uncemented, Open Approach

ØSRSØ3Z   Replacement of Left Hip Joint, Femoral Surface with Ceramic Synthetic Substitute, Open Approach

ØSRSØ7Z   Replacement of Left Hip Joint, Femoral Surface with Autologous Tissue Substitute, Open Approach

ØSRSØJ9   Replacement of Left Hip Joint, Femoral Surface with Synthetic Substitute, Cemented, Open Approach

ØSRSØJA   Replacement of Left Hip Joint, Femoral Surface with Synthetic Substitute, Uncemented, Open Approach

ØSRSØJZ   Replacement of Left Hip Joint, Femoral Surface with Synthetic Substitute, Open Approach

ØSRSØKZ   Replacement of Left Hip Joint, Femoral Surface with Nonautologous Tissue Substitute, Open Approach

ØSRTØ7Z   Replacement of Right Knee Joint, Femoral Surface with Autologous Tissue Substitute, Open Approach

Appendix I: Hospital Acquired Conditions

HAC 10: Deep Vein Thrombosis (DVT) or Pulmonary Embolism (PE) with Total Knee or Hip Replacement (continued)

ØSRTØJ9   Replacement of Right Knee Joint, Femoral Surface with Synthetic Substitute, Cemented, Open Approach

ØSRTØJA   Replacement of Right Knee Joint, Femoral Surface with Synthetic Substitute, Uncemented, Open Approach

ØSRTØJZ   Replacement of Right Knee Joint, Femoral Surface with Synthetic Substitute, Open Approach

ØSRTØKZ   Replacement of Right Knee Joint, Femoral Surface with Nonautologous Tissue Substitute, Open Approach

ØSRUØ7Z   Replacement of Left Knee Joint, Femoral Surface with Autologous Tissue Substitute, Open Approach

ØSRUØJ9   Replacement of Left Knee Joint, Femoral Surface with Synthetic Substitute, Cemented, Open Approach

ØSRUØJA   Replacement of Left Knee Joint, Femoral Surface with Synthetic Substitute, Uncemented, Open Approach

ØSRUØJZ   Replacement of Left Knee Joint, Femoral Surface with Synthetic Substitute, Open Approach

ØSRUØKZ   Replacement of Left Knee Joint, Femoral Surface with Nonautologous Tissue Substitute, Open Approach

ØSRVØ7Z   Replacement of Right Knee Joint, Tibial Surface with Autologous Tissue Substitute, Open Approach

ØSRVØJ9   Replacement of Right Knee Joint, Tibial Surface with Synthetic Substitute, Cemented, Open Approach

ØSRVØJA   Replacement of Right Knee Joint, Tibial Surface with Synthetic Substitute, Uncemented, Open Approach

ØSRVØJZ   Replacement of Right Knee Joint, Tibial Surface with Synthetic Substitute, Open Approach

ØSRVØKZ   Replacement of Right Knee Joint, Tibial Surface with Nonautologous Tissue Substitute, Open Approach

ØSRWØ7Z   Replacement of Left Knee Joint, Tibial Surface with Autologous Tissue Substitute, Open Approach

ØSRWØJ9   Replacement of Left Knee Joint, Tibial Surface with Synthetic Substitute, Cemented, Open Approach

ØSRWØJA   Replacement of Left Knee Joint, Tibial Surface with Synthetic Substitute, Uncemented, Open Approach

ØSRWØJZ   Replacement of Left Knee Joint, Tibial Surface with Synthetic Substitute, Open Approach

ØSRWØKZ   Replacement of Left Knee Joint, Tibial Surface with Nonautologous Tissue Substitute, Open Approach

ØSU9ØBZ   Supplement Right Hip Joint with Resurfacing Device, Open Approach

ØSUAØBZ   Supplement Right Hip Joint, Acetabular Surface with Resurfacing Device, Open Approach

ØSUBØBZ   Supplement Left Hip Joint with Resurfacing Device, Open Approach

ØSUEØBZ   Supplement Left Hip Joint, Acetabular Surface with Resurfacing Device, Open Approach

ØSURØBZ   Supplement Right Hip Joint, Femoral Surface with Resurfacing Device, Open Approach

ØSUSØBZ   Supplement Left Hip Joint, Femoral Surface with Resurfacing Device, Open Approach

HAC 11: Surgical Site Infection Following Bariatric Surgery

Principal diagnosis of:

  E66.Ø1

AND

Secondary diagnosis not POA:

  K68.11
  K95.Ø1
  K95.81
  T81.4XXA

AND

Any of the following procedures:

ØD16Ø79   Bypass Stomach to Duodenum with Autologous Tissue Substitute, Open Approach

ØD16Ø7A   Bypass Stomach to Jejunum with Autologous Tissue Substitute, Open Approach

ØD16Ø7B   Bypass Stomach to Ileum with Autologous Tissue Substitute, Open Approach

ØD16Ø7L   Bypass Stomach to Transverse Colon with Autologous Tissue Substitute, Open Approach

ØD16ØJ9   Bypass Stomach to Duodenum with Synthetic Substitute, Open Approach

ØD16ØJA   Bypass Stomach to Jejunum with Synthetic Substitute, Open Approach

ØD16ØJB   Bypass Stomach to Ileum with Synthetic Substitute, Open Approach

ØD16ØJL   Bypass Stomach to Transverse Colon with Synthetic Substitute, Open Approach

ØD16ØK9   Bypass Stomach to Duodenum with Nonautologous Tissue Substitute, Open Approach

ØD16ØKA   Bypass Stomach to Jejunum with Nonautologous Tissue Substitute, Open Approach

ØD16ØKB   Bypass Stomach to Ileum with Nonautologous Tissue Substitute, Open Approach

ØD16ØKL   Bypass Stomach to Transverse Colon with Nonautologous Tissue Substitute, Open Approach

ØD16ØZ9   Bypass Stomach to Duodenum, Open Approach

ØD16ØZA   Bypass Stomach to Jejunum, Open Approach

ØD16ØZB   Bypass Stomach to Ileum, Open Approach

ØD16ØZL   Bypass Stomach to Transverse Colon, Open Approach

ØD16479   Bypass Stomach to Duodenum with Autologous Tissue Substitute, Percutaneous Endoscopic Approach

ØD1647A   Bypass Stomach to Jejunum with Autologous Tissue Substitute, Percutaneous Endoscopic Approach

ØD1647B   Bypass Stomach to Ileum with Autologous Tissue Substitute, Percutaneous Endoscopic Approach

ØD1647L   Bypass Stomach to Transverse Colon with Autologous Tissue Substitute, Percutaneous Endoscopic Approach

ØD164J9   Bypass Stomach to Duodenum with Synthetic Substitute, Percutaneous Endoscopic Approach

ØD164JA   Bypass Stomach to Jejunum with Synthetic Substitute, Percutaneous Endoscopic Approach

ØD164JB   Bypass Stomach to Ileum with Synthetic Substitute, Percutaneous Endoscopic Approach

ØD164JL   Bypass Stomach to Transverse Colon with Synthetic Substitute, Percutaneous Endoscopic Approach

ØD164K9   Bypass Stomach to Duodenum with Nonautologous Tissue Substitute, Percutaneous Endoscopic Approach

ØD164KA   Bypass Stomach to Jejunum with Nonautologous Tissue Substitute, Percutaneous Endoscopic Approach

ØD164KB   Bypass Stomach to Ileum with Nonautologous Tissue Substitute, Percutaneous Endoscopic Approach

ØD164KL   Bypass Stomach to Transverse Colon with Nonautologous Tissue Substitute, Percutaneous Endoscopic Approach

ØD164Z9   Bypass Stomach to Duodenum, Percutaneous Endoscopic Approach

ØD164ZA   Bypass Stomach to Jejunum, Percutaneous Endoscopic Approach

ØD164ZB   Bypass Stomach to Ileum, Percutaneous Endoscopic Approach

ØD164ZL   Bypass Stomach to Transverse Colon, Percutaneous Endoscopic Approach

ØD16879   Bypass Stomach to Duodenum with Autologous Tissue Substitute, Via Natural or Artificial Opening Endoscopic

ØD1687A   Bypass Stomach to Jejunum with Autologous Tissue Substitute, Via Natural or Artificial Opening Endoscopic

ØD1687B   Bypass Stomach to Ileum with Autologous Tissue Substitute, Via Natural or Artificial Opening Endoscopic

ØD1687L   Bypass Stomach to Transverse Colon with Autologous Tissue Substitute, Via Natural or Artificial Opening Endoscopic

ØD168J9   Bypass Stomach to Duodenum with Synthetic Substitute, Via Natural or Artificial Opening Endoscopic

ØD168JA   Bypass Stomach to Jejunum with Synthetic Substitute, Via Natural or Artificial Opening Endoscopic

ØD168JB   Bypass Stomach to Ileum with Synthetic Substitute, Via Natural or Artificial Opening Endoscopic

ØD168JL   Bypass Stomach to Transverse Colon with Synthetic Substitute, Via Natural or Artificial Opening Endoscopic

ØD168K9   Bypass Stomach to Duodenum with Nonautologous Tissue Substitute, Via Natural or Artificial Opening Endoscopic

ØD168KA   Bypass Stomach to Jejunum with Nonautologous Tissue Substitute, Via Natural or Artificial Opening Endoscopic

ØD168KB   Bypass Stomach to Ileum with Nonautologous Tissue Substitute, Via Natural or Artificial Opening Endoscopic

ØD168KL   Bypass Stomach to Transverse Colon with Nonautologous Tissue Substitute, Via Natural or Artificial Opening Endoscopic

ØD168Z9   Bypass Stomach to Duodenum, Via Natural or Artificial Opening Endoscopic

ØD168ZA   Bypass Stomach to Jejunum, Via Natural or Artificial Opening Endoscopic

ØD168ZB   Bypass Stomach to Ileum, Via Natural or Artificial Opening Endoscopic

ØD168ZL   Bypass Stomach to Transverse Colon, Via Natural or Artificial Opening Endoscopic

ØDV64CZ   Restriction of Stomach with Extraluminal Device, Percutaneous Endoscopic Approach

HAC 12: Surgical Site Infection Following Certain Orthopedic Procedures of the Spine, Shoulder, and Elbow

Secondary diagnosis not POA:

- K68.11
- T81.4XXA
- T84.60XA
- T84.610A
- T84.611A
- T84.612A
- T84.613A
- T84.614A
- T84.615A
- T84.619A
- T84.63XA
- T84.69XA
- T84.7XXA

AND

Any of the following procedures:

- 0RG0070   Fusion of Occipital-cervical Joint with Autologous Tissue Substitute, Anterior Approach, Anterior Column, Open Approach
- 0RG0071   Fusion of Occipital-cervical Joint with Autologous Tissue Substitute, Posterior Approach, Posterior Column, Open Approach
- 0RG007J   Fusion of Occipital-cervical Joint with Autologous Tissue Substitute, Posterior Approach, Anterior Column, Open Approach
- 0RG00A0   Fusion of Occipital-cervical Joint with Interbody Fusion Device, Anterior Approach, Anterior Column, Open Approach
- 0RG00A1   Fusion of Occipital-cervical Joint with Interbody Fusion Device, Posterior Approach, Posterior Column, Open Approach
- 0RG00AJ   Fusion of Occipital-cervical Joint with Interbody Fusion Device, Posterior Approach, Anterior Column, Open Approach
- 0RG00J0   Fusion of Occipital-cervical Joint with Synthetic Substitute, Anterior Approach, Anterior Column, Open Approach
- 0RG00J1   Fusion of Occipital-cervical Joint with Synthetic Substitute, Posterior Approach, Posterior Column, Open Approach
- 0RG00JJ   Fusion of Occipital-cervical Joint with Synthetic Substitute, Posterior Approach, Anterior Column, Open Approach
- 0RG00K0   Fusion of Occipital-cervical Joint with Nonautologous Tissue Substitute, Anterior Approach, Anterior Column, Open Approach
- 0RG00K1   Fusion of Occipital-cervical Joint with Nonautologous Tissue Substitute, Posterior Approach, Posterior Column, Open Approach
- 0RG00KJ   Fusion of Occipital-cervical Joint with Nonautologous Tissue Substitute, Posterior Approach, Anterior Column, Open Approach
- 0RG00Z0   Fusion of Occipital-cervical Joint, Anterior Approach, Anterior Column, Open Approach
- 0RG00Z1   Fusion of Occipital-cervical Joint, Posterior Approach, Posterior Column, Open Approach
- 0RG00ZJ   Fusion of Occipital-cervical Joint, Posterior Approach, Anterior Column, Open Approach
- 0RG0370   Fusion of Occipital-cervical Joint with Autologous Tissue Substitute, Anterior Approach, Anterior Column, Percutaneous Approach
- 0RG0371   Fusion of Occipital-cervical Joint with Autologous Tissue Substitute, Posterior Approach, Posterior Column, Percutaneous Approach
- 0RG037J   Fusion of Occipital-cervical Joint with Autologous Tissue Substitute, Posterior Approach, Anterior Column, Percutaneous Approach
- 0RG03A0   Fusion of Occipital-cervical Joint with Interbody Fusion Device, Anterior Approach, Anterior Column, Percutaneous Approach
- 0RG03A1   Fusion of Occipital-cervical Joint with Interbody Fusion Device, Posterior Approach, Posterior Column, Percutaneous Approach
- 0RG03AJ   Fusion of Occipital-cervical Joint with Interbody Fusion Device, Posterior Approach, Anterior Column, Percutaneous Approach
- 0RG03J0   Fusion of Occipital-cervical Joint with Synthetic Substitute, Anterior Approach, Anterior Column, Percutaneous Approach
- 0RG03J1   Fusion of Occipital-cervical Joint with Synthetic Substitute, Posterior Approach, Posterior Column, Percutaneous Approach
- 0RG03JJ   Fusion of Occipital-cervical Joint with Synthetic Substitute, Posterior Approach, Anterior Column, Percutaneous Approach
- 0RG03K0   Fusion of Occipital-cervical Joint with Nonautologous Tissue Substitute, Anterior Approach, Anterior Column, Percutaneous Approach
- 0RG03K1   Fusion of Occipital-cervical Joint with Nonautologous Tissue Substitute, Posterior Approach, Posterior Column, Percutaneous Approach
- 0RG03KJ   Fusion of Occipital-cervical Joint with Nonautologous Tissue Substitute, Posterior Approach, Anterior Column, Percutaneous Approach
- 0RG03Z0   Fusion of Occipital-cervical Joint, Anterior Approach, Anterior Column, Percutaneous Approach
- 0RG03Z1   Fusion of Occipital-cervical Joint, Posterior Approach, Posterior Column, Percutaneous Approach
- 0RG03ZJ   Fusion of Occipital-cervical Joint, Posterior Approach, Anterior Column, Percutaneous Approach
- 0RG0470   Fusion of Occipital-cervical Joint with Autologous Tissue Substitute, Anterior Approach, Anterior Column, Percutaneous Endoscopic Approach
- 0RG0471   Fusion of Occipital-cervical Joint with Autologous Tissue Substitute, Posterior Approach, Posterior Column, Percutaneous Endoscopic Approach
- 0RG047J   Fusion of Occipital-cervical Joint with Autologous Tissue Substitute, Posterior Approach, Anterior Column, Percutaneous Endoscopic Approach
- 0RG04A0   Fusion of Occipital-cervical Joint with Interbody Fusion Device, Anterior Approach, Anterior Column, Percutaneous Endoscopic Approach
- 0RG04A1   Fusion of Occipital-cervical Joint with Interbody Fusion Device, Posterior Approach, Posterior Column, Percutaneous Endoscopic Approach
- 0RG04AJ   Fusion of Occipital-cervical Joint with Interbody Fusion Device, Posterior Approach, Anterior Column, Percutaneous Endoscopic Approach
- 0RG04J0   Fusion of Occipital-cervical Joint with Synthetic Substitute, Anterior Approach, Anterior Column, Percutaneous Endoscopic Approach
- 0RG04J1   Fusion of Occipital-cervical Joint with Synthetic Substitute, Posterior Approach, Posterior Column, Percutaneous Endoscopic Approach
- 0RG04JJ   Fusion of Occipital-cervical Joint with Synthetic Substitute, Posterior Approach, Anterior Column, Percutaneous Endoscopic Approach
- 0RG04K0   Fusion of Occipital-cervical Joint with Nonautologous Tissue Substitute, Anterior Approach, Anterior Column, Percutaneous Endoscopic Approach
- 0RG04K1   Fusion of Occipital-cervical Joint with Nonautologous Tissue Substitute, Posterior Approach, Posterior Column, Percutaneous Endoscopic Approach
- 0RG04KJ   Fusion of Occipital-cervical Joint with Nonautologous Tissue Substitute, Posterior Approach, Anterior Column, Percutaneous Endoscopic Approach
- 0RG04Z0   Fusion of Occipital-cervical Joint, Anterior Approach, Anterior Column, Percutaneous Endoscopic Approach
- 0RG04Z1   Fusion of Occipital-cervical Joint, Posterior Approach, Posterior Column, Percutaneous Endoscopic Approach
- 0RG04ZJ   Fusion of Occipital-cervical Joint, Posterior Approach, Anterior Column, Percutaneous Endoscopic Approach
- 0RG1070   Fusion of Cervical Vertebral Joint with Autologous Tissue Substitute, Anterior Approach, Anterior Column, Open Approach
- 0RG1071   Fusion of Cervical Vertebral Joint with Autologous Tissue Substitute, Posterior Approach, Posterior Column, Open Approach
- 0RG107J   Fusion of Cervical Vertebral Joint with Autologous Tissue Substitute, Posterior Approach, Anterior Column, Open Approach
- 0RG10A0   Fusion of Cervical Vertebral Joint with Interbody Fusion Device, Anterior Approach, Anterior Column, Open Approach
- 0RG10A1   Fusion of Cervical Vertebral Joint with Interbody Fusion Device, Posterior Approach, Posterior Column, Open Approach
- 0RG10AJ   Fusion of Cervical Vertebral Joint with Interbody Fusion Device, Posterior Approach, Anterior Column, Open Approach
- 0RG10J0   Fusion of Cervical Vertebral Joint with Synthetic Substitute, Anterior Approach, Anterior Column, Open Approach
- 0RG10J1   Fusion of Cervical Vertebral Joint with Synthetic Substitute, Posterior Approach, Posterior Column, Open Approach
- 0RG10JJ   Fusion of Cervical Vertebral Joint with Synthetic Substitute, Posterior Approach, Anterior Column, Open Approach
- 0RG10K0   Fusion of Cervical Vertebral Joint with Nonautologous Tissue Substitute, Anterior Approach, Anterior Column, Open Approach

HAC 12: Surgical Site Infection Following Certain Orthopedic Procedures of the Spine, Shoulder, and Elbow (continued)

ØRG1ØK1 Fusion of Cervical Vertebral Joint with Nonautologous Tissue Substitute, Posterior Approach, Posterior Column, Open Approach

ØRG1ØKJ Fusion of Cervical Vertebral Joint with Nonautologous Tissue Substitute, Posterior Approach, Anterior Column, Open Approach

ØRG1ØZØ Fusion of Cervical Vertebral Joint, Anterior Approach, Anterior Column, Open Approach

ØRG1ØZ1 Fusion of Cervical Vertebral Joint, Posterior Approach, Posterior Column, Open Approach

ØRG1ØZJ Fusion of Cervical Vertebral Joint, Posterior Approach, Anterior Column, Open Approach

ØRG137Ø Fusion of Cervical Vertebral Joint with Autologous Tissue Substitute, Anterior Approach, Anterior Column, Percutaneous Approach

ØRG1371 Fusion of Cervical Vertebral Joint with Autologous Tissue Substitute, Posterior Approach, Posterior Column, Percutaneous Approach

ØRG137J Fusion of Cervical Vertebral Joint with Autologous Tissue Substitute, Posterior Approach, Anterior Column, Percutaneous Approach

ØRG13AØ Fusion of Cervical Vertebral Joint with Interbody Fusion Device, Anterior Approach, Anterior Column, Percutaneous Approach

ØRG13A1 Fusion of Cervical Vertebral Joint with Interbody Fusion Device, Posterior Approach, Posterior Column, Percutaneous Approach

ØRG13AJ Fusion of Cervical Vertebral Joint with Interbody Fusion Device, Posterior Approach, Anterior Column, Percutaneous Approach

ØRG13JØ Fusion of Cervical Vertebral Joint with Synthetic Substitute, Anterior Approach, Anterior Column, Percutaneous Approach

ØRG13J1 Fusion of Cervical Vertebral Joint with Synthetic Substitute, Posterior Approach, Posterior Column, Percutaneous Approach

ØRG13JJ Fusion of Cervical Vertebral Joint with Synthetic Substitute, Posterior Approach, Anterior Column, Percutaneous Approach

ØRG13KØ Fusion of Cervical Vertebral Joint with Nonautologous Tissue Substitute, Anterior Approach, Anterior Column, Percutaneous Approach

ØRG13K1 Fusion of Cervical Vertebral Joint with Nonautologous Tissue Substitute, Posterior Approach, Posterior Column, Percutaneous Approach

ØRG13KJ Fusion of Cervical Vertebral Joint with Nonautologous Tissue Substitute, Posterior Approach, Anterior Column, Percutaneous Approach

ØRG13ZØ Fusion of Cervical Vertebral Joint, Anterior Approach, Anterior Column, Percutaneous Approach

ØRG13Z1 Fusion of Cervical Vertebral Joint, Posterior Approach, Posterior Column, Percutaneous Approach

ØRG13ZJ Fusion of Cervical Vertebral Joint, Posterior Approach, Anterior Column, Percutaneous Approach

ØRG147Ø Fusion of Cervical Vertebral Joint with Autologous Tissue Substitute, Anterior Approach, Anterior Column, Percutaneous Endoscopic Approach

ØRG1471 Fusion of Cervical Vertebral Joint with Autologous Tissue Substitute, Posterior Approach, Posterior Column, Percutaneous Endoscopic Approach

ØRG147J Fusion of Cervical Vertebral Joint with Autologous Tissue Substitute, Posterior Approach, Anterior Column, Percutaneous Endoscopic Approach

ØRG14AØ Fusion of Cervical Vertebral Joint with Interbody Fusion Device, Anterior Approach, Anterior Column, Percutaneous Endoscopic Approach

ØRG14A1 Fusion of Cervical Vertebral Joint with Interbody Fusion Device, Posterior Approach, Posterior Column, Percutaneous Endoscopic Approach

ØRG14AJ Fusion of Cervical Vertebral Joint with Interbody Fusion Device, Posterior Approach, Anterior Column, Percutaneous Endoscopic Approach

ØRG14JØ Fusion of Cervical Vertebral Joint with Synthetic Substitute, Anterior Approach, Anterior Column, Percutaneous Endoscopic Approach

ØRG14J1 Fusion of Cervical Vertebral Joint with Synthetic Substitute, Posterior Approach, Posterior Column, Percutaneous Endoscopic Approach

ØRG14JJ Fusion of Cervical Vertebral Joint with Synthetic Substitute, Posterior Approach, Anterior Column, Percutaneous Endoscopic Approach

ØRG14KØ Fusion of Cervical Vertebral Joint with Nonautologous Tissue Substitute, Anterior Approach, Anterior Column, Percutaneous Endoscopic Approach

ØRG14K1 Fusion of Cervical Vertebral Joint with Nonautologous Tissue Substitute, Posterior Approach, Posterior Column, Percutaneous Endoscopic Approach

ØRG14KJ Fusion of Cervical Vertebral Joint with Nonautologous Tissue Substitute, Posterior Approach, Anterior Column, Percutaneous Endoscopic Approach

ØRG14ZØ Fusion of Cervical Vertebral Joint, Anterior Approach, Anterior Column, Percutaneous Endoscopic Approach

ØRG14Z1 Fusion of Cervical Vertebral Joint, Posterior Approach, Posterior Column, Percutaneous Endoscopic Approach

ØRG14ZJ Fusion of Cervical Vertebral Joint, Posterior Approach, Anterior Column, Percutaneous Endoscopic Approach

ØRG2Ø7Ø Fusion of 2 or more Cervical Vertebral Joints with Autologous Tissue Substitute, Anterior Approach, Anterior Column, Open Approach

ØRG2Ø71 Fusion of 2 or more Cervical Vertebral Joints with Autologous Tissue Substitute, Posterior Approach, Posterior Column, Open Approach

ØRG2Ø7J Fusion of 2 or more Cervical Vertebral Joints with Autologous Tissue Substitute, Posterior Approach, Anterior Column, Open Approach

ØRG2ØAØ Fusion of 2 or more Cervical Vertebral Joints with Interbody Fusion Device, Anterior Approach, Anterior Column, Open Approach

ØRG2ØA1 Fusion of 2 or more Cervical Vertebral Joints with Interbody Fusion Device, Posterior Approach, Posterior Column, Open Approach

ØRG2ØAJ Fusion of 2 or more Cervical Vertebral Joints with Interbody Fusion Device, Posterior Approach, Anterior Column, Open Approach

ØRG2ØJØ Fusion of 2 or more Cervical Vertebral Joints with Synthetic Substitute, Anterior Approach, Anterior Column, Open Approach

ØRG2ØJ1 Fusion of 2 or more Cervical Vertebral Joints with Synthetic Substitute, Posterior Approach, Posterior Column, Open Approach

ØRG2ØJJ Fusion of 2 or more Cervical Vertebral Joints with Synthetic Substitute, Posterior Approach, Anterior Column, Open Approach

ØRG2ØKØ Fusion of 2 or more Cervical Vertebral Joints with Nonautologous Tissue Substitute, Anterior Approach, Anterior Column, Open Approach

ØRG2ØK1 Fusion of 2 or more Cervical Vertebral Joints with Nonautologous Tissue Substitute, Posterior Approach, Posterior Column, Open Approach

ØRG2ØKJ Fusion of 2 or more Cervical Vertebral Joints with Nonautologous Tissue Substitute, Posterior Approach, Anterior Column, Open Approach

ØRG2ØZØ Fusion of 2 or more Cervical Vertebral Joints, Anterior Approach, Anterior Column, Open Approach

ØRG2ØZ1 Fusion of 2 or more Cervical Vertebral Joints, Posterior Approach, Posterior Column, Open Approach

ØRG2ØZJ Fusion of 2 or more Cervical Vertebral Joints, Posterior Approach, Anterior Column, Open Approach

ØRG237Ø Fusion of 2 or more Cervical Vertebral Joints with Autologous Tissue Substitute, Anterior Approach, Anterior Column, Percutaneous Approach

ØRG2371 Fusion of 2 or more Cervical Vertebral Joints with Autologous Tissue Substitute, Posterior Approach, Posterior Column, Percutaneous Approach

ØRG237J Fusion of 2 or more Cervical Vertebral Joints with Autologous Tissue Substitute, Posterior Approach, Anterior Column, Percutaneous Approach

ØRG23AØ Fusion of 2 or more Cervical Vertebral Joints with Interbody Fusion Device, Anterior Approach, Anterior Column, Percutaneous Approach

ØRG23A1 Fusion of 2 or more Cervical Vertebral Joints with Interbody Fusion Device, Posterior Approach, Posterior Column, Percutaneous Approach

ØRG23AJ Fusion of 2 or more Cervical Vertebral Joints with Interbody Fusion Device, Posterior Approach, Anterior Column, Percutaneous Approach

ØRG23JØ Fusion of 2 or more Cervical Vertebral Joints with Synthetic Substitute, Anterior Approach, Anterior Column, Percutaneous Approach

ØRG23J1 Fusion of 2 or more Cervical Vertebral Joints with Synthetic Substitute, Posterior Approach, Posterior Column, Percutaneous Approach

ØRG23JJ Fusion of 2 or more Cervical Vertebral Joints with Synthetic Substitute, Posterior Approach, Anterior Column, Percutaneous Approach

ØRG23KØ Fusion of 2 or more Cervical Vertebral Joints with Nonautologous Tissue Substitute, Anterior Approach, Anterior Column, Percutaneous Approach

HAC 12: Surgical Site Infection Following Certain Orthopedic Procedures of the Spine, Shoulder, and Elbow (continued)

ØRG23K1　Fusion of 2 or more Cervical Vertebral Joints with Nonautologous Tissue Substitute, Posterior Approach, Posterior Column, Percutaneous Approach

ØRG23KJ　Fusion of 2 or more Cervical Vertebral Joints with Nonautologous Tissue Substitute, Posterior Approach, Anterior Column, Percutaneous Approach

ØRG23Z0　Fusion of 2 or more Cervical Vertebral Joints, Anterior Approach, Anterior Column, Percutaneous Approach

ØRG23Z1　Fusion of 2 or more Cervical Vertebral Joints, Posterior Approach, Posterior Column, Percutaneous Approach

ØRG23ZJ　Fusion of 2 or more Cervical Vertebral Joints, Posterior Approach, Anterior Column, Percutaneous Approach

ØRG2470　Fusion of 2 or more Cervical Vertebral Joints with Autologous Tissue Substitute, Anterior Approach, Anterior Column, Percutaneous Endoscopic Approach

ØRG2471　Fusion of 2 or more Cervical Vertebral Joints with Autologous Tissue Substitute, Posterior Approach, Posterior Column, Percutaneous Endoscopic Approach

ØRG247J　Fusion of 2 or more Cervical Vertebral Joints with Autologous Tissue Substitute, Posterior Approach, Anterior Column, Percutaneous Endoscopic Approach

ØRG24A0　Fusion of 2 or more Cervical Vertebral Joints with Interbody Fusion Device, Anterior Approach, Anterior Column, Percutaneous Endoscopic Approach

ØRG24A1　Fusion of 2 or more Cervical Vertebral Joints with Interbody Fusion Device, Posterior Approach, Posterior Column, Percutaneous Endoscopic Approach

ØRG24AJ　Fusion of 2 or more Cervical Vertebral Joints with Interbody Fusion Device, Posterior Approach, Anterior Column, Percutaneous Endoscopic Approach

ØRG24J0　Fusion of 2 or more Cervical Vertebral Joints with Synthetic Substitute, Anterior Approach, Anterior Column, Percutaneous Endoscopic Approach

ØRG24J1　Fusion of 2 or more Cervical Vertebral Joints with Synthetic Substitute, Posterior Approach, Posterior Column, Percutaneous Endoscopic Approach

ØRG24JJ　Fusion of 2 or more Cervical Vertebral Joints with Synthetic Substitute, Posterior Approach, Anterior Column, Percutaneous Endoscopic Approach

ØRG24K0　Fusion of 2 or more Cervical Vertebral Joints with Nonautologous Tissue Substitute, Anterior Approach, Anterior Column, Percutaneous Endoscopic Approach

ØRG24K1　Fusion of 2 or more Cervical Vertebral Joints with Nonautologous Tissue Substitute, Posterior Approach, Posterior Column, Percutaneous Endoscopic Approach

ØRG24KJ　Fusion of 2 or more Cervical Vertebral Joints with Nonautologous Tissue Substitute, Posterior Approach, Anterior Column, Percutaneous Endoscopic Approach

ØRG24Z0　Fusion of 2 or more Cervical Vertebral Joints, Anterior Approach, Anterior Column, Percutaneous Endoscopic Approach

ØRG24Z1　Fusion of 2 or more Cervical Vertebral Joints, Posterior Approach, Posterior Column, Percutaneous Endoscopic Approach

ØRG24ZJ　Fusion of 2 or more Cervical Vertebral Joints, Posterior Approach, Anterior Column, Percutaneous Endoscopic Approach

ØRG4070　Fusion of Cervicothoracic Vertebral Joint with Autologous Tissue Substitute, Anterior Approach, Anterior Column, Open Approach

ØRG4071　Fusion of Cervicothoracic Vertebral Joint with Autologous Tissue Substitute, Posterior Approach, Posterior Column, Open Approach

ØRG407J　Fusion of Cervicothoracic Vertebral Joint with Autologous Tissue Substitute, Posterior Approach, Anterior Column, Open Approach

ØRG40A0　Fusion of Cervicothoracic Vertebral Joint with Interbody Fusion Device, Anterior Approach, Anterior Column, Open Approach

ØRG40A1　Fusion of Cervicothoracic Vertebral Joint with Interbody Fusion Device, Posterior Approach, Posterior Column, Open Approach

ØRG40AJ　Fusion of Cervicothoracic Vertebral Joint with Interbody Fusion Device, Posterior Approach, Anterior Column, Open Approach

ØRG40J0　Fusion of Cervicothoracic Vertebral Joint with Synthetic Substitute, Anterior Approach, Anterior Column, Open Approach

ØRG40J1　Fusion of Cervicothoracic Vertebral Joint with Synthetic Substitute, Posterior Approach, Posterior Column, Open Approach

ØRG40JJ　Fusion of Cervicothoracic Vertebral Joint with Synthetic Substitute, Posterior Approach, Anterior Column, Open Approach

ØRG40K0　Fusion of Cervicothoracic Vertebral Joint with Nonautologous Tissue Substitute, Anterior Approach, Anterior Column, Open Approach

ØRG40K1　Fusion of Cervicothoracic Vertebral Joint with Nonautologous Tissue Substitute, Posterior Approach, Posterior Column, Open Approach

ØRG40KJ　Fusion of Cervicothoracic Vertebral Joint with Nonautologous Tissue Substitute, Posterior Approach, Anterior Column, Open Approach

ØRG40Z0　Fusion of Cervicothoracic Vertebral Joint, Anterior Approach, Anterior Column, Open Approach

ØRG40Z1　Fusion of Cervicothoracic Vertebral Joint, Posterior Approach, Posterior Column, Open Approach

ØRG40ZJ　Fusion of Cervicothoracic Vertebral Joint, Posterior Approach, Anterior Column, Open Approach

ØRG4370　Fusion of Cervicothoracic Vertebral Joint with Autologous Tissue Substitute, Anterior Approach, Anterior Column, Percutaneous Approach

ØRG4371　Fusion of Cervicothoracic Vertebral Joint with Autologous Tissue Substitute, Posterior Approach, Posterior Column, Percutaneous Approach

ØRG437J　Fusion of Cervicothoracic Vertebral Joint with Autologous Tissue Substitute, Posterior Approach, Anterior Column, Percutaneous Approach

ØRG43A0　Fusion of Cervicothoracic Vertebral Joint with Interbody Fusion Device, Anterior Approach, Anterior Column, Percutaneous Approach

ØRG43A1　Fusion of Cervicothoracic Vertebral Joint with Interbody Fusion Device, Posterior Approach, Posterior Column, Percutaneous Approach

ØRG43AJ　Fusion of Cervicothoracic Vertebral Joint with Interbody Fusion Device, Posterior Approach, Anterior Column, Percutaneous Approach

ØRG43J0　Fusion of Cervicothoracic Vertebral Joint with Synthetic Substitute, Anterior Approach, Anterior Column, Percutaneous Approach

ØRG43J1　Fusion of Cervicothoracic Vertebral Joint with Synthetic Substitute, Posterior Approach, Posterior Column, Percutaneous Approach

ØRG43JJ　Fusion of Cervicothoracic Vertebral Joint with Synthetic Substitute, Posterior Approach, Anterior Column, Percutaneous Approach

ØRG43K0　Fusion of Cervicothoracic Vertebral Joint with Nonautologous Tissue Substitute, Anterior Approach, Anterior Column, Percutaneous Approach

ØRG43K1　Fusion of Cervicothoracic Vertebral Joint with Nonautologous Tissue Substitute, Posterior Approach, Posterior Column, Percutaneous Approach

ØRG43KJ　Fusion of Cervicothoracic Vertebral Joint with Nonautologous Tissue Substitute, Posterior Approach, Anterior Column, Percutaneous Approach

ØRG43Z0　Fusion of Cervicothoracic Vertebral Joint, Anterior Approach, Anterior Column, Percutaneous Approach

ØRG43Z1　Fusion of Cervicothoracic Vertebral Joint, Posterior Approach, Posterior Column, Percutaneous Approach

ØRG43ZJ　Fusion of Cervicothoracic Vertebral Joint, Posterior Approach, Anterior Column, Percutaneous Approach

ØRG4470　Fusion of Cervicothoracic Vertebral Joint with Autologous Tissue Substitute, Anterior Approach, Anterior Column, Percutaneous Endoscopic Approach

ØRG4471　Fusion of Cervicothoracic Vertebral Joint with Autologous Tissue Substitute, Posterior Approach, Posterior Column, Percutaneous Endoscopic Approach

ØRG447J　Fusion of Cervicothoracic Vertebral Joint with Autologous Tissue Substitute, Posterior Approach, Anterior Column, Percutaneous Endoscopic Approach

ØRG44A0　Fusion of Cervicothoracic Vertebral Joint with Interbody Fusion Device, Anterior Approach, Anterior Column, Percutaneous Endoscopic Approach

ØRG44A1　Fusion of Cervicothoracic Vertebral Joint with Interbody Fusion Device, Posterior Approach, Posterior Column, Percutaneous Endoscopic Approach

ØRG44AJ　Fusion of Cervicothoracic Vertebral Joint with Interbody Fusion Device, Posterior Approach, Anterior Column, Percutaneous Endoscopic Approach

ØRG44J0　Fusion of Cervicothoracic Vertebral Joint with Synthetic Substitute, Anterior Approach, Anterior Column, Percutaneous Endoscopic Approach

ØRG44J1　Fusion of Cervicothoracic Vertebral Joint with Synthetic Substitute, Posterior Approach, Posterior Column, Percutaneous Endoscopic Approach

Appendix I: Hospital Acquired Conditions

HAC 12: Surgical Site Infection Following Certain Orthopedic Procedures of the Spine, Shoulder, and Elbow (continued)

ØRG44JJ Fusion of Cervicothoracic Vertebral Joint with Synthetic Substitute, Posterior Approach, Anterior Column, Percutaneous Endoscopic Approach

ØRG44KØ Fusion of Cervicothoracic Vertebral Joint with Nonautologous Tissue Substitute, Anterior Approach, Anterior Column, Percutaneous Endoscopic Approach

ØRG44K1 Fusion of Cervicothoracic Vertebral Joint with Nonautologous Tissue Substitute, Posterior Approach, Posterior Column, Percutaneous Endoscopic Approach

ØRG44KJ Fusion of Cervicothoracic Vertebral Joint with Nonautologous Tissue Substitute, Posterior Approach, Anterior Column, Percutaneous Endoscopic Approach

ØRG44ZØ Fusion of Cervicothoracic Vertebral Joint, Anterior Approach, Anterior Column, Percutaneous Endoscopic Approach

ØRG44Z1 Fusion of Cervicothoracic Vertebral Joint, Posterior Approach, Posterior Column, Percutaneous Endoscopic Approach

ØRG44ZJ Fusion of Cervicothoracic Vertebral Joint, Posterior Approach, Anterior Column, Percutaneous Endoscopic Approach

ØRG6Ø7Ø Fusion of Thoracic Vertebral Joint with Autologous Tissue Substitute, Anterior Approach, Anterior Column, Open Approach

ØRG6Ø71 Fusion of Thoracic Vertebral Joint with Autologous Tissue Substitute, Posterior Approach, Posterior Column, Open Approach

ØRG6Ø7J Fusion of Thoracic Vertebral Joint with Autologous Tissue Substitute, Posterior Approach, Anterior Column, Open Approach

ØRG6ØAØ Fusion of Thoracic Vertebral Joint with Interbody Fusion Device, Anterior Approach, Anterior Column, Open Approach

ØRG6ØA1 Fusion of Thoracic Vertebral Joint with Interbody Fusion Device, Posterior Approach, Posterior Column, Open Approach

ØRG6ØAJ Fusion of Thoracic Vertebral Joint with Interbody Fusion Device, Posterior Approach, Anterior Column, Open Approach

ØRG6ØJØ Fusion of Thoracic Vertebral Joint with Synthetic Substitute, Anterior Approach, Anterior Column, Open Approach

ØRG6ØJ1 Fusion of Thoracic Vertebral Joint with Synthetic Substitute, Posterior Approach, Posterior Column, Open Approach

ØRG6ØJJ Fusion of Thoracic Vertebral Joint with Synthetic Substitute, Posterior Approach, Anterior Column, Open Approach

ØRG6ØKØ Fusion of Thoracic Vertebral Joint with Nonautologous Tissue Substitute, Anterior Approach, Anterior Column, Open Approach

ØRG6ØK1 Fusion of Thoracic Vertebral Joint with Nonautologous Tissue Substitute, Posterior Approach, Posterior Column, Open Approach

ØRG6ØKJ Fusion of Thoracic Vertebral Joint with Nonautologous Tissue Substitute, Posterior Approach, Anterior Column, Open Approach

ØRG6ØZØ Fusion of Thoracic Vertebral Joint, Anterior Approach, Anterior Column, Open Approach

ØRG6ØZ1 Fusion of Thoracic Vertebral Joint, Posterior Approach, Posterior Column, Open Approach

ØRG6ØZJ Fusion of Thoracic Vertebral Joint, Posterior Approach, Anterior Column, Open Approach

ØRG637Ø Fusion of Thoracic Vertebral Joint with Autologous Tissue Substitute, Anterior Approach, Anterior Column, Percutaneous Approach

ØRG6371 Fusion of Thoracic Vertebral Joint with Autologous Tissue Substitute, Posterior Approach, Posterior Column, Percutaneous Approach

ØRG637J Fusion of Thoracic Vertebral Joint with Autologous Tissue Substitute, Posterior Approach, Anterior Column, Percutaneous Approach

ØRG63AØ Fusion of Thoracic Vertebral Joint with Interbody Fusion Device, Anterior Approach, Anterior Column, Percutaneous Approach

ØRG63A1 Fusion of Thoracic Vertebral Joint with Interbody Fusion Device, Posterior Approach, Posterior Column, Percutaneous Approach

ØRG63AJ Fusion of Thoracic Vertebral Joint with Interbody Fusion Device, Posterior Approach, Anterior Column, Percutaneous Approach

ØRG63JØ Fusion of Thoracic Vertebral Joint with Synthetic Substitute, Anterior Approach, Anterior Column, Percutaneous Approach

ØRG63J1 Fusion of Thoracic Vertebral Joint with Synthetic Substitute, Posterior Approach, Posterior Column, Percutaneous Approach

ØRG63JJ Fusion of Thoracic Vertebral Joint with Synthetic Substitute, Posterior Approach, Anterior Column, Percutaneous Approach

ØRG63KØ Fusion of Thoracic Vertebral Joint with Nonautologous Tissue Substitute, Anterior Approach, Anterior Column, Percutaneous Approach

ØRG63K1 Fusion of Thoracic Vertebral Joint with Nonautologous Tissue Substitute, Posterior Approach, Posterior Column, Percutaneous Approach

ØRG63KJ Fusion of Thoracic Vertebral Joint with Nonautologous Tissue Substitute, Posterior Approach, Anterior Column, Percutaneous Approach

ØRG63ZØ Fusion of Thoracic Vertebral Joint, Anterior Approach, Anterior Column, Percutaneous Approach

ØRG63Z1 Fusion of Thoracic Vertebral Joint, Posterior Approach, Posterior Column, Percutaneous Approach

ØRG63ZJ Fusion of Thoracic Vertebral Joint, Posterior Approach, Anterior Column, Percutaneous Approach

ØRG647Ø Fusion of Thoracic Vertebral Joint with Autologous Tissue Substitute, Anterior Approach, Anterior Column, Percutaneous Endoscopic Approach

ØRG6471 Fusion of Thoracic Vertebral Joint with Autologous Tissue Substitute, Posterior Approach, Posterior Column, Percutaneous Endoscopic Approach

ØRG647J Fusion of Thoracic Vertebral Joint with Autologous Tissue Substitute, Posterior Approach, Anterior Column, Percutaneous Endoscopic Approach

ØRG64AØ Fusion of Thoracic Vertebral Joint with Interbody Fusion Device, Anterior Approach, Anterior Column, Percutaneous Endoscopic Approach

ØRG64A1 Fusion of Thoracic Vertebral Joint with Interbody Fusion Device, Posterior Approach, Posterior Column, Percutaneous Endoscopic Approach

ØRG64AJ Fusion of Thoracic Vertebral Joint with Interbody Fusion Device, Posterior Approach, Anterior Column, Percutaneous Endoscopic Approach

ØRG64JØ Fusion of Thoracic Vertebral Joint with Synthetic Substitute, Anterior Approach, Anterior Column, Percutaneous Endoscopic Approach

ØRG64J1 Fusion of Thoracic Vertebral Joint with Synthetic Substitute, Posterior Approach, Posterior Column, Percutaneous Endoscopic Approach

ØRG64JJ Fusion of Thoracic Vertebral Joint with Synthetic Substitute, Posterior Approach, Anterior Column, Percutaneous Endoscopic Approach

ØRG64KØ Fusion of Thoracic Vertebral Joint with Nonautologous Tissue Substitute, Anterior Approach, Anterior Column, Percutaneous Endoscopic Approach

ØRG64K1 Fusion of Thoracic Vertebral Joint with Nonautologous Tissue Substitute, Posterior Approach, Posterior Column, Percutaneous Endoscopic Approach

ØRG64KJ Fusion of Thoracic Vertebral Joint with Nonautologous Tissue Substitute, Posterior Approach, Anterior Column, Percutaneous Endoscopic Approach

ØRG64ZØ Fusion of Thoracic Vertebral Joint, Anterior Approach, Anterior Column, Percutaneous Endoscopic Approach

ØRG64Z1 Fusion of Thoracic Vertebral Joint, Posterior Approach, Posterior Column, Percutaneous Endoscopic Approach

ØRG64ZJ Fusion of Thoracic Vertebral Joint, Posterior Approach, Anterior Column, Percutaneous Endoscopic Approach

ØRG7Ø7Ø Fusion of 2 to 7 Thoracic Vertebral Joints with Autologous Tissue Substitute, Anterior Approach, Anterior Column, Open Approach

ØRG7Ø71 Fusion of 2 to 7 Thoracic Vertebral Joints with Autologous Tissue Substitute, Posterior Approach, Posterior Column, Open Approach

ØRG7Ø7J Fusion of 2 to 7 Thoracic Vertebral Joints with Autologous Tissue Substitute, Posterior Approach, Posterior Column, Open Approach

ØRG7ØAØ Fusion of 2 to 7 Thoracic Vertebral Joints with Interbody Fusion Device, Anterior Approach, Anterior Column, Open Approach

ØRG7ØA1 Fusion of 2 to 7 Thoracic Vertebral Joints with Interbody Fusion Device, Posterior Approach, Posterior Column, Open Approach

ØRG7ØAJ Fusion of 2 to 7 Thoracic Vertebral Joints with Interbody Fusion Device, Posterior Approach, Anterior Column, Open Approach

ØRG7ØJØ Fusion of 2 to 7 Thoracic Vertebral Joints with Synthetic Substitute, Anterior Approach, Anterior Column, Open Approach

ØRG7ØJ1 Fusion of 2 to 7 Thoracic Vertebral Joints with Synthetic Substitute, Posterior Approach, Posterior Column, Open Approach

HAC 12: Surgical Site Infection Following Certain Orthopedic Procedures of the Spine, Shoulder, and Elbow (continued)

ØRG7ØJJ Fusion of 2 to 7 Thoracic Vertebral Joints with Synthetic Substitute, Posterior Approach, Anterior Column, Open Approach

ØRG7ØKØ Fusion of 2 to 7 Thoracic Vertebral Joints with Nonautologous Tissue Substitute, Anterior Approach, Anterior Column, Open Approach

ØRG7ØK1 Fusion of 2 to 7 Thoracic Vertebral Joints with Nonautologous Tissue Substitute, Posterior Approach, Posterior Column, Open Approach

ØRG7ØKJ Fusion of 2 to 7 Thoracic Vertebral Joints with Nonautologous Tissue Substitute, Posterior Approach, Anterior Column, Open Approach

ØRG7ØZØ Fusion of 2 to 7 Thoracic Vertebral Joints, Anterior Approach, Anterior Column, Open Approach

ØRG7ØZ1 Fusion of 2 to 7 Thoracic Vertebral Joints, Posterior Approach, Posterior Column, Open Approach

ØRG7ØZJ Fusion of 2 to 7 Thoracic Vertebral Joints, Posterior Approach, Anterior Column, Open Approach

ØRG737Ø Fusion of 2 to 7 Thoracic Vertebral Joints with Autologous Tissue Substitute, Anterior Approach, Anterior Column, Percutaneous Approach

ØRG7371 Fusion of 2 to 7 Thoracic Vertebral Joints with Autologous Tissue Substitute, Posterior Approach, Posterior Column, Percutaneous Approach

ØRG737J Fusion of 2 to 7 Thoracic Vertebral Joints with Autologous Tissue Substitute, Posterior Approach, Anterior Column, Percutaneous Approach

ØRG73AØ Fusion of 2 to 7 Thoracic Vertebral Joints with Interbody Fusion Device, Anterior Approach, Anterior Column, Percutaneous Approach

ØRG73A1 Fusion of 2 to 7 Thoracic Vertebral Joints with Interbody Fusion Device, Posterior Approach, Posterior Column, Percutaneous Approach

ØRG73AJ Fusion of 2 to 7 Thoracic Vertebral Joints with Interbody Fusion Device, Posterior Approach, Anterior Column, Percutaneous Approach

ØRG73JØ Fusion of 2 to 7 Thoracic Vertebral Joints with Synthetic Substitute, Anterior Approach, Anterior Column, Percutaneous Approach

ØRG73J1 Fusion of 2 to 7 Thoracic Vertebral Joints with Synthetic Substitute, Posterior Approach, Posterior Column, Percutaneous Approach

ØRG73JJ Fusion of 2 to 7 Thoracic Vertebral Joints with Synthetic Substitute, Posterior Approach, Anterior Column, Percutaneous Approach

ØRG73KØ Fusion of 2 to 7 Thoracic Vertebral Joints with Nonautologous Tissue Substitute, Anterior Approach, Anterior Column, Percutaneous Approach

ØRG73K1 Fusion of 2 to 7 Thoracic Vertebral Joints with Nonautologous Tissue Substitute, Posterior Approach, Posterior Column, Percutaneous Approach

ØRG73KJ Fusion of 2 to 7 Thoracic Vertebral Joints with Nonautologous Tissue Substitute, Posterior Approach, Anterior Column, Percutaneous Approach

ØRG73ZØ Fusion of 2 to 7 Thoracic Vertebral Joints, Anterior Approach, Anterior Column, Percutaneous Approach

ØRG73Z1 Fusion of 2 to 7 Thoracic Vertebral Joints, Posterior Approach, Posterior Column, Percutaneous Approach

ØRG73ZJ Fusion of 2 to 7 Thoracic Vertebral Joints, Posterior Approach, Anterior Column, Percutaneous Approach

ØRG747Ø Fusion of 2 to 7 Thoracic Vertebral Joints with Autologous Tissue Substitute, Anterior Approach, Anterior Column, Percutaneous Endoscopic Approach

ØRG7471 Fusion of 2 to 7 Thoracic Vertebral Joints with Autologous Tissue Substitute, Posterior Approach, Posterior Column, Percutaneous Endoscopic Approach

ØRG747J Fusion of 2 to 7 Thoracic Vertebral Joints with Autologous Tissue Substitute, Posterior Approach, Anterior Column, Percutaneous Endoscopic Approach

ØRG74AØ Fusion of 2 to 7 Thoracic Vertebral Joints with Interbody Fusion Device, Anterior Approach, Anterior Column, Percutaneous Endoscopic Approach

ØRG74A1 Fusion of 2 to 7 Thoracic Vertebral Joints with Interbody Fusion Device, Posterior Approach, Posterior Column, Percutaneous Endoscopic Approach

ØRG74AJ Fusion of 2 to 7 Thoracic Vertebral Joints with Interbody Fusion Device, Posterior Approach, Anterior Column, Percutaneous Endoscopic Approach

ØRG74JØ Fusion of 2 to 7 Thoracic Vertebral Joints with Synthetic Substitute, Anterior Approach, Anterior Column, Percutaneous Endoscopic Approach

ØRG74J1 Fusion of 2 to 7 Thoracic Vertebral Joints with Synthetic Substitute, Posterior Approach, Posterior Column, Percutaneous Endoscopic Approach

ØRG74JJ Fusion of 2 to 7 Thoracic Vertebral Joints with Synthetic Substitute, Posterior Approach, Anterior Column, Percutaneous Endoscopic Approach

ØRG74KØ Fusion of 2 to 7 Thoracic Vertebral Joints with Nonautologous Tissue Substitute, Anterior Approach, Anterior Column, Percutaneous Endoscopic Approach

ØRG74K1 Fusion of 2 to 7 Thoracic Vertebral Joints with Nonautologous Tissue Substitute, Posterior Approach, Posterior Column, Percutaneous Endoscopic Approach

ØRG74KJ Fusion of 2 to 7 Thoracic Vertebral Joints with Nonautologous Tissue Substitute, Posterior Approach, Anterior Column, Percutaneous Endoscopic Approach

ØRG74ZØ Fusion of 2 to 7 Thoracic Vertebral Joints, Anterior Approach, Anterior Column, Percutaneous Endoscopic Approach

ØRG74Z1 Fusion of 2 to 7 Thoracic Vertebral Joints, Posterior Approach, Posterior Column, Percutaneous Endoscopic Approach

ØRG74ZJ Fusion of 2 to 7 Thoracic Vertebral Joints, Posterior Approach, Anterior Column, Percutaneous Endoscopic Approach

ØRG8Ø7Ø Fusion of 8 or More Thoracic Vertebral Joints with Autologous Tissue Substitute, Anterior Approach, Anterior Column, Open Approach

ØRG8Ø71 Fusion of 8 or More Thoracic Vertebral Joints with Autologous Tissue Substitute, Posterior Approach, Posterior Column, Open Approach

ØRG8Ø7J Fusion of 8 or More Thoracic Vertebral Joints with Autologous Tissue Substitute, Posterior Approach, Anterior Column, Open Approach

ØRG8ØAØ Fusion of 8 or More Thoracic Vertebral Joints with Interbody Fusion Device, Anterior Approach, Anterior Column, Open Approach

ØRG8ØA1 Fusion of 8 or More Thoracic Vertebral Joints with Interbody Fusion Device, Posterior Approach, Posterior Column, Open Approach

ØRG8ØAJ Fusion of 8 or More Thoracic Vertebral Joints with Interbody Fusion Device, Posterior Approach, Anterior Column, Open Approach

ØRG8ØJØ Fusion of 8 or More Thoracic Vertebral Joints with Synthetic Substitute, Anterior Approach, Anterior Column, Open Approach

ØRG8ØJ1 Fusion of 8 or More Thoracic Vertebral Joints with Synthetic Substitute, Posterior Approach, Posterior Column, Open Approach

ØRG8ØJJ Fusion of 8 or More Thoracic Vertebral Joints with Synthetic Substitute, Posterior Approach, Anterior Column, Open Approach

ØRG8ØKØ Fusion of 8 or More Thoracic Vertebral Joints with Nonautologous Tissue Substitute, Anterior Approach, Anterior Column, Open Approach

ØRG8ØK1 Fusion of 8 or More Thoracic Vertebral Joints with Nonautologous Tissue Substitute, Posterior Approach, Posterior Column, Open Approach

ØRG8ØKJ Fusion of 8 or More Thoracic Vertebral Joints with Nonautologous Tissue Substitute, Posterior Approach, Anterior Column, Open Approach

ØRG8ØZØ Fusion of 8 or More Thoracic Vertebral Joints, Anterior Approach, Anterior Column, Open Approach

ØRG8ØZ1 Fusion of 8 or More Thoracic Vertebral Joints, Posterior Approach, Posterior Column, Open Approach

ØRG8ØZJ Fusion of 8 or More Thoracic Vertebral Joints, Posterior Approach, Anterior Column, Open Approach

ØRG837Ø Fusion of 8 or More Thoracic Vertebral Joints with Autologous Tissue Substitute, Anterior Approach, Anterior Column, Percutaneous Approach

ØRG8371 Fusion of 8 or More Thoracic Vertebral Joints with Autologous Tissue Substitute, Posterior Approach, Posterior Column, Percutaneous Approach

ØRG837J Fusion of 8 or More Thoracic Vertebral Joints with Autologous Tissue Substitute, Posterior Approach, Anterior Column, Percutaneous Approach

ØRG83AØ Fusion of 8 or More Thoracic Vertebral Joints with Interbody Fusion Device, Anterior Approach, Anterior Column, Percutaneous Approach

ØRG83A1 Fusion of 8 or More Thoracic Vertebral Joints with Interbody Fusion Device, Posterior Approach, Posterior Column, Percutaneous Approach

ØRG83AJ Fusion of 8 or More Thoracic Vertebral Joints with Interbody Fusion Device, Posterior Approach, Anterior Column, Percutaneous Approach

ØRG83JØ Fusion of 8 or More Thoracic Vertebral Joints with Synthetic Substitute, Anterior Approach, Anterior Column, Percutaneous Approach

HAC 12: Surgical Site Infection Following Certain Orthopedic Procedures of the Spine, Shoulder, and Elbow (continued)

ØRG83J1 Fusion of 8 or More Thoracic Vertebral Joints with Synthetic Substitute, Posterior Approach, Posterior Column, Percutaneous Approach

ØRG83JJ Fusion of 8 or More Thoracic Vertebral Joints with Synthetic Substitute, Posterior Approach, Anterior Column, Percutaneous Approach

ØRG83KØ Fusion of 8 or More Thoracic Vertebral Joints with Nonautologous Tissue Substitute, Anterior Approach, Anterior Column, Percutaneous Approach

ØRG83K1 Fusion of 8 or More Thoracic Vertebral Joints with Nonautologous Tissue Substitute, Posterior Approach, Posterior Column, Percutaneous Approach

ØRG83KJ Fusion of 8 or More Thoracic Vertebral Joints with Nonautologous Tissue Substitute, Posterior Approach, Anterior Column, Percutaneous Approach

ØRG83ZØ Fusion of 8 or More Thoracic Vertebral Joints, Anterior Approach, Anterior Column, Percutaneous Approach

ØRG83Z1 Fusion of 8 or More Thoracic Vertebral Joints, Posterior Approach, Posterior Column, Percutaneous Approach

ØRG83ZJ Fusion of 8 or More Thoracic Vertebral Joints, Posterior Approach, Anterior Column, Percutaneous Approach

ØRG847Ø Fusion of 8 or More Thoracic Vertebral Joints with Autologous Tissue Substitute, Anterior Approach, Anterior Column, Percutaneous Endoscopic Approach

ØRG8471 Fusion of 8 or More Thoracic Vertebral Joints with Autologous Tissue Substitute, Posterior Approach, Posterior Column, Percutaneous Endoscopic Approach

ØRG847J Fusion of 8 or More Thoracic Vertebral Joints with Autologous Tissue Substitute, Posterior Approach, Anterior Column, Percutaneous Endoscopic Approach

ØRG84AØ Fusion of 8 or More Thoracic Vertebral Joints with Interbody Fusion Device, Anterior Approach, Anterior Column, Percutaneous Endoscopic Approach

ØRG84A1 Fusion of 8 or More Thoracic Vertebral Joints with Interbody Fusion Device, Posterior Approach, Posterior Column, Percutaneous Endoscopic Approach

ØRG84AJ Fusion of 8 or More Thoracic Vertebral Joints with Interbody Fusion Device, Posterior Approach, Anterior Column, Percutaneous Endoscopic Approach

ØRG84JØ Fusion of 8 or More Thoracic Vertebral Joints with Synthetic Substitute, Anterior Approach, Anterior Column, Percutaneous Endoscopic Approach

ØRG84J1 Fusion of 8 or More Thoracic Vertebral Joints with Synthetic Substitute, Posterior Approach, Posterior Column, Percutaneous Endoscopic Approach

ØRG84JJ Fusion of 8 or More Thoracic Vertebral Joints with Synthetic Substitute, Posterior Approach, Anterior Column, Percutaneous Endoscopic Approach

ØRG84KØ Fusion of 8 or More Thoracic Vertebral Joints with Nonautologous Tissue Substitute, Anterior Approach, Anterior Column, Percutaneous Endoscopic Approach

ØRG84K1 Fusion of 8 or More Thoracic Vertebral Joints with Nonautologous Tissue Substitute, Posterior Approach, Posterior Column, Percutaneous Endoscopic Approach

ØRG84KJ Fusion of 8 or More Thoracic Vertebral Joints with Nonautologous Tissue Substitute, Posterior Approach, Anterior Column, Percutaneous Endoscopic Approach

ØRG84ZØ Fusion of 8 or More Thoracic Vertebral Joints, Anterior Approach, Anterior Column, Percutaneous Endoscopic Approach

ØRG84Z1 Fusion of 8 or More Thoracic Vertebral Joints, Posterior Approach, Posterior Column, Percutaneous Endoscopic Approach

ØRG84ZJ Fusion of 8 or More Thoracic Vertebral Joints, Posterior Approach, Anterior Column, Percutaneous Endoscopic Approach

ØRGAØ7Ø Fusion of Thoracolumbar Vertebral Joint with Autologous Tissue Substitute, Anterior Approach, Anterior Column, Open Approach

ØRGAØ71 Fusion of Thoracolumbar Vertebral Joint with Autologous Tissue Substitute, Posterior Approach, Posterior Column, Open Approach

ØRGAØ7J Fusion of Thoracolumbar Vertebral Joint with Autologous Tissue Substitute, Posterior Approach, Anterior Column, Open Approach

ØRGAØAØ Fusion of Thoracolumbar Vertebral Joint with Interbody Fusion Device, Anterior Approach, Anterior Column, Open Approach

ØRGAØA1 Fusion of Thoracolumbar Vertebral Joint with Interbody Fusion Device, Posterior Approach, Posterior Column, Open Approach

ØRGAØAJ Fusion of Thoracolumbar Vertebral Joint with Interbody Fusion Device, Posterior Approach, Anterior Column, Open Approach

ØRGAØJØ Fusion of Thoracolumbar Vertebral Joint with Synthetic Substitute, Anterior Approach, Anterior Column, Open Approach

ØRGAØJ1 Fusion of Thoracolumbar Vertebral Joint with Synthetic Substitute, Posterior Approach, Posterior Column, Open Approach

ØRGAØJJ Fusion of Thoracolumbar Vertebral Joint with Synthetic Substitute, Posterior Approach, Anterior Column, Open Approach

ØRGAØKØ Fusion of Thoracolumbar Vertebral Joint with Nonautologous Tissue Substitute, Anterior Approach, Anterior Column, Open Approach

ØRGAØK1 Fusion of Thoracolumbar Vertebral Joint with Nonautologous Tissue Substitute, Posterior Approach, Posterior Column, Open Approach

ØRGAØKJ Fusion of Thoracolumbar Vertebral Joint with Nonautologous Tissue Substitute, Posterior Approach, Anterior Column, Open Approach

ØRGAØZØ Fusion of Thoracolumbar Vertebral Joint, Anterior Approach, Anterior Column, Open Approach

ØRGAØZ1 Fusion of Thoracolumbar Vertebral Joint, Posterior Approach, Posterior Column, Open Approach

ØRGAØZJ Fusion of Thoracolumbar Vertebral Joint, Posterior Approach, Anterior Column, Open Approach

ØRGA37Ø Fusion of Thoracolumbar Vertebral Joint with Autologous Tissue Substitute, Anterior Approach, Anterior Column, Percutaneous Approach

ØRGA371 Fusion of Thoracolumbar Vertebral Joint with Autologous Tissue Substitute, Posterior Approach, Posterior Column, Percutaneous Approach

ØRGA37J Fusion of Thoracolumbar Vertebral Joint with Autologous Tissue Substitute, Posterior Approach, Anterior Column, Percutaneous Approach

ØRGA3AØ Fusion of Thoracolumbar Vertebral Joint with Interbody Fusion Device, Anterior Approach, Anterior Column, Percutaneous Approach

ØRGA3A1 Fusion of Thoracolumbar Vertebral Joint with Interbody Fusion Device, Posterior Approach, Posterior Column, Percutaneous Approach

ØRGA3AJ Fusion of Thoracolumbar Vertebral Joint with Interbody Fusion Device, Posterior Approach, Anterior Column, Percutaneous Approach

ØRGA3JØ Fusion of Thoracolumbar Vertebral Joint with Synthetic Substitute, Anterior Approach, Anterior Column, Percutaneous Approach

ØRGA3J1 Fusion of Thoracolumbar Vertebral Joint with Synthetic Substitute, Posterior Approach, Posterior Column, Percutaneous Approach

ØRGA3JJ Fusion of Thoracolumbar Vertebral Joint with Synthetic Substitute, Posterior Approach, Anterior Column, Percutaneous Approach

ØRGA3KØ Fusion of Thoracolumbar Vertebral Joint with Nonautologous Tissue Substitute, Anterior Approach, Anterior Column, Percutaneous Approach

ØRGA3K1 Fusion of Thoracolumbar Vertebral Joint with Nonautologous Tissue Substitute, Posterior Approach, Posterior Column, Percutaneous Approach

ØRGA3KJ Fusion of Thoracolumbar Vertebral Joint with Nonautologous Tissue Substitute, Posterior Approach, Anterior Column, Percutaneous Approach

ØRGA3ZØ Fusion of Thoracolumbar Vertebral Joint, Anterior Approach, Anterior Column, Percutaneous Approach

ØRGA3Z1 Fusion of Thoracolumbar Vertebral Joint, Posterior Approach, Posterior Column, Percutaneous Approach

ØRGA3ZJ Fusion of Thoracolumbar Vertebral Joint, Posterior Approach, Anterior Column, Percutaneous Approach

ØRGA47Ø Fusion of Thoracolumbar Vertebral Joint with Autologous Tissue Substitute, Anterior Approach, Anterior Column, Percutaneous Endoscopic Approach

ØRGA471 Fusion of Thoracolumbar Vertebral Joint with Autologous Tissue Substitute, Posterior Approach, Posterior Column, Percutaneous Endoscopic Approach

ØRGA47J Fusion of Thoracolumbar Vertebral Joint with Autologous Tissue Substitute, Posterior Approach, Anterior Column, Percutaneous Endoscopic Approach

ØRGA4AØ Fusion of Thoracolumbar Vertebral Joint with Interbody Fusion Device, Anterior Approach, Anterior Column, Percutaneous Endoscopic Approach

HAC 12: Surgical Site Infection Following Certain Orthopedic Procedures of the Spine, Shoulder, and Elbow (continued)

ØRGA4A1 Fusion of Thoracolumbar Vertebral Joint with Interbody Fusion Device, Posterior Approach, Posterior Column, Percutaneous Endoscopic Approach

ØRGA4AJ Fusion of Thoracolumbar Vertebral Joint with Interbody Fusion Device, Posterior Approach, Anterior Column, Percutaneous Endoscopic Approach

ØRGA4JØ Fusion of Thoracolumbar Vertebral Joint with Synthetic Substitute, Anterior Approach, Anterior Column, Percutaneous Endoscopic Approach

ØRGA4J1 Fusion of Thoracolumbar Vertebral Joint with Synthetic Substitute, Posterior Approach, Posterior Column, Percutaneous Endoscopic Approach

ØRGA4JJ Fusion of Thoracolumbar Vertebral Joint with Synthetic Substitute, Posterior Approach, Anterior Column, Percutaneous Endoscopic Approach

ØRGA4KØ Fusion of Thoracolumbar Vertebral Joint with Nonautologous Tissue Substitute, Anterior Approach, Anterior Column, Percutaneous Endoscopic Approach

ØRGA4K1 Fusion of Thoracolumbar Vertebral Joint with Nonautologous Tissue Substitute, Posterior Approach, Posterior Column, Percutaneous Endoscopic Approach

ØRGA4KJ Fusion of Thoracolumbar Vertebral Joint with Nonautologous Tissue Substitute, Posterior Approach, Anterior Column, Percutaneous Endoscopic Approach

ØRGA4ZØ Fusion of Thoracolumbar Vertebral Joint, Anterior Approach, Anterior Column, Percutaneous Endoscopic Approach

ØRGA4Z1 Fusion of Thoracolumbar Vertebral Joint, Posterior Approach, Posterior Column, Percutaneous Endoscopic Approach

ØRGA4ZJ Fusion of Thoracolumbar Vertebral Joint, Posterior Approach, Anterior Column, Percutaneous Endoscopic Approach

ØRGEØ4Z Fusion of Right Sternoclavicular Joint with Internal Fixation Device, Open Approach

ØRGEØ7Z Fusion of Right Sternoclavicular Joint with Autologous Tissue Substitute, Open Approach

ØRGEØJZ Fusion of Right Sternoclavicular Joint with Synthetic Substitute, Open Approach

ØRGEØKZ Fusion of Right Sternoclavicular Joint with Nonautologous Tissue Substitute, Open Approach

ØRGEØZZ Fusion of Right Sternoclavicular Joint, Open Approach

ØRGE34Z Fusion of Right Sternoclavicular Joint with Internal Fixation Device, Percutaneous Approach

ØRGE37Z Fusion of Right Sternoclavicular Joint with Autologous Tissue Substitute, Percutaneous Approach

ØRGE3JZ Fusion of Right Sternoclavicular Joint with Synthetic Substitute, Percutaneous Approach

ØRGE3KZ Fusion of Right Sternoclavicular Joint with Nonautologous Tissue Substitute, Percutaneous Approach

ØRGE3ZZ Fusion of Right Sternoclavicular Joint, Percutaneous Approach

ØRGE44Z Fusion of Right Sternoclavicular Joint with Internal Fixation Device, Percutaneous Endoscopic Approach

ØRGE47Z Fusion of Right Sternoclavicular Joint with Autologous Tissue Substitute, Percutaneous Endoscopic Approach

ØRGE4JZ Fusion of Right Sternoclavicular Joint with Synthetic Substitute, Percutaneous Endoscopic Approach

ØRGE4KZ Fusion of Right Sternoclavicular Joint with Nonautologous Tissue Substitute, Percutaneous Endoscopic Approach

ØRGE4ZZ Fusion of Right Sternoclavicular Joint, Percutaneous Endoscopic Approach

ØRGFØ4Z Fusion of Left Sternoclavicular Joint with Internal Fixation Device, Open Approach

ØRGFØ7Z Fusion of Left Sternoclavicular Joint with Autologous Tissue Substitute, Open Approach

ØRGFØJZ Fusion of Left Sternoclavicular Joint with Synthetic Substitute, Open Approach

ØRGFØKZ Fusion of Left Sternoclavicular Joint with Nonautologous Tissue Substitute, Open Approach

ØRGFØZZ Fusion of Left Sternoclavicular Joint, Open Approach

ØRGF34Z Fusion of Left Sternoclavicular Joint with Internal Fixation Device, Percutaneous Approach

ØRGF37Z Fusion of Left Sternoclavicular Joint with Autologous Tissue Substitute, Percutaneous Approach

ØRGF3JZ Fusion of Left Sternoclavicular Joint with Synthetic Substitute, Percutaneous Approach

ØRGF3KZ Fusion of Left Sternoclavicular Joint with Nonautologous Tissue Substitute, Percutaneous Approach

ØRGF3ZZ Fusion of Left Sternoclavicular Joint, Percutaneous Approach

ØRGF44Z Fusion of Left Sternoclavicular Joint with Internal Fixation Device, Percutaneous Endoscopic Approach

ØRGF47Z Fusion of Left Sternoclavicular Joint with Autologous Tissue Substitute, Percutaneous Endoscopic Approach

ØRGF4JZ Fusion of Left Sternoclavicular Joint with Synthetic Substitute, Percutaneous Endoscopic Approach

ØRGF4KZ Fusion of Left Sternoclavicular Joint with Nonautologous Tissue Substitute, Percutaneous Endoscopic Approach

ØRGF4ZZ Fusion of Left Sternoclavicular Joint, Percutaneous Endoscopic Approach

ØRGGØ4Z Fusion of Right Acromioclavicular Joint with Internal Fixation Device, Open Approach

ØRGGØ7Z Fusion of Right Acromioclavicular Joint with Autologous Tissue Substitute, Open Approach

ØRGGØJZ Fusion of Right Acromioclavicular Joint with Synthetic Substitute, Open Approach

ØRGGØKZ Fusion of Right Acromioclavicular Joint with Nonautologous Tissue Substitute, Open Approach

ØRGGØZZ Fusion of Right Acromioclavicular Joint, Open Approach

ØRGG34Z Fusion of Right Acromioclavicular Joint with Internal Fixation Device, Percutaneous Approach

ØRGG37Z Fusion of Right Acromioclavicular Joint with Autologous Tissue Substitute, Percutaneous Approach

ØRGG3JZ Fusion of Right Acromioclavicular Joint with Synthetic Substitute, Percutaneous Approach

ØRGG3KZ Fusion of Right Acromioclavicular Joint with Nonautologous Tissue Substitute, Percutaneous Approach

ØRGG3ZZ Fusion of Right Acromioclavicular Joint, Percutaneous Approach

ØRGG44Z Fusion of Right Acromioclavicular Joint with Internal Fixation Device, Percutaneous Endoscopic Approach

ØRGG47Z Fusion of Right Acromioclavicular Joint with Autologous Tissue Substitute, Percutaneous Endoscopic Approach

ØRGG4JZ Fusion of Right Acromioclavicular Joint with Synthetic Substitute, Percutaneous Endoscopic Approach

ØRGG4KZ Fusion of Right Acromioclavicular Joint with Nonautologous Tissue Substitute, Percutaneous Endoscopic Approach

ØRGG4ZZ Fusion of Right Acromioclavicular Joint, Percutaneous Endoscopic Approach

ØRGHØ4Z Fusion of Left Acromioclavicular Joint with Internal Fixation Device, Open Approach

ØRGHØ7Z Fusion of Left Acromioclavicular Joint with Autologous Tissue Substitute, Open Approach

ØRGHØJZ Fusion of Left Acromioclavicular Joint with Synthetic Substitute, Open Approach

ØRGHØKZ Fusion of Left Acromioclavicular Joint with Nonautologous Tissue Substitute, Open Approach

ØRGHØZZ Fusion of Left Acromioclavicular Joint, Open Approach

ØRGH34Z Fusion of Left Acromioclavicular Joint with Internal Fixation Device, Percutaneous Approach

ØRGH37Z Fusion of Left Acromioclavicular Joint with Autologous Tissue Substitute, Percutaneous Approach

ØRGH3JZ Fusion of Left Acromioclavicular Joint with Synthetic Substitute, Percutaneous Approach

ØRGH3KZ Fusion of Left Acromioclavicular Joint with Nonautologous Tissue Substitute, Percutaneous Approach

ØRGH3ZZ Fusion of Left Acromioclavicular Joint, Percutaneous Approach

ØRGH44Z Fusion of Left Acromioclavicular Joint with Internal Fixation Device, Percutaneous Endoscopic Approach

ØRGH47Z Fusion of Left Acromioclavicular Joint with Autologous Tissue Substitute, Percutaneous Endoscopic Approach

ØRGH4JZ Fusion of Left Acromioclavicular Joint with Synthetic Substitute, Percutaneous Endoscopic Approach

ØRGH4KZ Fusion of Left Acromioclavicular Joint with Nonautologous Tissue Substitute, Percutaneous Endoscopic Approach

ØRGH4ZZ Fusion of Left Acromioclavicular Joint, Percutaneous Endoscopic Approach

ØRGJØ4Z Fusion of Right Shoulder Joint with Internal Fixation Device, Open Approach

ØRGJØ7Z Fusion of Right Shoulder Joint with Autologous Tissue Substitute, Open Approach

ØRGJØJZ Fusion of Right Shoulder Joint with Synthetic Substitute, Open Approach

ØRGJØKZ Fusion of Right Shoulder Joint with Nonautologous Tissue Substitute, Open Approach

ØRGJØZZ Fusion of Right Shoulder Joint, Open Approach

ØRGJ34Z Fusion of Right Shoulder Joint with Internal Fixation Device, Percutaneous Approach

ØRGJ37Z Fusion of Right Shoulder Joint with Autologous Tissue Substitute, Percutaneous Approach

HAC 12: Surgical Site Infection Following Certain Orthopedic Procedures of the Spine, Shoulder, and Elbow (continued)

ØRGJ3JZ Fusion of Right Shoulder Joint with Synthetic Substitute, Percutaneous Approach

ØRGJ3KZ Fusion of Right Shoulder Joint with Nonautologous Tissue Substitute, Percutaneous Approach

ØRGJ3ZZ Fusion of Right Shoulder Joint, Percutaneous Approach

ØRGJ44Z Fusion of Right Shoulder Joint with Internal Fixation Device, Percutaneous Endoscopic Approach

ØRGJ47Z Fusion of Right Shoulder Joint with Autologous Tissue Substitute, Percutaneous Endoscopic Approach

ØRGJ4JZ Fusion of Right Shoulder Joint with Synthetic Substitute, Percutaneous Endoscopic Approach

ØRGJ4KZ Fusion of Right Shoulder Joint with Nonautologous Tissue Substitute, Percutaneous Endoscopic Approach

ØRGJ4ZZ Fusion of Right Shoulder Joint, Percutaneous Endoscopic Approach

ØRGKØ4Z Fusion of Left Shoulder Joint with Internal Fixation Device, Open Approach

ØRGKØ7Z Fusion of Left Shoulder Joint with Autologous Tissue Substitute, Open Approach

ØRGKØJZ Fusion of Left Shoulder Joint with Synthetic Substitute, Open Approach

ØRGKØKZ Fusion of Left Shoulder Joint with Nonautologous Tissue Substitute, Open Approach

ØRGKØZZ Fusion of Left Shoulder Joint, Open Approach

ØRGK34Z Fusion of Left Shoulder Joint with Internal Fixation Device, Percutaneous Approach

ØRGK37Z Fusion of Left Shoulder Joint with Autologous Tissue Substitute, Percutaneous Approach

ØRGK3JZ Fusion of Left Shoulder Joint with Synthetic Substitute, Percutaneous Approach

ØRGK3KZ Fusion of Left Shoulder Joint with Nonautologous Tissue Substitute, Percutaneous Approach

ØRGK3ZZ Fusion of Left Shoulder Joint, Percutaneous Approach

ØRGK44Z Fusion of Left Shoulder Joint with Internal Fixation Device, Percutaneous Endoscopic Approach

ØRGK47Z Fusion of Left Shoulder Joint with Autologous Tissue Substitute, Percutaneous Endoscopic Approach

ØRGK4JZ Fusion of Left Shoulder Joint with Synthetic Substitute, Percutaneous Endoscopic Approach

ØRGK4KZ Fusion of Left Shoulder Joint with Nonautologous Tissue Substitute, Percutaneous Endoscopic Approach

ØRGK4ZZ Fusion of Left Shoulder Joint, Percutaneous Endoscopic Approach

ØRGLØ4Z Fusion of Right Elbow Joint with Internal Fixation Device, Open Approach

ØRGLØ5Z Fusion of Right Elbow Joint with External Fixation Device, Open Approach

ØRGLØ7Z Fusion of Right Elbow Joint with Autologous Tissue Substitute, Open Approach

ØRGLØJZ Fusion of Right Elbow Joint with Synthetic Substitute, Open Approach

ØRGLØKZ Fusion of Right Elbow Joint with Nonautologous Tissue Substitute, Open Approach

ØRGLØZZ Fusion of Right Elbow Joint, Open Approach

ØRGL34Z Fusion of Right Elbow Joint with Internal Fixation Device, Percutaneous Approach

ØRGL35Z Fusion of Right Elbow Joint with External Fixation Device, Percutaneous Approach

ØRGL37Z Fusion of Right Elbow Joint with Autologous Tissue Substitute, Percutaneous Approach

ØRGL3JZ Fusion of Right Elbow Joint with Synthetic Substitute, Percutaneous Approach

ØRGL3KZ Fusion of Right Elbow Joint with Nonautologous Tissue Substitute, Percutaneous Approach

ØRGL3ZZ Fusion of Right Elbow Joint, Percutaneous Approach

ØRGL44Z Fusion of Right Elbow Joint with Internal Fixation Device, Percutaneous Endoscopic Approach

ØRGL45Z Fusion of Right Elbow Joint with External Fixation Device, Percutaneous Endoscopic Approach

ØRGL47Z Fusion of Right Elbow Joint with Autologous Tissue Substitute, Percutaneous Endoscopic Approach

ØRGL4JZ Fusion of Right Elbow Joint with Synthetic Substitute, Percutaneous Endoscopic Approach

ØRGL4KZ Fusion of Right Elbow Joint with Nonautologous Tissue Substitute, Percutaneous Endoscopic Approach

ØRGL4ZZ Fusion of Right Elbow Joint, Percutaneous Endoscopic Approach

ØRGMØ4Z Fusion of Left Elbow Joint with Internal Fixation Device, Open Approach

ØRGMØ5Z Fusion of Left Elbow Joint with External Fixation Device, Open Approach

ØRGMØ7Z Fusion of Left Elbow Joint with Autologous Tissue Substitute, Open Approach

ØRGMØJZ Fusion of Left Elbow Joint with Synthetic Substitute, Open Approach

ØRGMØKZ Fusion of Left Elbow Joint with Nonautologous Tissue Substitute, Open Approach

ØRGMØZZ Fusion of Left Elbow Joint, Open Approach

ØRGM34Z Fusion of Left Elbow Joint with Internal Fixation Device, Percutaneous Approach

ØRGM35Z Fusion of Left Elbow Joint with External Fixation Device, Percutaneous Approach

ØRGM37Z Fusion of Left Elbow Joint with Autologous Tissue Substitute, Percutaneous Approach

ØRGM3JZ Fusion of Left Elbow Joint with Synthetic Substitute, Percutaneous Approach

ØRGM3KZ Fusion of Left Elbow Joint with Nonautologous Tissue Substitute, Percutaneous Approach

ØRGM3ZZ Fusion of Left Elbow Joint, Percutaneous Approach

ØRGM44Z Fusion of Left Elbow Joint with Internal Fixation Device, Percutaneous Endoscopic Approach

ØRGM45Z Fusion of Left Elbow Joint with External Fixation Device, Percutaneous Endoscopic Approach

ØRGM47Z Fusion of Left Elbow Joint with Autologous Tissue Substitute, Percutaneous Endoscopic Approach

ØRGM4JZ Fusion of Left Elbow Joint with Synthetic Substitute, Percutaneous Endoscopic Approach

ØRGM4KZ Fusion of Left Elbow Joint with Nonautologous Tissue Substitute, Percutaneous Endoscopic Approach

ØRGM4ZZ Fusion of Left Elbow Joint, Percutaneous Endoscopic Approach

ØRQEØZZ Repair Right Sternoclavicular Joint, Open Approach

ØRQE3ZZ Repair Right Sternoclavicular Joint, Percutaneous Approach

ØRQE4ZZ Repair Right Sternoclavicular Joint, Percutaneous Endoscopic Approach

ØRQEXZZ Repair Right Sternoclavicular Joint, External Approach

ØRQFØZZ Repair Left Sternoclavicular Joint, Open Approach

ØRQF3ZZ Repair Left Sternoclavicular Joint, Percutaneous Approach

ØRQF4ZZ Repair Left Sternoclavicular Joint, Percutaneous Endoscopic Approach

ØRQFXZZ Repair Left Sternoclavicular Joint, External Approach

ØRQGØZZ Repair Right Acromioclavicular Joint, Open Approach

ØRQG3ZZ Repair Right Acromioclavicular Joint, Percutaneous Approach

ØRQG4ZZ Repair Right Acromioclavicular Joint, Percutaneous Endoscopic Approach

ØRQGXZZ Repair Right Acromioclavicular Joint, External Approach

ØRQHØZZ Repair Left Acromioclavicular Joint, Open Approach

ØRQH3ZZ Repair Left Acromioclavicular Joint, Percutaneous Approach

ØRQH4ZZ Repair Left Acromioclavicular Joint, Percutaneous Endoscopic Approach

ØRQHXZZ Repair Left Acromioclavicular Joint, External Approach

ØRQJØZZ Repair Right Shoulder Joint, Open Approach

ØRQJ3ZZ Repair Right Shoulder Joint, Percutaneous Approach

ØRQJ4ZZ Repair Right Shoulder Joint, Percutaneous Endoscopic Approach

ØRQJXZZ Repair Right Shoulder Joint, External Approach

ØRQKØZZ Repair Left Shoulder Joint, Open Approach

ØRQK3ZZ Repair Left Shoulder Joint, Percutaneous Approach

ØRQK4ZZ Repair Left Shoulder Joint, Percutaneous Endoscopic Approach

ØRQKXZZ Repair Left Shoulder Joint, External Approach

ØRQLØZZ Repair Right Elbow Joint, Open Approach

ØRQL3ZZ Repair Right Elbow Joint, Percutaneous Approach

ØRQL4ZZ Repair Right Elbow Joint, Percutaneous Endoscopic Approach

ØRQLXZZ Repair Right Elbow Joint, External Approach

ØRQMØZZ Repair Left Elbow Joint, Open Approach

ØRQM3ZZ Repair Left Elbow Joint, Percutaneous Approach

ØRQM4ZZ Repair Left Elbow Joint, Percutaneous Endoscopic Approach

ØRQMXZZ Repair Left Elbow Joint, External Approach

ØRUEØ7Z Supplement Right Sternoclavicular Joint with Autologous Tissue Substitute, Open Approach

ØRUEØJZ Supplement Right Sternoclavicular Joint with Synthetic Substitute, Open Approach

ØRUEØKZ Supplement Right Sternoclavicular Joint with Nonautologous Tissue Substitute, Open Approach

ØRUE37Z Supplement Right Sternoclavicular Joint with Autologous Tissue Substitute, Percutaneous Approach

HAC 12: Surgical Site Infection Following Certain Orthopedic Procedures of the Spine, Shoulder, and Elbow (continued)

ØRUE3JZ   Supplement Right Sternoclavicular Joint with Synthetic Substitute, Percutaneous Approach

ØRUE3KZ   Supplement Right Sternoclavicular Joint with Nonautologous Tissue Substitute, Percutaneous Approach

ØRUE47Z   Supplement Right Sternoclavicular Joint with Autologous Tissue Substitute, Percutaneous Endoscopic Approach

ØRUE4JZ   Supplement Right Sternoclavicular Joint with Synthetic Substitute, Percutaneous Endoscopic Approach

ØRUE4KZ   Supplement Right Sternoclavicular Joint with Nonautologous Tissue Substitute, Percutaneous Endoscopic Approach

ØRUF07Z   Supplement Left Sternoclavicular Joint with Autologous Tissue Substitute, Open Approach

ØRUF0JZ   Supplement Left Sternoclavicular Joint with Synthetic Substitute, Open Approach

ØRUF0KZ   Supplement Left Sternoclavicular Joint with Nonautologous Tissue Substitute, Open Approach

ØRUF37Z   Supplement Left Sternoclavicular Joint with Autologous Tissue Substitute, Percutaneous Approach

ØRUF3JZ   Supplement Left Sternoclavicular Joint with Synthetic Substitute, Percutaneous Approach

ØRUF3KZ   Supplement Left Sternoclavicular Joint with Nonautologous Tissue Substitute, Percutaneous Approach

ØRUF47Z   Supplement Left Sternoclavicular Joint with Autologous Tissue Substitute, Percutaneous Endoscopic Approach

ØRUF4JZ   Supplement Left Sternoclavicular Joint with Synthetic Substitute, Percutaneous Endoscopic Approach

ØRUF4KZ   Supplement Left Sternoclavicular Joint with Nonautologous Tissue Substitute, Percutaneous Endoscopic Approach

ØRUG07Z   Supplement Right Acromioclavicular Joint with Autologous Tissue Substitute, Open Approach

ØRUG0JZ   Supplement Right Acromioclavicular Joint with Synthetic Substitute, Open Approach

ØRUG0KZ   Supplement Right Acromioclavicular Joint with Nonautologous Tissue Substitute, Open Approach

ØRUG37Z   Supplement Right Acromioclavicular Joint with Autologous Tissue Substitute, Percutaneous Approach

ØRUG3JZ   Supplement Right Acromioclavicular Joint with Synthetic Substitute, Percutaneous Approach

ØRUG3KZ   Supplement Right Acromioclavicular Joint with Nonautologous Tissue Substitute, Percutaneous Approach

ØRUG47Z   Supplement Right Acromioclavicular Joint with Autologous Tissue Substitute, Percutaneous Endoscopic Approach

ØRUG4JZ   Supplement Right Acromioclavicular Joint with Synthetic Substitute, Percutaneous Endoscopic Approach

ØRUG4KZ   Supplement Right Acromioclavicular Joint with Nonautologous Tissue Substitute, Percutaneous Endoscopic Approach

ØRUH07Z   Supplement Left Acromioclavicular Joint with Autologous Tissue Substitute, Open Approach

ØRUH0JZ   Supplement Left Acromioclavicular Joint with Synthetic Substitute, Open Approach

ØRUH0KZ   Supplement Left Acromioclavicular Joint with Nonautologous Tissue Substitute, Open Approach

ØRUH37Z   Supplement Left Acromioclavicular Joint with Autologous Tissue Substitute, Percutaneous Approach

ØRUH3JZ   Supplement Left Acromioclavicular Joint with Synthetic Substitute, Percutaneous Approach

ØRUH3KZ   Supplement Left Acromioclavicular Joint with Nonautologous Tissue Substitute, Percutaneous Approach

ØRUH47Z   Supplement Left Acromioclavicular Joint with Autologous Tissue Substitute, Percutaneous Endoscopic Approach

ØRUH4JZ   Supplement Left Acromioclavicular Joint with Synthetic Substitute, Percutaneous Endoscopic Approach

ØRUH4KZ   Supplement Left Acromioclavicular Joint with Nonautologous Tissue Substitute, Percutaneous Endoscopic Approach

ØRUJ07Z   Supplement Right Shoulder Joint with Autologous Tissue Substitute, Open Approach

ØRUJ0JZ   Supplement Right Shoulder Joint with Synthetic Substitute, Open Approach

ØRUJ0KZ   Supplement Right Shoulder Joint with Nonautologous Tissue Substitute, Open Approach

ØRUJ37Z   Supplement Right Shoulder Joint with Autologous Tissue Substitute, Percutaneous Approach

ØRUJ3JZ   Supplement Right Shoulder Joint with Synthetic Substitute, Percutaneous Approach

ØRUJ3KZ   Supplement Right Shoulder Joint with Nonautologous Tissue Substitute, Percutaneous Approach

ØRUJ47Z   Supplement Right Shoulder Joint with Autologous Tissue Substitute, Percutaneous Endoscopic Approach

ØRUJ4JZ   Supplement Right Shoulder Joint with Synthetic Substitute, Percutaneous Endoscopic Approach

ØRUJ4KZ   Supplement Right Shoulder Joint with Nonautologous Tissue Substitute, Percutaneous Endoscopic Approach

ØRUK07Z   Supplement Left Shoulder Joint with Autologous Tissue Substitute, Open Approach

ØRUK0JZ   Supplement Left Shoulder Joint with Synthetic Substitute, Open Approach

ØRUK0KZ   Supplement Left Shoulder Joint with Nonautologous Tissue Substitute, Open Approach

ØRUK37Z   Supplement Left Shoulder Joint with Autologous Tissue Substitute, Percutaneous Approach

ØRUK3JZ   Supplement Left Shoulder Joint with Synthetic Substitute, Percutaneous Approach

ØRUK3KZ   Supplement Left Shoulder Joint with Nonautologous Tissue Substitute, Percutaneous Approach

ØRUK47Z   Supplement Left Shoulder Joint with Autologous Tissue Substitute, Percutaneous Endoscopic Approach

ØRUK4JZ   Supplement Left Shoulder Joint with Synthetic Substitute, Percutaneous Endoscopic Approach

ØRUK4KZ   Supplement Left Shoulder Joint with Nonautologous Tissue Substitute, Percutaneous Endoscopic Approach

ØRUL07Z   Supplement Right Elbow Joint with Autologous Tissue Substitute, Open Approach

ØRUL0JZ   Supplement Right Elbow Joint with Synthetic Substitute, Open Approach

ØRUL0KZ   Supplement Right Elbow Joint with Nonautologous Tissue Substitute, Open Approach

ØRUL37Z   Supplement Right Elbow Joint with Autologous Tissue Substitute, Percutaneous Approach

ØRUL3JZ   Supplement Right Elbow Joint with Synthetic Substitute, Percutaneous Approach

ØRUL3KZ   Supplement Right Elbow Joint with Nonautologous Tissue Substitute, Percutaneous Approach

ØRUL47Z   Supplement Right Elbow Joint with Autologous Tissue Substitute, Percutaneous Endoscopic Approach

ØRUL4JZ   Supplement Right Elbow Joint with Synthetic Substitute, Percutaneous Endoscopic Approach

ØRUL4KZ   Supplement Right Elbow Joint with Nonautologous Tissue Substitute, Percutaneous Endoscopic Approach

ØRUM07Z   Supplement Left Elbow Joint with Autologous Tissue Substitute, Open Approach

ØRUM0JZ   Supplement Left Elbow Joint with Synthetic Substitute, Open Approach

ØRUM0KZ   Supplement Left Elbow Joint with Nonautologous Tissue Substitute, Open Approach

ØRUM37Z   Supplement Left Elbow Joint with Autologous Tissue Substitute, Percutaneous Approach

ØRUM3JZ   Supplement Left Elbow Joint with Synthetic Substitute, Percutaneous Approach

ØRUM3KZ   Supplement Left Elbow Joint with Nonautologous Tissue Substitute, Percutaneous Approach

ØRUM47Z   Supplement Left Elbow Joint with Autologous Tissue Substitute, Percutaneous Endoscopic Approach

ØRUM4JZ   Supplement Left Elbow Joint with Synthetic Substitute, Percutaneous Endoscopic Approach

ØRUM4KZ   Supplement Left Elbow Joint with Nonautologous Tissue Substitute, Percutaneous Endoscopic Approach

ØSG0070   Fusion of Lumbar Vertebral Joint with Autologous Tissue Substitute, Anterior Approach, Anterior Column, Open Approach

ØSG0071   Fusion of Lumbar Vertebral Joint with Autologous Tissue Substitute, Posterior Approach, Posterior Column, Open Approach

ØSG007J   Fusion of Lumbar Vertebral Joint with Autologous Tissue Substitute, Posterior Approach, Anterior Column, Open Approach

ØSG00A0   Fusion of Lumbar Vertebral Joint with Interbody Fusion Device, Anterior Approach, Anterior Column, Open Approach

ØSG00A1   Fusion of Lumbar Vertebral Joint with Interbody Fusion Device, Posterior Approach, Posterior Column, Open Approach

ØSG00AJ   Fusion of Lumbar Vertebral Joint with Interbody Fusion Device, Posterior Approach, Anterior Column, Open Approach

HAC 12: Surgical Site Infection Following Certain Orthopedic Procedures of the Spine, Shoulder, and Elbow (continued)

0SG00J0 Fusion of Lumbar Vertebral Joint with Synthetic Substitute, Anterior Approach, Anterior Column, Open Approach

0SG00J1 Fusion of Lumbar Vertebral Joint with Synthetic Substitute, Posterior Approach, Posterior Column, Open Approach

0SG00JJ Fusion of Lumbar Vertebral Joint with Synthetic Substitute, Posterior Approach, Anterior Column, Open Approach

0SG00K0 Fusion of Lumbar Vertebral Joint with Nonautologous Tissue Substitute, Anterior Approach, Anterior Column, Open Approach

0SG00K1 Fusion of Lumbar Vertebral Joint with Nonautologous Tissue Substitute, Posterior Approach, Posterior Column, Open Approach

0SG00KJ Fusion of Lumbar Vertebral Joint with Nonautologous Tissue Substitute, Posterior Approach, Anterior Column, Open Approach

0SG00Z0 Fusion of Lumbar Vertebral Joint, Anterior Approach, Anterior Column, Open Approach

0SG00Z1 Fusion of Lumbar Vertebral Joint, Posterior Approach, Posterior Column, Open Approach

0SG00ZJ Fusion of Lumbar Vertebral Joint, Posterior Approach, Anterior Column, Open Approach

0SG0370 Fusion of Lumbar Vertebral Joint with Autologous Tissue Substitute, Anterior Approach, Anterior Column, Percutaneous Approach

0SG0371 Fusion of Lumbar Vertebral Joint with Autologous Tissue Substitute, Posterior Approach, Posterior Column, Percutaneous Approach

0SG037J Fusion of Lumbar Vertebral Joint with Autologous Tissue Substitute, Posterior Approach, Anterior Column, Percutaneous Approach

0SG03A0 Fusion of Lumbar Vertebral Joint with Interbody Fusion Device, Anterior Approach, Anterior Column, Percutaneous Approach

0SG03A1 Fusion of Lumbar Vertebral Joint with Interbody Fusion Device, Posterior Approach, Posterior Column, Percutaneous Approach

0SG03AJ Fusion of Lumbar Vertebral Joint with Interbody Fusion Device, Posterior Approach, Anterior Column, Percutaneous Approach

0SG03J0 Fusion of Lumbar Vertebral Joint with Synthetic Substitute, Anterior Approach, Anterior Column, Percutaneous Approach

0SG03J1 Fusion of Lumbar Vertebral Joint with Synthetic Substitute, Posterior Approach, Posterior Column, Percutaneous Approach

0SG03JJ Fusion of Lumbar Vertebral Joint with Synthetic Substitute, Posterior Approach, Anterior Column, Percutaneous Approach

0SG03K0 Fusion of Lumbar Vertebral Joint with Nonautologous Tissue Substitute, Anterior Approach, Anterior Column, Percutaneous Approach

0SG03K1 Fusion of Lumbar Vertebral Joint with Nonautologous Tissue Substitute, Posterior Approach, Posterior Column, Percutaneous Approach

0SG03KJ Fusion of Lumbar Vertebral Joint with Nonautologous Tissue Substitute, Posterior Approach, Anterior Column, Percutaneous Approach

0SG03Z0 Fusion of Lumbar Vertebral Joint, Anterior Approach, Anterior Column, Percutaneous Approach

0SG03Z1 Fusion of Lumbar Vertebral Joint, Posterior Approach, Posterior Column, Percutaneous Approach

0SG03ZJ Fusion of Lumbar Vertebral Joint, Posterior Approach, Anterior Column, Percutaneous Approach

0SG0470 Fusion of Lumbar Vertebral Joint with Autologous Tissue Substitute, Anterior Approach, Anterior Column, Percutaneous Endoscopic Approach

0SG0471 Fusion of Lumbar Vertebral Joint with Autologous Tissue Substitute, Posterior Approach, Posterior Column, Percutaneous Endoscopic Approach

0SG047J Fusion of Lumbar Vertebral Joint with Autologous Tissue Substitute, Posterior Approach, Anterior Column, Percutaneous Endoscopic Approach

0SG04A0 Fusion of Lumbar Vertebral Joint with Interbody Fusion Device, Anterior Approach, Anterior Column, Percutaneous Endoscopic Approach

0SG04A1 Fusion of Lumbar Vertebral Joint with Interbody Fusion Device, Posterior Approach, Posterior Column, Percutaneous Endoscopic Approach

0SG04AJ Fusion of Lumbar Vertebral Joint with Interbody Fusion Device, Posterior Approach, Anterior Column, Percutaneous Endoscopic Approach

0SG04J0 Fusion of Lumbar Vertebral Joint with Synthetic Substitute, Anterior Approach, Anterior Column, Percutaneous Endoscopic Approach

0SG04J1 Fusion of Lumbar Vertebral Joint with Synthetic Substitute, Posterior Approach, Posterior Column, Percutaneous Endoscopic Approach

0SG04JJ Fusion of Lumbar Vertebral Joint with Synthetic Substitute, Posterior Approach, Anterior Column, Percutaneous Endoscopic Approach

0SG04K0 Fusion of Lumbar Vertebral Joint with Nonautologous Tissue Substitute, Anterior Approach, Anterior Column, Percutaneous Endoscopic Approach

0SG04K1 Fusion of Lumbar Vertebral Joint with Nonautologous Tissue Substitute, Posterior Approach, Posterior Column, Percutaneous Endoscopic Approach

0SG04KJ Fusion of Lumbar Vertebral Joint with Nonautologous Tissue Substitute, Posterior Approach, Anterior Column, Percutaneous Endoscopic Approach

0SG04Z0 Fusion of Lumbar Vertebral Joint, Anterior Approach, Anterior Column, Percutaneous Endoscopic Approach

0SG04Z1 Fusion of Lumbar Vertebral Joint, Posterior Approach, Posterior Column, Percutaneous Endoscopic Approach

0SG04ZJ Fusion of Lumbar Vertebral Joint, Posterior Approach, Anterior Column, Percutaneous Endoscopic Approach

0SG1070 Fusion of 2 or More Lumbar Vertebral Joints with Autologous Tissue Substitute, Anterior Approach, Anterior Column, Open Approach

0SG1071 Fusion of 2 or More Lumbar Vertebral Joints with Autologous Tissue Substitute, Posterior Approach, Posterior Column, Open Approach

0SG107J Fusion of 2 or More Lumbar Vertebral Joints with Autologous Tissue Substitute, Posterior Approach, Anterior Column, Open Approach

0SG10A0 Fusion of 2 or More Lumbar Vertebral Joints with Interbody Fusion Device, Anterior Approach, Anterior Column, Open Approach

0SG10A1 Fusion of 2 or More Lumbar Vertebral Joints with Interbody Fusion Device, Posterior Approach, Posterior Column, Open Approach

0SG10AJ Fusion of 2 or More Lumbar Vertebral Joints with Interbody Fusion Device, Posterior Approach, Anterior Column, Open Approach

0SG10J0 Fusion of 2 or More Lumbar Vertebral Joints with Synthetic Substitute, Anterior Approach, Anterior Column, Open Approach

0SG10J1 Fusion of 2 or More Lumbar Vertebral Joints with Synthetic Substitute, Posterior Approach, Posterior Column, Open Approach

0SG10JJ Fusion of 2 or More Lumbar Vertebral Joints with Synthetic Substitute, Posterior Approach, Anterior Column, Open Approach

0SG10K0 Fusion of 2 or More Lumbar Vertebral Joints with Nonautologous Tissue Substitute, Anterior Approach, Anterior Column, Open Approach

0SG10K1 Fusion of 2 or More Lumbar Vertebral Joints with Nonautologous Tissue Substitute, Posterior Approach, Posterior Column, Open Approach

0SG10KJ Fusion of 2 or More Lumbar Vertebral Joints with Nonautologous Tissue Substitute, Posterior Approach, Anterior Column, Open Approach

0SG10Z0 Fusion of 2 or More Lumbar Vertebral Joints, Anterior Approach, Anterior Column, Open Approach

0SG10Z1 Fusion of 2 or More Lumbar Vertebral Joints, Posterior Approach, Posterior Column, Open Approach

0SG10ZJ Fusion of 2 or More Lumbar Vertebral Joints, Posterior Approach, Anterior Column, Open Approach

0SG1370 Fusion of 2 or More Lumbar Vertebral Joints with Autologous Tissue Substitute, Anterior Approach, Anterior Column, Percutaneous Approach

0SG1371 Fusion of 2 or More Lumbar Vertebral Joints with Autologous Tissue Substitute, Posterior Approach, Posterior Column, Percutaneous Approach

0SG137J Fusion of 2 or More Lumbar Vertebral Joints with Autologous Tissue Substitute, Posterior Approach, Anterior Column, Percutaneous Approach

0SG13A0 Fusion of 2 or More Lumbar Vertebral Joints with Interbody Fusion Device, Anterior Approach, Anterior Column, Percutaneous Approach

0SG13A1 Fusion of 2 or More Lumbar Vertebral Joints with Interbody Fusion Device, Posterior Approach, Posterior Column, Percutaneous Approach

0SG13AJ Fusion of 2 or More Lumbar Vertebral Joints with Interbody Fusion Device, Posterior Approach, Anterior Column, Percutaneous Approach

HAC 12: Surgical Site Infection Following Certain Orthopedic Procedures of the Spine, Shoulder, and Elbow (continued)

ØSG13JØ　Fusion of 2 or More Lumbar Vertebral Joints with Synthetic Substitute, Anterior Approach, Anterior Column, Percutaneous Approach

ØSG13J1　Fusion of 2 or More Lumbar Vertebral Joints with Synthetic Substitute, Posterior Approach, Posterior Column, Percutaneous Approach

ØSG13JJ　Fusion of 2 or More Lumbar Vertebral Joints with Synthetic Substitute, Posterior Approach, Anterior Column, Percutaneous Approach

ØSG13KØ　Fusion of 2 or More Lumbar Vertebral Joints with Nonautologous Tissue Substitute, Anterior Approach, Anterior Column, Percutaneous Approach

ØSG13K1　Fusion of 2 or More Lumbar Vertebral Joints with Nonautologous Tissue Substitute, Posterior Approach, Posterior Column, Percutaneous Approach

ØSG13KJ　Fusion of 2 or More Lumbar Vertebral Joints with Nonautologous Tissue Substitute, Posterior Approach, Anterior Column, Percutaneous Approach

ØSG13ZØ　Fusion of 2 or More Lumbar Vertebral Joints, Anterior Approach, Anterior Column, Percutaneous Approach

ØSG13Z1　Fusion of 2 or More Lumbar Vertebral Joints, Posterior Approach, Posterior Column, Percutaneous Approach

ØSG13ZJ　Fusion of 2 or More Lumbar Vertebral Joints, Posterior Approach, Anterior Column, Percutaneous Approach

ØSG147Ø　Fusion of 2 or More Lumbar Vertebral Joints with Autologous Tissue Substitute, Anterior Approach, Anterior Column, Percutaneous Endoscopic Approach

ØSG1471　Fusion of 2 or More Lumbar Vertebral Joints with Autologous Tissue Substitute, Posterior Approach, Posterior Column, Percutaneous Endoscopic Approach

ØSG147J　Fusion of 2 or More Lumbar Vertebral Joints with Autologous Tissue Substitute, Posterior Approach, Anterior Column, Percutaneous Endoscopic Approach

ØSG14AØ　Fusion of 2 or More Lumbar Vertebral Joints with Interbody Fusion Device, Anterior Approach, Anterior Column, Percutaneous Endoscopic Approach

ØSG14A1　Fusion of 2 or More Lumbar Vertebral Joints with Interbody Fusion Device, Posterior Approach, Posterior Column, Percutaneous Endoscopic Approach

ØSG14AJ　Fusion of 2 or More Lumbar Vertebral Joints with Interbody Fusion Device, Posterior Approach, Anterior Column, Percutaneous Endoscopic Approach

ØSG14JØ　Fusion of 2 or More Lumbar Vertebral Joints with Synthetic Substitute, Anterior Approach, Anterior Column, Percutaneous Endoscopic Approach

ØSG14J1　Fusion of 2 or More Lumbar Vertebral Joints with Synthetic Substitute, Posterior Approach, Posterior Column, Percutaneous Endoscopic Approach

ØSG14JJ　Fusion of 2 or More Lumbar Vertebral Joints with Synthetic Substitute, Posterior Approach, Anterior Column, Percutaneous Endoscopic Approach

ØSG14KØ　Fusion of 2 or More Lumbar Vertebral Joints with Nonautologous Tissue Substitute, Anterior Approach, Anterior Column, Percutaneous Endoscopic Approach

ØSG14K1　Fusion of 2 or More Lumbar Vertebral Joints with Nonautologous Tissue Substitute, Posterior Approach, Posterior Column, Percutaneous Endoscopic Approach

ØSG14KJ　Fusion of 2 or More Lumbar Vertebral Joints with Nonautologous Tissue Substitute, Posterior Approach, Anterior Column, Percutaneous Endoscopic Approach

ØSG14ZØ　Fusion of 2 or More Lumbar Vertebral Joints, Anterior Approach, Anterior Column, Percutaneous Endoscopic Approach

ØSG14Z1　Fusion of 2 or More Lumbar Vertebral Joints, Posterior Approach, Posterior Column, Percutaneous Endoscopic Approach

ØSG14ZJ　Fusion of 2 or More Lumbar Vertebral Joints, Posterior Approach, Anterior Column, Percutaneous Endoscopic Approach

ØSG3Ø7Ø　Fusion of Lumbosacral Joint with Autologous Tissue Substitute, Anterior Approach, Anterior Column, Open Approach

ØSG3Ø71　Fusion of Lumbosacral Joint with Autologous Tissue Substitute, Posterior Approach, Posterior Column, Open Approach

ØSG3Ø7J　Fusion of Lumbosacral Joint with Autologous Tissue Substitute, Posterior Approach, Anterior Column, Open Approach

ØSG3ØAØ　Fusion of Lumbosacral Joint with Interbody Fusion Device, Anterior Approach, Anterior Column, Open Approach

ØSG3ØA1　Fusion of Lumbosacral Joint with Interbody Fusion Device, Posterior Approach, Posterior Column, Open Approach

ØSG3ØAJ　Fusion of Lumbosacral Joint with Interbody Fusion Device, Posterior Approach, Anterior Column, Open Approach

ØSG3ØJØ　Fusion of Lumbosacral Joint with Synthetic Substitute, Anterior Approach, Anterior Column, Open Approach

ØSG3ØJ1　Fusion of Lumbosacral Joint with Synthetic Substitute, Posterior Approach, Posterior Column, Open Approach

ØSG3ØJJ　Fusion of Lumbosacral Joint with Synthetic Substitute, Posterior Approach, Anterior Column, Open Approach

ØSG3ØKØ　Fusion of Lumbosacral Joint with Nonautologous Tissue Substitute, Anterior Approach, Anterior Column, Open Approach

ØSG3ØK1　Fusion of Lumbosacral Joint with Nonautologous Tissue Substitute, Posterior Approach, Posterior Column, Open Approach

ØSG3ØKJ　Fusion of Lumbosacral Joint with Nonautologous Tissue Substitute, Posterior Approach, Anterior Column, Open Approach

ØSG3ØZØ　Fusion of Lumbosacral Joint, Anterior Approach, Anterior Column, Open Approach

ØSG3ØZ1　Fusion of Lumbosacral Joint, Posterior Approach, Posterior Column, Open Approach

ØSG3ØZJ　Fusion of Lumbosacral Joint, Posterior Approach, Anterior Column, Open Approach

ØSG337Ø　Fusion of Lumbosacral Joint with Autologous Tissue Substitute, Anterior Approach, Anterior Column, Percutaneous Approach

ØSG3371　Fusion of Lumbosacral Joint with Autologous Tissue Substitute, Posterior Approach, Posterior Column, Percutaneous Approach

ØSG337J　Fusion of Lumbosacral Joint with Autologous Tissue Substitute, Posterior Approach, Anterior Column, Percutaneous Approach

ØSG33AØ　Fusion of Lumbosacral Joint with Interbody Fusion Device, Anterior Approach, Anterior Column, Percutaneous Approach

ØSG33A1　Fusion of Lumbosacral Joint with Interbody Fusion Device, Posterior Approach, Posterior Column, Percutaneous Approach

ØSG33AJ　Fusion of Lumbosacral Joint with Interbody Fusion Device, Posterior Approach, Anterior Column, Percutaneous Approach

ØSG33JØ　Fusion of Lumbosacral Joint with Synthetic Substitute, Anterior Approach, Anterior Column, Percutaneous Approach

ØSG33J1　Fusion of Lumbosacral Joint with Synthetic Substitute, Posterior Approach, Posterior Column, Percutaneous Approach

ØSG33JJ　Fusion of Lumbosacral Joint with Synthetic Substitute, Posterior Approach, Anterior Column, Percutaneous Approach

ØSG33KØ　Fusion of Lumbosacral Joint with Nonautologous Tissue Substitute, Anterior Approach, Anterior Column, Percutaneous Approach

ØSG33K1　Fusion of Lumbosacral Joint with Nonautologous Tissue Substitute, Posterior Approach, Posterior Column, Percutaneous Approach

ØSG33KJ　Fusion of Lumbosacral Joint with Nonautologous Tissue Substitute, Posterior Approach, Anterior Column, Percutaneous Approach

ØSG33ZØ　Fusion of Lumbosacral Joint, Anterior Approach, Anterior Column, Percutaneous Approach

ØSG33Z1　Fusion of Lumbosacral Joint, Posterior Approach, Posterior Column, Percutaneous Approach

ØSG33ZJ　Fusion of Lumbosacral Joint, Posterior Approach, Anterior Column, Percutaneous Approach

ØSG347Ø　Fusion of Lumbosacral Joint with Autologous Tissue Substitute, Anterior Approach, Anterior Column, Percutaneous Endoscopic Approach

ØSG3471　Fusion of Lumbosacral Joint with Autologous Tissue Substitute, Posterior Approach, Posterior Column, Percutaneous Endoscopic Approach

ØSG347J　Fusion of Lumbosacral Joint with Autologous Tissue Substitute, Posterior Approach, Anterior Column, Percutaneous Endoscopic Approach

ØSG34AØ　Fusion of Lumbosacral Joint with Interbody Fusion Device, Anterior Approach, Anterior Column, Percutaneous Endoscopic Approach

ØSG34A1　Fusion of Lumbosacral Joint with Interbody Fusion Device, Posterior Approach, Posterior Column, Percutaneous Endoscopic Approach

Appendix I: Hospital Acquired Conditions

HAC 12: Surgical Site Infection Following Certain Orthopedic Procedures of the Spine, Shoulder, and Elbow (continued)

ØSG34AJ Fusion of Lumbosacral Joint with Interbody Fusion Device, Posterior Approach, Anterior Column, Percutaneous Endoscopic Approach

ØSG34JØ Fusion of Lumbosacral Joint with Synthetic Substitute, Anterior Approach, Anterior Column, Percutaneous Endoscopic Approach

ØSG34J1 Fusion of Lumbosacral Joint with Synthetic Substitute, Posterior Approach, Posterior Column, Percutaneous Endoscopic Approach

ØSG34JJ Fusion of Lumbosacral Joint with Synthetic Substitute, Posterior Approach, Anterior Column, Percutaneous Endoscopic Approach

ØSG34KØ Fusion of Lumbosacral Joint with Nonautologous Tissue Substitute, Anterior Approach, Anterior Column, Percutaneous Endoscopic Approach

ØSG34K1 Fusion of Lumbosacral Joint with Nonautologous Tissue Substitute, Posterior Approach, Posterior Column, Percutaneous Endoscopic Approach

ØSG34KJ Fusion of Lumbosacral Joint with Nonautologous Tissue Substitute, Posterior Approach, Anterior Column, Percutaneous Endoscopic Approach

ØSG34ZØ Fusion of Lumbosacral Joint, Anterior Approach, Anterior Column, Percutaneous Endoscopic Approach

ØSG34Z1 Fusion of Lumbosacral Joint, Posterior Approach, Posterior Column, Percutaneous Endoscopic Approach

ØSG34ZJ Fusion of Lumbosacral Joint, Posterior Approach, Anterior Column, Percutaneous Endoscopic Approach

ØSG7Ø4Z Fusion of Right Sacroiliac Joint with Internal Fixation Device, Open Approach

ØSG7Ø7Z Fusion of Right Sacroiliac Joint with Autologous Tissue Substitute, Open Approach

ØSG7ØJZ Fusion of Right Sacroiliac Joint with Synthetic Substitute, Open Approach

ØSG7ØKZ Fusion of Right Sacroiliac Joint with Nonautologous Tissue Substitute, Open Approach

ØSG7ØZZ Fusion of Right Sacroiliac Joint, Open Approach

ØSG734Z Fusion of Right Sacroiliac Joint with Internal Fixation Device, Percutaneous Approach

ØSG737Z Fusion of Right Sacroiliac Joint with Autologous Tissue Substitute, Percutaneous Approach

ØSG73JZ Fusion of Right Sacroiliac Joint with Synthetic Substitute, Percutaneous Approach

ØSG73KZ Fusion of Right Sacroiliac Joint with Nonautologous Tissue Substitute, Percutaneous Approach

ØSG73ZZ Fusion of Right Sacroiliac Joint, Percutaneous Approach

ØSG744Z Fusion of Right Sacroiliac Joint with Internal Fixation Device, Percutaneous Endoscopic Approach

ØSG747Z Fusion of Right Sacroiliac Joint with Autologous Tissue Substitute, Percutaneous Endoscopic Approach

ØSG74JZ Fusion of Right Sacroiliac Joint with Synthetic Substitute, Percutaneous Endoscopic Approach

ØSG74KZ Fusion of Right Sacroiliac Joint with Nonautologous Tissue Substitute, Percutaneous Endoscopic Approach

ØSG74ZZ Fusion of Right Sacroiliac Joint, Percutaneous Endoscopic Approach

ØSG8Ø4Z Fusion of Left Sacroiliac Joint with Internal Fixation Device, Open Approach

ØSG8Ø7Z Fusion of Left Sacroiliac Joint with Autologous Tissue Substitute, Open Approach

ØSG8ØJZ Fusion of Left Sacroiliac Joint with Synthetic Substitute, Open Approach

ØSG8ØKZ Fusion of Left Sacroiliac Joint with Nonautologous Tissue Substitute, Open Approach

ØSG8ØZZ Fusion of Left Sacroiliac Joint, Open Approach

ØSG834Z Fusion of Left Sacroiliac Joint with Internal Fixation Device, Percutaneous Approach

ØSG837Z Fusion of Left Sacroiliac Joint with Autologous Tissue Substitute, Percutaneous Approach

ØSG83JZ Fusion of Left Sacroiliac Joint with Synthetic Substitute, Percutaneous Approach

ØSG83KZ Fusion of Left Sacroiliac Joint with Nonautologous Tissue Substitute, Percutaneous Approach

ØSG83ZZ Fusion of Left Sacroiliac Joint, Percutaneous Approach

ØSG844Z Fusion of Left Sacroiliac Joint with Internal Fixation Device, Percutaneous Endoscopic Approach

ØSG847Z Fusion of Left Sacroiliac Joint with Autologous Tissue Substitute, Percutaneous Endoscopic Approach

ØSG84JZ Fusion of Left Sacroiliac Joint with Synthetic Substitute, Percutaneous Endoscopic Approach

ØSG84KZ Fusion of Left Sacroiliac Joint with Nonautologous Tissue Substitute, Percutaneous Endoscopic Approach

ØSG84ZZ Fusion of Left Sacroiliac Joint, Percutaneous Endoscopic Approach

XRGØØ92 Fusion of Occipital-cervical Joint using Nanotextured Surface Interbody Fusion Device, Open Approach, New Technology Group 2

XRG1Ø92 Fusion of Cervical Vertebral Joint using Nanotextured Surface Interbody Fusion Device, Open Approach, New Technology Group 2

XRG2Ø92 Fusion of 2 or more Cervical Vertebral Joints using Nanotextured Surface Interbody Fusion Device, Open Approach, New Technology Group 2

XRG4Ø92 Fusion of Cervicothoracic Vertebral Joint using Nanotextured Surface Interbody Fusion Device, Open Approach, New Technology Group 2

XRG6Ø92 Fusion of Thoracic Vertebral Joint using Nanotextured Surface Interbody Fusion Device, Open Approach, New Technology Group 2

XRG7Ø92 Fusion of 2 to 7 Thoracic Vertebral Joints using Nanotextured Surface Interbody Fusion Device, Open Approach, New Technology Group 2

XRG8Ø92 Fusion of 8 or more Thoracic Vertebral Joints using Nanotextured Surface Interbody Fusion Device, Open Approach, New Technology Group 2

XRGAØ92 Fusion of Thoracolumbar Vertebral Joint using Nanotextured Surface Interbody Fusion Device, Open Approach, New Technology Group 2

XRGBØ92 Fusion of Lumbar Vertebral Joint using Nanotextured Surface Interbody Fusion Device, Open Approach, New Technology Group 2

XRGCØ92 Fusion of 2 or more Lumbar Vertebral Joints using Nanotextured Surface Interbody Fusion Device, Open Approach, New Technology Group 2

XRGDØ92 Fusion of Lumbosacral Joint using Nanotextured Surface Interbody Fusion Device, Open Approach, New Technology Group 2

HAC 13: Surgical Site Infection (SSI) Following Cardiac Implantable Electronic Device (CIED) Procedures

Secondary diagnosis not POA:

K68.11
T81.4XXA
T82.6XXA
T82.7XXA

AND

Any of the following procedures:

Ø2H43JZ Insertion of Pacemaker Lead into Coronary Vein, Percutaneous Approach

Ø2H43KZ Insertion of Defibrillator Lead into Coronary Vein, Percutaneous Approach

Ø2H43MZ Insertion of Cardiac Lead into Coronary Vein, Percutaneous Approach

Ø2H63JZ Insertion of Pacemaker Lead into Right Atrium, Percutaneous Approach

Ø2H63MZ Insertion of Cardiac Lead into Right Atrium, Percutaneous Approach

Ø2H73JZ Insertion of Pacemaker Lead into Left Atrium, Percutaneous Approach

Ø2H73MZ Insertion of Cardiac Lead into Left Atrium, Percutaneous Approach

Ø2HK3JZ Insertion of Pacemaker Lead into Right Ventricle, Percutaneous Approach

Ø2HL3JZ Insertion of Pacemaker Lead into Left Ventricle, Percutaneous Approach

Ø2HNØJZ Insertion of Pacemaker Lead into Pericardium, Open Approach

Ø2HNØMZ Insertion of Cardiac Lead into Pericardium, Open Approach

Ø2HN3JZ Insertion of Pacemaker Lead into Pericardium, Percutaneous Approach

Ø2HN3MZ Insertion of Cardiac Lead into Pericardium, Percutaneous Approach

Ø2HN4JZ Insertion of Pacemaker Lead into Pericardium, Percutaneous Endoscopic Approach

Ø2HN4MZ Insertion of Cardiac Lead into Pericardium, Percutaneous Endoscopic Approach

Ø2PAØMZ Removal of Cardiac Lead from Heart, Open Approach

Ø2PA3MZ Removal of Cardiac Lead from Heart, Percutaneous Approach

Ø2PA4MZ Removal of Cardiac Lead from Heart, Percutaneous Endoscopic Approach

Ø2PAXMZ Removal of Cardiac Lead from Heart, External Approach

Ø2WAØMZ Revision of Cardiac Lead in Heart, Open Approach

Ø2WA3MZ Revision of Cardiac Lead in Heart, Percutaneous Approach

Ø2WA4MZ Revision of Cardiac Lead in Heart, Percutaneous Endoscopic Approach

ØJH6Ø4Z Insertion of Pacemaker, Single Chamber into Chest Subcutaneous Tissue and Fascia, Open Approach

ØJH6Ø5Z Insertion of Pacemaker, Single Chamber Rate Responsive into Chest Subcutaneous Tissue and Fascia, Open Approach

HAC 13: Surgical Site Infection (SSI) Following Cardiac Implantable Electronic Device (CIED) Procedures (continued)

ØJH6Ø6Z   Insertion of Pacemaker, Dual Chamber into Chest Subcutaneous Tissue and Fascia, Open Approach

ØJH6Ø7Z   Insertion of Cardiac Resynchronization Pacemaker Pulse Generator into Chest Subcutaneous Tissue and Fascia, Open Approach

ØJH6Ø8Z   Insertion of Defibrillator Generator into Chest Subcutaneous Tissue and Fascia, Open Approach

ØJH6Ø9Z   Insertion of Cardiac Resynchronization Defibrillator Pulse Generator into Chest Subcutaneous Tissue and Fascia, Open Approach

ØJH6ØPZ   Insertion of Cardiac Rhythm Related Device into Chest Subcutaneous Tissue and Fascia, Open Approach

ØJH634Z   Insertion of Pacemaker, Single Chamber into Chest Subcutaneous Tissue and Fascia, Percutaneous Approach

ØJH635Z   Insertion of Pacemaker, Single Chamber Rate Responsive into Chest Subcutaneous Tissue and Fascia, Percutaneous Approach

ØJH636Z   Insertion of Pacemaker, Dual Chamber into Chest Subcutaneous Tissue and Fascia, Percutaneous Approach

ØJH637Z   Insertion of Cardiac Resynchronization Pacemaker Pulse Generator into Chest Subcutaneous Tissue and Fascia, Percutaneous Approach

ØJH638Z   Insertion of Defibrillator Generator into Chest Subcutaneous Tissue and Fascia, Percutaneous Approach

ØJH639Z   Insertion of Cardiac Resynchronization Defibrillator Pulse Generator into Chest Subcutaneous Tissue and Fascia, Percutaneous Approach

ØJH63PZ   Insertion of Cardiac Rhythm Related Device into Chest Subcutaneous Tissue and Fascia, Percutaneous Approach

ØJH8Ø4Z   Insertion of Pacemaker, Single Chamber into Abdomen Subcutaneous Tissue and Fascia, Open Approach

ØJH8Ø5Z   Insertion of Pacemaker, Single Chamber Rate Responsive into Abdomen Subcutaneous Tissue and Fascia, Open Approach

ØJH8Ø6Z   Insertion of Pacemaker, Dual Chamber into Abdomen Subcutaneous Tissue and Fascia, Open Approach

ØJH8Ø7Z   Insertion of Cardiac Resynchronization Pacemaker Pulse Generator into Abdomen Subcutaneous Tissue and Fascia, Open Approach

ØJH8Ø8Z   Insertion of Defibrillator Generator into Abdomen Subcutaneous Tissue and Fascia, Open Approach

ØJH8Ø9Z   Insertion of Cardiac Resynchronization Defibrillator Pulse Generator into Abdomen Subcutaneous Tissue and Fascia, Open Approach

ØJH8ØPZ   Insertion of Cardiac Rhythm Related Device into Abdomen Subcutaneous Tissue and Fascia, Open Approach

ØJH834Z   Insertion of Pacemaker, Single Chamber into Abdomen Subcutaneous Tissue and Fascia, Percutaneous Approach

ØJH835Z   Insertion of Pacemaker, Single Chamber Rate Responsive into Abdomen Subcutaneous Tissue and Fascia, Percutaneous Approach

ØJH836Z   Insertion of Pacemaker, Dual Chamber into Abdomen Subcutaneous Tissue and Fascia, Percutaneous Approach

ØJH837Z   Insertion of Cardiac Resynchronization Pacemaker Pulse Generator into Abdomen Subcutaneous Tissue and Fascia, Percutaneous Approach

ØJH838Z   Insertion of Defibrillator Generator into Abdomen Subcutaneous Tissue and Fascia, Percutaneous Approach

ØJH839Z   Insertion of Cardiac Resynchronization Defibrillator Pulse Generator into Abdomen Subcutaneous Tissue and Fascia, Percutaneous Approach

ØJH83PZ   Insertion of Cardiac Rhythm Related Device into Abdomen Subcutaneous Tissue and Fascia, Percutaneous Approach

ØJPTØPZ   Removal of Cardiac Rhythm Related Device from Trunk Subcutaneous Tissue and Fascia, Open Approach

ØJPT3PZ   Removal of Cardiac Rhythm Related Device from Trunk Subcutaneous Tissue and Fascia, Percutaneous Approach

ØJWTØPZ   Revision of Cardiac Rhythm Related Device in Trunk Subcutaneous Tissue and Fascia, Open Approach

ØJWT3PZ   Revision of Cardiac Rhythm Related Device in Trunk Subcutaneous Tissue and Fascia, Percutaneous Approach

HAC 14: Iatrogenic Pneumothorax with Venous Catheterization

Secondary diagnosis not POA:

J95.811

AND

Any of the following procedures:

Ø2H633Z   Insertion of Infusion Device into Right Atrium, Percutaneous Approach

Ø2HK33Z   Insertion of Infusion Device into Right Ventricle, Percutaneous Approach

Ø2HS33Z   Insertion of Infusion Device into Right Pulmonary Vein, Percutaneous Approach

Ø2HS43Z   Insertion of Infusion Device into Right Pulmonary Vein, Percutaneous Endoscopic Approach

Ø2HT33Z   Insertion of Infusion Device into Left Pulmonary Vein, Percutaneous Approach

Ø2HT43Z   Insertion of Infusion Device into Left Pulmonary Vein, Percutaneous Endoscopic Approach

Ø2HV33Z   Insertion of Infusion Device into Superior Vena Cava, Percutaneous Approach

Ø2HV43Z   Insertion of Infusion Device into Superior Vena Cava, Percutaneous Endoscopic Approach

Ø5HØ33Z   Insertion of Infusion Device into Azygos Vein, Percutaneous Approach

Ø5HØ43Z   Insertion of Infusion Device into Azygos Vein, Percutaneous Endoscopic Approach

Ø5H133Z   Insertion of Infusion Device into Hemiazygos Vein, Percutaneous Approach

Ø5H143Z   Insertion of Infusion Device into Hemiazygos Vein, Percutaneous Endoscopic Approach

Ø5H333Z   Insertion of Infusion Device into Right Innominate Vein, Percutaneous Approach

Ø5H343Z   Insertion of Infusion Device into Right Innominate Vein, Percutaneous Endoscopic Approach

Ø5H433Z   Insertion of Infusion Device into Left Innominate Vein, Percutaneous Approach

Ø5H443Z   Insertion of Infusion Device into Left Innominate Vein, Percutaneous Endoscopic Approach

Ø5H533Z   Insertion of Infusion Device into Right Subclavian Vein, Percutaneous Approach

Ø5H543Z   Insertion of Infusion Device into Right Subclavian Vein, Percutaneous Endoscopic Approach

Ø5H633Z   Insertion of Infusion Device into Left Subclavian Vein, Percutaneous Approach

Ø5H643Z   Insertion of Infusion Device into Left Subclavian Vein, Percutaneous Endoscopic Approach

Ø5HM33Z   Insertion of Infusion Device into Right Internal Jugular Vein, Percutaneous Approach

Ø5HN33Z   Insertion of Infusion Device into Left Internal Jugular Vein, Percutaneous Approach

Ø5HP33Z   Insertion of Infusion Device into Right External Jugular Vein, Percutaneous Approach

Ø5HQ33Z   Insertion of Infusion Device into Left External Jugular Vein, Percutaneous Approach

ØJH63XZ   Insertion of Vascular Access Device into Chest Subcutaneous Tissue and Fascia, Percutaneous Approach

Appendix J: Centers for Medicare & Medicaid Services Hierarchical Condition Categories (CMS-HCC)

In the 1970s, Medicare began demonstration projects that contracted with health maintenance organizations (HMO) to provide care for Medicare beneficiaries in exchange for prospective payments. In 1985, this project changed from demonstration status to a regular part of the Medicare program, Medicare Part C. The Balanced Budget Act (BBA) of 1997 named Medicare's Part C managed care program Medicare+Choice, and the Medicare Modernization Act (MMA) of 2003 again renamed it to Medicare Advantage (MA).

Medicare is one of the world's largest health insurance programs, and about one-fourth of the beneficiaries on Medicare are enrolled in a MA private health care plan. Due to the great variance in the health status of Medicare beneficiaries, risk adjustment provides a means of adequately compensating those plans with large numbers of seriously ill patients while not overburdening other plans that have healthier individuals. Medicare Advantage (MA) plans have been using the HCC/risk adjustment model since 2004.

The Risk Adjustment Model

The primary purpose of a risk adjustment model is to predict (on average) the future health care costs for specific consortiums enrolled in Medicare Advantage (MA) health plans. CMS is then able to provide capitation payments to these private health plans. Capitation payments are an incentive for health plans to enroll not only healthier individuals but those with chronic conditions or who are more seriously ill by removing some of the financial burden.

The MA risk adjustment model uses hierarchical condition categories (HCC) to assess the disease burden of its enrollees. HCC diagnostic groupings were created after examining claims data so that enrollees with similar disease processes, and consequently similar health care expenditures, could be pooled into a larger data set in which an average expenditure rate could be determined. The medical conditions included in HCC categories are those that were determined to most predictably affect the health status and health care costs of any individual. Several important principles to the risk adjustment model and the development of the HCC categories include but are not limited to:

1. The HCC diagnostic categories should be clinically meaningful.
   - Diagnostic categories are well-defined.
   - Clinically specific diseases or medical conditions are grouped to each category.
2. The HCC diagnostic categories should predict medical expenditures.
   - The diagnoses grouped to a specific category should have as close to the same cost burden not only in the current year but also in the future.
3. The HCC diagnostic categories should have adequate sample sizes and discretionary categories excluded to be as accurate and stable in their estimate of costs as possible.
   - A diagnostic category that groups extremely rare diseases or conditions would not be reliably effective in determining current or future costs.
   - Codes that are not credible as cost predictors or may be subject to coding variation should be excluded, when possible.
4. The HCC diagnostic categories should be both hierarchical and accumulative.
   - Hierarchical measurement is used within a specific disease process.
   - Disease processes that are unrelated to each other are measured accumulatively.
5. The diagnostic classification should encourage specificity and should not reward coding proliferation.
   - More diagnosis codes and vague diagnosis codes do not equal greater disease burden.

More than 9,000 ICD-10-CM diagnosis codes map to 79 HCCs in the current risk adjustment model. Diagnoses are excluded from mapping when they do not predict future cost or are vague or variable in diagnosis, coding, or treatment, such as symptoms or osteoarthritis. Also excluded are diagnosis codes from laboratories, radiology, and home health claims.

Risk Adjustment Factors

The CMS-HCC risk adjustment model uses "risk adjustment factors" to calculate a risk score for each member. This score summarizes that particular patient's expected cost of care relative to other members'. Each member's risk score is based on demographic and health status information and is calculated as the sum of these demographic and health factors weighted by their estimated marginal contributions to total risk. The model also takes into account where the patient resides (community or institutional), Medicaid eligibility (full or partial benefits), the patient's Medicare enrollment status (new or established), age, disability status, whether the patient is frail or has end-stage renal disease (ESRD), and even prescription drug use.

No procedure codes, ICD-10-PCS or CPT, are included in the MA risk adjustment model. The model relies solely on diagnostic and demographic data. Not all ICD-10-CM diagnoses map to an HCC, and there is no specific code sequencing involved. The CMS-HCC model is accumulative as well as hierarchical. The accumulative functionality allows a patient to have more than one HCC category assigned, providing a more complete clinical picture and prediction of resource consumption. The hierarchical aspect of the model provides a means of ranking diagnoses that are similar in disease process, by severity. The hierarchy of the condition categories ensures the patient's conditions are classified to the most severe condition within the related group. Less severe conditions within a particular hierarchy are superseded by more severe diagnoses within the same group. The hierarchy and accumulative relationship permits this model to characterize the person's illness level within each disease process, while still allowing the effects of unrelated disease processes to be counted in the patient's overall score.

Certain combinations of coexisting diagnoses for an individual can increase medical costs. The CMS-HCC model adjusts for these higher costs by the addition of "disease interaction" factors. For each patient, multiple HCCs assigned, along with demographic and disease interaction factors, are used to calculate a single, combined risk adjustment factor (RAF). The RAF score for an individual member represents all of the HCCs that have been submitted from all sources for that member to CMS during the course of an entire calendar year.

There are separate CMS-HCC models for new enrollees and continuing enrollees. The new enrollee model uses demographic factors only, such as age, sex, and disability status, and is used when the enrollee has less than 12 months of medical history. The community model accounts for age, sex, original reason for Medicare entitlement (age or disability), Medicaid eligibility, and clinical conditions as measured by HCCs. In the second step, expected costs are adjusted for outliers based on the member's risk score and whether the patient has ESRD.

Demographic data (age, sex, eligibility) as well as health status (diagnoses codes submitted on claims to CMS) of an MA population are used to determine the reimbursement to the health plan to care for their members.

RAF scores, which range from 0.118 to 2.4888, indicate patient health status. A RAF score of 1.0 or below is the benchmark CMS uses to indicate the average healthy patient with the same demographic and diagnostic factors. These patients are expected to use average or lower-than-average resources. When the RAF score is higher than 1.0, CMS considers the patient to be sicker than the average patient with the same criteria and expects greater-than-average resource utilization.

A low RAF score may accurately indicate a healthier patient, but it may also falsely indicate a healthier patient due to incomplete or inaccurate coding, incomplete or insufficient record documentation, or patients who fail to complete an annual assessment.

A high RAF score may accurately indicate a sicker patient, or it may be falsely inflated from overcoding due to diagnoses that are reported but not documented, or from copying and pasting from previous encounters or problem lists of resolved conditions.

Documentation Requirements

Payment is made per HCC category (not per diagnosis code). No matter how many times in the year the diagnosis codes are reported, a single payment is made to the MA plan each year. Each year the list of HCCs and the RAF for each patient is "reset." This means the annual health assessment is extremely important, and adequate documentation is critical. Accurate risk adjustment payment relies on complete medical record documentation and diagnosis coding. CMS requires that all applicable diagnosis codes be reported and that all diagnoses be reported to the highest level of specificity and that these be substantiated by the medical record.

CMS's Guiding Principle:

The risk adjustment diagnosis must be based on clinical medical record documentation from a face-to-face encounter, coded according to the *ICD-10-CM Guidelines for Coding and Reporting*; assigned based on dates of service within the data collection period, submitted to the MA organization from an appropriate risk adjustment provider type and an appropriate risk adjustment physician data source.

A "face-to-face" health service encounter between a patient and healthcare provider describes an encounter between the patient and the provider (MD, DO), including qualified nonphysician practitioners (NPP) (e.g. nurse practitioner or physician's assistant), which is face-to-face with the patient. CMS provides a current listing of acceptable physician specialty types for risk adjustment data submission within the 2012 Regional Technical Assistance Participant Guide. The only exception to the face-to-face encounter requirement is pathology services (professional component only). Currently, CMS does not provide a listing of all services that are considered face-to-face visits for risk adjustment data, but does provide guidance on what types of services are not acceptable for risk adjustment in the Participant Guide. For example, diagnostic radiology does not qualify because diagnostic radiologists typically do not document confirmed diagnoses. Other examples of services that are not acceptable include diagnostic reports that have not been interpreted, such as laboratory reports.

It is essential that the medical record documentation show evidence by provider authentication that the direct face-to-face service was personally furnished by the physician or qualified NPP. Examples of these services include office visits, hospital visits, preoperative anesthesia assessment, and surgical and invasive procedures.

Risk adjustment relies on annual health information. Each enrollee is assigned an individual risk score based on the health status information obtained from the diagnosis codes on the claims. The CMS-HCC model relies on ICD-10-CM coding specificity for accurate risk adjustment by using the most specific code available that is substantiated by the documentation in the medical record. Providers should fully document and accurately code the evaluation and management of all severe and chronic conditions to ensure a full, complete, and accurate clinical record of the patient's condition and reflect the work involved in caring for the patient, particularly those with complex and challenging health issues. All conditions affecting the treatment or management of the patient's health should be documented at least once a year, as applicable to care provided, to accurately describe the true complexity and severity of the patient's health. If the diagnosis coding on the claim is not accurate or complete, the claim may indicate that the provider did much less medical decision-making, evaluation, and management than was actually performed.

Documentation for a valid reportable diagnosis must clearly indicate evidence of M.E.A.T., for each diagnosis:

M	managed
E	evaluated
A	assessed
T	treated

It is recommended that providers use the Subjective and Objective observation, Assessment and Plan (S.O.A.P.) format for progress notes to document evidence of M.E.A.T. A problem list, active condition list, past medical history list, etc., are not suitable examples of documentation of M.E.A.T. Diagnoses and documentation may not be captured from past encounters that have been copied and pasted. Each encounter must be unique and reflect only that visit as it occurred. Chronic conditions require long-term attention and management, and should be reported when treated but are often inadequately documented due to familiarity with the patient. Insufficient documentation influences the assignment of diagnosis codes and directly affects the patient's risk score.

Documentation should be concise, include the reason for the face-to-face visit, and support the need for the patient to be monitored, evaluated, assessed, and/or treated for the conditions listed through clinical rationale and/or plan of care described in clear (legible) notes. Each page of progress notes should be properly authenticated and include the patient's name and the date.

Providers should document each clinical diagnosis to the highest degree of specificity per encounter, including all complications and/or manifestations, including clear links to causal conditions. Only confirmed conditions should be documented—no rule-out conditions or abnormal findings without clinical significance. All known conditions, including chronic conditions, that affect the care and treatment of the patient at least once per year should be noted.

Providers should specifically document the condition and test or report results, and document the status of any changes to the condition, using terminology such as decreased, increased, worsening, improving, or unchanged. Documentation should include supporting evidence of the results or plan of care.

Documentation Tips

- Document all cause-and-effect relationships.
- Report the most specific diagnosis code available that is supported by the documentation.
- Include all current diagnoses as part of the current medical decision-making, and document for every visit.
- Identify diagnoses that are current or chronic problems rather than a past medical history or previous resolved condition.
- Document history of heart attack, status codes, etc., that affect the patient's care as "history of" or "PMH" when they no longer exist or are not current conditions.
- Ensure each progress note has the date, signature, and credentials/specialty.
- Document the thought processes used to assess each condition.
- Know high revenue HCCs that are often undiagnosed or undercoded.
- Avoid "unspecified" codes.
- Ensure the codes reported are accurate.
- Ensure each encounter is billed.
- Review rejection reports, and audit reports to assess risks.

Audits

Because reimbursement is by patient, rather than based on an average of the entire population, and is based upon documentation, there is the potential for upcoding. Audits are conducted by the MA plan and CMS recovery auditors.

Initial Validation Audit (IVA)

CMS requires that the MA plan validate HCCs. This is usually performed by an independent auditor working with the plan or a contracted vendor to validate the MA plan's data submitted to CMS.

The MA plan submits the one best medical record that supports each HCC identified for the beneficiary.

Risk Adjustment Data Validation Audit

Risk adjustment data validation (RADV) audits were introduced in 2011 and updated for 2015. They are performed by CMS to validate the integrity and accuracy of risk-adjusted payments by verifying that the diagnosis codes the MA plans submit are supported by the medical record documentation for a member.

MA plans can be selected by CMS for RADV audits annually and if chosen are required to submit their members' medical records to CMS. Providers are required to assist the MA plan by providing the medical record documentation included in the audit. Even though each diagnosis needs to be reported only once in a calendar year, during a RADV audit up to five dates of service may be submitted to support any one HCC.

To be validated, medical record documentation must meet certain criteria and standards. Even if the diagnosis is documented and coded correctly, any deficiency in the documentation can make the encounter and the HCC invalid. Diagnoses that cannot be validated are considered payment errors. The results of the audit are communicated to the MA plan, which then communicates these results to the provider. Under- and overpayments are subject to payment adjustment. The results of RADV audits can be extrapolated over the MA plan population to calculate potential payment errors and overpayments/recoupments. Regulations include a RADV appeal process, a document dispute process, and a procedure for obtaining physician-signature attestations.

The following items are reviewed during the validation process:

- The record is for the correct enrollee.
- The record is from the correct calendar year for the payment year being audited.
- The record is legible.
- The date of service is present on the records and is for a face-to-face visit.
- The record is from a valid provider type.

- Valid credentials and/or a valid physician specialty are documented on the record.
- The record contains a signature from an acceptable type of physician.
- There is a diagnosis on the record.
- The diagnosis supports an HCC.
- The diagnosis supports the submitted HCC.

Mitigate audit risk by coding each reportable diagnosis each time it meets reporting guidelines. Audit regularly to assess areas of risk and in need of improvement and to capture conditions documented but not coded. Check for additional qualifying HCCs. Ensure claims are submitted and that corrected claims are submitted when indicated. There are three claims submission deadlines: January, March, and September. CMS adjusts each member's risk score twice a year, with the final reconciliation in August of the year after the plan year.

If providers emphasize correct coding and documentation and perform internal audits to determine where the risks are and prepare for audits, incorrect payment is less likely.

Illustrations

Chapter 3. Diseases of the Blood and Blood-forming Organs and Certain Disorders Involving the Immune Mechanism (D50–D89)

Red Blood Cells

White Blood Cell

Platelet

Coagulation

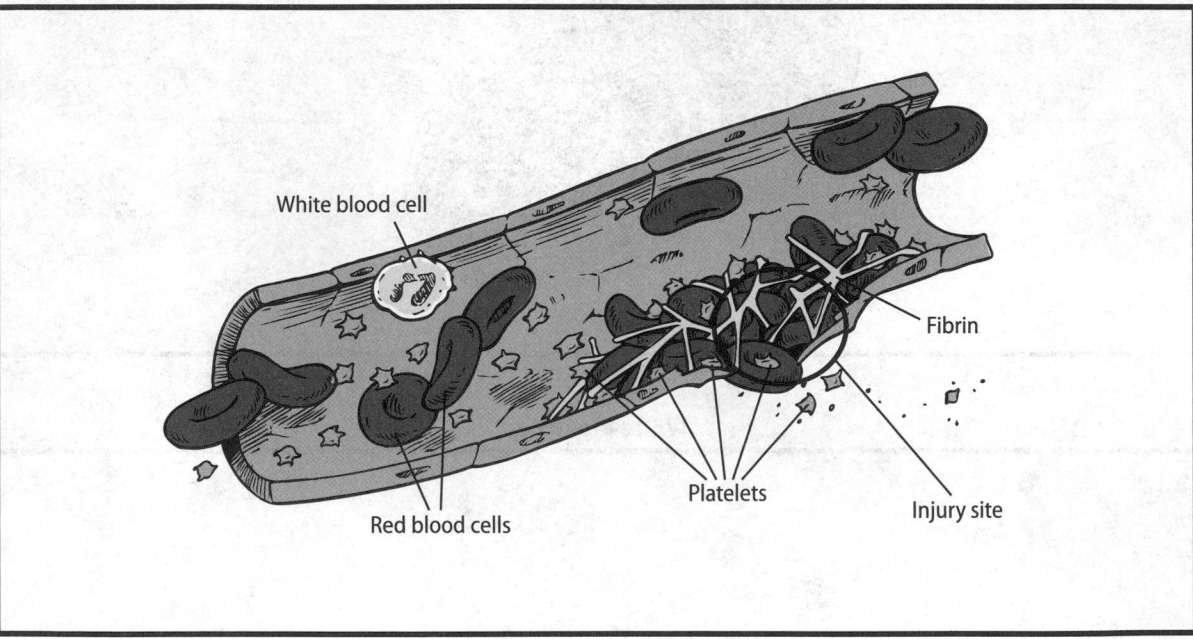

Spleen Anatomical Location and External Structures

Spleen Interior Structures

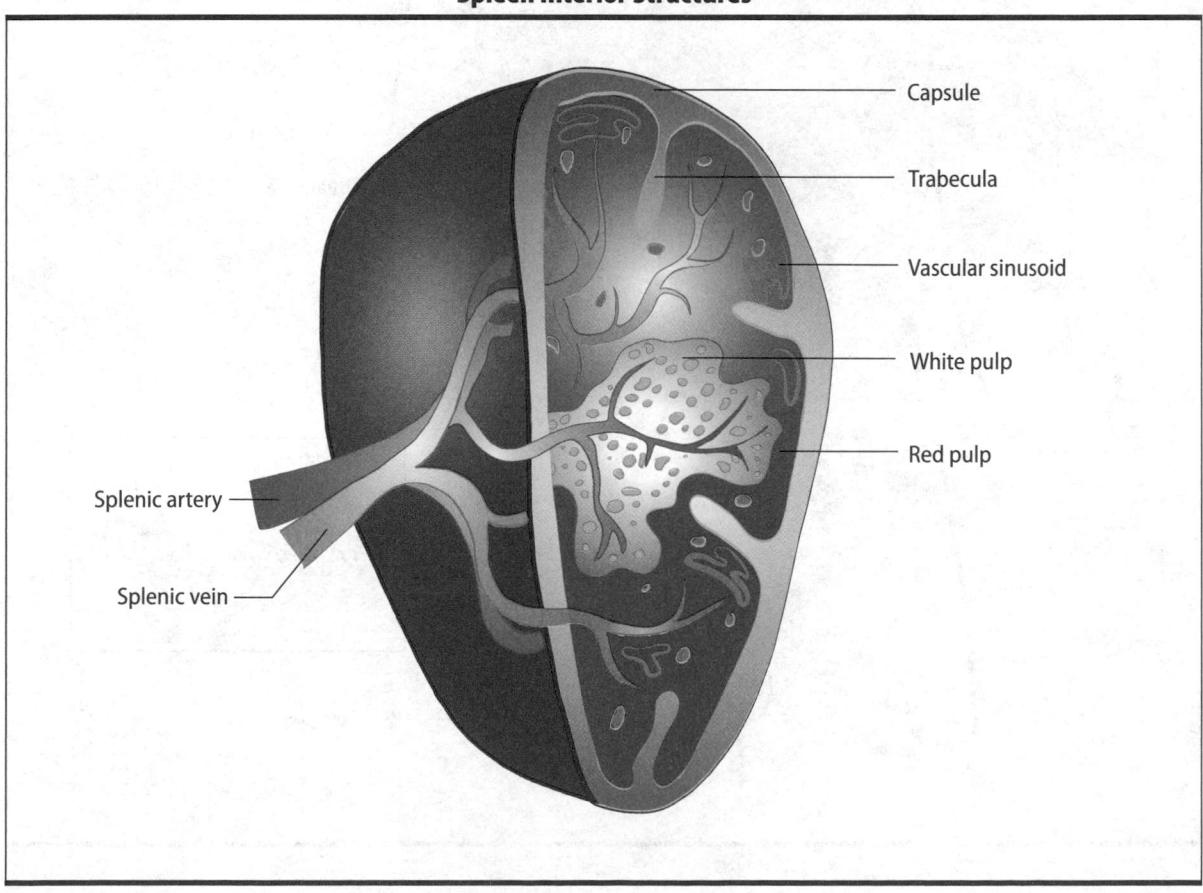

Chapter 4. Endocrine, Nutritional and Metabolic Diseases (E00–E89)

Endocrine System

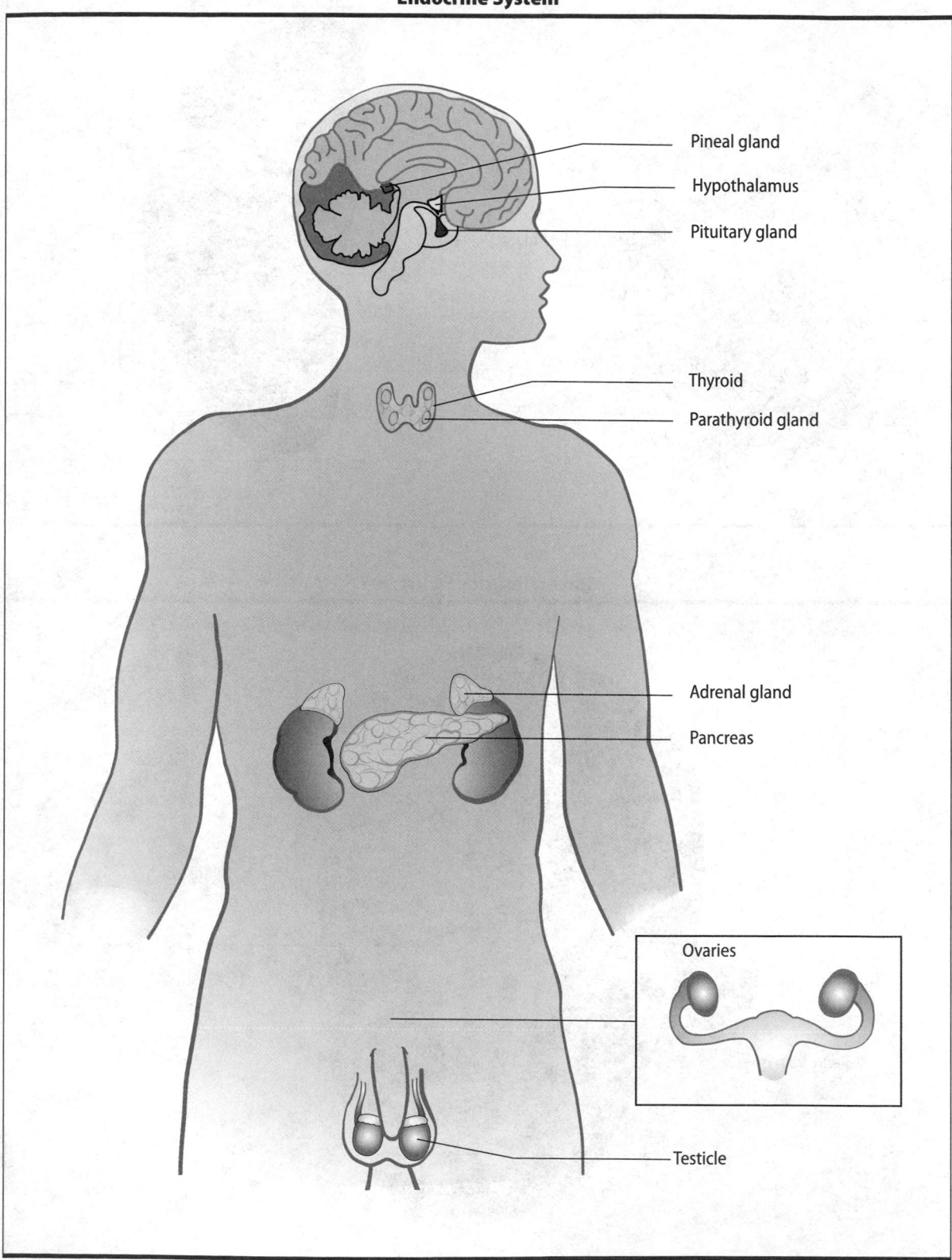

Pineal gland

Hypothalamus

Pituitary gland

Thyroid

Parathyroid gland

Adrenal gland

Pancreas

Ovaries

Testicle

Thyroid

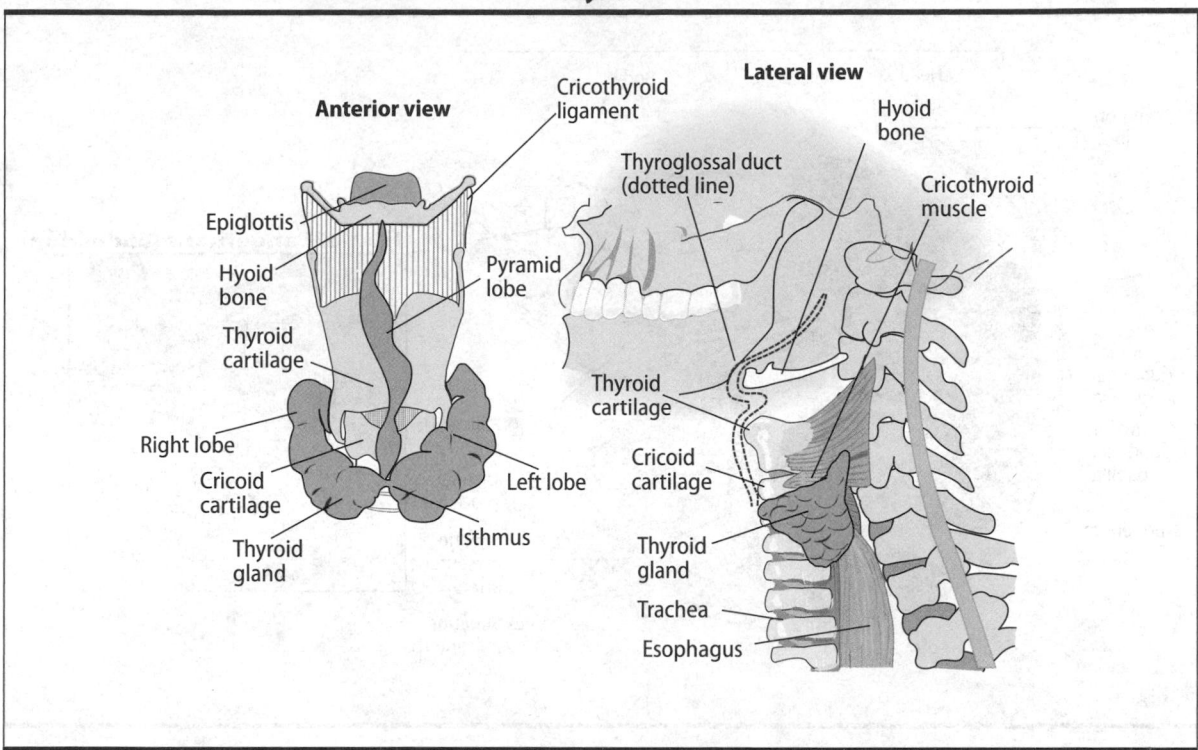

Thyroid and Parathyroid Glands

Pancreas

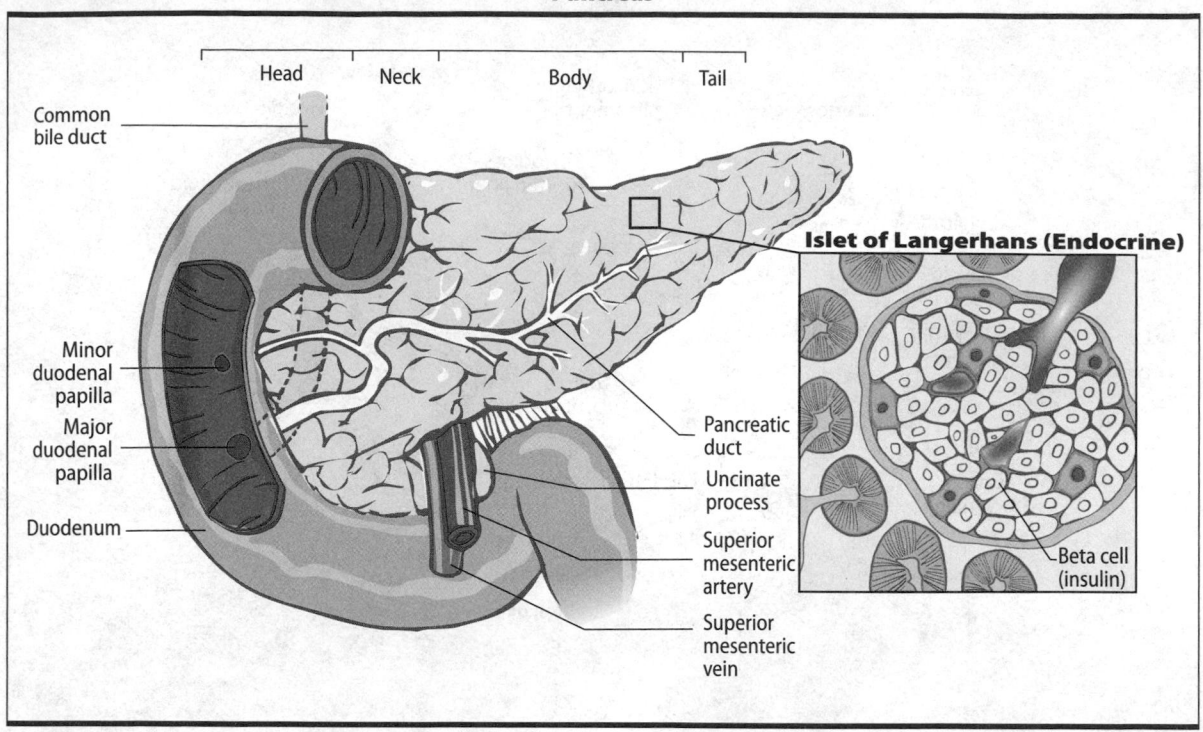

Head   Neck   Body   Tail

Common bile duct

Minor duodenal papilla

Major duodenal papilla

Duodenum

Pancreatic duct

Uncinate process

Superior mesenteric artery

Superior mesenteric vein

Islet of Langerhans (Endocrine)

Beta cell (insulin)

Anatomy of the Adrenal Gland

Adrenal glands

Kidney

Capsule

Cortex

Medulla

Structure of an Ovary

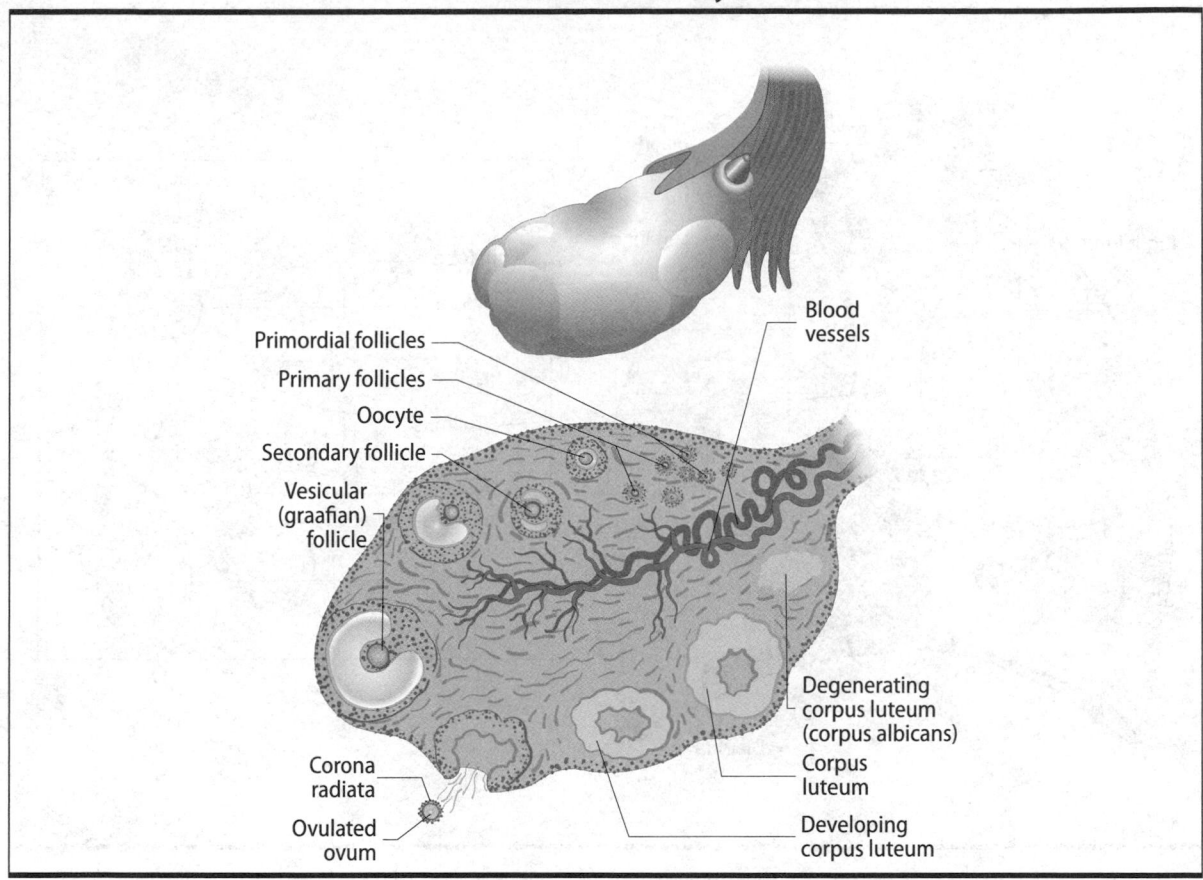

Testis and Associated Structures

Thymus

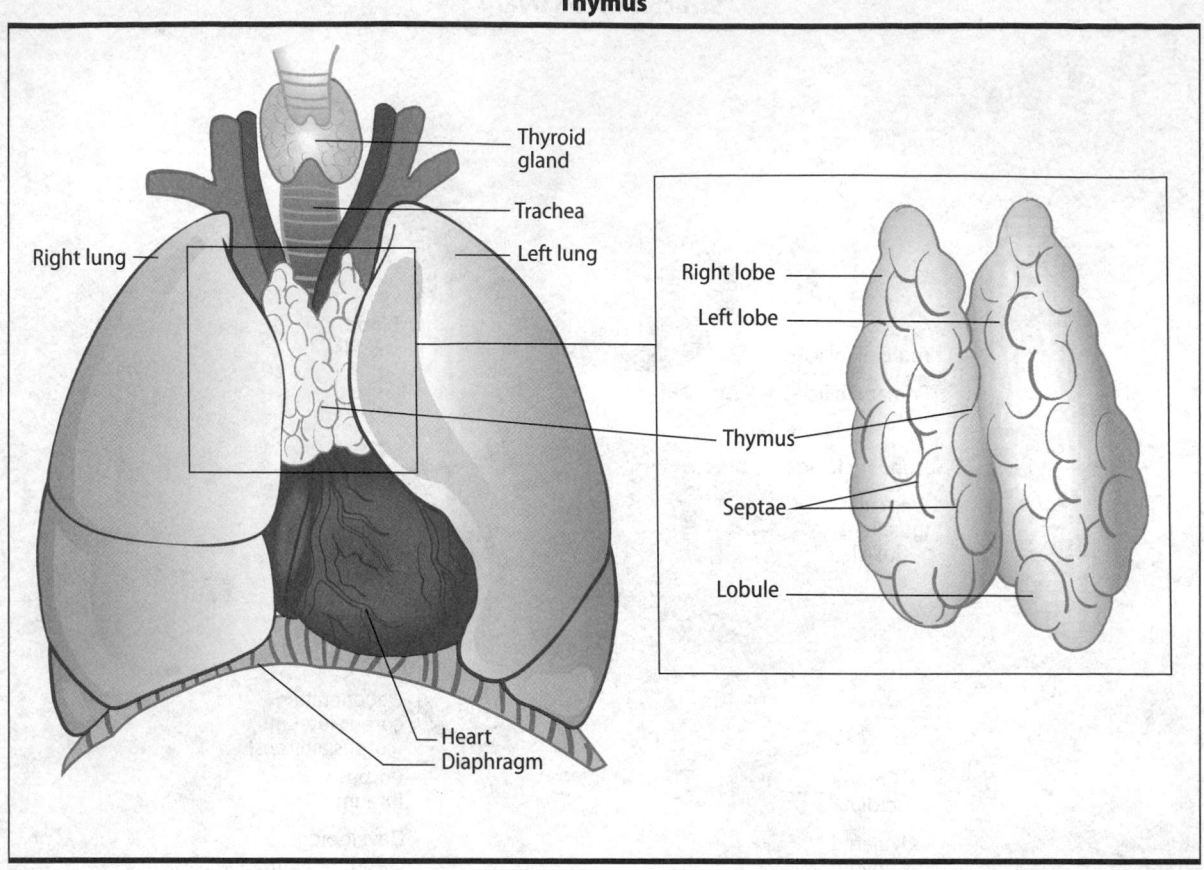

Chapter 6. Diseases of the Nervous System (G00–G99)

Brain

Cranial Nerves

Peripheral Nervous System

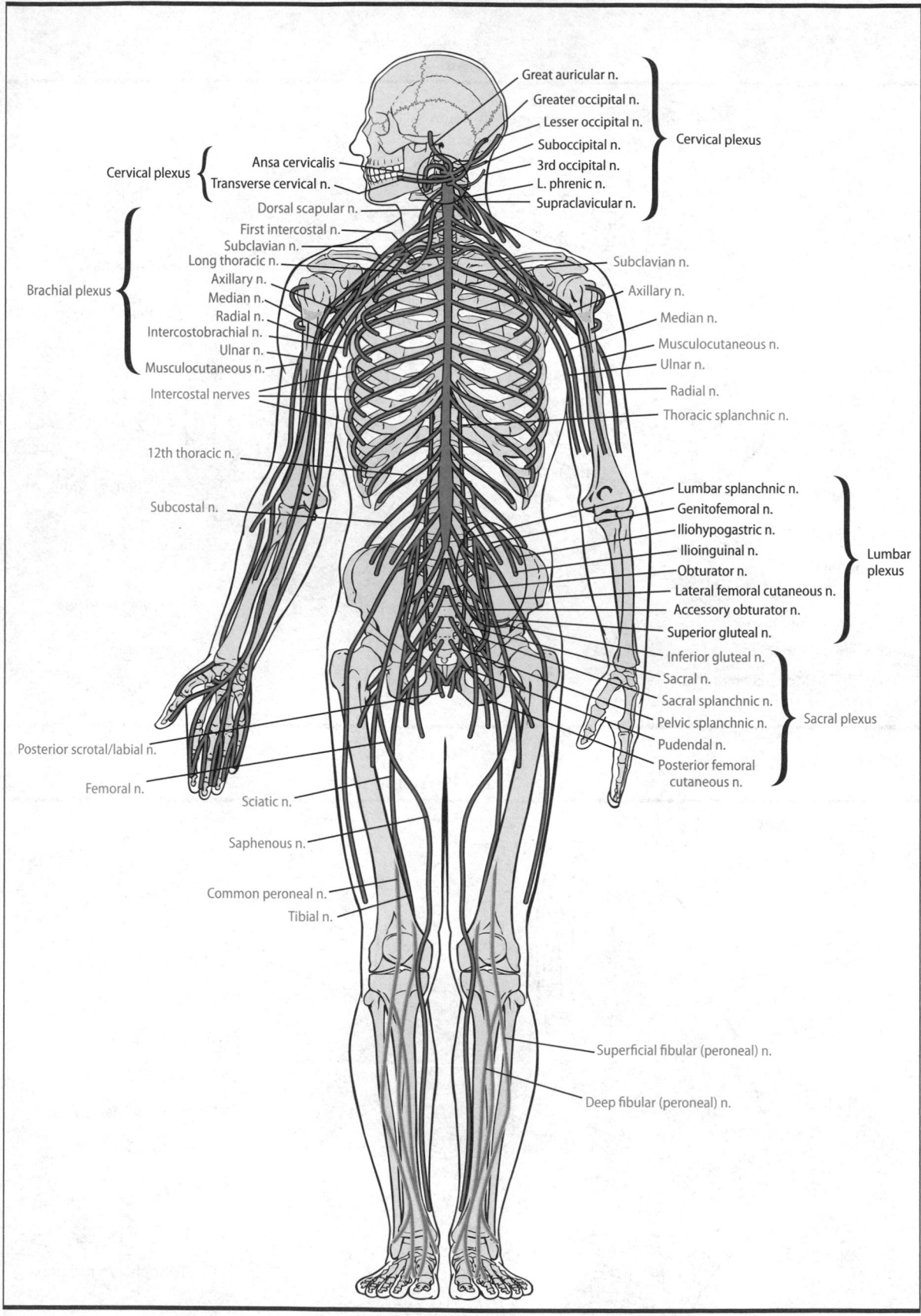

Spinal Cord and Spinal Nerves

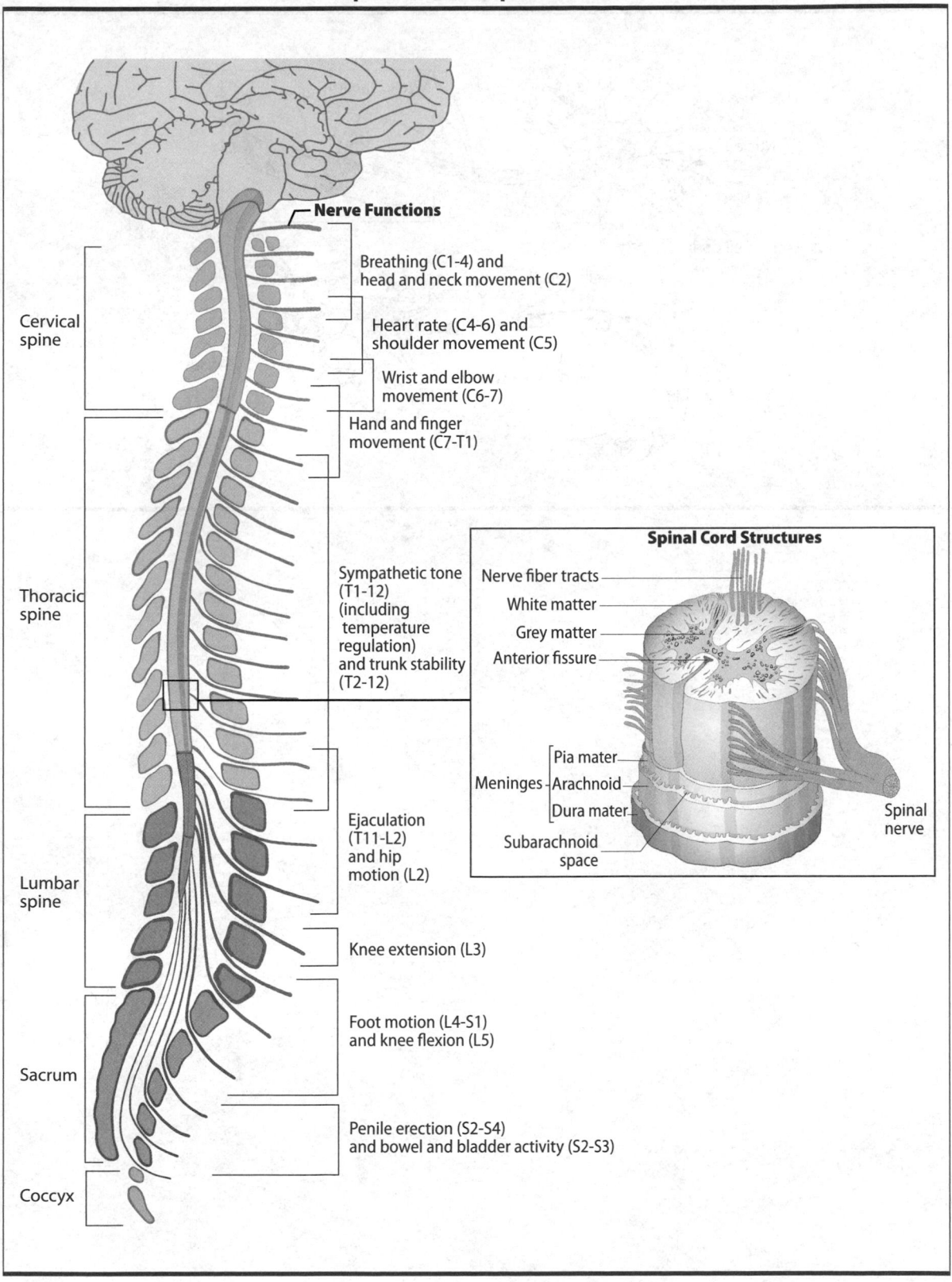

Nerve Functions

Breathing (C1-4) and
head and neck movement (C2)

Heart rate (C4-6) and
shoulder movement (C5)

Wrist and elbow
movement (C6-7)

Hand and finger
movement (C7-T1)

Cervical
spine

Thoracic
spine

Sympathetic tone
(T1-12)
(including
temperature
regulation)
and trunk stability
(T2-12)

Ejaculation
(T11-L2)
and hip
motion (L2)

Lumbar
spine

Knee extension (L3)

Foot motion (L4-S1)
and knee flexion (L5)

Sacrum

Penile erection (S2-S4)
and bowel and bladder activity (S2-S3)

Coccyx

Spinal Cord Structures

Nerve fiber tracts

White matter

Grey matter

Anterior fissure

Meninges
- Pia mater
- Arachnoid
- Dura mater

Subarachnoid
space

Spinal
nerve

Nerve Cell

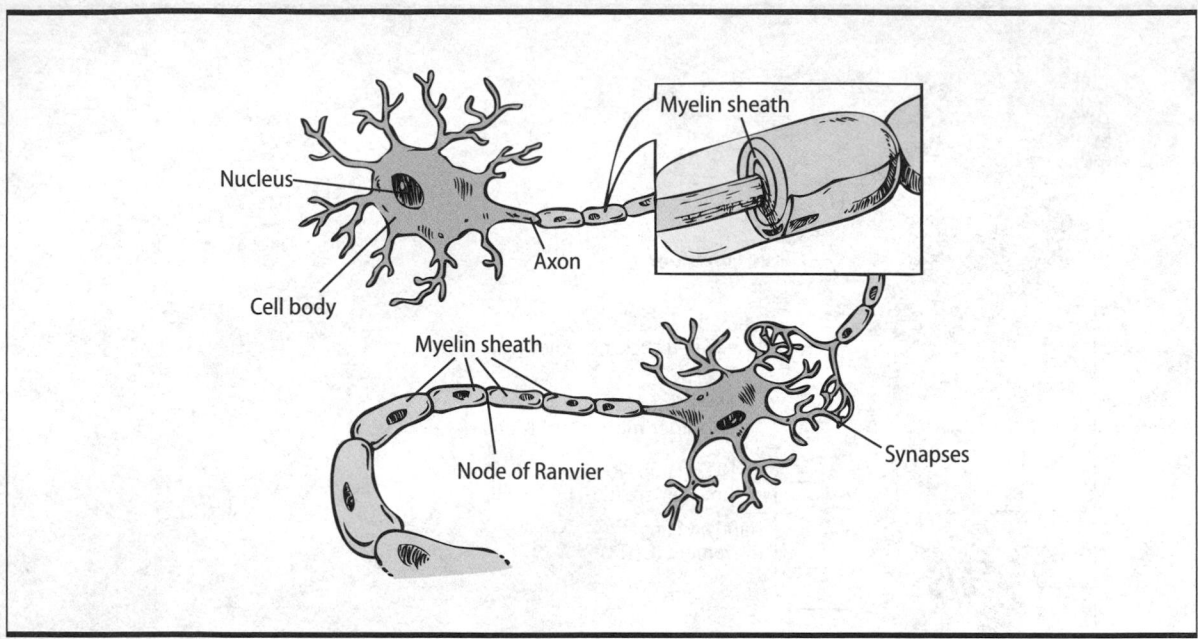

Chapter 7. Diseases of the Eye and Adnexa (H00–H59)

Eye

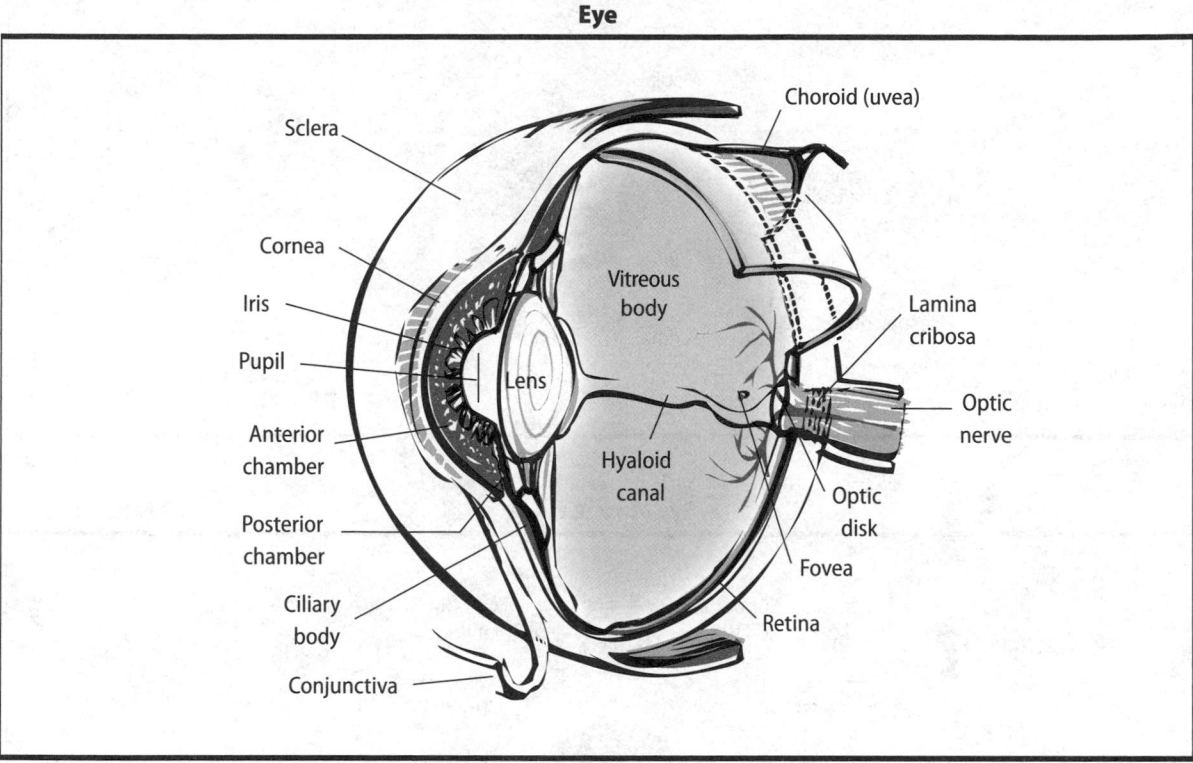

Posterior Pole of Globe/Flow of Aqueous Humor

Lacrimal System

Eye Musculature

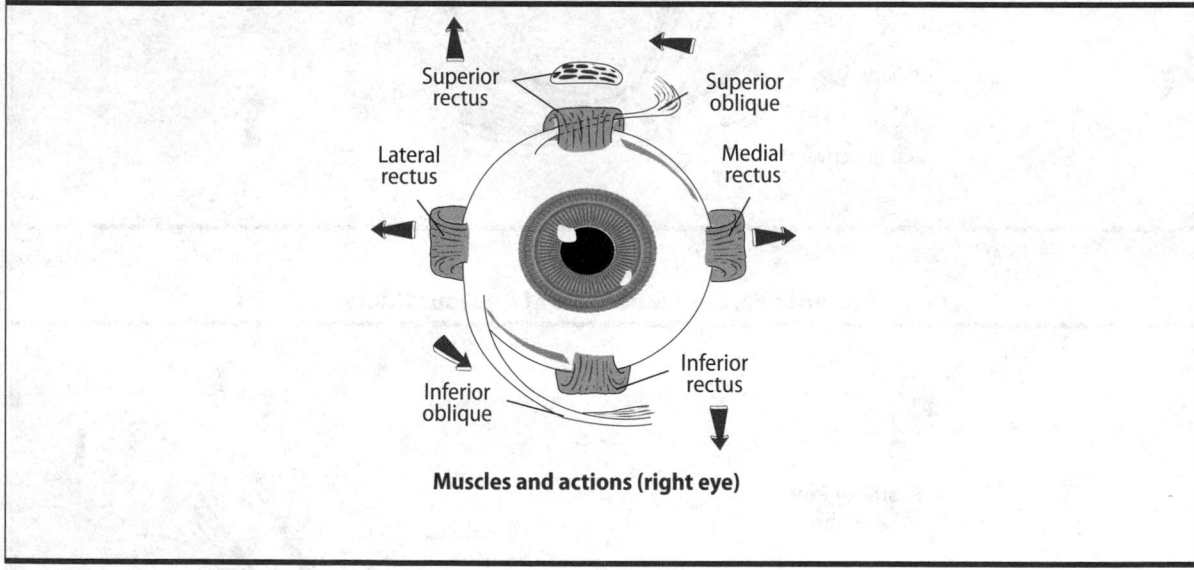

Muscles and actions (right eye)

Eyelid Structures

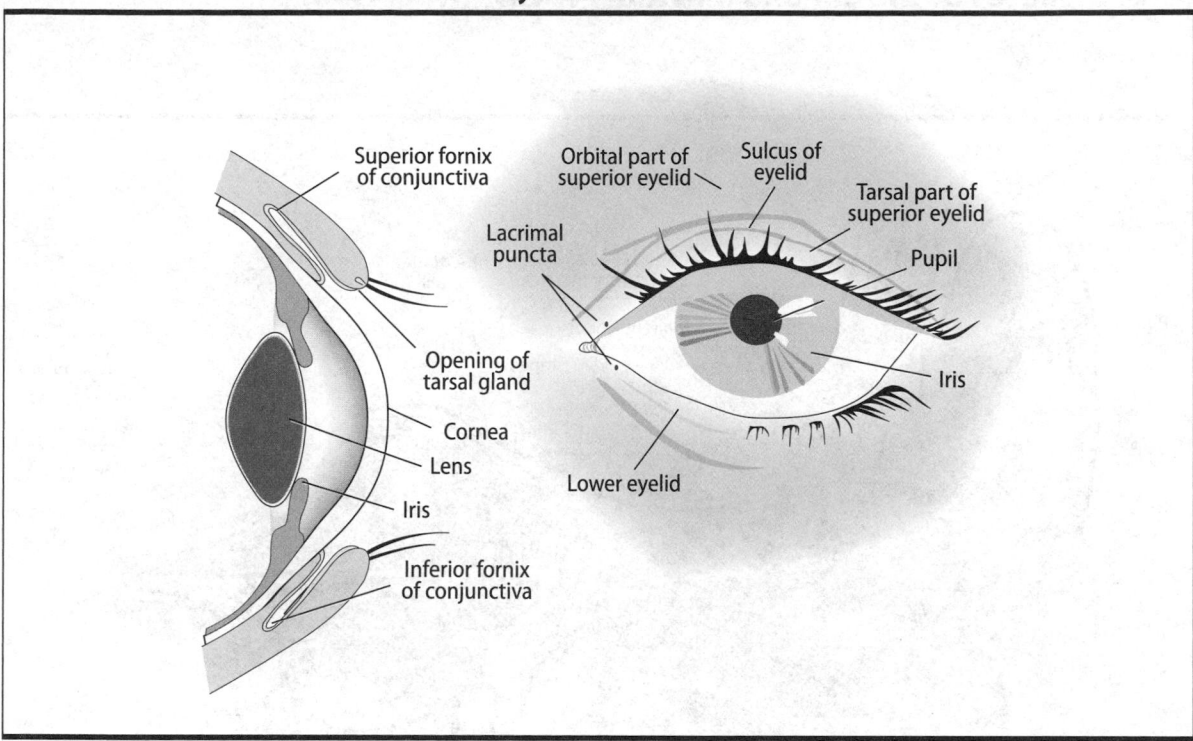

Chapter 8. Diseases of the Ear and Mastoid Process (H60–H95)

Ear Anatomy

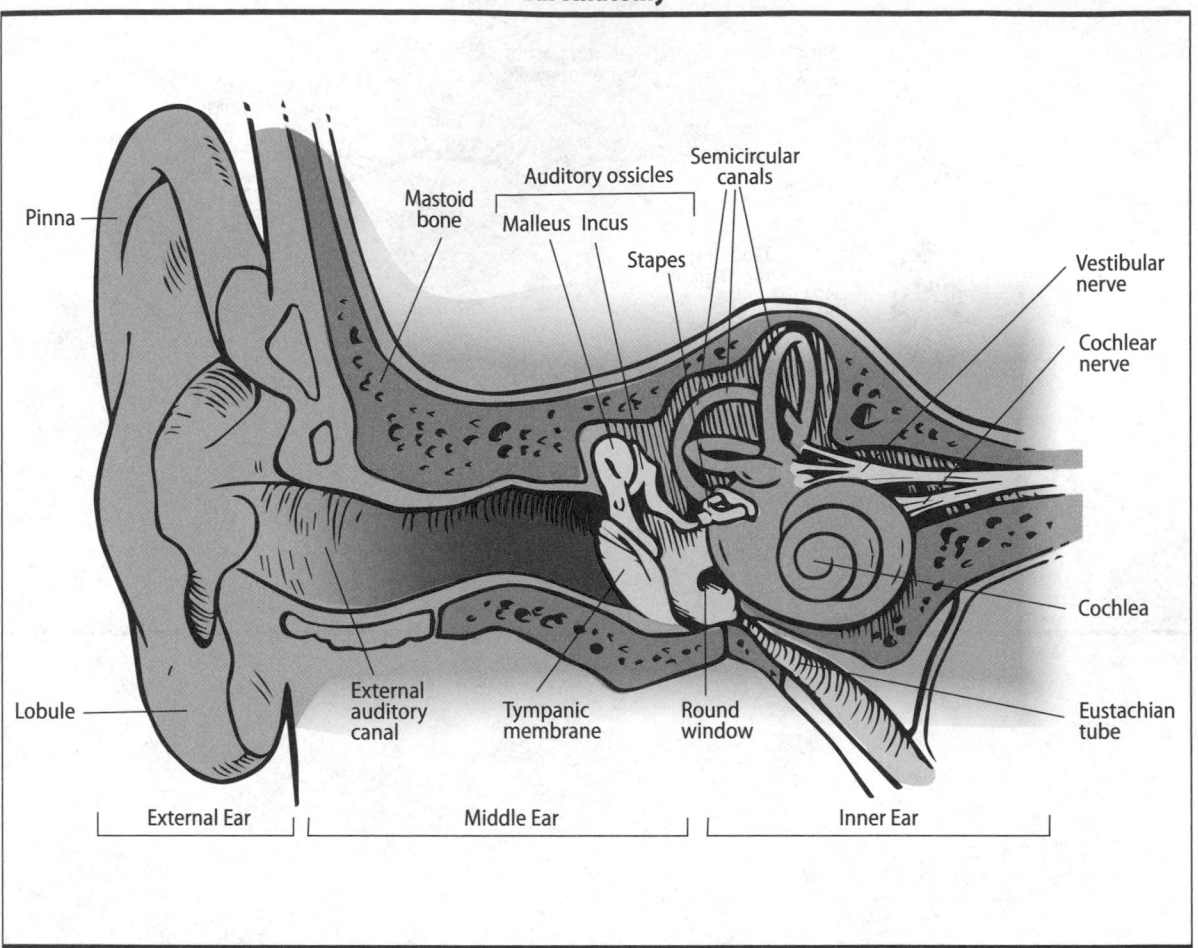

Chapter 9. Diseases of the Circulatory System (I00–I99)

Anatomy of the Heart

Aorta

Pulmonary artery

Pulmonary vein

Superior vena cava

Aortic valve

Pulmonary valve

Right atrium

Left atrium

Tricuspid valve

Mitral valve

Right ventricle

Chorda tendinae

Inferior vena cava

Left ventricle

Heart Cross Section

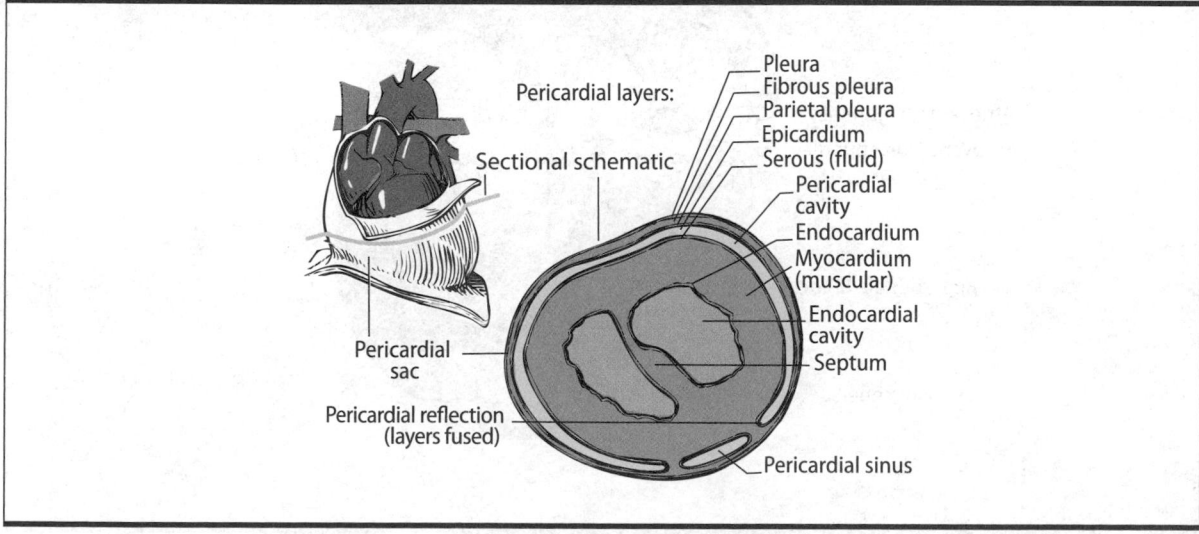

Pericardial layers:

Sectional schematic

Pleura
Fibrous pleura
Parietal pleura
Epicardium
Serous (fluid)
Pericardial cavity
Endocardium
Myocardium (muscular)
Endocardial cavity
Septum

Pericardial sac

Pericardial reflection (layers fused)

Pericardial sinus

Heart Valves

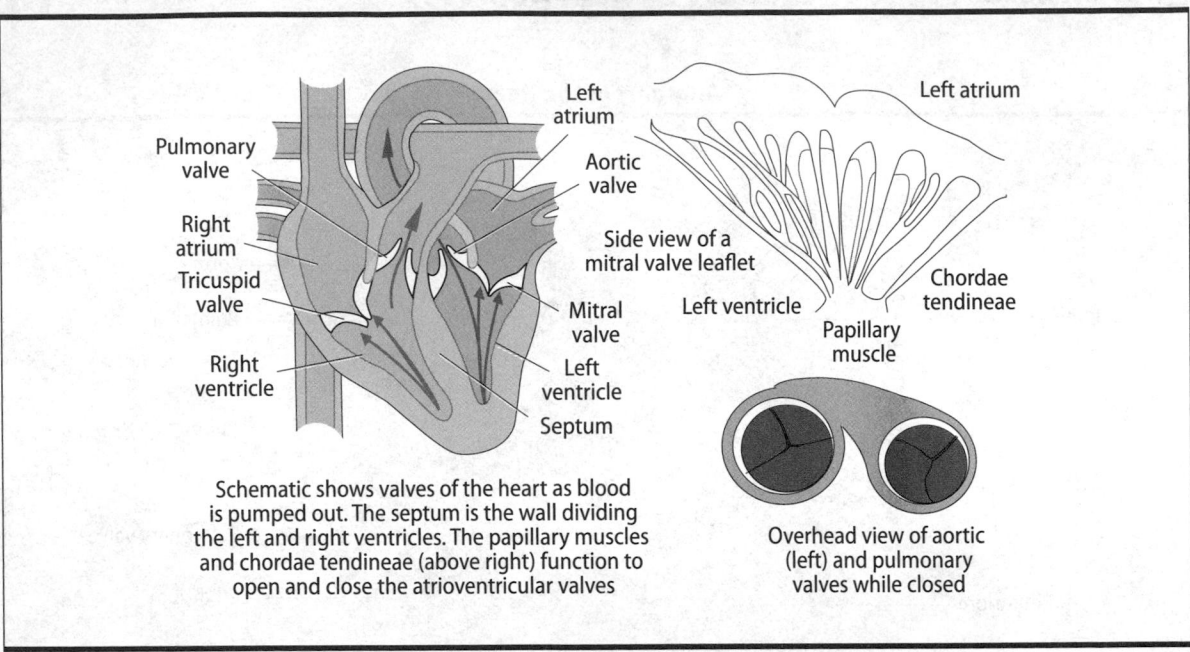

Schematic shows valves of the heart as blood is pumped out. The septum is the wall dividing the left and right ventricles. The papillary muscles and chordae tendineae (above right) function to open and close the atrioventricular valves

Overhead view of aortic (left) and pulmonary valves while closed

Heart Conduction System

Coronary Arteries

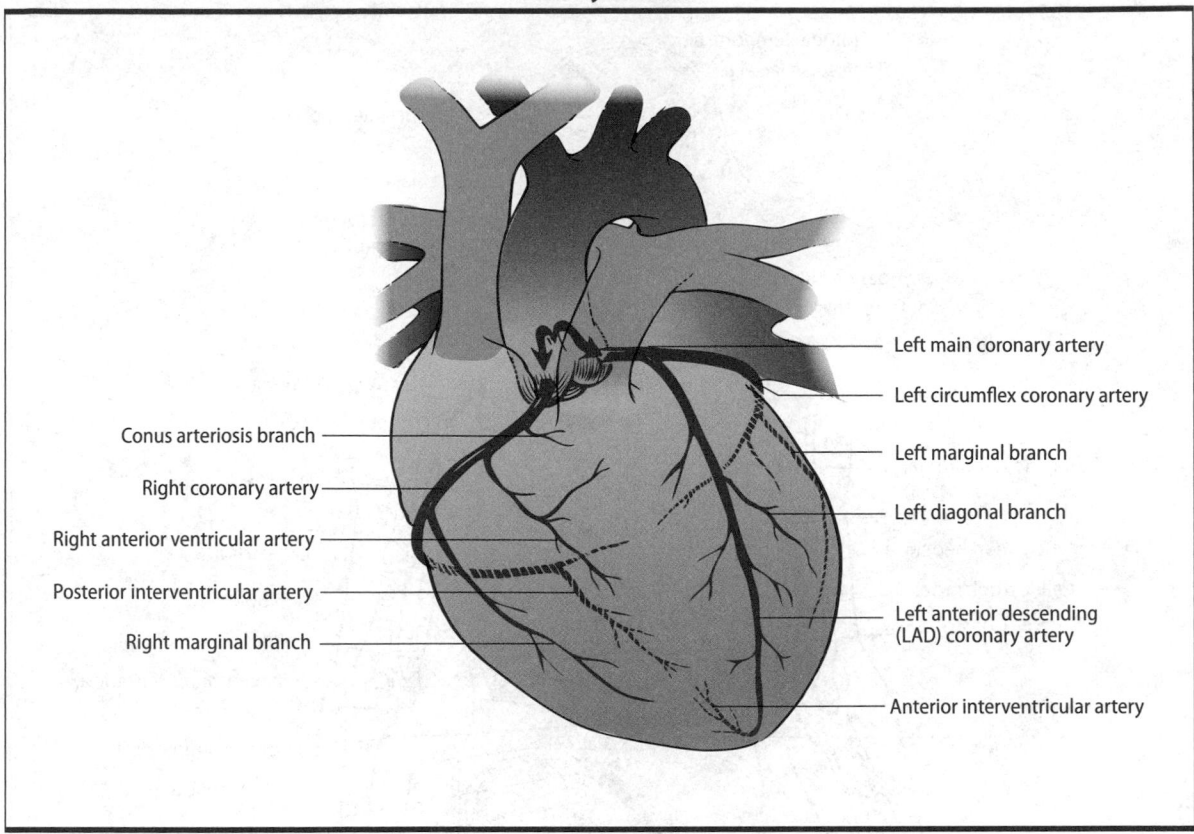

Conus arteriosis branch
Right coronary artery
Right anterior ventricular artery
Posterior interventricular artery
Right marginal branch

Left main coronary artery
Left circumflex coronary artery
Left marginal branch
Left diagonal branch
Left anterior descending (LAD) coronary artery
Anterior interventricular artery

Arteries

Veins

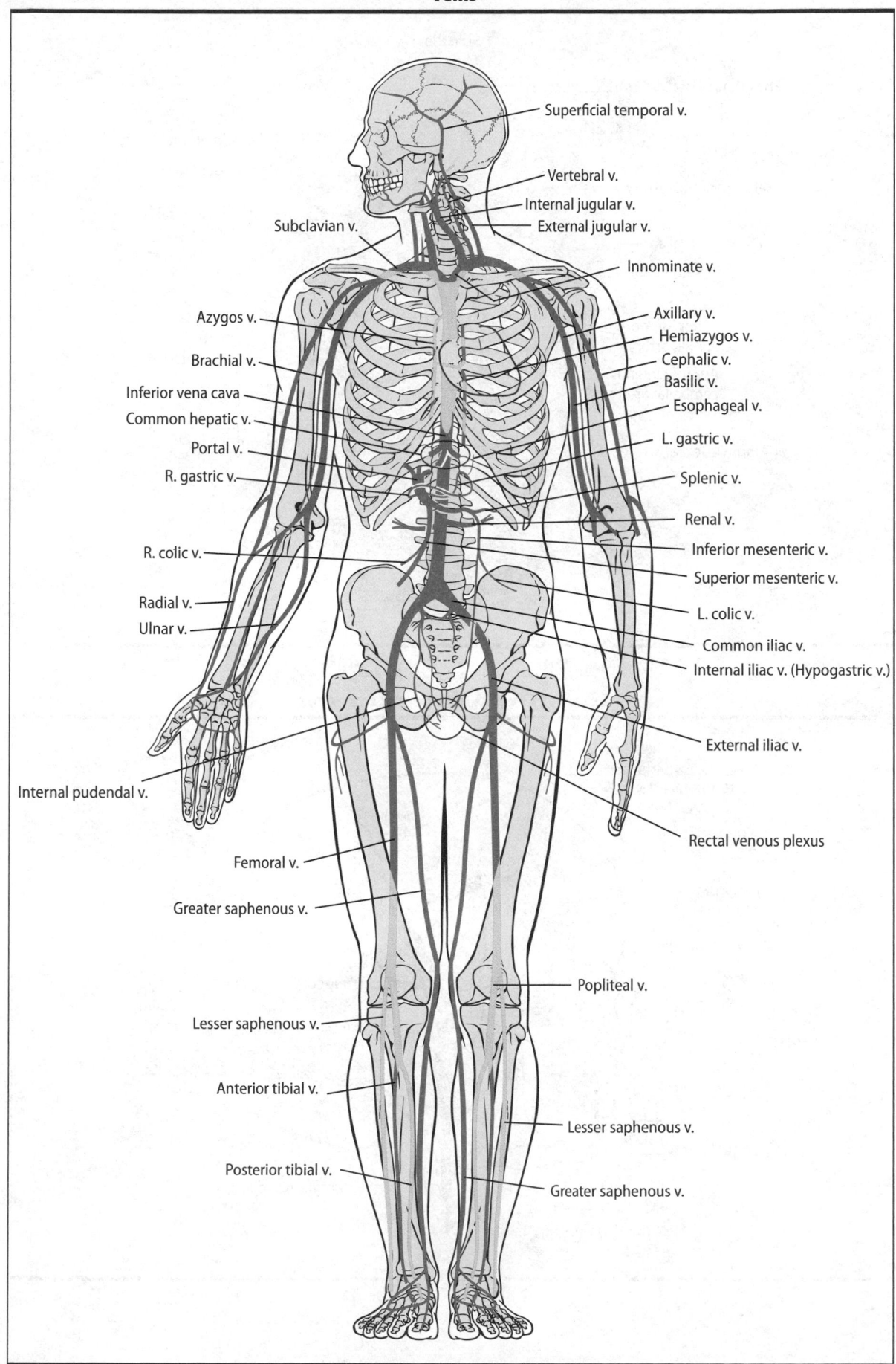

Superficial temporal v.
Vertebral v.
Internal jugular v.
External jugular v.
Subclavian v.
Innominate v.
Azygos v.
Axillary v.
Hemiazygos v.
Brachial v.
Cephalic v.
Inferior vena cava
Basilic v.
Common hepatic v.
Esophageal v.
Portal v.
L. gastric v.
R. gastric v.
Splenic v.
Renal v.
R. colic v.
Inferior mesenteric v.
Superior mesenteric v.
Radial v.
L. colic v.
Ulnar v.
Common iliac v.
Internal iliac v. (Hypogastric v.)
External iliac v.
Internal pudendal v.
Rectal venous plexus
Femoral v.
Greater saphenous v.
Popliteal v.
Lesser saphenous v.
Anterior tibial v.
Lesser saphenous v.
Posterior tibial v.
Greater saphenous v.

Internal Carotid and Vertebral Arteries and Branches

Side View

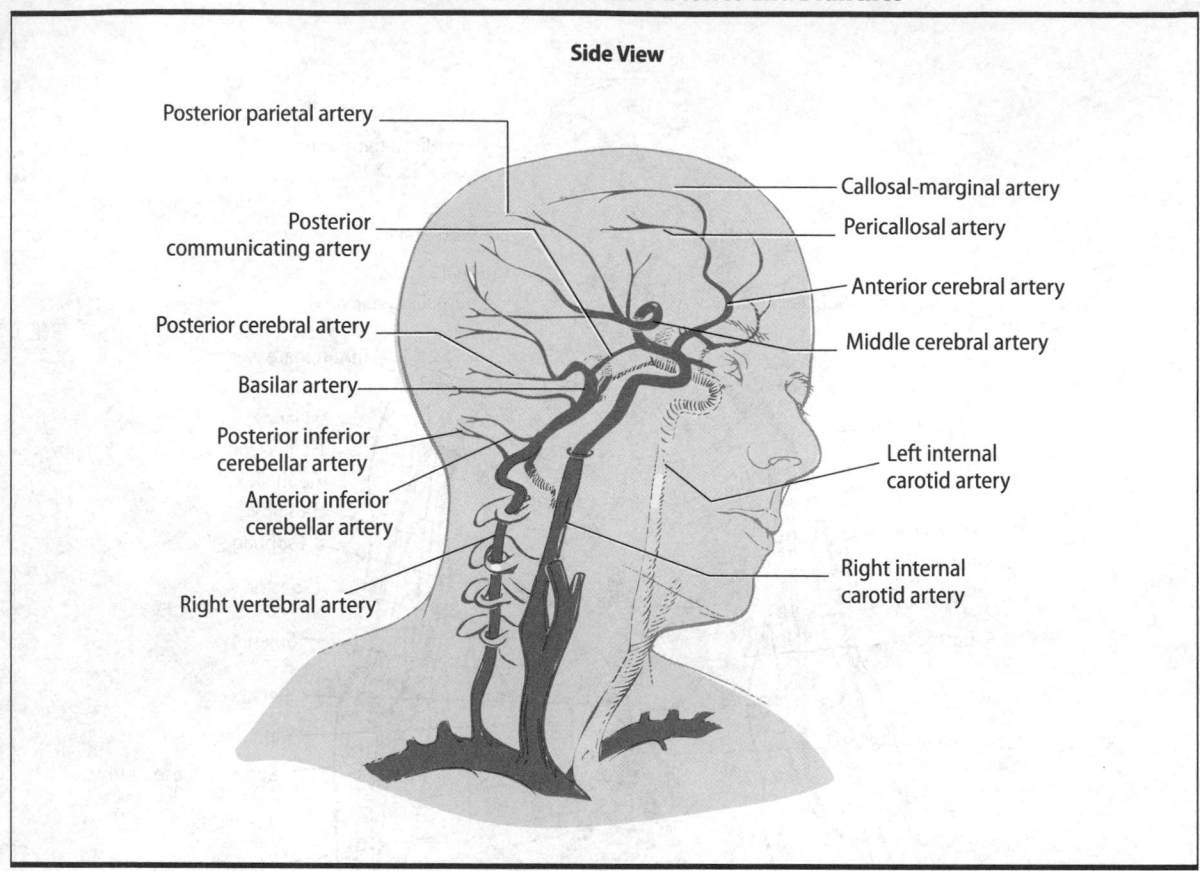

External Carotid Artery and Branches

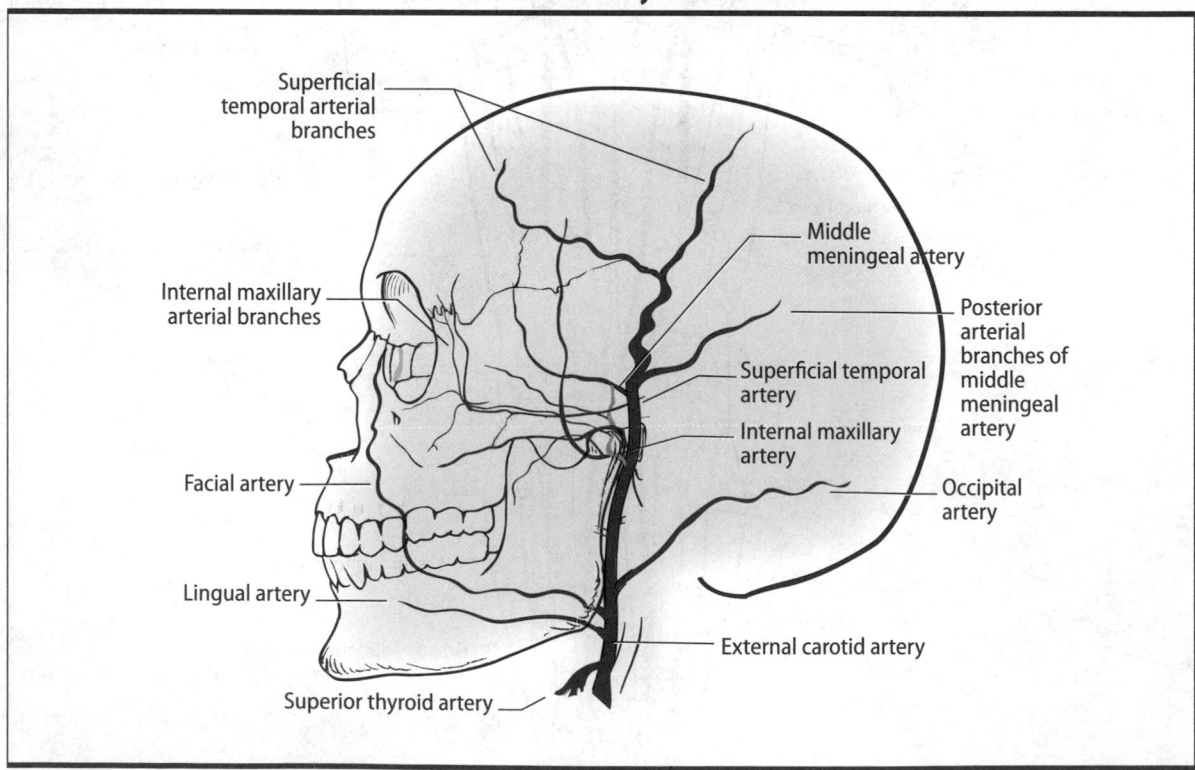

Branches of Abdominal Aorta

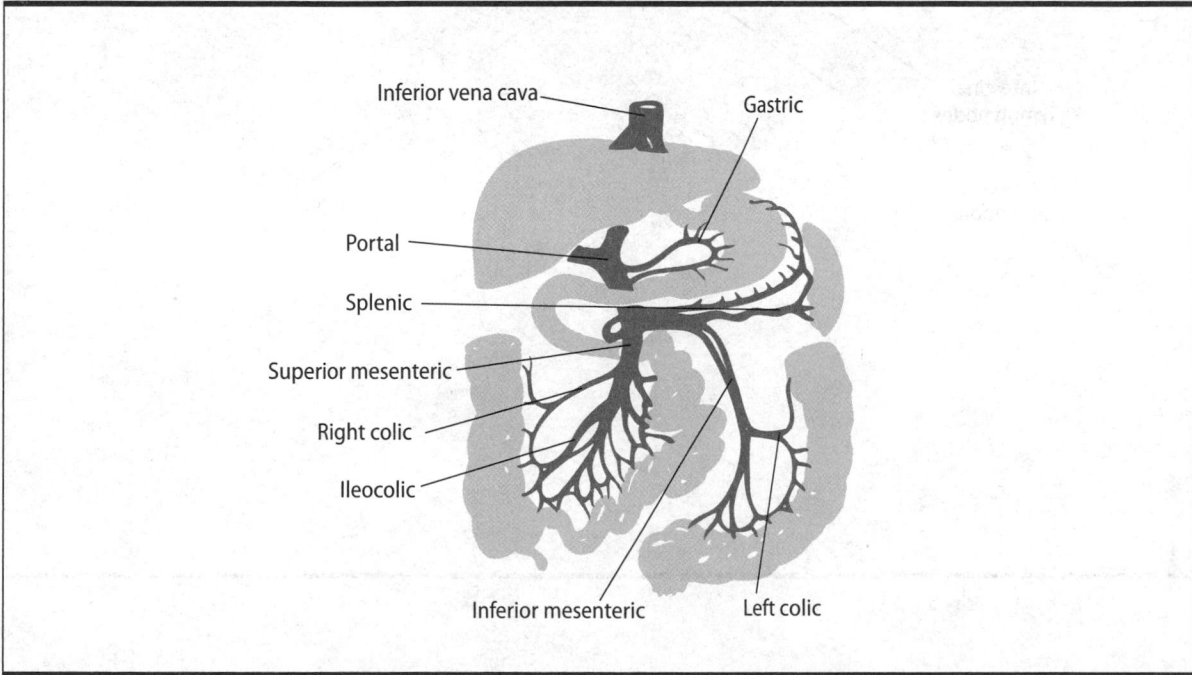

Portal Venous Circulation

Lymphatic System

Axillary Lymph Nodes

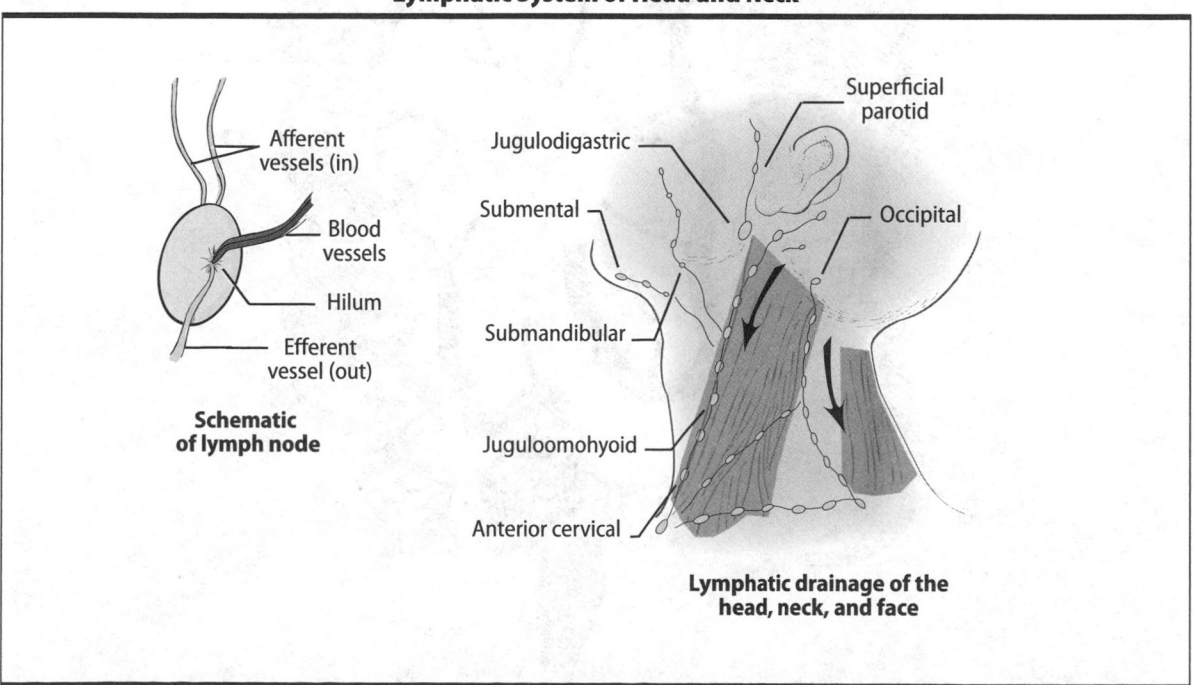

Lymphatic System of Head and Neck

**Schematic
of lymph node**

**Lymphatic drainage of the
head, neck, and face**

Lymphatic Capillaries

Schematic of lymphatic capillaries

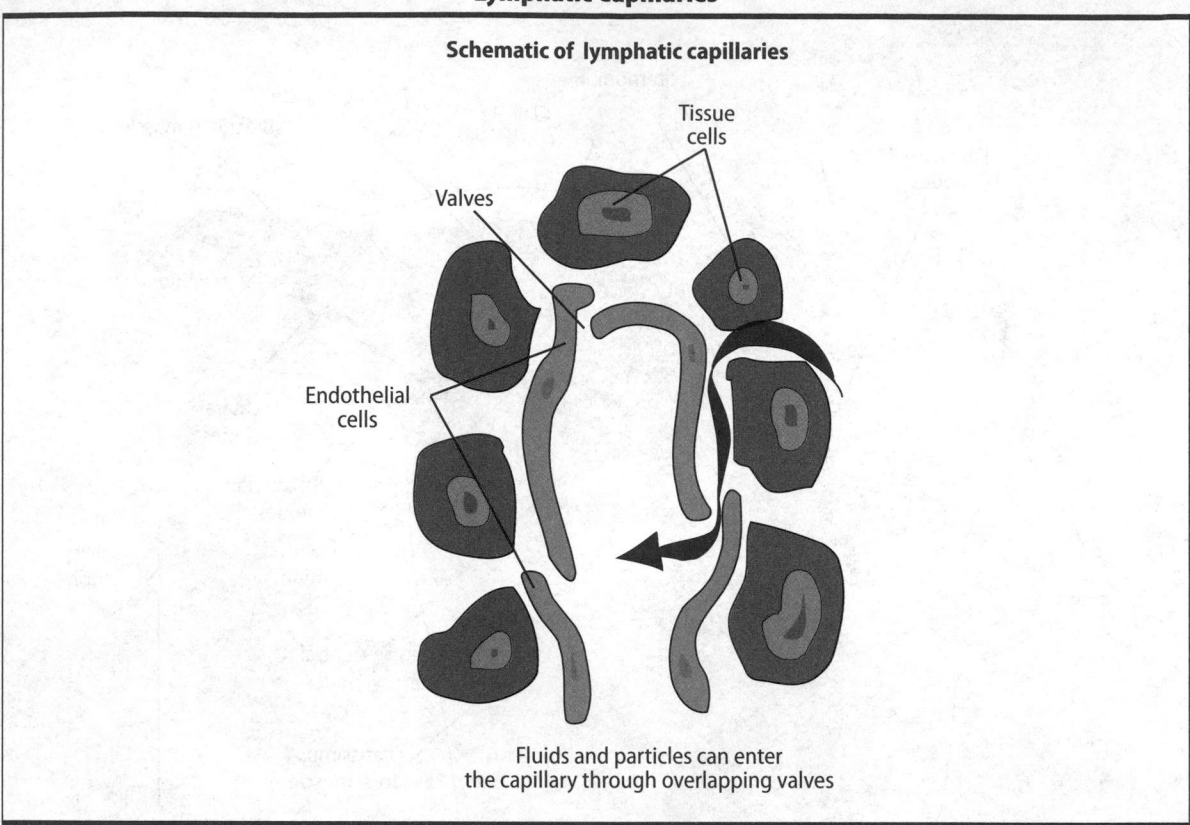

Tissue cells

Valves

Endothelial cells

Fluids and particles can enter the capillary through overlapping valves

Lymphatic Drainage

Lymphatic drainage of the colon follows blood supply

Middle colic nodes

Paracolic nodes

Left colic nodes

Ascending colon

Cecum

Rectum

Chapter 10. Diseases of the Respiratory System (JØØ–J99)

Respiratory System

Nasal cavity and paranasal sinuses

Nostril

Oral cavity

Pharynx

Larynx

Trachea

Pleura

Right lung

Left lung

Carina of trachea

Right main / primary bronchus

Left main/ primary bronchus

Secondary (lobar) bronchi

Tertiary (segmental) bronchi

Bronchioles

Alveoli

Diaphragm

Upper Respiratory System

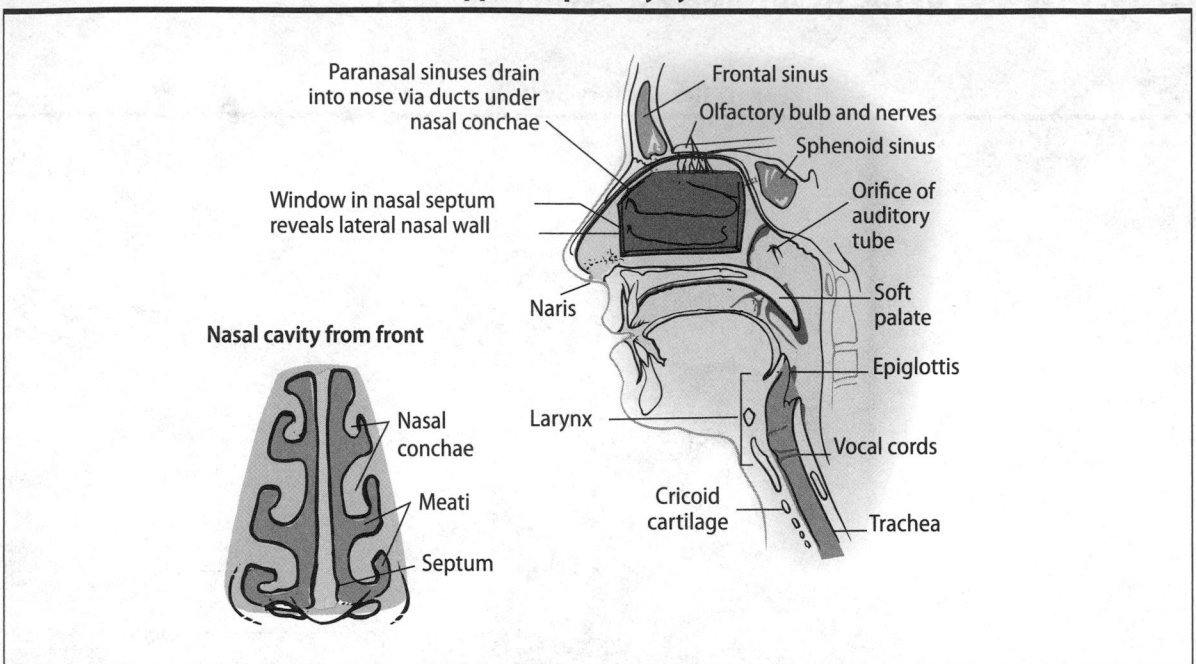

Paranasal sinuses drain into nose via ducts under nasal conchae

Window in nasal septum reveals lateral nasal wall

Nasal cavity from front

Nasal conchae

Meati

Septum

Naris

Larynx

Cricoid cartilage

Frontal sinus

Olfactory bulb and nerves

Sphenoid sinus

Orifice of auditory tube

Soft palate

Epiglottis

Vocal cords

Trachea

Lower Respiratory System

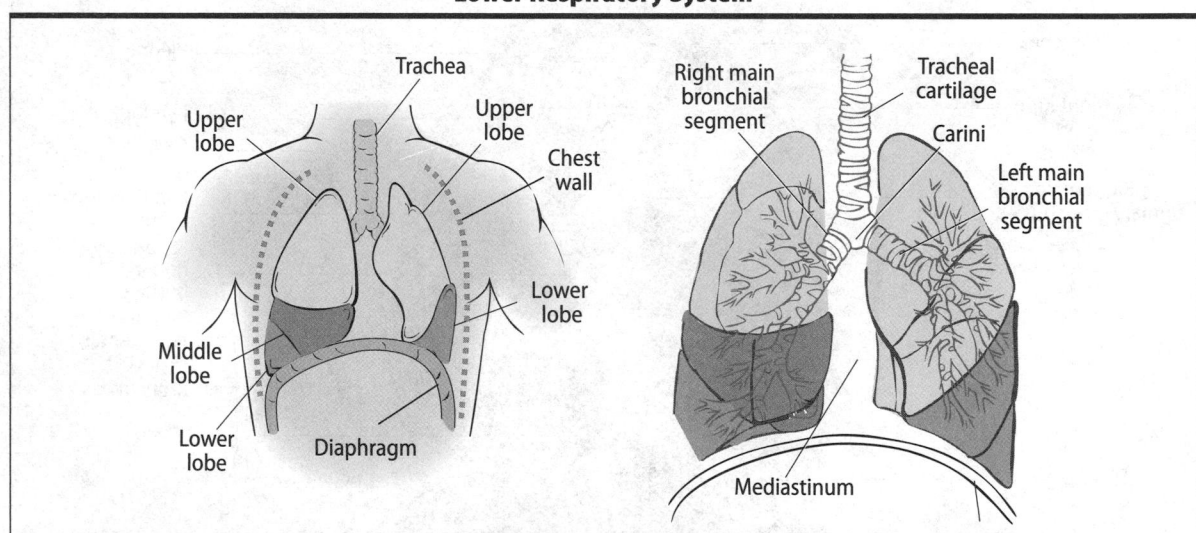

Trachea

Upper lobe

Upper lobe

Chest wall

Lower lobe

Middle lobe

Lower lobe

Diaphragm

Right main bronchial segment

Tracheal cartilage

Carini

Left main bronchial segment

Mediastinum

Paranasal Sinuses

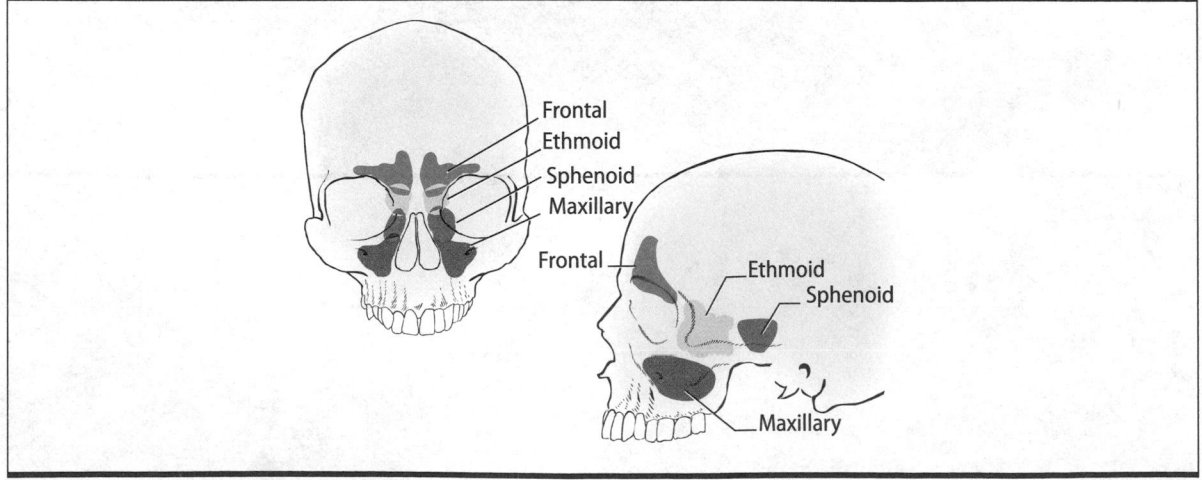

Frontal
Ethmoid
Sphenoid
Maxillary

Frontal

Ethmoid

Sphenoid

Maxillary

Lung Segments

Alveoli

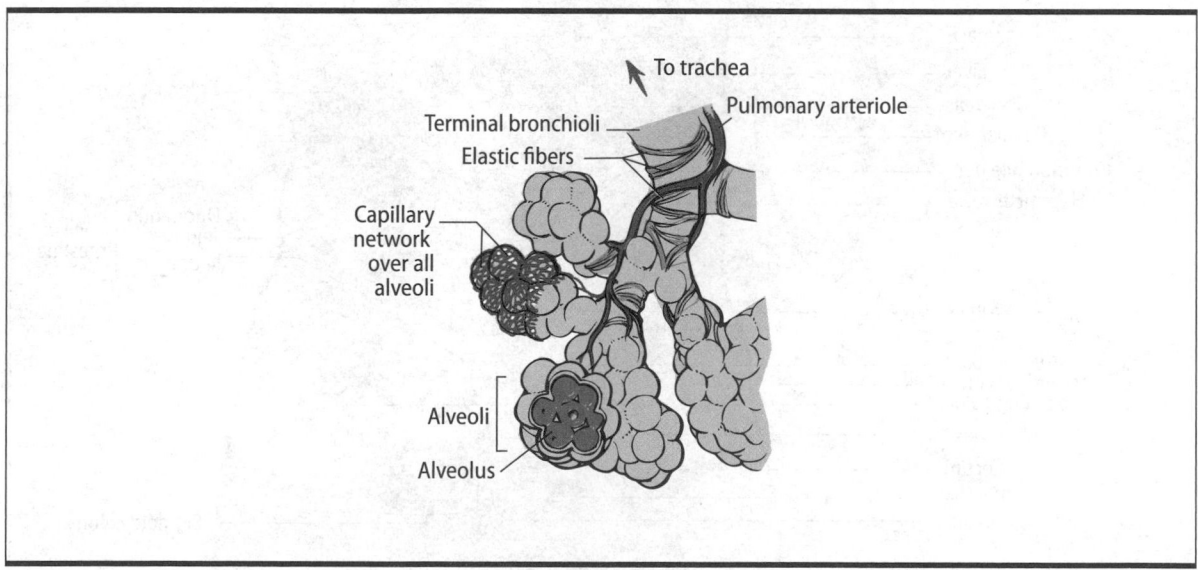

Chapter 11. Diseases of the Digestive System (K00–K95)

Digestive System

Omentum and Mesentery

Peritoneum and Retroperitoneum

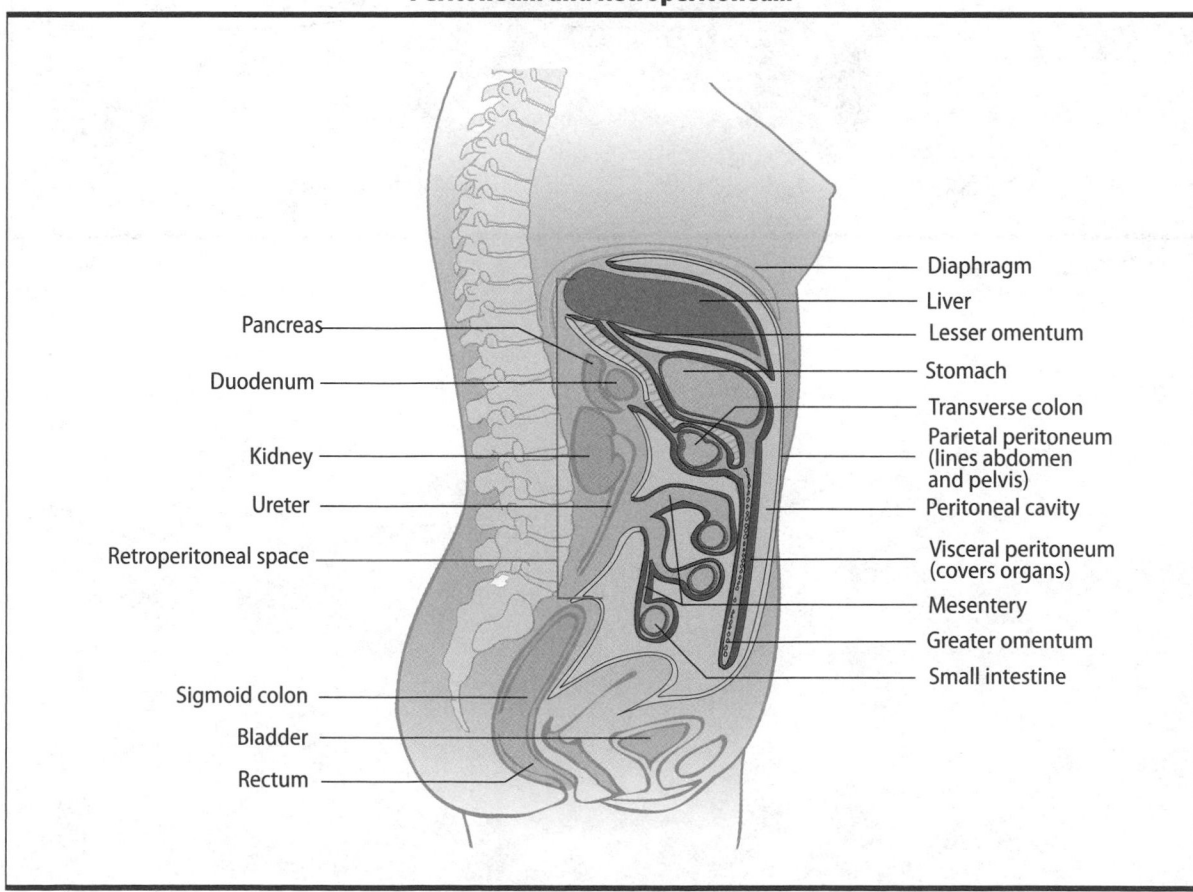

Chapter 12. Diseases of the Skin and Subcutaneous Tissue (L00–L99)

Nail Anatomy

Hyponychium

Cuticle

Nail plate

Nail Fold

Nail root

Nail Bed

Hyponychium

Matrix

Skin

Distal phalanx bone

Skin and Subcutaneous Tissue

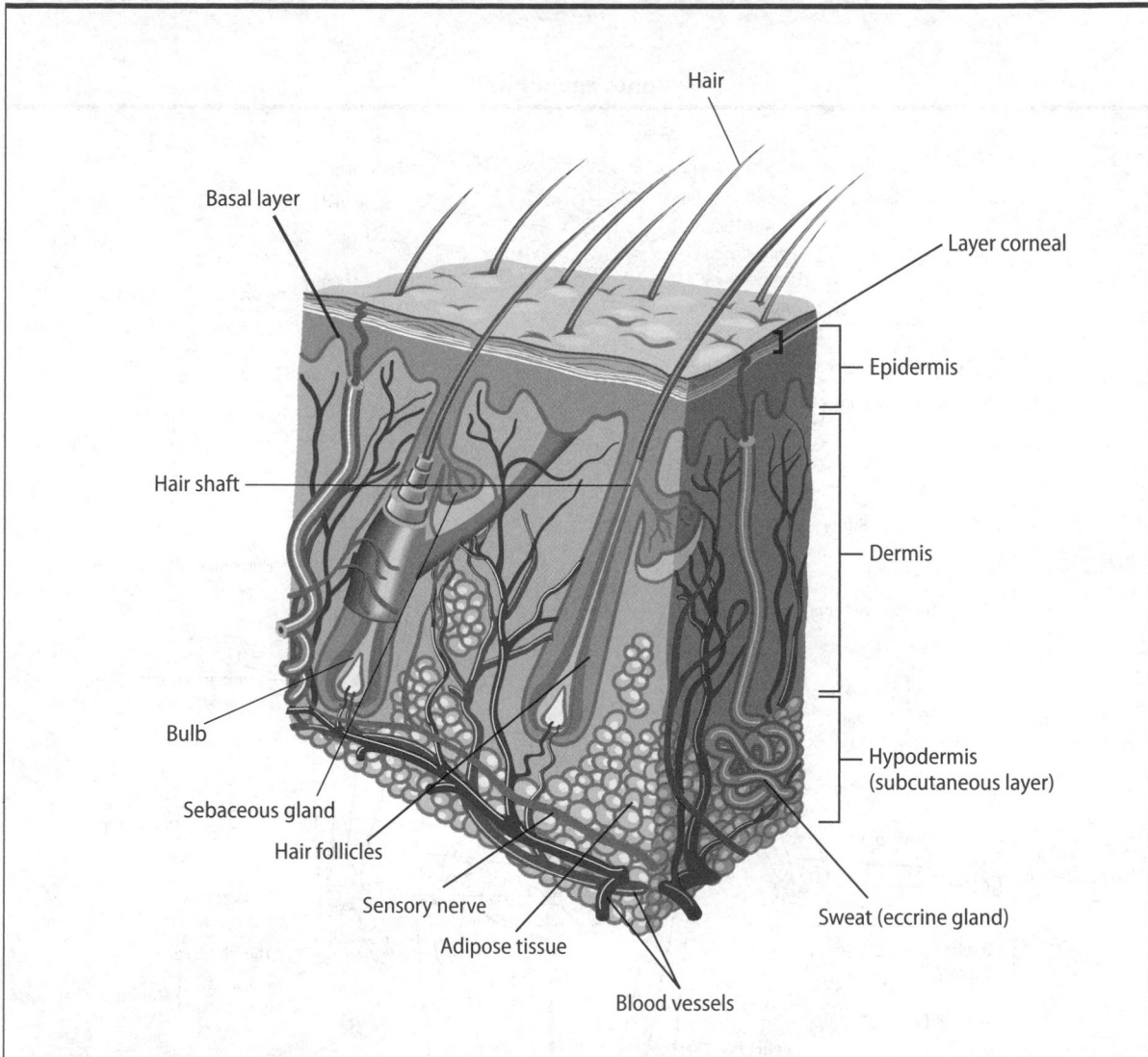

Chapter 13. Diseases of the Musculoskeletal System and Connective Tissue (MØØ–M99)

Bones and Joints

Shoulder Anterior View

Shoulder Posterior View

Elbow Anterior View

Elbow Posterior View

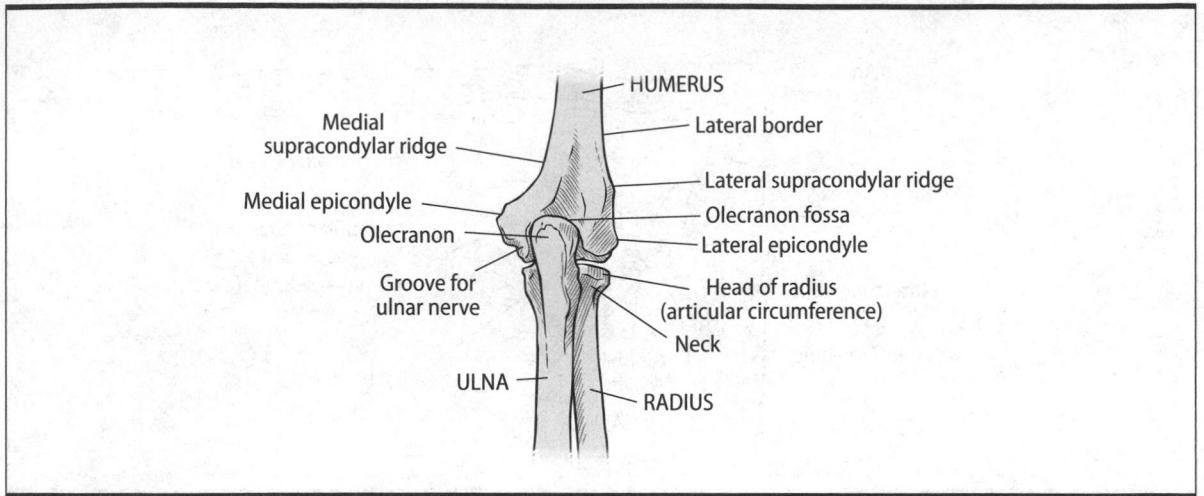

HUMERUS

Medial supracondylar ridge

Lateral border

Lateral supracondylar ridge

Medial epicondyle

Olecranon fossa

Olecranon

Lateral epicondyle

Groove for ulnar nerve

Head of radius (articular circumference)

Neck

ULNA

RADIUS

Hand

Distal phalanx

Middle phalanx

Proximal phalanx

Phalanges (digits)

Interphalangeal joints

Distal phalanx (thumb)

Metacarpophalangeal joint

Proximal phalanx (thumb)

Metacarpals

5 4 3 2

1

Carpometacarpal joint

Hamate

Pisiform

Carpals

Trapezium

Trapezoid

Scaphoid

Triquetral   Lunate   Cuboid

Hip Anterior View

Hip Posterior View

Knee Anterior View

Knee Posterior View

Foot

Muscles

Frontalis m.
Temporalis m.
Orbicularis oculi m.
Orbicularis oris m.
Masseter m.
Depressor labii inferioris m.
Zygomaticus major m.
Mentalis m.
Splenius m.
Sternocleidomastoid m. (clavicular head)
Omohyoid m.
Sternocleidomastoid m. (sternal head)
Levator scapulae m.
Platysma m.
Deltoid m.
Pectoralis major m.
Latissimus dorsi m.
Coracobrachialis m.
Biceps brachii m. (short head)
Serratus anterior m.
Biceps brachii m. (long head)
Biceps brachii m.
Triceps m.
Linea alba
Brachialis m.
Brachioradialis m.
Rectus abdominis m.
Extensor carpi radialis longus m.
Brachioradialis m.
Bicipital aponeurosis
Pronator teres m.
External oblique m.
Flexor carpi radialis m.
Flexor carpi radialis m.
Extensor carpi radialis longus m.
Palmaris longus m.
Flexor carpi ulnaris m.
Extensor carpi radialis brevis m.
Flexor digitorum superficialis m.
Extensor digitorum m.
Extensor digiti minimi m.
Extensor retinaculum
Anterior superior iliac spine
Extensor retinaculum
Iliopsoas m.
Pectineus m.
Pubic tubercle
Adductor longus m.
Sartorius m.
Gracilis m.
Tensor fascia latae m.
Rectus femoris m.
Vastus lateralis m.
Tensor fascia latae m.
Vastus medialis m.
Patella
Gastrocnemius m.
Tibia
Tibialis anterior m.
Peroneus longus m.
Soleus m.
Extensor digitorum longus m.
Superior extensor retinaculum
Medial maleolus
Lateral maleolus

Chapter 14. Diseases of the Genitourinary System (N00–N99)

Urinary System

Male Genitourinary System

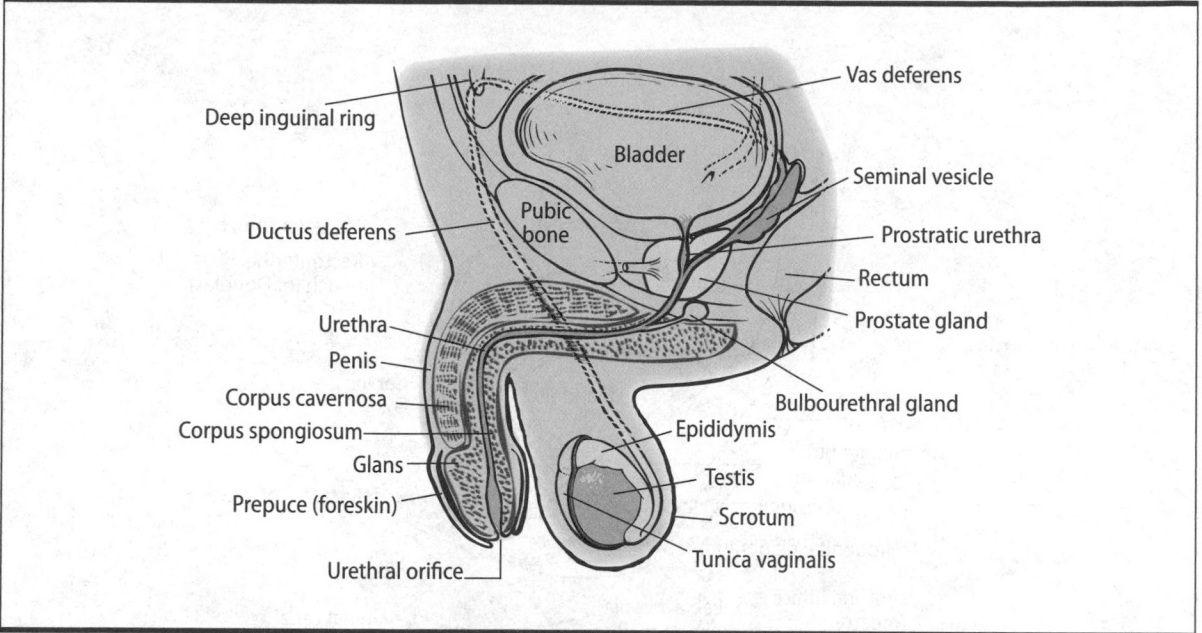

Deep inguinal ring
Ductus deferens
Urethra
Penis
Corpus cavernosa
Corpus spongiosum
Glans
Prepuce (foreskin)
Urethral orifice
Pubic bone
Bladder
Vas deferens
Seminal vesicle
Prostratic urethra
Rectum
Prostate gland
Bulbourethral gland
Epididymis
Testis
Scrotum
Tunica vaginalis

Female Internal Genitalia

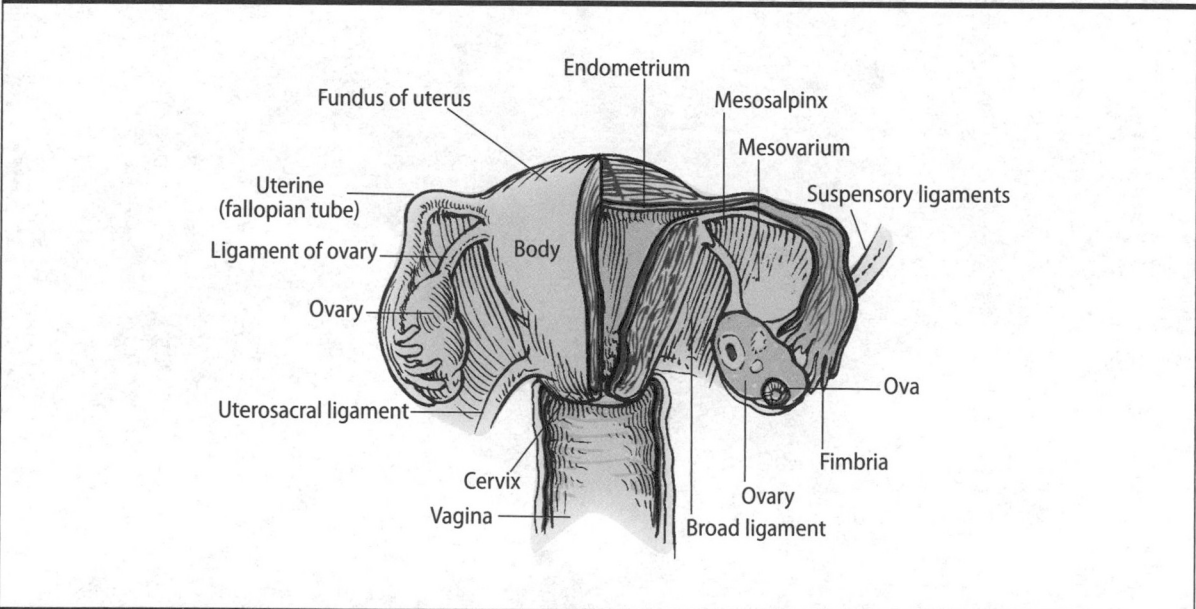

Fundus of uterus
Uterine (fallopian tube)
Ligament of ovary
Ovary
Uterosacral ligament
Cervix
Vagina
Body
Endometrium
Mesosalpinx
Mesovarium
Suspensory ligaments
Ova
Fimbria
Ovary
Broad ligament

Female Genitourinary Tract Lateral View

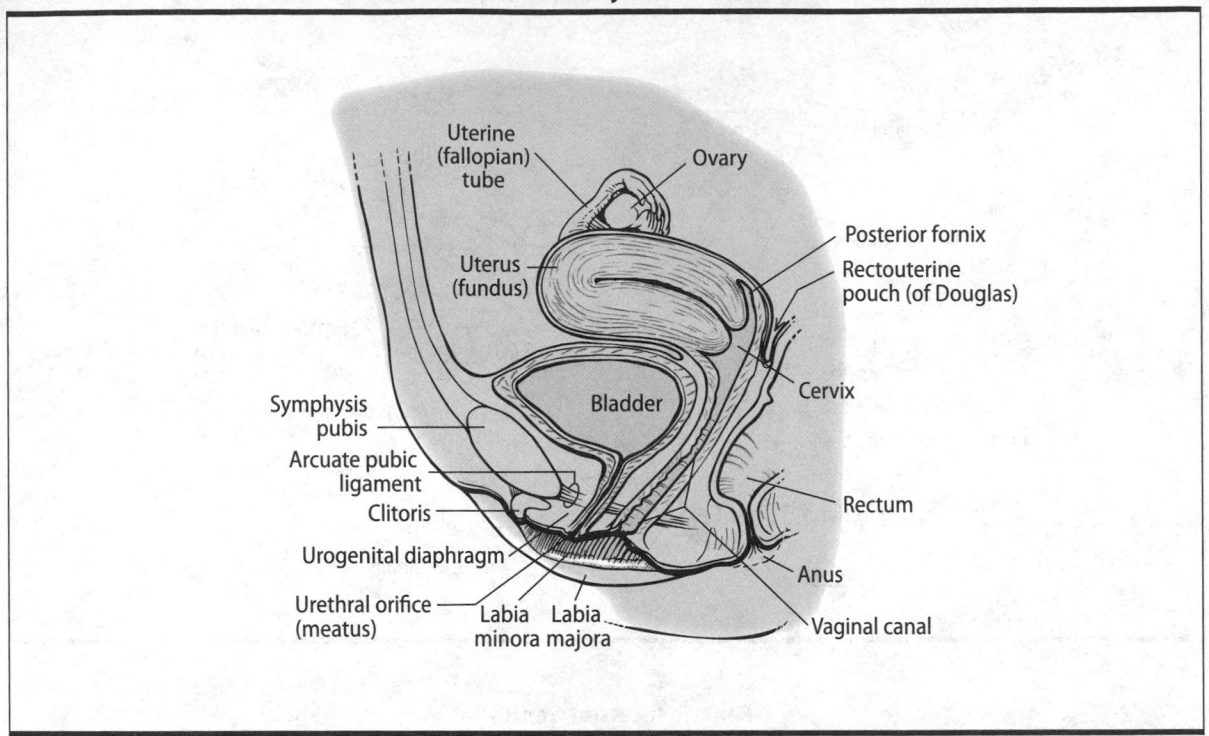

Chapter 15. Pregnancy, Childbirth and the Puerperium (O00–O9A)

Term Pregnancy – Single Gestation

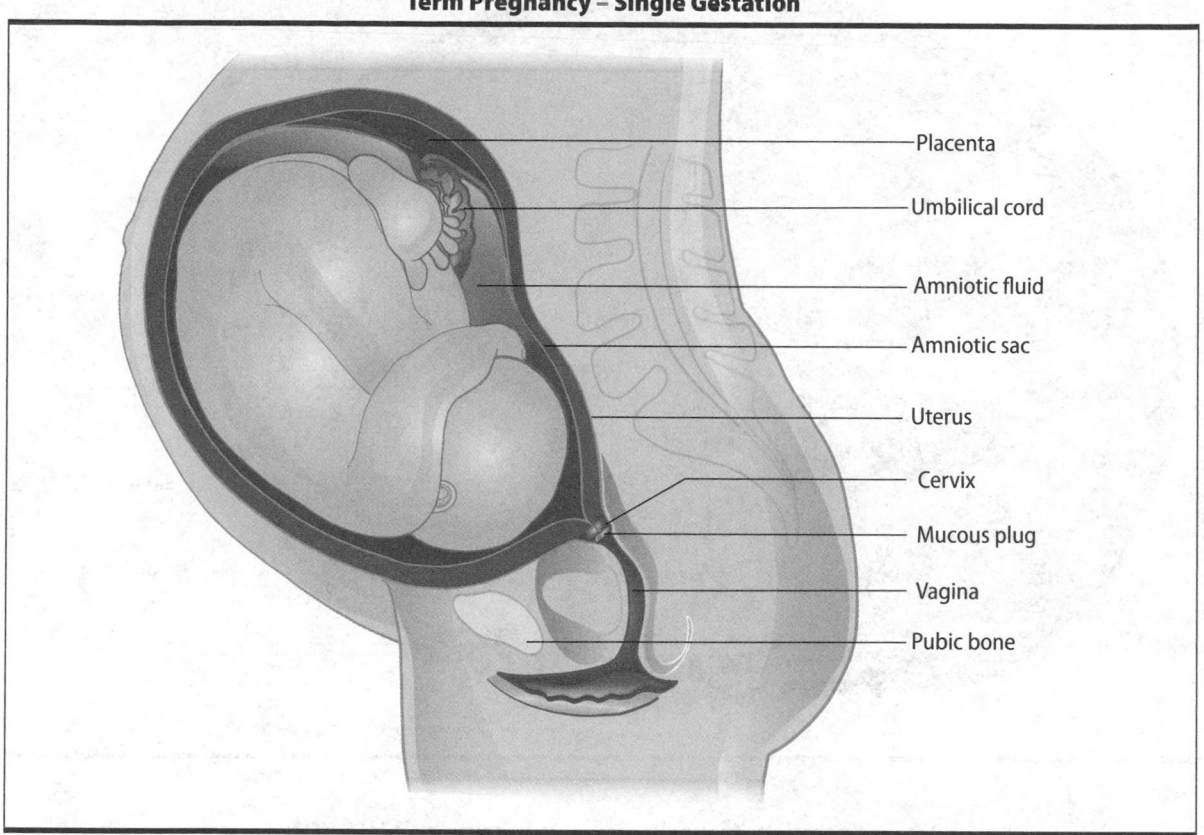

- Placenta
- Umbilical cord
- Amniotic fluid
- Amniotic sac
- Uterus
- Cervix
- Mucous plug
- Vagina
- Pubic bone

Twin Gestation–Dichorionic–Diamniotic (DI-DI)

- 2 Chorionic sacs
- 2 Amniotic sacs
- 2 Fetuses
- 2 Umbilical cords
- 2 Placentas

Twin Gestation–Monochorionic–Diamniotic (MO-DI)

1 Chorionic sac

2 Amniotic sacs

2 Fetuses

2 Umbilical cords

1 Placenta

Twin Gestation–Monochorionic–Monoamniotic (MO-MO)

1 Chorionic sac

1 Amniotic sac

2 Fetuses

2 Umbilical cords

1 Placenta

Chapter 19. Injury, Poisoning and Certain Other Consequences of External Causes (S00–T88)

Types of Fractures

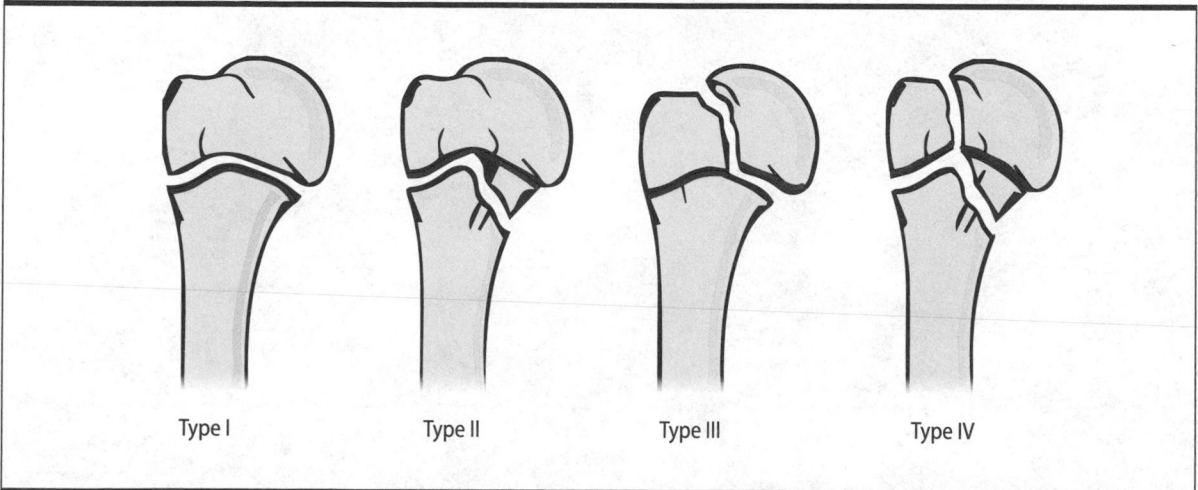

Normal	Transverse	Open/Compound	Oblique	Oblique displaced
Comminuted	Segmental	Avulsed	Spiral	Greenstick

Salter-Harris Fracture Types

Type I	Type II	Type III	Type IV